The MILLION WORD Crossword Answer Book

Books by Daniel Stark (Author/Editor)

The Million Word Crossword Dictionary (with Stanley Newman)
The Crossword Answer Book (with Stanley Newman)
Square One Crossword Dictionary (with Stanley Newman)
Random House Mega Crossword Omnibus
Crosswords Challenge (with Roslyn Stark)
Large-Print Crosswords Challenge (with Roslyn Stark)
The Ultimate Crosswords Omnibus (with Roslyn Stark)
The Ultimate Large-Print Crosswords Omnibus (with Roslyn Stark)

Books by Stanley Newman (Author/Editor)

Cruciverbalism: A Crossword Fanatic's Guide to Life in the Grid (with Mark Lasswell)
10,000 Answers: The Ultimate Trivia Encyclopedia (with Hal Fittipaldi)
Assorted Trifles: Thousands of Tantalizing Trivia Tidbits
Stanley Newman's Opus 100 Crosswords
Stanley Newman's Ultimate Trivia Crosswords
Stanley Newman's Movie Mania Crosswords
Stanley Newman's Screen Legend Crosswords
Stanley Newman's Sitcom Crosswords
Stanley Newman's Cartoon Crosswords
Stanley Newman's Comedy Legend Crosswords
Stanley Newman's What a Character! Crosswords
Stanley Newman's American Originals Crosswords
Stanley Newman's Literary Crosswords
Stan's Saturday Crosswords
Stanley Newman's Sunday Crosswords
Random House Vacation Crosswords
Random House Four Seasons Crossword Omnibus
Random House Masterpiece Crosswords
Random House Golf Crosswords
Random House Monster Sunday Crossword Omnibus
Random House Monster Crossword Omnibus
Random House Sunday Crossword Megamonster
Newsday Sunday Crossword Puzzles
Newsday Daily Crossword Puzzles

Acknowledgments

The suggestions, encouragement, and assistance of many people have made this book possible. The authors would especially like to thank:

- Joseph Vallely, our literary agent
- Toni Sciarra, our HarperCollins editor, who supported our second "Million Words" as enthusiastically as the first
- Kevin McCann and his outstanding "Crossword Community Center" Web site, www.cruciverb.com. Cruciverb is a cornucopia of useful crossword information, including the historical clue/answer database that we made frequent use of.
- Amy Reynaldo and two crossword colleagues who wish to remain anonymous, for their help in finding new words
- Sandy Fein, who proofread our master word-and-definition file
- Nawana Britenriker, for her suggestions on making the text more readable and accessible
- Roslyn Stark, for her assistance in compiling this manuscript and for her many valuable editorial suggestions

---

HarperCollins books may be purchased for educational, business, or sales promotional use. For information please write: Special Markets Department, HarperCollins Publishers, 10 East 53rd Street, New York, NY 10022.

First Collins paperback edition published 2008.

Text design and typography by Daniel Stark

The Library of Congress has catalogued the hardcover as follows:

Newman, Stanley, 1952–
The million word crossword answer book/Stanley Newman and Daniel Stark
p. cm.
Rev. ed. of: The crossword answer book. 1st ed. c1996.
ISBN 978-0-06-112590-4
1. Crossword puzzles—Glossaries, vocabularies, etc. I. Stark, Daniel. II. Newman, Stanley, 1952– Crossword answer book. III. Title.

GV1507.C7N444 2007
793.73'203—dc22 2006049683

ISBN 978-0-06-112591-1 (pbk.)

08 09 10 11 12 ❖/RRD 10 9 8 7 6 5 4 3 2 1

The MILLION WORD Crossword Answer Book

Stanley Newman and Daniel Stark

Collins
An Imprint of HarperCollinsPublishers

Introduction

Welcome to *The Million Word Crossword Answer Book*, your master key for unlocking any crossword puzzle.

The 1,060,000+ main entries in *The Million Word Crossword Answer Book* represent the most comprehensive listing ever assembled of contemporary crossword answers. They were individually selected by the authors, both full-time crossword professionals. They include not just "regular" words, but also phrases, slang, consumer products, celebrities from all eras and milieus, song, movie, and book titles, and the latest words from popular culture—all presented in a format specially designed to get you quickly to the answer you need.

This is a thoroughly updated and greatly expanded edition of *The Crossword Answer Book*, first published in 1996. This new edition has over 50 percent more entries, with new features added that will make the book easier and more educational to use.

To get the most out of the book, be sure to read all the material on the next few pages, especially "How to Use This Book."

May your puzzles be completely solved—with or without our help.

Stanley Newman
Daniel Stark

How to Use This Book

The Million Word Crossword Answer Book contains lists of possible crossword answers that are three to seven letters long, based upon all possible combinations of two known letters.

If you're stuck on a puzzle answer of three, four, five, six, or seven letters, and you know at least two of the letters in the answer, you'll find a list of possible answers in this book, no matter what those letters are.

The entries are arranged first by answer length (all the three-letters first, then the fours, fives, etc.), then alphabetically by the two known letters (AA through ZZ), then by position of the letters within the word (from the first two letters to the last two letters).

Here's how to get to the answer you're looking for most quickly. Let's say you're stuck on the clue "Christmas VIPs" that has a seven-letter answer, and you have this partial answer: __ H E __ __ G __.

Since you have three letters of the answer, you first select which two letters to look up. To give you the shortest list to select from, always select the two least common letters that you have. So we'll choose the H (2nd letter) and G (6th letter).

Finding the Pattern

Now, use the "thumb indexes" at the edge of each page to quickly find the list you're looking for: seven-letter words with 2nd letter H and 6th letter G.

Each thumb index has the number of letters on top, and the two key letters underneath. Thus, the main body of the book starts with "3 CC" and ends with "7 ZT." The thumb index on left-hand pages has the two key letters for the **first** pattern on the page; the thumb index on right-hand pages has the two key letters for the **last** pattern on the page (very much like the thumb index of a regular dictionary).

For this example, you're looking for "7 HG," so scan the thumb indexes until you find it, or something close to it (like "7 HF" or "7 HH"). That will bring you to page 723.

Another Way to Find the Pattern

Alternatively, you can use the information at the top of each page to locate the desired pattern. The top of every page in the main body of the book shows the number of letters in the answers on that page.

The guideword of every left-hand page shows the **first** pattern on the page and the guideword of every right-hand page shows the **last** pattern on the page (very much like the guidewords in a regular dictionary).

For this example, you're looking for • **H** • • • **G** •, so scan the guidewords until you find it, or something close to it (like **H** • • **H** • • •). This method will also bring you to page 723.

Zeroing in on Your Answer

Next, scan the boldface in-column headers (which are always preceded by a blank line) for the • **H** • • • **G** • list you're looking for.

The list for • **H** • • • **G** • has these nine answers: CHICAGO, OHFUDGE, PHOTOGS, THEBIGA, THEEDGE, THEHOGS, THEMAGI, THRONGS, THROUGH, ZHIVAGO.

Most of the time, the context of the clue will make it clear which of the answers is the correct one, in this case the two-word phrase THE MAGI.

Pattern Page Layout

7 Letter Words **H••H•••**

The guideword contains the last pattern on right-hand pages, and the first pattern on left-hand pages.

HAULOFF	THUSFAR	SYDHOFF	HUGGING	**H••••G•**	HODDING	PHRYGIA	GAHAGAN	MOSHING
HEADOFF	WHARFED	UNSHIFT	HUGGINS	HAULAGE	HOGGING	SHAGGED	JOHNGAY	MUSHING
HEAPSOF	WHATFOR	UPSHIFT	HYGELAC	HAVEAGO	HOLBERG	SHANGRI	LEHIGHU	NICHING
HEARDOF	WHIFFED	WASHOFF	HYGIEIA	HAYINGS	HOLDING	SHINGLE	MOHEGAN	NOSHING
HEARSOF	WHIFFER		HYGIENE	HAZINGS	HOMBURG	SHINGLY		NOTHING
HELDOFF	WHIFFLE	**•••H••F**	HYGINUS	HERBAGE	HONKING	SHOTGUN	**••H••G•**	PISHING
HENTOFF		BIGHALF		HEURIGE	HOODING	THEAGES	REHANGS	PITHING
HERSELF	**•H•••F•**	DASHOFF	**H••G•••**	HEXSIGN	HOOFING	THOUGHT	REHINGE	PUSHING
HIMSELF	CHOPOFF	INAHUFF	HAGGARD	HIDALGO	HOOKING	THURGAU	UNHINGE	RUCHING
HIPROOF	SHERIFF	ONEHALF	HAGGISH	HIDINGS	HOOPING	WHANGED		RUSHING
HITSOFF	SHERIFS	PUSHOFF	HAGGLED	HOSTAGE	HOOTING		**••H•••G**	SASHING
HIVEOFF	SHONUFF	RUSHOFF	HAGGLER	HOTDOGS	HOPPING	**•H•••G•**	ACHTUNG	SECHZIG
HOLDOFF	SHOOOFF	SAMHUFF	HAGGLES	HOWHIGH	HOPSING	CHICAGO	BEHRING	SIGHING
HOPSOFF	SHOWOFF	SYDHOFF	HANGARS	HUMBUGS	HORDING	OHFUDGE	ECHOING	TITHING
HUNGOFF	SHUTOFF	WASHOFF	HANGBYS		HORNING	PHOTOGS		WASHING
	THEGIFT		HANGDOG	**H•••••G**	HORNUNG	THEBIGA	**•••HG••**	WASHRAG
•HF••••	THELEFT	**••••H•F**	HANGERS	HACKING	HORSING	THEEDGE	LITHGOW	WISHING
OHFUDGE	WHATIFS	NORTHOF	HANGING	HAFTING	HOSTING	THEHOGS		
		SOUTHOF	HANGMAN	HAILING	HOUSING	THEMAGI	**•••H•G•**	**••••HG•**
•H•F•••	**•H••••F**		HANGMEN	HALFDUG	HOWLING	THRONGS	ACEHIGH	ROUGHGO
CHAFERS	AHEADOF	**HG•••••**	HANGOFF	HALOING	HOWLONG	THROUGH	AIMHIGH	
CHAFFED	AHOSTOF	HGWELLS	HANGOUT	HALTING	HUFFING	ZHIVAGO	BIGHUGS	**••••H•G**
CHAFFEE	CHOPOFF		HANGSBY	HALVING	HUGGING		FLYHIGH	BEARHUG
CHAFFER	SHERIFF	**H•G••••**	HANGSIN	HAMBURG	HULKING	**•H••••G**	GASHOGS	BUSHHOG
CHAFING	SHEWOLF	HAGERTY	HANGSON	HAMMING	HULLING	CHAFING	HOWHIGH	MALEHOG
CHEFING	SHONUFF	HAGGARD	HANGSUP	HANDBAG	HUMMING	CHARING	IMAHOGG	ROADHOG
CHIFFON	SHOOOFF	HAGGISH	HANGTEN	HANDING	HUNTING	CHASING	JIMHOGG	SANDHOG
CHUFFED	SHORTOF	HAGGLED	HANGUPS	HANGDOG	HURLING	CHAWING	MESHUGA	WARTHOG
SHAFFER	SHOWOFF	HAGGLER	HAUGHTY	HANGING	HURTING	CHEFING	ONTHEGO	
SHAFTED	SHUTOFF	HAGGLES	HEDGERS	HARBURG	HUSHING	CHEWING	QUAHOGS	**HH•••••**
SHEFFER	THEREOF	HAGLIKE	HEDGIER	HARDING	HUSKING	CHIDING	SKYHIGH	HHMUNRO
SHIFTED	THESELF	HEGIRAS	HEDGING	HARKING	HUTTING	CHIMING	THEHOGS	
SHIFTER	THINKOF	HIGGINS	HEIGHHO	HARMING	HYMNING	CHINWAG	TOOHIGH	**H•H••••**
SHOFARS	THYSELF	HIGGLED	HEIGHTS	HARPING	HYPOING	CHOKING		HAHNIUM

The in-column header displays the pattern.

The answers corresponding to the pattern are listed alphabetically.

7 HH

The thumb index displays the number of letters followed the two key letters.

How to Use the Crossword Answer Glossary

Use the Crossword Answer Glossary for assistance in deciding which of the answers listed is correct. The 24,000+ answers in the alphabetical Glossary, located at the back of the book, include factual references and less common or tricky words. When you find a answer on the list that you're not familiar with, chances are there will be an entry for it in the Glossary.

For clarity, boldface Glossary words include punctuation if any (hyphens, apostrophes, etc.), and multiple-word answers have spaces between the words.

To help you find the Glossary, each page has a shaded band at the outer edge that is visible when the book is closed. And the top of each Glossary page is clearly labeled.

Glossary Page Layout

Crossword Answer Glossary **BLIGE**

Guideword at the top of each page.

BIC: Pen brand
BICHON: Dog breed, for short
BICORN: Napoleon's hat
BICORNE: Napoleon's hat
BIDEN: Delaware senator
BID FAIR: Seem likely
BID IN: Try to buy your own stuff, at auction
BIDU: Soprano Sayao
BIEBER: Former UAW head
BIEHN: Actor Michael
BIEL: Actress Jessica
BIEN: Well: Spanish
BIENTOT: Soon: French
BIERCE: Journalist Ambrose
BIERE: Beer: French
BIERI: Actor Ramon
BIFF: Punch
BIFID: Cleft
BIG A: Aqueduct Racetrack, familiarly
BIG AIR: High jump in sports
BIG BAD: Like a toon wolf
BIG BEAR: California lake
BIG BEAT: Music genre
BIG BEND: Texas national park
BIKEL: Actor Theodore
BIKILA: Ethiopian runner
BIKO: Anti-apartheid activist
BIL: Cartoonist Keane
BILBAO: Spanish port
BILBO: "The Hobbit" character
BILDAD: "Moby-Dick" character
BILIOUS: Cranky
BILKO: Phil Silvers TV role
BILL G.: Microsoft head, familiarly
BILLIE: Actress Burke
BILLIS: "South Pacific" character
BILL NYE: "Science Guy" of TV
BILL W.: AA founder
BILLY: Police club
BILOBED: Type of leaf
BILOXI: Mississippi city
BILT: Constructed, in brand names
BIMBO: Knucklehead
BIMINIS: Bahama islands
BINACA: Breath-freshener brand
BINCHY: Author Maeve
BINDLE: Hobo's goods
BINE: Twining stem
BINET: IQ test developer
BINGHAM: Actress Traci
BISCAY: European bay
BISHKEK: Capital of Kirghizia
BISMUTH: Element #83
BISSAU: African capital
BISSELL: Vacuum brand
BISSET: Actress Jacqueline
BIST: "Bei Mir __ Du Schön"
BITMAP: Computer display
BITNET: Network of educational sites
BITT: Mooring post
BITTE: Please: German
BITTERN: Marsh bird
BIV: ROY G. __ (spectrum mnemonic)
BIWA: Japanese lake
BIX: Biederbecke of jazz
BIXBY: Actor Bill
BIZARRO: Newspaper cartoon
BIZET: French composer
BIZKIT: Limp __ (rock group)
BJORK: Icelandic singer
BJORN: Borg of tennis
BJ'S: Warehouse-club chain
B. KLIBAN: Cat cartoonist's signature

The **BOLDFACE** answer is followed by the definition.

The gray band makes it easy to find the Glossary whether the book is open or closed.

Questions?

Please let us know if you have any questions about how to use the book. Our contact information is on page x.

How the Words Were Chosen

The majority of the words and phrases are included in the book because they appeared in the nation's most popular crosswords sometime over the past ten years. These include the crosswords we edited or created ourselves.

The previous edition of the book (published in 1996) was assembled under similar criteria. But we were surprised to discover that many hundreds of obscure words in the previous edition, once common to puzzles, don't appear in crosswords anymore. So all those words, like GHARRY (horse-drawn cab of India) and TOURACO (African bird), were deleted.

Thanks to the sharper skills of crossword constructors and the vigilance of modern-day crossword editors, uninteresting obscurities have all but vanished from today's crosswords. Credit must also be given to the computer software that assists many constructors and editors.

As mentioned on the Introduction page, this new edition has over 50 percent more entries, more than 400,000, that weren't in the previous edition. Many months were spent ensuring we included not only those words that have appeared in crosswords recently, but also words that might reasonably be expected to appear but haven't as yet.

This "word gathering" task included checking the latest dictionaries, standard reference sources, and "popular culture" reference books, plus reading newspapers every day (including all the ads) in search of "the latest."

The process yielded such contemporary words as ALITO (2006 Supreme Court appointee), CSI: NY (CBS TV series), EGOSURF (to search the Internet for one's own name), GAG REEL (frequent DVD extra), KIA RIO (imported auto) and ROOMBA (robotic vacuum).

Two categories of words that were intentionally excluded from this book were plurals of names (like HARRYS and DAVISES) and multi-word partial phrases (like A HAT and IS MY). The book's word base goes up to seven letters because well over 90 percent of all crossword answers are seven letters long or less, and because adding eight-letter words would have required a book over 2,500 pages long!

One final point about the word selection. These words reflect the current usage of America's best-known crossword editors, but editors' individual tastes and preferences vary. There are some words listed in this book that not every editor would allow (including some that neither of us would use), and words that some solvers might think inappropriate for crosswords. The appearance of any word does not necessarily imply the endorsement of the authors, whose job is, as the compilers of any dictionary, merely to report its existence.

Write to Us!

In our ongoing effort to keep *The Million Word Crossword Answer Book* as useful and up-to-date as possible, we hope to hear from you. Please write us if you have questions, comments, quibbles, or suggestions. We would especially appreciate your sending along suggestions for new answers to include. (See below for more info on that.) Writing to us constitutes consent to publish your material without compensation.

Wanted—Puzzle Patrollers. Reward!

Professional lexicographers, who compile dictionaries for a living, depend on contributors to alert them to new words. For this reason, we've set up "Stan and Dan's Puzzle Patrol."

Please send us any "new" three-to-seven-letter answer words, phrases, slang terms, names, titles, etc. you encounter that aren't already in the book, so we can consider using them in future editions. They need not have appeared in a crossword. Each submission should include the answer and its meaning and, if it did appear in a crossword, the puzzle's source (newspaper, magazine, or Web site address, and date), along with your name, street address, and e-mail address (if any).

We will thank our 25 most prolific Puzzle Patrollers (the first senders of 50 or more new answers that we use in subsequent editions of the book) with a free copy of the next edition of *The Million Word Crossword Answer Book*.

How to Contact Us:

We can be reached in both low-tech and high-tech fashion.

Regular mail: Stanley Newman and Daniel Stark, P.O. Box 69, Massapequa Park, NY 11762. Please enclose a self-addressed stamped envelope if you'd like a reply.

E-mail: MillionXword@aol.com

3

AA• AAA AAH AAR AAS AAU

A•A AAA ABA ACA ADA AGA AHA AIA AJA AKA ALA AMA ANA APA ARA ASA AVA

•AA AAA BAA CAA FAA KAA MAA

AB• ABA ABC ABE ABM ABO ABR ABS ABT ABU ABY

A•B AFB ALB AMB APB ARB

•AB BAB CAB DAB FAB GAB HAB JAB LAB MAB NAB SAB TAB

AC• ACA ACC ACD ACE ACH ACK ACR ACS ACT ACU ACY

A•C ABC ACC ADC AEC AFC AIC AKC ALC AMC ANC ARC ASC ATC

•AC BAC CAC FAC JAC LAC MAC PAC SAC TAC VAC WAC ZAC

AD• ADA ADC ADD ADE ADJ ADL ADM ADO ADP ADS ADV ADZ

A•D ACD ADD AID ALD AND ARD AUD

•AD BAD CAD DAD EAD FAD GAD HAD LAD MAD PAD RAD SAD TAD WAD YAD

AE• AEC AEF AER AES

A•E ABE ACE ADE AGE ALE AME ANE APE ARE ASE ATE AVE AWE AXE AYE

•AE DAE GAE HAE LAE MAE NAE RAE SAE TAE UAE

AF• AFB AFC AFG AFL AFR AFS AFT

A•F AEF ALF AMF ARF ATF AUF

•AF GAF KAF OAF QAF RAF WAF

AG• AGA AGE AGI AGO AGR AGS AGT

A•G AFG AIG ALG ANG ARG AUG AVG

•AG BAG DAG GAG HAG JAG LAG MAG NAG RAG SAG TAG VAG WAG ZAG

AH• AHA AHH AHI AHN AHS

A•H AAH ACH AHH ASH

•AH AAH BAH DAH HAH LAH MAH NAH PAH RAH WAH YAH

AI• AIA AIC AID AIG AIL AIM AIN AIR AIS AIT AIX

A•I AGI AHI AJI ALI AMI ANI API ARI ATI AVI

•AI DAI GAI HAI JAI LAI MAI PAI RAI TAI

AJ• AJA AJI AJO AJS

A•J ADJ

•AJ HAJ MAJ RAJ TAJ

AK• AKA AKC AKU

A•K ACK ALK AOK ARK ASK AUK AWK

•AK DAK LAK OAK PAK YAK ZAK

AL• ALA ALB ALC ALD ALE ALF ALG ALI ALK ALL ALP ALS ALT ALW ALY

A•L ADL AFL AIL ALL AOL ASL ATL AWL AXL

•AL BAL CAL DAL GAL HAL IAL JAL LAL MAL NAL PAL RAL SAL TAL UAL VAL WAL ZAL

AM• AMA AMB AMC AME AMF AMI AMO AMP AMS AMT AMU AMY

A•M ABM ADM AIM ARM ATM

•AM BAM CAM DAM FAM GAM HAM IAM JAM KAM LAM MAM NAM PAM RAM SAM TAM YAM

AN• ANA ANC AND ANE ANG ANI ANN ANS ANT ANU ANY

A•N AHN AIN ANN ARN AWN AYN

•AN BAN CAN DAN FAN HAN IAN JAN KAN LAN MAN NAN PAN RAN SAN TAN VAN WAN YAN

AO• AOK AOL

A•O ABO ADO AGO AJO AMO APO ASO AVO AZO

•AO BAO FAO GAO HAO LAO MAO PAO RAO SAO TAO YAO

AP• APA APB APE API APO APP APR APT APU

A•P ADP ALP AMP APP ARP ASP ATP

•AP BAP CAP DAP EAP GAP HAP LAP MAP NAP PAP RAP SAP TAP YAP ZAP

•AQ FAQ JAQ

AR• ARA ARB ARC ARD ARE ARF ARG ARI ARK ARM ARN ARP ARR ARS ART ARU ARY

A•R AAR ABR ACR AER AFR AGR AIR APR ARR AUR AYR

•AR AAR BAR CAR DAR EAR FAR GAR HAR JAR LAR MAR NAR OAR PAR SAR TAR UAR VAR WAR YAR

AS• ASA ASC ASE ASH ASK ASL ASO ASP ASS AST ASU

A•S AAS ABS ACS ADS AES AFS AGS AHS AIS AJS ALS AMS ANS ARS ASS AUS AVS AWS AYS

•AS AAS BAS CAS DAS FAS GAS HAS JAS LAS MAS NAS OAS PAS RAS SAS TAS VAS WAS YAS ZAS

AT• ATC ATE ATF ATI ATL ATM ATP ATT ATV

A•T ABT ACT AFT AGT AIT ALT AMT ANT APT ART AST ATT AUT AZT

•AT BAT CAT DAT EAT FAT GAT HAT KAT LAT MAT NAT OAT PAT QAT RAT SAT TAT VAT WAT YAT

AU• AUD AUF AUG AUK AUR AUS AUT AUX

A•U AAU ABU ACU AKU AMU ANU APU ARU ASU

•AU AAU DAU EAU LAU OAU RAU TAU

AV• AVA AVE AVG AVI AVO AVS

A•V ADV ATV

•AV BAV CAV DAV LAV MAV NAV SAV TAV VAV

AW• AWE AWK AWL AWN AWS AWW

A•W ALW AWW

•AW CAW DAW HAW JAW LAW MAW NAW PAW RAW SAW TAW UAW WAW YAW

AX• AXE AXL

A•X AIX AUX

•AX BAX DAX FAX JAX LAX MAX PAX RAX SAX TAX VAX WAX ZAX

AY• AYE AYN AYR AYS

A•Y ABY ACY ALY AMY ANY ARY

•AY BAY CAY DAY FAY GAY HAY JAY KAY LAY MAY NAY PAY RAY SAY TAY WAY YAY

AZ• AZO AZT

A•Z ADZ

•AZ MAZ PAZ TAZ YAZ

BA• BAA BAB BAC BAD BAG BAH BAL BAM BAN BAO BAP BAR BAS BAT BAV BAX BAY

B•A BAA BBA BEA BFA BHA BOA BRA BSA

•BA ABA BBA DBA IBA MBA NBA PBA SBA TBA WBA

BB• BBA BBB BBC BBL BBQ BBS

B•B BAB BBB BIB BOB BUB

•BB BBB EBB

BC• BCC BCD BCE

B•C BAC BBC BCC BEC BIC BUC

•BC ABC BBC CBC NBC RBC WBC

BD• BDL BDS

B•D BAD BCD BED BID BOD BUD BVD

BE• BEA BEC BED BEE BEG BEI BEL BEM BEN BES BET BEV BEY

B•E BCE BEE BLE BME BYE

•BE ABE GBE MBE OBE

BF• BFA

BG• BGS

B•G BAG BEG BIG BOG BUG

BH• BHA BHT

B•H BAH BSH

BI• BIB BIC BID BIG BIL BIN BIO BIP BIS BIT BIV BIX BIZ

B•I BEI BMI BPI BWI

•BI FBI OBI RBI UBI

BJ• BJS

•BJ LBJ OBJ PBJ

BK• BKS

B•K BOK

BL• BLE BLS BLT BLU BLY

B•L BAL BBL BDL BEL BIL BOL

•BL BBL DBL OBL

BM• BME BMI BMT BMW BMX

B•M BAM BEM BOM BUM

•BM ABM IBM

B•N BAN BEN BIN BON BRN BUN

•BN EBN IBN

BO• BOA BOB BOD BOG BOK BOL BOM BON BOO BOP BOR BOS BOT BOW BOX BOY BOZ

B•O BAO BIO BOO BRO BYO

•BO ABO HBO IBO LBO

BP• BPI BPS

B•P BAP BIP BOP

B•Q BBQ

•BQ BBQ

BR• BRA BRN BRO BRR BRS

B•R BAR BOR BRR BUR

•BR ABR

BS• BSA BSH BSS

B•S BAS BBS BDS BES BGS BIS BJS BKS BLS BOS BPS BRS BSS BUS

•BS ABS BBS CBS FBS GBS LBS OBS PBS QBS TBS UBS VBS

BT• BTU BTW

B•T BAT BET BHT BIT BLT BMT BOT BUT

•BT ABT

BU• BUB BUC BUD BUG BUM BUN BUR BUS BUT BUY BUZ

B•U BLU BTU BYU

•BU ABU

BV• BVD

B•V BAV BEV BIV

•BV OBV

BW• BWI

B•W BMW BOW BTW

•BW EBW NBW

B•X BAX BIX BMX BOX

•BX PBX

BY• BYE BYO BYU

B•Y BAY BEY BLY BOY BUY

•BY ABY

B•Z BIZ BOZ BUZ

CA• CAA CAB CAC CAD CAL CAM CAN CAP CAR CAS CAT CAV CAW CAY

C•A CAA CEA CFA CHA CIA COA CPA CSA

•CA ACA MCA OCA RCA

CB• CBC CBS

C•B CAB CIB COB CUB

•CB PCB

CC• CCC

CCH CCI CCL CCR CCS CCU CCV CCX

C•C CAC CBC CCC CDC CFC CIC CXC

•CC ACC BCC CCC DCC FCC ICC MCC NCC OCC

CD• CDC CDE CDI CDL CDR CDS CDT CDV CDX

C•D CAD CID CMD COD CUD CYD

•CD ACD BCD LCD MCD RCD

CE• CEA CEE CEL CEN CEO CEP CER CES CET CEY

C•E CDE CEE CHE CIE CLE COE CUE

•CE ACE BCE ICE

CF• CFA CFC CFL CFO CFS

CG• CGM CGS

C•G CHG CIG COG

•CG ECG MCG

CH• CHA CHE CHG CHI CHK CHM CHO

C•H CCH

•CH ACH CCH HCH ICH OCH SCH

CI• CIA CIB CIC CID CIE CIG CII CIO CIR CIS CIT CIV CIX

C•I CCI CDI CHI CII CLI CMI CPI CRI CSI CUI CVI CXI

•CI CCI DCI ICI MCI SCI TCI XCI

•CJ ICJ

CK• CKS

C•K CHK CLK

•CK ACK ECK ICK OCK

CL• CLE CLI CLK CLR CLU CLV CLX CLY

C•L CAL CCL CDL CEL CFL CML COL CPL CUL CXL CYL

•CL CCL DCL HCL KCL MCL

CM• CMD CMI CML CMT CMV CMX

C•M CAM CGM CHM COM CUM CWM

•CM DCM LCM MCM TCM

CN• CNN CNO CNS

C•N CAN CEN CNN CON CTN

•CN RCN

CO• COA COB COD COE COG COL COM CON COO COP COQ COR COS COT COW COX COY COZ

C•O CEO CFO CHO CIO CNO COO CPO CRO CTO CWO CYO

•CO ECO NCO

CP• CPA CPI CPL CPO CPR CPT CPU

C•P CAP CEP COP CUP CWP

•CP MCP PCP

C•Q COQ

•CQ MCQ

CR• CRI CRO CRS CRT CRU CRV CRY

C•R CAR CCR CDR CER CIR CLR COR CPR CTR CUR

•CR ACR CCR NCR OCR VCR

CS• CSA CSI CST CSU

C•S CAS CBS CCS CDS CES CFS CGS CIS CKS CNS COS CRS CTS CUS CVS CYS

•CS ACS CCS ICS JCS MCS OCS PCS WCS

CT• CTN CTO CTR CTS

C•T CAT CDT CET CIT CMT COT CPT CRT CST CUT CWT

•CT ACT ECT JCT OCT PCT RCT

CU• CUB CUD CUE CUI CUL CUM CUP CUR CUS CUT CUZ

C•U CCU CLU CPU CRU CSU

•CU ACU CCU ECU ICU TCU

CV• CVI CVS

C•V CAV CCV CDV CIV CLV CMV CRV CXV

•CV CCV DCV MCV PCV XCV

CW• CWM CWO CWP CWT

C•W CAW COW

CX• CXC CXI CXL CXV CXX

C•X CCX CDX CIX CLX CMX COX CXX

•CX CCX DCX MCX

CY• CYD CYL CYO CYS

C•Y CAY CEY CLY COY CRY

•CY ACY ICY

C•Z COZ CUZ

DA• DAB DAD DAE DAG DAH DAI DAK DAL DAM DAN DAP DAR DAS DAT DAU DAV DAW DAX DAY

D•A DBA DEA DHA DIA DNA DOA

•DA ADA EDA FDA IDA ODA PDA RDA

DB• DBA DBL

D•B DAB DEB DOB DUB

•DB EDB

DC• DCC DCI DCL DCM DCV DCX

D•C DCC DEC DFC DMC DOC DSC DUC DXC

•DC ADC CDC MDC

DD• DDE DDS DDT

D•D DAD DID DMD DOD DUD DVD

•DD ADD EDD ODD

DE• DEA DEB DEC DEE DEF DEG DEI DEK DEL DEM DEN DEO DEP DER DES DET DEV DEW DEX DEY

D•E DAE DDE DEE DIE DOE DRE DUE DYE

•DE ADE CDE DDE EDE IDE ODE UDE

DF• DFC DFM

D•F DEF DIF

•DF PDF

D•G DAG DEG DIG DKG DOG DUG

•DG HDG

DH• DHA DHL DHS DHU

D•H DAH DOH DTH DUH

•DH EDH

DI• DIA DID DIE DIF DIG DII DIK DIL DIM DIN DIO DIP DIR DIS DIT DIU DIV DIX DIY

D•I DAI DCI DEI DII DLI DOI DPI DUI DVI DWI DXI

•DI CDI IDI MDI SDI

DJ• DJS

D•J DOJ DRJ

•DJ ADJ PDJ

DK• DKG DKL DKM

D•K DAK DEK DIK DRK

•DK TDK

DL• DLI DLO DLR DLS DLV DLX

D•L DAL DBL DCL DEL DHL DIL DKL DOL DPL DSL DXL

•DL ADL BDL CDL HDL LDL MDL

DM• DMC DMD DMV DMZ

D•M DAM DCM DEM DFM DIM DKM DOM DPM DSM DUM DVM

•DM ADM EDM

DN• DNA

D•N DAN DEN DIN DON DUN

DO• DOA DOB DOC DOD DOE DOG DOH DOI DOJ DOL DOM DON DOO DOR DOS DOT DOW DOZ

D•O DEO DIO DLO DOO DSO DUO DYO

•DO ADO EDO IDO ODO UDO

DP• DPI DPL DPM DPS DPT DPW

D•P DAP DEP DIP DUP

•DP ADP EDP

•DQ PDQ

DR• DRE DRJ DRK DRS DRT DRU DRX DRY

D•R DAR DER DIR DLR DOR

•DR CDR FDR GDR LDR PDR

DS• DSC DSL DSM DSO DST DSU

D•S DAS DDS DES DHS DIS DJS DLS DOS DPS DRS DTS DYS

•DS ADS BDS CDS DDS EDS FDS GDS HDS IDS JDS LDS MDS ODS PDS RDS SDS TDS WDS YDS

DT• DTH DTS

D•T DAT DDT DET DIT DOT DPT DRT DST DWT

•DT CDT DDT EDT MDT PDT VDT

DU• DUB DUC DUD DUE DUG DUH DUI DUM DUN DUO DUP DUZ

D•U DAU DHU DIU DRU DSU

•DU EDU NDU

DV• DVD DVI DVM

D•V DAV DCV DEV DIV DLV DMV DXV

•DV ADV CDV MDV

DW• DWI DWT

D•W DAW DEW DOW DPW

DX• DXC DXI DXL DXV DXX

D•X DAX DCX DEX DIX DLX DRX DXX

•DX CDX MDX

DY• DYE DYO DYS

D•Y DAY DEY DIY DRY

•DY EDY IDY

D•Z DMZ DOZ DUZ

•DZ ADZ

EA• EAD EAP EAR EAT EAU

E•A EDA EGA ELA ENA EPA ERA ESA ETA EVA EWA EXA

•EA BEA CEA DEA KEA LEA MEA NEA PEA REA SEA TEA YEA

EB• EBB EBN EBW

E•B EBB EDB EMB

•EB DEB FEB HEB JEB LEB NEB REB WEB

EC• ECG ECK ECO ECT ECU

E•C EEC ENC ESC ETC EXC

•EC AEC BEC DEC EEC FEC HEC JEC NEC PEC REC SEC TEC

ED• EDA EDB EDD EDE EDH EDM EDO EDP EDS EDT EDU EDY

E•D EAD EDD EID ELD END ESD ETD

•ED BED FED GED HED JED LED MED NED OED PED QED RED SED TED WED XED ZED

EE• EEC EEE EEG EEK EEL EEN EEO EER EES

E•E EDE EEE EKE EME ENE EOE ERE ESE ETE EVE EWE EXE EYE

•EE BEE CEE DEE EEE FEE GEE HEE LEE NEE PEE REE SEE TEE VEE WEE ZEE

EF• EFF EFG EFS EFT

E•F EFF ELF EMF

•EF AEF DEF HEF REF

EG• EGA EGG EGO

E•G ECG EEG EFG EGG EKG ELG ENG ERG ESG

•EG BEG DEG EEG KEG LEG MEG NEG PEG REG SEG VEG

EH• EHS

E•H EDH EPH ETH

•EH FEH HEH NEH VEH

EI• EID EIK EIN EIS

E•I ELI EMI EPI ERI ETI

•EI BEI DEI LEI NEI PEI REI SEI WEI

EK• EKE EKG

E•K ECK EEK EIK ELK EMK ESK

•EK DEK EEK LEK TEK

EL• ELA ELD ELF ELG ELI ELK ELL ELM ELO ELS ELU ELY

E•L EEL ELL ENL ERL ESL

•EL BEL CEL DEL EEL GEL HEL KEL MEL NEL REL SEL TEL VEL

EM• EMB EME EMF EMI EMK EMO EMP EMS EMT EMU

E•M EDM ELM EOM

•EM BEM DEM FEM GEM HEM JEM LEM MEM OEM REM SEM TEM

EN• ENA ENC END ENE ENG ENL ENO ENS ENT ENV ENZ

E•N EBN EEN EIN EON ERN

•EN BEN CEN DEN EEN FEN GEN HEN JEN KEN LEN MEN NEN OEN PEN REN SEN TEN VEN WEN YEN ZEN

EO• EOE EOM EON EOS

E•O ECO EDO EEO EGO ELO EMO ENO ERO ESO ETO EXO

•EO CEO DEO EEO GEO LEO NEO OEO REO TEO YEO

EP• EPA EPH EPI EPS

E•P EAP EDP EMP ESP EXP

•EP CEP DEP HEP PEP REP SEP YEP

E•Q ESQ

•EQ REQ SEQ

ER• ERA ERE ERG ERI ERL ERN ERO ERR ERS ERY

E•R EAR EER ERR EUR EWR EZR

•ER AER CER DER EER EER

FER GER HER IER JER KER LER MER NER OER PER SER TER VER XER YER

ES• ESA ESC ESD ESE ESG ESK ESL ESO ESP ESQ ESS EST ESV

E•S EDS EES EFS EHS EIS ELS EMS ENS EOS EPS ERS ESS ETS EVS EXS

•ES AES BES CES DES EES GES HES KES LES MES NES PES RES SES TES WES XES YES

ET• ETA ETC ETD ETE ETH ETI ETO ETS ETV

E•T EAT ECT EDT EFT EMT ENT EST EXT

•ET BET CET DET GET HET JET LET MET NET PET RET SET TET VET WET YET

EU• EUR

E•U EAU ECU EDU ELU EMU

•EU FEU JEU LEU NEU PEU

EV• EVA EVE EVS

E•V ENV ESV ETV

•EV BEV DEV KEV LEV NEV REV

EW• EWA EWE EWR EWW

E•W EBW EWW

•EW DEW FEW HEW JEW KEW LEW MEW NEW PEW REW SEW YEW

EX• EXA EXC EXE EXO EXP EXS EXT

•EX DEX HEX LEX MEX REX SEX TEX VEX

EY• EYE

E•Y EDY ELY ERY

•EY BEY CEY DEY FEY HEY KEY LEY NEY REY TEY UEY VEY

EZ• EZR

E•Z ENZ

•EZ FEZ NEZ PEZ SEZ VEZ ZEZ

FA• FAA FAB FAC FAD FAM FAN FAO FAQ FAR FAS FAT FAX FAY

F•A FAA FDA FHA FLA FPA FRA

•FA BFA CFA MFA

FB• FBI FBS

F•B FAB FEB FIB FOB FRB

•FB AFB RFB

FC• FCC

F•C FAC FCC FEC FIC FTC

•FC AFC CFC DFC KFC NFC PFC SFC

FD• FDA FDR FDS

F•D FAD FED FID FLD FTD FWD

•FD MFD NFD PFD RFD

FE• FEB FEC FED FEE FEH FEM FEN FER FEU FEW FEY FEZ

F•E FEE FIE FOE

FF• FFF

F•F FFF

•FF EFF FFF OFF

FG• FGH FGS

F•G FIG FOG

•FG AFG EFG MFG

FH• FHA

F•H FEH FGH

FI• FIB FIC FID FIE FIG FIL FIN FIR FIT FIX

F•I FBI FOI FRI FYI

•FK JFK RFK

FL• FLA FLD FLO FLU FLY

F•L FIL FOL FPL FUL

•FL AFL CFL NFL

FM• FMS

F•M FAM FEM FUM

•FM DFM

FN• FNS

F•N FAN FEN FIN FUN FYN

FO• FOB FOE FOG FOI FOL FOO FOP FOR FOU FOX FOY

F•O FAO FLO FOO FRO FTO

•FO CFO SFO UFO

FP• FPA FPL

F•P FOP

F•Q FAQ

FR• FRA FRB FRI FRO FRS FRT FRY

F•R FAR FDR FER FIR FOR FUR

•FR AFR MFR TFR

FS• FSU

F•S FAS FBS FDS FGS FMS FNS FRS FTS

•FS AFS CFS EFS IFS RFS

FT• FTC FTD FTO FTS

F•T FAT FIT FRT

•FT AFT EFT OFT UFT

FU• FUL FUM FUN FUR

F•U FEU FLU FOU FSU

•FU WFU

FW• FWD

F•W FEW

•FW UFW VFW

F•X FAX FIX FOX

FY• FYI FYN

F•Y FAY FEY FLY FOY FRY

•FY IFY

F•Z FEZ

GA• GAB GAD GAE GAF GAG GAI GAL GAM GAO GAP GAR GAS GAT GAY

G•A GIA GMA GOA GPA GSA

•GA AGA EGA IGA LGA OGA PGA VGA

GB• GBE GBS

G•B GAB GIB GOB

•GB KGB MGB

G•C GLC GMC GNC

GD• GDR GDS

G•D GAD GED GOD GTD

GE• GED GEE GEL GEM GEN GEO GER GES GET

G•E GAE GBE GEE GIE GRE GTE

•GE AGE LGE

G•F GAF GIF GRF

G•G GAG GIG GOG

•GG EGG IGG

GH• GHI GHZ

•GH FGH UGH WGH

GI• GIA GIB GIE GIF GIG GIL GIN GIS GIT

G•I GAI GHI GTI

•GI AGI

GL• GLC GLO

G•L GAL GEL GIL

GM• GMA GMC GMS GMT

G•M GAM GEM GUM GYM

•GM CGM MGM

GN• GNC GNP GNU

G•N GEN GIN GON GUN GYN

•GN IGN WGN

GO• GOA GOB GOD GOG GON GOO GOP GOR GOT GOV

G•O GAO GEO GLO GOO GPO GRO GSO GTO

•GO AGO EGO NGO UGO

GP• GPA GPO GPS

G•P GAP GNP GOP GRP GYP

GR• GRE GRF GRO GRP GRR

G•R GAR GDR GER GOR GRR GYR

•GR AGR MGR

GS• GSA GSO

G•S GAS GBS GDS GES GIS GMS GPS GUS

•GS AGS BGS CGS FGS LGS MGS RGS

GT• GTD GTE GTI GTO GTV GTX

G•T GAT GET GIT GMT GOT GUT

•GT AGT HGT MGT RGT SGT

GU• GUM GUN GUS GUT GUV GUY

G•U GNU GWU

GV• GVW

G•V GOV GTV GUV

GW• GWU

G•W GVW

•GW HGW

G•X GTX

GY• GYM GYN GYP GYR

G•Y GAY GUY

•GY IGY

G•Z GHZ

HA• HAB HAD HAE HAG HAH HAI HAJ HAL HAM HAN HAO HAP HAR HAS HAT HAW HAY

H•A HUA

•HA AHA BHA CHA DHA FHA KHA NHA SHA THA WHA

HB• HBO

H•B HAB HEB HOB HUB

•HB LHB RHB

HC• HCH HCL

H•C HEC HIC HOC

HD• HDG HDL HDS

H•D HAD HED HID HOD HUD

•HD LHD PHD THD

HE• HEB HEC HED HEE HEF HEH HEL HEM HEN HEP HER HES HET HEW HEX HEY

H•E HAE HEE HIE HOE HRE HUE

•HE CHE RHE SHE THE

H•F HEF HOF

•HF UHF VHF

HG• HGT HGW

H•G HAG HDG HOG HUG

•HG CHG

HH• HHH HHS

H•H HAH HCH HEH HHH HRH HUH

•HH AHH HHH SHH WHH

HI• HIC HID HIE HIJ HIM HIP HIQ HIS HIT HIX

H•I HAI HOI HSI

•HI AHI CHI GHI PHI THI

H•J HAJ HIJ

•HK CHK

H•L HAL HCL HDL HEL HOL

•HL DHL NHL

HM• HMM HMO HMS

H•M HAM HEM HIM HMM HOM HUM

•HM CHM OHM

H•N HAN HEN HON HSN HUN

•HN AHN IHN

HO• HOB HOC HOD HOE HOF HOG HOI HOL HOM HON HOO HOP HOR HOS HOT HOV HOW HOY

H•O HAO HBO HMO HOO

•HO CHO MHO OHO RHO SHO THO WHO

HP• HPS

H•P HAP HEP HIP HOP HUP HYP

HQ• HQS

H•Q HIQ

HR• HRE HRH HRS

H•R HAR HER HOR HUR

•HR IHR OHR PHR SHR

HS• HSI HSN HST

H•S HAS HDS HES HHS HIS HMS HOS HPS HQS HRS HTS HUS

•HS AHS DHS EHS HHS IHS JHS OHS PHS SHS UHS VHS

HT• HTS

H•T HAT HET HGT HIT HOT HST HUT

•HT BHT WHT

HU• HUA HUB HUD HUE HUG HUH HUM HUN HUP HUR HUS HUT

•HU DHU NHU PHU SHU THU

H•V HOV

HW• HWY

H•W HAW HEW HGW HOW

H•X HEX HIX

•HX THX

HY• HYP

H•Y HAY HEY HOY HWY

•HY SHY THY WHY

•HZ GHZ KHZ MHZ

IA• IAL IAM IAN

I•A IBA IDA IGA ILA IMA INA IPA IRA ITA IVA IZA

•IA AIA CIA DIA GIA KIA MIA NIA PIA RIA TIA VIA ZIA

IB• IBA IBM IBN IBO

•IB BIB CIB FIB GIB JIB LIB MIB NIB RIB SIB

IC• ICC ICE ICH ICI ICJ ICK ICS ICU ICY

I•C ICC INC IOC

•IC AIC BIC CIC FIC HIC LIC MIC NIC OIC PIC RIC SIC TIC VIC

ID• IDA IDE IDI IDO IDS IDY

I•D IND ITD

•ID AID BID CID DID EID FID HID KID LID MID OID QID RID SID TID VID

IE• IER

I•E ICE IDE IKE ILE INE IRE ISE ITE IVE IZE

•IE CIE DIE FIE GIE HIE LIE NIE OIE PIE SIE TIE VIE WIE

IF• IFS IFY

I•F IMF INF

•IF DIF GIF JIF RIF TIF

IG• IGA IGG IGN IGY

I•G IGG ING

•IG AIG BIG CIG DIG FIG GIG JIG MIG PIG RIG SIG TIG VIG WIG ZIG

IH• IHN IHR IHS

I•H ICH ISH

•IH NIH

II• III

I•I ICI IDI III

•II CII DII III LII MII VII WII XII

IJ• IJK

I•J ICJ

•IJ HIJ

IK• IKE

I•K ICK IJK ILK INK IRK

•IK DIK EIK

NIK
PIK
RIK

IL•
ILA
ILE
ILK
ILL
ILM
ILO
ILS

I•L
IAL
ILL
ISL

•IL
AIL
BIL
DIL
FIL
GIL
KIL
LIL
MIL
NIL
OIL
SIL
TIL
VIL
WIL
ZIL

IM•
IMA
IMF
IMP
IMS
IMU

I•M
IAM
IBM
ILM
ISM
IUM

•IM
AIM
DIM
HIM
JIM
KIM
LIM
MIM
NIM
PJM
RIM
SIM
TIM
VIM
WIM

IN•
INA
INC
IND
INE
INF
ING
INK
INN
INO
INQ
INS
INT
INU
INV

I•N
IAN
IBN
IGN
IHN
INN
ION

•IN
AIN
BIN
DIN
EIN
FIN
GIN
KIN
LIN
MIN
NIN
PIN
QIN
RIN
SIN
TIN
VIN
WIN
XIN
YIN
ZIN

IO•
IOC
ION
IOR
IOS
IOU

I•O
IBO
IDO
ILO
INO
IPO
IRO
ISO
ITO
IVO
IWO

•IO
BIO
CIO
DIO
MIO
PIO
RIO
TIO
ZIO

IP•
IPA
IPO
IPS

I•P
IMP
ISP

•IP
BIP
DIP
HIP
JIP
KIP
LIP
NIP
PIP
RIP
SIP
TIP
VIP
YIP
ZIP

IQ•
IQS

I•Q
INQ

•IQ
HIQ
LIQ

IR•
IRA
IRE
IRK
IRO
IRR
IRS
IRT
IRV

I•R
IER
IHR
IOR
IRR
ISR

•IR
AIR
CIR
DIR
FIR
KIR
MIR
OIR
SIR
VIR

IS•
ISE
ISH
ISL
ISM
ISO
ISP
ISR
ISS
IST
ISU

I•S
ICS
IDS
IFS
IHS
ILS
IMS
INS
IOS
IPS
IQS
IRS
ISS
ITS
IUS
IVS

•IS
AIS
BIS
CIS
DIS
EIS
GIS
HIS
LIS
MIS
PIS
RIS
SIS
TIS
VIS
WIS
XIS

IT•
ITA
ITD
ITE
ITO
ITS
ITT
ITV
ITY

I•T
INT
IRT
IST
ITT

•IT
AIT
BIT
CIT
DIT
FIT
GIT
HIT
KIT
LIT
MIT
NIT
PIT
RIT
SIT
TIT
VIT
WIT
ZIT

IU•
IUM
IUS

I•U
ICU
IMU
INU
IOU
ISU

•IU
DIU
LIU
PIU
TIU

IV•
IVA
IVE
IVO
IVS
IVY

I•V
INV
IRV
ITV

•IV
BIV
CIV
DIV
LIV
MIV
RIV
VIV
XIV

IW•
IWO
IWW

I•W
IWW

•IX
AIX
BIX
CIX
DIX
FIX
HIX
KIX
LIX
MIX
NIX
PIX
SIX
TIX
XIX

I•Y
ICY
IDY
IFY
IGY
ITY
IVY

•IY
DIY

IZ•
IZA
IZE
IZZ

I•Z
IZZ

•IZ
BIZ
LIZ
MIZ
VIZ
WIZ

JA•
JAB
JAC
JAG
JAI
JAL
JAM
JAN
JAQ
JAR
JAS
JAW
JAX
JAY

J•A
JQA

•JA
AJA

J•B
JAB
JEB
JIB
JOB

JC•
JCS
JCT

J•C
JAC
JEC
JVC

•JC
WJC

JD•
JDS

J•D
JED
JUD

JE•
JEB
JEC
JED
JEM
JEN
JER
JET
JEU
JEW

J•E
JOE

JF•
JFK

J•F
JIF

J•G
JAG
JIG
JOG
JPG
JUG

JH•
JHS

JI•
JIB
JIF
JIG
JIM
JIP

J•I
JAI
JOI

•JI
AJI

JK•
JKL
JKP

J•K
JFK

•JK
IJK

JL•
JLO

J•L
JAL
JKL
JUL

JM•
JMW

J•M
JAM
JEM
JIM

•JM
WJM

J•N
JAN
JEN
JON
JUN

JO•
JOB
JOE
JOG
JOI
JON
JOS
JOT
JOY

J•O
JLO

•JO
AJO
OJO

JP•
JPG
JPS

J•P
JIP
JKP

JQ•
JQA

J•Q
JAQ

JR•
JRR
JRS

J•R
JAR
JER
JRR

•JR
RJR

J•S
JAS
JCS
JDS
JHS
JOS
JPS
JRS
JUS
JVS

•JS
AJS
BJS
DJS
OJS
PJS
VJS
XJS

J•T
JCT
JET
JOT
JUT

JU•
JUD
JUG
JUL
JUN
JUS
JUT

J•U
JEU

JV•
JVC
JVS

•JV
KJV

J•W
JAW
JEW
JMW

J•X
JAX

J•Y
JAY
JOY

KA•
KAA
KAF
KAM
KAN
KAT
KAY

K•A
KAA
KEA
KHA
KIA
KOA
KRA
KWA

•KA
AKA
OKA
SKA
UKA

K•B
KGB
KOB

KC•
KCL

K•C
KFC

•KC
AKC

K•D
KID
KOD
KYD

•KD
OKD

KE•
KEA
KEG
KEL
KEN
KER
KES
KEV
KEW
KEY

•KE
EKE
IKE
OKE
UKE
XKE

KF•
KFC

K•F
KAF

KG•
KGB

K•G
KEG

•KG
DKG
EKG
PKG

KH•
KHA
KHZ

K•H
KOH
KPH
KWH

KI•
KIA
KID
KIL
KIM
KIN
KIP
KIR
KIT
KIX

K•I
KOI

•KI
SKI

KJ•
KJV

KK•
KKK

K•K
KKK

•KK
KKK

KL•
KLM

K•L
KCL
KEL
KIL
KOL

•KL
DKL
JKL

K•M
KAM
KIM
KLM

•KM
DKM

KN•
KNT

K•N
KAN
KEN
KIN
KON
KUN

KO•
KOA
KOB
KOD
KOH
KOI
KOL
KON
KOO
KOP
KOS
KOZ

K•O
KOO

•KO
RKO
TKO

KP•
KPH
KPS

K•P
KIP
KOP

•KP
JKP

KR•
KRA

K•R
KER
KIR

•KR
UKR
XKR

KS•
KSU

K•S
KES
KOS
KPS
KTS

•KS
BKS
CKS
OKS
WKS

KT•
KTS

K•T
KAT
KIT
KNT

•KT
MKT
TKT

KU•
KUN

K•U
KSU

•KU
AKU
SKU

K•V
KEV
KJV

KW•
KWA
KWH

K•W
KEW

K•X
KIX

KY•
KYD

K•Y
KAY
KEY

•KY
SKY

K•Z
KHZ
KOZ

LA•
LAB
LAC
LAD
LAE
LAG
LAH
LAI
LAK
LAL
LAM
LAN
LAO
LAP
LAR
LAS
LAT
LAU
LAV
LAW
LAX
LAY

L•A
LEA
LGA
LMA
LOA
LTA
LUA

•LA
ALA
ELA
FLA
ILA
OLA
SLA
TLA
ULA

LB•
LBJ
LBO
LBS

L•B
LAB
LEB
LHB
LIB
LLB
LOB
LUB
LVB

•LB
ALB
LLB
MLB

LC•
LCD
LCM

L•C
LAC
LIC
LLC
LOC
LUC

•LC
ALC
GLC
LLC
NLC
TLC

LD•
LDL
LDR
LDS

L•D
LAD
LCD
LED
LHD
LID
LLD
LOD
LSD
LTD

•LD
ALD
ELD
FLD
LLD
OLD
YLD

LE•
LEA
LEB
LED
LEE
LEG
LEI
LEK
LEM
LEN
LEO
LER
LES
LET
LEU
LEV
LEW
LEX
LEY

L•E
LAE
LEE
LGE
LIE
LYE

•LE
ALE
BLE
CLE
ILE
NLE
OLE
ULE

•LF
ALF
ELF
NLF
ULF
VLF

LG•
LGA
LGE
LGS

L•G
LAG
LEG
LNG
LOG
LPG
LUG

•LG
ALG
ELG

LH•
LHB
LHD

L•H
LAH

LI•
LIB
LIC
LID
LIE
LII
LIL
LIM
LIN
LIP
LIQ
LIS
LIT
LIU
LIV
LIX
LIZ

L•I
LAI
LEI
LII
LOI
LUI
LVI
LXI

•LI
ALI
CLI
DLI
ELI
MLI
XLI

L•J
LBJ

L•K
LAK
LEK

•LK
ALK
CLK
ELK
ILK
MLK

LL•
LLB
LLC
LLD
LLM

L•L
LAL
LDL
LIL
LOL

•LL
ALL
ELL
ILL

LM•
LMA
LMN

L•M
LAM
LCM
LEM
LIM
LLM
LOM
LUM

•LM
ELM
ILM
KLM
LLM
ULM

LN•
LNG

L•N
LAN
LEN
LIN
LMN
LON
LPN
LYN

LO•
LOA
LOB
LOC
LOD
LOG
LOI
LOL
LOM
LON
LOO
LOP
LOS
LOT
LOU
LOV
LOW
LOX
LOY

L•O
LAO
LBO
LEO
LOO

•LO
DLO
ELO
FLO
GLO
ILO
JLO
PLO
SLO

LP•
LPG
LPN
LPS

L•P
LAP
LIP
LOP

•LP
ALP

L•Q
LIQ

L•R
LAR
LDR
LER
LTR

•LR
CLR
DLR
SLR

LS•
LSD
LST
LSU

L•S
LAS
LBS
LDS
LES
LGS
LIS
LOS
LPS
LTS
LYS

•LS
ALS
BLS
DLS
ELS
ILS
MLS
PLS
RLS
WLS
XLS

LT•
LTA
LTD
LTR
LTS

L•T
LAT
LET
LIT
LOT
LST

•LT
ALT
BLT
ULT

LU•
LUA
LUB
LUC
LUG
LUI
LUM
LUV
LUX
LUZ

L•U
LAU
LEU
LIU
LOU
LSU

•LU
BLU
CLU
ELU
FLU
PLU
ULU

LV•
LVB
LVI

L•V
LAV
LEV
LIV
LOV
LUV
LXV

•LV
CLV
DLV
MLV
XLV

L•W
LAW
LEW
LOW

•LW
ALW
NLW

LX•
LXI
LXV
LXX

L•X
LAX
LEX
LIX
LOX
LUX
LXX

•LX
CLX
DLX
MLX
SLX

LY•
LYE
LYN
LYS

L•Y
LAY
LEY
LOY

•LY
ALY
BLY
CLY
ELY
FLY
PLY
SLY

L•Z
LIZ
LUZ

MA•
MAA
MAB
MAC
MAD
MAE
MAG
MAH
MAI
MAJ
MAL
MAM
MAN
MAO
MAP
MAR
MAS
MAT
MAV
MAW
MAX
MAY
MAZ

M•A
MAA
MBA
MCA
MEA
MFA
MIA
MOA
MTA

•MA
AMA
GMA
IMA
LMA
OMA
RMA
SMA
UMA
YMA

MB•
MBA
MBE

M•B
MAB
MGB
MIB
MLB
MOB
MRB

•MB
AMB
EMB
OMB

MC•
MCA
MCC
MCD
MCG
MCI
MCL
MCM
MCP
MCQ
MCS
MCV
MCX

M•C
MAC
MCC
MDC
MIC
MMC
MOC
MRC
MXC

•MC
AMC
DMC
GMC
MMC
TMC

MD•
MDC
MDI
MDL
MDS
MDT
MDV
MDX

M•D
MAD
MCD
MED
MFD
MID
MMD
MOD
MUD

•MD
CMD
DMD
MMD

ME•
MEA
MED
MEG
MEL
MEM
MEN
MER
MES
MET
MEW
MEX

M•E
MAE
MBE
MME
MOE
MRE

•ME
AME
BME
EME
MME
OME

MF•
MFA
MFD
MFG
MFR

•MF
AMF
EMF
IMF

MG•
MGB
MGM
MGR
MGS
MGT

M•G
MAG
MCG
MEG
MFG
MIG
MPG
MSG
MTG
MUG

MH• MHO MHZ

M•H MAH MPH

MI• MIA MIB MIC MID MIG MII MIL MIM MIN MIO MIR MIS MIT MIV MIX MIZ

M•I MAI MCI MDI MII MLI MMI MOI MRI MVI MXI

•MI AMI BMI CMI EMI MMI NMI OMI TMI VMI

M•J MAJ

MK• MKT

M•K MLK

•MK EMK PMK

ML• MLB MLI MLK MLS MLV MLX

M•L MAL MCL MDL MEL MIL MML MOL MXL

•ML CML MML SML

MM• MMC MMD MME MMI MML MMM MMV MMX

M•M MAM MCM MEM MGM MIM MMM MOM MTM MUM

•MM HMM MMM

MN• MNO

M•N MAN MEN MIN MON MSN MTN MUN

•MN LMN OMN RMN

MO• MOA MOB MOC MOD MOE MOI MOL MOM MON MOO MOP MOR MOS MOT MOW

M•O MAO MHO MIO MNO MOO MYO

•MO AMO EMO HMO

MP• MPG MPH MPS MPV

M•P MAP MCP MOP MVP

•MP AMP EMP IMP UMP

M•Q MCQ

MR• MRB MRC MRE MRI MRS MRT MRX

M•R MAR MER MFR MGR MIR MOR MUR

MS• MSG MSN MSS MST MSU

M•S MAS MCS MDS MES MGS MIS MLS MOS MPS MRS MSS MTS MUS

•MS AMS EMS FMS GMS HMS IMS OMS PMS RMS TMS UMS

MT• MTA MTG MTM MTN MTS MTV

M•T MAT MDT MET MGT MIT MKT MOT MRT MST

•MT AMT BMT CMT EMT GMT PMT

MU• MUD MUG MUM MUN MUR MUS MUY

M•U MSU

•MU AMU EMU IMU SMU

MV• MVI MVP

M•V MAV MCV MDV MIV MLV MMV MPV MTV MXV

•MV CMV DMV MMV

M•W MAW MEW MOW

•MW BMW JMW UMW

MX• MXC MXI MXL MXV MXX

M•X MAX MCX MDX MEX MIX MLX MMX MRX MXX

•MX BMX CMX MMX

MY• MYO

M•Y MAY MUY

•MY AMY

M•Z MAZ MHZ MIZ

•MZ DMZ

NA• NAB NAE NAG NAH NAL NAM NAN NAP NAR NAS NAT NAV NAW NAY

N•A NBA NEA NHA NIA NRA NSA

•NA ANA DNA ENA INA ONA RNA SNA UNA

NB• NBA NBC NBW

N•B NAB NEB NIB NOB NUB

NC• NCC NCO NCR

N•C NBC NCC NEC NFC NIC NLC NRC NSC NYC

•NC ANC ENC GNC INC RNC UNC

ND• NDU

N•D NED NFD NOD

•ND AND END IND RND UND

NE• NEA NEB NEC NED NEE NEG NEH NEI NEL NEN NEO NER NES NET NEU NEV NEW NEY NEZ

N•E NAE NEE NIE NLE NNE NOE NYE

•NE ANE ENE INE NNE ONE UNE

NF• NFC NFD NFL

N•F NLF NSF

•NF INF

NG• NGO

N•G NAG NEG NOG

•NG ANG ENG ING LNG

NH• NHA NHL NHU

N•H NAH NEH NIH NOH NTH

•NH UNH

NI• NIA NIB NIC NIE NIH NIK NIL NIM NIN NIP NIT NIX

N•I NEI NMI NUI

•NI ANI ONI UNI

N•K NIK NOK

•NK INK

NL• NLC NLE NLF NLW

N•L NAL NEL NFL NHL NIL NOL

•NL ENL SNL

NM• NMI

N•M NAM NIM NOM NYM

•NM UNM

NN• NNE NNW

N•N NAN NEN NIN NON NUN

•NN ANN CNN INN TNN

NO• NOB NOD NOE NOG NOH NOK NOL NOM NON NOP NOR NOS NOT NOV NOW

N•O NCO NEO NGO

•NO CNO ENO INO MNO ONO SNO UNO

NP• NPR NPS

N•P NAP NIP NOP

•NP GNP

•NQ INQ

NR• NRA NRC

N•R NAR NCR NER NOR NPR NUR

•NR SNR

NS• NSA NSC NSF NSW NSX

N•S NAS NES NOS NPS NUS NWS NYS

•NS ANS CNS ENS FNS INS ONS RNS TNS UNS

NT• NTH

N•T NAT NET NIT NOT NUT NWT NYT

•NT ANT ENT INT KNT ONT TNT

NU• NUB NUI NUN NUR NUS NUT

N•U NDU NEU NHU NYU

•NU ANU GNU INU UNU

N•V NAV NEV NOV

•NV ENV INV

NW• NWS NWT

N•W NAW NBW NEW NLW NNW NOW NSW

•NW NNW WNW

N•X NIX NSX NYX

NY• NYC NYE NYM NYS NYT NYU NYX NYY

N•Y NAY NEY NYY

•NY ANY

N•Z NEZ

•NZ ENZ

OA• OAF OAK OAR OAS OAT OAU

O•A OCA ODA OGA OKA OLA OMA ONA OPA ORA OSA OTA OVA

•OA BOA COA DOA GOA KOA LOA MOA ROA VOA ZOA

OB• OBE OBI OBJ OBL OBS OBV

O•B OMB ORB OTB

•OB BOB COB DOB FOB GOB HOB JOB KOB LOB MOB NOB POB ROB SOB YOB

OC• OCA OCC OCH OCK OCR OCS OCT

O•C OCC OIC ORC OTC

•OC DOC HOC IOC LOC MOC POC ROC SOC

OD• ODA ODD ODE ODO ODS

O•D ODD OED OID OKD OLD ORD OUD

•OD BOD COD DOD GOD HOD KOD LOD MOD NOD POD ROD SOD TOD YOD ZOD

OE• OED OEM OEN OEO OER

O•E OBE ODE OIE OKE OLE OME ONE OPE ORE OSE OTE OWE OYE

•OE COE DOE EOE FOE HOE JOE MOE NOE POE ROE TOE WOE ZOE

OF• OFF OFT

O•F OAF OFF OOF

•OF HOF OOF

OG• OGA

O•G ORG

•OG BOG COG DOG FOG GOG HOG JOG LOG NOG POG TOG ZOG

OH• OHM OHO OHR OHS

O•H OCH OOH OSH

•OH DOH KOH NOH OOH ROH

OI• OIC OID OIE OIL OIR

O•I OBI OMI ONI ORI OSI OUI OVI OWI

•OI DOI FOI HOI JOI KOI LOI MOI POI ROI SOI TOI

OJ• OJO OJS

O•J OBJ

•OJ DOJ

OK• OKA OKD OKE OKS

O•K OAK OCK ORK

•OK AOK BOK NOK ROK WOK

OL• OLA OLD OLE

O•L OBL OIL OWL OYL

•OL AOL BOL COL DOL FOL HOL KOL LOL MOL NOL POL SOL TOL VOL

OM• OMA OMB OME OMI OMN OMS

O•M OEM OHM OOM

•OM BOM COM DOM EOM HOM LOM MOM NOM OOM POM QOM ROM TOM YOM

ON• ONA ONE ONI ONO ONS ONT

O•N OEN OMN OON OWN

•ON BON CON DON EON GON HON ION JON KON LON MON NON OON RON SON TON VON WON YON

OO• OOF OOH OOM OON OOO OOP OOX

O•O ODO OEO OHO OJO ONO OOO ORO OSO OTO OVO OXO

•OO BOO COO DOO FOO GOO HOO KOO LOO MOO OOO POO ROO SOO TOO VOO WOO XOO YOO ZOO

OP• OPA OPE OPP OPQ OPS OPT

O•P OOP OPP

•OP BOP COP FOP GOP HOP KOP LOP MOP NOP OOP POP SOP TOP

O•Q OPQ

•OQ COQ

OR• ORA ORB ORC ORD ORE ORG ORI ORK ORO ORR ORS ORT ORV ORY

O•R OAR OCR OER OHR OIR ORR OUR

•OR BOR COR DOR FOR GOR HOR IOR MOR NOR POR SOR TOR

OS• OSA OSE OSH OSI OSO OSS OST OSU

O•S OAS OBS OCS ODS OHS OJS OKS OMS ONS OPS ORS OSS OTS OUS OWS OYS OZS

•OS BOS COS DOS EOS HOS IOS JOS KOS LOS MOS NOS POS ROS SOS TOS VOS YOS

OT• OTA OTB OTC OTE OTO OTS OTT

O•T OAT OCT OFT ONT OPT ORT OST OTT OUT

•OT BOT COT DOT GOT HOT JOT LOT MOT NOT POT ROT SOT TOT ZOT

OU• OUD OUI OUR OUS OUT

O•U OAU OSU

•OU FOU IOU LOU SOU YOU

OV• OVA OVI OVO

O•V OBV ORV

•OV GOV HOV LOV NOV POV SOV TOV

OW• OWE OWI OWL OWN OWS

•OW BOW COW DOW HOW LOW MOW NOW POW ROW SOW TOW VOW WOW YOW

OX• OXO OXX OXY

O•X OOX OXX

•OX BOX COX FOX LOX OOX POX ROX SOX TOX VOX XOX

OY• OYE OYL OYS

O•Y ORY OXY

•OY BOY COY FOY HOY JOY LOY ROY SOY TOY

OZ• OZS

•OZ BOZ COZ DOZ KOZ ROZ WOZ

PA• PAC PAD PAH PAI PAK PAL PAM PAN PAO PAP PAR PAS PAT PAW PAX PAY PAZ

P•A PBA PDA PEA PGA PIA PSA PTA PWA PYA

•PA APA CPA EPA FPA GPA IPA OPA SPA WPA

PB• PBA PBJ PBS PBX

P•B PCB POB PUB

•PB
APB

PC•
PCB
PCP
PCS
PCT
PCV

P•C
PAC
PEC
PFC
PIC
POC
PRC
PSC
PVC

•PC
UPC

PD•
PDA
PDF
PDJ
PDQ
PDR
PDS
PDT

P•D
PAD
PED
PFD
PHD
POD
PPD

•PD
PPD

PE•
PEA
PEC
PED
PEE
PEG
PEI
PEN
PEP
PER
PES
PET
PEU
PEW
PEZ

P•E
PEE
PIE
POE
PRE
PYE

•PE
APE
OPE

PF•
PFC
PFD

P•F
PDF
PSF
PUF

•PF
SPF

PG•
PGA

P•G
PEG
PIG
PKG
POG
PUG

•PG
JPG
LPG
MPG
ZPG

PH•
PHD
PHI
PHR
PHS
PHU

P•H
PAH

•PH
EPH
KPH
MPH

PI•
PIA
PIC
PIE
PIG
PIK
PIM
PIN
PIO
PIP
PIS
PIT
PIU
PIX

P•I
PAI
PEI
PHI
POI
PSI

•PI
API
BPI
CPI
DPI
EPI
RPI
UPI
VPI

PJ•
PJS

P•J
PBJ
PDJ

PK•
PKG

P•K
PAK
PIK
PMK

•PK
TPK

PL•
PLO
PLS
PLU
PLY

P•L
PAL
POL
PTL
PUL

•PL
CPL
DPL
FPL

PM•
PMK
PMS
PMT

P•M
PAM
PIM
POM
PPM
PYM

•PM
DPM
PPM
RPM
WPM

P•N
PAN
PEN
PIN
PRN
PUN

•PN
LPN
UPN

PO•
POB
POC
POD
POE
POG
POI
POL
POM
POO
POP
POR
POS
POT
POV
POW
POX

P•O
PAO
PIO
PLO
POO
PPO
PRO
PTO

•PO
APO
CPO
GPO
IPO
PPO

PP•
PPD
PPM
PPO
PPP
PPS
PPV

P•P
PAP
PCP
PEP
PIP
POP
PPM
PPP
PUP

•PP
APP
OPP
PPP

PQ•
PQR

P•Q
PDQ

•PQ
OPQ

PR•
PRC
PRE
PRN
PRO
PRS
PRU
PRY

P•R
PAR
PDR
PER
PHR
POR
PQR
PWR
PYR

•PR
APR
CPR
NPR
SPR

PS•
PSA
PSC
PSF
PSI
PSS
PST
PSU

P•S
PAS
PBS
PCS
PDS
PES
PHS
PIS
PJS
PLS
PMS
POS
PPS
PRS
PSS
PTS
PXS

•PS
BPS
DPS
EPS
GPS
HPS
IPS
JPS
KPS
LPS
MPS
NPS
OPS
PPS
RPS
TPS
UPS
VPS

PT•
PTA
PTL
PTO
PTS

P•T
PAT
PCT
PDT
PET
PIT
PMT
POT
PST
PUT
PVT
PWT
PYT

•PT
APT
CPT
DPT
OPT
RPT
SPT

PU•
PUB
PUF
PUG
PUL
PUN
PUP
PUT

P•U
PEU
PHU
PIU
PLU
PRU
PSU

•PU
APU
CPU

PV•
PVC
PVT

P•V
PCV
POV
PPV

•PV
MPV
PPV

PW•
PWA
PWR
PWT

P•W
PAW
PEW
POW

•PW
DPW

PX•
PXS

P•X
PAX
PBX
PIX
POX
PYX

PY•
PYA
PYE
PYM
PYR
PYT
PYX

P•Y
PAY
PLY
PRY

•PY
SPY

P•Z
PAZ
PEZ

QA•
QAF
QAT

•QA
JQA

QB•
QBS

Q•C
QVC

Q•D
QED
QID

QE•
QED

Q•E
QUE

Q•F
QAF

QI•
QID
QIN

Q•I
QUI

Q•M
QOM
QUM

Q•N
QIN

QO•
QOM

Q•O
QTO
QUO

QR•
QRS

Q•R
QTR

•QR
PQR
SQR

Q•S
QBS
QRS
QTS

•QS
HQS
IQS
SQS

QT•
QTO
QTR
QTS
QTY

Q•T
QAT

QU•
QUA
QUE
QUI
QUM
QUO

QV•
QVC

Q•Y
QTY

RA•
RAD
RAE
RAF
RAG
RAH
RAI
RAJ
RAL
RAM
RAN
RAO
RAP
RAS
RAT
RAU
RAW
RAX
RAY

R•A
RCA
RDA
REA
RIA
RMA
RNA
ROA
RSA
RYA
RZA

•RA
ARA
BRA
ERA
FRA
IRA
KRA
NRA
ORA
SRA
TRA

RB•
RBC
RBI

R•B
REB
RFB
RHB
RIB
ROB
RUB

•RB
ARB
FRB
MRB
ORB
URB

RC•
RCA
RCD
RCN
RCT

R•C
RBC
REC
RIC
RNC
ROC

•RC
ARC
MRC
NRC
ORC
PRC

RD•
RDA
RDS

R•D
RAD
RCD
RED
RFD
RID
RND
ROD

•RD
ARD
ORD

RE•
REA
REB
REC
RED
REE
REF
REG
REI
REL
REM
REN
REO
REP
REQ
RES
RET
REV
REW
REX
REY

R•E
RAE
REE
RHE
ROE
RTE
RUE
RWE
RYE

•RE
ARE
DRE
ERE
GRE
HRE
IRE
MRE
ORE
PRE
TRE
URE

RF•
RFB
RFD
RFK
RFS

R•F
RAF
REF
RIF

•RF
ARF
GRF

RG•
RGS
RGT

R•G
RAG
REG
RIG
RUG

•RG
ARG
ERG
ORG

RH•
RHB
RHE
RHO

R•H
RAH
ROH

•RH
HRH

RI•
RIA
RIB
RIC
RID
RIF
RIG
RIK
RIM
RIN
RIO
RIP
RIS
RIT
RIV

R•I
RAI
RBI
REI
ROI
RPI

•RI
ARI
CRI
ERI
FRI
MRI
ORI
SRI
TRI
URI

RJ•
RJR

R•J
RAJ

•RJ
DRJ

RK•
RKO

R•K
RFK
RIK
ROK

•RK
ARK
DRK
IRK
ORK

RL•
RLS

R•L
RAL
REL

•RL
ERL
URL

RM•
RMA
RMN
RMS

R•M
RAM
REM
RIM
ROM
RPM
RUM

•RM
ARM

RN•
RNA
RNC
RND
RNS

R•N
RAN
RCN
REN
RIN
RMN
RON
RUN
RYN

•RN
ARN
BRN
ERN
PRN
URN

RO•
ROA
ROB
ROC
ROD
ROE
ROH
ROI
ROK
ROM
RON
ROO
ROS
ROT
ROW
ROX
ROY
ROZ

R•O
RAO
REO
RHO
RIO
RKO
ROO

•RO
BRO
CRO
ERO
FRO
GRO
IRO
ORO
PRO
SRO
URO

RP•
RPI
RPM
RPS
RPT

R•P
RAP
REP
RIP

•RP
ARP
GRP

R•Q
REQ

RR•
RRR
RRS

R•R
RJR
RRR
RUR
RWR

•RR
ARR
BRR
ERR
GRR
IRR
JRR
ORR
RRR

RS•
RSA
RSS
RST
RSV
RSX

R•S
RAS
RDS
RES
RFS
RGS
RIS
RLS
RMS
RNS
ROS
RPS
RRS
RSS
RTS
RUS
RVS
RXS

•RS
ARS
BRS
CRS
DRS
ERS
FRS
HRS
IRS
JRS
MRS
ORS
PRS
QRS
RRS
SRS
TRS
YRS

RT•
RTE
RTS
RTW

R•T
RAT
RCT
RET
RGT
RIT
ROT
RPT
RST
RUT

•RT
ART
CRT
DRT
FRT
IRT
MRT
ORT

RU•
RUB
RUE
RUG
RUM
RUN
RUR
RUS
RUT
RUY

R•U
RAU

•RU
ARU
CRU
DRU
PRU
TRU
URU

RV•
RVS

R•V
REV
RIV
RSV

•RV
CRV
IRV
ORV

RW•
RWE
RWR
RWY

R•W
RAW
REW
ROW
RTW

•RW
TRW

RX•
RXS

R•X
RAX
REX
ROX
RSX

•RX
DRX
MRX
SRX
WRX

RY•
RYA
RYE
RYN

R•Y
RAY
REY
ROY
RUY
RWY

•RY
ARY
CRY
DRY
ERY
FRY
ORY
PRY
TRY
WRY

RZ•
RZA

R•Z
ROZ

SA•
SAB
SAC
SAD
SAE
SAG
SAL
SAM
SAN
SAO
SAP
SAR
SAS
SAT
SAV
SAW
SAX
SAY

S•A
SBA
SEA
SHA
SKA
SLA
SMA
SNA
SPA
SRA
SSA
STA
SWA

•SA
ASA
BSA
CSA
ESA
GSA
NSA
OSA
PSA
RSA
SSA
USA
ZSA

SB•
SBA

S•B
SAB
SIB
SOB
STB
SUB

•SB
USB

SC•
SCH
SCI

S•C
SAC
SEC
SFC
SIC
SOC

•SC
ASC
DSC
ESC
NSC
PSC
USC

SD•
SDI
SDS

S•D
SAD
SED
SID
SOD
STD
SUD
SYD

•SD
ESD
LSD
USD

SE•
SEA
SEC
SED
SEE
SEG
SEI
SEL
SEM
SEN
SEP
SEQ
SER
SES
SET
SEW
SEX
SEZ

S•E
SAE
SEE
SHE
SIE
SSE
STE
SUE
SWE

•SE
ASE
ESE
ISE
OSE
SSE
TSE
USE

SF•
SFC
SFO

S•F
SPF
SWF

•SF
NSF
PSF

SG•
SGT

S•G
SAG
SEG
SIG

•SG
ESG
MSG
USG

SH•
SHA
SHE
SHH
SHO
SHR
SHS
SHU
SHY

S•H
SCH
SHH
SSH

•SH
ASH
BSH
ISH
OSH
SSH
USH

SI•
SIB
SIC
SID
SIE
SIG
SIL
SIM
SIN
SIP
SIR
SIS
SIT
SIX

S•I
SCI
SDI
SEI
SKI
SOI
SRI
SSI
SUI

•SI
CSI
HSI
OSI
PSI
SSI

•SJ
WSJ

SK•
SKA
SKI
SKU
SKY

S•K
STK
SUK

•SK
ASK
ESK
TSK

SL•
SLA
SLO
SLR
SLX
SLY

S•L
SAL
SEL
SIL
SML
SNL
SOL
STL
SYL

•SL
ASL
DSL
ESL
ISL
YSL

SM•
SMA
SML
SMU

S•M
SAM
SEM
SIM
SUM
SWM
SYM

•SM
DSM
ISM
USM

SN•
SNA
SNL
SNO
SNR

S•N
SAN
SEN
SIN
SON
SSN
STN
SUN
SYN

•SN
HSN
MSN
SSN
USN

SO•
SOB
SOC
SOD
SOI
SOL
SON
SOO
SOP
SOR
SOS
SOT
SOU
SOV
SOW
SOX
SOY

S•O
SAO
SFO
SHO
SLO
SNO
SOO
SRO
STO

•SO
ASO
DSO
ESO
GSO
ISO
OSO
TSO
USO
VSO

SP•
SPA
SPF
SPR
SPT
SPY

S•P
SAP
SEP
SIP
SOP
STP
SUP

•SP
ASP
ESP
ISP
TSP

SQ•
SQR
SQS

S•Q
SEQ

•SQ
ESQ

SR•
SRA
SRI
SRO
SRS
SRX

S•R
SAR
SER
SHR
SIR
SLR
SNR
SOR
SPR
SQR
SSR
STR
SUR
SYR

•SR
ISR
SSR
TSR

SS•
SSA
SSE
SSH
SSI
SSN
SSR
SSS
SST
SSW

S•S
SAS
SDS
SES
SHS
SIS
SOS
SQS
SRS
SSS
STS
SYS

•SS ASS BSS ESS ISS MSS OSS PSS RSS SSS USS VSS

ST• STA STB STD STE STK STL STN STO STP STR STS STU STY

S•T SAT SET SGT SIT SOT SPT SST

•ST AST CST DST EST HST IST LST MST OST PST RST SST

SU• SUB SUD SUE SUI SUK SUM SUN SUP SUR SUV

S•U SHU SKU SMU SOU STU

•SU ASU CSU DSU FSU ISU KSU LSU MSU OSU PSU TSU

SV• SVX

S•V SAV SOV SUV

•SV ESV RSV

SW• SWA SWE SWF SWM

S•W SAW SEW SOW SSW

•SW NSW SSW WSW

S•X SAX SEX SIX SLX SOX SRX SVX

•SX NSX RSX TSX USX

SY• SYD SYL SYM SYN SYR SYS

S•Y SAY SHY SKY SLY SOY SPY STY

S•Z SEZ

TA• TAB TAC TAD TAE TAG TAI TAJ TAL TAM TAN TAO TAP TAR TAS TAT TAU TAV TAW TAX TAY TAZ

T•A TBA TEA THA TIA TLA TRA TVA TWA

•TA ETA ITA LTA MTA OTA PTA STA UTA

TB• TBA TBS

T•B TAB TUB

•TB OTB STB

TC• TCI TCM TCU

T•C TAC TEC TIC TLC TMC

•TC ATC ETC FTC OTC XTC

TD• TDK TDS

T•D TAD TED THD TID TOD

•TD ETD FTD GTD ITD LTD STD YTD

TE• TEA TEC TED TEE TEK TEL TEM TEN TEO TER TES TET TEX TEY

T•E TAE TEE THE TIE TOE TRE TSE TUE TYE TZE

•TE ATE ETE GTE ITE OTE RTE STE UTE

TF• TFR

T•F TIF

•TF ATF

T•G TAG TOG TUG TVG

•TG MTG

TH• THA THD THE THI THO THU THX THY

•TH DTH ETH NTH

TI• TIA TIC TID TIE TIF TIL TIM TIN TIO TIP TIS TIT TIU TIX

T•I TAI TCI THI TMI TOI TRI TUI TWI

•TI ATI ETI GTI

T•J TAJ

TK• TKO TKT

T•K TDK TEK TPK TSK

•TK STK

TL• TLA TLC

T•L TAL TEL TIL TOL

•TL ATL PTL STL

TM• TMC TMI TMS

T•M TAM TCM TEM TIM TOM TUM

•TM ATM MTM

TN• TNN TNS TNT

T•N TAN TEN TIN TNN TON TUN

•TN CTN MTN STN

TO• TOD TOE TOG TOI TOL TOM TON TOO TOP TOR TOS TOT TOV TOW TOX TOY

T•O TAO TEO THO TIO TKO TOO TSO TWO

•TO CTO ETO FTO GTO ITO OTO PTO QTO STO UTO

TP• TPK TPS

T•P TAP TIP TOP TSP TUP TWP TYP

•TP ATP STP

TR• TRA TRE TRI TRS TRU TRW TRY

T•R TAR TER TFR TOR TSR TYR

•TR CTR LTR QTR STR

TS• TSE TSK TSO TSP TSR TSU TSX

T•S TAS TBS TDS TES TIS TMS TNS TOS TPS TRS TVS TYS

•TS CTS DTS ETS FTS HTS ITS KTS LTS MTS OTS PTS QTS RTS STS UTS WTS

TT• TTU

T•T TAT TET TIT TKT TNT TOT TUT

•TT ATT ITT OTT

TU• TUB TUE TUG TUI TUM TUN TUP TUT TUV TUX

T•U TAU TCU THU TIU TRU TSU TTU TZU

•TU BTU STU TTU UTU

TV• TVA TVG TVS TVY

T•V TAV TOV TUV

•TV ATV ETV GTV ITV MTV

TW• TWA TWI TWO TWP

T•W TAW TOW TRW

•TW BTW RTW

T•X TAX TEX THX TIX TOX TSX TUX

•TX GTX

TY• TYE TYP TYR TYS

T•Y TAY TEY THY TOY TRY TVY

•TY ITY QTY STY

TZ• TZE TZU

T•Z TAZ

UA• UAE UAL UAR UAW

U•A UKA ULA UMA UNA USA UTA UVA

•UA HUA LUA QUA

UB• UBI UBS

U•B URB USB

•UB BUB CUB DUB HUB LUB NUB PUB RUB SUB TUB

U•C UNC UPC USC

•UC BUC DUC LUC

UD• UDE UDO

U•D UND USD

•UD AUD BUD CUD DUD HUD JUD MUD OUD SUD

UE• UEY

U•E UAE UDE UKE ULE UNE URE USE UTE UWE

•UE CUE DUE HUE QUE RUE SUE TUE VUE

UF• UFO UFT UFW

U•F UHF ULF

•UF AUF PUF

UG• UGH UGO

U•G USG

•UG AUG BUG DUG HUG JUG LUG MUG PUG RUG TUG VUG ZUG

UH• UHF UHS

U•H UGH UNH USH

•UH DUH HUH

U•I UBI UNI UPI URI UZI

•UI CUI DUI LUI NUI OUI QUI SUI TUI

UK• UKA UKE UKR

•UK AUK SUK YUK

UL• ULA ULE ULF ULM ULT ULU

U•L UAL URL

•UL CUL FUL JUL PUL VUL YUL

UM• UMA UMP UMS UMW

U•M ULM UNM USM

•UM BUM CUM DUM FUM GUM HUM IUM LUM MUM QUM RUM SUM TUM YUM

UN• UNA UNC UND UNE UNH UNI UNM UNO UNS UNU

U•N UPN URN USN

•UN BUN DUN FUN GUN HUN JUN KUN MUN NUN PUN RUN SUN TUN

U•O UDO UFO UGO UNO URO USO UTO

•UO DUO QUO

UP• UPC UPI UPN UPS

U•P UMP

•UP CUP DUP HUP PUP SUP TUP YUP

UR• URB URE URI URL URN URO URU

U•R UAR UKR

•UR AUR BUR CUR EUR FUR HUR MUR NUR OUR RUR SUR

US• USA USB USC USD USE USG USH USM USN USO USS USX

U•S UBS UHS UMS UNS UPS USS UTS

•US AUS BUS CUS GUS HUS IUS JUS MUS NUS OUS RUS

UT• UTA UTE UTO UTS UTU

U•T UFT ULT

•UT AUT BUT CUT GUT HUT JUT NUT OUT PUT RUT TUT ZUT

U•U ULU UNU URU UTU

UV• UVA UVW

•UV GUV LUV SUV TUV

UW• UWE

U•W UAW UFW UMW UVW

U•X USX

•UX AUX LUX TUX

U•Y UEY

•UY BUY GUY MUY RUY

UZ• UZI

•UZ BUZ CUZ DUZ LUZ WUZ

VA• VAC VAG VAL VAN VAR VAS VAT VAV VAX

V•A VGA VIA VOA

•VA AVA EVA IVA OVA TVA UVA WVA

VB• VBS

•VB LVB

VC• VCR

V•C VAC VIC

•VC JVC PVC QVC

VD• VDT

V•D VID

•VD BVD DVD

VE• VEE VEG VEH VEL VEN VER VET VEX VEY VEZ

V•E VEE VIE VUE VYE

•VE AVE EVE IVE

VF• VFW

V•F VHF VLF

VG• VGA

V•G VAG VEG VIG VUG

•VG AVG TVG

VH• VHF VHS

V•H VEH

VI• VIA VIC VID VIE VIG VII VIL VIM VIN VIP VIR VIS VIT VIV VIZ

V•I VII VMI VPI

•VI AVI CVI DVI LVI MVI OVI XVI

VJ• VJS

VL• VLF

V•L VAL VEL VIL VOL VUL

VM• VMI

V•M VIM

•VM DVM

V•N VAN VEN VIN VON

VO• VOA VOL VON VOO VOS VOW VOX

V•O VOO VSO

•VO AVO IVO OVO

VP• VPI VPS

V•P VIP

•VP MVP

V•R VAR VCR VER VIR

VS• VSO VSS

V•S VAS VBS VHS VIS VJS VOS VPS VSS VWS

•VS AVS CVS EVS IVS JVS RVS TVS

V•T VAT VDT VET VIT

•VT PVT

VU• VUE VUG VUL

•VU WVU

V•V VAV VIV

VW• VWS VWX

V•W VFW VOW

•VW GVW UVW

V•X VAX VEX VOX VWX

•VX SVX

VY• VYE

V•Y VEY

•VY IVY TVY

V•Z VEZ VIZ

WA• WAC WAD WAF WAG WAH WAL WAN WAR WAS WAT WAW WAX WAY

W•A WBA WHA WPA WVA

•WA EWA KWA PWA SWA TWA

WB• WBA WBC

W•B WEB

WC• WCS

W•C WAC WBC WJC

WD• WDS

W•D WAD WED

•WD FWD

WE• WEB WED WEE WEI WEN WES WET

W•E WEE WIE WOE WWE WYE

•WE AWE EWE OWE RWE SWE UWE WWE

WF• WFU

W•F WAF WWF

•WF SWF WWF

WG• WGH WGN

W•G WAG WIG

WH• WHA WHH WHO WHT WHY

W•H WAH WGH WHH

•WH KWH

WI• WIE WIG WII WIL WIM WIN WIS WIT WIZ

W•I WEI WII WWI

•WI BWI DWI OWI TWI WWI

WJ• WJC WJM

W•J WSJ

WK• WKS

W•K WOK

•WK AWK

WL• WLS

W•L	**WO•**	**W•R**	**W•T**	**W•W**	WXY	**XE•**	XXI	**•XO**	**X•V**	**XY•**	RYA	**•YE**	**Y•L**	FYN	YIP	**•YS**	**•YU**	ZAS	TZE	**ZO•**	**•ZS**
WAL	WOE	WAR	WAT	WAW		XED		EXO	XCV	XYZ		AYE	YSL	GYN	YUP	AYS	BYU	ZAX		ZOA	OZS
WIL	WOK		WET	WNW	**•WY**	XER	**XJ•**	OXO	XIV		**Y•B**	BYE	YUL	LYN		CYS	NYU		**Z•G**	ZOD	
	WON	**•WR**	WHT	WOW	HWY	XES	XJS	XXO	XLV	**•XY**	YOB	DYE		RYN	**•YP**	DYS		**Z•A**	ZAG	ZOE	**Z•T**
•WL	WOO	EWR	WIT	WSW	RWY				XXV	OXY		EYE	**•YL**	SYN	GYP	LYS	**Y•W**	ZIA	ZIG	ZOG	ZIT
AWL	WOW	PWR		WWW		**X•E**	**XK•**	**•XP**		WXY	**•YC**	LYE	CYL		HYP	NYS	YAW	ZOA	ZOG	ZOO	ZOT
OWL	WOZ	RWR	**•WT**		**W•Z**	XKE	XKE	EXP	**•XV**		NYC	NYE	OYL	**YO•**	TYP	OYS	YEW	ZSA	ZPG	ZOT	ZUT
			CWT	**•WW**	WIZ		XKR		CXV	**X•Z**		OYE	SYL	YOB		SYS	YOW		ZUG		
W•M	**W•O**	**WS•**	DWT	AWW	WOZ	**•XE**		**X•R**	DXV	XYZ	**YD•**	PYE		YOD	**YR•**	TYS		**•ZA**		**Z•O**	**•ZT**
WIM	WHO	WSJ	NWT	EWW	WUZ	AXE	**XL•**	XER	LXV		YDS	RYE	**YM•**	YOM	YRS		**•YX**	IZA	**ZI•**	ZIO	AZT
WJM	WOO	WSW	PWT	IWW		EXE	XLI	XKR	MXV	**YA•**		TYE	YMA	YON		**YT•**	NYX	RZA	ZIA	ZOO	
WPM	WYO			WWW	**•XA**		XLS		XXV	YAD	**Y•D**	VYE		YOO	**Y•R**	YTD	PYX		ZIG		**ZU•**
		W•S	**WU•**		EXA	**XI•**	XLV	**X•S**		YAH	YAD	WYE	**Y•M**	YOS	YAR			**Z•C**	ZIL	**•ZO**	ZUG
•WM	**•WO**	WAS	WUZ	**WX•**		XII		XES	**XX•**	YAK	YLD		YAM	YOU	YER	**Y•T**	**Y•Y**	ZAC	ZIN	AZO	ZUT
CWM	CWO	WCS		WXY	**XC•**	XIN	**•XL**	XIS	XXI	YAM	YOD	**Y•H**	YOM	YOW		YAT	YAY		ZIO		
SWM	IWO	WDS	**W•U**		XCI	XIS	AXL	XJS	XXO	YAN	YTD	YAH	YUM		**•YR**	YET		**Z•D**	ZIP	**ZP•**	**•ZU**
	TWO	WES	WFU	**W•X**	XCV	XIV	CXL	XLS	XXV	YAO				**Y•O**	AYR		**•YY**	ZED	ZIT	ZPG	TZU
WN•		WIS	WVU	WAX		XIX	DXL		XXX	YAP	**•YD**	**YI•**	**•YM**	YAO	GYR	**•YT**	NYY	ZOD			
WNW	**WP•**	WKS		WRX	**X•C**		MXL	**•XS**		YAR	CYD	YIN	GYM	YEO	PYR	NYT			**•ZI**	**Z•P**	**Z•X**
	WPA	WLS	**•WU**		XTC	**X•I**		EXS	**X•X**	YAS	KYD	YIP	NYM	YOO	SYR	PYT	**Y•Z**	**ZE•**	UZI	ZAP	ZAX
W•N	WPM	WTS	GWU	**•WX**		XCI	**X•N**	PXS	XIX	YAT	SYD		PYM		TYR		YAZ	ZED		ZIP	
WAN				VWX	**•XC**	XII	XIN	RXS	XOX	YAW		**•YI**	SYM	**•YO**		**YU•**		ZEE	**Z•K**		**ZZ•**
WEN	**•WP**	**•WS**	**WV•**		CXC	XLI			XXX	YAY	**YE•**	FYI		BYO	**YS•**	YUK	**•YZ**	ZEN	ZAK	**•ZR**	ZZZ
WGN	CWP	AWS	WVA	**WY•**	DXC	XVI	**XO•**	**XT•**		YAZ	YEA		**Y•N**	CYO	YSL	YUL	XYZ	ZEZ		EZR	
WIN	TWP	NWS	WVU	WYE	EXC	XXI	XOO	XTC	**•XX**		YEN	**Y•K**	YAN	DYO		YUM			**Z•L**		**Z•Z**
WON		OWS		WYO	MXC		XOX		CXX	**Y•A**	YEO	YAK	YEN	MYO	**Y•S**	YUP	**ZA•**	**Z•E**	ZAL	**ZS•**	ZEZ
	WR•	VWS	**WW•**			**•XI**		**•XT**	DXX	YEA	YEP	YUK	YIN	WYO	YAS		ZAC	ZEE	ZIL	ZSA	ZZZ
•WN	WRX		WWE	**W•Y**	**X•D**	CXI	**X•O**	EXT	LXX	YMA	YER		YON		YDS	**Y•U**	ZAG	ZOE			
AWN	WRY	**WT•**	WWF	WAY	XED	DXI	XOO		MXX		YES	**YL•**		**Y•P**	YES	YOU	ZAK		**Z•N**	**Z•S**	**•ZZ**
OWN		WTS	WWI	WHY		LXI	XXO	**XV•**	OXX	**•YA**	YET	YLD	**•YN**	YAP	YOS		ZAL	**•ZE**	ZEN	ZAS	IZZ
			WWW	WRY		MXI		XVI	XXX	PYA	YEW		AYN	YEP	YRS		ZAP	IZE	ZIN		ZZZ

4

AA••
AAAA AAAH AAAS AABA AAHS AARE AARP AASE

A•A•
AAAA AAAH AAAS ABAA ABAB ABAS ACAD ACAR ADAH ADAK ADAM ADAR ADAY AFAR AGAL AGAR AGAS AHAB AHAH AHAS AJAR AJAX AKAI AKAS ALAE ALAI ALAN ALAR ALAS AMAH AMAJ AMAS AMAT ANAG ANAS ANAT APAR ARAB ARAD ARAL ARAM ARAN ARAP ARAS ASAP ATAD ATAR AVAL AWAG AWAY AYAH AZAN

A••A
AAAA AABA ABAA ABBA ABRA ACTA ADIA AFTA AGFA AGHA AGRA AGUA AIDA AIEA AIWA ALBA ALDA ALEA ALFA ALGA ALIA ALKA ALLA ALMA ALTA ALVA ANGA ANKA ANNA ANOA ANSA ANTA ANYA APIA AQUA ARCA AREA ARIA ARMA AROA ARPA ARTA ASEA ASIA ASTA ATKA ATRA ATTA AURA AVIA AYLA

•AA•
AAAA AAAH AAAS BAAL BAAS CAAN HAAA HAAG HAAS KAAT MAAM MAAS PAAR RAAF SAAB SAAR TAAL WAAC

•A•A
AAAA AABA BABA BACA BAJA BALA BAMA BARA CAMA CANA CAPA CARA CASA CAVA DABA DADA DAMA DANA DARA DATA FAJA FALA FAMA FATA FAVA GAEA GAGA GAIA GALA GAMA GAZA HAAA HAHA HAMA HANA HARA HAVA IANA JADA JAJA JAMA JANA JAVA KABA KAIA KAMA KANA KARA KATA KAVA LADA LAMA LANA LARA LAVA MAIA MAJA MALA MAMA MARA MASA MATA MAYA NADA NAHA NALA NANA NAPA NARA NASA NAYA PABA PACA PAPA PARA PASA RAGA RAJA RAMA RANA RAPA RARA RASA RATA SABA SADA SAGA SALA SANA SARA TADA TAKA TALA TAMA TANA TAPA TARA TATA TAXA VACA VASA VAYA WAKA WAWA YADA ZARA ZAZA

••AA
AAAA ABAA HAAA MPAA NCAA NOAA RIAA

AB••
ABAA ABAB ABAS ABBA ABBE ABBR ABBY ABCD ABCS ABED ABEL ABER ABET ABIE ABIT ABLE ABLY ABMS ABOU ABRA ABRI ABUT

A•B•
AABA ABBA ABBE ABBR ABBY AFBS ALBA ALBS AMBI AMBO AMBS APBS ARBS AUBE

A••B
ABAB AHAB AORB ARAB

•AB•
AABA BABA BABE BABO BABS BABU BABY CABO CABS DABA DABO DABS FABI GABE GABS GABY HABS JABS KABA LABS NABE NABI NABS PABA RABE RABI SABA SABE SABO SABU TABI TABS TABU WABE

•A•B
BARB CARB DAUB GARB IAMB JAMB KALB LAMB SAAB SATB

••AB
ABAB AHAB ARAB BLAB CRAB DRAB FLAB GRAB JUAB MOAB SAAB SCAB SLAB STAB SWAB

AC••
ACAD ACAR ACCS ACCT ACDC ACED ACER ACES ACEY ACHE ACHT ACHY ACID ACIS ACLU ACME ACNE ACRE ACRO ACTA ACTE ACTH ACTI ACTO ACTS ACTV ACUP

A•C•
ABCD ABCS ACCS ACCT ADCS AGCY ALCS AMCS ANCE ANCY ARCA ARCH ARCO ARCS ASCH ASCI ATCO

A••C
ACDC ALEC AMIC APOC ATIC AVEC

•AC•
BACA BACH BACI BACK BACO BACS BACT CACO DACE EACH FACE FACP FACS FACT HACK JACK JACS LACE LACK LACS LACT LACY MACE MACH MACK MACR MACS MACY NACL PACA PACE PACK PACO PACS PACT RACE RACK RACY SACK SACO SACS TACH TACK TACO TACS TACT VACA VACS WACE WACK WACO WACS ZACH ZACK

•A•C
BANC CALC DARC HAEC LAIC LARC MARC MASC NARC PARC TALC WAAC

••AC
BOAC BRAC EVAC GMAC HUAC IMAC STAC TEAC TRAC WAAC

AD••
ADAH ADAK ADAM ADAR ADAY ADCS ADDL ADDN ADDR ADDS ADEN ADES ADIA ADIN ADIT ADJS ADJT ADMS ADOS ADUE ADZE

A•D•
ACDC ADDL ADDN ADDR ADDS AIDA AIDE AIDS ALDA ALDO ALDS ANDS ANDY AUDE AUDI AYDE

A••D
ABCD ABED ACAD ACED ACID AGED AHED AMID APED APOD ARAD ARID AROD ATAD AULD AVID AWED AXED

•AD•
BADD BADE BADS BADU CADE CADI CADS CADY DADA DADE DADO DADS EADS FADE FADO FADS GADS HADJ JADA JADE LADA LADD LADE LADS LADY MADD MADE MADS NADA PADS RADM RADO RADS SADA SADD SADE SADO SADR TADA TADS VADE VADM WADE WADI WADS YADA

•A•D
BADD BALD BAND BARD BAUD CARD CAUD FAHD GARD GAUD HAID HAND HARD LADD LAID LAND LAPD LARD LAUD LAWD MADD MAID MAUD NARD NASD PAID PARD QAID RAID RAND SADD SAID SAND SARD SAUD VAUD WALD WAND WARD YARD

••AD
ACAD ARAD ATAD BEAD BRAD CHAD CLAD DEAD DUAD DYAD EGAD FUAD GLAD GOAD GRAD HEAD HOAD JOAD LEAD LOAD MEAD NYAD OBAD ORAD QUAD READ ROAD SCAD SHAD SPAD STAD THAD TOAD TVAD VLAD WOAD

AE••
AEON AERI AERO AERY

A•E•
ABED ABEL ABER ABET ACED ACER ACES ACEY ADEN ADES AFEW AGED AGEE AGER AGES AHED AHEM AIEA ALEA ALEC ALEE ALEF ALEK ALEN ALER ALES ALEX AMEN AMER AMES AMEX ANES ANEW APED APER APES APEX AREA AREO ARES ASEA ASES ATEN ATES AUEL AUER AVEC AVER AVES AWED AWES AXED AXEL AXER AXES AYER AYES

A••E
AARE AASE ABBE ABIE ABLE ACHE ACME ACNE ACRE ACTE ADUE ADZE AGEE AGUE AHME AIDE AILE AIME AIRE ALAE ALEE ALLE ALOE ALPE ALTE AMIE ANCE ANGE ANKE ANNE ANSE ANTE AONE APSE ARIE ARME ARNE ARTE ARYE ASHE ASIE ATLE AUBE AUDE AXLE AYDE AYME

•AE•
BAER BAEZ CAEN GAEA GAEL HAEC KAEL NAES SAES TAEL

•A•E
AARE AASE BABE BADE BAIE BAKE BALE BANE BARE BASE BATE CADE CAFE CAGE CAKE CALE CAME CANE CAPE CARE CASE CATE CAVE DACE DADE DALE DAME DANE DARE DATE DAVE DAZE EASE EAVE FACE FADE FAKE FAME FANE FARE FATE FAVE FAYE FAZE GABE GAGE GALE GAME GAPE GARE GATE GAVE GAYE GAZE HAJE HAKE HALE HAME HARE HATE HAVE HAZE JADE JAKE JANE JAPE JAYE KALE KANE KATE KAYE LACE LADE LAKE LAME LANE LASE LATE LAUE LAVE LAZE MACE MADE MAGE MAKE MALE MAME MANE MARE MATE MAZE NABE NAME NAPE NATE NAVE PACE PAGE PALE PANE PARE PASE PATE PAVE RABE RACE RAGE RAKE RALE RARE RASE RATE RAVE RAYE RAZE SABE SADE SAFE SAGE SAKE SALE SAME SANE SASE SATE SAVE SAXE TAKE TALE TAME TAPE TARE TATE TAYE VADE VALE VANE VASE WABE WACE WADE WAGE WAKE WALE WANE WARE WAVE YALE YARE ZALE ZANE

••AE
ALAE BRAE FRAE IDAE IRAE ORAE QUAE THAE

AF••
AFAR AFBS AFEW AFGH AFIG AFRO AFTA AFTS

A•F•
AGFA ALFA AMFM ARFS

A••F
ALEF ALIF ASIF ASOF

•AF•
BAFF CAFE DAFT GAFF HAFT KAFS LAFF OAFS QAFS RAFF RAFT SAFE TAFT WAFS WAFT ZAFU

•A•F
BAFF BASF CALF GAFF HALF LAFF NAIF RAAF RAFF WAIF ZARF

••AF
DEAF GRAF LEAF LOAF OLAF PIAF RAAF RCAF USAF

AG••
AGAL AGAR AGAS AGCY AGED AGEE AGER AGES AGFA AGHA AGIN AGIO AGIS AGNI AGOG AGON AGRA AGRI AGRO AGST AGTS AGUA AGUE

A•G•
AFGH ALGA ANGA ANGE ARGO AUGS AVGS

A••G
AFIG AGOG ANAG AUNG AWAG

•AG•
BAGS CAGE CAGY GAGA GAGE GAGS HAGI HAGS IAGO JAGR JAGS LAGO LAGS MAGE MAGI MAGS NAGS NAGY PAGE PAGO RAGA RAGE RAGS RAGU SAGA SAGE SAGO SAGS SAGY TAGS VAGI VAGS WAGE WAGS ZAGS

•A•G
BANG DANG DAWG FANG GANG HAAG HAIG HANG HAWG KANG LANG MARG NANG PANG RANG SANG SARG

TANG WANG YANG

••AG
ANAG AWAG BRAG CRAG DIAG DRAG EMAG FLAG FRAG HAAG HOAG KNAG PHAG QUAG SHAG SLAG SNAG STAG SWAG

AH••
AHAB AHAH AHAS AHED AHEM AHME AHOY AHSO AHUM

A•H•
AAHS ACHE ACHT ACHY AGHA ASHE ASHY

A••H
AAAH ACTH ADAH AFGH AHAH ALPH AMAH ANKH ANTH ARCH ASCH AUTH AYAH

•AH•
AAHS BAHN BAHS BAHT CAHN DAHL DAHS FAHD FAHR HAHA HAHN HAHS JAHR KAHN LAHR MAHI NAHA NAHS OAHU PAHS RAHS SAHL WAHL WAHR WAHS ZAHN

•A•H
AAAH BACH BASH BATH BAYH CASH CATH DASH EACH FATH GASH HASH HATH KAPH LASH LATH MACH MASH MATH NAOH NASH OATH PASH PATH RAPH RASH SASH TACH TANH WASH ZACH

••AH
AAAH ADAH AHAH AMAH AYAH BEAH BLAH ETAH EVAH LEAH NOAH OLAH OPAH PTAH SHAH UTAH YEAH

AI••
AIDA AIDE AIDS AIEA AILE AILS AIME AIMS AINT AINU AIRE AIRS AIRY AITS AIWA

A•I•
ABIE ABIT ACID ACIS ADIA ADIN ADIT AFIG AGIN AGIO AGIS AJIS AKIM AKIN AKIO ALIA ALIF ALII ALIT ALIX AMIC AMID AMIE AMII AMIN AMIR AMIS ANIL ANIM ANIS APIA APIS ARIA ARID ARIE ARIL ARIZ ASIA ASIE ASIF ASIR ASIS ATIC ATIK ATIP ATIS ATIT AVIA AVID AVIS AVIV AXIL AXIS AYIN AZIZ

A••I
ABRI ACTI AERI AGNI AGRI AKAI ALAI ALII ALKI ALTI ALUI AMBI AMII AMOI ANNI ANTI AOKI AQUI ARTI ASCI ASTI ATLI ATOI ATRI AUDI AURI

•AI•
BAIE BAIL BAIN BAIO BAIT CAIN DAIL DAIN DAIS FAIL FAIM FAIN FAIR FAIT GAIA GAIL GAIN GAIT HAID HAIG HAIK HAIL HAIM HAIR JAIL JAIN KAIA LAIC LAID LAIN LAIR LAIS LAIT MAIA MAID MAIL MAIM MAIN MAIO MAIS NAIF NAIL NAIR PAID PAIL PAIN PAIR PAIS PAIX QAID RAID RAII RAIL RAIN SAID SAIL SAIS TAIL TAIS VAIL VAIN WAIF WAIL WAIN WAIT

•A•I
BACI BALI BANI BARI CADI CALI DALI DAVI FABI HAGI HAJI HALI HARI IASI JAMI KAKI KALI KAMI KARI KASI LANI LARI LAVI MAGI MAHI MALI MARI MAUI MAXI MAYI NABI NASI NAZI PALI PARI RABI RAII RAMI RANI RAVI SAKI SAMI SANI SARI SATI TABI TALI TAMI TATI TAVI TAXI VAGI WADI WASI

••AI
AKAI ALAI BNAI CHAI ESAI KWAI OJAI QUAI THAI VRAI

AJ••
AJAR AJAX AJIS AJOS

A•J•
ADJS ADJT

A••J
AMAJ

•AJ•
BAJA BAJO FAJA HAJE HAJI HAJJ JAJA MAJA MAJS RAJA TAJO

•A•J
HADJ HAJJ

••AJ
AMAJ BMAJ CMAJ DMAJ EMAJ FMAJ GMAJ

AK••
AKAI AKAS AKIM AKIN AKIO

A•K•
ALKA ALKI ALKY ANKA ANKE ANKH AOKI AOKS ARKS ARKY ASKS ATKA AUKS

A••K
ADAK ALEK AMOK ASOK ATIK

•AK•
BAKE BAKR BAKU CAKE CAKY FAKE HAKE JAKE KAKI LAKE LAKY MAKE MAKO OAKS OAKY RAKE RAKU SAKE SAKI SAKS TAKA TAKE WAKA WAKE YAKS

•A•K
BACK BALK BANK BARK BASK CALK CASK DANK DARK FALK GAWK HACK HAIK HANK HARK HAWK JACK LACK LANK LARK MACK MARK MASK NARK PACK PARK RACK RANK SACK SALK SANK SARK SASK SAUK TACK TALK TANK TASK WACK WALK YANK ZACK

••AK
ADAK BEAK DOAK FLAK ISAK LEAK NDAK PEAK SDAK SOAK SWAK TEAK WEAK

AL••
ALAE ALAI ALAN ALAR ALAS ALBA ALBS ALCS ALDA ALDO ALDS ALEA ALEC ALEE ALEF ALEK ALEN ALER ALES ALEX ALFA ALGA ALIA ALIF ALII ALIT ALIX ALKA ALKI ALKY ALLA ALLE ALLO ALLS ALLY ALMA ALMS ALOE ALOP ALOT ALOU ALOW ALPE ALPH ALPO ALPS ALSO ALTA ALTE ALTI ALTO ALTS ALUI ALUM ALVA ALVY ALYN

A•L•
ABLE ABLY ACLU AILE AILS ALLA ALLE ALLO ALLS ALLY ARLO ATLE ATLI AULD AWLS AXLE AYLA

A••L
ABEL ADDL AGAL AMUL AMYL ANIL APPL ARAL ARIL ARYL AUEL AVAL AWOL AXEL AXIL AZUL

•AL•
BALA BALD BALE BALI BALK BALL BALM BALS BALT CALC CALE CALF CALI CALK CALL CALM CALS CALX DALE DALI DALS DALY FALA FALK FALL GALA GALE GALL GALS GALT HALE HALF HALI HALL HALO HALS HALT KALB KALE KALI LALL LALO MALA MALE MALI MALL MALO MALT NALA PALE PALI PALL PALM PALO PALP PALS RALE RALL SALA SALE SALK SALS SALT TALA TALC TALE TALI TALK TALL VALE VALO WALD WALE WALK WALL WALT YALE YALL YALU ZALE

•A•L
BAAL BAIL BALL BAWL CALL CARL CAUL DAHL DAIL DANL EARL FAIL FALL GAEL GAIL GALL GAOL GAUL HAIL HALL HAUL JAIL KAEL KARL LALL MAIL MALL MARL MAUL NACL NAIL NASL NATL PAIL PALL PARL PAUL PAWL RAIL RALL RAUL SAHL SAIL SAML SAUL TAAL TAEL TAIL TALL VAIL WAHL WAIL WALL YALL YAWL

••AL
AGAL ARAL AVAL BAAL COAL CUAL DEAL DHAL DIAL DUAL EGAL ELAL ERAL ETAL EVAL FOAL GOAL HEAL ICAL ITAL KCAL LEAL MEAL NEAL OPAL ORAL OVAL PEAL REAL RIAL RYAL SEAL SIAL TAAL TEAL UCAL URAL VEAL VIAL WEAL ZEAL

AM••
AMAH AMAJ AMAS AMAT AMBI AMBO AMBS AMCS AMEN AMER AMES AMEX AMFM AMIC AMID AMIE AMII AMIN AMIR AMIS AMMO AMNT AMOI AMOK AMON AMOR AMOS AMOY AMPS AMSO AMTS AMUL AMUR AMYL

A•M•
ABMS ACME ADMS AHME AIME AIMS ALMA ALMS AMMO ARMA ARME ARMS ARMY ATMO ATMS AYME

A••M
ADAM AHEM AHUM AKIM ALUM AMFM ANIM ARAM ARUM ATOM

•AM•
BAMA BAMS CAMA CAME CAMO CAMP CAMS DAMA DAME DAMN DAMP DAMS FAMA FAME FAMS GAMA GAME GAMP GAMS GAMY HAMA HAME HAMM HAMP HAMS IAMB IAMS JAMA JAMB JAMI JAMS KAMA KAMI LAMA LAMB LAME LAMP LAMS MAMA MAME MAMS NAME NAMU RAMA RAMI RAMP RAMS SAME SAMI SAML SAMP SAMS TAMA TAME TAMI TAMP TAMS VAMP YAMS

•A•M
BALM BARM BAUM CALM FAIM FARM HAIM HAMM HARM MAAM MAIM MARM PALM RADM TASM VADM WARM

••AM
ADAM ARAM BEAM BLAM BRAM BYAM CLAM CRAM DIAM DRAM EDAM ELAM EXAM FLAM FOAM FRAM GLAM GRAM GUAM IMAM KIAM LIAM LOAM MAAM NOAM OGAM PRAM QUAM REAM ROAM SCAM SEAM SHAM SIAM SLAM SPAM SWAM TEAM TRAM WHAM

AN••
ANAG ANAS ANAT ANCE ANCY ANDS ANDY ANES ANEW ANGA ANGE ANIL ANIM ANIS ANKA ANKE ANKH ANNA ANNE ANNI ANNO ANNY ANOA ANON ANSA ANSE ANTA ANTE ANTH ANTI ANTS ANTZ ANYA

A•N•
ACNE AGNI AINT AINU AMNT ANNA ANNE ANNI ANNO ANNY AONE ARNE ARNO ATNO AUNG AUNT AWNS AWNY

A••N
ADDN ADEN ADIN AEON AGIN AGON AKIN ALAN ALEN ALYN AMEN AMIN AMON ANON ARAN ARON ASSN ATEN ATON ATTN AVON AXON AYIN AZAN

•AN•
BANC BAND BANE BANG BANI BANK BANO BANS CANA CANE CANS CANT CANY DANA DANE DANG DANK DANL DANO DANS FANE FANG FANS GANG GANN GANT HANA HAND HANG HANK HANS IANA JANA JANE JANN JANS KANA KANE KANG KANS KANT LANA LAND LANE LANG LANI LANK LANO LANS MANE MANN MANO MANS MANX MANY NANA NANG NANO NANU PANE PANG PANS PANT RANA RAND RANG RANI RANK RANN RANS RANT SANA SAND SANE SANG SANI SANK SANS SANT TANA TANG TANH TANK TANS VANE VANS WAND WANE WANG WANT WANY YANG YANK ZANE ZANT ZANY

•A•N
BAHN BAIN BARN CAAN CAEN CAHN CAIN CAPN DAIN DAMN DARN DAWN EARN FAIN FAUN FAWN GAIN GANN GARN HAHN HAWN JAIN JANN JAUN KAHN KAON KARN LAIN LAWN MAIN MANN PAIN PAON PAWN RAIN RANN SAWN TARN VAIN WAIN WARN YARN YAWN ZAHN

••AN
ALAN ARAN AZAN BEAN BRAN CAAN CHAN CLAN CRAN CYAN DEAN DIAN DWAN DYAN EBAN EGAN ELAN EOAN EVAN EWAN FLAN FRAN GIAN GMAN GRAN ICAN IMAN IRAN IVAN JEAN JOAN JUAN KEAN KHAN KLAN KOAN KWAN LEAN LOAN MCAN MEAN MOAN OBAN OLAN OMAN ONAN ORAN PLAN PRAN ROAN RYAN SCAN SEAN SHAN SIAN SPAN STAN SWAN THAN TMAN ULAN URAN WEAN XIAN YEAN YUAN

AO••
AOKI AOKS AONE AORB AORT AOUT

A•O•
ABOU ADOS AEON AGOG AGON AHOY AJOS ALOE ALOP ALOT ALOU ALOW AMOI AMOK AMON AMOR AMOS AMOY ANOA ANON APOC APOD APOP APOS AROA AROD ARON AROO AROW ASOF ASOK ASOR ATOI ATOM ATON ATOP ATOR ATOZ AVON AVOS AVOW AWOL AXON AZOV

A••O
ACRO ACTO AERO AFRO AGIO AGRO AHSO AKIO ALDO ALLO ALPO ALSO ALTO AMBO AMMO AMSO ANNO APSO ARCO AREO ARGO ARLO ARNO AROO ASTO ATCO ATMO ATNO ATTO AUTO

•AO•
GAOL HAOS KAON KAOS LAOS NAOH NAOS PAON TAOS

•A•O
BABO BACO BAIO BAJO BANO BARO CABO CACO CAMO CAPO CARO CATO DABO DADO DANO DATO DAYO FADO FARO FASO GARO GATO HALO IAGO JATO KARO KATO KAYO LAGO LALO LANO MAIO MAKO MALO MANO MATO MAYO MAZO NANO NASO NATO PACO PAGO PALO PASO PATO PAVO RADO SABO SACO SADO SAGO SATO TACO TAJO TARO TAXO VALO VARO VASO WACO

••AO
BIAO CHAO CIAO ISAO LIAO PIAO REAO

AP••
APAR APBS APED APER APES APEX APIA APIS APOC APOD APOP APOS APPL APPS APPT APRS APSE APSO APTS APUS

A•P•
ALPE ALPH ALPO ALPS AMPS APPL APPS APPT ARPA ARPS ASPS

A••P
AARP ACUP ALOP APOP ARAP ASAP ATIP ATOP

•AP•
BAPS BAPT CAPA CAPE CAPN CAPO CAPP CAPS CAPT DAPS GAPE GAPS HAPS JAPE KAPH LAPD LAPP LAPS MAPS NAPA NAPE NAPS PAPA PAPP PAPS RAPA RAPH RAPS RAPT SAPP SAPS TAPA TAPE TAPS YAPS ZAPS

•A•P
AARP CAMP CAPP CARP DAMP EARP FACP GAMP GARP GASP GAWP HAMP HARP HASP LAMP LAPP PALP PAPP RAMP RASP SAMP SAPP TAMP TARP VAMP WARP WASP YAWP

••AP
ARAP ASAP CHAP CLAP EVAP FLAP HEAP HRAP KNAP LEAP NEAP REAP RHAP SLAP SNAP SOAP SWAP TRAP WHAP WRAP

AQ••
AQUA AQUI

•AQ•
FAQS

••AQ
IRAQ SHAQ

AR••
ARAB ARAD ARAL ARAM ARAN ARAP ARAS ARBS ARCA ARCH ARCO ARCS AREA AREO ARES ARFS ARGO ARIA ARID ARIE ARIL ARIZ ARKS ARKY ARLO ARMA ARME ARMS ARMY ARNE ARNO AROA AROD ARON AROO AROW ARPA ARPS ARRS ARTA ARTE ARTI ARTS ARTY ARUM ARYE ARYL

A•R•
AARE AARP ABRA ABRI ACRE ACRO AERI AERO AERY AFRO AGRA AGRI AGRO AIRE AIRS AIRY AORB AORT APRS ARRS ATRA ATRI AURA AURI AWRY

A••R
ABBR ABER ACAR ACER ADAR ADDR AFAR AGAR AGER AJAR ALAR ALER AMER AMIR AMOR AMUR APAR APER ASIR ASOR ASTR ATAR ATOR AUER AVER AXER AYER AZUR

•AR•
AARE AARP BARA BARB BARD BARE BARI BARK BARM BARN BARO BARR BARS BART CARA CARB CARD CARE CARL CARO CARP CARR CARS CART CARY DARA DARC DARE DARK DARN DART EARL EARN EARP EARS FARE FARM FARO FARR GARB GARD GARE GARN GARO GARP GARR GARS GARY HARA HARD HARE HARI HARK HARM HARP HART HARZ JARS KARA KARI KARL KARN KARO KART LARA LARC LARD LARI LARK LARS LARY MARA MARC MARE MARG MARI MARK MARL MARM MARS MART MARU MARV MARX MARY MARZ NARA NARC NARD NARK NARY NARZ OARS PARA PARC PARD PARE PARI PARK PARL PARR PARS PART RARA RARE SARA SARD SARG SARI SARK TARA TARE TARN TARO TARP TARS TART VARO VARY WARD WARE WARM WARN WARP WARS WART WARY YARD YARE YARN ZARA ZARF

•A•R
BAER BAKR BARR CARR FAHR FAIR FARR GARR GAUR HAIR JAGR JAHR LAHR LAIR MACR MATR MAWR NAIR NATR PAAR PAIR PARR PATR SAAR SADR SAUR TAUR WAHR

••AR
ACAR ADAR AFAR AGAR AJAR ALAR APAR ATAR BEAR BOAR CHAR CLAR CZAR DEAR ESAR FEAR GEAR GNAR GUAR HBAR HEAR HOAR IBAR ISAR ITAR IVAR IYAR JBAR KCAR KEAR KNAR LBAR LEAR LIAR NCAR NEAR OMAR OSAR PAAR PEAR PHAR QUAR REAR ROAR SAAR SCAR SEAR SHAR SOAR SPAR STAR TBAR TEAR THAR TSAR TZAR ULAR USAR WEAR YEAR ZBAR

AS••
ASAP ASCH ASCI ASEA ASES ASHE ASHY ASIA ASIE ASIF ASIR ASIS ASKS ASOF ASOK ASOR ASPS ASSN ASST ASTA ASTI ASTO ASTR

A•S•
AASE AGST AHSO ALSO AMSO ANSA ANSE APSE APSO ASSN ASST AUST

A••S
AAAS AAHS ABAS ABCS ABMS ACCS ACES ACIS ACTS ADCS ADDS ADES ADJS ADMS ADOS AFBS AFTS AGAS AGES AGIS AGTS AHAS AIDS AILS AIMS AIRS AITS AJIS AJOS AKAS ALAS ALBS ALCS ALDS ALES ALLS ALMS ALPS ALTS AMAS AMBS AMCS AMES AMIS AMOS AMPS AMTS ANAS ANDS ANES ANIS ANTS AOKS APBS APES APIS APOS APPS APRS APTS APUS ARAS ARBS ARCS ARES ARFS ARKS ARMS ARPS ARRS ARTS ASES ASIS ASKS ASPS ATES ATIS ATMS ATTS ATVS AUGS AUKS AVES AVGS AVIS AVOS AWES AWLS AWNS AXES AXIS AYES

•AS•
AASE BASE BASF BASH BASK BASS BAST CASA CASE CASH CASK CASS CAST CASY DASH EASE EAST EASY FASO FAST GASH GASP GASX HASH HASP HAST IASI KASI LASE LASH LASS LAST MASA MASC MASH MASK MASS MAST NASA NASD NASH NASI NASL NASO NAST OAST PASA PASE PASH PASO PASS PAST RASA RASE RASH RASP SASE SASH SASK SASS TASK TASM TASS VASA VASE VASO VAST WASH WASI WASP WASS WAST ZASU

•A•S
AAAS AAHS BAAS BABS BACS BADS BAGS BAHS BALS BAMS BANS BAPS BARS BASS BATS BAYS CABS CADS CALS CAMS CANS CAPS CARS CASS CATS CAVS CAWS CAYS DABS DADS DAHS DAIS DALS DAMS DANS DAPS DAUS DAWS DAYS DAZS EADS EARS EATS FACS FADS FAMS FANS FAQS FATS FAYS GABS GADS GAGS GALS GAMS GAPS GARS GATS HAAS HABS HAGS HAHS HALS HAMS HANS HAOS HAPS HATS HAUS HAWS HAYS IAMS JABS JACS JAGS JAMS JANS JARS JAWS JAYS KAFS KANS KAOS KAYS LABS LACS LADS LAGS LAIS LAMS LANS LAOS LAPS LARS LASS LATS LAVS LAWS LAYS MAAS MACS MADS MAGS MAIS MAJS MAMS MANS MAPS MARS MASS MATS MAUS MAVS MAWS MAYS NABS NAES NAGS NAHS NAOS NAPS NATS NAYS OAFS OAKS OARS OATS PACS PADS PAHS PAIS PALS PANS PAPS PARS PASS PATS PAWS PAYS QAFS QATS RADS RAGS RAHS RAMS RANS RAPS RATS RAYS SACS SAES SAGS SAIS SAKS SALS SAMS SANS SAPS SASS SATS SAWS SAYS TABS TACS TADS TAGS TAIS TAMS TANS TAOS TAPS TARS TASS TATS TAUS TAVS TAWS VACS VAGS VANS VATS VAVS WACS WADS WAFS WAGS WAHS WARS WASS WATS WAWS WAYS YAKS YAMS YAPS YAWS YAYS ZAGS ZAPS

••AS
AAAS ABAS AGAS AHAS AKAS ALAS AMAS ANAS ARAS BAAS BBAS BFAS BIAS BLAS BOAS BRAS CHAS CPAS DBAS DIAS DNAS ELAS ERAS ESAS ETAS EVAS FRAS GOAS GPAS GRAS HAAS IRAS KEAS KHAS KIAS KOAS LEAS MAAS MBAS MEAS MFAS MIAS MOAS OCAS ODAS OLAS ORAS OSAS PDAS PEAS PSAS PTAS PYAS RCAS RDAS RIAS RNAS RYAS SEAS SOAS SPAS SRAS STAS TEAS TIAS TRAS TWAS UNAS XMAS YEAS

AT••
ATAD ATAR ATCO ATEN ATES ATIC ATIK ATIP ATIS ATIT ATKA ATLE ATLI ATMO ATMS ATNO ATOI ATOM ATON ATOP ATOR ATOZ ATRA ATRI ATTA ATTN ATTO ATTS ATTU ATTY ATVS ATWT

A•T•
ACTA ACTE ACTH ACTI ACTO ACTS ACTV AFTA AFTS AGTS AITS ALTA ALTE ALTI ALTO ALTS AMTS ANTA ANTE ANTH ANTI ANTS ANTZ APTS ARTA ARTE ARTI ARTS ARTY ASTA ASTI ASTO ASTR ATTA ATTN ATTO ATTS ATTU ATTY AUTH AUTO

A••T
ABET ABIT ABUT ACCT ACHT ADIT ADJT AGST AINT ALIT ALOT AMAT AMNT ANAT AORT AOUT APPT ASST ATIT ATWT AUNT AUST

•AT•
BATE BATH BATS BATT BATU CATE CATH CATO CATS CATT CATV DATA DATE DATO EATS FATA FATE FATH FATS GATE GATO GATS GATT HATE HATH HATS JATO KATA KATE KATO KATT KATY KATZ LATE LATH LATS MATA MATE MATH MATO MATR MATS MATT NATE NATL NATO NATR NATS OATH OATS OATY PATE PATH PATO PATR PATS QATS RATA RATE RATS SATB

SATE
SATI
SATO
SATS
TATA
TATE
TATI
TATS
VATS
VATU
WATS
WATT

•A•T
BACT
BAHT
BAIT
BALT
BAPT
BART
BAST
BATT
CANT
CAPT
CART
CAST
CATT
DAFT
DART
EAST
FACT
FAIT
FAST
FAUT
GAIT
GALT
GANT
GATT
HAFT
HALT
HART
HAST
HAUT
KAAT
KANT
KART
KATT
LACT
LAIT
LAST
MALT
MART
MAST
MATT
NAST
NAUT
OAST
PACT
PANT
PART
PAST
PAYT
RAFT
RANT
RAPT
SALT
SANT
TACT
TAFT
TART
TAUT
TAWT
VAST
WAFT
WAIT
WALT
WANT
WART
WAST
WATT
ZANT

••AT
AMAT
ANAT
BEAT
BHAT
BLAT
BOAT
BRAT
CHAT
COAT
CRAT
DRAT
ELAT
ERAT
ETAT
FEAT
FIAT
FLAT
FRAT
GHAT
GMAT
GNAT
GOAT
GUAT
HEAT
KAAT
KYAT
LIAT
LSAT
MCAT
MEAT
MOAT
NEAT
NHAT
NLAT
OMAT
PEAT
PHAT
PLAT
PRAT
PSAT
QUAT
SCAT
SEAT
SKAT
SLAT
SPAT
STAT
SWAT
TEAT
THAT
TOAT
WHAT

AU••
AUBE
AUDE
AUDI
AUEL
AUER
AUGS
AUKS
AULD
AUNG
AUNT
AURA
AURI
AUST
AUTH
AUTO

A•U•
ABUT
ACUP
ADUE
AGUA
AGUE
AHUM
ALUI
ALUM
AMUL
AMUR
AOUT
APUS
AQUA
AQUI
ARUM
AZUL
AZUR

A••U
ABOU
ACLU
AINU
ALOU
ATTU

•AU•
BAUD
BAUM
CAUD
CAUL
DAUB
DAUS
EAUX
FAUN
FAUT
FAUX
GAUD
GAUL
GAUR
HAUL
HAUS
HAUT
JAUN
LAUD
LAUE
MAUD
MAUI
MAUL
MAUS
NAUT
PAUL
RAUL
SAUD
SAUK
SAUL
SAUR
TAUR
TAUS
TAUT
VAUD
VAUX

•A•U
BABU
BADU
BAKU
BATU
MARU
NAMU
NANU
OAHU
RAGU
RAKU
SABU
TABU
VATU
YALU
ZAFU
ZASU

••AU
BEAU
BLAU
ESAU
FRAU
GRAU
LUAU
PEAU
SEAU
UNAU
VEAU

AV••
AVAL
AVEC
AVER
AVES
AVGS
AVIA
AVID
AVIS
AVIV
AVON
AVOS
AVOW

A•V•
ALVA
ALVY
ATVS

A••V
ACTV
AVIV
AZOV

•AV•
CAVA
CAVE
CAVS
CAVY
DAVE
DAVI
DAVY
EAVE
FAVA
FAVE
GAVE
HAVA
HAVE
JAVA
KAVA
LAVA
LAVE
LAVI
LAVS
MAVS
NAVE
NAVY
PAVE
PAVO
RAVE
RAVI
SAVE
TAVI
TAVS
VAVS
WAVE
WAVY

•A•V
CATV
MARV

••AV
BEAV
OLAV
SLAV

AW••
AWAG
AWAY
AWED
AWES
AWLS
AWNS
AWNY
AWOL
AWRY

A•W•
AIWA
ATWT

A••W
AFEW
ALOW
ANEW
AROW
AVOW

•AW•
BAWL
CAWS
DAWG
DAWN
DAWS
FAWN
GAWK
GAWP
HAWG
HAWK
HAWN
HAWS
JAWS
LAWD
LAWN
LAWS
MAWR
MAWS
PAWL
PAWN
PAWS
SAWN
SAWS
TAWS
TAWT
WAWA
WAWS
YAWL
YAWN
YAWP
YAWS

••AW
CHAW
CLAW
CRAW
DRAW
FLAW
GNAW
SHAW
SLAW
THAW

AX••
AXED
AXEL
AXER
AXES
AXIL
AXIS
AXLE
AXON

A••X
AJAX
ALEX
ALIX
AMEX
APEX

•AX•
MAXI
MAXX
SAXE
TAXA
TAXI
TAXO
TAXY
WAXY

•A•X
CALX
EAUX
FAUX
GASX
MANX
MARX
MAXX
PAIX
VAUX

••AX
AJAX
COAX
DRAX
EFAX
FLAX
HOAX
IMAX
KPAX
PLAX
SFAX
SNAX
TMAX
TRAX

AY••
AYAH
AYDE
AYER
AYES
AYIN
AYLA
AYME

A•Y•
ALYN
AMYL
ANYA
ARYE
ARYL

A••Y
ABBY
ABLY
ACEY
ACHY
ADAY
AERY
AGCY
AHOY
AIRY
ALKY
ALLY
ALVY
AMOY
ANCY
ANDY
ANNY
ARKY
ARMY
ARTY
ASHY
ATTY
AWAY
AWNY
AWRY

•AY•
BAYH
BAYS
CAYS
DAYO
DAYS
FAYE
FAYS
GAYE
HAYS
JAYE
JAYS
JAYZ
KAYE
KAYO
KAYS
LAYS
MAYA
MAYI
MAYO
MAYS
NAYA
NAYS
PAYS
PAYT
RAYE
RAYS
SAYS
TAYE
VAYA
WAYS
YAYS

•A•Y
BABY
CADY
CAGY
CAKY
CANY
CARY
CASY
CAVY
DALY
DAVY
EASY
GABY
GAMY
GARY
HAZY
KATY
LACY
LADY
LAKY
LARY
LAZY
MACY
MANY
MARY
MAZY
NAGY
NARY
NAVY
OAKY
OATY
RACY
SAGY
TAXY
VARY
WANY
WARY
WAVY
WAXY
ZANY

••AY
ADAY
AWAY
BDAY
BRAY
BWAY
CLAY
CRAY
DDAY
DRAY
EBAY
FLAY
FRAY
GDAY
GRAY
ISAY
ODAY
OKAY
OLAY
OTAY
PLAY
PRAY
QUAY
SHAY
SLAY
SPAY
STAY
SWAY
TRAY
TWAY
VDAY
WRAY
XRAY

AZ••
AZAN
AZIZ
AZOV
AZUL
AZUR

A•Z•
ADZE

A••Z
ANTZ
ARIZ
ATOZ
AZIZ

•AZ•
DAZE
DAZS
FAZE
GAZA
GAZE
HAZE
HAZY
JAZZ
LAZE
LAZY
MAZE
MAZO
MAZY
NAZI
RAZE
RAZZ
ZAZA

•A•Z
BAEZ
HARZ
JAYZ
JAZZ
KATZ
MARZ
NARZ
RAZZ

••AZ
BOAZ
BRAZ
DIAZ
GRAZ

BA••
BAAL
BAAS
BABA
BABE
BABO
BABS
BABU
BABY
BACA
BACH
BACI
BACK
BACO
BACS
BACT
BADD
BADE
BADS
BADU
BAER
BAEZ
BAFF
BAGS
BAHN
BAHS
BAHT
BAIE
BAIL
BAIN
BAIO
BAIT
BAJA
BAJO
BAKE
BAKR
BAKU
BALA
BALD
BALE
BALI
BALK
BALL
BALM
BALS
BALT
BAMA
BAMS
BANC
BAND
BANE
BANG
BANI
BANK
BANO
BANS
BAPS
BAPT
BARA
BARB
BARD
BARE
BARI
BARK
BARM
BARN
BARO
BARR
BARS
BART
BASE
BASF
BASH
BASK
BASS
BAST
BATE
BATH
BATS
BATT
BATU
BAUD
BAUM
BAWL
BAYH
BAYS

B•A•
BAAL
BAAS
BBAS
BDAY
BEAD
BEAH
BEAK
BEAM
BEAN
BEAR
BEAT
BEAU
BEAV
BFAS
BHAT
BIAO
BIAS
BLAB
BLAH
BLAM
BLAS
BLAT
BLAU
BMAJ
BNAI
BOAC
BOAR
BOAS
BOAT
BOAZ
BRAC
BRAD
BRAE
BRAG
BRAM
BRAN
BRAS
BRAT
BRAY
BRAZ
BWAY
BYAM

B••A
BABA
BACA
BAJA
BALA
BAMA
BARA
BEGA
BELA
BEMA
BETA
BIGA
BIWA
BOCA
BOLA
BONA
BORA
BOVA
BOWA
BREA
BUDA

•BA•
ABAA
ABAB
ABAS
BBAS
DBAS
EBAN
EBAY
HBAR
IBAR
JBAR
LBAR
MBAS
OBAD
OBAN
TBAR
ZBAR

•B•A
ABAA
ABBA
ABRA
OBRA

••BA
AABA
ABBA
ALBA
BABA
CUBA
DABA
ELBA
KABA
PABA
PEBA
REBA
SABA
SOBA
TUBA
WNBA
YUBA

BB••
BBAS
BBLS
BBOY
BBQS

B•B•
BABA
BABE
BABO
BABS
BABU
BABY
BEBE
BIBB
BIBI
BIBL
BIBS
BOBO
BOBS
BUBS

B••B
BARB
BEEB
BIBB
BLAB
BLEB
BLOB
BOMB
BOOB
BTOB
BULB
BURB
BYOB

•BB•
ABBA
ABBE
ABBR
ABBY
EBBS

•B•B
ABAB

••BB
BIBB
COBB
GIBB
HEBB
PIBB
ROBB
TUBB
WEBB

BC••
BCCS
BCDE
BCES
BCUP

B•C•
BACA
BACH
BACI
BACK
BACO
BACS
BACT
BCCS
BECH
BECK
BECS
BICS
BOCA
BOCK
BUCK
BUCO
BUCS

B••C
BANC
BLOC
BMOC
BOAC
BOSC
BRAC
BRIC

•BC•
ABCD
ABCS
RBCS

••BC
CNBC

BD••
BDAY
BDFT
BDLS
BDRM

B•D•
BADD
BADE
BADS
BADU
BCDE
BEDE
BEDS
BIDE
BIDS
BIDU
BLDG
BODE
BODS
BODY
BUDA
BUDD
BUDS
BVDS

B••D
BADD
BALD
BAND
BARD
BAUD
BEAD
BEND
BIGD
BIND
BIRD
BLED
BLVD
BOLD
BOND
BOYD
BRAD
BRED
BUDD
BUND
BYRD

•B•D
ABCD
ABED
IBID
OBAD

BE••
BEAD
BEAH
BEAK
BEAM
BEAN
BEAR
BEAT
BEAU
BEAV
BEBE
BECH
BECK
BECS
BEDE
BEDS
BEEB
BEEF
BEEM
BEEN
BEEP
BEER
BEES
BEET
BEGA
BEGS
BEIN
BELA
BELG
BELL
BELO
BELS
BELT
BELY
BEMA
BEMS
BEND
BENE
BENI
BENT
BENZ
BERG
BERM
BERN
BERT
BESO
BESS
BEST
BETA
BETE
BETH
BETS
BETZ
BEVS
BEVY
BEYS

B•E•
BAER
BAEZ
BCES
BEEB
BEEF
BEEM
BEEN
BEEP
BEER
BEES
BEET
BIEL
BIEN
BIER
BLEB
BLED
BLEU
BLEW
BMES
BNEG
BOER
BREA
BRED
BREE
BREI
BREL
BREN
BRER
BRET
BREW
BTEN
BYES

B••E
BABE
BADE
BAIE
BAKE
BALE
BANE
BARE
BASE
BATE
BCDE
BEBE
BEDE
BENE
BETE
BIDE
BIKE
BILE
BINE
BITE
BLUE
BODE
BOLE
BONE
BORE
BOSE
BOWE
BPOE
BRAE
BREE
BRIE
BYME
BYTE

•BE•
ABED
ABEL
ABER
ABET
CBER
EBEL
EBEN
GBES
IBET
IBEW
IBEX
MBES
OBER
OBES
OBEY
UBER

•B•E
ABBE
ABIE
ABLE
IBLE
OBIE
OBOE

••BE
ABBE
AUBE
BABE
BEBE
CUBE
ELBE
GABE
GIBE
HEBE
HOBE
JIBE
KOBE
LOBE
LUBE
NABE
RABE
ROBE
RUBE
SABE
TOBE
TUBE
VIBE
WABE

BF••
BFAS

B•F•
BAFF
BDFT
BIFF
BOFF
BUFF

B••F
BAFF
BASF
BEEF
BIFF
BOFF
BUFF

B•G•
BAGS
BEGA
BEGS
BIGA
BIGD
BIGO
BIGS
BOGS
BOGY
BUGS

B••G
BANG
BELG
BERG
BING
BIOG
BKPG
BLDG
BLOG
BNEG
BONG
BOOG
BORG
BRAG
BRIG
BULG
BUNG
BURG
BYNG

BH••
BHAT

B•H•
BAHN
BAHS
BAHT
BOHM
BOHO
BOHR

B••H
BACH
BASH
BATH
BAYH
BEAH
BECH
BETH
BLAH
BOSH
BOTH
BUSH

••BH
COBH

BI••
BIAO
BIAS
BIBB
BIBI
BIBL
BIBS
BICS
BIDE
BIDS
BIDU
BIEL
BIEN
BIER
BIFF
BIGA
BIGD
BIGO
BIGS
BIKE
BIKO
BILE
BILK
BILL
BILT
BIND
BINE
BING
BINS
BIOG
BIOL
BIOS
BIOT
BIRD
BIRL
BIRO
BIRR
BIST
BITE
BITS
BITT
BIWA

B•I•
BAIE
BAIL
BAIN
BAIO
BAIT
BEIN
BLIN
BLIP
BLIT
BOIL
BOIS
BRIC
BRIE
BRIG
BRIM

BRIO BRIT BRIX BSIX

B••I
BACI BALI BANI BARI BENI BIBI BNAI BREI

•BI•
ABIE ABIT IBID IBIS OBIE OBIS OBIT RBIS

•B•I
ABRI

••BI
AMBI BIBI DEBI FABI GOBI NABI RABI TABI

B•J•
BAJA BAJO

B••J
BMAJ

•BJ•
OBJS

••BJ
SUBJ

BK••
BKPG BKPR

B•K•
BAKE BAKR BAKU BIKE BIKO

B••K
BACK BALK BANK BARK BASK BEAK BECK BILK BLOK BOCK BONK BOOK BORK BUCK BULK BUNK BUSK

••BK
HDBK

BL••
BLAB BLAH BLAM BLAS BLAT BLAU BLDG BLEB BLED BLEU BLEW BLIN BLIP BLIT BLOB BLOC BLOG BLOK BLOT BLOW BLTS BLUE BLUM BLUR BLVD

B•L•
BALA BALD BALE BALI BALK BALL BALM BALS BALT BBLS BDLS BELA BELG BELL BELO BELS BELT BELY BILE BILK BILL BILT BOLA BOLD BOLE BOLL BOLO BOLT BULB BULG BULK BULL

B••L
BAAL BAIL BALL BAWL BELL BIBL BIEL BILL BIOL BIRL BOIL BOLL BOWL BREL BULL BURL

•BL•
ABLE ABLY BBLS DBLS IBLE IBLY

•B•L
ABEL EBEL OBOL

••BL
BIBL PUBL

BM••
BMAJ BMES BMOC BMUS BMWS

B•M•
BAMA BAMS BEMA BEMS BOMB BSMT BUMP BUMS BYME

B••M
BALM BARM BAUM BDRM BEAM BEEM BERM BLAM BLUM BOHM BOOM BRAM BRIM BROM BYAM

•BM•
ABMS IBMS

••BM
ICBM

BN••
BNAI BNEG

B•N•
BANC BAND BANE BANG BANI BANK BANO BANS BEND BENE BENI BENT BENZ BIND BINE BING BINS BONA BOND BONE BONG BONK BONN BONO BONT BONY BONZ BRNO BUND BUNG BUNK BUNS BUNT BYNG

B••N
BAHN BAIN BARN BEAN BEEN BEIN BERN BIEN BLIN BONN BOON BORN BOSN BRAN BREN BRON BRUN BRYN BTEN BUON BURN

•B•N
EBAN EBEN EBON OBAN

••BN
ISBN

BO••
BOAC BOAR BOAS BOAT BOAZ BOBO BOBS BOCA BOCK BODE BODS BODY BOER BOFF BOGS BOGY BOHM BOHO BOHR BOIL BOIS BOLA BOLD BOLE BOLL BOLO BOLT BOMB BONA BOND BONE BONG BONK BONN BONO BONT BONY BONZ BOOB BOOG BOOK BOOM BOON BOOP BOOR BOOS BOOT BOPP BOPS BORA BORE BORG BORK BORN BORO BORS BORU BOSC BOSE BOSH BOSN BOSS BOTH BOTS BOUT BOVA BOWA BOWE BOWL BOWS BOXY BOYD BOYO BOYS BOYZ BOZO

B•O•
BBOY BIOG BIOL BIOS BIOT BLOB BLOC BLOG BLOK BLOT BLOW BMOC BOOB BOOG BOOK BOOM BOON BOOP BOOR BOOS BOOT BPOE BROM BRON BROR BROS BROT BROW BROZ BTOB BUON BUOY BYOB

B••O
BABO BACO BAIO BAJO BANO BARO BELO BESO BIAO BIGO BIKO BIRO BOBO BOHO BOLO BONO BORO BOYO BOZO BRIO BRNO BTWO BUCO

•BO•
ABOU BBOY EBON IBOS LBOS OBOE OBOL XBOX YBOR

•B•O
EBRO

••BO
AMBO BABO BOBO CABO COBO DABO GOBO HOBO KOBO LOBO NEBO RIBO SABO

BP••
BPOE

B•P•
BAPS BAPT BKPG BKPR BOPP BOPS

B••P
BCUP BEEP BLIP BOOP BOPP BUMP BURP

•B•P
TBSP

B•Q•
BBQS

•BQ•
BBQS

BR••
BRAC BRAD BRAE BRAG BRAM BRAN BRAS BRAT BRAY BRAZ BREA BRED BREE BREI BREL BREN BRER BRET BREW BRIC BRIE BRIG BRIM BRIO BRIT BRIX BRNO BROM BRON BROR BROS BROT BROW BROZ BRRR BRUN BRUT BRUX BRYN

B•R•
BARA BARB BARD BARE BARI BARK BARM BARN BARO BARR BARS BART BDRM BERG BERM BERN BERT BIRD BIRL BIRO BIRR BORA BORE BORG BORK BORN BORO BORS BORU BRRR BURB BURG BURL BURN BURP BURR BURS BURT BURY BYRD

B••R
BAER BAKR BARR BEAR BEER BIER BIRR BKPR BLUR BOAR BOER BOHR BOOR BRER BROR BRRR BURR

•BR•
ABRA ABRI EBRO OBRA

•B•R
ABBR ABER CBER HBAR IBAR JBAR LBAR OBER TBAR UBER YBOR ZBAR

••BR
ABBR GRBR GTBR HEBR NEBR

BS••
BSIX BSMT

B•S•
BASE BASF BASH BASK BASS BAST BESO BESS BEST BIST BOSC BOSE BOSH BOSN BOSS BUSH BUSK BUSS BUST BUSY

B••S
BAAS BABS BACS BADS BAGS BAHS BALS BAMS BANS BAPS BARS BASS BATS BAYS BBAS BBLS BBQS BCCS BCES BDLS BECS BEDS BEES BEGS BELS BEMS BESS BETS BEVS BEYS BFAS BIAS BIBS BICS BIDS BIGS BINS BIOS BITS BLAS BLTS BMES BMUS BMWS BOAS BOBS BODS BOGS BOIS BOOS BOPS BORS BOSS BOTS BOWS BOYS BRAS BROS BTUS BUBS BUCS BUDS BUGS BUMS BUNS BURS BUSS BUTS BUYS BVDS BYES

•BS•
TBSP

•B•S
ABAS ABCS ABMS BBAS BBLS BBQS DBAS DBLS EBBS GBES IBIS IBMS IBOS LBOS MBAS MBES OBES OBIS OBJS RBCS RBIS

••BS
AFBS ALBS AMBS APBS ARBS BABS BIBS BOBS BUBS CABS COBS CUBS DABS DEBS DIBS DUBS EBBS EDBS FEBS FIBS FOBS GABS GIBS GOBS HABS HOBS HUBS JABS JIBS JOBS KOBS LABS LHBS LIBS LLBS LOBS MGBS MIBS MOBS NABS NEBS NIBS NOBS NUBS ORBS OTBS PCBS PUBS REBS RFBS RHBS RIBS ROBS RUBS SIBS SOBS SUBS TABS TUBS URBS USBS WEBS YOBS

BT••
BTEN BTOB BTUS BTWO

B•T•
BATE BATH BATS BATT BATU BETA BETE BETH BETS BETZ BITE BITS BITT BLTS BOTH BOTS BUTS BUTT BUTZ BYTE

B••T
BACT BAHT BAIT BALT BAPT BART BAST BATT BDFT BEAT BEET BELT BENT BERT BEST BHAT BILT BIOT BIST BITT BLAT BLIT BLOT BOAT BOLT BONT BOOT BOUT BRAT BRET BRIT BROT BRUT BSMT BUNT BURT BUST BUTT

•B•T
ABET ABIT ABUT IBET OBIT

••BT
DEBT ROBT

BU••
BUBS BUCK BUCO BUCS BUDA BUDD BUDS BUFF BUGS BULB BULG BULK BULL BUMP BUMS BUND BUNG BUNK BUNS BUNT BUON BUOY BURB BURG BURL BURN BURP BURR BURS BURT BURY BUSH BUSK BUSS BUST BUSY BUTS BUTT BUTZ BUYS BUZZ

B•U•
BAUD BAUM BCUP BLUE BLUM BLUR BMUS BOUT BRUN BRUT BRUX BTUS

B••U
BABU BADU BAKU BATU BEAU BIDU BLAU BLEU BORU

•BU•
ABUT

•B•U
ABOU

••BU
BABU CEBU FUBU SABU TABU ZEBU

BV••
BVDS

B•V•
BEVS BEVY BLVD BOVA

B••V
BEAV

BW••
BWAY

B•W•
BAWL BIWA BMWS BOWA BOWE BOWL BOWS BTWO

B••W
BLEW BLOW BREW BROW

•B•W
IBEW

B•X•
BOXY

B••X
BRIX BRUX BSIX

•B•X
IBEX XBOX

BY••
BYAM BYES BYME BYNG BYOB BYRD BYTE

B•Y•
BAYH BAYS BEYS BOYD BOYO BOYS BOYZ BRYN BUYS

B••Y
BABY BBOY BDAY BELY BEVY BODY BOGY BONY BOXY BRAY BUOY BURY BUSY BWAY

•B•Y
ABBY ABLY BBOY EBAY IBLY OBEY

••BY
ABBY BABY DOBY GABY GOBY IGBY MOBY NYBY RUBY TCBY TOBY

B•Z•
BOZO BUZZ

B••Z
BAEZ BENZ BETZ BOAZ BONZ BOYZ BRAZ BROZ BUTZ BUZZ

CA••
CAAN CABO CABS CACO CADE CADI CADS CADY CAEN CAFE CAGE CAGY CAHN CAIN CAKE CAKY CALC CALE CALF CALI CALK CALL CALM CALS CALX CAMA CAME CAMO CAMP CAMS CANA CANE CANS CANT CANY CAPA CAPE CAPN CAPO CAPP CAPS CAPT CARA CARB CARD CARE CARL CARO CARP CARR CARS CART CARY CASA CASE CASH CASK CASS CAST CASY CATE CATH CATO CATS CATT CATV CAUD CAUL CAVA CAVE CAVS CAVY CAWS CAYS

C•A•
CAAN CHAD CHAI CHAN CHAO CHAP CHAR CHAS CHAT CHAW CIAO CLAD CLAM CLAN CLAP CLAR CLAW CLAY CMAJ COAL COAT COAX CPAS CRAB CRAG CRAM CRAN CRAT CRAW CRAY CUAL CYAN CZAR

C••A
CAMA CANA CAPA CARA CASA CAVA CELA CENA CERA CETA CHIA CLEA COCA CODA COLA COMA COPA CORA COSA COXA CSEA CUBA CYMA

•CA•
ACAD ACAR ICAL ICAN KCAL KCAR MCAN MCAT NCAA NCAR OCAS RCAF RCAS SCAB SCAD SCAM SCAN SCAR SCAT UCAL

•C•A
ACTA ECUA NCAA OCTA UCLA

••CA
ARCA BACA BOCA COCA DECA FICA FUCA INCA LOCA MICA ORCA PACA PICA RICA ROCA SICA SOCA SPCA UNCA VACA YMCA YWCA

CB••
CBER

C•B•
CABO CABS CEBU CNBC COBB COBH COBO COBS CUBA CUBE CUBS

C••B
CARB
CHUB
CLUB
COBB
COMB
CRAB
CREB
CRIB
CURB

•CB•
ICBM
PCBS
TCBY

•C•B
SCAB

CC••
CCCI
CCCL
CCCP
CCCV
CCCX
CCED
CCII
CCIV
CCIX
CCLI
CCLV
CCLX
CCNY
CCUP
CCUS
CCVI
CCXC
CCXI
CCXL
CCXV
CCXX

C•C•
CACO
CCCI
CCCL
CCCP
CCCV
CCCX
CECE
CECI
CFCS
COCA
COCK
COCO
CXCI
CXCV
CYCL

C••C
CALC
CCXC
CDXC
CHIC
CHOC
CINC
CIRC
CMXC
CNBC
COFC
CONC
CROC

•CC•
ACCS
ACCT
BCCS
CCCI
CCCL
CCCP
CCCV
CCCX
DCCC
DCCI
DCCL
DCCV
DCCX
ECCE
ECCL
ECCO
MCCC
MCCI
MCCL
MCCV
MCCX

•C•C
ACDC
CCXC
DCCC
DCXC
MCCC
MCXC
SCLC

••CC
DCCC
MCCC
MDCC
MMCC
SNCC

CD••
CDEF
CDII
CDIV
CDIX
CDLI
CDLV
CDLX
CDRS
CDVI
CDXC
CDXI
CDXL
CDXV
CDXX

C•D•
CADE
CADI
CADS
CADY
CEDE
CEDI
CIDE
CMDG
CMDR
CODA
CODE
CODS
CODY
CUDS

C••D
CARD
CAUD
CCED
CHAD
CHID
CLAD
CLOD
COED
COLD
COND
CORD
CRED
CRUD
CUED
CURD
CUYD

•CD•
ACDC
BCDE
LCDS
MCDI
MCDL
MCDV
MCDX

•C•D
ACAD
ACED
ACID
CCED
ICED
SCAD
SCUD

••CD
ABCD
MMCD
ONCD
RECD

CE••
CEBU
CECE
CECI
CEDE
CEDI
CEES
CEIL
CELA
CELL
CELS
CELT
CENA
CENE
CENO
CENS
CENT
CEOS
CEPE
CEPS
CERA
CERE
CERF
CERO
CERT
CESS
CEST
CETA
CETE
CETO

C•E•
CAEN
CBER
CCED
CDEF
CEES
CHEE
CHEF
CHEM
CHEN
CHER
CHET
CHEW
CHEX
CHEZ
CIEL
CIEN
CLEA
CLEF
CLEM
CLEO
CLEW
COED
COEN
CREB
CRED
CREE
CREO
CREW
CSEA
CTEN
CUED
CUER
CUES

C••E
CADE
CAFE
CAGE
CAKE
CALE
CAME
CANE
CAPE
CARE
CASE
CATE
CAVE
CECE
CEDE
CENE
CEPE
CERE
CETE
CHEE
CIDE
CINE
CIRE
CITE
CLUE
CMTE
CODE
COKE
COLE
COME
CONE
COPE
CORE
COTE
COUE
COVE
CREE
CRUE
CUBE
CUKE
CULE
CUME
CURE
CUTE
CYME
CYTE

•CE•
ACED
ACER
ACES
ACEY
BCES
CCED
ICED
ICEE
ICEL
ICER
ICES
ICET

•C•E
ACHE
ACME
ACNE
ACRE
ACTE
BCDE
ECCE
ICEE

••CE
ANCE
CECE
DACE
DICE
DOCE
DUCE
DYCE
ECCE
ENCE
ESCE
FACE
FYCE
INCE
LACE
LICE
LUCE
MACE
MICE
NICE
ONCE
PACE
PICE
PUCE
RACE
RICE
VICE
VOCE
WACE

CF••
CFCS
CFOS

C•F•
CAFE
COFC
COFS
CUFF
CUFT

C••F
CALF
CDEF
CERF
CHEF
CLEF
COIF
CONF
CUFF

•C•F
RCAF

C•G•
CAGE
CAGY
CHGS
CIGS
COGS

C••G
CHUG
CLOG
CMDG
CONG
CRAG

•CG•
ECGS

••CG
USCG

CH••
CHAD
CHAI
CHAN
CHAO
CHAP
CHAR
CHAS
CHAT
CHAW
CHEE
CHEF
CHEM
CHEN
CHER
CHET
CHEW
CHEX
CHEZ
CHGS
CHIA
CHIC
CHID
CHIM
CHIN
CHIP
CHIS
CHIT
CHMN
CHOC
CHOL
CHON
CHOO
CHOP
CHOU
CHOW
CHOY
CHUB
CHUG
CHUM

C•H•
CAHN
COHN
COHO

C••H
CASH
CATH
COBH
COSH
CUSH

•CH•
ACHE
ACHT
ACHY
ECHO
ECHT
OCHO
OCHS
TCHR

•C•H
ACTH

••CH
ARCH
ASCH
BACH
BECH
EACH
ETCH
EXCH
FOCH
HOCH
INCH
ITCH
KOCH
LECH
LOCH
MACH
MECH
MICH
MUCH
ORCH
OUCH
RICH
SUCH
TACH
TECH
YECH
ZACH
ZECH

CI••
CIAO
CIDE
CIEL
CIEN
CIGS
CIII
CINC
CINE
CINQ
CION
CIRC
CIRE
CIST
CITE
CITO
CITY

C•I•
CAIN
CCII
CCIV
CCIX
CDII
CDIV
CDIX
CEIL
CHIA
CHIC
CHID
CHIM
CHIN
CHIP
CHIS
CHIT
CIII
CLII
CLIO
CLIP
CLIV
CLIX
CMII
CMIV
CMIX
COIF
COIL
COIN
COIR
COIT
CRIB
CRIN
CRIT
CUIN
CVII
CXII
CXIV
CXIX

C••I
CADI
CALI
CCCI
CCII
CCLI
CCVI
CCXI
CDII
CDLI
CDVI
CDXI
CECI
CEDI
CHAI
CIII
CLII
CLVI
CLXI
CMII
CMLI
CMVI
CMXI
COLI
CORI
COSI
CVII
CXCI
CXII
CXLI
CXVI
CXXI

•CI•
ACID
ACIS
CCII
CCIV
CCIX
DCII
DCIL
DCIV
DCIX
MCII
MCIV
MCIX
SCIS
XCII
XCIV
XCIX

•C•I
ACTI
CCCI
CCII
CCLI
CCVI
CCXI
DCCI
DCII
DCLI
DCVI
DCXI
MCCI
MCDI
MCII
MCLI
MCMI
MCVI
MCXI
XCII
XCVI

••CI
ASCI
BACI
CCCI
CECI
CXCI
DCCI
DECI
DXCI
FOCI
LOCI
LUCI
MCCI
MDCI
MMCI
MXCI
VICI

C•J•
CUJO

C••J
CMAJ
CONJ

C•K•
CAKE
CAKY
COKE
COKY
CUKE

C••K
CALK
CASK
COCK
CONK
COOK
CORK
CUSK

•CK•
ICKY

••CK
BACK
BECK
BOCK
BUCK
COCK
DECK
DICK
DOCK
DUCK
DYCK
EYCK
GUCK
HACK
HECK
HICK
HOCK
HUCK
JACK
JOCK
KICK
LACK
LICK
LOCK
LUCK
MACK
MICK
MOCK
MUCK
NECK
NICK
NOCK
PACK
PECK
PICK
PUCK
RACK
RECK
RICK
ROCK
RUCK
SACK
SICK
SOCK
SUCK
TACK
TICK
TOCK
TUCK
WACK
WICK
YUCK
ZACK

CL••
CLAD
CLAM
CLAN
CLAP
CLAR
CLAW
CLAY
CLEA
CLEF
CLEM
CLEO
CLEW
CLII
CLIO
CLIP
CLIV
CLIX
CLOD
CLOG
CLOP
CLOT
CLOY
CLUB
CLUE
CLVI
CLXI
CLXV
CLXX
CLYM

C•L•
CALC
CALE
CALF
CALI
CALK
CALL
CALM
CALS
CALX
CCLI
CCLV
CCLX
CDLI
CDLV
CDLX
CELA
CELL
CELS
CELT
CMLI
CMLV
CMLX
COLA
COLD
COLE
COLI
COLL
COLM
COLO
COLS
COLT
CPLS
CULE
CULL
CULP
CULT
CXLI
CXLV
CYLS

C••L
CALL
CARL
CAUL
CCCL
CCXL
CDXL
CEIL
CELL
CHOL
CIEL
CMXL
COAL
COIL
COLL
COOL
COWL
CTRL
CUAL
CULL
CURL
CYCL

•CL•
ACLU
CCLI
CCLV
CCLX
DCLI
DCLV
DCLX
MCLI
MCLV
MCLX
SCLC
UCLA

•C•L
CCCL
CCXL
DCCL
DCIL
DCXL
ECCL
ECOL
ICAL
ICEL
KCAL
MCCL
MCDL
MCML
MCXL
OCUL
UCAL

••CL
CCCL
CYCL
DCCL
ECCL
ENCL
EXCL
INCL
MCCL
MDCL
MMCL
NACL

CM••
CMAJ
CMDG
CMDR
CMII
CMIV
CMIX
CMLI
CMLV
CMLX
CMON
CMTE
CMVI
CMXC
CMXI
CMXL
CMXV
CMXX

C•M•
CAMA
CAME
CAMO
CAMP
CAMS
CHMN
COMA
COMB
COME
COMM
COMO
COMP
COMS
CUME
CWMS
CYMA
CYME

C••M
CALM
CHEM
CHIM
CHUM
CLAM
CLEM
CLYM
COLM
COMM
CORM
COSM
CRAM

•CM•
ACME
DCMS
LCMS
MCMI
MCML
MCMV
MCMX
RCMP

•C•M
ICBM
SCAM
SCUM

••CM
MMCM

CN••
CNBC
CNUT

C•N•
CANA
CANE
CANS
CANT
CANY
CCNY
CENA
CENE
CENO
CENS
CENT
CINC
CINE
CINQ
CONC
COND
CONE
CONF
CONG
CONJ
CONK
CONN
CONS
CONT
CONV
CONY
CTNS
CUNY
CYNO

C••N
CAAN
CAEN
CAHN
CAIN
CAPN
CHAN
CHEN
CHIN
CHMN
CHON
CIEN
CION
CLAN
CMON
COEN
COHN
COIN
CONN
COON
CORN
CRAN
CRIN
CTEN
CUIN
CYAN

•CN•
ACNE
CCNY

•C•N
DCON
ECON
ICAN
ICON
MCAN
SCAN

CO••
COAL
COAT
COAX
COBB
COBH
COBO
COBS
COCA
COCK
COCO
CODA
CODE
CODS
CODY
COED
COEN
COFC
COFS
COGS
COHN
COHO
COIF
COIL
COIN
COIR
COIT
COKE
COKY
COLA
COLD
COLE
COLI
COLL
COLM
COLO
COLS
COLT
COMA
COMB
COME
COMM
COMO
COMP
COMS
CONC
COND
CONE
CONF
CONG
CONJ
CONK
CONN
CONS
CONT
CONV
CONY
COOK
COOL
COON
COOP
COOS
COOT
COPA
COPE
COPS
COPT
COPY
COQS
CORA
CORD
CORE
CORI
CORK
CORM
CORN
CORP
CORR
CORS
CORT
CORY
COSA
COSH
COSI
COSM
COST
COSY
COTE
COTS
COTY
COUE
COUP
COVE
COWL
COWS
COWY
COXA
COZY

C•O•
CEOS
CFOS
CHOC
CHOL
CHON
CHOO
CHOP
CHOU
CHOW
CHOY
CION
CLOD
CLOG
CLOP
CLOT
CLOY
CMON
COOK
COOL
COON
COOP
COOS
COOT
CPOS
CROC
CROP
CROW
CWOS

C••O
CABO
CACO
CAMO
CAPO
CARO
CATO
CENO
CERO
CETO
CHAO
CHOO
CIAO
CITO
CLEO
CLIO
COBO
COCO
COHO
COLO
COMO
CREO
CRYO
CUJO
CYNO
CYTO

•CO•
DCON
ECOL
ECON
ICON
ICOS
NCOS
SCOT
SCOW

•C•O
ACRO
ACTO
ECCO
ECHO
ECTO
OCHO
OCTO

••CO
ARCO
ATCO
BACO
BUCO
CACO
COCO
DECO
DUCO
ECCO
EKCO
JUCO
LOCO
LYCO
MYCO
PACO
PICO
POCO
RICO
SACO
SECO
TACO
TICO
TYCO
VICO
WACO

CP••
CPAS
CPLS
CPOS
CPTS
CPUS

C•P•
CAPA
CAPE
CAPN
CAPO
CAPP
CAPS
CAPT
CEPE
CEPS
COPA
COPE
COPS
COPT
COPY
CUPR
CUPS

C••P
CAMP
CAPP
CARP
CCCP
CCUP
CHAP
CHIP
CHOP
CLAP
CLIP
CLOP
COMP
COOP
CORP
COUP
CROP
CULP
CUSP

•CP•
MCPS
PCPS
RCPT

•C•P
ACUP
BCUP
CCCP
CCUP
DCUP
RCMP
SCUP

••CP
CCCP
FACP

C•Q•
COQS

C••Q
CINQ

CR••
CRAB
CRAG
CRAM
CRAN
CRAT
CRAW
CRAY
CREB
CRED
CREE
CREO
CREW
CRIB
CRIN
CRIT

CROC
CROP
CROW
CRTS
CRUD
CRUE
CRUS
CRUX
CRUZ
CRVS
CRYO

C•R•
CARA
CARB
CARD
CARE
CARL
CARO
CARP
CARR
CARS
CART
CARY
CDRS
CERA
CERE
CERF
CERO
CERT
CIRC
CIRE
CORA
CORD
CORE
CORI
CORK
CORM
CORN
CORP
CORR
CORS
CORT
CORY
CTRL
CTRS
CURB
CURD
CURE
CURL
CURR
CURS
CURT

C••R
CARR
CBER
CHAR
CHER
CLAR
CMDR
COIR
CORR
CUER
CUPR
CURR
CZAR

•CR•
ACRE
ACRO
ECRU
VCRS

•C•R
ACAR
ACER
ICER
KCAR
NCAR
SCAR
TCHR

••CR
INCR
MACR
MICR

CS••
CSEA

C•S•
CASA
CASE
CASH
CASK
CASS
CAST
CASY
CESS
CEST
CIST
COSA
COSH
COSI
COSM
COST
COSY
CUSH
CUSK
CUSP
CUSS
CUST
CYST

C••S
CABS
CADS
CALS
CAMS
CANS
CAPS
CARS
CASS
CATS
CAVS
CAWS
CAYS
CCUS
CDRS
CEES
CELS
CENS
CEOS
CEPS
CESS
CFCS
CFOS
CHAS
CHGS
CHIS
CIGS
COBS
CODS
COFS
COGS
COLS
COMS
CONS
COOS
COPS
COQS
CORS
COTS
COWS
CPAS
CPLS
CPOS
CPTS
CPUS
CRTS
CRUS
CRVS
CTNS
CTRS
CUBS
CUDS
CUES
CUPS
CURS
CUSS
CUTS
CWMS
CWOS
CYLS

•C•S
ACCS
ACES
ACIS
ACTS
BCCS
BCES
CCUS
DCMS
ECGS
ECUS
ICES
ICOS
ICUS
LCDS
LCMS
MCPS
NCOS
OCAS
OCHS
OCTS
PCBS
PCPS
PCTS
RCAS
RCTS
SCIS
VCRS

••CS
ABCS
ACCS
ADCS
ALCS
AMCS
ARCS
BACS
BCCS
BECS
BICS
BUCS
CFCS
DECS
DFCS
DOCS
DSCS
ENCS
ESCS
ETCS
FACS
GLCS
GMCS
HICS
INCS
JACS
JVCS
LACS
LICS
MACS
MICS
MOCS
NLCS
ORCS
PACS
PECS
PFCS
PICS
POCS
RBCS
RECS
ROCS
SACS
SECS
SICS
SOCS
TACS
TECS
TICS
UPCS
VACS
WACS

CT••
CTEN
CTNS
CTRL
CTRS

C•T•
CATE
CATH
CATO
CATS
CATT
CATV
CETA
CETE
CETO
CITE
CITO
CITY
CMTE
COTE
COTS
COTY
CPTS
CRTS
CUTE
CUTS
CYTE
CYTO

C••T
CANT
CAPT
CART
CAST
CATT
CELT
CENT
CERT
CEST
CHAT
CHET
CHIT
CIST
CLOT
CNUT
COAT
COIT
COLT
CONT
COOT
COPT
CORT
COST
CRAT
CRIT
CUFT
CULT
CURT
CUST
CYST

•CT•
ACTA
ACTE
ACTH
ACTI
ACTO
ACTS
ACTV
ECTO
OCTA
OCTO
OCTS
PCTS
RCTS
SCTV
WCTU

•C•T
ACCT
ACHT
ECHT
ICET
MCAT
RCPT
SCAT
SCOT
SCUT

••CT
ACCT
BACT
DICT
DUCT
FACT
FICT
HECT
LACT
LECT
NOCT
NYCT
PACT
PICT
RECT
SECT
TACT

CU••
CUAL
CUBA
CUBE
CUBS
CUDS
CUED
CUER
CUES
CUFF
CUFT
CUIN
CUJO
CUKE
CULE
CULL
CULP
CULT
CUME
CUNY
CUPR
CUPS
CURB
CURD
CURE
CURL
CURR
CURS
CURT
CUSH
CUSK
CUSP
CUSS
CUST
CUTE
CUTS
CUYD

C•U•
CAUD
CAUL
CCUP
CCUS
CHUB
CHUG
CHUM
CLUB
CLUE
CNUT
COUE
COUP
CPUS
CRUD
CRUE
CRUS
CRUX
CRUZ

C••U
CEBU
CHOU

•CU•
ACUP
BCUP
CCUP
CCUS
DCUP
ECUA
ECUS
ICUS
OCUL
SCUD
SCUM
SCUP
SCUT

•C•U
ACLU
ECRU
WCTU

••CU
DOCU

CV••
CVII

C•V•
CAVA
CAVE
CAVS
CAVY
CCVI
CDVI
CLVI
CMVI
COVE
CRVS
CXVI

C••V
CATV
CCCV
CCIV
CCLV
CCXV
CDIV
CDLV
CDXV
CLIV
CLXV
CMIV
CMLV
CMXV
CONV
CXCV
CXIV
CXLV
CXXV

•CV•
CCVI
DCVI
MCVI
XCVI

•C•V
ACTV
CCCV
CCIV
CCLV
CCXV
DCCV
DCIV
DCLV
DCXV
MCCV
MCDV
MCIV
MCLV
MCMV
MCXV
SCTV
XCIV

••CV
CCCV
CXCV
DCCV
DXCV
MCCV
MDCV
MMCV
MXCV

CW••
CWMS
CWOS

C•W•
CAWS
COWL
COWS
COWY

C••W
CHAW
CHEW
CHOW
CLAW
CLEW
CRAW
CREW
CROW

•C•W
SCOW

CX••
CXCI
CXCV
CXII
CXIV
CXIX
CXLI
CXLV
CXVI
CXXI
CXXV
CXXX

C•X•
CCXC
CCXI
CCXL
CCXV
CCXX
CDXC
CDXI
CDXL
CDXV
CDXX
CLXI
CLXV
CLXX
CMXC
CMXI
CMXL
CMXV
CMXX
COXA
CXXI
CXXV
CXXX

C••X
CALX
CCCX
CCIX
CCLX
CCXX
CDIX
CDLX
CDXX
CHEX
CLIX
CLXX
CMIX
CMLX
CMXX
COAX
CRUX
CXIX
CXXX

•CX•
CCXC
CCXI
CCXL
CCXV
CCXX
DCXC
DCXI
DCXL
DCXV
DCXX
MCXC
MCXI
MCXL
MCXV
MCXX

•C•X
CCCX
CCIX
CCLX
CCXX
DCCX
DCIX
DCLX
DCXX
MCCX
MCDX
MCIX
MCLX
MCMX
MCXX
XCIX

••CX
CCCX
DCCX
MCCX
MDCX
MMCX

CY••
CYAN
CYCL
CYLS
CYMA
CYME
CYNO
CYST
CYTE
CYTO

C•Y•
CAYS
CLYM
CRYO
CUYD

C••Y
CADY
CAGY
CAKY
CANY
CARY
CASY
CAVY
CCNY
CHOY
CITY
CLAY
CLOY
CODY
COKY
CONY
COPY
CORY
COSY
COTY
COWY
COZY
CRAY
CUNY

•C•Y
ACEY
ACHY
CCNY
ICKY
TCBY

••CY
AGCY
ANCY
ENCY
LACY
LUCY
MACY
RACY
SECY

CZ••
CZAR

C•Z•
COZY

C••Z
CHEZ
CRUZ

DA••
DABA
DABO
DABS
DACE
DADA
DADE
DADO
DADS
DAFT
DAHL
DAHS
DAIL
DAIN
DAIS
DALE
DALI
DALS
DALY
DAMA
DAME
DAMN
DAMP
DAMS
DANA
DANE
DANG
DANK
DANL
DANO
DANS
DAPS
DARA
DARC
DARE
DARK
DARN
DART
DASH
DATA
DATE
DATO
DAUB
DAUS
DAVE
DAVI
DAVY
DAWG
DAWN
DAWS
DAYO
DAYS
DAZE
DAZS

D•A•
DBAS
DDAY
DEAD
DEAF
DEAL
DEAN
DEAR
DHAL
DIAG
DIAL
DIAM
DIAN
DIAS
DIAZ
DMAJ
DNAS
DOAK
DRAB
DRAG
DRAM
DRAT
DRAW
DRAX
DRAY
DUAD
DUAL
DWAN
DYAD
DYAN

D••A
DABA
DADA
DAMA
DANA
DARA
DATA
DECA
DEJA
DEKA
DENA
DEVA
DINA
DIVA
DJIA
DOHA
DONA
DOPA
DORA
DREA
DUMA
DUNA
DURA
DYNA

•DA•
ADAH
ADAK
ADAM
ADAR
ADAY
BDAY
DDAY
EDAM
GDAY
IDAE
NDAK
ODAS
ODAY
PDAS
RDAS
SDAK
VDAY

•D•A
ADIA
EDDA
EDNA
EDTA
IDEA
KDKA
ODEA
ODRA

••DA
AIDA
ALDA
BUDA
CODA
DADA
EDDA
ERDA
JADA
LADA
LEDA
LIDA
NADA
ONDA
PODA
REDA
SADA
SODA
TADA
USDA
VEDA
VIDA
YADA
YODA

DB••
DBAS
DBLS

D•B•
DABA
DABO
DABS
DEBI
DEBS
DEBT
DIBS
DOBY
DUBS

D••B
DAUB
DRAB
DRIB
DRUB
DUMB

•DB•
EDBS
HDBK

DC••
DCCC
DCCI
DCCL
DCCV
DCCX
DCII
DCIL
DCIV
DCIX
DCLI
DCLV
DCLX
DCMS
DCON
DCUP
DCVI
DCXC
DCXI
DCXL
DCXV
DCXX

D•C•
DACE
DCCC
DCCI
DCCL
DCCV
DCCX
DECA
DECI
DECK
DECO
DECS
DFCS
DICE
DICK
DICT
DOCE
DOCK
DOCS
DOCU
DSCS
DUCE
DUCK
DUCO
DUCT
DXCI
DXCV
DYCE
DYCK

D••C
DARC
DCCC
DCXC
DESC
DISC
DONC
DURC

•DC•
ADCS
MDCC
MDCI
MDCL
MDCV
MDCX

•D•C
CDXC
EDUC
FDIC
MDCC
MDXC
ODIC

••DC
ACDC
MMDC

DD••
DDAY
DDTS

D•D•
DADA
DADE
DADO
DADS
DEDE
DEDO
DIDI
DIDO
DIDY
DMDS
DODD
DODO
DODY
DUDE
DUDS
DVDS

D••D
DEAD
DEED
DHED
DIED
DODD
DOOD
DOUD
DOWD
DRED
DUAD
DYAD
DYED

•DD•
ADDL
ADDN
ADDR
ADDS
EDDA
EDDO
EDDS
EDDY
ODDS

•D•D
IDED
IDID
ODED

••DD
BADD
BUDD
DODD
FUDD
JUDD
KIDD
LADD
MADD
MUDD
REDD
RIDD
RODD
RUDD
SADD
TODD

DE••
DEAD
DEAF
DEAL
DEAN
DEAR
DEBI
DEBS
DEBT
DECA
DECI
DECK
DECO
DECS
DEDE
DEDO
DEED
DEEM
DEEP
DEER
DEES
DEET
DEFG
DEFS
DEFT
DEFY
DEGS
DEIL
DEJA
DEKA
DEKE
DELE
DELI
DELL
DELT
DEME
DEMI
DEMO
DEMS
DEMY
DENA
DENE
DENG
DENS
DENT
DENY
DEPP
DEPS
DEPT
DERE
DERM
DERN
DERR
DESC
DESE
DESI
DESK
DETS
DEUM
DEUS
DEUT
DEUX
DEVA
DEVI
DEVO
DEVS
DEWS
DEWY

D•E•
DEED
DEEM
DEEP
DEER
DEES
DEET
DHED
DIED
DIEM
DIEN
DIES
DIET
DIEU
DIEZ
DNET
DOER
DOES
DREA
DRED
DREG
DREI
DREK
DREW
DUEL
DUER
DUES
DUET
DYED
DYER
DYES

D••E
DACE
DADE
DALE
DAME
DANE
DARE
DATE
DAVE
DAZE
DEDE
DEKE
DELE
DEME
DENE
DERE
DESE
DICE
DIKE
DIME
DINE
DIRE
DIVE
DOCE
DOGE
DOKE
DOLE
DOME
DONE
DOPE
DORE
DOSE
DOTE
DOVE
DOZE
DUCE
DUDE
DUKE
DUNE
DUPE
DUSE
DUVE
DYCE
DYKE
DYNE

•DE•
ADEN
ADES
CDEF
EDEL
EDEN
EDER
IDEA
IDED
IDEE
IDEM
IDEO
IDES
ODEA
ODED
ODER
ODES

•D•E
ADUE
ADZE
EDGE
EDIE
IDAE
IDEE
IDLE
IDVE
KDOE
MDSE
ODIE

••DE
AIDE
AUDE
AYDE
BADE
BCDE
BEDE
BIDE
BODE
CADE
CEDE
CIDE
CODE
DADE
DEDE
DUDE
ENDE
ERDE
FADE
FIDE
GIDE
HIDE
HYDE
JADE
JUDE
LADE
LODE
MADE
MEDE
MODE
NIDE
NODE
NUDE
OLDE
ONDE
PEDE
REDE
RIDE
RODE
RUDE
SADE
SIDE
TIDE
TUDE
VADE
VIDE
WADE
WIDE

DF••
DFCS
DFMS

D•F•
DAFT
DEFG
DEFS
DEFT
DEFY
DIFF
DOFF

DUFF DUFY

D••F
DEAF DIFF DOFF DUFF

•DF•
BDFT PDFS

•D•F
CDEF

D•G•
DEGS DIGS DOGE DOGS

D••G
DANG DAWG DEFG DENG DIAG DING DONG DOUG DRAG DREG DRUG

•DG•
EDGE EDGY

•D•G
IDIG

••DG
BLDG CMDG

DH••
DHAL DHED DHOW

D•H•
DAHL DAHS DOHA DOHS DTHS DUHS

D••H
DASH DINH DISH DITH DOTH

•DH•
EDHS

•D•H
ADAH

••DH
YODH

DI••
DIAG DIAL DIAM DIAN DIAS DIAZ DIBS DICE DICK DICT DIDI DIDO DIDY DIED DIEM DIEN DIES DIET DIEU DIEZ DIFF DIGS DIII DIKE DILI DILL DIME DIMS DINA DINE DING DINH DINK DINO DINS DINT DION DIOR DIOS DIPL DIPS DIRE DIRK DIRS DIRT DISC DISH DISK DISS DIST DITH DITS DITZ DIVA DIVE DIVS DIXY

D•I•
DAIL DAIN DAIS DCII DCIL DCIV DCIX DEIL DIII DJIA DJIN DLII DLIT DLIV DLIX DMIN DOIN DOIS DOIT DRIB DRIN DRIP DRIQ DVII DXII DXIV DXIX

D••I
DALI DAVI DCCI DCII DCLI DCVI DCXI DEBI DECI DELI DEMI DESI DEVI DIDI DIII DILI DLII DLVI DLXI DREI DVII DXCI DXII DXLI DXVI DXXI

•DI•
ADIA ADIN ADIT CDII CDIV CDIX EDIE EDIT FDIC IDID IDIG IDIO MDII MDIV MDIX ODIC ODIE ODIN XDIN XDIV

•D•I
CDII CDLI CDVI CDXI MDCI MDII MDLI MDVI MDXI

••DI
AUDI CADI CEDI DIDI JEDI JUDI LODI MCDI MEDI MIDI MMDI MODI NIDI NODI PEDI REDI RIDI RUDI TODI VIDI WADI

DJ••
DJIA DJIN

D•J•
DEJA DOJO

D••J
DMAJ

•DJ•
ADJS ADJT

••DJ
HADJ

DK••
DKNY

D•K•
DEKA DEKE DIKE DOKE DUKE DYKE

D••K
DANK DARK DECK DESK DICK DINK DIRK DISK DOAK DOCK DOOK DORK DREK DUCK DUNK DUSK DYCK

•DK•
KDKA

•D•K
ADAK HDBK NDAK SDAK

DL••
DLII DLIT DLIV DLIX DLOS DLVI DLXI DLXV DLXX

D•L•
DALE DALI DALS DALY DBLS DCLI DCLV DCLX DELE DELI DELL DELT DILI DILL DOLE DOLL DOLT DULL DULY DXLI DXLV

D••L
DAHL DAIL DANL DCCL DCIL DCXL DEAL DEIL DELL DHAL DIAL DILL DIPL DOLL DUAL DUEL DULL

•DL•
BDLS CDLI CDLV CDLX IDLE IDLY MDLI MDLV MDLX

•D•L
ADDL CDXL EDEL IDOL IDYL MDCL MDXL

••DL
ADDL MCDL MMDL

DM••
DMAJ DMDS DMIN DMUS DMVS DMZS

D•M•
DAMA DAME DAMN DAMP DAMS DCMS DEME DEMI DEMO DEMS DEMY DFMS DIME DIMS DOME DOMO DOMS DPMS DSMS DUMA DUMB DUMP DVMS

D••M
DEEM DERM DEUM DIAM DIEM DOOM DORM DRAM DRUM

•DM•
ADMS EDMS

•D•M
ADAM BDRM EDAM EDOM IDEM ODOM

••DM
RADM VADM

DN••
DNAS DNET

D•N•
DANA DANE DANG DANK DANL DANO DANS DENA DENE DENG DENS DENT DENY DINA DINE DING DINH DINK DINO DINS DINT DKNY DONA DONC DONE DONG DONN DONS DONT DRNO DUNA DUNE DUNK DUNN DUNS DYNA DYNE

D••N
DAIN DAMN DARN DAWN DCON DEAN DERN DIAN DIEN DION DJIN DMIN DOIN DONN DOON DORN DOWN DRIN DUNN DURN DUUN DWAN DYAN

•DN•
EDNA FDNY

•D•N
ADDN ADEN ADIN EDEN ODIN ODON XDIN

••DN
ADDN

DO••
DOAK DOBY DOCE DOCK DOCS DOCU DODD DODO DODY DOER DOES DOFF DOGE DOGS DOHA DOHS DOIN DOIS DOIT DOJO DOKE DOLE DOLL DOLT DOME DOMO DOMS DONA DONC DONE DONG DONN DONS DONT DOOD DOOK DOOM DOON DOOR DOOS DOPA DOPE DOPY DORA DORE DORK DORM DORN DORO DORP DORS DORY DOSE DOSO DOSS DOST DOTE DOTH DOTO DOTS DOUD DOUG DOUP DOUR DOUW DOUX DOVE DOWD DOWN DOXY DOZE DOZO DOZY

D•O•
DCON DHOW DION DIOR DIOS DLOS DOOD DOOK DOOM DOON DOOR DOOS DROP DSOS DUOS

D••O
DABO DADO DANO DATO DAYO DECO DEDO DEMO DEVO DIDO DINO DODO DOJO DOMO DORO DOSO DOTO DOZO DRNO DUCO DURO

•DO•
ADOS EDOM IDOL IDOS KDOE ODOM ODON ODOR UDOS

•D•O
EDDO IDEO IDIO

••DO
ALDO DADO DEDO DIDO DODO EDDO ENDO FADO FIDO INDO IODO JUDO KUDO LIDO ORDO PEDO PODO RADO REDO SADO TODO UNDO UPDO

DP••
DPMS DPTS

D•P•
DAPS DEPP DEPS DEPT DIPL DIPS DOPA DOPE DOPY DUPE

D••P
DAMP DCUP DEEP DEPP DORP DOUP DRIP DROP DUMP

D••Q
DRIQ

DR••
DRAB DRAG DRAM DRAT DRAW DRAX DRAY DREA DRED DREG DREI DREK DREW DRIB DRIN DRIP DRIQ DRNO DROP DRUB DRUG DRUM DRYS

D•R•
DARA DARC DARE DARK DARN DART DERE DERM DERN DERR DIRE DIRK DIRS DIRT DORA DORE DORK DORM DORN DORO DORP DORS DORY DURA DURC DURN DURO

D••R
DEAR DEER DERR DIOR DOER DOOR DOUR DUER DYER

•DR•
BDRM CDRS LDRS ODRA PDRS

•D•R
ADAR ADDR EDER ODER ODOR

••DR
ADDR CMDR HYDR RMDR SADR

DS••
DSCS DSMS DSOS

D•S•
DASH DESC DESE DESI DESK DISC DISH DISK DISS DIST DOSE DOSO DOSS DOST DUSE DUSK DUST

D••S
DABS DADS DAHS DAIS DALS DAMS DANS DAPS DAUS DAWS DAYS DAZS DBAS DBLS DCMS DDTS DEBS DECS DEES DEFS DEGS DEMS DENS DEPS DETS DEUS DEVS DEWS DFCS DFMS DIAS DIBS DIES DIGS DIMS DINS DIOS DIPS DIRS DISS DITS DIVS DLOS DMDS DMUS DMVS DMZS DNAS DOCS DOES DOGS DOHS DOIS DOMS DONS DOOS DORS DOSS DOTS DPMS DPTS DRYS DSCS DSMS DSOS DTHS DUBS DUDS DUES DUHS DUNS DUOS DVDS DVMS DYES

•DS•
MDSE

•D•S
ADCS ADDS ADES ADJS ADMS ADOS BDLS CDRS DDTS EDBS EDDS EDHS EDMS EDYS IDES IDOS LDRS ODAS ODDS ODES PDAS PDFS PDRS RDAS UDOS VDTS

••DS
ADDS AIDS ALDS ANDS BADS BEDS BIDS BODS BUDS BVDS CADS CODS CUDS DADS DMDS DUDS DVDS EADS EDDS ENDS ETDS FADS FEDS FIDS GADS GEDS GODS HODS INDS KEDS KIDS LADS LCDS LEDS LIDS LLDS LTDS MADS MEDS MODS MUDS NODS ODDS OLDS OUDS PADS PEDS PHDS PODS RADS REDS RFDS RIDS RNDS RODS SJDS SODS STDS SUDS TADS TEDS THDS TODS VIDS WADS WEDS YODS ZEDS

DT••
DTHS

D•T•
DATA DATE DATO DDTS DETS DITH DITS DITZ DOTE DOTH DOTO DOTS DPTS DUTY

D••T
DAFT DART DEBT DEET DEFT DELT DENT DEPT DEUT DICT DIET DINT DIRT DIST DLIT DNET DOIT DOLT DONT DOST DRAT DUCT DUET DUST

•DT•
DDTS EDTA EDTV HDTV VDTS

•D•T
ADIT ADJT BDFT EDIT

••DT
USDT

DU••
DUAD DUAL DUBS DUCE DUCK DUCO DUCT DUDE DUDS DUEL DUER DUES DUET DUFF DUFY DUHS DUKE DULL DULY DUMA DUMB DUMP DUNA DUNE DUNK DUNN DUNS DUOS DUPE DURA DURC DURN DURO DUSE DUSK DUST DUTY DUUN DUVE

D•U•
DAUB DAUS DCUP DEUM DEUS DEUT DEUX DMUS DOUD DOUG DOUP DOUR DOUW DOUX DRUB DRUG DRUM DUUN

D••U
DIEU DOCU

•DU•
ADUE EDUC

••DU
BADU BIDU KUDU URDU

DV••
DVDS DVII DVMS

D•V•
DAVE DAVI DAVY DCVI DEVA DEVI DEVO DEVS DIVA DIVE DIVS DLVI DMVS DOVE DUVE DXVI

D••V
DCCV DCIV DCLV DCXV DLIV DLXV DXCV DXIV DXLV DXXV

•DV•
CDVI IDVE MDVI

•D•V
CDIV CDLV CDXV EDTV HDTV MDCV MDIV MDLV MDXV XDIV

••DV
MCDV MMDV

DW••
DWAN

D•W•
DAWG DAWN DAWS DEWS DEWY DOWD DOWN

D••W
DHOW DOUW DRAW DREW

DX••
DXCI DXCV DXII DXIV DXIX DXLI DXLV DXVI DXXI DXXV DXXX

D•X•
DCXC DCXI DCXL DCXV DCXX DIXY DLXI DLXV DLXX DOXY DXXI DXXV DXXX

D••X
DCCX DCIX DCLX DCXX DEUX DLIX DLXX DOUX DRAX DXIX DXXX

•DX•
CDXC CDXI CDXL CDXV CDXX MDXC MDXI MDXL MDXV MDXX

•D•X
CDIX CDLX CDXX MDCX MDIX MDLX MDXX

••DX
MCDX MMDX

DY••
DYAD DYAN DYCE DYCK DYED DYER DYES DYKE DYNA DYNE

D•Y•
DAYO DAYS DRYS

D••Y
DALY

DAVY DDAY DEFY DEMY DENY DEWY DIDY DIXY DKNY DOBY DODY DOPY DORY DOXY DOZY DRAY DUFY DULY DUTY

•DY•
EDYS IDYL

•D•Y
ADAY BDAY DDAY EDDY EDGY FDNY GDAY IDLY ODAY VDAY

••DY
ANDY BODY CADY CODY DIDY DODY EDDY HEDY INDY JODY JUDY LADY RUDY TIDY

D•Z•
DAZE DAZS DMZS DOZE DOZO DOZY

D••Z
DIAZ DIEZ DITZ

•DZ•
ADZE

••DZ
LODZ

EA••
EACH EADS EARL EARN EARP EARS EASE EAST EASY EATS EAUX EAVE

E•A•
EBAN EBAY EDAM EFAX EGAD EGAL EGAN ELAL ELAM ELAN ELAS ELAT EMAG EMAJ EOAN ERAL ERAS ERAT ESAI ESAR ESAS ESAU ETAH ETAL ETAS ETAT EVAC EVAH EVAL EVAN EVAP EVAS EWAN EXAM

E••A
ECUA EDDA EDNA EDTA ELBA ELEA ELIA ELLA ELSA EMIA EMMA ENNA ENYA EOLA EPHA EPPA ERDA ERIA ERMA ERNA ESSA ESTA ETNA ETTA EULA EYRA EZRA

•EA•
BEAD BEAH BEAK BEAM BEAN BEAR BEAT BEAU BEAV DEAD DEAF DEAL DEAN DEAR FEAR FEAT GEAR HEAD HEAL HEAP HEAR HEAT JEAN KEAN KEAR KEAS LEAD LEAF LEAH LEAK LEAL LEAN LEAP LEAR LEAS MEAD MEAL MEAN MEAS MEAT NEAL NEAP NEAR NEAT PEAK PEAL PEAR PEAS PEAT PEAU READ REAL REAM REAO REAP REAR SEAL SEAM SEAN SEAR SEAS SEAT SEAU TEAC TEAK TEAL TEAM TEAR TEAS TEAT VEAL VEAU WEAK WEAL WEAN WEAR YEAH YEAN YEAR YEAS ZEAL

•E•A
BEGA BELA BEMA BETA CELA CENA CERA CETA DECA DEJA DEKA DENA DEVA FEMA FETA GENA GETA HEMA HERA HEXA JENA LEDA LEIA LELA LEMA LENA LEVA MEGA MENA MESA META NENA NERA NEVA PEBA PENA PEPA PERA PETA REBA REDA RENA RETA REVA REZA SEGA SELA SERA SETA TEMA TENA TERA TEWA VEDA VEGA VELA VENA VERA VETA XENA ZETA

••EA
AIEA ALEA AREA ASEA BREA CLEA CSEA DREA ELEA FLEA GAEA IDEA IKEA ITEA ODEA OLEA ONEA OTEA PLEA RHEA SHEA TOEA UREA UVEA

EB••
EBAN EBAY EBBS EBEL EBEN EBON EBRO

E•B•
EBBS EDBS ELBA ELBE

•EB•
BEBE CEBU DEBI DEBS DEBT FEBS HEBB HEBE HEBR NEBO NEBR NEBS PEBA REBA REBS WEBB WEBS ZEBU

•E•B
BEEB FEEB HEBB HERB KERB SERB TENB VERB WEBB WEEB

••EB
BEEB BLEB CREB FEEB LIEB LOEB NHEB ONEB PLEB SHEB WEEB

EC••
ECCE ECCL ECCO ECGS ECHO ECHT ECOL ECON ECRU ECTO ECUA ECUS

E•C•
EACH ECCE ECCL ECCO EKCO ENCE ENCL ENCS ENCY ESCE ESCS ETCH ETCS EXCH EXCL EYCK

E••C
EDUC EEOC ELEC EPIC ERIC ETIC EVAC EXEC

•EC•
BECH BECK BECS CECE CECI DECA DECI DECK DECO DECS HECK HECT LECH LECT MECH NECK PECK PECS RECD RECK RECS RECT SECO SECS SECT SECY TECH TECS YECH ZECH

•E•C
DESC EEOC MERC PERC TEAC TENC

••EC
ALEC AVEC ELEC EXEC HAEC MSEC ONEC OPEC PREC SPEC

ED••
EDAM EDBS EDDA EDDO EDDS EDDY EDEL EDEN EDER EDGE EDGY EDHS EDIE EDIT EDMS EDNA EDOM EDTA EDTV EDUC EDYS

E•D•
EADS EDDA EDDO EDDS EDDY ENDE ENDO ENDS ERDA ERDE ETDS

E••D
EGAD EHUD EKED ENID ESTD EXED EXOD EYED

•ED•
BEDE BEDS CEDE CEDI DEDE DEDO FEDS GEDS HEDY JEDI KEDS LEDA LEDS MEDE MEDI MEDS PEDE PEDI PEDO PEDS REDA REDD REDE REDI REDO REDS TEDS VEDA WEDS ZEDS

•E•D
BEAD BEND DEAD DEED FEED FEND FEUD GEED GELD HEAD HEED HELD HERD LEAD LEND LEWD MEAD MELD MEND NEED NEJD NERD PEND READ RECD REDD REED REGD REID REND REQD RETD SEED SEND TEED TEND VELD VEND WEED WELD WEND ZEND

••ED
ABED ACED AGED AHED APED AWED AXED BLED BRED CCED COED CRED CUED DEED DHED DIED DRED DYED EKED EXED EYED FEED FLED FRED GEED GIED HEED HIED HOED HUED ICED IDED IRED JOED LIED MRED MSED NEED ODED OHED OKED ONED OPED OWED PIED PLED PRED REED RUED SEED SHED SKED SLED SPED SUED SWED TEED TIED TOED USED VIED WEED ZMED

EE••
EEEE EEES EEGS EEKS EELS EELY EENY EEOC EERO EERY

E•E•
EBEL EBEN EDEL EDEN EDER EEEE EEES EGER EIER EKED EKES ELEA ELEC ELEM ELEV EMER EMES EMEU ENES EPEE ERES EREV ESEL ETES EUER EVEL EVEN EVER EVES EWEN EWER EWES EXEC EXED EXEL EXES EYED EYER EYES EZEK EZER

E••E
EASE EAVE ECCE EDGE EDIE EEEE EHLE EHRE EILE EINE EIRE ELBE ELIE ELKE ELLE ELSE EMME ENCE ENDE ENKE ENNE ENSE EPEE ERDE ERIE ERLE ERNE ERSE ERTE ESCE ESME ESNE ESSE ESTE ETRE ETTE EURE EUWE EVIE EVOE EYRE

•EE•
BEEB BEEF BEEM BEEN BEEP BEER BEES BEET CEES DEED DEEM DEEP DEER DEES DEET EEEE EEES FEEB FEED FEEL FEES FEET GEED GEEK GEEP GEER GEES GEEZ HEED HEEL HEEP HEER HEET JEEP JEER JEEZ KEEL KEEN KEEP LEEJ LEEK LEER LEES MEEK MEER MEET NEED NEEL NEER NEET PEEK PEEL PEEN PEEP PEER PEES PEET REED REEF REEK REEL REES REET SEED SEEK SEEM SEEN SEEP SEER SEES TEED TEEM TEEN TEER TEES VEEP VEER VEES WEEB WEED WEEK WEEP WEER ZEES

•E•E
BEBE BEDE BENE BETE CECE CEDE CENE CEPE CERE CETE DEDE DEKE DELE DEME DENE DERE DESE EEEE FEME FETE GENE GERE HEBE HEHE HEME HERE JEFE JETE KEYE LESE MEDE MEME MENE MERE METE NENE NEUE NEVE PEDE PEKE PELE PEPE PERE PETE REDE RENE RETE REVE SENE SERE SESE SEVE TELE TENE TETE UELE VERE WERE WEVE ZEKE

••EE
AGEE ALEE BREE CHEE CREE EEEE EPEE FLEE FREE GHEE GLEE ICEE IDEE INEE ISEE JOEE KLEE KNEE OGEE ONEE OREE OSEE RHEE SKEE SMEE SNEE SPEE SWEE THEE TREE TWEE TYEE ULEE USEE WHEE

EF••
EFAX EFFS EFGH EFIK EFTS

E•F•
EFFS

E••F
ENIF ENUF

•EF•
DEFG DEFS DEFT DEFY HEFT JEFE JEFF LEFT NEFF REFI REFL REFS REFT WEFT

•E•F
BEEF CERF DEAF GENF JEFF KERF LEAF LEIF NEFF NERF NEUF NEWF OEUF PELF PERF REEF SELF SERF

••EF
ALEF BEEF CDEF CHEF CLEF FIEF LIEF ONEF PREF REEF TREF

EG••
EGAD EGAL EGAN EGER EGGO EGGS EGGY EGIS EGLI EGON EGOS

E•G•
ECGS EDGE EDGY EEGS EFGH EGGO EGGS EGGY EIGG EKGS ENGR ENGS ERGO ERGS ERGY EXGI

E••G
EIGG EMAG

•EG•
BEGA BEGS DEGS EEGS KEGS LEGG LEGO LEGS MEGA MEGS NEGS PEGS REGD REGO REGS REGT SEGA SEGO SEGS VEGA VEGS YEGG

•E•G
BELG BERG DEFG DENG FENG GEOG LEGG LEOG NENG PENG SENG TENG WENG YEGG

••EG
BNEG DREG GREG JPEG MPEG OLEG ONEG OREG ROEG SIEG SKEG

EH••
EHLE EHLO EHRE EHUD

E•H•
ECHO ECHT EDHS ELHI EPHA ETHN ETHS

E••H
EACH EFGH ESTH ETAH ETCH EVAH EXCH

•EH•
FEHR HEHE HEHS JEHU LEHI LEHN LEHR NEHI SEHR ZEHN

•E•H
BEAH BECH BETH HETH IEOH LEAH LECH MECH MESH METH NETH PENH RESH SETH TECH TESH TETH YEAH YECH YEOH ZECH ZEPH

••EH
ONEH

EI••
EIER EIGG EILE EIMI EINE EINS EIRE

E•I•
EDIE EDIT EFIK EGIS ELIA ELIE ELIO ELIS ELIZ EMIA EMIL EMIR EMIT ENID ENIF EPIC EPIS ERIA ERIC ERIE ERIK ERIN ERIQ ERIS ESIS ETIC EVIE EVIL EXIT EZIO

E••I
EGLI EIMI ELHI ELOI EQUI ESAI ESSI ETUI EXGI

•EI•
BEIN CEIL DEIL FEIN HEIN HEIR KEIR LEIA LEIF LEIS LEIX MEIN MEIR NEIL NEIN OEIL QEII REID REIN REIT SEIN SEIS VEIL VEIN WEIL WEIN WEIR WEIS ZEIT

•E•I
AERI BENI CECI CEDI DEBI DECI DELI DEMI DESI DEVI GERI HELI HEMI IERI JEDI JERI KEPI KERI LEHI LENI LEOI LEVI MEDI NEHI NERI NEVI PEDI PERI QEII REDI REFI REMI RENI SEMI SETI TERI VENI YETI

••EI
BREI DREI FREI LWEI OMEI ZWEI

E••J
EMAJ

4 EJ

•EJ• DEJA NEJD SEJM

•E•J LEEJ

••EJ LEEJ

EK•• EKCO EKED EKES EKGS

E•K• EEKS ELKE ELKO ELKS ENKE ESKS

E••K EFIK ERIK EWOK EYCK EZEK

•EK• DEKA DEKE EEKS LEKS PEKE SEKO ZEKE

•E•K BEAK BECK DECK DESK GEEK HECK JERK LEAK LEEK MEEK NECK PEAK PECK PEEK PERK RECK REEK SEEK TEAK TENK WEAK WEEK WELK

••EK ALEK DREK EZEK GEEK LEEK MEEK ONEK PEEK PREK REEK SEEK SHEK TREK WEEK

EL•• ELAL ELAM ELAN ELAS ELAT ELBA ELBE ELEA ELEC ELEM ELEV ELHI ELIA ELIE ELIO ELIS ELIZ ELKE ELKO ELKS ELLA ELLE ELLS ELLY ELMO ELMS ELMY ELOI ELON ELSA ELSE ELUL

E•L• EELS EELY EGLI EHLE EHLO EILE ELLA ELLE ELLS ELLY EMLY EOLA ERLE EULA

E••L EARL EBEL ECCL ECOL EDEL EGAL ELAL ELUL EMIL ENCL ENOL ERAL ESEL ETAL EVAL EVEL EVIL EXCL EXEL

•EL• BELA BELG BELL BELO BELS BELT BELY CELA CELL CELS CELT DELE DELI DELL DELT EELS EELY FELL FELS FELT GELD GELL GELS GELT HELD HELI HELL HELM HELO HELP JELL KELL KELP LELA LELY MELD MELL MELO MELS MELT NELL NELS PELE PELF PELL PELT RELO RELS RELY SELA SELF SELL TELE TELL TELS UELE VELA VELD VELO WELD WELK WELL WELT WELU YELL YELP ZELL

•E•L BELL CEIL CELL DEAL DEIL DELL FEEL FELL GELL GENL GEOL HEAL HEEL HELL JELL KEEL KELL LEAL MEAL MELL MERL MEWL NEAL NEEL NEIL NELL OEIL PEAL PEEL PELL REAL REEL REFL REPL SEAL SELL SEUL TEAL TELL VEAL VEIL WEAL WEIL WELL YELL ZEAL ZELL

••EL ABEL AUEL AXEL BIEL BREL CIEL DUEL EBEL EDEL ESEL EVEL EXEL FEEL FUEL GAEL HEEL ICEL JOEL KAEL KEEL KIEL KTEL MIEL NEEL NOEL ONEL OPEL OREL PEEL PIEL QUEL REEL RIEL SHEL TAEL

EM•• EMAG EMAJ EMER EMES EMEU EMIA EMIL EMIR EMIT EMLY EMMA EMME EMMY EMPS EMTS EMUS

E•M• EDMS EIMI ELMO ELMS ELMY EMMA EMME EMMY ERMA ESME

E••M EDAM EDOM ELAM ELEM ETUM ETYM EXAM

•EM• BEMA BEMS DEME DEMI DEMO DEMS DEMY FEMA FEME FEMS GEMS HEMA HEME HEMI HEMO HEMP HEMS KEMO KEMP LEMA LEMS MEME MEMO MEMS NEMO REMI REMO REMS REMY SEMI SEMS TEMA TEMP

•E•M BEAM BEEM BERM DEEM DERM DEUM GEOM GERM HELM MERM MEUM PERM REAM SEAM SEEM SEJM TEAM TEEM TERM YESM

••EM AHEM BEEM CHEM CLEM DEEM DIEM ELEM FLEM IDEM ITEM KLEM MNEM OREM POEM PREM QUEM SEEM SHEM STEM TEEM THEM YLEM

EN•• ENCE ENCL ENCS ENCY ENDE ENDO ENDS ENES ENGR ENGS ENID ENIF ENKE ENNA ENNE ENNS ENOL ENON ENOS ENOW ENRY ENSE ENTO ENTR ENTS ENUF ENVS ENVY ENYA ENYO ENZO

E•N• EDNA EENY EINE EINS ENNA ENNE ENNS EONS ERNA ERNE ERNO ERNS ESNE ETNA

E••N EARN EBAN EBEN EBON ECON EDEN EGAN EGON ELAN ELON ENON EOAN ERIN ESPN ETHN ETON EVAN EVEN EWAN EWEN EXON

•EN• BEND BENE BENI BENT BENZ CENA CENE CENO CENS CENT DENA DENE DENG DENS DENT DENY EENY FEND FENG FENN FENS GENA GENE GENF GENL GENO GENS GENT GENU GENX HENN HENS JENA JENS KENN KENO KENS KENT LENA LEND LENI LENO LENS LENT LENZ MENA MEND MENE MENS MENT MENU NENA NENE NENG OENO PENA PEND PENG PENH PENN PENS PENT RENA REND RENE RENI RENO RENT SEND SENE SENG SENS SENT TENA TENB TENC TEND TENE TENG TENK TENN TENS TENT VENA VEND VENI VENN VENO VENT WEND WENG WENS WENT XENA XENO YENS ZEND ZENO

•E•N AEON BEAN BEEN BEIN BERN DEAN DERN FEIN FENN FERN HEIN HENN HEWN JEAN JEON KEAN KEEN KENN KERN LEAN LEHN LEON MEAN MEIN NEIN NEON NEUN PEEN PENN PEON REIN SEAN SEEN SEIN SEWN TEEN TENN TERN VEIN VENN VERN WEAN WEIN XEON YEAN ZEHN

••EN ADEN ALEN AMEN ATEN BEEN BIEN BREN BTEN CAEN CHEN CIEN COEN CTEN DIEN EBEN EDEN EVEN EWEN GLEN GMEN GOEN GWEN ITEN KEEN LIEN MIEN MOEN OLEN OMEN OPEN OREN OVEN OWEN OXEN PEEN PHEN RIEN SEEN STEN SVEN TEEN THEN TMEN VTEN WHEN WIEN WREN XMEN

EO•• EOAN EOLA EONS EOUS

E•O• EBON ECOL ECON EDOM EEOC EGON EGOS ELOI ELON ENOL ENON ENOS ENOW EPOS EROO EROS ESOP ESOS ETON EVOE EWOK EXOD EXON

E••O EBRO ECCO ECHO ECTO EDDO EERO EGGO EHLO EKCO ELIO ELKO ELMO ENDO ENTO ENYO ENZO ERGO ERNO EROO ESPO ESSO ESTO EURO EXPO EZIO

•EO• AEON CEOS EEOC GEOG GEOL GEOM GEOS IEOH JEON KEOS LEOG LEOI LEON LEOV LEOX MEOW NEON NEOS PEON REOS XEON YEOH YEOW

•E•O AERO BELO BESO CENO CERO CETO DECO DEDO DEMO DEVO EERO GENO HELO HEMO HERO KEMO KENO LEGO LENO LETO LEVO MELO MEMO MESO NEBO NEMO NERO NEXO OENO PEDO PEPO PERO PESO PETO REAO REDO REGO RELO REMO RENO REPO SECO SEGO SEKO TERO VELO VENO VERO VETO XENO XERO ZENO ZERO

••EO AREO CLEO CREO IDEO OLEO OREO RHEO THEO

EP•• EPEE EPHA EPIC EPIS EPOS EPPA EPPS

E•P• EMPS EPPA EPPS ESPN ESPO ESPY EXPO EXPT

E••P EARP ESOP EVAP

•EP• CEPE CEPS DEPP DEPS DEPT HEPS HEPT KEPI KEPT PEPA PEPE PEPO PEPS REPL REPO REPP REPS REPT SEPT WEPT YEPS ZEPH

•E•P BEEP DEEP DEPP GEEP HEAP HEEP HELP HEMP JEEP KEEP KELP KEMP LEAP NEAP PEEP PERP REAP REPP RESP REUP SEEP TEMP TERP VEEP WEEP YELP

••EP BEEP DEEP GEEP HEEP JEEP KEEP PEEP PREP SEEP SHEP STEP UTEP VEEP WEEP

EQ•• EQUI

E•Q• ESQS

E••Q ERIQ

•EQ• REQD SEQS

••EQ FREQ

ER•• ERAL ERAS ERAT ERDA ERDE ERES EREV ERGO ERGS ERGY ERIA ERIC ERIE ERIK ERIN ERIQ ERIS ERLE ERMA ERNA ERNE ERNO ERNS EROO EROS ERRS ERSE ERST ERTE

E•R• EARL EARN EARP EARS EBRO ECRU EERO EERY EHRE EIRE ENRY ERRS ETRE EURE EURO EVRY EYRA EYRE EZRA

E••R EDER EGER EIER EMER EMIR ENGR ENTR ESAR EUER EVER EWER EYER EZER

•ER• AERI AERO AERY BERG BERM BERN BERT CERA CERE CERF CERO CERT DERE DERM DERN DERR EERO EERY FERN GERE GERI GERM GERT HERA HERB HERD HERE HERO HERR HERS IERI JERI JERK KERB KERF KERI KERN KERR KERT MERC MERE MERL MERM MERS MERV NERA NERD NERF NERI NERO PERA PERC PERE PERF PERI PERK PERM PERO PERP PERS PERT PERU SERA SERB SERE SERF SERS SERT TERA TERI TERM TERN TERO TERP TERR VERA VERB VERE VERN VERO VERS VERT VERY WERE WERT XERO ZERO

•E•R BEAR BEER DEAR DEER DERR FEAR FEHR GEAR GEER HEAR HEBR HEER HEIR HERR JEER KEAR KEIR KERR LEAR LEER LEHR LEUR MEER MEIR NEAR NEBR NEER NEUR PEAR PEER PEUR REAR SEAR SEER SEHR TEAR TEER TERR TETR VEER WEAR WEER WEIR YEAR

••ER ABER ACER AGER ALER AMER APER AUER AVER AXER AYER BAER BEER BIER BOER BRER CBER CHER CUER DEER DOER DUER DYER EDER EGER EIER EMER EUER EVER EWER EYER EZER GEER GOER HEER HIER HOER HUER HYER ICER IGER ILER ISER ITER JEER LEER MEER NEER NLER OBER ODER OMER ONER OPER OVER OWER OYER PEER PIER PTER PUER RUER RVER SEER STER SUER TEER TIER UBER USER VEER VIER WEER YSER

ES•• ESAI ESAR ESAS ESAU ESCE ESCS ESEL ESIS ESKS ESME ESNE ESOP ESOS ESPN ESPO ESPY ESQS ESSA ESSE ESSI ESSO ESTA ESTD ESTE ESTH ESTO ESTS ESVS

E•S• EASE EAST EASY ELSA ELSE ENSE ERSE ERST ESSA ESSE ESSI ESSO

E••S EADS EARS EATS EBBS ECGS ECUS EDBS EDDS EDHS EDMS EDYS EEES EEGS EEKS EELS EFFS

EFTS EGGS EGIS EGOS EINS EKES EKGS ELAS ELIS ELKS ELLS ELMS EMES EMPS EMTS EMUS ENCS ENDS ENES ENGS ENNS ENOS ENTS ENVS EONS EOUS EPIS EPOS EPPS ERAS ERES ERGS ERIS ERNS EROS ERRS ESAS ESCS ESIS ESKS ESOS ESQS ESTS ESVS ETAS ETCS ETDS ETES ETHS EVAS EVES EWES EXES EXTS EYES

•ES•
BESO BESS BEST CESS CEST DESC DESE DESI DESK FESS FEST GEST HESS HEST IEST JESS JEST JESU LESE LESS LEST MESA MESH MESO MESS NESS NEST PESO PEST RESH RESP REST SESE SESS TESH TESS TEST VEST WEST YESM ZEST

•E•S
BECS BEDS BEES BEGS BELS BEMS BESS BETS BEVS BEYS CEES CELS CENS CEOS CEPS CESS DEBS DECS DEES DEFS DEGS DEMS DENS DEPS DETS DEUS DEVS DEWS EEES EEGS EEKS EELS FEBS FEDS FEES FELS FEMS FENS FESS GEDS GEES GELS GEMS GENS GEOS GETS HEHS HEMS HENS HEPS HERS HESS HEWS HEYS JENS JESS JETS JEWS KEAS KEDS KEGS KENS KEOS KEYS LEAS LEDS LEES LEGS LEIS LEKS LEMS LENS LESS LETS MEAS MEDS MEGS MELS MEMS MENS MERS MESS METS MEWS NEBS NEGS NELS NEOS NESS NETS NEWS PEAS PECS PEDS PEES PEGS PENS PEPS PERS PETS PEWS REBS RECS REDS REES REFS REGS RELS REMS REOS REPS RETS REUS REVS SEAS SECS SEES SEGS SEIS SEMS SENS SEQS SERS SESS SETS SEWS TEAS TECS TEDS TEES TELS TENS TESS TETS UEYS VEES VEGS VERS VETS WEBS WEDS WEIS WENS WETS YEAS YENS YEPS YEWS ZEDS ZEES ZEUS

••ES
ACES ADES AGES ALES AMES ANES APES ARES ASES ATES AVES AWES AXES AYES BCES BEES BMES BYES CEES CUES DEES DIES DOES DUES DYES EEES EKES EMES ENES ERES ETES EVES EWES EXES EYES FEES FIES FOES GBES GEES GIES GOES GRES HIES HOES HUES ICES IDES ILES INES IRES ITES IVES JOES LEES LIES LYES MBES MIES MMES MOES NAES NOES OBES ODES OIES OLES OMES ONES OPES ORES OWES OXES PEES PIES PRES QUES REES RHES ROES RTES RUES RYES SAES SEES SHES STES SUES TEES THES TIES TOES TRES TUES TYES UKES UNES USES UTES VEES VIES VUES WOES WYES XKES YVES ZEES

ET••
ETAH ETAL ETAS ETAT ETCH ETCS ETDS ETES ETHN ETHS ETIC ETNA ETON ETRE ETTA ETTE ETTU ETUI ETUM ETYM

E•T•
EATS ECTO EDTA EDTV EFTS EMTS ENTO ENTR ENTS ERTE ESTA ESTD ESTE ESTH ESTO ESTS ETTA ETTE ETTU EXTS

E••T
EAST ECHT EDIT ELAT EMIT ERAT ERST ETAT EXIT EXPT

•ET•
BETA BETE BETH BETS BETZ CETA CETE CETO DETS FETA FETE FETT GETA GETS GETZ HETH JETE JETS JETT KETT KETZ LETO LETS LETT META METE METH METS METZ NETH NETS PETA PETE PETO PETS RETA RETD RETE RETS SETA SETH SETI SETS SETT TETE TETH TETR TETS VETA VETO VETS WETS YETI ZETA

•E•T
BEAT BEET BELT BENT BERT BEST CELT CENT CERT CEST DEBT DEET DEFT DELT DENT DEPT DEUT FEAT FEET FELT FEST FETT GELT GENT GERT GEST HEAT HECT HEET HEFT HEPT HEST IEST JEST JETT KENT KEPT KERT KETT LECT LEFT LENT LEST LETT MEAT MEET MELT MENT NEAT NEET NEST NEUT NEWT NEXT PEAT PEET PELT PENT PERT PEST PEUT RECT REET REFT REGT REIT RENT REPT REST SEAT SECT SENT SEPT SERT SETT TEAT TENT TEST TEUT TEXT VENT VERT VEST WEFT WELT WENT WEPT WERT WEST ZEIT ZEST

••ET
ABET BEET BRET CHET DEET DIET DNET DUET FEET FRET HEET HYET IBET ICET MEET MOET NEET NYET PEET PIET POET PRET REET RHET SPET STET SUET THET TRET VIET WHET

EU••
EUER EULA EURE EURO EUWE

E•U•
EAUX ECUA ECUS EDUC EHUD ELUL EMUS ENUF EOUS EQUI ETUI ETUM

E••U
ECRU EMEU ESAU ETTU

•EU•
DEUM DEUS DEUT DEUX FEUD FEUX JEUX LEUR MEUM NEUE NEUF NEUN NEUR NEUT OEUF PEUR PEUT REUP REUS SEUL TEUT YEUX ZEUS

•E•U
BEAU CEBU GENU JEHU JESU LEVU MENU PEAU PERU SEAU VEAU WELU ZEBU

••EU
BLEU DIEU EMEU LIEU

EV••
EVAC EVAH EVAL EVAN EVAP EVAS EVEL EVEN EVER EVES EVIE EVIL EVOE EVRY

E•V•
EAVE ENVS ENVY ESVS

E••V
EDTV ELEV EREV

•EV•
BEVS BEVY DEVA DEVI DEVO DEVS LEVA LEVI LEVO LEVU LEVY NEVA NEVE NEVI REVA REVE REVS SEVE WEVE

•E•V
BEAV LEOV MERV

••EV
ELEV EREV KIEV LIEV PREV

EW••
EWAN EWEN EWER EWES EWOK

E•W•
EUWE

E••W
ENOW

•EW•
DEWS DEWY HEWN HEWS JEWS LEWD MEWL MEWS NEWF NEWS NEWT PEWS SEWN SEWS TEWA YEWS

•E•W
MEOW YEOW

••EW
AFEW ANEW BLEW BREW CHEW CLEW CREW DREW FLEW GREW IBEW KNEW LOEW PHEW SHEW SKEW SLEW SMEW SPEW STEW THEW VIEW WHEW

EX••
EXAM EXCH EXCL EXEC EXED EXEL EXES EXGI EXIT EXOD EXON EXPO EXPT EXTS

E••X
EAUX EFAX

•EX•
HEXA NEXO NEXT SEXY TEXT

•E•X
DEUX FEUX GENX JEUX LEIX LEOX YEUX

••EX
ALEX AMEX APEX CHEX FLEX IBEX ILEX NMEX PLEX PREX SPEX TREX

EY••
EYCK EYED EYER EYES EYRA EYRE

E•Y•
EDYS ENYA ENYO ETYM

E••Y
EASY EBAY EDDY EDGY EELY EENY EERY EGGY ELLY ELMY EMLY EMMY ENCY ENRY ENVY ERGY ESPY EVRY

•EY•
BEYS HEYS KEYE KEYS UEYS

•E•Y
AERY BELY BEVY DEFY DEMY DENY DEWY EELY EENY EERY HEDY LELY LEVY RELY REMY SECY SEXY VERY

••EY
ACEY FREY GREY HUEY IVEY JOEY OBEY OKEY ONEY PREY SLEY SUEY THEY TREY UREY WHEY

EZ••
EZEK EZER EZIO EZRA

E•Z•
ENZO

E••Z
ELIZ

•EZ•
REZA

•E•Z
BENZ BETZ GEEZ GETZ JEEZ KETZ LENZ METZ

••EZ
BAEZ CHEZ DIEZ GEEZ INEZ JEEZ OYEZ PREZ SUEZ YNEZ

FA••
FABI FACE FACP FACS FACT FADE FADO FADS FAHD FAHR FAIL FAIM FAIN FAIR FAIT FAJA FAKE FALA FALK FALL FAMA FAME FAMS FANE FANG FANS FAQS FARE FARM FARO FARR FASO FAST FATA FATE FATH FATS FAUN FAUT FAUX FAVA FAVE FAWN FAYE FAYS FAZE

F•A•
FEAR FEAT FIAT FLAB FLAG FLAK FLAM FLAN FLAP FLAT FLAW FLAX FLAY FMAJ FOAL FOAM FRAE FRAG FRAM FRAN FRAS FRAT FRAU FRAY FUAD

F••A
FAJA FALA FAMA FATA FAVA FEMA FETA FICA FILA FINA FLEA FNMA FORA FRIA FUCA

•FA•
AFAR BFAS EFAX MFAS SFAX

•F•A
AFTA

••FA
AGFA ALFA SOFA

F•B•
FABI FEBS FIBS FOBS FUBU

F••B
FEEB FLAB FLUB FTLB

•FB•
AFBS RFBS

F•C•
FACE FACP FACS FACT FICA FICT FOCH FOCI FUCA FYCE

F••C
FDIC FISC FLIC

•FC•
CFCS DFCS PFCS

••FC
COFC KOFC

FD••
FDIC FDNY

F•D•
FADE FADO FADS FEDS FIDE FIDO FIDS FUDD

F••D
FAHD FEED FEND FEUD FIND FLED FOLD FOND FOOD FORD FRED FRID FUAD FUDD FUND

•FD•
RFDS

•F•D
NFLD SFPD

FE••
FEAR FEAT FEBS FEDS FEEB FEED FEEL FEES FEET FEHR FEIN FELL FELS FELT FEMA FEME FEMS FEND FENG FENN FENS FERN FESS FEST FETA FETE FETT FEUD FEUX

F•E•
FEEB FEED FEEL FEES FEET FIEF FIES FLEA FLED FLEE FLEM FLEW FLEX FOES FRED FREE FREI FREQ FRET FREY FUEL

F••E
FACE FADE FAKE FAME FANE FARE FATE FAVE FAYE FAZE FEME FETE FIDE FIFE FILE FINE FIRE FIVE FIXE FLEE FLOE FLUE FOIE FORE FRAE FREE FROE FRYE FUGE FUME FUSE FYCE

•FE•
AFEW

••FE
CAFE FIFE JEFE LIFE ORFE RIFE SAFE WIFE

F•F•
FIFE FIFI FIFO

F••F
FIEF FUNF

•FF•
EFFS IFFY OFFS PFFT

••FF
BAFF BIFF BOFF BUFF CUFF DIFF DOFF DUFF GAFF GUFF HOFF HUFF JEFF JIFF LAFF LUFF MIFF MUFF NEFF NUFF ORFF PUFF RAFF RIFF RUFF TIFF TOFF ZIFF

FG•• FGHI

F•G• FIGS FOGG FOGS FOGY FUGE FUGU

F••G FANG FENG FLAG FLOG FOGG FONG FRAG FRIG FROG FRUG

•FG• AFGH EFGH

•F•G AFIG

••FG DEFG

F•H• FAHD FAHR FEHR FGHI FOHN

F••H FATH FISH FOCH FROH

•F•H AFGH EFGH

FI•• FIAT FIBS FICA FICT FIDE FIDO FIDS FIEF FIES FIFE FIFI FIFO FIGS FIJI FILA FILE FILI FILL FILM FILO FILS FINA FIND FINE FINI FINK FINN FINO FINS FIRE FIRM FIRN FIRS FISC FISH FISK FIST FITS FIVE FIXE FIXX FIZZ

F•I• FAIL FAIM FAIN FAIR FAIT FDIC FEIN FLIC FLIM FLIP FLIR FLIT FLIX FOIE FOIL FRIA FRID FRIG FRIO FRIS FRIT FRIZ FWIW

F••I FABI FGHI FIFI FIJI FILI FINI FOCI FREI FUJI

•FI• AFIG EFIK

•F•I IFNI PFUI

••FI FIFI HIFI KOFI REFI SUFI WIFI

F•J• FAJA FIJI FUJI

F••J FMAJ

F•K• FAKE

F••K FALK FINK FISK FLAK FOLK FORK FUNK

•F•K EFIK

FL•• FLAB FLAG FLAK FLAM FLAN FLAP FLAT FLAW FLAX FLAY FLEA FLED FLEE FLEM FLEW FLEX FLIC FLIM FLIP FLIR FLIT FLIX FLOE FLOG FLON FLOP FLOR FLOW FLOY FLOZ FLUB FLUE FLUS FLUX

F•L• FALA FALK FALL FELL FELS FELT FILA FILE FILI FILL FILM FILO FILS FOLD FOLK FTLB FULL

F••L FAIL FALL FEEL FELL FILL FOAL FOIL FOOL FOUL FOWL FUEL FULL FURL

•FL• NFLD

••FL REFL USFL

FM•• FMAJ

F•M• FAMA FAME FAMS FEMA FEME FEMS FNMA FUME FUMY

F••M FAIM FARM FILM FIRM FLAM FLEM FLIM FOAM FORM FRAM FROM

•FM• DFMS

••FM AMFM UOFM

FN•• FNMA

F•N• FANE FANG FANS FDNY FEND FENG FENN FENS FINA FIND FINE FINI FINK FINN FINO FINS FOND FONG FONT FONZ FUND FUNF FUNK FUNS FUNT

F••N FAIN FAUN FAWN FEIN FENN FERN FINN FIRN FLAN FLON FOHN FRAN

•FN• IFNI

FO•• FOAL FOAM FOBS FOCH FOCI FOES FOGG FOGS FOGY FOHN FOIE FOIL FOLD FOLK FOND FONG FONT FONZ FOOD FOOL FOOT FOPS FORA FORD FORE FORK FORM FORS FORT FOSS FOTO FOUL FOUR FOWL FOXX FOXY FOYS FOYT

F•O• FLOE FLOG FLON FLOP FLOR FLOW FLOY FLOZ FOOD FOOL FOOT FROE FROG FROH FROM FROS FROW FTOS

F••O FADO FARO FASO FIDO FIFO FILO FINO FOTO FRIO FURO

•FO• CFOS UFOS

•F•O AFRO IFSO

••FO FIFO INFO LIFO

F•P• FOPS

F••P FACP FLAP FLIP FLOP

•FP• SFPD

••FP KOFP

F•Q• FAQS

F••Q FREQ

FR•• FRAE FRAG FRAM FRAN FRAS FRAT FRAU FRAY FRED FREE FREI FREQ FRET FREY FRIA FRID FRIG FRIO FRIS FRIT FRIZ FROE FROG FROH FROM FROS FROW FRUG FRYE

F•R• FARE FARM FARO FARR FERN FIRE FIRM FIRN FIRS FORA FORD FORE FORK FORM FORS FORT FURL FURO FURS FURY

F••R FAHR FAIR FARR FEAR FEHR FLIR FLOR FOUR

•FR• AFRO MFRS TFRS

•F•R AFAR

F•S• FASO FAST FESS FEST FISC FISH FISK FIST FOSS FUSE FUSS FUST

F••S FACS FADS FAMS FANS FAQS FATS FAYS FEBS FEDS FEES FELS FEMS FENS FESS FIBS FIDS FIES FIGS FILS FINS FIRS FITS FLUS FOBS FOES FOGS FOPS FORS FOSS FOYS FRAS FRIS FROS FTOS FUNS FURS FUSS

•FS• IFSO

•F•S AFBS AFTS BFAS CFCS CFOS DFCS DFMS EFFS EFTS MFAS MFRS OFFS PFCS RFBS RFDS TFRS UFOS

••FS ARFS COFS DEFS EFFS GIFS INFS KAFS OAFS OFFS OOFS PDFS QAFS REFS RIFS SPFS WAFS

FT•• FTLB FTOS

F•T• FATA FATE FATH FATS FETA FETE FETT FITS FOTO FUTZ

F••T FACT FAIT FAST FAUT FEAT FEET FELT FEST FETT FIAT FICT FIST FLAT FLIT FONT FOOT FORT FOYT FRAT FRET FRIT FUNT FUST

•FT• AFTA AFTS EFTS

•F•T PFFT

••FT BDFT CUFT DAFT DEFT GIFT HAFT HEFT LEFT LIFT LOFT LUFT PFFT RAFT REFT RIFT SIFT SOFT SQFT TAFT TOFT TUFT WAFT WEFT

FU•• FUAD FUBU FUCA FUDD FUEL FUGE FUGU FUJI FULL FUME FUMY FUND FUNF FUNK FUNS FUNT FURL FURO FURS FURY FUSE FUSS FUST FUTZ FUZZ

F•U• FAUN FAUT FAUX FEUD FEUX FLUB FLUE FLUS FLUX FOUL FOUR FRUG

F••U FRAU FUBU FUGU

•FU• PFUI

••FU TOFU ZAFU

F•V• FAVA FAVE FIVE

FW•• FWIW

F•W• FAWN FOWL

F••W FLAW FLEW FLOW FROW FWIW

•F•W AFEW

F•X• FIXE FIXX FOXX FOXY

F••X FAUX FEUX FIXX FLAX FLEX FLIX FLUX FOXX

•F•X EFAX SFAX

FY•• FYCE

F•Y• FAYE FAYS FOYS FOYT FRYE

F••Y FDNY FLAY FLOY FOGY FOXY FRAY FREY FUMY FURY

•F•Y IFFY

••FY DEFY DUFY IFFY

F•Z• FAZE FIZZ FUZZ

F••Z FIZZ FLOZ FONZ FRIZ FUTZ FUZZ

GA•• GABE GABS GABY GADS GAEA GAEL GAFF GAGA GAGE GAGS GAIA GAIL GAIN GAIT GALA GALE GALL GALS GALT GAMA GAME GAMP GAMS GAMY GANG GANN GANT GAOL GAPE GAPS GARB GARD GARE GARN GARO GARP GARR GARS GARY GASH GASP GASX GATE GATO GATS GATT GAUD GAUL GAUR GAVE GAWK GAWP GAYE GAZA GAZE

G•A• GDAY GEAR GHAT GIAN GLAD GLAM GMAC GMAJ GMAN GMAT GNAR GNAT GNAW GOAD GOAL GOAS GOAT GPAS GRAB GRAD GRAF GRAM GRAN GRAS GRAU GRAY GRAZ GUAM GUAR GUAT

G••A GAEA GAGA GAIA GALA GAMA GAZA GENA GETA GHIA GIGA GILA GINA GITA GIZA GLIA GNMA GOLA GOYA

•GA• AGAL AGAR AGAS EGAD EGAL EGAN OGAM

•G•A AGFA AGHA AGRA AGUA

••GA ALGA ANGA BEGA BIGA GAGA GIGA INGA LPGA MEGA OLGA RAGA RIGA SAGA SEGA TOGA USGA VEGA YOGA

GB•• GBES

G•B• GABE GABS GABY GIBB GIBE GIBS GOBI GOBO GOBS GOBY GRBR GTBR

G••B GARB GHWB GIBB GLIB GLOB GRAB GRUB

•GB• IGBY MGBS

G•C• GLCS GMCS GUCK

G••C GLUC GLYC GMAC

•GC• AGCY

GD•• GDAY

G•D• GADS GEDS GIDE GODS

G••D GARD GAUD GEED GELD GIED GILD GIRD GLAD GOAD GOLD GOOD GRAD GRID GUND

•G•D AGED EGAD OGOD

••GD BIGD REGD

GE•• GEAR GEDS GEED GEEK GEEP GEER GEES GEEZ GELD GELL GELS GELT GEMS GENA GENE GENF GENL GENO GENS GENT GENU GENX GEOG GEOL GEOM GEOS GERE GERI GERM GERT GEST GETA GETS GETZ

G•E• GAEA GAEL GBES GEED GEEK GEEP GEER GEES GEEZ GHEE GIED GIES GLEE GLEN GMEN GOEN GOER GOES GREG GRES GREW GREY GWEN

G••E GABE GAGE GALE GAME GAPE GARE GATE GAVE GAYE GAZE GENE GERE GHEE GIBE GIDE GIVE GLEE GLUE GONE GORE GRUE GUTE GYNE GYRE

•GE• AGED AGEE AGER AGES EGER IGER OGEE

•G•E AGEE AGUE OGEE OGLE OGRE

••GE ANGE CAGE DOGE EDGE FUGE GAGE HUGE INGE LOGE LUGE MAGE MTGE PAGE RAGE SAGE TIGE URGE WAGE

G•F• GAFF GIFS GIFT GUFF

G••F GAFF GENF GOLF GOOF GRAF GUFF GULF

•GF• AGFA

•G•F TGIF

G•G• GAGA GAGE GAGS GIGA GIGI GIGO GIGS GOGH GOGI GOGO

G••G GANG GEOG GLUG GONG GREG GRIG GROG GUNG

•GG• EGGO EGGS EGGY IGGS IGGY OGGI

•G•G AGOG

••GG EIGG FOGG HOGG LEGG RIGG YEGG

GH•• GHAT GHEE GHIA GHIJ GHWB

G••H GASH GISH GOGH GOSH GOTH GROH GUSH

•GH• AGHA FGHI UGHS

•G•H LGTH

••GH AFGH EFGH GOGH HIGH HUGH NIGH PUGH SIGH

GI•• GIAN GIBB GIBE GIBS GIDE GIED GIES GIFS GIFT GIGA GIGI GIGO GIGS GILA GILD GILL GILT GIMP GINA GINO GINS GIPP GIRD GIRL GIRO GIRT GISH GIST GITA GITS GIVE GIZA

G•I• GAIA GAIL GAIN GAIT GHIA GHIJ GLIA GLIB GLIM

GOIN
GRID
GRIG
GRIM
GRIN
GRIP
GRIS
GRIT
GTIS

G••I
GERI
GIGI
GOBI
GOGI
GYRI

•GI•
AGIN
AGIO
AGIS
EGIS
TGIF

•G•I
AGNI
AGRI
EGLI
FGHI
OGGI
UGLI

••GI
EXGI
GIGI
GOGI
HAGI
MAGI
OGGI
VAGI
YOGI
ZOGI

G••J
GHIJ
GMAJ

G••K
GAWK
GEEK
GOOK
GROK
GUCK
GUNK

GL••
GLAD
GLAM
GLCS
GLEE
GLEN
GLIA
GLIB
GLIM
GLOB
GLOM
GLOP
GLOT
GLOW
GLUC
GLUE
GLUG
GLUM
GLUT
GLYC
GLYN

G•L•
GALA
GALE
GALL
GALS
GALT
GELD
GELL
GELS
GELT
GILA
GILD
GILL
GILT
GOLA
GOLD
GOLF
GULF
GULL
GULP

G••L
GAEL
GAIL
GALL
GAOL
GAUL
GELL
GENL
GEOL
GILL
GIRL
GOAL
GRRL
GULL

•GL•
EGLI
IGLU
OGLE
UGLI
UGLY

•G•L
AGAL
EGAL

GM••
GMAC
GMAJ
GMAN
GMAT
GMCS
GMEN

G•M•
GAMA
GAME
GAMP
GAMS
GAMY
GEMS
GIMP
GNMA
GUMM
GUMP
GUMS
GYMS

G••M
GEOM
GERM
GLAM
GLIM
GLOM
GLUM
GORM
GRAM
GRIM
GUAM
GUMM

•GM•
MGMT

•G•M
OGAM

GN••
GNAR
GNAT
GNAW
GNMA
GNPS
GNUS

G•N•
GANG
GANN
GANT
GENA
GENE
GENF
GENL
GENO
GENS
GENT
GENU
GENX
GINA
GINO
GINS
GONE
GONG
GONY
GUND
GUNG
GUNK
GUNN
GUNS
GYNE
GYNT
GYNY

G••N
GAIN
GANN
GARN
GIAN
GLEN
GLYN
GMAN
GMEN
GOEN
GOIN
GOON
GOWN
GRAN
GRIN
GRUN
GUNN
GWEN
GWYN

•GN•
AGNI

•G•N
AGIN
AGON
EGAN
EGON

••GN
LIGN
SIGN

GO••
GOAD
GOAL
GOAS
GOAT
GOBI
GOBO
GOBS
GOBY
GODS
GOEN
GOER
GOES
GOGH
GOGI
GOGO
GOIN
GOLA
GOLD
GOLF
GONE
GONG
GONY
GOOD
GOOF
GOOK
GOON
GOOP
GOOS
GORE
GORM
GORO
GORP
GORT
GORY
GOSH
GOSS
GOTH
GOTO
GOTT
GOUP
GOUT
GOVS
GOVT
GOWN
GOYA

G•O•
GAOL
GEOG
GEOL
GEOM
GEOS
GLOB
GLOM
GLOP
GLOT
GLOW
GOOD
GOOF
GOOK
GOON
GOOP
GOOS
GPOS
GROG
GROH
GROK
GROS
GROT
GROW
GTOS

G••O
GARO
GATO
GENO
GIGO
GINO
GIRO
GOBO
GOGO
GORO
GOTO
GYRO

•GO•
AGOG
AGON
EGON
EGOS
IGOR
NGOR
OGOD
YGOR

•G•O
AGIO
AGRO
EGGO
OGRO

••GO
ARGO
BIGO
EGGO
ERGO
GIGO
GOGO
HUGO
IAGO
INGO
LAGO
LEGO
LOGO
NOGO
PAGO
POGO
REGO
SAGO
SEGO
TOGO
VIGO
YUGO

GP••
GPAS
GPOS

G•P•
GAPE
GAPS
GIPP
GNPS
GYPS

G••P
GAMP
GARP
GASP
GAWP
GEEP
GIMP
GIPP
GLOP
GOOP
GORP
GOUP
GRIP
GULP
GUMP

•GP•
OGPU

GR••
GRAB
GRAD
GRAF
GRAM
GRAN
GRAS
GRAU
GRAY
GRAZ
GRBR
GREG
GRES
GREW
GREY
GRID
GRIG
GRIM
GRIN
GRIP
GRIS
GRIT
GROG
GROH
GROK
GROS
GROT
GROW
GRRL
GRRR
GRRS
GRUB
GRUE
GRUN
GRUS
GRWT

G•R•
GARB
GARD
GARE
GARN
GARO
GARP
GARR
GARS
GARY
GERE
GERI
GERM
GERT
GIRD
GIRL
GIRO
GIRT
GORE
GORM
GORO
GORP
GORT
GORY
GRRL
GRRR
GRRS
GURU
GYRE
GYRI
GYRO

G••R
GARR
GAUR
GEAR
GEER
GNAR
GOER
GRBR
GRRR
GTBR
GUAR

•GR•
AGRA
AGRI
AGRO
MGRS
OGRE
OGRO

•G•R
AGAR
AGER
EGER
IGER
IGOR
NGOR
YGOR

••GR
ENGR
JAGR
MSGR

G•S•
GASH
GASP
GASX
GEST
GISH
GIST
GOSH
GOSS
GUSH
GUST

G••S
GABS
GADS
GAGS
GALS
GAMS
GAPS
GARS
GATS
GBES
GEDS
GEES
GELS
GEMS
GENS
GEOS
GETS
GIBS
GIES
GIFS
GIGS
GINS
GITS
GLCS
GMCS
GNPS
GNUS
GOAS
GOBS
GODS
GOES
GOOS
GOSS
GOVS
GPAS
GPOS
GRAS
GRES
GRIS
GROS
GRRS
GRUS
GTIS
GTOS
GTVS
GTXS
GUMS
GUNS
GUTS
GUVS
GUYS
GYMS
GYPS

•GS•
AGST

•G•S
AGAS
AGES
AGIS
AGTS
EGGS
EGIS
EGOS
HGTS
IGGS
MGBS
MGRS
RGTS
SGTS
UGHS

••GS
AUGS
AVGS
BAGS
BEGS
BIGS
BOGS
BUGS
CHGS
CIGS
COGS
DEGS
DIGS
DOGS
ECGS
EEGS
EGGS
EKGS
ENGS
ERGS
FIGS
FOGS
GAGS
GIGS
HAGS
HOGS
HUGS
IGGS
JAGS
JIGS
JOGS
JPGS
JUGS
KEGS
LAGS
LEGS
LOGS
LUGS
MAGS
MEGS
MIGS
MSGS
MTGS
MUGS
NAGS
NEGS
NOGS
ORGS
PEGS
PIGS
PKGS
POGS
PUGS
RAGS
REGS
RIGS
RUGS
SAGS
SEGS
SIGS
TAGS
TOGS
TUGS
VAGS
VEGS
VIGS
VUGS
WAGS
WIGS
ZAGS
ZIGS

GT••
GTBR
GTIS
GTOS
GTVS
GTXS

G•T•
GATE
GATO
GATS
GATT
GETA
GETS
GETZ
GITA
GITS
GOTH
GOTO
GOTT
GUTE
GUTS
GWTW

G••T
GAIT
GALT
GANT
GATT
GELT
GENT
GERT
GEST
GHAT
GIFT
GILT
GIRT
GIST
GLOT
GLUT
GMAT
GNAT
GOAT
GORT
GOTT
GOUT
GOVT
GRIT
GROT
GRWT
GUAT
GUST
GYNT

•GT•
AGTS
HGTS
HGTV
LGTH
RGTS
SGTS

•G•T
AGST
MGMT

••GT
MSGT
REGT
SSGT
TSGT

GU••
GUAM
GUAR
GUAT
GUCK
GUFF
GULF
GULL
GULP
GUMM
GUMP
GUMS
GUND
GUNG
GUNK
GUNN
GUNS
GURU
GUSH
GUST
GUTE
GUTS
GUVS
GUYS

G•U•
GAUD
GAUL
GAUR
GLUC
GLUE
GLUG
GLUM
GLUT
GNUS
GOUP
GOUT
GRUB
GRUE
GRUN
GRUS

G••U
GENU
GRAU
GURU

•GU•
AGUA
AGUE

•G•U
IGLU
OGPU

••GU
FUGU
RAGU

G•V•
GAVE
GIVE
GOVS
GOVT
GTVS
GUVS

•G•V
HGTV

GW••
GWEN
GWTW
GWYN

G•W•
GAWK
GAWP
GHWB
GOWN
GRWT

G••W
GLOW
GNAW
GREW
GROW
GWTW

•GW•
HGWY

G•X•
GTXS

G••X
GASX
GENX

GY••
GYMS
GYNE
GYNT
GYNY
GYPS
GYRE
GYRI
GYRO

G•Y•
GAYE
GLYC
GLYN
GOYA
GUYS
GWYN

G••Y
GABY
GAMY
GARY
GDAY
GOBY
GONY
GORY
GRAY
GREY
GYNY

•G•Y
AGCY
EGGY
HGWY
IGBY
IGGY
UGLY

••GY
BOGY
CAGY
EDGY
EGGY
ERGY
FOGY
IGGY
LOGY
NAGY
ORGY
SAGY
URGY

G•Z•
GAZA
GAZE
GIZA

G••Z
GEEZ
GETZ
GRAZ

HA••
HAAA
HAAG
HAAS
HABS
HACK
HADJ
HAEC
HAFT
HAGI
HAGS
HAHA
HAHN
HAHS
HAID
HAIG
HAIK
HAIL
HAIM
HAIR
HAJE
HAJI
HAJJ
HAKE
HALE
HALF
HALI
HALL
HALO
HALS
HALT
HAMA
HAME
HAMM
HAMP
HAMS
HANA
HAND
HANG
HANK
HANS
HAOS
HAPS
HARA
HARD
HARE
HARI
HARK
HARM
HARP
HART
HARZ
HASH
HASP
HAST
HATE
HATH
HATS
HAUL
HAUS
HAUT
HAVA
HAVE
HAWG
HAWK
HAWN
HAWS
HAYS
HAZE
HAZY

H•A•
HAAA
HAAG
HAAS
HBAR
HEAD
HEAL
HEAP
HEAR
HEAT
HOAD
HOAG
HOAR
HOAX
HRAP
HUAC

H••A
HAAA
HAHA
HAMA
HANA
HARA
HAVA
HEMA
HERA
HEXA
HIJA
HIVA
HIYA
HOLA
HORA
HOYA
HSIA
HULA
HYLA

•HA•
AHAB
AHAH
AHAS
BHAT
CHAD
CHAI
CHAN
CHAO
CHAP
CHAR
CHAS
CHAT
CHAW
DHAL
GHAT
KHAN
KHAS
NHAT
PHAG
PHAR
PHAT
RHAP
SHAD
SHAG
SHAH
SHAM
SHAN
SHAQ
SHAR
SHAW
SHAY
THAD
THAE
THAI
THAN
THAR
THAT
THAW
WHAM
WHAP
WHAT

•H•A
CHIA
GHIA
NHRA
RHEA
SHEA
WHOA

••HA
AGHA
DOHA
EPHA
HAHA
NAHA
OSHA
YMHA
YWHA

HB••
HBAR

H•B•
HABS
HDBK
HEBB
HEBE
HEBR
HOBE
HOBO
HOBS
HUBS

H••B
HEBB
HERB

•HB•
LHBS
RHBS

•H•B
AHAB
CHUB
GHWB
NHEB
SHEB

H•C•
HACK
HECK
HECT
HICK
HICS
HOCH
HOCK
HUCK

H••C
HAEC
HUAC

•H•C
CHIC
CHOC

HD••
HDBK
HDTV

H•D•
HADJ
HEDY
HIDE
HODS
HYDE
HYDR

H••D
HAID
HAND
HARD
HEAD
HEED
HELD
HERD
HIED
HIND
HOAD
HOED
HOLD
HOND
HOOD
HUED
HUND

•HD•
PHDS
THDS

•H•D
AHED
CHAD
CHID
DHED
EHUD
OHED
RHOD
SHAD
SHED
SHOD
THAD
THUD
WHOD
WHYD

••HD
FAHD

HE••
HEAD
HEAL
HEAP
HEAR
HEAT
HEBB
HEBE
HEBR
HECK
HECT
HEDY
HEED
HEEL
HEEP
HEER
HEET
HEFT
HEHE
HEHS
HEIN
HEIR
HELD
HELI
HELL
HELM
HELO
HELP
HEMA
HEME
HEMI
HEMO
HEMP
HEMS
HENN
HENS
HEPS
HEPT
HERA
HERB
HERD
HERE
HERO
HERR
HERS
HESS
HEST
HETH
HEWN
HEWS
HEXA
HEYS

H•E•
HAEC
HEED
HEEL
HEEP
HEER
HEET
HIED
HIER
HIES
HOED
HOER
HOES
HUED
HUER
HUES
HUEY
HYER
HYET

H••E
HAJE
HAKE
HALE
HAME
HARE
HATE
HAVE
HAZE
HEBE
HEHE
HEME
HERE
HIDE
HIKE
HIRE
HITE
HIVE
HOBE
HOKE
HOLE
HOME
HONE
HOPE
HOSE
HOTE
HOVE
HOWE
HUGE
HUME
HYDE
HYPE

•HE•
AHED
AHEM
CHEE
CHEF
CHEM
CHEN
CHER
CHET
CHEW
CHEX
CHEZ
DHED
GHEE
NHEB
OHED
PHEN
PHEW
RHEA
RHEE
RHEO
RHES
RHET
SHEA
SHEB
SHED
SHEK
SHEL
SHEM
SHEP
SHES
SHEW
THEE
THEM
THEN
THEO
THES

THET
THEW
THEY
WHEE
WHEN
WHET
WHEW
WHEY

•H•E
AHME
CHEE
EHLE
EHRE
GHEE
IHRE
OHME
OHNE
OHRE
RHEE
RHUE
SHOE
SHUE
THAE
THEE
WHEE

••HE
ACHE
ASHE
HEHE
ROHE

H•F•
HAFT
HEFT
HIFI
HOFF
HUFF

H••F
HALF
HOFF
HOOF
HUFF

•H•F
CHEF

HG••
HGTS
HGTV
HGWY

H•G•
HAGI
HAGS
HIGH
HOGG
HOGS
HUGE
HUGH
HUGO
HUGS

H••G
HAAG
HAIG
HANG
HAWG
HOAG
HOGG
HONG
HUNG

•HG•
CHGS

•H•G
CHUG
PHAG
SHAG
THUG
WHIG

H•H•
HAHA
HAHN
HAHS
HEHE
HEHS
HIHO
HOHO
HUHS

H••H
HASH
HATH
HETH
HIGH
HOCH
HOTH
HUGH
HUNH
HUSH

•HH•
OHHI
SHHH

•H•H
AHAH
OHOH
SHAH
SHHH
SHIH
UHOH
UHUH

••HH
SHHH

HI••
HICK
HICS
HIDE
HIED
HIER
HIES
HIFI
HIGH
HIHO
HIJA
HIJK
HIJO
HIKE
HILL
HILO
HILT
HIND
HINT
HIPS
HIRE
HIRT
HISN
HISS
HIST
HITE
HITS
HIVA
HIVE
HIYA
HIYO

H•I•
HAID
HAIG
HAIK
HAIL
HAIM
HAIR
HEIN
HEIR
HSIA
HUIS
HUIT

H••I
HAGI
HAJI
HALI
HARI
HELI
HEMI
HIFI
HONI
HOPI

•HI•
CHIA
CHIC
CHID
CHIM
CHIN
CHIP
CHIS
CHIT
GHIA
GHIJ
OHIO
PHIL
PHIS
PHIZ
RHIN
SHIH
SHIM
SHIN
SHIP
SHIV
THIN
THIS
WHIG
WHIM
WHIP
WHIR
WHIT
WHIZ

•H•I
CHAI
OHHI
SHUI
THAI

••HI
ELHI
FGHI
LEHI
MAHI
NEHI
OHHI

H•J•
HAJE
HAJI
HAJJ
HIJA
HIJK
HIJO
HOJO

H••J
HADJ
HAJJ

•H•J
GHIJ

H•K•
HAKE
HIKE
HOKE

H••K
HACK
HAIK
HANK
HARK
HAWK
HDBK
HECK
HICK
HIJK
HOCK
HONK
HOOK
HOUK
HUCK
HULK
HUNK
HUSK

•H•K
OHOK
SHEK

H•L•
HALE
HALF
HALI
HALL
HALO
HALS
HALT
HELD
HELI
HELL
HELM
HELO
HELP
HILL
HILO
HILT
HOLA
HOLD
HOLE
HOLM
HOLO
HOLS
HOLT
HOLY
HULA
HULK
HULL
HYLA

H••L
HAIL
HALL
HAUL
HEAL
HEEL
HELL
HILL
HOWL
HTML
HULL
HURL

•HL•
EHLE
EHLO

•H•L
CHOL
DHAL
PHIL
SHEL
SHUL

••HL
DAHL
KOHL
POHL
SAHL
WAHL
WUHL

HM••
HMMM
HMOS

H•M•
HAMA
HAME
HAMM
HAMP
HAMS
HEMA
HEME
HEMI
HEMO
HEMP
HEMS
HMMM
HOME
HOMO
HTML
HUME
HUMP
HUMS
HYMN

H••M
HAIM
HAMM
HARM
HELM
HMMM
HOLM
HOWM

•HM•
AHME
CHMN
OHME
OHMS
OHMY
SHMO

•H•M
AHEM
AHUM
CHEM
CHIM
CHUM
RHUM
SHAM
SHEM
SHIM
THEM
THOM
WHAM
WHIM
WHOM

••HM
BOHM

H•N•
HANA
HAND
HANG
HANK
HANS
HENN
HENS
HIND
HINT
HOND
HONE
HONG
HONI
HONK
HONS
HUND
HUNG
HUNH
HUNK
HUNS
HUNT

H••N
HAHN
HAWN
HEIN
HENN
HEWN
HISN
HORN
HYMN
HYPN

•HN•
OHNE
OHNO

•H•N
CHAN
CHEN
CHIN
CHMN
CHON
KHAN
PHEN
PHON
RHIN
SHAN
SHIN
SHUN
THAN
THEN
THIN
THON
WHEN

••HN
BAHN
CAHN
COHN
ETHN
FOHN
HAHN
JOHN
KAHN
KUHN
LEHN
ZAHN
ZEHN

HO••
HOAD
HOAG
HOAR
HOAX
HOBE
HOBO
HOBS
HOCH
HOCK
HODS
HOED
HOER
HOES
HOFF
HOGG
HOGS
HOHO
HOJO
HOKE
HOLA
HOLD
HOLE
HOLM
HOLO
HOLS
HOLT
HOLY
HOME
HOMO
HOND
HONE
HONG
HONI
HONK
HONS
HOOD
HOOF
HOOK
HOOP
HOOT
HOPE
HOPI
HOPS
HORA
HORN
HORS
HORT
HOSE
HOSP
HOSS
HOST
HOTE
HOTH
HOUK
HOUR
HOVE
HOWE
HOWL
HOWM
HOWS
HOYA
HOYT

H•O•
HAOS
HMOS
HOOD
HOOF
HOOK
HOOP
HOOT

H••O
HALO
HELO
HEMO
HERO
HIHO
HIJO
HILO
HIYO
HOBO
HOHO
HOJO
HOLO
HOMO
HUGO
HYPO

•HO•
AHOY
CHOC
CHOL
CHON
CHOO
CHOP
CHOU
CHOW
CHOY
DHOW
IHOP
MHOS
OHOH
OHOK
OHOS
PHON
PHOT
RHOD
RHOS
SHOD
SHOE
SHOO
SHOP
SHOR
SHOT
SHOW
THOM
THON
THOR
THOS
THOU
UHOH
WHOA
WHOD
WHOM
WHOP
WHOS
ZHOU

•H•O
AHSO
CHAO
CHOO
EHLO
OHIO
OHNO
OHSO
RHEO
SHMO
SHOO
THEO
THRO

••HO
BOHO
COHO
ECHO
HIHO
HOHO
IMHO
NOHO
OCHO
OTHO
SOHO
YOHO

H•P•
HAPS
HEPS
HEPT
HIPS
HOPE
HOPI
HOPS
HUPS
HYPE
HYPN
HYPO

H••P
HAMP
HARP
HASP
HEAP
HEEP
HELP
HEMP
HOOP
HOSP
HRAP
HTTP
HUMP

•H•P
CHAP
CHIP
CHOP
IHOP
RHAP
SHEP
SHIP
SHOP
WHAP
WHIP
WHOP
WHUP

•H•Q
SHAQ

HR••
HRAP

H•R•
HARA
HARD
HARE
HARI
HARK
HARM
HARP
HART
HARZ
HERA
HERB
HERD
HERE
HERO
HERR
HERS
HIRE
HIRT
HORA
HORN
HORS
HORT
HURL
HURT

H••R
HAIR
HBAR
HEAR
HEBR
HEER
HEIR
HERR
HIER
HOAR
HOER
HOUR
HUER
HYDR
HYER

•HR•
EHRE
IHRE
NHRA
OHRE
SHRS
THRO
THRU
UHRY

•H•R
CHAR
CHER
PHAR
SHAR
SHOR
THAR
THOR
THUR
WHIR

••HR
BOHR
FAHR
FEHR
JAHR
LAHR
LEHR
RUHR
SEHR
TCHR
WAHR

HS••
HSIA

H•S•
HASH
HASP
HAST
HESS
HEST
HISN
HISS
HIST
HOSE
HOSP
HOSS
HOST
HUSH
HUSK

H••S
HAAS
HABS
HAGS
HAHS
HALS
HAMS
HANS
HAOS
HAPS
HATS
HAUS
HAWS
HAYS
HEHS
HEMS
HENS
HEPS
HERS
HESS
HEWS
HEYS
HGTS
HICS
HIES
HIPS
HISS
HITS
HMOS
HOBS
HODS
HOES
HOGS
HOLS
HONS
HOPS
HORS
HOSS
HOWS
HUBS
HUES
HUGS
HUHS
HUIS
HUMS
HUNS
HUPS
HUTS
HWYS

•HS•
AHSO
OHSO

•H•S
AHAS
CHAS
CHGS
CHIS
KHAS
LHBS
MHOS
OHMS
OHOS
PHDS
PHIS
PHYS
RHBS
RHES
RHOS
RHYS
SHES
SHRS
THDS
THES
THIS
THOS
THUS
WHOS
WHYS

••HS
AAHS
BAHS
DAHS
DOHS
DTHS
DUHS
EDHS
ETHS
HAHS
HEHS
HUHS
MOHS
NAHS
OCHS
OOHS
PAHS
RAHS
UGHS
WAHS

HT••
HTML
HTTP

H•T•
HATE
HATH
HATS
HDTV
HETH
HGTS
HGTV
HITE
HITS
HOTE
HOTH
HTTP
HUTS
HUTT
HUTU

H••T
HAFT
HALT
HART
HAST
HAUT
HEAT
HECT
HEET
HEFT
HEPT
HEST
HILT
HINT
HIRT
HIST
HOLT
HOOT
HORT
HOST
HOYT
HUIT
HUNT
HURT
HUTT
HYET

•H•T
BHAT
CHAT
CHET
CHIT
GHAT
NHAT
PHAT
PHOT
PHYT
RHET
SHOT
SHUT
THAT
THET
WHAT
WHET
WHIT

••HT
ACHT
BAHT
ECHT

HU••
HUAC
HUBS
HUCK
HUED
HUER
HUES
HUEY
HUFF
HUGE
HUGH
HUGO
HUGS
HUHS
HUIS
HUIT
HULA
HULK
HULL
HUME
HUMP
HUMS
HUND
HUNG
HUNH
HUNK
HUNS
HUNT
HUPS
HURL
HURT
HUSH
HUSK
HUTS
HUTT
HUTU

H•U•
HAUL
HAUS
HAUT
HOUK
HOUR

H••U
HUTU

•HU•
AHUM
CHUB
CHUG
CHUM
EHUD
RHUE
RHUM
SHUE
SHUI
SHUL
SHUN
SHUT
THUD
THUG
THUR
THUS
UHUH
WHUP

•H•U
CHOU
THOU
THRU
ZHOU

••HU
JEHU
OAHU

H•V•
HAVA
HAVE
HIVA
HIVE
HOVE

H••V
HDTV
HGTV

•H•V
SHIV

HW••
HWYS

H•W•
HAWG
HAWK
HAWN
HAWS
HEWN
HEWS
HGWY
HOWE
HOWL
HOWM
HOWS

•HW•
GHWB

•H•W
CHAW
CHEW
CHOW
DHOW
PHEW
SHAW
SHEW
SHOW
THAW
THEW
WHEW

H•X•
HEXA

H••X
HOAX

•H•X
CHEX

HY••
HYDE
HYDR
HYER
HYET
HYLA
HYMN
HYPE
HYPN
HYPO

H•Y•
HAYS
HEYS
HIYA
HIYO
HOYA
HOYT
HWYS

H••Y
HAZY
HEDY
HGWY
HOLY
HUEY

•HY•
PHYS
PHYT
RHYS
WHYD
WHYS

•H•Y
AHOY
CHOY
OHMY
SHAY
THEY
UHRY
WHEY

••HY
ACHY
ASHY

H•Z•
HAZE
HAZY

H••Z
HARZ

•H•Z
CHEZ
PHIZ
WHIZ

IA••
IAGO
IAMB
IAMS
IANA
IASI

I•A•
IBAR
ICAL
ICAN
IDAE
IMAC
IMAM
IMAN
IMAX
IRAE
IRAN
IRAQ
IRAS
ISAK
ISAO
ISAR
ISAY
ITAL
ITAR
IVAN
IVAR
IYAR

I••A
IANA
IDEA
IKEA
ILIA
ILKA
ILLA
ILSA
ILYA
INCA
INGA
INKA
IOLA
IONA
IOTA
IOWA
IPSA
IRMA
IRRA
ISLA
ITEA
ITZA
IXIA

•IA•
BIAO
BIAS
CIAO
DIAG
DIAL
DIAM
DIAN
DIAS
DIAZ
FIAT
GIAN
KIAM
KIAS
LIAM
LIAO
LIAR
LIAT
MIAS
PIAF
PIAO
RIAA
RIAL
RIAS
SIAL
SIAM
SIAN
TIAS
VIAL
XIAN

•I•A
AIDA
AIEA
AIWA
BIGA
BIWA
DINA
DIVA
FICA
FILA
FINA
GIGA
GILA
GINA
GITA
GIZA
HIJA
HIVA
HIYA
JIMA
KINA
KIVA
LIDA
LILA
LIMA
LINA
LIRA
LISA
LITA
LIZA
MICA
MILA
MINA
MIRA
MITA
NIKA
NINA
NIPA
NITA
OITA
PICA
PIKA
PIMA
PINA
PISA
PITA
RIAA
RICA
RIGA
RIMA
RINA
RIPA
RITA
RIVA
SICA
SIKA
SIMA
SIVA
SIXA
TINA
TIWA
VIDA
VILA
VINA
VISA
VITA
VIVA
ZIMA
ZINA
ZIRA

••IA
ADIA
ALIA
APIA
ARIA
ASIA
AVIA
CHIA
DJIA
ELIA
EMIA
ERIA
FRIA

GAIA
GHIA
GLIA
HSIA
ILIA
IXIA
KAIA
LEIA
MAIA
NOIA
OPIA
USIA

IB••
IBAR
IBET
IBEW
IBEX
IBID
IBIS
IBLE
IBLY
IBMS
IBOS

I•B•
ICBM
IGBY
ISBN

I••B
IAMB

•IB•
BIBB
BIBI
BIBL
BIBS
DIBS
FIBS
GIBB
GIBE
GIBS
JIBE
JIBS
LIBS
MIBS
NIBS
PIBB
RIBO
RIBS
SIBS
VIBE

•I•B
BIBB
GIBB
LIEB
LIMB
LITB
PIBB
SIXB

••IB
CRIB
DRIB
GLIB
TRIB

IC••
ICAL
ICAN
ICBM
ICED
ICEE
ICEL
ICER
ICES
ICET
ICKY
ICON
ICOS
ICUS

I•C•
INCA
INCE
INCH
INCL
INCR
INCS
ITCH

I••C
IMAC
IROC
ITIC

•IC•
BICS
DICE
DICK
DICT
FICA
FICT
HICK
HICS
KICK
LICE
LICK
LICS
MICA
MICE
MICH
MICK
MICR
MICS
NICE
NICK
PICA
PICE
PICK
PICO
PICS
PICT
RICA
RICE
RICH
RICK
RICO
SICA
SICK
SICS
TICK
TICO
TICS
VICE
VICI
VICO
WICK

•I•C
CINC
CIRC
DISC
FISC
LINC
MISC
SIXC
VISC
WISC
ZINC

••IC
AMIC
ATIC
BRIC
CHIC
EPIC
ERIC
ETIC
FDIC
FLIC
ITIC
LAIC
ODIC
OLIC
ONIC
OTIC
SPIC
ZOIC

ID••
IDAE
IDEA
IDED
IDEE
IDEM
IDEO
IDES
IDID
IDIG
IDIO
IDLE
IDLY
IDOL
IDOS
IDVE
IDYL

I•D•
INDO
INDS
INDY
IODO

I••D
IBID
ICED
IDED
IDID
IPOD
IRED
IRID
IZOD

•ID•
AIDA
AIDE
AIDS
BIDE
BIDS
BIDU
CIDE
DIDI
DIDO
DIDY
FIDE
FIDO
FIDS
GIDE
HIDE
KIDD
KIDS
LIDA
LIDO
LIDS
MIDI
NIDE
NIDI
RIDD
RIDE
RIDI
RIDS
SIDE
TIDE
TIDY
VIDA
VIDE
VIDI
VIDS
WIDE

•I•D
BIGD
BIND
BIRD
DIED
FIND
GIED
GILD
GIRD
HIED
HIND
KIDD
KIND
LIED
LIND
LITD
MILD
MIND
PIED
RIDD
RIND
SIXD
TIED
VIED
WILD
WIND

••ID
ACID
AMID
ARID
AVID
CHID
ENID
FRID
GRID
HAID
IBID
IDID
IRID
LAID
LOID
MAID
NOID
OLID
OOID
OVID
PAID
QAID
QUID
RAID
REID
SAID
SKID
SLID
VOID

IE••
IEOH
IERI
IEST

I•E•
IBET
IBEW
IBEX
ICED
ICEE
ICEL
ICER
ICES
ICET
IDEA
IDED
IDEE
IDEM
IDEO
IDES
IGER
IKEA
ILER
ILES
ILEX
INEE
INES
INEZ
IRED
IRES
ISEE
ISER
ITEA
ITEM
ITEN
ITER
ITES
IVES
IVEY

I••E
IBLE
ICEE
IDAE
IDEE
IDLE
IDVE
IHRE
ILIE
ILLE
IMRE
INCE
INEE
INGE
INRE
IOLE
IONE
IPSE
IRAE
ISEE
ISLE
IVIE

•IE•
AIEA
BIEL
BIEN
BIER
CIEL
CIEN
DIED
DIEM
DIEN
DIES
DIET
DIEU
DIEZ
EIER
FIEF
FIES
GIED
GIES
HIED
HIER
HIES
KIEL
KIEV
LIEB
LIED
LIEF
LIEN
LIES
LIEU
LIEV
MIEL
MIEN
MIES
OIES
PIED
PIEL
PIER
PIES
PIET
RIEL
RIEN
SIEG
TIED
TIER
TIES
VIED
VIER
VIES
VIET
VIEW
WIEN

•I•E
AIDE
AILE
AIME
AIRE
BIDE
BIKE
BILE
BINE
BITE
CIDE
CINE
CIRE
CITE
DICE
DIKE
DIME
DINE
DIRE
DIVE
EILE
EINE
EIRE
FIDE
FIFE
FILE
FINE
FIRE
FIVE
FIXE
GIBE
GIDE
GIVE
HIDE
HIKE
HIRE
HITE
HIVE
JIBE
JIVE
KINE
KITE
LICE
LIFE
LIKE
LIME
LINE
LIRE
LITE
LIVE
MICE
MIKE
MILE
MIME
MINE
MIRE
MISE
MITE
MIZE
NICE
NIDE
NIKE
NILE
NINE
NITE
NIUE
OISE
PICE
PIKE
PILE
PINE
PIPE
PIRE
RICE
RIDE
RIFE
RILE
RIME
RIPE
RIRE
RISE
RITE
RIVE
SIDE
SINE
SIPE
SIRE
SITE
SIXE
SIZE
TIDE
TIGE
TIKE
TILE
TIME
TINE
TIRE
VIBE
VICE
VIDE
VILE
VINE
VISE
VITE
VIVE
WIDE
WIFE
WILE
WINE
WIPE
WIRE
WISE
WIVE
YIPE
ZINE

••IE
ABIE
AMIE
ARIE
ASIE
BAIE
BRIE
EDIE
ELIE
ERIE
EVIE
FOIE
ILIE
IVIE
JOIE
OBIE
ODIE
OKIE
OPIE
OWIE
PLIE
PRIE
SOIE
UNIE

IF••
IFFY
IFNI
IFSO

I•F•
IFFY
INFO
INFS

I••F
IMPF
IOOF

•IF•
BIFF
DIFF
FIFE
FIFI
FIFO
GIFS
GIFT
HIFI
JIFF
LIFE
LIFO
LIFT
MIFF
RIFE
RIFF
RIFS
RIFT
SIFT
TIFF
WIFE
WIFI
ZIFF

•I•F
BIFF
DIFF
FIEF
JIFF
LIEF
MIFF
PIAF
RIFF
TIFF
ZIFF

••IF
ALIF
ASIF
COIF
ENIF
LEIF
NAIF
TGIF
WAIF

IG••
IGBY
IGER
IGGS
IGGY
IGLU
IGOR

I•G•
IAGO
IGGS
IGGY
INGA
INGE
INGO

I••G
IDIG

•IG•
BIGA
BIGD
BIGO
BIGS
CIGS
DIGS
EIGG
FIGS
GIGA
GIGI
GIGO
GIGS
HIGH
JIGS
LIGN
MIGS
NIGH
PIGS
RIGA
RIGG
RIGS
SIGH
SIGN
SIGS
TIGE
VIGO
VIGS
WIGS
ZIGS

•I•G
BING
BIOG
DIAG
DING
EIGG
KING
LING
MING
PING
RIGG
RING
SIEG
SING
TING
VING
WING
XING
ZING

••IG
AFIG
BRIG
FRIG
GRIG
HAIG
IDIG
OLIG
ORIG
PRIG
PUIG
SWIG
TRIG
TWIG
WHIG

IH••
IHOP
IHRE

I•H•
IMHO

I••H
IEOH
INCH
IPOH
ISTH
ITCH

•IH•
HIHO

•I•H
DINH
DISH
DITH
FISH
GISH
HIGH
KITH
LITH
MICH
MINH
NIGH
NIMH
PISH
PITH
RICH
SIGH
SIKH
SINH
TISH
WISH
WITH

••IH
SHIH

II••
IIII

I•I•
IBID
IBIS
IDID
IDIG
IDIO
IIII
ILIA
ILIE
IMIN
IMIT
INIT
IRID
IRIS
ISIS
ITIC
ITIS
IVIE
IWIN
IXIA

I••I
IASI
IERI
IFNI
IIII
INRI

•II•
CIII
DIII
IIII
KIIL
LIII
MIII
RIIS
VIII
WIIS
XIII

•I•I
BIBI
CIII
DIDI
DIII
DILI
EIMI
FIFI
FIJI
FILI
FINI
GIGI
HIFI
IIII
JIMI
KIKI
KIRI
KIWI
LIII
LILI
LISI
MIDI
MIII
MIMI
MINI
NIDI
PILI
RIDI
SIMI
SISI
TIKI
TIPI
TITI
VICI
VIDI
VIII
VINI
VITI
VIVI
WIFI
WIKI
XIII
ZITI

••II
ALII
AMII
CCII
CDII
CIII
CLII
CMII
CVII
CXII
DCII
DIII
DLII
DVII
DXII
IIII
LIII
LVII
LXII
MCII
MDII
MIII
MLII
MMII
MVII
MXII
QEII
RAII
VIII
WWII
XCII
XIII
XLII
XVII
XXII

IJ••
IJKL

•IJ•
FIJI
HIJA
HIJK
HIJO
RIJN
RIJO

••IJ
GHIJ

IK••
IKEA
IKON

I•K•
ICKY
IJKL
ILKA
ILKS
INKA
INKS
INKY
IRKS

I••K
IMOK
ISAK

•IK•
BIKE
BIKO
DIKE
HIKE
KIKI
LIKE
MIKE
NIKA
NIKE
PIKA
PIKE
PIKS
SIKA
SIKH
TIKE
TIKI
WIKI

•I•K
BILK
DICK
DINK
DIRK
DISK
FINK
FISK
HICK
HIJK
KICK
KINK
KIRK
LICK
LINK
MICK
MILK
MINK
NICK
OINK
PICK
PINK
RICK
RINK
RISK
SICK
SILK
SINK
TICK
TINK
WICK
WINK
WISK

••IK
ATIK
EFIK
ERIK
HAIK
QUIK

IL••
ILER
ILES
ILEX
ILIA
ILIE
ILKA
ILKS
ILLA
ILLE
ILLS
ILLY
ILSA
ILUS
ILYA

I•L•
IBLE
IBLY
IDLE
IDLY
IGLU
ILLA
ILLE
ILLS
ILLY
INLY
IOLA
IOLE
ISLA
ISLE
ISLS
ITLL

I••L
ICAL
ICEL
IDOL
IDYL
IJKL
INCL
INTL
ITAL
ITLL
ITOL

•IL•
AILE
AILS
BILE
BILK
BILL
BILT
DILI
DILL
EILE
FILA
FILE
FILI
FILL
FILM
FILO
FILS
GILA
GILD
GILL
GILT
HILL
HILO
HILT
JILL
JILT
KILL
KILN
KILO
KILT
LILA
LILI
LILO
LILT
LILY
MILA
MILD
MILE
MILK
MILL
MILO
MILS
MILT
NILE
NILS
OILS
OILY
PILE
PILI
PILL
PILO
RILE
RILL
SILK
SILL
SILO
SILT
TILE
TILL
TILT
VILA
VILE
WILD
WILE
WILL
WILT
WILY
ZILL
ZILS

•I•L
BIBL
BIEL
BILL
BIOL
BIRL
CIEL
DIAL
DILL
DIPL
FILL
GILL
GIRL
HILL
JILL
KIEL
KIIL
KILL
MIEL
MILL
PIEL
PILL
RIAL
RIEL
RILL
SIAL
SILL
TILL
VIAL
VIOL
WILL
ZILL

••IL
ANIL
ARIL
AXIL
BAIL
BOIL
CEIL
COIL
DAIL
DCIL
DEIL
EMIL
EVIL
FAIL
FOIL
GAIL
HAIL
JAIL
KIIL
MAIL
MOIL
NAIL
NEIL
NOIL
OEIL
PAIL
PHIL
RAIL
ROIL
SAIL
SKIL
SOIL
TAIL
TOIL
UTIL
VAIL
VEIL
WAIL
WEIL

IM••
IMAC
IMAM
IMAN
IMAX
IMHO
IMIN
IMIT
IMOK
IMPF
IMPS
IMRE
IMUS

I•M•
IAMB
IAMS
IBMS
IRMA
ISMS

I••M
ICBM
IDEM
IMAM
ITEM

•IM•
AIME
AIMS
DIME
DIMS
EIMI
GIMP
JIMA
JIMI
LIMA
LIMB
LIME
LIMN
LIMO
LIMP
LIMY
MIME
MIMI
MIMS
NIMH
NIMS
PIMA
RIMA
RIME
RIMS
RIMY
SIMA
SIMI
SIMP
SIMS
TIME
VIMS
WIMP
ZIMA

•I•M
DIAM
DIEM
FILM
FIRM
KIAM
LIAM
LITM
SIAM

••IM
AKIM
ANIM
BRIM
CHIM
FAIM
FLIM
GLIM
GRIM
HAIM
MAIM
PRIM
SHIM
SKIM
SLIM
SWIM
TRIM
WHIM

IN••
INCA
INCE
INCH
INCL
INCR
INCS
INDO
INDS
INDY
INEE
INES
INEZ
INFO
INFS
INGA
INGE
INGO
INIT
INKA
INKS
INKY
INLY
INNS
INNY
INON
INQS
INRE
INRI
INRO
INSP
INST
INTL
INTO
INTR
INTS
INVS
INXS
INYO

I•N•
IANA
IFNI
INNS
INNY
IONA
IONE
IONO
IONS
ISNT

I••N
ICAN

ICON
IKON
IMAN
IMIN
INON
IRAN
IRON
ISBN
ITEN
IVAN
IWIN
IWON

•IN•
AINT
AINU
BIND
BINE
BING
BINS
CINC
CINE
CINQ
DINA
DINE
DING
DINH
DINK
DINO
DINS
DINT
EINE
EINS
FINA
FIND
FINE
FINI
FINK
FINN
FINO
FINS
GINA
GINO
GINS
HIND
HINT
JINN
JINX
KINA
KIND
KINE
KING
KINK
KINS
LINA
LINC
LIND
LINE
LING
LINK
LINN
LINO
LINT
LINY
LINZ
MINA
MIND
MINE
MING
MINH
MINI
MINK
MINN
MINS
MINT
MINX
NINA
NINE
NINO
OINK
PINA
PINE
PING
PINK
PINS
PINT
PINY
RINA
RIND
RING
RINK
SINE
SING
SINH
SINK
SINN
SINO
SINS
TINA
TINE
TING
TINK
TINO
TINS
TINT
TINY
VINA
VINE
VING
VINI
VINO
VINS
VINY
WIND
WINE
WING
WINK
WINN
WINS
WINY
XING
ZINA
ZINC
ZINE
ZING
ZINS

•I•N
BIEN
CIEN
CION
DIAN
DIEN
DION
FINN
FIRN
GIAN
HISN
JINN
KILN
LIEN
LIGN
LIMN
LINN
LION
MIEN
MINN
PION
PIRN
RIEN
RIJN
SIAN
SIGN
SINN
SION
TION
WIEN
WINN
XIAN
ZION

••IN
ADIN
AGIN
AKIN
AMIN
AYIN
BAIN
BEIN
BLIN
CAIN
CHIN
COIN
CRIN
CUIN
DAIN
DJIN
DMIN
DOIN
DRIN
ERIN
FAIN
FEIN
GAIN
GOIN
GRIN
HEIN
IMIN
IWIN
JAIN
JOIN
JUIN
LAIN
LOIN
LYIN
MAIN
MEIN
NEIN
ODIN
OLIN
ORIN
PAIN
PNIN
PRIN
RAIN
REIN
RHIN
RUIN
SEIN
SHIN
SKIN
SPIN
SQIN
THIN
TWIN
VAIN
VEIN
WAIN
WEIN
XDIN

IO••
IODO
IOLA
IOLE
IONA
IONE
IONO
IONS
IOOF
IOTA
IOUS
IOWA

I•O•
IBOS
ICON
ICOS
IDOL
IDOS
IEOH
IGOR
IHOP
IKON
IMOK
INON
IOOF
IPOD
IPOH
IPOS
IROC
IRON
ITOL
ITOO
IVOR
IWON
IZOD

I••O
IAGO
IDEO
IDIO
IFSO
IMHO
INDO
INFO
INGO
INRO
INTO
INYO
IODO
IONO
IPSO
ISAO
ISTO
ITOO

•IO•
BIOG
BIOL
BIOS
BIOT
CION
DION
DIOR
DIOS
LION
PION
RIOS
RIOT
SION
TION
TIOS
VIOL
ZION

•I•O
BIAO
BIGO
BIKO
BIRO
CIAO
CITO
DIDO
DINO
FIDO
FIFO
FILO
FINO
GIGO
GINO
GIRO
HIHO
HIJO
HILO
HIYO
KILO
LIAO
LIDO
LIFO
LILO
LIMO
LINO
LIPO
MILO
MIRO
MISO
NINO
NIRO
PIAO
PICO
PILO
RIBO
RICO
RIJO
SILO
SINO
TICO
TINO
TIRO
TITO
TIVO
VICO
VIGO
VINO
VITO
VIVO
XIXO
ZITO

••IO
AGIO
AKIO
BAIO
BRIO
CLIO
ELIO
EZIO
FRIO
IDIO
MAIO
OHIO
OLIO
TRIO

IP••
IPOD
IPOH
IPOS
IPSA
IPSE
IPSO

I•P•
IMPF
IMPS
ISPS
ISPY

I••P
IHOP
INSP

•IP•
DIPL
DIPS
GIPP
HIPS
KIPS
LIPO
LIPP
LIPS
MIPS
NIPA
NIPS
PIPE
PIPP
PIPS
PIPY
RIPA
RIPE
RIPS
SIPE
SIPS
TIPI
TIPS
VIPS
WIPE
YIPE
YIPS
ZIPS

•I•P
GIMP
GIPP
LIMP
LIPP
LISP
PIPP
SIMP
WIMP
WISP

••IP
ATIP
BLIP
CHIP
CLIP
DRIP
FLIP
GRIP
OSIP
QTIP
QUIP
SHIP
SKIP
SLIP
SNIP
TRIP
VOIP
WHIP

I•Q•
INQS

I••Q
IRAQ

•I•Q
CINQ

••IQ
DRIQ
ERIQ

IR••
IRAE
IRAN
IRAQ
IRAS
IRED
IRES
IRID
IRIS
IRKS
IRMA
IROC
IRON
IRRA
IRRS
IRUS

I•R•
IERI
IHRE
IMRE
INRE
INRI
INRO
IRRA
IRRS

I••R
IBAR
ICER
IGER
IGOR
ILER
INCR
INTR
ISAR
ISER
ITAR
ITER
IVAR
IVOR
IYAR

•IR•
AIRE
AIRS
AIRY
BIRD
BIRL
BIRO
BIRR
CIRC
CIRE
DIRE
DIRK
DIRS
DIRT
EIRE
FIRE
FIRM
FIRN
FIRS
GIRD
GIRL
GIRO
GIRT
HIRE
HIRT
KIRI
KIRK
KIRS
LIRA
LIRE
LIRR
MIRA
MIRE
MIRO
MIRS
MIRV
MIRY
NIRO
PIRE
PIRN
RIRE
SIRE
SIRS
TIRE
TIRO
WIRE
WIRY
ZIRA

•I•R
BIER
BIRR
DIOR
EIER
HIER
LIAR
LIRR
MICR
PIER
TIER
VIER
VITR

••IR
AMIR
ASIR
COIR
EMIR
FAIR
FLIR
HAIR
HEIR
KEIR
LAIR
MEIR
MUIR
NAIR
NOIR
PAIR
SOIR
STIR
VOIR
WEIR
WHIR
YMIR

IS••
ISAK
ISAO
ISAR
ISAY
ISBN
ISEE
ISER
ISIS
ISLA
ISLE
ISLS
ISMS
ISNT
ISPS
ISPY
ISSY
ISTH
ISTO
ISTS

I•S•
IASI
IEST
IFSO
ILSA
INSP
INST
IPSA
IPSE
IPSO
ISSY
ITSY

I••S
IAMS
IBIS
IBMS
IBOS
ICES
ICOS
ICUS
IDES
IDOS
IGGS
ILES
ILKS
ILLS
ILUS
IMPS
IMUS
INCS
INDS
INES
INFS
INKS
INNS
INQS
INTS
INVS
INXS
IONS
IOUS
IPOS
IRAS
IRES
IRIS
IRKS
IRRS
IRUS
ISIS
ISLS
ISMS
ISPS
ISTS
ITES
ITIS
IVES

•IS•
BIST
CIST
DISC
DISH
DISK
DISS
DIST
FISC
FISH
FISK
FIST
GISH
GIST
HISN
HISS
HIST
KISS
KIST
LISA
LISI
LISP
LIST
MISC
MISE
MISO
MISS
MIST
OISE
PISA
PISH
RISE
RISK
SISI
SISS
TISH
VISA
VISC
VISE
WISC
WISE
WISH
WISK
WISP

•I•S
AIDS
AILS
AIMS
AIRS
AITS
BIAS
BIBS
BICS
BIDS
BIGS
BINS
BIOS
BITS
CIGS
DIAS
DIBS
DIES
DIGS
DIMS
DINS
DIOS
DIPS
DIRS
DISS
DITS
DIVS
EINS
FIBS
FIDS
FIES
FIGS
FILS
FINS
FIRS
FITS
GIBS
GIES
GIFS
GIGS
GINS
GITS
HICS
HIES
HIPS
HISS
HITS
JIBS
JIGS
KIAS
KIDS
KINS
KIPS
KIRS
KISS
KITS
LIBS
LICS
LIDS
LIES
LIPS
LITS
MIAS
MIBS
MICS
MIES
MIGS
MILS
MIMS
MINS
MIPS
MIRS
MISS
NIBS
NILS
NIMS
NIPS
NITS
OIES
OILS
PICS
PIES
PIGS
PIKS
PINS
PIPS
PITS
PIUS
RIAS
RIBS
RIDS
RIFS
RIGS
RIIS
RIMS
RIOS
RIPS
RIVS
SIBS
SICS
SIGS
SIMS
SINS
SIPS
SIRS
SISS
SITS
TIAS
TICS
TIES
TINS
TIOS
TIPS
TITS
VIDS
VIES
VIGS
VIMS
VINS
VIPS
VITS
WIGS
WIIS
WINS
WITS
YIPS
ZIGS
ZILS
ZINS
ZIPS
ZITS

••IS
ACIS
AGIS
AJIS
AMIS
ANIS
APIS
ASIS
ATIS
AVIS
AXIS
BOIS
CHIS
DAIS
DOIS
EGIS
ELIS
EPIS
ERIS
ESIS
FRIS
GRIS
GTIS
HUIS
IBIS
IRIS
ISIS
ITIS
KOIS
KRIS
LAIS
LEIS
LOIS
LUIS
MAIS
MOIS
MRIS
OBIS
OPIS
OSIS
OTIS
OUIS
OVIS
PAIS
PHIS
POIS
PSIS
RBIS
RIIS
ROIS
SAIS
SCIS
SEIS
SKIS
SRIS
TAIS
THIS
TRIS
TUIS
UNIS
URIS
UZIS
WEIS
WIIS

IT••
ITAL
ITAR
ITCH
ITEA
ITEM
ITEN
ITER
ITES
ITIC
ITIS
ITLL
ITOL
ITOO
ITSY
ITTY
ITZA

I•T•
INTL
INTO
INTR
INTS
IOTA
ISTH
ISTO
ISTS
ITTY

I••T
IBET
ICET
IEST
IMIT
INIT
INST
ISNT

•IT•
AITS
BITE
BITS
BITT
CITE
CITO
CITY
DITH
DITS
DITZ
FITS
GITA
GITS
HITE
HITS
KITE
KITH
KITS
KITT
LITA
LITB
LITD
LITE
LITH
LITM
LITS
MITA
MITE
MITT
NITA
NITE
NITS
OITA
PITA
PITH
PITS
PITT
PITY
RITA
RITE
RITT
RITZ
SITE
SITS
SITU
SITZ
TITI
TITO
TITS
VITA
VITE
VITI
VITO
VITR
VITS
WITH
WITS
WITT
ZITI
ZITO
ZITS

•I•T
AINT
BILT
BIOT
BIST
BITT
CIST
DICT
DIET
DINT
DIRT
DIST
FIAT
FICT
FIST
GIFT
GILT
GIRT
GIST
HILT
HINT
HIRT
HIST
JILT
KILT
KIST
KITT
LIAT
LIFT
LILT
LINT
LIST
MILT
MINT
MIST
MITT
MIXT
PICT
PIET
PINT
PITT
RIFT
RIOT
RITT
SIFT
SILT
TILT
TINT
VIET
WILT
WITT

••IT
ABIT
ADIT
ALIT
ATIT
BAIT
BLIT
BRIT
CHIT
COIT
CRIT
DLIT
DOIT
EDIT
EMIT
EXIT
FAIT
FLIT
FRIT
GAIT
GRIT
HUIT
IMIT
INIT
KNIT
LAIT
NUIT
OBIT
OMIT
QUIT
REIT
SKIT
SLIT
SMIT
SNIT
SPIT
SUIT
SWIT
TWIT
UNIT
VOIT
WAIT
WHIT
WRIT
ZEIT

I•U•
ICUS
ILUS
IMUS
IOUS
IRUS

I••U
IGLU

•IU•
NIUE
PIUS

•I•U
AINU
BIDU
DIEU
LIEU
SITU

IV••
IVAN
IVAR
IVES
IVEY
IVIE
IVOR

I•V•
IDVE
INVS

•IV•
DIVA
DIVE
DIVS
FIVE
GIVE
HIVA
HIVE
JIVE
JIVY
KIVA
LIVE
LIVY
RIVA
RIVE
RIVS
SIVA
TIVO
VIVA
VIVE
VIVI
VIVO
WIVE

•I•V
KIEV
LIEV
MIRV

••IV
AVIV
CCIV
CDIV
CLIV
CMIV
CXIV
DCIV
DLIV
DXIV
LXIV
MCIV
MDIV
MLIV
MMIV
MXIV
PRIV
SHIV
UNIV
XCIV
XDIV
XLIV
XXIV

IW••
IWIN
IWON

I•W•
IOWA

I••W
IBEW

•IW•
AIWA
BIWA
KIWI
TIWA

•I•W
VIEW

••IW
FWIW

IX••
IXIA

I•X•
INXS

I••X
IBEX
ILEX
IMAX

•IX•
DIXY
FIXE
FIXX
MIXT
NIXY
PIXY
SIXA
SIXB
SIXC
SIXD
SIXE
XIXO

•I•X
FIXX
JINX
MINX

••IX
ALIX
BRIX
BSIX
CCIX
CDIX
CLIX
CMIX
CXIX
DCIX
DLIX
DXIX
FLIX
LEIX
LXIX
MCIX
MDIX
MLIX
MMIX
MXIX
PAIX
PRIX
TRIX
TWIX
UNIX
VOIX
VSIX
XCIX
XLIX
XXIX

IY••
IYAR

I•Y•
IDYL
ILYA
INYO

I••Y
IBLY
ICKY
IDLY
IFFY
IGBY
IGGY
ILLY
INDY
INKY

INLY INNY ISAY ISPY ISSY ITSY ITTY IVEY IZZY

•IY•
HIYA HIYO

•I•Y
AIRY CITY DIDY DIXY JIVY LILY LIMY LINY LIVY MIRY NIXY OILY PINY PIPY PITY PIXY RIMY TIDY TINY VINY WILY WINY WIRY

IZ••
IZOD IZZY

I•Z•
ITZA IZZY

I••Z
INEZ

•IZ•
FIZZ GIZA LIZA MIZE PIZZ SIZE ZIZZ

•I•Z
DIAZ DIEZ DITZ FIZZ LINZ PIZZ RITZ SITZ ZIZZ

••IZ
ARIZ AZIZ ELIZ FRIZ LUIZ PHIZ QUIZ WHIZ

JA••
JABS JACK JACS JADA JADE JAGR JAGS JAHR JAIL JAIN JAJA JAKE JAMA JAMB JAMI JAMS JANA JANE JANN JANS JAPE JARS JATO JAUN JAVA JAWS JAYE JAYS JAYZ JAZZ

J•A•
JBAR JEAN JOAD JOAN JUAB JUAN

J••A
JADA JAJA JAMA JANA JAVA JENA JIMA JOTA JURA

•JA•
AJAR AJAX OJAI

•J•A
DJIA

••JA
BAJA DEJA FAJA HIJA JAJA MAJA RAJA ROJA

JB••
JBAR

J•B•
JABS JIBE JIBS JOBS

J••B
JAMB JUAB

J•C•
JACK JACS JOCK JUCO JVCS

J••C
JUNC

J•D•
JADA JADE JEDI JODY JUDD JUDE JUDI JUDO JUDY

J••D
JOAD JOED JUDD

•JD•
SJDS

••JD
NEJD

JE••
JEAN JEDI JEEP JEER JEEZ JEFE JEFF JEHU JELL JENA JENS JEON JERI JERK JESS JEST JESU JETE JETS JETT JEUX JEWS

J•E•
JEEP JEER JEEZ JOED JOEE JOEL JOES JOEY JPEG

J••E
JADE JAKE JANE JAPE JAYE JEFE JETE JIBE JIVE JOEE JOIE JOKE JOSE JOVE JUDE JUKE JULE JUNE JURE JUTE

••JE
HAJE

J•F•
JEFE JEFF JIFF

J••F
JEFF JIFF

J•G•
JAGR JAGS JIGS JOGS JPGS JUGS

J••G
JONG JPEG JUNG

••JG
LTJG

J•H•
JAHR JEHU JOHN

J••H
JOSH

JI••
JIBE JIBS JIFF JIGS JILL JILT JIMA JIMI JINN JINX JIVE JIVY

J•I•
JAIL JAIN JOIE JOIN JUIN

J••I
JAMI JEDI JERI JIMI JOLI JONI JOVI JUDI JULI JUNI

•JI•
AJIS DJIA DJIN

•J•I
OJAI

••JI
FIJI FUJI HAJI KOJI

J•J•
JAJA JOJO JUJU

••JJ
HAJJ

JK••
JKLM

J•K•
JAKE JOKE JOKY JUKE

J••K
JACK JERK JOCK JUNK

•JK•
IJKL

••JK
HIJK

J•L•
JELL JILL JILT JKLM JOLI JOLT JULE JULI JULY

J••L
JAIL JELL JILL JOEL JOWL

•J•L
IJKL

J•M•
JAMA JAMB JAMI JAMS JIMA JIMI JOMO JUMP

J••M
JKLM

••JM
SEJM

J•N•
JANA JANE JANN JANS JENA JENS JINN JINX JONG JONI JUNC JUNE JUNG JUNI JUNK JUNO

J••N
JAIN JANN JAUN JEAN JEON JINN JOAN JOHN JOIN JOON JUAN JUIN

•J•N
DJIN

••JN
RIJN

JO••
JOAD JOAN JOBS JOCK JODY JOED JOEE JOEL JOES JOEY JOGS JOHN JOIE JOIN JOJO JOKE JOKY JOLI JOLT JOMO JONG JONI JOON JORY JOSE JOSH JOSS JOTA JOTS JOUR JOVE JOVI JOWL JOYS

J•O•
JEON JOON

J••O
JATO JOJO JOMO JUCO JUDO JUNO

•JO•
AJOS OJOS

••JO
BAJO CUJO DOJO HIJO HOJO JOJO MOJO RIJO ROJO TAJO TOJO WOJO

JP••
JPEG JPGS

J•P•
JAPE

J••P
JEEP JUMP

J•R•
JARS JERI JERK JORY JURA JURE JURY

J••R
JAGR JAHR JBAR JEER JOUR

•J•R
AJAR

J•S•
JESS JEST JESU JOSE JOSH JOSS JUST

J••S
JABS JACS JAGS JAMS JANS JARS JAWS JAYS JENS JESS JETS JEWS JIBS JIGS JOBS JOES JOGS JOSS JOTS JOYS JPGS JUGS JUTS JVCS

•J•S
AJIS AJOS OJOS SJDS

••JS
ADJS MAJS OBJS

J•T•
JATO JETE JETS JETT JOTA JOTS JUTE JUTS

J••T
JEST JETT JILT JOLT JUST

••JT
ADJT

JU••
JUAB JUAN JUCO JUDD JUDE JUDI JUDO JUDY JUGS JUIN JUJU JUKE JULE JULI JULY JUMP JUNC JUNE JUNG JUNI JUNK JUNO JURA JURE JURY JUST JUTE JUTS

J•U•
JAUN JEUX JOUR

J••U
JEHU JESU JUJU

••JU
JUJU

JV••
JVCS

J•V•
JAVA JIVE JIVY JOVE JOVI

J•W•
JAWS JEWS JOWL

J••X
JEUX JINX

•J•X
AJAX

J•Y•
JAYE JAYS JAYZ JOYS

J••Y
JIVY JODY JOEY JOKY JORY JUDY JULY JURY

J•Z•
JAZZ

J••Z
JAYZ JAZZ JEEZ

KA••
KAAT KABA KAEL KAFS KAHN KAIA KAKI KALB KALE KALI KAMA KAMI KANA KANE KANG KANS KANT KAON KAOS KAPH KARA KARI KARL KARN KARO KART KASI KATA KATE KATO KATT KATY KATZ KAVA KAYE KAYO KAYS

K•A•
KAAT KCAL KCAR KEAN KEAR KEAS KHAN KHAS KIAM KIAS KLAN KNAG KNAP KNAR KOAN KOAS KPAX KWAI KWAN KYAT

K••A
KABA KAIA KAMA KANA KARA KATA KAVA KDKA KINA KIVA KOLA KONA KYRA

•KA•
AKAI AKAS OKAY SKAT

•K•A
IKEA OKLA OKRA SKUA

••KA
ALKA ANKA ATKA DEKA ILKA INKA KDKA LUKA NIKA PIKA PUKA SIKA TAKA WAKA

K•B•
KABA KOBE KOBO KOBS

K••B
KALB KERB KNOB

KC••
KCAL KCAR

K•C•
KICK KOCH

K••C
KOFC KROC

•KC•
EKCO

KD••
KDKA KDOE

K•D•
KEDS KIDD KIDS KUDO KUDU

K••D
KIDD KIND KURD

•K•D
EKED NKVD OKED SKED SKID TKOD

KE••
KEAN KEAR KEAS KEDS KEEL KEEN KEEP KEGS KEIR KELL KELP KEMO KEMP KENN KENO KENS KENT KEOS KEPI KEPT KERB KERF KERI KERN KERR KERT KETT KETZ KEYE KEYS

K•E•
KAEL KEEL KEEN KEEP KIEL KIEV KLEE KLEM KNEE KNEW KTEL

K••E
KALE KANE KATE KAYE KDOE KEYE KINE KITE KLEE KNEE KOBE KYLE

•KE•
EKED EKES IKEA OKED OKEY SKED SKEE SKEG SKEW UKES XKES

•K•E
OKIE SKEE SKYE

••KE
ANKE BAKE BIKE CAKE COKE CUKE DEKE DIKE DOKE DUKE DYKE ELKE ENKE FAKE HAKE HIKE HOKE JAKE JOKE JUKE LAKE LIKE LUKE MAKE MIKE NIKE NUKE PEKE PIKE POKE PYKE RAKE SAKE TAKE TIKE TOKE TPKE TYKE WAKE WOKE YOKE ZEKE

K•F•
KAFS KOFC KOFI KOFP

K••F
KERF KOPF

K•G•
KEGS

K••G
KANG KING KNAG KONG KUNG

•KG•
EKGS PKGS

•K•G
BKPG MKTG SKEG

KH••
KHAN KHAS

K•H•
KAHN KOHL KUHN

K••H
KAPH KITH KOCH KOPH

••KH
ANKH SIKH

KI••
KIAM KIAS KICK KIDD KIDS KIEL KIEV KIIL KIKI KILL KILN KILO KILT KINA KIND KINE KING KINK KINS KIPS KIRI KIRK KIRS KISS KIST KITE KITH KITS KITT KIVA KIWI

K•I•
KAIA KEIR KIIL KNIT KOIS KRIS

K••I
KAKI KALI KAMI KARI KASI KEPI KERI KIKI KIRI KIWI KOFI KOJI KWAI

•KI•
AKIM AKIN AKIO OKIE SKID SKIL SKIM SKIN SKIP SKIS SKIT

•K•I
AKAI

••KI
ALKI AOKI KAKI KIKI LOKI SAKI TIKI WIKI

K•J•
KOJI

K•K•
KAKI KDKA KIKI KOKO

K••K
KICK KINK KIRK KOOK KRUK

•K•K
OKOK

KL••
KLAN KLEE KLEM KLMN KLUM

K•L•
KALB KALE KALI KELL KELP KILL KILN KILO KILT KOLA KOLN KULP KYLE

K••L
KAEL KARL KCAL KEEL KELL KIEL KIIL KILL KOHL KOOL KTEL

•KL•
JKLM OKLA WKLY

•K•L
SKIL

••KL
IJKL

K•M•
KAMA KAMI KEMO KEMP KLMN

K••M
KIAM KLEM KLUM

•K•M
AKIM JKLM SKIM

KN••
KNAG KNAP KNAR KNEE KNEW KNIT KNOB KNOT KNOW KNOX KNTS KNUR KNUT

K•N•
KANA KANE KANG KANS KANT KENN KENO KENS KENT KINA KIND KINE KING KINK KINS KONA KONG KUNG

K••N
KAHN KAON KARN KEAN KEEN KENN KERN KHAN KILN KLAN KLMN KOAN KOLN KORN KUHN KWAN KWON

•KN•
DKNY

•K•N
AKIN IKON SKIN

KO••
KOAN KOAS KOBE KOBO KOBS KOCH KOFC KOFI KOFP KOHL KOIS KOJI KOKO KOLA KOLN KONA KONG KOOK KOOL KOOP KOPF KOPH KOPS KORN KORS KOSS KOTO

K•O•
KAON KAOS KDOE KEOS KNOB KNOT KNOW KNOX KOOK KOOL KOOP KROC KWON

K••O
KARO KATO KAYO KEMO KENO KILO KOBO KOKO KOTO

KTWO
KUDO

•KO•
IKON
OKOK
RKOS
TKOD
TKOS

•K•O
AKIO
EKCO

••KO
BIKO
ELKO
KOKO
MAKO
MOKO
SEKO
YOKO

KP••
KPAX

K•P•
KAPH
KEPI
KEPT
KIPS
KOPF
KOPH
KOPS

K••P
KEEP
KELP
KEMP
KNAP
KOFP
KOOP
KULP

•KP•
BKPG
BKPR

•K•P
SKIP
WKRP

••KP
ONKP

KR••
KRIS
KROC
KRUK

K•R•
KARA
KARI
KARL
KARN
KARO
KART
KERB
KERF
KERI
KERN
KERR
KERT
KIRI
KIRK
KIRS
KORN
KORS
KURD
KURT
KYRA

K••R
KCAR
KEAR
KEIR
KERR
KNAR
KNUR

•KR•
OKRA
WKRP
XKRS

•K•R
BKPR

••KR
BAKR

K•S•
KASI
KISS
KIST
KOSS

K••S
KAFS
KANS
KAOS
KAYS
KEAS
KEDS
KEGS
KENS
KEOS
KEYS
KHAS
KIAS
KIDS
KINS
KIPS
KIRS
KISS
KITS
KNTS
KOAS
KOBS
KOIS
KOPS
KORS
KOSS
KRIS

•K•S
AKAS
EKES
EKGS
MKTS
PKGS
RKOS
SKIS
SKUS
SKYS
TKOS
TKTS
UKES
XKES
XKRS

••KS
AOKS
ARKS
ASKS
AUKS
EEKS
ELKS
ESKS
ILKS
INKS
IRKS
LEKS
LUKS
OAKS
PIKS
PMKS
ROKS
SAKS
STKS
SUKS
TPKS
TSKS
WOKS
YAKS
YUKS

KT••
KTEL
KTWO

K•T•
KATA
KATE
KATO
KATT
KATY
KATZ
KETT
KETZ
KITE
KITH
KITS
KITT
KNTS
KOTO

K••T
KAAT
KANT
KART
KATT
KENT
KEPT
KERT
KETT
KILT
KIST
KITT
KNIT
KNOT
KNUT
KURT
KYAT

•KT•
MKTG
MKTS
TKTS

•K•T
SKAT
SKIT

KU••
KUDO
KUDU
KUHN
KULP
KUNG
KURD
KURT

K•U•
KLUM
KNUR
KNUT
KRUK

K••U
KUDU

•KU•
SKUA
SKUS

••KU
BAKU
RAKU

K•V•
KAVA
KIVA

K••V
KIEV

•KV•
NKVD

KW••
KWAI
KWAN
KWON

K•W•
KIWI
KTWO

K••W
KNEW
KNOW

•KW•
PKWY

•K•W
SKEW

K••X
KNOX
KPAX

KY••
KYAT
KYLE
KYRA

K•Y•
KAYE
KAYO
KAYS
KEYE
KEYS

K••Y
KATY

•KY•
SKYE
SKYS

•K•Y
DKNY
OKAY
OKEY
PKWY
WKLY

••KY
ALKY
ARKY
CAKY
COKY
ICKY
INKY
JOKY
LAKY
OAKY
OOKY
POKY

K••Z
KATZ
KETZ

LA••
LABS
LACE
LACK
LACS
LACT
LACY
LADA
LADD
LADE
LADS
LADY
LAFF
LAGO
LAGS
LAHR
LAIC
LAID
LAIN
LAIR
LAIS
LAIT
LAKE
LAKY
LALL
LALO
LAMA
LAMB
LAME
LAMP
LAMS
LANA
LAND
LANE
LANG
LANI
LANK
LANO
LANS
LAOS
LAPD
LAPP
LAPS
LARA
LARC
LARD
LARI
LARK
LARS
LARY
LASE
LASH
LASS
LAST
LATE
LATH
LATS
LAUD
LAUE
LAVA
LAVE
LAVI
LAVS
LAWD
LAWN
LAWS
LAYS
LAZE
LAZY

L•A•
LBAR
LEAD
LEAF
LEAH
LEAK
LEAL
LEAN
LEAP
LEAR
LEAS
LIAM
LIAO
LIAR
LIAT
LOAD
LOAF
LOAM
LOAN
LSAT
LUAU

L••A
LADA
LAMA
LANA
LARA
LAVA
LEDA
LEIA
LELA
LEMA
LENA
LEVA
LIDA
LILA
LIMA
LINA
LIRA
LISA
LITA
LIZA
LOCA
LOLA
LOMA
LPGA
LUKA
LULA
LUMA
LUNA
LYRA

•LA•
ALAE
ALAI
ALAN
ALAR
ALAS
BLAB
BLAH
BLAM
BLAS
BLAT
BLAU
CLAD
CLAM
CLAN
CLAP
CLAR
CLAW
CLAY
ELAL
ELAM
ELAN
ELAS
ELAT
FLAB
FLAG
FLAK
FLAM
FLAN
FLAP
FLAT
FLAW
FLAX
FLAY
GLAD
GLAM
KLAN
NLAT
OLAF
OLAH
OLAN
OLAS
OLAV
OLAY
PLAN
PLAT
PLAX
PLAY
SLAB
SLAG
SLAM
SLAP
SLAT
SLAV
SLAW
SLAY
ULAN
ULAR
VLAD

•L•A
ALBA
ALDA
ALEA
ALFA
ALGA
ALIA
ALKA
ALLA
ALMA
ALTA
ALVA
CLEA
ELBA
ELEA
ELIA
ELLA
ELSA
FLEA
GLIA
ILIA
ILKA
ILLA
ILSA
ILYA
OLEA
OLGA
OLLA
PLEA
ULLA
ULNA

••LA
ALLA
AYLA
BALA
BELA
BOLA
CELA
COLA
ELLA
EOLA
EULA
FALA
FILA
GALA
GILA
GOLA
HOLA
HULA
HYLA
ILLA
IOLA
ISLA
KOLA
LELA
LILA
LOLA
LULA
MALA
MILA
NALA
NOLA
OKLA
OLLA
OOLA
POLA
PULA
RULA
SALA
SELA
SOLA
SULA
TALA
TULA
UCLA
ULLA
VELA
VILA
ZOLA

LB••
LBAR
LBOS

L•B•
LABS
LHBS
LIBS
LLBS
LOBE
LOBO
LOBS
LUBE

L••B
LAMB
LIEB
LIMB
LITB
LOEB
LOMB

•LB•
ALBA
ALBS
ELBA
ELBE
LLBS

•L•B
BLAB
BLEB
BLOB
CLUB
FLAB
FLUB
GLIB
GLOB
NLRB
PLEB
SLAB
SLOB

••LB
BULB
FTLB
KALB

LC••
LCDS
LCMS

L•C•
LACE
LACK
LACS
LACT
LACY
LECH
LECT
LICE
LICK
LICS
LOCA
LOCH
LOCI
LOCK
LOCO
LUCE
LUCI
LUCK
LUCY
LYCO

L••C
LAIC
LARC
LINC

•LC•
ALCS
GLCS
NLCS

•L•C
ALEC
BLOC
ELEC
FLIC
GLUC
GLYC
OLIC

••LC
CALC
SCLC
TALC

LD••
LDRS

L•D•
LADA
LADD
LADE
LADS
LADY
LCDS
LEDA
LEDS
LIDA
LIDO
LIDS
LLDS
LODE
LODI
LODZ
LTDS

L••D
LADD
LAID
LAND
LAPD
LARD
LAUD
LAWD
LEAD
LEND
LEWD
LIED
LIND
LITD
LOAD
LOID
LORD
LOUD
LOYD
LUND
LYND

•LD•
ALDA
ALDO
ALDS
BLDG
LLDS
OLDE
OLDS

•L•D
BLED
BLVD
CLAD
CLOD
FLED
GLAD
OLID
PLED
PLOD
SLED
SLID
VLAD

••LD
AULD
BALD
BOLD
COLD
FOLD
GELD
GILD
GOLD
HELD
HOLD
MELD
MILD
MOLD
NFLD
SOLD
TOLD
VELD
WALD
WELD
WILD

LE••
LEAD
LEAF
LEAH
LEAK
LEAL
LEAN
LEAP
LEAR
LEAS
LECH
LECT
LEDA
LEDS
LEEJ
LEEK
LEER
LEES
LEFT
LEGG
LEGO
LEGS
LEHI
LEHN
LEHR
LEIA
LEIF
LEIS
LEIX
LEKS
LELA
LELY
LEMA
LEMS
LENA
LEND
LENI
LENO
LENS
LENT
LENZ
LEOG
LEOI
LEON
LEOV
LEOX
LESE
LESS
LEST
LETO
LETS
LETT
LEUR
LEVA
LEVI
LEVO
LEVU
LEVY
LEWD

L•E•
LEEJ
LEEK
LEER
LEES
LIEB
LIED
LIEF
LIEN
LIES
LIEU
LIEV
LOEB
LOEW
LWEI
LYES

L••E
LACE
LADE
LAKE
LAME
LANE
LASE
LATE
LAUE
LAVE
LAZE
LESE
LICE
LIFE
LIKE
LIME
LINE
LIRE
LITE
LIVE
LOBE
LODE
LOGE
LOME
LONE
LOPE
LORE
LOSE
LOVE
LOWE
LUBE
LUCE
LUGE
LUKE
LUNE
LUPE
LURE
LUTE
LUXE
LYLE
LYME
LYNE
LYRE
LYSE
LYTE

•LE•
ALEA
ALEC
ALEE
ALEF
ALEK
ALEN
ALER
ALES
ALEX
BLEB
BLED
BLEU
BLEW
CLEA
CLEF
CLEM
CLEO
CLEW
ELEA
ELEC
ELEM
ELEV
FLEA
FLED
FLEE
FLEM
FLEW
FLEX
GLEE
GLEN
ILER
ILES
ILEX
KLEE
KLEM
NLER
OLEA
OLEG
OLEN
OLEO
OLES
PLEA
PLEB
PLED
PLEX
SLED
SLEW
SLEY
ULEE
YLEM

•L•E
ALAE
ALEE
ALLE
ALOE
ALPE
ALTE
BLUE
CLUE
ELBE
ELIE
ELKE
ELLE
ELSE
FLEE
FLOE
FLUE
GLEE
GLUE
ILIE
ILLE
KLEE
MLLE
OLDE
OLPE
PLIE
SLOE
SLUE
SLYE
ULEE

••LE
ABLE
AILE
ALLE
ATLE
AXLE
BALE
BILE
BOLE
CALE
COLE
CULE
DALE
DELE
DOLE
EHLE
EILE
ELLE
ERLE
FILE
GALE
HALE
HOLE
IBLE
IDLE
ILLE
IOLE
ISLE
JULE
KALE
KYLE
LYLE
MALE
MILE
MLLE
MOLE
MULE
NILE
NOLE
OGLE
ORLE
PALE
PELE
PILE
POLE
PULE
PYLE
RALE
RILE
ROLE
RULE
RYLE
SALE
SOLE
TALE
TELE
TILE
TOLE
TULE
UELE
VALE
VILE
VOLE
WALE
WILE
WOLE
WYLE
YALE
YULE
ZALE

L•F•
LAFF
LEFT
LIFE
LIFO
LIFT
LOFT
LUFF
LUFT

L••F
LAFF
LEAF
LEIF
LIEF
LOAF
LUFF

•LF•
ALFA

•L•F
ALEF
ALIF
CLEF
OLAF
OLOF

••LF
CALF
GOLF
GULF
HALF
PELF
ROLF
SELF
WOLF

LG••
LGTH

L•G•
LAGO
LAGS
LEGG
LEGO
LEGS
LIGN
LOGE
LOGO
LOGS
LOGY
LPGA
LUGE
LUGS

L••G
LANG
LEGG
LEOG
LING
LONG
LTJG
LUNG
LYNG

•LG•
ALGA
OLGA

•L•G
BLDG
BLOG
CLOG
FLAG
FLOG
GLUG
OLEG
OLIG
PLUG
SLAG
SLOG
SLUG

••LG
BELG
BULG
VULG

LH••
LHBS

L•H•
LAHR
LEHI
LEHN
LEHR

L••H
LASH
LATH
LEAH
LECH
LGTH
LITH
LOCH
LUSH
LUTH

•LH•
ELHI

•L•H
ALPH
BLAH
OLAH

LI••
LIAM
LIAO
LIAR
LIAT
LIBS
LICE
LICK
LICS
LIDA
LIDO
LIDS
LIEB
LIED
LIEF
LIEN
LIES
LIEU
LIEV
LIFE
LIFO
LIFT
LIGN
LIII
LIKE
LILA
LILI
LILO
LILT
LILY
LIMA
LIMB
LIME
LIMN
LIMO
LIMP
LIMY
LINA
LINC
LIND
LINE
LING
LINK
LINN
LINO
LINT
LINY
LINZ
LION
LIPO
LIPP
LIPS
LIRA
LIRE
LIRR
LISA
LISI
LISP
LIST
LITA
LITB
LITD
LITE
LITH
LITM
LITS
LIVE
LIVY
LIZA

L•I•
LAIC
LAID
LAIN
LAIR
LAIS
LAIT
LEIA
LEIF
LEIS
LEIX
LIII
LOID
LOIN
LOIS
LUIS
LUIZ
LVII
LXII
LXIV
LXIX
LYIN

L••I
LANI
LARI
LAVI
LEHI
LENI
LEOI
LEVI
LIII
LILI
LISI
LOCI
LODI
LOKI
LONI
LORI
LOTI
LUCI
LVII
LWEI
LXII
LXVI
LXXI

•LI•
ALIA
ALIF
ALII

ALIT ALIX BLIN BLIP BLIT CLII CLIO CLIP CLIV CLIX DLII DLIT DLIV DLIX ELIA ELIE ELIO ELIS ELIZ FLIC FLIM FLIP FLIR FLIT FLIX GLIA GLIB GLIM ILIA ILIE MLII MLIV MLIX OLIC OLID OLIG OLIN OLIO PLIE SLID SLIM SLIP SLIT XLII XLIV XLIX

•L•I
ALAI ALII ALKI ALTI ALUI CLII CLVI CLXI DLII DLVI DLXI ELHI ELOI MLII MLVI MLXI XLII XLVI

••LI
ATLI BALI CALI CCLI CDLI CMLI COLI CXLI DALI DCLI DELI DILI DXLI EGLI FILI HALI HELI JOLI JULI KALI LILI MALI MCLI MDLI MMLI MXLI NOLI PALI PILI POLI PULI SOLI TALI UGLI

L•J•
LTJG

L••J
LEEJ

L•K•
LAKE LAKY LEKS LIKE LOKI LUKA LUKE LUKS

L••K
LACK LANK LARK LEAK LEEK LICK LINK LOCK LOOK LUCK LUNK LURK

•LK•
ALKA ALKI ALKY ELKE ELKO ELKS ILKA ILKS

•L•K
ALEK BLOK FLAK

••LK
BALK BILK BULK CALK FALK FOLK HULK MILK POLK SALK SILK SULK TALK VOLK WALK WELK YOLK

LL••
LLBS LLDS LLMS

L•L•
LALL LALO LELA LELY LILA LILI LILO LILT LILY LOLA LOLL LULA LULL LULU LYLE LYLY

L••L
LALL LEAL LOLL LULL

•LL•
ALLA ALLE ALLO ALLS ALLY ELLA ELLE ELLS ELLY ILLA ILLE ILLS ILLY MLLE OLLA ULLA

•L•L
ELAL ELUL

••LL
BALL BELL BILL BOLL BULL CALL CELL COLL CULL DELL DILL DOLL DULL FALL FELL FILL FULL GALL GELL GILL GULL HALL HELL HILL HULL ITLL JELL JILL KELL KILL LALL LOLL LULL MALL MELL MILL MOLL MULL NELL NOLL NULL PALL PELL PILL POLL PULL RALL RILL ROLL SELL SILL SYLL TALL TELL TILL TOLL TULL WALL WELL WILL YALL YELL ZELL ZILL

LM••
LMNO

L•M•
LAMA LAMB LAME LAMP LAMS LCMS LEMA LEMS LIMA LIMB LIME LIMN LIMO LIMP LIMY LLMS LOMA LOMB LOME LUMA LUMP LYME

L••M
LIAM LITM LOAM LOOM

•LM•
ALMA ALMS ELMO ELMS ELMY KLMN LLMS

•L•M
ALUM BLAM BLUM CLAM CLEM CLYM ELAM ELEM FLAM FLEM FLIM GLAM GLIM GLOM GLUM KLEM KLUM PLUM SLAM SLIM SLUM YLEM

••LM
BALM CALM COLM FILM HELM HOLM JKLM PALM

L•N•
LANA LAND LANE LANG LANI LANK LANO LANS LENA LEND LENI LENO LENS LENT LENZ LINA LINC LIND LINE LING LINK LINN LINO LINT LINY LINZ LMNO LONE LONG LONI LPNS LUNA LUND LUNE LUNG LUNK LUNN LUNT LYND LYNE LYNG LYNN LYNX

L••N
LAIN LAWN LEAN LEHN LEON LIEN LIGN LIMN LINN LION LOAN LOIN LOON LORN LRON LUNN LYIN LYNN LYON

•LN•
ULNA

•L•N
ALAN ALEN ALYN BLIN CLAN ELAN ELON FLAN FLON GLEN GLYN KLAN KLMN OLAN OLEN OLIN PLAN ULAN

••LN
KILN KOLN

LO••
LOAD LOAF LOAM LOAN LOBE LOBO LOBS LOCA LOCH LOCI LOCK LOCO LODE LODI LODZ LOEB LOEW LOFT LOGE LOGO LOGS LOGY LOID LOIN LOIS LOKI LOLA LOLL LOMA LOMB LOME LONE LONG LONI LOOK LOOM LOON LOOP LOOS LOOT LOPE LOPS LORD LORE LORI LORN LORY LOSE LOSS LOST LOTI LOTS LOTT LOUD LOUP LOUR LOUT LOVE LOWE LOWS LOXY LOYD

L•O•
LAOS LBOS LEOG LEOI LEON LEOV LEOX LION LOOK LOOM LOON LOOP LOOS LOOT LRON LVOV LYON

L••O
LAGO LALO LANO LEGO LENO LETO LEVO LIAO LIDO LIFO LILO LIMO LINO LIPO LMNO LOBO LOCO LOGO LYCO

•LO•
ALOE ALOP ALOT ALOU ALOW BLOB BLOC BLOG BLOK BLOT BLOW CLOD CLOG CLOP CLOT CLOY DLOS ELOI ELON FLOE FLOG FLON FLOP FLOR FLOW FLOY FLOZ GLOB GLOM GLOP GLOT GLOW OLOF OLOR PLOD PLOP PLOT PLOW PLOY SLOB SLOE SLOG SLOP SLOT SLOW

•L•O
ALDO ALLO ALPO ALSO ALTO CLEO CLIO ELIO ELKO ELMO OLEO OLIO

••LO
ALLO ARLO BELO BOLO COLO EHLO FILO HALO HELO HILO HOLO KILO LALO LILO MALO MELO MILO NOLO ORLO OSLO PALO PILO POLO RELO ROLO SILO SOLO STLO TYLO VALO VELO XYLO

LP••
LPGA LPNS

L•P•
LAPD LAPP LAPS LIPO LIPP LIPS LOPE LOPS LUPE

L••P
LAMP LAPP LEAP LIMP LIPP LISP LOOP LOUP LUMP

•LP•
ALPE ALPH ALPO ALPS OLPE

•L•P
ALOP BLIP CLAP CLIP CLOP FLAP FLIP FLOP GLOP PLOP SLAP SLIP SLOP

••LP
CULP GULP HELP KELP KULP PALP PULP YELP

LR••
LRON

L•R•
LARA LARC LARD LARI LARK LARS LARY LDRS LIRA LIRE LIRR LORD LORE LORI LORN LORY LTRS LURE LURK LYRA LYRE

L••R
LAHR LAIR LBAR LEAR LEER LEHR LEUR LIAR LIRR LOUR LTYR

•LR•
NLRB SLRS

•L•R
ALAR ALER BLUR CLAR FLIR FLOR ILER NLER OLOR PLUR SLUR ULAR

LS••
LSAT LSTS

L•S•
LASE LASH LASS LAST LESE LESS LEST LISA LISI LISP LIST LOSE LOSS LOST LUSH LUST LYSE

L••S
LABS LACS LADS LAGS LAIS LAMS LANS LAOS LAPS LARS LASS LATS LAVS LAWS LAYS LBOS LCDS LCMS LDRS LEAS LEDS LEES LEGS LEIS LEKS LEMS LENS LESS LETS LHBS LIBS LICS LIDS LIES LIPS LITS LLBS LLDS LLMS LOBS LOGS LOIS LOOS LOPS LOSS LOTS LOWS LPNS LSTS LTDS LTRS LUGS LUIS LUKS LUVS LYES

•LS•
ALSO ELSA ELSE ILSA

•L•S
ALAS ALBS ALCS ALDS ALES ALLS ALMS ALPS ALTS BLAS BLTS DLOS ELAS ELIS ELKS ELLS ELMS FLUS GLCS ILES ILKS ILLS ILUS LLBS LLDS LLMS NLCS OLAS OLDS OLES PLUS SLRS SLXS ULUS

••LS
AILS ALLS AWLS BALS BBLS BDLS BELS CALS CELS COLS CPLS CYLS DALS DBLS EELS ELLS FELS FILS GALS GELS HALS HOLS ILLS ISLS MELS MILS MOLS NELS NILS OILS OWLS PALS POLS PULS RELS SALS SOLS SYLS TELS URLS VOLS ZILS

LT••
LTDS LTJG LTRS LTYR

L•T•
LATE LATH LATS LETO LETS LETT LGTH LITA LITB LITD LITE LITH LITM LITS LOTI LOTS LOTT LSTS LUTE LUTH LUTZ LYTE

L••T
LACT LAIT LAST LECT LEFT LENT LEST LETT LIAT LIFT LILT LINT LIST LOFT LOOT LOST LOTT LOUT LSAT LUFT LUNT LUST

•LT•
ALTA ALTE ALTI ALTO ALTS BLTS

•L•T
ALIT ALOT BLAT BLIT BLOT CLOT DLIT ELAT FLAT FLIT GLOT GLUT NLAT PLAT PLOT PLUT SLAT SLIT SLOT

••LT
BALT BELT BILT BOLT CELT COLT CULT DELT DOLT FELT GALT GELT GILT HALT HILT HOLT JILT JOLT KILT LILT MALT MELT MILT MOLT PELT SALT SILT TILT VOLT WALT WELT WILT

LU••
LUAU LUBE LUCE LUCI LUCK LUCY LUFF LUFT LUGE LUGS LUIS LUIZ LUKA LUKE LUKS LULA LULL LULU LUMA LUMP LUNA LUND LUNE LUNG LUNK LUNN LUNT LUPE LURE LURK LUSH LUST LUTE LUTH LUTZ LUVS LUXE

L•U•
LAUD LAUE LEUR LOUD LOUP LOUR LOUT

L••U
LEVU LIEU LUAU LULU

•LU•
ALUI ALUM BLUE BLUM BLUR CLUB CLUE ELUL FLUB FLUE FLUS FLUX GLUC GLUE GLUG GLUM GLUT ILUS KLUM PLUG PLUM PLUR PLUS PLUT SLUE SLUG SLUM SLUR ULUS

•L•U
ALOU BLAU BLEU

••LU
ACLU IGLU LULU OULU SULU WELU YALU ZULU

LV••
LVII LVOV

L•V•
LAVA LAVE LAVI LAVS LEVA LEVI LEVO LEVU LEVY LIVE LIVY LOVE LUVS LXVI

L••V
LEOV LIEV LVOV LXIV LXXV

•LV•
ALVA ALVY BLVD CLVI DLVI MLVI XLVI

•L•V
CLIV CLXV DLIV DLXV ELEV MLIV MLXV OLAV SLAV XLIV

••LV
CCLV CDLV CMLV CXLV DCLV DXLV MCLV MDLV MMLV MXLV UNLV

LW••
LWEI

L•W•
LAWD LAWN LAWS LEWD LOWE LOWS

L••W
LOEW

•L•W
ALOW BLEW BLOW CLAW CLEW FLAW FLEW FLOW GLOW PLOW SLAW SLEW SLOW

LX••
LXII LXIV LXIX LXVI LXXI LXXV LXXX

L•X•
LOXY LUXE LXXI LXXV LXXX

L••X
LEIX LEOX LXIX LXXX LYNX

•LX•
CLXI CLXV CLXX DLXI DLXV DLXX MLXI MLXV MLXX SLXS

•L•X
ALEX ALIX CLIX CLXX DLIX DLXX FLAX FLEX FLIX FLUX ILEX MLIX

MLXX
PLAX
PLEX
XLIX

••LX
CALX
CCLX
CDLX
CMLX
DCLX
MCLX
MDLX
MMLX

LY••
LYCO
LYES
LYIN
LYLE
LYLY
LYME
LYND
LYNE
LYNG
LYNN
LYNX
LYON
LYRA
LYRE
LYSE
LYTE

L•Y•
LAYS
LOYD
LTYR

L••Y
LACY
LADY
LAKY
LARY
LAZY
LELY
LEVY
LILY
LIMY
LINY
LIVY
LOGY
LORY
LOXY
LUCY
LYLY

•LY•
ALYN
CLYM
GLYC
GLYN
ILYA
SLYE

•L•Y
ALKY
ALLY
ALVY
CLAY
CLOY
ELLY
ELMY
FLAY
FLOY
ILLY
OLAY
PLAY
PLOY
SLAY
SLEY

••LY
ABLY
ALLY
BELY
DALY
DULY
EELY
ELLY
EMLY
HOLY
IBLY
IDLY
ILLY
INLY
JULY
LELY
LILY
LYLY
MOLY
OILY
ONLY
ORLY
OWLY
POLY
RELY
ROLY
RULY
UGLY
WILY
WKLY

L•Z•
LAZE
LAZY
LIZA

L••Z
LENZ
LINZ
LODZ
LUIZ
LUTZ

•L•Z
ELIZ
FLOZ

MA••
MAAM
MAAS
MACE
MACH
MACK
MACR
MACS
MACY
MADD
MADE
MADS
MAGE
MAGI
MAGS
MAHI
MAIA
MAID
MAIL
MAIM
MAIN
MAIO
MAIS
MAJA
MAJS
MAKE
MAKO
MALA
MALE
MALI
MALL
MALO
MALT
MAMA
MAME
MAMS
MANE
MANN
MANO
MANS
MANX
MANY
MAPS
MARA
MARC
MARE
MARG
MARI
MARK
MARL
MARM
MARS
MART
MARU
MARV
MARX
MARY
MARZ
MASA
MASC
MASH
MASK
MASS
MAST
MATA
MATE
MATH
MATO
MATR
MATS
MATT
MAUD
MAUI
MAUL
MAUS
MAVS
MAWR
MAWS
MAXI
MAXX
MAYA
MAYI
MAYO
MAYS
MAZE
MAZO
MAZY

M•A•
MAAM
MAAS
MBAS
MCAN
MCAT
MEAD
MEAL
MEAN
MEAS
MEAT
MFAS
MIAS
MOAB
MOAN
MOAS
MOAT
MPAA

M••A
MAIA
MAJA
MALA
MAMA
MARA
MASA
MATA
MAYA
MEGA
MENA
MESA
META
MICA
MILA
MINA
MIRA
MITA
MOMA
MONA
MORA
MOTA
MPAA
MYNA
MYRA

•MA•
AMAH
AMAJ
AMAS
AMAT
BMAJ
CMAJ
DMAJ
EMAG
EMAJ
FMAJ
GMAC
GMAJ
GMAN
GMAT
IMAC
IMAM
IMAN
IMAX
OMAN
OMAR
OMAT
TMAN
TMAX
XMAS

•M•A
EMIA
EMMA
YMCA
YMHA

••MA
ALMA
ARMA
BAMA
BEMA
CAMA
COMA
CYMA
DAMA
DUMA
EMMA
ERMA
FAMA
FEMA
FNMA
GAMA
GNMA
HAMA
HEMA
IRMA
JAMA
JIMA
KAMA
LAMA
LEMA
LIMA
LOMA
LUMA
MAMA
MOMA
OZMA
PIMA
PUMA
RAMA
RIMA
ROMA
SIMA
SOMA
TAMA
TEMA
TOMA
TVMA
USMA
YUMA
ZIMA

MB••
MBAS
MBES

M•B•
MGBS
MIBS
MOBS
MOBY

M••B
MOAB
MYOB

•MB•
AMBI
AMBO
AMBS

••MB
BOMB
COMB
DUMB
IAMB
JAMB
LAMB
LIMB
LOMB
NUMB
TOMB
WOMB

MC••
MCAN
MCAT
MCCC
MCCI
MCCL
MCCV
MCCX
MCDI
MCDL
MCDV
MCDX
MCII
MCIV
MCIX
MCLI
MCLV
MCLX
MCMI
MCML
MCMV
MCMX
MCPS
MCVI
MCXC
MCXI
MCXL
MCXV
MCXX

M•C•
MACE
MACH
MACK
MACR
MACS
MACY
MCCC
MCCI
MCCL
MCCV
MCCX
MDCC
MDCI
MDCL
MDCV
MDCX
MECH
MICA
MICE
MICH
MICK
MICR
MICS
MMCC
MMCD
MMCI
MMCL
MMCM
MMCV
MMCX
MOCK
MOCS
MUCH
MUCK
MXCI
MXCV
MYCO

M••C
MARC
MASC
MCCC
MCXC
MDCC
MDXC
MERC
MISC
MMCC
MMDC
MMMC
MMXC
MRSC
MSEC

•MC•
AMCS
GMCS
MMCC
MMCD
MMCI
MMCL
MMCM
MMCV
MMCX
YMCA

•M•C
AMIC
BMOC
CMXC
GMAC
IMAC
MMCC
MMDC
MMMC
MMXC

••MC
MMMC
USMC

MD••
MDCC
MDCI
MDCL
MDCV
MDCX
MDII
MDIV
MDIX
MDLI
MDLV
MDLX
MDSE
MDVI
MDXC
MDXI
MDXL
MDXV
MDXX

M•D•
MADD
MADE
MADS
MCDI
MCDL
MCDV
MCDX
MEDE
MEDI
MEDS
MIDI
MMDC
MMDI
MMDL
MMDV
MMDX
MODE
MODI
MODS
MUDD
MUDS

M••D
MADD
MAID
MAUD
MEAD
MELD
MEND
MILD
MIND
MMCD
MMMD
MOLD
MOOD
MRED
MSED
MUDD

•MD•
CMDG
CMDR
DMDS
MMDC
MMDI
MMDL
MMDV
MMDX
RMDR

•M•D
AMID
MMCD
MMMD
ZMED

••MD
MMMD

ME••
MEAD
MEAL
MEAN
MEAS
MEAT
MECH
MEDE
MEDI
MEDS
MEEK
MEER
MEET
MEGA
MEGS
MEIN
MEIR
MELD
MELL
MELO
MELS
MELT
MEME
MEMO
MEMS
MENA
MEND
MENE
MENS
MENT
MENU
MEOW
MERC
MERE
MERL
MERM
MERS
MERV
MESA
MESH
MESO
MESS
META
METE
METH
METS
METZ
MEUM
MEWL
MEWS

M•E•
MBES
MEEK
MEER
MEET
MIEL
MIEN
MIES
MMES
MNEM
MOEN
MOES
MOET
MPEG
MRED
MSEC
MSED

M••E
MACE
MADE
MAGE
MAKE
MALE
MAME
MANE
MARE
MATE
MAZE
MDSE
MEDE
MEME
MENE
MERE
METE
MICE
MIKE
MILE
MIME
MINE
MIRE
MISE
MITE
MIZE
MLLE
MODE
MOLE
MOME
MOPE
MORE
MOSE
MOTE
MOUE
MOVE
MTGE
MULE
MUSE
MUTE

•ME•
AMEN
AMER
AMES
AMEX
BMES
EMER
EMES
EMEU
GMEN
MMES
NMEX
OMEI
OMEN
OMER
OMES
SMEE
SMEW
TMEN
XMEN
ZMED

•M•E
AMIE
CMTE
EMME
IMRE
SMEE

••ME
ACME
AHME
AIME
ARME
AYME
BYME
CAME
COME
CUME
CYME
DAME
DEME
DIME
DOME
EMME
ESME
FAME
FEME
FUME
GAME
HAME
HEME
HOME
HUME
LAME
LIME
LOME
LYME
MAME
MEME
MIME
MOME
NAME
NOME
OHME
POME
RIME
ROME
SAME
SOME
TAME
TIME
TOME

MF••
MFAS
MFRS

M•F•
MIFF
MUFF

M••F
MIFF
MUFF

•MF•
AMFM

•M•F
IMPF

MG••
MGBS
MGMT
MGRS

M•G•
MAGE
MAGI
MAGS
MEGA
MEGS
MIGS
MSGR
MSGS
MSGT
MTGE
MTGS
MUGS

M••G
MARG
MING
MKTG
MOOG
MPEG
MUNG

•M•G
CMDG
EMAG
SMOG
SMUG

MH••
MHOS

M•H•
MAHI
MOHS

M••H
MACH
MASH
MATH
MECH
MESH
METH
MICH
MINH
MOSH
MOTH
MUCH
MUSH
MYTH

•MH•
IMHO
YMHA

•M•H
AMAH
UMPH

••MH
NIMH

MI••
MIAS
MIBS
MICA
MICE
MICH
MICK
MICR
MICS
MIDI
MIEL
MIEN
MIES
MIFF
MIGS
MIII
MIKE
MILA
MILD
MILE
MILK
MILL
MILO
MILS
MILT
MIME
MIMI
MIMS
MINA
MIND
MINE
MING
MINH
MINI
MINK
MINN
MINS
MINT
MINX
MIPS
MIRA
MIRE
MIRO
MIRS
MIRV
MIRY
MISC
MISE
MISO
MISS
MIST
MITA
MITE
MITT
MIXT
MIZE

M•I•
MAIA
MAID
MAIL
MAIM
MAIN
MAIO
MAIS
MCII
MCIV
MCIX
MDII
MDIV
MDIX
MEIN
MEIR
MIII
MLII
MLIV
MLIX
MMII
MMIV
MMIX
MOIL
MOIS
MRIS
MUIR
MVII
MXII
MXIV
MXIX

M••I
MAGI
MAHI
MALI
MARI
MAUI
MAXI
MAYI
MCCI
MCDI
MCII
MCLI
MCMI
MCVI
MCXI
MDCI
MDII
MDLI
MDVI
MDXI
MEDI
MIDI
MIII
MIMI
MINI
MLII
MLVI
MLXI
MMCI
MMDI
MMII
MMLI
MMMI
MMVI
MMXI
MODI
MOMI
MUNI
MUTI
MVII
MXCI
MXII
MXLI
MXVI
MXXI

•MI•
AMIC
AMID
AMIE
AMII
AMIN
AMIR
AMIS
CMII
CMIV
CMIX
DMIN
EMIA
EMIL
EMIR
EMIT
IMIN
IMIT
MMII
MMIV
MMIX
OMIT
SMIT
YMIR

•M•I
AMBI
AMII
AMOI
CMII
CMLI
CMVI
CMXI
MMCI
MMDI
MMII
MMLI
MMMI
MMVI
MMXI
OMEI
OMNI
OMRI

••MI
DEMI
EIMI
HEMI
JAMI
JIMI
KAMI
MCMI
MIMI
MMMI
MOMI
RAMI
REMI
SAMI
SEMI
SIMI
SOMI
TAMI

M•J•
MAJA
MAJS
MOJO

•M•J
AMAJ
BMAJ
CMAJ
DMAJ
EMAJ
FMAJ
GMAJ

MK••
MKTG
MKTS

M•K•
MAKE
MAKO
MIKE
MOKO

M••K
MACK
MARK
MASK
MEEK
MICK
MILK
MINK
MOCK
MONK
MORK
MUCK
MURK
MUSK

•MK•
PMKS

•M•K
AMOK
IMOK
OMSK

ML••
MLII
MLIV
MLIX
MLLE
MLVI
MLXI
MLXV
MLXX

M•L•
MALA
MALE
MALI
MALL
MALO
MALT
MCLI
MCLV
MCLX
MDLI
MDLV
MDLX
MELD
MELL
MELO
MELS
MELT
MILA
MILD
MILE
MILK
MILL
MILO
MILS
MILT
MLLE
MMLI
MMLV
MMLX
MOLD
MOLE
MOLL
MOLS
MOLT
MOLY
MULE
MULL
MXLI
MXLV

M••L
MAIL
MALL
MARL
MAUL
MCCL
MCDL
MCML
MCXL
MDCL
MDXL
MEAL
MELL
MERL
MEWL
MIEL
MILL
MMCL
MMDL
MMML
MMXL
MOIL
MOLL
MULL

•ML•
CMLI
CMLV
CMLX
EMLY
MMLI
MMLV
MMLX

•M•L
AMUL
AMYL
CMXL
EMIL
MMCL
MMDL
MMML
MMXL

••ML
HTML
MCML
MMML
SAML

MM••
MMCC
MMCD
MMCI
MMCL
MMCM
MMCV
MMCX
MMDC
MMDI
MMDL
MMDV
MMDX
MMES
MMII
MMIV
MMIX
MMLI
MMLV
MMLX
MMMC
MMMD
MMMI
MMML
MMMM
MMMV
MMMX
MMVI
MMXC
MMXI
MMXL
MMXV
MMXX

M•M•
MAMA
MAME
MAMS
MCMI
MCML
MCMV
MCMX
MEME
MEMO
MEMS
MGMT
MIME
MIMI
MIMS
MMMC
MMMD
MMMI
MMML
MMMM
MMMV
MMMX
MOMA
MOME
MOMI
MOMS
MUMM
MUMS
MYMY

M••M
MAAM
MAIM
MARM
MERM
MEUM
MMCM
MMMM
MNEM
MUMM

•MM•
AMMO
EMMA
EMME
EMMY
HMMM
MMMC
MMMD
MMMI
MMML
MMMM
MMMV
MMMX

•M•M
AMFM
HMMM
IMAM
MMCM
MMMM

••MM
COMM
GUMM
HAMM
HMMM
MMMM
MUMM

MN••
MNEM
MNOP

M•N•
MANE
MANN
MANO
MANS

MANX
MANY
MENA
MEND
MENE
MENS
MENT
MENU
MINA
MIND
MINE
MING
MINH
MINI
MINK
MINN
MINS
MINT
MINX
MONA
MONK
MONO
MONS
MONT
MONY
MTNS
MUNG
MUNI
MYNA

M••N
MAIN
MANN
MCAN
MEAN
MEIN
MIEN
MINN
MOAN
MOEN
MOON
MORN
MOWN
MUON

•MN•
AMNT
LMNO
OMNI

•M•N
AMEN
AMIN
AMON
CMON
DMIN
GMAN
GMEN
IMAN
IMIN
OMAN
OMEN
TMAN
TMEN
XMEN

••MN
CHMN
DAMN
HYMN
KLMN
LIMN

MO••
MOAB
MOAN
MOAS
MOAT
MOBS
MOBY
MOCK
MOCS
MODE
MODI
MODS
MOEN
MOES
MOET
MOHS
MOIL
MOIS
MOJO
MOKO
MOLD
MOLE
MOLL
MOLS
MOLT
MOLY
MOMA
MOME
MOMI
MOMS
MONA
MONK
MONO
MONS
MONT
MONY
MOOD
MOOG
MOON
MOOR
MOOS
MOOT
MOPE
MOPS
MOPY
MORA
MORE
MORK
MORN
MORO
MORT
MOSE
MOSH
MOSS
MOST
MOTA
MOTE
MOTH
MOTO
MOTS
MOTT
MOUE
MOVE
MOWN
MOWS
MOZO

M•O•
MEOW
MHOS
MNOP
MOOD
MOOG
MOON
MOOR
MOOS
MOOT
MUON
MYOB

M••O
MAIO
MAKO
MALO
MANO
MATO
MAYO
MAZO
MELO
MEMO
MESO
MILO
MIRO
MISO
MOJO
MOKO
MONO
MORO
MOTO
MOZO
MYCO

•MO•
AMOI
AMOK
AMON
AMOR
AMOS
AMOY
BMOC
CMON
HMOS
IMOK
OMOO
SMOG

•M•O
AMBO
AMMO
AMSO
IMHO
LMNO
OMOO

••MO
AMMO
ATMO
CAMO
COMO
DEMO
DOMO
ELMO
HEMO
HOMO
JOMO
KEMO
LIMO
MEMO
NEMO
NOMO
POMO
REMO
SHMO
SUMO
UOMO

MP••
MPAA
MPEG
MPVS

M•P•
MAPS
MCPS
MIPS
MOPE
MOPS
MOPY
MVPS

M••P
MNOP
MSRP

•MP•
AMPS
EMPS
IMPF
IMPS
UMPH
UMPS

••MP
BUMP
CAMP
COMP
DAMP
DUMP
GAMP
GIMP
GUMP
HAMP
HEMP
HUMP
JUMP
KEMP
LAMP
LIMP
LUMP
POMP
PUMP
RAMP
RCMP
ROMP
RUMP
SAMP
SIMP
SUMP
TAMP
TEMP
VAMP
WIMP

MR••
MRED
MRIS
MRSC

M•R•
MARA
MARC
MARE
MARG
MARI
MARK
MARL
MARM
MARS
MART
MARU
MARV
MARX
MARY
MARZ
MERC
MERE
MERL
MERM
MERS
MERV
MFRS
MGRS
MIRA
MIRE
MIRO
MIRS
MIRV
MIRY
MORA
MORE
MORK
MORN
MORO
MORT
MSRP
MURK
MURS
MYRA

M••R
MACR
MATR
MAWR
MEER
MEIR
MICR
MOOR
MSGR
MUIR

•MR•
IMRE
OMRI

•M•R
AMER
AMIR
AMOR
AMUR
CMDR
EMER
EMIR
OMAR
OMER
RMDR
YMIR

MS••
MSEC
MSED
MSGR
MSGS
MSGT
MSRP

M•S•
MASA
MASC
MASH
MASK
MASS
MAST
MDSE
MESA
MESH
MESO
MESS
MISC
MISE
MISO
MISS
MIST
MOSE
MOSH
MOSS
MOST
MRSC
MUSE
MUSH
MUSK
MUSS
MUST
MYST

M••S
MAAS
MACS
MADS
MAGS
MAIS
MAJS
MAMS
MANS
MAPS
MARS
MASS
MATS
MAUS
MAVS
MAWS
MAYS
MBAS
MBES
MCPS
MEAS
MEDS
MEGS
MELS
MEMS
MENS
MERS
MESS
METS
MEWS
MFAS
MFRS
MGBS
MGRS
MHOS
MIAS
MIBS
MICS
MIES
MIGS
MILS
MIMS
MINS
MIPS
MIRS
MISS
MKTS
MMES
MOAS
MOBS
MOCS
MODS
MOES
MOHS
MOIS
MOLS
MOMS
MONS
MOOS
MOPS
MOSS
MOTS
MOWS
MPVS
MRIS
MSGS
MTGS
MTNS
MUDS
MUGS
MUMS
MURS
MUSS
MVPS

•MS•
AMSO
OMSK

•M•S
AMAS
AMBS
AMCS
AMES
AMIS
AMOS
AMPS
AMTS
BMES
BMUS
BMWS
DMDS
DMUS
DMVS
DMZS
EMES
EMPS
EMTS
EMUS
GMCS
HMOS
IMPS
IMUS
MMES
OMES
PMKS
PMTS
UMPS
XMAS

••MS
ABMS
ADMS
AIMS
ALMS
ARMS
ATMS
BAMS
BEMS
BUMS
CAMS
COMS
CWMS
DAMS
DCMS
DEMS
DFMS
DIMS
DOMS
DPMS
DSMS
DVMS
EDMS
ELMS
FAMS
FEMS
GAMS
GEMS
GUMS
GYMS
HAMS
HEMS
HUMS
IAMS
IBMS
ISMS
JAMS
LAMS
LCMS
LEMS
LLMS
MAMS
MEMS
MIMS
MOMS
MUMS
NIMS
NOMS
OHMS
POMS
RAMS
REMS
RIMS
ROMS
RPMS
RUMS
SAMS
SEMS
SIMS
SUMS
SYMS
TAMS
TOMS
TUMS
VIMS
YAMS

MT••
MTGE
MTGS
MTNS

M•T•
MATA
MATE
MATH
MATO
MATR
MATS
MATT
META
METE
METH
METS
METZ
MITA
MITE
MITT
MKTG
MKTS
MOTA
MOTE
MOTH
MOTO
MOTS
MOTT
MUTE
MUTI
MUTT
MYTH

M••T
MALT
MART
MAST
MATT
MCAT
MEAT
MEET
MELT
MENT
MGMT
MILT
MINT
MIST
MITT
MIXT
MOAT
MOET
MOLT
MONT
MOOT
MORT
MOST
MOTT
MSGT
MUST
MUTT
MYST

•MT•
AMTS
CMTE
EMTS
PMTS

•M•T
AMAT
AMNT
EMIT
GMAT
IMIT
OMAT
OMIT
SMIT
SMUT

••MT
BSMT
MGMT
STMT
TOMT

MU••
MUCH
MUCK
MUDD
MUDS
MUFF
MUGS
MUIR
MULE
MULL
MUMM
MUMS
MUNG
MUNI
MUON
MURK
MURS
MUSE
MUSH
MUSK
MUSS
MUST
MUTE
MUTI
MUTT

M•U•
MAUD
MAUI
MAUL
MAUS
MEUM
MOUE

M••U
MARU
MENU

•MU•
AMUL
AMUR
BMUS
DMUS
EMUS
IMUS
SMUG
SMUT

•M•U
EMEU

••MU
NAMU

MV••
MVII
MVPS

M•V•
MAVS
MCVI
MDVI
MLVI
MMVI
MOVE
MPVS
MXVI

M••V
MARV
MCCV
MCDV
MCIV
MCLV
MCMV
MCXV
MDCV
MDIV
MDLV
MDXV
MERV
MIRV
MLIV
MLXV
MMCV
MMDV
MMIV
MMLV
MMMV
MMXV
MXCV
MXIV
MXLV
MXXV

•MV•
CMVI
DMVS
MMVI

•M•V
CMIV
CMLV
CMXV
MMCV
MMDV
MMIV
MMLV
MMMV
MMXV

••MV
MCMV
MMMV

M•W•
MAWR
MAWS
MEWL
MEWS
MOWN
MOWS

M••W
MEOW

•MW•
BMWS

•M•W
SMEW

MX••
MXCI
MXCV
MXII
MXIV
MXIX
MXLI
MXLV
MXVI
MXXI
MXXV
MXXX

M•X•
MAXI
MAXX
MCXC
MCXI
MCXL
MCXV
MCXX
MDXC
MDXI
MDXL
MDXV
MDXX
MIXT
MLXI
MLXV
MLXX
MMXC
MMXI
MMXL
MMXV
MMXX
MXXI
MXXV
MXXX

M••X
MANX
MARX
MAXX
MCCX
MCDX
MCIX
MCLX
MCMX
MCXX
MDCX
MDIX
MDLX
MDXX
MINX
MLIX
MLXX
MMCX
MMDX
MMIX
MMLX
MMMX
MMXX
MXIX
MXXX

•MX•
CMXC
CMXI
CMXL
CMXV
CMXX
MMXC
MMXI
MMXL
MMXV
MMXX

•M•X
AMEX
CMIX
CMLX
CMXX
IMAX
MMCX
MMDX
MMIX
MMLX
MMMX
MMXX
NMEX
TMAX

••MX
MCMX
MMMX

MY••
MYCO
MYMY
MYNA
MYOB
MYRA
MYST
MYTH

M•Y•
MAYA
MAYI
MAYO
MAYS

M••Y
MACY
MANY
MARY
MAZY
MIRY
MOBY
MOLY
MONY
MOPY
MYMY

•MY•
AMYL

•M•Y
AMOY
EMLY
EMMY

••MY
ARMY
DEMY
ELMY
EMMY
FUMY
GAMY
LIMY
MYMY
NOMY
OHMY
REMY
RIMY
ROMY

M•Z•
MAZE
MAZO
MAZY
MIZE
MOZO

M••Z
MARZ
METZ

•MZ•
DMZS

NA••
NABE
NABI
NABS
NACL
NADA
NAES
NAGS
NAGY
NAHA
NAHS
NAIF
NAIL
NAIR
NALA
NAME
NAMU
NANA
NANG
NANO
NANU
NAOH
NAOS
NAPA
NAPE
NAPS
NARA
NARC
NARD
NARK
NARY
NARZ
NASA
NASD
NASH
NASI
NASL
NASO
NAST
NATE
NATL
NATO
NATR
NATS
NAUT
NAVE
NAVY
NAYA
NAYS
NAZI

N•A•
NCAA
NCAR
NDAK
NEAL
NEAP
NEAR
NEAT
NHAT
NLAT
NOAA
NOAH
NOAM
NYAD

N••A
NADA
NAHA
NALA
NANA
NAPA
NARA
NASA
NAYA
NCAA
NENA
NERA
NEVA
NHRA
NIKA
NINA
NIPA
NITA
NOAA
NOIA
NOLA
NORA
NOTA
NOVA

•NA•
ANAG
ANAS
ANAT
BNAI
DNAS
GNAR
GNAT
GNAW
KNAG
KNAP
KNAR
ONAN
RNAS
SNAG
SNAP
SNAX
UNAS
UNAU

•N•A
ANGA
ANKA
ANNA
ANOA
ANSA
ANTA
ANYA
ENNA
ENYA
FNMA
GNMA
INCA
INGA
INKA
ONDA
ONEA
ONNA
UNCA
WNBA

••NA
ANNA
BONA
CANA
CENA
DANA
DENA
DINA
DONA
DUNA
DYNA
EDNA
ENNA
ERNA
ETNA
FINA
GENA
GINA
HANA
IANA
IONA
JANA
JENA
KANA
KINA
KONA
LANA
LENA
LINA
LUNA
MENA
MINA
MONA
MYNA
NANA
NENA
NINA
ONNA
OONA
PENA
PINA
RANA
RENA
RINA
RONA
SANA
TANA
TENA
TINA
TUNA
ULNA
USNA
VENA
VINA
XENA
ZINA
ZONA

N•B•
NABE
NABI
NABS
NEBO
NEBR
NEBS
NIBS
NOBS
NUBS
NYBY

N••B
NHEB
NLRB
NTSB
NUMB

•NB•
CNBC
WNBA

•N•B
KNOB
ONEB
SNOB
SNUB

••NB
TENB

NC••
NCAA
NCAR
NCOS

N•C•
NACL
NECK
NICE
NICK
NLCS
NOCK
NOCT
NYCT

N••C
NARC
NUNC

•NC•
ANCE
ANCY
ENCE
ENCL
ENCS
ENCY
INCA
INCE
INCH
INCL
INCR
INCS
ONCD
ONCE
SNCC
UNCA

•N•C
CNBC
ONEC
ONIC
SNCC
UNPC

••NC
BANC
CINC
CONC
DONC
JUNC
LINC
NUNC
SYNC
TENC
ZINC

ND••
NDAK

N•D•
NADA
NIDE
NIDI
NODE
NODI
NODS
NUDE

N••D
NARD
NASD
NEED
NEJD
NERD
NFLD
NKVD
NOID
NORD
NYAD
NYPD

•ND•
ANDS
ANDY
ENDE
ENDO
ENDS
INDO
INDS
INDY
ONDA
ONDE
RNDS
UNDO

•N•D
ENID
ONCD
ONED

••ND
BAND
BEND
BIND
BOND
BUND
COND
FEND
FIND
FOND
FUND
GUND
HAND
HIND
HOND
HUND
KIND
LAND
LEND
LIND
LUND
LYND
MEND
MIND
PEND
POND
RAND
REND
RIND

4 NE

SAND SEND TEND VEND WAND WEND WIND YOND ZEND

NE••
NEAL NEAP NEAR NEAT NEBO NEBR NEBS NECK NEED NEEL NEER NEET NEFF NEGS NEHI NEIL NEIN NEJD NELL NELS NEMO NENA NENE NENG NEON NEOS NERA NERD NERF NERI NERO NESS NEST NETH NETS NEUE NEUF NEUN NEUR NEUT NEVA NEVE NEVI NEWF NEWS NEWT NEXO NEXT

N•E•
NAES NEED NEEL NEER NEET NHEB NLER NMEX NOEL NOES NYET

N••E
NABE NAME NAPE NATE NAVE NENE NEUE NEVE NICE NIDE NIKE NILE NINE NITE NIUE NODE NOLE NOME NONE NOPE NOSE NOTE NOVE NUDE NUKE NYSE

•NE•
ANES ANEW BNEG DNET ENES INEE INES INEZ KNEE KNEW MNEM ONEA ONEB ONEC ONED ONEE ONEF ONEG ONEH ONEK ONEL ONER ONES ONEY SNEE UNES YNEZ

•N•E
ANCE ANGE ANKE ANNE ANSE ANTE ENCE ENDE ENKE ENNE ENSE INCE INEE INGE INRE KNEE ONCE ONDE ONEE ONZE SNEE UNIE

••NE
ACNE ANNE AONE ARNE BANE BENE BINE BONE CANE CENE CINE CONE DANE DENE DINE DONE DUNE DYNE EINE ENNE ERNE ESNE FANE FINE GENE GONE GYNE HONE IONE JANE JUNE KANE KINE LANE LINE LONE LUNE LYNE MANE MENE MINE NENE NINE NONE OHNE ORNE PANE PINE PONE PYNE RENE RUNE RYNE SANE SENE SINE SONE SYNE TENE TINE TONE TUNE TYNE URNE UTNE VANE VINE WANE WINE ZANE ZINE ZONE

NF••
NFLD

N•F•
NEFF NUFF

N••F
NAIF NEFF NERF NEUF NEWF NUFF

•NF•
INFO INFS

•N•F
ENIF ENUF ONEF

••NF
CONF FUNF GENF

NG••
NGOR

N•G•
NAGS NAGY NEGS NIGH NOGO NOGS

N••G
NANG NENG

•NG•
ANGA ANGE ENGR ENGS INGA INGE INGO

•N•G
ANAG BNEG KNAG ONEG SNAG SNUG

••NG
AUNG BANG BING BONG BUNG BYNG CONG DANG DENG DING DONG FANG FENG FONG GANG GONG GUNG HANG HONG HUNG JONG JUNG KANG KING KONG KUNG LANG LING LONG LUNG LYNG MING MUNG NANG NENG PANG PENG PING PONG PUNG RANG RING RUNG SANG SENG SING SONG SUNG TANG TENG TING TONG TUNG VING WANG WENG WING WONG XING YANG YONG YUNG ZING

NH••
NHAT NHEB NHRA

N•H•
NAHA NAHS NEHI NOHO

N••H
NAOH NASH NETH NIGH NIMH NOAH NOSH NOTH

•N•H
ANKH ANTH INCH ONEH

••NH
DINH HUNH MINH PENH SINH TANH

NI••
NIBS NICE NICK NIDE NIDI NIGH NIKA NIKE NILE NILS NIMH NIMS NINA NINE NINO NIPA NIPS NIRO NITA NITE NITS NIUE NIXY

N•I•
NAIF NAIL NAIR NEIL NEIN NOIA NOID NOIL NOIR NUIT

N••I
NABI NASI NAZI NEHI NERI NEVI NIDI NODI NOLI NORI NOTI

•NI•
ANIL ANIM ANIS ENID ENIF INIT KNIT ONIC PNIN SNIP SNIT UNIE UNIS UNIT UNIV UNIX

•N•I
ANNI ANTI BNAI INRI

••NI
AGNI ANNI BANI BENI FINI HONI IFNI JONI JUNI LANI LENI LONI MINI MUNI OMNI RANI RENI RONI SANI TONI VENI VINI ZUNI

N•J•
NEJD

••NJ
CONJ

NK••
NKVD

N•K•
NIKA NIKE NUKE

N••K
NARK NDAK NECK NICK NOCK NOOK NYUK

•NK•
ANKA ANKE ANKH ENKE INKA INKS INKY ONKP

•N•K
ONEK TNPK

••NK
BANK BONK BUNK CONK DANK DINK DUNK FINK FUNK GUNK HANK HONK HUNK JUNK KINK LANK LINK LUNK MINK MONK OINK PINK PUNK RANK RINK SANK SINK SUNK TANK TENK TINK TONK WINK WONK YANK ZONK

NL••
NLAT NLCS NLER NLRB

N•L•
NALA NELL NELS NFLD NILE NILS NOLA NOLE NOLI NOLL NOLO NULL

N••L
NACL NAIL NASL NATL NEAL NEEL NEIL NELL NOEL NOIL NOLL NULL

•NL•
INLY ONLY UNLV

•N•L
ANIL ENCL ENOL INCL INTL ONEL

••NL
DANL GENL

NM••
NMEX

N•M•
NAME NAMU NEMO NIMH NIMS NOME NOMO NOMS NOMY NUMB

N••M
NOAM NORM

•NM•
FNMA GNMA

•N•M
ANIM MNEM ONYM PNOM UNUM

N•N•
NANA NANG NANO NANU NENA NENE NENG NINA NINE NINO NONE NONO NONS NONU NUNC NUNN NUNS NYNY

N••N
NEIN NEON NEUN NOON NORN NOUN NUNN

•NN•
ANNA ANNE ANNI ANNO ANNY ENNA ENNE ENNS INNS INNY ONNA

•N•N
ANON ENON INON ONAN PNIN

••NN
BONN CONN DONN DUNN FENN FINN GANN GUNN HENN JANN JINN KENN LINN LUNN LYNN MANN MINN NUNN PENN RANN SINN TENN VENN WINN WYNN

NO••
NOAA NOAH NOAM NOBS NOCK NOCT NODE NODI NODS NOEL NOES NOGO NOGS NOHO NOIA NOID NOIL NOIR NOLA NOLE NOLI NOLL NOLO NOME NOMO NOMS NOMY NONE NONO NONS NONU NOOK NOON NOOR NOPE NOPQ NORA NORD NORI NORM NORN NORW NOSE NOSH NOSY NOTA NOTE NOTH NOTI NOTS NOTV NOUN NOUS NOVA NOVE NOVO

N•O•
NAOH NAOS NCOS NEON NEOS NGOR NOOK NOON NOOR

N••O
NANO NASO NATO NEBO NEMO NERO NEXO NINO NIRO NOGO NOHO NOLO NOMO NONO NOVO NYRO

•NO•
ANOA ANON ENOL ENON ENOS ENOW INON KNOB KNOT KNOW KNOX MNOP PNOM SNOB SNOW UNOS

•N•O
ANNO ENDO ENTO ENYO ENZO INDO INFO INGO INRO INTO INYO ONTO UNDO UNTO

••NO
ANNO ARNO ATNO BANO BONO BRNO CENO CYNO DANO DINO DRNO ERNO FINO GENO GINO IONO JUNO KENO LANO LENO LINO LMNO MANO MONO NANO NINO NONO OENO OHNO RENO SINO TINO TONO VENO VINO XENO ZENO

N•P•
NAPA NAPE NAPS NIPA NIPS NOPE NOPQ NYPD

N••P
NEAP

•NP•
GNPS TNPK UNPC

•N•P
INSP KNAP MNOP ONKP SNAP SNIP

N••Q
NOPQ

•NQ•
INQS

••NQ
CINQ

N•R•
NARA NARC NARD NARK NARY NARZ NERA NERD NERF NERI NERO NHRA NIRO NLRB NORA NORD NORI NORM NORN NORW NYRO

N••R
NAIR NATR NCAR NEAR NEBR NEER NEUR NGOR NLER NOIR NOOR

•NR•
ENRY INRE INRI INRO

•N•R
ENGR ENTR GNAR INCR INTR KNAR KNUR ONER

••NR
USNR

NS••
NSXS

N•S•
NASA NASD NASH NASI NASL NASO NAST NESS NEST NOSE NOSH NOSY NTSB NYSE

N••S
NABS NAES NAGS NAHS NAOS NAPS NATS NAYS NCOS NEBS NEGS NELS NEOS NESS NETS NEWS NIBS NILS NIMS NIPS NITS NLCS NOBS NODS NOES NOGS NOMS NONS NOTS NOUS NSXS NUBS NUNS NUTS NUYS

•NS•
ANSA ANSE ENSE INSP INST

•N•S
ANAS ANDS ANES ANIS ANTS DNAS ENCS ENDS ENES ENGS ENNS ENOS ENTS ENVS GNPS GNUS INCS INDS INES INFS INKS INNS INQS INTS INVS INXS KNTS ONES ONUS RNAS RNDS TNTS UNAS UNES UNIS UNOS

••NS
AWNS BANS BINS BUNS CANS CENS CONS CTNS DANS DENS DINS DONS DUNS EINS ENNS EONS ERNS FANS FENS FINS FUNS GENS GINS GUNS HANS HENS HONS HUNS INNS IONS JANS JENS KANS KENS KINS LANS LENS LPNS MANS MENS MINS MONS MTNS NONS NUNS OWNS PANS PENS PINS PONS PUNS RANS RUNS SANS SENS SINS SONS SSNS STNS SUNS SYNS TANS TENS TINS TONS TUNS URNS VANS VINS WENS WINS YENS ZINS

NT••
NTSB NTWT

N•T•
NATE NATL NATO NATR NATS NETH NETS NITA NITE NITS NOTA NOTE NOTH NOT1 NOTS NOTV NUTS

N••T
NAST NAUT NEAT NEET NEST NEUT NEWT NEXT NHAT NLAT NOCT NTWT NUIT NYCT NYET

•NT•
ANTA ANTE ANTH ANTI ANTS ANTZ ENTO ENTR ENTS INTL INTO INTR INTS KNTS ONTO ONTV TNTS UNTO

•N•T
ANAT CNUT DNET GNAT INIT INST KNIT KNOT KNUT SNIT TNUT UNIT

••NT
AINT AMNT AUNT BENT BONT BUNT CANT CENT CONT DENT DINT DONT FONT FUNT GANT GENT GYNT HINT HUNT ISNT KANT KENT LENT LINT LUNT MENT MINT MONT PANT PENT PINT PONT PUNT RANT RENT RUNT SANT SENT TENT TINT VENT WANT WENT WONT ZANT

NU••
NUBS NUDE NUFF NUIT NUKE NULL NUMB NUNC NUNN NUNS NUTS NUYS

N•U•
NAUT NEUE NEUF NEUN NEUR NEUT NIUE NOUN NOUS

NYUK

N••U
NAMU
NANU
NONU

•NU•
CNUT
ENUF
GNUS
KNUR
KNUT
ONUS
SNUB
SNUG
TNUT
UNUM

•N•U
UNAU

••NU
AINU
GENU
MENU
NANU
NONU

N•V•
NAVE
NAVY
NEVA
NEVE
NEVI
NKVD
NOVA
NOVE
NOVO

N••V
NOTV

•NV•
ENVS
ENVY
INVS

•N•V
ONTV
UNIV
UNLV

••NV
CONV

N•W•
NEWF
NEWS
NEWT
NTWT

N••W
NORW

•N•W
ANEW
ENOW
GNAW
KNEW
KNOW
SNOW

N•X•
NEXO
NEXT
NIXY
NSXS

N••X
NMEX

•NX•
INXS

•N•X
KNOX
ONYX
SNAX
UNIX

••NX
GENX
JINX
LYNX
MANX
MINX

NY••
NYAD
NYBY
NYCT
NYET
NYNY
NYPD
NYRO
NYSE
NYUK

N•Y•
NAYA
NAYS
NUYS

N••Y
NAGY
NARY
NAVY
NIXY
NOMY
NOSY
NYBY
NYNY

•NY•
ANYA
ENYA
ENYO
INYO
ONYM
ONYX

•N•Y
ANCY
ANDY
ANNY
ENCY
ENRY
ENVY
INDY
INKY
INLY
INNY
ONEY
ONLY

••NY
ANNY
AWNY
BONY
CANY
CCNY
CONY
CUNY
DENY
DKNY
EENY
FDNY
GONY
GYNY
INNY
LINY
MANY
MONY
NYNY
PINY
PONY
PUNY
SONY
SUNY
TINY
TONY
VINY
WANY
WINY
ZANY

N•Z•
NAZI

N••Z
NARZ

•NZ•
ENZO
ONZE

•N•Z
ANTZ
INEZ
YNEZ

••NZ
BENZ
BONZ
FONZ
LENZ
LINZ

OA••
OAFS
OAHU
OAKS
OAKY
OARS
OAST
OATH
OATS
OATY

O•A•
OBAD
OBAN
OCAS
ODAS
ODAY
OGAM
OJAI
OKAY
OLAF
OLAH
OLAN
OLAS
OLAV
OLAY
OMAN
OMAR
OMAT
ONAN
OPAH
OPAL
ORAD
ORAE
ORAL
ORAN
ORAS
OSAR
OSAS
OTAY
OVAL

O••A
OBRA
OCTA
ODEA
ODRA
OITA
OKLA
OKRA
OLEA
OLGA
OLLA
ONDA
ONEA
ONNA
OOLA
OONA
OPIA
ORCA
ORRA
OSHA
OSSA
OTEA
OTRA
OZMA

•OA•
BOAC
BOAR
BOAS
BOAT
BOAZ
COAL
COAT
COAX
DOAK
EOAN
FOAL
FOAM
GOAD
GOAL
GOAS
GOAT
HOAD
HOAG
HOAR
HOAX
JOAD
JOAN
KOAN
KOAS
LOAD
LOAF
LOAM
LOAN
MOAB
MOAN
MOAS
MOAT
NOAA
NOAH
NOAM
ROAD
ROAM
ROAN
ROAR
SOAK
SOAP
SOAR
SOAS
TOAD
TOAT
WOAD

•O•A
BOCA
BOLA
BONA
BORA
BOVA
BOWA
COCA
CODA
COLA
COMA
COPA
CORA
COSA
COXA
DOHA
DONA
DOPA
DORA
EOLA
FORA
GOLA
GOYA
HOLA
HORA
HOYA
IOLA
IONA
IOTA
IOWA
JOTA
KOLA
KONA
LOCA
LOLA
LOMA
MOMA
MONA
MORA
MOTA
NOAA
NOIA
NOLA
NORA
NOTA
NOVA
OOLA
OONA
PODA
POLA
ROCA
ROJA
ROMA
RONA
ROPA
ROSA
ROTA
ROWA
SOBA
SOCA
SODA
SOFA
SOLA
SOMA
SORA
SOSA
SOYA
TOEA
TOGA
TOMA
TORA
TOYA
VORA
YODA
YOGA
ZOLA
ZONA
ZORA

••OA
ANOA
AROA
PROA
STOA
TWOA
WHOA

OB••
OBAD
OBAN
OBER
OBES
OBEY
OBIE
OBIS
OBIT
OBJS
OBOE
OBOL
OBRA

O•B•
ORBS
OTBS

O••B
ONEB

•OB•
BOBO
BOBS
COBB
COBH
COBO
COBS
DOBY
FOBS
GOBI
GOBO
GOBS
GOBY
HOBE
HOBO
HOBS
JOBS
KOBE
KOBO
KOBS
LOBE
LOBO
LOBS
MOBS
MOBY
NOBS
ROBB
ROBE
ROBS
ROBT
SOBA
SOBS
TOBE
TOBY
YOBS

•O•B
AORB
BOMB
BOOB
COBB
COMB
LOEB
LOMB
MOAB
ROBB
ROWB
SORB
TOMB
WOMB

••OB
BLOB
BOOB
BTOB
BYOB
GLOB
KNOB
MYOB
PROB
SLOB
SNOB
TWOB

OC••
OCAS
OCHO
OCHS
OCTA
OCTO
OCTS
OCUL

O•C•
ONCD
ONCE
ORCA
ORCH
ORCS
OUCH

O••C
ODIC
OLIC
ONEC
ONIC
OPEC
OTIC

•OC•
BOCA
BOCK
COCA
COCK
COCO
DOCE
DOCK
DOCS
DOCU
FOCH
FOCI
HOCH
HOCK
JOCK
KOCH
LOCA
LOCH
LOCI
LOCK
LOCO
MOCK
MOCS
NOCK
NOCT
POCO
POCS
ROCA
ROCK
ROCS
SOCA
SOCK
SOCS
TOCK
VOCE

•O•C
BOAC
BOSC
COFC
CONC
DONC
KOFC
PORC
ROTC
ROWC
ZOIC

••OC
APOC
BLOC
BMOC
CHOC
CROC
EEOC
IROC
KROC
PROC
TWOC
USOC

OD••
ODAS
ODAY
ODDS
ODEA
ODED
ODER
ODES
ODIC
ODIE
ODIN
ODOM
ODON
ODOR
ODRA

O•D•
ODDS
OLDE
OLDS
ONDA
ONDE
ORDO
OUDS

O••D
OBAD
ODED
OGOD
OHED
OKED
OLID
ONCD
ONED
OOID
OPED
ORAD
OVID
OWED

•OD•
BODE
BODS
BODY
CODA
CODE
CODS
CODY
DODD
DODO
DODY
GODS
HODS
IODO
JODY
LODE
LODI
LODZ
MODE
MODI
MODS
NODE
NODI
NODS
PODA
PODO
PODS
RODD
RODE
RODS
SODA
SODS
TODD
TODI
TODO
TODS
YODA
YODH
YODS

•O•D
BOLD
BOND
BOYD
COED
COLD
COND
CORD
DODD
DOOD
DOUD
DOWD
FOLD
FOND
FOOD
FORD
GOAD
GOLD
GOOD
HOAD
HOED
HOLD
HOND
HOOD
JOAD
JOED
LOAD
LOID
LORD
LOUD
LOYD
MOLD
MOOD
NOID
NORD
OOID
POND
ROAD
RODD
ROOD
ROWD
SOLD
TOAD
TODD
TOED
TOLD
VOID
WOAD
WOOD
WORD
YOND
YOUD

••OD
APOD
AROD
CLOD
DOOD
EXOD
FOOD
GOOD
HOOD
IPOD
IZOD
MOOD
OGOD
PLOD
PROD
QUOD
RHOD
ROOD
SHOD
TKOD
TROD
TWOD
WHOD
WOOD

OE••
OEIL
OENO
OEUF

O•E•
OBER
OBES
OBEY
ODEA
ODED
ODER
ODES
OGEE
OHED
OIES
OKED
OKEY
OLEA
OLEG
OLEN
OLEO
OLES
OMEI
OMEN
OMER
OMES
ONEA
ONEB
ONEC
ONED
ONEE
ONEF
ONEG
ONEH
ONEK
ONEL
ONER
ONES
ONEY
OPEC
OPED
OPEL
OPEN
OPER
OPES
OREE
OREG
OREL
OREM
OREN
OREO
ORES
OSEE
OTEA
OVEN
OVER
OWED
OWEN
OWER
OWES
OXEN
OXES
OYER
OYEZ

O••E
OBIE
OBOE
ODIE
OGEE
OGLE
OGRE
OHME
OHNE
OHRE
OISE
OKIE
OLDE
OLPE
ONCE
ONDE
ONEE
ONZE
OOZE
OPIE
ORAE
OREE
ORFE
ORLE
ORNE
ORSE
OSEE
OSTE
OTOE
OUSE
OWIE

•OE•
BOER
COED
COEN
DOER
DOES
FOES
GOEN
GOER
GOES
HOED
HOER
HOES
JOED
JOEE
JOEL
JOES
JOEY
LOEB
LOEW
MOEN
MOES
MOET
NOEL
NOES
POEM
POET
ROEG
ROES
TOEA
TOED
TOES
WOES

•O•E
AONE
BODE
BOLE
BONE
BORE
BOSE
BOWE
CODE
COKE
COLE
COME
CONE
COPE
CORE
COTE
COUE
COVE
DOCE
DOGE
DOKE
DOLE
DOME
DONE
DOPE
DORE
DOSE
DOTE
DOVE
DOZE
FOIE
FORE
GONE
GORE
HOBE
HOKE
HOLE
HOME
HONE
HOPE
HOSE
HOTE
HOVE
HOWE
IOLE
IONE
JOEE
JOIE
JOKE
JOSE
JOVE
KOBE
LOBE
LODE
LOGE
LOME
LONE
LOPE
LORE
LOSE
LOVE
LOWE
MODE
MOLE
MOME
MOPE
MORE
MOSE
MOTE
MOUE
MOVE
NODE
NOLE
NOME
NONE
NOPE
NOSE
NOTE
NOVE
OOZE
POKE
POLE
POME
PONE
POPE
PORE
POSE
ROBE
RODE
ROHE
ROLE
ROME
ROPE
ROSE
ROTE
ROUE
ROVE
ROWE
SOIE
SOLE
SOME
SONE
SORE
TOBE
TOKE
TOLE
TOME
TONE
TOPE
TORE
TOTE
TOVE
VOCE
VOLE
VORE
VOTE
WOKE
WOLE
WORE
WOVE
YOKE
YORE
ZONE

••OE
ALOE
BPOE
EVOE
FLOE
FROE
KDOE
OBOE
OTOE
SHOE
SLOE
TWOE

OF••
OFFS

O•F•
OAFS
OFFS
OOFS
ORFE
ORFF

O••F
OEUF
OLAF
OLOF
ONEF
ORFF

•OF•
BOFF
COFC
COFS
DOFF
HOFF
KOFC
KOFI
KOFP
LOFT
OOFS
SOFA
SOFT
TOFF
TOFT
TOFU
UOFM

•O•F
BOFF
COIF
CONF
DOFF
GOLF
GOOF
HOFF
HOOF
IOOF
KOPF
LOAF
POOF
POUF
ROLF
ROOF
ROWF
TOFF
WOLF
WOOF
WORF

••OF
ASOF
GOOF
HOOF
IOOF
OLOF
POOF
PROF
ROOF
WOOF

OG••
OGAM
OGEE
OGGI
OGLE
OGOD
OGPU
OGRE
OGRO

O•G•
OGGI
OLGA
ORGS
ORGY

O••G
OLEG
OLIG
ONEG
OREG
ORIG

•OG•
BOGS
BOGY
COGS
DOGE
DOGS
FOGG
FOGS
FOGY
GOGH
GOGI
GOGO
HOGG
HOGS
JOGS
LOGE
LOGO
LOGS
LOGY
NOGO
NOGS
POGO
POGS
TOGA
TOGO
TOGS
YOGA
YOGI
ZOGI

•O•G
BONG
BOOG
BORG
CONG
DONG
DOUG
FOGG
FONG
GONG
HOAG
HOGG
HONG
JONG
KONG
LONG
MOOG
PONG
ROEG
ROWG
ROYG
SONG
TONG
WONG
YONG

••OG
AGOG
BIOG
BLOG
BOOG
CLOG
FLOG
FROG
GEOG
GROG
LEOG
MOOG
PROG
SLOG
SMOG

OH••
OHED
OHHI
OHIO
OHME
OHMS
OHMY
OHNE
OHNO
OHOH
OHOK
OHOS
OHRE
OHSO

O•H•
OAHU
OCHO
OCHS
OHHI
OOHS
OSHA
OTHO

O••H
OATH
OHOH
OLAH
ONEH
OOOH
OPAH
ORCH
ORTH
OUCH

•OH•
BOHM
BOHO
BOHR
COHN
COHO
DOHA
DOHS
FOHN
HOHO
JOHN
KOHL
MOHS
NOHO
OOHS
POHL
ROHE
SOHO
YOHO

•O•H
BOSH
BOTH
COBH
COSH
DOTH
FOCH
GOGH
GOSH
GOTH
HOCH
HOTH
JOSH
KOCH
KOPH
LOCH
MOSH
MOTH
NOAH
NOSH
NOTH
OOOH
POOH
POSH
QOPH
ROSH
ROTH
ROWH
SOPH
TOSH
YODH

••OH
FROH
GROH
IEOH
IPOH
NAOH
OHOH
OOOH
POOH
UHOH
YEOH

OI••
OIES
OILS
OILY
OINK
OISE
OITA

O•I•
OBIE
OBIS
OBIT
ODIC
ODIE
ODIN
OEIL
OHIO
OKIE
OLIC
OLID
OLIG
OLIN
OLIO
OMIT
ONIC
OOID
OPIA
OPIE
OPIS
ORIG
ORIN

4 OI

OSIP OSIS OTIC OTIS OUIS OVID OVIS OWIE

O••I
OGGI OHHI OJAI OMEI OMNI OMRI OSSI

•OI•
BOIL BOIS COIF COIL COIN COIR COIT DOIN DOIS DOIT FOIE FOIL GOIN JOIE JOIN KOIS LOID LOIN LOIS MOIL MOIS NOIA NOID NOIL NOIR OOID POIS ROIL ROIS SOIE SOIL SOIR TOIL VOID VOIP VOIR VOIT VOIX ZOIC

•O•I
AOKI COLI CORI COSI FOCI GOBI GOGI HONI HOPI JOLI JONI JOVI KOFI KOJI LOCI LODI LOKI LONI LORI LOTI MODI MOMI NODI NOLI NORI NOTI POLI POPI RONI ROTI ROWI SOLI TODI TONI TOPI TORI YOGI ZOGI ZORI

••OI
AMOI ATOI ELOI LEOI QUOI TROI

OJ••
OJAI OJOS

O•J•
OBJS

•OJ•
DOJO HOJO JOJO KOJI MOJO ROJA ROJO TOJO WOJO

•O•J
CONJ ROWJ

OK••
OKAY OKED OKEY OKIE OKLA OKOK OKRA

O•K•
OAKS OAKY ONKP OOKY

O••K
OHOK OINK OKOK OMSK ONEK ORSK

•OK•
AOKI AOKS COKE COKY DOKE HOKE JOKE JOKY KOKO LOKI MOKO OOKY POKE POKY ROKS TOKE WOKE WOKS YOKE YOKO

•O•K
BOCK BONK BOOK BORK COCK CONK COOK CORK DOAK DOCK DOOK DORK FOLK FORK GOOK HOCK HONK HOOK HOUK JOCK KOOK LOCK LOOK MOCK MONK MORK NOCK NOOK POLK PORK ROCK ROOK ROWK SOAK SOCK TOCK TONK TOOK TORK VOLK WONK WORK WOUK YOLK YORK ZONK ZOUK

••OK
AMOK ASOK BLOK BOOK COOK DOOK EWOK GOOK GROK HOOK IMOK KOOK LOOK NOOK OHOK OKOK ROOK TOOK

OL••
OLAF OLAH OLAN OLAS OLAV OLAY OLDE OLDS OLEA OLEG OLEN OLEO OLES OLGA OLIC OLID OLIG OLIN OLIO OLLA OLOF OLOR OLPE

O•L•
OGLE OILS OILY OKLA OLLA ONLY OOLA ORLE ORLO ORLY OSLO OULU OWLS OWLY

O••L
OBOL OCUL OEIL ONEL OPAL OPEL ORAL OREL OVAL

•OL•
BOLA BOLD BOLE BOLL BOLO BOLT COLA COLD COLE COLI COLL COLM COLO COLS COLT DOLE DOLL DOLT EOLA FOLD FOLK GOLA GOLD GOLF HOLA HOLD HOLE HOLM HOLO HOLS HOLT HOLY IOLA IOLE JOLI JOLT KOLA KOLN LOLA LOLL MOLD MOLE MOLL MOLS MOLT MOLY NOLA NOLE NOLI NOLL NOLO OOLA POLA POLE POLI POLK POLL POLO POLS POLY ROLE ROLF ROLL ROLO ROLY SOLA SOLD SOLE SOLI SOLO SOLS TOLD TOLE TOLL VOLE VOLK VOLS VOLT WOLE WOLF YOLK ZOLA

•O•L
BOIL BOLL BOWL COAL COIL COLL COOL COWL DOLL FOAL FOIL FOOL FOUL FOWL GOAL HOWL JOEL JOWL KOHL KOOL LOLL MOIL MOLL NOEL NOIL NOLL POHL POLL POOL ROIL ROLL ROTL ROWL SOIL SOUL TOIL TOLL TOOL WOOL YOWL ZOOL

••OL
AWOL BIOL CHOL COOL ECOL ENOL FOOL GAOL GEOL IDOL ITOL KOOL OBOL POOL STOL TOOL VIOL VTOL WOOL ZOOL

OM••
OMAN OMAR OMAT OMEI OMEN OMER OMES OMIT OMNI OMOO OMRI OMSK

O•M•
OHME OHMS OHMY OZMA

O••M
ODOM OGAM ONYM OREM OVUM

•OM•
BOMB COMA COMB COME COMM COMO COMP COMS DOME DOMO DOMS HOME HOMO JOMO LOMA LOMB LOME MOMA MOME MOMI MOMS NOME NOMO NOMS NOMY POME POMO POMP POMS ROMA ROME ROMP ROMS ROMY SOMA SOME TOMA TOMB TOME TOMS TOMT UOMO WOMB

•O•M
BOHM BOOM COLM COMM CORM COSM DOOM DORM FOAM FORM GORM HOLM HOWM LOAM LOOM NOAM NORM POEM ROAM ROOM ROWM UOFM VOOM WORM ZOOM

••OM
ATOM BOOM BROM DOOM EDOM FROM GEOM GLOM LOOM ODOM PNOM PROM ROOM THOM VOOM WHOM ZOOM

ON••
ONAN ONCD ONCE ONDA ONDE ONEA ONEB ONEC ONED ONEE ONEF ONEG ONEH ONEK ONEL ONER ONES ONEY ONIC ONKP ONLY ONNA ONTO ONTV ONUS ONYM ONYX ONZE

O•N•
OENO OHNE OHNO OINK OMNI ONNA OONA ORNE OWNS

O••N
OBAN ODIN ODON OLAN OLEN OLIN OMAN OMEN ONAN OPEN ORAN OREN ORIN OVEN OWEN OXEN OXON

•ON•
AONE BONA BOND BONE BONG BONK BONN BONO BONT BONY BONZ CONC COND CONE CONF CONG CONJ CONK CONN CONS CONT CONV CONY DONA DONC DONE DONG DONN DONS DONT EONS FOND FONG FONT FONZ GONE GONG GONY HOND HONE HONG HONI HONK HONS IONA IONE IONO IONS JONG JONI KONA KONG LONE LONG LONI MONA MONK MONO MONS MONT MONY NONE NONO NONS NONU OONA POND PONE PONG PONS PONT PONY RONA RONI SONE SONG SONS SONY TONE TONG TONI TONK TONO TONS TONY WONG WONK WONT YOND YONG ZONA ZONE ZONK

•O•N
BONN BOON BORN BOSN COEN COHN COIN CONN COON CORN DOIN DONN DOON DORN DOWN EOAN FOHN GOEN GOIN GOON GOWN HORN JOAN JOHN JOIN JOON KOAN KOLN KORN LOAN LOIN LOON LORN MOAN MOEN MOON MORN MOWN NOON NORN NOUN PORN ROAN ROWN SOON SOWN TOON TORN TOWN WORN YORN ZORN

••ON
AEON AGON AMON ANON ARON ATON AVON AXON BOON BRON BUON CHON CION CMON COON DCON DION DOON EBON ECON EGON ELON ENON ETON EXON FLON GOON ICON IKON INON IRON IWON JEON JOON KAON KWON LEON LION LOON LRON LYON MOON MUON NEON NOON ODON OXON PAON PEON PHON PION PRON SION SOON THON TION TOON TRON UPON XEON ZION

OO••
OOFS OOHS OOID OOKY OOLA OONA OOOH OOOO OOPS OORT OOZE OOZY

O•O•
OBOE OBOL ODOM ODON ODOR OGOD OHOH OHOK OHOS OJOS OKOK OLOF OLOR OMOO OOOH OOOO OROS OSOS OTOE OTOS OXON

O••O
OCHO OCTO OENO OGRO OHIO OHNO OHSO OLEO OLIO OMOO ONTO OOOO OPTO ORDO OREO ORLO ORZO OSLO OSSO OTHO OTRO OTTO OUZO

•OO•
BOOB BOOG BOOK BOOM BOON BOOP BOOR BOOS BOOT COOK COOL COON COOP COOS COOT DOOD DOOK DOOM DOON DOOR DOOS FOOD FOOL FOOT GOOD GOOF GOOK GOON GOOP GOOS HOOD HOOF HOOK HOOP HOOT IOOF JOON KOOK KOOL KOOP LOOK LOOM LOON LOOP LOOS LOOT MOOD MOOG MOON MOOR MOOS MOOT NOOK NOON NOOR OOOH OOOO POOF POOH POOL POOP POOR ROOD ROOF ROOK ROOM ROOS ROOT SOON SOOT TOOK TOOL TOON TOOT VOOM WOOD WOOF WOOL WOOS ZOOL ZOOM ZOOS ZOOT

•O•O
BOBO BOHO BOLO BONO BORO BOYO BOZO COBO COCO COHO COLO COMO DODO DOJO DOMO DORO DOSO DOTO DOZO FOTO GOBO GOGO GORO GOTO HOBO HOHO HOJO HOLO HOMO IODO IONO JOJO JOMO KOBO KOKO KOTO LOBO LOCO LOGO MOJO MOKO MONO MORO MOTO MOZO NOGO NOHO NOLO NOMO NONO NOVO OOOO POCO PODO POGO POLO POMO ROJO ROLO ROTO ROWO SOHO SOLO SOSO SOTO TODO TOGO TOJO TONO TOPO TORO TOTO TOXO TOYO UOMO UOVO WOJO YOHO YOKO YOYO

••OO
AROO CHOO EROO ITOO OMOO OOOO SHOO

OP••
OPAH OPAL OPEC OPED OPEL OPEN OPER OPES OPIA OPIE OPIS OPPS OPQR OPRY OPTO OPTS OPUS

O•P•
OGPU OLPE OOPS OPPS

O••P
ONKP OSIP

•OP•
BOPP BOPS COPA COPE COPS COPT COPY DOPA DOPE DOPY FOPS HOPE HOPI HOPS KOPF KOPH KOPS LOPE LOPS MOPE MOPS MOPY NOPE NOPQ OOPS POPE POPI POPP POPS QOPH ROPA ROPE ROPY SOPH SOPS TOPE TOPI TOPO TOPS

•O•P
BOOP BOPP COMP COOP CORP COUP DORP DOUP GOOP GORP GOUP HOOP HOSP KOFP KOOP LOOP LOUP POMP POOP POPP ROMP ROWP SOAP SOUP VOIP

••OP
ALOP APOP ATOP BOOP CHOP CLOP COOP CROP DROP ESOP FLOP GLOP GOOP HOOP IHOP KOOP LOOP MNOP PLOP POOP PROP SHOP SLOP STOP TROP TTOP VSOP WHOP

O•Q•
OPQR

•OQ•
COQS

•O•Q
NOPQ ROWQ

OR••
ORAD ORAE ORAL ORAN ORAS ORBS ORCA ORCH ORCS ORDO OREE OREG OREL OREM OREN OREO ORES ORFE ORFF ORGS ORGY ORIG ORIN ORLE ORLO ORLY ORNE OROS ORRA ORSE ORSK ORTH ORTS ORVS ORYX ORZO

O•R•
OARS OBRA ODRA OGRE OGRO OHRE OKRA OMRI OORT OPRY ORRA OTRA OTRO OURS

O••R
OBER ODER ODOR OLOR OMAR OMER ONER OPER OPQR OSAR OVER OWER OYER

•OR•
AORB AORT BORA BORE BORG BORK BORN BORO BORS BORU CORA CORD

CORE CORI CORK CORM CORN CORP CORR CORS CORT CORY DORA DORE DORK DORM DORN DORO DORP DORS DORY FORA FORD FORE FORK FORM FORS FORT GORE GORM GORO GORP GORT GORY HORA HORN HORS HORT JORY KORN KORS LORD LORE LORI LORN LORY MORA MORE MORK MORN MORO MORT NORA NORD NORI NORM NORN NORW OORT PORC PORE PORK PORN PORT RORY SORA SORB SORE SORT TORA TORE TORI TORK TORN TORO TORR TORS TORT TORY VORA VORE WORD WORE WORF WORK WORM WORN WORT XORY YORE YORK YORN ZORA ZORI ZORN

•O•R

BOAR BOER BOHR BOOR COIR CORR DOER DOOR DOUR FOUR GOER HOAR HOER HOUR JOUR LOUR MOOR NOIR NOOR POOR POUR ROAR ROWR SOAR SOIR SOUR TORR TOUR VOIR YOUR

••OR

AMOR ASOR ATOR BOOR BROR DIOR DOOR FLOR IGOR IVOR MOOR NGOR NOOR ODOR OLOR POOR SHOR THOR UXOR YBOR YGOR

OS••

OSAR OSAS OSEE OSHA OSIP OSIS OSLO OSOS OSSA OSSI OSSO OSTE

O•S•

OAST OHSO OISE OMSK ORSE ORSK OSSA OSSI OSSO OUSE OUST

O••S

OAFS OAKS OARS OATS OBES OBIS OBJS OCAS OCHS OCTS ODAS ODDS ODES OFFS OHMS OHOS OIES OILS OJOS OLAS OLDS OLES OMES ONES ONUS OOFS OOHS OOPS OPES OPIS OPPS OPTS OPUS ORAS ORBS ORCS ORES ORGS OROS ORTS ORVS OSAS OSIS OSOS OTBS OTIS OTOS OUDS OUIS OURS OUTS OVIS OWES OWLS OWNS OXES OXUS

•OS•

BOSC BOSE BOSH BOSN BOSS COSA COSH COSI COSM COST COSY DOSE DOSO DOSS DOST FOSS GOSH GOSS HOSE HOSP HOSS HOST JOSE JOSH JOSS KOSS LOSE LOSS LOST MOSE MOSH MOSS MOST NOSE NOSH NOSY POSE POSH POST POSY ROSA ROSE ROSH ROSS ROSY SOSA SOSO TOSH TOSS VOSS YOST

•O•S

AOKS BOAS BOBS BODS BOGS BOIS BOOS BOPS BORS BOSS BOTS BOWS BOYS COBS CODS COFS COGS COLS COMS CONS COOS COPS COQS CORS COTS COWS DOCS DOES DOGS DOHS DOIS DOMS DONS DOOS DORS DOSS DOTS EONS EOUS FOBS FOES FOGS FOPS FORS FOSS FOYS GOAS GOBS GODS GOES GOOS GOSS GOVS HOBS HODS HOES HOGS HOLS HONS HOPS HORS HOSS HOWS IONS IOUS JOBS JOES JOGS JOSS JOTS JOYS KOAS KOBS KOIS KOPS KORS KOSS LOBS LOGS LOIS LOOS LOPS LOSS LOTS LOWS MOAS MOBS MOCS MODS MOES MOHS MOIS MOLS MOMS MONS MOOS MOPS MOSS MOTS MOWS NOBS NODS NOES NOGS NOMS NONS NOTS NOUS OOFS OOHS OOPS POCS PODS POGS POIS POLS POMS PONS POPS POTS POVS POWS ROBS ROCS RODS ROES ROIS ROKS ROMS ROOS ROSS ROTS ROUS ROWS SOAS SOBS SOCS SODS SOLS SONS SOPS SOTS SOUS SOVS SOWS SOYS TODS TOES TOGS TOMS TONS TOPS TORS TOSS TOTS TOWS TOYS UOUS VOLS VOSS VOUS VOWS WOES WOKS WOOS WOWS YOBS YODS ZOOS

••OS

ADOS AJOS AMOS APOS AVOS BIOS BOOS BROS CEOS CFOS COOS CPOS CWOS DIOS DLOS DOOS DSOS DUOS EGOS ENOS EPOS EROS ESOS FROS FTOS GEOS GOOS GPOS GROS GTOS HAOS HMOS IBOS ICOS IDOS IPOS KAOS KEOS LAOS LBOS LOOS MHOS MOOS NAOS NCOS NEOS OHOS OJOS OROS OSOS OTOS PROS REOS RHOS RIOS RKOS ROOS SROS TAOS THOS TIOS TKOS TSOS TWOS UDOS UFOS UNOS USOS WHOS WOOS ZOOS

OT••

OTAY OTBS OTEA OTHO OTIC OTIS OTOE OTOS OTRA OTRO OTTO

O•T•

OATH OATS OATY OCTA OCTO OCTS OITA ONTO ONTV OPTO OPTS ORTH ORTS OSTE OTTO OUTS

O••T

OAST OBIT OMAT OMIT OORT OUST

•OT•

BOTH BOTS COTE COTS COTY DOTE DOTH DOTO DOTS FOTO GOTH GOTO GOTT HOTE HOTH IOTA JOTA JOTS KOTO LOTI LOTS LOTT MOTA MOTE MOTH MOTO MOTS MOTT NOTA NOTE NOTH NOTI NOTS NOTV POTS ROTA ROTC ROTE ROTH ROTI ROTL ROTO ROTS SOTO SOTS TOTE TOTO TOTS VOTE ZOTZ

•O•T

AORT AOUT BOAT BOLT BONT BOOT BOUT COAT COIT COLT CONT COOT COPT CORT COST DOIT DOLT DONT DOST FONT FOOT FORT FOYT GOAT GORT GOTT GOUT GOVT HOLT HOOT HORT HOST HOYT JOLT LOFT LOOT LOST LOTT LOUT MOAT MOET MOLT MONT MOOT MORT MOST MOTT NOCT OORT POET PONT PORT POST POUT ROBT ROOT ROUT ROWT SOFT SOOT SORT TOAT TOFT TOMT TOOT TORT TOUT VOIT VOLT WONT WORT XOUT YOST ZOOT

••OT

ALOT BIOT BLOT BOOT BROT CLOT COOT FOOT GLOT GROT HOOT KNOT LOOT MOOT PHOT PLOT PROT QUOT RIOT ROOT SCOT SHOT SLOT SOOT SPOT TOOT TROT ZOOT

OU••

OUCH OUDS OUIS OULU OURS OUSE OUST OUTS OUZO

O•U•

OCUL OEUF ONUS OPUS OVUM OXUS

O••U

OAHU OGPU OULU

•OU•

AOUT BOUT COUE COUP DOUD DOUG DOUP DOUR DOUW DOUX EOUS FOUL FOUR GOUP GOUT HOUK HOUR IOUS JOUR LOUD LOUP LOUR LOUT MOUE NOUN NOUS POUF POUR POUT ROUE ROUS ROUT ROUX SOUL SOUP SOUR SOUS TOUR TOUT UOUS VOUS WOUK XOUT YOUD YOUR ZOUK

•O•U

BORU DOCU NONU ROWU TOFU

••OU

ABOU ALOU CHOU THOU ZHOU

OV••

OVAL OVEN OVER OVID OVIS OVUM

O•V•

ORVS

O••V

OLAV ONTV

•OV•

BOVA COVE DOVE GOVS GOVT HOVE JOVE JOVI LOVE MOVE NOVA NOVE NOVO POVS ROVE SOVS TOVE UOVO WOVE

•O•V

CONV NOTV ROWV

••OV

AZOV LEOV LVOV PROV

OW••

OWED OWEN OWER OWES OWIE OWLS OWLY OWNS

•OW•

BOWA BOWE BOWL BOWS COWL COWS COWY DOWD DOWN FOWL GOWN HOWE HOWL HOWM HOWS IOWA JOWL LOWE LOWS MOWN MOWS POWS ROWA ROWB ROWC ROWD ROWE ROWF ROWG ROWH ROWI ROWJ ROWK ROWL ROWM ROWN ROWO ROWP ROWQ ROWR ROWS ROWT ROWU ROWV ROWW ROWX ROWY ROWZ SOWN SOWS TOWN TOWS VOWS WOWS YOWL

•O•W

DOUW LOEW NORW ROWW

••OW

ALOW AROW AVOW BLOW BROW CHOW CROW DHOW ENOW FLOW FROW GLOW GROW KNOW MEOW PLOW PROW SCOW SHOW SLOW SNOW STOW TROW YEOW

OX••

OXEN OXES OXON OXUS

O••X

ONYX ORYX

•OX•

BOXY COXA DOXY FOXX FOXY LOXY ROXY TOXO

•O•X

COAX DOUX FOXX HOAX ROUX ROWX VOIX

••OX

KNOX LEOX XBOX

OY••

OYER OYEZ

O•Y•

ONYM ONYX ORYX

O••Y

OAKY OATY OBEY ODAY OHMY OILY OKAY OKEY OLAY ONEY ONLY OOKY OOZY OPRY ORGY ORLY OTAY OWLY OZZY

•OY•

BOYD BOYO BOYS BOYZ FOYS FOYT GOYA HOYA HOYT JOYS LOYD ROYG SOYA SOYS TOYA TOYO TOYS YOYO

•O•Y

BODY BOGY BONY BOXY CODY COKY CONY COPY CORY COSY COTY COWY COZY DOBY DODY DOPY DORY DOXY DOZY FOGY FOXY GOBY GONY GORY HOLY JODY JOEY JOKY JORY LOGY LORY LOXY MOBY MOLY MONY MOPY NOMY NOSY OOKY OOZY POKY POLY PONY POSY ROLY ROMY ROPY RORY ROSY ROWY ROXY SONY TOBY TONY TORY XORY

••OY

AHOY AMOY BBOY BUOY CHOY CLOY FLOY PLOY TROY

OZ••

OZMA OZZY

O•Z•

ONZE OOZE OOZY ORZO OUZO OZZY

O••Z

OYEZ

•OZ•

BOZO COZY DOZE DOZO DOZY MOZO OOZE OOZY

•O•Z

BOAZ BONZ BOYZ FONZ LODZ ROWZ ZOTZ

••OZ

ATOZ BROZ FLOZ

PA••

PAAR PABA PACA PACE PACK PACO PACS PACT PADS PAGE PAGO PAHS PAID PAIL PAIN PAIR PAIS PAIX PALE PALI PALL PALM PALO PALP PALS PANE PANG PANS PANT PAON PAPA PAPP PAPS PARA PARC PARD PARE PARI PARK PARL PARR PARS PART PASA PASE PASH PASO PASS PAST PATE PATH PATO PATR PATS PAUL PAVE PAVO PAWL PAWN PAWS PAYS PAYT

P•A•

PAAR PDAS PEAK PEAL PEAR PEAS PEAT PEAU PHAG PHAR PHAT PIAF PIAO PLAN PLAT PLAX PLAY PRAM PRAN PRAT PRAY PSAS PSAT PTAH PTAS PYAS

P••A

PABA PACA PAPA PARA PASA PEBA PENA PEPA PERA PETA PICA PIKA PIMA PINA PISA PITA PLEA PODA POLA PROA PUKA PULA PUMA PUPA PURA

•PA•

APAR CPAS GPAS KPAX MPAA OPAH OPAL SPAD SPAM SPAN SPAR SPAS SPAT SPAY

•P•A

APIA EPHA

EPPA
IPSA
LPGA
MPAA
OPIA
SPCA
UPSA

••PA
ARPA
CAPA
COPA
DOPA
EPPA
NAPA
NIPA
PAPA
PEPA
PUPA
RAPA
RIPA
ROPA
TAPA

P•B•
PABA
PCBS
PEBA
PIBB
PUBL
PUBS

P••B
PIBB
PLEB
PROB

•PB•
APBS

PC••
PCBS
PCPS
PCTS

P•C•
PACA
PACE
PACK
PACO
PACS
PACT
PECK
PECS
PFCS
PICA
PICE
PICK
PICO
PICS
PICT
POCO
POCS
PUCE
PUCK

P••C
PARC
PERC
PORC
PREC
PROC

•PC•
SPCA
UPCS

•P•C
APOC
EPIC
OPEC
SPEC
SPIC

••PC
UNPC

PD••
PDAS
PDFS
PDRS

P•D•
PADS
PEDE
PEDI
PEDO
PEDS
PHDS
PODA
PODO
PODS

P••D
PAID
PARD
PEND
PIED
PLED
PLOD
POND
PRED
PROD

•PD•
UPDO

•P•D
APED
APOD
IPOD
OPED
SPAD
SPED
SPUD

••PD
LAPD
NYPD
SFPD

PE••
PEAK
PEAL
PEAR
PEAS
PEAT
PEAU
PEBA
PECK
PECS
PEDE
PEDI
PEDO
PEDS
PEEK
PEEL
PEEN
PEEP
PEER
PEES
PEET
PEGS
PEKE
PELE
PELF
PELL
PELT
PENA
PEND
PENG
PENH
PENN
PENS
PENT
PEON
PEPA
PEPE
PEPO
PEPS
PERA
PERC
PERE
PERF
PERI
PERK
PERM
PERO
PERP
PERS
PERT
PERU
PESO
PEST
PETA
PETE
PETO
PETS
PEUR
PEUT
PEWS

P•E•
PEEK
PEEL
PEEN
PEEP
PEER
PEES
PEET
PHEN
PHEW
PIED
PIEL
PIER
PIES
PIET
PLEA
PLEB
PLED
PLEX
POEM
POET
PREC
PRED
PREF
PREK
PREM
PREP
PRES
PRET
PREV
PREX
PREY
PREZ
PTER
PUER

P••E
PACE
PAGE
PALE
PANE
PARE
PASE
PATE
PAVE
PEDE
PEKE
PELE
PEPE
PERE
PETE
PICE
PIKE
PILE
PINE
PIPE
PIRE
PLIE
POKE
POLE
POME
PONE
POPE
PORE
POSE
PRIE
PUCE
PULE
PURE
PYKE
PYLE
PYNE
PYRE

•PE•
APED
APER
APES
APEX
EPEE
JPEG
MPEG
OPEC
OPED
OPEL
OPEN
OPER
OPES
SPEC
SPED
SPEE
SPET
SPEW
SPEX

•P•E
APSE
BPOE
EPEE
IPSE
OPIE
SPEE
TPKE

••PE
ALPE
CAPE
CEPE
COPE
DOPE
DUPE
GAPE
HOPE
HYPE
JAPE
LOPE
LUPE
MOPE
NAPE
NOPE
OLPE
PEPE
PIPE
POPE
RIPE
ROPE
SIPE
SUPE
TAPE
TOPE
TYPE
WIPE
YIPE

PF••
PFCS
PFFT
PFUI

P•F•
PDFS
PFFT
PUFF

P••F
PELF
PERF
PIAF
POOF
POUF
PREF
PROF
PUFF

•PF•
SPFS

••PF
IMPF
KOPF

P•G•
PAGE
PAGO
PEGS
PIGS
PKGS
POGO
POGS
PUGH
PUGS

P••G
PANG
PENG
PHAG
PING
PLUG
PONG
PRIG
PROG
PUIG
PUNG

•PG•
JPGS
LPGA

•P•G
JPEG
MPEG

••PG
BKPG
TVPG

PH••
PHAG
PHAR
PHAT
PHDS
PHEN
PHEW
PHIL
PHIS
PHIZ
PHON
PHOT
PHYS
PHYT

P•H•
PAHS
POHL

P••H
PASH
PATH
PENH
PISH
PITH
POOH
POSH
PTAH
PUGH
PUSH

•PH•
EPHA

•P•H
IPOH
OPAH

••PH
ALPH
KAPH
KOPH
QOPH
RAPH
SOPH
UMPH
ZEPH

PI••
PIAF
PIAO
PIBB
PICA
PICE
PICK
PICO
PICS
PICT
PIED
PIEL
PIER
PIES
PIET
PIGS
PIKA
PIKE
PIKS
PILE
PILI
PILL
PILO
PIMA
PINA
PINE
PING
PINK
PINS
PINT
PINY
PION
PIPE
PIPP
PIPS
PIPY
PIRE
PIRN
PISA
PISH
PITA
PITH
PITS
PITT
PITY
PIUS
PIXY
PIZZ

P•I•
PAID
PAIL
PAIN
PAIR
PAIS
PAIX
PHIL
PHIS
PHIZ
PLIE
PNIN
POIS
PRIE
PRIG
PRIM
PRIN
PRIV
PRIX
PSIS
PUIG

P••I
PALI
PARI
PEDI
PERI
PFUI
PILI
POLI
POPI
PTUI
PULI
PUYI

•PI•
APIA
APIS
EPIC
EPIS
OPIA
OPIE
OPIS
SPIC
SPIN
SPIT

••PI
HOPI
KEPI
POPI
TIPI
TOPI

PK••
PKGS
PKWY

P•K•
PEKE
PIKA
PIKE
PIKS
PMKS
POKE
POKY
PUKA
PYKE

P••K
PACK
PARK
PEAK
PECK
PEEK
PERK
PICK
PINK
POLK
PORK
PREK
PUCK
PUNK

•PK•
TPKE
TPKS

••PK
TNPK

PL••
PLAN
PLAT
PLAX
PLAY
PLEA
PLEB
PLED
PLEX
PLIE
PLOD
PLOP
PLOT
PLOW
PLOY
PLUG
PLUM
PLUR
PLUS
PLUT

P•L•
PALE
PALI
PALL
PALM
PALO
PALP
PALS
PELE
PELF
PELL
PELT
PILE
PILI
PILL
PILO
POLA
POLE
POLI
POLK
POLL
POLO
POLS
POLY
PULA
PULE
PULI
PULL
PULP
PULS
PYLE

P••L
PAIL
PALL
PARL
PAUL
PAWL
PEAL
PEEL
PELL
PHIL
PIEL
PILL
POHL
POLL
POOL
PUBL
PULL
PURL

•PL•
CPLS

•P•L
APPL
OPAL
OPEL

••PL
APPL
DIPL
REPL

PM••
PMKS
PMTS

P•M•
PIMA
POME
POMO
POMP
POMS
PUMA
PUMP

P••M
PALM
PERM
PLUM
PNOM
POEM
PRAM
PREM
PRIM
PROM

•PM•
DPMS
RPMS

•P•M
SPAM

PN••
PNIN
PNOM

P•N•
PANE
PANG
PANS
PANT
PENA
PEND
PENG
PENH
PENN
PENS
PENT
PINA
PINE
PING
PINK
PINS
PINT
PINY
POND
PONE
PONG
PONS
PONT
PONY
PUNG
PUNK
PUNS
PUNT
PUNY
PYNE

P••N
PAIN
PAON
PAWN
PEEN
PENN
PEON
PHEN
PHON
PION
PIRN
PLAN
PNIN
PORN
PRAN
PRIN
PRON

•PN•
LPNS

•P•N
OPEN
SPAN
SPIN
SPUN
UPON

••PN
CAPN
ESPN
HYPN

PO••
POCO
POCS
PODA
PODO
PODS
POEM
POET
POGO
POGS
POHL
POIS
POKE
POKY
POLA
POLE
POLI
POLK
POLL
POLO
POLS
POLY
POME
POMO
POMP
POMS
POND
PONE
PONG
PONS
PONT
PONY
POOF
POOH
POOL
POOP
POOR
POPE
POPI
POPP
POPS
PORC
PORE
PORK
PORN
PORT
POSE
POSH
POST
POSY
POTS
POUF
POUR
POUT
POVS
POWS

P•O•
PAON
PEON
PHON
PHOT
PION
PLOD
PLOP
PLOT
PLOW
PLOY
PNOM
POOF
POOH
POOL
POOP
POOR
PROA
PROB
PROC
PROD
PROF
PROG
PROM
PRON
PROP
PROS
PROT
PROV
PROW

P••O
PACO
PAGO
PALO
PASO
PATO
PAVO
PEDO
PEPO
PERO
PESO
PETO
PIAO
PICO
PILO
POCO
PODO
POGO
POLO
POMO
PURO
PUZO
PYRO

•PO•
APOC
APOD
APOP
APOS
BPOE
CPOS
EPOS
GPOS
IPOD
IPOH
IPOS
SPOT
UPON

•P•O
APSO
IPSO
OPTO
UPDO
UPTO

••PO
ALPO
CAPO
ESPO
EXPO
HYPO
LIPO
PEPO
REPO
TOPO
TYPO

P•P•
PAPA
PAPP
PAPS
PCPS
PEPA
PEPE
PEPO
PEPS
PIPE
PIPP
PIPS
PIPY
POPE
POPI
POPP
POPS
PUPA
PUPP
PUPS
PUPU

P••P
PALP
PAPP
PEEP
PERP
PIPP
PLOP
POMP
POOP
POPP
PREP
PROP
PULP
PUMP
PUPP

•PP•
APPL
APPS
APPT
EPPA
EPPS
OPPS

•P•P
APOP

••PP
BOPP
CAPP
DEPP
GIPP
LAPP
LIPP
PAPP
PIPP
POPP
PUPP
REPP
SAPP

PQ••
PQRS

•PQ•
OPQR
SPQR

••PQ
NOPQ

PR••
PRAM
PRAN
PRAT
PRAY
PREC
PRED
PREF
PREK
PREM
PREP
PRES
PRET
PREV
PREX
PREY
PREZ
PRIE
PRIG
PRIM
PRIN
PRIV
PRIX
PROA
PROB
PROC
PROD
PROF
PROG
PROM
PRON
PROP
PROS
PROT
PROV
PROW

P•R•
PARA
PARC
PARD
PARE
PARI
PARK
PARL
PARR
PARS
PART
PDRS
PERA
PERC
PERE
PERF
PERI
PERK
PERM
PERO
PERP
PERS
PERT
PERU
PIRE
PIRN
PORC
PORE
PORK
PORN
PORT
PQRS
PURA
PURE
PURL
PURO
PURR
PYRE
PYRO

P••R
PAAR
PAIR
PARR
PATR
PEAR
PEER
PEUR
PHAR
PIER
PLUR
POOR
POUR
PTER
PUER
PURR

•PR•
APRS
OPRY
SPRY

•P•R
APAR
APER
OPER
OPQR
SPAR
SPQR
SPUR

••PR
BKPR
CUPR

PS••
PSAS
PSAT
PSIS
PSST

P•S•
PASA
PASE
PASH
PASO
PASS
PAST
PESO
PEST
PISA
PISH
POSE
POSH
POST
POSY
PSST
PUSH
PUSS

P••S
PACS
PADS
PAHS
PAIS
PALS
PANS
PAPS
PARS
PASS
PATS
PAWS
PAYS
PCBS
PCPS
PCTS
PDAS
PDFS
PDRS
PEAS
PECS
PEDS
PEES
PEGS
PENS
PEPS
PERS
PETS
PEWS
PFCS
PHDS
PHIS
PHYS
PICS
PIES
PIGS
PIKS
PINS
PIPS
PITS
PIUS
PKGS
PLUS
PMKS
PMTS
POCS
PODS
POGS
POIS
POLS
POMS
PONS
POPS
POTS
POVS
POWS
PQRS
PRES
PROS
PSAS
PSIS
PTAS
PUBS
PUGS
PULS
PUNS
PUPS
PUSS
PUTS
PVTS
PWTS
PYAS

•PS•
APSE
APSO
IPSA
IPSE
IPSO
UPSA
UPSY

•P•S
APBS
APES
APIS
APOS
APPS
APRS
APTS
APUS
CPAS
CPLS
CPOS
CPTS
CPUS
DPMS
DPTS
EPIS
EPOS
EPPS
GPAS
GPOS
IPOS
JPGS
LPNS
MPVS
OPES
OPIS
OPPS
OPTS
OPUS
RPMS
RPTS
SPAS
SPFS
SPYS
TPKS
UPCS

••PS
ALPS
AMPS
APPS
ARPS
ASPS
BAPS
BOPS
CAPS
CEPS
COPS
CUPS
DAPS
DEPS
DIPS
EMPS
EPPS
FOPS
GAPS
GNPS
GYPS
HAPS
HEPS
HIPS
HOPS
HUPS
IMPS
ISPS
KIPS
KOPS
LAPS
LIPS
LOPS
MAPS
MCPS
MIPS
MOPS
MVPS
NAPS
NIPS
OOPS
OPPS
PAPS
PCPS
PEPS
PIPS
POPS
PUPS
RAPS
REPS
RIPS
SAPS

SIPS SOPS SUPS TAPS TIPS TOPS TSPS TWPS UMPS USPS VIPS YAPS YEPS YIPS ZAPS ZIPS

PT••
PTAH PTAS PTER PTUI

P•T•
PATE PATH PATO PATR PATS PCTS PETA PETE PETO PETS PITA PITH PITS PITT PITY PMTS POTS PUTS PUTT PVTS PWTS

P••T
PACT PANT PART PAST PAYT PEAT PEET PELT PENT PERT PEST PEUT PFFT PHAT PHOT PHYT PICT PIET PINT PITT PLAT PLOT PLUT POET PONT PORT POST POUT PRAT PRET PROT PSAT PSST PUNT PUTT

•PT•
APTS CPTS DPTS OPTO OPTS RPTS UPTO

•P•T
APPT SPAT SPET SPIT SPOT

••PT
APPT BAPT CAPT COPT DEPT EXPT HEPT KEPT RAPT RCPT REPT SEPT SUPT WEPT

PU••
PUBL PUBS PUCE PUCK PUER PUFF PUGH PUGS PUIG PUKA PULA PULE PULI PULL PULP PULS PUMA PUMP PUNG PUNK PUNS PUNT PUNY PUPA PUPP PUPS PUPU PURA PURE PURL PURO PURR PUSH PUSS PUTS PUTT PUYI PUZO

P•U•
PAUL PEUR PEUT PFUI PIUS PLUG PLUM PLUR PLUS PLUT POUF POUR POUT PTUI

P••U
PEAU PERU PUPU

•PU•
APUS CPUS OPUS SPUD SPUN SPUR

••PU
OGPU PUPU

P•V•
PAVE PAVO POVS

P••V
PREV PRIV PROV

•PV•
MPVS

PW••
PWTS

P•W•
PAWL PAWN PAWS PEWS PKWY POWS

P••W
PHEW PLOW PROW

•P•W
SPEW

P•X•
PIXY

P••X
PAIX PLAX PLEX PREX PRIX

•P•X
APEX KPAX SPEX

PY••
PYAS PYKE PYLE PYNE PYRE PYRO

P•Y•
PAYS PAYT PHYS PHYT PUYI

P••Y
PINY PIPY PITY PIXY PKWY PLAY PLOY POKY POLY PONY POSY PRAY PREY PUNY

•PY•
SPYS

•P•Y
OPRY SPAY SPRY UPSY

••PY
COPY DOPY ESPY ISPY MOPY PIPY ROPY

P•Z•
PIZZ PUZO

P••Z
PHIZ PIZZ PREZ

QA••
QAFS QAID QATS

Q•A•
QUAD QUAE QUAG QUAI QUAM QUAR QUAT QUAY

•Q•A
AQUA

Q••D
QAID QUAD QUID QUOD

•Q•D
SQYD

••QD
REQD

QE••
QEII

Q•E•
QUEL QUEM QUES

Q••E
QUAE

Q•F•
QAFS

•QF•
SQFT

Q••G
QUAG

Q••H
QOPH

Q•I•
QAID QEII QTIP QUID QUIK QUIP QUIT QUIZ

Q••I
QEII QUAI QUOI

•QI•
SQIN

•Q•I
AQUI EQUI SQMI

Q••K
QUIK

Q••L
QUEL

Q••M
QUAM QUEM

•QM•
SQMI

•Q•N
SQIN

QO••
QOPH

Q•O•
QUOD QUOI QUOT

Q•P•
QOPH

Q••P
QTIP QUIP

QR••
QRST

Q•R•
QTRS

Q••R
QUAR

•QR•
PQRS

••QR
OPQR SPQR

Q•S•
QRST

Q••S
QAFS QATS QTRS QTYS QUES

•Q•S
PQRS

••QS
BBQS COQS ESQS FAQS INQS SEQS

QT••
QTIP QTRS QTYS

Q•T•
QATS

Q••T
QRST QUAT QUIT QUOT

•Q•T
SQFT

QU••
QUAD QUAE QUAG QUAI QUAM QUAR QUAT QUAY QUEL QUEM QUES QUID QUIK QUIP QUIT QUIZ QUOD QUOI QUOT

•QU•
AQUA AQUI EQUI

Q•Y•
QTYS

Q••Y
QUAY

•QY•
SQYD

Q••Z
QUIZ

RA••
RAAF RABE RABI RACE RACK RACY RADM RADO RADS RAFF RAFT RAGA RAGE RAGS RAGU RAHS RAID RAII RAIL RAIN RAJA RAKE RAKU RALE RALL RAMA RAMI RAMP RAMS RANA RAND RANG RANI RANK RANN RANS RANT RAPA RAPH RAPS RAPT RARA RARE RASA RASE RASH RASP RATA RATE RATS RAUL RAVE RAVI RAYE RAYS RAZE RAZZ

R•A•
RAAF RCAF RCAS RDAS READ REAL REAM REAO REAP REAR RHAP RIAA RIAL RIAS RNAS ROAD ROAM ROAN ROAR RYAL RYAN RYAS

R••A
RAGA RAJA RAMA RANA RAPA RARA RASA RATA REBA REDA RENA RETA REVA REZA RHEA RIAA RICA RIGA RIMA RINA RIPA RITA RIVA ROCA ROJA ROMA RONA ROPA ROSA ROTA ROWA RULA RUTA

•RA•
ARAB ARAD ARAL ARAM ARAN ARAP ARAS BRAC BRAD BRAE BRAG BRAM BRAN BRAS BRAT BRAY BRAZ CRAB CRAG CRAM CRAN CRAT CRAW CRAY DRAB DRAG DRAM DRAT DRAW DRAX DRAY ERAL ERAS ERAT FRAE FRAG FRAM FRAN FRAS FRAT FRAU FRAY GRAB GRAD GRAF GRAM GRAN GRAS GRAU GRAY GRAZ HRAP IRAE IRAN IRAQ IRAS ORAD ORAE ORAL ORAN ORAS PRAM PRAN PRAT PRAY SRAS TRAC TRAM TRAP TRAS TRAX TRAY URAL URAN VRAI WRAP WRAY XRAY

•R•A
ARCA AREA ARIA ARMA AROA ARPA ARTA BREA DREA ERDA ERIA ERMA ERNA FRIA IRMA IRRA ORCA ORRA PROA SRTA UREA URSA

••RA
ABRA AGRA ATRA AURA BARA BORA CARA CERA CORA DARA DORA DURA EYRA EZRA FORA HARA HERA HORA IRRA JURA KARA KYRA LARA LIRA LYRA MARA MIRA MORA MYRA NARA NERA NHRA NORA OBRA ODRA OKRA ORRA OTRA PARA PERA PURA RARA SARA SERA SORA SURA TARA TERA TORA TYRA VERA VORA XTRA ZARA ZIRA ZORA ZURA ZYRA

RB••
RBCS RBIS

R•B•
RABE RABI REBA REBS RFBS RHBS RIBO RIBS ROBB ROBE ROBS ROBT RUBE RUBS RUBY

R••B
ROBB ROWB

•RB•
ARBS GRBR ORBS URBS

•R•B
ARAB CRAB CREB CRIB DRAB DRIB DRUB GRAB GRUB PROB TRIB

••RB
AORB BARB BURB CARB CURB GARB HERB KERB NLRB SERB SORB VERB

RC••
RCAF RCAS RCMP RCPT RCTS

R•C•
RACE RACK RACY RBCS RECD RECK RECS RECT RICA RICE RICH RICK RICO ROCA ROCK ROCS RUCK

R••C
ROTC ROWC

•RC•
ARCA ARCH ARCO ARCS ORCA ORCH ORCS

•R•C
BRAC BRIC CROC ERIC IROC KROC MRSC PREC PROC TRAC

••RC
CIRC DARC DURC LARC MARC MERC NARC PARC PERC PORC

RD••
RDAS

R•D•
RADM RADO RADS REDA REDD REDE REDI REDO REDS RFDS RIDD RIDE RIDI RIDS RMDR RNDS RODD RODE RODS RUDD RUDE RUDI RUDY

R••D
RAID RAND READ RECD REDD REED REGD REID REND REQD RETD RHOD RIDD RIND ROAD RODD ROOD ROWD RUDD RUED

•RD•
ERDA ERDE ORDO URDU

•R•D
ARAD ARID AROD BRAD BRED CRED CRUD DRED FRED FRID GRAD GRID IRED IRID MRED ORAD PRED PROD TROD

••RD
BARD BIRD BYRD CARD CORD CURD FORD GARD GIRD HARD HERD KURD LARD LORD NARD NERD NORD PARD SARD WARD WORD YARD

RE••
READ REAL REAM REAO REAP REAR REBA REBS RECD RECK RECS RECT REDA REDD REDE REDI REDO REDS REED REEF REEK REEL REES REET REFI REFL REFS REFT REGD REGO REGS REGT REID REIN REIT RELO RELS RELY REMI REMO REMS REMY RENA REND RENE RENI RENO RENT REOS REPL REPO REPP REPS REPT REQD RESH RESP REST RETA RETD RETE RETS REUP REUS REVA REVE REVS REZA

R•E•
REED REEF REEK REEL REES REET RHEA RHEE RHEO RHES RHET RIEL RIEN ROEG ROES RTES RUED RUER RUES RVER RYES

R••E
RABE RACE RAGE RAKE RALE RARE RASE RATE RAVE RAYE RAZE REDE RENE RETE REVE RHEE RHUE RICE RIDE RIFE RILE RIME RIPE RIRE RISE RITE RIVE ROBE RODE ROHE ROLE ROME ROPE ROSE ROTE ROUE ROVE ROWE RUBE RUDE RULE RUNE RUSE RYLE RYNE

•RE•
AREA AREO ARES BREA BRED BREE BREI BREL BREN BRER BRET BREW CREB CRED CREE CREO CREW DREA DRED DREG DREI DREK DREW ERES EREV FRED FREE FREI FREQ FRET FREY GREG GRES GREW GREY IRED IRES MRED OREE OREG OREL OREM OREN OREO ORES PREC PRED PREF PREK PREM PREP PRES PRET PREV PREX PREY PREZ TREE TREF TREK TRES TRET TREX TREY UREA UREY WREN

•R•E
ARIE ARME ARNE ARTE ARYE BRAE BREE BRIE CREE CRUE ERDE ERIE ERLE ERNE ERSE ERTE FRAE FREE FROE FRYE GRUE IRAE ORAE OREE ORFE ORLE ORNE ORSE PRIE TREE TRUE URGE URNE

••RE
AARE ACRE AIRE BARE BORE CARE CERE CIRE CORE CURE DARE DERE DIRE DORE EHRE EIRE ETRE EURE EYRE FARE FIRE FORE GARE GERE GORE GYRE HARE HERE HIRE IHRE IMRE INRE JURE LIRE LORE LURE LYRE MARE MERE MIRE MORE OGRE OHRE PARE PERE PIRE PORE PURE PYRE RARE

RIRE SERE SIRE SORE SURE TARE TIRE TORE TYRE VERE VORE WARE WERE WIRE WORE YARE YORE

RF••
RFBS RFDS

R•F•
RAFF RAFT REFI REFL REFS REFT RIFE RIFF RIFS RIFT RUFF

R••F
RAAF RAFF RCAF REEF RIFF ROLF ROOF ROWF RUFF

•RF•
ARFS ORFE ORFF

•R•F
GRAF ORFF PREF PROF TREF

••RF
CERF KERF NERF PERF SERF SURF TURF WORF ZARF

RG••
RGTS

R•G•
RAGA RAGE RAGS RAGU REGD REGO REGS REGT RIGA RIGG RIGS RUGS

R••G
RANG RIGG RING ROEG ROWG ROYG RUNG

•RG•
ARGO ERGO ERGS ERGY ORGS ORGY URGE URGY

•R•G
BRAG BRIG CRAG DRAG DREG DRUG FRAG FRIG FROG FRUG GREG GRIG GROG OREG ORIG PRIG PROG TRIG

••RG
BERG BORG BURG MARG SARG SURG

RH••
RHAP RHBS RHEA RHEE RHEO RHES RHET RHIN RHOD RHOS RHUE RHUM RHYS

R•H•
RAHS ROHE RUHR

R••H
RAPH RASH RESH RICH ROSH ROTH ROWH RUSH RUTH

•R•H
ARCH FROH GROH ORCH ORTH

RI••
RIAA RIAL RIAS RIBO RIBS RICA RICE RICH RICK RICO RIDD RIDE RIDI RIDS RIEL RIEN RIFE RIFF RIFS RIFT RIGA RIGG RIGS RIIS RIJN RIJO RILE RILL RIMA RIME RIMS RIMY RINA RIND RING RINK RIOS RIOT RIPA RIPE RIPS RIRE RISE RISK RITA RITE RITT RITZ RIVA RIVE RIVS

R•I•
RAID RAII RAIL RAIN RBIS REID REIN REIT RHIN RIIS ROIL ROIS RUIN

R••I
RABI RAII RAMI RANI RAVI REDI REFI REMI RENI RIDI RONI ROTI ROWI RUDI

•RI•
ARIA ARID ARIE ARIL ARIZ BRIC BRIE BRIG BRIM BRIO BRIT BRIX CRIB CRIN CRIT DRIB DRIN DRIP DRIQ ERIA ERIC ERIE ERIK ERIN ERIQ ERIS FRIA FRID FRIG FRIO FRIS FRIT FRIZ GRID GRIG GRIM GRIN GRIP GRIS GRIT IRID IRIS KRIS MRIS ORIG ORIN PRIE PRIG PRIM PRIN PRIV PRIX SRIS TRIB TRIG TRIM TRIO TRIP TRIS TRIX URIS WRIT

•R•I
ARTI BREI DREI FREI TROI VRAI

••RI
ABRI AERI AGRI ATRI AURI BARI CORI GERI GYRI HARI IERI INRI JERI KARI KERI KIRI LARI LORI MARI NERI NORI OMRI PARI PERI SARI TERI TORI YURI ZORI

R•J•
RAJA RIJN RIJO ROJA ROJO

R••J
ROWJ

RK••
RKOS

R•K•
RAKE RAKU ROKS

R••K
RACK RANK RECK REEK RICK RINK RISK ROCK ROOK ROWK RUCK RUSK

•RK•
ARKS ARKY IRKS

•R•K
DREK ERIK GROK KRUK ORSK PREK TREK TRUK

••RK
BARK BORK CORK DARK DIRK DORK FORK HARK JERK KIRK LARK LURK MARK MORK MURK NARK PARK PERK PORK SARK TORK TURK WORK YORK

R•L•
RALE RALL RELO RELS RELY RILE RILL ROLE ROLF ROLL ROLO ROLY RULA RULE RULY RYLE

R••L
RAIL RALL RAUL REAL REEL REFL REPL RIAL RIEL RILL ROIL ROLL ROTL ROWL RYAL

•RL•
ARLO ERLE ORLE ORLO ORLY URLS

•R•L
ARAL ARIL ARYL BREL ERAL GRRL ORAL OREL URAL

••RL
BIRL BURL CARL CTRL CURL EARL FURL GIRL GRRL HURL KARL MARL MERL PARL PURL

RM••
RMDR

R•M•
RAMA RAMI RAMP RAMS RCMP REMI REMO REMS REMY RIMA RIME RIMS RIMY ROMA ROME ROMP ROMS ROMY RPMS RUMP RUMS

R••M
RADM REAM RHUM ROAM ROOM ROWM

•RM•
ARMA ARME ARMS ARMY ERMA IRMA

•R•M
ARAM ARUM BRAM BRIM BROM CRAM DRAM DRUM FRAM FROM GRAM GRIM OREM PRAM PREM PRIM PROM TRAM TRIM

••RM
BARM BDRM BERM CORM DERM DORM FARM FIRM FORM GERM GORM HARM MARM MERM NORM PERM TERM WARM WORM

RN••
RNAS RNDS

R•N•
RANA RAND RANG RANI RANK RANN RANS RANT RENA REND RENE RENI RENO RENT RINA RIND RING RINK RONA RONI RUNE RUNG RUNS RUNT RYNE

R••N
RAIN RANN REIN RHIN RIEN RIJN ROAN ROWN RUIN RYAN RYUN

•RN•
ARNE ARNO BRNO DRNO ERNA ERNE ERNO ERNS ORNE URNE URNS

•R•N
ARAN ARON BRAN BREN BRON BRUN BRYN CRAN CRIN DRIN ERIN FRAN GRAN GRIN GRUN IRAN IRON LRON ORAN OREN ORIN PRAN PRIN PRON TRON URAN WREN

••RN
BARN BERN BORN BURN CORN DARN DERN DORN DURN EARN FERN FIRN GARN HORN KARN KERN KORN LORN MORN NORN PIRN PORN TARN TERN TORN TURN VERN WARN WORN YARN YORN ZORN

RO••
ROAD ROAM ROAN ROAR ROBB ROBE ROBS ROBT ROCA ROCK ROCS RODD RODE RODS ROEG ROES ROHE ROIL ROIS ROJA ROJO ROKS ROLE ROLF ROLL ROLO ROLY ROMA ROME ROMP ROMS ROMY RONA RONI ROOD ROOF ROOK ROOM ROOS ROOT ROPA ROPE ROPY RORY ROSA ROSE ROSH ROSS ROSY ROTA ROTC ROTE ROTH ROTI ROTL ROTO ROTS ROUE ROUS ROUT ROUX ROVE ROWA ROWB ROWC ROWD ROWE ROWF ROWG ROWH ROWI ROWJ ROWK ROWL ROWM ROWN ROWO ROWP ROWQ ROWR ROWS ROWT ROWU ROWV ROWW ROWX ROWY ROWZ ROXY ROYG

R•O•
REOS RHOD RHOS RIOS RIOT RKOS ROOD ROOF ROOK ROOM ROOS ROOT

R••O
RADO REAO REDO REGO RELO REMO RENO REPO RHEO RIBO RICO RIJO ROJO ROLO ROTO ROWO

•RO•
AROA AROD ARON AROO AROW BROM BRON BROR BROS BROT BROW BROZ CROC CROP CROW DROP EROO EROS FROE FROG FROH FROM FROS FROW GROG GROH GROK GROS GROT GROW IROC IRON KROC LRON OROS PROA PROB PROC PROD PROF PROG PROM PRON PROP PROS PROT PROV PROW SROS TROD TROI TRON TROP TROT TROW TROY

•R•O
ARCO AREO ARGO ARLO ARNO AROO BRIO BRNO CREO CRYO DRNO ERGO ERNO EROO FRIO ORDO OREO ORLO ORZO TRIO URSO

••RO
ACRO AERO AFRO AGRO BARO BIRO BORO CARO CERO DORO DURO EBRO EERO EURO FARO FURO GARO GIRO GORO GYRO HERO INRO KARO MIRO MORO NERO NIRO NYRO OGRO OTRO PERO PURO PYRO STRO TARO TERO THRO TIRO TORO TYRO VARO VERO XERO ZERO

RP••
RPMS RPTS

R•P•
RAPA RAPH RAPS RAPT RCPT REPL REPO REPP REPS REPT RIPA RIPE RIPS ROPA ROPE ROPY

R••P
RAMP RASP RCMP REAP REPP RESP REUP RHAP ROMP ROWP RSVP RUMP

•RP•
ARPA ARPS

•R•P
ARAP CROP DRIP DROP GRIP HRAP PREP PROP TRAP TRIP TROP WRAP

••RP
AARP BURP CARP CORP DORP EARP GARP GORP HARP MSRP PERP TARP TERP WARP WKRP

R•Q•
REQD

R••Q
ROWQ

•R•Q
DRIQ ERIQ FREQ IRAQ

R•R•
RARA RARE RIRE RORY

R••R
REAR RMDR ROAR ROWR RUER RUHR RVER

•RR•
ARRS BRRR ERRS GRRL GRRR GRRS IRRA IRRS ORRA

•R•R
BRER BROR BRRR GRBR GRRR

••RR
BARR BIRR BRRR BURR CARR CORR CURR DERR FARR GARR GRRR HERR KERR LIRR PARR PURR TERR TORR

RS••
RSTU RSVP RSXS

R•S•
RASA RASE RASH RASP RESH RESP REST RISE RISK ROSA ROSE ROSH ROSS ROSY RUSE RUSH RUSK RUSS RUST

R••S
RADS RAGS RAHS RAMS RANS RAPS RATS RAYS RBCS RBIS RCAS RCTS RDAS REBS RECS REDS REES REFS REGS RELS REMS REOS REPS RETS REUS REVS RFBS RFDS RGTS RHBS RHES RHOS RHYS RIAS RIBS RIDS RIFS RIGS RIIS RIMS RIOS RIPS RIVS RKOS RNAS RNDS ROBS ROCS RODS ROES ROIS ROKS ROMS ROOS ROSS ROTS ROUS ROWS RPMS RPTS RSXS RTES RUBS RUES RUGS RUMS RUNS RUSS RUTS RWYS RYAS RYES

•RS•
ERSE ERST MRSC ORSE ORSK ORST URSA URSO

•R•S
ARAS ARBS ARCS ARES ARFS ARKS ARMS ARPS ARRS ARTS BRAS BROS CRTS CRUS CRVS DRYS ERAS ERES ERGS ERIS ERNS EROS ERRS FRAS FRIS FROS GRAS GRES GRIS GROS GRRS GRUS IRAS IRES IRIS IRKS IRRS IRUS KRIS MRIS ORAS ORBS ORCS ORES ORGS OROS ORTS ORVS PRES PROS SRAS SRIS SROS SRXS TRAS TRES TRIS URBS URIS URLS URNS WRXS

••RS
AIRS APRS ARRS BARS BORS BURS CARS CDRS CORS CTRS CURS DIRS DORS EARS ERRS FIRS FORS FURS GARS GRRS HERS HORS IRRS JARS

KIRS
KORS
LARS
LDRS
LTRS
MARS
MERS
MFRS
MGRS
MIRS
MURS
OARS
OURS
PARS
PDRS
PERS
PQRS
QTRS
SERS
SHRS
SIRS
SLRS
SSRS
STRS
TARS
TFRS
TORS
VCRS
VERS
WARS
XKRS

RT••
RTES

R•T•
RATA
RATE
RATS
RCTS
RETA
RETD
RETE
RETS
RGTS
RITA
RITE
RITT
RITZ
ROTA
ROTC
ROTE
ROTH
ROTI
ROTL
ROTO
ROTS
RPTS
RSTU
RUTA
RUTH
RUTS

R••T
RAFT
RANT
RAPT
RCPT
RECT
REET
REFT
REGT
REIT
RENT
REPT
REST
RHET
RIFT
RIOT
RITT
ROBT
ROOT
ROUT
ROWT
RUNT
RUST

•RT•
ARTA
ARTE
ARTI
ARTS
ARTY
CRTS
ERTE
ORTH
ORTS
SRTA

•R•T
BRAT
BRET
BRIT
BROT
BRUT
CRAT
CRIT
DRAT
ERAT
ERST
FRAT
FRET
FRIT
GRIT
GROT
GRWT
PRAT
PRET
PROT
QRST
TRET
TROT
WRIT

••RT
AORT
BART
BERT
BURT
CART
CERT
CORT
CURT
DART
DIRT
FORT
GERT
GIRT
GORT
HART
HIRT
HORT
HURT
KART
KERT
KURT
MART
MORT
OORT
PART
PERT
PORT
SERT
SORT
TART
TORT
VERT
WART
WERT
WORT
YURT

RU••
RUBE
RUBS
RUBY
RUCK
RUDD
RUDE
RUDI
RUDY
RUED
RUER
RUES
RUFF
RUGS
RUHR
RUIN
RULA
RULE
RULY
RUMP
RUMS
RUNE
RUNG
RUNS
RUNT
RUSE
RUSH
RUSK
RUSS
RUST
RUTA
RUTH
RUTS

R•U•
RAUL
REUP
REUS
RHUE
RHUM
ROUE
ROUS
ROUT
ROUX
RYUN

R••U
RAGU
RAKU
ROWU
RSTU

•RU•
ARUM
BRUN
BRUT
BRUX
CRUD
CRUE
CRUS
CRUX
CRUZ
DRUB
DRUG
DRUM
FRUG
GRUB
GRUE
GRUN
GRUS
IRUS
KRUK
TRUE
TRUK

•R•U
FRAU
GRAU
URDU

••RU
BORU
ECRU
GURU
MARU
PERU
THRU

RV••
RVER

R•V•
RAVE
RAVI
REVA
REVE
REVS
RIVA
RIVE
RIVS
ROVE
RSVP

R••V
ROWV

•RV•
CRVS
ORVS

•R•V
EREV
PREV
PRIV
PROV

••RV
MARV
MERV
MIRV

RW••
RWYS

R•W•
ROWA
ROWB
ROWC
ROWD
ROWE
ROWF
ROWG
ROWH
ROWI
ROWJ
ROWK
ROWL
ROWM
ROWN
ROWO
ROWP
ROWQ
ROWR
ROWS
ROWT
ROWU
ROWV
ROWW
ROWX
ROWY
ROWZ

R••W
ROWW

•RW•
GRWT

•R•W
AROW
BREW
BROW
CRAW
CREW
CROW
DRAW
DREW
FROW
GREW
GROW
PROW
TROW

••RW
NORW

R•X•
ROXY
RSXS

R••X
ROUX
ROWX

•RX•
SRXS
WRXS

•R•X
BRIX
BRUX
CRUX
DRAX
ORYX
PREX
PRIX
TRAX
TREX
TRIX

••RX
MARX

RY••
RYAL
RYAN
RYAS
RYES
RYLE
RYNE
RYUN

R•Y•
RAYE
RAYS
RHYS
ROYG
RWYS

R••Y
RACY
RELY
REMY
RIMY
ROLY
ROMY
ROPY
RORY
ROSY
ROWY
ROXY
RUBY
RUDY
RULY

•RY•
ARYE
ARYL
BRYN
CRYO
DRYS
FRYE
ORYX

•R•Y
ARKY
ARMY
ARTY
BRAY
CRAY
DRAY
ERGY
FRAY
FREY
GRAY
GREY
ORGY
ORLY
PRAY
PREY
TRAY
TREY
TROY
UREY
URGY
WRAY
XRAY

••RY
AERY
AIRY
AWRY
BURY
CARY
CORY
DORY
EERY
ENRY
EVRY
FURY
GARY
GORY
JORY
JURY
LARY
LORY
MARY
MIRY
NARY
OPRY
RORY
SPRY
TORY
UHRY
VARY
VERY
WARY
WIRY
XORY

R•Z•
RAZE
RAZZ
REZA

R••Z
RAZZ
RITZ
ROWZ

•RZ•
ORZO

•R•Z
ARIZ
BRAZ
BROZ
CRUZ
FRIZ
GRAZ
PREZ

••RZ
HARZ
MARZ
NARZ

SA••
SAAB
SAAR
SABA
SABE
SABO
SABU
SACK
SACO
SACS
SADA
SADD
SADE
SADO
SADR
SAES
SAFE
SAGA
SAGE
SAGO
SAGS
SAGY
SAHL
SAID
SAIL
SAIS
SAKE
SAKI
SAKS
SALA
SALE
SALK
SALS
SALT
SAME
SAMI
SAML
SAMP
SAMS
SANA
SAND
SANE
SANG
SANI
SANK
SANS
SANT
SAPP
SAPS
SARA
SARD
SARG
SARI
SARK
SASE
SASH
SASK
SASS
SATB
SATE
SATI
SATO
SATS
SAUD
SAUK
SAUL
SAUR
SAVE
SAWN
SAWS
SAXE
SAYS

S•A•
SAAB
SAAR
SCAB
SCAD
SCAM
SCAN
SCAR
SCAT
SDAK
SEAL
SEAM
SEAN
SEAR
SEAS
SEAT
SEAU
SFAX
SHAD
SHAG
SHAH
SHAM
SHAN
SHAQ
SHAR
SHAW
SHAY
SIAL
SIAM
SIAN
SKAT
SLAB
SLAG
SLAM
SLAP
SLAT
SLAV
SLAW
SLAY
SNAG
SNAP
SNAX
SOAK
SOAP
SOAR
SOAS
SPAD
SPAM
SPAN
SPAR
SPAS
SPAT
SPAY
SRAS
STAB
STAC
STAD
STAG
STAN
STAR
STAS
STAT
STAY
SWAB
SWAG
SWAK
SWAM
SWAN
SWAP
SWAT
SWAY

S••A
SABA
SADA
SAGA
SALA
SANA
SARA
SEGA
SELA
SERA
SETA
SHEA
SICA
SIKA
SIMA
SIVA
SIXA
SKUA
SOBA
SOCA
SODA
SOFA
SOLA
SOMA
SORA
SOSA
SOYA
SPCA
SRTA
STOA
SULA
SURA
SUVA

•SA•
ASAP
ESAI
ESAR
ESAS
ESAU
ISAK
ISAO
ISAR
ISAY
LSAT
OSAR
OSAS
PSAS
PSAT
TSAR
USAF
USAR

•S•A
ASEA
ASIA
ASTA
CSEA
ESSA
ESTA
HSIA
ISLA
OSHA
OSSA
USDA
USGA
USIA
USMA
USNA
USTA

••SA
ANSA
CASA
COSA
ELSA
ESSA
ILSA
IPSA
LISA
MASA
MESA
NASA
OSSA
PASA
PISA
RASA
ROSA
SOSA
UPSA
URSA
VASA
VISA
WUSA

S•B•
SABA
SABE
SABO
SABU
SIBS
SOBA
SOBS
SUBJ
SUBS

S••B
SAAB
SATB
SCAB
SERB
SHEB
SIXB
SLAB
SLOB
SNOB
SNUB
SORB
STAB
STUB
SWAB

•SB•
ISBN
USBS

••SB
NTSB

SC••
SCAB
SCAD
SCAM
SCAN
SCAR
SCAT
SCIS
SCLC
SCOT
SCOW
SCTV
SCUD
SCUM
SCUP
SCUT

S•C•
SACK
SACO
SACS
SECO
SECS
SECT
SECY
SICA
SICK
SICS
SNCC
SOCA
SOCK
SOCS
SPCA
SUCH
SUCK

S••C
SCLC
SIXC
SNCC
SPEC
SPIC
STAC
SYNC

•SC•
ASCH
ASCI
DSCS
ESCE
ESCS
USCG

•S•C
MSEC
USMC
USOC

••SC
BOSC
DESC
DISC
FISC
MASC
MISC
MRSC
VISC
WISC

SD••
SDAK

S•D•
SADA
SADD
SADE
SADO
SADR
SIDE
SJDS
SODA
SODS
STDS
SUDS

S••D
SADD
SAID
SAND
SARD
SAUD
SCAD
SCUD
SEED
SEND
SFPD
SHAD
SHED
SHOD
SIXD
SKED
SKID
SLED
SLID
SOLD
SPAD
SPED
SPUD
SQYD
STAD
STUD
SUED
SWED

•SD•
USDA
USDT

•S•D
ESTD
MSED
USED

••SD
NASD

SE••
SEAL
SEAM
SEAN
SEAR
SEAS
SEAT
SEAU
SECO
SECS
SECT
SECY
SEED
SEEK
SEEM
SEEN
SEEP
SEER
SEES
SEGA
SEGO
SEGS
SEHR
SEIN
SEIS
SEJM
SEKO
SELA
SELF
SELL
SEMI
SEMS
SEND
SENE
SENG
SENS
SENT
SEPT
SEQS
SERA
SERB
SERE
SERF
SERS
SERT
SESE
SESS
SETA
SETH
SETI
SETS
SETT
SEUL
SEVE
SEWN
SEWS
SEXY

S•E•
SAES
SEED
SEEK
SEEM
SEEN
SEEP
SEER
SEES
SHEA
SHEB
SHED
SHEK
SHEL
SHEM
SHEP
SHES
SHEW
SIEG
SKED
SKEE
SKEG
SKEW
SLED
SLEW
SLEY
SMEE
SMEW
SNEE
SPEC
SPED
SPEE
SPET
SPEW
SPEX
STEM
STEN
STEP
STER
STES
STET
STEW
SUED
SUER
SUES
SUET
SUEY
SUEZ
SVEN
SWED
SWEE

S••E
SABE
SADE
SAFE
SAGE
SAKE
SALE
SAME
SANE
SASE
SATE
SAVE
SAXE
SENE
SERE
SESE
SEVE
SHOE
SHUE
SIDE
SINE
SIPE
SIRE
SITE
SIXE
SIZE
SKEE
SKYE
SLOE
SLUE
SLYE
SMEE
SNEE
SOIE
SOLE
SOME
SONE
SORE
SPEE
STYE
SUPE
SURE
SUZE
SWEE
SYNE

•SE•
ASEA
ASES
CSEA
ESEL
ISEE
ISER
MSEC
MSED
OSEE
USED
USEE
USER
USES
YSER

•S•E
ASHE
ASIE
ESCE
ESME
ESNE
ESSE
ESTE
ISEE
ISLE
OSEE
OSTE
USEE

••SE
AASE
ANSE
APSE
BASE
BOSE
CASE
DESE
DOSE
DUSE
EASE
ELSE
ENSE
ERSE
ESSE
FUSE
HOSE
IPSE
JOSE
LASE
LESE
LOSE
LYSE
MDSE
MISE
MOSE
MUSE
NOSE
NYSE
OISE
ORSE
OUSE
PASE
POSE
RASE
RISE
ROSE
RUSE
SASE
SESE
VASE
VISE
VYSE
WISE

SF••
SFAX
SFPD

S•F•
SAFE
SIFT
SOFA
SOFT
SPFS
SQFT
SUFI

S••F
SELF
SERF
SURF

•SF•
USFL

•S•F
ASIF
ASOF
USAF

••SF
BASF

SG••
SGTS

S•G•
SAGA
SAGE
SAGO
SAGS
SAGY
SEGA
SEGO
SEGS
SIGH
SIGN
SIGS
SSGT

S••G
SANG
SARG
SENG
SHAG
SIEG
SING
SKEG
SLAG
SLOG
SLUG
SMOG
SMUG
SNAG
SNUG
SONG
STAG
SUNG
SURG
SWAG
SWIG

•SG•
MSGR
MSGS
MSGT
SSGT
TSGT
USGA

•S•G
USCG

SH••
SHAD
SHAG
SHAH
SHAM
SHAN
SHAQ
SHAR
SHAW
SHAY
SHEA
SHEB
SHED
SHEK
SHEL
SHEM
SHEP
SHES
SHEW
SHHH
SHIH
SHIM
SHIN
SHIP
SHIV
SHMO
SHOD
SHOE
SHOO
SHOP
SHOR
SHOT
SHOW
SHRS
SHUE
SHUI
SHUL
SHUN
SHUT

S•H•
SAHL
SEHR
SHHH
SOHO

S••H
SASH
SETH
SHAH
SHHH
SHIH
SIGH
SIKH
SINH
SOPH
SUCH

•SH•
ASHE
ASHY
OSHA

•S•H
ASCH
ESTH
ISTH

••SH
BASH
BOSH
BUSH
CASH
COSH
CUSH
DASH
DISH
FISH
GASH
GISH
GOSH
GUSH
HASH
HUSH
JOSH
LASH
LUSH
MASH
MESH
MOSH
MUSH
NASH
NOSH

PASH
PISH
POSH
PUSH
RASH
RESH
ROSH
RUSH
SASH
TESH
TISH
TOSH
TUSH
WASH
WISH

SI••
SIAL
SIAM
SIAN
SIBS
SICA
SICK
SICS
SIDE
SIEG
SIFT
SIGH
SIGN
SIGS
SIKA
SIKH
SILK
SILL
SILO
SILT
SIMA
SIMI
SIMP
SIMS
SINE
SING
SINH
SINK
SINN
SINO
SINS
SION
SIPE
SIPS
SIRE
SIRS
SISI
SISS
SITE
SITS
SITU
SITZ
SIVA
SIXA
SIXB
SIXC
SIXD
SIXE
SIZE

S•I•
SAID
SAIL
SAIS
SCIS
SEIN
SEIS
SHIH
SHIM
SHIN
SHIP
SHIV
SKID
SKIL
SKIM
SKIN
SKIP
SKIS
SKIT
SLID
SLIM
SLIP
SLIT
SMIT
SNIP
SNIT
SOIE
SOIL
SOIR
SPIC
SPIN
SPIT
SQIN
SRIS
STIR
SUIT
SWIG
SWIM
SWIT

S••I
SAKI
SAMI
SANI
SARI
SATI
SEMI
SETI
SHUI
SIMI
SISI
SOLI
SQMI
SUFI
SUZI

•SI•
ASIA
ASIE
ASIF
ASIR
ASIS
BSIX
ESIS
HSIA
ISIS
OSIP
OSIS
PSIS
USIA
VSIX

•S•I
ASCI
ASTI
ESAI
ESSI
OSSI

••SI
COSI
DESI
ESSI
IASI
KASI
LISI
NASI
OSSI
SISI
WASI

SJ••
SJDS

S•J•
SEJM

S••J
SUBJ

SK••
SKAT
SKED
SKEE
SKEG
SKEW
SKID
SKIL
SKIM
SKIN
SKIP
SKIS
SKIT
SKUA
SKUS
SKYE
SKYS

S•K•
SAKE
SAKI
SAKS
SEKO
SIKA
SIKH
STKS
SUKS

S••K
SACK
SALK
SANK
SARK
SASK
SAUK
SDAK
SEEK
SHEK
SICK
SILK
SINK
SOAK
SOCK
SUCK
SULK
SUNK
SWAK

•SK•
ASKS
ESKS
TSKS

•S•K
ASOK
ISAK

••SK
BASK
BUSK
CASK
CUSK
DESK
DISK
DUSK
FISK
HUSK
MASK
MUSK
OMSK
ORSK
RISK
RUSK
SASK
TASK
TUSK
WISK

SL••
SLAB
SLAG
SLAM
SLAP
SLAT
SLAV
SLAW
SLAY
SLED
SLEW
SLEY
SLID
SLIM
SLIP
SLIT
SLOB
SLOE
SLOG
SLOP
SLOT
SLOW
SLRS
SLUE
SLUG
SLUM
SLUR
SLXS
SLYE

S•L•
SALA
SALE
SALK
SALS
SALT
SCLC
SELA
SELF
SELL
SILK
SILL
SILO
SILT
SOLA
SOLD
SOLE
SOLI
SOLO
SOLS
STLO
SULA
SULK
SULU
SYLL
SYLS

S••L
SAHL
SAIL
SAML
SAUL
SEAL
SELL
SEUL
SHEL
SHUL
SIAL
SILL
SKIL
SOIL
SOUL
STOL
SYLL

•SL•
ISLA
ISLE
ISLS
OSLO

•S•L
ESEL
USFL

••SL
NASL

SM••
SMEE
SMEW
SMIT
SMOG
SMUG
SMUT

S•M•
SAME
SAMI
SAML
SAMP
SAMS
SEMI
SEMS
SHMO
SIMA
SIMI
SIMP
SIMS
SOMA
SOME
SQMI
STMT
SUMO
SUMP
SUMS
SYMS

S••M
SCAM
SCUM
SEAM
SEEM
SEJM
SHAM
SHEM
SHIM
SIAM
SKIM
SLAM
SLIM
SLUM
SPAM
STEM
SWAM
SWIM
SWUM

•SM•
BSMT
DSMS
ESME
ISMS
USMA
USMC

••SM
COSM
TASM
YESM

SN••
SNAG
SNAP
SNAX
SNCC
SNEE
SNIP
SNIT
SNOB
SNOW
SNUB
SNUG

S•N•
SANA
SAND
SANE
SANG
SANI
SANK
SANS
SANT
SEND
SENE
SENG
SENS
SENT
SINE
SING
SINH
SINK
SINN
SINO
SINS
SONE
SONG
SONS
SONY
SSNS
STNS
SUNG
SUNK
SUNS
SUNY
SYNC
SYNE
SYNS

S••N
SAWN
SCAN
SEAN
SEEN
SEIN
SEWN
SHAN
SHIN
SHUN
SIAN
SIGN
SINN
SION
SKIN
SOON
SOWN
SPAN
SPIN
SPUN
SQIN
STAN
STEN
STUN
SVEN
SWAN

•SN•
ESNE
ISNT
SSNS
USNA
USNR

•S•N
ASSN
ESPN
ISBN

••SN
ASSN
BOSN
HISN

SO••
SOAK
SOAP
SOAR
SOAS
SOBA
SOBS
SOCA
SOCK
SOCS
SODA
SODS
SOFA
SOFT
SOHO
SOIE
SOIL
SOIR
SOLA
SOLD
SOLE
SOLI
SOLO
SOLS
SOMA
SOME
SONE
SONG
SONS
SONY
SOON
SOOT
SOPH
SOPS
SORA
SORB
SORE
SORT
SOSA
SOSO
SOTO
SOTS
SOUL
SOUP
SOUR
SOUS
SOVS
SOWN
SOWS
SOYA
SOYS

S•O•
SCOT
SCOW
SHOD
SHOE
SHOO
SHOP
SHOR
SHOT
SHOW
SION
SLOB
SLOE
SLOG
SLOP
SLOT
SLOW
SMOG
SNOB
SNOW
SOON
SOOT
SPOT
SROS
STOA
STOL
STOP
STOW

S••O
SABO
SACO
SADO
SAGO
SATO
SECO
SEGO
SEKO
SHMO
SHOO
SILO
SINO
SOHO
SOLO
SOSO
SOTO
STLO
STRO
SUMO

•SO•
ASOF
ASOK
ASOR
DSOS
ESOP
ESOS
OSOS
TSOS
USOC
USOS
VSOP

•S•O
ASTO
ESPO
ESSO
ESTO
ISAO
ISTO
OSLO
OSSO

••SO
AHSO
ALSO
AMSO
APSO
BESO
DOSO
ESSO
FASO
IFSO
IPSO
MESO
MISO
NASO
OHSO
OSSO
PASO
PESO
SOSO
URSO
VASO

SP••
SPAD
SPAM
SPAN
SPAR
SPAS
SPAT
SPAY
SPCA
SPEC
SPED
SPEE
SPET
SPEW
SPEX
SPFS
SPIC
SPIN
SPIT
SPOT
SPQR
SPRY
SPUD
SPUN
SPUR
SPYS

S•P•
SAPP
SAPS
SEPT
SFPD
SIPE
SIPS
SOPH
SOPS
SUPE
SUPS
SUPT

S••P
SAMP
SAPP
SCUP
SEEP
SHEP
SHIP
SHOP
SIMP
SKIP
SLAP
SLIP
SLOP
SNAP
SNIP
SOAP
SOUP
STEP
STOP
SUMP
SWAP

•SP•
ASPS
ESPN
ESPO
ESPY
ISPS
ISPY
TSPS
USPS

•S•P
ASAP
ESOP
MSRP
OSIP
RSVP
VSOP

••SP
CUSP
GASP
HASP
HOSP
INSP
LISP
RASP
RESP
TBSP
WASP
WISP

SQ••
SQFT
SQIN
SQMI
SQYD

S•Q•
SEQS
SPQR

S••Q
SHAQ

•SQ•
ESQS

SR••
SRAS
SRIS
SROS
SRTA
SRXS

S•R•
SARA
SARD
SARG
SARI
SARK
SERA
SERB
SERE
SERF
SERS
SERT
SHRS
SIRE
SIRS
SLRS
SORA
SORB
SORE
SORT
SPRY
SSRS
STRO
STRS
SURA
SURE
SURF
SURG

S••R
SAAR
SADR
SAUR
SCAR
SEAR
SEER
SEHR
SHAR
SHOR
SLUR
SOAR
SOIR
SOUR
SPAR
SPQR
SPUR
STAR
STER
STIR
SUER

•SR•
MSRP
SSRS

•S•R
ASIR
ASOR
ASTR
ESAR
ISAR
ISER
MSGR
OSAR
TSAR
USAR
USER
USNR
USSR
YSER

••SR
USSR

SS••
SSGT
SSNS
SSRS
SSSS
SSTS

S•S•
SASE
SASH
SASK
SASS
SESE
SESS
SISI
SISS
SOSA
SOSO
SSSS
SUSS
SYST

S••S
SACS
SAES
SAGS
SAIS
SAKS
SALS
SAMS
SANS
SAPS
SASS
SATS
SAWS
SAYS
SCIS
SEAS
SECS
SEES
SEGS
SEIS
SEMS
SENS
SEQS
SERS
SESS
SETS
SEWS
SGTS
SHES
SHRS
SIBS
SICS
SIGS
SIMS
SINS
SIPS
SIRS
SISS
SITS
SJDS
SKIS
SKUS
SKYS
SLRS
SLXS
SOAS
SOBS
SOCS
SODS
SOLS
SONS
SOPS
SOTS
SOUS
SOVS
SOWS
SOYS
SPAS
SPFS
SPYS
SRAS
SRIS
SROS
SRXS
SSNS
SSRS
SSSS
SSTS
STAS
STDS
STES
STKS
STNS
STRS
SUBS
SUDS
SUES
SUKS
SUMS
SUNS
SUPS
SUSS
SUVS
SVXS
SYLS
SYMS
SYNS

•SS•
ASSN
ASST
ESSA
ESSE
ESSI
ESSO
ISSY
OSSA
OSSI
OSSO
PSST
SSSS
USSR

•S•S
ASES
ASIS
ASKS
ASPS
DSCS
DSMS
DSOS
ESAS
ESCS
ESIS
ESKS
ESOS
ESQS
ESTS
ESVS
ISIS
ISLS
ISMS
ISPS
ISTS
LSTS
MSGS
NSXS
OSAS
OSIS
OSOS
PSAS
PSIS
RSXS
SSNS
SSRS
SSSS
SSTS
TSKS
TSOS
TSPS
TSXS
USBS
USES
USOS
USPS

••SS
BASS
BESS
BOSS
BUSS
CASS
CESS
CUSS
DISS
DOSS
FESS
FOSS
FUSS
GOSS
HESS
HISS
HOSS
JESS
JOSS
KISS
KOSS
LASS
LESS
LOSS
MASS
MESS
MISS
MOSS
MUSS
NESS
PASS
PUSS
ROSS
RUSS
SASS
SESS
SISS
SSSS
SUSS
TASS
TESS
TOSS
VOSS
WASS
WUSS
WYSS

ST••
STAB
STAC
STAD
STAG
STAN
STAR
STAS
STAT
STAY
STDS
STEM
STEN
STEP
STER
STES
STET
STEW
STIR
STKS
STLO
STMT
STNS
STOA
STOL
STOP
STOW
STRO
STRS
STUB
STUD
STUN
STUV
STYE
STYX

S•T•
SATB
SATE
SATI
SATO
SATS
SCTV
SETA
SETH
SETI
SETS
SETT
SGTS
SITE
SITS
SITU
SITZ
SOTO
SOTS
SRTA
SSTS

S••T
SALT
SANT
SCAT
SCOT
SCUT
SEAT
SECT
SENT
SEPT
SERT
SETT
SHOT
SHUT
SIFT
SILT
SKAT
SKIT
SLAT
SLIT
SLOT
SMIT
SMUT
SNIT
SOFT
SOOT
SORT
SPAT
SPET
SPIT
SPOT
SQFT
SSGT
STAT
STET
STMT
SUET
SUIT
SUPT
SWAT
SWIT
SYST

•ST•
ASTA
ASTI
ASTO
ASTR
ESTA
ESTD
ESTE
ESTH
ESTO
ESTS
ISTH
ISTO
ISTS
LSTS
OSTE
RSTU
SSTS
USTA

•S•T
ASST
BSMT
ISNT
LSAT
MSGT
PSAT
PSST
SSGT
TSGT
USDT

••ST
AGST
ASST
AUST
BAST
BEST
BIST
BUST
CAST
CEST
CIST
COST
CUST
CYST
DIST
DOST
DUST
EAST
ERST
FAST
FEST
FIST
FUST
GEST
GIST
GUST
HAST
HEST
HIST
HOST
IEST
INST
JEST
JUST
KIST
LAST
LEST
LIST
LOST
LUST
MAST
MIST
MOST
MUST
MYST
NAST
NEST
OAST
OUST
PAST
PEST
POST
PSST
QRST
REST
RUST
SYST
TEST
VAST
VEST
WAST
WEST
XYST
YOST
ZEST

SU••
SUBJ
SUBS
SUCH
SUCK
SUDS
SUED
SUER
SUES
SUET
SUEY
SUEZ
SUFI
SUIT
SUKS
SULA
SULK
SULU
SUMO
SUMP
SUMS
SUNG
SUNK
SUNS
SUNY
SUPE
SUPS
SUPT
SURA
SURE
SURF
SURG
SUSS
SUVA
SUVS
SUZE
SUZI
SUZY

S•U•
SAUD
SAUK
SAUL
SAUR
SCUD
SCUM
SCUP
SCUT
SEUL
SHUE
SHUI
SHUL
SHUN
SHUT

SKUA SKUS SLUE SLUG SLUM SLUR SMUG SMUT SNUB SNUG SOUL SOUP SOUR SOUS SPUD SPUN SPUR STUB STUD STUN STUV SWUM

S••U
SABU SEAU SITU SULU

•S•U
ESAU RSTU

••SU
JESU ZASU

SV••
SVEN SVXS

S•V•
SAVE SEVE SIVA SOVS SUVA SUVS

S••V
SCTV SHIV SLAV STUV

•SV•
ESVS RSVP

SW••
SWAB SWAG SWAK SWAM SWAN SWAP SWAT SWAY SWED SWEE SWIG SWIM SWIT SWUM

S•W•
SAWN SAWS SEWN SEWS SOWN SOWS

S••W
SCOW SHAW SHEW SHOW SKEW SLAW SLEW SLOW SMEW SNOW SPEW STEW STOW

S•X•
SAXE SEXY SIXA SIXB SIXC SIXD SIXE SLXS SRXS SVXS

S••X
SFAX SNAX SPEX STYX

•SX•
NSXS RSXS TSXS

•S•X
BSIX VSIX

••SX
GASX

SY••
SYLL SYLS SYMS SYNC SYNE SYNS SYST

S•Y•
SAYS SKYE SKYS SLYE SOYA SOYS SPYS SQYD STYE STYX

S••Y
SAGY SECY SEXY SHAY SLAY SLEY SONY SPAY SPRY STAY SUEY SUNY SUZY SWAY

•S•Y
ASHY ESPY ISAY ISPY ISSY

••SY
BUSY CASY COSY EASY ISSY ITSY NOSY POSY ROSY UPSY

S•Z•
SIZE SUZE SUZI SUZY

S••Z
SITZ SUEZ

T•A•

TA••
TAAL TABI TABS TABU TACH TACK TACO TACS TACT TADA TADS TAEL TAFT TAGS TAIL TAIS TAJO TAKA TAKE TALA TALC TALE TALI TALK TALL TAMA TAME TAMI TAMP TAMS TANA TANG TANH TANK TANS TAOS TAPA TAPE TAPS TARA TARE TARN TARO TARP TARS TART TASK TASM TASS TATA TATE TATI TATS TAUR TAUS TAUT TAVI TAVS TAWS TAWT TAXA TAXI TAXO TAXY TAYE

TAAL TBAR TEAC TEAK TEAL TEAM TEAR TEAS TEAT THAD THAE THAI THAN THAR THAT THAW TIAS TMAN TMAX TOAD TOAT TRAC TRAM TRAP TRAS TRAX TRAY TSAR TVAD TWAS TWAY TZAR

T••A
TADA TAKA TALA TAMA TANA TAPA TARA TATA TAXA TEMA TENA TERA TEWA TINA TIWA TOEA TOGA TOMA TORA TOYA TUBA TULA TUNA TVMA TWOA TYRA

•TA•
ATAD ATAR ETAH ETAL ETAS ETAT ITAL ITAR OTAY PTAH PTAS STAB STAC STAD STAG STAN STAR STAS STAT STAY UTAH

•T•A
ATKA ATRA ATTA ETNA ETTA ITEA ITZA OTEA OTRA STOA XTRA

••TA
ACTA AFTA ALTA ANTA ARTA ASTA ATTA BETA CETA DATA EDTA ESTA ETTA FATA FETA GETA GITA IOTA JOTA KATA LITA MATA META MITA MOTA NITA NOTA OCTA OITA PETA PITA RATA RETA RITA ROTA RUTA SETA SRTA TATA USTA VETA VITA ZETA

TB••
TBAR TBSP

T•B•
TABI TABS TABU TCBY TOBE TOBY TUBA TUBB TUBE TUBS

T••B
TENB TOMB TRIB TUBB TWOB

•TB•
GTBR OTBS

•T•B
BTOB FTLB NTSB STAB STUB

••TB
LITB SATB

TC••
TCBY TCHR

T•C•
TACH TACK TACO TACS TACT TECH TECS TICK TICO TICS TOCK TUCK TYCO

T••C
TALC TEAC TENC TRAC TWOC

•TC•
ATCO ETCH ETCS ITCH

•T•C
ATIC ETIC ITIC OTIC STAC

••TC
ROTC

T•D•
TADA TADS TEDS THDS TIDE TIDY TODD TODI TODO TODS TUDE

T••D
TEED TEND THAD THUD TIED TKOD TOAD TODD TOED TOLD TROD TVAD TWOD

•TD•
ETDS LTDS STDS

•T•D
ATAD STAD STUD

••TD
ESTD LITD RETD

TE••
TEAC TEAK TEAL TEAM TEAR TEAS TEAT TECH TECS TEDS TEED TEEM TEEN TEER TEES TELE TELL TELS TEMA TEMP TENA TENB TENC TEND TENE TENG TENK TENN TENS TENT TERA TERI TERM TERN TERO TERP TERR TESH TESS TEST TETE TETH TETR TETS TEUT TEWA TEXT

T•E•
TAEL TEED TEEM TEEN TEER TEES THEE THEM THEN THEO THES THET THEW THEY TIED TIER TIES TMEN TOEA TOED TOES TREE TREF TREK TRES TRET TREX TREY TUES TWEE TYEE TYES

T••E
TAKE TALE TAME TAPE TARE TATE TAYE TELE TENE TETE THAE THEE TIDE TIGE TIKE TILE TIME TINE TIRE TOBE TOKE TOLE TOME TONE TOPE TORE TOTE TOVE TPKE TREE TRUE TUBE TUDE TULE TUNE TWEE TWOE TYEE TYKE TYNE TYPE TYRE

•TE•
ATEN ATES BTEN CTEN ETES ITEA ITEM ITEN ITER ITES KTEL OTEA PTER RTES STEM STEN STEP STER STES STET STEW UTEP UTES VTEN

•T•E
ATLE ETRE ETTE MTGE OTOE STYE UTNE

••TE
ACTE ALTE ANTE ARTE BATE BETE BITE BYTE CATE CETE CITE CMTE COTE CUTE CYTE DATE DOTE ERTE ESTE ETTE FATE FETE GATE GUTE HATE HITE HOTE JETE JUTE KATE KITE LATE LITE LUTE LYTE MATE METE MITE MOTE MUTE NATE NITE NOTE OSTE PATE PETE RATE RETE RITE ROTE SATE SITE TATE TETE TOTE VITE VOTE

TF••
TFRS

T•F•
TAFT TIFF TOFF TOFT TOFU TUFT

T••F
TGIF TIFF TOFF TREF TURF

TG••
TGIF

T•G•
TAGS TIGE TOGA TOGO TOGS TSGT TUGS

T••G
TANG TENG THUG TING TONG TRIG TUNG TVPG TWIG

•TG•
MTGE MTGS

•T•G
LTJG STAG

••TG
MKTG

TH••
THAD THAE THAI THAN THAR THAT THAW THDS THEE THEM THEN THEO THES THET THEW THEY THIN THIS THOM THON THOR THOS THOU THRO THRU THUD THUG THUR THUS

T•H•
TCHR

T••H
TACH TANH TECH TESH TETH TISH TOSH TUSH

•TH•
DTHS ETHN ETHS OTHO

•T•H
ETAH ETCH ITCH PTAH UTAH

••TH
ACTH ANTH AUTH BATH BETH BOTH CATH DITH DOTH ESTH FATH GOTH HATH HETH HOTH ISTH KITH LATH LGTH LITH LUTH MATH METH MOTH MYTH NETH NOTH OATH ORTH PATH PITH ROTH RUTH SETH TETH WITH

TI••
TIAS TICK TICO TICS TIDE TIDY TIED TIER TIES TIFF TIGE TIKE TIKI TILE TILL TILT TIME TINA TINE TING TINK TINO TINS TINT TINY TION TIOS TIPI TIPS TIRE TIRO TISH TITI TITO TITS TIVO TIWA

T•I•
TAIL TAIS TGIF THIN THIS TOIL TRIB TRIG TRIM TRIO TRIP TRIS TRIX TUIS TWIG TWIN TWIT TWIX

T••I
TABI TALI TAMI TATI TAVI TAXI TERI THAI TIKI TIPI TITI TODI TONI TOPI TORI TROI

•TI•
ATIC ATIK ATIP ATIS ATIT ETIC GTIS ITIC ITIS OTIC OTIS QTIP STIR UTIL

•T•I
ATLI ATOI ATRI ETUI PTUI

••TI
ACTI ALTI ANTI ARTI ASTI LOTI MUTI NOTI ROTI SATI SETI TATI TITI VITI YETI ZITI

T•J•
TAJO TOJO

•TJ•
LTJG

TK••
TKOD TKOS TKTS

T•K•
TAKA TAKE TIKE TIKI TOKE TPKE TPKS TSKS TYKE

T••K
TACK TALK TANK TASK TEAK TENK TICK TINK TNPK TOCK TONK TOOK TORK TREK TRUK TUCK TURK TUSK

•TK•
ATKA STKS

•T•K
ATIK

T•L•
TALA TALC TALE TALI TALK TALL TELE TELL TELS TILE TILL TILT TOLD TOLE TOLL TULA TULE TULL TYLO

T••L
TAAL TAEL TAIL TALL TEAL TELL TILL TOIL TOLL TOOL TULL

•TL•
ATLE ATLI FTLB ITLL STLO

•T•L
CTRL ETAL HTML ITAL ITLL ITOL KTEL STOL UTIL VTOL

••TL
INTL NATL ROTL

TM••
TMAN TMAX TMEN

T•M•
TAMA TAME TAMI TAMP TAMS TEMA TEMP TIME TOMA TOMB TOME TOMS TOMT TUMS TVMA

T••M
TASM TEAM TEEM TERM THEM THOM TRAM TRIM

•TM•
ATMO ATMS HTML STMT

•T•M
ATOM ETUM ETYM ITEM STEM

••TM
LITM

TN••
TNPK TNTS TNUT

T•N•
TANA TANG TANH TANK TANS TENA TENB TENC TEND TENE TENG TENK TENN TENS TENT TINA TINE TING TINK TINO TINS TINT TINY TONE TONG TONI TONK TONO TONS TONY TUNA TUNE TUNG TUNS TYNE

T••N
TARN TEEN TENN TERN THAN THEN THIN THON TION TMAN TMEN TOON TORN TOWN TRON TURN TWIN

•TN•
ATNO CTNS ETNA MTNS STNS UTNE

•T•N
ATEN ATON ATTN BTEN CTEN ETHN ETON ITEN STAN STEN STUN VTEN

••TN
ATTN

TO••
TOAD TOAT TOBE TOBY TOCK TODD TODI TODO TODS TOEA TOED TOES TOFF TOFT TOFU TOGA TOGO TOGS TOIL TOJO TOKE TOLD TOLE TOLL TOMA TOMB TOME TOMS TOMT TONE TONG TONI TONK TONO TONS TONY

TOOK TOOL TOON TOOT TOPE TOPI TOPO TOPS TORA TORE TORI TORK TORN TORO TORR TORS TORT TORY TOSH TOSS TOTE TOTO TOTS TOUR TOUT TOVE TOWN TOWS TOXO TOYA TOYO TOYS

T•O•
TAOS THOM THON THOR THOS THOU TION TIOS TKOD TKOS TOOK TOOL TOON TOOT TROD TROI TRON TROP TROT TROW TROY TSOS TTOP TWOA TWOB TWOC TWOD TWOE TWOS

T••O
TACO TAJO TARO TAXO TERO THEO THRO TICO TINO TIRO TITO TIVO TODO TOGO TOJO TONO TOPO TORO TOTO TOXO TOYO TRIO TYCO TYLO TYPO TYRO

•TO•
ATOI ATOM ATON ATOP ATOR ATOZ BTOB ETON FTOS GTOS ITOL ITOO OTOE OTOS STOA STOL STOP STOW TTOP VTOL

•T•O
ATCO ATMO ATNO ATTO BTWO ITOO KTWO OTHO OTRO OTTO STLO STRO UTWO WTWO

••TO
ACTO ALTO ASTO ATTO AUTO CATO CETO CITO CYTO DATO DOTO ECTO ENTO ESTO FOTO GATO GOTO INTO ISTO JATO KATO KOTO LETO MATO MOTO NATO OCTO ONTO OPTO OTTO PATO PETO ROTO SATO SOTO TITO TOTO UNTO UPTO VETO VITO ZITO

TP••
TPKE TPKS

T•P•
TAPA TAPE TAPS TIPI TIPS TNPK TOPE TOPI TOPO TOPS TSPS TVPG TWPS TYPE TYPO

T••P
TAMP TARP TBSP TEMP TERP TRAP TRIP TROP TTOP

•T•P
ATIP ATOP HTTP QTIP STEP STOP TTOP UTEP

••TP
HTTP

TR••
TRAC TRAM TRAP TRAS TRAX TRAY TREE TREF TREK TRES TRET TREX TREY TRIB TRIG TRIM TRIO TRIP TRIS TRIX TROD TROI TRON TROP TROT TROW TROY TRUE TRUK

T•R•
TARA TARE TARN TARO TARP TARS TART TERA TERI TERM TERN TERO TERP TERR TFRS THRO THRU TIRE TIRO TORA TORE TORI TORK TORN TORO TORR TORS TORT TORY TURF TURK TURN TYRA TYRE TYRO

T••R
TAUR TBAR TCHR TEAR TEER TERR TETR THAR THOR THUR TIER TORR TOUR TSAR TZAR

•TR•
ATRA ATRI CTRL CTRS ETRE LTRS OTRA OTRO QTRS STRO STRS XTRA

•T•R
ATAR ATOR GTBR ITAR ITER LTYR PTER STAR STER STIR

••TR
ASTR ENTR INTR MATR NATR PATR TETR VITR

TS••
TSAR TSGT TSKS TSOS TSPS TSXS

T•S•
TASK TASM TASS TBSP TESH TESS TEST TISH TOSH TOSS TUSH TUSK

T••S
TABS TACS TADS TAGS TAIS TAMS TANS TAOS TAPS TARS TASS TATS TAUS TAVS TAWS TEAS TECS TEDS TEES TELS TENS TESS TETS TFRS THDS THES THIS THOS THUS TIAS TICS TIES TINS TIOS TIPS TITS TKOS TKTS TNTS TODS TOES TOGS TOMS TONS TOPS TORS TOSS TOTS TOWS TOYS TPKS TRAS TRES TRIS TSKS TSOS TSPS TSXS TUBS TUES TUGS TUIS TUMS TUNS TUTS TWAS TWOS TWPS TYES TYUS TZUS

•TS•
ITSY NTSB

•T•S
ATES ATIS ATMS ATTS ATVS BTUS CTNS CTRS DTHS ETAS ETCS ETDS ETES ETHS FTOS GTIS GTOS GTVS GTXS ITES ITIS LTDS LTRS MTGS MTNS OTBS OTIS OTOS PTAS QTRS QTYS RTES STAS STDS STES STKS STNS STRS UTES

••TS
ACTS AFTS AGTS AITS ALTS AMTS ANTS APTS ARTS ATTS BATS BETS BITS BLTS BOTS BUTS CATS COTS CPTS CRTS CUTS DDTS DETS DITS DOTS DPTS EATS EFTS EMTS ENTS ESTS EXTS FATS FITS GATS GETS GITS GUTS HATS HGTS HITS HUTS INTS ISTS JETS JOTS JUTS KITS KNTS LATS LETS LITS LOTS LSTS MATS METS MKTS MOTS NATS NETS NITS NOTS NUTS OATS OCTS OPTS ORTS OUTS PATS PCTS PETS PITS PMTS POTS PUTS PVTS PWTS QATS RATS RCTS RETS RGTS ROTS RPTS RUTS SATS SETS SGTS SITS SOTS SSTS TATS TETS TITS TKTS TNTS TOTS TUTS VATS VDTS VETS VITS WATS WETS WITS ZITS

TT••
TTOP

T•T•
TATA TATE TATI TATS TETE TETH TETR TETS TITI TITO TITS TKTS TNTS TOTE TOTO TOTS TUTS TUTU

T••T
TACT TAFT TART TAUT TAWT TEAT TENT TEST TEUT TEXT THAT THET TILT TINT TNUT TOAT TOFT TOMT TOOT TORT TOUT TRET TROT TSGT TUFT TWIT

•TT•
ATTA ATTN ATTO ATTS ATTU ATTY ETTA ETTE ETTU HTTP ITTY OTTO

•T•T
ATIT ATWT ETAT NTWT STAT STET STMT

••TT
BATT BITT BUTT CATT FETT GATT GOTT HUTT JETT KATT KETT KITT LETT LOTT MATT MITT MOTT MUTT PITT PUTT RITT SETT WATT WITT

TU••
TUBA TUBB TUBE TUBS TUCK TUDE TUES TUFT TUGS TUIS TULA TULE TULL TUMS TUNA TUNE TUNG TUNS TURF TURK TURN TUSH TUSK TUTS TUTU TUVW

T•U•
TAUR TAUS TAUT TEUT THUD THUG THUR THUS TNUT TOUR TOUT TRUE TRUK TYUS TZUS

T••U
TABU THOU THRU TOFU TUTU

•TU•
BTUS ETUI ETUM PTUI STUB STUD STUN STUV

•T•U
ATTU ETTU

••TU
ATTU BATU ETTU HUTU RSTU SITU TUTU VATU WCTU

TV••
TVAD TVMA TVPG

T•V•
TAVI TAVS TIVO TOVE TUVW

•TV•
ATVS GTVS

•T•V
STUV

••TV
ACTV CATV EDTV HDTV HGTV NOTV ONTV SCTV

TW••
TWAS TWAY TWEE TWIG TWIN TWIT TWIX TWOA TWOB TWOC TWOD TWOE TWOS TWPS

T•W•
TAWS TAWT TEWA TIWA TOWN TOWS

T••W
THAW THEW TROW TUVW

•TW•
ATWT BTWO KTWO NTWT UTWO WTWO

•T•W
STEW STOW

••TW
GWTW

T•X•
TAXA TAXI TAXO TAXY TEXT TOXO TSXS

T••X
TMAX TRAX TREX TRIX TWIX

•TX•
GTXS

•T•X
STYX

TY••
TYCO TYEE TYES TYKE TYLO TYNE TYPE TYPO TYRA TYRE TYRO TYUS

T•Y•
TAYE TOYA TOYO TOYS

T••Y
TAXY TCBY THEY TIDY TINY TOBY TONY TORY TRAY TREY TROY TWAY

•TY•
ETYM LTYR QTYS STYE STYX

•T•Y
ATTY ITSY ITTY OTAY STAY

••TY
ARTY ATTY CITY COTY DUTY ITTY KATY OATY PITY

TZ••
TZAR TZUS

•TZ•
ITZA

•T•Z
ATOZ

••TZ
ANTZ BETZ BUTZ DITZ FUTZ GETZ KATZ KETZ LUTZ METZ RITZ SITZ YUTZ ZOTZ

U•A•
UCAL ULAN ULAR UNAS UNAU URAL URAN USAF USAR UTAH

U••A
UCLA ULLA ULNA UNCA UPSA UREA URSA USDA USGA USIA USMA USNA USTA UVEA

•UA•
CUAL DUAD DUAL FUAD GUAM GUAR GUAT HUAC JUAB JUAN LUAU QUAD QUAE QUAG QUAI QUAM QUAR QUAT QUAY YUAN

•U•A
AURA BUDA CUBA DUMA DUNA DURA EULA FUCA HULA JURA LUKA LULA LUMA LUNA PUKA PULA PUMA PUPA PURA RULA RUTA SULA SURA SUVA TUBA TULA TUNA WUSA YUBA YUMA ZURA

••UA
AGUA AQUA ECUA SKUA

UB••
UBER

U•B•
URBS USBS

•UB•
AUBE BUBS CUBA CUBE CUBS DUBS FUBU HUBS LUBE NUBS PUBL PUBS RUBE RUBS RUBY SUBJ SUBS TUBA TUBB TUBE TUBS YUBA

•U•B
BULB BURB CURB DUMB JUAB NUMB TUBB

••UB
CHUB CLUB DAUB DRUB FLUB GRUB SNUB STUB

UC••
UCAL UCLA

U•C•
UNCA UPCS USCG

U••C
UNPC USMC USOC

•UC•
BUCK BUCO BUCS DUCE DUCK DUCO DUCT FUCA GUCK HUCK JUCO LUCE LUCI LUCK LUCY MUCH MUCK OUCH PUCE PUCK RUCK SUCH SUCK TUCK YUCK

•U•C
DURC HUAC JUNC NUNC

••UC
EDUC GLUC

UD••
UDOS

U•D•
UNDO UPDO URDU USDA USDT

U••D
USED

•UD•
AUDE AUDI BUDA BUDD BUDS CUDS DUDE DUDS FUDD JUDD JUDE JUDI JUDO JUDY KUDO KUDU MUDD MUDS NUDE OUDS RUDD RUDE RUDI RUDY SUDS TUDE

•U•D
AULD BUDD BUND CUED CURD CUYD DUAD FUAD FUDD FUND GUND HUED HUND JUDD KURD LUND MUDD QUAD QUID QUOD RUDD RUED SUED

••UD
BAUD CAUD CRUD DOUD EHUD FEUD GAUD LAUD LOUD MAUD SAUD SCUD SPUD STUD THUD VAUD YOUD

UE••
UELE UEYS

U•E•
UBER UKES ULEE UNES UREA UREY USED USEE USER USES UTEP UTES UVEA

U••E
UELE ULEE UNIE URGE URNE USEE UTNE

•UE•
AUEL AUER CUED CUER CUES DUEL DUER DUES DUET EUER FUEL HUED HUER HUES HUEY PUER QUEL QUEM QUES RUED RUER RUES SUED SUER SUES SUET SUEY SUEZ TUES VUES

•U•E
AUBE AUDE CUBE CUKE CULE CUME CURE CUTE DUCE

DUDE DUKE DUNE DUPE DUSE DUVE EURE EUWE FUGE FUME FUSE GUTE HUGE HUME JUDE JUKE JULE JUNE JURE JUTE LUBE LUCE LUGE LUKE LUNE LUPE LURE LUTE LUXE MULE MUSE MUTE NUDE NUKE OUSE PUCE PULE PURE QUAE RUBE RUDE RULE RUNE RUSE SUPE SURE SUZE TUBE TUDE TULE TUNE YULE

••UE
ADUE AGUE BLUE CLUE COUE CRUE FLUE GLUE GRUE LAUE MOUE NEUE NIUE RHUE ROUE SHUE SLUE TRUE

UF••
UFOS

U•F•
UOFM USFL

U••F
USAF

•UF•
BUFF CUFF CUFT DUFF DUFY GUFF HUFF LUFF LUFT MUFF NUFF PUFF RUFF SUFI TUFT

•U•F
BUFF CUFF DUFF FUNF GUFF GULF HUFF LUFF MUFF NUFF PUFF RUFF SURF TURF

••UF
ENUF NEUF OEUF POUF

UG••
UGHS UGLI UGLY

U•G•
URGE URGY USGA

U••G
USCG

•UG•
AUGS BUGS FUGE FUGU HUGE HUGH HUGO HUGS JUGS LUGE LUGS MUGS PUGH PUGS RUGS TUGS VUGS YUGO

•U•G
AUNG BULG BUNG BURG GUNG HUNG JUNG KUNG LUNG MUNG PUIG PUNG QUAG RUNG SUNG SURG TUNG VULG YUNG

••UG
CHUG DOUG DRUG FRUG GLUG PLUG SLUG SMUG SNUG THUG

UH••
UHOH UHRY UHUH

U•H•
UGHS

U••H
UHOH UHUH UMPH UTAH

•UH•
DUHS HUHS KUHN RUHR WUHL

•U•H
AUTH BUSH CUSH GUSH HUGH HUNH HUSH LUSH LUTH MUCH MUSH OUCH PUGH PUSH RUSH RUTH SUCH TUSH

••UH
UHUH

U•I•
UNIE UNIS UNIT UNIV UNIX URIS USIA UTIL UZIS

U••I
UGLI

•UI•
CUIN HUIS HUIT JUIN LUIS LUIZ MUIR NUIT OUIS PUIG QUID QUIK QUIP QUIT QUIZ RUIN SUIT TUIS

•U•I
AUDI AURI FUJI JUDI JULI JUNI LUCI MUNI MUTI PULI PUYI QUAI QUOI RUDI SUFI SUZI YURI ZUNI

••UI
ALUI AQUI EQUI ETUI MAUI PFUI PTUI SHUI

•UJ•
CUJO FUJI JUJU

•U•J
SUBJ

UK••
UKES

•UK•
AUKS CUKE DUKE JUKE LUKA LUKE LUKS NUKE PUKA SUKS YUKS

•U•K
BUCK BULK BUNK BUSK CUSK DUCK DUNK DUSK FUNK GUCK GUNK HUCK HULK HUNK HUSK JUNK LUCK LUNK LURK MUCK MURK MUSK PUCK PUNK QUIK RUCK RUSK SUCK SULK SUNK TUCK TURK TUSK YUCK

••UK
HOUK KRUK NYUK SAUK TRUK WOUK ZOUK

UL••
ULAN ULAR ULEE ULLA ULNA ULUS

U•L•
UCLA UELE UGLI UGLY ULLA UNLV URLS

U••L
UCAL URAL USFL UTIL

•UL•
AULD BULB BULG BULK BULL CULE CULL CULP CULT DULL DULY EULA FULL GULF GULL GULP HULA HULK HULL JULE JULI JULY KULP LULA LULL LULU MULE MULL NULL OULU PULA PULE PULI PULL PULP PULS RULA RULE RULY SULA SULK SULU TULA TULE TULL VULG YULE ZULU

•U•L
AUEL BULL BURL CUAL CULL CURL DUAL DUEL DULL FUEL FULL FURL GULL HULL HURL LULL MULL NULL PUBL PULL PURL QUEL TULL WUHL

••UL
AMUL AZUL CAUL ELUL FOUL GAUL HAUL MAUL OCUL PAUL RAUL SAUL SEUL SHUL SOUL

UM••
UMPH UMPS

U•M•
UOMO USMA USMC

U••M
UNUM UOFM

•UM•
BUMP BUMS CUME DUMA DUMB DUMP FUME FUMY GUMM GUMP GUMS HUME HUMP HUMS JUMP LUMA LUMP MUMM MUMS NUMB PUMA PUMP RUMP RUMS SUMO SUMP SUMS TUMS YUMA

•U•M
GUAM GUMM MUMM QUAM QUEM

••UM
AHUM ALUM ARUM BAUM BLUM CHUM DEUM DRUM ETUM GLUM KLUM MEUM OVUM PLUM RHUM SCUM SLUM SWUM UNUM

UN••
UNAS UNAU UNCA UNDO UNES UNIE UNIS UNIT UNIV UNIX UNLV UNOS UNPC UNTO UNUM

U•N•
ULNA URNE URNS USNA USNR UTNE

U••N
ULAN UPON URAN

•UN•
AUNG AUNT BUND BUNG BUNK BUNS BUNT CUNY DUNA DUNE DUNK DUNN DUNS FUND FUNF FUNK FUNS FUNT GUND GUNG GUNK GUNN GUNS HUND HUNG HUNH HUNK HUNS HUNT JUNC JUNE JUNG JUNI JUNK JUNO KUNG LUNA LUND LUNE LUNG LUNK LUNN LUNT MUNG MUNI NUNC NUNN NUNS PUNG PUNK PUNS PUNT PUNY RUNE RUNG RUNS RUNT SUNG SUNK SUNS SUNY TUNA TUNE TUNG TUNS YUNG ZUNI

•U•N
BUON BURN CUIN DUNN DURN DUUN GUNN JUAN JUIN KUHN LUNN MUON NUNN RUIN TURN YUAN

••UN
BRUN DUUN FAUN GRUN JAUN NEUN NOUN RYUN SHUN SPUN STUN

UO••
UOFM UOMO UOUS UOVO

U•O•
UDOS UFOS UHOH UNOS UPON USOC USOS UXOR

U••O
UNDO UNTO UOMO UOVO UPDO UPTO URSO UTWO

•UO•
BUON BUOY DUOS MUON QUOD QUOI QUOT

•U•O
AUTO BUCO CUJO DUCO DURO EURO FURO HUGO JUCO JUDO JUNO KUDO OUZO PURO PUZO SUMO YUGO

UP••
UPCS UPDO UPON UPSA UPSY UPTO

U•P•
UMPH UMPS UNPC USPS

U••P
UTEP

•UP•
CUPR CUPS DUPE HUPS LUPE PUPA PUPP PUPS PUPU SUPE SUPS SUPT

•U•P
BUMP BURP CULP CUSP DUMP GULP GUMP HUMP JUMP KULP LUMP PULP PUMP PUPP QUIP RUMP SUMP

••UP
ACUP BCUP CCUP COUP DCUP DOUP GOUP LOUP REUP SCUP SOUP WHUP

UR••
URAL URAN URBS URDU UREA UREY URGE URGY URIS URLS URNE URNS URSA URSO

U•R•
UHRY

U••R
UBER ULAR USAR USER USNR USSR UXOR

•UR•
AURA AURI BURB BURG BURL BURN BURP BURR BURS BURT BURY CURB CURD CURE CURL CURR CURS CURT DURA DURC DURN DURO EURE EURO FURL FURO FURS FURY GURU HURL HURT JURA JURE JURY KURD KURT LURE LURK MURK MURS OURS PURA PURE PURL PURO PURR SURA SURE SURF SURG TURF TURK TURN YURI YURT ZURA

•U•R
AUER BURR CUER CUPR CURR DUER EUER GUAR HUER MUIR PUER PURR QUAR RUER RUHR SUER

••UR
AMUR AZUR BLUR DOUR FOUR GAUR HOUR JOUR KNUR LEUR LOUR NEUR PEUR PLUR POUR SAUR SLUR SOUR SPUR TAUR THUR TOUR YOUR

US••
USAF USAR USBS USCG USDA USDT USED USEE USER USES USFL USGA USIA USMA USMC USNA USNR USOC USOS USPS USSR USTA

U•S•
UPSA UPSY URSA URSO USSR

U••S
UDOS UEYS UFOS UGHS UKES ULUS UMPS UNAS UNES UNIS UNOS UOUS UPCS URBS URIS URLS URNS USBS USES USOS USPS UTES UZIS

•US•
AUST BUSH BUSK BUSS BUST BUSY CUSH CUSK CUSP CUSS CUST DUSE DUSK DUST FUSE FUSS FUST GUSH GUST HUSH HUSK JUST LUSH LUST MUSE MUSH MUSK MUSS MUST OUSE OUST PUSH PUSS RUSE RUSH RUSK RUSS RUST SUSS TUSH TUSK WUSA WUSS

•U•S
AUGS AUKS BUBS BUCS BUDS BUGS BUMS BUNS BURS BUSS BUTS BUYS CUBS CUDS CUES CUPS CURS CUSS CUTS DUBS DUDS DUES DUHS DUNS DUOS FUNS FURS FUSS GUMS GUNS GUTS GUVS GUYS HUBS HUES HUGS HUHS HUIS HUMS HUNS HUPS HUTS JUGS JUTS LUGS LUIS LUKS LUVS MUDS MUGS MUMS MURS MUSS NUBS NUNS NUTS NUYS OUDS OUIS OURS OUTS PUBS PUGS PULS PUNS PUPS PUSS PUTS QUES RUBS RUES RUGS RUMS RUNS RUSS RUTS SUBS SUDS SUES SUKS SUMS SUNS SUPS SUSS SUVS TUBS TUES TUGS TUIS TUMS TUNS TUTS VUES VUGS WUSS YUKS

••US
APUS BMUS BTUS CCUS CPUS CRUS DAUS DEUS DMUS ECUS EMUS EOUS FLUS GNUS GRUS HAUS ICUS ILUS IMUS IOUS IRUS MAUS NOUS ONUS OPUS OXUS PIUS PLUS REUS ROUS SKUS SOUS TAUS THUS TYUS TZUS ULUS UOUS VOUS ZEUS

UT••
UTAH UTEP UTES UTIL UTNE UTWO

U•T•
UNTO UPTO USTA

U••T
UNIT USDT

•UT•
AUTH AUTO BUTS BUTT BUTZ CUTE CUTS DUTY FUTZ GUTE GUTS HUTS HUTT HUTU JUTE JUTS LUTE LUTH LUTZ MUTE MUTI MUTT NUTS OUTS PUTS PUTT RUTA RUTH RUTS TUTS TUTU YUTZ

•U•T
AUNT AUST BUNT BURT BUST BUTT CUFT CULT CURT CUST DUCT DUET DUST FUNT FUST GUAT GUST HUIT HUNT HURT HUTT JUST KURT LUFT LUNT LUST MUST MUTT NUIT OUST PUNT PUTT QUAT QUIT QUOT RUNT RUST SUET SUIT SUPT TUFT YURT

••UT
ABUT AOUT BOUT BRUT CNUT DEUT FAUT GLUT GOUT HAUT KNUT LOUT NAUT NEUT PEUT PLUT POUT ROUT SCUT SHUT SMUT TAUT TEUT

TNUT
TOUT
XOUT

U•U•
UHUH
ULUS
UNUM
UOUS

U••U
UNAU
URDU

•UU•
DUUN

•U•U
FUBU
FUGU
GURU
HUTU
JUJU
KUDU
LUAU
LULU
OULU
PUPU
SULU
TUTU
ZULU

UV••
UVEA
UVWX

U•V•
UOVO

U••V
UNIV
UNLV

•UV•
DUVE
GUVS
LUVS
SUVA
SUVS
TUVW

••UV
STUV

U•W•
UTWO
UVWX

•UW•
EUWE

•U•W
TUVW

••UW
DOUW

UX••
UXOR

U••X
UNIX
UVWX

•UX•
LUXE

••UX
BRUX
CRUX
DEUX
DOUX
EAUX
FAUX
FEUX
FLUX
JEUX
ROUX
VAUX
YEUX

U•Y•
UEYS

U••Y
UGLY
UHRY
UPSY
UREY
URGY

•UY•
BUYS
CUYD
GUYS
NUYS
PUYI

•U•Y
BUOY
BURY
BUSY
CUNY
DUFY
DULY
DUTY
FUMY
FURY
HUEY
JUDY
JULY
JURY
LUCY
PUNY
QUAY
RUBY
RUDY
RULY
SUEY
SUNY
SUZY

UZ••
UZIS

•UZ•
BUZZ
FUZZ
OUZO
PUZO
SUZE
SUZI
SUZY

•U•Z
BUTZ
BUZZ
FUTZ
FUZZ
LUIZ
LUTZ
QUIZ
SUEZ
YUTZ

••UZ
CRUZ

VA••
VACA
VACS
VADE
VADM
VAGI
VAGS
VAIL
VAIN
VALE
VALO
VAMP
VANE
VANS
VARO
VARY
VASA
VASE
VASO
VAST
VATS
VATU
VAUD
VAUX
VAVS
VAYA

V•A•
VDAY
VEAL
VEAU
VIAL
VLAD
VRAI

V••A
VACA
VASA
VAYA
VEDA
VEGA
VELA
VENA
VERA
VETA
VIDA
VILA
VINA
VISA
VITA
VIVA
VORA

•VA•
AVAL
EVAC
EVAH
EVAL
EVAN
EVAP
EVAS
IVAN
IVAR
OVAL
TVAD

•V•A
AVIA
TVMA
UVEA

••VA
ALVA
BOVA
CAVA
DEVA
DIVA
FAVA
HAVA
HIVA
JAVA
KAVA
KIVA
LAVA
LEVA
NEVA
NOVA
REVA
RIVA
SIVA
SUVA
VIVA

V•B•
VIBE

V••B
VERB

VC••
VCRS

V•C•
VACA
VACS
VICE
VICI
VICO
VOCE

V••C
VISC

•VC•
JVCS

•V•C
AVEC
EVAC

VD••
VDAY
VDTS

V•D•
VADE
VADM
VEDA
VIDA
VIDE
VIDI
VIDS

V••D
VAUD
VELD
VEND
VIED
VLAD
VOID

•VD•
BVDS
DVDS

•V•D
AVID
OVID
TVAD

••VD
BLVD
NKVD

VE••
VEAL
VEAU
VEDA
VEEP
VEER
VEES
VEGA
VEGS
VEIL
VEIN
VELA
VELD
VELO
VENA
VEND
VENI
VENN
VENO
VENT
VERA
VERB
VERE
VERN
VERO
VERS
VERT
VERY
VEST
VETA
VETO
VETS

V•E•
VEEP
VEER
VEES
VIED
VIER
VIES
VIET
VIEW
VTEN
VUES

V••E
VADE
VALE
VANE
VASE
VERE
VIBE
VICE
VIDE
VILE
VINE
VISE
VITE
VIVE
VOCE
VOLE
VORE
VOTE
VYSE

•VE•
AVEC
AVER
AVES
EVEL
EVEN
EVER
EVES
IVES
IVEY
OVEN
OVER
RVER
SVEN
UVEA
YVES

•V•E
EVIE
EVOE
IVIE

••VE
CAVE
COVE
DAVE
DIVE
DOVE
DUVE
EAVE
FAVE
FIVE
GAVE
GIVE
HAVE
HIVE
HOVE
IDVE
JIVE
JOVE
LAVE
LIVE
LOVE
MOVE
NAVE
NEVE
NOVE
PAVE
RAVE
REVE
RIVE
ROVE
SAVE
SEVE
TOVE
VIVE
WAVE
WEVE
WIVE
WOVE

V•G•
VAGI
VAGS
VEGA
VEGS
VIGO
VIGS
VUGS

V••G
VING
VULG

•VG•
AVGS

•V•G
TVPG

•V•H
EVAH

VI••
VIAL
VIBE
VICE
VICI
VICO
VIDA
VIDE
VIDI
VIDS
VIED
VIER
VIES
VIET
VIEW
VIGO
VIGS
VIII
VILA
VILE
VIMS
VINA
VINE
VING
VINI
VINO
VINS
VINY
VIOL
VIPS
VISA
VISC
VISE
VITA
VITE
VITI
VITO
VITR
VITS
VIVA
VIVE
VIVI
VIVO

V•I•
VAIL
VAIN
VEIL
VEIN
VIII
VOID
VOIP
VOIR
VOIT
VOIX
VSIX

V••I
VAGI
VENI
VICI
VIDI
VIII
VINI
VITI
VIVI
VRAI

•VI•
AVIA
AVID
AVIS
AVIV
CVII
DVII
EVIE
EVIL
IVIE
LVII
MVII
OVID
OVIS
XVII

•V•I
CVII
DVII
LVII
MVII
XVII

••VI
CCVI
CDVI
CLVI
CMVI
CXVI
DAVI
DCVI
DEVI
DLVI
DXVI
JOVI
LAVI
LEVI
LXVI
MCVI
MDVI
MLVI
MMVI
MXVI
NEVI
RAVI
TAVI
VIVI
XCVI
XLVI
XXVI

V••K
VOLK

VL••
VLAD

V•L•
VALE
VALO
VELA
VELD
VELO
VILA
VILE
VOLE
VOLK
VOLS
VOLT
VULG

V••L
VAIL
VEAL
VEIL
VIAL
VIOL
VTOL

•V•L
AVAL
EVAL
EVEL
EVIL
OVAL

V•M•
VAMP
VIMS

V••M
VADM
VOOM

•VM•
DVMS
TVMA

•V•M
OVUM

V•N•
VANE
VANS
VENA
VEND
VENI
VENN
VENO
VENT
VINA
VINE
VING
VINI
VINO
VINS
VINY

V••N
VAIN
VEIN
VENN
VERN
VTEN

•V•N
AVON
EVAN
EVEN
IVAN
OVEN
SVEN

VO••
VOCE
VOID
VOIP
VOIR
VOIT
VOIX
VOLE
VOLK
VOLS
VOLT
VOOM
VORA
VORE
VOSS
VOTE
VOUS
VOWS

V•O•
VIOL
VOOM
VSOP
VTOL

V••O
VALO
VARO
VASO
VELO
VENO
VERO
VETO
VICO
VIGO
VINO
VITO
VIVO

•VO•
AVON
AVOS
AVOW
EVOE
IVOR
LVOV

••VO
DEVO
LEVO
NOVO
PAVO
TIVO
UOVO
VIVO

V•P•
VIPS

V••P
VAMP
VEEP
VOIP
VSOP

•VP•
MVPS
TVPG

•V•P
EVAP

••VP
RSVP

VR••
VRAI

V•R•
VARO
VARY
VCRS
VERA
VERB
VERE
VERN
VERO
VERS
VERT
VERY
VORA
VORE

V••R
VEER
VIER
VITR
VOIR

•VR•
EVRY

•V•R
AVER
EVER
IVAR
IVOR
OVER
RVER

VS••
VSIX
VSOP

V•S•
VASA
VASE
VASO
VAST
VEST
VISA
VISC
VISE
VOSS
VYSE

V••S
VACS
VAGS
VANS
VATS
VAVS
VCRS
VDTS
VEES
VEGS
VERS
VETS
VIDS
VIES
VIGS
VIMS
VINS
VIPS
VITS
VOLS
VOSS
VOUS
VOWS
VUES
VUGS

•V•S
AVES
AVGS
AVIS
AVOS
BVDS
DVDS
DVMS
EVAS
EVES
IVES
JVCS
MVPS
OVIS
PVTS
SVXS
YVES

••VS
ATVS
BEVS
CAVS
CRVS
DEVS
DIVS
DMVS
ENVS
ESVS
GOVS
GTVS
GUVS
INVS
LAVS
LUVS
MAVS
MPVS
ORVS
POVS
REVS
RIVS
SOVS
SUVS
TAVS
VAVS

VT••
VTEN
VTOL

V•T•
VATS
VATU
VDTS
VETA
VETO
VETS
VITA
VITE
VITI
VITO
VITR
VITS
VOTE

V••T
VAST
VENT
VERT
VEST
VIET
VOIT
VOLT

•VT•
PVTS

••VT
GOVT

VU••
VUES
VUGS
VULG

V•U•
VAUD
VAUX
VOUS

V••U
VATU
VEAU

•VU•
OVUM

••VU
LEVU

V•V•
VAVS
VIVA
VIVE
VIVI
VIVO

•V•V
AVIV
LVOV

VW••
VWXY

V•W•
VOWS

V••W
VIEW

•VW•
UVWX

•V•W
AVOW

••VW
TUVW

V•X•
VWXY

V••X
VAUX
VOIX
VSIX

•VX•
SVXS

•V•X
UVWX

VY••
VYSE

V•Y•
VAYA

V••Y
VARY
VDAY
VERY
VINY
VWXY

•V•Y
EVRY
IVEY

••VY
ALVY
BEVY
CAVY
DAVY
ENVY
JIVY
LEVY
LIVY
NAVY
WAVY

WA••
WAAC
WABE
WACE
WACK
WACO
WACS
WADE
WADI
WADS
WAFS
WAFT
WAGE
WAGS
WAHL
WAHR
WAHS
WAIF
WAIL
WAIN
WAIT
WAKA
WAKE
WALD
WALE
WALK
WALL
WALT
WAND
WANE
WANG
WANT
WANY
WARD
WARE
WARM
WARN
WARP
WARS
WART
WARY
WASH
WASI
WASP
WASS
WAST
WATS
WATT
WAVE
WAVY
WAWA
WAWS
WAXY
WAYS

W•A•
WAAC
WEAK
WEAL
WEAN
WEAR
WHAM
WHAP
WHAT
WOAD
WRAP
WRAY

W••A
WAKA
WAWA
WHOA
WNBA
WUSA

•WA•
AWAG
AWAY
BWAY
DWAN
EWAN
KWAI
KWAN
SWAB
SWAG
SWAK
SWAM
SWAN
SWAP
SWAT
SWAY
TWAS
TWAY

•W•A
TWOA
YWCA
YWHA

••WA
AIWA
BIWA
BOWA
IOWA
ROWA
TEWA
TIWA
WAWA

W•B•
WABE
WEBB
WEBS
WNBA

W••B
WEBB
WEEB
WOMB

•W•B
SWAB
TWOB

••WB
GHWB
ROWB

WC••
WCTU

W•C•
WACE
WACK
WACO
WACS
WICK

W••C
WAAC
WISC

•WC•
YWCA

•W•C
TWOC

••WC
ROWC

W•D•
WADE
WADI
WADS
WEDS
WIDE

W••D
WALD
WAND
WARD
WEED
WELD
WEND
WHOD
WHYD
WILD
WIND
WOAD
WOOD
WORD

•W•D
AWED
OWED
SWED
TWOD

••WD
DOWD
LAWD
LEWD
ROWD

WE••
WEAK
WEAL
WEAN
WEAR
WEBB
WEBS
WEDS
WEEB
WEED
WEEK
WEEP
WEER
WEFT
WEIL
WEIN
WEIR
WEIS
WELD
WELK
WELL
WELT
WELU
WEND
WENG
WENS
WENT
WEPT
WERE
WERT
WEST
WETS
WEVE

W•E•
WEEB
WEED
WEEK
WEEP
WEER
WHEE
WHEN
WHET
WHEW
WHEY
WIEN
WOES
WREN
WYES

W••E
WABE
WACE
WADE
WAGE
WAKE
WALE
WANE
WARE
WAVE
WERE
WEVE
WHEE
WIDE
WIFE
WILE
WINE
WIPE
WIRE
WISE
WIVE
WOKE
WOLE
WORE
WOVE
WYLE

•WE•
AWED
AWES
EWEN
EWER
EWES
GWEN
LWEI
OWED
OWEN
OWER
OWES
SWED
SWEE
TWEE
ZWEI

•W•E
OWIE
SWEE
TWEE
TWOE

••WE
BOWE
EUWE
HOWE
LOWE
ROWE

W•F•
WAFS
WAFT
WEFT
WIFE
WIFI

W••F
WAIF
WOLF
WOOF
WORF

••WF
NEWF
ROWF

W•G•
WAGE
WAGS
WIGS

W••G
WANG
WENG
WHIG
WING
WONG

•W•G
AWAG
SWAG
SWIG
TWIG

••WG
DAWG
HAWG
ROWG

WH••
WHAM
WHAP
WHAT
WHEE
WHEN
WHET
WHEW
WHEY
WHIG
WHIM
WHIP
WHIR
WHIT
WHIZ
WHOA
WHOD
WHOM
WHOP
WHOS
WHUP
WHYD
WHYS

W•H•
WAHL
WAHR
WAHS
WUHL

W••H
WASH
WISH
WITH

•WH•
YWHA

••WH
ROWH

WI••
WICK
WIDE
WIEN
WIFE
WIFI
WIGS
WIIS
WIKI
WILD
WILE
WILL
WILT
WILY
WIMP
WIND
WINE
WING
WINK
WINN
WINS
WINY
WIPE
WIRE
WIRY
WISC
WISE
WISH
WISK
WISP
WITH
WITS
WITT
WIVE

W•I•
WAIF
WAIL
WAIN
WAIT
WEIL
WEIN
WEIR
WEIS
WHIG
WHIM
WHIP
WHIR
WHIT
WHIZ
WIIS
WRIT
WWII

W••I
WADI
WASI
WIFI
WIKI
WWII
WWII

•W•I
KWAI
LWEI
WWII
ZWEI

••WI
KIWI
ROWI

•WI•
FWIW
IWIN
OWIE
SWIG
SWIM
SWIT
TWIG
TWIN
TWIT
TWIX

W•J•
WOJO

••WJ
ROWJ

WK••
WKLY
WKRP

W•K•
WAKA
WAKE
WIKI
WOKE
WOKS

W••K
WACK
WALK
WEAK
WEEK
WELK
WICK
WINK
WISK
WONK
WORK
WOUK

•W•K
EWOK
SWAK

••WK
GAWK
HAWK
ROWK

W•L•
WALD
WALE
WALK
WALL
WALT
WELD
WELK
WELL
WELT
WELU
WILD
WILE
WILL
WILT
WILY
WKLY
WOLE
WOLF
WYLE

W••L
WAHL
WAIL
WALL
WEAL
WEIL
WELL
WILL
WOOL
WUHL

•WL•
AWLS
OWLS
OWLY

•W•L
AWOL

••WL
BAWL
BOWL
COWL
FOWL
HOWL
JOWL
MEWL
PAWL
ROWL
YAWL
YOWL

W•M•
WIMP
WOMB

W••M
WARM
WHAM
WHIM
WHOM
WORM

•WM•
CWMS

•W•M
SWAM
SWIM
SWUM

••WM
HOWM
ROWM

WN••
WNBA

W•N•
WAND
WANE
WANG
WANT
WANY
WEND
WENG
WENS
WENT
WIND
WINE
WING
WINK
WINN
WINS
WINY
WONG
WONK
WONT
WYNN

W••N
WAIN
WARN
WEAN
WEIN
WHEN
WIEN
WINN
WORN
WREN
WYNN

•WN•
AWNS
AWNY
OWNS

•W•N
DWAN
EWAN
EWEN
GWEN
GWYN
IWIN
IWON
KWAN
KWON
OWEN
SWAN
TWIN

••WN
DAWN
DOWN
FAWN
GOWN
HAWN
HEWN
LAWN
MOWN
PAWN
ROWN
SAWN
SEWN
SOWN
TOWN
YAWN

WO••
WOAD
WOES
WOJO
WOKE
WOKS
WOLE
WOLF
WOMB
WONG
WONK
WONT
WOOD
WOOF
WOOL
WOOS
WORD
WORE
WORF
WORK
WORM
WORN
WORT
WOUK
WOVE
WOWS

W•O•
WHOA
WHOD
WHOM
WHOP
WHOS
WOOD
WOOF
WOOL
WOOS

W••O
WACO
WOJO
WTWO

•WO•
AWOL
CWOS
EWOK
IWON
KWON
TWOA
TWOB
TWOC
TWOD
TWOE
TWOS

••WO
BTWO
KTWO
ROWO
UTWO
WTWO

W•P•
WEPT
WIPE

W••P
WARP
WASP
WEEP
WHAP
WHIP
WHOP
WHUP
WIMP
WISP
WKRP
WRAP

•WP•
TWPS

•W•P
SWAP

••WP
GAWP
ROWP
YAWP

••WQ
ROWQ

WR••
WRAP
WRAY
WREN
WRIT
WRXS

W•R•
WARD
WARE
WARM
WARN
WARP
WARS
WART
WARY
WERE
WERT
WIRE
WIRY
WKRP
WORD
WORE
WORF
WORK
WORM
WORN
WORT

W••R
WAHR
WEAR
WEER
WEIR
WHIR

•WR•
AWRY

•W•R
EWER
OWER

••WR
MAWR
ROWR

W•S•
WASH
WASI
WASP
WASS
WAST
WEST
WISC
WISE
WISH
WISK
WISP
WUSA
WUSS
WYSS

W••S
WACS
WADS
WAFS
WAGS
WAHS
WARS
WASS
WATS
WAWS
WAYS
WEBS
WEDS
WEIS
WENS
WETS
WHOS
WHYS
WIGS
WIIS
WINS
WITS
WOES
WOKS
WOOS
WOWS
WRXS
WUSS
WYES
WYSS

•W•S
AWES
AWLS
AWNS
CWMS
CWOS
EWES
HWYS
OWES
OWLS
OWNS
PWTS
RWYS
TWAS
TWOS
TWPS

••WS
BMWS
BOWS
CAWS
COWS
DAWS
DEWS
HAWS
HEWS
HOWS
JAWS
JEWS
LAWS
LOWS
MAWS
MEWS
MOWS
NEWS
PAWS
PEWS
POWS
ROWS
SAWS
SEWS
SOWS
TAWS
TOWS
VOWS
WAWS
WOWS
YAWS
YEWS

WT••
WTWO

W•T•
WATS
WATT
WCTU
WETS
WITH
WITS
WITT

W••T
WAFT
WAIT
WALT
WANT
WART
WAST
WATT
WEFT
WELT
WENT
WEPT
WERT
WEST
WHAT
WHET
WHIT
WILT
WITT
WONT
WORT
WRIT

•WT•
GWTW
PWTS

•W•T
SWAT
SWIT
TWIT

••WT
ATWT
GRWT
NEWT
NTWT
ROWT
TAWT

WU••
WUHL
WUSA
WUSS

W•U•
WHUP
WOUK

W••U
WCTU
WELU

•WU•
SWUM

••WU
ROWU

W•V•
WAVE
WAVY
WEVE
WIVE
WOVE

••WV
ROWV

WW••
WWII

W•W•
WAWA
WAWS
WOWS
WTWO

W••W
WHEW

•W•W
FWIW
GWTW

••WW
ROWW

WX••
WXYZ

W•X•
WAXY
WRXS

•WX•
VWXY

•W•X
TWIX

••WX
ROWX
UVWX

WY••
WYES
WYLE
WYNN
WYSS

W•Y•
WAYS
WHYD
WHYS
WXYZ

W••Y
WANY
WARY
WAVY
WAXY
WHEY
WILY
WINY
WIRY
WKLY
WRAY

•WY•
GWYN
HWYS
RWYS

•W•Y
AWAY
AWNY
AWRY
BWAY
OWLY
SWAY
TWAY
VWXY

••WY
COWY
DEWY
HGWY
PKWY
ROWY

W••Z
WHIZ
WXYZ

••WZ
ROWZ

X•A•
XIAN
XMAS
XRAY

X••A
XENA
XTRA

•XA•
EXAM

•X•A
IXIA

••XA
COXA
HEXA
SIXA
TAXA

XB••
XBOX

••XB
SIXB

XC••
XCII
XCIV
XCIX
XCVI

•XC•
CXCI
CXCV
DXCI
DXCV
EXCH
EXCL
MXCI
MXCV

•X•C
EXEC

••XC
CCXC
CDXC
CMXC
DCXC
MCXC
MDXC
MMXC
SIXC

XD••
XDIN
XDIV

•X•D
AXED
EXED
EXOD

••XD
SIXD

XE••
XENA
XENO
XEON
XERO

X•E•
XKES
XMEN

•XE•
AXED
AXEL
AXER
AXES
EXEC
EXED
EXEL
EXES
OXEN
OXES

•X•E
AXLE

••XE
FIXE
LUXE
SAXE
SIXE

X••G
XING

•XG•
EXGI

•X•H
EXCH

XI••
XIAN
XIII
XING
XIXO

X•I•
XCII
XCIV
XCIX
XDIN
XDIV
XIII
XLII
XLIV
XLIX
XVII
XXII
XXIV
XXIX

X••I
XCII
XCVI
XIII
XLII
XLVI
XVII
XXII
XXVI
XXXI

•XI•
AXIL
AXIS
CXII
CXIV
CXIX
DXII
DXIV
DXIX
EXIT
IXIA
LXII
LXIV
LXIX
MXII
MXIV
MXIX
XXII
XXIV
XXIX

•X•I
CXCI
CXII
CXLI
CXVI
CXXI
DXCI
DXII
DXLI
DXVI
DXXI
EXGI
LXII
LXVI
LXXI
MXCI
MXII
MXLI
MXVI
MXXI
XXII
XXVI
XXXI

••XI
CCXI
CDXI
CLXI
CMXI
CXXI
DCXI
DLXI
DXXI
LXXI
MAXI
MCXI
MDXI
MLXI
MMXI
MXXI
TAXI
XXXI

XK••
XKES
XKRS

XL••
XLII
XLIV
XLIX
XLVI

X•L•
XYLO

•XL•
AXLE
CXLI
CXLV
DXLI
DXLV
MXLI
MXLV

•X•L
AXEL
AXIL
EXCL
EXEL

••XL
CCXL
CDXL
CMXL
DCXL
MCXL
MDXL
MMXL

XM••
XMAS
XMEN

•X•M
EXAM

X•N•
XENA
XENO
XING

X••N
XDIN
XEON
XIAN
XMEN

•X•N
AXON
EXON
OXEN
OXON

XO••
XORY
XOUT

X•O•
XBOX
XEON

X••O
XENO
XERO
XIXO
XYLO

•XO•
AXON
EXOD
EXON
OXON
UXOR

•X•O
EXPO

••XO
NEXO
TAXO
TOXO
XIXO

•XP•
EXPO
EXPT

XR••
XRAY

X•R•
XERO
XKRS
XORY
XTRA

•X•R
AXER
UXOR

X•S•
XYST

X••S
XKES
XKRS
XMAS

•X•S
AXES
AXIS
EXES
EXTS
OXES
OXUS

••XS
GTXS
INXS
NSXS
RSXS
SLXS
SRXS
SVXS
TSXS
WRXS

XT••
XTRA

X••T
XOUT
XYST

•XT•
EXTS

•X•T
EXIT
EXPT

••XT
MIXT
NEXT
TEXT

X•U•
XOUT

•XU•
OXUS

XV••
XVII

X•V•
XCVI
XLVI
XXVI

X••V
XCIV
XDIV
XLIV
XXIV
XXXV

•XV•
CXVI
DXVI
LXVI
MXVI
XXVI

•X•V
CXCV
CXIV
CXLV
CXXV
DXCV
DXIV
DXLV
DXXV
LXIV
LXXV
MXCV
MXIV
MXLV
MXXV
XXIV
XXXV

••XV
CCXV
CDXV
CLXV
CMXV
CXXV
DCXV
DLXV
DXXV
LXXV
MCXV
MDXV
MLXV
MMXV
MXXV
XXXV

XX••
XXII
XXIV
XXIX
XXVI
XXXI
XXXV
XXXX

X•X•
XIXO
XXXI
XXXV
XXXX

X••X
XBOX
XCIX
XLIX
XXIX
XXXX

•XX•
CXXI
CXXV
CXXX
DXXI
DXXV
DXXX
LXXI
LXXV
LXXX
MXXI
MXXV
MXXX
XXXI
XXXV
XXXX

•X•X
CXIX
CXXX
DXIX
DXXX
LXIX
LXXX
MXIX
MXXX
XXIX
XXXX

••XX
CCXX
CDXX
CLXX
CMXX
CXXX
DCXX
DLXX
DXXX
FIXX
FOXX
LXXX
MAXX
MCXX
MDXX
MLXX
MMXX
MXXX
XXXX

XY••
XYLO
XYST

X••Y
XORY
XRAY

•XY•
WXYZ

••XY
BOXY
DIXY
DOXY
FOXY
LOXY
NIXY
PIXY
ROXY
SEXY
TAXY
VWXY
WAXY

•X•Z
WXYZ

YA••
YADA
YAKS
YALE
YALL
YALU
YAMS
YANG
YANK
YAPS
YARD
YARE
YARN
YAWL
YAWN
YAWP
YAWS
YAYS

Y•A•
YEAH
YEAN
YEAR
YEAS
YUAN

Y••A
YADA
YMCA
YMHA

YODA YOGA YUBA YUMA YWCA YWHA

•YA• AYAH BYAM CYAN DYAD DYAN IYAR KYAT NYAD PYAS RYAL RYAN RYAS

•Y•A AYLA CYMA DYNA EYRA HYLA KYRA LYRA MYNA MYRA TYRA ZYRA

••YA ANYA ENYA GOYA HIYA HOYA ILYA MAYA NAYA SOYA TOYA VAYA

YB•• YBOR

Y•B• YOBS YUBA

•YB• NYBY

•Y•B BYOB MYOB

Y•C• YECH YMCA YUCK YWCA

•YC• CYCL DYCE DYCK EYCK FYCE LYCO MYCO NYCT TYCO

•Y•C SYNC

••YC GLYC

Y•D• YADA YODA YODH YODS

Y••D YARD YOND YOUD

•YD• AYDE HYDE HYDR

•Y•D BYRD DYAD DYED EYED LYND NYAD NYPD

••YD BOYD CUYD LOYD SOYD WHYD

YE•• YEAH YEAN YEAR YEAS YECH YEGG YELL YELP YENS YEOH YEOW YEPS YESM YETI YEUX YEWS

Y•E• YLEM YNEZ YSER YVES

Y••E YALE YARE YIPE YOKE YORE YULE

•YE• AYER AYES BYES DYED DYER DYES EYED EYER EYES HYER HYET LYES NYET OYER OYEZ RYES TYEE TYES WYES

•Y•E AYDE AYME BYME BYTE CYME CYTE DYCE DYKE DYNE EYRE FYCE GYNE GYRE HYDE HYPE KYLE LYLE LYME LYNE LYRE LYSE LYTE NYSE PYKE PYLE PYNE PYRE RYLE RYNE SYNE TYEE TYKE TYNE TYPE TYRE VYSE WYLE

••YE ARYE FAYE FRYE GAYE JAYE KAYE KEYE RAYE SKYE SLYE STYE TAYE

YG•• YGOR

Y•G• YEGG YOGA YOGI YUGO

Y••G YANG YEGG YONG YUNG

•Y•G BYNG LYNG

••YG ROYG

Y•H• YMHA YOHO YWHA

Y••H YEAH YECH YEOH YODH

•Y•H AYAH MYTH

••YH BAYH

YI•• YIPE YIPS

Y•I• YMIR

Y••I YETI YOGI YURI

•YI• AYIN LYIN

•Y•I GYRI

••YI MAYI PUYI

Y•K• YAKS YOKE YOKO YUKS

Y••K YANK YOLK YORK YUCK

•YK• DYKE PYKE TYKE

•Y•K DYCK EYCK NYUK

YL•• YLEM

Y•L• YALE YALL YALU YELL YELP YOLK YULE

Y••L YALL YAWL YELL YOWL

•YL• AYLA CYLS HYLA KYLE LYLE LYLY PYLE RYLE SYLL SYLS TYLO WYLE XYLO

•Y•L CYCL RYAL SYLL

••YL AMYL ARYL IDYL

YM•• YMCA YMHA YMIR

Y•M• YAMS YUMA

Y••M YESM YLEM

•YM• AYME BYME CYMA CYME GYMS HYMN LYME MYMY SYMS

•Y•M BYAM

••YM CLYM ETYM ONYM

YN•• YNEZ

Y•N• YANG YANK YENS YOND YONG YUNG

Y••N YARN YAWN YEAN YORN YUAN

•YN• BYNG CYNO DYNA DYNE GYNE GYNT GYNY LYND LYNE LYNG LYNN LYNX MYNA NYNY PYNE RYNE SYNC SYNE SYNS TYNE WYNN

•Y•N AYIN CYAN DYAN HYMN LYIN LYNN LYON RYAN RYUN WYNN

••YN ALYN BRYN GLYN GWYN

YO•• YOBS YODA YODH YODS YOGA YOGI YOHO YOKE YOKO YOLK YOND YONG YORE YORK YORN YOST YOUD YOUR YOWL YOYO

Y•O• YBOR YEOH YEOW YGOR

Y••O YOHO YOKO YOYO YUGO

•YO• BYOB LYON MYOB

•Y•O CYNO CYTO GYRO HYPO LYCO MYCO NYRO PYRO TYCO TYLO TYPO TYRO XYLO

••YO BOYO CRYO DAYO ENYO HIYO INYO KAYO MAYO TOYO YOYO

Y•P• YAPS YEPS YIPE YIPS

Y••P YAWP YELP

•YP• GYPS HYPE HYPN HYPO NYPD TYPE TYPO

Y•R• YARD YARE YARN YORE YORK YORN YURI YURT

Y••R YBOR YEAR YGOR YMIR YOUR YSER

•YR• BYRD EYRA EYRE GYRE GYRI GYRO KYRA LYRA LYRE MYRA NYRO PYRE PYRO TYRA TYRE TYRO ZYRA

•Y•R AYER DYER EYER HYDR HYER IYAR OYER

••YR LTYR

YS•• YSER

Y•S• YESM YOST

Y••S YAKS YAMS YAPS YAWS YAYS YEAS YENS YEPS YEWS YIPS YOBS YODS YUKS YVES

•YS• CYST LYSE MYST NYSE SYST VYSE WYSS XYST

•Y•S AYES BYES CYLS DYES EYES GYMS GYPS LYES PYAS RYAS RYES SYLS SYMS SYNS TYES TYUS WYES WYSS

••YS BAYS BEYS BOYS BUYS CAYS DAYS DRYS EDYS FAYS FOYS GUYS HAYS HEYS HWYS JAYS JOYS KAYS KEYS LAYS MAYS NAYS NUYS PAYS PHYS QTYS RAYS RHYS RWYS SAYS SKYS SOYS SPYS TOYS UEYS WAYS WHYS YAYS

Y•T• YETI YUTZ

Y••T YOST YURT

•YT• BYTE CYTE CYTO LYTE MYTH

•Y•T CYST GYNT HYET KYAT MYST NYCT NYET SYST XYST

••YT FOYT HOYT PAYT PHYT

YU•• YUAN YUBA YUCK YUGO YUKS YULE YUMA YUNG YURI YURT YUTZ

Y•U• YEUX YOUD YOUR

Y••U YALU

•YU• NYUK RYUN TYUS

YV•• YVES

YW•• YWCA YWHA

Y•W• YAWL YAWN YAWP YAWS YEWS YOWL

Y••W YEOW

Y••X YEUX

•Y•X LYNX

••YX ONYX ORYX STYX

Y•Y• YAYS YOYO

•Y•Y GYNY LYLY MYMY NYBY NYNY

Y••Z YNEZ YUTZ

•Y•Z OYEZ

••YZ BOYZ JAYZ WXYZ

ZA•• ZACH ZACK ZAFU ZAGS ZAHN ZALE ZANE ZANT ZANY ZAPS ZARA ZARF ZASU ZAZA

Z•A• ZBAR ZEAL

Z••A ZARA ZAZA ZETA ZIMA ZINA ZIRA ZOLA ZONA ZORA ZURA ZYRA

•ZA• AZAN CZAR TZAR

•Z•A EZRA OZMA

••ZA GAZA GIZA ITZA LIZA REZA ZAZA

ZB•• ZBAR

Z•B• ZEBU

Z•C• ZACH ZACK ZECH

Z••C ZINC ZOIC

Z•D• ZEDS

Z••D ZEND ZMED

•Z•D IZOD

ZE•• ZEAL ZEBU ZECH ZEDS ZEES ZEHN ZEIT ZEKE ZELL ZEND ZENO ZEPH ZERO ZEST ZETA ZEUS

Z•E• ZEES ZMED ZWEI

Z••E ZALE ZANE ZEKE ZINE ZONE

•ZE• EZEK EZER

••ZE ADZE DAZE DOZE FAZE GAZE HAZE LAZE MAZE MIZE ONZE OOZE RAZE SIZE SUZE

Z•F• ZAFU ZIFF

Z••F ZARF ZIFF

Z•G• ZAGS ZIGS ZOGI

Z••G ZING

ZH•• ZHOU

Z•H• ZAHN ZEHN

Z••H ZACH ZECH ZEPH

ZI•• ZIFF ZIGS ZILL ZILS ZIMA ZINA ZINC ZINE ZING ZINS ZION ZIPS ZIRA ZITI ZITO ZITS ZIZZ

Z•I• ZEIT ZOIC

Z••I ZITI ZOGI ZORI ZUNI ZWEI

•ZI• AZIZ EZIO UZIS

••ZI NAZI SUZI

Z•K• ZEKE

Z••K ZACK ZONK ZOUK

•Z•K EZEK

Z•L• ZALE ZELL ZILL ZILS ZOLA ZULU

Z••L ZEAL ZELL ZILL ZOOL

•Z•L AZUL

ZM•• ZMED

Z•M• ZIMA

Z••M ZOOM

•ZM• OZMA

Z•N• ZANE ZANT ZANY ZEND ZENO ZINA ZINC ZINE ZING ZINS ZONA ZONE ZONK ZUNI

Z••N ZAHN ZEHN ZION ZORN

•Z•N AZAN

ZO•• ZOGI ZOIC ZOLA ZONA ZONE ZONK ZOOL ZOOM ZOOS ZOOT ZORA ZORI ZORN ZOTZ ZOUK

Z•O• ZHOU ZION ZOOL ZOOM ZOOS ZOOT

Z••O ZENO ZERO ZITO

•ZO• AZOV IZOD

•Z•O EZIO

••ZO BOZO DOZO ENZO MAZO MOZO ORZO OUZO PUZO

Z•P• ZAPS ZEPH ZIPS

Z•R• ZARA ZARF ZERO ZIRA ZORA ZORI ZORN ZURA ZYRA

Z••R ZBAR

•ZR• EZRA

•Z•R AZUR CZAR EZER TZAR

Z•S• ZASU ZEST

Z••S ZAGS ZAPS ZEDS ZEES ZEUS ZIGS ZILS ZINS ZIPS ZITS ZOOS

••ZS DAZS DMZS

•Z•S TZUS UZIS

Z•T• ZETA ZITI ZITO ZITS ZOTZ

Z••T ZANT ZEIT ZEST ZOOT

ZU•• ZULU ZUNI ZURA

Z•U• ZEUS ZOUK

Z••U ZAFU ZASU ZEBU ZHOU ZULU

•ZU• AZUL AZUR TZUS

•Z•V AZOV

ZW•• ZWEI

ZY•• ZYRA

Z••Y ZANY

•Z•Y IZZY OZZY

••ZY COZY DOZY HAZY IZZY LAZY MAZY OOZY OZZY SUZY

Z•Z• ZAZA ZIZZ

Z••Z ZIZZ ZOTZ

•ZZ• IZZY OZZY

•Z•Z AZIZ

••ZZ BUZZ FIZZ FUZZ JAZZ PIZZ RAZZ ZIZZ

5

AA•••
AABBA
AAHED
AALTO
AAMCO
AAMES
AANDE
AANDM
AANDP
AANDW
AARAU
AARGH
AARON

A•A••
ABABA
ABACA
ABACI
ABACK
ABACO
ABAFT
ABAJO
ABASE
ABASH
ABATE
ACADS
ADAGE
ADAIR
ADAMA
ADAMS
ADANA
ADANO
ADAOK
ADAPT
ADARN
ADARS
AEAEA
AFARS
AGAIN
AGALS
AGAMA
AGAME
AGANA
AGAPE
AGARN
AGARS
AGASP
AGATE
AGAVE
AGAZE
AHAIR
AHANG
AKAIS
ALACK
ALADO
ALAIN
ALAIS
ALALA
ALAMO
ALANA
ALARM
ALATE
ALAVA
AMADA
AMADO
AMAHL
AMAHS
AMAIN
AMANA
AMAND
AMANT
AMAPA
AMARA
AMARE
AMASS
AMATI
AMATO
AMAZE
ANAGS
ANAIS
ANANA
ANAND
APACE
APAIN
APARS
APART
AQABA
ARABS
ARABY
ARADO
ARAME
ARANS
ARARA
ASAGI
ASAHI
ASAMI
ASANA
ATALA
ATALL
ATARI
ATARS
AVAIL
AVANT
AVAST
AWACS
AWAIT
AWAKE
AWARD
AWARE
AWASH
AWAVE
AYAHS
AYAKO
AZANS

A••A•
AARAU
ABBAS
ABEAM
ABEAR
ABFAB
ABRAM
ACTAS
ADDAX
ADLAI
ADMAN
ADNAN
ADWAR
AFLAC
AFLAT
AGHAS
AGUAS
AGWAY
AHEAD
AHEAP
AHMAD
AIDAN
AIMAT
AIWAS
AKBAR
ALBAN
ALBAS
ALCAN
ALEAK
ALFAS
ALGAE
ALGAL
ALGAS
ALIAS
ALKAB
ALLAH
ALLAN
ALLAY
ALMAY
ALSAB
ALTAI
ALTAR
ALVAR
ALWAY
AMMAN
AMPAS
AMRAM
AMWAY
AMYAS
ANNAL
ANNAM
ANNAN
ANNAS
ANOAS
ANSAE
ANTAE
ANTAL
ANTAS
ANWAR
ANZAC
AOKAY
APEAK
APIAN
APPAL
AQUAE
AQUAS
ARCAE
AREAL
AREAR
AREAS
ARHAT
ARIAL
ARIAN
ARIAS
ARMAH
ARMAS
ARNAZ
AROAR
ARPAD
ARRAH
ARRAN
ARRAS
ARRAU
ARRAY
ARYAN
ASCAP
ASFAT
ASIAN
ASLAK
ASLAN
ASMAD
ASNAP
ASSAD
ASSAI
ASSAM
ASSAY
ASWAN
ASWAY
ATBAR
ATBAT
ATBAY
ATEAM
ATEAT
ATLAS
ATMAN
ATPAR
ATRAS
ATTAR
ATWAR
AURAE
AURAL
AURAR
AURAS
AVGAS
AVIAN
AVIAS
AXIAL
AXMAN
AYEAR

A•••A
AABBA
ABABA
ABACA
ABOMA
ABUJA
ACCRA
ACELA
ACQUA
ACURA
ADAMA
ADANA
ADELA
ADYTA
AEAEA
AECIA
AETNA
AFTRA
AGAMA
AGANA
AGENA
AGITA
AGORA
AGURA
AHORA
AISHA
AKELA
AKIRA
AKITA
ALALA
ALANA
ALAVA
ALCOA
ALETA
ALEXA
ALGIA
ALIDA
ALISA
ALOHA
ALPHA
ALULA
AMADA
AMANA
AMAPA
AMARA
AMEBA
AMICA
AMIGA
AMNIA
ANANA
ANIMA
ANITA
ANOKA
ANTRA
AORTA
AOSTA
APNEA
APPIA
AQABA
ARARA
ARECA
ARENA
ARICA
AROMA
ARUBA
ASANA
ASPCA
ASTRA
ASYLA
ATALA
ATRIA
ATSEA
AUDRA
AVENA
AVILA
AZERA
AZUSA

•AA••
BAAED
BAALS
MAAMS
NAACP
PAAVO
RAABE
SAABS
WAACS
WAALS
WAART

•A•A•
AARAU
BABAR
BABAS
BADAT
BAHAI
BALAS
BANAL
BARAK
BASAL
BAYAR
BAYAT
CABAL
CACAO
CALAF
CAMAS
CAMAY
CANAL
CAPAS
CARAT
CARAY
CASAS
CAVAE
CAVAN
DABAT
DADAS
DAGAN
DAKAR
DALAI
DAMAS
DANAE
DAVAO
DAYAN
EAGAN
EATAT
EAVAN
FAJAS
FARAD
FARAH
FATAL
GAHAN
GALAS
GALAX
GAMAL
GAMAY
HADAT
HAGAR
HAHAS
HALAL
HALAS
HAMAN
HAMAS
HASAT
HAZAN
JACAL
JAFAR
JAHAN
JAMAL
JAPAN
JAVAN
JAVAS
JAWAT
KABAS
KADAR
KANAR
KANAS
KARAN
KARAS
KARAT
KATAS
KAUAI
KAVAS
KAYAK
KAZAN
LABAN
LADAS
LALAW
LAMAR
LAMAS
LANAI
LAPAT
LAPAZ
LARAM
LARAS
LAVAL
LAVAS
LAZAR
MACAO
MACAW
MADAM
MADAT
MAHAL
MAHAN
MALAR
MALAY
MAMAS
MANAT
MARAT
MASAI
MASAS
MAYAN
MAYAS
MAZAR
NAGAT
NAIAD
NANAK
NANAS
NARAS
NASAL
NATAL
NATAN
NAVAL
OASAL
PACAS
PAEAN
PAGAN
PALAR
PALAU
PANAM
PANAY
PAPAL
PAPAS
PAPAW
PARAS
PAWAT
QATAR
RABAT
RADAR
RAGAS
RAHAL
RAJAB
RAJAH
RAJAS
RAMAN
RAMAR
RAMAS
RANAS
RANAT
RARAE
RASAE
RAZAF
SABAL
SADAT
SAFAR
SAGAL
SAGAN
SAGAS
SAJAK
SAKAI
SALAD
SALAS
SAMAR
SANAA
SARAH
SARAI
SARAN
SATAN
SATAT
SATAY
SAYAH
TADAS
TAKAS
TALAS
TAMAR
TAPAS
TARAS
TATAR
TATAS
VACAS
WAKAS
WASAT
WAWAS
YAPAT
YAYAS
ZADAR
ZAGAT
ZAYAK

•A••A
AABBA
BABKA
BAEDA
BAEZA
BAHIA
BAISA
BAIZA
BALSA
BAMBA
BANCA
BANDA
BANTA
BARBA
BARCA
BASIA
BASRA
BASTA
BATNA
CALLA
CANEA
CANNA
CAPRA
CARLA
CARTA
CASCA
CASTA
DABBA
DACCA
DACHA
DACIA
DAIWA
DANIA
DANZA
DARIA
DARLA
DARYA
EASYA
FACIA
FACTA
FAENA
FALLA
FANTA
FATHA
FATWA
FAUNA
GAETA
GALBA
GALEA
GAMBA
GAMMA
GARDA
HABLA
HAEMA
HAIDA
HAIFA
HALVA
HANNA
HANSA
HANYA
HASTA
HATHA
JABBA
JAFFA
JALPA
JAMBA
KAFKA
KANGA
KANSA
KAPPA
KARLA
KARMA
KASHA
LABIA
LAIKA
LAILA
LALIA
LALLA
LAMIA
LANKA
LANZA
LARVA
LATKA
LAUDA
LAURA
LAYLA
MAFIA
MAGDA
MAGMA
MAGNA
MAGUA
MALTA
MAMBA
MAMMA
MANGA
MANIA
MANNA
MANTA
MARCA
MARIA
MARKA
MARLA
MARTA
MARYA
MASHA
MASSA
MAUNA
MAURA
MAZDA
NADIA
NADJA
NAFTA
NAIMA
NAINA
NAIRA
NAKFA
NAMPA
NANNA
NARDA
NATTA
PADUA
PAISA
PALEA
PALMA
PAMPA
PANDA
PANTA
PANZA
PAPUA
PARCA
PARKA
PARMA
PARRA
PARTA
PASHA
PASTA
PATNA
PAULA
PAVIA
QANDA
RAISA
RAITA
RANDA
RASPA
RASTA
SABRA
SACRA
SALMA
SALSA
SAMBA
SAMOA
SAMSA
SANAA
SANKA
SANTA
SASHA
SAUNA
TABLA
TAIGA
TAINA
TALIA
TAMPA
TANIA
TANKA
TANNA
TANYA
TARGA
TATRA
VACUA
VAMPA
VANNA
VANUA
VANYA
VARDA
VARIA
VARNA
VARYA
WAJDA
WALLA
WANDA
WANNA
YABBA
YADDA
YALTA
YARRA
YASHA
ZAPPA

••AA•
ISAAC
ISAAK
IZAAK
KRAAL
SPAAK

••A•A
ABABA
ABACA
ADAMA
ADANA
AEAEA
AGAMA
AGANA
ALALA
ALANA
ALAVA
AMADA
AMANA
AMAPA
AMARA
ANANA
AQABA
ARARA
ASANA
ATALA
BRAGA
BRAVA
BWANA
CEARA
CHAKA
CHAVA
CLARA
DEANA
DHAKA
DIANA
DRAMA
DRAVA
ELARA
FLAVA
GHANA
GRATA
GUAPA
GUAVA
IPANA
IVANA
KOALA
KUALA
LHASA
LIANA
LLAMA
LUANA
MEARA
MIATA
NGANA
NWAPA
NYALA
NYASA
OBAMA
OCALA
OHARA
OKARA
OMAHA
ORAMA
OSAKA
OXANA
OZAWA
PLANA
PLATA
PLAYA
PLAZA
PRADA
PRAHA
PRAIA
PRANA
REATA
RIATA
SCALA
SCAPA
SHANA
TIARA
TRALA
TZARA
URAWA
USAFA
XSARA

•••AA
BEKAA
SANAA

AB•••
ABABA
ABACA
ABACI
ABACK
ABACO
ABAFT
ABAJO
ABASE
ABASH
ABATE
ABBAS
ABBES
ABBEY
ABBIE
ABBOT
ABBRS
ABCDE
ABCTV
ABDEL
ABDUL
ABEAM
ABEAR
ABELE
ABEND
ABETS
ABFAB
ABHOR
ABIDE
ABIES
ABLED
ABLER
ABMHO
ABNER
ABODE
ABOHM
ABOIL
ABOMA
ABOMB
ABORT
ABOUT
ABOVE
ABOVO
ABRAM
ABRIL
ABRIM
ABRIS
ABUJA
ABUSE
ABUTS
ABUZZ
ABYSM
ABYSS
ABZUG

A•B••
AABBA
ABBAS
ABBES
ABBEY
ABBIE
ABBOT
ABBRS
ADBIZ
AKBAR
ALBAN
ALBAS
ALBEE
ALBEN
ALBOM
ALBUM
AMBER
AMBIT
AMBLE
AMBOS
AMBOY
AMBRY
ARBER
ARBIL
ARBOL
ARBOR
ARBRE
ARBUS
ARBYS
ASBIG
ATBAR
ATBAT
ATBAY
AUBER

A••B•
AABBA
ABABA
ADOBE
ADOBO
ALIBI
AMEBA
AQABA
ARABS
ARABY
ARUBA
ASHBY

A•••B
ABFAB
ABOMB
ACERB
ADLIB
ALKAB
ALSAB

•AB••
AABBA
BABAR
BABAS
BABEL
BABES
BABKA
BABOO
BABUS
BABYS
CABAL
CABBY
CABER
CABIN
CABLE
CABOB
CABOT
DABAT
DABBA
DABIH
DABON
FABER
FABIO
FABLE
FABRE
GABBY
GABEL
GABIN
GABLE
GABON
GABOR
HABER
HABIB
HABIT
HABLA
JABBA
JABOT
KABAS
KABOB
KABUL
LABAN
LABEL
LABIA
LABOR
MABEL
NABES
NABOB
NABOO
PABLO
PABST
RABAT
RABBI
RABID
RABIN
SABAL
SABER
SABIN
SABLE
SABOT
SABRA
SABRE
TABBY
TABIS
TABLA
TABLE
TABOO
TABOR
TABUS
YABBA

•A•B•
AABBA
BALBO
BAMBA
BAMBI
BARBA
BARBI
BARBQ
BARBS
CABBY
CAMBS
CANBY
CARBO
CARBS
CASBY
DABBA
DARBY
DAUBE
DAUBS
GABBY
GALBA
GAMBA
GARBO
GARBS
IAMBI
IAMBS
JABBA
JAMBA
JAMBE
JAMBS
LAMBS
LAYBY
MAMBA
MAMBO
MAYBE
NAMBY
NASBY
PAMBY
RAABE
RABBI
RAMBO
RANBY
SAABS
SAMBA
SATBY
TABBY
TAEBO
YABBA

•A••B
BANDB
CABOB
CALEB
CARIB

CAROB
HABIB
JACOB
JAKOB
JANDB
KABOB
NABOB
NAMIB
PARTB
RAJAB
RANDB
SAHIB

••AB•

ABABA
AQABA
ARABS
ARABY
BLABS
CRABS
DHABI
DRABS
GRABS
IRABU
PEABO
RAABE
SAABS
SCABS
SLABS
STABS
SWABS

••A•B

ORALB
PLANB
STAUB

•••AB

ABFAB
ALKAB
ALSAB
BYCAB
COHAB
DCCAB
ESTAB
GETAB
GOTAB
KEBAB
MCNAB
PCLAB
RAJAB
REHAB
SQUAB
VOCAB

AC•••

ACADS
ACCEL
ACCRA
ACCTS
ACEIT
ACELA
ACERB
ACERS
ACETO
ACHED
ACHER
ACHES
ACHOO
ACIDS
ACIDY
ACING
ACMES
ACNES
ACORN
ACQUA
ACRED
ACRES
ACRID
ACTAS
ACTED
ACTER
ACTES
ACTII
ACTIN
ACTIV
ACTON
ACTOR
ACTOS
ACTUP
ACUFF
ACUPS
ACURA
ACUTE

A•C••

ABCDE
ABCTV
ACCEL
ACCRA
ACCTS
AECIA
ALCAN
ALCOA
ALCOR
ANCHO
ANCON
ARCAE
ARCED
ARCHE
ARCHI
ARCHY
ASCAP
ASCII
ASCOT
ASCUS

A••C•

AAMCO
ABACA
ABACI
ABACK
ABACO
AITCH
ALACK
ALECK
ALICE
ALYCE
AMICA
AMICE
AMICI
AMICK
AMICO
AMOCO
AMUCK
APACE
ARECA
ARICA
ASICS
ASPCA
AWACS

A•••C

ADHOC
AFLAC
AFRIC
AGRIC
ANTIC
ANZAC
ASDIC
ASPIC
ASSOC
ATTIC
AURIC
AZOIC
AZTEC

•AC••

BACIO
BACKS
BACON
BACOS
CACAO
CACHE
CACTI
DACCA
DACES
DACHA
DACHE
DACIA
FACED
FACER
FACES
FACET
FACIA
FACIE
FACIL
FACTA
FACTO
FACTS
HACEK
HACKL
HACKS
HACKY
JACAL
JACET
JACEY
JACKO
JACKS
JACKY
JACOB
LACED
LACER
LACES
LACEY
LACIE
LACKS
LACTI
LACTO
MACAO
MACAW
MACED
MACER
MACES
MACHE
MACHO
MACHU
MACHY
MACKE
MACKS
MACLE
MACON
MACRO
MACYS
NACHO
NACHT
NACIO
NACRE
PACAS
PACED
PACEM
PACER
PACES
PACEY
PACHY
PACKS
PACTS
RACED
RACER
RACES
RACKS
SACCO
SACHS
SACKS
SACRA
SACRE
SACRO
TACET
TACHO
TACHS
TACIT
TACKS
TACKY
TACOS
VACAS
VACHE
VACUA
WACKO
WACKY
XACTO
YACHT
YACKS

•A•C•

AAMCO
BALCH
BANCA
BANCO
BANCS
BARCA
BARCO
BATCH
CASCA
CASCO
CATCH
CAYCE
DACCA
DANCE
DARCI
DARCY
FALCO
FANCY
FARCE
FARCI
GANCE
HATCH
LAICS
LANCE
LARCH
LATCH
MANCY
MARCA
MARCH
MARCI
MARCO
MARCY
MATCH
NAACP
NANCE
NANCI
NANCY
NARCO
NARCS
NATCH
PARCA
PARCH
PARCS
PASCH
PASCO
PATCH
PATCO
RANCH
SACCO
SATCH
SAUCE
SAUCY
TALCS
TAXCO
VANCE
VASCO
WAACS
WASCO
WATCH
YANCY

•A••C

BARIC
BASIC
HARDC
HAVOC
MADOC
MAGIC
MALIC
MANIC
NARIC
PANIC
PARTC
SALIC
VATIC

••AC•

ABACA
ABACI
ABACK
ABACO
ALACK
APACE
AWACS
BEACH
BLACK
BRACE
BRACH
BRACK
BRACT
CHACO
CLACK
COACH
COACT
CRACK
CRACY
DBACK
DRACO
ENACT
EPACT
EXACT
FLACK
GLACE
GRACE
IMACS
KEACH
KNACK
KVACK
LEACH
NAACP
NYACK
ORACH
ORACY
PEACE
PEACH
PLACE
POACH
QUACK
REACH
REACT
ROACH
SHACK
SLACK
SMACK
SNACK
SPACE
SPACY
STACK
STACY
TEACH
TRACE
TRACI
TRACK
TRACT
TRACY
WAACS
WHACK
WRACK

••A•C

BLANC
FRANC
ISAAC

•••AC

AFLAC
ANZAC
DIRAC
DIVAC
ENIAC
GETAC
GOTAC
ILEAC
ILIAC
ISAAC
LILAC
SERAC
SUMAC
TUPAC

AD•••

ADAGE
ADAIR
ADAMA
ADAMS
ADANA
ADANO
ADAOK
ADAPT
ADARN
ADARS
ADBIZ
ADDAX
ADDED
ADDER
ADDIE
ADDIN
ADDIO
ADDIS
ADDLE
ADDNL
ADDON
ADDRS
ADDTO
ADDUP
ADEEM
ADELA
ADELE
ADENI
ADENO
ADEPT
ADEUX
ADFEE
ADHEM
ADHOC
ADIEU
ADIGE
ADINS
ADIOS
ADITS
ADJTS
ADLAI
ADLER
ADLIB
ADMAN
ADMEN
ADMIN
ADMIT
ADMIX
ADNAN
ADOBE
ADOBO
ADOLF
ADOPT
ADORE
ADORN
ADOUT
ADOZE
ADREM
ADREP
ADRIP
ADULT
ADUST
ADVIL
ADWAR
ADYTA
ADZED
ADZES

A•D••

ABDEL
ABDUL
ADDAX
ADDED
ADDER
ADDIE
ADDIN
ADDIO
ADDIS
ADDLE
ADDNL
ADDON
ADDRS
ADDTO
ADDUP
AEDES
AIDAN
AIDED
AIDER
AIDES
AIDOO
ALDEN
ALDER
ANDES
ANDIE
ANDOR
ANDRE
ANDRO
ANDRY
ANDSO
ANDUP
ANDYS
ARDEN
ARDOR
ASDIC
ASDRY
AUDEN
AUDIE
AUDIO
AUDIS
AUDIT
AUDRA

A••D•

AANDE
AANDM
AANDP
AANDW
ABCDE
ABIDE
ABODE
ACADS
ACIDS
ACIDY
ALADO
ALIDA
AMADA
AMADO
AMIDE
ANODE
APODS
ARADO
ASIDE
AVIDE
AZIDE

A•••D

AAHED
ABEND
ABLED
ACHED
ACRED
ACRID
ACTED
ADDED
ADZED
AHEAD
AHMAD
AHMED
AHOLD
AIDED
AILED
AIMED
AIRED
ALGID
ALKYD
ALOUD
AMAND
AMEND
AMPED
ANAND
ANTED
APHID
APIED
APTED
ARCED
ARMED
AROID
ARPAD
ARRID
ASHED
ASKED
ASMAD
ASOLD
ASRED
ASSAD
ASSTD
AVOID
AWARD
AWNED
AXLED

•AD••

BADAT
BADDY
BADEN
BADER
BADGE
BADLY
BADUN
CADDY
CADET
CADGE
CADIS
CADIZ
CADRE
DADAS
DADDY
DADOS
EADIE
FADDY
FADED
FADER
FADES
FADOS
GADDI
HADAT
HADES
HADIN
HADIT
HADJI
HADNO
HADNT
HADON
HADST
HADTO
HADUP
JADED
JADES
KADAR
LADAS
LADED
LADEN
LADER
LADES
LADLE
LADYL
LADYS
MADAM
MADAT
MADGE
MADLY
MADOC
MADOX
MADRE
MADTV
NADER
NADIA
NADIR
NADJA
PADDY
PADRE
PADUA
RADAR
RADER
RADII
RADIO
RADIX
RADON
SADAT
SADHE
SADHU
SADIE
SADLY
TADAS
VADER
VADIM
VADIS
VADUZ
WADED
WADER
WADES
WADIS
WADUP
YADDA
YADIM
ZADAR
ZADIE
ZADIG

•A•D•

AANDE
AANDM
AANDP
AANDW
BADDY
BAEDA
BALDS
BALDY
BANDA
BANDB
BANDO
BANDS
BANDW
BANDY
BARDS
BAUDS
BAWDY
CADDY
CANDO
CANDW
CANDY
CARDI
CARDS
CAUDI
CAUDO
DADDY
DANDD
DANDY
DARDY
FADDY
FALDO
GADDI
GANDT
GANDY
GARDA
GARDE
GAUDI
GAUDS
GAUDY
HAIDA
HANDI
HANDS
HANDY
HARDC
HARDG
HARDY
HAYDN
JANDB
JANDJ
KANDY
LANDI
LANDO
LANDS
LARDS
LARDY
LAUDA
LAUDE
LAUDS
MAGDA
MAHDI
MAIDS
MANDY
MARDI
MAUDE
MAZDA
NALDI
NARDA
NARDO
NARDS
PADDY
PANDA
PANDL
PARDO
PARDS
QAIDS
QANDA
RAIDS
RANDA
RANDB
RANDD
RANDI
RANDR
RANDS
RANDY
SANDE
SANDH
SANDL
SANDP
SANDS
SANDY
SARDI
SARDS
SAUDI
TANDY
TARDE
TARDO
TARDY
VARDA
WAJDA
WALDO
WANDA
WANDS
WARDS
XANDO
XANDY
YADDA
YARDS

•A••D

AAHED
BAAED
BAIRD
BAKED
BALED
BARED
BASED
BATED
BAYED
CAGED
CAKED
CANED
CANID
CAPED
CARED
CASED
CAVED
CAWED
DANDD
DARED
DATED
DAVID
DAZED
EARED
EASED
EAVED
FACED
FADED
FAKED
FAMED
FARAD
FARED
FATED
FAXED
FAZED
GAGED
GALED
GAMED
GAPED
GATED
GAZED
HALED
HARED
HASID
HATED
HAWED
HAYED
HAZED
JADED
JAPED
JARED
JAWED
LACED
LADED
LAIRD
LAMED
LANED
LASED
LAVED
LAWED
LAZED
MACED
MANED
MATED
MAXED
MAZED
NAIAD
NAKED
NAMED
OARED
PACED
PAGED
PALED
PANED
PARED
PATED
PAVED
PAVID
PAWED
RABID
RACED
RAGED
RAKED
RANDD
RANID
RAPID
RASED
RATED
RAVED
RAXED
RAYED
RAZED
SALAD
SALUD
SAPID
SATED
SAVED
SAWED
TAMED
TAPED
TARED
TAXED
VALID
VANED
VAPID
WADED
WAGED
WAKED
WALED
WANED
WARED
WAVED
WAXED
YAWED
ZAHND

••AD•

ACADS
ALADO
AMADA
AMADO
ARADO
BEADS
BEADY
BLADE
BRADS
BRADY
CHADS
CLADS
DUADS
DYADS
EGADI
EGADS
EVADE
FUADI
GLADE
GLADS
GOADS
GRADE
GRADS
HEADS
HEADY
JOADS
LEADS
LEADY
LOADS
MEADE
MEADS
PRADA
PRADO
QUADR
QUADS
READD
READE
READS
READY
ROADS
SCADS
SHADE
SHADS
SHADY
SLADE
SPADE
SPADS
STADE
STADS
STADT
TOADS
TOADY
TRADE
TSADE
TSADI
TVADS
VLADE
WOADS

••A•D

AMAND
ANAND
AWARD
BAAED
BEARD
BLAND
BOARD
BRAID
BRAND
CHARD
CHAUD
ECARD
ELAND
EWALD
FRAUD
GLAND
GRAND
GUARD
HEALD
HEARD
HOARD
ISAID
LEAUD
OLAND
PLAID
QUAID
QUAND
READD
ROALD
SCALD
SHARD
SKALD
STAID
STAND
SWARD
USAID
VIAND
WEALD
WHATD

•••AD

AHEAD
AHMAD
ARPAD
ASMAD
ASSAD
BEBAD
BEMAD
BREAD
BROAD
CURAD
CYCAD
DECAD
DOBAD
DREAD
DRYAD
ECTAD
ENTAD
FARAD
GETAD
GOBAD
GOMAD
GOTAD
HEXAD
HODAD
ILIAD
IMBAD
IMMAD
INBAD
JIHAD
KNEAD
MONAD
MYBAD
MYDAD
NAIAD
NICAD
NOMAD
NORAD
OCTAD
ONEAD
OREAD
PLEAD
REPAD
SALAD
SIXAD
SNEAD
SOBAD
SOSAD
SQUAD
STEAD
STRAD
TENAD
TREAD
TRIAD
TWOAD
UNMAD
UNSAD
WEBAD

AE•••

AEAEA
AECIA
AEDES
AEGIR
AEGIS
AEIOU
AEONS
AEREO
AERIE
AERIO
AEROS
AESIR
AESOP
AETNA

A•E••

ABEAM
ABEAR
ABELE
ABEND
ABETS
ACEIT
ACELA
ACERB
ACERS
ACETO
ADEEM
ADELA
ADELE
ADENI
ADENO
ADEPT
ADEUX
AGENA
AGENT
AGERS
AHEAD
AHEAP
AHEMS
AKEEM
AKELA
AKENE
AKERS
ALEAK
ALECK
ALEFS
ALENE
ALEPH
ALERO
ALERS
ALERT
ALETA
ALEUT
ALEVE
ALEXA
ALEXI
AMEBA
AMEER
AMEND
AMENS
AMENT
AMERY
ANELE
ANEMO
ANENT
ANETO
APEAK
APEEK
APEEP
APERS
APERY
AREAL
AREAR
AREAS
ARECA
AREEL
ARENA
ARENS
ARENT
ARESO
ARETE
ATEAM
ATEAT
ATEIN
ATEIT

ATEOF
ATEST
ATEUP
AVENA
AVERS
AVERT
AVERY
AWEEK
AXELF
AXELS
AXERS
AYEAR
AYERS
AZERA
AZERI

A••E•

AAHED
AAMES
ABBES
ABBEY
ABDEL
ABIES
ABLED
ABLER
ABNER
ACCEL
ACHED
ACHER
ACHES
ACMES
ACNES
ACRED
ACRES
ACTED
ACTER
ACTES
ADDED
ADDER
ADEEM
ADFEE
ADHEM
ADIEU
ADLER
ADMEN
ADREM
ADREP
ADZED
ADZES
AEAEA
AEDES
AEREO
AFTER
AGLET
AGLEY
AGNES
AGNEW
AGREE
AGUES
AHMED
AHYES
AIDED
AIDER
AIDES
AIKEN
AILED
AILES
AILEY
AIMED
AIMEE
AIMER
AIRED
AIRER
AIRES
AKEEM
ALBEE
ALBEN
ALDEN
ALDER
ALGER
ALIEN
ALLEE
ALLEN
ALLER
ALLES
ALLEY
ALLEZ
ALOES
ALPEN
ALPES
ALTER
AMBER
AMEER
AMIEL
AMIES
AMPED
AMVET
ANDES
ANGEL
ANGER
ANGES
ANNEE
ANNEX
ANSEL
ANSER
ANTED
ANTES
AOLER
AONES
APEEK
APEEP
APFEL
APIED
APLEY
APNEA
APPEL
APRES
APSES
APTED
APTER
ARBER
ARCED
ARDEN
AREEL
ARIEL
ARIES
ARLEN
ARLES
ARMED
ARMEE
ARMEN
ARMER
ARMES
ARMET
ARMEY
ARNEL
ARPEL
ARRET
ARSES
ARTEL
ARWEN
ASHED
ASHEN
ASHER
ASHES
ASKED
ASKER
ASKEW
ASNER
ASNEW
ASPEN
ASPER
ASRED
ASSER
ASSES
ASSET
ASSEZ
ASTER
ASYET
ATLES
ATSEA
ATTEN
AUBER
AUDEN
AUGER
AVNET
AWEEK
AWGEE
AWNED
AXLED
AXLES
AXMEN
AYRES
AZTEC
AZTEK

A•••E

AANDE
ABASE
ABATE
ABBIE
ABCDE
ABELE
ABIDE
ABODE
ABOVE
ABUSE
ACUTE
ADAGE
ADDIE
ADDLE
ADELE
ADFEE
ADIGE
ADOBE
ADORE
ADOZE
AERIE
AFIRE
AFORE
AGAME
AGAPE
AGATE
AGAVE
AGAZE
AGGIE
AGILE
AGREE
AIMEE
AINGE
AISLE
AISNE
AKENE
ALATE
ALBEE
ALENE
ALEVE
ALFIE
ALFRE
ALGAE
ALICE
ALIKE
ALINE
ALIVE
ALLEE
ALLIE
ALONE
ALYCE
AMARE
AMAZE
AMBLE
AMICE
AMIDE
AMINE
AMITE
AMOLE
AMORE
AMPLE
AMUSE
ANDIE
ANDRE
ANELE
ANGIE
ANGLE
ANILE
ANIME
ANISE
ANKLE
ANNEE
ANNIE
ANODE
ANOLE
ANSAE
ANTAE
ANTRE
APACE
APPLE
AQUAE
ARAME
ARBRE
ARCAE
ARCHE
ARETE
ARGUE
ARISE
ARMEE
ARNIE
AROSE
ARTIE
ASIDE
ASKME
ASONE
ASTRE
ATILE
ATIVE
ATONE
ATQUE
AUDIE
AUGIE
AURAE
AUTRE
AVIDE
AWAKE
AWARE
AWAVE
AWGEE
AWOKE
AXONE
AZIDE
AZOLE
AZORE
AZURE

•AE••

BAEDA
BAEZA
FAENA
FAERY
GAELS
GAETA
HAEMA
MAEVE
PAEAN
PAESE
SAENS
TAEBO
TAEGU
TAELS

•A•E•

AAHED
AAMES
BAAED
BABEL
BABES
BADEN
BADER
BAGEL
BAIES
BAJER
BAKED
BAKER
BAKES
BALED
BALER
BALES
BANES
BARED
BARER
BARES
BASED
BASEL
BASER
BASES
BATED
BATES
BAUER
BAYED
BAYER
BAYES
CABER
CADET
CAFES
CAGED
CAGER
CAGES
CAGEY
CAKED
CAKES
CAKEY
CALEB
CAMEL
CAMEO
CANEA
CANED
CANEM
CANER
CANES
CAPED
CAPEK
CAPER
CAPES
CAPET
CARED
CARER
CARES
CARET
CAREW
CAREY
CASED
CASER
CASES
CASEY
CATER
CATES
CAVED
CAVER
CAVES
CAWED
DACES
DALEN
DALES
DALET
DALEY
DAMEN
DAMES
DANES
DARED
DARER
DARES
DATED
DATER
DATES
DAVEN
DAVES
DAVEY
DAWES
DAZED
DAZER
DAZES
EAGER
EAMES
EARED
EASED
EASEL
EASER
EASES
EATEN
EATER
EAVED
EAVES
FABER
FACED
FACER
FACES
FACET
FADED
FADER
FADES
FAHEY
FAKED
FAKER
FAKES
FAMED
FAMER
FAMES
FANES
FARED
FARER
FARES
FATED
FATES
FAVES
FAXED
FAXER
FAXES
FAZED
FAZES
GABEL
GAGED
GAGES
GALEA
GALED
GALEN
GALES
GAMED
GAMER
GAMES
GANEF
GAPED
GAPER
GAPES
GARES
GASES
GATED
GATER
GATES
GAVEL
GAYER
GAZED
GAZER
GAZES
HABER
HACEK
HADES
HAGEN
HAKES
HALED
HALEN
HALER
HALES
HALEY
HAMEL
HAMER
HAMES
HANES
HANEY
HARED
HAREM
HARES
HASEK
HATED
HATER
HATES
HAUER
HAVEL
HAVEN
HAVER
HAVES
HAWED
HAWER
HAYED
HAYEK
HAYER
HAYES
HAYEY
HAZED
HAZEL
HAZER
HAZES
JACET
JACEY
JADED
JADES
JAKES
JAMES
JANET
JAPED
JAPER
JAPES
JARED
JAWED
JAWER
KALEL
KALES
KAMEN
KAREL
KAREN
KASEM
KATEY
LABEL
LACED
LACER
LACES
LACEY
LADED
LADEN
LADER
LADES
LAFEU
LAGER
LAKER
LAKES
LAMED
LAMER
LAMES
LANED
LANES
LAPEL
LAREE
LARES
LASED
LASER
LASES
LATEN
LATER
LATEX
LAUER
LAVED
LAVER
LAVES
LAWED
LAWES
LAXER
LAYER
LAZED
LAZES
MABEL
MACED
MACER
MACES
MAGEE
MAGES
MAHER
MAKEM
MAKER
MAKES
MALES
MALEV
MAMET
MANED
MANES
MANET
MAPES
MAREK
MARES
MASER
MATED
MATEO
MATER
MATES
MATEY
MAVEN
MAXED
MAXES
MAYER
MAZED
MAZEL
MAZES
NABES
NADER
NAGEL
NAKED
NAMED
NAMER
NAMES
NAPES
NARES
NAVEE
NAVEL
NAVES
OAKEN
OAKES
OARED
OARER
OASES
OATEN
OATER
OATES
PACED
PACEM
PACER
PACES
PACEY
PAGED
PAGER
PAGES
PAGET
PALEA
PALED
PALEO
PALER
PALES
PALEY
PANED
PANEL
PANES
PAPEL
PAPER
PARED
PAREE
PAREN
PARER
PARES
PAREU
PASEO
PASES
PATED
PATEK
PATEN
PATER
PATES
PAVED
PAVEL
PAVER
PAVES
PAWED
PAWER
PAYEE
PAYER
RACED
RACER
RACES
RADER
RAFER
RAGED
RAGER
RAGES
RAKED
RAKER
RAKES
RALES
RAMEN
RAMET
RAMEY
RANEE
RAPEE
RAREE
RARER
RASED
RASER
RASES
RATED
RATEL
RATER
RATES
RAVED
RAVEL
RAVEN
RAVER
RAVES
RAWER
RAXED
RAXES
RAYED
RAZED
RAZER
RAZES
SABER
SAFER
SAFES
SAGER
SAGES
SAGET
SAHEL
SAKES
SALEM
SALEP
SALES
SANER
SAREE
SAREK
SASES
SATED
SATES
SAVED
SAVER
SAVES
SAWED
SAWER
SAXES
SAYER
TACET
TAKEI
TAKEN
TAKER
TAKES
TALER
TALES
TAMED
TAMER
TAMES
TANEY
TAPED
TAPER
TAPES
TARED
TARES
TASER
TATER
TATES
TAVEL
TAXED
TAXER
TAXES
VADER
VALES
VALET
VANED
VANES
VASES
VATER
VAXES
WADED
WADER
WADES
WAFER
WAGED
WAGER
WAGES
WAKED
WAKEN
WAKER
WAKES
WALED
WALES
WANED
WANER
WANES
WARED
WARES
WATER
WAVED
WAVER
WAVES
WAXED
WAXEN
WAXER
WAXES
XAXES
YALEU
YARER
YATES
YAWED
YAXES
ZALES
ZAXES
ZAZEN

•A••E

AANDE
BADGE
BAIZE
BARGE
BARRE
BASIE
BASLE
BASSE
BASTE
BATHE
BAUME
BAYLE
CABLE
CACHE
CADGE
CADRE
CAFFE
CAINE
CALLE
CALME
CALVE
CANOE
CARLE
CARME
CARNE
CARPE
CARRE
CARTE
CARVE
CASTE
CAUSE
CAVAE
CAYCE
DACHE
DAFOE
DAMME
DANAE
DANCE
DANKE
DANSE
DANTE
DARTE
DAUBE
DAVIE
DAYNE
EADIE
EAGLE
EAGRE
EAPOE
EARLE
EATME
EAZYE
FABLE
FABRE
FACIE
FAIRE
FALKE
FALSE
FAMKE
FARCE
FAROE
FAURE
FAUTE
FAUVE
FAVRE
GABLE
GAFFE
GANCE
GARDE
GASPE
GAUGE
GAUZE
GAYLE
HAGUE
HAILE
HAISE
HALLE
HALVE
HANSE
HAOLE
HARTE
HASTE
HAUTE
HAVRE
HAWKE
HAWSE
JAFFE
JAHRE
JAIME
JAMBE
JAMIE
JANIE
JARRE
JAUNE
JAYNE
KANYE
KARLE
KATHE
KATIE
KATZE
LACIE
LADLE
LAINE
LAKME
LANCE
LANGE
LAPSE
LAREE
LARGE
LARUE
LASSE
LATHE
LATKE
LATTE
LAUDE
LAVIE
LAYNE
MACHE
MACKE
MACLE
MADGE
MADRE
MAEVE
MAGEE
MAHRE
MAINE
MAIRE
MAIZE
MALLE
MAMIE
MANGE
MANNE
MANSE
MAPLE
MARGE
MARIE
MARNE
MASSE
MATTE
MAUDE
MAUVE
MAXIE
MAYBE
MAYLE
NACRE
NAIVE
NANCE
NAPPE
NASHE
NAVEE
OAKIE
PADRE
PAESE
PAIGE
PAINE
PAISE
PALME
PANNE
PAREE
PARGE
PARLE
PARSE
PARTE
PASSE
PASTE
PATHE
PAUSE
PAYEE
PAYNE
RAABE
RAINE
RAISE
RAMIE
RANEE
RANGE
RANKE
RAPEE
RARAE
RAREE
RASAE
RASPE
RASSE
SABLE
SABRE
SACRE
SADHE
SADIE
SALLE
SALVE
SANDE
SANTE
SAONE
SAREE
SARGE
SATIE
SAUCE
SAUTE
TABLE
TAHOE
TANTE
TARDE
TARTE
TASSE
TASTE
TAUPE
VACHE
VAGUE
VALLE
VALSE
VALUE
VALVE
VANCE
WAITE
WAIVE
WASTE
WAYNE
YALIE
YAYME
ZADIE
ZAIRE

••AE•

AEAEA
BAAED
BHAER
BRAES
CLAES
NBAER
SHAEF
STAEL

••A•E

ABASE
ABATE
ADAGE
AGAME
AGAPE
AGATE
AGAVE
AGAZE
ALATE
AMARE
AMAZE
APACE
ARAME
AWAKE
AWARE
AWAVE
BEALE
BEAME
BLADE
BLAKE
BLAME
BLANE
BLARE
BLASE
BLAZE
BRACE
BRAHE
BRAKE
BRAVE
BYAGE
CEASE
CHAFE
CHASE
CLARE
CLASE
CLAVE
COASE
CRAKE
CRANE
CRAPE
CRATE
CRAVE
CRAZE
DEANE
DEARE
DIANE
DNASE
DOANE
DRAKE
DRAPE
DUANE
EGALE
ELATE
ENARE
ENATE
ERASE
ETAGE
ETAPE
EVADE
FLAKE
FLAME
FLARE
FRAME
GLACE
GLADE
GLARE
GLAZE
GOAPE
GRACE
GRADE
GRAPE
GRATE
GRAVE
GRAZE
GUARE
HEAVE
HOARE
ICAME
ICARE
IMAGE
INAGE
INANE
INAWE
IRATE
JEANE
KEANE
KNAVE
KWAME
LEAKE
LEASE
LEAVE
LIANE
LWAVE
MEADE
NEALE
NEAME
OFAGE
OHARE
ONATE
ORALE
ORATE
OSAGE
OVATE
PEACE
PEALE
PEASE
PHAGE
PHASE
PIAVE
PLACE
PLAGE
PLANE
PLATE
PRATE
QUAKE
QUARE
RAABE
READE
REAVE
RNASE
SCALE
SCAPE
SCARE
SEALE
SHADE
SHAKE
SHALE
SHAME
SHANE
SHAPE
SHARE
SHAVE
SKATE
SLADE
SLAKE
SLATE
SLAVE
SMAZE
SNAKE
SNARE
SOAVE
SPACE
SPADE
SPAKE

SPARE
SPATE
STADE
STAGE
STAKE
STALE
STARE
STATE
STAVE
SUAVE
SWALE
TEASE
THANE
TRACE
TRADE
TRANE
TRAVE
TSADE
UKASE
USAGE
VEALE
VLADE
WEAVE
WHALE
YSAYE

•••AE
ALGAE
ANSAE
ANTAE
AQUAE
ARCAE
AURAE
CAVAE
COMAE
COXAE
CYMAE
DANAE
DIRAE
HORAE
MCRAE
NOVAE
OLPAE
PUPAE
RARAE
RASAE
SETAE
STOAE
TOGAE
ULNAE
URSAE
VENAE
VITAE

AF•••
AFARS
AFFIX
AFIRE
AFLAC
AFLAT
AFOFL
AFOOT
AFORE
AFOUL
AFRIC
AFROS
AFTER
AFTON
AFTRA

A•F••
ABFAB
ADFEE
AFFIX
ALFAS
ALFIE
ALFIO
ALFRE
APFEL
ASFAT
ASFIT
ASFOR
AWFUL

A••F•
ABAFT
ACUFF
AFOFL
ALEFS
ALIFS
ALOFT

A•••F
ACUFF
ADOLF
ALLOF
ALOOF
ASKOF
ATEOF
AXELF

•AF••
BAFFS
BAFFY
CAFES
CAFFE
DAFFY
DAFOE
GAFFE
GAFFS
HAFIZ
HAFTS
JAFAR
JAFFA
JAFFE
KAFKA
LAFEU
LAFFS
MAFJA
NAFTA
RAFER
RAFFI
RAFKO
RAFTS
SAFAR
SAFER
SAFES
SAFFI
SAFIN
TAFFY
TAFTS
WAFER
WAFTS
ZAFUS

•A•F•
BAFFS
BAFFY
BANFF
BARFY
CAFFE
DAFFY
GAFFE
GAFFS
HAIFA
HANFF
JAFFA
JAFFE
LAFFS
NAIFS
NAKFA
RAFFI
SAFFI
TAFFY
WAIFS
ZARFS

•A••F
BANFF
CALAF
CALIF
EATOF
GANEF
HANFF
RAZAF

••AF•
ABAFT
BLAFF
CHAFE
CHAFF
CRAFT
DRAFT
GOAFT
GRAFF
GRAFT
KRAFT
LEAFS
LEAFY
LOAFS
OLAFI
OLAFV
QUAFF
SHAFT
SNAFU
STAFF
USAFA

••A•F
BLAFF
CHAFF
DWARF
GRAFF
QUAFF
SCARF
SHAEF
SNARF
STAFF
WHARF

•••AF
CALAF
DECAF
PILAF
RAZAF
SHEAF

AG•••
AGAIN
AGALS
AGAMA
AGAME
AGANA
AGAPE
AGARN
AGARS
AGASP
AGATE
AGAVE
AGAZE
AGENA
AGENT
AGERS
AGGIE
AGHAS
AGILE
AGING
AGIOS
AGITA
AGLET
AGLEY
AGLOW
AGNES
AGNEW
AGNON
AGNUS
AGOGO
AGONY
AGORA
AGREE
AGRIC
AGRIN
AGRON
AGUAS
AGUES
AGURA
AGUSH
AGWAY

A•G••
AEGIR
AEGIS
AGGIE
ALGAE
ALGAL
ALGAS
ALGER
ALGIA
ALGID
ALGOL
ANGEL
ANGER
ANGES
ANGIE
ANGIO
ANGLE
ANGLO
ANGRY
ANGST
ANGUS
ARGON
ARGOS
ARGOT
ARGUE
ARGUS
AUGER
AUGHT
AUGIE
AUGUR
AVGAS
AWGEE

A••G•
AARGH
ADAGE
ADIGE
AGOGO
AINGE
ALIGN
AMIGA
AMIGO
ANAGS
ANIGH
ASAGI

A•••G
ABZUG
ACING
AGING
AHANG
AHING
ALONG
AMONG
APING
ASBIG
AWING
AXING

•AG••
BAGEL
BAGGY
BAGIT
CAGED
CAGER
CAGES
CAGEY
DAGAN
EAGAN
EAGER
EAGLE
EAGRE
FAGIN
FAGOT
GAGED
GAGES
HAGAR
HAGEN
HAGIO
HAGUE
JAGGY
LAGER
LAGOS
MAGDA
MAGEE
MAGES
MAGIC
MAGMA
MAGNA
MAGOG
MAGOO
MAGUA
MAGUS
NAGAT
NAGEL
NAGGY
PAGAN
PAGED
PAGER
PAGES
PAGET
RAGAS
RAGED
RAGER
RAGES
RAGGY
RAGON
SAGAL
SAGAN
SAGAS
SAGER
SAGES
SAGET
SAGGY
SAGOS
TAGON
TAGUP
TAGUS
VAGUE
VAGUS
WAGED
WAGER
WAGES
WAGON
ZAGAT

•A•G•
AARGH
BADGE
BAGGY
BANGS
BARGE
BAUGH
CADGE
CARGO
DANGS
FANGS
FARGO
GANGS
GAUGE
HANGS
HAWGS
JAGGY
KANGA
KANGS
LANGE
LARGE
LARGO
LAUGH
MADGE
MANGA
MANGE
MANGO
MANGY
MARGE
MARGO
MARGY
NAGGY
PAIGE
PANGS
PARGE
RAGGY
RANGE
RANGO
RANGY
SAGGY
SARGE
TAEGU
TAIGA
TANGO
TANGS
TANGY
TARGA
WAUGH

•A••G
HAING
HARDG
LAING
MAGOG
NAVIG
VARIG
ZADIG

••AG•
ADAGE
ANAGS
ASAGI
BRAGA
BRAGG
BRAGH
BRAGS
BYAGE
CRAGS
DRAGO
DRAGS
EMAGS
ETAGE
FLAGG
FLAGS
FRAGS
HOAGY
IMAGE
IMAGO
INAGE
OFAGE
OSAGE
PHAGE
PHAGO
PHAGY
PLAGE
QUAGS
SHAGS
SLAGS
SNAGS
SPAGO
STAGE
STAGG
STAGS
STAGY
SWAGS
TIAGO
TRAGG
USAGE

••A•G
AHANG
BHANG
BRAGG
BRANG
CHANG
CLANG
CRAIG
DRANG
FLAGG
GRAIG
HUANG
JIANG
LIANG
LUANG
ORANG
QUANG
SHANG
SLANG
SMAUG
SPANG
STAGG
STANG
TRAGG
TWANG
WHANG

•••AG
DEBAG
DIMAG
DORAG
GULAG
IDTAG
REBAG
RETAG
SCRAG
UNBAG
UNGAG

AH•••
AHAIR
AHANG
AHEAD
AHEAP
AHEMS
AHING
AHMAD
AHMED
AHOLD
AHOOT
AHORA
AHOYS
AHSIN
AHYES

A•H••
AAHED
ABHOR
ACHED
ACHER
ACHES
ACHOO
ADHEM
ADHOC
AGHAS
APHID
APHIS
ARHAT
ASHBY
ASHED
ASHEN
ASHER
ASHES
ASHOT
ASHUR
ATHOL
ATHON
ATHOS
AWHIT

A••H•
ABMHO
ABOHM
AISHA
ALOHA
ALPHA
ALTHO
AMAHL
AMAHS
AMPHI
ANCHO
ANKHS
ARCHE
ARCHI
ARCHY
ASAHI
AUGHT
AYAHS

A•••H
AARGH
ABASH
AGUSH
AITCH
ALEPH
ALLAH
AMISH
ANIGH
APISH
ARITH
ARMAH
ARRAH
AWASH
AZOTH

•AH••
AAHED
BAHAI
BAHIA
BAHTS
FAHEY
GAHAN
HAHAS
JAHAN
JAHRE
KAHLO
KAHNS
LAHTI
MAHAL
MAHAN
MAHDI
MAHER
MAHON
MAHRE
NAHUM
RAHAL
SAHEL
SAHIB
TAHOE
WAHOO
YAHOO
ZAHND

•A•H•
BASHO
BATHE
BATHO
BATHS
BATHY
CACHE
CATHS
CATHY
DACHA
DACHE
DASHI
DASHY
FATHA
HATHA
HATHI
KAPHS
KASHA
KASHI
KATHE
KATHY
LATHE
LATHS
LATHY
MACHE
MACHO
MACHU
MACHY
MASHA
MATHS
NACHO
NACHT
NASHE
OATHS
PACHY
PASHA
PATHE
PATHO
PATHS
PATHY
RASHI
RASHT
RATHS
SACHS
SADHE
SADHU
SASHA
SAYHI
TACHO
TACHS
TASHI
VACHE
WASHO
WASHY
YACHT
YASHA

•A••H
AARGH
BALCH
BALPH
BARTH
BATCH
BAUGH
DABIH
DARTH
EARTH
FAITH
FARAH
GARTH
HARSH
HATCH
KARSH
LARCH
LATCH
LAUGH
MALPH
MARCH
MARSH
MATCH
NAISH
NATCH
PARCH
PASCH
PATCH
RAJAH
RALPH
RANCH
SAITH
SANDH
SARAH
SATCH
SAYAH
WALSH
WATCH
WAUGH

••AH•
AMAHL
AMAHS
ASAHI
AYAHS
BLAHS
BRAHE
ICAHN
IDAHO
LEAHY
OMAHA
OPAHS
PRAHA
SHAHN
SHAHS
SPAHN
STAHL
STAHR
UTAHN
YEAHS

••A•H
ABASH
AWASH
BEACH
BRACH
BRAGH
BRASH
CLASH
COACH
CRASH
DEATH
ECASH
ELATH
FLASH
GNASH
GRAPH
HEATH
KEACH
LEACH
LEASH
LOATH
MEATH
NEATH
ORACH
PEACH
PLASH
PLATH
POACH
QUASH
REACH
ROACH
SLASH
SMASH
SNATH
STAPH
STASH
SWASH
SWATH
TEACH
TRASH
WRATH

•••AH
ALLAH
ARMAH
ARRAH
BORAH
DINAH
EPHAH
FARAH
ISIAH
JONAH
JUDAH
MICAH
MYNAH
NORAH
NOTAH
OBEAH
OPRAH
ORPAH
RAJAH
SARAH
SAYAH
SELAH
SURAH
TORAH
TOVAH
UKIAH
URIAH

AI•••
AIDAN
AIDED
AIDER
AIDES
AIDOO
AIKEN
AILED
AILES
AILEY
AILUR
AIMAT
AIMED
AIMEE
AIMER
AINGE
AINSI
AINUS
AIOLI
AIRED
AIRER
AIRES
AIRUP
AISHA
AISLE
AISNE
AITCH
AIWAS

A•I••
ABIDE
ABIES
ACIDS
ACIDY
ACING
ADIEU
ADIGE
ADINS
ADIOS
ADITS
AEIOU
AFIRE
AGILE
AGING
AGIOS
AGITA
AHING
AKINS
AKIRA
AKITA
ALIAS
ALIBI
ALICE
ALIDA
ALIEN
ALIFS
ALIGN
ALIKE
ALINE
ALIOS
ALISA
ALIST
ALITO
ALITY
ALIVE
AMICA
AMICE
AMICI
AMICK
AMICO
AMIDE
AMIEL
AMIES
AMIGA
AMIGO
AMINE
AMINO
AMIRI
AMIRS
AMISH
AMISS
AMITE
AMITY
ANIGH
ANILE
ANILS
ANIMA
ANIME
ANIMO
ANION
ANISE
ANITA
APIAN
APIED
APING
APISH
ARIAL
ARIAN
ARIAS
ARICA
ARIEL
ARIES
ARILS
ARION
ARIOT
ARISE
ARITH
ARIUM
ASIAN
ASICS
ASIDE
ATILE
ATILT
ATION
ATIVE
AVIAN
AVIAS
AVIDE
AVILA
AVION
AVIOR
AVISO
AWING
AXIAL
AXILS
AXING
AXIOM
AXION
AYINS
AZIDE

A••I•
ABBIE
ABOIL
ABRIL
ABRIM
ABRIS
ACEIT
ACRID
ACTII
ACTIN
ACTIV
ADAIR
ADBIZ
ADDIE
ADDIN
ADDIO
ADDIS
ADLIB
ADMIN
ADMIT
ADMIX
ADRIP
ADVIL
AECIA
AEGIR
AEGIS
AERIE
AERIO
AESIR
AFFIX
AFRIC
AGAIN
AGGIE
AGRIC
AGRIN
AHAIR
AHSIN
AKAIS
ALAIN
ALAIS
ALFIE
ALFIO
ALGIA
ALGID
ALLIE
ALLIN
ALLIS
ALOIS
ALVIN
AMAIN
AMBIT
AMLIT
AMNIA
AMNIO
ANAIS
ANDIE
ANGIE
ANGIO
ANNIE
ANNIV
ANTIC
ANTIQ
ANTIS
ANVIL
ANZIO
APAIN
APHID
APHIS
APPIA
APRIL
APSIS
ARBIL
ARKIN
ARMIN
ARNIE
AROID
ARRID
ARRIS
ARSIS
ARTIE
ARTIS
ASBIG
ASCII
ASDIC
ASFIT
ASKIN
ASPIC
ASPIN
ASTIN
ASTIR
ASWIM
ATEIN
ATEIT
ATRIA
ATRIP
ATSIX
ATTIC
AUDIE
AUDIO
AUDIS
AUDIT
AUGIE
AULIS
AURIC
AUVIN
AVAIL
AVOID
AVOIR
AVRIL
AWAIT
AWHIT
AZOIC

A•••I
ABACI
ACTII
ADENI
ADLAI
AINSI
AIOLI
ALEXI
ALIBI
ALTAI
AMATI
AMICI
AMIRI
AMPHI
ARCHI
ARONI
ASAGI
ASAHI
ASAMI
ASCII
ASSAI
ATARI
AUSSI
AZERI
AZUKI

•AI••
BAIES
BAILS
BAIRD
BAIRN
BAISA
BAITS
BAIUL
BAIZA
BAIZE
CAINE
CAINT
CAIRN
CAIRO
CAIUS
DAILY
DAIRY
DAISY
DAIWA
FAILS
FAIMS
FAINT
FAIRE
FAIRS
FAIRY
FAITH
GAILY
GAINS
GAITS
GAIUS
HAIDA
HAIFA
HAIKS
HAIKU
HAILE
HAILS
HAING
HAIRS
HAIRY
HAISE
HAITI
JAILS
JAIME
JAINS
LAICS
LAIKA
LAILA
LAINE
LAING
LAIRD
LAIRS
LAITS
LAITY
LAIUS
MAIDS
MAILS
MAIMS
MAINE
MAINS
MAINZ
MAIRE
MAIZE
NAIAD
NAIFS
NAILS
NAIMA
NAINA
NAIRA
NAISH
NAIVE
PAIGE
PAILS
PAINE
PAINS
PAINT
PAIRS
PAISA
PAISE

QAIDS RAIDS RAILS RAIMI RAINE RAINS RAINY RAISA RAISE RAITA RAITT SAILS SAINT SAIRY SAITH TAIGA TAILS TAINA TAINT TAITO WAIFS WAILS WAINS WAIST WAITE WAITS WAITZ WAIVE ZAIRE

•A•I•

BACIO BAGIT BAHIA BALIN BARIC BARIT BASIA BASIC BASIE BASIL BASIN BASIS BATIK BATIN CABIN CADIS CADIZ CALIF CALIX CANID CANIO CANIS CANIT CARIB CASIO CAVIL DABIH DACIA DALIS DAMIS DANIA DANIO DARIA DARIN DARIO DAVID DAVIE DAVIS DAVIT EADIE EATIN EATIT FABIO FACIA FACIE FACIL FAGIN FAKIR FAQIR FARIS GABIN GAMIN GAVIN HABIB HABIT HADIN HADIT HAFIZ HAGIO HAJIS HAKIM HASID HASIN HASIT JAMIE JAMIN JANIE JANIS KANIN KATIE KAZIN LABIA LACIE LALIA LAMIA LAMIT LANIN LAPIN LAPIS LARIS LASIK LATIN LAVIE LAVIN LAYIN MAFIA MAGIC MAKIN MALIC MAMIE MANIA MANIC MAOII MARIA MARIE MARIN MARIO MARIS MATIN MAVIN MAVIS MAXIE MAXIM MAXIS NACIO NADIA NADIR NAMIB NARIC NARIS NAVIG NAVIS NAZIS OAKIE OASIS PALIN PANIC PANIN PANIS PARIS PATIO PAVIA PAVID PAVIN PAYIN RABID RABIN RADII RADIO RADIX RAJIV RAMIE RAMIN RAMIS RANID RANIN RANIS RAPID RATIO SABIN SADIE SAFIN SAHIB SAKIS SALIC SAMIS SAPID SARIS SATIE SATII SATIN SAWII SAWIN SAYIT TABIS TACIT TAKIN TALIA TAMIL TANIA TANIS TAPIN TAPIR TAPIS TARIQ TATIS TAVIS TAXIS VADIM VADIS VALID VAPID VARIA VARIG VATIC WADIS WASIN WASIT WAYIN XAXIS YADIM YALIE YASIR YAXIS ZADIE ZADIG ZAXIS ZAYIN

•A••I

BAHAI BALKI BAMBI BARBI BASSI CACTI CALLI CAPRI CARDI CARPI CAUDI DALAI DARCI DASHI FARCI FARSI GADDI GALLI GARNI GAUDI HADJI HAITI HAJJI HANDI HANOI HATHI IAMBI KALKI KANJI KASHI KAUAI LACTI LAHTI LANAI LANDI LASKI MAHDI MAOII MAORI MAQUI MARCI MARDI MARKI MARNI MARTI MARYI MASAI MATRI NALDI NANCI NANKI NAOMI PAOLI PARSI PARTI PATRI PATTI PAULI RABBI RADII RAFFI RAIMI RANDI RASHI SAFFI SAKAI SALMI SALTI SAMMI SARAI SARDI SATII SAUDI SAWII SAYHI TAKEI TAMMI TARSI TASHI TAURI VALLI VARSI VASTI YANNI YAQUI

••AI•

ADAIR AGAIN AHAIR AKAIS ALAIN ALAIS AMAIN ANAIS APAIN AVAIL AWAIT BLAIR BLAIS BRAID BRAIN BYAIR CHAIM CHAIN CHAIR CHAIS CLAIM CLAIR CRAIG CRAIK CRAIN DEAIR DRAIN EMAIL ETAIL FLAIL FLAIR FRAIL FRAIS GHAIN GRAIG GRAIL GRAIN ISAID KRAIT NGAIO OHAIR ONAIR PHAIR PLAID PLAIN PLAIT PRAIA QUAID QUAIL QUAIS REAIM REAIR SLAIN SNAIL SPAIN STAID STAIN STAIR SWAIN THAIS TRAIL TRAIN TRAIT TWAIN USAID USAIR YVAIN YWAIN

••A•I

ABACI AMATI ASAGI ASAHI ASAMI ATARI COATI CRANI DHABI EGADI ENAMI ESAKI FUADI GHALI GHAZI GRANI GRAVI IMARI INARI IRANI IRAQI IVANI KHAKI MIAMI OKAPI OLAFI OLAVI OMANI ORANI PIANI PIAUI PLANI QUASI SHARI SOAMI STASI SWAMI SWAZI TRACI TSADI UNAMI

•••AI

ADLAI ALTAI ASSAI BAHAI DALAI DESAI DOUAI DUBAI ENLAI ESSAI KAUAI KENAI LANAI MASAI SAKAI SARAI SERAI SINAI

A•J••

ADJTS ANJOU AUJUS

A••J•

ABAJO ABUJA

•AJ••

BAJER CAJON CAJUN FAJAS HAJIS HAJJI MAJOR RAJAB RAJAH RAJAS RAJIV SAJAK WAJDA

•A•J•

BANJO HADJI HAJJI KANJI NADJA

•A••J

JANDJ MARYJ

••AJ•

ABAJO

AK•••

AKAIS AKBAR AKEEM AKELA AKENE AKERS AKINS AKIRA AKITA AKRON

A•K••

AIKEN ALKAB ALKYD ALKYL ANKHS ANKLE AOKAY ARKIN ASKED ASKER ASKEW ASKIN ASKME ASKOF ASKUP

A••K•

ALIKE ALUKO ANOKA AWAKE AWOKE AYAKO AZUKI

A•••K

ABACK ADAOK ALACK ALEAK ALECK ALLOK AMICK AMUCK ANOUK APEAK APEEK ASLAK AWEEK AZTEK

•AK••

BAKED BAKER BAKES BAKST CAKED CAKES CAKEY DAKAR FAKED FAKER FAKES FAKIR HAKES HAKIM JAKES JAKOB LAKER LAKES LAKME MAKEM MAKER MAKES MAKIN MAKOS NAKED NAKFA OAKEN OAKES OAKIE OAKUM RAKED RAKER RAKES RAKUS SAKAI SAKES SAKIS TAKAS TAKEI TAKEN TAKER TAKES TAKIN WAKAS WAKED WAKEN WAKER WAKES WAKKO YAKOV YAKUT

•A•K•

BABKA BACKS BALKI BALKS BALKY BANKS BANKY BARKS BARKY BASKS CALKS CASKS DANKE DARKS FALKE FAMKE GAWKS GAWKY HACKL HACKS HACKY HAIKS HAIKU HANKS HANKY HARKS HAWKE HAWKS JACKO JACKS JACKY KAFKA KALKI LACKS LAIKA LANKA LANKY LARKS LARKY LASKI LASKY LATKA LATKE MACKE MACKS MARKA MARKI MARKS MARKV MASKS NANKI NARKS PACKS PANKY PARKA PARKS RACKS RAFKO RANKE RANKS SACKS SANKA SAUKS TACKS TACKY TALKS TALKY TANKA TANKS TASKS WACKO WACKY WAKKO WALKS WARKS YACKS YANKS

•A••K

BARAK BATIK BAULK CAPEK CAULK FARUK HACEK HASEK HAYEK KAPOK KAYAK LASIK MAREK NANAK PATEK SAJAK SAREK SAYOK ZAYAK

••AK•

AWAKE AYAKO BEAKS BLAKE BRAKE CHAKA CRAKE DHAKA DRAKE ESAKI FLAKE FLAKY KHAKI LEAKE LEAKS LEAKY OSAKA PEAKS QUAKE QUAKY SHAKE SHAKO SHAKY SLAKE SNAKE SNAKY SOAKS SPAKE STAKE TEAKS

••A•K

ABACK ADAOK ALACK BLACK BLANK BRACK CHALK CLACK CLANK CLARK CRACK CRAIK CRANK DBACK DMARK DRANK EBANK FLACK FLANK FLASK FRANK GOASK ISAAK IZAAK KNACK KVACK NYACK OZARK PLANK PRANK QUACK QUARK REASK ROARK RUARK SHACK SHANK SHARK SKANK SLACK SMACK SNACK SNARK SPAAK SPANK SPARK STACK STALK STANK STARK SWANK THANK TRACK TRASK WHACK WRACK

•••AK

ALEAK APEAK ASLAK BARAK BLEAK BREAK CLOAK CREAK CROAK FREAK HUSAK ISAAK IZAAK KAYAK KODAK KOJAK KULAK MUZAK NANAK NOVAK SAJAK SNEAK SPAAK SPEAK STEAK TILAK TWEAK UHNAK UMIAK WREAK ZAYAK

AL•••

ALACK ALADO ALAIN ALAIS ALALA ALAMO ALANA ALARM ALATE ALAVA ALBAN ALBAS ALBEE ALBEN ALBOM ALBUM ALCAN ALCOA ALCOR ALDEN ALDER ALEAK ALECK ALEFS ALENE ALEPH ALERO ALERS ALERT ALETA ALEUT ALEVE ALEXA ALEXI ALFAS ALFIE ALFIO ALFRE ALGAE ALGAL ALGAS ALGER ALGIA ALGID ALGOL ALIAS ALIBI ALICE ALIDA ALIEN ALIFS ALIGN ALIKE ALINE ALIOS ALISA ALIST ALITO ALITY ALIVE ALKAB ALKYD ALKYL ALLAH ALLAN ALLAY ALLEE ALLEN ALLER ALLES ALLEY ALLEZ ALLIE ALLIN ALLIS ALLOF ALLOK ALLOT ALLOW ALLOY ALLYL ALLYN ALMAY ALMVP ALOES ALOFT ALOHA ALOIS ALONE ALONG ALOOF ALORS ALOUD ALPEN ALPES ALPHA ALROY ALSAB ALSOP ALTAI ALTAR ALTER ALTHO ALTON ALTOS ALTUS ALUKO ALULA ALUMS ALVAR ALVIN ALWAY ALYCE

A•L••

AALTO ABLED ABLER ADLAI ADLER ADLIB AFLAC AFLAT AGLET AGLEY AGLOW AILED AILES AILEY AILUR ALLAH ALLAN ALLAY ALLEE ALLEN ALLER ALLES ALLEY ALLEZ ALLIE ALLIN ALLIS ALLOF ALLOK ALLOT ALLOW ALLOY ALLYL ALLYN AMLIT AOLER APLEY APLUS ARLEN ARLES ASLAK ASLAN ATLAS ATLES AULIS AULUS AXLED AXLES

A••L•

ABELE ACELA ADDLE ADELA ADELE ADOLF ADULT AGALS AGILE AHOLD AIOLI AISLE AKELA ALALA ALULA AMBLE AMOLE AMPLE AMPLY AMYLO AMYLS ANELE ANGLE ANGLO ANILE ANILS ANKLE ANOLE APPLE APPLY APTLY ARILS ARYLS ASOLD ASYLA ATALA ATALL ATILE ATILT ATOLL AVILA AWOLS AXELF AXELS AXILS AZOLE

A•••L

ABDEL ABDUL ABOIL ABRIL ACCEL ADDNL ADVIL AFOFL AFOUL ALGAL ALGOL ALKYL ALLYL AMAHL AMIEL ANGEL ANNAL ANNUL ANSEL ANTAL ANVIL APFEL APPAL APPEL APRIL ARBIL ARBOL AREAL AREEL ARIAL ARIEL ARNEL ARPEL ARTEL ASOUL ATALL ATHOL ATOLL AURAL AVAIL AVRIL AWFUL AXIAL

•AL••

AALTO BALAS BALBO BALCH BALDS BALDY BALED BALER BALES BALIN BALKI BALKS BALKY BALLO BALLS BALLY BALMS BALMY BALON BALOO BALPH BALSA BALTO BALTS CALAF CALEB CALIF CALIX CALKS CALLA CALLE CALLI CALLS CALME CALMS CALOR CALVE CALYX DALAI DALEN DALES DALET DALEY DALIS DALLY FALCO FALDO FALKE FALLA FALLS FALSE GALAS GALAX GALBA GALEA GALED GALEN GALES GALLI GALLO GALLS GALOP HALAL HALAS HALED HALEN HALER HALES HALEY HALLE HALLO HALLS HALOP HALOS HALTS HALVA HALVE JALPA KALEL KALES KALKI LALAW LALIA LALLA MALAR MALAY MALES MALEV

MALIC MALLE MALLS MALMO MALPH MALTA MALTS MALTY NALDI PALAR PALAU PALEA PALED PALEO PALER PALES PALEY PALIN PALLS PALLY PALMA PALME PALMS PALMY PALOS PALPS PALSY RALES RALLY RALPH SALAD SALAS SALEM SALEP SALES SALIC SALLE SALLY SALMA SALMI SALON SALOP SALSA SALTI SALTS SALTY SALUD SALUT SALVE SALVO TALAS TALCS TALER TALES TALIA TALKS TALKY TALLS TALLY TALON TALUS VALES VALET VALID VALLE VALLI VALOR VALSE VALUE VALVE WALDO WALED WALES WALKS WALLA WALLS WALLY WALSH WALSY WALTZ YALEU YALIE YALOW YALTA ZALES

•A•L•

BAALS BADLY BAILS BALLO BALLS BALLY BASLE BAULK BAWLS BAYLE CABLE CALLA CALLE CALLI CALLS CARLA CARLE CARLO CARLY CAULK DAILY DALLY DARLA EAGLE EARLE EARLS EARLY FABLE FAILS FALLA FALLS FATLY FAULT GABLE GAELS GAILY GALLI GALLO GALLS GAOLS GAULS GAYLE GAYLY HABLA HAILE HAILS HALLE HALLO HALLS HAOLE HAPLY HATLO HAULS JAILS KAHLO KARLA KARLE LADLE LAILA LALLA LAXLY LAYLA MACLE MADLY MAILS MALLE MALLS MANLY MAPLE MARLA MARLO MARLS MARLY MAULS MAYLE NAILS PABLO PAILS PALLS PALLY PAOLI PAOLO PARLE PATLY PAULA PAULI PAULO PAULV PAWLS RAILS RALLY RAWLS RAWLY SABLE SADLY SAILS SALLE SALLY SAULT TABLA TABLE TAELS TAILS TALLS TALLY VALLE VALLI VAULT WAALS WAILS WALLA WALLS WALLY WANLY YAWLS

•A••L

BABEL BAGEL BAIUL BANAL BASAL BASEL BASIL CABAL CAMEL CANAL CAROL CAVIL DARYL EASEL FACIL FATAL GABEL GAMAL GASOL GAVEL HACKL HALAL HAMEL HAVEL HAZEL JACAL JAMAL KABUL KALEL KAREL KAROL LABEL LADYL LAPEL LAVAL MABEL MAHAL MAZEL NAGEL NASAL NATAL NAVAL NAVEL OASAL PANDL PANEL PAPAL PAPEL PAROL PAVEL RAHAL RAOUL RATEL RAVEL SABAL SAGAL SAHEL SANDL TAMIL TAVEL TAXOL

••AL•

AGALS ALALA ATALA ATALL BAALS BBALL BEALE BEALL BEALS BIALY CHALK COALS DEALS DEALT DHALS DIALO DIALS DOALL DUALS EGALE EGALS EMALL EWALD EXALT FOALS GHALI GOALS HEALD HEALS HEALY ICALL INALL ITALO ITALS ITALY KOALA KUALA MEALS MEALY NEALE NEALY NYALA OCALA OPALS ORALB ORALE ORALS OVALS PEALE PEALS PSALM QUALM REALM REALS RIALS ROALD RYALS SCALA SCALD SCALE SCALP SCALY SEALE SEALS SEALY SHALE SHALL SHALT SKALD SMALL STALE STALK STALL SWALE TBALL TEALS TRALA UDALL URALS VEALE VEALS VEALY VIALS WAALS WEALD WEALS WHALE ZEALS

••A•L

AMAHL ATALL AVAIL BBALL BEALL BRAWL CRAWL DOALL DRAWL EMAIL EMALL ETAIL FLAIL FRAIL GNARL GRAIL ICALL INALL JPAUL KRAAL PEARL QUAIL SHALL SHAWL SMALL SNAIL SNARL STAEL STAHL STALL TBALL TRAIL TRAWL UDALL UHAUL

•••AL

ALGAL ANNAL ANTAL APPAL AREAL ARIAL AURAL AXIAL BANAL BASAL BINAL CABAL CANAL COPAL CORAL DECAL DORAL DOTAL DUCAL DUVAL ECTAL EQUAL FATAL FERAL FETAL FINAL FOCAL FUGAL GAMAL GLIAL GYRAL HALAL HEMAL HORAL IDEAL IGUAL ILEAL IQBAL JACAL JAMAL JUBAL JUGAL JURAL KEMAL KRAAL LAVAL LEGAL LOCAL LOYAL MAHAL MEDAL METAL MODAL MORAL MURAL NASAL NATAL NAVAL NEPAL NIVAL NOCAL NODAL NOPAL OASAL OCTAL OFFAL OIDAL ONEAL ORVAL PAPAL PEDAL PENAL PETAL PHIAL PODAL PUPAL RAHAL REGAL RENAL RIVAL RIYAL RIZAL ROYAL RURAL SABAL SAGAL SEGAL SEPAL SERAL SHOAL SISAL SKOAL SMEAL SOCAL SONAL STEAL TICAL TIDAL TONAL TOTAL TRIAL TUBAL TYPAL USUAL UVEAL UXMAL VENAL VIDAL VIRAL VITAL VOCAL ZONAL

AM•••

AMADA AMADO AMAHL AMAHS AMAIN AMANA AMAND AMANT AMAPA AMARA AMARE AMASS AMATI AMATO AMAZE AMBER AMBIT AMBLE AMBOS AMBOY AMBRY AMEBA AMEER AMEND AMENS AMENT AMERY AMICA AMICE AMICI AMICK AMICO AMIDE AMIEL AMIES AMIGA AMIGO AMINE AMINO AMIRI AMIRS AMISH AMISS AMITE AMITY AMLIT AMMAN AMMOS AMNIA AMNIO AMOCO AMOLE AMONG AMORE AMORS AMORT AMORY AMOUR AMPAS AMPED AMPHI AMPLE AMPLY AMPUP AMRAM AMTOO AMUCK AMUSE AMUST AMVET AMWAY AMYAS AMYLO AMYLS

A•M••

AAMCO AAMES ABMHO ACMES ADMAN ADMEN ADMIN ADMIT ADMIX AHMAD AHMED AIMAT AIMED AIMEE AIMER ALMAY ALMVP AMMAN AMMOS ARMAH ARMAS ARMED ARMEE ARMEN ARMER ARMES ARMET ARMEY ARMIN ARMOR ASMAD ATMAN ATMOS AXMAN AXMEN

A••M•

ABOMA ABOMB ADAMA ADAMS AGAMA AGAME AHEMS ALAMO ALUMS ANEMO ANIMA ANIME ANIMO ANOMY ARAME AROMA ARUMS ASAMI ASKME ATOMS ATOMY

A•••M

AANDM ABEAM ABOHM ABRAM ABRIM ABYSM ADEEM ADHEM ADREM AKEEM ALARM ALBOM ALBUM AMRAM ANNAM ANNUM ARIUM ASSAM ASWIM ATEAM AURUM AXIOM

•AM••

AAMCO AAMES BAMBA BAMBI BAMMY CAMAS CAMAY CAMBS CAMEL CAMEO CAMOS CAMPO CAMPS CAMPY CAMRY CAMUS DAMAS DAMEN DAMES DAMIS DAMME DAMNS DAMON DAMPS DAMUP EAMES EAMON FAMED FAMER FAMES FAMKE GAMAL GAMAY GAMBA GAMED GAMER GAMES GAMIN GAMMA GAMOW GAMPS GAMUT HAMAN HAMAS HAMEL HAMER HAMES HAMMS HAMMY HAMUP IAMBI IAMBS IAMSO JAMAL JAMBA JAMBE JAMBS JAMES JAMIE JAMIN JAMON JAMUP KAMEN LAMAR LAMAS LAMBS LAMED LAMER LAMES LAMIA LAMIT LAMPS MAMAS MAMBA MAMBO MAMET MAMIE MAMMA MAMMY NAMBY NAMED NAMER NAMES NAMIB NAMPA NAMUR PAMBY PAMPA RAMAN RAMAR RAMAS RAMBO RAMEN RAMET RAMEY RAMIE RAMIN RAMIS RAMON RAMOS RAMPS RAMUS RAMUZ SAMAR SAMBA SAMIS SAMMI SAMMS SAMMY SAMOA SAMOS SAMPS SAMSA TAMAR TAMED TAMER TAMES TAMIL TAMMI TAMMY TAMPA TAMPS VAMOS VAMPA VAMPS VAMPY

•A•M•

BALMS BALMY BAMMY BARMS BARMY BAUME CALME CALMS CARME DAMME EATME FAIMS FARMS GAMMA HAEMA HAMMS HAMMY HARMS JAIME KARMA LAKME MAAMS MAGMA MAIMS MALMO MAMMA MAMMY MARMS NAIMA NAOMI PALMA PALME PALMS PALMY PARMA RAIMI SALMA SALMI SAMMI SAMMS SAMMY TAMMI TAMMY WARMS YAYME

•A••M

AANDM CANEM CAROM DATUM HAKIM HAREM HARUM KASEM LARAM MADAM MAKEM MAXIM NAHUM OAKUM PACEM PANAM SALEM TATUM VADIM YADIM

••AM•

ADAMA ADAMS AGAMA AGAME ALAMO ARAME ASAMI BEAME BEAMS BEAMY BLAME BLAMS CHAMP CLAMP CLAMS CRAMP CRAMS DIAMS DRAMA DRAMS EDAMS ENAMI EXAMS FLAME FLAMS FLAMY FOAMS FOAMY FRAME GLAMS GRAMM GRAMO GRAMP GRAMS HYAMS ICAME IMAMS IMAMU ISAMU KLAMM KWAME LLAMA LOAMS LOAMY MAAMS MIAMI NEAME OBAMA OGAMS ORAMA PRAMS REAMS ROAMS SCAMP SCAMS SEAMS SEAMY SHAME SHAMS SHAMU SLAMS SOAMI SPAMS STAMP SWAMI SWAMP TEAMO TEAMS TIAMO TRAMP TRAMS UNAMI WHAMO WHAMS

••A•M

ALARM CHAIM CHARM CHASM CLAIM ENARM GRAMM KLAMM PHARM PLASM PSALM QUALM REAIM REALM REARM SMARM SPASM SWARM UNARM

•••AM

ABEAM ABRAM AMRAM ANNAM ASSAM ATEAM BREAM BTEAM CERAM CREAM DIRAM DREAM DRIAM EGHAM GLEAM GLOAM HBEAM HIRAM IBEAM ISHAM ISLAM LARAM LBEAM MADAM OCCAM OGHAM ONEAM OXFAM PANAM PRIAM PROAM SCRAM SIXAM STEAM STRAM TENAM TWOAM UNDAM UNJAM VITAM

AN•••

ANAGS ANAIS ANANA ANAND ANCHO ANCON ANDES ANDIE ANDOR ANDRE ANDRO ANDRY ANDSO ANDUP ANDYS ANELE ANEMO ANENT ANETO ANGEL ANGER ANGES ANGIE ANGIO ANGLE ANGLO ANGRY ANGST ANGUS ANIGH ANILE ANILS ANIMA ANIME ANIMO ANION ANISE ANITA ANJOU ANKHS ANKLE ANNAL ANNAM ANNAN ANNAS ANNEE ANNEX ANNIE ANNIV ANNOY ANNUL ANNUM ANNUS ANOAS ANODE ANOKA ANOLE ANOMY ANOUK ANSAE ANSEL ANSER ANSON ANTAE ANTAL ANTAS ANTED ANTES ANTIC ANTIQ ANTIS ANTON ANTRA ANTRE ANTSY ANVIL ANWAR ANYON ANZAC ANZIO ANZUS

A•N••

AANDE AANDM AANDP AANDW ABNER ACNES ADNAN AGNES AGNEW AGNON AGNUS AINGE AINSI AINUS AMNIA AMNIO ANNAL ANNAM ANNAN ANNAS ANNEE ANNEX ANNIE ANNIV ANNOY ANNUL ANNUM ANNUS AONES APNEA ARNAZ ARNEL ARNIE ASNAP ASNER ASNEW ATNOS AUNTS AUNTY AVNET AWNED

A••N•

ABEND ACING ADANA ADANO ADDNL ADENI ADENO ADINS AEONS AETNA AGANA AGENA AGENT AGING AGONY AHANG AHING AISNE AKENE AKINS ALANA ALENE ALINE ALONE

ALONG AMANA AMAND AMANT AMEND AMENS AMENT AMINE AMINO AMONG ANANA ANAND ANENT APING ARANS ARENA ARENS ARENT ARONI ARUNS ASANA ASONE ASSNS ATONE ATONY AVANT AVENA AWING AXING AXONE AXONS AYINS AZANS

A•••N

AARON ACORN ACTIN ACTON ADARN ADDIN ADDON ADMAN ADMEN ADMIN ADNAN ADORN AFTON AGAIN AGARN AGNON AGRIN AGRON AHSIN AIDAN AIKEN AKRON ALAIN ALBAN ALBEN ALCAN ALDEN ALIEN ALIGN ALLAN ALLEN ALLIN ALLYN ALPEN ALTON ALVIN AMAIN AMMAN ANCON ANION ANNAN ANSON ANTON ANYON APAIN APIAN APRON ARDEN ARGON ARIAN ARION ARKIN ARLEN ARMEN ARMIN ARRAN ARSON ARWEN ARYAN ASHEN ASIAN ASKIN ASLAN ASPEN ASPIN ASTIN ASTON ASWAN ATEIN ATHON ATION ATMAN ATTEN AUDEN AUVIN AVIAN AVION AXION AXMAN AXMEN AXTON

•AN••

AANDE AANDM AANDP AANDW BANAL BANCA BANCO BANCS BANDA BANDB BANDO BANDS BANDW BANDY BANES BANFF BANGS BANJO BANKS BANKY BANNS BANON BANOS BANTA BANTU CANAL CANBY CANDO CANDW CANDY CANEA CANED CANEM CANER CANES CANID CANIO CANIS CANIT CANNA CANNY CANOE CANON CANSO CANST CANTO CANTS CANTY DANAE DANCE DANDD DANDY DANES DANGS DANIA DANIO DANKE DANNO DANNY DANSE DANTE DANZA FANCY FANES FANGS FANNY FANON FANTA GANCE GANDT GANDY GANEF GANGS GANSU HANDI HANDS HANDY HANES HANEY HANFF HANGS HANKS HANKY HANNA HANOI HANSA HANSE HANTS HANYA JANDB JANDJ JANET JANIE JANIS JANOS JANUS KANAR KANAS KANDY KANGA KANGS KANIN KANJI KANSA KANYE LANAI LANCE LANDI LANDO LANDS LANED LANES LANGE LANIN LANKA LANKY LANNY LANOS LANTZ LANZA MANAT MANCY MANDY MANED MANES MANET MANGA MANGE MANGO MANGY MANIA MANIC MANLY MANNA MANNE MANNY MANON MANOR MANOS MANSE MANTA MANUS NANAK NANAS NANCE NANCI NANCY NANKI NANNA NANNO NANNY NANON NANTZ PANAM PANAY PANDA PANDL PANED PANEL PANES PANGS PANIC PANIN PANIS PANKY PANNE PANSY PANTA PANTO PANTS PANTY PANZA QANDA RANAS RANAT RANBY RANCH RANDA RANDB RANDD RANDI RANDR RANDS RANDY RANEE RANGE RANGO RANGY RANID RANIN RANIS RANKE RANKS RANON RANTO RANTS RANUP SANAA SANDE SANDH SANDL SANDP SANDS SANDY SANER SANKA SANTA SANTE SANTO SANYO TANDY TANEY TANGO TANGS TANGY TANIA TANIS TANKA TANKS TANNA TANSY TANTE TANTO TANYA VANCE VANED VANES VANNA VANUA VANYA WANDA WANDS WANED WANER WANES WANLY WANNA WANTS XANDO XANDY YANCY YANKS YANNI

•A•N•

BANNS BARNS BATNA CAINE CAINT CANNA CANNY CARNE CARNY DAMNS DANNO DANNY DARNS DASNT DAUNT DAWNN DAWNS DAYNE EARNS FAENA FAINT FANNY FAUNA FAUNS FAWNS GAINS GARNI GAUNT HADNO HADNT HAING HANNA HASNO HASNT HAUNT JAINS JAUNE JAUNT JAYNE KAHNS KAONS KARNS LAINE LAING LANNY LAWNS LAWNY LAYNE MAGNA MAINE MAINS MAINZ MANNA MANNE MANNY MARNE MARNI MAUNA MAYNT NAINA NANNA NANNO NANNY PAINE PAINS PAINT PANNE PAONS PATNA PAWNS PAYNE RAINE RAINS RAINY SAENS SAINT SAONE SAUNA SAYNO TAINA TAINT TANNA TARNS TAUNT TAWNY VANNA VARNA VAUNT WAINS WANNA WARNS WASNT WAYNE YANNI YARNS YAWNS YAWNY ZAHND

•A••N

AARON BACON BADEN BADUN BAIRN BALIN BALON BANON BARON BASIN BATIN BATON CABIN CAIRN CAJON CAJUN CANON CAPON CARON CAVAN DABON DAGAN DALEN DAMEN DAMON DARIN DAVEN DAWNN DAYAN EAGAN EAMON EATEN EATIN EATON EAVAN FAGIN FANON FARON GABIN GABON GAHAN GALEN GAMIN GATUN GAVIN HADIN HADON HAGEN HALEN HAMAN HASIN HASON HAVEN HAYDN HAZAN JAHAN JAMIN JAMON JAPAN JASON JAVAN KAMEN KANIN KARAN KAREN KARYN KAZAN KAZIN LABAN LADEN LANIN LAPIN LATEN LATIN LAVIN LAYIN LAYON MACON MAHAN MAHON MAKIN MANON MARIN MASON MATIN MAVEN MAVIN MAYAN NANON NATAN OAKEN OATEN PAEAN PAGAN PALIN PANIN PAREN PATEN PATON PAVIN PAYIN RABIN RADON RAGON RAMAN RAMEN RAMIN RAMON RANIN RANON RAPON RATON RAVEN RAYON SABIN SAFIN SAGAN SALON SARAN SATAN SATIN SATON SAWIN SAXON TAGON TAKEN TAKIN TALON TAPIN TAPON TAUON TAXON WAGON WAKEN WASIN WASON WAXEN WAYIN ZAYIN ZAZEN

••AN•

ADANA ADANO AGANA AHANG ALANA AMANA AMAND AMANT ANANA ANAND ARANS ASANA AVANT AZANS BEANO BEANS BEANY BHANG BLANC BLAND BLANE BLANK BRAND BRANG BRANS BRANT BWANA CHANG CHANT CIANO CLANG CLANK CLANS CRANE CRANI CRANK CYANO CYANS DEANA DEANE DEANS DIANA DIANE DOANE DOANS DRANG DRANK DRANO DUANE EBANK ELAND EVANS FLANK FLANN FLANS FRANC FRANK FRANN FRANS FRANZ GHANA GIANT GLAND GRAND GRANI GRANT GUANO HUANG ICANT INANE IPANA IRANI IVANA IVANI IVANV IWANT JEANE JEANS JIANG JUANO KEANE KEANU KHANS KOANS LEANN LEANS LEANT LIANA LIANE LIANG LLANO LOANS LUANA LUANG LUANN MEANS MEANT MEANY MOANS NGANA OLAND OMANI ORANG ORANI ORANT OXANA PEANO PHANY PIANI PIANO PLANA PLANB PLANE PLANI PLANK PLANO PLANS PLANT PRANA PRANK QUAND QUANG QUANT RIANT ROANS RYANS SCANS SCANT SEANN SHANA SHANE SHANG SHANK SHANT SKANK SLANG SLANT SPANG SPANK SPANO SPANS STAND STANG STANK STANS SWANK SWANN SWANS THANE THANK THANT THANX TIANT TRANE TRANS TWANG URANO VIAND WEANS WHANG YEANS YUANS

••A•N

ADARN AGAIN AGARN ALAIN AMAIN APAIN BRAIN BRAUN BRAWN CHAIN CRAIN DRAIN DRAWN FLANN FRANN FRAYN GHAIN GNAWN GRAIN HEARN ICAHN LEANN LEARN LUANN PLAIN PRAWN SEANN SHAHN SHAUN SHAWN SLAIN SPAHN SPAIN SPAWN STAIN SWAIN SWANN TRAIN TWAIN UTAHN YEARN YVAIN YWAIN

•••AN

ADMAN ADNAN AIDAN ALBAN ALCAN ALLAN AMMAN ANNAN APIAN ARIAN ARRAN ARYAN ASIAN ASLAN ASWAN ATMAN AVIAN AXMAN BEGAN BEHAN BEMAN BOGAN BRIAN BRYAN CAVAN CLEAN COHAN CONAN COTAN CSPAN CUBAN DAGAN DAYAN DIVAN DORAN DUGAN DURAN DYLAN EAGAN EAVAN ELMAN ESTAN ETHAN EVIAN GAHAN GLEAN GOLAN GOMAN GORAN GROAN HAMAN HAZAN HEMAN HOBAN HOGAN HONAN HUMAN HUNAN HYMAN IMEAN INCAN IOWAN JAHAN JAPAN JAVAN JEHAN JIHAN JOHAN JOVAN JURAN KARAN KAZAN KORAN LABAN LEMAN LEXAN LIMAN LOGAN LOHAN LOMAN LORAN LUCAN LUJAN LUMAN LYMAN MAHAN MAYAN MEGAN MIKAN MILAN MORAN MULAN MYMAN NATAN NEMAN NISAN NOLAN NUMAN NYMAN OCEAN OCTAN OHMAN OLEAN ORGAN ORKAN ORMAN OSCAN OSMAN PAEAN PAGAN PECAN PERAN PISAN PRMAN PUSAN QURAN RAMAN RECAN REDAN REGAN REHAN REMAN RENAN RERAN RETAN RICAN RIGAN RODAN ROMAN RONAN ROWAN RUMAN SAGAN SARAN SATAN SEDAN SHEAN SIVAN SLOAN SOLAN SUDAN SUSAN TEXAN TITAN TVMAN TYNAN UCLAN UHLAN UNMAN URBAN VEGAN WOMAN WOTAN WUHAN WYMAN YUBAN YUMAN

AO•••

AOKAY AOLER AONES AORTA AOSTA AOUTS

A•O••

ABODE ABOHM ABOIL ABOMA ABOMB ABORT ABOUT ABOVE ABOVO ACORN ADOBE ADOBO ADOLF ADOPT ADORE ADORN ADOUT ADOZE AEONS AFOFL AFOOT AFORE AFOUL AGOGO AGONY AGORA AHOLD AHOOT AHORA AHOYS AIOLI ALOES ALOFT ALOHA ALOIS ALONE ALONG ALOOF ALORS ALOUD AMOCO AMOLE AMONG AMORE AMORS AMORT AMORY AMOUR ANOAS ANODE ANOKA ANOLE ANOMY ANOUK APODS APORT AROAR AROID AROMA ARONI AROSE ASOLD ASONE ASORS ASOUL ATOLL ATOMS ATOMY ATONE ATONY ATORY AVOID AVOIR AVOWS AWOKE AWOLS AXONE AXONS AZOIC AZOLE AZORE AZOTH

A••O•

AARON ABBOT ABHOR ACHOO ACTON ACTOR ACTOS ADAOK ADDON ADHOC ADIOS AEIOU AEROS AESOP AFOOT AFROS AFTON AGIOS AGLOW AGNON AGRON AHOOT AIDOO AKRON ALBOM ALCOA ALCOR ALGOL ALIOS ALLOF ALLOK ALLOT ALLOW ALLOY ALOOF ALROY ALSOP ALTON ALTOS AMBOS AMBOY AMMOS AMTOO ANCON ANDOR ANION ANJOU ANNOY ANSON ANTON ANYON APRON APSOS ARBOL ARBOR ARDOR ARGON ARGOS ARGOT ARION ARIOT ARMOR ARROW ARROZ ARSON ARTOO ASCOT ASFOR ASHOT ASKOF ASSOC ASTON ASTOR ATEOF ATHOL ATHON ATHOS ATION ATMOS ATNOS AUTOS AVION AVIOR AXIOM AXION AXTON

A•••O

AALTO AAMCO ABACO

5
AO

ABAJO
ABMHO
ABOVO
ACETO
ACHOO
ADANO
ADDIO
ADDTO
ADENO
ADOBO
AEREO
AERIO
AGOGO
AIDOO
ALADO
ALAMO
ALERO
ALFIO
ALITO
ALTHO
ALUKO
AMADO
AMATO
AMICO
AMIGO
AMINO
AMNIO
AMOCO
AMTOO
AMYLO
ANCHO
ANDRO
ANDSO
ANEMO
ANETO
ANGIO
ANGLO
ANIMO
ANZIO
ARADO
ARESO
ARTOO
ASTRO
ATTWO
AUDIO
AVISO
AYAKO

•AO••
GAOLS
HAOLE
KAONS
MAOII
MAORI
NAOMI
PAOLI
PAOLO
PAONS
RAOUL
SAONE

•A•O•
AARON
BABOO
BACON
BACOS
BALON
BALOO
BANON
BANOS
BARON
BASOV
BATON
BATOR
BAYOU
BAZOO
CABOB
CABOT
CAJON
CALOR
CAMOS
CANOE
CANON
CAPON
CAPOS
CAROB
CAROL
CAROM
CARON
DABON
DADOS
DAFOE
DAMON
DATOS
DAVOS
EAMON
EAPOE
EATOF
EATON
FADOS
FAGOT
FANON
FAROE
FARON
FAROS
FAVOR
GABON
GABOR
GALOP
GAMOW
GAROU
GASOL
GATOR
GATOS
GAVOT
HADON
HALOP
HALOS
HANOI
HASON
HAVOC
JABOT
JACOB
JAKOB
JAMON
JANOS
JASON
JATOS
KABOB
KAPOK
KAPOW
KAROL
KAYOS
KAZOO
LABOR
LAGOS
LANOS
LAYON
MACON
MADOC
MADOX
MAGOG
MAGOO
MAHON
MAJOR
MAKOS
MANON
MANOR
MANOS
MAROT
MASON
MAYOR
MAYOS
NABOB
NABOO
NANON
NAXOS
PALOS
PAROL
PAROO
PAROS
PASOS
PATON
PATOS
PAXOS
PAYOR
RADON
RAGON
RAMON
RAMOS
RANON
RAPON
RATON
RAYON
RAZOR
SABOT
SAGOS
SALON
SALOP
SAMOA
SAMOS
SAPOR
SAROS
SATON
SAVOR
SAVOY
SAXON
SAYOK
TABOO
TABOR
TACOS
TAGON
TAHOE
TALON
TAPON
TAROS
TAROT
TAUON
TAXOL
TAXON
VALOR
VAMOS
VAPOR
WAGON
WAHOO
WASON
YAHOO
YAKOV
YALOW
YAZOO

•A••O
AALTO
AAMCO
BABOO
BACIO
BALBO
BALLO
BALOO
BALTO
BANCO
BANDO
BANJO
BARCO
BASHO
BASSO
BATHO
BAZOO
CACAO
CAIRO
CAMEO
CAMPO
CANDO
CANIO
CANSO
CANTO
CARBO
CARGO
CARLO
CARPO
CASCO
CASIO
CAUDO
DANIO
DANNO
DARIO
DAVAO
FABIO
FACTO
FALCO
FALDO
FARGO
FATSO
GALLO
GARBO
GATTO
HADNO
HADTO
HAGIO
HALLO
HARPO
HASNO
HASSO
HASTO
HATLO
IAMSO
IATRO
JACKO
KAHLO
KAZOO
LACTO
LANDO
LARGO
LASSO
LAURO
LAYTO
MACAO
MACHO
MACRO
MAGOO
MALMO
MAMBO
MANGO
MARCO
MARGO
MARIO
MARLO
MARZO
MATEO
MATRO
MATZO
MAYPO
NABOO
NACHO
NACIO
NANNO
NARCO
NARDO
NATRO
PAAVO
PABLO
PALEO
PANTO
PAOLO
PARDO
PAROO
PASCO
PASEO
PASTO
PATCO
PATHO
PATIO
PATRO
PAULO
PAYTO
RADIO
RAFKO
RAMBO
RANGO
RANTO
RATIO
RATSO
SACCO
SACRO
SALVO
SANTO
SANYO
SARTO
SAURO
SAWTO
SAYNO
SAYSO
TABOO
TACHO
TAEBO
TAITO
TANGO
TANTO
TARDO
TARSO
TASSO
TAURO
TAUTO
TAXCO
VARRO
VASCO
WACKO
WAHOO
WAKKO
WALDO
WASCO
WASHO
WASSO
XACTO
XANDO
YAHOO
YAZOO

••AO•
ADAOK
CHAOS
CIAOS
MIAOU
MIAOW

••A•O
ABACO
ABAJO
ADANO
ALADO
ALAMO
AMADO
AMATO
ARADO
AYAKO
BEANO
BRAVO
BRAZO
CHACO
CHARO
CIANO
CLARO
CYANO
DIALO
DRACO
DRAGO
DRANO
ERATO
GLAXO
GRAMO
GUANO
GUAPO
IDAHO
IMAGO
ITALO
JUANO
LLANO
MTAPO
NEATO
NGAIO
OHAYO
PAAVO
PEABO
PEANO
PHAGO
PIANO
PLANO
PLATO
PRADO
PRATO
QUAXO
SEATO
SHAKO
SPAGO
SPANO
TEAMO
TIAGO
TIAMO
TSAVO
URANO
WHAMO

•••AO
CACAO
DAVAO
DRLAO
MACAO

AP•••
APACE
APAIN
APARS
APART
APEAK
APEEK
APEEP
APERS
APERY
APFEL
APHID
APHIS
APIAN
APIED
APING
APISH
APLEY
APLUS
APNEA
APODS
APORT
APPAL
APPEL
APPIA
APPLE
APPLY
APPTS
APRES
APRIL
APRON
APSES
APSIS
APSOS
APTED
APTER
APTLY

A•P••
ALPEN
ALPES
ALPHA
AMPAS
AMPED
AMPHI
AMPLE
AMPLY
AMPUP
APPAL
APPEL
APPIA
APPLE
APPLY
APPTS
ARPAD
ARPEL
ASPCA
ASPEN
ASPER
ASPIC
ASPIN
ATPAR

A••P•
ACUPS
ADAPT
ADEPT
ADOPT
AGAPE
ALEPH
AMAPA

A•••P
AANDP
ACTUP
ADDUP
ADREP
ADRIP
AESOP
AGASP
AHEAP
AIRUP
ALMVP
ALSOP
AMPUP
ANDUP
APEEP
ASCAP
ASKUP
ASNAP
ATEUP
ATRIP

•AP••
CAPAS
CAPED
CAPEK
CAPER
CAPES
CAPET
CAPON
CAPOS
CAPRA
CAPRI
CAPTS
CAPUT
EAPOE
GAPED
GAPER
GAPES
HAPLY
HAPPY
JAPAN
JAPED
JAPER
JAPES
KAPHS
KAPOK
KAPOW
KAPPA
KAPUT
LAPAT
LAPAZ
LAPEL
LAPIN
LAPIS
LAPPS
LAPSE
LAPUP
MAPES
MAPLE
NAPES
NAPPE
NAPPY
PAPAL
PAPAS
PAPAW
PAPEL
PAPER
PAPPY
PAPUA
RAPEE
RAPID
RAPON
SAPID
SAPOR
SAPPY
TAPAS
TAPED
TAPER
TAPES
TAPIN
TAPIR
TAPIS
TAPON
VAPID
VAPOR
YAPAT
ZAPPA
ZAPPY

•A•P•
BALPH
CAMPO
CAMPS
CAMPY
CARPE
CARPI
CARPO
CARPS
DAMPS
EARPS
GAMPS
GASPE
GASPS
GAWPS
HARPO
HARPS
HARPY
HASPS
JALPA
KAPPA
LAMPS
LAPPS
MALPH
MAYPO
NAMPA
NAPPE
NAPPY
PALPS
PAMPA
PAPPY
RALPH
RAMPS
RASPA
RASPE
RASPS
RASPY
SAMPS
SAPPY
TAMPA
TAMPS
TARPS
TAUPE
VAMPA
VAMPS
VAMPY
WARPS
WASPS
WASPY
YAWPS
ZAPPA
ZAPPY

•A••P
AANDP
DAMUP
EATUP
GALOP
GASUP
HADUP
HALOP
HAMUP
HASUP
JAMUP
LAPUP
LAYUP
NAACP
PAYUP
RANUP
SALEP
SALOP
SANDP
SATUP
SAWUP
TAGUP
WADUP
WASUP
WAXUP
WAYUP

••AP•
ADAPT
AGAPE
AMAPA
CHAPS
CLAPS
COAPT
CRAPE
CRAPS
DRAPE
ETAPE
FLAPS
GOAPE
GRAPE
GRAPH
GRAPY
GUAPA
GUAPO
HEAPS
HEAPY
INAPT
LEAPS
LEAPT
MTAPO
NEAPS
NWAPA
OKAPI
REAPS
SCAPA
SCAPE
SHAPE
SLAPS
SNAPS
SOAPS
SOAPY
STAPH
SWAPS
TRAPP
TRAPS
UNAPT
WHAPS
WRAPS
WRAPT

••A•P
AGASP
CHAMP
CLAMP
CLASP
CRAMP
GRAMP
GRASP
NAACP
SCALP
SCAMP
SCARP
SHARP
STAMP
SWAMP
THARP
TRAMP
TRAPP

•••AP
AHEAP
ASCAP
ASNAP
CHEAP
DECAP
ONTAP
PTRAP
RECAP
RELAP
REMAP
RETAP
SCRAP
STRAP
UNCAP

AQ•••
AQABA
AQUAE
AQUAS

A•Q••
ACQUA
ATQUE

A•••Q
ANTIQ

•AQ••
FAQIR
MAQUI
YAQUI

•A•Q•
BARQS

•A••Q
BARBQ
TARIQ

••AQ•
IRAQI

AR•••
ARABS
ARABY
ARADO
ARAME
ARANS
ARARA
ARBER
ARBIL
ARBOL
ARBOR
ARBRE
ARBUS
ARBYS
ARCAE
ARCED
ARCHE
ARCHI
ARCHY
ARDEN
ARDOR
AREAL
AREAR
AREAS
ARECA
AREEL
ARENA
ARENS
ARENT
ARESO
ARETE
ARGON
ARGOS
ARGOT
ARGUE
ARGUS
ARHAT
ARIAL
ARIAN
ARIAS
ARICA
ARIEL
ARIES
ARILS
ARION
ARIOT
ARISE
ARITH
ARIUM
ARKIN
ARLEN
ARLES
ARMAH
ARMAS
ARMED
ARMEE
ARMEN
ARMER
ARMES
ARMET
ARMEY
ARMIN
ARMOR
ARNAZ
ARNEL
ARNIE
AROAR
AROID
AROMA
ARONI
AROSE
ARPAD
ARPEL
ARRAH
ARRAN
ARRAS
ARRAU
ARRAY
ARRET
ARRID
ARRIS
ARROW
ARROZ
ARSES
ARSIS
ARSON
ARTEL
ARTIE
ARTIS
ARTOO
ARTSY
ARTUR
ARUBA
ARUMS
ARUNS
ARWEN
ARYAN
ARYLS

A•R••
AARAU
AARGH
AARON
ABRAM
ABRIL
ABRIM
ABRIS
ACRED
ACRES
ACRID
ADREM
ADREP
ADRIP
AEREO
AERIE
AERIO
AEROS
AFRIC
AFROS
AGREE
AGRIC
AGRIN
AGRON
AIRED
AIRER
AIRES
AIRUP
AKRON
ALROY
AMRAM
AORTA
APRES
APRIL
APRON
ARRAH
ARRAN
ARRAS
ARRAU
ARRAY
ARRET
ARRID
ARRIS
ARROW
ARROZ
ASRED
ATRAS
ATRIA
ATRIP
AURAE
AURAL
AURAR
AURAS
AURIC
AURUM
AVRIL
AYRES

A••R•
ABBRS
ABORT
ACCRA
ACERB
ACERS
ACORN
ACURA
ADARN
ADARS
ADDRS
ADORE
ADORN
AFARS
AFIRE
AFORE
AFTRA
AGARN
AGARS
AGERS
AGORA
AGURA
AHORA
AKERS
AKIRA
ALARM
ALERO
ALERS
ALERT
ALFRE
ALORS
AMARA
AMARE
AMBRY
AMERY
AMIRI
AMIRS
AMORE
AMORS
AMORT
AMORY
ANDRE
ANDRO
ANDRY
ANGRY
ANTRA
ANTRE
APARS
APART
APERS
APERY
APORT
ARARA
ARBRE
ASDRY
ASORS
ASTRA
ASTRE
ASTRO
ATARI
ATARS
ATORY
AUDRA
AUTRE
AUTRY
AVERS
AVERT
AVERY
AWARD
AWARE
AXERS
AYERS
AZERA
AZERI
AZORE
AZURE

A•••R
ABEAR
ABHOR
ABLER
ABNER
ACHER
ACTER
ACTOR
ADAIR
ADDER
ADLER
ADWAR
AEGIR
AESIR
AFTER
AHAIR
AIDER
AILUR
AIMER
AIRER
AKBAR
ALCOR
ALDER
ALGER
ALLER
ALTAR
ALTER
ALVAR
AMBER
AMEER
AMOUR
ANDOR
ANGER
ANSER
ANWAR
AOLER
APTER
ARBER
ARBOR
ARDOR
AREAR
ARMER
ARMOR
AROAR
ARTUR
ASFOR
ASHER
ASHUR
ASKER
ASNER
ASPER
ASSER
ASSYR
ASTER
ASTIR
ASTOR
ATBAR
ATPAR
ATTAR
ATWAR
AUBER
AUGER
AUGUR
AURAR
AUSTR
AVIOR
AVOIR
AYEAR

•AR••
AARAU
AARGH
AARON
BARAK
BARBA
BARBI
BARBQ
BARBS
BARCA
BARCO
BARDS
BARED
BARER
BARES
BARFY
BARGE
BARIC
BARIT
BARKS
BARKY
BARMS
BARMY
BARNS
BARON
BARQS
BARRE
BARRY
BARTH
BARTY
CARAT
CARAY
CARBO
CARBS
CARDI
CARDS
CARED
CARER
CARES
CARET
CAREW
CAREY
CARGO
CARIB
CARLA
CARLE
CARLO
CARLY
CARME
CARNE
CARNY
CAROB
CAROL
CAROM
CARON
CARPE
CARPI
CARPO
CARPS
CARRE
CARRY
CARTA
CARTE
CARTS
CARVE
DARBY
DARCI
DARCY
DARDY
DARED
DARER
DARES
DARIA
DARIN
DARIO
DARKS
DARLA
DARNS

DARTE
DARTH
DARTS
DARYA
DARYL
EARED
EARLE
EARLS
EARLY
EARNS
EARPS
EARTH
FARAD
FARAH
FARCE
FARCI
FARED
FARER
FARES
FARGO
FARIS
FARMS
FAROE
FARON
FAROS
FARSI
FARUK
GARBO
GARBS
GARDA
GARDE
GARES
GARNI
GAROU
GARRY
GARTH
HARDC
HARDG
HARDY
HARED
HAREM
HARES
HARKS
HARMS
HARPO
HARPS
HARPY
HARRY
HARSH
HARTE
HARUM
JARED
JARRE
KARAN
KARAS
KARAT
KAREL
KAREN
KARLA
KARLE
KARMA
KARNS
KAROL
KARSH
KARST
KARTS
KARUS
KARYN

LARAM
LARAS
LARCH
LARDS
LARDY
LAREE
LARES
LARGE
LARGO
LARIS
LARKS
LARKY
LARRY
LARUE
LARVA
MARAT
MARCA
MARCH
MARCI
MARCO
MARCY
MARDI
MAREK
MARES
MARGE
MARGO
MARGY
MARIA
MARIE
MARIN
MARIO
MARIS
MARKA
MARKI
MARKS
MARKV
MARLA
MARLO
MARLS
MARLY
MARMS
MARNE
MARNI
MAROT
MARRY
MARSH
MARTA
MARTI
MARTS
MARTY
MARVY
MARYA
MARYI
MARYJ
MARYS
MARZO
NARAS
NARCO
NARCS
NARDA
NARDO
NARDS
NARES
NARIC
NARIS
NARKS
OARED
OARER

PARAS
PARCA
PARCH
PARCS
PARDO
PARDS
PARED
PAREE
PAREN
PARER
PARES
PAREU
PARGE
PARIS
PARKA
PARKS
PARLE
PARMA
PAROL
PAROO
PAROS
PARRA
PARRS
PARRY
PARSE
PARSI
PARTA
PARTB
PARTC
PARTE
PARTI
PARTS
PARTV
PARTY
RARAE
RAREE
RARER
SARAH
SARAI
SARAN
SARDI
SARDS
SAREE
SAREK
SARGE
SARIS
SAROS
SARTO
TARAS
TARDE
TARDO
TARDY
TARED
TARES
TARGA
TARIQ
TARNS
TAROS
TAROT
TARPS
TARRY
TARSI
TARSO
TARTE
TARTS
TARTU
TARTY
VARDA

VARIA
VARIG
VARNA
VARRO
VARSI
VARYA
WARDS
WARED
WARES
WARKS
WARMS
WARNS
WARPS
WARTS
WARTY
YARDS
YARER
YARNS
YARRA
ZARFS

•A•R•

BAIRD
BAIRN
BARRE
BARRY
BASRA
CADRE
CAIRN
CAIRO
CAMRY
CAPRA
CAPRI
CARRE
CARRY
DAIRY
EAGRE
FABRE
FAERY
FAIRE
FAIRS
FAIRY
FAURE
FAVRE
GARRY
GAURS
HAIRS
HAIRY
HARRY
HAVRE
IATRO
IATRY
JAHRE
JARRE
LAIRD
LAIRS
LARRY
LAURA
LAURO
MACRO
MADRE
MAHRE
MAIRE
MAORI
MARRY
MATRI
MATRO
MAURA

MAURY
NACRE
NAIRA
NATRO
NAURU
PADRE
PAIRS
PARRA
PARRS
PARRY
PATRI
PATRO
SABRA
SABRE
SACRA
SACRE
SACRO
SAIRY
SAURO
TARRY
TATRA
TAURI
TAURO
VARRO
WAART
YARRA
ZAIRE

•A••R

BABAR
BADER
BAJER
BAKER
BALER
BARER
BASER
BATOR
BAUER
BAYAR
BAYER
CABER
CAGER
CALOR
CANER
CAPER
CARER
CASER
CATER
CAVER
DAKAR
DARER
DATER
DAZER
DAZUR
EAGER
EASER
EATER
FABER
FACER
FADER
FAKER
FAKIR
FAMER
FAQIR
FARER
FAVOR
FAXER
GABOR

GAMER
GAPER
GASTR
GATER
GATOR
GAYER
GAZER
HABER
HAGAR
HALER
HAMER
HATER
HAUER
HAVER
HAWER
HAYER
HAZER
JAFAR
JAPER
JAWER
KADAR
KANAR
LABOR
LACER
LADER
LAGER
LAKER
LAMAR
LAMER
LASER
LATER
LAUER
LAVER
LAXER
LAYER
LAZAR
MACER
MAHER
MAJOR
MAKER
MALAR
MANOR
MASER
MASUR
MATER
MAYER
MAYOR
MAZAR
NADER
NADIR
NAMER
NAMUR
OARER
OATER
PACER
PAGER
PALAR
PALER
PAPER
PARER
PATER
PAVER
PAWER
PAYER
PAYOR
QATAR
RACER
RADAR

RADER
RAFER
RAGER
RAKER
RAMAR
RANDR
RARER
RASER
RATER
RAVER
RAWER
RAZER
RAZOR
SABER
SAFAR
SAFER
SAGER
SAMAR
SANER
SAPOR
SATYR
SAVER
SAVOR
SAWER
SAYER
TABOR
TAKER
TALER
TAMAR
TAMER
TAPER
TAPIR
TASER
TATAR
TATER
TAXER
VADER
VALOR
VAPOR
VATER
WADER
WAFER
WAGER
WAKER
WANER
WATER
WAVER
WAXER
YARER
YASIR
ZADAR

••AR•

ADARN
ADARS
AFARS
AGARN
AGARS
ALARM
AMARA
AMARE
APARS
APART
ARARA
ATARI
ATARS
AWARD
AWARE

BEARD
BEARS
BEART
BLARE
BOARD
BOARS
CEARA
CHARD
CHARM
CHARO
CHARS
CHART
CHARY
CLARA
CLARE
CLARK
CLARO
CLARY
CZARS
DEARE
DEARS
DEARY
DIARY
DMARK
DWARF
ECARD
ELARA
ENARE
ENARM
EWART
FEARS
FLARE
GEARS
GEARY
GLARE
GLARY
GNARL
GNARS
GUARD
GUARE
GUARS
HBARS
HEARD
HEARN
HEARS
HEART
HOARD
HOARE
HOARS
HOARY
IBARS
ICARE
IMARI
INARI
IYARS
JBARS
KCARS
KMART
KNARS
LBARS
LEARN
LEARS
LEARY
LIARS
MEARA
MEARS
NEARS
OHARA

OHARE
OKARA
OMARR
OPART
OTARU
OTARY
OVARY
OZARK
PEARL
PEARS
PEARY
PHARM
QUARE
QUARK
QUART
REARM
REARS
ROARK
ROARS
RUARK
SCARE
SCARF
SCARP
SCARS
SCARY
SEARS
SHARD
SHARE
SHARI
SHARK
SHARP
SMARM
SMART
SNARE
SNARF
SNARK
SNARL
SOARS
SPARE
SPARK
SPARS
STARE
STARK
STARR
STARS
START
STARZ
SWARD
SWARM
TBARS
TEARS
TEARY
THARP
TIARA
TSARS
TZARA
TZARS
UNARM
UNARY
WAART
WEARS
WEARY
WHARF
XSARA
YEARN
YEARS
ZBARS

••A•R

ADAIR
AHAIR
BHAER
BLAIR
BYAIR
CHAIR
CLAIR
DEAIR
FLAIR
NBAER
OHAIR
OMARR
ONAIR
PHAIR
QUADR
REAIR
STAHR
STAIR
STARR
USAIR

•••AR

ABEAR
ADWAR
AKBAR
ALTAR
ALVAR
ANWAR
AREAR
AROAR
ATBAR
ATPAR
ATTAR
ATWAR
AURAR
AYEAR
BABAR
BAYAR
BEHAR
BEXAR
BLEAR
BOLAR
BONAR
BRIAR
BSTAR
BYCAR
BYEAR
BYFAR
CEDAR
CESAR
CIGAR
CLEAR
CSTAR
DAKAR
DEBAR
DENAR
DETAR
DEWAR
DINAR
DREAR
EDGAR
EDMAR
EGGAR
ELCAR
ELGAR
ELMAR
EMBAR

ESTAR
FILAR
FRIAR
FSTAR
GOFAR
GSTAR
HAGAR
HOWAR
IHEAR
JAFAR
KADAR
KANAR
KOSAR
KSTAR
LAMAR
LAZAR
LECAR
LEHAR
LEVAR
LIDAR
LIFAR
LOBAR
LUGAR
LUNAR
MALAR
MAZAR
MIZAR
MOLAR
MSTAR
MYLAR
MYWAR
NOEAR
NOMAR
NOPAR
NSTAR
ONPAR
OSCAR
OSKAR
OSTAR
PALAR
PILAR
PIXAR
POLAR
QATAR
RADAR
RAMAR
REBAR
RETAR
SAFAR
SAMAR
SEGAR
SHEAR
SITAR
SMEAR
SOFAR
SOLAR
SONAR
SPEAR
SSTAR
SUGAR
SWEAR
TAMAR
TATAR
TELAR
TOLAR
TOMAR
TOWAR
ULNAR

UNBAR
UNFAR
UNGAR
UTTAR
VELAR
VICAR
VOLAR
ZADAR

AS•••

ASAGI
ASAHI
ASAMI
ASANA
ASBIG
ASCAP
ASCII
ASCOT
ASCUS
ASDIC
ASDRY
ASFAT
ASFIT
ASFOR
ASHBY
ASHED
ASHEN
ASHER
ASHES
ASHOT
ASHUR
ASIAN
ASICS
ASIDE
ASKED
ASKER
ASKEW
ASKIN
ASKME
ASKOF
ASKUP
ASLAK
ASLAN
ASMAD
ASNAP
ASNER
ASNEW
ASOLD
ASONE
ASORS
ASOUL
ASPCA
ASPEN
ASPER
ASPIC
ASPIN
ASRED
ASSAD
ASSAI
ASSAM
ASSAY
ASSER
ASSES
ASSET
ASSEZ
ASSNS
ASSOC
ASSTD

ASSTS
ASSYR
ASTER
ASTIN
ASTIR
ASTON
ASTOR
ASTRA
ASTRE
ASTRO
ASWAN
ASWAY
ASWIM
ASYET
ASYLA

A•S••

AESIR
AESOP
AHSIN
AISHA
AISLE
AISNE
ALSAB
ALSOP
ANSAE
ANSEL
ANSER
ANSON
AOSTA
APSES
APSIS
APSOS
ARSES
ARSIS
ARSON
ASSAD
ASSAI
ASSAM
ASSAY
ASSER
ASSES
ASSET
ASSEZ
ASSNS
ASSOC
ASSTD
ASSTS
ASSYR
ATSEA
ATSIX
AUSSI
AUSTR

A••S•

ABASE
ABASH
ABUSE
ABYSM
ABYSS
ADUST
AGASP
AGUSH
AINSI
ALISA
ALIST
AMASS
AMISH

AMISS
AMUSE
AMUST
ANDSO
ANGST
ANISE
ANTSY
APISH
ARESO
ARISE
AROSE
ARTSY
ATEST
AUSSI
AVAST
AVISO
AWASH
AZUSA

A•••S

AAMES
ABBAS
ABBES
ABBRS
ABETS
ABIES
ABRIS
ABUTS
ABYSS
ACADS
ACCTS
ACERS
ACHES
ACIDS
ACMES
ACNES
ACRES
ACTAS
ACTES
ACTOS
ACUPS
ADAMS
ADARS
ADDIS
ADDRS
ADINS
ADIOS
ADITS
ADJTS
ADZES
AEDES
AEGIS
AEONS
AEROS
AFARS
AFROS
AGALS
AGARS
AGERS
AGHAS
AGIOS
AGNES
AGNUS
AGUAS
AGUES
AHEMS
AHOYS
AHYES

AIDES
AILES
AINUS
AIRES
AIWAS
AKAIS
AKERS
AKINS
ALAIS
ALBAS
ALEFS
ALERS
ALFAS
ALGAS
ALIAS
ALIFS
ALIOS
ALLES
ALLIS
ALOES
ALOIS
ALORS
ALPES
ALTOS
ALTUS
ALUMS
AMAHS
AMASS
AMBOS
AMENS
AMIES
AMIRS
AMISS
AMMOS
AMORS
AMPAS
AMYAS
AMYLS
ANAGS
ANAIS
ANDES
ANDYS
ANGES
ANGUS
ANILS
ANKHS
ANNAS
ANNUS
ANOAS
ANTAS
ANTES
ANTIS
ANZUS
AONES
AOUTS
APARS
APERS
APHIS
APLUS
APODS
APPTS
APRES
APSES
APSIS
APSOS
AQUAS
ARABS
ARANS

ARBUS
ARBYS
AREAS
ARENS
ARGOS
ARGUS
ARIAS
ARIES
ARILS
ARLES
ARMAS
ARMES
ARRAS
ARRIS
ARSES
ARSIS
ARTIS
ARUMS
ARUNS
ARYLS
ASCUS
ASHES
ASICS
ASORS
ASSES
ASSNS
ASSTS
ATARS
ATHOS
ATLAS
ATLES
ATMOS
ATNOS
ATOMS
ATRAS
ATTYS
AUDIS
AUJUS
AULIS
AULUS
AUNTS
AURAS
AUTOS
AVERS
AVGAS
AVIAS
AVOWS
AWACS
AWOLS
AXELS
AXERS
AXILS
AXLES
AXONS
AYAHS
AYERS
AYINS
AYRES
AZANS

•AS••

BASAL
BASED
BASEL
BASER
BASES
BASHO
BASIA

BASIC
BASIE
BASIL
BASIN
BASIS
BASKS
BASLE
BASOV
BASRA
BASSE
BASSI
BASSO
BASSY
BASTA
BASTE
BASTS
CASAS
CASBY
CASCA
CASCO
CASED
CASER
CASES
CASEY
CASIO
CASKS
CASTA
CASTE
CASTS
CASUS
DASHI
DASHY
DASNT
EASED
EASEL
EASER
EASES
EASTS
EASYA
FASTS
GASES
GASOL
GASPE
GASPS
GASSY
GASTR
GASUP
HASAT
HASEK
HASID
HASIN
HASIT
HASNO
HASNT
HASON
HASPS
HASSO
HASTA
HASTE
HASTO
HASTY
HASUP
JASON
KASEM
KASHA
KASHI
LASED
LASER

LASES LASIK LASKI LASKY LASSE LASSO LASTS MASAI MASAS MASER MASHA MASKS MASON MASSA MASSE MASSY MASTS MASUR NASAL NASBY NASHE NASTY OASAL OASES OASIS OASTS PASCH PASCO PASEO PASES PASHA PASOS PASSE PASSU PASSY PASTA PASTE PASTO PASTS PASTY RASAE RASED RASER RASES RASHI RASHT RASPA RASPE RASPS RASPY RASSE RASTA SASES SASHA SASSY TASER TASHI TASKS TASSE TASSO TASTE TASTY VASCO VASES VASTI VASTS VASTY WASAT

WASCO WASHO WASHY WASIN WASIT WASNT WASON WASPS WASPY WASSO WASTE WASUP YASHA YASIR

•A•S•

BAISA BAKST BALSA BASSE BASSI BASSO BASSY CANSO CANST CAUSE DAISY DANSE FALSE FARSI FATSO FAUSS FAUST GANSU GASSY GAUSS HADST HAISE HANSA HANSE HARSH HASSO HAWSE IAMSO KANSA KARSH KARST LAPSE LASSE LASSO MANSE MARSH MASSA MASSE MASSY MATSU MAYST NAISH PABST PAESE PAISA PAISE PALSY PANSY PARSE PARSI PASSE PASSU

PASSY PATSY PAUSE RAISA RAISE RASSE RATSO SALSA SAMSA SASSY SAYSO TANSY TARSI TARSO TASSE TASSO VALSE VARSI WAIST WALSH WALSY WASSO

•A••S

AAMES BAALS BABAS BABES BABUS BABYS BACKS BACOS BAFFS BAHTS BAIES BAILS BAITS BAKES BALAS BALDS BALES BALKS BALLS BALMS BALTS BANCS BANDS BANES BANGS BANKS BANNS BANOS BARBS BARDS BARES BARKS BARMS BARNS BARQS BASES BASIS BASKS BASTS BATES BATHS BATTS BAUDS BAWLS

BAYES CADIS CAFES CAGES CAIUS CAKES CALKS CALLS CALMS CAMAS CAMBS CAMOS CAMPS CAMUS CANES CANIS CANTS CAPAS CAPES CAPOS CAPTS CARBS CARDS CARES CARPS CARTS CASAS CASES CASKS CASTS CASUS CATES CATHS CAVES DACES DADAS DADOS DALES DALIS DAMAS DAMES DAMIS DAMNS DAMPS DANES DANGS DARES DARKS DARNS DARTS DATES DATOS DAUBS DAVES DAVIS DAVOS DAWES DAWNS DAZES EAMES EARLS EARNS EARPS EASES EASTS EAVES FACES FACTS

FADES FADOS FAILS FAIMS FAIRS FAJAS FAKES FALLS FAMES FANES FANGS FARES FARIS FARMS FAROS FASTS FATES FAUNS FAUSS FAVES FAWNS FAXES FAZES GAELS GAFFS GAGES GAINS GAITS GAIUS GALAS GALES GALLS GAMES GAMPS GANGS GAOLS GAPES GARBS GARES GASES GASPS GATES GATOS GAUDS GAULS GAURS GAUSS GAWKS GAWPS GAZES HACKS HADES HAFTS HAHAS HAIKS HAILS HAIRS HAJIS HAKES HALAS HALES HALLS HALOS HALTS HAMAS HAMES HAMMS HANDS

HANES HANGS HANKS HANTS HARES HARKS HARMS HARPS HASPS HATES HAULS HAVES HAWGS HAWKS HAYES HAZES IAMBS JACKS JADES JAILS JAINS JAKES JAMBS JAMES JANIS JANOS JANUS JAPES JATOS JAVAS KABAS KAHNS KALES KANAS KANGS KAONS KAPHS KARAS KARNS KARTS KARUS KATAS KAVAS KAYOS LACES LACKS LADAS LADES LADYS LAFFS LAGOS LAICS LAIRS LAITS LAIUS LAKES LAMAS LAMBS LAMES LAMPS LANDS LANES LANOS LAPIS LAPPS LARAS LARDS LARES

LARIS LARKS LASES LASTS LATHS LAUDS LAVAS LAVES LAWES LAWNS LAZES MAAMS MACES MACKS MACYS MAGES MAGUS MAIDS MAILS MAIMS MAINS MAKES MAKOS MALES MALLS MALTS MAMAS MANES MANOS MANUS MAPES MARES MARIS MARKS MARLS MARMS MARTS MARYS MASAS MASKS MASTS MATES MATHS MAULS MAVIS MAXES MAXIS MAYAS MAYOS MAZES NABES NAIFS NAILS NAMES NANAS NAPES NARAS NARCS NARDS NARES NARIS NARKS NAVES NAVIS NAXOS NAZIS OAKES OASES

OASIS OASTS OATES OATHS PACAS PACES PACKS PACTS PAGES PAILS PAINS PAIRS PALES PALLS PALMS PALOS PALPS PANES PANGS PANIS PANTS PAONS PAPAS PARAS PARCS PARDS PARES PARIS PARKS PAROS PARRS PARTS PASES PASOS PASTS PATES PATHS PATOS PAVES PAWLS PAWNS PAXOS QAIDS RACES RACKS RAFTS RAGAS RAGES RAIDS RAILS RAINS RAJAS RAKES RAKUS RALES RAMAS RAMIS RAMOS RAMPS RAMUS RANAS RANDS RANIS RANKS RANTS RASES RASPS RATES

RATHS RAVES RAWLS RAXES RAZES SAABS SACHS SACKS SAENS SAFES SAGAS SAGES SAGOS SAILS SAKES SAKIS SALAS SALES SALTS SAMIS SAMMS SAMOS SAMPS SANDS SARDS SARIS SAROS SASES SATES SAUKS SAVES SAXES TABIS TABUS TACHS TACKS TACOS TADAS TAELS TAFTS TAGUS TAILS TAKAS TAKES TALAS TALCS TALES TALKS TALLS TALUS TAMES TAMPS TANGS TANIS TANKS TAPAS TAPES TAPIS TARAS TARES TARNS TAROS TARPS TARTS TASKS TATAS TATES TATIS

TAVIS TAXES TAXIS VACAS VADIS VAGUS VALES VAMOS VAMPS VANES VASES VASTS VATUS VAXES WAACS WAALS WADES WADIS WAFTS WAGES WAIFS WAILS WAINS WAITS WAKAS WAKES WALES WALKS WALLS WANDS WANES WANTS WARDS WARES WARKS WARMS WARNS WARPS WARTS WASPS WATTS WAVES WAWAS WAXES XAXES XAXIS YACKS YANKS YARDS YARNS YATES YAWLS YAWNS YAWPS YAXES YAXIS YAYAS ZAFUS ZALES ZARFS ZAXES ZAXIS

••AS•

ABASE ABASH AGASP AMASS

AVAST AWASH BEAST BLASE BLASS BLAST BOAST BRASH BRASS CEASE CHASE CHASM CHAST CLASE CLASH CLASP CLASS COASE COAST CRASH CRASS DNASE ECASH ERASE FEAST FLASH FLASK GLASS GNASH GOASK GRASP GRASS IPASS KVASS LEASE LEASH LEAST LHASA NYASA PEASE PHASE PLASH PLASM PLAST QUASH QUASI REASK RNASE ROAST SLASH SMASH SPASM STASH STASI SWASH TEASE TOAST TRASH TRASK UKASE UMASS YEAST

••A•S

ACADS ADAMS ADARS AFARS

AGALS AGARS AKAIS ALAIS AMAHS AMASS ANAGS ANAIS APARS ARABS ARANS ATARS AWACS AYAHS AZANS BAALS BDAYS BEADS BEAKS BEALS BEAMS BEANS BEARS BEATS BEAUS BHATS BLABS BLAHS BLAIS BLAMS BLASS BLATS BOARS BOATS BRADS BRAES BRAGS BRANS BRASS BRATS BRAYS CHADS CHAIS CHAOS CHAPS CHARS CHATS CHAWS CIAOS CLADS CLAES CLAMS CLANS CLAPS CLASS CLAUS CLAWS CLAYS COALS COATS CRABS CRAGS CRAMS CRAPS CRASS CRAWS CRAYS CYANS

CZARS DDAYS DEALS DEANS DEARS DHALS DIALS DIAMS DOANS DOATS DRABS DRAGS DRAMS DRATS DRAWS DRAYS DUADS DUALS DYADS EDAMS EGADS EGALS EMAGS ETATS EVANS EXAMS FEARS FEATS FIATS FLAGS FLAMS FLANS FLAPS FLATS FLAWS FLAYS FOALS FOAMS FRAGS FRAIS FRANS FRATS FRAYS GEARS GHATS GLADS GLAMS GLASS GMATS GNARS GNATS GNAWS GOADS GOALS GOATS GRABS GRADS GRAMS GRASS GRAYS GUARS HBARS HEADS HEALS HEAPS HEARS HEATS HOARS

HYAMS IBARS IMACS IMAMS IPASS ITALS IYARS JBARS JEANS JOADS KCARS KEATS KHANS KLAUS KNARS KOANS KRAUS KVASS KYATS LBARS LEADS LEAFS LEAKS LEANS LEAPS LEARS LIARS LOADS LOAFS LOAMS LOANS LSATS LUAUS MAAMS MCATS MEADS MEALS MEANS MEARS MEATS MOANS MOATS NEAPS NEARS NEATS OGAMS OJAYS OKAYS OPAHS OPALS ORALS OVALS PEAKS PEALS PEARS PEATS PLANS PLATS PLAYS PRAMS PRAYS PSATS QUADS QUAGS QUAIS QUAYS READS REALS

REAMS REAPS REARS RIALS ROADS ROAMS ROANS ROARS RYALS RYANS SAABS SCABS SCADS SCAMS SCANS SCARS SCATS SEALS SEAMS SEARS SEATS SHADS SHAGS SHAHS SHAMS SHAYS SLABS SLAGS SLAMS SLAPS SLATS SLAVS SLAWS SLAYS SNAGS SNAPS SOAKS SOAPS SOARS SPADS SPAMS SPANS SPARS SPATS SPAYS STABS STADS STAGS STANS STARS STATS STAYS SWABS SWAGS SWANS SWAPS SWATS SWAYS TBARS TEAKS TEALS TEAMS TEARS TEATS THAIS THATS THAWS TOADS

TRAMS TRANS TRAPS TRAYS TSARS TVADS TZARS UMASS UNAUS URALS VDAYS VEALS VIALS WAACS WAALS WEALS WEANS WEARS WHAMS WHAPS WHATS WOADS WRAPS XRAYS YEAHS YEANS YEARS YEATS YUANS ZBARS ZEALS

•••AS

ABBAS ACTAS AGHAS AGUAS AIWAS ALBAS ALFAS ALGAS ALIAS AMPAS AMYAS ANNAS ANOAS ANTAS AQUAS AREAS ARIAS ARMAS ARRAS ATLAS ATRAS AURAS AVGAS AVIAS BABAS BALAS BEMAS BETAS BOCAS BOLAS BORAS CAMAS CAPAS CASAS CENAS

CHIAS COCAS CODAS COLAS COMAS CYMAS DADAS DAMAS DEGAS DEVAS DIMAS DIVAS DONAS DOPAS DUKAS DUMAS DURAS EDDAS ELIAS ELSAS ENBAS EPHAS ERIAS ERMAS ESTAS ETNAS EYRAS FAJAS FETAS FILAS FLEAS GALAS GETAS GILAS GLIAS GOYAS HAHAS HALAS HAMAS HIJAS HORAS HOYAS HULAS HYLAS IDEAS INCAS IOTAS IOWAS ISLAS ITEAS JAVAS JONAS JOTAS JUDAS KABAS KANAS KARAS KATAS KAVAS KINAS KIVAS KOLAS KONAS LADAS LAMAS LARAS LAVAS LIMAS

LIRAS
LOMAS
LPGAS
LUCAS
LUKAS
LUMAS
LUNAS
LYRAS
MAMAS
MASAS
MAYAS
MENAS
MESAS
MICAS
MIDAS
MINAS
MITAS
MORAS
MYNAS
NANAS
NARAS
NINAS
NIPAS
NOGAS
NOMAS
NOVAS
OBRAS
OKRAS
OLLAS
ONDAS
ORCAS
OTRAS
PACAS
PAPAS
PARAS
PEBAS
PERAS
PICAS
PIKAS
PIMAS
PITAS
PLEAS
PROAS
PUKAS
PULAS
PUMAS
PUPAS
RAGAS
RAJAS
RAMAS
RANAS
RHEAS
ROJAS
ROTAS
SAGAS
SALAS
SEEAS
SIKAS
SILAS
SKUAS
SOBAS
SOCAS
SODAS
SOFAS
SOMAS
SORAS
SOYAS
SRTAS
STOAS
SURAS
TADAS
TAKAS
TALAS
TAPAS
TARAS
TATAS
TEMAS
TEWAS
TEXAS
THEAS
TIWAS
TOEAS
TOGAS
TOMAS
TORAS
TREAS
TUBAS
TUNAS
ULNAS
UNCAS
UREAS
USEAS
UVEAS
VACAS
VEDAS
VEGAS
VIDAS
VILAS
VINAS
VISAS
VITAS
VIVAS
WAKAS
WAWAS
YAYAS
YMCAS
YMHAS
YOGAS
YUMAS
YWCAS
YWHAS
ZETAS

AT•••

ATALA
ATALL
ATARI
ATARS
ATBAR
ATBAT
ATBAY
ATEAM
ATEAT
ATEIN
ATEIT
ATEOF
ATEST
ATEUP
ATHOL
ATHON
ATHOS
ATILE
ATILT
ATION
ATIVE
ATLAS
ATLES
ATMAN
ATMOS
ATNOS
ATOLL
ATOMS
ATOMY
ATONE
ATONY
ATORY
ATPAR
ATQUE
ATRAS
ATRIA
ATRIP
ATSEA
ATSIX
ATTAR
ATTEN
ATTIC
ATTWO
ATTYS
ATWAR

A•T••

ACTAS
ACTED
ACTER
ACTES
ACTII
ACTIN
ACTIV
ACTON
ACTOR
ACTOS
ACTUP
AETNA
AFTER
AFTON
AFTRA
AITCH
ALTAI
ALTAR
ALTER
ALTHO
ALTON
ALTOS
ALTUS
AMTOO
ANTAE
ANTAL
ANTAS
ANTED
ANTES
ANTIC
ANTIQ
ANTIS
ANTON
ANTRA
ANTRE
ANTSY
APTED
APTER
APTLY
ARTEL
ARTIE
ARTIS
ARTOO
ARTSY
ARTUR
ASTER
ASTIN
ASTIR
ASTON
ASTOR
ASTRA
ASTRE
ASTRO
ATTAR
ATTEN
ATTIC
ATTWO
ATTYS
AUTOS
AUTRE
AUTRY
AXTON
AZTEC
AZTEK

A••T•

AALTO
ABATE
ABCTV
ABETS
ABUTS
ACCTS
ACETO
ACUTE
ADDTO
ADITS
ADJTS
ADYTA
AGATE
AGITA
AKITA
ALATE
ALETA
ALITO
ALITY
AMATI
AMATO
AMITE
AMITY
ANETO
ANITA
AORTA
AOSTA
AOUTS
APPTS
ARETE
ARITH
ASSTD
ASSTS
AUNTS
AUNTY
AUSTR
AZOTH

A•••T

ABAFT
ABBOT
ABORT
ABOUT
ACEIT
ADAPT
ADEPT
ADMIT
ADOPT
ADOUT
ADULT
ADUST
AFLAT
AFOOT
AGENT
AGLET
AHOOT
AIMAT
ALERT
ALEUT
ALIST
ALLOT
ALOFT
AMANT
AMBIT
AMENT
AMLIT
AMORT
AMUST
AMVET
ANENT
ANGST
APART
APORT
ARENT
ARGOT
ARHAT
ARIOT
ARMET
ARRET
ASCOT
ASFAT
ASFIT
ASHOT
ASSET
ASYET
ATBAT
ATEAT
ATEIT
ATEST
ATILT
AUDIT
AUGHT
AVANT
AVAST
AVERT
AVNET
AWAIT
AWHIT

•AT••

BATCH
BATED
BATES
BATHE
BATHO
BATHS
BATHY
BATIK
BATIN
BATNA
BATON
BATOR
BATTS
BATTY
CATCH
CATER
CATES
CATHS
CATHY
CATTY
DATED
DATER
DATES
DATOS
DATUM
EATAT
EATEN
EATER
EATIN
EATIT
EATME
EATOF
EATON
EATUP
FATAL
FATED
FATES
FATHA
FATLY
FATSO
FATTY
FATWA
GATED
GATER
GATES
GATOR
GATOS
GATTO
GATUN
HATCH
HATED
HATER
HATES
HATHA
HATHI
HATLO
IATRO
IATRY
JATOS
KATAS
KATEY
KATHE
KATHY
KATIE
KATZE
LATCH
LATEN
LATER
LATEX
LATHE
LATHS
LATHY
LATIN
LATKA
LATKE
LATTE
MATCH
MATED
MATEO
MATER
MATES
MATEY
MATHS
MATIN
MATRI
MATRO
MATSU
MATTE
MATTY
MATZO
NATAL
NATAN
NATCH
NATRO
NATTA
NATTY
OATEN
OATER
OATES
OATHS
PATCH
PATCO
PATED
PATEK
PATEN
PATER
PATES
PATHE
PATHO
PATHS
PATHY
PATIO
PATLY
PATNA
PATON
PATOS
PATRI
PATRO
PATSY
PATTI
PATTY
QATAR
RATED
RATEL
RATER
RATES
RATHS
RATIO
RATON
RATSO
RATTY
SATAN
SATAT
SATAY
SATBY
SATCH
SATED
SATES
SATIE
SATII
SATIN
SATON
SATUP
SATYR
TATAR
TATAS
TATER
TATES
TATIS
TATRA
TATTY
TATUM
VATER
VATIC
VATUS
WATCH
WATER
WATTS
YATES

•A•T•

AALTO
BAHTS
BAITS
BALTO
BALTS
BANTA
BANTU
BARTH
BARTY
BASTA
BASTE
BASTS
BATTS
BATTY
CACTI
CANTO
CANTS
CANTY
CAPTS
CARTA
CARTE
CARTS
CASTA
CASTE
CASTS
CATTY
DANTE
DARTE
DARTH
DARTS
EARTH
EASTS
FACTA
FACTO
FACTS
FAITH
FANTA
FASTS
FATTY
FAUTE
GAETA
GAITS
GARTH
GASTR
GATTO
HADTO
HAFTS
HAITI
HALTS
HANTS
HARTE
HASTA
HASTE
HASTO
HASTY
HAUTE
KARTS
LACTI
LACTO
LAHTI
LAITS
LAITY
LANTZ
LASTS
LATTE
LAYTO
MADTV
MALTA
MALTS
MALTY
MANTA
MARTA
MARTI
MARTS
MARTY
MASTS
MATTE
MATTY
NAFTA
NANTZ
NASTY
NATTA
NATTY
OASTS
PACTS
PANTA
PANTO
PANTS
PANTY
PARTA
PARTB
PARTC
PARTE
PARTI
PARTS
PARTV
PARTY
PASTA
PASTE
PASTO
PASTS
PASTY
PATTI
PATTY
PAYTO
PAYTV
RAFTS
RAITA
RAITT
RANTO
RANTS
RASTA
RATTY
SAITH
SALTI
SALTS
SALTY
SANTA
SANTE
SANTO
SARTO
SAUTE
SAWTO
TAFTS
TAITO
TANTE
TANTO
TARTE
TARTS
TARTU
TARTY
TASTE
TASTY
TATTY
TAUTO
VASTI
VASTS
VASTY
WAFTS
WAITE
WAITS
WAITZ
WALTZ
WANTS
WARTS
WARTY
WASTE
WATTS
XACTO
YALTA

•A••T

BADAT
BAGIT
BAKST
BARIT
BAYAT
CABOT
CADET
CAINT
CANIT
CANST
CAPET
CAPUT
CARAT
CARET
DABAT
DALET
DASNT
DAUNT
DAVIT
EATAT
EATIT
FACET
FAGOT
FAINT
FAULT
FAUST
GAMUT
GANDT
GAUNT
GAVOT
HABIT
HADAT
HADIT
HADNT
HADST
HASAT
HASIT
HASNT
HAUNT
JABOT
JACET
JANET
JAUNT
JAWAT
KAPUT
KARAT
KARST
LAMIT
LAPAT
MADAT
MAMET
MANAT
MANET
MARAT
MAROT
MAYNT
MAYST
NACHT
NAGAT
PABST
PAGET
PAINT
PAWAT
RABAT
RAITT
RAMET
RANAT
RASHT
SABOT
SADAT
SAGET
SAINT
SALUT
SATAT
SAULT
SAYIT
TACET
TACIT
TAINT
TAROT
TAUNT
VALET
VAULT
VAUNT
WAART
WAIST
WASAT
WASIT
WASNT
YACHT
YAKUT
YAPAT
ZAGAT

••AT•

ABATE
AGATE
ALATE
AMATI
AMATO
BEATS
BEATY
BHATS
BLATS
BLATZ
BOATS
BRATS
BRATT
BYATT
CHATS
COATI
COATS
CRATE
DEATH
DOATS
DRATS
ELATE
ELATH
ENATE
ERATO
ETATS
FEATS
FIATS
FLATS
FLATT
FRATS
GHATS
GLATT
GMATS
GNATS
GOATS
GRATA
GRATE
HEATH
HEATS
HYATT
IRATE
KEATS
KYATS
LOATH
LSATS
MCATS
MEATH
MEATS
MEATY
MIATA
MOATS
NEATH
NEATO
NEATS
ONATE
ORATE
OVATE
PEATS
PEATY
PLATA
PLATE
PLATH
PLATO
PLATS
PLATT
PLATY
PRATE
PRATO
PRATT
PSATS
REATA
RIATA
SCATS
SEATO
SEATS
SHATT
SKATE
SLATE
SLATS
SLATY
SNATH
SPATE
SPATS
STATE
STATS
SWATH
SWATS
TEATS
THATS
WHATD
WHATS
WRATH
WYATT
YEATS

••A•T

ABAFT
ADAPT
AMANT
APART
AVANT
AVAST
AWAIT
BEART
BEAST
BEAUT
BLAST
BOAST
BRACT
BRANT
BRATT
BYATT
CHANT
CHART
CHAST
COACT
COAPT
COAST
CRAFT
DEALT
DRAFT
ENACT
EPACT
EWART
EXACT
EXALT
FEAST
FLATT
GIANT
GLATT
GOAFT
GRAFT
GRANT
HEART
HYATT
ICANT
INAPT
IWANT
KMART
KRAFT
KRAIT
KRAUT
LEANT
LEAPT
LEAST
MEANT
OPART
ORANT
PLAIT
PLANT
PLAST
PLATT
PRATT
QUANT
QUART
REACT
RIANT
ROAST
SCANT
SHAFT
SHALT
SHANT
SHATT
SLANT
SMART
STADT
START
THANT
TIANT
TOAST
TRACT
TRAIT
UNAPT
WAART
WRAPT
WYATT
YEAST

•••AT

AFLAT
AIMAT
ARHAT
ASFAT
ATBAT
ATEAT
BADAT
BAYAT
BEGAT
BFLAT
BLEAT
BLOAT
BOOAT
BUYAT
CARAT
CERAT
CFLAT
CHEAT
CLEAT
CROAT
CUGAT
DABAT
DEFAT
DERAT
DETAT
DFLAT
DIGAT
DITAT
DONAT
DUCAT
DUGAT
EATAT
EBOAT
ECLAT
EFLAT
EILAT
ENDAT
ESBAT
EXPAT
FFLAT
FLOAT
FLYAT
GETAT
GFLAT
GLOAT
GOBAT
GOTAT
GREAT
GROAT
HADAT
HASAT
HEMAT
HEPAT
HERAT
HIHAT
HITAT
JAWAT
KARAT
KORAT
LAPAT
LEMAT
LETAT
LOFAT
LOPAT
MADAT
MANAT
MARAT
MOWAT
MURAT
NAGAT
NEWAT
NIPAT
NODAT
NOFAT
OCRAT
PAWAT
PLEAT
RABAT
RANAT
REMAT
RESAT
RIPAT
RUNAT
SADAT
SATAT
SCRAT
SENAT
SETAT
SHOAT
SITAT
SOMAT
SPLAT
SPRAT
SQUAT
STOAT
STPAT
STRAT
SWEAT
TERAT
TREAT
TUGAT
UBOAT
UNHAT
UNIAT
WASAT
WHEAT
WINAT
WOFAT
WONAT
WOPAT
YAPAT
ZAGAT

AU•••

AUBER
AUDEN
AUDIE
AUDIO
AUDIS
AUDIT
AUDRA
AUGER
AUGHT
AUGIE
AUGUR
AUJUS
AULIS
AULUS
AUNTS
AUNTY
AURAE
AURAL
AURAR
AURAS
AURIC
AURUM
AUSSI
AUSTR
AUTOS
AUTRE
AUTRY
AUVIN

A•U••

ABUJA
ABUSE
ABUTS
ABUZZ
ACUFF
ACUPS
ACURA
ACUTE
ADULT
ADUST
AGUAS
AGUES
AGURA
AGUSH
ALUKO
ALULA
ALUMS
AMUCK
AMUSE
AMUST
AOUTS
AQUAE
AQUAS
ARUBA
ARUMS
ARUNS
AZUKI
AZURE
AZUSA

A••U•

ABDUL
ABOUT
ABZUG
ACQUA
ACTUP
ADDUP
ADEUX
ADOUT
AFOUL
AGNUS
AILUR
AINUS
AIRUP
ALBUM
ALEUT
ALOUD
ALTUS
AMOUR
AMPUP
ANDUP
ANGUS
ANNUL
ANNUM
ANNUS
ANOUK
ANZUS
APLUS
ARBUS
ARGUE
ARGUS
ARIUM
ARTUR
ASCUS
ASHUR
ASKUP
ASOUL
ATEUP
ATQUE
AUGUR
AUJUS
AULUS
AURUM
AWFUL

A•••U

AARAU
ADIEU
AEIOU
ANJOU
ARRAU

•AU••

BAUDS
BAUER
BAUGH
BAULK
BAUME
CAUDI
CAUDO
CAULK
CAUSE
DAUBE
DAUBS
DAUNT
FAULT
FAUNA
FAUNS

FAURE FAUSS FAUST FAUTE FAUVE GAUDI GAUDS GAUDY GAUGE GAULS GAUNT GAURS GAUSS GAUZE GAUZY HAUER HAULS HAUNT HAUTE JAUNE JAUNT KAUAI LAUDA LAUDE LAUDS LAUER LAUGH LAURA LAURO MAUDE MAULS MAUNA MAURA MAURY MAUVE NAURU PAULA PAULI PAULO PAULV PAUSE SAUCE SAUCY SAUDI SAUKS SAULT SAUNA SAURO SAUTE TAUNT TAUON TAUPE TAURI TAURO TAUTO VAULT VAUNT WAUGH

•A•U•

BABUS BADUN BAIUL CAIUS CAJUN CAMUS CAPUT CASUS DAMUP DATUM DAZUR EATUP FARUK GAIUS GAMUT GASUP GATUN HADUP HAGUE HAMUP HARUM HASUP JAMUP JANUS KABUL KAPUT KARUS LAIUS LAPUP LARUE LAYUP MAGUA MAGUS MANUS MAQUI MASUR NAHUM NAMUR OAKUM PADUA PAPUA PAYUP RAKUS RAMUS RAMUZ RANUP RAOUL SALUD SALUT SATUP SAWUP TABUS TAGUP TAGUS TALUS TATUM VACUA VADUZ VAGUE VAGUS VALUE VANUA VATUS WADUP WASUP WAXUP WAYUP YAKUT YAQUI ZAFUS

•A••U

AARAU BANTU BAYOU GANSU GAROU HAIKU LAFEU MACHU MATSU NAURU PALAU PAREU PASSU SADHU TAEGU TARTU YALEU

••AU•

BEAUS BEAUT BEAUX BRAUN CHAUD CLAUS FRAUD JPAUL KLAUS KRAUS KRAUT LEAUD LUAUS PIAUI SHAUN SMAUG STAUB UHAUL UNAUS

••A•U

IMAMU IRABU ISAMU KEANU MIAOU OTARU SHAMU SNAFU

•••AU

AARAU ARRAU BELAU DONAU IOWAU PALAU PILAU

AV•••

AVAIL AVANT AVAST AVENA AVERS AVERT AVERY AVGAS AVIAN AVIAS AVIDE AVILA AVION AVIOR AVISO AVNET AVOID AVOIR AVOWS AVRIL

A•V••

ADVIL ALVAR ALVIN AMVET ANVIL AUVIN

A••V•

ABOVE ABOVO AGAVE ALAVA ALEVE ALIVE ALMVP ATIVE AWAVE

A•••V

ABCTV ACTIV ANNIV

•AV••

CAVAE CAVAN CAVED CAVER CAVES CAVIL DAVAO DAVEN DAVES DAVEY DAVID DAVIE DAVIS DAVIT DAVOS EAVAN EAVED EAVES FAVES FAVOR FAVRE GAVEL GAVIN GAVOT HAVEL HAVEN HAVER HAVES HAVOC HAVRE JAVAN JAVAS KAVAS LAVAL LAVAS LAVED LAVER LAVES LAVIE LAVIN MAVEN MAVIN MAVIS NAVAL NAVEE NAVEL NAVES NAVIG NAVIS PAVED PAVEL PAVER PAVES PAVIA PAVID PAVIN RAVED RAVEL RAVEN RAVER RAVES SAVED SAVER SAVES SAVOR SAVOY SAVVY TAVEL TAVIS WAVED WAVER WAVES

•A•V•

CALVE CARVE FAUVE HALVA HALVE LARVA MAEVE MARVY MAUVE NAIVE PAAVO SALVE SALVO SAVVY VALVE WAIVE

•A••V

BASOV MADTV MALEV MARKV PARTV PAULV PAYTV RAJIV YAKOV

••AV•

AGAVE ALAVA AWAVE BRAVA BRAVE BRAVO CHAVA CLAVE CRAVE DRAVA FLAVA GRAVE GRAVI GRAVY GUAVA HEAVE HEAVY KNAVE LEAVE LWAVE OLAVI OLAVV PAAVO PIAVE REAVE SHAVE SLAVE SLAVS SOAVE STAVE SUAVE TRAVE TSAVO WEAVE

••A•V

IVANV OLAFV OLAVV

•••AV

SCHAV

AW•••

AWACS AWAIT AWAKE AWARD AWARE AWASH AWAVE AWEEK AWFUL AWGEE AWHIT AWING AWNED AWOKE AWOLS

A•W••

ADWAR AGWAY AIWAS ALWAY AMWAY ANWAR ARWEN ASWAN ASWAY ASWIM ATWAR

A••W•

ATTWO AVOWS

A•••W

AANDW AGLOW AGNEW ALLOW ARROW ASKEW ASNEW

•AW••

BAWDY BAWLS CAWED DAWES DAWNN DAWNS FAWNS GAWKS GAWKY GAWPS HAWED HAWER HAWGS HAWKE HAWKS HAWSE JAWAT JAWED JAWER LAWED LAWES LAWNS LAWNY PAWAT PAWED PAWER PAWLS PAWNS RAWER RAWLS RAWLY SAWED SAWER SAWII SAWIN SAWTO SAWUP TAWNY WAWAS YAWED YAWLS YAWNS YAWNY YAWPS

•A•W•

DAIWA FATWA

•A••W

AANDW BANDW CANDW CAREW GAMOW KAPOW LALAW MACAW PAPAW YALOW

••AW•

BRAWL BRAWN CHAWS CLAWS CRAWL CRAWS DRAWL DRAWN DRAWS FLAWS FLAWY GNAWN GNAWS INAWE OZAWA PRAWN SHAWL SHAWN SLAWS SPAWN THAWS TRAWL URAWA

••A•W

MIAOW

•••AW

BYLAW INLAW LALAW MACAW PAPAW PSHAW RESAW SQUAW STRAW

AX•••

AXELF AXELS AXERS AXIAL AXILS AXING AXIOM AXION AXLED AXLES AXMAN AXMEN AXONE AXONS AXTON

A••X•

ALEXA ALEXI

A•••X

ADDAX ADEUX ADMIX AFFIX ANNEX ATSIX

•AX••

FAXED FAXER FAXES LAXER LAXLY MAXED MAXES MAXIE MAXIM MAXIS NAXOS PAXOS RAXED RAXES SAXES SAXON TAXCO TAXED TAXER TAXES TAXIS TAXOL TAXON VAXES WAXED WAXEN WAXER WAXES WAXUP XAXES XAXIS YAXES YAXIS ZAXES ZAXIS

•A••X

CALIX CALYX GALAX LATEX MADOX RADIX

••AX•

FLAXY GLAXO QUAXO

••A•X

BEAUX THANX

•••AX

ADDAX BORAX BYFAX DEWAX GALAX HYRAX ICEAX LOMAX LORAX NOTAX REFAX RELAX REMAX RETAX REWAX THEAX UNLAX UNTAX

AY•••

AYAHS AYAKO AYEAR AYERS AYINS AYRES

A•Y••

ABYSM ABYSS ADYTA AHYES ALYCE AMYAS AMYLO AMYLS ANYON ARYAN ARYLS ASYET ASYLA

A••Y•

AHOYS ALKYD ALKYL ALLYL ALLYN ANDYS ARBYS ASSYR ATTYS

A•••Y

ABBEY ACIDY AGLEY AGONY AGWAY AILEY ALITY ALLAY ALLEY ALLOY ALMAY ALROY ALWAY AMBOY AMBRY AMERY AMITY AMORY AMPLY AMWAY ANDRY ANGRY ANNOY ANOMY ANTSY AOKAY APERY APLEY APPLY APTLY ARABY ARCHY ARMEY ARRAY ARTSY ASDRY ASHBY ASSAY ASWAY ATBAY ATOMY ATONY ATORY AUNTY AUTRY AVERY

•AY••

BAYAR BAYAT BAYED BAYER BAYES BAYLE BAYOU CAYCE DAYAN DAYNE GAYER GAYLE GAYLY HAYDN HAYED HAYEK HAYER HAYES HAYEY JAYNE KAYAK KAYOS LAYBY LAYER LAYIN LAYLA LAYNE LAYON LAYTO LAYUP MAYAN MAYAS MAYBE MAYER MAYLE MAYNT MAYOR MAYOS MAYPO MAYST PAYEE PAYER PAYIN PAYNE PAYOR PAYTO PAYTV PAYUP RAYED RAYON SAYAH SAYER SAYHI SAYIT SAYNO SAYOK SAYSO WAYIN WAYNE WAYUP YAYAS YAYME ZAYAK ZAYIN

•A•Y•

BABYS CALYX DARYA DARYL EASYA EAZYE HANYA KANYE KARYN LADYL LADYS MACYS MARYA MARYI MARYJ MARYS SANYO SATYR TANYA VANYA VARYA

•A••Y

BADDY BADLY BAFFY BAGGY BALDY BALKY BALLY BALMY BAMMY BANDY BANKY BARFY BARKY BARMY BARRY BARTY BASSY BATHY BATTY BAWDY CABBY CADDY CAGEY CAKEY CAMAY CAMPY CAMRY CANBY CANDY CANNY CANTY CARAY CAREY CARLY CARNY CARRY CASBY CASEY CATHY CATTY DADDY DAFFY DAILY DAIRY DAISY DALEY DALLY DANDY DANNY DARBY DARCY DARDY DASHY DAVEY DAZZY EARLY FADDY FAERY FAHEY FAIRY FANCY FANNY FATLY FATTY GABBY GAILY GAMAY GANDY GARRY GASSY GAUDY GAUZY GAWKY GAYLY HACKY HAIRY HALEY HAMMY HANDY HANEY HANKY HAPLY HAPPY HARDY HARPY HARRY HASTY HAYEY IATRY JACEY JACKY JAGGY JAZZY KANDY KATEY KATHY LACEY LAITY LANKY LANNY LARDY LARKY LARRY LASKY LATHY LAWNY LAXLY LAYBY MACHY MADLY MALAY MALTY MAMMY MANCY MANDY MANGY MANLY MANNY MARCY MARGY MARLY MARRY MARTY MARVY MASSY MATEY MATTY MAURY NAGGY NAMBY NANCY NANNY NAPPY NASBY NASTY NATTY PACEY PACHY PADDY PALEY PALLY PALMY PALSY PAMBY PANAY PANKY PANSY PANTY PAPPY PARRY PARTY PASSY PASTY PATHY PATLY PATSY PATTY RAGGY RAINY RALLY RAMEY RANBY RANDY RANGY RASPY RATTY RAWLY SADLY SAGGY SAIRY SALLY SALTY SAMMY SANDY SAPPY SASSY SATAY SATBY SAUCY SAVOY SAVVY TABBY TACKY TAFFY TALKY TALLY TAMMY TANDY TANEY TANGY TANSY TARDY TARRY TARTY TASTY TATTY TAWNY VAMPY VASTY WACKY WALLY WALSY WANLY WARTY WASHY WASPY XANDY YANCY YAWNY ZAPPY

••AY•

BDAYS BRAYS CLAYS CRAYS DDAYS DRAYS FLAYS FRAYN FRAYS GRAYS OHAYO OJAYS OKAYS PLAYA PLAYS PRAYS QUAYS SHAYS SLAYS SPAYS STAYS SWAYS TRAYS VDAYS XRAYS YSAYE

••A•Y

ARABY BEADY BEAMY BEANY BEATY BIALY BRADY CHARY CLARY CRACY CRAZY DEARY DIARY FLAKY FLAMY FLAWY FLAXY FOAMY FRAZY GEARY GLARY GLAZY GRAPY GRAVY HEADY HEALY HEAPY HEAVY HOAGY HOARY ITALY KRAZY LEADY LEAFY LEAHY LEAKY LEARY LOAMY MEALY MEANY MEATY NEALY ORACY OTARY OVARY PEARY PEATY PHAGY PHANY PLATY QUAKY READY SCALY SCARY SEALY SEAMY SHADY SHAKY SLATY SNAKY SOAPY SPACY STACY STAGY TEARY TOADY TRACY UNARY VEALY WEARY

•••AY

AGWAY ALLAY ALMAY ALWAY AMWAY AOKAY ARRAY ASSAY ASWAY ATBAY BEGAY BELAY BOHAY BYWAY CAMAY CARAY COPAY DECAY DELAY DOSAY DOUAY DUFAY ELWAY EMBAY ESSAY FORAY GAMAY IFSAY INLAY INMAY IOWAY IPRAY IXNAY LEFAY LEMAY LURAY MALAY MCKAY MORAY MYDAY MYWAY NOWAY

OHKAY ONLAY ORSAY OSHAY OTWAY OURAY PANAY POWAY RELAY RENAY REPAY RESAY SATAY SFBAY SPLAY SPRAY STRAY TODAY TOKAY UNDAY UNLAY UNSAY UVRAY VEDAY VIJAY VJDAY

AZ•••
AZANS AZERA AZERI AZIDE AZOIC AZOLE AZORE AZOTH AZTEC AZTEK AZUKI AZURE AZUSA

A•Z••
ABZUG ADZED ADZES ANZAC ANZIO ANZUS

A••Z•
ABUZZ ADOZE AGAZE AMAZE

A•••Z
ABUZZ ADBIZ ALLEZ ARNAZ ARROZ ASSEZ

•AZ••
BAZOO DAZED DAZER DAZES DAZUR DAZZY EAZYE FAZED FAZES GAZED GAZER GAZES HAZAN HAZED HAZEL HAZER HAZES JAZZY KAZAN KAZIN KAZOO LAZAR LAZED LAZES MAZAR MAZDA MAZED MAZEL MAZES NAZIS RAZAF RAZED RAZER RAZES RAZOR YAZOO ZAZEN

•A•Z•
BAEZA BAIZA BAIZE DANZA DAZZY GAUZE GAUZY JAZZY KATZE LANZA MAIZE MARZO MATZO PANZA

•A••Z
CADIZ HAFIZ LANTZ LAPAZ MAINZ NANTZ RAMUZ VADUZ WAITZ WALTZ

••AZ•
AGAZE AMAZE BLAZE BRAZO CHAZZ CRAZE CRAZY FRAZY GHAZI GLAZE GLAZY GRAZE KRAZY PLAZA SMAZE SNAZZ SWAZI

••A•Z
BLATZ CHAZZ FRANZ SNAZZ STARZ

•••AZ
ARNAZ LAPAZ TOPAZ

BA•••
BAAED BAALS BABAR BABAS BABEL BABES BABKA BABOO BABUS BABYS BACIO BACKS BACON BACOS BADAT BADDY BADEN BADER BADGE BADLY BADUN BAEDA BAEZA BAFFS BAFFY BAGEL BAGGY BAGIT BAHAI BAHIA BAHTS BAIES BAILS BAIRD BAIRN BAISA BAITS BAIUL BAIZA BAIZE BAJER BAKED BAKER BAKES BAKST BALAS BALBO BALCH BALDS BALDY BALED BALER BALES BALIN BALKI BALKS BALKY BALLO BALLS BALLY BALMS BALMY BALON BALOO BALPH BALSA BALTO BALTS BAMBA BAMBI BAMMY BANAL BANCA BANCO BANCS BANDA BANDB BANDO BANDS BANDW BANDY BANES BANFF BANGS BANJO BANKS BANKY BANNS BANON BANOS BANTA BANTU BARAK BARBA BARBI BARBQ BARBS BARCA BARCO BARDS BARED BARER BARES BARFY BARGE BARIC BARIT BARKS BARKY BARMS BARMY BARNS BARON BARQS BARRE BARRY BARTH BARTY BASAL BASED BASEL BASER BASES BASHO BASIA BASIC BASIE BASIL BASIN BASIS BASKS BASLE BASOV BASRA BASSE BASSI BASSO BASSY BASTA BASTE BASTS BATCH BATED BATES BATHE BATHO BATHS BATHY BATIK BATIN BATNA BATON BATOR BATTS BATTY BAUDS BAUER BAUGH BAULK BAUME BAWDY BAWLS BAYAR BAYAT BAYED BAYER BAYES BAYLE BAYOU BAZOO

B•A••
BAAED BAALS BBALL BDAYS BEACH BEADS BEADY BEAKS BEALE BEALL BEALS BEAME BEAMS BEAMY BEANO BEANS BEANY BEARD BEARS BEART BEAST BEATS BEATY BEAUS BEAUT BEAUX BHAER BHANG BHATS BIALY BLABS BLACK BLADE BLAFF BLAHS BLAIR BLAIS BLAKE BLAME BLAMS BLANC BLAND BLANE BLANK BLARE BLASE BLASS BLAST BLATS BLATZ BLAZE BOARD BOARS BOAST BOATS BRACE BRACH BRACK BRACT BRADS BRADY BRAES BRAGA BRAGG BRAGH BRAGS BRAHE BRAID BRAIN BRAKE BRAND BRANG BRANS BRANT BRASH BRASS BRATS BRATT BRAUN BRAVA BRAVE BRAVO BRAWL BRAWN BRAYS BRAZO BWANA BYAGE BYAIR BYATT

B••A•
BABAR BABAS BADAT BAHAI BALAS BANAL BARAK BASAL BAYAR BAYAT BEBAD BEGAN BEGAT BEGAY BEHAN BEHAR BEKAA BELAU BELAY BEMAD BEMAN BEMAS BETAS BEXAR BFLAT BINAL BLEAK BLEAR BLEAT BLOAT BOCAS BOGAN BOHAY BOLAR BOLAS BONAR BOOAT BORAH BORAS BORAX BREAD BREAK BREAM BRIAN BRIAR BROAD BRYAN BSTAR BTEAM BUYAT BYCAB BYCAR BYEAR BYFAR BYFAX BYLAW BYWAY

B•••A
BABKA BAEDA BAEZA BAHIA BAISA BAIZA BALSA BAMBA BANCA BANDA BANTA BARBA BARCA BASIA BASRA BASTA BATNA BECCA BEIRA BEKAA BELLA BELVA BEREA BERIA BERRA BERTA BETTA BIOTA BIRRA BOHEA BOLLA BOMBA BOOLA BOPHA BORSA BOSSA BOTHA BRAGA BRAVA BRECA BREDA BROCA BUBBA BUBKA BUENA BUFFA BULBA BULLA BUONA BURKA BURMA BURSA BUSTA BWANA BYSEA

•BA••
ABABA ABACA ABACI ABACK ABACO ABAFT ABAJO ABASE ABASH ABATE BBALL DBACK EBANK HBARS IBARS JBARS LBARS NBAER OBAMA TBALL TBARS ZBARS

•B•A•
ABBAS ABEAM ABEAR ABFAB ABRAM EBOAT HBEAM IBEAM LBEAM OBEAH OBRAS UBOAT

•B••A
ABABA ABACA ABOMA ABUJA EBOLA IBIZA OBAMA

••BA•
ABBAS AKBAR ALBAN ALBAS ATBAR ATBAT ATBAY BABAR BABAS BEBAD CABAL CUBAN DABAT DEBAG DEBAR DOBAD DUBAI EMBAR EMBAY ENBAS ESBAT GOBAD GOBAT HOBAN IMBAD INBAD IQBAL JUBAL KABAS KEBAB LABAN LOBAR MYBAD PEBAS RABAT REBAG REBAR SABAL SFBAY SOBAD SOBAS TUBAL TUBAS UNBAG UNBAR URBAN WEBAD YUBAN

••B•A
AABBA BABKA BUBBA BUBKA COBRA DABBA DEBRA DUBYA HABLA JABBA KUBLA LABIA LIBRA LIBYA NUBIA SABRA TABLA TIBIA UMBRA YABBA ZEBRA

•••BA
AABBA ABABA AMEBA AQABA ARUBA BAMBA BARBA BOMBA BUBBA BULBA CEIBA DABBA GALBA GAMBA JABBA JAMBA KIMBA MAMBA MELBA PEMBA RUMBA SAMBA SCUBA SHEBA SIMBA TOMBA YABBA YERBA YOOBA YORBA ZORBA

BB•••
BBALL BBGUN BBOYS

B•B••
BABAR BABAS BABEL BABES BABKA BABOO BABUS BABYS BEBAD BEBOP BIBBS BIBLE BOBBY BOBUP BUBBA BUBER BUBKA BYBUS

B••B•
BALBO BAMBA BAMBI BARBA BARBI BARBQ BARBS BEEBE BELBY BIBBS BILBO BIMBO BIXBY BLABS BLEBS BLOBS BOBBY BOMBA BOMBE BOMBS BOOBS BOOBY BRIBE BUBBA BULBA BULBS BURBS BUSBY

B•••B
BANDB BLURB BYCAB

•BB••
ABBAS ABBES ABBEY ABBIE ABBOT ABBRS EBBED

•B•B•
ABABA

•B••B
ABFAB ABOMB HBOMB NBOMB

••BB•
AABBA BIBBS BOBBY BUBBA CABBY CUBBY DABBA DEBBE DEBBI DEBBY DOBBS GABBY GIBBS HOBBS HOBBY HUBBY JABBA LIBBY LOBBY NOBBY NUBBY RABBI REBBE RIBBY ROBBE ROBBY TABBY TIBBS TUBBS TUBBY WEBBY YABBA

••B•B
CABOB CUBEB HABIB KABOB KEBAB NABOB

•••BB
CHUBB

BC•••
BCCED BCDEF BCELL BCUPS

B•C••
BACIO BACKS BACON BACOS BCCED BECCA BECKS BECKY BICEP BOCAS BOCCE BOCCI BOCHY BOCKS BUCCO BUCKO BUCKS BUCKY BYCAB BYCAR

B••C•
BALCH BANCA BANCO BANCS BARCA BARCO BATCH BEACH BECCA BEECH BELCH BENCH BERCY BIRCH BLACK BLOCH BLOCK BLOCS BMOCS BOCCE BOCCI BOSCH BOSCO BOSCS BOTCH BRACE BRACH BRACK BRACT BRECA BRECK BRICE BRICK BROCA BROCK BRUCE BRUCH BRYCE BUCCO BUICK BUNCH BUNCO BUSCH BUTCH

B•••C
BARIC BASIC BLANC BORIC BRONC

•BC••
ABCDE ABCTV NBCTV

•B•C•
ABACA ABACI ABACK ABACO DBACK

•B••C
IBMPC

••B•C
CUBIC ORBIC REBEC SUBIC XEBEC

•••BC
MSNBC ONEBC SIXBC TENBC TWOBC

BD•••
BDAYS

B•D••
BADAT BADDY BADEN BADER BADGE BADLY BADUN BCDEF BEDDY BEDEW BEDIM BEDNY BEDOG BIDDY BIDED BIDEN BIDER BIDES BIDET BIDIN BIDON BIDUP BLDGS BODDY BODED BODEL BODES BUDDY BUDGE

B••D•
BADDY BAEDA BALDS BALDY BANDA BANDB BANDO BANDS BANDW BANDY BARDS BAUDS BAWDY BEADS BEADY BEDDY BENDS BENDY BIDDY BIGDO BINDS BIRDS BIRDY BLADE BLVDS BODDY BOLDS BONDI BONDS BRADS BRADY BREDA BREDE BRIDE BRODY BSIDE BUDDY BUNDS BUNDT BUNDY BYRDS

B•••D
BAAED BAIRD BAKED BALED BARED BASED BATED BAYED BCCED BEARD BEBAD BEMAD BIDED BIFID BIKED BIPED BIPOD BLAND BLEED BLEND BLIND BLOND BLOOD BLUED BOARD BODED BONED BOOED BORED BOUND BOVID BOWED BOXED BRAID BRAND BREAD BREED BROAD BROOD BROUD BUILD BUSED BYGOD

•BD••
ABDEL ABDUL

•B•D•
ABCDE ABIDE ABODE

•B••D
ABEND ABLED EBBED EBOND TBIRD TBOND

••BD•
EGBDF

••B•D
BEBAD CUBED DOBAD EBBED EMBED GIBED GOBAD IMBAD IMBED INBAD INBED JIBED LOBED LUBED MYBAD NOBID ORBED RABID REBID ROBED SOBAD TUBED UNBID UNBUD WEBAD

BE•••
BEACH BEADS BEADY BEAKS BEALE BEALL BEALS BEAME BEAMS BEAMY BEANO BEANS BEANY BEARD BEARS BEART BEAST BEATS BEATY BEAUS BEAUT BEAUX BEBAD BEBOP BECCA BECKS BECKY BEDDY BEDEW BEDIM BEDNY BEDOG BEEBE BEECH BEEFS BEEFY BEENE BEENS BEEPS BEERS BEERY BEETS BEETY BEFIT BEFOG BEFOR BEGAN BEGAT BEGAY BEGEM BEGET BEGIN BEGOT BEGUM BEGUN BEHAN BEHAR

BEIGE
BEING
BEINS
BEIRA
BEKAA
BELAU
BELAY
BELBY
BELCH
BELEM
BELIE
BELLA
BELLE
BELLI
BELLO
BELLS
BELLY
BELON
BELOW
BELTS
BELVA
BEMAD
BEMAN
BEMAS
BENCH
BENDS
BENDY
BENES
BENET
BENIN
BENJI
BENNY
BENTO
BENTS
BEOFF
BEPPE
BEPPO
BERCY
BEREA
BERET
BERGS
BERIA
BERKS
BERLE
BERMS
BERNE
BERNI
BERRA
BERRY
BERTA
BERTH
BERYL
BESES
BESET
BESOM
BESOS
BESOT
BESTS
BETAS
BETEL
BETES
BETHS
BETON
BETSY
BETTA
BETTE
BETTI
BETTY
BEVEL
BEVIN
BEWIG
BEXAR
BEYLE
BEZEL
BEZOS

B•E••
BAEDA
BAEZA
BCELL
BEEBE
BEECH
BEEFS
BEEFY
BEENE
BEENS
BEEPS
BEERS
BEERY
BEETS
BEETY
BIEHN
BIERE
BIERI
BIERS
BLEAK
BLEAR
BLEAT
BLEBS
BLEED
BLEEP
BLEND
BLENT
BLESS
BLEST
BLEUS
BOERS
BOEUF
BREAD
BREAK
BREAM
BRECA
BRECK
BREDA
BREDE
BREED
BREEN
BREES
BRENS
BRENT
BRERS
BREST
BRETT
BREVE
BREVI
BREWS
BTEAM
BUELL
BUENA
BUENO
BYEAR

B••E•
BAAED
BABEL
BABES
BADEN
BADER
BAGEL
BAIES
BAJER
BAKED
BAKER
BAKES
BALED
BALER
BALES
BANES
BARED
BARER
BARES
BASED
BASEL
BASER
BASES
BATED
BATES
BAUER
BAYED
BAYER
BAYES
BCCED
BCDEF
BEDEW
BEGEM
BEGET
BELEM
BENES
BENET
BEREA
BERET
BESES
BESET
BETEL
BETES
BEVEL
BEZEL
BHAER
BICEP
BIDED
BIDEN
BIDER
BIDES
BIDET
BIKED
BIKEL
BIKER
BIKES
BILES
BINES
BINET
BIPED
BITER
BITES
BIZET
BLEED
BLEEP
BLUED
BLUER
BLUES
BLUET
BODED
BODEL
BODES
BOGEY
BOHEA
BOJER
BOLES
BOLET
BONED
BONER
BONES
BONET
BONEY
BOOED
BOOER
BORED
BOREL
BOREN
BORER
BORES
BOTEL
BOVET
BOWED
BOWEL
BOWEN
BOWER
BOWES
BOXED
BOXER
BOXES
BOYER
BRAES
BREED
BREEN
BREES
BRIEF
BRIER
BRIES
BUBER
BUREN
BURET
BUSED
BUSES
BUSEY
BUTEO
BUYER
BYNER
BYSEA
BYTES

B•••E
BADGE
BAIZE
BARGE
BARRE
BASIE
BASLE
BASSE
BASTE
BATHE
BAUME
BAYLE
BEALE
BEAME
BEEBE
BEENE
BEIGE
BELIE
BELLE
BEPPE
BERLE
BERNE
BETTE
BEYLE
BFIVE
BIBLE
BIERE
BILGE
BINGE
BIOME
BIORE
BIRSE
BITTE
BLADE
BLAKE
BLAME
BLANE
BLARE
BLASE
BLAZE
BLIGE
BLOKE
BLORE
BLUME
BNINE
BOCCE
BOGIE
BOGLE
BOIRE
BOISE
BOITE
BOMBE
BONNE
BONZE
BOOLE
BOONE
BOOZE
BORGE
BORNE
BOTHE
BOULE
BOWIE
BOYLE
BRACE
BRAHE
BRAKE
BRAVE
BREDE
BREVE
BRIBE
BRICE
BRIDE
BRINE
BRISE
BRITE
BROKE
BRUCE
BRULE
BRUME
BRUTE
BRYCE
BSIDE
BTILE
BUDGE
BUGLE
BULGE
BURKE
BUTTE
BYAGE
BYONE
BYRNE

•BE••
ABEAM
ABEAR
ABELE
ABEND
ABETS
CBERS
EBELS
EBERT
HBEAM
IBEAM
IBERT
LBEAM
MBEKI
OBEAH
OBELI
OBESE
OBEYS
QBERT

•B•E•
ABBES
ABBEY
ABDEL
ABIES
ABLED
ABLER
ABNER
EBBED
EBSEN
IBSEN
NBAER
OBIES
OBJET
OBOES

•B••E
ABASE
ABATE
ABBIE
ABCDE
ABELE
ABIDE
ABODE
ABOVE
ABUSE
OBESE
OBOTE
TBONE

••BE•
ABBES
ABBEY
ALBEE
ALBEN
AMBER
ARBER
AUBER
BABEL
BABES
BUBER
CABER
CUBEB
CUBED
CUBER
CUBES
CYBER
DOBEE
EBBED
EMBED
EMBER
FABER
FIBER
GABEL
GIBED
GIBER
GIBES
GOBEL
HABER
HOBEY
HRBEK
HUBEL
HUBER
IMBED
INBED
JIBED
JIBES
KUBEK
LABEL
LIBEL
LIBER
LOBED
LOBES
LUBED
LUBES
MABEL
NABES
NOBEL
NOBET
OMBER
ORBED
REBEC
REBEL
REBER
REBET
ROBED
ROBER
ROBES
RUBEL
RUBEN
RUBES
SABER
SOBER
TEBET
TIBER
TIBET
TOBEY
TUBED
TUBER
TUBES
UMBEL
UMBER
UNBET
UZBEK
VIBES
WEBER
XEBEC

••B•E
ABBIE
ALBEE
AMBLE
ARBRE
BIBLE
CABLE
DEBBE
DEBYE
DOBEE
DOBIE
DOBLE
DUBHE
EUBIE
FABLE
FABRE
FIBRE
GABLE
HOBIE
HUBIE
IMBUE
LIBRE
NOBLE
OMBRE
POBRE
REBBE
ROBBE
ROBLE
RUBLE
SABLE
SABRE
TABLE
UMBLE

•••BE
ADOBE
BEEBE
BOMBE
BRIBE
DAUBE
DEBBE
FROBE
GLOBE
GREBE
HERBE
ILLBE
JAMBE
LETBE
LIEBE
MAYBE
NIOBE
PHEBE
PHOBE
PLEBE
PROBE
RAABE
REBBE
ROBBE
THEBE
TOMBE
TRIBE
UTUBE
WIEBE
ZERBE

BF•••
BFIVE
BFLAT
BFOUR

B•F••
BAFFS
BAFFY
BEFIT
BEFOG
BEFOR
BIFFS
BIFID
BOFFO
BOFFS
BUFFA
BUFFI
BUFFO
BUFFS
BUFFY
BYFAR
BYFAX

B••F•
BAFFS
BAFFY
BANFF
BARFY
BEEFS
BEEFY
BEOFF
BIFFS
BLAFF
BLUFF
BOFFO
BOFFS
BUFFA
BUFFI
BUFFO
BUFFS
BUFFY

B•••F
BANFF
BCDEF
BEOFF
BLAFF
BLUFF
BOEUF
BRIEF

•BF••
ABFAB

•B•F•
ABAFT

••B•F
EGBDF
ROBOF

BG•••
BGIRL
BGOSH

B•G••
BAGEL
BAGGY
BAGIT
BBGUN
BEGAN
BEGAT
BEGAY
BEGEM
BEGET
BEGIN
BEGOT
BEGUM
BEGUN
BIGDO
BIGGS
BIGGY
BIGHT
BIGLY
BIGMO
BIGON
BIGOT
BOGAN
BOGEY
BOGGS
BOGGY
BOGIE
BOGLE
BOGUS
BUGGY
BUGLE
BUGSY
BYGOD
BYGUM

B••G•
BADGE
BAGGY
BANGS
BARGE
BAUGH
BEIGE
BERGS
BIGGS
BIGGY
BILGE
BILGY
BINGE
BINGO
BINGS
BIOGS
BLDGS
BLIGE
BLIGH
BLOGS
BOGGS
BOGGY
BONGO
BONGS
BORGE
BORGS
BOUGH
BRAGA
BRAGG
BRAGH
BRAGS
BRIGS
BUDGE
BUGGY
BULGE
BULGY
BUNGS
BURGH
BURGS
BYAGE

B•••G
BEDOG
BEFOG
BEING
BEWIG
BHANG
BILLG
BLING
BOING
BOURG
BRAGG
BRANG
BRING
BRUNG

•BG••
BBGUN
OBGYN

•B••G
ABZUG

••B•G
ASBIG
DEBAG
DEBUG
EMBOG
INBIG
MRBIG
REBAG
SOBIG
UNBAG
VWBUG

BH•••
BHAER
BHANG
BHATS

B•H••
BAHAI
BAHIA
BAHTS
BEHAN
BEHAR
BOHAY
BOHEA
BOHOS

B••H•
BASHO
BATHE
BATHO
BATHS
BATHY
BETHS
BIEHN
BIGHT
BLAHS
BOCHY
BOPHA
BOTHA
BOTHE
BRAHE
BRUHL
BRUHN
BUSHY

B•••H
BALCH
BALPH
BARTH
BATCH
BAUGH
BEACH
BEECH
BELCH
BENCH
BERTH
BGOSH
BIRCH
BIRTH
BLIGH
BLISH
BLOCH
BLUSH
BLUTH
BLYTH
BOOTH
BORAH
BOSCH
BOTCH
BOUGH
BRACH
BRAGH
BRASH
BRITH
BROTH
BRUCH
BRUSH
BUNCH
BURGH
BUSCH
BUTCH

•BH••
ABHOR

•B•H•
ABMHO
ABOHM

•B••H
ABASH
OBEAH

••BH•
DUBHE

••B•H
DABIH

BI•••
BIALY
BIBBS
BIBLE
BICEP
BIDDY
BIDED
BIDEN
BIDER
BIDES
BIDET
BIDIN
BIDON
BIDUP
BIEHN
BIERE
BIERI
BIERS
BIFFS
BIFID
BIGDO
BIGGS
BIGGY
BIGHT
BIGLY
BIGMO
BIGON
BIGOT
BIJOU
BIKED
BIKEL
BIKER
BIKES
BILBO
BILES
BILGE
BILGY
BILKO
BILKS
BILLG
BILLS
BILLW
BILLY
BIMBO
BINAL
BINDS
BINES
BINET
BINGE
BINGO
BINGS
BIOGS
BIOME
BIONT
BIORE
BIOTA
BIPED
BIPOD
BIPPY
BIRCH
BIRDS
BIRDY
BIRLS
BIROS
BIRRA
BIRRI
BIRRS
BIRSE
BIRTH
BISON
BITER
BITES
BITIN
BITON
BITSY
BITTE
BITTS
BITTY
BITUP
BIXBY
BIZET

B•I••
BAIES
BAILS
BAIRD
BAIRN
BAISA
BAITS
BAIUL
BAIZA
BAIZE
BEIGE
BEING
BEINS
BEIRA
BFIVE
BGIRL
BLIGE
BLIGH
BLIMP
BLIND
BLING
BLINI
BLINK
BLIPS
BLISH
BLISS
BLIST
BLITT
BLITZ
BNINE
BOILS
BOING
BOIRE
BOISE
BOITE
BOITO
BRIAN
BRIAR
BRIBE
BRICE
BRICK
BRIDE
BRIEF
BRIER
BRIES
BRIGS
BRILL
BRIMS
BRINE
BRING
BRINK
BRINY
BRISE
BRISK
BRITE
BRITH
BRITS
BRITT
BRITZ
BSIDE
BTILE
BUICK
BUILD
BUILT

B••I•
BACIO
BAGIT
BAHIA
BALIN
BARIC
BARIT
BASIA
BASIC
BASIE
BASIL
BASIN
BASIS
BATIK
BATIN
BEDIM
BEFIT
BEGIN
BELIE
BENIN
BERIA
BEVIN
BEWIG
BIDIN
BIFID
BITIN
BLAIR
BLAIS
BLOIS
BOGIE
BORIC
BORIS
BOVID
BOWIE
BOXIN
BRAID
BRAIN
BROIL
BRUIN
BRUIT
BUNIN
BURIN
BUYIN
BUYIT
BYAIR

B•••I
BAHAI
BALKI
BAMBI
BARBI
BASSI
BELLI
BENJI
BERNI
BETTI
BIERI
BIRRI
BLINI
BOCCI
BONDI
BOOKI
BREVI
BRUNI
BUFFI
BUZZI

•BI••
ABIDE
ABIES
IBIZA
OBIES
OBITS
TBILL
TBIRD

•B•I•
ABBIE
ABOIL
ABRIL
ABRIM
ABRIS
QBVII

•B••I
ABACI
EBOLI
MBEKI
OBELI
OBOLI
QBVII

••BI•
ABBIE
ADBIZ
AMBIT
ARBIL
ASBIG
CABIN
CUBIC
CUBIT
DABIH
DEBIT
DOBIE
DUBIN
ERBIL
EUBIE
FABIO
GABIN
HABIB
HABIT
HOBIE
HUBIE
INBIG
LABIA
LUBIN
MOBIL
MRBIG
NOBID
NOBIS
NUBIA
ORBIC
ORBIT
RABID
RABIN
REBID
ROBIN
RUBIK
RUBIN
SABIN
SOBIG
SUBIC
SYBIL
TABIS
TIBIA
TOBIT
UNBID
UNBIT
ZUBIN

••B•I
DEBBI
DUBAI
LIBRI
RABBI

•••BI
ALIBI
BAMBI
BARBI
DEBBI
DHABI
IAMBI
NIMBI
ORIBI
RABBI

BJ•••
BJORK
BJORN

B•J••
BAJER
BIJOU
BOJER

B••J•
BANJO
BENJI

•BJ••
OBJET

•B•J•
ABAJO
ABUJA

B•K••
BAKED
BAKER
BAKES
BAKST
BEKAA
BIKED
BIKEL
BIKER
BIKES

B••K•
BABKA
BACKS
BALKI
BALKS
BALKY
BANKS
BANKY
BARKS
BARKY
BASKS
BEAKS
BECKS
BECKY
BERKS
BILKO
BILKS
BLAKE
BLOKE
BOCKS
BONKS
BOOKI

BOOKS BOOKV BOOKX BORKS BRAKE BROKE BUBKA BUCKO BUCKS BUCKY BULKS BULKY BUNKO BUNKS BURKA BURKE BUSKS

B•••K
BARAK BATIK BAULK BJORK BLACK BLANK BLEAK BLINK BLOCK BRACK BREAK BRECK BRICK BRINK BRISK BROCK BROOK BRUSK BUICK

•B•K•
MBEKI

•B••K
ABACK DBACK EBANK EBOOK IBOOK PBOOK

••BK•
BABKA BUBKA

••B•K
HRBEK KUBEK RUBIK UZBEK

BL•••
BLABS BLACK BLADE BLAFF BLAHS BLAIR BLAIS BLAKE BLAME BLAMS BLANC BLAND BLANE BLANK BLARE BLASE BLASS BLAST BLATS BLATZ BLAZE BLDGS BLEAK BLEAR BLEAT BLEBS BLEED BLEEP BLEND BLENT BLESS BLEST BLEUS BLIGE BLIGH BLIMP BLIND BLING BLINI BLINK BLIPS BLISH BLISS BLIST BLITT BLITZ BLOAT BLOBS BLOCH BLOCK BLOCS BLOGS BLOIS BLOKE BLOND BLOOD BLOOM BLOOP BLORE BLOTS BLOWN BLOWS BLOWY BLUED BLUER BLUES BLUET BLUFF BLUME BLUNT BLURB BLURS BLURT BLUSH BLUTH BLUTO BLVDS BLYTH

B•L••
BALAS BALBO BALCH BALDS BALDY BALED BALER BALES BALIN BALKI BALKS BALKY BALLO BALLS BALLY BALMS BALMY BALON BALOO BALPH BALSA BALTO BALTS BELAU BELAY BELBY BELCH BELEM BELIE BELLA BELLE BELLI BELLO BELLS BELLY BELON BELOW BELTS BELVA BFLAT BILBO BILES BILGE BILGY BILKO BILKS BILLG BILLS BILLW BILLY BOLAR BOLAS BOLDS BOLES BOLET BOLLA BOLLS BOLOS BOLTS BOLUS BPLUS BULBA BULBS BULGE BULGY BULKS BULKY BULLA BULLS BULLY BULOW BYLAW BYLOT

B••L•
BAALS BADLY BAILS BALLO BALLS BALLY BASLE BAULK BAWLS BAYLE BBALL BCELL BEALE BEALL BEALS BELLA BELLE BELLI BELLO BELLS BELLY BERLE BEYLE BIALY BIBLE BIGLY BILLG BILLS BILLW BILLY BIRLS BOGLE BOILS BOLLA BOLLS BOOLA BOOLE BOULE BOULT BOWLS BOYLE BRILL BRULE BTILE BUELL BUGLE BUILD BUILT BULLA BULLS BULLY BURLS BURLY

B•••L
BABEL BAGEL BAIUL BANAL BASAL BASEL BASIL BBALL BCELL BEALL BERYL BETEL BEVEL BEZEL BGIRL BIKEL BINAL BODEL BOREL BOTEL BOWEL BRAWL BRILL BROIL BRUHL BUELL BUTYL

•BL••
ABLED ABLER

•B•L•
ABELE BBALL EBELS EBOLA EBOLI OBELI OBOLI OBOLS TBALL TBILL UBOLT

•B••L
ABDEL ABDUL ABOIL ABRIL BBALL TBALL TBILL

••BL•
AMBLE BIBLE CABLE DOBLE FABLE GABLE HABLA KUBLA NIBLO NOBLE NOBLY PABLO ROBLE RUBLE SABLE TABLA TABLE UMBLE

••B•L
ARBIL ARBOL BABEL CABAL COBOL ERBIL GABEL GOBEL HUBEL IQBAL JUBAL KABUL LABEL LIBEL MABEL MOBIL NOBEL REBEL RUBEL SABAL SIBYL SYBIL TUBAL UMBEL

BM•••
BMOCS

B•M••
BAMBA BAMBI BAMMY BEMAD BEMAN BEMAS BIMBO BOMBA BOMBE BOMBS BUMPS BUMPY

B••M•
BALMS BALMY BAMMY BARMS BARMY BAUME BEAME BEAMS BEAMY BERMS BIGMO BIOME BLAME BLAMS BLIMP BLUME BOOMS BOOMY BRIMS BROMO BRUME BURMA

B•••M
BEDIM BEGEM BEGUM BELEM BESOM BLOOM BONUM BOSOM BREAM BROOM BTEAM BUXOM BYGUM

•BM••
ABMHO IBMPC

•B•M•
ABOMA ABOMB HBOMB NBOMB OBAMA

•B••M
ABEAM ABOHM ABRAM ABRIM ABYSM HBEAM IBEAM LBEAM

••BM•
ICBMS

••B•M
ALBOM ALBUM

BN•••
BNINE

B•N••
BANAL BANCA BANCO BANCS BANDA BANDB BANDO BANDS BANDW BANDY BANES BANFF BANGS BANJO BANKS BANKY BANNS BANON BANOS BANTA BANTU BENCH BENDS BENDY BENES BENET BENIN BENJI BENNY BENTO BENTS BINAL BINDS BINES BINET BINGE BINGO BINGS BONAR BONDI BONDS BONED BONER BONES BONET BONEY BONGO BONGS BONKS BONNE BONNY BONUM BONUS BONZE BONZO BUNCH BUNCO BUNDS BUNDT BUNDY BUNGS BUNIN BUNKO BUNKS BUNNY BUNTS BYNER BYNOW

B••N•
BANNS BARNS BATNA BEANO BEANS BEANY BEDNY BEENE BEENS BEING BEINS BENNY BERNE BERNI BHANG BIONT BLANC BLAND BLANE BLANK BLEND BLENT BLIND BLING BLINI BLINK BLOND BLUNT BNINE BOING BONNE BONNY BOONE BOONS BORNE BOSNS BOUND BRAND BRANG BRANS BRANT BRENS BRENT BRINE BRING BRINK BRINY BRONC BRONX BRUNG BRUNI BRUNO BRUNT BUENA BUENO BUNNY BUONA BUONO BURNS BURNT BUTNO BWANA BYONE BYRNE

B•••N
BACON BADEN BADUN BAIRN BALIN BALON BANON BARON BASIN BATIN BATON BBGUN BEGAN BEGIN BEGUN BEHAN BELON BEMAN BENIN BETON BEVIN BIDEN BIDIN BIDON BIEHN BIGON BISON BITIN BITON BJORN BLOWN BOGAN BOREN BORON BOSON BOSUN BOWEN BOXIN BRAIN BRAUN BRAWN BREEN BRIAN BROUN BROWN BRUHN BRUIN BRYAN BUNIN BUREN BURIN BUSON BUYIN BYRON

•BN••
ABNER

•B•N•
ABEND EBANK EBOND EBONS EBONY TBOND TBONE

•B••N
BBGUN EBSEN IBSEN OBGYN

••BN•
ISBNS

••B•N
ALBAN ALBEN CABIN CUBAN DABON DUBIN GABIN GABON HOBAN LABAN LUBIN RABIN ROBIN ROBYN RUBEN RUBIN RUBON SABIN URBAN YUBAN ZUBIN

BO•••
BOARD BOARS BOAST BOATS BOBBY BOBUP BOCAS BOCCE BOCCI BOCHY BOCKS BODDY BODED BODEL BODES BOERS BOEUF BOFFO BOFFS BOGAN BOGEY BOGGS BOGGY BOGIE BOGLE BOGUS BOHAY BOHEA BOHOS BOILS BOING BOIRE BOISE BOITE BOITO BOJER BOLAR BOLAS BOLDS BOLES BOLET BOLLA BOLLS BOLOS BOLTS BOLUS BOMBA BOMBE BOMBS BONAR BONDI BONDS BONED BONER BONES BONET BONEY BONGO BONGS BONKS BONNE BONNY BONUM BONUS BONZE BONZO BOOAT BOOBS BOOBY BOOED BOOER BOOKI BOOKS BOOKV BOOKX BOOLA BOOLE BOOMS BOOMY BOONE BOONS BOORS BOOST BOOTH BOOTS BOOTY BOOZE BOPHA BORAH BORAS BORAX BORED BOREL BOREN BORER BORES BORGE BORGS BORIC BORIS BORKS BORNE BORON BOROS BORSA BOSCH BOSCO BOSCS BOSNS BOSOM BOSON BOSOX BOSSA BOSSY BOSUN BOTCH BOTEL BOTHA BOTHE BOTOX BOTTS BOUGH BOULE BOULT BOUND BOURG BOUTS BOVET BOVID BOWED BOWEL BOWEN BOWER BOWES BOWIE BOWLS BOWTO BOXED BOXER BOXES BOXIN BOXUP BOYER BOYLE BOYOS BOZOS

B•O••
BBOYS BEOFF BFOUR BGOSH BIOGS BIOME BIONT BIORE BIOTA BJORK BJORN BLOAT BLOBS BLOCH BLOCK BLOCS BLOGS BLOIS BLOKE BLOND BLOOD BLOOM BLOOP BLORE BLOTS BLOWN BLOWS BLOWY BMOCS BOOAT BOOBS BOOBY BOOED BOOER BOOKI BOOKS BOOKV BOOKX BOOLA BOOLE BOOMS BOOMY BOONE BOONS BOORS BOOST BOOTH BOOTS BOOTY BOOZE BROAD BROCA BROCK BRODY BROIL BROKE BROMO BRONC BRONX BROOD BROOK BROOM BROTH BROUD BROUN BROWN BROWS BUONA BUONO BUOYS BYONE

B••O•
BABOO BACON BACOS BALON BALOO BANON BANOS BARON BASOV BATON BATOR BAYOU BAZOO BEBOP BEDOG BEFOG BEFOR BEGOT BELON BELOW BESOM BESOS BESOT BETON BEZOS BIDON BIGON BIGOT BIJOU BIPOD BIROS BISON BITON BLOOD BLOOM BLOOP BOHOS BOLOS BORON BOROS BOSOM BOSON BOSOX BOTOX BOYOS BOZOS BROOD BROOK BROOM BULOW BUSON BUXOM BYGOD BYLOT BYNOW BYRON

B•••O
BABOO BACIO BALBO BALLO BALOO BALTO BANCO BANDO BANJO BARCO BASHO BASSO BATHO BAZOO BEANO BELLO BENTO BEPPO BIGDO BIGMO BILBO BILKO BIMBO BINGO BLUTO BOFFO BOITO BONGO BONZO BOSCO BOWTO BRAVO BRAZO BROMO BRUNO BUCCO BUCKO BUENO BUFFO BUNCO BUNKO BUONO BURRO BUTEO BUTNO BYTWO

•BO••
ABODE ABOHM ABOIL ABOMA ABOMB ABORT ABOUT ABOVE ABOVO BBOYS EBOAT EBOLA EBOLI EBOND EBONS EBONY EBOOK HBOMB IBOOK NBOMB OBOES OBOLI OBOLS OBOTE PBOOK TBOND TBONE UBOAT UBOLT

•B•O•
ABBOT ABHOR EBOOK IBOOK PBOOK

•B••O
ABACO ABAJO ABMHO ABOVO

••BO•
ABBOT ALBOM AMBOS AMBOY ARBOL ARBOR BABOO BEBOP CABOB CABOT COBOL DABON ELBOW EMBOG GABON GABOR GOBOS GOBOT HOBOS INBOX JABOT KABOB KOBOS LABOR LOBOS MYBOY NABOB NABOO OHBOY OXBOW POBOX POBOY REBOP REBOX ROBOF ROBOT RUBON SABOT TABOO TABOR UNBOX UPBOW

••B•O
BABOO DOBRO FABIO FIBRO LIBRO NABOO NIBLO PABLO TABOO

•••BO
ADOBO BALBO BILBO BIMBO CARBO COMBO DUMBO GARBO GUMBO JUMBO LIMBO MAMBO MUMBO PEABO PHOBO RAMBO SERBO SORBO TAEBO TURBO

BP•••
BPLUS

B•P••
BEPPE BEPPO BIPED BIPOD BIPPY BOPHA

B••P•
BALPH BCUPS BEEPS

BEPPE
BEPPO
BIPPY
BLIPS
BUMPS
BUMPY
BURPS

B•••P
BEBOP
BICEP
BIDUP
BITUP
BLEEP
BLIMP
BLOOP
BOBUP
BOXUP
BUYUP

•B•P•
IBMPC
TBSPS

••B•P
BEBOP
BOBUP
REBOP
RUBUP

B••Q•
BARQS

B•••Q
BARBQ

•••BQ
BARBQ

BR•••
BRACE
BRACH
BRACK
BRACT
BRADS
BRADY
BRAES
BRAGA
BRAGG
BRAGH
BRAGS
BRAHE
BRAID
BRAIN
BRAKE
BRAND
BRANG
BRANS
BRANT
BRASH
BRASS
BRATS
BRATT
BRAUN
BRAVA
BRAVE
BRAVO
BRAWL
BRAWN
BRAYS
BRAZO
BREAD
BREAK
BREAM
BRECA
BRECK
BREDA
BREDE
BREED
BREEN
BREES
BRENS
BRENT
BRERS
BREST
BRETT
BREVE
BREVI
BREWS
BRIAN
BRIAR
BRIBE
BRICE
BRICK
BRIDE
BRIEF
BRIER
BRIES
BRIGS
BRILL
BRIMS
BRINE
BRING
BRINK
BRINY
BRISE
BRISK
BRITE
BRITH
BRITS
BRITT
BRITZ
BROAD
BROCA
BROCK
BRODY
BROIL
BROKE
BROMO
BRONC
BRONX
BROOD
BROOK
BROOM
BROTH
BROUD
BROUN
BROWN
BROWS
BRUCE
BRUCH
BRUHL
BRUHN
BRUIN
BRUIT
BRULE
BRUME
BRUNG
BRUNI
BRUNO
BRUNT
BRUSH
BRUSK
BRUTE
BRUTS
BRYAN
BRYCE

B•R••
BARAK
BARBA
BARBI
BARBQ
BARBS
BARCA
BARCO
BARDS
BARED
BARER
BARES
BARFY
BARGE
BARIC
BARIT
BARKS
BARKY
BARMS
BARMY
BARNS
BARON
BARQS
BARRE
BARRY
BARTH
BARTY
BERCY
BEREA
BERET
BERGS
BERIA
BERKS
BERLE
BERMS
BERNE
BERNI
BERRA
BERRY
BERTA
BERTH
BERYL
BIRCH
BIRDS
BIRDY
BIRLS
BIROS
BIRRA
BIRRI
BIRRS
BIRSE
BIRTH
BORAH
BORAS
BORAX
BORED
BOREL
BOREN
BORER
BORES
BORGE
BORGS
BORIC
BORIS
BORKS
BORNE
BORON
BOROS
BORSA
BURBS
BUREN
BURET
BURGH
BURGS
BURIN
BURKA
BURKE
BURLS
BURLY
BURMA
BURNS
BURNT
BURPS
BURRO
BURRS
BURRY
BURSA
BURST
BYRDS
BYRNE
BYRON

B••R•
BAIRD
BAIRN
BARRE
BARRY
BASRA
BEARD
BEARS
BEART
BEERS
BEERY
BEIRA
BERRA
BERRY
BGIRL
BIERE
BIERI
BIERS
BIORE
BIRRA
BIRRI
BIRRS
BJORK
BJORN
BLARE
BLORE
BLURB
BLURS
BLURT
BOARD
BOARS
BOERS
BOIRE
BOORS
BOURG
BRERS
BURRO
BURRS
BURRY

B•••R
BABAR
BADER
BAJER
BAKER
BALER
BARER
BASER
BATOR
BAUER
BAYAR
BAYER
BEFOR
BEHAR
BEXAR
BFOUR
BHAER
BIDER
BIKER
BITER
BLAIR
BLEAR
BLUER
BOJER
BOLAR
BONAR
BONER
BOOER
BORER
BOWER
BOXER
BOYER
BRIAR
BRIER
BSTAR
BUBER
BUYER
BYAIR
BYCAR
BYEAR
BYFAR
BYNER

•BR••
ABRAM
ABRIL
ABRIM
ABRIS
OBRAS

•B•R•
ABBRS
ABORT
CBERS
EBERT
HBARS
IBARS
IBERT
JBARS
LBARS
QBERT
TBARS
TBIRD
ZBARS

•B••R
ABEAR
ABHOR
ABLER
ABNER
NBAER

••BR•
ABBRS
AMBRY
ARBRE
COBRA
DEBRA
DOBRO
FABRE
FIBRE
FIBRO
LIBRA
LIBRE
LIBRI
LIBRO
OMBRE
POBRE
SABRA
SABRE
UMBRA
ZEBRA

••B•R
AKBAR
AMBER
ARBER
ARBOR
ATBAR
AUBER
BABAR
BUBER
CABER
CUBER
CYBER
DEBAR
EMBAR
EMBER
FABER
FIBER
GABOR
GIBER
HABER
HUBER
LABOR
LIBER
LOBAR
OMBER
REBAR
REBER
ROBER
SABER
SOBER
TABOR
TIBER
TUBER
UMBER
UNBAR
WEBER

BS•••
BSIDE
BSTAR

B•S••
BASAL
BASED
BASEL
BASER
BASES
BASHO
BASIA
BASIC
BASIE
BASIL
BASIN
BASIS
BASKS
BASLE
BASOV
BASRA
BASSE
BASSI
BASSO
BASSY
BASTA
BASTE
BASTS
BESES
BESET
BESOM
BESOS
BESOT
BESTS
BISON
BOSCH
BOSCO
BOSCS
BOSNS
BOSOM
BOSON
BOSOX
BOSSA
BOSSY
BOSUN
BUSBY
BUSCH
BUSED
BUSES
BUSEY
BUSHY
BUSKS
BUSON
BUSTA
BUSTS
BYSEA

B••S•
BAISA
BAKST
BALSA
BASSE
BASSI
BASSO
BASSY
BEAST
BETSY
BGOSH
BIRSE
BITSY
BLASE
BLASS
BLAST
BLESS
BLEST
BLISH
BLISS
BLIST
BLUSH
BOAST
BOISE
BOOST
BORSA
BOSSA
BOSSY
BRASH
BRASS
BREST
BRISE
BRISK
BRUSH
BRUSK
BUGSY
BURSA
BURST

B•••S
BAALS
BABAS
BABES
BABUS
BABYS
BACKS
BACOS
BAFFS
BAHTS
BAIES
BAILS
BAITS
BAKES
BALAS
BALDS
BALES
BALKS
BALLS
BALMS
BALTS
BANCS
BANDS
BANES
BANGS
BANKS
BANNS
BANOS
BARBS
BARDS
BARES
BARKS
BARMS
BARNS
BARQS
BASES
BASIS
BASKS
BASTS
BATES
BATHS
BATTS
BAUDS
BAWLS
BAYES
BBOYS
BCUPS
BDAYS
BEADS
BEAKS
BEALS
BEAMS
BEANS
BEARS
BEATS
BEAUS
BECKS
BEEFS
BEENS
BEEPS
BEERS
BEETS
BEINS
BELLS
BELTS
BEMAS
BENDS
BENES
BENTS
BERGS
BERKS
BERMS
BESES
BESOS
BESTS
BETAS
BETES
BETHS
BEZOS
BHATS
BIBBS
BIDES
BIERS
BIFFS
BIGGS
BIKES
BILES
BILKS
BILLS
BINDS
BINES
BINGS
BIOGS
BIRDS
BIRLS
BIROS
BIRRS
BITES
BITTS
BLABS
BLAHS
BLAIS
BLAMS
BLASS
BLATS
BLDGS
BLEBS
BLESS
BLEUS
BLIPS
BLISS
BLOBS
BLOCS
BLOGS
BLOIS
BLOTS
BLOWS
BLUES
BLURS
BLVDS
BMOCS
BOARS
BOATS
BOCAS
BOCKS
BODES
BOERS
BOFFS
BOGGS
BOGUS
BOHOS
BOILS
BOLAS
BOLDS
BOLES
BOLLS
BOLOS
BOLTS
BOLUS
BOMBS
BONDS
BONES
BONGS
BONKS
BONUS
BOOBS
BOOKS
BOOMS
BOONS
BOORS
BOOTS
BORAS
BORES
BORGS
BORIS
BORKS
BOROS
BOSCS
BOSNS
BOTTS
BOUTS
BOWES
BOWLS
BOXES
BOYOS
BOZOS
BPLUS
BRADS
BRAES
BRAGS
BRANS
BRASS
BRATS
BRAYS
BREES
BRENS
BRERS
BREWS
BRIES
BRIGS
BRIMS
BRITS
BROWS
BRUTS
BUCKS
BUFFS
BULBS
BULKS
BULLS
BUMPS
BUNDS
BUNGS
BUNKS
BUNTS
BUOYS
BURBS
BURGS
BURLS
BURNS
BURPS
BURRS
BUSES
BUSKS
BUSTS
BUTTS
BYBUS
BYRDS
BYTES

•BS••
CBSTV
EBSEN
IBSEN
TBSPS

•B•S•
ABASE
ABASH
ABUSE
ABYSM
ABYSS
OBESE

•B••S
ABBAS
ABBES
ABBRS
ABETS
ABIES
ABRIS
ABUTS
ABYSS
BBOYS
CBERS
EBELS
EBONS
HBARS
IBARS
JBARS
LBARS
OBEYS
OBIES
OBITS
OBOES
OBOLS
OBRAS
TBARS
TBSPS
ZBARS

••BS•
FUBSY
PABST

••B•S
ABBAS
ABBES
ABBRS
ALBAS
AMBOS
ARBUS
ARBYS
BABAS
BABES
BABUS
BABYS
BIBBS
BYBUS
CUBES
DEBTS
DEBUS
DOBBS
ENBAS
GIBBS
GIBES
GIBUS
GOBOS
HOBBS
HOBOS
ICBMS
ISBNS
JIBES
KABAS
KOBOS
LOBES
LOBOS
LUBES
NABES
NOBIS
PEBAS
REBUS
ROBES
RUBES
SOBAS
TABIS
TABUS
TIBBS
TUBAS
TUBBS
TUBES
VIBES
ZEBUS

•••BS
ARABS
BARBS
BIBBS
BLABS
BLEBS
BLOBS
BOMBS
BOOBS
BULBS
BURBS
CAMBS
CARBS
CHUBS
CLUBS
COMBS
CRABS
CRIBS
CURBS
DAUBS
DOBBS
DOUBS
DRABS
DRIBS
DRUBS
DUMBS
FEEBS
FLUBS
FTLBS
GARBS
GIBBS
GLOBS
GRABS
GRUBS
HERBS
HOBBS
IAMBS
JAMBS
KERBS
KNOBS
KREBS
LAMBS
LIMBS
NUMBS
PLEBS
PROBS
SAABS
SCABS
SERBS
SLABS
SLOBS
SNOBS
SNUBS
SORBS
STABS
STUBS
SWABS
TIBBS
TOMBS
TUBBS
VERBS
WOMBS

BT•••
BTEAM
BTILE

B•T••
BATCH
BATED
BATES
BATHE
BATHO
BATHS
BATHY
BATIK
BATIN
BATNA
BATON
BATOR
BATTS
BATTY
BETAS
BETEL
BETES
BETHS
BETON
BETSY
BETTA
BETTE
BETTI
BETTY
BITER
BITES
BITIN
BITON
BITSY
BITTE
BITTS
BITTY
BITUP
BOTCH
BOTEL
BOTHA
BOTHE
BOTOX
BOTTS
BSTAR
BUTCH
BUTEO
BUTNO
BUTTE
BUTTS
BUTUT
BUTYL
BYTES
BYTWO

B••T•
BAHTS
BAITS
BALTO
BALTS
BANTA
BANTU
BARTH
BARTY
BASTA
BASTE
BASTS
BATTS
BATTY
BEATS
BEATY
BEETS
BEETY
BELTS
BENTO
BENTS
BERTA
BERTH
BESTS
BETTA
BETTE
BETTI
BETTY
BHATS
BIOTA
BIRTH
BITTE
BITTS
BITTY
BLATS
BLATZ
BLITT
BLITZ
BLOTS
BLUTH
BLUTO
BLYTH
BOATS
BOITE
BOITO
BOLTS
BOOTH
BOOTS
BOOTY
BOTTS
BOUTS
BOWTO
BRATS
BRATT
BRETT
BRITE
BRITH
BRITS
BRITT
BRITZ
BROTH
BRUTE
BRUTS
BUNTS
BUSTA
BUSTS
BUTTE
BUTTS
BYATT

B•••T
BADAT
BAGIT
BAKST
BARIT
BAYAT
BEART
BEAST
BEAUT
BEFIT
BEGAT
BEGET
BEGOT
BENET
BERET
BESET
BESOT
BFLAT
BIDET
BIGHT
BIGOT
BINET
BIONT
BIZET
BLAST
BLEAT
BLENT
BLEST
BLIST
BLITT
BLOAT
BLUET
BLUNT
BLURT
BOAST
BOLET
BONET
BOOAT
BOOST
BOULT
BOVET
BRACT
BRANT
BRATT
BRENT
BREST
BRETT
BRITT
BRUIT
BRUNT
BUILT
BUNDT
BURET
BURNT
BURST
BUTUT
BUYAT
BUYIT
BYATT
BYLOT

•B•T•
ABATE
ABCTV
ABETS
ABUTS
CBSTV
NBCTV
OBITS
OBOTE

•B••T
ABAFT
ABBOT
ABORT
ABOUT
EBERT
EBOAT
IBERT
OBJET
QBERT
UBOAT
UBOLT

••BT•
DEBTS
WEBTV

••B•T
ABBOT
AMBIT
ATBAT
CABOT
CUBIT
DABAT
DEBIT
DEBUT
ESBAT
GOBAT
GOBOT
HABIT
JABOT
NOBET
ORBIT
PABST
RABAT
REBET
REBUT
ROBOT
SABOT
TEBET
TIBET
TOBIT
UNBET
UNBIT

•••BT
DOUBT

BU•••
BUBBA
BUBER
BUBKA
BUCCO
BUCKO
BUCKS
BUCKY
BUDDY
BUDGE
BUELL
BUENA
BUENO
BUFFA
BUFFI
BUFFO
BUFFS
BUFFY
BUGGY
BUGLE
BUGSY
BUICK
BUILD
BUILT
BULBA
BULBS
BULGE
BULGY
BULKS
BULKY
BULLA
BULLS
BULLY
BULOW
BUMPS
BUMPY
BUNCH
BUNCO
BUNDS
BUNDT

BUNDY BUNGS BUNIN BUNKO BUNKS BUNNY BUNTS BUONA BUONO BUOYS BURBS BUREN BURET BURGH BURGS BURIN BURKA BURKE BURLS BURLY BURMA BURNS BURNT BURPS BURRO BURRS BURRY BURSA BURST BUSBY BUSCH BUSED BUSES BUSEY BUSHY BUSKS BUSON BUSTA BUSTS BUTCH BUTEO BUTNO BUTTE BUTTS BUTUT BUTYL BUXOM BUYAT BUYER BUYIN BUYIT BUYUP BUZZI BUZZY

B•U••
BAUDS BAUER BAUGH BAULK BAUME BCUPS BLUED BLUER BLUES BLUET BLUFF BLUME BLUNT BLURB BLURS BLURT BLUSH BLUTH BLUTO BOUGH BOULE BOULT BOUND BOURG BOUTS BRUCE BRUCH BRUHL BRUHN BRUIN BRUIT BRULE BRUME BRUNG BRUNI BRUNO BRUNT BRUSH BRUSK BRUTE BRUTS

B••U•
BABUS BADUN BAIUL BBGUN BEAUS BEAUT BEAUX BEGUM BEGUN BFOUR BIDUP BITUP BLEUS BOBUP BOEUF BOGUS BOLUS BONUM BONUS BOSUN BOXUP BPLUS BRAUN BROUD BROUN BUTUT BUYUP BYBUS BYGUM

B•••U
BANTU BAYOU BELAU BIJOU

•BU••
ABUJA ABUSE ABUTS ABUZZ EBUZZ

•B•U•
ABDUL ABOUT ABZUG BBGUN

••BU•
ALBUM ARBUS BABUS BOBUP BYBUS DEBUG DEBUS DEBUT GIBUS IMBUE KABUL REBUS REBUT REBUY RUBUP TABUS UNBUD VWBUG ZEBUS

•••BU
IRABU KOMBU

B•V••
BEVEL BEVIN BLVDS BOVET BOVID

B••V•
BELVA BFIVE BRAVA BRAVE BRAVO BREVE BREVI

B•••V
BASOV BOOKV

•BV••
QBVII

•B•V•
ABOVE ABOVO

•B••V
ABCTV CBSTV NBCTV

••B•V
WEBTV

BW•••
BWANA

B•W••
BAWDY BAWLS BEWIG BOWED BOWEL BOWEN BOWER BOWES BOWIE BOWLS BOWTO BYWAY

B••W•
BLOWN BLOWS BLOWY BRAWL BRAWN BREWS BROWN BROWS BYTWO

B•••W
BANDW BEDEW BELOW BILLW BULOW BYLAW BYNOW

••B•W
ELBOW OXBOW UPBOW

B•X••
BEXAR BIXBY BOXED BOXER BOXES BOXIN BOXUP BUXOM

B•••X
BEAUX BOOKX BORAX BOSOX BOTOX BRONX BYFAX

••B•X
INBOX POBOX REBOX UNBOX

BY•••
BYAGE BYAIR BYATT BYBUS BYCAB BYCAR BYEAR BYFAR BYFAX BYGOD BYGUM BYLAW BYLOT BYNER BYNOW BYONE BYRDS BYRNE BYRON BYSEA BYTES BYTWO BYWAY

B•Y••
BAYAR BAYAT BAYED BAYER BAYES BAYLE BAYOU BEYLE BLYTH BOYER BOYLE BOYOS BRYAN BRYCE BUYAT BUYER BUYIN BUYIT BUYUP

B••Y•
BABYS BBOYS BDAYS BERYL BRAYS BUOYS BUTYL

B•••Y
BADDY BADLY BAFFY BAGGY BALDY BALKY BALLY BALMY BAMMY BANDY BANKY BARFY BARKY BARMY BARRY BARTY BASSY BATHY BATTY BAWDY BEADY BEAMY BEANY BEATY BECKY BEDDY BEDNY BEEFY BEERY BEETY BEGAY BELAY BELBY BELLY BENDY BENNY BERCY BERRY BETSY BETTY BIALY BIDDY BIGGY BIGLY BILGY BILLY BIPPY BIRDY BITSY BITTY BIXBY BLOWY BOBBY BOCHY BODDY BOGEY BOGGY BOHAY BONEY BONNY BOOBY BOOMY BOOTY BOSSY BRADY BRINY BRODY BUCKY BUDDY BUFFY BUGGY BUGSY BULGY BULKY BULLY BUMPY BUNDY BUNNY BURLY BURRY BUSBY BUSEY BUSHY BUZZY BYWAY

•BY••
ABYSM ABYSS

•B•Y•
BBOYS OBEYS OBGYN

•B••Y
ABBEY EBONY

••BY•
ARBYS BABYS DEBYE DUBYA LIBYA ROBYN SIBYL

••B•Y
ABBEY AMBOY AMBRY ATBAY BOBBY CABBY CUBBY DEBBY EMBAY FUBSY GABBY HOBBY HOBEY HUBBY LIBBY LOBBY MYBOY NOBBY NOBLY NUBBY OHBOY POBOY REBUY RIBBY ROBBY SFBAY TABBY TOBEY TUBBY WEBBY

•••BY
ARABY ASHBY BELBY BIXBY BOBBY BOOBY BUSBY CABBY CANBY CASBY COLBY CORBY COSBY CUBBY DARBY DEBBY DERBY DIDBY DIGBY DOLBY EKEBY FLYBY FURBY GABBY GETBY GORBY GOTBY GUMBY HERBY HOBBY HUBBY KILBY KIRBY LAYBY LETBY LIBBY LIEBY LOBBY LOOBY NAMBY NASBY NIMBY NOBBY NUBBY PAMBY POPBY PUTBY RANBY RIBBY RIGBY ROBBY RUGBY RUNBY SATBY SETBY SITBY TABBY TUBBY USEBY WEBBY WELBY WILBY WINBY WONBY ZIPBY

B•Z••
BAZOO BEZEL BEZOS BIZET BOZOS BUZZI BUZZY

B••Z•
BAEZA BAIZA BAIZE BLAZE BONZE BONZO BOOZE BRAZO BUZZI BUZZY

B•••Z
BLATZ BLITZ BRITZ

•BZ••
ABZUG

•B•Z•
ABUZZ EBUZZ IBIZA

•B••Z
ABUZZ EBUZZ

••B•Z
ADBIZ

CA•••
CABAL CABBY CABER CABIN CABLE CABOB CABOT CACAO CACHE CACTI CADDY CADET CADGE CADIS CADIZ CADRE CAFES CAFFE CAGED CAGER CAGES CAGEY CAINE CAINT CAIRN CAIRO CAIUS CAJON CAJUN CAKED CAKES CAKEY CALAF CALEB CALIF CALIX CALKS CALLA CALLE CALLI CALLS CALME CALMS CALOR CALVE CALYX CAMAS CAMAY CAMBS CAMEL CAMEO CAMOS CAMPO CAMPS CAMPY CAMRY CAMUS CANAL CANBY CANDO CANDW CANDY CANEA CANED CANEM CANER CANES CANID CANIO CANIS CANIT CANNA CANNY CANOE CANON CANSO CANST CANTO CANTS CANTY CAPAS CAPED CAPEK CAPER CAPES CAPET CAPON CAPOS CAPRA CAPRI CAPTS CAPUT CARAT CARAY CARBO CARBS CARDI CARDS CARED CARER CARES CARET CAREW CAREY CARGO CARIB CARLA CARLE CARLO CARLY CARME CARNE CARNY CAROB CAROL CAROM CARON CARPE CARPI CARPO CARPS CARRE CARRY CARTA CARTE CARTS CARVE CASAS CASBY CASCA CASCO CASED CASER CASES CASEY CASIO CASKS CASTA CASTE CASTS CASUS CATCH CATER CATES CATHS CATHY CATTY CAUDI CAUDO CAULK CAUSE CAVAE CAVAN CAVED CAVER CAVES CAVIL CAWED CAYCE

C•A••
CEARA CEASE CHACO CHADS CHAFE CHAFF CHAIM CHAIN CHAIR CHAIS CHAKA CHALK CHAMP CHANG CHANT CHAOS CHAPS CHARD CHARM CHARO CHARS CHART CHARY CHASE CHASM CHAST CHATS CHAUD CHAVA CHAWS CHAZZ CIANO CIAOS CLACK CLADS CLAES CLAIM CLAIR CLAMP CLAMS CLANG CLANK CLANS CLAPS CLARA CLARE CLARK CLARO CLARY CLASE CLASH CLASP CLASS CLAUS CLAVE CLAWS CLAYS COACH COACT COALS COAPT COASE COAST COATI COATS CRABS CRACK CRACY CRAFT CRAGS CRAIG CRAIK CRAIN CRAKE CRAMP CRAMS CRANE CRANI CRANK CRAPE CRAPS CRASH CRASS CRATE CRAVE CRAWL CRAWS CRAYS CRAZE CRAZY CYANO CYANS CZARS

C••A•
CABAL CACAO CALAF CAMAS CAMAY CANAL CAPAS CARAT CARAY CASAS CAVAE CAVAN CEDAR CENAS CERAM CERAT CESAR CFLAT CHEAP CHEAT CHIAS CIGAR CLEAN CLEAR CLEAT CLOAK COCAS CODAS COHAB COHAN COLAS COMAE COMAS CONAN COPAL COPAY CORAL COTAN COXAE CREAK CREAM CROAK CROAT CSPAN CSTAR CUBAN CUGAT CURAD CYCAD CYMAE CYMAS

C•••A
CALLA CANEA CANNA CAPRA CARLA CARTA CASCA CASTA CEARA CEIBA CELIA CELLA CERIA CESTA CEUTA CHAKA CHAVA CHEKA CHELA CHETA CHICA CHINA CHITA CHULA CIERA CIGNA CILIA CILLA CINNA CIRCA CLARA COBRA COCOA COMMA CONGA COOSA COPIA COPRA CORDA COREA CORIA CORSA COSTA COTTA CREMA CRURA CUICA CULPA CUPPA CURIA CURSA

•CA••
ACADS ECARD ECASH ICAHN ICALL ICAME ICANT ICARE KCARS MCATS OCALA SCABS SCADS SCALA SCALD SCALE SCALP SCALY SCAMP SCAMS SCANS SCANT SCAPA SCAPE SCARE SCARF SCARP SCARS SCARY SCATS

•C•A•
ACTAS DCCAB ECLAT ECTAD ECTAL ICEAX MCKAY MCNAB MCRAE OCCAM OCEAN OCRAT OCTAD OCTAL OCTAN PCLAB SCHAV SCRAG SCRAM SCRAP SCRAT UCLAN

•C••A
ACCRA ACELA ACQUA ACURA ICOSA OCALA OCHOA SCALA SCAPA SCENA SCHWA SCUBA SCUSA

••CA•
ALCAN ARCAE ASCAP BOCAS BYCAB BYCAR CACAO COCAS CYCAD DCCAB DECAD DECAF DECAL DECAP DECAY DUCAL DUCAT ELCAR FOCAL INCAN INCAS JACAL LECAR LOCAL LUCAN LUCAS MACAO MACAW MICAH MICAS NICAD NOCAL OCCAM ORCAS OSCAN OSCAR PACAS PECAN PICAS RECAN RECAP RICAN SOCAL SOCAS TICAL UNCAP UNCAS VACAS VICAR VOCAB VOCAL YMCAS YWCAS

••C•A
ACCRA AECIA ALCOA BECCA COCOA DACCA DACHA DACIA DECCA DICTA FACIA FACTA LICIA LOCKA LUCCA LUCIA LYCRA MECCA MICRA MOCHA MUCHA NUCHA RECTA SACRA USCGA VACUA WICCA YUCCA

•••CA
ABACA AMICA ARECA ARICA ASPCA BANCA BARCA BECCA BRECA BROCA CASCA CHICA CIRCA CUICA DACCA DECCA ERICA FINCA LEICA LORCA LUCCA MARCA MECCA MUSCA NUNCA PARCA PONCA SPICA TOSCA UTICA WICCA YUCCA

CB•••
CBERS CBSTV

C•B••
CABAL CABBY CABER CABIN CABLE CABOB CABOT COBOL COBRA CUBAN CUBBY CUBEB CUBED CUBER CUBES CUBIC CUBIT CYBER

5 CB

C••B•

CABBY CAMBS CANBY CARBO CARBS CASBY CEIBA CHUBB CHUBS CLUBS COLBY COMBO COMBS CORBY COSBY CRABS CRIBS CUBBY CURBS

C•••B

CABOB CALEB CARIB CAROB CELEB CHUBB CLIMB COHAB CRUMB CUBEB

•CB••

ICBMS

•C•B•

SCABS SCUBA

•C••B

ACERB DCCAB MCJOB MCNAB PCLAB SCRUB

••C•B

BYCAB DCCAB EXCUB JACOB MRCUB VOCAB

CC•••

CCCII CCCIV CCCIX CCCLI CCCLV CCCLX CCCVI CCCXC CCCXI CCCXL CCCXV CCCXX CCELL CCIII CCING CCLEF CCLII CCLIV CCLIX CCLVI CCLXI CCLXV CCLXX CCUPS CCVII CCXCI CCXCV CCXII CCXIV CCXIX CCXLI CCXLV CCXVI CCXXI CCXXV CCXXX

C•C••

CACAO CACHE CACTI CCCII CCCIV CCCIX CCCLI CCCLV CCCLX CCCVI CCCXC CCCXI CCCXL CCCXV CCCXX CECIL CECUM COCAS COCCI COCKS COCKY COCOA COCOS CXCII CXCIV CXCIX CXCVI CYCAD CYCLE CYCLO

C••C•

CASCA CASCO CATCH CAYCE CCXCI CCXCV CDXCI CDXCV CHACO CHECK CHICA CHICK CHICO CHICS CHOCK CHOCO CHUCK CINCH CINCO CINCY CIRCA CIRCE CIRCS CISCO CLACK CLICK CLOCK CLUCK CMXCI CMXCV COACH COACT COCCI CONCH COUCH CRACK CRACY CRECY CRICK CROCE CROCI CROCK CROCS CUICA CULCH CUZCO CZECH

C•••C

CCCXC CERIC CIVIC COLIC COMIC CONIC COSEC CRESC CUBIC CUSEC CYNIC

•CC••

ACCEL ACCRA ACCTS BCCED CCCII CCCIV CCCIX CCCLI CCCLV CCCLX CCCVI CCCXC CCCXI CCCXL CCCXV CCCXX DCCAB DCCCI DCCCL DCCCV DCCCX DCCII DCCIV DCCIX DCCLI DCCLV DCCLX DCCVI DCCXC DCCXI DCCXL DCCXV DCCXX MCCCI MCCCL MCCCV MCCCX MCCII MCCIV MCCIX MCCLI MCCLV MCCLX MCCOO MCCOY MCCVI MCCXC MCCXI MCCXL MCCXV MCCXX OCCAM OCCUR

•C•C•

CCXCI CCXCV DCCCI DCCCL DCCCV DCCCX DCXCI DCXCV MCCCI MCCCL MCCCV MCCCX MCXCI MCXCV

•C••C

CCCXC DCCXC MCCXC MCDXC MCMXC

••CC•

BECCA BOCCE BOCCI BUCCO COCCI DACCA DCCCI DCCCL DCCCV DCCCX DECCA GUCCI LUCCA LUCCI MCCCI MCCCL MCCCV MCCCX MDCCC MDCCI MDCCL MDCCV MDCCX MECCA MMCCC MMCCI MMCCL MMCCV MMCCX PUCCI RICCI ROCCO SACCO TUCCI WICCA YECCH YUCCA ZUCCO

••C•C

CCCXC DCCXC ENCYC MCCXC MDCCC MDCXC MMCCC MMCXC

•••CC

MDCCC MMCCC MMDCC MMMCC TENCC

CD•••

CDEFG CDIII CDLII CDLIV CDLIX CDLVI CDLXI CDLXV CDLXX CDROM CDVII CDXCI CDXCV CDXII CDXIV CDXIX CDXLI CDXLV CDXVI CDXXI CDXXV CDXXX

C•D••

CADDY CADET CADGE CADIS CADIZ CADRE CEDAR CEDED CEDER CEDES CEDIS CIDER CMDRS CODAS CODED CODER CODES CODEX CODON CUDDY CYDER

C••D•

CADDY CANDO CANDW CANDY CARDI CARDS CAUDI CAUDO CHADS CHIDE CINDY CLADS CLODS CLYDE COEDS COLDS COMDR CONDE CONDI CONDO CONDS COODY CORDA CORDS CREDO CREDS CRUDE CRUDS CUDDY CURDS CURDY CUYDS CYNDI

C•••D

CAGED CAKED CANED CANID CAPED CARED CASED CAVED CAWED CEDED CHARD CHAUD CHILD CHORD CITED CLOUD CLUED CLWYD CODED COKED CONED CONTD COOED COPED CORED COULD COVED COWED COXED CREED CRIED CROWD CUBED CUPID CURAD CURED CYCAD

•CD••

BCDEF MCDII MCDIV MCDIX MCDLI MCDLV MCDLX MCDVI MCDXC MCDXI MCDXL MCDXV MCDXX

•C•D•

ACADS ACIDS ACIDY SCADS SCUDS

•C••D

ACHED ACRED ACRID ACTED BCCED ECARD ECTAD OCTAD SCALD SCHED SCOLD SCROD

••CD•

ABCDE MMCDI MMCDL MMCDV MMCDX

••C•D

ARCED BCCED CYCAD DECAD DICED ELCID FACED LACED LECID LUCID MACED NICAD PACED RACED RICED

•••CD

MMMCD SPECD

CE•••

CEARA CEASE CECIL CECUM CEDAR CEDED CEDER CEDES CEDIS CEIBA CEILS CELEB CELIA CELIE CELLA CELLE CELLI CELLO CELLS CELTS CENAS CENSE CENTI CENTO CENTR CENTS CENTU CEORL CEPES CERAM CERAT CERES CERIA CERIC CEROS CERRO CERTS CESAR CESTA CESTI CETTE CETUS CEUTA

C•E••

CBERS CCELL CDEFG CHEAP CHEAT CHECK CHEEK CHEEP CHEER CHEEZ CHEFS CHEKA CHELA CHELY CHEMO CHERE CHERI CHERT CHESS CHEST CHETA CHEVY CHEWS CHEWY CHEXX CIELO CIELS CIENS CIERA CLEAN CLEAR CLEAT CLEEF CLEEK CLEFS CLEFT CLEON CLEPT CLERK CLETE CLEVE CLEWS COEDS COEUR CREAK CREAM CRECY CREDO CREDS CREED CREEK CREEL CREEP CREES CREMA CREME CREON CREPE CREPT CRESC CRESS CREST CRETE CREVE CREWS CTENO CUEIN CUERS CUEUP CZECH

C••E•

CABER CADET CAFES CAGED CAGER CAGES CAGEY CAKED CAKES CAKEY CALEB CAMEL CAMEO CANEA CANED CANEM CANER CANES CAPED CAPEK CAPER CAPES CAPET CARED CARER CARES CARET CAREW CAREY CASED CASER CASES CASEY CATER CATES CAVED CAVER CAVES CAWED CCLEF CEDED CEDER CEDES CELEB CEPES CERES CHEEK CHEEP CHEER CHEEZ CHIEF CHIEN CIDER CINES CIRES CITED CITEE CITER CITES CIVET CLAES CLEEF CLEEK CLUED CLUER CLUES CODED CODER CODES CODEX COHEN COKED COKER COKES COLES COMER COMES COMET COMEX CONED CONER CONES CONEY COOED COOEE COOER COPED COPER COPES COREA CORED CORER CORES COREY COSEC COSET COTES COVED COVEN COVER COVES COVET COVEY COWED COWER COWES COXED COXES COYER COZEN COZES CREED CREEK CREEL CREEP CREES CRIED CRIER CRIES CRUEL CRUET CRYER CUBEB CUBED CUBER CUBES CUKES CULET CUMES CUNEO CUPEL CURED CUREL CURER CURES CURET CUSEC CUTER CUTES CUTEX CUTEY CUVEE CYBER CYDER CYMES

C•••E

CABLE CACHE CADGE CADRE CAFFE CAINE CALLE CALME CALVE CANOE CARLE CARME CARNE CARPE CARRE CARTE CARVE CASTE CAUSE CAVAE CAYCE CEASE CELIE CELLE CENSE CETTE CHAFE CHASE CHERE CHIDE CHILE CHIME CHINE CHIVE CHLOE CHOKE CHOLE CHORE CHOSE CHUTE CIRCE CITEE CLARE CLASE CLAVE CLETE CLEVE CLIME CLINE CLIVE CLONE CLOSE CLOVE CLYDE CNOTE COASE COKIE COMAE COMME COMTE CONDE CONGE CONTE COOEE COOKE COOTE COPSE COUPE COXAE CRAKE CRANE CRAPE CRATE CRAVE CRAZE CREME CREPE CRETE CREVE CRIME CROCE CRONE CRORE CROWE CRUDE CRUSE CTILE CUIRE CUORE CURIE CURSE CURVE CUTIE CUVEE CYCLE CYMAE

•CE••

ACEIT ACELA ACERB ACERS ACETO BCELL CCELL DCELL ICEAX ICEES ICEIN ICEIT ICENI ICERS ICEUP OCEAN SCENA SCENE SCENT TCELL

•C•E•

ACCEL ACHED ACHER ACHES ACMES ACNES ACRED ACRES ACTED ACTER ACTES BCCED BCDEF CCLEF FCLEF GCLEF ICEES ICIER ICKES JCREW MCGEE MCKEE OCHER OCTET SCHED SCREE SCREW

•C••E

ACUTE ECOLE ICAME ICARE MCGEE MCKEE MCRAE MCVIE OCHRE SCALE SCAPE SCARE SCENE SCIRE SCONE SCOPE SCORE SCREE

••CE•

ACCEL ARCED BCCED BICEP DACES DECEM DICED DICER DICES DICEY DOCES DUCES EMCEE EXCEL FACED FACER FACES FACET HACEK JACET JACEY LACED LACER LACES LACEY LYCEE MACED MACER MACES NICER PACED PACEM PACER PACES PACEY PUCES RACED RACER RACES RICED RICER RICES RICEU SICEM TACET ULCER VICES

••C•E

ABCDE ARCAE ARCHE BOCCE CACHE CYCLE DACHE EMCEE ENCRE FACIE FICHE HECHE LACIE LECHE LOCKE LUCIE LUCRE LYCEE MACHE MACKE MACLE NACRE NICHE NOCHE ONCLE ONCUE PECHE RECUE RICHE ROCHE RUCHE SACRE SOCLE SUCRE TYCHE UNCLE VACHE

•••CE

ALICE ALYCE AMICE APACE BOCCE BRACE BRICE BRUCE BRYCE CAYCE CIRCE CROCE DANCE DEICE DEUCE DOLCE DOUCE DOYCE DULCE DUNCE EDUCE FARCE FENCE FORCE GANCE GLACE GRACE HENCE HULCE INICE JOYCE JUICE LANCE MERCE MINCE NANCE NIECE NONCE NOYCE ONICE OUNCE PEACE PENCE PERCE PESCE PIECE PINCE PLACE PLOCE PONCE PRICE PRYCE REECE REICE ROYCE SAUCE SINCE SLICE SPACE SPICE TERCE TRACE TRECE TRICE TRUCE TWICE UNICE VANCE VINCE VOICE WINCE

CF•••

CFLAT

C•F••

CAFES CAFFE CUFFS

C••F•

CAFFE CDEFG CHAFE CHAFF CHEFS CHUFF CLEFS CLEFT CLIFF CLIFT COIFS COMFY CORFU CRAFT CROFT CUFFS

C•••F

CALAF CALIF CCLEF CHAFF CHIEF CHUFF CLEEF CLIFF

•CF••

MCFLY

•C•F•

ACUFF SCIFI SCOFF SCUFF

•C••F

ACUFF BCDEF CCLEF FCLEF GCLEF SCARF SCOFF SCUFF

••C•F
DECAF

C•G••
CAGED
CAGER
CAGES
CAGEY
CIGAR
CIGGY
CIGNA
CUGAT
CYGNI

C••G•
CADGE
CARGO
CHUGS
CIGGY
CITGO
CLOGS
COIGN
CONGA
CONGE
CONGO
CORGI
COUGH
CRAGS

C•••G
CCING
CDEFG
CHANG
CHING
CHONG
CHUNG
CLANG
CLING
CLUNG
CRAIG
CUING

•CG••
MCGEE

•C••G
ACING
CCING
ICING
SCRAG

••CG•
USCGA

••C•G
INCOG

CH•••
CHACO
CHADS
CHAFE
CHAFF
CHAIM
CHAIN
CHAIR
CHAIS
CHAKA
CHALK
CHAMP
CHANG
CHANT
CHAOS
CHAPS
CHARD
CHARM
CHARO
CHARS
CHART
CHARY
CHASE
CHASM
CHAST
CHATS
CHAUD
CHAVA
CHAWS
CHAZZ
CHEAP
CHEAT
CHECK
CHEEK
CHEEP
CHEER
CHEEZ
CHEFS
CHEKA
CHELA
CHELY
CHEMO
CHERE
CHERI
CHERT
CHESS
CHEST
CHETA
CHEVY
CHEWS
CHEWY
CHEXX
CHIAS
CHICA
CHICK
CHICO
CHICS
CHIDE
CHIEF
CHIEN
CHILD
CHILE
CHILI
CHILL
CHIME
CHIMP
CHINA
CHINE
CHING
CHINK
CHINO
CHINS
CHIOS
CHIPS
CHIRO
CHIRP
CHIRR
CHITA
CHITS
CHIVE
CHIVY
CHLOE
CHLOR
CHOCK
CHOCO
CHOIR
CHOKE
CHOKY
CHOLE
CHOLO
CHOMP
CHONG
CHOPS
CHORD
CHORE
CHORO
CHOSE
CHOWS
CHRIS
CHROM
CHRON
CHUBB
CHUBS
CHUCK
CHUFF
CHUGS
CHULA
CHUMP
CHUMS
CHUNG
CHUNK
CHURL
CHURN
CHUTE

C•H••
COHAB
COHAN
COHEN
COHOS

C••H•
CACHE
CATHS
CATHY
CUSHY

C•••H
CATCH
CINCH
CLASH
CLOTH
COACH
CONCH
COUCH
COUGH
COUTH
CRASH
CRUSH
CRWTH
CULCH
CZECH

•CH••
ACHED
ACHER
ACHES
ACHOO
ECHOS
ICHOR
OCHER
OCHOA
OCHOS
OCHRE
SCHAV
SCHED
SCHMO
SCHON
SCHWA
VCHIP

•C•H•
ICAHN

•C••H
ECASH

••CH•
ANCHO
ARCHE
ARCHI
ARCHY
BOCHY
CACHE
DACHA
DACHE
DICHO
DUCHY
FICHE
FICHU
FUCHS
HECHE
HECHT
ITCHY
LECHE
LICHT
LOCHS
MACHE
MACHO
MACHU
MACHY
MOCHA
MUCHA
MUCHO
NACHO
NACHT
NICHE
NICHT
NOCHE
NUCHA
ORCHS
PACHY
PECHE
RICHE
ROCHE
RUCHE
SACHS
SECHS
TACHO
TACHS
TECHS
TYCHE
TYCHO
VACHE
VICHY
YACHT

••C•H
MICAH
RICOH
YECCH

•••CH
AITCH
BALCH
BATCH
BEACH
BEECH
BELCH
BENCH
BIRCH
BLOCH
BOSCH
BOTCH
BRACH
BRUCH
BUNCH
BUSCH
BUTCH
CATCH
CINCH
COACH
CONCH
COUCH
CULCH
CZECH
DENCH
DITCH
DUTCH
ENOCH
EPOCH
ERICH
FETCH
FILCH
FINCH
FITCH
GOOCH
GULCH
HATCH
HENCH
HITCH
HOOCH
HUNCH
HUTCH
ILICH
KEACH
KETCH
KOTCH
KUSCH
LARCH
LATCH
LEACH
LEECH
LUNCH
LURCH
LYNCH
MARCH
MATCH
MERCH
MITCH
MOOCH
MOUCH
MULCH
MUNCH
NATCH
NOTCH
ORACH
PARCH
PASCH
PATCH
PEACH
PERCH
PINCH
PITCH
POACH
PONCH
POOCH
PORCH
POUCH
PSYCH
PUNCH
RANCH
REACH
REICH
ROACH
SATCH
STICH
SYNCH
TEACH
TENCH
TISCH
TORCH
TOUCH
URICH
VETCH
VOUCH
WATCH
WELCH
WENCH
WHICH
WINCH
WITCH
YECCH
ZILCH

CI•••
CIANO
CIAOS
CIDER
CIELO
CIELS
CIENS
CIERA
CIGAR
CIGGY
CIGNA
CILIA
CILLA
CINCH
CINCO
CINCY
CINDY
CINES
CINNA
CIONS
CIRCA
CIRCE
CIRCS
CIRES
CIRRI
CIRRO
CISCO
CISSY
CISTS
CITED
CITEE
CITER
CITES
CITGO
CITRI
CITRO
CIVET
CIVIC
CIVIL

C•I••
CAINE
CAINT
CAIRN
CAIRO
CAIUS
CCIII
CCING
CDIII
CEIBA
CEILS
CHIAS
CHICA
CHICK
CHICO
CHICS
CHIDE
CHIEF
CHIEN
CHILD
CHILE
CHILI
CHILL
CHIME
CHIMP
CHINA
CHINE
CHING
CHINK
CHINO
CHINS
CHIOS
CHIPS
CHIRO
CHIRP
CHIRR
CHITA
CHITS
CHIVE
CHIVY
CLICK
CLIFF
CLIFT
CLIII
CLIMB
CLIME
CLINE
CLING
CLINK
CLINT
CLIOS
CLIPS
CLIPT
CLIVE
CMIII
COIFS
COIGN
COILS
COINS
COIRS
CRIBS
CRICK
CRIED
CRIER
CRIES
CRIME
CRIMP
CRISP
CRIST
CRITS
CRIUS
CSINY
CTILE
CUICA
CUING
CUIRE
CVIII
CXIII

C••I•
CABIN
CADIS
CADIZ
CALIF
CALIX
CANID
CANIO
CANIS
CANIT
CARIB
CASIO
CAVIL
CCCII
CCCIV
CCCIX
CCIII
CCLII
CCLIV
CCLIX
CCVII
CCXII
CCXIV
CCXIX
CDIII
CDLII
CDLIV
CDLIX
CDVII
CDXII
CDXIV
CDXIX
CECIL
CEDIS
CELIA
CELIE
CERIA
CERIC
CHAIM
CHAIN
CHAIR
CHAIS
CHOIR
CHRIS
CILIA
CIVIC
CIVIL
CLAIM
CLAIR
CLIII
CLVII
CLXII
CLXIV
CLXIX
CMIII
CMLII
CMLIV
CMLIX
CMVII
CMXII
CMXIV
CMXIX
COKIE
COLIC
COLIN
COMIC
COMIN
COMIX
CONIC
COPIA
COPIT
CORIA
CRAIG
CRAIK
CRAIN
CROIX
CUBIC
CUBIT
CUEIN
CUMIN
CUPID
CURIA
CURIE
CURIO
CUTIE
CUTIN
CUTIS
CUTIT
CVIII
CXCII
CXCIV
CXCIX
CXIII
CXLII
CXLIV
CXLIX
CXVII
CXXII
CXXIV
CXXIX
CYNIC
CYRIL

C•••I
CACTI
CALLI
CAPRI
CARDI
CARPI
CAUDI
CCCII
CCCLI
CCCVI
CCCXI
CCIII
CCLII
CCLVI
CCLXI
CCVII
CCXCI
CCXII
CCXLI
CCXVI
CCXXI
CDIII
CDLII
CDLVI
CDLXI
CDVII
CDXCI
CDXII
CDXLI
CDXVI
CDXXI
CELLI
CENTI
CESTI
CHERI
CHILI
CIRRI
CITRI
CLIII
CLVII
CLXII
CLXVI
CLXXI
CMIII
CMLII
CMLVI
CMLXI
CMVII
CMXCI
CMXII
CMXLI
CMXVI
CMXXI
COATI
COCCI
CONDI
CONTI
COQUI
CORGI
CORNI
CORRI
CRANI
CROCI
CULTI
CUPRI
CURVI
CVIII
CXCII
CXCVI
CXIII
CXLII
CXLVI
CXVII
CXXII
CXXVI
CXXXI
CYGNI
CYNDI

•CI••
ACIDS
ACIDY
ACING
CCIII
CCING
DCIII
ICIER
ICILY
ICING
MCIII
SCIFI
SCION
SCIRE
XCIII

•C•I•
ACEIT
ACRID
ACTII
ACTIN
ACTIV
CCCII
CCCIV
CCCIX
CCIII
CCLII
CCLIV
CCLIX
CCVII
CCXII
CCXIV
CCXIX
DCCII
DCCIV
DCCIX
DCIII
DCLII
DCLIV
DCLIX
DCVII
DCXII
DCXIV
DCXIX
ICEIN
ICEIT
MCCII
MCCIV
MCCIX
MCDII
MCDIV
MCDIX
MCIII
MCKIM
MCLII
MCLIV
MCLIX
MCMII
MCMIV
MCMIX
MCVIE
MCVII
MCXII
MCXIV
MCXIX
SCRIM
SCRIP
VCHIP
XCIII
XCVII

•C••I
ACTII
CCCII
CCCLI
CCCVI
CCCXI
CCIII
CCLII
CCLVI
CCLXI
CCVII
CCXCI
CCXII
CCXLI
CCXVI
CCXXI
DCCCI
DCCII
DCCLI
DCCVI
DCCXI
DCIII
DCLII
DCLVI
DCLXI
DCVII
DCXCI
DCXII
DCXLI
DCXVI
DCXXI
ECOLI
ICENI
ICOSI
MCCCI
MCCII
MCCLI
MCCVI
MCCXI
MCDII
MCDLI
MCDVI
MCDXI
MCIII
MCLII
MCLVI
MCLXI
MCMII
MCMLI
MCMVI
MCMXI
MCVII
MCXCI
MCXII
MCXLI
MCXVI
MCXXI
OCULI
SCIFI
SCUSI
XCIII
XCVII

••CI•
AECIA
ASCII
BACIO
CCCII
CCCIV
CCCIX
CECIL
CXCII
CXCIV
CXCIX
DACIA
DCCII
DCCIV
DCCIX
DECIR
DXCII
DXCIV
DXCIX
ELCID
FACIA
FACIE
FACIL
LACIE
LECID
LICIA
LICIT
LUCIA
LUCID
LUCIE
LUCIO
MCCII
MCCIV
MCCIX
MDCII
MDCIV
MDCIX
MMCII
MMCIV
MMCIX
MXCII
MXCIV
MXCIX
MYCIN
NACIO
OPCIT
RECIP
SOCIO
TACIT

••C•I
ARCHI
ASCII
BOCCI
CACTI
CCCII
CCCLI
CCCVI
CCCXI
COCCI
CXCII
CXCVI
DCCCI
DCCII
DCCLI
DCCVI
DCCXI
DXCII
DXCVI
GUCCI
LACTI
LUCCI
MCCCI
MCCII
MCCLI
MCCVI
MCCXI
MDCCI
MDCII
MDCLI
MDCVI
MDCXI
MMCCI
MMCDI
MMCII
MMCLI
MMCMI
MMCVI
MMCXI
MXCII
MXCVI
NOCTI
NYCTI
PUCCI
RECTI
RICCI
RICKI
TUCCI
VICKI

•••CI
ABACI
AMICI
BOCCI
CCXCI
CDXCI
CMXCI
COCCI
CROCI
DARCI
DCCCI
DCXCI
DIECI
DISCI
DOLCI
FARCI
GUCCI
LUCCI
MARCI
MCCCI
MCXCI
MDCCI
MDXCI
MERCI
MMCCI
MMDCI
MMMCI
MMXCI
NANCI
PESCI
PISCI
PUCCI
RICCI
SOUCI
TRACI
TUCCI
VINCI
VOICI

C•J••
CAJON
CAJUN

•CJ••
MCJOB

C•K••
CAKED
CAKES
CAKEY
COKED
COKER
COKES
COKIE
CUKES
CUKOR

C••K•
CALKS
CASKS
CHAKA
CHEKA
CHOKE
CHOKY
COCKS
COCKY
CONKS
COOKE
COOKS
COOKY
CORKS
CORKY
CRAKE
CUSKS

C•••K
CAPEK
CAULK
CHALK
CHECK
CHEEK
CHICK
CHINK
CHOCK
CHUCK
CHUNK
CLACK
CLANK
CLARK
CLEEK
CLERK
CLICK
CLINK
CLOAK
CLOCK
CLONK
CLUCK
CLUNK
CRACK
CRAIK
CRANK
CREAK
CREEK
CRICK
CROAK
CROCK
CROOK

•CK••
ICKES
MCKAY
MCKEE
MCKIM

••CK•
BACKS
BECKS
BECKY
BOCKS
BUCKO
BUCKS
BUCKY
COCKS
COCKY
DECKS
DICKS
DICKY
DOCKS
DUCKS
DUCKY
GECKO
GUCKS
GUCKY
HACKL
HACKS
HACKY
HECKS
HICKS
HOCKS
JACKO
JACKS
JACKY
JOCKO
JOCKS
KICKS
KICKY
LACKS
LECKY
LICKS
LOCKA
LOCKE
LOCKS
LUCKS
LUCKY
MACKE
MACKS
MICKY
MOCKS
MUCKS
MUCKY
NECKS
NICKS
NICKY
NOCKS
PACKS
PECKS
PICKS
PICKY
PUCKS
RACKS
RECKS
RICKI
RICKS
RICKY
ROCKS
ROCKY
RUCKS
SACKS
SICKO
SOCKO
SOCKS
SUCKS
SUCKY
TACKS
TACKY
TICKS
TICKY
TUCKS
VICKI
VICKS
VICKY
WACKO
WACKY
WICKS
YACKS
YUCKY

••C•K
HACEK

•••CK
ABACK
ALACK
ALECK
AMICK
AMUCK
BLACK
BLOCK
BRACK
BRECK
BRICK
BROCK
BUICK
CHECK
CHICK
CHOCK
CHUCK
CLACK
CLICK
CLOCK
CLUCK
CRACK
CRICK
CROCK
DBACK
DRECK
ERICK
FLACK
FLECK
FLICK
FLOCK
FRICK
FROCK
GLICK
GLOCK
GLUCK
KLICK
KNACK
KNICK
KNOCK

5
CL

KROCK
KVACK
MERCK
NYACK
ORECK
OZICK
PLUCK
PRICK
QUACK
QUICK
SHACK
SHOCK
SHUCK
SLACK
SLICK
SMACK
SMOCK
SNACK
SNICK
SNUCK
SPECK
SPOCK
STACK
STICK
STOCK
STUCK
THICK
TRACK
TRICK
TRUCK
VEECK
VLECK
VNECK
WHACK
WRACK
WRECK
ZWICK

CL•••
CLACK
CLADS
CLAES
CLAIM
CLAIR
CLAMP
CLAMS
CLANG
CLANK
CLANS
CLAPS
CLARA
CLARE
CLARK
CLARO
CLARY
CLASE
CLASH
CLASP
CLASS
CLAUS
CLAVE
CLAWS
CLAYS
CLEAN
CLEAR
CLEAT
CLEEF
CLEEK
CLEFS
CLEFT
CLEON
CLEPT
CLERK
CLETE
CLEVE
CLEWS
CLICK
CLIFF
CLIFT
CLIII
CLIMB
CLIME
CLINE
CLING
CLINK
CLINT
CLIOS
CLIPS
CLIPT
CLIVE
CLOAK
CLOCK
CLODS
CLOGS
CLOMP
CLONE
CLONK
CLOPS
CLOSE
CLOTH
CLOTS
CLOUD
CLOUT
CLOVE
CLOWN
CLOYS
CLUBS
CLUCK
CLUED
CLUER
CLUES
CLUMP
CLUNG
CLUNK
CLUNY
CLVII
CLWYD
CLXII
CLXIV
CLXIX
CLXVI
CLXXI
CLXXV
CLXXX
CLYDE

C•L••
CALAF
CALEB
CALIF
CALIX
CALKS
CALLA
CALLE
CALLI
CALLS
CALME
CALMS
CALOR
CALVE
CALYX
CCLEF
CCLII
CCLIV
CCLIX
CCLVI
CCLXI
CCLXV
CCLXX
CDLII
CDLIV
CDLIX
CDLVI
CDLXI
CDLXV
CDLXX
CELEB
CELIA
CELIE
CELLA
CELLE
CELLI
CELLO
CELLS
CELTS
CFLAT
CHLOE
CHLOR
CILIA
CILLA
CMLII
CMLIV
CMLIX
CMLVI
CMLXI
CMLXV
CMLXX
COLAS
COLBY
COLDS
COLES
COLIC
COLIN
COLON
COLOR
COLTS
COLUM
CPLUS
CULCH
CULET
CULLS
CULLY
CULPA
CULTI
CULTS
CXLII
CXLIV
CXLIX
CXLVI

C••L•
CABLE
CALLA
CALLE
CALLI
CALLS
CARLA
CARLE
CARLO
CARLY
CAULK
CCCLI
CCCLV
CCCLX
CCELL
CCXLI
CCXLV
CDXLI
CDXLV
CEILS
CELLA
CELLE
CELLI
CELLO
CELLS
CHALK
CHELA
CHELY
CHILD
CHILE
CHILI
CHILL
CHOLE
CHOLO
CHULA
CIELO
CIELS
CILLA
CMXLI
CMXLV
COALS
COILS
COOLS
COULD
COWLS
COYLY
CTILE
CULLS
CULLY
CURLS
CURLY
CYCLE
CYCLO

C•••L
CABAL
CAMEL
CANAL
CAROL
CAVIL
CCCXL
CCELL
CECIL
CEORL
CHILL
CHURL
CIVIL
COBOL
COPAL
CORAL
CRAWL
CREEL
CRUEL
CUMUL
CUPEL
CUREL
CYRIL

•CL••
CCLEF
CCLII
CCLIV
CCLIX
CCLVI
CCLXI
CCLXV
CCLXX
DCLII
DCLIV
DCLIX
DCLVI
DCLXI
DCLXV
DCLXX
ECLAT
FCLEF
GCLEF
MCLII
MCLIV
MCLIX
MCLVI
MCLXI
MCLXV
MCLXX
PCLAB
UCLAN

•C•L•
ACELA
BCELL
CCCLI
CCCLV
CCCLX
CCELL
CCXLI
CCXLV
DCCLI
DCCLV
DCCLX
DCELL
DCXLI
DCXLV
ECOLE
ECOLI
ICALL
ICILY
MCCLI
MCCLV
MCCLX
MCDLI
MCDLV
MCDLX
MCFLY
MCMLI
MCMLV
MCMLX
MCXLI
MCXLV
OCALA
OCULI
OCULO
SCALA
SCALD
SCALE
SCALP
SCALY
SCOLD
SCULL
TCELL

•C••L
ACCEL
BCELL
CCCXL
CCELL

•••CL
DCCCL
DCCXL
DCELL
ECTAL
ICALL
MCCCL
MCCXL
MCDXL
MCMXL
OCTAL
SCOWL
SCULL
TCELL

••CL•
CCCLI
CCCLV
CCCLX
CYCLE
CYCLO
DCCLI
DCCLV
DCCLX
ENCLS
MACLE
MCCLI
MCCLV
MCCLX
MDCLI
MDCLV
MDCLX
MMCLI
MMCLV
MMCLX
ONCLE
SOCLE
UNCLE

••C•L
ACCEL
CCCXL
CECIL
DCCCL
DCCXL
DECAL
DUCAL
EXCEL
FACIL
FOCAL
HACKL
JACAL
LOCAL
LTCOL
MCCCL
MCCXL
MDCCL
MDCXL
MMCCL
MMCDL
MMCML
MMCXL
NICOL
NOCAL
SOCAL
TICAL
VOCAL
DCCCL
MCCCL
MDCCL
MMCCL
MMDCL
MMMCL

CM•••
CMDRS
CMIII
CMLII
CMLIV
CMLIX
CMLVI
CMLXI
CMLXV
CMLXX
CMVII
CMXCI
CMXCV
CMXII
CMXIV
CMXIX
CMXLI
CMXLV
CMXVI
CMXXI
CMXXV
CMXXX

C•M••
CAMAS
CAMAY
CAMBS
CAMEL
CAMEO
CAMOS
CAMPO
CAMPS
CAMPY
CAMRY
CAMUS
COMAE
COMAS
COMBO
COMBS
COMDR
COMER
COMES
COMET
COMEX
COMFY
COMIC
COMIN
COMIX
COMMA
COMME
COMPS
COMTE
COMUS
CUMES
CUMIN
CUMUL
CYMAE
CYMAS
CYMES
CYMRY

C••M•
CALME
CALMS
CARME
CHAMP
CHEMO
CHIME
CHIMP
CHOMP
CHUMP
CHUMS
CLAMP
CLAMS
CLIMB
CLIME
CLOMP
CLUMP
COMMA
COMME
CORMS
COSMO
CRAMP
CRAMS
CREMA
CREME
CRIME
CRIMP
CRUMB
CRUMP
CUOMO

C•••M
CANEM
CAROM
CDROM
CECUM
CERAM
CHAIM
CHARM
CHASM
CHROM
CLAIM
COLUM
CREAM

•CM••
ACMES
MCMII
MCMIV
MCMIX
MCMLI
MCMLV
MCMLX
MCMVI
MCMXC
MCMXI
MCMXL
MCMXV
MCMXX

•C•M•
ICAME
ICBMS
SCAMP
SCAMS
SCHMO
SCUMS

•C••M
MCKIM
OCCAM
SCRAM
SCRIM
SCRUM

••CM•
MMCMI
MMCML
MMCMV
MMCMX

••C•M
CECUM
DECEM
LOCUM
LTCOM
MECUM
OCCAM
PACEM
SICEM

•••CM
MMMCM

CN•••
CNOTE

C•N••
CANAL
CANBY
CANDO
CANDW
CANDY
CANEA
CANED
CANEM
CANER
CANES
CANID
CANIO
CANIS
CANIT
CANNA
CANNY
CANOE
CANON
CANSO
CANST
CANTO
CANTS
CANTY
CENAS
CENSE
CENTI
CENTO
CENTR
CENTS
CENTU
CINCH
CINCO
CINCY
CINDY
CINES
CINNA
CONAN
CONCH
CONDE
CONDI
CONDO
CONDS
CONED
CONER
CONES
CONEY
CONGA
CONGE
CONGO
CONIC
CONKS
CONNS
CONON
CONST
CONTD
CONTE
CONTI
CONTR
CONTS
CONUS
CONVY
CUNEO
CYNDI
CYNIC

C••N•
CAINE
CAINT
CANNA
CANNY
CARNE
CARNY
CCING
CHANG
CHANT
CHINA
CHINE
CHING
CHINK
CHINO
CHINS
CHONG
CHUNG
CHUNK
CIANO
CIENS
CIGNA
CINNA
CIONS
CLANG
CLANK
CLANS
CLINE
CLING
CLINK
CLINT
CLONE
CLONK
CLUNG
CLUNK
CLUNY
COINS
CONNS
COONS
CORNI
CORNO
CORNS
CORNU
CORNY
COUNT
CRANE
CRANI
CRANK
CRONE
CRONY
CSINY
CTENO
CUING
CYANO
CYANS
CYGNI

C•••N
CABIN
CAIRN
CAJON
CAJUN
CANON
CAPON
CARON
CAVAN
CHAIN
CHIEN
CHRON
CHURN
CLEAN
CLEON
CLOWN
CODON
COHAN
COHEN
COIGN
COLIN
COLON
COMIN
CONAN
CONON
COOWN
COTAN
COVEN
COZEN
CRAIN
CREON
CROON
CROWN
CSPAN
CUBAN
CUEIN
CUMIN
CUTIN

•CN••
ACNES
MCNAB

•C•N•
ACING
CCING
ECONO
ECONS
ICANT
ICENI
ICING
ICONO
ICONS
SCANS
SCANT
SCENA
SCENE
SCENT
SCONE
UCONN

•C••N
ACORN
ACTIN
ACTON
ICAHN
ICEIN
OCEAN
OCTAN
SCHON
SCION
SCORN
UCLAN
UCONN

••C•N
ALCAN
ANCON
BACON
EXCON
INCAN
LECON
LUCAN
MACON
MYCIN
OSCAN
PECAN
PICON
RECAN
RECON
RICAN

CO•••
COACH
COACT
COALS
COAPT
COASE
COAST
COATI
COATS
COBOL
COBRA
COCAS
COCCI
COCKS
COCKY
COCOA
COCOS
CODAS
CODED
CODER
CODES
CODEX
CODON
COEDS
COEUR
COHAB
COHAN
COHEN
COHOS
COIFS
COIGN
COILS
COINS
COIRS
COKED
COKER
COKES
COKIE
COLAS
COLBY
COLDS
COLES
COLIC
COLIN
COLON
COLOR
COLTS
COLUM
COMAE
COMAS
COMBO
COMBS
COMDR
COMER
COMES
COMET
COMEX
COMFY
COMIC
COMIN
COMIX
COMMA
COMME
COMPS
COMTE
COMUS
CONAN
CONCH
CONDE
CONDI
CONDO
CONDS
CONED
CONER
CONES
CONEY
CONGA
CONGE
CONGO
CONIC
CONKS
CONNS
CONON
CONST
CONTD
CONTE
CONTI
CONTR
CONTS
CONUS
CONVY
COODY
COOED
COOEE
COOER
COOKE
COOKS
COOKY
COOLS
COONS
COOPS
COOPT
COORS
COOSA
COOTE
COOTS
COOTY
COOWN
COPAL
COPAY
COPED
COPER
COPES
COPIA
COPIT
COPRA
COPSE
COPTO
COPTS
COQUI
CORAL
CORBY
CORDA
CORDS
COREA
CORED
CORER
CORES
COREY
CORFU
CORGI
CORIA
CORKS
CORKY
CORMS
CORNI
CORNO
CORNS
CORNU
CORNY
COROT
CORPS
CORRI
CORSA
CORSO
CORVO
COSBY
COSEC
COSET
COSMO
COSTA
COSTS
COTAN
COTES
COTTA
COUCH
COUGH
COULD
COUNT
COUPE
COUPS
COURT
COURU
COUSY
COUTH
COVED
COVEN
COVER
COVES
COVET
COVEY
COWED
COWER
COWES
COWLS
COWRY
COXAE
COXED
COXES
COYER
COYLY
COYPU
COZEN
COZES

C•O••
CEORL
CHOCK
CHOCO
CHOIR
CHOKE
CHOKY
CHOLE
CHOLO
CHOMP
CHONG
CHOPS
CHORD
CHORE
CHORO
CHOSE
CHOWS
CIONS
CLOAK
CLOCK
CLODS
CLOGS
CLOMP
CLONE
CLONK
CLOPS
CLOSE
CLOTH
CLOTS
CLOUD
CLOUT
CLOVE
CLOWN
CLOYS
CNOTE
COODY
COOED
COOEE
COOER
COOKE
COOKS
COOKY
COOLS
COONS
COOPS
COOPT
COORS
COOSA
COOTE
COOTS
COOTY
COOWN
CROAK
CROAT
CROCE
CROCI
CROCK
CROCS
CROFT
CROIX
CRONE
CRONY
CROOK
CROON
CROPS
CRORE
CROSS
CROUP
CROWD
CROWE
CROWN
CROWS
CUOMO
CUORE

C••O•
CABOB
CABOT
CAJON
CALOR
CAMOS
CANOE
CANON
CAPON
CAPOS
CAROB
CAROL
CAROM
CARON
CDROM
CEROS
CHAOS
CHIOS
CHLOE
CHLOR
CHROM
CHRON
CIAOS
CLEON
CLIOS
COBOL
COCOA
COCOS
CODON
COHOS
COLON
COLOR
CONON
COROT
CREON
CROOK
CROON
CRUOR
CSPOT
CUKOR

C•••O
CACAO
CAIRO
CAMEO
CAMPO
CANDO
CANIO
CANSO
CANTO
CARBO
CARGO
CARLO
CARPO
CASCO
CASIO
CAUDO
CELLO
CENTO
CERRO
CHACO
CHARO
CHEMO
CHICO
CHINO
CHIRO
CHOCO
CHOLO
CHORO
CIANO
CIELO
CINCO
CIRRO
CISCO
CITGO
CITRO
CLARO
COMBO
CONDO
CONGO
COPTO
CORNO
CORSO
CORVO
COSMO
CREDO
CTENO
CUNEO
CUOMO
CUPRO
CURIO
CUZCO
CYANO

CYCLO

•CO••
ACORN
ECOLE
ECOLI
ECONO
ECONS
ICONO
ICONS
ICOSA
ICOSI
SCOFF
SCOLD
SCONE
SCOOP
SCOOT
SCOPE
SCORE
SCORN
SCOTS
SCOTT
SCOUR
SCOUT
SCOWL
SCOWS
UCONN

•C•O•
ACHOO
ACTON
ACTOR
ACTOS
ECHOS
ECTOR
ICHOR
MCCOO
MCCOY
MCJOB
OCHOA
OCHOS
SCHON
SCION
SCOOP
SCOOT
SCROD

•C••O
ACETO
ACHOO
ECONO
ICONO
MCCOO
OCULO
SCHMO

••CO•
ALCOA
ALCOR
ANCON
ASCOT
BACON
BACOS
COCOA
COCOS
DECOR
DECOY
DICOT
EPCOT
EXCON
EXCOP
INCOG
JACOB
JUCOS
LECON
LOCOS
LTCOL
LTCOM
LYCOS
MACON
MCCOO
MCCOY
NICOL
PECOS
PICON
PICOT
RECON
RICOH
TACOS
TICOS
UNCOY

••C•O
ANCHO
BACIO
BUCCO
BUCKO
CACAO
CYCLO
DICHO
FACTO
GECKO
HECTO
JACKO
JOCKO
LACTO
LUCIO
MACAO
MACHO
MACRO
MCCOO
MICRO
MUCHO
NACHO
NACIO
NYCTO
PICTO
RECTO
ROCCO
SACCO
SACRO
SICKO
SOCIO
SOCKO
TACHO
TYCHO
WACKO
XACTO
YOCTO
ZUCCO

•••CO
AAMCO
ABACO
AMICO
AMOCO
BANCO
BARCO
BOSCO
BUCCO
BUNCO
CASCO
CHACO
CHICO
CHOCO
CINCO
CISCO
CUZCO
DELCO
DISCO
DRACO
FALCO
FUOCO
GEICO
GLUCO
GLYCO
GRECO
JUNCO
MARCO
NARCO
PASCO
PATCO
PETCO
ROCCO
RONCO
SACCO
SYSCO
TAXCO
TELCO
TURCO
VASCO
VESCO
WASCO
WILCO
ZUCCO

CP•••
CPLUS

C•P••
CAPAS
CAPED
CAPEK
CAPER
CAPES
CAPET
CAPON
CAPOS
CAPRA
CAPRI
CAPTS
CAPUT
CEPES
COPAL
COPAY
COPED
COPER
COPES
COPIA
COPIT
COPRA
COPSE
COPTO
COPTS
CSPAN
CSPOT
CUPEL
CUPID
CUPPA
CUPPY
CUPRI
CUPRO

C••P•
CAMPO
CAMPS
CAMPY
CARPE
CARPI
CARPO
CARPS
CCUPS
CHAPS
CHIPS
CHOPS
CLAPS
CLEPT
CLIPS
CLIPT
CLOPS
COAPT
COMPS
COOPS
COOPT
CORPS
COUPE
COUPS
COYPU
CRAPE
CRAPS
CREPE
CREPT
CROPS
CRYPT
CULPA
CUPPA
CUPPY
CUSPS

C•••P
CHAMP
CHEAP
CHEEP
CHIMP
CHIRP
CHOMP
CHUMP
CLAMP
CLASP
CLOMP
CLUMP
CRAMP
CREEP
CRIMP
CRISP
CROUP
CRUMP
CRYUP
CUEUP
CUTUP

•C•P•
ACUPS
BCUPS
CCUPS
DCUPS
SCAPA
SCAPE
SCOPE
SCUPS

•C••P
ACTUP
ICEUP
SCALP
SCAMP
SCARP
SCOOP
SCRAP
SCRIP
VCHIP

••C•P
ASCAP
BICEP
DECAP
EXCOP
RECAP
RECIP
UNCAP

•••CP
NAACP

C•Q••
COQUI

•CQ••
ACQUA

CR•••
CRABS
CRACK
CRACY
CRAFT
CRAGS
CRAIG
CRAIK
CRAIN
CRAKE
CRAMP
CRAMS
CRANE
CRANI
CRANK
CRAPE
CRAPS
CRASH
CRASS
CRATE
CRAVE
CRAWL
CRAWS
CRAYS
CRAZE
CRAZY
CREAK
CREAM
CRECY
CREDO
CREDS
CREED
CREEK
CREEL
CREEP
CREES
CREMA
CREME
CREON
CREPE
CREPT
CRESC
CRESS
CREST
CRETE
CREVE
CREWS
CRIBS
CRICK
CRIED
CRIER
CRIES
CRIME
CRIMP
CRISP
CRIST
CRITS
CRIUS
CROAK
CROAT
CROCE
CROCI
CROCK
CROCS
CROFT
CROIX
CRONE
CRONY
CROOK
CROON
CROPS
CRORE
CROSS
CROUP
CROWD
CROWE
CROWN
CROWS
CRUDE
CRUDS
CRUEL
CRUET
CRUMB
CRUMP
CRUOR
CRURA
CRUSE
CRUSH
CRUST
CRWTH
CRYER
CRYPT
CRYUP

C•R••
CARAT
CARAY
CARBO
CARBS
CARDI
CARDS
CARED
CARER
CARES
CARET
CAREW
CAREY
CARGO
CARIB
CARLA
CARLE
CARLO
CARLY
CARME
CARNE
CARNY
CAROB
CAROL
CAROM
CARON
CARPE
CARPI
CARPO
CARPS
CARRE
CARRY
CARTA
CARTE
CARTS
CARVE
CDROM
CERAM
CERAT
CERES
CERIA
CERIC
CEROS
CERRO
CERTS
CHRIS
CHROM
CHRON
CIRCA
CIRCE
CIRCS
CIRES
CIRRI
CIRRO
CORAL
CORBY
CORDA
CORDS
COREA
CORED
CORER
CORES
COREY
CORFU
CORGI
CORIA
CORKS
CORKY
CORMS
CORNI
CORNO
CORNS
CORNU
CORNY
COROT
CORPS
CORRI
CORSA
CORSO
CORVO
CURAD
CURBS
CURDS
CURDY
CURED
CUREL
CURER
CURES
CURET
CURIA
CURIE
CURIO
CURLS
CURLY
CURRS
CURRY
CURSA
CURSE
CURST
CURVE
CURVI
CURVY
CYRIL
CYRUS

C••R•
CADRE
CAIRN
CAIRO
CAMRY
CAPRA
CAPRI
CARRE
CARRY
CBERS
CEARA
CEORL
CERRO
CHARD
CHARM
CHARO
CHARS
CHART
CHARY
CHERE
CHERI
CHERT
CHIRO
CHIRP
CHIRR
CHORD
CHORE
CHORO
CHURL
CHURN
CIERA
CIRRI
CIRRO
CITRI
CITRO
CLARA
CLARE
CLARK
CLARO
CLARY
CLERK
CMDRS
COBRA
COIRS
COORS
COPRA
CORRI
COURT
COURU
COWRY
CRORE
CRURA
CUERS
CUIRE
CUORE
CUPRI
CUPRO
CURRS
CURRY
CYMRY
CZARS

C•••R
CABER
CAGER
CALOR
CANER
CAPER
CARER
CASER
CATER
CAVER
CEDAR
CEDER
CENTR
CESAR
CHAIR
CHEER
CHIRR
CHLOR
CHOIR
CIDER
CIGAR
CITER
CLAIR
CLEAR
CLUER
CODER
COEUR
COKER
COLOR
COMDR
COMER
CONER
CONTR
COOER
COPER
CORER
COVER
COWER
COYER
CRIER
CRUOR
CRYER
CSTAR
CUBER
CUKOR
CURER
CUTER
CYBER
CYDER

•CR••
ACRED
ACRES
ACRID
ECRUS
JCREW
MCRAE
OCRAT
SCRAG
SCRAM
SCRAP
SCRAT
SCREE
SCREW
SCRIM
SCRIP
SCROD
SCRUB
SCRUM

•C•R•
ACCRA
ACERB
ACERS
ACORN
ACURA
ECARD
ICARE
ICERS
KCARS
OCHRE
SCARE
SCARF
SCARP
SCARS
SCARY
SCIRE
SCORE
SCORN

•C••R
ACHER
ACTER
ACTOR
ECTOR
ICHOR
ICIER
OCCUR
OCHER
SCOUR

••CR•
ACCRA
DECRY
ENCRE
INCRS
LUCRE
LYCRA
MACRO
MICRA
MICRO
NACRE
SACRA
SACRE
SACRO
SUCRE

••C•R
ALCOR
BYCAR
DECIR
DECOR
DICER
ELCAR
FACER
INCUR
LACER
LECAR
MACER
NICER
OCCUR
OSCAR
PACER
RACER
RECUR
RICER
ULCER
VICAR

•••CR
TVVCR

CS•••
CSINY
CSPAN
CSPOT
CSTAR

C•S••
CASAS
CASBY
CASCA
CASCO
CASED
CASER
CASES
CASEY
CASIO
CASKS
CASTA
CASTE
CASTS
CASUS
CBSTV
CESAR
CESTA
CESTI
CISCO
CISSY
CISTS
COSBY
COSEC
COSET
COSMO
COSTA
COSTS
CUSEC
CUSHY
CUSKS
CUSPS
CYSTS

C••S•
CANSO
CANST
CAUSE
CEASE
CENSE
CHASE
CHASM
CHAST
CHESS
CHEST
CHOSE
CISSY
CLASE
CLASH
CLASP
CLASS
CLOSE
COASE
COAST
CONST
COOSA
COPSE
CORSA
CORSO
COUSY
CRASH
CRASS
CRESC
CRESS
CREST
CRISP
CRIST
CROSS
CRUSE
CRUSH
CRUST
CURSA
CURSE
CURST

C•••S
CADIS
CAFES
CAGES
CAIUS
CAKES
CALKS
CALLS
CALMS
CAMAS
CAMBS
CAMOS
CAMPS
CAMUS
CANES
CANIS
CANTS
CAPAS
CAPES
CAPOS
CAPTS
CARBS
CARDS
CARES
CARPS
CARTS
CASAS
CASES
CASKS
CASTS
CASUS
CATES
CATHS
CAVES
CBERS
CCUPS
CEDES
CEDIS
CEILS
CELLS
CELTS
CENAS
CENTS
CEPES
CERES
CEROS
CERTS
CETUS
CHADS
CHAIS
CHAOS
CHAPS
CHARS
CHATS
CHAWS
CHEFS
CHESS
CHEWS
CHIAS
CHICS
CHINS
CHIOS
CHIPS
CHITS
CHOPS
CHOWS
CHRIS
CHUBS
CHUGS
CHUMS
CIAOS
CIELS
CIENS
CINES
CIONS
CIRCS
CIRES
CISTS
CITES
CLADS
CLAES
CLAMS
CLANS
CLAPS
CLASS
CLAUS
CLAWS
CLAYS
CLEFS
CLEWS
CLIOS
CLIPS
CLODS
CLOGS
CLOPS
CLOTS
CLOYS
CLUBS
CLUES
CMDRS
COALS
COATS
COCAS
COCKS
COCOS
CODAS
CODES
COEDS
COHOS
COIFS
COILS
COINS
COIRS
COKES
COLAS
COLDS
COLES
COLTS
COMAS
COMBS
COMES
COMPS
COMUS
CONDS
CONES
CONKS
CONNS
CONTS
CONUS
COOKS
COOLS
COONS
COOPS
COORS
COOTS
COPES
COPTS
CORDS
CORES
CORKS
CORMS
CORNS
CORPS
COSTS
COTES
COUPS
COVES
COWES
COWLS
COXES
COZES
CPLUS
CRABS
CRAGS
CRAMS
CRAPS
CRASS
CRAWS
CRAYS
CREDS
CREES
CRESS
CREWS
CRIBS
CRIES
CRITS
CRIUS
CROCS
CROPS
CROSS
CROWS
CRUDS
CUBES
CUERS
CUFFS
CUKES
CULLS
CULTS
CUMES
CURBS
CURDS
CURES
CURLS
CURRS
CUSKS
CUSPS
CUTES
CUTIS
CUYDS
CYANS
CYMAS
CYMES
CYRUS
CYSTS
CZARS

•C•S•
ECASH
ICOSA
ICOSI
SCUSA
SCUSI

•C••S
ACADS
ACCTS
ACERS
ACHES
ACIDS
ACMES
ACNES
ACRES
ACTAS
ACTES
ACTOS
ACUPS
BCUPS
CCUPS
DCUPS
ECHOS
ECONS
ECRUS
ICBMS
ICEES
ICERS
ICKES
ICONS
ICTUS
KCARS
MCATS
OCHOS
SCABS
SCADS
SCAMS
SCANS
SCARS
SCATS
SCOTS
SCOWS
SCUDS
SCUMS
SCUPS
SCUTS

••C•S
ACCTS
ASCUS
BACKS
BACOS
BECKS
BOCAS
BOCKS
BUCKS
COCAS
COCKS
COCOS
DACES
DECKS
DICES
DICKS
DICTS
DOCES
DOCKS
DUCES
DUCKS
DUCTS
ENCLS
FACES
FACTS
FICUS
FOCUS
FUCHS
GUCKS
HACKS
HECKS
HICKS
HOCKS
HOCUS
INCAS
INCRS
INCUS
JACKS
JOCKS
JUCOS
KICKS
LACES
LACKS
LECTS
LICKS
LOCHS
LOCKS
LOCOS
LOCUS
LUCAS
LUCKS
LYCOS
MACES
MACKS
MACYS
MICAS
MOCKS
MUCKS
NECKS
NICKS
NOCKS
ORCAS
ORCHS
ORCUS
PACAS
PACES
PACKS
PACTS
PECKS
PECOS
PICAS
PICKS
PICTS
POCUS
PUCES
PUCKS
RACES
RACKS
RECKS
RECTS
RICES
RICKS
ROCKS
RUCKS
SACHS
SACKS
SECHS
SECTS
SOCAS
SOCKS
SUCKS
TACHS
TACKS
TACOS
TECHS
TICKS
TICOS
TUCKS
UNCAS
VACAS
VICES
VICKS
WICKS
YACKS
YMCAS
YWCAS

•••CS
ASICS
AWACS
BANCS
BLOCS
BMOCS
BOSCS
CHICS
CIRCS
CROCS

DISCS EPICS EXECS FISCS FLICS IMACS IROCS LAICS LINCS MERCS NARCS PARCS PERCS PORCS ROTCS SPECS SYNCS TALCS WAACS ZINCS

CT•••
CTENO CTILE

C•T••
CATCH CATER CATES CATHS CATHY CATTY CETTE CETUS CITED CITEE CITER CITES CITGO CITRI CITRO COTAN COTES COTTA CSTAR CUTER CUTES CUTEX CUTEY CUTIE CUTIN CUTIS CUTIT CUTTY CUTUP

C••T•
CACTI CANTO CANTS CANTY CAPTS CARTA CARTE CARTS CASTA CASTE CASTS CATTY CBSTV CELTS CENTI CENTO CENTR CENTS CENTU CERTS CESTA CESTI CETTE CEUTA CHATS CHETA CHITA CHITS CHUTE CISTS CLETE CLOTH CLOTS CNOTE COATI COATS COLTS COMTE CONTD CONTE CONTI CONTR CONTS COOTE COOTS COOTY COPTO COPTS COSTA COSTS COTTA COUTH CRATE CRETE CRITS CRWTH CULTI CULTS CUTTY CYSTS

C•••T
CABOT CADET CAINT CANIT CANST CAPET CAPUT CARAT CARET CERAT CFLAT CHANT CHART CHAST CHEAT CHERT CHEST CIVET CLEAT CLEFT CLEPT CLIFT CLINT CLIPT CLOUT COACT COAPT COAST COMET CONST COOPT COPIT COROT COSET COUNT COURT COVET CRAFT CREPT CREST CRIST CROAT CROFT CRUET CRUST CRYPT CSPOT CUBIT CUGAT CULET CURET CURST CUTIT

•CT••
ACTAS ACTED ACTER ACTES ACTII ACTIN ACTIV ACTON ACTOR ACTOS ACTUP ECTAD ECTAL ECTOR ICTUS OCTAD OCTAL OCTAN OCTET

•C•T•
ACCTS ACETO ACUTE MCATS SCATS SCOTS SCOTT SCUTS

•C••T
ACEIT ECLAT ICANT ICEIT OCRAT OCTET SCANT SCENT SCOOT SCOTT SCOUT SCRAT

••CT•
ABCTV ACCTS CACTI DICTA DICTS DICTU DUCTS FACTA FACTO FACTS HECTO LACTI LACTO LECTS NBCTV NOCTI NYCTI NYCTO PACTS PICTO PICTS RECTA RECTI RECTO RECTS SECTS XACTO YOCTO

••C•T
ASCOT DICOT DUCAT EPCOT FACET HECHT JACET LICHT LICIT NACHT NICHT NOCUT OPCIT PICOT RECUT TACET TACIT UNCUT YACHT

•••CT
BRACT COACT EDICT EDUCT EJECT ELECT ENACT EPACT ERECT ERUCT EVICT EXACT FRUCT MULCT REACT TINCT TRACT

CU•••
CUBAN CUBBY CUBEB CUBED CUBER CUBES CUBIC CUBIT CUDDY CUEIN CUERS CUEUP CUFFS CUGAT CUICA CUING CUIRE CUKES CUKOR CULCH CULET CULLS CULLY CULPA CULTI CULTS CUMES CUMIN CUMUL CUNEO CUOMO CUORE CUPEL CUPID CUPPA CUPPY CUPRI CUPRO CURAD CURBS CURDS CURDY CURED CUREL CURER CURES CURET CURIA CURIE CURIO CURLS CURLY CURRS CURRY CURSA CURSE CURST CURVE CURVI CURVY CUSEC CUSHY CUSKS CUSPS CUTER CUTES CUTEX CUTEY CUTIE CUTIN CUTIS CUTIT CUTTY CUTUP CUVEE CUYDS CUZCO

C•U••
CAUDI CAUDO CAULK CAUSE CCUPS CEUTA CHUBB CHUBS CHUCK CHUFF CHUGS CHULA CHUMP CHUMS CHUNG CHUNK CHURL CHURN CHUTE CLUBS CLUCK CLUED CLUER CLUES CLUMP CLUNG CLUNK CLUNY COUCH COUGH COULD COUNT COUPE COUPS COURT COURU COUSY COUTH CRUDE CRUDS CRUEL CRUET CRUMB CRUMP CRUOR CRURA CRUSE CRUSH CRUST

C••U•
CAIUS CAJUN CAMUS CAPUT CASUS CECUM CETUS CHAUD CLAUS CLOUD CLOUT COEUR COLUM COMUS CONUS COQUI CPLUS CRIUS CROUP CRYUP CUEUP CUMUL CUTUP CYRUS

C•••U
CENTU CORFU CORNU COURU COYPU

•CU••
ACUFF ACUPS ACURA ACUTE BCUPS CCUPS DCUPS OCULI OCULO SCUBA SCUDS SCUFF SCULL SCUMS SCUPS SCUSA SCUSI SCUTS SCUZZ

•C•U•
ACQUA ACTUP ECRUS ICEUP ICTUS OCCUR SCOUR SCOUT SCRUB SCRUM

••CU•
ASCUS CECUM EXCUB FICUS FOCUS HOCUS INCUR INCUS LOCUM LOCUS MECUM MRCUB NOCUT OCCUR ONCUE ORCUS POCUS RECUE RECUR RECUT UNCUT VACUA

••C•U
DICTU FICHU MACHU RICEU

CV•••
CVIII

C•V••
CAVAE CAVAN CAVED CAVER CAVES CAVIL CCVII CDVII CIVET CIVIC CIVIL CLVII CMVII COVED COVEN COVER COVES COVET COVEY CUVEE CXVII

C••V•
CALVE CARVE CCCVI CCLVI CCXVI CDLVI CDXVI CHAVA CHEVY CHIVE CHIVY CLAVE CLEVE CLIVE CLOVE CLXVI CMLVI CMXVI CONVY CORVO CRAVE CREVE CURVE CURVI CURVY CXCVI CXLVI CXXVI

C•••V
CBSTV CCCIV CCCLV CCCXV CCLIV CCLXV CCXCV CCXIV CCXLV CCXXV CDLIV CDLXV CDXCV CDXIV CDXLV CDXXV CLXIV CLXXV CMLIV CMLXV CMXCV CMXIV CMXLV CMXXV CXCIV CXLIV CXXIV CXXXV

•CV••
CCVII DCVII MCVIE MCVII XCVII

•C•V•
CCCVI CCLVI CCXVI DCCVI DCLVI DCXVI MCCVI MCDVI MCLVI MCMVI MCXVI

•C••V
ACTIV CCCIV CCCLV CCCXV CCLIV CCLXV CCXCV CCXIV CCXLV CCXXV DCCCV DCCIV DCCLV DCCXV DCLIV DCLXV DCXCV DCXIV DCXLV DCXXV MCCCV MCCIV MCCLV MCCXV MCDIV MCDLV MCDXV MCLIV MCLXV MCMIV MCMLV MCMXV MCXCV MCXIV MCXLV MCXXV SCHAV

••CV•
CCCVI CXCVI DCCVI DXCVI MCCVI MDCVI MMCVI MXCVI

••C•V
ABCTV CCCIV CCCLV CCCXV CXCIV DCCCV DCCIV DCCLV DCCXV DXCIV MCCCV MCCIV MCCLV MCCXV MDCCV MDCIV MDCLV MDCXV MMCCV MMCDV MMCIV MMCLV MMCMV MMCXV MXCIV NBCTV

•••CV
CCXCV CDXCV CMXCV DCCCV DCXCV MCCCV MCXCV MDCCV MDXCV MMCCV MMDCV MMMCV MMXCV

C•W••
CAWED CLWYD COWED COWER COWES COWLS COWRY CRWTH

C••W•
CHAWS CHEWS CHEWY CHOWS CLAWS CLEWS CLOWN COOWN CRAWL CRAWS CREWS CROWD CROWE CROWN CROWS

C•••W
CANDW CAREW

•C•W•
SCHWA SCOWL SCOWS

•C••W
JCREW SCREW

••C•W
MACAW

CX•••
CXCII CXCIV CXCIX CXCVI CXIII CXLII CXLIV CXLIX CXLVI CXVII CXXII CXXIV CXXIX CXXVI CXXXI CXXXV

C•X••
CCXCI CCXCV CCXII CCXIV CCXIX CCXLI CCXLV CCXVI CCXXI CCXXV CCXXX CDXCI CDXCV CDXII CDXIV CDXIX CDXLI CDXLV CDXVI CDXXI CDXXV CDXXX CLXII CLXIV CLXIX CLXVI CLXXI CLXXV CLXXX CMXCI CMXCV CMXII CMXIV CMXIX CMXLI CMXLV CMXVI CMXXI CMXXV CMXXX COXAE COXED COXES CXXII CXXIV CXXIX CXXVI CXXXI CXXXV

C••X•
CCCXC CCCXI CCCXL CCCXV CCCXX CCLXI CCLXV CCLXX CCXXI CCXXV CCXXX CDLXI CDLXV CDLXX CDXXI CDXXV CDXXX CHEXX CLXXI CLXXV CLXXX CMLXI CMLXV CMLXX CMXXI CMXXV CMXXX CXXXI CXXXV

C•••X
CALIX CALYX CCCIX CCCLX CCCXX CCLIX CCLXX CCXIX CCXXX CDLIX CDLXX CDXIX CDXXX CHEXX CLXIX CLXXX CMLIX CMLXX CMXIX CMXXX CODEX COMEX COMIX CROIX CUTEX CXCIX CXLIX CXXIX

•CX••
CCXCI CCXCV CCXII CCXIV CCXIX CCXLI CCXLV CCXVI CCXXI CCXXV CCXXX DCXCI DCXCV DCXII DCXIV DCXIX DCXLI DCXLV DCXVI DCXXI DCXXV DCXXX MCXCI MCXCV MCXII MCXIV MCXIX MCXLI MCXLV MCXVI MCXXI MCXXV MCXXX

•C•X•
CCCXC CCCXI CCCXL CCCXV CCCXX CCLXI CCLXV CCLXX CCXXI CCXXV CCXXX DCCXC DCCXI DCCXL DCCXV DCCXX DCLXI DCLXV DCLXX DCXXI DCXXV DCXXX MCCXC MCCXI MCCXL MCCXV MCCXX MCDXC MCDXI MCDXL MCDXV MCDXX MCLXI MCLXV MCLXX MCMXC MCMXI MCMXL MCMXV MCMXX MCXXI MCXXV MCXXX

•C••X
CCCIX CCCLX CCCXX CCLIX CCLXX CCXIX CCXXX DCCCX DCCIX DCCLX DCCXX DCLIX DCLXX DCXIX DCXXX ICEAX MCCCX MCCIX MCCLX MCCXX MCDIX MCDLX MCDXX MCLIX MCLXX MCMIX MCMLX MCMXX MCXIX MCXXX

••CX•
CCCXC CCCXI CCCXL CCCXV CCCXX DCCXC DCCXI DCCXL DCCXV DCCXX MCCXC MCCXI MCCXL MCCXV MCCXX MDCXC MDCXI MDCXL MDCXV MDCXX MMCXC MMCXI MMCXL MMCXV MMCXX

••C•X
CCCIX CCCLX CCCXX CXCIX DCCCX DCCIX DCCLX DCCXX DXCIX MCCCX MCCIX MCCLX MCCXX MDCCX MDCIX MDCLX MDCXX MMCCX MMCDX MMCIX MMCLX MMCMX MMCXX MXCIX

•••CX
DCCCX MCCCX MDCCX MMCCX MMDCX MMMCX

CY•••
CYANO CYANS CYBER CYCAD CYCLE CYCLO CYDER CYGNI CYMAE CYMAS CYMES CYMRY CYNDI CYNIC CYRIL CYRUS CYSTS

C•Y••
CAYCE CLYDE COYER COYLY COYPU CRYER CRYPT CRYUP CUYDS

C••Y•
CALYX CLAYS CLOYS CLWYD CRAYS

C•••Y
CABBY CADDY CAGEY CAKEY CAMAY CAMPY CAMRY CANBY CANDY CANNY CANTY CARAY CAREY CARLY CARNY CARRY CASBY CASEY CATHY CATTY CHARY CHELY CHEVY CHEWY CHIVY CHOKY CIGGY CINCY CINDY CISSY CLARY CLUNY COCKY COLBY COMFY CONEY CONVY COODY COOKY COOTY COPAY CORBY COREY CORKY CORNY COSBY COUSY COVEY COWRY COYLY CRACY CRAZY CRECY CRONY CSINY CUBBY CUDDY CULLY CUPPY CURDY

CURLY
CURRY
CURVY
CUSHY
CUTEY
CUTTY
CYMRY

•C••Y
ACIDY
ICILY
MCCOY
MCFLY
MCKAY
SCALY
SCARY

••CY•
ENCYC
MACYS

••C•Y
ARCHY
BECKY
BOCHY
BUCKY
COCKY
DECAY
DECOY
DECRY
DICEY
DICKY
DUCHY
DUCKY
GUCKY
HACKY
ITCHY
JACEY
JACKY
KICKY
LACEY
LECKY
LUCKY
MACHY
MCCOY
MICKY
MUCKY
NICKY
ORCZY
PACEY
PACHY
PICKY
RICKY
ROCKY
SUCKY
TACKY
TICKY
UNCOY
VICHY
VICKY
WACKY
YUCKY

•••CY
BERCY
CINCY
CRACY
CRECY
DARCY
DEUCY
FANCY
JUICY
MANCY
MARCY
MERCY
NANCY
ORACY
PERCY
PRICY
SAUCY
SPACY
SPICY
STACY
TRACY
VINCY
YANCY
ZINCY

CZ•••
CZARS
CZECH

C•Z••
COZEN
COZES
CUZCO

C••Z•
CHAZZ
CRAZE
CRAZY

C•••Z
CADIZ
CHAZZ
CHEEZ

•C•Z•
SCUZZ

•C••Z
SCUZZ

••CZ•
ORCZY

DA•••
DABAT
DABBA
DABIH
DABON
DACCA
DACES
DACHA
DACHE
DACIA
DADAS
DADDY
DADOS
DAFFY
DAFOE
DAGAN
DAILY
DAIRY
DAISY
DAIWA
DAKAR
DALAI
DALEN
DALES
DALET
DALEY
DALIS
DALLY
DAMAS
DAMEN
DAMES
DAMIS
DAMME
DAMNS
DAMON
DAMPS
DAMUP
DANAE
DANCE
DANDD
DANDY
DANES
DANGS
DANIA
DANIO
DANKE
DANNO
DANNY
DANSE
DANTE
DANZA
DARBY
DARCI
DARCY
DARDY
DARED
DARER
DARES
DARIA
DARIN
DARIO
DARKS
DARLA
DARNS
DARTE
DARTH
DARTS
DARYA
DARYL
DASHI
DASHY
DASNT
DATED
DATER
DATES
DATOS
DATUM
DAUBE
DAUBS
DAUNT
DAVAO
DAVEN
DAVES
DAVEY
DAVID
DAVIE
DAVIS
DAVIT
DAVOS
DAWES
DAWNN
DAWNS
DAYAN
DAYNE
DAZED
DAZER
DAZES
DAZUR
DAZZY

D•A••
DBACK
DDAYS
DEAIR
DEALS
DEALT
DEANA
DEANE
DEANS
DEARE
DEARS
DEARY
DEATH
DHABI
DHAKA
DHALS
DIALO
DIALS
DIAMS
DIANA
DIANE
DIARY
DMARK
DNASE
DOALL
DOANE
DOANS
DOATS
DRABS
DRACO
DRAFT
DRAGO
DRAGS
DRAIN
DRAKE
DRAMA
DRAMS
DRANG
DRANK
DRANO
DRAPE
DRATS
DRAVA
DRAWL
DRAWN
DRAWS
DRAYS
DUADS
DUALS
DUANE
DWARF
DYADS

D••A•
DABAT
DADAS
DAGAN
DAKAR
DALAI
DAMAS
DANAE
DAVAO
DAYAN
DCCAB
DEBAG
DEBAR
DECAD
DECAF
DECAL
DECAP
DECAY
DEFAT
DEGAS
DELAY
DENAR
DERAT
DESAI
DETAR
DETAT
DEVAS
DEWAR
DEWAX
DFLAT
DIGAT
DIMAG
DIMAS
DINAH
DINAR
DIRAC
DIRAE
DIRAM
DITAT
DIVAC
DIVAN
DIVAS
DOBAD
DONAS
DONAT
DONAU
DOPAS
DORAG
DORAL
DORAN
DOSAY
DOTAL
DOUAI
DOUAY
DREAD
DREAM
DREAR
DRIAM
DRLAO
DRYAD
DUBAI
DUCAL
DUCAT
DUFAY
DUGAN
DUGAT
DUKAS
DUMAS
DURAN
DURAS
DUVAL
DYLAN

D•••A
DABBA
DACCA
DACHA
DACIA
DAIWA
DANIA
DANZA
DARIA
DARLA
DARYA
DEANA
DEBRA
DECCA
DELIA
DELLA
DELTA
DERMA
DESNA
DHAKA
DIANA
DICTA
DINKA
DITKA
DJUNA
DOGMA
DOLMA
DONNA
DORIA
DORSA
DOULA
DRAMA
DRAVA
DRINA
DUBYA
DUENA
DURRA
DVINA

•DA••
ADAGE
ADAIR
ADAMA
ADAMS
ADANA
ADANO
ADAOK
ADAPT
ADARN
ADARS
BDAYS
DDAYS
EDAMS
IDAHO
UDALL
VDAYS

•D•A•
ADDAX
ADLAI
ADMAN
ADNAN
ADWAR
EDDAS
EDGAR
EDMAR
IDEAL
IDEAS
IDTAG

•D••A
ADAMA
ADANA
ADELA
ADYTA
EDEMA
EDINA
IDOLA
LDOPA
ODESA

••DA•
ADDAX
AIDAN
BADAT
CEDAR
CODAS
DADAS
EDDAS
ENDAT
HADAT
HODAD
JUDAH
JUDAS
KADAR
KODAK
LADAS
LIDAR
MADAM
MADAT
MEDAL
MIDAS
MODAL
MYDAD
MYDAY
NODAL
NODAT
OIDAL
ONDAS
PEDAL
PODAL
RADAR
REDAN
RODAN
SADAT
SEDAN
SODAS
SUDAN
TADAS
TIDAL
TODAY
UNDAM
UNDAY
VEDAS
VEDAY
VIDAL
VIDAS
VJDAY
ZADAR

••D•A
AUDRA
HEDDA
HYDRA
INDIA
INDRA
JIDDA
JUDEA
LYDIA
MEDEA
MEDIA
NADIA
NADJA
NEDDA
NEDRA
NYDIA
PADUA
PODIA
RODYA
SIDEA
VODKA
YADDA

•••DA
ALIDA
AMADA
BAEDA
BANDA
BREDA
CORDA
FONDA
FREDA
FRIDA
FULDA
GARDA
GILDA
GOLDA
GOUDA
HAIDA
HEDDA
HILDA
HONDA
JIDDA
KINDA
KORDA
LAUDA
LINDA
LYNDA
MAGDA
MAZDA
MTIDA
NARDA
NEDDA
OJEDA
OUIDA
PANDA
PRADA
QANDA
RANDA
RHODA
SUNDA
THEDA
TILDA
USRDA
VARDA
VELDA
VONDA
WAJDA
WANDA
YADDA
ZELDA
ZENDA

DB•••
DBACK

D•B••
DABAT
DABBA
DABIH
DABON
DEBAG
DEBAR
DEBBE
DEBBI
DEBBY
DEBIT
DEBRA
DEBTS
DEBUG
DEBUS
DEBUT
DEBYE
DOBAD
DOBBS
DOBEE
DOBIE
DOBLE
DOBRO
DUBAI
DUBHE
DUBIN
DUBYA

D••B•
DABBA
DARBY
DAUBE
DAUBS
DEBBE
DEBBI
DEBBY
DERBY
DHABI
DIDBY
DIGBY
DOBBS
DOLBY
DOUBS
DOUBT
DRABS
DRIBS
DRUBS
DUMBO
DUMBS

D•••B
DCCAB
DEMOB
DENEB
DWEEB

•DB••
ADBIZ

•D•B•
ADOBE
ADOBO

•D••B
ADLIB

••DB•
DIDBY

••D•B
REDUB
SIDEB

•••DB
BANDB
JANDB
RANDB

DC•••
DCCAB
DCCCI
DCCCL
DCCCV
DCCCX
DCCII
DCCIV
DCCIX
DCCLI
DCCLV
DCCLX
DCCVI
DCCXC
DCCXI
DCCXL
DCCXV
DCCXX
DCELL
DCIII
DCLII
DCLIV
DCLIX
DCLVI
DCLXI
DCLXV
DCLXX
DCUPS
DCVII
DCXCI
DCXCV
DCXII
DCXIV
DCXIX
DCXLI
DCXLV
DCXVI
DCXXI
DCXXV
DCXXX

D•C••
DACCA
DACES
DACHA
DACHE
DACIA
DCCAB
DCCCI
DCCCL
DCCCV
DCCCX
DCCII
DCCIV
DCCIX
DCCLI
DCCLV
DCCLX
DCCVI
DCCXC
DCCXI
DCCXL
DCCXV
DCCXX
DECAD
DECAF
DECAL
DECAP
DECAY
DECCA
DECEM
DECIR
DECKS
DECOR
DECOY
DECRY
DICED
DICER
DICES
DICEY
DICHO
DICKS
DICKY
DICOT
DICTA
DICTS
DICTU
DOCES
DOCKS
DUCAL
DUCAT
DUCES
DUCHY
DUCKS
DUCKY
DUCTS
DXCII
DXCIV
DXCIX
DXCVI

D••C•
DACCA
DANCE
DARCI
DARCY
DBACK
DCCCI
DCCCL
DCCCV
DCCCX
DCXCI
DCXCV
DECCA
DEICE
DELCO
DENCH
DEUCE
DEUCY
DIECI
DISCI
DISCO
DISCS
DITCH
DOLCE
DOLCI
DOUCE
DOYCE
DRACO
DRECK
DULCE
DUNCE
DUTCH

D•••C
DCCXC
DIRAC
DIVAC
DODEC
DORIC
DUROC

•DC••
MDCCC
MDCCI
MDCCL
MDCCV
MDCCX
MDCII
MDCIV
MDCIX
MDCLI
MDCLV
MDCLX
MDCVI
MDCXC
MDCXI
MDCXL
MDCXV
MDCXX

•D•C•
CDXCI
CDXCV
EDICT
EDUCE
EDUCT
MDCCC
MDCCI
MDCCL
MDCCV
MDCCX
MDXCI
MDXCV

•D••C
ADHOC
EDDIC
MDCCC
MDCXC

••DC•
MMDCC
MMDCI
MMDCL
MMDCV
MMDCX

••D•C
ASDIC
DODEC
EDDIC
INDIC
IODIC
LUDIC
MADOC
MCDXC
MEDIC
MEDOC
MMDCC
MMDXC
UNDEC
VEDIC

•••DC
HARDC
MMMDC

DD•••
DDAYS

D•D••
DADAS
DADDY
DADOS
DEDOS
DIDBY
DIDIN
DIDIT
DIDNT
DIDOK
DIDOS
DIDSO
DIDST
DIDTO
DIDUP
DODEC
DODGE
DODGY
DODIE
DODOS
DRDRE
DUDDY
DUDED
DUDEK
DUDES

D••D•
DADDY
DANDD
DANDY
DARDY
DEEDS
DENDR
DESDE
DINDY
DIODE
DOIDO
DONDE
DONDI
DOODY
DOWDY
DREDD
DUADS
DUDDY
DYADS

D•••D
DANDD
DARED
DATED
DAVID
DAZED
DECAD
DEKED
DELED
DESOD
DEWED
DICED
DIKED
DIMED
DINED
DIVED
DOBAD
DOLED
DOMED
DOPED
DOSED
DOTED
DOZED
DREAD
DREDD
DRIED
DROID
DROOD
DRUID
DRYAD
DUDED
DUKED
DUPED

•DD••
ADDAX
ADDED
ADDER
ADDIE
ADDIN
ADDIO
ADDIS
ADDLE
ADDNL
ADDON
ADDRS
ADDTO
ADDUP
EDDAS
EDDIC
EDDIE
ODDER
ODDLY
UDDER

•D••D
ADDED
ADZED
EDGED
EDRED
IDLED

••DD•
BADDY
BEDDY
BIDDY
BODDY
BUDDY
CADDY
CUDDY
DADDY
DUDDY
FADDY
FUDDY
GADDI
GIDDY
HEDDA
JIDDA
JUDDS
KIDDO
KIDDY
LIDDY
MIDDY
MUDDY
NEDDA
NODDY
PADDY
PUDDY
REDDI
REDDY
RODDY
RUDDY
SODDY
TEDDY
TODDY
YADDA

••D•D
ADDED
AIDED
BIDED
BODED
CEDED
CODED
DUDED
ENDED
FADED
HODAD
JADED
LADED
MYDAD
ONDVD
REDED
REDID
SIDED
TIDED
TVDVD
UNDID
WADED

•••DD
DANDD
DREDD
RANDD
READD

DE•••
DEAIR
DEALS
DEALT
DEANA
DEANE
DEANS
DEARE
DEARS
DEARY
DEATH
DEBAG
DEBAR
DEBBE
DEBBI
DEBBY
DEBIT
DEBRA
DEBTS
DEBUG
DEBUS
DEBUT
DEBYE
DECAD
DECAF
DECAL
DECAP
DECAY
DECCA
DECEM
DECIR
DECKS
DECOR
DECOY
DECRY
DEDOS
DEEDS
DEEMS
DEEPS
DEERE
DEERS
DEFAT
DEFER
DEFGH
DEFOE
DEFOG
DEGAS
DEGEL
DEGUM
DEHEX
DEICE
DEIFY
DEIGN
DEILS
DEION
DEISM
DEIST
DEITY
DEKED
DEKES
DEKKO
DELAY
DELCO
DELED
DELES
DELFT
DELHI
DELIA
DELIS
DELLA
DELLO
DELLS
DELON
DELOS
DELPY
DELTA
DELTS
DELVE
DEMES
DEMIT
DEMME
DEMOB
DEMON
DEMOS
DEMUR
DENAR
DENCH
DENDR
DENEB
DENES
DENIM
DENIS
DENNY
DENOM
DENSE
DENTE
DENTI
DENTO
DENTS
DENYS
DEOXY
DEPEW
DEPOT
DEPTH
DEPTS
DERAT
DERBY
DEREK
DERIV
DERMA
DERMO
DERRY
DESAI
DESDE
DESEX
DESKS
DESNA
DESOD
DESTE
DETAR
DETAT
DETER
DETOO
DETOX
DETRE
DETTE
DEUCE
DEUCY
DEUEL
DEUTO
DEVAS
DEVIL
DEVOL
DEVON
DEVRY
DEWAR
DEWAX
DEWED
DEWEY
DEXTR

D•E••
DCELL
DEEDS
DEEMS
DEEPS
DEERE
DEERS
DIECI

DIEGO DIELS DIEMS DIENE DIETE DIETS DIETZ DIEUX DNEPR DNETS DOERR DOERS DOEST DOETH DREAD DREAM DREAR DRECK DREDD DREFT DREGS DREKS DRESS DREWU DUEIN DUELS DUENA DUENO DUETO DUETS DUEUP DWEEB DWELL DWELT DYERS DYESS

D••E•

DACES DALEN DALES DALET DALEY DAMEN DAMES DANES DARED DARER DARES DATED DATER DATES DAVEN DAVES DAVEY DAWES DAZED DAZER DAZES DECEM DEFER DEGEL DEHEX DEKED DEKES DELED DELES DEMES DENEB DENES DEPEW DEREK DESEX DETER DEUEL DEWED DEWEY DICED DICER DICES DICEY DIGEL DIGEM DIKED DIKER DIKES DIMED DIMES DINED DINER DINES DIRER DIVED DIVER DIVES DIYER DOBEE DOCES DODEC DOGES DOKEY DOLED DOLES DOMED DOMES DONEE DONEN DOPED DOPER DOPES DOPEY DOREN DOSED DOSER DOSES DOTED DOTER DOTES DOVER DOVES DOVEY DOWEL DOYEN DOZED DOZEN DOZER DOZES DRIED DRIER DRIES DRYER DUCES DUDED DUDEK DUDES DUKED DUKES DUNES DUPED DUPER DUPES DUREN DURER DUVET DWEEB DYKER DYNEL DYNES

D•••E

DACHE DAFOE DAMME DANAE DANCE DANKE DANSE DANTE DARTE DAUBE DAVIE DAYNE DEANE DEARE DEBBE DEBYE DEERE DEFOE DEICE DELVE DEMME DENSE DENTE DESDE DESTE DETRE DETTE DEUCE DHOLE DHOTE DIANE DIENE DIETE DINGE DIODE DIONE DIRAE DIRGE DISME DIXIE DNASE DOANE DOBEE DOBIE DOBLE DODGE DODIE DOGIE DOLCE DONDE DONEE DONNE DOONE DOUCE DOUSE DOUTE DOUZE DOWSE DOXIE DOYCE DOYLE DRAKE DRAPE DRDRE DRIVE DROLE DROME DRONE DROVE DRUPE DRUSE DRUZE DTILE DUANE DUBHE DULCE DUNCE DUNNE DUPLE DUPRE

•DE••

ADEEM ADELA ADELE ADENI ADENO ADEPT ADEUX CDEFG EDEMA EDENS IDEAL IDEAS IDEES IDENT IDEST ODELL ODEON ODESA ODETS ODEUM

•D•E•

ADDED ADDER ADEEM ADFEE ADHEM ADIEU ADLER ADMEN ADREM ADREP ADZED ADZES EDGED EDGER EDGES EDIES EDRED EDSEL IDEES IDLED IDLER IDLES ODDER UDDER

•D••E

ADAGE ADDIE ADDLE ADELE ADFEE ADIGE ADOBE ADORE ADOZE EDDIE EDILE EDUCE ODILE UDINE

••DE•

ABDEL ADDED ADDER AEDES AIDED AIDER AIDES ALDEN ALDER ANDES ARDEN AUDEN BADEN BADER BCDEF BEDEW BIDED BIDEN BIDER BIDES BIDET BODED BODEL BODES CADET CEDED CEDER CEDES CIDER CODED CODER CODES CODEX CYDER DODEC DUDED DUDEK DUDES EIDER ELDER EMDEN ENDED ENDER FADED FADER FADES FEDEX FIDEL FIDES GODEL GODET GODEY HADES HIDEO HIDER HIDES HIDEY INDEF INDEX JADED JADES JUDEA JUDEO JUDES KIDEO KODEL KODES LADED LADEN LADER LADES LEDEE LEDER LODEN LODER LODES MEDEA MEDEE MEDES MODEL MODEM MODES NADER NODES NUDER NUDES ODDER OGDEN OLDEN OLDER ONDES ORDER PEDER RADER REDED REDES RIDER RIDES RODEO RUDEL RUDER RYDER SEDER SIDEA SIDEB SIDED SIDES TIDED TIDES UDDER UNDEC UNDER VADER VIDEO WADED WADER WADES WEDEL WIDEN WIDER WODEN YODEL

••D•E

ADDIE ADDLE ANDIE ANDRE AUDIE BADGE BUDGE CADGE CADRE DODGE DODIE DRDRE EADIE EDDIE ENDUE EYDIE FUDGE HEDGE INDIE INDRE INDUE JODIE JUDGE KEDGE LADLE LEDEE LEDGE LODGE MADGE MADRE MEDEE MIDGE NIDRE NUDGE OLDIE PADRE REDYE RIDGE RUDGE SADHE SADIE SEDGE SIDLE UNDUE WEDGE ZADIE

•••DE

AANDE ABCDE ABIDE ABODE AMIDE ANODE ASIDE AVIDE AZIDE BLADE BREDE BRIDE BSIDE CHIDE CLYDE CONDE CRUDE DESDE DIODE DONDE ELIDE ELUDE ÉPODE EREDE ERODE ETUDE EVADE EXUDE FERDE GARDE GEODE GLADE GLIDE GOLDE GOODE GRADE GRIDE GUIDE HORDE HYNDE IMIDE LAUDE LYNDE MAUDE MEADE MONDE NOLDE OXIDE PRIDE PRUDE READE RHODE RONDE SANDE SHADE SLADE SLIDE SNIDE SONDE SPADE SPODE STADE SUEDE SWEDE TARDE TILDE TRADE TSADE VERDE VLADE WILDE

DF•••

DFLAT

D•F••

DAFFY DAFOE DEFAT DEFER DEFGH DEFOE DEFOG DIFFS DOFFS DOFOR DUFAY DUFFY DUFUS DUFYS

D••F•

DAFFY DEIFY DELFT DIFFS DOFFS DORFF DRAFT DREFT DRIFT DUFFY

D•••F

DECAF DORFF DWARF

•DF••

ADFEE

•D•F•

CDEFG EDIFY

•D••F

ADOLF

••D•F

BCDEF INDEF RIDOF

•••DF

EGBDF

D•G••

DAGAN DEGAS DEGEL DEGUM DIGAT DIGBY DIGEL DIGEM DIGGS DIGIN DIGIT DIGUP DOGES DOGGO DOGGY DOGIE DOGIT DOGMA DOGON DUGAN DUGAT DUGIN DUGIT DUGUP

D••G•

DANGS DEFGH DEIGN DIEGO DIGGS DINGE DINGO DINGS DINGY DIRGE DODGE DODGY DOGGO DOGGY DONGS DOUGH DRAGO DRAGS DREGS DRIGO DRUGS

D•••G

DEBAG DEBUG DEFOG DHING DIMAG DOING DORAG DRANG DRHUG DRING DYING

•DG••

EDGAR EDGED EDGER EDGES

•D•G•

ADAGE ADIGE

•D••G

CDEFG IDING IDTAG ODING

••DG•

BADGE BLDGS BUDGE CADGE DODGE DODGY FUDGE HEDGE HEDGY JUDGE KEDGE LEDGE LEDGY LODGE MADGE MIDGE NUDGE PUDGY RIDGE RIDGY RUDGE SEDGE SEDGY WEDGE WEDGY

••D•G

BEDOG REDIG REDUG UNDUG ZADIG

•••DG

HARDG

DH•••

DHABI DHAKA DHALS DHING DHOLE DHOTE DHOTI DHOWS

D•H••

DEHEX DRHUG

D••H•

DACHA DACHE DASHI DASHY DELHI DICHO DISHY DONHO DRWHO DUBHE DUCHY

D•••H

DABIH DARTH DEATH DEFGH DENCH DEPTH DINAH DITCH DOETH DOLPH DOUGH DUTCH

•DH••

ADHEM ADHOC

•D•H•

IDAHO

•D••H

EDITH

••DH•

SADHE SADHU YODHS

••D•H

JUDAH NODUH NUDZH WIDTH

•••DH

SANDH

DI•••

DIALO DIALS DIAMS DIANA DIANE DIARY DICED DICER DICES DICEY DICHO DICKS DICKY DICOT DICTA DICTS DICTU DIDBY DIDIN DIDIT DIDNT DIDOK DIDOS DIDSO DIDST DIDTO DIDUP DIECI DIEGO DIELS DIEMS DIENE DIETE DIETS DIETZ DIEUX DIFFS DIGAT DIGBY DIGEL DIGEM DIGGS DIGIN DIGIT DIGUP DIJON DIKED DIKER DIKES DILLS DILLY DIMAG DIMAS DIMED DIMES DIMIN DIMLY DINAH DINAR DINDY DINED DINER DINES DINGE DINGO DINGS DINGY DINKA DINKS DINKY DINNY DINOS DINTS DINTY DIODE DIONE DIORS DIPIN DIPLO DIPPY DIPSO DIPSY DIRAC DIRAE DIRAM DIRER DIRGE DIRKS DIRTS DIRTY DISCI DISCO DISCS DISHY DISKO DISKS DISME DISTS DITAT DITCH DITKA DITSY DITTO DITTY DITZY DIVAC DIVAN DIVAS DIVED DIVER DIVES DIVOT DIVVY DIXIE DIXIT DIXON DIYER DIZZY

D•I••

DAILY DAIRY DAISY DAIWA DCIII DEICE DEIFY DEIGN DEILS DEION DEISM DEIST DEITY DHING DJINN DJINS DLIII DOIDO DOILY DOING DOISY DOITS DRIAM DRIBS DRIED DRIER DRIES DRIFT DRIGO DRILL DRILY DRINA DRING DRINK DRIPS DRIVE DTILE DUINO DVIII DVINA DXIII DYING

D••I•

DABIH DACIA DALIS DAMIS DANIA DANIO DARIA DARIN DARIO DAVID DAVIE DAVIS DAVIT DCCII DCCIV DCCIX DCIII DCLII DCLIV DCLIX DCVII DCXII DCXIV DCXIX DEAIR DEBIT DECIR DELIA DELIS DEMIT DENIM DENIS DERIV DEVIL DIDIN DIDIT DIGIN DIGIT DIMIN DIPIN DIXIE DIXIT DLIII DLVII DLXII DLXIV DLXIX DOBIE DODIE DOGIE DOGIT DOLIN DORIA DORIC DORIS DOXIE DRAIN DROID DROIT DRUID DUBIN DUEIN DUGIN DUGIT DUPIN DVIII DXCII DXCIV DXCIX DXIII DXLII DXLIV DXLIX DXVII DXXII DXXIV DXXIX

D•••I

DALAI DARCI DASHI DCCCI DCCII DCCLI DCCVI DCCXI DCIII DCLII DCLVI DCLXI DCVII DCXCI DCXII DCXLI DCXVI DCXXI DEBBI DELHI DENTI DESAI DHABI DHOTI DIECI DISCI DLIII DLVII DLXII DLXVI DLXXI DOLCI DONDI DORSI DOUAI DUBAI DUOMI DVIII DXCII DXCVI DXIII DXLII DXLVI DXVII DXXII DXXVI DXXXI

•DI••

ADIEU ADIGE ADINS ADIOS ADITS CDIII EDICT EDIES EDIFY EDILE EDINA EDIPO EDITH EDITS IDING IDIOM IDIOT MDIII ODILE ODING ODIST ODIUM UDINE

•D•I•

ADAIR ADBIZ ADDIE ADDIN ADDIO ADDIS ADLIB ADMIN ADMIT ADMIX ADRIP ADVIL CDIII CDLII CDLIV CDLIX CDVII CDXII CDXIV CDXIX EDDIC EDDIE EDWIN MDCII MDCIV MDCIX MDIII MDLII MDLIV MDLIX MDVII MDXII MDXIV MDXIX

•D••I

ADENI ADLAI CDIII CDLII CDLVI CDLXI CDVII CDXCI CDXII CDXLI CDXVI CDXXI MDCCI MDCII MDCLI MDCVI MDCXI MDIII MDLII MDLVI MDLXI MDVII MDXCI MDXII MDXLI MDXVI MDXXI

••DI•
ADDIE ADDIN ADDIO ADDIS ANDIE ASDIC AUDIE AUDIO AUDIS AUDIT BEDIM BIDIN CADIS CADIZ CEDIS DIDIN DIDIT DODIE EADIE EDDIC EDDIE ELDIN ENDIN ENDIT EXDIV EYDIE FEDIN FTDIX HADIN HADIT HEDIN INDIA INDIC INDIE INDIO INDIV IODIC JODIE JUDIT LEDIN LUDIC LYDIA MCDII MCDIV MCDIX MEDIA MEDIC MEDII MEDIO MEDIT MIDIS MMDII MMDIV MMDIX NADIA NADIR NYDIA OLDIE ONDIT PODIA RADII RADIO RADIX REDID REDIG REDIP RODIN SADIE UNDID UNDIM VADIM VADIS VEDIC WADIS XEDIN YADIM ZADIE ZADIG

••D•I
GADDI HADJI MCDII MCDLI MCDVI MCDXI MEDII MMDCI MMDII MMDLI MMDVI MMDXI RADII REDDI SODOI

•••DI
BONDI CARDI CAUDI CONDI CYNDI DONDI EGADI FENDI FUADI GADDI GAUDI HANDI HEIDI HINDI JEUDI LANDI LUNDI MAHDI MARDI MMCDI MMMDI MUNDI NALDI RANDI REDDI SARDI SAUDI SOLDI TONDI TSADI VERDI

DJ•••
DJINN DJINS DJUNA

D•J••
DIJON DOJOS

•DJ••
ADJTS

••DJ•
HADJI NADJA

•••DJ
JANDJ

D•K••
DAKAR DEKED DEKES DEKKO DIKED DIKER DIKES DOKEY DUKAS DUKED DUKES DYKER

D••K•
DANKE DARKS DECKS DEKKO DESKS DHAKA DICKS DICKY DINKA DINKS DINKY DIRKS DISKO DISKS DITKA DOCKS DORKS DORKY DRAKE DREKS DUCKS DUCKY DUNKS DUSKS DUSKY

D•••K
DBACK DEREK DIDOK DMARK DRANK DRECK DRINK DRUNK DUDEK

•D••K
ADAOK

••DK•
VODKA

••D•K
DIDOK DUDEK KODAK

DL•••
DLIII DLVII DLXII DLXIV DLXIX DLXVI DLXXI DLXXV DLXXX

D•L••
DALAI DALEN DALES DALET DALEY DALIS DALLY DCLII DCLIV DCLIX DCLVI DCLXI DCLXV DCLXX DELAY DELCO DELED DELES DELFT DELHI DELIA DELIS DELLA DELLO DELLS DELON DELOS DELPY DELTA DELTS DELVE DFLAT DILLS DILLY DOLBY DOLCE DOLCI DOLED DOLES DOLIN DOLLS DOLLY DOLMA DOLON DOLOR DOLPH DOLTS DPLUS DRLAO DULCE DULLS DULLY DXLII DXLIV DXLIX DXLVI DYLAN

D••L•
DAILY DALLY DARLA DCCLI DCCLV DCCLX DCELL DCXLI DCXLV DEALS DEALT DEILS DELLA DELLO DELLS DHALS DHOLE DIALO DIALS DIELS DILLS DILLY DIMLY DIPLO DOALL DOBLE DOILY DOLLS DOLLY DOULA DOYLE DOYLY DRILL DRILY DROLE DROLL DRYLY DTILE DUALS DUELS DULLS DULLY DUPLE DUPLO DWELL DWELT

D•••L
DARYL DCCCL DCCXL DCELL DECAL DEGEL DEUEL DEVIL DEVOL DIGEL DOALL DORAL DOTAL DOWEL DRAWL DRILL DROLL DROOL DUCAL DUVAL DWELL DYNEL

•DL••
ADLAI ADLER ADLIB CDLII CDLIV CDLIX CDLVI CDLXI CDLXV CDLXX IDLED IDLER IDLES MDLII MDLIV MDLIX MDLVI MDLXI MDLXV MDLXX

•D•L•
ADDLE ADELA ADELE ADOLF ADULT CDXLI CDXLV EDILE IDOLA IDOLS IDYLL IDYLS MDCLI MDCLV MDCLX MDXLI MDXLV ODDLY ODELL ODILE UDALL

•D••L
ADDNL ADVIL EDSEL IDEAL IDYLL MDCCL MDCXL ODELL ODOUL UDALL

••DL•
ADDLE BADLY GODLY LADLE MADLY MCDLI MCDLV MCDLX MMDLI MMDLV MMDLX ODDLY REDLY SADLY SIDLE

••D•L
ABDEL ABDUL ADDNL BODEL FIDEL GODEL KODEL LADYL MCDXL MEDAL MMDCL MMDXL MODAL MODEL NODAL OIDAL PEDAL PODAL RUDEL TIDAL VIDAL WEDEL YODEL

•••DL
LENDL MMCDL MMMDL PANDL PRNDL SANDL

DM•••
DMARK

D•M••
DAMAS DAMEN DAMES DAMIS DAMME DAMNS DAMON DAMPS DAMUP DEMES DEMIT DEMME DEMOB DEMON DEMOS DEMUR DIMAG DIMAS DIMED DIMES DIMIN DIMLY DOMED DOMES DOMOS DUMAS DUMBO DUMBS DUMMY DUMPS DUMPY

D••M•
DAMME DEEMS DEMME DERMA DERMO DIAMS DIEMS DISME DOGMA DOLMA DOOMS DOOMY DORMS DORMY DRAMA DRAMS DROME DRUMS DUMMY DUOMI DUOMO

D•••M
DATUM DECEM DEGUM DEISM DENIM DENOM DIGEM DIRAM DREAM DRIAM DURUM

•DM••
ADMAN ADMEN ADMIN ADMIT ADMIX EDMAR

•D•M•
ADAMA ADAMS EDAMS EDEMA

•D••M
ADEEM ADHEM ADREM CDROM IDIOM ODEUM ODIUM

••D•M
BEDIM MADAM MODEM SEDUM SODOM UNDAM UNDIM VADIM YADIM

•••DM
AANDM

DN•••
DNASE DNEPR DNETS

D•N••
DANAE DANCE DANDD DANDY DANES DANGS DANIA DANIO DANKE DANNO DANNY DANSE DANTE DANZA DENAR DENCH DENDR DENEB DENES DENIM DENIS DENNY DENOM DENSE DENTE DENTI DENTO DENTS DENYS DINAH DINAR DINDY DINED DINER DINES DINGE DINGO DINGS DINGY DINKA DINKS DINKY DINNY DINOS DINTS DINTY DONAS DONAT DONAU DONDE DONDI DONEE DONEN DONGS DONHO DONNA DONNE DONNY DONOR DONOT DONOW DONTS DONUS DONUT DUNCE DUNES DUNKS DUNNE DUNNO DUNST DYNEL DYNES

D••N•
DAMNS DANNO DANNY DARNS DASNT DAUNT DAWNN DAWNS DAYNE DEANA DEANE DEANS DENNY DESNA DHING DIANA DIANE DIDNT DIENE DINNY DIONE DJINN DJINS DJUNA DOANE DOANS DOING DONNA DONNE DONNY DOONE DOWNS DOWNY DRANG DRANK DRANO DRINA DRING DRINK DRONE DRUNK DUANE DUENA DUENO DUINO DUNNE DUNNO DURNS DVINA DYING

D•••N
DABON DAGAN DALEN DAMEN DAMON DARIN DAVEN DAWNN DAYAN DEIGN DEION DELON DEMON DEVON DIDIN DIGIN DIJON DIMIN DIPIN DIVAN DIXON DJINN DOGON DOLIN DOLON DONEN DOORN DORAN DOREN DOYEN DOZEN DRAIN DRAWN DROWN DRUON DUBIN DUEIN DUGAN DUGIN DUPIN DURAN DUREN DYLAN DYSON

•DN••
ADNAN

•D•N•
ADANA ADANO ADDNL ADENI ADENO ADINS EDENS EDINA IDENT IDING IDONT ODING ODONT UDINE

•D••N
ADARN ADDIN ADDON ADMAN ADMEN ADMIN ADNAN ADORN EDSON EDWIN ODEON

••DN•
ADDNL BEDNY DIDNT HADNO HADNT

••D•N
ADDIN ADDON AIDAN ALDEN ARDEN AUDEN BADEN BADUN BIDEN BIDIN BIDON CODON DIDIN EGDON ELDIN ELDON EMDEN ENDIN ENDON FEDIN FEDON HADIN HADON HEDIN LADEN LEDIN LEDON LODEN LYDON MIDON OGDEN OLDEN RADON REDAN REDON RODAN RODIN SEDAN SIDON SUDAN WIDEN WODEN XEDIN

•••DN
HAYDN

DO•••
DOALL DOANE DOANS DOATS DOBAD DOBBS DOBEE DOBIE DOBLE DOBRO DOCES DOCKS DODEC DODGE DODGY DODIE DODOS DOERR DOERS DOEST DOETH DOFFS DOFOR DOGES DOGGO DOGGY DOGIE DOGIT DOGMA DOGON DOIDO DOILY DOING DOISY DOITS DOJOS DOKEY DOLBY DOLCE DOLCI DOLED DOLES DOLIN DOLLS DOLLY DOLMA DOLON DOLOR DOLPH DOLTS DOMED DOMES DOMOS DONAS DONAT DONAU DONDE DONDI DONEE DONEN DONGS DONHO DONNA DONNE DONNY DONOR DONOT DONOW DONTS DONUS DONUT DOODY DOOMS DOOMY DOONE DOORN DOORS DOOZY DOPAS DOPED DOPER DOPES DOPEY DORAG DORAL DORAN DOREN DORFF DORIA DORIC DORIS DORKS DORKY DORMS DORMY DORPS DORSA DORSI DORSO DOSAY DOSED DOSER DOSES DOTAL DOTED DOTER DOTES DOTTO DOTTY DOUAI DOUAY DOUBS DOUBT DOUCE DOUGH DOULA DOURO DOUSE DOUTE DOUZE DOVER DOVES DOVEY DOWDY DOWEL DOWNS DOWNY DOWRY DOWSE DOXIE DOYCE DOYEN DOYLE DOYLY DOZED DOZEN DOZER DOZES

D•O••
DEOXY DHOLE DHOTE DHOTI DHOWS DIODE DIONE DIORS DOODY DOOMS DOOMY DOONE DOORN DOORS DOOZY DROID DROIT DROLE DROLL DROME DRONE DROOD DROOL DROOP DROPO DROPS DROPT DROSS DROVE DROWN DUOMI DUOMO

D••O•
DABON DADOS DAFOE DAMON DATOS DAVOS DECOR DECOY DEDOS DEFOE DEFOG DEION DELON DELOS DEMOB DEMON DEMOS DENOM DEPOT DESOD DETOO DETOX DEVOL DEVON DICOT DIDOK DIDOS DIJON DINOS DIVOT DIXON DODOS DOFOR DOGON DOJOS DOLON DOLOR DOMOS DONOR DONOT DONOW DROOD DROOL DROOP DRUON DUROC DUROS DYSON

D•••O
DANIO DANNO DARIO DAVAO DEKKO DELCO DELLO DENTO DERMO DETOO DEUTO DIALO DICHO DIDSO DIDTO DIEGO DINGO DIPLO DIPSO DISCO DISKO DITTO DOBRO DOGGO DOIDO DONHO DORSO DOTTO DOURO DRACO DRAGO DRANO DRIGO DRLAO DROPO DRWHO DUENO DUETO DUINO DUMBO DUNNO DUOMO DUPLO

•DO••
ADOBE ADOBO ADOLF ADOPT ADORE ADORN ADOUT ADOZE IDOLA IDOLS IDONT LDOPA ODONT ODORS ODOUL ODOUR XDOUT

•D•O•
ADAOK ADDON ADHOC ADIOS CDROM EDSON IDIOM IDIOT ODEON

•D••O
ADANO ADDIO ADDTO ADENO ADOBO EDIPO IDAHO

••DO•
ADDON AIDOO ANDOR ARDOR BEDOG BIDON CODON DADOS DEDOS DIDOK DIDOS DODOS

5 DO

EGDON ELDON ENDON ENDOR ENDOW ERDOS FADOS FEDON FODOR GODOT HADON JUDOS KUDOS LEDON LIDOS LYDON MADOC MADOX MEDOC MIDON MSDOS NODOZ RADON REDON REDOS REDOX RIDOF SIDON SODOI SODOM SYDOW TODOS TUDOR UPDOS VIDOR WIDOW

••D•O

ADDIO ADDTO AIDOO ANDRO ANDSO AUDIO DIDSO DIDTO FEDTO HADNO HADTO HIDEO HYDRO INDIO JUDEO KIDDO KIDEO LEDTO MEDIO NODTO PEDRO RADIO RODEO VIDEO WEDTO

•••DO

ALADO AMADO ARADO BANDO BIGDO CANDO CAUDO CONDO CREDO DOIDO EJIDO FALDO FORDO FREDO FRODO GORDO GUIDO HONDO HOWDO IRIDO KENDO KIDDO LANDO LINDO MISDO MONDO NARDO NOTDO OUTDO PARDO PRADO RHODO RONDO SOLDO TARDO TONDO WALDO XANDO ZENDO

DP•••

DPLUS

D•P••

DEPEW DEPOT DEPTH DEPTS DIPIN DIPLO DIPPY DIPSO DIPSY DOPAS DOPED DOPER DOPES DOPEY DUPED DUPER DUPES DUPIN DUPLE DUPLO DUPRE

D••P•

DAMPS DCUPS DEEPS DELPY DIPPY DNEPR DOLPH DORPS DRAPE DRIPS DROPO DROPS DROPT DRUPE DUMPS DUMPY

D•••P

DAMUP DECAP DIDUP DIGUP DROOP DRYUP DUEUP DUGUP

•D•P•

ADAPT ADEPT ADOPT EDIPO LDOPA

•D••P

ADDUP ADREP ADRIP

••D•P

ADDUP ANDUP BIDUP DIDUP ENDUP FEDUP HADUP REDIP WADUP

•••DP

AANDP SANDP

DR•••

DRABS DRACO DRAFT DRAGO DRAGS DRAIN DRAKE DRAMA DRAMS DRANG DRANK DRANO DRAPE DRATS DRAVA DRAWL DRAWN DRAWS DRAYS DRDRE DREAD DREAM DREAR DRECK DREDD DREFT DREGS DREKS DRESS DREWU DRHUG DRIAM DRIBS DRIED DRIER DRIES DRIFT DRIGO DRILL DRILY DRINA DRING DRINK DRIPS DRIVE DRLAO DROID DROIT DROLE DROLL DROME DRONE DROOD DROOL DROOP DROPO DROPS DROPT DROSS DROVE DROWN DRUBS DRUGS DRUID DRUMS DRUNK DRUON DRUPE DRURY DRUSE DRUZE DRWHO DRYAD DRYER DRYLY DRYUP

D•R••

DARBY DARCI DARCY DARDY DARED DARER DARES DARIA DARIN DARIO DARKS DARLA DARNS DARTE DARTH DARTS DARYA DARYL DERAT DERBY DEREK DERIV DERMA DERMO DERRY DIRAC DIRAE DIRAM DIRER DIRGE DIRKS DIRTS DIRTY DORAG DORAL DORAN DOREN DORFF DORIA DORIC DORIS DORKS DORKY DORMS DORMY DORPS DORSA DORSI DORSO DURAN DURAS DUREN DURER DURNS DUROC DUROS DURRA DURST DURUM

D••R•

DAIRY DEARE DEARS DEARY DEBRA DECRY DEERE DEERS DERRY DETRE DEVRY DIARY DIORS DMARK DOBRO DOERR DOERS DOORN DOORS DOURO DOWRY DRDRE DRURY DUPRE DURRA DWARF DYERS

D•••R

DAKAR DARER DATER DAZER DAZUR DEAIR DEBAR DECIR DECOR DEFER DEMUR DENAR DENDR DETAR DETER DEWAR DEXTR DICER DIKER DINAR DINER DIRER DIVER DIYER DNEPR DOERR DOFOR DOLOR DONOR DOPER DOSER DOTER DOVER DOZER DREAR DRIER DRYER DUPER DURER DYKER

•DR••

ADREM ADREP ADRIP CDROM EDRED

•D•R•

ADARN ADARS ADDRS ADORE ADORN ODORS

•D••R

ADAIR ADDER ADLER ADWAR EDGAR EDGER EDMAR IDLER ODDER ODOUR UDDER

••DR•

ADDRS ANDRE ANDRO ANDRY ASDRY AUDRA CADRE CMDRS DRDRE HYDRA HYDRO INDRA INDRE MADRE NEDRA NIDRE PADRE PEDRO REDRY UNDRY UPDRY

••D•R

ADDER AIDER ALDER ANDOR ARDOR BADER BIDER CEDAR CEDER CIDER CODER CYDER EIDER ELDER ENDER ENDOR FADER FODOR HIDER KADAR LADER LEDER LIDAR LODER NADER NADIR NUDER ODDER OLDER ORDER PEDER RADAR RADER RIDER RUDER RYDER SEDER TUDOR UDDER UNDER VADER VIDOR WADER WIDER ZADAR

•••DR

COMDR DENDR QUADR RANDR

D•S••

DASHI DASHY DASNT DESAI DESDE DESEX DESKS DESNA DESOD DESTE DISCI DISCO DISCS DISHY DISKO DISKS DISME DISTS DOSAY DOSED DOSER DOSES DUSKS DUSKY DUSTS DUSTY DYSON

D••S•

DAISY DANSE DEISM DEIST DENSE DIDSO DIDST DIPSO DIPSY DITSY DNASE DOEST DOISY DORSA DORSI DORSO DOUSE DOWSE DRESS DROSS DRUSE DUNST DURST DYESS

D•••S

DACES DADAS DADOS DALES DALIS DAMAS DAMES DAMIS DAMNS DAMPS DANES DANGS DARES DARKS DARNS DARTS DATES DATOS DAUBS DAVES DAVIS DAVOS DAWES DAWNS DAZES DCUPS DDAYS DEALS DEANS DEARS DEBTS DEBUS DECKS DEDOS DEEDS DEEMS DEEPS DEERS DEGAS DEILS DEKES DELES DELIS DELLS DELOS DELTS DEMES DEMOS DENES DENIS DENTS DENYS DEPTS DESKS DEVAS DHALS DHOWS DIALS DIAMS DICES DICKS DICTS DIDOS DIELS DIEMS DIETS DIFFS DIGGS DIKES DILLS DIMAS DIMES DINES DINGS DINKS DINOS DINTS DIORS DIRKS DIRTS DISCS DISKS DISTS DIVAS DIVES DJINS DNETS DOANS DOATS DOBBS DOCES DOCKS DODOS DOERS DOFFS DOGES DOITS DOJOS DOLES DOLLS DOLTS DOMES DOMOS DONAS DONGS DONTS DONUS DOOMS DOORS DOPAS DOPES DORIS DORKS DORMS DORPS DOSES DOTES DOUBS DOVES DOWNS DOZES DPLUS DRABS DRAGS DRAMS DRATS DRAWS DRAYS DREGS DREKS DRESS DRIBS DRIES DRIPS DROPS DROSS DRUBS DRUGS DRUMS DUADS DUALS DUCES DUCKS DUCTS DUDES DUELS DUETS DUFUS DUFYS DUKAS DUKES DULLS DUMAS DUMBS DUMPS DUNES DUNKS DUPES DURAS DURNS DUROS DUSKS DUSTS DYADS DYERS DYESS DYNES

•DS••

EDSEL EDSON

•D•S•

ADUST IDEST ODESA ODIST

•D••S

ADAMS ADARS ADDIS ADDRS ADINS ADIOS ADITS ADJTS ADZES BDAYS DDAYS EDAMS EDDAS EDENS EDGES EDIES EDITS HDTVS IDEAS IDEES IDLES IDOLS IDYLS ODETS ODORS VDAYS

••DS•

ANDSO DIDSO DIDST HADST MIDST SUDSY

••D•S

ADDIS ADDRS AEDES AIDES ANDES ANDYS AUDIS BIDES BLDGS BODES CADIS CEDES CEDIS CMDRS CODAS CODES DADAS DADOS DEDOS DIDOS DODOS DUDES EDDAS ERDOS FADES FADOS FIDES HADES HIDES INDUS INDYS JADES JUDAS JUDDS JUDES JUDOS KODES KUDOS KUDUS LADAS LADES LADYS LIDOS LODES MEDES MIDAS MIDIS MODES MODUS MSDOS NIDUS NODES NODUS NUDES ONDAS ONDES REDES REDOS RIDES SIDES SODAS TADAS TIDES TODOS UPDOS VADIS VEDAS VIDAS WADES WADIS YODHS

•••DS

ACADS ACIDS APODS BALDS BANDS BARDS BAUDS BEADS BENDS BINDS BIRDS BLVDS BOLDS BONDS BRADS BUNDS BYRDS CARDS CHADS CLADS CLODS COEDS COLDS CONDS CORDS CREDS CRUDS CURDS CUYDS DEEDS DUADS DYADS EGADS FEEDS FENDS FEUDS FINDS FOLDS FOODS FORDS FUNDS GAUDS GELDS GILDS GIRDS GLADS GOADS GOLDS GOODS GRADS GRIDS HANDS HEADS HEEDS HERDS HINDS HOLDS HOODS IPODS IRIDS IZODS JOADS JUDDS KINDS KURDS LANDS LARDS LAUDS LEADS LEEDS LENDS LOADS LOIDS LORDS MAIDS MEADS MELDS MENDS MINDS MOLDS MOODS NARDS NEEDS NERDS OPEDS PARDS PENDS PIEDS PLODS PONDS PRODS QAIDS QUADS QUIDS RAIDS RANDS READS REEDS RENDS RINDS ROADS ROODS SANDS SARDS SCADS SCUDS SEEDS SENDS SHADS SHEDS SKEDS SKIDS SLEDS SPADS SPUDS STADS STUDS SYNDS TENDS THUDS TOADS TVADS VELDS VENDS VOIDS WANDS WARDS WEEDS WELDS WENDS WILDS WINDS WOADS WOODS WORDS YARDS ZENDS

DT•••

DTILE

D•T••

DATED DATER DATES DATOS DATUM DETAR DETAT DETER DETOO DETOX DETRE DETTE DITAT DITCH DITKA DITSY DITTO DITTY DITZY DOTAL DOTED DOTER DOTES DOTTO DOTTY DUTCH

D••T•

DANTE DARTE DARTH DARTS DEATH DEBTS DEITY DELTA DELTS DENTE DENTI DENTO DENTS DEPTH DEPTS DESTE DETTE DEUTO DEXTR DHOTE DHOTI DICTA DICTS DICTU DIDTO DIETE DIETS DIETZ DINTS DINTY DIRTS DIRTY DISTS DITTO DITTY DNETS DOATS DOETH DOITS DOLTS DONTS DOTTO DOTTY DOUTE DRATS DUCTS DUETO DUETS DUSTS DUSTY

D•••T

DABAT DALET DASNT DAUNT DAVIT DEALT DEBIT DEBUT DEFAT DEIST DELFT DEMIT DEPOT DERAT DETAT DFLAT DICOT DIDIT DIDNT DIDST DIGAT DIGIT DITAT DIVOT DIXIT DOEST DOGIT DONAT DONOT DONUT DOUBT DRAFT DREFT DRIFT DROIT DROPT DUCAT DUGAT DUGIT DUNST DURST DUVET DWELT

•DT••

HDTVS IDTAG

•D•T•

ADDTO ADITS ADJTS ADYTA EDITH EDITS ODETS

•D••T

ADAPT ADEPT ADMIT ADOPT ADOUT ADULT ADUST EDICT EDUCT IDENT IDEST IDIOT IDONT ODIST ODONT XDOUT

••DT•

ADDTO DIDTO FEDTO HADTO LEDTO MADTV NODTO WEDTO WIDTH

••D•T

AUDIT BADAT BIDET

CADET DIDIT DIDNT DIDST ENDAT ENDIT GODET GODOT HADAT HADIT HADNT HADST JUDIT MADAT MEDIT MIDST NODAT ONDIT SADAT

•••DT
BUNDT GANDT HEIDT LINDT STADT VEIDT VELDT WENDT WUNDT

DU•••
DUADS DUALS DUANE DUBAI DUBHE DUBIN DUBYA DUCAL DUCAT DUCES DUCHY DUCKS DUCKY DUCTS DUDDY DUDED DUDEK DUDES DUEIN DUELS DUENA DUENO DUETO DUETS DUEUP DUFAY DUFFY DUFUS DUFYS DUGAN DUGAT DUGIN DUGIT DUGUP DUINO DUKAS DUKED DUKES DULCE DULLS DULLY DUMAS DUMBO DUMBS DUMMY DUMPS DUMPY DUNCE DUNES DUNKS DUNNE DUNNO DUNST DUOMI DUOMO DUPED DUPER DUPES DUPIN DUPLE DUPLO DUPRE DURAN DURAS DUREN DURER DURNS DUROC DUROS DURRA DURST DURUM DUSKS DUSKY DUSTS DUSTY DUTCH DUVAL DUVET

D•U••
DAUBE DAUBS DAUNT DCUPS DEUCE DEUCY DEUEL DEUTO DJUNA DOUAI DOUAY DOUBS DOUBT DOUCE DOUGH DOULA DOURO DOUSE DOUTE DOUZE DRUBS DRUGS DRUID DRUMS DRUNK DRUON DRUPE DRURY DRUSE DRUZE

D••U•
DAMUP DATUM DAZUR DEBUG DEBUS DEBUT DEGUM DEMUR DIDUP DIEUX DIGUP DONUS DONUT DPLUS DRHUG DRYUP DUEUP DUFUS DUGUP DURUM

D•••U
DICTU DONAU DREWU

•DU••
ADULT ADUST EDUCE EDUCT

•D•U•
ADDUP ADEUX ADOUT ODEUM ODIUM ODOUL ODOUR XDOUT

•D••U
ADIEU

••DU•
ABDUL ADDUP ANDUP BADUN BIDUP DIDUP ENDUE ENDUP FEDUP HADUP INDUE INDUS KUDUS MODUS NIDUS NODUH NODUS PADUA REDUB REDUG REDUX SEDUM UNDUE UNDUG VADUZ WADUP

••D•U
KUDZU SADHU

•••DU
FONDU HINDU PERDU TENDU

DV•••
DVIII DVINA

D•V••
DAVAO DAVEN DAVES DAVEY DAVID DAVIE DAVIS DAVIT DAVOS DCVII DEVAS DEVIL DEVOL DEVON DEVRY DIVAC DIVAN DIVAS DIVED DIVER DIVES DIVOT DIVVY DLVII DOVER DOVES DOVEY DUVAL DUVET DXVII

D••V•
DCCVI DCLVI DCXVI DELVE DIVVY DLXVI DRAVA DRIVE DROVE DXCVI DXLVI DXXVI

D•••V
DCCCV DCCIV DCCLV DCCXV DCLIV DCLXV DCXCV DCXIV DCXLV DCXXV DERIV DLXIV DLXXV DXCIV DXLIV DXXIV DXXXV

•DV••
ADVIL CDVII MDVII

•D•V•
CDLVI CDXVI HDTVS MDCVI MDLVI MDXVI

•D••V
CDLIV CDLXV CDXCV CDXIV CDXLV CDXXV MDCCV MDCIV MDCLV MDCXV MDLIV MDLXV MDXCV MDXIV MDXLV MDXXV

••DV•
MCDVI MMDVI ONDVD TVDVD

••D•V
EXDIV INDIV MADTV MCDIV MCDLV MCDXV MMDCV MMDIV MMDLV MMDXV

•••DV
MMCDV MMMDV

DW•••
DWARF DWEEB DWELL DWELT

D•W••
DAWES DAWNN DAWNS DEWAR DEWAX DEWED DEWEY DOWDY DOWEL DOWNS DOWNY DOWRY DOWSE DRWHO

D••W•
DAIWA DHOWS DRAWL DRAWN DRAWS DREWU DROWN

D•••W
DEPEW DONOW

•DW••
ADWAR EDWIN

••D•W
BEDEW ENDOW SYDOW WIDOW

•••DW
AANDW BANDW CANDW

DX•••
DXCII DXCIV DXCIX DXCVI DXIII DXLII DXLIV DXLIX DXLVI DXVII DXXII DXXIV DXXIX DXXVI DXXXI DXXXV

D•X••
DCXCI DCXCV DCXII DCXIV DCXIX DCXLI DCXLV DCXVI DCXXI DCXXV DCXXX DEXTR DIXIE DIXIT DIXON DLXII DLXIV DLXIX DLXVI DLXXI DLXXV DLXXX DOXIE DXXII DXXIV DXXIX DXXVI DXXXI DXXXV

D••X•
DCCXC DCCXI DCCXL DCCXV DCCXX DCLXI DCLXV DCLXX DCXXI DCXXV DCXXX DEOXY DLXXI DLXXV DLXXX DXXXI DXXXV

D•••X
DCCCX DCCIX DCCLX DCCXX DCLIX DCLXX DCXIX DCXXV DEHEX DESEX DETOX DEWAX DIEUX DLXIX DLXXX DXCIX DXLIX DXXIX

•DX••
CDXCI CDXCV CDXII CDXIV CDXIX CDXLI CDXLV CDXVI CDXXI CDXXV CDXXX MDXCI MDXCV MDXII MDXIV MDXIX MDXLI MDXLV MDXVI MDXXI MDXXV MDXXX

•D•X•
CDLXI CDLXV CDLXX CDXXI CDXXV CDXXX MDCXC MDCXI MDCXL MDCXV MDCXX MDLXI MDLXV MDLXX MDXXI MDXXV MDXXX

•D••X
ADDAX ADEUX ADMIX CDLIX CDLXX CDXIX CDXXX MDCCX MDCIX MDCLX MDCXX MDLIX MDLXX MDXIX MDXXX

••DX•
MCDXC MCDXI MCDXL MCDXV MCDXX MMDXC MMDXI MMDXL MMDXV MMDXX

••D•X
ADDAX CODEX FEDEX FTDIX INDEX MADOX MCDIX MCDLX MCDXX MMDCX MMDIX MMDLX MMDXX RADIX REDOX REDUX

•••DX
MMCDX MMMDX

DY•••
DYADS DYERS DYESS DYING DYKER DYLAN DYNEL DYNES DYSON

D•Y••
DAYAN DAYNE DIYER DOYCE DOYEN DOYLE DOYLY DRYAD DRYER DRYLY DRYUP

D••Y•
DARYA DARYL DDAYS DEBYE DENYS DRAYS DUBYA DUFYS

D•••Y
DADDY DAFFY DAILY DAIRY DAISY DALEY DALLY DANDY DANNY DARBY DARCY DARDY DASHY DAVEY DAZZY DEARY DEBBY DECAY DECOY DECRY DEIFY DEITY DELAY DELPY DENNY DEOXY DERBY DERRY DEUCY DEVRY DEWEY DIARY DICEY DICKY DIDBY DIGBY DILLY DIMLY DINDY DINGY DINKY DINNY DINTY DIPPY DIPSY DIRTY DISHY DITSY DITTY DITZY DIVVY DIZZY DODGY DOGGY DOILY DOISY DOKEY DOLBY DOLLY DONNY DOODY DOOMY DOOZY DOPEY DORKY DORMY DOSAY DOTTY DOUAY DOVEY DOWDY DOWNY DOWRY DOYLY DRILY DRURY DRYLY DUCHY DUCKY DUDDY DUFAY DUFFY DULLY DUMMY DUMPY DUSKY DUSTY

•DY••
ADYTA IDYLL IDYLS

•D•Y•
BDAYS DDAYS VDAYS

•D••Y
EDIFY ODDLY

••DY•
ANDYS INDYS LADYL LADYS REDYE RODYA

••D•Y
ANDRY ASDRY BADDY BADLY BEDDY BEDNY BIDDY BODDY BUDDY CADDY CUDDY DADDY DIDBY DODGY DUDDY FADDY FUDDY GIDDY GODEY GODLY HEDGY HIDEY KIDDY LEDGY LIDDY MADLY MIDDY MUDDY MYDAY NODDY ODDLY PADDY PUDDY PUDGY REDDY REDLY REDRY RIDGY RODDY RUDDY SADLY SEDGY SODDY SUDSY TEDDY TODAY TODDY UNDAY UNDRY UPDRY VEDAY VJDAY WEDGY

•••DY
ACIDY BADDY BALDY BANDY BAWDY BEADY BEDDY BENDY BIDDY BIRDY BODDY BRADY BRODY BUDDY BUNDY CADDY CANDY CINDY COODY CUDDY CURDY DADDY DANDY DARDY DINDY DOODY DOWDY DUDDY FADDY FUDDY FUNDY GANDY GAUDY GIDDY GOODY GORDY GOUDY GOWDY GRODY GURDY HANDY HARDY HEADY HOODY HOWDY HURDY KANDY KIDDY LARDY LEADY LIDDY LINDY LORDY LUNDY MANDY MIDDY MINDY MOLDY MOODY MTIDY MUDDY NEEDY NERDY NODDY PADDY PUDDY PURDY RANDY READY REDDY REEDY RHODY RINDY RODDY ROWDY RUDDY SANDY SEEDY SHADY SODDY STUDY TANDY TARDY TEDDY TOADY TODDY TOODY TRUDY WEEDY WENDY WINDY WOODY WORDY XANDY

D•Z••
DAZED DAZER DAZES DAZUR DAZZY DIZZY DOZED DOZEN DOZER DOZES

D••Z•
DANZA DAZZY DITZY DIZZY DOOZY DOUZE DRUZE

D•••Z
DIETZ

•DZ••
ADZED ADZES

•D•Z•
ADOZE

•D••Z
ADBIZ

••DZ•
KUDZU NUDZH

••D•Z
CADIZ NODOZ VADUZ

EA•••
EADIE EAGAN EAGER EAGLE EAGRE EAMES EAMON EAPOE EARED EARLE EARLS EARLY EARNS EARPS EARTH EASED EASEL EASER EASES EASTS EASYA EATAT EATEN EATER EATIN EATIT EATME EATOF EATON EATUP EAVAN EAVED EAVES EAZYE

E•A••
EBANK ECARD ECASH EDAMS EGADI EGADS EGALE EGALS ELAND ELARA ELATE ELATH EMAGS EMAIL EMALL ENACT ENAMI ENARE ENARM ENATE EPACT ERASE ERATO ESAKI ETAGE ETAIL ETAPE ETATS EVADE EVANS EWALD EWART EXACT EXALT EXAMS

E••A•
EAGAN EATAT EAVAN EBOAT ECLAT ECTAD ECTAL EDDAS EDGAR EDMAR EFLAT EGGAR EGHAM EILAT ELCAR ELGAR ELIAS ELMAN ELMAR ELSAS ELWAY EMBAR EMBAY ENBAS ENDAT ENIAC ENLAI ENTAD EPHAH EPHAS EQUAL ERIAS ERMAS ESBAT ESSAI ESSAY ESTAB ESTAN ESTAR ESTAS ETHAN ETNAS EVIAN EXPAT EYRAS

E•••A
EASYA EBOLA EDEMA EDINA ELARA ELENA ELISA ELIZA ELURA EMESA ENNEA ENOLA EOLIA ERICA ERIKA ERISA ETYMA EVITA EVORA EXTRA EXUMA

•EA••
AEAEA BEACH BEADS BEADY BEAKS BEALE BEALL BEALS BEAME BEAMS BEAMY BEANO BEANS BEANY BEARD BEARS BEART BEAST BEATS BEATY BEAUS BEAUT BEAUX CEARA CEASE DEAIR DEALS DEALT DEANA DEANE DEANS DEARE DEARS DEARY DEATH FEARS FEAST FEATS GEARS GEARY HEADS HEADY HEALD HEALS HEALY HEAPS HEAPY HEARD HEARN HEARS HEART HEATH HEATS HEAVE HEAVY JEANE JEANS KEACH KEANE KEANU KEATS LEACH LEADS LEADY LEAFS LEAFY LEAHY LEAKE LEAKS LEAKY LEANN LEANS LEANT LEAPS LEAPT LEARN LEARS LEARY LEASE LEASH LEAST LEAUD LEAVE MEADE MEADS MEALS MEALY MEANS MEANT MEANY MEARA

MEARS
MEATH
MEATS
MEATY
NEALE
NEALY
NEAME
NEAPS
NEARS
NEATH
NEATO
NEATS
PEABO
PEACE
PEACH
PEAKS
PEALE
PEALS
PEANO
PEARL
PEARS
PEARY
PEASE
PEATS
PEATY
REACH
REACT
READD
READE
READS
READY
REAIM
REAIR
REALM
REALS
REAMS
REAPS
REARM
REARS
REASK
REATA
REAVE
SEALE
SEALS
SEALY
SEAMS
SEAMY
SEANN
SEARS
SEATO
SEATS
TEACH
TEAKS
TEALS
TEAMO
TEAMS
TEARS
TEARY
TEASE
TEATS
VEALE
VEALS
VEALY
WEALD
WEALS
WEANS
WEARS
WEARY
WEAVE
YEAHS
YEANS
YEARN
YEARS
YEAST
YEATS
ZEALS

•E•A•

BEBAD
BEGAN
BEGAT
BEGAY
BEHAN
BEHAR
BEKAA
BELAU
BELAY
BEMAD
BEMAN
BEMAS
BETAS
BEXAR
CEDAR
CENAS
CERAM
CERAT
CESAR
DEBAG
DEBAR
DECAD
DECAF
DECAL
DECAP
DECAY
DEFAT
DEGAS
DELAY
DENAR
DERAT
DESAI
DETAR
DETAT
DEVAS
DEWAR
DEWAX
FERAL
FETAL
FETAS
GETAB
GETAC
GETAD
GETAS
GETAT
HEMAL
HEMAN
HEMAT
HEPAT
HERAT
HEXAD
JEHAN
KEBAB
KEMAL
KENAI
LECAR
LEFAY
LEGAL
LEHAR
LEMAN
LEMAT
LEMAY
LETAT
LEVAR
LEXAN
MEDAL
MEGAN
MENAS
MESAS
METAL
NEMAN
NEPAL
NEWAT
PEBAS
PECAN
PEDAL
PENAL
PERAN
PERAS
PETAL
REBAG
REBAR
RECAN
RECAP
REDAN
REFAX
REGAL
REGAN
REHAB
REHAN
RELAP
RELAX
RELAY
REMAN
REMAP
REMAT
REMAX
RENAL
RENAN
RENAY
REPAD
REPAY
RERAN
RESAT
RESAW
RESAY
RETAG
RETAN
RETAP
RETAR
RETAX
REWAX
SEDAN
SEEAS
SEGAL
SEGAR
SELAH
SENAT
SEPAL
SERAC
SERAI
SERAL
SETAE
SETAT
TELAR
TEMAS
TENAD
TENAM
TERAT
TEWAS
TEXAN
TEXAS
VEDAS
VEDAY
VEGAN
VEGAS
VELAR
VENAE
VENAL
WEBAD
ZETAS

•E••A

AEAEA
AECIA
AETNA
BECCA
BEIRA
BEKAA
BELLA
BELVA
BEREA
BERIA
BERRA
BERTA
BETTA
CEARA
CEIBA
CELIA
CELLA
CERIA
CESTA
CEUTA
DEANA
DEBRA
DECCA
DELIA
DELLA
DELTA
DERMA
DESNA
FELLA
FERIA
FESTA
GEENA
GEMMA
GENOA
HEDDA
HELGA
HENNA
HEPTA
JENNA
JETTA
KEIRA
KENYA
LEEZA
LEHUA
LEICA
LEILA
LELIA
LEMMA
LENYA
LEONA
LEORA
MEARA
MECCA
MEDEA
MEDIA
MEHTA
MEKKA
MELBA
MENSA
MESTA
NEDDA
NEDRA
NEMEA
NERVA
NESIA
PEKKA
PELLA
PEMBA
PENNA
PENTA
PEPLA
PERMA
PETRA
REATA
RECTA
REGIA
REGNA
REINA
RENGA
RETIA
REZIA
SEEYA
SELMA
SENNA
SENTA
SEPIA
SEPTA
SERIA
SERRA
SERTA
TEENA
TELMA
TERIA
TERRA
TERZA
TESLA
TESSA
TESTA
TETRA
VELDA
VELMA
VELVA
VENTA
VERNA
VERSA
VESPA
VESTA
WEENA
WELLA
XENIA
YENTA
YERBA
YETTA
ZEBRA
ZEENA
ZELDA
ZENDA
ZESTA
ZETTA

••EA•

ABEAM
ABEAR
AHEAD
AHEAP
ALEAK
APEAK
AREAL
AREAR
AREAS
ATEAM
ATEAT
AYEAR
BLEAK
BLEAR
BLEAT
BREAD
BREAK
BREAM
BTEAM
BYEAR
CHEAP
CHEAT
CLEAN
CLEAR
CLEAT
CREAK
CREAM
DREAD
DREAM
DREAR
FLEAS
FREAK
GLEAM
GLEAN
GREAT
HBEAM
IBEAM
ICEAX
IDEAL
IDEAS
IHEAR
ILEAC
ILEAL
IMEAN
ITEAS
KNEAD
LBEAM
NOEAR
OBEAH
OCEAN
OLEAN
ONEAD
ONEAL
ONEAM
OREAD
PAEAN
PLEAD
PLEAS
PLEAT
RHEAS
SEEAS
SHEAF
SHEAN
SHEAR
SMEAL
SMEAR
SNEAD
SNEAK
SPEAK
SPEAR
STEAD
STEAK
STEAL
STEAM
SWEAR
SWEAT
THEAS
THEAX
TOEAS
TREAD
TREAS
TREAT
TWEAK
UREAS
USEAS
UVEAL
UVEAS
WHEAT
WREAK

••E•A

ACELA
ADELA
AGENA
AKELA
ALETA
ALEXA
AMEBA
ARECA
ARENA
AVENA
AZERA
BAEDA
BAEZA
BRECA
BREDA
BUENA
CHEKA
CHELA
CHETA
CIERA
CREMA
DUENA
EDEMA
ELENA
EMESA
FAENA
FREDA
FREIA
FRENA
FREYA
GAETA
GEENA
GRETA
HAEMA
HYENA
IRENA
LEEZA
NIETA
NUEVA
ODESA
OJEDA
OLETA
OMEGA
ONEGA
ONELA
ONERA
OPERA
ORENA
OVETA
PIETA
PLENA
PRESA
SCENA
SEEYA
SHEBA
SHERA
SIENA
SNEVA
STELA
TEENA
THEDA
THEMA
THERA
THETA
VIEJA
WEENA
YREKA
ZEENA

•••EA

AEAEA
APNEA
ATSEA
BEREA
BOHEA
BYSEA
CANEA
COREA
ENNEA
FIVEA
GALEA
HOSEA
JUDEA
KOREA
LINEA
LULEA
MEDEA
NEMEA
NINEA
NIVEA
OSHEA
PALEA
PILEA
RRHEA
SIDEA
SOLEA
TINEA
TOSEA
TYPEA

EB•••

EBANK
EBBED
EBELS
EBERT
EBOAT
EBOLA
EBOLI
EBOND
EBONS
EBONY
EBOOK
EBSEN
EBUZZ

E•B••

EBBED
EGBDF
ELBOW
EMBAR
EMBAY
EMBED
EMBER
EMBOG
ENBAS
ERBIL
ESBAT
EUBIE

E••B•

EKEBY

E•••B

ESTAB
EXCUB
EXLIB
EXURB

•EB••

BEBAD
BEBOP
DEBAG
DEBAR
DEBBE
DEBBI
DEBBY
DEBIT
DEBRA
DEBTS
DEBUG
DEBUS
DEBUT
DEBYE
KEBAB
PEBAS
REBAG
REBAR
REBBE
REBEC
REBEL
REBER
REBET
REBID
REBOP
REBOX
REBUS
REBUT
REBUY
TEBET
WEBAD
WEBBY
WEBER
WEBTV
XEBEC
ZEBRA
ZEBUS

•E•B•

BEEBE
BELBY
CEIBA
DEBBE
DEBBI
DEBBY
DERBY
FEEBS
GETBY
HERBE
HERBS
HERBY
KERBS
LETBE
LETBY
MELBA
PEABO
PEMBA
REBBE
SERBO
SERBS
SETBY
TENBC
VERBS
WEBBY
WELBY
YERBA
ZERBE

•E••B

CELEB
DEMOB
DENEB
GETAB
KEBAB
NEGEB
REDUB
REHAB
REPUB
TENLB

••EB•

AMEBA
BEEBE
BLEBS
EKEBY
FEEBS
GREBE
KREBS
LIEBE
LIEBY
ONEBC
PHEBE
PLEBE
PLEBS
SHEBA
TAEBO
THEBE
USEBY
WIEBE

••E•B

ACERB
DWEEB
ONELB
PRESB
THEWB

•••EB

CALEB
CELEB
CUBEB
DENEB
DWEEB
FIVEB
HOREB
LINEB
NEGEB
NINEB
PHLEB
SIDEB
STIEB
TYPEB

EC•••

ECARD
ECASH
ECHOS
ECLAT
ECOLE
ECOLI
ECONO
ECONS
ECRUS
ECTAD
ECTAL
ECTOR

E•C••

ELCAR
ELCID
EMCEE
ENCLS
ENCRE
ENCYC
EPCOT
EXCEL
EXCON
EXCOP
EXCUB

E••C•

EDICT
EDUCE
EDUCT
EJECT
ELECT
ENACT
ENOCH
EPACT
EPICS
EPOCH
ERECT
ERICA
ERICH
ERICK
ERUCT
EVICT
EXACT
EXECS

E•••C

EDDIC
ENCYC
ENIAC
EOLIC
EPISC
ESTOC
ETHIC

•EC••

AECIA
BECCA
BECKS
BECKY
CECIL
CECUM
DECAD
DECAF
DECAL
DECAP
DECAY
DECCA
DECEM
DECIR
DECKS
DECOR
DECOY
DECRY
GECKO
HECHE
HECHT
HECKS
HECTO
LECAR
LECHE
LECID
LECKY
LECON
LECTS
MECCA
MECUM
NECKS
PECAN
PECHE
PECKS
PECOS
RECAN
RECAP
RECIP
RECKS
RECON
RECTA
RECTI
RECTO
RECTS
RECUE
RECUR
RECUT
SECHS
SECTS
TECHS
YECCH

•E•C•

BEACH
BECCA
BEECH
BELCH
BENCH
BERCY
DECCA
DEICE
DELCO
DENCH
DEUCE
DEUCY
FENCE
FETCH
GEICO
HENCE
HENCH
KEACH
KETCH
LEACH
LEECH
LEICA
MECCA
MERCE
MERCH
MERCI
MERCK
MERCS
MERCY
PEACE
PEACH
PENCE
PERCE
PERCH
PERCS
PERCY
PESCE
PESCI
PETCO
REACH
REACT
REECE
REICE
REICH
TEACH
TELCO
TENCC
TENCH
TERCE
VEECK
VESCO
VETCH
WELCH
WENCH
YECCH

•E••C

CERIC
GENIC
GETAC
HELIC
HEMIC
MEDIC
MEDOC
MELIC
NEMEC
REBEC
RELIC
SERAC
TELIC
TENBC
TENCC
VEDIC
XEBEC
XERIC
ZENIC

••EC•

ALECK
ARECA
BEECH
BRECA
BRECK
CHECK
CRECY
CZECH
DIECI
DRECK
EJECT
ELECT
ERECT
EXECS
FLECK
GRECO
LEECH
NIECE
ORECK
PIECE
REECE
SPECD
SPECK
SPECS
TRECE
VEECK
VLECK
VNECK
WRECK

••E•C

CRESC
ILEAC
OLEIC
ONEBC
THEOC

•••EC

AZTEC
COSEC
CUSEC
DODEC
FIVEC
GYNEC
LINEC
NEMEC
NINEC
OLMEC
REBEC
UNDEC
XEBEC

ED•••

EDAMS
EDDAS
EDDIC
EDDIE
EDEMA
EDENS
EDGAR
EDGED
EDGER
EDGES
EDICT
EDIES
EDIFY
EDILE
EDINA
EDIPO
EDITH
EDITS
EDMAR
EDRED
EDSEL
EDSON
EDUCE
EDUCT
EDWIN

E•D••

EADIE
EDDAS
EDDIC
EDDIE
EGDON
EIDER
ELDER
ELDIN
ELDON
EMDEN
ENDAT
ENDED
ENDER
ENDIN
ENDIT
ENDON
ENDOR
ENDOW
ENDUE
ENDUP
ERDOS
EXDIV
EYDIE

E••D•

EGADI
EGADS
EGBDF
EJIDO
ELIDE
ELUDE
EPODE
EREDE
ERODE
ETUDE
EVADE
EXUDE

E•••D

EARED
EASED
EAVED
EBBED
EBOND
ECARD
ECTAD
EDGED
EDRED
EELED
EGGED
ELAND
ELCID
EMBED
EMEND
ENDED
ENTAD
EPHOD
ERRED
EWALD

•ED••

AEDES
BEDDY
BEDEW
BEDIM
BEDNY
BEDOG
CEDAR
CEDED
CEDER
CEDES
CEDIS
DEDOS
FEDEX
FEDIN
FEDON
FEDTO
FEDUP
HEDDA
HEDGE
HEDGY
HEDIN
KEDGE
LEDEE
LEDER
LEDGE
LEDGY
LEDIN
LEDON
LEDTO
MEDAL
MEDEA
MEDEE
MEDES
MEDIA
MEDIC
MEDII
MEDIO
MEDIT
MEDOC
NEDDA
NEDRA
PEDAL
PEDER
PEDRO
REDAN
REDDI
REDDY
REDED
REDES
REDID
REDIG
REDIP
REDLY
REDON
REDOS
REDOX
REDRY
REDUB
REDUG
REDUX
REDYE
SEDAN
SEDER
SEDGE
SEDGY
SEDUM
TEDDY
VEDAS
VEDAY
VEDIC
WEDEL
WEDGE
WEDGY
WEDTO
XEDIN

•E•D•

BEADS
BEADY
BEDDY
BENDS
BENDY
DEEDS
DENDR
DESDE
FEEDS
FENDI
FENDS
FERDE
FEUDS
GELDS
GEODE
HEADS
HEADY
HEDDA
HEEDS
HEIDI
HEIDT
HERDS
JEUDI
KENDO
LEADS
LEADY
LEEDS
LENDL
LENDS
MEADE
MEADS
MELDS
MENDS
NEDDA
NEEDS
NEEDY
NERDS
NERDY
PENDS
PERDU
READD
READE
READS
READY
REDDI
REDDY
REEDS
REEDY
RENDS
SEEDS
SEEDY
SENDS
TEDDY
TENDS
TENDU

VEIDT
VELDA
VELDS
VELDT
VENDS
VERDE
VERDI
WEEDS
WEEDY
WELDS
WENDS
WENDT
WENDY
ZELDA
ZENDA
ZENDO
ZENDS

•E••D
BEARD
BEBAD
BEMAD
CEDED
DECAD
DEKED
DELED
DESOD
DEWED
EELED
FELID
FETED
FETID
GELID
GETAD
HEALD
HEARD
HEROD
HEWED
HEXAD
HEXED
KEYED
LEAUD
LECID
METED
MEWED
NEFUD
READD
REBID
REDED
REDID
REFED
REHID
RELED
REPAD
RESOD
REWED
SEWED
SEXED
TENAD
TEPID
VEXED
WEALD
WEBAD
WEIRD

••ED•
BAEDA
BREDA
BREDE
COEDS
CREDO
CREDS
DEEDS
DREDD
EREDE
FEEDS
FREDA
FREDO
HEEDS
LEEDS
NEEDS
NEEDY
OJEDA
OPEDS
PIEDS
REEDS
REEDY
SEEDS
SEEDY
SHEDS
SKEDS
SLEDS
SUEDE
SWEDE
THEDA
WEEDS
WEEDY

••E•D
ABEND
AHEAD
AMEND
BLEED
BLEND
BREAD
BREED
CREED
DREAD
DREDD
EMEND
FIELD
FIEND
FREED
FREUD
GREED
KNEAD
KNEED
NOEND
ONEAD
ONEND
OREAD
PFERD
PLEAD
PSEUD
SNEAD
SNERD
SPECD
SPEED
SPEND
STEAD
STEED
THEYD
TREAD
TREED
TREND
TWEED
UPEND
WIELD
YIELD

•••ED
AAHED
ABLED
ACHED
ACRED
ACTED
ADDED
ADZED
AHMED
AIDED
AILED
AIMED
AIRED
AMPED
ANTED
APIED
APTED
ARCED
ARMED
ASHED
ASKED
ASRED
AWNED
AXLED
BAAED
BAKED
BALED
BARED
BASED
BATED
BAYED
BCCED
BIDED
BIKED
BIPED
BLEED
BLUED
BODED
BONED
BOOED
BORED
BOWED
BOXED
BREED
BUSED
CAGED
CAKED
CANED
CAPED
CARED
CASED
CAVED
CAWED
CEDED
CITED
CLUED
CODED
COKED
CONED
COOED
COPED
CORED
COVED
COWED
COXED
CREED
CRIED
CUBED
CURED
DARED
DATED
DAZED
DEKED
DELED
DEWED
DICED
DIKED
DIMED
DINED
DIVED
DOLED
DOMED
DOPED
DOSED
DOTED
DOZED
DRIED
DUDED
DUKED
DUPED
EARED
EASED
EAVED
EBBED
EDGED
EDRED
EELED
EGGED
EMBED
ENDED
ERRED
FACED
FADED
FAKED
FAMED
FARED
FATED
FAXED
FAZED
FETED
FIFED
FILED
FINED
FIRED
FIVED
FIXED
FLIED
FOXED
FREED
FRIED
FUMED
FUSED
GAGED
GALED
GAMED
GAPED
GATED
GAZED
GIBED
GLUED
GORED
GREED
GRUED
GUYED
GYRED
HALED
HARED
HATED
HAWED
HAYED
HAZED
HEWED
HEXED
HIKED
HIRED
HIVED
HOKED
HOLED
HOMED
HONED
HOPED
HOSED
HYPED
IDLED
IGGED
ILIED
IMBED
INBED
INKED
INRED
IRKED
IVIED
JADED
JAPED
JARED
JAWED
JIBED
JIVED
JOKED
JOYED
JUKED
KEYED
KITED
KNEED
LACED
LADED
LAMED
LANED
LASED
LAVED
LAWED
LAZED
LIKED
LIMED
LINED
LIVED
LOBED
LOPED
LOVED
LOWED
LUBED
LUGED
LURED
LUTED
LYSED
MACED
MANED
MATED
MAXED
MAZED
METED
MEWED
MIKED
MIMED
MINED
MIRED
MIXED
MOOED
MOPED
MOVED
MOWED
MUSED
MUTED
NAKED
NAMED
NINED
NIXED
NOSED
NOTED
NUKED
OARED
OFFED
OGLED
OILED
OOHED
OOZED
OPTED
ORBED
OUTED
OWNED
PACED
PAGED
PALED
PANED
PARED
PATED
PAVED
PAWED
PIKED
PILED
PINED
PIPED
PLIED
POKED
POLED
PORED
POSED
PRIED
PULED
RACED
RAGED
RAKED
RASED
RATED
RAVED
RAXED
RAYED
RAZED
REDED
REFED
RELED
REWED
RICED
RILED
RIMED
RIVED
ROBED
ROPED
ROVED
ROWED
RULED
SATED
SAVED
SAWED
SCHED
SEWED
SEXED
SHIED
SHOED
SHRED
SIDED
SIRED
SITED
SIXED
SIZED
SKIED
SLUED
SOLED
SOWED
SPEED
SPIED
STEED
STIED
TAMED
TAPED
TARED
TAXED
TIDED
TILED
TIMED
TINED
TIRED
TOKED
TONED
TOPED
TOTED
TOWED
TOYED
TREED
TRIED
TRUED
TSKED
TUBED
TUNED
TWEED
TYPED
UMPED
UNFED
UNLED
UNWED
UPPED
URGED
USHED
USTED
VANED
VEXED
VINED
VISED
VOTED
VOWED
WADED
WAGED
WAKED
WALED
WANED
WARED
WAVED
WAXED
WILED
WINED
WIPED
WIRED
WISED
WIVED
WOOED
WOWED
YAWED
YOKED
ZONED

EE•••
EELED
EELER
EENSY
EERIE

E•E••
EBELS
EBERT
EDEMA
EDENS
EGEST
EGEUS
EIEIO
EJECT
EKEBY
ELECT
ELEGY
ELEMI
ELEMS
ELENA
ELENI
ELEVE
ELEVS
EMEER
EMEND
EMERY
EMESA
EMEUS
ENEMY
ENERO
EPEES
ERECT
EREDE
ERETZ
EREVS
EUELL
EVENS
EVENT
EVERS
EVERT
EVERY
EWEEK
EWELL
EWERS
EWERY
EXECS
EXERT
EYERS
EYEUP

E••E•
EAGER
EAMES
EARED
EASED
EASEL
EASER
EASES
EATEN
EATER
EAVED
EAVES
EBBED
EBSEN
EDGED
EDGER
EDGES
EDIES
EDRED
EDSEL
EELED
EELER
EFREM
EGGED
EGGER
EGRET
EHREN
EIDER
EIGEN
EIGER
EINEN
EINER
EINES
EISEN
ELDER
ELIEL
ELLEN
ELLER
ELLES
ELMER
ELREY
ELSES
ELVER
ELVES
ELWES
EMBED
EMBER
EMCEE
EMDEN
EMEER
EMLEN
EMMER
EMMET
ENDED
ENDER
ENGEL
ENNEA
ENTER
ENVER
EPEES
ERIES
ERNES
EROES
ERRED
ERTES
ESKER
ESNES
ESSEN
ESSES
ESSEX
ESTEE
ESTER
ESTES
ETHEL
ETHER
ETRES
ETSEQ
ETTES
EULER
EWEEK
EXCEL
EXMET
EXPEL

E•••E
EADIE
EAGLE
EAGRE
EAPOE
EARLE
EATME
EAZYE
ECOLE
EDDIE
EDILE
EDUCE
EERIE
EFFIE
EFILE
EGALE
ELATE
ELEVE
ELIDE
ELISE
ELITE
ELLIE
ELOGE
ELOPE
ELSIE
ELUDE
ELUTE
ELYSE
EMCEE
EMILE
EMOTE
ENARE
ENATE
ENCRE
ENDUE
ENGLE
ENOTE
ENSUE
ENTRE
ENURE
EPODE
EPPIE
ERASE
EREDE
ERNIE
ERODE
EROSE
ESQUE
ESSIE
ESTEE
ETAGE
ETAPE
ETILE
ETUDE
EUBIE
EVADE
EVITE
EVOKE
EXILE
EXUDE
EYDIE
EYRIE
EZINE

•EE••
BEEBE
BEECH
BEEFS
BEEFY
BEENE
BEENS
BEEPS
BEERS
BEERY
BEETS
BEETY
DEEDS
DEEMS
DEEPS
DEERE
DEERS
FEEBS
FEEDS
FEELS
FEELY
FEETS
GEEKS
GEEKY
GEENA
GEEPS
GEESE
HEEDS
HEELS
JEEPS
JEERS
JEERY
KEEFE
KEELS
KEELY
KEENE
KEENS
KEEPS
LEECH
LEEDS
LEEKS
LEERS
LEERY
LEEZA
MEENY
MEESE
MEETS
NEEDS
NEEDY
NEELY
NEEME
PEEKS
PEELE
PEELS
PEENS
PEEPS
PEERS
PEETE
PEEVE
REECE
REEDS
REEDY
REEFS
REEFY
REEGE
REEKS
REEKY
REELS
REESE
REEVE
SEEAS
SEEDS
SEEDY
SEEIN
SEEKS
SEEME
SEEMS
SEEPS
SEEPY
SEERS
SEEST
SEETH
SEETO
SEEUP
SEEYA
TEEMS
TEENA
TEENS
TEENY
TEERS
TEETH
TEEUP
VEECK
VEEPS
VEERS
VEERY
WEEDS
WEEDY
WEEKS
WEEMS
WEENA
WEENY
WEEPS
WEEPY
WEEST
WEEUN
ZEENA

•E•E•
AEAEA
AEDES
AEREO
BEDEW
BEGEM
BEGET
BELEM
BENES
BENET
BEREA
BERET
BESES
BESET
BETEL
BETES
BEVEL
BEZEL
CEDED
CEDER
CEDES
CELEB
CEPES
CERES
DECEM
DEFER
DEGEL
DEHEX
DEKED
DEKES
DELED
DELES
DEMES
DENEB
DENES
DEPEW
DEREK
DESEX
DETER
DEUEL
DEWED
DEWEY
EELED
EELER
FEDEX
FEMES
FETED
FETES
FEUER
FEVER
FEWER
FEYER
FEZES
GELEE
GENES
GENET
HEGEL
HEHES
HELEN
HEMEN
HEMES
HEMET
HEREK
HERES
HETER
HEUER
HEWED
HEWER
HEXED
HEXER
HEXES
HEYER
JEFES
JEREZ
JETER
JETES
JEWEL
KESEY
KEYED
KEYES
LEDEE
LEDER
LEGER
LENES
LEPEN
LEPER
LEPEW
LEVEE
LEVEL
LEVER
LEWES
MEDEA
MEDEE
MEDES
MEIER
MELEE
MENES
MERER
MERES
MESES
METED
METER
METES
MEWED
MEWER
MEYER
NEGEB
NEGEV
NEHER
NEMEA
NEMEC
NENEH
NENES
NEVER
NEVES
NEWEL
NEWER
PEDER
PEKES
PELEE
PELEG
PERES
PEREZ
PETER
PETES
PETEY
PEWEE
REBEC
REBEL
REBER
REBET
REDED
REDES
REFED
REFER
REGEL
REGER
REGES
REHEM
REKEY
RELED
RELEE
RELET
REMET
RENEE
RENEW
REPEG
REPEL
REPEN
RESEE
RESET
RESEW
REUEL
REVEL
REVES
REVET
REWED
REWET
REXES
REYES
SEDER
SEGER
SELES
SEVEN
SEVER
SEWED
SEWER
SEXED
SEXER
SEXES
TEBET
TEHEE
TEKEL
TELES
TELEX
TENEE
TENET
TEPEE
TETES
TEVET
TEWES
VEGES
VELEZ
VENEZ
VEXED
VEXER
VEXES
VEZES
WEBER
WEDEL
WESER
WEZEN
XEBEC
XEMEX
YEMEN
YESES
ZENER

•E••E
AERIE
BEALE
BEAME
BEEBE
BEENE
BEIGE
BELIE
BELLE
BEPPE
BERLE
BERNE
BETTE
BEYLE
CEASE
CELIE
CELLE
CENSE
CETTE
DEANE
DEARE
DEBBE
DEBYE
DEERE
DEFOE
DEICE
DELVE
DEMME
DENSE
DENTE
DESDE
DESTE
DETRE
DETTE
DEUCE
EERIE
FEMME
FENCE
FERDE
FESTE
GEESE
GELEE
GENIE
GENRE
GENTE
GEODE
GESTE
GETME
HEAVE
HECHE
HEDGE
HEINE
HENCE
HENGE
HENIE
HENZE
HERBE
HERNE
HERVE
HESHE
HESSE
HEURE
HEYSE
JEANE
JERNE
JESSE
JEUNE
KEANE
KEDGE
KEEFE
KEENE
KERNE
LEAKE
LEASE
LEAVE
LECHE
LEDEE
LEDGE
LEMME
LENTE
LEONE
LEPKE
LETBE
LETHE
LETME
LEVEE
LEYTE
MEADE
MEDEE
MEESE
MEINE
MELEE
MERCE
MERGE
MERLE
MEROE
MESNE
MESSE
METRE
MEUSE
NEALE
NEAME
NEEME
NEIGE
NELLE
NELSE
NERVE
NEWIE
OESTE
PEACE
PEALE
PEASE
PECHE
PEELE
PEETE
PEEVE
PEKOE
PELEE
PELLE
PENCE
PENNE
PENTE
PERCE
PERLE
PERSE
PESCE
PETRE
PEWEE
READE
REAVE
REBBE
RECUE
REDYE
REECE
REEGE
REESE
REEVE
REGLE
REHOE
REICE
REINE
RELEE
RENEE
RENTE
RESEE
RESTE
RETIE
REUNE
REUSE
REVUE
SEALE
SEDGE
SEEME
SEGRE
SEGUE
SEINE
SEIZE
SENSE
SENTE
SERGE
SERVE

SETAE SETTE SEULE TEASE TEHEE TEMPE TENEE TENGE TENSE TEPEE TERCE TERME TERNE TERRE TERSE TEVYE VEALE VENAE VENUE VERDE VERGE VERNE VERRE VERSE VERTE VERVE VETTE WEAVE WEDGE YENTE ZEILE ZERBE

••EE•

ADEEM AKEEM AMEER APEEK APEEP AREEL AWEEK BLEED BLEEP BREED BREEN BREES CHEEK CHEEP CHEER CHEEZ CLEEF CLEEK CREED CREEK CREEL CREEP CREES DWEEB EMEER EPEES EWEEK FLEER FLEES FLEET FREED FREEH FREER FREES GHEES GLEEM GLEES GREED GREEK GREEN GREER GREET ICEES IDEES IFEEL INEES KNEED KNEEL KNEES OGEES ONEEE PREEN QUEEG QUEEN QUEER RHEEM SHEEN SHEEP SHEER SHEET SKEET SLEEK SLEEP SLEET SMEES SNEER SNEES SPEED SPEER STEED STEEL STEEN STEEP STEER SWEEP SWEET TREED TREEN TREES TWEED TWEEN TWEET TYEES ULEES USEES WHEEL WHEES

••E•E

ABELE ADELE AKENE ALENE ALEVE ANELE ARETE BEEBE BEENE BIERE BREDE BREVE CHERE CLETE CLEVE CREME CREPE CRETE CREVE DEERE DIENE DIÈTE ELEVE EREDE FRERE GEESE GREBE GRETE ILENE IRENE ISERE KEEFE KEENE KREME KREWE LIEBE LIEGE LOEWE MAEVE MEESE MIELE MNEME MYEYE NEEME NIECE NIEVE NUEVE OBESE ONEEE OPERE OXEYE PAESE PEELE PEETE PEEVE PHEBE PIECE PLEBE POEME POETE PRESE QUEUE REECE REEGE REESE REEVE RHEME SCENE SEEME SHERE SIEGE SIETE SIEVE SPEKE STELE STERE STEVE SUEDE SUEME SWEDE THEBE THEME THERE THESE TIENE TRECE TWERE ULENE USEME WHERE WIEBE

•••EE

ADFEE AGREE AIMEE ALBEE ALLEE ANNEE ARMEE AWGEE CITEE COOEE CUVEE DOBEE DONEE EMCEE ESTEE FIVEE FTLEE FUSEE GELEE GOSEE GUMEE HIREE LAREE LEDEE LEVEE LYCEE MAGEE MCGEE MCKEE MEDEE MELEE MRLEE MUSEE NAVEE NGWEE NINEE NOFEE OHGEE ONEEE PAREE PAYEE PELEE PEWEE PUREE RANEE RAPEE RAREE RELEE RENEE RESEE RONEE RUPEE SAREE SCREE SIREE SIXEE SPREE TEHEE TENEE TEPEE THREE TOPEE TUTEE TWOEE TYPEE WILEE WOWEE

EF•••

EFFIE EFGHI EFIKS EFILE EFLAT EFREM

E•F••

EFFIE ELFIN ENFIN EOFOR

E••F•

EDIFY

E•••F

EATOF EGBDF

•EF••

BEFIT BEFOG BEFOR DEFAT DEFER DEFGH DEFOE DEFOG HEFTI HEFTS HEFTY JEFES JEFFY KEFIR LEFAY LEFTS LEFTY NEFUD REFAX REFED REFER REFIS REFIT REFIX REFLY REFRY WEFTS

•E•F•

BEEFS BEEFY BEOFF DEIFY DELFT FEOFF JEFFY KEEFE KERFS LEAFS LEAFY MELFI NERFS OEUFS PELFS PERFS REEFS REEFY REIFY SERFS

•E••F

BEOFF DECAF FEOFF SERIF TENOF

••EF•

ALEFS BEEFS BEEFY CDEFG CHEFS CLEFS CLEFT DREFT FIEFS KEEFE REEFS REEFY THEFT TOEFL ZIEFF

••E•F

ATEOF AXELF BOEUF CLEEF SHEAF SHELF USEOF ZIEFF

•••EF

BCDEF BRIEF CCLEF CHIEF CLEEF FCLEF GANEF GCLEF GRIEF INDEF JOSEF SHAEF THIEF

EG•••

EGADI EGADS EGALE EGALS EGBDF EGDON EGEST EGEUS EGGAR EGGED EGGER EGGON EGGOS EGHAM EGLIN EGRET EGYPT

E•G••

EAGAN EAGER EAGLE EAGRE EDGAR EDGED EDGER EDGES EFGHI EGGAR EGGED EGGER EGGON EGGOS EIGEN EIGER EIGHT ELGAR ELGIN ENGEL ENGLE ENGRS ERGOT EXGIS EXGOV

E••G•

ELEGY ELOGE EMAGS ETAGE

E•••G

EKING EMBOG ERING EWING EXING EYING

•EG••

AEGIR AEGIS BEGAN BEGAT BEGAY BEGEM BEGET BEGIN BEGOT BEGUM BEGUN DEGAS DEGEL DEGUM HEGEL LEGAL LEGER LEGGS LEGGY LEGIT LEGNO LEGOS LEGUP MEGAN NEGEB NEGEV NEGRI NEGRO NEGUS PEGGY PEGUY REGAL REGAN REGEL REGER REGES REGIA REGIS REGLE REGNA REGTS REGUM SEGAL SEGAR SEGER SEGNI SEGNO SEGOS SEGRE SEGUE VEGAN VEGAS VEGES YEGGS

•E•G•

BEIGE BERGS DEFGH DEIGN FEIGN GETGO HEDGE HEDGY HEIGH HEIGL HELGA HENGE KEDGE KEOGH LEDGE LEDGY LEGGS LEGGY LEIGH LETGO MERGE NEIGE NEIGH PEGGY REEGE REIGN RENGA SEDGE SEDGY SENGI SERGE TENGE TENGO VERGE WEDGE WEDGY WEIGH YEGGS

•E••G

BEDOG BEFOG BEING BEWIG DEBAG DEBUG DEFOG GEORG PELEG REBAG REDIG REDUG REJIG RELIG RELOG REPEG RERIG RETAG SELIG ZELIG ZEROG

••EG•

DIEGO DREGS ELEGY FUEGO GREGG JPEGS JUEGO LIEGE LUEGO MPEGS OMEGA ONEGA PREGL PREGO REEGE SIEGE SKEGS TAEGU TIEGS

••E•G

CDEFG GREGG QUEEG STEIG ZWEIG

•••EG

GRIEG IRREG KLIEG KRIEG PELEG QUEEG REPEG UNPEG

EH•••

EHREN

E•H••

ECHOS EGHAM EPHAH EPHAS EPHOD EPHOR ETHAN ETHEL ETHER ETHIC ETHNO ETHOS ETHYL

E••H•

EFGHI EIGHT ELIHU ESTHS

E•••H

EARTH ECASH EDITH ELATH ENOCH EPHAH EPOCH ERICH

•EH••

BEHAN BEHAR DEHEX HEHES JEHAN LEHAR LEHRS LEHUA MEHTA NEHER NEHIS NEHRU REHAB REHAN REHEM REHID REHIT REHOE TEHEE

•E•H•

BETHS DELHI HECHE HECHT HESHE HETHS LEAHY LECHE LETHE MEKHI MESHY NEPHR PECHE RESHT SECHS TECHS TETHS YEAHS

•E••H

BEACH BEECH BELCH BENCH BERTH DEATH DEFGH DENCH DEPTH FETCH HEATH HEIGH HENCH HERSH KEACH KEITH KEOGH KERSH KETCH LEACH LEASH LEECH LEIGH LEITH MEATH MERCH NEATH NEIGH NENEH PEACH PERCH PERTH REACH REICH SEETH SELAH TEACH TEETH TENCH TENTH VETCH WEIGH WELCH WELSH WENCH YECCH

••EH•

BIEHN RUEHL

••E•H

ALEPH BEECH CZECH DOETH FLESH FREEH FRESH GOETH LEECH OBEAH SEETH TEETH WYETH

•••EH

FREEH HOPEH NENEH

EI•••

EIDER EIEIO EIGEN EIGER EIGHT EILAT EINEN EINER EINES EISEN

E•I••

EDICT EDIES EDIFY EDILE EDINA EDIPO EDITH EDITS EFIKS EFILE EJIDO EKING ELIAS ELIDE ELIEL ELIHU ELION ELIOT ELISA ELISE ELIST ELITE ELIZA EMILE EMILY EMIRS EMITS ENIAC EPICS EPISC ERIAS ERICA ERICH ERICK ERIES ERIKA ERING ERISA ERITU ESIST ETILE EVIAN EVICT EVILS EVITA EVITE EWING EXILE EXING EXIST EXITS EYING EZINE

E••I•

EADIE EATIN EATIT EDDIC EDDIE EDWIN EERIE EFFIE EGLIN EIEIO ELCID ELDIN ELFIN ELGIN ELKIN ELLIE ELLIN ELLIS ELPIS ELSIE ELVIN ELVIS EMAIL ENDIN ENDIT ENFIN ENNIO ENNIS ENOIL EOLIA EOLIC EOSIN EPPIE EQUIP EQUIS EQUIV ERBIL ERNIE ERVIN ERWIN ESPIO ESSIE ETAIL ETHIC ETUIS EUBIE EXDIV EXGIS EXLIB EYDIE EYRIE EYRIR

E•••I

EBOLI ECOLI EFGHI EGADI ELEMI ELENI ENAMI ENLAI ENNUI ENOKI ENVOI ESAKI ESSAI ETMOI

•EI••

AEIOU BEIGE BEING BEINS BEIRA CEIBA CEILS DEICE DEIFY DEIGN DEILS DEION DEISM DEIST DEITY FEIGN FEINT GEICO GEIST HEIDI HEIDT HEIGH HEIGL HEINE HEINZ HEIRS HEISS HEIST KEINO KEIRA KEITH LEICA LEIGH LEILA LEITH MEIER MEIJI MEINE NEIGE NEIGH NEILL REICE REICH REIFY REIGN REIMS REINA REINE REINK REINS REISZ REITS SEIJI SEIKO SEINE SEISM SEIZE VEIDT VEILS VEINS VEINY WEIGH WEILL WEIRD WEIRS WEISS WEISZ WEITZ ZEILE ZEISS ZEIST

•E•I•

AECIA AEGIR AEGIS AERIE AERIO AESIR BEDIM BEFIT BEGIN BELIE BENIN BERIA BEVIN BEWIG CECIL CEDIS CELIA CELIE CERIA CERIC DEAIR DEBIT DECIR DELIA DELIS DEMIT DENIM DENIS DERIV DEVIL EERIE FEDIN FELID FELIS FELIX FELIZ FERIA FETID GELID GENIC GENIE GENII GETIN GETIT HEDIN HELIC HELIO HELIX HEMIC HEMIN HENIE KEFIR KEPIS KEVIN KEYIN LECID LEDIN LEGIT LELIA LENIN LENIS LEOII LEOIV LEOIX LETIN LEVIN LEVIS LEVIT LEWIS LEXIS MEDIA MEDIC MEDII MEDIO MEDIT MELIC MELIS MERIT METIS NEHIS NESIA NEVIL NEVIN NEVIS NEWIE NEXIS PEKIN PENIN PEPIN PERIL PERIS PETIT PEWIT REAIM REAIR REBID RECIP REDID REDIG REDIP REFIS REFIT REFIX REGIA REGIS REHID REHIT REJIG RELIC RELIG RELIT REMIT REMIX RENIN REOIL REPIN RERIG RESIN RESIT RETIA RETIE RETIN RETIP REWIN REZIA REZIP SEEIN SELIG SEMIS SEPIA SERIA SERIF SERIN SERIO SETIN SEWIN TELIC TEPID TERIA VEDIC VENIN XEDIN XENIA XERIC XESIN YETIS ZELIG ZENIC

•E••I

BELLI BENJI BERNI BETTI CELLI CENTI CESTI DEBBI DELHI DENTI DESAI FENDI FERMI FERRI GENII HEFTI HEIDI HENRI JETLI JEUDI KELLI KENAI KERRI KETTI LENNI LEOII LEONI

LEOVI
LEOXI
LEROI
LEUMI
MEDII
MEIJI
MEKHI
MELFI
MERCI
NEGRI
PELLI
PENNI
PEPSI
PESCI
PETRI
PETTI
RECTI
REDDI
SEGNI
SEIJI
SENGI
SERAI
TEMPI
TERRI
TETRI
VENTI
VERDI
VERMI
VESTI

••EI•
ACEIT
ATEIN
ATEIT
CUEIN
DUEIN
EIEIO
FREIA
ICEIN
ICEIT
KLEIN
LIEIN
LOEIL
LWEIS
OLEIC
OLEIN
ONEIL
ONEIR
RHEIN
SEEIN
SHEIK
SKEIN
STEIG
STEIN
THEIR
TIEIN
TOEIN
USEIN
USEIT
ZWEIG

••E•I
ADENI
ALEXI
AZERI
BIERI
BREVI
CHERI
DIECI
ELEMI
ELENI
FRENI
ICENI
LOEWI
MBEKI
OBELI
OTERI
RIETI
TREVI
UMEKI

•••EI
IMPEI
ISSEI
NISEI
PILEI
SOLEI
TAKEI
TOMEI

EJ•••
EJECT
EJIDO

E•J••
ENJOY

•EJ••
REJIG

•E•J•
BENJI
MEIJI
SEIJI

••EJ•
VIEJA
VIEJO

EK•••
EKEBY
EKING

E•K••
ELKIN
ESKER

E••K•
EFIKS
ENOKI
ENSKY
ERIKA
ESAKI
EVOKE
EWOKS

E•••K
EBANK
EBOOK
ERICK
EWEEK

•EK••
BEKAA
DEKED
DEKES
DEKKO
GEKKO
MEKHI
MEKKA
PEKES
PEKIN
PEKKA
PEKOE
REKEY
TEKEL

•E•K•
BEAKS
BECKS
BECKY
BERKS
DECKS
DEKKO
DESKS
GECKO
GEEKS
GEEKY
GEKKO
HECKS
HERKY
JERKS
JERKY
LEAKE
LEAKS
LEAKY
LECKY
LEEKS
LEPKE
LEUKO
MEKKA
NECKS
PEAKS
PECKS
PEEKS
PEKKA
PERKS
PERKY
PESKY
RECKS
REEKS
REEKY
SEEKS
SEIKO
TEAKS
TENKS
WEEKS

•E••K
DEREK
HEREK
MERCK
REASK
REINK
VEECK

••EK•
CHEKA
DREKS
GEEKS
GEEKY
LEEKS
MBEKI
ONEKS
PEEKS
REEKS
REEKY
SEEKS
SPEKE
TREKS
UMEKI
WEEKS
YREKA

••E•K
ALEAK
ALECK
APEAK
APEEK
AWEEK
BLEAK
BREAK
BRECK
CHECK
CHEEK
CLEEK
CLERK
CREAK
CREEK
DRECK
EWEEK
FLECK
FREAK
GREEK
KREUK
ORECK
SHEIK
SLEEK
SNEAK
SPEAK
SPECK
STEAK
THEOK
TWEAK
VEECK
VLECK
VNECK
WHELK
WREAK
WRECK

•••EK
APEEK
AWEEK
AZTEK
CAPEK
CHEEK
CLEEK
CREEK
DEREK
DUDEK
EWEEK
GREEK
HACEK
HASEK
HAYEK
HEREK
HRBEK
KOPEK
KUBEK
MAREK
PATEK
SAREK
SHREK
SLEEK
TYVEK
UZBEK

EL•••
ELAND
ELARA
ELATE
ELATH
ELBOW
ELCAR
ELCID
ELDER
ELDIN
ELDON
ELECT
ELEGY
ELEMI
ELEMS
ELENA
ELENI
ELEVE
ELEVS
ELFIN
ELGAR
ELGIN
ELIAS
ELIDE
ELIEL
ELIHU
ELION
ELIOT
ELISA
ELISE
ELIST
ELITE
ELIZA
ELKIN
ELLEN
ELLER
ELLES
ELLIE
ELLIN
ELLIS
ELLOS
ELMAN
ELMAR
ELMER
ELMOS
ELMST
ELOGE
ELOPE
ELORO
ELPIS
ELREY
ELROY
ELSAS
ELSES
ELSIE
ELSOL
ELTON
ELUDE
ELULS
ELURA
ELUTE
ELVER
ELVES
ELVIN
ELVIS
ELWAY
ELWES
ELYNV
ELYOT
ELYSE

E•L••
ECLAT
EELED
EELER
EFLAT
EGLIN
EILAT
ELLEN
ELLER
ELLES
ELLIE
ELLIN
ELLIS
ELLOS
EMLEN
EMLYN
ENLAI
EOLIA
EOLIC
EOLUS
EULER
EXLIB

E••L•
EAGLE
EARLE
EARLS
EARLY
EBELS
EBOLA
EBOLI
ECOLE
ECOLI
EDILE
EFILE
EGALE
EGALS
ELULS
EMALL
EMILE
EMILY
ENCLS
ENGLE
ENOLA
ENOLS
ETILE
EUELL
EVILS
EWALD
EWELL
EXALT
EXILE
EXULT

E•••L
EASEL
ECTAL
EDSEL
ELIEL
ELSOL
EMAIL
EMALL
ENGEL
ENOIL
ENROL
EQUAL
ERBIL
ERROL
ETAIL
ETHEL
ETHYL
EUELL
EWELL
EXCEL
EXPEL
EXTOL

•EL••
BELAU
BELAY
BELBY
BELCH
BELEM
BELIE
BELLA
BELLE
BELLI
BELLO
BELLS
BELLY
BELON
BELOW
BELTS
BELVA
CELEB
CELIA
CELIE
CELLA
CELLE
CELLI
CELLO
CELLS
CELTS
DELAY
DELCO
DELED
DELES
DELFT
DELHI
DELIA
DELIS
DELLA
DELLO
DELLS
DELON
DELOS
DELPY
DELTA
DELTS
DELVE
EELED
EELER
FELID
FELIS
FELIX
FELIZ
FELLA
FELLS
FELON
FELTS
GELDS
GELEE
GELID
GELTS
HELEN
HELGA
HELIC
HELIO
HELIX
HELLO
HELLS
HELMS
HELOS
HELOT
HELPS
JELLO
JELLS
JELLY
KELLI
KELLY
KELPS
KELSO
LELIA
MELBA
MELDS
MELEE
MELFI
MELIC
MELIS
MELLO
MELON
MELOS
MELOT
MELTS
NELLE
NELLO
NELLY
NELSE
PELEE
PELEG
PELFS
PELLA
PELLE
PELLI
PELTS
RELAP
RELAX
RELAY
RELED
RELEE
RELET
RELIC
RELIG
RELIT
RELOG
SELAH
SELES
SELIG
SELLS
SELMA
TELAR
TELCO
TELES
TELEX
TELIC
TELLS
TELLY
TELMA
VELAR
VELDA
VELDS
VELDT
VELEZ
VELMA
VELOX
VELUM
VELVA
WELBY
WELCH
WELDS
WELLA
WELLS
WELSH
WELTS
WELTY
YELLO
YELLS
YELPS
ZELDA
ZELIG

•E•L•
BEALE
BEALL
BEALS
BELLA
BELLE
BELLI
BELLO
BELLS
BELLY
BERLE
BEYLE
CEILS
CELLA
CELLE
CELLI
CELLO
CELLS
DEALS
DEALT
DEILS
DELLA
DELLO
DELLS
FEELS
FEELY
FELLA
FELLS
FEYLY
HEALD
HEALS
HEALY
HEELS
HELLO
HELLS
JELLO
JELLS
JELLY
JETLI
KEELS
KEELY
KELLI
KELLY
LEILA
MEALS
MEALY
MELLO
MENLO
MERLE
MERLS
MEWLS
NEALE
NEALY
NEELY
NEILL
NELLE
NELLO
NELLY
NEWLY
PEALE
PEALS
PEELE
PEELS
PELLA
PELLE
PELLI
PEPLA
PERLE
REALM
REALS
REDLY
REELS
REFLY
REGLE
REPLY
SEALE
SEALS
SEALY
SELLS
SEULE
TEALS
TELLS
TELLY
TENLB
TESLA
VEALE
VEALS
VEALY
VEILS
VENLO
WEALD
WEALS
WEILL
WELLA
WELLS
WETLY
YELLO
YELLS
ZEALS
ZEILE

•E••L
BEALL
BERYL
BETEL
BEVEL
BEZEL
CECIL
CEORL
DECAL
DEGEL
DEUEL
DEVIL
DEVOL
FERAL
FETAL
HEGEL
HEIGL
HEMAL
HERZL
JEWEL
KEMAL
LEGAL
LENDL
LEVEL
MEDAL
MERYL
METAL
NEILL
NEPAL
NEROL
NEVIL
NEWEL
PEARL
PEDAL
PENAL
PERIL
PETAL
REBEL
REGAL
REGEL
RENAL
REOIL
REPEL
REUEL
REVEL
SEGAL
SEOUL
SEPAL
SERAL
TEKEL
VENAL
WEDEL
WEILL
YENTL

••EL•
ABELE
ACELA
ADELA
ADELE
AKELA
ANELE
AXELF
AXELS
BCELL
BUELL
CCELL
CHELA
CHELY
CIELO
CIELS
DCELL
DIELS
DUELS
DWELL
DWELT
EBELS
EUELL
EWELL
FEELS
FEELY
FIELD
FUELS
GAELS
HEELS
KEELS
KEELY
KNELL
KNELT
KVELL
LYELL
MIELE
MIELS
MTELY
NEELY
NIELS
NOELS
OBELI
ODELL
ONELA
ONELB
ONELS
OPELS
PEELE
PEELS
PIELS
PRELL
QUELL
REELS
RIELS
SHELF
SHELL
SMELL
SMELT
SNELL
SPELL
SPELT
STELA
STELE
SWELL
SZELL
TAELS
TCELL
WHELK
WHELM
WHELP
WIELD
YIELD

••E•L
AREAL
AREEL
BCELL
BUELL
CCELL
CREEL
DCELL
DWELL
EUELL
EWELL
IDEAL
IFEEL
ILEAL
KNEEL
KNELL
KVELL
LIESL
LOEIL
LYELL
ODELL
ONEAL
ONEIL
PREGL
PRELL
QUELL
RUEHL
SHELL
SMEAL
SMELL
SNELL
SPELL
STEAL
STEEL
SWELL
SZELL
TCELL
THEOL
TOEFL
UVEAL
WHEEL

•••EL
ABDEL
ACCEL
AMIEL
ANGEL
ANSEL
APFEL
APPEL
AREEL
ARIEL
ARNEL
ARPEL
ARTEL
BABEL
BAGEL
BASEL
BETEL
BEVEL
BEZEL
BIKEL
BODEL
BOREL
BOTEL
BOWEL
CAMEL
CREEL
CRUEL
CUPEL
CUREL
DEGEL
DEUEL
DIGEL
DOWEL
DYNEL
EASEL
EDSEL
ELIEL
ENGEL
ETHEL
EXCEL
EXPEL
FIDEL
FOGEL
FRIEL
GABEL
GAVEL
GIMEL
GOBEL
GODEL
GRUEL
HAMEL
HAVEL
HAZEL
HEGEL
HOSEL
HOTEL
HOVEL
HUBEL
IFEEL
IMPEL
INTEL
ISSEL
JEWEL
JOREL
KALEL
KAREL
KNEEL
KODEL
KUGEL
LABEL
LAPEL
LEVEL
LIBEL
LITEL
MABEL
MAZEL
MODEL
MONEL
MOREL
MOSEL
MOTEL
NAGEL
NAVEL
NEWEL
NIGEL
NOBEL
NOVEL
ORIEL
OUSEL
OUZEL
PANEL
PAPEL
PAVEL
PIXEL
RATEL
RAVEL
REBEL
REGEL
REPEL
REUEL
REVEL
RIGEL
ROWEL
RUBEL
RUDEL
SAHEL
SOREL
SPIEL
STAEL
STEEL
TAVEL
TEKEL
TOWEL
UMBEL
URIEL
URKEL
VOGEL
VOWEL
WEDEL
WHEEL
YODEL
YOKEL
ZOREL

EM•••
EMAGS
EMAIL
EMALL
EMBAR
EMBAY
EMBED
EMBER
EMBOG
EMCEE
EMDEN
EMEER
EMEND
EMERY
EMESA
EMEUS
EMILE
EMILY
EMIRS
EMITS
EMLEN
EMLYN
EMMER
EMMET
EMMYS
EMORY
EMOTE
EMPTY

E•M••
EAMES
EAMON
EDMAR
ELMAN
ELMAR
ELMER
ELMOS
ELMST
EMMER
EMMET
EMMYS
ERMAS
ETMOI
EXMET

E••M•
EATME
EDAMS
EDEMA
ELEMI
ELEMS
ENAMI
ENEMY
ETYMA
EXAMS
EXUMA

E•••M
EFREM
EGHAM
ENARM
ENORM
ENTOM
EPROM
EPSOM

•EM••
BEMAD
BEMAN
BEMAS
DEMES
DEMIT
DEMME
DEMOB
DEMON
DEMOS
DEMUR
FEMES
FEMME
FEMTO
FEMUR
GEMMA
GEMMY
HEMAL
HEMAN
HEMAT
HEMEN
HEMES
HEMET
HEMIC
HEMIN
HEMON
HEMPS
HEMPY
KEMAL
KEMPT
LEMAN
LEMAT
LEMAY
LEMMA
LEMME
LEMON
LEMUR
MEMOS
NEMAN
NEMEA
NEMEC
NEMOS
PEMBA
REMAN
REMAP
REMAT
REMAX
REMET
REMIT
REMIX
REMOP
REMOW
REMUS
SEMIS
TEMAS
TEMPE
TEMPI
TEMPO
TEMPS
TEMPT
XEMEX
YEMEN

•E•M•
BEAME
BEAMS
BEAMY
BERMS
DEEMS
DEMME
DERMA
DERMO
FEMME
FERMI
GEMMA
GEMMY
GERMS
GERMY
GETME
HELMS
LEMMA
LEMME
LETME
LEUMI
NEAME
NEEME
PERMA
PERMS
REAMS
REIMS
SEAMS
SEAMY
SEEME
SEEMS
SELMA
TEAMO
TEAMS
TEEMS
TELMA
TERME
TERMS
VELMA
VERMI
WEEMS

•E••M
BEDIM
BEGEM
BEGUM
BELEM
BESOM
CECUM
CERAM
DECEM
DEGUM
DEISM
DENIM
DENOM
MECUM
REAIM
REALM
REARM
REGUM
REHEM

5 EM

SEDUM SEISM SERUM TENAM TENPM VELUM VENOM

• • EM •

AHEMS ANEMO CHEMO CREMA CREME DEEMS DIEMS EDEMA ELEMI ELEMS ENEMY HAEMA ITEMS KREME MNEME MNEMO NEEME OKEMO POEME POEMS RHEME SEEME SEEMS SHEMP STEMS SUEME TEEMS THEMA THEME THEMS USEME WEEMS

• • E • M

ABEAM ADEEM AKEEM ATEAM BREAM BTEAM CREAM DREAM GLEAM GLEEM HBEAM IBEAM ILEUM LBEAM ODEUM OLEUM ONEAM ONEPM PNEUM RHEEM RHEUM SHERM SPERM STEAM THERM

WHELM

• • • EM

ADEEM ADHEM ADREM AKEEM BEGEM BELEM CANEM DECEM DIGEM EFREM GLEEM GOLEM HAREM INREM KASEM MAKEM MODEM NOVEM PACEM PROEM REHEM RHEEM ROREM SALEM SICEM TOTEM TWOEM WOWEM XYLEM

EN • • •

ENACT ENAMI ENARE ENARM ENATE ENBAS ENCLS ENCRE ENCYC ENDAT ENDED ENDER ENDIN ENDIT ENDON ENDOR ENDOW ENDUE ENDUP ENEMY ENERO ENFIN ENGEL ENGLE ENGRS ENIAC ENJOY ENLAI ENNEA ENNIO ENNIS ENNUI ENOCH ENOIL ENOKI ENOLA ENOLS ENORM ENOTE ENROL ENRON ENSKY ENSOR ENSUE ENTAD ENTER ENTOM ENTRE ENTRY ENURE ENVER ENVOI ENVOY

E • N • •

EENSY EINEN EINER EINES ENNEA ENNIO ENNIS ENNUI ERNES ERNIE ERNST ESNES ETNAS

E • • N •

EARNS EBANK EBOND EBONS EBONY ECONO ECONS EDENS EDINA EKING ELAND ELENA ELENI ELYNV EMEND ERING ETHNO ETONS EVANS EVENS EVENT EWING EXING EXONS EYING EZINE

E • • • N

EAGAN EAMON EATEN EATIN EATON EAVAN EBSEN EDSON EDWIN EGDON EGGON EGLIN EHREN EIGEN EINEN EISEN ELDIN ELDON ELFIN ELGIN ELION ELKIN ELLEN ELLIN ELMAN ELTON ELVIN EMDEN EMLEN EMLYN ENDIN ENDON ENFIN ENRON EOSIN EPSON ERVIN ERWIN ESSEN ESTAN ETHAN EVIAN EXCON EXXON

• EN • •

BENCH BENDS BENDY BENES BENET BENIN BENJI BENNY BENTO BENTS CENAS CENSE CENTI CENTO CENTR CENTS CENTU DENAR DENCH DENDR DENEB DENES DENIM DENIS DENNY DENOM DENSE DENTE DENTI DENTO DENTS DENYS EENSY FENCE FENDI FENDS FENNY GENES GENET GENIC GENIE GENII GENOA GENRE GENTE GENTS GENUS GENXS HENCE HENCH HENGE HENIE HENNA HENNY HENRI HENRY HENZE JENNA JENNY JENOS KENAI KENDO KENNY KENOS KENYA LENDL LENDS LENES LENIN LENIS LENNI LENNY LENOS LENOX LENTE LENTO LENTS LENYA MENAS MENDS MENES MENLO MENOS MENSA MENUS NENEH NENES PENAL PENCE PENDS PENIN PENNA PENNE PENNI PENNY PENTA PENTE PENUP RENAL RENAN RENAY RENDS RENEE RENEW RENGA RENIN RENNY RENTE RENTS SENAT SENDS SENGI SENNA SENOR SENSE SENTA SENTE TENAD TENAM TENBC TENCC TENCH TENDS TENDU TENEE TENET TENGE TENGO TENKS TENLB TENOF TENON TENOR TENPM TENSE TENTH TENTO TENTS TENUP VENAE VENAL VENDS VENEZ VENIN VENLO VENOM VENTA VENTI VENTO VENTS VENUE VENUS WENCH WENDS WENDT WENDY XENIA XENON YENTA YENTE YENTL ZENDA ZENDO ZENDS ZENER ZENIC ZENOS

• E • N •

AEONS AETNA BEANO BEANS BEANY BEDNY BEENE BEENS BEING BEINS BENNY BERNE BERNI DEANA DEANE DEANS DENNY DESNA FEINT FENNY FERNS FERNY GEENA HEINE HEINZ HENNA HENNY HERNE JEANE JEANS JENNA JENNY JERNE JEUNE KEANE KEANU KEENE KEENS KEINO KENNY KERNE KERNS LEANN LEANS LEANT LEGNO LENNI LENNY LEONA LEONE LEONI MEANS MEANT MEANY MEENY MEINE MESNE NEONS PEANO PEENS PENNA PENNE PENNI PENNY PEONS PEONY REGNA REINA REINE REINK REINS RENNY REUNE SEANN SEGNI SEGNO SEINE SENNA TEENA TEENS TEENY TERNE TERNS VEINS VEINY VERNA VERNE WEANS WEENA WEENY XEONS YEANS YESNO ZEENA

• E • • N

BEGAN BEGIN BEGUN BEHAN BELON BEMAN BENIN BETON BEVIN DEIGN DEION DELON DEMON DEVON FEDIN FEDON FEIGN FELON GETIN GETON HEARN HEDIN HELEN HEMAN HEMEN HEMIN HEMON HERON HESON JEHAN KEVIN KEVON KEYIN KEYON LEANN LEARN LECON LEDIN LEDON LEMAN LEMON LENIN LEPEN LETIN LETON LEVIN LEVON LEXAN MEGAN MELON MESON NEMAN NEVIN PECAN PEKIN PENIN PEPIN PERAN PERON RECAN RECON REDAN REDON REGAN REHAN REIGN REMAN RENAN RENIN REOWN REPEN REPIN RERAN RERUN RESIN RETAN RETIN REWIN REWON SEANN SEDAN SEEIN SERIN SETIN SETON SEVEN SEWIN SEWON TENON TETON TEXAN VEGAN VENIN WEEUN WEWON WEZEN XEDIN XENON XESIN YEARN YEMEN ZEVON

• • EN •

ABEND ADENI ADENO AGENA AGENT AKENE ALENE AMEND AMENS AMENT ANENT ARENA ARENS ARENT AVENA BEENE BEENS BLEND BLENT BRENS BRENT BUENA BUENO CIENS CTENO DIENE DUENA DUENO EDENS ELENA ELENI EMEND EVENS EVENT FAENA FIEND FRENA FRENI GEENA GHENT GLENN GLENS GWENN HYENA ICENI IDENT ILENE IRENA IRENE KEENE KEENS LIENS MEENY MIENS NOEND OMENS ONEND ONENO OPENS ORENA OVENS OWENS PEENS PHENO PLENA RIENS SAENS SCENA SCENE SCENT SIENA SPEND SPENT STENO STENS STENT SUENO TEENA TEENS TEENY TIENE TREND TRENT ULENE ULENT UPEND UPENN VTENS WEENA WEENY WHENS WRENS ZEENA

• • E • N

ATEIN BIEHN BREEN CLEAN CLEON CREON CUEIN DUEIN FREON GLEAN GLENN GREEN GWENN ICEIN IMEAN KLEIN LIEIN LIEON OCEAN ODEON OLEAN OLEIN ONEON OWEON PAEAN PREEN QUEEN RHEIN SEEIN SHEAN SHEEN SKEIN STEEN STEIN STERN THEUN TIEIN TIEON TOEIN TREEN TWEEN UPENN USEIN USEON WEEUN

• • • EN

ADMEN AIKEN ALBEN ALDEN ALIEN ALLEN ALPEN ARDEN ARLEN ARMEN ARWEN ASHEN ASPEN ATTEN AUDEN AXMEN BADEN BIDEN BOREN BOWEN BREEN BUREN CHIEN COHEN COVEN COZEN DALEN DAMEN DAVEN DONEN DOREN DOYEN DOZEN DUREN EATEN EBSEN EHREN EIGEN EINEN EISEN ELLEN EMDEN EMLEN ESSEN GALEN GIVEN GOREN GOYEN GREEN GUTEN HAGEN HALEN HAVEN HELEN HEMEN HIKEN HOSEN IBSEN INPEN KAMEN KAREN LADEN LATEN LEPEN LIKEN LINEN LIVEN LODEN LOREN LTGEN LUMEN LYNEN MAVEN MOGEN MOWEN NIVEN NOMEN NOREN NUMEN NUYEN OAKEN OATEN OFTEN OGDEN OLDEN OLSEN ORREN PAREN PATEN PIMEN PIVEN PLZEN PREEN PRMEN QUEEN QUIEN RAMEN RAVEN REPEN RIPEN RISEN RIVEN ROLEN ROSEN ROUEN ROWEN RUBEN SEVEN SHEEN SIREN SOREN STEEN TAKEN TOKEN TREEN TVMEN TWEEN UNPEN USTEN VIXEN WAKEN WAXEN WEZEN WIDEN WIZEN WODEN WOKEN WOMEN WOVEN YEMEN ZAZEN

EO • • •

EOFOR EOLIA EOLIC EOLUS EOSIN

E • O • •

EBOAT EBOLA EBOLI EBOND EBONS EBONY EBOOK ECOLE ECOLI ECONO ECONS ELOGE ELOPE ELORO EMORY EMOTE ENOCH ENOIL ENOKI ENOLA ENOLS ENORM ENOTE EPOCH EPODE EPOXY ERODE EROES EROSE ESOPS ETONS EVOKE EVORA EWOKS EXONS

E • • O •

EAMON EAPOE EATOF EATON EBOOK ECHOS ECTOR EDSON EGDON EGGON EGGOS ELBOW ELDON ELION ELIOT ELLOS ELMOS ELROY ELSOL ELTON ELYOT EMBOG ENDON ENDOR ENDOW ENJOY ENROL ENRON ENSOR ENTOM ENVOI ENVOY EOFOR EPCOT EPHOD EPHOR EPROM EPSOM EPSON ERDOS ERGOT ERROL ERROR ESPOO ESTOC ESTOP ESTOS ETHOS ETMOI EUROS EXCON EXCOP EXGOV EXPOS EXTOL EXXON

E • • • O

ECONO EDIPO EIEIO EJIDO ELORO ENERO ENNIO ERATO ESPIO ESPOO ETHNO EXTRO

• EO • •

AEONS BEOFF CEORL DEOXY FEOFF GEODE GEORG KEOGH LEOII LEOIV LEOIX LEONA LEONE LEONI LEORA LEOVI LEOXI MEOWS NEONS PEONS PEONY REOIL REOWN SEOUL XEONS YEOWS

• E • O •

AEIOU AEROS AESOP BEBOP BEDOG BEFOG BEFOR BEGOT BELON BELOW BESOM BESOS BESOT BETON BEZOS CEROS DECOR DECOY DEDOS DEFOE DEFOG DEION DELON DELOS DEMOB DEMON DEMOS DENOM DEPOT DESOD DETOO DETOX DEVOL DEVON FEDON FELON FETOR GENOA GETON HELOS HELOT HEMON HEROD HERON HEROS HESON JENOS KENOS KEVON KEYON LECON LEDON LEGOS LEMON LENOS LENOX LEROI LEROS LEROY LETON LEVON MEDOC MELON MELOS MELOT MEMOS MENOS MEROE MESON METOO NEMOS NEPOS NEROL PECOS PEKOE PEPOS PERON PEROT PESOS PETOS REBOP REBOX RECON REDON REDOS REDOX REHOE RELOG REMOP REMOW REPOS REPOT RESOD RESOW RETOP RETOW REWON SEGOS SENOR SEPOY SETON SEWON TENOF TENON TENOR TETON VELOX VENOM WEWON XENON XEROX YESOR ZENOS ZEROG ZEROS ZEVON

• E • • O

AEREO AERIO BEANO BELLO

BENTO
BEPPO
CELLO
CENTO
CERRO
DEKKO
DELCO
DELLO
DENTO
DERMO
DETOO
DEUTO
FEDTO
FEMTO
FERRO
GECKO
GEICO
GEKKO
GESSO
GETGO
GETTO
HECTO
HELIO
HELLO
HEPTO
HEWTO
JELLO
KEINO
KELSO
KENDO
LEDTO
LEGNO
LENTO
LETGO
LEUKO
MEDIO
MELLO
MENLO
METOO
METRO
MEZZO
NEATO
NEGRO
NELLO
NERVO
NEURO
NEWTO
PEABO
PEANO
PEDRO
PEPTO
PERRO
PESTO
PETCO
PETRO
RECTO
REPRO
RETRO
SEATO
SEETO
SEGNO
SEIKO
SERBO
SERIO
SERVO
SETTO
TEAMO
TELCO

TEMPO
TENGO
TENTO
VENLO
VENTO
VERSO
VESCO
WEDTO
YELLO
YESNO
ZENDO
ZEPPO
ZEPTO

••EO•
ATEOF
CLEON
CREON
FREON
LIEON
ODEON
OLEOS
ONEON
OREOS
OWEON
PREOP
THEOC
THEOK
THEOL
TIEON
USEOF
USEON

••E•O
ACETO
ADENO
ALERO
ANEMO
ANETO
ARESO
BUENO
CHEMO
CIELO
CREDO
CTENO
DIEGO
DUENO
DUETO
EIEIO
ENERO
FIERO
FREDO
FUEGO
GRECO
HIERO
HUEVO
HYETO
JUEGO
LIETO
LUEGO
MNEMO
NIETO
NUEVO
OKEMO
ONENO
OTERO
PHENO
PREGO

PTERO
QUESO
SEETO
SPERO
STENO
SUENO
TAEBO
THEPO
TIETO
USETO
VIEJO

•••EO
AEREO
BUTEO
CAMEO
CUNEO
FIVEO
HIDEO
HOMEO
JUDEO
KIDEO
MATEO
MIMEO
MINEO
MUSEO
ORFEO
OSSEO
OSTEO
PALEO
PASEO
RODEO
ROLEO
ROMEO
STLEO
TYPEO
VIDEO
VIREO

EP•••
EPACT
EPCOT
EPEES
EPHAH
EPHAS
EPHOD
EPHOR
EPICS
EPISC
EPOCH
EPODE
EPOXY
EPPIE
EPROM
EPSOM
EPSON

E•P••
EAPOE
ELPIS
EMPTY
EPPIE
ESPIO
ESPOO
ESPYS
EXPAT
EXPEL
EXPOS

E••P•
EARPS
EDIPO
EGYPT
ELOPE
ERUPT
ESOPS
ETAPE

E•••P
EATUP
ENDUP
EQUIP
ESTOP
EXCOP
EYEUP

•EP••
BEPPE
BEPPO
CEPES
DEPEW
DEPOT
DEPTH
DEPTS
HEPAT
HEPTA
HEPTO
KEPIS
LEPEN
LEPER
LEPEW
LEPKE
LEPUS
NEPAL
NEPHR
NEPOS
PEPIN
PEPLA
PEPOS
PEPPY
PEPSI
PEPTO
PEPUP
PEPYS
REPAD
REPAY
REPEG
REPEL
REPEN
REPIN
REPLY
REPOS
REPOT
REPPS
REPRO
REPUB
SEPAL
SEPIA
SEPOY
SEPTA
SEPTS
TEPEE
TEPID
ZEPPO
ZEPTO

•E•P•
BEEPS
BEPPE
BEPPO
DEEPS
DELPY
GEEPS
HEAPS
HEAPY
HELPS
HEMPS
HEMPY
JEEPS
KEEPS
KELPS
KEMPT
LEAPS
LEAPT
NEAPS
PEEPS
PEPPY
PERPS
REAPS
REPPS
REUPS
SEEPS
SEEPY
TEMPE
TEMPI
TEMPO
TEMPS
TEMPT
TENPM
TERPS
VEEPS
VESPA
WEEPS
WEEPY
YELPS
ZEPPO

•E••P
AESOP
BEBOP
DECAP
FEDUP
GETUP
HETUP
KEYUP
LEGUP
LETUP
METUP
PENUP
PEPUP
REBOP
RECAP
RECIP
REDIP
RELAP
REMAP
REMOP
RETAP
RETIP
RETOP
REVUP
REZIP
SEEUP
SETUP

SEWUP
TEEUP
TENUP

••EP•
ADEPT
ALEPH
BEEPS
CLEPT
CREPE
CREPT
DEEPS
DNEPR
GEEPS
INEPT
JEEPS
KEEPS
KREPS
ONEPM
PEEPS
PREPS
SEEPS
SEEPY
SLEPT
STEPS
SWEPT
THEPO
VEEPS
WEEPS
WEEPY

••E•P
AHEAP
APEEP
ATEUP
BLEEP
CHEAP
CHEEP
CREEP
CUEUP
DUEUP
EYEUP
ICEUP
LIEUP
ONEUP
PREOP
SEEUP
SHEEP
SHEMP
SLEEP
STEEP
SWEEP
TEEUP
THESP
TIEUP
TWERP
USEUP
WHELP

•••EP
ADREP
APEEP
BICEP
BLEEP
CHEEP
CREEP
JULEP
SALEP

SHEEP
SHLEP
SLEEP
STEEP
STREP
SWEEP

EQ•••
EQUAL
EQUIP
EQUIS
EQUIV
EQUUS

E•Q••
ESQUE

E•••Q
ETSEQ

•••EQ
ETSEQ

ER•••
ERASE
ERATO
ERBIL
ERDOS
ERECT
EREDE
ERETZ
EREVS
ERGOT
ERIAS
ERICA
ERICH
ERICK
ERIES
ERIKA
ERING
ERISA
ERITU
ERMAS
ERNES
ERNIE
ERNST
ERODE
EROES
EROSE
ERRED
ERROL
ERROR
ERTES
ERUCT
ERUPT
ERVIN
ERWIN

E•R••
EARED
EARLE
EARLS
EARLY
EARNS
EARPS
EARTH
ECRUS
EDRED

EERIE
EFREM
EGRET
EHREN
ELREY
ELROY
ENROL
ENRON
EPROM
ERRED
ERROL
ERROR
ETRES
EUROS
EURUS
EYRAS
EYRIE
EYRIR

E••R•
EAGRE
EBERT
ECARD
ELARA
ELORO
ELURA
EMERY
EMIRS
EMORY
ENARE
ENARM
ENCRE
ENERO
ENGRS
ENORM
ENTRE
ENTRY
ENURE
EVERS
EVERT
EVERY
EVORA
EWART
EWERS
EWERY
EXERT
EXTRA
EXTRO
EXURB
EYERS

E•••R
EAGER
EASER
EATER
ECTOR
EDGAR
EDGER
EDMAR
EELER
EGGAR
EGGER
EIDER
EIGER
EINER
ELCAR
ELDER
ELGAR

ELLER
ELMAR
ELMER
ELVER
EMBAR
EMBER
EMEER
EMMER
ENDER
ENDOR
ENSOR
ENTER
ENVER
EOFOR
EPHOR
ERROR
ESKER
ESTAR
ESTER
ETHER
EULER
EYRIR

•ER••
AEREO
AERIE
AERIO
AEROS
BERCY
BEREA
BERET
BERGS
BERIA
BERKS
BERLE
BERMS
BERNE
BERNI
BERRA
BERRY
BERTA
BERTH
BERYL
CERAM
CERAT
CERES
CERIA
CERIC
CEROS
CERRO
CERTS
DERAT
DERBY
DEREK
DERIV
DERMA
DERMO
DERRY
EERIE
FERAL
FERDE
FERIA
FERMI
FERNS
FERNY
FERRI
FERRO
FERRY

GERMS
GERMY
GERRY
GERTZ
HERAT
HERBE
HERBS
HERBY
HERDS
HEREK
HERES
HERKY
HERNE
HEROD
HERON
HEROS
HERSH
HERTS
HERTZ
HERVE
HERZL
JEREZ
JERKS
JERKY
JERNE
JERRY
JERZY
KERBS
KERFS
KERNE
KERNS
KERRI
KERRY
KERSH
LEROI
LEROS
LEROY
MERCE
MERCH
MERCI
MERCK
MERCS
MERCY
MERER
MERES
MERGE
MERIT
MERLE
MERLS
MEROE
MERRY
MERTZ
MERYL
NERDS
NERDY
NERFS
NEROL
NERTS
NERTZ
NERVA
NERVE
NERVO
NERVY
PERAN
PERAS
PERCE
PERCH
PERCS

PERCY
PERDU
PERES
PEREZ
PERFS
PERIL
PERIS
PERKS
PERKY
PERLE
PERMA
PERMS
PERON
PEROT
PERPS
PERRO
PERRY
PERSE
PERTH
RERAN
RERIG
RERUN
SERAC
SERAI
SERAL
SERBO
SERBS
SERFS
SERGE
SERIA
SERIF
SERIN
SERIO
SERRA
SERTA
SERTS
SERUM
SERVE
SERVO
TERAT
TERCE
TERIA
TERME
TERMS
TERNE
TERNS
TERPS
TERRA
TERRE
TERRI
TERRS
TERRY
TERSE
TERZA
VERBS
VERDE
VERDI
VERGE
VERMI
VERNA
VERNE
VERRE
VERSA
VERSE
VERSO
VERST
VERTE
VERTS

VERVE
XERIC
XEROX
YERBA
ZERBE
ZEROG
ZEROS

•E•R•
BEARD
BEARS
BEART
BEERS
BEERY
BEIRA
BERRA
BERRY
CEARA
CEORL
CERRO
DEARE
DEARS
DEARY
DEBRA
DECRY
DEERE
DEERS
DERRY
DETRE
DEVRY
FEARS
FERRI
FERRO
FERRY
GEARS
GEARY
GENRE
GEORG
GERRY
HEARD
HEARN
HEARS
HEART
HEIRS
HENRI
HENRY
HEURE
JEERS
JEERY
JERRY
JEWRY
KEIRA
KERRI
KERRY
LEARN
LEARS
LEARY
LEERS
LEERY
LEHRS
LEORA
LEURS
MEARA
MEARS
MERRY
METRE
METRO
METRY

NEARS
NEDRA
NEGRI
NEGRO
NEHRU
NEURO
PEARL
PEARS
PEARY
PEDRO
PEERS
PERRO
PERRY
PETRA
PETRE
PETRI
PETRO
PEURS
REARM
REARS
REDRY
REFRY
REPRO
RETRO
RETRY
SEARS
SEERS
SEGRE
SERRA
TEARS
TEARY
TEERS
TERRA
TERRE
TERRI
TERRS
TERRY
TETRA
TETRI
VEERS
VEERY
VERRE
WEARS
WEARY
WEIRD
WEIRS
YEARN
YEARS
ZEBRA

•E••R
AEGIR
AESIR
BEFOR
BEHAR
BEXAR
CEDAR
CEDER
CENTR
CESAR
DEAIR
DEBAR
DECIR
DECOR
DEFER
DEMUR
DENAR
DENDR

DETAR
DETER
DEWAR
DEXTR
EELER
FEMUR
FETOR
FEUER
FEVER
FEWER
FEYER
HETER
HEUER
HEWER
HEXER
HEYER
JETER
KEFIR
LECAR
LEDER
LEGER
LEHAR
LEMUR
LEPER
LEVAR
LEVER
MEIER
MERER
METER
MEWER
MEYER
NEHER
NEPHR
NEVER
NEWER
PEDER
PETER
REAIR
REBAR
REBER
RECUR
REFER
REGER
RETAR
SEDER
SEGAR
SEGER
SENOR
SEVER
SEWER
SEXER
TELAR
TENOR
VELAR
VEXER
WEBER
WESER
YESOR
ZENER

••ER•
ACERB
ACERS
AGERS
AKERS
ALERO
ALERS
ALERT

AMERY
APERS
APERY
AVERS
AVERT
AVERY
AXERS
AYERS
AZERA
AZERI
BEERS
BEERY
BIERE
BIERI
BIERS
BOERS
BRERS
CBERS
CHERE
CHERI
CHERT
CIERA
CLERK
CUERS
DEERE
DEERS
DOERR
DOERS
DYERS
EBERT
EMERY
ENERO
EVERS
EVERT
EVERY
EWERS
EWERY
EXERT
EYERS
FAERY
FIERO
FIERS
FIERY
FRERE
GOERS
HIERO
HOERS
HUERS
IBERT
ICERS
INERT
ISERE
ITERS
JEERS
JEERY
LEERS
LEERY
MIERS
MYERS
NLERS
OMERS
ONERA
ONERS
OPERA
OPERE
OTERI
OTERO
OVERS

OVERT
OWERS
OYERS
PEERS
PFERD
PIERS
PTERO
QBERT
QUERY
RUERS
RVERS
SEERS
SHERA
SHERE
SHERM
SNERD
SNERT
SPERM
SPERO
STERE
STERN
SUERS
TEERS
THERA
THERE
THERM
TIERS
TWERE
TWERP
USERS
VEERS
VEERY
VIERS
WHERE

••E•R
ABEAR
AMEER
AREAR
AYEAR
BLEAR
BYEAR
CHEER
CLEAR
COEUR
DNEPR
DOERR
DREAR
EMEER
FLEER
FLEUR
FREER
GREER
IHEAR
NOEAR
ONEIR
QUEER
SHEAR
SHEER
SMEAR
SNEER
SOEUR
SPEAR
SPEER
STEER
SWEAR
THEIR

•••ER
ABLER
ABNER
ACHER
ACTER
ADDER
ADLER
AFTER
AIDER
AIMER
AIRER
ALDER
ALGER
ALLER
ALTER
AMBER
AMEER
ANGER
ANSER
AOLER
APTER
ARBER
ARMER
ASHER
ASKER
ASNER
ASPER
ASSER
ASTER
AUBER
AUGER
BADER
BAJER
BAKER
BALER
BARER
BASER
BAUER
BAYER
BHAER
BIDER
BIKER
BITER
BLUER
BOJER
BONER
BOOER
BORER
BOWER
BOXER
BOYER
BRIER
BUBER
BUYER
BYNER
CABER
CAGER
CANER
CAPER
CARER
CASER
CATER
CAVER
CEDER
CHEER
CIDER
CITER
CLUER

5
ES

CODER COKER COMER CONER COOER COPER CORER COVER COWER COYER CRIER CRYER CUBER CURER CUTER CYBER CYDER DARER DATER DAZER DEFER DETER DICER DIKER DINER DIRER DIVER DIYER DOPER DOSER DOTER DOVER DOZER DRIER DRYER DUPER DURER DYKER EAGER EASER EATER EDGER EELER EGGER EIDER EIGER EINER ELDER ELLER ELMER ELVER EMBER EMEER EMMER ENDER ENTER ENVER ESKER ESTER ETHER EULER FABER FACER FADER FAKER FAMER FARER FAXER

FEUER FEVER FEWER FEYER FIBER FIFER FILER FINER FIRER FIVER FIXER FLEER FLIER FLYER FOYER FREER FRIER FRYER FUMER GAMER GAPER GATER GAYER GAZER GIBER GIVER GLUER GOFER GOMER GONER GOWER GREER GRIER HABER HALER HAMER HATER HAUER HAVER HAWER HAYER HAZER HETER HEUER HEWER HEXER HEYER HIDER HIKER HIRER HIVER HOLER HOMER HONER HOPER HOSER HOVER HUBER HUGER HYPER HYSER ICIER IDLER ILLER INFER INGER INKER INNER

INTER INVER IRKER JAPER JAWER JETER JIVER JOKER KHMER KINER KISER KITER KYSER LACER LADER LAGER LAKER LAMER LASER LATER LAUER LAVER LAXER LAYER LEDER LEGER LEPER LEVER LIBER LIFER LIGER LIKER LINER LITER LIVER LODER LONER LOPER LOSER LOVER LOWER LUGER LUNER LURER MACER MAHER MAKER MASER MATER MAYER MEIER MERER METER MEWER MEYER MILER MIMER MINER MISER MITER MIXER MOOER MOPER MOVER MOWER MUJER MUSER MUTER

NADER NAMER NBAER NEHER NEVER NEWER NFLER NHLER NICER NIGER NINER NITER NIXER NIZER NOSER NOTER NUDER OARER OATER OCHER ODDER OFFER OGIER OGLER OILER OLDER OMBER OPPER ORDER ORSER OSIER OSLER OSTER OTHER OTTER OUTER OWNER PACER PAGER PALER PAPER PARER PATER PAVER PAWER PAYER PEDER PETER PIKER PILER PINER PIPER PLIER PLYER POKER POLER PORER POSER POWER PRIER PRYER PULER PURER QUEER RACER RADER RAFER RAGER

RAKER RARER RASER RATER RAVER RAWER RAZER REBER REFER REGER RICER RIDER RIFER RIKER RIMER RIPER RISER RIVER ROBER ROGER ROKER ROPER ROVER ROWER RUDER RULER RUMER RYDER SABER SAFER SAGER SANER SAVER SAWER SAYER SEDER SEGER SEVER SEWER SEXER SHEER SHIER SHOER SHYER SIXER SIZER SKIER SLIER SLYER SNEER SOBER SOFER SOLER SORER SOWER SPEER SPIER STEER SUMER SUPER SURER TAKER TALER TAMER TAPER TASER TATER TAXER

TIBER TIGER TILER TIMER TITER TOLER TONER TOOER TOPER TOTER TOWER TOYER TRIER TRUER TUBER TUNER TYGER TYLER TYNER TYPER UDDER ULCER UMBER UNDER UNGER UNSER UNTER UPPER URGER USHER UTHER UTTER VADER VATER VEXER VILER VINER VIPER VOMER VOTER VOWER WADER WAFER WAGER WAKER WANER WATER WAVER WAXER WEBER WESER WIDER WIPER WIRER WISER WOOER WRIER WRYER WYLER YARER ZENER ZONER

ES•••

ESAKI ESBAT ESIST ESKER ESNES ESOPS ESPIO ESPOO ESPYS ESQUE ESSAI ESSAY ESSEN ESSES ESSEX ESSIE ESTAB ESTAN ESTAR ESTAS ESTEE ESTER ESTES ESTHS ESTOC ESTOP ESTOS

E•S••

EASED EASEL EASER EASES EASTS EASYA EBSEN EDSEL EDSON EISEN ELSAS ELSES ELSIE ELSOL ENSKY ENSOR ENSUE EOSIN EPSOM EPSON ESSAI ESSAY ESSEN ESSES ESSEX ESSIE ETSEQ

E••S•

ECASH EENSY EGEST ELISA ELISE ELIST ELMST ELYSE EMESA EPISC ERASE ERISA ERNST EROSE ESIST EXIST

E•••S

EAMES EARLS EARNS EARPS EASES EASTS EAVES EBELS EBONS ECHOS ECONS ECRUS EDAMS EDDAS EDENS EDGES EDIES EDITS EFIKS EGADS EGALS EGEUS EGGOS EINES ELEMS ELEVS ELIAS ELLES ELLIS ELLOS ELMOS ELPIS ELSAS ELSES ELULS ELVES ELVIS ELWES EMAGS EMEUS EMIRS EMITS EMMYS ENBAS ENCLS ENGRS ENNIS ENOLS EOLUS EPEES EPHAS EPICS EQUIS EQUUS ERDOS EREVS ERIAS ERIES ERMAS ERNES EROES ERTES ESNES ESOPS ESPYS ESSES ESTAS ESTES ESTHS ESTOS ETATS ETHOS ETNAS ETONS ETRES ETTES ETUIS EUROS EURUS EVANS EVENS EVERS EVILS EWERS EWOKS EXAMS EXECS EXGIS EXITS EXONS EXPOS EYERS EYRAS

•ES••

AESIR AESOP BESES BESET BESOM BESOS BESOT BESTS CESAR CESTA CESTI DESAI DESDE DESEX DESKS DESNA DESOD DESTE FESTA FESTE FESTS GESSO GESTE GESTS HESHE HESON HESSE HESTS JESSE JESSY JESTS JESUS KESEY MESAS MESES MESHY MESNE MESON MESSE MESSY MESTA NESIA NESTS NESTY OESTE PESCE PESCI PESKY PESOS PESTO PESTS RESAT RESAW RESAY RESEE RESET RESEW RESHT RESIN RESIT RESOD RESOW RESTE RESTS TESLA TESSA TESTA TESTS TESTY VESCO VESPA VESTA VESTI VESTS WESER WESTS XESIN YESES YESNO YESOR ZESTA ZESTS ZESTY

•E•S•

BEAST BETSY CEASE CENSE DEISM DEIST DENSE EENSY FEAST GEESE GEIST GESSO HEISS HEIST HERSH HESSE HEYSE JESSE JESSY KELSO KERSH LEASE LEASH LEAST MEESE MENSA MESSE MESSY MEUSE NELSE NEUSS NEWSY PEASE PEPSI PERSE REASK REESE REISZ REUSE REUSS SEEST SEISM SENSE SEUSS TEASE TENSE TERSE TESSA VERSA VERSE VERSO VERST WEEST WEISS WEISZ WELSH YEAST ZEISS ZEIST

•E••S

AEDES AEGIS AEONS AEROS BEADS BEAKS BEALS BEAMS BEANS BEARS BEATS BEAUS BECKS BEEFS BEENS BEEPS BEERS BEETS BEINS BELLS BELTS BEMAS BENDS BENES BENTS BERGS BERKS BERMS BESES BESOS BESTS BETAS BETES BETHS BEZOS CEDES CEDIS CEILS CELLS CELTS CENAS CENTS CEPES CERES CEROS CERTS CETUS DEALS DEANS DEARS DEBTS DEBUS DECKS DEDOS DEEDS DEEMS DEEPS DEERS DEGAS DEILS DEKES DELES DELIS DELLS DELOS DELTS DEMES DEMOS DENES DENIS DENTS DENYS DEPTS DESKS DEVAS FEARS FEATS FEEBS FEEDS FEELS FEETS FELIS FELLS FELTS FEMES FENDS FERNS FESTS FETAS FETES FETUS FEUDS FEZES GEARS GEEKS GEEPS GELDS GELTS GENES GENTS GENUS GENXS GERMS GESTS GETAS HEADS HEALS HEAPS HEARS HEATS HECKS HEEDS HEELS HEFTS HEHES HEIRS HEISS HELLS HELMS HELOS HELPS HEMES HEMPS HERBS HERDS HERES HEROS HERTS HESTS HETHS HEXES JEANS JEEPS JEERS JEFES JELLS JENOS JERKS JESTS JESUS JETES KEATS KEELS KEENS KEEPS KELPS KENOS KEPIS KERBS KERFS KERNS KEYES LEADS LEAFS LEAKS LEANS LEAPS LEARS LECTS LEEDS LEEKS LEERS LEFTS LEGGS LEGOS LEHRS LENDS LENES LENIS LENOS LENTS LEPUS LEROS LETTS LEURS LEVIS LEWES LEWIS LEXIS LEXUS MEADS MEALS MEANS MEARS MEATS MEDES MEETS MELDS MELIS MELOS MELTS MEMOS MENAS MENDS MENES MENOS MENUS MEOWS MERCS MERES MERLS MESAS MESES METES METIS MEWLS NEAPS NEARS NEATS NECKS NEEDS NEGUS NEHIS NEMOS NENES NEONS NEPOS NERDS NERFS NERTS NESTS NEUSS NEVES NEVIS NEVUS NEWTS NEXIS NEXUS OEUFS PEAKS PEALS PEARS PEATS PEBAS PECKS PECOS PEEKS PEELS PEENS PEEPS PEERS PEKES PELFS PELTS PENDS PEONS PEPOS PEPYS PERAS PERCS PERES PERFS PERIS PERKS PERMS PERPS PESOS PESTS PETES PETOS PEURS READS REALS REAMS REAPS REARS REBUS RECKS RECTS REDES REDOS REEDS REEFS REEKS REELS REFIS REGES REGIS REGTS REIMS REINS REITS REMUS RENDS RENTS REPOS REPPS RESTS REUPS REUSS REVES REXES REYES SEALS SEAMS SEARS SEATS SECHS SECTS SEEAS SEEDS SEEKS SEEMS SEEPS SEERS SEGOS SELES SELLS SEMIS SENDS SEPTS SERBS SERFS SERTS SETTS SEUSS SEXES TEAKS TEALS TEAMS TEARS TEATS TECHS TEEMS TEENS TEERS TELES TELLS TEMAS TEMPS TENDS TENKS TENTS TERMS TERNS TERPS TERRS TESTS TETES TETHS TEWAS TEWES TEXAS TEXTS VEALS VEDAS VEEPS VEERS VEGAS VEGES VEILS VEINS VELDS VENDS VENTS VENUS VERBS VERTS VESTS VEXES VEZES WEALS WEANS WEARS WEEDS WEEKS WEEMS WEEPS WEFTS WEIRS WEISS WELDS WELLS WELTS WENDS WESTS XEONS YEAHS YEANS YEARS YEATS YEGGS YELLS YELPS YEOWS YESES YETIS ZEALS ZEBUS ZEISS ZENDS ZENOS ZEROS ZESTS ZETAS

••ES•

ARESO ATEST BLESS BLEST BREST CHESS CHEST CRESC CRESS CREST DOEST DRESS DYESS EGEST EMESA FLESH FRESH FRESS GEESE GLESS GOEST GUESS GUEST HOEST HTEST IDEST KRESS LIESL LIEST LOESS MEESE NTEST OBESE ODESA OUEST PAESE POESY PRESA

PRESB PRESE PRESS QUESO QUEST QWEST REESE RLESS SEEST THESE THESP TRESS WEEST WIEST WREST

••E•S

ABETS ACERS AGERS AHEMS AKERS ALEFS ALERS AMENS APERS AREAS ARENS AVERS AXELS AXERS AYERS BEEFS BEENS BEEPS BEERS BEETS BIERS BLEBS BLESS BLEUS BOERS BREES BRENS BRERS BREWS CBERS CHEFS CHESS CHEWS CIELS CIENS CLEFS CLEWS COEDS CREDS CREES CRESS CREWS CUERS DEEDS DEEMS DEEPS DEERS DIELS DIEMS DIETS DNETS

DOERS DREGS DREKS DRESS DUELS DUETS DYERS DYESS EBELS EDENS EGEUS ELEMS ELEVS EMEUS EPEES EREVS EVENS EVERS EWERS EXECS EYERS FEEBS FEEDS FEELS FEETS FIEFS FIERS FLEAS FLEES FREES FRESS FRETS FUELS GAELS GEEKS GEEPS GHEES GLEES GLENS GLESS GOERS GREYS GUESS HEEDS HEELS HOERS HUERS HUEYS ICEES ICERS IDEAS IDEES INEES ITEAS ITEMS ITERS JEEPS JEERS JOEYS JPEGS KEELS KEENS KEEPS KNEES KREBS KREPS KRESS LEEDS

LEEKS LEERS LIENS LIEUS LOESS LOEWS LWEIS MEETS MIELS MIENS MIERS MPEGS MYERS NEEDS NIELS NLERS NOELS NYETS OBEYS ODETS OGEES OLEOS OMENS OMERS ONEKS ONELS ONERS OPEDS OPELS OPENS OREOS OVENS OVERS OWENS OWERS OYERS PEEKS PEELS PEENS PEEPS PEERS PIEDS PIELS PIERS PLEAS PLEBS POEMS POETS PREPS PRESS PREYS REEDS REEFS REEKS REELS RHEAS RIELS RIENS RLESS RUERS RVERS SAENS SEEAS SEEDS SEEKS SEEMS SEEPS SEERS

SHEDS SKEDS SKEGS SKEWS SLEDS SLEWS SLEYS SMEES SMEWS SNEES SPECS SPETS SPEWS STEMS STENS STEPS STETS STEWS SUERS SUETS TAELS TEEMS TEENS TEERS THEAS THEMS THEWS TIEGS TIERS TOEAS TREAS TREES TREKS TRESS TRETS TREWS TREYS TYEES ULEES UREAS USEAS USEES USERS UVEAS VEEPS VEERS VIERS VIEWS VTENS WEEDS WEEKS WEEMS WEEPS WHEES WHENS WHETS WHEWS WHEYS WRENS

•••ES

AAMES ABBES ABIES ACHES ACMES ACNES ACRES ACTES ADZES AEDES AGNES AGUES AHYES AIDES AILES AIRES ALLES ALOES ALPES AMIES ANDES ANGES ANTES AONES APRES APSES ARIES ARLES ARMES ARSES ASHES ASSES ATLES AXLES AYRES BABES BAIES BAKES BALES BANES BARES BASES BATES BAYES BENES BESES BETES BIDES BIKES BILES BINES BITES BLUES BODES BOLES BONES BORES BOWES BOXES BRAES BREES BRIES BUSES BYTES CAFES CAGES CAKES CANES CAPES CARES CASES CATES CAVES CEDES CEPES

CERES CINES CIRES CITES CLAES CLUES CODES COKES COLES COMES CONES COPES CORES COTES COVES COWES COXES COZES CREES CRIES CUBES CUKES CUMES CURES CUTES CYMES DACES DALES DAMES DANES DARES DATES DAVES DAWES DAZES DEKES DELES DEMES DENES DICES DIKES DIMES DINES DIVES DOCES DOGES DOLES DOMES DOPES DOSES DOTES DOVES DOZES DRIES DUCES DUDES DUKES DUNES DUPES DYNES EAMES EASES EAVES EDGES EDIES EINES ELLES ELSES

ELVES ELWES EPEES ERIES ERNES EROES ERTES ESNES ESSES ESTES ETRES ETTES FACES FADES FAKES FAMES FANES FARES FATES FAVES FAXES FAZES FEMES FETES FEZES FIDES FIFES FILES FINES FIRES FIVES FIXES FLEES FLIES FLOES FLUES FOIES FORES FOXES FREES FRIES FROES FUMES FUSES GAGES GALES GAMES GAPES GARES GASES GATES GAZES GENES GHEES GIBES GILES GIVES GLEES GLUES GORES GRUES GYRES HADES HAKES HALES HAMES HANES HARES

HATES HAVES HAYES HAZES HEHES HEMES HERES HEXES HIDES HIKES HIMES HINES HIRES HIVES HOKES HOLES HOMES HONES HOPES HOSES HOWES HYPES ICEES ICKES IDEES IDLES IGNES INEES INNES ISLES IVIES JADES JAKES JAMES JAPES JEFES JETES JIBES JIVES JOKES JONES JUDES JUKES JULES JUNES JUTES KALES KEYES KITES KNEES KODES LACES LADES LAKES LAMES LANES LARES LASES LAVES LAWES LAZES LENES LEWES LIKES LIMES LINES LITES LIVES

LOBES LODES LOGES LOPES LORES LOSES LOVES LOWES LOXES LUBES LUGES LUNES LURES LUTES LUXES LYRES LYSES MACES MAGES MAKES MALES MANES MAPES MARES MATES MAXES MAZES MEDES MENES MERES MESES METES MIKES MILES MIMES MINES MIRES MITES MIXES MLLES MODES MOLES MOPES MORES MOSES MOTES MOUES MOVES MTGES MULES MURES MUSES MUTES MYLES NABES NAMES NAPES NARES NAVES NENES NEVES NIKES NILES NIMES NINES NITES NIXES NODES

NOLES NONES NOPES NOSES NOTES NOYES NUDES NUKES OAKES OASES OATES OBIES OBOES OGEES OGLES OGRES OHYES OKIES OLPES OMNES ONDES ONNES OOZES ORFES ORLES ORSES OTOES OWIES PACES PAGES PALES PANES PARES PASES PATES PAVES PEKES PERES PETES PIKES PILES PINES PIPES PLIES POKES POLES POMES PONES POPES PORES POSES POXES PRIES PUCES PULES PYRES PYXES RACES RAGES RAKES RALES RASES RATES RAVES RAXES RAZES REDES REGES

REVES REXES REYES RICES RIDES RILES RIMES RISES RITES RIVES ROBES ROLES ROMES ROPES ROSES ROTES ROUES ROVES RUBES RULES RUNES RUSES SAFES SAGES SAKES SALES SASES SATES SAVES SAXES SELES SEXES SHIES SHOES SIDES SIKES SINES SIRES SITES SIXES SIZES SKIES SKYES SLOES SLUES SMEES SNEES SOLES SONES SORES SPIES STIES STYES SUPES TAKES TALES TAMES TAPES TARES TATES TAXES TELES TETES TEWES TIDES TIKES TILES TIMES

TINES TIRES TOKES TOLES TOMES TONES TOPES TOTES TOVES TPKES TREES TRIES TRUES TUBES TULES TUNES TUXES TYEES TYKES TYPES TYRES ULEES URGES URNES USEES USHES VALES VANES VASES VAXES VEGES VEXES VEZES VIBES VICES VIKES VINES VISES VOLES VOTES WADES WAGES WAKES WALES WANES WARES WAVES WAXES WHEES WILES WINES WIPES WIRES WISES WIVES WIZES XAXES YATES YAXES YESES YIKES YIPES YOKES YORES YPRES YULES ZALES ZAXES

ZINES ZONES

ET•••

ETAGE ETAIL ETAPE ETATS ETHAN ETHEL ETHER ETHIC ETHNO ETHOS ETHYL ETILE ETMOI ETNAS ETONS ETRES ETSEQ ETTES ETUDE ETUIS ETYMA

E•T••

EATAT EATEN EATER EATIN EATIT EATME EATOF EATON EATUP ECTAD ECTAL ECTOR ELTON ENTAD ENTER ENTOM ENTRE ENTRY ERTES ESTAB ESTAN ESTAR ESTAS ESTEE ESTER ESTES ESTHS ESTOC ESTOP ESTOS ETTES EXTOL EXTRA EXTRO

E••T•

EARTH EASTS EDITH EDITS ELATE ELATH ELITE ELUTE EMITS EMOTE EMPTY ENATE ENOTE ERATO ERETZ ERITU ETATS EVITA EVITE EXITS

E•••T

EATAT EATIT EBERT EBOAT ECLAT EDICT EDUCT EFLAT EGEST EGRET EGYPT EIGHT EILAT EJECT ELECT ELIOT ELIST ELMST ELYOT EMMET ENACT ENDAT ENDIT EPACT EPCOT ERECT ERGOT ERNST ERUCT ERUPT ESBAT ESIST EVENT EVERT EVICT EWART EXACT EXALT EXERT EXIST EXMET EXPAT EXULT

•ET••

AETNA BETAS BETEL BETES BETHS BETON BETSY BETTA BETTE BETTI BETTY CETTE CETUS DETAR DETAT DETER DETOO DETOX DETRE DETTE FETAL FETAS FETCH FETED FETES FETID FETOR FETUS GETAB GETAC GETAD GETAS GETAT GETBY GETGO GETIN GETIT GETME GETON GETTO GETTY GETUP HETER HETHS HETTY HETUP JETER JETES JETLI JETTA JETTY KETCH KETTI KETTY LETAT LETBE LETBY LETGO LETHE LETIN LETME LETON LETTS LETTY LETUP METAL METED METER METES METIS METOO METRE METRO METRY METUP NETTY NETWT PETAL PETCO PETER PETES PETEY PETIT PETOS PETRA PETRE PETRI PETRO PETTI PETTY RETAG RETAN RETAP RETAR RETAX RETIA RETIE RETIN RETIP RETOP RETOW RETRO RETRY RETTY SETAE SETAT SETBY SETIN SETON SETTE SETTO SETTS SETUP TETES TETHS TETON TETRA TETRI VETCH VETTE WETLY YETIS YETTA ZETAS ZETTA

•E•T•

BEATS BEATY BEETS BEETY BELTS BENTO BENTS BERTA BERTH BESTS BETTA BETTE BETTI BETTY CELTS CENTI CENTO CENTR CENTS CENTU CERTS CESTA CESTI CETTE CEUTA DEATH DEBTS DEITY DELTA DELTS DENTE DENTI DENTO DENTS DEPTH DEPTS DESTE DETTE DEUTO DEXTR FEATS FEDTO FEETS FELTS FEMTO FESTA FESTE FESTS GELTS GENTE GENTS GERTZ GESTE GESTS GETTO GETTY HEATH HEATS HECTO HEFTI HEFTS HEFTY HEPTA HEPTO HERTS HERTZ HESTS HETTY HEWTO JESTS JETTA JETTY KEATS KEITH KETTI KETTY LECTS LEDTO LEFTS LEFTY LEITH LENTE LENTO

5 ET

LENTS LETTS LETTY LEYTE MEATH MEATS MEATY MEETS MEHTA MELTS MERTZ MESTA NEATH NEATO NEATS NERTS NERTZ NESTS NESTY NETTY NEWTO NEWTS OESTE PEATS PEATY PEETE PELTS PENTA PENTE PEPTO PERTH PESTO PESTS PETTI PETTY REATA RECTA RECTI RECTO RECTS REGTS REITS RENTE RENTS RESTE RESTS RETTY SEATO SEATS SECTS SEETH SEETO SENTA SENTE SEPTA SEPTS SERTA SERTS SETTE SETTO SETTS TEATS TEETH TENTH TENTO TENTS TESTA TESTS TESTY TEXTS VENTA VENTI VENTO VENTS VERTE VERTS VESTA VESTI VESTS VETTE WEBTV WEDTO WEFTS WEITZ WELTS WELTY WESTS YEATS YENTA YENTE YENTL YETTA ZEPTO ZESTA ZESTS ZESTY ZETTA

•E••T

BEART BEAST BEAUT BEFIT BEGAT BEGET BEGOT BENET BERET BESET BESOT CERAT DEALT DEBIT DEBUT DEFAT DEIST DELFT DEMIT DEPOT DERAT DETAT FEAST FEINT GEIST GENET GETAT GETIT HEART HECHT HEIDT HEIST HELOT HEMAT HEMET HEPAT HERAT KEMPT LEANT LEAPT LEAST LEGIT LEMAT LETAT LEVIT MEANT MEDIT. MELOT MERIT NETWT NEWAT PEROT PETIT PEWIT REACT REBET REBUT RECUT REFIT REHIT RELET RELIT REMAT REMET REMIT REPOT RESAT RESET RESHT RESIT REVET REWET SEEST SENAT SETAT TEBET TEMPT TENET TERAT TEVET VEIDT VELDT VERST WEEST WENDT YEAST ZEIST

••ET•

ABETS ACETO ALETA ANETO ARETE BEETS BEETY BRETT CHETA CLETE CRETE DIETE DIETS DIETZ DNETS DOETH DUETO DUETS ERETZ FEETS FRETS GAETA GOETH GRETA GRETE HYETO LIETO MEETS NIETA NIETO NYETS ODETS OLETA OVETA OVETT PEETE PIETA PIETY POETE POETS RHETT RIETI SEETH SEETO SIETE SPETS STETS SUETS SUETY TEETH THETA TIETO TRETS USETO WHETS WYETH

••E•T

ACEIT ADEPT AGENT ALERT ALEUT AMENT ANENT ARENT ATEAT ATEIT ATEST AVERT BLEAT BLENT BLEST BRENT BREST BRETT CHEAT CHERT CHEST CLEAT CLEFT CLEPT CREPT CREST DOEST DREFT DWELT EBERT EGEST EJECT ELECT ERECT EVENT EVERT EXERT FLEET GHENT GOEST GREAT GREET GUEST HOEST HTEST IBERT ICEIT IDENT IDEST INEPT INERT KNELT LIEST LIEUT NTEST OUEST OVERT OVETT PLEAT QBERT QUEST QWEST RHETT SCENT SEEST SHEET SKEET SLEET SLEPT SMELT SNERT SPELT SPENT STENT SWEAT SWEET SWEPT THEFT TREAT TRENT TWEET ULENT USEIT WEEST WHEAT WIEST WREST

•••ET

AGLET AMVET ARMET ARRET ASSET ASYET AVNET BEGET BENET BERET BESET BIDET BINET BIZET BLUET BOLET BONET BOVET BURET CADET CAPET CARET CIVET COMET COSET COVET CRUET CULET CURET DALET DUVET EGRET EMMET EXMET FACET FILET FLEET FUMET GENET GODET GOGET GREET HEMET IMSET INLET INSET ISLET JACET JANET LOTET LUMET MAMET MANET MONET MOTET MRMET NOBET NONET NYJET NYMET OBJET OCTET ONSET OSSET OWLET PAGET PIPET PUGET QUIET RAMET REBET RELET REMET RESET REVET REWET RIVET ROGET SAGET SHEET SKEET SLEET SWEET TACET TEBET TENET TEVET TIBET TOLET TVSET TWEET UNBET UNLET UNMET UNSET UNWET UPSET VALET

EU•••

EUBIE EUELL EULER EUROS EURUS

E•U••

EBUZZ EDUCE EDUCT ELUDE ELULS ELURA ELUTE ENURE EQUAL EQUIP EQUIS EQUIV EQUUS ERUCT ERUPT ETUDE ETUIS EXUDE EXULT EXUMA EXURB

E••U•

EATUP ECRUS EGEUS EMEUS ENDUE ENDUP ENNUI ENSUE EOLUS EQUUS ESQUE EURUS EXCUB EYEUP

E•••U

ELIHU ERITU

•EU••

CEUTA DEUCE DEUCY DEUEL DEUTO FEUDS FEUER HEUER HEURE JEUDI JEUNE LEUKO LEUMI LEURS MEUSE NEURO NEUSS OEUFS PEURS REUEL REUNE REUPS REUSE REUSS SEULE SEUSS

•E•U•

BEAUS BEAUT BEAUX BEGUM BEGUN CECUM CETUS DEBUG DEBUS DEBUT DEGUM DEMUR FEDUP FEMUR FETUS GENUS GETUP HETUP JESUS KEYUP LEAUD LEGUP LEHUA LEMUR LEPUS LETUP LEXUS MECUM MENUS METUP NEFUD NEGUS NEVUS NEXUS PEGUY PENUP PEPUP REBUS REBUT REBUY RECUE RECUR RECUT REDUB REDUG REDUX REGUM REMUS REPUB RERUN REVUE REVUP SEDUM SEEUP SEGUE SEOUL SERUM SETUP SEWUP TEEUP TENUP VELUM VENUE VENUS WEEUN ZEBUS

•E••U

AEIOU BELAU CENTU KEANU NEHRU PERDU TENDU

••EU•

ADEUX ALEUT ATEUP BLEUS BOEUF COEUR CUEUP DIEUX DUEUP EGEUS EMEUS EYEUP FLEUR FREUD ICEUP ILEUM KREUK LIEUP LIEUS LIEUT MIEUX NIEUW ODEUM OLEUM ONEUP PNEUM PSEUD QUEUE RHEUM SEEUP SOEUR TEEUP THEUN TIEUP USEUP VIEUX WEEUN

••E•U

DREWU TAEGU

•••EU

ADIEU LAFEU PAREU RICEU THIEU YALEU

EV•••

EVADE EVANS EVENS EVENT EVERS EVERT EVERY EVIAN EVICT EVILS EVITA EVITE EVOKE EVORA

E•V••

EAVAN EAVED EAVES ELVER ELVES ELVIN ELVIS ENVER ENVOI ENVOY ERVIN

E••V•

ELEVE ELEVS EREVS

E•••V

ELYNV EQUIV EXDIV EXGOV

•EV••

BEVEL BEVIN DEVAS DEVIL DEVOL DEVON DEVRY FEVER KEVIN KEVON LEVAR LEVEE LEVEL LEVER LEVIN LEVIS LEVIT LEVON NEVER NEVES NEVIL NEVIN NEVIS NEVUS REVEL REVES REVET REVUE REVUP SEVEN SEVER TEVET TEVYE ZEVON

•E•V•

BELVA DELVE HEAVE HEAVY HERVE LEAVE LEOVI NERVA NERVE NERVO NERVY PEEVE REAVE REEVE SERVE SERVO VELVA VERVE WEAVE

•E••V

DERIV LEOIV NEGEV WEBTV

••EV•

ALEVE BREVE BREVI CHEVY CLEVE CREVE ELEVE ELEVS EREVS HUEVO MAEVE NIEVE NUEVA NUEVE NUEVO PEEVE REEVE SIEVE SNEVA STEVE TREVI

•••EV

MALEV NEGEV RTREV

EW•••

EWALD EWART EWEEK EWELL EWERS EWERY EWING EWOKS

E•W••

EDWIN ELWAY ELWES ERWIN

E•••W

ELBOW ENDOW

•EW••

BEWIG DEWAR DEWAX DEWED DEWEY FEWER HEWED HEWER HEWTO JEWEL JEWRY LEWES LEWIS MEWED MEWER MEWLS NEWAT NEWEL NEWER NEWIE NEWLY NEWSY NEWTO NEWTS PEWEE PEWIT REWAX REWED REWET REWIN REWON SEWED SEWER SEWIN SEWON SEWUP TEWAS TEWES WEWON

•E•W•

MEOWS NETWT REOWN YEOWS

•E••W

BEDEW BELOW DEPEW LEPEW REMOW RENEW RESAW RESEW RESOW RETOW

••EW•

BREWS CHEWS CHEWY CLEWS CREWS DREWU KREWE LOEWE LOEWI LOEWS LOEWY SKEWS SLEWS SMEWS SPEWS STEWS STEWY THEWB THEWS THEWY TREWS VIEWS VIEWY WHEWS

••E•W

NIEUW

•••EW

AGNEW ASKEW ASNEW BEDEW CAREW DEPEW JCREW LEPEW RENEW RESEW SCREW SHREW SINEW SOFEW STREW THREW UNMEW UNNEW UNSEW

EX•••

EXACT EXALT EXAMS EXCEL EXCON EXCOP EXCUB EXDIV EXECS EXERT EXGIS EXGOV EXILE EXING EXIST EXITS EXLIB EXMET EXONS EXPAT EXPEL EXPOS EXTOL EXTRA EXTRO EXUDE EXULT EXUMA EXURB EXXON

E•X••

EXXON

E••X•

EPOXY

E•••X

ESSEX

•EX••

BEXAR DEXTR HEXAD HEXED HEXER HEXES LEXAN LEXIS LEXUS NEXIS NEXUS REXES SEXED SEXER SEXES TEXAN TEXAS TEXTS VEXED VEXER VEXES

•E•X•

DEOXY GENXS LEOXI

•E••X

BEAUX DEHEX DESEX DETOX DEWAX FEDEX FELIX HELIX LENOX LEOIX REBOX REDOX REDUX REFAX REFIX RELAX REMAX REMIX RETAX REWAX TELEX VELOX XEMEX XEROX

••EX•

ALEXA ALEXI CHEXX PREXY

••E•X

ADEUX CHEXX DIEUX ICEAX MIEUX THEAX VIEUX

•••EX

ANNEX CODEX COMEX CUTEX DEHEX DESEX ESSEX FEDEX INDEX LATEX LUREX MRHEX NYNEX PUREX PYREX ROLEX SILEX SINEX TELEX TILEX TIMEX XEMEX YONEX

EY•••

EYDIE EYERS EYEUP EYING EYRAS EYRIE EYRIR

E•Y••

EGYPT ELYNV ELYOT ELYSE ETYMA

E••Y•

EASYA EAZYE EMLYN EMMYS ENCYC ESPYS ETHYL

E•••Y

EARLY EBONY EDIFY EENSY EKEBY ELEGY ELREY ELROY ELWAY EMBAY EMERY EMILY EMORY EMPTY ENEMY ENJOY ENSKY ENTRY ENVOY EPOXY ESSAY EVERY EWERY

•EY••

BEYLE FEYER FEYLY HEYER HEYSE KEYED KEYES KEYIN KEYON KEYUP LEYTE MEYER REYES

•E•Y•

BERYL DEBYE DENYS KENYA LENYA MERYL PEPYS REDYE SEEYA TEVYE

•E••Y

BEADY BEAMY BEANY BEATY BECKY BEDDY BEDNY BEEFY BEERY BEETY BEGAY BELAY BELBY BELLY BENDY BENNY BERCY BERRY BETSY BETTY DEARY DEBBY DECAY DECOY DECRY DEIFY DEITY DELAY DELPY DENNY DEOXY DERBY DERRY DEUCY DEVRY DEWEY EENSY FEELY FENNY FERNY FERRY FEYLY FEZZY

GEARY GEEKY GEMMY GERMY GERRY GETBY GETTY HEADY HEALY HEAPY HEAVY HEDGY HEFTY HEMPY HENNY HENRY HERBY HERKY HETTY JEERY JEFFY JELLY JENNY JERKY JERRY JERZY JESSY JETTY JEWRY KEELY KELLY KENNY KERRY KESEY KETTY LEADY LEAFY LEAHY LEAKY LEARY LECKY LEDGY LEERY LEFAY LEFTY LEGGY LEMAY LENNY LEROY LETBY LETTY MEALY MEANY MEATY MEENY MERCY MERRY MESHY MESSY METRY NEALY NEEDY NEELY NELLY NERDY NERVY NESTY NETTY

NEWLY NEWSY PEARY PEATY PEGGY PEGUY PENNY PEONY PEPPY PERCY PERKY PERRY PESKY PETEY PETTY READY REBUY REDDY REDLY REDRY REEDY REEFY REEKY REFLY REFRY REIFY REKEY RELAY RENAY RENNY REPAY REPLY RESAY RETRY RETTY SEALY SEAMY SEDGY SEEDY SEEPY SEPOY SETBY TEARY TEDDY TEENY TELLY TERRY TESTY VEALY VEDAY VEERY VEINY WEARY WEBBY WEDGY WEEDY WEENY WEEPY WELBY WELTY WENDY WETLY ZESTY

••EY•
FREYA GREYS HUEYS JOEYS MYEYE OBEYS OXEYE PREYS SEEYA SLEYS THEYD TREYS WHEYS

••E•Y
AMERY APERY AVERY BEEFY BEERY BEETY CHELY CHEVY CHEWY CRECY EKEBY ELEGY EMERY ENEMY EVERY EWERY FAERY FEELY FIERY GEEKY JEERY KEELY LEERY LIEBY LOEWY MEENY MTELY NEEDY NEELY PIETY POESY PREXY QUERY REEDY REEFY REEKY SEEDY SEEPY STEWY SUETY TEENY THEWY USEBY VEERY VIEWY WEEDY WEENY WEEPY

•••EY
ABBEY AGLEY AILEY ALLEY APLEY ARMEY BOGEY BONEY BUSEY CAGEY CAKEY CAREY CASEY CONEY COREY COVEY CUTEY DALEY DAVEY DEWEY DICEY DOKEY DOPEY DOVEY ELREY FAHEY FOGEY FOLEY GLUEY GODEY GOOEY GOREY HALEY HANEY HAYEY HIDEY HOBEY HOKEY HOLEY HOMEY HONEY HOOEY HOVEY INKEY ISLEY JACEY JIVEY JOKEY JOSEY JULEY KATEY KESEY KILEY LACEY LOOEY LOSEY LOVEY MATEY MIKEY MINEY MONEY MOPEY MOREY MOSEY MULEY NOSEY ONKEY OYVEY PACEY PALEY PETEY PINEY POKEY POSEY RAMEY REKEY RILEY RIXEY ROSEY SKYEY SOOEY TANEY TOBEY UTLEY WIFEY WILEY ZOOEY

EZ•••
EZINE

E•Z••
EAZYE

E••Z•
EBUZZ ELIZA

E•••Z
EBUZZ ERETZ

•EZ••
BEZEL BEZOS FEZES FEZZY MEZZO REZIA REZIP VEZES WEZEN

•E•Z•
FEZZY HENZE HERZL JERZY LEEZA MEZZO SEIZE TERZA

•E••Z
FELIZ GERTZ HEINZ HERTZ JEREZ MERTZ NERTZ PEREZ REISZ VELEZ VENEZ WEISZ WEITZ

••EZ•
BAEZA LEEZA

••E•Z
CHEEZ DIETZ ERETZ

•••EZ
ALLEZ ASSEZ CHEEZ GOMEZ JEREZ LOPEZ NUNEZ PEREZ VELEZ VENEZ

FA•••
FABER FABIO FABLE FABRE FACED FACER FACES FACET FACIA FACIE FACIL FACTA FACTO FACTS FADDY FADED FADER FADES FADOS FAENA FAERY FAGIN FAGOT FAHEY FAILS FAIMS FAINT FAIRE FAIRS FAIRY FAITH FAJAS FAKED FAKER FAKES FAKIR FALCO FALDO FALKE FALLA FALLS FALSE FAMED FAMER FAMES FAMKE FANCY FANES FANGS FANNY FANON FANTA FAQIR FARAD FARAH FARCE FARCI FARED FARER FARES FARGO FARIS FARMS FAROE FARON FAROS FARSI FARUK FASTS FATAL FATED FATES FATHA FATLY FATSO FATTY FATWA FAULT FAUNA FAUNS FAURE FAUSS FAUST FAUTE FAUVE FAVES FAVOR FAVRE FAWNS FAXED FAXER FAXES FAZED FAZES

F•A••
FEARS FEAST FEATS FIATS FLACK FLAGG FLAGS FLAIL FLAIR FLAKE FLAKY FLAME FLAMS FLAMY FLANK FLANN FLANS FLAPS FLARE FLASH FLASK FLATS FLATT FLAVA FLAWS FLAWY FLAXY FLAYS FOALS FOAMS FOAMY FRAGS FRAIL FRAIS FRAME FRANC FRANK FRANN FRANS FRANZ FRATS FRAUD FRAYN FRAYS FRAZY FUADI

F••A•
FAJAS FARAD FARAH FATAL FERAL FETAL FETAS FFLAT FILAR FILAS FINAL FLEAS FLOAT FLYAT FOCAL FORAY FREAK FRIAR FSTAR FUGAL

F•••A
FACIA FACTA FAENA FALLA FANTA FATHA FATWA FAUNA FELLA FERIA FESTA FINCA FIONA FIRMA FIVEA FLAVA FLORA FOLIA FONDA FORMA FORZA FOSSA FOURA FREDA FREIA FRENA FREYA FRIDA FRITA FULDA

•FA••
AFARS OFAGE

•F•A•
AFLAC AFLAT BFLAT CFLAT DFLAT EFLAT FFLAT GFLAT IFSAY OFFAL SFBAY

•F••A
AFTRA

••FA•
ABFAB ALFAS ASFAT BYFAR BYFAX DEFAT DUFAY GOFAR JAFAR LEFAY LIFAR LOFAT NOFAT OFFAL OXFAM REFAX SAFAR SOFAR SOFAS UNFAR WOFAT

••F•A
BUFFA HOFFA INFRA JAFFA KAFKA MAFIA NAFTA SOFIA

•••FA
BUFFA HAIFA HOFFA JAFFA LOOFA NAKFA SULFA USAFA USOFA

F•B••
FABER FABIO FABLE FABRE FIBER FIBRE FIBRO FUBSY

F••B•
FEEBS FLUBS FLYBY FROBE FTLBS FURBY

F•••B
FIVEB FOURB

•FB••
SFBAY

••F•B
ABFAB

FC•••
FCLEF

F•C••
FACED FACER FACES FACET FACIA FACIE FACIL FACTA FACTO FACTS FICHE FICHU FICUS FOCAL FOCUS FUCHS

F••C•
FALCO FANCY FARCE FARCI FENCE FETCH FILCH FINCA FINCH FISCS FITCH FLACK FLECK FLICK FLICS FLOCK FORCE FRICK FROCK FRUCT FUOCO

F•••C
FIVEC FOLIC FOURC FRANC FSLIC

•F••C
AFLAC AFRIC

••F•C
SOFTC

F•D••
FADDY FADED FADER FADES FADOS FEDEX FEDIN FEDON FEDTO FEDUP FIDEL FIDES FODOR FTDIX FUDDY FUDGE

F••D•
FADDY FALDO FEEDS FENDI FENDS FERDE FEUDS FINDS FOLDS FONDA FONDU FOODS FORDO FORDS FREDA FREDO FRIDA FRODO FUADI FUDDY FULDA FUNDS FUNDY

F•••D
FACED FADED FAKED FAMED FARAD FARED FATED FAXED FAZED FELID FETED FETID FIELD FIEND FIFED FILED FINED FIORD FIRED FIVED FIXED FJORD FLIED FLOOD FLOYD FLUID FOUND FOURD FOXED FRAUD FREED FREUD FRIED FROID FROND FTORD FUMED FUSED

•F••D
IFOLD OFFED PFERD

••F•D
BIFID FIFED NEFUD OFFED REFED UNFED

FE•••
FEARS FEAST FEATS FEDEX FEDIN FEDON FEDTO FEDUP FEEBS FEEDS FEELS FEELY FEETS FEIGN FEINT FELID FELIS FELIX FELIZ FELLA FELLS FELON FELTS FEMES FEMME FEMTO FEMUR FENCE FENDI FENDS FENNY FEOFF FERAL FERDE FERIA FERMI FERNS FERNY FERRI FERRO FERRY FESTA FESTE FESTS FETAL FETAS FETCH FETED FETES FETID FETOR FETUS FEUDS FEUER FEVER FEWER FEYER FEYLY FEZES FEZZY

F•E••
FAENA FAERY FEEBS FEEDS FEELS FEELY FEETS FIEFS FIELD FIEND FIERO FIERS FIERY FLEAS FLECK FLEER FLEES FLEET FLESH FLEUR FREAK FREDA FREDO FREED FREEH FREER FREES FREIA FRENA FRENI FREON FRERE FRESH FRESS FRETS FREUD FREYA FUEGO FUELS

F••E•
FABER FACED FACER FACES FACET FADED FADER FADES FAHEY FAKED FAKER FAKES FAMED FAMER FAMES FANES FARED FARER FARES FATED FATES FAVES FAXED FAXER FAXES FAZED FAZES FCLEF FEDEX FEMES FETED FETES FEUER FEVER FEWER FEYER FEZES FIBER FIDEL FIDES FIFED FIFER FIFES FILED FILER FILES FILET FINED FINER FINES FIRED FIRER FIRES FIVEA FIVEB FIVEC FIVED FIVEE FIVEO FIVER FIVES FIXED FIXER FIXES FLEER FLEES FLEET FLIED FLIER FLIES FLOES FLUES FLYER FOGEL FOGEY FOIES FOLEY FORES FOXED FOXES FOYER FREED FREEH FREER FREES FRIED FRIEL FRIER FRIES FROES FRYER FTLEE FUMED FUMER FUMES FUMET FUSED FUSEE FUSES

F•••E
FABLE FABRE FACIE FAIRE FALKE FALSE FAMKE FARCE FAROE FAURE FAUTE FAUVE FAVRE FEMME FENCE FERDE FESTE FHOLE FIBRE FICHE FILLE FIORE FISKE FIVEE FLAKE FLAME FLARE FLUKE FLUME FLUTE FLYME FOOTE FORCE FORGE FORTE FOSSE FOURE FOYLE FRAME FRERE FRISE FRITE FROBE FROME FROZE FTILE FTLEE FUDGE FUGUE FURIE FURZE FUSEE

•FE••
IFEEL PFERD

•F•E•
AFTER EFREM IFEEL NFLER OFFED OFFER OFTEN

•F••E
AFIRE AFORE BFIVE EFFIE EFILE IFIVE MFUME OFAGE OFUSE XFILE

••FE•
ADFEE APFEL CAFES DEFER FIFED FIFER FIFES GOFER INFER JEFES LAFEU LIFER NOFEE OFFED OFFER ORFEO ORFES RAFER REFED REFER RIFER SAFER SAFES SOFER SOFEW UNFED WAFER WIFEY

••F•E
ADFEE ALFIE ALFRE CAFFE DAFOE DEFOE EFFIE GAFFE JAFFE JOFFE NOFEE RIFLE SOFIE

•••FE
CAFFE CHAFE GAFFE GROFE JAFFE JOFFE KEEFE KNIFE KOPFE MLIFE PHYFE ROLFE WOLFE

FF•••
FFLAT

F•F••
FIFED FIFER FIFES FIFTH FIFTY

F••F•
FEOFF

FIEFS
FLUFF

F•••F
FCLEF
FEOFF
FLUFF
FOURF

•FF••
AFFIX
EFFIE
OFFAL
OFFED
OFFER
OFFOF
PFFFT

•F•F•
AFOFL
PFFFT

•F••F
OFFOF

••FF•
BAFFS
BAFFY
BIFFS
BOFFO
BOFFS
BUFFA
BUFFI
BUFFO
BUFFS
BUFFY
CAFFE
CUFFS
DAFFY
DIFFS
DOFFS
DUFFY
GAFFE
GAFFS
GUFFS
HOFFA
HUFFS
HUFFY
JAFFA
JAFFE
JEFFY
JIFFS
JIFFY
JOFFE
LAFFS
LUFFS
MIFFS
MIFFY
MOFFO
MUFFS
PFFFT
PHFFT
PUFFS
PUFFY
RAFFI
RIFFS
RUFFS
SAFFI
TAFFY
TIFFS
TOFFS

••F•F
OFFOF

•••FF
ACUFF
BANFF
BEOFF
BLAFF
BLUFF
CHAFF
CHUFF
CLIFF
DORFF
FEOFF
FLUFF
GOOFF
GRAFF
GRUFF
HANFF
IMOFF
LWOFF
ONOFF
QUAFF
SCOFF
SCUFF
SKIFF
SNIFF
SNUFF
SPIFF
STAFF
STIFF
STUFF
WHIFF
WOLFF
ZIEFF

FG•••
FGHIJ

F•G••
FAGIN
FAGOT
FIGHT
FOGEL
FOGEY
FOGGY
FOGIN
FOGUP
FUGAL
FUGIT
FUGUE
FUGUS

F••G•
FANGS
FARGO
FEIGN
FLAGG
FLAGS
FLOGS
FOGGY
FORGE
FORGO
FRAGS
FRIGG
FROGS
FRUGS
FUDGE
FUEGO
FUNGI
FUNGO

F•••G
FLAGG
FLING
FLUNG
FRIGG

•FG••
EFGHI

•F•G•
OFAGE

•F••G
PFLUG

••FG•
DEFGH

••F•G
BEFOG
DEFOG
SOFTG

•••FG
CDEFG

FH•••
FHOLE

F•H••
FAHEY
FGHIJ
FOHNS

F••H•
FATHA
FICHE
FICHU
FIGHT
FISHY
FUCHS

F•••H
FAITH
FARAH
FETCH
FIFTH
FILCH
FILTH
FINCH
FIRTH
FITCH
FLASH
FLESH
FLUSH
FORTH
FOURH
FREEH
FRESH
FROSH
FROTH

•F•H•
EFGHI

••F•H
DEFGH

FI•••
FIATS
FIBER
FIBRE
FIBRO
FICHE
FICHU
FICUS
FIDEL
FIDES
FIEFS
FIELD
FIEND
FIERO
FIERS
FIERY
FIFED
FIFER
FIFES
FIFTH
FIFTY
FIGHT
FILAR
FILAS
FILCH
FILED
FILER
FILES
FILET
FILLE
FILLS
FILLY
FILMS
FILMY
FILOS
FILTH
FILUM
FINAL
FINCA
FINCH
FINDS
FINED
FINER
FINES
FINIS
FINKS
FINNO
FINNS
FINNY
FINOS
FIONA
FIORD
FIORE
FIORI
FIRED
FIRER
FIRES
FIRMA
FIRMS
FIRNS
FIRPO
FIRRY
FIRST
FIRTH
FISCS
FISHY
FISKE
FISTS
FITCH
FITIN
FITLY
FITON
FITUP
FIVEA
FIVEB
FIVEC
FIVED
FIVEE
FIVEO
FIVER
FIVES
FIXED
FIXER
FIXES
FIXIT
FIXON
FIXUP
FIZZY

F•I••
FAILS
FAIMS
FAINT
FAIRE
FAIRS
FAIRY
FAITH
FEIGN
FEINT
FLICK
FLICS
FLIED
FLIER
FLIES
FLING
FLINT
FLIPS
FLIRS
FLIRT
FLITS
FOIES
FOILS
FOIST
FRIAR
FRICK
FRIDA
FRIED
FRIEL
FRIER
FRIES
FRIGG
FRILL
FRIML
FRISE
FRISK
FRIST
FRITA
FRITE
FRITO
FRITS
FRITZ
FRIZZ
FTILE

F••I•
FABIO
FACIA
FACIE
FACIL
FAGIN
FAKIR
FAQIR
FARIS
FEDIN
FELID
FELIS
FELIX
FELIZ
FERIA
FETID
FGHIJ
FINIS
FITIN
FIXIT
FLAIL
FLAIR
FLUID
FLYIN
FOGIN
FOLIA
FOLIC
FOLIO
FRAIL
FRAIS
FREIA
FROID
FRUIT
FSLIC
FTDIX
FUGIT
FUJIS
FURIE
FUSIL

F•••I
FARCI
FARSI
FENDI
FERMI
FERRI
FIORI
FLORI
FRENI
FUADI
FUNGI

•FI••
AFIRE
BFIVE
EFIKS
EFILE
IFILL
IFIVE
XFILE

•F•I•
AFFIX
AFRIC
EFFIE

•F••I
EFGHI

••FI•
AFFIX
ALFIE
ALFIO
ASFIT
BEFIT
BIFID
EFFIE
ELFIN
ENFIN
HAFIZ
HIFIS
INFIX
KEFIR
MAFIA
REFIS
REFIT
REFIX
SAFIN
SOFIA
SOFIE
SUFIS
UNFIT
UNFIX

••F•I
BUFFI
HEFTI
MUFTI
RAFFI
SAFFI

•••FI
BUFFI
MELFI
OLAFI
RAFFI
SAFFI
SCIFI

FJ•••
FJORD

F•J••
FAJAS
FUJIS

F••J•
FLOJO

F•••J
FGHIJ

•F•J•
JFKJR

F•K••
FAKED
FAKER
FAKES
FAKIR

F••K•
FALKE
FAMKE
FINKS
FISKE
FLAKE
FLAKY
FLUKE
FLUKY
FOLKS
FOLKY
FORKS
FORKY
FUNKS
FUNKY

F•••K
FARUK
FLACK
FLANK
FLASK
FLECK
FLICK
FLOCK
FLUNK
FRANK
FREAK
FRICK
FRISK
FROCK

•FK••
JFKJR

•F•K•
EFIKS

••FK•
KAFKA
RAFKO

FL•••
FLACK
FLAGG
FLAGS
FLAIL
FLAIR
FLAKE
FLAKY
FLAME
FLAMS
FLAMY
FLANK
FLANN
FLANS
FLAPS
FLARE
FLASH
FLASK
FLATS
FLATT
FLAVA
FLAWS
FLAWY
FLAXY
FLAYS
FLEAS
FLECK
FLEER
FLEES
FLEET
FLESH
FLEUR
FLICK
FLICS
FLIED
FLIER
FLIES
FLING
FLINT
FLIPS
FLIRS
FLIRT
FLITS
FLOAT
FLOCK
FLOES
FLOGS
FLOJO
FLOOD
FLOOR
FLOPS
FLORA
FLORI
FLORY
FLOSS
FLOUR
FLOUT
FLOWN
FLOWS
FLOYD
FLUBS
FLUES
FLUFF
FLUID
FLUKE
FLUKY
FLUME
FLUNG
FLUNK
FLUOR
FLUSH
FLUTE
FLUTY
FLYAT
FLYBY
FLYER
FLYIN
FLYME
FLYNN
FLYON
FLYTO
FLYUP

F•L••
FALCO
FALDO
FALKE
FALLA
FALLS
FALSE
FCLEF
FELID
FELIS
FELIX
FELIZ
FELLA
FELLS
FELON
FELTS
FFLAT
FILAR
FILAS
FILCH
FILED
FILER
FILES
FILET
FILLE
FILLS
FILLY
FILMS
FILMY
FILOS
FILTH
FILUM
FOLDS
FOLEY
FOLIA
FOLIC
FOLIO
FOLKS
FOLKY
FOLLY
FSLIC
FTLBS
FTLEE
FULDA
FULLS
FULLY

F••L•
FABLE
FAILS
FALLA
FALLS
FATLY
FAULT
FEELS
FEELY
FELLA
FELLS
FEYLY
FHOLE
FIELD
FILLE
FILLS
FILLY
FITLY
FOALS
FOILS
FOLLY
FOOLS
FOULS
FOWLS
FOYLE
FRILL
FTILE
FUELS
FULLS
FULLY
FURLS

F•••L
FACIL
FATAL
FERAL
FETAL
FIDEL
FINAL
FLAIL
FOCAL
FOGEL
FRAIL
FRIEL
FRILL
FRIML
FUGAL
FUSIL

•FL••
AFLAC
AFLAT
BFLAT
CFLAT
DFLAT
EFLAT
FFLAT
GFLAT
NFLER
PFLUG

•F•L•
EFILE
IFILL
IFOLD
XFILE

•F••L
AFOFL
AFOUL
IFEEL
IFILL
OFFAL

••FL•
MCFLY
NUFLO
REFLY
RIFLE

••F•L
APFEL
AWFUL
OFFAL

•••FL
AFOFL
TOEFL

F•M••
FAMED
FAMER
FAMES
FAMKE
FEMES
FEMME
FEMTO
FEMUR
FUMED
FUMER
FUMES
FUMET

F••M•
FAIMS
FARMS
FEMME
FERMI
FILMS
FILMY
FIRMA
FIRMS
FLAME
FLAMS
FLAMY
FLUME
FLYME
FOAMS
FOAMY
FORMA
FORMS
FRAME
FRIML
FROME
FROMM
FRUMP

F•••M
FILUM
FORUM
FROMM

•F•M•
MFUME

•F••M
EFREM

••F•M
OXFAM

F•N••
FANCY
FANES
FANGS
FANNY
FANON
FANTA
FENCE
FENDI
FENDS
FENNY
FINAL
FINCA
FINCH
FINDS
FINED
FINER
FINES
FINIS
FINKS
FINNO
FINNS
FINNY
FINOS
FONDA
FONDU
FONTS
FUNDS
FUNDY
FUNGI
FUNGO
FUNKS
FUNKY
FUNNY

F••N•
FAENA
FAINT
FANNY
FAUNA
FAUNS
FAWNS
FEINT
FENNY
FERNS
FERNY
FIEND
FINNO
FINNS
FINNY
FIONA
FIRNS
FLANK
FLANN
FLANS
FLING
FLINT
FLUNG
FLUNK
FLYNN
FOHNS
FOUND
FOUNT
FRANC
FRANK
FRANN
FRANS
FRANZ
FRENA
FRENI
FROND
FRONT
FUNNY

F•••N
FAGIN
FANON
FARON
FEDIN
FEDON
FEIGN
FELON
FITIN
FITON
FIXON
FLANN
FLOWN
FLYIN
FLYNN
FLYON
FOGIN
FRANN
FRAYN
FREON
FROWN
FUTON

•FN••
IFNOT

•F••N
AFTON
OFTEN

••F•N
ELFIN
ENFIN
INFUN
NOFUN
SAFIN
UNFUN

FO•••
FOALS
FOAMS
FOAMY
FOCAL
FOCUS
FODOR
FOGEL
FOGEY
FOGGY
FOGIN
FOGUP
FOHNS
FOIES
FOILS
FOIST
FOLDS
FOLEY
FOLIA
FOLIC
FOLIO
FOLKS
FOLKY
FOLLY
FONDA
FONDU
FONTS
FOODS
FOOLS
FOOTE
FOOTS
FOOZY
FORAY
FORCE
FORDO
FORDS
FORES
FORGE
FORGO
FORKS
FORKY
FORMA
FORMS
FORTE
FORTH
FORTS
FORTY
FORUM
FORZA
FOSSA
FOSSE
FOULS
FOUND
FOUNT
FOURA
FOURB
FOURC
FOURD
FOURE
FOURF
FOURH
FOURS
FOUTS
FOWLS
FOXED
FOXES
FOXTV
FOYER
FOYLE

F•O••
FEOFF
FHOLE
FIONA
FIORD
FIORE
FIORI
FJORD
FLOAT
FLOCK
FLOES
FLOGS
FLOJO
FLOOD
FLOOR
FLOPS
FLORA
FLORI
FLORY
FLOSS
FLOUR
FLOUT
FLOWN
FLOWS
FLOYD
FOODS
FOOLS
FOOTE
FOOTS
FOOZY
FROBE
FROCK
FRODO
FROES
FROGS
FROID
FROME
FROMM
FROND
FRONT
FROOT
FROSH
FROST
FROTH
FROWN
FROWS
FROYO
FROZE
FTORD
FUOCO

F••O•
FADOS
FAGOT
FANON
FAROE
FARON
FAROS
FAVOR
FEDON
FELON
FETOR
FILOS
FINOS
FITON
FIXON
FLOOD
FLOOR
FLUOR
FLYON
FODOR
FREON
FROOT
FSTOP
FUROR
FUROS
FUTON

F•••O
FABIO
FACTO
FALCO
FALDO
FARGO
FATSO
FEDTO
FEMTO
FERRO
FIBRO
FIERO
FINNO
FIRPO
FIVEO
FLOJO
FLYTO
FOLIO
FORDO
FORGO
FREDO
FRITO
FRODO
FROYO
FUEGO
FUNGO
FUOCO

•FO••
AFOFL
AFOOT
AFORE
AFOUL
BFOUR
IFOLD
IFOUR
VFOUR

•F•O•
AFOOT
AFROS
AFTON
IFNOT
OFFOF

••FO•
ASFOR
BEFOG
BEFOR
DAFOE
DEFOE
DEFOG
DEFOR
DOFOR
EOFOR
GOFOR
INFOR
MRFOX
OFFOF
UPFOR

••F•O
ALFIO
BOFFO
BUFFO
MOFFO
NUFLO
ORFEO
RAFKO

•••FO
BOFFO
BUFFO
MOFFO
RULFO

F••P•
FIRPO
FLAPS
FLIPS
FLOPS

F•••P
FEDUP
FITUP
FIXUP
FLYUP
FOGUP
FRUMP
FRYUP
FSTOP

F•Q••
FAQIR

FR•••
FRAGS
FRAIL
FRAIS
FRAME
FRANC
FRANK
FRANN
FRANS
FRANZ
FRATS
FRAUD

FRAYN
FRAYS
FRAZY
FREAK
FREDA
FREDO
FREED
FREEH
FREER
FREES
FREIA
FRENA
FRENI
FREON
FRERE
FRESH
FRESS
FRETS
FREUD
FREYA
FRIAR
FRICK
FRIDA
FRIED
FRIEL
FRIER
FRIES
FRIGG
FRILL
FRIML
FRISE
FRISK
FRIST
FRITA
FRITE
FRITO
FRITS
FRITZ
FRIZZ
FROBE
FROCK
FRODO
FROES
FROGS
FROID
FROME
FROMM
FROND
FRONT
FROOT
FROSH
FROST
FROTH
FROWN
FROWS
FROYO
FROZE
FRUCT
FRUGS
FRUIT
FRUMP
FRYER
FRYUP

F•R••
FARAD
FARAH
FARCE
FARCI
FARED
FARER
FARES
FARGO
FARIS
FARMS
FAROE
FARON
FAROS
FARSI
FARUK
FERAL
FERDE
FERIA
FERMI
FERNS
FERNY
FERRI
FERRO
FERRY
FIRED
FIRER
FIRES
FIRMA
FIRMS
FIRNS
FIRPO
FIRRY
FIRST
FIRTH
FORAY
FORCE
FORDO
FORDS
FORES
FORGE
FORGO
FORKS
FORKY
FORMA
FORMS
FORTE
FORTH
FORTS
FORTY
FORUM
FORZA
FURBY
FURIE
FURLS
FUROR
FUROS
FURRY
FURST
FURZE

F••R•
FABRE
FAERY
FAIRE
FAIRS
FAIRY
FAURE
FAVRE
FEARS
FERRI
FERRO
FERRY
FIBRE
FIBRO
FIERO
FIERS
FIERY
FIORD
FIORE
FIORI
FIRRY
FJORD
FLARE
FLIRS
FLIRT
FLORA
FLORI
FLORY
FOURA
FOURB
FOURC
FOURD
FOURE
FOURF
FOURH
FOURS
FRERE
FTORD
FURRY

F•••R
FABER
FACER
FADER
FAKER
FAKIR
FAMER
FAQIR
FARER
FAVOR
FAXER
FEMUR
FETOR
FEUER
FEVER
FEWER
FEYER
FIBER
FIFER
FILAR
FILER
FINER
FIRER
FIVER
FIXER
FLAIR
FLEER
FLEUR
FLIER
FLOOR
FLOUR
FLUOR
FLYER
FODOR
FOYER
FREER
FRIAR
FRIER
FRYER
FSTAR
FUMER
FUROR

•FR••
AFRIC
AFROS
EFREM

•F•R•
AFARS
AFIRE
AFORE
AFTRA
PFERD

•F••R
AFTER
BFOUR
IFOUR
JFKJR
NFLER
OFFER
VFOUR

••FR•
ALFRE
INFRA
REFRY

••F•R
ASFOR
BEFOR
BYFAR
DEFER
DOFOR
EOFOR
FIFER
GOFAR
GOFER
GOFOR
INFER
INFOR
JAFAR
KEFIR
LIFAR
LIFER
OFFER
RAFER
REFER
RIFER
RSFSR
SAFAR
SAFER
SOFAR
SOFER
UNFAR
UPFOR
WAFER

FS•••
FSLIC
FSTAR
FSTOP

F•S••
FASTS
FESTA
FESTE
FESTS
FISCS
FISHY
FISKE
FISTS
FOSSA
FOSSE
FUSED
FUSEE
FUSES
FUSIL
FUSSY
FUSTY

F••S•
FALSE
FARSI
FATSO
FAUSS
FAUST
FEAST
FIRST
FLASH
FLASK
FLESH
FLOSS
FLUSH
FOIST
FOSSA
FOSSE
FRESH
FRESS
FRISE
FRISK
FRIST
FROSH
FROST
FUBSY
FURST
FUSSY

F•••S
FACES
FACTS
FADES
FADOS
FAILS
FAIMS
FAIRS
FAJAS
FAKES
FALLS
FAMES
FANES
FANGS
FARES
FARIS
FARMS
FAROS
FASTS
FATES
FAUNS
FAUSS
FAVES
FAWNS
FAXES
FAZES
FEARS
FEATS
FEEBS
FEEDS
FEELS
FEETS
FELIS
FELLS
FELTS
FEMES
FENDS
FERNS
FESTS
FETAS
FETES
FETUS
FEUDS
FEZES
FIATS
FICUS
FIDES
FIEFS
FIERS
FIFES
FILAS
FILES
FILLS
FILMS
FILOS
FINDS
FINES
FINIS
FINKS
FINNS
FINOS
FIRES
FIRMS
FIRNS
FISCS
FISTS
FIVES
FIXES
FLAGS
FLAMS
FLANS
FLAPS
FLATS
FLAWS
FLAYS
FLEAS
FLEES
FLICS
FLIES
FLIPS
FLIRS
FLITS
FLOES
FLOGS
FLOPS
FLOSS
FLOWS
FLUBS
FLUES
FOALS
FOAMS
FOCUS
FOHNS
FOIES
FOILS
FOLDS
FOLKS
FONTS
FOODS
FOOLS
FOOTS
FORDS
FORES
FORKS
FORMS
FORTS
FOULS
FOURS
FOUTS
FOWLS
FOXES
FRAGS
FRAIS
FRANS
FRATS
FRAYS
FREES
FRESS
FRETS
FRIES
FRITS
FROES
FROGS
FROWS
FRUGS
FTLBS
FUCHS
FUELS
FUGUS
FUJIS
FULLS
FUMES
FUNDS
FUNKS
FURLS
FUROS
FUSES

•FS••
IFSAY

•F•S•
OFUSE

•F••S
AFARS
AFROS
EFIKS

••FS•
RSFSR

••F•S
ALFAS
BAFFS
BIFFS
BOFFS
BUFFS
CAFES
CUFFS
DIFFS
DOFFS
DUFUS
DUFYS
FIFES
GAFFS
GIFTS
GUFFS
HAFTS
HEFTS
HIFIS
HUFFS
JEFES
JIFFS
LAFFS
LEFTS
LIFTS
LOFTS
LUFFS
MIFFS
MUFFS
ORFES
PUFFS
RAFTS
REFIS
RIFFS
RIFTS
RUFFS
RUFUS
SAFES
SIFTS
SOFAS
SUFIS
TAFTS
TIFFS
TOFFS
TOFTS
TOFUS
TUFTS
WAFTS
WEFTS
ZAFUS

•••FS
ALEFS
ALIFS
BAFFS
BEEFS
BIFFS
BOFFS
BUFFS
CHEFS
CLEFS
COIFS
CUFFS
DIFFS
DOFFS
FIEFS
GAFFS
GOLFS
GOOFS
GUFFS
GULFS
HOOFS
HUFFS
JIFFS
KERFS
LAFFS
LEAFS
LOAFS
LUFFS
MIFFS
MUFFS
NAIFS
NERFS
OEUFS
PELFS
PERFS
POUFS
PROFS
PUFFS
REEFS
RIFFS
ROLFS
ROOFS
RUFFS
SERFS
SURFS
TIFFS
TOFFS
TURFS
WAIFS
WOLFS
WOOFS
ZARFS

FT•••
FTDIX
FTILE
FTLBS
FTLEE
FTORD

F•T••
FATAL
FATED
FATES
FATHA
FATLY
FATSO
FATTY
FATWA
FETAL
FETAS
FETCH
FETED
FETES
FETID
FETOR
FETUS
FITCH
FITIN
FITLY
FITON
FITUP
FSTAR
FSTOP
FUTON

F••T•
FACTA
FACTO
FACTS
FAITH
FANTA
FASTS
FATTY
FAUTE
FEATS
FEDTO
FEETS
FELTS
FEMTO
FESTA
FESTE
FESTS
FIATS
FIFTH
FIFTY
FILTH
FIRTH
FISTS
FLATS
FLATT
FLITS
FLUTE
FLUTY
FLYTO
FONTS
FOOTE
FOOTS
FORTE
FORTH
FORTS
FORTY
FOUTS
FOXTV
FRATS
FRETS
FRITA
FRITE
FRITO
FRITS
FRITZ
FROTH
FUSTY

F•••T
FACET
FAGOT
FAINT
FAULT
FAUST
FEAST
FEINT
FFLAT
FIGHT
FILET
FIRST
FIXIT
FLATT
FLEET
FLINT
FLIRT
FLOAT
FLOUT
FLYAT
FOIST
FOUNT
FRIST
FRONT
FROOT
FROST
FRUCT
FRUIT
FUGIT
FUMET
FURST

•FT••
AFTER
AFTON
AFTRA
OFTEN

•F••T
AFLAT
AFOOT
BFLAT
CFLAT
DFLAT
EFLAT
FFLAT
GFLAT
IFNOT
PFFFT

••FT•
FIFTH
FIFTY
GIFTS
HAFTS
HEFTI
HEFTS
HEFTY
LEFTS
LEFTY
LIFTS
LOFTS
LOFTY
MUFTI
NAFTA
NIFTY
RAFTS
RIFTS
SIFTS
SOFTC
SOFTG
SOFTY
TAFTS
TOFTS
TUFTS
TUFTY
WAFTS
WEFTS

••F•T
ASFAT
ASFIT
BEFIT
DEFAT
LOFAT
NOFAT
PFFFT
PHFFT
REFIT
UNFIT
WOFAT

•••FT
ABAFT
ALOFT
CLEFT
CLIFT
CRAFT
CROFT
DELFT
DRAFT
DREFT
DRIFT
GOAFT
GRAFT
GRIFT
KRAFT
KROFT
LINFT
PFFFT
PHFFT
SHAFT
SHIFT
SWIFT
THEFT

FU•••
FUADI
FUBSY
FUCHS
FUDDY
FUDGE
FUEGO
FUELS
FUGAL
FUGIT
FUGUE
FUGUS
FUJIS
FULDA
FULLS
FULLY
FUMED
FUMER
FUMES
FUMET
FUNDS
FUNDY
FUNGI
FUNGO
FUNKS
FUNKY
FUNNY
FUOCO
FURBY
FURIE
FURLS
FUROR
FUROS
FURRY
FURST
FURZE
FUSED
FUSEE
FUSES
FUSIL
FUSSY
FUSTY
FUTON
FUZZY

F•U••
FAULT
FAUNA
FAUNS
FAURE
FAUSS
FAUST
FAUTE
FAUVE
FEUDS
FEUER
FLUBS
FLUES
FLUFF
FLUID
FLUKE
FLUKY
FLUME
FLUNG
FLUNK
FLUOR
FLUSH
FLUTE
FLUTY
FOULS
FOUND
FOUNT
FOURA
FOURB
FOURC
FOURD
FOURE
FOURF
FOURH
FOURS
FOUTS
FRUCT
FRUGS
FRUIT
FRUMP

F••U•
FARUK
FEDUP
FEMUR
FETUS
FICUS
FILUM
FITUP
FIXUP
FLEUR
FLOUR
FLOUT
FLYUP
FOCUS
FOGUP
FORUM
FRAUD
FREUD
FRYUP
FUGUE
FUGUS

F•••U
FICHU
FONDU

•FU••
MFUME
OFUSE

•F•U•
AFOUL
BFOUR
IFOUR
PFLUG
VFOUR

••FU•
AWFUL
DUFUS
INFUN
NEFUD
NOFUN
RUFUS
TOFUS
UNFUN
ZAFUS

••F•U
LAFEU

•••FU
CORFU
KHUFU
SNAFU

F•V••
FAVES
FAVOR
FAVRE
FEVER
FIVEA
FIVEB
FIVEC
FIVED
FIVEE
FIVEO
FIVER
FIVES

F••V•
FAUVE
FLAVA

F•••V
FOXTV

•F•V•
BFIVE
IFIVE

•••FV
OLAFV

F•W••
FAWNS
FEWER
FOWLS

F••W•
FATWA
FLAWS
FLAWY
FLOWN
FLOWS
FROWN
FROWS

••F•W
SOFEW

F•X••
FAXED
FAXER
FAXES
FIXED
FIXER
FIXES
FIXIT
FIXON
FIXUP
FOXED
FOXES
FOXTV

F••X•
FLAXY

F•••X
FEDEX
FELIX
FTDIX

•F••X
AFFIX

••F•X
AFFIX
BYFAX
INFIX
MRFOX
REFAX
REFIX
UNFIX

F•Y••
FEYER
FEYLY
FLYAT
FLYBY
FLYER
FLYIN
FLYME
FLYNN
FLYON
FLYTO
FLYUP
FOYER
FOYLE
FRYER
FRYUP

F••Y•
FLAYS
FLOYD
FRAYN
FRAYS
FREYA
FROYO

F•••Y
FADDY
FAERY
FAHEY
FAIRY
FANCY
FANNY
FATLY
FATTY
FEELY
FENNY
FERNY
FERRY
FEYLY
FEZZY
FIERY
FIFTY
FILLY
FILMY
FINNY
FIRRY
FISHY
FITLY
FIZZY
FLAKY
FLAMY
FLAWY
FLAXY
FLORY
FLUKY
FLUTY
FLYBY
FOAMY
FOGEY
FOGGY
FOLEY
FOLKY
FOLLY
FOOZY
FORAY
FORKY
FORTY
FRAZY
FUBSY
FUDDY
FULLY
FUNDY
FUNKY
FUNNY
FURBY
FURRY
FUSSY
FUSTY
FUZZY

•F••Y
IFSAY
SFBAY

••FY•
DUFYS

••F•Y
BAFFY
BUFFY
DAFFY
DUFAY
DUFFY
FIFTY
HEFTY
HUFFY
JEFFY
JIFFY
LEFAY
LEFTY
LOFTY
MCFLY
MIFFY
NIFTY
PUFFY
REFLY
REFRY
SOFTY
TAFFY
TUFTY
WIFEY

•••FY
BAFFY
BARFY
BEEFY
BUFFY
COMFY
DAFFY
DEIFY
DUFFY
EDIFY
GOOFY
HUFFY
JEFFY
JIFFY
LEAFY
MIFFY
PUFFY
REEFY
REIFY
SURFY
TAFFY
TURFY
UNIFY

F•Z••
FAZED
FAZES
FEZES
FEZZY
FIZZY
FUZZY

F••Z•
FEZZY
FIZZY
FOOZY
FORZA
FRAZY
FRIZZ
FROZE
FURZE
FUZZY

F•••Z
FELIZ
FRANZ
FRITZ
FRIZZ

••F•Z
HAFIZ

GA•••
GABBY
GABEL

GABIN
GABLE
GABON
GABOR
GADDI
GAELS
GAETA
GAFFE
GAFFS
GAGED
GAGES
GAHAN
GAILY
GAINS
GAITS
GAIUS
GALAS
GALAX
GALBA
GALEA
GALED
GALEN
GALES
GALLI
GALLO
GALLS
GALOP
GAMAL
GAMAY
GAMBA
GAMED
GAMER
GAMES
GAMIN
GAMMA
GAMOW
GAMPS
GAMUT
GANCE
GANDT
GANDY
GANEF
GANGS
GANSU
GAOLS
GAPED
GAPER
GAPES
GARBO
GARBS
GARDA
GARDE
GARES
GARNI
GAROU
GARRY
GARTH
GASES
GASOL
GASPE
GASPS
GASSY
GASTR
GASUP
GATED
GATER
GATES
GATOR
GATOS
GATTO
GATUN
GAUDI
GAUDS
GAUDY
GAUGE
GAULS
GAUNT
GAURS
GAUSS
GAUZE
GAUZY
GAVEL
GAVIN
GAVOT
GAWKS
GAWKY
GAWPS
GAYER
GAYLE
GAYLY
GAZED
GAZER
GAZES

G•A••

GEARS
GEARY
GHAIN
GHALI
GHANA
GHATS
GHAZI
GIANT
GLACE
GLADE
GLADS
GLAMS
GLAND
GLARE
GLARY
GLASS
GLATT
GLAXO
GLAZE
GLAZY
GMATS
GNARL
GNARS
GNASH
GNATS
GNAWN
GNAWS
GOADS
GOAFT
GOALS
GOAPE
GOASK
GOATS
GRABS
GRACE
GRADE
GRADS
GRAFF
GRAFT
GRAIG
GRAIL
GRAIN
GRAMM
GRAMO
GRAMP
GRAMS
GRAND
GRANI
GRANT
GRAPE
GRAPH
GRAPY
GRASP
GRASS
GRATA
GRATE
GRAVE
GRAVI
GRAVY
GRAYS
GRAZE
GUAPA
GUANO
GUAPA
GUAPO
GUARD
GUARE
GUARS
GUAVA

G••A•

GAHAN
GALAS
GALAX
GAMAL
GAMAY
GETAB
GETAC
GETAD
GETAS
GETAT
GFLAT
GILAS
GLEAM
GLEAN
GLIAL
GLIAS
GLOAM
GLOAT
GOBAD
GOBAT
GOFAR
GOLAN
GOMAD
GOMAN
GORAN
GOTAB
GOTAC
GOTAD
GOTAT
GOYAS
GREAT
GROAN
GROAT
GSTAR
GULAG
GYRAL

G•••A

GAETA
GALBA
GALEA
GAMBA
GAMMA
GARDA
GEENA
GEMMA
GENOA
GHANA
GILDA
GINZA
GOLDA
GONNA
GOTHA
GOTTA
GOUDA
GRATA
GRETA
GROZA
GUAPA
GUAVA
GUNGA
GYOZA

•GA••

AGAIN
AGALS
AGAMA
AGAME
AGANA
AGAPE
AGARN
AGARS
AGASP
AGATE
AGAVE
AGAZE
EGADI
EGADS
EGALE
EGALS
NGAIO
NGANA
OGAMS

•G•A•

AGHAS
AGUAS
AGWAY
EGGAR
EGHAM
IGUAL
OGHAM

•G••A

AGAMA
AGANA
AGENA
AGITA
AGORA
AGURA
NGANA

••GA•

ALGAE
ALGAL
ALGAS
AVGAS
BEGAN
BEGAT
BEGAY
BOGAN
CIGAR
CUGAT
DAGAN
DEGAS
DIGAT
DUGAN
DUGAT
EAGAN
EDGAR
EGGAR
ELGAR
FUGAL
HAGAR
HOGAN
JUGAL
LEGAL
LOGAN
LPGAS
LUGAR
MEGAN
NAGAT
NOGAS
ORGAN
PAGAN
RAGAS
REGAL
REGAN
RIGAN
SAGAL
SAGAN
SAGAS
SEGAL
SEGAR
SUGAR
TOGAE
TOGAS
TUGAT
UNGAG
UNGAR
VEGAN
VEGAS
YOGAS
ZAGAT

••G•A

ALGIA
CIGNA
DOGMA
LOGIA
LYGIA
MAGDA
MAGMA
MAGNA
MAGUA
REGIA
REGNA
SIGMA
VIGIA

•••GA

AMIGA
BRAGA
CONGA
GUNGA
HELGA
KANGA
LONGA
MANGA
OMEGA
ONEGA
RENGA
TAIGA
TARGA
TIOGA
TONGA
USCGA
VIRGA
VOLGA

G•B••

GABBY
GABEL
GABIN
GABLE
GABON
GABOR
GIBBS
GIBED
GIBER
GIBES
GIBUS
GOBAD
GOBAT
GOBEL
GOBOS
GOBOT

G••B•

GABBY
GALBA
GAMBA
GARBO
GARBS
GETBY
GIBBS
GLOBE
GLOBS
GORBY
GOTBY
GRABS
GREBE
GRUBS
GUMBO
GUMBY

G•••B

GETAB
GOTAB

•GB••

EGBDF

••GB•

DIGBY
RIGBY
RUGBY

••G•B

NEGEB

GC•••

GCLEF

G•C••

GECKO
GUCCI
GUCKS
GUCKY

G••C•

GANCE
GEICO
GLACE
GLICK
GLOCK
GLUCK
GLUCO
GLYCO
GOOCH
GRACE
GRECO
GUCCI
GULCH

G•••C

GENIC
GETAC
GOTAC
GYNEC

•G••C

AGRIC
UGRIC

••G•C

HIGHC
LOGIC
MAGIC
YOGIC

G•D••

GADDI
GIDDY
GODEL
GODET
GODEY
GODLY
GODOT

G••D•

GADDI
GANDT
GANDY
GARDA
GARDE
GAUDI
GAUDS
GAUDY
GELDS
GEODE
GIDDY
GILDA
GILDS
GIRDS
GLADE
GLADS
GLIDE
GOADS
GOLDA
GOLDE
GOLDS
GOODE
GOODS
GOODY
GORDO
GORDY
GOUDA
GOUDY
GOWDY
GRADE
GRADS
GRIDE
GRIDS
GRODY
GUIDE
GUIDO
GURDY

G•••D

GAGED
GALED
GAMED
GAPED
GATED
GAZED
GELID
GETAD
GIBED
GLAND
GLUED
GOBAD
GOMAD
GORED
GOTAD
GOULD
GOURD
GRAND
GREED
GRIND
GRUED
GUARD
GUILD
GUYED
GYRED

•GD••

EGDON
OGDEN

•G•D•

EGADI
EGADS
EGBDF

•G••D

EGGED
IGGED
OGLED

••GD•

BIGDO
MAGDA

••G•D

ALGID
BYGOD
CAGED
EDGED
EGGED
GAGED
IGGED
LUGED
MYGOD
OHGOD
PAGED
RAGED
RIGID
URGED
WAGED

GE•••

GEARS
GEARY
GECKO
GEEKS
GEEKY
GEENA
GEEPS
GEESE
GEICO
GEIST
GEKKO
GELDS
GELEE
GELID
GELTS
GEMMA
GEMMY
GENES
GENET
GENIC
GENIE
GENII
GENOA
GENRE
GENTE
GENTS
GENUS
GENXS
GEODE
GEORG
GERMS
GERMY
GERRY
GERTZ
GESSO
GESTE
GESTS
GETAB
GETAC
GETAD
GETAS
GETAT
GETBY
GETGO
GETIN
GETIT
GETME
GETON
GETTO
GETTY
GETUP

G•E••

GAELS
GAETA
GEEKS
GEEKY
GEENA
GEEPS
GEESE
GHEES
GHENT
GLEAM
GLEAN
GLEEM
GLEES
GLENN
GLENS
GLESS
GOERS
GOEST
GOETH
GREAT
GREBE
GRECO
GREED
GREEK
GREEN
GREER
GREET
GREGG
GRETA
GRETE
GREYS
GUESS
GUEST
GWENN

G••E•

GABEL
GAGED
GAGES
GALEA
GALED
GALEN
GALES
GAMED
GAMER
GAMES
GANEF
GAPED
GAPER
GAPES
GARES
GASES
GATED
GATER
GATES
GAVEL
GAYER
GAZED
GAZER
GAZES
GCLEF
GELEE
GENES
GENET
GHEES
GIBED
GIBER
GIBES
GILES
GIMEL
GIVEN
GIVER
GIVES
GLEEM
GLEES
GLUED
GLUER
GLUES
GLUEY
GOBEL
GODEL
GODET
GODEY
GOFER
GOGET
GOLEM
GOMER
GOMEZ
GONER
GOOEY
GORED
GOREN
GORES
GOREY
GOSEE
GOWER
GOYEN
GREED
GREEK
GREEN
GREER
GREET
GRIEF
GRIEG
GRIER
GRUED
GRUEL
GRUES
GUMEE
GUTEN
GUYED
GYNEC
GYRED
GYRES

G•••E

GABLE
GAFFE
GANCE
GARDE
GASPE
GAUGE
GAUZE
GAYLE
GEESE
GELEE
GENIE
GENRE
GENTE
GEODE
GESTE
GETME
GIGUE
GIJOE
GIMME
GLACE
GLADE
GLARE
GLAZE
GLIDE
GLOBE
GLOVE
GLUTE
GNOME
GNOTE
GOAPE
GOLDE
GOODE
GOOSE
GORGE
GORME
GORSE
GOSEE
GOSSE
GOTME
GOUGE
GRACE
GRADE
GRAPE
GRATE
GRAVE
GRAZE
GREBE
GRETE
GRIDE
GRIME
GRIPE
GRISE
GROFE
GROPE
GROTE
GROVE
GTILE
GUARE
GUIDE
GUILE
GUISE
GUMEE

•GE••

AGENA
AGENT
AGERS
EGEST
EGEUS
OGEES

•G•E•

AGLET
AGLEY
AGNES
AGNEW
AGREE
AGUES
EGGED
EGGER
EGRET
IGGED
IGNES
NGWEE
OGDEN
OGEES
OGIER
OGLED
OGLER
OGLES
OGRES

•G••E

AGAME
AGAPE
AGATE
AGAVE
AGAZE
AGGIE
AGILE
AGREE
EGALE
IGIVE
NGWEE
OGIVE

••GE•

ALGER
ANGEL
ANGER
ANGES
AUGER
AWGEE
BAGEL
BEGEM
BEGET
BOGEY
CAGED
CAGER
CAGES
CAGEY
DEGEL
DIGEL
DIGEM
DOGES
EAGER
EDGED
EDGER
EDGES
EGGED
EGGER
EIGEN
EIGER
ENGEL
FOGEL
FOGEY
GAGED
GAGES
GOGET
HAGEN
HEGEL
HUGER
IGGED
INGER
KUGEL
LAGER
LEGER
LIGER
LOGES
LTGEN
LUGED
LUGER
LUGES
MAGEE
MAGES
MCGEE
MOGEN
MTGES
NAGEL
NEGEB
NEGEV
NIGEL
NIGER
OHGEE
PAGED
PAGER
PAGES
PAGET
PUGET
RAGED
RAGER
RAGES
REGEL
REGER
REGES
RIGEL
ROGER
ROGET
SAGER
SAGES
SAGET
SEGER
TIGER
TYGER
UNGER
URGED
URGER
URGES
VEGES
VOGEL
WAGED
WAGER
WAGES

••G•E

AGGIE
ALGAE
ANGIE
ANGLE
ARGUE
AUGIE
AWGEE
BOGIE
BOGLE
BUGLE
DOGIE
EAGLE
EAGRE
ENGLE
FUGUE
GIGUE
HAGUE
INGLE
LIGNE
LOGUE
MAGEE
MCGEE
OHGEE
REGLE
ROGUE
SEGRE
SEGUE
SIGNE
TIGRE
TOGAE
TOGUE
VAGUE
VOGUE

•••GE

ADAGE
ADIGE
AINGE
BADGE
BARGE
BEIGE
BILGE
BINGE
BLIGE
BORGE
BUDGE
BULGE
BYAGE
CADGE
CONGE
DINGE
DIRGE
DODGE
ELOGE
ETAGE
FORGE
FUDGE
GAUGE
GORGE
GOUGE
HEDGE
HENGE
HINGE
IMAGE
INAGE
JORGE
JUDGE
KEDGE
KRIGE
LANGE
LARGE
LEDGE
LIEGE
LODGE
LONGE
LUNGE
MADGE
MANGE
MARGE
MERGE
MIDGE
NEIGE
NORGE
NUDGE
OFAGE
OSAGE
PAIGE
PARGE
PHAGE
PLAGE
PURGE
RANGE
REEGE
RIDGE
ROUGE
RUDGE
SARGE
SEDGE
SERGE
SIEGE
SINGE
STAGE
SURGE
SYNGE
TENGE
TINGE
USAGE
VERGE
WEDGE

GF•••

GFLAT

G•F••

GAFFE
GAFFS
GIFTS
GOFAR
GOFER
GOFOR
GUFFS

G••F•

GAFFE
GAFFS
GOAFT
GOLFS
GOOFF
GOOFS
GOOFY
GRAFF
GRAFT
GRIFT
GROFE
GRUFF
GUFFS
GULFS

G•••F

GANEF
GCLEF
GOOFF
GRAFF
GRIEF
GRUFF

•G••F

EGBDF

G•G••

GAGED
GAGES
GIGIO
GIGLI
GIGOT
GIGUE
GOGET
GOGOL
GOGOS

G••G•

GANGS
GAUGE
GETGO
GITGO
GLOGG
GLUGS
GOLGI
GONGS
GORGE
GOUGE
GREGG
GRIGS
GROGS
GUNGA

G•••G

GEORG
GLOGG
GOING
GRAIG
GREGG
GRIEG
GULAG

•GG••

AGGIE
EGGAR
EGGED
EGGER
EGGON
EGGOS
IGGED

•G•G•

AGOGO

•G••G

AGING

••GG•

BAGGY
BIGGS
BIGGY
BOGGS
BOGGY
BUGGY
CIGGY
DIGGS
DOGGO
DOGGY
FOGGY
JAGGY
JIGGS
JIGGY
LEGGS
LEGGY
MUGGS
MUGGY
NAGGY
NOGGS
PEGGY
PIGGY
PUGGY
RAGGY
RIGGS
SAGGY
SOGGY
VIGGO
VUGGY
WIGGY
YEGGS
ZIGGY

••G•G

MAGOG
UNGAG

•••GG
BRAGG
FLAGG
FRIGG
GLOGG
GREGG
JONGG
STAGG
TRAGG

GH•••
GHAIN
GHALI
GHANA
GHATS
GHAZI
GHEES
GHENT
GHIJK
GHOST
GHOUL

G•H••
GAHAN

G••H•
GOTHA
GOTHS
GUSHY

G•••H
GARTH
GIRSH
GIRTH
GLYPH
GNASH
GOETH
GOOCH
GRAPH
GULCH
GURSH

•GH••
AGHAS
EGHAM
FGHIJ
OGHAM

•G••H
AGUSH
BGOSH

••GH•
AUGHT
BIGHT
EFGHI
EIGHT
FIGHT
HIGHC
HIGHS
LIGHT
MIGHT
NIGHT
OUGHT
RIGHT
SIGHS
SIGHT
TIGHT
WIGHT

•••GH
AARGH
ANIGH
BAUGH
BLIGH
BOUGH
BRAGH
BURGH
COUGH
DEFGH
DOUGH
HEIGH
HOUGH
KEOGH
KLUGH
KROGH
LAUGH
LEIGH
NEIGH
ROUGH
SINGH
THIGH
TOUGH
WAUGH
WEIGH

GI•••
GIANT
GIBBS
GIBED
GIBER
GIBES
GIBUS
GIDDY
GIFTS
GIGIO
GIGLI
GIGOT
GIGUE
GIJOE
GILAS
GILDA
GILDS
GILES
GILLS
GILTS
GIMEL
GIMLI
GIMME
GIMPS
GIMPY
GINNY
GINSU
GINUP
GINZA
GIONO
GIPSY
GIRDS
GIRLS
GIRLY
GIROS
GIRSH
GIRTH
GIRTS
GISMO
GISTS
GITGO
GITMO
GIVEN
GIVER
GIVES
GIZMO

G•I••
GAILY
GAINS
GAITS
GAIUS
GEICO
GEIST
GHIJK
GLIAL
GLIAS
GLICK
GLIDE
GLIMS
GLINT
GLITZ
GOING
GRIDE
GRIDS
GRIEF
GRIEG
GRIER
GRIFT
GRIGS
GRILL
GRIME
GRIMM
GRIMY
GRIND
GRINS
GRINT
GRIOT
GRIPE
GRIPS
GRIPY
GRISE
GRIST
GRITS
GTILE
GUIDE
GUIDO
GUILD
GUILE
GUILT
GUISE

G••I•
GABIN
GAMIN
GAVIN
GELID
GENIC
GENIE
GENII
GETIN
GETIT
GHAIN
GIGIO
GOPIK
GOSIT
GOTIN
GOTIT
GRAIG
GRAIL
GRAIN
GROIN
GSUIT
GUNIT

G•••I
GADDI
GALLI
GARNI
GAUDI
GENII
GHALI
GHAZI
GIGLI
GIMLI
GOLGI
GORKI
GOTTI
GOZZI
GRANI
GRAVI
GUCCI
GUMMI

•GI••
AGILE
AGING
AGIOS
AGITA
BGIRL
IGIVE
OGIER
OGIVE

•G•I•
AGAIN
AGGIE
AGRIC
AGRIN
EGLIN
FGHIJ
IGNIS
NGAIO
UGLIS
UGRIC

•G••I
EGADI

••GI•
AEGIR
AEGIS
AGGIE
ALGIA
ALGID
ANGIE
ANGIO
AUGIE
BAGIT
BEGIN
BOGIE
DIGIN
DIGIT
DOGIE
DOGIT
DUGIN
DUGIT
ELGIN
EXGIS
FAGIN
FOGIN
FUGIT
GIGIO
HAGIO
LEGIT
LOGIA
LOGIC
LOGIN
LYGIA
MAGIC
PIGIT
REGIA
REGIS
RIGID
SIGIL
VIGIA
VIGIL
YOGIC
YOGIS

••G•I
CYGNI
EFGHI
GIGLI
LIGNI
NEGRI
SEGNI

•••GI
ASAGI
CORGI
FUNGI
GOLGI
LONGI
LUIGI
SENGI
SHOGI

G•J••
GIJOE

G••J•
GHIJK

•G••J
FGHIJ

G•K••
GEKKO

G••K•
GAWKS
GAWKY
GECKO
GEEKS
GEEKY
GEKKO
GOOKS
GORKI
GORKY
GROKS
GUCKS
GUCKY
GUNKS
GUNKY

G•••K
GHIJK
GLICK
GLOCK
GLUCK
GLUNK
GOASK
GOPIK
GREEK

GL•••
GLACE
GLADE
GLADS
GLAMS
GLAND
GLARE
GLARY
GLASS
GLATT
GLAXO
GLAZE
GLAZY
GLEAM
GLEAN
GLEEM
GLEES
GLENN
GLENS
GLESS
GLIAL
GLIAS
GLICK
GLIDE
GLIMS
GLINT
GLITZ
GLOAM
GLOAT
GLOBE
GLOBS
GLOCK
GLOGG
GLOMS
GLOOM
GLOPS
GLORY
GLOSS
GLOTT
GLOVE
GLOWS
GLUCK
GLUCO
GLUED
GLUER
GLUES
GLUEY
GLUGS
GLUMS
GLUNK
GLUON
GLUTE
GLUTS
GLYCO
GLYPH
GLYPT

G•L••
GALAS
GALAX
GALBA
GALEA
GALED
GALEN
GALES
GALLI
GALLO
GALLS
GALOP
GCLEF
GELDS
GELEE
GELID
GELTS
GFLAT
GILAS
GILDA
GILDS
GILES
GILLS
GILTS
GOLAN
GOLDA
GOLDE
GOLDS
GOLEM
GOLFS
GOLGI
GOLLY
GULAG
GULCH
GULFS
GULLS
GULLY
GULPS
GULPY

G••L•
GABLE
GAELS
GAILY
GALLI
GALLO
GALLS
GAOLS
GAULS
GAYLE
GAYLY
GHALI
GIGLI
GILLS
GIMLI
GIRLS
GIRLY
GOALS
GODLY
GOLLY
GOULD
GRILL
GRRLS
GTILE
GUILD
GUILE
GUILT
GULLS
GULLY

G•••L
GABEL
GAMAL
GASOL
GAVEL
GHOUL
GIMEL
GLIAL
GNARL
GOBEL
GODEL
GOGOL
GRAIL
GRILL
GROWL
GRRRL
GRUEL
GYRAL

•GL••
AGLET
AGLEY
AGLOW
EGLIN
IGLOO
IGLUS
OGLED
OGLER
OGLES
UGLIS

•G•L•
AGALS
AGILE
EGALE
EGALS

•G••L
BGIRL
IGUAL

••GL•
ANGLE
ANGLO
BIGLY
BOGLE
BUGLE
EAGLE
ENGLE
GIGLI
INGLE
REGLE

••G•L
ALGAL
ALGOL
ANGEL
BAGEL
DEGEL
DIGEL
ENGEL
FOGEL
FUGAL
GOGOL
HEGEL
JUGAL
KUGEL
LEGAL
MOGUL
NAGEL
NIGEL
REGAL
REGEL
RIGEL
SAGAL
SEGAL
SIGIL
VIGIL
VOGEL

•••GL
HEIGL
PREGL

GM•••
GMATS

G•M••
GAMAL
GAMAY
GAMBA
GAMED
GAMER
GAMES
GAMIN
GAMMA
GAMOW
GAMPS
GAMUT
GEMMA
GEMMY
GIMEL
GIMLI
GIMME
GIMPS
GIMPY
GOMAD
GOMAN
GOMER
GOMEZ
GUMBO
GUMBY
GUMEE
GUMMI
GUMMO
GUMMY
GUMUP
GYMNO

G••M•
GAMMA
GEMMA
GEMMY
GERMS
GERMY
GETME
GIMME
GISMO
GITMO
GIZMO
GLAMS
GLIMS
GLOMS
GLUMS
GNOME
GNOMY
GORME
GORMS
GOTME
GRAMM
GRAMO
GRAMP
GRAMS
GRIME
GRIMM
GRIMY
GRUMP
GUMMI
GUMMO
GUMMY

G•••M
GLEAM
GLEEM
GLOAM
GLOOM
GOLEM
GRAMM
GRIMM
GROOM

•G•M•
AGAMA
AGAME
OGAMS

•G••M
EGHAM
OGHAM

••GM•
BIGMO
DOGMA
MAGMA
PYGMY
SIGMA

••G•M
BEGEM
BEGUM
BYGUM
DEGUM
DIGEM
REGUM

GN•••
GNARL
GNARS
GNASH
GNATS
GNAWN
GNAWS
GNOME
GNOMY
GNOTE

G•N••
GANCE
GANDT
GANDY
GANEF
GANGS
GANSU
GENES
GENET
GENIC
GENIE
GENII
GENOA
GENRE
GENTE
GENTS
GENUS
GENXS
GINNY
GINSU
GINUP
GINZA
GONER
GONGS
GONNA
GONOW
GONZO
GUNGA
GUNIT
GUNKS
GUNKY
GUNNY
GYNEC

G••N•
GAINS
GARNI
GAUNT
GEENA
GHANA
GHENT
GIANT
GINNY
GIONO
GLAND
GLENN
GLENS
GLINT
GLUNK
GOING
GONNA
GOONS
GOONY
GOWNS
GRAND
GRANI
GRANT
GRIND
GRINS
GRINT
GRUNT
GUANO
GUNNY
GWENN
GWYNN
GYMNO

G•••N
GABIN
GABON
GAHAN
GALEN
GAMIN
GATUN
GAVIN
GETIN
GETON
GHAIN
GIVEN
GLEAN
GLENN
GLUON
GNAWN
GOLAN
GOMAN
GORAN
GOREN
GOTIN
GOTON
GOYEN
GRAIN
GREEN
GROAN
GROIN
GROWN
GUTEN
GUYON
GWENN
GWYNN

•GN••
AGNES
AGNEW
AGNON
AGNUS
IGNES
IGNIS

•G•N•
AGANA
AGENA
AGENT
AGING
AGONY
NGANA

•G••N
AGAIN
AGARN
AGNON
AGRIN
AGRON
EGDON
EGGON
EGLIN
OGDEN

••GN•
CIGNA
CYGNI
LEGNO
LIGNE
LIGNI
LIGNO
MAGNA
REGNA
SEGNI
SEGNO
SIGNE
SIGNS
VIGNY

••G•N
ARGON
BBGUN
BEGAN
BEGIN
BEGUN
BIGON
BOGAN
DAGAN
DIGIN
DOGON
DUGAN
DUGIN
EAGAN
EGGON
EIGEN
ELGIN
FAGIN
FOGIN
HAGEN
HOGAN
LOGAN
LOGIN
LOGON
LTGEN
MEGAN
MOGEN
OBGYN
ORGAN
ORGON
PAGAN
RAGON
REGAN
RIGAN
SAGAN
TAGON
TIGON
TUGON
VEGAN
WAGON

•••GN
ALIGN
COIGN
DEIGN
FEIGN
REIGN
VSIGN

GO•••
GOADS
GOAFT
GOALS
GOAPE
GOASK
GOATS
GOBAD
GOBAT
GOBEL
GOBOS
GOBOT
GODEL
GODET
GODEY
GODLY
GODOT
GOERS
GOEST
GOETH
GOFAR
GOFER
GOFOR
GOGET
GOGOL
GOGOS
GOING
GOLAN
GOLDA
GOLDE
GOLDS
GOLEM
GOLFS
GOLGI
GOLLY
GOMAD
GOMAN
GOMER
GOMEZ
GONER
GONGS
GONNA
GONOW
GONZO
GOOCH
GOODE
GOODS
GOODY
GOOEY
GOOFF
GOOFS
GOOFY
GOOKS
GOONS
GOONY
GOOPS
GOOPY
GOOSE
GOOSY
GOOUT
GOPIK
GOPRO
GORAN
GORBY
GORDO
GORDY
GORED
GOREN
GORES
GOREY
GORGE
GORKI
GORKY
GORME
GORMS
GORPS
GORSE
GORSY
GOSEE
GOSIT
GOSSE
GOTAB
GOTAC
GOTAD
GOTAT
GOTBY
GOTHA
GOTHS
GOTIN
GOTIT
GOTME
GOTON
GOTTA
GOTTI
GOTTO
GOTUP
GOUDA
GOUDY
GOUGE
GOULD
GOURD
GOUTS
GOUTY
GOVTS
GOWDY
GOWER
GOWNS
GOYAS
GOYEN
GOZZI

G•O••
GAOLS
GEODE
GEORG
GHOST
GHOUL
GIONO
GLOAM
GLOAT
GLOBE
GLOBS
GLOCK
GLOGG
GLOMS
GLOOM
GLOPS
GLORY
GLOSS
GLOTT
GLOVE
GLOWS
GNOME
GNOMY
GNOTE
GOOCH
GOODE
GOODS
GOODY
GOOEY
GOOFF
GOOFS
GOOFY
GOOKS
GOONS
GOONY
GOOPS
GOOPY
GOOSE
GOOSY
GOOUT
GROAN
GROAT
GRODY
GROFE
GROGS
GROIN
GROKS
GROOM
GROPE
GROSS
GROSZ
GROTE
GROTS
GROUP
GROUT
GROVE
GROWL
GROWN
GROWS
GROZA
GYOZA

G••O•
GABON
GABOR
GALOP
GAMOW
GAROU
GASOL
GATOR
GATOS
GAVOT
GENOA
GETON
GIGOT
GIJOE
GIROS
GLOOM
GLUON
GOBOS
GOBOT
GODOT
GOFOR
GOGOL
GOGOS
GONOW
GOTON
GRIOT
GROOM
GUYON
GYROS

G•••O
GALLO
GARBO
GATTO
GECKO
GEICO
GEKKO
GESSO
GETGO
GETTO
GIGIO
GIONO
GISMO
GITGO
GITMO
GIZMO
GLAXO
GLUCO
GLYCO
GONZO
GOPRO
GORDO
GOTTO
GRAMO
GRECO
GUANO
GUAPO
GUIDO
GUMBO
GUMMO
GUSTO
GYMNO

•GO••
AGOGO
AGONY
AGORA
BGOSH

•G•O•
AGIOS
AGLOW
AGNON
AGRON
EGDON
EGGON
EGGOS
IGLOO
OGROS

•G••O
AGOGO
IGLOO
NGAIO

••GO•
ALGOL
ARGON
ARGOS
ARGOT
BEGOT
BIGON
BIGOT
BYGOD
DOGON
EGGON
EGGOS
ERGOT
EXGOV
FAGOT
GIGOT
GOGOL
GOGOS
HUGOS
INGOT
LAGOS
LEGOS
LOGON
LOGOS
LTGOV
MAGOG
MAGOO
MYGOD
NOGOS
OHGOD
ORGON
RAGON
RIGOR

SAGOS
SEGOS
TAGON
TIGON
TUGON
UNGOT
VIGOR
WAGON
YUGOS

••G•O
ANGIO
ANGLO
BIGDO
BIGMO
DOGGO
GIGIO
HAGIO
HYGRO
LEGNO
LIGNO
MAGOO
NEGRO
SEGNO
VIGGO

•••GO
AGOGO
AMIGO
BINGO
BONGO
CARGO
CITGO
CONGO
DIEGO
DINGO
DOGGO
DRAGO
DRIGO
FARGO
FORGO
FUEGO
FUNGO
GETGO
GITGO
ILLGO
IMAGO
INIGO
JINGO
JUEGO
LARGO
LETGO
LINGO
LONGO
LUEGO
MANGO
MARGO
MONGO
OINGO
OLIGO
OUTGO
PHAGO
PONGO
PREGO
RANGO
RINGO
SLIGO
SPAGO
TANGO
TENGO
TIAGO
VIGGO
VIRGO

G•P••
GAPED
GAPER
GAPES
GIPSY
GOPIK
GOPRO
GUPPY
GYPSY

G••P•
GAMPS
GASPE
GASPS
GAWPS
GEEPS
GIMPS
GIMPY
GLOPS
GLYPH
GLYPT
GOAPE
GOOPS
GOOPY
GORPS
GRAPE
GRAPH
GRAPY
GRIPE
GRIPS
GRIPY
GROPE
GUAPA
GUAPO
GULPS
GULPY
GUPPY

G•••P
GALOP
GASUP
GETUP
GINUP
GOTUP
GRAMP
GRASP
GROUP
GRUMP
GUMUP

•G•P•
AGAPE
EGYPT

•G••P
AGASP

••G•P
DIGUP
DUGUP
FOGUP
LEGUP
RIGUP
TAGUP
TOGUP

GR•••
GRABS
GRACE
GRADE
GRADS
GRAFF
GRAFT
GRAIG
GRAIL
GRAIN
GRAMM
GRAMO
GRAMP
GRAMS
GRAND
GRANI
GRANT
GRAPE
GRAPH
GRAPY
GRASP
GRASS
GRATA
GRATE
GRAVE
GRAVI
GRAVY
GRAYS
GRAZE
GREAT
GREBE
GRECO
GREED
GREEK
GREEN
GREER
GREET
GREGG
GRETA
GRETE
GREYS
GRIDE
GRIDS
GRIEF
GRIEG
GRIER
GRIFT
GRIGS
GRILL
GRIME
GRIMM
GRIMY
GRIND
GRINS
GRINT
GRIOT
GRIPE
GRIPS
GRIPY
GRISE
GRIST
GRITS
GROAN
GROAT
GRODY
GROFE
GROGS
GROIN
GROKS
GROOM
GROPE
GROSS
GROSZ
GROTE
GROTS
GROUP
GROUT
GROVE
GROWL
GROWN
GROWS
GROZA
GRRLS
GRRRL
GRRRS
GRUBS
GRUED
GRUEL
GRUES
GRUFF
GRUMP
GRUNT

G•R••
GARBO
GARBS
GARDA
GARDE
GARES
GARNI
GAROU
GARRY
GARTH
GERMS
GERMY
GERRY
GERTZ
GIRDS
GIRLS
GIRLY
GIROS
GIRSH
GIRTH
GIRTS
GORAN
GORBY
GORDO
GORDY
GORED
GOREN
GORES
GOREY
GORGE
GORKI
GORKY
GORME
GORMS
GORPS
GORSE
GORSY
GRRLS
GRRRL
GRRRS
GURDY
GURSH
GURUS
GYRAL
GYRED
GYRES
GYROS

G••R•
GARRY
GAURS
GEARS
GEARY
GENRE
GEORG
GERRY
GLARE
GLARY
GLORY
GNARL
GNARS
GOERS
GOPRO
GOURD
GRRRL
GRRRS
GUARD
GUARE
GUARS

G•••R
GABOR
GAMER
GAPER
GASTR
GATER
GATOR
GAYER
GAZER
GIBER
GIVER
GLUER
GOFAR
GOFER
GOFOR
GOMER
GONER
GOWER
GREER
GRIER
GSTAR

•GR••
AGREE
AGRIC
AGRIN
AGRON
EGRET
OGRES
OGROS
UGRIC

•G•R•
AGARN
AGARS
AGERS
AGORA
AGURA
BGIRL

•G••R
EGGAR
EGGER
OGIER
OGLER

••GR•
ANGRY
EAGRE
ENGRS
HYGRO
NEGRI
NEGRO
SEGRE
TIGRE

••G•R
AEGIR
ALGER
ANGER
AUGER
AUGUR
CAGER
CIGAR
EAGER
EDGAR
EDGER
EGGAR
EGGER
EIGER
ELGAR
HAGAR
HUGER
INGER
LAGER
LEGER
LIGER
LUGAR
LUGER
NIGER
PAGER
RAGER
REGER
RIGOR
ROGER
SAGER
SEGAR
SEGER
SUGAR
TIGER
TYGER
UNGAR
UNGER
URGER
VIGOR
WAGER

GS•••
GSTAR
GSUIT

G•S••
GASES
GASOL
GASPE
GASPS
GASSY
GASTR
GASUP
GESSO
GESTE
GESTS
GISMO
GISTS
GOSEE
GOSIT
GOSSE
GUSHY
GUSSY
GUSTO
GUSTS
GUSTY

G••S•
GANSU
GASSY
GAUSS
GEESE
GEIST
GESSO
GHOST
GINSU
GIPSY
GIRSH
GLASS
GLESS
GLOSS
GNASH
GOASK
GOEST
GOOSE
GOOSY
GORSE
GORSY
GOSSE
GRASP
GRASS
GRISE
GRIST
GROSS
GROSZ
GUESS
GUEST
GUISE
GURSH
GUSSY
GUTSY
GYPSY

G•••S
GAELS
GAFFS
GAGES
GAINS
GAITS
GAIUS
GALAS
GALES
GALLS
GAMES
GAMPS
GANGS
GAOLS
GAPES
GARBS
GARES
GASES
GASPS
GATES
GATOS
GAUDS
GAULS
GAURS
GAUSS
GAWKS
GAWPS
GAZES
GEARS
GEEKS
GEEPS
GELDS
GELTS
GENES
GENTS
GENUS
GENXS
GERMS
GESTS
GETAS
GHATS
GHEES
GIBBS
GIBES
GIBUS
GIFTS
GILAS
GILDS
GILES
GILLS
GILTS
GIMPS
GIRDS
GIRLS
GIROS
GIRTS
GISTS
GIVES
GLADS
GLAMS
GLASS
GLEES
GLENS
GLESS
GLIAS
GLIMS
GLOBS
GLOMS
GLOPS
GLOSS
GLOWS
GLUES
GLUGS
GLUMS
GLUTS
GMATS
GNARS
GNATS
GNAWS
GOADS
GOALS
GOATS
GOBOS
GOERS
GOGOS
GOLDS
GOLFS
GONGS
GOODS
GOOFS
GOOKS
GOONS
GOOPS
GORES
GORMS
GORPS
GOTHS
GOUTS
GOVTS
GOWNS
GOYAS
GRABS
GRADS
GRAMS
GRASS
GRAYS
GREYS
GRIDS
GRIGS
GRINS
GRIPS
GRITS
GROGS
GROKS
GROSS
GROTS
GROWS
GRRLS
GRRRS
GRUBS
GRUES
GUARS
GUCKS
GUESS
GUFFS
GULFS
GULLS
GULPS
GUNKS
GURUS
GUSTS
GYRES
GYROS

•G•S•
AGASP
AGUSH
BGOSH
EGEST

•G••S
AGALS
AGARS
AGERS
AGHAS
AGIOS
AGNES
AGNUS
AGUAS
AGUES
EGADS
EGALS
EGEUS
EGGOS
IGLUS
IGNES
IGNIS
OGAMS
OGEES
OGLES
OGRES
OGROS
UGLIS

••GS•
ANGST
BUGSY

••G•S
AEGIS
ALGAS
ANGES
ANGUS
ARGOS
ARGUS
AVGAS
BIGGS
BOGGS
BOGUS
CAGES
DEGAS
DIGGS
DOGES
EDGES
EGGOS
ENGRS
EXGIS
FUGUS
GAGES
GOGOS
HIGHS
HUGOS
JIGGS
LAGOS
LEGGS
LEGOS
LOGES
LOGOS
LPGAS
LUGES
MAGES
MAGUS
MSGTS
MTGES
MUGGS
NEGUS
NOGAS
NOGGS
NOGOS
PAGES
RAGAS
RAGES
REGES
REGIS
REGTS
RIGGS
SAGAS
SAGES
SAGOS
SEGOS
SIGHS
SIGNS
SSGTS
TAGUS
TOGAS
TSGTS
URGES
VAGUS
VEGAS
VEGES
WAGES
YEGGS
YOGAS
YOGIS
YUGOS

•••GS
ANAGS
BANGS
BERGS
BIGGS
BINGS
BIOGS
BLDGS
BLOGS
BOGGS
BONGS
BORGS
BRAGS
BRIGS
BUNGS
BURGS
CHUGS
CLOGS
CRAGS
DANGS
DIGGS
DINGS
DONGS
DRAGS
DREGS
DRUGS
EMAGS
FANGS
FLAGS
FLOGS
FRAGS
FROGS
FRUGS
GANGS
GLUGS
GONGS
GRIGS
GROGS
HANGS
HAWGS
JIGGS
JPEGS
KANGS
KINGS
LEGGS
LINGS
LONGS
LUNGS
MOOGS
MPEGS
MUGGS
NOGGS
PANGS
PINGS
PLUGS
PONGS
PRIGS
PROGS
PUNGS
QUAGS
RIGGS
RINGS
RUNGS
SHAGS
SINGS
SKEGS
SLAGS
SLOGS
SLUGS
SMOGS
SNAGS
SNUGS
SONGS
STAGS
SWAGS
SWIGS
TANGS
THUGS
TIEGS
TINGS
TONGS
TWIGS
WHIGS
WINGS
YEGGS
ZINGS

GT•••
GTILE

G•T••
GATED
GATER
GATES
GATOR
GATOS
GATTO
GATUN
GETAB
GETAC
GETAD
GETAS
GETAT
GETBY
GETGO
GETIN
GETIT
GETME
GETON
GETTO
GETTY
GETUP
GITGO
GITMO
GOTAB
GOTAC
GOTAD
GOTAT
GOTBY
GOTHA
GOTHS
GOTIN
GOTIT
GOTME
GOTON
GOTTA
GOTTI
GOTTO
GOTUP
GSTAR
GUTEN
GUTSY
GUTTY

G••T•
GAETA
GAITS
GARTH
GASTR
GATTO
GELTS
GENTE
GENTS
GERTZ
GESTE
GESTS
GETTO
GETTY
GHATS
GIFTS
GILTS
GIRTH
GIRTS
GISTS
GLATT
GLITZ
GLOTT
GLUTE
GLUTS
GMATS
GNATS
GNOTE
GOATS
GOETH
GOTTA
GOTTI
GOTTO
GOUTS
GOUTY
GOVTS
GRATA
GRATE
GRETA
GRETE
GRITS
GROTE
GROTS
GUSTO
GUSTS
GUSTY
GUTTY

G•••T
GAMUT
GANDT
GAUNT
GAVOT
GEIST
GENET
GETAT
GETIT
GFLAT
GHENT
GHOST
GIANT
GIGOT
GLATT
GLINT
GLOAT
GLOTT
GLYPT
GOAFT
GOBAT
GOBOT
GODET
GODOT
GOEST
GOGET
GOOUT
GOSIT
GOTAT
GOTIT
GRAFT
GRANT
GREAT
GREET
GRIFT
GRINT
GRIOT
GRIST
GROAT
GROUT
GRUNT
GSUIT
GUEST
GUILT
GUNIT

•G•T•
AGATE
AGITA

•G••T
AGENT
AGLET
EGEST
EGRET
EGYPT

••GT•
MSGTS
REGTS
SSGTS
TSGTS

••G•T
ANGST
ARGOT
AUGHT
BAGIT
BEGAT
BEGET
BEGOT
BIGHT
BIGOT
CUGAT
DIGAT
DIGIT
DOGIT
DUGAT
DUGIT
EIGHT
ERGOT
FAGOT
FIGHT
FUGIT
GIGOT
GOGET
INGOT
LEGIT
LIGHT
MIGHT
NAGAT
NIGHT
OUGHT
PAGET
PIGIT
PUGET
RIGHT
ROGET
SAGET
SIGHT
TIGHT
TUGAT
UNGOT
WIGHT
ZAGAT

•••GT
VINGT

GU•••
GUANO
GUAPA
GUAPO
GUARD
GUARE
GUARS
GUAVA
GUCCI
GUCKS
GUCKY
GUESS
GUEST
GUFFS
GUIDE
GUIDO
GUILD
GUILE
GUILT
GUISE
GULAG
GULCH
GULFS
GULLS
GULLY
GULPS
GULPY
GUMBO
GUMBY
GUMEE
GUMMI
GUMMO
GUMMY
GUMUP
GUNGA
GUNIT
GUNKS
GUNKY
GUNNY
GUPPY
GURDY
GURSH
GURUS
GUSHY
GUSSY
GUSTO
GUSTS
GUSTY
GUTEN
GUTSY
GUTTY
GUYED
GUYON

G•U••
GAUDI
GAUDS
GAUDY
GAUGE
GAULS
GAUNT
GAURS
GAUSS
GAUZE
GAUZY
GLUCK
GLUCO
GLUED
GLUER
GLUES
GLUEY
GLUGS
GLUMS
GLUNK
GLUON
GLUTE
GLUTS
GOUDA
GOUDY
GOUGE
GOULD
GOURD
GOUTS
GOUTY
GRUBS
GRUED
GRUEL
GRUES
GRUFF
GRUMP
GRUNT
GSUIT

G••U•
GAIUS
GAMUT
GASUP
GATUN
GENUS
GETUP
GHOUL
GIBUS
GIGUE
GINUP
GOOUT
GOTUP
GROUP
GROUT
GUMUP
GURUS

G•••U
GANSU
GAROU
GINSU

•GU••
AGUAS
AGUES
AGURA
AGUSH
IGUAL

•G•U•
AGNUS
EGEUS
IGLUS

••GU•
ANGUS
ARGUE
ARGUS
AUGUR
BBGUN
BEGUM
BEGUN
BOGUS
BYGUM
DEGUM
DIGUP
DUGUP
FOGUP
FUGUE
FUGUS
GIGUE
HAGUE
LEGUP
LOGUE
MAGUA
MAGUS
MOGUL
MYGUY
NEGUS
PEGUY
REGUM
RIGUP
ROGUE
SEGUE
TAGUP
TAGUS
TOGUE
TOGUP
VAGUE
VAGUS
VOGUE

••G•U
ILGWU

•••GU
LINGU
LONGU
TAEGU

G•V••
GAVEL
GAVIN
GAVOT
GIVEN
GIVER
GIVES
GOVTS

G••V•
GLOVE
GRAVE
GRAVI
GRAVY
GROVE
GUAVA

•G•V•
AGAVE
IGIVE
OGIVE

••G•V
EXGOV
LTGOV
NEGEV

GW•••
GWENN
GWYNN

G•W••
GAWKS
GAWKY
GAWPS
GOWDY
GOWER
GOWNS

G••W•
GLOWS
GNAWN
GNAWS
GROWL
GROWN
GROWS

G•••W
GAMOW
GONOW

•GW••
AGWAY
NGWEE

•G••W
AGLOW
AGNEW

••GW•
ILGWU

G••X•
GENXS
GLAXO

G•••X
GALAX

GY•••
GYMNO
GYNEC
GYOZA
GYPSY
GYRAL
GYRED
GYRES
GYROS

G•Y••
GAYER
GAYLE
GAYLY
GLYCO
GLYPH
GLYPT
GOYAS
GOYEN
GUYED
GUYON
GWYNN

G••Y•
GRAYS
GREYS

G•••Y
GABBY
GAILY
GAMAY
GANDY
GARRY
GASSY
GAUDY
GAUZY
GAWKY
GAYLY
GEARY
GEEKY
GEMMY
GERMY
GERRY
GETBY
GETTY
GIDDY
GIMPY
GINNY
GIPSY
GIRLY
GLARY
GLAZY
GLORY
GLUEY
GNOMY
GODEY
GODLY
GOLLY
GOODY
GOOEY
GOOFY
GOONY
GOOPY
GOOSY
GORBY
GORDY
GOREY
GORKY
GORSY
GOTBY
GOUDY
GOUTY
GOWDY
GRAPY
GRAVY
GRIMY
GRIPY
GRODY
GUCKY
GULLY
GULPY
GUMBY
GUMMY
GUNKY
GUNNY
GUPPY
GURDY
GUSHY
GUSSY
GUSTY
GUTSY
GUTTY
GYPSY

•GY••
EGYPT

•G••Y
AGLEY
AGONY
AGWAY

••GY•
OBGYN

••G•Y
ANGRY
BAGGY
BEGAY
BIGGY
BIGLY
BOGEY
BOGGY
BUGGY
BUGSY
CAGEY
CIGGY
DIGBY
DOGGY
FOGEY
FOGGY
JAGGY
JIGGY
LEGGY
MUGGY
MYGUY
NAGGY
PEGGY
PEGUY
PIGGY
PUGGY
PYGMY
RAGGY
RIGBY
RUGBY
SAGGY
SOGGY
VIGNY
VUGGY
WIGGY
ZIGGY

•••GY
BAGGY
BIGGY
BILGY
BOGGY
BUGGY
BULGY
CIGGY
DINGY
DODGY
DOGGY
ELEGY
FOGGY
HEDGY
HOAGY
JAGGY
JIGGY
LEDGY
LEGGY
MANGY
MARGY
MINGY
MUGGY
NAGGY
OLOGY
PEGGY
PHAGY
PIGGY
PORGY
PUDGY
PUGGY
RAGGY
RANGY
RIDGY
SAGGY
SEDGY
SOGGY
STAGY
STOGY
TANGY
VUGGY
WEDGY
WIGGY
WINGY
ZIGGY
ZINGY

G•Z••
GAZED
GAZER
GAZES
GIZMO
GOZZI

G••Z•
GAUZE
GAUZY
GHAZI
GINZA
GLAZE
GLAZY
GONZO
GOZZI
GRAZE
GROZA
GYOZA

G•••Z
GERTZ
GLITZ
GOMEZ
GROSZ

•G•Z•
AGAZE

HA•••
HABER
HABIB
HABIT
HABLA
HACEK
HACKL
HACKS
HACKY
HADAT
HADES
HADIN
HADIT
HADJI
HADNO
HADNT
HADON
HADST
HADTO
HADUP
HAEMA
HAFIZ
HAFTS
HAGAR
HAGEN
HAGIO
HAGUE
HAHAS
HAIDA
HAIFA
HAIKS
HAIKU
HAILE
HAILS
HAING
HAIRS
HAIRY
HAISE
HAITI
HAJIS
HAJJI
HAKES
HAKIM
HALAL
HALAS
HALED
HALEN
HALER
HALES
HALEY
HALLE
HALLO
HALLS
HALOP
HALOS
HALTS
HALVA
HALVE
HAMAN
HAMAS
HAMEL
HAMER
HAMES
HAMMS
HAMMY
HAMUP
HANDI
HANDS
HANDY
HANES
HANEY
HANFF
HANGS
HANKS
HANKY
HANNA
HANOI
HANSA
HANSE
HANTS
HANYA
HAOLE
HAPLY
HAPPY
HARDC
HARDG
HARDY
HARED
HAREM
HARES
HARKS
HARMS
HARPO
HARPS
HARPY
HARRY
HARSH
HARTE
HARUM
HASAT
HASEK
HASID
HASIN
HASIT
HASNO
HASNT
HASON
HASPS
HASSO
HASTA
HASTE
HASTO
HASTY
HASUP
HATCH
HATED
HATER
HATES
HATHA
HATHI
HATLO
HAUER
HAULS
HAUNT
HAUTE
HAVEL
HAVEN
HAVER
HAVES
HAVOC
HAVRE
HAWED
HAWER
HAWGS
HAWKE
HAWKS
HAWSE
HAYDN
HAYED
HAYEK
HAYER
HAYES
HAYEY
HAZAN
HAZED
HAZEL
HAZER
HAZES

H•A••
HBARS
HEADS
HEADY
HEALD
HEALS
HEALY
HEAPS
HEAPY
HEARD
HEARN
HEARS
HEART
HEATH
HEATS
HEAVE
HEAVY
HOAGY
HOARD
HOARE
HOARS
HOARY
HUANG
HYAMS
HYATT

H••A•
HADAT
HAGAR
HAHAS
HALAL
HALAS
HAMAN
HAMAS
HASAT
HAZAN
HBEAM
HEMAL
HEMAN
HEMAT
HEPAT
HERAT
HEXAD
HIHAT
HIJAS
HIRAM
HITAT
HOBAN
HODAD
HOGAN
HONAN
HORAE
HORAL
HORAS
HOWAR
HOYAS
HULAS
HUMAN
HUNAN
HUSAK
HYLAS
HYMAN
HYRAX

H•••A
HABLA
HAEMA
HAIDA
HAIFA
HALVA
HANNA
HANSA
HANYA
HASTA
HATHA
HEDDA
HELGA
HENNA
HEPTA
HILDA
HOFFA
HONDA
HOOHA
HOOKA
HOSEA
HOSTA
HOUMA
HOXHA
HYDRA
HYENA

•HA••
AHAIR
AHANG
BHAER
BHANG
BHATS
CHACO
CHADS
CHAFE
CHAFF
CHAIM
CHAIN
CHAIR
CHAIS
CHAKA
CHALK
CHAMP
CHANG
CHANT
CHAOS
CHAPS
CHARD
CHARM
CHARO
CHARS
CHART
CHARY
CHASE
CHASM
CHAST
CHATS
CHAUD
CHAVA
CHAWS
CHAZZ
DHABI
DHAKA
DHALS
GHAIN
GHALI
GHANA
GHATS
GHAZI
KHAKI
KHANS
LHASA
OHAIR
OHARA
OHARE
OHAYO
PHAGE
PHAGO
PHAGY
PHAIR
PHANY
PHARM
PHASE
SHACK
SHADE
SHADS
SHADY
SHAEF
SHAFT
SHAGS
SHAHN
SHAHS
SHAKE
SHAKO
SHAKY
SHALE
SHALL
SHALT
SHAME
SHAMS
SHAMU
SHANA
SHANE
SHANG
SHANK
SHANT
SHAPE
SHARD
SHARE
SHARI
SHARK
SHARP
SHATT
SHAUN
SHAVE
SHAWL
SHAWN
SHAYS
THAIS
THANE
THANK
THANT
THANX
THARP
THATS
THAWS
UHAUL
WHACK
WHALE
WHAMO
WHAMS
WHANG
WHAPS
WHARF
WHATD
WHATS

•H•A•
AHEAD
AHEAP
AHMAD
CHEAP
CHEAT
CHIAS
IHEAR
OHKAY
OHMAN
PHIAL
RHEAS
SHEAF
SHEAN
SHEAR
SHOAL
SHOAT
THEAS
THEAX
UHLAN
UHNAK
WHEAT

•H••A
AHORA
CHAKA
CHAVA
CHEKA
CHELA
CHETA
CHICA
CHINA
CHITA
CHULA
DHAKA
GHANA
LHASA
OHARA
PHYLA
RHODA
SHANA
SHEBA
SHERA
SHIVA
SHULA
THEDA
THEMA
THERA
THETA
THORA
UHURA
XHOSA

••HA•
AGHAS
ARHAT
BAHAI
BEHAN
BEHAR
BOHAY
COHAB
COHAN
EGHAM
EPHAH
EPHAS
ETHAN
GAHAN
HAHAS
HIHAT
ISHAM
JAHAN
JEHAN
JIHAD
JIHAN
JOHAN
LEHAR
LOHAN
MAHAL
MAHAN
OGHAM
OSHAY
PSHAW
RAHAL
REHAB
REHAN
SCHAV
UNHAT
WUHAN
YMHAS
YWHAS

••H•A
BAHIA
BOHEA
LEHUA
MEHTA
OCHOA
OSHEA
RRHEA
SCHWA

•••HA
AISHA
ALOHA
ALPHA
BOPHA
BOTHA
DACHA
FATHA
GOTHA
HATHA
HOOHA
HOXHA
KASHA
MASHA
MISHA
MOCHA
MUCHA
NUCHA
OMAHA
PASHA
PRAHA
SASHA
TISHA
YASHA

HB•••
HBARS
HBEAM
HBOMB

H•B••
HABER
HABIB
HABIT
HABLA
HOBAN
HOBBS
HOBBY
HOBEY
HOBIE
HOBOS
HRBEK
HUBBY
HUBEL
HUBER
HUBIE

H••B•
HERBE
HERBS
HERBY
HOBBS
HOBBY
HUBBY

H•••B
HABIB
HBOMB
HOREB

•HB••
OHBOY

•H•B•
CHUBB
CHUBS
DHABI
PHEBE
PHOBE
PHOBO
SHEBA
THEBE

•H••B
CHUBB
OHROB
PHLEB
RHOMB
RHUMB
SHRUB
THEWB
THROB
THUMB
ZHLOB
ZHLUB

••HB•
ASHBY

••H•B
COHAB
REHAB
SAHIB

H•C••
HACEK
HACKL
HACKS
HACKY
HECHE
HECHT
HECKS
HECTO
HICKS
HOCKS
HOCUS

H••C•
HATCH
HENCE
HENCH
HITCH
HOOCH
HULCE
HUNCH
HUTCH

H•••C
HARDC
HAVOC
HELIC
HEMIC
HIGHC
HOLIC

•H•C•
CHACO
CHECK
CHICA
CHICK
CHICO
CHICS
CHOCK
CHOCO
CHUCK
SHACK
SHOCK
SHUCK
THICK
WHACK
WHICH

•H••C
OHMIC
THEOC

••H•C
ADHOC
ETHIC
INHOC
JOHNC

•••HC
HIGHC

HD•••
HDTVS

H•D••
HADAT
HADES
HADIN
HADIT
HADJI
HADNO
HADNT
HADON
HADST
HADTO
HADUP
HEDDA
HEDGE
HEDGY
HEDIN
HIDEO
HIDER
HIDES
HIDEY
HODAD
HYDRA
HYDRO

H••D•
HAIDA
HANDI
HANDS
HANDY
HARDC
HARDG
HARDY
HAYDN
HEADS
HEADY
HEDDA
HEEDS
HEIDI
HEIDT
HERDS
HILDA
HINDI
HINDS
HINDU
HOLDS
HONDA
HONDO
HOODS
HOODY
HORDE
HOWDO
HOWDY
HURDY
HYNDE

H•••D
HALED
HARED
HASID
HATED
HAWED
HAYED
HAZED
HEALD
HEARD
HEROD
HEWED
HEXAD
HEXED
HIKED
HIRED
HIVED
HOARD
HODAD
HOKED
HOLED
HOMED
HONED
HOPED
HOSED
HOUND
HUMID
HYOID
HYPED

•H•D•
CHADS
CHIDE
RHODA
RHODE
RHODO
RHODY
SHADE
SHADS
SHADY
SHEDS
THEDA
THUDS

•H••D
AHEAD
AHMAD
AHMED
AHOLD
CHARD
CHAUD
CHILD
CHORD
OHGOD
SHARD
SHIED
SHOED
SHRED
THEYD
THIRD
WHATD

••HD•
MAHDI

••H•D
AAHED
ACHED
APHID
ASHED
EPHOD
JIHAD
JOHND
OOHED
REHID
SCHED
UNHID
USHED
ZAHND

HE•••
HEADS
HEADY
HEALD
HEALS
HEALY
HEAPS
HEAPY
HEARD
HEARN
HEARS
HEART
HEATH
HEATS
HEAVE
HEAVY
HECHE
HECHT
HECKS
HECTO
HEDDA
HEDGE
HEDGY
HEDIN
HEEDS
HEELS
HEFTI
HEFTS
HEFTY
HEGEL
HEHES
HEIDI
HEIDT
HEIGH
HEIGL
HEINE
HEINZ
HEIRS
HEISS
HEIST
HELEN
HELGA
HELIC
HELIO
HELIX
HELLO
HELLS
HELMS
HELOS
HELOT
HELPS
HEMAL
HEMAN
HEMAT
HEMEN
HEMES
HEMET
HEMIC
HEMIN
HEMON
HEMPS
HEMPY
HENCE
HENCH
HENGE
HENIE
HENNA
HENNY
HENRI
HENRY
HENZE
HEPAT
HEPTA
HEPTO
HERAT
HERBE
HERBS
HERBY
HERDS
HEREK
HERES
HERKY
HERNE
HEROD
HERON
HEROS
HERSH
HERTS
HERTZ
HERVE
HERZL
HESHE
HESON
HESSE
HESTS
HETER
HETHS
HETTY
HETUP
HEUER
HEURE
HEWED
HEWER
HEWTO
HEXAD
HEXED
HEXER
HEXES
HEYER
HEYSE

H•E••
HAEMA
HBEAM
HEEDS

HEELS
HIERO
HOERS
HOEST
HTEST
HUERS
HUEVO
HUEYS
HYENA
HYETO

H••E•
HABER
HACEK
HADES
HAGEN
HAKES
HALED
HALEN
HALER
HALES
HALEY
HAMEL
HAMER
HAMES
HANES
HANEY
HARED
HAREM
HARES
HASEK
HATED
HATER
HATES
HAUER
HAVEL
HAVEN
HAVER
HAVES
HAWED
HAWER
HAYED
HAYEK
HAYER
HAYES
HAYEY
HAZED
HAZEL
HAZER
HAZES
HEGEL
HEHES
HELEN
HEMEN
HEMES
HEMET
HEREK
HERES
HETER
HEUER
HEWED
HEWER
HEXED
HEXER
HEXES
HEYER
HIDEO
HIDER
HIDES
HIDEY
HIKED
HIKEN
HIKER
HIKES
HIMES
HINES
HIRED
HIREE
HIRER
HIRES
HIVED
HIVER
HIVES
HOBEY
HOKED
HOKES
HOKEY
HOLED
HOLER
HOLES
HOLEY
HOMED
HOMEO
HOMER
HOMES
HOMEY
HONED
HONER
HONES
HONEY
HOOEY
HOPED
HOPEH
HOPER
HOPES
HOREB
HOSEA
HOSED
HOSEL
HOSEN
HOSER
HOSES
HOTEL
HOVEL
HOVER
HOVEY
HOWES
HRBEK
HUBEL
HUBER
HUGER
HYPED
HYPER
HYPES
HYSER

H•••E
HAGUE
HAILE
HAISE
HALLE
HALVE
HANSE
HAOLE
HARTE
HASTE
HAUTE
HAVRE
HAWKE
HAWSE
HEAVE
HECHE
HEDGE
HEINE
HENCE
HENGE
HENIE
HENZE
HERBE
HERNE
HERVE
HESHE
HESSE
HEURE
HEYSE
HINGE
HIREE
HITME
HOARE
HOBIE
HOKIE
HOMIE
HOMME
HOOKE
HOPPE
HORAE
HORDE
HORNE
HORSE
HOUSE
HOWIE
HOYLE
HTILE
HUBIE
HULCE
HULME
HYNDE

•HE••
AHEAD
AHEAP
AHEMS
CHEAP
CHEAT
CHECK
CHEEK
CHEEP
CHEER
CHEEZ
CHEFS
CHEKA
CHELA
CHELY
CHEMO
CHERE
CHERI
CHERT
CHESS
CHEST
CHETA
CHEVY
CHEWS
CHEWY
CHEXX
GHEES
GHENT
IHEAR
PHEBE
PHENO
RHEAS
RHEEM
RHEIN
RHEME
RHETT
RHEUM
SHEAF
SHEAN
SHEAR
SHEBA
SHEDS
SHEEN
SHEEP
SHEER
SHEET
SHEIK
SHELF
SHELL
SHEMP
SHERA
SHERE
SHERM
THEAS
THEAX
THEBE
THEDA
THEFT
THEIR
THEMA
THEME
THEMS
THEOC
THEOK
THEOL
THEPO
THERA
THERE
THERM
THESE
THESP
THETA
THEUN
THEWB
THEWS
THEWY
THEYD
WHEAT
WHEEL
WHEES
WHELK
WHELM
WHELP
WHENS
WHERE
WHETS
WHEWS
WHEYS

•H•E•
AHMED
AHYES
BHAER
CHEEK
CHEEP
CHEER
CHEEZ
CHIEF
CHIEN
EHREN
GHEES
KHMER
NHLER
OHGEE
OHYES
PHLEB
RHEEM
SHAEF
SHEEN
SHEEP
SHEER
SHEET
SHIED
SHIER
SHIES
SHLEP
SHOED
SHOER
SHOES
SHRED
SHREK
SHREW
SHYER
THIEF
THIEU
THREE
THREW
WHEEL
WHEES

•H••E
CHAFE
CHASE
CHERE
CHIDE
CHILE
CHIME
CHINE
CHIVE
CHLOE
CHOKE
CHOLE
CHORE
CHOSE
CHUTE
DHOLE
DHOTE
FHOLE
IHOPE
OHARE
OHGEE
PHAGE
PHASE
PHEBE
PHILE
PHOBE
PHONE
PHYFE
PHYTE
RHEME
RHINE
RHODE
RHONE
RHYME
SHADE
SHAKE
SHALE
SHAME
SHANE
SHAPE
SHARE
SHAVE
SHERE
SHINE
SHIRE
SHONE
SHORE
SHOVE
SHUTE
THANE
THEBE
THEME
THERE
THESE
THINE
THOLE
THOSE
THREE
THROE
THULE
THYME
VHONE
WHALE
WHERE
WHILE
WHINE
WHITE
WHOLE
WHOME
WHOSE
WHYME
WHYRE
WHYTE

••HE•
AAHED
ACHED
ACHER
ACHES
ADHEM
ASHED
ASHEN
ASHER
ASHES
BOHEA
COHEN
DEHEX
ETHEL
ETHER
FAHEY
HEHES
MAHER
MRHEX
NEHER
OCHER
OOHED
OSHEA
OTHER
REHEM
RRHEA
SAHEL
SCHED
TEHEE
USHED
USHER
USHES
UTHER

••H•E
JAHRE
MAHRE
OCHRE
REHOE
TAHOE
TEHEE

•••HE
ARCHE
BATHE
BOTHE
BRAHE
CACHE
DACHE
DUBHE
FICHE
HECHE
HESHE
KATHE
LATHE
LECHE
LETHE
LITHE
MACHE
MOSHE
NASHE
NICHE
NOCHE
PATHE
PECHE
RICHE
ROCHE
RUCHE
SADHE
TITHE
TYCHE
VACHE
WYTHE

H•F••
HAFIZ
HAFTS
HEFTI
HEFTS
HEFTY
HIFIS
HOFFA
HUFFS
HUFFY

H••F•
HAIFA
HANFF
HOFFA
HOOFS
HUFFS
HUFFY

H•••F
HANFF

•HF••
PHFFT

•H•F•
CHAFE
CHAFF
CHEFS
CHUFF
KHUFU
PHFFT
PHYFE
SHAFT
SHIFT
THEFT
WHIFF

•H••F
CHAFF
CHIEF
CHUFF
SHAEF
SHEAF
SHELF
SHYOF
THIEF
WHARF
WHIFF

••H•F
JOHNF

H•G••
HAGAR
HAGEN
HAGIO
HAGUE
HEGEL
HIGHC
HIGHS
HOGAN
HUGER
HUGOS
HYGRO

H••G•
HANGS
HAWGS
HEDGE
HEDGY
HEIGH
HEIGL
HELGA
HENGE
HINGE
HOAGY
HOUGH

H•••G
HAING
HARDG
HMONG
HUANG
HYING

•HG••
OHGEE
OHGOD

•H•G•
CHUGS
PHAGE
PHAGO
PHAGY
SHAGS
SHOGI
THIGH
THUGS
WHIGS

•H••G
AHANG
AHING
BHANG
CHANG
CHING
CHONG
CHUNG
DHING
OHING
SHANG
SHRUG
THING
THONG
WHANG

••H•G
DRHUG

HH•••
HHOUR

H•H••
HAHAS
HEHES
HIHAT
HIHOS
HOHOS
HOHUM

H••H•
HATHA
HATHI
HECHE
HECHT
HESHE
HETHS
HIGHC
HIGHS
HOOHA
HOXHA

H•••H
HARSH
HATCH
HEATH
HEIGH
HENCH
HERSH
HITCH
HOOCH
HOPEH
HOUGH
HUMPH
HUNCH
HUTCH

•HH••
SHHHH
UHHUH

•H•H•
OHOHS
SHAHN
SHAHS
SHHHH

•H••H
PHISH
SHHHH
SHISH
SHUSH
THIGH
UHHUH
WHICH
WHISH

••HH•
SHHHH

••H•H
EPHAH
SHHHH
UHHUH

•••HH
SHHHH

HI•••
HICKS
HIDEO
HIDER
HIDES
HIDEY
HIERO
HIFIS
HIGHC
HIGHS
HIHAT
HIHOS
HIJAS
HIJKL
HIJOS
HIKED
HIKEN
HIKER
HIKES
HILDA
HILLS
HILLY
HILTS
HILUM
HIMES
HIMOM
HINDI
HINDS
HINDU
HINES
HINGE
HINKY
HINNY
HINTS
HIPLY
HIPPO
HIPPY
HIPTO
HIRAM
HIRED
HIREE
HIRER
HIRES
HISSY
HISTO
HITAT
HITCH
HITIN
HITIT
HITME
HITON
HITUP
HIVED
HIVER
HIVES

H•I••
HAIDA
HAIFA
HAIKS
HAIKU
HAILE
HAILS
HAING
HAIRS
HAIRY
HAISE
HAITI
HEIDI
HEIDT
HEIGH
HEIGL
HEINE
HEINZ
HEIRS
HEISS
HEIST
HOIST
HOITY
HTILE
HUITS
HYING

H••I•
HABIB
HABIT
HADIN
HADIT
HAFIZ
HAGIO
HAJIS
HAKIM
HASID
HASIN
HASIT
HEDIN
HELIC
HELIO
HELIX
HEMIC
HEMIN
HENIE
HIFIS
HITIN
HITIT
HOBIE
HOKIE
HOLIC
HOMIE
HOPIN
HOPIS
HOVIS
HOWIE
HUBIE
HUMID
HYOID

H•••I
HADJI
HAITI
HAJJI
HANDI
HANOI
HATHI
HEFTI
HEIDI
HENRI
HINDI
HOSNI
HOURI

•HI••
AHING
CHIAS
CHICA
CHICK
CHICO
CHICS
CHIDE
CHIEF
CHIEN
CHILD
CHILE
CHILI
CHILL
CHIME
CHIMP
CHINA
CHINE
CHING
CHINK
CHINO
CHINS
CHIOS
CHIPS
CHIRO
CHIRP
CHIRR
CHITA
CHITS
CHIVE
CHIVY
DHING
GHIJK
OHING
OHIOU
PHIAL
PHILE
PHILO
PHISH
RHINE
RHINO
SHIED
SHIER
SHIES
SHIFT
SHILL
SHIMS
SHINE
SHINS
SHINY
SHIPS
SHIRE
SHIRK
SHIRR
SHIRT
SHISH
SHIVA
SHIVS
THICK
THIEF
THIEU
THIGH
THILL
THINE
THING
THINK
THINS
THIRD
WHICH
WHIFF
WHIGS
WHILE
WHIMS
WHINE
WHINY
WHIPS
WHIPT
WHIRL
WHIRR
WHIRS
WHISH
WHISK
WHIST
WHITE
WHITS

•H•I•
AHAIR
AHSIN
CHAIM
CHAIN
CHAIR
CHAIS
CHOIR
CHRIS
GHAIN
OHAIR
OHLIN
OHMIC
PHAIR
RHEIN
SHEIK
THAIS
THEIR

•H••I
CHERI
CHILI
DHABI
DHOTI
GHALI
GHAZI
KHAKI
SHARI
SHOGI
SHOJI

••HI•
APHID
APHIS
AWHIT
BAHIA
ETHIC
FGHIJ
IMHIP
NEHIS
NIHIL
NOHIT
OPHIR
REHID
REHIT
SAHIB
TVHIT
UNHID
UNHIP
UNHIT
VCHIP

••H•I
BAHAI
JOHNI
LAHTI
MAHDI

•••HI
AMPHI
ARCHI
ASAHI
DASHI
DELHI
EFGHI
HATHI
KASHI
MEKHI
RASHI
RISHI
ROSHI
SAYHI
SUSHI
TASHI

H•J••
HAJIS
HAJJI
HIJAS
HIJKL
HIJOS
HOJOS

H••J•
HADJI
HAJJI

•HJ••
OHJOY

•H•J•
GHIJK
SHOJI

••H•J
FGHIJ
JOHNJ

H•K••
HAKES
HAKIM
HIKED
HIKEN
HIKER
HIKES
HOKED
HOKES
HOKEY
HOKIE
HOKUM

H••K•
HACKL
HACKS
HACKY
HAIKS
HAIKU
HANKS
HANKY
HARKS
HAWKE
HAWKS
HECKS
HERKY
HICKS
HIJKL
HINKY
HOCKS
HONKS
HONKY
HOOKA
HOOKE
HOOKS
HOOKY
HULKS
HULKY
HUNKS
HUNKY
HUSKS
HUSKY

H•••K
HACEK
HASEK
HAYEK
HEREK
HRBEK
HUROK
HUSAK

•HK••
OHKAY

•H•K•
CHAKA
CHEKA
CHOKE
CHOKY
DHAKA
KHAKI
SHAKE
SHAKO
SHAKY

•H••K
CHALK
CHECK
CHEEK
CHICK
CHINK
CHOCK
CHUCK
CHUNK
GHIJK
SHACK
SHANK
SHARK
SHEIK
SHIRK
SHOCK
SHOOK
SHREK
SHUCK
THANK
THEOK
THICK
THINK
THUNK
UHNAK
WHACK
WHELK
WHISK

H•L••
HALAL
HALAS
HALED
HALEN
HALER
HALES
HALEY
HALLE
HALLO
HALLS
HALOP
HALOS
HALTS
HALVA
HALVE
HELEN
HELGA
HELIC
HELIO
HELIX
HELLO
HELLS
HELMS
HELOS
HELOT
HELPS
HILDA
HILLS
HILLY
HILTS
HILUM
HOLDS
HOLED
HOLER
HOLES
HOLEY
HOLIC
HOLLY
HOLMS
HOLST
HOLTZ
HULAS
HULCE
HULKS
HULKY
HULLO
HULLS
HULLY
HULME
HULOT
HYLAS

H••L•
HABLA
HAILE
HAILS
HALLE
HALLO
HALLS
HAOLE
HAPLY
HATLO
HAULS
HEALD
HEALS
HEALY
HEELS
HELLO
HELLS
HILLS
HILLY
HIPLY
HOLLY
HOTLY
HOWLS
HOYLE
HTILE
HULLO
HULLS
HULLY
HURLS
HURLY

H•••L
HACKL
HALAL
HAMEL
HAVEL
HAZEL
HEGEL
HEIGL
HEMAL
HERZL
HIJKL
HORAL
HOSEL
HOTEL

HOVEL
HUBEL

•HL••
CHLOE
CHLOR
NHLER
OHLIN
PHLEB
PHLOX
SHLEP
UHLAN
ZHLOB
ZHLUB

•H•L•
AHOLD
CHALK
CHELA
CHELY
CHILD
CHILE
CHILI
CHILL
CHOLE
CHOLO
CHULA
DHALS
DHOLE
FHOLE
GHALI
PHILE
PHILO
PHYLA
PHYLL
PHYLO
SHALE
SHALL
SHALT
SHELF
SHELL
SHILL
SHULA
SHULS
SHYLY
THILL
THOLE
THULE
WHALE
WHELK
WHELM
WHELP
WHILE
WHOLE
WHOLL
WHYLL

•H••L
CHILL
CHURL
GHOUL
PHIAL
PHYLL
SHALL
SHAWL
SHELL
SHILL
SHOAL

THEOL
THILL
UHAUL
WHEEL
WHIRL
WHOLL
WHORL
WHYLL

••HL•
KAHLO
KOHLS

••H•L
ATHOL
ETHEL
ETHYL
JOHNL
MAHAL
NIHIL
RAHAL
SAHEL

•••HL
AMAHL
BRUHL
RUEHL
STAHL

HM•••
HMONG

H•M••
HAMAN
HAMAS
HAMEL
HAMER
HAMES
HAMMS
HAMMY
HAMUP
HEMAL
HEMAN
HEMAT
HEMEN
HEMES
HEMET
HEMIC
HEMIN
HEMON
HEMPS
HEMPY
HIMES
HIMOM
HOMED
HOMEO
HOMER
HOMES
HOMEY
HOMIE
HOMME
HUMAN
HUMID
HUMOR
HUMPH
HUMPS
HUMPY
HUMUS

HYMAN
HYMNS

H••M•
HAEMA
HAMMS
HAMMY
HARMS
HBOMB
HELMS
HITME
HOLMS
HOMME
HOUMA
HULME
HYAMS

H•••M
HAKIM
HAREM
HARUM
HBEAM
HILUM
HIMOM
HIRAM
HOHUM
HOKUM

•HM••
AHMAD
AHMED
KHMER
OHMAN
OHMIC
SHMOO

•H•M•
AHEMS
CHAMP
CHEMO
CHIME
CHIMP
CHOMP
CHUMP
CHUMS
RHEME
RHOMB
RHUMB
RHYME
SHAME
SHAMS
SHAMU
SHEMP
SHIMS
THEMA
THEME
THEMS
THUMB
THUMP
THYME
THYMY
WHAMO
WHAMS
WHIMS
WHOME
WHOMP
WHYME

•H••M
CHAIM
CHARM
CHASM
CHROM
PHARM
PHNOM
RHEEM
RHEUM
SHERM
THERM
THRUM
WHELM

••HM•
SCHMO

••H•M
ADHEM
EGHAM
HOHUM
ISHAM
NAHUM
OGHAM
REHEM

•••HM
ABOHM

H•N••
HANDI
HANDS
HANDY
HANES
HANEY
HANFF
HANGS
HANKS
HANKY
HANNA
HANOI
HANSA
HANSE
HANTS
HANYA
HENCE
HENCH
HENGE
HENIE
HENNA
HENNY
HENRI
HENRY
HENZE
HINDI
HINDS
HINDU
HINES
HINGE
HINKY
HINNY
HINTS
HONAN
HONDA
HONDO
HONED
HONER
HONES
HONEY
HONKS
HONKY
HONOR
HONUS
HUNAN
HUNCH
HUNKS
HUNKY
HUNTS
HUNTZ
HYNDE

H••N•
HADNO
HADNT
HAING
HANNA
HASNO
HASNT
HAUNT
HEINE
HEINZ
HENNA
HENNY
HERNE
HINNY
HMONG
HORNE
HORNS
HORNY
HOSNI
HOUND
HUANG
HYENA
HYING
HYMNS
HYPNO

H•••N
HADIN
HADON
HAGEN
HALEN
HAMAN
HASIN
HASON
HAVEN
HAYDN
HAZAN
HEARN
HEDIN
HELEN
HEMAN
HEMEN
HEMIN
HEMON
HERON
HESON
HIKEN
HITIN
HITON
HOBAN
HOGAN
HONAN
HOPIN
HOPON
HOSEN
HOTON
HUMAN
HUNAN
HURON
HYMAN
HYSON

•HN••
PHNOM
UHNAK

•H•N•
AHANG
AHING
BHANG
CHANG
CHANT
CHINA
CHINE
CHING
CHINK
CHINO
CHINS
CHONG
CHUNG
CHUNK
DHING
GHANA
GHENT
KHANS
OHING
PHANY
PHENO
PHONE
PHONO
PHONS
PHONY
RHINE
RHINO
RHONE
SHANA
SHANE
SHANG
SHANK
SHANT
SHINE
SHINS
SHINY
SHONE
SHUNS
SHUNT
THANE
THANK
THANT
THANX
THINE
THING
THINK
THINS
THONG
THUNK
VHONE
WHANG
WHENS
WHINE
WHINY

•H••N
AHSIN
CHAIN
CHIEN
CHRON
CHURN
EHREN
GHAIN
OHLIN
OHMAN
RHEIN
SHAHN
SHAUN
SHAWN
SHEAN
SHEEN
SHORN
SHOWN
THEUN
THORN
UHLAN

••HN•
ETHNO
FOHNS
JOHNC
JOHND
JOHNF
JOHNI
JOHNJ
JOHNL
JOHNP
JOHNQ
JOHNS
JOHNV
JOHNX
KAHNS
ZAHND

••H•N
ASHEN
ATHON
BEHAN
COHAN
COHEN
ETHAN
GAHAN
JAHAN
JEHAN
JIHAN
JOHAN
LOHAN
MAHAN
MAHON
NIHON
OTHON
REHAN
SCHON
WUHAN

•••HN
BIEHN
BRUHN
ICAHN
IJOHN
SHAHN
SPAHN
UTAHN

HO•••
HOAGY
HOARD
HOARE
HOARS
HOARY
HOBAN
HOBBS
HOBBY
HOBEY
HOBIE
HOBOS
HOCKS
HOCUS
HODAD
HOERS
HOEST
HOFFA
HOGAN
HOHOS
HOHUM
HOIST
HOITY
HOJOS
HOKED
HOKES
HOKEY
HOKIE
HOKUM
HOLDS
HOLED
HOLER
HOLES
HOLEY
HOLIC
HOLLY
HOLMS
HOLST
HOLTZ
HOMED
HOMEO
HOMER
HOMES
HOMEY
HOMIE
HOMME
HONAN
HONDA
HONDO
HONED
HONER
HONES
HONEY
HONKS
HONKY
HONOR
HONUS
HOOCH
HOODS
HOODY
HOOEY
HOOFS
HOOHA
HOOKA
HOOKE
HOOKS
HOOKY
HOOPS
HOOTS
HOPED
HOPEH
HOPER
HOPES
HOPIN
HOPIS
HOPON
HOPPE
HOPPY
HOPTO
HOPUP
HORAE
HORAL
HORAS
HORDE
HOREB
HORNE
HORNS
HORNY
HORSE
HORST
HORSY
HORUS
HOSEA
HOSED
HOSEL
HOSEN
HOSER
HOSES
HOSNI
HOSPS
HOSTA
HOSTS
HOTEL
HOTLY
HOTON
HOTSY
HOUGH
HOUMA
HOUND
HOURI
HOURS
HOUSE
HOVEL
HOVER
HOVEY
HOVIS
HOWAR
HOWDO
HOWDY
HOWES
HOWIE
HOWLS
HOWSO
HOWTO
HOXHA
HOYAS
HOYLE

H•O••
HAOLE
HBOMB
HHOUR
HMONG
HOOCH
HOODS
HOODY
HOOEY
HOOFS
HOOHA
HOOKA
HOOKE
HOOKS
HOOKY
HOOPS
HOOTS
HROSS
HYOID

H••O•
HADON
HALOP
HALOS
HANOI
HASON
HAVOC
HELOS
HELOT
HEMON
HEROD
HERON
HEROS
HESON
HIHOS
HIJOS
HIMOM
HITON
HOBOS
HOHOS
HOJOS
HONOR
HOPON
HOTON
HUGOS
HULOT
HUMOR
HUROK
HURON
HYPOS
HYSON

H•••O
HADNO
HADTO
HAGIO
HALLO
HARPO
HASNO
HASSO
HASTO
HATLO
HECTO
HELIO
HELLO
HEPTO
HEWTO
HIDEO
HIERO
HIPPO
HIPTO
HISTO
HOMEO
HONDO
HOPTO
HOWDO
HOWSO
HOWTO
HUEVO
HULLO
HUTTO
HYDRO
HYETO
HYGRO
HYPNO

•HO••
AHOLD
AHOOT
AHORA
AHOYS
CHOCK
CHOCO
CHOIR
CHOKE
CHOKY
CHOLE
CHOLO
CHOMP
CHONG
CHOPS
CHORD
CHORE
CHORO
CHOSE
CHOWS
DHOLE
DHOTE
DHOTI
DHOWS
FHOLE
GHOST
GHOUL
HHOUR
IHOPE
IHOPS
OHOHS
PHOBE
PHOBO
PHONE
PHONO
PHONS
PHONY
PHOTO
PHOTS
RHODA
RHODE
RHODO
RHODY
RHOMB
RHONE
SHOAL
SHOAT
SHOCK
SHOED
SHOER
SHOES
SHOGI
SHOJI
SHONE
SHOOK
SHOOS
SHOOT
SHOPS
SHORE
SHORN
SHORT
SHOTS
SHOUT
SHOVE
SHOWN
SHOWS
SHOWY
THOLE
THONG
THORA
THORN
THORO
THOSE
THOUS
VHONE
WHOLE
WHOLL
WHOME
WHOMP
WHOOP
WHOPS
WHORL
WHOSE
WHOSO
XHOSA

•H•O•
AHOOT
CHAOS
CHIOS
CHLOE
CHLOR
CHROM
CHRON
OHBOY
OHGOD
OHIOU
OHJOY
OHROB
OHWOW
OHYOU
PHLOX
PHNOM
SHMOO
SHOOK
SHOOS
SHOOT
SHYOF
THEOC
THEOK
THEOL
THROB
THROE
THROW
WHOOP
ZHLOB

•H••O
CHACO
CHARO
CHEMO
CHICO
CHINO
CHIRO
CHOCO
CHOLO
CHORO
OHAYO
PHAGO
PHENO
PHILO
PHOBO
PHONO
PHOTO
PHYLO
PHYTO
RHINO
RHODO
SHAKO
SHMOO
THEPO
THORO
WHAMO
WHOSO

••HO•
ABHOR
ACHOO
ADHOC
ASHOT
ATHOL
ATHON
ATHOS
BOHOS
COHOS
ECHOS
EPHOD
EPHOR
ETHOS
HIHOS
HOHOS
ICHOR
IMHOT
INHOC
MAHON
NIHON
NOHOW
OCHOA
OCHOS
OTHON
REHOE
SCHON
TAHOE
UNHOT
WAHOO
YAHOO

••H•O
ACHOO
ETHNO
KAHLO
SCHMO
WAHOO
YAHOO

•••HO
ABMHO
ALTHO
ANCHO
BASHO
BATHO
DICHO
DONHO
DRWHO
IDAHO
LITHO
MACHO
MINHO
MUCHO
NACHO
ORTHO
PATHO
TACHO
TYCHO
WASHO

H•P••
HAPLY
HAPPY
HEPAT
HEPTA
HEPTO
HIPLY
HIPPO
HIPPY
HIPTO
HOPED
HOPEH
HOPER
HOPES
HOPIN
HOPIS
HOPON
HOPPE
HOPPY
HOPTO
HOPUP
HYPED
HYPER
HYPES
HYPNO
HYPOS

H••P•
HAPPY
HARPO
HARPS
HARPY
HASPS
HEAPS
HEAPY
HELPS
HEMPS
HEMPY
HIPPO
HIPPY
HOOPS
HOPPE
HOPPY
HOSPS
HUMPH
HUMPS
HUMPY

H•••P
HADUP
HALOP
HAMUP
HASUP
HETUP
HITUP
HOPUP

•H•P•
CHAPS
CHIPS
CHOPS
IHOPE
IHOPS
SHAPE
SHIPS
SHOPS
THEPO
WHAPS
WHIPS
WHIPT
WHOPS
WHUPS

•H••P
AHEAP
CHAMP
CHEAP
CHEEP
CHIMP
CHIRP
CHOMP
CHUMP
SHARP
SHEEP
SHEMP
SHLEP
THARP
THESP
THUMP
WHELP
WHOMP
WHOOP

••H•P
IMHIP
JOHNP
UNHIP
VCHIP

••H•Q
JOHNQ

HR•••
HRBEK
HROSS

H•R••
HARDC
HARDG
HARDY
HARED
HAREM
HARES
HARKS
HARMS
HARPO
HARPS
HARPY
HARRY
HARSH
HARTE
HARUM
HERAT
HERBE
HERBS
HERBY
HERDS
HEREK
HERES
HERKY
HERNE
HEROD
HERON
HEROS
HERSH
HERTS
HERTZ
HERVE
HERZL
HIRAM
HIRED
HIREE
HIRER
HIRES
HORAE
HORAL
HORAS
HORDE
HOREB
HORNE
HORNS
HORNY
HORSE
HORST
HORSY
HORUS
HURDY
HURLS
HURLY
HUROK
HURON
HURRY
HURST
HURTS
HYRAX

H••R•
HAIRS
HAIRY
HARRY
HAVRE
HBARS
HEARD
HEARN
HEARS
HEART
HEIRS
HENRI
HENRY
HEURE
HIERO
HOARD
HOARE
HOARS
HOARY
HOERS
HOURI
HOURS
HUERS
HURRY
HYDRA
HYDRO
HYGRO

H•••R
HABER
HAGAR
HALER
HAMER
HATER
HAUER
HAVER
HAWER
HAYER
HAZER
HETER
HEUER
HEWER
HEXER
HEYER
HHOUR
HIDER
HIKER
HIRER
HIVER
HOLER
HOMER
HONER
HONOR
HOPER
HOSER
HOVER
HOWAR
HUBER
HUGER
HUMOR
HYPER
HYSER

•HR••
CHRIS
CHROM
CHRON
EHREN
OHROB
SHRED
SHREK
SHREW
SHRUB
SHRUG
THREE
THREW
THROB
THROE
THROW
THRUM

•H•R•
AHORA
CHARD
CHARM
CHARO
CHARS
CHART
CHARY
CHERE
CHERI
CHERT
CHIRO
CHIRP
CHIRR
CHORD

CHORE CHORO CHURL CHURN OHARA OHARE PHARM SHARD SHARE SHARI SHARK SHARP SHERA SHERE SHERM SHIRE SHIRK SHIRR SHIRT SHORE SHORN SHORT THARP THERA THERE THERM THIRD THORA THORN THORO THURS UHURA UHURU WHARF WHERE WHIRL WHIRR WHIRS WHORL WHYRE

•H••R

AHAIR BHAER CHAIR CHEER CHIRR CHLOR CHOIR HHOUR IHEAR KHMER NHLER OHAIR PHAIR SHEAR SHEER SHIER SHIRR SHOER SHYER THEIR WHIRR

••HR•

JAHRE LEHRS MAHRE NEHRU OCHRE

••H•R

ABHOR ACHER ASHER ASHUR BEHAR EPHOR ETHER ICHOR LEHAR MAHER NEHER OCHER OPHIR OTHER USHER UTHER

•••HR

NEPHR STAHR

H•S••

HASAT HASEK HASID HASIN HASIT HASNO HASNT HASON HASPS HASSO HASTA HASTE HASTO HASTY HASUP HESHE HESON HESSE HESTS HISSY HISTO HOSEA HOSED HOSEL HOSEN HOSER HOSES HOSNI HOSPS HOSTA HOSTS HUSAK HUSKS HUSKY HUSSY HYSER HYSON

H••S•

HADST HAISE HANSA HANSE HARSH HASSO HAWSE HEISS HEIST HERSH HESSE HEYSE HISSY HOEST HOIST HOLST HORSE HORST HORSY HOTSY HOUSE HOWSO HROSS HTEST HURST HUSSY

H•••S

HACKS HADES HAFTS HAHAS HAIKS HAILS HAIRS HAJIS HAKES HALAS HALES HALLS HALOS HALTS HAMAS HAMES HAMMS HANDS HANES HANGS HANKS HANTS HARES HARKS HARMS HARPS HASPS HATES HAULS HAVES HAWGS HAWKS HAYES HAZES HBARS HDTVS HEADS HEALS HEAPS HEARS HEATS HECKS HEEDS HEELS HEFTS HEHES HEIRS HEISS HELLS HELMS HELOS HELPS HEMES HEMPS HERBS HERDS HERES HEROS HERTS HESTS HETHS HEXES HICKS HIDES HIFIS HIGHS HIHOS HIJAS HIJOS HIKES HILLS HILTS HIMES HINDS HINES HINTS HIRES HIVES HOARS HOBBS HOBOS HOCKS HOCUS HOERS HOHOS HOJOS HOKES HOLDS HOLES HOLMS HOMES HONES HONKS HONUS HOODS HOOFS HOOKS HOOPS HOOTS HOPES HOPIS HORAS HORNS HORUS HOSES HOSPS HOSTS HOURS HOVIS HOWES HOWLS HOYAS HROSS HUERS HUEYS HUFFS HUGOS HUITS HULAS HULKS HULLS HUMPS HUMUS HUNKS HUNTS HURLS HURTS HUSKS HUTUS HYAMS HYLAS HYMNS HYPES HYPOS

•HS••

AHSIN

•H•S•

CHASE CHASM CHAST CHESS CHEST CHOSE GHOST LHASA PHASE PHISH SHISH SHUSH THESE THESP THOSE WHISH WHISK WHIST WHOSE WHOSO XHOSA

•H••S

AHEMS AHOYS AHYES BHATS CHADS CHAIS CHAOS CHAPS CHARS CHATS CHAWS CHEFS CHESS CHEWS CHIAS CHICS CHINS CHIOS CHIPS CHITS CHOPS CHOWS CHRIS CHUBS CHUGS CHUMS DHALS DHOWS GHATS GHEES IHOPS KHANS OHOHS OHYES PHONS PHOTS RHEAS SHADS SHAGS SHAHS SHAMS SHAYS SHEDS SHIES SHIMS SHINS SHIPS SHIVS SHOES SHOOS SHOPS SHOTS SHOWS SHULS SHUNS SHUTS THAIS THATS THAWS THEAS THEMS THEWS THINS THOUS THUDS THUGS THURS WHAMS WHAPS WHATS WHEES WHENS WHETS WHEWS WHEYS WHIGS WHIMS WHIPS WHIRS WHITS WHOPS WHUPS

••H•S

ACHES AGHAS APHIS ASHES ATHOS BAHTS BOHOS COHOS ECHOS EPHAS ETHOS FOHNS HAHAS HEHES HIHOS HOHOS JOHNS KAHNS KOHLS LEHRS NEHIS OCHOS USHES YMHAS YWHAS

•••HS

AMAHS ANKHS AYAHS BATHS BETHS BLAHS CATHS ESTHS FUCHS GOTHS HETHS HIGHS KAPHS KOPHS LATHS LOCHS MATHS MOTHS MYTHS OATHS OHOHS OPAHS ORCHS PATHS PITHS POOHS QOPHS RATHS ROTHS RUTHS SACHS SECHS SHAHS SIGHS SIKHS SOPHS TACHS TECHS TETHS YEAHS YODHS

HT•••

HTEST HTILE

H•T••

HATCH HATED HATER HATES HATHA HATHI HATLO HDTVS HETER HETHS HETTY HETUP HITAT HITCH HITIN HITIT HITME HITON HITUP HOTEL HOTLY HOTON HOTSY HUTCH HUTTO HUTUS

H••T•

HADTO HAFTS HAITI HALTS HANTS HARTE HASTA HASTE HASTO HASTY HAUTE HEATH HEATS HECTO HEFTI HEFTS HEFTY HEPTA HEPTO HERTS HERTZ HESTS HETTY HEWTO HILTS HINTS HIPTO HISTO HOITY HOLTZ HOOTS HOPTO HOSTA HOSTS HOWTO HUITS HUNTS HUNTZ HURTS HUTTO HYATT HYETO

H•••T

HABIT HADAT HADIT HADNT HADST HASAT HASIT HASNT HAUNT HEART HECHT HEIDT HEIST HELOT HEMAT HEMET HEPAT HERAT HIHAT HITAT HITIT HOEST HOIST HOLST HORST HTEST HULOT HURST HYATT

•H•T•

BHATS CHATS CHETA CHITA CHITS CHUTE DHOTE DHOTI GHATS PHOTO PHOTS PHYTE PHYTO RHETT SHATT SHOTS SHUTE SHUTS THATS THETA WHATD WHATS WHETS WHITE WHITS WHYTE

•H••T

AHOOT CHANT CHART CHAST CHEAT CHERT CHEST GHENT GHOST PHFFT RHETT SHAFT SHALT SHANT SHATT SHEET SHIFT SHIRT SHOAT SHOOT SHORT SHOUT SHUNT THANT THEFT WHEAT WHIPT WHIST

••HT•

BAHTS LAHTI MEHTA

••H•T

ARHAT ASHOT AWHIT HIHAT IMHOT NOHIT REHIT TVHIT UNHAT UNHIT UNHOT

•••HT

AUGHT BIGHT EIGHT FIGHT HECHT LICHT LIGHT MIGHT NACHT NICHT NIGHT OUGHT RASHT RESHT RIGHT SIGHT TIGHT WIGHT YACHT

HU•••

HUANG HUBBY HUBEL HUBER HUBIE HUERS HUEVO HUEYS HUFFS HUFFY HUGER HUGOS HUITS HULAS HULCE HULKS HULKY HULLO HULLS HULLY HULME HULOT HUMAN HUMID HUMOR HUMPH HUMPS HUMPY HUMUS HUNAN HUNCH HUNKS HUNKY HUNTS HUNTZ HURDY HURLS HURLY HUROK HURON HURRY HURST HURTS HUSAK HUSKS HUSKY HUSSY HUTCH HUTTO HUTUS

H•U••

HAUER HAULS HAUNT HAUTE HEUER HEURE HOUGH HOUMA HOUND HOURI HOURS HOUSE

H••U•

HADUP HAGUE HAMUP HARUM HASUP HETUP HHOUR HILUM HITUP HOCUS HOHUM HOKUM HONUS HOPUP HORUS HUMUS HUTUS

H•••U

HAIKU HINDU

•HU••

CHUBB CHUBS CHUCK CHUFF CHUGS CHULA CHUMP CHUMS CHUNG CHUNK CHURL CHURN CHUTE KHUFU RHUMB SHUCK SHULA SHULS SHUNS SHUNT SHUSH SHUTE SHUTS THUDS THUGS THULE THUMB THUMP THUNK THURS UHURA UHURU WHUPS

•H•U•

CHAUD GHOUL HHOUR RHEUM SHAUN SHOUT SHRUB SHRUG THEUN THOUS THRUM UHAUL UHHUH ZHLUB

•H••U

KHUFU OHIOU OHYOU SHAMU THIEU UHURU

••HU•

ASHUR DRHUG HOHUM LEHUA NAHUM UHHUH

••H•U

NEHRU

•••HU

ELIHU FICHU MACHU MUSHU SADHU WUSHU

H•V••

HAVEL HAVEN HAVER HAVES HAVOC HAVRE HIVED HIVER HIVES HOVEL HOVER HOVEY HOVIS

H••V•

HALVA HALVE HDTVS HEAVE HEAVY HERVE HUEVO

•H•V•

CHAVA CHEVY CHIVE CHIVY SHAVE SHIVA SHIVS SHOVE

••H•V

JOHNV SCHAV

H•W••

HAWED HAWER HAWGS HAWKE HAWKS HAWSE HEWED HEWER HEWTO HOWAR HOWDO HOWDY HOWES HOWIE HOWLS HOWSO HOWTO

•HW••

OHWOW

•H•W•

CHAWS CHEWS CHEWY CHOWS DHOWS SHAWL SHAWN SHOWN SHOWS SHOWY THAWS THEWB THEWS THEWY WHEWS

•H••W

OHWOW SHREW THREW THROW

••HW•

SCHWA

••H•W

NOHOW PSHAW

H•X••

HEXAD HEXED HEXER HEXES HOXHA

H•••X

HELIX HYRAX

•H•X•

CHEXX

•H••X

CHEXX PHLOX THANX THEAX

••H•X

DEHEX JOHNX MRHEX

HY•••

HYAMS HYATT HYDRA HYDRO HYENA HYETO HYGRO HYING HYLAS HYMAN HYMNS HYNDE HYOID HYPED HYPER HYPES HYPNO HYPOS HYRAX HYSER HYSON

H•Y••

HAYDN HAYED HAYEK HAYER HAYES HAYEY HEYER HEYSE HOYAS HOYLE

H••Y•

HANYA HUEYS

H•••Y

HACKY HAIRY HALEY HAMMY HANDY HANEY HANKY HAPLY HAPPY HARDY HARPY HARRY HASTY HAYEY HEADY HEALY HEAPY HEAVY HEDGY HEFTY HEMPY HENNY HENRY HERBY HERKY HETTY HIDEY HILLY HINKY HINNY HIPLY HIPPY HISSY HOAGY HOARY HOBBY HOBEY HOITY HOKEY HOLEY HOLLY HOMEY HONEY HONKY HOODY HOOEY HOOKY HOPPY HORNY HORSY HOTLY HOTSY HOVEY HOWDY HUBBY HUFFY HULKY HULLY HUMPY HUNKY HURDY HURLY HURRY HUSKY HUSSY

•HY••

AHYES OHYES OHYOU PHYFE PHYLA PHYLL PHYLO PHYTE PHYTO RHYME SHYER SHYLY SHYOF THYME THYMY WHYLL WHYME WHYRE WHYTE

•H•Y•

AHOYS OHAYO SHAYS THEYD WHEYS

•H••Y

CHARY CHELY CHEVY CHEWY CHIVY CHOKY OHBOY OHJOY OHKAY PHAGY PHANY PHONY RHODY SHADY SHAKY SHINY SHOWY SHYLY THEWY THYMY WHINY

••HY•

ETHYL

••H•Y

ASHBY BOHAY FAHEY OSHAY

•••HY

ARCHY BATHY BOCHY BUSHY CATHY CUSHY DASHY DISHY DUCHY FISHY GUSHY ITCHY KATHY LATHY LEAHY LUSHY MACHY MESHY MOTHY MUSHY PACHY PATHY PITHY PUSHY RUSHY TUSHY UNSHY VICHY

WASHY
WISHY

H•Z••
HAZAN
HAZED
HAZEL
HAZER
HAZES

H••Z•
HENZE
HERZL

H•••Z
HAFIZ
HEINZ
HERTZ
HOLTZ
HUNTZ

•H•Z•
CHAZZ
GHAZI

•H••Z
CHAZZ
CHEEZ

IA•••
IAMBI
IAMBS
IAMSO
IATRO
IATRY

I•A••
IBARS
ICAHN
ICALL
ICAME
ICANT
ICARE
IDAHO
IMACS
IMAGE
IMAGO
IMAMS
IMAMU
IMARI
INAGE
INALL
INANE
INAPT
INARI
INAWE
IPANA
IPASS
IRABU
IRANI
IRAQI
IRATE
ISAAC
ISAAK
ISAID
ISAMU
ITALO
ITALS
ITALY
IVANA
IVANI
IVANV
IWANT
IYARS
IZAAK

I••A•
IBEAM
ICEAX
IDEAL
IDEAS
IDTAG
IFSAY
IGUAL
IHEAR
ILEAC
ILEAL
ILIAC
ILIAD
IMBAD
IMEAN
IMMAD
INBAD
INCAN
INCAS
INLAW
INLAY
INMAY
IOTAS
IOWAN
IOWAS
IOWAU
IOWAY
IPRAY
IQBAL
ISAAC
ISAAK
ISHAM
ISIAH
ISLAM
ISLAS
ITEAS
IXNAY
IZAAK

I•••A
IBIZA
ICOSA
IDOLA
ILLYA
ILONA
INDIA
INDRA
INFRA
INTRA
IONIA
IPANA
IRENA
IRINA
ISOLA
ITINA
IVANA

•IA••
BIALY
CIANO
CIAOS
DIALO
DIALS
DIAMS
DIANA
DIANE
DIARY
FIATS
GIANT
JIANG
LIANA
LIANE
LIANG
LIARS
MIAMI
MIAOU
MIAOW
MIATA
PIANI
PIANO
PIAUI
PIAVE
RIALS
RIANT
RIATA
TIAGO
TIAMO
TIANT
TIARA
VIALS
VIAND

•I•A•
AIDAN
AIMAT
AIWAS
BINAL
CIGAR
DIGAT
DIMAG
DIMAS
DINAH
DINAR
DIRAC
DIRAE
DIRAM
DITAT
DIVAC
DIVAN
DIVAS
EILAT
FILAR
FILAS
FINAL
GILAS
HIHAT
HIJAS
HIRAM
HITAT
JIHAD
JIHAN
KINAS
KIVAS
LIDAR
LIFAR
LILAC
LIMAN
LIMAS
LIRAS
MICAH
MICAS
MIDAS
MIKAN
MILAN
MINAS
MITAS
MIZAR
NICAD
NINAS
NIPAS
NIPAT
NISAN
NIVAL
OIDAL
PICAS
PIKAS
PILAF
PILAR
PILAU
PIMAS
PISAN
PITAS
PIXAR
RICAN
RIGAN
RIPAT
RIVAL
RIYAL
RIZAL
SIKAS
SILAS
SINAI
SISAL
SITAR
SITAT
SIVAN
SIXAD
SIXAM
TICAL
TIDAL
TILAK
TITAN
TIWAS
VICAR
VIDAL
VIDAS
VIJAY
VILAS
VINAS
VIRAL
VISAS
VITAE
VITAL
VITAM
VITAS
VIVAS
WINAT

•I••A
AISHA
BIOTA
BIRRA
CIERA
CIGNA
CILIA
CILLA
CINNA
CIRCA
DIANA
DICTA
DINKA
DITKA
FINCA
FIONA
FIRMA
FIVEA
GILDA
GINZA
HILDA
JIDDA
KIMBA
KINDA
KIOWA
KISKA
LIANA
LIBRA
LIBYA
LICIA
LILIA
LINDA
LINEA
LIVIA
MIATA
MICRA
MISHA
MISSA
MITLA
MITYA
NIETA
NILLA
NINEA
NINJA
NIVEA
PIETA
PILEA
PINNA
PINTA
PINZA
PIPPA
PIZZA
RIATA
RIOJA
SIDEA
SIENA
SIGMA
SILVA
SIMBA
SITKA
TIARA
TIBIA
TIKKA
TILDA
TINEA
TIOGA
TISHA
UINTA
VIEJA
VIGIA
VILLA
VILMA
VILNA
VIOLA
VIRGA
VIRNA
VISTA
WICCA
WILLA
WILMA
ZILLA

••IA•
ALIAS
APIAN
ARIAL
ARIAN
ARIAS
ASIAN
AVIAN
AVIAS
AXIAL
BRIAN
BRIAR
CHIAS
DRIAM
ELIAS
ENIAC
ERIAS
EVIAN
FRIAR
GLIAL
GLIAS
ILIAC
ILIAD
ISIAH
NAIAD
PHIAL
PRIAM
TRIAD
TRIAL
UKIAH
UMIAK
UNIAT
URIAH

••I•A
AGITA
AKIRA
AKITA
ALIDA
ALISA
AMICA
AMIGA
ANIMA
ANITA
ARICA
AVILA
BAISA
BAIZA
BEIRA
CEIBA
CHICA
CHINA
CHITA
CUICA
DAIWA
DRINA
DVINA
EDINA
ELISA
ELIZA
ERICA
ERIKA
ERISA
EVITA
FRIDA
FRITA
HAIDA
HAIFA
IBIZA
IRINA
ITINA
KEIRA
LAIKA
LAILA
LEICA
LEILA
LUISA
MOIRA
MTIDA
NAIMA
NAINA
NAIRA
OLIVA
OUIDA
OUIJA
PAISA
PRIMA
RAISA
RAITA
REINA
SHIVA
SLIWA
SPICA
TAIGA
TAINA
TRINA
UNITA
UTICA
VOILA

•••IA
AECIA
ALGIA
AMNIA
APPIA
ATRIA
BAHIA
BASIA
BERIA
CELIA
CERIA
CILIA
COPIA
CORIA
CURIA
DACIA
DANIA
DARIA
DELIA
DORIA
EOLIA
FACIA
FERIA
FOLIA
FREIA
INDIA
IONIA
JULIA
LABIA
LALIA
LAMIA
LELIA
LICIA
LILIA
LIVIA
LOGIA
LUCIA
LURIA
LYDIA
LYGIA
MAFIA
MANIA
MARIA
MEDIA
MYRIA
NADIA
NESIA
NOKIA
NORIA
NOVIA
NUBIA
NYDIA
OMNIA
OSSIA
OSTIA
PAVIA
PODIA
PRAIA
REGIA
RETIA
REZIA
SEPIA
SERIA
SOFIA
SONIA
STRIA
SYRIA
TALIA
TANIA
TERIA
TIBIA
VARIA
VIGIA
WUXIA
XENIA

IB•••
IBARS
IBEAM
IBERT
IBIZA
IBMPC
IBOOK
IBSEN

I•B••
ICBMS
IMBAD
IMBED
IMBUE
INBAD
INBED
INBIG
INBOX
IQBAL
ISBNS

I••B•
IAMBI
IAMBS
ILLBE
IRABU

•IB••
BIBBS
BIBLE
FIBER
FIBRE
FIBRO
GIBBS
GIBED
GIBER
GIBES
GIBUS
JIBED
JIBES
LIBBY
LIBEL
LIBER
LIBRA
LIBRE
LIBRI
LIBRO
LIBYA
NIBLO
RIBBY
SIBYL
TIBBS
TIBER
TIBET
TIBIA
VIBES

•I•B•
BIBBS
BILBO
BIMBO
BIXBY
DIDBY
DIGBY
GIBBS
KILBY
KIMBA
KIRBY
LIBBY
LIEBE
LIEBY
LIMBO
LIMBS
NIMBI
NIMBY
NIOBE
RIBBY
RIGBY
SIMBA
SITBY
SIXBC
TIBBS
WIEBE
WILBY
WINBY
ZIPBY

•I••B
FIVEB
LINEB
LITTB
NINEB
SIDEB

••IB•
ALIBI
BRIBE
CEIBA
CRIBS
DRIBS
ORIBI
TRIBE

••I•B
CLIMB
STIEB

•••IB
ADLIB
CARIB
EXLIB
HABIB
NAMIB
SAHIB
SQUIB

IC•••
ICAHN
ICALL
ICAME
ICANT
ICARE
ICBMS
ICEAX
ICEES
ICEIN
ICEIT
ICENI
ICERS
ICEUP
ICHOR
ICIER
ICILY
ICING
ICKES
ICONO
ICONS
ICOSA
ICOSI
ICTUS

I•C••
INCAN
INCAS
INCOG
INCRS
INCUR
INCUS
ITCHY

I••C•
ILICH
IMACS
INICE
IROCS

I•••C
IBMPC
ILEAC
ILIAC
INDIC
INHOC
IODIC
IONIC
ISAAC
ISTIC

•IC••
BICEP
DICED
DICER
DICES
DICEY
DICHO
DICKS
DICKY
DICOT
DICTA
DICTS
DICTU
FICHE
FICHU
FICUS
HICKS
KICKS
KICKY
LICHT
LICIA
LICIT
LICKS
MICAH
MICAS
MICKY
MICRA
MICRO
NICAD
NICER
NICHE
NICHT
NICKS
NICKY
NICOL
PICAS
PICKS
PICKY
PICON
PICOT
PICTO
PICTS
RICAN
RICCI
RICED
RICER
RICES
RICEU
RICHE
RICKI
RICKS
RICKY
RICOH
SICEM
SICKO
TICAL
TICKS
TICKY
TICOS
VICAR
VICES
VICHY
VICKI
VICKS
VICKY
WICCA
WICKS

•I•C•
AITCH
BIRCH
CINCH
CINCO
CINCY
CIRCA
CIRCE
CIRCS
CISCO
DIECI
DISCI
DISCO
DISCS
DITCH
FILCH
FINCA
FINCH
FISCS
FITCH
HITCH
LINCS
MINCE
MITCH
NIECE
PIECE
PINCE
PINCH
PISCI
PITCH
RICCI
SINCE
TINCT
TISCH
VINCE
VINCI
VINCY
WICCA
WILCO
WINCE
WINCH
WITCH
ZILCH
ZINCS
ZINCY

•I••C
CIVIC
DIRAC
DIVAC
FIVEC
HIGHC
LILAC
LINEC
MIMIC
NINEC
SIXBC
VINIC

••IC•
ALICE
AMICA
AMICE
AMICI
AMICK
AMICO
ARICA
ASICS
BRICE
BRICK
BUICK
CHICA
CHICK
CHICO
CHICS
CLICK
CRICK
CUICA
DEICE
EDICT
EPICS
ERICA
ERICH
ERICK
EVICT
FLICK
FLICS
FRICK
GEICO
GLICK
ILICH
INICE
JUICE
JUICY
KLICK
KNICK
LAICS
LEICA
ONICE
OZICK
PRICE
PRICK
PRICY
QUICK
REICE
REICH
SLICE
SLICK
SNICK
SPICA
SPICE
SPICY
STICH
STICK
THICK
TRICE
TRICK
TWICE
UNICE
URICH
UTICA
VOICE
VOICI
WHICH
ZWICK

••I•C
ENIAC
EPISC
ILIAC

•••IC
AFRIC
AGRIC
ANTIC
ASDIC
ASPIC
ATTIC
AURIC
AZOIC
BARIC
BASIC
BORIC
CERIC
CIVIC
COLIC
COMIC
CONIC
CUBIC
CYNIC
DORIC
EDDIC
EOLIC
ETHIC
FOLIC
FSLIC
GENIC
HELIC
HEMIC
HOLIC
INDIC
IODIC
IONIC
ISTIC
KOVIC
LOGIC
LUDIC
LYRIC
MAGIC
MALIC
MANIC
MEDIC
MELIC
MIMIC
MONIC
MUSIC
NARIC
NUMIC
OHMIC
OLEIC
OPTIC
ORBIC
OSMIC
OSRIC
PANIC
PUNIC
RELIC
RUNIC
SALIC
SONIC
STOIC
SUBIC
TELIC
TONIC
TOPIC
TORIC
TOXIC
TUNIC
TYPIC
UGRIC
ULRIC
VATIC
VEDIC
VINIC
XERIC
YOGIC
ZENIC

ID•••
IDAHO
IDEAL
IDEAS
IDEES
IDENT
IDEST
IDING
IDIOM
IDIOT
IDLED
IDLER
IDLES
IDOLA
IDOLS
IDONT
IDTAG
IDYLL
IDYLS

I•D••
INDEF
INDEX
INDIA
INDIC
INDIE
INDIO
INDIV
INDRA
INDRE
INDUE
INDUS
INDYS
IODIC

I••D•
IMIDE
IPODS
IRIDO
IRIDS
IZODS

I•••D
IDLED
IFOLD
IGGED
ILIAD
ILIED
IMBAD
IMBED
IMMAD
INBAD
INBED
INKED
INRED
IRKED
ISAID
IVIED

•ID••
AIDAN
AIDED
AIDER
AIDES
AIDOO
BIDDY
BIDED
BIDEN
BIDER
BIDES
BIDET
BIDIN
BIDON
BIDUP
CIDER
DIDBY
DIDIN
DIDIT
DIDNT
DIDOK
DIDOS
DIDSO
DIDST
DIDTO
DIDUP
EIDER
FIDEL
FIDES
GIDDY
HIDEO
HIDER
HIDES
HIDEY
JIDDA
KIDDO
KIDDY
KIDEO
LIDAR
LIDDY
LIDOS
MIDAS
MIDDY
MIDGE
MIDIS
MIDON
MIDST
NIDRE
NIDUS
OIDAL
RIDER
RIDES
RIDGE
RIDGY
RIDOF
SIDEA
SIDEB
SIDED
SIDES
SIDLE
SIDON
TIDAL
TIDED
TIDES
VIDAL
VIDAS
VIDEO
VIDOR
WIDEN
WIDER
WIDOW
WIDTH

•I•D•
BIDDY
BIGDO
BINDS
BIRDS
BIRDY
CINDY
DINDY
DIODE
FINDS
GIDDY
GILDA
GILDS
GIRDS
HILDA
HINDI
HINDS
HINDU
JIDDA
KIDDO
KIDDY
KINDA
KINDS
LIDDY
LINDA
LINDO
LINDT
LINDY
MIDDY
MINDS
MINDY
MISDO
PIEDS
RINDS
RINDY
TILDA
TILDE
WILDE
WILDS
WINDS
WINDY

•I••D
AIDED
AILED
AIMED
AIRED
BIDED
BIFID
BIKED
BIPED
BIPOD
CITED
DICED
DIKED
DIMED
DINED
DIVED

FIELD
FIEND
FIFED
FILED
FINED
FIORD
FIRED
FIVED
FIXED
GIBED
HIKED
HIRED
HIVED
JIBED
JIHAD
JIVED
KITED
LIKED
LIKUD
LIMED
LINED
LIPID
LITTD
LIVED
LIVID
MIKED
MIMED
MINED
MIRED
MIXED
NICAD
NINED
NITID
NIXED
OILED
PIKED
PILED
PINED
PIPED
RICED
RIGID
RILED
RIMED
RIVED
SIDED
SIRED
SITED
SIXAD
SIXED
SIZED
TIDED
TILED
TIMED
TIMID
TINED
TIRED
VIAND
VINED
VIRID
VISED
VIVID
WIELD
WILED
WINED
WIPED
WIRED
WISED
WIVED
YIELD

••ID•

ABIDE
ACIDS
ACIDY
ALIDA
AMIDE
ASIDE
AVIDE
AZIDE
BRIDE
BSIDE
CHIDE
DOIDO
EJIDO
ELIDE
FRIDA
GLIDE
GRIDE
GRIDS
GUIDE
GUIDO
HAIDA
HEIDI
HEIDT
IMIDE
IRIDO
IRIDS
LOIDS
MAIDS
MTIDA
MTIDY
OUIDA
OXIDE
PRIDE
QAIDS
QUIDS
RAIDS
SKIDS
SLIDE
SNIDE
VEIDT
VOIDS

••I•D

APIED
BAIRD
BLIND
BUILD
CHILD
CRIED
DRIED
FLIED
FRIED
GRIND
GUILD
ILIAD
ILIED
IVIED
LAIRD
NAIAD
PLIED
PRIED
SHIED
SKIED
SPIED
STIED
TBIRD
THIRD
TRIAD
TRIED
WEIRD

•••ID

ACRID
ALGID
APHID
AROID
ARRID
AVOID
BIFID
BOVID
BRAID
CANID
CUPID
DAVID
DROID
DRUID
ELCID
FELID
FETID
FLUID
FROID
GELID
HASID
HUMID
HYOID
ISAID
LECID
LIPID
LIVID
LUCID
LURID
LYRID
NITID
NOBID
OOTID
OVOID
PAVID
PLAID
QUAID
RABID
RANID
RAPID
REBID
REDID
REHID
RIGID
SAPID
SOLID
SQUID
STAID
TEPID
TIMID
TUMID
UNBID
UNDID
UNHID
URSID
USAID
VALID
VAPID
VIRID
VIVID
ZOOID

I•E••

IBEAM
IBERT
ICEAX
ICEES
ICEIN
ICEIT
ICENI
ICERS
ICEUP
IDEAL
IDEAS
IDEES
IDENT
IDEST
IFEEL
IHEAR
ILEAC
ILEAL
ILENE
ILEUM
IMEAN
INEES
INEPT
INERT
IRENA
IRENE
ISERE
ITEAS
ITEMS
ITERS

I••E•

IBSEN
ICEES
ICIER
ICKES
IDEES
IDLED
IDLER
IDLES
IFEEL
IGGED
IGNES
ILIED
ILLER
IMBED
IMPEI
IMPEL
IMSET
INBED
INDEF
INDEX
INEES
INFER
INGER
INKED
INKER
INKEY
INLET
INNER
INNES
INPEN
INRED
INREM
INSET
INTEL
INTER
INVER
IRKED
IRKER
IRREG
ISLES
ISLET
ISLEY
ISSEI
ISSEL
IVIED
IVIES

I•••E

ICAME
ICARE
IFIVE
IGIVE
IHOPE
ILENE
ILLBE
ILOSE
ILOVE
IMAGE
IMBUE
IMIDE
IMINE
IMMIE
IMOVE
INAGE
INANE
INAWE
INDIE
INDRE
INDUE
INGLE
INICE
INKLE
INNIE
INURE
INUSE
IRATE
IRENE
ISERE
ISSUE
ISTLE
ITILE
ITSME

•IE••

BIEHN
BIERE
BIERI
BIERS
CIELO
CIELS
CIENS
CIERA
DIECI
DIEGO
DIELS
DIEMS
DIENE
DIETE
DIETS
DIETZ
DIEUX
EIEIO
FIEFS
FIELD
FIEND
FIERO
FIERS
FIERY
HIERO
LIEBE
LIEBY
LIEGE
LIEIN
LIENS
LIEON
LIESL
LIEST
LIETO
LIEUP
LIEUS
LIEUT
MIELE
MIELS
MIENS
MIERS
MIEUX
NIECE
NIELS
NIETA
NIETO
NIEUW
NIEVE
PIECE
PIEDS
PIELS
PIERS
PIETA
PIETY
RIELS
RIENS
RIETI
SIEGE
SIENA
SIETE
SIEVE
TIEGS
TIEIN
TIENE
TIEON
TIERS
TIETO
TIEUP
VIEJA
VIEJO
VIERS
VIEUX
VIEWS
VIEWY
WIEBE
WIELD
WIEST
YIELD
ZIEFF

•I•E•

AIDED
AIDER
AIDES
AIKEN
AILED
AILES
AILEY
AIMED
AIMEE
AIMER
AIRED
AIRER
AIRES
BICEP
BIDED
BIDEN
BIDER
BIDES
BIDET
BIKED
BIKEL
BIKER
BIKES
BILES
BINES
BINET
BIPED
BITER
BITES
BIZET
CIDER
CINES
CIRES
CITED
CITEE
CITER
CITES
CIVET
DICED
DICER
DICES
DICEY
DIGEL
DIGEM
DIKED
DIKER
DIKES
DIMED
DIMES
DINED
DINER
DINES
DIRER
DIVED
DIVER
DIVES
DIYER
EIDER
EIGEN
EIGER
EINEN
EINER
EINES
EISEN
FIBER
FIDEL
FIDES
FIFED
FIFER
FIFES
FILED
FILER
FILES
FILET
FINED
FINER
FINES
FIRED
FIRER
FIRES
FIVEA
FIVEB
FIVEC
FIVED
FIVEE
FIVEO
FIVER
FIVES
FIXED
FIXER
FIXES
GIBED
GIBER
GIBES
GILES
GIMEL
GIVEN
GIVER
GIVES
HIDEO
HIDER
HIDES
HIDEY
HIKED
HIKEN
HIKER
HIKES
HIMES
HINES
HIRED
HIREE
HIRER
HIRES
HIVED
HIVER
HIVES
JIBED
JIBES
JIVED
JIVER
JIVES
JIVEY
KIDEO
KILEY
KINER
KISER
KITED
KITER
KITES
LIBEL
LIBER
LIFER
LIGER
LIKED
LIKEN
LIKER
LIKES
LIMED
LIMES
LINEA
LINEB
LINEC
LINED
LINEN
LINER
LINES
LITEL
LITER
LITES
LIVED
LIVEN
LIVER
LIVES
MIKED
MIKES
MIKEY
MILER
MILES
MIMED
MIMEO
MIMER
MIMES
MINED
MINEO
MINER
MINES
MINEY
MIRED
MIRES
MISER
MITER
MITES
MIXED
MIXER
MIXES
NICER
NIGEL
NIGER
NIKES
NILES
NIMES
NINEA
NINEB
NINEC
NINED
NINEE
NINER
NINES
NISEI
NITER
NITES
NIVEA
NIVEN
NIXED
NIXER
NIXES
NIZER
OILED
OILER
PIKED
PIKER
PIKES
PILEA
PILED
PILEI
PILER
PILES
PIMEN
PINED
PINER
PINES
PINEY
PIPED
PIPER
PIPES
PIPET
PIVEN
PIXEL
RICED
RICER
RICES
RICEU
RIDER
RIDES
RIFER
RIGEL
RIKER
RILED
RILES
RILEY
RIMED
RIMER
RIMES
RIPEN
RIPER
RISEN
RISER
RISES
RITES
RIVED
RIVEN
RIVER
RIVES
RIVET
RIXEY
SICEM
SIDEA
SIDEB
SIDED
SIDES
SIKES
SILEX
SINES
SINEW
SINEX
SIRED
SIREE
SIREN
SIRES
SITED
SITES
SIXED
SIXEE
SIXER
SIXES
SIZED
SIZER
SIZES
TIBER
TIBET
TIDED
TIDES
TIGER
TIKES
TILED
TILER
TILES
TILEX
TIMED
TIMER
TIMES
TIMEX
TINEA
TINED
TINES
TIRED
TIRES
TITER
VIBES
VICES
VIDEO
VIKES
VILER
VINED
VINER
VINES
VIPER
VIREO
VISED
VISES
VIXEN
WIDEN
WIDER
WIFEY
WILED
WILEE
WILES
WILEY
WINED
WINES
WIPED
WIPER
WIPES
WIRED
WIRER
WIRES
WISED
WISER
WISES
WIVED
WIVES
WIZEN
WIZES
YIKES
YIPES
ZINES

•I••E

AIMEE
AINGE
AISLE
AISNE
BIBLE
BIERE
BILGE
BINGE
BIOME
BIORE
BIRSE
BITTE
CIRCE
CITEE
DIANE
DIENE
DIETE
DINGE
DIODE
DIONE
DIRAE
DIRGE
DISME
DIXIE
FIBRE
FICHE
FILLE
FIORE
FISKE
FIVEE
GIGUE
GIJOE
GIMME
HINGE
HIREE
HITME
KINTE
LIANE
LIBRE
LIEBE
LIEGE
LIGNE
LILLE
LISLE
LISSE
LITHE
LITRE
LIVRE
MIDGE
MIELE
MILLE
MILNE
MINCE
MITRE
NICHE
NIDRE
NIECE
NIEVE
NINEE
NIOBE
NITRE
NIXIE
PIAVE
PIECE
PINCE
PIQUE
PISTE
PIUTE
PIXIE
RICHE
RIDGE
RIFLE
RILKE
RILLE
RINSE
SIDLE
SIEGE
SIETE
SIEVE
SIGNE
SINCE
SINGE
SIREE
SIXEE
TIENE
TIGRE
TILDE
TINGE
TITHE
TITLE
TITRE
VILLE
VINCE
VITAE
VIVRE
WIEBE
WILDE
WILEE
WINCE
WITTE

••IE•

ABIES
ADIEU
ALIEN
AMIEL
AMIES
APIED
ARIEL
ARIES
BAIES
BRIEF
BRIER
BRIES
CHIEF
CHIEN
CRIED
CRIER
CRIES
DRIED
DRIER
DRIES
EDIES
ELIEL
ERIES
FLIED
FLIER
FLIES
FOIES
FRIED
FRIEL
FRIER
FRIES
GRIEF
GRIEG
GRIER
ICIER
ILIED
IVIED
IVIES
KLIEG
KRIEG
MEIER
OBIES
OGIER
OKIES
ORIEL
OSIER
OWIES
PLIED
PLIER
PLIES
PRIED
PRIER
PRIES
QUIEN
QUIET
SHIED
SHIER
SHIES
SKIED
SKIER
SKIES
SLIER
SPIED
SPIEL
SPIER
SPIES
STIEB
STIED
STIES
THIEF
THIEU
TRIED
TRIER
TRIES
URIEL
WRIER

••I•E

ABIDE
ADIGE
AFIRE
AGILE
ALICE
ALIKE
ALINE
ALIVE
AMICE
AMIDE
AMINE
AMITE
ANILE
ANIME
ANISE
ARISE
ASIDE
ATILE
ATIVE
AVIDE
AZIDE
BAIZE
BEIGE
BFIVE
BLIGE
BNINE
BOIRE
BOISE
BOITE
BRIBE
BRICE
BRIDE
BRINE
BRISE
BRITE
BSIDE
BTILE
CAINE
CHIDE
CHILE
CHIME
CHINE
CHIVE
CLIME
CLINE
CLIVE
CRIME
CTILE
CUIRE
DEICE
DRIVE
DTILE
EDILE
EFILE
ELIDE
ELISE
ELITE
EMILE
ETILE
EVITE
EXILE
EZINE
FAIRE
FRISE
FRITE
FTILE
GLIDE
GRIDE
GRIME
GRIPE
GRISE
GTILE
GUIDE
GUILE
GUISE
HAILE
HAISE
HEINE
HTILE
IFIVE
IGIVE
IMIDE
IMINE
INICE
ITILE
JAIME
JTILE
JUICE
KLINE
KNIFE
KRIGE
KTILE
LAINE
LOIRE
LTILE
LUISE
MAINE
MAIRE
MAIZE
MEINE
MLIFE
MOIRE
MTILE
NAIVE
NEIGE
NOIRE
NOISE
NTILE
ODILE
OGIVE
OLIVE
ONICE
OPINE
OTILE
OVINE
OXIDE
PAIGE
PAINE
PAISE
PHILE
POIRE
POISE
PRICE
PRIDE
PRIME
PRINE
PRIZE
PTILE
QTILE
QUINE
QUIRE
QUITE
RAINE
RAISE
REICE
REINE
RHINE
RTILE
SCIRE
SEINE
SEIZE
SHINE
SHIRE
SLICE
SLIDE
SLIME
SMILE
SMITE
SNIDE
SNIPE
SPICE
SPIKE
SPILE
SPINE
SPIRE
SPITE
STILE
STINE
STIPE
SUITE
SWINE
SWIPE
THINE
TOILE
TRIBE
TRICE
TRIKE
TRINE
TRIPE
TRITE
TTILE
TWICE
TWINE
UDINE
UNICE
UNITE
UTILE
VOICE
VOILE
VTILE
WAITE
WAIVE
WHILE
WHINE
WHITE
WRITE
WTILE
XFILE
XTILE
YLIKE
YTILE
ZAIRE
ZEILE
ZTILE

•••IE

ABBIE
ADDIE
AERIE
AGGIE
ALFIE
ALLIE
ANDIE
ANGIE
ANNIE
ARNIE
ARTIE
AUDIE
AUGIE
BASIE
BELIE
BOGIE
BOWIE
CELIE
COKIE
CURIE
CUTIE
DAVIE
DIXIE
DOBIE
DODIE
DOGIE
DOXIE
EADIE
EDDIE
EERIE
EFFIE
ELLIE
ELSIE
EPPIE
ERNIE
ESSIE
EUBIE
EYDIE
EYRIE
FACIE
FURIE
GENIE
HENIE
HOBIE
HOKIE
HOMIE
HOWIE
HUBIE
IMMIE
INDIE

INNIE
JAMIE
JANIE
JODIE
JOLIE
JOSIE
JULIE
KATIE
KYLIE
KYRIE
LACIE
LAVIE
LOOIE
LOUIE
LUCIE
LURIE
MAMIE
MARIE
MAXIE
MCVIE
MOVIE
MOXIE
NEWIE
NIXIE
NOLIE
NOTIE
OAKIE
OLDIE
OLLIE
OSSIE
OUTIE
OZZIE
PIXIE
PLUIE
RAMIE
RETIE
ROSIE
ROXIE
SADIE
SATIE
SOFIE
SUSIE
SUZIE
TOTIE
UNTIE
WOWIE
WYLIE
YALIE
YOWIE
ZADIE
ZOWIE

IF•••
IFEEL
IFILL
IFIVE
IFNOT
IFOLD
IFOUR
IFSAY

I•F••
INFER
INFIX
INFOR
INFRA
INFUN

I••F•
IMOFF

I•••F
IMOFF
INDEF

•IF••
BIFFS
BIFID
DIFFS
FIFED
FIFER
FIFES
FIFTH
FIFTY
GIFTS
HIFIS
JIFFS
JIFFY
LIFAR
LIFER
LIFTS
MIFFS
MIFFY
NIFTY
RIFER
RIFFS
RIFLE
RIFTS
SIFTS
TIFFS
WIFEY

•I•F•
BIFFS
DIFFS
FIEFS
JIFFS
JIFFY
LINFT
MIFFS
MIFFY
RIFFS
TIFFS
ZIEFF

•I••F
PILAF
RIDOF
ZIEFF

••IF•
ALIFS
CLIFF
CLIFT
COIFS
DEIFY
DRIFT
EDIFY
GRIFT
HAIFA
KNIFE
MLIFE
NAIFS
REIFY
SCIFI
SHIFT
SKIFF
SNIFF
SPIFF
STIFF
SWIFT
UNIFY
WAIFS
WHIFF

••I•F
BRIEF
CHIEF
CLIFF
GRIEF
SKIFF
SNIFF
SPIFF
STIFF
THIEF
WHIFF

•••IF
CALIF
MOTIF
SERIF

IG•••
IGGED
IGIVE
IGLOO
IGLUS
IGNES
IGNIS
IGUAL

I•G••
IGGED
ILGWU
INGER
INGLE
INGOT

I••G•
ILLGO
IMAGE
IMAGO
INAGE
INIGO

I•••G
ICING
IDING
IDTAG
INBIG
INCOG
INORG
IRREG

•IG••
BIGDO
BIGGS
BIGGY
BIGHT
BIGLY
BIGMO
BIGON
BIGOT
CIGAR
CIGGY
CIGNA
DIGAT
DIGBY
DIGEL
DIGEM
DIGGS
DIGIN
DIGIT
DIGUP
EIGEN
EIGER
EIGHT
FIGHT
GIGIO
GIGLI
GIGOT
GIGUE
HIGHC
HIGHS
JIGGS
JIGGY
LIGER
LIGHT
LIGNE
LIGNI
LIGNO
MIGHT
NIGEL
NIGER
NIGHT
PIGGY
PIGIT
RIGAN
RIGBY
RIGEL
RIGGS
RIGHT
RIGID
RIGOR
RIGUP
SIGHS
SIGHT
SIGIL
SIGMA
SIGNE
SIGNS
TIGER
TIGHT
TIGON
TIGRE
VIGGO
VIGIA
VIGIL
VIGNY
VIGOR
WIGGY
WIGHT
ZIGGY

•I•G•
AINGE
BIGGS
BIGGY
BILGE
BILGY
BINGE
BINGO
BINGS
BIOGS
CIGGY
CITGO
DIEGO
DIGGS
DINGE
DINGO
DINGS
DINGY
DIRGE
GITGO
HINGE
JIGGS
JIGGY
JINGO
KINGS
LIEGE
LINGO
LINGS
LINGU
MIDGE
MINGY
OINGO
PIGGY
PINGS
RIDGE
RIDGY
RIGGS
RINGO
RINGS
SIEGE
SINGE
SINGH
SINGS
TIAGO
TIEGS
TINGE
TINGS
TIOGA
VIGGO
VINGT
VIRGA
VIRGO
WIGGY
WINGS
WINGY
ZIGGY
ZINGS
ZINGY

•I••G
BILLG
DIMAG
JIANG
LIANG

••IG•
ADIGE
ALIGN
AMIGA
AMIGO
ANIGH
BEIGE
BLIGE
BLIGH
BRIGS
COIGN
DEIGN
DRIGO
FEIGN
FRIGG
GRIGS
HEIGH
HEIGL
INIGO
KRIGE
LEIGH
LUIGI
NEIGE
NEIGH
OLIGO
PAIGE
PRIGS
REIGN
SLIGO
SWIGS
TAIGA
THIGH
TWIGS
VSIGN
WEIGH
WHIGS

••I•G
ACING
AGING
AHING
APING
AWING
AXING
BEING
BLING
BOING
BRING
CCING
CHING
CLING
CUING
DHING
DOING
DRING
DYING
EKING
ERING
EWING
EXING
EYING
FLING
FRIGG
GOING
GRIEG
HAING
HYING
ICING
IDING
KLIEG
KOING
KRIEG
LAING
LYING
ODING
OHING
OKING
OPING
ORING
OWING
RUING
RVING
SLING
STING
SUING
SWING
THING
TYING
USING
VYING
WRING

•••IG
ASBIG
BEWIG
CRAIG
GRAIG
INBIG
MRBIG
NAVIG
REDIG
REJIG
RELIG
RERIG
SELIG
SOBIG
SPRIG
STEIG
UNRIG
UNWIG
VARIG
ZADIG
ZELIG
ZWEIG

IH•••
IHEAR
IHOPE
IHOPS

I•H••
ICHOR
IMHIP
IMHOT
INHOC
ISHAM

I••H•
ICAHN
IDAHO
IJOHN
ITCHY

I•••H
ILICH
IRISH
ISIAH
IWISH

•IH••
HIHAT
HIHOS
JIHAD
JIHAN
NIHIL
NIHON

•I•H•
AISHA
BIEHN
BIGHT
DICHO
DISHY
EIGHT
FICHE
FICHU
FIGHT
FISHY
HIGHC
HIGHS
LICHT
LIGHT
LITHE
LITHO
MIGHT
MINHO
MISHA
NICHE
NICHT
NIGHT
PITHS
PITHY
RICHE
RIGHT
RISHI
SIGHS
SIGHT
SIKHS
TIGHT
TISHA
TITHE
VICHY
WIGHT
WISHY

•I••H
AITCH
BIRCH
BIRTH
CINCH
DINAH
DITCH
FIFTH
FILCH
FILTH
FINCH
FIRTH
FITCH
GIRSH
GIRTH
HITCH
MICAH
MIRTH
MITCH
NINTH
PINCH
PITCH
QIRSH
RICOH
SINGH
SIXTH
TILTH
TISCH
WIDTH
WINCH
WIRTH
WITCH
ZILCH

••IH•
ELIHU

••I•H
AMISH
ANIGH
APISH
ARITH
BLIGH
BLISH
BRITH
EDITH
ERICH
FAITH
HEIGH
ILICH
IRISH
ISIAH
IWISH
KEITH
KNISH
LEIGH
LEITH
NAISH
NEIGH
PHISH
REICH
SAITH
SHISH
SMITH
STICH
SWISH
THIGH
TRISH
UKIAH
URIAH
URICH
WEIGH
WHICH
WHISH

•••IH
DABIH

I•I••
IBIZA
ICIER
ICILY
ICING
IDING
IDIOM
IDIOT
IFILL
IFIVE
IGIVE
ILIAC
ILIAD
ILICH
ILIED
ILION
ILIUM
IMIDE
IMINE
INICE
INIGO
INIKI
ININK
INION
INITS
IRIDO
IRIDS
IRINA
IRISH
ISIAH
ITILE
ITINA
IVIED
IVIES
IVINS
IWILL
IWISH
IXION

I••I•
ICEIN
ICEIT
IGNIS
ILLIN
IMHIP
IMMIE
IMMIX
INBIG
INDIA
INDIC
INDIE
INDIO
INDIV
INFIX
INKIN
INNIE
INNIS
INOIL
INUIT
IODIC
IONIA
IONIC
IQUIT
IRVIN
IRWIN
ISAID
ISLIP
ISTIC
IZMIR

I•••I
IAMBI
ICENI
ICOSI
IMARI
IMPEI
INARI
INIKI
IRANI
IRAQI
ISSEI
IVANI

•I•I•
BIDIN
BIFID
BITIN
CILIA
CIVIC
CIVIL
DIDIN
DIDIT
DIGIN
DIGIT
DIMIN
DIPIN
DIXIE
DIXIT
EIEIO
FINIS
FITIN
FIXIT
GIGIO
HIFIS
HITIN
HITIT
KILIM
KIRIN
KIWIS
LICIA
LICIT
LIEIN
LILIA
LIMIT
LIPID
LIVIA
LIVID
LIVIN
MIDIS
MIMIC
MINIM
MINIS
MIRIN
MIXIN
NIHIL
NITID
NIXIE
PIGIT
PIPIT
PIXIE
RIGID
SIGIL
SITIN
TIBIA
TIEIN
TIKIS
TIMID
TIPIN
TIPIS
TITIS
VIGIA
VIGIL
VINIC
VIRID
VISIT
VIVID
VIZIR
WIKIS
ZIPIN
ZIPIT
ZITIS

•I••I
AINSI
AIOLI
BIERI
BIRRI
CIRRI
CITRI
DIECI
DISCI
FIORI
GIGLI
GIMLI
HINDI
JINNI
LIBRI
LIGNI
LILLI
LIPPI
LIZZI
MIAMI
MILLI
MISTI
MITZI
NIKKI
NIMBI
NISEI
NITTI
PIANI
PIAUI
PILEI
PIPPI
PISCI
PITTI
PIUSI
RICCI
RICKI
RIETI
RIKKI
RISHI
SINAI
TIKKI
TIPPI
VICKI
VIKKI
VILLI
VINCI
VITRI

••II•
CCIII
CDIII
CLIII
CMIII
CVIII
CXIII
DCIII
DLIII
DVIII
DXIII
LVIII
LXIII
MCIII
MDIII
MLIII
MMIII
MVIII
MXIII
XCIII
XLIII
XVIII
XXIII

••I•I
ALIBI
AMICI
AMIRI
BLINI
CCIII
CDIII
CHILI
CLIII
CMIII
CVIII
CXIII
DCIII
DLIII
DVIII
DXIII
HAITI
HEIDI
INIKI
LUIGI
LVIII
LXIII
MCIII
MDIII
MEIJI
MLIII
MMIII
MVIII
MXIII
ORIBI
RAIMI
SCIFI
SEIJI
TRINI
UJIJI
VOICI
XCIII
XLIII
XVIII
XXIII

•••II
ACTII
ASCII
CCCII
CCIII
CCLII
CCVII
CCXII
CDIII
CDLII
CDVII
CDXII
CLIII
CLVII
CLXII
CMIII
CMLII
CMVII
CMXII
CVIII
CXCII
CXIII
CXLII
CXVII
CXXII
DCCII
DCIII
DCLII
DCVII
DCXII
DLIII
DLVII
DLXII
DVIII
DXCII
DXIII
DXLII
DXVII
DXXII
GENII
LEOII
LVIII
LXIII
LXVII
LXXII
MAOII
MCCII
MCDII
MCIII
MCLII
MCMII
MCVII
MCXII
MDCII
MDIII
MDLII
MDVII
MDXII
MEDII
MLIII
MLVII
MLXII
MMCII
MMDII
MMIII
MMLII
MMMII
MMVII
MMXII
MVIII
MXCII
MXIII
MXLII
MXVII
MXXII
QBVII
RADII
SATII
SAWII
TORII
XCIII
XCVII
XLIII
XLVII
XVIII
XXIII
XXVII
XXXII

IJ•••
IJKLM
IJOHN

I•J••
INJUN

•IJ••
BIJOU
DIJON
GIJOE
HIJAS
HIJKL
HIJOS
VIJAY

•I•J•
NINJA
RIOJA
VIEJA
VIEJO

••IJ•
GHIJK
MEIJI
OUIJA
SEIJI
UJIJI

•••IJ
FGHIJ

IK•••
IKNOW

I•K••
ICKES
IJKLM
INKED
INKER
INKEY
INKIN
INKLE
IRKED
IRKER

I••K•
INIKI

I•••K
IBOOK
ININK
ISAAK
ITSOK
IZAAK

•IK••
AIKEN
BIKED
BIKEL
BIKER
BIKES
DIKED
DIKER
DIKES
HIKED
HIKEN
HIKER
HIKES
LIKED
LIKEN
LIKER
LIKES
LIKUD
MIKAN
MIKED
MIKES
MIKEY
NIKES
NIKKI
NIKON
PIKAS
PIKED
PIKER
PIKES
RIKER
RIKKI
SIKAS
SIKES
SIKHS
TIKES
TIKIS
TIKKA
TIKKI
VIKES
VIKKI
WIKIS
YIKES

•I•K•
BILKO
BILKS
DICKS
DICKY
DINKA
DINKS
DINKY
DIRKS
DISKO
DISKS
DITKA
FINKS
FISKE
HICKS
HIJKL
HINKY
JINKS
KICKS
KICKY
KINKO
KINKS
KINKY
KIRKS
KISKA
LICKS
LINKS
MICKY
MILKS
MILKY
MINKS
NICKS
NICKY
NIKKI
OINKS
PICKS
PICKY
PINKO
PINKS
PINKY
RICKI
RICKS
RICKY
RIKKI
RILKE
RINKS
RINKY
RISKS
RISKY
SICKO
SILKS
SILKY
SINKS
SITKA
TICKS
TICKY
TIKKA
TIKKI
VICKI
VICKS
VICKY
VIKKI
WICKS
WINKS
ZINKY

•I••K
DIDOK
KIOSK
MINSK
PINSK
TILAK

••IK•
ALIKE
EFIKS
ERIKA
HAIKS
HAIKU
INIKI
LAIKA
SEIKO
SPIKE
SPIKY
TRIKE
YLIKE

••I•K
AMICK
BLINK
BRICK
BRINK
BRISK
BUICK
CHICK
CHINK
CLICK
CLINK
CRICK
DRINK
ERICK
FLICK
FRICK
FRISK
GHIJK
GLICK
ININK
KLICK
KLINK
KNICK
OZICK
PLINK

PRICK
PRINK
QUICK
QUIRK
REINK
SHIRK
SKINK
SLICK
SLINK
SMIRK
SNICK
STICK
STINK
THICK
THINK
TRICK
UMIAK
WHISK
ZWICK

•••IK
BATIK
CRAIK
GOPIK
KULIK
LASIK
LUNIK
PULIK
RUBIK
RURIK
SHEIK

IL•••
ILEAC
ILEAL
ILENE
ILEUM
ILGWU
ILIAC
ILIAD
ILICH
ILIED
ILION
ILIUM
ILLBE
ILLER
ILLGO
ILLIN
ILLUS
ILLYA
ILONA
ILOSE
ILOVE

I•L••
IDLED
IDLER
IDLES
IGLOO
IGLUS
ILLBE
ILLER
ILLGO
ILLIN
ILLUS
ILLYA
INLAW
INLAY
INLET
INLOW
ISLAM
ISLAS
ISLES
ISLET
ISLEY
ISLIP

I••L•
ICALL
ICILY
IDOLA
IDOLS
IDYLL
IDYLS
IFILL
IFOLD
IJKLM
IMPLY
INALL
INGLE
INKLE
ISOLA
ISOLT
ISTLE
ITALO
ITALS
ITALY
ITILE
IWILL

I•••L
ICALL
IDEAL
IDYLL
IFEEL
IFILL
IGUAL
ILEAL
IMPEL
INALL
INOIL
INTEL
IQBAL
ISSEL
IWILL

•IL••
AILED
AILES
AILEY
AILUR
BILBO
BILES
BILGE
BILGY
BILKO
BILKS
BILLG
BILLS
BILLW
BILLY
CILIA
CILLA
DILLS
DILLY
EILAT
FILAR
FILAS
FILCH
FILED
FILER
FILES
FILET
FILLE
FILLS
FILLY
FILMS
FILMY
FILOS
FILTH
FILUM
GILAS
GILDA
GILDS
GILES
GILLS
GILTS
HILDA
HILLS
HILLY
HILTS
HILUM
JILTS
KILBY
KILEY
KILIM
KILLS
KILLY
KILNS
KILOS
KILTS
LILAC
LILIA
LILLE
LILLI
LILLY
LILTS
MILAN
MILER
MILES
MILKS
MILKY
MILLE
MILLI
MILLO
MILLS
MILNE
MILOS
NILES
NILLA
NILLY
OILED
OILER
PILAF
PILAR
PILAU
PILEA
PILED
PILEI
PILER
PILES
PILLS
PILON
PILOT
PILUS
RILED
RILES
RILEY
RILKE
RILLE
RILLS
SILAS
SILEX
SILKS
SILKY
SILLS
SILLY
SILOS
SILTS
SILTY
SILVA
TILAK
TILDA
TILDE
TILED
TILER
TILES
TILEX
TILLS
TILLY
TILTH
TILTS
VILAS
VILER
VILLA
VILLE
VILLI
VILMA
VILNA
WILBY
WILCO
WILDE
WILDS
WILED
WILEE
WILES
WILEY
WILLA
WILLS
WILLY
WILMA
WILTS
ZILCH
ZILLA
ZILLS

•I•L•
AIOLI
AISLE
BIALY
BIBLE
BIGLY
BILLG
BILLS
BILLW
BILLY
BIRLS
CIELO
CIELS
CILLA
DIALO
DIALS
DIELS
DILLS
DILLY
DIMLY
DIPLO
FIELD
FILLE
FILLS
FILLY
FITLY
GIGLI
GILLS
GIMLI
GIRLS
GIRLY
HILLS
HILLY
HIPLY
KILLS
KILLY
LILLE
LILLI
LILLY
LISLE
MIELE
MIELS
MILLE
MILLI
MILLO
MILLS
MITLA
NIBLO
NIELS
NILLA
NILLY
PIELS
PILLS
RIALS
RIELS
RIFLE
RILLE
RILLS
SIDLE
SILLS
SILLY
TILLS
TILLY
TITLE
TIXLS
VIALS
VILLA
VILLE
VILLI
VIOLA
VIOLS
WIELD
WILLA
WILLS
WILLY
YIELD
ZILLA
ZILLS

•I••L
BIKEL
BINAL
CIVIL
DIGEL
FIDEL
FINAL
GIMEL
HIJKL
LIBEL
LIESL
LITEL
NICOL
NIGEL
NIHIL
NIVAL
OIDAL
PIXEL
RIGEL
RIVAL
RIYAL
RIZAL
SIBYL
SIGIL
SISAL
TICAL
TIDAL
TIROL
VIDAL
VIGIL
VINYL
VIRAL
VITAL

••IL•
AGILE
ANILE
ANILS
ARILS
ATILE
ATILT
AVILA
AXILS
BAILS
BOILS
BRILL
BTILE
BUILD
BUILT
CEILS
CHILD
CHILE
CHILI
CHILL
COILS
CTILE
DAILY
DEILS
DOILY
DRILL
DRILY
DTILE
EDILE
EFILE
EMILE
EMILY
ETILE
EVILS
EXILE
FAILS
FOILS
FRILL
FTILE
GAILY
GRILL
GTILE
GUILD
GUILE
GUILT
HAILE
HAILS
HTILE
ICILY
IFILL
ITILE
IWILL
JAILS
JTILE
KRILL
KTILE
LAILA
LEILA
LTILE
MAILS
MOILS
MTILE
NAILS
NEILL
NOILS
NOILY
NTILE
ODILE
OTILE
PAILS
PHILE
PHILO
POILU
PTILE
QTILE
QUILL
QUILP
QUILT
RAILS
ROILS
ROILY
RTILE
SAILS
SHILL
SKILL
SMILE
SOILS
SPILE
SPILL
SPILT
STILE
STILL
STILT
SWILL
TAILS
TBILL
THILL
TOILE
TOILS
TRILL
TTILE
TWILL
UTILE
UTILS
VEILS
VOILA
VOILE
VTILE
WAILS
WEILL
WHILE
WTILE
XFILE
XTILE
YTILE
ZEILE
ZTILE

••I•L
AMIEL
ARIAL
ARIEL
AXIAL
BAIUL
BGIRL
BRILL
CHILL
DRILL
ELIEL
FRIEL
FRILL
FRIML
GLIAL
GRILL
HEIGL
IFILL
IWILL
KRILL
NEILL
ORIEL
PHIAL
QUILL
SHILL
SKILL
SKIRL
SPIEL
SPILL
STILL
SWILL
SWIRL
TBILL
THILL
TRIAL
TRILL
TWILL
TWIRL
URIEL
WEILL
WHIRL

•••IL
ABOIL
ABRIL
ADVIL
ANVIL
APRIL
ARBIL
AVAIL
AVRIL
BASIL
BROIL
CAVIL
CECIL
CIVIL
CYRIL
DEVIL
EMAIL
ENOIL
ERBIL
ETAIL
FACIL
FLAIL
FRAIL
FUSIL
GRAIL
INOIL
LOEIL
MOBIL
MUSIL
NEVIL
NIHIL
NOOIL
ONEIL
PERIL
PUPIL
QUAIL
REOIL
SIGIL
SNAIL
SPOIL
SYBIL
TAMIL
TRAIL
UNTIL
VIGIL

IM•••
IMACS
IMAGE
IMAGO
IMAMS
IMAMU
IMARI
IMBAD
IMBED
IMBUE
IMEAN
IMHIP
IMHOT
IMIDE
IMINE
IMMAD
IMMIE
IMMIX
IMOFF
IMOUT
IMOVE
IMPEI
IMPEL
IMPLY
IMSET

I•M••
IAMBI
IAMBS
IAMSO
IBMPC
IMMAD
IMMIE
IMMIX
INMAY
IZMIR

I••M•
ICAME
ICBMS
IMAMS
IMAMU
ISAMU
ITEMS
ITSME

I•••M
IBEAM
IDIOM
IJKLM
ILEUM
ILIUM
INREM
INSUM
ISHAM
ISLAM

•IM••
AIMAT
AIMED
AIMEE
AIMER
BIMBO
DIMAG
DIMAS
DIMED
DIMES
DIMIN
DIMLY
GIMEL
GIMLI
GIMME
GIMPS
GIMPY
HIMES
HIMOM
JIMMY
KIMBA
KIMPO
LIMAN
LIMAS
LIMBO
LIMBS
LIMED
LIMES
LIMIT
LIMNS
LIMON
LIMOS
LIMPS
LIMPY
MIMED
MIMEO
MIMER
MIMES
MIMIC
MIMSY
NIMBI
NIMBY
NIMES
NIMOY
PIMAS
PIMEN
RIMED
RIMER
RIMES
SIMBA
SIMMS
SIMON
SIMPS
TIMED
TIMER
TIMES
TIMEX
TIMID
TIMMY
TIMON
TIMOR
WIMPS
WIMPY

•I•M•
BIGMO
BIOME
DIAMS
DIEMS
DISME
FILMS
FILMY
FIRMA
FIRMS
GIMME
GISMO
GITMO
GIZMO
HITME
JIMMY
MIAMI
PISMO
SIGMA
SIMMS
TIAMO
TIMMY
VILMA
WILMA

•I••M
DIGEM
DIRAM
FILUM
HILUM
HIMOM
HIRAM
KILIM
MINIM
MISSM
SICEM
SIXAM
SIXPM
VITAM

••IM•
ANIMA
ANIME
ANIMO
BLIMP
BRIMS
CHIME
CHIMP
CLIMB
CLIME
CRIME
CRIMP
FAIMS
FRIML
GLIMS
GRIME
GRIMM
GRIMY
JAIME
KLIMT
MAIMS
NAIMA
PRIMA
PRIME
PRIMO
PRIMP
PRIMS
RAIMI
REIMS
SHIMS
SKIMP
SKIMS
SLIME
SLIMS
SLIMY
SWIMS
TRIMS
WHIMS

••I•M
ARIUM
AXIOM
DEISM
DRIAM
GRIMM
IDIOM
ILIUM
ODIUM
OPIUM
ORIUM
PRIAM
PRISM
PRIZM
SEISM

•••IM
ABRIM
ASWIM
BEDIM
CHAIM
CLAIM
DENIM
HAKIM
KILIM
MAXIM
MCKIM
MINIM
PURIM
REAIM
SCRIM
UNDIM
VADIM
YADIM

IN•••
INAGE
INALL
INANE
INAPT
INARI
INAWE
INBAD
INBED
INBIG
INBOX
INCAN
INCAS
INCOG
INCRS
INCUR
INCUS
INDEF
INDEX
INDIA
INDIC
INDIE
INDIO
INDIV
INDRA
INDRE
INDUE
INDUS
INDYS
INEES
INEPT
INERT
INFER
INFIX
INFOR
INFRA
INFUN
INGER
INGLE
INGOT
INHOC
INICE
INIGO
INIKI
ININK
INION
INITS
INJUN
INKED
INKER
INKEY
INKIN
INKLE
INLAW
INLAY
INLET
INLOW
INMAY
INNER
INNES
INNIE
INNIS
INOIL
INONU
INORG
INPEN
INPUT
INRED
INREM
INRUN
INSET
INSTR
INSTS
INSUM
INTEL
INTER
INTOW
INTRA
INTRO
INTWO
INUIT
INURE
INUSE
INVER

I•N••
IFNOT
IGNES
IGNIS
IKNOW
INNER
INNES
INNIE
INNIS
IONIA
IONIC
IXNAY

I••N•
ICANT
ICENI
ICING
ICONO
ICONS
IDENT
IDING
IDONT
ILENE
ILONA
IMINE
INANE
ININK
INONU
IPANA
IRANI
IRENA
IRENE
IRINA
IRONS
IRONY
ISBNS
ITINA
IVANA
IVANI
IVANV
IVINS
IWANT
IWONT

I•••N
IBSEN
ICAHN
ICEIN
IJOHN
ILION
ILLIN
IMEAN
INCAN
INFUN
INION
INJUN
INKIN
INPEN
INRUN
IOWAN
IRVIN
IRWIN
IXION

•IN••
AINGE
AINSI
AINUS
BINAL
BINDS
BINES
BINET
BINGE
BINGO
BINGS
CINCH
CINCO
CINCY
CINDY
CINES
CINNA
DINAH
DINAR
DINDY
DINED
DINER
DINES
DINGE
DINGO
DINGS
DINGY
DINKA
DINKS
DINKY
DINNY
DINOS
DINTS
DINTY
EINEN
EINER
EINES
FINAL
FINCA
FINCH
FINDS
FINED
FINER
FINES
FINIS
FINKS
FINNO
FINNS
FINNY
FINOS
GINNY
GINSU
GINUP
GINZA
HINDI
HINDS
HINDU
HINES
HINGE
HINKY
HINNY
HINTS
JINGO
JINKS
JINNJ
JINNS
KINAS
KINDA
KINDS
KINER
KINGS
KINKO
KINKS
KINKY
KINTE
LINCS
LINDA
LINDO
LINDT
LINDY
LINEA
LINEB
LINEC
LINED
LINEN
LINER
LINES
LINFT
LINGO
LINGS
LINGU
LINKS
LINOS
LINTS
LINTY
LINUS
LINUX
MINAS
MINCE
MINDS
MINDY
MINED
MINEO
MINER
MINES
MINEY
MINGY
MINHO
MINIM
MINIS
MINKS
MINOR
MINOS
MINOT
MINOW
MINSK
MINTS
MINTY
MINUS
NINAS
NINEA
NINEB
NINEC
NINED
NINEE
NINER
NINES
NINJA
NINNY
NINON
NINOS
NINTH
OINGO
OINKS
PINCE
PINCH
PINED
PINER
PINES
PINEY
PINGS
PINKO
PINKS
PINKY
PINNA
PINON
PINOT
PINSK
PINTA
PINTO
PINTS
PINUP
PINZA
RINDS
RINDY
RINGO
RINGS
RINKS
RINKY
RINSE
RINSO
RINTY
SINAI
SINCE
SINES
SINEW
SINEX
SINGE
SINGH
SINGS
SINKS
SINUS
TINCT
TINEA
TINED
TINES
TINGE
TINGS
TINNY
TINTS
UINTA
VINAS
VINCE
VINCI
VINCY
VINED
VINER
VINES
VINGT
VINIC
VINNY
VINOS
VINYL
WINAT
WINBY
WINCE
WINCH

WINDS WINDY WINED WINES WINGS WINGY WINKS ZINCS ZINCY ZINES ZINGS ZINGY ZINKY

•I•N•

AISNE BIONT CIANO CIENS CIGNA CINNA CIONS DIANA DIANE DIDNT DIENE DINNY DIONE FIEND FINNO FINNS FINNY FIONA FIRNS GIANT GINNY GIONO HINNY JIANG JINNI JINNS KILNS LIANA LIANE LIANG LIENS LIGNE LIGNI LIGNO LIMNS LIONS MIENS MILNE NINNY PIANI PIANO PINNA PIONS PIRNS RIANT RIENS SIENA SIGNE SIGNS SIXNO TIANT TIENE TINNY TISNT VIAND VIGNY VILNA VINNY VIRNA

•I••N

AIDAN AIKEN BIDEN BIDIN BIDON BIEHN BIGON BISON BITIN BITON DIDIN DIGIN DIJON DIMIN DIPIN DIVAN DIXON EIGEN EINEN EISEN FITIN FITON FIXON GIVEN HIKEN HITIN HITON JIHAN KIRIN LIEIN LIEON LIKEN LIMAN LIMON LINEN LITON LIVEN LIVIN MIDON MIKAN MILAN MIRIN MIXIN NIHON NIKON NINON NISAN NITON NIVEN NIXON PICON PILON PIMEN PINON PISAN PITON PIVEN RICAN RIGAN RIPEN RIPON RISEN RIVEN SIDON SIMON SIPON SIREN SITIN SITON SIVAN TIEIN TIEON TIGON TIMON TIPIN TITAN VIXEN WIDEN WIZEN ZIPIN ZIPON

••IN•

ACING ADINS AGING AHING AKINS ALINE AMINE AMINO APING AWING AXING AYINS BEING BEINS BLIND BLING BLINI BLINK BNINE BOING BRINE BRING BRINK BRINY CAINE CAINT CCING CHINA CHINE CHING CHINK CHINO CHINS CLINE CLING CLINK CLINT COINS CSINY CUING DHING DJINN DJINS DOING DRINA DRING DRINK DUINO DVINA DYING EDINA EKING ERING EWING EXING EYING EZINE FAINT FEINT FLING FLINT GAINS GLINT GOING GRIND GRINS GRINT HAING HEINE HEINZ HYING ICING IDING IMINE ININK IRINA ITINA IVINS JAINS JOINS JOINT JUINS KEINO KLINE KLINK KOING LAINE LAING LOINS LYING MAINE MAINS MAINZ MEINE NAINA ODING OHING OKING OPINE OPING ORING OVINE OWING PAINE PAINS PAINT PLINK PLINY POINT PRINE PRINK PRINT QUINE QUINN QUINO QUINT RAINE RAINS RAINY REINA REINE REINK REINS RHINE RHINO RUING RUINS RVING SAINT SEINE SHINE SHINS SHINY SKINK SKINS SLING SLINK SPINE SPINS SPINY STINE STING STINK STINT SUING SWINE SWING TAINA TAINT THINE THING THINK THINS TRINA TRINE TRINI TWINE TWINS TWINY TYING UDINE USING VEINS VEINY VYING WAINS WHINE WHINY WRING

••I•N

ALIEN ALIGN ANION APIAN ARIAN ARION ASIAN ATION AVIAN AVION AXION BAIRN BRIAN CAIRN CHIEN COIGN DEIGN DEION DJINN ELION EVIAN FEIGN ILION INION IXION ONION ORION QUIEN QUINN REIGN SCION TYIYN UNION VSIGN

•••IN

ACTIN ADDIN ADMIN AGAIN AGRIN AHSIN ALAIN ALLIN ALVIN AMAIN APAIN ARKIN ARMIN ASKIN ASPIN ASTIN ATEIN AUVIN BALIN BASIN BATIN BEGIN BENIN BEVIN BIDIN BITIN BOXIN BRAIN BRUIN BUNIN BURIN BUYIN CABIN CHAIN COLIN COMIN CRAIN CUEIN CUMIN CUTIN DARIN DIDIN DIGIN DIMIN DIPIN DOLIN DRAIN DUBIN DUEIN DUGIN DUPIN EATIN EDWIN EGLIN ELDIN ELFIN ELGIN ELKIN ELLIN ELVIN ENDIN ENFIN EOSIN ERVIN ERWIN FAGIN FEDIN FITIN FLYIN FOGIN GABIN GAMIN GAVIN GETIN GHAIN GOTIN GRAIN GROIN HADIN HASIN HEDIN HEMIN HITIN HOPIN ICEIN ILLIN INKIN IRVIN IRWIN JAMIN KANIN KAZIN KEVIN KEYIN KIRIN KLEIN KUMIN LANIN LAPIN LATIN LAVIN LAYIN LEDIN LENIN LETIN LEVIN LIEIN LIVIN LOGIN LORIN LOSIN LOVIN LUBIN LUPIN MAKIN MARIN MATIN MAVIN MIRIN MIXIN MOVIN MYCIN MYSIN NEVIN NOTIN NOWIN OHLIN OLEIN OPTIN ORKIN ORRIN OSLIN PALIN PANIN PAVIN PAYIN PEKIN PENIN PEPIN PLAIN POPIN PUPIN PUTIN QUOIN RABIN RAMIN RANIN RENIN REPIN RESIN RETIN REWIN RHEIN ROBIN RODIN RONIN ROSIN RUBIN RUNIN RUTIN SABIN SAFIN SATIN SAWIN SEEIN SERIN SETIN SEWIN SITIN SKEIN SLAIN SPAIN STAIN STEIN SWAIN TAKIN TAPIN TIEIN TIPIN TOEIN TOWIN TOXIN TRAIN TURIN TWAIN UNPIN USEIN VENIN WASIN WAYIN XEDIN XESIN YULIN YVAIN YWAIN ZAYIN ZIPIN ZUBIN

IO•••

IODIC IONIA IONIC IOTAS IOWAN IOWAS IOWAU IOWAY

I•O••

IBOOK ICONO ICONS ICOSA ICOSI IDOLA IDOLS IDONT IFOLD IFOUR IHOPE IHOPS IJOHN ILONA ILOSE ILOVE IMOFF IMOUT IMOVE INOIL INONU INORG IPODS IROCS IRONS IRONY ISOLA ISOLT IVORY IWONT IZODS

I••O•

IBOOK ICHOR IDIOM IDIOT IFNOT IGLOO IKNOW ILION IMHOT INBOX INCOG INFOR INGOT INHOC INION INLOW INTOW ISTOO ITSOK IXION

I•••O

IAMSO IATRO ICONO IDAHO IGLOO ILLGO IMAGO INDIO INIGO INTRO INTWO IRIDO ISTOO ITALO

•IO••

AIOLI BIOGS BIOME BIONT BIORE BIOTA CIONS DIODE DIONE DIORS FIONA FIORD FIORE FIORI GIONO KIOSK KIOWA LIONS NIOBE NIORT PIONS PIOUS RIOJA RIOTS SIOUX TIOGA TIOUS VIOLA VIOLS

•I•O•

AIDOO BIDON BIGON BIGOT BIJOU BIPOD BIROS BISON BITON CIAOS DICOT DIDOK DIDOS DIJON DINOS DIVOT DIXON FILOS FINOS FITON FIXON GIGOT GIJOE GIROS HIHOS HIJOS HIMOM HITON KILOS KIROV LIDOS LIEON LIMON LIMOS LINOS LITON MIAOU MIAOW MIDON MILOS MINOR MINOS MINOT MINOW MIROS MISOS NICOL NIHON NIKON NIMOY NINON NINOS NITON NIXON PICON PICOT PILON PILOT PINON PINOT PITON PITOT PIVOT RICOH RIDOF RIGOR RIPON SIDON SILOS SIMON SIPON SITON TICOS TIEON TIGON TIMON TIMOR TIROL TIROS TITOV TIVOS VIDOR VIGOR VINOS VISOR VIZOR WIDOW ZIPON

•I••O

AIDOO BIGDO BIGMO BILBO BILKO BIMBO BINGO CIANO CIELO CINCO CIRRO CISCO CITGO CITRO DIALO DICHO DIDSO DIDTO DIEGO DINGO DIPLO DIPSO DISCO DISKO DITTO EIEIO FIBRO FIERO FINNO FIRPO FIVEO GIGIO GIONO GISMO GITGO GITMO GIZMO HIDEO HIERO HIPPO HIPTO HISTO JINGO KIDDO KIDEO KIMPO KINKO LIBRO LIETO LIGNO LIMBO LINDO LINGO LIPPO LITHO MICRO MILLO MIMEO MINEO MINHO MIRRO MISDO NIBLO NIETO NITRO OINGO PIANO PICTO PINKO PINTO PISMO RINGO RINSO RIZZO SICKO SISQO SIXNO TIAGO TIAMO TIETO VIDEO VIEJO VIGGO VIREO VIRGO VITRO WILCO ZIPPO

••IO•

ADIOS AEIOU AGIOS ALIOS ANION ARION ARIOT ATION AVION AVIOR AXIOM AXION CHIOS CLIOS DEION ELION ELIOT GRIOT IDIOM IDIOT ILION INION IXION OHIOU OLIOS ONION ORION PRIOR SCION TRIOS UNION

••I•O

ALITO AMICO AMIGO AMINO ANIMO AVISO BOITO CAIRO CHICO CHINO CHIRO DOIDO DRIGO DUINO EDIPO EJIDO FRITO GEICO GUIDO INIGO IRIDO KEINO OLIGO PHILO PRIMO QUINO QUITO RHINO SEIKO SLIGO SPIRO TAITO

•••IO

ADDIO AERIO ALFIO AMNIO ANGIO ANZIO AUDIO BACIO CANIO CASIO CURIO DANIO DARIO EIEIO ENNIO ESPIO FABIO FOLIO GIGIO HAGIO HELIO INDIO JULIO JUNIO LUCIO MARIO MEDIO NACIO NGAIO NOVIO PATIO POLIO RADIO RATIO SERIO SOCIO TONIO YUKIO

IP•••

IPANA IPASS IPODS IPRAY

I•P••

IMPEI IMPEL IMPLY INPEN INPUT

I••P•

IBMPC IHOPE IHOPS INAPT INEPT

I•••P

ICEUP IMHIP ISLIP

•IP••

BIPED BIPOD BIPPY DIPIN DIPLO DIPPY DIPSO DIPSY GIPSY HIPLY HIPPO HIPPY HIPTO LIPID LIPPI LIPPO LIPPY NIPAS NIPAT NIPPY NIPUP PIPED PIPER PIPES PIPET PIPIT PIPPA PIPPI RIPAT RIPEN RIPER RIPON RIPUP SIPON TIPIN TIPIS TIPPI TIPPY TIPSY TIPUP VIPER WIPED WIPER WIPES YIPES ZIPBY ZIPIN ZIPIT ZIPON ZIPPO ZIPPY ZIPUP

•I•P•

BIPPY DIPPY FIRPO GIMPS GIMPY HIPPO HIPPY KIMPO LIMPS LIMPY LIPPI LIPPO LIPPY LISPS NIPPY PIPPA PIPPI SIMPS SIXPM TIPPI TIPPY WIMPS WIMPY WISPS WISPY ZIPPO ZIPPY

•I••P

AIRUP BICEP BIDUP BITUP DIDUP DIGUP FITUP FIXUP GINUP HITUP LIEUP LITUP MIXUP NIPUP PINUP RIGUP RIPUP SIRUP SITUP SIXUP TIEUP TIPUP ZIPUP

••IP•

BLIPS CHIPS CLIPS CLIPT DRIPS EDIPO FLIPS GRIPE GRIPS GRIPY KRIPS QTIPS QUIPS QUIPU SHIPS SKIPS SLIPS SNIPE SNIPS STIPE SWIPE TRIPE TRIPP TRIPS VOIPS WHIPS WHIPT

••I•P

BLIMP CHIMP CHIRP CRIMP CRISP PRIMP QUILP QUISP SKIMP TRIPP TWIRP

•••IP

ADRIP ATRIP EQUIP IMHIP ISLIP JOSIP NOTIP OXLIP RECIP REDIP RETIP REZIP SCRIP STRIP TULIP UNHIP

UNRIP UNZIP VCHIP

IQ•••
IQBAL IQUIT

I••Q•
IRAQI

5 IQ

•IQ••
PIQUE

•I•Q•
SISQO

•••IQ
ANTIQ LOWIQ TARIQ

IR•••
IRABU IRANI IRAQI IRATE IRENA IRENE IRIDO IRIDS IRINA IRISH IRKED IRKER IROCS IRONS IRONY IRREG IRVIN IRWIN

I•R••
INRED INREM INRUN IPRAY IRREG

I••R•
IATRO IATRY IBARS IBERT ICARE ICERS IMARI INARI INCRS INDRA INDRE INERT INFRA INORG INTRA INTRO INURE ISERE ITERS IVORY IYARS

I•••R
ICHOR ICIER IDLER IFOUR IHEAR ILLER INCUR INFER INFOR INGER INKER INNER INSTR INTER INVER IRKER IZMIR

•IR••
AIRED AIRER AIRES AIRUP BIRCH BIRDS BIRDY BIRLS BIROS BIRRA BIRRI BIRRS BIRSE BIRTH CIRCA CIRCE CIRCS CIRES CIRRI CIRRO DIRAC DIRAE DIRAM DIRER DIRGE DIRKS DIRTS DIRTY FIRED FIRER FIRES FIRMA FIRMS FIRNS FIRPO FIRRY FIRST FIRTH GIRDS GIRLS GIRLY GIROS GIRSH GIRTH GIRTS HIRAM HIRED HIREE HIRER HIRES KIRBY KIRIN KIRKS KIROV LIRAS MIRED MIRES MIRIN MIROS MIRRO MIRTH MIRVS PIRNS QIRSH SIRED SIREE SIREN SIRES SIRUP TIRED TIRES TIROL TIROS VIRAL VIREO VIRGA VIRGO VIRID VIRNA VIRTU VIRUS WIRED WIRER WIRES WIRTH

•I•R•
BIERE BIERI BIERS BIORE BIRRA BIRRI BIRRS CIERA CIRRI CIRRO CITRI CITRO DIARY DIORS FIBRE FIBRO FIERO FIERS FIERY FIORD FIORE FIORI FIRRY HIERO LIARS LIBRA LIBRE LIBRI LIBRO LITRE LIVRE MICRA MICRO MIERS MIRRO MITRE NIDRE NIORT NITRE NITRO PIERS TIARA TIERS TIGRE TITRE VIERS VITRI VITRO VIVRE

•I••R
AIDER AILUR AIMER AIRER BIDER BIKER BITER CIDER CIGAR CITER DICER DIKER DINAR DINER DIRER DIVER DIYER EIDER EIGER EINER FIBER FIFER FILAR FILER FINER FIRER FIVER FIXER GIBER GIVER HIDER HIKER HIRER HIVER JIVER KINER KISER KITER LIBER LIDAR LIFAR LIFER LIGER LIKER LINER LITER LIVER MILER MIMER MINER MINOR MISER MITER MIXER MIZAR NICER NIGER NINER NITER NIXER NIZER OILER PIKER PILAR PILER PINER PIPER PIXAR RICER RIDER RIFER RIGOR RIKER RIMER RIPER RISER RIVER SITAR SIXER SIZER TIBER TIGER TILER TIMER TIMOR TITER VICAR VIDOR VIGOR VILER VINER VIPER VISOR VIZIR VIZOR WIDER WIPER WIRER WISER

••IR•
AFIRE AKIRA AMIRI AMIRS BAIRD BAIRN BEIRA BGIRL BOIRE CAIRN CAIRO CHIRO CHIRP CHIRR COIRS CUIRE DAIRY EMIRS FAIRE FAIRS FAIRY FLIRS FLIRT HAIRS HAIRY HEIRS KEIRA LAIRD LAIRS LOIRE MAIRE MOIRA MOIRE NAIRA NOIRE NOIRS PAIRS POIRE QUIRE QUIRK QUIRT SAIRY SCIRE SHIRE SHIRK SHIRR SHIRT SKIRL SKIRT SMIRK SOIRS SPIRE SPIRO SPIRY STIRS SWIRL TBIRD THIRD TWIRL TWIRP WEIRD WEIRS WHIRL WHIRR WHIRS ZAIRE

••I•R
AVIOR BRIAR BRIER CHIRR CRIER DRIER FLIER FRIAR FRIER GRIER ICIER MEIER OGIER OSIER PLIER PRIER PRIOR SHIER SHIRR SKIER SLIER SPIER TRIER WHIRR WRIER

•••IR
ADAIR AEGIR AESIR AHAIR ASTIR AVOIR BLAIR BYAIR CHAIR CHOIR CLAIR DEAIR DECIR EYRIR FAKIR FAQIR FLAIR IZMIR KEFIR NADIR NOSIR OHAIR ONAIR ONEIR OPHIR PHAIR REAIR STAIR TAPIR THEIR USAIR VIZIR YASIR

IS•••
ISAAC ISAAK ISAID ISAMU ISBNS ISERE ISHAM ISIAH ISLAM ISLAS ISLES ISLET ISLEY ISLIP ISOLA ISOLT ISSEI ISSEL ISSUE ISSUS ISTIC ISTLE ISTOO ISUZU

I•S••
IBSEN IFSAY IMSET INSET INSTR INSTS INSUM ISSEI ISSEL ISSUE ISSUS ITSME ITSOK

I••S•
IAMSO ICOSA ICOSI IDEST ILOSE INUSE IPASS IRISH IWISH

I•••S
IAMBS IBARS ICBMS ICEES ICERS ICKES ICONS ICTUS IDEAS IDEES IDLES IDOLS IDYLS IGLUS IGNES IGNIS IHOPS ILLUS IMACS IMAMS INCAS INCRS INCUS INDUS INDYS INEES INITS INNES INNIS INSTS IOTAS IOWAS IPASS IPODS IRIDS IROCS IRONS ISBNS ISLAS ISLES ISSUS ITALS ITEAS ITEMS ITERS IVIES IVINS IYARS IZODS

•IS••
AISHA AISLE AISNE BISON CISCO CISSY CISTS DISCI DISCO DISCS DISHY DISKO DISKS DISME DISTS EISEN FISCS FISHY FISKE FISTS GISMO GISTS HISSY HISTO KISER KISKA KISSY LISLE LISPS LISSE LISTS LISZT MISDO MISER MISHA MISOS MISSA MISSM MISSY MISTI MISTS MISTY NISAN NISEI NISUS PISAN PISCI PISMO PISTE RISEN RISER RISES RISHI RISKS RISKY SISAL SISQO SISSY TISCH TISHA TISNT VISAS VISED VISES VISIT VISOR VISTA WISED WISER WISES WISHY WISPS WISPY

•I•S•
AINSI BIRSE BITSY CISSY DIDSO DIDST DIPSO DIPSY DITSY FIRST GINSU GIPSY GIRSH HISSY KIOSK KISSY LIESL LIEST LISSE MIDST MIMSY MINSK MISSA MISSM MISSY PINSK PIUSI PIUSV PIUSX QIRSH RINSE RINSO SISSY TIPSY WIEST

•I••S
AIDES AILES AINUS AIRES AIWAS BIBBS BIDES BIERS BIFFS BIGGS BIKES BILES BILKS BILLS BINDS BINES BINGS BIOGS BIRDS BIRLS BIROS BIRRS BITES BITTS CIAOS CIELS CIENS CINES CIONS CIRCS CIRES CISTS CITES DIALS DIAMS DICES DICKS DICTS DIDOS DIELS DIEMS DIETS DIFFS DIGGS DIKES DILLS DIMAS DIMES DINES DINGS DINKS DINOS DINTS DIORS DIRKS DIRTS DISCS DISKS DISTS DIVAS DIVES EINES FIATS FICUS FIDES FIEFS FIERS FIFES FILAS FILES FILLS FILMS FILOS FINDS FINES FINIS FINKS FINNS FINOS FIRES FIRMS FIRNS FISCS FISTS FIVES FIXES GIBBS GIBES GIBUS GIFTS GILAS GILDS GILES GILLS GILTS GIMPS GIRDS GIRLS GIROS GIRTS GISTS GIVES HICKS HIDES HIFIS HIGHS HIHOS HIJAS HIJOS HIKES HILLS HILTS HIMES HINDS HINES HINTS HIRES HIVES JIBES JIFFS JIGGS JILTS JINKS JINNS JIVES KICKS KILLS KILNS KILOS KILTS KINAS KINDS KINGS KINKS KIRKS KITES KITTS KIVAS KIWIS LIARS LICKS LIDOS LIENS LIEUS LIFTS LIKES LILTS LIMAS LIMBS LIMES LIMNS LIMOS LIMPS LINCS LINES LINGS LINKS LINOS LINTS LINUS LIONS LIRAS LISPS LISTS LITES LIVES MICAS MIDAS MIDIS MIELS MIENS MIERS MIFFS MIKES MILES MILKS MILLS MILOS MIMES MINAS MINDS MINES MINIS MINKS MINOS MINTS MINUS MIRES MIROS MIRVS MISOS MISTS MITAS MITES MITTS MIXES NICKS NIDUS NIELS NIKES NILES NIMES NINAS NINES NINOS NIPAS NISUS NITES NIXES OINKS PICAS PICKS PICTS PIEDS PIELS PIERS PIKAS PIKES PILES PILLS PILUS PIMAS PINES PINGS PINKS PINTS PIONS PIOUS PIPES PIRNS PITAS PITHS PITTS PITYS RIALS RICES RICKS RIDES RIELS RIENS RIFFS RIFTS RIGGS RILES RILLS RIMES RINDS RINGS RINKS RIOTS RISES RISKS RITES RIVES SIDES SIFTS SIGHS SIGNS SIKAS SIKES SIKHS SILAS SILKS SILLS SILOS SILTS SIMMS SIMPS SINES SINGS SINKS SINUS SIRES SITES SIXES SIZES TIBBS TICKS TICOS TIDES TIEGS TIERS TIFFS TIKES TIKIS TILES TILLS TILTS TIMES TINES TINGS TINTS TIOUS TIPIS TIRES TIROS TITIS TITUS TIVOS TIWAS TIXLS VIALS VIBES VICES VICKS VIDAS VIERS VIEWS VIKES VILAS VINAS VINES VINOS VIOLS VIRUS VISAS VISES VITAS VITUS VIVAS WICKS WIKIS WILDS WILES WILLS WILTS WIMPS WINDS WINES WINGS WINKS WIPES WIRES WISES WISPS WIVES WIZES YIKES YIPES ZILLS ZINCS ZINES ZINGS ZITIS

••IS•
ALISA ALIST AMISH AMISS ANISE APISH ARISE AVISO BAISA BLISH BLISS BLIST BOISE BRISE BRISK CRISP CRIST DAISY DEISM DEIST DOISY ELISA ELISE ELIST EPISC ERISA ESIST EXIST FOIST FRISE FRISK FRIST GEIST GRISE GRIST GUISE HAISE HEISS HEIST HOIST IRISH IWISH JOIST KNISH KRISS LUISA LUISE MOIST NAISH NOISE NOISY ODIST PAISA PAISE PHISH POISE PRISM PRISS QUISP RAISA RAISE REISZ SEISM SHISH SWISH SWISS TRISH TWIST WAIST WEISS WEISZ WHISH WHISK WHIST WRIST ZEISS ZEIST

••I•S
ABIES ACIDS ADINS ADIOS ADITS AGIOS AKINS ALIAS ALIFS ALIOS AMIES AMIRS AMISS ANILS ARIAS ARIES ARILS ASICS AVIAS AXILS AYINS BAIES BAILS BAITS BEINS BLIPS BLISS BOILS BRIES BRIGS BRIMS BRITS CAIUS CEILS CHIAS CHICS CHINS CHIOS CHIPS CHITS CLIOS CLIPS COIFS COILS COINS COIRS CRIBS CRIES CRITS CRIUS DEILS DJINS DOITS DRIBS DRIES DRIPS

EDIES
EDITS
EFIKS
ELIAS
EMIRS
EMITS
EPICS
ERIAS
ERIES
EVILS
EXITS
FAILS
FAIMS
FAIRS
FLICS
FLIES
FLIPS
FLIRS
FLITS
FOIES
FOILS
FRIES
FRITS
GAINS
GAITS
GAIUS
GLIAS
GLIMS
GRIDS
GRIGS
GRINS
GRIPS
GRITS
HAIKS
HAILS
HAIRS
HEIRS
HEISS
HUITS
INITS
IRIDS
IVIES
IVINS
JAILS
JAINS
JOINS
JUINS
KNITS
KRIPS
KRISS
LAICS
LAIRS
LAITS
LAIUS
LOIDS
LOINS
MAIDS
MAILS
MAIMS
MAINS
MOILS
NAIFS
NAILS
NOILS
NOIRS
NUITS
OBIES
OBITS
OKIES
OLIOS
OMITS
OWIES
PAILS
PAINS
PAIRS
PLIES
PRIES
PRIGS
PRIMS
PRISS
PRIUS
QAIDS
QTIPS
QUIDS
QUIPS
QUITS
RAIDS
RAILS
RAINS
REIMS
REINS
REITS
ROILS
RUINS
SAILS
SHIES
SHIMS
SHINS
SHIPS
SHIVS
SKIDS
SKIES
SKIMS
SKINS
SKIPS
SKITS
SLIMS
SLIPS
SLITS
SMITS
SNIPS
SNITS
SOILS
SOIRS
SPIES
SPINS
SPITS
STIES
STIRS
SUITS
SWIGS
SWIMS
SWISS
TAILS
THINS
TOILS
TRIES
TRIMS
TRIOS
TRIPS
TWIGS
TWINS
TWITS
UNITS
UNIVS
UTILS
VEILS
VEINS
VOIDS
VOIPS
WAIFS
WAILS
WAINS
WAITS
WEIRS
WEISS
WHIGS
WHIMS
WHIPS
WHIRS
WHITS
WRITS
ZEISS

•••IS

ABRIS
ADDIS
AEGIS
AKAIS
ALAIS
ALLIS
ALOIS
ANAIS
ANTIS
APHIS
APSIS
ARRIS
ARSIS
ARTIS
AUDIS
AULIS
BASIS
BLAIS
BLOIS
BORIS
CADIS
CANIS
CEDIS
CHAIS
CHRIS
CUTIS
DALIS
DAMIS
DAVIS
DELIS
DENIS
DORIS
ELLIS
ELPIS
ELVIS
ENNIS
EQUIS
ETUIS
EXGIS
FARIS
FELIS
FINIS
FRAIS
FUJIS
HAJIS
HIFIS
HOPIS
HOVIS
IGNIS
INNIS
JANIS
JURIS
KEPIS
KIWIS
KOJIS
LAPIS
LARIS
LENIS
LEVIS
LEWIS
LEXIS
LORIS
LOUIS
LWEIS
LYSIS
MARIS
MAVIS
MAXIS
MELIS
METIS
MIDIS
MINIS
MOWIS
MUNIS
NARIS
NAVIS
NAZIS
NEHIS
NEVIS
NEXIS
NOBIS
NORIS
OASIS
OMNIS
ORNIS
ORRIS
ORVIS
OTTIS
PANIS
PARIS
PERIS
POLIS
PULIS
QUAIS
RAMIS
RANIS
REFIS
REGIS
SAKIS
SAMIS
SARIS
SEMIS
SUFIS
TABIS
TANIS
TAPIS
TATIS
TAVIS
TAXIS
THAIS
TIKIS
TIPIS
TITIS
TOPIS
TROIS
TUNIS
UGLIS
VADIS
WADIS
WIKIS
XAXIS
YAXIS
YETIS
YOGIS
YURIS
ZAXIS
ZITIS
ZORIS
ZUNIS

IT•••

ITALO
ITALS
ITALY
ITCHY
ITEAS
ITEMS
ITERS
ITILE
ITINA
ITSME
ITSOK

I•T••

IATRO
IATRY
ICTUS
IDTAG
INTEL
INTER
INTOW
INTRA
INTRO
INTWO
IOTAS
ISTIC
ISTLE
ISTOO

I••T•

INITS
INSTR
INSTS
IRATE

I•••T

IBERT
ICANT
ICEIT
IDENT
IDEST
IDIOT
IDONT
IFNOT
IMHOT
IMOUT
IMSET
INAPT
INEPT
INERT
INGOT
INLET
INPUT
INSET
INUIT
IQUIT
ISLET
ISOLT
IWANT
IWONT

•IT••

AITCH
BITER
BITES
BITIN
BITON
BITSY
BITTE
BITTS
BITTY
BITUP
CITED
CITEE
CITER
CITES
CITGO
CITRI
CITRO
DITAT
DITCH
DITKA
DITSY
DITTO
DITTY
DITZY
FITCH
FITIN
FITLY
FITON
FITUP
GITGO
GITMO
HITAT
HITCH
HITIN
HITIT
HITME
HITON
HITUP
KITED
KITER
KITES
KITTS
KITTY
LITEL
LITER
LITES
LITHE
LITHO
LITON
LITRE
LITTB
LITTD
LITUP
MITAS
MITCH
MITER
MITES
MITLA
MITRE
MITTS
MITTY
MITYA
MITZI
NITER
NITES
NITID
NITON
NITRE
NITRO
NITTI
NITTY
PITAS
PITCH
PITHS
PITHY
PITON
PITOT
PITTI
PITTS
PITYS
RITES
RITZY
SITAR
SITAT
SITBY
SITED
SITES
SITIN
SITKA
SITON
SITUP
TITAN
TITER
TITHE
TITIS
TITLE
TITOV
TITRE
TITUS
VITAE
VITAL
VITAM
VITAS
VITRI
VITRO
VITUS
WITCH
WITTE
WITTY
ZITIS

•I•T•

BIOTA
BIRTH
BITTE
BITTS
BITTY
CISTS
DICTA
DICTS
DICTU
DIDTO
DIETE
DIETS
DIETZ
DINTS
DINTY
DIRTS
DIRTY
DISTS
DITTO
DITTY
FIATS
FIFTH
FIFTY
FILTH
FIRTH
FISTS
GIFTS
GILTS
GIRTH
GIRTS
GISTS
HILTS
HINTS
HIPTO
HISTO
JILTS
KILTS
KINTE
KITTS
KITTY
LIETO
LIFTS
LILTS
LINTS
LINTY
LISTS
LITTB
LITTD
MIATA
MINTS
MINTY
MIRTH
MISTI
MISTS
MISTY
MITTS
MITTY
NIETA
NIETO
NIFTY
NINTH
NITTI
NITTY
PICTO
PICTS
PIETA
PIETY
PINTA
PINTO
PINTS
PISTE
PITTI
PITTS
PIUTE
RIATA
RIETI
RIFTS
RINTY
RIOTS
SIETE
SIFTS
SILTS
SILTY
SIXTH
SIXTY
TIETO
TILTH
TILTS
TINTS
UINTA
VIRTU
VISTA
WIDTH
WILTS
WIRTH
WITTE
WITTY

•I••T

AIMAT
BIDET
BIGHT
BIGOT
BINET
BIONT
BIZET
CIVET
DICOT
DIDIT
DIDNT
DIDST
DIGAT
DIGIT
DITAT
DIVOT
DIXIT
EIGHT
EILAT
FIGHT
FILET
FIRST
FIXIT
GIANT
GIGOT
HIHAT
HITAT
HITIT
LICHT
LICIT
LIEST
LIEUT
LIGHT
LIMIT
LINDT
LINFT
LISZT
MIDST
MIGHT
MINOT
NICHT
NIGHT
NIORT
NIPAT
PICOT
PIGIT
PILOT
PINOT
PIPET
PIPIT
PITOT
PIVOT
RIANT
RIGHT
RIPAT
RIVET
SIGHT
SITAT
TIANT
TIBET
TIGHT
TINCT
TISNT
VINGT
VISIT
WIEST
WIGHT
WINAT
ZIPIT

••IT•

ADITS
AGITA
AKITA
ALITO
ALITY
AMITE
AMITY
ANITA
ARITH
BAITS
BLITT
BLITZ
BOITE
BOITO
BRITE
BRITH
BRITS
BRITT
BRITZ
CHITA
CHITS
CRITS
DEITY
DOITS
EDITH
EDITS
ELITE
EMITS
ERITU
EVITA
EVITE
EXITS
FAITH
FLITS
FRITA
FRITE
FRITO
FRITS
FRITZ
GAITS
GLITZ
GRITS
HAITI
HOITY
HUITS
INITS
KEITH
KNITS
LAITS
LAITY
LEITH
NUITS
OBITS
OMITS
OVITZ
QUITE
QUITO
QUITS
RAITA
RAITT
REITS
SAITH
SKITS
SLITS
SMITE
SMITH
SMITS
SNITS
SPITE
SPITS
SPITZ
SUITE
SUITS
TAITO
TOITY
TRITE
TRITT
TWITS
UNITA
UNITE
UNITS
UNITY
WAITE
WAITS
WAITZ
WEITZ
WHITE
WHITS
WRITE
WRITS

••I•T

ALIST
ARIOT
ATILT
BLIST
BLITT
BRITT
BUILT
CAINT
CLIFT
CLINT
CLIPT
CRIST
DEIST
DRIFT
EDICT
ELIOT
ELIST
ESIST
EVICT
EXIST
FAINT
FEINT
FLINT
FLIRT
FOIST
FRIST
GEIST
GLINT
GRIFT
GRINT
GRIOT
GRIST
GUILT
HEIDT
HEIST
HOIST
IDIOT
JOINT
JOIST
KLIMT
MOIST
ODIST
PAINT
POINT
PRINT
QUIET
QUILT
QUINT
QUIRT
RAITT
SAINT
SHIFT
SHIRT
SKIRT
SPILT
STILT
STINT
SWIFT
TAINT
TRITT
TWIST
TWIXT
UNIAT
VEIDT
WAIST
WHIPT
WHIST
WRIST
ZEIST

•••IT

ACEIT
ADMIT
AMBIT
AMLIT
ASFIT
ATEIT
AUDIT
AWAIT
AWHIT
BAGIT
BARIT
BEFIT
BRUIT
BUYIT
CANIT
COPIT
CUBIT
CUTIT
DAVIT
DEBIT
DEMIT
DIDIT
DIGIT
DIXIT
DOGIT
DROIT
DUGIT
EATIT
ENDIT
FIXIT
FRUIT
FUGIT
GETIT
GOSIT
GOTIT
GSUIT
GUNIT
HABIT
HADIT
HASIT
HITIT
ICEIT
INUIT
IQUIT
JUDIT
KOPIT
KRAIT
LAMIT
LEGIT
LEVIT
LICIT
LIMIT
MEDIT
MERIT
NOHIT
NOTIT
ONDIT
OPCIT
ORBIT
PETIT
PEWIT
PIGIT
PIPIT
PLAIT
POLIT
POSIT
QUOIT
REFIT
REHIT
RELIT
REMIT
RESIT
SAYIT
SPLIT
SPRIT
TACIT
TOBIT
TOWIT
TRAIT
TRYIT
TVHIT
UNBIT
UNFIT
UNHIT
UNLIT
UPLIT
USEIT
VISIT
WASIT
ZIPIT

I•U••

IGUAL
INUIT
INURE
INUSE
IQUIT
ISUZU

I••U•

ICEUP
ICTUS
IFOUR
IGLUS
ILEUM
ILIUM
ILLUS
IMBUE
IMOUT
INCUR
INCUS
INDUE
INDUS
INFUN
INJUN
INPUT
INRUN
INSUM
ISSUE
ISSUS

I•••U

ILGWU
IMAMU
INONU
IOWAU
IRABU
ISAMU
ISUZU

•IU••

PIUSI
PIUSV
PIUSX
PIUTE

•I•U•

AILUR
AINUS
AIRUP
BIDUP
BITUP
DIDUP
DIEUX
DIGUP
FICUS
FILUM
FITUP
FIXUP
GIBUS
GIGUE
GINUP
HILUM
HITUP
LIEUP
LIEUS
LIEUT
LIKUD
LINUS
LINUX
LITUP
MIEUX
MINUS
MIXUP
NIDUS
NIEUW
NIPUP
NISUS
PIAUI
PILUS
PINUP
PIOUS
PIQUE
RIGUP
RIPUP
SINUS
SIOUX
SIRUP
SITUP
SIXUP
TIEUP
TIOUS
TIPUP
TITUS
VIEUX
VIRUS
VITUS
ZIPUP

•I••U

BIJOU
DICTU
FICHU
GINSU
HINDU
LINGU
MIAOU
PILAU
RICEU
VIRTU

••IU•

ARIUM
BAIUL
CAIUS
CRIUS
GAIUS
ILIUM
LAIUS
ODIUM
OPIUM
ORIUM
PRIUS

••I•U

ADIEU
AEIOU
ELIHU
ERITU
HAIKU
OHIOU
POILU
QUIPU
THIEU

IV•••

IVANA
IVANI
IVANV
IVIED
IVIES
IVINS
IVORY

I•V••

INVER
IRVIN

I••V•

IFIVE
IGIVE
ILOVE
IMOVE

I•••V

INDIV
IVANV

•IV••

CIVET
CIVIC
CIVIL
DIVAC
DIVAN
DIVAS
DIVED
DIVER
DIVES
DIVOT
DIVVY
FIVEA
FIVEB
FIVEC
FIVED
FIVEE
FIVEO
FIVER
FIVES
GIVEN
GIVER
GIVES
HIVED
HIVER
HIVES
JIVED
JIVER
JIVES
JIVEY
KIVAS
LIVED
LIVEN
LIVER
LIVES
LIVIA
LIVID
LIVIN
LIVRE
NIVAL
NIVEA
NIVEN
PIVEN
PIVOT
RIVAL
RIVED
RIVEN
RIVER
RIVES
RIVET
SIVAN
TIVOS
VIVAS
VIVID
VIVRE
WIVED
WIVES

•I•V•

DIVVY
MIRVS
NIEVE
PIAVE
SIEVE
SILVA

•I••V

KIROV
PIUSV
TITOV

••IV•

ALIVE
ATIVE
BFIVE
CHIVE
CHIVY
CLIVE
DRIVE
IFIVE
IGIVE
NAIVE
OGIVE
OLIVA
OLIVE
PRIVY
SHIVA
SHIVS
UNIVS
WAIVE

•••IV

ACTIV
ANNIV
CCCIV
CCLIV
CCXIV
CDLIV
CDXIV
CLXIV
CMLIV
CMXIV
CXCIV
CXLIV
CXXIV
DCCIV
DCLIV
DCXIV
DERIV
DLXIV
DXCIV
DXLIV
DXXIV
EQUIV
EXDIV

INDIV
LEOIV
LXXIV
MCCIV
MCDIV
MCLIV
MCMIV
MCXIV
MDCIV
MDLIV
MDXIV
MLXIV
MMCIV
MMDIV
MMLIV
MMMIV
MMXIV
MXCIV
MXLIV
MXXIV
RAJIV
XXXIV

IW•••
IWANT
IWILL
IWISH
IWONT

I•W••
IOWAN
IOWAS
IOWAU
IOWAY
IRWIN

I••W•
ILGWU
INAWE
INTWO

I•••W
IKNOW
INLAW
INLOW
INTOW

•IW••
AIWAS
KIWIS
TIWAS

•I•W•
KIOWA
VIEWS
VIEWY

•I••W
BILLW
MIAOW
MINOW
NIEUW
SINEW
WIDOW

••IW•
DAIWA
SLIWA

IX•••
IXION
IXNAY

I•••X
ICEAX
IMMIX
INBOX
INDEX
INFIX

•IX••
BIXBY
DIXIE
DIXIT
DIXON
FIXED
FIXER
FIXES
FIXIT
FIXON
FIXUP
MIXED
MIXER
MIXES
MIXIN
MIXUP
NIXED
NIXER
NIXES
NIXIE
NIXON
PIXAR
PIXEL
PIXIE
RIXEY
SIXAD
SIXAM
SIXBC
SIXED
SIXEE
SIXER
SIXES
SIXNO
SIXPM
SIXTH
SIXTY
SIXUP
TIXLS
VIXEN

•I••X
DIEUX
LINUX
MIEUX
PIUSX
SILEX
SINEX
SIOUX
TILEX
TIMEX
VIEUX

••IX•
TWIXT

•••IX
ADMIX
AFFIX
ATSIX
CALIX
CCCIX
CCLIX
CCXIX
CDLIX
CDXIX
CLXIX
CMLIX
CMXIX
COMIX
CROIX
CXCIX
CXLIX
CXXIX
DCCIX
DCLIX
DCXIX
DLXIX
DXCIX
DXLIX
DXXIX
FELIX
FTDIX
HELIX
IMMIX
INFIX
LEOIX
LXXIX
MCCIX
MCDIX
MCLIX
MCMIX
MCXIX
MDCIX
MDLIX
MDXIX
MLXIX
MMCIX
MMDIX
MMLIX
MMMIX
MMXIX
MXCIX
MXLIX
MXXIX
RADIX
REFIX
REMIX
UNFIX
UNMIX
XXXIX

IY•••
IYARS

I•Y••
IDYLL
IDYLS

I••Y•
ILLYA
INDYS

I•••Y
IATRY
ICILY
IFSAY
IMPLY
INKEY
INLAY
INMAY
IOWAY
IPRAY
IRONY
ISLEY
ITALY
ITCHY
IVORY
IXNAY

•IY••
DIYER
RIYAL

•I•Y•
LIBYA
MITYA
PITYS
SIBYL
VINYL

•I••Y
AILEY
BIALY
BIDDY
BIGGY
BIGLY
BILGY
BILLY
BIPPY
BIRDY
BITSY
BITTY
BIXBY
CIGGY
CINCY
CINDY
CISSY
DIARY
DICEY
DICKY
DIDBY
DIGBY
DILLY
DIMLY
DINDY
DINGY
DINKY
DINNY
DINTY
DIPPY
DIPSY
DIRTY
DISHY
DITSY
DITTY
DITZY
DIVVY
DIZZY
FIERY
FIFTY
FILLY
FILMY
FINNY
FIRRY
FISHY
FITLY
FIZZY
GIDDY
GIMPY
GINNY
GIPSY
GIRLY
HIDEY
HILLY
HINKY
HINNY
HIPLY
HIPPY
HISSY
JIFFY
JIGGY
JIMMY
JIVEY
KICKY
KIDDY
KILBY
KILEY
KILLY
KINKY
KIRBY
KISSY
KITTY
LIBBY
LIDDY
LIEBY
LILLY
LIMPY
LINDY
LINTY
LIPPY
MICKY
MIDDY
MIFFY
MIKEY
MILKY
MIMSY
MINDY
MINEY
MINGY
MINTY
MISSY
MISTY
MITTY
NICKY
NIFTY
NILLY
NIMBY
NIMOY
NINNY
NIPPY
NITTY
PICKY
PIETY
PIGGY
PINEY
PINKY
PITHY
RIBBY
RICKY
RIDGY
RIGBY
RILEY
RINDY
RINKY
RINTY
RISKY
RITZY
RIXEY
SILKY
SILLY
SILTY
SISSY
SITBY
SIXTY
TICKY
TILLY
TIMMY
TINNY
TIPPY
TIPSY
TIZZY
VICHY
VICKY
VIEWY
VIGNY
VIJAY
VINCY
VINNY
WIFEY
WIGGY
WILBY
WILEY
WILLY
WIMPY
WINBY
WINDY
WINGY
WISHY
WISPY
WITTY
ZIGGY
ZINCY
ZINGY
ZINKY
ZIPBY
ZIPPY

••IY•
TYIYN

••I•Y
ACIDY
ALITY
AMITY
BRINY
CHIVY
CSINY
DAILY
DAIRY
DAISY
DEIFY
DEITY
DOILY
DOISY
DRILY
EDIFY
EMILY
FAIRY
GAILY
GRIMY
GRIPY
HAIRY
HOITY
ICILY
JUICY
LAITY
MTIDY
NOILY
NOISY
PLINY
PRICY
PRIVY
RAINY
REIFY
ROILY
SAIRY
SHINY
SLIMY
SPICY
SPIKY
SPINY
SPIRY
TOITY
TWINY
UNIFY
UNITY
VEINY
WHINY

IZ•••
IZAAK
IZMIR
IZODS

I••Z•
IBIZA
ISUZU

•IZ••
BIZET
DIZZY
FIZZY
GIZMO
LIZZI
MIZAR
NIZER
PIZZA
RIZAL
RIZZO
SIZED
SIZER
SIZES
TIZZY
VIZIR
VIZOR
WIZEN
WIZES

•I•Z•
DITZY
DIZZY
FIZZY
GINZA
LISZT
LIZZI
MITZI
PINZA
PIZZA
RITZY
RIZZO
TIZZY

•I••Z
DIETZ

••IZ•
BAIZA
BAIZE
ELIZA
FRIZZ
IBIZA
MAIZE
PRIZE
PRIZM
SEIZE

••I•Z
BLITZ
BRITZ
FRITZ
FRIZZ
GLITZ
HEINZ
MAINZ
OVITZ
REISZ
SPITZ
WAITZ
WEISZ
WEITZ

•••IZ
ADBIZ
CADIZ
FELIZ
HAFIZ
MONIZ
ORTIZ

JA•••
JABBA
JABOT
JACAL
JACET
JACEY
JACKO
JACKS
JACKY
JACOB
JADED
JADES
JAFAR
JAFFA
JAFFE
JAGGY
JAHAN
JAHRE
JAILS
JAIME
JAINS
JAKES
JAKOB
JALPA
JAMAL
JAMBA
JAMBE
JAMBS
JAMES
JAMIE
JAMIN
JAMON
JAMUP
JANDB
JANDJ
JANET
JANIE
JANIS
JANOS
JANUS
JAPAN
JAPED
JAPER
JAPES
JARED
JARRE
JASON
JATOS
JAUNE
JAUNT
JAVAN
JAVAS
JAWAT
JAWED
JAWER
JAYNE
JAZZY

J•A••
JBARS
JEANE
JEANS
JIANG
JOADS
JPAUL
JUANO

J••A•
JACAL
JAFAR
JAHAN
JAMAL
JAPAN
JAVAN
JAVAS
JAWAT
JEHAN
JIHAD
JIHAN
JOHAN
JONAH
JONAS
JOTAS
JOVAN
JUBAL
JUDAH
JUDAS
JUGAL
JURAL
JURAN

J•••A
JABBA
JAFFA
JALPA
JAMBA
JENNA
JETTA
JIDDA
JOLLA
JUDEA
JULIA
JUMNA
JUNTA

•JA••
OJAYS

•J•A•
VJDAY

•J••A
DJUNA
OJEDA

••JA•
FAJAS
HIJAS
KOJAK
LUJAN
RAJAB
RAJAH
RAJAS
ROJAS
SAJAK
UNJAM
VIJAY

••J•A
WAJDA

•••JA
ABUJA
NADJA
NINJA
OUIJA
RIOJA
SONJA
VIEJA

JB•••
JBARS

J•B••
JABBA
JABOT
JIBED
JIBES
JUBAL

J••B•
JABBA
JAMBA
JAMBE
JAMBS
JUMBO

J•••B
JACOB
JAKOB
JANDB

••J•B
MCJOB
RAJAB

JC•••
JCREW

J•C••
JACAL
JACET
JACEY
JACKO
JACKS
JACKY
JACOB
JOCKO
JOCKS
JUCOS

J••C•
JOYCE
JUICE
JUICY
JUNCO

J•••C
JOHNC
JROTC

•J•C•
EJECT

J•D••
JADED
JADES
JIDDA
JODIE
JUDAH
JUDAS
JUDDS
JUDEA
JUDEO
JUDES
JUDGE
JUDIT
JUDOS

J••D•
JANDB
JANDJ
JEUDI
JIDDA
JOADS
JUDDS

J•••D
JADED
JAPED
JARED
JAWED
JIBED
JIHAD
JIVED
JOHND
JOKED
JOYED
JUKED

•JD••
VJDAY

•J•D•
EJIDO
OJEDA

•J••D
FJORD

••JD•
WAJDA

JE•••
JEANE
JEANS
JEEPS
JEERS
JEERY
JEFES
JEFFY
JEHAN
JELLO
JELLS
JELLY
JENNA
JENNY
JENOS
JEREZ
JERKS
JERKY
JERNE
JERRY
JERZY
JESSE
JESSY
JESTS
JESUS
JETER
JETES
JETLI
JETTA
JETTY
JEUDI
JEUNE
JEWEL
JEWRY

J•E••
JEEPS
JEERS
JEERY
JOEYS
JPEGS
JUEGO

J••E•
JACET
JACEY
JADED
JADES
JAKES
JAMES
JANET
JAPED
JAPER
JAPES
JARED
JAWED
JAWER
JCREW
JEFES
JEREZ
JETER
JETES
JEWEL
JIBED
JIBES
JIVED
JIVER
JIVES
JIVEY
JOKED
JOKER
JOKES
JOKEY
JONES
JOREL
JOSEF
JOSEY
JOYED
JUDEA
JUDEO
JUDES
JUKED
JUKES
JULEP
JULES
JULEY
JUNES
JUTES

J•••E
JAFFE
JAHRE
JAIME
JAMBE
JAMIE
JANIE
JARRE
JAUNE
JAYNE
JEANE
JERNE
JESSE
JEUNE
JODIE
JOFFE
JOLIE
JONZE
JORGE
JOSIE
JOULE
JOUVE
JOYCE
JTILE
JUDGE
JUICE
JULIE
JUSTE

•JE••
EJECT
OJEDA

••JE•
BAJER
BOJER
MUJER
NYJET
OBJET

••J•E
GIJOE
STJOE

•••JE
KOPJE

JF•••
JFKJR

J•F••
JAFAR
JAFFA
JAFFE
JEFES
JEFFY
JIFFS
JIFFY
JOFFE

J••F•
JAFFA
JAFFE
JEFFY
JIFFS
JIFFY
JOFFE

J•••F
JOHNF
JOSEF

J•G••
JAGGY
JIGGS
JIGGY
JUGAL

J••G•
JAGGY
JIGGS
JIGGY
JINGO
JONGG
JORGE
JPEGS
JUDGE
JUEGO

J•••G
JIANG
JONGG

••J•G
REJIG

J•H••
JAHAN
JAHRE
JEHAN
JIHAD
JIHAN
JOHAN
JOHNC
JOHND
JOHNF
JOHNI
JOHNJ
JOHNL
JOHNP
JOHNQ
JOHNS
JOHNV
JOHNX

J•••H
JONAH
JUDAH

•J•H•
IJOHN

••J•H
RAJAH

JI•••
JIANG
JIBED
JIBES
JIDDA
JIFFS
JIFFY
JIGGS
JIGGY
JIHAD
JIHAN
JILTS
JIMMY
JINGO
JINKS
JINNI
JINNS
JIVED
JIVER
JIVES
JIVEY

J•I••
JAILS
JAIME
JAINS
JOINS
JOINT
JOIST
JTILE
JUICE
JUICY
JUINS

J••I•
JAMIE
JAMIN
JANIE
JANIS
JODIE
JOLIE
JOSIE
JOSIP
JUDIT
JULIA
JULIE
JULIO
JUNIO
JURIS

J•••I
JETLI
JEUDI
JINNI
JOHNI

•JI••
DJINN
DJINS
EJIDO
UJIJI

•J••I
UJIJI

••JI•
FUJIS
HAJIS
KOJIS
RAJIV
REJIG

••J•I
HAJJI

•••JI
BENJI
HADJI
HAJJI
KANJI
MEIJI
SEIJI
SHOJI
UJIJI

J•J••
JUJUS

J••J•
JFKJR

J•••J
JANDJ
JOHNJ

•J•J•
UJIJI

••JJ•
HAJJI

JK•••
JKLMN

J•K••
JAKES
JAKOB
JFKJR
JOKED
JOKER
JOKES
JOKEY
JUKED
JUKES

J••K•
JACKO
JACKS
JACKY
JERKS
JERKY
JINKS
JOCKO
JOCKS
JUNKS
JUNKY

•JK••
IJKLM

•J••K
BJORK

••JK•
HIJKL

••J•K
KOJAK
SAJAK

•••JK
GHIJK

J•L••
JALPA
JELLO
JELLS
JELLY
JILTS
JKLMN
JOLIE
JOLLA
JOLLY
JOLTS
JOLTY
JULEP
JULES
JULEY
JULIA
JULIE
JULIO
JULYS

J••L•
JAILS
JELLO
JELLS
JELLY
JETLI
JOLLA
JOLLY
JOULE
JOWLS
JOWLY
JTILE

J•••L
JACAL
JAMAL
JEWEL

JOHNL
JOREL
JPAUL
JUBAL
JUGAL
JURAL

•J•L•
IJKLM

••J•L
HIJKL

J•M••
JAMAL
JAMBA
JAMBE
JAMBS
JAMES
JAMIE
JAMIN
JAMON
JAMUP
JIMMY
JUMBO
JUMNA
JUMPS
JUMPY

J••M•
JAIME
JIMMY
JKLMN

J•••M
JORUM

•J••M
IJKLM

••J•M
UNJAM

J•N••
JANDB
JANDJ
JANET
JANIE
JANIS
JANOS
JANUS
JENNA
JENNY
JENOS
JINGO
JINKS
JINNI
JINNS
JONAH
JONAS
JONES
JONGG
JONNY
JONZE
JUNCO
JUNES
JUNIO
JUNKS
JUNKY
JUNTA
JUNTO

J••N•
JAINS
JAUNE
JAUNT
JAYNE
JEANE
JEANS
JENNA
JENNY
JERNE
JEUNE
JIANG
JINNI
JINNS
JOHNC
JOHND
JOHNF
JOHNI
JOHNJ
JOHNL
JOHNP
JOHNQ
JOHNS
JOHNV
JOHNX
JOINS
JOINT
JONNY
JUANO
JUINS
JUMNA

J•••N
JAHAN
JAMIN
JAMON
JAPAN
JASON
JAVAN
JEHAN
JIHAN
JKLMN
JOHAN
JOVAN
JURAN

•J•N•
DJINN
DJINS
DJUNA

•J••N
BJORN
DJINN
IJOHN

••J•N
CAJON
CAJUN
DIJON
INJUN
LUJAN

JO•••
JOADS
JOCKO
JOCKS
JODIE
JOEYS
JOFFE
JOHAN
JOHNC
JOHND
JOHNF
JOHNI
JOHNJ
JOHNL
JOHNP
JOHNQ
JOHNS
JOHNV
JOHNX
JOINS
JOINT
JOIST
JOKED
JOKER
JOKES
JOKEY
JOLIE
JOLLA
JOLLY
JOLTS
JOLTY
JONAH
JONAS
JONES
JONGG
JONNY
JONZE
JOOSS
JOREL
JORGE
JORUM
JOSEF
JOSEY
JOSIE
JOSIP
JOTAS
JOTTO
JOULE
JOURS
JOUST
JOUVE
JOVAN
JOWLS
JOWLY
JOYCE
JOYED

J•O••
JOOSS
JROTC

J••O•
JABOT
JACOB
JAKOB
JAMON
JANOS
JASON
JATOS
JENOS
JUCOS
JUDOS
JUROR

J•••O
JACKO
JELLO
JINGO
JOCKO
JOTTO
JUANO
JUDEO
JUEGO
JULIO
JUMBO
JUNCO
JUNIO
JUNTO

•JO••
BJORK
BJORN
FJORD
IJOHN

•J••O
EJIDO

••JO•
ANJOU
BIJOU
CAJON
DIJON
DOJOS
ENJOY
GIJOE
HIJOS
HOJOS
MAJOR
MCJOB
MOJOS
OHJOY
STJOE

•••JO
ABAJO
BANJO
FLOJO
VIEJO

JP•••
JPAUL
JPEGS

J•P••
JAPAN
JAPED
JAPER
JAPES

J••P•
JALPA
JEEPS
JUMPS
JUMPY

J•••P
JAMUP
JOHNP
JOSIP
JULEP

J•••Q
JOHNQ

JR•••
JROTC

J•R••
JARED
JARRE
JCREW
JEREZ
JERKS
JERKY
JERNE
JERRY
JERZY
JOREL
JORGE
JORUM
JURAL
JURAN
JURIS
JUROR

J••R•
JAHRE
JARRE
JBARS
JEERS
JEERY
JERRY
JEWRY
JOURS

J•••R
JAFAR
JAPER
JAWER
JETER
JFKJR
JIVER
JOKER
JUROR

•J•R•
BJORK
BJORN
FJORD

••J•R
BAJER
BOJER
MAJOR
MUJER

•••JR
JFKJR

J•S••
JASON
JESSE
JESSY
JESTS
JESUS
JOSEF
JOSEY
JOSIE
JOSIP
JUSTE
JUSTY

J••S•
JESSE
JESSY
JOIST
JOOSS
JOUST

J•••S
JACKS
JADES
JAILS
JAINS
JAKES
JAMBS
JAMES
JANIS
JANOS
JANUS
JAPES
JATOS
JAVAS
JBARS
JEANS
JEEPS
JEERS
JEFES
JELLS
JENOS
JERKS
JESTS
JESUS
JETES
JIBES
JIFFS
JIGGS
JILTS
JINKS
JINNS
JIVES
JOADS
JOCKS
JOEYS
JOHNS
JOINS
JOKES
JOLTS
JONAS
JONES
JOOSS
JOTAS
JOURS
JOWLS
JPEGS
JUCOS
JUDAS
JUDDS
JUDES
JUDOS
JUINS
JUJUS
JUKES
JULES
JULYS
JUMPS
JUNES
JUNKS
JURIS
JUTES

•J••S
DJINS
OJAYS

••J•S
ADJTS
AUJUS
DOJOS
FAJAS
FUJIS
HAJIS
HIJAS
HIJOS
HOJOS
JUJUS
KOJIS
MOJOS
RAJAS
ROJAS

JT•••
JTILE

J•T••
JATOS
JETER
JETES
JETLI
JETTA
JETTY
JOTAS
JOTTO
JUTES

J••T•
JESTS
JETTA
JETTY
JILTS
JOLTS
JOLTY
JOTTO
JROTC
JUNTA
JUNTO
JUSTE
JUSTY

J•••T
JABOT
JACET
JANET
JAUNT
JAWAT
JOINT
JOIST
JOUST
JUDIT

•J••T
EJECT

••JT•
ADJTS

••J•T
NYJET
OBJET

JU•••
JUANO
JUBAL
JUCOS
JUDAH
JUDAS
JUDDS
JUDEA
JUDEO
JUDES
JUDGE
JUDIT
JUDOS
JUEGO
JUGAL
JUICE
JUICY
JUINS
JUJUS
JUKED
JUKES
JULEP
JULES
JULEY
JULIA
JULIE
JULIO
JULYS
JUMBO
JUMNA
JUMPS
JUMPY
JUNCO
JUNES
JUNIO
JUNKS
JUNKY
JUNTA
JUNTO
JURAL
JURAN
JURIS
JUROR
JUSTE
JUSTY
JUTES

J•U••
JAUNE
JAUNT
JEUDI
JEUNE
JOULE
JOURS
JOUST
JOUVE

J••U•
JAMUP
JANUS
JESUS
JORUM
JPAUL
JUJUS

•JU••
DJUNA

••JU•
AUJUS
CAJUN
INJUN
JUJUS

••J•U
ANJOU
BIJOU

J•V••
JAVAN
JAVAS
JIVED
JIVER
JIVES
JIVEY
JOVAN

J••V•
JOUVE

J•••V
JOHNV

••J•V
RAJIV

J•W••
JAWAT
JAWED
JAWER
JEWEL
JEWRY
JOWLS
JOWLY

J•••W
JCREW

J•••X
JOHNX

J•Y••
JAYNE
JOYCE
JOYED

J••Y•
JOEYS
JULYS

J•••Y
JACEY
JACKY
JAGGY
JAZZY
JEERY
JEFFY
JELLY
JENNY
JERKY
JERRY
JERZY
JESSY
JETTY
JEWRY
JIFFY
JIGGY
JIMMY
JIVEY
JOKEY
JOLLY
JOLTY
JONNY
JOSEY
JOWLY
JUICY
JULEY
JUMPY
JUNKY
JUSTY

•J•Y•
OJAYS

•J••Y
VJDAY

••J•Y
ENJOY
OHJOY
VIJAY

J•Z••
JAZZY

J••Z•
JAZZY
JERZY
JONZE

J•••Z
JEREZ

KA•••
KABAS
KABOB
KABUL
KADAR
KAFKA
KAHLO
KAHNS
KALEL
KALES
KALKI
KAMEN
KANAR
KANAS
KANDY
KANGA
KANGS
KANIN
KANJI
KANSA
KANYE
KAONS
KAPHS
KAPOK
KAPOW
KAPPA
KAPUT
KARAN
KARAS
KARAT
KAREL
KAREN
KARLA
KARLE
KARMA
KARNS
KAROL
KARSH
KARST
KARTS
KARUS
KARYN
KASEM
KASHA
KASHI
KATAS
KATEY
KATHE
KATHY
KATIE
KATZE
KAUAI
KAVAS
KAYAK
KAYOS
KAZAN
KAZIN
KAZOO

K•A••
KCARS
KEACH
KEANE
KEANU
KEATS
KHAKI
KHANS
KLAMM
KLAUS
KMART
KNACK
KNARS
KNAVE
KOALA
KOANS
KRAAL
KRAFT
KRAIT
KRAUS
KRAUT
KRAZY
KUALA
KVACK
KVASS
KWAME
KYATS

K••A•
KABAS
KADAR
KANAR
KANAS
KARAN
KARAS
KARAT
KATAS
KAUAI
KAVAS
KAYAK
KAZAN
KEBAB
KEMAL
KENAI
KINAS
KIVAS
KNEAD
KODAK
KOJAK
KOLAS
KONAS
KORAN
KORAT
KOSAR
KRAAL
KSTAR
KULAK

K•••A
KAFKA
KANGA
KANSA
KAPPA
KARLA
KARMA
KASHA
KEIRA
KENYA
KIMBA
KINDA
KIOWA
KISKA
KOALA
KORDA
KOREA
KRONA
KRUPA
KUALA
KUBLA
KUKLA
KUNTA

•KA••
AKAIS
OKAPI
OKARA
OKAYS
SKALD
SKANK
SKATE
UKASE

•K•A•
AKBAR
OKRAS
SKOAL
SKUAS
UKIAH

•K••A
AKELA
AKIRA
AKITA
OKARA

••KA•
ALKAB
AOKAY
BEKAA
DAKAR
DUKAS
LUKAS
MCKAY
MIKAN
OHKAY
ORKAN
OSKAR
PIKAS
PUKAS
SAKAI
SIKAS
TAKAS
TOKAY
WAKAS

••K•A
BEKAA
KUKLA
MEKKA
NAKFA
NOKIA
PEKKA
PUKKA
TIKKA

•••KA
ANOKA
BABKA
BUBKA
BURKA
CHAKA
CHEKA
DHAKA
DINKA
DITKA
ERIKA
HOOKA
KAFKA
KISKA
LAIKA
LANKA
LATKA
LOCKA
MARKA
MEKKA
OSAKA
PARKA
PEKKA
POLKA
PUKKA
PUNKA
RUSKA
SANKA
SITKA
STUKA
TANKA
TIKKA
TONKA
VODKA
WONKA
YREKA
YULKA

K•B••
KABAS
KABOB
KABUL
KEBAB
KOBOS
KUBEK
KUBLA

K••B•
KERBS
KILBY
KIMBA
KIRBY
KNOBS
KOMBU
KREBS

K•••B
KABOB
KEBAB

•KB••
AKBAR

•K•B•
EKEBY

••K•B
ALKAB
JAKOB

KC•••
KCARS

K•C••
KICKS
KICKY

K••C•
KEACH
KETCH
KLICK
KNACK
KNICK
KNOCK
KOTCH
KROCK
KUSCH
KVACK

K•••C
KOVIC

K•D••
KADAR
KEDGE
KIDDO
KIDDY
KIDEO
KODAK
KODEL
KODES
KUDOS
KUDUS
KUDZU

K••D•
KANDY
KENDO
KIDDO
KIDDY
KINDA
KINDS
KORDA
KURDS

K•••D
KEYED
KITED
KNEAD
KNEED

•K•D•
SKEDS
SKIDS

•K••D
SKALD
SKIED

••K•D
ALKYD
ASKED
BAKED
BIKED
CAKED
COKED
DEKED
DIKED
DUKED
FAKED
HIKED
HOKED
INKED
IRKED
JOKED
JUKED
LIKED
LIKUD
MIKED
NAKED
NUKED
PIKED
POKED
RAKED
TOKED
TSKED
WAKED
YOKED

KE•••
KEACH
KEANE
KEANU
KEATS
KEBAB
KEDGE
KEEFE
KEELS
KEELY
KEENE
KEENS
KEEPS
KEFIR
KEINO
KEIRA
KEITH
KELLI
KELLY
KELPS
KELSO
KEMAL
KEMPT
KENAI
KENDO
KENNY
KENOS
KENYA
KEOGH
KEPIS
KERBS
KERFS
KERNE
KERNS
KERRI
KERRY
KERSH
KESEY
KETCH
KETTI
KETTY
KEVIN
KEVON
KEYED
KEYES
KEYIN
KEYON
KEYUP

K•E••
KEEFE
KEELS
KEELY
KEENE
KEENS
KEEPS
KLEIN
KNEAD
KNEED
KNEEL
KNEES
KNELL
KNELT
KREBS
KREME
KREPS
KRESS
KREUK
KREWE
KVELL

K••E•
KALEL
KALES
KAMEN
KAREL
KAREN
KASEM
KATEY
KESEY
KEYED
KEYES
KHMER
KIDEO
KILEY
KINER
KISER
KITED
KITER
KITES
KLIEG
KNEED
KNEEL
KNEES
KODEL
KODES
KOPEK
KOREA
KRIEG
KUBEK
KUGEL
KYSER

K•••E
KANYE
KARLE
KATHE
KATIE
KATZE
KEANE
KEDGE
KEEFE
KEENE
KERNE
KINTE
KLINE
KLUTE
KNAVE
KNIFE
KNUTE
KOPFE
KOPJE
KREME
KREWE
KRIGE
KRONE
KTILE
KWAME
KYLIE
KYRIE

•KE••
AKEEM
AKELA
AKENE
AKERS
EKEBY
OKEMO
SKEDS
SKEET
SKEGS
SKEIN

SKEWS

•K•E•
AKEEM OKIES SKEET SKIED SKIER SKIES SKYES SKYEY

•K••E
AKENE SKATE SKYPE UKASE

••KE•
AIKEN ASKED ASKER ASKEW BAKED BAKER BAKES BIKED BIKEL BIKER BIKES CAKED CAKES CAKEY COKED COKER COKES CUKES DEKED DEKES DIKED DIKER DIKES DOKEY DUKED DUKES DYKER ESKER FAKED FAKER FAKES HAKES HIKED HIKEN HIKER HIKES HOKED HOKES HOKEY ICKES INKED INKER INKEY IRKED IRKER JAKES JOKED JOKER JOKES JOKEY JUKED JUKES LAKER LAKES LIKED LIKEN LIKER LIKES MAKEM MAKER MAKES MCKEE MIKED MIKES MIKEY NAKED NIKES NUKED NUKES OAKEN OAKES ONKEY PEKES PIKED PIKER PIKES POKED POKER POKES POKEY RAKED RAKER RAKES REKEY RIKER ROKER SAKES SIKES TAKEI TAKEN TAKER TAKES TEKEL TIKES TOKED TOKEN TOKES TPKES TSKED TYKES URKEL VIKES WAKED WAKEN WAKER WAKES WOKEN YIKES YOKED YOKEL YOKES

••K•E
ANKLE ASKME COKIE HOKIE INKLE LAKME MCKEE OAKIE PEKOE

•••KE
ALIKE AWAKE AWOKE BLAKE BLOKE BRAKE BROKE BURKE CHOKE COOKE CRAKE DANKE DRAKE EVOKE FALKE FAMKE FISKE FLAKE FLUKE HAWKE HOOKE LATKE LEAKE LEPKE LOCKE MACKE QUAKE RANKE RILKE SHAKE SLAKE SLYKE SMOKE SNAKE SPAKE SPEKE SPIKE SPOKE STAKE STOKE TRIKE YLIKE

K•F••
KAFKA KEFIR

K••F•
KEEFE KERFS KHUFU KNIFE KOPFE KRAFT KROFT

K•••F
KNOPF

•K•F•
SKIFF

•K••F
SKIFF

••KF•
NAKFA

••K•F
ASKOF

K•G••
KUGEL

K••G•
KANGA KANGS KEDGE KEOGH KINGS KLUGH KRIGE KROGH

K•••G
KLIEG KOING KRIEG

•K•G•
SKEGS

•K••G
EKING OKING

KH•••
KHAKI KHANS KHMER KHUFU

K•H••
KAHLO KAHNS KOHLS

K••H•
KAPHS KASHA KASHI KATHE KATHY KOPHS

K•••H
KARSH KEACH KEITH KEOGH KERSH KETCH KLUGH KNISH KOOSH KOTCH KROGH KUSCH

•K••H
SKOSH UKIAH

••KH•
ANKHS MEKHI SIKHS

KI•••
KICKS KICKY KIDDO KIDDY KIDEO KILBY KILEY KILIM KILLS KILLY KILNS KILOS KILTS KIMBA KIMPO KINAS KINDA KINDS KINER KINGS KINKO KINKS KINKY KINTE KIOSK KIOWA KIRBY KIRIN KIRKS KIROV KISER KISKA KISSY KITED KITER KITES KITTS KITTY KIVAS KIWIS

K•I••
KEINO KEIRA KEITH KLICK KLIEG KLIMT KLINE KLINK KNICK KNIFE KNISH KNITS KOING KRIEG KRIGE KRILL KRIPS KRISS KTILE

K••I•
KANIN KATIE KAZIN KEFIR KEPIS KEVIN KEYIN KILIM KIRIN KIWIS KLEIN KOJIS KOPIT KOVIC KRAIT KULIK KUMIN KYLIE KYRIE

K•••I
KALKI KANJI KASHI KAUAI KELLI KENAI KERRI KETTI KHAKI

•KI••
AKINS AKIRA AKITA EKING OKIES OKING SKIDS SKIED SKIER SKIES SKIFF SKILL SKIMP SKIMS SKINK SKINS SKIPS SKIRL SKIRT SKITS UKIAH

•K•I•
AKAIS SKEIN

•K••I
OKAPI

••KI•
ARKIN ASKIN COKIE ELKIN FAKIR HAKIM HOKIE INKIN MAKIN MCKIM NOKIA OAKIE ORKIN PEKIN SÁKIS TAKIN TIKIS WIKIS YUKIO

••K•I
MEKHI NIKKI RIKKI SAKAI TAKEI TIKKI VIKKI

•••KI
AZUKI BALKI BOOKI ENOKI ESAKI GORKI INIKI KALKI KHAKI LASKI MARKI MBEKI NANKI NIKKI RICKI RIKKI TIKKI UMEKI VICKI VIKKI

K•J••
KOJAK KOJIS

K••J•
KANJI KOPJE

••KJ•
JFKJR

K•K••
KUKLA

K••K•
KAFKA KALKI KHAKI KICKS KICKY KINKO KINKS KINKY KIRKS KISKA KOOKS KOOKY

K•••K
KAPOK KAYAK KIOSK KLICK KLINK KNACK KNICK KNOCK KODAK KOJAK KOPEK KREUK KROCK KUBEK KULAK KULIK KVACK

•K••K
SKANK SKINK SKULK SKUNK

••KK•
DEKKO GEKKO MEKKA NIKKI PEKKA PUKKA RIKKI TIKKA TIKKI VIKKI WAKKO

KL•••
KLAMM KLAUS KLEIN KLICK KLIEG KLIMT KLINE KLINK KLMNO KLUGH KLUMP KLUTE KLUTZ

K•L••
KALEL KALES KALKI KELLI KELLY KELPS KELSO KILBY KILEY KILIM KILLS KILLY KILNS KILOS KILTS KOLAS KULAK KULIK KYLIE

K••L•
KAHLO KARLA KARLE KEELS KEELY KELLI KELLY KILLS KILLY KNELL KNELT KNOLL KOALA KOHLS KRILL KRULL KTILE KUALA KUBLA KUKLA KVELL

K•••L
KABUL KALEL KAREL KAROL KEMAL KNEEL KNELL KNOLL KNURL KODEL KRAAL KRILL KRULL KUGEL KVELL KYZYL

•KL••
JKLMN

•K•L•
AKELA SKALD SKILL SKULK SKULL

•K••L
SKILL SKIRL SKOAL SKULL

••KL•
ANKLE IJKLM INKLE KUKLA

••K•L
ALKYL BIKEL TEKEL URKEL YOKEL

•••KL
HACKL HIJKL

KM•••
KMART

K•M••
KAMEN KEMAL KEMPT KHMER KIMBA KIMPO KLMNO KOMBU KUMIN

K••M•
KARMA KLAMM KLIMT KLUMP KREME KWAME

K•••M
KASEM KILIM KLAMM

•K•M•
JKLMN OKEMO SKIMP SKIMS

•K••M
AKEEM

••KM•
ASKME LAKME

••K•M
HAKIM HOKUM IJKLM MAKEM MCKIM OAKUM YOKUM

KN•••
KNACK KNARS KNAVE KNEAD KNEED KNEEL KNEES KNELL KNELT KNICK KNIFE KNISH KNITS KNOBS KNOCK KNOLL KNOPF KNORR KNOTS KNOTT KNOUT KNOWN KNOWS KNURL KNURS KNUTE

K•N••
KANAR KANAS KANDY KANGA KANGS KANIN KANJI KANSA KANYE KENAI KENDO KENNY KENOS KENYA KINAS KINDA KINDS KINER KINGS KINKO KINKS KINKY KINTE KONAS KUNTA

K••N•
KAHNS KAONS KARNS KEANE KEANU KEENE KEENS KEINO KENNY KERNE KERNS KHANS KILNS KLINE KLINK KLMNO KOANS KOING KRONA KRONE

K•••N
KAMEN KANIN KARAN KAREN KARYN KAZAN KAZIN KEVIN KEVON KEYIN KEYON KIRIN KLEIN KNOWN KORAN KROON KUMIN

•KN••
IKNOW SKNXX YKNOW

•K•N•
AKENE AKINS EKING OKING SKANK SKINK SKINS SKUNK

•K••N
AKRON JKLMN SKEIN

••K•N
AIKEN ARKIN ASKIN ELKIN HIKEN INKIN LIKEN MAKIN MIKAN NIKON OAKEN ORKAN ORKIN PEKIN TAKEN TAKIN TOKEN WAKEN WOKEN YUKON

KO•••
KOALA KOANS KOBOS KODAK KODEL KODES KOHLS KOING KOJAK KOJIS KOLAS KOMBU KONAS KOOKS KOOKY KOOSH KOPEK KOPFE KOPHS KOPIT KOPJE KORAN KORAT KORDA KOREA KOSAR KOTCH KOTOS KOTTO KOVIC

K•O••
KAONS KEOGH KIOSK KIOWA KNOBS KNOCK KNOLL KNOPF KNORR KNOTS KNOTT KNOUT KNOWN KNOWS KOOKS KOOKY KOOSH KROCK KROFT KROGH KRONA KRONE KROON KROTO KYOTO

K••O•
KABOB KAPOK KAPOW KAROL KAYOS KAZOO KENOS KEVON KEYON KILOS KIROV KOBOS KOTOS KROON KUDOS

K•••O
KAHLO KAZOO KEINO KELSO KENDO KIDDO KIDEO KIMPO KINKO KLMNO KOTTO KROTO KYOTO

•KO••
SKOAL SKORT SKOSH

•K•O•
AKRON IKNOW YKNOW

•K••O
OKEMO

••KO•
ASKOF CUKOR JAKOB MAKOS NIKON PEKOE YAKOV YUKON YUKOS ZUKOR

••K•O
DEKKO GEKKO ONKYO TOKYO WAKKO YUKIO

•••KO
ALUKO AYAKO BILKO BUCKO BUNKO DEKKO DISKO GECKO GEKKO JACKO JOCKO KINKO LEUKO PINKO RAFKO ROYKO SEIKO SHAKO SICKO SOCKO WACKO WAKKO

K•P••
KAPHS KAPOK KAPOW KAPPA KAPUT KEPIS KOPEK KOPFE KOPHS KOPIT KOPJE

K••P•
KAPPA KEEPS KELPS KEMPT KIMPO KNOPF KREPS KRIPS KRUPA KRUPP KRUPS

K•••P
KEYUP KLUMP KRUPP

•K•P•
OKAPI SKIPS SKYPE

•K••P
SKIMP

••K•P
ASKUP

KR•••
KRAAL KRAFT KRAIT KRAUS KRAUT KRAZY KREBS KREME KREPS KRESS KREUK KREWE KRIEG KRIGE KRILL KRIPS KRISS KROCK KROFT KROGH KRONA KRONE KROON KROTO KRULL KRUPA KRUPP KRUPS

K•R••
KARAN KARAS KARAT KAREL KAREN KARLA KARLE KARMA KARNS KAROL KARSH KARST KARTS KARUS KARYN KERBS KERFS KERNE KERNS KERRI KERRY KERSH KIRBY KIRIN KIRKS KIROV KORAN KORAT KORDA KOREA KURDS KURTZ KURUS KURYS KYRIE

K••R•
KCARS KEIRA KERRI KERRY KMART KNARS KNORR KNURL KNURS

K•••R
KADAR KANAR KEFIR KHMER KINER KISER KITER KNORR KOSAR KSTAR KYSER

•KR••
AKRON OKRAS

•K•R•
AKERS AKIRA OKARA SKIRL SKIRT SKORT

•K••R
AKBAR SKIER

••K•R
ASKER BAKER BIKER COKER CUKOR DAKAR DIKER DYKER ESKER FAKER FAKIR HIKER INKER IRKER JFKJR JOKER LAKER LIKER MAKER OSKAR PIKER POKER RAKER RIKER ROKER TAKER WAKER ZUKOR

KS•••
KSTAR

K•S••
KASEM KASHA KASHI

KESEY KISER KISKA KISSY KOSAR KUSCH KYSER

K••S•
KANSA KARSH KARST KELSO KERSH KIOSK KISSY KNISH KOOSH KRESS KRISS KVASS

K•••S
KABAS KAHNS KALES KANAS KANGS KAONS KAPHS KARAS KARNS KARTS KARUS KATAS KAVAS KAYOS KCARS KEATS KEELS KEENS KEEPS KELPS KENOS KEPIS KERBS KERFS KERNS KEYES KHANS KICKS KILLS KILNS KILOS KILTS KINAS KINDS KINGS KINKS KIRKS KITES KITTS KIVAS KIWIS KLAUS KNARS KNEES KNITS KNOBS KNOTS KNOWS KNURS KOANS KOBOS KODES KOHLS KOJIS KOLAS KONAS KOOKS KOPHS KOTOS KRAUS KREBS KREPS KRESS KRIPS KRISS KRUPS KUDOS KUDUS KURDS KURUS KURYS KVASS KYATS

•K•S•
SKOSH UKASE

•K••S
AKAIS AKERS AKINS OKAYS OKIES OKRAS SKEDS SKEGS SKEWS SKIDS SKIES SKIMS SKINS SKIPS SKITS SKUAS SKYES

••KS•
BAKST

••K•S
ANKHS BAKES BIKES CAKES COKES CUKES DEKES DIKES DUKAS DUKES FAKES HAKES HIKES HOKES ICKES JAKES JOKES JUKES LAKES LIKES LUKAS MAKES MAKOS MIKES NIKES NUKES OAKES PEKES PIKAS PIKES POKES PUKAS RAKES RAKUS SAKES SAKIS SIKAS SIKES SIKHS TAKAS TAKES TIKES TIKIS TOKES TPKES TYKES VIKES WAKAS WAKES WIKIS YIKES YOKES YUKOS

•••KS
BACKS BALKS BANKS BARKS BASKS BEAKS BECKS BERKS BILKS BOCKS BONKS BOOKS BORKS BUCKS BULKS BUNKS BUSKS CALKS CASKS COCKS CONKS COOKS CORKS CUSKS DARKS DECKS DESKS DICKS DINKS DIRKS DISKS DOCKS DORKS DREKS DUCKS DUNKS DUSKS EFIKS EWOKS FINKS FOLKS FORKS FUNKS GAWKS GEEKS GOOKS GROKS GUCKS GUNKS HACKS HAIKS HANKS HARKS HAWKS HECKS HICKS HOCKS HONKS HOOKS HULKS HUNKS HUSKS JACKS JERKS JINKS JOCKS JUNKS KICKS KINKS KIRKS KOOKS LACKS LARKS LEAKS LEEKS LICKS LINKS LOCKS LOOKS LUCKS LURKS MACKS MARKS MASKS MILKS MINKS MOCKS MONKS MUCKS MUSKS NARKS NECKS NICKS NOCKS NOOKS OINKS ONEKS PACKS PARKS PEAKS PECKS PEEKS PERKS PICKS PINKS POLKS PORKS PUCKS PUNKS RACKS RANKS RECKS REEKS RICKS RINKS RISKS ROCKS ROOKS RUCKS RUSKS SACKS SAUKS SEEKS SILKS SINKS SOAKS SOCKS SUCKS SULKS TACKS TALKS TANKS TASKS TEAKS TENKS TICKS TREKS TUCKS TURKS TUSKS VICKS WALKS WARKS WEEKS WICKS WINKS WONKS WORKS YACKS YANKS YOLKS YORKS ZONKS ZOUKS

KT•••
KTILE

K•T••
KATAS KATEY KATHE KATHY KATIE KATZE KETCH KETTI KETTY KITED KITER KITES KITTS KITTY KOTCH KOTOS KOTTO KSTAR

K••T•
KARTS KEATS KEITH KETTI KETTY KILTS KINTE KITTS KITTY KLUTE KLUTZ KNITS KNOTS KNOTT KNUTE KOTTO KROTO KUNTA KURTZ KYATS KYOTO

K•••T
KAPUT KARAT KARST KEMPT KLIMT KMART KNELT KNOTT KNOUT KOPIT KORAT KRAFT KRAIT KRAUT KROFT

•K•T•
AKITA SKATE SKITS

•K••T
SKEET SKIRT SKORT

••K•T
BAKST YAKUT

KU•••
KUALA KUBEK KUBLA KUDOS KUDUS KUDZU KUGEL KUKLA KULAK KULIK KUMIN KUNTA KURDS KURTZ KURUS KURYS KUSCH

K•U••
KAUAI KHUFU KLUGH KLUMP KLUTE KLUTZ KNURL KNURS KNUTE KRULL KRUPA KRUPP KRUPS

K••U•
KABUL KAPUT KARUS KEYUP KLAUS KNOUT KRAUS KRAUT KREUK KUDUS KURUS

K•••U
KEANU KHUFU KOMBU KUDZU

•KU••
SKUAS SKULK SKULL SKUNK

••KU•
ASKUP HOKUM LIKUD OAKUM RAKUS YAKUT YOKUM

•••KU
HAIKU TURKU

KV•••
KVACK KVASS KVELL

K•V••
KAVAS KEVIN KEVON KIVAS KOVIC

K••V•
KNAVE

K•••V
KIROV

••K•V
YAKOV

•••KV
BOOKV MARKV

KW•••
KWAME

K•W••
KIWIS

K••W•
KIOWA KNOWN KNOWS KREWE

K•••W
KAPOW

•K•W•
SKEWS

•K••W
IKNOW YKNOW

••K•W
ASKEW

•K•X•
SKNXX

•K••X
SKNXX

•••KX
BOOKX

KY•••
KYATS KYLIE KYOTO KYRIE KYSER KYZYL

K•Y••
KAYAK KAYOS KEYED KEYES KEYIN KEYON KEYUP

K••Y•
KANYE KARYN KENYA KURYS KYZYL

K•••Y
KANDY KATEY KATHY KEELY KELLY KENNY KERRY KESEY KETTY KICKY KIDDY KILBY KILEY KILLY KINKY KIRBY KISSY KITTY KOOKY KRAZY

•KY••
SKYES SKYEY SKYPE

•K•Y•
OKAYS

•K••Y
EKEBY SKYEY

••KY•
ALKYD ALKYL ONKYO TOKYO

••K•Y
AOKAY CAKEY DOKEY HOKEY INKEY JOKEY MCKAY MIKEY OHKAY ONKEY POKEY REKEY TOKAY

•••KY
BALKY BANKY BARKY BECKY BUCKY BULKY CHOKY COCKY COOKY CORKY DICKY DINKY DORKY DUCKY DUSKY ENSKY FLAKY FLUKY FOLKY FORKY FUNKY GAWKY GEEKY GORKY GUCKY GUNKY HACKY HANKY HERKY HINKY HONKY HOOKY HULKY HUNKY HUSKY JACKY JERKY JUNKY KICKY KINKY KOOKY LANKY LARKY LASKY LEAKY LECKY LOOKY LUCKY MICKY MILKY MUCKY MURKY MUSKY NICKY PANKY PERKY PESKY PICKY PINKY PORKY PUNKY QUAKY REEKY RICKY RINKY RISKY ROCKY ROOKY SHAKY SILKY SMOKY SNAKY SPIKY SUCKY SULKY TACKY TALKY TICKY VICKY WACKY YOLKY YUCKY ZINKY

K•Z••
KAZAN KAZIN KAZOO KYZYL

K••Z•
KATZE KRAZY KUDZU

K•••Z
KLUTZ KURTZ

LA•••
LABAN LABEL LABIA LABOR LACED LACER LACES LACEY LACIE LACKS LACTI LACTO LADAS LADED LADEN LADER LADES LADLE LADYL LADYS LAFEU LAFFS LAGER LAGOS LAHTI LAICS LAIKA LAILA LAINE LAING LAIRD LAIRS LAITS LAITY LAIUS LAKER LAKES LAKME LALAW LALIA LALLA LAMAR LAMAS LAMBS LAMED LAMER LAMES LAMIA LAMIT LAMPS LANAI LANCE LANDI LANDO LANDS LANED LANES LANGE LANIN LANKA LANKY LANNY LANOS LANTZ LANZA LAPAT LAPAZ LAPEL LAPIN LAPIS LAPPS LAPSE LAPUP LARAM LARAS LARCH LARDS LARDY LAREE LARES LARGE LARGO LARIS LARKS LARKY LARRY LARUE LARVA LASED LASER LASES LASIK LASKI LASKY LASSE LASSO LASTS LATCH LATEN LATER LATEX LATHE LATHS LATHY LATIN LATKA LATKE LATTE LAUDA LAUDE LAUDS LAUER LAUGH LAURA LAURO LAVAL LAVAS LAVED LAVER LAVES LAVIE LAVIN LAWED LAWES LAWNS LAWNY LAXER LAXLY LAYBY LAYER LAYIN LAYLA LAYNE LAYON LAYTO LAYUP LAZAR LAZED LAZES

L•A••
LBARS LEACH LEADS LEADY LEAFS LEAFY LEAHY LEAKE LEAKS LEAKY LEANN LEANS LEANT LEAPS LEAPT LEARN LEARS LEARY LEASE LEASH LEAST LEAUD LEAVE LHASA LIANA LIANE LIANG LIARS LLAMA LLANO LOADS LOAFS LOAMS LOAMY LOANS LOATH LSATS LUANA LUANG LUANN LUAUS LWAVE

L••A•
LABAN LADAS LALAW LAMAR LAMAS LANAI LAPAT LAPAZ LARAM LARAS LAVAL LAVAS LAZAR LBEAM LECAR LEFAY LEGAL LEHAR LEMAN LEMAT LEMAY LETAT LEVAR LEXAN LIDAR LIFAR LILAC LIMAN LIMAS LIRAS LOBAR LOCAL LOFAT LOGAN LOHAN LOMAN LOMAS LOMAX LOPAT LORAN LORAX LOYAL LPGAS LUCAN LUCAS LUGAR LUJAN LUKAS LUMAN LUMAS LUNAR LUNAS LURAY LYMAN LYRAS

L•••A
LABIA LAIKA LAILA LALIA LALLA LAMIA LANKA LANZA LARVA LATKA LAUDA LAURA LAYLA LDOPA LEEZA LEHUA LEICA LEILA LELIA LEMMA LENYA LEONA LEORA LHASA LIANA LIBRA LIBYA LICIA LILIA LINDA LINEA LIVIA LLAMA LLOSA LOCKA LOGIA LONGA LOOFA LORCA LORNA LOTSA LOTTA LOUMA LUANA LUCCA LUCIA LUISA LULEA LURIA LYCRA LYDIA LYGIA LYNDA

•LA••
ALACK ALADO ALAIN ALAIS ALALA ALAMO ALANA ALARM ALATE ALAVA BLABS BLACK BLADE BLAFF BLAHS BLAIR BLAIS BLAKE BLAME BLAMS BLANC BLAND BLANE BLANK BLARE BLASE BLASS BLAST BLATS BLATZ BLAZE CLACK CLADS CLAES CLAIM CLAIR CLAMP CLAMS CLANG CLANK CLANS CLAPS CLARA CLARE CLARK CLARO CLARY CLASE CLASH CLASP CLASS CLAUS CLAVE CLAWS CLAYS ELAND ELARA ELATE ELATH FLACK FLAGG FLAGS FLAIL FLAIR FLAKE FLAKY FLAME FLAMS FLAMY FLANK FLANN FLANS FLAPS FLARE FLASH FLASK FLATS FLATT FLAVA FLAWS FLAWY FLAXY FLAYS GLACE GLADE GLADS GLAMS GLAND GLARE GLARY GLASS GLATT GLAXO GLAZE GLAZY KLAMM KLAUS LLAMA LLANO OLAFI OLAFV OLAND OLAVI OLAVV PLACE PLAGE PLAID PLAIN PLAIT PLANA PLANB PLANE PLANI PLANK PLANO PLANS PLANT PLASH PLASM PLAST PLATA PLATE PLATH PLATO PLATS PLATT PLATY PLAYA PLAYS PLAZA SLABS SLACK SLADE SLAGS SLAIN

SLAKE
SLAMS
SLANG
SLANT
SLAPS
SLASH
SLATE
SLATS
SLATY
SLAVE
SLAVS
SLAWS
SLAYS
VLADE

•L•A•
ALBAN
ALBAS
ALCAN
ALEAK
ALFAS
ALGAE
ALGAL
ALGAS
ALIAS
ALKAB
ALLAH
ALLAN
ALLAY
ALMAY
ALSAB
ALTAI
ALTAR
ALVAR
ALWAY
BLEAK
BLEAR
BLEAT
BLOAT
CLEAN
CLEAR
CLEAT
CLOAK
ELCAR
ELGAR
ELIAS
ELMAN
ELMAR
ELSAS
ELWAY
FLEAS
FLOAT
FLYAT
GLEAM
GLEAN
GLIAL
GLIAS
GLOAM
GLOAT
ILEAC
ILEAL
ILIAC
ILIAD
OLEAN
OLLAS
OLPAE
PLEAD
PLEAS
PLEAT
SLOAN
ULNAE
ULNAR
ULNAS

•L••A
ALALA
ALANA
ALAVA
ALCOA
ALETA
ALEXA
ALGIA
ALIDA
ALISA
ALOHA
ALPHA
ALULA
CLARA
ELARA
ELENA
ELISA
ELIZA
ELURA
FLAVA
FLORA
ILLYA
ILONA
LLAMA
LLOSA
OLETA
OLIVA
PLANA
PLATA
PLAYA
PLAZA
PLENA
SLIWA
ULTRA

••LA•
ADLAI
AFLAC
AFLAT
ALLAH
ALLAN
ALLAY
ASLAK
ASLAN
ATLAS
BALAS
BELAU
BELAY
BFLAT
BOLAR
BOLAS
BYLAW
CALAF
CFLAT
COLAS
DALAI
DELAY
DFLAT
DRLAO
DYLAN
ECLAT
EFLAT
EILAT
ENLAI
FFLAT
FILAR
FILAS
GALAS
GALAX
GFLAT
GILAS
GOLAN
GULAG
HALAL
HALAS
HULAS
HYLAS
INLAW
INLAY
ISLAM
ISLAS
KOLAS
KULAK
LALAW
LILAC
MALAR
MALAY
MILAN
MOLAR
MULAN
MYLAR
NOLAN
OLLAS
ONLAY
PALAR
PALAU
PCLAB
PILAF
PILAR
PILAU
POLAR
PULAS
RELAP
RELAX
RELAY
SALAD
SALAS
SELAH
SILAS
SOLAN
SOLAR
SPLAT
SPLAY
TALAS
TELAR
TILAK
TOLAR
UCLAN
UHLAN
UNLAX
UNLAY
VELAR
VILAS
VOLAR

••L•A
BALSA
BELLA
BELVA
BOLLA
BULBA
BULLA
CALLA
CELIA
CELLA
CILIA
CILLA
CULPA
DELIA
DELLA
DELTA
DOLMA
EOLIA
FALLA
FELLA
FOLIA
FULDA
GALBA
GALEA
GILDA
GOLDA
HALVA
HELGA
HILDA
ILLYA
JALPA
JOLLA
JULIA
LALIA
LALLA
LELIA
LILIA
LULEA
MALTA
MELBA
MULLA
NILLA
NULLA
PALEA
PALMA
PELLA
PILEA
POLKA
SALMA
SALSA
SELMA
SILVA
SOLEA
SOLLA
SULFA
SULLA
TALIA
TELMA
TILDA
TULSA
USLTA
VELDA
VELMA
VELVA
VILLA
VILMA
VILNA
VOLGA
VOLTA
WALLA
WELLA
WILLA
WILMA
YALTA
YULKA
ZELDA
ZILLA

•••LA
ACELA
ADELA
AKELA
ALALA
ALULA
ASYLA
ATALA
AVILA
BELLA
BOLLA
BOOLA
BULLA
CALLA
CARLA
CELLA
CHELA
CHULA
CILLA
DARLA
DELLA
DOULA
EBOLA
ENOLA
FALLA
FELLA
HABLA
IDOLA
ISOLA
JOLLA
KARLA
KOALA
KUALA
KUBLA
KUKLA
LAILA
LALLA
LAYLA
LEILA
MARLA
MITLA
MOOLA
MULLA
NILLA
NULLA
NYALA
OCALA
ONELA
OOOLA
PAULA
PELLA
PEPLA
PHYLA
SCALA
SHULA
SOLLA
STELA
STOLA
SULLA
TABLA
TESLA
TRALA
TWYLA
UVULA
VILLA
VIOLA
VOILA
WALLA
WELLA
WILLA
ZILLA

LB•••
LBARS
LBEAM

L•B••
LABAN
LABEL
LABIA
LABOR
LIBBY
LIBEL
LIBER
LIBRA
LIBRE
LIBRI
LIBRO
LIBYA
LOBAR
LOBBY
LOBED
LOBES
LOBOS
LUBED
LUBES
LUBIN

L••B•
LAMBS
LAYBY
LETBE
LETBY
LIBBY
LIEBE
LIEBY
LIMBO
LIMBS
LOBBY
LOOBY

L•••B
LINEB
LITTB

•LB••
ALBAN
ALBAS
ALBEE
ALBEN
ALBOM
ALBUM
ELBOW

•L•B•
ALIBI
BLABS
BLEBS
BLOBS
CLUBS
FLUBS
FLYBY
GLOBE
GLOBS
ILLBE
PLEBE
PLEBS
SLABS
SLOBS

•L••B
ALKAB
ALSAB
BLURB
CLIMB
PLANB
PLUMB

••LB•
BALBO
BELBY
BILBO
BULBA
BULBS
COLBY
DOLBY
FTLBS
GALBA
ILLBE
KILBY
MELBA
WELBY
WILBY

••L•B
ADLIB
CALEB
CELEB
EXLIB
PCLAB
PHLEB
ZHLOB
ZHLUB

•••LB
ONELB
ORALB
TENLB

L•C••
LACED
LACER
LACES
LACEY
LACIE
LACKS
LACTI
LACTO
LECAR
LECHE
LECID
LECKY
LECON
LECTS
LICHT
LICIA
LICIT
LICKS
LOCAL
LOCHS
LOCKA
LOCKE
LOCKS
LOCOS
LOCUM
LOCUS
LTCOL
LTCOM
LUCAN
LUCAS
LUCCA
LUCCI
LUCIA
LUCID
LUCIE
LUCIO
LUCKS
LUCKY
LUCRE
LYCEE
LYCOS
LYCRA

L••C•
LAICS
LANCE
LARCH
LATCH
LEACH
LEECH
LEICA
LINCS
LORCA
LUCCA
LUCCI
LUNCH
LURCH
LYNCH

L•••C
LILAC
LINEC
LOGIC
LUDIC
LYRIC

•LC••
ALCAN
ALCOA
ALCOR
ELCAR
ELCID
ULCER

•L•C•
ALACK
ALECK
ALICE
ALYCE
BLACK
BLOCH
BLOCK
BLOCS
CLACK
CLICK
CLOCK
CLUCK
ELECT
FLACK
FLECK
FLICK
FLICS
FLOCK
GLACE
GLICK
GLOCK
GLUCK
GLUCO
GLYCO
ILICH
KLICK
PLACE
PLOCE
PLUCK
SLACK
SLICE
SLICK
VLECK

•L••C
BLANC
ILEAC
ILIAC
OLEIC
OLMEC
ULRIC

••LC•
BALCH
BELCH
CULCH
DELCO
DOLCE
DOLCI
DULCE
FALCO
FILCH
GULCH
HULCE
MULCH
MULCT
TALCS
TELCO
WELCH
WILCO
ZILCH

••L•C
AFLAC
COLIC
EOLIC
FOLIC
FSLIC
HELIC
HOLIC
LILAC
MALIC
MELIC
RELIC
SALIC
TELIC

LD•••
LDOPA

L•D••
LADAS
LADED
LADEN
LADER
LADES
LADLE
LADYL
LADYS
LEDEE
LEDER
LEDGE
LEDGY
LEDIN
LEDON
LEDTO
LIDAR
LIDDY
LIDOS
LODEN
LODER
LODES
LODGE
LUDIC
LYDIA
LYDON

L••D•
LANDI
LANDO
LANDS
LARDS
LARDY
LAUDA
LAUDE
LAUDS
LEADS
LEADY
LEEDS
LENDL
LENDS
LIDDY
LINDA
LINDO
LINDT
LINDY
LOADS
LOIDS
LORDS
LORDY
LUNDI
LUNDY
LYNDA
LYNDE

L•••D
LACED
LADED
LAIRD
LAMED
LANED
LASED
LAVED
LAWED
LAZED
LEAUD
LECID
LIKED
LIKUD
LIMED
LINED
LIPID
LITTD
LIVED
LIVID
LLOYD
LOBED
LOPED
LOVED
LOWED
LUBED
LUCID
LUGED
LURED
LURID
LUTED
LYRID
LYSED

•LD••
ALDEN
ALDER
BLDGS
ELDER
ELDIN
ELDON
OLDEN
OLDER
OLDIE

•L•D•
ALADO
ALIDA
BLADE
BLVDS
CLADS
CLODS
CLYDE
ELIDE
ELUDE
GLADE
GLADS
GLIDE
PLODS
SLADE
SLEDS
SLIDE
VLADE

•L••D
ALGID
ALKYD
ALOUD
BLAND
BLEED
BLEND
BLIND
BLOND
BLOOD
BLUED
CLOUD
CLUED
CLWYD
ELAND
ELCID
FLIED
FLOOD
FLOYD
FLUID
GLAND
GLUED
ILIAD
ILIED
LLOYD
OLAND
PLAID
PLEAD
PLIED
SLUED

••LD•
BALDS
BALDY
BOLDS
COLDS
FALDO
FOLDS
FULDA
GELDS
GILDA
GILDS
GOLDA
GOLDE
GOLDS
HILDA
HOLDS
MELDS
MOLDS
MOLDY
NALDI
NOLDE
SOLDI
SOLDO
TILDA
TILDE
VELDA
VELDS
VELDT
WALDO
WELDS
WILDE
WILDS
ZELDA

••L•D
ABLED
AILED
AXLED
BALED
DELED
DOLED
EELED
FELID
FILED
GALED
GELID
HALED
HOLED
IDLED
OGLED
OILED
PALED
PILED
POLED
PULED
RELED
RILED
RULED
SALAD
SALUD
SOLED
SOLID
TILED
UNLED
VALID
WALED
WILED

•••LD
AHOLD
ASOLD
BUILD
CHILD
COULD
EWALD
FIELD
GOULD
GUILD
HEALD
IFOLD
MOULD
ROALD
SCALD
SCOLD
SKALD
WEALD
WIELD
WORLD
WOULD
YIELD

LE•••
LEACH
LEADS
LEADY
LEAFS
LEAFY
LEAHY
LEAKE
LEAKS
LEAKY
LEANN
LEANS
LEANT
LEAPS
LEAPT
LEARN
LEARS
LEARY
LEASE
LEASH
LEAST
LEAUD
LEAVE
LECAR
LECHE
LECID
LECKY
LECON
LECTS
LEDEE
LEDER
LEDGE
LEDGY
LEDIN
LEDON
LEDTO
LEECH
LEEDS
LEEKS
LEERS
LEERY
LEEZA
LEFAY
LEFTS
LEFTY
LEGAL
LEGER
LEGGS
LEGGY
LEGIT
LEGNO
LEGOS
LEGUP
LEHAR
LEHRS
LEHUA
LEICA
LEIGH
LEILA
LEITH
LELIA
LEMAN
LEMAT
LEMAY
LEMMA
LEMME
LEMON
LEMUR
LENDL
LENDS
LENES
LENIN
LENIS
LENNI
LENNY
LENOS
LENOX
LENTE
LENTO
LENTS
LENYA
LEOII
LEOIV
LEOIX
LEONA
LEONE
LEONI
LEORA
LEOVI
LEOXI
LEPEN
LEPER
LEPEW
LEPKE
LEPUS
LEROI
LEROS
LEROY
LETAT
LETBE
LETBY
LETGO
LETHE
LETIN
LETME
LETON
LETTS
LETTY
LETUP
LEUKO
LEUMI
LEURS
LEVAR
LEVEE
LEVEL
LEVER
LEVIN
LEVIS
LEVIT
LEVON
LEWES
LEWIS
LEXAN
LEXIS
LEXUS
LEYTE

L•E••
LBEAM
LEECH
LEEDS
LEEKS
LEERS
LEERY
LEEZA
LIEBE
LIEBY
LIEGE
LIEIN
LIENS
LIEON
LIESL
LIEST
LIETO
LIEUP
LIEUS
LIEUT
LOEIL
LOESS
LOEWE
LOEWI
LOEWS
LOEWY
LUEGO
LWEIS
LYELL

L••E•
LABEL
LACED
LACER
LACES
LACEY
LADED
LADEN
LADER
LADES
LAFEU
LAGER
LAKER
LAKES
LAMED
LAMER
LAMES
LANED
LANES
LAPEL
LAREE
LARES
LASED
LASER
LASES
LATEN
LATER
LATEX
LAUER
LAVED
LAVER
LAVES
LAWED
LAWES
LAXER
LAYER
LAZED
LAZES
LEDEE
LEDER
LEGER
LENES
LEPEN
LEPER
LEPEW
LEVEE
LEVEL
LEVER
LEWES
LIBEL
LIBER
LIFER
LIGER
LIKED
LIKEN
LIKER
LIKES
LIMED
LIMES
LINEA
LINEB
LINEC
LINED
LINEN
LINER
LINES
LITEL
LITER
LITES
LIVED
LIVEN
LIVER
LIVES
LOBED
LOBES
LODEN
LODER
LODES
LOGES
LONER
LOOEY
LOPED
LOPER
LOPES
LOPEZ
LOREN
LORES
LOSER
LOSES
LOSEY
LOTET
LOVED
LOVER
LOVES
LOVEY
LOWED
LOWER
LOWES
LOXES
LTGEN
LUBED
LUBES
LUGED
LUGER
LUGES
LULEA
LUMEN
LUMET
LUNER
LUNES
LURED
LURER
LURES
LUREX
LUTED
LUTES
LUXES
LYCEE
LYNEN
LYRES
LYSED
LYSES

L•••E
LACIE
LADLE
LAINE
LAKME
LANCE
LANGE
LAPSE
LAREE
LARGE
LARUE
LASSE
LATHE
LATKE
LATTE
LAUDE
LAVIE
LAYNE
LEAKE
LEASE
LEAVE
LECHE
LEDEE

LEDGE
LEMME
LENTE
LEONE
LEPKE
LETBE
LETHE
LETME
LEVEE
LEYTE
LIANE
LIBRE
LIEBE
LIEGE
LIGNE
LILLE
LISLE
LISSE
LITHE
LITRE
LIVRE
LOCKE
LODGE
LOEWE
LOGUE
LOIRE
LONGE
LOOIE
LOOSE
LORNE
LORRE
LOTTE
LOUIE
LOUPE
LOUSE
LTILE
LUCIE
LUCRE
LUISE
LUNGE
LURIE
LWAVE
LYCEE
LYNDE
LYNNE

•LE••

ALEAK
ALECK
ALEFS
ALENE
ALEPH
ALERO
ALERS
ALERT
ALETA
ALEUT
ALEVE
ALEXA
ALEXI
BLEAK
BLEAR
BLEAT
BLEBS
BLEED
BLEEP
BLEND
BLENT
BLESS
BLEST
BLEUS
CLEAN
CLEAR
CLEAT
CLEEF
CLEEK
CLEFS
CLEFT
CLEON
CLEPT
CLERK
CLETE
CLEVE
CLEWS
ELECT
ELEGY
ELEMI
ELEMS
ELENA
ELENI
ELEVE
ELEVS
FLEAS
FLECK
FLEER
FLEES
FLEET
FLESH
FLEUR
GLEAM
GLEAN
GLEEM
GLEES
GLENN
GLENS
GLESS
ILEAC
ILEAL
ILENE
ILEUM
KLEIN
NLERS
OLEAN
OLEIC
OLEIN
OLEOS
OLETA
OLEUM
PLEAD
PLEAS
PLEAT
PLEBE
PLEBS
PLENA
RLESS
SLEDS
SLEEK
SLEEP
SLEET
SLEPT
SLEWS
SLEYS
ULEES
ULENE
ULENT
VLECK

•L•E•

ALBEE
ALBEN
ALDEN
ALDER
ALGER
ALIEN
ALLEE
ALLEN
ALLER
ALLES
ALLEY
ALLEZ
ALOES
ALPEN
ALPES
ALTER
BLEED
BLEEP
BLUED
BLUER
BLUES
BLUET
CLAES
CLEEF
CLEEK
CLUED
CLUER
CLUES
ELDER
ELIEL
ELLEN
ELLER
ELLES
ELMER
ELREY
ELSES
ELVER
ELVES
ELWES
FLEER
FLEES
FLEET
FLIED
FLIER
FLIES
FLOES
FLUES
FLYER
GLEEM
GLEES
GLUED
GLUER
GLUES
GLUEY
ILIED
ILLER
KLIEG
MLLES
OLDEN
OLDER
OLMEC
OLPES
OLSEN
PLIED
PLIER
PLIES
PLYER
PLZEN
SLEEK
SLEEP
SLEET
SLIER
SLOES
SLUED
SLUES
SLYER
ULCER
ULEES

•L••E

ALATE
ALBEE
ALENE
ALEVE
ALFIE
ALFRE
ALGAE
ALICE
ALIKE
ALINE
ALIVE
ALLEE
ALLIE
ALONE
ALYCE
BLADE
BLAKE
BLAME
BLANE
BLARE
BLASE
BLAZE
BLIGE
BLOKE
BLORE
BLUME
CLARE
CLASE
CLAVE
CLETE
CLEVE
CLIME
CLINE
CLIVE
CLONE
CLOSE
CLOVE
CLYDE
ELATE
ELEVE
ELIDE
ELISE
ELITE
ELLIE
ELOGE
ELOPE
ELSIE
ELUDE
ELUTE
ELYSE
FLAKE
FLAME
FLARE
FLUKE
FLUME
FLUTE
FLYME
GLACE
GLADE
GLARE
GLAZE
GLIDE
GLOBE
GLOVE
GLUTE
ILENE
ILLBE
ILOSE
ILOVE
KLINE
KLUTE
MLIFE
OLDIE
OLIVE
OLLIE
OLPAE
PLACE
PLAGE
PLANE
PLATE
PLEBE
PLOCE
PLUIE
PLUME
SLADE
SLAKE
SLATE
SLAVE
SLICE
SLIDE
SLIME
SLOPE
SLYKE
ULENE
ULNAE
VLADE
YLIKE

••LE•

ABLED
ABLER
ADLER
AGLET
AGLEY
AILED
AILES
AILEY
ALLEE
ALLEN
ALLER
ALLES
ALLEY
ALLEZ
AOLER
APLEY
ARLEN
ARLES
ATLES
AXLED
AXLES
BALED
BALER
BALES
BELEM
BILES
BOLES
BOLET
CALEB
CCLEF
CELEB
COLES
CULET
DALEN
DALES
DALET
DALEY
DELED
DELES
DOLED
DOLES
EELED
EELER
ELLEN
ELLER
ELLES
EMLEN
EULER
FCLEF
FILED
FILER
FILES
FILET
FOLEY
FTLEE
GALEA
GALED
GALEN
GALES
GCLEF
GELEE
GILES
GOLEM
HALED
HALEN
HALER
HALES
HALEY
HELEN
HOLED
HOLER
HOLES
HOLEY
IDLED
IDLER
IDLES
ILLER
INLET
ISLES
ISLET
ISLEY
JULEP
JULES
JULEY
KALEL
KALES
KILEY
LULEA
MALES
MALEV
MELEE
MILER
MILES
MLLES
MOLES
MRLEE
MULES
MULEY
MYLES
NFLER
NHLER
NILES
NOLES
OGLED
OGLER
OGLES
OILED
OILER
ORLES
OSLER
OWLET
PALEA
PALED
PALEO
PALER
PALES
PALEY
PELEE
PELEG
PHLEB
PILEA
PILED
PILEI
PILER
PILES
POLED
POLER
POLES
PULED
PULER
PULES
RALES
RELED
RELEE
RELET
RILED
RILES
RILEY
ROLEN
ROLEO
ROLES
ROLEX
RULED
RULER
RULES
SALEM
SALEP
SALES
SELES
SHLEP
SILEX
SOLEA
SOLED
SOLEI
SOLER
SOLES
STLEO
TALER
TALES
TELES
TELEX
TILED
TILER
TILES
TILEX
TOLER
TOLES
TOLET
TULES
TYLER
UNLED
UNLET
UTLEY
VALES
VALET
VELEZ
VILER
VOLES
WALED
WALES
WILED
WILEE
WILES
WILEY
WYLER
XYLEM
YALEU
YULES
ZALES

••L•E

ALLEE
ALLIE
BELIE
BELLE
BILGE
BULGE
CALLE
CALME
CALVE
CELIE
CELLE
CHLOE
DELVE
DOLCE
DULCE
ELLIE
FALKE
FALSE
FILLE
FTLEE
GELEE
GOLDE
HALLE
HALVE
HULCE
HULME
ILLBE
JOLIE
JULIE
KYLIE
LILLE
MALLE
MELEE
MILLE
MILNE
MRLEE
NELLE
NELSE
NOLDE
NOLIE
NOLLE
NOLTE
OLLIE
PALME
PELEE
PELLE
PULSE
RELEE
RILKE
RILLE
ROLFE
ROLLE
SALLE
SALVE
SOLVE
TILDE
TULLE
VALLE
VALSE
VALUE
VALVE
VILLE
VOLPE
VOLTE
WILDE
WILEE
WOLFE
WYLIE
YALIE

•••LE

ABELE
ADDLE
ADELE
AGILE
AISLE
AMBLE
AMOLE
AMPLE
ANELE
ANGLE
ANILE
ANKLE
ANOLE
APPLE
ATILE
AZOLE
BASLE
BAYLE
BEALE
BELLE
BERLE
BEYLE
BIBLE
BOGLE
BOOLE
BOULE
BOYLE
BRULE
BTILE
BUGLE
CABLE
CALLE
CARLE
CELLE
CHILE
CHOLE
CTILE
CYCLE
DHOLE
DOBLE
DOYLE
DROLE
DTILE
DUPLE
EAGLE
EARLE
ECOLE
EDILE
EFILE
EGALE
EMILE
ENGLE
ETILE
EXILE
FABLE
FHOLE
FILLE
FOYLE
FTILE
GABLE
GAYLE
GTILE
GUILE
HAILE
HALLE
HAOLE
HOYLE
HTILE
INGLE
INKLE
ISTLE
ITILE
JOULE
JTILE
KARLE
KTILE
LADLE
LILLE
LISLE
LTILE
MACLE
MALLE
MAPLE
MAYLE
MERLE
MIELE
MILLE
MTILE
NEALE
NELLE
NOBLE
NOLLE
NTILE
ODILE
ONCLE
ORALE
OTILE
OVULE
PARLE
PEALE
PEELE
PELLE
PERLE
PHILE
POOLE
POPLE
POULE
PROLE
PTILE
QTILE
REGLE
RIFLE
RILLE
ROBLE
ROLLE
RTILE
RUBLE
SABLE
SALLE
SCALE
SEALE
SEULE
SHALE
SIDLE
SMILE
SOCLE
SPILE
STALE
STELE
STILE
STOLE
STYLE
SWALE
TABLE
THOLE
THULE
TITLE
TOILE
TOOLE
TTILE
TULLE
UMBLE
UNCLE
UTILE
VALLE
VEALE
VILLE
VOILE
VTILE
WHALE
WHILE
WHOLE
WTILE
XFILE
XTILE
YTILE
ZEILE
ZTILE

L•F••

LAFEU
LAFFS
LEFAY
LEFTS
LEFTY
LIFAR
LIFER
LIFTS
LOFAT
LOFTS
LOFTY
LUFFS

L••F•

LAFFS
LEAFS
LEAFY
LINFT
LOAFS
LOOFA
LUFFS
LWOFF

L•••F

LWOFF

•LF••

ALFAS
ALFIE
ALFIO
ALFRE
ELFIN

•L•F•

ALEFS
ALIFS
ALOFT
BLAFF
BLUFF
CLEFS
CLEFT
CLIFF
CLIFT
FLUFF
MLIFE
OLAFI
OLAFV

•L••F

ALLOF
ALOOF
BLAFF
BLUFF
CLEEF
CLIFF
FLUFF

••LF•

DELFT
GOLFS
GULFS
MELFI
PELFS
ROLFE
ROLFS
RULFO
SULFA
WOLFE
WOLFF
WOLFS

••L•F

ALLOF
CALAF
CALIF
CCLEF
FCLEF
GCLEF
PILAF
WOLFF

•••LF

ADOLF
AXELF
ROWLF
SHELF
WOOLF
ZWOLF

L•G••

LAGER
LAGOS
LEGAL
LEGER
LEGGS
LEGGY
LEGIT
LEGNO
LEGOS
LEGUP
LIGER
LIGHT
LIGNE
LIGNI
LIGNO
LOGAN
LOGES
LOGIA
LOGIC
LOGIN
LOGON
LOGOS
LOGUE
LPGAS
LTGEN
LTGOV
LUGAR
LUGED
LUGER
LUGES
LYGIA

L••G•

LANGE
LARGE
LARGO
LAUGH
LEDGE
LEDGY
LEGGS
LEGGY
LEIGH
LETGO
LIEGE
LINGO
LINGS
LINGU
LODGE
LONGA
LONGE
LONGI
LONGO
LONGS
LONGU
LUEGO
LUIGI
LUNGE
LUNGS

L•••G

LAING
LIANG
LUANG
LYING

•LG••

ALGAE
ALGAL
ALGAS
ALGER
ALGIA
ALGID
ALGOL
ELGAR
ELGIN
ILGWU

•L•G•

ALIGN
BLDGS
BLIGE
BLIGH
BLOGS
CLOGS
ELEGY
ELOGE
FLAGG
FLAGS
FLOGS
GLOGG
GLUGS
ILLGO
KLUGH
OLIGO
OLOGY
PLAGE
PLUGS
SLAGS
SLIGO
SLOGS
SLUGS

•L••G

ALONG
BLING
CLANG
CLING
CLUNG
FLAGG
FLING
FLUNG
GLOGG
KLIEG
SLANG
SLING
SLUNG

••LG•

BILGE
BILGY
BULGE
BULGY
GOLGI
HELGA
ILLGO
VOLGA

••L•G

BILLG
GULAG
PELEG
PFLUG
RELIG
RELOG
SELIG
ZELIG

•••LG

BILLG

LH•••

LHASA

L•H••

LAHTI
LEHAR
LEHRS
LEHUA
LOHAN

L••H•

LATHE
LATHS
LATHY
LEAHY
LECHE
LETHE
LICHT
LIGHT
LITHE
LITHO
LOCHS
LUSHY

L•••H

LARCH
LATCH
LAUGH
LEACH
LEASH
LEECH
LEIGH
LEITH
LOATH
LOUTH
LOWPH
LUNCH
LURCH
LYMPH
LYNCH

•L•H•

ALOHA
ALPHA
ALTHO
BLAHS
ELIHU

•L••H

ALEPH
ALLAH
BLIGH
BLISH
BLOCH
BLUSH
BLUTH
BLYTH
CLASH
CLOTH
ELATH
FLASH
FLESH
FLUSH
GLYPH
ILICH
KLUGH
PLASH
PLATH
PLUSH
SLASH
SLOSH
SLOTH
SLUSH

••LH•

DELHI

••L•H

ALLAH
BALCH
BALPH
BELCH
CULCH
DOLPH
FILCH
FILTH
GULCH
MALPH
MULCH
RALPH
SELAH
SYLPH
TILTH
WALSH
WELCH
WELSH
ZILCH

LI•••

LIANA
LIANE
LIANG
LIARS
LIBBY
LIBEL
LIBER
LIBRA
LIBRE
LIBRI
LIBRO
LIBYA
LICHT
LICIA
LICIT
LICKS
LIDAR
LIDDY
LIDOS
LIEBE
LIEBY
LIEGE
LIEIN
LIENS
LIEON
LIESL
LIEST
LIETO
LIEUP
LIEUS
LIEUT
LIFAR
LIFER
LIFTS
LIGER
LIGHT
LIGNE
LIGNI
LIGNO
LIKED
LIKEN
LIKER
LIKES
LIKUD
LILAC
LILIA
LILLE
LILLI
LILLY
LILTS
LIMAN
LIMAS
LIMBO
LIMBS
LIMED
LIMES
LIMIT
LIMNS
LIMON
LIMOS
LIMPS
LIMPY
LINCS
LINDA
LINDO
LINDT
LINDY
LINEA
LINEB
LINEC
LINED
LINEN
LINER
LINES
LINFT
LINGO
LINGS
LINGU
LINKS
LINOS
LINTS
LINTY
LINUS
LINUX
LIONS
LIPID
LIPPI
LIPPO
LIPPY

LIRAS LISLE LISPS LISSE LISTS LISZT LITEL LITER LITES LITHE LITHO LITON LITRE LITTB LITTD LITUP LIVED LIVEN LIVER LIVES LIVIA LIVID LIVIN LIVRE LIZZI

L•I••

LAICS LAIKA LAILA LAINE LAING LAIRD LAIRS LAITS LAITY LAIUS LEICA LEIGH LEILA LEITH LOIDS LOINS LOIRE LTILE LUIGI LUISA LUISE LVIII LXIII LYING

L••I•

LABIA LACIE LALIA LAMIA LAMIT LANIN LAPIN LAPIS LARIS LASIK LATIN LAVIE LAVIN LAYIN LECID LEDIN LEGIT LELIA LENIN LENIS LEOII LEOIV LEOIX LETIN LEVIN LEVIS LEVIT LEWIS LEXIS LICIA LICIT LIEIN LILIA LIMIT LIPID LIVIA LIVID LIVIN LOEIL LOGIA LOGIC LOGIN LOOIE LORIN LORIS LOSIN LOUIE LOUIS LOVIN LOWIQ LUBIN LUCIA LUCID LUCIE LUCIO LUDIC LUNIK LUPIN LURIA LURID LURIE LVIII LWEIS LXIII LXVII LXXII LXXIV LXXIX LYDIA LYGIA LYRIC LYRID LYSIS

L•••I

LACTI LAHTI LANAI LANDI LASKI LENNI LEOII LEONI LEOVI LEOXI LEROI LEUMI LIBRI LIGNI LILLI LIPPI LIZZI LOEWI LONGI LUCCI LUIGI LUNDI LVIII LXIII LXVII LXXII LXXVI LXXXI

•LI••

ALIAS ALIBI ALICE ALIDA ALIEN ALIFS ALIGN ALIKE ALINE ALIOS ALISA ALIST ALITO ALITY ALIVE BLIGE BLIGH BLIMP BLIND BLING BLINI BLINK BLIPS BLISH BLISS BLIST BLITT BLITZ CLICK CLIFF CLIFT CLIII CLIMB CLIME CLINE CLING CLINK CLINT CLIOS CLIPS CLIPT CLIVE DLIII ELIAS ELIDE ELIEL ELIHU ELION ELIOT ELISA ELISE ELIST ELITE ELIZA FLICK FLICS FLIED FLIER FLIES FLING FLINT FLIPS FLIRS FLIRT FLITS GLIAL GLIAS GLICK GLIDE GLIMS GLINT GLITZ ILIAC ILIAD ILICH ILIED ILION ILIUM KLICK KLIEG KLIMT KLINE KLINK MLIFE MLIII OLIGO OLIOS OLIVA OLIVE PLIED PLIER PLIES PLINK PLINY SLICE SLICK SLIDE SLIER SLIGO SLIME SLIMS SLIMY SLING SLINK SLIPS SLITS SLIWA XLIII YLIKE

•L•I•

ALAIN ALAIS ALFIE ALFIO ALGIA ALGID ALLIE ALLIN ALLIS ALOIS ALVIN BLAIR BLAIS BLOIS CLAIM CLAIR CLIII CLVII CLXII CLXIV CLXIX DLIII DLVII DLXII DLXIV DLXIX ELCID ELDIN ELFIN ELGIN ELKIN ELLIE ELLIN ELLIS ELPIS ELSIE ELVIN ELVIS FLAIL FLAIR FLUID FLYIN ILLIN KLEIN MLIII MLVII MLXII MLXIV MLXIX OLDIE OLEIC OLEIN OLLIE PLAID PLAIN PLAIT PLUIE SLAIN ULRIC XLIII XLVII

•L••I

ALEXI ALIBI ALTAI BLINI CLIII CLVII CLXII CLXVI CLXXI DLIII DLVII DLXII DLXVI DLXXI ELEMI ELENI FLORI MLIII MLVII MLXII MLXVI MLXXI OLAFI OLAVI PLANI PLURI PLUVI XLIII XLVII

••LI•

ADLIB ALLIE ALLIN ALLIS AMLIT AULIS BALIN BELIE CALIF CALIX CCLII CCLIV CCLIX CDLII CDLIV CDLIX CELIA CELIE CILIA CMLII CMLIV CMLIX COLIC COLIN CXLII CXLIV CXLIX DALIS DCLII DCLIV DCLIX DELIA DELIS DOLIN DXLII DXLIV DXLIX EGLIN ELLIE ELLIN ELLIS EOLIA EOLIC EXLIB FELID FELIS FELIX FELIZ FOLIA FOLIC FOLIO FSLIC GELID HELIC HELIO HELIX HOLIC ILLIN ISLIP JOLIE JULIA JULIE JULIO KILIM KULIK KYLIE LALIA LELIA LILIA MALIC MCLII MCLIV MCLIX MDLII MDLIV MDLIX MELIC MELIS MMLII MMLIV MMLIX MXLII MXLIV MXLIX NOLIE OHLIN OLLIE OSLIN OXLIP PALIN POLIO POLIS POLIT PULIK PULIS RELIC RELIG RELIT SALIC SELIG SOLID SPLIT TALIA TELIC TULIP UGLIS UNLIT UPLIT VALID WYLIE YALIE YULIN ZELIG

••L•I

ADLAI BALKI BELLI CALLI CCLII CCLVI CCLXI CDLII CDLVI CDLXI CELLI CMLII CMLVI CMLXI CULTI CXLII CXLVI DALAI DCLII DCLVI DCLXI DELHI DOLCI DXLII DXLVI ENLAI GALLI GOLGI KALKI KELLI LILLI MCLII MCLVI MCLXI MDLII MDLVI MDLXI MELFI MILLI MMLII MMLVI MMLXI MULTI MXLII MXLVI NALDI PELLI PILEI SALMI SALTI SOLDI SOLEI SOLTI VALLI VILLI

•••LI

AIOLI BELLI CALLI CCCLI CCXLI CDXLI CELLI CHILI CMXLI DCCLI DCXLI EBOLI ECOLI GALLI GHALI GIGLI GIMLI JETLI KELLI LILLI MCCLI MCDLI MCMLI MCXLI MDCLI MDXLI MILLI MMCLI MMDLI MMMLI MMXLI OBELI OBOLI OCULI OVOLI PAOLI PAULI PELLI STOLI STYLI VALLI VILLI

L•J••

LUJAN

•L•J•

FLOJO

L•K••

LAKER LAKES LAKME LIKED LIKEN LIKER LIKES LIKUD LUKAS

L••K•

LACKS LAIKA LANKA LANKY LARKS LARKY LASKI LASKY LATKA LATKE LEAKE LEAKS LEAKY LECKY LEEKS LEPKE LEUKO LICKS LINKS LOCKA LOCKE LOCKS LOOKS LOOKY LUCKS LUCKY LURKS

L•••K

LASIK LUNIK LUTSK

•LK••

ALKAB ALKYD ALKYL ELKIN

•L•K•

ALIKE ALUKO BLAKE BLOKE FLAKE FLAKY FLUKE FLUKY SLAKE SLYKE YLIKE

•L••K

ALACK ALEAK ALECK ALLOK BLACK BLANK BLEAK BLINK BLOCK CLACK CLANK CLARK CLEEK CLERK CLICK CLINK CLOAK CLOCK CLONK CLUCK CLUNK FLACK FLANK FLASK FLECK FLICK FLOCK FLUNK GLICK GLOCK GLUCK GLUNK KLICK KLINK PLANK PLINK PLONK PLUCK PLUNK SLACK SLEEK SLICK SLINK SLUNK VLECK

••LK•

BALKI BALKS BALKY BILKO BILKS BULKS BULKY CALKS FALKE FOLKS FOLKY HULKS HULKY KALKI MILKS MILKY POLKA POLKS RILKE SILKS SILKY SULKS SULKY TALKS TALKY WALKS YOLKS YOLKY YULKA

••L•K

ALLOK ASLAK KULAK KULIK PULIK TILAK

•••LK

BAULK CAULK CHALK SKULK STALK WHELK

LL•••

LLAMA LLANO LLOSA LLOYD

L•L••

LALAW LALIA LALLA LELIA LILAC LILIA LILLE LILLI LILLY LILTS LOLLS LOLLY LULEA LULLS LULLY LULUS

L••L•

LADLE LAILA LALLA LAXLY LAYLA LEILA LILLE LILLI LILLY LISLE LOLLS LOLLY LOWLY LTILE LULLS LULLY LYELL

L•••L

LABEL LADYL LAPEL LAVAL LEGAL LENDL LEVEL LIBEL LIESL LITEL LOCAL LOEIL LOYAL LTCOL LYELL LYSOL

•LL••

ALLAH ALLAN ALLAY ALLEE ALLEN ALLER ALLES ALLEY ALLEZ ALLIE ALLIN ALLIS ALLOF ALLOK ALLOT ALLOW ALLOY ALLYL ALLYN ELLEN ELLER ELLES ELLIE ELLIN ELLIS ELLOS ILLBE ILLER ILLGO ILLIN ILLUS ILLYA MLLES OLLAS OLLIE

•L•L•

ALALA ALULA ELULS SLYLY

•L••L

ALGAL ALGOL ALKYL ALLYL ELIEL ELSOL FLAIL GLIAL ILEAL

••LL•

BALLO BALLS BALLY BELLA BELLE BELLI BELLO BELLS BELLY BILLG BILLS BILLW BILLY BOLLA BOLLS BULLA BULLS BULLY CALLA CALLE CALLI CALLS CELLA CELLE CELLI CELLO CELLS CILLA CULLS CULLY DALLY DELLA DELLO DELLS DILLS DILLY DOLLS DOLLY DULLS DULLY FALLA FALLS FELLA FELLS FILLE FILLS FILLY FOLLY FULLS FULLY GALLI GALLO GALLS GILLS GOLLY GULLS GULLY HALLE HALLO HALLS HELLO HELLS HILLS HILLY HOLLY HULLO HULLS HULLY JELLO JELLS JELLY JOLLA JOLLY KELLI KELLY KILLS KILLY LALLA LILLE LILLI LILLY LOLLS LOLLY LULLS LULLY MALLE MALLS MELLO MILLE MILLI MILLO MILLS MOLLS MOLLY MULLA MULLS NELLE NELLO NELLY NILLA NILLY NOLLE NULLA NULLO NULLS PALLS PALLY PELLA PELLE PELLI PILLS POLLO POLLS POLLY PULLS RALLY RILLE RILLS ROLLE ROLLO ROLLS SALLE SALLY SELLS SILLS SILLY SOLLA SULLA SULLY TALLS TALLY TELLS TELLY TILLS TILLY TOLLS TULLE TULLY VALLE VALLI VILLA VILLE VILLI WALLA WALLS WALLY WELLA WELLS WILLA WILLS WILLY YELLO YELLS ZILLA ZILLS

••L•L

ALLYL HALAL KALEL

•••LL

ATALL ATOLL BBALL BCELL BEALL BRILL BUELL CCELL CHILL DCELL DOALL DRILL DROLL DWELL EMALL EUELL EWELL FRILL GRILL ICALL IDYLL IFILL INALL IWILL KNELL KNOLL KRILL KRULL KVELL LYELL NEILL ODELL PHYLL PRELL QUELL QUILL SCULL SHALL SHELL SHILL SKILL SKULL SMALL SMELL SNELL SPELL SPILL STALL STILL SWELL SWILL SZELL TBALL TBILL TCELL THILL TRILL TROLL TWILL UDALL WEILL WHOLL WHYLL YOULL

LM•••

LMNOP

L•M••

LAMAR LAMAS LAMBS LAMED LAMER LAMES LAMIA LAMIT LAMPS LEMAN LEMAT LEMAY LEMMA LEMME LEMON LEMUR LIMAN LIMAS LIMBO LIMBS LIMED LIMES LIMIT LIMNS LIMON LIMOS LIMPS LIMPY LOMAN LOMAS LOMAX LUMAN LUMAS LUMEN LUMET LUMPS LUMPY LYMAN LYMON LYMPH

L••M•

LAKME LEMMA LEMME LETME LEUMI LLAMA LOAMS LOAMY LOOMS LOUMA

L•••M

LARAM LBEAM LOCUM LTCOM

•LM••

ALMAY ALMVP ELMAN ELMAR ELMER ELMOS ELMST

KLMNO NLMVP OLMEC OLMOS

•L•M•
ALAMO ALUMS BLAME BLAMS BLIMP BLUME CLAMP CLAMS CLIMB CLIME CLOMP CLUMP ELEMI ELEMS FLAME FLAMS FLAMY FLUME FLYME GLAMS GLIMS GLOMS GLUMS KLAMM KLIMT KLUMP LLAMA PLUMB PLUME PLUMP PLUMR PLUMS PLUMY SLAMS SLIME SLIMS SLIMY SLOMO SLUMP SLUMS

•L••M
ALARM ALBOM ALBUM BLOOM CLAIM GLEAM GLEEM GLOAM GLOOM ILEUM ILIUM KLAMM OLEUM PLASM

••LM•
BALMS BALMY CALME CALMS DOLMA FILMS FILMY HELMS HOLMS HULME JKLMN MALMO PALMA PALME PALMS PALMY PULMO SALMA SALMI SELMA TELMA VELMA VILMA WILMA

••L•M
BELEM COLUM FILUM GOLEM HILUM ISLAM KILIM SALEM VELUM XYLEM

•••LM
IJKLM PSALM QUALM REALM WHELM

L•N••
LANAI LANCE LANDI LANDO LANDS LANED LANES LANGE LANIN LANKA LANKY LANNY LANOS LANTZ LANZA LENDL LENDS LENES LENIN LENIS LENNI LENNY LENOS LENOX LENTE LENTO LENTS LENYA LINCS LINDA LINDO LINDT LINDY LINEA LINEB LINEC LINED LINEN LINER LINES LINFT LINGO LINGS LINGU LINKS LINOS LINTS LINTY LINUS LINUX LMNOP LONER LONGA LONGE LONGI LONGO LONGS LONGU LUNAR LUNAS LUNCH LUNDI LUNDY LUNER LUNES LUNGE LUNGS LUNIK LUNNS LUNTS LYNCH LYNDA LYNDE LYNEN LYNNE

L••N•
LAINE LAING LANNY LAWNS LAWNY LAYNE LEANN LEANS LEANT LEGNO LENNI LENNY LEONA LEONE LEONI LIANA LIANE LIANG LIENS LIGNE LIGNI LIGNO LIMNS LIONS LLANO LOANS LOINS LOONS LOONY LORNA LORNE LOTNO LUANA LUANG LUANN LUNNS LYING LYNNE LYONS

L•••N
LABAN LADEN LANIN LAPIN LATEN LATIN LAVIN LAYIN LAYON LEANN LEARN LECON LEDIN LEDON LEMAN LEMON LENIN LEPEN LETIN LETON LEVIN LEVON LEXAN LIEIN LIEON LIKEN LIMAN LIMON LINEN LITON LIVEN LIVIN LODEN LOGAN LOGIN LOGON LOHAN LOMAN LORAN LOREN LORIN LOSIN LOVIN LOWON LTGEN LUANN LUBIN LUCAN LUJAN LUMAN LUMEN LUPIN LUZON LYDON LYMAN LYMON LYNEN

•LN••
ULNAE ULNAR ULNAS

•L•N•
ALANA ALENE ALINE ALONE ALONG BLANC BLAND BLANE BLANK BLEND BLENT BLIND BLING BLINI BLINK BLOND BLUNT CLANG CLANK CLANS CLINE CLING CLINK CLINT CLONE CLONK CLUNG CLUNK CLUNY ELAND ELENA ELENI ELYNV FLANK FLANN FLANS FLING FLINT FLUNG FLUNK FLYNN GLAND GLENN GLENS GLINT GLUNK ILENE ILONA KLINE KLINK KLMNO LLANO OLAND PLANA PLANB PLANE PLANI PLANK PLANO PLANS PLANT PLENA PLINK PLINY PLONK PLUNK SLANG SLANT SLING SLINK SLUNG SLUNK ULENE ULENT

•L••N
ALAIN ALBAN ALBEN ALCAN ALDEN ALIEN ALIGN ALLAN ALLEN ALLIN ALLYN ALPEN ALTON ALVIN BLOWN CLEAN CLEON CLOWN ELDIN ELDON ELFIN ELGIN ELION ELKIN ELLEN ELLIN ELMAN ELTON ELVIN FLANN FLOWN FLYIN FLYNN FLYON GLEAN GLENN GLUON ILION ILLIN KLEIN OLDEN OLEAN OLEIN OLSEN OLSON PLAIN PLZEN SLAIN SLOAN

••LN•
KILNS MILNE VILNA

••L•N
ALLAN ALLEN ALLIN ALLYN ARLEN ASLAN BALIN BALON BELON COLIN COLON DALEN DELON DOLIN DOLON DYLAN EGLIN ELLEN ELLIN EMLEN EMLYN FELON GALEN GOLAN HALEN HELEN ILLIN JKLMN MELON MILAN MULAN NOLAN NYLON OHLIN ORLON OSLIN PALIN PILON PYLON ROLEN SALON SOLAN SOLON TALON UCLAN UHLAN YULIN

LO•••
LOADS LOAFS LOAMS LOAMY LOANS LOATH LOBAR LOBBY LOBED LOBES LOBOS LOCAL LOCHS LOCKA LOCKE LOCKS LOCOS LOCUM LOCUS LODEN LODER LODES LODGE LOEIL LOESS LOEWE LOEWI LOEWS LOEWY LOFAT LOFTS LOFTY LOGAN LOGES LOGIA LOGIC LOGIN LOGON LOGOS LOGUE LOHAN LOIDS LOINS LOIRE LOLLS LOLLY LOMAN LOMAS LOMAX LONER LONGA LONGE LONGI LONGO LONGS LONGU LOOBY LOOEY LOOFA LOOIE LOOKS LOOKY LOOMS LOONS LOONY LOOPS LOOPY LOOSE LOOTS LOPAT LOPED LOPER LOPES LOPEZ LOPPY LORAN LORAX LORCA LORDS LORDY LOREN LORES LORIN LORIS LORNA LORNE LORRE LORRY LORUS LOSER LOSES LOSEY LOSIN LOTET LOTNO LOTOS LOTSA LOTTA LOTTE LOTTO LOTUS LOUIE LOUIS LOUMA LOUPE LOUPS LOURS LOURY LOUSE LOUSY LOUTH LOUTS LOVED LOVER LOVES LOVEY LOVIN LOWED LOWER LOWES LOWIQ LOWLY LOWON LOWPH LOWRY LOXES LOYAL

L•O••
LDOPA LEOII LEOIV LEOIX LEONA LEONE LEONI LEORA LEOVI LEOXI LIONS LLOSA LLOYD LOOBY LOOEY LOOFA LOOIE LOOKS LOOKY LOOMS LOONS LOONY LOOPS LOOPY LOOSE LOOTS LWOFF LYONS

L••O•
LABOR LAGOS LANOS LAYON LECON LEDON LEGOS LEMON LENOS LENOX LEROI LEROS LEROY LETON LEVON LIDOS LIEON LIMON LIMOS LINOS LITON LMNOP LOBOS LOCOS LOGON LOGOS LOTOS LOWON LTCOL LTCOM LTGOV LUXOR LUZON LYCOS LYDON LYMON LYSOL

L•••O
LACTO LANDO LARGO LASSO LAURO LAYTO LEDTO LEGNO LENTO LETGO LEUKO LIBRO LIETO LIGNO LIMBO LINDO LINGO LIPPO LITHO LLANO LONGO LOTNO LOTTO LUCIO LUEGO

•LO••
ALOES ALOFT ALOHA ALOIS ALONE ALONG ALOOF ALORS ALOUD BLOAT BLOBS BLOCH BLOCK BLOCS BLOGS BLOIS BLOKE BLOND BLOOD BLOOM BLOOP BLORE BLOTS BLOWN BLOWS BLOWY CLOAK CLOCK CLODS CLOGS CLOMP CLONE CLONK CLOPS CLOSE CLOTH CLOTS CLOUD CLOUT CLOVE CLOWN CLOYS ELOGE ELOPE ELORO FLOAT FLOCK FLOES FLOGS FLOJO FLOOD FLOOR FLOPS FLORA FLORI FLORY FLOSS FLOUR FLOUT FLOWN FLOWS FLOYD GLOAM GLOAT GLOBE GLOBS GLOCK GLOGG GLOMS GLOOM GLOPS GLORY GLOSS GLOTT GLOVE GLOWS ILONA ILOSE ILOVE LLOSA LLOYD OLOGY PLOCE PLODS PLONK PLOPS PLOTS PLOTZ PLOWS PLOYS SLOAN SLOBS SLOES SLOGS SLOMO SLOOP SLOPE SLOPS SLOSH SLOTH SLOTS SLOWS ULOUS ZLOTY

•L•O•
ALBOM ALCOA ALCOR ALGOL ALIOS ALLOF ALLOK ALLOT ALLOW ALLOY ALOOF ALROY ALSOP ALTON ALTOS BLOOD BLOOM BLOOP CLEON CLIOS ELBOW ELDON ELION ELIOT ELLOS ELMOS ELROY ELSOL ELTON ELYOT FLOOD FLOOR FLUOR FLYON GLOOM GLUON ILION OLEOS OLIOS OLMOS OLSON SLOOP

•L••O
ALADO ALAMO ALERO ALFIO ALITO ALTHO ALUKO BLUTO CLARO ELORO FLOJO FLYTO GLAXO GLUCO GLYCO ILLGO KLMNO LLANO OLIGO PLANO PLATO PLUTO SLIGO SLOMO

••LO•
AGLOW ALLOF ALLOK ALLOT ALLOW ALLOY BALON BALOO BELON BELOW BOLOS BULOW BYLOT CALOR CHLOE CHLOR COLON COLOR DELON DELOS DOLON DOLOR ELLOS FELON FILOS GALOP HALOP HALOS HELOS HELOT HULOT IGLOO INLOW KILOS MELON MELOS MELOT MILOS NOLOS NYLON ONLOW ORLON ORLOP ORLOS PALOS PHLOX PILON PILOT POLOS PYLON RELOG ROLOS RVLOT SALON SALOP SILOS SOLON SOLOS TALON VALOR VELOX YALOW ZHLOB

••L•O
AALTO BALBO BALLO BALOO BALTO BELLO BILBO BILKO CELLO DELCO DELLO DRLAO FALCO FALDO FOLIO GALLO HALLO HELIO HELLO HULLO IGLOO ILLGO JELLO JULIO KELSO MALMO MELLO MILLO MOLTO NELLO NULLO PALEO POLIO POLLO PULMO ROLEO ROLLO RULFO SALVO SOLDO STLEO TELCO VOLVO WALDO WILCO YELLO

•••LO
AMYLO ANGLO BALLO BELLO CARLO CELLO CHOLO CIELO CYCLO DELLO DIALO DIPLO DUPLO GALLO HALLO HATLO HELLO HULLO ITALO JELLO KAHLO MARLO MELLO MENLO MILLO NELLO NIBLO NUFLO NULLO OCULO OVOLO PABLO PAOLO PAULO PHILO PHYLO POLLO ROLLO VENLO YELLO

LP•••
LPGAS

L•P••
LAPAT LAPAZ LAPEL LAPIN LAPIS LAPPS LAPSE LAPUP LEPEN LEPER LEPEW LEPKE LEPUS LIPID LIPPI LIPPO LIPPY LOPAT LOPED LOPER LOPES LOPEZ LOPPY LUPIN LUPUS

L••P•
LAMPS LAPPS LDOPA LEAPS LEAPT LIMPS LIMPY LIPPI LIPPO LIPPY LISPS LOOPS LOOPY LOPPY LOUPE LOUPS LOWPH LUMPS LUMPY LYMPH

L•••P
LAPUP LAYUP LEGUP LETUP LIEUP LITUP LMNOP

•LP••
ALPEN ALPES ALPHA ELPIS OLPAE OLPES

•L•P•
ALEPH BLIPS CLAPS CLEPT CLIPS CLIPT CLOPS ELOPE FLAPS FLIPS FLOPS GLOPS GLYPH GLYPT PLOPS SLAPS SLEPT SLIPS SLOPE SLOPS

•L••P
ALMVP ALSOP BLEEP BLIMP BLOOP CLAMP CLASP CLOMP CLUMP FLYUP KLUMP NLMVP PLUMP SLEEP SLOOP SLUMP SLURP

••LP•
BALPH CULPA DELPY DOLPH GULPS GULPY HELPS JALPA KELPS MALPH PALPS PULPS PULPY RALPH SYLPH VOLPE YELPS

••L•P
GALOP
HALOP
ISLIP
JULEP
ORLOP
OXLIP
POLYP
RELAP
SALEP
SALOP
SHLEP
TULIP

•••LP
QUILP
SCALP
WHELP

L•••Q
LOWIQ

L•R••
LARAM
LARAS
LARCH
LARDS
LARDY
LAREE
LARES
LARGE
LARGO
LARIS
LARKS
LARKY
LARRY
LARUE
LARVA
LEROI
LEROS
LEROY
LIRAS
LORAN
LORAX
LORCA
LORDS
LORDY
LOREN
LORES
LORIN
LORIS
LORNA
LORNE
LORRE
LORRY
LORUS
LURAY
LURCH
LURED
LURER
LURES
LUREX
LURIA
LURID
LURIE
LURKS
LYRAS
LYRES
LYRIC
LYRID

L••R•
LAIRD
LAIRS
LARRY
LAURA
LAURO
LBARS
LEARN
LEARS
LEARY
LEERS
LEERY
LEHRS
LEORA
LEURS
LIARS
LIBRA
LIBRE
LIBRI
LIBRO
LITRE
LIVRE
LOIRE
LORRE
LORRY
LOURS
LOURY
LOWRY
LUCRE
LYCRA

L•••R
LABOR
LACER
LADER
LAGER
LAKER
LAMAR
LAMER
LASER
LATER
LAUER
LAVER
LAXER
LAYER
LAZAR
LECAR
LEDER
LEGER
LEHAR
LEMUR
LEPER
LEVAR
LEVER
LIBER
LIDAR
LIFAR
LIFER
LIGER
LIKER
LINER
LITER
LIVER
LOBAR
LODER
LONER
LOPER
LOSER
LOVER
LOWER
LUGAR
LUGER
LUNAR
LUNER
LURER
LUXOR

•LR••
ALROY
ELREY
ELROY
ULRIC

•L•R•
ALARM
ALERO
ALERS
ALERT
ALFRE
ALORS
BLARE
BLORE
BLURB
BLURS
BLURT
CLARA
CLARE
CLARK
CLARO
CLARY
CLERK
ELARA
ELORO
ELURA
FLARE
FLIRS
FLIRT
FLORA
FLORI
FLORY
GLARE
GLARY
GLORY
NLERS
PLURI
SLURP
SLURS
ULTRA

•L••R
ALCOR
ALDER
ALGER
ALLER
ALTAR
ALTER
ALVAR
BLAIR
BLEAR
BLUER
CLAIR
CLEAR
CLUER
ELCAR
ELDER
ELGAR
ELLER
ELMAR
ELMER
ELVER
FLAIR
FLEER
FLEUR
FLIER
FLOOR
FLOUR
FLUOR
FLYER
GLUER
ILLER
OLDER
PLIER
PLUMR
PLYER
SLIER
SLYER
ULCER
ULNAR

••L•R
ABLER
ADLER
AILUR
ALLER
AOLER
BALER
BOLAR
CALOR
CHLOR
COLOR
DOLOR
EELER
ELLER
EULER
FILAR
FILER
HALER
HOLER
IDLER
ILLER
MALAR
MILER
MOLAR
MYLAR
NFLER
NHLER
OGLER
OILER
OSLER
PALAR
PALER
PILAR
PILER
POLAR
POLER
PULER
RULER
SOLAR
SOLER
TALER
TELAR
TILER
TOLAR
TOLER
TYLER
VALOR
VELAR
VILER
VOLAR
WYLER

LS•••
LSATS

L•S••
LASED
LASER
LASES
LASIK
LASKI
LASKY
LASSE
LASSO
LASTS
LISLE
LISPS
LISSE
LISTS
LISZT
LOSER
LOSES
LOSEY
LOSIN
LUSHY
LUSTS
LUSTY
LYSED
LYSES
LYSIS
LYSOL

L••S•
LAPSE
LASSE
LASSO
LEASE
LEASH
LEAST
LHASA
LIESL
LIEST
LISSE
LLOSA
LOESS
LOOSE
LOTSA
LOUSE
LOUSY
LUISA
LUISE
LUTSK

L•••S
LACES
LACKS
LADAS
LADES
LADYS
LAFFS
LAGOS
LAICS
LAIRS
LAITS
LAIUS
LAKES
LAMAS
LAMBS
LAMES
LAMPS
LANDS
LANES
LANOS
LAPIS
LAPPS
LARAS
LARDS
LARES
LARIS
LARKS
LASES
LASTS
LATHS
LAUDS
LAVAS
LAVES
LAWES
LAWNS
LAZES
LBARS
LEADS
LEAFS
LEAKS
LEANS
LEAPS
LEARS
LECTS
LEEDS
LEEKS
LEERS
LEFTS
LEGGS
LEGOS
LEHRS
LENDS
LENES
LENIS
LENOS
LENTS
LEPUS
LEROS
LETTS
LEURS
LEVIS
LEWES
LEWIS
LEXIS
LEXUS
LIARS
LICKS
LIDOS
LIENS
LIEUS
LIFTS
LIKES
LILTS
LIMAS
LIMBS
LIMES
LIMNS
LIMOS
LIMPS
LINCS
LINES
LINGS
LINKS
LINOS
LINTS
LINUS
LIONS
LIRAS
LISPS
LISTS
LITES
LIVES
LOADS
LOAFS
LOAMS
LOANS
LOBES
LOBOS
LOCHS
LOCKS
LOCOS
LOCUS
LODES
LOESS
LOEWS
LOFTS
LOGES
LOGOS
LOIDS
LOINS
LOLLS
LOMAS
LONGS
LOOKS
LOOMS
LOONS
LOOPS
LOOTS
LOPES
LORDS
LORES
LORIS
LORUS
LOSES
LOTOS
LOTUS
LOUIS
LOUPS
LOURS
LOUTS
LOVES
LOWES
LOXES
LPGAS
LSATS
LUAUS
LUBES
LUCAS
LUCKS
LUFFS
LUGES
LUKAS
LULLS
LULUS
LUMAS
LUMPS
LUNAS
LUNES
LUNGS
LUNNS
LUNTS
LUPUS
LURES
LURKS
LUSTS
LUTES
LUXES
LWEIS
LYCOS
LYONS
LYRAS
LYRES
LYSES
LYSIS

•LS••
ALSAB
ALSOP
ELSAS
ELSES
ELSIE
ELSOL
OLSEN
OLSON

•L•S•
ALISA
ALIST
BLASE
BLASS
BLAST
BLESS
BLEST
BLISH
BLISS
BLIST
BLUSH
CLASE
CLASH
CLASP
CLASS
CLOSE
ELISA
ELISE
ELIST
ELMST
ELYSE
FLASH
FLASK
FLESH
FLOSS
FLUSH
GLASS
GLESS
GLOSS
ILOSE
LLOSA
PLASH
PLASM
PLAST
PLUSH
RLESS
SLASH
SLOSH
SLUSH

•L••S
ALAIS
ALBAS
ALEFS
ALERS
ALFAS
ALGAS
ALIAS
ALIFS
ALIOS
ALLES
ALLIS
ALOES
ALOIS
ALORS
ALPES
ALTOS
ALTUS
ALUMS
BLABS
BLAHS
BLAIS
BLAMS
BLASS
BLATS
BLDGS
BLEBS
BLESS
BLEUS
BLIPS
BLISS
BLOBS
BLOCS
BLOGS
BLOIS
BLOTS
BLOWS
BLUES
BLURS
BLVDS
CLADS
CLAES
CLAMS
CLANS
CLAPS
CLASS
CLAUS
CLAWS
CLAYS
CLEFS
CLEWS
CLIOS
CLIPS
CLODS
CLOGS
CLOPS
CLOTS
CLOYS
CLUBS
CLUES
ELEMS
ELEVS
ELIAS
ELLES
ELLIS
ELLOS
ELMOS
ELPIS
ELSAS
ELSES
ELULS
ELVES
ELVIS
ELWES
FLAGS
FLAMS
FLANS
FLAPS
FLATS
FLAWS
FLAYS
FLEAS
FLEES
FLICS
FLIES
FLIPS
FLIRS
FLITS
FLOES
FLOGS
FLOPS
FLOSS
FLOWS
FLUBS
FLUES
GLADS
GLAMS
GLASS
GLEES
GLENS
GLESS
GLIAS
GLIMS
GLOBS
GLOMS
GLOPS
GLOSS
GLOWS
GLUES
GLUGS
GLUMS
GLUTS
ILLUS
KLAUS
MLLES
NLERS
OLEOS
OLIOS
OLLAS
OLMOS
OLPES
PLANS
PLATS
PLAYS
PLEAS
PLEBS
PLIES
PLODS
PLOPS
PLOTS
PLOWS
PLOYS
PLUGS
PLUMS
RLESS
SLABS
SLAGS
SLAMS
SLAPS
SLATS
SLAVS
SLAWS
SLAYS
SLEDS
SLEWS
SLEYS
SLIMS
SLIPS
SLITS
SLOBS
SLOES
SLOGS
SLOPS
SLOTS
SLOWS
SLUES
SLUGS
SLUMS
SLURS
ULEES
ULNAS
ULOUS

••LS•
BALSA
FALSE
HOLST
KELSO
NELSE
PALSY
PULSE
SALSA
TULSA
VALSE
WALSH
WALSY
WELSH

••L•S
AILES
ALLES
ALLIS
APLUS
ARLES
ATLAS
ATLES
AULIS
AULUS
AXLES
BALAS
BALDS
BALES
BALKS
BALLS
BALMS
BALTS
BELLS
BELTS
BILES
BILKS
BILLS
BOLAS
BOLDS
BOLES
BOLLS
BOLOS
BOLTS
BOLUS
BPLUS
BULBS
BULKS
BULLS
CALKS
CALLS
CALMS
CELLS
CELTS
COLAS
COLDS
COLES
COLTS
CPLUS
CULLS
CULTS
DALES
DALIS
DELES
DELIS
DELLS
DELOS
DELTS
DILLS
DOLES
DOLLS
DOLTS
DPLUS
DULLS
ELLES
ELLIS
ELLOS
EOLUS
FALLS
FELIS
FELLS
FELTS
FILAS
FILES
FILLS
FILMS
FILOS
FOLDS
FOLKS
FTLBS
FULLS
GALAS
GALES
GALLS
GELDS
GELTS
GILAS
GILDS
GILES
GILLS
GILTS
GOLDS
GOLFS
GULFS
GULLS
GULPS
HALAS
HALES
HALLS
HALOS
HALTS
HELLS
HELMS
HELOS
HELPS
HILLS
HILTS
HOLDS
HOLES
HOLMS
HULAS
HULKS
HULLS
HYLAS
IDLES
IGLUS
ILLUS
ISLAS
ISLES
JELLS
JILTS
JOLTS
JULES
JULYS
KALES
KELPS
KILLS
KILNS
KILOS
KILTS
KOLAS
LILTS
LOLLS
LULLS
LULUS
MALES
MALLS
MALTS
MELDS
MELIS
MELOS
MELTS
MILES
MILKS
MILLS
MILOS
MLLES
MOLDS
MOLES
MOLLS
MOLTS
MULES
MULLS
MYLES
NILES
NOLES
NOLOS
NULLS
OGLES
OLLAS
ORLES
ORLOS
PALES
PALLS
PALMS
PALOS
PALPS
PELFS
PELTS
PILES
PILLS
PILUS
POLES
POLIS
POLKS
POLLS
POLOS
PULAS
PULES
PULIS
PULLS
PULPS
RALES
RILES
RILLS
ROLES
ROLFS
ROLLS
ROLOS
RULES
SALAS
SALES
SALTS
SELES
SELLS
SILAS
SILKS
SILLS
SILOS
SILTS
SOLES
SOLOS
SULKS
TALAS
TALCS
TALES
TALKS
TALLS
TALUS
TELES
TELLS
TILES
TILLS
TILTS
TOLES
TOLLS
TULES
UGLIS
VALES
VELDS
VILAS
VOLES
VOLTS
WALES
WALKS
WALLS
WELDS
WELLS
WELTS
WILDS
WILES
WILLS
WILTS
WOLFS
YELLS
YELPS
YOLKS
YULES
ZALES
ZILLS
ZULUS

•••LS
AGALS
AMYLS
ANILS
ARILS
ARYLS
AWOLS
AXELS
AXILS
BAALS
BAILS
BALLS
BAWLS
BEALS
BELLS
BILLS
BIRLS
BOILS
BOLLS
BOWLS
BULLS
BURLS
CALLS
CEILS
CELLS
CIELS
COALS
COILS
COOLS
COWLS
CULLS
CURLS
DEALS
DEILS
DELLS
DHALS
DIALS
DIELS
DILLS
DOLLS
DUALS
DUELS
DULLS
EARLS
EBELS
EGALS
ELULS
ENCLS
ENOLS
EVILS
FAILS
FALLS
FEELS
FELLS
FILLS
FOALS
FOILS
FOOLS
FOULS
FOWLS
FUELS
FULLS
FURLS
GAELS
GALLS
GAOLS
GAULS
GILLS
GIRLS
GOALS
GRRLS
GULLS
HAILS
HALLS
HAULS
HEALS
HEELS
HELLS
HILLS
HOWLS
HULLS
HURLS
IDOLS
IDYLS
ITALS
JAILS
JELLS
JOWLS
KEELS
KILLS
KOHLS
LOLLS
LULLS
MAILS
MALLS
MARLS
MAULS
MEALS
MERLS
MEWLS
MIELS
MILLS
MOILS
MOLLS
MULLS
NAILS
NIELS
NOELS
NOILS
NULLS
OBOLS
ONELS
OPALS
OPELS
ORALS
OVALS
PAILS
PALLS
PAWLS
PEALS
PEELS
PIELS
PILLS
POLLS
POOLS
PULLS
PURLS
RAILS
RAWLS
REALS
REELS
RIALS
RIELS
RILLS
ROILS
ROLLS
ROTLS
RYALS
SAILS
SEALS
SELLS
SHULS
SILLS
SOILS
SOULS
STOLS
TAELS
TAILS
TALLS
TEALS
TELLS
TILLS
TIXLS
TOILS
TOLLS
TOOLS
URALS
UTILS
VEALS
VEILS
VIALS
VIOLS
VTOLS
WAALS
WAILS
WALLS
WEALS
WELLS
WILLS
WOOLS
YAWLS
YELLS
YOWLS
ZEALS
ZILLS

LT•••
LTCOL
LTCOM
LTGEN
LTGOV
LTILE

L•T••
LATCH
LATEN
LATER
LATEX
LATHE
LATHS
LATHY
LATIN

LATKA
LATKE
LATTE
LETAT
LETBE
LETBY
LETGO
LETHE
LETIN
LETME
LETON
LETTS
LETTY
LETUP
LITEL
LITER
LITES
LITHE
LITHO
LITON
LITRE
LITTB
LITTD
LITUP
LOTET
LOTNO
LOTOS
LOTSA
LOTTA
LOTTE
LOTTO
LOTUS
LUTED
LUTES
LUTSK

L••T•

LACTI
LACTO
LAHTI
LAITS
LAITY
LANTZ
LASTS
LATTE
LAYTO
LECTS
LEDTO
LEFTS
LEFTY
LEITH
LENTE
LENTO
LENTS
LETTS
LETTY
LEYTE
LIETO
LIFTS
LILTS
LINTS
LINTY
LISTS
LITTB
LITTD
LOATH
LOFTS
LOFTY
LOOTS
LOTTA
LOTTE
LOTTO
LOUTH
LOUTS
LSATS
LUNTS
LUSTS
LUSTY

L•••T

LAMIT
LAPAT
LEANT
LEAPT
LEAST
LEGIT
LEMAT
LETAT
LEVIT
LICHT
LICIT
LIEST
LIEUT
LIGHT
LIMIT
LINDT
LINFT
LISZT
LOFAT
LOPAT
LOTET
LUMET

•LT••

ALTAI
ALTAR
ALTER
ALTHO
ALTON
ALTOS
ALTUS
ELTON
ULTRA

•L•T•

ALATE
ALETA
ALITO
ALITY
BLATS
BLATZ
BLITT
BLITZ
BLOTS
BLUTH
BLUTO
BLYTH
CLETE
CLOTH
CLOTS
ELATE
ELATH
ELITE
ELUTE
FLATS
FLATT
FLITS
FLUTE
FLUTY
FLYTO
GLATT
GLITZ
GLOTT
GLUTE
GLUTS
KLUTE
KLUTZ
OLETA
PLATA
PLATE
PLATH
PLATO
PLATS
PLATT
PLATY
PLOTS
PLOTZ
PLUTO
SLATE
SLATS
SLATY
SLITS
SLOTH
SLOTS
ZLOTY

•L••T

ALERT
ALEUT
ALIST
ALLOT
ALOFT
BLAST
BLEAT
BLENT
BLEST
BLIST
BLITT
BLOAT
BLUET
BLUNT
BLURT
CLEAT
CLEFT
CLEPT
CLIFT
CLINT
CLIPT
CLOUT
ELECT
ELIOT
ELIST
ELMST
ELYOT
FLATT
FLEET
FLINT
FLIRT
FLOAT
FLOUT
FLYAT
GLATT
GLINT
GLOAT
GLOTT
GLYPT
KLIMT
PLAIT
PLANT
PLAST
PLATT
PLEAT
SLANT
SLEET
SLEPT
ULENT

••LT•

AALTO
BALTO
BALTS
BELTS
BOLTS
CELTS
COLTS
CULTI
CULTS
DELTA
DELTS
DOLTS
FELTS
FILTH
GELTS
GILTS
HALTS
HILTS
HOLTZ
JILTS
JOLTS
JOLTY
KILTS
LILTS
MALTA
MALTS
MALTY
MELTS
MOLTO
MOLTS
MULTI
NOLTE
PELTS
SALTI
SALTS
SALTY
SILTS
SILTY
SOLTI
TILTH
TILTS
USLTA
VOLTA
VOLTE
VOLTS
WALTZ
WELTS
WELTY
WILTS
YALTA

••L•T

AFLAT
AGLET
ALLOT
AMLIT
BFLAT
BOLET
BYLOT
CFLAT
CULET
DALET
DELFT
DFLAT
ECLAT
EFLAT
EILAT
FFLAT
FILET
GFLAT
HELOT
HOLST
HULOT
INLET
ISLET
MELOT
MULCT
OWLET
PILOT
POLIT
RELET
RELIT
RVLOT
SALUT
SPLAT
SPLIT
TOLET
UNLET
UNLIT
UPLIT
VALET
VELDT

•••LT

ADULT
ATILT
BOULT
BUILT
DEALT
DWELT
EXALT
EXULT
FAULT
GUILT
ISOLT
KNELT
MOULT
POULT
QUILT
SAULT
SHALT
SMELT
SMOLT
SPELT
SPILT
STILT
UBOLT
VAULT

LU•••

LUANA
LUANG
LUANN
LUAUS
LUBED
LUBES
LUBIN
LUCAN
LUCAS
LUCCA
LUCCI
LUCIA
LUCID
LUCIE
LUCIO
LUCKS
LUCKY
LUCRE
LUDIC
LUEGO
LUFFS
LUGAR
LUGED
LUGER
LUGES
LUIGI
LUISA
LUISE
LUJAN
LUKAS
LULEA
LULLS
LULLY
LULUS
LUMAN
LUMAS
LUMEN
LUMET
LUMPS
LUMPY
LUNAR
LUNAS
LUNCH
LUNDI
LUNDY
LUNER
LUNES
LUNGE
LUNGS
LUNIK
LUNNS
LUNTS
LUPIN
LUPUS
LURAY
LURCH
LURED
LURER
LURES
LUREX
LURIA
LURID
LURIE
LURKS
LUSHY
LUSTS
LUSTY
LUTED
LUTES
LUTSK
LUXES
LUXOR
LUZON

L•U••

LAUDA
LAUDE
LAUDS
LAUER
LAUGH
LAURA
LAURO
LEUKO
LEUMI
LEURS
LOUIE
LOUIS
LOUMA
LOUPE
LOUPS
LOURS
LOURY
LOUSE
LOUSY
LOUTH
LOUTS

L••U•

LAIUS
LAPUP
LARUE
LAYUP
LEAUD
LEGUP
LEHUA
LEMUR
LEPUS
LETUP
LEXUS
LIEUP
LIEUS
LIEUT
LIKUD
LINUS
LINUX
LITUP
LOCUM
LOCUS
LOGUE
LORUS
LOTUS
LUAUS
LULUS
LUPUS

L•••U

LAFEU
LINGU
LONGU

•LU••

ALUKO
ALULA
ALUMS
BLUED
BLUER
BLUES
BLUET
BLUFF
BLUME
BLUNT
BLURB
BLURS
BLURT
BLUSH
BLUTH
BLUTO
CLUBS
CLUCK
CLUED
CLUER
CLUES
CLUMP
CLUNG
CLUNK
CLUNY
ELUDE
ELULS
ELURA
ELUTE
FLUBS
FLUES
FLUFF
FLUID
FLUKE
FLUKY
FLUME
FLUNG
FLUNK
FLUOR
FLUSH
FLUTE
FLUTY
GLUCK
GLUCO
GLUED
GLUER
GLUES
GLUEY
GLUGS
GLUMS
GLUNK
GLUON
GLUTE
GLUTS
KLUGH
KLUMP
KLUTE
KLUTZ
PLUCK
PLUGS
PLUIE
PLUMB
PLUME
PLUMP
PLUMR
PLUMS
PLUMY
PLUNK
PLURI
PLUSH
PLUTO
PLUVI
SLUED
SLUES
SLUGS
SLUMP
SLUMS
SLUNG
SLUNK
SLURP
SLURS
SLUSH

•L•U•

ALBUM
ALEUT
ALOUD
ALTUS
BLEUS
CLAUS
CLOUD
CLOUT
FLEUR
FLOUR
FLOUT
FLYUP
ILEUM
ILIUM
ILLUS
KLAUS
OLEUM
ULOUS

•L••U

ELIHU
ILGWU

••LU•

AILUR
APLUS
AULUS
BOLUS
BPLUS
COLUM
CPLUS
DPLUS
EOLUS
FILUM
HILUM
IGLUS
ILLUS
LULUS
PFLUG
PILUS
SALUD
SALUT
TALUS
VALUE
VELUM
ZHLUB
ZULUS

••L•U

BELAU
PALAU
PILAU
YALEU

•••LU

POILU
UPOLU

LV•••

LVIII

L•V••

LAVAL
LAVAS
LAVED
LAVER
LAVES
LAVIE
LAVIN
LEVAR
LEVEE
LEVEL
LEVER
LEVIN
LEVIS
LEVIT
LEVON
LIVED
LIVEN
LIVER
LIVES
LIVIA
LIVID
LIVIN
LIVRE
LOVED
LOVER
LOVES
LOVEY
LOVIN
LXVII

L••V•

LARVA
LEAVE
LEOVI
LWAVE
LXXVI

L•••V

LEOIV
LTGOV
LXXIV
LXXXV

•LV••

ALVAR
ALVIN
BLVDS
CLVII
DLVII
ELVER
ELVES
ELVIN
ELVIS
MLVII
XLVII

•L•V•

ALAVA
ALEVE
ALIVE
ALMVP
CLAVE
CLEVE
CLIVE
CLOVE
CLXVI
DLXVI
ELEVE
ELEVS
FLAVA
GLOVE
ILOVE
MLXVI
NLMVP
OLAVI
OLAVV
OLIVA
OLIVE
PLUVI
SLAVE
SLAVS

•L••V

CLXIV
CLXXV
DLXIV
DLXXV
ELYNV
MLXIV
MLXXV
OLAFV
OLAVV

••LV•

BELVA
CALVE
CCLVI
CDLVI
CMLVI
CXLVI
DCLVI
DELVE
DXLVI
HALVA
HALVE
MCLVI
MDLVI
MMLVI
MXLVI
SALVE
SALVO
SILVA
SOLVE
VALVE
VELVA
VOLVO

••L•V

CCLIV
CCLXV
CDLIV
CDLXV
CMLIV
CMLXV
CXLIV
DCLIV
DCLXV
DXLIV
MALEV
MCLIV
MCLXV
MDLIV
MDLXV
MMLIV
MMLXV
MXLIV

•••LV

CCCLV
CCXLV
CDXLV
CMXLV
DCCLV
DCXLV
MCCLV
MCDLV
MCMLV
MCXLV
MDCLV
MDXLV
MMCLV
MMDLV
MMMLV
MMXLV
PAULV

LW•••

LWAVE
LWEIS
LWOFF

L•W••

LAWED
LAWES
LAWNS
LAWNY
LEWES
LEWIS
LOWED
LOWER
LOWES
LOWIQ
LOWLY
LOWON
LOWPH
LOWRY

L••W•

LOEWE
LOEWI
LOEWS
LOEWY

L•••W

LALAW
LEPEW

•LW••

ALWAY
CLWYD
ELWAY
ELWES

•L•W•

BLOWN
BLOWS
BLOWY
CLAWS
CLEWS
CLOWN
FLAWS
FLAWY
FLOWN
FLOWS
GLOWS
ILGWU
PLOWS
SLAWS
SLEWS
SLIWA
SLOWS

•L••W

ALLOW
ELBOW

••L•W

AGLOW
ALLOW
BELOW
BILLW
BULOW
BYLAW
INLAW
INLOW
LALAW
ONLOW
YALOW

•••LW

BILLW

LX•••

LXIII
LXVII
LXXII
LXXIV
LXXIX
LXXVI
LXXXI
LXXXV

L•X••

LAXER
LAXLY
LEXAN
LEXIS
LEXUS
LOXES
LUXES
LUXOR
LXXII
LXXIV
LXXIX
LXXVI
LXXXI
LXXXV

L••X•

LEOXI
LXXXI
LXXXV

L•••X

LATEX
LENOX
LEOIX
LINUX
LOMAX
LORAX
LUREX
LXXIX

•LX••

CLXII
CLXIV
CLXIX
CLXVI
CLXXI
CLXXV
CLXXX
DLXII
DLXIV
DLXIX
DLXVI
DLXXI
DLXXV
DLXXX
MLXII
MLXIV
MLXIX
MLXVI
MLXXI
MLXXV
MLXXX

•L•X•

ALEXA
ALEXI
CLXXI
CLXXV
CLXXX
DLXXI
DLXXV
DLXXX
FLAXY
GLAXO
MLXXI
MLXXV
MLXXX

•L••X

CLXIX
CLXXX
DLXIX
DLXXX
MLXIX
MLXXX

••LX•

CCLXI
CCLXV
CCLXX
CDLXI
CDLXV
CDLXX
CMLXI
CMLXV
CMLXX
DCLXI
DCLXV
DCLXX
MCLXI
MCLXV
MCLXX
MDLXI
MDLXV
MDLXX
MMLXI
MMLXV
MMLXX

••L•X

CALIX
CALYX
CCLIX
CCLXX
CDLIX
CDLXX
CMLIX
CMLXX
CXLIX
DCLIX
DCLXX
DXLIX
FELIX
GALAX
HELIX
MCLIX
MCLXX
MDLIX
MDLXX
MMLIX
MMLXX
MXLIX
PHLOX
RELAX
ROLEX
SILEX
TELEX
TILEX
UNLAX
VELOX

•••LX

CCCLX
DCCLX
MCCLX
MCDLX
MCMLX
MDCLX
MMCLX
MMDLX
MMMLX

LY•••

LYCEE
LYCOS
LYCRA
LYDIA
LYDON
LYELL
LYGIA
LYING
LYMAN
LYMON
LYMPH
LYNCH
LYNDA
LYNDE
LYNEN
LYNNE
LYONS
LYRAS
LYRES
LYRIC
LYRID
LYSED
LYSES
LYSIS
LYSOL

L•Y••

LAYBY
LAYER
LAYIN
LAYLA
LAYNE
LAYON
LAYTO
LAYUP
LEYTE
LOYAL

L••Y•

LADYL
LADYS
LENYA
LIBYA
LLOYD

L•••Y

LACEY
LAITY
LANKY
LANNY
LARDY
LARKY
LARRY
LASKY
LATHY
LAWNY
LAXLY
LAYBY
LEADY
LEAFY
LEAHY
LEAKY
LEARY
LECKY
LEDGY
LEERY
LEFAY
LEFTY
LEGGY
LEMAY
LENNY
LEROY
LETBY
LETTY
LIBBY
LIDDY
LIEBY
LILLY
LIMPY
LINDY
LINTY
LIPPY
LOAMY
LOBBY
LOEWY
LOFTY
LOLLY
LOOBY
LOOEY
LOOKY
LOONY
LOOPY
LOPPY
LORDY
LORRY
LOSEY
LOURY
LOUSY
LOVEY
LOWLY
LOWRY
LUCKY
LULLY
LUMPY
LUNDY
LURAY
LUSHY
LUSTY

•LY••

ALYCE
BLYTH
CLYDE
ELYNV
ELYOT
ELYSE
FLYAT
FLYBY
FLYER
FLYIN
FLYME
FLYNN
FLYON
FLYTO
FLYUP
GLYCO
GLYPH
GLYPT
PLYER
SLYER
SLYKE
SLYLY

•L•Y•

ALKYD
ALKYL
ALLYL
ALLYN
CLAYS
CLOYS
CLWYD
FLAYS
FLOYD
ILLYA
LLOYD
PLAYA
PLAYS
PLOYS
SLAYS
SLEYS

•L••Y

ALITY
ALLAY

ALLEY
ALLOY
ALMAY
ALROY
ALWAY
BLOWY
CLARY
CLUNY
ELEGY
ELREY
ELROY
ELWAY
FLAKY
FLAMY
FLAWY
FLAXY
FLORY
FLUKY
FLUTY
FLYBY
GLARY
GLAZY
GLORY
GLUEY
OLOGY
PLATY
PLINY
PLUMY
SLATY
SLIMY
SLYLY
ZLOTY

••LY•
ALLYL
ALLYN
CALYX
EMLYN
ILLYA
JULYS
POLYP

••L•Y
AGLEY
AILEY
ALLAY
ALLEY
ALLOY
APLEY
BALDY
BALKY
BALLY
BALMY
BELAY
BELBY
BELLY
BILGY
BILLY
BULGY
BULKY
BULLY
COLBY
CULLY
DALEY
DALLY
DELAY
DELPY
DILLY
DOLBY
DOLLY
DULLY
FILLY
FILMY
FOLEY
FOLKY
FOLLY
FULLY
GOLLY
GULLY
GULPY
HALEY
HILLY
HOLEY
HOLLY
HULKY
HULLY
INLAY
ISLEY
JELLY
JOLLY
JOLTY
JULEY
KELLY
KILBY
KILEY
KILLY
LILLY
LOLLY
LULLY
MALAY
MALTY
MILKY
MOLDY
MOLLY
MULEY
NELLY
NILLY
ONLAY
PALEY
PALLY
PALMY
PALSY
POLLY
PULPY
RALLY
RELAY
RILEY
SALLY
SALTY
SILKY
SILLY
SILTY
SPLAY
SULKY
SULLY
TALKY
TALLY
TELLY
TILLY
TULLY
UNLAY
UTLEY
WALLY
WALSY
WELBY
WELTY
WILBY
WILEY
WILLY
YOLKY

•••LY
AMPLY
APPLY
APTLY
BADLY
BALLY
BELLY
BIALY
BIGLY
BILLY
BULLY
BURLY
CARLY
CHELY
COYLY
CULLY
CURLY
DAILY
DALLY
DILLY
DIMLY
DOILY
DOLLY
DOYLY
DRILY
DRYLY
DULLY
EARLY
EMILY
FATLY
FEELY
FEYLY
FILLY
FITLY
FOLLY
FULLY
GAILY
GAYLY
GIRLY
GODLY
GOLLY
GULLY
HAPLY
HEALY
HILLY
HIPLY
HOLLY
HOTLY
HULLY
HURLY
ICILY
IMPLY
ITALY
JELLY
JOLLY
JOWLY
KEELY
KELLY
KILLY
LAXLY
LILLY
LOLLY
LOWLY
LULLY
MADLY
MANLY
MARLY
MCFLY
MEALY
MOLLY
MTELY
NEALY
NEELY
NELLY
NEWLY
NILLY
NOBLY
NOILY
ODDLY
PALLY
PATLY
POLLY
RALLY
RAWLY
REDLY
REFLY
REPLY
ROILY
SADLY
SALLY
SCALY
SEALY
SHYLY
SILLY
SLYLY
SULLY
SURLY
TALLY
TELLY
TILLY
TRULY
TULLY
UNSLY
VEALY
WALLY
WANLY
WETLY
WILLY
WOOLY
WRYLY

L•Z••
LAZAR
LAZED
LAZES
LIZZI
LUZON

L••Z•
LANZA
LEEZA
LISZT
LIZZI

L•••Z
LANTZ
LAPAZ
LOPEZ

•LZ••
PLZEN

•L•Z•
BLAZE
ELIZA
GLAZE
GLAZY
PLAZA

•L••Z
ALLEZ
BLATZ
BLITZ
GLITZ
KLUTZ
PLOTZ

••L•Z
ALLEZ
FELIZ
HOLTZ
VELEZ
WALTZ

MA•••
MAAMS
MABEL
MACAO
MACAW
MACED
MACER
MACES
MACHE
MACHO
MACHU
MACHY
MACKE
MACKS
MACLE
MACON
MACRO
MACYS
MADAM
MADAT
MADGE
MADLY
MADOC
MADOX
MADRE
MADTV
MAEVE
MAFIA
MAGDA
MAGEE
MAGES
MAGIC
MAGMA
MAGNA
MAGOG
MAGOO
MAGUA
MAGUS
MAHAL
MAHAN
MAHDI
MAHER
MAHON
MAHRE
MAIDS
MAILS
MAIMS
MAINE
MAINS
MAINZ
MAIRE
MAIZE
MAJOR
MAKEM
MAKER
MAKES
MAKIN
MAKOS
MALAR
MALAY
MALES
MALEV
MALIC
MALLE
MALLS
MALMO
MALPH
MALTA
MALTS
MALTY
MAMAS
MAMBA
MAMBO
MAMET
MAMIE
MAMMA
MAMMY
MANAT
MANCY
MANDY
MANED
MANES
MANET
MANGA
MANGE
MANGO
MANGY
MANIA
MANIC
MANLY
MANNA
MANNE
MANNY
MANON
MANOR
MANOS
MANSE
MANTA
MANUS
MAOII
MAORI
MAPES
MAPLE
MAQUI
MARAT
MARCA
MARCH
MARCI
MARCO
MARCY
MARDI
MAREK
MARES
MARGE
MARGO
MARGY
MARIA
MARIE
MARIN
MARIO
MARIS
MARKA
MARKI
MARKS
MARKV
MARLA
MARLO
MARLS
MARLY
MARMS
MARNE
MARNI
MAROT
MARRY
MARSH
MARTA
MARTI
MARTS
MARTY
MARVY
MARYA
MARYI
MARYJ
MARYS
MARZO
MASAI
MASAS
MASER
MASHA
MASKS
MASON
MASSA
MASSE
MASSY
MASTS
MASUR
MATCH
MATED
MATEO
MATER
MATES
MATEY
MATHS
MATIN
MATRI
MATRO
MATSU
MATTE
MATTY
MATZO
MAUDE
MAULS
MAUNA
MAURA
MAURY
MAUVE
MAVEN
MAVIN
MAVIS
MAXED
MAXES
MAXIE
MAXIM
MAXIS
MAYAN
MAYAS
MAYBE
MAYER
MAYLE
MAYNT
MAYOR
MAYOS
MAYPO
MAYST
MAZAR
MAZDA
MAZED
MAZEL
MAZES

M•A••
MAAMS
MCATS
MEADE
MEADS
MEALS
MEALY
MEANS
MEANT
MEANY
MEARA
MEARS
MEATH
MEATS
MEATY
MIAMI
MIAOU
MIAOW
MIATA
MOANS
MOATS
MTAPO

M••A•
MACAO
MACAW
MADAM
MADAT
MAHAL
MAHAN
MALAR
MALAY
MAMAS
MANAT
MARAT
MASAI
MASAS
MAYAN
MAYAS
MAZAR
MCKAY
MCNAB
MCRAE
MEDAL
MEGAN
MENAS
MESAS
METAL
MICAH
MICAS
MIDAS
MIKAN
MILAN
MINAS
MITAS
MIZAR
MODAL
MOLAR
MONAD
MORAL
MORAN
MORAS
MORAY
MOWAT
MSTAR
MULAN
MURAL
MURAT
MUZAK
MYBAD
MYDAD
MYDAY
MYLAR
MYMAN
MYNAH
MYNAS
MYWAR
MYWAY

M•••A
MAFIA
MAGDA
MAGMA
MAGNA
MAGUA
MALTA
MAMBA
MAMMA
MANGA
MANIA
MANNA
MANTA
MARCA
MARIA
MARKA
MARLA
MARTA
MARYA
MASHA
MASSA
MAUNA
MAURA
MAZDA
MEARA
MECCA
MEDEA
MEDIA
MEHTA
MEKKA
MELBA
MENSA
MESTA
MIATA
MICRA
MISHA
MISSA
MITLA
MITYA
MOCHA
MOIRA
MOMMA
MONZA
MOOLA
MORRA
MTIDA
MUCHA
MULLA
MUNNA
MUSCA
MYRIA
MYRNA

•MA••
AMADA
AMADO
AMAHL
AMAHS
AMAIN
AMANA
AMAND
AMANT
AMAPA
AMARA
AMARE
AMASS
AMATI
AMATO
AMAZE
DMARK
EMAGS
EMAIL
EMALL
GMATS
IMACS
IMAGE
IMAGO
IMAMS
IMAMU
IMARI
KMART
OMAHA
OMANI
OMARR
SMACK
SMALL
SMARM
SMART
SMASH
SMAUG
SMAZE
UMASS

•M•A•
AMMAN
AMPAS
AMRAM
AMWAY
AMYAS
EMBAR
EMBAY
IMBAD
IMEAN
IMMAD
SMEAL
SMEAR
UMIAK
YMCAS
YMHAS

•M••A
AMADA
AMANA
AMAPA
AMARA
AMEBA
AMICA
AMIGA
AMNIA
EMESA
OMAHA
OMEGA
OMNIA
UMBRA

••MA•
ADMAN
AHMAD
AIMAT
ALMAY
AMMAN
ARMAH
ARMAS
ASMAD
ATMAN
AXMAN
BEMAD
BEMAN
BEMAS
CAMAS
CAMAY
COMAE
COMAS
CYMAE
CYMAS
DAMAS
DIMAG
DIMAS
DUMAS
EDMAR
ELMAN
ELMAR
ERMAS
GAMAL
GAMAY
GOMAD
GOMAN
HAMAN
HAMAS
HEMAL
HEMAN
HEMAT
HUMAN
HYMAN
IMMAD
INMAY
JAMAL
KEMAL
LAMAR
LAMAS
LEMAN
LEMAT
LEMAY
LIMAN
LIMAS
LOMAN
LOMAS
LOMAX
LUMAN
LUMAS
LYMAN
MAMAS
MYMAN
NEMAN
NOMAD
NOMAR
NOMAS
NUMAN
NYMAN
OHMAN
ORMAN
OSMAN
PIMAS
PRMAN
PUMAS
RAMAN
RAMAR
RAMAS
REMAN
REMAP
REMAT
REMAX
ROMAN
RUMAN
SAMAR
SOMAS
SOMAT
SUMAC
TAMAR
TEMAS
TOMAR
TOMAS
TVMAN
UNMAD
UNMAN
UXMAL
WOMAN
WYMAN
YUMAN
YUMAS

••M•A
BAMBA
BOMBA
COMMA
GAMBA
GAMMA
GEMMA
JAMBA
JUMNA
KIMBA
LAMIA
LEMMA
MAMBA
MAMMA
MOMMA
NAMPA
NEMEA
OOMPA
PAMPA
PEMBA
RUMBA
SAMBA
SAMOA
SAMSA
SIMBA
SUMMA
TAMPA
TOMBA
VAMPA

•••MA
ABOMA
ADAMA
AGAMA
ANIMA
AROMA
BURMA
COMMA
CREMA
DERMA
DOGMA
DOLMA
DRAMA
EDEMA
ETYMA
EXUMA
FIRMA
FORMA
GAMMA
GEMMA
HAEMA
HOUMA
KARMA
LEMMA
LLAMA
LOUMA
MAGMA
MAMMA
MOMMA
NAIMA
NORMA
OBAMA
ORAMA
PALMA
PARMA
PERMA
PRIMA
SALMA
SELMA
SIGMA
STOMA
SUMMA
TELMA
THEMA
VELMA
VILMA
WILMA
ZOSMA

MB•••
MBEKI

M•B••
MABEL
MOBIL
MRBIG
MYBAD
MYBOY

M••B•
MAMBA
MAMBO
MAYBE
MELBA
MSNBC
MUMBO

M•••B
MCJOB
MCNAB
MRCUB

•MB••
AMBER
AMBIT
AMBLE
AMBOS
AMBOY
AMBRY
EMBAR
EMBAY
EMBED
EMBER
EMBOG
IMBAD
IMBED
IMBUE
OMBER
OMBRE
UMBEL
UMBER
UMBLE
UMBRA

•M•B•
AMEBA

••MB•
BAMBA
BAMBI
BIMBO
BOMBA
BOMBE
BOMBS
CAMBS
COMBO
COMBS
DUMBO
DUMBS
GAMBA
GUMBO
GUMBY
IAMBI
IAMBS
JAMBA
JAMBE
JAMBS
JUMBO
KIMBA
KOMBU
LAMBS
LIMBO
LIMBS
MAMBA
MAMBO
MUMBO
NAMBY
NIMBI
NIMBY
NUMBS
PAMBY
PEMBA
RAMBO
RUMBA
SAMBA
SIMBA
TOMBA
TOMBE
TOMBS
WOMBS

••M•B
DEMOB
NAMIB

•••MB
ABOMB
CLIMB
CRUMB
HBOMB
NBOMB
PLUMB
RHOMB
RHUMB
THUMB

MC•••
MCATS
MCCCI
MCCCL
MCCCV
MCCCX
MCCII
MCCIV
MCCIX
MCCLI
MCCLV
MCCLX
MCCOO
MCCOY
MCCVI
MCCXC
MCCXI
MCCXL
MCCXV
MCCXX
MCDII
MCDIV
MCDIX
MCDLI
MCDLV
MCDLX
MCDVI
MCDXC
MCDXI
MCDXL
MCDXV
MCDXX
MCFLY
MCGEE
MCIII
MCJOB
MCKAY
MCKEE
MCKIM
MCLII
MCLIV
MCLIX
MCLVI
MCLXI
MCLXV
MCLXX
MCMII
MCMIV
MCMIX
MCMLI
MCMLV
MCMLX
MCMVI
MCMXC
MCMXI
MCMXL
MCMXV
MCMXX
MCNAB
MCRAE
MCVIE
MCVII
MCXCI
MCXCV
MCXII
MCXIV
MCXIX
MCXLI
MCXLV
MCXVI
MCXXI
MCXXV
MCXXX

M•C••
MACAO
MACAW
MACED
MACER
MACES
MACHE
MACHO
MACHU
MACHY
MACKE
MACKS
MACLE
MACON
MACRO
MACYS
MCCCI
MCCCL
MCCCV
MCCCX
MCCII
MCCIV
MCCIX
MCCLI
MCCLV
MCCLX
MCCOO
MCCOY
MCCVI
MCCXC
MCCXI
MCCXL
MCCXV
MCCXX
MDCCC
MDCCI
MDCCL
MDCCV
MDCCX
MDCII
MDCIV
MDCIX
MDCLI
MDCLV
MDCLX
MDCVI
MDCXC
MDCXI
MDCXL
MDCXV
MDCXX
MECCA
MECUM
MICAH
MICAS
MICKY
MICRA
MICRO
MMCCC
MMCCI
MMCCL
MMCCV
MMCCX
MMCDI
MMCDL
MMCDV
MMCDX
MMCII
MMCIV
MMCIX
MMCLI
MMCLV
MMCLX
MMCMI
MMCML
MMCMV
MMCMX
MMCVI
MMCXC
MMCXI
MMCXL
MMCXV
MMCXX
MOCHA
MOCKS
MRCUB
MUCHA
MUCHO
MUCKS
MUCKY
MXCII
MXCIV
MXCIX
MXCVI
MYCIN

M••C•
MANCY
MARCA
MARCH
MARCI

5 LY

MARCO MARCY MATCH MCCCI MCCCL MCCCV MCCCX MCXCI MCXCV MDCCC MDCCI MDCCL MDCCV MDCCX MDXCI MDXCV MECCA MERCE MERCH MERCI MERCK MERCS MERCY MINCE MITCH MMCCC MMCCI MMCCL MMCCV MMCCX MMDCC MMDCI MMDCL MMDCV MMDCX MMMCC MMMCD MMMCI MMMCL MMMCM MMMCV MMMCX MMXCI MMXCV MOOCH MOUCH MULCH MULCT MUNCH MUSCA

M•••C

MADOC MAGIC MALIC MANIC MCCXC MCDXC MCMXC MDCCC MDCXC MEDIC MEDOC MELIC MIMIC MMCCC MMCXC MMDCC MMDXC MMMCC MMMDC MMMXC MONIC MSNBC MUSIC

•MC••

EMCEE MMCCC MMCCI MMCCL MMCCV MMCCX MMCDI MMCDL MMCDV MMCDX MMCII MMCIV MMCIX MMCLI MMCLV MMCLX MMCMI MMCML MMCMV MMCMX MMCVI MMCXC MMCXI MMCXL MMCXV MMCXX YMCAS

•M•C•

AMICA AMICE AMICI AMICK AMICO AMOCO AMUCK BMOCS CMXCI CMXCV IMACS MMCCC MMCCI MMCCL MMCCV MMCCX MMDCC MMDCI MMDCL MMDCV MMDCX MMMCC MMMCD MMMCI MMMCL MMMCM MMMCV MMMCX MMXCI MMXCV SMACK SMOCK

•M••C

MMCCC MMCXC MMDCC MMDXC MMMCC MMMDC MMMXC

••MC•

AAMCO MMMCC MMMCD MMMCI MMMCL MMMCM MMMCV MMMCX

••M•C

COMIC HEMIC IBMPC MCMXC MIMIC MMMCC MMMDC MMMXC NEMEC NUMIC OHMIC OLMEC OSMIC SUMAC

MD•••

MDCCC MDCCI MDCCL MDCCV MDCCX MDCII MDCIV MDCIX MDCLI MDCLV MDCLX MDCVI MDCXC MDCXI MDCXL MDCXV MDCXX MDIII MDLII MDLIV MDLIX MDLVI MDLXI MDLXV MDLXX MDVII MDXCI MDXCV MDXII MDXIV MDXIX MDXLI MDXLV MDXVI MDXXI MDXXV MDXXX

M•D••

MADAM MADAT MADGE MADLY MADOC MADOX MADRE MADTV MCDII MCDIV MCDIX MCDLI MCDLV MCDLX MCDVI MCDXC MCDXI MCDXL MCDXV MCDXX MEDAL MEDEA MEDEE MEDES MEDIA MEDIC MEDII MEDIO MEDIT MEDOC MIDAS MIDDY MIDGE MIDIS MIDON MIDST MMDCC MMDCI MMDCL MMDCV MMDCX MMDII MMDIV MMDIX MMDLI MMDLV MMDLX MMDVI MMDXC MMDXI MMDXL MMDXV MMDXX MODAL MODEL MODEM MODES MODUS MSDOS MUDDY MYDAD MYDAY

M••D•

MAGDA MAHDI MAIDS MANDY MARDI MAUDE MAZDA MEADE MEADS MELDS MENDS MIDDY MINDS MINDY MISDO MMCDI MMCDL MMCDV MMCDX MMMDC MMMDI MMMDL MMMDV MMMDX MOLDS MOLDY MONDE MONDO MOODS MOODY MTIDA MTIDY MUDDY MUNDI

M•••D

MACED MANED MATED MAXED MAZED METED MEWED MIKED MIMED MINED MIRED MIXED MMMCD MONAD MONOD MOOED MOPED MOULD MOUND MOVED MOWED MUSED MUTED MYBAD MYDAD MYGOD

•MD••

CMDRS EMDEN MMDCC MMDCI MMDCL MMDCV MMDCX MMDII MMDIV MMDIX MMDLI MMDLV MMDLX MMDVI MMDXC MMDXI MMDXL MMDXV MMDXX

•M•D•

AMADA AMADO AMIDE IMIDE MMCDI MMCDL MMCDV MMCDX MMMDC MMMDI MMMDL MMMDV MMMDX

•M••D

AMAND AMEND AMPED EMBED EMEND IMBAD IMBED IMMAD MMMCD UMPED

••MD•

COMDR MMMDC MMMDI MMMDL MMMDV MMMDX

••M•D

AHMAD AHMED AIMED ARMED ASMAD BEMAD DIMED DOMED FAMED FUMED GAMED GOMAD HOMED HUMID IMMAD LAMED LIMED MIMED MMMCD NAMED NOMAD RIMED TAMED TIMED TIMID TUMID UNMAD

ME•••

MEADE MEADS MEALS MEALY MEANS MEANT MEANY MEARA MEARS MEATH MEATS MEATY MECCA MECUM MEDAL MEDEA MEDEE MEDES MEDIA MEDIC MEDII MEDIO MEDIT MEDOC MEENY MEESE MEETS MEGAN MEHTA MEIER MEIJI MEINE MEKHI MEKKA MELBA MELDS MELEE MELFI MELIC MELIS MELLO MELON MELOS MELOT MELTS MEMOS MENAS MENDS MENES MENLO MENOS MENSA MENUS MEOWS MERCE MERCH MERCI MERCK MERCS MERCY MERER MERES MERGE MERIT MERLE MERLS MEROE MERRY MERTZ MERYL MESAS MESES MESHY MESNE MESON MESSE MESSY MESTA METAL METED METER METES METIS METOO METRE METRO METRY METUP MEUSE MEWED MEWER MEWLS MEYER MEZZO

M•E••

MAEVE MBEKI MEENY MEESE MEETS MIELE MIELS MIENS MIERS MIEUX MNEME MNEMO MPEGS MTELY MYERS MYEYE

M••E•

MABEL MACED MACER MACES MAGEE MAGES MAHER MAKEM MAKER MAKES MALES MALEV MAMET MANED MANES MANET MAPES MAREK MARES MASER MATED MATEO MATER MATES MATEY MAVEN MAXED MAXES MAYER MAZED MAZEL MAZES MCGEE MCKEE MEDEA MEDEE MEDES MEIER MELEE MENES MERER MERES MESES METED METER METES MEWED MEWER MEYER MIKED MIKES MIKEY MILER MILES MIMED MIMEO MIMER MIMES MINED MINEO MINER MINES MINEY MIRED MIRES MISER MITER MITES MIXED MIXER MIXES MLLES MODEL MODEM MODES MOGEN MOLES MONEL MONET MONEY MOOED MOOER MOPED MOPER MOPES MOPEY MOREL MORES MOREY MOSEL MOSES MOSEY MOTEL MOTES MOTET MOUES MOVED MOVER MOVES MOWED MOWEN MOWER MRHEX MRLEE MRMET MTGES MUJER MULES MULEY MURES MUSED MUSEE MUSEO MUSER MUSES MUTED MUTER MUTES MYLES

M•••E

MACHE MACKE MACLE MADGE MADRE MAEVE MAGEE MAHRE MAINE MAIRE MAIZE MALLE MAMIE MANGE MANNE MANSE MAPLE MARGE MARIE MARNE MASSE MATTE MAUDE MAUVE MAXIE MAYBE MAYLE MCGEE MCKEE MCRAE MCVIE MEADE MEDEE MEESE MEINE MELEE MERCE MERGE MERLE MEROE MESNE MESSE METRE MEUSE MFUME MIDGE MIELE MILLE MILNE MINCE MITRE MLIFE MNEME MOIRE MONDE MONTE MOORE MOOSE MORSE MORTE MOSHE MOUSE MOVIE MOXIE MRLEE MTILE MURRE MUSEE MYEYE MYOPE

•ME••

AMEBA AMEER AMEND AMENS AMENT AMERY EMEER EMEND EMERY EMESA EMEUS IMEAN OMEGA OMENS OMERS SMEAL SMEAR SMEES SMELL SMELT SMEWS UMEKI

•M•E•

AMBER AMEER AMIEL AMIES AMPED AMVET EMBED EMBER EMCEE EMDEN EMEER EMLEN EMMER EMMET IMBED IMPEI IMPEL IMSET OMBER OMNES SMEES UMBEL UMBER UMPED

•M••E

AMARE AMAZE AMBLE AMICE AMIDE AMINE AMITE AMOLE AMORE AMPLE AMUSE EMCEE EMILE EMOTE IMAGE IMBUE IMIDE IMINE IMMIE IMOVE OMBRE SMAZE SMILE SMITE SMOKE SMORE SMOTE UMBLE

••ME•

AAMES ACMES ADMEN AHMED AIMED AIMEE AIMER ARMED ARMEE ARMEN ARMER ARMES ARMET ARMEY AXMEN CAMEL CAMEO COMER COMES COMET COMEX CUMES CYMES DAMEN DAMES DEMES DIMED DIMES DOMED DOMES EAMES ELMER EMMER EMMET EXMET FAMED FAMER FAMES FEMES FUMED FUMER FUMES FUMET GAMED GAMER GAMES GIMEL GOMER GOMEZ GUMEE HAMEL HAMER HAMES HEMEN HEMES HEMET HIMES HOMED HOMEO HOMER HOMES HOMEY JAMES KAMEN KHMER LAMED LAMER LAMES LIMED LIMES LUMEN LUMET MAMET MIMED MIMEO MIMER MIMES MRMET NAMED NAMER NAMES NEMEA NEMEC NIMES NOMEN NUMEN NYMET OLMEC PIMEN POMES PRMEN RAMEN RAMET RAMEY REMET RIMED RIMER RIMES ROMEO ROMES RUMER SUMER TAMED TAMER TAMES TIMED TIMER TIMES TIMEX TOMEI TOMES TVMEN UNMET UNMEW VOMER WOMEN XEMEX YEMEN

••M•E

AIMEE ARMEE BOMBE COMAE COMME COMTE CYMAE DAMME DEMME FAMKE FEMME GIMME GUMEE HOMIE HOMME IMMIE JAMBE JAMIE LEMME MAMIE POMME RAMIE SOMME TEMPE TOMBE

•••ME

AGAME ANIME ARAME ASKME BAUME BEAME BIOME BLAME BLUME BRUME CALME CARME CHIME CLIME COMME CREME CRIME DAMME DEMME DISME DROME EATME FEMME FLAME FLUME FLYME FRAME FROME GETME GIMME GNOME GORME GOTME GRIME HITME HOMME HULME ICAME ITSME JAIME KREME KWAME LAKME LEMME LETME MFUME MNEME NEAME NEEME NOTME PALME PLUME POEME POMME PRIME RHEME RHYME SEEME SHAME SLIME SOMME SPUME SUEME TERME THEME THYME TORME TRYME USEME WHOME WHYME YAYME

MF•••

MFUME

M•F••

MAFIA MCFLY MIFFS MIFFY MOFFO MRFOX MUFFS MUFTI

M••F•

MELFI MIFFS MIFFY MLIFE MOFFO MUFFS

M•••F

MOTIF MTWTF

•M•F•

IMOFF

•M••F

IMOFF SMURF

••MF•

COMFY

M•G••

MAGDA MAGEE MAGES MAGIC MAGMA MAGNA MAGOG MAGOO MAGUA MAGUS MCGEE MEGAN MIGHT MOGEN MOGUL MSGTS MTGES MUGGS MUGGY MYGOD MYGUY

M••G•

MADGE MANGA MANGE MANGO MANGY MARGE MARGO MARGY MERGE MIDGE MINGY MONGO MOOGS MPEGS MUGGS MUGGY

M•••G

MAGOG MRBIG MYUNG

•M•G•

AMIGA AMIGO EMAGS IMAGE IMAGO OMEGA SMOGS

•M••G

AMONG EMBOG HMONG SMAUG

••M•G

DIMAG NOMSG

M•H••

MAHAL MAHAN MAHDI MAHER MAHON MAHRE MEHTA MRHEX

M••H•

MACHE MACHO MACHU MACHY MASHA MATHS MEKHI MESHY MIGHT MINHO MISHA MOCHA

MOSHE
MOTHS
MOTHY
MUCHA
MUCHO
MUSHU
MUSHY
MYTHS

M•••H
MALPH
MARCH
MARSH
MATCH
MEATH
MERCH
MICAH
MIRTH
MITCH
MONTH
MOOCH
MORPH
MOUCH
MOUTH
MULCH
MUNCH
MYNAH
MYRRH

•MH••
IMHIP
IMHOT
YMHAS

•M•H•
AMAHL
AMAHS
AMPHI
OMAHA

•M••H
AMISH
SMASH
SMITH
SMUSH
SMYTH

••MH•
ABMHO

••M•H
ARMAH
HUMPH
LYMPH
NYMPH
OOMPH

MI•••
MIAMI
MIAOU
MIAOW
MIATA
MICAH
MICAS
MICKY
MICRA
MICRO
MIDAS
MIDDY
MIDGE
MIDIS
MIDON
MIDST
MIELE
MIELS
MIENS
MIERS
MIEUX
MIFFS
MIFFY
MIGHT
MIKAN
MIKED
MIKES
MIKEY
MILAN
MILER
MILES
MILKS
MILKY
MILLE
MILLI
MILLO
MILLS
MILNE
MILOS
MIMED
MIMEO
MIMER
MIMES
MIMIC
MIMSY
MINAS
MINCE
MINDS
MINDY
MINED
MINEO
MINER
MINES
MINEY
MINGY
MINHO
MINIM
MINIS
MINKS
MINOR
MINOS
MINOT
MINOW
MINSK
MINTS
MINTY
MINUS
MIRED
MIRES
MIRIN
MIROS
MIRRO
MIRTH
MIRVS
MISDO
MISER
MISHA
MISOS
MISSA
MISSM
MISSY
MISTI
MISTS
MISTY
MITAS
MITCH
MITER
MITES
MITLA
MITRE
MITTS
MITTY
MITYA
MITZI
MIXED
MIXER
MIXES
MIXIN
MIXUP
MIZAR

M•I••
MAIDS
MAILS
MAIMS
MAINE
MAINS
MAINZ
MAIRE
MAIZE
MCIII
MDIII
MEIER
MEIJI
MEINE
MLIFE
MLIII
MMIII
MOILS
MOIRA
MOIRE
MOIST
MTIDA
MTIDY
MTILE
MVIII
MXIII

M••I•
MAFIA
MAGIC
MAKIN
MALIC
MAMIE
MANIA
MANIC
MAOII
MARIA
MARIE
MARIN
MARIO
MARIS
MATIN
MAVIN
MAVIS
MAXIE
MAXIM
MAXIS
MCCII
MCCIV
MCCIX
MCDII
MCDIV
MCDIX
MCIII
MCKIM
MCLII
MCLIV
MCLIX
MCMII
MCMIV
MCMIX
MCVIE
MCVII
MCXII
MCXIV
MCXIX
MDCII
MDCIV
MDCIX
MDIII
MDLII
MDLIV
MDLIX
MDVII
MDXII
MDXIV
MDXIX
MEDIA
MEDIC
MEDII
MEDIO
MEDIT
MELIC
MELIS
MERIT
METIS
MIDIS
MIMIC
MINIM
MINIS
MIRIN
MIXIN
MLIII
MLVII
MLXII
MLXIV
MLXIX
MMCII
MMCIV
MMCIX
MMDII
MMDIV
MMDIX
MMIII
MMLII
MMLIV
MMLIX
MMMII
MMMIV
MMMIX
MMVII
MMXII
MMXIV
MMXIX
MOBIL
MONIC
MONIZ
MOTIF
MOVIE
MOVIN
MOWIS
MOXIE
MRBIG
MUNIS
MUSIC
MUSIL
MVIII
MXCII
MXCIV
MXCIX
MXIII
MXLII
MXLIV
MXLIX
MXVII
MXXII
MXXIV
MXXIX
MYCIN
MYRIA
MYSIN

M•••I
MAHDI
MAOII
MAORI
MAQUI
MARCI
MARDI
MARKI
MARNI
MARTI
MARYI
MASAI
MATRI
MBEKI
MCCCI
MCCII
MCCLI
MCCVI
MCCXI
MCDII
MCDLI
MCDVI
MCDXI
MCIII
MCLII
MCLVI
MCLXI
MCMII
MCMLI
MCMVI
MCMXI
MCVII
MCXCI
MCXII
MCXLI
MCXVI
MCXXI
MDCCI
MDCII
MDCLI
MDCVI
MDCXI
MDIII
MDLII
MDLVI
MDLXI
MDVII
MDXCI
MDXII
MDXLI
MDXVI
MDXXI
MEDII
MEIJI
MEKHI
MELFI
MERCI
MIAMI
MILLI
MISTI
MITZI
MLIII
MLVII
MLXII
MLXVI
MLXXI
MMCCI
MMCDI
MMCII
MMCLI
MMCMI
MMCVI
MMCXI
MMDCI
MMDII
MMDLI
MMDVI
MMDXI
MMIII
MMLII
MMLVI
MMLXI
MMMCI
MMMDI
MMMII
MMMLI
MMMVI
MMMXI
MMVII
MMXCI
MMXII
MMXLI
MMXVI
MMXXI
MUFTI
MULTI
MUNDI
MVIII
MXCII
MXCVI
MXIII
MXLII
MXLVI
MXVII
MXXII
MXXVI
MXXXI

•MI••
AMICA
AMICE
AMICI
AMICK
AMICO
AMIDE
AMIEL
AMIES
AMIGA
AMIGO
AMINE
AMINO
AMIRI
AMIRS
AMISH
AMISS
AMITE
AMITY
CMIII
EMILE
EMILY
EMIRS
EMITS
IMIDE
IMINE
MMIII
OMITS
SMILE
SMIRK
SMITE
SMITH
SMITS
UMIAK

•M•I•
AMAIN
AMBIT
AMLIT
AMNIA
AMNIO
CMIII
CMLII
CMLIV
CMLIX
CMVII
CMXII
CMXIV
CMXIX
EMAIL
IMHIP
IMMIE
IMMIX
MMCII
MMCIV
MMCIX
MMDII
MMDIV
MMDIX
MMIII
MMLII
MMLIV
MMLIX
MMMII
MMMIV
MMMIX
MMVII
MMXII
MMXIV
MMXIX
OMNIA
OMNIS

•M••I
AMATI
AMICI
AMIRI
AMPHI
CMIII
CMLII
CMLVI
CMLXI
CMVII
CMXCI
CMXII
CMXLI
CMXVI
CMXXI
IMARI
IMPEI
MMCCI
MMCDI
MMCII
MMCLI
MMCMI
MMCVI
MMCXI
MMDCI
MMDII
MMDLI
MMDVI
MMDXI
MMIII
MMLII
MMLVI
MMLXI
MMMCI
MMMDI
MMMII
MMMLI
MMMVI
MMMXI
MMVII
MMXCI
MMXII
MMXLI
MMXVI
MMXXI
OMANI
UMEKI

••MI•
ADMIN
ADMIT
ADMIX
ARMIN
COMIC
COMIN
COMIX
CUMIN
DAMIS
DEMIT
DIMIN
GAMIN
HEMIC
HEMIN
HOMIE
HUMID
IMMIE
IMMIX
IZMIR
JAMIE
JAMIN
KUMIN
LAMIA
LAMIT
LIMIT
MAMIE
MCMII
MCMIV
MCMIX
MIMIC
MMMII
MMMIV
MMMIX
NAMIB
NUMIC
OHMIC
OSMIC
RAMIE
RAMIN
RAMIS
REMIT
REMIX
SAMIS
SEMIS
TAMIL
TIMID
TUMID
UNMIX

••M•I
BAMBI
ETMOI
GIMLI
GUMMI
IAMBI
MCMII
MCMLI
MCMVI
MCMXI
MMMCI
MMMDI
MMMII
MMMLI
MMMVI
MMMXI
NIMBI
SAMMI
SOMNI
TAMMI
TEMPI
TOMEI

•••MI
ASAMI
DUOMI
ELEMI
ENAMI
FERMI
GUMMI
LEUMI
MIAMI
MMCMI
NAOMI
NURMI
OTOMI
RAIMI
SALMI
SAMMI
SOAMI
SUOMI
SWAMI
TAMMI
UNAMI
VERMI

M•J••
MAJOR
MCJOB
MOJOS
MUJER

M••J•
MEIJI

M•••J
MARYJ
MTVVJ

M•K••
MAKEM
MAKER
MAKES
MAKIN
MAKOS
MCKAY
MCKEE
MCKIM
MEKHI
MEKKA
MIKAN
MIKED
MIKES
MIKEY

M••K•
MACKE
MACKS
MARKA
MARKI
MARKS
MARKV
MASKS
MBEKI
MEKKA
MICKY
MILKS
MILKY
MINKS
MOCKS
MONKS
MUCKS
MUCKY
MURKY
MUSKS
MUSKY

M•••K
MAREK
MERCK
MINSK
MRYUK
MUZAK

•M•K•
SMOKE
SMOKY
UMEKI

•M••K
AMICK
AMUCK
DMARK
SMACK
SMIRK
SMOCK
UMIAK

••MK•
FAMKE

••M•K
TOMSK

ML•••
MLIFE
MLIII
MLLES
MLVII
MLXII
MLXIV
MLXIX
MLXVI
MLXXI
MLXXV
MLXXX

M•L••
MALAR
MALAY
MALES
MALEV
MALIC
MALLE
MALLS
MALMO
MALPH
MALTA
MALTS
MALTY
MCLII
MCLIV
MCLIX
MCLVI
MCLXI
MCLXV
MCLXX
MDLII
MDLIV
MDLIX
MDLVI
MDLXI
MDLXV
MDLXX
MELBA
MELDS
MELEE
MELFI
MELIC
MELIS
MELLO
MELON
MELOS
MELOT
MELTS
MILAN
MILER
MILES
MILKS
MILKY
MILLE
MILLI
MILLO
MILLS
MILNE
MILOS
MLLES
MMLII
MMLIV
MMLIX
MMLVI
MMLXI
MMLXV
MMLXX
MOLAR
MOLDS
MOLDY
MOLES
MOLLS
MOLLY
MOLTO
MOLTS
MRLEE
MULAN
MULCH
MULCT
MULES
MULEY
MULLA
MULLS
MULTI
MXLII
MXLIV
MXLIX
MXLVI
MYLAR
MYLES

M••L•
MACLE
MADLY
MAILS
MALLE
MALLS
MANLY
MAPLE
MARLA
MARLO
MARLS
MARLY
MAULS
MAYLE
MCCLI
MCCLV
MCCLX
MCDLI
MCDLV
MCDLX
MCFLY
MCMLI
MCMLV
MCMLX
MCXLI
MCXLV
MDCLI
MDCLV
MDCLX
MDXLI
MDXLV
MEALS
MEALY
MELLO
MENLO
MERLE
MERLS
MEWLS
MIELE
MIELS
MILLE
MILLI
MILLO
MILLS
MITLA
MMCLI
MMCLV
MMCLX
MMDLI
MMDLV
MMDLX
MMMLI
MMMLV
MMMLX
MMXLI
MMXLV
MOILS
MOLLS
MOLLY
MOOLA
MOULD
MOULT
MTELY
MTILE
MULLA
MULLS

M•••L
MABEL
MAHAL
MAZEL
MCCCL
MCCXL
MCDXL
MCMXL
MDCCL
MDCXL
MEDAL
MERYL
METAL
MMCCL
MMCDL
MMCML
MMCXL
MMDCL
MMDXL
MMMCL
MMMDL
MMMXL
MOBIL
MODAL
MODEL
MOGUL
MONEL
MORAL
MOREL
MOSEL
MOSUL
MOTEL
MURAL
MUSIL

•ML••
AMLIT
CMLII
CMLIV
CMLIX
CMLVI
CMLXI
CMLXV
CMLXX
EMLEN
EMLYN
MMLII
MMLIV
MMLIX
MMLVI
MMLXI
MMLXV
MMLXX

•M•L•
AMBLE
AMOLE
AMPLE
AMPLY
AMYLO
AMYLS
CMXLI
CMXLV
EMALL
EMILE
EMILY
IMPLY
MMCLI
MMCLV
MMCLX
MMDLI
MMDLV
MMDLX
MMMLI
MMMLV
MMMLX
MMXLI
MMXLV
SMALL
SMELL
SMELT
SMILE
SMOLT
UMBLE

•M••L
AMAHL
AMIEL
EMAIL
EMALL
IMPEL
MMCCL
MMCDL
MMCML
MMCXL
MMDCL
MMDXL
MMMCL
MMMDL
MMMXL
SMALL
SMEAL
SMELL
UMBEL

••ML•
DIMLY
GIMLI
MCMLI
MCMLV
MCMLX
MMMLI
MMMLV
MMMLX

••M•L
CAMEL
CUMUL
GAMAL
GIMEL
HAMEL
HEMAL
JAMAL
KEMAL
MCMXL
MMMCL
MMMDL
MMMXL
TAMIL
UXMAL

•••ML
FRIML
MMCML

MM•••
MMCCC
MMCCI
MMCCL
MMCCV
MMCCX
MMCDI
MMCDL
MMCDV
MMCDX
MMCII
MMCIV
MMCIX
MMCLI
MMCLV
MMCLX
MMCMI
MMCML
MMCMV
MMCMX
MMCVI
MMCXC
MMCXI
MMCXL
MMCXV
MMCXX
MMDCC
MMDCI
MMDCL
MMDCV
MMDCX
MMDII
MMDIV
MMDIX
MMDLI
MMDLV
MMDLX
MMDVI
MMDXC
MMDXI
MMDXL
MMDXV
MMDXX
MMIII
MMLII
MMLIV
MMLIX
MMLVI
MMLXI
MMLXV
MMLXX
MMMCC
MMMCD
MMMCI
MMMCL
MMMCM
MMMCV
MMMCX
MMMDC
MMMDI
MMMDL
MMMDV
MMMDX
MMMII
MMMIV
MMMIX
MMMLI
MMMLV
MMMLX
MMMVI
MMMXC
MMMXI
MMMXL
MMMXV
MMMXX
MMVII
MMXCI
MMXCV
MMXII
MMXIV
MMXIX
MMXLI
MMXLV
MMXVI
MMXXI
MMXXV
MMXXX

M•M••
MAMAS
MAMBA
MAMBO
MAMET
MAMIE
MAMMA
MAMMY
MCMII
MCMIV
MCMIX
MCMLI
MCMLV
MCMLX
MCMVI
MCMXC
MCMXI
MCMXL
MCMXV
MCMXX
MEMOS
MIMED
MIMEO
MIMER
MIMES
MIMIC
MIMSY
MMMCC
MMMCD
MMMCI
MMMCL
MMMCM
MMMCV
MMMCX
MMMDC
MMMDI
MMMDL
MMMDV
MMMDX
MMMII
MMMIV
MMMIX
MMMLI
MMMLV
MMMLX
MMMVI
MMMXC
MMMXI
MMMXL
MMMXV
MMMXX
MOMMA
MOMMY
MOMUS
MRMET
MRMOM
MUMBO
MUMMS
MUMMY
MUMPS
MYMAN

M••M•
MAAMS
MAGMA
MAIMS
MALMO
MAMMA

5 MH

MAMMY
MARMS
MFUME
MIAMI
MMCMI
MMCML
MMCMV
MMCMX
MNEME
MNEMO
MOMMA
MOMMY
MUMMS
MUMMY

M•••M
MADAM
MAKEM
MAXIM
MCKIM
MECUM
MINIM
MISSM
MMMCM
MODEM
MRMOM

•MM••
AMMAN
AMMOS
EMMER
EMMET
EMMYS
IMMAD
IMMIE
IMMIX
MMMCC
MMMCD
MMMCI
MMMCL
MMMCM
MMMCV
MMMCX
MMMDC
MMMDI
MMMDL
MMMDV
MMMDX
MMMII
MMMIV
MMMIX
MMMLI
MMMLV
MMMLX
MMMVI
MMMXC
MMMXI
MMMXL
MMMXV
MMMXX

•M•M•
IMAMS
IMAMU
MMCMI
MMCML
MMCMV
MMCMX

•M••M
AMRAM
MMMCM
SMARM

••MM•
BAMMY
COMMA
COMME
DAMME
DEMME
DUMMY
FEMME
GAMMA
GEMMA
GEMMY
GIMME
GUMMI
GUMMO
GUMMY
HAMMS
HAMMY
HOMME
JIMMY
LEMMA
LEMME
MAMMA
MAMMY
MOMMA
MOMMY
MUMMS
MUMMY
POMME
RUMMY
SAMMI
SAMMS
SAMMY
SIMMS
SOMME
SUMMA
TAMMI
TAMMY
TIMMY
TOMMY
TUMMY
YUMMY

••M•M
HIMOM
MMMCM
MRMOM

•••MM
FROMM
GRAMM
GRIMM
KLAMM

MN•••
MNEME
MNEMO
MNOPQ

M•N••
MANAT
MANCY
MANDY
MANED
MANES
MANET
MANGA
MANGE
MANGO
MANGY
MANIA
MANIC
MANLY
MANNA
MANNE
MANNY
MANON
MANOR
MANOS
MANSE
MANTA
MANUS
MCNAB
MENAS
MENDS
MENES
MENLO
MENOS
MENSA
MENUS
MINAS
MINCE
MINDS
MINDY
MINED
MINEO
MINER
MINES
MINEY
MINGY
MINHO
MINIM
MINIS
MINKS
MINOR
MINOS
MINOT
MINOW
MINSK
MINTS
MINTY
MINUS
MONAD
MONDE
MONDO
MONEL
MONET
MONEY
MONGO
MONIC
MONIZ
MONKS
MONOD
MONOS
MONRO
MONTE
MONTH
MONTS
MONTY
MONZA
MSNBC
MUNCH
MUNDI
MUNIS
MUNNA
MUNRO
MYNAH
MYNAS

M••N•
MAGNA
MAINE
MAINS
MAINZ
MANNA
MANNE
MANNY
MARNE
MARNI
MAUNA
MAYNT
MEANS
MEANT
MEANY
MEENY
MEINE
MESNE
MIENS
MILNE
MOANS
MOONS
MOONY
MORNS
MOUND
MOUNT
MUNNA
MUONS
MYRNA
MYUNG

M•••N
MACON
MAHAN
MAHON
MAKIN
MANON
MARIN
MASON
MATIN
MAVEN
MAVIN
MAYAN
MEGAN
MELON
MESON
MIDON
MIKAN
MILAN
MIRIN
MIXIN
MOGEN
MORAN
MORON
MOURN
MOVIN
MOWEN
MULAN
MUTON
MYCIN
MYMAN
MYRON
MYSIN

•MN••
AMNIA
AMNIO
LMNOP
OMNES
OMNIA
OMNIS

•M•N•
AMANA
AMAND
AMANT
AMEND
AMENS
AMENT
AMINE
AMINO
AMONG
EMEND
HMONG
IMINE
OMANI
OMENS

•M••N
AMAIN
AMMAN
EMDEN
EMLEN
EMLYN
IMEAN

••MN•
DAMNS
GYMNO
HYMNS
JUMNA
KLMNO
LIMNS
SOMNI

••M•N
ADMAN
ADMEN
ADMIN
AMMAN
ARMEN
ARMIN
ATMAN
AXMAN
AXMEN
BEMAN
COMIN
CUMIN
DAMEN
DAMON
DEMON
DIMIN
EAMON
ELMAN
GAMIN
GOMAN
HAMAN
HEMAN
HEMEN
HEMIN
HEMON
HUMAN
HYMAN
JAMIN
JAMON
KAMEN
KUMIN
LEMAN
LEMON
LIMAN
LIMON
LOMAN
LUMAN
LUMEN
LYMAN
LYMON
MYMAN
NEMAN
NOMEN
NUMAN
NUMEN
NYMAN
OHMAN
ORMAN
OSMAN
PIMEN
PRMAN
PRMEN
RAMAN
RAMEN
RAMIN
RAMON
REMAN
ROMAN
RUMAN
SIMON
TIMON
TVMAN
TVMEN
UNMAN
WOMAN
WOMEN
WOMYN
WYMAN
YEMEN
YUMAN

•••MN
JKLMN

MO•••
MOANS
MOATS
MOBIL
MOCHA
MOCKS
MODAL
MODEL
MODEM
MODES
MODUS
MOFFO
MOGEN
MOGUL
MOILS
MOIRA
MOIRE
MOIST
MOJOS
MOLAR
MOLDS
MOLDY
MOLES
MOLLS
MOLLY
MOLTO
MOLTS
MOMMA
MOMMY
MOMUS
MONAD
MONDE
MONDO
MONEL
MONET
MONEY
MONGO
MONIC
MONIZ
MONKS
MONOD
MONOS
MONRO
MONTE
MONTH
MONTS
MONTY
MONZA
MOOCH
MOODS
MOODY
MOOED
MOOER
MOOGS
MOOLA
MOONS
MOONY
MOORE
MOORS
MOORY
MOOSE
MOOTS
MOPED
MOPER
MOPES
MOPEY
MOPSY
MOPUP
MORAL
MORAN
MORAS
MORAY
MOREL
MORES
MOREY
MORNS
MORON
MOROS
MORPH
MORRA
MORRO
MORSE
MORTE
MORTY
MOSEL
MOSES
MOSEY
MOSHE
MOSSO
MOSSY
MOSUL
MOTEL
MOTES
MOTET
MOTHS
MOTHY
MOTIF
MOTOR
MOTTO
MOTTS
MOUCH
MOUES
MOULD
MOULT
MOUND
MOUNT
MOURN
MOUSE
MOUSY
MOUTH
MOVED
MOVER
MOVES
MOVIE
MOVIN
MOWAT
MOWED
MOWEN
MOWER
MOWIS
MOXIE
MOZOS

M•O••
MAOII
MAORI
MEOWS
MNOPQ
MOOCH
MOODS
MOODY
MOOED
MOOER
MOOGS
MOOLA
MOONS
MOONY
MOORE
MOORS
MOORY
MOOSE
MOOTS
MUONS
MYOPE

M••O•
MACON
MADOC
MADOX
MAGOG
MAGOO
MAHON
MAJOR
MAKOS
MANON
MANOR
MANOS
MAROT
MASON
MAYOR
MAYOS
MCCOO
MCCOY
MCJOB
MEDOC
MELON
MELOS
MELOT
MEMOS
MENOS
MEROE
MESON
METOO
MIAOU
MIAOW
MIDON
MILOS
MINOR
MINOS
MINOT
MINOW
MIROS
MISOS
MOJOS
MONOD
MONOS
MORON
MOROS
MOTOR
MOZOS
MRFOX
MRMOM
MSDOS
MUTON
MYBOY
MYGOD
MYRON

M•••O
MACAO
MACHO
MACRO
MAGOO
MALMO
MAMBO
MANGO
MARCO
MARGO
MARIO
MARLO
MARZO
MATEO
MATRO
MATZO
MAYPO
MCCOO
MEDIO
MELLO
MENLO
METOO
METRO
MEZZO
MICRO
MILLO
MIMEO
MINEO
MINHO
MIRRO
MISDO
MNEMO
MOFFO
MOLTO
MONDO
MONGO
MONRO
MORRO
MOSSO
MOTTO
MTAPO
MUCHO
MUMBO
MUNRO
MUSEO

•MO••
AMOCO
AMOLE
AMONG
AMORE
AMORS
AMORT
AMORY
AMOUR
BMOCS
EMORY
EMOTE
HMONG
IMOFF
IMOUT
IMOVE
SMOCK
SMOGS
SMOKE
SMOKY
SMOLT
SMOOT
SMORE
SMOTE

•M•O•
AMBOS
AMBOY
AMMOS
AMTOO
EMBOG
IMHOT
LMNOP
SMOOT

•M••O
AMADO
AMATO
AMICO
AMIGO
AMINO
AMNIO
AMOCO
AMTOO
AMYLO
IMAGO

••MO•
AMMOS
ARMOR
ATMOS
CAMOS
DAMON
DEMOB
DEMON
DEMOS
DOMOS
EAMON
ELMOS
ETMOI
GAMOW
HEMON
HIMOM
HUMOR
JAMON
LEMON
LIMON
LIMOS
LYMON
MEMOS
MRMOM
NEMOS
NIMOY
OLMOS
POMOS
RAMON
RAMOS
REMOP
REMOW
RUMOR
SAMOA
SAMOS
SHMOO
SIMON
SUMOS
TIMON
TIMOR
VAMOS

••M•O
AAMCO
ABMHO
BIMBO
CAMEO
CAMPO
COMBO
DUMBO
FEMTO
GUMBO
GUMMO
GYMNO
HOMEO
IAMSO
JUMBO
KIMPO
KLMNO
LIMBO
MAMBO
MIMEO
MUMBO
RAMBO
ROMEO
SHMOO
TEMPO

•••MO
ALAMO
ANEMO
ANIMO
BIGMO
BROMO
CHEMO
COSMO
CUOMO
DERMO
DUOMO
GISMO
GITMO
GIZMO
GRAMO
GUMMO
MALMO
MNEMO
OKEMO
PISMO
PRIMO
PROMO
PULMO
SCHMO
SLOMO
TEAMO
TIAMO
WHAMO

MP•••
MPEGS

M•P••
MAPES
MAPLE
MOPED
MOPER
MOPES
MOPEY
MOPSY
MOPUP

M••P•
MALPH
MAYPO
MNOPQ
MORPH
MSRPS
MTAPO
MUMPS
MYOPE

M•••P
METUP
MIXUP
MOPUP

•MP••
AMPAS
AMPED
AMPHI
AMPLE
AMPLY
AMPUP
EMPTY
IMPEI
IMPEL
IMPLY
UMPED

•M•P•
AMAPA

•M••P
AMPUP
IMHIP
LMNOP

••MP•
BUMPS
BUMPY
CAMPO
CAMPS
CAMPY
COMPS
DAMPS
DUMPS
DUMPY
GAMPS
GIMPS
GIMPY
HEMPS
HEMPY
HUMPH
HUMPS
HUMPY
IBMPC
JUMPS
JUMPY
KEMPT
KIMPO
LAMPS
LIMPS
LIMPY
LUMPS
LUMPY
LYMPH
MUMPS
NAMPA
NYMPH
OOMPA
OOMPH
PAMPA
PUMPS
RAMPS
ROMPS
RUMPS
SAMPS
SIMPS
SUMPS
TAMPA
TAMPS
TEMPE
TEMPI
TEMPO
TEMPS
TEMPT
VAMPA
VAMPS
VAMPY
WIMPS
WIMPY

••M•P
ALMVP
DAMUP
GUMUP
HAMUP
JAMUP
NLMVP
REMAP
REMOP
SUMUP

•••MP
BLIMP
CHAMP
CHIMP
CHOMP
CHUMP
CLAMP
CLOMP
CLUMP
CRAMP
CRIMP
CRUMP
FRUMP
GRAMP
GRUMP
KLUMP
PLUMP
PRIMP
SCAMP
SHEMP
SKIMP
SLUMP
STAMP
STOMP
STUMP
SWAMP
THUMP
TRAMP
TROMP
TRUMP
WHOMP

M•Q••
MAQUI

M•••Q
MNOPQ

MR•••
MRBIG
MRCUB
MRFOX
MRHEX
MRLEE
MRMET
MRMOM
MRYUK

M•R••
MARAT
MARCA
MARCH
MARCI
MARCO
MARCY
MARDI
MAREK
MARES
MARGE
MARGO
MARGY
MARIA
MARIE
MARIN
MARIO
MARIS
MARKA
MARKI
MARKS
MARKV
MARLA
MARLO
MARLS
MARLY
MARMS
MARNE
MARNI
MAROT
MARRY
MARSH
MARTA
MARTI
MARTS
MARTY
MARVY
MARYA
MARYI
MARYJ
MARYS
MARZO
MCRAE
MERCE
MERCH
MERCI
MERCK
MERCS
MERCY
MERER
MERES
MERGE
MERIT
MERLE
MERLS
MEROE
MERRY
MERTZ
MERYL
MIRED
MIRES
MIRIN
MIROS
MIRRO
MIRTH
MIRVS
MORAL
MORAN
MORAS
MORAY
MOREL
MORES
MOREY
MORNS
MORON
MOROS
MORPH
MORRA
MORRO
MORSE
MORTE
MORTY
MSRPS
MURAL
MURAT
MURES
MURKY
MURRE
MYRIA
MYRNA
MYRON
MYRRH

M••R•
MACRO
MADRE
MAHRE
MAIRE
MAORI
MARRY
MATRI
MATRO
MAURA
MAURY
MEARA
MEARS
MERRY
METRE
METRO
METRY
MICRA
MICRO
MIERS
MIRRO
MITRE
MOIRA
MOIRE
MONRO
MOORE
MOORS
MOORY
MORRA
MORRO
MOURN
MUNRO
MURRE
MYERS
MYRRH

M•••R
MACER
MAHER
MAJOR
MAKER
MALAR
MANOR
MASER
MASUR
MATER
MAYER
MAYOR
MAZAR
MEIER
MERER
METER
MEWER
MEYER
MILER
MIMER
MINER
MINOR
MISER
MITER
MIXER
MIZAR
MOLAR
MOOER
MOPER
MOTOR
MOVER
MOWER
MSTAR
MUJER
MUSER
MUTER
MYLAR
MYWAR

•MR••
AMRAM

•M•R•
AMARA
AMARE
AMBRY
AMERY
AMIRI
AMIRS
AMORE
AMORS
AMORT
AMORY
CMDRS
DMARK
EMERY
EMIRS
EMORY
IMARI
KMART
OMARR
OMBRE
OMERS
SMARM
SMART
SMIRK
SMORE
SMURF
UMBRA

•M••R
AMBER
AMEER
AMOUR
EMBAR
EMBER
EMEER
EMMER
OMARR
OMBER
SMEAR
UMBER

••MR•
CAMRY
CYMRY

••M•R
AIMER
ARMER
ARMOR
COMDR
COMER
DEMUR
EDMAR
ELMAR
ELMER
EMMER
FAMER
FEMUR
FUMER
GAMER
GOMER
HAMER
HOMER
HUMOR
IZMIR
KHMER
LAMAR
LAMER
LEMUR
MIMER
NAMER
NAMUR
NOMAR
RAMAR
RIMER
RUMER
RUMOR
SAMAR
SUMER
TAMAR
TAMER
TIMER
TIMOR
TOMAR
VOMER

•••MR
PLUMR

MS•••
MSDOS
MSGTS
MSNBC
MSRPS
MSTAR

M•S••
MASAI
MASAS
MASER
MASHA
MASKS
MASON
MASSA
MASSE
MASSY
MASTS
MASUR
MESAS
MESES
MESHY
MESNE
MESON
MESSE
MESSY
MESTA
MISDO
MISER
MISHA
MISOS
MISSA
MISSM
MISSY
MISTI
MISTS
MISTY
MOSEL
MOSES
MOSEY
MOSHE
MOSSO
MOSSY
MOSUL
MUSCA
MUSED
MUSEE
MUSEO
MUSER
MUSES
MUSHU
MUSHY
MUSIC
MUSIL
MUSKS
MUSKY
MUSSY
MUSTS
MUSTY
MYSIN

M••S•
MANSE
MARSH
MASSA
MASSE
MASSY
MATSU
MAYST
MEESE
MENSA
MESSE
MESSY
MEUSE
MIDST
MIMSY
MINSK
MISSA
MISSM
MISSY
MOIST
MOOSE
MOPSY
MORSE
MOSSO
MOSSY
MOUSE
MOUSY
MUSSY

M•••S
MAAMS
MACES
MACKS
MACYS
MAGES
MAGUS
MAIDS
MAILS
MAIMS
MAINS
MAKES
MAKOS
MALES
MALLS
MALTS
MAMAS
MANES
MANOS
MANUS
MAPES
MARES
MARIS
MARKS
MARLS
MARMS
MARTS
MARYS
MASAS
MASKS
MASTS
MATES
MATHS
MAULS
MAVIS
MAXES
MAXIS
MAYAS
MAYOS
MAZES
MCATS
MEADS
MEALS
MEANS
MEARS
MEATS
MEDES
MEETS
MELDS
MELIS
MELOS
MELTS
MEMOS
MENAS
MENDS
MENES
MENOS
MENUS
MEOWS
MERCS
MERES
MERLS
MESAS
MESES
METES
METIS
MEWLS
MICAS
MIDAS
MIDIS
MIELS
MIENS
MIERS
MIFFS
MIKES
MILES
MILKS
MILLS
MILOS
MIMES
MINAS
MINDS
MINES
MINIS
MINKS
MINOS
MINTS
MINUS
MIRES
MIROS
MIRVS
MISOS
MISTS
MITAS
MITES
MITTS
MIXES
MLLES
MOANS
MOATS
MOCKS
MODES
MODUS
MOILS
MOJOS
MOLDS
MOLES
MOLLS
MOLTS
MOMUS
MONKS
MONOS
MONTS
MOODS
MOOGS
MOONS
MOORS
MOOTS
MOPES
MORAS
MORES
MORNS
MOROS
MOSES
MOTES
MOTHS
MOTTS
MOUES
MOVES
MOWIS
MOZOS
MPEGS
MSDOS
MSGTS
MSRPS
MTGES
MUCKS
MUFFS
MUGGS
MULES
MULLS
MUMMS
MUMPS
MUNIS
MUONS
MURES
MUSES
MUSKS
MUSTS
MUTES
MUTTS
MYERS
MYLES
MYNAS
MYTHS

•MS••
IMSET

•M•S•
AMASS
AMISH
AMISS
AMUSE
AMUST
EMESA
SMASH
SMUSH
UMASS

•M••S
AMAHS
AMASS
AMBOS
AMENS
AMIES
AMIRS
AMISS
AMMOS
AMORS
AMPAS
AMYAS
AMYLS
BMOCS
CMDRS
EMAGS
EMEUS
EMIRS
EMITS
EMMYS
GMATS
IMACS
IMAMS
OMENS
OMERS
OMITS
OMNES
OMNIS
SMEES
SMEWS
SMITS
SMOGS
SMUTS
UMASS
YMCAS
YMHAS

••MS•
ELMST
IAMSO
MIMSY
NOMSG
SAMSA
TOMSK

••M•S
AAMES
ACMES
AMMOS
ARMAS
ARMES
ATMOS
BEMAS
BOMBS
BUMPS
CAMAS
CAMBS
CAMOS
CAMPS
CAMUS
COMAS
COMBS
COMES
COMPS
COMUS
CUMES
CYMAS
CYMES
DAMAS
DAMES
DAMIS
DAMNS
DAMPS
DEMES
DEMOS
DIMAS
DIMES
DOMES
DOMOS
DUMAS
DUMBS
DUMPS
EAMES
ELMOS
EMMYS
ERMAS
FAMES
FEMES
FUMES
GAMES
GAMPS
GIMPS
HAMAS
HAMES
HAMMS
HEMES
HEMPS
HIMES
HOMES
HUMPS
HUMUS
HYMNS
IAMBS
JAMBS
JAMES
JUMPS
LAMAS
LAMBS
LAMES
LAMPS
LIMAS
LIMBS
LIMES
LIMNS
LIMOS
LIMPS
LOMAS
LUMAS
LUMPS
MAMAS
MEMOS
MIMES
MOMUS
MUMMS
MUMPS
NAMES
NEMOS
NIMES
NOMAS
NUMBS
OLMOS
PIMAS
POMES
POMOS
PUMAS
PUMPS
RAMAS
RAMIS
RAMOS
RAMPS
RAMUS
REMUS
RIMES
ROMES
ROMPS
RUMPS
SAMIS
SAMMS
SAMOS
SAMPS
SEMIS
SIMMS
SIMPS
SOMAS
SUMOS
SUMPS
TAMES
TAMPS
TEMAS
TEMPS
TIMES
TOMAS
TOMBS
TOMES
VAMOS
VAMPS
WIMPS
WOMBS
YUMAS

•••MS
ADAMS
AHEMS
ALUMS
ARUMS
ATOMS
BALMS
BARMS
BEAMS
BERMS
BLAMS
BOOMS
BRIMS
CALMS
CHUMS
CLAMS
CORMS
CRAMS
DEEMS
DIAMS
DIEMS
DOOMS
DORMS
DRAMS
DRUMS
EDAMS
ELEMS
EXAMS
FAIMS
FARMS
FILMS
FIRMS
FLAMS
FOAMS
FORMS
GERMS
GLAMS
GLIMS
GLOMS
GLUMS
GORMS
GRAMS
HAMMS
HARMS
HELMS
HOLMS
HYAMS
ICBMS
IMAMS
ITEMS
LOAMS
LOOMS
MAAMS
MAIMS
MARMS
MUMMS
NORMS
OGAMS
PALMS
PERMS
PLUMS
POEMS
PRAMS
PRIMS
PROMS
REAMS
REIMS
ROAMS
ROOMS
SAMMS
SCAMS
SCUMS
SEAMS
SEEMS
SHAMS
SHIMS
SIMMS
SKIMS
SLAMS
SLIMS
SLUMS
SPAMS
STEMS
SWIMS
TEAMS
TEEMS
TERMS
THEMS
TRAMS
TRIMS
WARMS
WEEMS
WHAMS
WHIMS
WORMS
ZOOMS

MT•••
MTAPO
MTELY
MTGES
MTIDA
MTIDY
MTILE
MTVVJ
MTWTF

M•T••
MATCH
MATED
MATEO
MATER
MATES
MATEY
MATHS
MATIN
MATRI
MATRO
MATSU
MATTE
MATTY
MATZO
METAL
METED
METER
METES
METIS
METOO
METRE
METRO
METRY
METUP
MITAS
MITCH
MITER
MITES
MITLA
MITRE
MITTS
MITTY
MITYA
MITZI
MOTEL
MOTES
MOTET
MOTHS
MOTHY
MOTIF
MOTOR
MOTTO
MOTTS
MSTAR
MUTED
MUTER
MUTES
MUTON
MUTTS
MYTHS

M••T•
MADTV
MALTA
MALTS
MALTY
MANTA
MARTA
MARTI
MARTS
MARTY
MASTS
MATTE
MATTY
MCATS
MEATH
MEATS
MEATY
MEETS
MEHTA
MELTS
MERTZ
MESTA
MIATA
MINTS
MINTY
MIRTH
MISTI
MISTS
MISTY
MITTS
MITTY
MOATS
MOLTO
MOLTS
MONTE
MONTH
MONTS
MONTY
MOOTS
MORTE
MORTY
MOTTO
MOTTS
MOUTH
MSGTS
MTWTF
MUFTI
MULTI
MUSTS
MUSTY
MUTTS

M•••T
MADAT
MAMET
MANAT
MANET
MARAT
MAROT
MAYNT
MAYST
MEANT
MEDIT
MELOT
MERIT
MIDST
MIGHT
MINOT
MOIST
MONET
MOTET
MOULT
MOUNT
MOWAT
MRMET
MULCT
MURAT

•MT••
AMTOO

•M•T•
AMATI
AMATO
AMITE
AMITY
EMITS
EMOTE
EMPTY
GMATS
OMITS
SMITE
SMITH
SMITS
SMOTE
SMUTS
SMYTH

•M••T
AMANT
AMBIT
AMENT
AMLIT
AMORT
AMUST
AMVET
EMMET
IMHOT
IMOUT
IMSET
KMART
SMART
SMELT
SMOLT
SMOOT

••MT•
COMTE
FEMTO

••M•T
ADMIT
AIMAT
ARMET
COMET
DEMIT
ELMST
EMMET
EXMET
FUMET
GAMUT
HEMAT
HEMET
KEMPT
LAMIT
LEMAT
LIMIT
LUMET
MAMET
MRMET
NYMET
RAMET
REMAT
REMET
REMIT
SOMAT
TEMPT
UNMET

•••MT
KLIMT

MU•••
MUCHA
MUCHO
MUCKS
MUCKY
MUDDY
MUFFS
MUFTI
MUGGS
MUGGY
MUJER
MULAN
MULCH
MULCT
MULES
MULEY
MULLA
MULLS
MULTI
MUMBO
MUMMS
MUMMY
MUMPS
MUNCH
MUNDI
MUNIS
MUNNA
MUNRO
MUONS
MURAL
MURAT
MURES
MURKY
MURRE
MUSCA
MUSED
MUSEE
MUSEO
MUSER
MUSES
MUSHU
MUSHY
MUSIC
MUSIL
MUSKS
MUSKY
MUSSY
MUSTS
MUSTY
MUTED
MUTER
MUTES
MUTON
MUTTS
MUZAK
MUZZY

M•U••
MAUDE
MAULS
MAUNA
MAURA
MAURY
MAUVE
MEUSE
MFUME
MOUCH
MOUES
MOULD
MOULT
MOUND
MOUNT
MOURN
MOUSE
MOUSY
MOUTH
MYUNG

M••U•
MAGUA
MAGUS
MANUS
MAQUI
MASUR
MECUM
MENUS
METUP
MIEUX
MINUS
MIXUP
MODUS
MOGUL
MOMUS
MOPUP
MOSUL
MRCUB
MRYUK
MYGUY

M•••U
MACHU
MATSU
MIAOU
MUSHU

•MU••
AMUCK
AMUSE
AMUST
SMURF
SMUSH
SMUTS

•M•U•
AMOUR
AMPUP
EMEUS
IMBUE
IMOUT
SMAUG

•M••U
IMAMU

••MU•
CAMUS
COMUS
CUMUL
DAMUP
DEMUR
FEMUR
GAMUT
GUMUP
HAMUP
HUMUS
JAMUP
LEMUR
MOMUS
NAMUR
RAMUS
RAMUZ
REMUS
SUMUP

••M•U
KOMBU

•••MU
IMAMU
ISAMU
SHAMU

MV•••
MVIII

M•V••
MAVEN
MAVIN
MAVIS
MCVIE
MCVII
MDVII
MLVII
MMVII
MOVED
MOVER
MOVES
MOVIE
MOVIN
MTVVJ
MXVII

M••V•
MAEVE
MARVY
MAUVE
MCCVI
MCDVI
MCLVI
MCMVI
MCXVI
MDCVI
MDLVI
MDXVI
MIRVS
MLXVI
MMCVI
MMDVI
MMLVI
MMMVI
MMXVI
MTVVJ
MXCVI
MXLVI
MXXVI

M•••V
MADTV
MALEV
MARKV
MCCCV
MCCIV
MCCLV
MCCXV
MCDIV
MCDLV
MCDXV
MCLIV
MCLXV
MCMIV
MCMLV
MCMXV
MCXCV
MCXIV
MCXLV
MCXXV
MDCCV
MDCIV
MDCLV
MDCXV
MDLIV
MDLXV
MDXCV
MDXIV
MDXLV
MDXXV
MLXIV
MLXXV
MMCCV
MMCDV
MMCIV
MMCLV
MMCMV
MMCXV
MMDCV
MMDIV
MMDLV
MMDXV
MMLIV
MMLXV
MMMCV
MMMDV
MMMIV
MMMLV
MMMXV
MMXCV
MMXIV
MMXLV
MMXXV
MXCIV
MXLIV
MXXIV
MXXXV

•MV••
AMVET
CMVII
MMVII

•M•V•
CMLVI
CMXVI
IMOVE
MMCVI
MMDVI
MMLVI
MMMVI
MMXVI

•M••V
CMLIV
CMLXV
CMXCV
CMXIV
CMXLV
CMXXV
MMCCV
MMCDV
MMCIV
MMCLV
MMCMV
MMCXV
MMDCV
MMDIV
MMDLV
MMDXV
MMLIV
MMLXV
MMMCV
MMMDV
MMMIV
MMMLV
MMMXV
MMXCV
MMXIV
MMXLV
MMXXV

••MV•
ALMVP
MCMVI
MMMVJ
NLMVP

••M•V
MCMIV
MCMLV
MCMXV
MMMCV
MMMDV
MMMIV
MMMLV
MMMXV

•••MV
MMCMV

M•W••
MEWED
MEWER
MEWLS
MOWAT
MOWED
MOWEN
MOWER
MOWIS
MTWTF
MYWAR
MYWAY

M••W•
MEOWS

M•••W
MACAW
MIAOW
MINOW

•MW••
AMWAY

•M•W•
SMEWS

••M•W
GAMOW
REMOW
UNMEW

MX•••
MXCII
MXCIV
MXCIX
MXCVI
MXIII
MXLII
MXLIV
MXLIX
MXLVI
MXVII
MXXII
MXXIV
MXXIX
MXXVI
MXXXI
MXXXV

M•X••
MAXED MAXES MAXIE MAXIM MAXIS MCXCI MCXCV MCXII MCXIV MCXIX MCXLI MCXLV MCXVI MCXXI MCXXV MCXXX MDXCI MDXCV MDXII MDXIV MDXIX MDXLI MDXLV MDXVI MDXXI MDXXV MDXXX MIXED MIXER MIXES MIXIN MIXUP MLXII MLXIV MLXIX MLXVI MLXXI MLXXV MLXXX MMXCI MMXCV MMXII MMXIV MMXIX MMXLI MMXLV MMXVI MMXXI MMXXV MMXXX MOXIE MXXII MXXIV MXXIX MXXVI MXXXI MXXXV

M••X•
MCCXC MCCXI MCCXL MCCXV MCCXX MCDXC MCDXI MCDXL MCDXV MCDXX MCLXI MCLXV MCLXX MCMXC MCMXI MCMXL MCMXV MCMXX MCXXI MCXXV MCXXX MDCXC MDCXI MDCXL MDCXV MDCXX MDLXI MDLXV MDLXX MDXXI MDXXV MDXXX MLXXI MLXXV MLXXX MMCXC MMCXI MMCXL MMCXV MMCXX MMDXC MMDXI MMDXL MMDXV MMDXX MMLXI MMLXV MMLXX MMMXC MMMXI MMMXL MMMXV MMMXX MMXXI MMXXV MMXXX MXXXI MXXXV

M•••X
MADOX MCCCX MCCIX MCCLX MCCXX MCDIX MCDLX MCDXX MCLIX MCLXX MCMIX MCMLX MCMXX MCXIX MCXXX MDCCX MDCIX MDCLX MDCXX MDLIX MDLXX MDXIX MDXXX MIEUX MLXIX MLXXX MMCCX MMCDX MMCIX MMCLX MMCMX MMCXX MMDCX MMDIX MMDLX MMDXX MMLIX MMLXX MMMCX MMMDX MMMIX MMMLX MMMXX MMXIX MMXXX MRFOX MRHEX MXCIX MXLIX MXXIX

•MX••
CMXCI CMXCV CMXII CMXIV CMXIX CMXLI CMXLV CMXVI CMXXI CMXXV CMXXX MMXCI MMXCV MMXII MMXIV MMXIX MMXLI MMXLV MMXVI MMXXI MMXXV MMXXX

•M•X•
CMLXI CMLXV CMLXX CMXXI CMXXV CMXXX MMCXC MMCXI MMCXL MMCXV MMCXX MMDXC MMDXI MMDXL MMDXV MMDXX MMLXI MMLXV MMLXX MMMXC MMMXI MMMXL MMMXV MMMXX MMXXI MMXXV MMXXX

•M••X
CMLIX CMLXX CMXIX CMXXX IMMIX MMCCX MMCDX MMCIX MMCLX MMCMX MMCXX MMDCX MMDIX MMDLX MMDXX MMLIX MMLXX MMMCX MMMDX MMMIX MMMLX MMMXX MMXIX MMXXX

••MX•
MCMXC MCMXI MCMXL MCMXV MCMXX MMMXC MMMXI MMMXL MMMXV MMMXX

••M•X
ADMIX COMEX COMIX IMMIX LOMAX MCMIX MCMLX MCMXX MMMCX MMMDX MMMIX MMMLX MMMXX REMAX REMIX TIMEX UNMIX XEMEX

•••MX
MMCMX

MY•••
MYBAD MYBOY MYCIN MYDAD MYDAY MYERS MYEYE MYGOD MYGUY MYLAR MYLES MYMAN MYNAH MYNAS MYOPE MYRIA MYRNA MYRON MYRRH MYSIN MYTHS MYUNG MYWAR MYWAY

M•Y••
MAYAN MAYAS MAYBE MAYER MAYLE MAYNT MAYOR MAYOS MAYPO MAYST MEYER MRYUK

M••Y•
MACYS MARYA MARYI MARYJ MARYS MERYL MITYA MYEYE

M•••Y
MACHY MADLY MALAY MALTY MAMMY MANCY MANDY MANGY MANLY MANNY MARCY MARGY MARLY MARRY MARTY MARVY MASSY MATEY MATTY MAURY MCCOY MCFLY MCKAY MEALY MEANY MEATY MEENY MERCY MERRY MESHY MESSY METRY MICKY MIDDY MIFFY MIKEY MILKY MIMSY MINDY MINEY MINGY MINTY MISSY MISTY MITTY MOLDY MOLLY MOMMY MONEY MONTY MOODY MOONY MOORY MOPEY MOPSY MORAY MOREY MORTY MOSEY MOSSY MOTHY MOUSY MTELY MTIDY MUCKY MUDDY MUGGY MULEY MUMMY MURKY MUSHY MUSKY MUSSY MUSTY MUZZY MYBOY MYDAY MYGUY MYWAY

•MY••
AMYAS AMYLO AMYLS SMYTH

•M•Y•
EMLYN EMMYS

•M••Y
AMBOY AMBRY AMERY AMITY AMORY AMPLY AMWAY EMBAY EMERY EMILY EMORY EMPTY IMPLY SMOKY

••MY•
EMMYS WOMYN

••M•Y
ALMAY ARMEY BAMMY BUMPY CAMAY CAMPY CAMRY COMFY CYMRY DIMLY DUMMY DUMPY GAMAY GEMMY GIMPY GUMBY GUMMY HAMMY HEMPY HOMEY HUMPY INMAY JIMMY JUMPY LEMAY LIMPY LUMPY MAMMY MIMSY MOMMY MUMMY NAMBY NIMBY NIMOY PAMBY RAMEY RUMMY SAMMY TAMMY TIMMY TOMMY TUMMY VAMPY WIMPY YUMMY

•••MY
ANOMY ATOMY BALMY BAMMY BARMY BEAMY BOOMY DOOMY DORMY DUMMY ENEMY FILMY FLAMY FOAMY GEMMY GERMY GNOMY GRIMY GUMMY HAMMY JIMMY LOAMY MAMMY MOMMY MUMMY PALMY PLUMY PYGMY ROOMY RUMMY SAMMY SEAMY SLIMY SPUMY TAMMY THYMY TIMMY TOMMY TUMMY WORMY YUMMY

M•Z••
MAZAR MAZDA MAZED MAZEL MAZES MEZZO MIZAR MOZOS MUZAK MUZZY

M••Z•
MAIZE MARZO MATZO MEZZO MITZI MONZA MUZZY

M•••Z
MAINZ MERTZ MONIZ

•M•Z•
AMAZE SMAZE

••M•Z
GOMEZ RAMUZ

NA•••
NAACP NABES NABOB NABOO NACHO NACHT NACIO NACRE NADER NADIA NADIR NADJA NAFTA NAGAT NAGEL NAGGY NAHUM NAIAD NAIFS NAILS NAIMA NAINA NAIRA NAISH NAIVE NAKED NAKFA NALDI NAMBY NAMED NAMER NAMES NAMIB NAMPA NAMUR NANAK NANAS NANCE NANCI NANCY NANKI NANNA NANNO NANNY NANON NANTZ NAOMI NAPES NAPPE NAPPY NARAS NARCO NARCS NARDA NARDO NARDS NARES NARIC NARIS NARKS NASAL NASBY NASHE NASTY NATAL NATAN NATCH NATRO NATTA NATTY NAURU NAVAL NAVEE NAVEL NAVES NAVIG NAVIS NAXOS NAZIS

N•A••
NAACP NBAER NEALE NEALY NEAME NEAPS NEARS NEATH NEATO NEATS NGAIO NGANA NWAPA NYACK NYALA NYASA

N••A•
NAGAT NAIAD NANAK NANAS NARAS NASAL NATAL NATAN NAVAL NEMAN NEPAL NEWAT NICAD NINAS NIPAS NIPAT NISAN NIVAL NOCAL NODAL NODAT NOEAR NOFAT NOGAS NOLAN NOMAD NOMAR NOMAS NOPAL NOPAR NORAD NORAH NOTAH NOTAX NOVAE NOVAK NOVAS NOWAY NSTAR NUMAN NYMAN

N•••A
NADIA NADJA NAFTA NAIMA NAINA NAIRA NAKFA NAMPA NANNA NARDA NATTA NEDDA NEDRA NEMEA NERVA NESIA NGANA NIETA NILLA NINEA NINJA NIVEA NOKIA NORIA NORMA NOVIA NUBIA NUCHA NUEVA NULLA NUNCA NUOVA NWAPA NYALA NYASA NYDIA

•NA••
ANAGS ANAIS ANANA ANAND DNASE ENACT ENAMI ENARE ENARM ENATE GNARL GNARS GNASH GNATS GNAWN GNAWS INAGE INALL INANE INAPT INARI INAWE KNACK KNARS KNAVE ONAIR ONATE RNASE SNACK SNAFU SNAGS SNAIL SNAKE SNAKY SNAPS SNARE SNARF SNARK SNARL SNATH SNAZZ UNAMI UNAPT UNARM UNARY UNAUS

•N•A•
ANNAL ANNAM ANNAN ANNAS ANOAS ANSAE ANTAE ANTAL ANTAS ANWAR ANZAC ENBAS ENDAT ENIAC ENLAI ENTAD INBAD INCAN INCAS INLAW INLAY INMAY KNEAD ONDAS ONEAD ONEAL ONEAM ONLAY ONPAR ONTAP SNEAD SNEAK UNBAG UNBAR UNCAP UNCAS UNDAM UNDAY UNFAR UNGAG UNGAR UNHAT UNIAT UNJAM UNLAX UNLAY UNMAD UNMAN UNSAD UNSAY UNTAX

•N••A
ANANA ANIMA ANITA ANOKA ANTRA ENNEA ENOLA INDIA INDRA INFRA INTRA ONEGA ONELA ONERA SNEVA UNITA

••NA•
ADNAN ANNAL ANNAM ANNAN ANNAS ARNAZ ASNAP BANAL BINAL BONAR CANAL CENAS CONAN DANAE DENAR DINAH DINAR DONAS DONAT DONAU ETNAS FINAL HONAN HUNAN IXNAY JONAH JONAS KANAR KANAS KENAI KINAS KONAS LANAI LUNAR LUNAS MANAT MCNAB MENAS MINAS MONAD MYNAH MYNAS NANAK NANAS NINAS PANAM PANAY PENAL RANAS RANAT RENAL RENAN RENAY RONAN RUNAT SANAA SENAT SINAI SONAL SONAR TENAD TENAM TONAL TUNAS TYNAN UHNAK ULNAE ULNAR ULNAS VENAE VENAL VINAS WINAT WONAT ZONAL

••N•A
AMNIA APNEA BANCA BANDA BANTA CANEA CANNA CINNA CONGA DANIA DANZA DINKA DONNA ENNEA FANTA FINCA FONDA GENOA GINZA GONNA GUNGA HANNA HANSA HANYA HENNA HONDA IONIA JENNA JUNTA KANGA KANSA KENYA KINDA KUNTA LANKA LANZA LENYA LINDA LINEA LONGA LYNDA MANGA MANIA MANNA MANTA MENSA MONZA MUNNA NANNA NINEA NINJA NUNCA OMNIA PANDA PANTA PANZA PENNA PENTA PINNA PINTA PINZA PONCA PONTA PUNKA PUNTA QANDA RANDA RENGA SANAA SANKA SANTA SENNA SENTA SONIA SONJA SONYA SUNDA SUNNA TANIA TANKA TANNA TANYA TINEA TONGA TONKA TONYA UINTA VANNA VANUA VANYA VENTA VONDA WANDA WANNA WONKA XENIA YENTA ZENDA

•••NA
ADANA AETNA AGANA AGENA ALANA AMANA ANANA ARENA ASANA AVENA BATNA BUENA BUONA BWANA CANNA CHINA CIGNA CINNA DEANA DESNA DIANA DJUNA DONNA DRINA DUENA DVINA EDINA ELENA FAENA FAUNA FIONA FRENA GEENA GHANA GONNA HANNA HENNA HYENA ILONA IPANA IRENA IRINA ITINA IVANA JENNA JUMNA KRONA LEONA LIANA LORNA LUANA MAGNA MANNA MAUNA MUNNA MYRNA NAINA NANNA NGANA ORENA OXANA PATNA PENNA PINNA PLANA PLENA POONA PRANA REGNA REINA SAUNA SCENA SENNA SHANA SIENA SUNNA TAINA TANNA TEENA TRINA VANNA VARNA VERNA VILNA VIRNA WANNA WEENA ZEENA

NB•••
NBAER NBCTV NBOMB

N•B••
NABES NABOB NABOO NIBLO NOBBY NOBEL NOBET NOBID NOBIS NOBLE NOBLY NUBBY NUBIA

N••B•
NAMBY
NASBY
NIMBI
NIMBY
NIOBE
NOBBY
NUBBY
NUMBS

N•••B
NABOB
NAMIB
NBOMB
NEGEB
NINEB

•NB••
ENBAS
INBAD
INBED
INBIG
INBOX
UNBAG
UNBAR
UNBET
UNBID
UNBIT
UNBOX
UNBUD

•N•B•
KNOBS
ONEBC
SNOBS
SNUBS

•N••B
ONELB

••NB•
CANBY
MSNBC
RANBY
RUNBY
TENBC
WINBY
WONBY

••N•B
BANDB
DENEB
JANDB
LINEB
MCNAB
NINEB
RANDB
TENLB

•••NB
PLANB

N•C••
NACHO
NACHT
NACIO
NACRE
NBCTV
NECKS
NICAD
NICER
NICHE
NICHT
NICKS
NICKY
NICOL
NOCAL
NOCHE
NOCKS
NOCTI
NOCUT
NUCHA
NYCTI
NYCTO

N••C•
NAACP
NANCE
NANCI
NANCY
NARCO
NARCS
NATCH
NIECE
NONCE
NOTCH
NOYCE
NUNCA
NYACK

N•••C
NARIC
NEMEC
NINEC
NROTC
NSYNC
NUMIC

•NC••
ANCHO
ANCON
ENCLS
ENCRE
ENCYC
INCAN
INCAS
INCOG
INCRS
INCUR
INCUS
ONCLE
ONCUE
UNCAP
UNCAS
UNCLE
UNCOY
UNCUT

•N•C•
ENACT
ENOCH
INICE
KNACK
KNICK
KNOCK
ONICE
SNACK
SNICK
SNUCK
UNICE
VNECK

•N••C
ANTIC
ANZAC
ENCYC
ENIAC
INDIC
INHOC
ONEBC
UNDEC

••NC•
BANCA
BANCO
BANCS
BENCH
BUNCH
BUNCO
CINCH
CINCO
CINCY
CONCH
DANCE
DENCH
DUNCE
FANCY
FENCE
FINCA
FINCH
GANCE
HENCE
HENCH
HUNCH
JUNCO
LANCE
LINCS
LUNCH
LYNCH
MANCY
MINCE
MUNCH
NANCE
NANCI
NANCY
NONCE
NUNCA
OUNCE
PENCE
PINCE
PINCH
PONCA
PONCE
PONCH
PUNCH
RANCH
RONCO
SINCE
SYNCH
SYNCS
TENCC
TENCH
TINCT
VANCE
VINCE
VINCI
VINCY
WENCH
WINCE
WINCH
YANCY
ZINCS
ZINCY

••N•C
CONIC
CYNIC
GENIC
GYNEC
IONIC
LINEC
MANIC
MONIC
MSNBC
NINEC
PANIC
PUNIC
RUNIC
SONIC
TENBC
TENCC
TONIC
TUNIC
VINIC
ZENIC

•••NC
BLANC
BRONC
FRANC
JOHNC
NSYNC

N•D••
NADER
NADIA
NADIR
NADJA
NEDDA
NEDRA
NIDRE
NIDUS
NODAL
NODAT
NODDY
NODES
NODOZ
NODTO
NODUH
NODUS
NUDER
NUDES
NUDGE
NUDZH
NYDIA

N••D•
NALDI
NARDA
NARDO
NARDS
NEDDA
NEEDS
NEEDY
NERDS
NERDY
NODDY
NOLDE
NOTDO

N•••D
NAIAD
NAKED
NAMED
NEFUD
NICAD
NINED
NITID
NIXED
NOBID
NOEND
NOMAD
NORAD
NOSED
NOTED
NUKED

•ND••
ANDES
ANDIE
ANDOR
ANDRE
ANDRO
ANDRY
ANDSO
ANDUP
ANDYS
ENDAT
ENDED
ENDER
ENDIN
ENDIT
ENDON
ENDOR
ENDOW
ENDUE
ENDUP
INDEF
INDEX
INDIA
INDIC
INDIE
INDIO
INDIV
INDRA
INDRE
INDUE
INDUS
INDYS
ONDAS
ONDES
ONDIT
ONDVD
UNDAM
UNDAY
UNDEC
UNDER
UNDID
UNDIM
UNDRY
UNDUE
UNDUG

•N•D•
ANODE
SNIDE

•N••D
ANAND
ANTED
ENDED
ENTAD
INBAD
INBED
INKED
INRED
KNEAD
KNEED
ONDVD
ONEAD
ONEND
SNEAD
SNERD
SNOOD
UNBID
UNBUD
UNDID
UNFED
UNHID
UNLED
UNMAD
UNSAD
UNWED

••ND•
AANDE
AANDM
AANDP
AANDW
BANDA
BANDB
BANDO
BANDS
BANDW
BANDY
BENDS
BENDY
BINDS
BONDI
BONDS
BUNDS
BUNDT
BUNDY
CANDO
CANDW
CANDY
CINDY
CONDE
CONDI
CONDO
CONDS
CYNDI
DANDD
DANDY
DENDR
DINDY
DONDE
DONDI
FENDI
FENDS
FINDS
FONDA
FONDU
FUNDS
FUNDY
GANDT
GANDY
HANDI
HANDS
HANDY
HINDI
HINDS
HINDU
HONDA
HONDO
HYNDE
JANDB
JANDJ
KANDY
KENDO
KINDA
KINDS
LANDI
LANDO
LANDS
LENDL
LENDS
LINDA
LINDO
LINDT
LINDY
LUNDI
LUNDY
LYNDA
LYNDE
MANDY
MENDS
MINDS
MINDY
MONDE
MONDO
MUNDI
PANDA
PANDL
PENDS
PONDS
PRNDL
QANDA
RANDA
RANDB
RANDD
RANDI
RANDR
RANDS
RANDY
RENDS
RINDS
RINDY
RONDE
RONDO
SANDE
SANDH
SANDL
SANDP
SANDS
SANDY
SENDS
SONDE
SUNDA
SYNDS
TANDY
TENDS
TENDU
TONDI
TONDO
VENDS
VONDA
WANDA
WANDS
WENDS
WENDT
WENDY
WINDS
WINDY
WUNDT
XANDO
XANDY
ZENDA
ZENDO
ZENDS

••N•D
AWNED
BONED
CANED
CANID
CONED
CONTD
DANDD
DINED
FINED
HONED
LANED
LINED
MANED
MINED
MONAD
MONOD
NINED
OWNED
PANED
PINED
RANDD
RANID
SYNOD
TENAD
TINED
TONED
TUNED
VANED
VINED
WANED
WINED
ZONED

•••ND
ABEND
AMAND
AMEND
ANAND
BLAND
BLEND
BLIND
BLOND
BOUND
BRAND
EBOND
ELAND
EMEND
FIEND
FOUND
FROND
GLAND
GRAND
GRIND
HOUND
JOHND
MOUND
NOEND
OLAND
ONEND
POUND
QUAND
ROUND
SOUND
SPEND
STAND
TBOND
TREND
UPEND
VIAND
WOUND
ZAHND

NE•••
NEALE
NEALY
NEAME
NEAPS
NEARS
NEATH
NEATO
NEATS
NECKS
NEDDA
NEDRA
NEEDS
NEEDY
NEELY
NEEME
NEFUD
NEGEB
NEGEV
NEGRI
NEGRO
NEGUS
NEHER
NEHIS
NEHRU
NEIGE
NEIGH
NEILL
NELLE
NELLO
NELLY
NELSE
NEMAN
NEMEA
NEMEC
NEMOS
NENEH
NENES
NEONS
NEPAL
NEPHR
NEPOS
NERDS
NERDY
NERFS
NEROL
NERTS
NERTZ
NERVA
NERVE
NERVO
NERVY
NESIA
NESTS
NESTY
NETTY
NETWT
NEURO
NEUSS
NEVER
NEVES
NEVIL
NEVIN
NEVIS
NEVUS
NEWAT
NEWEL
NEWER
NEWIE
NEWLY
NEWSY
NEWTO
NEWTS
NEXIS
NEXUS

N•E••
NEEDS
NEEDY
NEELY
NEEME
NIECE
NIELS
NIETA
NIETO
NIEUW
NIEVE
NLERS
NOEAR
NOELS
NOEND
NTEST
NUEVA
NUEVE
NUEVO
NYETS

N••E•
NABES
NADER
NAGEL
NAKED
NAMED
NAMER
NAMES
NAPES
NARES
NAVEE
NAVEL
NAVES
NBAER
NEGEB
NEGEV
NEHER
NEMEA
NEMEC
NENEH
NENES
NEVER
NEVES
NEWEL
NEWER
NFLER
NGWEE
NHLER
NICER
NIGEL
NIGER
NIKES
NILES
NIMES
NINEA
NINEB
NINEC
NINED
NINEE
NINER
NINES
NISEI
NITER
NITES
NIVEA
NIVEN
NIXED
NIXER
NIXES
NIZER
NOBEL
NOBET
NODES
NOFEE
NOLES
NOMEN
NONES
NONET
NOPES
NOREN
NOSED
NOSER
NOSES
NOSEY
NOTED
NOTER
NOTES
NOVEL
NOVEM
NOYES
NUDER
NUDES
NUKED
NUKES
NUMEN
NUNEZ
NUYEN
NYJET
NYMET
NYNEX

N•••E
NACRE
NAIVE
NANCE
NAPPE
NASHE
NAVEE
NEALE
NEAME
NEEME
NEIGE
NELLE
NELSE
NERVE
NEWIE
NGWEE
NICHE
NIDRE
NIECE
NIEVE
NINEE
NIOBE
NITRE
NIXIE
NOBLE
NOCHE
NOFEE
NOIRE
NOISE
NOLDE
NOLIE
NOLLE
NOLTE
NONCE
NOONE
NOOSE
NORGE
NORSE
NORTE
NOTIE
NOTME
NOTRE
NOTTE
NOUSE
NOVAE
NOYCE
NTILE
NUDGE
NUEVE
NURSE

•NE••
ANELE
ANEMO
ANENT
ANETO
DNEPR
DNETS
ENEMY
ENERO
INEES
INEPT
INERT
KNEAD
KNEED
KNEEL
KNEES
KNELL
KNELT
MNEME
MNEMO
ONEAD
ONEAL
ONEAM
ONEBC
ONEEE
ONEGA
ONEIL
ONEIR
ONEKS
ONELA
ONELB
ONELS
ONEND
ONENO
ONEON
ONEPM
ONERA
ONERS
ONEUP
PNEUM
SNEAD
SNEAK
SNEER
SNEES
SNELL
SNERD
SNERT
SNEVA
VNECK

•N•E•
ANDES
ANGEL
ANGER
ANGES
ANNEE
ANNEX
ANSEL
ANSER
ANTED
ANTES
ENDED
ENDER
ENGEL
ENNEA
ENTER
ENVER
INBED
INDEF
INDEX
INEES
INFER
INGER
INKED
INKER
INKEY
INLET
INNER
INNES
INPEN
INRED
INREM
INSET
INTEL
INTER
INVER
KNEED
KNEEL
KNEES
ONDES
ONEEE
ONKEY
ONNES
ONSET
SNEER
SNEES
UNBET
UNDEC
UNDER
UNFED
UNGER
UNLED
UNLET
UNMET
UNMEW
UNNEW
UNPEG
UNPEN
UNSER
UNSET
UNSEW
UNTER
UNWED
UNWET

•N••E
ANDIE
ANDRE
ANELE
ANGIE
ANGLE
ANILE
ANIME
ANISE
ANKLE
ANNEE
ANNIE
ANODE
ANOLE
ANSAE
ANTAE
ANTRE
BNINE
CNOTE
DNASE
ENARE
ENATE
ENCRE
ENDUE
ENGLE
ENOTE
ENSUE
ENTRE
ENURE
GNOME
GNOTE
INAGE
INANE
INAWE
INDIE
INDRE
INDUE
INGLE
INICE
INKLE
INNIE
INURE
INUSE
KNAVE
KNIFE
KNUTE
MNEME
ONATE
ONCLE
ONCUE
ONEEE
ONICE
ONONE
ONRYE
RNASE
SNAKE
SNARE
SNIDE
SNIPE
SNORE
SNOWE
TNOTE
UNCLE
UNDUE
UNICE
UNITE
UNTIE

••NE•
ABNER
ACNES
AGNES
AGNEW
ANNEE
ANNEX
AONES
APNEA
ARNEL
ASNER
ASNEW
AVNET
AWNED
BANES
BENES
BENET
BINES
BINET
BONED
BONER
BONES
BONET
BONEY
BYNER
CANEA
CANED
CANEM
CANER
CANES
CINES
CONED
CONER
CONES
CONEY
CUNEO
DANES
DENEB
DENES
DINED
DINER
DINES
DONEE
DONEN
DUNES
DYNEL
DYNES
EINEN
EINER
EINES
ENNEA
ERNES
ESNES
FANES
FINED
FINER
FINES
GANEF
GENES
GENET
GONER
GYNEC
HANES
HANEY
HINES
HONED
HONER
HONES
HONEY
IGNES
INNER
INNES
JANET
JONES
JUNES
KINER
LANED
LANES
LENES
LINEA
LINEB
LINEC
LINED
LINEN
LINER
LINES
LONER
LUNER
LUNES
LYNEN
MANED
MANES
MANET
MENES
MINED
MINEO
MINER
MINES
MINEY
MONEL
MONET
MONEY
NENEH
NENES
NINEA
NINEB
NINEC
NINED
NINEE
NINER
NINES
NONES
NONET
NUNEZ
NYNEX
OMNES
ONNES
OWNED
OWNER
PANED
PANEL
PANES
PINED
PINER
PINES
PINEY
PONES
RANEE
RENEE
RENEW
RONEE
RUNES
SANER
SINES
SINEW
SINEX
SONES
TANEY
TENEE
TENET
TINEA
TINED
TINES
TONED
TONER
TONES
TUNED
TUNER
TUNES
TYNER
UNNEW
URNES
VANED
VANES
VENEZ
VINED
VINER
VINES
WANED
WANER
WANES
WINED
WINES
YONEX
ZENER
ZINES
ZONED
ZONER
ZONES

••N•E
AANDE
AINGE
ANNEE
ANNIE
ARNIE
BINGE
BONNE
BONZE
CANOE
CENSE
CONDE
CONGE
CONTE
DANAE
DANCE
DANKE
DANSE
DANTE
DENSE
DENTE
DINGE
DONDE
DONEE
DONNE
DUNCE
DUNNE
ERNIE
FENCE
GANCE
GENIE
GENRE
GENTE
HANSE
HENCE
HENGE
HENIE
HENZE
HINGE
HYNDE
INNIE
JANIE
JONZE
KANYE
KINTE
LANCE
LANGE
LENTE
LONGE
LUNGE
LYNDE
LYNNE
MANGE
MANNE
MANSE
MINCE
MONDE
MONTE
NANCE
NINEE
NONCE
OUNCE
PANNE
PENCE
PENNE
PENTE
PINCE
PONCE
PONTE
RANEE
RANGE
RANKE
RENEE
RENTE
RINSE
RONDE
RONEE
SANDE
SANTE
SENSE
SENTE
SINCE
SINGE
SONDE
SYNGE
TANTE
TENEE
TENGE
TENSE
TINGE
TONNE
ULNAE
VANCE
VENAE
VENUE
VINCE
WINCE
WYNNE
YENTE
YONNE

•••NE
AISNE
AKENE
ALENE
ALINE
ALONE
AMINE
ASONE
ATONE
AXONE
BEENE
BERNE
BLANE
BNINE
BONNE
BOONE
BORNE
BRINE
BYONE
BYRNE
CAINE
CARNE
CHINE
CLINE
CLONE
CRANE
CRONE
DAYNE
DEANE
DIANE
DIENE
DIONE
DOANE
DONNE
DOONE
DRONE
DUANE
DUNNE
EZINE
HEINE
HERNE
HORNE
ILENE
IMINE
INANE
IRENE
JAUNE
JAYNE
JEANE
JERNE
JEUNE
KEANE
KEENE
KERNE
KLINE
KRONE
LAINE
LAYNE
LEONE
LIANE
LIGNE
LORNE
LYNNE
MAINE
MANNE
MARNE
MEINE
MESNE
MILNE
NOONE
ONONE
OPINE
OVINE
OZONE
PAINE
PANNE
PAYNE
PENNE
PHONE
PLANE
PRINE
PRONE
PRUNE
QUINE
RAINE
REINE
REUNE
RHINE
RHONE
ROONE
SAONE
SCENE
SCONE
SEINE
SHANE
SHINE
SHONE
SIGNE
SPINE
STINE
STONE
STYNE
SWINE
TBONE
TERNE
THANE
THINE
TIENE
TONNE
TOWNE
TRANE
TRINE
TWINE
UDINE
ULENE
UPONE
USONE
VERNE
VHONE
WAYNE
WHINE
WYNNE
YONNE

NF•••
NFLER

N•F••
NAFTA
NEFUD
NIFTY
NOFAT
NOFEE
NOFUN
NUFLO

N••F•
NAIFS
NAKFA
NERFS

•NF••
ENFIN
INFER
INFIX
INFOR
INFRA
INFUN
UNFAR
UNFED
UNFIT
UNFIX
UNFUN

•N•F•
KNIFE
ONOFF
SNAFU
SNIFF
SNUFF
UNIFY

•N••F
INDEF
KNOPF
ONOFF
SNARF
SNIFF
SNUFF

••NF•
BANFF
HANFF
LINFT

••N•F
BANFF
GANEF
HANFF
TENOF

•••NF
JOHNF

NG•••
NGAIO
NGANA
NGWEE

N•G••
NAGAT
NAGEL
NAGGY
NEGEB
NEGEV
NEGRI
NEGRO
NEGUS
NIGEL
NIGER
NIGHT
NOGAS
NOGGS
NOGOS

N••G•
NAGGY
NEIGE
NEIGH
NOGGS
NORGE
NUDGE

N•••G
NAVIG
NOMSG

•NG••
ANGEL
ANGER
ANGES
ANGIE
ANGIO
ANGLE
ANGLO
ANGRY
ANGST
ANGUS
ENGEL
ENGLE
ENGRS
INGER
INGLE
INGOT
UNGAG
UNGAR
UNGER
UNGOT

•N•G•
ANAGS
ANIGH
INAGE
INIGO
ONEGA
SNAGS
SNUGS

•N••G
INBIG
INCOG
INORG
UNBAG
UNDUG
UNGAG
UNPEG
UNRIG
UNWIG

••NG•
AINGE
BANGS
BINGE
BINGO
BINGS
BONGO
BONGS
BUNGS
CONGA
CONGE
CONGO
DANGS
DINGE
DINGO
DINGS
DINGY
DONGS
FANGS
FUNGI
FUNGO
GANGS
GONGS
GUNGA
HANGS
HENGE
HINGE
JINGO
JONGG
KANGA
KANGS
KINGS
LANGE
LINGO
LINGS
LINGU
LONGA
LONGE
LONGI
LONGO
LONGS
LONGU
LUNGE
LUNGS
MANGA
MANGE
MANGO
MANGY
MINGY
MONGO
OINGO
PANGS
PINGS
PONGO
PONGS
PUNGS
RANGE
RANGO
RANGY
RENGA
RINGO
RINGS
RUNGS
SENGI
SINGE
SINGH
SINGS
SONGS
SYNGE
TANGO
TANGS
TANGY
TENGE
TENGO
TINGE
TINGS
TONGA
TONGS
VINGT
WINGS
WINGY
ZINGS
ZINGY

••N•G
JONGG

•••NG
ACING
AGING
AHANG
AHING
ALONG
AMONG
APING
AWING
AXING
BEING
BHANG
BLING
BOING
BRANG
BRING
BRUNG
CCING
CHANG
CHING
CHONG
CHUNG
CLANG
CLING
CLUNG
CUING
DHING
DOING
DRANG
DRING
DYING
EKING
ERING
EWING
EXING
EYING
FLING
FLUNG
GOING
HAING
HMONG
HUANG
HYING
ICING
IDING
JIANG
KOING
LAING
LIANG
LUANG
LYING
MYUNG
ODING
OHING
OKING
OPING
ORANG
ORING
OWING
PRONG
QUANG
RUING
RVING
SHANG
SLANG
SLING
SLUNG
SPANG
STANG
STING
STUNG
SUING
SWING
SWUNG
THING
THONG
TWANG
TYING
USING
VYING
WHANG
WRING
WRONG
WRUNG
YOUNG

NH•••
NHLER

N•H••
NAHUM
NEHER
NEHIS
NEHRU
NIHIL
NIHON
NOHIT
NOHOW

N••H•
NACHO
NACHT
NASHE
NEPHR
NICHE
NICHT
NIGHT
NOCHE
NUCHA

N•••H
NAISH
NATCH
NEATH
NEIGH
NENEH
NINTH
NODUH
NORAH
NORTH
NOTAH
NOTCH
NUDZH
NYMPH

•NH••
INHOC
UNHAT
UNHID
UNHIP
UNHIT
UNHOT

•N•H•
ANCHO
ANKHS
UNSHY

•N••H
ANIGH
ENOCH
GNASH
KNISH
SNATH

••NH•
DONHO
MINHO

••N•H
BENCH
BUNCH
CINCH
CONCH
DENCH
DINAH
FINCH
HENCH
HUNCH
JONAH
LUNCH
LYNCH
MONTH
MUNCH
MYNAH
NENEH
NINTH
PINCH
PONCH
PUNCH
RANCH
SANDH
SINGH
SYNCH
SYNTH
TENCH
TENTH
WENCH
WINCH

NI•••
NIBLO
NICAD
NICER
NICHE
NICHT
NICKS
NICKY
NICOL
NIDRE
NIDUS
NIECE
NIELS
NIETA
NIETO
NIEUW
NIEVE
NIFTY
NIGEL
NIGER
NIGHT
NIHIL
NIHON
NIKES
NIKKI
NIKON
NILES
NILLA
NILLY
NIMBI
NIMBY
NIMES
NIMOY
NINAS
NINEA
NINEB
NINEC
NINED
NINEE
NINER
NINES
NINJA
NINNY
NINON
NINOS
NINTH
NIOBE
NIORT
NIPAS
NIPAT
NIPPY
NIPUP
NISAN
NISEI
NISUS
NITER
NITES
NITID
NITON
NITRE
NITRO
NITTI
NITTY
NIVAL
NIVEA
NIVEN
NIXED
NIXER
NIXES
NIXIE
NIXON
NIZER

N•I••
NAIAD
NAIFS
NAILS
NAIMA
NAINA
NAIRA
NAISH
NAIVE
NEIGE
NEIGH
NEILL
NOILS
NOILY
NOIRE
NOIRS
NOISE
NOISY
NTILE
NUITS

N••I•
NACIO
NADIA
NADIR
NAMIB
NARIC
NARIS
NAVIG
NAVIS
NAZIS
NEHIS
NESIA
NEVIL
NEVIN
NEVIS
NEWIE
NEXIS
NGAIO
NIHIL
NITID
NIXIE
NOBID
NOBIS
NOHIT
NOKIA
NOLIE
NOOIL
NORIA
NORIS
NOSIR
NOTIE
NOTIN
NOTIP
NOTIT
NOVIA
NOVIO
NOWIN
NUBIA
NUMIC
NYDIA

N•••I
NALDI
NANCI
NANKI
NAOMI
NEGRI
NIKKI
NIMBI
NISEI
NITTI
NOCTI
NOTTI
NOURI
NURMI
NYCTI

•NI••
ANIGH
ANILE
ANILS
ANIMA
ANIME
ANIMO
ANION
ANISE
ANITA
BNINE
ENIAC
INICE
INIGO
INIKI
ININK
INION
INITS
KNICK
KNIFE
KNISH
KNITS
ONICE
ONION
SNICK
SNIDE
SNIFF
SNIPE
SNIPS
SNITS
UNIAT
UNICE
UNIFY
UNION
UNITA
UNITE
UNITS
UNITY
UNIVS

•N•I•
ANAIS
ANDIE
ANGIE
ANGIO
ANNIE
ANNIV
ANTIC
ANTIQ
ANTIS
ANVIL
ANZIO
ENDIN
ENDIT
ENFIN
ENNIO
ENNIS
ENOIL
INBIG
INDIA
INDIC
INDIE
INDIO
INDIV
INFIX
INKIN
INNIE
INNIS
INOIL
INUIT
ONAIR
ONDIT
ONEIL
ONEIR
SNAIL
UNBID
UNBIT
UNDID
UNDIM
UNFIT
UNFIX
UNHID
UNHIP
UNHIT
UNLIT
UNMIX
UNPIN
UNRIG
UNRIP
UNTIE
UNTIL
UNWIG
UNZIP

•N••I
ENAMI
ENLAI
ENNUI
ENOKI
ENVOI
INARI
INIKI
UNAMI

••NI•
AMNIA
AMNIO
ANNIE
ANNIV
ARNIE
BENIN
BUNIN
CANID
CANIO
CANIS
CANIT
CONIC
CYNIC
DANIA
DANIO
DENIM
DENIS
ENNIO
ENNIS
ERNIE
FINIS
GENIC
GENIE
GENII
GUNIT
HENIE
IGNIS
INNIE
INNIS
IONIA
IONIC
JANIE
JANIS
JUNIO
KANIN
LANIN
LENIN
LENIS
LUNIK
MANIA
MANIC
MINIM
MINIS
MONIC
MONIZ
MUNIS
OMNIA
OMNIS
ORNIS
PANIC
PANIN
PANIS
PENIN
PUNIC
RANID
RANIN
RANIS
RENIN
RONIN
RUNIC
RUNIN
SONIA
SONIC
TANIA
TANIS
TONIC
TONIO
TUNIC
TUNIS
VENIN
VINIC
XENIA
ZENIC
ZUNIS

••N•I
AINSI
BENJI
BONDI
CENTI
CONDI
CONTI
CYNDI
DENTI
DONDI
ENNUI
FENDI
FUNGI
GENII
HANDI
HANOI
HENRI
HINDI
JINNI
KANJI
KENAI
LANAI
LANDI
LENNI
LONGI
LUNDI
MUNDI
NANCI
NANKI
PENNI
PONTI
PONZI
RANDI
SENGI
SINAI
SUNNI
TONDI
VENTI
VINCI
YANNI

•••NI
ADENI
ARONI
BERNI
BLINI
BRUNI
CORNI
CRANI
CYGNI
ELENI
FRENI
GARNI
GRANI
HOSNI
ICENI
IRANI
IVANI
JINNI
JOHNI
LENNI
LEONI
LIGNI
MARNI
OMANI
ORANI
PENNI
PIANI
PLANI
SEGNI
SOMNI
SUNNI
TRINI
YANNI

N•J••
NYJET

N••J•
NADJA
NINJA

•NJ••
ANJOU
ENJOY
INJUN
UNJAM

••NJ•
BANJO
BENJI
KANJI
NINJA
SONJA

••N•J
JANDJ

•••NJ
JOHNJ

N•K••
NAKED
NAKFA
NIKES
NIKKI
NIKON
NOKIA
NUKED
NUKES

N••K•
NANKI
NARKS
NECKS
NICKS
NICKY
NIKKI
NOCKS
NOOKS

N•••K
NANAK
NORSK
NOTOK
NOVAK
NYACK

•NK••
ANKHS
ANKLE
INKED
INKER
INKEY
INKIN
INKLE
ONKEY
ONKYO

•N•K•
ANOKA
ENOKI
ENSKY
INIKI
ONEKS
SNAKE
SNAKY

•N••K
ANOUK
ININK
KNACK
KNICK
KNOCK
SNACK
SNARK
SNEAK
SNICK
SNOOK
SNUCK
VNECK

••NK•
BANKS
BANKY
BONKS
BUNKO
BUNKS
CONKS
DANKE
DINKA
DINKS
DINKY
DUNKS
FINKS
FUNKS
FUNKY
GUNKS
GUNKY
HANKS
HANKY
HINKY
HONKS
HONKY
HUNKS
HUNKY
JINKS
JUNKS
JUNKY
KINKO
KINKS
KINKY
LANKA
LANKY
LINKS
MINKS
MONKS
NANKI

OINKS
PANKY
PINKO
PINKS
PINKY
PUNKA
PUNKS
PUNKY
RANKE
RANKS
RINKS
RINKY
SANKA
SINKS
TANKA
TANKS
TENKS
TONKA
WINKS
WONKA
WONKS
YANKS
ZINKY
ZONKS

••N•K

LUNIK
MINSK
NANAK
PINSK
UHNAK

•••NK

BLANK
BLINK
BRINK
CHINK
CHUNK
CLANK
CLINK
CLONK
CLUNK
CRANK
DRANK
DRINK
DRUNK
EBANK
FLANK
FLUNK
FRANK
GLUNK
ININK
KLINK
PLANK
PLINK
PLONK
PLUNK
PRANK
PRINK
REINK
SHANK
SKANK
SKINK
SKUNK
SLINK
SLUNK
SPANK
SPUNK
STANK
STINK
STUNK
SWANK
THANK
THINK
THUNK
TRUNK

NL•••

NLERS
NLMVP

N•L••

NALDI
NELLE
NELLO
NELLY
NELSE
NFLER
NHLER
NILES
NILLA
NILLY
NOLAN
NOLDE
NOLES
NOLIE
NOLLE
NOLOS
NOLTE
NULLA
NULLO
NULLS
NYLON

N••L•

NAILS
NEALE
NEALY
NEELY
NEILL
NELLE
NELLO
NELLY
NEWLY
NIBLO
NIELS
NILLA
NILLY
NOBLE
NOBLY
NOELS
NOILS
NOILY
NOLLE
NTILE
NUFLO
NULLA
NULLO
NULLS
NYALA

N•••L

NAGEL
NASAL
NATAL
NAVAL
NAVEL
NEILL
NEPAL
NEROL
NEVIL
NEWEL
NICOL
NIGEL
NIHIL
NIVAL
NOBEL
NOCAL
NODAL
NOOIL
NOPAL
NOVEL
NYTOL

•NL••

ENLAI
INLAW
INLAY
INLET
INLOW
ONLAY
ONLOW
UNLAX
UNLAY
UNLED
UNLET
UNLIT

•N•L•

ANELE
ANGLE
ANGLO
ANILE
ANILS
ANKLE
ANOLE
ENCLS
ENGLE
ENOLA
ENOLS
INALL
INGLE
INKLE
KNELL
KNELT
KNOLL
ONCLE
ONELA
ONELB
ONELS
SNELL
UNCLE
UNSLY

•N••L

ANGEL
ANNAL
ANNUL
ANSEL
ANTAL
ANVIL
ENGEL
ENOIL
ENROL
GNARL
INALL
INOIL
INTEL
KNEEL
KNELL
KNOLL
KNURL
ONEAL
ONEIL
SNAIL
SNARL
SNELL
UNTIL

••NL•

MANLY
MENLO
TENLB
VENLO
WANLY

••N•L

ANNAL
ANNUL
ARNEL
BANAL
BINAL
CANAL
DYNEL
FINAL
LENDL
MONEL
PANDL
PANEL
PENAL
PRNDL
RENAL
SANDL
SONAL
TONAL
VENAL
VINYL
YENTL
ZONAL

•••NL

ADDNL
JOHNL

N•M••

NAMBY
NAMED
NAMER
NAMES
NAMIB
NAMPA
NAMUR
NEMAN
NEMEA
NEMEC
NEMOS
NIMBI
NIMBY
NIMES
NIMOY
NLMVP
NOMAD
NOMAR
NOMAS
NOMEN
NOMSG
NUMAN
NUMBS
NUMEN
NUMIC
NYMAN
NYMET
NYMPH

N••M•

NAIMA
NAOMI
NBOMB
NEAME
NEEME
NORMA
NORMS
NOTME
NURMI

N•••M

NAHUM
NOVEM

•NM••

INMAY
UNMAD
UNMAN
UNMET
UNMEW
UNMIX

•N•M•

ANEMO
ANIMA
ANIME
ANIMO
ANOMY
ENAMI
ENEMY
GNOME
GNOMY
MNEME
MNEMO
UNAMI

•N••M

ANNAM
ANNUM
ENARM
ENORM
ENTOM
INREM
INSUM
ONEAM
ONEPM
PNEUM
UNARM
UNDAM
UNDIM
UNJAM

••N•M

AANDM
ANNAM
ANNUM
BONUM
CANEM
DENIM
DENOM
MINIM
PANAM
PHNOM
TENAM
TENPM
VENOM

N•N••

NANAK
NANAS
NANCE
NANCI
NANCY
NANKI
NANNA
NANNO
NANNY
NANON
NANTZ
NENEH
NENES
NINAS
NINEA
NINEB
NINEC
NINED
NINEE
NINER
NINES
NINJA
NINNY
NINON
NINOS
NINTH
NONCE
NONES
NONET
NONNO
NONOS
NUNCA
NUNEZ
NYNEX

N••N•

NAINA
NANNA
NANNO
NANNY
NEONS
NGANA
NINNY
NOEND
NONNO
NOONE
NOONS
NORNS
NOUNS
NSYNC

N•••N

NANON
NATAN
NEMAN
NEVIN
NIHON
NIKON
NINON
NISAN
NITON
NIVEN
NIXON
NOFUN
NOLAN
NOMEN
NOREN
NORUN
NOTIN
NOTON
NOWIN
NUMAN
NUMEN
NUYEN
NYLON
NYMAN

•NN••

ANNAL
ANNAM
ANNAN
ANNAS
ANNEE
ANNEX
ANNIE
ANNIV
ANNOY
ANNUL
ANNUM
ANNUS
ENNEA
ENNIO
ENNIS
ENNUI
INNER
INNES
INNIE
INNIS
ONNES
UNNEW

•N•N•

ANANA
ANAND
ANENT
BNINE
INANE
ININK
INONU
ONEND
ONENO
ONONE

•N••N

ANCON
ANION
ANNAN
ANSON
ANTON
ANYON
ENDIN
ENDON
ENFIN
ENRON
GNAWN
INCAN
INFUN
INION
INJUN
INKIN
INPEN
INRUN
KNOWN
ONEON
ONION
UNFUN
UNION
UNMAN
UNPEN
UNPIN
UNRUN
UNWON

••NN•

BANNS
BENNY
BONNE
BONNY
BUNNY
CANNA
CANNY
CINNA
CONNS
DANNO
DANNY
DENNY
DINNY
DONNA
DONNE
DONNY
DUNNE
DUNNO
FANNY
FENNY
FINNO
FINNS
FINNY
FUNNY
GINNY
GONNA
GUNNY
HANNA
HENNA
HENNY
HINNY
JENNA
JENNY
JINNI
JINNS
JONNY
KENNY
LANNY
LENNI
LENNY
LUNNS
LYNNE
MANNA
MANNE
MANNY
MUNNA
NANNA
NANNO
NANNY
NINNY
NONNO
PANNE
PENNA
PENNE
PENNI
PENNY
PINNA
PUNNY
RENNY
RONNY
RUNNY
SENNA
SONNY
SUNNA
SUNNI
SUNNY
TANNA
TINNY
TONNE
VANNA
VINNY
WANNA
WYNNE
YANNI
YONNE

••N•N

ADNAN
AGNON
ANNAN
BANON
BENIN
BUNIN
CANON
CONAN
CONON
DONEN
EINEN
FANON
HONAN
HUNAN
KANIN
LANIN
LENIN
LINEN
LYNEN
MANON
NANON
NINON
PANIN
PENIN
PINON
RANIN
RANON
RENAN
RENIN
RONAN
RONIN
RUNIN
RUNON
TENON
TYNAN
VENIN
XENON

•••NN

DAWNN
DJINN
FLANN
FLYNN
FRANN
GLENN
GWENN
GWYNN
LEANN
LUANN
QUINN
SEANN
SWANN
UCONN
UPENN

NO•••

NOBBY
NOBEL
NOBET
NOBID
NOBIS
NOBLE
NOBLY
NOCAL
NOCHE
NOCKS
NOCTI
NOCUT
NODAL
NODAT
NODDY
NODES
NODOZ
NODTO
NODUH
NODUS
NOEAR
NOELS
NOEND
NOFAT
NOFEE
NOFUN
NOGAS
NOGGS
NOGOS
NOHIT
NOHOW
NOILS
NOILY
NOIRE
NOIRS
NOISE
NOISY
NOKIA
NOLAN
NOLDE
NOLES
NOLIE
NOLLE
NOLOS
NOLTE
NOMAD
NOMAR
NOMAS
NOMEN
NOMSG
NONCE
NONES
NONET
NONNO
NONOS
NOOIL
NOOKS
NOONE
NOONS
NOORT
NOOSE
NOPAL
NOPAR
NOPES
NOPQR
NORAD
NORAH
NOREN
NORGE
NORIA
NORIS
NORMA
NORMS
NORNS
NORSE
NORSK
NORTE
NORTH
NORUN
NORVO
NOSED
NOSER
NOSES
NOSEY
NOSIR
NOTAH
NOTAX
NOTCH
NOTDO
NOTED
NOTER
NOTES
NOTIE
NOTIN
NOTIP
NOTIT
NOTME
NOTOK
NOTON
NOTRE
NOTSO
NOTTE
NOTTI
NOTUP
NOTUS
NOUNS
NOURI
NOUSE
NOVAE
NOVAK
NOVAS
NOVEL
NOVEM
NOVIA
NOVIO
NOVUS
NOWAY
NOWIN
NOYCE
NOYES

N•O••

NAOMI
NBOMB
NEONS
NIOBE
NIORT
NOOIL
NOOKS
NOONE
NOONS
NOORT
NOOSE
NROTC
NUOVA
NUOVO

N••O•

NABOB
NABOO
NANON
NAXOS
NEMOS
NEPOS
NEROL
NICOL
NIHON
NIKON
NIMOY
NINON
NINOS
NITON
NIXON
NODOZ
NOGOS
NOHOW
NOLOS
NONOS
NOTOK
NOTON
NYLON
NYTOL

N•••O

NABOO
NACHO
NACIO
NANNO
NARCO
NARDO
NATRO
NEATO
NEGRO
NELLO
NERVO
NEURO
NEWTO
NGAIO
NIBLO
NIETO
NITRO
NODTO
NONNO
NORVO
NOTDO
NOTSO
NOVIO
NUEVO
NUFLO
NULLO
NUOVO
NUTRO
NYCTO

•NO••

ANOAS
ANODE
ANOKA
ANOLE
ANOMY
ANOUK
CNOTE
ENOCH
ENOIL
ENOKI
ENOLA
ENOLS
ENORM
ENOTE
GNOME
GNOMY
GNOTE
INOIL
INONU
INORG
KNOBS
KNOCK
KNOLL
KNOPF
KNORR
KNOTS
KNOTT
KNOUT
KNOWN
KNOWS
MNOPQ
ONOFF
ONONE
SNOBS
SNOOD
SNOOK
SNOOP
SNOOT
SNORE
SNORT
SNOUT
SNOWE
SNOWS
SNOWY
TNOTE

•N•O•

ANCON
ANDOR
ANION
ANJOU
ANNOY
ANSON
ANTON
ANYON
ENDON
ENDOR
ENDOW
ENJOY
ENROL
ENRON
ENSOR
ENTOM
ENVOI
ENVOY
INBOX
INCOG
INFOR
INGOT
INHOC
INION
INLOW
INTOW
ONEON
ONION
ONLOW
ONTOP
SNOOD
SNOOK
SNOOP
SNOOT
UNBOX
UNCOY
UNGOT
UNHOT
UNION
UNPOT
UNWON

•N••O

ANCHO
ANDRO
ANDSO
ANEMO
ANETO
ANGIO
ANGLO
ANIMO
ANZIO
ENERO
ENNIO
INDIO
INIGO
INTRO
INTWO
MNEMO
ONENO
ONKYO
ONTWO

••NO•

AGNON
ANNOY
ATNOS
BANON
BANOS
BYNOW
CANOE
CANON
CONON
DENOM
DINOS
DONOR
DONOT
DONOW
FANON
FINOS
GENOA
GONOW
HANOI
HONOR
IFNOT
IKNOW
JANOS
JENOS
KENOS
LANOS
LENOS
LENOX
LINOS
LMNOP
MANON
MANOR
MANOS
MENOS
MINOR
MINOS
MINOT
MINOW
MONOD
MONOS
NANON
NINON
NINOS
NONOS
PHNOM
PINON
PINOT
RANON
RUNON
SENOR
SYNOD
TENOF
TENON
TENOR
TONOW
VENOM
VINOS
XENON
YKNOW
ZENOS

••N•O

AMNIO
BANCO
BANDO
BANJO
BENTO
BINGO
BONGO
BONZO
BUNCO
BUNKO
CANDO
CANIO
CANSO
CANTO
CENTO
CINCO
CONDO
CONGO
CUNEO
DANIO
DANNO
DENTO
DINGO
DONHO
DUNNO
ENNIO
FINNO
FUNGO
GONZO
HONDO
JINGO
JUNCO
JUNIO
JUNTO
KENDO
KINKO
LANDO
LENTO
LINDO
LINGO
LONGO
MANGO
MENLO
MINEO
MINHO
MONDO
MONGO
MONRO
MUNRO
NANNO
NONNO
OINGO
PANTO
PINKO
PINTO
PONGO
RANGO
RANTO
RINGO
RINSO
RONCO
RONDO
RUNTO
SANTO
SANYO
TANGO
TANTO
TENGO
TENTO
TONDO
TONIO
TONTO
VENLO
VENTO
XANDO
ZENDO

•••NO

ADANO
ADENO
AMINO
BEANO
BRUNO
BUENO
BUONO
BUTNO
CHINO
CIANO
CORNO
CTENO
CYANO
DANNO
DRANO
DUENO
DUINO
DUNNO
ECONO
ETHNO
FINNO
GIONO
GUANO
GYMNO
HADNO
HASNO
HYPNO
ICONO
JUANO
KEINO
KLMNO
LEGNO
LIGNO
LLANO
LOTNO
NANNO
NONNO
ONENO
ORONO
OTONO
PEANO
PHENO
PHONO
PIANO
PLANO
PORNO
QUINO
RHINO
SAYNO
SEGNO
SIXNO
SPANO
STENO
SUENO
URANO
YESNO

N•P••

NAPES
NAPPE
NAPPY
NEPAL
NEPHR
NEPOS
NIPAS
NIPAT
NIPPY
NIPUP
NOPAL
NOPAR
NOPES
NOPQR

N••P•

NAMPA
NAPPE
NAPPY
NEAPS
NIPPY
NWAPA

NYMPH

N•••P
NAACP
NIPUP
NLMVP
NOTIP
NOTUP

•NP••
INPEN
INPUT
ONPAR
UNPEG
UNPEN
UNPIN
UNPOT

•N•P•
DNEPR
INAPT
INEPT
KNOPF
MNOPQ
ONEPM
SNAPS
SNIPE
SNIPS
UNAPT

•N••P
ANDUP
ENDUP
ONEUP
ONTAP
ONTOP
SNOOP
UNCAP
UNHIP
UNRIP
UNZIP

••NP•
TENPM

••N•P
AANDP
ASNAP
GINUP
LMNOP
OWNUP
PENUP
PINUP
RANUP
RUNUP
SANDP
SUNUP
TENUP

•••NP
JOHNP

N••Q•
NOPQR

•N••Q
ANTIQ
MNOPQ

•••NQ
JOHNQ

NR•••
NROTC

N•R••
NARAS
NARCO
NARCS
NARDA
NARDO
NARDS
NARES
NARIC
NARIS
NARKS
NERDS
NERDY
NERFS
NEROL
NERTS
NERTZ
NERVA
NERVE
NERVO
NERVY
NORAD
NORAH
NOREN
NORGE
NORIA
NORIS
NORMA
NORMS
NORNS
NORSE
NORSK
NORTE
NORTH
NORUN
NORVO
NURMI
NURSE

N••R•
NACRE
NAIRA
NATRO
NAURU
NEARS
NEDRA
NEGRI
NEGRO
NEHRU
NEURO
NIDRE
NIORT
NITRE
NITRO
NLERS
NOIRE
NOIRS
NOORT
NOTRE
NOURI
NUTRO

N•••R
NADER
NADIR
NAMER
NAMUR
NBAER
NEHER
NEPHR
NEVER
NEWER
NFLER
NHLER
NICER
NIGER
NINER
NITER
NIXER
NIZER
NOEAR
NOMAR
NOPAR
NOPQR
NOSER
NOSIR
NOTER
NSTAR
NUDER

•NR••
ENROL
ENRON
INRED
INREM
INRUN
ONRYE
UNRIG
UNRIP
UNRUN

•N•R•
ANDRE
ANDRO
ANDRY
ANGRY
ANTRA
ANTRE
ENARE
ENARM
ENCRE
ENERO
ENGRS
ENORM
ENTRE
ENTRY
ENURE
GNARL
GNARS
INARI
INCRS
INDRA
INDRE
INERT
INFRA
INORG
INTRA
INTRO
INURE
KNARS
KNORR
KNURL
KNURS
ONERA
ONERS
SNARE
SNARF
SNARK
SNARL
SNERD
SNERT
SNORE
SNORT
UNARM
UNARY
UNDRY

•N••R
ANDOR
ANGER
ANSER
ANWAR
DNEPR
ENDER
ENDOR
ENSOR
ENTER
ENVER
INCUR
INFER
INFOR
INGER
INKER
INNER
INSTR
INTER
INVER
KNORR
ONAIR
ONEIR
ONPAR
SNEER
UNBAR
UNDER
UNFAR
UNGAR
UNGER
UNSER
UNTER

••NR•
GENRE
HENRI
HENRY
MONRO
MUNRO

••N•R
ABNER
ASNER
BONAR
BONER
BYNER
CANER
CENTR
CONER
CONTR
DENAR
DENDR
DINAR
DINER
DONOR
EINER
FINER
GONER
HONER
HONOR
INNER
KANAR
KINER
LINER
LONER
LUNAR
LUNER
MANOR
MINER
MINOR
NINER
OWNER
PINER
RANDR
SANER
SENOR
SONAR
TENOR
TONER
TUNER
TYNER
ULNAR
VINER
WANER
ZENER
ZONER

NS•••
NSTAR
NSYNC

N•S••
NASAL
NASBY
NASHE
NASTY
NESIA
NESTS
NESTY
NISAN
NISEI
NISUS
NOSED
NOSER
NOSES
NOSEY
NOSIR

N••S•
NAISH
NELSE
NEUSS
NEWSY
NOISE
NOISY
NOMSG
NOOSE
NORSE
NORSK
NOTSO
NOUSE
NTEST
NURSE
NUTSY
NYASA

N•••S
NABES
NAIFS
NAILS
NAMES
NANAS
NAPES
NARAS
NARCS
NARDS
NARES
NARIS
NARKS
NAVES
NAVIS
NAXOS
NAZIS
NEAPS
NEARS
NEATS
NECKS
NEEDS
NEGUS
NEHIS
NEMOS
NENES
NEONS
NEPOS
NERDS
NERFS
NERTS
NESTS
NEUSS
NEVES
NEVIS
NEVUS
NEWTS
NEXIS
NEXUS
NICKS
NIDUS
NIELS
NIKES
NILES
NIMES
NINAS
NINES
NINOS
NIPAS
NISUS
NITES
NIXES
NLERS
NOBIS
NOCKS
NODES
NODUS
NOELS
NOGAS
NOGGS
NOGOS
NOILS
NOIRS
NOLES
NOLOS
NOMAS
NONES
NONOS
NOOKS
NOONS
NOPES
NORIS
NORMS
NORNS
NOSES
NOTES
NOTUS
NOUNS
NOVAS
NOVUS
NOYES
NUDES
NUITS
NUKES
NULLS
NUMBS
NYETS

•NS••
ANSAE
ANSEL
ANSER
ANSON
ENSKY
ENSOR
ENSUE
INSET
INSTR
INSTS
INSUM
ONSET
UNSAD
UNSAY
UNSER
UNSET
UNSEW
UNSHY
UNSLY

•N•S•
ANDSO
ANGST
ANISE
ANTSY
DNASE
GNASH
INUSE
KNISH
RNASE

•N••S
ANAGS
ANAIS
ANDES
ANDYS
ANGES
ANGUS
ANILS
ANKHS
ANNAS
ANNUS
ANOAS
ANTAS
ANTES
ANTIS
ANZUS
DNETS
ENBAS
ENCLS
ENGRS
ENNIS
ENOLS
GNARS
GNATS
GNAWS
INCAS
INCRS
INCUS
INDUS
INDYS
INEES
INITS
INNES
INNIS
INSTS
KNARS
KNEES
KNITS
KNOBS
KNOTS
KNOWS
KNURS
ONDAS
ONDES
ONEKS
ONELS
ONERS
ONNES
SNAGS
SNAPS
SNEES
SNIPS
SNITS
SNOBS
SNOWS
SNUBS
SNUGS
TNUTS
UNAUS
UNCAS
UNITS
UNIVS

••NS•
AINSI
CANSO
CANST
CENSE
CONST
DANSE
DENSE
DUNST
EENSY
ERNST
GANSU
GINSU
HANSA
HANSE
KANSA
MANSE
MENSA
MINSK
PANSY
PINSK
RINSE
RINSO
SENSE
TANSY
TENSE

••N•S
ACNES
AGNES
AGNUS
AINUS
ANNAS
ANNUS
AONES
ATNOS
AUNTS
BANCS
BANDS
BANES
BANGS
BANKS
BANNS
BANOS
BENDS
BENES
BENTS
BINDS
BINES
BINGS
BONDS
BONES
BONGS
BONKS
BONUS
BUNDS
BUNGS
BUNKS
BUNTS
CANES
CANIS
CANTS
CENAS
CENTS
CINES
CONDS
CONES
CONKS
CONNS
CONTS
CONUS
DANES
DANGS
DENES
DENIS
DENTS
DENYS
DINES
DINGS
DINKS
DINOS
DINTS
DONAS
DONGS
DONTS
DONUS
DUNES
DUNKS
DYNES
EINES
ENNIS
ERNES
ESNES
ETNAS
FANES
FANGS
FENDS
FINDS
FINES
FINIS
FINKS
FINNS
FINOS
FONTS
FUNDS
FUNKS
GANGS
GENES
GENTS
GENUS
GENXS
GONGS
GUNKS
HANDS
HANES
HANGS
HANKS
HANTS
HINDS
HINES
HINTS
HONES
HONKS
HONUS
HUNKS
HUNTS
IGNES
IGNIS
INNES
INNIS
JANIS
JANOS
JANUS
JENOS
JINKS
JINNS
JONAS
JONES
JUNES
JUNKS
KANAS
KANGS
KENOS
KINAS
KINDS
KINGS
KINKS
KONAS
LANDS
LANES
LANOS
LENDS
LENES
LENIS
LENOS
LENTS
LINCS
LINES
LINGS
LINKS
LINOS
LINTS
LINUS
LONGS
LUNAS
LUNES
LUNGS
LUNNS
LUNTS
MANES
MANOS
MANUS
MENAS
MENDS
MENES
MENOS
MENUS
MINAS
MINDS
MINES
MINIS
MINKS
MINOS
MINTS
MINUS
MONKS
MONOS
MONTS
MUNIS
MYNAS
NANAS
NENES
NINAS
NINES
NINOS
NONES
NONOS
OINKS
OMNES
OMNIS
ONNES
ORNIS
PANES
PANGS
PANIS
PANTS
PENDS
PINES
PINGS
PINKS
PINTS
PONDS
PONES
PONGS
PONTS
PUNGS
PUNKS
PUNTS
RANAS
RANDS
RANIS
RANKS
RANTS
RENDS
RENTS
RINDS
RINGS
RINKS
RUNES
RUNGS
RUNTS
SANDS
SENDS
SINES
SINGS
SINKS
SINUS
SONES
SONGS
SONYS
SYNCS
SYNDS
TANGS
TANIS
TANKS
TENDS
TENKS
TENTS
TINES
TINGS
TINTS
TONES
TONGS
TONUS
TONYS
TUNAS
TUNES
TUNIS
ULNAS
URNES
VANES
VENDS
VENTS
VENUS
VINAS
VINES
VINOS
WANDS
WANES
WANTS
WENDS
WINDS
WINES
WINGS
WINKS
WONKS
WONTS
YANKS
ZENDS
ZENOS
ZINCS
ZINES
ZINGS
ZONES
ZONKS
ZUNIS

•••NS
ADINS
AEONS
AKINS
AMENS
ARANS
ARENS
ARUNS
ASSNS
AXONS
AYINS
AZANS
BANNS
BARNS
BEANS
BEENS
BEINS
BOONS
BOSNS
BRANS
BRENS
BURNS
CHINS
CIENS
CIONS
CLANS
COINS
CONNS
COONS
CORNS
CYANS
DAMNS
DARNS
DAWNS
DEANS
DJINS
DOANS
DOWNS
DURNS
EARNS
EBONS
ECONS
EDENS
ETONS
EVANS
EVENS
EXONS
FAUNS
FAWNS
FERNS
FINNS
FIRNS
FLANS
FOHNS
FRANS
GAINS
GLENS
GOONS
GOWNS
GRINS
HORNS
HYMNS
ICONS
IRONS
ISBNS
IVINS
JAINS
JEANS
JINNS
JOHNS
JOINS
JUINS
KAHNS
KAONS
KARNS
KEENS
KERNS
KHANS
KILNS
KOANS
LAWNS
LEANS
LIENS
LIMNS
LIONS
LOANS
LOINS
LOONS
LUNNS
LYONS
MAINS
MEANS
MIENS
MOANS
MOONS
MORNS
MUONS
NEONS
NOONS
NORNS
NOUNS
OMENS
OPENS
OVENS
OWENS
PAINS
PAONS
PAWNS
PEENS
PEONS
PHONS
PIONS
PIRNS
PLANS
RAINS
REINS
RIENS
ROANS
RUINS
RYANS
SAENS
SCANS
SHINS
SHUNS
SIGNS
SKINS
SPANS
SPINS
STANS
STENS
STUNS
SWANS
TARNS
TEENS
TERNS
THINS
TOONS
TOWNS
TRANS
TURNS
TWINS
VEINS
VTENS
WAINS
WARNS
WEANS
WHENS
WRENS
XEONS
YARNS
YAWNS
YEANS
YUANS

NT•••
NTEST
NTILE

N•T••
NATAL
NATAN
NATCH
NATRO
NATTA
NATTY
NETTY
NETWT
NITER
NITES
NITID
NITON
NITRE
NITRO
NITTI
NITTY
NOTAH
NOTAX
NOTCH
NOTDO
NOTED
NOTER
NOTES
NOTIE
NOTIN
NOTIP
NOTIT
NOTME
NOTOK
NOTON
NOTRE
NOTSO
NOTTE
NOTTI
NOTUP
NOTUS
NSTAR
NUTRO
NUTSY
NUTTY
NYTOL

N••T•
NAFTA
NANTZ
NASTY
NATTA
NATTY
NBCTV
NEATH
NEATO
NEATS
NERTS
NERTZ
NESTS
NESTY
NETTY
NEWTO
NEWTS
NIETA
NIETO
NIFTY
NINTH
NITTI
NITTY
NOCTI
NODTO
NOLTE
NORTE
NORTH
NOTTE
NOTTI
NROTC
NUITS
NUTTY
NYCTI
NYCTO
NYETS

N•••T
NACHT
NAGAT
NETWT
NEWAT
NICHT
NIGHT
NIORT
NIPAT
NOBET
NOCUT
NODAT
NOFAT
NOHIT
NONET
NOORT
NOTIT
NTEST
NYJET
NYMET

•NT••
ANTAE
ANTAL
ANTAS
ANTED
ANTES
ANTIC
ANTIQ
ANTIS
ANTON
ANTRA
ANTRE
ANTSY
ENTAD
ENTER
ENTOM
ENTRE
ENTRY
INTEL
INTER
INTOW
INTRA
INTRO
INTWO
ONTAP
ONTOP
ONTWO
UNTAX
UNTER
UNTIE
UNTIL

•N•T•
ANETO
ANITA
CNOTE
DNETS
ENATE
ENOTE
GNATS
GNOTE
INITS
INSTR
INSTS
KNITS
KNOTS
KNOTT
KNUTE
ONATE
SNATH
SNITS
TNOTE
TNUTS
UNITA
UNITE
UNITS
UNITY

•N••T
ANENT
ANGST
ENACT
ENDAT
ENDIT
INAPT
INEPT
INERT
INGOT
INLET
INPUT
INSET
INUIT
KNELT
KNOTT
KNOUT
ONDIT
ONSET
SNERT
SNOOT
SNORT
SNOUT

UNAPT
UNBET
UNBIT
UNCUT
UNFIT
UNGOT
UNHAT
UNHIT
UNHOT
UNIAT
UNLET
UNLIT
UNMET
UNPOT
UNSET
UNWET

••NT•
AUNTS
AUNTY
BANTA
BANTU
BENTO
BENTS
BUNTS
CANTO
CANTS
CANTY
CENTI
CENTO
CENTR
CENTS
CENTU
CONTD
CONTE
CONTI
CONTR
CONTS
DANTE
DENTE
DENTI
DENTO
DENTS
DINTS
DINTY
DONTS
FANTA
FONTS
GENTE
GENTS
HANTS
HINTS
HUNTS
HUNTZ
JUNTA
JUNTO
KINTE
KUNTA
LANTZ
LENTE
LENTO
LENTS
LINTS
LINTY
LUNTS
MANTA
MINTS
MINTY
MONTE
MONTH
MONTS
MONTY
NANTZ
NINTH
PANTA
PANTO
PANTS
PANTY
PENTA
PENTE
PINTA
PINTO
PINTS
PONTA
PONTE
PONTI
PONTS
PUNTA
PUNTS
RANTO
RANTS
RENTE
RENTS
RINTY
RUNTO
RUNTS
RUNTY
SANTA
SANTE
SANTO
SENTA
SENTE
SYNTH
TANTE
TANTO
TENTH
TENTO
TENTS
TINTS
TONTO
UINTA
VENTA
VENTI
VENTO
VENTS
WANTS
WONTS
YENTA
YENTE
YENTL

••N•T
AVNET
BENET
BINET
BONET
BUNDT
CANIT
CANST
CONST
DONAT
DONOT
DONUT
DUNST
ERNST
GANDT
GENET
GUNIT
IFNOT
JANET
LINDT
LINFT
MANAT
MANET
MINOT
MONET
NONET
PINOT
RANAT
RUNAT
SENAT
TENET
TINCT
VINGT
WENDT
WINAT
WONAT
WUNDT

•••NT
AGENT
AMANT
AMENT
ANENT
ARENT
AVANT
BIONT
BLENT
BLUNT
BRANT
BRENT
BRUNT
BURNT
CAINT
CHANT
CLINT
COUNT
DASNT
DAUNT
DIDNT
EVENT
FAINT
FEINT
FLINT
FOUNT
FRONT
GAUNT
GHENT
GIANT
GLINT
GRANT
GRINT
GRUNT
HADNT
HASNT
HAUNT
ICANT
IDENT
IDONT
IWANT
IWONT
JAUNT
JOINT
LEANT
MAYNT
MEANT
MOUNT
ODONT
ORANT
PAINT
PLANT
POINT
PRINT
QUANT
QUINT
RIANT
SAINT
SCANT
SCENT
SHANT
SHUNT
SLANT
SPENT
STENT
STINT
STUNT
TAINT
TAUNT
THANT
TIANT
TISNT
TRENT
ULENT
VAUNT
WASNT
YOUNT

NU•••
NUBBY
NUBIA
NUCHA
NUDER
NUDES
NUDGE
NUDZH
NUEVA
NUEVE
NUEVO
NUFLO
NUITS
NUKED
NUKES
NULLA
NULLO
NULLS
NUMAN
NUMBS
NUMEN
NUMIC
NUNCA
NUNEZ
NUOVA
NUOVO
NURMI
NURSE
NUTRO
NUTSY
NUTTY
NUYEN

N•U••
NAURU
NEURO
NEUSS
NOUNS
NOURI
NOUSE

N••U•
NAHUM
NAMUR
NEFUD
NEGUS
NEVUS
NEXUS
NIDUS
NIEUW
NIPUP
NISUS
NOCUT
NODUH
NODUS
NOFUN
NORUN
NOTUP
NOTUS
NOVUS

N•••U
NAURU
NEHRU

•NU••
ENURE
INUIT
INURE
INUSE
KNURL
KNURS
KNUTE
SNUBS
SNUCK
SNUFF
SNUGS
TNUTS

•N•U•
ANDUP
ANGUS
ANNUL
ANNUM
ANNUS
ANOUK
ANZUS
ENDUE
ENDUP
ENNUI
ENSUE
INCUR
INCUS
INDUE
INDUS
INFUN
INJUN
INPUT
INRUN
INSUM
KNOUT
ONCUE
ONEUP
PNEUM
SNOUT
UNAUS
UNBUD
UNCUT
UNDUE
UNDUG
UNFUN
UNRUN

•N••U
ANJOU
INONU
SNAFU

••NU•
AGNUS
AINUS
ANNUL
ANNUM
ANNUS
BONUM
BONUS
CONUS
DONUS
DONUT
ENNUI
GENUS
GINUP
HONUS
JANUS
LINUS
LINUX
MANUS
MENUS
MINUS
OWNUP
PENUP
PINUP
RANUP
RUNUP
SINUS
SUNUP
TENUP
TONUS
VANUA
VENUE
VENUS

••N•U
BANTU
CENTU
DONAU
FONDU
GANSU
GINSU
HINDU
LINGU
LONGU
PONZU
TENDU

•••NU
CORNU
INONU
KEANU

N•V••
NAVAL
NAVEE
NAVEL
NAVES
NAVIG
NAVIS
NEVER
NEVES
NEVIL
NEVIN
NEVIS
NEVUS
NIVAL
NIVEA
NIVEN
NOVAE
NOVAK
NOVAS
NOVEL
NOVEM
NOVIA
NOVIO
NOVUS

N••V•
NAIVE
NERVA
NERVE
NERVO
NERVY
NIEVE
NLMVP
NORVO
NUEVA
NUEVE
NUEVO
NUOVA
NUOVO

N•••V
NBCTV
NEGEV

•NV••
ANVIL
ENVER
ENVOI
ENVOY
INVER

•N•V•
KNAVE
ONDVD
SNEVA
UNIVS

•N••V
ANNIV
INDIV

••NV•
CONVY

••N•V
ANNIV

•••NV
ELYNV
IVANV
JOHNV

NW•••
NWAPA

N•W••
NEWAT
NEWEL
NEWER
NEWIE
NEWLY
NEWSY
NEWTO
NEWTS
NGWEE
NOWAY
NOWIN

N••W•
NETWT

N•••W
NIEUW
NOHOW

•NW••
ANWAR
UNWED
UNWET
UNWIG
UNWON

•N•W•
GNAWN
GNAWS
INAWE
INTWO
KNOWN
KNOWS
ONTWO
SNOWE
SNOWS
SNOWY

•N••W
ENDOW
INLAW
INLOW
INTOW
ONLOW
UNMEW
UNNEW
UNSEW

••N•W
AANDW
AGNEW
ASNEW
BANDW
BYNOW
CANDW
DONOW
GONOW
IKNOW
MINOW
RENEW
SINEW
TONOW
UNNEW
YKNOW

N•X••
NAXOS
NEXIS
NEXUS
NIXED
NIXER
NIXES
NIXIE
NIXON

N•••X
NOTAX
NYNEX

•N••X
ANNEX
INBOX
INDEX
INFIX
UNBOX
UNFIX
UNLAX
UNMIX
UNTAX

••NX•
GENXS
SKNXX

••N•X
ANNEX
LENOX
LINUX
NYNEX
SINEX
SKNXX
YONEX

•••NX
BRONX
JOHNX
THANX

NY•••
NYACK
NYALA
NYASA
NYCTI
NYCTO
NYDIA
NYETS
NYJET
NYLON
NYMAN
NYMET
NYMPH
NYNEX
NYTOL

N•Y••
NOYCE
NOYES
NSYNC
NUYEN

N•••Y
NAGGY
NAMBY
NANCY
NANNY
NAPPY
NASBY
NASTY
NATTY
NEALY
NEEDY
NEELY
NELLY
NERDY
NERVY
NESTY
NETTY
NEWLY
NEWSY
NICKY
NIFTY
NILLY
NIMBY
NIMOY
NINNY
NIPPY
NITTY
NOBBY
NOBLY
NODDY
NOILY
NOISY
NOSEY
NOWAY
NUBBY
NUTSY
NUTTY

•NY••
ANYON

•N•Y•
ANDYS
ENCYC
INDYS
ONKYO
ONRYE

•N••Y
ANDRY
ANGRY
ANNOY
ANOMY
ANTSY
ENEMY
ENJOY
ENSKY
ENTRY
ENVOY
GNOMY
INKEY
INLAY
INMAY
ONKEY
ONLAY
SNAKY
SNOWY
UNARY
UNCOY
UNDAY
UNDRY
UNIFY
UNITY
UNLAY
UNSAY
UNSHY
UNSLY

••NY•
DENYS
HANYA
KANYE
KENYA
LENYA
SANYO
SONYA
SONYS
TANYA
TONYA
TONYS
VANYA
VINYL

••N•Y
ANNOY
AUNTY
BANDY
BANKY
BENDY
BENNY
BONEY
BONNY
BUNDY
BUNNY
CANBY
CANDY
CANNY
CANTY
CINCY
CINDY
CONEY
CONVY
DANDY
DANNY
DENNY
DINDY
DINGY
DINKY
DINNY
DINTY
DONNY
EENSY
FANCY
FANNY
FENNY
FINNY
FUNDY
FUNKY
FUNNY
GANDY
GINNY
GUNKY
GUNNY
HANDY
HANEY
HANKY
HENNY
HENRY
HINKY
HINNY
HONEY
HONKY
HUNKY
IXNAY
JENNY
JONNY
JUNKY
KANDY
KENNY
KINKY
LANKY
LANNY
LENNY
LINDY
LINTY
LUNDY
MANCY
MANDY
MANGY
MANLY
MANNY
MINDY
MINEY
MINGY
MINTY
MONEY
MONTY
NANCY
NANNY
NINNY
PANAY
PANKY
PANSY
PANTY
PENNY
PINEY
PINKY
PUNKY
PUNNY
RANBY
RANDY
RANGY
RENAY
RENNY
RINDY
RINKY
RINTY
RONNY
RUNBY
RUNNY
RUNTY
SANDY
SONNY
SUNNY
TANDY
TANEY
TANGY
TANSY
TINNY
VINCY
VINNY
WANLY
WENDY
WINBY
WINDY
WINGY
WONBY
XANDY
YANCY
ZINCY
ZINGY
ZINKY

•••NY
AGONY
ATONY
BEANY
BEDNY
BENNY
BONNY
BRINY
BUNNY
CANNY
CARNY
CLUNY
CORNY
CRONY
CSINY
DANNY
DENNY
DINNY
DONNY
DOWNY
EBONY
FANNY
FENNY
FERNY
FINNY
FUNNY
GINNY
GOONY
GUNNY
HENNY
HINNY
HORNY
IRONY
JENNY
JONNY
KENNY
LANNY
LAWNY
LENNY
LOONY
MANNY
MEANY
MEENY
MOONY
NANNY
NINNY
PENNY
PEONY
PHANY
PHONY
PLINY
PUNNY
RAINY
RENNY
RONNY
RUNNY
SHINY
SONNY
SPINY
STONY
SUNNY
TAWNY
TEENY
TINNY
TWINY
VEINY
VIGNY
VINNY
WEENY
WHINY
YAWNY

N•Z••
NAZIS
NIZER

N••Z•
NUDZH

N•••Z
NANTZ
NERTZ
NODOZ
NUNEZ

•NZ••
ANZAC
ANZIO
ANZUS
UNZIP

•N•Z•
SNAZZ

•N••Z
SNAZZ

••NZ•
BONZE
BONZO
DANZA
GINZA
GONZO
HENZE
JONZE
LANZA
MONZA
PANZA
PINZA
PONZI
PONZU

••N•Z
ARNAZ
HUNTZ
LANTZ
MONIZ
NANTZ
NUNEZ
VENEZ

•••NZ
FRANZ
HEINZ
MAINZ

OA•••
OAKEN
OAKES
OAKIE
OAKUM
OARED
OARER
OASAL
OASES
OASIS
OASTS
OATEN
OATER
OATES
OATHS

O•A••
OBAMA
OCALA
OFAGE
OGAMS
OHAIR
OHARA
OHARE
OHAYO
OJAYS
OKAPI
OKARA
OKAYS
OLAFI
OLAFV
OLAND
OLAVI
OLAVV
OMAHA
OMANI
OMARR
ONAIR
ONATE
OPAHS
OPALS
OPART
ORACH
ORACY
ORALB
ORALE
ORALS
ORAMA
ORANG
ORANI
ORANT
ORATE
OSAGE
OSAKA
OTARU
OTARY
OVALS
OVARY
OVATE
OXANA
OZARK
OZAWA

O••A•
OASAL
OBEAH
OBRAS
OCCAM
OCEAN
OCRAT
OCTAD
OCTAL
OCTAN
OFFAL
OGHAM
OHKAY
OHMAN
OIDAL
OKRAS
OLEAN
OLLAS
OLPAE
ONDAS
ONEAD
ONEAL
ONEAM
ONLAY
ONPAR
ONTAP
OPRAH
ORCAS
OREAD
ORGAN
ORKAN
ORMAN
ORPAH
ORSAY
ORVAL
OSCAN
OSCAR
OSHAY
OSKAR
OSMAN
OSTAR
OTRAS
OTWAY
OURAY
OXFAM

O•••A
OBAMA
OCALA
OCHOA
ODESA
OHARA
OJEDA
OKARA
OLETA
OLIVA
OMAHA
OMEGA
OMNIA
ONEGA
ONELA
ONERA
OOMPA
OOOLA
OPERA
ORAMA
ORENA
OSAKA
OSHEA
OSSIA
OSTIA
OUIDA
OUIJA
OUTTA
OVETA
OXANA
OZAWA

•OA••
BOARD
BOARS
BOAST
BOATS
COACH
COACT
COALS
COAPT
COASE
COAST
COATI
COATS
DOALL
DOANE
DOANS
DOATS
FOALS
FOAMS
FOAMY
GOADS
GOAFT
GOALS
GOAPE
GOASK
GOATS
HOAGY
HOARD
HOARE
HOARS
HOARY
JOADS
KOALA
KOANS
LOADS
LOAFS
LOAMS
LOAMY
LOANS
LOATH
MOANS
MOATS
POACH
ROACH
ROADS
ROALD
ROAMS
ROANS
ROARK
ROARS
ROAST
SOAKS
SOAMI
SOAPS
SOAPY
SOARS
SOAVE
TOADS
TOADY
TOAST
WOADS

•O•A•

AOKAY BOCAS BOGAN BOHAY BOLAR BOLAS BONAR BOOAT BORAH BORAS BORAX COCAS CODAS COHAB COHAN COLAS COMAE COMAS CONAN COPAL COPAY CORAL COTAN COXAE DOBAD DONAS DONAT DONAU DOPAS DORAG DORAL DORAN DOSAY DOTAL DOUAI DOUAY FOCAL FORAY GOBAD GOBAT GOFAR GOLAN GOMAD GOMAN GORAN GOTAB GOTAC GOTAD GOTAT GOYAS HOBAN HODAD HOGAN HONAN HORAE HORAL HORAS HOWAR HOYAS IOTAS IOWAN IOWAS IOWAU IOWAY JOHAN JONAH JONAS JOTAS JOVAN KODAK KOJAK KOLAS KONAS KORAN KORAT KOSAR LOBAR LOCAL LOFAT LOGAN LOHAN LOMAN LOMAS LOMAX LOPAT LORAN LORAX LOYAL MODAL MOLAR MONAD MORAL MORAN MORAS MORAY MOWAT NOCAL NODAL NODAT NOEAR NOFAT NOGAS NOLAN NOMAD NOMAR NOMAS NOPAL NOPAR NORAD NORAH NOTAH NOTAX NOVAE NOVAK NOVAS NOWAY PODAL POLAR POWAY RODAN ROJAS ROMAN RONAN ROTAS ROWAN ROYAL SOBAD SOBAS SOCAL SOCAS SODAS SOFAR SOFAS SOLAN SOLAR SOMAS SOMAT SONAL SONAR SORAS SOSAD SOYAS TODAY TOEAS TOGAE TOGAS TOKAY TOLAR TOMAR TOMAS TONAL TOPAZ TORAH TORAS TOTAL TOVAH TOWAR VOCAB VOCAL VOLAR WOFAT WOMAN WONAT WOPAT WOTAN YOGAS ZONAL

•O••A

AORTA AOSTA BOHEA BOLLA BOMBA BOOLA BOPHA BORSA BOSSA BOTHA COBRA COCOA COMMA CONGA COOSA COPIA COPRA CORDA COREA CORIA CORSA COSTA COTTA DOGMA DOLMA DONNA DORIA DORSA DOULA EOLIA FOLIA FONDA FORMA FORZA FOSSA FOURA GOLDA GONNA GOTHA GOTTA GOUDA HOFFA HONDA HOOHA HOOKA HOSEA HOSTA HOUMA HOXHA IONIA JOLLA KOALA KORDA KOREA LOCKA LOGIA LONGA LOOFA LORCA LORNA LOTSA LOTTA LOUMA MOCHA MOIRA MOMMA MONZA MOOLA MORRA NOKIA NORIA NORMA NOVIA OOMPA OOOLA PODIA POLKA PONCA PONTA POONA POPPA PORTA RODYA ROOSA ROSSA SOFIA SOLEA SOLLA SONIA SONJA SONYA SORTA SOUSA TOMBA TONGA TONKA TONYA TORTA TOSCA TOSEA VODKA VOILA VOLGA VOLTA VONDA WONKA YOOBA YORBA YOWZA ZORBA ZOSMA

••OA•

ANOAS AROAR BLOAT BOOAT BROAD CLOAK CROAK CROAT EBOAT FLOAT GLOAM GLOAT GROAN GROAT PROAM PROAS SHOAL SHOAT SKOAL SLOAN STOAE STOAS STOAT TWOAD TWOAM UBOAT

••O•A

ABOMA AGORA AHORA ALOHA ANOKA AROMA BIOTA BOOLA BROCA BUONA COOSA EBOLA ENOLA EVORA FIONA FLORA GROZA GYOZA HOOHA HOOKA ICOSA IDOLA ILONA ISOLA KIOWA KRONA LDOPA LEONA LEORA LLOSA LOOFA MOOLA NUOVA OOOLA POONA QUOTA RHODA RIOJA ROOSA SPOSA STOLA STOMA THORA TIOGA USOFA VIOLA XHOSA YOOBA

•••OA

ALCOA COCOA GENOA OCHOA SAMOA

OB•••

OBAMA OBEAH OBELI OBESE OBEYS OBGYN OBIES OBITS OBJET OBOES OBOLI OBOLS OBOTE OBRAS

O•B••

OHBOY OMBER OMBRE ORBED ORBIC ORBIT OXBOW

O••B•

ONEBC ORIBI

O•••B

OHROB ONELB ORALB

•OB••

BOBBY BOBUP COBOL COBRA DOBAD DOBBS DOBEE DOBIE DOBLE DOBRO GOBAD GOBAT GOBEL GOBOS GOBOT HOBAN HOBBS HOBBY HOBEY HOBIE HOBOS KOBOS LOBAR LOBBY LOBED LOBES LOBOS MOBIL NOBBY NOBEL NOBET NOBID NOBIS NOBLE NOBLY POBOX POBOY POBRE ROBBE ROBBY ROBED ROBER ROBES ROBIN ROBLE ROBOF ROBOT ROBYN SOBAD SOBAS SOBER SOBIG TOBEY TOBIT

•O•B•

BOBBY BOMBA BOMBE BOMBS BOOBS BOOBY COLBY COMBO COMBS CORBY COSBY DOBBS DOLBY DOUBS DOUBT GORBY GOTBY HOBBS HOBBY KOMBU LOBBY LOOBY NOBBY POPBY ROBBE ROBBY SORBO SORBS TOMBA TOMBE TOMBS WOMBS WONBY YOOBA YORBA ZORBA

•O••B

COHAB FOURB GOTAB HOREB VOCAB

••OB•

ADOBE ADOBO BLOBS BOOBS BOOBY FROBE GLOBE GLOBS KNOBS LOOBY NIOBE PHOBE PHOBO PROBE PROBS SLOBS SNOBS TWOBC YOOBA

••O•B

ABOMB HBOMB NBOMB RHOMB

•••OB

CABOB CAROB DEMOB JACOB JAKOB KABOB MCJOB NABOB OHROB THROB ZHLOB

OC•••

OCALA OCCAM OCCUR OCEAN OCHER OCHOA OCHOS OCHRE OCRAT OCTAD OCTAL OCTAN OCTET OCULI OCULO

O•C••

OCCAM OCCUR ONCLE ONCUE OPCIT ORCAS ORCHS ORCUS ORCZY OSCAN OSCAR

O••C•

ONICE ORACH ORACY ORECK OUNCE OZICK

O•••C

OHMIC OLEIC OLMEC ONEBC OPTIC ORBIC OSMIC OSRIC

•OC••

BOCAS BOCCE BOCCI BOCHY BOCKS COCAS COCCI COCKS COCKY COCOA COCOS DOCES DOCKS FOCAL FOCUS HOCKS HOCUS JOCKO JOCKS LOCAL LOCHS LOCKA LOCKE LOCKS LOCOS LOCUM LOCUS MOCHA MOCKS NOCAL NOCHE NOCKS NOCTI NOCUT POCUS ROCCO ROCHE ROCKS ROCKY SOCAL SOCAS SOCIO SOCKO SOCKS SOCLE VOCAB VOCAL YOCTO

•O•C•

BOCCE BOCCI BOSCH BOSCO BOSCS BOTCH COACH COACT COCCI CONCH COUCH DOLCE DOLCI DOUCE DOYCE FORCE GOOCH HOOCH JOYCE KOTCH LORCA MOOCH MOUCH NONCE NOTCH NOYCE POACH PONCA PONCE PONCH POOCH PORCH PORCS POUCH ROACH ROCCO RONCO ROTCS ROYCE SOUCI TORCH TOSCA TOUCH VOICE VOICI VOUCH

•O••C

BORIC COLIC COMIC CONIC COSEC DODEC DORIC EOLIC FOLIC FOURC GOTAC HOLIC IODIC IONIC JOHNC KOVIC LOGIC MONIC SOFTC SONIC TONIC TOPIC TORIC TOXIC YOGIC

••OC•

AMOCO BLOCH BLOCK BLOCS BMOCS BROCA BROCK CHOCK CHOCO CLOCK CROCE CROCI CROCK CROCS ENOCH EPOCH FLOCK FROCK FUOCO GLOCK GOOCH HOOCH IROCS KNOCK KROCK MOOCH PLOCE POOCH SHOCK SMOCK SPOCK STOCK

••O•C

AZOIC BRONC JROTC NROTC STOIC TWOBC

•••OC

ADHOC ASSOC DUROC ESTOC HAVOC INHOC MADOC MEDOC THEOC

OD•••

ODDER ODDLY ODELL ODEON ODESA ODETS ODEUM ODILE ODING ODIST ODIUM ODONT ODORS ODOUL ODOUR

O•D••

ODDER ODDLY OGDEN OIDAL OLDEN OLDER OLDIE ONDAS ONDES ONDIT ONDVD ORDER

O••D•

OJEDA OPEDS OUIDA OUTDO OXIDE

O•••D

OARED OCTAD OFFED OGLED OHGOD OILED OLAND ONDVD ONEAD ONEND OOHED OOPOD OOTID OOZED OPTED ORBED OREAD OUTED OVOID OWNED

•OD••

BODDY BODED BODEL BODES CODAS CODED CODER CODES CODEX CODON DODEC DODGE DODGY DODIE DODOS FODOR GODEL GODET GODEY GODLY GODOT HODAD IODIC JODIE KODAK KODEL KODES LODEN LODER LODES LODGE MODAL MODEL MODEM MODES MODUS NODAL NODAT NODDY NODES NODOZ NODTO NODUH NODUS PODAL PODIA RODAN RODDY RODEO RODIN RODYA SODAS SODDY SODOI SODOM TODAY TODDY TODOS VODKA WODEN YODEL YODHS

•O•D•

BODDY BOLDS BONDI BONDS COEDS COLDS COMDR CONDE CONDI CONDO CONDS COODY CORDA CORDS DOIDO DONDE DONDI DOODY DOWDY FOLDS FONDA FONDU FOODS FORDO FORDS GOADS GOLDA GOLDE GOLDS GOODE GOODS GOODY GORDO GORDY GOUDA GOUDY GOWDY HOLDS HONDA HONDO HOODS HOODY HORDE HOWDO HOWDY JOADS KORDA LOADS LOIDS LORDS LORDY MOLDS MOLDY MONDE MONDO MOODS MOODY NODDY NOLDE NOTDO PONDS ROADS RODDY RONDE RONDO ROODS ROWDY SODDY SOLDI SOLDO SONDE TOADS TOADY TODDY TONDI TONDO TOODY VOIDS VONDA WOADS WOODS WOODY WORDS WORDY

•O••D

BOARD BODED BONED BOOED BORED BOUND BOVID BOWED BOXED CODED COKED CONED CONTD COOED COPED CORED COULD COVED COWED COXED DOBAD DOLED DOMED DOPED DOSED DOTED DOZED FOUND FOURD FOXED GOBAD GOMAD GORED GOTAD GOULD GOURD HOARD HODAD HOKED HOLED HOMED HONED HOPED HOSED HOUND JOHND JOKED JOYED LOBED LOPED LOVED LOWED MONAD MONOD MOOED MOPED MOULD MOUND MOVED MOWED NOBID NOEND NOMAD NORAD NOSED NOTED OOHED OOPOD OOTID OOZED POKED POLED PORED POSED POUND ROALD ROBED ROPED ROUND ROVED ROWED SOBAD SOLED SOLID SOSAD SOUND SOWED TOKED TONED TOPED TOTED TOWED TOYED VOTED VOWED WOOED WORLD WOULD WOUND WOWED YOKED ZONED ZOOID

••OD•

ABODE ANODE APODS BRODY CLODS COODY DIODE DOODY EPODE ERODE FOODS FRODO GEODE GOODE GOODS GOODY GRODY HOODS HOODY IPODS IZODS MOODS MOODY PLODS PRODS RHODA RHODE RHODO RHODY ROODS SPODE TOODY WOODS WOODY

••O•D

AHOLD ALOUD AROID ASOLD AVOID BLOND BLOOD BOOED BROAD BROOD BROUD CHORD CLOUD COOED CROWD DROID DROOD EBOND FIORD FJORD FLOOD FLOYD FROID FROND FTORD HYOID IFOLD LLOYD MOOED OVOID PROUD SCOLD SHOED SNOOD STOOD SWORD TBOND

TWOAD
WOOED
ZOOID

•••OD
BIPOD
BLOOD
BROOD
BYGOD
DESOD
DROOD
EPHOD
FLOOD
HEROD
MONOD
MYGOD
OHGOD
OOPOD
RESOD
SCROD
SNOOD
STOOD
SYNOD

OE•••
OESTE
OEUFS

O•E••
OBEAH
OBELI
OBESE
OBEYS
OCEAN
ODELL
ODEON
ODESA
ODETS
ODEUM
OGEES
OJEDA
OKEMO
OLEAN
OLEIC
OLEIN
OLEOS
OLETA
OLEUM
OMEGA
OMENS
OMERS
ONEAD
ONEAL
ONEAM
ONEBC
ONEEE
ONEGA
ONEIL
ONEIR
ONEKS
ONELA
ONELB
ONELS
ONEND
ONENO
ONEON
ONEPM
ONERA
ONERS
ONEUP
OPEDS
OPELS
OPENS
OPERA
OPERE
OREAD
ORECK
ORENA
OREOS
OTERI
OTERO
OUEST
OVENS
OVERS
OVERT
OVETA
OVETT
OWENS
OWEON
OWERS
OXEYE
OYERS

O••E•
OAKEN
OAKES
OARED
OARER
OASES
OATEN
OATER
OATES
OBIES
OBJET
OBOES
OCHER
OCTET
ODDER
OFFED
OFFER
OFTEN
OGDEN
OGEES
OGIER
OGLED
OGLER
OGLES
OGRES
OHGEE
OHYES
OILED
OILER
OKIES
OLDEN
OLDER
OLMEC
OLPES
OLSEN
OMBER
OMNES
ONDES
ONEEE
ONKEY
ONNES
ONSET
OOHED
OOZED
OOZES
OPPER
OPTED
ORBED
ORDER
ORFEO
ORFES
ORIEL
ORLES
ORREN
ORSER
ORSES
OSHEA
OSIER
OSLER
OSSEO
OSSET
OSTEO
OSTER
OTHER
OTOES
OTTER
OUSEL
OUTED
OUTER
OUZEL
OWIES
OWLET
OWNED
OWNER
OYVEY

O•••E
OAKIE
OBESE
OBOTE
OCHRE
ODILE
OESTE
OFAGE
OFUSE
OGIVE
OHARE
OHGEE
OLDIE
OLIVE
OLLIE
OLPAE
OMBRE
ONATE
ONCLE
ONCUE
ONEEE
ONICE
ONONE
ONRYE
OPERE
OPINE
ORALE
ORATE
OSAGE
OSSIE
OTILE
OUNCE
OUTIE
OUTRE
OVATE
OVINE
OVULE
OXEYE
OXIDE
OZONE
OZZIE

•OE••
BOERS
BOEUF
COEDS
COEUR
DOERR
DOERS
DOEST
DOETH
GOERS
GOEST
GOETH
HOERS
HOEST
JOEYS
LOEIL
LOESS
LOEWE
LOEWI
LOEWS
LOEWY
NOEAR
NOELS
NOEND
POEME
POEMS
POESY
POETE
POETS
SOEUR
TOEAS
TOEFL
TOEIN

•O•E•
AOLER
AONES
BODED
BODEL
BODES
BOGEY
BOHEA
BOJER
BOLES
BOLET
BONED
BONER
BONES
BONET
BONEY
BOOED
BOOER
BORED
BOREL
BOREN
BORER
BORES
BOTEL
BOVET
BOWED
BOWEL
BOWEN
BOWER
BOWES
BOXED
BOXER
BOXES
BOYER
CODED
CODER
CODES
CODEX
COHEN
COKED
COKER
COKES
COLES
COMER
COMES
COMET
COMEX
CONED
CONER
CONES
CONEY
COOED
COOEE
COOER
COPED
COPER
COPES
COREA
CORED
CORER
CORES
COREY
COSEC
COSET
COTES
COVED
COVEN
COVER
COVES
COVET
COVEY
COWED
COWER
COWES
COXED
COXES
COYER
COZEN
COZES
DOBEE
DOCES
DODEC
DOGES
DOKEY
DOLED
DOLES
DOMED
DOMES
DONEE
DONEN
DOPED
DOPER
DOPES
DOPEY
DOREN
DOSED
DOSER
DOSES
DOTED
DOTER
DOTES
DOVER
DOVES
DOVEY
DOWEL
DOYEN
DOZED
DOZEN
DOZER
DOZES
FOGEL
FOGEY
FOIES
FOLEY
FORES
FOXED
FOXES
FOYER
GOBEL
GODEL
GODET
GODEY
GOFER
GOGET
GOLEM
GOMER
GOMEZ
GONER
GOOEY
GORED
GOREN
GORES
GOREY
GOSEE
GOWER
GOYEN
HOBEY
HOKED
HOKES
HOKEY
HOLED
HOLER
HOLES
HOLEY
HOMED
HOMEO
HOMER
HOMES
HOMEY
HONED
HONER
HONES
HONEY
HOOEY
HOPED
HOPEH
HOPER
HOPES
HOREB
HOSEA
HOSED
HOSEL
HOSEN
HOSER
HOSES
HOTEL
HOVEL
HOVER
HOVEY
HOWES
JOKED
JOKER
JOKES
JOKEY
JONES
JOREL
JOSEF
JOSEY
JOYED
KODEL
KODES
KOPEK
KOREA
LOBED
LOBES
LODEN
LODER
LODES
LOGES
LONER
LOOEY
LOPED
LOPER
LOPES
LOPEZ
LOREN
LORES
LOSER
LOSES
LOSEY
LOTET
LOVED
LOVER
LOVES
LOVEY
LOWED
LOWER
LOWES
LOXES
MODEL
MODEM
MODES
MOGEN
MOLES
MONEL
MONET
MONEY
MOOED
MOOER
MOPED
MOPER
MOPES
MOPEY
MOREL
MORES
MOREY
MOSEL
MOSES
MOSEY
MOTEL
MOTES
MOTET
MOUES
MOVED
MOVER
MOVES
MOWED
MOWEN
MOWER
NOBEL
NOBET
NODES
NOFEE
NOLES
NOMEN
NONES
NONET
NOPES
NOREN
NOSED
NOSER
NOSES
NOSEY
NOTED
NOTER
NOTES
NOVEL
NOVEM
NOYES
OOHED
OOZED
OOZES
POKED
POKER
POKES
POKEY
POLED
POLER
POLES
POMES
PONES
POPES
PORED
PORER
PORES
POSED
POSER
POSES
POSEY
POWER
POXES
ROBED
ROBER
ROBES
RODEO
ROGER
ROGET
ROKER
ROLEN
ROLEO
ROLES
ROLEX
ROMEO
ROMES
RONEE
ROPED
ROPER
ROPES
ROREM
ROSEN
ROSES
ROSEY
ROTES
ROUEN
ROUES
ROVED
ROVER
ROVES
ROWED
ROWEL
ROWEN
ROWER
SOBER
SOFER
SOFEW
SOLEA
SOLED
SOLEI
SOLER
SOLES
SONES
SOOEY
SOREL
SOREN
SORER
SORES
SOWED
SOWER
TOBEY
TOKED
TOKEN
TOKES
TOLER
TOLES
TOLET
TOMEI
TOMES
TONED
TONER
TONES
TOOER
TOPED
TOPEE
TOPER
TOPES
TOSEA
TOTED
TOTEM
TOTER
TOTES
TOVES
TOWED
TOWEL
TOWER
TOYED
TOYER
VOGEL
VOLES
VOMER
VOTED
VOTER
VOTES
VOWED
VOWEL
VOWER
WODEN
WOKEN
WOMEN
WOOED
WOOER
WOVEN
WOWED
WOWEE
WOWEM
YODEL
YOKED
YOKEL
YOKES
YONEX
YORES
ZONED
ZONER
ZONES
ZOOEY
ZOREL

•O••E
BOCCE
BOGIE
BOGLE
BOIRE
BOISE
BOITE
BOMBE
BONNE
BONZE
BOOLE
BOONE
BOOZE
BORGE
BORNE
BOTHE
BOULE
BOWIE
BOYLE
COASE
COKIE
COMAE
COMME
COMTE
CONDE
CONGE
CONTE
COOEE
COOKE
COOTE
COPSE
COUPE
COXAE
DOANE
DOBEE
DOBIE
DOBLE
DODGE
DODIE
DOGIE
DOLCE
DONDE
DONEE
DONNE
DOONE
DOUCE
DOUSE
DOUTE
DOUZE
DOWSE
DOXIE
DOYCE
DOYLE
FOOTE
FORCE
FORGE
FORTE
FOSSE
FOURE
FOYLE
GOAPE
GOLDE
GOODE
GOOSE
GORGE
GORME
GORSE
GOSEE
GOSSE
GOTME
GOUGE
HOARE
HOBIE
HOKIE
HOMIE
HOMME
HOOKE
HOPPE
HORAE
HORDE
HORNE
HORSE
HOUSE
HOWIE
HOYLE
JODIE
JOFFE
JOLIE
JONZE
JORGE
JOSIE
JOULE
JOUVE
JOYCE
KOPFE
KOPJE
LOCKE
LODGE
LOEWE
LOGUE
LOIRE
LONGE
LOOIE
LOOSE
LORNE
LORRE
LOTTE
LOUIE
LOUPE
LOUSE
MOIRE
MONDE
MONTE
MOORE
MOOSE
MORSE
MORTE
MOSHE
MOUSE
MOVIE
MOXIE
NOBLE
NOCHE
NOFEE
NOIRE
NOISE
NOLDE
NOLIE
NOLLE
NOLTE
NONCE
NOONE
NOOSE
NORGE
NORSE
NORTE
NOTIE
NOTME
NOTRE
NOTTE
NOUSE
NOVAE
NOYCE
POBRE
POEME
POETE
POIRE
POISE
POMME
PONCE
PONTE
POOLE
POPLE
PORTE
POSSE
POSTE
POULE
ROBBE
ROBLE
ROCHE
ROGUE
ROLFE
ROLLE
RONDE
RONEE
ROONE
ROQUE
ROSIE
ROUGE
ROUSE
ROUTE
ROWSE
ROXIE
ROYCE
SOAVE
SOCLE
SOFIE
SOLVE
SOMME
SONDE
SOUSE
TOGAE
TOGUE
TOILE
TOMBE
TONNE
TOOLE
TOPEE
TOQUE
TORME
TORRE
TORTE
TOTIE
TOUTE
TOWNE
VOGUE
VOICE
VOILE
VOLPE
VOLTE
VOTRE
WOLFE
WORSE
WOWEE
WOWIE
YONNE
YOURE
YOUSE
YOUVE
YOWIE
ZOWIE

••OE•
ALOES
BOOED
BOOER
COOED
COOEE
COOER
EROES
FLOES
FROES
GOOEY
HOOEY
LOOEY
MOOED
MOOER
OBOES
OTOES
PROEM
SHOED
SHOER
SHOES
SLOES
SOOEY
TOOER
TWOEE
TWOEM
WOOED
WOOER
ZOOEY

••O•E
ABODE
ABOVE
ADOBE
ADORE
ADOZE
AFORE
ALONE
AMOLE
AMORE
ANODE
ANOLE
AROSE
ASONE
ATONE
AWOKE
AXONE
AZOLE
AZORE
BIOME
BIORE
BLOKE
BLORE
BOOLE
BOONE
BOOZE
BROKE
BYONE
CHOKE
CHOLE
CHORE
CHOSE
CLONE
CLOSE
CLOVE
CNOTE
COOEE
COOKE
COOTE
CROCE
CRONE
CRORE
CROWE
CUORE
DHOLE
DHOTE
DIODE
DIONE
DOONE
DROLE
DROME
DRONE
DROVE
ECOLE
ELOGE
ELOPE
EMOTE
ENOTE
EPODE
ERODE
EROSE
EVOKE
FHOLE
FIORE
FOOTE
FROBE
FROME
FROZE
GEODE
GLOBE
GLOVE
GNOME
GNOTE
GOODE
GOOSE
GROFE
GROPE
GROTE
GROVE
HAOLE
HOOKE
IHOPE
ILOSE
ILOVE
IMOVE
KRONE
LEONE
LOOIE
LOOSE
MOORE
MOOSE
MYOPE
NIOBE
NOONE
NOOSE
OBOTE
ONONE
OZONE
PHOBE
PHONE
PLOCE
POOLE
PROBE
PROLE
PRONE
PROSE
PROVE
QUOTE
RHODE
RHONE
ROONE
SAONE
SCONE
SCOPE
SCORE
SHONE
SHORE
SHOVE
SLOPE
SMOKE
SMORE
SMOTE
SNORE
SNOWE
SPODE
SPOKE
SPORE
SPOSE
STOAE
STOKE
STOLE
STONE
STORE
STOVE
STOWE
SWORE
TBONE
THOLE
THOSE
TNOTE
TOOLE
TROPE
TROVE
TROWE
TWOEE
UPONE
USONE
VHONE
WHOLE
WHOME
WHOSE
WROTE

•••OE
CANOE
CHLOE
DAFOE
DEFOE
EAPOE
FAROE
GIJOE
MEROE
PEKOE
REHOE
STJOE
TAHOE
THROE

OF•••
OFAGE
OFFAL
OFFED
OFFER
OFFOF
OFTEN
OFUSE

O•F••
OFFAL
OFFED
OFFER
OFFOF
ORFEO
ORFES
OXFAM

O••F•
OEUFS
OLAFI
OLAFV
ONOFF

O•••F
OFFOF
ONOFF
OUTOF

•OF••
BOFFO
BOFFS
DOFFS
DOFOR
EOFOR
GOFAR
GOFER
GOFOR
HOFFA
JOFFE
LOFAT
LOFTS
LOFTY
MOFFO
NOFAT
NOFEE
NOFUN
SOFAR
SOFAS
SOFER
SOFEW
SOFIA
SOFIE
SOFTC
SOFTG
SOFTY
TOFFS
TOFTS
TOFUS
WOFAT

•O•F•
BOFFO
BOFFS
COIFS
COMFY
CORFU
DOFFS
DORFF
GOAFT
GOLFS
GOOFF
GOOFS
GOOFY
HOFFA
HOOFS
JOFFE
KOPFE
LOAFS
LOOFA
MOFFO
POUFS
ROLFE
ROLFS
ROOFS
TOEFL
TOFFS
WOLFE
WOLFF
WOLFS
WOOFS

•O••F
BOEUF
DORFF
FOURF
GOOFF
JOHNF
JOSEF
MOTIF
ROBOF
ROWLF
WOLFF
WOOLF

••OF•
AFOFL
ALOFT
BEOFF
CROFT
FEOFF
GOOFF
GOOFS
GOOFY
GROFE

HOOFS
IMOFF
KROFT
LOOFA
LWOFF
ONOFF
PROFS
ROOFS
SCOFF
USOFA
WOOFS

••O•F
ADOLF
ALOOF
BEOFF
FEOFF
GOOFF
IMOFF
KNOPF
LWOFF
ONOFF
PROOF
SCOFF
SPOOF
WOOLF
ZWOLF

•••OF
ALLOF
ALOOF
ASKOF
ATEOF
EATOF
OFFOF
OUTOF
PROOF
RIDOF
ROBOF
SHYOF
SPOOF
TENOF
USEOF

OG•••
OGAMS
OGDEN
OGEES
OGHAM
OGIER
OGIVE
OGLED
OGLER
OGLES
OGRES
OGROS

O•G••
OBGYN
OHGEE
OHGOD
ORGAN
ORGON
OUGHT

O••G•
OFAGE
OINGO
OLIGO
OLOGY
OMEGA
ONEGA
OSAGE
OUTGO

O•••G
ODING
OHING
OKING
OPING
ORANG
ORING
OWING

•OG••
BOGAN
BOGEY
BOGGS
BOGGY
BOGIE
BOGLE
BOGUS
DOGES
DOGGO
DOGGY
DOGIE
DOGIT
DOGMA
DOGON
FOGEL
FOGEY
FOGGY
FOGIN
FOGUP
GOGET
GOGOL
GOGOS
HOGAN
LOGAN
LOGES
LOGIA
LOGIC
LOGIN
LOGON
LOGOS
LOGUE
MOGEN
MOGUL
NOGAS
NOGGS
NOGOS
ROGER
ROGET
ROGUE
SOGGY
TOGAE
TOGAS
TOGUE
TOGUP
VOGEL
VOGUE
YOGAS
YOGIC
YOGIS

•O•G•
BOGGS
BOGGY
BONGO
BONGS
BORGE
BORGS
BOUGH
COIGN
CONGA
CONGE
CONGO
CORGI
COUGH
DODGE
DODGY
DOGGO
DOGGY
DONGS
DOUGH
FOGGY
FORGE
FORGO
GOLGI
GONGS
GORGE
GOUGE
HOAGY
HOUGH
JONGG
JORGE
LODGE
LONGA
LONGE
LONGI
LONGO
LONGS
LONGU
MONGO
MOOGS
NOGGS
NORGE
PONGO
PONGS
PORGY
ROUGE
ROUGH
SOGGY
SONGS
TONGA
TONGS
TOUGH
VOLGA

•O••G
BOING
BOURG
DOING
DORAG
GOING
JONGG
KOING
NOMSG
SOBIG
SOFTG
TOPOG
YOUNG

••OG•
AGOGO
BIOGS
BLOGS
CLOGS
ELOGE
FLOGS
FROGS
GLOGG
GROGS
KEOGH
KROGH
MOOGS
OLOGY
PROGS
SHOGI
SLOGS
SMOGS
STOGY
TIOGA

••O•G
ALONG
AMONG
CHONG
GEORG
GLOGG
HMONG
INORG
PRONG
THONG
WRONG

•••OG
BEDOG
BEFOG
DEFOG
EMBOG
INCOG
MAGOG
RELOG
TOPOG
ZEROG

OH•••
OHAIR
OHARA
OHARE
OHAYO
OHBOY
OHGEE
OHGOD
OHING
OHIOU
OHJOY
OHKAY
OHLIN
OHMAN
OHMIC
OHOHS
OHROB
OHWOW
OHYES
OHYOU

O•H••
OCHER
OCHOA
OCHOS
OCHRE
OGHAM
OOHED
OPHIR
OSHAY
OSHEA
OTHER
OTHON

O••H•
OATHS
OHOHS
OMAHA
OPAHS
ORCHS
ORTHO
OUGHT

O•••H
OBEAH
OOMPH
OPRAH
ORACH
ORPAH

•OH••
BOHAY
BOHEA
BOHOS
COHAB
COHAN
COHEN
COHOS
FOHNS
HOHOS
HOHUM
JOHAN
JOHNC
JOHND
JOHNF
JOHNI
JOHNJ
JOHNL
JOHNP
JOHNQ
JOHNS
JOHNV
JOHNX
KOHLS
LOHAN
NOHIT
NOHOW
OOHED

•O•H•
BOCHY
BOPHA
BOTHA
BOTHE
DONHO
GOTHA
GOTHS
HOOHA
HOXHA
KOPHS
LOCHS
MOCHA
MOSHE
MOTHS
MOTHY
NOCHE
POOHS
QOPHS
ROCHE
ROSHI
ROTHS
SOPHS
YODHS

•O••H
BOOTH
BORAH
BOSCH
BOTCH
BOUGH
COACH
CONCH
COUCH
COUGH
COUTH
DOETH
DOLPH
DOUGH
FORTH
FOURH
GOETH
GOOCH
HOOCH
HOPEH
HOUGH
JONAH
KOOSH
KOTCH
LOATH
LOUTH
LOWPH
MONTH
MOOCH
MORPH
MOUCH
MOUTH
NODUH
NORAH
NORTH
NOTAH
NOTCH
OOMPH
POACH
PONCH
POOCH
PORCH
POUCH
ROACH
ROUGH
ROUSH
SOOTH
SOUTH
TOOTH
TORAH
TORCH
TOUCH
TOUGH
TOVAH
VOUCH
WOOSH
WORTH
YOUTH

••OH•
ABOHM
ALOHA
HOOHA
IJOHN
OHOHS
POOHS

••O•H
AZOTH
BGOSH
BLOCH
BOOTH
BROTH
CLOTH
ENOCH
EPOCH
FROSH
FROTH
GOOCH
HOOCH
KEOGH
KOOSH
KROGH
MOOCH
POOCH
QUOTH
SKOSH
SLOSH
SLOTH
SOOTH
TOOTH
TROTH
WOOSH
WROTH

•••OH
RICOH
STROH

OI•••
OIDAL
OILED
OILER
OINGO
OINKS

O•I••
OBIES
OBITS
ODILE
ODING
ODIST
ODIUM
OGIER
OGIVE
OHING
OHIOU
OKIES
OKING
OLIGO
OLIOS
OLIVA
OLIVE
OMITS
ONICE
ONION
OPINE
OPING
OPIUM
ORIBI
ORIEL
ORING
ORION
ORIUM
OSIER
OTILE
OUIDA
OUIJA
OVINE
OVITZ
OWIES
OWING
OXIDE
OZICK

O••I•
OAKIE
OASIS
OHAIR
OHLIN
OHMIC
OLDIE
OLEIC
OLEIN
OLLIE
OMNIA
OMNIS
ONAIR
ONDIT
ONEIL
ONEIR
OOTID
OPCIT
OPHIR
OPTIC
OPTIN
ORBIC
ORBIT
ORKIN
ORNIS
ORRIN
ORRIS
ORTIZ
ORVIS
OSLIN
OSMIC
OSRIC
OSSIA
OSSIE
OSTIA
OTTIS
OUTIE
OVOID
OXLIP
OZZIE

O•••I
OBELI
OBOLI
OCULI
OKAPI
OLAFI
OLAVI
OMANI
ORANI
ORIBI
OTERI
OTOMI
OTTOI
OVOLI

•OI••
BOILS
BOING
BOIRE
BOISE
BOITE
BOITO
COIFS
COIGN
COILS
COINS
COIRS
DOIDO
DOILY
DOING
DOISY
DOITS
FOIES
FOILS
FOIST
GOING
HOIST
HOITY
JOINS
JOINT
JOIST
KOING
LOIDS
LOINS
LOIRE
MOILS
MOIRA
MOIRE
MOIST
NOILS
NOILY
NOIRE
NOIRS
NOISE
NOISY
POILU
POINT
POIRE
POISE
ROILS
ROILY
SOILS
SOIRS
TOILE
TOILS
TOITY
VOICE
VOICI
VOIDS
VOILA
VOILE
VOIPS

•O•I•
BOGIE
BORIC
BORIS
BOVID
BOWIE
BOXIN
COKIE
COLIC
COLIN
COMIC
COMIN
COMIX
CONIC
COPIA
COPIT
CORIA
DOBIE
DODIE
DOGIE
DOGIT
DOLIN
DORIA
DORIC
DORIS
DOXIE
EOLIA
EOLIC
EOSIN
FOGIN
FOLIA
FOLIC
FOLIO
GOPIK
GOSIT
GOTIN
GOTIT
HOBIE
HOKIE
HOLIC
HOMIE
HOPIN
HOPIS
HOVIS
HOWIE
IODIC
IONIA
IONIC
JODIE
JOLIE
JOSIE
JOSIP
KOJIS
KOPIT
KOVIC
LOEIL
LOGIA
LOGIC
LOGIN
LOOIE
LORIN
LORIS
LOSIN
LOUIE
LOUIS
LOVIN
LOWIQ
MOBIL
MONIC
MONIZ
MOTIF
MOVIE
MOVIN
MOWIS
MOXIE
NOBID
NOBIS
NOHIT
NOKIA
NOLIE
NOOIL
NORIA
NORIS
NOSIR
NOTIE
NOTIN
NOTIP
NOTIT
NOVIA
NOVIO
NOWIN
OOTID
PODIA
POLIO
POLIS
POLIT
POPIN
POSIT
ROBIN
RODIN
RONIN
ROSIE
ROSIN
ROXIE
SOBIG
SOCIO
SOFIA
SOFIE
SOLID
SONIA
SONIC
TOBIT
TOEIN
TONIC
TONIO
TOPIC
TOPIS
TORIC
TORII
TOTIE
TOWIN
TOWIT
TOXIC
TOXIN
WOWIE
YOGIC
YOGIS
YOWIE
ZOOID
ZORIS
ZOWIE

•O••I
BOCCI
BONDI
BOOKI
COATI
COCCI
CONDI
CONTI
COQUI
CORGI
CORNI
CORRI
DOLCI
DONDI
DORSI
DOUAI
GOLGI
GORKI
GOTTI
GOZZI
HOSNI
HOURI
JOHNI
LOEWI
LONGI
NOCTI
NOTTI
NOURI
PONTI
PONZI
POORI
ROSHI
ROSSI
SOAMI
SODOI
SOLDI
SOLEI
SOLTI
SOMNI
SOUCI
TOMEI
TONDI
TORII
TORSI
VOICI

••OI•
ABOIL
ALOIS
AROID
AVOID
AVOIR
AZOIC
BLOIS
BROIL
CHOIR
CROIX
DROID
DROIT
ENOIL
FROID
GROIN
HYOID
INOIL
LEOII
LEOIV
LEOIX
LOOIE
MAOII
NOOIL
OVOID
QUOIN
QUOIT
REOIL
SPOIL
STOIC
TROIS
ZOOID

••O•I
AIOLI
ARONI
BOOKI
CROCI
DHOTI
DUOMI
EBOLI
ECOLI
ENOKI
FIORI
FLORI
ICOSI
LEOII
LEONI
LEOVI
LEOXI
MAOII
MAORI
NAOMI
OBOLI
OTOMI
OVOLI
PAOLI
POORI
SHOGI
SHOJI
STOLI
SUOMI

•••OI
ENVOI
ETMOI
HANOI
LEROI
OTTOI
SODOI

OJ•••
OJAYS
OJEDA

O•J••
OBJET
OHJOY

O••J•
OUIJA

•OJ••
BOJER
DOJOS
HOJOS
KOJAK
KOJIS
MOJOS
ROJAS

•O•J•
KOPJE
SONJA

•O••J
JOHNJ

••OJ•
FLOJO
RIOJA
SHOJI

OK•••
OKAPI
OKARA
OKAYS
OKEMO
OKIES
OKING
OKRAS

O•K••
OAKEN
OAKES
OAKIE
OAKUM
OHKAY
ONKEY
ONKYO
ORKAN
ORKIN
OSKAR

O••K•
OINKS
ONEKS
OSAKA

O•••K
ORECK
OZARK
OZICK

•OK••
AOKAY
COKED
COKER
COKES
COKIE
DOKEY
HOKED
HOKES
HOKEY
HOKIE
HOKUM
JOKED
JOKER
JOKES
JOKEY
NOKIA
POKED
POKER
POKES
POKEY
ROKER
TOKAY
TOKED
TOKEN
TOKES
TOKYO
WOKEN
YOKED
YOKEL
YOKES
YOKUM

•O•K•
BOCKS
BONKS
BOOKI
BOOKS
BOOKV
BOOKX
BORKS
COCKS
COCKY
CONKS
COOKE
COOKS
COOKY
CORKS
CORKY
DOCKS
DORKS
DORKY
FOLKS
FOLKY
FORKS
FORKY
GOOKS
GORKI
GORKY
HOCKS
HONKS
HONKY
HOOKA
HOOKE
HOOKS
HOOKY
JOCKO
JOCKS
KOOKS
KOOKY
LOCKA
LOCKE
LOCKS
LOOKS
LOOKY
MOCKS
MONKS
NOCKS
NOOKS
POLKA
POLKS
PORKS
PORKY
ROCKS
ROCKY
ROOKS
ROOKY
ROYKO
SOAKS
SOCKO
SOCKS
TONKA
VODKA
WONKA
WONKS
WORKS
YOLKS
YOLKY
YORKS
ZONKS
ZOUKS

•O••K
GOASK
GOPIK
KODAK
KOJAK
KOPEK
NORSK
NOTOK
NOVAK
POTOK
ROARK
TOMSK

••OK•
ANOKA
AWOKE
BLOKE
BOOKI
BOOKS
BOOKV
BOOKX
BROKE
CHOKE
CHOKY
COOKE
COOKS
COOKY
ENOKI
EVOKE
EWOKS
GOOKS
GROKS
HOOKA
HOOKE
HOOKS
HOOKY
KOOKS
KOOKY
LOOKS
LOOKY
NOOKS
ROOKS
ROOKY
SMOKE
SMOKY
SPOKE
STOKE

••O•K
ANOUK
BJORK
BLOCK
BROCK
BROOK
CHOCK
CLOAK
CLOCK
CLONK
CROAK
CROCK
CROOK
EBOOK
FLOCK
FROCK
GLOCK
IBOOK
KIOSK
KNOCK
KROCK
PBOOK
PLONK
SHOCK
SHOOK
SMOCK
SNOOK
SPOCK
SPOOK
SPORK
STOCK
STORK

•••OK
ADAOK
ALLOK
BROOK
CROOK
DIDOK
EBOOK
HUROK
IBOOK
ITSOK
KAPOK
NOTOK
PBOOK
POTOK
SAYOK
SHOOK
SNOOK
SPOOK
THEOK

OL•••
OLAFI
OLAFV
OLAND
OLAVI
OLAVV
OLDEN
OLDER
OLDIE
OLEAN
OLEIC
OLEIN
OLEOS
OLETA
OLEUM
OLIGO
OLIOS
OLIVA
OLIVE
OLLAS
OLLIE
OLMEC
OLMOS
OLOGY
OLPAE
OLPES
OLSEN
OLSON

O•L••
OGLED OGLER OGLES OHLIN OILED OILER OLLAS OLLIE ONLAY ONLOW ORLES ORLON ORLOP ORLOS OSLER OSLIN OWLET OXLIP

O••L•
OBELI OBOLI OBOLS OCALA OCULI OCULO ODDLY ODELL ODILE ONCLE ONELA ONELB ONELS OOOLA OPALS OPELS ORALB ORALE ORALS OTILE OVALS OVOLI OVOLO OVULE

O•••L
OASAL OCTAL ODELL ODOUL OFFAL OIDAL ONEAL ONEIL ORIEL ORVAL OUSEL OUZEL

•OL••
AOLER BOLAR BOLAS BOLDS BOLES BOLET BOLLA BOLLS BOLOS BOLTS BOLUS COLAS COLBY COLDS COLES COLIC COLIN COLON COLOR COLTS COLUM DOLBY DOLCE DOLCI DOLED DOLES DOLIN DOLLS DOLLY DOLMA DOLON DOLOR DOLPH DOLTS EOLIA EOLIC EOLUS FOLDS FOLEY FOLIA FOLIC FOLIO FOLKS FOLKY FOLLY GOLAN GOLDA GOLDE GOLDS GOLEM GOLFS GOLGI GOLLY HOLDS HOLED HOLER HOLES HOLEY HOLIC HOLLY HOLMS HOLST HOLTZ JOLIE JOLLA JOLLY JOLTS JOLTY KOLAS LOLLS LOLLY MOLAR MOLDS MOLDY MOLES MOLLS MOLLY MOLTO MOLTS NOLAN NOLDE NOLES NOLIE NOLLE NOLOS NOLTE POLAR POLED POLER POLES POLIO POLIS POLIT POLKA POLKS POLLO POLLS POLLY POLOS POLYP ROLEN ROLEO ROLES ROLEX ROLFE ROLFS ROLLE ROLLO ROLLS ROLOS SOLAN SOLAR SOLDI SOLDO SOLEA SOLED SOLEI SOLER SOLES SOLID SOLLA SOLON SOLOS SOLTI SOLVE TOLAR TOLER TOLES TOLET TOLLS VOLAR VOLES VOLGA VOLPE VOLTA VOLTE VOLTS VOLVO WOLFE WOLFF WOLFS YOLKS YOLKY

•O•L•
BOGLE BOILS BOLLA BOLLS BOOLA BOOLE BOULE BOULT BOWLS BOYLE COALS COILS COOLS COULD COWLS COYLY DOALL DOBLE DOILY DOLLS DOLLY DOULA DOYLE DOYLY FOALS FOILS FOLLY FOOLS FOULS FOWLS FOYLE GOALS GODLY GOLLY GOULD HOLLY HOTLY HOWLS HOYLE JOLLA JOLLY JOULE JOWLS JOWLY KOALA KOHLS LOLLS LOLLY LOWLY MOILS MOLLS MOLLY MOOLA MOULD MOULT NOBLE NOBLY NOELS NOILS NOILY NOLLE OOOLA POILU POLLO POLLS POLLY POOLE POOLS POPLE POULE POULT ROALD ROBLE ROILS ROILY ROLLE ROLLO ROLLS ROTLS ROWLF SOCLE SOILS SOLLA SOULS TOILE TOILS TOLLS TOOLE TOOLS VOILA VOILE WOOLF WOOLS WOOLY WORLD WOULD YOULL YOWLS

•O••L
BODEL BOREL BOTEL BOWEL COBOL COPAL CORAL DOALL DORAL DOTAL DOWEL FOCAL FOGEL GOBEL GODEL GOGOL HORAL HOSEL HOTEL HOVEL JOHNL JOREL KODEL LOCAL LOEIL LOYAL MOBIL MODAL MODEL MOGUL MONEL MORAL MOREL MOSEL MOSUL MOTEL NOBEL NOCAL NODAL NOOIL NOPAL NOVEL PODAL ROWEL ROYAL SOCAL SONAL SOREL TOEFL TONAL TOPOL TOTAL TOWEL VOCAL VOGEL VOWEL YODEL YOKEL YOULL ZONAL ZOREL

••OL•
ADOLF AHOLD AIOLI AMOLE ANOLE ASOLD ATOLL AWOLS AZOLE BOOLA BOOLE CHOLE CHOLO COOLS DHOLE DROLE DROLL EBOLA EBOLI ECOLE ECOLI ENOLA ENOLS FHOLE FOOLS GAOLS HAOLE IDOLA IDOLS IFOLD ISOLA ISOLT KNOLL MOOLA OBOLI OBOLS OOOLA OVOLI OVOLO PAOLI PAOLO POOLE POOLS PROLE SCOLD SMOLT STOLA STOLE STOLI STOLS THOLE TOOLE TOOLS TROLL UBOLT UPOLU VIOLA VIOLS VTOLS WHOLE WHOLL WOOLF WOOLS WOOLY ZWOLF

••O•L
ABOIL AFOFL AFOUL ASOUL ATOLL BROIL CEORL DROLL DROOL ENOIL GHOUL GROWL INOIL KNOLL NOOIL ODOUL PROWL RAOUL REOIL SCOWL SEOUL SHOAL SKOAL SPOIL SPOOL STOOL TROLL WHOLL WHORL

•••OL
ALGOL ARBOL ATHOL CAROL COBOL DEVOL DROOL ELSOL ENROL ERROL EXTOL GASOL GOGOL KAROL LTCOL LYSOL NEROL NICOL NYTOL PAROL SPOOL STOOL TAXOL THEOL TIROL TOPOL TYROL

OM•••
OMAHA OMANI OMARR OMBER OMBRE OMEGA OMENS OMERS OMITS OMNES OMNIA OMNIS

O•M••
OHMAN OHMIC OLMEC OLMOS OOMPA OOMPH ORMAN OSMAN OSMIC

O••M•
OBAMA OGAMS OKEMO ORAMA OTOMI

O•••M
OAKUM OCCAM ODEUM ODIUM OGHAM OLEUM ONEAM ONEPM OPIUM ORIUM OXFAM

•OM••
BOMBA BOMBE BOMBS COMAE COMAS COMBO COMBS COMDR COMER COMES COMET COMEX COMFY COMIC COMIN COMIX COMMA COMME COMPS COMTE COMUS DOMED DOMES DOMOS GOMAD GOMAN GOMER GOMEZ HOMED HOMEO HOMER HOMES HOMEY HOMIE HOMME KOMBU LOMAN LOMAS LOMAX MOMMA MOMMY MOMUS NOMAD NOMAR NOMAS NOMEN NOMSG OOMPA OOMPH POMES POMME POMOS ROMAN ROMEO ROMES ROMPS SOMAS SOMAT SOMME SOMNI TOMAR TOMAS TOMBA TOMBE TOMBS TOMEI TOMES TOMMY TOMSK VOMER WOMAN WOMBS WOMEN WOMYN

•O•M•
BOOMS BOOMY COMMA COMME CORMS COSMO DOGMA DOLMA DOOMS DOOMY DORMS DORMY FOAMS FOAMY FORMA FORMS GORME GORMS GOTME HOLMS HOMME HOUMA LOAMS LOAMY LOOMS LOUMA MOMMA MOMMY NORMA NORMS NOTME POEME POEMS POMME ROAMS ROOMS ROOMY SOAMI SOMME TOMMY TORME WORMS WORMY ZOOMS ZOSMA

•O••M
BONUM BOSOM COLUM FORUM GOLEM HOHUM HOKUM JORUM LOCUM MODEM NOVEM ROREM SODOM TOTEM WOWEM YOKUM

••OM•
ABOMA ABOMB ANOMY AROMA ATOMS ATOMY BIOME BOOMS BOOMY BROMO CHOMP CLOMP CUOMO DOOMS DOOMY DROME DUOMI DUOMO FROME FROMM GLOMS GNOME GNOMY HBOMB LOOMS NAOMI NBOMB OTOMI PROMO PROMS RHOMB ROOMS ROOMY SLOMO STOMA STOMP SUOMI TROMP WHOME WHOMP ZOOMS

••O•M
ABOHM BLOOM BROOM ENORM FROMM GLOAM GLOOM GROOM PROAM PROEM STORM TWOAM TWOEM TWOPM VROOM

•••OM
ALBOM AXIOM BESOM BLOOM BOSOM BROOM BUXOM CAROM CDROM CHROM DENOM ENTOM EPROM EPSOM GLOOM GROOM HIMOM IDIOM LTCOM MRMOM PHNOM SODOM STROM VENOM VROOM

ON•••
ONAIR ONATE ONCLE ONCUE ONDAS ONDES ONDIT ONDVD ONEAD ONEAL ONEAM ONEBC ONEEE ONEGA ONEIL ONEIR ONEKS ONELA ONELB ONELS ONEND ONENO ONEON ONEPM ONERA ONERS ONEUP ONICE ONION ONKEY ONKYO ONLAY ONLOW ONNES ONOFF ONONE ONPAR ONRYE ONSET ONTAP ONTOP ONTWO

O•N••
OINGO OINKS OMNES OMNIA OMNIS ONNES ORNIS OUNCE OWNED OWNER OWNUP

O••N•
ODING ODONT OHING OKING OLAND OMANI OMENS ONEND ONENO ONONE OPENS OPINE OPING ORANG ORANI ORANT ORENA ORING ORONO OTONO OVENS OVINE OWENS OWING OXANA OZONE

O•••N
OAKEN OATEN OBGYN OCEAN OCTAN ODEON OFTEN OGDEN OHLIN OHMAN OLDEN OLEAN OLEIN OLSEN OLSON ONEON ONION OPTIN ORGAN ORGON ORION ORKAN ORKIN ORLON ORMAN ORREN ORRIN ORSON ORTON OSCAN OSLIN OSMAN OTHON OTOWN OUTON OWEON

•ON••
AONES BONAR BONDI BONDS BONED BONER BONES BONET BONEY BONGO BONGS BONKS BONNE BONNY BONUM BONUS BONZE BONZO CONAN CONCH CONDE CONDI CONDO CONDS CONED CONER CONES CONEY CONGA CONGE CONGO CONIC CONKS CONNS CONON CONST CONTD CONTE CONTI CONTR CONTS CONUS CONVY DONAS DONAT DONAU DONDE DONDI DONEE DONEN DONGS DONHO DONNA DONNE DONNY DONOR DONOT DONOW DONTS DONUS DONUT FONDA FONDU FONTS GONER GONGS GONNA GONOW GONZO HONAN HONDA HONDO HONED HONER HONES HONEY HONKS HONKY HONOR HONUS IONIA IONIC JONAH JONAS JONES JONGG JONNY JONZE KONAS LONER LONGA LONGE LONGI LONGO LONGS LONGU MONAD MONDE MONDO MONEL MONET MONEY MONGO MONIC MONIZ MONKS MONOD MONOS MONRO MONTE MONTH MONTS MONTY MONZA NONCE NONES NONET NONNO NONOS PONCA PONCE PONCH PONDS PONES PONGO PONGS PONTA PONTE PONTI PONTS PONZI PONZU RONAN RONCO RONDE RONDO RONEE RONIN RONNY SONAL SONAR SONDE SONES SONGS SONIA SONIC SONJA SONNY SONYA SONYS TONAL TONDI TONDO TONED TONER TONES TONGA TONGS TONIC TONIO TONKA TONNE TONOW TONTO TONUS TONYA TONYS VONDA WONAT WONBY WONKA WONKS WONTS YONEX YONNE ZONAL ZONED ZONER ZONES ZONKS

•O•N•
BOING BONNE BONNY BOONE BOONS BORNE BOSNS BOUND COINS CONNS COONS CORNI CORNO CORNS CORNU CORNY COUNT DOANE DOANS DOING DONNA DONNE DONNY DOONE DOWNS DOWNY FOHNS FOUND FOUNT GOING GONNA GOONS GOONY GOWNS HORNE HORNS HORNY HOSNI HOUND JOHNC JOHND JOHNF JOHNI JOHNJ JOHNL JOHNP JOHNQ JOHNS JOHNV JOHNX JOINS JOINT JONNY KOANS KOING LOANS LOINS LOONS LOONY LORNA LORNE LOTNO MOANS MOONS MOONY MORNS MOUND MOUNT NOEND NONNO NOONE NOONS NORNS NOUNS POINT POONA PORNO POUND ROANS RONNY ROONE ROUND SOMNI

SONNY
SOUND
TONNE
TOONS
TOWNE
TOWNS
WOUND
YONNE
YOUNG
YOUNT

•O••N
BOGAN
BOREN
BORON
BOSON
BOSUN
BOWEN
BOXIN
CODON
COHAN
COHEN
COIGN
COLIN
COLON
COMIN
CONAN
CONON
COOWN
COTAN
COVEN
COZEN
DOGON
DOLIN
DOLON
DONEN
DOORN
DORAN
DOREN
DOYEN
DOZEN
EOSIN
FOGIN
GOLAN
GOMAN
GORAN
GOREN
GOTIN
GOTON
GOYEN
HOBAN
HOGAN
HONAN
HOPIN
HOPON
HOSEN
HOTON
IOWAN
JOHAN
JOVAN
KORAN
LODEN
LOGAN
LOGIN
LOGON
LOHAN
LOMAN
LORAN
LOREN
LORIN
LOSIN
LOVIN
LOWON
MOGEN
MORAN
MORON
MOURN
MOVIN
MOWEN
NOFUN
NOLAN
NOMEN
NOREN
NORUN
NOTIN
NOTON
NOWIN
POPIN
ROBIN
ROBYN
RODAN
RODIN
ROLEN
ROMAN
RONAN
RONIN
ROSEN
ROSIN
ROUEN
ROWAN
ROWEN
SOLAN
SOLON
SOREN
TOEIN
TOKEN
TOWIN
TOXIN
TOYON
WODEN
WOKEN
WOMAN
WOMEN
WOMYN
WOTAN
WOVEN
YOURN

••ON•
AEONS
AGONY
ALONE
ALONG
AMONG
ARONI
ASONE
ATONE
ATONY
AXONE
AXONS
BIONT
BLOND
BOONE
BOONS
BRONC
BRONX
BUONA
BUONO
BYONE
CHONG
CIONS
CLONE
CLONK
COONS
CRONE
CRONY
DIONE
DOONE
DRONE
EBOND
EBONS
EBONY
ECONO
ECONS
ETONS
EXONS
FIONA
FROND
FRONT
GIONO
GOONS
GOONY
HMONG
ICONO
ICONS
IDONT
ILONA
INONU
IRONS
IRONY
IWONT
KAONS
KRONA
KRONE
LEONA
LEONE
LEONI
LIONS
LOONS
LOONY
LYONS
MOONS
MOONY
MUONS
NEONS
NOONE
NOONS
ODONT
ONONE
ORONO
OTONO
OZONE
PAONS
PEONS
PEONY
PHONE
PHONO
PHONS
PHONY
PIONS
PLONK
POONA
PRONE
PRONG
RHONE
ROONE
SAONE
SCONE
SHONE
STONE
STONY
TBOND
TBONE
THONG
TOONS
UCONN
UPONE
USONE
VHONE
WRONG
XEONS

••O•N
ACORN
ADORN
BJORN
BLOWN
BROUN
BROWN
CLOWN
COOWN
CROON
CROWN
DOORN
DROWN
FLOWN
FROWN
GROAN
GROIN
GROWN
IJOHN
KNOWN
KROON
OTOWN
QUOIN
REOWN
SCORN
SHORN
SHOWN
SLOAN
SPOON
SWOON
SWORN
THORN
TROON
TWOON
UCONN

•••ON
AARON
ACTON
ADDON
AFTON
AGNON
AGRON
AKRON
ALTON
ANCON
ANION
ANSON
ANTON
ANYON
APRON
ARGON
ARION
ARSON
ASTON
ATHON
ATION
AVION
AXION
AXTON
BACON
BALON
BANON
BARON
BATON
BELON
BETON
BIDON
BIGON
BISON
BITON
BORON
BOSON
BUSON
BYRON
CAJON
CANON
CAPON
CARON
CHRON
CLEON
CODON
COLON
CONON
CREON
CROON
DABON
DAMON
DEION
DELON
DEMON
DEVON
DIJON
DIXON
DOGON
DOLON
DRUON
DYSON
EAMON
EATON
EDSON
EGDON
EGGON
ELDON
ELION
ELTON
ENDON
ENRON
EPSON
EXCON
EXXON
FANON
FARON
FEDON
FELON
FITON
FIXON
FLYON
FREON
FUTON
GABON
GETON
GLUON
GOTON
GUYON
HADON
HASON
HEMON
HERON
HESON
HITON
HOPON
HOTON
HURON
HYSON
ILION
INION
IXION
JAMON
JASON
KEVON
KEYON
KROON
LAYON
LECON
LEDON
LEMON
LETON
LEVON
LIEON
LIMON
LITON
LOGON
LOWON
LUZON
LYDON
LYMON
MACON
MAHON
MANON
MASON
MELON
MESON
MIDON
MORON
MUTON
MYRON
NANON
NIHON
NIKON
NINON
NITON
NIXON
NOTON
NYLON
ODEON
OLSON
ONEON
ONION
ORGON
ORION
ORLON
ORSON
ORTON
OTHON
OUTON
OWEON
PATON
PERON
PICON
PILON
PINON
PITON
PUTON
PYLON
RADON
RAGON
RAMON
RANON
RAPON
RATON
RAYON
RECON
REDON
REWON
RIPON
RUBON
RUNON
SALON
SATON
SAXON
SCHON
SCION
SETON
SEWON
SIDON
SIMON
SIPON
SITON
SOLON
SPOON
SPYON
SWOON
TAGON
TALON
TAPON
TAUON
TAXON
TENON
TETON
TIEON
TIGON
TIMON
TOYON
TROON
TRYON
TUGON
TWOON
TYSON
UNION
UNWON
UPTON
USEON
WAGON
WASON
WEWON
XENON
YUKON
ZEVON
ZIPON

OO•••
OOHED
OOMPA
OOMPH
OOOLA
OOOOO
OOPOD
OOTID
OOZED
OOZES

O•O••
OBOES
OBOLI
OBOLS
OBOTE
ODONT
ODORS
ODOUL
ODOUR
OHOHS
OLOGY
ONOFF
ONONE
OOOLA
OOOOO
ORONO
ORORY
OTOES
OTOMI
OTONO
OTOWN
OVOID
OVOLI
OVOLO
OZONE

O••O•
OCHOA
OCHOS
ODEON
OFFOF
OGROS
OHBOY
OHGOD
OHIOU
OHJOY
OHROB
OHWOW
OHYOU
OLEOS
OLIOS
OLMOS
OLSON
ONEON
ONION
ONLOW
ONTOP
OOOOO
OOPOD
OREOS
ORGON
ORION
ORLON
ORLOP
ORLOS
ORSON
ORTON
ORZOS
OTHON
OTROS
OTTOI
OUTOF
OUTON
OUZOS
OWEON
OXBOW

O•••O
OCULO
OHAYO
OINGO
OKEMO
OLIGO
ONENO
ONKYO
ONTWO
OOOOO
OPTTO
ORFEO
ORONO
ORTHO
ORURO
OSSEO
OSTEO
OTERO
OTONO
OUTDO
OUTGO
OVOLO

•OO••
BOOAT
BOOBS
BOOBY
BOOED
BOOER
BOOKI
BOOKS
BOOKV
BOOKX
BOOLA
BOOLE
BOOMS
BOOMY
BOONE
BOONS
BOORS
BOOST
BOOTH
BOOTS
BOOTY
BOOZE
COODY
COOED
COOEE
COOER
COOKE
COOKS
COOKY
COOLS
COONS
COOPS
COOPT
COORS
COOSA
COOTE
COOTS
COOTY
COOWN
DOODY
DOOMS
DOOMY
DOONE
DOORN
DOORS
DOOZY
FOODS
FOOLS
FOOTE
FOOTS
FOOZY
GOOCH
GOODE
GOODS
GOODY
GOOEY
GOOFF
GOOFS
GOOFY
GOOKS
GOONS
GOONY
GOOPS
GOOPY
GOOSE
GOOSY
GOOUT
HOOCH
HOODS
HOODY
HOOEY
HOOFS
HOOHA
HOOKA
HOOKE
HOOKS
HOOKY
HOOPS
HOOTS
JOOSS
KOOKS
KOOKY
KOOSH
LOOBY
LOOEY
LOOFA
LOOIE
LOOKS
LOOKY
LOOMS
LOONS
LOONY
LOOPS
LOOPY
LOOSE
LOOTS
MOOCH
MOODS
MOODY
MOOED
MOOER
MOOGS
MOOLA
MOONS
MOONY
MOORE
MOORS
MOORY
MOOSE
MOOTS
NOOIL
NOOKS
NOONE
NOONS
NOORT
NOOSE
OOOLA
OOOOO
POOCH
POOHS
POOLE
POOLS
POONA
POOPS
POORI
POORS
ROODS
ROOFS
ROOKS
ROOKY
ROOMS
ROOMY
ROONE
ROOSA
ROOST
ROOTS
ROOTY
SOOEY
SOOTH
SOOTS
SOOTY
TOODY
TOOER
TOOLE
TOOLS
TOONS
TOOTH
TOOTS
WOODS
WOODY
WOOED
WOOER
WOOFS
WOOLF
WOOLS
WOOLY
WOOSH
WOOZY
YOOBA
ZOOEY
ZOOID
ZOOMS

•O•O•
BOHOS
BOLOS
BORON
BOROS
BOSOM
BOSON
BOSOX
BOTOX
BOYOS
BOZOS
COBOL
COCOA
COCOS
CODON
COHOS
COLON
COLOR
CONON
COROT
DODOS
DOFOR
DOGON
DOJOS
DOLON
DOLOR
DOMOS
DONOR
DONOT
DONOW
EOFOR
FODOR
GOBOS
GOBOT
GODOT
GOFOR
GOGOL
GOGOS
GONOW
GOTON
HOBOS
HOHOS
HOJOS
HONOR
HOPON
HOTON
KOBOS
KOTOS
LOBOS
LOCOS
LOGON
LOGOS
LOTOS
LOWON
MOJOS
MONOD
MONOS
MORON
MOROS
MOTOR
MOZOS
NODOZ
NOGOS
NOHOW
NOLOS
NONOS
NOTOK
NOTON
OOOOO
OOPOD
POBOX
POBOY
POLOS
POMOS
POPOV
POTOK
ROBOF
ROBOT
ROLOS
ROTOR
ROTOS
SODOI
SODOM
SOLON
SOLOS
SOPOR
SOROS
TODOS
TONOW
TOPOG
TOPOL
TOROS
TOYON
TOYOS
TOYOU
XOXOX
YOSOY
YOYOS

•O••O
BOFFO
BOITO
BONGO
BONZO
BOSCO
BOWTO
COMBO
CONDO
CONGO
COPTO
CORNO
CORSO
CORVO
COSMO
DOBRO
DOGGO
DOIDO
DONHO
DORSO
DOTTO
DOURO
FOLIO
FORDO
FORGO
GONZO
GOPRO
GORDO
GOTTO
HOMEO
HONDO
HOPTO
HOWDO
HOWSO
HOWTO
JOCKO
JOTTO
KOTTO
LONGO
LOTNO
LOTTO
MOFFO
MOLTO
MONDO
MONGO
MONRO
MORRO
MOSSO
MOTTO
NODTO
NONNO
NORVO
NOTDO
NOTSO
NOVIO
OOOOO
POLIO
POLLO
PONGO
PORNO
PORTO
POTTO
POZZO
ROCCO
RODEO
ROLEO
ROLLO
ROMEO
RONCO
RONDO
ROSSO
ROYKO
SOCIO
SOCKO
SOLDO
SORBO
SOTTO
TOKYO
TONDO
TONIO
TONTO
TORSO
TOURO
VOLVO
YOCTO
YOTTO
ZORRO

••OO•
AFOOT
AHOOT
ALOOF
BLOOD
BLOOM
BLOOP
BROOD
BROOK
BROOM
CROOK
CROON
DROOD
DROOL
DROOP
EBOOK
FLOOD
FLOOR
FROOT
GLOOM
GROOM
IBOOK
KROON
OOOOO
PBOOK
PROOF
SCOOP
SCOOT
SHOOK
SHOOS
SHOOT
SLOOP
SMOOT
SNOOD
SNOOK
SNOOP
SNOOT
SPOOF
SPOOK
SPOOL
SPOON
SPOOR
STOOD
STOOL
STOOP
SWOON
SWOOP
TROON
TROOP
TWOON
VROOM
WHOOP

••O•O
ABOVO
ADOBO
AGOGO
AMOCO
BROMO
BUONO
CHOCO
CHOLO
CHORO
CUOMO
DROPO
DUOMO
ECONO
ELORO
FLOJO
FRODO
FROYO
FUOCO
GIONO
ICONO
KROTO
KYOTO
NUOVO
OOOOO
ORONO
OTONO
OVOLO
PAOLO
PHOBO
PHONO
PHOTO
PROMO
PROTO
PROVO
RHODO
SLOMO
SPOSO
THORO
TROPO
WHOSO

•••OO
ACHOO
AIDOO
AMTOO
ARTOO
BABOO
BALOO
BAZOO
DETOO
ESPOO
IGLOO
ISTOO
KAZOO
MAGOO
MCCOO
METOO
NABOO
OOOOO
PAROO
SHMOO
TABOO
WAHOO
YAHOO
YAZOO

OP•••
OPAHS
OPALS
OPART
OPCIT
OPEDS
OPELS
OPENS
OPERA
OPERE
OPHIR
OPINE
OPING
OPIUM
OPPER
OPQRS
OPRAH
OPTED
OPTIC
OPTIN
OPTTO

O•P••
OLPAE
OLPES
ONPAR
OOPOD
OPPER
ORPAH

O••P•
OKAPI
ONEPM
OOMPA
OOMPH

O•••P
ONEUP
ONTAP
ONTOP
ORLOP
OWNUP
OXLIP

•OP••
BOPHA
COPAL
COPAY
COPED
COPER
COPES
COPIA
COPIT
COPRA
COPSE
COPTO
COPTS
DOPAS
DOPED
DOPER
DOPES
DOPEY
GOPIK
GOPRO
HOPED
HOPEH
HOPER
HOPES
HOPIN
HOPIS
HOPON
HOPPE
HOPPY
HOPTO
HOPUP
KOPEK
KOPFE
KOPHS
KOPIT
KOPJE
LOPAT
LOPED
LOPER
LOPES
LOPEZ
LOPPY
MOPED
MOPER
MOPES
MOPEY
MOPSY
MOPUP
NOPAL
NOPAR
NOPES
NOPQR
OOPOD
POPBY
POPES
POPIN
POPLE
POPOV
POPPA
POPPY
POPUP
QOPHS
ROPED
ROPER
ROPES
SOPHS
SOPOR
SOPPY

SOPUP
TOPAZ
TOPED
TOPEE
TOPER
TOPES
TOPIC
TOPIS
TOPOG
TOPOL
TOPPS
TOPSY
TOPUP
WOPAT

•O•P•

COAPT
COMPS
COOPS
COOPT
CORPS
COUPE
COUPS
COYPU
DOLPH
DORPS
GOAPE
GOOPS
GOOPY
GORPS
HOOPS
HOPPE
HOPPY
HOSPS
LOOPS
LOOPY
LOPPY
LOUPE
LOUPS
LOWPH
MORPH
OOMPA
OOMPH
POOPS
POPPA
POPPY
ROMPS
SOAPS
SOAPY
SOPPY
SOUPS
SOUPY
TOPPS
VOIPS
VOLPE

•O••P

BOBUP
BOXUP
FOGUP
GOTUP
HOPUP
JOHNP
JOSIP
MOPUP
NOTIP
NOTUP
POLYP
POPUP
SOPUP
TOGUP
TOPUP
TOTUP

••OP•

ADOPT
CHOPS
CLOPS
COOPS
COOPT
CROPS
DROPO
DROPS
DROPT
ELOPE
ESOPS
FLOPS
GLOPS
GOOPS
GOOPY
GROPE
HOOPS
IHOPE
IHOPS
KNOPF
LDOPA
LOOPS
LOOPY
MNOPQ
MYOPE
PLOPS
POOPS
PROPS
SCOPE
SHOPS
SLOPE
SLOPS
STOPS
TROPE
TROPO
TTOPS
TWOPM
WHOPS

••O•P

BLOOP
CHOMP
CLOMP
CROUP
DROOP
GROUP
SCOOP
SLOOP
SNOOP
STOMP
STOOP
SWOOP
TROMP
TROOP
TROUP
TWOUP
WHOMP
WHOOP

•••OP

AESOP
ALSOP
BEBOP
BLOOP
DROOP
ESTOP
EXCOP
FSTOP
GALOP
HALOP
LMNOP
ONTOP
ORLOP
PREOP
REBOP
REMOP
RETOP
SALOP
SCOOP
SLOOP
SNOOP
STOOP
STROP
SWOOP
SYSOP
TROOP
TSTOP
UPTOP
WHOOP
ZZTOP

O•Q••

OPQRS

•OQ••

COQUI
ROQUE
TOQUE

•O•Q•

NOPQR

•O••Q

JOHNQ
LOWIQ

••O•Q

MNOPQ

OR•••

ORACH
ORACY
ORALB
ORALE
ORALS
ORAMA
ORANG
ORANI
ORANT
ORATE
ORBED
ORBIC
ORBIT
ORCAS
ORCHS
ORCUS
ORCZY
ORDER
OREAD
ORECK
ORENA
OREOS
ORFEO
ORFES
ORGAN
ORGON
ORIBI
ORIEL
ORING
ORION
ORIUM
ORKAN
ORKIN
ORLES
ORLON
ORLOP
ORLOS
ORMAN
ORNIS
ORONO
ORORY
ORPAH
ORREN
ORRIN
ORRIS
ORSAY
ORSER
ORSES
ORSON
ORTHO
ORTIZ
ORTON
ORURO
ORVAL
ORVIS
ORZOS

O•R••

OARED
OARER
OBRAS
OCRAT
OGRES
OGROS
OHROB
OKRAS
ONRYE
OPRAH
ORREN
ORRIN
ORRIS
OSRIC
OTRAS
OTROS
OURAY

O••R•

OCHRE
ODORS
OHARA
OHARE
OKARA
OMARR
OMBRE
OMERS
ONERA
ONERS
OPART
OPERA
OPERE
OPQRS
ORORY
ORURO
OTARU
OTARY
OTERI
OTERO
OUTRE
OVARY
OVERS
OVERT
OWERS
OYERS
OZARK

O•••R

OARER
OATER
OCCUR
OCHER
ODDER
ODOUR
OFFER
OGIER
OGLER
OHAIR
OILER
OLDER
OMARR
OMBER
ONAIR
ONEIR
ONPAR
OPHIR
OPPER
ORDER
ORSER
OSCAR
OSIER
OSKAR
OSLER
OSTAR
OSTER
OTHER
OTTER
OUTER
OWNER

•OR••

AORTA
BORAH
BORAS
BORAX
BORED
BOREL
BOREN
BORER
BORES
BORGE
BORGS
BORIC
BORIS
BORKS
BORNE
BORON
BOROS
BORSA
CORAL
CORBY
CORDA
CORDS
COREA
CORED
CORER
CORES
COREY
CORFU
CORGI
CORIA
CORKS
CORKY
CORMS
CORNI
CORNO
CORNS
CORNU
CORNY
COROT
CORPS
CORRI
CORSA
CORSO
CORVO
DORAG
DORAL
DORAN
DOREN
DORFF
DORIA
DORIC
DORIS
DORKS
DORKY
DORMS
DORMY
DORPS
DORSA
DORSI
DORSO
FORAY
FORCE
FORDO
FORDS
FORES
FORGE
FORGO
FORKS
FORKY
FORMA
FORMS
FORTE
FORTH
FORTS
FORTY
FORUM
FORZA
GORAN
GORBY
GORDO
GORDY
GORED
GOREN
GORES
GOREY
GORGE
GORKI
GORKY
GORME
GORMS
GORPS
GORSE
GORSY
HORAE
HORAL
HORAS
HORDE
HOREB
HORNE
HORNS
HORNY
HORSE
HORST
HORSY
HORUS
JOREL
JORGE
JORUM
KORAN
KORAT
KORDA
KOREA
LORAN
LORAX
LORCA
LORDS
LORDY
LOREN
LORES
LORIN
LORIS
LORNA
LORNE
LORRE
LORRY
LORUS
MORAL
MORAN
MORAS
MORAY
MOREL
MORES
MOREY
MORNS
MORON
MOROS
MORPH
MORRA
MORRO
MORSE
MORTE
MORTY
NORAD
NORAH
NOREN
NORGE
NORIA
NORIS
NORMA
NORMS
NORNS
NORSE
NORSK
NORTE
NORTH
NORUN
NORVO
PORCH
PORCS
PORED
PORER
PORES
PORGY
PORKS
PORKY
PORNO
PORTA
PORTE
PORTO
PORTS
ROREM
SORAS
SORBO
SORBS
SOREL
SOREN
SORER
SORES
SOROS
SORRY
SORTA
SORTS
TORAH
TORAS
TORCH
TORIC
TORII
TORME
TOROS
TORRE
TORRS
TORSI
TORSO
TORTA
TORTE
TORTS
TORUS
WORDS
WORDY
WORKS
WORLD
WORMS
WORMY
WORRY
WORSE
WORST
WORTH
WORTS
YORBA
YORES
YORKS
YORTY
ZORBA
ZOREL
ZORIS
ZORRO

•O•R•

BOARD
BOARS
BOERS
BOIRE
BOORS
BOURG
COBRA
COIRS
COORS
COPRA
CORRI
COURT
COURU
COWRY
DOBRO
DOERR
DOERS
DOORN
DOORS
DOURO
DOWRY
FOURA
FOURB
FOURC
FOURD
FOURE
FOURF
FOURH
FOURS
GOERS
GOPRO
GOURD
HOARD
HOARE
HOARS
HOARY
HOERS
HOURI
HOURS
JOURS
LOIRE
LORRE
LORRY
LOURS
LOURY
LOWRY
MOIRA
MOIRE
MONRO
MOORE
MOORS
MOORY
MORRA
MORRO
MOURN
NOIRE
NOIRS
NOORT
NOTRE
NOURI
POBRE
POIRE
POORI
POORS
POURS
ROARK
ROARS
SOARS
SOIRS
SORRY
SOURS
TORRE
TORRS
TOURO
TOURS
VOTRE
WORRY
YOURE
YOURN
YOURS
ZORRO

•O••R

AOLER
BOJER
BOLAR
BONAR
BONER
BOOER
BORER
BOWER
BOXER
BOYER
CODER
COEUR
COKER
COLOR
COMDR
COMER
CONER
CONTR
COOER
COPER
CORER
COVER
COWER
COYER
DOERR
DOFOR
DOLOR
DONOR
DOPER
DOSER
DOTER
DOVER
DOZER
EOFOR
FODOR
FOYER
GOFAR
GOFER
GOFOR
GOMER
GONER
GOWER
HOLER
HOMER
HONER
HONOR
HOPER
HOSER
HOVER
HOWAR
JOKER
KOSAR
LOBAR
LODER
LONER
LOPER
LOSER
LOVER
LOWER
MOLAR
MOOER
MOPER
MOTOR
MOVER
MOWER
NOEAR
NOMAR
NOPAR
NOPQR
NOSER
NOSIR
NOTER
POKER
POLAR
POLER
PORER
POSER
POWER
ROBER
ROGER
ROKER
ROPER
ROTOR
ROVER
ROWER
SOBER
SOEUR
SOFAR
SOFER
SOLAR
SOLER
SONAR
SOPOR
SORER
SOWER
TOLAR
TOLER
TOMAR
TONER
TOOER
TOPER
TOTER
TOWAR
TOWER
TOYER
VOLAR
VOMER
VOTER
VOWER
WOOER
ZONER

••OR•

ABORT
ACORN
ADORE
ADORN
AFORE
AGORA
AHORA
ALORS
AMORE
AMORS
AMORT
AMORY
APORT
ASORS
ATORY
AZORE
BIORE
BJORK
BJORN
BLORE
BOORS
CEORL
CHORD
CHORE
CHORO
COORS
CRORE
CUORE
DIORS
DOORN
DOORS
ELORO
EMORY
ENORM
EVORA
FIORD
FIORE
FIORI
FJORD
FLORA
FLORI
FLORY
FTORD
GEORG
GLORY
INORG
IVORY
KNORR
LEORA
MAORI
MOORE
MOORS
MOORY
NIORT
NOORT
ODORS
ORORY
POORI
POORS
SCORE
SCORN
SHORE
SHORN
SHORT
SKORT
SMORE
SNORE
SNORT
SPORE
SPORK
SPORT
STORE
STORK
STORM
STORY
SWORD
SWORE
SWORN
THORA
THORN
THORO
WHORL

••O•R

AMOUR
AROAR
AVOIR
BFOUR
BOOER
CHOIR
COOER
FLOOR
FLOUR
HHOUR
IFOUR
KNORR
MOOER
ODOUR
SCOUR
SHOER
SPOOR
TOOER
VFOUR
WOOER

•••OR

ABHOR
ACTOR
ALCOR
ANDOR
ARBOR
ARDOR
ARMOR
ASFOR
ASTOR
AVIOR
BATOR
BEFOR
CALOR
CHLOR
COLOR
CRUOR
CUKOR
DECOR
DOFOR
DOLOR
DONOR
ECTOR
ENDOR
ENSOR
EOFOR
EPHOR
ERROR
FAVOR
FETOR
FLOOR
FLUOR
FODOR
FUROR
GABOR
GATOR
GOFOR
HONOR
HUMOR
ICHOR
INFOR
JUROR
LABOR
LUXOR
MAJOR
MANOR
MAYOR
MINOR
MOTOR
PAYOR
PRIOR
PRYOR
RAZOR
RIGOR
ROTOR
RUMOR
SAPOR
SAVOR
SENOR
SOPOR
SPOOR
TABOR
TENOR
TIMOR
TUDOR
TUTOR
UPFOR
VALOR
VAPOR
VIDOR
VIGOR
VISOR
VIZOR
YESOR
ZUKOR

OS•••

OSAGE
OSAKA
OSCAN
OSCAR
OSHAY
OSHEA
OSIER
OSKAR
OSLER
OSLIN
OSMAN
OSMIC
OSRIC
OSSEO
OSSET
OSSIA
OSSIE
OSTAR
OSTEO
OSTER
OSTIA

O•S••

OASAL
OASES
OASIS
OASTS
OESTE
OLSEN
OLSON
ONSET
ORSAY
ORSER
ORSES
ORSON
OSSEO
OSSET
OSSIA
OSSIE
OUSEL
OUSTS

O••S•

OBESE
ODESA
ODIST
OFUSE
OUEST

O•••S

OAKES
OASES
OASIS
OASTS
OATES
OATHS
OBEYS
OBIES
OBITS
OBOES
OBOLS
OBRAS
OCHOS
ODETS
ODORS
OEUFS
OGAMS
OGEES
OGLES
OGRES
OGROS
OHOHS
OHYES
OINKS
OJAYS
OKAYS
OKIES
OKRAS
OLEOS
OLIOS
OLLAS
OLMOS
OLPES
OMENS
OMERS
OMITS
OMNES
OMNIS
ONDAS
ONDES
ONEKS
ONELS
ONERS
ONNES
OOZES
OPAHS
OPALS
OPEDS
OPELS
OPENS
OPQRS
ORALS
ORCAS
ORCHS
ORCUS
OREOS
ORFES
ORLES
ORLOS
ORNIS
ORRIS
ORSES
ORVIS
ORZOS
OTOES
OTRAS
OTROS
OTTIS
OUSTS
OUZOS
OVALS
OVENS
OVERS
OWENS
OWERS
OWIES
OYERS

•OS••

AOSTA
BOSCH
BOSCO
BOSCS
BOSNS
BOSOM
BOSON
BOSOX
BOSSA
BOSSY
BOSUN
COSBY
COSEC
COSET
COSMO
COSTA
COSTS
DOSAY
DOSED
DOSER
DOSES
EOSIN
FOSSA
FOSSE
GOSEE
GOSIT
GOSSE
HOSEA
HOSED
HOSEL
HOSEN
HOSER
HOSES
HOSNI
HOSPS
HOSTA
HOSTS
JOSEF
JOSEY
JOSIE
JOSIP
KOSAR
LOSER
LOSES
LOSEY
LOSIN
MOSEL
MOSES
MOSEY
MOSHE
MOSSO
MOSSY
MOSUL
NOSED
NOSER
NOSES
NOSEY
NOSIR
POSED
POSER
POSES
POSEY
POSIT
POSSE
POSTE
POSTS
ROSEN
ROSES
ROSEY
ROSHI
ROSIE
ROSIN
ROSSA
ROSSI
ROSSO
SOSAD
TOSCA
TOSEA
YOSOY
ZOSMA

•O•S•

BOAST
BOISE
BOOST
BORSA
BOSSA
BOSSY
COASE
COAST
CONST
COOSA
COPSE
CORSA
CORSO
COUSY
DOEST
DOISY
DORSA
DORSI
DORSO
DOUSE
DOWSE
FOIST
FOSSA
FOSSE
GOASK

GOEST GOOSE GOOSY GORSE GORSY GOSSE HOEST HOIST HOLST HORSE HORST HORSY HOTSY HOUSE HOWSO JOIST JOOSS JOUST KOOSH LOESS LOOSE LOTSA LOUSE LOUSY MOIST MOOSE MOPSY MORSE MOSSO MOSSY MOUSE MOUSY NOISE NOISY NOMSG NOOSE NORSE NORSK NOTSO NOUSE POESY POISE POSSE POTSY ROAST ROOSA ROOST ROSSA ROSSI ROSSO ROUSE ROUSH ROUST ROWSE SOUSA SOUSE TOAST TOMSK TOPSY TORSI TORSO TOTSY WOOSH WORSE WORST YOUSE

•O••S

AONES AOUTS BOARS BOATS BOCAS BOCKS BODES BOERS BOFFS BOGGS BOGUS BOHOS BOILS BOLAS BOLDS BOLES BOLLS BOLOS BOLTS BOLUS BOMBS BONDS BONES BONGS BONKS BONUS BOOBS BOOKS BOOMS BOONS BOORS BOOTS BORAS BORES BORGS BORIS BORKS BOROS BOSCS BOSNS BOTTS BOUTS BOWES BOWLS BOXES BOYOS BOZOS COALS COATS COCAS COCKS COCOS CODAS CODES COEDS COHOS COIFS COILS COINS COIRS COKES COLAS COLDS COLES COLTS COMAS COMBS

COMES COMPS COMUS CONDS CONES CONKS CONNS CONTS CONUS COOKS COOLS COONS COOPS COORS COOTS COPES COPTS CORDS CORES CORKS CORMS CORNS CORPS COSTS COTES COUPS COVES COWES COWLS COXES COZES DOANS DOATS DOBBS DOCES DOCKS DODOS DOERS DOFFS DOGES DOITS DOJOS DOLES DOLLS DOLTS DOMES DOMOS DONAS DONGS DONTS DONUS DOOMS DOORS DOPAS DOPES DORIS DORKS DORMS DORPS DOSES DOTES DOUBS DOVES DOWNS DOZES EOLUS FOALS FOAMS

FOCUS FOHNS FOIES FOILS FOLDS FOLKS FONTS FOODS FOOLS FOOTS FORDS FORES FORKS FORMS FORTS FOULS FOURS FOUTS FOWLS FOXES GOADS GOALS GOATS GOBOS GOERS GOGOS GOLDS GOLFS GONGS GOODS GOOFS GOOKS GOONS GOOPS GORES GORMS GORPS GOTHS GOUTS GOVTS GOWNS GOYAS HOARS HOBBS HOBOS HOCKS HOCUS HOERS HOHOS HOJOS HOKES HOLDS HOLES HOLMS HOMES HONES HONKS HONUS HOODS HOOFS HOOKS HOOPS HOOTS HOPES HOPIS HORAS HORNS HORUS

HOSES HOSPS HOSTS HOURS HOVIS HOWES HOWLS HOYAS IOTAS IOWAS JOADS JOCKS JOEYS JOHNS JOINS JOKES JOLTS JONAS JONES JOOSS JOTAS JOURS JOWLS KOANS KOBOS KODES KOHLS KOJIS KOLAS KONAS KOOKS KOPHS KOTOS LOADS LOAFS LOAMS LOANS LOBES LOBOS LOCHS LOCKS LOCOS LOCUS LODES LOESS LOEWS LOFTS LOGES LOGOS LOIDS LOINS LOLLS LOMAS LONGS LOOKS LOOMS LOONS LOOPS LOOTS LOPES LORDS LORES LORIS LORUS LOSES LOTOS LOTUS LOUIS

LOUPS LOURS LOUTS LOVES LOWES LOXES MOANS MOATS MOCKS MODES MODUS MOILS MOJOS MOLDS MOLES MOLLS MOLTS MOMUS MONKS MONOS MONTS MOODS MOOGS MOONS MOORS MOOTS MOPES MORAS MORES MORNS MOROS MOSES MOTES MOTHS MOTTS MOUES MOVES MOWIS MOZOS NOBIS NOCKS NODES NODUS NOELS NOGAS NOGGS NOGOS NOILS NOIRS NOLES NOLOS NOMAS NONES NONOS NOOKS NOONS NOPES NORIS NORMS NORNS NOSES NOTES NOTUS NOUNS NOVAS NOVUS NOYES OOZES

POCUS POEMS POETS POKES POLES POLIS POLKS POLLS POLOS POMES POMOS PONDS PONES PONGS PONTS POOHS POOLS POOPS POORS POPES PORCS PORES PORKS PORTS POSES POSTS POTTS POTUS POUFS POURS POUTS POWYS POXES QOPHS ROADS ROAMS ROANS ROARS ROBES ROCKS ROILS ROJAS ROLES ROLFS ROLLS ROLOS ROMES ROMPS ROODS ROOFS ROOKS ROOMS ROOTS ROPES ROSES ROTAS ROTCS ROTES ROTHS ROTLS ROTOS ROUES ROUTS ROVES SOAKS SOAPS SOARS SOBAS

SOCAS SOCKS SODAS SOFAS SOILS SOIRS SOLES SOLOS SOMAS SONES SONGS SONYS SOOTS SOPHS SORAS SORBS SORES SOROS SORTS SOULS SOUPS SOURS SOYAS TOADS TODOS TOEAS TOFFS TOFTS TOFUS TOGAS TOILS TOKES TOLES TOLLS TOMAS TOMBS TOMES TONES TONGS TONUS TONYS TOOLS TOONS TOOTS TOPES TOPIS TOPPS TORAS TOROS TORRS TORTS TORUS TOTES TOURS TOUTS TOVES TOWNS TOYOS VOIDS VOIPS VOLES VOLTS VOTES WOADS WOLFS WOMBS WONKS WONTS

WOODS WOOFS WOOLS WORDS WORKS WORMS WORTS XOUTS YODHS YOGAS YOGIS YOKES YOLKS YORES YORKS YOURS YOWLS YOYOS ZONES ZONKS ZOOMS ZORIS ZOUKS

••OS•

AROSE BGOSH BOOST CHOSE CLOSE COOSA CROSS DROSS EROSE FLOSS FROSH FROST GHOST GLOSS GOOSE GOOSY GROSS GROSZ HROSS ICOSA ICOSI ILOSE JOOSS KIOSK KOOSH LLOSA LOOSE MOOSE NOOSE PROSE PROSS PROST PROSY ROOSA ROOST SKOSH SLOSH SPOSA SPOSE SPOSO THOSE WHOSE WHOSO

WOOSH XHOSA

••O•S

AEONS AHOYS ALOES ALOIS ALORS AMORS ANOAS APODS ASORS ATOMS AVOWS AWOLS AXONS BBOYS BIOGS BLOBS BLOCS BLOGS BLOIS BLOTS BLOWS BMOCS BOOBS BOOKS BOOMS BOONS BOORS BOOTS BROWS BUOYS CHOPS CHOWS CIONS CLODS CLOGS CLOPS CLOTS CLOYS COOKS COOLS COONS COOPS COORS COOTS CROCS CROPS CROSS CROWS DHOWS DIORS DOOMS DOORS DROPS DROSS EBONS ECONS ENOLS EROES ESOPS ETONS EWOKS EXONS FLOES FLOGS

FLOPS FLOSS FLOWS FOODS FOOLS FOOTS FROES FROGS FROWS GAOLS GLOBS GLOMS GLOPS GLOSS GLOWS GOODS GOOFS GOOKS GOONS GOOPS GROGS GROKS GROSS GROTS GROWS HOODS HOOFS HOOKS HOOPS HOOTS HROSS ICONS IDOLS IHOPS IPODS IROCS IRONS IZODS JOOSS KAONS KNOBS KNOTS KNOWS KOOKS LIONS LOOKS LOOMS LOONS LOOPS LOOTS LYONS MEOWS MOODS MOOGS MOONS MOORS MOOTS MUONS NEONS NOOKS NOONS OBOES OBOLS ODORS OHOHS OTOES PAONS PEONS

PHONS PHOTS PIONS PIOUS PLODS PLOPS PLOTS PLOWS PLOYS POOHS POOLS POOPS POORS PROAS PROBS PRODS PROFS PROGS PROMS PROPS PROSS PROTS PROVS PROWS RIOTS ROODS ROOFS ROOKS ROOMS ROOTS SCOTS SCOWS SHOES SHOOS SHOPS SHOTS SHOWS SLOBS SLOES SLOGS SLOPS SLOTS SLOWS SMOGS SNOBS SNOWS SOOTS SPOTS STOAS STOLS STOPS STOWS THOUS TIOUS TOOLS TOONS TOOTS TROIS TROTS TROWS TTOPS ULOUS UROUS VIOLS VTOLS WHOPS WOODS WOOFS

WOOLS XEONS YEOWS ZOOMS

•••OS

ACTOS ADIOS AEROS AFROS AGIOS ALIOS ALTOS AMBOS AMMOS APSOS ARGOS ATHOS ATMOS ATNOS AUTOS BACOS BANOS BESOS BEZOS BIROS BOHOS BOLOS BOROS BOYOS BOZOS CAMOS CAPOS CEROS CHAOS CHIOS CIAOS CLIOS COCOS COHOS DADOS DATOS DAVOS DEDOS DELOS DEMOS DIDOS DINOS DODOS DOJOS DOMOS DUROS ECHOS EGGOS ELLOS ELMOS ERDOS ESTOS ETHOS EUROS EXPOS FADOS FAROS FILOS FINOS FUROS GATOS GIROS

GOBOS GOGOS GYROS HALOS HELOS HEROS HIHOS HIJOS HOBOS HOHOS HOJOS HUGOS HYPOS JANOS JATOS JENOS JUCOS JUDOS KAYOS KENOS KILOS KOBOS KOTOS KUDOS LAGOS LANOS LEGOS LENOS LEROS LIDOS LIMOS LINOS LOBOS LOCOS LOGOS LOTOS LYCOS MAKOS MANOS MAYOS MELOS MEMOS MENOS MILOS MINOS MIROS MISOS MOJOS MONOS MOROS MOZOS MSDOS NAXOS NEMOS NEPOS NINOS NOGOS NOLOS NONOS OCHOS OGROS OLEOS OLIOS OLMOS OREOS ORLOS ORZOS OTROS

OUZOS PALOS PAROS PASOS PATOS PAXOS PECOS PEPOS PESOS PETOS POLOS POMOS PYROS RAMOS REDOS REPOS ROLOS ROTOS SAGOS SAMOS SAROS SEGOS SHOOS SILOS SOLOS SOROS STROS SUMOS TACOS TAROS TICOS TIROS TIVOS TODOS TOROS TOYOS TRIOS TYPOS TYROS UPDOS VAMOS VINOS YOYOS YUGOS YUKOS ZENOS ZEROS

OT•••

OTARU OTARY OTERI OTERO OTHER OTHON OTILE OTOES OTOMI OTONO OTOWN OTRAS OTROS OTTER OTTIS OTTOI OTWAY

O•T••

OATEN OATER OATES OATHS OCTAD OCTAL OCTAN OCTET OFTEN ONTAP ONTOP ONTWO OOTID OPTED OPTIC OPTIN OPTTO ORTHO ORTIZ ORTON OSTAR OSTEO OSTER OSTIA OTTER OTTIS OTTOI OUTDO OUTED OUTER OUTGO OUTIE OUTOF OUTON OUTRE OUTTA

O••T•

OASTS OBITS OBOTE ODETS OESTE OLETA OMITS ONATE OPTTO ORATE OUSTS OUTTA OVATE OVETA OVETT OVITZ

O•••T

OBJET OCRAT OCTET ODIST ODONT ONDIT ONSET OPART OPCIT ORANT ORBIT

OSSET OUEST OUGHT OVERT OVETT OWLET

•OT••

BOTCH BOTEL BOTHA BOTHE BOTOX BOTTS COTAN COTES COTTA DOTAL DOTED DOTER DOTES DOTTO DOTTY GOTAB GOTAC GOTAD GOTAT GOTBY GOTHA GOTHS GOTIN GOTIT GOTME GOTON GOTTA GOTTI GOTTO GOTUP HOTEL HOTLY HOTON HOTSY IOTAS JOTAS JOTTO KOTCH KOTOS KOTTO LOTET LOTNO LOTOS LOTSA LOTTA LOTTE LOTTO LOTUS MOTEL MOTES MOTET MOTHS MOTHY MOTIF MOTOR MOTTO MOTTS NOTAH NOTAX NOTCH

NOTDO
NOTED
NOTER
NOTES
NOTIE
NOTIN
NOTIP
NOTIT
NOTME
NOTOK
NOTON
NOTRE
NOTSO
NOTTE
NOTTI
NOTUP
NOTUS
OOTID
POTOK
POTSY
POTTO
POTTS
POTTY
POTUS
ROTAS
ROTCS
ROTES
ROTHS
ROTLS
ROTOR
ROTOS
SOTTO
TOTAL
TOTED
TOTEM
TOTER
TOTES
TOTIE
TOTSY
TOTUP
VOTED
VOTER
VOTES
VOTRE
WOTAN
YOTTO

•O•T•

AORTA
AOSTA
AOUTS
BOATS
BOITE
BOITO
BOLTS
BOOTH
BOOTS
BOOTY
BOTTS
BOUTS
BOWTO
COATI
COATS
COLTS
COMTE
CONTD
CONTE
CONTI
CONTR
CONTS
COOTE
COOTS
COOTY
COPTO
COPTS
COSTA
COSTS
COTTA
COUTH
DOATS
DOETH
DOITS
DOLTS
DONTS
DOTTO
DOTTY
DOUTE
FONTS
FOOTE
FOOTS
FORTE
FORTH
FORTS
FORTY
FOUTS
FOXTV
GOATS
GOETH
GOTTA
GOTTI
GOTTO
GOUTS
GOUTY
GOVTS
HOITY
HOLTZ
HOOTS
HOPTO
HOSTA
HOSTS
HOWTO
JOLTS
JOLTY
JOTTO
KOTTO
LOATH
LOFTS
LOFTY
LOOTS
LOTTA
LOTTE
LOTTO
LOUTH
LOUTS
MOATS
MOLTO
MOLTS
MONTE
MONTH
MONTS
MONTY
MOOTS
MORTE
MORTY
MOTTO
MOTTS
MOUTH
NOCTI
NODTO
NOLTE
NORTE
NORTH
NOTTE
NOTTI
POETE
POETS
PONTA
PONTE
PONTI
PONTS
PORTA
PORTE
PORTO
PORTS
POSTE
POSTS
POTTO
POTTS
POTTY
POUTS
POUTY
ROOTS
ROOTY
ROUTE
ROUTS
SOFTC
SOFTG
SOFTY
SOLTI
SOOTH
SOOTS
SOOTY
SORTA
SORTS
SOTTO
SOUTH
TOFTS
TOITY
TONTO
TOOTH
TOOTS
TORTA
TORTE
TORTS
TOUTE
TOUTS
VOLTA
VOLTE
VOLTS
WONTS
WORTH
WORTS
XOUTS
YOCTO
YORTY
YOTTO
YOUTH

•O••T

BOAST
BOLET
BONET
BOOAT
BOOST
BOULT
BOVET
COACT
COAPT
COAST
COMET
CONST
COOPT
COPIT
COROT
COSET
COUNT
COURT
COVET
DOEST
DOGIT
DONAT
DONOT
DONUT
DOUBT
FOIST
FOUNT
GOAFT
GOBAT
GOBOT
GODET
GODOT
GOEST
GOGET
GOOUT
GOSIT
GOTAT
GOTIT
HOEST
HOIST
HOLST
HORST
JOINT
JOIST
JOUST
KOPIT
KORAT
LOFAT
LOPAT
LOTET
MOIST
MONET
MOTET
MOULT
MOUNT
MOWAT
NOBET
NOCUT
NODAT
NOFAT
NOHIT
NONET
NOORT
NOTIT
POINT
POLIT
POSIT
POULT
ROAST
ROBOT
ROGET
ROOST
ROUST
SOMAT
TOAST
TOBIT
TOLET
TOWIT
WOFAT
WONAT
WOPAT
WORST
YOUNT

••OT•

AZOTH
BIOTA
BLOTS
BOOTH
BOOTS
BOOTY
BROTH
CLOTH
CLOTS
CNOTE
COOTE
COOTS
COOTY
DHOTE
DHOTI
EMOTE
ENOTE
FOOTE
FOOTS
FROTH
GLOTT
GNOTE
GROTE
GROTS
HOOTS
JROTC
KNOTS
KNOTT
KROTO
KYOTO
LOOTS
MOOTS
NROTC
OBOTE
PHOTO
PHOTS
PLOTS
PLOTZ
PROTO
PROTS
QUOTA
QUOTE
QUOTH
RIOTS
ROOTS
ROOTY
SCOTS
SCOTT
SHOTS
SLOTH
SLOTS
SMOTE
SOOTH
SOOTS
SOOTY
SPOTS
TNOTE
TOOTH
TOOTS
TROTH
TROTS
WROTE
WROTH
ZLOTY

••O•T

ABORT
ABOUT
ADOPT
ADOUT
AFOOT
AHOOT
ALOFT
AMORT
APORT
BIONT
BLOAT
BOOAT
BOOST
CLOUT
COOPT
CROAT
CROFT
DROIT
DROPT
EBOAT
FLOAT
FLOUT
FRONT
FROOT
FROST
GHOST
GLOAT
GLOTT
GOOUT
GROAT
GROUT
IDONT
IMOUT
ISOLT
IWONT
KNOTT
KNOUT
KROFT
NIORT
NOORT
ODONT
PROST
QUOIT
ROOST
SCOOT
SCOTT
SCOUT
SHOAT
SHOOT
SHORT
SHOUT
SKORT
SMOLT
SMOOT
SNOOT
SNORT
SNOUT
SPORT
SPOUT
STOAT
STOUT
TROUT
UBOAT
UBOLT
XDOUT
XSOUT

•••OT

ABBOT
AFOOT
AHOOT
ALLOT
ARGOT
ARIOT
ASCOT
ASHOT
BEGOT
BESOT
BIGOT
BYLOT
CABOT
COROT
CSPOT
DEPOT
DICOT
DIVOT
DONOT
ELIOT
ELYOT
EPCOT
ERGOT
FAGOT
FROOT
GAVOT
GIGOT
GOBOT
GODOT
GRIOT
HELOT
HULOT
IDIOT
IFNOT
IMHOT
INGOT
JABOT
MAROT
MELOT
MINOT
PEROT
PICOT
PILOT
PINOT
PITOT
PIVOT
REPOT
ROBOT
RVLOT
SABOT
SCOOT
SHOOT
SMOOT
SNOOT
TAROT
UNGOT
UNHOT
UNPOT

OU•••

OUEST
OUGHT
OUIDA
OUIJA
OUNCE
OURAY
OUSEL
OUSTS
OUTDO
OUTED
OUTER
OUTGO
OUTIE
OUTOF
OUTON
OUTRE
OUTTA
OUZEL
OUZOS

O•U••

OCULI
OCULO
OEUFS
OFUSE
ORURO
OVULE

O••U•

OAKUM
OCCUR
ODEUM
ODIUM
ODOUL
ODOUR
OLEUM
ONCUE
ONEUP
OPIUM
ORCUS
ORIUM
OWNUP

O•••U

OHIOU
OHYOU
OTARU

•OU••

AOUTS
BOUGH
BOULE
BOULT
BOUND
BOURG
BOUTS
COUCH
COUGH
COULD
COUNT
COUPE
COUPS
COURT
COURU
COUSY
COUTH
DOUAI
DOUAY
DOUBS
DOUBT
DOUCE
DOUGH
DOULA
DOURO
DOUSE
DOUTE
DOUZE
FOULS
FOUND
FOUNT
FOURA
FOURB
FOURC
FOURD
FOURE
FOURF
FOURH
FOURS
FOUTS
GOUDA
GOUDY
GOUGE
GOULD
GOURD
GOUTS
GOUTY
HOUGH
HOUMA
HOUND
HOURI
HOURS
HOUSE
JOULE
JOURS
JOUST
JOUVE
LOUIE
LOUIS
LOUMA
LOUPE
LOUPS
LOURS
LOURY
LOUSE
LOUSY
LOUTH
LOUTS
MOUCH
MOUES
MOULD
MOULT
MOUND
MOUNT
MOURN
MOUSE
MOUSY
MOUTH
NOUNS
NOURI
NOUSE
POUCH
POUFS
POULE
POULT
POUND
POURS
POUTS
POUTY
ROUEN
ROUES
ROUGE
ROUGH
ROUND
ROUSE
ROUSH
ROUST
ROUTE
ROUTS
SOUCI
SOULS
SOUND
SOUPS
SOUPY
SOURS
SOUSA
SOUSE
SOUTH
TOUCH
TOUGH
TOURO
TOURS
TOUTE
TOUTS
VOUCH
WOULD
WOUND
XOUTS
YOULL
YOUNG
YOUNT
YOURE
YOURN
YOURS
YOUSE
YOUTH
YOUVE
ZOUKS

•O•U•

BOBUP
BOEUF
BOGUS
BOLUS
BONUM
BONUS
BOSUN
BOXUP
COEUR
COLUM
COMUS
CONUS
COQUI
DONUS
DONUT
EOLUS
FOCUS
FOGUP
FORUM
GOOUT
GOTUP
HOCUS
HOHUM
HOKUM
HONUS
HOPUP
HORUS
JORUM
LOCUM
LOCUS
LOGUE
LORUS
LOTUS
MODUS
MOGUL
MOMUS
MOPUP
MOSUL
NOCUT
NODUH
NODUS
NOFUN
NORUN
NOTUP
NOTUS
NOVUS
POCUS
POPUP
POTUS
ROGUE
ROQUE
SOEUR
SOPUP
SOYUZ
TOFUS
TOGUE
TOGUP
TONUS
TOPUP
TOQUE
TORUS
TOTUP
VOGUE
YOKUM

•O••U

CORFU
CORNU
COURU
COYPU
DONAU
FONDU
IOWAU
KOMBU
LONGU
POILU
PONZU
TOYOU

••OU•

ABOUT
ADOUT
AFOUL
ALOUD
AMOUR
ANOUK
ASOUL
BFOUR
BROUD
BROUN
CLOUD
CLOUT
CROUP
FLOUR
FLOUT
GHOUL
GOOUT
GROUP
GROUT
HHOUR
IFOUR
IMOUT
KNOUT
ODOUL
ODOUR
PIOUS
PROUD
RAOUL
SCOUR
SCOUT
SEOUL
SHOUT
SIOUX
SNOUT
SPOUT
STOUT
THOUS
TIOUS
TROUP
TROUT
TWOUP
ULOUS
UROUS
VFOUR
XDOUT
XSOUT

••O•U

INONU
UPOLU

•••OU

AEIOU
ANJOU
BAYOU
BIJOU
GAROU
MIAOU
OHIOU
OHYOU
TOYOU

OV•••

OVALS
OVARY
OVATE
OVENS
OVERS
OVERT
OVETA
OVETT
OVINE
OVITZ
OVOID
OVOLI
OVOLO
OVULE

O•V••

ORVAL
ORVIS
OYVEY

O••V•

OGIVE
OLAVI
OLAVV
OLIVA
OLIVE
ONDVD

O•••V

OLAFV
OLAVV

•OV••

BOVET
BOVID
COVED
COVEN
COVER
COVES
COVET
COVEY
DOVER
DOVES
DOVEY
GOVTS
HOVEL
HOVER
HOVEY
HOVIS
JOVAN
KOVIC
LOVED
LOVER
LOVES
LOVEY
LOVIN
MOVED
MOVER
MOVES
MOVIE
MOVIN
NOVAE
NOVAK
NOVAS
NOVEL
NOVEM
NOVIA
NOVIO
NOVUS
ROVED
ROVER
ROVES
TOVAH
TOVES
WOVEN

•O•V•

CONVY
CORVO
JOUVE
NORVO
SOAVE
SOLVE
VOLVO
YOUVE

•O••V

BOOKV
FOXTV
JOHNV
POPOV

••OV•

ABOVE
ABOVO
CLOVE
DROVE
GLOVE
GROVE
ILOVE
IMOVE
LEOVI
NUOVA
NUOVO
PROVE
PROVO
PROVS
SHOVE
STOVE
TROVE

••O•V

BOOKV
LEOIV

•••OV

BASOV
EXGOV
KIROV
LTGOV
POPOV
TITOV
YAKOV

OW•••

OWENS
OWEON
OWERS
OWIES
OWING
OWLET
OWNED
OWNER
OWNUP

O•W••

OHWOW
OTWAY

O••W•

ONTWO
OTOWN
OZAWA

O•••W

OHWOW
ONLOW
OXBOW

•OW••

BOWED
BOWEL
BOWEN
BOWER
BOWES
BOWIE
BOWLS
BOWTO
COWED
COWER
COWES
COWLS
COWRY
DOWDY
DOWEL
DOWNS
DOWNY
DOWRY
DOWSE
FOWLS
GOWDY
GOWER
GOWNS
HOWAR
HOWDO
HOWDY
HOWES
HOWIE
HOWLS
HOWSO
HOWTO
IOWAN
IOWAS
IOWAU
IOWAY
JOWLS
JOWLY
LOWED
LOWER
LOWES
LOWIQ
LOWLY
LOWON
LOWPH
LOWRY
MOWAT
MOWED
MOWEN
MOWER
MOWIS
NOWAY
NOWIN
POWAY
POWER
POWYS
ROWAN
ROWDY
ROWED
ROWEL
ROWEN
ROWER
ROWLF
ROWSE
SOWED
SOWER
TOWAR
TOWED
TOWEL
TOWER
TOWIN
TOWIT
TOWNE
TOWNS
VOWED
VOWEL
VOWER
WOWED
WOWEE
WOWEM
WOWIE
YOWIE
YOWLS
YOWZA
ZOWIE

•O•W•

COOWN
LOEWE
LOEWI
LOEWS
LOEWY

•O••W

DONOW
GONOW
NOHOW
SOFEW
TONOW

••OW•

AVOWS
BLOWN
BLOWS
BLOWY
BROWN
BROWS
CHOWS
CLOWN
COOWN
CROWD
CROWE
CROWN
CROWS
DHOWS
DROWN
FLOWN
FLOWS
FROWN
FROWS
GLOWS
GROWL
GROWN
GROWS
KIOWA
KNOWN
KNOWS
MEOWS
OTOWN
PLOWS
PROWL
PROWS
REOWN
SCOWL
SCOWS
SHOWN
SHOWS
SHOWY
SLOWS
SNOWE
SNOWS
SNOWY
STOWE
STOWS
TROWE
TROWS
YEOWS

•••OW

AGLOW
ALLOW
ARROW
BELOW
BULOW
BYNOW
DONOW
ELBOW
ENDOW
GAMOW
GONOW
IKNOW
INLOW
INTOW
KAPOW
MIAOW
MINOW
NOHOW
OHWOW
ONLOW
OXBOW
REMOW
RESOW
RETOW
SYDOW
THROW
TONOW
TUROW
UPBOW
WIDOW
YALOW
YKNOW

OX•••

OXANA
OXBOW
OXEYE
OXFAM
OXIDE
OXLIP

•OX••

BOXED
BOXER
BOXES
BOXIN
BOXUP
COXAE
COXED
COXES
DOXIE
FOXED
FOXES
FOXTV
HOXHA
LOXES
MOXIE
POXES
ROXIE
TOXIC

TOXIN
XOXOX

•O••X
BOOKX
BORAX
BOSOX
BOTOX
CODEX
COMEX
COMIX
JOHNX
LOMAX
LORAX
NOTAX
POBOX
ROLEX
XOXOX
YONEX

••OX•
DEOXY
EPOXY
LEOXI
PROXY

••O•X
BOOKX
BRONX
CROIX
LEOIX
SIOUX

•••OX
BOSOX
BOTOX
DETOX
INBOX
LENOX
MADOX
MRFOX
PHLOX
POBOX
REBOX
REDOX
UNBOX
VELOX
XEROX
XOXOX

OY•••
OYERS
OYVEY

O•Y••
OHYES
OHYOU

O••Y•
OBEYS
OBGYN
OHAYO
OJAYS
OKAYS
ONKYO
ONRYE
OXEYE

O•••Y
ODDLY
OHBOY
OHJOY
OHKAY
OLOGY
ONKEY
ONLAY
ORACY
ORCZY
ORORY
ORSAY
OSHAY
OTARY
OTWAY
OURAY
OVARY
OYVEY

•OY••
BOYER
BOYLE
BOYOS
COYER
COYLY
COYPU
DOYCE
DOYEN
DOYLE
DOYLY
FOYER
FOYLE
GOYAS
GOYEN
HOYAS
HOYLE
JOYCE
JOYED
LOYAL
NOYCE
NOYES
ROYAL
ROYCE
ROYKO
SOYAS
SOYUZ
TOYED
TOYER
TOYON
TOYOS
TOYOU
YOYOS

•O•Y•
JOEYS
POLYP
POWYS
ROBYN
RODYA
SONYA
SONYS
TOKYO
TONYA
TONYS
WOMYN

•O••Y
AOKAY
BOBBY
BOCHY
BODDY
BOGEY
BOGGY
BOHAY
BONEY
BONNY
BOOBY
BOOMY
BOOTY
BOSSY
COCKY
COLBY
COMFY
CONEY
CONVY
COODY
COOKY
COOTY
COPAY
CORBY
COREY
CORKY
CORNY
COSBY
COUSY
COVEY
COWRY
COYLY
DODGY
DOGGY
DOILY
DOISY
DOKEY
DOLBY
DOLLY
DONNY
DOODY
DOOMY
DOOZY
DOPEY
DORKY
DORMY
DOSAY
DOTTY
DOUAY
DOVEY
DOWDY
DOWNY
DOWRY
DOYLY
FOAMY
FOGEY
FOGGY
FOLEY
FOLKY
FOLLY
FOOZY
FORAY
FORKY
FORTY
GODEY
GODLY
GOLLY
GOODY
GOOEY
GOOFY
GOONY
GOOPY
GOOSY
GORBY
GORDY
GOREY
GORKY
GORSY
GOTBY
GOUDY
GOUTY
GOWDY
HOAGY
HOARY
HOBBY
HOBEY
HOITY
HOKEY
HOLEY
HOLLY
HOMEY
HONEY
HONKY
HOODY
HOOEY
HOOKY
HOPPY
HORNY
HORSY
HOTLY
HOTSY
HOVEY
HOWDY
IOWAY
JOKEY
JOLLY
JOLTY
JONNY
JOSEY
JOWLY
KOOKY
LOAMY
LOBBY
LOEWY
LOFTY
LOLLY
LOOBY
LOOEY
LOOKY
LOONY
LOOPY
LOPPY
LORDY
LORRY
LOSEY
LOURY
LOUSY
LOVEY
LOWLY
LOWRY
MOLDY
MOLLY
MOMMY
MONEY
MONTY
MOODY
MOONY
MOORY
MOPEY
MOPSY
MORAY
MOREY
MORTY
MOSEY
MOSSY
MOTHY
MOUSY
NOBBY
NOBLY
NODDY
NOILY
NOISY
NOSEY
NOWAY
POBOY
POESY
POKEY
POLLY
POPBY
POPPY
PORGY
PORKY
POSEY
POTSY
POTTY
POUTY
POWAY
ROBBY
ROCKY
RODDY
ROILY
RONNY
ROOKY
ROOMY
ROOTY
ROSEY
ROWDY
SOAPY
SODDY
SOFTY
SOGGY
SONNY
SOOEY
SOOTY
SOPPY
SORRY
SOUPY
TOADY
TOBEY
TODAY
TODDY
TOITY
TOKAY
TOMMY
TOODY
TOPSY
TOTSY
WONBY
WOODY
WOOLY
WOOZY
WORDY
WORMY
WORRY
YOLKY
YORTY
YOSOY
ZOOEY

••OY•
AHOYS
BBOYS
BUOYS
CLOYS
FLOYD
FROYO
LLOYD
PLOYS

••O•Y
AGONY
AMORY
ANOMY
ATOMY
ATONY
ATORY
BLOWY
BOOBY
BOOMY
BOOTY
BRODY
CHOKY
COODY
COOKY
COOTY
CRONY
DEOXY
DOODY
DOOMY
DOOZY
EBONY
EMORY
EPOXY
FLORY
FOOZY
GLORY
GNOMY
GOODY
GOOEY
GOOFY
GOONY
GOOPY
GOOSY
GRODY
HOODY
HOOEY
HOOKY
IRONY
IVORY
KOOKY
LOOBY
LOOEY
LOOKY
LOONY
LOOPY
MOODY
MOONY
MOORY
OLOGY
ORORY
PEONY
PHONY
PROSY
PROXY
RHODY
ROOKY
ROOMY
ROOTY
SHOWY
SMOKY
SNOWY
SOOEY
SOOTY
STOGY
STONY
STORY
TOODY
WOODY
WOOLY
WOOZY
ZLOTY
ZOOEY

•••OY
ALLOY
ALROY
AMBOY
ANNOY
DECOY
ELROY
ENJOY
ENVOY
LEROY
MCCOY
MYBOY
NIMOY
OHBOY
OHJOY
POBOY
SAVOY
SEPOY
UNCOY
YOSOY

OZ•••
OZARK
OZAWA
OZICK
OZONE
OZZIE

O•Z••
OOZED
OOZES
ORZOS
OUZEL
OUZOS
OZZIE

O••Z•
ORCZY

O•••Z
ORTIZ
OVITZ

•OZ••
BOZOS
COZEN
COZES
DOZED
DOZEN
DOZER
DOZES
GOZZI
MOZOS
OOZED
OOZES
POZZO

•O•Z•
BONZE
BONZO
BOOZE
DOOZY
DOUZE
FOOZY
FORZA
GONZO
GOZZI
JONZE
MONZA
PONZI
PONZU
POZZO
WOOZY
YOWZA

•O••Z
GOMEZ
HOLTZ
LOPEZ
MONIZ
NODOZ
SOYUZ
TOPAZ

••OZ•
ADOZE
BOOZE
DOOZY
FOOZY
FROZE
GROZA
GYOZA
WOOZY

••O•Z
GROSZ
PLOTZ

•••OZ
ARROZ
NODOZ

PA•••
PAAVO
PABLO
PABST
PACAS
PACED
PACEM
PACER
PACES
PACEY
PACHY
PACKS
PACTS
PADDY
PADRE
PADUA
PAEAN
PAESE
PAGAN
PAGED
PAGER
PAGES
PAGET
PAIGE
PAILS
PAINE
PAINS
PAINT
PAIRS
PAISA
PAISE
PALAR
PALAU
PALEA
PALED
PALEO
PALER
PALES
PALEY
PALIN
PALLS
PALLY
PALMA
PALME
PALMS
PALMY
PALOS
PALPS
PALSY
PAMBY
PAMPA
PANAM
PANAY
PANDA
PANDL
PANED
PANEL
PANES
PANGS
PANIC
PANIN
PANIS
PANKY
PANNE
PANSY
PANTA
PANTO
PANTS
PANTY
PANZA
PAOLI
PAOLO
PAONS
PAPAL
PAPAS
PAPAW
PAPEL
PAPER
PAPPY
PAPUA
PARAS
PARCA
PARCH
PARCS
PARDO
PARDS
PARED
PAREE
PAREN
PARER
PARES
PAREU
PARGE
PARIS
PARKA
PARKS
PARLE
PARMA
PAROL
PAROO
PAROS
PARRA
PARRS
PARRY
PARSE
PARSI
PARTA
PARTB
PARTC
PARTE
PARTI
PARTS
PARTV
PARTY
PASCH
PASCO
PASEO
PASES
PASHA
PASOS
PASSE
PASSU
PASSY
PASTA
PASTE
PASTO
PASTS
PASTY
PATCH
PATCO
PATED
PATEK
PATEN
PATER
PATES
PATHE
PATHO
PATHS
PATHY
PATIO
PATLY
PATNA
PATON
PATOS
PATRI
PATRO
PATSY
PATTI
PATTY
PAULA
PAULI
PAULO
PAULV
PAUSE
PAVED
PAVEL
PAVER
PAVES
PAVIA
PAVID
PAVIN
PAWAT
PAWED
PAWER
PAWLS
PAWNS
PÁXOS
PAYEE
PAYER
PAYIN
PAYNE
PAYOR
PAYTO
PAYTV
PAYUP

P•A••
PAAVO
PEABO
PEACE
PEACH
PEAKS
PEALE
PEALS
PEANO
PEARL
PEARS
PEARY
PEASE
PEATS
PEATY
PHAGE
PHAGO
PHAGY
PHAIR
PHANY
PHARM
PHASE
PIANI
PIANO
PIAUI
PIAVE
PLACE
PLAGE
PLAID
PLAIN
PLAIT
PLANA
PLANB
PLANE
PLANI
PLANK
PLANO
PLANS
PLANT
PLASH
PLASM
PLAST
PLATA
PLATE
PLATH
PLATO
PLATS
PLATT
PLATY
PLAYA
PLAYS
PLAZA
POACH
PRADA
PRADO
PRAHA
PRAIA
PRAMS
PRANA
PRANK
PRATE
PRATO
PRATT
PRAWN
PRAYS
PSALM
PSATS

P••A•
PACAS
PAEAN
PAGAN
PALAR
PALAU
PANAM
PANAY
PAPAL
PAPAS
PAPAW
PARAS
PAWAT
PCLAB
PEBAS
PECAN
PEDAL
PENAL
PERAN
PERAS
PETAL
PHIAL
PICAS
PIKAS
PILAF
PILAR
PILAU
PIMAS
PISAN
PITAS
PIXAR
PLEAD
PLEAS
PLEAT
PODAL
POLAR
POWAY
PRIAM
PRMAN
PROAM
PROAS
PSHAW
PTRAP
PUKAS
PULAS
PUMAS
PUPAE
PUPAL
PUPAS
PUSAN

P•••A
PADUA
PAISA
PALEA
PALMA
PAMPA
PANDA
PANTA
PANZA
PAPUA
PARCA
PARKA
PARMA
PARRA
PARTA
PASHA
PASTA
PATNA
PAULA
PAVIA
PEKKA
PELLA
PEMBA
PENNA
PENTA
PEPLA
PERMA
PETRA
PHYLA
PIETA
PILEA
PINNA
PINTA
PINZA
PIPPA
PIZZA
PLANA
PLATA
PLAYA
PLAZA
PLENA
PODIA
POLKA
PONCA
PONTA
POONA
POPPA
PORTA
PRADA
PRAHA
PRAIA
PRANA
PRESA
PRIMA
PUKKA
PUNKA
PUNTA

•PA••
APACE
APAIN
APARS
APART
EPACT
IPANA
IPASS
JPAUL
OPAHS
OPALS
OPART
SPAAK
SPACE
SPACY
SPADE
SPADS
SPAGO
SPAHN
SPAIN
SPAKE
SPAMS
SPANG
SPANK
SPANO
SPANS
SPARE
SPARK
SPARS
SPASM
SPATE
SPATS
SPAWN
SPAYS

•P•A•
APEAK
APIAN
APPAL
EPHAH
EPHAS
IPRAY
LPGAS
OPRAH
SPAAK
SPEAK
SPEAR
SPLAT
SPLAY
SPRAT
SPRAY

•P••A
APNEA
APPIA
IPANA
OPERA
SPICA
SPOSA

••PA•
AMPAS
APPAL
ARPAD
ATPAR
CAPAS
COPAL
COPAY
CSPAN
DOPAS
EXPAT
HEPAT
JAPAN
LAPAT
LAPAZ
LOPAT
NEPAL
NIPAS
NIPAT
NOPAL
NOPAR
OLPAE
ONPAR
ORPAH
PAPAL
PAPAS
PAPAW
PUPAE
PUPAL
PUPAS
REPAD
REPAY
RIPAT
SEPAL
STPAT
TAPAS
TOPAZ
TUPAC
TYPAL
WOPAT
YAPAT

••P•A
ALPHA
APPIA
ASPCA
BOPHA
CAPRA
COPIA
COPRA
CUPPA
HEPTA
KAPPA
PAPUA
PEPLA
PIPPA
POPPA
SEPIA
SEPTA
SUPRA
TYPEA
ZAPPA
ZUPPA

•••PA
AMAPA
CULPA
CUPPA
GUAPA
JALPA
KAPPA
KRUPA
LDOPA
NAMPA
NWAPA
OOMPA
PAMPA
PIPPA
POPPA
RASPA
SCAPA
STUPA
TAMPA
VAMPA
VESPA
ZAPPA
ZUPPA

PB•••
PBOOK

P•B••
PABLO
PABST
PEBAS
POBOX
POBOY
POBRE

P••B•
PAMBY
PEABO
PEMBA
PHEBE
PHOBE
PHOBO
PLEBE
PLEBS
POPBY
PROBE
PROBS
PUTBY

P•••B
PARTB
PCLAB
PHLEB
PLANB
PLUMB
PRESB

•PB••
UPBOW

••PB•
POPBY
ZIPBY

••P•B
REPUB
TYPEB

PC•••
PCLAB

P•C••
PACAS
PACED
PACEM
PACER
PACES
PACEY
PACHY
PACKS
PACTS
PECAN
PECHE
PECKS
PECOS
PICAS
PICKS
PICKY
PICON
PICOT
PICTO
PICTS
POCUS
PUCCI
PUCES
PUCKS

P••C•
PARCA
PARCH
PARCS
PASCH
PASCO
PATCH
PATCO
PEACE
PEACH
PENCE
PERCE
PERCH
PERCS
PERCY
PESCE
PESCI
PETCO
PIECE
PINCE
PINCH
PISCI
PITCH
PLACE
PLOCE
PLUCK
POACH
PONCA
PONCE
PONCH
POOCH
PORCH
PORCS
POUCH
PRICE
PRICK
PRICY
PRYCE
PSYCH
PUCCI
PUNCH

P•••C
PANIC
PARTC
PUNIC

•PC••
EPCOT
OPCIT

•P•C•
APACE

EPACT EPICS EPOCH SPACE SPACY SPECD SPECK SPECS SPICA SPICE SPICY SPOCK

•P••C
EPISC OPTIC

••PC•
ASPCA

••P•C
ASPIC TOPIC TUPAC TYPIC

•••PC
IBMPC

P•D••
PADDY PADRE PADUA PEDAL PEDER PEDRO PODAL PODIA PUDDY PUDGY

P••D•
PADDY PANDA PANDL PARDO PARDS PENDS PERDU PIEDS PLODS PONDS PRADA PRADO PRIDE PRNDL PRODS PRUDE PUDDY PURDY

P•••D
PACED PAGED PALED PANED PARED PATED PAVED PAVID PAWED PFERD PIKED PILED PINED PIPED PLAID PLEAD PLIED POKED POLED PORED POSED POUND PRIED PROUD PSEUD PULED

•PD••
UPDOS UPDRY

•P•D•
APODS EPODE IPODS OPEDS SPADE SPADS SPODE SPUDS

•P••D
APHID APIED APTED EPHOD OPTED SPECD SPEED SPEND SPIED UPEND UPPED

••P•D
AMPED ARPAD BIPED BIPOD CAPED COPED CUPID DOPED DUPED GAPED HOPED HYPED JAPED LIPID LOPED MOPED OOPOD PIPED RAPID REPAD ROPED SAPID TAPED TEPID TOPED TYPED UMPED UPPED VAPID WIPED

•••PD
RSVPD

PE•••
PEABO PEACE PEACH PEAKS PEALE PEALS PEANO PEARL PEARS PEARY PEASE PEATS PEATY PEBAS PECAN PECHE PECKS PECOS PEDAL PEDER PEDRO PEEKS PEELE PEELS PEENS PEEPS PEERS PEETE PEEVE PEGGY PEGUY PEKES PEKIN PEKKA PEKOE PELEE PELEG PELFS PELLA PELLE PELLI PELTS PEMBA PENAL PENCE PENDS PENIN PENNA PENNE PENNI PENNY PENTA PENTE PENUP PEONS PEONY PEPIN PEPLA PEPOS PEPPY PEPSI PEPTO PEPUP PEPYS PERAN PERAS PERCE PERCH PERCS PERCY PERDU PERES PEREZ PERFS PERIL PERIS PERKS PERKY PERLE PERMA PERMS PERON PEROT PERPS PERRO PERRY PERSE PERTH PESCE PESCI PESKY PESOS PESTO PESTS PETAL PETCO PETER PETES PETEY PETIT PETOS PETRA PETRE PETRI PETRO PETTI PETTY PEURS PEWEE PEWIT

P•E••
PAEAN PAESE PEEKS PEELE PEELS PEENS PEEPS PEERS PEETE PEEVE PFERD PHEBE PHENO PIECE PIEDS PIELS PIERS PIETA PIETY PLEAD PLEAS PLEAT PLEBE PLEBS PLENA PNEUM POEME POEMS POESY POETE POETS PREEN PREGL PREGO PRELL PREOP PREPS PRESA PRESB PRESE PRESS PREXY PREYS PSEUD PTERO

P••E•
PACED PACEM PACER PACES PACEY PAGED PAGER PAGES PAGET PALEA PALED PALEO PALER PALES PALEY PANED PANEL PANES PAPEL PAPER PARED PAREE PAREN PARER PARES PAREU PASEO PASES PATED PATEK PATEN PATER PATES PAVED PAVEL PAVER PAVES PAWED PAWER PAYEE PAYER PEDER PEKES PELEE PELEG PERES PEREZ PETER PETES PETEY PEWEE PHLEB PIKED PIKER PIKES PILEA PILED PILEI PILER PILES PIMEN PINED PINER PINES PINEY PIPED PIPER PIPES PIPET PIVEN PIXEL PLIED PLIER PLIES PLYER PLZEN POKED POKER POKES POKEY POLED POLER POLES POMES PONES POPES PORED PORER PORES POSED POSER POSES POSEY POWER POXES PREEN PRIED PRIER PRIES PRMEN PROEM PRYER PUCES PUGET PULED PULER PULES PUREE PURER PUREX PYRES PYREX PYXES

P•••E
PADRE PAESE PAIGE PAINE PAISE PALME PANNE PAREE PARGE PARLE PARSE PARTÉ PASSE PASTE PATHE PAUSE PAYEE PAYNE PEACE PEALE PEASE PECHE PEELE PEETE PEEVE PEKOE PELEE PELLE PENCE PENNE PENTE PERCE PERLE PERSE PESCE PETRE PEWEE PHAGE PHASE PHEBE PHILE PHOBE PHONE PHYFE PHYTE PIAVE PIECE PINCE PIQUE PISTE PIUTE PIXIE PLACE PLAGE PLANE PLATE PLEBE PLOCE PLUIE PLUME POBRE POEME POETE POIRE POISE POMME PONCE PONTE POOLE POPLE PORTE POSSE POSTE POULE PRATE PRESE PRICE PRIDE PRIME PRINE PRIZE PROBE PROLE PRONE PROSE PROVE PRUDE PRUNE PRYCE PTILE PULSE PUPAE PUREE PURGE PURSE

•PE••
APEAK APEEK APEEP APERS APERY EPEES JPEGS MPEGS OPEDS OPELS OPENS OPERA OPERE SPEAK SPEAR SPECD SPECK SPECS SPEED SPEER SPEKE SPELL SPELT SPEND SPENT SPERM SPERO SPETS SPEWS UPEND UPENN

•P•E•
APEEK APEEP APFEL APIED APLEY APNEA APPEL APRES APSES APTED APTER EPEES OPPER OPTED SPEED SPEER SPIED SPIEL SPIER SPIES SPREE TPKES UPPED UPPER UPSET YPRES

•P••E
APACE APPLE EPODE EPPIE OPERE OPINE SPACE SPADE SPAKE SPARE SPATE SPEKE SPICE SPIKE SPILE SPINE SPIRE SPITE SPODE SPOKE SPORE SPOSE SPREE SPUME UPONE

••PE•
ALPEN ALPES AMPED APPEL ARPEL ASPEN ASPER BIPED CAPED CAPEK CAPER CAPES CAPET CEPES COPED COPER COPES CUPEL DEPEW DOPED DOPER DOPES DOPEY DUPED DUPER DUPES EXPEL GAPED GAPER GAPES HOPED HOPEH HOPER HOPES HYPED HYPER HYPES IMPEI IMPEL INPEN JAPED JAPER JAPES KOPEK LAPEL LEPEN LEPER LEPEW LOPED LOPER LOPES LOPEZ MAPES MOPED MOPER MOPES MOPEY NAPES NOPES OLPES OPPER PAPEL PAPER PIPED PIPER PIPES PIPET POPES RAPEE REPEG REPEL REPEN RIPEN RIPER ROPED ROPER ROPES RUPEE SUPER SUPES TAPED TAPER TAPES TEPEE TOPED TOPEE TOPER TOPES TYPEA TYPEB TYPED TYPEE TYPEO TYPER TYPES UMPED UNPEG UNPEN UPPED UPPER VIPER WIPED WIPER WIPES YIPES

••P•E
AMPLE APPLE BEPPE COPSE DUPLE DUPRE EAPOE EPPIE HOPPE KOPFE KOPJE LAPSE LEPKE MAPLE NAPPE OLPAE POPLE PUPAE RAPEE RUPEE SUPPE TEPEE TOPEE TYPEE

•••PE
AGAPE BEPPE CARPE COUPE CRAPE CREPE DRAPE DRUPE ELOPE ETAPE GASPE GOAPE GRAPE GRIPE GROPE HOPPE IHOPE LOUPE MYOPE NAPPE RASPE SCAPE SCOPE SHAPE SKYPE SLOPE SNIPE STIPE STUPE SUPPE SWIPE TAUPE TEMPE TRIPE TROPE VOLPE VTYPE XTYPE

PF•••
PFERD PFFFT PFLUG

P•F••
PFFFT PHFFT PUFFS PUFFY

P••F•
PELFS PERFS PFFFT PHFFT PHYFE POUFS PROFS PUFFS PUFFY

P•••F
PILAF PROOF

•PF••
APFEL UPFOR

•P•F•
SPIFF

•P••F
SPIFF SPOOF

••PF•
KOPFE

•••PF
KNOPF

P•G••
PAGAN PAGED PAGER PAGES PAGET PEGGY PEGUY PIGGY PIGIT PUGET PUGGY PYGMY

P••G•
PAIGE PANGS PARGE PEGGY PHAGE PHAGO PHAGY PIGGY PINGS PLAGE PLUGS PONGO PONGS PORGY PREGL PREGO PRIGS PROGS PUDGY PUGGY PUNGS PURGE

P•••G
PELEG PFLUG PRONG

•PG••
LPGAS

•P•G•
JPEGS MPEGS SPAGO

•P••G
APING OPING SPANG SPRIG

••P•G
REPEG TOPOG UNPEG

PH•••
PHAGE PHAGO PHAGY PHAIR PHANY PHARM PHASE PHEBE PHENO PHFFT PHIAL PHILE PHILO PHISH PHLEB PHLOX PHNOM PHOBE PHOBO PHONE PHONO PHONS PHONY PHOTO PHOTS PHYFE PHYLA PHYLL PHYLO PHYTE PHYTO

P•H••
PSHAW

P••H•
PACHY PASHA PATHE PATHO PATHS PATHY PECHE PITHS PITHY POOHS PRAHA PUSHY

P•••H
PARCH PASCH PATCH PEACH PERCH PERTH PHISH PINCH PITCH PLASH PLATH PLUSH POACH PONCH POOCH PORCH POUCH PSYCH PUNCH

•PH••
APHID APHIS EPHAH EPHAS EPHOD EPHOR OPHIR

•P•H•
OPAHS SPAHN

•P••H
APISH EPHAH EPOCH OPRAH

••PH•
ALPHA AMPHI BOPHA KAPHS KOPHS NEPHR OOPHS SOPHS

••P•H
DEPTH HOPEH ORPAH

•••PH
ALEPH BALPH DOLPH GLYPH GRAPH HUMPH LOWPH LYMPH MALPH MORPH NYMPH OOMPH RALPH STAPH SYLPH

PI•••
PIANI PIANO PIAUI PIAVE PICAS PICKS PICKY PICON PICOT PICTO PICTS PIECE PIEDS PIELS PIERS PIETA PIETY PIGGY PIGIT PIKAS PIKED PIKER PIKES PILAF PILAR PILAU PILEA PILED PILEI PILER PILES PILLS PILON PILOT PILUS PIMAS PIMEN PINCE PINCH PINED PINER PINES PINEY PINGS PINKO PINKS PINKY PINNA PINON PINOT PINSK PINTA PINTO PINTS PINUP PINZA PIONS PIOUS PIPED PIPER PIPES PIPET PIPIT PIPPA PIPPI PIQUE PIRNS PISAN PISCI PISMO PISTE PITAS PITCH PITHS PITHY PITON PITOT PITTI PITTS PITYS PIUSI PIUSV PIUSX PIUTE PIVEN PIVOT PIXAR PIXEL PIXIE PIZZA

P•I••
PAIGE PAILS PAINE PAINS PAINT PAIRS PAISA PAISE PHIAL PHILE PHILO PHISH PLIED PLIER PLIES PLINK PLINY POILU POINT POIRE POISE PRIAM PRICE PRICK PRICY PRIDE PRIED PRIER PRIES PRIGS PRIMA PRIME PRIMO PRIMP PRIMS PRINE PRINK PRINT PRIOR PRISM PRISS PRIUS PRIVY PRIZE PRIZM PTILE

P••I•
PALIN PANIC PANIN PANIS

PARIS
PATIO
PAVIA
PAVID
PAVIN
PAYIN
PEKIN
PENIN
PEPIN
PERIL
PERIS
PETIT
PEWIT
PHAIR
PIGIT
PIPIT
PIXIE
PLAID
PLAIN
PLAIT
PLUIE
PODIA
POLIO
POLIS
POLIT
POPIN
POSIT
PRAIA
PULIK
PULIS
PUNIC
PUPIL
PUPIN
PURIM
PUTIN

P•••I
PAOLI
PARSI
PARTI
PATRI
PATTI
PAULI
PELLI
PENNI
PEPSI
PESCI
PETRI
PETTI
PIANI
PIAUI
PILEI
PIPPI
PISCI
PITTI
PIUSI
PLANI
PLURI
PLUVI
PONTI
PONZI
POORI
PUCCI

•PI••
APIAN
APIED
APING
APISH
EPICS
EPISC
OPINE
OPING
OPIUM
SPICA
SPICE
SPICY
SPIED
SPIEL
SPIER
SPIES
SPIFF
SPIKE
SPIKY
SPILE
SPILL
SPILT
SPINE
SPINS
SPINY
SPIRE
SPIRO
SPIRY
SPITE
SPITS
SPITZ

•P•I•
APAIN
APHID
APHIS
APPIA
APRIL
APSIS
EPPIE
OPCIT
OPHIR
OPTIC
OPTIN
SPAIN
SPLIT
SPOIL
SPRIG
SPRIT
UPLIT

•P••I
SPYRI

••PI•
APPIA
ASPIC
ASPIN
COPIA
COPIT
CUPID
DIPIN
DUPIN
ELPIS
EPPIE
ESPIO
GOPIK
HOPIN
HOPIS
KEPIS
KOPIT
LAPIN
LAPIS
LIPID
LUPIN
PEPIN
PIPIT
POPIN
PUPIL
PUPIN
RAPID
REPIN
SAPID
SEPIA
TAPIN
TAPIR
TAPIS
TEPID
TIPIN
TIPIS
TOPIC
TOPIS
TYPIC
UNPIN
VAPID
ZIPIN
ZIPIT

••P•I
AMPHI
CAPRI
CUPRI
IMPEI
LIPPI
PEPSI
PIPPI
TIPPI

•••PI
CARPI
LIPPI
OKAPI
PIPPI
TEMPI
TIPPI

••PJ•
KOPJE

P•K••
PEKES
PEKIN
PEKKA
PEKOE
PIKAS
PIKED
PIKER
PIKES
POKED
POKER
POKES
POKEY
PUKAS
PUKKA

P••K•
PACKS
PANKY
PARKA
PARKS
PEAKS
PECKS
PEEKS
PEKKA
PERKS
PERKY
PESKY
PICKS
PICKY
PINKO
PINKS
PINKY
POLKA
POLKS
PORKS
PORKY
PUCKS
PUKKA
PUNKA
PUNKS
PUNKY

P•••K
PATEK
PBOOK
PINSK
PLANK
PLINK
PLONK
PLUCK
PLUNK
POTOK
PRANK
PRICK
PRINK
PULIK

•PK••
TPKES

•P•K•
SPAKE
SPEKE
SPIKE
SPIKY
SPOKE

•P••K
APEAK
APEEK
SPAAK
SPANK
SPARK
SPEAK
SPECK
SPOCK
SPOOK
SPORK
SPUNK

••PK•
LEPKE

••P•K
CAPEK
GOPIK
KAPOK
KOPEK

PL•••
PLACE
PLAGE
PLAID
PLAIN
PLAIT
PLANA
PLANB
PLANE
PLANI
PLANK
PLANO
PLANS
PLANT
PLASH
PLASM
PLAST
PLATA
PLATE
PLATH
PLATO
PLATS
PLATT
PLATY
PLAYA
PLAYS
PLAZA
PLEAD
PLEAS
PLEAT
PLEBE
PLEBS
PLENA
PLIED
PLIER
PLIES
PLINK
PLINY
PLOCE
PLODS
PLONK
PLOPS
PLOTS
PLOTZ
PLOWS
PLOYS
PLUCK
PLUGS
PLUIE
PLUMB
PLUME
PLUMP
PLUMR
PLUMS
PLUMY
PLUNK
PLURI
PLUSH
PLUTO
PLUVI
PLYER
PLZEN

P•L••
PALAR
PALAU
PALEA
PALED
PALEO
PALER
PALES
PALEY
PALIN
PALLS
PALLY
PALMA
PALME
PALMS
PALMY
PALOS
PALPS
PALSY
PCLAB
PELEE
PELEG
PELFS
PELLA
PELLE
PELLI
PELTS
PFLUG
PHLEB
PHLOX
PILAF
PILAR
PILAU
PILEA
PILED
PILEI
PILER
PILES
PILLS
PILON
PILOT
PILUS
POLAR
POLED
POLER
POLES
POLIO
POLIS
POLIT
POLKA
POLKS
POLLO
POLLS
POLLY
POLOS
POLYP
PULAS
PULED
PULER
PULES
PULIK
PULIS
PULLS
PULMO
PULPS
PULPY
PULSE
PYLON

P••L•
PABLO
PAILS
PALLS
PALLY
PAOLI
PAOLO
PARLE
PATLY
PAULA
PAULI
PAULO
PAULV
PAWLS
PEALE
PEALS
PEELE
PEELS
PELLA
PELLE
PELLI
PEPLA
PERLE
PHILE
PHILO
PHYLA
PHYLL
PHYLO
PIELS
PILLS
POILU
POLLO
POLLS
POLLY
POOLE
POOLS
POPLE
POULE
POULT
PRELL
PROLE
PSALM
PTILE
PULLS
PURLS

P•••L
PANDL
PANEL
PAPAL
PAPEL
PAROL
PAVEL
PEARL
PEDAL
PENAL
PERIL
PETAL
PHIAL
PHYLL
PIXEL
PODAL
PREGL
PRELL
PRNDL
PROWL
PUPAL
PUPIL

•PL••
APLEY
APLUS
BPLUS
CPLUS
DPLUS
SPLAT
SPLAY
SPLIT
UPLIT

•P•L•
APPLE
APPLY
APTLY
OPALS
OPELS
SPELL
SPELT
SPILE
SPILL
SPILT
UPOLU

•P••L
APFEL
APPAL
APPEL
APRIL
JPAUL
SPELL
SPIEL
SPILL
SPOIL
SPOOL

••PL•
AMPLE
AMPLY
APPLE
APPLY
DIPLO
DUPLE
DUPLO
HAPLY
HIPLY
IMPLY
MAPLE
PEPLA
POPLE
REPLY

••P•L
APPAL
APPEL
ARPEL
COPAL
CUPEL
EXPEL
IMPEL
LAPEL
NEPAL
NOPAL
PAPAL
PAPEL
PUPAL
PUPIL
REPEL
SEPAL
TOPOL
TYPAL

P•M••
PAMBY
PAMPA
PEMBA
PIMAS
PIMEN
POMES
POMME
POMOS
PRMAN
PRMEN
PUMAS
PUMPS

P••M•
PALMA
PALME
PALMS
PALMY
PARMA
PERMA
PERMS
PISMO
PLUMB
PLUME
PLUMP
PLUMR
PLUMS
PLUMY
POEME
POEMS
POMME
PRAMS
PRIMA
PRIME
PRIMO
PRIMP
PRIMS
PROMO
PROMS
PULMO
PYGMY

P•••M
PACEM
PANAM
PHARM
PHNOM
PLASM
PNEUM
PRIAM
PRISM
PRIZM
PROAM
PROEM
PSALM
PURIM

•P•M•
SPAMS
SPUME
SPUMY

•P••M
EPROM
EPSOM
OPIUM
SPASM
SPERM

•••PM
ONEPM
SIXPM
TENPM
TWOPM

PN•••
PNEUM

P•N••
PANAM
PANAY
PANDA
PANDL
PANED
PANEL
PANES
PANGS
PANIC
PANIN
PANIS
PANKY
PANNE
PANSY
PANTA
PANTO
PANTS
PANTY
PANZA
PENAL
PENCE
PENDS
PENIN
PENNA
PENNE
PENNI
PENNY
PENTA
PENTE
PENUP
PHNOM
PINCE
PINCH
PINED
PINER
PINES
PINEY
PINGS
PINKO
PINKS
PINKY
PINNA
PINON
PINOT
PINSK
PINTA
PINTO
PINTS
PINUP
PINZA
PONCA
PONCE
PONCH
PONDS
PONES
PONGO
PONGS
PONTA
PONTE
PONTI
PONTS
PONZI
PONZU
PRNDL
PUNCH
PUNGS
PUNIC
PUNKA
PUNKS
PUNKY
PUNNY
PUNTA
PUNTS

P••N•
PAINE
PAINS
PAINT
PANNE
PAONS
PATNA
PAWNS
PAYNE
PEANO
PEENS
PENNA
PENNE
PENNI
PENNY
PEONS
PEONY
PHANY
PHENO
PHONE
PHONO
PHONS
PHONY
PIANI
PIANO
PINNA
PIONS
PIRNS
PLANA
PLANB
PLANE
PLANI
PLANK
PLANO
PLANS
PLANT
PLENA
PLINK
PLINY
PLONK
PLUNK
POINT
POONA
PORNO
POUND
PRANA
PRANK
PRINE
PRINK
PRINT
PRONE
PRONG
PRUNE
PUNNY

P•••N
PAEAN
PAGAN
PALIN
PANIN
PAREN
PATEN
PATON
PAVIN
PAYIN
PECAN
PEKIN
PENIN
PEPIN
PERAN
PERON
PICON
PILON
PIMEN
PINON
PISAN
PITON
PIVEN
PLAIN
PLZEN
POPIN
PRAWN
PREEN
PRMAN
PRMEN
PUPIN
PUSAN
PUTIN
PUTON
PYLON

•PN••
APNEA

•P•N•
APING
IPANA
OPENS
OPINE
OPING
SPANG
SPANK
SPANO
SPANS
SPEND
SPENT
SPINE
SPINS
SPINY
SPUNK
UPEND
UPENN
UPONE

•P••N
APAIN
APIAN
APRON
EPSON
OPTIN
SPAHN
SPAIN
SPAWN
SPOON
SPURN
SPYON
UPENN
UPTON

••PN•
HYPNO

••P•N
ALPEN
ASPEN
ASPIN
CAPON
CSPAN
DIPIN
DUPIN
HOPIN
HOPON
INPEN
JAPAN
LAPIN
LEPEN
LUPIN
PEPIN
POPIN
PUPIN
RAPON
REPEN
REPIN
RIPEN
RIPON
SIPON
TAPIN
TAPON
TIPIN
UNPEN
UNPIN
ZIPIN
ZIPON

PO•••
POACH
POBOX
POBOY
POBRE
POCUS
PODAL
PODIA
POEME
POEMS
POESY
POETE
POETS
POILU
POINT
POIRE
POISE
POKED
POKER
POKES
POKEY
POLAR
POLED
POLER
POLES
POLIO
POLIS
POLIT
POLKA
POLKS
POLLO
POLLS
POLLY
POLOS
POLYP
POMES
POMME
POMOS
PONCA
PONCE
PONCH
PONDS
PONES
PONGO
PONGS
PONTA
PONTE
PONTI
PONTS
PONZI
PONZU
POOCH
POOHS
POOLE
POOLS
POONA
POOPS
POORI
POORS
POPBY
POPES
POPIN
POPLE
POPOV
POPPA
POPPY
POPUP
PORCH
PORCS
PORED
PORER
PORES
PORGY
PORKS
PORKY
PORNO
PORTA
PORTE
PORTO
PORTS
POSED
POSER
POSES
POSEY
POSIT
POSSE
POSTE
POSTS
POTOK
POTSY
POTTO
POTTS
POTTY
POTUS
POUCH
POUFS
POULE
POULT
POUND
POURS
POUTS
POUTY
POWAY
POWER
POWYS
POXES
POZZO

P•O••
PAOLI
PAOLO
PAONS
PBOOK
PEONS
PEONY
PHOBE
PHOBO
PHONE
PHONO
PHONS
PHONY
PHOTO
PHOTS
PIONS
PIOUS
PLOCE
PLODS
PLONK
PLOPS
PLOTS
PLOTZ
PLOWS
PLOYS
POOCH
POOHS
POOLE
POOLS
POONA
POOPS
POORI
POORS
PROAM
PROAS
PROBE
PROBS
PRODS
PROEM
PROFS
PROGS
PROLE
PROMO
PROMS
PRONE
PRONG
PROOF
PROPS
PROSE
PROSS
PROST
PROSY
PROTO
PROTS
PROUD
PROVE
PROVO
PROVS
PROWL
PROWS
PROXY

P••O•
PALOS
PAROL
PAROO
PAROS
PASOS
PATON
PATOS
PAXOS
PAYOR
PBOOK
PECOS
PEKOE
PEPOS
PERON
PEROT
PESOS
PETOS
PHLOX
PHNOM
PICON
PICOT
PILON
PILOT
PINON
PINOT
PITON
PITOT
PIVOT
POBOX
POBOY
POLOS
POMOS
POPOV
POTOK
PREOP
PRIOR
PROOF
PRYOR
PUTON
PYLON
PYROS

P•••O
PAAVO
PABLO
PALEO
PANTO
PAOLO
PARDO
PAROO
PASCO
PASEO
PASTO
PATCO
PATHO
PATIO
PATRO
PAULO
PAYTO
PEABO
PEANO
PEDRO
PEPTO
PERRO
PESTO
PETCO
PETRO
PHAGO
PHENO
PHILO
PHOBO
PHONO
PHOTO
PHYLO
PHYTO
PIANO
PICTO
PINKO
PINTO
PISMO
PLANO
PLATO
PLUTO
POLIO
POLLO
PONGO
PORNO
PORTO
POTTO
POZZO
PRADO
PRATO
PREGO
PRIMO
PROMO
PROTO
PROVO
PTERO
PULMO
PUTTO

•PO••
APODS
APORT
EPOCH
EPODE
EPOXY
IPODS
SPOCK
SPODE
SPOIL
SPOKE
SPOOF
SPOOK
SPOOL
SPOON
SPOOR
SPORE
SPORK

SPORT SPOSA SPOSE SPOSO SPOTS SPOUT UPOLU UPONE

•P•O•

APRON APSOS EPCOT EPHOD EPHOR EPROM EPSOM EPSON SPOOF SPOOK SPOOL SPOON SPOOR SPYON UPBOW UPDOS UPFOR UPTON UPTOP

•P••O

OPTTO SPAGO SPANO SPERO SPIRO SPOSO SPYRO

••PO•

BIPOD CAPON CAPOS CSPOT DEPOT EAPOE ESPOO EXPOS HOPON HYPOS KAPOK KAPOW NEPOS OOPOD PEPOS POPOV RAPON REPOS REPOT RIPON SAPOR SEPOY SIPON SOPOR TAPON TOPOG TOPOL TYPOS UNPOT VAPOR ZIPON

••P•O

BEPPO COPTO CUPRO DIPLO DIPSO DUPLO ESPIO ESPOO GOPRO HEPTO HIPPO HIPTO HOPTO HYPNO LIPPO PEPTO REPRO TYPEO ZEPPO ZEPTO ZIPPO

•••PO

BEPPO CAMPO CARPO DROPO EDIPO FIRPO GUAPO HARPO HIPPO KIMPO LIPPO MAYPO MTAPO TEMPO THEPO TROPO ZEPPO ZIPPO

P•P••

PAPAL PAPAS PAPAW PAPEL PAPER PAPPY PAPUA PEPIN PEPLA PEPOS PEPPY PEPSI PEPTO PEPUP PEPYS PIPED PIPER PIPES PIPET PIPIT PIPPA PIPPI POPBY POPES POPIN POPLE POPOV POPPA POPPY POPUP PUPAE PUPAL PUPAS PUPIL PUPIN PUPPY PUPUS

P••P•

PALPS PAMPA PAPPY PEEPS PEPPY PERPS PIPPA PIPPI PLOPS POOPS POPPA POPPY PREPS PROPS PULPS PULPY PUMPS PUPPY

P•••P

PAYUP PENUP PEPUP PINUP PLUMP POLYP POPUP PREOP PRIMP PTRAP PUTUP

•PP••

APPAL APPEL APPIA APPLE APPLY APPTS EPPIE OPPER UPPED UPPER

•P••P

APEEP UPTOP

••PP•

BEPPE BEPPO BIPPY CUPPA CUPPY DIPPY GUPPY HAPPY HIPPO HIPPY HOPPE HOPPY KAPPA LAPPS LIPPI LIPPO LIPPY LOPPY NAPPE NAPPY NIPPY PAPPY PEPPY PIPPA PIPPI POPPA POPPY PUPPY REPPS SAPPY SOPPY SUPPE TIPPI TIPPY TOPPS ZAPPA ZAPPY ZEPPO ZIPPO ZIPPY ZUPPA

••P•P

AMPUP HOPUP LAPUP MOPUP NIPUP PEPUP POPUP RIPUP SOPUP TIPUP TOPUP ZIPUP

•••PP

KRUPP TRAPP TRIPP

PQ•••

PQRST

P•Q••

PIQUE

•PQ••

OPQRS

••PQ•

NOPQR

•••PQ

MNOPQ

PR•••

PRADA PRADO PRAHA PRAIA PRAMS PRANA PRANK PRATE PRATO PRATT PRAWN PRAYS PREEN PREGL PREGO PRELL PREOP PREPS PRESA PRESB PRESE PRESS PREXY PREYS PRIAM PRICE PRICK PRICY PRIDE PRIED PRIER PRIES PRIGS PRIMA PRIME PRIMO PRIMP PRIMS PRINE PRINK PRINT PRIOR PRISM PRISS PRIUS PRIVY PRIZE PRIZM PRMAN PRMEN PRNDL PROAM PROAS PROBE PROBS PRODS PROEM PROFS PROGS PROLE PROMO PROMS PRONE PRONG PROOF PROPS PROSE PROSS PROST PROSY PROTO PROTS PROUD PROVE PROVO PROVS PROWL PROWS PROXY PRUDE PRUNE PRYCE PRYER PRYOR

P•R••

PARAS PARCA PARCH PARCS PARDO PARDS PARED PAREE PAREN PARER PARES PAREU PARGE PARIS PARKA PARKS PARLE PARMA PAROL PAROO PAROS PARRA PARRS PARRY PARSE PARSI PARTA PARTB PARTC PARTE PARTI PARTS PARTV PARTY PERAN PERAS PERCE PERCH PERCS PERCY PERDU PERES PEREZ PERFS PERIL PERIS PERKS PERKY PERLE PERMA PERMS PERON PEROT PERPS PERRO PERRY PERSE PERTH PIRNS PORCH PORCS PORED PORER PORES PORGY PORKS PORKY PORNO PORTA PORTE PORTO PORTS PQRST PTRAP PURDY PUREE PURER PUREX PURGE PURIM PURLS PURRS PURSE PURSY PURTY PYRES PYREX PYROS

P••R•

PADRE PAIRS PARRA PARRS PARRY PATRI PATRO PEARL PEARS PEARY PEDRO PEERS PERRO PERRY PETRA PETRE PETRI PETRO PEURS PFERD PHARM PIERS PLURI POBRE POIRE POORI POORS POURS PTERO PURRS

P•••R

PACER PAGER PALAR PALER PAPER PARER PATER PAVER PAWER PAYER PAYOR PEDER PETER PHAIR PIKER PILAR PILER PINER PIPER PIXAR PLIER PLUMR PLYER POKER POLAR POLER PQRER POSER POWER PRIER PRIOR PRYER PRYOR PULER PURER

•PR••

APRES APRIL APRON EPROM IPRAY OPRAH SPRAT SPRAY SPREE SPRIG SPRIT YPRES

•P•R•

APARS APART APERS APERY APORT OPART OPERA OPERE OPQRS SPARE SPARK SPARS SPERM SPERO SPIRE SPIRO SPIRY SPORE SPORK SPORT SPURN SPURS SPURT SPYRI SPYRO UPDRY

•P••R

APTER EPHOR OPHIR OPPER SPEAR SPEER SPIER SPOOR UPFOR UPPER

••PR•

CAPRA CAPRI COPRA CUPRI CUPRO DUPRE GOPRO REPRO SUPRA

••P•R

ASPER ATPAR CAPER COPER DOPER DUPER GAPER HOPER HYPER JAPER LEPER LOPER MOPER NEPHR NOPAR NOPQR ONPAR OPPER PAPER PIPER RIPER ROPER SAPOR SOPOR SUPER TAPER TAPIR TOPER TYPER UPPER VAPOR VIPER WIPER

•••PR

DNEPR

PS•••

PSALM PSATS PSEUD PSHAW PSSST PSSTS PSYCH

P•S••

PASCH PASCO PASEO PASES PASHA PASOS PASSE PASSU PASSY PASTA PASTE PASTO PASTS PASTY PESCE PESCI PESKY PESOS PESTO PESTS PISAN PISCI PISMO PISTE POSED POSER POSES POSEY POSIT POSSE POSTE POSTS PSSST PSSTS PUSAN PUSHY PUSSY

P••S•

PABST PAESE PAISA PAISE PALSY PANSY PARSE PARSI PASSE PASSU PASSY PATSY PAUSE PEASE PEPSI PERSE PHASE PHISH PINSK PIUSI PIUSV PIUSX PLASH PLASM PLAST PLUSH POESY POISE POSSE POTSY PQRST PRESA PRESB PRESE PRESS PRISM PRISS PROSE PROSS PROST PROSY PSSST PULSE PURSE PURSY PUSSY

P•••S

PACAS PACES PACKS PACTS PAGES PAILS PAINS PAIRS PALES PALLS PALMS PALOS PALPS PANES PANGS PANIS PANTS PAONS PAPAS PARAS PARCS PARDS PARES PARIS PARKS PAROS PARRS PARTS PASES PASOS PASTS PATES PATHS PATOS PAVES PAWLS PAWNS PAXOS PEAKS PEALS PEARS PEATS PEBAS PECKS PECOS PEEKS PEELS PEENS PEEPS PEERS PEKES PELFS PELTS PENDS PEONS PEPOS PEPYS PERAS PERCS PERES PERFS PERIS PERKS PERMS PERPS PESOS PESTS PETES PETOS PEURS PHONS PHOTS PICAS PICKS PICTS PIEDS PIELS PIERS PIKAS PIKES PILES PILLS PILUS PIMAS PINES PINGS PINKS PINTS PIONS PIOUS PIPES PIRNS PITAS PITHS PITTS PITYS PLANS PLATS PLAYS PLEAS PLEBS PLIES PLODS PLOPS PLOTS PLOWS PLOYS PLUGS PLUMS POCUS POEMS POETS POKES POLES POLIS POLKS POLLS POLOS POMES POMOS PONDS PONES PONGS PONTS POOHS POOLS POOPS POORS POPES PORCS PORES PORKS PORTS POSES POSTS POTTS POTUS POUFS POURS POUTS POWYS POXES PRAMS PRAYS PREPS PRESS PREYS PRIES PRIGS PRIMS PRISS PRIUS PROAS PROBS PRODS PROFS PROGS PROMS PROPS PROSS PROTS PROVS PROWS PSATS PSSTS PUCES PUCKS PUFFS PUKAS PULAS PULES PULIS PULLS PULPS PUMAS PUMPS PUNGS PUNKS PUNTS PUPAS PUPUS PURLS PURRS PUTTS PYRES PYROS PYXES

•PS••

APSES APSIS APSOS EPSOM EPSON UPSET

•P•S•

APISH EPISC IPASS SPASM SPOSA SPOSE SPOSO

•P••S

APARS APERS APHIS APLUS APODS APPTS APRES APSES APSIS APSOS BPLUS CPLUS DPLUS EPEES EPHAS EPICS IPASS IPODS JPEGS LPGAS MPEGS OPAHS OPALS OPEDS OPELS OPENS OPQRS SPADS SPAMS SPANS SPARS SPATS SPAYS SPECS SPETS SPEWS SPIES SPINS SPITS SPOTS SPUDS SPURS TPKES UPDOS YPRES

••PS•

COPSE DIPSO DIPSY GIPSY GYPSY LAPSE MOPSY PEPSI TIPSY TOPSY

••P•S

ALPES AMPAS APPTS CAPAS CAPES CAPOS CAPTS CEPES COPES COPTS DEPTS DOPAS DOPES DUPES ELPIS ESPYS EXPOS GAPES HOPES HOPIS HYPES HYPOS JAPES KAPHS KEPIS KOPHS LAPIS LAPPS LEPUS LOPES LUPUS MAPES MOPES NAPES NEPOS NIPAS NOPES OLPES PAPAS PEPOS PEPYS PIPES POPES PUPAS PUPUS QOPHS REPOS REPPS ROPES SEPTS SOPHS SUPES SUPTS TAPAS TAPES TAPIS TIPIS TOPES TOPIS TOPPS TYPES TYPOS WIPES YIPES

•••PS

ACUPS BCUPS BEEPS BLIPS BUMPS BURPS CAMPS CARPS CCUPS CHAPS CHIPS CHOPS CLAPS CLIPS CLOPS COMPS COOPS CORPS COUPS CRAPS CROPS CUSPS DAMPS DCUPS DEEPS DORPS DRIPS DROPS DUMPS EARPS ESOPS FLAPS FLIPS FLOPS GAMPS GASPS GAWPS GEEPS GIMPS GLOPS GOOPS GORPS GRIPS GULPS HARPS HASPS HEAPS HELPS HEMPS HOOPS HOSPS HUMPS IHOPS JEEPS JUMPS KEEPS KELPS KREPS KRIPS KRUPS LAMPS LAPPS LEAPS LIMPS LISPS LOOPS LOUPS LUMPS MSRPS MUMPS NEAPS PALPS PEEPS PERPS PLOPS POOPS PREPS PROPS PULPS PUMPS QTIPS QUIPS RAMPS RASPS REAPS REPPS REUPS ROMPS RSVPS RUMPS SAMPS SCUPS SEEPS SHIPS SHOPS SIMPS SKIPS SLAPS SLIPS

SLOPS
SNAPS
SNIPS
SOAPS
SOUPS
STEPS
STOPS
SUMPS
SWAPS
TAMPS
TARPS
TBSPS
TEMPS
TERPS
TOPPS
TRAPS
TRIPS
TTOPS
VAMPS
VEEPS
VOIPS
WARPS
WASPS
WEEPS
WHAPS
WHIPS
WHOPS
WHUPS
WIMPS
WISPS
WRAPS
YAWPS
YELPS

PT•••
PTERO
PTILE
PTRAP

P•T••
PATCH
PATCO
PATED
PATEK
PATEN
PATER
PATES
PATHE
PATHO
PATHS
PATHY
PATIO
PATLY
PATNA
PATON
PATOS
PATRI
PATRO
PATSY
PATTI
PATTY
PETAL
PETCO
PETER
PETES
PETEY
PETIT
PETOS
PETRA
PETRE
PETRI
PETRO
PETTI
PETTY
PITAS
PITCH
PITHS
PITHY
PITON
PITOT
PITTI
PITTS
PITYS
POTOK
POTSY
POTTO
POTTS
POTTY
POTUS
PUTBY
PUTIN
PUTON
PUTTO
PUTTS
PUTTY
PUTUP

P••T•
PACTS
PANTA
PANTO
PANTS
PANTY
PARTA
PARTB
PARTC
PARTE
PARTI
PARTS
PARTV
PARTY
PASTA
PASTE
PASTO
PASTS
PASTY
PATTI
PATTY
PAYTO
PAYTV
PEATS
PEATY
PEETE
PELTS
PENTA
PENTE
PEPTO
PERTH
PESTO
PESTS
PETTI
PETTY
PHOTO
PHOTS
PHYTE
PHYTO
PICTO
PICTS
PIETA
PIETY
PINTA
PINTO
PINTS
PISTE
PITTI
PITTS
PIUTE
PLATA
PLATE
PLATH
PLATO
PLATS
PLATT
PLATY
PLOTS
PLOTZ
PLUTO
POETE
POETS
PONTA
PONTE
PONTI
PONTS
PORTA
PORTE
PORTO
PORTS
POSTE
POSTS
POTTO
POTTS
POTTY
POUTS
POUTY
PRATE
PRATO
PRATT
PROTO
PROTS
PSATS
PSSTS
PUNTA
PUNTS
PURTY
PUTTO
PUTTS
PUTTY

P•••T
PABST
PAGET
PAINT
PAWAT
PEROT
PETIT
PEWIT
PFFFT
PHFFT
PICOT
PIGIT
PILOT
PINOT
PIPET
PIPIT
PITOT
PIVOT
PLAIT
PLANT
PLAST
PLATT
PLEAT
POINT
POLIT
POSIT
POULT
PQRST
PRATT
PRINT
PROST
PSSST
PUGET

•PT••
APTED
APTER
APTLY
OPTED
OPTIC
OPTIN
OPTTO
UPTON
UPTOP

•P•T•
APPTS
OPTTO
SPATE
SPATS
SPETS
SPITE
SPITS
SPITZ
SPOTS

•P••T
APART
APORT
EPACT
EPCOT
OPART
OPCIT
SPELT
SPENT
SPILT
SPLAT
SPLIT
SPORT
SPOUT
SPRAT
SPRIT
SPURT
UPLIT
UPSET

••PT•
APPTS
CAPTS
COPTO
COPTS
DEPTH
DEPTS
EMPTY
HEPTA
HEPTO
HIPTO
HOPTO
PEPTO
SEPTA
SEPTS
SUPTS
ZEPTO

••P•T
CAPET
CAPUT
COPIT
CSPOT
DEPOT
EXPAT
HEPAT
INPUT
KAPUT
KOPIT
LAPAT
LOPAT
NIPAT
PIPET
PIPIT
REPOT
RIPAT
STPAT
UNPOT
WOPAT
YAPAT
ZIPIT

•••PT
ADAPT
ADEPT
ADOPT
CLEPT
CLIPT
COAPT
COOPT
CREPT
CRYPT
DROPT
EGYPT
ERUPT
GLYPT
INAPT
INEPT
KEMPT
LEAPT
SLEPT
SWEPT
TEMPT
UNAPT
WHIPT
WRAPT

PU•••
PUCCI
PUCES
PUCKS
PUDDY
PUDGY
PUFFS
PUFFY
PUGET
PUGGY
PUKAS
PUKKA
PULAS
PULED
PULER
PULES
PULIK
PULIS
PULLS
PULMO
PULPS
PULPY
PULSE
PUMAS
PUMPS
PUNCH
PUNGS
PUNIC
PUNKA
PUNKS
PUNKY
PUNNY
PUNTA
PUNTS
PUPAE
PUPAL
PUPAS
PUPIL
PUPIN
PUPPY
PUPUS
PURDY
PUREE
PURER
PUREX
PURGE
PURIM
PURLS
PURRS
PURSE
PURSY
PURTY
PUSAN
PUSHY
PUSSY
PUTBY
PUTIN
PUTON
PUTTO
PUTTS
PUTTY
PUTUP

P•U••
PAULA
PAULI
PAULO
PAULV
PAUSE
PEURS
PIUSI
PIUSV
PIUSX
PIUTE
PLUCK
PLUGS
PLUIE
PLUMB
PLUME
PLUMP
PLUMR
PLUMS
PLUMY
PLUNK
PLURI
PLUSH
PLUTO
PLUVI
POUCH
POUFS
POULE
POULT
POUND
POURS
POUTS
POUTY
PRUDE
PRUNE

P••U•
PADUA
PAPUA
PAYUP
PEGUY
PENUP
PEPUP
PFLUG
PIAUI
PILUS
PINUP
PIOUS
PIQUE
PNEUM
POCUS
POPUP
POTUS
PRIUS
PROUD
PSEUD
PUPUS
PUTUP

P•••U
PALAU
PAREU
PASSU
PERDU
PILAU
POILU
PONZU

•PU••
SPUDS
SPUME
SPUMY
SPUNK
SPURN
SPURS
SPURT

•P•U•
APLUS
BPLUS
CPLUS
DPLUS
JPAUL
OPIUM
SPOUT

•P••U
UPOLU

••PU•
AMPUP
CAPUT
HOPUP
INPUT
KAPUT
LAPUP
LEPUS
LUPUS
MOPUP
NIPUP
PAPUA
PEPUP
POPUP
PUPUS
REPUB
RIPUP
SOPUP
TIPUP
TOPUP
ZIPUP

•••PU
COYPU
QUIPU

P•V••
PAVED
PAVEL
PAVER
PAVES
PAVIA
PAVID
PAVIN
PIVEN
PIVOT

P••V•
PAAVO
PEEVE
PIAVE
PLUVI
PRIVY
PROVE
PROVO
PROVS

P•••V
PARTV
PAULV
PAYTV
PIUSV
POPOV

••P•V
POPOV

P•W••
PAWAT
PAWED
PAWER
PAWLS
PAWNS
PEWEE
PEWIT
POWAY
POWER
POWYS

P••W•
PLOWS
PRAWN
PROWL
PROWS

P•••W
PAPAW
PSHAW

•P•W•
SPAWN
SPEWS

•P••W
UPBOW

••P•W
DEPEW
KAPOW
LEPEW
PAPAW

P•X••
PAXOS
PIXAR
PIXEL
PIXIE
POXES
PYXES

P••X•
PREXY
PROXY

P•••X
PHLOX
PIUSX
POBOX
PUREX
PYREX

•P•X•
EPOXY

PY•••
PYGMY
PYLON
PYRES
PYREX
PYROS
PYXES

P•Y••
PAYEE
PAYER
PAYIN
PAYNE
PAYOR
PAYTO
PAYTV
PAYUP
PHYFE
PHYLA
PHYLL
PHYLO
PHYTE
PHYTO
PLYER
PRYCE
PRYER
PRYOR
PSYCH

P••Y•
PEPYS
PITYS
PLAYA
PLAYS
PLOYS
POLYP
POWYS
PRAYS
PREYS

P•••Y
PACEY
PACHY
PADDY
PALEY
PALLY
PALMY
PALSY
PAMBY
PANAY
PANKY
PANSY
PANTY
PAPPY
PARRY
PARTY
PASSY
PASTY
PATHY
PATLY
PATSY
PATTY
PEARY
PEATY
PEGGY
PEGUY
PENNY
PEONY
PEPPY
PERCY
PERKY
PERRY
PESKY
PETEY
PETTY
PHAGY
PHANY
PHONY
PICKY
PIETY
PIGGY
PINEY
PINKY
PITHY
PLATY
PLINY
PLUMY
POBOY
POESY
POKEY
POLLY
POPBY
POPPY
PORGY
PORKY
POSEY
POTSY
POTTY
POUTY
POWAY
PREXY
PRICY
PRIVY
PROSY
PROXY
PUDDY
PUDGY
PUFFY
PUGGY
PULPY
PUNKY
PUNNY
PUPPY
PURDY
PURSY
PURTY
PUSHY
PUSSY
PUTBY
PUTTY
PYGMY

•PY••
SPYON
SPYRI
SPYRO

•P•Y•
SPAYS

•P••Y
APERY
APLEY
APPLY
APTLY
EPOXY
IPRAY
SPACY
SPICY
SPIKY
SPINY
SPIRY
SPLAY
SPRAY
SPUMY
UPDRY

••PY•
ESPYS
PEPYS

••P•Y
AMPLY
APPLY
BIPPY
COPAY
CUPPY
DIPPY
DIPSY
DOPEY
EMPTY
GIPSY
GUPPY
GYPSY
HAPLY
HAPPY
HIPLY
HIPPY
HOPPY
IMPLY
LIPPY
LOPPY
MOPEY
MOPSY
NAPPY
NIPPY
PAPPY
PEPPY
POPBY
POPPY
PUPPY
REPAY
REPLY
SAPPY
SEPOY
SOPPY
TIPPY
TIPSY
TOPSY
ZAPPY
ZIPBY
ZIPPY

•••PY
BIPPY
BUMPY
CAMPY
CUPPY
DELPY
DIPPY
DUMPY
GIMPY
GOOPY
GRAPY
GRIPY
GULPY
GUPPY
HAPPY
HARPY
HEAPY
HEMPY
HIPPY
HOPPY
HUMPY
JUMPY
LIMPY
LIPPY
LOOPY
LOPPY
LUMPY
NAPPY
NIPPY
PAPPY
PEPPY
POPPY
PULPY
PUPPY
RASPY
SAPPY
SEEPY
SOAPY
SOPPY
SOUPY
TIPPY
VAMPY
WASPY
WEEPY
WIMPY
WISPY
ZAPPY
ZIPPY

P•Z••
PIZZA
PLZEN
POZZO

P••Z•
PANZA
PINZA
PIZZA
PLAZA
PONZI
PONZU
POZZO
PRIZE
PRIZM

P•••Z
PEREZ
PLOTZ

•P••Z
SPITZ

••P•Z
LAPAZ
LOPEZ
TOPAZ

QA•••
QAIDS
QANDA
QATAR

Q•A••
QUACK
QUADR
QUADS
QUAFF
QUAGS
QUAID
QUAIL
QUAIS
QUAKE
QUAKY
QUALM
QUAND
QUANG
QUANT
QUARE
QUARK
QUART
QUASH
QUASI
QUAXO
QUAYS

Q••A•
QATAR
QURAN

Q•••A
QANDA
QUOTA

•QA••
AQABA

•Q•A•
AQUAE
AQUAS
EQUAL
IQBAL
SQUAB
SQUAD
SQUAT
SQUAW

•Q••A
AQABA

••Q•A
ACQUA

QB•••
QBERT
QBVII

•QB••
IQBAL

•Q•B•
AQABA

•Q••B
SQUAB
SQUIB

Q••C•
QUACK
QUICK

Q••D•
QAIDS
QANDA
QUADR
QUADS
QUIDS

Q•••D
QUAID
QUAND

•Q••D
SQUAD
SQUID

Q•E••
QBERT
QUEEG
QUEEN
QUEER
QUELL
QUERY
QUESO
QUEST
QUEUE
QWEST

Q••E•
QUEEG
QUEEN
QUEER
QUIEN
QUIET

Q•••E
QTILE
QUAKE
QUARE
QUEUE
QUINE
QUIRE
QUITE
QUOTE

•Q••E
AQUAE

••Q•E
ATQUE
ESQUE
PIQUE
ROQUE
TOQUE
TUQUE

Q••F•
QUAFF

Q•••F
QUAFF

Q••G•
QUAGS

Q•••G
QUANG
QUEEG

Q••H•
QOPHS

Q•••H
QIRSH
QUASH
QUOTH

QI•••
QIRSH

Q•I••
QAIDS
QTILE
QTIPS
QUICK
QUIDS
QUIEN
QUIET
QUILL
QUILP
QUILT
QUINE
QUINN
QUINO
QUINT
QUIPS
QUIPU
QUIRE
QUIRK
QUIRT
QUISP
QUITE
QUITO
QUITS

Q••I•
QBVII
QUAID
QUAIL
QUAIS
QUOIN
QUOIT

Q•••I
QBVII
QUASI

•Q•I•
EQUIP
EQUIS
EQUIV
IQUIT
SQUIB
SQUID

••QI•
FAQIR

••Q•I
COQUI
MAQUI
YAQUI

•••QI
IRAQI

Q••K•
QUAKE
QUAKY

Q•••K
QUACK
QUARK
QUICK
QUIRK

Q••L•
QTILE
QUALM
QUELL
QUILL
QUILP
QUILT

Q•••L
QUAIL
QUELL
QUILL

•Q••L
EQUAL
IQBAL

Q•••M
QUALM

Q•N••
QANDA

Q••N•
QUAND
QUANG
QUANT
QUINE
QUINN
QUINO
QUINT

Q•••N
QUEEN
QUIEN
QUINN
QUOIN
QURAN

QO•••
QOPHS

Q•O••
QUOIN
QUOIT
QUOTA
QUOTE
QUOTH

Q•••O
QUAXO
QUESO
QUINO
QUITO

•••QO
SISQO

Q•P••
QOPHS

Q••P•
QTIPS
QUIPS
QUIPU

Q•••P
QUILP
QUISP

•Q••P
EQUIP

QR•••
QRSTU

Q•R••
QIRSH QURAN

Q••R•
QBERT QUARE QUARK QUART QUERY QUIRE QUIRK QUIRT

Q•••R
QATAR QUADR QUEER

•QR••
PQRST

••QR•
OPQRS

••Q•R
FAQIR

•••QR
NOPQR

Q•S••
QRSTU

Q••S•
QIRSH QUASH QUASI QUESO QUEST QUISP QWEST

Q•••S
QAIDS QOPHS QTIPS QUADS QUAGS QUAIS QUAYS QUIDS QUIPS QUITS

•Q•S•
PQRST

•Q••S
AQUAS EQUIS EQUUS

••Q•S
OPQRS

•••QS
BARQS

QT•••
QTILE QTIPS

Q•T••
QATAR

Q••T•
QRSTU QUITE QUITO QUITS QUOTA QUOTE QUOTH

Q•••T
QBERT QUANT QUART QUEST QUIET QUILT QUINT QUIRT QUOIT QWEST

•Q••T
IQUIT PQRST SQUAT

QU•••
QUACK QUADR QUADS QUAFF QUAGS QUAID QUAIL QUAIS QUAKE QUAKY QUALM QUAND QUANG QUANT QUARE QUARK QUART QUASH QUASI QUAXO QUAYS QUEEG QUEEN QUEER QUELL QUERY QUESO QUEST QUEUE QUICK QUIDS QUIEN QUIET QUILL QUILP QUILT QUINE QUINN QUINO QUINT QUIPS QUIPU QUIRE QUIRK QUIRT QUISP QUITE QUITO QUITS QUOIN QUOIT QUOTA QUOTE QUOTH QURAN

Q••U•
QUEUE

Q•••U
QRSTU QUIPU

•QU••
AQUAE AQUAS EQUAL EQUIP EQUIS EQUIV EQUUS IQUIT SQUAB SQUAD SQUAT SQUAW SQUIB SQUID

•Q•U•
EQUUS

••QU•
ACQUA ATQUE COQUI ESQUE MAQUI PIQUE ROQUE TOQUE TUQUE YAQUI

Q•V••
QBVII

•Q••V
EQUIV

QW•••
QWEST

•Q••W
SQUAW

Q••X•
QUAXO

Q••Y•
QUAYS

Q•••Y
QUAKY QUERY

RA•••
RAABE RABAT RABBI RABID RABIN RACED RACER RACES RACKS RADAR RADER RADII RADIO RADIX RADON RAFER RAFFI RAFKO RAFTS RAGAS RAGED RAGER RAGES RAGGY RAGON RAHAL RAIDS RAILS RAIMI RAINE RAINS RAINY RAISA RAISE RAITA RAITT RAJAB RAJAH RAJAS RAJIV RAKED RAKER RAKES RAKUS RALES RALLY RALPH RAMAN RAMAR RAMAS RAMBO RAMEN RAMET RAMEY RAMIE RAMIN RAMIS RAMON RAMOS RAMPS RAMUS RAMUZ RANAS RANAT RANBY RANCH RANDA RANDB RANDD RANDI RANDR RANDS RANDY RANEE RANGE RANGO RANGY RANID RANIN RANIS RANKE RANKS RANON RANTO RANTS RANUP RAOUL RAPEE RAPID RAPON RARAE RAREE RARER RASAE RASED RASER RASES RASHI RASHT RASPA RASPE RASPS RASPY RASSE RASTA RATED RATEL RATER RATES RATHS RATIO RATON RATSO RATTY RAVED RAVEL RAVEN RAVER RAVES RAWER RAWLS RAWLY RAXED RAXES RAYED RAYON RAZAF RAZED RAZER RAZES RAZOR

R•A••
RAABE REACH REACT READD READE READS READY REAIM REAIR REALM REALS REAMS REAPS REARM REARS REASK REATA REAVE RIALS RIANT RIATA RNASE ROACH ROADS ROALD ROAMS ROANS ROARK ROARS ROAST RUARK RYALS RYANS

R••A•
RABAT RADAR RAGAS RAHAL RAJAB RAJAH RAJAS RAMAN RAMAR RAMAS RANAS RANAT RARAE RASAE RAZAF REBAG REBAR RECAN RECAP REDAN REFAX REGAL REGAN REHAB REHAN RELAP RELAX RELAY REMAN REMAP REMAT REMAX RENAL RENAN RENAY REPAD REPAY RERAN RESAT RESAW RESAY RETAG RETAN RETAP RETAR RETAX REWAX RHEAS RICAN RIGAN RIPAT RIVAL RIYAL RIZAL RODAN ROJAS ROMAN RONAN ROTAS ROWAN ROYAL RUMAN RUNAT RURAL

R•••A
RAISA RAITA RANDA RASPA RASTA REATA RECTA REGIA REGNA REINA RENGA RETIA REZIA RHODA RIATA RIOJA RODYA ROOSA ROSSA RRHEA RUMBA RUSKA RUSSA

•RA••
ARABS ARABY ARADO ARAME ARANS ARARA BRACE BRACH BRACK BRACT BRADS BRADY BRAES BRAGA BRAGG BRAGH BRAGS BRAHE BRAID BRAIN BRAKE BRAND BRANG BRANS BRANT BRASH BRASS BRATS BRATT BRAUN BRAVA BRAVE BRAVO BRAWL BRAWN BRAYS BRAZO CRABS CRACK CRACY CRAFT CRAGS CRAIG CRAIK CRAIN CRAKE CRAMP CRAMS CRANE CRANI CRANK CRAPE CRAPS CRASH CRASS CRATE CRAVE CRAWL CRAWS CRAYS CRAZE CRAZY DRABS DRACO DRAFT DRAGO DRAGS DRAIN DRAKE DRAMA DRAMS DRANG DRANK DRANO DRAPE DRATS DRAVA DRAWL DRAWN DRAWS DRAYS ERASE ERATO FRAGS FRAIL FRAIS FRAME FRANC FRANK FRANN FRANS FRANZ FRATS FRAUD FRAYN FRAYS FRAZY GRABS GRACE GRADE GRADS GRAFF GRAFT GRAIG GRAIL GRAIN GRAMM GRAMO GRAMP GRAMS GRAND GRANI GRANT GRAPE GRAPH GRAPY GRASP GRASS GRATA GRATE GRAVE GRAVI GRAVY GRAYS GRAZE IRABU IRANI IRAQI IRATE KRAAL KRAFT KRAIT KRAUS KRAUT KRAZY ORACH ORACY ORALB ORALE ORALS ORAMA ORANG ORANI ORANT ORATE PRADA PRADO PRAHA PRAIA PRAMS PRANA PRANK PRATE PRATO PRATT PRAWN PRAYS TRACE TRACI TRACK TRACT TRACY TRADE TRAGG TRAIL TRAIN TRAIT TRALA TRAMP TRAMS TRANE TRANS TRAPP TRAPS TRASH TRASK TRAVE TRAWL TRAYS URALS URANO URAWA WRACK WRAPS WRAPT WRATH XRAYS

•R•A•
ARCAE AREAL AREAR AREAS ARHAT ARIAL ARIAN ARIAS ARMAH ARMAS ARNAZ AROAR ARPAD ARRAH ARRAN ARRAS ARRAU ARRAY ARYAN BREAD BREAK BREAM BRIAN BRIAR BROAD BRYAN CREAK CREAM CROAK CROAT DREAD DREAM DREAR DRIAM DRLAO DRYAD ERIAS ERMAS FREAK FRIAR GREAT GROAN GROAT KRAAL ORCAS OREAD ORGAN ORKAN ORMAN ORPAH ORSAY ORVAL PRIAM PRMAN PROAM PROAS SRTAS TREAD TREAS TREAT TRIAD TRIAL URBAN UREAS URIAH URSAE WREAK

•R••A
ARARA ARECA ARENA ARICA AROMA ARUBA BRAGA BRAVA BRECA BREDA BROCA CREMA CRURA DRAMA DRAVA DRINA ERICA ERIKA ERISA FREDA FREIA FRENA FREYA FRIDA FRITA GRATA GRETA GROZA IRENA IRINA KRONA KRUPA ORAMA ORENA PRADA PRAHA PRAIA PRANA PRESA PRIMA RRHEA TRALA TRINA URAWA YREKA

••RA•
AARAU ABRAM AMRAM ARRAH ARRAN ARRAS ARRAU ARRAY ATRAS AURAE AURAL AURAR AURAS BARAK BORAH BORAS BORAX CARAT CARAY CERAM CERAT CORAL CURAD DERAT DIRAC DIRAE DIRAM DORAG DORAL DORAN DURAN DURAS EYRAS FARAD FARAH FERAL FORAY GORAN GYRAL HERAT HIRAM HORAE HORAL HORAS HYRAX IPRAY JURAL JURAN KARAN KARAS KARAT KORAN KORAT LARAM LARAS LIRAS LORAN LORAX LURAY LYRAS MARAT MCRAE MORAL MORAN MORAS MORAY MURAL MURAT NARAS NORAD NORAH OBRAS OCRAT OKRAS OPRAH OTRAS OURAY PARAS PERAN PERAS PTRAP QURAN RARAE RERAN RURAL SARAH SARAI SARAN SCRAG SCRAM SCRAP SCRAT SERAC SERAI SERAL SORAS SPRAT SPRAY STRAD STRAM STRAP STRAT STRAW STRAY SURAH SURAS TARAS TERAT TORAH TORAS UVRAY VIRAL

••R•A
AORTA ATRIA BARBA BARCA BEREA BERIA BERRA BERTA BIRRA BORSA BURKA BURMA BURSA CARLA CARTA CERIA CIRCA CORDA COREA CORIA CORSA CURIA CURSA DARIA DARLA DARYA DERMA DORIA DORSA DURRA FERIA FIRMA FORMA FORZA GARDA KARLA KARMA KORDA KOREA LARVA LORCA LORNA LURIA MARCA MARIA MARKA MARLA MARTA MARYA MORRA MYRIA MYRNA NARDA NERVA NORIA NORMA PARCA PARKA PARMA PARRA PARTA PERMA PORTA SERIA SERRA SERTA SORTA STRIA SYRIA TARGA TERIA TERRA TERZA TORTA USRDA VARDA VARIA VARNA VARYA VERNA VERSA VIRGA VIRNA YARRA YERBA YORBA ZORBA

•••RA
ACCRA ACURA AFTRA AGORA AGURA AHORA AKIRA AMARA ANTRA ARARA ASTRA AUDRA AZERA BASRA BEIRA BERRA BIRRA CAPRA CEARA CIERA CLARA COBRA COPRA CRURA DEBRA DURRA ELARA ELURA EVORA EXTRA FLORA FOURA HYDRA INDRA INFRA INTRA KEIRA LAURA LEORA LIBRA LYCRA MAURA MEARA MICRA MOIRA MORRA NAIRA NEDRA OHARA OKARA ONERA OPERA PARRA PETRA SABRA SACRA SERRA SHERA SUPRA SUTRA TATRA TERRA TETRA THERA THORA TIARA TZARA UHURA ULTRA UMBRA XSARA YARRA ZEBRA

R•B••
RABAT RABBI RABID RABIN REBAG REBAR REBBE REBEC REBEL REBER REBET REBID REBOP REBOX REBUS REBUT REBUY RIBBY ROBBE ROBBY ROBED ROBER ROBES ROBIN ROBLE ROBOF ROBOT ROBYN RUBEL RUBEN RUBES RUBIK RUBIN RUBLE RUBON RUBUP

R••B•
RAABE RABBI RAMBO RANBY REBBE RIBBY RIGBY ROBBE ROBBY RUGBY RUMBA RUNBY

R•••B
RAJAB RANDB REDUB REHAB REPUB RHOMB RHUMB

•RB••
ARBER ARBIL ARBOL ARBOR ARBRE ARBUS ARBYS ERBIL HRBEK MRBIG ORBED ORBIC ORBIT URBAN

•R•B•
ARABS ARABY ARUBA BRIBE CRABS CRIBS DRABS DRIBS DRUBS FROBE GRABS GREBE GRUBS

IRABU KREBS ORIBI PROBE PROBS TRIBE

•R••B
CRUMB MRCUB ORALB PRESB

••RB•
BARBA BARBI BARBQ BARBS BURBS CARBO CARBS CORBY CURBS DARBY DERBY FURBY GARBO GARBS GORBY HERBE HERBS HERBY KERBS KIRBY SERBO SERBS SORBO SORBS TURBO VERBS YERBA YORBA ZERBE ZORBA

••R•B
CARIB CAROB HOREB OHROB PARTB SCRUB SHRUB THROB

•••RB
ACERB BLURB EXURB FOURB

R•C••
RACED RACER RACES RACKS RECAN RECAP RECIP RECKS RECON RECTA RECTI RECTO RECTS RECUE RECUR RECUT RICAN RICCI RICED RICER RICES RICEU RICHE RICKI RICKS RICKY RICOH ROCCO ROCHE ROCKS ROCKY RUCHE RUCKS

R••C•
RANCH REACH REACT REECE REICE REICH RICCI ROACH ROCCO RONCO ROTCS ROYCE

R•••C
REBEC RELIC RUNIC

•RC••
ARCAE ARCED ARCHE ARCHI ARCHY MRCUB ORCAS ORCHS ORCUS ORCZY

•R•C•
ARECA ARICA BRACE BRACH BRACK BRACT BRECA BRECK BRICE BRICK BROCA BROCK BRUCE BRUCH BRYCE CRACK CRACY CRECY CRICK CROCE CROCI CROCK CROCS DRACO DRECK ERECT ERICA ERICH ERICK ERUCT FRICK FROCK FRUCT GRACE GRECO IROCS KROCK ORACH ORACY ORECK PRICE PRICK PRICY PRYCE TRACE TRACI TRACK TRACT TRACY TRECE TRICE TRICK TRUCE TRUCK URICH WRACK WRECK

•R••C
BRONC CRESC FRANC JROTC NROTC ORBIC

••RC•
BARCA BARCO BERCY BIRCH CIRCA CIRCE CIRCS DARCI DARCY FARCE FARCI FORCE LARCH LORCA LURCH MARCA MARCH MARCI MARCO MARCY MERCE MERCH MERCI MERCK MERCS MERCY NARCO NARCS PARCA PARCH PARCS PERCE PERCH PERCS PERCY PORCH PORCS TERCE TORCH TURCO

••R•C
AFRIC AGRIC AURIC BARIC BORIC CERIC DIRAC DORIC DUROC HARDC LYRIC NARIC OSRIC PARTC SERAC TORIC UGRIC ULRIC XERIC

•••RC
FOURC

R•D••
RADAR RADER RADII RADIO RADIX RAĐON REDAN REDDI REDDY REDED REDES REDID REDIG REDIP REDLY REDON REDOS REDOX REDRY REDUB REDUG REDUX REDYE RIDER RIDES RIDGE RIDGY RIDOF RODAN RODDY RODEO RODIN RODYA RUDDY RUDEL RUDER RUDGE RYDER

R••D•
RAIDS RANDA RANDB RANDD RANDI RANDR RANDS RANDY READD READE READS READY REDDI REDDY REEDS REEDY RENDS RHODA RHODE RHODO RHODY RINDS RINDY ROADS RODDY RONDE RONDO ROODS ROWDY RUDDY

R•••D
RABID RACED RAGED RAKED RANDD RANID RAPID RASED RATED RAVED RAXED RAYED RAZED READD REBID REDED REDID REFED REHID RELED REPAD RESOD REWED RICED RIGID RILED RIMED RIVED ROALD ROBED ROPED ROUND ROVED ROWED RSVPD RULED

•RD••
ARDEN ARDOR DRDRE ERDOS ORDER

•R•D•
ARADO BRADS BRADY BREDA BREDE BRIDE BRODY CREDO CREDS CRUDE CRUDS DREDD EREDE ERODE FREDA FREDO FRIDA FRODO GRADE GRADS GRIDE GRIDS GRODY IRIDO IRIDS PRADA PRADO PRIDE PRNDL PRODS PRUDE TRADE TRUDY

•R••D
ARCED ARMED AROID ARPAD ARRID BRAID BRAND BREAD BREED BROAD BROOD BROUD CREED CRIED CROWD DREAD DREDD DRIED DROID DROOD DRUID DRYAD ERRED FRAUD FREED FREUD FRIED FROID FROND GRAND GREED GRIND GRUED IRKED ORBED OREAD PRIED PROUD TREAD TREED TREND TRIAD TRIED TRUED URGED URSID

••RD•
BARDS BIRDS BIRDY BYRDS CARDI CARDS CORDA CORDS CURDS CURDY DARDY FERDE FORDO FORDS GARDA GARDE GIRDS GORDO GORDY GURDY HARDC HARDG HARDY HERDS HORDE HURDY KORDA KURDS LARDS LARDY LORDS LORDY MARDI NARDA NARDO NARDS NERDS NERDY PARDO PARDS PERDU PURDY SARDI SARDS TARDE TARDO TARDY USRDA VARDA VERDE VERDI WARDS WORDS WORDY YARDS

••R•D
ACRED ACRID AIRED ARRID ASRED BARED BORED CARED CORED CURAD CURED DARED EARED EDRED ERRED FARAD FARED FIRED GORED GYRED HARED HEROD HIRED INRED JARED LURED LURID LYRID MIRED NORAD OARED PARED PORED SCROD SHRED SIRED STRAD TARED TIRED VIRID WARED WIRED WORLD

•••RD
AWARD BAIRD BEARD BOARD CHARD CHORD ECARD FIORD FJORD FOURD FTORD GOURD GUARD HEARD HOARD LAIRD PFERD SHARD SNERD SWARD SWORD TBIRD THIRD WEIRD

RE•••
REACH REACT READD READE READS READY REAIM REAIR REALM REALS REAMS REAPS REARM REARS REASK REATA REAVE REBAG REBAR REBBE REBEC REBEL REBER REBET REBID REBOP REBOX REBUS REBUT REBUY RECAN RECAP RECIP RECKS RECON RECTA RECTI RECTO RECTS RECUE RECUR RECUT REDAN REDDI REDDY REDED REDES REDID REDIG REDIP REDLY REDON REDOS REDOX REDRY REDUB REDUG REDUX REDYE REECE REEDS REEDY REEFS REEFY REEGE REEKS REEKY REELS REESE REEVE REFAX REFED REFER REFIS REFIT REFIX REFLY REFRY REGAL REGAN REGEL REGER REGES REGIA REGIS REGLE REGNA REGTS REGUM REHAB REHAN REHEM REHID REHIT REHOE REICE REICH REIFY REIGN REIMS REINA REINE REINK REINS REISZ REITS REJIG REKEY RELAP RELAX RELAY RELED RELEE RELET RELIC RELIG RELIT RELOG REMAN REMAP REMAT REMAX REMET REMIT REMIX REMOP REMOW REMUS RENAL RENAN RENAY RENDS RENEE RENEW RENGA RENIN RENNY RENTE RENTS REOIL REOWN REPAD REPAY REPEG REPEL REPEN REPIN REPLY REPOS REPOT REPPS REPRO REPUB RERAN RERIG RERUN RESAT RESAW RESAY RESEE RESET RESEW RESHT RESIN RESIT RESOD RESOW RESTE RESTS RETAG RETAN RETAP RETAR RETAX RETIA RETIE RETIN RETIP RETOP RETOW RETRO RETRY RETTY REUEL REUNE REUPS REUSE REUSS REVEL REVES REVET REVUE REVUP REWAX REWED REWET REWIN REWON REXES REYES REZIA REZIP

R•E••
REECE REEDS REEDY REEFS REEFY REEGE REEKS REEKY REELS REESE REEVE RHEAS RHEEM RHEIN RHEME RHETT RHEUM RIELS RIENS RIETI RLESS RUEHL RUERS RVERS

R••E•
RACED RACER RACES RADER RAFER RAGED RAGER RAGES RAKED RAKER RAKES RALES RAMEN RAMET RAMEY RANEE RAPEE RAREE RARER RASED RASER RASES RATED RATEL RATER RATES RAVED RAVEL RAVEN RAVER RAVES RAWER RAXED RAXES RAYED RAZED RAZER RAZES REBEC REBEL REBER REBET REDED REDES REFED REFER REGEL REGER REGES REHEM REKEY RELED RELEE RELET REMET RENEE RENEW REPEG REPEL REPEN RESEE RESET RESEW REUEL REVEL REVES REVET REWED REWET REXES REYES RHEEM RICED RICER RICES RICEU RIDER RIDES RIFER RIGEL RIKER RILED RILES RILEY RIMED RIMER RIMES RIPEN RIPER RISEN RISER RISES RITES RIVED RIVEN RIVER RIVES RIVET RIXEY ROBED ROBER ROBES RODEO ROGER ROGET ROKER ROLEN ROLEO ROLES ROLEX ROMEO ROMES RONEE ROPED ROPER ROPES ROREM ROSEN ROSES ROSEY ROTES ROUEN ROUES ROVED ROVER ROVES ROWED ROWEL ROWEN ROWER RRHEA RTREV RUBEL RUBEN RUBES RUDEL RUDER RULED RULER RULES RUMER RUNES RUPEE RUSES RYDER

R•••E
RAABE RAINE RAISE RAMIE RANEE RANGE RANKE RAPEE RARAE RAREE RASAE RASPE RASSE READE REAVE REBBE RECUE REDYE REECE REEGE REESE REEVE REGLE REHOE REICE REINE RELEE RENEE RENTE RESEE RESTE RETIE REUNE REUSE REVUE RHEME RHINE RHODE RHONE RHYME RICHE RIDGE RIFLE RILKE RILLE RINSE RNASE ROBBE ROBLE ROCHE ROGUE ROLFE ROLLE RONDE RONEE ROONE ROQUE ROSIE ROUGE ROUSE ROUTE ROWSE ROXIE ROYCE RTILE RUBLE RUCHE RUDGE RUPEE RUSSE

•RE••
AREAL AREAR AREAS ARECA AREEL ARENA ARENS ARENT ARESO ARETE BREAD BREAK BREAM BRECA BRECK BREDA BREDE BREED BREEN BREES BRENS BRENT BRERS BREST BRETT BREVE BREVI BREWS CREAK CREAM CRECY CREDO CREDS CREED CREEK CREEL CREEP CREES CREMA CREME CREON CREPE CREPT CRESC CRESS CREST CRETE CREVE CREWS DREAD DREAM DREAR DRECK DREDD DREFT DREGS DREKS DRESS DREWU ERECT EREDE ERETZ EREVS FREAK FREDA FREDO FREED FREEH FREER FREES FREIA FRENA FRENI FREON FRERE FRESH FRESS FRETS FREUD FREYA GREAT GREBE GRECO GREED GREEK GREEN GREER GREET GREGG GRETA GRETE GREYS IRENA IRENE KREBS KREME KREPS KRESS KREUK KREWE OREAD ORECK ORENA OREOS PREEN PREGL PREGO PRELL PREOP PREPS PRESA PRESB PRESE PRESS PREXY PREYS TREAD TREAS

TREAT TRECE TREED TREEN TREES TREKS TREND TRENT TRESS TRETS TREVI TREWS TREYS UREAS WREAK WRECK WRENS WREST YREKA

•R•E•

ARBER ARCED ARDEN AREEL ARIEL ARIES ARLEN ARLES ARMED ARMEE ARMEN ARMER ARMES ARMET ARMEY ARNEL ARPEL ARRET ARSES ARTEL ARWEN BRAES BREED BREEN BREES BRIEF BRIER BRIES CREED CREEK CREEL CREEP CREES CRIED CRIER CRIES CRUEL CRUET CRYER DRIED DRIER DRIES DRYER ERIES ERNES EROES ERRED ERTES FREED FREEH FREER FREES FRIED FRIEL FRIER FRIES FROES FRYER GREED GREEK GREEN GREER GREET GRIEF GRIEG GRIER GRUED GRUEL GRUES HRBEK IRKED IRKER IRREG KRIEG MRHEX MRLEE MRMET ORBED ORDER ORFEO ORFES ORIEL ORLES ORREN ORSER ORSES PREEN PRIED PRIER PRIES PRMEN PROEM PRYER RRHEA TREED TREEN TREES TRIED TRIER TRIES TRUED TRUER TRUES URGED URGER URGES URIEL URKEL URNES WRIER WRYER

•R••E

ARAME ARBRE ARCAE ARCHE ARETE ARGUE ARISE ARMEE ARNIE AROSE ARTIE BRACE BRAHE BRAKE BRAVE BREDE BREVE BRIBE BRICE BRIDE BRINE BRISE BRITE BROKE BRUCE BRULE BRUME BRUTE BRYCE CRAKE CRANE CRAPE CRATE CRAVE CRAZE CREME CREPE CRETE CREVE CRIME CROCE CRONE CRORE CROWE CRUDE CRUSE DRAKE DRAPE DRDRE DRIVE DROLE DROME DRONE DROVE DRUPE DRUSE DRUZE ERASE EREDE ERNIE ERODE EROSE FRAME FRERE FRISE FRITE FROBE FROME FROZE GRACE GRADE GRAPE GRATE GRAVE GRAZE GREBE GRETE GRIDE GRIME GRIPE GRISE GROFE GROPE GROTE GROVE IRATE IRENE KREME KREWE KRIGE KRONE MRLEE ORALE ORATE PRATE PRESE PRICE PRIDE PRIME PRINE PRIZE PROBE PROLE PRONE PROSE PROVE PRUDE PRUNE PRYCE TRACE TRADE TRANE TRAVE TRECE TRIBE TRICE TRIKE TRINE TRIPE TRITE TROPE TROVE TROWE TRUCE TRYME URSAE WRITE WROTE

••RE•

ACRED ACRES ADREM ADREP AEREO AGREE AIRED AIRER AIRES APRES ARRET ASRED AYRES BARED BARER BARES BEREA BERET BORED BOREL BOREN BORER BORES BUREN BURET CARED CARER CARES CARET CAREW CAREY CERES CIRES COREA CORED CORER CORES COREY CURED CUREL CURER CURES CURET DARED DARER DARES DEREK DIRER DOREN DUREN DURER EARED EDRED EFREM EGRET EHREN ELREY ERRED ETRES FARED FARER FARES FIRED FIRER FIRES FORES GARES GORED GOREN GORES GOREY GYRED GYRES HARED HAREM HARES HEREK HERES HIRED HIREE HIRER HIRES HOREB INRED INREM IRREG JARED JCREW JEREZ JOREL KAREL KAREN KOREA LAREE LARES LOREN LORES LURED LURER LURES LUREX LYRES MAREK MARES MERER MERES MIRED MIRES MOREL MORES MOREY MURES NARES NOREN OARED OARER OGRES ORREN PARED PAREE PAREN PARER PARES PAREU PERES PEREZ PORED PORER PORES PUREE PURER PUREX PYRES PYREX RAREE RARER ROREM RTREV SAREE SAREK SCREE SCREW SHRED SHREK SHREW SIRED SIREE SIREN SIRES SOREL SOREN SORER SORES SPREE STREP STREW SURER TARED TARES THREE THREW TIRED TIRES TYRES VIREO WARED WARES WIRED WIRER WIRES YARER YORES YPRES ZOREL

••R•E

AERIE AGREE AURAE BARGE BARRE BERLE BERNE BIRSE BORGE BORNE BURKE BYRNE CARLE CARME CARNE CARPE CARRE CARTE CARVE CIRCE CURIE CURSE CURVE DARTE DIRAE DIRGE EARLE EERIE EYRIE FARCE FAROE FERDE FORCE FORGE FORTE FURIE FURZE GARDE GORGE GORME GORSE HARTE HERBE HERNE HERVE HIREE HORAE HORDE HORNE HORSE JARRE JERNE JORGE KARLE KERNE KYRIE LAREE LARGE LARUE LORNE LORRE LURIE MARGE MARIE MARNE MCRAE MERCE MERGE MERLE MEROE MORSE MORTE MURRE NERVE NORGE NORSE NORTE NURSE ONRYE PAREE PARGE PARLE PARSE PARTE PERCE PERLE PERSE PORTE PUREE PURGE PURSE RARAE RAREE SAREE SARGE SCREE SERGE SERVE SIREE SPREE SURGE TARDE TARTE TERCE TERME TERNE TERRE TERSE THREE THROE TORME TORRE TORTE VERDE VERGE VERNE VERRE VERSE VERTE VERVE WORSE ZERBE

•••RE

ADORE AFIRE AFORE ALFRE AMARE AMORE ANDRE ANTRE ARBRE ASTRE AUTRE AWARE AZORE AZURE BARRE BIERE BIORE BLARE BLORE BOIRE CADRE CARRE CHERE CHORE CLARE CRORE CUIRE CUORE DEARE DEERE DETRE DRDRE DUPRE EAGRE ENARE ENCRE ENTRE ENURE FABRE FAIRE FAURE FAVRE FIBRE FIORE FLARE FOURE FRERE GENRE GLARE GUARE HAVRE HEURE HOARE ICARE INDRE INURE ISERE JAHRE JARRE LIBRE LITRE LIVRE LOIRE LORRE LUCRE MADRE MAHRE MAIRE METRE MITRE MOIRE MOORE MURRE NACRE NIDRE NITRE NOIRE NOTRE OCHRE OHARE OMBRE OPERE OUTRE PADRE PETRE POBRE POIRE QUARE QUIRE SABRE SACRE SCARE SCIRE SCORE SEGRE SHARE SHERE SHIRE SHORE SMORE SNARE SNORE SPARE SPIRE SPORE STARE STERE STORE SUCRE SWORE TERRE THERE TIGRE TITRE TORRE TWERE VERRE VIVRE VOTRE WHERE WHYRE YOURE ZAIRE

R•F••

RAFER RAFFI RAFKO RAFTS REFAX REFED REFER REFIS REFIT REFIX REFLY REFRY RIFER RIFFS RIFLE RIFTS RSFSR RUFFS RUFUS

R••F•

RAFFI REEFS REEFY REIFY RIFFS ROLFE ROLFS ROOFS RUFFS RULFO

R•••F

RAZAF RIDOF ROBOF ROWLF

•RF••

MRFOX ORFEO ORFES

•R•F•

CRAFT CROFT DRAFT DREFT DRIFT GRAFF GRAFT GRIFT GROFE GRUFF KRAFT KROFT PROFS

•R••F

BRIEF GRAFF GRIEF GRUFF PROOF

••RF•

BARFY CORFU DORFF KERFS NERFS PERFS SERFS SURFS SURFY TURFS TURFY ZARFS

••R•F

DORFF SERIF

•••RF

DWARF FOURF SCARF SMURF SNARF WHARF

R•G••

RAGAS RAGED RAGER RAGES RAGGY RAGON REGAL REGAN REGEL REGER REGES REGIA REGIS REGLE REGNA REGTS REGUM RIGAN RIGBY RIGEL RIGGS RIGHT RIGID RIGOR RIGUP ROGER ROGET ROGUE RUGBY

R••G•

RAGGY RANGE RANGO RANGY REEGE REIGN RENGA RIDGE RIDGY RIGGS RINGO RINGS ROUGE ROUGH RUDGE RUNGS

R•••G

REBAG REDIG REDUG REJIG RELIG RELOG REPEG RERIG RETAG RUING RVING

•RG••

ARGON ARGOS ARGOT ARGUE ARGUS ERGOT ORGAN ORGON URGED URGER URGES

•R•G•

BRAGA BRAGG BRAGH BRAGS BRIGS CRAGS DRAGO DRAGS DREGS DRIGO DRUGS FRAGS FRIGG FROGS FRUGS GREGG GRIGS GROGS KRIGE KROGH PREGL PREGO PRIGS PROGS TRAGG

•R••G

BRAGG BRANG BRING BRUNG CRAIG DRANG DRHUG DRING ERING FRIGG GRAIG GREGG GRIEG IRREG KRIEG MRBIG ORANG ORING PRONG TRAGG WRING WRONG WRUNG

••RG•

AARGH BARGE BERGS BORGE BORGS BURGH BURGS CARGO CORGI DIRGE FARGO FORGE FORGO GORGE JORGE LARGE LARGO MARGE MARGO MARGY MERGE NORGE PARGE PORGY PURGE SARGE SERGE SURGE TARGA VERGE VIRGA VIRGO

••R•G

DORAG HARDG IRREG RERIG SCRAG SHRUG SPRIG STRUG UNRIG VARIG ZEROG

•••RG

BOURG GEORG INORG

RH•••

RHEAS RHEEM RHEIN RHEME RHETT RHEUM RHINE RHINO RHODA RHODE RHODO RHODY RHOMB RHONE RHUMB RHYME

R•H••

RAHAL REHAB REHAN REHEM REHID REHIT REHOE RRHEA

R••H•

RASHI RASHT RATHS RESHT RICHE RIGHT RISHI ROCHE ROSHI ROTHS RUCHE RUEHL RUSHY RUTHS

R•••H

RAJAH RALPH RANCH REACH REICH RICOH ROACH ROUGH ROUSH

•RH••

ARHAT DRHUG MRHEX RRHEA

•R•H•

ARCHE ARCHI ARCHY BRAHE BRUHL BRUHN DRWHO ORCHS ORTHO PRAHA

•R••H

ARITH ARMAH ARRAH BRACH BRAGH BRASH BRITH BROTH BRUCH BRUSH CRASH CRUSH CRWTH ERICH FREEH FRESH FROSH FROTH GRAPH IRISH KROGH ORACH ORPAH TRASH TRISH TROTH TRUTH URIAH URICH WRATH WROTH

••R•H

AARGH ARRAH BARTH BERTH BIRCH BIRTH BORAH BURGH DARTH EARTH FARAH FIRTH FORTH GARTH GIRSH GIRTH GURSH HARSH HERSH KARSH KERSH LARCH LURCH MARCH MARSH MERCH MIRTH MORPH MYRRH NORAH NORTH OPRAH PARCH PERCH PERTH PORCH QIRSH SARAH STROH SURAH TORAH TORCH WIRTH WORTH

•••RH

FOURH MYRRH

RI•••

RIALS RIANT RIATA RIBBY RICAN RICCI RICED RICER RICES RICEU RICHE RICKI RICKS RICKY RICOH RIDER RIDES RIDGE RIDGY RIDOF RIELS RIENS RIETI RIFER RIFFS RIFLE RIFTS RIGAN RIGBY RIGEL RIGGS RIGHT RIGID RIGOR RIGUP RIKER RIKKI RILED

RILES
RILEY
RILKE
RILLE
RILLS
RIMED
RIMER
RIMES
RINDS
RINDY
RINGO
RINGS
RINKS
RINKY
RINSE
RINSO
RINTY
RIOJA
RIOTS
RIPAT
RIPEN
RIPER
RIPON
RIPUP
RISEN
RISER
RISES
RISHI
RISKS
RISKY
RITES
RITZY
RIVAL
RIVED
RIVEN
RIVER
RIVES
RIVET
RIXEY
RIYAL
RIZAL
RIZZO

R•I••
RAIDS
RAILS
RAIMI
RAINE
RAINS
RAINY
RAISA
RAISE
RAITA
RAITT
REICE
REICH
REIFY
REIGN
REIMS
REINA
REINE
REINK
REINS
REISZ
REITS
RHINE
RHINO
ROILS
ROILY
RTILE
RUING
RUINS
RVING

R••I•
RABID
RABIN
RADII
RADIO
RADIX
RAJIV
RAMIE
RAMIN
RAMIS
RANID
RANIN
RANIS
RAPID
RATIO
REAIM
REAIR
REBID
RECIP
REDID
REDIG
REDIP
REFIS
REFIT
REFIX
REGIA
REGIS
REHID
REHIT
REJIG
RELIC
RELIG
RELIT
REMIT
REMIX
RENIN
REOIL
REPIN
RERIG
RESIN
RESIT
RETIA
RETIE
RETIN
RETIP
REWIN
REZIA
REZIP
RHEIN
RIGID
ROBIN
RODIN
RONIN
ROSIE
ROSIN
ROXIE
RUBIK
RUBIN
RUNIC
RUNIN
RURIK
RUTIN

R•••I
RABBI
RADII
RAFFI
RAIMI
RANDI
RASHI
RECTI
REDDI
RICCI
RICKI
RIETI
RIKKI
RISHI
ROSHI
ROSSI

•RI••
ARIAL
ARIAN
ARIAS
ARICA
ARIEL
ARIES
ARILS
ARION
ARIOT
ARISE
ARITH
ARIUM
BRIAN
BRIAR
BRIBE
BRICE
BRICK
BRIDE
BRIEF
BRIER
BRIES
BRIGS
BRILL
BRIMS
BRINE
BRING
BRINK
BRINY
BRISE
BRISK
BRITE
BRITH
BRITS
BRITT
BRITZ
CRIBS
CRICK
CRIED
CRIER
CRIES
CRIME
CRIMP
CRISP
CRIST
CRITS
CRIUS
DRIAM
DRIBS
DRIED
DRIER
DRIES
DRIFT
DRIGO
DRILL
DRILY
DRINA
DRING
DRINK
DRIPS
DRIVE
ERIAS
ERICA
ERICH
ERICK
ERIES
ERIKA
ERING
ERISA
ERITU
FRIAR
FRICK
FRIDA
FRIED
FRIEL
FRIER
FRIES
FRIGG
FRILL
FRIML
FRISE
FRISK
FRIST
FRITA
FRITE
FRITO
FRITS
FRITZ
FRIZZ
GRIDE
GRIDS
GRIEF
GRIEG
GRIER
GRIFT
GRIGS
GRILL
GRIME
GRIMM
GRIMY
GRIND
GRINS
GRINT
GRIOT
GRIPE
GRIPS
GRIPY
GRISE
GRIST
GRITS
IRIDO
IRIDS
IRINA
IRISH
KRIEG
KRIGE
KRILL
KRIPS
KRISS
ORIBI
ORIEL
ORING
ORION
ORIUM
PRIAM
PRICE
PRICK
PRICY
PRIDE
PRIED
PRIER
PRIES
PRIGS
PRIMA
PRIME
PRIMO
PRIMP
PRIMS
PRINE
PRINK
PRINT
PRIOR
PRISM
PRISS
PRIUS
PRIVY
PRIZE
PRIZM
TRIAD
TRIAL
TRIBE
TRICE
TRICK
TRIED
TRIER
TRIES
TRIKE
TRILL
TRIMS
TRINA
TRINE
TRINI
TRIOS
TRIPE
TRIPP
TRIPS
TRISH
TRITE
TRITT
URIAH
URICH
URIEL
WRIER
WRING
WRIST
WRITE
WRITS

•R•I•
ARBIL
ARKIN
ARMIN
ARNIE
AROID
ARRID
ARRIS
ARSIS
ARTIE
ARTIS
BRAID
BRAIN
BROIL
BRUIN
BRUIT
CRAIG
CRAIK
CRAIN
CROIX
DRAIN
DROID
DROIT
DRUID
ERBIL
ERNIE
ERVIN
ERWIN
FRAIL
FRAIS
FREIA
FROID
FRUIT
GRAIG
GRAIL
GRAIN
GROIN
IRVIN
IRWIN
KRAIT
MRBIG
ORBIC
ORBIT
ORKIN
ORNIS
ORRIN
ORRIS
ORTIZ
ORVIS
PRAIA
TRAIL
TRAIN
TRAIT
TROIS
TRYIT
URSID

•R••I
ARCHI
ARONI
BREVI
BRUNI
CRANI
CROCI
FRENI
GRANI
GRAVI
IRANI
IRAQI
ORANI
ORIBI
TRACI
TREVI
TRINI

••RI•
ABRIL
ABRIM
ABRIS
ACRID
ADRIP
AERIE
AERIO
AFRIC
AGRIC
AGRIN
APRIL
ARRID
ARRIS
ATRIA
ATRIP
AURIC
AVRIL
BARIC
BARIT
BERIA
BORIC
BORIS
BURIN
CARIB
CERIA
CERIC
CHRIS
CORIA
CURIA
CURIE
CURIO
CYRIL
DARIA
DARIN
DARIO
DERIV
DORIA
DORIC
DORIS
EERIE
EYRIE
EYRIR
FARIS
FERIA
FURIE
JURIS
KIRIN
KYRIE
LARIS
LORIN
LORIS
LURIA
LURID
LURIE
LYRIC
LYRID
MARIA
MARIE
MARIN
MARIO
MARIS
MERIT
MIRIN
MYRIA
NARIC
NARIS
NORIA
NORIS
ORRIN
ORRIS
OSRIC
PARIS
PERIL
PERIS
PURIM
RERIG
RURIK
SARIS
SCRIM
SCRIP
SERIA
SERIF
SERIN
SERIO
SPRIG
SPRIT
STRIA
STRIP
SYRIA
TARIQ
TERIA
TORIC
TORII
TURIN
UGRIC
ULRIC
UNRIG
UNRIP
VARIA
VARIG
VIRID
XERIC
YURIS
ZORIS

••R•I
BARBI
BERNI
BIRRI
CARDI
CARPI
CIRRI
CORGI
CORNI
CORRI
CURVI
DARCI
DORSI
FARCI
FARSI
FERMI
FERRI
GARNI
GORKI
KERRI
LEROI
MARCI
MARDI
MARKI
MARNI
MARTI
MARYI
MERCI
NURMI
PARSI
PARTI
SARAI
SARDI
SERAI
TARSI
TERRI
TORII
TORSI
VARSI
VERDI
VERMI

•••RI
AMIRI
ATARI
AZERI
BIERI
BIRRI
CAPRI
CHERI
CIRRI
CITRI
CORRI
CUPRI
FERRI
FIORI
FLORI
HENRI
HOURI
IMARI
INARI
KERRI
LIBRI
MAORI
MATRI
NEGRI
NOURI
OTERI
PATRI
PETRI
PLURI
POORI
SHARI
SPYRI
TAURI
TERRI
TETRI
VITRI

R•J••
RAJAB
RAJAH
RAJAS
RAJIV
REJIG
ROJAS

R••J•
RIOJA

••R•J
MARYJ

R•K••
RAKED
RAKER
RAKES
RAKUS
REKEY
RIKER
RIKKI
ROKER

R••K•
RACKS
RAFKO
RANKE
RANKS
RECKS
REEKS
REEKY
RICKI
RICKS
RICKY
RIKKI
RILKE
RINKS
RINKY
RISKS
RISKY
ROCKS
ROCKY
ROOKS
ROOKY
ROYKO
RUCKS
RUSKA
RUSKS

R•••K
REASK
REINK
ROARK
RUARK
RUBIK
RURIK

•RK••
ARKIN
IRKED
IRKER
ORKAN
ORKIN
URKEL

•R•K•
BRAKE
BROKE
CRAKE
DRAKE
DREKS
ERIKA
GROKS
TREKS
TRIKE
YREKA

•R••K
BRACK
BREAK
BRECK
BRICK
BRINK
BRISK
BROCK
BROOK
BRUSK
CRACK
CRAIK
CRANK
CREAK
CREEK
CRICK
CROAK
CROCK
CROOK
DRANK
DRECK
DRINK
DRUNK
ERICK
FRANK
FREAK
FRICK
FRISK
FROCK
GREEK
HRBEK
KREUK
KROCK
MRYUK
ORECK
PRANK
PRICK
PRINK
TRACK
TRASK
TRICK
TRUCK
TRUNK
WRACK
WREAK
WRECK

••RK•
BARKS
BARKY
BERKS
BORKS
BURKA
BURKE
CORKS
CORKY
DARKS
DIRKS
DORKS
DORKY
FORKS
FORKY
GORKI
GORKY
HARKS
HERKY
JERKS
JERKY
KIRKS
LARKS
LARKY
LURKS
MARKA
MARKI
MARKS
MARKV
MURKY
NARKS
PARKA
PARKS
PERKS
PERKY
PORKS
PORKY
TURKS
TURKU
WARKS
WORKS
YORKS

••R•K
BARAK
DEREK
FARUK
HEREK
HUROK
MAREK
MERCK
NORSK
RURIK
SAREK
SHREK

•••RK
BJORK
CLARK
CLERK
DMARK
OZARK
QUARK
QUIRK
ROARK
RUARK
SHARK
SHIRK
SMIRK
SNARK
SPARK
SPORK
STARK
STORK

RL•••
RLESS

R•L••
RALES
RALLY
RALPH
RELAP
RELAX
RELAY
RELED
RELEE
RELET
RELIC
RELIG
RELIT
RELOG
RILED
RILES
RILEY
RILKE
RILLE
RILLS
ROLEN
ROLEO
ROLES
ROLEX
ROLFE
ROLFS
ROLLE
ROLLO
ROLLS
ROLOS
RULED
RULER
RULES
RULFO
RVLOT

R••L•
RAILS
RALLY
RAWLS
RAWLY
REALM
REALS
REDLY
REELS
REFLY
REGLE
REPLY
RIALS
RIELS
RIFLE
RILLE
RILLS
ROALD
ROBLE
ROILS
ROILY
ROLLE
ROLLO
ROLLS
ROTLS
ROWLF
RTILE
RUBLE
RYALS

R•••L
RAHAL
RAOUL
RATEL
RAVEL
REBEL
REGAL
REGEL
RENAL
REOIL
REPEL
REUEL
REVEL
RIGEL
RIVAL
RIYAL
RIZAL
ROWEL
ROYAL
RUBEL
RUDEL
RUEHL
RURAL

•RL••
ARLEN
ARLES
DRLAO
MRLEE
ORLES
ORLON
ORLOP
ORLOS

•R•L•
ARILS
ARYLS
BRILL
BRULE
DRILL
DRILY
DROLE
DROLL
DRYLY
FRILL
GRILL
GRRLS
KRILL
KRULL
ORALB
ORALE
ORALS
PRELL
PROLE
TRALA
TRILL
TROLL
TRULY
URALS
WRYLY

•R••L
ARBIL
ARBOL
AREAL
AREEL
ARIAL
ARIEL
ARNEL
ARPEL
ARTEL
BRAWL
BRILL
BROIL
BRUHL
CRAWL
CREEL
CRUEL
DRAWL
DRILL
DROLL
DROOL
ERBIL
ERROL
FRAIL
FRIEL
FRILL
FRIML
GRAIL
GRILL
GROWL
GRRRL
GRUEL
KRAAL
KRILL
KRULL
ORIEL
ORVAL
PREGL
PRELL
PRNDL
PROWL
TRAIL
TRAWL
TRIAL
TRILL
TROLL
URIEL
URKEL

••RL•
BERLE
BIRLS
BURLS
BURLY
CARLA
CARLE
CARLO
CARLY
CURLS
CURLY
DARLA
EARLE
EARLS
EARLY
FURLS
GIRLS
GIRLY
GRRLS
HURLS
HURLY
KARLA
KARLE
MARLA
MARLO
MARLS
MARLY
MERLE
MERLS
PARLE
PERLE
PURLS
SURLY
WORLD

••R•L
ABRIL
APRIL
AURAL
AVRIL
BERYL
BOREL
CAROL
CORAL
CUREL
CYRIL
DARYL
DORAL
ENROL
ERROL
FERAL
GRRRL
GYRAL
HERZL
HORAL
JOREL
JURAL
KAREL
KAROL
MERYL
MORAL
MOREL
MURAL
NEROL
PAROL
PERIL
RURAL
SERAL
SOREL
TIROL
TYROL
VIRAL
ZOREL

•••RL
BGIRL
CEORL
CHURL
GNARL
GRRRL
KNURL
PEARL
SKIRL
SNARL
SWIRL
TWIRL
WHIRL
WHORL

R•M••
RAMAN
RAMAR
RAMAS
RAMBO
RAMEN
RAMET
RAMEY
RAMIE
RAMIN
RAMIS
RAMON
RAMOS
RAMPS
RAMUS
RAMUZ
REMAN
REMAP
REMAT
REMAX
REMET
REMIT
REMIX
REMOP
REMOW
REMUS
RIMED
RIMER
RIMES
ROMAN
ROMEO
ROMES
ROMPS
RUMAN
RUMBA
RUMER
RUMMY
RUMOR
RUMPS

R••M•
RAIMI
REAMS
REIMS
RHEME
RHOMB
RHUMB
RHYME
ROAMS
ROOMS
ROOMY
RUMMY

R•••M
REAIM
REALM
REARM
REGUM
REHEM
RHEEM
RHEUM
ROREM

•RM••
ARMAH
ARMAS
ARMED
ARMEE
ARMEN
ARMER
ARMES
ARMET
ARMEY
ARMIN
ARMOR
ERMAS
MRMET
MRMOM
ORMAN
PRMAN
PRMEN

•R•M•
ARAME
AROMA
ARUMS
BRIMS
BROMO
BRUME
CRAMP
CRAMS
CREMA
CREME
CRIME
CRIMP
CRUMB
CRUMP

DRAMA
DRAMS
DROME
DRUMS
FRAME
FRIML
FROME
FROMM
FRUMP
GRAMM
GRAMO
GRAMP
GRAMS
GRIME
GRIMM
GRIMY
GRUMP
KREME
ORAMA
PRAMS
PRIMA
PRIME
PRIMO
PRIMP
PRIMS
PROMO
PROMS
TRAMP
TRAMS
TRIMS
TROMP
TRUMP
TRYME

•R••M

ARIUM
BREAM
BROOM
CREAM
DREAM
DRIAM
FROMM
GRAMM
GRIMM
GROOM
MRMOM
ORIUM
PRIAM
PRISM
PRIZM
PROAM
PROEM
VROOM

••RM•

BARMS
BARMY
BERMS
BURMA
CARME
CORMS
DERMA
DERMO
DORMS
DORMY
FARMS
FERMI
FIRMA
FIRMS
FORMA
FORMS
GERMS
GERMY
GORME
GORMS
HARMS
KARMA
MARMS
NORMA
NORMS
NURMI
PARMA
PERMA
PERMS
TERME
TERMS
TORME
VERMI
WARMS
WORMS
WORMY

••R•M

ABRAM
ABRIM
ADREM
AMRAM
AURUM
CAROM
CDROM
CERAM
CHROM
DIRAM
DURUM
EFREM
EPROM
FORUM
HAREM
HARUM
HIRAM
INREM
JORUM
LARAM
PURIM
ROREM
SCRAM
SCRIM
SCRUM
SERUM
STRAM
STROM
STRUM
THRUM

•••RM

ALARM
CHARM
ENARM
ENORM
PHARM
REARM
SHERM
SMARM
SPERM
STORM
STURM
SWARM
THERM
UNARM

RN•••

RNASE

R•N••

RANAS
RANAT
RANBY
RANCH
RANDA
RANDB
RANDD
RANDI
RANDR
RANDS
RANDY
RANEE
RANGE
RANGO
RANGY
RANID
RANIN
RANIS
RANKE
RANKS
RANON
RANTO
RANTS
RANUP
RENAL
RENAN
RENAY
RENDS
RENEE
RENEW
RENGA
RENIN
RENNY
RENTE
RENTS
RINDS
RINDY
RINGO
RINGS
RINKS
RINKY
RINSE
RINSO
RINTY
RONAN
RONCO
RONDE
RONDO
RONEE
RONIN
RONNY
RUNAT
RUNBY
RUNES
RUNGS
RUNIC
RUNIN
RUNNY
RUNON
RUNTO
RUNTS
RUNTY
RUNUP

R••N•

RAINE
RAINS
RAINY
REGNA
REINA
REINE
REINK
REINS
RENNY
REUNE
RHINE
RHINO
RHONE
RIANT
RIENS
ROANS
RONNY
ROONE
ROUND
RUING
RUINS
RUNNY
RVING
RYANS

R•••N

RABIN
RADON
RAGON
RAMAN
RAMEN
RAMIN
RAMON
RANIN
RANON
RAPON
RATON
RAVEN
RAYON
RECAN
RECON
REDAN
REDON
REGAN
REHAN
REIGN
REMAN
RENAN
RENIN
REOWN
REPEN
REPIN
RERAN
RERUN
RESIN
RETAN
RETIN
REWIN
REWON
RHEIN
RICAN
RIGAN
RIPEN
RIPON
RISEN
RIVEN
ROBIN
ROBYN
RODAN
RODIN
ROLEN
ROMAN
RONAN
RONIN
ROSEN
ROSIN
ROUEN
ROWAN
ROWEN
RUBEN
RUBIN
RUBON
RUMAN
RUNIN
RUNON
RUTIN

•RN••

ARNAZ
ARNEL
ARNIE
ERNES
ERNIE
ERNST
ORNIS
PRNDL
URNES

•R•N•

ARANS
ARENA
ARENS
ARENT
ARONI
ARUNS
BRAND
BRANG
BRANS
BRANT
BRENS
BRENT
BRINE
BRING
BRINK
BRINY
BRONC
BRONX
BRUNG
BRUNI
BRUNO
BRUNT
CRANE
CRANI
CRANK
CRONE
CRONY
DRANG
DRANK
DRANO
DRINA
DRING
DRINK
DRONE
DRUNK
ERING
FRANC
FRANK
FRANN
FRANS
FRANZ
FRENA
FRENI
FROND
FRONT
GRAND
GRANI
GRANT
GRIND
GRINS
GRINT
GRUNT
IRANI
IRENA
IRENE
IRINA
IRONS
IRONY
KRONA
KRONE
ORANG
ORANI
ORANT
ORENA
ORING
ORONO
PRANA
PRANK
PRINE
PRINK
PRINT
PRONE
PRONG
PRUNE
TRANE
TRANS
TREND
TRENT
TRINA
TRINE
TRINI
TRUNK
URANO
WRENS
WRING
WRONG
WRUNG

•R••N

ARDEN
ARGON
ARIAN
ARION
ARKIN
ARLEN
ARMEN
ARMIN
ARRAN
ARSON
ARWEN
ARYAN
BRAIN
BRAUN
BRAWN
BREEN
BRIAN
BROUN
BROWN
BRUHN
BRUIN
BRYAN
CRAIN
CREON
CROON
CROWN
DRAIN
DRAWN
DROWN
DRUON
ERVIN
ERWIN
FRANN
FRAYN
FREON
FROWN
GRAIN
GREEN
GROAN
GROIN
GROWN
IRVIN
IRWIN
KROON
ORGAN
ORGON
ORION
ORKAN
ORKIN
ORLON
ORMAN
ORREN
ORRIN
ORSON
ORTON
PRAWN
PREEN
PRMAN
PRMEN
TRAIN
TREEN
TROON
TRYON
URBAN

••RN•

BARNS
BERNE
BERNI
BORNE
BURNS
BURNT
BYRNE
CARNE
CARNY
CORNI
CORNO
CORNS
CORNU
CORNY
DARNS
DURNS
EARNS
FERNS
FERNY
FIRNS
GARNI
HERNE
HORNE
HORNS
HORNY
JERNE
KARNS
KERNE
KERNS
LORNA
LORNE
MARNE
MARNI
MORNS
MYRNA
NORNS
PIRNS
PORNO
TARNS
TERNE
TERNS
TURNS
VARNA
VERNA
VERNE
VIRNA
WARNS
YARNS

••R•N

AARON
AGRIN
AGRON
AKRON
APRON
ARRAN
BARON
BOREN
BORON
BUREN
BURIN
BYRON
CARON
CHRON
DARIN
DORAN
DOREN
DURAN
DUREN
EHREN
ENRON
FARON
GORAN
GOREN
HERON
HURON
INRUN
JURAN
KARAN
KAREN
KARYN
KIRIN
KORAN
LORAN
LOREN
LORIN
MARIN
MIRIN
MORAN
MORON
MYRON
NOREN
NORUN
ORREN
ORRIN
PAREN
PERAN
PERON
QURAN
RERAN
RERUN
SARAN
SERIN
SIREN
SOREN
TURIN
UNRUN

•••RN

ACORN
ADARN
ADORN
AGARN
BAIRN
BJORN
CAIRN
CHURN
DOORN
HEARN
LEARN
MOURN
SCORN
SHORN
SPURN
STERN
SWORN
THORN
UTURN
YEARN
YOURN

RO•••

ROACH
ROADS
ROALD
ROAMS
ROANS
ROARK
ROARS
ROAST
ROBBE
ROBBY
ROBED
ROBER
ROBES
ROBIN
ROBLE
ROBOF
ROBOT
ROBYN
ROCCO
ROCHE
ROCKS
ROCKY
RODAN
RODDY
RODEO
RODIN
RODYA
ROGER
ROGET
ROGUE
ROILS
ROILY
ROJAS
ROKER
ROLEN
ROLEO
ROLES
ROLEX
ROLFE
ROLFS
ROLLE
ROLLO
ROLLS
ROLOS
ROMAN
ROMEO
ROMES
ROMPS
RONAN
RONCO
RONDE
RONDO
RONEE
RONIN
RONNY
ROODS
ROOFS
ROOKS
ROOKY
ROOMS
ROOMY
ROONE
ROOSA
ROOST
ROOTS
ROOTY
ROPED
ROPER
ROPES
ROQUE
ROREM
ROSEN
ROSES
ROSEY
ROSHI
ROSIE
ROSIN
ROSSA
ROSSI
ROSSO
ROTAS
ROTCS
ROTES
ROTHS
ROTLS
ROTOR
ROTOS
ROUEN
ROUES
ROUGE
ROUGH
ROUND
ROUSE
ROUSH
ROUST
ROUTE
ROUTS
ROVED
ROVER
ROVES
ROWAN
ROWDY
ROWED
ROWEL
ROWEN
ROWER
ROWLF
ROWSE
ROXIE
ROYAL
ROYCE
ROYKO

R•O••

RAOUL
REOIL
REOWN
RHODA
RHODE
RHODO
RHODY
RHOMB
RHONE
RIOJA
RIOTS
ROODS
ROOFS
ROOKS
ROOKY
ROOMS
ROOMY
ROONE
ROOSA
ROOST
ROOTS
ROOTY

R••O•

RADON
RAGON
RAMON
RAMOS
RANON
RAPON
RATON
RAYON
RAZOR
REBOP
REBOX
RECON
REDON
REDOS
REDOX
REHOE
RELOG
REMOP
REMOW
REPOS
REPOT
RESOD
RESOW
RETOP
RETOW
REWON
RICOH
RIDOF
RIGOR
RIPON
ROBOF
ROBOT
ROLOS
ROTOR
ROTOS
RUBON
RUMOR
RUNON
RVLOT

R•••O

RADIO
RAFKO
RAMBO
RANGO
RANTO
RATIO
RATSO
RECTO
REPRO
RETRO
RHINO
RHODO
RINGO
RINSO
RIZZO
ROCCO
RODEO
ROLEO
ROLLO
ROMEO
RONCO
RONDO
ROSSO
ROYKO
RULFO
RUNTO
RUSSO

•RO••

AROAR
AROID
AROMA
ARONI
AROSE
BROAD
BROCA
BROCK
BRODY
BROIL
BROKE
BROMO
BRONC
BRONX
BROOD
BROOK
BROOM
BROTH
BROUD
BROUN
BROWN
BROWS
CROAK
CROAT
CROCE
CROCI
CROCK
CROCS
CROFT
CROIX
CRONE
CRONY
CROOK
CROON
CROPS
CRORE
CROSS
CROUP
CROWD
CROWE
CROWN
CROWS
DROID
DROIT
DROLE
DROLL
DROME
DRONE
DROOD
DROOL
DROOP
DROPO
DROPS
DROPT
DROSS
DROVE
DROWN
ERODE
EROES
EROSE
FROBE
FROCK
FRODO
FROES
FROGS
FROID
FROME
FROMM
FROND
FRONT
FROOT
FROSH
FROST
FROTH
FROWN
FROWS
FROYO
FROZE
GROAN
GROAT
GRODY
GROFE
GROGS
GROIN
GROKS
GROOM
GROPE
GROSS
GROSZ
GROTE
GROTS
GROUP
GROUT
GROVE
GROWL
GROWN
GROWS
GROZA
HROSS
IROCS
IRONS
IRONY
JROTC
KROCK
KROFT
KROGH
KRONA
KRONE
KROON
KROTO
NROTC
ORONO
ORORY
PROAM
PROAS
PROBE
PROBS
PRODS
PROEM
PROFS
PROGS
PROLE
PROMO
PROMS
PRONE
PRONG
PROOF
PROPS
PROSE
PROSS
PROST
PROSY
PROTO
PROTS
PROUD
PROVE
PROVO
PROVS
PROWL
PROWS
PROXY
TROIS
TROLL
TROMP
TROON
TROOP
TROPE
TROPO
TROTH
TROTS
TROUP
TROUT
TROVE
TROWE
TROWS
UROUS
VROOM
WRONG
WROTE
WROTH

•R•O•

ARBOL
ARBOR
ARDOR
ARGON
ARGOS
ARGOT
ARION
ARIOT
ARMOR
ARROW
ARROZ
ARSON
ARTOO
BROOD
BROOK
BROOM
CREON
CROOK
CROON
CRUOR
DROOD
DROOL
DROOP
DRUON
ERDOS
ERGOT
ERROL
ERROR
FREON
FROOT
GRIOT
GROOM
KROON
MRFOX
MRMOM
OREOS
ORGON
ORION
ORLON
ORLOP
ORLOS
ORSON
ORTON
ORZOS
PREOP
PRIOR
PROOF
PRYOR
TRIOS
TROON
TROOP
TRYON
VROOM

•R••O

ARADO
ARESO
ARTOO
BRAVO
BRAZO
BROMO
BRUNO
CREDO
DRACO
DRAGO
DRANO
DRIGO
DRLAO
DROPO
DRWHO
ERATO
FREDO
FRITO
FRODO
FROYO
GRAMO
GRECO
IRIDO
KROTO
ORFEO
ORONO
ORTHO
ORURO
PRADO
PRATO
PREGO
PRIMO
PROMO
PROTO
PROVO
TROPO
TRURO
TRYTO
URANO

••RO•

AARON
AEROS
AFROS
AGRON
AKRON
ALROY
APRON
ARROW
ARROZ
BARON
BIROS
BORON
BOROS
BYRON
CAROB
CAROL
CAROM
CARON
CDROM
CEROS
CHROM
CHRON
COROT
DUROC
DUROS
ELROY
ENROL
ENRON
EPROM
ERROL
ERROR
EUROS
FAROE
FARON
FAROS
FUROR
FUROS
GAROU
GIROS
GYROS
HEROD
HERON
HEROS
HUROK
HURON
JUROR
KAROL
KIROV
LEROI
LEROS
LEROY
MAROT
MEROE
MIROS
MORON
MOROS
MYRON
NEROL
OGROS
OHROB
OTROS
PAROL
PAROO
PAROS
PERON
PEROT
PYROS
SAROS
SCROD
SOROS
STROH
STROM
STROP
STROS
TAROS
TAROT
THROB
THROE
THROW
TIROL
TIROS
TOROS
TUROW
TYROL
TYROS
XEROX
ZEROG
ZEROS

••R•O

AEREO
AERIO
BARCO
BURRO

CARBO
CARGO
CARLO
CARPO
CERRO
CIRRO
CORNO
CORSO
CORVO
CURIO
DARIO
DERMO
DORSO
FARGO
FERRO
FIRPO
FORDO
FORGO
GARBO
GORDO
HARPO
LARGO
MARCO
MARGO
MARIO
MARLO
MARZO
MIRRO
MORRO
NARCO
NARDO
NERVO
NORVO
PARDO
PAROO
PERRO
PORNO
PORTO
SARTO
SERBO
SERIO
SERVO
SORBO
TARDO
TARSO
TORSO
TURBO
TURCO
VARRO
VERSO
VIREO
VIRGO
ZORRO

•••RO

ALERO
ANDRO
ASTRO
BURRO
CAIRO
CERRO
CHARO
CHIRO
CHORO
CIRRO
CITRO
CLARO
CUPRO
DOBRO
DOURO
ELORO
ENERO
EXTRO
FERRO
FIBRO
FIERO
GOPRO
HIERO
HYDRO
HYGRO
IATRO
INTRO
LAURO
LIBRO
MACRO
MATRO
METRO
MICRO
MIRRO
MONRO
MORRO
MUNRO
NATRO
NEGRO
NEURO
NITRO
NUTRO
ORURO
OTERO
PATRO
PEDRO
PERRO
PETRO
PTERO
REPRO
RETRO
SACRO
SAURO
SPERO
SPIRO
SPYRO
STYRO
TAURO
THORO
TOURO
TRURO
VARRO
VITRO
ZORRO

R•P••

RAPEE
RAPID
RAPON
REPAD
REPAY
REPEG
REPEL
REPEN
REPIN
REPLY
REPOS
REPOT
REPPS
REPRO
REPUB
RIPAT
RIPEN
RIPER
RIPON
RIPUP
ROPED
ROPER
ROPES
RUPEE

R••P•

RALPH
RAMPS
RASPA
RASPE
RASPS
RASPY
REAPS
REPPS
REUPS
ROMPS
RSVPD
RSVPS
RUMPS

R•••P

RANUP
REBOP
RECAP
RECIP
REDIP
RELAP
REMAP
REMOP
RETAP
RETIP
RETOP
REVUP
REZIP
RIGUP
RIPUP
RUBUP
RUNUP

•RP••

ARPAD
ARPEL
ORPAH

•R•P•

CRAPE
CRAPS
CREPE
CREPT
CROPS
CRYPT
DRAPE
DRIPS
DROPO
DROPS
DROPT
DRUPE
ERUPT
GRAPE
GRAPH
GRAPY
GRIPE
GRIPS
GRIPY
GROPE
KREPS
KRIPS
KRUPA
KRUPP
KRUPS
PREPS
PROPS
TRAPP
TRAPS
TRIPE
TRIPP
TRIPS
TROPE
TROPO
WRAPS
WRAPT

•R••P

CRAMP
CREEP
CRIMP
CRISP
CROUP
CRUMP
CRYUP
DROOP
DRYUP
FRUMP
FRYUP
GRAMP
GRASP
GROUP
GRUMP
KRUPP
ORLOP
PREOP
PRIMP
TRAMP
TRAPP
TRIPP
TROMP
TROOP
TROUP
TRUMP

••RP•

BURPS
CARPE
CARPI
CARPO
CARPS
CORPS
DORPS
EARPS
FIRPO
GORPS
HARPO
HARPS
HARPY
MORPH
MSRPS
PERPS
TARPS
TERPS
WARPS

••R•P

ADREP
ADRIP
AIRUP
ATRIP
PTRAP
SCRAP
SCRIP
SIRUP
STRAP
STREP
STRIP
STROP
SYRUP
UNRIP

•••RP

CHIRP
SCARP
SHARP
SLURP
THARP
TWERP
TWIRP
USURP

R•Q••

ROQUE

•R•Q•

IRAQI

••RQ•

BARQS

••R•Q

BARBQ
TARIQ

RR•••

RRHEA

R•R••

RARAE
RAREE
RARER
RERAN
RERIG
RERUN
ROREM
RTREV
RURAL
RURIK

R••R•

REARM
REARS
REDRY
REFRY
REPRO
RETRO
RETRY
ROARK
ROARS
RUARK
RUERS
RVERS

R•••R

RACER
RADAR
RADER
RAFER
RAGER
RAKER
RAMAR
RANDR
RARER
RASER
RATER
RAVER
RAWER
RAZER
RAZOR
REAIR
REBAR
REBER
RECUR
REFER
REGER
RETAR
RICER
RIDER
RIFER
RIGOR
RIKER
RIMER
RIPER
RISER
RIVER
ROBER
ROGER
ROKER
ROPER
ROTOR
ROVER
ROWER
RSFSR
RUDER
RULER
RUMER
RUMOR
RYDER

•RR••

ARRAH
ARRAN
ARRAS
ARRAU
ARRAY
ARRET
ARRID
ARRIS
ARROW
ARROZ
ERRED
ERROL
ERROR
GRRLS
GRRRL
GRRRS
IRREG
ORREN
ORRIN
ORRIS

•R•R•

ARARA
ARBRE
BRERS
CRORE
CRURA
DRDRE
DRURY
FRERE
GRRRL
GRRRS
ORORY
ORURO
GRRRL
GRRRS
TRURO

•R••R

ARBER
ARBOR
ARDOR
AREAR
ARMER
ARMOR
AROAR
ARTUR
BRIAR
BRIER
CRIER
CRUOR
CRYER
DREAR
DRIER
DRYER
ERROR
FREER
FRIAR
FRIER
FRYER
GREER
GRIER
IRKER
ORDER
ORSER
PRIER
PRIOR
PRYER
PRYOR
TRIER
TRUER
URGER
WRIER
WRYER

••RR•

BARRE
BARRY
BERRA
BERRY
BIRRA
BIRRI
BIRRS
BURRO
BURRS
BURRY
CARRE
CARRY
CERRO
CIRRI
CIRRO
CORRI
CURRS
CURRY
DERRY
DURRA
FERRI
FERRO
FERRY
FIRRY
FURRY
GARRY
GERRY
GRRRL
GRRRS
HARRY
HURRY
JARRE
JERRY
KERRI
KERRY
LARRY
LORRE
LORRY
MARRY
MERRY
MIRRO
MORRA
MORRO
MURRE
MYRRH
PARRA
PARRS
PARRY
PERRO
PERRY
PURRS
SERRA
SORRY
TARRY
TERRA
TERRE
TERRI
TERRS
TERRY
TORRE
TORRS
VARRO
VERRE
WORRY
YARRA
ZORRO

••R•R

AIRER
AURAR
BARER
BORER
CARER
CORER
CURER
DARER
DIRER
DURER
ERROR
EYRIR
FARER
FIRER
FUROR
HIRER
JUROR
LURER
MERER
OARER
PARER
PORER
PURER
RARER
SORER
SURER
WIRER
YARER

•••RR

CHIRR
DOERR
KNORR
OMARR
SHIRR
STARR
WHIRR

RS•••

RSFSR
RSTUV
RSVPD
RSVPS

R•S••

RASAE
RASED
RASER
RASES
RASHI
RASHT
RASPA
RASPE
RASPS
RASPY
RASSE
RASTA
RESAT
RESAW
RESAY
RESEE
RESET
RESEW
RESHT
RESIN
RESIT
RESOD
RESOW
RESTE
RESTS
RISEN
RISER
RISES
RISHI
RISKS
RISKY
ROSEN
ROSES
ROSEY
ROSHI
ROSIE
ROSIN
ROSSA
ROSSI
ROSSO
RUSES
RUSHY
RUSKA
RUSKS
RUSSA
RUSSE
RUSSO
RUSTS
RUSTY

R••S•

RAISA
RAISE
RASSE
RATSO
REASK
REESE
REISZ
REUSE
REUSS
RINSE
RINSO
RLESS
RNASE
ROAST
ROOSA
ROOST
ROSSA
ROSSI
ROSSO
ROUSE
ROUSH
ROUST
ROWSE
RSFSR
RUSSA
RUSSE
RUSSO

R•••S

RACES
RACKS
RAFTS
RAGAS
RAGES
RAIDS
RAILS
RAINS
RAJAS
RAKES
RAKUS
RALES
RAMAS
RAMIS
RAMOS
RAMPS
RAMUS
RANAS
RANDS
RANIS
RANKS
RANTS
RASES
RASPS
RATES
RATHS
RAVES
RAWLS
RAXES
RAZES
READS
REALS
REAMS
REAPS
REARS
REBUS
RECKS
RECTS
REDES
REDOS
REEDS
REEFS
REEKS
REELS
REFIS
REGES
REGIS
REGTS
REIMS
REINS
REITS
REMUS
RENDS
RENTS
REPOS
REPPS
RESTS
REUPS
REUSS
REVES
REXES
REYES
RHEAS
RIALS
RICES
RICKS
RIDES
RIELS
RIENS
RIFFS
RIFTS
RIGGS
RILES
RILLS
RIMES
RINDS
RINGS
RINKS
RIOTS
RISES
RISKS
RITES
RIVES
RLESS
ROADS
ROAMS
ROANS
ROARS
ROBES
ROCKS
ROILS
ROJAS
ROLES
ROLFS
ROLLS
ROLOS
ROMES
ROMPS
ROODS
ROOFS
ROOKS
ROOMS
ROOTS
ROPES
ROSES
ROTAS
ROTCS
ROTES
ROTHS
ROTLS
ROTOS
ROUES
ROUTS
ROVES
RSVPS
RUBES
RUCKS
RUERS
RUFFS
RUFUS
RUINS
RULES
RUMPS
RUNES
RUNGS
RUNTS
RUSES
RUSKS
RUSTS
RUTHS
RVERS
RYALS
RYANS

•RS••

ARSES
ARSIS
ARSON
ORSAY
ORSER
ORSES
ORSON
QRSTU
URSAE
URSID
URSUS

•R•S•

ARESO
ARISE
AROSE
ARTSY
BRASH
BRASS
BREST
BRISE
BRISK
BRUSH
BRUSK
CRASH
CRASS
CRESC
CRESS
CREST
CRISP
CRIST
CROSS
CRUSE
CRUSH
CRUST
DRESS
DROSS
DRUSE
ERASE
ERISA
ERNST
EROSE
FRESH
FRESS
FRISE
FRISK
FRIST
FROSH
FROST
GRASP
GRASS
GRISE
GRIST
GROSS
GROSZ
HROSS
IRISH
KRESS
KRISS
PRESA
PRESB
PRESE
PRESS
PRISM
PRISS
PROSE
PROSS
PROST
PROSY
TRASH
TRASK
TRESS
TRISH
TRUSS
TRUST
TRYST
WREST
WRIST

•R••S

ARABS
ARANS
ARBUS
ARBYS
AREAS
ARENS
ARGOS
ARGUS
ARIAS
ARIES
ARILS
ARLES
ARMAS
ARMES
ARRAS
ARRIS
ARSES
ARSIS
ARTIS
ARUMS
ARUNS
ARYLS
BRADS
BRAES
BRAGS
BRANS
BRASS
BRATS
BRAYS
BREES
BRENS
BRERS
BREWS
BRIES
BRIGS
BRIMS
BRITS
BROWS
BRUTS
CRABS
CRAGS
CRAMS
CRAPS
CRASS
CRAWS
CRAYS
CREDS
CREES
CRESS
CREWS
CRIBS
CRIES
CRITS
CRIUS
CROCS
CROPS
CROSS
CROWS
CRUDS
DRABS
DRAGS
DRAMS
DRATS
DRAWS
DRAYS
DREGS
DREKS
DRESS
DRIBS
DRIES
DRIPS
DROPS
DROSS
DRUBS
DRUGS
DRUMS
ERDOS
EREVS
ERIAS
ERIES
ERMAS
ERNES
EROES
ERTES
FRAGS
FRAIS
FRANS
FRATS
FRAYS
FREES
FRESS
FRETS
FRIES
FRITS
FROES
FROGS
FROWS
FRUGS
GRABS
GRADS
GRAMS
GRASS
GRAYS
GREYS
GRIDS
GRIGS
GRINS
GRIPS
GRITS
GROGS
GROKS
GROSS
GROTS
GROWS
GRRLS
GRRRS
GRUBS
GRUES
HROSS
IRIDS
IROCS
IRONS
KRAUS
KREBS
KREPS
KRESS
KRIPS
KRISS
KRUPS
ORALS
ORCAS
ORCHS
ORCUS
OREOS
ORFES
ORLES
ORLOS
ORNIS
ORRIS
ORSES
ORVIS
ORZOS
PRAMS
PRAYS
PREPS
PRESS
PREYS
PRIES
PRIGS
PRIMS
PRISS
PRIUS
PROAS
PROBS
PRODS
PROFS
PROGS
PROMS
PROPS
PROSS
PROTS
PROVS
PROWS
SRTAS
TRAMS
TRANS
TRAPS
TRAYS
TREAS
TREES
TREKS
TRESS
TRETS
TREWS
TREYS
TRIES
TRIMS
TRIOS
TRIPS
TROIS
TROTS
TROWS
TRUES
TRUSS
URALS
UREAS
URGES
URNES
UROUS
URSUS
WRAPS
WRENS
WRITS
XRAYS

••RS•

BIRSE
BORSA
BURSA
BURST
CORSA
CORSO
CURSA
CURSE
CURST
DORSA
DORSI
DORSO
DURST
FARSI
FIRST
FURST
GIRSH
GORSE
GORSY
GURSH
HARSH
HERSH
HORSE
HORST
HORSY
HURST
KARSH
KARST
KERSH
MARSH
MORSE
NORSE
NORSK
NURSE
PARSE
PARSI
PERSE
PQRST
PURSE
PURSY
QIRSH
TARSI
TARSO
TERSE
TORSI
TORSO
VARSI
VERSA
VERSE
VERSO
VERST
WORSE
WORST
WURST

••R•S

ABRIS
ACRES
AEROS
AFROS
AIRES
APRES
ARRAS
ARRIS
ATRAS
AURAS
AYRES
BARBS
BARDS
BARES
BARKS
BARMS
BARNS
BARQS
BERGS
BERKS
BERMS
BIRDS
BIRLS
BIROS
BIRRS
BORAS
BORES
BORGS
BORIS
BORKS
BOROS
BURBS
BURGS
BURLS
BURNS

BURPS BURRS BYRDS CARBS CARDS CARES CARPS CARTS CERES CEROS CERTS CHRIS CIRCS CIRES CORDS CORES CORKS CORMS CORNS CORPS CURBS CURDS CURES CURLS CURRS CYRUS DARES DARKS DARNS DARTS DIRKS DIRTS DORIS DORKS DORMS DORPS DURAS DURNS DUROS EARLS EARNS EARPS ECRUS ETRES EUROS EURUS EYRAS FARES FARIS FARMS FAROS FERNS FIRES FIRMS FIRNS FORDS FORES FORKS FORMS FORTS FURLS FUROS GARBS GARES GERMS GIRDS GIRLS GIROS

GIRTS GORES GORMS GORPS GRRLS GRRRS GURUS GYRES GYROS HARES HARKS HARMS HARPS HERBS HERDS HERES HEROS HERTS HIRES HORAS HORNS HORUS HURLS HURTS JERKS JURIS KARAS KARNS KARTS KARUS KERBS KERFS KERNS KIRKS KURDS KURUS KURYS LARAS LARDS LARES LARIS LARKS LEROS LIRAS LORDS LORES LORIS LORUS LURES LURKS LYRAS LYRES MARES MARIS MARKS MARLS MARMS MARTS MARYS MERCS MERES MERLS MIRES MIROS MIRVS MORAS MORES MORNS

MOROS MSRPS MURES NARAS NARCS NARDS NARES NARIS NARKS NERDS NERFS NERTS NORIS NORMS NORNS OBRAS OGRES OGROS OKRAS ORRIS OTRAS OTROS PARAS PARCS PARDS PARES PARIS PARKS PAROS PARRS PARTS PERAS PERCS PERES PERFS PERIS PERKS PERMS PERPS PIRNS PORCS PORES PORKS PORTS PURLS PURRS PYRES PYROS SARDS SARIS SAROS SERBS SERFS SERTS SIRES SORAS SORBS SORES SOROS SORTS STROS SURAS SURFS TARAS TARES TARNS TAROS TARPS

TARTS TERMS TERNS TERPS TERRS TIRES TIROS TORAS TOROS TORRS TORTS TORUS TURFS TURKS TURNS TYRES TYROS TYRUS VERBS VERTS VIRUS WARDS WARES WARKS WARMS WARNS WARPS WARTS WIRES WORDS WORKS WORMS WORTS YARDS YARNS YORES YORKS YPRES YURIS YURTS ZARFS ZEROS ZORIS

•••RS

ABBRS ACERS ADARS ADDRS AFARS AGARS AGERS AKERS ALERS ALORS AMIRS AMORS APARS APERS ASORS ATARS AVERS AXERS AYERS BEARS BEERS BIERS BIRRS

BLURS BOARS BOERS BOORS BRERS BURRS CBERS CHARS CMDRS COIRS COORS CUERS CURRS CZARS DEARS DEERS DIORS DOERS DOORS DYERS EMIRS ENGRS EVERS EWERS EYERS FAIRS FEARS FIERS FLIRS FOURS GAURS GEARS GNARS GOERS GRRRS GUARS HAIRS HBARS HEARS HEIRS HOARS HOERS HOURS HUERS IBARS ICERS INCRS ITERS IYARS JBARS JEERS JOURS KCARS KNARS KNURS LAIRS LBARS LEARS LEERS LEHRS LEURS LIARS LOURS MEARS MIERS MOORS MYERS NEARS

NLERS NOIRS ODORS OMERS ONERS OPQRS OVERS OWERS OYERS PAIRS PARRS PEARS PEERS PEURS PIERS POORS POURS PURRS REARS ROARS RUERS RVERS SCARS SEARS SEERS SLURS SOARS SOIRS SOURS SPARS SPURS STARS STIRS SUERS TBARS TEARS TEERS TERRS THURS TIERS TORRS TOURS TSARS TZARS USERS VEERS VIERS WEARS WEIRS WHIRS YEARS YOURS ZBARS

RT•••

RTILE RTREV

R•T••

RATED RATEL RATER RATES RATHS RATIO RATON RATSO RATTY

RETAG RETAN RETAP RETAR RETAX RETIA RETIE RETIN RETIP RETOP RETOW RETRO RETRY RETTY RITES RITZY ROTAS ROTCS ROTES ROTHS ROTLS ROTOR ROTOS RSTUV RUTHS RUTIN RUTTY

R••T•

RAFTS RAITA RAITT RANTO RANTS RASTA RATTY REATA RECTA RECTI RECTO RECTS REGTS REITS RENTE RENTS RESTE RESTS RETTY RHETT RIATA RIETI RIFTS RINTY RIOTS ROOTS ROOTY ROUTE ROUTS RUNTO RUNTS RUNTY RUSTS RUSTY RUTTY

R•••T

RABAT RAITT

RAMET RANAT RASHT REACT REBET REBUT RECUT REFIT REHIT RELET RELIT REMAT REMET REMIT REPOT RESAT RESET RESHT RESIT REVET REWET RHETT RIANT RIGHT RIPAT RIVET ROAST ROBOT ROGET ROOST ROUST RUNAT RVLOT

•RT••

ARTEL ARTIE ARTIS ARTOO ARTSY ARTUR ERTES ORTHO ORTIZ ORTON SRTAS

•R•T•

ARETE ARITH BRATS BRATT BRETT BRITE BRITH BRITS BRITT BRITZ BROTH BRUTE BRUTS CRATE CRETE CRITS CRWTH DRATS ERATO ERETZ

ERITU FRATS FRETS FRITA FRITE FRITO FRITS FRITZ FROTH GRATA GRATE GRETA GRETE GRITS GROTE GROTS IRATE JROTC KROTO NROTC ORATE PRATE PRATO PRATT PROTO PROTS QRSTU TRETS TRITE TRITT TROTH TROTS TRUTH TRYTO WRATH WRITE WRITS WROTE WROTH

•R••T

ARENT ARGOT ARHAT ARIOT ARMET ARRET BRACT BRANT BRATT BRENT BREST BRETT BRITT BRUIT BRUNT CRAFT CREPT CREST CRIST CROAT CROFT CRUET CRUST CRYPT DRAFT DREFT DRIFT

DROIT DROPT ERECT ERGOT ERNST ERUCT ERUPT FRIST FRONT FROOT FROST FRUCT FRUIT GRAFT GRANT GREAT GREET GRIFT GRINT GRIOT GRIST GROAT GROUT GRUNT KRAFT KRAIT KRAUT KROFT MRMET ORANT ORBIT PRATT PRINT PROST TRACT TRAIT TREAT TRENT TRITT TROUT TRUST TRYIT TRYST WRAPT WREST WRIST

••RT•

AORTA BARTH BARTY BERTA BERTH BIRTH CARTA CARTE CARTS CERTS DARTE DARTH DARTS DIRTS DIRTY EARTH FIRTH FORTE FORTH FORTS

FORTY GARTH GERTZ GIRTH GIRTS HARTE HERTS HERTZ HURTS KARTS KURTZ MARTA MARTI MARTS MARTY MERTZ MIRTH MORTE MORTY NERTS NERTZ NORTE NORTH PARTA PARTB PARTC PARTE PARTI PARTS PARTV PARTY PERTH PORTA PORTE PORTO PORTS PURTY SARTO SERTA SERTS SORTA SORTS TARTE TARTS TARTU TARTY TORTA TORTE TORTS VERTE VERTS VIRTU WARTS WARTY WIRTH WORTH WORTS YORTY YURTS

••R•T

ARRET BARIT BERET BURET BURNT BURST CARAT

CARET CERAT COROT CURET CURST DERAT DURST EGRET FIRST FURST HERAT HORST HURST KARAT KARST KORAT MARAT MAROT MERIT MURAT OCRAT PEROT PQRST SCRAT SPRAT SPRIT STRAT STRUT TAROT TERAT VERST WORST WURST

•••RT

ABORT ALERT AMORT APART APORT AVERT BEART BLURT CHART CHERT COURT EBERT EVERT EWART EXERT FLIRT HEART IBERT INERT KMART NIORT NOORT OPART OVERT QBERT QUART QUIRT SHIRT SHORT SKIRT SKORT SMART SNERT

SNORT SPORT SPURT START WAART

RU•••

RUARK RUBEL RUBEN RUBES RUBIK RUBIN RUBLE RUBON RUBUP RUCHE RUCKS RUDDY RUDEL RUDER RUDGE RUEHL RUERS RUFFS RUFUS RUGBY RUING RUINS RULED RULER RULES RULFO RUMAN RUMBA RUMER RUMMY RUMOR RUMPS RUNAT RUNBY RUNES RUNGS RUNIC RUNIN RUNNY RUNON RUNTO RUNTS RUNTY RUNUP RUPEE RURAL RURIK RUSES RUSHY RUSKA RUSKS RUSSA RUSSE RUSSO RUSTS RUSTY RUTHS RUTIN RUTTY

R•U••

REUEL REUNE REUPS REUSE REUSS RHUMB ROUEN ROUES ROUGE ROUGH ROUND ROUSE ROUSH ROUST ROUTE ROUTS

R••U•

RAKUS RAMUS RAMUZ RANUP RAOUL REBUS REBUT REBUY RECUE RECUR RECUT REDUB REDUG REDUX REGUM REMUS REPUB RERUN REVUE REVUP RHEUM RIGUP RIPUP ROGUE ROQUE RSTUV RUBUP RUFUS RUNUP

R•••U

RICEU

•RU••

ARUBA ARUMS ARUNS BRUCE BRUCH BRUHL BRUHN BRUIN BRUIT BRULE BRUME BRUNG BRUNI BRUNO BRUNT

BRUSH BRUSK BRUTE BRUTS CRUDE CRUDS CRUEL CRUET CRUMB CRUMP CRUOR CRURA CRUSE CRUSH CRUST DRUBS DRUGS DRUID DRUMS DRUNK DRUON DRUPE DRURY DRUSE DRUZE ERUCT ERUPT FRUCT FRUGS FRUIT FRUMP GRUBS GRUED GRUEL GRUES GRUFF GRUMP GRUNT KRULL KRUPA KRUPP KRUPS ORURO PRUDE PRUNE TRUCE TRUCK TRUDY TRUED TRUER TRUES TRULY TRUMP TRUNK TRURO TRUSS TRUST TRUTH WRUNG

•R•U•

ARBUS ARGUE ARGUS ARIUM ARTUR BRAUN BROUD

BROUN CRIUS CROUP CRYUP DRHUG DRYUP FRAUD FREUD FRYUP GROUP GROUT KRAUS KRAUT KREUK MRCUB MRYUK ORCUS ORIUM PRIUS PROUD TROUP TROUT UROUS URSUS

•R••U

ARRAU DREWU ERITU IRABU QRSTU

••RU•

AIRUP AURUM CYRUS DURUM ECRUS EURUS FARUK FORUM GURUS HARUM HORUS INRUN JORUM KARUS KURUS LARUE LORUS NORUN RERUN SCRUB SCRUM SERUM SHRUB SHRUG SIRUP STRUG STRUM STRUT SYRUP THRUM TORUS TYRUS UNRUN VIRUS

••R•U

AARAU ARRAU CORFU CORNU GAROU PAREU PERDU TARTU TURKU VIRTU

•••RU

COURU NAURU NEHRU OTARU UHURU

RV•••

RVERS RVING RVLOT

R•V••

RAVED RAVEL RAVEN RAVER RAVES REVEL REVES REVET REVUE REVUP RIVAL RIVED RIVEN RIVER RIVES RIVET ROVED ROVER ROVES RSVPD RSVPS

R••V•

REAVE REEVE

R•••V

RAJIV RSTUV RTREV

•RV••

ERVIN IRVIN ORVAL ORVIS

•R•V•

BRAVA BRAVE BRAVO BREVE BREVI

CRAVE
CREVE
DRAVA
DRIVE
DROVE
EREVS
GRAVE
GRAVI
GRAVY
GROVE
PRIVY
PROVE
PROVO
PROVS
TRAVE
TREVI
TROVE

••RV•
CARVE
CORVO
CURVE
CURVI
CURVY
HERVE
LARVA
MARVY
MIRVS
NERVA
NERVE
NERVO
NERVY
NORVO
SERVE
SERVO
TURVY
VERVE

••R•V
DERIV
KIROV
MARKV
PARTV
RTREV

R•W••
RAWER
RAWLS
RAWLY
REWAX
REWED
REWET
REWIN
REWON
ROWAN
ROWDY
ROWED
ROWEL
ROWEN
ROWER
ROWLF
ROWSE

R••W•
REOWN

R•••W
REMOW

RENEW
RESAW
RESEW
RESOW
RETOW

•RW••
ARWEN
CRWTH
DRWHO
ERWIN
IRWIN

•R•W•
BRAWL
BRAWN
BREWS
BROWN
BROWS
CRAWL
CRAWS
CREWS
CROWD
CROWE
CROWN
CROWS
DRAWL
DRAWN
DRAWS
DREWU
DROWN
FROWN
FROWS
GROWL
GROWN
GROWS
KREWE
PRAWN
PROWL
PROWS
TRAWL
TREWS
TROWE
TROWS
URAWA

•R••W
ARROW

••R•W
ARROW
CAREW
JCREW
SCREW
SHREW
STRAW
STREW
THREW
THROW
TUROW

R•X••
RAXED
RAXES
REXES
RIXEY
ROXIE

R•••X
RADIX
REBOX
REDOX
REDUX
REFAX
REFIX
RELAX
REMAX
REMIX
RETAX
REWAX
ROLEX

•R•X•
PREXY
PROXY

•R••X
BRONX
CROIX
MRFOX
MRHEX

••R•X
BORAX
HYRAX
LORAX
LUREX
PUREX
PYREX
XEROX

RY•••
RYALS
RYANS
RYDER

R•Y••
RAYED
RAYON
REYES
RHYME
RIYAL
ROYAL
ROYCE
ROYKO

R••Y•
REDYE
ROBYN
RODYA

R•••Y
RAGGY
RAINY
RALLY
RAMEY
RANBY
RANDY
RANGY
RASPY
RATTY
RAWLY
READY
REBUY
REDDY
REDLY
REDRY
REEDY
REEFY
REEKY
REFLY
REFRY
REIFY
REKEY
RELAY
RENAY
RENNY
REPAY
REPLY
RESAY
RETRY
RETTY
RHODY
RIBBY
RICKY
RIDGY
RIGBY
RILEY
RINDY
RINKY
RINTY
RISKY
RITZY
RIXEY
ROBBY
ROCKY
RODDY
ROILY
RONNY
ROOKY
ROOMY
ROOTY
ROSEY
ROWDY
RUDDY
RUGBY
RUMMY
RUNBY
RUNNY
RUNTY
RUSHY
RUSTY
RUTTY

•RY••
ARYAN
ARYLS
BRYAN
BRYCE
CRYER
CRYPT
CRYUP
DRYAD
DRYER
DRYLY
DRYUP
FRYER
FRYUP
MRYUK
PRYCE
PRYER
PRYOR
TRYIT
TRYME
TRYON
TRYST
TRYTO
WRYER
WRYLY

•R•Y•
ARBYS
BRAYS
CRAYS
DRAYS
FRAYN
FRAYS
FREYA
FROYO
GRAYS
GREYS
PRAYS
PREYS
TRAYS
TREYS
XRAYS

•R••Y
ARABY
ARCHY
ARMEY
ARRAY
ARTSY
BRADY
BRINY
BRODY
CRACY
CRAZY
CRECY
CRONY
DRILY
DRURY
DRYLY
FRAZY
GRAPY
GRAVY
GRIMY
GRIPY
GRODY
IRONY
KRAZY
ORACY
ORCZY
ORORY
ORSAY
PREXY
PRICY
PRIVY
PROSY
PROXY
TRACY
TRUDY
TRULY
WRYLY

••RY•
BERYL
DARYA
DARYL
KARYN
KURYS
MARYA
MARYI
MARYJ
MARYS
MERYL
ONRYE
VARYA

••R•Y
ALROY
ARRAY
BARFY
BARKY
BARMY
BARRY
BARTY
BERCY
BERRY
BIRDY
BURLY
BURRY
CARAY
CAREY
CARLY
CARNY
CARRY
CORBY
COREY
CORKY
CORNY
CURDY
CURLY
CURRY
CURVY
DARBY
DARCY
DARDY
DERBY
DERRY
DIRTY
DORKY
DORMY
EARLY
ELREY
ELROY
FERNY
FERRY
FIRRY
FORAY
FORKY
FORTY
FURBY
FURRY
GARRY
GERMY
GERRY
GIRLY
GORBY
GORDY
GOREY
GORKY
GORSY
GURDY
HARDY
HARPY
HARRY
HERBY
HERKY
HORNY
HORSY
HURDY
HURLY
HURRY
IPRAY
JERKY
JERRY
JERZY
KERRY
KIRBY
LARDY
LARKY
LARRY
LEROY
LORDY
LORRY
LURAY
MARCY
MARGY
MARLY
MARRY
MARTY
MARVY
MERCY
MERRY
MORAY
MOREY
MORTY
MURKY
NERDY
NERVY
OURAY
PARRY
PARTY
PERCY
PERKY
PERRY
PORGY
PORKY
PURDY
PURSY
PURTY
SORRY
SPRAY
STRAY
SURFY
SURLY
TARDY
TARRY
TARTY
TERRY
TURFY
TURVY
UVRAY
WARTY
WORDY
WORMY
WORRY
YORTY

•••RY
AMBRY
AMERY
AMORY
ANDRY
ANGRY
APERY
ASDRY
ATORY
AUTRY
AVERY
BARRY
BEERY
BERRY
BURRY
CAMRY
CARRY
CHARY
CLARY
COWRY
CURRY
CYMRY
DAIRY
DEARY
DECRY
DERRY
DEVRY
DIARY
DOWRY
DRURY
EMERY
EMORY
ENTRY
EVERY
EWERY
FAERY
FAIRY
FERRY
FIERY
FIRRY
FLORY
FURRY
GARRY
GEARY
GERRY
GLARY
GLORY
HAIRY
HARRY
HENRY
HOARY
HURRY
IATRY
IVORY
JEERY
JERRY
JEWRY
KERRY
LARRY
LEARY
LEERY
LORRY
LOURY
LOWRY
MARRY
MAURY
MERRY
METRY
MOORY
ORORY
OTARY
OVARY
PARRY
PEARY
PERRY
QUERY
REDRY
REFRY
RETRY
SAIRY
SCARY
SORRY
SPIRY
STORY
TARRY
TEARY
TERRY
UNARY
UNDRY
UPDRY
USURY
VEERY
WEARY
WORRY

R•Z••
RAZAF
RAZED
RAZER
RAZES
RAZOR
REZIA
REZIP
RIZAL
RIZZO

R••Z•
RITZY
RIZZO

R•••Z
RAMUZ
REISZ

•RZ••
ORZOS

•R•Z•
BRAZO
CRAZE
CRAZY
DRUZE
FRAZY
FRIZZ
FROZE
GRAZE
GROZA
KRAZY
ORCZY
PRIZE
PRIZM

•R••Z
ARNAZ
ARROZ
BRITZ
ERETZ
FRANZ
FRITZ
FRIZZ
GROSZ
ORTIZ

••RZ•
FORZA
FURZE
HERZL
JERZY
MARZO
TERZA

••R•Z
ARROZ
GERTZ
HERTZ
JEREZ
KURTZ
MERTZ
NERTZ
PEREZ

•••RZ
STARZ

SA•••
SAABS
SABAL
SABER
SABIN
SABLE
SABOT
SABRA
SABRE
SACCO
SACHS
SACKS
SACRA
SACRE
SACRO
SADAT
SADHE
SADHU
SADIE
SADLY
SAENS
SAFAR
SAFER
SAFES
SAFFI
SAFIN
SAGAL
SAGAN
SAGAS
SAGER
SAGES
SAGET
SAGGY
SAGOS
SAHEL
SAHIB
SAILS
SAINT
SAIRY
SAITH
SAJAK
SAKAI
SAKES
SAKIS
SALAD
SALAS
SALEM
SALEP
SALES
SALIC
SALLE
SALLY
SALMA
SALMI
SALON
SALOP
SALSA
SALTI
SALTS
SALTY
SALUD
SALUT
SALVE
SALVO
SAMAR
SAMBA
SAMIS
SAMMI
SAMMS
SAMMY
SAMOA
SAMOS
SAMPS
SAMSA
SANAA
SANDE
SANDH
SANDL
SANDP
SANDS
SANDY
SANER
SANKA
SANTA
SANTE
SANTO
SANYO
SAONE
SAPID
SAPOR
SAPPY
SARAH
SARAI
SARAN
SARDI
SARDS
SAREE
SAREK
SARGE
SARIS
SAROS
SARTO
SASES
SASHA
SASSY
SATAN
SATAT
SATAY
SATBY
SATCH
SATED
SATES
SATIE
SATII
SATIN
SATON
SATUP
SATYR
SAUCE
SAUCY
SAUDI
SAUKS
SAULT
SAUNA
SAURO
SAUTE
SAVED
SAVER
SAVES
SAVOR
SAVOY
SAVVY
SAWED
SAWER
SAWII
SAWIN
SAWTO
SAWUP
SAXES
SAXON
SAYAH
SAYER
SAYHI
SAYIT
SAYNO
SAYOK
SAYSO

S•A••
SAABS
SCABS
SCADS
SCALA
SCALD
SCALE
SCALP
SCALY
SCAMP
SCAMS
SCANS
SCANT
SCAPA
SCAPE
SCARE
SCARF
SCARP
SCARS
SCARY
SCATS
SEALE
SEALS
SEALY
SEAMS
SEAMY
SEANN
SEARS
SEATO
SEATS
SHACK
SHADE
SHADS
SHADY
SHAEF
SHAFT
SHAGS
SHAHN
SHAHS
SHAKE
SHAKO
SHAKY
SHALE
SHALL
SHALT
SHAME
SHAMS
SHAMU
SHANA
SHANE
SHANG
SHANK
SHANT
SHAPE
SHARD
SHARE
SHARI
SHARK
SHARP
SHATT
SHAUN
SHAVE
SHAWL
SHAWN
SHAYS
SKALD
SKANK
SKATE
SLABS
SLACK
SLADE
SLAGS
SLAIN
SLAKE
SLAMS
SLANG
SLANT
SLAPS
SLASH
SLATE
SLATS
SLATY
SLAVE
SLAVS
SLAWS
SLAYS
SMACK
SMALL
SMARM
SMART
SMASH
SMAUG
SMAZE
SNACK
SNAFU
SNAGS
SNAIL
SNAKE
SNAKY
SNAPS
SNARE
SNARF
SNARK
SNARL
SNATH
SNAZZ
SOAKS
SOAMI
SOAPS
SOAPY
SOARS
SOAVE
SPAAK
SPACE
SPACY
SPADE
SPADS
SPAGO
SPAHN
SPAIN
SPAKE
SPAMS
SPANG
SPANK
SPANO
SPANS
SPARE
SPARK
SPARS
SPASM
SPATE
SPATS
SPAWN
SPAYS
STABS
STACK
STACY
STADE
STADS
STADT
STAEL
STAFF
STAGE
STAGG
STAGS
STAGY
STAHL
STAHR
STAID
STAIN
STAIR
STAKE
STALE
STALK
STALL
STAMP
STAND
STANG
STANK
STANS
STAPH
STARE
STARK
STARR
STARS
START
STARZ
STASH
STASI
STATE
STATS
STAUB
STAVE
STAYS
SUAVE
SWABS
SWAGS
SWAIN
SWALE
SWAMI
SWAMP
SWANK
SWANN
SWANS
SWAPS
SWARD
SWARM
SWASH
SWATH
SWATS
SWAYS
SWAZI

S••A•
SABAL
SADAT
SAFAR
SAGAL
SAGAN
SAGAS
SAJAK
SAKAI
SALAD
SALAS
SAMAR
SANAA
SARAH
SARAI
SARAN
SATAN
SATAT
SATAY
SAYAH
SCHAV
SCRAG
SCRAM
SCRAP
SCRAT
SEDAN
SEEAS
SEGAL
SEGAR
SELAH
SENAT
SEPAL
SERAC
SERAI
SERAL
SETAE
SETAT
SFBAY
SHEAF
SHEAN
SHEAR
SHOAL
SHOAT
SIKAS
SILAS
SINAI
SISAL
SITAR
SITAT
SIVAN
SIXAD
SIXAM
SKOAL
SKUAS
SLOAN
SMEAL
SMEAR
SNEAD
SNEAK
SOBAD
SOBAS
SOCAL
SOCAS
SODAS
SOFAR
SOFAS
SOLAN
SOLAR
SOMAS
SOMAT
SONAL
SONAR
SORAS
SOSAD
SOYAS
SPAAK
SPEAK
SPEAR
SPLAT
SPLAY
SPRAT
SPRAY
SQUAB
SQUAD
SQUAT
SQUAW
SRTAS
SSTAR
STEAD
STEAK
STEAL
STEAM
STOAE
STOAS
STOAT
STPAT
STRAD
STRAM
STRAP
STRAT
STRAW
STRAY
SUDAN
SUGAR
SUMAC
SURAH
SURAS
SUSAN
SWEAR
SWEAT

S•••A
SABRA
SACRA
SALMA
SALSA
SAMBA
SAMOA
SAMSA
SANAA
SANKA
SANTA
SASHA
SAUNA
SCALA
SCAPA
SCENA
SCHWA
SCUBA
SCUSA
SEEYA
SELMA
SENNA
SENTA
SEPIA
SEPTA
SERIA
SERRA
SERTA
SHANA
SHEBA
SHERA
SHIVA
SHULA
SIDEA
SIENA
SIGMA
SILVA
SIMBA
SITKA
SLIWA
SNEVA
SOFIA
SOLEA
SOLLA
SONIA
SONJA
SONYA
SORTA
SOUSA
SPICA
SPOSA
STELA
STOLA
STOMA
STRIA
STUKA
STUPA
SULFA
SULLA
SUMMA
SUNDA
SUNNA
SUPRA
SUTRA
SYRIA

•SA••
ASAGI
ASAHI
ASAMI
ASANA

ESAKI
ISAAC
ISAAK
ISAID
ISAMU
LSATS
OSAGE
OSAKA
PSALM
PSATS
TSADE
TSADI
TSARS
TSAVO
USAFA
USAGE
USAID
USAIR
XSARA
YSAYE

•S•A•
ASCAP
ASFAT
ASIAN
ASLAK
ASLAN
ASMAD
ASNAP
ASSAD
ASSAI
ASSAM
ASSAY
ASWAN
ASWAY
BSTAR
CSPAN
CSTAR
ESBAT
ESSAI
ESSAY
ESTAB
ESTAN
ESTAR
ESTAS
FSTAR
GSTAR
ISAAC
ISAAK
ISHAM
ISIAH
ISLAM
ISLAS
KSTAR
MSTAR
NSTAR
OSCAN
OSCAR
OSHAY
OSKAR
OSMAN
OSTAR
PSHAW
SSTAR
USEAS
USUAL

•S••A
ASANA
ASPCA
ASTRA
ASYLA
ISOLA
OSAKA
OSHEA
OSSIA
OSTIA
USAFA
USCGA
USLTA
USOFA
USRDA
XSARA

••SA•
ALSAB
ANSAE
ASSAD
ASSAI
ASSAM
ASSAY
BASAL
CASAS
CESAR
DESAI
DOSAY
ELSAS
ESSAI
ESSAY
HASAT
HUSAK
IFSAY
KOSAR
MASAI
MASAS
MESAS
NASAL
NISAN
OASAL
ORSAY
PISAN
PUSAN
RASAE
RESAT
RESAW
RESAY
SISAL
SOSAD
SUSAN
UNSAD
UNSAY
URSAE
VISAS
WASAT

••S•A
AISHA
AOSTA
ATSEA
BASIA
BASRA
BASTA
BOSSA
BUSTA
BYSEA
CASCA
CASTA
CESTA
COSTA
DESNA
EASYA
FESTA
FOSSA
HASTA
HOSEA
HOSTA
KASHA
KISKA
MASHA
MASSA
MESTA
MISHA
MISSA
MUSCA
NESIA
OSSIA
PASHA
PASTA
RASPA
RASTA
ROSSA
RUSKA
RUSSA
SASHA
TESLA
TESSA
TESTA
TISHA
TOSCA
TOSEA
VESPA
VESTA
VISTA
YASHA
ZESTA
ZOSMA

•••SA
ALISA
AZUSA
BAISA
BALSA
BORSA
BOSSA
BURSA
COOSA
CORSA
CURSA
DORSA
ELISA
EMESA
ERISA
FOSSA
HANSA
ICOSA
KANSA
LHASA
LLOSA
LOTSA
LUISA
MASSA
MENSA
MISSA
NYASA
ODESA
PAISA
PRESA
RAISA
ROOSA
ROSSA
RUSSA
SALSA
SAMSA
SCUSA
SOUSA
SPOSA
TESSA
TULSA
VERSA
XHOSA

S•B••
SABAL
SABER
SABIN
SABLE
SABOT
SABRA
SABRE
SFBAY
SIBYL
SOBAD
SOBAS
SOBER
SOBIG
SUBIC
SYBIL

S••B•
SAABS
SAMBA
SATBY
SCABS
SCUBA
SERBO
SERBS
SETBY
SHEBA
SIMBA
SITBY
SIXBC
SLABS
SLOBS
SNOBS
SNUBS
SORBO
SORBS
STABS
STUBS
SWABS

S•••B
SAHIB
SCRUB
SHRUB
SIDEB
SQUAB
SQUIB
STAUB
STIEB

•SB••
ASBIG
ESBAT
ISBNS

•S•B•
ASHBY
MSNBC
USEBY

•S••B
ESTAB

••SB•
BUSBY
CASBY
COSBY
NASBY

••S•B
ALSAB

•••SB
PRESB

SC•••
SCABS
SCADS
SCALA
SCALD
SCALE
SCALP
SCALY
SCAMP
SCAMS
SCANS
SCANT
SCAPA
SCAPE
SCARE
SCARF
SCARP
SCARS
SCARY
SCATS
SCENA
SCENE
SCENT
SCHAV
SCHED
SCHMO
SCHON
SCHWA
SCIFI
SCION
SCIRE
SCOFF
SCOLD
SCONE
SCOOP
SCOOT
SCOPE
SCORE
SCORN
SCOTS
SCOTT
SCOUR
SCOUT
SCOWL
SCOWS
SCRAG
SCRAM
SCRAP
SCRAT
SCREE
SCREW
SCRIM
SCRIP
SCROD
SCRUB
SCRUM
SCUBA
SCUDS
SCUFF
SCULL
SCUMS
SCUPS
SCUSA
SCUSI
SCUTS
SCUZZ

S•C••
SACCO
SACHS
SACKS
SACRA
SACRE
SACRO
SECHS
SECTS
SICEM
SICKO
SOCAL
SOCAS
SOCIO
SOCKO
SOCKS
SOCLE
SUCKS
SUCKY
SUCRE

S••C•
SACCO
SATCH
SAUCE
SAUCY
SHACK
SHOCK
SHUCK
SINCE
SLACK
SLICE
SLICK
SMACK
SMOCK
SNACK
SNICK
SNUCK
SOUCI
SPACE
SPACY
SPECD
SPECK
SPECS
SPICA
SPICE
SPICY
SPOCK
STACK
STACY
STICH
STICK
STOCK
STUCK
SYNCH
SYNCS
SYSCO

S•••C
SALIC
SERAC
SIXBC
SOFTC
SONIC
STOIC
SUBIC
SUMAC

•SC••
ASCAP
ASCII
ASCOT
ASCUS
OSCAN
OSCAR
USCGA

•S•C•
ASICS
ASPCA
PSYCH

•S••C
ASDIC
ASPIC
ASSOC
ESTOC
FSLIC
ISAAC
ISTIC
MSNBC
NSYNC
OSMIC
OSRIC

••SC•
BOSCH
BOSCO
BOSCS
BUSCH
CASCA
CASCO
CISCO
DISCI
DISCO
DISCS
FISCS
KUSCH
MUSCA
PASCH
PASCO
PESCE
PESCI
PISCI
SYSCO
TISCH
TOSCA
VASCO
VESCO
WASCO

••S•C
ASSOC
BASIC
COSEC
CUSEC
MUSIC

•••SC
CRESC
EPISC

S•D••
SADAT
SADHE
SADHU
SADIE
SADLY
SEDAN
SEDER
SEDGE
SEDGY
SEDUM
SIDEA
SIDEB
SIDED
SIDES
SIDLE
SIDON
SODAS
SODDY
SODOI
SODOM
SUDAN
SUDSY
SYDOW

S••D•
SANDE
SANDH
SANDL
SANDP
SANDS
SANDY
SARDI
SARDS
SAUDI
SCADS
SCUDS
SEEDS
SEEDY
SENDS
SHADE
SHADS
SHADY
SHEDS
SKEDS
SKIDS
SLADE
SLEDS
SLIDE
SNIDE
SODDY
SOLDI
SOLDO
SONDE
SPADE
SPADS
SPODE
SPUDS
STADE
STADS
STADT
STUDS
STUDY
SUEDE
SUNDA
SWEDE
SYNDS

S•••D
SALAD
SALUD
SAPID
SATED
SAVED
SAWED
SCALD
SCHED
SCOLD
SCROD
SEWED
SEXED
SHARD
SHIED
SHOED
SHRED
SIDED
SIRED
SITED
SIXAD
SIXED
SIZED
SKALD
SKIED
SLUED
SNEAD
SNERD
SNOOD
SOBAD
SOLED
SOLID
SOSAD
SOUND
SOWED
SPECD
SPEED
SPEND
SPIED
SQUAD
SQUID
STAID
STAND
STEAD
STEED
STIED
STOOD
STRAD
SWARD
SWORD
SYNOD

•SD••
ASDIC
ASDRY
MSDOS

•S•D•
ASIDE
BSIDE
TSADE
TSADI
USRDA

•S••D
ASHED
ASKED
ASMAD
ASOLD
ASRED
ASSAD
ASSTD
ISAID
PSEUD
RSVPD
TSKED
USAID
USHED
USTED

••SD•
DESDE
MISDO

••S•D
ASSAD
ASSTD
BASED
BUSED
CASED
DESOD
DOSED
EASED
FUSED
HASID
HOSED
LASED
LYSED
MUSED
NOSED
POSED
RASED
RESOD
SOSAD
UNSAD
URSID
VISED
WISED

SE•••
SEALE
SEALS
SEALY
SEAMS
SEAMY
SEANN
SEARS
SEATO
SEATS
SECHS
SECTS
SEDAN
SEDER
SEDGE
SEDGY
SEDUM
SEEAS
SEEDS
SEEDY
SEEIN
SEEKS
SEEME
SEEMS
SEEPS
SEEPY
SEERS
SEEST
SEETH
SEETO
SEEUP
SEEYA
SEGAL
SEGAR
SEGER
SEGNI
SEGNO
SEGOS
SEGRE
SEGUE
SEIJI
SEIKO
SEINE
SEISM
SEIZE
SELAH
SELES
SELIG
SELLS
SELMA
SEMIS
SENAT
SENDS
SENGI
SENNA
SENOR
SENSE
SENTA
SENTE
SEOUL
SEPAL
SEPIA
SEPOY
SEPTA
SEPTS
SERAC
SERAI
SERAL
SERBO
SERBS
SERFS
SERGE
SERIA
SERIF
SERIN
SERIO
SERRA
SERTA
SERTS
SERUM
SERVE
SERVO
SETAE
SETAT
SETBY
SETIN
SETON
SETTE
SETTO
SETTS
SETUP
SEULE
SEUSS
SEVEN
SEVER
SEWED
SEWER
SEWIN
SEWON
SEWUP
SEXED
SEXER
SEXES

S•E••
SAENS
SCENA
SCENE
SCENT
SEEAS
SEEDS
SEEDY
SEEIN
SEEKS
SEEME
SEEMS
SEEPS
SEEPY
SEERS
SEEST
SEETH
SEETO
SEEUP
SEEYA
SHEAF
SHEAN
SHEAR
SHEBA
SHEDS
SHEEN
SHEEP
SHEER
SHEET
SHEIK
SHELF
SHELL
SHEMP
SHERA
SHERE
SHERM
SIEGE
SIENA
SIETE
SIEVE
SKEDS
SKEET
SKEGS
SKEIN
SKEWS
SLEDS
SLEEK
SLEEP
SLEET
SLEPT
SLEWS
SLEYS
SMEAL
SMEAR
SMEES
SMELL
SMELT
SMEWS
SNEAD
SNEAK
SNEER
SNEES
SNELL
SNERD
SNERT
SNEVA
SOEUR
SPEAK
SPEAR
SPECD
SPECK
SPECS
SPEED
SPEER
SPEKE
SPELL
SPELT
SPEND
SPENT
SPERM
SPERO
SPETS
SPEWS
STEAD
STEAK
STEAL
STEAM
STEED
STEEL
STEEN
STEEP
STEER
STEIG
STEIN
STELA
STELE
STEMS
STENO
STENS
STENT
STEPS
STERE
STERN
STETS
STEVE
STEWS
STEWY
SUEDE
SUEME
SUENO
SUERS
SUETS
SUETY
SWEAR
SWEAT
SWEDE
SWEEP
SWEET
SWELL
SWEPT
SZELL

S••E•
SABER
SAFER
SAFES
SAGER
SAGES
SAGET
SAHEL
SAKES
SALEM
SALEP
SALES
SANER
SAREE
SAREK
SASES
SATED
SATES
SAVED
SAVER
SAVES
SAWED
SAWER
SAXES
SAYER
SCHED
SCREE
SCREW
SEDER
SEGER
SELES
SEVEN
SEVER
SEWED
SEWER
SEXED
SEXER
SEXES
SHAEF
SHEEN
SHEEP
SHEER
SHEET
SHIED
SHIER
SHIES
SHLEP
SHOED
SHOER
SHOES
SHRED
SHREK
SHREW
SHYER
SICEM
SIDEA
SIDEB
SIDED
SIDES
SIKES
SILEX
SINES
SINEW
SINEX
SIRED
SIREE
SIREN
SIRES
SITED
SITES
SIXED
SIXEE
SIXER
SIXES
SIZED
SIZER
SIZES
SKEET
SKIED
SKIER
SKIES
SKYES
SKYEY
SLEEK
SLEEP
SLEET
SLIER
SLOES
SLUED
SLUES
SLYER
SMEES
SNEER
SNEES
SOBER
SOFER
SOFEW
SOLEA
SOLED
SOLEI
SOLER
SOLES
SONES
SOOEY
SOREL
SOREN
SORER
SORES
SOWED
SOWER
SPEED
SPEER
SPIED
SPIEL
SPIER
SPIES
SPREE
STAEL
STEED
STEEL
STEEN
STEEP
STEER
STIEB
STIED
STIES
STLEO
STREP
STREW
STYES
SUMER
SUPER
SUPES
SURER
SWEEP
SWEET

S•••E
SABLE
SABRE
SACRE
SADHE
SADIE
SALLE
SALVE
SANDE
SANTE
SAONE
SAREE
SARGE
SATIE
SAUCE
SAUTE
SCALE
SCAPE
SCARE
SCENE
SCIRE
SCONE
SCOPE
SCORE
SCREE
SEALE
SEDGE
SEEME
SEGRE
SEGUE
SEINE
SEIZE
SENSE
SENTE
SERGE
SERVE
SETAE
SETTE
SEULE
SHADE
SHAKE
SHALE
SHAME
SHANE
SHAPE
SHARE
SHAVE
SHERE
SHINE
SHIRE
SHONE
SHORE
SHOVE
SHUTE
SIDLE
SIEGE
SIETE
SIEVE
SIGNE
SINCE
SINGE
SIREE
SIXEE
SKATE
SKYPE
SLADE
SLAKE
SLATE
SLAVE
SLICE
SLIDE
SLIME
SLOPE
SLYKE
SMAZE
SMILE
SMITE
SMOKE
SMORE
SMOTE
SNAKE
SNARE
SNIDE
SNIPE
SNORE
SNOWE
SOAVE
SOCLE
SOFIE
SOLVE
SOMME
SONDE
SOUSE
SPACE
SPADE
SPAKE
SPARE
SPATE
SPEKE
SPICE
SPIKE
SPILE
SPINE
SPIRE
SPITE
SPODE
SPOKE
SPORE
SPOSE
SPREE
SPUME
STADE
STAGE
STAKE
STALE
STARE
STATE
STAVE
STELE
STERE

STEVE STILE STINE STIPE STJOE STOAE STOKE STOLE STONE STORE STOVE STOWE STUPE STYLE STYNE SUAVE SUCRE SUEDE SUEME SUITE SUPPE SURGE SUSIE SUZIE SWALE SWEDE SWINE SWIPE SWORE SYNGE

•SE••

ISERE PSEUD USEAS USEBY USEES USEIN USEIT USEME USEOF USEON USERS USETO USEUP

•S•E•

ASHED ASHEN ASHER ASHES ASKED ASKER ASKEW ASNER ASNEW ASPEN ASPER ASRED ASSER ASSES ASSET ASSEZ ASTER ASYET ESKER ESNES ESSEN ESSES ESSEX ESTEE ESTER ESTES ISLES ISLET ISLEY ISSEI ISSEL OSHEA OSIER OSLER OSSEO OSSET OSTEO OSTER TSKED USEES USHED USHER USHES USTED USTEN

•S••E

ASIDE ASKME ASONE ASTRE BSIDE ESQUE ESSIE ESTEE ISERE ISSUE ISTLE OSAGE OSSIE TSADE USAGE USEME USONE YSAYE

••SE•

ANSEL ANSER APSES ARSES ASSER ASSES ASSET ASSEZ ATSEA BASED BASEL BASER BASES BESES BESET BUSED BUSES BUSEY BYSEA CASED CASER CASES CASEY COSEC COSET CUSEC DESEX DOSED DOSER DOSES EASED EASEL EASER EASES EBSEN EDSEL EISEN ELSES ESSEN ESSES ESSEX ETSEQ FUSED FUSEE FUSES GASES GOSEE HASEK HOSEA HOSED HOSEL HOSEN HOSER HOSES HYSER IBSEN IMSET INSET ISSEI ISSEL JOSEF JOSEY KASEM KESEY KISER KYSER LASED LASER LASES LOSER LOSES LOSEY LYSED LYSES MASER MESES MISER MOSEL MOSES MOSEY MUSED MUSEE MUSEO MUSER MUSES NISEI NOSED NOSER NOSES NOSEY OASES OLSEN ONSET ORSER ORSES OSSEO OSSET OUSEL PASEO PASES POSED POSER POSES POSEY RASED RASER RASES RESEE RESET RESEW RISEN RISER RISES ROSEN ROSES ROSEY RUSES SASES TASER TOSEA TVSET UNSER UNSET UNSEW UPSET VASES VISED VISES WESER WISED WISER WISES YESES

••S•E

AISLE AISNE ANSAE BASIE BASLE BASSE BASTE CASTE DESDE DESTE DISME ELSIE ENSUE ESSIE FESTE FISKE FOSSE FUSEE GASPE GESTE GOSEE GOSSE HASTE HESHE HESSE ISSUE ITSME JESSE JOSIE JUSTE LASSE LISLE LISSE MASSE MESNE MESSE MOSHE MUSEE NASHE OESTE OSSIE PASSE PASTE PESCE PISTE POSSE POSTE RASAE RASPE RASSE RESEE RESTE ROSIE RUSSE SUSIE TASSE TASTE URSAE WASTE

•••SE

ABASE ABUSE AMUSE ANISE ARISE AROSE BASSE BIRSE BLASE BOISE BRISE CAUSE CEASE CENSE CHASE CHOSE CLASE CLOSE COASE COPSE CRUSE CURSE DANSE DENSE DNASE DOUSE DOWSE DRUSE ELISE ELYSE ERASE EROSE FALSE FOSSE FRISE GEESE GOOSE GORSE GOSSE GRISE GUISE HAISE HANSE HAWSE HESSE HEYSE HORSE HOUSE ILOSE INUSE JESSE LAPSE LASSE LEASE LISSE LOOSE LOUSE LUISE MANSE MASSE MEESE MESSE MEUSE MOOSE MORSE MOUSE NELSE NOISE NOOSE NORSE NOUSE NURSE OBESE OFUSE PAESE PAISE PARSE PASSE PAUSE PEASE PERSE PHASE POISE POSSE PRESE PROSE PULSE PURSE RAISE RASSE REESE REUSE RINSE RNASE ROUSE ROWSE RUSSE SENSE SOUSE SPOSE TASSE TEASE TENSE TERSE THESE THOSE UKASE VALSE VERSE WHOSE WORSE YOUSE

SF•••

SFBAY

S•F••

SAFAR SAFER SAFES SAFFI SAFIN SIFTS SOFAR SOFAS SOFER SOFEW SOFIA SOFIE SOFTC SOFTG SOFTY SUFIS

S••F•

SAFFI SCIFI SCOFF SCUFF SERFS SHAFT SHIFT SKIFF SNAFU SNIFF SNUFF SPIFF STAFF STIFF STUFF SULFA SURFS SURFY SWIFT

S•••F

SCARF SCOFF SCUFF SERIF SHAEF SHEAF SHELF SHYOF SKIFF SMURF SNARF SNIFF SNUFF SPIFF SPOOF STAFF STIFF STUFF

•SF••

ASFAT ASFIT ASFOR RSFSR

•S•F•

USAFA USOFA

•S••F

ASKOF USEOF

••S•F

JOSEF

S•G••

SAGAL SAGAN SAGAS SAGER SAGES SAGET SAGGY SAGOS SEGAL SEGAR SEGER SEGNI SEGNO SEGOS SEGRE SEGUE SIGHS SIGHT SIGIL SIGMA SIGNE SIGNS SOGGY SSGTS SUGAR

S••G•

SAGGY SARGE SEDGE SEDGY SENGI SERGE SHAGS SHOGI SIEGE SINGE SINGH SINGS SKEGS SLAGS SLIGO SLOGS SLUGS SMOGS SNAGS SNUGS SOGGY SONGS SPAGO STAGE STAGG STAGS STAGY STOGY SURGE SWAGS SWIGS SYNGE

S•••G

SCRAG SELIG SHANG SHRUG SLANG SLING SLUNG SMAUG SOBIG SOFTG SPANG SPRIG STAGG STANG STEIG STING STRUG STUNG SUING SWING SWUNG

•SG••

MSGTS SSGTS TSGTS

•S•G•

ASAGI OSAGE USAGE USCGA VSIGN

•S••G

ASBIG USING

•••SG

NOMSG

SH•••

SHACK SHADE SHADS SHADY SHAEF SHAFT SHAGS SHAHN SHAHS SHAKE SHAKO SHAKY SHALE SHALL SHALT SHAME SHAMS SHAMU SHANA SHANE SHANG SHANK SHANT SHAPE SHARD SHARE SHARI SHARK SHARP SHATT SHAUN SHAVE SHAWL SHAWN SHAYS SHEAF SHEAN SHEAR SHEBA SHEDS SHEEN SHEEP SHEER SHEET SHEIK SHELF SHELL SHEMP SHERA SHERE SHERM SHHHH SHIED SHIER SHIES SHIFT SHILL SHIMS SHINE SHINS SHINY SHIPS SHIRE SHIRK SHIRR SHIRT SHISH SHIVA SHIVS SHLEP SHMOO SHOAL SHOAT SHOCK SHOED SHOER SHOES SHOGI SHOJI SHONE SHOOK SHOOS SHOOT SHOPS SHORE SHORN SHORT SHOTS SHOUT SHOVE SHOWN SHOWS SHOWY SHRED SHREK SHREW SHRUB SHRUG SHUCK SHULA SHULS SHUNS SHUNT SHUSH SHUTE SHUTS SHYER SHYLY SHYOF

S•H••

SAHEL SAHIB SCHAV SCHED SCHMO SCHON SCHWA SHHHH

S••H•

SACHS SADHE SADHU SASHA SAYHI SECHS SHAHN SHAHS SHHHH SIGHS SIGHT SIKHS SOPHS SPAHN STAHL STAHR SUSHI

S•••H

SAITH SANDH SARAH SATCH SAYAH SEETH SELAH SHHHH SHISH SHUSH SINGH SIXTH SKOSH SLASH SLOSH SLOTH SLUSH SMASH SMITH SMUSH SMYTH SNATH SOOTH SOUTH STAPH STASH STICH STROH SURAH SWASH SWATH SWISH SYLPH SYNCH SYNTH

•SH••

ASHBY ASHED ASHEN ASHER ASHES ASHOT ASHUR ISHAM OSHAY OSHEA PSHAW USHED USHER USHES

•S•H•

ASAHI ESTHS

•S••H

ISIAH PSYCH

••SH•

AISHA BASHO BUSHY CUSHY DASHI DASHY DISHY FISHY GUSHY HESHE KASHA KASHI LUSHY MASHA MESHY MISHA MOSHE MUSHU MUSHY NASHE PASHA PUSHY RASHI RASHT RESHT RISHI ROSHI RUSHY SASHA SUSHI TASHI TISHA TUSHY UNSHY WASHO WASHY WISHY WUSHU YASHA

••S•H

BOSCH BUSCH KUSCH PASCH TISCH

•••SH

ABASH AGUSH AMISH APISH AWASH BGOSH BLISH BLUSH BRASH BRUSH CLASH CRASH CRUSH ECASH FLASH FLESH FLUSH FRESH FROSH GIRSH GNASH GURSH HARSH HERSH IRISH IWISH KARSH KERSH KNISH KOOSH LEASH MARSH NAISH PHISH PLASH PLUSH QIRSH QUASH ROUSH SHISH SHUSH SKOSH SLASH SLOSH SLUSH SMASH SMUSH STASH SWASH SWISH TRASH TRISH WALSH WELSH WHISH WOOSH

SI•••

SIBYL SICEM SICKO SIDEA SIDEB SIDED SIDES SIDLE SIDON SIEGE SIENA SIETE SIEVE SIFTS SIGHS SIGHT SIGIL SIGMA SIGNE SIGNS SIKAS SIKES SIKHS SILAS SILEX SILKS SILKY SILLS SILLY SILOS SILTS SILTY SILVA SIMBA SIMMS SIMON SIMPS SINAI SINCE SINES SINEW SINEX SINGE SINGH SINGS SINKS SINUS SIOUX SIPON SIRED SIREE SIREN SIRES SIRUP SISAL SISQO SISSY SITAR SITAT SITBY SITED SITES SITIN SITKA SITON SITUP SIVAN SIXAD SIXAM SIXBC SIXED SIXEE SIXER SIXES SIXNO SIXPM SIXTH SIXTY SIXUP SIZED SIZER SIZES

S•I••

SAILS SAINT SAIRY SAITH SCIFI SCION SCIRE SEIJI SEIKO SEINE SEISM SEIZE SHIED SHIER SHIES SHIFT SHILL SHIMS SHINE SHINS SHINY SHIPS SHIRE SHIRK SHIRR SHIRT SHISH SHIVA SHIVS SKIDS SKIED SKIER SKIES SKIFF SKILL SKIMP SKIMS SKINK SKINS SKIPS SKIRL SKIRT SKITS SLICE SLICK SLIDE SLIER SLIGO SLIME SLIMS SLIMY SLING SLINK SLIPS SLITS SLIWA SMILE SMIRK SMITE SMITH SMITS SNICK SNIDE SNIFF SNIPE SNIPS SNITS SOILS SOIRS SPICA SPICE SPICY SPIED SPIEL SPIER SPIES SPIFF SPIKE SPIKY SPILE SPILL SPILT SPINE SPINS SPINY SPIRE SPIRO SPIRY SPITE SPITS SPITZ STICH STICK STIEB STIED STIES STIFF STILE STILL STILT STINE STING STINK STINT STIPE STIRS SUING SUITE SUITS SWIFT SWIGS SWILL SWIMS SWINE SWING SWIPE SWIRL SWISH SWISS

S••I•

SABIN SADIE SAFIN SAHIB SAKIS SALIC SAMIS SAPID SARIS SATIE SATII SATIN SAWII SAWIN SAYIT SCRIM SCRIP SEEIN SELIG SEMIS SEPIA SERIA SERIF SERIN SERIO SETIN SEWIN SHEIK SIGIL SITIN SKEIN SLAIN SNAIL SOBIG SOCIO SOFIA SOFIE SOLID

5 SI

SONIA SONIC SPAIN SPLIT SPOIL SPRIG SPRIT SQUIB SQUID STAID STAIN STAIR STEIG STEIN STOIC STRIA STRIP SUBIC SUFIS SUSIE SUZIE SWAIN SYBIL SYRIA

S•••I

SAFFI SAKAI SALMI SALTI SAMMI SARAI SARDI SATII SAUDI SAWII SAYHI SCIFI SCUSI SEGNI SEIJI SENGI SERAI SHARI SHOGI SHOJI SINAI SOAMI SODOI SOLDI SOLEI SOLTI SOMNI SOUCI SPYRI STASI STOLI STYLI SUNNI SUOMI SUSHI SWAMI SWAZI

•SI••

ASIAN ASICS ASIDE BSIDE CSINY ESIST ISIAH OSIER USING VSIGN

•S•I•

ASBIG ASCII ASDIC ASFIT ASKIN ASPIC ASPIN ASTIN ASTIR ASWIM ESPIO ESSIE FSLIC GSUIT ISAID ISLIP ISTIC OSLIN OSMIC OSRIC OSSIA OSSIE OSTIA USAID USAIR USEIN USEIT

•S••I

ASAGI ASAHI ASAMI ASCII ASSAI ESAKI ESSAI ISSEI TSADI

••SI•

AESIR AHSIN APSIS ARSIS ATSIX BASIA BASIC BASIE BASIL BASIN BASIS CASIO ELSIE EOSIN ESSIE FUSIL GOSIT HASID HASIN HASIT JOSIE JOSIP LASIK LOSIN LYSIS MUSIC MUSIL MYSIN NESIA NOSIR OASIS OSSIA OSSIE POSIT RESIN RESIT ROSIE ROSIN SUSIE URSID VISIT WASIN WASIT XESIN YASIR

••S•I

ASSAI AUSSI BASSI CESTI DASHI DESAI DISCI ESSAI HOSNI ISSEI KASHI LASKI MASAI MISTI NISEI PESCI PISCI RASHI RISHI ROSHI ROSSI SUSHI TASHI VASTI VESTI

•••SI

AINSI AUSSI BASSI DORSI FARSI ICOSI PARSI PEPSI PIUSI QUASI ROSSI SCUSI STASI TARSI TORSI TUTSI VARSI

S•J••

SAJAK STJOE

S••J•

SEIJI SHOJI SONJA

SK•••

SKALD SKANK SKATE SKEDS SKEET SKEGS SKEIN SKEWS SKIDS SKIED SKIER SKIES SKIFF SKILL SKIMP SKIMS SKINK SKINS SKIPS SKIRL SKIRT SKITS SKNXX SKOAL SKORT SKOSH SKUAS SKULK SKULL SKUNK SKYES SKYEY SKYPE

S•K••

SAKAI SAKES SAKIS SIKAS SIKES SIKHS

S••K•

SACKS SANKA SAUKS SEEKS SEIKO SHAKE SHAKO SHAKY SICKO SILKS SILKY SINKS SITKA SLAKE SLYKE SMOKE SMOKY SNAKE SNAKY SOAKS SOCKO SOCKS SPAKE SPEKE SPIKE SPIKY SPOKE STAKE STOKE STUKA SUCKS SUCKY SULKS SULKY

S•••K

SAJAK SAREK SAYOK SHACK SHANK SHARK SHEIK SHIRK SHOCK SHOOK SHREK SHUCK SKANK SKINK SKULK SKUNK SLACK SLEEK SLICK SLINK SLUNK SMACK SMIRK SMOCK SNACK SNARK SNEAK SNICK SNOOK SNUCK SPAAK SPANK SPARK SPEAK SPECK SPOCK SPOOK SPORK SPUNK STACK STALK STANK STARK STEAK STICK STINK STOCK STORK STUCK STUNK SWANK

•SK••

ASKED ASKER ASKEW ASKIN ASKME ASKOF ASKUP ESKER OSKAR TSKED

•S•K•

ESAKI OSAKA

•S••K

ASLAK ISAAK

••SK•

BASKS BUSKS CASKS CUSKS DESKS DISKO DISKS DUSKS DUSKY ENSKY FISKE HUSKS HUSKY KISKA LASKI LASKY MASKS MUSKS MUSKY PESKY RISKS RISKY RUSKA RUSKS TASKS TUSKS

••S•K

HASEK HUSAK ITSOK LASIK

•••SK

BRISK BRUSK FLASK FRISK GOASK KIOSK LUTSK MINSK NORSK PINSK REASK TOMSK TRASK WHISK

SL•••

SLABS SLACK SLADE SLAGS SLAIN SLAKE SLAMS SLANG SLANT SLAPS SLASH SLATE SLATS SLATY SLAVE SLAVS SLAWS SLAYS SLEDS SLEEK SLEEP SLEET SLEPT SLEWS SLEYS SLICE SLICK SLIDE SLIER SLIGO SLIME SLIMS SLIMY SLING SLINK SLIPS SLITS SLIWA SLOAN SLOBS SLOES SLOGS SLOMO SLOOP SLOPE SLOPS SLOSH SLOTH SLOTS SLOWS SLUED SLUES SLUGS SLUMP SLUMS SLUNG SLUNK SLURP SLURS SLUSH SLYER SLYKE SLYLY

S•L••

SALAD SALAS SALEM SALEP SALES SALIC SALLE SALLY SALMA SALMI SALON SALOP SALSA SALTI SALTS SALTY SALUD SALUT SALVE SALVO SELAH SELES SELIG SELLS SELMA SHLEP SILAS SILEX SILKS SILKY SILLS SILLY SILOS SILTS SILTY SILVA SOLAN SOLAR SOLDI SOLDO SOLEA SOLED SOLEI SOLER SOLES SOLID SOLLA SOLON SOLOS SOLTI SOLVE SPLAT SPLAY SPLIT STLEO SULFA SULKS SULKY SULLA SULLY SYLPH

S••L•

SABLE SADLY SAILS SALLE SALLY SAULT SCALA SCALD SCALE SCALP SCALY SCOLD SCULL SEALE SEALS SEALY SELLS SEULE SHALE SHALL SHALT SHELF SHELL SHILL SHULA SHULS SHYLY SIDLE SILLS SILLY SKALD SKILL SKULK SKULL SLYLY SMALL SMELL SMELT SMILE SMOLT SNELL SOCLE SOILS SOLLA SOULS SPELL SPELT SPILE SPILL SPILT STALE STALK STALL STELA STELE STILE STILL STILT STOLA STOLE STOLI STOLS STYLE STYLI SULLA SULLY SURLY SWALE SWELL SWILL SZELL

S•••L

SABAL SAGAL SAHEL SANDL SCOWL SCULL SEGAL SEOUL SEPAL SERAL SHALL SHAWL SHELL SHILL SHOAL SIBYL SIGIL SISAL SKILL SKIRL SKOAL SKULL SMALL SMEAL SMELL SNAIL SNARL SNELL SOCAL SONAL SOREL SPELL SPIEL SPILL SPOIL SPOOL STAEL STAHL STALL STEAL STEEL STILL STOOL SWELL SWILL SWIRL SYBIL SZELL

•SL••

ASLAK ASLAN FSLIC ISLAM ISLAS ISLES ISLET ISLEY ISLIP OSLER OSLIN USLTA

•S•L•

ASOLD ASYLA ISOLA ISOLT ISTLE PSALM

•S••L

ASOUL ISSEL USUAL

••SL•

AISLE BASLE LISLE TESLA UNSLY

••S•L

ANSEL BASAL BASEL BASIL EASEL EDSEL ELSOL FUSIL GASOL HOSEL ISSEL LYSOL MOSEL MOSUL MUSIL NASAL OASAL OUSEL SISAL

•••SL

LIESL

SM•••

SMACK SMALL SMARM SMART SMASH SMAUG SMAZE SMEAL SMEAR SMEES SMELL SMELT SMEWS SMILE SMIRK SMITE SMITH SMITS SMOCK SMOGS SMOKE SMOKY SMOLT SMOOT SMORE SMOTE SMURF SMUSH SMUTS SMYTH

S•M••

SAMAR SAMBA SAMIS SAMMI SAMMS SAMMY SAMOA SAMOS SAMPS SAMSA SEMIS SHMOO SIMBA SIMMS SIMON SIMPS SOMAS SOMAT SOMME SOMNI SUMAC SUMER SUMMA SUMOS SUMPS SUMUP

S••M•

SALMA SALMI SAMMI SAMMS SAMMY SCAMP SCAMS SCHMO SCUMS SEAMS SEAMY SEEME SEEMS SELMA SHAME SHAMS SHAMU SHEMP SHIMS SIGMA SIMMS SKIMP SKIMS SLAMS SLIME SLIMS SLIMY SLOMO SLUMP SLUMS SOAMI SOMME SPAMS SPUME SPUMY STAMP STEMS STOMA STOMP STUMP SUEME SUMMA SUOMI SWAMI SWAMP SWIMS

S•••M

SALEM SCRAM SCRIM SCRUM SEDUM SEISM SERUM SHERM SICEM SIXAM SIXPM SMARM SODOM SPASM SPERM STEAM STORM STRAM STROM STRUM STURM SWARM

•SM••

ASMAD OSMAN OSMIC

•S•M•

ASAMI ASKME ISAMU USEME

•S••M

ASSAM ASWIM ISHAM ISLAM PSALM

••SM•

COSMO DISME GISMO ITSME PISMO ZOSMA

••S•M

ASSAM BESOM BOSOM EPSOM INSUM KASEM MISSM

•••SM

ABYSM CHASM DEISM MISSM PLASM PRISM SEISM SPASM

SN•••

SNACK SNAFU SNAGS SNAIL SNAKE SNAKY SNAPS SNARE SNARF SNARK SNARL SNATH SNAZZ SNEAD SNEAK SNEER SNEES SNELL SNERD SNERT SNEVA SNICK SNIDE SNIFF SNIPE SNIPS SNITS SNOBS SNOOD SNOOK SNOOP SNOOT SNORE SNORT SNOUT SNOWE SNOWS SNOWY SNUBS SNUCK SNUFF SNUGS

S•N••

SANAA SANDE SANDH SANDL SANDP SANDS SANDY SANER SANKA SANTA SANTE SANTO SANYO SENAT SENDS SENGI SENNA SENOR SENSE SENTA SENTE SINAI SINCE SINES SINEW SINEX SINGE SINGH SINGS SINKS SINUS SKNXX SONAL SONAR SONDE SONES SONGS SONIA SONIC SONJA SONNY SONYA SONYS SUNDA SUNNA SUNNI SUNNY SUNUP SYNCH SYNCS SYNDS SYNGE SYNOD SYNTH

S••N•

SAENS SAINT SAONE SAUNA SAYNO SCANS SCANT SCENA SCENE SCENT SCONE SEANN SEGNI SEGNO SEINE SENNA SHANA SHANE SHANG SHANK SHANT SHINE SHINS SHINY SHONE SHUNS SHUNT SIENA SIGNE SIGNS SIXNO SKANK SKINK SKINS SKUNK SLANG SLANT SLING SLINK SLUNG SLUNK SOMNI SONNY SOUND SPANG SPANK SPANO SPANS SPEND SPENT SPINE SPINS SPINY SPUNK STAND STANG STANK STANS STENO STENS STENT STINE STING STINK STINT STONE STONY STUNG STUNK STUNS STUNT STYNE SUENO SUING SUNNA SUNNI SUNNY SWANK SWANN SWANS SWINE SWING SWUNG

S•••N

SABIN SAFIN SAGAN SALON SARAN SATAN SATIN SATON SAWIN SAXON SCHON SCION SCORN SEANN SEDAN SEEIN SERIN SETIN SETON SEVEN SEWIN SEWON SHAHN SHAUN SHAWN SHEAN SHEEN SHORN SHOWN SIDON SIMON SIPON SIREN SITIN SITON SIVAN SKEIN SLAIN SLOAN SOLAN SOLON SOREN SPAHN SPAIN SPAWN SPOON SPURN SPYON STAIN STEEN STEIN STERN SUDAN SUSAN SWAIN SWANN SWOON SWORN

•SN••

ASNAP ASNER ASNEW ESNES

MSNBC

•S•N•
ASANA
ASONE
ASSNS
CSINY
ISBNS
NSYNC
USING
USONE

•S••N
ASHEN
ASIAN
ASKIN
ASLAN
ASPEN
ASPIN
ASTIN
ASTON
ASWAN
CSPAN
ESSEN
ESTAN
OSCAN
OSLIN
OSMAN
USEIN
USEON
USTEN
VSIGN

••SN•
AISNE
ASSNS
BOSNS
DASNT
DESNA
HASNO
HASNT
HOSNI
MESNE
TISNT
WASNT
YESNO

••S•N
AHSIN
ANSON
ARSON
BASIN
BISON
BOSON
BOSUN
BUSON
DYSON
EBSEN
EDSON
EISEN
EOSIN
EPSON
ESSEN
HASIN
HASON
HESON
HOSEN
HYSON
IBSEN
JASON
LOSIN
MASON
MESON
MYSIN
NISAN
OLSEN
OLSON
ORSON
PISAN
PUSAN
RESIN
RISEN
ROSEN
ROSIN
SUSAN
TYSON
WASIN
WASON
XESIN

SO•••
SOAKS
SOAMI
SOAPS
SOAPY
SOARS
SOAVE
SOBAD
SOBAS
SOBER
SOBIG
SOCAL
SOCAS
SOCIO
SOCKO
SOCKS
SOCLE
SODAS
SODDY
SODOI
SODOM
SOEUR
SOFAR
SOFAS
SOFER
SOFEW
SOFIA
SOFIE
SOFTC
SOFTG
SOFTY
SOGGY
SOILS
SOIRS
SOLAN
SOLAR
SOLDI
SOLDO
SOLEA
SOLED
SOLEI
SOLER
SOLES
SOLID
SOLLA
SOLON
SOLOS
SOLTI
SOLVE
SOMAS
SOMAT
SOMME
SOMNI
SONAL
SONAR
SONDE
SONES
SONGS
SONIA
SONIC
SONJA
SONNY
SONYA
SONYS
SOOEY
SOOTH
SOOTS
SOOTY
SOPHS
SOPOR
SOPPY
SOPUP
SORAS
SORBO
SORBS
SOREL
SOREN
SORER
SORES
SOROS
SORRY
SORTA
SORTS
SOSAD
SOTTO
SOUCI
SOULS
SOUND
SOUPS
SOUPY
SOURS
SOUSA
SOUSE
SOUTH
SOWED
SOWER
SOYAS
SOYUZ

S•O••
SAONE
SCOFF
SCOLD
SCONE
SCOOP
SCOOT
SCOPE
SCORE
SCORN
SCOTS
SCOTT
SCOUR
SCOUT
SCOWL
SCOWS
SEOUL
SHOAL
SHOAT
SHOCK
SHOED
SHOER
SHOES
SHOGI
SHOJI
SHONE
SHOOK
SHOOS
SHOOT
SHOPS
SHORE
SHORN
SHORT
SHOTS
SHOUT
SHOVE
SHOWN
SHOWS
SHOWY
SIOUX
SKOAL
SKORT
SKOSH
SLOAN
SLOBS
SLOES
SLOGS
SLOMO
SLOOP
SLOPE
SLOPS
SLOSH
SLOTH
SLOTS
SLOWS
SMOCK
SMOGS
SMOKE
SMOKY
SMOLT
SMOOT
SMORE
SMOTE
SNOBS
SNOOD
SNOOK
SNOOP
SNOOT
SNORE
SNORT
SNOUT
SNOWE
SNOWS
SNOWY
SOOEY
SOOTH
SOOTS
SOOTY
SPOCK
SPODE
SPOIL
SPOKE
SPOOF
SPOOK
SPOOL
SPOON
SPOOR
SPORE
SPORK
SPORT
SPOSA
SPOSE
SPOSO
SPOTS
SPOUT
STOAE
STOAS
STOAT
STOCK
STOGY
STOIC
STOKE
STOLA
STOLE
STOLI
STOLS
STOMA
STOMP
STONE
STONY
STOOD
STOOL
STOOP
STOPS
STORE
STORK
STORM
STORY
STOUT
STOVE
STOWE
STOWS
SUOMI
SWOON
SWOOP
SWORD
SWORE
SWORN

S••O•
SABOT
SAGOS
SALON
SALOP
SAMOA
SAMOS
SAPOR
SAROS
SATON
SAVOR
SAVOY
SAXON
SAYOK
SCHON
SCION
SCOOP
SCOOT
SCROD
SEGOS
SENOR
SEPOY
SETON
SEWON
SHMOO
SHOOK
SHOOS
SHOOT
SHYOF
SIDON
SILOS
SIMON
SIPON
SITON
SLOOP
SMOOT
SNOOD
SNOOK
SNOOP
SNOOT
SODOI
SODOM
SOLON
SOLOS
SOPOR
SOROS
SPOOF
SPOOK
SPOOL
SPOON
SPOOR
SPYON
STJOE
STOOD
STOOL
STOOP
STROH
STROM
STROP
STROS
SUMOS
SWOON
SWOOP
SYDOW
SYNOD
SYSOP

S•••O
SACCO
SACRO
SALVO
SANTO
SANYO
SARTO
SAURO
SAWTO
SAYNO
SAYSO
SCHMO
SEATO
SEETO
SEGNO
SEIKO
SERBO
SERIO
SERVO
SETTO
SHAKO
SHMOO
SICKO
SISQO
SIXNO
SLIGO
SLOMO
SOCIO
SOCKO
SOLDO
SORBO
SOTTO
SPAGO
SPANO
SPERO
SPIRO
SPOSO
SPYRO
STENO
STLEO
STYRO
SUENO
SYSCO

•SO••
ASOLD
ASONE
ASORS
ASOUL
ESOPS
ISOLA
ISOLT
USOFA
USONE
XSOUT

•S•O•
ASCOT
ASFOR
ASHOT
ASKOF
ASSOC
ASTON
ASTOR
CSPOT
ESPOO
ESTOC
ESTOP
ESTOS
FSTOP
ISTOO
MSDOS
TSTOP
USEOF
USEON

•S••O
ASTRO
ESPIO
ESPOO
ISTOO
OSSEO
OSTEO
TSAVO
USETO

••SO•
AESOP
ALSOP
ANSON
APSOS
ARSON
ASSOC
BASOV
BESOM
BESOS
BESOT
BISON
BOSOM
BOSON
BOSOX
BUSON
DESOD
DYSON
EDSON
ELSOL
ENSOR
EPSOM
EPSON
GASOL
HASON
HESON
HYSON
ITSOK
JASON
LYSOL
MASON
MESON
MISOS
OLSON
ORSON
PASOS
PESOS
RESOD
RESOW
SYSOP
TYSON
VISOR
WASON
YESOR
YOSOY

••S•O
BASHO
BASSO
BOSCO
CASCO
CASIO
CISCO
COSMO
DISCO
DISKO
GESSO
GISMO
GUSTO
HASNO
HASSO
HASTO
HISTO
LASSO
MISDO
MOSSO
MUSEO
OSSEO
PASCO
PASEO
PASTO
PESTO
PISMO
ROSSO
RUSSO
SISQO
SYSCO
TASSO
VASCO
VESCO
WASCO
WASHO
WASSO
YESNO

•••SO
ANDSO
ARESO
AVISO
BASSO
CANSO
CORSO
DIDSO
DIPSO
DORSO
FATSO
GESSO
HASSO
HOWSO
IAMSO
KELSO
LASSO
MOSSO
NOTSO
QUESO
RATSO
RINSO
ROSSO
RUSSO
SAYSO
SPOSO
TARSO
TASSO
TORSO
VERSO
WASSO
WHOSO

SP•••
SPAAK
SPACE
SPACY
SPADE
SPADS
SPAGO
SPAHN
SPAIN
SPAKE
SPAMS
SPANG
SPANK
SPANO
SPANS
SPARE
SPARK
SPARS
SPASM
SPATE
SPATS
SPAWN
SPAYS
SPEAK
SPEAR
SPECD
SPECK
SPECS
SPEED
SPEER
SPEKE
SPELL
SPELT
SPEND
SPENT
SPERM
SPERO
SPETS
SPEWS
SPICA
SPICE
SPICY
SPIED
SPIEL
SPIER
SPIES
SPIFF
SPIKE
SPIKY
SPILE
SPILL
SPILT
SPINE
SPINS
SPINY
SPIRE
SPIRO
SPIRY
SPITE
SPITS
SPITZ
SPLAT
SPLAY
SPLIT
SPOCK
SPODE
SPOIL
SPOKE
SPOOF
SPOOK
SPOOL
SPOON
SPOOR
SPORE
SPORK
SPORT
SPOSA
SPOSE
SPOSO
SPOTS
SPOUT
SPRAT
SPRAY
SPREE
SPRIG
SPRIT
SPUDS
SPUME
SPUMY
SPUNK
SPURN
SPURS
SPURT
SPYON
SPYRI
SPYRO

S•P••
SAPID
SAPOR
SAPPY
SEPAL
SEPIA
SEPOY
SEPTA
SEPTS
SIPON
SOPHS
SOPOR
SOPPY
SOPUP
STPAT
SUPER
SUPES
SUPPE
SUPRA
SUPTS

S••P•
SAMPS
SAPPY
SCAPA
SCAPE
SCOPE
SCUPS
SEEPS
SEEPY
SHAPE
SHIPS
SHOPS
SIMPS
SIXPM
SKIPS
SKYPE
SLAPS
SLEPT
SLIPS
SLOPE
SLOPS
SNAPS
SNIPE
SNIPS
SOAPS
SOAPY
SOPPY
SOUPS
SOUPY
STAPH
STEPS
STIPE
STOPS
STUPA
STUPE
SUMPS
SUPPE
SWAPS
SWEPT
SWIPE
SYLPH

S•••P
SALEP
SALOP
SANDP
SATUP
SAWUP
SCALP
SCAMP
SCARP
SCOOP
SCRAP
SCRIP
SEEUP
SETUP
SEWUP
SHARP
SHEEP
SHEMP
SHLEP
SIRUP
SITUP
SIXUP
SKIMP
SLEEP
SLOOP
SLUMP
SLURP
SNOOP
SOPUP
STAMP
STEEP
STOMP
STOOP
STRAP
STREP
STRIP
STROP
STUMP
SUMUP
SUNUP
SWAMP
SWEEP
SWOOP
SYRUP
SYSOP

•SP••
ASPCA
ASPEN
ASPER
ASPIC
ASPIN
CSPAN
CSPOT
ESPIO
ESPOO
ESPYS

•S•P•
ESOPS
MSRPS
RSVPD
RSVPS

•S••P
ASCAP
ASKUP
ASNAP
ESTOP
FSTOP
ISLIP
TSTOP
USEUP
USURP

••SP•
CUSPS
GASPE
GASPS
HASPS
HOSPS
LISPS
RASPA
RASPE
RASPS
RASPY
TBSPS
VESPA
WASPS
WASPY
WISPS
WISPY

••S•P
AESOP
ALSOP
GASUP
HASUP
JOSIP
SYSOP
WASUP

•••SP
AGASP
CLASP
CRISP
GRASP
QUISP
THESP

SQ•••
SQUAB
SQUAD
SQUAT
SQUAW
SQUIB
SQUID

S••Q•
SISQO

S•••Q
SUZYQ

•SQ••
ESQUE

••SQ•
SISQO

••S•Q
ETSEQ

SR•••
SRTAS

S•R••
SARAH
SARAI
SARAN
SARDI
SARDS
SAREE
SAREK
SARGE
SARIS
SAROS
SARTO
SCRAG
SCRAM
SCRAP
SCRAT
SCREE
SCREW
SCRIM
SCRIP
SCROD
SCRUB
SCRUM
SERAC
SERAI
SERAL
SERBO
SERBS
SERFS
SERGE
SERIA
SERIF
SERIN
SERIO
SERRA
SERTA
SERTS
SERUM
SERVE
SERVO
SHRED
SHREK
SHREW
SHRUB
SHRUG
SIRED
SIREE
SIREN
SIRES
SIRUP
SORAS
SORBO
SORBS
SOREL
SOREN
SORER
SORES
SOROS
SORRY
SORTA
SORTS
SPRAT
SPRAY
SPREE
SPRIG
SPRIT
STRAD
STRAM
STRAP
STRAT
STRAW
STRAY
STREP
STREW
STRIA
STRIP
STROH
STROM
STROP
STROS
STRUG
STRUM
STRUT
SURAH
SURAS
SURER
SURFS
SURFY
SURGE
SURLY
SYRIA
SYRUP

S••R•
SABRA
SABRE
SACRA
SACRE
SACRO
SAIRY
SAURO
SCARE
SCARF
SCARP
SCARS
SCARY
SCIRE
SCORE
SCORN
SEARS
SEERS
SEGRE
SERRA
SHARD
SHARE
SHARI
SHARK
SHARP
SHERA
SHERE
SHERM
SHIRE
SHIRK
SHIRR
SHIRT
SHORE
SHORN
SHORT
SKIRL
SKIRT
SKORT
SLURP
SLURS
SMARM
SMART
SMIRK
SMORE
SMURF
SNARE
SNARF
SNARK
SNARL
SNERD
SNERT
SNORE
SNORT
SOARS
SOIRS
SORRY
SOURS
SPARE
SPARK
SPARS
SPERM
SPERO
SPIRE
SPIRO
SPIRY
SPORE
SPORK
SPORT
SPURN
SPURS
SPURT
SPYRI
SPYRO
STARE
STARK
STARR
STARS
START
STARZ
STERE
STERN
STIRS
STORE
STORK
STORM
STORY
STURM
STYRO
SUCRE
SUERS
SUPRA
SUTRA
SWARD
SWARM
SWIRL
SWORD
SWORE
SWORN

S•••R
SABER
SAFAR
SAFER
SAGER
SAMAR
SANER
SAPOR
SATYR
SAVER
SAVOR
SAWER
SAYER
SCOUR
SEDER
SEGAR
SEGER
SENOR
SEVER
SEWER
SEXER
SHEAR
SHEER
SHIER
SHIRR
SHOER
SHYER
SITAR
SIXER
SIZER
SKIER
SLIER
SLYER
SMEAR
SNEER
SOBER
SOEUR
SOFAR
SOFER
SOLAR
SOLER
SONAR
SOPOR
SORER
SOWER
SPEAR
SPEER
SPIER
SPOOR
SSTAR
STAHR
STAIR
STARR
STEER
SUGAR
SUMER
SUPER
SURER
SWEAR

•SR••
ASRED
MSRPS
OSRIC
USRDA

•S•R•
ASDRY
ASORS
ASTRA
ASTRE
ASTRO
ISERE
TSARS
USERS
USURP
USURY
XSARA

5 SR

•S••R

ASFOR ASHER ASHUR ASKER ASNER ASPER ASSER ASSYR ASTER ASTIR ASTOR BSTAR CSTAR ESKER ESTAR ESTER FSTAR GSTAR KSTAR MSTAR NSTAR OSCAR OSIER OSKAR OSLER OSTAR OSTER RSFSR SSTAR USAIR USHER

••SR•

BASRA

••S•R

AESIR ANSER ASSER ASSYR AUSTR BASER CASER CESAR DOSER EASER ENSOR GASTR HOSER HYSER INSTR KISER KOSAR KYSER LASER LOSER MASER MASUR MISER MUSER NOSER NOSIR ORSER POSER RASER RISER TASER UNSER VISOR WESER WISER YASIR YESOR

•••SR

RSFSR

SS•••

SSGTS SSTAR

S•S••

SASES SASHA SASSY SISAL SISQO SISSY SOSAD SUSAN SUSHI SUSIE SYSCO SYSOP SYSTS

S••S•

SALSA SAMSA SASSY SAYSO SCUSA SCUSI SEEST SEISM SENSE SEUSS SHISH SHUSH SISSY SKOSH SLASH SLOSH SLUSH SMASH SMUSH SOUSA SOUSE SPASM SPOSA SPOSE SPOSO STASH STASI SUDSY SWASH SWISH SWISS

S•••S

SAABS SACHS SACKS SAENS SAFES SAGAS SAGES SAGOS SAILS SAKES SAKIS SALAS SALES SALTS SAMIS SAMMS SAMOS SAMPS SANDS SARDS SARIS SAROS SASES SATES SAUKS SAVES SAXES SCABS SCADS SCAMS SCANS SCARS SCATS SCOTS SCOWS SCUDS SCUMS SCUPS SCUTS SEALS SEAMS SEARS SEATS SECHS SECTS SEEAS SEEDS SEEKS SEEMS SEEPS SEERS SEGOS SELES SELLS SEMIS SENDS SEPTS SERBS SERFS SERTS SETTS SEUSS SEXES SHADS SHAGS SHAHS SHAMS SHAYS SHEDS SHIES SHIMS SHINS SHIPS SHIVS SHOES SHOOS SHOPS SHOTS SHOWS SHULS SHUNS SHUTS SIDES SIFTS SIGHS SIGNS SIKAS SIKES SIKHS SILAS SILKS SILLS SILOS SILTS SIMMS SIMPS SINES SINGS SINKS SINUS SIRES SITES SIXES SIZES SKEDS SKEGS SKEWS SKIDS SKIES SKIMS SKINS SKIPS SKITS SKUAS SKYES SLABS SLAGS SLAMS SLAPS SLATS SLAVS SLAWS SLAYS SLEDS SLEWS SLEYS SLIMS SLIPS SLITS SLOBS SLOES SLOGS SLOPS SLOTS SLOWS SLUES SLUGS SLUMS SLURS SMEES SMEWS SMITS SMOGS SMUTS SNAGS SNAPS SNEES SNIPS SNITS SNOBS SNOWS SNUBS SNUGS SOAKS SOAPS SOARS SOBAS SOCAS SOCKS SODAS SOFAS SOILS SOIRS SOLES SOLOS SOMAS SONES SONGS SONYS SOOTS SOPHS SORAS SORBS SORES SOROS SORTS SOULS SOUPS SOURS SOYAS SPADS SPAMS SPANS SPARS SPATS SPAYS SPECS SPETS SPEWS SPIES SPINS SPITS SPOTS SPUDS SPURS SRTAS SSGTS STABS STADS STAGS STANS STARS STATS STAYS STEMS STENS STEPS STETS STEWS STIES STIRS STOAS STOLS STOPS STOWS STROS STUBS STUDS STUNS STYES SUCKS SUERS SUETS SUFIS SUITS SULKS SUMOS SUMPS SUPES SUPTS SURAS SURFS SWABS SWAGS SWANS SWAPS SWATS SWAYS SWIGS SWIMS SWISS SYNCS SYNDS SYSTS

•SS••

ASSAD ASSAI ASSAM ASSAY ASSER ASSES ASSET ASSEZ ASSNS ASSOC ASSTD ASSTS ASSYR ESSAI ESSAY ESSEN ESSES ESSEX ESSIE ISSEI ISSEL ISSUE ISSUS OSSEO OSSET OSSIA OSSIE PSSST PSSTS

•S•S•

ESIST PSSST RSFSR

•S••S

ASCUS ASHES ASICS ASORS ASSES ASSNS ASSTS ESNES ESOPS ESPYS ESSES ESTAS ESTES ESTHS ESTOS ISBNS ISLAS ISLES ISSUS LSATS MSDOS MSGTS MSRPS PSATS PSSTS RSVPS SSGTS TSARS TSGTS USEAS USEES USERS USHES

••SS•

AUSSI BASSE BASSI BASSO BASSY BOSSA BOSSY CISSY FOSSA FOSSE FUSSY GASSY GESSO GOSSE GUSSY HASSO HESSE HISSY HUSSY JESSE JESSY KISSY LASSE LASSO LISSE MASSA MASSE MASSY MESSE MESSY MISSA MISSM MISSY MOSSO MOSSY MUSSY PASSE PASSU PASSY POSSE PSSST PUSSY RASSE ROSSA ROSSI ROSSO RUSSA RUSSE RUSSO SASSY SISSY TASSE TASSO TESSA WASSO

••S•S

APSES APSIS APSOS ARSES ARSIS ASSES ASSNS ASSTS BASES BASIS BASKS BASTS BESES BESOS BESTS BOSCS BOSNS BUSES BUSKS BUSTS CASAS CASES CASKS CASTS CASUS CISTS COSTS CUSKS CUSPS CYSTS DESKS DISCS DISKS DISTS DOSES DUSKS DUSTS EASES EASTS ELSAS ELSES ESSES FASTS FESTS FISCS FISTS FUSES GASES GASPS GESTS GISTS GUSTS HASPS HESTS HOSES HOSPS HOSTS HUSKS INSTS ISSUS JESTS JESUS LASES LASTS LISPS LISTS LOSES LUSTS LYSES LYSIS MASAS MASKS MASTS MESAS MESES MISOS MISTS MOSES MUSES MUSKS MUSTS NESTS NISUS NOSES OASES OASIS OASTS ORSES OUSTS PASES PASOS PASTS PESOS PESTS POSES POSTS PSSTS RASES RASPS RESTS RISES RISKS ROSES RUSES RUSKS RUSTS SASES SYSTS TASKS TBSPS TESTS TUSKS URSUS VASES VASTS VESTS VISAS VISES WASPS WESTS WISES WISPS XYSTS YESES ZESTS

•••SS

ABYSS AMASS AMISS BLASS BLESS BLISS BRASS CHESS CLASS CRASS CRESS CROSS DRESS DROSS DYESS FAUSS FLOSS FRESS GAUSS GLASS GLESS GLOSS GRASS GROSS GUESS HEISS HROSS IPASS JOOSS KRESS KRISS KVASS LOESS NEUSS PRESS PRISS PROSS REUSS RLESS SEUSS SWISS TRESS TRUSS UMASS WEISS ZEISS

ST•••

STABS STACK STACY STADE STADS STADT STAEL STAFF STAGE STAGG STAGS STAGY STAHL STAHR STAID STAIN STAIR STAKE STALE STALK STALL STAMP STAND STANG STANK STANS STAPH STARE STARK STARR STARS START STARZ STASH STASI STATE STATS STAUB STAVE STAYS STEAD STEAK STEAL STEAM STEED STEEL STEEN STEEP STEER STEIG STEIN STELA STELE STEMS STENO STENS STENT STEPS STERE STERN STETS STEVE STEWS STEWY STICH STICK STIEB STIED STIES STIFF STILE STILL STILT STINE STING STINK STINT STIPE STIRS STJOE STLEO STOAE STOAS STOAT STOCK STOGY STOIC STOKE STOLA STOLE STOLI STOLS STOMA STOMP STONE STONY STOOD STOOL STOOP STOPS STORE STORK STORM STORY STOUT STOVE STOWE STOWS STPAT STRAD STRAM STRAP STRAT STRAW STRAY STREP STREW STRIA STRIP STROH STROM STROP STROS STRUG STRUM STRUT STUBS STUCK STUDS STUDY STUFF STUKA STUMP STUNG STUNK STUNS STUNT STUPA STUPE STURM STUTZ STUVW STYES STYLE STYLI STYNE STYRO

S•T••

SATAN SATAT SATAY SATBY SATCH SATED SATES SATIE SATII SATIN SATON SATUP SATYR SETAE SETAT SETBY SETIN SETON SETTE SETTO SETTS SETUP SITAR SITAT SITBY SITED SITES SITIN SITKA SITON SITUP SOTTO SRTAS SSTAR SUTRA

S••T•

SAITH SALTI SALTS SALTY SANTA SANTE SANTO SARTO SAUTE SAWTO SCATS SCOTS SCOTT SCUTS SEATO SEATS SECTS SEETH SEETO SENTA SENTE SEPTA SEPTS SERTA SERTS SETTE SETTO SETTS SHATT SHOTS SHUTE SHUTS SIETE SIFTS SILTS SILTY SIXTH SIXTY SKATE SKITS SLATE SLATS SLATY SLITS SLOTH SLOTS SMITE SMITH SMITS SMOTE SMUTS SMYTH SNATH SNITS SOFTC SOFTG SOFTY SOLTI SOOTH SOOTS SOOTY SORTA SORTS SOTTO SOUTH SPATE SPATS SPETS SPITE SPITS SPITZ SPOTS SSGTS STATE STATS STETS STUTZ SUETS SUETY SUITE SUITS SUPTS SWATH SWATS SYNTH SYSTS

S•••T

SABOT SADAT SAGET SAINT SALUT SATAT SAULT SAYIT SCANT SCENT SCOOT SCOTT SCOUT SCRAT SEEST SENAT SETAT SHAFT SHALT SHANT SHATT SHEET SHIFT SHIRT SHOAT SHOOT SHORT SHOUT SHUNT SIGHT SITAT SKEET SKIRT SKORT SLANT SLEET SLEPT SMART SMELT SMOLT SMOOT SNERT SNOOT SNORT SNOUT SOMAT SPELT SPENT SPILT SPLAT SPLIT SPORT SPOUT SPRAT SPRIT SPURT SQUAT STADT START STENT STILT STINT STOAT STOUT STPAT STRAT STRUT STUNT SWEAT SWEET SWEPT SWIFT

•ST••

ASTER ASTIN ASTIR ASTON ASTOR ASTRA ASTRE ASTRO BSTAR CSTAR ESTAB ESTAN ESTAR ESTAS ESTEE ESTER ESTES ESTHS ESTOC ESTOP ESTOS FSTAR FSTOP GSTAR ISTIC ISTLE ISTOO KSTAR MSTAR NSTAR OSTAR OSTEO OSTER OSTIA RSTUV SSTAR TSTOP USTED USTEN

•S•T•

ASSTD ASSTS LSATS MSGTS PSATS PSSTS SSGTS TSGTS USETO USLTA

•S••T

ASCOT ASFAT ASFIT ASHOT ASSET ASYET CSPOT ESBAT ESIST GSUIT ISLET ISOLT OSSET PSSST USEIT XSOUT

••ST•

AOSTA ASSTD ASSTS AUSTR BASTA BASTE BASTS BESTS BUSTA BUSTS CASTA CASTE CASTS CBSTV CESTA CESTI CISTS COSTA COSTS CYSTS DESTE DISTS DUSTS DUSTY EASTS FASTS FESTA FESTE FESTS FISTS FUSTY GASTR GESTE GESTS GISTS GUSTO GUSTS GUSTY HASTA HASTE HASTO HASTY HESTS HISTO HOSTA HOSTS INSTR INSTS JESTS JUSTE JUSTY LASTS LISTS LUSTS LUSTY MASTS

MESTA MISTI MISTS MISTY MUSTS MUSTY NASTY NESTS NESTY OASTS OESTE OUSTS PASTA PASTE PASTO PASTS PASTY PESTO PESTS PISTE POSTE POSTS PSSTS QRSTU RASTA RESTE RESTS RUSTS RUSTY SYSTS TASTE TASTY TESTA TESTS TESTY VASTI VASTS VASTY VESTA VESTI VESTS VISTA WASTE WESTS XYSTS ZESTA ZESTS ZESTY

••S•T

ASSET BESET BESOT COSET DASNT GOSIT HASAT HASIT HASNT IMSET INSET LISZT ONSET OSSET POSIT PSSST RASHT RESAT RESET RESHT RESIT TISNT TVSET UNSET UPSET VISIT WASAT WASIT WASNT

•••ST

ADUST ALIST AMUST ANGST ATEST AVAST BAKST BEAST BLAST BLEST BLIST BOAST BOOST BREST BURST CANST CHAST CHEST COAST CONST CREST CRIST CRUST CURST DEIST DIDST DOEST DUNST DURST EGEST ELIST ELMST ERNST ESIST EXIST FAUST FEAST FIRST FOIST FRIST FROST FURST GEIST GHOST GOEST GRIST GUEST HADST HEIST HOEST HOIST HOLST HORST HTEST HURST IDEST JOIST JOUST KARST LEAST LIEST MAYST MIDST MOIST NTEST ODIST OUEST PABST PLAST PQRST PROST PSSST QUEST QWEST ROAST ROOST ROUST SEEST TOAST TRUST TRYST TWIST VERST WAIST WEEST WHIST WIEST WORST WREST WRIST WURST YEAST ZEIST

SU•••

SUAVE SUBIC SUCKS SUCKY SUCRE SUDAN SUDSY SUEDE SUEME SUENO SUERS SUETS SUETY SUFIS SUGAR SUING SUITE SUITS SULFA SULKS SULKY SULLA SULLY SUMAC SUMER SUMMA SUMOS SUMPS SUMUP SUNDA SUNNA SUNNI SUNNY SUNUP SUOMI SUPER SUPES SUPPE SUPRA SUPTS SURAH SURAS SURER SURFS SURFY SURGE SURLY SUSAN SUSHI SUSIE SUTRA SUZIE SUZYQ

S•U••

SAUCE SAUCY SAUDI SAUKS SAULT SAUNA SAURO SAUTE SCUBA SCUDS SCUFF SCULL SCUMS SCUPS SCUSA SCUSI SCUTS SCUZZ SEULE SEUSS SHUCK SHULA SHULS SHUNS SHUNT SHUSH SHUTE SHUTS SKUAS SKULK SKULL SKUNK SLUED SLUES SLUGS SLUMP SLUMS SLUNG SLUNK SLURP SLURS SLUSH SMURF SMUSH SMUTS SNUBS SNUCK SNUFF SNUGS SOUCI SOULS SOUND SOUPS SOUPY SOURS SOUSA SOUSE SOUTH SPUDS SPUME SPUMY SPUNK SPURN SPURS SPURT SQUAB SQUAD SQUAT SQUAW SQUIB SQUID STUBS STUCK STUDS STUDY STUFF STUKA STUMP STUNG STUNK STUNS STUNT STUPA STUPE STURM STUTZ STUVW SWUNG

S••U•

SALUD SALUT SATUP SAWUP SCOUR SCOUT SCRUB SCRUM SEDUM SEEUP SEGUE SEOUL SERUM SETUP SEWUP SHAUN SHOUT SHRUB SHRUG SINUS SIOUX SIRUP SITUP SIXUP SMAUG SNOUT SOEUR SOPUP SOYUZ SPOUT STAUB STOUT STRUG STRUM STRUT SUMUP SUNUP SYRUP

S•••U

SADHU SHAMU SNAFU

•SU••

GSUIT ISUZU USUAL USURP USURY

•S•U•

ASCUS ASHUR ASKUP ASOUL ESQUE ISSUE ISSUS PSEUD RSTUV USEUP XSOUT

•S••U

ISAMU ISUZU

••SU•

BOSUN CASUS ENSUE GASUP HASUP INSUM ISSUE ISSUS JESUS MASUR MOSUL NISUS URSUS WASUP

••S•U

MUSHU PASSU QRSTU WUSHU

•••SU

GANSU GINSU MATSU PASSU

S•V••

SAVED SAVER SAVES SAVOR SAVOY SAVVY SEVEN SEVER SIVAN

S••V•

SALVE SALVO SAVVY SERVE SERVO SHAVE SHIVA SHIVS SHOVE SIEVE SILVA SLAVE SLAVS SNEVA SOAVE SOLVE STAVE STEVE STOVE STUVW SUAVE

S•••V

SCHAV

•SV••

RSVPD RSVPS

•S•V•

TSAVO

•S••V

RSTUV

••S•V

BASOV CBSTV

•••SV

PIUSV

SW•••

SWABS SWAGS SWAIN SWALE SWAMI SWAMP SWANK SWANN SWANS SWAPS SWARD SWARM SWASH SWATH SWATS SWAYS SWAZI SWEAR SWEAT SWEDE SWEEP SWEET SWELL SWEPT SWIFT SWIGS SWILL SWIMS SWINE SWING SWIPE SWIRL SWISH SWISS SWOON SWOOP SWORD SWORE SWORN SWUNG

S•W••

SAWED SAWER SAWII SAWIN SAWTO SAWUP SEWED SEWER SEWIN SEWON SEWUP SOWED SOWER

S••W•

SCHWA SCOWL SCOWS SHAWL SHAWN SHOWN SHOWS SHOWY SKEWS SLAWS SLEWS SLIWA SLOWS SMEWS SNOWE SNOWS SNOWY SPAWN SPEWS STEWS STEWY STOWE STOWS

S•••W

SCREW SHREW SINEW SOFEW SQUAW STRAW STREW STUVW SYDOW

•SW••

ASWAN ASWAY ASWIM

•S••W

ASKEW ASNEW PSHAW

••S•W

RESAW RESEW RESOW UNSEW

S•X••

SAXES SAXON SEXED SEXER SEXES SIXAD SIXAM SIXBC SIXED SIXEE SIXER SIXES SIXNO SIXPM SIXTH SIXTY SIXUP

S••X•

SKNXX

S•••X

SILEX SINEX SIOUX SKNXX

•S••X

ESSEX

••S•X

ATSIX BOSOX DESEX ESSEX

•••SX

PIUSX

SY•••

SYBIL SYDOW SYLPH SYNCH SYNCS SYNDS SYNGE SYNOD SYNTH SYRIA SYRUP SYSCO SYSOP SYSTS

S•Y••

SAYAH SAYER SAYHI SAYIT SAYNO SAYOK SAYSO SHYER SHYLY SHYOF SKYES SKYEY SKYPE SLYER SLYKE SLYLY SMYTH SOYAS SOYUZ SPYON SPYRI SPYRO STYES STYLE STYLI STYNE STYRO

S••Y•

SANYO SATYR SEEYA SHAYS SIBYL SLAYS SLEYS SONYA SONYS SPAYS STAYS SUZYQ SWAYS

S•••Y

SADLY SAGGY SAIRY SALLY SALTY SAMMY SANDY SAPPY SASSY SATAY SATBY SAUCY SAVOY SAVVY SCALY SCARY SEALY SEAMY SEDGY SEEDY SEEPY SEPOY SETBY SFBAY SHADY SHAKY SHINY SHOWY SHYLY SILKY SILLY SILTY SISSY SITBY SIXTY SKYEY SLATY SLIMY SLYLY SMOKY SNAKY SNOWY SOAPY SODDY SOFTY SOGGY SONNY SOOEY SOOTY SOPPY SORRY SOUPY SPACY SPICY SPIKY SPINY SPIRY SPLAY SPRAY SPUMY STACY STAGY STEWY STOGY STONY STORY STRAY STUDY SUCKY SUDSY SUETY SULKY SULLY SUNNY SURFY SURLY

•SY••

ASYET ASYLA NSYNC PSYCH

•S•Y•

ASSYR ESPYS YSAYE

•S••Y

ASDRY ASHBY ASSAY ASWAY CSINY ESSAY ISLEY OSHAY USEBY USURY

••SY•

ASSYR EASYA

••S•Y

ASSAY BASSY BOSSY BUSBY BUSEY BUSHY CASBY CASEY CISSY COSBY CUSHY DASHY DISHY DOSAY DUSKY DUSTY ENSKY ESSAY FISHY FUSSY FUSTY GASSY GUSHY GUSSY GUSTY HASTY HISSY HUSKY HUSSY IFSAY JESSY JOSEY JUSTY KESEY KISSY LASKY LOSEY LUSHY LUSTY MASSY MESHY MESSY MISSY MISTY MOSEY MOSSY MUSHY MUSKY MUSSY MUSTY NASBY NASTY NESTY NOSEY ORSAY PASSY PASTY PESKY POSEY PUSHY PUSSY RASPY RESAY RISKY ROSEY RUSHY RUSTY SASSY SISSY TASTY TESTY TUSHY UNSAY UNSHY UNSLY VASTY WASHY WASPY WISHY WISPY YOSOY ZESTY

•••SY

ANTSY ARTSY BASSY BETSY BITSY BOSSY BUGSY CISSY COUSY DAISY DIPSY DITSY DOISY EENSY FUBSY FUSSY GASSY GIPSY GOOSY GORSY GUSSY GUTSY GYPSY HISSY HORSY HOTSY HUSSY JESSY KISSY LOUSY MASSY MESSY MIMSY MISSY MOPSY MOSSY MOUSY MUSSY NEWSY NOISY NUTSY PALSY PANSY PASSY PATSY POESY POTSY PROSY PURSY PUSSY SASSY SISSY SUDSY TANSY TIPSY TOPSY TOTSY WALSY

SZ•••

SZELL

S•Z••

SIZED SIZER SIZES SUZIE SUZYQ

S••Z•

SCUZZ SEIZE SMAZE SNAZZ SWAZI

S•••Z

SCUZZ SNAZZ SOYUZ SPITZ STARZ STUTZ

•S•Z•

ISUZU

•S••Z

ASSEZ

••SZ•

LISZT

••S•Z

ASSEZ

•••SZ

GROSZ REISZ WEISZ

TA•••

TABBY TABIS TABLA TABLE TABOO TABOR TABUS TACET TACHO TACHS TACIT TACKS TACKY TACOS TADAS TAEBO TAEGU TAELS TAFFY TAFTS TAGON TAGUP TAGUS TAHOE TAIGA TAILS TAINA TAINT TAITO TAKAS TAKEI TAKEN TAKER TAKES TAKIN TALAS TALCS TALER TALES TALIA TALKS TALKY TALLS TALLY TALON TALUS TAMAR TAMED TAMER TAMES TAMIL TAMMI TAMMY TAMPA TAMPS TANDY TANEY TANGO TANGS TANGY TANIA TANIS TANKA TANKS TANNA TANSY TANTE TANTO TANYA TAPAS TAPED TAPER TAPES TAPIN TAPIR TAPIS TAPON TARAS TARDE TARDO TARDY TARED TARES TARGA TARIQ TARNS TAROS TAROT TARPS TARRY TARSI TARSO TARTE TARTS TARTU TARTY TASER TASHI TASKS TASSE TASSO TASTE TASTY TATAR TATAS TATER TATES TATIS TATRA TATTY TATUM TAUNT TAUON TAUPE TAURI TAURO TAUTO TAVEL TAVIS TAWNY TAXCO TAXED TAXER TAXES TAXIS TAXOL TAXON

T•A••

TBALL TBARS TEACH TEAKS TEALS TEAMO TEAMS TEARS TEARY TEASE TEATS THAIS THANE THANK THANT THANX THARP THATS THAWS TIAGO TIAMO TIANT TIARA TOADS TOADY TOAST TRACE TRACI TRACK TRACT TRACY TRADE TRAGG TRAIL TRAIN TRAIT TRALA TRAMP TRAMS TRANE TRANS TRAPP TRAPS TRASH TRASK TRAVE TRAWL TRAYS TSADE TSADI TSARS TSAVO TVADS TWAIN TWANG

TZARA TZARS

T••A•

TADAS TAKAS TALAS TAMAR TAPAS TARAS TATAR TATAS TELAR TEMAS TENAD TENAM TERAT TEWAS TEXAN TEXAS THEAS THEAX TICAL TIDAL TILAK TITAN TIWAS TODAY TOEAS TOGAE TOGAS TOKAY TOLAR TOMAR TOMAS TONAL TOPAZ TORAH TORAS TOTAL TOVAH TOWAR TREAD TREAS TREAT TRIAD TRIAL TUBAL TUBAS TUGAT TUNAS TUPAC TVMAN TWEAK TWOAD TWOAM TYNAN TYPAL

T•••A

TABLA TAIGA TAINA TALIA TAMPA TANIA TANKA TANNA TANYA TARGA TATRA TEENA TELMA TERIA TERRA TERZA TESLA TESSA TESTA TETRA THEDA THEMA THERA THETA THORA TIARA TIBIA TIKKA TILDA TINEA TIOGA TISHA TOMBA TONGA TONKA TONYA TORTA TOSCA TOSEA TRALA TRINA TULSA TWYLA TYPEA TZARA

•TA••

ATALA ATALL ATARI ATARS ETAGE ETAIL ETAPE ETATS ITALO ITALS ITALY MTAPO OTARU OTARY STABS STACK STACY STADE STADS STADT STAEL STAFF STAGE STAGG STAGS STAGY STAHL STAHR STAID STAIN STAIR STAKE STALE STALK STALL STAMP STAND STANG STANK STANS STAPH STARE STARK STARR STARS START STARZ STASH STASI STATE STATS STAUB STAVE STAYS UTAHN

•T•A•

ATBAR ATBAT ATBAY ATEAM ATEAT ATLAS ATMAN ATPAR ATRAS ATTAR ATWAR BTEAM ETHAN ETNAS ITEAS OTRAS OTWAY PTRAP STEAD STEAK STEAL STEAM STOAE STOAS STOAT STPAT STRAD STRAM STRAP STRAT STRAW STRAY UTTAR

•T••A

ATALA ATRIA ATSEA ETYMA ITINA MTIDA STELA STOLA STOMA STRIA STUKA STUPA UTICA

••TA•

ACTAS ALTAI ALTAR ANTAE ANTAL ANTAS ATTAR BETAS BSTAR COTAN CSTAR DETAR DETAT DITAT DOTAL EATAT ECTAD ECTAL ENTAD ESTAB ESTAN ESTAR ESTAS FATAL FETAL FETAS FSTAR GETAB GETAC GETAD GETAS GETAT GOTAB GOTAC GOTAD GOTAT GSTAR HITAT IDTAG IOTAS JOTAS KATAS KSTAR LETAT METAL MITAS MSTAR NATAL NATAN NOTAH NOTAX NSTAR OCTAD OCTAL OCTAN ONTAP OSTAR PETAL PITAS QATAR RETAG RETAN RETAP RETAR RETAX ROTAS SATAN SATAT SATAY SETAE SETAT SITAR SITAT SRTAS SSTAR TATAR TATAS TITAN TOTAL UNTAX UTTAR VITAE VITAL VITAM VITAS WOTAN ZETAS

••T•A

AETNA AFTRA ANTRA ASTRA BATNA BETTA BOTHA COTTA DITKA EXTRA FATHA FATWA GOTHA GOTTA HATHA INTRA JETTA LATKA LOTSA LOTTA MITLA MITYA NATTA OSTIA OUTTA PATNA PETRA RETIA SITKA SUTRA TATRA TETRA ULTRA YETTA ZETTA

•••TA

ADYTA AGITA AKITA ALETA ANITA AORTA AOSTA BANTA BASTA BERTA BETTA BIOTA BUSTA CARTA CASTA CESTA CEUTA CHETA CHITA COSTA COTTA DELTA DICTA EVITA FACTA FANTA FESTA FRITA GAETA GOTTA GRATA GRETA HASTA HEPTA HOSTA JETTA JUNTA KUNTA LOTTA MALTA MANTA MARTA MEHTA MESTA MIATA NAFTA NATTA NIETA OLETA OUTTA OVETA PANTA PARTA PASTA PENTA PIETA PINTA PLATA PONTA PORTA PUNTA QUOTA RAITA RASTA REATA RECTA RIATA SANTA SENTA SEPTA SERTA SORTA TESTA THETA TORTA UINTA UNITA USLTA VENTA VESTA VISTA VOLTA YALTA YENTA YETTA ZESTA ZETTA

TB•••

TBALL TBARS TBILL TBIRD TBOND TBONE TBSPS

T•B••

TABBY TABIS TABLA TABLE TABOO TABOR TABUS TEBET TIBBS TIBER TIBET TIBIA TOBEY TOBIT TUBAL TUBAS TUBBS TUBBY TUBED TUBER TUBES

T••B•

TABBY TAEBO TENBC THEBE TIBBS TOMBA TOMBE TOMBS TRIBE TUBBS TUBBY TURBO TWOBC

T•••B

TENLB THEWB THROB THUMB TYPEB

•TB••

ATBAR ATBAT ATBAY

•T•B•

FTLBS STABS STUBS UTUBE

•T••B

STAUB STIEB

••TB•

GETBY GOTBY LETBE LETBY PUTBY SATBY SETBY SITBY

••T•B

ESTAB GETAB GOTAB LITTB

•••TB

LITTB PARTB

TC•••

TCELL

T•C••

TACET TACHO TACHS TACIT TACKS TACKY TACOS TECHS TICAL TICKS TICKY TICOS TUCCI TUCKS TYCHE TYCHO

T••C•

TALCS TAXCO TEACH TELCO TENCC TENCH TERCE THICK TINCT TISCH TORCH TOSCA TOUCH TRACE TRACI TRACK TRACT TRACY TRECE TRICE TRICK TRUCE TRUCK TUCCI TURCO TVVCR TWICE

T•••C

TELIC TENBC TENCC THEOC TONIC TOPIC TORIC TOXIC TUNIC TUPAC TWOBC TYPIC

•TC••

ITCHY LTCOL LTCOM

•T•C•

STACK STACY STICH STICK STOCK STUCK UTICA

•T••C

ATTIC ETHIC STOIC

••TC•

AITCH BATCH BOTCH BUTCH CATCH DITCH DUTCH FETCH FITCH HATCH HITCH HUTCH KETCH KOTCH LATCH MATCH MITCH NATCH NOTCH PATCH PATCO PETCO PITCH ROTCS SATCH VETCH WATCH WITCH

••T•C

ANTIC ATTIC AZTEC ESTOC GETAC GOTAC ISTIC OPTIC VATIC

•••TC

JROTC NROTC PARTC SOFTC

T•D••

TADAS TEDDY TIDAL TIDED TIDES TODAY TODDY TODOS TUDOR TVDVD

T••D•

TANDY TARDE TARDO TARDY TEDDY TENDS TENDU THEDA THUDS TILDA TILDE TOADS TOADY TODDY TONDI TONDO TOODY TRADE TRUDY TSADE TSADI TVADS

T•••D

TAMED TAPED TARED TAXED TBIRD TBOND TENAD TEPID THEYD THIRD TIDED TILED TIMED TIMID TINED TIRED TOKED TONED TOPED TOTED TOWED TOYED TREAD TREED TREND TRIAD TRIED TRUED TSKED TUBED TUMID TUNED TVDVD TWEED TWOAD TYPED

•TD••

FTDIX

•T•D•

ETUDE MTIDA MTIDY STADE STADS STADT STUDS STUDY

•T••D

FTORD STAID STAND STEAD STEED STIED STOOD STRAD

••TD•

NOTDO OUTDO

••T•D

ACTED ANTED APTED BATED CITED DATED DOTED ECTAD ENTAD FATED FETED FETID GATED GETAD GOTAD HATED KITED LITTD LUTED MATED METED MUTED NITID NOTED OCTAD OOTID OPTED OUTED PATED RATED SATED SITED TOTED USTED VOTED

•••TD

ASSTD CONTD LITTD WHATD

TE•••

TEACH TEAKS TEALS TEAMO TEAMS TEARS TEARY TEASE TEATS TEBET TECHS TEDDY TEEMS TEENA TEENS TEENY TEERS TEETH TEEUP TEHEE TEKEL TELAR TELCO TELES TELEX TELIC TELLS TELLY TELMA TEMAS TEMPE TEMPI TEMPO TEMPS TEMPT TENAD TENAM TENBC TENCC TENCH TENDS TENDU TENEE TENET TENGE TENGO TENKS TENLB TENOF TENON TENOR TENPM TENSE TENTH TENTO TENTS TENUP TEPEE TEPID TERAT TERCE TERIA TERME TERMS TERNE TERNS TERPS TERRA TERRE TERRI TERRS TERRY TERSE TERZA TESLA TESSA TESTA TESTS TESTY TETES TETHS TETON TETRA TETRI TEVET TEVYE TEWAS TEWES TEXAN TEXAS TEXTS

T•E••

TAEBO TAEGU TAELS TCELL TEEMS TEENA TEENS TEENY TEERS TEETH TEEUP THEAS THEAX THEBE THEDA THEFT THEIR THEMA THEME THEMS THEOC THEOK THEOL THEPO THERA THERE THERM THESE THESP THETA THEUN THEWB THEWS THEWY THEYD TIEGS TIEIN TIENE TIEON TIERS TIETO TIEUP TOEAS TOEFL TOEIN TREAD TREAS TREAT TRECE TREED TREEN TREES TREKS TREND TRENT TRESS TRETS TREVI TREWS TREYS TWEAK TWEED TWEEN TWEET TWERE TWERP TYEES

T••E•

TACET TAKEI TAKEN TAKER TAKES TALER TALES TAMED TAMER TAMES TANEY TAPED TAPER TAPES TARED TARES TASER TATER TATES TAVEL TAXED TAXER TAXES TEBET TEHEE TEKEL TELES TELEX TENEE TENET TEPEE TETES TEVET TEWES THIEF THIEU THREE THREW TIBER TIBET TIDED TIDES TIGER TIKES TILED TILER TILES TILEX TIMED TIMER TIMES TIMEX TINEA TINED TINES TIRED TIRES TITER TOBEY TOKED TOKEN TOKES TOLER TOLES TOLET TOMEI TOMES TONED TONER TONES TOOER TOPED TOPEE TOPER TOPES TOSEA TOTED TOTEM TOTER TOTES TOVES TOWED TOWEL TOWER TOYED TOYER TPKES TREED TREEN TREES TRIED TRIER TRIES TRUED TRUER TRUES TSKED TUBED TUBER TUBES TULES TUNED TUNER TUNES TUTEE TUXES TVMEN TVSET TWEED TWEEN TWEET TWOEE TWOEM TYEES TYGER TYKES TYLER TYNER TYPEA TYPEB TYPED TYPEE TYPEO TYPER TYPES TYRES TYVEK

T•••E

TABLE TAHOE TANTE TARDE TARTE TASSE TASTE TAUPE TBONE TEASE TEHEE TEMPE TENEE TENGE TENSE TEPEE TERCE TERME TERNE TERRE TERSE TEVYE THANE THEBE THEME THERE THESE THINE THOLE THOSE THREE THROE THULE THYME TIENE TIGRE TILDE TINGE TITHE TITLE TITRE TNOTE TOGAE TOGUE TOILE TOMBE TONNE TOOLE TOPEE TOQUE TORME TORRE TORTE TOTIE TOUTE TOWNE TRACE TRADE TRANE TRAVE TRECE TRIBE TRICE TRIKE TRINE TRIPE TRITE TROPE TROVE TROWE TRUCE TRYME TSADE TTILE

TULLE
TUQUE
TUTEE
TUTTE
TWERE
TWICE
TWINE
TWOEE
TYCHE
TYPEE

•TE••

ATEAM
ATEAT
ATEIN
ATEIT
ATEOF
ATEST
ATEUP
BTEAM
CTENO
HTEST
ITEAS
ITEMS
ITERS
MTELY
NTEST
OTERI
OTERO
PTERO
STEAD
STEAK
STEAL
STEAM
STEED
STEEL
STEEN
STEEP
STEER
STEIG
STEIN
STELA
STELE
STEMS
STENO
STENS
STENT
STEPS
STERE
STERN
STETS
STEVE
STEWS
STEWY
VTENS

•T•E•

ATLES
ATSEA
ATTEN
ETHEL
ETHER
ETRES
ETSEQ
ETTES
FTLEE
LTGEN
MTGES
OTHER
OTOES
OTTER
RTREV
STAEL
STEED
STEEL
STEEN
STEEP
STEER
STIEB
STIED
STIES
STLEO
STREP
STREW
STYES
UTHER
UTLEY
UTTER

•T••E

ATILE
ATIVE
ATONE
ATQUE
BTILE
CTILE
DTILE
ETAGE
ETAPE
ETILE
ETUDE
FTILE
FTLEE
GTILE
HTILE
ITILE
ITSME
JTILE
KTILE
LTILE
MTILE
NTILE
OTILE
PTILE
QTILE
RTILE
STADE
STAGE
STAKE
STALE
STARE
STATE
STAVE
STELE
STERE
STEVE
STILE
STINE
STIPE
STJOE
STOAE
STOKE
STOLE
STONE
STORE
STOVE
STOWE
STUPE
STYLE
STYNE
TTILE
UTILE
UTUBE
VTILE
VTYPE
WTILE
XTILE
XTYPE
YTILE
ZTILE

••TE•

ACTED
ACTER
ACTES
AFTER
ALTER
ANTED
ANTES
APTED
APTER
ARTEL
ASTER
ATTEN
AZTEC
AZTEK
BATED
BATES
BETEL
BETES
BITER
BITES
BOTEL
BUTEO
BYTES
CATER
CATES
CITED
CITEE
CITER
CITES
COTES
CUTER
CUTES
CUTEX
CUTEY
DATED
DATER
DATES
DETER
DOTED
DOTER
DOTES
EATEN
EATER
ENTER
ERTES
ESTEE
ESTER
ESTES
ETTES
FATED
FATES
FETED
FETES
GATED
GATER
GATES
GUTEN
HATED
HATER
HATES
HETER
HOTEL
INTEL
INTER
JETER
JETES
JUTES
KATEY
KITED
KITER
KITES
LATEN
LATER
LATEX
LITEL
LITER
LITES
LOTET
LUTED
LUTES
MATED
MATEO
MATER
MATES
MATEY
METED
METER
METES
MITER
MITES
MOTEL
MOTES
MOTET
MUTED
MUTER
MUTES
NITER
NITES
NOTED
NOTER
NOTES
OATEN
OATER
OATES
OCTET
OFTEN
OPTED
OSTEO
OSTER
OTTER
OUTED
OUTER
PATED
PATEK
PATEN
PATER
PATES
PETER
PETES
PETEY
RATED
RATEL
RATER
RATES
RITES
ROTES
SATED
SATES
SITED
SITES
TATER
TATES
TETES
TITER
TOTED
TOTEM
TOTER
TOTES
TUTEE
UNTER
USTED
USTEN
UTTER
VATER
VOTED
VOTER
VOTES
WATER
YATES

••T•E

ANTAE
ANTRE
ARTIE
ASTRE
AUTRE
BATHE
BETTE
BITTE
BOTHE
BUTTE
CETTE
CITEE
CUTIE
DETRE
DETTE
EATME
ENTRE
ESTEE
GETME
GOTME
HITME
ISTLE
KATHE
KATIE
KATZE
LATHE
LATKE
LATTE
LETBE
LETHE
LETME
LITHE
LITRE
LOTTE
MATTE
METRE
MITRE
NITRE
NOTIE
NOTME
NOTRE
NOTTE
OUTIE
OUTRE
PATHE
PETRE
RETIE
SATIE
SETAE
SETTE
TITHE
TITLE
TITRE
TOTIE
TUTEE
TUTTE
UNTIE
VETTE
VITAE
VOTRE
WITTE
WYTHE

•••TE

ABATE
ACUTE
AGATE
ALATE
AMITE
ARETE
BASTE
BETTE
BITTE
BOITE
BRITE
BRUTE
BUTTE
CARTE
CASTE
CETTE
CHUTE
CLETE
CNOTE
COMTE
CONTE
COOTE
CRATE
CRETE
DANTE
DARTE
DENTE
DESTE
DETTE
DHOTE
DIETE
DOUTE
ELATE
ELITE
ELUTE
EMOTE
ENATE
ENOTE
EVITE
FAUTE
FESTE
FLUTE
FOOTE
FORTE
FRITE
GENTE
GESTE
GLUTE
GNOTE
GRATE
GRETE
GROTE
HARTE
HASTE
HAUTE
IRATE
JUSTE
KINTE
KLUTE
KNUTE
LATTE
LENTE
LEYTE
LOTTE
MATTE
MONTE
MORTE
NOLTE
NORTE
NOTTE
OBOTE
OESTE
ONATE
ORATE
OVATE
PARTE
PASTE
PEETE
PENTE
PHYTE
PISTE
PIUTE
PLATE
POETE
PONTE
PORTE
POSTE
PRATE
QUITE
QUOTE
RENTE
RESTE
ROUTE
SANTE
SAUTE
SENTE
SETTE
SHUTE
SIETE
SKATE
SLATE
SMITE
SMOTE
SPATE
SPITE
STATE
SUITE
TANTE
TARTE
TASTE
TNOTE
TORTE
TOUTE
TRITE
TUTTE
UNITE
VERTE
VETTE
VOLTE
WAITE
WASTE
WHITE
WHYTE
WITTE
WRITE
WROTE
YENTE

T•F••

TAFFY
TAFTS
TIFFS
TOFFS
TOFTS
TOFUS
TUFTS
TUFTY

T••F•

TAFFY
THEFT
TIFFS
TOEFL
TOFFS
TURFS
TURFY

T•••F

TENOF
THIEF

•T•F•

STAFF
STIFF
STUFF

•T••F

ATEOF
MTWTF
STAFF
STIFF
STUFF

••T•F

EATOF
MOTIF
OUTOF

•••TF

MTWTF

T•G••

TAGON
TAGUP
TAGUS
TIGER
TIGHT
TIGON
TIGRE
TOGAE
TOGAS
TOGUE
TOGUP
TSGTS
TUGAT
TUGON
TYGER

T••G•

TAEGU
TAIGA
TANGO
TANGS
TANGY
TARGA
TENGE
TENGO
THIGH
THUGS
TIAGO
TIEGS
TINGE
TINGS
TIOGA
TONGA
TONGS
TOUGH
TRAGG
TWIGS

T•••G

THING
THONG
TOPOG
TRAGG
TWANG
TYING

•TG••

LTGEN
LTGOV
MTGES

•T•G•

ETAGE
STAGE
STAGG
STAGS
STAGY
STOGY

•T••G

STAGG
STANG
STEIG
STING
STRUG
STUNG

••TG•

CITGO
GETGO
GITGO
LETGO
OUTGO

••T•G

IDTAG
RETAG

•••TG

SOFTG

TH•••

THAIS
THANE
THANK
THANT
THANX
THARP
THATS
THAWS
THEAS
THEAX
THEBE
THEDA
THEFT
THEIR
THEMA
THEME
THEMS
THEOC
THEOK
THEOL
THEPO
THERA
THERE
THERM
THESE
THESP
THETA
THEUN
THEWB
THEWS
THEWY
THEYD
THICK
THIEF
THIEU
THIGH
THILL
THINE
THING
THINK
THINS
THIRD
THOLE
THONG
THORA
THORN
THORO
THOSE
THOUS
THREE
THREW
THROB
THROE
THROW
THRUM
THUDS
THUGS
THULE
THUMB
THUMP
THUNK
THURS
THYME
THYMY

T•H••

TAHOE
TEHEE
TVHIT

T••H•

TACHO
TACHS
TASHI
TECHS
TETHS
TIGHT
TISHA
TITHE
TUSHY
TYCHE
TYCHO

T•••H

TEACH
TEETH
TENCH
TENTH
THIGH
TILTH
TISCH
TOOTH
TORAH
TORCH
TOUCH
TOUGH
TOVAH
TRASH
TRISH
TROTH
TRUTH

•TH••

ATHOL
ATHON
ATHOS
ETHAN
ETHEL
ETHER
ETHIC
ETHNO
ETHOS
ETHYL
OTHER
OTHON
UTHER

•T•H•

ITCHY
STAHL
STAHR
UTAHN

•T••H

STAPH
STASH
STICH
STROH

••TH•

ALTHO
BATHE
BATHO
BATHS
BATHY
BETHS
BOTHA
BOTHE
CATHS
CATHY
ESTHS
FATHA
GOTHA
GOTHS
HATHA
HATHI
HETHS
KATHE
KATHY
LATHE
LATHS
LATHY
LETHE
LITHE
LITHO
MATHS
MOTHS
MOTHY
MYTHS
OATHS
ORTHO
PATHE
PATHO
PATHS
PATHY
PITHS
PITHY
RATHS
ROTHS
RUTHS
TETHS
TITHE
WYTHE

••T•H

AITCH
BATCH
BOTCH
BUTCH
CATCH
DITCH
DUTCH
FETCH
FITCH
HATCH
HITCH
HUTCH
KETCH
KOTCH
LATCH
MATCH
MITCH
NATCH
NOTAH
NOTCH
PATCH
PITCH
SATCH
VETCH
WATCH
WITCH

•••TH

ARITH
AZOTH
BARTH
BERTH
BIRTH
BLUTH
BLYTH
BOOTH
BRITH
BROTH
CLOTH
COUTH
CRWTH
DARTH
DEATH
DEPTH
DOETH
EARTH
EDITH
ELATH
FAITH
FIFTH
FILTH
FIRTH
FORTH
FROTH
GARTH
GIRTH
GOETH
HEATH
KEITH
LEITH
LOATH
LOUTH
MEATH
MIRTH
MONTH
MOUTH
NEATH
NINTH
NORTH
PERTH
PLATH
QUOTH
SAITH
SEETH
SIXTH
SLOTH
SMITH
SMYTH
SNATH
SOOTH
SOUTH
SWATH
SYNTH
TEETH
TENTH
TILTH
TOOTH
TROTH
TRUTH
WIDTH
WIRTH
WORTH
WRATH
WROTH
WYETH
YOUTH

TI•••

TIAGO
TIAMO
TIANT
TIARA
TIBBS
TIBER
TIBET
TIBIA
TICAL
TICKS
TICKY
TICOS
TIDAL
TIDED
TIDES
TIEGS
TIEIN
TIENE
TIEON
TIERS
TIETO
TIEUP
TIFFS
TIGER
TIGHT
TIGON
TIGRE
TIKES
TIKIS
TIKKA
TIKKI
TILAK
TILDA
TILDE
TILED
TILER
TILES
TILEX
TILLS
TILLY
TILTH
TILTS
TIMED
TIMER
TIMES
TIMEX
TIMID
TIMMY
TIMON
TIMOR
TINCT
TINEA
TINED
TINES
TINGE
TINGS
TINNY
TINTS
TIOGA
TIOUS
TIPIN
TIPIS
TIPPI
TIPPY
TIPSY
TIPUP
TIRED
TIRES
TIROL
TIROS
TISCH
TISHA
TISNT
TITAN
TITER
TITHE
TITIS
TITLE
TITOV
TITRE
TITUS
TIVOS
TIWAS
TIXLS
TIZZY

T•I••

TAIGA
TAILS
TAINA
TAINT
TAITO
TBILL
TBIRD
THICK
THIEF
THIEU
THIGH
THILL
THINE
THING
THINK
THINS
THIRD
TOILE
TOILS
TOITY
TRIAD
TRIAL
TRIBE
TRICE
TRICK
TRIED
TRIER
TRIES
TRIKE
TRILL
TRIMS
TRINA
TRINE
TRINI
TRIOS
TRIPE
TRIPP
TRIPS
TRISH
TRITE
TRITT
TTILE
TWICE
TWIGS
TWILL
TWINE
TWINS
TWINY
TWIRL
TWIRP
TWIST
TWITS
TWIXT
TYING
TYIYN

T••I•

TABIS
TACIT
TAKIN
TALIA
TAMIL
TANIA
TANIS
TAPIN
TAPIR
TAPIS
TARIQ
TATIS
TAVIS
TAXIS
TELIC
TEPID
TERIA
THAIS
THEIR
TIBIA
TIEIN
TIKIS
TIMID
TIPIN
TIPIS
TITIS
TOBIT
TOEIN
TONIC
TONIO
TOPIC
TOPIS
TORIC
TORII
TOTIE
TOWIN
TOWIT
TOXIC
TOXIN
TRAIL
TRAIN
TRAIT
TROIS
TRYIT
TULIP
TUMID
TUNIC
TUNIS
TURIN
TVHIT
TWAIN
TYPIC

T•••I

TAKEI
TAMMI
TARSI
TASHI
TAURI
TEMPI
TERRI
TETRI
TIKKI
TIPPI
TOMEI
TONDI
TORII
TORSI
TRACI
TREVI
TRINI
TSADI
TUCCI
TUTSI
TUTTI

•TI••

ATILE
ATILT
ATION
ATIVE
BTILE
CTILE
DTILE
ETILE
FTILE
GTILE
HTILE
ITILE
ITINA
JTILE
KTILE
LTILE
MTIDA
MTIDY
MTILE
NTILE
OTILE
PTILE
QTILE
QTIPS
RTILE
STICH
STICK
STIEB
STIED
STIES
STIFF
STILE
STILL
STILT
STINE
STING
STINK
STINT
STIPE
STIRS
TTILE
UTICA
UTILE
UTILS

VTILE WTILE XTILE YTILE ZTILE

•T•I•
ATEIN ATEIT ATRIA ATRIP ATSIX ATTIC ETAIL ETHIC ETUIS FTDIX OTTIS STAID STAIN STAIR STEIG STEIN STOIC STRIA STRIP

•T••I
ATARI ETMOI OTERI OTOMI OTTOI STASI STOLI STYLI

••TI•
ACTII ACTIN ACTIV ANTIC ANTIQ ANTIS ARTIE ARTIS ASTIN ASTIR ATTIC BATIK BATIN BITIN CUTIE CUTIN CUTIS CUTIT EATIN EATIT FETID FITIN GETIN GETIT GOTIN GOTIT HITIN HITIT ISTIC KATIE LATIN LETIN MATIN METIS MOTIF NITID NOTIE NOTIN NOTIP NOTIT OOTID OPTIC OPTIN ORTIZ OSTIA OTTIS OUTIE PATIO PETIT PUTIN RATIO RETIA RETIE RETIN RETIP RUTIN SATIE SATII SATIN SETIN SITIN TATIS TITIS TOTIE UNTIE UNTIL VATIC YETIS ZITIS

••T•I
ACTII ALTAI BETTI CITRI GOTTI HATHI JETLI KETTI MATRI MITZI NITTI NOTTI OTTOI PATRI PATTI PETRI PETTI PITTI SATII TETRI TUTSI TUTTI VITRI

•••TI
AMATI BETTI CACTI CENTI CESTI COATI CONTI CULTI DENTI DHOTI GOTTI HAITI HEFTI KETTI LACTI LAHTI MARTI MISTI MUFTI MULTI NITTI NOCTI NOTTI NYCTI PARTI PATTI PETTI PITTI PONTI RECTI RIETI SALTI SOLTI TUTTI VASTI VENTI VESTI

•TJ••
STJOE

•T••J
MTVVJ

T•K••
TAKAS TAKEI TAKEN TAKER TAKES TAKIN TEKEL TIKES TIKIS TIKKA TIKKI TOKAY TOKED TOKEN TOKES TOKYO TPKES TSKED TYKES

T••K•
TACKS TACKY TALKS TALKY TANKA TANKS TASKS TEAKS TENKS TICKS TICKY TIKKA TIKKI TONKA TREKS TRIKE TUCKS TURKS TURKU TUSKS

T•••K
THANK THEOK THICK THINK THUNK TILAK TOMSK TRACK TRASK TRICK TRUCK TRUNK TWEAK TYVEK

•T•K•
STAKE STOKE STUKA

•T••K
ITSOK STACK STALK STANK STARK STEAK STICK STINK STOCK STORK STUCK STUNK

••TK•
DITKA LATKA LATKE SITKA

••T•K
AZTEK BATIK LUTSK NOTOK PATEK POTOK

T•L••
TALAS TALCS TALER TALES TALIA TALKS TALKY TALLS TALLY TALON TALUS TELAR TELCO TELES TELEX TELIC TELLS TELLY TELMA TILAK TILDA TILDE TILED TILER TILES TILEX TILLS TILLY TILTH TILTS TOLAR TOLER TOLES TOLET TOLLS TULES TULIP TULLE TULLY TULSA TYLER

T••L•
TABLA TABLE TAELS TAILS TALLS TALLY TBALL TBILL TCELL TEALS TELLS TELLY TENLB TESLA THILL THOLE THULE TILLS TILLY TITLE TIXLS TOILE TOILS TOLLS TOOLE TOOLS TRALA TRILL TROLL TRULY TTILE TULLE TULLY TWILL TWYLA

T•••L
TAMIL TAVEL TAXOL TBALL TBILL TCELL TEKEL THEOL THILL TICAL TIDAL TIROL TOEFL TONAL TOPOL TOTAL TOWEL TRAIL TRAWL TRIAL TRILL TROLL TUBAL TWILL TWIRL TYPAL TYROL

•TL••
ATLAS ATLES FTLBS FTLEE STLEO UTLEY

•T•L•
ATALA ATALL ATILE ATILT ATOLL BTILE CTILE DTILE ETILE FTILE GTILE HTILE ITALO ITALS ITALY ITILE JTILE KTILE LTILE MTELY MTILE NTILE OTILE PTILE QTILE RTILE STALE STALK STALL STELA STELE STILE STILL STILT STOLA STOLE STOLI STOLS STYLE STYLI TTILE UTILE UTILS VTILE VTOLS WTILE XTILE YTILE ZTILE

•T••L
ATALL ATHOL ATOLL ETAIL ETHEL ETHYL LTCOL STAEL STAHL STALL STEAL STEEL STILL STOOL

••TL•
APTLY FATLY FITLY HATLO HOTLY ISTLE JETLI MITLA PATLY ROTLS TITLE WETLY

••T•L
ANTAL ARTEL BETEL BOTEL BUTYL DOTAL ECTAL EXTOL FATAL FETAL HOTEL INTEL LITEL METAL MOTEL NATAL NYTOL OCTAL PETAL RATEL TOTAL UNTIL VITAL

•••TL
YENTL

T•M••
TAMAR TAMED TAMER TAMES TAMIL TAMMI TAMMY TAMPA TAMPS TEMAS TEMPE TEMPI TEMPO TEMPS TEMPT TIMED TIMER TIMES TIMEX TIMID TIMMY TIMON TIMOR TOMAR TOMAS TOMBA TOMBE TOMBS TOMEI TOMES TOMMY TOMSK TUMID TUMMY TVMAN TVMEN

T••M•
TAMMI TAMMY TEAMO TEAMS TEEMS TELMA TERME TERMS THEMA THEME THEMS THUMB THUMP THYME THYMY TIAMO TIMMY TOMMY TORME TRAMP TRAMS TRIMS TROMP TRUMP TRYME TUMMY

T•••M
TATUM TENAM TENPM THERM THRUM TOTEM TWOAM TWOEM TWOPM

•TM••
ATMAN ATMOS ETMOI

•T•M•
ATOMS ATOMY ETYMA ITEMS ITSME OTOMI STAMP STEMS STOMA STOMP STUMP

•T••M
ATEAM BTEAM LTCOM STEAM STORM STRAM STROM STRUM STURM

••TM•
EATME GETME GITMO GOTME HITME LETME NOTME

••T•M
DATUM ENTOM TATUM TOTEM VITAM

TN•••
TNOTE TNUTS

T•N••
TANDY TANEY TANGO TANGS TANGY TANIA TANIS TANKA TANKS TANNA TANSY TANTE TANTO TANYA TENAD TENAM TENBC TENCC TENCH TENDS TENDU TENEE TENET TENGE TENGO TENKS TENLB TENOF TENON TENOR TENPM TENSE TENTH TENTO TENTS TENUP TINCT TINEA TINED TINES TINGE TINGS TINNY TINTS TONAL TONDI TONDO TONED TONER TONES TONGA TONGS TONIC TONIO TONKA TONNE TONOW TONTO TONUS TONYA TONYS TUNAS TUNED TUNER TUNES TUNIC TUNIS TYNAN TYNER

T••N•
TAINA TAINT TANNA TARNS TAUNT TAWNY TBOND TBONE TEENA TEENS TEENY TERNE TERNS THANE THANK THANT THANX THINE THING THINK THINS THONG THUNK TIANT TIENE TINNY TISNT TONNE TOONS TOWNE TOWNS TRANE TRANS TREND TRENT TRINA TRINE TRINI TRUNK TURNS TWANG TWINE TWINS TWINY TYING

T•••N
TAGON TAKEN TAKIN TALON TAPIN TAPON TAUON TAXON TENON TETON TEXAN THEUN THORN TIEIN TIEON TIGON TIMON TIPIN TITAN TOEIN TOKEN TOWIN TOXIN TOYON TRAIN TREEN TROON TRYON TUGON TURIN TVMAN TVMEN TWAIN TWEEN TWOON TYIYN TYNAN TYSON

•TN••
ATNOS ETNAS

•T•N•
ATONE ATONY CTENO ETHNO ETONS ITINA OTONO STAND STANG STANK STANS STENO STENS STENT STINE STING STINK STINT STONE STONY STUNG STUNK STUNS STUNT STYNE VTENS

•T••N
ATEIN ATHON ATION ATMAN ATTEN ETHAN LTGEN OTHON OTOWN STAIN STEEN STEIN STERN UTAHN UTURN

••TN•
AETNA BATNA BUTNO LOTNO PATNA

••T•N
ACTIN ACTON AFTON ALTON ANTON ASTIN ASTON ATTEN AXTON BATIN BATON BETON BITIN BITON COTAN CUTIN EATEN EATIN EATON ELTON ESTAN FITIN FITON FUTON GATUN GETIN GETON GOTIN GOTON GUTEN HITIN HITON HOTON LATEN LATIN LETIN LETON LITON MATIN MUTON NATAN NITON NOTIN NOTON OATEN OCTAN OFTEN OPTIN ORTON OUTON PATEN PATON PITON PUTIN PUTON RATON RETAN RETIN RUTIN SATAN SATIN SATON SETIN SETON SITIN SITON TETON TITAN UPTON USTEN WOTAN

TO•••
TOADS TOADY TOAST TOBEY TOBIT TODAY TODDY TODOS TOEAS TOEFL TOEIN TOFFS TOFTS TOFUS TOGAE TOGAS TOGUE TOGUP TOILE TOILS TOITY TOKAY TOKED TOKEN TOKES TOKYO TOLAR TOLER TOLES TOLET TOLLS TOMAR TOMAS TOMBA TOMBE TOMBS TOMEI TOMES TOMMY TOMSK TONAL TONDI TONDO TONED TONER TONES TONGA TONGS TONIC TONIO TONKA TONNE TONOW TONTO TONUS TONYA TONYS TOODY TOOER TOOLE TOOLS TOONS TOOTH TOOTS TOPAZ TOPED TOPEE TOPER TOPES TOPIC TOPIS TOPOG TOPOL TOPPS TOPSY TOPUP TOQUE TORAH TORAS TORCH TORIC TORII TORME TOROS TORRE TORRS TORSI TORSO TORTA TORTE TORTS TORUS TOSCA TOSEA TOTAL TOTED TOTEM TOTER TOTES TOTIE TOTSY TOTUP TOUCH TOUGH TOURO TOURS TOUTE TOUTS TOVAH TOVES TOWAR TOWED TOWEL TOWER TOWIN TOWIT TOWNE TOWNS TOXIC TOXIN TOYED TOYER TOYON TOYOS TOYOU

T•O••
TBOND TBONE THOLE THONG THORA THORN THORO THOSE THOUS TIOGA TIOUS TNOTE TOODY TOOER TOOLE TOOLS TOONS TOOTH TOOTS TROIS TROLL TROMP TROON TROOP TROPE TROPO TROTH TROTS TROUP TROUT TROVE TROWE TROWS TTOPS TWOAD TWOAM TWOBC TWOEE TWOEM TWOON TWOPM TWOUP

T••O•
TABOO TABOR TACOS TAGON TAHOE TALON TAPON TAROS TAROT TAUON TAXOL TAXON TENOF TENON TENOR TETON THEOC THEOK THEOL THROB THROE THROW TICOS TIEON TIGON TIMON TIMOR TIROL TIROS TITOV TIVOS TODOS TONOW TOPOG TOPOL TOROS TOYON TOYOS TOYOU TRIOS TROON TROOP TRYON TSTOP TUDOR TUGON TUROW TUTOR TWOON TYPOS TYROL TYROS TYSON

T•••O
TABOO TACHO TAEBO TAITO TANGO TANTO TARDO TARSO TASSO TAURO TAUTO TAXCO TEAMO TELCO TEMPO TENGO TENTO THEPO THORO

5 TI

TIAGO
TIAMO
TIETO
TOKYO
TONDO
TONIO
TONTO
TORSO
TOURO
TROPO
TRURO
TRYTO
TSAVO
TURBO
TURCO
TUTTO
TYCHO
TYPEO

•TO••

ATOLL
ATOMS
ATOMY
ATONE
ATONY
ATORY
ETONS
FTORD
OTOES
OTOMI
OTONO
OTOWN
STOAE
STOAS
STOAT
STOCK
STOGY
STOIC
STOKE
STOLA
STOLE
STOLI
STOLS
STOMA
STOMP
STONE
STONY
STOOD
STOOL
STOOP
STOPS
STORE
STORK
STORM
STORY
STOUT
STOVE
STOWE
STOWS
TTOPS
VTOLS

•T•O•

ATEOF
ATHOL
ATHON
ATHOS
ATION
ATMOS
ATNOS
ETHOS
ETMOI
ITSOK
LTCOL
LTCOM
LTGOV
OTHON
OTROS
OTTOI
STJOE
STOOD
STOOL
STOOP
STROH
STROM
STROP
STROS

•T••O

ATTWO
CTENO
ETHNO
ITALO
MTAPO
OTERO
OTONO
PTERO
STENO
STLEO
STYRO

••TO•

ACTON
ACTOR
ACTOS
AFTON
ALTON
ALTOS
AMTOO
ANTON
ARTOO
ASTON
ASTOR
AUTOS
AXTON
BATON
BATOR
BETON
BITON
BOTOX
DATOS
DETOO
DETOX
EATOF
EATON
ECTOR
ELTON
ENTOM
ESTOC
ESTOP
ESTOS
EXTOL
FETOR
FITON
FSTOP
FUTON
GATOR
GATOS
GETON
GOTON
HITON
HOTON
INTOW
ISTOO
JATOS
KOTOS
LETON
LITON
LOTOS
METOO
MOTOR
MUTON
NITON
NOTOK
NOTON
NYTOL
ONTOP
ORTON
OTTOI
OUTOF
OUTON
PATON
PATOS
PETOS
PITON
PITOT
POTOK
PUTON
RATON
RETOP
RETOW
ROTOR
ROTOS
SATON
SETON
SITON
TETON
TITOV
TSTOP
TUTOR
UPTON
UPTOP
ZZTOP

••T•O

ALTHO
AMTOO
ARTOO
ASTRO
ATTWO
BATHO
BUTEO
BUTNO
BYTWO
CITGO
CITRO
DETOO
DITTO
DOTTO
EXTRO
FATSO
GATTO
GETGO
GETTO
GITGO
GITMO
GOTTO
HATLO
HUTTO
IATRO
INTRO
INTWO
ISTOO
JOTTO
KOTTO
LETGO
LITHO
LOTNO
LOTTO
MATEO
MATRO
MATZO
METOO
METRO
MOTTO
NATRO
NITRO
NOTDO
NOTSO
NUTRO
ONTWO
OPTTO
ORTHO
OSTEO
OUTDO
OUTGO
PATCO
PATHO
PATIO
PATRO
PETCO
PETRO
POTTO
PUTTO
RATIO
RATSO
RETRO
SETTO
SOTTO
TUTTO
VITRO
YOTTO

•••TO

AALTO
ACETO
ADDTO
ALITO
AMATO
ANETO
BALTO
BENTO
BLUTO
BOITO
BOWTO
CANTO
CENTO
COPTO
DENTO
DEUTO
DIDTO
DITTO
DOTTO
DUETO
ERATO
FACTO
FEDTO
FEMTO
FLYTO
FRITO
GATTO
GETTO
GOTTO
GUSTO
HADTO
HASTO
HECTO
HEPTO
HEWTO
HIPTO
HISTO
HOPTO
HOWTO
HUTTO
HYETO
JOTTO
JUNTO
KOTTO
KROTO
KYOTO
LACTO
LAYTO
LEDTO
LENTO
LIETO
LOTTO
MOLTO
MOTTO
NEATO
NEWTO
NIETO
NODTO
NYCTO
OPTTO
PANTO
PASTO
PAYTO
PEPTO
PESTO
PHOTO
PHYTO
PICTO
PINTO
PLATO
PLUTO
PORTO
POTTO
PRATO
PROTO
PUTTO
QUITO
RANTO
RECTO
RUNTO
SANTO
SARTO
SAWTO
SEATO
SEETO
SETTO
SOTTO
TAITO
TANTO
TAUTO
TENTO
TIETO
TONTO
TRYTO
TUTTO
USETO
VENTO
WEDTO
XACTO
YOCTO
YOTTO
ZEPTO

TP•••

TPKES

T•P••

TAPAS
TAPED
TAPER
TAPES
TAPIN
TAPIR
TAPIS
TAPON
TEPEE
TEPID
TIPIN
TIPIS
TIPPI
TIPPY
TIPSY
TIPUP
TOPAZ
TOPED
TOPEE
TOPER
TOPES
TOPIC
TOPIS
TOPOG
TOPOL
TOPPS
TOPSY
TOPUP
TUPAC
TYPAL
TYPEA
TYPEB
TYPED
TYPEE
TYPEO
TYPER
TYPES
TYPIC
TYPOS

T••P•

TAMPA
TAMPS
TARPS
TAUPE
TBSPS
TEMPE
TEMPI
TEMPO
TEMPS
TEMPT
TENPM
TERPS
THEPO
TIPPI
TIPPY
TOPPS
TRAPP
TRAPS
TRIPE
TRIPP
TRIPS
TROPE
TROPO
TTOPS
TWOPM

T•••P

TAGUP
TEEUP
TENUP
THARP
THESP
THUMP
TIEUP
TIPUP
TOGUP
TOPUP
TOTUP
TRAMP
TRAPP
TRIPP
TROMP
TROOP
TROUP
TRUMP
TSTOP
TULIP
TWERP
TWIRP
TWOUP

•TP••

ATPAR
STPAT

•T•P•

ETAPE
MTAPO
QTIPS
STAPH
STEPS
STIPE
STOPS
STUPA
STUPE
TTOPS
VTYPE
XTYPE

•T••P

ATEUP
ATRIP
PTRAP
STAMP
STEEP
STOMP
STOOP
STRAP
STREP
STRIP
STROP
STUMP

••T•P

ACTUP
BITUP
CUTUP
EATUP
ESTOP
FITUP
FSTOP
GETUP
GOTUP
HETUP
HITUP
LETUP
LITUP
METUP
NOTIP
NOTUP
ONTAP
ONTOP
PUTUP
RETAP
RETIP
RETOP
SATUP
SETUP
SITUP
TOTUP
TSTOP
UPTOP
ZZTOP

T•Q••

TOQUE
TUQUE

T•••Q

TARIQ

•TQ••

ATQUE

•T••Q

ETSEQ

••T•Q

ANTIQ

TR•••

TRACE
TRACI
TRACK
TRACT
TRACY
TRADE
TRAGG
TRAIL
TRAIN
TRAIT
TRALA
TRAMP
TRAMS
TRANE
TRANS
TRAPP
TRAPS
TRASH
TRASK
TRAVE
TRAWL
TRAYS
TREAD
TREAS
TREAT
TRECE
TREED
TREEN
TREES
TREKS
TREND
TRENT
TRESS
TRETS
TREVI
TREWS
TREYS
TRIAD
TRIAL
TRIBE
TRICE
TRICK
TRIED
TRIER
TRIES
TRIKE
TRILL
TRIMS
TRINA
TRINE
TRINI
TRIOS
TRIPE
TRIPP
TRIPS
TRISH
TRITE
TRITT
TROIS
TROLL
TROMP
TROON
TROOP
TROPE
TROPO
TROTH
TROTS
TROUP
TROUT
TROVE
TROWE
TROWS
TRUCE
TRUCK
TRUDY
TRUED
TRUER
TRUES
TRULY
TRUMP
TRUNK
TRURO
TRUSS
TRUST
TRUTH
TRYIT
TRYME
TRYON
TRYST
TRYTO

T•R••

TARAS
TARDE
TARDO
TARDY
TARED
TARES
TARGA
TARIQ
TARNS
TAROS
TAROT
TARPS
TARRY
TARSI
TARSO
TARTE
TARTS
TARTU
TARTY
TERAT
TERCE
TERIA
TERME
TERMS
TERNE
TERNS
TERPS
TERRA
TERRE
TERRI
TERRS
TERRY
TERSE
TERZA
THREE
THREW
THROB
THROE
THROW
THRUM
TIRED
TIRES
TIROL
TIROS
TORAH
TORAS
TORCH
TORIC
TORII
TORME
TOROS
TORRE
TORRS
TORSI
TORSO
TORTA
TORTE
TORTS
TORUS
TURBO
TURCO
TURFS
TURFY
TURIN
TURKS
TURKU
TURNS
TUROW
TURVY
TYRES
TYROL
TYROS
TYRUS

T••R•

TARRY
TATRA
TAURI
TAURO
TBARS
TBIRD
TEARS
TEARY
TEERS
TERRA
TERRE
TERRI
TERRS
TERRY
TETRA
TETRI
THARP
THERA
THERE
THERM
THIRD
THORA
THORN
THORO
THURS
TIARA
TIERS
TIGRE
TITRE
TORRE
TORRS
TOURO
TOURS
TRURO
TSARS
TWERE
TWERP
TWIRL
TWIRP
TZARA
TZARS

T•••R

TABOR
TAKER
TALER
TAMAR
TAMER
TAPER
TAPIR
TASER
TATAR
TATER
TAXER
TELAR
TENOR
THEIR
TIBER
TIGER
TILER
TIMER
TIMOR
TITER
TOLAR
TOLER
TOMAR
TONER
TOOER
TOPER
TOTER
TOWAR
TOWER
TOYER
TRIER
TRUER
TUBER
TUDOR
TUNER
TUTOR
TVVCR
TYGER
TYLER
TYNER
TYPER

•TR••

ATRAS
ATRIA
ATRIP
ETRES
OTRAS
OTROS
PTRAP
RTREV
STRAD
STRAM
STRAP
STRAT
STRAW
STRAY
STREP
STREW
STRIA
STRIP
STROH
STROM
STROP
STROS
STRUG
STRUM
STRUT

•T•R•

ATARI
ATARS
ATORY
FTORD
ITERS
OTARU
OTARY
OTERI
OTERO
PTERO
STARE
STARK
STARR
STARS
START
STARZ
STERE
STERN
STIRS
STORE
STORK
STORM
STORY
STURM
STYRO
UTURN

•T••R

ATBAR
ATPAR
ATTAR
ATWAR
ETHER
OTHER
OTTER
STAHR
STAIR
STARR
STEER
UTHER
UTTAR
UTTER

••TR•

AFTRA
ANTRA
ANTRE
ASTRA
ASTRE
ASTRO
AUTRE
AUTRY
CITRI
CITRO
DETRE
ENTRE
ENTRY
EXTRA
EXTRO
IATRO
IATRY
INTRA
INTRO
LITRE
MATRI
MATRO
METRE
METRO
METRY
MITRE
NATRO
NITRE
NITRO
NOTRE
NUTRO
OUTRE
PATRI
PATRO
PETRA
PETRE
PETRI
PETRO
RETRO
RETRY
SUTRA
TATRA
TETRA
TETRI
TITRE
ULTRA
VITRI
VITRO
VOTRE

••T•R

ACTER
ACTOR
AFTER
ALTAR
ALTER
APTER
ARTUR
ASTER
ASTIR
ASTOR
ATTAR
BATOR
BITER
BSTAR
CATER
CITER
CSTAR
CUTER
DATER
DETAR
DETER
DOTER
EATER
ECTOR
ENTER
ESTAR
ESTER
FETOR
FSTAR
GATER
GATOR
GSTAR
HATER
HETER
INTER
JETER
KITER
KSTAR
LATER
LITER
MATER
METER
MITER
MOTOR
MSTAR
MUTER
NITER
NOTER
NSTAR
OATER
OSTAR
OSTER
OTTER
OUTER
PATER
PETER
QATAR
RATER
RETAR
ROTOR
SATYR
SITAR
SSTAR
TATAR
TATER
TITER
TOTER
TUTOR
UNTER
UTTAR
UTTER
VATER
VOTER
WATER

•••TR

AUSTR
CENTR
CONTR
DEXTR
GASTR
INSTR

TS•••

TSADE
TSADI
TSARS
TSAVO
TSGTS
TSKED
TSTOP

T•S••

TASER
TASHI
TASKS
TASSE
TASSO
TASTE
TASTY
TBSPS
TESLA
TESSA
TESTA
TESTS
TESTY
TISCH
TISHA
TISNT
TOSCA
TOSEA
TUSHY
TUSKS
TVSET
TYSON

T••S•

TANSY
TARSI
TARSO
TASSE
TASSO
TEASE
TENSE
TERSE
TESSA
THESE
THESP
THOSE
TIPSY
TOAST
TOMSK
TOPSY
TORSI
TORSO
TOTSY
TRASH
TRASK
TRESS
TRISH
TRUSS
TRUST
TRYST
TULSA
TUTSI
TWIST

T•••S

TABIS
TABUS
TACHS
TACKS
TACOS
TADAS
TAELS
TAFTS
TAGUS
TAILS
TAKAS
TAKES
TALAS
TALCS
TALES
TALKS
TALLS
TALUS
TAMES
TAMPS
TANGS
TANIS
TANKS
TAPAS
TAPES
TAPIS
TARAS
TARES
TARNS
TAROS
TARPS
TARTS
TASKS
TATAS
TATES
TATIS
TAVIS
TAXES
TAXIS
TBARS
TBSPS
TEAKS
TEALS
TEAMS
TEARS
TEATS
TECHS
TEEMS
TEENS
TEERS
TELES
TELLS
TEMAS
TEMPS
TENDS
TENKS
TENTS
TERMS
TERNS
TERPS
TERRS
TESTS
TETES
TETHS
TEWAS
TEWES
TEXAS
TEXTS
THAIS
THATS
THAWS
THEAS
THEMS
THEWS
THINS
THOUS
THUDS
THUGS
THURS
TIBBS
TICKS
TICOS
TIDES
TIEGS
TIERS
TIFFS
TIKES
TIKIS
TILES
TILLS
TILTS
TIMES
TINES
TINGS
TINTS
TIOUS
TIPIS
TIRES
TIROS
TITIS

TITUS TIVOS TIWAS TIXLS TNUTS TOADS TODOS TOEAS TOFFS TOFTS TOFUS TOGAS TOILS TOKES TOLES TOLLS TOMAS TOMBS TOMES TONES TONGS TONUS TONYS TOOLS TOONS TOOTS TOPES TOPIS TOPPS TORAS TOROS TORRS TORTS TORUS TOTES TOURS TOUTS TOVES TOWNS TOYOS TPKES TRAMS TRANS TRAPS TRAYS TREAS TREES TREKS TRESS TRETS TREWS TREYS TRIES TRIMS TRIOS TRIPS TROIS TROTS TROWS TRUES TRUSS TSARS TSGTS TTOPS TUBAS TUBBS TUBES TUCKS

TUFTS TULES TUNAS TUNES TUNIS TURFS TURKS TURNS TUSKS TUTUS TUXES TVADS TWIGS TWINS TWITS TYEES TYKES TYPES TYPOS TYRES TYROS TYRUS TZARS

•TS••

ATSEA ATSIX ETSEQ ITSME ITSOK

•T•S•

ATEST HTEST NTEST STASH STASI

•T••S

ATARS ATHOS ATLAS ATLES ATMOS ATNOS ATOMS ATRAS ATTYS ETATS ETHOS ETNAS ETONS ETRES ETTES ETUIS FTLBS ITALS ITEAS ITEMS ITERS MTGES OTOES OTRAS OTROS OTTIS QTIPS STABS STADS

STAGS STANS STARS STATS STAYS STEMS STENS STEPS STETS STEWS STIES STIRS STOAS STOLS STOPS STOWS STROS STUBS STUDS STUNS STYES TTOPS UTILS VTENS VTOLS

••TS•

ANTSY ARTSY BETSY BITSY DITSY FATSO GUTSY HOTSY LOTSA LUTSK MATSU NOTSO NUTSY PATSY POTSY RATSO TOTSY TUTSI

••T•S

ACTAS ACTES ACTOS ALTOS ALTUS ANTAS ANTES ANTIS ARTIS ATTYS AUTOS BATES BATHS BATTS BETAS BETES BETHS BITES BITTS BOTTS BUTTS

BYTES CATES CATHS CETUS CITES COTES CUTES CUTIS DATES DATOS DOTES ERTES ESTAS ESTES ESTHS ESTOS ETTES FATES FETAS FETES FETUS GATES GATOS GETAS GOTHS HATES HDTVS HETHS HUTUS ICTUS IOTAS JATOS JETES JOTAS JUTES KATAS KITES KITTS KOTOS LATHS LETTS LITES LOTOS LOTUS LUTES MATES MATHS METES METIS MITAS MITES MITTS MOTES MOTHS MOTTS MUTES MUTTS MYTHS NITES NOTES NOTUS OATES OATHS OTTIS PATES PATHS PATOS PETES

PETOS PITAS PITHS PITTS PITYS POTTS POTUS PUTTS RATES RATHS RITES ROTAS ROTCS ROTES ROTHS ROTLS ROTOS RUTHS SATES SETTS SITES SRTAS TATAS TATES TATIS TETES TETHS TITIS TITUS TOTES TUTUS VATUS VITAS VITUS VOTES WATTS YATES YETIS ZETAS ZITIS

•••TS

ABETS ABUTS ACCTS ADITS ADJTS AOUTS APPTS ASSTS AUNTS BAHTS BAITS BALTS BASTS BATTS BEATS BEETS BELTS BENTS BESTS BHATS BITTS BLATS BLOTS BOATS BOLTS BOOTS

BOTTS BOUTS BRATS BRITS BRUTS BUNTS BUSTS BUTTS CANTS CAPTS CARTS CASTS CELTS CENTS CERTS CHATS CHITS CISTS CLOTS COATS COLTS CONTS COOTS COPTS COSTS CRITS CULTS CYSTS DARTS DEBTS DELTS DENTS DEPTS DICTS DIETS DINTS DIRTS DISTS DNETS DOATS DOITS DOLTS DONTS DRATS DUCTS DUETS DUSTS EASTS EDITS EMITS ETATS EXITS FACTS FASTS FEATS FEETS FELTS FESTS FIATS FISTS FLATS FLITS FONTS FOOTS FORTS FOUTS FRATS FRETS

FRITS GAITS GELTS GENTS GESTS GHATS GIFTS GILTS GIRTS GISTS GLUTS GMATS GNATS GOATS GOUTS GOVTS GRITS GROTS GUSTS HAFTS HALTS HANTS HEATS HEFTS HERTS HESTS HILTS HINTS HOOTS HOSTS HUITS HUNTS HURTS INITS INSTS JESTS JILTS JOLTS KARTS KEATS KILTS KITTS KNITS KNOTS KYATS LAITS LASTS LECTS LEFTS LENTS LETTS LIFTS LILTS LINTS LISTS LOFTS LOOTS LOUTS LSATS LUNTS LUSTS MALTS MARTS MASTS MCATS MEATS MEETS MELTS

MINTS MISTS MITTS MOATS MOLTS MONTS MOOTS MOTTS MSGTS MUSTS MUTTS NEATS NERTS NESTS NEWTS NUITS NYETS OASTS OBITS ODETS OMITS OUSTS PACTS PANTS PARTS PASTS PEATS PELTS PESTS PHOTS PICTS PINTS PITTS PLATS PLOTS POETS PONTS PORTS POSTS POTTS POUTS PROTS PSATS PSSTS PUNTS PUTTS QUITS RAFTS RANTS RECTS REGTS REITS RENTS RESTS RIFTS RIOTS ROOTS ROUTS RUNTS RUSTS SALTS SCATS SCOTS SCUTS SEATS SECTS SEPTS SERTS

SETTS SHOTS SHUTS SIFTS SILTS SKITS SLATS SLITS SLOTS SMITS SMUTS SNITS SOOTS SORTS SPATS SPETS SPITS SPOTS SSGTS STATS STETS SUETS SUITS SUPTS SWATS SYSTS TAFTS TARTS TEATS TENTS TESTS TEXTS THATS TILTS TINTS TNUTS TOFTS TOOTS TORTS TOUTS TRETS TROTS TSGTS TUFTS TWITS UNITS VASTS VENTS VERTS VESTS VOLTS WAFTS WAITS WANTS WARTS WATTS WEFTS WELTS WESTS WHATS WHETS WHITS WILTS WONTS WORTS WRITS XOUTS XYSTS

YEATS YURTS ZESTS

TT•••

TTILE TTOPS

T•T••

TATAR TATAS TATER TATES TATIS TATRA TATTY TATUM TETES TETHS TETON TETRA TETRI TITAN TITER TITHE TITIS TITLE TITOV TITRE TITUS TOTAL TOTED TOTEM TOTER TOTES TOTIE TOTSY TOTUP TSTOP TUTEE TUTOR TUTSI TUTTE TUTTI TUTTO TUTUS

T••T•

TAFTS TAITO TANTE TANTO TARTE TARTS TARTU TARTY TASTE TASTY TATTY TAUTO TEATS TEETH TENTH TENTO TENTS TESTA TESTS TESTY

TEXTS THATS THETA TIETO TILTH TILTS TINTS TNOTE TNUTS TOFTS TOITY TONTO TOOTH TOOTS TORTA TORTE TORTS TOUTE TOUTS TRETS TRITE TRITT TROTH TROTS TRUTH TRYTO TSGTS TUFTS TUFTY TUTTE TUTTI TUTTO TWITS

T•••T

TACET TACIT TAINT TAROT TAUNT TEBET TEMPT TENET TERAT TEVET THANT THEFT TIANT TIBET TIGHT TINCT TISNT TOAST TOBIT TOLET TOWIT TRACT TRAIT TREAT TRENT TRITT TROUT TRUST TRYIT TRYST TUGAT TVHIT TVSET

TWEET TWIST TWIXT

•TT••

ATTAR ATTEN ATTIC ATTWO ATTYS ETTES OTTER OTTIS OTTOI UTTAR UTTER

•T•T•

ETATS MTWTF STATE STATS STETS STUTZ

•T••T

ATBAT ATEAT ATEIT ATEST ATILT HTEST NTEST STADT START STENT STILT STINT STOAT STOUT STPAT STRAT STRUT STUNT

••TT•

BATTS BATTY BETTA BETTE BETTI BETTY BITTE BITTS BITTY BOTTS BUTTE BUTTS CATTY CETTE COTTA CUTTY DETTE DITTO DITTY DOTTO DOTTY FATTY

GATTO GETTO GETTY GOTTA GOTTI GOTTO GUTTY HETTY HUTTO JETTA JETTY JOTTO KETTI KETTY KITTS KITTY KOTTO LATTE LETTS LETTY LITTB LITTD LOTTA LOTTE LOTTO MATTE MATTY MITTS MITTY MOTTO MOTTS MUTTS NATTA NATTY NETTY NITTI NITTY NOTTE NOTTI NUTTY OPTTO OUTTA PATTI PATTY PETTI PETTY PITTI PITTS POTTO POTTS POTTY PUTTO PUTTS PUTTY RATTY RETTY RUTTY SETTE SETTO SETTS SOTTO TATTY TUTTE TUTTI TUTTO VETTE WATTS WITTE

WITTY YETTA YOTTO ZETTA

••T•T

BUTUT CUTIT DETAT DITAT EATAT EATIT GETAT GETIT GOTAT GOTIT HITAT HITIT LETAT LOTET MOTET NETWT NOTIT OCTET PETIT PITOT SATAT SETAT SITAT

•••TT

BLITT BRATT BRETT BRITT BYATT FLATT GLATT GLOTT HYATT KNOTT OVETT PLATT PRATT RAITT RHETT SCOTT SHATT TRITT WYATT

TU•••

TUBAL TUBAS TUBBS TUBBY TUBED TUBER TUBES TUCCI TUCKS TUDOR TUFTS TUFTY TUGAT TUGON TULES TULIP

TULLE TULLY TULSA TUMID TUMMY TUNAS TUNED TUNER TUNES TUNIC TUNIS TUPAC TUQUE TURBO TURCO TURFS TURFY TURIN TURKS TURKU TURNS TUROW TURVY TUSHY TUSKS TUTEE TUTOR TUTSI TUTTE TUTTI TUTTO TUTUS TUVWX TUXES

T•U••

TAUNT TAUON TAUPE TAURI TAURO TAUTO THUDS THUGS THULE THUMB THUMP THUNK THURS TNUTS TOUCH TOUGH TOURO TOURS TOUTE TOUTS TRUCE TRUCK TRUDY TRUED TRUER TRUES TRULY TRUMP TRUNK TRURO TRUSS TRUST

TRUTH

T••U•

TABUS TAGUP TAGUS TALUS TATUM TEEUP TENUP THEUN THOUS THRUM TIEUP TIOUS TIPUP TITUS TOFUS TOGUE TOGUP TONUS TOPUP TOQUE TORUS TOTUP TROUP TROUT TUQUE TUTUS TWOUP TYRUS

T•••U

TAEGU TARTU TENDU THIEU TOYOU TURKU

•TU••

ETUDE ETUIS STUBS STUCK STUDS STUDY STUFF STUKA STUMP STUNG STUNK STUNS STUNT STUPA STUPE STURM STUTZ STUVW UTUBE UTURN

•T•U•

ATEUP ATQUE STAUB STOUT STRUG

STRUM STRUT

•T••U

OTARU

••TU•

ACTUP ALTUS ARTUR BITUP BUTUT CETUS CUTUP DATUM EATUP FETUS FITUP GATUN GETUP GOTUP HETUP HITUP HUTUS ICTUS LETUP LITUP LOTUS METUP NOTUP NOTUS POTUS PUTUP RSTUV SATUP SETUP SITUP TATUM TITUS TOTUP TUTUS VATUS VITUS

••T•U

MATSU

•••TU

BANTU CENTU DICTU ERITU QRSTU TARTU VIRTU

TV•••

TVADS TVDVD TVHIT TVMAN TVMEN TVSET TVVCR

T•V••

TAVEL TAVIS

TEVET
TEVYE
TIVOS
TOVAH
TOVES
TUVWX
TVVCR
TYVEK

T••V•
TRAVE
TREVI
TROVE
TSAVO
TURVY
TVDVD

T•••V
TITOV

•TV••
MTVVJ

•T•V•
ATIVE
MTVVJ
STAVE
STEVE
STOVE
STUVW

•T••V
LTGOV
RTREV

••TV•
HDTVS

••T•V
ACTIV
RSTUV
TITOV

•••TV
ABCTV
CBSTV
FOXTV
MADTV
NBCTV
PARTV
PAYTV
WEBTV

TW•••
TWAIN
TWANG
TWEAK
TWEED
TWEEN
TWEET
TWERE
TWERP
TWICE
TWIGS
TWILL
TWINE
TWINS
TWINY

TWIRL
TWIRP
TWIST
TWITS
TWIXT
TWOAD
TWOAM
TWOBC
TWOEE
TWOEM
TWOON
TWOPM
TWOUP
TWYLA

T•W••
TAWNY
TEWAS
TEWES
TIWAS
TOWAR
TOWED
TOWEL
TOWER
TOWIN
TOWIT
TOWNE
TOWNS

T••W•
THAWS
THEWB
THEWS
THEWY
TRAWL
TREWS
TROWE
TROWS
TUVWX

T•••W
THREW
THROW
TONOW
TUROW

•TW••
ATWAR
MTWTF
OTWAY

•T•W•
ATTWO
OTOWN
STEWS
STEWY
STOWE
STOWS

•T••W
STRAW
STREW
STUVW

••TW•
ATTWO
BYTWO
FATWA

INTWO
NETWT
ONTWO

••T•W
INTOW
RETOW

T•X••
TAXCO
TAXED
TAXER
TAXES
TAXIS
TAXOL
TAXON
TEXAN
TEXAS
TEXTS
TIXLS
TOXIC
TOXIN
TUXES

T••X•
TWIXT

T•••X
TELEX
THANX
THEAX
TILEX
TIMEX
TUVWX

•T••X
ATSIX
FTDIX

••T•X
BOTOX
CUTEX
DETOX
LATEX
NOTAX
RETAX
UNTAX

TY•••
TYCHE
TYCHO
TYEES
TYGER
TYING
TYIYN
TYKES
TYLER
TYNAN
TYNER
TYPAL
TYPEA
TYPEB
TYPED
TYPEE
TYPEO
TYPER
TYPES
TYPIC

TYPOS
TYRES
TYROL
TYROS
TYRUS
TYSON
TYVEK

T•Y••
THYME
THYMY
TOYED
TOYER
TOYON
TOYOS
TOYOU
TRYIT
TRYME
TRYON
TRYST
TRYTO
TWYLA

T••Y•
TANYA
TEVYE
THEYD
TOKYO
TONYA
TONYS
TRAYS
TREYS
TYIYN

T•••Y
TABBY
TACKY
TAFFY
TALKY
TALLY
TAMMY
TANDY
TANEY
TANGY
TANSY
TARDY
TARRY
TARTY
TASTY
TATTY
TAWNY
TEARY
TEDDY
TEENY
TELLY
TERRY
TESTY
THEWY
THYMY
TICKY
TILLY
TIMMY
TINNY
TIPPY
TIPSY
TIZZY
TOADY
TOBEY

TODAY
TODDY
TOITY
TOKAY
TOMMY
TOODY
TOPSY
TOTSY
TRACY
TRUDY
TRULY
TUBBY
TUFTY
TULLY
TUMMY
TURFY
TURVY
TUSHY
TWINY

•TY••
ETYMA
STYES
STYLE
STYLI
STYNE
STYRO
VTYPE
XTYPE

•T•Y•
ATTYS
ETHYL
STAYS

•T••Y
ATBAY
ATOMY
ATONY
ATORY
ITALY
ITCHY
MTELY
MTIDY
OTARY
OTWAY
STACY
STAGY
STEWY
STOGY
STONY
STORY
STRAY
STUDY
UTLEY

••TY•
ATTYS
BUTYL
MITYA
PITYS
SATYR

••T•Y
ANTSY
APTLY
ARTSY
AUTRY

BATHY
BATTY
BETSY
BETTY
BITSY
BITTY
CATHY
CATTY
CUTEY
CUTTY
DITSY
DITTY
DITZY
DOTTY
ENTRY
FATLY
FATTY
FITLY
GETBY
GETTY
GOTBY
GUTSY
GUTTY
HETTY
HOTLY
HOTSY
IATRY
JETTY
KATEY
KATHY
KETTY
KITTY
LATHY
LETBY
LETTY
MATEY
MATTY
METRY
MITTY
MOTHY
NATTY
NETTY
NITTY
NUTSY
NUTTY
PATHY
PATLY
PATSY
PATTY
PETEY
PETTY
PITHY
POTSY
POTTY
PUTBY
PUTTY
RATTY
RETRY
RETTY
RITZY
RUTTY
SATAY
SATBY
SETBY
SITBY
TATTY
TOTSY
WETLY

WITTY

•••TY
ALITY
AMITY
AUNTY
BARTY
BATTY
BEATY
BEETY
BETTY
BITTY
BOOTY
CANTY
CATTY
COOTY
CUTTY
DEITY
DINTY
DIRTY
DITTY
DOTTY
DUSTY
EMPTY
FATTY
FIFTY
FLUTY
FORTY
FUSTY
GETTY
GOUTY
GUSTY
GUTTY
HASTY
HEFTY
HETTY
HOITY
JETTY
JOLTY
JUSTY
KETTY
KITTY
LAITY
LEFTY
LETTY
LINTY
LOFTY
LUSTY
MALTY
MARTY
MATTY
MEATY
MINTY
MISTY
MITTY
MONTY
MORTY
MUSTY
NASTY
NATTY
NESTY
NETTY
NIFTY
NITTY
NUTTY
PANTY
PARTY
PASTY

PATTY
PEATY
PETTY
PIETY
PLATY
POTTY
POUTY
PURTY
PUTTY
RATTY
RETTY
RINTY
ROOTY
RUNTY
RUSTY
RUTTY
SALTY
SILTY
SIXTY
SLATY
SOFTY
SOOTY
SUETY
TARTY
TASTY
TATTY
TESTY
TOITY
TUFTY
UNITY
VASTY
WARTY
WELTY
WITTY
YORTY
ZESTY
ZLOTY

TZ•••
TZARA
TZARS

T•Z••
TIZZY

T••Z•
TERZA
TIZZY

T•••Z
TOPAZ

•T••Z
STARZ
STUTZ

••TZ•
DITZY
KATZE
MATZO
MITZI
RITZY

••T•Z
ORTIZ

•••TZ
BLATZ

BLITZ
BRITZ
DIETZ
ERETZ
FRITZ
GERTZ
GLITZ
HERTZ
HOLTZ
HUNTZ
KLUTZ
KURTZ
LANTZ
MERTZ
NANTZ
NERTZ
OVITZ
PLOTZ
SPITZ
STUTZ
WAITZ
WALTZ
WEITZ

U•A••
UDALL
UHAUL
UKASE
UMASS
UNAMI
UNAPT
UNARM
UNARY
UNAUS
URALS
URANO
URAWA
USAFA
USAGE
USAID
USAIR
UTAHN

U••A•
UBOAT
UCLAN
UHLAN
UHNAK
UKIAH
ULNAE
ULNAR
ULNAS
UMIAK
UNBAG
UNBAR
UNCAP
UNCAS
UNDAM
UNDAY
UNFAR
UNGAG
UNGAR
UNHAT
UNIAT
UNJAM
UNLAX
UNLAY
UNMAD

UNMAN
UNSAD
UNSAY
UNTAX
URBAN
UREAS
URIAH
URSAE
USEAS
USUAL
UTTAR
UVEAL
UVEAS
UVRAY
UXMAL

U•••A
UHURA
UINTA
ULTRA
UMBRA
UNITA
URAWA
USAFA
USCGA
USLTA
USOFA
USRDA
UTICA
UVULA

•UA••
DUADS
DUALS
DUANE
FUADI
GUANO
GUAPA
GUAPO
GUARD
GUARE
GUARS
GUAVA
HUANG
JUANO
KUALA
LUANA
LUANG
LUANN
LUAUS
QUACK
QUADR
QUADS
QUAFF
QUAGS
QUAID
QUAIL
QUAIS
QUAKE
QUAKY
QUALM
QUAND
QUANG
QUANT
QUARE
QUARK
QUART
QUASH

QUASI
QUAXO
QUAYS
RUARK
SUAVE
YUANS

•U•A•
AURAE
AURAL
AURAR
AURAS
BUYAT
CUBAN
CUGAT
CURAD
DUBAI
DUCAL
DUCAT
DUFAY
DUGAN
DUGAT
DUKAS
DUMAS
DURAN
DURAS
DUVAL
FUGAL
GULAG
HULAS
HUMAN
HUNAN
HUSAK
JUBAL
JUDAH
JUDAS
JUGAL
JURAL
JURAN
KULAK
LUCAN
LUCAS
LUGAR
LUJAN
LUKAS
LUMAN
LUMAS
LUNAR
LUNAS
LURAY
MULAN
MURAL
MURAT
MUZAK
NUMAN
OURAY
PUKAS
PULAS
PUMAS
PUPAE
PUPAL
PUPAS
PUSAN
QURAN
RUMAN
RUNAT
RURAL
SUDAN

SUGAR
SUMAC
SURAH
SURAS
SUSAN
TUBAL
TUBAS
TUGAT
TUNAS
TUPAC
WUHAN
YUBAN
YUMAN
YUMAS

•U••A
AUDRA
BUBBA
BUBKA
BUENA
BUFFA
BULBA
BULLA
BUONA
BURKA
BURMA
BURSA
BUSTA
CUICA
CULPA
CUPPA
CURIA
CURSA
DUBYA
DUENA
DURRA
FULDA
GUAPA
GUAVA
GUNGA
JUDEA
JULIA
JUMNA
JUNTA
KUALA
KUBLA
KUKLA
KUNTA
LUANA
LUCCA
LUCIA
LUISA
LULEA
LURIA
MUCHA
MULLA
MUNNA
MUSCA
NUBIA
NUCHA
NUEVA
NULLA
NUNCA
NUOVA
OUIDA
OUIJA
OUTTA
PUKKA

PUNKA
PUNTA
QUOTA
RUMBA
RUSKA
RUSSA
SULFA
SULLA
SUMMA
SUNDA
SUNNA
SUPRA
SUTRA
TULSA
WUXIA
YUCCA
YULKA
ZUPPA

••UA•
AGUAS
AQUAE
AQUAS
DOUAI
DOUAY
EQUAL
IGUAL
KAUAI
SKUAS
SQUAB
SQUAD
SQUAT
SQUAW
USUAL

••U•A
ABUJA
ACURA
AGURA
ALULA
ARUBA
AZUSA
CEUTA
CHULA
CRURA
DJUNA
DOULA
ELURA
EXUMA
FAUNA
FOURA
GOUDA
HOUMA
KRUPA
LAUDA
LAURA
LOUMA
MAUNA
MAURA
PAULA
SAUNA
SCUBA
SCUSA
SHULA
SOUSA
STUKA
STUPA
UHURA

UVULA

•••UA
ACQUA
LEHUA
MAGUA
PADUA
PAPUA
VACUA
VANUA

UB•••
UBOAT
UBOLT

U•B••
UMBEL
UMBER
UMBLE
UMBRA
UNBAG
UNBAR
UNBET
UNBID
UNBIT
UNBOX
UNBUD
UPBOW
URBAN
UZBEK

U••B•
USEBY
UTUBE

•UB••
AUBER
BUBBA
BUBER
BUBKA
CUBAN
CUBBY
CUBEB
CUBED
CUBER
CUBES
CUBIC
CUBIT
DUBAI
DUBHE
DUBIN
DUBYA
EUBIE
FUBSY
HUBBY
HUBEL
HUBER
HUBIE
JUBAL
KUBEK
KUBLA
LUBED
LUBES
LUBIN
NUBBY
NUBIA
RUBEL
RUBEN

RUBES
RUBIK
RUBIN
RUBLE
RUBON
RUBUP
SUBIC
TUBAL
TUBAS
TUBBS
TUBBY
TUBED
TUBER
TUBES
YUBAN
ZUBIN

•U•B•
BUBBA
BULBA
BULBS
BURBS
BUSBY
CUBBY
CURBS
DUMBO
DUMBS
FURBY
GUMBO
GUMBY
HUBBY
JUMBO
MUMBO
NUBBY
NUMBS
PUTBY
RUGBY
RUMBA
RUNBY
TUBBS
TUBBY
TURBO

•U••B
CUBEB

••UB•
ARUBA
CHUBB
CHUBS
CLUBS
DAUBE
DAUBS
DOUBS
DOUBT
DRUBS
FLUBS
GRUBS
SCUBA
SNUBS
STUBS
UTUBE

••U•B
BLURB
CHUBB
CRUMB
EXURB

FOURB
PLUMB
RHUMB
SQUAB
SQUIB
THUMB

•••UB
EXCUB
MRCUB
REDUB
REPUB
SCRUB
SHRUB
STAUB
ZHLUB

UC•••
UCLAN
UCONN

U•C••
ULCER
UNCAP
UNCAS
UNCLE
UNCOY
UNCUT
USCGA

U••C•
UNICE
URICH
UTICA

U•••C
UGRIC
ULRIC
UNDEC

•UC••
BUCCO
BUCKO
BUCKS
BUCKY
DUCAL
DUCAT
DUCES
DUCHY
DUCKS
DUCKY
DUCTS
FUCHS
GUCCI
GUCKS
GUCKY
JUCOS
LUCAN
LUCAS
LUCCA
LUCCI
LUCIA
LUCID
LUCIE
LUCIO
LUCKS
LUCKY
LUCRE

MUCHA
MUCHO
MUCKS
MUCKY
NUCHA
PUCCI
PUCES
PUCKS
RUCHE
RUCKS
SUCKS
SUCKY
SUCRE
TUCCI
TUCKS
YUCCA
YUCKY
ZUCCO

•U•C•
BUCCO
BUICK
BUNCH
BUNCO
BUSCH
BUTCH
CUICA
CULCH
CUZCO
DULCE
DUNCE
DUTCH
FUOCO
GUCCI
GULCH
HULCE
HUNCH
HUTCH
JUICE
JUICY
JUNCO
KUSCH
LUCCA
LUCCI
LUNCH
LURCH
MULCH
MULCT
MUNCH
MUSCA
NUNCA
OUNCE
PUCCI
PUNCH
QUACK
QUICK
TUCCI
TURCO
YUCCA
ZUCCO

•U••C
AURIC
CUBIC
CUSEC
DUROC
LUDIC
MUSIC

NUMIC
PUNIC
RUNIC
SUBIC
SUMAC
TUNIC
TUPAC

••UC•
AMUCK
BRUCE
BRUCH
CHUCK
CLUCK
COUCH
DEUCE
DEUCY
DOUCE
EDUCE
EDUCT
ERUCT
FRUCT
GLUCK
GLUCO
MOUCH
PLUCK
POUCH
SAUCE
SAUCY
SHUCK
SNUCK
SOUCI
STUCK
TOUCH
TRUCE
TRUCK
VOUCH

••U•C
FOURC

UD•••
UDALL
UDDER
UDINE

U•D••
UDDER
UNDAM
UNDAY
UNDEC
UNDER
UNDID
UNDIM
UNDRY
UNDUE
UNDUG
UPDOS
UPDRY

U••D•
USRDA

U•••D
UMPED
UNBID
UNBUD
UNDID
UNFED
UNHID
UNLED
UNMAD
UNSAD
UNWED
UPEND
UPPED
URGED
URSID
USAID
USHED
USTED

•UD••
AUDEN
AUDIE
AUDIO
AUDIS
AUDIT
AUDRA
BUDDY
BUDGE
CUDDY
DUDDY
DUDED
DUDEK
DUDES
FUDDY
FUDGE
JUDAH
JUDAS
JUDDS
JUDEA
JUDEO
JUDES
JUDGE
JUDIT
JUDOS
KUDOS
KUDUS
KUDZU
LUDIC
MUDDY
NUDER
NUDES
NUDGE
NUDZH
PUDDY
PUDGY
RUDDY
RUDEL
RUDER
RUDGE
SUDAN
SUDSY
TUDOR

•U•D•
BUDDY
BUNDS
BUNDT
BUNDY
CUDDY
CURDS
CURDY
CUYDS
DUADS
DUDDY
FUADI
FUDDY
FULDA
FUNDS
FUNDY
GUIDE
GUIDO
GURDY
HURDY
JUDDS
KURDS
LUNDI
LUNDY
MUDDY
MUNDI
OUIDA
OUTDO
PUDDY
PURDY
QUADR
QUADS
QUIDS
RUDDY
SUEDE
SUNDA
WUNDT

•U••D
BUILD
BUSED
CUBED
CUPID
CURAD
CURED
DUDED
DUKED
DUPED
FUMED
FUSED
GUARD
GUILD
GUYED
HUMID
JUKED
LUBED
LUCID
LUGED
LURED
LURID
LUTED
MUSED
MUTED
NUKED
OUTED
PULED
QUAID
QUAND
RULED
TUBED
TUMID
TUNED

••UD•
BAUDS
CAUDI
CAUDO
CRUDE
CRUDS
ELUDE
ETUDE
EXUDE
FEUDS
GAUDI
GAUDS
GAUDY
GOUDA
GOUDY
JEUDI
LAUDA
LAUDE
LAUDS
MAUDE
PRUDE
SAUDI
SCUDS
SPUDS
STUDS
STUDY
THUDS
TRUDY

••U•D
BLUED
BOUND
CLUED
COULD
DRUID
FLUID
FOUND
FOURD
GLUED
GOULD
GOURD
GRUED
HOUND
MOULD
MOUND
POUND
ROUND
SLUED
SOUND
SQUAD
SQUID
TRUED
WOULD
WOUND

•••UD
ALOUD
BROUD
CHAUD
CLOUD
FRAUD
FREUD
LEAUD
LIKUD
NEFUD
PROUD
PSEUD
SALUD
UNBUD

U•E••
ULEES
ULENE
ULENT
UMEKI
UPEND
UPENN
UREAS
USEAS
USEBY
USEES
USEIN
USEIT
USEME
USEOF
USEON
USERS
USETO
USEUP
UVEAL
UVEAS

U••E•
UDDER
ULCER
ULEES
UMBEL
UMBER
UMPED
UNBET
UNDEC
UNDER
UNFED
UNGER
UNLED
UNLET
UNMET
UNMEW
UNNEW
UNPEG
UNPEN
UNSER
UNSET
UNSEW
UNTER
UNWED
UNWET
UPPED
UPPER
UPSET
URGED
URGER
URGES
URIEL
URKEL
URNES
USEES
USHED
USHER
USHES
USTED
USTEN
UTHER
UTLEY
UTTER
UZBEK

U•••E
UDINE
UKASE
ULENE
ULNAE
UMBLE
UNCLE
UNDUE
UNICE
UNITE
UNTIE
UPONE
URSAE
USAGE
USEME
USONE
UTILE
UTUBE

•UE••
BUELL
BUENA
BUENO
CUEIN
CUERS
CUEUP
DUEIN
DUELS
DUENA
DUENO
DUETO
DUETS
DUEUP
EUELL
FUEGO
FUELS
GUESS
GUEST
HUERS
HUEVO
HUEYS
JUEGO
LUEGO
NUEVA
NUEVE
NUEVO
OUEST
QUEEG
QUEEN
QUEER
QUELL
QUERY
QUESO
QUEST
QUEUE
RUEHL
RUERS
SUEDE
SUEME
SUENO
SUERS
SUETS
SUETY

•U•E•
AUBER
AUDEN
AUGER
BUBER
BUREN
BURET
BUSED
BUSES
BUSEY
BUTEO
BUYER
CUBEB
CUBED
CUBER
CUBES
CUKES
CULET
CUMES
CUNEO
CUPEL
CURED
CUREL
CURER
CURES
CURET
CUSEC
CUTER
CUTES
CUTEX
CUTEY
CUVEE
DUCES
DUDED
DUDEK
DUDES
DUKED
DUKES
DUNES
DUPED
DUPER
DUPES
DUREN
DURER
DUVET
EULER
FUMED
FUMER
FUMES
FUMET
FUSED
FUSEE
FUSES
GUMEE
GUTEN
GUYED
HUBEL
HUBER
HUGER
JUDEA
JUDEO
JUDES
JUKED
JUKES
JULEP
JULES
JULEY
JUNES
JUTES
KUBEK
KUGEL
LUBED
LUBES
LUGED
LUGER
LUGES
LULEA
LUMEN
LUMET
LUNER
LUNES
LURED
LURER
LURES
LUREX
LUTED
LUTES
LUXES
MUJER
MULES
MULEY
MURES
MUSED
MUSEE
MUSEO
MUSER
MUSES
MUTED
MUTER
MUTES
NUDER
NUDES
NUKED
NUKES
NUMEN
NUNEZ
NUYEN
OUSEL
OUTED
OUTER
OUZEL
PUCES
PUGET
PULED
PULER
PULES
PUREE
PURER
PUREX
QUEEG
QUEEN
QUEER
QUIEN
QUIET
RUBEL
RUBEN
RUBES
RUDEL
RUDER
RULED
RULER
RULES
RUMER
RUNES
RUPEE
RUSES
SUMER
SUPER
SUPES
SURER
TUBED
TUBER
TUBES
TULES
TUNED
TUNER
TUNES
TUTEE
TUXES
YULES

•U••E
AUDIE
AUGIE
AURAE
AUTRE
BUDGE
BUGLE
BULGE
BURKE
BUTTE
CUIRE
CUORE
CURIE
CURSE
CURVE
CUTIE
CUVEE
DUANE
DUBHE
DULCE
DUNCE
DUNNE
DUPLE
DUPRE
EUBIE
FUDGE
FUGUE
FURIE
FURZE
FUSEE
GUARE
GUIDE
GUILE
GUISE
GUMEE
HUBIE
HULCE
HULME
JUDGE
JUICE
JULIE
JUSTE
LUCIE
LUCRE
LUISE
LUNGE
LURIE
MURRE
MUSEE
NUDGE
NUEVE
NURSE
OUNCE
OUTIE
OUTRE
PULSE
PUPAE
PUREE
PURGE
PURSE
QUAKE
QUARE
QUEUE
QUINE
QUIRE
QUITE
QUOTE
RUBLE
RUCHE
RUDGE
RUPEE
RUSSE
SUAVE
SUCRE
SUEDE
SUEME
SUITE
SUPPE
SURGE
SUSIE
SUZIE
TULLE
TUQUE
TUTEE
TUTTE

••UE•
AGUES
BAUER
BLUED
BLUER
BLUES
BLUET
CLUED
CLUER
CLUES
CRUEL
CRUET
DEUEL
FEUER
FLUES
GLUED
GLUER
GLUES
GLUEY
GRUED
GRUEL
GRUES
HAUER
HEUER
LAUER
MOUES
REUEL
ROUEN
ROUES
SLUED
SLUES
TRUED
TRUER
TRUES

••U•E
ABUSE
ACUTE
AMUSE
AQUAE
AZURE
BAUME
BLUME
BOULE
BRUCE
BRULE
BRUME
BRUTE
CAUSE
CHUTE
COUPE
CRUDE
CRUSE
DAUBE
DEUCE
DOUCE
DOUSE
DOUTE
DOUZE
DRUPE
DRUSE
DRUZE
EDUCE
ELUDE
ELUTE
ENURE
ETUDE
EXUDE
FAURE
FAUTE
FAUVE
FLUKE
FLUME
FLUTE
FOURE
GAUGE
GAUZE
GLUTE
GOUGE
HAUTE
HEURE
HOUSE
INURE
INUSE
JAUNE
JEUNE
JOULE
JOUVE
KLUTE
KNUTE
LAUDE
LOUIE
LOUPE
LOUSE
MAUDE
MAUVE
MEUSE
MFUME
MOUSE
NOUSE
OFUSE
OVULE
PAUSE
PIUTE
PLUIE
PLUME
POULE
PRUDE
PRUNE
REUNE
REUSE
ROUGE
ROUSE
ROUTE
SAUCE
SAUTE
SEULE
SHUTE
SOUSE
SPUME
STUPE
TAUPE
THULE
TOUTE
TRUCE
UTUBE
YOURE
YOUSE
YOUVE

•••UE
ARGUE
ATQUE
ENDUE
ENSUE
ESQUE
FUGUE
GIGUE
HAGUE
IMBUE
INDUE
ISSUE
LARUE
LOGUE
ONCUE
PIQUE
QUEUE
RECUE
REVUE
ROGUE
ROQUE
SEGUE
TOGUE
TOQUE
TUQUE
UNDUE
VAGUE
VALUE
VENUE
VOGUE

U•F••
UNFAR
UNFED
UNFIT
UNFIX
UNFUN
UPFOR

U••F•
UNIFY
USAFA
USOFA

U•••F
USEOF

•UF••
BUFFA
BUFFI
BUFFO
BUFFS
BUFFY
CUFFS
DUFAY
DUFFY
DUFUS
DUFYS
GUFFS
HUFFS
HUFFY
LUFFS
MUFFS
MUFTI
NUFLO
PUFFS
PUFFY
RUFFS
RUFUS
SUFIS
TUFTS
TUFTY

•U•F•
BUFFA
BUFFI
BUFFO
BUFFS
BUFFY
CUFFS
DUFFY
GUFFS
GULFS
HUFFS
HUFFY
LUFFS
MUFFS
PUFFS
PUFFY
QUAFF
RUFFS
RULFO
SULFA
SURFS
SURFY
TURFS
TURFY

•U••F
OUTOF
QUAFF

••UF•
ACUFF
BLUFF
CHUFF
FLUFF
GRUFF
KHUFU
OEUFS
POUFS
SCUFF
SNUFF
STUFF

••U•F
ACUFF
BLUFF
CHUFF
FLUFF
FOURF
GRUFF
SCUFF
SMURF
SNUFF
STUFF

•••UF
BOEUF

UG•••
UGLIS
UGRIC

U•G••
UNGAG
UNGAR
UNGER
UNGOT
URGED
URGER
URGES

U••G•
USAGE
USCGA

U•••G
UNBAG
UNDUG
UNGAG
UNPEG
UNRIG
UNWIG
USING

•UG••
AUGER
AUGHT
AUGIE
AUGUR
BUGGY
BUGLE
BUGSY
CUGAT
DUGAN
DUGAT
DUGIN
DUGIT
DUGUP
FUGAL
FUGIT
FUGUE
FUGUS
HUGER
HUGOS
JUGAL
KUGEL
LUGAR
LUGED
LUGER
LUGES
MUGGS
MUGGY
OUGHT
PUGET
PUGGY
RUGBY
SUGAR
TUGAT
TUGON
VUGGY
YUGOS

•U•G•
BUDGE
BUGGY
BULGE
BULGY
BUNGS
BURGH
BURGS
FUDGE
FUEGO
FUNGI
FUNGO
GUNGA
JUDGE
JUEGO
LUEGO
LUIGI
LUNGE
LUNGS
MUGGS
MUGGY
NUDGE
OUTGO
PUDGY
PUGGY
PUNGS
PURGE
QUAGS
RUDGE
RUNGS
SURGE
VUGGY

•U••G
CUING
GULAG
HUANG
LUANG
QUANG
QUEEG
RUING
SUING

••UG•
BAUGH
BOUGH
CHUGS
COUGH
DOUGH
DRUGS
FRUGS
GAUGE
GLUGS
GOUGE
HOUGH
KLUGH
LAUGH
PLUGS
ROUGE
ROUGH
SLUGS
SNUGS
THUGS
TOUGH
WAUGH

••U•G
BOURG
BRUNG
CHUNG
CLUNG
FLUNG
MYUNG
SLUNG
STUNG
SWUNG
WRUNG
YOUNG

•••UG
ABZUG
DEBUG
DRHUG
PFLUG
REDUG
SHRUG
SMAUG
STRUG
UNDUG
VWBUG

UH•••
UHAUL
UHHUH
UHLAN
UHNAK
UHURA
UHURU

U•H••
UHHUH
UNHAT
UNHID
UNHIP
UNHIT
UNHOT
USHED
USHER
USHES
UTHER

U••H•
UNSHY
UTAHN

U•••H
UHHUH
UKIAH
URIAH
URICH

•UH••
WUHAN

•U•H•
AUGHT
BUSHY
CUSHY
DUBHE
DUCHY
FUCHS
GUSHY
LUSHY
MUCHA
MUCHO
MUSHU
MUSHY
NUCHA
OUGHT
PUSHY
RUCHE
RUEHL
RUSHY
RUTHS
SUSHI
TUSHY
WUSHU

•U••H
BUNCH
BURGH
BUSCH
BUTCH
CULCH
DUTCH
GULCH
GURSH
HUMPH
HUNCH
HUTCH
JUDAH
KUSCH
LUNCH
LURCH
MULCH
MUNCH
NUDZH
PUNCH
QUASH
QUOTH
SURAH

••UH•
BRUHL
BRUHN

••U•H
AGUSH
BAUGH
BLUSH
BLUTH
BOUGH
BRUCH
BRUSH
COUCH
COUGH
COUTH
CRUSH
DOUGH
FLUSH
FOURH
HOUGH
KLUGH
LAUGH
LOUTH

MOUCH
MOUTH
PLUSH
POUCH
ROUGH
ROUSH
SHUSH
SLUSH
SMUSH
SOUTH
TOUCH
TOUGH
TRUTH
VOUCH
WAUGH
YOUTH

•••UH
NODUH
UHHUH

UI•••
UINTA

U•I••
UDINE
UJIJI
UKIAH
UMIAK
UNIAT
UNICE
UNIFY
UNION
UNITA
UNITE
UNITS
UNITY
UNIVS
URIAH
URICH
URIEL
USING
UTICA
UTILE
UTILS

U••I•
UGLIS
UGRIC
ULRIC
UNBID
UNBIT
UNDID
UNDIM
UNFIT
UNFIX
UNHID
UNHIP
UNHIT
UNLIT
UNMIX
UNPIN
UNRIG
UNRIP
UNTIE
UNTIL
UNWIG
UNZIP
UPLIT
URSID
USAID
USAIR
USEIN
USEIT

U•••I
UJIJI
UMEKI
UNAMI

•UI••
BUICK
BUILD
BUILT
CUICA
CUING
CUIRE
DUINO
GUIDE
GUIDO
GUILD
GUILE
GUILT
GUISE
HUITS
JUICE
JUICY
JUINS
LUIGI
LUISA
LUISE
NUITS
OUIDA
OUIJA
QUICK
QUIDS
QUIEN
QUIET
QUILL
QUILP
QUILT
QUINE
QUINN
QUINO
QUINT
QUIPS
QUIPU
QUIRE
QUIRK
QUIRT
QUISP
QUITE
QUITO
QUITS
RUING
RUINS
SUING
SUITE
SUITS

•U•I•
AUDIE
AUDIO
AUDIS
AUDIT
AUGIE
AULIS
AURIC
AUVIN
BUNIN
BURIN
BUYIN
BUYIT
CUBIC
CUBIT
CUEIN
CUMIN
CUPID
CURIA
CURIE
CURIO
CUTIE
CUTIN
CUTIS
CUTIT
DUBIN
DUEIN
DUGIN
DUGIT
DUPIN
EUBIE
FUGIT
FUJIS
FURIE
FUSIL
GUNIT
HUBIE
HUMID
JUDIT
JULIA
JULIE
JULIO
JUNIO
JURIS
KULIK
KUMIN
LUBIN
LUCIA
LUCID
LUCIE
LUCIO
LUDIC
LUNIK
LUPIN
LURIA
LURID
LURIE
MUNIS
MUSIC
MUSIL
NUBIA
NUMIC
OUTIE
PULIK
PULIS
PUNIC
PUPIL
PUPIN
PURIM
PUTIN
QUAID
QUAIL
QUAIS
QUOIN
QUOIT
RUBIK
RUBIN
RUNIC
RUNIN
RURIK
RUTIN
SUBIC
SUFIS
SUSIE
SUZIE
TULIP
TUMID
TUNIC
TUNIS
TURIN
WUXIA
YUKIO
YULIN
YURIS
ZUBIN
ZUNIS

•U••I
AUSSI
BUFFI
BUZZI
CULTI
CUPRI
CURVI
DUBAI
DUOMI
FUADI
FUNGI
GUCCI
GUMMI
LUCCI
LUIGI
LUNDI
MUFTI
MULTI
MUNDI
NURMI
PUCCI
QUASI
SUNNI
SUOMI
SUSHI
TUCCI
TUTSI
TUTTI

••UI•
BRUIN
BRUIT
DRUID
EQUIP
EQUIS
EQUIV
ETUIS
FLUID
FRUIT
GSUIT
INUIT
IQUIT
LOUIE
LOUIS
PLUIE
SQUIB
SQUID

••U•I
AZUKI
BRUNI
CAUDI
DOUAI
GAUDI
HOURI
JEUDI
KAUAI
LEUMI
NOURI
OCULI
PAULI
PIUSI
PLURI
PLUVI
SAUDI
SCUSI
SOUCI
TAURI

•••UI
COQUI
ENNUI
MAQUI
PIAUI
YAQUI

UJ•••
UJIJI

U•J••
UNJAM

U••J•
UJIJI

•UJ••
AUJUS
FUJIS
JUJUS
LUJAN
MUJER

•U•J•
OUIJA

••UJ•
ABUJA

UK•••
UKASE
UKIAH

U•K••
URKEL

U••K•
UMEKI

U•••K
UHNAK
UMIAK
UZBEK

•UK••
CUKES
CUKOR
DUKAS
DUKED
DUKES
JUKED
JUKES
KUKLA
LUKAS
NUKED
NUKES
PUKAS
PUKKA
YUKIO
YUKON
YUKOS
ZUKOR

•U•K•
BUBKA
BUCKO
BUCKS
BUCKY
BULKS
BULKY
BUNKO
BUNKS
BURKA
BURKE
BUSKS
CUSKS
DUCKS
DUCKY
DUNKS
DUSKS
DUSKY
FUNKS
FUNKY
GUCKS
GUCKY
GUNKS
GUNKY
HULKS
HULKY
HUNKS
HUNKY
HUSKS
HUSKY
JUNKS
JUNKY
LUCKS
LUCKY
LURKS
MUCKS
MUCKY
MURKY
MUSKS
MUSKY
PUCKS
PUKKA
PUNKA
PUNKS
PUNKY
QUAKE
QUAKY
RUCKS
RUSKA
RUSKS
SUCKS
SUCKY
SULKS
SULKY
TUCKS
TURKS
TURKU
TUSKS
YUCKY
YULKA

•U••K
BUICK
DUDEK
HUROK
HUSAK
KUBEK
KULAK
KULIK
LUNIK
LUTSK
MUZAK
PULIK
QUACK
QUARK
QUICK
QUIRK
RUARK
RUBIK
RURIK

••UK•
ALUKO
AZUKI
FLUKE
FLUKY
LEUKO
SAUKS
STUKA
ZOUKS

••U•K
AMUCK
BAULK
BRUSK
CAULK
CHUCK
CHUNK
CLUCK
CLUNK
DRUNK
FLUNK
GLUCK
GLUNK
PLUCK
PLUNK
SHUCK
SKULK
SKUNK
SLUNK
SNUCK
SPUNK
STUCK
STUNK
THUNK
TRUCK
TRUNK

•••UK
ANOUK
FARUK
KREUK
MRYUK

UL•••
ULCER
ULEES
ULENE
ULENT
ULNAE
ULNAR
ULNAS
ULOUS
ULRIC
ULTRA

U•L••
UCLAN
UGLIS
UHLAN
UNLAX
UNLAY
UNLED
UNLET
UNLIT
UPLIT
USLTA
UTLEY

U••L•
UBOLT
UDALL
UMBLE
UNCLE
UNSLY
UPOLU
URALS
UTILE
UTILS
UVULA

U•••L
UDALL
UHAUL
UMBEL
UNTIL
URIEL
URKEL
USUAL
UVEAL
UXMAL

•UL••
AULIS
AULUS
BULBA
BULBS
BULGE
BULGY
BULKS
BULKY
BULLA
BULLS
BULLY
BULOW
CULCH
CULET
CULLS
CULLY
CULPA
CULTI
CULTS
DULCE
DULLS
DULLY
EULER
FULDA
FULLS
FULLY
GULAG
GULCH
GULFS
GULLS
GULLY
GULPS
GULPY
HULAS
HULCE
HULKS
HULKY
HULLO
HULLS
HULLY
HULME
HULOT
JULEP
JULES
JULEY
JULIA
JULIE
JULIO
JULYS
KULAK
KULIK
LULEA
LULLS
LULLY
LULUS
MULAN
MULCH
MULCT
MULES
MULEY
MULLA
MULLS
MULTI
NULLA
NULLO
NULLS
PULAS
PULED
PULER
PULES
PULIK
PULIS
PULLS
PULMO
PULPS
PULPY
PULSE
RULED
RULER
RULES
RULFO
SULFA
SULKS
SULKY
SULLA
SULLY
TULES
TULIP
TULLE
TULLY
TULSA
YULES
YULIN
YULKA
ZULUS

•U•L•
BUELL
BUGLE
BUILD
BUILT
BULLA
BULLS
BULLY
BURLS
BURLY
CULLS
CULLY
CURLS
CURLY
DUALS
DUELS
DULLS
DULLY
DUPLE
DUPLO
EUELL
FUELS
FULLS
FULLY
FURLS
GUILD
GUILE
GUILT
GULLS
GULLY
HULLO
HULLS
HULLY
HURLS
HURLY
KUALA
KUBLA
KUKLA
LULLS
LULLY
MULLA
MULLS
NUFLO
NULLA
NULLO
NULLS
PULLS
PURLS
QUALM
QUELL
QUILL
QUILP
QUILT
RUBLE
SULLA
SULLY
SURLY
TULLE
TULLY

•U••L
AURAL
BUELL
BUTYL
CUMUL
CUPEL
CUREL
DUCAL
DUVAL
EUELL
FUGAL
FUSIL
HUBEL
JUBAL
JUGAL
JURAL
KUGEL
MURAL
MUSIL
OUSEL
OUZEL
PUPAL
PUPIL
QUAIL
QUELL
QUILL
RUBEL
RUDEL
RUEHL
RURAL
TUBAL

••UL•
ADULT
ALULA
BAULK
BOULE
BOULT
BRULE
CAULK
CHULA
COULD
DOULA
ELULS
EXULT
FAULT
FOULS
GAULS
GOULD
HAULS
JOULE
KRULL
MAULS
MOULD
MOULT
OCULI
OCULO
OVULE
PAULA
PAULI
PAULO
PAULV
POULE
POULT
SAULT
SCULL
SEULE
SHULA
SHULS
SKULK
SKULL
SOULS
THULE
TRULY
UVULA
VAULT
WOULD
YOULL

••U•L
BRUHL
CHURL
CRUEL
DEUEL
EQUAL
GRUEL
IGUAL
KNURL
KRULL
REUEL
SCULL
SKULL
USUAL
YOULL

•••UL
ABDUL
AFOUL
ANNUL
ASOUL
AWFUL
BAIUL
CUMUL
GHOUL
JPAUL
KABUL
MOGUL
MOSUL
ODOUL
RAOUL
SEOUL
UHAUL

UM•••
UMASS
UMBEL
UMBER
UMBLE
UMBRA
UMEKI
UMIAK
UMPED

U•M••
UNMAD
UNMAN
UNMET
UNMEW
UNMIX
UXMAL

U••M•
UNAMI
USEME

U•••M
UNARM
UNDAM
UNDIM
UNJAM

•UM••
BUMPS
BUMPY
CUMES
CUMIN
CUMUL
DUMAS
DUMBO
DUMBS
DUMMY
DUMPS
DUMPY
FUMED
FUMER
FUMES
FUMET
GUMBO
GUMBY
GUMEE
GUMMI
GUMMO
GUMMY
GUMUP
HUMAN
HUMID
HUMOR
HUMPH
HUMPS
HUMPY
HUMUS
JUMBO
JUMNA
JUMPS
JUMPY
KUMIN
LUMAN
LUMAS
LUMEN
LUMET
LUMPS
LUMPY
MUMBO
MUMMS
MUMMY
MUMPS
NUMAN
NUMBS
NUMEN
NUMIC
PUMAS
PUMPS
RUMAN
RUMBA
RUMER
RUMMY
RUMOR
RUMPS
SUMAC
SUMER
SUMMA
SUMOS
SUMPS
SUMUP
TUMID
TUMMY
YUMAN
YUMAS
YUMMY

•U•M•
BURMA
CUOMO
DUMMY
DUOMI
DUOMO
GUMMI
GUMMO
GUMMY
HULME
MUMMS
MUMMY
NURMI
PULMO
RUMMY
SUEME
SUMMA
SUOMI
TUMMY
YUMMY

•U••M
AURUM
BUXOM
DURUM
PURIM
QUALM

••UM•
ALUMS
ARUMS
BAUME
BLUME
BRUME
CHUMP
CHUMS
CLUMP
CRUMB
CRUMP
DRUMS
EXUMA
FLUME
FRUMP
GLUMS
GRUMP
HOUMA
KLUMP
LEUMI
LOUMA
MFUME
PLUMB
PLUME
PLUMP
PLUMR
PLUMS
PLUMY
RHUMB
SCUMS
SLUMP
SLUMS
SPUME
SPUMY
STUMP
THUMB
THUMP
TRUMP

••U•M
STURM

•••UM
ALBUM
ANNUM
ARIUM
AURUM
BEGUM
BONUM
BYGUM
CECUM
COLUM
DATUM
DEGUM
DURUM
FILUM
FORUM
HARUM
HILUM
HOHUM
HOKUM
ILEUM
ILIUM
INSUM
JORUM
LOCUM
MECUM
NAHUM
OAKUM
ODEUM
ODIUM
OLEUM
OPIUM
ORIUM
PNEUM
REGUM
RHEUM
SCRUM
SEDUM
SERUM
STRUM
TATUM
THRUM
VELUM
YOKUM

UN•••
UNAMI
UNAPT
UNARM
UNARY
UNAUS
UNBAG
UNBAR
UNBET
UNBID
UNBIT
UNBOX
UNBUD
UNCAP
UNCAS
UNCLE
UNCOY
UNCUT
UNDAM
UNDAY
UNDEC
UNDER
UNDID
UNDIM
UNDRY
UNDUE
UNDUG
UNFAR
UNFED
UNFIT
UNFIX
UNFUN
UNGAG
UNGAR
UNGER
UNGOT
UNHAT
UNHID
UNHIP
UNHIT
UNHOT
UNIAT
UNICE
UNIFY
UNION
UNITA
UNITE
UNITS
UNITY
UNIVS
UNJAM
UNLAX
UNLAY
UNLED
UNLET
UNLIT
UNMAD
UNMAN
UNMET
UNMEW
UNMIX
UNNEW
UNPEG
UNPEN
UNPIN
UNPOT
UNRIG
UNRIP
UNRUN
UNSAD
UNSAY
UNSER
UNSET
UNSEW
UNSHY
UNSLY
UNTAX
UNTER
UNTIE
UNTIL
UNWED
UNWET
UNWIG
UNWON
UNZIP

U•N••
UHNAK
UINTA
ULNAE
ULNAR
ULNAS
UNNEW
URNES

U••N•
UCONN
UDINE
ULENE
ULENT
UPEND
UPENN
UPONE
URANO
USING
USONE

U•••N
UCLAN
UCONN
UHLAN
UNFUN
UNION
UNMAN
UNPEN
UNPIN
UNRUN
UNWON
UPENN
UPTON
URBAN
USEIN
USEON
USTEN
UTAHN
UTURN

•UN••
AUNTS
AUNTY
BUNCH
BUNCO
BUNDS
BUNDT
BUNDY
BUNGS
BUNIN
BUNKO
BUNKS
BUNNY
BUNTS
CUNEO
DUNCE
DUNES
DUNKS

DUNNE DUNNO DUNST FUNDS FUNDY FUNGI FUNGO FUNKS FUNKY FUNNY GUNGA GUNIT GUNKS GUNKY GUNNY HUNAN HUNCH HUNKS HUNKY HUNTS HUNTZ JUNCO JUNES JUNIO JUNKS JUNKY JUNTA JUNTO KUNTA LUNAR LUNAS LUNCH LUNDI LUNDY LUNER LUNES LUNGE LUNGS LUNIK LUNNS LUNTS MUNCH MUNDI MUNIS MUNNA MUNRO NUNCA NUNEZ OUNCE PUNCH PUNGS PUNIC PUNKA PUNKS PUNKY PUNNY PUNTA PUNTS RUNAT RUNBY RUNES RUNGS RUNIC RUNIN RUNNY RUNON RUNTO RUNTS RUNTY RUNUP SUNDA SUNNA SUNNI SUNNY SUNUP TUNAS TUNED TUNER TUNES TUNIC TUNIS WUNDT ZUNIS

•U•N•

BUENA BUENO BUNNY BUONA BUONO BURNS BURNT BUTNO CUING DUANE DUENA DUENO DUINO DUNNE DUNNO DURNS FUNNY GUANO GUNNY HUANG JUANO JUINS JUMNA LUANA LUANG LUANN LUNNS MUNNA MUONS PUNNY QUAND QUANG QUANT QUINE QUINN QUINO QUINT RUING RUINS RUNNY SUENO SUING SUNNA SUNNI SUNNY TURNS YUANS

•U••N

AUDEN AUVIN BUNIN BUREN BURIN BUSON BUYIN CUBAN CUEIN CUMIN CUTIN DUBIN DUEIN DUGAN DUGIN DUPIN DURAN DUREN FUTON GUTEN GUYON HUMAN HUNAN HURON JURAN KUMIN LUANN LUBIN LUCAN LUJAN LUMAN LUMEN LUPIN LUZON MULAN MUTON NUMAN NUMEN NUYEN OUTON PUPIN PUSAN PUTIN PUTON QUEEN QUIEN QUINN QUOIN QURAN RUBEN RUBIN RUBON RUMAN RUNIN RUNON RUTIN SUDAN SUSAN TUGON TURIN WUHAN YUBAN YUKON YULIN YUMAN ZUBIN

••UN•

ARUNS BLUNT BOUND BRUNG BRUNI BRUNO BRUNT CHUNG CHUNK CLUNG CLUNK CLUNY COUNT DAUNT DJUNA DRUNK FAUNA FAUNS FLUNG FLUNK FOUND FOUNT GAUNT GLUNK GRUNT HAUNT HOUND JAUNE JAUNT JEUNE MAUNA MOUND MOUNT MYUNG NOUNS PLUNK POUND PRUNE REUNE ROUND SAUNA SHUNS SHUNT SKUNK SLUNG SLUNK SOUND SPUNK STUNG STUNK STUNS STUNT SWUNG TAUNT THUNK TRUNK VAUNT WOUND WRUNG YOUNG YOUNT

••U•N

BRUHN BRUIN CHURN DRUON GLUON MOURN ROUEN SPURN TAUON UTURN YOURN

•••UN

BADUN BBGUN BEGUN BOSUN BRAUN BROUN CAJUN GATUN INFUN INJUN INRUN NOFUN NORUN RERUN SHAUN THEUN UNFUN UNRUN WEEUN

U•O••

UBOAT UBOLT UCONN ULOUS UPOLU UPONE UROUS USOFA USONE

U••O•

UNBOX UNCOY UNGOT UNHOT UNION UNPOT UNWON UPBOW UPDOS UPFOR UPTON UPTOP USEOF USEON

U•••O

URANO USETO

•UO••

BUONA BUONO BUOYS CUOMO CUORE DUOMI DUOMO FUOCO MUONS NUOVA NUOVO QUOIN QUOIT QUOTA QUOTE QUOTH SUOMI

•U•O•

AUTOS BULOW BUSON BUXOM CUKOR DUROC DUROS EUROS FUROR FUROS FUTON GUYON HUGOS HULOT HUMOR HUROK HURON JUCOS JUDOS JUROR KUDOS LUXOR LUZON MUTON OUTOF OUTON OUZOS PUTON RUBON RUMOR RUNON SUMOS TUDOR TUGON TUROW TUTOR YUGOS YUKON YUKOS ZUKOR

•U••O

AUDIO BUCCO BUCKO BUENO BUFFO BUNCO BUNKO BUONO BURRO BUTEO BUTNO CUNEO CUOMO CUPRO CURIO CUZCO DUENO DUETO DUINO DUMBO DUNNO DUOMO DUPLO FUEGO FUNGO FUOCO GUANO GUAPO GUIDO GUMBO GUMMO GUSTO HUEVO HULLO HUTTO JUANO JUDEO JUEGO JULIO JUMBO JUNCO JUNIO JUNTO LUCIO LUEGO MUCHO MUMBO MUNRO MUSEO NUEVO NUFLO NULLO NUOVO NUTRO OUTDO OUTGO PULMO PUTTO QUAXO QUESO QUINO QUITO RULFO RUNTO RUSSO SUENO TURBO TURCO TUTTO YUKIO ZUCCO

••UO•

CRUOR DRUON FLUOR GLUON TAUON

••U•O

ALUKO BLUTO BRUNO CAUDO DEUTO DOURO GLUCO LAURO LEUKO NEURO OCULO ORURO PAULO PLUTO SAURO TAURO TAUTO TOURO TRURO

UP•••

UPBOW UPDOS UPDRY UPEND UPENN UPFOR UPLIT UPOLU UPONE UPPED UPPER UPSET UPTON UPTOP

U•P••

UMPED UNPEG UNPEN UNPIN UNPOT UPPED UPPER

U••P•

UNAPT

U•••P

UNCAP UNHIP UNRIP UNZIP UPTOP USEUP USURP

•UP••

CUPEL CUPID CUPPA CUPPY CUPRI CUPRO DUPED DUPER DUPES DUPIN DUPLE DUPLO DUPRE GUPPY LUPIN LUPUS PUPAE PUPAL PUPAS PUPIL PUPIN PUPPY PUPUS RUPEE SUPER SUPES SUPPE SUPRA SUPTS TUPAC ZUPPA

•U•P•

BUMPS BUMPY BURPS CULPA CUPPA CUPPY CUSPS DUMPS DUMPY GUAPA GUAPO GULPS GULPY GUPPY HUMPH HUMPS HUMPY JUMPS JUMPY LUMPS LUMPY MUMPS PULPS PULPY PUMPS PUPPY QUIPS QUIPU RUMPS SUMPS SUPPE ZUPPA

•U••P

BUYUP CUEUP CUTUP DUEUP DUGUP GUMUP JULEP PUTUP QUILP QUISP RUBUP RUNUP SUMUP SUNUP TULIP

••UP•

ACUPS BCUPS CCUPS COUPE COUPS DCUPS DRUPE ERUPT KRUPA KRUPP KRUPS LOUPE LOUPS REUPS SCUPS SOUPS SOUPY STUPA STUPE TAUPE WHUPS

••U•P

CHUMP CLUMP CRUMP EQUIP FRUMP GRUMP KLUMP KRUPP PLUMP SLUMP SLURP STUMP THUMP TRUMP USURP

•••UP

ACTUP ADDUP AIRUP AMPUP ANDUP ASKUP ATEUP BIDUP BITUP BOBUP BOXUP BUYUP CROUP CRYUP CUEUP CUTUP DAMUP DIDUP DIGUP DRYUP DUEUP DUGUP EATUP ENDUP EYEUP FEDUP FITUP FIXUP FLYUP FOGUP FRYUP GASUP GETUP GINUP GOTUP GROUP GUMUP HADUP HAMUP HASUP HETUP HITUP HOPUP ICEUP JAMUP KEYUP LAPUP LAYUP LEGUP LETUP LIEUP LITUP METUP MIXUP MOPUP NIPUP NOTUP ONEUP OWNUP PAYUP PENUP PEPUP PINUP POPUP PUTUP RANUP REVUP RIGUP RIPUP RUBUP RUNUP SATUP SAWUP SEEUP SETUP SEWUP SIRUP SITUP SIXUP SOPUP SUMUP SUNUP SYRUP TAGUP TEEUP TENUP TIEUP TIPUP TOGUP TOPUP TOTUP TROUP TWOUP USEUP WADUP WASUP WAXUP WAYUP ZIPUP

•UQ••

TUQUE

•U••Q

SUZYQ

UR•••

URALS URANO URAWA URBAN UREAS URGED URGER URGES URIAH URICH URIEL URKEL URNES UROUS URSAE URSID URSUS

U•R••

UGRIC ULRIC UNRIG UNRIP UNRUN USRDA UVRAY

U••R•

UHURA UHURU ULTRA UMBRA UNARM UNARY UNDRY UPDRY USERS USURP USURY UTURN

U•••R

UDDER ULCER ULNAR UMBER UNBAR UNDER UNFAR UNGAR UNGER UNSER UNTER UPFOR UPPER URGER USAIR USHER UTHER UTTAR UTTER

•UR••

AURAE AURAL AURAR AURAS AURIC AURUM BURBS BUREN BURET BURGH BURGS BURIN BURKA BURKE BURLS BURLY BURMA BURNS BURNT BURPS BURRO BURRS BURRY BURSA BURST CURAD CURBS CURDS CURDY CURED CUREL CURER CURES CURET CURIA CURIE CURIO CURLS CURLY CURRS CURRY CURSA CURSE CURST CURVE CURVI CURVY DURAN DURAS DUREN DURER DURNS DUROC DUROS DURRA DURST DURUM EUROS EURUS FURBY FURIE FURLS FUROR FUROS FURRY FURST FURZE GURDY GURSH GURUS HURDY HURLS HURLY HUROK HURON HURRY HURST HURTS JURAL JURAN JURIS JUROR KURDS KURTZ KURUS KURYS LURAY LURCH LURED LURER LURES LUREX LURIA LURID LURIE LURKS MURAL MURAT MURES MURKY MURRE NURMI NURSE OURAY PURDY PUREE PURER PUREX PURGE PURIM PURLS PURRS PURSE PURSY PURTY QURAN RURAL RURIK SURAH SURAS SURER SURFS SURFY SURGE SURLY TURBO TURCO TURFS TURFY TURIN TURKS TURKU TURNS TUROW TURVY WURST YURIS YURTS

•U•R•

AUDRA AUTRE AUTRY BURRO BURRS BURRY CUERS CUIRE CUORE CUPRI CUPRO CURRS CURRY DUPRE DURRA FURRY GUARD GUARE GUARS HUERS HURRY LUCRE MUNRO MURRE NUTRO OUTRE PURRS QUARE QUARK QUART QUERY QUIRE QUIRK QUIRT RUARK RUERS SUCRE SUERS SUPRA SUTRA

•U••R

AUBER AUGER AUGUR AURAR AUSTR BUBER BUYER CUBER CUKOR CURER CUTER DUPER DURER EULER FUMER FUROR HUBER HUGER HUMOR JUROR LUGAR LUGER LUNAR LUNER LURER LUXOR MUJER MUSER MUTER NUDER OUTER PULER PURER QUADR QUEER RUDER RULER RUMER RUMOR SUGAR SUMER SUPER SURER TUBER TUDOR TUNER TUTOR ZUKOR

••UR•

ACURA AGURA AZURE BLURB BLURS BLURT BOURG CHURL CHURN COURT COURU CRURA DOURO DRURY ELURA ENURE EXURB FAURE FOURA FOURB FOURC FOURD FOURE FOURF FOURH FOURS GAURS GOURD HEURE HOURI HOURS INURE JOURS KNURL KNURS LAURA LAURO LEURS LOURS LOURY MAURA MAURY MOURN NAURU NEURO NOURI ORURO PEURS PLURI POURS SAURO SLURP SLURS SMURF SOURS SPURN SPURS SPURT STURM TAURI TAURO THURS TOURO TOURS TRURO UHURA UHURU USURP USURY UTURN YOURE YOURN YOURS

••U•R

BAUER BLUER CLUER CRUOR FEUER FLUOR GLUER HAUER HEUER LAUER PLUMR TRUER

•••UR

AILUR AMOUR ARTUR ASHUR AUGUR BFOUR COEUR DAZUR DEMUR FEMUR FLEUR FLOUR

HHOUR
IFOUR
INCUR
LEMUR
MASUR
NAMUR
OCCUR
ODOUR
RECUR
SCOUR
SOEUR
VFOUR

US•••
USAFA
USAGE
USAID
USAIR
USCGA
USEAS
USEBY
USEES
USEIN
USEIT
USEME
USEOF
USEON
USERS
USETO
USEUP
USHED
USHER
USHES
USING
USLTA
USOFA
USONE
USRDA
USTED
USTEN
USUAL
USURP
USURY

U•S••
UNSAD
UNSAY
UNSER
UNSET
UNSEW
UNSHY
UNSLY
UPSET
URSAE
URSID
URSUS

U••S•
UKASE
UMASS

U•••S
UGLIS
ULEES
ULNAS
ULOUS
UMASS
UNAUS
UNCAS
UNITS
UNIVS
UPDOS
URALS
UREAS
URGES
URNES
UROUS
URSUS
USEAS
USEES
USERS
USHES
UTILS
UVEAS

•US••
AUSSI
AUSTR
BUSBY
BUSCH
BUSED
BUSES
BUSEY
BUSHY
BUSKS
BUSON
BUSTA
BUSTS
CUSEC
CUSHY
CUSKS
CUSPS
DUSKS
DUSKY
DUSTS
DUSTY
FUSED
FUSEE
FUSES
FUSIL
FUSSY
FUSTY
GUSHY
GUSSY
GUSTO
GUSTS
GUSTY
HUSAK
HUSKS
HUSKY
HUSSY
JUSTE
JUSTY
KUSCH
LUSHY
LUSTS
LUSTY
MUSCA
MUSED
MUSEE
MUSEO
MUSER
MUSES
MUSHU
MUSHY
MUSIC
MUSIL
MUSKS
MUSKY
MUSSY
MUSTS
MUSTY
OUSEL
OUSTS
PUSAN
PUSHY
PUSSY
RUSES
RUSHY
RUSKA
RUSKS
RUSSA
RUSSE
RUSSO
RUSTS
RUSTY
SUSAN
SUSHI
SUSIE
TUSHY
TUSKS
WUSHU

•U•S•
AUSSI
BUGSY
BURSA
BURST
CURSA
CURSE
CURST
DUNST
DURST
FUBSY
FURST
FUSSY
GUESS
GUEST
GUISE
GURSH
GUSSY
GUTSY
HURST
HUSSY
LUISA
LUISE
LUTSK
MUSSY
NURSE
NUTSY
OUEST
PULSE
PURSE
PURSY
PUSSY
QUASH
QUASI
QUESO
QUEST
QUISP
RUSSA
RUSSE
RUSSO
SUDSY
TULSA
TUTSI
WURST

•U••S
AUDIS
AUJUS
AULIS
AULUS
AUNTS
AURAS
AUTOS
BUCKS
BUFFS
BULBS
BULKS
BULLS
BUMPS
BUNDS
BUNGS
BUNKS
BUNTS
BUOYS
BURBS
BURGS
BURLS
BURNS
BURPS
BURRS
BUSES
BUSKS
BUSTS
BUTTS
CUBES
CUERS
CUFFS
CUKES
CULLS
CULTS
CUMES
CURBS
CURDS
CURES
CURLS
CURRS
CUSKS
CUSPS
CUTES
CUTIS
CUYDS
DUADS
DUALS
DUCES
DUCKS
DUCTS
DUDES
DUELS
DUETS
DUFUS
DUFYS
DUKAS
DUKES
DULLS
DUMAS
DUMBS
DUMPS
DUNES
DUNKS
DUPES
DURAS
DURNS
DUROS
DUSKS
DUSTS
EUROS
EURUS
FUCHS
FUELS
FUGUS
FUJIS
FULLS
FUMES
FUNDS
FUNKS
FURLS
FUROS
FUSES
GUARS
GUCKS
GUESS
GUFFS
GULFS
GULLS
GULPS
GUNKS
GURUS
GUSTS
HUERS
HUEYS
HUFFS
HUGOS
HUITS
HULAS
HULKS
HULLS
HUMPS
HUMUS
HUNKS
HUNTS
HURLS
HURTS
HUSKS
HUTUS
JUCOS
JUDAS
JUDDS
JUDES
JUDOS
JUINS
JUJUS
JUKES
JULES
JULYS
JUMPS
JUNES
JUNKS
JURIS
JUTES
KUDOS
KUDUS
KURDS
KURUS
KURYS
LUAUS
LUBES
LUCAS
LUCKS
LUFFS
LUGES
LUKAS
LULLS
LULUS
LUMAS
LUMPS
LUNAS
LUNES
LUNGS
LUNNS
LUNTS
LUPUS
LURES
LURKS
LUSTS
LUTES
LUXES
MUCKS
MUFFS
MUGGS
MULES
MULLS
MUMMS
MUMPS
MUNIS
MUONS
MURES
MUSES
MUSKS
MUSTS
MUTES
MUTTS
NUDES
NUITS
NUKES
NULLS
NUMBS
OUSTS
OUZOS
PUCES
PUCKS
PUFFS
PUKAS
PULAS
PULES
PULIS
PULLS
PULPS
PUMAS
PUMPS
PUNGS
PUNKS
PUNTS
PUPAS
PUPUS
PURLS
PURRS
PUTTS
QUADS
QUAGS
QUAIS
QUAYS
QUIDS
QUIPS
QUITS
RUBES
RUCKS
RUERS
RUFFS
RUFUS
RUINS
RULES
RUMPS
RUNES
RUNGS
RUNTS
RUSES
RUSKS
RUSTS
RUTHS
SUCKS
SUERS
SUETS
SUFIS
SUITS
SULKS
SUMOS
SUMPS
SUPES
SUPTS
SURAS
SURFS
TUBAS
TUBBS
TUBES
TUCKS
TUFTS
TULES
TUNAS
TUNES
TUNIS
TURFS
TURKS
TURNS
TUSKS
TUTUS
TUXES
YUANS
YUGOS
YUKOS
YULES
YUMAS
YURIS
YURTS
ZULUS
ZUNIS

••US•
ABUSE
ADUST
AGUSH
AMUSE
AMUST
AZUSA
BLUSH
BRUSH
BRUSK
CAUSE
COUSY
CRUSE
CRUSH
CRUST
DOUSE
DRUSE
FAUSS
FAUST
FLUSH
GAUSS
HOUSE
INUSE
JOUST
LOUSE
LOUSY
MEUSE
MOUSE
MOUSY
NEUSS
NOUSE
OFUSE
PAUSE
PIUSI
PIUSV
PIUSX
PLUSH
REUSE
REUSS
ROUSE
ROUSH
ROUST
SCUSA
SCUSI
SEUSS
SHUSH
SLUSH
SMUSH
SOUSA
SOUSE
TRUSS
TRUST
YOUSE

••U•S
ABUTS
ACUPS
AGUAS
AGUES
ALUMS
AOUTS
AQUAS
ARUMS
ARUNS
BAUDS
BCUPS
BLUES
BLURS
BOUTS
BRUTS
CCUPS
CHUBS
CHUGS
CHUMS
CLUBS
CLUES
COUPS
CRUDS
DAUBS
DCUPS
DOUBS
DRUBS
DRUGS
DRUMS
ELULS
EQUIS
EQUUS
ETUIS
FAUNS
FAUSS
FEUDS
FLUBS
FLUES
FOULS
FOURS
FOUTS
FRUGS
GAUDS
GAULS
GAURS
GAUSS
GLUES
GLUGS
GLUMS
GLUTS
GOUTS
GRUBS
GRUES
HAULS
HOURS
JOURS
KNURS
KRUPS
LAUDS
LEURS
LOUIS
LOUPS
LOURS
LOUTS
MAULS
MOUES
NEUSS
NOUNS
OEUFS
PEURS
PLUGS
PLUMS
POUFS
POURS
POUTS
REUPS
REUSS
ROUES
ROUTS
SAUKS
SCUDS
SCUMS
SCUPS
SCUTS
SEUSS
SHULS
SHUNS
SHUTS
SKUAS
SLUES
SLUGS
SLUMS
SLURS
SMUTS
SNUBS
SNUGS
SOULS
SOUPS
SOURS
SPUDS
SPURS
STUBS
STUDS
STUNS
THUDS
THUGS
THURS
TNUTS
TOURS
TOUTS
TRUES
TRUSS
WHUPS
XOUTS
YOURS
ZOUKS

•••US
AGNUS
AINUS
ALTUS
ANGUS
ANNUS
ANZUS
APLUS
ARBUS
ARGUS
ASCUS
AUJUS
AULUS
BABUS
BEAUS
BLEUS
BOGUS
BOLUS
BONUS
BPLUS
BYBUS
CAIUS
CAMUS
CASUS
CETUS
CLAUS
COMUS
CONUS
CPLUS
CRIUS
CYRUS
DEBUS
DONUS
DPLUS
DUFUS
ECRUS
EGEUS
EMEUS
EOLUS
EQUUS
EURUS
FETUS
FICUS
FOCUS
FUGUS
GAIUS
GENUS
GIBUS
GURUS
HOCUS
HONUS
HORUS
HUMUS
HUTUS
ICTUS
IGLUS
ILLUS
INCUS
INDUS
ISSUS
JANUS
JESUS
JUJUS
KARUS
KLAUS
KRAUS
KUDUS
KURUS
LAIUS
LEPUS
LEXUS
LIEUS
LINUS
LOCUS
LORUS
LOTUS
LUAUS
LULUS
LUPUS
MAGUS
MANUS
MENUS
MINUS
MODUS
MOMUS
NEGUS
NEVUS
NEXUS
NIDUS
NISUS
NODUS
NOTUS
NOVUS
ORCUS
PILUS
PIOUS
POCUS
POTUS
PRIUS
PUPUS
RAKUS
RAMUS
REBUS
REMUS
RUFUS
SINUS
TABUS
TAGUS
TALUS
THOUS
TIOUS
TITUS
TOFUS
TONUS
TORUS
TUTUS
TYRUS
ULOUS
UNAUS
UROUS
URSUS
VAGUS
VATUS
VENUS
VIRUS
VITUS
ZAFUS
ZEBUS
ZULUS

UT•••
UTAHN
UTHER
UTICA
UTILE
UTILS
UTLEY
UTTAR
UTTER
UTUBE
UTURN

U•T••
ULTRA
UNTAX
UNTER
UNTIE
UNTIL
UPTON
UPTOP
USTED
USTEN
UTTAR
UTTER

U••T•
UINTA
UNITA
UNITE
UNITS
UNITY
USETO
USLTA

U•••T
UBOAT
UBOLT
ULENT
UNAPT
UNBET
UNBIT
UNCUT
UNFIT
UNGOT
UNHAT
UNHIT
UNHOT
UNIAT
UNLET
UNLIT
UNMET
UNPOT
UNSET
UNWET
UPLIT
UPSET
USEIT

•UT••
AUTOS
AUTRE
AUTRY
BUTCH
BUTEO
BUTNO
BUTTE
BUTTS
BUTUT
BUTYL
CUTER
CUTES
CUTEX
CUTEY
CUTIE
CUTIN
CUTIS
CUTIT
CUTTY
CUTUP
DUTCH
FUTON
GUTEN
GUTSY
GUTTY
HUTCH
HUTTO
HUTUS
JUTES
LUTED
LUTES
LUTSK
MUTED
MUTER
MUTES
MUTON
MUTTS
NUTRO
NUTSY
NUTTY
OUTDO
OUTED
OUTER
OUTGO
OUTIE
OUTOF
OUTON
OUTRE
OUTTA
PUTBY
PUTIN
PUTON
PUTTO
PUTTS
PUTTY
PUTUP
RUTHS
RUTIN
RUTTY
SUTRA
TUTEE
TUTOR
TUTSI
TUTTE
TUTTI
TUTTO
TUTUS

•U•T•
AUNTS
AUNTY
AUSTR
BUNTS
BUSTA
BUSTS
BUTTE
BUTTS
CULTI
CULTS
CUTTY
DUCTS
DUETO
DUETS
DUSTS
DUSTY
FUSTY
GUSTO
GUSTS
GUSTY
GUTTY
HUITS
HUNTS
HUNTZ
HURTS
HUTTO
JUNTA
JUNTO
JUSTE
JUSTY
KUNTA
KURTZ
LUNTS
LUSTS
LUSTY
MUFTI
MULTI
MUSTS
MUSTY
MUTTS
NUITS
NUTTY
OUSTS
OUTTA
PUNTA
PUNTS
PURTY
PUTTO
PUTTS
PUTTY
QUITE
QUITO
QUITS
QUOTA
QUOTE
QUOTH
RUNTO
RUNTS
RUNTY
RUSTS
RUSTY
RUTTY
SUETS
SUETY
SUITE
SUITS
SUPTS
TUFTS
TUFTY
TUTTE
TUTTI
TUTTO
YURTS

•U••T
AUDIT
AUGHT
BUILT
BUNDT
BURET
BURNT
BURST
BUTUT
BUYAT
BUYIT
CUBIT
CUGAT
CULET
CURET
CURST
CUTIT
DUCAT
DUGAT
DUGIT
DUNST
DURST
DUVET
FUGIT
FUMET
FURST
GUEST
GUILT
GUNIT
HULOT
HURST
JUDIT
LUMET
MULCT
MURAT
OUEST
OUGHT
PUGET
QUANT
QUART
QUEST
QUIET
QUILT
QUINT
QUIRT
QUOIT
RUNAT
TUGAT
WUNDT
WURST

••UT•
ABUTS
ACUTE
AOUTS
BLUTH
BLUTO
BOUTS
BRUTE
BRUTS
CEUTA
CHUTE
COUTH
DEUTO
DOUTE
ELUTE
FAUTE
FLUTE
FLUTY
FOUTS
GLUTE
GLUTS
GOUTS
GOUTY
HAUTE
KLUTE
KLUTZ
KNUTE
LOUTH
LOUTS
MOUTH
PIUTE
PLUTO
POUTS
POUTY
ROUTE
ROUTS
SAUTE
SCUTS
SHUTE
SHUTS
SMUTS
SOUTH
STUTZ
TAUTO
TNUTS
TOUTE
TOUTS
TRUTH
XOUTS
YOUTH

••U•T
ADULT
ADUST
AMUST
BLUET
BLUNT
BLURT
BOULT
BRUIT
BRUNT
COUNT
COURT
CRUET
CRUST
DAUNT
DOUBT
EDUCT
ERUCT
ERUPT
EXULT
FAULT
FAUST
FOUNT
FRUCT
FRUIT
GAUNT
GRUNT
GSUIT
HAUNT
INUIT
IQUIT
JAUNT
JOUST
MOULT
MOUNT
POULT
ROUST
SAULT
SHUNT
SPURT
SQUAT
STUNT
TAUNT
TRUST
VAULT
VAUNT
YOUNT

•••UT
ABOUT
ADOUT
ALEUT
BEAUT
BUTUT
CAPUT
CLOUT
DEBUT
DONUT
FLOUT
GAMUT
GOOUT
GROUT
IMOUT
INPUT
KAPUT
KNOUT
KRAUT
LIEUT
NOCUT
REBUT
RECUT
SALUT
SCOUT
SHOUT
SNOUT
SPOUT
STOUT
STRUT
TROUT
UNCUT
XDOUT
XSOUT
YAKUT

U•U••
UHURA
UHURU
USUAL
USURP
USURY
UTUBE

UTURN
UVULA

U••U•
UHAUL
UHHUH
ULOUS
UNAUS
UNBUD
UNCUT
UNDUE
UNDUG
UNFUN
UNRUN
UROUS
URSUS
USEUP

U•••U
UHURU
UPOLU

•U•U•
AUGUR
AUJUS
AULUS
AURUM
BUTUT
BUYUP
CUEUP
CUMUL
CUTUP
DUEUP
DUFUS
DUGUP
DURUM
EURUS
FUGUE
FUGUS
GUMUP
GURUS
HUMUS
HUTUS
JUJUS
KUDUS
KURUS
LUAUS
LULUS
LUPUS
PUPUS
PUTUP
QUEUE
RUBUP
RUFUS
RUNUP
SUMUP
SUNUP
TUQUE
TUTUS
ZULUS

•U••U
KUDZU
MUSHU
QUIPU
TURKU
WUSHU

••UU•
EQUUS

••U•U
COURU
ISUZU
KHUFU
NAURU
UHURU

UV•••
UVEAL
UVEAS
UVRAY
UVULA
UVWXY

U••V•
UNIVS

•UV••
AUVIN
CUVEE
DUVAL
DUVET
TUVWX

•U•V•
CURVE
CURVI
CURVY
GUAVA
HUEVO
NUEVA
NUEVE
NUEVO
NUOVA
NUOVO
SUAVE
TURVY

••UV•
FAUVE
JOUVE
MAUVE
PLUVI
STUVW
YOUVE

••U•V
EQUIV
PAULV
PIUSV

•••UV
RSTUV

U•W••
UNWED
UNWET
UNWIG
UNWON
UVWXY

U••W•
URAWA

U•••W
UNMEW
UNNEW
UNSEW
UPBOW

•U•W•
TUVWX

•U••W
BULOW
TUROW

••U•W
SQUAW
STUVW

•••UW
NIEUW

UX•••
UXMAL

U••X•
UVWXY

U•••X
UNBOX
UNFIX
UNLAX
UNMIX
UNTAX

•UX••
BUXOM
LUXES
LUXOR
TUXES
WUXIA

•U•X•
QUAXO

•U••X
CUTEX
LUREX
PUREX
TUVWX

••U•X
PIUSX

•••UX
ADEUX
BEAUX
DIEUX
LINUX
MIEUX
REDUX
SIOUX
VIEUX

U•••Y
UNARY
UNCOY
UNDAY
UNDRY
UNIFY
UNITY
UNLAY
UNSAY
UNSHY
UNSLY
UPDRY
USEBY
USURY
UTLEY
UVRAY
UVWXY

•UY••
BUYAT
BUYER
BUYIN
BUYIT
BUYUP
CUYDS
GUYED
GUYON
NUYEN

•U•Y•
BUOYS
BUTYL
DUBYA
DUFYS
HUEYS
JULYS
KURYS
QUAYS
SUZYQ

•U••Y
AUNTY
AUTRY
BUCKY
BUDDY
BUFFY
BUGGY
BUGSY
BULGY
BULKY
BULLY
BUMPY
BUNDY
BUNNY
BURLY
BURRY
BUSBY
BUSEY
BUSHY
BUZZY
CUBBY
CUDDY
CULLY
CUPPY
CURDY
CURLY
CURRY
CURVY
CUSHY
CUTEY
CUTTY
DUCHY
DUCKY
DUDDY
DUFAY
DUFFY
DULLY
DUMMY
DUMPY
DUSKY
DUSTY
FUBSY
FUDDY
FULLY
FUNDY
FUNKY
FUNNY
FURBY
FURRY
FUSSY
FUSTY
FUZZY
GUCKY
GULLY
GULPY
GUMBY
GUMMY
GUNKY
GUNNY
GUPPY
GURDY
GUSHY
GUSSY
GUSTY
GUTSY
GUTTY
HUBBY
HUFFY
HULKY
HULLY
HUMPY
HUNKY
HURDY
HURLY
HURRY
HUSKY
HUSSY
JUICY
JULEY
JUMPY
JUNKY
JUSTY
LUCKY
LULLY
LUMPY
LUNDY
LURAY
LUSHY
LUSTY
MUCKY
MUDDY
MUGGY
MULEY
MUMMY
MURKY
MUSHY
MUSKY
MUSSY
MUSTY
MUZZY
NUBBY
NUTSY
NUTTY
OURAY
PUDDY
PUDGY
PUFFY
PUGGY
PULPY
PUNKY
PUNNY
PUPPY
PURDY
PURSY
PURTY
PUSHY
PUSSY
PUTBY
PUTTY
QUAKY
QUERY
RUDDY
RUGBY
RUMMY
RUNBY
RUNNY
RUNTY
RUSHY
RUSTY
RUTTY
SUCKY
SUDSY
SUETY
SULKY
SULLY
SUNNY
SURFY
SURLY
TUBBY
TUFTY
TULLY
TUMMY
TURFY
TURVY
TUSHY
VUGGY
YUCKY
YUMMY

••U•Y
CLUNY
COUSY
DEUCY
DOUAY
DRURY
FLUKY
FLUTY
GAUDY
GAUZY
GLUEY
GOUDY
GOUTY
LOURY
LOUSY
MAURY
MOUSY
PLUMY
POUTY
SAUCY
SOUPY
SPUMY
STUDY
TRUDY
TRULY
USURY

•••UY
MYGUY
PEGUY
REBUY

UZ•••
UZBEK

U•Z••
UNZIP

•UZ••
BUZZI
BUZZY
CUZCO
FUZZY
LUZON
MUZAK
MUZZY
OUZEL
OUZOS
SUZIE
SUZYQ

•U•Z•
BUZZI
BUZZY
FURZE
FUZZY
KUDZU
MUZZY
NUDZH

•U••Z
HUNTZ
KURTZ
NUNEZ

••UZ•
ABUZZ
DOUZE
DRUZE
EBUZZ
GAUZE
GAUZY
ISUZU
SCUZZ

••U•Z
ABUZZ
EBUZZ
KLUTZ
SCUZZ
STUTZ

•••UZ
RAMUZ
SOYUZ
VADUZ

VA•••
VACAS
VACHE
VACUA
VADER
VADIM
VADIS
VADUZ
VAGUE
VAGUS
VALES
VALET
VALID
VALLE
VALLI
VALOR
VALSE
VALUE
VALVE
VAMOS
VAMPA
VAMPS
VAMPY
VANCE
VANED
VANES
VANNA
VANUA
VANYA
VAPID
VAPOR
VARDA
VARIA
VARIG
VARNA
VARRO
VARSI
VARYA
VASCO
VASES
VASTI
VASTS
VASTY
VATER
VATIC
VATUS
VAULT
VAUNT
VAXES

V•A••
VDAYS
VEALE
VEALS
VEALY
VIALS
VIAND
VLADE

V••A•
VACAS
VEDAS
VEDAY
VEGAN
VEGAS
VELAR
VENAE
VENAL
VICAR
VIDAL
VIDAS
VIJAY
VILAS
VINAS
VIRAL
VISAS
VITAE
VITAL
VITAM
VITAS
VIVAS
VJDAY
VOCAB
VOCAL
VOLAR

V•••A
VACUA
VAMPA
VANNA
VANUA
VANYA
VARDA
VARIA
VARNA
VARYA
VELDA
VELMA
VELVA
VENTA
VERNA
VERSA
VESPA
VESTA
VIEJA
VIGIA
VILLA
VILMA
VILNA
VIOLA
VIRGA
VIRNA
VISTA
VODKA
VOILA
VOLGA
VOLTA
VONDA

•VA••
AVAIL
AVANT
AVAST
EVADE
EVANS
IVANA
IVANI
IVANV
KVACK
KVASS
OVALS
OVARY
OVATE
TVADS
YVAIN

•V•A•
AVGAS
AVIAN
AVIAS
EVIAN
TVMAN
UVEAL
UVEAS
UVRAY

•V••A
AVENA
AVILA
DVINA
EVITA
EVORA
IVANA
OVETA
UVULA

••VA•
ALVAR
CAVAE
CAVAN
DAVAO
DEVAS
DIVAC
DIVAN
DIVAS
DUVAL
EAVAN
JAVAN
JAVAS
JOVAN
KAVAS
KIVAS
LAVAL
LAVAS
LEVAR
NAVAL
NIVAL
NOVAE
NOVAK
NOVAS
ORVAL
RIVAL
SIVAN
TOVAH
VIVAS

••V•A
FIVEA
LIVIA
NIVEA
NOVIA
PAVIA

•••VA
ALAVA
BELVA
BRAVA
CHAVA
DRAVA
FLAVA
GUAVA
HALVA
LARVA
NERVA
NUEVA
NUOVA
OLIVA
SHIVA
SILVA
SNEVA
VELVA

V•B••
VIBES
VWBUG

V••B•
VERBS

V•••B
VOCAB

••V•B
FIVEB

VC•••
VCHIP

V•C••
VACAS
VACHE
VACUA
VICAR
VICES
VICHY
VICKI
VICKS
VICKY
VOCAB
VOCAL

V••C•
VANCE
VASCO
VEECK
VESCO
VETCH
VINCE
VINCI
VINCY
VLECK
VNECK
VOICE
VOICI
VOUCH

V•••C
VATIC
VEDIC
VINIC

•V•C•
EVICT
KVACK
TVVCR

••VC•
TVVCR

••V•C
CIVIC
DIVAC
FIVEC
HAVOC
KOVIC

VD•••
VDAYS

V•D••
VADER
VADIM
VADIS
VADUZ
VEDAS
VEDAY
VEDIC
VIDAL
VIDAS
VIDEO
VIDOR
VJDAY
VODKA

V••D•
VARDA
VEIDT
VELDA
VELDS
VELDT
VENDS
VERDE
VERDI
VLADE
VOIDS
VONDA

V•••D
VALID
VANED
VAPID
VEXED
VIAND
VINED
VIRID
VISED
VIVID
VOTED
VOWED

•VD••
TVDVD

•V•D•
AVIDE
EVADE
TVADS

•V••D
AVOID
IVIED
OVOID
TVDVD

••VD•
BLVDS

••V•D
BOVID
CAVED
COVED
DAVID
DIVED
EAVED
FIVED
HIVED
JIVED
LAVED
LIVED
LIVID
LOVED
MOVED
PAVED
PAVID
RAVED
RIVED
ROVED
RSVPD
SAVED
VIVID
WAVED
WIVED

•••VD
ONDVD
TVDVD

VE•••
VEALE
VEALS
VEALY
VEDAS
VEDAY
VEDIC
VEECK
VEEPS
VEERS
VEERY
VEGAN
VEGAS
VEGES
VEIDT
VEILS
VEINS
VEINY
VELAR
VELDA
VELDS
VELDT
VELEZ
VELMA
VELOX
VELUM
VELVA
VENAE
VENAL
VENDS
VENEZ
VENIN
VENLO
VENOM
VENTA
VENTI
VENTO
VENTS
VENUE
VENUS
VERBS
VERDE
VERDI
VERGE
VERMI
VERNA
VERNE
VERRE
VERSA
VERSE
VERSO
VERST
VERTE
VERTS
VERVE
VESCO
VESPA
VESTA
VESTI
VESTS
VETCH
VETTE
VEXED
VEXER
VEXES
VEZES

V•E••
VEECK
VEEPS
VEERS
VEERY
VIEJA
VIEJO
VIERS
VIEUX
VIEWS
VIEWY
VLECK
VNECK
VTENS

V••E•
VADER
VALES
VALET
VANED
VANES
VASES
VATER
VAXES
VEGES
VELEZ
VENEZ
VEXED
VEXER
VEXES
VEZES
VIBES
VICES
VIDEO
VIKES
VILER
VINED
VINER
VINES
VIPER
VIREO
VISED
VISES
VIXEN
VOGEL
VOLES
VOMER
VOTED
VOTER
VOTES
VOWED
VOWEL
VOWER

V•••E
VACHE
VAGUE
VALLE
VALSE
VALUE
VALVE
VANCE
VEALE
VENAE
VENUE
VERDE
VERGE
VERNE
VERRE
VERSE
VERTE
VERVE
VETTE
VHONE
VILLE
VINCE
VITAE
VIVRE
VLADE
VOGUE
VOICE
VOILE
VOLPE
VOLTE
VOTRE
VTILE
VTYPE

•VE••
AVENA
AVERS
AVERT
AVERY
EVENS
EVENT
EVERS
EVERT
EVERY
KVELL
OVENS
OVERS
OVERT
OVETA
OVETT
RVERS
UVEAL
UVEAS

•V•E•
AVNET
IVIED
IVIES
TVMEN
TVSET

•V••E
AVIDE
EVADE
EVITE
EVOKE
OVATE
OVINE
OVULE

••VE•
AMVET
BEVEL
BOVET
CAVED
CAVER
CAVES
CIVET
COVED
COVEN
COVER
COVES
COVET
COVEY
CUVEE
DAVEN
DAVES
DAVEY
DIVED
DIVER
DIVES
DOVER
DOVES
DOVEY
DUVET
EAVED
EAVES
ELVER
ELVES
ENVER
FAVES
FEVER
FIVEA
FIVEB
FIVEC
FIVED
FIVEE
FIVEO
FIVER
FIVES
GAVEL
GIVEN
GIVER
GIVES
HAVEL
HAVEN
HAVER
HAVES
HIVED
HIVER
HIVES
HOVEL
HOVER
HOVEY
INVER
JIVED
JIVER
JIVES
JIVEY
LAVED
LAVER
LAVES
LEVEE
LEVEL
LEVER
LIVED
LIVEN
LIVER
LIVES
LOVED
LOVER
LOVES
LOVEY
MAVEN
MOVED
MOVER
MOVES
NAVEE
NAVEL
NAVES
NEVER
NEVES
NIVEA
NIVEN
NOVEL
NOVEM
OYVEY
PAVED
PAVEL
PAVER
PAVES
PIVEN
RAVED
RAVEL
RAVEN
RAVER
RAVES
REVEL
REVES
REVET
RIVED
RIVEN
RIVER
RIVES
RIVET
ROVED
ROVER
ROVES
SAVED
SAVER
SAVES
SEVEN
SEVER
TAVEL
TEVET
TOVES
TYVEK
WAVED
WAVER
WAVES
WIVED
WIVES
WOVEN

••V•E
CAVAE CUVEE DAVIE FAVRE FIVEE HAVRE LAVIE LEVEE LIVRE MCVIE MOVIE NAVEE NOVAE REVUE TEVYE VIVRE

•••VE
ABOVE AGAVE ALEVE ALIVE ATIVE AWAVE BFIVE BRAVE BREVE CALVE CARVE CHIVE CLAVE CLEVE CLIVE CLOVE CRAVE CREVE CURVE DELVE DRIVE DROVE ELEVE FAUVE GLOVE GRAVE GROVE HALVE HEAVE HERVE IFIVE IGIVE ILOVE IMOVE JOUVE KNAVE LEAVE LWAVE MAEVE MAUVE NAIVE NERVE NIEVE NUEVE OGIVE OLIVE PEEVE PIAVE PROVE REAVE REEVE SALVE SERVE SHAVE SHOVE SIEVE SLAVE SOAVE SOLVE STAVE STEVE STOVE SUAVE TRAVE TROVE VALVE VERVE WAIVE WEAVE YOUVE

VF•••
VFOUR

V•G••
VAGUE VAGUS VEGAN VEGAS VEGES VIGGO VIGIA VIGIL VIGNY VIGOR VOGEL VOGUE VUGGY

V••G•
VERGE VIGGO VINGT VIRGA VIRGO VOLGA VSIGN VUGGY

V•••G
VARIG VWBUG VYING

•VG••
AVGAS

•V••G
RVING

••V•G
NAVIG

VH•••
VHONE

V•H••
VCHIP

V••H•
VACHE VICHY

V•••H
VETCH VOUCH

•VH••
TVHIT

••V•H
TOVAH

VI•••
VIALS VIAND VIBES VICAR VICES VICHY VICKI VICKS VICKY VIDAL VIDAS VIDEO VIDOR VIEJA VIEJO VIERS VIEUX VIEWS VIEWY VIGGO VIGIA VIGIL VIGNY VIGOR VIJAY VIKES VIKKI VILAS VILER VILLA VILLE VILLI VILMA VILNA VINAS VINCE VINCI VINCY VINED VINER VINES VINGT VINIC VINNY VINOS VINYL VIOLA VIOLS VIPER VIRAL VIREO VIRGA VIRGO VIRID VIRNA VIRTU VIRUS VISAS VISED VISES VISIT VISOR VISTA VITAE VITAL VITAM VITAS VITRI VITRO VITUS VIVAS VIVID VIVRE VIXEN VIZIR VIZOR

V•I••
VEIDT VEILS VEINS VEINY VOICE VOICI VOIDS VOILA VOILE VOIPS VSIGN VTILE VYING

V••I•
VADIM VADIS VALID VAPID VARIA VARIG VATIC VCHIP VEDIC VENIN VIGIA VIGIL VINIC VIRID VISIT VIVID VIZIR

V•••I
VALLI VARSI VASTI VENTI VERDI VERMI VESTI VICKI VIKKI VILLI VINCI VITRI VOICI

•VI••
AVIAN AVIAS AVIDE AVILA AVION AVIOR AVISO CVIII DVIII DVINA EVIAN EVICT EVILS EVITA EVITE IVIED IVIES IVINS LVIII MVIII OVINE OVITZ RVING XVIII

•V•I•
AVAIL AVOID AVOIR AVRIL CVIII DVIII LVIII MVIII OVOID TVHIT XVIII YVAIN

•V••I
CVIII DVIII IVANI LVIII MVIII OVOLI XVIII

••VI•
ADVIL ALVIN ANVIL AUVIN BEVIN BOVID CAVIL CCVII CDVII CIVIC CIVIL CLVII CMVII CXVII DAVID DAVIE DAVIS DAVIT DCVII DEVIL DLVII DXVII ELVIN ELVIS ERVIN GAVIN HOVIS IRVIN KEVIN KOVIC LAVIE LAVIN LEVIN LEVIS LEVIT LIVIA LIVID LIVIN LOVIN LXVII MAVIN MAVIS MCVIE MCVII MDVII MLVII MMVII MOVIE MOVIN MXVII NAVIG NAVIS NEVIL NEVIN NEVIS NOVIA NOVIO ORVIS PAVIA PAVID PAVIN QBVII TAVIS VIVID XCVII XLVII XXVII

••V•I
CCVII CDVII CLVII CMVII CXVII DCVII DLVII DXVII ENVOI LXVII MCVII MDVII MLVII MMVII MXVII QBVII XCVII XLVII XXVII

•••VI
BREVI CCCVI CCLVI CCXVI CDLVI CDXVI CLXVI CMLVI CMXVI CURVI CXCVI CXLVI CXXVI DCCVI DCLVI DCXVI DLXVI DXCVI DXLVI DXXVI GRAVI LEOVI LXXVI MCCVI MCDVI MCLVI MCMVI MCXVI MDCVI MDLVI MDXVI MLXVI MMCVI MMDVI MMLVI MMMVI MMXVI MXCVI MXLVI MXXVI OLAVI PLUVI TREVI XXXVI

VJ•••
VJDAY

V•J••
VIJAY

V••J•
VIEJA VIEJO

••V•J
MTVVJ

•••VJ
MTVVJ

V•K••
VIKES VIKKI

V••K•
VICKI VICKS VICKY VIKKI VODKA

V•••K
VEECK VLECK VNECK

•V•K•
EVOKE

•V••K
KVACK

••V•K
NOVAK TYVEK

VL•••
VLADE VLECK

V•L••
VALES VALET VALID VALLE VALLI VALOR VALSE VALUE VALVE VELAR VELDA VELDS VELDT VELEZ VELMA VELOX VELUM VELVA VILAS VILER VILLA VILLE VILLI VILMA VILNA VOLAR VOLES VOLGA VOLPE VOLTA VOLTE VOLTS VOLVO

V••L•
VALLE VALLI VAULT VEALE VEALS VEALY VEILS VENLO VIALS VILLA VILLE VILLI VIOLA VIOLS VOILA VOILE VTILE VTOLS

V•••L
VENAL VIDAL VIGIL VINYL VIRAL VITAL VOCAL VOGEL VOWEL

•VL••
RVLOT

•V•L•
AVILA EVILS KVELL OVALS OVOLI OVOLO OVULE UVULA

•V••L
AVAIL AVRIL KVELL UVEAL

••V•L
ADVIL ANVIL BEVEL CAVIL CIVIL DEVIL DEVOL DUVAL GAVEL HAVEL HOVEL LAVAL LEVEL NAVAL NAVEL NEVIL NIVAL NOVEL ORVAL PAVEL RAVEL REVEL RIVAL TAVEL

V•M••
VAMOS VAMPA VAMPS VAMPY VOMER

V••M•
VELMA VERMI VILMA

V•••M
VADIM VELUM VENOM VITAM VROOM

•VM••
TVMAN TVMEN

••V•M
NOVEM

VN•••
VNECK

V•N••
VANCE VANED VANES VANNA VANUA VANYA VENAE VENAL VENDS VENEZ VENIN VENLO VENOM VENTA VENTI VENTO VENTS VENUE VENUS VINAS VINCE VINCI VINCY VINED VINER VINES VINGT VINIC VINNY VINOS VINYL VONDA

V••N•
VANNA VARNA VAUNT VEINS VEINY VERNA VERNE VHONE VIAND VIGNY VILNA VINNY VIRNA VTENS VYING

V•••N
VEGAN VENIN VIXEN VSIGN

•VN••
AVNET

•V•N•
AVANT AVENA DVINA EVANS EVENS EVENT IVANA IVANI IVANV IVINS OVENS OVINE RVING

•V••N
AVIAN AVION EVIAN TVMAN TVMEN YVAIN

••V•N
ALVIN AUVIN BEVIN CAVAN COVEN DAVEN DEVON DIVAN EAVAN ELVIN ERVIN GAVIN GIVEN HAVEN IRVIN JAVAN JOVAN KEVIN KEVON LAVIN LEVIN LEVON LIVEN LIVIN LOVIN MAVEN MAVIN MOVIN NEVIN NIVEN PAVIN PIVEN RAVEN RIVEN SEVEN SIVAN WOVEN ZEVON

VO•••
VOCAB VOCAL VODKA VOGEL VOGUE VOICE VOICI VOIDS VOILA VOILE VOIPS VOLAR VOLES VOLGA VOLPE VOLTA VOLTE VOLTS VOLVO VOMER VONDA VOTED VOTER VOTES VOTRE VOUCH VOWED VOWEL VOWER

V•O••
VFOUR VHONE VIOLA VIOLS VROOM VTOLS

V••O•
VALOR VAMOS VAPOR VELOX VENOM VIDOR VIGOR VINOS VISOR VIZOR VROOM

V•••O
VARRO VASCO VENLO VENTO VERSO VESCO VIDEO VIEJO VIGGO VIREO VIRGO VITRO VOLVO

•VO••
AVOID AVOIR AVOWS EVOKE EVORA IVORY OVOID OVOLI OVOLO

•V•O•
AVION AVIOR RVLOT

•V••O
AVISO OVOLO

••VO•
DAVOS DEVOL DEVON DIVOT ENVOI ENVOY FAVOR GAVOT HAVOC KEVON LEVON PIVOT SAVOR SAVOY TIVOS ZEVON

••V•O
DAVAO FIVEO NOVIO

•••VO
ABOVO BRAVO CORVO HUEVO NERVO NORVO NUEVO NUOVO PAAVO PROVO SALVO SERVO TSAVO VOLVO

V•P••
VAPID VAPOR VIPER

V••P•
VAMPA VAMPS VAMPY VEEPS VESPA VOIPS VOLPE VTYPE

V•••P
VCHIP

••VP•
RSVPD RSVPS

••V•P
REVUP

•••VP
ALMVP NLMVP

VR•••
VROOM

V•R••
VARDA VARIA VARIG VARNA VARRO VARSI VARYA VERBS VERDE VERDI VERGE VERMI VERNA VERNE VERRE VERSA VERSE VERSO VERST VERTE VERTS VERVE VIRAL VIREO VIRGA VIRGO VIRID VIRNA VIRTU VIRUS

V••R•
VARRO VEERS VEERY VERRE VIERS VITRI VITRO VIVRE VOTRE

V•••R
VADER VALOR VAPOR VATER VELAR VEXER VFOUR VICAR VIDOR VIGOR VILER VINER VIPER VISOR VIZIR VIZOR VOLAR VOMER VOTER VOWER

•VR••
AVRIL UVRAY

•V•R•
AVERS AVERT AVERY EVERS EVERT EVERY EVORA IVORY OVARY OVERS OVERT RVERS

•V••R
AVIOR AVOIR TVVCR

••VR•
DEVRY FAVRE HAVRE LIVRE VIVRE

••V•R
ALVAR CAVER COVER DIVER DOVER ELVER ENVER FAVOR FEVER FIVER GIVER HAVER HIVER HOVER INVER JIVER LAVER LEVAR LEVER LIVER LOVER MOVER NEVER PAVER RAVER RIVER ROVER SAVER SAVOR SEVER TVVCR WAVER

VS•••
VSIGN

V•S••
VASCO VASES VASTI VASTS VASTY VESCO VESPA VESTA VESTI VESTS VISAS VISED VISES VISIT VISOR VISTA

V••S•
VALSE VARSI VERSA VERSE VERSO VERST

V•••S
VACAS VADIS VAGUS VALES VAMOS VAMPS VANES VASES VASTS VATUS VAXES VDAYS VEALS VEDAS VEEPS VEERS VEGAS VEGES VEILS VEINS VELDS VENDS VENTS VENUS VERBS VERTS VESTS VEXES VEZES VIALS VIBES VICES VICKS VIDAS VIERS VIEWS VIKES VILAS VINAS VINES VINOS VIOLS VIRUS VISAS VISES VITAS VITUS VIVAS VOIDS VOIPS VOLES VOLTS VOTES VTENS VTOLS

•VS••
TVSET

•V•S•
AVAST AVISO KVASS

5 VS

•V••S
AVERS
AVGAS
AVIAS
AVOWS
EVANS
EVENS
EVERS
EVILS
IVIES
IVINS
KVASS
OVALS
OVENS
OVERS
RVERS
TVADS
UVEAS

••V•S
BLVDS
CAVES
COVES
DAVES
DAVIS
DAVOS
DEVAS
DIVAS
DIVES
DOVES
EAVES
ELVES
ELVIS
FAVES
FIVES
GIVES
GOVTS
HAVES
HIVES
HOVIS
JAVAS
JIVES
KAVAS
KIVAS
LAVAS
LAVES
LEVIS
LIVES
LOVES
MAVIS
MOVES
NAVES
NAVIS
NEVES
NEVIS
NEVUS
NOVAS
NOVUS
ORVIS
PAVES
RAVES
REVES
RIVES
ROVES
RSVPS
SAVES
TAVIS
TIVOS
TOVES
VIVAS
WAVES
WIVES

•••VS
ELEVS
EREVS
HDTVS
MIRVS
PROVS
SHIVS
SLAVS
UNIVS

VT•••
VTENS
VTILE
VTOLS
VTYPE

V•T••
VATER
VATIC
VATUS
VETCH
VETTE
VITAE
VITAL
VITAM
VITAS
VITRI
VITRO
VITUS
VOTED
VOTER
VOTES
VOTRE

V••T•
VASTI
VASTS
VASTY
VENTA
VENTI
VENTO
VENTS
VERTE
VERTS
VESTA
VESTI
VESTS
VETTE
VIRTU
VISTA
VOLTA
VOLTE
VOLTS

V•••T
VALET
VAULT
VAUNT
VEIDT
VELDT
VERST
VINGT
VISIT

•V•T•
EVITA
EVITE
OVATE
OVETA
OVETT
OVITZ

•V••T
AVANT
AVAST
AVERT
AVNET
EVENT
EVERT
EVICT
OVERT
OVETT
RVLOT
TVHIT
TVSET

••VT•
GOVTS

••V•T
AMVET
BOVET
CIVET
COVET
DAVIT
DIVOT
DUVET
GAVOT
LEVIT
PIVOT
REVET
RIVET
TEVET

VU•••
VUGGY

V•U••
VAULT
VAUNT
VOUCH

V••U•
VACUA
VADUZ
VAGUE
VAGUS
VALUE
VANUA
VATUS
VELUM
VENUE
VENUS
VFOUR
VIEUX
VIRUS
VITUS
VOGUE
VWBUG

V•••U
VIRTU

•VU••
OVULE
UVULA

••VU•
NEVUS
NOVUS
REVUE
REVUP

V•V••
VIVAS
VIVID
VIVRE

V••V•
VALVE
VELVA
VERVE
VOLVO

•VV••
TVVCR

•V•V•
TVDVD

•V••V
IVANV

••VV•
DIVVY
MTVVJ
SAVVY

•••VV
OLAVV

VW•••
VWBUG
VWXYZ

V•W••
VOWED
VOWEL
VOWER

V••W•
VIEWS
VIEWY

•VW••
UVWXY

•V•W•
AVOWS

••VW•
TUVWX

•••VW
STUVW

V•X••
VAXES
VEXED
VEXER
VEXES
VIXEN
VWXYZ

V•••X
VELOX
VIEUX

•V•X•
UVWXY

••V•X
TUVWX

VY•••
VYING

V•Y••
VTYPE

V••Y•
VANYA
VARYA
VDAYS
VINYL
VWXYZ

V•••Y
VAMPY
VASTY
VEALY
VEDAY
VEERY
VEINY
VICHY
VICKY
VIEWY
VIGNY
VIJAY
VINCY
VINNY
VJDAY
VUGGY

•V••Y
AVERY
EVERY
IVORY
OVARY
UVRAY
UVWXY

••VY•
TEVYE

••V•Y
COVEY
DAVEY
DEVRY
DIVVY
DOVEY
ENVOY
HOVEY
JIVEY
LOVEY
OYVEY
SAVOY
SAVVY

•••VY
CHEVY
CHIVY
CONVY
CURVY
DIVVY
GRAVY
HEAVY
MARVY
NERVY
PRIVY
SAVVY
TURVY

V•Z••
VEZES
VIZIR
VIZOR

V•••Z
VADUZ
VELEZ
VENEZ
VWXYZ

•V••Z
OVITZ

WA•••
WAACS
WAALS
WAART
WACKO
WACKY
WADED
WADER
WADES
WADIS
WADUP
WAFER
WAFTS
WAGED
WAGER
WAGES
WAGON
WAHOO
WAIFS
WAILS
WAINS
WAIST
WAITE
WAITS
WAITZ
WAIVE
WAJDA
WAKAS
WAKED
WAKEN
WAKER
WAKES
WAKKO
WALDO
WALED
WALES
WALKS
WALLA
WALLS
WALLY
WALSH
WALSY
WALTZ
WANDA
WANDS
WANED
WANER
WANES
WANLY
WANNA
WANTS
WARDS
WARED
WARES
WARKS
WARMS
WARNS
WARPS
WARTS
WARTY
WASAT
WASCO
WASHO
WASHY
WASIN
WASIT
WASNT
WASON
WASPS
WASPY
WASSO
WASTE
WASUP
WATCH
WATER
WATTS
WAUGH
WAVED
WAVER
WAVES
WAWAS
WAXED
WAXEN
WAXER
WAXES
WAXUP
WAYIN
WAYNE
WAYUP

W•A••
WAACS
WAALS
WAART
WEALD
WEALS
WEANS
WEARS
WEARY
WEAVE
WHACK
WHALE
WHAMO
WHAMS
WHANG
WHAPS
WHARF
WHATD
WHATS
WOADS
WRACK
WRAPS
WRAPT
WRATH
WYATT

W••A•
WAKAS
WASAT
WAWAS
WEBAD
WHEAT
WINAT
WOFAT
WOMAN
WONAT
WOPAT
WOTAN
WREAK
WUHAN
WYMAN

W•••A
WAJDA
WALLA
WANDA
WANNA
WEENA
WELLA
WICCA
WILLA
WILMA
WONKA
WUXIA

•WA••
AWACS
AWAIT
AWAKE
AWARD
AWARE
AWASH
AWAVE
BWANA
DWARF
EWALD
EWART
IWANT
KWAME
LWAVE
NWAPA
SWABS
SWAGS
SWAIN
SWALE
SWAMI
SWAMP
SWANK
SWANN
SWANS
SWAPS
SWARD
SWARM
SWASH
SWATH
SWATS
SWAYS
SWAZI
TWAIN
TWANG
YWAIN

•W•A•
SWEAR
SWEAT
TWEAK
TWOAD
TWOAM
YWCAS
YWHAS

•W••A
BWANA
NWAPA
TWYLA

••WA•
ADWAR
AGWAY
AIWAS
ALWAY
AMWAY
ANWAR
ASWAN
ASWAY
ATWAR
BYWAY
DEWAR
DEWAX
ELWAY
HOWAR
IOWAN
IOWAS
IOWAU
IOWAY
JAWAT
MOWAT
MYWAR
MYWAY
NEWAT
NOWAY
OTWAY
PAWAT
POWAY
REWAX
ROWAN
TEWAS
TIWAS
TOWAR
WAWAS

••W•A
YOWZA

•••WA
DAIWA
FATWA
KIOWA
OZAWA
SCHWA
SLIWA
URAWA

W•B••
WEBAD
WEBBY
WEBER
WEBTV

W••B•
WEBBY
WELBY
WIEBE
WILBY
WINBY
WOMBS
WONBY

•WB••
VWBUG

•W•B•
SWABS
TWOBC

•W••B
DWEEB

•••WB
THEWB

W•C••
WACKO
WACKY
WICCA
WICKS

W••C•
WAACS
WASCO
WATCH
WELCH
WENCH
WHACK
WHICH
WICCA
WILCO
WINCE
WINCH
WITCH
WRACK
WRECK

•WC••
YWCAS

•W•C•
AWACS
TWICE
ZWICK

•W••C
TWOBC

W•D••
WADED
WADER
WADES
WADIS
WADUP
WEDEL
WEDGE
WEDGY
WEDTO
WIDEN
WIDER
WIDOW
WIDTH
WODEN

W••D•
WAJDA
WALDO
WANDA
WANDS
WARDS
WEEDS
WEEDY
WELDS
WENDS
WENDT
WENDY
WILDE
WILDS
WINDS
WINDY
WOADS
WOODS
WOODY
WORDS
WORDY
WUNDT

W•••D
WADED
WAGED
WAKED
WALED
WANED
WARED
WAVED
WAXED
WEBAD
WEIRD
WHATD
WIELD
WILED
WINED
WIPED
WIRED
WISED
WIVED
WOOED
WORLD
WOULD
WOUND
WOWED

•W•D•
SWEDE

•W••D
AWARD
AWNED
EWALD
OWNED
SWARD
SWORD
TWEED
TWOAD

••WD•
BAWDY
DOWDY
GOWDY
HOWDO
HOWDY
ROWDY

••W•D
BOWED
CAWED
CLWYD
COWED
DEWED
HAWED
HEWED
JAWED
LAWED
LOWED
MEWED
MOWED
PAWED
REWED
ROWED
SAWED
SEWED
SOWED
TOWED
UNWED
VOWED
WOWED
YAWED

•••WD
CROWD

WE•••
WEALD
WEALS
WEANS
WEARS
WEARY
WEAVE
WEBAD
WEBBY
WEBER
WEBTV
WEDEL
WEDGE
WEDGY
WEDTO
WEEDS
WEEDY
WEEKS
WEEMS
WEENA
WEENY
WEEPS
WEEPY
WEEST
WEEUN
WEFTS
WEIGH
WEILL
WEIRD
WEIRS
WEISS
WEISZ
WEITZ
WELBY
WELCH
WELDS
WELLA
WELLS
WELSH
WELTS
WELTY
WENCH
WENDS
WENDT
WENDY
WESER
WESTS
WETLY
WEWON
WEZEN

W•E••
WEEDS
WEEDY
WEEKS
WEEMS
WEENA
WEENY
WEEPS
WEEPY
WEEST
WEEUN
WHEAT
WHEEL
WHEES
WHELK
WHELM
WHELP
WHENS
WHERE
WHETS
WHEWS
WHEYS
WIEBE
WIELD
WIEST
WREAK
WRECK
WRENS
WREST
WYETH

W••E•
WADED
WADER
WADES
WAFER
WAGED
WAGER
WAGES
WAKED
WAKEN
WAKER
WAKES
WALED
WALES
WANED
WANER
WANES
WARED
WARES
WATER
WAVED
WAVER
WAVES
WAXED
WAXEN
WAXER
WAXES
WEBER
WEDEL
WESER
WEZEN
WHEEL
WHEES
WIDEN
WIDER
WIFEY
WILED
WILEE
WILES
WILEY
WINED
WINES
WIPED
WIPER
WIPES
WIRED
WIRER
WIRES
WISED
WISER
WISES
WIVED
WIVES
WIZEN
WIZES
WODEN
WOKEN
WOMEN
WOOED
WOOER
WOVEN
WOWED
WOWEE
WOWEM
WRIER
WRYER
WYLER

W•••E
WAITE
WAIVE
WASTE
WAYNE
WEAVE
WEDGE
WHALE
WHERE
WHILE
WHINE
WHITE
WHOLE
WHOME
WHOSE
WHYME
WHYRE
WHYTE
WIEBE
WILDE
WILEE
WINCE
WITTE
WOLFE
WORSE
WOWEE
WOWIE
WRITE
WROTE
WTILE
WYLIE
WYNNE
WYTHE

•WE••
AWEEK
DWEEB
DWELL
DWELT
EWEEK
EWELL
EWERS
EWERY
GWENN
LWEIS
OWENS
OWEON
OWERS
QWEST
SWEAR
SWEAT
SWEDE
SWEEP
SWEET
SWELL
SWEPT
TWEAK
TWEED
TWEEN
TWEET
TWERE
TWERP
ZWEIG

•W•E•
AWEEK
AWGEE
AWNED
DWEEB
EWEEK
OWIES
OWLET
OWNED
OWNER
SWEEP
SWEET
TWEED
TWEEN
TWEET
TWOEE
TWOEM

•W••E
AWAKE
AWARE
AWAVE
AWGEE
AWOKE
KWAME
LWAVE
SWALE
SWEDE
SWINE
SWIPE
SWORE
TWERE
TWICE
TWINE
TWOEE

••WE•
ARWEN
BOWED
BOWEL
BOWEN
BOWER
BOWES
CAWED
COWED
COWER
COWES
DAWES
DEWED
DEWEY
DOWEL
ELWES
FEWER
GOWER
HAWED
HAWER
HEWED
HEWER
HOWES
JAWED
JAWER
JEWEL
LAWED
LAWES
LEWES
LOWED
LOWER
LOWES
MEWED
MEWER
MOWED
MOWEN
MOWER
NEWEL
NEWER
NGWEE
PAWED
PAWER
PEWEE
POWER
RAWER
REWED
REWET
ROWED
ROWEL
ROWEN
ROWER
SAWED
SAWER
SEWED
SEWER
SOWED
SOWER
TEWES
TOWED
TOWEL
TOWER
UNWED
UNWET
VOWED
VOWEL
VOWER
WOWED
WOWEE
WOWEM
YAWED

••W•E
BOWIE
DOWSE
HAWKE
HAWSE
HOWIE
NEWIE
NGWEE
PEWEE
ROWSE
TOWNE
WOWEE
WOWIE
YOWIE
ZOWIE

•••WE
CROWE
INAWE
KREWE
LOEWE
SNOWE
STOWE
TROWE

W•F••
WAFER
WAFTS
WEFTS
WIFEY
WOFAT

W••F•
WAIFS
WHIFF
WOLFE
WOLFF
WOLFS
WOOFS

W•••F
WHARF
WHIFF
WOLFF
WOOLF

•WF••
AWFUL

•W•F•
LWOFF SWIFT

•W••F
DWARF LWOFF ZWOLF

••W•F
MTWTF ROWLF

W•G••
WAGED WAGER WAGES WAGON WIGGY WIGHT

W••G•
WAUGH WEDGE WEDGY WEIGH WHIGS WIGGY WINGS WINGY

W•••G
WHANG WRING WRONG WRUNG

•WG••
AWGEE

•W•G•
SWAGS SWIGS TWIGS

•W••G
AWING EWING OWING SWING SWUNG TWANG VWBUG ZWEIG

••WG•
HAWGS

••W•G
BEWIG UNWIG

WH•••
WHACK WHALE WHAMO WHAMS WHANG WHAPS WHARF WHATD WHATS WHEAT WHEEL WHEES WHELK WHELM WHELP WHENS WHERE WHETS WHEWS WHEYS WHICH WHIFF WHIGS WHILE WHIMS WHINE WHINY WHIPS WHIPT WHIRL WHIRR WHIRS WHISH WHISK WHIST WHITE WHITS WHOLE WHOLL WHOME WHOMP WHOOP WHOPS WHORL WHOSE WHOSO WHUPS WHYLL WHYME WHYRE WHYTE

W•H••
WAHOO WUHAN

W••H•
WASHO WASHY WIGHT WISHY WUSHU WYTHE

W•••H
WALSH WATCH WAUGH WEIGH WELCH WELSH WENCH WHICH WHISH WIDTH WINCH WIRTH WITCH WOOSH WORTH WRATH WROTH WYETH

•WH••
AWHIT YWHAS

•W••H
AWASH IWISH SWASH SWATH SWISH

••WH•
DRWHO

••W•H
CRWTH LOWPH

WI•••
WICCA WICKS WIDEN WIDER WIDOW WIDTH WIEBE WIELD WIEST WIFEY WIGGY WIGHT WIKIS WILBY WILCO WILDE WILDS WILED WILEE WILES WILEY WILLA WILLS WILLY WILMA WILTS WIMPS WIMPY WINAT WINBY WINCE WINCH WINDS WINDY WINED WINES WINGS WINGY WINKS WIPED WIPER WIPES WIRED WIRER WIRES WIRTH WISED WISER WISES WISHY WISPS WISPY WITCH WITTE WITTY WIVED WIVES WIZEN WIZES

W•I••
WAIFS WAILS WAINS WAIST WAITE WAITS WAITZ WAIVE WEIGH WEILL WEIRD WEIRS WEISS WEISZ WEITZ WHICH WHIFF WHIGS WHILE WHIMS WHINE WHINY WHIPS WHIPT WHIRL WHIRR WHIRS WHISH WHISK WHIST WHITE WHITS WRIER WRING WRIST WRITE WRITS WTILE

W••I•
WADIS WASIN WASIT WAYIN WIKIS WOWIE WUXIA WYLIE

•WI••
AWING EWING IWILL IWISH OWIES OWING SWIFT SWIGS SWILL SWIMS SWINE SWING SWIPE SWIRL SWISH SWISS TWICE TWIGS TWILL TWINE TWINS TWINY TWIRL TWIRP TWIST TWITS TWIXT ZWICK

•W•I•
AWAIT AWHIT LWEIS SWAIN TWAIN YWAIN ZWEIG

•W••I
SWAMI SWAZI

••WI•
ASWIM BEWIG BOWIE EDWIN ERWIN HOWIE IRWIN KIWIS LEWIS LOWIQ MOWIS NEWIE NOWIN PEWIT REWIN SAWII SAWIN SEWIN TOWIN TOWIT UNWIG WOWIE YOWIE ZOWIE

••W•I
SAWII

•••WI
LOEWI

W•J••
WAJDA

W•K••
WAKAS WAKED WAKEN WAKER WAKES WAKKO WIKIS WOKEN

W••K•
WACKO WACKY WAKKO WALKS WARKS WEEKS WICKS WINKS WONKA WONKS WORKS

W•••K
WHACK WHELK WHISK WRACK WREAK WRECK

•W•K•
AWAKE AWOKE EWOKS

•W••K
AWEEK EWEEK SWANK TWEAK ZWICK

••WK•
GAWKS GAWKY HAWKE HAWKS

W•L••
WALDO WALED WALES WALKS WALLA WALLS WALLY WALSH WALSY WALTZ WELBY WELCH WELDS WELLA WELLS WELSH WELTS WELTY WILBY WILCO WILDE WILDS WILED WILEE WILES WILEY WILLA WILLS WILLY WILMA WILTS WOLFE WOLFF WOLFS WYLER WYLIE

W••L•
WAALS WAILS WALLA WALLS WALLY WANLY WEALD WEALS WEILL WELLA WELLS WETLY WHALE WHELK WHELM WHELP WHILE WHOLE WHOLL WHYLL WIELD WILLA WILLS WILLY WOOLF WOOLS WOOLY WORLD WOULD WRYLY WTILE

W•••L
WEDEL WEILL WHEEL WHIRL WHOLL WHORL WHYLL

•WL••
OWLET

•W•L•
AWOLS DWELL DWELT EWALD EWELL IWILL SWALE SWELL SWILL TWILL TWYLA ZWOLF

•W••L
AWFUL DWELL EWELL IWILL SWELL SWILL SWIRL TWILL TWIRL

••WL•
BAWLS BOWLS COWLS FOWLS HOWLS JOWLS JOWLY LOWLY MEWLS NEWLY PAWLS RAWLS RAWLY ROWLF YAWLS YOWLS

••W•L
BOWEL DOWEL JEWEL NEWEL ROWEL TOWEL VOWEL

•••WL
BRAWL CRAWL DRAWL GROWL PROWL SCOWL SHAWL TRAWL

W•M••
WIMPS WIMPY WOMAN WOMBS WOMEN WOMYN WYMAN

W••M•
WARMS WEEMS WHAMO WHAMS WHIMS WHOME WHOMP WHYME WILMA WORMS WORMY

W•••M
WHELM WOWEM

•W•M•
KWAME SWAMI SWAMP SWIMS

•W••M
SWARM TWOAM TWOEM TWOPM

••W•M
ASWIM WOWEM

W•N••
WANDA WANDS WANED WANER WANES WANLY WANNA WANTS WENCH WENDS WENDT WENDY WINAT WINBY WINCE WINCH WINDS WINDY WINED WINES WINGS WINGY WINKS WONAT WONBY WONKA WONKS WONTS WUNDT WYNNE

W••N•
WAINS WANNA WARNS WASNT WAYNE WEANS WEENA WEENY WHANG WHENS WHINE WHINY WOUND WRENS WRING WRONG WRUNG WYNNE

W•••N
WAGON WAKEN WASIN WASON WAXEN WAYIN WEEUN WEWON WEZEN WIDEN WIZEN WODEN WOKEN WOMAN WOMEN WOMYN WOTAN WOVEN WUHAN WYMAN

•WN••
AWNED OWNED OWNER OWNUP

•W•N•
AWING BWANA EWING GWENN GWYNN IWANT IWONT OWENS OWING SWANK SWANN SWANS SWINE SWING SWUNG TWANG TWINE TWINS TWINY

•W••N
GWENN GWYNN OWEON SWAIN SWANN SWOON SWORN TWAIN TWEEN TWOON YWAIN

••WN•
DAWNN DAWNS DOWNS DOWNY FAWNS GOWNS LAWNS LAWNY PAWNS TAWNY TOWNE TOWNS YAWNS YAWNY

••W•N
ARWEN ASWAN BOWEN DAWNN EDWIN ERWIN IOWAN IRWIN LOWON MOWEN NOWIN REWIN REWON ROWAN ROWEN SAWIN SEWIN SEWON TOWIN UNWON WEWON

•••WN
BLOWN BRAWN BROWN CLOWN COOWN CROWN DRAWN DROWN FLOWN FROWN GNAWN GROWN KNOWN OTOWN PRAWN REOWN SHAWN SHOWN SPAWN

WO•••
WOADS WODEN WOFAT WOKEN WOLFE WOLFF WOLFS WOMAN WOMBS WOMEN WOMYN WONAT WONBY WONKA WONKS WONTS WOODS WOODY WOOED WOOER WOOFS WOOLF WOOLS WOOLY WOOSH WOOZY WOPAT WORDS WORDY WORKS WORLD WORMS WORMY WORRY WORSE WORST WORTH WORTS WOTAN WOULD WOUND WOVEN WOWED WOWEE WOWEM WOWIE

W•O••
WHOLE WHOLL WHOME WHOMP WHOOP WHOPS WHORL WHOSE WHOSO WOODS WOODY WOOED WOOER WOOFS WOOLF WOOLS WOOLY WOOSH WOOZY WRONG WROTE WROTH

W••O•
WAGON WAHOO WASON WEWON WHOOP WIDOW

W•••O
WACKO WAHOO WAKKO WALDO WASCO WASHO WASSO WEDTO WHAMO WHOSO WILCO

•WO••
AWOKE AWOLS EWOKS IWONT LWOFF SWOON SWOOP SWORD SWORE SWORN TWOAD TWOAM TWOBC TWOEE TWOEM TWOON TWOPM TWOUP ZWOLF

•W•O•
OWEON SWOON SWOOP TWOON

••WO•
LOWON OHWOW REWON SEWON UNWON WEWON

••W•O
BOWTO DRWHO HEWTO HOWDO HOWSO HOWTO NEWTO SAWTO

•••WO
ATTWO BYTWO INTWO ONTWO

W•P••
WIPED WIPER WIPES WOPAT

W••P•
WARPS WASPS WASPY WEEPS WEEPY WHAPS WHIPS WHIPT WHOPS WHUPS WIMPS WIMPY WISPS WISPY WRAPS WRAPT

W•••P
WADUP WASUP WAXUP WAYUP WHELP WHOMP WHOOP

•W•P•
NWAPA SWAPS SWEPT SWIPE TWOPM

•W••P
OWNUP SWAMP SWEEP SWOOP TWERP TWIRP TWOUP

••WP•
GAWPS LOWPH YAWPS

••W•P
SAWUP SEWUP

••W•Q
LOWIQ

WR•••
WRACK WRAPS WRAPT WRATH WREAK WRECK WRENS WREST WRIER WRING WRIST WRITE WRITS WRONG WROTE WROTH WRUNG WRYER WRYLY

W•R••
WARDS WARED WARES WARKS WARMS WARNS WARPS WARTS WARTY WIRED WIRER WIRES WIRTH WORDS WORDY WORKS WORLD WORMS WORMY WORRY WORSE WORST WORTH WORTS WURST

W••R•
WAART WEARS WEARY WEIRD WEIRS WHARF WHERE WHIRL WHIRR WHIRS WHORL WHYRE WORRY

W•••R
WADER WAFER WAGER WAKER WANER WATER WAVER WAXER WEBER WESER WHIRR WIDER WIPER WIRER WISER WOOER WRIER WRYER WYLER

•W•R•
AWARD AWARE DWARF EWART EWERS EWERY OWERS SWARD SWARM SWIRL SWORD SWORE SWORN TWERE TWERP TWIRL TWIRP

•W••R
OWNER SWEAR

••WR•
COWRY DOWRY JEWRY LOWRY

••W•R
ADWAR ANWAR ATWAR BOWER COWER DEWAR FEWER GOWER HAWER HEWER HOWAR JAWER LOWER MEWER MOWER MYWAR NEWER PAWER POWER RAWER ROWER SAWER SEWER SOWER TOWAR TOWER VOWER

W•S••
WASAT WASCO WASHO WASHY WASIN WASIT WASNT WASON WASPS WASPY WASSO WASTE WASUP WESER WESTS WISED WISER WISES WISHY WISPS WISPY WUSHU

W••S•
WAIST WALSH WALSY WASSO WEEST WEISS WEISZ WELSH WHISH WHISK WHIST WHOSE WHOSO WIEST WOOSH WORSE WORST

WREST
WRIST
WURST

W•••S
WAACS
WAALS
WADES
WADIS
WAFTS
WAGES
WAIFS
WAILS
WAINS
WAITS
WAKAS
WAKES
WALES
WALKS
WALLS
WANDS
WANES
WANTS
WARDS
WARES
WARKS
WARMS
WARNS
WARPS
WARTS
WASPS
WATTS
WAVES
WAWAS
WAXES
WEALS
WEANS
WEARS
WEEDS
WEEKS
WEEMS
WEEPS
WEFTS
WEIRS
WEISS
WELDS
WELLS
WELTS
WENDS
WESTS
WHAMS
WHAPS
WHATS
WHEES
WHENS
WHETS
WHEWS
WHEYS
WHIGS
WHIMS
WHIPS
WHIRS
WHITS
WHOPS
WHUPS
WICKS
WIKIS
WILDS
WILES
WILLS
WILTS
WIMPS
WINDS
WINES
WINGS
WINKS
WIPES
WIRES
WISES
WISPS
WIVES
WIZES
WOADS
WOLFS
WOMBS
WONKS
WONTS
WOODS
WOOFS
WOOLS
WORDS
WORKS
WORMS
WORTS
WRAPS
WRENS
WRITS

•W•S•
AWASH
IWISH
QWEST
SWASH
SWISH
SWISS
TWIST

•W••S
AWACS
AWOLS
EWERS
EWOKS
LWEIS
OWENS
OWERS
OWIES
SWABS
SWAGS
SWANS
SWAPS
SWATS
SWAYS
SWIGS
SWIMS
SWISS
TWIGS
TWINS
TWITS
YWCAS
YWHAS

••WS•
DOWSE
HAWSE
HOWSO
NEWSY
ROWSE

••W•S
AIWAS
BAWLS
BOWES
BOWLS
COWES
COWLS
DAWES
DAWNS
DOWNS
ELWES
FAWNS
FOWLS
GAWKS
GAWPS
GOWNS
HAWGS
HAWKS
HOWES
HOWLS
IOWAS
JOWLS
KIWIS
LAWES
LAWNS
LEWES
LEWIS
LOWES
MEWLS
MOWIS
NEWTS
PAWLS
PAWNS
POWYS
RAWLS
TEWAS
TEWES
TIWAS
TOWNS
WAWAS
YAWLS
YAWNS
YAWPS
YOWLS

•••WS
AVOWS
BLOWS
BREWS
BROWS
CHAWS
CHEWS
CHOWS
CLAWS
CLEWS
CRAWS
CREWS
CROWS
DHOWS
DRAWS
FLAWS
FLOWS
FROWS
GLOWS
GNAWS
GROWS
KNOWS
LOEWS
MEOWS
PLOWS
PROWS
SCOWS
SHOWS
SKEWS
SLAWS
SLEWS
SLOWS
SMEWS
SNOWS
SPEWS
STEWS
STOWS
THAWS
THEWS
TREWS
TROWS
VIEWS
WHEWS
YEOWS

WT•••
WTILE

W•T••
WATCH
WATER
WATTS
WETLY
WITCH
WITTE
WITTY
WOTAN
WYTHE

W••T•
WAFTS
WAITE
WAITS
WAITZ
WALTZ
WANTS
WARTS
WARTY
WASTE
WATTS
WEBTV
WEDTO
WEFTS
WEITZ
WELTS
WELTY
WESTS
WHATD
WHATS
WHETS
WHITE
WHITS
WHYTE
WIDTH
WILTS
WIRTH
WITTE
WITTY
WONTS
WORTH
WORTS
WRATH
WRITE
WRITS
WROTE
WROTH
WYATT
WYETH

W•••T
WAART
WAIST
WASAT
WASIT
WASNT
WEEST
WENDT
WHEAT
WHIPT
WHIST
WIEST
WIGHT
WINAT
WOFAT
WONAT
WOPAT
WORST
WRAPT
WREST
WRIST
WUNDT
WURST
WYATT

•W•T•
SWATH
SWATS
TWITS

•W••T
AWAIT
AWHIT
DWELT
EWART
IWANT
IWONT
OWLET
QWEST
SWEAT
SWEET
SWEPT
SWIFT
TWEET
TWIST
TWIXT

••WT•
BOWTO
CRWTH
HEWTO
HOWTO
MTWTF
NEWTO
NEWTS
SAWTO

••W•T
JAWAT
MOWAT
NEWAT
PAWAT
PEWIT
REWET
TOWIT
UNWET

•••WT
NETWT

WU•••
WUHAN
WUNDT
WURST
WUSHU
WUXIA

W•U••
WAUGH
WHUPS
WOULD
WOUND
WRUNG

W••U•
WADUP
WASUP
WAXUP
WAYUP
WEEUN

W•••U
WUSHU

•WU••
SWUNG

•W•U•
AWFUL
OWNUP
TWOUP
VWBUG

••WU•
SAWUP
SEWUP

••W•U
IOWAU

•••WU
DREWU
ILGWU

W•V••
WAVED
WAVER
WAVES
WIVED
WIVES
WOVEN

W••V•
WAIVE
WEAVE

W•••V
WEBTV

•W•V•
AWAVE
LWAVE

W•W••
WAWAS
WEWON
WOWED
WOWEE
WOWEM
WOWIE

W••W•
WHEWS

W•••W
WIDOW

••W•W
OHWOW

W•X••
WAXED
WAXEN
WAXER
WAXES
WAXUP
WAXUP
WUXIA

•WX••
VWXYZ

•W•X•
TWIXT

••WX•
UVWXY

••W•X
DEWAX
REWAX

•••WX
TUVWX

WY•••
WYATT
WYETH
WYLER
WYLIE
WYMAN
WYNNE
WYTHE

W•Y••
WAYIN
WAYNE
WAYUP
WHYLL
WHYME
WHYRE
WHYTE
WRYER
WRYLY

W••Y•
WHEYS
WOMYN

W•••Y
WACKY
WALLY
WALSY
WANLY
WARTY
WASHY
WASPY
WEARY
WEBBY
WEDGY
WEEDY
WEENY
WEEPY
WELBY
WELTY
WENDY
WETLY
WHINY
WIFEY
WIGGY
WILBY
WILEY
WILLY
WIMPY
WINBY
WINDY
WINGY
WISHY
WISPY
WITTY
WONBY
WOODY
WOOLY
WOOZY
WORDY
WORMY
WORRY
WRYLY

•WY••
GWYNN
TWYLA

•W•Y•
SWAYS
VWXYZ

•W••Y
EWERY
TWINY

••WY•
CLWYD
POWYS

••W•Y
AGWAY
ALWAY
AMWAY
ASWAY
BAWDY
BYWAY
COWRY
DEWEY
DOWDY
DOWNY
DOWRY
ELWAY
GAWKY
GOWDY
HOWDY
IOWAY
JEWRY
JOWLY
LAWNY
LOWLY
LOWRY
MYWAY
NEWLY
NEWSY
NOWAY
OTWAY
POWAY
RAWLY
ROWDY
TAWNY
UVWXY
YAWNY

•••WY
BLOWY
CHEWY
FLAWY
LOEWY
SHOWY
SNOWY
STEWY
THEWY
VIEWY

W•Z••
WEZEN
WIZEN
WIZES

W••Z•
WOOZY

W•••Z
WAITZ
WALTZ
WEISZ
WEITZ

•W•Z•
SWAZI

•W••Z
VWXYZ

••WZ•
YOWZA

XA•••
XACTO
XANDO
XANDY
XAXES
XAXIS

X•A••
XRAYS
XSARA

X•••A
XENIA
XHOSA
XSARA

•XA••
EXACT
EXALT
EXAMS
OXANA

•X•A•
AXIAL
AXMAN
EXPAT
IXNAY
OXFAM
UXMAL

•X••A
EXTRA
EXUMA
OXANA

••XA•
BEXAR
COXAE
HEXAD
LEXAN
PIXAR
SIXAD
SIXAM
TEXAN
TEXAS

••X•A
HOXHA
WUXIA

•••XA
ALEXA

X•B••
XEBEC

•XB••
OXBOW

•X••B
EXCUB
EXLIB
EXURB

••XB•
BIXBY
SIXBC

XC•••
XCIII
XCVII

X•C••
XACTO

X•••C
XEBEC
XERIC

•XC••
CXCII
CXCIV
CXCIX
CXCVI
DXCII
DXCIV
DXCIX
DXCVI
EXCEL
EXCON
EXCOP
EXCUB
MXCII
MXCIV
MXCIX
MXCVI

•X•C•
EXACT
EXECS

••XC•
CCXCI
CCXCV
CDXCI
CDXCV
CMXCI
CMXCV
DCXCI
DCXCV
MCXCI
MCXCV
MDXCI
MDXCV
MMXCI
MMXCV
TAXCO

••X•C
SIXBC
TOXIC

•••XC
CCCXC
DCCXC
MCCXC
MCDXC
MCMXC
MDCXC
MMCXC
MMDXC
MMMXC

XD•••
XDOUT

X•D••
XEDIN

X••D•
XANDO
XANDY

•XD••
EXDIV

•X•D•
EXUDE
OXIDE

•X••D
AXLED

••X•D
BOXED
COXED
FAXED
FIXED
FOXED
HEXAD
HEXED
MAXED
MIXED
NIXED
RAXED
SEXED
SIXAD
SIXED
TAXED
VEXED
WAXED

XE•••
XEBEC
XEDIN
XEMEX
XENIA
XENON
XEONS
XERIC
XEROX
XESIN

X••E•
XAXES
XEBEC
XEMEX
XYLEM

X•••E
XFILE
XTILE
XTYPE

•XE••
AXELF
AXELS
AXERS
EXECS
EXERT
OXEYE

•X•E•
AXLED
AXLES
AXMEN
EXCEL
EXMET
EXPEL

•X••E
AXONE
EXILE
EXUDE
OXEYE
OXIDE

••XE•
BOXED
BOXER
BOXES
COXED
COXES
FAXED
FAXER
FAXES
FIXED
FIXER
FIXES
FOXED
FOXES
HEXED
HEXER
HEXES
LAXER
LOXES
LUXES
MAXED
MAXES
MIXED
MIXER
MIXES
NIXED
NIXER
NIXES
PIXEL
POXES
PYXES
RAXED
RAXES
REXES
RIXEY
SAXES
SEXED
SEXER
SEXES
SIXED
SIXEE
SIXER
SIXES
TAXED
TAXER
TAXES
TUXES
VAXES
VEXED
VEXER
VEXES
VIXEN
WAXED
WAXEN
WAXER
WAXES
XAXES
YAXES
ZAXES

••X•E
COXAE
DIXIE
DOXIE
MAXIE
MOXIE
NIXIE
PIXIE
ROXIE
SIXEE

XF•••
XFILE

•XF••
OXFAM

•X••F
AXELF

•XG••
EXGIS
EXGOV

•X••G
AXING
EXING

XH•••
XHOSA

••XH•
HOXHA

••X•H
SIXTH

X•I••
XCIII
XFILE
XLIII
XTILE
XVIII
XXIII

X••I•
XAXIS
XCIII
XCVII
XEDIN
XENIA
XERIC
XESIN
XLIII
XLVII
XVIII
XXIII
XXVII
XXXII
XXXIV
XXXIX

X•••I
XCIII
XCVII
XLIII
XLVII
XVIII
XXIII
XXVII
XXXII
XXXVI

•XI••
AXIAL
AXILS
AXING
AXIOM
AXION
CXIII
DXIII
EXILE
EXING
EXIST
EXITS
IXION
LXIII
MXIII
OXIDE
XXIII

•X•I•
CXCII
CXCIV
CXCIX
CXIII
CXLII
CXLIV
CXLIX
CXVII
CXXII
CXXIV
CXXIX
DXCII
DXCIV
DXCIX
DXIII
DXLII
DXLIV
DXLIX
DXVII
DXXII
DXXIV
DXXIX
EXDIV
EXGIS
EXLIB
LXIII
LXVII
LXXII
LXXIV
LXXIX
MXCII
MXCIV
MXCIX
MXIII
MXLII
MXLIV
MXLIX
MXVII
MXXII
MXXIV
MXXIX
OXLIP
XXIII
XXVII
XXXII
XXXIV
XXXIX

•X••I
CXCII
CXCVI
CXIII
CXLII
CXLVI
CXVII
CXXII
CXXVI
CXXXI
DXCII
DXCVI
DXIII
DXLII
DXLVI
DXVII
DXXII
DXXVI
DXXXI
LXIII
LXVII
LXXII
LXXVI
LXXXI
MXCII
MXCVI
MXIII
MXLII
MXLVI
MXVII
MXXII
MXXVI
MXXXI
XXIII
XXVII
XXXII
XXXVI

••XI•
BOXIN
CCXII
CCXIV
CCXIX
CDXII
CDXIV
CDXIX
CLXII
CLXIV
CLXIX
CMXII
CMXIV
CMXIX
CXXII
CXXIV
CXXIX
DCXII
DCXIV
DCXIX
DIXIE
DIXIT
DLXII
DLXIV
DLXIX
DOXIE
DXXII
DXXIV
DXXIX
FIXIT
LEXIS
LXXII
LXXIV
LXXIX
MAXIE
MAXIM
MAXIS
MCXII
MCXIV
MCXIX
MDXII
MDXIV
MDXIX
MIXIN
MLXII
MLXIV
MLXIX
MMXII
MMXIV
MMXIX
MOXIE
MXXII
MXXIV
MXXIX
NEXIS
NIXIE
PIXIE
ROXIE
TAXIS
TOXIC
TOXIN
WUXIA
XAXIS
XXXII
XXXIV
XXXIX
YAXIS
ZAXIS

••X•I
CCXCI
CCXII
CCXLI
CCXVI
CCXXI
CDXCI
CDXII
CDXLI
CDXVI
CDXXI
CLXII
CLXVI
CLXXI
CMXCI
CMXII
CMXLI
CMXVI
CMXXI
CXXII
CXXVI
CXXXI
DCXCI
DCXII
DCXLI

DCXVI
DCXXI
DLXII
DLXVI
DLXXI
DXXII
DXXVI
DXXXI
LXXII
LXXVI
LXXXI
MCXCI
MCXII
MCXLI
MCXVI
MCXXI
MDXCI
MDXII
MDXLI
MDXVI
MDXXI
MLXII
MLXVI
MLXXI
MMXCI
MMXII
MMXLI
MMXVI
MMXXI
MXXII
MXXVI
MXXXI
XXXII
XXXVI

•••XI
ALEXI
CCCXI
CCLXI
CCXXI
CDLXI
CDXXI
CLXXI
CMLXI
CMXXI
CXXXI
DCCXI
DCLXI
DCXXI
DLXXI
DXXXI
LEOXI
LXXXI
MCCXI
MCDXI
MCLXI
MCMXI
MCXXI
MDCXI
MDLXI
MDXXI
MLXXI
MMCXI
MMDXI
MMLXI
MMMXI
MMXXI
MXXXI

XL•••
XLIII
XLVII

X•L••
XYLEM

X••L•
XFILE
XTILE

•XL••
AXLED
AXLES
CXLII
CXLIV
CXLIX
CXLVI
DXLII
DXLIV
DXLIX
DXLVI
EXLIB
MXLII
MXLIV
MXLIX
MXLVI
OXLIP

•X•L•
AXELF
AXELS
AXILS
EXALT
EXILE
EXULT

•X••L
AXIAL
EXCEL
EXPEL
EXTOL
UXMAL

••XL•
CCXLI
CCXLV
CDXLI
CDXLV
CMXLI
CMXLV
DCXLI
DCXLV
LAXLY
MCXLI
MCXLV
MDXLI
MDXLV
MMXLI
MMXLV
TIXLS

••X•L
PIXEL
TAXOL

•••XL
CCCXL
DCCXL
MCCXL
MCDXL
MCMXL
MDCXL
MMCXL
MMDXL
MMMXL

X•M••
XEMEX

X•••M
XYLEM

•XM••
AXMAN
AXMEN
EXMET
UXMAL

•X•M•
EXAMS
EXUMA

•X••M
AXIOM
OXFAM

••X•M
BUXOM
MAXIM
SIXAM
SIXPM

X•N••
XANDO
XANDY
XENIA
XENON

X••N•
XEONS

X•••N
XEDIN
XENON
XESIN

•XN••
IXNAY

•X•N•
AXING
AXONE
AXONS
EXING
EXONS
OXANA

•X••N
AXION
AXMAN
AXMEN
AXTON
EXCON
EXXON
IXION

••XN•
SIXNO

••X•N
BOXIN
DIXON
EXXON
FIXON
LEXAN
MIXIN
NIXON
SAXON
TAXON
TEXAN
TOXIN
VIXEN
WAXEN

XO•••
XOUTS
XOXOX

X•O••
XDOUT
XEONS
XHOSA
XSOUT

X••O•
XENON
XEROX
XOXOX

X•••O
XACTO
XANDO

•XO••
AXONE
AXONS
EXONS

•X•O•
AXIOM
AXION
AXTON
EXCON
EXCOP
EXGOV
EXPOS
EXTOL
EXXON
IXION
OXBOW

•X••O
EXTRO

••XO•
BUXOM
DIXON
EXXON
FIXON
LUXOR
NAXOS
NIXON
PAXOS
SAXON
TAXOL
TAXON
XOXOX

••X•O
SIXNO
TAXCO

•••XO
GLAXO
QUAXO

X••P•
XTYPE

•XP••
EXPAT
EXPEL
EXPOS

•X••P
EXCOP
OXLIP

••XP•
SIXPM

••X•P
BOXUP
FIXUP
MIXUP
SIXUP
WAXUP

XR•••
XRAYS

X•R••
XERIC
XEROX

X••R•
XSARA

•X•R•
AXERS
EXERT
EXTRA
EXTRO
EXURB

••X•R
BEXAR
BOXER
DEXTR
FAXER
FIXER
HEXER
LAXER
LUXOR
MIXER
NIXER
PIXAR
SEXER
SIXER
TAXER
VEXER
WAXER

XS•••
XSARA
XSOUT

X•S••
XESIN
XYSTS

X••S•
XHOSA

X•••S
XAXES
XAXIS
XEONS
XOUTS
XRAYS
XYSTS

•X•S•
EXIST

•X••S
AXELS
AXERS
AXILS
AXLES
AXONS
EXAMS
EXECS
EXGIS
EXITS
EXONS
EXPOS

••X•S
BOXES
COXES
FAXES
FIXES
FOXES
HEXES
LEXIS
LEXUS
LOXES
LUXES
MAXES
MAXIS
MIXES
NAXOS
NEXIS
NEXUS
NIXES
PAXOS
POXES
PYXES
RAXES
REXES
SAXES
SEXES
SIXES
TAXES
TAXIS
TEXAS
TEXTS
TIXLS
TUXES
VAXES
VEXES
WAXES
XAXES
XAXIS
YAXES
YAXIS
ZAXES
ZAXIS

•••XS
GENXS

XT•••
XTILE
XTYPE

X••T•
XACTO
XOUTS
XYSTS

X•••T
XDOUT
XSOUT

•XT••
AXTON
EXTOL
EXTRA
EXTRO

•X•T•
EXITS

•X••T
EXACT
EXALT
EXERT
EXIST
EXMET
EXPAT
EXULT

••XT•
DEXTR
FOXTV
SIXTH
SIXTY
TEXTS

••X•T
DIXIT
FIXIT

•••XT
TWIXT

X•U••
XOUTS

X••U•
XDOUT
XSOUT

•XU••
EXUDE
EXULT
EXUMA
EXURB

•X•U•
EXCUB

••XU•
BOXUP
FIXUP
LEXUS
MIXUP
NEXUS
SIXUP
WAXUP

XV•••
XVIII

X•V••
XCVII
XLVII
XXVII

X••V•
XXXVI

X•••V
XXXIV

•XV••
CXVII
DXVII
LXVII
MXVII
XXVII

•X•V•
CXCVI
CXLVI
CXXVI
DXCVI
DXLVI
DXXVI
LXXVI
MXCVI
MXLVI
MXXVI
XXXVI

•X••V
CXCIV
CXLIV
CXXIV
CXXXV
DXCIV
DXLIV
DXXIV
DXXXV
EXDIV
EXGOV
LXXIV
LXXXV
MXCIV
MXLIV
MXXIV
MXXXV
XXXIV

••XV•
CCXVI
CDXVI
CLXVI
CMXVI
CXXVI
DCXVI
DLXVI
DXXVI
LXXVI
MCXVI
MDXVI
MLXVI
MMXVI
MXXVI
XXXVI

••X•V
CCXCV
CCXIV
CCXLV
CCXXV
CDXCV
CDXIV
CDXLV
CDXXV
CLXIV
CLXXV
CMXCV
CMXIV
CMXLV
CMXXV
CXXIV
CXXXV
DCXCV
DCXIV
DCXLV
DCXXV
DLXIV
DLXXV
DXXIV
DXXXV
FOXTV
LXXIV
LXXXV
MCXCV
MCXIV
MCXLV
MCXXV
MDXCV
MDXIV
MDXLV
MDXXV
MLXIV
MLXXV
MMXCV
MMXIV
MMXLV
MMXXV
MXXIV
MXXXV
XXXIV

•••XV
CCCXV
CCLXV
CCXXV
CDLXV
CDXXV
CLXXV
CMLXV
CMXXV
CXXXV
DCCXV
DCLXV
DCXXV
DLXXV
DXXXV
LXXXV
MCCXV
MCDXV
MCLXV
MCMXV
MCXXV
MDCXV
MDLXV
MDXXV
MLXXV
MMCXV
MMDXV
MMLXV
MMMXV
MMXXV
MXXXV

•X••W
OXBOW

XX•••
XXIII
XXVII
XXXII
XXXIV
XXXIX
XXXVI

X•X••
XAXES
XAXIS
XOXOX
XXXII
XXXIV
XXXIX
XXXVI

X•••X
XEMEX
XEROX
XOXOX
XXXIX

•XX••
CXXII
CXXIV
CXXIX
CXXVI
CXXXI
CXXXV
DXXII
DXXIV
DXXIX
DXXVI
DXXXI
DXXXV
EXXON
LXXII
LXXIV
LXXIX
LXXVI
LXXXI
LXXXV
MXXII
MXXIV
MXXIX
MXXVI
MXXXI
MXXXV
XXXII
XXXIV
XXXIX
XXXVI

•X•X•
CXXXI
CXXXV
DXXXI
DXXXV
LXXXI
LXXXV
MXXXI
MXXXV

•X••X
CXCIX
CXLIX
CXXIX
DXCIX
DXLIX
DXXIX
LXXIX
MXCIX
MXLIX
MXXIX
XXXIX

••XX•
CCXXI
CCXXV
CCXXX
CDXXI
CDXXV
CDXXX
CLXXI
CLXXV
CLXXX
CMXXI
CMXXV
CMXXX
CXXXI
CXXXV
DCXXI
DCXXV
DCXXX
DLXXI
DLXXV
DLXXX
DXXXI
DXXXV
LXXXI
LXXXV
MCXXI
MCXXV
MCXXX
MDXXI
MDXXV
MDXXX
MLXXI
MLXXV
MLXXX
MMXXI
MMXXV
MMXXX
MXXXI
MXXXV

••X•X
CCXIX
CCXXX
CDXIX
CDXXX
CLXIX
CLXXX
CMXIX
CMXXX
CXXIX
DCXIX
DCXXX
DLXIX
DLXXX
DXXIX
LXXIX
MCXIX
MCXXX
MDXIX
MDXXX
MLXIX
MLXXX
MMXIX
MMXXX
MXXIX
XOXOX
XXXIX

•••XX
CCCXX
CCLXX
CCXXX
CDLXX
CDXXX
CHEXX
CLXXX
CMLXX
CMXXX
DCCXX
DCLXX
DCXXX
DLXXX
MCCXX
MCDXX
MCLXX
MCMXX
MCXXX
MDCXX
MDLXX
MDXXX
MLXXX
MMCXX
MMDXX
MMLXX
MMMXX
MMXXX
SKNXX

XY•••
XYLEM
XYSTS

X•Y••
XTYPE

X••Y•
XRAYS

X•••Y
XANDY

•X•Y•
OXEYE

•X••Y
IXNAY

••XY•
VWXYZ

••X•Y
BIXBY
LAXLY
RIXEY
SIXTY

•••XY
DEOXY
EPOXY
FLAXY
PREXY
PROXY
UVWXY

••X•Z
VWXYZ

YA•••
YABBA
YACHT
YACKS
YADDA
YADIM
YAHOO
YAKOV
YAKUT
YALEU
YALIE
YALOW
YALTA
YANCY
YANKS
YANNI
YAPAT
YAQUI
YARDS
YARER
YARNS
YARRA
YASHA
YASIR
YATES
YAWED
YAWLS
YAWNS
YAWNY
YAWPS
YAXES
YAXIS
YAYAS
YAYME
YAZOO

Y•A••
YEAHS
YEANS
YEARN
YEARS
YEAST
YEATS
YSAYE
YUANS
YVAIN
YWAIN

Y••A•
YAPAT
YAYAS
YMCAS
YMHAS
YOGAS
YUBAN
YUMAN
YUMAS
YWCAS
YWHAS

Y•••A
YABBA
YADDA
YALTA
YARRA
YASHA
YENTA
YERBA
YETTA
YOOBA
YORBA
YOWZA
YREKA
YUCCA
YULKA

•YA••
AYAHS
AYAKO
BYAGE
BYAIR
BYATT
CYANO
CYANS
DYADS
HYAMS
HYATT
IYARS
KYATS
NYACK
NYALA
NYASA
RYALS
RYANS
WYATT

•Y•A•
AYEAR
BYCAB
BYCAR
BYEAR
BYFAR
BYFAX
BYLAW
BYWAY
CYCAD
CYMAE
CYMAS
DYLAN
EYRAS
GYRAL
HYLAS
HYMAN
HYRAX
LYMAN
LYRAS
MYBAD
MYDAD
MYDAY
MYLAR
MYMAN
MYNAH
MYNAS
MYWAR
MYWAY
NYMAN
TYNAN
TYPAL
WYMAN

•Y••A
BYSEA
GYOZA
HYDRA
HYENA
LYCRA
LYDIA
LYGIA
LYNDA
MYRIA
MYRNA
NYALA
NYASA
NYDIA
SYRIA
TYPEA

••YA•
AMYAS
ARYAN
BAYAR
BAYAT
BRYAN
BUYAT
DAYAN
DRYAD
FLYAT
GOYAS
HOYAS
KAYAK
LOYAL
MAYAN
MAYAS
RIYAL
ROYAL
SAYAH
SOYAS
YAYAS
ZAYAK

••Y•A
ADYTA
ASYLA
ETYMA
LAYLA
PHYLA
TWYLA

•••YA
DARYA
DUBYA
EASYA
FREYA
HANYA
ILLYA
KENYA
LENYA
LIBYA
MARYA
MITYA
PLAYA
RODYA
SEEYA
SONYA
TANYA
TONYA
VANYA
VARYA

Y•B••
YABBA
YUBAN

Y••B•
YABBA
YERBA
YOOBA
YORBA

•YB••
BYBUS
CYBER
MYBAD
MYBOY
SYBIL

•Y••B
BYCAB
TYPEB

••YB•
FLYBY
LAYBY
MAYBE

Y•C••
YACHT
YACKS
YECCH
YMCAS
YOCTO
YUCCA
YUCKY
YWCAS

Y••C•
YANCY
YECCH
YUCCA

Y•••C
YOGIC

•YC••
BYCAB
BYCAR
CYCAD
CYCLE
CYCLO
LYCEE
LYCOS
LYCRA
MYCIN
NYCTI
NYCTO
TYCHE
TYCHO

•Y•C•
LYNCH
NYACK
SYNCH
SYNCS
SYSCO

•Y••C
CYNIC
GYNEC
LYRIC
TYPIC

••YC•
ALYCE
BRYCE
CAYCE
DOYCE
GLYCO
JOYCE
NOYCE
PRYCE
PSYCH
ROYCE

••Y•C
NSYNC

•••YC
ENCYC

Y•D••
YADDA
YADIM
YODEL
YODHS

Y••D•
YADDA
YARDS

Y•••D
YAWED YIELD YOKED

•YD••
CYDER EYDIE HYDRA HYDRO LYDIA LYDON MYDAD MYDAY NYDIA RYDER SYDOW

•Y•D•
BYRDS CYNDI DYADS HYNDE LYNDA LYNDE SYNDS

•Y••D
BYGOD CYCAD GYRED HYOID HYPED LYRID LYSED MYBAD MYDAD MYGOD SYNOD TYPED

••YD•
CLYDE CUYDS HAYDN

••Y•D
BAYED DRYAD GUYED HAYED JOYED KEYED RAYED TOYED

•••YD
ALKYD CLWYD FLOYD LLOYD THEYD

YE•••
YEAHS YEANS YEARN YEARS YEAST YEATS YECCH YEGGS YELLO YELLS YELPS YEMEN YENTA YENTE YENTL YEOWS YERBA YESES YESNO YESOR YETIS YETTA

Y•E••
YIELD YREKA

Y••E•
YALEU YARER YATES YAWED YAXES YEMEN YESES YIKES YIPES YODEL YOKED YOKEL YOKES YONEX YORES YPRES YULES

Y•••E
YALIE YAYME YENTE YLIKE YONNE YOURE YOUSE YOUVE YOWIE YSAYE YTILE

•YE••
AYEAR AYERS BYEAR DYERS DYESS EYERS EYEUP HYENA HYETO LYELL MYERS MYEYE NYETS OYERS TYEES WYETH

•Y•E•
AYRES BYNER BYSEA BYTES CYBER CYDER CYMES DYKER DYNEL DYNES GYNEC GYRED GYRES HYPED HYPER HYPES HYSER KYSER LYCEE LYNEN LYRES LYSED LYSES MYLES NYJET NYMET NYNEX OYVEY PYRES PYREX PYXES RYDER TYEES TYGER TYKES TYLER TYNER TYPEA TYPEB TYPED TYPEE TYPEO TYPER TYPES TYRES TYVEK WYLER XYLEM

•Y••E
BYAGE BYONE BYRNE CYCLE CYMAE EYDIE EYRIE HYNDE KYLIE KYRIE LYCEE LYNDE LYNNE MYEYE MYOPE SYNGE TYCHE TYPEE WYLIE WYNNE WYTHE

••YE•
AHYES ASYET BAYED BAYER BAYES BOYER BUYER COYER CRYER DIYER DOYEN DRYER FEYER FLYER FOYER FRYER GAYER GOYEN GUYED HAYED HAYEK HAYER HAYES HAYEY HEYER JOYED KEYED KEYES LAYER MAYER MEYER NOYES NUYEN OHYES PAYEE PAYER PLYER PRYER RAYED REYES SAYER SHYER SKYES SKYEY SLYER STYES TOYED TOYER WRYER

••Y•E
ALYCE BAYLE BEYLE BOYLE BRYCE CAYCE CLYDE DAYNE DOYCE DOYLE ELYSE FLYME FOYLE GAYLE HEYSE HOYLE JAYNE JOYCE LAYNE LEYTE MAYBE MAYLE NOYCE PAYEE PAYNE PHYFE PHYTE PRYCE RHYME ROYCE SKYPE SLYKE STYLE STYNE THYME TRYME VTYPE WAYNE WHYME WHYRE WHYTE XTYPE YAYME

•••YE
DEBYE EAZYE KANYE MYEYE ONRYE OXEYE REDYE TEVYE YSAYE

•YF••
BYFAR BYFAX

••YF•
PHYFE

••Y•F
SHYOF

Y•G••
YEGGS YOGAS YOGIC YOGIS YUGOS

Y••G•
YEGGS

Y•••G
YOUNG

•YG••
BYGOD BYGUM CYGNI HYGRO LYGIA MYGOD MYGUY PYGMY TYGER

•Y•G•
BYAGE SYNGE

•Y••G
DYING EYING HYING LYING MYUNG TYING VYING

Y•H••
YAHOO YMHAS YWHAS

Y••H•
YACHT YASHA YEAHS YODHS

Y•••H
YECCH YOUTH

•Y•H•
AYAHS MYTHS TYCHE TYCHO WYTHE

•Y••H
LYMPH LYNCH MYNAH MYRRH NYMPH SYLPH SYNCH SYNTH WYETH

••YH•
SAYHI

••Y•H
BLYTH GLYPH PSYCH SAYAH SMYTH

YI•••
YIELD YIKES YIPES

Y•I••
YLIKE YTILE

Y••I•
YADIM YALIE YASIR YAXIS YETIS YOGIC YOGIS YOWIE YUKIO YULIN YURIS YVAIN YWAIN

Y•••I
YANNI YAQUI

•YI••
AYINS DYING EYING HYING LYING TYING TYIYN VYING

•Y•I•
BYAIR CYNIC CYRIL EYDIE EYRIE EYRIR HYOID KYLIE KYRIE LYDIA LYGIA LYRIC LYRID LYSIS MYCIN MYRIA MYSIN NYDIA SYBIL SYRIA TYPIC WYLIE

•Y••I
CYGNI CYNDI NYCTI

••YI•
BUYIN BUYIT FLYIN KEYIN LAYIN PAYIN SAYIT TRYIT WAYIN ZAYIN

••Y•I
SAYHI SPYRI STYLI

•••YI
MARYI

•YJ••
NYJET

•••YJ
MARYJ

YK•••
YKNOW

Y•K••
YAKOV YAKUT YIKES YOKED YOKEL YOKES YOKUM YUKIO YUKON YUKOS

Y••K•
YACKS YANKS YLIKE YOLKS YOLKY YORKS YREKA YUCKY YULKA

•YK••
DYKER TYKES

•Y•K•
AYAKO

•Y••K
NYACK TYVEK

••YK•
ROYKO SLYKE

••Y•K
HAYEK KAYAK MRYUK SAYOK ZAYAK

YL•••
YLIKE

Y•L••
YALEU YALIE YALOW YALTA YELLO YELLS YELPS YOLKS YOLKY YULES YULIN YULKA

Y••L•
YAWLS YELLO YELLS YIELD YOULL YOWLS YTILE

Y•••L
YENTL YODEL YOKEL YOULL

•YL••
BYLAW BYLOT DYLAN HYLAS KYLIE MYLAR MYLES NYLON PYLON SYLPH TYLER WYLER WYLIE XYLEM

•Y•L•
CYCLE CYCLO LYELL NYALA RYALS

•Y••L
CYRIL DYNEL GYRAL KYZYL LYELL LYSOL NYTOL SYBIL TYPAL TYROL

••YL•
AMYLO AMYLS ARYLS ASYLA BAYLE BEYLE BOYLE COYLY DOYLE DOYLY DRYLY FEYLY FOYLE GAYLE GAYLY HOYLE IDYLL IDYLS LAYLA MAYLE PHYLA PHYLL PHYLO SHYLY SLYLY STYLE STYLI TWYLA WHYLL WRYLY

••Y•L
IDYLL LOYAL PHYLL RIYAL ROYAL WHYLL

•••YL
ALKYL ALLYL BERYL BUTYL DARYL ETHYL KYZYL LADYL MERYL SIBYL VINYL

YM•••
YMCAS YMHAS

Y•M••
YEMEN YUMAN YUMAS YUMMY

Y••M•
YAYME YUMMY

Y•••M
YADIM YOKUM

•YM••
CYMAE CYMAS CYMES CYMRY GYMNO HYMAN HYMNS LYMAN LYMON LYMPH MYMAN NYMAN NYMET NYMPH WYMAN

•Y•M•
HYAMS PYGMY

•Y••M
BYGUM XYLEM

••YM•
ETYMA FLYME RHYME THYME THYMY TRYME WHYME YAYME

••Y•M
ABYSM

Y•N••
YANCY YANKS YANNI YENTA YENTE YENTL YKNOW YONEX YONNE

Y••N•
YANNI YARNS YAWNS YAWNY YEANS YESNO YONNE YOUNG YOUNT YUANS

Y•••N
YEARN YEMEN YOURN YUBAN YUKON YULIN YUMAN YVAIN YWAIN

•YN••
BYNER BYNOW CYNDI CYNIC DYNEL DYNES GYNEC HYNDE LYNCH LYNDA LYNDE LYNEN LYNNE MYNAH MYNAS NYNEX SYNCH SYNCS SYNDS SYNGE SYNOD SYNTH TYNAN TYNER WYNNE

•Y•N•
AYINS BYONE BYRNE CYANO CYANS CYGNI DYING EYING GYMNO HYENA HYING HYMNS HYPNO LYING LYNNE LYONS MYRNA MYUNG RYANS TYING VYING WYNNE

•Y••N
BYRON DYLAN DYSON HYMAN HYSON LYDON LYMAN LYMON LYNEN MYCIN MYMAN MYRON MYSIN NYLON NYMAN PYLON TYIYN TYNAN TYSON WYMAN

••YN•
DAYNE ELYNV FLYNN GWYNN JAYNE LAYNE MAYNT NSYNC PAYNE SAYNO STYNE WAYNE

••Y•N
ANYON ARYAN BRYAN BUYIN DAYAN DOYEN FLYIN FLYNN FLYON GOYEN GUYON GWYNN HAYDN KEYIN KEYON LAYIN LAYON MAYAN NUYEN PAYIN RAYON SPYON TOYON TRYON WAYIN ZAYIN

•••YN
ALLYN EMLYN FRAYN KARYN OBGYN ROBYN TYIYN WOMYN

YO•••
YOCTO YODEL YODHS YOGAS YOGIC YOGIS YOKED YOKEL YOKES YOKUM YOLKS YOLKY YONEX YONNE YOOBA YORBA YORES YORKS YORTY YOSOY YOTTO YOULL YOUNG YOUNT YOURE YOURN YOURS YOUSE YOUTH YOUVE YOWIE YOWLS YOWZA YOYOS

Y•O••
YEOWS YOOBA

Y••O•
YAHOO YAKOV YALOW YAZOO YESOR YKNOW YOSOY YOYOS YUGOS YUKON YUKOS

Y•••O
YAHOO YAZOO YELLO YESNO YOCTO YOTTO YUKIO

•YO••
BYONE GYOZA HYOID KYOTO LYONS MYOPE

•Y•O•
BYGOD BYLOT BYNOW BYRON DYSON GYROS HYPOS HYSON LYCOS LYDON LYMON LYSOL MYBOY MYGOD MYRON NYLON NYTOL PYLON PYROS SYDOW SYNOD SYSOP TYPOS TYROL TYROS TYSON

•Y••O
AYAKO BYTWO CYANO CYCLO GYMNO HYDRO HYETO HYGRO HYPNO KYOTO NYCTO SYSCO TYCHO TYPEO

••YO•
ANYON BAYOU BOYOS ELYOT FLYON GUYON KAYOS KEYON LAYON MAYOR MAYOS OHYOU PAYOR PRYOR RAYON SAYOK SHYOF SPYON TOYON TOYOS TOYOU TRYON YOYOS

••Y•O
AMYLO FLYTO GLYCO LAYTO MAYPO PAYTO PHYLO PHYTO ROYKO SAYNO SAYSO SPYRO STYRO TRYTO

•••YO
FROYO OHAYO ONKYO SANYO TOKYO

YP•••
YPRES

Y•P••
YAPAT YIPES

Y••P•
YAWPS YELPS

•YP••
GYPSY HYPED HYPER HYPES HYPNO HYPOS TYPAL TYPEA TYPEB TYPED TYPEE TYPEO TYPER TYPES TYPIC TYPOS

•Y•P•
LYMPH MYOPE NYMPH SYLPH

•Y••P
EYEUP SYRUP SYSOP

••YP•
COYPU CRYPT EGYPT GLYPH GLYPT MAYPO SKYPE VTYPE XTYPE

••Y•P
BUYUP CRYUP DRYUP FLYUP FRYUP KEYUP LAYUP PAYUP WAYUP

•••YP
POLYP

Y•Q••
YAQUI

•••YQ
SUZYQ

YR•••
YREKA

Y•R••
YARDS YARER YARNS YARRA YERBA YORBA YORES YORKS YORTY YPRES YURIS YURTS

Y••R•
YARRA YEARN YEARS YOURE YOURN YOURS

Y•••R
YARER YASIR YESOR

•YR••
AYRES BYRDS BYRNE BYRON CYRIL CYRUS EYRAS EYRIE

EYRIR
GYRAL
GYRED
GYRES
GYROS
HYRAX
KYRIE
LYRAS
LYRES
LYRIC
LYRID
MYRIA
MYRNA
MYRON
MYRRH
PYRES
PYREX
PYROS
SYRIA
SYRUP
TYRES
TYROL
TYROS
TYRUS

•Y•R•
AYERS
CYMRY
DYERS
EYERS
HYDRA
HYDRO
HYGRO
IYARS
LYCRA
MYERS
MYRRH
OYERS

•Y••R
AYEAR
BYAIR
BYCAR
BYEAR
BYFAR
BYNER
CYBER
CYDER
DYKER
EYRIR
HYPER
HYSER
KYSER
MYLAR
MYWAR
RYDER
TYGER
TYLER
TYNER
TYPER
WYLER

••YR•
SPYRI
SPYRO
STYRO
WHYRE

••Y•R
BAYAR
BAYER
BOYER
BUYER
COYER
CRYER
DIYER
DRYER
FEYER
FLYER
FOYER
FRYER
GAYER
HAYER
HEYER
LAYER
MAYER
MAYOR
MEYER
PAYER
PAYOR
PLYER
PRYER
PRYOR
SAYER
SHYER
SLYER
TOYER
WRYER

•••YR
ASSYR
SATYR

YS•••
YSAYE

Y•S••
YASHA
YASIR
YESES
YESNO
YESOR
YOSOY

Y••S•
YEAST
YOUSE

Y•••S
YACKS
YANKS
YARDS
YARNS
YATES
YAWLS
YAWNS
YAWPS
YAXES
YAXIS
YAYAS
YEAHS
YEANS
YEARS
YEATS
YEGGS
YELLS
YELPS
YEOWS
YESES
YETIS
YIKES
YIPES
YMCAS
YMHAS
YODHS
YOGAS
YOGIS
YOKES
YOLKS
YORES
YORKS
YOURS
YOWLS
YOYOS
YPRES
YUANS
YUGOS
YUKOS
YULES
YUMAS
YURIS
YURTS
YWCAS
YWHAS

•YS••
BYSEA
CYSTS
DYSON
HYSER
HYSON
KYSER
LYSED
LYSES
LYSIS
LYSOL
MYSIN
SYSCO
SYSOP
SYSTS
TYSON
XYSTS

•Y•S•
DYESS
GYPSY
NYASA

•Y••S
AYAHS
AYERS
AYINS
AYRES
BYBUS
BYRDS
BYTES
CYANS
CYMAS
CYMES
CYRUS
CYSTS
DYADS
DYERS
DYESS
DYNES
EYERS
EYRAS
GYRES
GYROS
HYAMS
HYLAS
HYMNS
HYPES
HYPOS
IYARS
KYATS
LYCOS
LYONS
LYRAS
LYRES
LYSES
LYSIS
MYERS
MYLES
MYNAS
MYTHS
NYETS
OYERS
PYRES
PYROS
PYXES
RYALS
RYANS
SYNCS
SYNDS
SYSTS
TYEES
TYKES
TYPES
TYPOS
TYRES
TYROS
TYRUS
XYSTS

••YS•
ABYSM
ABYSS
ELYSE
HEYSE
MAYST
SAYSO
TRYST

••Y•S
ABYSS
AHYES
AMYAS
AMYLS
ARYLS
BAYES
BOYOS
CUYDS
GOYAS
HAYES
HOYAS
IDYLS
KAYOS
KEYES
MAYAS
MAYOS
NOYES
OHYES
REYES
SKYES
SOYAS
STYES
TOYOS
YAYAS
YOYOS

•••YS
AHOYS
ANDYS
ARBYS
ATTYS
BABYS
BBOYS
BDAYS
BRAYS
BUOYS
CLAYS
CLOYS
CRAYS
DDAYS
DENYS
DRAYS
DUFYS
EMMYS
ESPYS
FLAYS
FRAYS
GRAYS
GREYS
HUEYS
INDYS
JOEYS
JULYS
KURYS
LADYS
MACYS
MARYS
OBEYS
OJAYS
OKAYS
PEPYS
PITYS
PLAYS
PLOYS
POWYS
PRAYS
PREYS
QUAYS
SHAYS
SLAYS
SLEYS
SONYS
SPAYS
STAYS
SWAYS
TONYS
TRAYS
TREYS
VDAYS
WHEYS
XRAYS

YT•••
YTILE

Y•T••
YATES
YETIS
YETTA
YOTTO

Y••T•
YALTA
YEATS
YENTA
YENTE
YENTL
YETTA
YOCTO
YORTY
YOTTO
YOUTH
YURTS

Y•••T
YACHT
YAKUT
YAPAT
YEAST
YOUNT

•YT••
BYTES
BYTWO
MYTHS
NYTOL
WYTHE

•Y•T•
BYATT
CYSTS
HYATT
HYETO
KYATS
KYOTO
NYCTI
NYCTO
NYETS
SYNTH
SYSTS
WYATT
WYETH
XYSTS

•Y••T
BYATT
BYLOT
HYATT
NYJET
NYMET
WYATT

••YT•
ADYTA
BLYTH
FLYTO
LAYTO
LEYTE
PAYTO
PAYTV
PHYTE
PHYTO
SMYTH
TRYTO
WHYTE

••Y•T
ASYET
BAYAT
BUYAT
BUYIT
CRYPT
EGYPT
ELYOT
FLYAT
GLYPT
MAYNT
MAYST
SAYIT
TRYIT
TRYST

YU•••
YUANS
YUBAN
YUCCA
YUCKY
YUGOS
YUKIO
YUKON
YUKOS
YULES
YULIN
YULKA
YUMAN
YUMAS
YUMMY
YURIS
YURTS

Y•U••
YOULL
YOUNG
YOUNT
YOURE
YOURN
YOURS
YOUSE
YOUTH
YOUVE

Y••U•
YAKUT
YAQUI
YOKUM

Y•••U
YALEU

•YU••
MYUNG

•Y•U•
BYBUS
BYGUM
CYRUS
EYEUP
MYGUY
SYRUP
TYRUS

••YU•
BUYUP
CRYUP
DRYUP
FLYUP
FRYUP
KEYUP
LAYUP
MRYUK
PAYUP
SOYUZ
WAYUP

••Y•U
BAYOU
COYPU
OHYOU
TOYOU

YV•••
YVAIN

Y••V•
YOUVE

Y•••V
YAKOV

•YV••
OYVEY
TYVEK

••Y•V
ELYNV
PAYTV

YW•••
YWAIN
YWCAS
YWHAS

Y•W••
YAWED
YAWLS
YAWNS
YAWNY
YAWPS
YOWIE
YOWLS
YOWZA

Y••W•
YEOWS

Y•••W
YALOW
YKNOW

•YW••
BYWAY
MYWAR
MYWAY

•Y•W•
BYTWO

•Y••W
BYLAW
BYNOW
SYDOW

Y•X••
YAXES
YAXIS

Y•••X
YONEX

•YX••
PYXES

•Y••X
BYFAX
HYRAX
NYNEX
PYREX

•••YX
CALYX

Y•Y••
YAYAS
YAYME
YOYOS

Y••Y•
YSAYE

Y•••Y
YANCY
YAWNY
YOLKY
YORTY
YOSOY
YUCKY
YUMMY

•Y•Y•
KYZYL
MYEYE
TYIYN

•Y••Y
BYWAY
CYMRY
GYPSY
MYBOY
MYDAY
MYGUY
MYWAY
OYVEY
PYGMY

••Y•Y
COYLY
DOYLY
DRYLY
FEYLY
FLYBY
GAYLY
HAYEY
LAYBY
SHYLY
SKYEY
SLYLY
THYMY
WRYLY

Y•Z••
YAZOO

Y••Z•
YOWZA

•YZ••
KYZYL

•Y•Z•
GYOZA

••Y•Z
SOYUZ

•••YZ
VWXYZ

ZA•••
ZADAR
ZADIE
ZADIG
ZAFUS
ZAGAT
ZAHND
ZAIRE
ZALES
ZAPPA
ZAPPY
ZARFS
ZAXES
ZAXIS
ZAYAK
ZAYIN
ZAZEN

Z•A••
ZBARS
ZEALS

Z••A•
ZADAR
ZAGAT
ZAYAK
ZETAS
ZONAL

Z•••A
ZAPPA
ZEBRA
ZEENA
ZELDA
ZENDA
ZESTA
ZETTA
ZILLA
ZORBA
ZOSMA
ZUPPA

•ZA••
AZANS
CZARS
IZAAK
OZARK
OZAWA
TZARA
TZARS

•Z•A•
IZAAK

•Z••A
AZERA
AZUSA
OZAWA
TZARA

••ZA•
ANZAC
HAZAN
KAZAN
LAZAR
MAZAR
MIZAR
MUZAK
RAZAF
RIZAL

••Z•A
MAZDA
PIZZA
REZIA

•••ZA
BAEZA
BAIZA
DANZA
ELIZA
FORZA
GINZA
GROZA
GYOZA
IBIZA
LANZA
LEEZA
MONZA
PANZA
PINZA
PIZZA
PLAZA
TERZA
YOWZA

ZB•••
ZBARS

Z•B••
ZEBRA
ZEBUS
ZUBIN

Z••B•
ZERBE
ZIPBY
ZORBA

Z•••B
ZHLOB
ZHLUB

•ZB••
UZBEK

Z•C••
ZUCCO

Z••C•
ZILCH
ZINCS
ZINCY
ZUCCO
ZWICK

Z•••C
ZENIC

•Z•C•
CZECH
OZICK

•Z••C
AZOIC
AZTEC

••ZC•
CUZCO

••Z•C
ANZAC

Z•D••
ZADAR
ZADIE
ZADIG

Z••D•
ZELDA
ZENDA
ZENDO
ZENDS

Z•••D
ZAHND
ZONED
ZOOID

•Z•D•
AZIDE
IZODS

••ZD•
MAZDA

••Z•D
ADZED
DAZED
DOZED
FAZED
GAZED
HAZED
LAZED
MAZED
OOZED
RAZED
SIZED

ZE•••
ZEALS
ZEBRA
ZEBUS
ZEENA
ZEILE
ZEISS
ZEIST
ZELDA
ZELIG
ZENDA
ZENDO
ZENDS
ZENER
ZENIC
ZENOS
ZEPPO
ZEPTO
ZERBE
ZEROG
ZEROS
ZESTA
ZESTS
ZESTY
ZETAS
ZETTA
ZEVON

Z•E••
ZEENA
ZIEFF
ZWEIG

Z••E•
ZALES
ZAXES
ZAZEN
ZENER
ZINES
ZONED
ZONER
ZONES
ZOOEY
ZOREL

Z•••E
ZADIE
ZAIRE
ZEILE
ZERBE
ZOWIE
ZTILE

•ZE••
AZERA
AZERI
CZECH
SZELL

•Z•E•
AZTEC
AZTEK
UZBEK

•Z••E
AZIDE
AZOLE
AZORE
AZURE
EZINE
OZONE
OZZIE

••ZE•
ADZED
ADZES
BEZEL
BIZET
COZEN
COZES
DAZED
DAZER
DAZES
DOZED
DOZEN
DOZER
DOZES
FAZED
FAZES
FEZES
GAZED
GAZER
GAZES
HAZED
HAZEL
HAZER
HAZES
LAZED
LAZES
MAZED
MAZEL
MAZES
NIZER
OOZED
OOZES
OUZEL
PLZEN
RAZED
RAZER
RAZES
SIZED
SIZER
SIZES
VEZES
WEZEN
WIZEN
WIZES
ZAZEN

••Z•E
EAZYE
OZZIE
SUZIE

•••ZE
ADOZE
AGAZE
AMAZE
BAIZE
BLAZE
BONZE
BOOZE
CRAZE
DOUZE
DRUZE
FROZE
FURZE
GAUZE
GLAZE
GRAZE
HENZE
JONZE
KATZE
MAIZE
PRIZE
SEIZE
SMAZE

Z•F••
ZAFUS

Z••F•
ZARFS
ZIEFF

Z•••F
ZIEFF
ZWOLF

••Z•F
RAZAF

Z•G••
ZAGAT
ZIGGY

Z••G•
ZIGGY
ZINGS
ZINGY

Z•••G
ZADIG
ZELIG
ZEROG
ZWEIG

••Z•G
ABZUG

ZH•••
ZHLOB
ZHLUB

Z•H••
ZAHND

Z•••H
ZILCH

•Z••H
AZOTH
CZECH

•••ZH
NUDZH

ZI•••
ZIEFF
ZIGGY
ZILCH
ZILLA
ZILLS
ZINCS
ZINCY
ZINES
ZINGS
ZINGY
ZINKY
ZIPBY
ZIPIN
ZIPIT
ZIPON
ZIPPO
ZIPPY
ZIPUP
ZITIS

Z•I••
ZAIRE
ZEILE
ZEISS
ZEIST
ZTILE
ZWICK

Z••I•
ZADIE
ZADIG
ZAXIS
ZAYIN
ZELIG
ZENIC
ZIPIN
ZIPIT
ZITIS
ZOOID
ZORIS
ZOWIE
ZUBIN
ZUNIS
ZWEIG

•ZI••
AZIDE
EZINE
OZICK

•Z•I•
AZOIC
IZMIR
OZZIE

•Z••I
AZERI
AZUKI

••ZI•
ANZIO
KAZIN
NAZIS
OZZIE
REZIA
REZIP
SUZIE
UNZIP
VIZIR

••Z•I
BUZZI
GOZZI
LIZZI

•••ZI
BUZZI
GHAZI
GOZZI
LIZZI
MITZI
PONZI
SWAZI

Z•K••
ZUKOR

Z••K•
ZINKY
ZONKS
ZOUKS

Z•••K
ZAYAK
ZWICK

•Z•K•
AZUKI

•Z••K
AZTEK
IZAAK
OZARK
OZICK
UZBEK

••Z•K
MUZAK

ZL•••
ZLOTY

Z•L••
ZALES
ZELDA
ZELIG
ZHLOB
ZHLUB
ZILCH
ZILLA
ZILLS
ZULUS

Z••L•
ZEALS
ZEILE
ZILLA
ZILLS
ZTILE
ZWOLF

Z•••L
ZONAL
ZOREL

•Z•L•
AZOLE
SZELL

•Z••L
SZELL

••Z•L
BEZEL
HAZEL
KYZYL
MAZEL

OUZEL
RIZAL

•••ZL
HERZL

Z••M•
ZOOMS
ZOSMA

•ZM••
IZMIR

••ZM•
GIZMO

•••ZM
PRIZM

Z•N••
ZENDA
ZENDO
ZENDS
ZENER
ZENIC
ZENOS
ZINCS
ZINCY
ZINES
ZINGS
ZINGY
ZINKY
ZONAL
ZONED
ZONER
ZONES
ZONKS
ZUNIS

Z••N•
ZAHND
ZEENA

Z•••N
ZAYIN
ZAZEN
ZEVON
ZIPIN
ZIPON
ZUBIN

•Z•N•
AZANS
EZINE
OZONE

••Z•N
COZEN
DOZEN
HAZAN
KAZAN
KAZIN
LUZON
PLZEN
WEZEN
WIZEN
ZAZEN

ZO•••
ZONAL
ZONED
ZONER
ZONES
ZONKS
ZOOEY
ZOOID
ZOOMS
ZORBA
ZOREL
ZORIS
ZORRO
ZOSMA
ZOUKS
ZOWIE

Z•O••
ZLOTY
ZOOEY
ZOOID
ZOOMS
ZWOLF

Z••O•
ZENOS
ZEROG
ZEROS
ZEVON
ZHLOB
ZIPON
ZUKOR
ZZTOP

Z•••O
ZENDO
ZEPPO
ZEPTO
ZIPPO
ZORRO
ZUCCO

•ZO••
AZOIC
AZOLE
AZORE
AZOTH
IZODS
OZONE

•Z•O•
ZZTOP

••ZO•
BAZOO
BEZOS
BOZOS
KAZOO
LUZON
MOZOS
ORZOS
OUZOS
RAZOR
VIZOR
YAZOO

••Z•O
ANZIO
BAZOO
CUZCO
GIZMO
KAZOO
MEZZO
POZZO
RIZZO
YAZOO

•••ZO
BONZO
BRAZO
GONZO
MARZO
MATZO
MEZZO
POZZO
RIZZO

Z•P••
ZAPPA
ZAPPY
ZEPPO
ZEPTO
ZIPBY
ZIPIN
ZIPIT
ZIPON
ZIPPO
ZIPPY
ZIPUP
ZUPPA

Z••P•
ZAPPA
ZAPPY
ZEPPO
ZIPPO
ZIPPY
ZUPPA

Z•••P
ZIPUP
ZZTOP

•Z••P
ZZTOP

••Z•P
REZIP
UNZIP

••Z•Q
SUZYQ

Z•R••
ZARFS
ZERBE
ZEROG
ZEROS
ZORBA
ZOREL
ZORIS
ZORRO

Z••R•
ZAIRE
ZBARS
ZEBRA
ZORRO

Z•••R
ZADAR
ZENER
ZONER
ZUKOR

•Z•R•
AZERA
AZERI
AZORE
AZURE
CZARS
OZARK
TZARA
TZARS

•Z••R
IZMIR

••Z•R
DAZER
DAZUR
DOZER
GAZER
HAZER
LAZAR
MAZAR
MIZAR
NIZER
RAZER
RAZOR
SIZER
VIZIR
VIZOR

Z•S••
ZESTA
ZESTS
ZESTY
ZOSMA

Z••S•
ZEISS
ZEIST

Z•••S
ZAFUS
ZALES
ZARFS
ZAXES
ZAXIS
ZBARS
ZEALS
ZEBUS
ZEISS
ZENDS
ZENOS
ZEROS
ZESTS
ZETAS
ZILLS
ZINCS
ZINES
ZINGS
ZITIS
ZONES
ZONKS
ZOOMS
ZORIS
ZOUKS
ZULUS
ZUNIS

•Z•S•
AZUSA

•Z••S
AZANS
CZARS
IZODS
TZARS

••Z•S
ADZES
ANZUS
BEZOS
BOZOS
COZES
DAZES
DOZES
FAZES
FEZES
GAZES
HAZES
LAZES
MAZES
MOZOS
NAZIS
OOZES
ORZOS
OUZOS
RAZES
SIZES
VEZES
WIZES

ZT•••
ZTILE

Z•T••
ZETAS
ZETTA
ZITIS
ZZTOP

Z••T•
ZEPTO
ZESTA
ZESTS
ZESTY
ZETTA
ZLOTY

Z•••T
ZAGAT
ZEIST
ZIPIT

•ZT••
AZTEC
AZTEK
ZZTOP

•Z•T•
AZOTH

••Z•T
BIZET

•••ZT
LISZT

ZU•••
ZUBIN
ZUCCO
ZUKOR
ZULUS
ZUNIS
ZUPPA

Z•U••
ZOUKS

Z••U•
ZAFUS
ZEBUS
ZHLUB
ZIPUP
ZULUS

•ZU••
AZUKI
AZURE
AZUSA

••ZU•
ABZUG
ANZUS
DAZUR

•••ZU
ISUZU
KUDZU
PONZU

Z•V••
ZEVON

ZW•••
ZWEIG
ZWICK
ZWOLF

Z•W••
ZOWIE

•Z•W•
OZAWA

Z•X••
ZAXES
ZAXIS

Z•Y••
ZAYAK
ZAYIN

Z•••Y
ZAPPY
ZESTY
ZIGGY
ZINCY
ZINGY
ZINKY
ZIPBY
ZIPPY
ZLOTY
ZOOEY

••ZY•
EAZYE
KYZYL
SUZYQ

••Z•Y
BUZZY
DAZZY
DIZZY
FEZZY
FIZZY
FUZZY
JAZZY
MUZZY
TIZZY

•••ZY
BUZZY
CRAZY
DAZZY
DITZY
DIZZY
DOOZY
FEZZY
FIZZY
FOOZY
FRAZY
FUZZY
GAUZY
GLAZY
JAZZY
JERZY
KRAZY
MUZZY
ORCZY
RITZY
TIZZY
WOOZY

ZZ•••
ZZTOP

Z•Z••
ZAZEN

•ZZ••
OZZIE

••ZZ•
BUZZI
BUZZY
DAZZY
DIZZY
FEZZY
FIZZY
FUZZY
GOZZI
JAZZY
LIZZI
MEZZO
MUZZY
PIZZA
POZZO
RIZZO
TIZZY

•••ZZ
ABUZZ
CHAZZ
EBUZZ
FRIZZ
SCUZZ
SNAZZ

6

AA••••
AAAMAP
AAAUGH
AACELL
AACHEN
AAFAIR
AAHING
AARGAU
AARHUS

A•A•••
AAAMAP
AAAUGH
ABACAB
ABACAS
ABACUS
ABASED
ABASER
ABASES
ABATED
ABATER
ABATES
ABATIS
ABATOR
ACACIA
ACADIA
ACARID
ADAGES
ADAGIO
ADAPTS
AGADIR
AGAMAS
AGAMES
AGARIC
AGASSI
AGATES
AGATHA
AGAVES
AGAWAM
ALABAM
ALAINA
ALALAS
ALAMOS
ALANIS
ALANON
ALARIC
ALARMS
ALARUM
ALASKA
ALATED
AMADEO
AMADIS
AMAJOR
AMALFI
AMALIA
AMALIE
AMANAS
AMANDA
AMANTI
AMANTS
AMARNA
AMATIS
AMATOL
AMAZED
AMAZES
AMAZIN
AMAZON
ANACIN
ANADEM
ANAKIN
ANALOG
ANANAS
ANANKE
ANARCH
ANATTO
APACHE
APATHY
ARABIA
ARABIC
ARABLE
ARADOS
ARAFAT
ARAGON
ARAMES
ARAMID
ARAMIS
ARARAS
ARARAT
ASANAS
ASANTE
ASARCO
ATALOW
ATAMAN
ATARIS
ATAVIC
ATAXIA
ATAXIC
AVAILS
AVALON
AVANTI
AVATAR
AVAUNT
AWAITS
AWAKED
AWAKEN
AWAKER
AWAKES
AWARDS
AWARER
AZALEA
AZANIA
AZARIA

A••A••
AAFAIR
ABBACY
ABBADO
ABLARE
ABLATE
ABLAZE
ABOARD
ABRADE
ABRAMS
ACKACK
ACUATE
ADDAMS
ADJANI
ADNATE
ADRATE
ADWARE
ADWARS
AERATE
AFEARD
AFFAIR
AFLAME
AFLARE
AFLATS
AFRAID
AFRAME
AGHAST
AGLAIA
AGLARE
AGNAIL
AGNATE
AIRACE
AIRARM
AKUAKU
ALBANO
ALBANS
ALBANY
ALCAPP
ALEAST
ALHAIG
ALKAID
ALKALI
ALLAIS
ALLAYS
ALMAAZ
ALMACH
ALMATY
ALNASL
ALPACA
ALSACE
ALTAIC
ALTAIR
ALTARF
ALTARS
ALVARO
ALWAYS
ALZADO
AMBAND
ANKARA
ANNALS
ANSARA
ANSATE
ANTAWN
ANWANG
ANZACS
APIARY
APPALL
APPALS
AQUAKE
ARCADE
ARCANA
ARCANE
ARCARO
ARFARF
ARGALI
ARHATS
ARIANA
ARIANE
ARIARY
ARMADA
ARMAGH
ARMAND
ARMANI
ARNALL
ARRACK
ARRANT
ARRAYS
ARTAUD
ARVADA
ARYANS
ASCALE
ASEASY
ASFAST
ASGARD
ASHADE
ASHAME
ASHARP
ASIAGO
ASIANS
ASKAMY
ASKANT
ASLANT
ASMANY
ASMARA
ASRARE
ASSAIL
ASSAYS
ASTALL
ASTANA
ASTARE
ASTART
ASWARM
ATBATS
ATDAWN
ATEAMS
ATEASE
ATHAND
ATLAST
ATMANS
ATRAIN
ATTACH
ATTACK
ATTAIN
ATTARS
ATYALE
AUBADE
AUFAIT
AULAIT
AUPAIR
AURATE
AVIANS
AVIARY
AVIATE
AWEARY
AYEAYE
AZRAEL

A•••A•
AAAMAP
AARGAU
ABACAB
ABACAS
ABOMAS
ABORAL
ABROAD
ABSCAM
ACELAS
ACETAL
ACTSAS
ACTUAL
ACURAS
ADIDAS
ADONAI
ADRIAN
AEGEAN
AENEAS
AERIAL
AFFRAY
AFGHAN
AFLOAT
AGAMAS
AGAWAM
AGENAS
AGITAS
AGLEAM
AGORAE
AGORAS
AIDMAN
AIKMAN
AIMSAT
AIRBAG
AIRDAM
AIRMAN
AIRSAC
AIRWAR
AIRWAY
AJOWAN
AKELAS
AKITAS
ALABAM
ALALAS
ALEGAR
ALEMAN
ALETAP
ALEXAS
ALIYAH
ALLDAY
ALLMAN
ALMAAZ
ALOHAS
ALOMAR
ALPHAS
ALTMAN
ALTTAB
ALULAE
ALULAR
ALYDAR
AMANAS
AMEBAE
AMEBAS
AMICAL
AMIDAS
AMIGAS
AMORAL
AMTRAC
AMTRAK
AMYTAN
ANANAS
ANDEAN
ANDRAE
ANIMAL
ANIMAS
ANNEAL
ANNUAL
ANODAL
ANORAK
ANTRAL
ANYDAY
ANYMAN
ANYWAY
AORTAE
AORTAL
AORTAS
AOUDAD
APEMAN
APICAL
APNEAS
APODAL
APPEAL
APPEAR
APPIAN
ARAFAT
ARARAS
ARARAT
ARCTAN
ARECAS
ARENAS
AROMAS
ARREAR
ARTCAR
ARUBAN
ASANAS
ASFLAT
ASHCAN
ASHLAR
ASHMAN
ASHPAN
ASHRAM
ASNEAR
ASNEAT
ASOSAN
ASTEAL
ASTRAL
ASTRAY
ATAMAN
ATONAL
ATPLAY
ATRIAL
ATTHAT
AUDIAL
AUGEAN
AUGEAS
AVATAR
AVOWAL
AXEMAN
AXHEAD
AXONAL
AZERAS
AZONAL

A••••A
ABOLLA
ACACIA
ACADIA
ACEDIA
ACTIVA
AEOLIA
AFRICA
AGATHA
AGENDA
AGLAIA
AHIMSA
AIRSEA
ALAINA
ALASKA
ALCINA
ALEXIA
ALHENA
ALICIA
ALOGIA
ALPACA
ALTHEA
ALTIMA
ALTRIA
ALUDRA
ALUMNA
ALYSSA
ALZIRA
AMALIA
AMANDA
AMARNA
AMELIA
AMENRA
AMESIA
AMINTA
AMOEBA
AMONRA
AMRITA
ANDREA
ANEMIA
ANGELA
ANGLIA
ANGOLA
ANGORA
ANITRA
ANKARA
ANNIKA
ANNINA
ANOMIA
ANOXIA
ANSARA
ANTLIA
APOPKA
APULIA
AQUILA
ARABIA
ARBELA
ARCANA
AREOLA
ARETHA
ARIANA
ARISTA
ARJUNA
ARLOVA
ARMADA
ARNICA
ARRIBA
ARVADA
ASMARA
ASONIA
ASPERA
ASSTDA
ASTANA
ASTHMA
ATAXIA
ATHENA
ATONIA
ATTICA
ATTILA
AURIGA
AURORA
AVESTA
AXILLA
AYESHA
AZALEA
AZANIA
AZARIA
AZELMA
AZTECA
AZUELA

•AA•••
AAAMAP
AAAUGH
BAABAA
BAAING
BAALIM
HAAGEN
HAAKON
LAALAA
MAALOX
MAAZEL
PAANGA

•A•A••
AAFAIR
BABALU
BACALL
BAHAMA
BALAAM
BALATA
BAMAKO
BANANA
BANANE
BARACK
BARADA
BARAKA
BARANY
BARATA
BARATO
BASALT
BATAAN
BAYARD
BAZAAR
CABALA
CABALS
CABANA
CACAOS
CALAIS
CALASH
CAMARO
CANAAN
CANADA
CANALS
CANAPE
CANARD
CANARY
CARAFE
CARATS
CASABA
CASALS
CASAVA
CATALO
CATANO
CAVAFY
CAZALE
DACAPO
DAGAMA
DALAND
DALASI
DAMAGE
DAMASK
DAMATO
DANANG
DATARY
FACADE
FALALA
FALANA
FARACY
FARADS
FARAHS
FATALE
FAYARD
GALANT
GALAXY
GAMAYS
GARAGE
GAWAIN
HABANA
HADAGO
HAHAHA
HALALA
HAMATE
HARALD
HARARE
HARASS
HASAGO
HATARI
HAVANA
HAVASU
HAWAII
HAZANS
HAZARD
JACALS
JALAPA
JAMAAL
JAMAIS
JAPANS
JARABE
KAGAWA
KAKAPO
KAMALI
KANAKA
KANALY
KANATA
KANAWA
KARATE
KARATS
KAYAKS
LABATT
LACAGE
LACASA
LACAVA
LALALA
LAMARR
LAMAZE
LANAIS
LANARK
LANATE
LARAMS
LARAZA
LAVABO
LAVAGE
LAVAIN
LAXALT
MACACO
MACAPA
MACAWS
MADAMA
MADAME
MADAMS
MAHALO
MALABO
MALADY
MALAGA
MALARS
MALAWI
MALAYA
MALAYS
MANAGE
MANAMA
MANANA
MANAOS
MANAPE
MANATS
MARACA
MARAUD
MASADA
MASAIS
MASALA
MAYANS
NAGANO
NAIADS
NAMATH
NAPACA
NAPALM
NARADA
NASALS
NATALE
NATANT
NAVAHO
NAVAID
NAVAJO
OARAGE
OAXACA
PAEANS
PAGANS
PAJAMA
PALACE
PALADE
PALAIS
PALATE
PANADA
PANAMA
PAPACY
PAPAGO
PAPAWS
PAPAYA
PARADE
PARANA
PARAPH
PATACA
PATAKI
PAVANE
QABALA
QATARI
RADARS
RAFAEL
RAJABS
RAJAHS
RAMADA
RAMAPO
RAMATE
RAVAGE
SABADO
SABALS
SABATO
SAFARI
SAHARA
SALAAM
SALADA
SALADE
SALADS
SALAMI
SALARY
SAMARA
SARANS
SATAYS
SAVAGE
SAVAII
SAVANA
SAVANT
SAVATE
SAWALL
SAYAAH
SAYAYE
TABARD
TAMALE
TAMARA
TAMAYO
TANAKA
TANANA
TARAWA
TATAMI
TATARS
VACANT
VACATE
VAGARY
VALAIS
VANARK
WABASH
WAKAME
WASABI
WAYANS
XANADU
YAMAHA
YAMANI
YATATA
ZAPATA

•A••A•
AAAMAP
AARGAU
BAABAA
BABKAS
BADDAY
BADHAM
BADHAT
BADMAN
BADRAP
BAGDAD
BAGMAN
BAHIAN
BAIKAL
BAISAS
BAIZAS
BALAAM
BALKAN
BALKAT
BALLAD
BALSAM
BALSAS
BALZAC
BANTAM
BANYAN
BANZAI
BAOBAB
BARBAN
BARCAR
BARKAT
BARMAN
BARTAB
BASIAL
BASRAH
BATAAN
BATDAY
BATEAU
BATMAN
BATYAM
BAUMAN
BAYMAN
BAYSAT
BAZAAR
CABMAN
CABRAL
CADEAU
CAESAR
CAFTAN
CAGUAS
CAIMAN
CALLAN
CALLAO
CALLAS
CAMEAS
CAMEAT
CANAAN
CANCAN
CANNAS
CANTAB
CANTAL
CANVAS
CARMAN
CARNAC
CARNAL
CARNAP
CARPAL
CARPAT
CARWAX
CASBAH
CASPAR
CASUAL
CATHAY
CATMAN
CATNAP
CATSAT
CAUDAD
CAUDAL
CAUSAL
CAVEAT
CAVIAR
CAWCAW
CAYMAN
DABRAT
DABSAT
DACHAS
DAEDAL
DAGMAR
DALLAS
DANNAY
DARNAY
DATHAN
EARLAP
EARTAB
EARTAG
EARWAX
EASYAS
EATSAT
FABIAN
FABRAY
FACIAE
FACIAL
FACIAS
FAENAS
FAIMAN
FAISAL
FALLAL
FANTAN
FANTAS
FARRAH
FARRAR
FATCAT
FATMAN
FATWAS
FAUNAE
FAUNAL
FAUNAS
GAGLAW
GAGMAN
GALEAE
GALEAO
GALPAL
GALWAY
GAMMAS
GAPEAT
GARGAN
GASBAG
GASCAN
GASCAP
GASMAN
GASPAR
GASTAX
GASWAR
GATEAU
GAVIAL
GAVRAS
GAWKAT
GAZEAT
HABEAS
HABLAR
HADEAN
HAGGAI
HAGMAN
HAIDAS
HAIKAI
HALLAM
HALVAH
HALVAS
HANDAX
HANGAR
HANNAH
HANSAS
HARHAR
HARLAN
HARRAD
HARRAH
HASSAM
HASSAN
HAVEAT
HAWHAW
HAZMAT
IAMSAM
JABBAR
JACKAL
JAGUAR
JALPAS
JAMAAL
JAMCAM
JANUAR
JARJAR
JAWSAT
KALKAN
KALMAR
KANSAN
KANSAS
KAPLAN
KAPPAS
KARMAS
KARNAK
KARRAS
KASBAH
KASDAN
KASHAS
KATMAI
KAUNAS
LAALAA
LABIAL
LABRAT

LAGEAR
LAICAL
LAMIAE
LAMIAS
LANDAT
LANDAU
LANVAL
LAPCAT
LAPHAM
LAPSAT
LARIAT
LARVAE
LARVAL
LARVAS
LASCAR
LAULAU
LAWMAN
LAYMAN
MACRAE
MADCAP
MADMAN
MADMAX
MADRAS
MAENAD
MAFIAS
MAGIAN
MAGMAS
MAGYAR
MAITAI
MAJOAD
MALIAN
MAMBAS
MAMMAL
MAMMAS
MANDAN
MANDAY
MANGAS
MANIAC
MANIAS
MANNAS
MANRAY
MANTAS
MANUAL
MAOTAI
MARIAH
MARIAN
MARIAS
MARKAS
MARYAM
MATMAN
MAUMAU
MAYDAY
MAYHAP
MAYTAG
MAZDAS
NACHAS
NADSAT
NAGNAG
NAGSAT
NAIRAS
NAKFAS
NARIAL
NASCAR
NASDAQ
NASSAU
NATHAN
NAYSAY
OAHUAN
OAKTAG
OARMAN
PACMAN
PADUAN
PAIDAD
PAISAN
PAJOAD
PALEAE
PALLAS
PALMAR
PALMAS
PAMPAS
PANDAS
PAPPAS
PAPUAN
PARCAE
PARIAH
PARKAS
PARKAV
PARKAY
PARLAY
PASCAL
PASDAR
PASHAS
PASSAS
PASSAT
PASTAS
PATDAY
PATHAN
PAUSAL
PAWPAW
PAWSAT
PAYDAY
PAYPAL
QANTAS
RACIAL
RADIAL
RADIAN
RAGBAG
RAGLAN
RAGMAN
RAGNAR
RAGTAG
RAHRAH
RAHWAY
RAILAT
RAITAS
RAMEAU
RAMFAN
RAMPAL
RAMSAY
RANDAL
RANTAT
RASCAL
RASHAD
RASPAS
RASTAS
RATTAN
RATTAT
RAVEAT
RAWBAR
RAYBAN
SABRAS
SADDAM
SADDAY
SAIDAH
SAIPAN
SALAAM
SALMAN
SALSAS
SAMBAS
SAMEAS
SAMIAM
SAMOAN
SAMPAN
SANDAL
SANKAS
SANTAS
SASHAY
SATPAT
SATRAP
SAUNAS
SAVEAS
SAYAAH
SAYNAY
SAYSAH
TABLAS
TAGDAY
TAIGAS
TAIPAN
TAIWAN
TALKAT
TAMTAM
TANKAS
TANOAK
TAPPAN
TARGAS
TARMAC
TARSAL
TARTAN
TARTAR
TARZAN
TASMAN
TATRAS
TAXLAW
TAXMAN
VACLAV
VANDAL
VARGAS
VARIAS
VARNAS
VASLAV
VASSAL
VASSAR
WAHWAH
WANTAD
WARSAW
WASHAD
WAUSAU
WAVEAT
WAYLAY
YANKAT
YAPSAT
ZANTAC

•A•••A

BAABAA
BAERGA
BAHAMA
BAKULA
BALATA
BALBOA
BANANA
BARADA
BARAKA
BARATA
BARBRA
BARKLA
BAROJA
BASTIA
CABALA
CABANA
CABEZA
CAMERA
CANADA
CANCHA
CANDIA
CANOLA
CANOVA
CANULA
CAPITA
CARBRA
CARDIA
CARINA
CASABA
CASAVA
CASITA
CASSIA
CATENA
CATERA
CAYUGA
DAGAMA
DAHLIA
DAKOTA
DAMITA
DANOVA
DAOSTA
DAYSPA
EARTHA
EASTLA
FACULA
FAJITA
FALALA
FALANA
FARINA
FASCIA
FATIMA
GALENA
GALLIA
GAMBIA
GARCIA
HABANA
HAHAHA
HALALA
HAVANA
JALAPA
JAMESA
JAMOCA
JASCHA
KAGAWA
KAHLUA
KAHUNA
KAILUA
KANAKA
KANATA
KANAWA
KARINA
KAUNDA
LAALAA
LABREA
LACASA
LACAVA
LACTEA
LACUNA
LADIDA
LADOGA
LAGUNA
LAKOTA
LALALA
LAMBDA
LAMESA
LAMINA
LANCIA
LANINA
LAONZA
LAPUTA
LARAZA
LAROSA
LASTRA
LATINA
LATOYA
LATRIA
LATVIA
LAURIA
LAVIDA
MACAPA
MACULA
MADAMA
MADERA
MAKEBA
MAKUTA
MALAGA
MALAYA
MANAMA
MANANA
MANCHA
MANILA
MANTRA
MANTUA
MARACA
MARCIA
MARIDA
MARINA
MARISA
MARKKA
MARSHA
MARTHA
MASADA
MASALA
MATTEA
MAXIMA
MAZOLA
MAZUMA
NAGOYA
NAPACA
NAPHTA
NARADA
NARITA
NARNIA
NASHUA
NAUSEA
OAXACA
PAANGA
PACULA
PADOVA
PAELLA
PAGLIA
PAGODA
PAJAMA
PAKULA
PALOMA
PAMELA
PAMINA
PANADA
PANAMA
PAPAYA
PARANA
PASCUA
PATACA
PATINA
PATRIA
PAYOLA
QABALA
RAFFIA
RAGUSA
RAMADA
RAMONA
RATEDA
SABENA
SABINA
SAHARA
SALADA
SALINA
SALIVA
SAMARA
SAMOSA
SANCTA
SANDIA
SANDRA
SANTHA
SARNIA
SAVANA
TABULA
TACOMA
TALISA
TAMARA
TANAKA
TANANA
TANTRA
TARAWA
VALERA
VALOVA
WADENA
WALESA
WASECA
YAKIMA
YAKUZA
YAMAHA
YAMUNA
YATATA
ZADORA
ZAMBIA
ZAMORA
ZAPATA

••AA••

DNAASE
GRAAFF
ISAACS
KLAATU
KRAALS
RNAASE
SCAASI
SEAAIR
SEAARM
TEAACT

••A•A•

AAAMAP
ABACAB
ABACAS
AGAMAS
AGAWAM
ALABAM
ALALAS
AMANAS
ANANAS
ARAFAT
ARARAS
ARARAT
ASANAS
ATAMAN
AVATAR
BAABAA
BEAMAN
BEAPAL
BEATAT
BRAMAH
BRAVAS
BWANAS
CHAZAN
CLAWAT
COAXAL
CRAVAT
DNALAB
DRAMAS
FRACAS
GNAWAT
GOAWAY
GRABAT
GRAHAM
GRATAE
GRAVAS
GUAVAS
HIATAL
IBADAN
IMAMAN
INADAY
INAJAM
INARAY
INAWAY
ISAIAH
ISAIAN
KOALAS
LAALAA
LEAPAT
LHASAN
LIANAS
LLAMAS
MEATAX
MIATAS
NYALAS
ODAMAE
OMAHAN
OMAHAS
ONAJAG
ONAPAR
OSAKAN
PLAKAT
PLANAR
PLANAS
PLAYAS
PLAYAT
PLAZAS
PRADAS
PRANAS
QUAPAW
QUASAR
REAGAN
REATAS
RIATAS
ROARAT
SCALAR
SCARAB
SEABAG
SEACAT
SEAGAL
SEAHAG
SEALAB
SEAMAN
SEAMAP
SEATAC
SEAWAY
SHAMAN
SHAZAM
SNAPAT
STABAT
STALAG
STAYAT
SWATAT
TEABAG
TEARAT
TIARAS
TOAMAN
TRAJAN
TRALAS
UTAHAN
VEADAR
XSARAS
YOAKAM

••A••A

ACACIA
ACADIA
AGATHA
ALAINA
ALASKA
AMALIA
AMANDA
AMARNA
ARABIA
ATAXIA
AZALEA
AZANIA
AZARIA
BAABAA
BIAFRA
BIANCA
BLANCA
BLANDA
BRAHMA
BRANCA
BRAZZA
CHACHA
CHAKRA
CHARTA
CLAMMA
CLASSA
CRANIA
DCAREA
DEANNA
DHARMA
ETALIA
EXACTA
FLAUTA
FLAVIA
FRANCA
GRADEA
GRAMPA
GRANPA
GRAPPA
GRATIA
IBARRA
ICARIA
INAREA
ITALIA
ITASCA
IVANKA
IWANNA
JOANNA
KRASNA
KWACHA
KWANZA
LAALAA
LUANDA
MIASMA
OJAICA
PAANGA
PHAGIA
PIAZZA
PLASMA
PRAVDA
QUAGGA
QUANTA
REALIA
REATTA
RUANDA
RWANDA
SCALIA
SHANIA
SHASTA
SMALLA
SPARTA
STADIA
STANZA
THALIA
TRAUMA
UGANDA
URANIA
USAUSA
VIAGRA
ZSAZSA

•••AA•

ALMAAZ
BALAAM
BATAAN
BAZAAR
CANAAN
GSTAAD
JAMAAL
MESAAZ
NOMAAM
SALAAM
SAYAAH
SCHAAP
YUMAAZ

•••A•A

AGLAIA
ALPACA
ANKARA
ANSARA
ARCANA
ARIANA
ARMADA
ARVADA
ASMARA
ASTANA
BAHAMA
BALATA
BANANA
BARADA
BARAKA
BARATA
BEMATA
BINACA
BRIANA
BROADA
BURANA
CABALA
CABANA
CANADA
CASABA
CASAVA
CICADA
COLADA
DAGAMA
DENADA
ERRATA
ESPANA
FALALA
FALANA
GEMARA
GETANA
GOTAMA
GOTANA
GUIANA
GUYANA
HABANA
HAHAHA
HALALA
HAVANA
HIVAOA
IGUANA
ILEANA
IMPALA
INSANA
ITHACA
JALAPA
JICAMA
JUDAEA
JUMADA
KAGAWA
KANAKA
KANATA
KANAWA
KERALA
LACASA
LACAVA
LALALA
LARAZA
LUSAKA
MACAPA
MADAMA
MALAGA
MALAYA
MANAMA
MANANA
MARACA
MASADA
MASALA
MEDAKA
MIKASA
MIRADA
MUFASA
NAPACA
NARADA
NEVADA
OAXACA
OGLALA
OKSANA
OMEARA
OOLALA
ORGANA
ORIANA
OSHAWA
OTTAVA
OTTAWA
PAJAMA
PANADA
PANAMA
PAPAYA
PARANA
PATACA
PICARA
PINATA
PIRANA
PITAYA
POEANA
POLARA
POSADA
QABALA
RAMADA
RENATA
ROXANA
SAHARA
SALADA
SAMARA
SAVANA
SECADA
SEDAKA
SEMANA
SOLARA
SOMATA
SONATA
STRADA
STRATA
TAMARA
TANAKA
TANANA
TARAWA
TEJANA
TIRANA
TOYAMA
TUCANA
UMTATA
UNGAVA
UPSALA
URBANA
VIHARA
VITARA
YAMAHA
YATATA
YEMANA
YUKATA
YUKAWA
ZAPATA
ZENANA

••••AA

BAABAA
FIVEAA
FOURAA
LAALAA

AB••••

ABACAB
ABACAS
ABACUS
ABASED
ABASER
ABASES
ABATED
ABATER
ABATES
ABATIS
ABATOR
ABBACY
ABBADO
ABBESS
ABBEYS
ABBOTS
ABBOTT
ABBREV
ABCDEF
ABDIEL
ABDUCE
ABDUCT
ABELES
ABHORS
ABIDED
ABIDER
ABIDES
ABITOF
ABJECT
ABJURE
ABLARE
ABLATE
ABLAZE
ABLEST
ABLOOM
ABLUSH
ABMHOS
ABOARD
ABODES
ABOHMS
ABOLLA
ABOMAS
ABOMBS
ABORAL
ABORTS
ABOUND
ABRADE
ABRAMS
ABROAD
ABRUPT
ABSCAM
ABSENT
ABSORB
ABSURD
ABUSED
ABUSER
ABUSES
ABUTON
ABYSMS

A•B•••

ABBACY
ABBADO
ABBESS
ABBEYS
ABBOTS
ABBOTT
ABBREV
ALBANO
ALBANS
ALBANY
ALBEDO
ALBEIT
ALBERS
ALBERT
ALBINE
ALBINO
ALBION
ALBORG
ALBUMS
AMBAND
AMBERS
AMBERY
AMBIEN
AMBITS
AMBLED
AMBLER
AMBLES
AMBLIN
AMBUSH
ARBELA
ARBORS
ARBOUR
ARBRES
ASBURY
ATBATS
ATBEST
AUBADE
AUBREY
AUBURN

A••B••

ADOBES
ADOBOS
AIRBAG
AIRBUD
AIRBUS
ALABAM
ALIBIS
ALIBLE
ALLBUT
AMEBAE
AMEBAS
AMEBIC
ANUBIS
ARABIA
ARABIC
ARABLE
ARUBAN
ASHBIN

A•••B•

ABOMBS
ACHEBE
ADLIBS
AEROBE
AKIMBO
AMOEBA
ARRIBA

A••••B

ABACAB
ABSORB
ADSORB
ADVERB
ALICEB
ALTTAB
APLOMB
ATHROB

•AB•••

BABALU
BABBLE
BABBLY
BABELS
BABIED
BABIER
BABIES
BABKAS
BABOON
BABOOS
BABSON
CABALA
CABALS
CABANA
CABBED
CABBIE
CABELL
CABERS
CABEZA
CABINS
CABLED
CABLER
CABLES
CABLET
CABMAN
CABMEN
CABRAL
CABRIO
DABBED
DABBER
DABBLE
DABNEY
DABRAT
DABSAT
FABBER
FABIAN
FABLED
FABLER
FABLES
FABRAY
FABRIC
GABBED
GABBER
GABBLE
GABBRO
GABLED
GABLER
GABLES
HABANA
HABEAS
HABILE
HABITS
HABLAR
JABBAR
JABBED
JABBER
JABOTS
KABOBS
KABOOM
KABUKI
LABATT
LABELS
LABFEE
LABIAL
LABILE
LABINE
LABIUM
LABORS
LABOUR
LABRAT
LABREA
MABELL
MABLEY
NABBED
NABBER
NABOBS
NABORS
PABLUM
PABSTS
QABALA
RABBET
RABBIS
RABBIT
RABBLE
RABIES
SABADO
SABALS
SABATO
SABENA
SABERS
SABINA
SABINE
SABLES
SABOTS
SABRAS
SABRES
TABARD
TABBED
TABKEY
TABLAS
TABLED
TABLES
TABLET
TABOOS
TABORS
TABRIZ
TABSET
TABUED
TABULA
WABASH
WABBIT
ZABRZE

•A•B••

BAABAA
BABBLE
BABBLY
BADBOY
BAGBOY
BALBOA
BAMBIS
BAMBOO
BAOBAB

BARBAN BARBED BARBER BARBET BARBIE BARBRA BATBOY BAUBLE CABBED CABBIE CAMBER CAMBOY CARBON CARBOS CARBOY CARBRA CASBAH CATBED DABBED DABBER DABBLE DAUBED DAUBER DAUBES DAWBER DAYBED EARBUD FABBER GABBED GABBER GABBLE GABBRO GAMBIA GAMBIT GAMBLE GAMBOL GARBED GARBER GARBLE GASBAG HARBIN HARBOR HASBRO HATBOX IAMBIC IAMBUS JABBAR JABBED JABBER JAMBES KASBAH LAMBDA LAMBED LAYBYS LAZBOY MAMBAS MAMBOS MARBLE MARBLY MAYBES NABBED NABBER RABBET RABBIS RABBIT RABBLE RAGBAG RAMBLE RAMBOS RAWBAR RAYBAN SAMBAS SAYBOO TABBED TAMBOR WABBIT WAMBLE WAMBLY WARBLE ZAMBIA

•A••B•

CAMEBY CANTBE CARIBE CARIBS CAROBS CASABA DANUBE EASEBY GATSBY GAZEBO HANGBY HARDBY JACOBI JACOBY JARABE JAZZBO KABOBS LAIDBY LAVABO LAYSBY MAKEBA MALABO MALIBU MALTBY NABOBS NASEBY PASSBY RACEBY RAJABS SAHIBS SASEBO WALKBY WASABI

•A•••B

BAGJOB BAOBAB BARTAB CANTAB DAYJOB EARTAB MACOMB RAGHIB ZAGREB

••AB••

ALABAM ARABIA ARABIC ARABLE BAABAA BLABBY CRABBE CRABBY DIABLE DIABLO DIABOL DOABLE DRABEK DRABLY ENABLE FLABBY GRABAT GRABBY GRABLE INABIT INABOX ISABEL LIABLE ONABUN SEABAG SEABED SEABEE SHABBY STABAT STABLE STABLY SUABLE SWABBY TEABAG UNABLE UNABLY USABLE USABLY VIABLE VIABLY YEABIG

••A•B•

BLABBY CRABBE CRABBY CRAMBO FLABBY FLAMBE GIAMBI GOALBY GRABBY GRANBY NEARBY PLANBS PLAYBY SHABBY SWABBY

••A••B

ABACAB DNALAB GRADEB INATUB SCARAB SEALAB SMALLB

•••AB•

CASABA COHABS JARABE KEBABS LAVABO MALABO MCCABE MCNABB MESABI MUGABE MYBABY OHBABY PCLABS PICABO RAJABS REHABS SQUABS VOCABS WASABI

•••A•B

BEDAUB BICARB DEKALB MCNABB STRAUB SUSANB

••••AB

ABACAB ALTTAB BAOBAB BARTAB BIOLAB CANTAB CONFAB DNALAB EARTAB ECOLAB GETSAB PREFAB PUNJAB REDTAB REGRAB RESTAB SCARAB SCHWAB SEALAB SKYLAB TYPEAB

AC••••

ACACIA ACADIA ACARID ACCEDE ACCENT ACCEPT ACCESS ACCORD ACCOST ACCRUE ACCTNO ACCUSE ACEDIA ACEDIT ACELAS ACEOUT ACESIT ACESUP ACETAL ACETIC ACETYL ACHEBE ACHENE ACHERS ACHIER ACHING ACIDIC ACIDLY ACKACK ACORNS ACQUIT ACROSS ACTFOR ACTIII ACTING ACTION ACTIUM ACTIVA ACTIVE ACTNOW ACTONE ACTORS ACTOUT ACTSAS ACTSIN ACTSON ACTSUP ACTTWO ACTUAL ACUATE ACUITY ACUMEN ACURAS ACUTER ACUTES

A•C•••

AACELL AACHEN ABCDEF ACCEDE ACCENT ACCEPT ACCESS ACCORD ACCOST ACCRUE ACCTNO ACCUSE AECIUM AHCHOO ALCAPP ALCINA ALCOTT ALCOVE ANCHOR ANCHOS ANCIEN ARCADE ARCANA ARCANE ARCARO ARCCOS ARCHED ARCHER ARCHES ARCHIE ARCHLY ARCHON ARCING ARCSEC ARCSIN ARCTAN ARCTIC ASCALE ASCEND ASCENT ASCOLD ASCOOL ASCOTS ATCOST AWCMON

A••C••

ABACAB ABACAS ABACUS ABSCAM ACACIA AFLCIO ALECKS ALECKY ALECTO ALICEB ALICES ALICIA AMECHE AMICAL AMICES AMICUS ANACIN ANTCOW APACHE APICAL APICES ARCCOS ARECAS ARTCAR ASHCAN AVOCET

A•••C•

ABBACY ABDUCE ABDUCT ABJECT ACKACK ADDICT ADDUCE ADDUCT ADVICE AFFECT AFRICA AGENCE AGENCY AIRACE ALLYCE ALMACH ALNICO ALPACA ALSACE AMERCE ANARCH ANTICS ANZACS APERCU APIECE ARNICA ARRACK ASARCO ASDICS ASMUCH ASPECT ASPICS ASSUCH ATONCE ATTACH ATTACK ATTICA ATTICS AVOUCH AWHECK AZTECA AZTECS

A••••C

ACETIC ACIDIC ADONIC AGARIC AHOLIC AIRSAC AJIJIC ALARIC ALTAIC AMEBIC AMTRAC ANDRIC ANEMIC ANGLIC ANODIC ANOMIC ANOXIC AORTIC ARABIC ARCSEC ARCTIC ATAVIC ATAXIC ATOMIC ATONIC ATOXIC ATYPIC AXENIC AZONIC

•AC•••

AACELL AACHEN BACALL BACHED BACHES BACHIT BACKED BACKER BACKIN BACKUP BACKUS BACONS CACAOS CACHED CACHES CACHET CACKLE CACTUS DACAPO DACHAS DACRON DACTYL FACADE FACEIT FACEON FACERS FACETS FACEUP FACIAE FACIAL FACIAS FACIES FACILE FACING FACTOR FACTUM FACULA HACEKS HACHOO HACKED HACKER HACKIE HACKIT HACKLE HACKLY HACKUP JACALS JACKAL JACKED JACKET JACKIE JACKUP JACLYN JACOBI JACOBY LACAGE LACASA LACAVA LACEON LACERS LACEUP LACHEY LACHOY LACIER LACILY LACING LACKED LACKEY LACLOS LACTEA LACTIC LACUNA MACACO MACAPA MACAWS MACERS MACHOS MACKIE MACLEN MACLES MACNEE MACOMB MACOUN MACRAE MACRON MACROS MACULA NACHAS NACHOS NACION NACRED NACRES PACERS PACHIN PACIER PACIFY PACING PACINO PACKED PACKER PACKET PACKIN PACKON PACKUP PACMAN PACTEN PACULA RACEBY RACEIN RACEME RACERS RACETO RACEUP RACHEL RACIAL RACIER RACILY RACINE RACING RACINO RACISM RACIST RACKED RACKER RACKET RACKUP SACFLY SACHEM SACHER SACHET SACKED SACKER SACKUP SACQUE SACRED SACRUM TACKED TACKER TACKLE TACKON TACKUP TACOMA TACTEL TACTIC VACANT VACATE VACHEL VACHES VACLAV VACUUM WACKER WACKOS WACOTX YACHTS

•A•C••

BADCOP BANCOS BARCAR BARCOS CAICOS CANCAN CANCEL CANCER CANCHA CANCUN CATCHY CAUCHY CAUCUS CAWCAW DANCED DANCER DANCES DANCIN DARCEL FALCON FARCED FARCES FARCRY FASCES FASCIA FATCAT FAUCET GARCIA GARCON GASCAN GASCAP GASCON GAUCHE GAUCHO JAMCAM JASCHA JAYCEE LAICAL LANCED LANCER LANCES LANCET LANCIA LANCIE LAPCAT LASCAR MADCAP MANCHA MANCHE MANCHU MARCEL MARCHE MARCIA MARCIE MARCIL MARCIX MARCOS MARCUS MASCOT NARCOS NASCAR PANCHO PANCKS PARCAE PARCEL PASCAL PASCHS PASCUA PATCHY PAYCUT RANCHO RANCID RANCOR RASCAL RASCHE SANCHO SANCTA SATCOM SAUCED SAUCER SAUCES TAICHI TALCED TALCUM TAXCUT WARCRY

•A••C•

BARACK BARUCH BASICS BAUSCH CALICO CANUCK FARACY HAUNCH HAVOCS JAMOCA JANICE LAUNCH MACACO MAGICS MALICE MALICK MARACA NAPACA NATICK OAXACA PALACE PANICS PAPACY PATACA PAUNCH RAUNCH SAFECO VAILCO WASECA ZANUCK

•A•••C

BALTIC BALZAC BARDIC CADMIC CARNAC FABRIC FANFIC GAELIC GALLIC GARLIC IAMBIC IATRIC KAONIC KARMIC LACTIC LAURIC MALEIC MANIAC MANTIC MASTIC PARSEC PATHIC PATRIC TACTIC TANNIC TARMAC TAURIC ZANTAC

••AC••

ABACAB ABACAS ABACUS ACACIA ANACIN APACHE BEACHY BEACON BLACKS BRACCO BRACED BRACER BRACES BRACHS BRACTS CHACEL CHACHA CHACHI CHACUN CLACKS COACTS CRACKD CRACKS CRACOW DBACKS DEACON ENACTS EPACTS EXACTA EXACTS FIACRE FLACKS FLACON FRACAS FRACTO GLACES GLACIS GRACED GRACES GRACIE IMACOP KNACKS KWACHA LEACHY NIACIN ORACHS ORACLE PEACHY PLACED PLACER PLACES PLACID POACHY QUACKS QUACKY REACTS SEACAT SEACOW SHACKS SLACKS SMACKS SNACKS SPACED SPACEK SPACER SPACES SPACEY STACEY STACKS TEACUP TRACED TRACER TRACES TRACEY TRACHE TRACII TRACKS TRACTS URACIL VIACOM WHACKS WRACKS

••A•C•

ANARCH ASARCO BIANCA BIANCO BLANCA BLANCH BLANCO BRACCO BRANCA BRANCH BRASCO CHANCE CHANCY CLANCY DRANCY ELANCE EPARCH EXARCH FIANCE FIASCO FRANCA FRANCE FRANCK FRANCO FRANCS GLANCE GRAECO INARCH ISAACS ITASCA KLATCH NUANCE OJAICA PEARCE PLAICE PLANCK PRANCE SCARCE SEAICE SEANCE SEARCH SNATCH STANCE STANCH STARCH SWATCH TEAACT THATCH TRANCE USANCE

••A••C

AGARIC ALARIC ARABIC ATAVIC ATAXIC CYANIC DYADIC INASEC ITALIC OXALIC PHASIC SEATAC SLAVIC SMALLC STATIC TRAGIC URALIC URANIC VLASIC

•••AC•

ABBACY ACKACK AIRACE ALMACH ALPACA ALSACE ANZACS ARRACK ATTACH ATTACK BARACK BINACA BLEACH BONACI BREACH BROACH CDRACK CORACI CURACY CUSACK DEFACE DETACH DIDACT EFFACE ENFACE ENIACS ENLACE FARACY GOBACK HIJACK HORACE IGNACE IMBACK IMPACT INBACK INFACT INTACT ISAACS ITHACA JSBACH KOVACS LEGACY LILACS LUNACY MACACO MARACA MENACE MISACT MONACO NAPACA OAXACA ONEACT ORBACH OUTACT PALACE PAPACY PATACA PESACH PIRACY PREACH PREACT REDACE REDACT REFACE RELACE REPACK RERACK RETACK SERACS SOLACE SPRACH SUMACS TEAACT TENACE TEXACO THEACT THRACE THWACK TWOACT UNFACT UNLACE UNPACK UNRACK UNTACK VIVACE WOMACK

•••A•C

ALTAIC EDDAIC ENBANC INCAIC JUDAIC MOSAIC ROMAIC VEDAIC

••••AC

AIRSAC AMTRAC

BALZAC BIGMAC CARNAC CHIRAC COGNAC CONTAC EGGSAC GETSAC HOOSAC INKSAC IPECAC MANIAC MELMAC MICMAC OVISAC PROZAC RICRAC SEATAC TARMAC TICTAC TIETAC TIRIAC UNIVAC ZANTAC ZODIAC

AD••••

ADAGES ADAGIO ADAPTS ADDAMS ADDEND ADDERS ADDICT ADDING ADDINS ADDLED ADDLES ADDONS ADDSIN ADDSON ADDSTO ADDSUP ADDUCE ADDUCT ADEEMS ADELEH ADELIE ADELLE ADENIS ADEPTS ADESTE ADFEES ADHERE ADIDAS ADIEUS ADIEUX ADJANI ADJOIN ADJURE ADJUST ADLIBS ADMINS ADMIRE ADMITS ADNATE ADNOUN ADOBES ADOBOS ADOLFO ADOLPH ADONAI ADONIC ADONIS ADOPTS ADORED ADOREE ADORER ADORES ADORNS ADOUTS ADRATE ADRENO ADREPS ADRIAN ADRIEN ADRIFT ADRIVE ADROIT ADSORB ADULTS ADVENT ADVERB ADVERT ADVICE ADVILS ADVISE ADWARE ADWARS ADWEEK ADYTUM ADZING ADZUKI

A•D•••

ABDIEL ABDUCE ABDUCT ADDAMS ADDEND ADDERS ADDICT ADDING ADDINS ADDLED ADDLES ADDONS ADDSIN ADDSON ADDSTO ADDSUP ADDUCE ADDUCT AEDILE AIDERS AIDFUL AIDING AIDMAN AIDMEN ALDERS ALDINE ALDISS ALDOUS ALDRIN ANDEAN ANDERS ANDHOW ANDRAE ANDREA ANDREI ANDRES ANDREW ANDREY ANDRIC ANDROS ANDYET ARDENT ARDORS ARDOUR ASDEEP ASDICS ASDULL ATDAWN ATDUSK AUDIAL AUDILE AUDIOS AUDITS AUDREY

A••D••

ABCDEF ABIDED ABIDER ABIDES ABODES ACADIA ACEDIA ACEDIT ACIDIC ACIDLY ADIDAS AGADIR AGEDLY AIRDAM AIRDRY ALLDAY ALUDEL ALUDRA ALYDAR AMADEO AMADIS AMEDEE AMEDEO AMIDAS AMIDES AMIDOL AMIDST ANADEM ANODAL ANODES ANODIC ANYDAY AOUDAD APODAL ARADOS ARIDER ARIDLY ASHDOD ASIDES ATODDS AVEDON AVIDER AVIDLY AWEDLY AZIDES AZODYE

A•••D•

ABBADO ABRADE ACCEDE AGENDA AIKIDO ALBEDO ALGEDI ALKYDS ALLUDE ALZADO AMANDA AMENDS APHIDS ARCADE ARENDT ARMADA AROIDS ARVADA ASHADE ASSTDA ATODDS AUBADE AVOIDS AWARDS

A••••D

ABASED ABATED ABIDED ABOARD ABOUND ABROAD ABSURD ABUSED ACARID ACCORD ADDEND ADDLED ADORED AENEID AFEARD AFFORD AFIELD AFRAID AGEOLD AGREED AIRBUD AISLED ALATED ALFRED ALINED ALIPED ALKAID ALLIED ALMOND ALTOID AMAZED AMBAND AMBLED AMUSED ANELED ANGLED ANKLED ANTEED ANYOLD AOUDAD APPEND ARAMID ARCHED ARGUED ARMAND ARNOLD AROUND ARTAUD ASCEND ASCOLD ASGARD ASGOOD ASHDOD ASTRID ASTRUD ATHAND ATONED ATSTUD ATTEND ATWOOD AUFOND AUGEND AUTOED AVOWED AWAKED AXHEAD AXSEED AZURED

•AD•••

BADBOY BADCOP BADDAY BADDER BADDIE BADDOG BADEGG BADEMS BADEND BADFIT BADGER BADGES BADGUY BADHAM BADHAT BADLIE BADLOT BADMAN BADMEN BADOFF BADRAP BADUNS CADDIE CADEAU CADENT CADETS CADGED CADGER CADGES CADMIC CADMUS CADRES DADDYO DADDYS DADGUM DADOED DADOES FADDLE FADEIN FADERS FADING GADDED GADDER GADDIS GADFLY GADGET HADAGO HADDEN HADDIE HADDIX HADEAN HADFUN HADJES HADJIS HADONE HADOUT HADRON JADING JADISH KADEEM KADETT LADDER LADDIE LADERS LADIDA LADIES LADING LADINO LADLED LADLER LADLES LADOGA LADUKE LADYDI MADAMA MADAME MADAMS MADCAP MADDED MADDEN MADDER MADDIE MADDOG MADDOX MADDUX MADEDO MADEGO MADEIT MADEOF MADERA MADERO MADEUP MADFOR MADLYN MADMAN MADMAX MADMEN MADRAS MADRES MADRID MADSEN MADURO MADVIG NADINE NADIRS NADSAT PADDED PADDER PADDLE PADOVA PADRES PADUAN RADARS RADIAL RADIAN RADIOS RADISH RADIUM RADIUS RADLEY RADNER RADNOR RADOME SADDAM SADDAY SADDEN SADDER SADDLE SADHES SADHUS SADISM SADIST SADLER WADDED WADDER WADDLE WADDLY WADEIN WADENA WADERS WADING WADSUP ZADDIK ZADORA

•A•D••

BADDAY BADDER BADDIE BADDOG BAGDAD BALDED BALDER BALDIE BALDLY BALDUR BANDED BANDER BANDIT BARDIC BARDOT BATDAY CADDIE CALDER CAMDEN CANDIA CANDID CANDLE CANDOR CARDED CARDER CARDIA CARDIN CARDIO CATDOM CAUDAD CAUDAL CAWDOR DADDYO DADDYS DAEDAL DANDER DANDIE DANDLE DANDYL DAUDET DAWDLE FADDLE FANDOM GADDED GADDER GADDIS GANDER GANDHI GARDEN HADDEN HADDIE HADDIX HAIDAS HAIDEE HAMDEN HANDAX HANDED HANDEL HANDER HANDIN HANDKE HANDLE HANDON HANDUP HARDBY HARDEN HARDER HARDIN HARDLY HARDUP HAYDEN JARDIN KANDEL KANDER KASDAN LADDER LADDIE LAIDBY LAIDIN LAIDON LAIDTO LAIDUP LANDAT LANDAU LANDED LANDER LANDHO LANDIS LANDON LANDOR LANDRY LANDUP LANDUS LAPDOG LARDED LARDER LARDON LAUDED LAUDER MADDED MADDEN MADDER MADDIE MADDOG MADDOX MADDUX MAHDIS MAIDEN MALDEN MANDAN MANDAY MANDEL MANDMS MARDEN MARDIS MAYDAY MAZDAS NASDAQ PADDED PADDER PADDLE PAIDAD PAIDIN PAIDUP PANDAS PANDER PANDIT PANDLS PARDON PASDAR PATDAY PATDRY PAYDAY RAIDED RAIDER RANDAL RANDOM RANDRY RAWDON SADDAM SADDAY SADDEN SADDER SADDLE SAIDAH SAIDHI SAIDNO SAIDOK SAIDSO SAIDTO SANDAL SANDED SANDER SANDIA SANDRA SANDRO SARDIS SARDOU SAUDIS SAYDIE TAGDAY TANDEM TARDES TAWDRY VALDEZ VANDAL VARDEN VATDYE WADDED WADDER WADDLE WADDLY WALDEN WANDER WARDED WARDEN WARDER YARDED YARDER ZADDIK

•A••D•

BARADA CANADA CANIDS DAVIDE DAVIDI DAVIDL DAVIDO FACADE FALUDI FARADS HAIRDO HALIDE KAUNDA LADIDA LADYDI LAIRDS LAMBDA LAMEDS LAREDO LAVIDA MADEDO MAKEDO MALADY MARIDA MARIDO MASADA MAUNDY NAIADS NARADA PAGODA PALADE PANADA PARADE PARODY RAMADA RANIDS RAPIDO RAPIDS RATEDA RATEDG RATEDR RATEDX SABADO SALADA SALADE SALADS SAMEDI SAYIDO XANADU

•A•••D

BABIED BACHED BACKED BADEND BAFFED BAGDAD BAGEND BAGGED BAILED BAITED BALDED BALKED BALLAD BANDED BANGED BANKED BANNED BARBED BARGED BARKED BARNED BARRED BASHED BASKED BASTED BATHED BATTED BAWLED BAYARD CABBED CABLED CACHED CADGED CALKED CALLED CALMED CALVED CAMPED CANARD CANDID CANNED CANOED CANTED CAPPED CAPRID CARDED CARPED CARTED CARVED CASHED CASKED CASTED CATBED CAUDAD CAUSED DABBED DADOED DALAND DAMMED DAMNED DAMPED DANCED DANGED DAPPED DARNED DARTED DASHED DAUBED DAWNED DAYBED DAYOLD EAGLED EARBUD EARNED FABLED FAGEND FAILED FAIRED FAKEID FANGED FANNED FARCED FARMED FASTED FATTED FAWNED FAYARD GABBED GABLED GADDED GAFFED GAGGED GAINED GAITED GALLED GAMMED GANGED GAOLED GAPPED GARBED GASHED GASPED GASSED GAUGED GAWKED GAWPED HACKED HAFTED HAILED HAIRED HALOED HALOID HALTED HALVED HAMMED HANDED HANGED HARALD HARKED HARMED HAROLD HARPED HARRAD HASHED HASPED HASSID HASTED HATRED HATTED HAULED HAWKED HAZARD JABBED JACKED JAGGED JAILED JAMMED JARRED JAZZED KAYOED LACKED LADLED LAGGED LAIRED LALLED LAMBED LAMMED LANCED LANDED LAPPED LAPSED LARDED LARKED LASHED LASTED LATHED LAUDED MADDED MADRID MAENAD MAILED MAIMED MAJOAD MALTED MANNED MAPPED MARAUD MARKED MARLED MARRED MASHED MASKED MASSED MASTED MATTED MAULED NABBED NACRED NAGGED NAILED NAPPED NAVAID PACKED PADDED PAIDAD PAINED PAIRED PAJOAD PALLED PALLID PALMED PANNED PANTED PARGED PARKED PARRED PARSED PARTED PASSED PASTED PATTED PAUSED PAWNED RACKED RAFTED RAGGED RAIDED RAILED RAINED RAISED RAMMED RAMPED RAMROD RANCID RANGED RANKED RANTED RAPPED RASHAD RASHID RASPED RATTED RAZZED SACKED SACRED SAGGED SAILED SALTED SALVED SANDED SAPPED SASHED SASSED SAUCED SAWRED TABARD TABBED TABLED TABUED TACKED TAGEND TAGGED TAILED TALCED TALKED TALMUD TAMPED TANGED TANKED TANNED TAPPED TARRED TARTED TASKED TASTED TATTED TAXIED VALUED VALVED VAMPED VANNED VARIED VATTED WADDED WAFTED WAGGED WAILED WAITED WAIVED WALKED WALLED WANNED WANTAD WANTED WARDED WARGOD WARMED WARNED WARPED WARRED WARTED WASHAD WASHED WASLED WASOLD WASTED YAKKED YANKED YAPPED YARDED YARNED YAWNED YAWPED ZAGGED ZAPPED

••AD••

ACADIA AGADIR AMADEO AMADIS ANADEM ARADOS BEADED BEADER BEADLE BEADUP BLADED BLADER BLADES CLADIN CRADLE DEADEN DEADER DEADLY DEADON DIADEM DYADIC ELADIO EVADED EVADER EVADES GLADES GLADLY GLADTO GLADYS GOADED GRADEA GRADEB GRADED GRADER GRADES HEADED HEADER HEADIN HEADON

6 AD

HEADTO
HEADUP
HYADES
IBADAN
INADAY
LEADED
LEADEN
LEADER
LEADIN
LEADON
LEADTO
LEADUP
LLADRO
LOADED
LOADER
LOADIN
LOADUP
MCADOO
MEADER
MEADOW
PRADAS
QUADRI
READDS
READER
READIN
README
READON
READTO
READUP
ROADEO
ROADER
ROADIE
SEADOG
SHADED
SHADER
SHADES
SHADOW
SPADED
SPADER
SPADES
STADIA
TRADED
TRADER
TRADES
TSADES
TSADIS
VEADAR

••A•D•

AMANDA
AWARDS
BEARDS
BLANDA
BOARDS
BRAIDS
BRANDI
BRANDO
BRANDS
BRANDT
BRANDX
BRANDY
CHANDU
CHARDS
CIARDI
CLAUDE
CUANDO
ECARDS
ELANDS
FRAIDY
FRAUDS
GLANDS
GRANDE
GRANDS
GRANDY
GUARDS
HOARDS
LUANDA
PBANDJ
PLAIDS
PRAVDA
READDS
RUANDA
RWANDA
SCALDS
SHANDY
SHARDS
SKALDS
STANDS
SWARDS
UGANDA
UVALDE
VIANDS
WEALDS
XYANDZ

••A••D

ABASED
ABATED
ACARID
ALATED
AMAZED
ARAMID
AWAKED
BEADED
BEAKED
BEAMED
BEANED
BIASED
BLADED
BLAMED
BLARED
BLAZED
BOATED
BRACED
BRAKED
BRAVED
BRAYED
CEASED
CHAFED
CHASED
CHAWED
CLAWED
COALED
COATED
COAXED
CRACKD
CRANED
CRAPED
CRATED
CRAVED
CRAZED
CYANID
DIALED
DRAPED
DRAYED
ELAPID
ELATED
ERASED
EVADED
FEARED
FLAKED
FLAMED
FLARED
FLAWED
FLAYED
FOALED
FOAMED
FRAMED
FRAYED
GEARED
GLARED
GLAZED
GNAWED
GOADED
GRACED
GRADED
GRATED
GRAVED
GRAVID
GRAYED
GRAZED
HEADED
HEALED
HEAPED
HEATED
HEAVED
HOAXED
IDARED
IMAGED
INAPOD
JEANED
KHALID
LEADED
LEAFED
LEAKED
LEANED
LEAPED
LEASED
LEAVED
LOADED
LOAFED
LOAMED
LOANED
MOANED
MOATED
NEARED
OKAYED
ORATED
PEAKED
PEALED
PEAPOD
PHASED
PLACED
PLACID
PLANED
PLATED
PLAYED
PRATED
PRAYED
QUAKED
REAMED
REAPED
REARED
REAVED
ROAMED
ROARED
RRATED
SCALED
SCARED
SEABED
SEAGOD
SEALED
SEAMED
SEARED
SEATED
SHADED
SHAMED
SHAPED
SHARED
SHAVED
SKATED
SLAKED
SLATED
SLAVED
SLAYED
SMALLD
SNAKED
SNARED
SOAKED
SOAPED
SOARED
SPACED
SPADED
SPARED
SPAYED
STAGED
STAKED
STALED
STARED
STATED
STAVED
STAYED
SWAYED
TEAMED
TEARED
TEASED
THAWED
TRACED
TRADED
UNAGED
UNAVID
UNAWED
UNAXED
VIALED
WEANED
WEAVED
WHALED
XRATED
XRAYED
YEANED

•••AD•

ABBADO
ABRADE
ALZADO
ARCADE
ARMADA
ARVADA
ASHADE
AUBADE
BARADA
BREADS
BROADA
CANADA
CICADA
COLADA
CURADS
CYCADS
DECADE
DECADS
DENADA
DESADE
DORADO
DOSADO
DREADS
DRYADS
ESTADO
ETRADE
FACADE
FARADS
HEXADS
HODADS
ILIADS
INVADE
JIHADS
JUMADA
JURADO
KNEADS
LEVADE
MALADY
MASADA
MIKADO
MILADY
MIRADA
MISADD
MONADS
MOVADO
MYLADY
NAIADS
NARADA
NEVADA
NICADS
NOMADS
OBLADI
OCTADS
OGRADY
OREADS
OUTADD
PALADE
PANADA
PARADE
PESADE
PLEADS
POMADE
POSADA
RAMADA
REMADE
REPADS
RIYADH
SABADO
SALADA
SALADE
SALADS
SECADA
SQUADS
STEADS
STEADY
STRADA
STRADS
TIRADE
TREADS
TRIADS
UNLADE
UNMADE
WEBADS
XANADU

•••A•D

ABOARD
AFEARD
AFRAID
ALKAID
AMBAND
ARMAND
ARTAUD
ASGARD
ATHAND
BAYARD
BRIAND
BRIARD
BYHAND
BYLAND
CANARD
COWARD
CUNARD
DALAND
DELAND
DEMAND
DONALD
DOTARD
DUGALD
DUGARD
EDGARD
EDUARD
EDVARD
EDWARD
EKLAND
ELUARD
ERHARD
ERRAND
EXPAND
EZZARD
FAYARD
FMBAND
FUGARD
GERALD
GERARD
GODARD
GSTAAD
HARALD
HAZARD
HERALD
HOWARD
IDCARD
INHAND
INLAID
INLAND
INWARD
ISLAND
LELAND
LENARD
LIGAND
LIZARD
MARAUD
MISADD
NAVAID
ONHAND
ONLAID
ONLAND
ONWARD
OSWALD
OUTADD
OXNARD
PETARD
PICARD
POLAND
REGARD
RELAID
RELAND
REMAND
RENARD
REPAID
RESAID
RESAND
RETARD
REWARD
RIBALD
RIBAND
RITARD
ROLAND
RONALD
SEWARD
STRAND
TABARD
TOGAED
TOWARD
TVLAND
UNHAND
UNLAID
UNPAID
UNSAID
UPCARD
UPLAND
UPWARD
VISAED
WIGAND
WIZARD

••••AD

ABROAD
AOUDAD
AXHEAD
BAGDAD
BALLAD
BEHEAD
BIGBAD
BILDAD
BYROAD
CAUDAD
CIUDAD
CONRAD
DELEAD
DIDBAD
DOODAD
DORSAD
EMQUAD
ENNEAD
ENQUAD
ERSTAD
FIVEAD
FORBAD
FOURAD
GETMAD
GETSAD
GILEAD
GODEAD
GOTMAD
GSTAAD
HARRAD
HEPTAD
HOWSAD
IMGLAD
INKPAD
INROAD
JOYPAD
KEYPAD
KONRAD
MAENAD
MAJOAD
MOSSAD
MSQUAD
MYRIAD
NEXRAD
NIKEAD
NINEAD
NOLEAD
NOLOAD
NOTBAD
OGDOAD
ONLOAD
PAIDAD
PAJOAD
PENTAD
PLEIAD
RASHAD
RECLAD
RELEAD
RELOAD
REREAD
RIBPAD
SINBAD
SINEAD
SOSPAD
SPREAD
TETRAD
THREAD
TOOBAD
UNCLAD
UNDEAD
UNGLAD
UNLEAD
UNLOAD
UNREAD
UPLOAD
WANTAD
WASHAD

AE••••

AECIUM
AEDILE
AEGEAN
AENEAS
AENEID
AEOLIA
AEOLUS
AERATE
AERIAL
AERIER
AERIES
AERIFY
AERILY
AERIOS
AEROBE
AESOPS
AETHER

A•E•••

ABELES
ACEDIA
ACEDIT
ACELAS
ACEOUT
ACESIT
ACESUP
ACETAL
ACETIC
ACETYL
ADEEMS
ADELEH
ADELIE
ADELLE
ADENIS
ADEPTS
ADESTE
AFEARD
AGEDLY
AGEING
AGEISM
AGEIST
AGENAS
AGENCE
AGENCY
AGENDA
AGENTJ
AGENTK
AGENTS
AGEOLD
AGEONE
AGEOUT
AGESIX
AGETEN
AGETWO
AHERNE
AIELLO
AKELAS
AKENES
ALEAST
ALECKS
ALECKY
ALECTO
ALEGAR
ALEGRE
ALEGUP
ALEKEG
ALEMAN
ALEPHS
ALEPPO
ALEROS
ALERTS
ALETAP
ALETTE
ALEUTS
ALEVEL
ALEVES
ALEXAS
ALEXEI
ALEXEY
ALEXIA
ALEXIS
AMEBAE
AMEBAS
AMEBIC
AMECHE
AMEDEE
AMEDEO
AMEERS
AMELIA
AMELIE
AMENDS
AMENRA
AMENTS
AMERCE
AMESIA
ANELED
ANELES
ANEMIA
ANEMIC
ANERGY
APELET
APEMAN
APEMEN
APERCU
APEXES
ARECAS
ARENAS
ARENDT
AREOLA
AREOLE
ARETES
ARETHA
ARETOO
AREZZO
ASEASY
ASEVER
ATEAMS
ATEASE
ATEMPO
ATENTH
ATEOUT
ATERRE
ATESTS
AVEDON
AVEENO
AVENGE
AVENUE
AVERSE
AVERTS
AVESTA
AWEARY
AWEDLY
AWEIGH
AXEMAN
AXEMEN
AXENIC
AYEAYE
AYESHA
AYESIR
AZELMA
AZERAS
AZERIS

A••E••

AACELL
ABBESS
ABBEYS
ABJECT
ABLEST
ABSENT
ACCEDE
ACCENT
ACCEPT
ACCESS
ACHEBE
ACHENE
ACHERS
ADDEND
ADDERS
ADEEMS
ADFEES
ADHERE
ADIEUS
ADIEUX
ADRENO
ADREPS
ADVENT
ADVERB
ADVERT
ADWEEK
AEGEAN
AENEAS
AENEID
AFFECT
AFIELD
AFRESH
AFTERS
AGLEAM
AGLETS
AGREED
AGREER
AGREES
AIDERS
AILEEN
AIMERS
AIRERS
ALBEDO
ALBEIT
ALBERS
ALBERT
ALDERS
ALGEDI
ALHENA
ALIENS
ALKENE
ALLEES
ALLEGE
ALLELE
ALLEYN
ALLEYS
ALPERT
ALTERS
ALWEST
AMBERS
AMBERY
AMEERS
AMIENS
AMOEBA
AMPERE
AMVETS
ANDEAN
ANDERS
ANGELA
ANGELI
ANGELL
ANGELO
ANGELS
ANGERS
ANNEAL
ANNEES
ANSEIS
ANSELM
ANTEED
ANTERO
ANTEUP
AOLERS
APIECE
APNEAS
APPEAL
APPEAR
APPELS
APPEND
APPERT
APTEST
ARBELA
ARDENT
ARGENT
ARIEGE
ARLENE
ARMERS
ARMETS
ARNEIS
ARNESS
ARNETT
ARPEGE
ARPELS
ARREAR
ARREST
ARRETE
ARSENE
ARSENO
ARTELS
ARTERY
ARTEST
ASCEND
ASCENT
ASDEEP
ASKERS
ASLEEP
ASNEAR
ASNEAT
ASPECT
ASPENS
ASPERA
ASSENT
ASSERT
ASSESS
ASSETS
ASTEAL
ASTEEP
ASTERN
ASTERO
ASTERS
ASWELL
ATBEST
ATHEEL
ATHENA
ATHENE
ATHENS
ATREST
ATREUS
ATTEND
ATTEST
AUGEAN
AUGEAS
AUGEND
AUGERS
AUTEUR
AVEENO
AWHECK
AWLESS
AXHEAD
AXSEED
AZTECA
AZTECS
AZTEKS
AZUELA

A•••E•

AACHEN
ABASED
ABASER
ABASES
ABATED
ABATER
ABATES
ABBREV
ABCDEF
ABDIEL
ABELES
ABIDED
ABIDER
ABIDES
ABODES
ABUSED
ABUSER
ABUSES
ACHIER
ACUMEN
ACUTER
ACUTES
ADAGES
ADDLED
ADDLES
ADELEH
ADFEES
ADOBES
ADORED
ADOREE
ADORER
ADORES
ADRIEN
ADWEEK
AERIER
AERIES
AETHER
AGAMES
AGATES
AGAVES
AGETEN
AGGIES
AGILER
AGONES
AGREED
AGREER
AGREES
AIDMEN
AIGLET
AIGRET
AILEEN
AIRIER
AIRMEN
AIRSEA
AISLED
AISLES
AKENES
ALATED
ALEKEG
ALEVEL
ALEVES
ALEXEI
ALEXEY
ALFRED
ALFVEN
ALGREN
ALICEB
ALICES
ALIKES
ALINED
ALINER
ALINES
ALIPED
ALIVEO
ALKIES
ALLEES
ALLIED
ALLIES
ALLMEN
ALLNEW
ALLSET
ALLWET
ALTHEA
ALTKEY
ALUDEL
AMADEO
AMAZED
AMAZES
AMBIEN
AMBLED
AMBLER
AMBLES
AMEDEE
AMEDEO
AMICES
AMIDES
AMINES
AMOLES
AMORES
AMORET
AMPLER
AMSTEL
AMULET
AMUSED
AMUSER
AMUSES
ANADEM
ANCIEN
ANDREA
ANDREI
ANDRES
ANDREW
ANDREY
ANDYET
ANELED
ANELES
ANGLED
ANGLEE
ANGLER
ANGLES
ANIMES
ANISES
ANKLED
ANKLES
ANKLET
ANNEES
ANNIES
ANNLEE
ANODES
ANOLES
ANSWER
ANTEED
ANTHEM
ANTHER
ANTLER
ANTRES
APELET
APEMEN
APEXES
APICES
APOGEE
APPLES
APPLET
ARAMES
ARBRES
ARCHED
ARCHER
ARCHES
ARCSEC
ARETES
ARGUED
ARGUER
ARGUES
ARIDER
ARISEN
ARISES
ARMIES
ARMLET
ARNHEM
ARNIES
AROUET
ARTIER
ASDEEP
ASEVER
ASFREE
ASHIER
ASHLEE
ASHLEY
ASHMEN
ASIDES
ASLEEP
ASTEEP
ASTHER
ASTLEY
ASTRES
ATHEEL
ATILES
ATISES
ATMFEE
ATONED
ATONER
ATONES
ATTLEE
AUBREY
AUDREY
AUKLET
AUNTEM
AUSPEX
AUSTEN
AUSTER
AUTOED
AVIDER
AVOCET

AVOWED
AVOWER
AWAKED
AWAKEN
AWAKER
AWAKES
AWARER
AWOKEN
AXEMEN
AXISES
AXONES
AXSEED
AZALEA
AZIDES
AZOLES
AZORES
AZRAEL
AZURED
AZURES

A••••E

ABDUCE
ABJURE
ABLARE
ABLATE
ABLAZE
ABRADE
ACCEDE
ACCRUE
ACCUSE
ACHEBE
ACHENE
ACTIVE
ACTONE
ACUATE
ADDUCE
ADELIE
ADELLE
ADESTE
ADHERE
ADJURE
ADMIRE
ADNATE
ADOREE
ADRATE
ADRIVE
ADVICE
ADVISE
ADWARE
AEDILE
AERATE
AEROBE
AFFINE
AFLAME
AFLARE
AFRAME
AGENCE
AGEONE
AGLARE
AGNATE
AGORAE
AHERNE
AHORSE
AIRACE
ALBINE
ALCOVE
ALDINE
ALEGRE
ALETTE
ALFINE
ALGORE
ALIBLE
ALKENE
ALLEGE
ALLELE
ALLUDE
ALLURE
ALLYCE
ALPINE
ALSACE
ALULAE
AMALIE
AMEBAE
AMECHE
AMEDEE
AMELIE
AMERCE
AMITIE
AMPERE
AMPULE
ANANKE
ANDRAE
ANGLEE
ANNLEE
ANOMIE
ANSATE
ANTONE
ANYONE
AORTAE
APACHE
APIECE
APLITE
APOGEE
APPOSE
APRILE
AQUAKE
ARABLE
ARCADE
ARCANE
ARCHIE
AREOLE
ARGIVE
ARGYLE
ARIANE
ARIEGE
ARIOSE
ARLENE
AROUSE
ARPEGE
ARRETE
ARRIVE
ARSENE
ASANTE
ASCALE
ASFREE
ASHADE
ASHAME
ASHINE
ASHLEE
ASHORE
ASLOPE
ASPIRE
ASPURE
ASRARE
ASSIZE
ASSUME
ASSURE
ASTARE
ASTUTE
ATEASE
ATERRE
ATFIVE
ATHENE
ATHOME
ATMFEE
ATNINE
ATONCE
ATTIRE
ATTLEE
ATTUNE
ATYALE
AUBADE
AUDILE
AUGITE
AUNTIE
AURATE
AUSSIE
AVENGE
AVENUE
AVERSE
AVIATE
AVULSE
AWHILE
AXLIKE
AYEAYE
AZODYE

•AE•••

BAERGA
BAEYER
CAESAR
DAEDAL
DAEMON
DAEWOO
FAENAS
FAERIE
FAEROE
GAELIC
JAEGER
KAETHE
MAENAD
PAEANS
PAELLA

•A•E••

AACELL
BABELS
BADEGG
BADEMS
BADEND
BAGELS
BAGEND
BAKERS
BAKERY
BALEEN
BALERS
BAREGE
BARELY
BAREST
BASELY
BASEST
BATEAU
BAYERN
BAYEUX
CABELL
CABERS
CABEZA
CADEAU
CADENT
CADETS
CAGEIN
CAGERS
CAGEUP
CAKEUP
CAMEAS
CAMEAT
CAMEBY
CAMEIN
CAMELS
CAMEON
CAMEOS
CAMERA
CAMETO
CAMEUP
CANERS
CAPERS
CAREEN
CAREER
CAREOF
CARERS
CARESS
CARETO
CARETS
CASEFY
CASEIN
CASERN
CASERS
CATENA
CATERA
CATERS
CAVEAT
CAVEIN
CAVELL
CAVERN
CAVERS
CAVETT
DALENE
DALETH
DALETS
DAREME
DARENT
DARERS
DAREST
DARETO
DATERS
DAVENS
DAZERS
EASEBY
EASEIN
EASELS
EASEON
EASERS
EASEUP
EATERS
EATERY
FACEIT
FACEON
FACERS
FACETS
FACEUP
FADEIN
FADERS
FAGEND
FAKEID
FAKEIT
FAKERS
FAKERY
FARERS
FAXERS
GAIETY
GALEAE
GALEAO
GALENA
GAMELY
GAMERS
GAMEST
GAMETE
GANEFS
GAPEAT
GAPERS
GARETH
GATEAU
GATERS
GAVEIN
GAVELS
GAVEOF
GAVEON
GAVETO
GAVEUP
GAYEST
GAZEAT
GAZEBO
GAZEON
GAZERS
HABEAS
HACEKS
HADEAN
HAKEEM
HALEST
HALEVY
HAMELN
HAREMS
HATEIT
HATERS
HATETO
HAVEAT
HAVEIN
HAVEIT
HAVENO
HAVENS
HAVENT
HAVEON
HAVETO
HAVEUP
HAYERS
HAZELS
HAZERS
JAMESA
JAMESI
JAMESJ
JAMESK
JAMESM
JAMESS
JAMEST
JAMESV
JAPERS
JAPERY
JAVERT
KADEEM
KADETT
KAPELL
KAREEM
LABELS
LACEON
LACERS
LACEUP
LADERS
LAGEAR
LAGERS
LAKERS
LAMEDS
LAMELY
LAMENT
LAMESA
LAMEST
LAPELS
LAPERI
LAPERM
LAREDO
LAREES
LASERS
LATEEN
LATELY
LATENE
LATENS
LATENT
LATEOF
LATEON
LATERI
LATERO
LATEST
LATETO
LAVERN
LAVERS
LAXEST
LAYERS
MABELL
MACERS
MADEDO
MADEGO
MADEIT
MADEOF
MADERA
MADERO
MADEUP
MAKEBA
MAKEDO
MAKEGO
MAKEIT
MAKEME
MAKEOF
MAKERS
MAKEUP
MALEIC
MANEGE
MANERO
MANETS
MASERS
MASERU
MATERS
MATEYS
MAVENS
MAXELL
MAXENE
MAYEST
NAMEIT
NAMELY
NAMERS
NAPERY
NASEBY
NAVELS
OARERS
OATERS
PACERS
PAGERS
PAGEUP
PALEAE
PALELY
PALEST
PAMELA
PANELS
PAPERS
PAPERY
PARENS
PARENT
PARERS
PARETO
PAREUS
PAREVE
PASEOS
PATENS
PATENT
PATERS
PAVERS
PAVESE
PAWERS
PAYEES
PAYERS
RACEBY
RACEIN
RACEME
RACERS
RACETO
RACEUP
RAGERS
RAKEIN
RAKERS
RAKEUP
RAMEAU
RAMENS
RAMETS
RANEES
RAREES
RAREFY
RARELY
RAREST
RASERS
RATEDA
RATEDG
RATEDR
RATEDX
RATELS
RATERS
RAVEAT
RAVELS
RAVENS
RAVEON
RAVERS
RAVEUP
RAWEGG
RAWEST
RAZERS
SABENA
SABERS
SAFECO
SAFELY
SAFEST
SAFETY
SAGELY
SAGEST
SALEPS
SAMEAS
SAMEDI
SAMEKH
SANELY
SANEST
SAREES
SASEBO
SATEEN
SAVEAS
SAVEIT
SAVEME
SAVEON
SAVERS
SAVEUP
SAWERS
SAYERS
SAYEST
TAGEND
TAKEIN
TAKEIT
TAKEON
TAKERS
TAKETH
TAKETO
TAKEUP
TALENT
TALERS
TALESE
TAMELY
TAMERS
TAMEST
TAPEON
TAPERS
TAPEUP
TASERS
TATERS
TAVELS
TAVERN
TAXERS
VALENE
VALENS
VALENT
VALERA
VALERE
VALERO
VALERY
VALETS
VARESE
WADEIN
WADENA
WADERS
WAFERS
WAFERY
WAGERS
WAKENS
WAKERS
WAKEUP
WALESA
WASECA
WATERS
WATERY
WAVEAT
WAVEIN
WAVERS
WAVERY
WAVETO
WAXERS
YARELY
YAREST
ZAZENS

•A••E•

AACHEN
BABIED
BABIER
BABIES
BACHED
BACHES
BACKED
BACKER
BADDER
BADGER
BADGES
BADMEN
BAEYER
BAFFED
BAFFER
BAGGED
BAGGER
BAGMEN
BAHNEN
BAILED
BAILEE
BAILER
BAILEY
BAINES
BAITED
BAITER
BAIZES
BAKKER
BALDED
BALDER
BALEEN
BALKED
BALKER
BALLET
BALMER
BANDED
BANDER
BANGED
BANGER
BANKED
BANKER
BANNED
BANNEN
BANNER
BANTER
BARBED
BARBER
BARBET
BARGED
BARGER
BARGES
BARKED
BARKER
BARLEY
BARMEN
BARNED
BARNES
BARNET
BARNEY
BARRED
BARREL
BARREN
BARRES
BARRET
BARTEL
BARTER
BASHED
BASHER
BASHES
BASKED
BASKER
BASKET
BASSES
BASSET
BASSEY
BASTED
BASTER
BASTES
BATHED
BATHER
BATHES
BATLEY
BATMEN
BATTED
BATTEN
BATTER
BAUMER
BAVIER
BAWLED
BAWLER
BAXTER
BAYMEN
CABBED
CABLED
CABLER
CABLES
CABLET
CABMEN
CACHED
CACHES
CACHET
CADGED
CADGER
CADGES
CADRES
CAGIER
CAGNEY
CAHIER
CAKIER
CALDER
CALKED
CALKER
CALLED
CALLEE
CALLER
CALLES
CALMED
CALMER
CALMEX
CALVED
CALVES
CALVET
CALXES
CAMBER
CAMDEN
CAMOES
CAMPED
CAMPER
CANCEL
CANCER
CANIER
CANKER
CANNED
CANNEL
CANNER
CANNES
CANOED
CANOER
CANOES
CANTED
CANTER
CAPLET
CAPPED
CAPPER
CARDED
CARDER
CAREEN
CAREER
CARIES
CARKEY
CARMEL
CARMEN
CARNER
CARNES
CARNET
CARNEY
CARPED
CARPEL
CARPER
CARPET
CARREL
CARREY
CARSEY
CARTED
CARTEL
CARTER
CARTES
CARVED
CARVEL
CARVER
CARVES
CARVEY
CASHED
CASHES
CASHEW
CASKED
CASKET
CASPER
CASTED
CASTEL
CASTER
CASTES
CATBED
CATHER
CATMEN
CAUSED
CAUSER
CAUSES
CAVIES
DABBED
DABBER
DABNEY
DADOED
DADOES
DAFTER
DAGGER
DAILEY
DAISES
DALLES
DAMIEN
DAMMED
DAMMER
DAMNED
DAMNER
DAMPED
DAMPEN
DAMPER
DAMSEL
DANCED
DANCER
DANCES
DANDER
DANGED
DANGER
DANIEL
DANKER
DANNER
DANSES
DANTEI
DANTES
DAPPED
DAPPER
DARCEL
DARIEN
DARKEN
DARKER
DARNED
DARNER
DARREN
DARTED
DARTER
DASHED
DASHER
DASHES
DAUBED
DAUBER
DAUBES
DAUDET
DAVIES
DAWBER
DAWNED
DAYBED
EAGLED
EAGLES
EAGLET
EAGRES
EARLET
EARNED
EARNER
EASIER
EASLEY
EASTER
FABBER
FABLED
FABLER
FABLES
FACIES
FAFNER
FAILED
FAINER
FAIRED
FAIRER
FAITES
FALLEN
FALLER
FALSER
FALTER
FANGED
FANJET
FANNED
FANNER
FARCED
FARCES
FARFEL
FARLEY
FARMED
FARMER
FAROES
FASCES
FASTED
FASTEN
FASTER
FATHER
FATTED
FATTEN
FATTER
FAUCET
FAUTES
FAUVES
FAWKES
FAWNED
FAWNER
FAYLEN
GABBED
GABBER
GABLED
GABLER
GABLES
GADDED
GADDER
GADGET
GAFFED
GAFFER
GAFFES
GAGGED
GAGGER
GAGMEN
GAINED
GAINER
GAINES
GAITED
GAITER
GALLED
GALLEY
GAMGEE
GAMIER
GAMMED
GAMMER
GANDER
GANGED
GANGER
GANGES
GANNET
GAOLED
GAOLER
GAPPED
GARBED
GARBER
GARDEN
GARNER
GARNET
GARRET
GARTER
GARVEY
GASHED
GASHES
GASJET
GASKET
GASMEN
GASPED
GASPER
GASSED
GASSER
GASSES
GASTER
GATHER
GAUGED
GAUGER
GAUGES
GAUZES
GAWKED
GAWKER
GAWPED
GAWPER
GAYNES
HAAGEN
HACKED
HACKER
HADDEN
HADJES
HAFTED
HAGLER
HAIDEE
HAILED
HAILER
HAILEY
HAINES
HAIRED
HAJJES
HAKEEM
HALLEL
HALLEY
HALOED
HALOES
HALSEY
HALTED
HALTER
HALVED
HALVER
HALVES
HAMDEN
HAMLET
HAMMED
HAMMER
HAMPER
HANDED
HANDEL
HANDER
HANGED
HANGER
HANKER
HANLEY
HANSEL
HANSES
HAOLES
HAPPEN
HARDEN
HARDER
HARKED
HARKEN
HARKER
HARLEM
HARLEY
HARMED
HARMER
HARNEY
HARPED
HARPER
HARVEY
HASHED
HASHES
HASPED
HASSEL
HASTED
HASTEN
HASTES
HATRED
HATTED
HATTER
HAULED
HAULER
HAWKED
HAWKER
HAWSER
HAWSES
HAYDEN
HAYLEY
HAYMES
HAYNES
HAZIER
IAGREE
JABBED
JABBER
JACKED
JACKET
JAEGER
JAFFEE
JAGGED
JAGGER
JAILED
JAILER
JAMBES
JAMMED
JAMMER
JANNEY
JANSEN
JANZEN
JARRED
JASPER
JAUNES
JAURES
JAVIER
JAYCEE
JAYMES
JAYVEE
JAZZED
JAZZER
JAZZES
KADEEM
KAISER
KALLEN
KANDEL
KANDER
KAREEM
KARLEN
KARRER
KATZEN

KAVNER KAYOED LABFEE LABREA LACHEY LACIER LACKED LACKEY LACTEA LADDER LADIES LADLED LADLER LADLES LAFFER LAGGED LAGGER LAIRED LAKIER LALLED LAMBED LAMMED LANCED LANCER LANCES LANCET LANDED LANDER LANGER LANIER LANKER LAPPED LAPPER LAPPET LAPSED LAPSER LAPSES LAPTEV LARDED LARDER LAREES LARGER LARGES LARKED LARKER LARMEN LARSEN LARTER LARTET LASHED LASHER LASHES LASKER LASSEN LASSER LASSES LASTED LASTEX LATEEN LATHED LATHEN LATHER LATHES LATKES LATTER LATTES LAUDED LAUDER

LAUPER LAUREL LAUREN LAUREY LAUTER LAWMEN LAWYER LAYMEN LAZIER MAAZEL MABLEY MACLEN MACLES MACNEE MADDED MADDEN MADDER MADMEN MADRES MADSEN MAGLEV MAGNET MAHLER MAIDEN MAILED MAILER MAIMED MAIMER MAINER MAIRES MAIZES MAJGEN MALDEN MALLEI MALLET MALTED MANDEL MANGER MANLEY MANNED MANNER MANSES MANTEE MANTEL MANUEL MAPLES MAPPED MAPPER MARCEL MARDEN MARIEL MARKED MARKER MARKET MARKEY MARLED MARLEE MARLEY MARMEE MARNER MARRED MARRER MARTEL MARTEN MARTES MARVEL MARXES MASHED

MASHER MASHES MASKED MASKER MASSED MASSES MASSEY MASTED MASTER MATHER MATHEW MATJES MATMEN MATTEA MATTED MATTEL MATTER MATTES MAULED MAULER MAUMEE MAUSER MAUVES MAYBES MAYHEM MAZIER NABBED NABBER NACRED NACRES NAGGED NAGGER NAILED NAILER NAIVER NANSEN NANTES NAPIER NAPLES NAPPED NAPPER NAPPES NASHES NASSER NATTER NAUSEA NAUTES NAVIES OAKIER OAKLEY OARMEN OATIER PACIER PACKED PACKER PACKET PACTEN PADDED PADDER PADRES PAINED PAIRED PAISES PALLED PALLET PALMED PALMER PALTER

PAMPER PANDER PANIER PANNED PANNER PANNES PANTED PANTER PANZER PAPIER PARCEL PARGED PARGER PARGES PARKED PARKER PARKES PARLEY PARLEZ PARRED PARSEC PARSED PARSEE PARSER PARSES PARTED PASSED PASSEL PASSER PASSES PASTED PASTEL PASTER PASTES PATTED PATTEN PATTER PATZER PAULEY PAUPER PAUSED PAUSER PAUSES PAWNED PAWNEE PAWNER PAYEES RABBET RABIES RACHEL RACIER RACKED RACKER RACKET RADLEY RADNER RAFAEL RAFTED RAFTER RAGGED RAGMEN RAIDED RAIDER RAILED RAILER RAINED RAINER RAINES

RAINEY RAISED RAISER RAISES RAMIES RAMJET RAMMED RAMMER RAMPED RAMSES RAMSEY RANEES RANGED RANGEL RANGER RANGES RANKED RANKER RANTED RANTER RAPIER RAPPED RAPPEL RAPPER RAPTER RAQUEL RAREES RASHER RASHES RASPED RASPER RASSES RASTER RATHER RATNER RATTED RATTER RAZZED RAZZES SABLES SABRES SACHEM SACHER SACHET SACKED SACKER SACRED SADDEN SADDER SADHES SADLER SAGGED SAGIER SAILED SAILER SAITEK SALLES SALTED SALTEN SALTER SALVED SALVER SALVES SAMLET SAMUEL SANDED SANDER SANGER

SANSEI SANTEE SAPPED SAPPER SAREES SARGES SASHED SASHES SASSED SASSER SASSES SATEEN SAUCED SAUCER SAUCES SAUTES SAWRED SAWYER SAYHEY SAYLES SAYYES TABBED TABKEY TABLED TABLES TABLET TABSET TABUED TACKED TACKER TACTEL TAGGED TAGGER TAHNEE TAHOES TAILED TAILER TAIPEI TALCED TALKED TALKER TALLER TAMPED TAMPER TANDEM TANGED TANKED TANKER TANNED TANNER TANTES TAPPED TAPPER TAPPET TARDES TARGET TARLEK TARRED TARTED TARTER TARTES TASKED TASKET TASSEL TASSES TASTED TASTEE TASTER

TASTES TATLER TATTED TATTER TAUPES TAUTEN TAUTER TAXIED TAXIES TAXMEN VACHEL VACHES VAGUER VAINER VALDEZ VALLEE VALLEY VALSES VALUED VALUER VALUES VALVED VALVES VAMPED VAMPER VANIER VANNED VANNES VARDEN VARIED VARIER VARIES VARLET VARNEY VASTER VATTED WACKER WADDED WADDER WAFTED WAFTER WAGGED WAGGER WAGNER WAILED WAILER WAITED WAITER WAIVED WAIVER WAIVES WALDEN WALKED WALKEN WALKER WALLED WALLER WALLET WALTER WANDER WANIER WANKEL WANNED WANNER WANTED WANTER WAPNER WARDED

WARDEN WARDER WARIER WARMED WARMER WARNED WARNER WARNES WARPED WARPER WARRED WARREN WARTED WARVET WASHED WASHER WASHES WASLED WASMET WASSER WASTED WASTER WASTES WATNEY WAVIER WAXIER WAYNES XAVIER YAKKED YAKKER YALIES YAMMER YANKED YANKEE YANKER YAPHET YAPPED YAPPER YARDED YARDER YARNED YASSER YATSEN YATTER YAWKEY YAWNED YAWNER YAWPED YAWPER ZAGGED ZAGREB ZAIRES ZANIER ZANIES ZAPPED ZAPPER

•A•••E

BABBLE BADDIE BADLIE BAFFLE BAGGIE BAILEE BALDIE BALINE BANANE BANGLE

BANQUE BARBIE BAREGE BARITE BARONE BARQUE BARRIE BARTLE BASQUE BATTLE BAUBLE CABBIE CACKLE CADDIE CAJOLE CALLEE CALLME CAMISE CAMMIE CANAPE CANDLE CANINE CANTBE CANTLE CANUTE CAPONE CAPOTE CARAFE CARIBE CAROLE CARRIE CASQUE CASSIE CASTLE CATTLE CAYUSE CAZALE DABBLE DALENE DAMAGE DAMONE DAMORE DANDIE DANDLE DANGLE DANGME DANITE DANUBE DAPHNE DAPPLE DAREME DARKLE DARTLE DATIVE DAVIDE DAWDLE DAYONE DAZZLE EANNIE EARNIE FACADE FACIAE FACILE FADDLE FAERIE FAEROE FAILLE FALINE

FAMINE FANNIE FATALE FATONE FAUNAE GABBLE GAGGLE GALEAE GALORE GAMBLE GAMETE GAMGEE GAMINE GARAGE GARBLE GARGLE GAUCHE GAULLE HABILE HACKIE HACKLE HADDIE HADONE HAGGLE HAIDEE HALIDE HALITE HALLIE HAMATE HAMITE HANDKE HANDLE HANKIE HARARE HASONE HASSLE HATTIE HAYNIE IAGREE JACKIE JAFFEE JAMOKE JANGLE JANICE JANINE JARABE JARULE JAYCEE JAYVEE KAETHE KALINE KARATE KARRIE KATHIE LABFEE LABILE LABINE LACAGE LADDIE LADUKE LAHORE LAINIE LAJOIE LAMAZE LAMIAE LANATE LANCIE LANOSE

LAOTSE LARINE LARVAE LASSIE LATENE LAURIE LAVAGE MACKIE MACNEE MACRAE MADAME MADDIE MAGGIE MAGLIE MAGPIE MAISIE MAITRE MAKEME MALICE MALONE MANAGE MANAPE MANCHE MANEGE MANGLE MANQUE MANTEE MANTLE MANURE MANUTE MAPPLE MARBLE MARCHE MARCIE MARGIE MARINE MARJOE MARKIE MARLEE MARMEE MARNIE MARPLE MARQUE MARTHE MASHIE MASQUE MATTIE MATURE MAUMEE MAXENE MAXINE MAXIXE NADINE NANINE NANNIE NAPPIE NARINE NATALE NATIVE NATURE OARAGE PADDLE PAIUTE PALACE PALADE PALATE PALEAE PANOPE

PANTIE PARADE PARCAE PAREVE PAROLE PARSEE PARURE PATINE PATRIE PATTIE PAVANE PAVESE PAWNEE RABBLE RACEME RACINE RADOME RAFFLE RALLYE RAMATE RAMBLE RAMONE RAMOSE RANINE RANKLE RAPINE RASCHE RASSLE RASURE RATINE RATITE RATTLE RAVAGE RAVINE RAZZIE RAZZLE SABINE SACQUE SADDLE SAFIRE SAINTE SALADE SALINE SALLIE SALOME SALUTE SAMPLE SANGRE SANTEE SARTRE SATIRE SAVAGE SAVATE SAVEME SAVOIE SAYAYE SAYDIE TACKLE TAGORE TAHNEE TALESE TALKIE TAMALE TANGLE TASTEE TATTLE VACATE VALENE

VALERE VALINE VALISE VALLEE VARESE VATDYE WADDLE WAFFLE WAGGLE WAHINE WAKAME WALKIE WAMBLE WANGLE WARBLE WASHME WASHOE WATTLE YANKEE ZABRZE

••AE••

GRAECO NBAERS SEAEEL URAEUS

••A•E•

ABASED ABASER ABASES ABATED ABATER ABATES ADAGES AGAMES AGATES AGAVES ALATED AMADEO AMAZED AMAZES ANADEM ARAMES AWAKED AWAKEN AWAKER AWAKES AWARER AZALEA BEADED BEADER BEAKED BEAKER BEAMED BEAMER BEANED BEARER BEATEN BEATER BEAVER BIASED BIASES BLADED BLADER BLADES BLAKEY BLAMED

BLAMER BLAMES BLARED BLARES BLAZED BLAZER BLAZES BOATED BOATEL BOATER BRACED BRACER BRACES BRAKED BRAKES BRAVED BRAVER BRAVES BRAYED BRAYER BRAZEN CEASED CEASES CHACEL CHAFED CHAFER CHAFES CHALET CHANEL CHANEY CHAPEL CHASED CHASER CHASES CHAVEZ CHAWED CLARET CLAVES CLAWED CLAWER CLAYEY COALED COALER COATED COATEE COATER COATES COAXED COAXER COAXES CRAKES CRAMER CRANED CRANES CRAPED CRAPES CRATED CRATER CRATES CRAVED CRAVEN CRAVER CRAVES CRAZED CRAZES DCAREA DEADEN DEADER

DEAFEN DEAFER DEALER DEARER DIADEM DIALED DIALER DIAPER DLAYER DNASES DOAKES DOASET DRABEK DRAGEE DRAKES DRAKEU DRAPED DRAPER DRAPES DRAWEE DRAWER DRAYED EBATES EBAYER EDAMES EGALES ELANET ELATED ELATER ELATES ELAYER ENAMEL ENATES ERASED ERASER ERASES ESALEN ETAGES ETAPES EVADED EVADER EVADES FEARED FEARER FLAKED FLAKER FLAKES FLAMED FLAMER FLAMES FLARED FLARES FLAWED FLAXEN FLAXES FLAYED FLAYER FOALED FOAMED FOAMER FRAKES FRAMED FRAMER FRAMES FRASER FRATER FRAUEN FRAYED

FRAZER
GEARED
GLACES
GLADES
GLARED
GLARES
GLASER
GLAZED
GLAZER
GLAZES
GNAWED
GNAWER
GOADED
GOATEE
GRACED
GRACES
GRADEA
GRADEB
GRADED
GRADER
GRADES
GRAPES
GRAPEY
GRATED
GRATER
GRATES
GRAVED
GRAVEL
GRAVEN
GRAVER
GRAVES
GRAYED
GRAYER
GRAZED
GRAZER
GRAZES
HAAGEN
HEADED
HEADER
HEALED
HEALER
HEALEY
HEANEY
HEAPED
HEAPER
HEARER
HEATED
HEATER
HEAVED
HEAVEN
HEAVER
HEAVES
HOAXED
HOAXER
HOAXES
HYADES
IBANEZ
IDARED
IMAGED
IMAGER
IMAGES
IMARET
IMAXES
INAFEW
INAGES
INANER
INAPET
INAREA
INASEC
IRATER
ISABEL
JEANED
JUAREZ
KNAVES
KRAKEN
KRAMER
LEADED
LEADEN
LEADER
LEAFED
LEAKED
LEAKER
LEAKEY
LEANED
LEANER
LEAPED
LEAPER
LEASED
LEASER
LEASES
LEAVED
LEAVEN
LEAVER
LEAVES
LIANES
LOADED
LOADER
LOAFED
LOAFER
LOAMED
LOANED
LOANER
LOAVES
LWAVES
MAAZEL
MCAFEE
MEADER
MEAGER
MEANER
MEANEY
MOANED
MOANER
MOATED
NEARED
NEARER
NEATEN
NEATER
NIAMEY
OCASEK
OCASEY
OKAYED
OLAKES
ONAGER
ORAJEL
ORALES
ORATED
ORATES
OSAGES
PEAHEN
PEAKED
PEALED
PEALER
PEALES
PHASED
PHASER
PHASES
PIAGET
PLACED
PLACER
PLACES
PLAGES
PLANED
PLANER
PLANES
PLANET
PLATED
PLATEN
PLATER
PLATES
PLAYED
PLAYER
PRATED
PRATER
PRATES
PRAWER
PRAXES
PRAYED
PRAYER
QUAKED
QUAKER
QUAKES
QUALES
QUAVER
READER
REALER
REALES
REAMED
REAMER
REAPED
REAPER
REARED
REARER
REAVED
REAVER
REAVES
RHAMES
ROADEO
ROADER
ROAMED
ROAMER
ROARED
ROARER
RRATED
SCALED
SCALER
SCALES
SCARED
SCARER
SCARES
SEABED
SEABEE
SEAEEL
SEALED
SEALER
SEAMED
SEAMEN
SEAMER
SEARED
SEARER
SEATED
SEATER
SEAVER
SHADED
SHADER
SHADES
SHAKEN
SHAKER
SHAKES
SHALES
SHALEY
SHAMED
SHAMES
SHAPED
SHAPER
SHAPES
SHARED
SHARER
SHARES
SHAVED
SHAVEN
SHAVER
SHAVES
SKATED
SKATER
SKATES
SLAKED
SLAKER
SLAKES
SLATED
SLATER
SLATES
SLAVED
SLAVER
SLAVES
SLAYED
SLAYER
SMAZES
SNAKED
SNAKER
SNAKES
SNARED
SNARER
SNARES
SOAKED
SOAKER
SOAPED
SOAPER
SOARED
SOARER
SOAVES
SPACED
SPACEK
SPACER
SPACES
SPACEY
SPADED
SPADER
SPADES
SPARED
SPARER
SPARES
SPATES
SPAYED
SPAYER
STACEY
STAGED
STAGER
STAGES
STAGEY
STAKED
STAKES
STALED
STALER
STALES
STAMEN
STAPES
STARED
STARER
STARES
STASES
STATED
STATEN
STATER
STATES
STAVED
STAVES
STAYED
STAYER
SUAVER
SWALES
SWANEE
SWAYED
SWAYER
TEAMED
TEARED
TEARER
TEASED
TEASEL
TEASER
TEASES
TEASET
THALER
THALES
THAMES
THANES
THAWED
THAWER
THAYER
TOATEE
TRACED
TRACER
TRACES
TRACEY
TRADED
TRADER
TRADES
TRALEE
TRANES
TRAVEL
TRAVEN
TRAVES
TSADES
UKASES
UNAGED
UNAWED
UNAXED
USAGES
VIALED
WEAKEN
WEAKER
WEANED
WEANER
WEARER
WEASEL
WEAVED
WEAVER
WEAVES
WHALED
WHALER
WHALES
WHALEY
XGAMES
XMASES
XRATED
XRAYED
YEAGER
YEANED

••A••E

AMALIE
ANANKE
APACHE
ARABLE
ASANTE
BEADLE
BEAGLE
BEANIE
BEARSE
BEATLE
BLAINE
BLAISE
BRAISE
BRAQUE
CHAINE
CHAISE
CHANCE
CHANGE
CHANTE
CHARGE
CHASSE
CHASTE
CLAIRE
CLAQUE
CLARKE
CLASSE
CLAUDE
CLAUSE
COARSE
COATEE
CRABBE
CRADLE
DEARIE
DEARME
DIABLE
DIANNE
DNAASE
DOABLE
DRAGEE
DRAWEE
DUARTE
DWAYNE
ECARTE
ELAINE
ELANCE
ELAPSE
ELAYNE
ENABLE
EWAINE
FIACRE
FIANCE
FLAMBE
FLANGE
FRAISE
FRANCE
FRAPPE
GLANCE
GOALIE
GOATEE
GRABLE
GRACIE
GRAMME
GRANDE
GRANGE
GRATAE
GRAZIE
HEARSE
HEARYE
HOAGIE
HOARSE
INAPIE
INATIE
IRAISE
JEANIE
JEANNE
JOANIE
JOANNE
LEAGUE
LEANNE
LIABLE
LIAISE
LOATHE
MCAFEE
MEAGRE
MEALIE
MEANIE
MEASLE
NUANCE
ODAMAE
OGAUGE
OLATHE
OPAQUE
ORACLE
ORANGE
PEARCE
PEARLE
PIAFFE
PLAGUE
PLAICE
PLANTE
PLAQUE
PLATTE
PRAGUE
PRAISE
PRANCE
QUAKIE
QUARTE
QUATRE
QUAYLE
README
RNAASE
ROADIE
RVALUE
SCARCE
SCARNE
SCATHE
SEABEE
SEAICE
SEANCE
SEARLE
SHARPE
SHAYNE
SMALLE
SPARSE
SPATHE
STABLE
STANCE
STAPLE
STARVE
STATUE
SUABLE
SWANEE
SWATHE
SWAYZE
TOATEE
TRACHE
TRALEE
TRANCE
UGARTE
UNABLE
USABLE
USANCE
UVALDE
UVALUE
VIABLE
WHATVE
WRASSE
XLARGE

•••AE•

AZRAEL
ISRAEL
JUDAEA
KITAEN
RAFAEL
TOGAED
VISAED

•••A•E

ABLARE
ABLATE
ABLAZE
ABRADE
ACUATE
ADNATE
ADRATE
ADWARE
AERATE
AFLAME
AFLARE
AFRAME
AGLARE
AGNATE
AIRACE
ALSACE
ANSATE
AQUAKE
ARCADE
ARCANE
ARIANE
ASCALE
ASHADE
ASHAME
ASRARE
ASTARE
ATEASE
ATYALE
AUBADE
AURATE
AVIATE
AYEAYE
BANANE
BECAME
BEDAZE
BEHAVE
BELATE
BERATE
BESAME
BETAKE
BEWARE
BIGAPE
BINATE
BORATE
BSCALE
BUTANE
BYDATE
BYNAME
CANAPE
CARAFE
CAZALE
CDCASE
CDRATE
CERATE
CESARE
CETANE
CHOATE
CLEAVE
COMATE
CREASE
CREATE
CSCALE
CUBAGE
CURARE
CURATE
DAMAGE
DEBASE
DEBATE
DECADE
DECARE
DEFACE
DEFAME
DEGAGE
DERATE
DESADE
DEVANE
DILATE
DIMAGE
DNAASE
DOGAPE
DONATE
DOSAGE
DOTAGE
DOUANE
DSCALE
EFFACE
ELUATE
EMPALE
ENCAGE
ENCASE
ENFACE
ENGAGE
ENLACE
ENRAGE
ENSATE
EQUATE
ERRARE
ESCALE
ESCAPE
ESTATE
ETHANE
ETRADE
EXHALE
EXMATE
FACADE
FATALE
FEMALE
FINALE
FIXATE
FOLATE
FORAGE
FSCALE
GARAGE
GELATE
GIJANE
GOLAME
GREASE
GREAVE
GSCALE
GYRATE
HAMATE
HARARE
HECATE
HEXANE
HOMAGE
HORACE
HUMANE
ICEAGE
ICEAXE
IDEATE
IGNACE
IMGAME
IMLATE
IMPALE
INCASE
INGATE
INHALE
INMATE
INNAGE
INNATE
INSANE
INTAKE
INVADE
IODATE
ISLATE
JARABE
KARATE
LACAGE
LAMAZE
LANATE
LAVAGE
LEGATE
LENAPE
LESAGE
LEVADE
LIGATE
LINAGE
LIPASE
LOBATE
LOCALE
LOCANE
LOCATE
LOVAGE
LOYALE
LUNATE
LUXATE
MADAME
MANAGE
MANAPE
MCCABE
MCHALE
MEGANE
MENACE
MENAGE
METATE
MIRAGE
MOHAVE
MOJAVE
MORALE
MUGABE
MUTATE
NATALE
NEGATE
NEWAGE
NOBAKE
NONAGE
NONAME
NOSALE
NOTATE
NUTATE
OARAGE
OBLATE
OCTANE
OCTAVE
OFLATE
OHMAGE
OLDAGE
OLEATE
ONBASE
ONLATE
ONSALE
ONTAPE
OPIATE
ORNATE
OUTAGE
OUTATE
OUTAWE
PALACE
PALADE
PALATE
PARADE
PAVANE
PEDATE
PELAGE
PESADE
PETALE
PHRASE
PILATE
PIPAGE
PIRATE
PLEASE
POMADE
POTAGE
PREAGE
PUPATE
RAMATE
RAVAGE
REBAKE
REBALE
REBATE
RECAGE
RECANE
RECASE
REDACE
REDARE
REDATE
REFACE
REGALE
REGAVE
RELACE
RELATE
REMADE
REMAKE
REMATE
RENAME
REPAGE
REPANE
REPAVE
RERAKE
RERATE
RESALE
RESAVE
RETAKE
RETAME
RETAPE
REWAKE
RIMATE
RNAASE
RODALE
ROTATE
ROXANE
ROYALE
SALADE
SAVAGE
SAVATE
SAYAYE
SCRAPE
SEDATE
SENATE
SERAPE
SESAME
SEWAGE
SHEAVE
SILAGE
SLEAZE
SLOANE
SOLACE
SPEARE
SQUARE
STRAFE
SUEANE
TAMALE
TECATE
TENACE
THEAGE
THEAPE
THEAXE
THRACE
TIRADE
TIRANE
TISANE
TODATE
TOWAGE
TRIAGE
TSHAPE
TUBAGE
TUBATE
TULANE
TULARE
TVGAME
TVTAPE
ULLAGE
UNBALE
UNBARE
UNCAGE
UNCAKE
UNCASE
UNEASE
UNHALE
UNIATE
UNLACE
UNLADE
UNMADE
UNMAKE
UNMATE
UNPALE
UNSAFE
UNSAGE
UNTAME
UNTAPE
UPDATE
UPGAZE
UPLATE
UPRATE
UPTAKE
URBANE
USHAPE
VACATE
VISAGE
VITALE
VIVACE
VOLARE
VOYAGE
VSHAPE
WAKAME
WECARE
YSHAPE
ZYMASE

••••AE

AGORAE
ALULAE
AMEBAE
ANDRAE
AORTAE
BELGAE
BULLAE
BURSAE
CELLAE
CHELAE
COSTAE
COTTAE
CURIAE
FACIAE
FAUNAE
FLORAE
FOSSAE
GALEAE
GEMMAE
GESTAE
GRATAE
HYDRAE
LAMIAE
LARVAE
LIBRAE
MACRAE
MCCRAE
MOERAE
NUCHAE
ODAMAE
PALEAE
PARCAE
PINNAE
REGGAE
STOLAE
STRIAE
SUNDAE
TERRAE
TESTAE
TIBIAE
UMBRAE
UVULAE

AF••••

AFEARD
AFFAIR
AFFECT
AFFINE
AFFIRM
AFFORD
AFFRAY
AFGHAN
AFIELD
AFIFTH
AFLAME
AFLARE
AFLATS
AFLCIO
AFLOAT
AFRAID
AFRAME
AFRESH
AFRICA
AFTERS

A•F•••

AAFAIR
ADFEES
AFFAIR
AFFECT
AFFINE
AFFIRM
AFFORD
AFFRAY
AJFOYT
ALFINE
ALFRED
ALFVEN
ARFARF
ASFAST
ASFLAT
ASFREE
ATFIVE
ATFOUR
AUFAIT
AUFOND

A••F••

ACTFOR
AFIFTH
AIDFUL
AIMFOR
AIMFUL
ALLFOR
ARAFAT
ARMFUL
ARTFUL
ASKFOR
ATMFEE

A•••F•

ADOLFO
ADRIFT
AERIFY
AMALFI
ARGUFY
ASSOFT
AURIFY

A••••F

ABCDEF
ABITOF
ALOTOF
ALTARF
ARFARF
ASKSOF
ATONOF

•AF•••

AAFAIR
BAFFED
BAFFER
BAFFIN
BAFFLE
CAFTAN
DAFTER
DAFTLY
FAFNER
FAFNIR
GAFFED
GAFFER
GAFFES
HAFTED
JAFFEE
LAFFER
MAFIAS
OAFISH
RAFAEL
RAFFIA
RAFFIN
RAFFLE
RAFTED
RAFTER
SAFARI
SAFECO
SAFELY
SAFEST
SAFETY
SAFIRE
WAFERS
WAFERY
WAFFLE
WAFFLY
WAFTED
WAFTER
ZAFTIG

•A•F••

BADFIT
BAFFED
BAFFER
BAFFIN
BAFFLE
BAGFUL
BARFLY
BATFOR
CANFUL
CAPFUL
CARFUL
CATFIT
EARFUL
FANFIC

FARFEL
GADFLY
GAFFED
GAFFER
GAFFES
HADFUN
HASFUN
HATFUL
JAFFEE
JARFUL
LABFEE
LAFFER
LAPFUL
LAWFUL
LAYFOR
MADFOR
MANFUL
MAYFLY
NAKFAS
PANFRY
PANFUL
PARFUM
PAYFOR
RAFFIA
RAFFIN
RAFFLE
RAMFAN
RAMFIS
RANFOR
SACFLY
SATFOR
SAWFIT
VATFUL
WAFFLE
WAFFLY
WASFUN

•A••F•

BADOFF
BASIFY
CALIFS
CANIFF
CARAFE
CASEFY
CAVAFY
DAYOFF
FAROFF
GANEFS
GASIFY
LAYOFF
MANOFF
PACIFY
PAYOFF
RAMIFY
RANOFF
RAREFY
RATIFY
RATOFF
SALIFY
SAWOFF
TAPOFF
TARIFF
WASOFF
WAYOFF

•A•••F

BADOFF
CANIFF
CAREOF
DAYOFF
EATSOF
FAROFF
GAVEOF
LATEOF
LAYOFF
MADEOF
MAKEOF
MANOFF
MASSIF
PARTOF
PAYOFF
RANOFF
RATOFF
SAWOFF
TALKOF
TAPOFF
TARIFF
WARNOF
WASOFF
WAYOFF

••AF••

ARAFAT
BIAFRA
BLAFFS
CHAFED
CHAFER
CHAFES
CHAFFS
CHAFFY
CRAFTS
CRAFTY
DEAFEN
DEAFER
DEAFLY
DEAFTO
DRAFTS
DRAFTY
GRAFTS
INAFEW
INAFIX
INAFOG
LEAFED
LOAFED
LOAFER
MCAFEE
OLAFII
OLAFIV
PIAFFE
QUAFFS
SEAFOX
SHAFTS
SNAFUS
STAFFS

••A•F•

AMALFI
BLAFFS
CHAFFS
CHAFFY
DWARFS
GRAAFF
PIAFFE
QUAFFS
SCARFS
SNARFS
STAFFS
WHARFS

••A••F

GRAAFF
HEAROF
SHARIF
SMALLF
STAPUF
WHATIF

•••AF•

CARAFE
CAVAFY
DECAFS
GRAAFF
PILAFS
SCLAFF
STRAFE
UNHAFT
UNSAFE
UPWAFT

•••A•F

ALTARF
ARFARF
BEHALF
BYHALF
GETANF
GOTANF
GRAAFF
INHALF
SCLAFF

••••AF

INLEAF
STOLAF
UNLEAF

AG••••

AGADIR
AGAMAS
AGAMES
AGARIC
AGASSI
AGATES
AGATHA
AGAVES
AGAWAM
AGEDLY
AGEING
AGEISM
AGEIST
AGENAS
AGENCE
AGENCY
AGENDA
AGENTJ
AGENTK
AGENTS
AGEOLD
AGEONE
AGEOUT
AGESIX
AGETEN
AGETWO
AGGIES
AGHAST
AGILER
AGITAS
AGLAIA
AGLARE
AGLEAM
AGLETS
AGLINT
AGNAIL
AGNATE
AGONES
AGORAE
AGORAS
AGOROT
AGOSTO
AGOUTI
AGREED
AGREER
AGREES
AGUISH

A•G•••

AEGEAN
AFGHAN
AGGIES
AIGLET
AIGRET
ALGEDI
ALGORE
ALGREN
ANGELA
ANGELI
ANGELL
ANGELO
ANGELS
ANGERS
ANGKOR
ANGLED
ANGLEE
ANGLER
ANGLES
ANGLIA
ANGLIC
ANGLOS
ANGOLA
ANGORA
ANGSTS
ARGALI
ARGENT
ARGIVE
ARGOSY
ARGOTS
ARGUED
ARGUER
ARGUES
ARGUFY
ARGYLE
ARGYLL
ASGARD
ASGOOD
AUGEAN
AUGEAS
AUGEND
AUGERS
AUGHTS
AUGITE
AUGURS
AUGURY
AUGUST

A••G••

AARGAU
ADAGES
ADAGIO
AIRGUN
ALEGAR
ALEGRE
ALEGUP
ALIGHT
ALIGNS
ALOGIA
AMIGAS
AMIGOS
APOGEE
ARAGON
ARIGHT
ARTGUM

A•••G•

AAAUGH
ALLEGE
ALONGS
ANERGY
ANTIGO
ARIEGE
ARMAGH
ARPEGE
ASIAGO
ASSIGN
ATSIGN
AURIGA
AVENGE
AWEIGH

A••••G

AAHING
ACHING
ACTING
ADDING
ADZING
AGEING
AIDING
AILING
AIMING
AIRBAG
AIRING
AIRLOG
ALBORG
ALEKEG
ALHAIG
ALVING
AMPING
ANALOG
ANWANG
ARCING
ARMING
ASHING
ASKING
ATHING
AWNING

•AG•••

BAGBOY
BAGDAD
BAGELS
BAGEND
BAGFUL
BAGGED
BAGGER
BAGGIE
BAGJOB
BAGMAN
BAGMEN
BAGNIO
BAGSIT
BAGWIG
CAGEIN
CAGERS
CAGEUP
CAGIER
CAGILY
CAGING
CAGNEY
CAGUAS
DAGAMA
DAGGER
DAGGOO
DAGMAR
EAGLED
EAGLES
EAGLET
EAGRES
FAGEND
FAGINS
FAGOTS
GAGGED
GAGGER
GAGGLE
GAGING
GAGLAW
GAGMAN
GAGMEN
HAGGAI
HAGGIS
HAGGLE
HAGLER
HAGMAN
IAGREE
JAGGED
JAGGER
JAGLOM
JAGUAR
KAGAWA
LAGEAR
LAGERS
LAGGED
LAGGER
LAGOON
LAGUNA
MAGGIE
MAGGIO
MAGGOT
MAGIAN
MAGICS
MAGLEV
MAGLIE
MAGMAS
MAGNET
MAGNOL
MAGNON
MAGNUM
MAGNUS
MAGPIE
MAGYAR
NAGANO
NAGGED
NAGGER
NAGNAG
NAGOYA
NAGSAT
PAGANS
PAGERS
PAGEUP
PAGING
PAGLIA
PAGNOL
PAGODA
RAGBAG
RAGERS
RAGGED
RAGHIB
RAGING
RAGLAN
RAGMAN
RAGMEN
RAGMOP
RAGNAR
RAGOUT
RAGRUG
RAGSON
RAGTAG
RAGTOP
RAGUSA
SAGELY
SAGEST
SAGGED
SAGIER
TAGDAY
TAGEND
TAGGED
TAGGER
TAGORE
TAGOUT
TAGSON
TAGSUP
VAGARY
VAGUER
WAGERS
WAGGED
WAGGER
WAGGLE
WAGGLY
WAGING
WAGNER
WAGONS
ZAGGED
ZAGNUT
ZAGREB

•A•G••

AARGAU
BADGER
BADGES
BADGUY
BAGGED
BAGGER
BAGGIE
BANGED
BANGER
BANGLE
BANGON
BANGOR
BANGUI
BANGUP
BARGED
BARGER
BARGES
CADGED
CADGER
CADGES
CALGON
CAPGUN
CARGOS
CATGUT
CAUGHT
DADGUM
DAGGER
DAGGOO
DANGED
DANGER
DANGIT
DANGLE
DANGLY
DANGME
DAYGLO
FANGED
FANGIO
GADGET
GAGGED
GAGGER
GAGGLE
GAMGEE
GANGED
GANGER
GANGES
GANGLY
GANGUP
GARGAN
GARGLE
GAUGED
GAUGER
GAUGES
HAAGEN
HAGGAI
HAGGIS
HAGGLE
HAIGHT
HANGAR
HANGBY
HANGED
HANGER
HANGIN
HANGON
HANGUL
HANGUP
JAEGER
JAGGED
JAGGER
JANGLE
JANGLY
JARGON
LAGGED
LAGGER
LANGER
LARGER
LARGES
LARGOS
LAUGHS
MAGGIE
MAGGIO
MAGGOT
MAJGEN
MANGAS
MANGER
MANGLE
MANGOS
MARGIE
MARGIN
MARGOT
NAGGED
NAGGER
NAUGHT
PARGED
PARGER
PARGES
RAGGED
RANGED
RANGEL
RANGER
RANGES
RANGIN
RANGUP
RAYGUN
SAGGED
SAIGON
SANGER
SANGRE
SANGTO
SARGES
SARGON
TAGGED
TAGGER
TAIGAS
TANGED
TANGLE
TANGLY
TANGOS
TANGUY
TARGAS
TARGET
TAUGHT
VARGAS
VAUGHN
WAGGED
WAGGER
WAGGLE
WAGGLY
WANGLE
WARGOD
YANGON
YASGUR
ZAGGED

•A••G•

AAAUGH
BADEGG
BAERGA
BAREGE
CAYUGA
DAMAGE
EASYGO
GARAGE
HADAGO
HASAGO
LACAGE
LADOGA
LATIGO
LAVAGE
MADEGO
MAKEGO
MALAGA
MALIGN
MANAGE
MANEGE
MAYIGO
OARAGE
PAANGA
PAPAGO
PASSGO
RAVAGE
RAWEGG
SAVAGE

•A•••G

AAHING
BAAING
BADDOG
BADEGG
BAGWIG
BAKING
BALING
BARING
BASING
BATING
BAYING
CAGING
CAKING
CANING
CARING
CASING
CATRIG
CAVING
CAWING
DANANG
DANZIG
DARING
DATING
DAZING
EALING
EARING
EARTAG
EARWIG
EASING
EATING
FACING
FADING
FAKING
FAMING
FARING
FAXING
FAZING
GAGING
GAMING
GAPING
GASBAG
GASHOG
GASLOG
GATING
GAZING
HALING
HARING
HATING
HAVING
HAWING
HAYING
HAZING
JADING
JAPING
JAWING
LACING
LADING
LAMING
LAPDOG
LASING
LAVING
LAWING
LAYING
LAZING
MADDOG
MADVIG
MAKING
MATING
MAXING
MAYING
MAYTAG
MAZING
NAGNAG
NAMING
OAKTAG
OARING
PACING
PAGING
PALING
PARING
PAVING
PAWING
PAYING
RACING
RAGBAG
RAGING
RAGRUG
RAGTAG
RAKING
RARING
RASING
RATEDG
RATING
RAVING
RAWEGG
RAXING
RAYING
RAZING
SARONG
SATING
SAVING
SAWING
SAWLOG
SAYING
TAKING
TAMING
TAPING
TARING
TAUROG
TAXING
WADING
WAGING
WAKING
WALING
WANING
WARING
WAVING
WAXING
YAWING
ZAFTIG

••AG••

ADAGES
ADAGIO
ARAGON
BEAGLE
CRAGGY
DRAGEE
DRAGGY
DRAGIN
DRAGON
DRAGUP
ETAGES
FLAGGY
FLAGON
HAAGEN
HOAGIE
IMAGED
IMAGER
IMAGES
IMAGOS
INAGES
LEAGUE
MEAGER
MEAGRE
ONAGER
OSAGES
PHAGIA
PIAGET
PLAGES
PLAGUE
PRAGUE
QUAGGA
QUAGGY
REAGAN
SCAGGS
SEAGAL
SEAGOD
SHAGGY
SKAGGS
SNAGGY
SNAGUP
STAGED
STAGER
STAGES
STAGEY
TRAGIC
TRAGUS
UNAGED
USAGES
VIAGRA
YEAGER

••A•G•

AAAUGH
BHANGS
CHANGE
CHANGO
CHARGE
CLANGS
CRAGGY
CRAIGT
DRAGGY
FLAGGY
FLANGE
GRANGE
LIANGS
OGAUGE
ORANGE
ORANGS
ORANGY
PAANGA
QUAGGA
QUAGGY
SCAGGS
SHAGGY
SKAGGS
SLANGS
SLANGY
SNAGGY
TWANGS
TWANGY
UBANGI
WHANGS
XLARGE

••A••G

ANALOG
BAAING
DIALOG
INAFOG
INARUG
ONAJAG
QUAHOG
SEABAG
SEADOG
SEAHAG
SMALLG
STALAG
TEABAG
YEABIG

•••AG•

ARMAGH
ASIAGO
CUBAGE
DAMAGE
DEBAGS
DEGAGE
DIMAGE
DORAGS
DOSAGE
DOTAGE
ENCAGE
ENGAGE
ENRAGE
FORAGE
GARAGE
GULAGS
HADAGO
HASAGO
HOMAGE
ICEAGE
IDTAGS
INNAGE
INRAGS
ITSAGO
LACAGE
LAVAGE
LESAGE
LINAGE
LOVAGE
MALAGA
MANAGE
MENAGE
MIRAGE
NEWAGE
NONAGE
OARAGE
OHMAGE
OLDAGE
OUTAGE
PAPAGO
PELAGE
PIPAGE
POTAGE
PREAGE
RAVAGE
REBAGS
RECAGE
REPAGE
RETAGS
SAVAGE
SCRAGS
SEWAGE
SILAGE
THEAGE
TOBAGO
TOWAGE
TRIAGE
TUBAGE
ULLAGE
UNBAGS
UNCAGE
UNGAGS
UNSAGE
VIRAGO
VISAGE
VOYAGE

•••A•G

ALHAIG
ANWANG
CHIANG
DANANG
DEFANG
ERLANG
GOBANG
KDLANG
MCHARG
REHANG
RESANG
SPRANG
YUTANG

••••AG

AIRBAG
DEFRAG
DOGTAG
EARTAG
GASBAG
GIGBAG
GOSTAG
GYMBAG
ICEBAG
JETLAG
KITBAG
MAYTAG
MITTAG
MONTAG
NAGNAG
OAKTAG
OLDGAG
ONAJAG
RAGBAG
RAGTAG
REDRAG
REDTAG
REFLAG
SEABAG
SEAHAG
SONTAG
STALAG
TEABAG
UNSNAG
USFLAG
WETRAG
WIGWAG
ZIGZAG

AH••••

AHCHOO
AHERNE
AHIMSA
AHOLIC
AHORSE

A•H•••

AAHING
ABHORS
ACHEBE
ACHENE
ACHERS
ACHIER
ACHING
ADHERE
AGHAST
ALHAIG
ALHENA
ALHIRT
APHIDS
ARHATS
ASHADE
ASHAME
ASHARP
ASHBIN
ASHCAN
ASHDOD
ASHIER
ASHINE
ASHING
ASHLAR
ASHLEE
ASHLEY
ASHMAN
ASHMEN
ASHORE
ASHPAN
ASHPIT
ASHRAM
ASHTON
ATHAND
ATHEEL
ATHENA
ATHENE
ATHENS
ATHING
ATHOME
ATHROB
ATHROW
AWHECK
AWHILE
AWHIRL

AXHEAD

A••H••
AACHEN
AARHUS
ABMHOS
ABOHMS
AETHER
AFGHAN
AHCHOO
ALOHAS
ALPHAS
ALTHEA
ANCHOR
ANCHOS
ANDHOW
ANTHEM
ANTHER
ANYHOW
ARCHED
ARCHER
ARCHES
ARCHIE
ARCHLY
ARCHON
ARNHEM
ARTHRO
ARTHUR
ASTHER
ASTHMA
ATTHAT
AUGHTS
AUTHOR

A•••H•
AGATHA
ALEPHS
ALIGHT
AMECHE
APACHE
APATHY
ARETHA
ARIGHT
AYESHA

A••••H
AAAUGH
ABLUSH
ADELEH
ADOLPH
AFIFTH
AFRESH
AGUISH
ALIOTH
ALIYAH
ALMACH
AMBUSH
AMONTH
ANARCH
ARMAGH
ASLOSH
ASMUCH
ASPISH
ASSUCH
ATENTH
ATTACH
AVOUCH
AWEIGH

•AH•••
AAHING
BAHAMA
BAHIAN
BAHNEN
CAHIER
CAHILL
CAHOOT
DAHLIA
HAHAHA
KAHLIL
KAHLUA
KAHUNA
LAHORE
MAHALO
MAHDIS
MAHLER
MAHOUT
MAHZOR
OAHUAN
RAHRAH
RAHWAY
SAHARA
SAHIBS
TAHINI
TAHITI
TAHNEE
TAHOES
WAHINE
WAHLOO
WAHOOS
WAHWAH
YAHOOS

•A•H••
AACHEN
AARHUS
BACHED
BACHES
BACHIT
BADHAM
BADHAT
BARHOP
BASHED
BASHER
BASHES
BASHIN
BATHED
BATHER
BATHES
BATHOS
CACHED
CACHES
CACHET
CARHOP
CASHED
CASHES
CASHEW
CASHIN
CATHAY
CATHER
CATHYS
DACHAS
DAPHNE
DASHED
DASHER
DASHES
DASHIS
DASHIT
DATHAN
DAYHOP
FATHER
FATHOM
GASHED
GASHES
GASHOG
GATHER
HACHOO
HARHAR
HASHED
HASHES
HATHOR
HAWHAW
JANHUS
KASHAS
KATHIE
LACHEY
LACHOY
LAPHAM
LASHED
LASHER
LASHES
LASHTO
LASHUP
LATHED
LATHEN
LATHER
LATHES
MACHOS
MASHED
MASHER
MASHES
MASHIE
MASHUP
MATHER
MATHEW
MATHIS
MAYHAP
MAYHEM
NACHAS
NACHOS
NAPHTA
NASHES
NASHUA
NATHAN
PACHIN
PASHAS
PASHTO
PATHAN
PATHIC
PATHOS
RACHEL
RAGHIB
RASHAD
RASHER
RASHES
RASHID
RASHLY
RATHER
SACHEM
SACHER
SACHET
SADHES
SADHUS
SASHAY
SASHED
SASHES
SAYHEY
VACHEL
VACHES
VASHTI
WARHOL
WASHAD
WASHED
WASHER
WASHES
WASHME
WASHOE
WASHOS
WASHUP
YACHTS
YAPHET
YASHIN

•A••H•
BAKSHI
CANCHA
CATCHY
CAUCHY
CAUGHT
EARTHA
EARTHS
EARTHY
FAITHS
FARAHS
GANDHI
GAUCHE
GAUCHO
HAHAHA
HAIGHT
JASCHA
JAWOHL
KAETHE
LANDHO
LAUGHS
MANCHA
MANCHE
MANCHU
MARCHE
MARSHA
MARSHY
MARTHA
MARTHE
NAUGHT
NAVAHO
PANCHO
PASCHS
PATCHY
RAJAHS
RALPHJ
RANCHO
RASCHE
SAIDHI
SANCHO
SANTHA
SAPPHO
SAYSHI
TAICHI
TAUGHT
VAUGHN
YAMAHA

•A•••H
AAAUGH
BANISH
BARUCH
BASRAH
BAUSCH
CALASH
CALIPH
CASBAH
DALETH
DANISH
FAMISH
FARRAH
GALOSH
GARETH
GARISH
HALVAH
HANNAH
HARRAH
HAUNCH
JADISH
KASBAH
LATISH
LAUNCH
LAVISH
MANUSH
MARIAH
MATZOH
NAMATH
OAFISH
PALISH
PARAPH
PARIAH
PARISH
PAUNCH
RADISH
RAHRAH
RAKISH
RAUNCH
RAVISH
RAWISH
SAIDAH
SALISH
SAMEKH
SAYAAH
SAYSAH
TAKETH
VANISH
WABASH
WAHWAH
WARMTH

••AH••
BRAHMA
BRAHMS
GRAHAM
IDAHOS
OMAHAN
OMAHAS
ONAHOP
PEAHEN
QUAHOG
SEAHAG
UTAHAN
UTAHNS

••A•H•
AGATHA
APACHE
APATHY
BEACHY
BRACHS
BRASHY
CHACHA
CHACHI
DEATHS
FLASHY
GRAPHO
GRAPHS
GRAPHY
HEATHS
HEATHY
KWACHA
LEACHY
LOATHE
OLATHE
ORACHS
PEACHY
PLASHY
POACHY
SCATHE
SNATHS
SPATHE
STAPHS
SWATHE
SWATHS
TRACHE
TRASHY
WRATHS

••A••H
AAAUGH
ANARCH
BLANCH
BRAMAH
BRANCH
DEARTH
EPARCH
EXARCH
HEALTH
HEARTH
INARCH
ISAIAH
KLATCH
SEARCH
SMALLH
SNATCH
STANCH
STARCH
SWATCH
THATCH
WEALTH
WRAITH

•••AH•
CUDAHY
EPHAHS
FARAHS
HAHAHA
JONAHS
MYNAHS
NAVAHO
OBEAHS
OPRAHS
RAJAHS
SURAHS
TORAHS
YAMAHA

•••A•H
ALMACH
ARMAGH
ATTACH
BLEACH
BREACH
BREATH
BROACH
BYPATH
CALASH
DETACH
DONATH
ELNATH
EMDASH
EMPATH
ENDASH
FLYASH
INCASH
INDASH
JSBACH
MORATH
NAMATH
ORBACH
PARAPH
PESACH
POTASH
PREACH
REHASH
REWASH
RIYADH
SAYAAH
SERAPH
SHEATH
SPLASH
SPRACH
SQUASH
THRASH
UNLASH
UNRASH
WABASH
WREATH

••••AH
ALIYAH
BASRAH
BEULAH
BRAMAH
CASBAH
DEBRAH
DOODAH
ELIJAH
ERYKAH
FARRAH
FELLAH
GULLAH
HALVAH
HANNAH
HARRAH
HOOHAH
HOOKAH
HOORAH
HOWDAH
HUPPAH
HURRAH
HUZZAH
ISAIAH
JOSIAH
KASBAH
LOOFAH
MARIAH
MOOLAH
MULLAH
NEENAH
OHYEAH
OOMPAH
PARIAH
PISGAH
RAHRAH
RUPIAH
SAIDAH
SAYAAH
SAYSAH
SIRRAH
WAHWAH
YOWZAH

AI••••
AIDERS
AIDFUL
AIDING
AIDMAN
AIDMEN
AIELLO
AIGLET
AIGRET
AIKIDO
AIKMAN
AILEEN
AILING
AILURO
AIMERS
AIMFOR
AIMFUL
AIMING
AIMSAT
AINTSO
AIOLIS
AIRACE
AIRARM
AIRBAG
AIRBUD
AIRBUS
AIRDAM
AIRDRY
AIRERS
AIRGUN
AIRIER
AIRILY
AIRING
AIRLOG
AIRMAN
AIRMEN
AIROUT
AIRPOP
AIRPOT
AIRSAC
AIRSEA
AIRSUP
AIRWAR
AIRWAY
AISLED
AISLES

A•I•••
ABIDED
ABIDER
ABIDES
ABITOF
ACIDIC
ACIDLY
ADIDAS
ADIEUS
ADIEUX
AFIELD
AFIFTH
AGILER
AGITAS
AHIMSA
AJIJIC
AKIMBO
AKINTO
AKITAS
ALIBIS
ALIBLE
ALICEB
ALICES
ALICIA
ALIENS
ALIGHT
ALIGNS
ALIKES
ALINED
ALINER
ALINES
ALIOTH
ALIOTO
ALIPED
ALISON
ALISTS
ALIVEO
ALIYAH
ALIYOT
AMICAL
AMICES
AMICUS
AMIDAS
AMIDES
AMIDOL
AMIDST
AMIENS
AMIGAS
AMIGOS
AMINES
AMINOR
AMINOS
AMINTA
AMINUS
AMITIE
ANIMAL
ANIMAS
ANIMES
ANIMUS
ANIONS
ANISES
ANITRA
APIARY
APICAL
APICES
APIECE
ARIANA
ARIANE
ARIARY
ARIDER
ARIDLY
ARIEGE
ARIGHT
ARIOSE
ARIOSI
ARIOSO
ARISEN
ARISES
ARISTA
ARISTO
ASIAGO
ASIANS
ASIDES
ASIMOV
ATILES
ATISES
AVIANS
AVIARY
AVIATE
AVIDER
AVIDLY
AVISON
AVISOS
AXILLA
AXIOMS
AXIONS
AXISES
AZIDES

A••I••
AAHING
ABDIEL
ACHIER
ACHING
ACTIII
ACTING
ACTION
ACTIUM
ACTIVA
ACTIVE
ACUITY
ADDICT
ADDING
ADDINS
ADLIBS
ADMINS
ADMIRE
ADMITS
ADRIAN
ADRIEN
ADRIFT
ADRIVE
ADVICE
ADVILS
ADVISE
ADZING
AECIUM
AEDILE
AERIAL
AERIER
AERIES
AERIFY
AERILY
AERIOS
AFFINE
AFFIRM
AFRICA
AGEING
AGEISM
AGEIST
AGGIES
AGLINT
AGUISH
AIDING
AIKIDO
AILING
AIMING
AIRIER
AIRILY
AIRING
ALAINA
ALBINE
ALBINO
ALBION
ALCINA
ALDINE
ALDISS
ALFINE
ALHIRT
ALKIES
ALLIED
ALLIES
ALLIUM
ALNICO
ALPINE
ALRITZ
ALTIMA
ALTIUS
ALVING
ALVINO
ALZIRA
AMBIEN
AMBITS
AMNION
AMNIOS
AMPING
AMRITA
ANCIEN
ANNIES
ANNIKA
ANNINA
ANOINT
ANTICS
ANTIGO
ANVILS
APHIDS
APLITE
APPIAN
APRILE
APRILS
AQUILA
AQUINO
ARCING
ARGIVE
ARLISS
ARMIES
ARMING
ARNICA
ARNIES
AROIDS
AROINT
ARRIBA
ARRIVE
ARTIER
ARTILY
ARTIST
ASDICS
ASHIER
ASHINE
ASHING
ASKING
ASPICS
ASPIRE
ASPISH
ASSIGN
ASSISI
ASSIST
ASSIZE
ASWIRL
ATFIVE
ATHING
ATKINS
ATNINE
ATRIAL
ATRISK
ATRIUM
ATSIGN
ATTICA
ATTICS
ATTILA
ATTIRE
ATWILL
ATWIST
AUDIAL
AUDILE
AUDIOS
AUDITS
AUGITE
AURIFY
AURIGA
AURIST
AUTISM
AUTIST
AVAILS
AVOIDS
AVRILS
AWAITS
AWEIGH
AWHILE
AWHIRL
AWNING
AXLIKE

A•••I•
AAFAIR
ABATIS
ACACIA
ACADIA
ACARID
ACEDIA
ACEDIT
ACESIT
ACETIC
ACIDIC
ACQUIT
ACTIII
ACTSIN
ADAGIO
ADDSIN
ADELIE
ADENIS
ADJOIN
ADONIC
ADONIS
ADROIT
AENEID
AEOLIA
AFFAIR
AFLCIO
AFRAID
AGADIR
AGARIC
AGESIX
AGLAIA
AGNAIL
AHOLIC
AIOLIS
AJIJIC
ALANIS
ALARIC
ALBEIT
ALDRIN
ALEXIA
ALEXIS
ALHAIG
ALIBIS
ALICIA
ALKAID
ALLAIS
ALOGIA
ALTAIC
ALTAIR
ALTOID
ALTRIA
AMADIS
AMALIA
AMALIE
AMATIS
AMAZIN
AMBLIN
AMEBIC
AMELIA
AMELIE
AMESIA
AMITIE
ANACIN
ANAKIN
ANDRIC
ANEMIA
ANEMIC
ANGLIA
ANGLIC
ANNUIT
ANODIC
ANOMIA
ANOMIC
ANOMIE
ANOXIA
ANOXIC
ANSEIS
ANTLIA
ANTRIM
ANUBIS
AORTIC
APULIA
ARABIA
ARABIC
ARAMID
ARAMIS
ARCHIE
ARCSIN
ARCTIC
ARMPIT
ARNEIS
ARTOIS
ASHBIN
ASHPIT
ASKSIN
ASONIA
ASSAIL
ASTRID
ATARIS
ATAVIC
ATAXIA
ATAXIC
ATOMIC
ATONIA
ATONIC
ATOXIC
ATRAIN
ATROIS
ATTAIN
ATTRIT
ATYPIC
AUFAIT
AULAIT
AUNTIE
AUPAIR
AUSSIE
AUSTIN
AXENIC
AYESIR
AZANIA
AZARIA
AZERIS
AZONIC
AZORIN
AZUKIS

A••••I
ACTIII
ADJANI
ADONAI
ADZUKI
AGASSI
AGOUTI
ALEXEI
ALGEDI
ALKALI
ALUMNI
AMALFI
AMANTI
ANDREI
ANGELI
ANNULI
ARGALI
ARIOSI
ARMANI
ASSISI
AVANTI

•AI•••
BAIKAL
BAILED
BAILEE
BAILER
BAILEY
BAILON
BAILOR
BAINES
BAIRNS
BAISAS
BAITED
BAITER
BAIZAS
BAIZES
CAICOS
CAIMAN
CAIRNS
DAILEY
DAINTY
DAISES
FAILED
FAILLE
FAILTO
FAIMAN
FAINER
FAINTS
FAIRED
FAIRER
FAIRLY
FAIRUP
FAISAL
FAITES
FAITHS
GAIETY
GAIJIN
GAINED
GAINER
GAINES
GAINLY
GAINON
GAINST
GAITED
GAITER
HAIDAS
HAIDEE
HAIGHT
HAIKAI
HAIKUS
HAILED
HAILER
HAILEY
HAINES
HAIRDO
HAIRED
JAILED
JAILER
JAILOR
JAIPUR
KAILUA
KAISER
LAICAL
LAIDBY
LAIDIN
LAIDON
LAIDTO
LAIDUP
LAINIE
LAIRDS
LAIRED
MAIDEN
MAILED
MAILER
MAILIN
MAILTO
MAIMED
MAIMER
MAINER

MAINLY
MAINST
MAIRES
MAIRZY
MAISIE
MAISON
MAITAI
MAITRE
MAIZES
NAIADS
NAILED
NAILER
NAILIN
NAILIT
NAILUP
NAIRAS
NAIVER
PAIDAD
PAIDIN
PAIDUP
PAINED
PAINTS
PAINTY
PAIRED
PAIRUP
PAISAN
PAISES
PAIUTE
RAIDED
RAIDER
RAILAT
RAILED
RAILER
RAILON
RAINED
RAINER
RAINES
RAINEY
RAININ
RAINON
RAIPUR
RAISED
RAISER
RAISES
RAISIN
RAISON
RAITAS
SAIDAH
SAIDHI
SAIDNO
SAIDOK
SAIDSO
SAIDTO
SAIGON
SAILED
SAILER
SAILON
SAILOR
SAILTO
SAINTE
SAINTS
SAIPAN
SAISON
SAITEK
TAICHI
TAIGAS
TAILED
TAILER

TAILOR
TAINTS
TAIPAN
TAIPEI
TAIWAN
VAILCO
VAINER
VAINLY
WAILED
WAILER
WAISTS
WAITED
WAITER
WAITON
WAITUP
WAIVED
WAIVER
WAIVES
ZAIRES

•A•I••

AAHING
BAAING
BABIED
BABIER
BABIES
BAHIAN
BAKING
BALINE
BALING
BANISH
BARING
BARITE
BARIUM
BASIAL
BASICS
BASIFY
BASILS
BASING
BASINS
BATIKS
BATING
BAVIER
BAYING
CABINS
CAGIER
CAGILY
CAGING
CAHIER
CAHILL
CAKIER
CAKING
CALICO
CALIFS
CALIPH
CAMINO
CAMION
CAMISE
CANIDS
CANIER
CANIFF
CANINE
CANING
CAPITA
CARIBE
CARIBS
CARIES
CARINA

CARING
CARIOU
CASING
CASINO
CASIOS
CASITA
CATION
CAVIAR
CAVIES
CAVILS
CAVING
CAVITY
CAWING
DAMIEN
DAMITA
DANIEL
DANILO
DANIOS
DANISH
DANITE
DARIEN
DARING
DARIUS
DATING
DATIVE
DAVIDE
DAVIDI
DAVIDL
DAVIDO
DAVIES
DAVITS
DAZING
EAKINS
EALING
EARING
EASIER
EASILY
EASING
EATING
FABIAN
FACIAE
FACIAL
FACIAS
FACIES
FACILE
FACING
FADING
FAGINS
FAJITA
FAKING
FAKIRS
FALINE
FAMILY
FAMINE
FAMING
FAMISH
FANION
FAQIRS
FARINA
FARING
FATIMA
FAXING
FAZING
GAGING
GAMIER
GAMILY
GAMINE
GAMING

GAMINS
GAPING
GARISH
GASIFY
GATING
GAVIAL
GAZING
HABILE
HABITS
HAKIMS
HALIDE
HALING
HALITE
HAMILL
HAMITE
HARING
HATING
HAVING
HAWING
HAYING
HAZIER
HAZILY
HAZING
JADING
JADISH
JANICE
JANINE
JAPING
JAVIER
JAVITS
JAWING
KALINE
KARINA
LABIAL
LABILE
LABINE
LABIUM
LACIER
LACILY
LACING
LADIDA
LADIES
LADING
LADINO
LAKIER
LAKIST
LAMIAE
LAMIAS
LAMINA
LAMING
LANIER
LANINA
LAPINS
LARIAT
LARINE
LASING
LATIGO
LATINA
LATINI
LATINO
LATINS
LATISH
LAVIDA
LAVING
LAVISH
LAWING
LAXITY
LAYING

LAYINS
LAZIER
LAZILY
LAZING
MAFIAS
MAGIAN
MAGICS
MAKING
MALIAN
MALIBU
MALICE
MALICK
MALIGN
MANIAC
MANIAS
MANILA
MAOISM
MAOIST
MARIAH
MARIAN
MARIAS
MARIDA
MARIDO
MARIEL
MARIKO
MARILU
MARINA
MARINE
MARINO
MARION
MARISA
MARIST
MATING
MATINS
MAVINS
MAXIMA
MAXIMS
MAXINE
MAXING
MAXIXE
MAYIGO
MAYING
MAZIER
MAZILY
MAZING
NACION
NADINE
NADIRS
NAJIMY
NAMING
NANINE
NAPIER
NARIAL
NARINE
NARITA
NATICK
NATION
NATIVE
NAVIES
OAFISH
OAKIER
OARING
OATIER
PACIER
PACIFY
PACING
PACINO
PAGING

PALING
PALISH
PAMINA
PAMIRS
PANICS
PANIER
PANINI
PANINO
PAPIER
PAPIST
PARIAH
PARING
PARINI
PARISH
PARITY
PATINA
PATINE
PATIOS
PAVING
PAVIOR
PAWING
PAYING
RABIES
RACIAL
RACIER
RACILY
RACINE
RACING
RACINO
RACISM
RACIST
RADIAL
RADIAN
RADIOS
RADISH
RADIUM
RADIUS
RAGING
RAKING
RAKISH
RAMIES
RAMIFY
RANIDS
RANINE
RAPIDO
RAPIDS
RAPIER
RAPINE
RAPINI
RARING
RARITY
RASING
RATIFY
RATINE
RATING
RATION
RATIOS
RATITE
RAVINE
RAVING
RAVISH
RAWISH
RAWIST
RAXING
RAYING
RAZING
SABINA
SABINE

SADISM
SADIST
SAFIRE
SAGIER
SAHIBS
SALIFY
SALINA
SALINE
SALISH
SALIVA
SAMIAM
SANITY
SATING
SATINS
SATINY
SATIRE
SAVING
SAVIOR
SAWING
SAYIDO
SAYING
TAHINI
TAHITI
TAKING
TALISA
TAMILS
TAMING
TAOISM
TAOIST
TAPING
TAPINS
TAPIRS
TARIFF
TARING
TAVIST
TAXIED
TAXIES
TAXING
VALINE
VALISE
VALIUM
VANIER
VANISH
VANITY
VARIAS
VARIED
VARIER
VARIES
VASILY
WADING
WAGING
WAHINE
WAKING
WALING
WANIER
WANING
WAPITI
WARIER
WARILY
WARING
WAVIER
WAVILY
WAVING
WAXIER
WAXILY
WAXING
XAVIER
YAKIMA

YALIES
YAWING
ZANIER
ZANIES
ZANILY
ZAYINS

•A••I•

AAFAIR
BAALIM
BACHIT
BACKIN
BADDIE
BADFIT
BADLIE
BAFFIN
BAGGIE
BAGNIO
BAGSIT
BAGWIG
BALDIE
BALLIN
BALTIC
BAMBIS
BANDIT
BANKIT
BARBIE
BARDIC
BARKIN
BARRIE
BARRIO
BARRIS
BASHIN
BASKIN
BASTIA
BATSIN
CABBIE
CABRIO
CADDIE
CADMIC
CAGEIN
CALAIS
CALLIN
CALLIT
CALVIN
CAMEIN
CAMMIE
CANDIA
CANDID
CANLIT
CAPRID
CAPRIS
CARDIA
CARDIN
CARDIO
CARLIN
CARRIE
CARTIN
CASEIN
CASHIN
CASSIA
CASSIE
CASSIM
CASSIN
CASSIO
CASSIS
CATFIT
CATKIN

CATLIN
CATNIP
CATRIG
CATSIT
CAVEIN
DAHLIA
DANCIN
DANDIE
DANGIT
DANZIG
DARLIN
DARNIT
DARRIN
DARWIN
DASHIS
DASHIT
DASSIN
DATRIL
DAYLIT
EANNIE
EARNIE
EARNIT
EARVIN
EARWIG
EASEIN
EATSIN
EATSIT
FABRIC
FACEIT
FADEIN
FAERIE
FAFNIR
FAKEID
FAKEIT
FALLIN
FANFIC
FANGIO
FANNIE
FARRIS
FASCIA
FATLIP
FATSIS
GADDIS
GAELIC
GAIJIN
GALLIA
GALLIC
GALOIS
GAMBIA
GAMBIT
GARCIA
GARLIC
GARYIN
GASLIT
GASOIL
GATLIN
GAVEIN
GAWAIN
HACKIE
HACKIT
HADDIE
HADDIX
HADJIS
HAGGIS
HAJJIS
HALLIE
HALOID
HALPIN

HAMLIN
HANDIN
HANGIN
HANKIE
HARBIN
HARDIN
HARLIN
HARRIS
HASSID
HATEIT
HATPIN
HATTIE
HAULIN
HAVEIN
HAVEIT
HAWAII
HAYNIE
IAMBIC
IATRIC
JACKIE
JAMAIS
JAMSIN
JARDIN
JARVIK
JASMIN
KAHLIL
KANJIS
KAOLIN
KAONIC
KARMIC
KARRIE
KATHIE
KATRIN
LACTIC
LADDIE
LAIDIN
LAINIE
LAJOIE
LAMSIT
LANAIS
LANCIA
LANCIE
LANDIS
LANVIN
LARKIN
LASSIE
LATRIA
LATVIA
LAURIA
LAURIC
LAURIE
LAVAIN
LAYSIN
MACKIE
MADDIE
MADEIT
MADRID
MADVIG
MAGGIE
MAGGIO
MAGLIE
MAGPIE
MAHDIS
MAILIN
MAISIE
MAJLIS
MAKEIT
MAKSIM

MALEIC
MALTIN
MANNIX
MANTIC
MANTIS
MAORIS
MAQUIS
MARCIA
MARCIE
MARCIL
MARCIX
MARDIS
MARGIE
MARGIN
MARKIE
MARKII
MARKIV
MARKIX
MARLIN
MARNIE
MARTIN
MARVIN
MARVIS
MARYII
MASAIS
MASHIE
MASLIN
MASSIF
MASTIC
MATHIS
MATLIN
MATRIX
MATTIE
NAILIN
NAILIT
NAMEIT
NANNIE
NAPKIN
NAPPIE
NARNIA
NARVIK
NAVAID
PACHIN
PACKIN
PAGLIA
PAIDIN
PALAIS
PALLID
PANDIT
PANSIN
PANTIE
PAQUIN
PARKIT
PARNIS
PARRIS
PARTII
PARTIV
PASSIM
PASTIS
PASTIT
PATHIC
PATOIS
PATRIA
PATRIC
PATRIE
PATTIE
PAULII
PAULIV

PAYSIN
RABBIS
RABBIT
RACEIN
RAFFIA
RAFFIN
RAGHIB
RAININ
RAISIN
RAKEIN
RAMFIS
RAMSIN
RANCID
RANGIN
RANKIN
RASHID
RASKIN
RATLIN
RAZZIE
SALLIE
SALMIS
SALTII
SANDIA
SANKIN
SARDIS
SARNIA
SAUDIS
SAVAII
SAVEIT
SAVOIE
SAVOIR
SAWFIT
SAWPIT
SAYDIE
TABRIZ
TACTIC
TAKEIN
TAKEIT
TALKIE
TALKIN
TANNIC
TANNIN
TAPSIN
TAROIL
TARPIT
TAUPIN
TAURIC
VALAIS
VALOIS
WABBIT
WADEIN
WALKIE
WALKIN
WALLIN
WALLIS
WANTIN
WAVEIN
WAYSIN
YAQUIS
YASHIN
YASMIN
ZADDIK
ZAFTIG
ZAMBIA

•A•••I

BAKSHI
BANGUI

BANZAI
BARONI
CAPONI
CAROLI
CARONI
DALASI
DANTEI
DAVIDI
FALUDI
FAMULI
FARUKI
GANDHI
HAGGAI
HAIKAI
HAMULI
HATARI
HAWAII
JACOBI
JAMESI
KABUKI
KAMALI
KATMAI
LADYDI
LAPERI
LATERI
LATINI
LAZULI
MAITAI
MALAWI
MALLEI
MALOTI
MAOTAI
MARKII
MARKVI
MARYII
MATSUI
NAPOLI
PANINI
PAPYRI
PARINI
PARTII
PASMOI
PATAKI
PAULII
PAULVI
QATARI
RAPINI
SAFARI
SAIDHI
SALAMI
SALTII
SALUKI
SAMEDI
SANSEI
SATORI
SAVAII
SAYSHI
TAHINI
TAHITI
TAICHI
TAIPEI
TATAMI
VASHTI
WAPITI
WASABI
WATUSI
YAMANI
YANQUI

ZANONI

••AI••

ALAINA
AVAILS
AWAITS
BAAING
BLAINE
BLAISE
BRAIDS
BRAINS
BRAINY
BRAISE
CHAINE
CHAINS
CHAIRS
CHAISE
CLAIMS
CLAIRE
CLAIRS
CRAIGT
CRAINS
DEAIRS
DRAINS
ELAINE
EMAILS
ETAILS
EWAINE
FLAILS
FLAIRS
FRAIDY
FRAISE
GHAINS
GRAILS
GRAINS
GRAINY
IRAISE
ISAIAH
ISAIAN
KRAITS
LIAISE
MTAIRY
OJAICA
PLAICE
PLAIDS
PLAINS
PLAINT
PLAITS
PRAISE
QUAILS
QUAINT
REAIMS
REAIRS
SEAICE
SNAILS
STAINS
STAIRS
SWAINS
TRAILS
TRAINS
TRAITS
TWAINS
WRAITH

••A•I•

ABATIS
ACACIA
ACADIA
ACARID
ADAGIO
AGADIR
AGARIC
ALANIS
ALARIC
AMADIS
AMALIA
AMALIE
AMATIS
AMAZIN
ANACIN
ANAKIN
ARABIA
ARABIC
ARAMID
ARAMIS
ATARIS
ATAVIC
ATAXIA
ATAXIC
AZANIA
AZARIA
BAALIM
BEANIE
BEATIT
BEAVIS
BIALIK
BRASIL
BRAZIL
CHAPIN
CLADIN
CLAVIN
COATIS
CRAMIN
CRANIA
CRANIO
CYANIC
CYANID
DEALIN
DEARIE
DEASIL
DIALIN
DIARIO
DRAGIN
DRATIT
DRAWIN
DYADIC
ELADIO
ELAPID
ETALIA
ETALII
ETAOIN
FLAVIA
GHAZIS
GLACIS
GOALIE
GOATIT
GRACIE
GRANIT
GRATIA
GRATIN
GRATIS
GRAVID
GRAZIE
HEADIN
HOAGIE
ICARIA

INABIT
INAFIX
INAPIE
INATIE
IRANIS
IRAQIS
ITALIA
ITALIC
IVANIV
JEANIE
JOANIE
KHAKIS
KHALID
KIARIO
KRAVIS
LEADIN
LEAKIN
LEANIN
LEAPIN
LOADIN
MEALIE
MEANIE
MEANIT
MIAMIS
MIAMIU
NIACIN
OKAPIS
OLAFII
OLAFIV
OLAVII
OLAVIV
OMANIS
ORANIS
OXALIC
OXALIS
PHAGIA
PHASIC
PLACID
PLAYIT
PRAXIS
QRATIO
QUAKIE
READIN
REALIA
ROADIE
ROAMIN
SCALIA
SEAAIR
SEALIN
SHAKIN
SHALIT
SHAMIR
SHANIA
SHARIF
SLAVIC
SOAKIN
STADIA
STALIN
STARIN
STASIS
STATIC
STATIN
STAYIN
SWAMIS
TEARIT
THALIA
THATIS
TRACII
TRAGIC
TRAVIS
TSADIS
UNAKIN
UNAMIS
UNAVID
URACIL
URALIC
URANIA
URANIC
VLASIC
WHATIF
YEABIG

••A••I

AGASSI
AMALFI
AMANTI
AVANTI
BRANDI
BRAZZI
CHACHI
CIARDI
ETALII
GIAMBI
GIANNI
ISANTI
IVANVI
OLAFII
OLAVII
PIAZZI
QUADRI
SCAASI
SCAMPI
SHALLI
SMALLI
TRACII
UBANGI

•••AI•

AAFAIR
AFFAIR
AFRAID
AGLAIA
AGNAIL
ALHAIG
ALKAID
ALLAIS
ALTAIC
ALTAIR
ASSAIL
ATRAIN
ATTAIN
AUFAIT
AULAIT
AUPAIR
BEFAIR
BEHAIM
BELAIR
BEWAIL
BIGAIR
BYMAIL
CALAIS
COBAIN
CONAIR
DEHAIR
DEMAIN
DERAIL
DERAIN
DETAIL
DETAIN
DIZAIN
DOMAIN
ECLAIR
EDDAIC
ELPAIS
ENFAIT
ENTAIL
ESSAIS
EURAIL
GAWAIN
HAWAII
HOTAIR
IMPAIR
INCAIC
INJAIL
INLAID
INVAIN
ISMAIL
ISRAIR
JAMAIS
JUDAIC
KUWAIT
LANAIS
LAVAIN
LCHAIM
LECAIN
LENAIN
LORAIN
MASAIS
MCBAIN
MCCAIN
MCLAIN
MCNAIR
MIDAIR
MISAIM
MOHAIR
MOSAIC
NAVAID
NOFAIR
NORAIN
NOTAIL
NOWAIT
OBTAIN
ONBAIL
ONLAID
ORDAIN
OXTAIL
PALAIS
PETAIN
REBAIT
REGAIN
REJAIL
RELAID
REMAIL
REMAIN
RENAIL
REPAID
REPAIR
RESAID
RETAIL
RETAIN
ROMAIC
ROMAIN
SAVAII
SEAAIR
SERAIS
SPRAIN
STRAIN
STRAIT
UNBAIT
UNFAIR
UNHAIR
UNLAID
UNNAIL
UNPAID
UNSAID
UNVAIN
USMAIL
VALAIS
VEDAIC

•••A•I

ADJANI
ALKALI
ARGALI
ARMANI
BONACI
BONAMI
BYTAXI
CORACI
DALASI
DENALI
DENARI
DITALI
DOMANI
DORATI
ERNANI
GELATI
HATARI
HAWAII
IOLANI
KAMALI
KIGALI
LIPARI
MALAWI
MESABI
MONAMI
NEPALI
OBLADI
ORIANI
PATAKI
QATARI
RIGATI
ROMAJI
ROMANI
RUBATI
RUMAKI
SAFARI
SALAMI
SAVAII
SCAASI
SOCANI
SOLATI
SOMALI
STRATI
SUVARI
TATAMI
URBANI
WASABI
WHOAMI
YAMANI

••••AI

ADONAI
BANZAI
BOLYAI
BONSAI
CENTAI
HAGGAI
HAIKAI
KATMAI
KUBLAI
MAITAI
MAOTAI
MUMBAI
SHUMAI

AJ••••

AJFOYT
AJIJIC
AJOWAN

A•J•••

ABJECT
ABJURE
ADJANI
ADJOIN
ADJURE
ADJUST
ANJOUS
ARJUNA

A••J••

AJIJIC
AMAJOR

A••••J

AGENTJ

•AJ•••

CAJOLE
CAJUNS
FAJITA
HAJJES
HAJJIS
LAJOIE
MAJGEN
MAJLIS
MAJOAD
MAJORS
NAJIMY
PAJAMA
PAJOAD
RAJABS
RAJAHS

•A•J••

BAGJOB
BANJOS
BANJUL
DAYJOB
FANJET
GAIJIN
GASJET
HADJES
HADJIS
HAJJES
HAJJIS
JARJAR
KANJIS
MARJOE
MATJES
RAMJET

•A••J•

BAROJA
MARYJO
NAVAJO

•A•••J

JAMESJ
RALPHJ

••AJ••

AMAJOR
BMAJOR
CMAJOR
DMAJOR
EMAJOR
FMAJOR
GMAJOR
INAJAM
ONAJAG
ORAJEL
TRAJAN

••A••J

PBANDJ
SMALLJ

•••AJ•

NAVAJO
ROMAJI

••••AJ

SGTMAJ
THEHAJ

AK••••

AKELAS
AKENES
AKIMBO
AKINTO
AKITAS
AKUAKU

A•K•••

ACKACK
AIKIDO
AIKMAN
ALKAID
ALKALI
ALKENE
ALKIES
ALKYDS
ALKYLS
ANKARA
ANKLED
ANKLES
ANKLET
ASKAMY
ASKANT
ASKERS
ASKFOR
ASKING
ASKOUT
ASKSIN
ASKSOF
ASKSUP
ATKINS
AUKLET

A••K••

ALEKEG
ALIKES
ALTKEY
ANAKIN
ANGKOR
AWAKED
AWAKEN
AWAKER
AWAKES
AWOKEN
AZUKIS

A•••K•

ADZUKI
AKUAKU
ALASKA
ALECKS
ALECKY
ANANKE
ANNIKA
APOPKA
AQUAKE
AXLIKE
AZTEKS

A••••K

ACKACK
ADWEEK
AGENTK
AMTRAK
ANORAK
ARMONK
ARRACK
ATDUSK
ATRISK
ATTACK
ATWORK
AWHECK

•AK•••

BAKERS
BAKERY
BAKING
BAKKER
BAKSHI
BAKULA
CAKEUP
CAKIER
CAKING
DAKOTA
EAKINS
FAKEID
FAKEIT
FAKERS
FAKERY
FAKING
FAKIRS
HAKEEM
HAKIMS
KAKAPO
KAKURO
LAKERS
LAKIER
LAKIST
LAKOTA
MAKEBA
MAKEDO
MAKEGO
MAKEIT
MAKEME
MAKEOF
MAKERS
MAKEUP
MAKING
MAKSIM
MAKUTA
NAKFAS
OAKIER
OAKLEY
OAKTAG
OAKUMS
PAKULA
RAKEIN
RAKERS
RAKEUP
RAKING
RAKISH
TAKEIN
TAKEIT
TAKEON
TAKERS
TAKETH
TAKETO
TAKEUP
TAKING
WAKAME
WAKENS
WAKERS
WAKEUP
WAKING
YAKIMA
YAKKED
YAKKER
YAKUTS
YAKUZA

•A•K••

BABKAS
BACKED
BACKER
BACKIN
BACKUP
BACKUS
BAIKAL
BAKKER
BALKAN
BALKAT
BALKED
BALKER
BANKED
BANKER
BANKIT
BANKON
BANKUP
BARKAT
BARKED
BARKER
BARKIN
BARKLA
BASKED
BASKER
BASKET
BASKIN
CACKLE
CALKED
CALKER
CANKER
CARKEY
CASKED
CASKET
CATKIN
DANKER
DANKLY
DARKEN
DARKER
DARKLE
DARKLY
FAWKES
GASKET
GAWKAT
GAWKED
GAWKER
HAAKON
HACKED
HACKER
HACKIE
HACKIT
HACKLE
HACKLY
HACKUP
HAIKAI
HAIKUS
HANKER
HANKIE
HARKED
HARKEN
HARKER
HAWKED
HAWKER
JACKAL
JACKED
JACKET
JACKIE
JACKUP
KALKAN
KARKOV
LACKED
LACKEY
LANKER
LANKLY
LARKED
LARKER
LARKIN
LASKER
LATKES
MACKIE
MARKAS
MARKED
MARKER
MARKET
MARKEY
MARKIE
MARKII
MARKIV
MARKIX
MARKKA
MARKOV
MARKUP
MARKVI
MASKED
MASKER
NAPKIN
PACKED
PACKER
PACKET
PACKIN
PACKON
PACKUP
PARKAS
PARKAV
PARKAY
PARKED
PARKER
PARKES
PARKIT
RACKED
RACKER
RACKET
RACKUP
RANKED
RANKER
RANKIN
RANKLE
RANKLY
RASKIN
SACKED
SACKER
SACKUP
SANKAS
SANKIN
TABKEY
TACKED
TACKER
TACKLE
TACKON
TACKUP
TALKAT
TALKED
TALKER
TALKIE
TALKIN
TALKOF
TALKON
TALKTO
TALKUP
TANKAS
TANKED
TANKER
TANKUP
TASKED
TASKET
WACKER
WACKOS
WALKBY
WALKED
WALKEN
WALKER
WALKIE
WALKIN
WALKON
WALKTO
WALKUP
WANKEL
YAKKED
YAKKER
YANKAT
YANKED
YANKEE
YANKER
YANKON
YAWKEY
ZARKOV

•A••K•

BAMAKO
BARAKA
BATIKS
BAULKS
CAULKS
FARUKI
HACEKS
HANDKE
JAMOKE
KABUKI
KANAKA
KAPOKS
KAYAKS
LADUKE
LANSKY
MARIKO
MARKKA
PANCKS
PATAKI
SALUKI
SAMEKH
TANAKA

•A•••K

BARACK
BARTOK
CANUCK
DAMASK
FAROUK
JAMESK
JARVIK
KARNAK
LANARK
MALICK
NANOOK
NARVIK
NATICK
SAIDOK
SAITEK
SAYSOK
TANOAK
TARLEK
VANARK
ZADDIK
ZANUCK

••AK••

ANAKIN
AWAKED
AWAKEN
AWAKER
AWAKES
BEAKED
BEAKER
BLAKEY
BRAKED
BRAKES
CHAKRA
CRAKES
DOAKES
DRAKES
DRAKEU
FLAKED
FLAKER
FLAKES
FRAKES
HAAKON
KHAKIS
KRAKEN
KRAKOW
LEAKED
LEAKER
LEAKEY
LEAKIN
OLAKES
OSAKAN
PEAKED
PLAKAT
QUAKED
QUAKER
QUAKES
QUAKIE
SHAKEN
SHAKER
SHAKES
SHAKIN
SHAKOS
SHAKUR
SLAKED
SLAKER
SLAKES
SNAKED
SNAKER
SNAKES
SOAKED
SOAKER
SOAKIN
SOAKUP
STAKED
STAKES
UNAKIN
WEAKEN
WEAKER
WEAKLY
WEAKON
YOAKAM

••A•K•

ALASKA
ANANKE
BLACKS
BLANKS
CHALKS
CHALKY
CLACKS
CLANKS
CLANKY
CLARKE
CRACKD
CRACKS
CRANKS
CRANKY
DBACKS
DMARKS
EBANKS
FLACKS
FLANKS
FLASKS
FRANKS
IVANKA
KNACKS
OZARKS
PLANKS
PRANKS
QUACKS
QUACKY
QUARKS
REASKS
SHACKS
SHANKS
SHARKS
SKANKS
SKANKY
SLACKS
SMACKS
SNACKS
SNARKS
SNARKY
SPANKS
SPANKY
SPARKS
SPARKY
STACKS
STALKS
STALKY
SWANKY
THANKS
TRACKS
WHACKS
WRACKS

••A••K

BIALIK
BRATSK
DRABEK
FRANCK
GDANSK
OCASEK
PLANCK
SMALLK
SPACEK
URALSK

•••AK•

AKUAKU
AQUAKE
BAMAKO
BARAKA
BETAKE
BLEAKS
BREAKS
BUGAKU
CLOAKS
CREAKS
CREAKY
CROAKS
CROAKY
FREAKS
FREAKY
INTAKE
KANAKA
KAYAKS
KODAKS
KULAKS
LUSAKA
MEDAKA
NOBAKE
PATAKI
REBAKE
REMAKE
RERAKE
RETAKE
REWAKE
RUMAKI
SEDAKA
SNEAKS
SNEAKY
SPEAKS
STEAKS
TANAKA
TILAKS
TWEAKS
TWEAKY
UMIAKS
UNCAKE
UNMAKE
UPTAKE
WREAKS

•••A•K

ACKACK
ARRACK
ATTACK
BARACK
BYTALK
CDRACK
CUSACK
DAMASK
DEBARK
DEMARK
EMBANK
EMBARK
ENRANK
EWBANK
EXYANK
GOBACK
GODARK
HIJACK
IMBACK
INBACK
INPARK
LANARK
LFRANK
MOHAWK
NEWARK
NYYANK
OUTASK
REBANK
REMARK
REPACK
REPARK
RERACK
RERANK
RETACK
RVPARK
SHRANK
SQUAWK
STMARK
THWACK
UNCASK
UNMASK
UNPACK
UNRACK
UNTACK
UPTALK
UQUARK
USBANK
VANARK
WOMACK

••••AK

AMTRAK
ANORAK
BUROAK
DEEPAK
DVORAK
HODIAK
ITZHAK
KARNAK
KODIAK
LITVAK
NOMEAK
PINOAK
POLLAK
REDOAK
RESOAK
SCREAK
SENDAK
SLEZAK
SLOVAK
SPIVAK
SQUEAK
STREAK
TANOAK

AL••••

ALABAM
ALAINA
ALALAS
ALAMOS
ALANIS
ALANON
ALARIC
ALARMS
ALARUM
ALASKA
ALATED
ALBANO
ALBANS
ALBANY
ALBEDO
ALBEIT
ALBERS
ALBERT
ALBINE
ALBINO
ALBION
ALBORG
ALBUMS
ALCAPP
ALCINA
ALCOTT
ALCOVE
ALDERS
ALDINE
ALDISS
ALDOUS
ALDRIN
ALEAST
ALECKS
ALECKY
ALECTO
ALEGAR

ALEGRE
ALEGUP
ALEKEG
ALEMAN
ALEPHS
ALEPPO
ALEROS
ALERTS
ALETAP
ALETTE
ALEUTS
ALEVEL
ALEVES
ALEXAS
ALEXEI
ALEXEY
ALEXIA
ALEXIS
ALFINE
ALFRED
ALFVEN
ALGEDI
ALGORE
ALGREN
ALHAIG
ALHENA
ALHIRT
ALIBIS
ALIBLE
ALICEB
ALICES
ALICIA
ALIENS
ALIGHT
ALIGNS
ALIKES
ALINED
ALINER
ALINES
ALIOTH
ALIOTO
ALIPED
ALISON
ALISTS
ALIVEO
ALIYAH
ALIYOT
ALKAID
ALKALI
ALKENE
ALKIES
ALKYDS
ALKYLS
ALLAIS
ALLAYS
ALLBUT
ALLDAY
ALLEES
ALLEGE
ALLELE
ALLEYN
ALLEYS
ALLFOR
ALLIED
ALLIES
ALLIUM
ALLMAN
ALLMEN
ALLNEW
ALLOTS
ALLOUT
ALLOWS
ALLOYS
ALLPRO
ALLSET
ALLUDE
ALLURE
ALLWET
ALLYCE
ALLYLS
ALMAAZ
ALMACH
ALMATY
ALMOND
ALMOST
ALMVPS
ALNASL
ALNICO
ALOGIA
ALOHAS
ALOMAR
ALONGS
ALONSO
ALONZO
ALOTOF
ALPACA
ALPERT
ALPHAS
ALPINE
ALRITZ
ALSACE
ALSTON
ALTAIC
ALTAIR
ALTARF
ALTARS
ALTERS
ALTHEA
ALTIMA
ALTIUS
ALTKEY
ALTMAN
ALTOID
ALTRIA
ALTTAB
ALUDEL
ALUDRA
ALULAE
ALULAR
ALUMNA
ALUMNI
ALVARO
ALVING
ALVINO
ALWAYS
ALWEST
ALYDAR
ALYSSA
ALZADO
ALZIRA

A•L•••

ABLARE
ABLATE
ABLAZE
ABLEST
ABLOOM
ABLUSH
ADLIBS
AFLAME
AFLARE
AFLATS
AFLCIO
AFLOAT
AGLAIA
AGLARE
AGLEAM
AGLETS
AGLINT
AILEEN
AILING
AILURO
ALLAIS
ALLAYS
ALLBUT
ALLDAY
ALLEES
ALLEGE
ALLELE
ALLEYN
ALLEYS
ALLFOR
ALLIED
ALLIES
ALLIUM
ALLMAN
ALLMEN
ALLNEW
ALLOTS
ALLOUT
ALLOWS
ALLOYS
ALLPRO
ALLSET
ALLUDE
ALLURE
ALLWET
ALLYCE
ALLYLS
AOLERS
APLITE
APLOMB
ARLENE
ARLISS
ARLOVA
ASLANT
ASLEEP
ASLOPE
ASLOSH
ATLAST
AULAIT
AWLESS
AXLIKE

A••L••

ABELES
ABOLLA
ACELAS
ADDLED
ADDLES
ADELEH
ADELIE
ADELLE
ADOLFO
ADOLPH
ADULTS
AEOLIA
AEOLUS
AGILER
AHOLIC
AIELLO
AIGLET
AIOLIS
AIRLOG
AISLED
AISLES
AKELAS
ALALAS
ALULAE
ALULAR
AMALFI
AMALIA
AMALIE
AMBLED
AMBLER
AMBLES
AMBLIN
AMELIA
AMELIE
AMOLES
AMPLER
AMULET
ANALOG
ANELED
ANELES
ANGLED
ANGLEE
ANGLER
ANGLES
ANGLIA
ANGLIC
ANGLOS
ANKLED
ANKLES
ANKLET
ANNLEE
ANOLES
ANTLER
ANTLIA
APELET
APOLLO
APPLES
APPLET
APULIA
ARMLET
ASFLAT
ASHLAR
ASHLEE
ASHLEY
ASSLOW
ASTLEY
ASYLUM
ATALOW
ATILES
ATOLLS
ATPLAY
ATTLEE
AUKLET
AVALON
AVULSE
AXILLA
AZALEA
AZELMA
AZOLES

A•••L•

AACELL
ABOLLA
ACIDLY
ADELLE
ADVILS
AEDILE
AERILY
AFIELD
AGEDLY
AGEOLD
AIELLO
AIRILY
ALIBLE
ALKALI
ALKYLS
ALLELE
ALLYLS
AMPULE
ANGELA
ANGELI
ANGELL
ANGELO
ANGELS
ANGOLA
ANNALS
ANNULI
ANNULS
ANSELM
ANVILS
ANYOLD
APOLLO
APPALL
APPALS
APPELS
APRILE
APRILS
AQUILA
ARABLE
ARBELA
ARCHLY
AREOLA
AREOLE
ARGALI
ARGYLE
ARGYLL
ARIDLY
ARNALL
ARNOLD
ARPELS
ARTELS
ARTILY
ASCALE
ASCOLD
ASDULL
ASTALL
ASWELL
ATOLLS
ATTILA
ATWILL
ATYALE
AUDILE
AVAILS
AVIDLY
AVRILS
AWEDLY
AWHILE
AXILLA
AZUELA

A••••L

AACELL
ABDIEL
ABORAL
ACETAL
ACETYL
ACTUAL
AERIAL
AGNAIL
AIDFUL
AIMFUL
ALEVEL
ALNASL
ALUDEL
AMATOL
AMICAL
AMIDOL
AMORAL
AMSTEL
ANGELL
ANIMAL
ANNEAL
ANNUAL
ANODAL
ANTRAL
AORTAL
APICAL
APODAL
APPALL
APPEAL
ARGYLL
ARMFUL
ARNALL
ARTFUL
ASCOOL
ASDULL
ASSAIL
ASTALL
ASTEAL
ASTRAL
ASWELL
ASWIRL
ATHEEL
ATONAL
ATRIAL
ATWILL
AUDIAL
AVOWAL
AWHIRL
AXONAL
AZONAL
AZRAEL

•AL•••

BALAAM
BALATA
BALBOA
BALDED
BALDER
BALDIE
BALDLY
BALDUR
BALEEN
BALERS
BALINE
BALING
BALKAN
BALKAT
BALKED
BALKER
BALLAD
BALLET
BALLIN
BALLON
BALLOT
BALLOU
BALLST
BALLUP
BALLYS
BALMER
BALSAM
BALSAS
BALTIC
BALZAC
CALAIS
CALASH
CALDER
CALGON
CALICO
CALIFS
CALIPH
CALKED
CALKER
CALLAN
CALLAO
CALLAS
CALLED
CALLEE
CALLER
CALLES
CALLIN
CALLIT
CALLME
CALLON
CALLOW
CALLTO
CALLUP
CALLUS
CALMED
CALMER
CALMEX
CALMLY
CALORY
CALVED
CALVES
CALVET
CALVIN
CALXES
DALAND
DALASI
DALENE
DALETH
DALETS
DALLAS
DALLES
DALTON
EALING
FALALA
FALANA
FALCON
FALINE
FALLAL
FALLEN
FALLER
FALLIN
FALLON
FALLOW
FALLTO
FALSER
FALTER
FALUDI
GALANT
GALAXY
GALEAE
GALEAO
GALENA
GALLED
GALLEY
GALLIA
GALLIC
GALLON
GALLOP
GALLUP
GALOIS
GALOOT
GALOPS
GALORE
GALOSH
GALPAL
GALTON
GALWAY
HALALA
HALEST
HALEVY
HALIDE
HALING
HALITE
HALLAM
HALLEL
HALLEY
HALLIE
HALLOO
HALLOS
HALLOW
HALLUX
HALOED
HALOES
HALOID
HALPIN
HALSEY
HALTED
HALTER
HALVAH
HALVAS
HALVED
HALVER
HALVES
JALAPA
JALOPY
JALPAS
KALINE
KALKAN
KALLEN
KALMAR
LALALA
LALLED
MALABO
MALADY
MALAGA
MALARS
MALAWI
MALAYA
MALAYS
MALDEN
MALEIC
MALIAN
MALIBU
MALICE
MALICK
MALIGN
MALLEI
MALLET
MALLON
MALLOW
MALONE
MALORY
MALOTI
MALTBY
MALTED
MALTIN
PALACE
PALADE
PALAIS
PALATE
PALEAE
PALELY
PALEST
PALING
PALISH
PALLAS
PALLED
PALLET
PALLID
PALLOR
PALMAR
PALMAS
PALMED
PALMER
PALOMA
PALTER
PALTRY
RALLYE
RALPHJ
SALAAM
SALADA
SALADE
SALADS
SALAMI
SALARY
SALEPS
SALIFY
SALINA
SALINE
SALISH
SALIVA
SALLES
SALLIE
SALLOW
SALMAN
SALMIS
SALMON
SALOME
SALONS
SALOON
SALSAS
SALTED
SALTEN
SALTER
SALTII
SALTON
SALUKI
SALUTE
SALUTO
SALVED
SALVER
SALVES
SALVOR
SALVOS
SALYUT
TALCED
TALCUM
TALENT
TALERS
TALESE
TALISA
TALKAT
TALKED
TALKER
TALKIE
TALKIN
TALKOF
TALKON
TALKTO
TALKUP
TALLER
TALLOW
TALMUD
TALONS
TALTOS
VALAIS
VALDEZ
VALENE
VALENS
VALENT
VALERA
VALERE
VALERO
VALERY
VALETS
VALINE
VALISE
VALIUM
VALLEE
VALLEY
VALOIS
VALORS
VALOUR
VALOVA
VALSES
VALUED
VALUER
VALUES
VALVED
VALVES
WALDEN
WALESA
WALING
WALKBY
WALKED
WALKEN
WALKER
WALKIE
WALKIN
WALKON
WALKTO
WALKUP
WALLED
WALLER
WALLET
WALLIN
WALLIS
WALLOP
WALLOW
WALLST
WALLUP
WALNUT
WALRUS
WALTER
WALTON
YALIES

•A•L••

BAALIM
BADLIE
BADLOT
BAILED
BAILEE
BAILER
BAILEY
BAILON
BAILOR
BALLAD
BALLET
BALLIN
BALLON
BALLOT
BALLOU
BALLST
BALLUP
BALLYS
BANLON
BARLEY
BARLOW
BATLEY
BAULKS
BAWLED
BAWLER
BAYLOR
CABLED
CABLER
CABLES
CABLET
CALLAN
CALLAO
CALLAS
CALLED
CALLEE
CALLER
CALLES
CALLIN
CALLIT
CALLME
CALLON
CALLOW
CALLTO
CALLUP
CALLUS
CANLIT
CAPLET
CARLIN
CARLOS
CARLOT
CARLOW
CATLIN
CAULKS
DAHLIA
DAILEY
DALLAS
DALLES
DARLIN
DAYLIT
EAGLED
EAGLES
EAGLET
EARLAP
EARLET
EASLEY
FABLED
FABLER
FABLES
FAILED
FAILLE
FAILTO
FALLAL
FALLEN
FALLER
FALLIN
FALLON
FALLOW
FALLTO
FARLEY
FARLOW
FATLIP
FAULTS
FAULTY
FAWLTY
FAYLEN
GABLED
GABLER
GABLES
GAELIC
GAGLAW
GALLED
GALLEY
GALLIA
GALLIC
GALLON
GALLOP
GALLUP
GAOLED
GAOLER
GARLIC
GASLIT
GASLOG
GATLIN
GAULLE
HABLAR
HAGLER
HAILED
HAILER
HAILEY
HALLAM
HALLEL
HALLEY
HALLIE
HALLOO
HALLOS
HALLOW
HALLUX
HAMLET
HAMLIN
HANLEY
HANLON
HAOLES
HARLAN
HARLEM
HARLEY
HARLIN
HARLOT
HARLOW
HAULED
HAULER
HAULIN
HAULUP
HAYLEY
JACLYN
JAGLOM
JAILED
JAILER
JAILOR
KAHLIL
KAHLUA
KAILUA
KALLEN
KAOLIN
KAPLAN
KARLEN
LAALAA
LACLOS
LADLED
LADLER
LADLES
LALLED
LAULAU
LAYLOW
MAALOX
MABLEY
MACLEN
MACLES
MADLYN
MAGLEV
MAGLIE
MAHLER
MAILED
MAILER
MAILIN
MAILTO
MAJLIS
MALLEI
MALLET
MALLON
MALLOW
MANLEY
MAPLES
MARLED
MARLEE
MARLEY
MARLIN
MARLON
MASLIN
MATLIN
MAULED
MAULER
NAILED
NAILER
NAILIN
NAILIT
NAILUP
NAPLES
OAKLEY
PABLUM
PAELLA
PAGLIA
PALLAS
PALLED
PALLET
PALLID
PALLOR
PARLAY
PARLEY
PARLEZ
PARLOR
PAULEY
PAULII
PAULIV
PAULVI
PAVLOV
RADLEY
RAGLAN
RAILAT
RAILED
RAILER
RAILON
RALLYE
RANLOW
RATLIN
SABLES
SADLER
SAILED
SAILER
SAILON
SAILOR
SAILTO
SALLES
SALLIE
SALLOW
SAMLET
SAULTS
SAWLOG
SAYLES
TABLAS
TABLED
TABLES
TABLET
TAILED
TAILER
TAILOR
TALLER
TALLOW
TARLEK
TATLER
TAXLAW
TAYLOR
VACLAV
VAILCO
VALLEE
VALLEY
VARLET
VASLAV
VAULTS
VAULTY
WAHLOO
WAILED
WAILER
WALLED
WALLER
WALLET
WALLIN
WALLIS
WALLOP
WALLOW
WALLST
WALLUP
WASLED
WAYLAY
WAYLON

•A••L•

AACELL
BABALU
BABBLE
BABBLY
BABELS
BACALL
BAFFLE
BAGELS
BAKULA
BALDLY
BANGLE
BARELY
BARFLY
BARKLA
BAROLO
BARTLE
BASALT
BASELY
BASILS
BASSLY
BATTLE
BAUBLE
CABALA
CABALS
CABELL
CACKLE
CAGILY
CAHILL
CAJOLE
CALMLY
CAMELS
CANALS
CANDLE
CANOLA
CANTLE
CANULA
CAROLE
CAROLI
CAROLL
CAROLS
CASALS
CASTLE
CATALO
CATTLE
CAVELL
CAVILS
CAZALE
DABBLE
DAFTLY
DAMPLY
DANDLE
DANGLE
DANGLY
DANILO
DANKLY
DAPPLE
DARKLE

DARKLY
DARTLE
DAWDLE
DAYGLO
DAYOLD
DAZZLE
EASELS
EASILY
EASTLA
FACILE
FACULA
FADDLE
FAILLE
FAIRLY
FALALA
FAMILY
FAMULI
FATALE
GABBLE
GADFLY
GAGGLE
GAINLY
GAMBLE
GAMELY
GAMILY
GANGLY
GARBLE
GARGLE
GAULLE
GAVELS
HABILE
HACKLE
HACKLY
HAGGLE
HALALA
HAMELN
HAMILL
HAMULI
HANDLE
HARALD
HARDLY
HAROLD
HASSLE
HAZELS
HAZILY
JACALS
JANGLE
JANGLY
JARULE
KAMALI
KANALY
KAPELL
LABELS
LABILE
LACILY
LALALA
LAMELY
LANKLY
LAPELS
LASTLY
LASZLO
LATELY
LAXALT
LAZILY
LAZULI
MABELL
MACULA
MAHALO
MAINLY
MANGLE
MANILA
MANTLE
MAPPLE
MARBLE
MARBLY
MARILU
MARPLE
MASALA
MAXELL
MAYFLY
MAZILY
MAZOLA
NAMELY
NAPALM
NAPOLI
NASALS
NATALE
NAVELS
PACULA
PADDLE
PAELLA
PAKULA
PALELY
PAMELA
PANDLS
PANELS
PAROLE
PAROLS
PARTLY
PAYOLA
QABALA
RABBLE
RACILY
RAFFLE
RAMBLE
RANKLE
RANKLY
RAPTLY
RARELY
RASHLY
RASSLE
RATELS
RATTLE
RATTLY
RAVELS
RAZZLE
SABALS
SACFLY
SADDLE
SAFELY
SAGELY
SAMPLE
SANELY
SAWALL
TABULA
TACKLE
TAMALE
TAMELY
TAMILS
TANGLE
TANGLY
TARTLY
TATTLE
TAUTLY
TAVELS
TAXOLS
VAINLY
VASILY
VASTLY
WADDLE
WADDLY
WAFFLE
WAFFLY
WAGGLE
WAGGLY
WAMBLE
WAMBLY
WANGLE
WARBLE
WARILY
WARMLY
WASOLD
WATTLE
WAVILY
WAXILY
YARELY
ZANILY

•A•••L

AACELL
BACALL
BAGFUL
BAIKAL
BANJUL
BARREL
BARTEL
BASIAL
CABELL
CABRAL
CAHILL
CANCEL
CANFUL
CANNEL
CANTAL
CAPFUL
CARFUL
CARMEL
CARNAL
CAROLL
CARPAL
CARPEL
CARREL
CARROL
CARTEL
CARVEL
CASTEL
CASUAL
CAUDAL
CAUSAL
CAVELL
DACTYL
DAEDAL
DAMSEL
DANDYL
DANIEL
DARCEL
DARRYL
DATRIL
DAVIDL
EARFUL
FACIAL
FAISAL
FALLAL
FARFEL
FAUNAL
FAZOOL
GALPAL
GAMBOL
GASOIL
GAVIAL
HALLEL
HAMILL
HANDEL
HANGUL
HANSEL
HASSEL
HATFUL
JACKAL
JAMAAL
JARFUL
JAWOHL
KAHLIL
KANDEL
KAPELL
LABIAL
LAICAL
LANVAL
LAPFUL
LARVAL
LAUREL
LAURYL
LAWFUL
MAAZEL
MABELL
MAGNOL
MAMMAL
MANDEL
MANFUL
MANTEL
MANUAL
MANUEL
MARCEL
MARCIL
MARIEL
MARTEL
MARVEL
MATTEL
MAXELL
NARIAL
PAGNOL
PANFUL
PARCEL
PASCAL
PASSEL
PASTEL
PATROL
PAUSAL
PAYPAL
RACHEL
RACIAL
RADIAL
RAFAEL
RAMPAL
RANDAL
RANGEL
RAPPEL
RAQUEL
RASCAL
SAMUEL
SANDAL
SAWALL
TACTEL
TAROIL
TARSAL
TASSEL
VACHEL
VANDAL
VASSAL
VATFUL
WANKEL
WARHOL

••AL••

ALALAS
AMALFI
AMALIA
AMALIE
ANALOG
ATALOW
AVALON
AZALEA
BAALIM
BEALLS
BIALIK
CHALET
CHALKS
CHALKY
COALED
COALER
DEALER
DEALIN
DEALTO
DEALUP
DIALED
DIALER
DIALIN
DIALOG
DIALSO
DIALUP
DNALAB
DOALLS
DUALLY
EGALES
EMALLS
ESALEN
ETALIA
ETALII
EXALTS
FEALTY
FOALED
GOALBY
GOALIE
HEALED
HEALER
HEALEY
HEALTH
HEALUP
ICALLY
ITALIA
ITALIC
KHALID
KOALAS
LAALAA
LEALTY
MAALOX
MEALIE
NEALON
NYALAS
ORALES
ORALLY
OVALLY
OXALIC
OXALIS
PEALED
PEALER
PEALES
PSALMS
QUALES
QUALMS
REALER
REALES
REALIA
REALLY
REALMS
REALTY
RIALTO
RVALUE
SCALAR
SCALDS
SCALED
SCALER
SCALES
SCALIA
SCALPS
SEALAB
SEALED
SEALER
SEALIN
SEALUP
SEALYS
SHALES
SHALEY
SHALIT
SHALLI
SHALLY
SHALOM
SKALDS
SLALOM
SMALLA
SMALLB
SMALLC
SMALLD
SMALLE
SMALLF
SMALLG
SMALLH
SMALLI
SMALLJ
SMALLK
SMALLL
SMALLM
SMALLN
SMALLO
SMALLP
SMALLQ
SMALLR
SMALLS
SMALLT
SMALLU
SMALLV
SMALLW
SMALLX
SMALLY
SMALLZ
STALAG
STALED
STALER
STALES
STALIN
STALKS
STALKY
STALLS
SWALES
THALER
THALES
THALIA
TRALAS
TRALEE
URALIC
URALSK
UVALDE
UVALUE
VIALED
WEALDS
WEALTH
WHALED
WHALER
WHALES
WHALEY
ZEALOT

••A•L•

ARABLE
AVAILS
BEADLE
BEAGLE
BEALLS
BEATLE
BRAWLS
CHARLY
CRADLE
CRAWLS
CRAWLY
DEADLY
DEAFLY
DEARLY
DIABLE
DIABLO
DOABLE
DOALLS
DRABLY
DRAWLS
DRAWLY
DUALLY
EMAILS
EMALLS
ENABLE
ETAILS
FLAILS
FLATLY
GLADLY
GNARLS
GNARLY
GRABLE
GRAILS
GRAYLY
ICALLY
KRAALS
LEANLY
LIABLE
MEANLY
MEASLE
MEASLY
NEARLY
NEATLY
ORACLE
ORALLY
OVALLY
PEARLE
PEARLS
PEARLY
QUAILS
QUAYLE
REALLY
SEARLE
SHALLI
SHALLY
SHAWLS
SMALLA
SMALLB
SMALLC
SMALLD
SMALLE
SMALLF
SMALLG
SMALLH
SMALLI
SMALLJ
SMALLK
SMALLL
SMALLM
SMALLN
SMALLO
SMALLP
SMALLQ
SMALLR
SMALLS
SMALLT
SMALLU
SMALLV
SMALLW
SMALLX
SMALLY
SMALLZ
SNAILS
SNARLS
SNARLY
STABLE
STABLY
STALLS
STAPLE
SUABLE
THATLL
TRAILS
TRAWLS
UHAULS
UNABLE
UNABLY
USABLE
USABLY
VIABLE
VIABLY
WEAKLY
WHATLL
YEARLY

••A••L

AMATOL
BEAPAL
BOATEL
BRASIL
BRAZIL
CHACEL
CHANEL
CHAPEL
COAXAL
DEASIL
DIABOL
ENAMEL
GOAWOL
GRAVEL
HIATAL
ISABEL
MAAZEL
ORAJEL
SEAEEL
SEAGAL
SMALLL
TEASEL
THATLL
TRAVEL
URACIL
WEASEL
WHATLL

•••AL•

ALKALI
ANNALS
APPALL
APPALS
ARGALI
ARNALL
ASCALE
ASTALL
ATYALE
BABALU
BACALL
BASALT
BECALM
BEFALL
BEHALF
BSCALE
BYHALF
BYTALK
CABALA
CABALS
CANALS
CASALS
CATALO
CAZALE
COBALT
COPALS
CORALS
CSCALE
DECALS
DEKALB
DENALI
DESALT
DITALI
DONALD
DSCALE
DUGALD
DUVALL
EMBALM
EMPALE
ENDALL
ENHALO
EQUALS
ESCALE
EXHALE
FALALA
FATALE
FEMALE
FERALS
FINALE
FINALS
FSCALE
GERALD
GSCALE
HALALA
HARALD
HERALD
HIYALL
IDEALS
IMPALA
IMPALE
INFALL
INHALE
INHALF
JACALS
KAMALI
KANALY
KERALA
KIGALI
KODALY
KRAALS
KURALT
LALALA
LAXALT
LEGALS
LIZALU
LOCALE
LOCALS
LOYALE
MAHALO
MASALA
MCHALE
MEDALS
MEGALO
METALS
MODALS
MORALE
MORALS
MURALS
NAPALM
NASALS
NATALE
NEPALI
NOBALL
NOPALS
NOSALE
NOSALT
NOTALL
OFFALS
OFFALY
OGLALA
ONCALL
ONEALL
ONSALE
OOLALA
OSWALD
PEDALS
PETALE
PETALS
PHIALS
QABALA
REBALE
RECALL
REFALL
REGALE
RESALE
RESALT
REXALL
RIBALD
RIVALS
RIYALS
RODALE
RONALD
ROYALE
ROYALS
SABALS
SAWALL
SEEALL
SEPALS
SHOALS
SHOALY
SISALS
SKOALS
SOMALI
SQUALL
STEALS
STMALO
TAMALE
THRALL
TICALS
TOTALS
TRIALS
TUVALU
TYBALT
UNBALE
UNCALM
UNHALE
UNPALE
UNWALL
UPSALA
UPTALK
USUALS
VITALE
VITALS
VOCALS
YOUALL
ZOCALO

•••A•L

AGNAIL
ALNASL
APPALL
ARNALL
ASSAIL
ASTALL
AZRAEL
BACALL
BEFALL
BEWAIL
BYMAIL
DEPAUL
DERAIL
DETAIL
DUVALL
ENDALL
ENTAIL
EURAIL
HIYALL
INFALL
INJAIL
ISMAIL
ISRAEL
JAMAAL
NOBALL
NOTAIL
NOTALL
ONBAIL
ONCALL
ONEALL
OXTAIL
RAFAEL
RECALL
REFALL
REHAUL
REJAIL
REMAIL
RENAIL
RETAIL
REXALL
SAWALL
SCRAWL
SEEALL
SPRAWL
SQUALL
STPAUL
THRALL
UNNAIL
UNWALL
USMAIL
YOUALL

••••AL

ABORAL
ACETAL
ACTUAL
AERIAL
AMICAL
AMORAL
ANIMAL
ANNEAL
ANNUAL
ANODAL
ANTRAL
AORTAL
APICAL
APODAL
APPEAL
ASTEAL
ASTRAL
ATONAL
ATRIAL
AUDIAL
AVOWAL
AXONAL
AZONAL
BAIKAL
BASIAL
BEAPAL
BELIAL
BENGAL
BHOPAL
BOMBAL
BOREAL
BRIDAL
BRUMAL
BRUTAL
BUCCAL
BURIAL
BURSAL
CABRAL
CANTAL
CARNAL
CARPAL
CASUAL
CAUDAL
CAUSAL
CENTAL
CEPHAL
CEREAL
CHEVAL
CHORAL
CLONAL
COAXAL
COEVAL
CORRAL
COSTAL
CRURAL
CUNEAL
CUSPAL
CYMBAL
DAEDAL
DENIAL
DENTAL
DERMAL
DISMAL
DISTAL
DORSAL
DOSSAL
DOUGAL
DUCTAL
ENSEAL
ENTIAL
EPICAL
EPINAL
ESPIAL
FACIAL
FAISAL
FALLAL
FAUNAL
FESTAL
FEUDAL
FILIAL
FINIAL
FISCAL
FLORAL
FONTAL
FORMAL
FRUGAL
FUNGAL
GALPAL
GAVIAL
GENIAL
GENUAL
GIMBAL
GLOBAL
HEDRAL
HERBAL
HIATAL
HIEMAL
HYETAL
HYMNAL
INGOAL
INSTAL
IRREAL
JACKAL
JAMAAL
JOVIAL
KEYPAL
LABIAL
LAICAL
LANVAL
LARVAL
LETHAL
LINEAL
LOREAL
LOWCAL
MAMMAL
MANUAL
MCBEAL
MEDIAL
MENIAL
MENSAL
MENTAL
MESCAL
MESIAL
MISSAL
MITRAL
MORTAL
MUSIAL
MUTUAL
MYRDAL
NARIAL
NERMAL
NERVAL
NEURAL
NODEAL
NOMIAL
NORMAL
NORVAL
NOUNAL
NUCHAL
OGIVAL
OLDPAL
OMPHAL
ORDEAL
OSTEAL
PASCAL
PAUSAL
PAYPAL
PENPAL
PINEAL
PLEXAL
PLURAL
PORTAL
POSTAL
PRIMAL
RACIAL
RADIAL
RAMPAL
RANDAL
RASCAL
RECOAL
REDEAL
REDIAL
REGNAL
REHEAL
RENTAL
REPEAL
RESEAL
RETIAL
RETRAL
REVEAL
RHINAL
RICTAL
RITUAL
SANDAL
SEAGAL
SEPTAL
SERIAL
SIGNAL
SOCIAL
SPINAL
SPIRAL
SQUEAL
TARSAL
TIBIAL
TIMBAL
TINEAL
TRIBAL
TRINAL
TUSSAL
UMBRAL
UNCIAL
UNGUAL
UNOCAL
UNORAL
UNREAL
UNSEAL
VANDAL
VASSAL
VEINAL
VENIAL
VERBAL
VERNAL
VESTAL
VISUAL
VORPAL
WITHAL

AM••••

AMADEO
AMADIS
AMAJOR
AMALFI
AMALIA
AMALIE
AMANAS
AMANDA
AMANTI
AMANTS
AMARNA
AMATIS
AMATOL
AMAZED
AMAZES
AMAZIN
AMAZON
AMBAND
AMBERS
AMBERY
AMBIEN
AMBITS
AMBLED
AMBLER
AMBLES
AMBLIN
AMBUSH
AMEBAE
AMEBAS
AMEBIC
AMECHE
AMEDEE
AMEDEO
AMEERS
AMELIA

AMELIE AMENDS AMENRA AMENTS AMERCE AMESIA AMICAL AMICES AMICUS AMIDAS AMIDES AMIDOL AMIDST AMIENS AMIGAS AMIGOS AMINES AMINOR AMINOS AMINTA AMINUS AMITIE AMNION AMNIOS AMOEBA AMOLES AMONRA AMONTH AMORAL AMORES AMORET AMOSOZ AMOUNT AMOURS AMPERE AMPING AMPLER AMPSUP AMPULE AMRITA AMSTEL AMTRAC AMTRAK AMULET AMUSED AMUSER AMUSES AMVETS AMYTAN

A•M•••

ABMHOS ADMINS ADMIRE ADMITS AIMERS AIMFOR AIMFUL AIMING AIMSAT ALMAAZ ALMACH ALMATY ALMOND ALMOST ALMVPS ARMADA ARMAGH ARMAND ARMANI ARMERS ARMETS ARMFUL ARMIES ARMING ARMLET ARMONK ARMORS ARMORY ARMOUR ARMPIT ASMANY ASMARA ASMUCH ATMANS ATMFEE ATMOST AUMONT

A••M••

AAAMAP ABOMAS ABOMBS ACUMEN AGAMAS AGAMES AHIMSA AIDMAN AIDMEN AIKMAN AIRMAN AIRMEN AKIMBO ALAMOS ALEMAN ALLMAN ALLMEN ALOMAR ALTMAN ALUMNA ALUMNI ANEMIA ANEMIC ANIMAL ANIMAS ANIMES ANIMUS ANOMIA ANOMIC ANOMIE ANYMAN APEMAN APEMEN ARAMES ARAMID ARAMIS AROMAS ASHMAN ASHMEN ASIMOV ATAMAN ATEMPO ATOMIC AWCMON AXEMAN AXEMEN

A•••M•

ABOHMS ABRAMS ABYSMS ADDAMS ADEEMS AFLAME AFRAME ALARMS ALBUMS ALTIMA APLOMB ASHAME ASKAMY ASSUME ASTHMA ATEAMS ATHOME AUTUMN AXIOMS AZELMA

A••••M

ABLOOM ABSCAM ACTIUM ADYTUM AECIUM AFFIRM AGAWAM AGEISM AGLEAM AIRARM AIRDAM ALABAM ALARUM ALLIUM ANADEM ANONYM ANSELM ANTHEM ANTRIM ANTRUM ARNHEM ARTGUM ASHRAM ASWARM ASYLUM ATRIUM AUNTEM AUTISM

•AM•••

BAMAKO BAMBIS BAMBOO CAMARO CAMBER CAMBOY CAMDEN CAMEAS CAMEAT CAMEBY CAMEIN CAMELS CAMEON CAMEOS CAMERA CAMETO CAMEUP CAMINO CAMION CAMISE CAMMIE CAMOES CAMPED CAMPER CAMPOS CAMPUP CAMPUS CAMRYN CAMRYS DAMAGE DAMASK DAMATO DAMIEN DAMITA DAMMED DAMMER DAMNED DAMNER DAMONE DAMORE DAMOUR DAMPED DAMPEN DAMPER DAMPLY DAMSEL DAMSON DAMSUP EAMONN FAMILY FAMINE FAMING FAMISH FAMOUS FAMULI GAMAYS GAMBIA GAMBIT GAMBLE GAMBOL GAMELY GAMERS GAMEST GAMETE GAMGEE GAMIER GAMILY GAMINE GAMING GAMINS GAMMAS GAMMED GAMMER GAMMON GAMOUS GAMUTS HAMATE HAMDEN HAMELN HAMILL HAMITE HAMLET HAMLIN HAMMED HAMMER HAMPER HAMSUN HAMSUP HAMULI IAMBIC IAMBUS IAMNOT IAMSAM IAMTOO JAMAAL JAMAIS JAMBES JAMCAM JAMESA JAMESI JAMESJ JAMESK JAMESM JAMESS JAMEST JAMESV JAMMED JAMMER JAMOCA JAMOKE JAMSIN JAMSUP JAMUPS KAMALI LAMARR LAMAZE LAMBDA LAMBED LAMEDS LAMELY LAMENT LAMESA LAMEST LAMIAE LAMIAS LAMINA LAMING LAMMED LAMONT LAMOUR LAMSIT MAMBAS MAMBOS MAMMAL MAMMAS MAMMON NAMATH NAMEIT NAMELY NAMERS NAMING PAMELA PAMINA PAMIRS PAMPAS PAMPER RAMADA RAMAPO RAMATE RAMBLE RAMBOS RAMEAU RAMENS RAMETS RAMFAN RAMFIS RAMIES RAMIFY RAMJET RAMMED RAMMER RAMONA RAMONE RAMOSE RAMPAL RAMPED RAMPUP RAMROD RAMSAY RAMSES RAMSEY RAMSIN RAMSON SAMARA SAMBAS SAMEAS SAMEDI SAMEKH SAMIAM SAMLET SAMOAN SAMOSA SAMPAN SAMPLE SAMSON SAMUEL TAMALE TAMARA TAMAYO TAMBOR TAMELY TAMERS TAMEST TAMILS TAMING TAMMUZ TAMPED TAMPER TAMTAM VAMPED VAMPER WAMBLE WAMBLY WAMPUM YAMAHA YAMANI YAMMER YAMUNA ZAMBIA ZAMORA

•A•M••

AAAMAP BADMAN BADMEN BAGMAN BAGMEN BALMER BARMAN BARMEN BATMAN BATMEN BAUMAN BAUMER BAYMAN BAYMEN CABMAN CABMEN CADMIC CADMUS CAIMAN CALMED CALMER CALMEX CALMLY CAMMIE CARMAN CARMEL CARMEN CATMAN CATMEN CAYMAN DAEMON DAGMAR DAMMED DAMMER FAIMAN FARMED FARMER FATMAN GAGMAN GAGMEN GAMMAS GAMMED GAMMER GAMMON GASMAN GASMEN HAGMAN HAMMED HAMMER HARMED HARMER HARMON HAYMES HAYMOW HAZMAT JAMMED JAMMER JASMIN JAYMES KALMAR KARMAS KARMIC KATMAI LAMMED LARMEN LARMOR LAWMAN LAWMEN LAYMAN LAYMEN MADMAN MADMAX MADMEN MAGMAS MAIMED MAIMER MAMMAL MAMMAS MAMMON MARMEE MARMOT MATMAN MATMEN MAUMAU MAUMEE OARMAN OARMEN PACMAN PALMAR PALMAS PALMED PALMER PASMOI PATMOS RAGMAN RAGMEN RAGMOP RAMMED RAMMER SALMAN SALMIS SALMON TALMUD TAMMUZ TARMAC TASMAN TAXMAN TAXMEN VARMUS WARMED WARMER WARMLY WARMTH WARMTO WARMUP WASMET YAMMER YASMIN

•A••M•

BADEMS BAHAMA CALLME CAROMS DAGAMA DANGME DAREME FATIMA HAKIMS HAREMS LARAMS MACOMB MADAMA MADAME MADAMS MAKEME MANAMA MANDMS MAXIMA MAXIMS MAZUMA NAJIMY OAKUMS PAJAMA PALOMA PANAMA RACEME RADOME SALAMI SALOME SAVEME TACOMA TATAMI WAKAME WASHME YAKIMA

•A•••M

BAALIM BADHAM BALAAM BALSAM BANTAM BARIUM BARNUM BATYAM BAYRUM CASSIM CATDOM DADGUM FACTUM FANDOM FARNUM FATHOM HAKEEM HALLAM HANSOM HARLEM HASSAM IAMSAM JAGLOM JAMCAM JAMESM KABOOM KADEEM KAREEM LABIUM LAPERM LAPHAM MAGNUM MAKSIM MAOISM MARYAM MAYHEM NAPALM PABLUM PARFUM PASSIM RACISM RADIUM RANDOM RANSOM SACHEM SACRUM SADDAM SADISM SALAAM SAMIAM SATCOM TALCUM TAMTAM TANDEM TAOISM TAOSNM VACUUM VALIUM WAMPUM

••AM••

AAAMAP AGAMAS AGAMES ALAMOS ARAMES ARAMID ARAMIS ATAMAN BEAMAN BEAMED BEAMER BEAMON BEAMUP BLAMED BLAMER BLAMES BRAMAH CHAMMY CHAMPS CLAMMA CLAMMY CLAMOR CLAMPS CLAMUP CRAMBO CRAMER CRAMIN CRAMPS CRAMPY DRAMAS EDAMES ENAMEL ENAMOR FLAMBE FLAMED FLAMER FLAMES FOAMED FOAMER FRAMED FRAMER FRAMES GIAMBI GLAMOR GLAMUP GRAMME GRAMMY GRAMPA GRAMPS IMAMAN KRAMER LLAMAS LOAMED MIAMIS MIAMIU NIAMEY ODAMAE REAMED REAMER RHAMES ROAMED ROAMER ROAMIN SCAMPI SCAMPS SEAMAN SEAMAP SEAMED SEAMEN SEAMER SEAMUS SHAMAN SHAMED SHAMES SHAMIR SHAMMY SHAMUS SLAMON STAMEN STAMOS STAMPS SWAMIS SWAMPS SWAMPY SWAMUP TEAMED TEAMUP THAMES TOAMAN TRAMPS TRAMPY UNAMIS WHAMMO WHAMMY XGAMES

••A•M•

ALARMS BRAHMA BRAHMS CHAMMY CHARMS CHASMS CLAIMS CLAMMA CLAMMY DEARME DHARMA ENARMS GRAMME GRAMMY MIASMA PLASMA PLASMO PSALMS QUALMS README REAIMS REALMS REARMS SHAMMY SMARMY SPASMS SWARMS TRAUMA UNARMS USARMY WHAMMO WHAMMY

••A••M

AGAWAM ALABAM ALARUM ANADEM BAALIM DIADEM DIATOM GRAHAM INAJAM OMASUM SCARUM SEAARM SHALOM SHAZAM SLALOM SMALLM VIACOM YOAKAM

•••AM•

ABRAMS ADDAMS AFLAME AFRAME ASHAME ASKAMY ATEAMS BAHAMA BECAME BESAME BIGAMY BONAMI BREAMS BTEAMS BYNAME CCLAMP CREAMS CREAMY DAGAMA DECAMP DEFAME DIGAMY DIRAMS DREAMS DREAMT DREAMY DYNAMO ENCAMP GLEAMS GLEAMY GOLAME GOTAMA HBEAMS IBEAMS IMGAME INFAMY JICAMA LARAMS LBEAMS MADAMA MADAME MADAMS MANAMA MONAMI NONAME OCCAMS OGHAMS ONRAMP PAJAMA PANAMA PREAMP PROAMS RENAME RETAME REVAMP SALAMI SCRAMS SESAME STEAMS STEAMY TATAMI TOYAMA TVGAME UGGAMS UNDAMS UNGAMY UNJAMS UNTAME WAKAME WHOAMI

•••A•M

AIRARM ASWARM BALAAM BECALM BEHAIM DISARM EMBALM LCHAIM MISAIM NAPALM NOMAAM ONEARM PREARM REWARM SALAAM SEAARM UNCALM

••••AM

ABSCAM AGAWAM AGLEAM AIRDAM ALABAM ASHRAM BADHAM BALAAM BALSAM BANTAM BATYAM BEDLAM BELDAM BONHAM COBHAM CORFAM DEDHAM DEFJAM DEFOAM DENHAM DIGRAM DIRHAM DUNHAM DURHAM ENGRAM FIVEAM FOURAM GORHAM GOTEAM GOTHAM GRAHAM HALLAM HASSAM HICKAM IAMSAM ICEDAM INAJAM INGRAM INSEAM JAMCAM JETSAM LAPHAM LOGJAM MARYAM MIRIAM NINEAM NOMAAM OLDHAM PELHAM PELLAM PUTNAM RESEAM RESWAM RODHAM SADDAM SALAAM SAMIAM SCREAM SHAZAM SKYCAM SPYCAM STREAM SUREAM TAMTAM THERAM UNSEAM VIBRAM WEBCAM WIGWAM YESIAM YOAKAM

AN••••

ANACIN ANADEM ANAKIN ANALOG ANANAS ANANKE ANARCH ANATTO ANCHOR ANCHOS ANCIEN ANDEAN ANDERS ANDHOW ANDRAE ANDREA ANDREI ANDRES ANDREW ANDREY ANDRIC ANDROS ANDYET ANELED ANELES ANEMIA ANEMIC ANERGY ANGELA ANGELI ANGELL ANGELO ANGELS ANGERS ANGKOR ANGLED ANGLEE ANGLER ANGLES ANGLIA ANGLIC ANGLOS ANGOLA ANGORA ANGSTS ANIMAL ANIMAS ANIMES ANIMUS ANIONS ANISES ANITRA ANJOUS ANKARA ANKLED ANKLES ANKLET ANNALS ANNEAL ANNEES ANNIES ANNIKA ANNINA ANNLEE ANNOYS ANNUAL ANNUIT ANNULI ANNULS ANODAL ANODES ANODIC ANOINT ANOLES ANOMIA ANOMIC ANOMIE ANONYM ANORAK ANOXIA ANOXIC ANSARA ANSATE ANSEIS ANSELM

ANSWER
ANTAWN
ANTCOW
ANTEED
ANTERO
ANTEUP
ANTHEM
ANTHER
ANTICS
ANTIGO
ANTLER
ANTLIA
ANTONE
ANTONY
ANTRAL
ANTRES
ANTRIM
ANTRON
ANTRUM
ANUBIS
ANVILS
ANWANG
ANYDAY
ANYHOW
ANYMAN
ANYOLD
ANYONE
ANYONS
ANYWAY
ANZACS

A•N•••

ADNATE
ADNOUN
AENEAS
AENEID
AGNAIL
AGNATE
AINTSO
ALNASL
ALNICO
AMNION
AMNIOS
ANNALS
ANNEAL
ANNEES
ANNIES
ANNIKA
ANNINA
ANNLEE
ANNOYS
ANNUAL
ANNUIT
ANNULI
ANNULS
APNEAS
ARNALL
ARNEIS
ARNESS
ARNETT
ARNHEM
ARNICA
ARNIES
ARNOLD
ASNEAR
ASNEAT
ATNINE
ATNOON
AUNTEM
AUNTIE
AWNING

A••N••

ACTNOW
ADENIS
ADONAI
ADONIC
ADONIS
AGENAS
AGENCE
AGENCY
AGENDA
AGENTJ
AGENTK
AGENTS
AGONES
AKENES
AKINTO
ALANIS
ALANON
ALINED
ALINER
ALINES
ALLNEW
ALONGS
ALONSO
ALONZO
AMANAS
AMANDA
AMANTI
AMANTS
AMENDS
AMENRA
AMENTS
AMINES
AMINOR
AMINOS
AMINTA
AMINUS
AMONRA
AMONTH
ANANAS
ANANKE
ANONYM
ARENAS
ARENDT
ASANAS
ASANTE
ASONIA
ATENTH
ATONAL
ATONCE
ATONED
ATONER
ATONES
ATONIA
ATONIC
ATONOF
AVANTI
AVENGE
AVENUE
AXENIC
AXONAL
AXONES
AZANIA
AZONAL
AZONIC

A•••N•

AAHING
ABOUND
ABSENT
ACCENT
ACCTNO
ACHENE
ACHING
ACORNS
ACTING
ACTONE
ADDEND
ADDING
ADDINS
ADDONS
ADJANI
ADMINS
ADORNS
ADRENO
ADVENT
ADZING
AFFINE
AGEING
AGEONE
AGLINT
AHERNE
AIDING
AILING
AIMING
AIRING
ALAINA
ALBANO
ALBANS
ALBANY
ALBINE
ALBINO
ALCINA
ALDINE
ALFINE
ALHENA
ALIENS
ALIGNS
ALKENE
ALMOND
ALPINE
ALUMNA
ALUMNI
ALVING
ALVINO
AMARNA
AMBAND
AMIENS
AMOUNT
AMPING
ANIONS
ANNINA
ANOINT
ANTONE
ANTONY
ANWANG
ANYONE
ANYONS
APPEND
APRONS
AQUINO
ARCANA
ARCANE
ARCING
ARDENT
ARGENT
ARIANA
ARIANE
ARJUNA
ARLENE
ARMAND
ARMANI
ARMING
ARMONK
AROINT
AROUND
ARRANT
ARSENE
ARSENO
ARSONS
ARYANS
ASCEND
ASCENT
ASHINE
ASHING
ASIANS
ASKANT
ASKING
ASLANT
ASMANY
ASPENS
ASSENT
ASTANA
ATHAND
ATHENA
ATHENE
ATHENS
ATHING
ATKINS
ATMANS
ATNINE
ATTEND
ATTUNE
AUFOND
AUGEND
AUMONT
AVAUNT
AVEENO
AVIANS
AWNING
AXIONS

A••••N

AACHEN
ABUTON
ACTION
ACTSIN
ACTSON
ACUMEN
ADDSIN
ADDSON
ADJOIN
ADNOUN
ADRIAN
ADRIEN
AEGEAN
AFGHAN
AGETEN
AIDMAN
AIDMEN
AIKMAN
AILEEN
AIRGUN
AIRMAN
AIRMEN
AJOWAN
ALANON
ALBION
ALDRIN
ALEMAN
ALFVEN
ALGREN
ALISON
ALLEYN
ALLMAN
ALLMEN
ALSTON
ALTMAN
AMAZIN
AMAZON
AMBIEN
AMBLIN
AMNION
AMYTAN
ANACIN
ANAKIN
ANCIEN
ANDEAN
ANTAWN
ANTRON
ANYMAN
APEMAN
APEMEN
APPIAN
ARAGON
ARCHON
ARCSIN
ARCTAN
ARISEN
ARUBAN
ASHBIN
ASHCAN
ASHMAN
ASHMEN
ASHPAN
ASHTON
ASKSIN
ASOSAN
ASSIGN
ASTERN
ASWOON
ATAMAN
ATDAWN
ATNOON
ATRAIN
ATSIGN
ATTAIN
AUBURN
AUGEAN
AUSTEN
AUSTIN
AUTUMN
AVALON
AVEDON
AVISON
AWAKEN
AWCMON
AWOKEN
AXEMAN
AXEMEN
AYRTON
AZORIN

•AN•••

BANANA
BANANE
BANCOS
BANDED
BANDER
BANDIT
BANGED
BANGER
BANGLE
BANGON
BANGOR
BANGUI
BANGUP
BANISH
BANJOS
BANJUL
BANKED
BANKER
BANKIT
BANKON
BANKUP
BANLON
BANNED
BANNEN
BANNER
BANONS
BANQUE
BANQUO
BANTAM
BANTER
BANTUS
BANYAN
BANZAI
CANAAN
CANADA
CANALS
CANAPE
CANARD
CANARY
CANCAN
CANCEL
CANCER
CANCHA
CANCUN
CANDIA
CANDID
CANDLE
CANDOR
CANERS
CANFUL
CANIDS
CANIER
CANIFF
CANINE
CANING
CANKER
CANLIT
CANNAS
CANNED
CANNEL
CANNER
CANNES
CANNON
CANNOT
CANOED
CANOER
CANOES
CANOLA
CANONS
CANOPY
CANOVA
CANTAB
CANTAL
CANTBE
CANTED
CANTER
CANTLE
CANTON
CANTOO
CANTOR
CANTOS
CANUCK
CANULA
CANUTE
CANVAS
CANYON
DANANG
DANCED
DANCER
DANCES
DANCIN
DANDER
DANDIE
DANDLE
DANDYL
DANGED
DANGER
DANGIT
DANGLE
DANGLY
DANGME
DANIEL
DANILO
DANIOS
DANISH
DANITE
DANKER
DANKLY
DANNAY
DANNER
DANNON
DANNYS
DANOVA
DANSES
DANSON
DANTEI
DANTES
DANTON
DANUBE
DANZIG
EANNIE
FANDOM
FANFIC
FANGED
FANGIO
FANION
FANJET
FANNED
FANNER
FANNIE
FANONS
FANOUT
FANTAN
FANTAS
GANDER
GANDHI
GANEFS
GANGED
GANGER
GANGES
GANGLY
GANGUP
GANNET
GANNON
GANTRY
HANDAX
HANDED
HANDEL
HANDER
HANDIN
HANDKE
HANDLE
HANDON
HANDUP
HANGAR
HANGBY
HANGED
HANGER
HANGIN
HANGON
HANGUL
HANGUP
HANKER
HANKIE
HANLEY
HANLON
HANNAH
HANSAS
HANSEL
HANSES
HANSOM
HANSON
JANGLE
JANGLY
JANHUS
JANICE
JANINE
JANNEY
JANSEN
JANUAR
JANZEN
KANAKA
KANALY
KANATA
KANAWA
KANDEL
KANDER
KANJIS
KANSAN
KANSAS
KANTOR
LANAIS
LANARK
LANATE
LANCED
LANCER
LANCES
LANCET
LANCIA
LANCIE
LANDAT
LANDAU
LANDED
LANDER
LANDHO
LANDIS
LANDON
LANDOR
LANDRY
LANDUP
LANDUS
LANGER
LANIER
LANINA
LANKER
LANKLY
LANOSE
LANSKY
LANSON
LANTOS
LANVAL
LANVIN
MANAGE
MANAMA
MANANA
MANAOS
MANAPE
MANATS
MANCHA
MANCHE
MANCHU
MANDAN
MANDAY
MANDEL
MANDMS
MANEGE
MANERO
MANETS
MANFUL
MANGAS
MANGER
MANGLE
MANGOS
MANIAC
MANIAS
MANILA
MANLEY
MANNAS
MANNED
MANNER
MANNIX
MANNON
MANOFF
MANORS
MANQUE
MANRAY
MANSES
MANTAS
MANTEE
MANTEL
MANTIC
MANTIS
MANTLE
MANTRA
MANTUA
MANUAL
MANUEL
MANURE
MANUSH
MANUTE
MANZON
NANINE
NANNIE
NANOOK
NANSEN
NANTES
PANADA
PANAMA
PANCHO
PANCKS
PANDAS
PANDER
PANDIT
PANDLS
PANELS
PANFRY
PANFUL
PANICS
PANIER
PANINI
PANINO
PANNED
PANNER
PANNES
PANOPE
PANOUT
PANSIN
PANTED
PANTER
PANTIE
PANTOS
PANTRY
PANZER
QANTAS
RANCHO
RANCID
RANCOR
RANDAL
RANDOM
RANDRY
RANEES
RANFOR
RANGED
RANGEL
RANGER
RANGES
RANGIN
RANGUP
RANIDS
RANINE
RANKED
RANKER
RANKIN
RANKLE
RANKLY
RANLOW
RANOFF
RANOUT
RANSOM
RANTAT
RANTED
RANTER
SANCHO
SANCTA
SANDAL
SANDED
SANDER
SANDIA
SANDRA
SANDRO
SANELY
SANEST
SANGER
SANGRE
SANGTO
SANITY
SANKAS
SANKIN
SANSEI
SANTAS
SANTEE
SANTHA
SANTOS
SANYOS
TANAKA
TANANA
TANDEM
TANGED
TANGLE
TANGLY
TANGOS
TANGUY
TANKAS
TANKED
TANKER
TANKUP
TANNED
TANNER
TANNIC
TANNIN
TANOAK
TANTES
TANTRA
VANARK
VANDAL
VANIER
VANISH
VANITY
VANNED
VANNES
VANRYN
WANDER
WANGLE
WANIER
WANING
WANKEL
WANNED
WANNER
WANTAD
WANTED
WANTER
WANTIN
WANTON
WANTTO
XANADU
YANGON
YANKAT
YANKED
YANKEE
YANKER
YANKON
YANQUI
ZANIER
ZANIES
ZANILY
ZANONI
ZANTAC
ZANUCK

•A•N••

BAGNIO
BAHNEN
BAINES
BANNED
BANNEN
BANNER
BARNED
BARNES
BARNET
BARNEY
BARNUM
CAGNEY
CANNAS
CANNED
CANNEL
CANNER
CANNES
CANNON
CANNOT
CAPNUT
CARNAC
CARNAL
CARNAP
CARNER
CARNES
CARNET
CARNEY
CATNAP
CATNIP
DABNEY
DAINTY
DAMNED
DAMNER
DANNAY
DANNER
DANNON
DANNYS
DARNAY
DARNED
DARNER
DARNIT
DAUNTS
DAWNED
DAWNON
EANNIE
EARNED
EARNER
EARNIE
EARNIT
FAENAS
FAFNER
FAFNIR
FAINER
FAINTS
FANNED
FANNER
FANNIE
FARNUM
FAUNAE
FAUNAL
FAUNAS
FAUNUS
FAWNED
FAWNER
FAWNON
GAINED
GAINER
GAINES
GAINLY
GAINON
GAINST
GANNET
GANNON
GARNER
GARNET
GAYNES
GAYNOR
HAINES
HANNAH
HARNEY
HAUNCH
HAUNTS
HAYNES
HAYNIE
IAMNOT
JANNEY
JAUNES
JAUNTS
JAUNTY
KAONIC
KARNAK
KAUNAS
KAUNDA
KAVNER
LAINIE
LAONZA
LAUNCH
MACNEE
MAENAD
MAGNET
MAGNOL
MAGNON
MAGNUM
MAGNUS
MAINER
MAINLY
MAINST
MANNAS
MANNED
MANNER
MANNIX
MANNON
MARNER
MARNIE
MAUNDY
NAGNAG
NANNIE
NARNIA
PAANGA
PAGNOL
PAINED
PAINTS
PAINTY
PANNED
PANNER
PANNES
PARNIS
PAUNCH
PAWNED
PAWNEE
PAWNER
PAYNOW
RADNER
RADNOR
RAGNAR
RAINED
RAINER
RAINES
RAINEY
RAININ
RAINON
RATNER
RAUNCH
SAINTE
SAINTS
SARNIA
SAUNAS
SAYNAY
TAHNEE
TAINTS
TANNED
TANNER
TANNIC
TANNIN
TAUNTS
VAINER
VAINLY
VANNED
VANNES
VARNAS
VARNEY
VAUNTS
VAUNTY
WAGNER
WALNUT
WANNED
WANNER
WAPNER
WARNED
WARNER
WARNES
WARNOF
WATNEY
WAYNES
YARNED
YAWNED
YAWNER
ZAGNUT

•A••N•

AAHING
BAAING
BACONS
BADEND
BADUNS
BAGEND
BAIRNS
BAKING
BALINE
BALING
BANANA
BANANE
BANONS
BARANY
BARING
BARONE
BARONI
BARONS
BARONY
BASING
BASINS
BATING
BATONS
BAYING
CABANA
CABINS
CADENT
CAGING
CAIRNS
CAJUNS
CAKING
CAMINO
CANINE
CANING
CANONS
CAPONE
CAPONI
CAPONS
CARINA
CARING
CARONI
CASING
CASINO
CATANO
CATENA
CAVING
CAWING
DALAND
DALENE
DAMONE
DANANG
DAPHNE
DARENT
DARING
DATING
DAVENS
DAYONE
DAZING
EAKINS
EALING
EAMONN
EARING
EASING
EATING
FACING
FADING
FAGEND
FAGINS
FAKING
FALANA
FALINE
FAMINE
FAMING
FANONS
FARINA
FARING
FATONE
FAXING
FAZING
GAGING
GALANT
GALENA
GAMINE
GAMING

GAMINS
GAPING
GATING
GAZING
HABANA
HADONE
HALING
HARING
HASONE
HATING
HAVANA
HAVENO
HAVENS
HAVENT
HAVING
HAWING
HAYING
HAZANS
HAZING
JADING
JANINE
JAPANS
JAPING
JAWING
KAHUNA
KALINE
KARINA
LABINE
LACING
LACUNA
LADING
LADINO
LAGUNA
LAMENT
LAMINA
LAMING
LAMONT
LANINA
LAPINS
LARINE
LARYNX
LASING
LATENE
LATENS
LATENT
LATINA
LATINI
LATINO
LATINS
LAVING
LAWING
LAYING
LAYINS
LAZING
MAKING
MALONE
MANANA
MARINA
MARINE
MARINO
MASONS
MATING
MATINS
MAVENS
MAVINS
MAXENE
MAXINE
MAXING
MAYANS
MAYING
MAZING
NADINE
NAGANO
NAMING
NANINE
NARINE
NATANT
OARING
PACING
PACINO
PAEANS
PAGANS
PAGING
PALING
PAMINA
PANINI
PANINO
PARANA
PARENS
PARENT
PARING
PARINI
PATENS
PATENT
PATINA
PATINE
PAVANE
PAVING
PAWING
PAYING
RACINE
RACING
RACINO
RAGING
RAKING
RAMENS
RAMONA
RAMONE
RANINE
RAPINE
RAPINI
RARING
RASING
RATINE
RATING
RAVENS
RAVINE
RAVING
RAXING
RAYING
RAYONS
RAZING
SABENA
SABINA
SABINE
SAIDNO
SALINA
SALINE
SALONS
SARANS
SARONG
SATING
SATINS
SATINY
SAVANA
SAVANT
SAVING
SAWING
SAXONS
SAXONY
SAYING
SAYSNO
TAGEND
TAHINI
TAKING
TALENT
TALONS
TAMING
TANANA
TAOSNM
TAPING
TAPINS
TARING
TAUONS
TAXING
VACANT
VALENE
VALENS
VALENT
VALINE
WADENA
WADING
WAGING
WAGONS
WAHINE
WAKENS
WAKING
WALING
WANING
WARING
WAVING
WAXING
WAYANS
YAMANI
YAMUNA
YAWING
ZANONI
ZAYINS
ZAZENS

•A•••N

AACHEN
BABOON
BABSON
BACKIN
BADMAN
BADMEN
BAFFIN
BAGMAN
BAGMEN
BAHIAN
BAHNEN
BAILON
BALEEN
BALKAN
BALLIN
BALLON
BANGON
BANKON
BANLON
BANNEN
BANYAN
BARBAN
BARKIN
BARMAN
BARMEN
BARREN
BARRON
BARTON
BARYON
BARZUN
BASHIN
BASKIN
BATAAN
BATMAN
BATMEN
BATSIN
BATSON
BATTEN
BAUMAN
BAYERN
BAYMAN
BAYMEN
CABMAN
CABMEN
CAFTAN
CAGEIN
CAIMAN
CALGON
CALLAN
CALLIN
CALLON
CALVIN
CAMDEN
CAMEIN
CAMEON
CAMION
CAMRYN
CANAAN
CANCAN
CANCUN
CANNON
CANTON
CANYON
CAPGUN
CARBON
CARDIN
CAREEN
CARLIN
CARMAN
CARMEN
CARSON
CARTIN
CARTON
CASEIN
CASERN
CASHIN
CASSIN
CASTON
CATION
CATKIN
CATLIN
CATMAN
CATMEN
CATTON
CAVEIN
CAVERN
CAYMAN
DACRON
DAEMON
DALTON
DAMIEN
DAMPEN
DAMSON
DANCIN
DANNON
DANSON
DANTON
DARIEN
DARKEN
DARLIN
DARREN
DARRIN
DARWIN
DASSIN
DATHAN
DATSUN
DAWNON
DAWSON
DAYTON
EAMONN
EARVIN
EASEIN
EASEON
EASTON
EATSIN
FABIAN
FACEON
FADEIN
FAIMAN
FALCON
FALLEN
FALLIN
FALLON
FANION
FANTAN
FASTEN
FATMAN
FATTEN
FAWNON
FAYLEN
GAGMAN
GAGMEN
GAIJIN
GAINON
GALLON
GALTON
GAMMON
GANNON
GARCON
GARDEN
GARGAN
GARSON
GARYIN
GASCAN
GASCON
GASMAN
GASMEN
GASTON
GATLIN
GAVEIN
GAVEON
GAWAIN
GAZEON
HAAGEN
HAAKON
HADDEN
HADEAN
HADFUN
HADRON
HAGMAN
HALPIN
HAMDEN
HAMELN
HAMLIN
HAMSUN
HANDIN
HANDON
HANGIN
HANGON
HANLON
HANSON
HAPPEN
HARBIN
HARDEN
HARDIN
HARKEN
HARLAN
HARLIN
HARMON
HARPON
HASFUN
HASSAN
HASTEN
HATPIN
HAULIN
HAVEIN
HAVEON
HAYDEN
JACLYN
JAMSIN
JANSEN
JANZEN
JARDIN
JARGON
JASMIN
KALKAN
KALLEN
KANSAN
KAOLIN
KAPLAN
KARLEN
KASDAN
KATRIN
KATZEN
LACEON
LAGOON
LAIDIN
LAIDON
LANDON
LANSON
LANVIN
LARDON
LARKIN
LARMEN
LARSEN
LARSON
LASSEN
LATEEN
LATEON
LATHEN
LAUREN
LAURYN
LAVAIN
LAVERN
LAWMAN
LAWMEN
LAWSON
LAWTON
LAYMAN
LAYMEN
LAYSIN
LAYSON
MACLEN
MACOUN
MACRON
MADDEN
MADLYN
MADMAN
MADMEN
MADSEN
MAGIAN
MAGNON
MAIDEN
MAILIN
MAISON
MAJGEN
MALDEN
MALIAN
MALIGN
MALLON
MALTIN
MAMMON
MANDAN
MANNON
MANZON
MARDEN
MARGIN
MARIAN
MARION
MARLIN
MARLON
MAROON
MARRON
MARTEN
MARTIN
MARVIN
MASLIN
MASSON
MATLIN
MATMAN
MATMEN
MATRON
MATSON
MAWSON
MAXSON
MAYRON
NACION
NAILIN
NANSEN
NAPKIN
NATHAN
NATION
NATRON
OAHUAN
OARMAN
OARMEN
PACHIN
PACKIN
PACKON
PACMAN
PACTEN
PADUAN
PAIDIN
PAISAN
PANSIN
PAPUAN
PAQUIN
PARDON
PARSON
PARTON
PASSON
PATHAN
PATRON
PATTEN
PATTON
PAXTON
PAYSIN
PAYSON
PAYTON
RACEIN
RADIAN
RAFFIN
RAGLAN
RAGMAN
RAGMEN
RAGSON
RAILON
RAININ
RAINON
RAISIN
RAISON
RAKEIN
RAMFAN
RAMSIN
RAMSON
RANGIN
RANKIN
RAPSON
RASKIN
RATION
RATLIN
RATSON
RATTAN
RAVEON
RAWDON
RAYBAN
RAYGUN
SADDEN
SAIGON
SAILON
SAIPAN
SAISON
SALMAN
SALMON
SALOON
SALTEN
SALTON
SAMOAN
SAMPAN
SAMSON
SANKIN
SARGON
SARTON
SASSON
SATEEN
SATURN
SAURON
SAVEON
TACKON
TAGSON
TAIPAN
TAIWAN
TAKEIN
TAKEON
TALKIN
TALKON
TANNIN
TAPEON
TAPPAN
TAPSIN
TAPSON
TARPON
TARTAN
TARZAN
TASMAN
TAUPIN
TAUTEN
TAVERN
TAXMAN
TAXMEN
VANRYN
VARDEN
VAUGHN
WADEIN
WAITON
WALDEN
WALKEN
WALKIN
WALKON
WALLIN
WALTON
WANTIN
WANTON
WARDEN
WARREN
WASFUN
WATSON
WAVEIN
WAYLON
WAYSIN
YANGON
YANKON
YASHIN
YASMIN
YATSEN

••AN••

ALANIS
ALANON
AMANAS
AMANDA
AMANTI
AMANTS
ANANAS
ANANKE
ASANAS
ASANTE
AVANTI
AZANIA
BEANED
BEANIE
BEANOS
BHANGS
BIANCA
BIANCO
BLANCA
BLANCH
BLANCO
BLANDA
BLANKS
BRANCA
BRANCH
BRANDI
BRANDO
BRANDS
BRANDT
BRANDX
BRANDY
BRANNY
BRANTS
BWANAS
CHANCE
CHANCY
CHANDU
CHANEL
CHANEY
CHANGE
CHANGO
CHANTE
CHANTS
CHANTY
CLANCY
CLANGS
CLANKS
CLANKY
CRANED
CRANES
CRANIA
CRANIO
CRANKS
CRANKY
CRANNY
CUANDO
CUANTO
CYANIC
CYANID
DEANNA
DIANNE
DRANCY
EBANKS
ELANCE
ELANDS
ELANET
FIANCE
FLANGE
FLANKS
FRANCA
FRANCE
FRANCK
FRANCO
FRANCS
FRANKS
FRANNY
FRANTZ
GDANSK
GIANNI
GIANTS
GLANCE
GLANDS
GRANBY
GRANDE
GRANDS
GRANDY
GRANGE
GRANIT
GRANNY
GRANPA
GRANTS
GUANOS
HEANEY
IBANEZ
ICANSO
INANER
IRANIS
ISANTI
IVANIV
IVANKA
IVANOV
IVANVI
IWANNA
JEANED
JEANIE
JEANNE
JOANIE
JOANNA
JOANNE
JOANOU
KRANTZ
KWANZA
LEANED
LEANER
LEANIN
LEANLY
LEANNE
LEANON
LEANTO
LIANAS
LIANES
LIANGS
LLANOS
LOANED
LOANER
LUANDA
MEANER
MEANEY
MEANIE
MEANIT
MEANLY
MEANTO
MOANED
MOANER
NUANCE
OMANIS
ORANGE
ORANGS
ORANGY
ORANIS
ORANTS
PAANGA
PBANDJ
PEANUT
PIANOS
PLANAR
PLANAS
PLANBS
PLANCK
PLANED
PLANER
PLANES
PLANET
PLANKS
PLANON
PLANTE
PLANTO
PLANTS
PRANAS
PRANCE
PRANKS
QUANTA
RUANDA
RWANDA
SCANTS
SCANTY
SEANCE
SHANDY
SHANIA
SHANKS
SHANTY
SKANKS
SKANKY
SLANGS
SLANGY
SLANTS
SPANKS
SPANKY
STANCE
STANCH
STANDS
STANZA
SWANEE
SWANKY
SWANNS
THANES
THANKS
TRANCE
TRANES
TRANNY
TWANGS
TWANGY
UBANGI
UGANDA
URANIA
URANIC
URANUS
USANCE
VIANDS
WEANED
WEANER
WHANGS
XYANDZ
YEANED

••A•N•

ALAINA
AMARNA
AVAUNT
BAAING
BLAINE
BRAINS
BRAINY
BRANNY
BRAWNY
CHAINE
CHAINS
CRAINS
CRANNY
DEANNA
DIANNE
DRAINS
DWAYNE
ELAINE
ELAYNE
EWAINE
FLAUNT
FRANNY
GHAINS
GIANNI
GRAINS
GRAINY
GRANNY
HEARNS
ISAYNO
IWANNA
JEANNE
JOANNA
JOANNE
KEARNS
KEARNY
KRASNA
LEANNE
LEARNS
LEARNT
PLAINS
PLAINT
PRAWNS
QUAINT
SCARNE
SHAYNE
SPAWNS
STAINS
SWAINS
SWANNS
TRAINS
TRANNY
TWAINS
UTAHNS
YEARNS

••A••N

ALANON
AMAZIN
AMAZON
ANACIN
ANAKIN
ARAGON
ATAMAN
AVALON
AWAKEN
BEACON
BEAMAN
BEAMON
BEARON
BEATEN
BEATON
BLAZON
BRAZEN
CHACUN
CHAPIN
CHARON
CHAZAN
CLADIN
CLAVIN
CRAMIN
CRAVEN
CRAYON
DEACON
DEADEN
DEADON
DEAFEN
DEALIN
DIALIN
DRAGIN
DRAGON
DRAWIN
DRAWON
ESALEN
ETAOIN
FLACON
FLAGON
FLAXEN
FRAUEN
GNAWON
GRATIN
GRAVEN
HAAGEN
HAAKON
HEADIN
HEADON
HEAPON
HEATON
HEAVEN
IBADAN
IMAMAN
ISAIAN
KEATON
KLAXON
KRAKEN
LEADEN
LEADIN
LEADON
LEAKIN
LEANIN
LEANON
LEAPIN
LEAPON
LEAVEN
LHASAN
LOADIN
NEALON
NEATEN
NIACIN
OMAHAN
ONABUN
OSAKAN
PEAHEN
PLANON
PLATEN
PLAYON
READIN
READON
REAGAN
REASON
ROAMIN
SEALIN
SEAMAN
SEAMEN
SEASON
SEATON
SHAKEN
SHAKIN
SHAMAN
SHARON
SHARYN
SHAVEN
SLAMON
SLAPON
SMALLN
SNAPON
SOAKIN
STALIN
STAMEN
STARIN
STATEN
STATIN
STAYIN
STAYON
TEAURN
TOAMAN
TRAJAN
TRAVEN
UNAKIN
UTAHAN
WEAKEN
WEAKON
WEAPON
WEARON

•••AN•

ADJANI
ALBANO
ALBANS
ALBANY
AMBAND
ANWANG
ARCANA
ARCANE
ARIANA
ARIANE
ARMAND
ARMANI
ARRANT
ARYANS
ASIANS
ASKANT
ASLANT
ASMANY
ASTANA
ATHAND
ATMANS
AVIANS
BANANA
BANANE
BARANY
BESANT
BEVANS
BOTANY
BRIANA
BRIAND
BRYANT
BURANA
BUTANE
BYHAND
BYLAND
CABANA
CATANO
CETANE
CHIANG
CLEANS
CONANT
COTANS
CUBANS
CYRANO
DALAND
DANANG
DECANT
DEDANS
DEFANG
DELAND
DELANO

DELANY
DEMAND
DEVANE
DISANT
DIVANS
DOMANI
DOUANE
DUNANT
DURANT
EKLAND
ELUANT
EMBANK
ENBANC
ENFANT
ENRANK
ERLANG
ERNANI
ERRAND
ERRANT
ESPANA
ETHANE
EWBANK
EXPAND
EXTANT
EXYANK
FALANA
FMBAND
GALANT
GETANA
GETANF
GIJANE
GITANO
GLEANS
GOBANG
GOTANA
GOTANF
GROANS
GUIANA
GUYANA
HABANA
HAVANA
HAZANS
HEXANE
HOGANS
HUMANE
HUMANS
IGUANA
ILEANA
IMEANT
INCANS
INCANT
INFANT
INHAND
INLAND
INSANA
INSANE
INWANT
IOLANI
IOWANS
ISLAND
JAPANS
JOHANN
KDLANG
KORANS
LEEANN
LELAND
LEMANS
LEVANT
LFRANK
LIGAND
LIMANS
LITANY
LOCANE
LOGANS
LORANS
LOUANN
MANANA
MAYANS
MCCANN
MEGANE
MILANO
MILANS
MORANT
MURANO
MUTANT
NAGANO
NATANT
NISANS
NOHANT
NOTANY
NYYANK
OCEANS
OCTANE
OCTANS
OCTANT
OKSANA
ONHAND
ONLAND
ORGANA
ORGANS
ORIANA
ORIANI
ORKANS
OSCANS
PAEANS
PAGANS
PARANA
PAVANE
PECANS
PEDANT
PIRANA
PISANO
PISANS
PLIANT
POEANA
POLAND
REBANK
RECANE
RECANS
RECANT
REDANS
REDANT
REHANG
RELAND
REMAND
REMANS
REPANE
RERANK
RESAND
RESANG
RETANS
RIBAND
RICANS
RIGANS
ROLAND
ROMANI
ROMANO
ROMANS
ROMANY
ROWANS
ROXANA
ROXANE
SARANS
SAVANA
SAVANT
SECANT
SEDANS
SEMANA
SHRANK
SIVANS
SLOANE
SOCANI
SOLANO
SOLANS
SOMANY
SONANT
SPRANG
STRAND
SUEANE
SUEANN
SUSANB
SUSANN
TANANA
TEJANA
TEJANO
TENANT
TEXANS
TIRANA
TIRANE
TISANE
TITANS
TRUANT
TUCANA
TULANE
TVLAND
TYRANT
UCLANS
UHLANS
UNHAND
UNMANS
UPLAND
URBANA
URBANE
URBANI
URBANV
USBANK
UTHANT
VACANT
VEGANS
VIVANT
VOLANS
VOLANT
WAYANS
WIGAND
WINANS
WOMANS
YAMANI
YEMANA
YOSANO
YUMANS
YUTANG
ZENANA

•••A•N

ANTAWN
ATDAWN
ATRAIN
ATTAIN
BATAAN
CANAAN
CEDARN
COBAIN
DEMAIN
DERAIN
DETAIN
DIZAIN
DOMAIN
GAWAIN
INPAWN
INVAIN
JOHANN
KITAEN
LAVAIN
LECAIN
LEEANN
LENAIN
LORAIN
LOUANN
MCBAIN
MCCAIN
MCCANN
MCLAIN
NORAIN
OBTAIN
OHDARN
ORDAIN
PETAIN
REDARN
REEARN
REGAIN
REMAIN
RESAWN
RETAIN
REWARN
ROMAIN
SPRAIN
STRAIN
SUEANN
SUSANN
UNPAWN
UNSAWN
UNVAIN

••••AN

ADRIAN
AEGEAN
AFGHAN
AIDMAN
AIKMAN
AIRMAN
AJOWAN
ALEMAN
ALLMAN
ALTMAN
AMYTAN
ANDEAN
ANYMAN
APEMAN
APPIAN
ARCTAN
ARUBAN
ASHCAN
ASHMAN
ASHPAN
ASOSAN
ATAMAN
AUGEAN
AXEMAN
BADMAN
BAGMAN
BAHIAN
BALKAN
BANYAN
BARBAN
BARMAN
BATAAN
BATMAN
BAUMAN
BAYMAN
BEAMAN
BEMOAN
BERMAN
BHUTAN
BIGFAN
BIGMAN
BIRMAN
BORMAN
BOWMAN
BROGAN
BUCHAN
BUNYAN
BURMAN
BUSMAN
CABMAN
CAFTAN
CAIMAN
CALLAN
CANAAN
CANCAN
CARMAN
CATMAN
CAYMAN
CERNAN
CHAZAN
COLMAN
CONLAN
CONMAN
COOGAN
CORMAN
COWMAN
CRETAN
CRUZAN
CTSCAN
CUBFAN
DATHAN
DELIAN
DEMEAN
DOLMAN
DOOHAN
DORIAN
DOTHAN
DUNCAN
DURBAN
EGOYAN
ELFMAN
ENDMAN
ENDRAN
EOLIAN
EONIAN
ERDMAN
EREVAN
ERIVAN
FABIAN
FAIMAN
FANTAN
FATMAN
FBIMAN
FIJIAN
FINIAN
FINNAN
FLYMAN
FOEMAN
FORMAN
FRYPAN
FURMAN
GAGMAN
GARGAN
GASCAN
GASMAN
GENOAN
GERMAN
GIBRAN
GILLAN
GILMAN
GROBAN
GUINAN
GUNMAN
GUTMAN
GUZMAN
HADEAN
HAGMAN
HARLAN
HASSAN
HERMAN
HERNAN
HEYMAN
HITMAN
HODMAN
HOLMAN
HORGAN
IBADAN
IBIZAN
ICEMAN
IFICAN
IMAMAN
INDIAN
INSPAN
IONIAN
ISAIAN
JETFAN
JORDAN
JOVIAN
JUDEAN
JULIAN
KALKAN
KANSAN
KAPLAN
KASDAN
KEENAN
KENNAN
KENYAN
KEYMAN
KIDMAN
KIERAN
KINNAN
KIOWAN
KIRMAN
KLIBAN
KOREAN
KORMAN
LAWMAN
LAYMAN
LEGMAN
LEHMAN
LESHAN
LHASAN
LIBRAN
LIBYAN
LILIAN
LLBEAN
LOWMAN
LUCIAN
LYDIAN
MADMAN
MAGIAN
MALIAN
MANDAN
MARIAN
MATMAN
MCEWAN
MCKEAN
MCLEAN
MECCAN
MEDIAN
MENSAN
MERMAN
METFAN
MIDIAN
MINOAN
MINYAN
MORGAN
MRBEAN
NATHAN
NEIMAN
NEMEAN
NEPEAN
NETMAN
NEUMAN
NEWMAN
NISSAN
NONFAN
NONMAN
NONTAN
NOONAN
NORMAN
NOWLAN
NUBIAN
OAHUAN
OARMAN
OBIWAN
OBRIAN
ODDMAN
OHIOAN
OILCAN
OILMAN
OILPAN
OLDMAN
OMAHAN
ONEMAN
ONLOAN
ORPHAN
OSAKAN
OSSIAN
OUTBAN
OUTMAN
OUTRAN
PACMAN
PADUAN
PAISAN
PAPUAN
PATHAN
PENMAN
PIEMAN
PIEPAN
PIGMAN
PITMAN
POZNAN
RADIAN
RAGLAN
RAGMAN
RAMFAN
RATTAN
RAYBAN
RBIMAN
REAGAN
RELOAN
REPLAN
RESCAN
RESPAN
RIOPAN
RODMAN
RUDMAN
RUTTAN
RYOKAN
SAIPAN
SALMAN
SAMOAN
SAMPAN
SEAMAN
SHAMAN
SIMIAN
SIOUAN
SKYMAN
SLOGAN
SOXFAN
STEFAN
STJOAN
SULTAN
SUNFAN
SUNTAN
SYLVAN
SYRIAN
TAIPAN
TAIWAN
TAPPAN
TARTAN
TARZAN
TASMAN
TAXMAN
TEHRAN
TERRAN
THEBAN
THECAN
THEFAN
THEMAN
TINCAN
TINIAN
TINMAN
TINPAN
TITIAN
TOAMAN
TODMAN
TONGAN
TOPMAN
TOUCAN
TRAJAN
TREPAN
TROJAN
TRUMAN
TUBMAN
TULSAN
TURBAN
TURHAN
TUSCAN
TWOMAN
TWYMAN
ULLMAN
UNLEAN
UNPLAN
UNSPAN
UTAHAN
UTICAN
VIVIAN
VULCAN
WHELAN
WICCAN
WIEMAN
WYSTAN
YEOMAN
YESMAN
ZEEMAN
ZOLTAN
ZONIAN
ZUNIAN

AO••••

AOLERS
AORTAE
AORTAL
AORTAS
AORTIC
AOUDAD

A•O•••

ABOARD
ABODES
ABOHMS
ABOLLA
ABOMAS
ABOMBS
ABORAL
ABORTS
ABOUND
ACORNS
ADOBES
ADOBOS
ADOLFO
ADOLPH
ADONAI
ADONIC
ADONIS
ADOPTS
ADORED
ADOREE
ADORER
ADORES
ADORNS
ADOUTS
AEOLIA
AEOLUS
AGONES
AGORAE
AGORAS
AGOROT
AGOSTO
AGOUTI
AHOLIC
AHORSE
AIOLIS
AJOWAN
ALOGIA
ALOHAS
ALOMAR
ALONGS
ALONSO
ALONZO
ALOTOF
AMOEBA
AMOLES
AMONRA
AMONTH
AMORAL
AMORES
AMORET
AMOSOZ
AMOUNT
AMOURS
ANODAL
ANODES
ANODIC
ANOINT
ANOLES
ANOMIA
ANOMIC
ANOMIE
ANONYM
ANORAK
ANOXIA
ANOXIC
APODAL
APOGEE
APOLLO
APOPKA
AROIDS
AROINT
AROMAS
AROUET
AROUND
AROUSE
ASONIA
ASOSAN
ATODDS
ATOLLS
ATOMIC
ATONAL
ATONCE
ATONED
ATONER
ATONES
ATONIA
ATONIC
ATONOF
ATOXIC
AVOCET
AVOIDS
AVOUCH
AVOWAL
AVOWED
AVOWER
AWOKEN
AXONAL
AXONES
AZODYE
AZOLES
AZONAL
AZONIC
AZORES
AZORIN

A••O••

ABBOTS
ABBOTT
ABHORS
ABLOOM
ABROAD
ABSORB
ACCORD
ACCOST
ACEOUT
ACROSS
ACTONE
ACTORS
ACTOUT
ADDONS
ADJOIN
ADNOUN
ADROIT
ADSORB
AEROBE
AESOPS
AFFORD
AFLOAT
AGEOLD
AGEONE
AGEOUT
AIROUT
AJFOYT
ALBORG
ALCOTT
ALCOVE
ALDOUS
ALGORE
ALIOTH
ALIOTO
ALLOTS
ALLOUT
ALLOWS
ALLOYS
ALMOND
ALMOST
ALTOID
ANGOLA
ANGORA
ANIONS
ANJOUS
ANNOYS
ANTONE
ANTONY
ANYOLD
ANYONE
ANYONS
APLOMB
APPOSE
APRONS
ARBORS
ARBOUR
ARDORS
ARDOUR
AREOLA
AREOLE
ARGOSY
ARGOTS
ARIOSE
ARIOSI
ARIOSO
ARLOVA
ARMONK
ARMORS
ARMORY
ARMOUR
ARNOLD
ARROWS
ARROYO
ARSONS
ARTOIS
ASCOLD
ASCOOL
ASCOTS
ASGOOD
ASHORE
ASKOUT
ASLOPE
ASLOSH
ASSOFT
ASSORT
ASTOOP
ASWOON
ATCOST
ATEOUT
ATFOUR
ATHOME
ATMOST
ATNOON
ATROIS
ATWOOD
ATWORK
AUFOND
AUMONT
AURORA
AUROUS
AUTOED
AXIOMS
AXIONS

A•••O•

ABATOR
ABITOF
ABLOOM
ABMHOS
ABUTON
ACTFOR
ACTION
ACTNOW
ACTSON
ADDSON
ADOBOS
AERIOS
AGOROT
AHCHOO
AIMFOR
AIRLOG
AIRPOP
AIRPOT
ALAMOS
ALANON
ALBION
ALEROS
ALISON
ALIYOT
ALLFOR
ALOTOF
ALSTON
AMAJOR
AMATOL
AMAZON
AMIDOL
AMIGOS
AMINOR
AMINOS
AMNION
AMNIOS
AMOSOZ
ANALOG
ANCHOR
ANCHOS
ANDHOW
ANDROS
ANGKOR
ANGLOS
ANTCOW
ANTRON
ANYHOW
APPROX
ARADOS
ARAGON
ARCCOS
ARCHON
ARETOO
ASCOOL
ASGOOD
ASHDOD
ASHTON
ASIMOV
ASKFOR
ASKSOF
ASSLOW
ASTOOP
ASTROS
ASTROV
ASWOON
ATALOW
ATHROB
ATHROW
ATNOON
ATONOF
ATWOOD
AUDIOS
AUTHOR
AVALON
AVEDON
AVISON
AVISOS
AWCMON
AYRTON

A••••O

ABBADO
ACCTNO
ACTTWO
ADAGIO
ADDSTO
ADOLFO
ADRENO
AFLCIO
AGETWO
AGOSTO
AHCHOO
AIELLO
AIKIDO
AILURO
AINTSO
AKIMBO
AKINTO
ALBANO
ALBEDO
ALBINO
ALECTO
ALEPPO
ALIOTO
ALIVEO
ALLPRO
ALNICO
ALONSO
ALONZO
ALVARO
ALVINO
ALZADO
AMADEO
AMEDEO
ANATTO
ANGELO
ANTERO
ANTIGO
APOLLO
AQUINO
ARCARO
ARETOO
AREZZO
ARIOSO
ARISTO
ARROYO
ARSENO
ARTHRO
ARTURO
ASARCO
ASIAGO
ASTERO
ATEMPO
AUSTRO
AVEENO

•AO•••

BAOBAB
DAOSTA
GAOLED
GAOLER
HAOLES
KAOLIN
KAONIC
LAONZA
LAOTSE
LAOTZU
MAOISM
MAOIST
MAORIS
MAOTAI
TAOISM
TAOIST
TAOSNM

•A•O••

BABOON
BABOOS
BACONS
BADOFF
BANONS
BAROJA
BAROLO
BARONE
BARONI
BARONS
BARONY
BATONS
BAYOUS
BAZOOS
CAHOOT
CAJOLE
CALORY
CAMOES
CANOED
CANOER
CANOES
CANOLA
CANONS
CANOPY
CANOVA
CAPONE
CAPONI
CAPONS
CAPOTE
CAROBS
CAROLE
CAROLI
CAROLL
CAROLS
CAROMS
CARONI
CAVORT
DADOED
DADOES
DAKOTA
DAMONE
DAMORE
DAMOUR
DANOVA
DAYOFF
DAYOLD
DAYONE
EAMONN
EATOUT
FAGOTS
FAMOUS
FANONS
FANOUT
FAROES
FAROFF
FAROUK
FAROUT
FATONE
FAVORS
FAVOUR
FAZOOL
GALOIS
GALOOT
GALOPS
GALORE
GALOSH
GAMOUS

GASOIL
GATORS
GAVOTS
HADONE
HADOUT
HALOED
HALOES
HALOID
HAROLD
HASONE
HASOUT
HAVOCS
JABOTS
JACOBI
JACOBY
JALOPY
JAMOCA
JAMOKE
JAWOHL
KABOBS
KABOOM
KAPOKS
KAYOED
KAZOOS
LABORS
LABOUR
LADOGA
LAGOON
LAHORE
LAJOIE
LAKOTA
LAMONT
LAMOUR
LANOSE
LAROSA
LATOUR
LATOYA
LAYOFF
LAYOUT
MACOMB
MACOUN
MAHOUT
MAJOAD
MAJORS
MALONE
MALORY
MALOTI
MANOFF
MANORS
MAPOUT
MAROON
MASONS
MAXOUT
MAYORS
MAZOLA
NABOBS
NABORS
NAGOYA
NANOOK
NAPOLI
PADOVA
PAGODA
PAJOAD
PALOMA
PANOPE
PANOUT
PARODY
PAROLE
PAROLS
PATOIS
PAYOFF
PAYOLA
PAYOUT
RADOME
RAGOUT
RAMONA
RAMONE
RAMOSE
RANOFF
RANOUT
RATOFF
RATOUT
RAYONS
RAZORS
SABOTS
SALOME
SALONS
SALOON
SAMOAN
SAMOSA
SAPORS
SARONG
SATORI
SATOUT
SAVOIE
SAVOIR
SAVORS
SAVORY
SAVOUR
SAWOFF
SAWOUT
SAXONS
SAXONY
TABOOS
TABORS
TACOMA
TAGORE
TAGOUT
TAHOES
TALONS
TANOAK
TAPOFF
TAPOUT
TAROIL
TAROTS
TAUONS
TAXOLS
VALOIS
VALORS
VALOUR
VALOVA
VAPORS
VAPORY
VAPOUR
WACOTX
WAGONS
WAHOOS
WASOFF
WASOLD
WAYOFF
WAYOUT
YAHOOS
ZADORA
ZAMORA
ZANONI

•A••O•

BABOON
BABOOS
BABSON
BADBOY
BADCOP
BADDOG
BADLOT
BAGBOY
BAGJOB
BAILON
BAILOR
BALBOA
BALLON
BALLOT
BALLOU
BAMBOO
BANCOS
BANGON
BANGOR
BANJOS
BANKON
BANLON
BARCOS
BARDOT
BARHOP
BARLOW
BARRON
BARROW
BARTOK
BARTON
BARYON
BASSOS
BATBOY
BATFOR
BATHOS
BATSON
BAYLOR
BAZOOS
CACAOS
CAHOOT
CAICOS
CALGON
CALLON
CALLOW
CAMBOY
CAMEON
CAMEOS
CAMION
CAMPOS
CANDOR
CANNON
CANNOT
CANTON
CANTOO
CANTOR
CANTOS
CANYON
CAPTOR
CARBON
CARBOS
CARBOY
CAREOF
CARGOS
CARHOP
CARIOU
CARLOS
CARLOT
CARLOW
CARROL
CARROT
CARSON
CARTON
CARTOP
CASIOS
CASTON
CASTOR
CATDOM
CATION
CATTON
CATTOY
CAWDOR
DACRON
DAEMON
DAEWOO
DAGGOO
DALTON
DAMSON
DANIOS
DANNON
DANSON
DANTON
DARROW
DAWNON
DAWSON
DAYHOP
DAYJOB
DAYTON
EASEON
EASTON
EATSOF
FACEON
FACTOR
FAEROE
FALCON
FALLON
FALLOW
FANDOM
FANION
FARLOW
FARROW
FATHOM
FAWNON
FAZOOL
GAINON
GALLON
GALLOP
GALOOT
GALTON
GAMBOL
GAMMON
GANNON
GARCON
GARSON
GASCON
GASHOG
GASLOG
GASTON
GAVEOF
GAVEON
GAYNOR
GAZEON
HAAKON
HACHOO
HADRON
HALLOO
HALLOS
HALLOW
HANDON
HANGON
HANLON
HANSOM
HANSON
HARBOR
HARLOT
HARLOW
HARMON
HARPON
HARROW
HATBOX
HATHOR
HAVEON
HAYMOW
IAMNOT
IAMTOO
JAGLOM
JAILOR
JARGON
KABOOM
KANTOR
KARKOV
KARPOV
KAYYOW
KAZOOS
LACEON
LACHOY
LACLOS
LAGOON
LAIDON
LANDON
LANDOR
LANSON
LANTOS
LAPDOG
LAPTOP
LARDON
LARGOS
LARMOR
LARSON
LASSOS
LATEOF
LATEON
LAWSON
LAWTON
LAYFOR
LAYLOW
LAYSON
LAZBOY
MAALOX
MACHOS
MACRON
MACROS
MADDOG
MADDOX
MADEOF
MADFOR
MAGGOT
MAGNOL
MAGNON
MAHZOR
MAISON
MAKEOF
MALLON
MALLOW
MAMBOS
MAMMON
MANAOS
MANGOS
MANNON
MANZON
MARCOS
MARGOT
MARION
MARJOE
MARKOV
MARLON
MARMOT
MAROON
MARRON
MARROW
MASCOT
MASSON
MATRON
MATSON
MATZOH
MATZOS
MAWSON
MAXSON
MAYRON
NACHOS
NACION
NANOOK
NARCOS
NARROW
NATION
NATRON
PACKON
PAGNOL
PALLOR
PANTOS
PARDON
PARLOR
PARROT
PARSON
PARTOF
PARTON
PASEOS
PASMOI
PASSON
PASSOS
PASTOR
PATHOS
PATIOS
PATMOS
PATROL
PATRON
PATTON
PAVIOR
PAVLOV
PAXTON
PAYFOR
PAYNOW
PAYSON
PAYTON
RADIOS
RADNOR
RAGMOP
RAGSON
RAGTOP
RAILON
RAINON
RAISON
RAMBOS
RAMROD
RAMSON
RANCOR
RANDOM
RANFOR
RANLOW
RANSOM
RAPSON
RAPTOR
RATION
RATIOS
RATSON
RAVEON
RAWDON
SAIDOK
SAIGON
SAILON
SAILOR
SAISON
SALLOW
SALMON
SALOON
SALTON
SALVOR
SALVOS
SAMSON
SANTOS
SANYOS
SARDOU
SARGON
SARTON
SARTOR
SASSON
SATCOM
SATFOR
SAURON
SAVEON
SAVIOR
SAWLOG
SAYBOO
SAYSOK
SAYSOS
TABOOS
TACKON
TAGSON
TAILOR
TAKEON
TALKOF
TALKON
TALLOW
TALTOS
TAMBOR
TANGOS
TAPEON
TAPSON
TARPON
TATTOO
TAUROG
TAYLOR
WACKOS
WAHLOO
WAHOOS
WAITON
WALKON
WALLOP
WALLOW
WALTON
WANTON
WARGOD
WARHOL
WARNOF
WASHOE
WASHOS
WATSON
WAYLON
YAHOOS
YANGON
YANKON
YARROW
ZARKOV

•A•••O

BAGNIO
BAMAKO
BAMBOO
BANQUO
BARATO
BAROLO
BARRIO
CABRIO
CALICO
CALLAO
CALLTO
CAMARO
CAMETO
CAMINO
CANTOO
CARDIO
CARETO
CARUSO
CASINO
CASSIO
CASTRO
CATALO
CATANO
DACAPO
DADDYO
DAEWOO
DAGGOO
DAMATO
DANILO
DARETO
DAVIDO
DAYGLO
EASYGO
FAILTO
FALLTO
FANGIO
GABBRO
GALEAO
GASTRO
GAUCHO
GAVETO
GAZEBO
HACHOO
HADAGO
HAIRDO
HALLOO
HARRYO
HASAGO
HASBRO
HATETO
HAVENO
HAVETO
IAMTOO
JAZZBO
KAKAPO
KAKURO
LADINO
LAIDTO
LANDHO
LAREDO
LASHTO
LASZLO
LATERO
LATETO
LATIGO
LATINO
LAVABO
LAYSTO
MACACO
MADEDO
MADEGO
MADERO
MADURO
MAGGIO
MAHALO
MAILTO
MAKEDO
MAKEGO
MALABO
MANERO
MAPUTO
MARIDO
MARIKO
MARINO
MARYJO
MATSUO
MAYIGO
NAGANO
NAVAHO
NAVAJO
PACINO
PANCHO
PANINO
PAPAGO
PARETO
PASHTO
PASSGO
PASSTO
RACETO
RACINO
RAMAPO
RANCHO
RAPIDO
SABADO
SABATO
SAFECO
SAIDNO
SAIDSO
SAIDTO
SAILTO
SALUTO
SANCHO
SANDRO
SANGTO
SAPPHO
SASEBO
SAYBOO
SAYIDO
SAYSNO
SAYSSO
TAKETO
TALKTO
TAMAYO
TATTOO
VAILCO
VALERO
WAHLOO
WALKTO
WANTTO
WARMTO
WAVETO

••AO••

ETAOIN
MIAOUS
MIAOWS

••A•O•

ABATOR
ALAMOS
ALANON
AMAJOR
AMATOL
AMAZON
ANALOG
ARADOS
ARAGON
ATALOW
AVALON
BEACON
BEAMON
BEANOS
BEARON
BEATON
BLAZON
BMAJOR
BRASOV
BRAVOS
BRAZOS
CHARON
CLAMOR
CLAROS
CMAJOR
CRACOW
CRAYON
DEACON
DEADON
DIABOL
DIALOG
DIATOM
DMAJOR
DRAGON
DRAWON
EMAJOR
ENAMOR
FLACON
FLAGON
FLAVOR
FMAJOR
GLAMOR
GMAJOR
GNAWON
GOAWOL
GUANOS
HAAKON
HEADON
HEAPON
HEAROF
HEATON
IDAHOS
IMACOP
IMAGOS
INABOX
INAFOG
INAPOD
INAROW
IVANOV
JOANOU
KEATON
KLAXON
KRAKOW
LEADON
LEANON
LEAPON
LLANOS
MAALOX
MCADOO
MCAVOY
MEADOW
NEALON
ONAHOP
ORATOR
PEAPOD
PHAROS
PIANOS
PLANON
PLATOS
PLAYON
QUAHOG
READON
REASON
REAVOW
SEACOW
SEADOG
SEAFOX
SEAGOD
SEASON
SEATON
SHADOW
SHAKOS
SHALOM
SHARON
SLALOM
SLAMON
SLAPON
SNAPON
STAMOS
STATOR
STAYON
TEAPOT
TEAPOY
VIACOM
VIATOR
WEAKON
WEAPON
WEARON
ZEALOT

••A••O

ADAGIO
AMADEO
ANATTO
ASARCO
BIANCO
BLANCO
BRACCO
BRANDO
BRASCO
CHANGO
CHARRO
CRAMBO
CRANIO
CUANDO
CUANTO
CUATRO
DEAFTO
DEALTO
DEARTO
DIABLO
DIALSO
DIARIO
DRAWTO
ELADIO
FIASCO
FRACTO
FRANCO
GEARTO
GLADTO
GRAECO
GRAPHO
GRASSO
HEADTO
ICANSO
ISAYNO
KIARIO
LEADTO
LEANTO
LLADRO
MCADOO
MEANTO
NEARTO
ONAUTO
PGAPRO
PLANTO
PLASMO
PLAYTO
PRAYTO
QRATIO
QUARTO
READTO
RIALTO
ROADEO
SBARRO
SMALLO
SNAPTO
SOASTO
TEATRO
WHAMMO

•••AO•

CACAOS
HIVAOA
MANAOS

•••A•O

ABBADO
ALBANO
ALVARO
ALZADO
ARCARO
ASIAGO
BAMAKO
BARATO
BORAXO
CAMARO
CATALO
CATANO
CERATO
CHEAPO
CYRANO
DACAPO
DAMATO
DELANO
DORADO
DOSADO
DYNAMO
ELPASO
ENHALO
ESTADO
FIGARO
FUGATO
GELATO
GITANO
HADAGO
HASAGO
HEMATO
HEPATO
ITSAGO
JURADO
KAKAPO
LAVABO
LEGATO
MACACO
MAHALO
MALABO
MEGALO
MIKADO
MILANO
MONACO
MOVADO
MURANO
NAGANO
NAVAHO
NAVAJO
NOMAYO
NOVATO
OCTAVO
PAPAGO
PICABO
PICARO
PISANO
POTATO
RAMAPO
RENATO
ROMANO
RUBATO
SABADO
SABATO
SOLANO
STMALO
STRATO
TAMAYO
TEJANO
TERATO
TEXACO
TOBAGO
TOMATO
VIRAGO
YOSANO
ZOCALO

••••AO

BILBAO
CALLAO
FERNAO
GALEAO
TODDAO

AP••••

APACHE
APATHY
APELET
APEMAN
APEMEN
APERCU
APEXES
APHIDS
APIARY
APICAL
APICES
APIECE
APLITE
APLOMB
APNEAS
APODAL
APOGEE
APOLLO
APOPKA
APPALL
APPALS
APPEAL
APPEAR
APPELS
APPEND
APPERT
APPIAN
APPLES
APPLET
APPOSE
APPROX
APRILE
APRILS
APRONS
APTEST
APULIA

A•P•••

ALPACA
ALPERT
ALPHAS
ALPINE
AMPERE
AMPING
AMPLER
AMPSUP
AMPULE
APPALL
APPALS
APPEAL
APPEAR
APPELS
APPEND
APPERT
APPIAN
APPLES
APPLET
APPOSE
APPROX
ARPEGE
ARPELS
ASPECT
ASPENS
ASPERA
ASPICS
ASPIRE
ASPISH
ASPURE
ATPLAY
AUPAIR

A••P••

ADAPTS
ADEPTS
ADOPTS
AIRPOP
AIRPOT
ALEPHS
ALEPPO
ALIPED
ALLPRO
APOPKA
ARMPIT
ASHPAN
ASHPIT
ATYPIC
AUSPEX

A•••P•

ABRUPT
ACCEPT
ADOLPH
ADREPS
AESOPS
ALCAPP
ALEPPO
ALMVPS
ASLOPE
ATEMPO

A••••P

AAAMAP
ACESUP
ACTSUP
ADDSUP
AIRPOP
AIRSUP
ALCAPP
ALEGUP
ALETAP
AMPSUP
ANTEUP
ASDEEP
ASHARP
ASKSUP
ASLEEP
ASTEEP
ASTOOP

•AP•••

CAPERS
CAPFUL
CAPGUN
CAPITA
CAPLET
CAPNUT
CAPONE
CAPONI
CAPONS
CAPOTE

CAPPED
CAPPER
CAPRID
CAPRIS
CAPTOR
DAPHNE
DAPPED
DAPPER
DAPPLE
GAPEAT
GAPERS
GAPING
GAPPED
HAPPEN
JAPANS
JAPERS
JAPERY
JAPING
KAPELL
KAPLAN
KAPOKS
KAPPAS
KAPUTT
LAPCAT
LAPDOG
LAPELS
LAPERI
LAPERM
LAPFUL
LAPHAM
LAPINS
LAPPED
LAPPER
LAPPET
LAPSAT
LAPSED
LAPSER
LAPSES
LAPSUP
LAPSUS
LAPTEV
LAPTOP
LAPUTA
MAPLES
MAPOUT
MAPPED
MAPPER
MAPPLE
MAPUTO
NAPACA
NAPALM
NAPERY
NAPHTA
NAPIER
NAPKIN
NAPLES
NAPOLI
NAPPED
NAPPER
NAPPES
NAPPIE
PAPACY
PAPAGO
PAPAWS
PAPAYA
PAPERS
PAPERY
PAPIER
PAPIST
PAPPAS
PAPUAN
PAPYRI
RAPIDO
RAPIDS
RAPIER
RAPINE
RAPINI
RAPPED
RAPPEL
RAPPER
RAPSON
RAPTER
RAPTLY
RAPTOR
RAPTUS
SAPORS
SAPPED
SAPPER
SAPPHO
TAPEON
TAPERS
TAPEUP
TAPING
TAPINS
TAPIRS
TAPOFF
TAPOUT
TAPPAN
TAPPED
TAPPER
TAPPET
TAPSIN
TAPSON
VAPORS
VAPORY
VAPOUR
WAPITI
WAPNER
YAPHET
YAPPED
YAPPER
YAPSAT
ZAPATA
ZAPPED
ZAPPER

•A•P••

CAMPED
CAMPER
CAMPOS
CAMPUP
CAMPUS
CAPPED
CAPPER
CARPAL
CARPAT
CARPED
CARPEL
CARPER
CARPET
CARPUS
CASPAR
CASPER
DAMPED
DAMPEN
DAMPER
DAMPLY
DAPPED
DAPPER
DAPPLE
GALPAL
GAPPED
GASPAR
GASPED
GASPER
GAWPED
GAWPER
HALPIN
HAMPER
HAPPEN
HARPED
HARPER
HARPON
HASPED
HATPIN
JAIPUR
JALPAS
JASPER
KAPPAS
KARPOV
LAPPED
LAPPER
LAPPET
LAUPER
MAGPIE
MAPPED
MAPPER
MAPPLE
MARPLE
NAPPED
NAPPER
NAPPES
NAPPIE
PAMPAS
PAMPER
PAPPAS
PAUPER
PAWPAW
PAYPAL
RAIPUR
RALPHJ
RAMPAL
RAMPED
RAMPUP
RAPPED
RAPPEL
RAPPER
RASPAS
RASPED
RASPER
SAIPAN
SAMPAN
SAMPLE
SAPPED
SAPPER
SAPPHO
SATPAT
SAWPIT
TAIPAN
TAIPEI
TAMPED
TAMPER
TAPPAN
TAPPED
TAPPER
TAPPET
TARPIT
TARPON
TAUPES
TAUPIN
VAMPED
VAMPER
WAMPUM
WARPED
WARPER
YAPPED
YAPPER
YAWPED
YAWPER
ZAPPED
ZAPPER

•A••P•

CALIPH
CANAPE
CANOPY
DACAPO
DAYSPA
GALOPS
JALAPA
JALOPY
JAMUPS
KAKAPO
LAYUPS
MACAPA
MANAPE
PANOPE
PARAPH
RAMAPO
SALEPS

•A•••P

AAAMAP
BACKUP
BADCOP
BADRAP
BALLUP
BANGUP
BANKUP
BARHOP
CAGEUP
CAKEUP
CALLUP
CAMEUP
CAMPUP
CARHOP
CARNAP
CARTOP
CASTUP
CATNAP
CATNIP
CATSUP
DAMSUP
DAYHOP
EARLAP
EASEUP
EATSUP
FACEUP
FAIRUP
FATLIP
GALLOP
GALLUP
GANGUP
GASCAP
GAVEUP
HACKUP
HAMSUP
HANDUP
HANGUP
HARDUP
HAULUP
HAVEUP
JACKUP
JAMSUP
JAZZUP
LACEUP
LAIDUP
LANDUP
LAPSUP
LAPTOP
LARRUP
LASHUP
LASTUP
LAYSUP
MADCAP
MADEUP
MAKEUP
MARKUP
MASHUP
MAYHAP
NAILUP
PACKUP
PAGEUP
PAIDUP
PAIRUP
PASSUP
PAYSUP
RACEUP
RACKUP
RAGMOP
RAGTOP
RAKEUP
RAMPUP
RANGUP
RAVEUP
SACKUP
SATRAP
SAVEUP
SAWSUP
TACKUP
TAGSUP
TAKEUP
TALKUP
TANKUP
TAPEUP
TARTUP
WADSUP
WAITUP
WAKEUP
WALKUP
WALLOP
WALLUP
WARMUP
WASHUP

••AP••

ADAPTS
BEAPAL
CHAPEL
CHAPIN
COAPTS
CRAPED
CRAPES
DIAPER
DRAPED
DRAPER
DRAPES
ELAPID
ELAPSE
ETAPES
FLAPPY
FRAPPE
GRAPES
GRAPEY
GRAPHO
GRAPHS
GRAPHY
GRAPPA
HEAPED
HEAPER
HEAPON
HEAPUP
INAPET
INAPIE
INAPOD
LEAPAT
LEAPED
LEAPER
LEAPIN
LEAPON
LEAPUP
OKAPIS
ONAPAR
PEAPOD
PGAPRO
QUAPAW
REAPED
REAPER
SHAPED
SHAPER
SHAPES
SLAPON
SLAPPY
SNAPAT
SNAPON
SNAPPY
SNAPTO
SNAPUP
SOAPED
SOAPER
SOAPUP
STAPES
STAPHS
STAPLE
STAPUF
TEAPOT
TEAPOY
TRAPPY
WEAPON
WRAPUP

••A•P•

CHAMPS
CIASPY
CLAMPS
CLASPS
CRAMPS
CRAMPY
FLAPPY
FRAPPE
GRAMPA
GRAMPS
GRANPA
GRAPPA
GRASPS
SCALPS
SCAMPI
SCAMPS
SCARPS
SHARPE
SHARPS
SHARPY
SLAPPY
SNAPPY
STAMPS
SWAMPS
SWAMPY
TRAMPS
TRAMPY
TRAPPY

••A••P

AAAMAP
BEADUP
BEAMUP
BEARUP
BEATUP
CHATUP
CLAMUP
DEALUP
DIALUP
DRAGUP
DRAWUP
GEARUP
GLAMUP
HEADUP
HEALUP
HEAPUP
HEATUP
IMACOP
LEADUP
LEAPUP
LOADUP
ONAHOP
PLAYUP
READUP
REARUP
SEALUP
SEAMAP
SMALLP
SNAGUP
SNAPUP
SOAKUP
SOAPUP
STAYUP
SWAMUP
TEACUP
TEAMUP
TEARUP
WRAPUP

•••AP•

ALCAPP
BIGAPE
CANAPE
CHEAPO
DACAPO
DECAPS
DOGAPE
DOLAPS
ENRAPT
ESCAPE
INCAPS
JALAPA
KAKAPO
LENAPE
MACAPA
MANAPE
ONTAPE
PARAPH
PTRAPS
RAMAPO
RECAPS
RELAPS
REMAPS
RETAPE
RETAPS
SCRAPE
SCRAPS
SERAPE
SERAPH
STRAPS
THEAPE
TSHAPE
TVTAPE
UNCAPS
UNTAPE
USHAPE
VSHAPE
YSHAPE

•••A•P

ALCAPP
ASHARP
BSHARP
CCLAMP
CSHARP
DECAMP
DSHARP
ENCAMP
ESCARP
ESHARP
FSHARP
GSHARP
ONRAMP
PREAMP
REVAMP
SCHAAP
THEASP
TSGARP
UNHASP

••••AP

AAAMAP
ALETAP
BADRAP
BITMAP
BUMRAP
BURLAP
CARNAP
CATNAP
DEWLAP
DOGNAP
DUNLAP
EARLAP
ENTRAP
ENWRAP
GASCAP
GELCAP
GIDDAP
GUNLAP
HOTCAP
HUBCAP
ICECAP
KIDNAP
MADCAP
MAYHAP
MIDCAP
MILSAP
MISHAP
NOSOAP
ONELAP
OUTRAP
PETNAP
REDCAP
RELEAP
RESNAP
RESOAP
RETRAP
REWRAP
RIPRAP
SATRAP
SCHAAP
SEAMAP
SKICAP
SKYCAP
SKYMAP
THEGAP
THERAP
TOECAP
TOETAP
TSTRAP
UNSNAP
UNTRAP
UNWRAP
UPHEAP
UPLEAP
WETNAP

AQ••••

AQUAKE
AQUILA
AQUINO

A•Q•••

ACQUIT

•AQ•••

FAQIRS
MAQUIS
PAQUIN
RAQUEL
YAQUIS

•A•Q••

BANQUE
BANQUO
BARQUE
BASQUE
CASQUE
MANQUE
MARQUE
MASQUE
SACQUE
YANQUI

•A•••Q

NASDAQ

••AQ••

BRAQUE
CLAQUE
IRAQIS
OPAQUE
PLAQUE

••A••Q

SMALLQ

••••AQ

COMPAQ
NASDAQ

AR••••

ARABIA
ARABIC
ARABLE
ARADOS
ARAFAT
ARAGON
ARAMES
ARAMID
ARAMIS
ARARAS
ARARAT
ARBELA
ARBORS
ARBOUR
ARBRES
ARCADE
ARCANA
ARCANE
ARCARO
ARCCOS
ARCHED
ARCHER
ARCHES
ARCHIE
ARCHLY
ARCHON
ARCING
ARCSEC
ARCSIN
ARCTAN
ARCTIC
ARDENT
ARDORS
ARDOUR
ARECAS
ARENAS
ARENDT
AREOLA
AREOLE
ARETES
ARETHA
ARETOO
AREZZO
ARFARF
ARGALI
ARGENT
ARGIVE
ARGOSY
ARGOTS
ARGUED
ARGUER
ARGUES
ARGUFY
ARGYLE
ARGYLL
ARHATS
ARIANA
ARIANE
ARIARY
ARIDER
ARIDLY
ARIEGE
ARIGHT
ARIOSE
ARIOSI
ARIOSO
ARISEN
ARISES
ARISTA
ARISTO
ARJUNA
ARLENE
ARLISS
ARLOVA
ARMADA
ARMAGH
ARMAND
ARMANI
ARMERS
ARMETS
ARMFUL
ARMIES
ARMING
ARMLET
ARMONK
ARMORS
ARMORY
ARMOUR
ARMPIT
ARNALL
ARNEIS
ARNESS
ARNETT
ARNHEM
ARNICA
ARNIES
ARNOLD
AROIDS
AROINT
AROMAS
AROUET
AROUND
AROUSE
ARPEGE
ARPELS
ARRACK
ARRANT
ARRAYS
ARREAR
ARREST
ARRETE
ARRIBA
ARRIVE
ARROWS
ARROYO
ARSENE
ARSENO
ARSONS
ARTAUD
ARTCAR
ARTELS
ARTERY
ARTEST
ARTFUL
ARTGUM
ARTHRO
ARTHUR
ARTIER
ARTILY
ARTIST
ARTOIS
ARTURO
ARUBAN
ARVADA
ARYANS

A•R•••

AARGAU
AARHUS
ABRADE
ABRAMS
ABROAD
ABRUPT
ACROSS
ADRATE
ADRENO
ADREPS
ADRIAN
ADRIEN
ADRIFT
ADRIVE
ADROIT
AERATE
AERIAL
AERIER
AERIES
AERIFY
AERILY
AERIOS
AEROBE
AFRAID
AFRAME
AFRESH
AFRICA
AGREED
AGREER
AGREES
AIRACE
AIRARM
AIRBAG
AIRBUD
AIRBUS
AIRDAM
AIRDRY
AIRERS
AIRGUN
AIRIER
AIRILY
AIRING
AIRLOG
AIRMAN
AIRMEN
AIROUT
AIRPOP
AIRPOT
AIRSAC
AIRSEA
AIRSUP
AIRWAR
AIRWAY
ALRITZ
AMRITA
AORTAE
AORTAL
AORTAS
AORTIC
APRILE
APRILS
APRONS
ARRACK
ARRANT
ARRAYS
ARREAR
ARREST
ARRETE
ARRIBA
ARRIVE
ARROWS
ARROYO
ASRARE
ATRAIN
ATREST
ATREUS
ATRIAL
ATRISK
ATRIUM
ATROIS
AURATE
AURIFY
AURIGA
AURIST
AURORA
AUROUS
AVRILS
AYRTON
AZRAEL

A••R••

ABBREV
ABORAL
ABORTS
ACARID
ACCRUE
ACORNS
ACURAS
ADORED
ADOREE
ADORER
ADORES
ADORNS
AFFRAY
AGARIC
AGORAE
AGORAS
AGOROT
AHERNE
AHORSE
AIGRET
ALARIC
ALARMS
ALARUM
ALDRIN
ALEROS
ALERTS
ALFRED
ALGREN
ALTRIA
AMARNA
AMERCE
AMORAL
AMORES
AMORET
AMTRAC
AMTRAK
ANARCH
ANDRAE
ANDREA
ANDREI
ANDRES
ANDREW
ANDREY
ANDRIC
ANDROS
ANERGY
ANORAK
ANTRAL
ANTRES
ANTRIM
ANTRON
ANTRUM
APERCU
APPROX
ARARAS
ARARAT
ARBRES
ASARCO
ASFREE
ASHRAM
ASTRAL
ASTRAY
ASTRES
ASTRID
ASTROS
ASTROV
ASTRUD
ATARIS
ATERRE
ATHROB
ATHROW
ATTRIT
AUBREY
AUDREY
AVERSE
AVERTS
AWARDS
AWARER
AZARIA
AZERAS
AZERIS
AZORES
AZORIN
AZURED
AZURES

A•••R•

ABHORS
ABJURE
ABLARE
ABOARD
ABSORB
ABSURD
ACCORD
ACHERS
ACTORS
ADDERS
ADHERE
ADJURE
ADMIRE
ADSORB
ADVERB
ADVERT
ADWARE
ADWARS
AFEARD
AFFIRM
AFFORD
AFLARE
AFTERS
AGLARE
AIDERS
AILURO
AIMERS
AIRARM
AIRDRY
AIRERS
ALBERS
ALBERT
ALBORG
ALDERS
ALEGRE
ALGORE
ALHIRT
ALLPRO
ALLURE
ALPERT
ALTARF
ALTARS
ALTERS
ALUDRA
ALVARO
ALZIRA
AMBERS
AMBERY
AMEERS
AMENRA
AMONRA
AMOURS
AMPERE
ANDERS
ANGERS
ANGORA
ANITRA
ANKARA
ANSARA
ANTERO
AOLERS
APIARY
APPERT
ARBORS
ARCARO
ARDORS
ARFARF
ARIARY
ARMERS
ARMORS
ARMORY

ARTERY
ARTHRO
ARTURO
ASBURY
ASGARD
ASHARP
ASHORE
ASKERS
ASMARA
ASPERA
ASPIRE
ASPURE
ASRARE
ASSERT
ASSORT
ASSURE
ASTARE
ASTART
ASTERN
ASTERO
ASTERS
ASWARM
ASWIRL
ATERRE
ATTARS
ATTIRE
ATWORK
AUBURN
AUGERS
AUGURS
AUGURY
AURORA
AUSTRO
AVIARY
AWEARY
AWHIRL

A••••R

AAFAIR
ABASER
ABATER
ABATOR
ABIDER
ABUSER
ACHIER
ACTFOR
ACUTER
ADORER
AERIER
AETHER
AFFAIR
AGADIR
AGILER
AGREER
AIMFOR
AIRIER
AIRWAR
ALEGAR
ALINER
ALLFOR
ALOMAR
ALTAIR
ALULAR
ALYDAR
AMAJOR
AMBLER
AMINOR
AMPLER
AMUSER
ANCHOR
ANGKOR
ANGLER
ANSWER
ANTHER
ANTLER
APPEAR
ARBOUR
ARCHER
ARDOUR
ARGUER
ARIDER
ARMOUR
ARREAR
ARTCAR
ARTHUR
ARTIER
ASEVER
ASHIER
ASHLAR
ASKFOR
ASNEAR
ASTHER
ATFOUR
ATONER
AUPAIR
AUSTER
AUTEUR
AUTHOR
AVATAR
AVIDER
AVOWER
AWAKER
AWARER
AYESIR

•AR•••

AARGAU
AARHUS
BARACK
BARADA
BARAKA
BARANY
BARATA
BARATO
BARBAN
BARBED
BARBER
BARBET
BARBIE
BARBRA
BARCAR
BARCOS
BARDIC
BARDOT
BAREGE
BARELY
BAREST
BARFLY
BARGED
BARGER
BARGES
BARHOP
BARING
BARITE
BARIUM
BARKAT
BARKED
BARKER
BARKIN
BARKLA
BARLEY
BARLOW
BARMAN
BARMEN
BARNED
BARNES
BARNET
BARNEY
BARNUM
BAROJA
BAROLO
BARONE
BARONI
BARONS
BARONY
BARQUE
BARRED
BARREL
BARREN
BARRES
BARRET
BARRIE
BARRIO
BARRIS
BARRON
BARROW
BARTAB
BARTEL
BARTER
BARTLE
BARTOK
BARTON
BARUCH
BARYON
BARZUN
CARAFE
CARATS
CARBON
CARBOS
CARBOY
CARBRA
CARDED
CARDER
CARDIA
CARDIN
CARDIO
CAREEN
CAREER
CAREOF
CARERS
CARESS
CARETO
CARETS
CARFUL
CARGOS
CARHOP
CARIBE
CARIBS
CARIES
CARINA
CARING
CARIOU
CARKEY
CARLIN
CARLOS
CARLOT
CARLOW
CARMAN
CARMEL
CARMEN
CARNAC
CARNAL
CARNAP
CARNER
CARNES
CARNET
CARNEY
CAROBS
CAROLE
CAROLI
CAROLL
CAROLS
CAROMS
CARONI
CARPAL
CARPAT
CARPED
CARPEL
CARPER
CARPET
CARPUS
CARREL
CARREY
CARRIE
CARROL
CARROT
CARSEY
CARSON
CARTED
CARTEL
CARTER
CARTES
CARTIN
CARTON
CARTOP
CARUSO
CARVED
CARVEL
CARVER
CARVES
CARVEY
CARWAX
DARCEL
DAREME
DARENT
DARERS
DAREST
DARETO
DARIEN
DARING
DARIUS
DARKEN
DARKER
DARKLE
DARKLY
DARLIN
DARNAY
DARNED
DARNER
DARNIT
DARREN
DARRIN
DARROW
DARRYL
DARTED
DARTER
DARTLE
DARWIN
EARBUD
EARFUL
EARING
EARLAP
EARLET
EARNED
EARNER
EARNIE
EARNIT
EARTAB
EARTAG
EARTHA
EARTHS
EARTHY
EARVIN
EARWAX
EARWIG
FARACY
FARADS
FARAHS
FARCED
FARCES
FARCRY
FARERS
FARFEL
FARINA
FARING
FARLEY
FARLOW
FARMED
FARMER
FARNUM
FAROES
FAROFF
FAROUK
FAROUT
FARRAH
FARRAR
FARRIS
FARROW
FARUKI
GARAGE
GARBED
GARBER
GARBLE
GARCIA
GARCON
GARDEN
GARETH
GARGAN
GARGLE
GARISH
GARLIC
GARNER
GARNET
GARRET
GARSON
GARTER
GARVEY
GARYIN
HARALD
HARARE
HARASS
HARBIN
HARBOR
HARDBY
HARDEN
HARDER
HARDIN
HARDLY
HARDUP
HAREMS
HARHAR
HARING
HARKED
HARKEN
HARKER
HARLAN
HARLEM
HARLEY
HARLIN
HARLOT
HARLOW
HARMED
HARMER
HARMON
HARNEY
HAROLD
HARPED
HARPER
HARPON
HARRAD
HARRAH
HARRIS
HARROW
HARRYO
HARRYS
HARVEY
JARABE
JARDIN
JARFUL
JARGON
JARJAR
JARRED
JARULE
JARVIK
KARATE
KARATS
KAREEM
KARINA
KARKOV
KARLEN
KARMAS
KARMIC
KARNAK
KARPOV
KARRAS
KARRER
KARRIE
KARSTS
LARAMS
LARAZA
LARDED
LARDER
LARDON
LAREDO
LAREES
LARGER
LARGES
LARGOS
LARIAT
LARINE
LARKED
LARKER
LARKIN
LARMEN
LARMOR
LAROSA
LARRUP
LARSEN
LARSON
LARTER
LARTET
LARVAE
LARVAL
LARVAS
LARYNX
MARACA
MARAUD
MARBLE
MARBLY
MARCEL
MARCHE
MARCIA
MARCIE
MARCIL
MARCIX
MARCOS
MARCUS
MARDEN
MARDIS
MARGIE
MARGIN
MARGOT
MARIAH
MARIAN
MARIAS
MARIDA
MARIDO
MARIEL
MARIKO
MARILU
MARINA
MARINE
MARINO
MARION
MARISA
MARIST
MARJOE
MARKAS
MARKED
MARKER
MARKET
MARKEY
MARKIE
MARKII
MARKIV
MARKIX
MARKKA
MARKOV
MARKUP
MARKVI
MARLED
MARLEE
MARLEY
MARLIN
MARLON
MARMEE
MARMOT
MARNER
MARNIE
MAROON
MARPLE
MARQUE
MARRED
MARRER
MARRON
MARROW
MARSHA
MARSHY
MARTEL
MARTEN
MARTES
MARTHA
MARTHE
MARTIN
MARTYR
MARVEL
MARVIN
MARVIS
MARXES
MARYAM
MARYII
MARYJO
NARADA
NARCOS
NARIAL
NARINE
NARITA
NARNIA
NARROW
NARVIK
OARAGE
OARERS
OARING
OARMAN
OARMEN
PARADE
PARANA
PARAPH
PARCAE
PARCEL
PARDON
PARENS
PARENT
PARERS
PARETO
PAREUS
PAREVE
PARFUM
PARGED
PARGER
PARGES
PARIAH
PARING
PARINI
PARISH
PARITY
PARKAS
PARKAV
PARKAY
PARKED
PARKER
PARKES
PARKIT
PARLAY
PARLEY
PARLEZ
PARLOR
PARNIS
PARODY
PAROLE
PAROLS
PARRED
PARRIS
PARROT
PARSEC
PARSED
PARSEE
PARSER
PARSES
PARSON
PARTED
PARTII
PARTIV
PARTLY
PARTOF
PARTON
PARTYS
PARURE
RAREES
RAREFY
RARELY
RAREST
RARING
RARITY
SARANS
SARDIS
SARDOU
SAREES
SARGES
SARGON
SARNIA
SARONG
SARTON
SARTOR
SARTRE
TARAWA
TARDES
TARGAS
TARGET
TARIFF
TARING
TARLEK
TARMAC
TAROIL
TAROTS
TARPIT
TARPON
TARRED
TARSAL
TARSUS
TARTAN
TARTAR
TARTED
TARTER
TARTES
TARTLY
TARTUP
TARZAN
VARDEN
VARESE
VARGAS
VARIAS
VARIED
VARIER
VARIES
VARLET
VARMUS
VARNAS
VARNEY
WARBLE
WARCRY
WARDED
WARDEN
WARDER
WARGOD
WARHOL
WARIER
WARILY
WARING
WARMED
WARMER
WARMLY
WARMTH
WARMTO
WARMUP
WARNED
WARNER
WARNES
WARNOF
WARPED
WARPER
WARRED
WARREN
WARSAW
WARTED
WARVET
YARDED
YARDER
YARELY
YAREST
YARNED
YARROW
ZARKOV

•A•R••

BADRAP
BAERGA
BAIRNS
BARRED
BARREL
BARREN
BARRES
BARRET
BARRIE
BARRIO
BARRIS
BARRON
BARROW
BASRAH
BAYRUM
CABRAL
CABRIO
CADRES
CAIRNS
CAMRYN
CAMRYS
CAPRID
CAPRIS
CARREL
CARREY
CARRIE
CARROL
CARROT
CATRIG
DABRAT
DACRON
DARREN
DARRIN
DARROW
DARRYL
DATRIL
EAGRES
FABRAY
FABRIC
FAERIE
FAEROE
FAIRED
FAIRER
FAIRLY
FAIRUP
FARRAH
FARRAR
FARRIS
FARROW
GARRET
GAVRAS
HADRON
HAIRDO
HAIRED
HARRAD
HARRAH
HARRIS
HARROW
HARRYO
HARRYS
HATRED
IAGREE
IATRIC
JARRED
JAURES
KARRAS
KARRER
KARRIE
KATRIN
LABRAT
LABREA
LAIRDS
LAIRED
LARRUP
LATRIA
LAUREL
LAUREN
LAUREY
LAURIA
LAURIC
LAURIE
LAURYL
LAURYN
MACRAE
MACRON
MACROS
MADRAS
MADRES
MADRID
MAIRES
MAIRZY
MANRAY
MAORIS
MARRED
MARRER
MARRON
MARROW
MATRIX
MATRON
MAYRON
NACRED
NACRES
NAIRAS
NARROW
NATRON
PADRES
PAIRED
PAIRUP
PARRED
PARRIS
PARROT
PATRIA
PATRIC
PATRIE
PATROL
PATRON
RAGRUG
RAHRAH
RAMROD
SABRAS
SABRES
SACRED
SACRUM
SATRAP
SAURON
SAURUS
SAWRED
TABRIZ
TARRED
TATRAS
TAURIC
TAUROG
TAURUS
VANRYN
WALRUS
WARRED
WARREN
YARROW
ZABRZE
ZAGREB
ZAIRES

•A••R•

BAKERS
BAKERY
BALERS
BARBRA
BAYARD
BAYERN
CABERS
CAGERS
CALORY
CAMARO
CAMERA
CANARD
CANARY
CANERS
CAPERS
CARBRA
CARERS
CASERN
CASERS
CASTRO
CATERA
CATERS
CAVERN
CAVERS
CAVORT
DAMORE
DARERS
DATARY
DATERS
DAZERS
EASERS
EATERS
EATERY
FACERS
FADERS
FAKERS
FAKERY
FAKIRS
FAQIRS
FARCRY
FARERS
FAVORS
FAXERS
FAYARD
GABBRO
GALORE
GAMERS
GANTRY
GAPERS
GASTRO
GATERS
GATORS
GAZERS
HARARE
HASBRO
HATARI
HATERS
HAYERS
HAZARD
HAZERS
JAPERS
JAPERY
JAVERT
KAKURO
LABORS
LACERS
LADERS
LAGERS
LAHORE
LAKERS
LAMARR
LANARK
LANDRY
LAPERI
LAPERM
LASERS
LASTRA
LATERI
LATERO
LAVERN
LAVERS
LAYERS
MACERS
MADERA
MADERO
MADURO
MAITRE
MAJORS
MAKERS
MALARS
MALORY
MANERO
MANORS
MANTRA
MANURE
MASERS
MASERU
MATERS
MATURE
MAYORS
NABORS
NADIRS
NAMERS
NAPERY
NATURE
OARERS
OATERS
PACERS
PAGERS
PALTRY
PAMIRS
PANFRY
PANTRY
PAPERS
PAPERY
PAPYRI
PARERS
PARURE
PASTRY
PATDRY
PATERS
PAVERS
PAWERS
PAYERS
QATARI
RACERS
RADARS
RAGERS
RAKERS
RANDRY
RASERS
RASURE
RATERS
RAVERS
RAZERS
RAZORS
SABERS
SAFARI
SAFIRE
SAHARA
SALARY
SAMARA
SANDRA
SANDRO
SANGRE
SAPORS
SARTRE
SATIRE
SATORI
SATURN
SATYRS
SAVERS
SAVORS
SAVORY
SAWERS
SAYERS
TABARD
TABORS
TAGORE
TAKERS
TALERS
TAMARA
TAMERS
TANTRA
TAPERS
TAPIRS
TASERS
TATARS
TATERS
TAVERN
TAWDRY
TAXERS
VAGARY
VALERA
VALERE
VALERO
VALERY
VALORS
VANARK
VAPORS
VAPORY
WADERS
WAFERS
WAFERY
WAGERS
WAKERS
WARCRY
WATERS
WATERY
WAVERS
WAVERY
WAXERS
ZADORA
ZAMORA

•A•••R

AAFAIR
BABIER
BACKER
BADDER
BADGER
BAEYER
BAFFER
BAGGER
BAILER
BAILOR
BAITER
BAKKER
BALDER
BALDUR
BALKER
BALMER
BANDER
BANGER
BANGOR
BANKER
BANNER
BANTER
BARBER
BARCAR
BARGER
BARKER

BARTER
BASHER
BASKER
BASTER
BATFOR
BATHER
BATTER
BAUMER
BAVIER
BAWLER
BAXTER
BAYLOR
BAZAAR
CABLER
CADGER
CAESAR
CAGIER
CAHIER
CAKIER
CALDER
CALKER
CALLER
CALMER
CAMBER
CAMPER
CANCER
CANDOR
CANIER
CANKER
CANNER
CANOER
CANTER
CANTOR
CAPPER
CAPTOR
CARDER
CAREER
CARNER
CARPER
CARTER
CARVER
CASPAR
CASPER
CASTER
CASTOR
CATHER
CAUSER
CAVIAR
CAWDOR
DABBER
DAFTER
DAGGER
DAGMAR
DAMMER
DAMNER
DAMOUR
DAMPER
DANCER
DANDER
DANGER
DANKER
DANNER
DAPPER
DARKER
DARNER
DARTER
DASHER
DAUBER
DAWBER
EARNER
EASIER
EASTER
FABBER
FABLER
FACTOR
FAFNER
FAFNIR
FAINER
FAIRER
FALLER
FALSER
FALTER
FANNER
FARMER
FARRAR
FASTER
FATHER
FATTER
FAVOUR
FAWNER
GABBER
GABLER
GADDER
GAFFER
GAGGER
GAINER
GAITER
GAMIER
GAMMER
GANDER
GANGER
GAOLER
GARBER
GARNER
GARTER
GASPAR
GASPER
GASSER
GASTER
GASWAR
GATHER
GAUGER
GAWKER
GAWPER
GAYNOR
HABLAR
HACKER
HAGLER
HAILER
HALTER
HALVER
HAMMER
HAMPER
HANDER
HANGAR
HANGER
HANKER
HARBOR
HARDER
HARHAR
HARKER
HARMER
HARPER
HATHOR
HATTER
HAULER
HAWKER
HAWSER
HAZIER
JABBAR
JABBER
JAEGER
JAGGER
JAGUAR
JAILER
JAILOR
JAIPUR
JAMMER
JANUAR
JARJAR
JASPER
JAVIER
JAZZER
KAISER
KALMAR
KANDER
KANTOR
KARRER
KAVNER
LABOUR
LACIER
LADDER
LADLER
LAFFER
LAGEAR
LAGGER
LAKIER
LAMARR
LAMOUR
LANCER
LANDER
LANDOR
LANGER
LANIER
LANKER
LAPPER
LAPSER
LARDER
LARGER
LARKER
LARMOR
LARTER
LASCAR
LASHER
LASKER
LASSER
LATHER
LATOUR
LATTER
LAUDER
LAUPER
LAUTER
LAWYER
LAYFOR
LAZIER
MADDER
MADFOR
MAGYAR
MAHLER
MAHZOR
MAILER
MAIMER
MAINER
MANGER
MANNER
MAPPER
MARKER
MARNER
MARRER
MARTYR
MASHER
MASKER
MASTER
MATHER
MATTER
MAULER
MAUSER
MAZIER
NABBER
NAGGER
NAILER
NAIVER
NAPIER
NAPPER
NASCAR
NASSER
NATTER
OAKIER
OATIER
PACIER
PACKER
PADDER
PALLOR
PALMAR
PALMER
PALTER
PAMPER
PANDER
PANIER
PANNER
PANTER
PANZER
PAPIER
PARGER
PARKER
PARLOR
PARSER
PASDAR
PASSER
PASTER
PASTOR
PATTER
PATZER
PAUPER
PAUSER
PAVIOR
PAWNER
PAYFOR
RACIER
RACKER
RADNER
RADNOR
RAFTER
RAGNAR
RAIDER
RAILER
RAINER
RAIPUR
RAISER
RAMMER
RANCOR
RANFOR
RANGER
RANKER
RANTER
RAPIER
RAPPER
RAPTER
RAPTOR
RASHER
RASPER
RASTER
RATEDR
RATHER
RATNER
RATTER
RAWBAR
SACHER
SACKER
SADDER
SADLER
SAGIER
SAILER
SAILOR
SALTER
SALVER
SALVOR
SANDER
SANGER
SAPPER
SARTOR
SASSER
SATFOR
SAUCER
SAVIOR
SAVOIR
SAVOUR
SAWYER
TACKER
TAGGER
TAILER
TAILOR
TALKER
TALLER
TAMBOR
TAMPER
TANKER
TANNER
TAPPER
TARTAR
TARTER
TASTER
TATLER
TATTER
TAUTER
TAYLOR
VAGUER
VAINER
VALOUR
VALUER
VAMPER
VANIER
VAPOUR
VARIER
VASSAR
VASTER
WACKER
WADDER
WAFTER
WAGGER
WAGNER
WAILER
WAITER
WAIVER
WALKER
WALLER
WALTER
WANDER
WANIER
WANNER
WANTER
WAPNER
WARDER
WARIER
WARMER
WARNER
WARPER
WASHER
WASSER
WASTER
WAVIER
WAXIER
XAVIER
YAKKER
YAMMER
YANKER
YAPPER
YARDER
YASGUR
YASSER
YATTER
YAWNER
YAWPER
ZANIER
ZAPPER

••AR••

ACARID
AGARIC
ALARIC
ALARMS
ALARUM
AMARNA
ANARCH
ARARAS
ARARAT
ASARCO
ATARIS
AWARDS
AWARER
AZARIA
BEARDS
BEARER
BEARON
BEARSE
BEARUP
BLARED
BLARES
BOARDS
CHARDS
CHARGE
CHARLY
CHARMS
CHARON
CHARRO
CHARTA
CHARTS
CIARDI
CLARET
CLARKE
CLAROS
COARSE
DCAREA
DEARER
DEARIE
DEARLY
DEARME
DEARTH
DEARTO
DHARMA
DIARIO
DMARKS
DUARTE
DWARFS
ECARDS
ECARTE
ENARMS
EPARCH
EXARCH
FEARED
FEARER
FLARED
FLARES
GEARED
GEARTO
GEARUP
GLARED
GLARES
GLARUS
GNARLS
GNARLY
GNARRS
GUARDS
HEARER
HEARNS
HEAROF
HEARSE
HEARST
HEARTH
HEARTS
HEARTY
HEARYE
HOARDS
HOARSE
IBARRA
ICARIA
ICARUS
IDARED
IMARET
INARAY
INARCH
INAREA
INAROW
INARUG
INARUT
JUAREZ
KEARNS
KEARNY
KIARIO
KMARTS
KNARRS
KNARRY
LEARNS
LEARNT
NEARBY
NEARED
NEARER
NEARLY
NEARTO
OZARKS
PEARCE
PEARLE
PEARLS
PEARLY
PHAROS
QUARKS
QUARRY
QUARTE
QUARTO
QUARTS
QUARTZ
REARED
REARER
REARMS
REARUP
ROARAT
ROARED
ROARER
SBARRO
SCARAB
SCARCE
SCARED
SCARER
SCARES
SCARFS
SCARNE
SCARPS
SCARRY
SCARUM
SEARCH
SEARED
SEARER
SEARLE
SHARDS
SHARED
SHARER
SHARES
SHARIF
SHARKS
SHARON
SHARPE
SHARPS
SHARPY
SHARYN
SMARMY
SMARTS
SMARTY
SNARED
SNARER
SNARES
SNARFS
SNARKS
SNARKY
SNARLS
SNARLY
SOARED
SOARER
SPARED
SPARER
SPARES
SPARKS
SPARKY
SPARSE
SPARTA
STARCH
STARED
STARER
STARES
STARIN
STARRY
STARTS
STARVE
STARZZ
SWARDS
SWARMS
TEARAT
TEARED
TEARER
TEARIT
TEARUP
TIARAS
UGARTE
UNARMS
USARMY
WEARER
WEARON
WHARFS
XLARGE
XSARAS
YEARLY
YEARNS

••A•R•

BIAFRA
CHAIRS
CHAKRA
CHARRO
CLAIRE
CLAIRS
CUATRO
DEAIRS
FIACRE
FLAIRS
GNARRS
GOAWRY
IBARRA
KNARRS
KNARRY
LLADRO
MEAGRE
MTAIRY
NBAERS
PGAPRO
QUADRI
QUARRY
QUATRE
REAIRS
SBARRO
SCARRY
SEAARM
STAIRS
STARRY
TEATRO
TEAURN
VIAGRA

••A••R

ABASER
ABATER
ABATOR
AGADIR
AMAJOR
AVATAR
AWAKER
AWARER
BEADER
BEAKER
BEAMER
BEARER
BEATER
BEAVER
BLADER
BLAMER
BLAZER
BMAJOR
BOATER
BRACER
BRAVER
BRAYER
CHAFER
CHASER
CLAMOR
CLAWER
CMAJOR
COALER
COATER
COAXER
CRAMER
CRATER
CRAVER
DEADER
DEAFER
DEALER
DEARER
DIALER
DIAPER
DLAYER
DMAJOR
DRAPER
DRAWER
EBAYER
ELATER
ELAYER
EMAJOR
ENAMOR
ERASER
EVADER
FEARER
FLAKER
FLAMER
FLAVOR
FLAYER
FMAJOR
FOAMER
FRAMER
FRASER
FRATER
FRAZER
GLAMOR
GLASER
GLAZER
GMAJOR
GNAWER
GRADER
GRATER
GRAVER
GRAYER
GRAZER
HEADER
HEALER
HEAPER
HEARER
HEATER
HEAVER
HOAXER
IMAGER
INANER
IRATER
KRAMER
LEADER
LEAKER
LEANER
LEAPER
LEASER
LEAVER
LOADER
LOAFER
LOANER
MEADER
MEAGER
MEANER
MOANER
NEARER
NEATER
ONAGER
ONAPAR
ORATOR
PEALER
PHASER
PLACER
PLANAR
PLANER
PLATER
PLAYER
PRATER
PRAWER
PRAYER
QUAKER
QUASAR
QUAVER
READER
REALER
REAMER
REAPER
REARER
REAVER
ROADER
ROAMER
ROARER
SCALAR
SCALER
SCARER
SEAAIR
SEALER
SEAMER
SEARER
SEATER
SEAVER
SHADER
SHAKER
SHAKUR
SHAMIR
SHAPER
SHARER
SHAVER
SKATER
SLAKER
SLATER
SLAVER
SLAYER
SMALLR
SNAKER
SNARER
SOAKER
SOAPER
SOARER
SPACER
SPADER
SPARER
SPAYER
STAGER
STALER
STARER
STATER
STATOR
STAYER
SUAVER
SWAYER
TEARER
TEASER
THALER
THAWER
THAYER
TRACER
TRADER
VEADAR
VIATOR
WEAKER
WEANER
WEARER
WEAVER
WHALER
YEAGER

•••AR•

ABLARE
ABOARD
ADWARE
ADWARS
AFEARD
AFLARE
AGLARE
AIRARM
ALTARF
ALTARS
ALVARO
ANKARA
ANSARA
APIARY
ARCARO
ARFARF
ARIARY
ASGARD
ASHARP
ASMARA
ASRARE
ASTARE
ASTART
ASWARM
ATTARS
AVIARY
AWEARY
BAYARD
BEJART
BEWARE
BEWARY
BICARB
BINARY
BLEARS
BLEARY
BOGART
BOVARY
BOYARS
BRIARD
BRIARS
BRIARY
BSHARP
BSTARS
CAMARO
CANARD
CANARY
CEDARN
CEDARS
CEDARY
CESARE
CESARS
CIGARS
CLEARS
CLEARY
COWARD
CSHARP
CSTARS
CUNARD
CURARE
DATARY
DEBARK
DEBARS
DECARE
DEMARK
DENARI
DENARS
DENARY
DEPART
DETARS
DEWARS
DINARS
DISARM
DOTARD
DREARY
DSHARP
DUGARD
DYSART
ECKART
EDGARD
EDGARS
EDUARD
EDVARD
EDWARD
ELGART
ELUARD
EMBARK
EMBARS
ERHARD
ERRARE
ESCARP
ESHARP
EZZARD
FAYARD
FIGARO
FRIARS
FRIARY
FSHARP
FSTARS
FUGARD
GEMARA
GERARD
GOCART
GODARD
GODARK
GOKART
GSHARP
GSTARS
HARARE
HATARI
HAZARD
HILARY
HOBART
HOWARD
IDCARD
IMPART
INPARK
INPART
INWARD
KSTARS
LAMARR
LANARK
LEGART
LENARD
LIPARI
LIZARD
MALARS
MCHARG
MOLARS
MOZART
MSTARS
MYLARS
NEWARK
NONART
NONARY
NOTARY
NSTARS
OHDARN
OLEARY
OMEARA
ONEARM
ONWARD
OSCARS
OSTARS
OXCART
OXNARD
PETARD
PICARA
PICARD
PICARO
POLARA
POPART
PREARM
PROART
QATARI
RADARS
REBARS
REDARE
REDARN
REEARN
REGARD
REMARK
RENARD
REPARK
RETARD
RETARS
REWARD
REWARM
REWARN
RITARD
ROSARY
ROTARY
RVPARK
SAFARI
SAHARA
SALARY
SAMARA
SEAARM
SENARY
SEWARD
SHEARS
SITARS
SMEARS
SMEARY
SOLARA
SONARS
SPEARE
SPEARS
SQUARE
SSTARS
STMARK
STMARY
STUART
SUBARU
SUGARS
SUGARY
SUVARI
SWEARS
TABARD
TAMARA
TATARS
THWART
TOLARS
TOWARD
TSGARP
TULARE
UNBARE
UNBARS
UNWARY
UPCARD
UPDART
UPWARD
UQUARK
VAGARY
VANARK
VELARS
VICARS
VIHARA
VITARA
VOLARE
VOTARY
WECARE
WIZARD

•••A•R

AAFAIR
AFFAIR
ALTAIR
AUPAIR
BAZAAR
BEFAIR
BELAIR
BIGAIR
CONAIR
DEHAIR
ECLAIR

HOTAIR
IMPAIR
ISRAIR
LAMARR
MCNAIR
MIDAIR
MOHAIR
NOFAIR
REPAIR
SEAAIR
UNFAIR
UNHAIR

••••AR

AIRWAR
ALEGAR
ALOMAR
ALULAR
ALYDAR
APPEAR
ARREAR
ARTCAR
ASHLAR
ASNEAR
AVATAR
BARCAR
BAZAAR
BEGGAR
BIGCAR
BIGEAR
BOWOAR
BOXCAR
BULGAR
BURSAR
CAESAR
CASPAR
CAVIAR
CELLAR
COLLAR
COLMAR
COPCAR
COSTAR
COUGAR
DAGMAR
DELMAR
DEODAR
DILLAR
DISBAR
DJEBAR
DOGEAR
DOLLAR
DUNBAR
ENDEAR
FARRAR
FIGBAR
FOLIAR
FULMAR
GASPAR
GASWAR
GELLAR
GETFAR
GONEAR
GOTFAR
GUITAR
GUNNAR
HABLAR
HANGAR
HARHAR
HOTCAR
HOTWAR
HOWFAR
HUSSAR
INFEAR
INGEAR
INGMAR
ISHTAR
ISOBAR
ISWEAR
JABBAR
JAGUAR
JANUAR
JARJAR
JEDGAR
JOBJAR
KALMAR
KCSTAR
KEVLAR
LAGEAR
LASCAR
LINEAR
LOTHAR
LOWTAR
LUMBAR
MAGYAR
MEDGAR
MOLNAR
MORTAR
MYDEAR
NASCAR
NECTAR
NEWCAR
NEWMAR
NODEAR
NONPAR
NONWAR
NOTFAR
OCEDAR
OCULAR
OHDEAR
OLDCAR
ONAPAR
ONECAR
ONSTAR
OTHMAR
OUTWAR
OVULAR
PALMAR
PASDAR
PILLAR
PINDAR
PLANAR
POLGAR
POPLAR
PREWAR
PROWAR
PSYWAR
PULSAR
QINTAR
QUASAR
RAGNAR
RAWBAR
REGEAR
REHEAR
RETEAR
REWEAR
SCALAR
SHOFAR
STELAR
SUBPAR
SUBWAR
TARTAR
TEKWAR
THEBAR
THECAR
TIEBAR
TINEAR
TIPJAR
TOOFAR
TOWBAR
TOWCAR
TOYCAR
TVSTAR
TWOCAR
UPBEAR
UPREAR
UPROAR
UPSOAR
UPTEAR
UVULAR
VASSAR
VEADAR
VULGAR
WEIMAR
WETBAR

AS••••

ASANAS
ASANTE
ASARCO
ASBURY
ASCALE
ASCEND
ASCENT
ASCOLD
ASCOOL
ASCOTS
ASDEEP
ASDICS
ASDULL
ASEASY
ASEVER
ASFAST
ASFLAT
ASFREE
ASGARD
ASGOOD
ASHADE
ASHAME
ASHARP
ASHBIN
ASHCAN
ASHDOD
ASHIER
ASHINE
ASHING
ASHLAR
ASHLEE
ASHLEY
ASHMAN
ASHMEN
ASHORE
ASHPAN
ASHPIT
ASHRAM
ASHTON
ASIAGO
ASIANS
ASIDES
ASIMOV
ASKAMY
ASKANT
ASKERS
ASKFOR
ASKING
ASKOUT
ASKSIN
ASKSOF
ASKSUP
ASLANT
ASLEEP
ASLOPE
ASLOSH
ASMANY
ASMARA
ASMUCH
ASNEAR
ASNEAT
ASONIA
ASOSAN
ASPECT
ASPENS
ASPERA
ASPICS
ASPIRE
ASPISH
ASPURE
ASRARE
ASSAIL
ASSAYS
ASSENT
ASSERT
ASSESS
ASSETS
ASSIGN
ASSISI
ASSIST
ASSIZE
ASSLOW
ASSOFT
ASSORT
ASSTDA
ASSUCH
ASSUME
ASSURE
ASTALL
ASTANA
ASTARE
ASTART
ASTEAL
ASTEEP
ASTERN
ASTERO
ASTERS
ASTHER
ASTHMA
ASTLEY
ASTOOP
ASTRAL
ASTRAY
ASTRES
ASTRID
ASTROS
ASTROV
ASTRUD
ASTUTE
ASWARM
ASWELL
ASWIRL
ASWOON
ASYLUM

A•S•••

ABSCAM
ABSENT
ABSORB
ABSURD
ADSORB
AESOPS
AISLED
AISLES
ALSACE
ALSTON
AMSTEL
ANSARA
ANSATE
ANSEIS
ANSELM
ANSWER
ARSENE
ARSENO
ARSONS
ASSAIL
ASSAYS
ASSENT
ASSERT
ASSESS
ASSETS
ASSIGN
ASSISI
ASSIST
ASSIZE
ASSLOW
ASSOFT
ASSORT
ASSTDA
ASSUCH
ASSUME
ASSURE
ATSIGN
ATSTUD
AUSPEX
AUSSIE
AUSTEN
AUSTER
AUSTIN
AUSTRO
AXSEED

A••S••

ABASED
ABASER
ABASES
ABUSED
ABUSER
ABUSES
ABYSMS
ACESIT
ACESUP
ACTSAS
ACTSIN
ACTSON
ACTSUP
ADDSIN
ADDSON
ADDSTO
ADDSUP
ADESTE
AGASSI
AGESIX
AGOSTO
AIMSAT
AIRSAC
AIRSEA
AIRSUP
ALASKA
ALISON
ALISTS
ALLSET
ALYSSA
AMESIA
AMOSOZ
AMPSUP
AMUSED
AMUSER
AMUSES
ANGSTS
ANISES
ARCSEC
ARCSIN
ARISEN
ARISES
ARISTA
ARISTO
ASKSIN
ASKSOF
ASKSUP
ASOSAN
ATESTS
ATISES
AUSSIE
AVESTA
AVISON
AVISOS
AXISES
AYESHA
AYESIR

A•••S•

ABBESS
ABLEST
ABLUSH
ACCESS
ACCOST
ACCUSE
ACROSS
ADJUST
ADVISE
AFRESH
AGASSI
AGEISM
AGEIST
AGHAST
AGUISH
AHIMSA
AHORSE
AINTSO
ALDISS
ALEAST
ALMOST
ALNASL
ALONSO
ALWEST
ALYSSA
AMBUSH
AMIDST
APPOSE
APTEST
ARGOSY
ARIOSE
ARIOSI
ARIOSO
ARLISS
ARNESS
AROUSE
ARREST
ARTEST
ARTIST
ASEASY
ASFAST
ASLOSH
ASPISH
ASSESS
ASSISI
ASSIST
ATBEST
ATCOST
ATDUSK
ATEASE
ATLAST
ATMOST
ATREST
ATRISK
ATTEST
ATWIST
AUGUST
AURIST
AUTISM
AUTIST
AVERSE
AVULSE
AWLESS

A••••S

AARHUS
ABACAS
ABACUS
ABASES
ABATES
ABATIS
ABBESS
ABBEYS
ABBOTS
ABELES
ABHORS
ABIDES
ABMHOS
ABODES
ABOHMS
ABOMAS
ABOMBS
ABORTS
ABRAMS
ABUSES
ABYSMS
ACCESS
ACELAS
ACHERS
ACORNS
ACROSS
ACTORS
ACTSAS
ACURAS
ACUTES
ADAGES
ADAPTS
ADDAMS
ADDERS
ADDINS
ADDLES
ADDONS
ADEEMS
ADENIS
ADEPTS
ADFEES
ADIDAS
ADIEUS
ADLIBS
ADMINS
ADMITS
ADOBES
ADOBOS
ADONIS
ADOPTS
ADORES
ADORNS
ADOUTS
ADREPS
ADULTS
ADVILS
ADWARS
AENEAS
AEOLUS
AERIES
AERIOS
AESOPS
AFLATS
AFTERS
AGAMAS
AGAMES
AGATES
AGAVES
AGENAS
AGENTS
AGGIES
AGITAS
AGLETS
AGONES
AGORAS
AGREES
AIDERS
AIMERS
AIOLIS
AIRBUS
AIRERS
AISLES
AKELAS
AKENES
AKITAS
ALALAS
ALAMOS
ALANIS
ALARMS
ALBANS
ALBERS
ALBUMS
ALDERS
ALDISS
ALDOUS
ALECKS
ALEPHS
ALEROS
ALERTS
ALEUTS
ALEVES
ALEXAS
ALEXIS
ALIBIS
ALICES
ALIENS
ALIGNS
ALIKES
ALINES
ALISTS
ALKIES
ALKYDS
ALKYLS
ALLAIS
ALLAYS
ALLEES
ALLEYS
ALLIES
ALLOTS
ALLOWS
ALLOYS
ALLYLS
ALMVPS
ALOHAS
ALONGS
ALPHAS
ALTARS
ALTERS
ALTIUS
ALWAYS
AMADIS
AMANAS
AMANTS
AMATIS
AMAZES
AMBERS
AMBITS
AMBLES
AMEBAS
AMEERS
AMENDS
AMENTS
AMICES
AMICUS
AMIDAS
AMIDES
AMIENS
AMIGAS
AMIGOS
AMINES
AMINOS
AMINUS
AMNIOS
AMOLES
AMORES
AMOURS
AMUSES
AMVETS
ANANAS
ANCHOS
ANDERS
ANDRES
ANDROS
ANELES
ANGELS
ANGERS
ANGLES
ANGLOS
ANGSTS
ANIMAS
ANIMES
ANIMUS
ANIONS
ANISES
ANJOUS
ANKLES
ANNALS
ANNEES
ANNIES
ANNOYS
ANNULS
ANODES
ANOLES
ANSEIS
ANTICS
ANTRES
ANUBIS
ANVILS
ANYONS
ANZACS
AOLERS
AORTAS
APEXES
APHIDS
APICES
APNEAS
APPALS
APPELS
APPLES
APRILS
APRONS
ARADOS
ARAMES
ARAMIS
ARARAS
ARBORS
ARBRES
ARCCOS
ARCHES
ARDORS
ARECAS
ARENAS
ARETES
ARGOTS
ARGUES
ARHATS
ARISES
ARLISS
ARMERS
ARMETS
ARMIES
ARMORS
ARNEIS
ARNESS
ARNIES
AROIDS
AROMAS
ARPELS
ARRAYS
ARROWS
ARSONS
ARTELS
ARTOIS
ARYANS
ASANAS
ASCOTS
ASDICS
ASIANS
ASIDES
ASKERS
ASPENS
ASPICS
ASSAYS
ASSESS
ASSETS
ASTERS
ASTRES
ASTROS
ATARIS
ATBATS
ATEAMS
ATESTS
ATHENS
ATILES
ATISES
ATKINS
ATMANS
ATODDS
ATOLLS
ATONES
ATREUS
ATROIS
ATTARS
ATTICS
AUDIOS
AUDITS
AUGEAS
AUGERS
AUGHTS
AUGURS
AUROUS
AVAILS
AVERTS
AVIANS
AVISOS
AVOIDS
AVRILS
AWAITS
AWAKES
AWARDS
AWLESS
AXIOMS
AXIONS
AXISES
AXONES
AZERAS
AZERIS
AZIDES
AZOLES
AZORES
AZTECS
AZTEKS
AZUKIS
AZURES

•AS•••

BASALT
BASELY
BASEST
BASHED
BASHER
BASHES
BASHIN
BASIAL
BASICS
BASIFY
BASILS
BASING
BASINS
BASKED
BASKER
BASKET
BASKIN
BASQUE
BASRAH
BASSES
BASSET
BASSEY
BASSLY
BASSOS
BASTED
BASTER
BASTES
BASTIA
CASABA
CASALS
CASAVA
CASBAH
CASEFY
CASEIN
CASERN
CASERS
CASHED
CASHES
CASHEW
CASHIN
CASING
CASINO
CASIOS
CASITA
CASKED
CASKET
CASPAR
CASPER
CASQUE
CASSIA
CASSIE
CASSIM
CASSIN
CASSIO
CASSIS
CASTED
CASTEL
CASTER
CASTES
CASTLE
CASTON
CASTOR
CASTRO
CASTUP
CASUAL
DASHED
DASHER
DASHES
DASHIS
DASHIT
DASSIN
EASEBY
EASEIN
EASELS
EASEON
EASERS
EASEUP
EASIER
EASILY
EASING
EASLEY
EASTER
EASTLA
EASTON
EASYAS
EASYGO
FASCES
FASCIA
FASTED
FASTEN
FASTER
GASBAG
GASCAN
GASCAP
GASCON
GASHED
GASHES
GASHOG
GASIFY
GASJET
GASKET
GASLIT
GASLOG
GASMAN
GASMEN
GASOIL
GASPAR
GASPED
GASPER
GASSED
GASSER
GASSES
GASTAX
GASTER
GASTON
GASTRO
GASWAR
HASAGO
HASBRO
HASFUN
HASHED
HASHES
HASONE
HASOUT
HASPED
HASSAM
HASSAN
HASSEL
HASSID
HASSLE
HASTED
HASTEN
HASTES
JASCHA
JASMIN
JASPER
KASBAH
KASDAN
KASHAS
LASCAR
LASERS
LASHED
LASHER
LASHES
LASHTO
LASHUP
LASING
LASKER
LASSEN
LASSER
LASSES
LASSIE
LASSOS
LASTED
LASTEX
LASTLY
LASTRA
LASTUP
LASZLO
MASADA
MASAIS
MASALA
MASCOT
MASERS
MASERU
MASHED
MASHER
MASHES
MASHIE
MASHUP
MASKED
MASKER
MASLIN
MASONS
MASQUE
MASSED
MASSES
MASSEY
MASSIF
MASSON
MASSYS
MASTED
MASTER
MASTIC
NASALS
NASCAR
NASDAQ
NASEBY
NASHES
NASHUA
NASSAU
NASSER
PASCAL
PASCHS
PASCUA
PASDAR
PASEOS
PASHAS
PASHTO
PASMOI
PASSAS
PASSAT
PASSBY
PASSED
PASSEL
PASSER
PASSES
PASSGO
PASSIM
PASSON
PASSOS
PASSTO
PASSUP
PASTAS
PASTED
PASTEL
PASTER
PASTES
PASTIS
PASTIT
PASTOR
PASTRY
RASCAL
RASCHE
RASERS
RASHAD
RASHER
RASHES
RASHID
RASHLY
RASING
RASKIN
RASPAS
RASPED
RASPER
RASSES
RASSLE
RASTAS
RASTER
RASURE
SASEBO
SASHAY
SASHED
SASHES
SASSED
SASSER
SASSES
SASSON
TASERS
TASKED
TASKET
TASMAN
TASSEL
TASSES
TASTED
TASTEE
TASTER
TASTES
VASHTI
VASILY
VASLAV
VASSAL
VASSAR
VASTER
VASTLY
VASTUS
WASABI
WASECA
WASFUN
WASHAD
WASHED

WASHER
WASHES
WASHME
WASHOE
WASHOS
WASHUP
WASLED
WASMET
WASOFF
WASOLD
WASSER
WASTED
WASTER
WASTES
YASGUR
YASHIN
YASMIN
YASSER

•A•S••

BABSON
BAGSIT
BAISAS
BAKSHI
BALSAM
BALSAS
BASSES
BASSET
BASSEY
BASSLY
BASSOS
BATSIN
BATSON
BAUSCH
BAYSAT
CAESAR
CARSEY
CARSON
CASSIA
CASSIE
CASSIM
CASSIN
CASSIO
CASSIS
CATSAT
CATSIT
CATSUP
CAUSAL
CAUSED
CAUSER
CAUSES
DABSAT
DAISES
DAMSEL
DAMSON
DAMSUP
DANSES
DANSON
DAOSTA
DASSIN
DATSUN
DAWSON
DAYSPA
EATSAT
EATSIN
EATSIT
EATSOF
EATSUP
FAISAL
FALSER
FATSIS
GARSON
GASSED
GASSER
GASSES
GATSBY
HALSEY
HAMSUN
HAMSUP
HANSAS
HANSEL
HANSES
HANSOM
HANSON
HASSAM
HASSAN
HASSEL
HASSID
HASSLE
HAWSER
HAWSES
IAMSAM
JAMSIN
JAMSUP
JANSEN
JAWSAT
KAISER
KANSAN
KANSAS
KARSTS
LAMSIT
LANSKY
LANSON
LAPSAT
LAPSED
LAPSER
LAPSES
LAPSUP
LAPSUS
LARSEN
LARSON
LASSEN
LASSER
LASSES
LASSIE
LASSOS
LAWSON
LAYSBY
LAYSIN
LAYSON
LAYSTO
LAYSUP
MADSEN
MAISIE
MAISON
MAKSIM
MANSES
MARSHA
MARSHY
MASSED
MASSES
MASSEY
MASSIF
MASSON
MASSYS
MATSON
MATSUI
MATSUO
MAUSER
MAWSON
MAXSON
NADSAT
NAGSAT
NANSEN
NASSAU
NASSER
NAUSEA
NAYSAY
PABSTS
PAISAN
PAISES
PANSIN
PARSEC
PARSED
PARSEE
PARSER
PARSES
PARSON
PASSAS
PASSAT
PASSBY
PASSED
PASSEL
PASSER
PASSES
PASSGO
PASSIM
PASSON
PASSOS
PASSTO
PASSUP
PAUSAL
PAUSED
PAUSER
PAUSES
PAWSAT
PAYSIN
PAYSON
PAYSUP
RAGSON
RAISED
RAISER
RAISES
RAISIN
RAISON
RAMSAY
RAMSES
RAMSEY
RAMSIN
RAMSON
RANSOM
RAPSON
RASSES
RASSLE
RATSON
SAISON
SALSAS
SAMSON
SANSEI
SASSED
SASSER
SASSES
SASSON
SAWSUP
SAYSAH
SAYSHI
SAYSNO
SAYSOK
SAYSOS
SAYSSO
TABSET
TAGSON
TAGSUP
TAOSNM
TAPSIN
TAPSON
TARSAL
TARSUS
TASSEL
TASSES
VALSES
VASSAL
VASSAR
WADSUP
WAISTS
WARSAW
WASSER
WATSON
WAUSAU
WAYSIN
YAPSAT
YASSER
YATSEN

•A••S•

BALLST
BANISH
BAREST
BASEST
CALASH
CAMISE
CARESS
CARUSO
CAYUSE
DALASI
DAMASK
DANISH
DAREST
FAMISH
GAINST
GALOSH
GAMEST
GARISH
GAYEST
HALEST
HARASS
HAVASU
JADISH
JAMESA
JAMESI
JAMESJ
JAMESK
JAMESM
JAMESS
JAMEST
JAMESV
LACASA
LAKIST
LAMESA
LAMEST
LANOSE
LAOTSE
LAROSA
LATEST
LATISH
LAVISH
LAXEST
MAINST
MANUSH
MAOISM
MAOIST
MARISA
MARIST
MAYEST
OAFISH
PALEST
PALISH
PAPIST
PARISH
PAVESE
RACISM
RACIST
RADISH
RAGUSA
RAKISH
RAMOSE
RAREST
RAVISH
RAWEST
RAWISH
RAWIST
SADISM
SADIST
SAFEST
SAGEST
SAIDSO
SALISH
SAMOSA
SANEST
SAYEST
SAYSSO
TALESE
TALISA
TAMEST
TAOISM
TAOIST
TAVIST
VALISE
VANISH
VARESE
WABASH
WALESA
WALLST
WATUSI
YAREST

•A•••S

AARHUS
BABELS
BABIES
BABKAS
BABOOS
BACHES
BACKUS
BACONS
BADEMS
BADGES
BADUNS
BAGELS
BAINES
BAIRNS
BAISAS
BAIZAS
BAIZES
BAKERS
BALERS
BALLYS
BALSAS
BAMBIS
BANCOS
BANJOS
BANONS
BANTUS
BARCOS
BARGES
BARNES
BARONS
BARRES
BARRIS
BASHES
BASICS
BASILS
BASINS
BASSES
BASSOS
BASTES
BATHES
BATHOS
BATIKS
BATONS
BAULKS
BAYOUS
BAZOOS
CABALS
CABERS
CABINS
CABLES
CACAOS
CACHES
CACTUS
CADETS
CADGES
CADMUS
CADRES
CAGERS
CAGUAS
CAICOS
CAIRNS
CAJUNS
CALAIS
CALIFS
CALLAS
CALLES
CALLUS
CALVES
CALXES
CAMEAS
CAMELS
CAMEOS
CAMOES
CAMPOS
CAMPUS
CAMRYS
CANALS
CANERS
CANIDS
CANNAS
CANNES
CANOES
CANONS
CANTOS
CANVAS
CAPERS
CAPONS
CAPRIS
CARATS
CARBOS
CARERS
CARESS
CARETS
CARGOS
CARIBS
CARIES
CARLOS
CARNES
CAROBS
CAROLS
CAROMS
CARPUS
CARTES
CARVES
CASALS
CASERS
CASHES
CASIOS
CASSIS
CASTES
CATERS
CATHYS
CAUCUS
CAULKS
CAUSES
CAVERS
CAVIES
CAVILS
DACHAS
DADDYS
DADOES
DAISES
DALETS
DALLAS
DALLES
DANCES
DANIOS
DANNYS
DANSES
DANTES
DARERS
DARIUS
DASHES
DASHIS
DATERS
DAUBES
DAUNTS
DAVENS
DAVIES
DAVITS
DAZERS
EAGLES
EAGRES
EAKINS
EARTHS
EASELS
EASERS
EASYAS
EATERS
FABLES
FACERS
FACETS
FACIAS
FACIES
FADERS
FAENAS
FAGINS
FAGOTS
FAINTS
FAITES
FAITHS
FAKERS
FAKIRS
FAMOUS
FANONS
FANTAS
FAQIRS
FARADS
FARAHS
FARCES
FARERS
FAROES
FARRIS
FASCES
FATSIS
FATWAS
FAULTS
FAUNAS
FAUNUS
FAUTES
FAUVES
FAVORS
FAWKES
FAXERS
GABLES
GADDIS
GAFFES
GAINES
GALOIS
GALOPS
GAMAYS
GAMERS
GAMINS
GAMMAS
GAMOUS
GAMUTS
GANEFS
GANGES
GAPERS
GASHES
GASSES
GATERS
GATORS
GAUGES
GAUZES
GAVELS
GAVOTS
GAVRAS
GAYNES
GAZERS
HABEAS
HABITS
HACEKS
HADJES
HADJIS
HAGGIS
HAIDAS
HAIKUS
HAINES
HAJJES
HAJJIS
HAKIMS
HALLOS
HALOES
HALVAS
HALVES
HANSAS
HANSES
HAOLES
HARASS
HAREMS
HARRIS
HARRYS
HASHES
HASTES
HATERS
HAUNTS
HAVENS
HAVOCS
HAWSES
HAYERS
HAYMES
HAYNES
HAZANS
HAZELS
HAZERS
IAMBUS
JABOTS
JACALS
JALPAS
JAMAIS
JAMBES
JAMESS
JAMUPS
JANHUS
JAPANS
JAPERS
JAUNES
JAUNTS
JAURES
JAVITS
JAYMES
JAZZES
KABOBS
KANJIS
KANSAS
KAPOKS
KAPPAS
KARATS
KARMAS
KARRAS
KARSTS
KASHAS
KAUNAS
KAYAKS
KAZOOS
LABELS
LABORS
LACERS
LACLOS
LADERS
LADIES
LADLES
LAGERS
LAIRDS
LAKERS
LAMEDS
LAMIAS
LANAIS
LANCES
LANDIS
LANDUS
LANTOS
LAPELS
LAPINS
LAPSES
LAPSUS
LARAMS
LAREES
LARGES
LARGOS
LARVAS
LASERS
LASHES
LASSES
LASSOS
LATENS
LATHES
LATINS
LATKES
LATTES
LAUGHS
LAVERS
LAYBYS
LAYERS
LAYINS
LAYUPS
MACAWS
MACERS
MACHOS
MACLES
MACROS
MADAMS
MADRAS
MADRES
MAFIAS
MAGICS
MAGMAS
MAGNUS
MAHDIS
MAIRES
MAIZES
MAJLIS
MAJORS
MAKERS
MALARS
MALAYS
MAMBAS
MAMBOS
MAMMAS
MANAOS
MANATS
MANDMS
MANETS
MANGAS
MANGOS
MANIAS
MANNAS
MANORS
MANSES
MANTAS
MANTIS
MAORIS
MAPLES
MAQUIS
MARCOS
MARCUS
MARDIS
MARIAS
MARKAS
MARTES
MARVIS
MARXES
MASAIS
MASERS
MASHES
MASONS
MASSES
MASSYS
MATERS
MATEYS
MATHIS
MATINS
MATJES
MATTES
MATZOS
MAUVES
MAVENS
MAVINS
MAXIMS
MAYANS
MAYBES
MAYORS
MAZDAS
NABOBS
NABORS
NACHAS
NACHOS
NACRES
NADIRS
NAIADS
NAIRAS
NAKFAS
NAMERS
NANTES
NAPLES
NAPPES
NARCOS
NASALS
NASHES
NAUTES
NAVELS
NAVIES
OAKUMS
OARERS
OATERS
PABSTS
PACERS
PADRES
PAEANS
PAGANS
PAGERS
PAINTS
PAISES
PALAIS
PALLAS
PALMAS
PAMIRS
PAMPAS
PANCKS
PANDAS
PANDLS
PANELS
PANICS
PANNES
PANTOS
PAPAWS
PAPERS
PAPPAS
PARENS
PARERS
PAREUS
PARGES
PARKAS
PARKES
PARNIS
PAROLS
PARRIS
PARSES
PARTYS
PASCHS
PASEOS
PASHAS
PASSAS
PASSES
PASSOS
PASTAS
PASTES
PASTIS
PATENS
PATERS
PATHOS
PATIOS
PATMOS
PATOIS
PAUSES
PAVERS
PAWERS
PAYEES
PAYERS
QANTAS
RABBIS
RABIES
RACERS
RADARS
RADIOS
RADIUS
RAGERS
RAINES
RAISES
RAITAS
RAJABS
RAJAHS
RAKERS
RAMBOS
RAMENS
RAMETS
RAMFIS
RAMIES
RAMSES
RANEES
RANGES
RANIDS
RAPIDS
RAPTUS
RAREES
RASERS
RASHES
RASPAS
RASSES
RASTAS
RATELS
RATERS
RATIOS
RAVELS
RAVENS
RAVERS
RAYONS
RAZERS
RAZORS
RAZZES
SABALS
SABERS
SABLES
SABOTS
SABRAS
SABRES
SADHES
SADHUS
SAHIBS
SAINTS
SALADS
SALEPS
SALLES
SALMIS
SALONS
SALSAS
SALVES
SALVOS
SAMBAS
SAMEAS
SANKAS
SANTAS
SANTOS
SANYOS
SAPORS
SARANS
SARDIS
SAREES
SARGES
SASHES
SASSES
SATAYS
SATINS
SATYRS
SAUCES
SAUDIS
SAULTS
SAUNAS
SAURUS
SAUTES
SAVEAS
SAVERS
SAVORS
SAWERS
SAXONS
SAYERS
SAYLES
SAYSOS
SAYYES
TABLAS
TABLES
TABOOS
TABORS
TAHOES
TAIGAS
TAINTS
TAKERS
TALERS
TALONS
TALTOS
TAMERS
TAMILS
TANGOS
TANKAS
TANTES
TAPERS
TAPINS
TAPIRS
TARDES
TARGAS
TAROTS
TARSUS
TARTES
TASERS
TASSES
TASTES
TATARS
TATERS
TATRAS
TAUNTS
TAUONS
TAUPES
TAURUS
TAVELS
TAXERS
TAXIES
TAXOLS
VACHES
VALAIS
VALENS
VALETS
VALOIS
VALORS
VALSES
VALUES
VALVES
VANNES
VAPORS
VARGAS
VARIAS
VARIES
VARMUS
VARNAS
VASTUS
VAULTS
VAUNTS
WACKOS
WADERS
WAFERS
WAGERS
WAGONS
WAHOOS
WAISTS
WAIVES
WAKENS
WAKERS
WALLIS
WALRUS
WARNES
WASHES
WASHOS
WASTES
WATERS
WAVERS
WAXERS
WAYANS
WAYNES
YACHTS
YAHOOS
YAKUTS
YALIES
YAQUIS
ZAIRES
ZANIES
ZAYINS
ZAZENS

••AS••

ABASED
ABASER
ABASES
AGASSI
ALASKA
BEASTS
BIASED
BIASES
BLASTS
BOASTS
BRASCO
BRASHY
BRASIL
BRASOV
BRASSY
CEASED
CEASES
CHASED
CHASER
CHASES
CHASMS
CHASSE
CHASTE
CIASPY
CLASPS
CLASSA
CLASSE
CLASSY
COASTS
DEASIL
DNASES
DOASET
ERASED
ERASER
ERASES
FEASTS
FIASCO
FLASHY
FLASKS
FRASER
GLASER
GLASSY
GRASPS
GRASSO
GRASSY
INASEC
ITASCA
KRASNA
LEASED
LEASER
LEASES
LEASTS
LHASAN
MEASLE

MEASLY
MIASMA
OCASEK
OCASEY
OMASUM
PHASED
PHASER
PHASES
PHASIC
PLASHY
PLASMA
PLASMO
QUASAR
REASKS
REASON
ROASTS
SEASON
SHASTA
SOASTO
SPASMS
STASES
STASIS
TEASED
TEASEL
TEASER
TEASES
TEASET
TOASTS
TOASTY
TRASHY
UKASES
VLASIC
WEASEL
WRASSE
XMASES
YEASTS
YEASTY

••A•S•

AGASSI
BEARSE
BLAISE
BRAISE
BRASSY
BRATSK
CHAISE
CHASSE
CLASSA
CLASSE
CLASSY
CLAUSE
COARSE
DIALSO
DNAASE
ELAPSE
FRAISE
GDANSK
GLASSY
GRASSO
GRASSY
HEARSE
HEARST
HOARSE
ICANSO
IRAISE
KRAUSS
LIAISE
PRAISE
RNAASE
SCAASI
SPARSE
URALSK
USAUSA
WRASSE
ZSAZSA

••A••S

ABACAS
ABACUS
ABASES
ABATES
ABATIS
ADAGES
ADAPTS
AGAMAS
AGAMES
AGATES
AGAVES
ALALAS
ALAMOS
ALANIS
ALARMS
AMADIS
AMANAS
AMANTS
AMATIS
AMAZES
ANANAS
ARADOS
ARAMES
ARAMIS
ARARAS
ASANAS
ATARIS
AVAILS
AWAITS
AWAKES
AWARDS
BEALLS
BEANOS
BEARDS
BEASTS
BEAUTS
BEAVIS
BHANGS
BIASES
BLACKS
BLADES
BLAFFS
BLAMES
BLANKS
BLARES
BLASTS
BLAZES
BOARDS
BOASTS
BRACES
BRACHS
BRACTS
BRAHMS
BRAIDS
BRAINS
BRAKES
BRANDS
BRANTS
BRAVAS
BRAVES
BRAVOS
BRAWLS
BRAZOS
BWANAS
CEASES
CHAFES
CHAFFS
CHAINS
CHAIRS
CHALKS
CHAMPS
CHANTS
CHARDS
CHARMS
CHARTS
CHASES
CHASMS
CLACKS
CLAIMS
CLAIRS
CLAMPS
CLANGS
CLANKS
CLAROS
CLASPS
CLAVES
COACTS
COAPTS
COASTS
COATES
COATIS
COAXES
CRACKS
CRAFTS
CRAINS
CRAKES
CRAMPS
CRANES
CRANKS
CRAPES
CRATES
CRAVES
CRAWLS
CRAZES
DBACKS
DEAIRS
DEATHS
DMARKS
DNASES
DOAKES
DOALLS
DRAFTS
DRAINS
DRAKES
DRAMAS
DRAPES
DRAWLS
DWARFS
EBANKS
EBATES
ECARDS
EDAMES
EGALES
ELANDS
ELATES
EMAILS
EMALLS
ENACTS
ENARMS
ENATES
EPACTS
ERASES
ETAGES
ETAILS
ETAPES
EVADES
EXACTS
EXALTS
FEASTS
FLACKS
FLAILS
FLAIRS
FLAKES
FLAMES
FLANKS
FLARES
FLASKS
FLAXES
FRACAS
FRAKES
FRAMES
FRANCS
FRANKS
FRAUDS
GHAINS
GHAZIS
GIANTS
GLACES
GLACIS
GLADES
GLADYS
GLANDS
GLARES
GLARUS
GLAZES
GNARLS
GNARRS
GRACES
GRADES
GRAFTS
GRAILS
GRAINS
GRAMPS
GRANDS
GRANTS
GRAPES
GRAPHS
GRASPS
GRATES
GRATIS
GRAVAS
GRAVES
GRAZES
GUANOS
GUARDS
GUAVAS
HEARNS
HEARTS
HEATHS
HEAVES
HIATUS
HOARDS
HOAXES
HYADES
HYATTS
ICARUS
IDAHOS
IMAGES
IMAGOS
IMAXES
INAGES
IRANIS
IRAQIS
ISAACS
KEARNS
KHAKIS
KMARTS
KNACKS
KNARRS
KNAVES
KOALAS
KRAALS
KRAITS
KRAUSS
KRAVIS
LEARNS
LEASES
LEASTS
LEAVES
LIANAS
LIANES
LIANGS
LLAMAS
LLANOS
LOAVES
LWAVES
MEATUS
MIAMIS
MIAOUS
MIAOWS
MIATAS
NBAERS
NYALAS
OKAPIS
OLAKES
OMAHAS
OMANIS
ORACHS
ORALES
ORANGS
ORANIS
ORANTS
ORATES
OSAGES
OXALIS
OZARKS
PEALES
PEARLS
PHAROS
PHASES
PIANOS
PLACES
PLAGES
PLAIDS
PLAINS
PLAITS
PLANAS
PLANBS
PLANES
PLANKS
PLANTS
PLATES
PLATOS
PLATYS
PLAYAS
PLAZAS
PRADAS
PRANAS
PRANKS
PRATES
PRAWNS
PRAXES
PRAXIS
PSALMS
QUACKS
QUAFFS
QUAILS
QUAKES
QUALES
QUALMS
QUARKS
QUARTS
REACTS
READDS
REAIMS
REAIRS
REALES
REALMS
REARMS
REASKS
REATAS
REAVES
RHAMES
RIATAS
ROASTS
SCAGGS
SCALDS
SCALES
SCALPS
SCAMPS
SCANTS
SCARES
SCARFS
SCARPS
SEALYS
SEAMUS
SHACKS
SHADES
SHAFTS
SHAKES
SHAKOS
SHALES
SHAMES
SHAMUS
SHANKS
SHAPES
SHARDS
SHARES
SHARKS
SHARPS
SHAVES
SHAWLS
SKAGGS
SKALDS
SKANKS
SKATES
SLACKS
SLAKES
SLANGS
SLANTS
SLATES
SLAVES
SMACKS
SMALLS
SMARTS
SMAZES
SNACKS
SNAFUS
SNAILS
SNAKES
SNARES
SNARFS
SNARKS
SNARLS
SNATHS
SOAVES
SPACES
SPADES
SPANKS
SPARES
SPARKS
SPASMS
SPATES
SPAWNS
STACKS
STAFFS
STAGES
STAINS
STAIRS
STAKES
STALES
STALKS
STALLS
STAMOS
STAMPS
STANDS
STAPES
STAPHS
STARES
STARTS
STASES
STASIS
STATES
STATUS
STAVES
SWAINS
SWALES
SWAMIS
SWAMPS
SWANNS
SWARDS
SWARMS
SWATHS
TEASES
THALES
THAMES
THANES
THANKS
THATIS
TIARAS
TOASTS
TRACES
TRACKS
TRACTS
TRADES
TRAGUS
TRAILS
TRAINS
TRAITS
TRALAS
TRAMPS
TRANES
TRAVES
TRAVIS
TRAWLS
TSADES
TSADIS
TWAINS
TWANGS
UHAULS
UKASES
UNAMIS
UNARMS
URAEUS
URANUS
USAGES
UTAHNS
VIANDS
WEALDS
WEAVES
WHACKS
WHALES
WHANGS
WHARFS
WRACKS
WRATHS
XGAMES
XMASES
XSARAS
YEARNS
YEASTS

•••AS•

AGHAST
ALEAST
ALNASL
ASEASY
ASFAST
ATEASE
ATLAST
BREAST
BROAST
BYPASS
BYPAST
CALASH
CDCASE
CREASE
CREASY
DALASI
DAMASK
DEBASE
DEMAST
DNAASE
DYNAST
ECLASS
ELPASO
EMDASH
ENCASE
ENDASH
EZPASS
FLYASH
GOEASY
GOFAST
GOLAST
GOPAST
GREASE
GREASY
HARASS
HAVASU
IMEASY
INCASE
INCASH
INDASH
KUVASZ
LACASA
LIPASE
MIKASA
MORASS
MUFASA
NLEAST
OBLAST
ONBASE
OUTASK
PHRASE
PLEASE
POTASH
QUEASY
RECASE
RECAST
REHASH
REPASS
REPAST
REWASH
RNAASE
SCAASI
SPLASH
SQUASH
THEASP
THRASH
TOLAST
UNCASE
UNCASK
UNCAST
UNEASE
UNEASY
UNHASP
UNLASH
UNMASK
UNMAST
UNRASH
UPCAST
UPLAST
WABASH
ZYMASE

•••A•S

ABRAMS
ADDAMS
ADWARS
AFLATS
ALBANS
ALLAIS
ALLAYS
ALTARS
ALWAYS
ANNALS
ANZACS
APPALS
ARHATS
ARRAYS
ARYANS
ASIANS
ASSAYS
ATBATS
ATEAMS
ATMANS
ATTARS
AVIANS
BELAYS
BEVANS
BFLATS
BLEAKS
BLEARS
BLEATS
BLOATS
BOYARS
BREADS
BREAKS
BREAMS
BRIARS
BSTARS
BTEAMS
BYLAWS
BYPASS
BYWAYS
CABALS
CACAOS
CALAIS
CANALS
CARATS
CASALS
CEDARS
CESARS
CFLATS
CHEATS
CIGARS
CLEANS
CLEARS
CLEATS
CLOAKS
COHABS
COPALS
COPAYS
CORALS
COTANS
CREAKS
CREAMS
CROAKS
CROATS
CSTARS
CUBANS
CURADS
CYCADS
DEBAGS
DEBARS
DECADS
DECAFS
DECALS
DECAPS
DECAYS
DEDANS
DEFATS
DELAYS
DENARS
DERATS
DETARS
DEWARS
DFLATS
DINARS
DIRAMS
DIVANS
DOLAPS
DORAGS
DREADS
DREAMS
DRYADS
DUCATS
EBOATS
ECLASS
ECLATS
EDGARS
EFLATS
ELPAIS
EMBARS
EMBAYS
EMMAUS
ENIACS
EPHAHS
EQUALS
ESBATS
ESSAIS
ESSAYS
EXPATS
EZPASS
FARADS
FARAHS
FERALS
FFLATS
FINALS
FLOATS
FORAYS
FREAKS
FRIARS
FSTARS
GAMAYS
GFLATS
GLEAMS
GLEANS
GLOATS
GREATS
GROANS
GROATS
GSTARS
GULAGS
HARASS
HAZANS
HBEAMS
HEXADS
HIHATS
HODADS
HOGANS
HUMANS
IBEAMS
IDEALS
IDTAGS
ILIADS
INCANS
INCAPS
INLAWS
INLAYS
INRAGS
IOWANS
ISAACS
JACALS
JAMAIS
JAPANS
JIHADS
JONAHS
KARATS
KAYAKS
KEBABS
KNEADS
KODAKS
KORANS
KORATS
KOVACS
KRAALS
KSTARS
KULAKS
LANAIS
LARAMS
LBEAMS
LEGALS
LEMANS
LILACS
LIMANS
LOCALS
LOGANS
LORANS
MACAWS
MADAMS
MALARS
MALAYS
MANAOS
MANATS
MASAIS
MAYANS
MEDALS
METALS
MILANS
MODALS
MOLARS
MONADS
MORALS
MORASS
MORAYS
MRPAWS
MSTARS
MURALS
MYLARS
MYNAHS
NAIADS
NASALS
NICADS
NISANS
NOMADS
NOPALS
NOWAYS
NSTARS
OBEAHS
OCCAMS
OCEANS
OCTADS
OCTANS
OFFALS
OGHAMS
ONLAYS
OPRAHS
OREADS
ORGANS
ORKANS
OSCANS
OSCARS
OSTARS
PAEANS
PAGANS
PALAIS
PAPAWS
PCLABS
PECANS
PEDALS
PETALS
PHIALS
PILAFS
PILAUS
PISANS
PLEADS
PLEATS
PROAMS
PSHAWS
PTRAPS
RADARS
RAJABS
RAJAHS
REBAGS
REBARS
RECANS
RECAPS
REDANS
REHABS
RELAPS
RELAYS
REMANS
REMAPS
REMATS
REPADS
REPASS
REPAYS
RESAWS
RESAYS
RETAGS
RETANS
RETAPS
RETARS
RICANS
RIGANS
RIVALS
RIYALS
ROMANS
ROWANS
ROYALS
SABALS
SALADS
SARANS
SATAYS
SCHAVS
SCRAGS
SCRAMS
SCRAPS
SEDANS
SENATS
SEPALS
SERACS
SERAIS
SHEARS
SHOALS
SHOATS
SISALS
SITARS
SIVANS
SKOALS
SMEARS
SNEAKS
SOLANS
SONARS
SPEAKS
SPEARS
SPLATS
SPLAYS
SPRATS
SPRAYS
SQUABS
SQUADS
SQUATS
SSTARS
STEADS
STEAKS
STEALS
STEAMS
STOATS
STPATS
STRADS
STRAPS
STRATS
STRAWS
STRAYS
SUGARS
SUMACS
SURAHS
SWEARS
SWEATS
TATARS
TEXANS
TICALS
TILAKS
TITANS
TODAYS
TOKAYS
TOLARS
TORAHS
TOTALS
TREADS
TREATS
TRIADS
TRIALS
TWEAKS
UBOATS
UCLANS
UGGAMS
UHLANS
UMIAKS
UNBAGS
UNBARS
UNCAPS
UNDAMS
UNGAGS
UNHATS
UNIATS
UNJAMS
UNLAYS
UNMANS
UNSAYS
USUALS
UVRAYS
VALAIS
VEGANS
VELARS
VICARS
VITALS
VOCABS
VOCALS
VOLANS
WAYANS
WEBADS
WHEATS
WINANS
WOMANS
WREAKS
YUMANS

••••AS

ABACAS
ABOMAS
ACELAS
ACTSAS
ACURAS
ADIDAS
AENEAS
AGAMAS
AGENAS
AGITAS
AGORAS
AKELAS
AKITAS
ALALAS
ALEXAS
ALOHAS
ALPHAS
AMANAS
AMEBAS
AMIDAS
AMIGAS
ANANAS
ANIMAS
AORTAS
APNEAS
ARARAS
ARECAS
ARENAS
AROMAS
ASANAS
AUGEAS
AZERAS
BABKAS
BAISAS
BAIZAS
BALSAS
BETTAS
BIOGAS
BIOTAS
BOLLAS
BOREAS
BRAVAS
BROCAS
BUBBAS
BUENAS
BURKAS
BURSAS
BWANAS
CAGUAS
CALLAS
CAMEAS
CANNAS
CANVAS
CEIBAS
CENTAS
CESTAS
CHICAS
CHINAS
CHIVAS
CIERAS
COBRAS
COCOAS

COMEAS
COMMAS
COMPAS
CONGAS
COPRAS
CORSAS
COSMAS
COSTAS
COTTAS
CUICAS
CUPPAS
DACHAS
DALLAS
DELTAS
DERMAS
DINKAS
DISMAS
DJILAS
DOGMAS
DOLMAS
DORCAS
DOULAS
DRAMAS
DUENAS
DUNDAS
DURRAS
EASYAS
EDEMAS
ERICAS
ESDRAS
EVENAS
EXTRAS
FACIAS
FAENAS
FANTAS
FATWAS
FAUNAS
FELLAS
FERIAS
FESTAS
FINCAS
FLORAS
FONDAS
FORTAS
FRACAS
FRITAS
GAMMAS
GAVRAS
GENOAS
GOUDAS
GRAVAS
GUAVAS
GYOZAS
HABEAS
HAIDAS
HALVAS
HANSAS
HELLAS
HENNAS
HONDAS
HOOHAS
HOSTAS
HYDRAS
HYENAS
JALPAS
JETTAS
JUNTAS
JUSTAS

KANSAS
KAPPAS
KARMAS
KARRAS
KASHAS
KAUNAS
KIOWAS
KOALAS
LAMIAS
LARVAS
LEHUAS
LEICAS
LEMMAS
LIANAS
LIBRAS
LLAMAS
LOOFAS
LOUMAS
LYCRAS
MADRAS
MAFIAS
MAGMAS
MAMBAS
MAMMAS
MANGAS
MANIAS
MANNAS
MANTAS
MARIAS
MARKAS
MAZDAS
MECCAS
MEDIAS
MIATAS
MOCHAS
MOMMAS
MONZAS
MUCHAS
MULLAS
NACHAS
NAIRAS
NAKFAS
NICIAS
NIETAS
NINJAS
NOKIAS
NONGAS
NORIAS
NOVIAS
NYALAS
OMAHAS
OMEGAS
OPERAS
OUIJAS
OUTGAS
PALLAS
PALMAS
PAMPAS
PANDAS
PAPPAS
PARKAS
PASHAS
PASSAS
PASTAS
PIETAS
PINNAS
PIZZAS
PLANAS

PLAYAS
PLAZAS
POLKAS
PONCAS
POPPAS
POSEAS
PRADAS
PRANAS
PROYAS
PUNKAS
PUNTAS
QANTAS
QUOTAS
RAITAS
RASPAS
RASTAS
REATAS
REINAS
RENGAS
RIATAS
RIOJAS
RUMBAS
SABRAS
SALSAS
SAMBAS
SAMEAS
SANKAS
SANTAS
SAUNAS
SAVEAS
SCENAS
SCHWAS
SCUBAS
SEENAS
SEESAS
SENNAS
SEPIAS
SERTAS
SIGMAS
SILVAS
SOLEAS
SOONAS
STELAS
STOLAS
STOMAS
STUKAS
STUPAS
SUCHAS
SULFAS
SUNDAS
SUPRAS
SUTRAS
TABLAS
TAIGAS
TANKAS
TARGAS
TATRAS
TESLAS
TETRAS
THETAS
THOMAS
TIARAS
TIBIAS
TIKKAS
TOBIAS
TOKLAS
TONKAS
TORTAS

TRALAS
TYPEAS
UINTAS
ULTRAS
UMBRAS
UNITAS
UVULAS
VARGAS
VARIAS
VARNAS
VENTAS
VESPAS
VESTAS
VIGIAS
VILLAS
VIOLAS
VIRGAS
VISTAS
VODKAS
XHOSAS
XSARAS
YENTAS
YUCCAS
ZEBRAS
ZESTAS

AT••••

ATALOW
ATAMAN
ATARIS
ATAVIC
ATAXIA
ATAXIC
ATBATS
ATBEST
ATCOST
ATDAWN
ATDUSK
ATEAMS
ATEASE
ATEMPO
ATENTH
ATEOUT
ATERRE
ATESTS
ATFIVE
ATFOUR
ATHAND
ATHEEL
ATHENA
ATHENE
ATHENS
ATHING
ATHOME
ATHROB
ATHROW
ATILES
ATISES
ATKINS
ATLAST
ATMANS
ATMFEE
ATMOST
ATNINE
ATNOON
ATODDS
ATOLLS
ATOMIC
ATONAL
ATONCE
ATONED
ATONER
ATONES
ATONIA
ATONIC
ATONOF
ATOXIC
ATPLAY
ATRAIN
ATREST
ATREUS
ATRIAL
ATRISK
ATRIUM
ATROIS
ATSIGN
ATSTUD
ATTACH
ATTACK
ATTAIN
ATTARS
ATTEND
ATTEST
ATTHAT
ATTICA
ATTICS
ATTILA
ATTIRE
ATTLEE
ATTRIT
ATTUNE
ATWILL
ATWIST
ATWOOD
ATWORK
ATYALE
ATYPIC

A•T•••

ACTFOR
ACTIII
ACTING
ACTION
ACTIUM
ACTIVA
ACTIVE
ACTNOW
ACTONE
ACTORS
ACTOUT
ACTSAS
ACTSIN
ACTSON
ACTSUP
ACTTWO
ACTUAL
AETHER
AFTERS
ALTAIC
ALTAIR
ALTARF
ALTARS
ALTERS
ALTHEA
ALTIMA
ALTIUS
ALTKEY
ALTMAN
ALTOID
ALTRIA
ALTTAB
AMTRAC
AMTRAK
ANTAWN
ANTCOW
ANTEED
ANTERO
ANTEUP
ANTHEM
ANTHER
ANTICS
ANTIGO
ANTLER
ANTLIA
ANTONE
ANTONY
ANTRAL
ANTRES
ANTRIM
ANTRON
ANTRUM
APTEST
ARTAUD
ARTCAR
ARTELS
ARTERY
ARTEST
ARTFUL
ARTGUM
ARTHRO
ARTHUR
ARTIER
ARTILY
ARTIST
ARTOIS
ARTURO
ASTALL
ASTANA
ASTARE
ASTART
ASTEAL
ASTEEP
ASTERN
ASTERO
ASTERS
ASTHER
ASTHMA
ASTLEY
ASTOOP
ASTRAL
ASTRAY
ASTRES
ASTRID
ASTROS
ASTROV
ASTRUD
ASTUTE
ATTACH
ATTACK
ATTAIN
ATTARS
ATTEND
ATTEST
ATTHAT
ATTICA
ATTICS
ATTILA
ATTIRE
ATTLEE
ATTRIT
ATTUNE
AUTEUR
AUTHOR
AUTISM
AUTIST
AUTOED
AUTUMN
AZTECA
AZTECS
AZTEKS

A••T••

ABATED
ABATER
ABATES
ABATIS
ABATOR
ABITOF
ABUTON
ACCTNO
ACETAL
ACETIC
ACETYL
ACTTWO
ACUTER
ACUTES
ADYTUM
AGATES
AGATHA
AGETEN
AGETWO
AGITAS
AINTSO
AKITAS
ALATED
ALETAP
ALETTE
ALOTOF
ALSTON
ALTTAB
AMATIS
AMATOL
AMITIE
AMSTEL
AMYTAN
ANATTO
ANITRA
AORTAE
AORTAL
AORTAS
AORTIC
APATHY
ARCTAN
ARCTIC
ARETES
ARETHA
ARETOO
ASHTON
ASSTDA
ATSTUD
AUNTEM
AUNTIE
AUSTEN
AUSTER
AUSTIN
AUSTRO
AVATAR
AYRTON

A•••T•

ABBOTS
ABBOTT
ABLATE
ABORTS
ACUATE
ACUITY
ADAPTS
ADDSTO
ADEPTS
ADESTE
ADMITS
ADNATE
ADOPTS
ADOUTS
ADRATE
ADULTS
AERATE
AFIFTH
AFLATS
AGENTJ
AGENTK
AGENTS
AGLETS
AGNATE
AGOSTO
AGOUTI
AKINTO
ALCOTT
ALECTO
ALERTS
ALETTE
ALEUTS
ALIOTH
ALIOTO
ALISTS
ALLOTS
ALMATY
ALRITZ
AMANTI
AMANTS
AMBITS
AMENTS
AMINTA
AMONTH
AMRITA
AMVETS
ANATTO
ANGSTS
ANSATE
APLITE
ARGOTS
ARHATS
ARISTA
ARISTO
ARMETS
ARNETT
ARRETE
ASANTE
ASCOTS
ASSETS
ASTUTE
ATBATS
ATENTH
ATESTS
AUDITS
AUGHTS
AUGITE
AURATE
AVANTI
AVERTS
AVESTA
AVIATE
AWAITS

A••••T

ABBOTT
ABDUCT
ABJECT
ABLEST
ABRUPT
ABSENT
ACCENT
ACCEPT
ACCOST
ACEDIT
ACEOUT
ACESIT
ACQUIT
ACTOUT
ADDICT
ADDUCT
ADJUST
ADRIFT
ADROIT
ADVENT
ADVERT
AFFECT
AFLOAT
AGEIST
AGEOUT
AGHAST
AGLINT
AGOROT
AIGLET
AIGRET
AIMSAT
AIROUT
AIRPOT
AJFOYT
ALBEIT
ALBERT
ALCOTT
ALEAST
ALHIRT
ALIGHT
ALIYOT
ALLBUT
ALLOUT
ALLSET
ALLWET
ALMOST
ALPERT
ALWEST
AMIDST
AMORET
AMOUNT
AMULET
ANDYET
ANKLET
ANNUIT
ANOINT
APELET
APPERT
APPLET
APTEST
ARAFAT
ARARAT
ARDENT
ARENDT
ARGENT
ARIGHT
ARMLET
ARMPIT
ARNETT
AROINT
AROUET
ARRANT
ARREST
ARTEST
ARTIST
ASCENT
ASFAST
ASFLAT
ASHPIT
ASKANT
ASKOUT
ASLANT
ASNEAT
ASPECT
ASSENT
ASSERT
ASSIST
ASSOFT
ASSORT
ASTART
ATBEST
ATCOST
ATEOUT
ATLAST
ATMOST
ATREST
ATTEST
ATTHAT
ATTRIT
ATWIST
AUFAIT
AUGUST
AUKLET
AULAIT
AUMONT
AURIST
AUTIST
AVAUNT
AVOCET

•AT•••

BATAAN
BATBOY
BATDAY
BATEAU
BATFOR
BATHED
BATHER
BATHES
BATHOS
BATIKS
BATING
BATLEY
BATMAN
BATMEN
BATONS
BATSIN
BATSON
BATTED
BATTEN
BATTER
BATTLE
BATYAM
CATALO
CATANO
CATBED
CATCHY
CATDOM
CATENA
CATERA
CATERS
CATFIT
CATGUT
CATHAY
CATHER
CATHYS
CATION
CATKIN
CATLIN
CATMAN
CATMEN
CATNAP
CATNIP
CATRIG
CATSAT
CATSIT
CATSUP
CATTLE
CATTON
CATTOY
DATARY
DATERS
DATHAN
DATING
DATIVE
DATRIL
DATSUN
EATERS
EATERY
EATING
EATOUT
EATSAT
EATSIN
EATSIT
EATSOF
EATSUP
FATALE
FATCAT
FATHER
FATHOM
FATIMA
FATLIP
FATMAN
FATONE
FATSIS
FATTED
FATTEN
FATTER
FATWAS
GATEAU
GATERS
GATHER
GATING
GATLIN
GATORS
GATSBY
HATARI
HATBOX
HATEIT
HATERS
HATETO
HATFUL
HATHOR
HATING
HATPIN
HATRED
HATTED
HATTER
HATTIE
IATRIC
KATHIE
KATMAI
KATRIN
KATZEN
LATEEN
LATELY
LATENE
LATENS
LATENT
LATEOF
LATEON
LATERI
LATERO
LATEST
LATETO
LATHED
LATHEN
LATHER
LATHES
LATIGO
LATINA
LATINI
LATINO
LATINS
LATISH
LATKES
LATOUR
LATOYA
LATRIA
LATTER
LATTES
LATVIA
MATERS
MATEYS
MATHER
MATHEW
MATHIS
MATING
MATINS
MATJES
MATLIN
MATMAN
MATMEN
MATRIX
MATRON
MATSON
MATSUI
MATSUO
MATTEA
MATTED
MATTEL
MATTER
MATTES
MATTIE
MATURE
MATZOH
MATZOS
NATALE
NATANT
NATHAN
NATICK
NATION
NATIVE
NATRON
NATTER
NATURE
OATERS
OATIER
PATACA
PATAKI
PATCHY
PATDAY
PATDRY
PATENS
PATENT
PATERS
PATHAN
PATHIC
PATHOS
PATINA
PATINE
PATIOS
PATMOS
PATOIS
PATRIA
PATRIC
PATRIE
PATROL
PATRON
PATTED
PATTEN
PATTER
PATTIE
PATTON
PATZER
QATARI
RATEDA
RATEDG
RATEDR
RATEDX
RATELS
RATERS
RATHER
RATIFY
RATINE
RATING
RATION
RATIOS
RATITE
RATLIN
RATNER
RATOFF
RATOUT
RATSON
RATTAN
RATTAT
RATTED
RATTER
RATTLE
RATTLY
SATAYS
SATCOM
SATEEN
SATFOR
SATING
SATINS
SATINY
SATIRE
SATORI
SATOUT
SATPAT
SATRAP
SATURN
SATYRS
TATAMI
TATARS
TATERS
TATLER
TATRAS
TATTED
TATTER
TATTLE
TATTOO
VATDYE
VATFUL
VATTED
WATERS
WATERY
WATNEY
WATSON
WATTLE
WATUSI
YATATA
YATSEN
YATTER

•A•T••

BAITED
BAITER
BALTIC
BANTAM
BANTER
BANTUS
BARTAB
BARTEL
BARTER
BARTLE
BARTOK
BARTON
BASTED
BASTER
BASTES
BASTIA
BATTED
BATTEN
BATTER
BATTLE
BAXTER
CACTUS
CAFTAN
CANTAB
CANTAL
CANTBE
CANTED
CANTER
CANTLE
CANTON
CANTOO
CANTOR
CANTOS
CAPTOR
CARTED
CARTEL
CARTER
CARTES
CARTIN
CARTON
CARTOP
CASTED
CASTEL
CASTER
CASTES
CASTLE
CASTON
CASTOR
CASTRO
CASTUP
CATTLE
CATTON
CATTOY
DACTYL
DAFTER
DAFTLY
DALTON
DANTEI
DANTES
DANTON
DARTED
DARTER
DARTLE
DAYTON
EARTAB
EARTAG
EARTHA
EARTHS
EARTHY
EASTER
EASTLA
EASTON
FACTOR
FACTUM
FAITES
FAITHS
FALTER
FANTAN
FANTAS
FASTED
FASTEN
FASTER
FATTED
FATTEN
FATTER
FAUTES
GAITED
GAITER
GALTON
GANTRY
GARTER
GASTAX
GASTER
GASTON

GASTRO
HAFTED
HALTED
HALTER
HASTED
HASTEN
HASTES
HATTED
HATTER
HATTIE
IAMTOO
KAETHE
KANTOR
LACTEA
LACTIC
LANTOS
LAOTSE
LAOTZU
LAPTEV
LAPTOP
LARTER
LARTET
LASTED
LASTEX
LASTLY
LASTRA
LASTUP
LATTER
LATTES
LAUTER
LAWTON
MAITAI
MAITRE
MALTBY
MALTED
MALTIN
MANTAS
MANTEE
MANTEL
MANTIC
MANTIS
MANTLE
MANTRA
MANTUA
MAOTAI
MARTEL
MARTEN
MARTES
MARTHA
MARTHE
MARTIN
MARTYR
MASTED
MASTER
MASTIC
MATTEA
MATTED
MATTEL
MATTER
MATTES
MATTIE
MAYTAG
NANTES
NATTER
NAUTES
OAKTAG
PACTEN
PALTER

PALTRY
PANTED
PANTER
PANTIE
PANTOS
PANTRY
PARTED
PARTII
PARTIV
PARTLY
PARTOF
PARTON
PARTYS
PASTAS
PASTED
PASTEL
PASTER
PASTES
PASTIS
PASTIT
PASTOR
PASTRY
PATTED
PATTEN
PATTER
PATTIE
PATTON
PAXTON
PAYTON
QANTAS
RAFTED
RAFTER
RAGTAG
RAGTOP
RAITAS
RANTAT
RANTED
RANTER
RAPTER
RAPTLY
RAPTOR
RAPTUS
RASTAS
RASTER
RATTAN
RATTAT
RATTED
RATTER
RATTLE
RATTLY
SAITEK
SALTED
SALTEN
SALTER
SALTII
SALTON
SANTAS
SANTEE
SANTHA
SANTOS
SARTON
SARTOR
SARTRE
SAUTES
TACTEL
TACTIC
TALTOS
TAMTAM

TANTES
TANTRA
TARTAN
TARTAR
TARTED
TARTER
TARTES
TARTLY
TARTUP
TASTED
TASTEE
TASTER
TASTES
TATTED
TATTER
TATTLE
TATTOO
TAUTEN
TAUTER
TAUTLY
VASTER
VASTLY
VASTUS
VATTED
WAFTED
WAFTER
WAITED
WAITER
WAITON
WAITUP
WALTER
WALTON
WANTAD
WANTED
WANTER
WANTIN
WANTON
WANTTO
WARTED
WASTED
WASTER
WASTES
WATTLE
YATTER
ZAFTIG
ZANTAC

•A••T•

BALATA
BARATA
BARATO
BARITE
CADETS
CALLTO
CAMETO
CANUTE
CAPITA
CAPOTE
CARATS
CARETO
CARETS
CASITA
CAVETT
CAVITY
DAINTY
DAKOTA
DALETH
DALETS

DAMATO
DAMITA
DANITE
DAOSTA
DARETO
DAUNTS
DAVITS
FACETS
FAGOTS
FAILTO
FAINTS
FAJITA
FALLTO
FAULTS
FAULTY
FAWLTY
GAIETY
GAMETE
GAMUTS
GARETH
GAVETO
GAVOTS
HABITS
HALITE
HAMATE
HAMITE
HATETO
HAUNTS
HAVETO
JABOTS
JAUNTS
JAUNTY
JAVITS
KADETT
KANATA
KAPUTT
KARATE
KARATS
KARSTS
LABATT
LAIDTO
LAKOTA
LANATE
LAPUTA
LASHTO
LATETO
LAXITY
LAYSTO
MAILTO
MAKUTA
MALOTI
MANATS
MANETS
MANUTE
MAPUTO
NAMATH
NAPHTA
NARITA
PABSTS
PAINTS
PAINTY
PAIUTE
PALATE
PARETO
PARITY
PASHTO
PASSTO
RACETO

RAMATE
RAMETS
RARITY
RATITE
SABATO
SABOTS
SAFETY
SAIDTO
SAILTO
SAINTE
SAINTS
SALUTE
SALUTO
SANCTA
SANGTO
SANITY
SAULTS
SAVATE
TAHITI
TAINTS
TAKETH
TAKETO
TALKTO
TAROTS
TAUNTS
VACATE
VALETS
VANITY
VASHTI
VAULTS
VAULTY
VAUNTS
VAUNTY
WACOTX
WAISTS
WALKTO
WANTTO
WAPITI
WARMTH
WARMTO
WAVETO
YACHTS
YAKUTS
YATATA
ZAPATA

•A•••T

BACHIT
BADFIT
BADHAT
BADLOT
BAGSIT
BALKAT
BALLET
BALLOT
BALLST
BANDIT
BANKIT
BARBET
BARDOT
BAREST
BARKAT
BARNET
BARRET
BASALT
BASEST
BASKET
BASSET

BAYSAT
CABLET
CACHET
CADENT
CAHOOT
CALLIT
CALVET
CAMEAT
CANLIT
CANNOT
CAPLET
CAPNUT
CARLOT
CARNET
CARPAT
CARPET
CARROT
CASKET
CATFIT
CATGUT
CATSAT
CATSIT
CAUGHT
CAVEAT
CAVETT
CAVORT
DABRAT
DABSAT
DANGIT
DARENT
DAREST
DARNIT
DASHIT
DAUDET
DAYLIT
EAGLET
EARLET
EARNIT
EATOUT
EATSAT
EATSIT
FACEIT
FAKEIT
FANJET
FANOUT
FAROUT
FATCAT
FAUCET
GADGET
GAINST
GALANT
GALOOT
GAMBIT
GAMEST
GANNET
GAPEAT
GARNET
GARRET
GASJET
GASKET
GASLIT
GAWKAT
GAYEST
GAZEAT
HACKIT
HADOUT
HAIGHT
HALEST

HAMLET
HARLOT
HASOUT
HATEIT
HAVEAT
HAVEIT
HAVENT
HAZMAT
IAMNOT
JACKET
JAMEST
JAVERT
JAWSAT
KADETT
KAPUTT
LABATT
LABRAT
LAKIST
LAMENT
LAMEST
LAMONT
LAMSIT
LANCET
LANDAT
LAPCAT
LAPPET
LAPSAT
LARIAT
LARTET
LATENT
LATEST
LAXALT
LAXEST
LAYOUT
MADEIT
MAGGOT
MAGNET
MAHOUT
MAINST
MAKEIT
MALLET
MAOIST
MAPOUT
MARGOT
MARIST
MARKET
MARMOT
MASCOT
MAXOUT
MAYEST
NADSAT
NAGSAT
NAILIT
NAMEIT
NATANT
NAUGHT
PACKET
PALEST
PALLET
PANDIT
PANOUT
PAPIST
PARENT
PARKIT
PARROT
PASSAT
PASTIT
PATENT

PAWSAT
PAYCUT
PAYOUT
RABBET
RABBIT
RACIST
RACKET
RAGOUT
RAILAT
RAMJET
RANOUT
RANTAT
RAREST
RATOUT
RATTAT
RAVEAT
RAWEST
RAWIST
SACHET
SADIST
SAFEST
SAGEST
SALYUT
SAMLET
SANEST
SATOUT
SATPAT
SAVANT
SAVEIT
SAWFIT
SAWOUT
SAWPIT
SAYEST
TABLET
TABSET
TAGOUT
TAKEIT
TALENT
TALKAT
TAMEST
TAOIST
TAPOUT
TAPPET
TARGET
TARPIT
TASKET
TAUGHT
TAVIST
TAXCUT
VACANT
VALENT
VARLET
WABBIT
WALLET
WALLST
WALNUT
WARVET
WASMET
WAVEAT
WAYOUT
YANKAT
YAPHET
YAPSAT
YAREST
ZAGNUT

••AT••

ABATED

ABATER
ABATES
ABATIS
ABATOR
AGATES
AGATHA
ALATED
AMATIS
AMATOL
ANATTO
APATHY
AVATAR
BEATAT
BEATEN
BEATER
BEATIT
BEATLE
BEATON
BEATTY
BEATUP
BLATTY
BOATED
BOATEL
BOATER
BRATSK
BRATTY
CHATTY
CHATUP
COATED
COATEE
COATER
COATES
COATIS
CRATED
CRATER
CRATES
CUATRO
DEATHS
DIATOM
DRATIT
EBATES
ELATED
ELATER
ELATES
ENATES
FLATLY
FLATTV
FRATER
GNATTY
GOATEE
GOATIT
GRATAE
GRATED
GRATER
GRATES
GRATIA
GRATIN
GRATIS
HEATED
HEATER
HEATHS
HEATHY
HEATON
HEATUP
HIATAL
HIATUS
HYATTS
INATIE

INATUB
IRATER
KEATON
KLATCH
LOATHE
MEATAX
MEATUS
MIATAS
MOATED
NEATEN
NEATER
NEATLY
OLATHE
ORATED
ORATES
ORATOR
PLATED
PLATEN
PLATER
PLATES
PLATOS
PLATTE
PLATYS
PRATED
PRATER
PRATES
QRATIO
QUATRE
REATAS
REATTA
RIATAS
RRATED
SCATHE
SEATAC
SEATED
SEATER
SEATON
SKATED
SKATER
SKATES
SLATED
SLATER
SLATES
SNATCH
SNATHS
SPATES
SPATHE
STATED
STATEN
STATER
STATES
STATIC
STATIN
STATOR
STATUE
STATUS
SWATAT
SWATCH
SWATHE
SWATHS
TEATRO
THATCH
THATIS
THATLL
TOATEE
VIATOR
WHATIF
WHATLL

WHATVE
WRATHS
XRATED

••A•T•

ADAPTS
AMANTI
AMANTS
ANATTO
ASANTE
AVANTI
AWAITS
BEASTS
BEATTY
BEAUTS
BEAUTY
BLASTS
BLATTY
BOASTS
BRACTS
BRANTS
BRATTY
CHANTE
CHANTS
CHANTY
CHARTA
CHARTS
CHASTE
CHATTY
COACTS
COAPTS
COASTS
CRAFTS
CRAFTY
CUANTO
DEAFTO
DEALTO
DEARTH
DEARTO
DRAFTS
DRAFTY
DRAWTO
DUARTE
ECARTE
ENACTS
EPACTS
EXACTA
EXACTS
EXALTS
FEALTY
FEASTS
FLATTV
FLAUTA
FRACTO
FRANTZ
GEARTO
GIANTS
GLADTO
GNATTY
GRAFTS
GRANTS
HEADTO
HEALTH
HEARTH
HEARTS
HEARTY
HYATTS
ISANTI

KLAATU
KMARTS
KRAITS
KRANTZ
LEADTO
LEALTY
LEANTO
LEASTS
MEANTO
NEARTO
ONAUTO
ORANTS
PLAITS
PLANTE
PLANTO
PLANTS
PLATTE
PLAYTO
PRAYTO
QUANTA
QUARTE
QUARTO
QUARTS
QUARTZ
REACTS
READTO
REALTY
REATTA
RIALTO
ROASTS
SCANTS
SCANTY
SHAFTS
SHANTY
SHASTA
SLANTS
SMARTS
SMARTY
SNAPTO
SOASTO
SPARTA
STARTS
TOASTS
TOASTY
TRACTS
TRAITS
UGARTE
WEALTH
WRAITH
YEASTS
YEASTY

••A••T

ARAFAT
ARARAT
AVAUNT
BEATAT
BEATIT
BRANDT
CHALET
CLARET
CLAWAT
CRAIGT
CRAVAT
DOASET
DRATIT
ELANET
FLAUNT

GNAWAT
GOATIT
GRABAT
GRANIT
HEARST
IMARET
INABIT
INAPET
INARUT
LEAPAT
LEARNT
MEANIT
PEANUT
PIAGET
PLAINT
PLAKAT
PLANET
PLAYAT
PLAYIT
QUAINT
ROARAT
SEACAT
SHALIT
SMALLT
SNAPAT
STABAT
STAYAT
SWATAT
TEAACT
TEAPOT
TEARAT
TEARIT
TEASET
ZEALOT

•••AT•

ABLATE
ACUATE
ADNATE
ADRATE
AERATE
AFLATS
AGNATE
ALMATY
ANSATE
ARHATS
ATBATS
AURATE
AVIATE
BALATA
BARATA
BARATO
BELATE
BEMATA
BERATE
BFLATS
BINATE
BLEATS
BLOATS
BORATE
BREATH
BYDATE
BYPATH
CARATS
CDRATE
CERATE
CERATO
CFLATS

CHEATS
CHOATE
CLEATS
COMATE
CREATE
CROATS
CURATE
DAMATO
DEBATE
DEFATS
DERATE
DERATS
DFLATS
DILATE
DONATE
DONATH
DORATI
DUCATS
EBOATS
ECLATS
EFLATS
ELNATH
ELUATE
EMPATH
ENSATE
EQUATE
ERRATA
ERSATZ
ESBATS
ESTATE
EXMATE
EXPATS
FFLATS
FIXATE
FLOATS
FLOATY
FOLATE
FUGATO
GELATE
GELATI
GELATO
GFLATS
GLOATS
GREATS
GROATS
GYRATE
HAMATE
HECATE
HEMATO
HEPATO
HIHATS
IDEATE
IGNATZ
IMLATE
INGATE
INMATE
INNATE
IODATE
ISLATE
KANATA
KARATE
KARATS
KLAATU
KORATS
LABATT
LANATE
LEGATE
LEGATO

LIGATE
LOBATE
LOCATE
LUNATE
LUXATE
MANATS
METATE
MORATH
MUTATE
NAMATH
NEGATE
NOTATE
NOVATO
NUTATE
OBLATE
OFLATE
OLEATE
ONLATE
OPIATE
ORNATE
OUTATE
PALATE
PEDATE
PILATE
PINATA
PIRATE
PLEATS
POTATO
PUPATE
RAMATE
REBATE
REDATE
RELATE
REMATE
REMATS
RENATA
RENATO
RERATE
RIGATI
RIMATE
ROTATE
RUBATI
RUBATO
SABATO
SAVATE
SEDATE
SENATE
SENATS
SHEATH
SHOATS
SOLATI
SOMATA
SONATA
SPLATS
SPRATS
SQUATS
STOATS
STPATS
STRATA
STRATI
STRATO
STRATS
SWEATS
SWEATY
TECATE
TERATO
TODATE
TOMATO

TREATS TREATY TUBATE UBOATS UMTATA UNHATS UNIATE UNIATS UNMATE UPDATE UPLATE UPRATE VACATE WHEATS WREATH YATATA YUKATA ZAPATA

6•••A•T

AGHAST ALEAST ARRANT ASFAST ASKANT ASLANT ASTART ATLAST AUFAIT AULAIT BASALT BEJART BESANT BOGART BREAST BROAST BRYANT BYPAST COBALT CONANT DECANT DEMAST DEPART DESALT DIDACT DISANT DREAMT DUNANT DURANT DYNAST DYSART ECKART ELGART ELUANT ENFAIT ENFANT ENHAUT ENRAPT ERRANT ESCAUT EXTANT GALANT GOCART GOFAST GOKART GOLAST GOPAST HOBART

IMEANT IMPACT IMPART INCANT INFACT INFANT INPART INTACT INWANT KURALT KUWAIT LABATT LAXALT LEGART LEVANT MISACT MORANT MOZART MUTANT NATANT NLEAST NOHANT NONART NOSALT NOWAIT OBLAST OCTANT ONEACT OUTACT OXCART PEDANT PLIANT POPART PREACT PROART REBAIT RECANT RECAST REDACT REDANT REPAST RESALT SAVANT SECANT SONANT STRAIT STUART TEAACT TENANT THEACT THWART TOLAST TRUANT TWOACT TYBALT TYRANT UMLAUT UNBAIT UNCAST UNFACT UNHAFT UNMAST UNTAUT UPCAST UPDART UPLAST UPWAFT UTHANT

VACANT VIVANT VOLANT

••••AT

AFLOAT AIMSAT ARAFAT ARARAT ASFLAT ASNEAT ATTHAT BADHAT BALKAT BARKAT BAYSAT BEATAT BEEPAT BIGCAT BOBCAT BOOSAT BUYSAT CAMEAT CARPAT CATSAT CAVEAT CLAWAT CLIMAT COLLAT COMBAT COMEAT COMSAT CRAVAT DABRAT DABSAT DEFEAT DERMAT DIGSAT DIKTAT DINEAT DOGSAT DOTOAT DYEVAT EATSAT ENDSAT ENSEAT FATCAT FERMAT FIREAT FLEWAT FORMAT FRETAT FUMEAT FUSSAT GAPEAT GAWKAT GAZEAT GETSAT GIBEAT GNAWAT GOESAT GOFLAT GONEAT GOODAT GRABAT GRINAT GYMRAT HAVEAT

HAZMAT HEGOAT HEPCAT HEREAT HINTAT HISSAT HITSAT HONKAT HOOTAT HOWLAT IMBEAT INTHAT ITSPAT JAWSAT JEERAT JIBEAT JUMPAT KEEPAT KEPTAT KITKAT KOMBAT LABRAT LANDAT LAPCAT LAPSAT LARIAT LEAPAT LEERAT LESTAT LETSAT LIVEAT LOOKAT LOQUAT LOWFAT MUDCAT MUSCAT NADSAT NAGSAT NEWHAT NIPSAT NODSAT NOMEAT NONFAT NOUGAT NUMBAT OCICAT OHDRAT OLDBAT OLDHAT ORGEAT ORWHAT OUTBAT OUTEAT OUTSAT PASSAT PAWSAT PECKAT PEEKAT PEEPAT PEERAT PETCAT PETRAT PETSAT PICKAT PLAKAT PLAYAT POKEAT POORAT

PTBOAT RAILAT RANTAT RATTAT RAVEAT RECOAT REDBAT REDHAT REGNAT REHEAT REPEAT RESEAT REXCAT ROARAT ROCHAT RUGRAT RUNSAT RUSHAT SATPAT SEACAT SETSAT SEURAT SHEBAT SHEVAT SHOPAT SHOTAT SIGHAT SITPAT SITSAT SKIHAT SNAPAT SNOCAT SOREAT SOTHAT SOWHAT STABAT STAYAT STOPAT SUNHAT SWATAT TALKAT TEARAT THERAT THREAT THROAT TILTAT TINHAT TOILAT TOMCAT TOOTAT TOPCAT TOPHAT TOREAT TOYHAT TUGSAT UNFLAT UNNEAT UNSEAT UPBEAT WAVEAT WENTAT WHODAT WINKAT WINSAT WOMBAT WORKAT YANKAT YAPSAT

YELLAT

AU••••

AUBADE AUBREY AUBURN AUDIAL AUDILE AUDIOS AUDITS AUDREY AUFAIT AUFOND AUGEAN AUGEAS AUGEND AUGERS AUGHTS AUGITE AUGURS AUGURY AUGUST AUKLET AULAIT AUMONT AUNTEM AUNTIE AUPAIR AURATE AURIFY AURIGA AURIST AURORA AUROUS AUSPEX AUSSIE AUSTEN AUSTER AUSTIN AUSTRO AUTEUR AUTHOR AUTISM AUTIST AUTOED AUTUMN

A•U•••

ABUSED ABUSER ABUSES ABUTON ACUATE ACUITY ACUMEN ACURAS ACUTER ACUTES ADULTS AGUISH AKUAKU ALUDEL ALUDRA ALULAE ALULAR ALUMNA ALUMNI AMULET

AMUSED AMUSER AMUSES ANUBIS AOUDAD APULIA AQUAKE AQUILA AQUINO ARUBAN AVULSE AZUELA AZUKIS AZURED AZURES

A••U••

AAAUGH ABDUCE ABDUCT ABJURE ABLUSH ABOUND ABRUPT ABSURD ACCUSE ACQUIT ACTUAL ADDUCE ADDUCT ADJURE ADJUST ADOUTS ADZUKI AGOUTI AILURO ALBUMS ALEUTS ALLUDE ALLURE AMBUSH AMOUNT AMOURS AMPULE ANNUAL ANNUIT ANNULI ANNULS ARGUED ARGUER ARGUES ARGUFY ARJUNA AROUET AROUND AROUSE ARTURO ASBURY ASDULL ASMUCH ASPURE ASSUCH ASSUME ASSURE ASTUTE ATDUSK ATTUNE AUBURN

AUGURS AUGURY AUGUST AUTUMN AVAUNT AVOUCH

A•••U•

AARHUS ABACUS ACCRUE ACEOUT ACESUP ACTIUM ACTOUT ACTSUP ADDSUP ADIEUS ADIEUX ADNOUN ADYTUM AECIUM AEOLUS AGEOUT AIDFUL AIMFUL AIRBUD AIRBUS AIRGUN AIROUT AIRSUP ALARUM ALDOUS ALEGUP ALLBUT ALLIUM ALLOUT ALTIUS AMICUS AMINUS AMPSUP ANIMUS ANJOUS ANTEUP ANTRUM ARBOUR ARDOUR ARMFUL ARMOUR ARTAUD ARTFUL ARTGUM ARTHUR ASKOUT ASKSUP ASTRUD ASYLUM ATEOUT ATFOUR ATREUS ATRIUM ATSTUD AUROUS AUTEUR AVENUE

A••••U

AARGAU

AKUAKU APERCU

•AU•••

BAUBLE BAULKS BAUMAN BAUMER BAUSCH CAUCHY CAUCUS CAUDAD CAUDAL CAUGHT CAULKS CAUSAL CAUSED CAUSER CAUSES DAUBED DAUBER DAUBES DAUDET DAUNTS FAUCET FAULTS FAULTY FAUNAE FAUNAL FAUNAS FAUNUS FAUTES FAUVES GAUCHE GAUCHO GAUGED GAUGER GAUGES GAULLE GAUZES HAULED HAULER HAULIN HAULUP HAUNCH HAUNTS JAUNES JAUNTS JAUNTY JAURES KAUNAS KAUNDA LAUDED LAUDER LAUGHS LAULAU LAUNCH LAUPER LAUREL LAUREN LAUREY LAURIA LAURIC LAURIE LAURYL LAURYN LAUTER MAULED

MAULER MAUMAU MAUMEE MAUNDY MAUSER MAUVES NAUGHT NAUSEA NAUTES PAULEY PAULII PAULIV PAULVI PAUNCH PAUPER PAUSAL PAUSED PAUSER PAUSES RAUNCH SAUCED SAUCER SAUCES SAUDIS SAULTS SAUNAS SAURON SAURUS SAUTES TAUGHT TAUNTS TAUONS TAUPES TAUPIN TAURIC TAUROG TAURUS TAUTEN TAUTER TAUTLY VAUGHN VAULTS VAULTY VAUNTS VAUNTY WAUSAU

•A•U••

AAAUGH BADUNS BAKULA BARUCH CAGUAS CAJUNS CANUCK CANULA CANUTE CARUSO CASUAL CAYUGA CAYUSE DANUBE FACULA FALUDI FAMULI FARUKI GAMUTS HAMULI

JAGUAR JAMUPS JANUAR JARULE KABUKI KAHUNA KAKURO KAPUTT LACUNA LADUKE LAGUNA LAPUTA LAYUPS LAZULI MACULA MADURO MAKUTA MANUAL MANUEL MANURE MANUSH MANUTE MAPUTO MAQUIS MATURE MAZUMA NATURE OAHUAN OAKUMS PACULA PADUAN PAIUTE PAKULA PAPUAN PAQUIN PARURE RAGUSA RAQUEL RASURE SALUKI SALUTE SALUTO SAMUEL SATURN TABUED TABULA VACUUM VAGUER VALUED VALUER VALUES WATUSI YAKUTS YAKUZA YAMUNA YAQUIS ZANUCK

•A••U•

AARHUS BACKUP BACKUS BADGUY BAGFUL BALDUR BALLUP BANGUI BANGUP

BANJUL BANKUP BANQUE BANQUO BANTUS BARIUM BARNUM BARQUE BARZUN BASQUE BAYEUX BAYOUS BAYRUM CACTUS CADMUS CAGEUP CAKEUP CALLUP CALLUS CAMEUP CAMPUP CAMPUS CANCUN CANFUL CAPFUL CAPGUN CAPNUT CARFUL CARPUS CASQUE CASTUP CATGUT CATSUP CAUCUS DADGUM DAMOUR DAMSUP DARIUS DATSUN EARBUD EARFUL EASEUP EATOUT EATSUP FACEUP FACTUM FAIRUP FAMOUS FANOUT FARNUM FAROUK FAROUT FAUNUS FAVOUR GALLUP GAMOUS GANGUP GAVEUP HACKUP HADFUN HADOUT HAIKUS HALLUX HAMSUN HAMSUP HANDUP HANGUL HANGUP

HARDUP HASFUN HASOUT HATFUL HAULUP HAVEUP IAMBUS JACKUP JAIPUR JAMSUP JANHUS JARFUL JAZZUP KAHLUA KAILUA LABIUM LABOUR LACEUP LAIDUP LAMOUR LANDUP LANDUS LAPFUL LAPSUP LAPSUS LARRUP LASHUP LASTUP LATOUR LAWFUL LAYOUT LAYSUP MACOUN MADDUX MADEUP MAGNUM MAGNUS MAHOUT MAKEUP MANFUL MANQUE MANTUA MAPOUT MARAUD MARCUS MARKUP MARQUE MASHUP MASQUE MATSUI MATSUO MAXOUT NAILUP NASHUA PABLUM PACKUP PAGEUP PAIDUP PAIRUP PANFUL PANOUT PAREUS PARFUM PASCUA PASSUP PAYCUT PAYOUT PAYSUP

RACEUP RACKUP RADIUM RADIUS RAGOUT RAGRUG RAIPUR RAKEUP RAMPUP RANGUP RANOUT RAPTUS RATOUT RAVEUP RAYGUN SACKUP SACQUE SACRUM SADHUS SALYUT SATOUT SAURUS SAVEUP SAVOUR SAWOUT SAWSUP TACKUP TAGOUT TAGSUP TAKEUP TALCUM TALKUP TALMUD TAMMUZ TANGUY TANKUP TAPEUP TAPOUT TARSUS TARTUP TAURUS TAXCUT VACUUM VALIUM VALOUR VAPOUR VARMUS VASTUS VATFUL WADSUP WAITUP WAKEUP WALKUP WALLUP WALNUT WALRUS WAMPUM WARMUP WASFUN WASHUP WAYOUT YANQUI YASGUR ZAGNUT

•A•••U

AARGAU BABALU

BALLOU BATEAU CADEAU CARIOU GATEAU HAVASU LANDAU LAOTZU LAULAU MALIBU MANCHU MARILU MASERU MAUMAU NASSAU RAMEAU SARDOU WAUSAU XANADU

••AU••

AAAUGH AVAUNT BEAUTS BEAUTY CLAUDE CLAUSE FLAUNT FLAUTA FRAUDS FRAUEN KRAUSS OGAUGE ONAUTO TEAURN TRAUMA UHAULS USAUSA

••A•U•

ABACUS ALARUM BEADUP BEAMUP BEARUP BEATUP BRAQUE CHACUN CHATUP CLAMUP CLAQUE DEALUP DIALUP DRAGUP DRAWUP GEARUP GLAMUP GLARUS HEADUP HEALUP HEAPUP HEATUP HIATUS ICARUS INARUG INARUT INATUB LEADUP

LEAGUE
LEAPUP
LOADUP
MEATUS
MIAOUS
OMASUM
ONABUN
OPAQUE
PEANUT
PLAGUE
PLAQUE
PLAYUP
PRAGUE
READUP
REARUP
RVALUE
SCARUM
SEALUP
SEAMUS
SHAKUR
SHAMUS
SNAFUS
SNAGUP
SNAPUP
SOAKUP
SOAPUP
STAPUF
STATUE
STATUS
STAYUP
SWAMUP
TEACUP
TEAMUP
TEARUP
TRAGUS
URAEUS
URANUS
UVALUE
WRAPUP

••A••U
CHANDU
DRAKEU
JOANOU
KLAATU
MIAMIU
SMALLU

•••AU•
ARTAUD
BEDAUB
DEPAUL
DEPAUW
EMMAUS
ENHAUT
ESCAUT
MARAUD
PILAUS
REHAUL
STPAUL
STRAUB
UMLAUT
UNTAUT

•••A•U
AKUAKU
BABALU
BUGAKU
BUKAVU
DEJAVU
HAVASU
KLAATU
LIZALU
SUBARU
TUVALU
XANADU

••••AU
AARGAU
BATEAU
BISSAU
BUREAU
CADEAU
DESSAU
GATEAU
JUNEAU
LANDAU
LAULAU
LEBEAU
MAUMAU
MOLDAU
MOREAU
NASSAU
NIIHAU
OISEAU
RAMEAU
RESEAU
ROSEAU
WAUSAU

AV••••
AVAILS
AVALON
AVANTI
AVATAR
AVAUNT
AVEDON
AVEENO
AVENGE
AVENUE
AVERSE
AVERTS
AVESTA
AVIANS
AVIARY
AVIATE
AVIDER
AVIDLY
AVISON
AVISOS
AVOCET
AVOIDS
AVOUCH
AVOWAL
AVOWED
AVOWER
AVRILS
AVULSE

A•V•••
ADVENT
ADVERB
ADVERT
ADVICE
ADVILS
ADVISE
ALVARO
ALVING
ALVINO
AMVETS
ANVILS
ARVADA

A••V••
AGAVES
ALEVEL
ALEVES
ALFVEN
ALIVEO
ALMVPS
ASEVER
ATAVIC

A•••V•
ACTIVA
ACTIVE
ADRIVE
ALCOVE
ARGIVE
ARLOVA
ARRIVE
ATFIVE

A••••V
ABBREV
ASIMOV
ASTROV

•AV•••
BAVIER
CAVAFY
CAVEAT
CAVEIN
CAVELL
CAVERN
CAVERS
CAVETT
CAVIAR
CAVIES
CAVILS
CAVING
CAVITY
CAVORT
DAVENS
DAVIDE
DAVIDI
DAVIDL
DAVIDO
DAVIES
DAVITS
FAVORS
FAVOUR
GAVEIN
GAVELS
GAVEOF
GAVEON
GAVETO
GAVEUP
GAVIAL
GAVOTS
GAVRAS
HAVANA
HAVASU
HAVEAT
HAVEIN
HAVEIT
HAVENO
HAVENS
HAVENT
HAVEON
HAVETO
HAVEUP
HAVING
HAVOCS
JAVERT
JAVIER
JAVITS
KAVNER
LAVABO
LAVAGE
LAVAIN
LAVERN
LAVERS
LAVIDA
LAVING
LAVISH
MAVENS
MAVINS
NAVAHO
NAVAID
NAVAJO
NAVELS
NAVIES
PAVANE
PAVERS
PAVESE
PAVING
PAVIOR
PAVLOV
RAVAGE
RAVEAT
RAVELS
RAVENS
RAVEON
RAVERS
RAVEUP
RAVINE
RAVING
RAVISH
SAVAGE
SAVAII
SAVANA
SAVANT
SAVATE
SAVEAS
SAVEIT
SAVEME
SAVEON
SAVERS
SAVEUP
SAVING
SAVIOR
SAVOIE
SAVOIR
SAVORS
SAVORY
SAVOUR
TAVELS
TAVERN
TAVIST
WAVEAT
WAVEIN
WAVERS
WAVERY
WAVETO
WAVIER
WAVILY
WAVING
XAVIER

•A•V••
CALVED
CALVES
CALVET
CALVIN
CANVAS
CARVED
CARVEL
CARVER
CARVES
CARVEY
EARVIN
FAUVES
GARVEY
HALVAH
HALVAS
HALVED
HALVER
HALVES
HARVEY
JARVIK
JAYVEE
LANVAL
LANVIN
LARVAE
LARVAL
LARVAS
LATVIA
MADVIG
MARVEL
MARVIN
MARVIS
MAUVES
NAIVER
NARVIK
SALVED
SALVER
SALVES
SALVOR
SALVOS
VALVED
VALVES
WAIVED
WAIVER
WAIVES
WARVET

•A••V•
CANOVA
CASAVA
DANOVA
DATIVE
HALEVY
LACAVA
MARKVI
NATIVE
PADOVA
PAREVE
PAULVI
SALIVA
VALOVA

•A•••V
JAMESV
KARKOV
KARPOV
LAPTEV
MAGLEV
MARKIV
MARKOV
PARKAV
PARTIV
PAULIV
PAVLOV
VACLAV
VASLAV
ZARKOV

••AV••
AGAVES
ATAVIC
BEAVER
BEAVIS
BRAVAS
BRAVED
BRAVER
BRAVES
BRAVOS
CHAVEZ
CLAVES
CLAVIN
CRAVAT
CRAVED
CRAVEN
CRAVER
CRAVES
FLAVIA
FLAVOR
GRAVAS
GRAVED
GRAVEL
GRAVEN
GRAVER
GRAVES
GRAVID
GUAVAS
HEAVED
HEAVEN
HEAVER
HEAVES
KNAVES
KRAVIS
LEAVED
LEAVEN
LEAVER
LEAVES
LOAVES
LWAVES
MCAVOY
OLAVII
OLAVIV
PRAVDA
QUAVER
REAVED
REAVER
REAVES
REAVOW
SEAVER
SHAVED
SHAVEN
SHAVER
SHAVES
SLAVED
SLAVER
SLAVES
SLAVIC
SOAVES
STAVED
STAVES
SUAVER
TRAVEL
TRAVEN
TRAVES
TRAVIS
UNAVID
WEAVED
WEAVER
WEAVES

••A•V•
IVANVI
STARVE
WHATVE

••A••V
BRASOV
FLATTV
IVANIV
IVANOV
OLAFIV
OLAVIV
SMALLV

•••AV•
BEHAVE
BUKAVU
CASAVA
CLEAVE
DEJAVU
GREAVE
LACAVA
MOHAVE
MOJAVE
OCTAVE
OCTAVO
OTTAVA
REGAVE
REPAVE
RESAVE
SCHAVS
SHEAVE
UNGAVA
USNAVY

•••A•V
URBANV

••••AV
GUSTAV
MOSHAV
PARKAV
VACLAV
VASLAV

AW••••
AWAITS
AWAKED
AWAKEN
AWAKER
AWAKES
AWARDS
AWARER
AWCMON
AWEARY
AWEDLY
AWEIGH
AWHECK
AWHILE
AWHIRL
AWLESS
AWNING
AWOKEN

A•W•••
ADWARE
ADWARS
ADWEEK
ALWAYS
ALWEST
ANWANG
ASWARM
ASWELL
ASWIRL
ASWOON
ATWILL
ATWIST
ATWOOD
ATWORK

A••W••
AGAWAM
AIRWAR
AIRWAY
AJOWAN
ALLWET
ANSWER
ANYWAY
AVOWAL
AVOWED
AVOWER

A•••W•
ACTTWO
AGETWO
ALLOWS
ANTAWN
ARROWS
ATDAWN

A••••W
ACTNOW
ALLNEW
ANDHOW
ANDREW
ANTCOW
ANYHOW
ASSLOW
ATALOW
ATHROW

•AW•••
BAWLED
BAWLER
CAWCAW
CAWDOR
CAWING
DAWBER
DAWDLE
DAWNED
DAWNON
DAWSON
FAWKES
FAWLTY
FAWNED
FAWNER
FAWNON
GAWAIN
GAWKAT
GAWKED
GAWKER
GAWPED
GAWPER
HAWAII
HAWHAW
HAWING
HAWKED
HAWKER
HAWSER
HAWSES
JAWING
JAWOHL
JAWSAT
LAWFUL
LAWING
LAWMAN
LAWMEN
LAWSON
LAWTON
LAWYER
MAWSON
PAWERS
PAWING
PAWNED
PAWNEE
PAWNER
PAWPAW
PAWSAT
RAWBAR
RAWDON
RAWEGG
RAWEST
RAWISH
RAWIST
SAWALL
SAWERS
SAWFIT
SAWING
SAWLOG
SAWOFF
SAWOUT
SAWPIT
SAWRED
SAWSUP
SAWYER
TAWDRY
YAWING
YAWKEY
YAWNED
YAWNER
YAWPED
YAWPER

•A•W••
BAGWIG
CARWAX
DAEWOO
DARWIN
EARWAX
EARWIG
FATWAS
GALWAY
GASWAR
RAHWAY
TAIWAN
WAHWAH

•A••W•
KAGAWA
KANAWA
MACAWS
MALAWI
PAPAWS
TARAWA

•A•••W
BARLOW
BARROW
CALLOW
CARLOW
CASHEW
CAWCAW
DARROW
FALLOW
FARLOW
FARROW
GAGLAW
HALLOW
HARLOW
HARROW
HAWHAW
HAYMOW
KAYYOW
LAYLOW
MALLOW
MARROW
MATHEW
NARROW
PAWPAW
PAYNOW
RANLOW
SALLOW
TALLOW
TAXLAW
WALLOW
WARSAW
YARROW

••AW••
AGAWAM
BRAWLS
BRAWNY
CHAWED
CLAWAT
CLAWED
CLAWER
CRAWLS
CRAWLY
DRAWEE
DRAWER
DRAWIN
DRAWLS
DRAWLY
DRAWON
DRAWTO
DRAWUP
FLAWED
GNAWAT
GNAWED
GNAWER
GNAWON
GOAWAY
GOAWOL
GOAWRY
INAWAY
PRAWER
PRAWNS
SEAWAY
SHAWLS
SPAWNS
THAWED
THAWER
TRAWLS
UNAWED

••A•W•
MIAOWS

••A••W
ATALOW
CRACOW
INAFEW
INAROW
KRAKOW
MEADOW
QUAPAW
REAVOW
SEACOW
SHADOW
SMALLW

•••AW•
ANTAWN
ATDAWN
BYLAWS
INLAWS
INPAWN
KAGAWA
KANAWA
MACAWS
MALAWI
MOHAWK
MRPAWS
OSHAWA
OTTAWA
OUTAWE
PAPAWS
PSHAWS
RESAWN
RESAWS
SCRAWL
SPRAWL
SQUAWK
STRAWS
TARAWA
UNPAWN
UNSAWN
YUKAWA

•••A•W
DEPAUW

••••AW
BOWSAW
BROKAW
CAWCAW
CUSHAW
DECLAW
DRCLAW
ECOLAW
GAGLAW
GEEGAW
GEWGAW
GUFFAW
GUNLAW
HAWHAW
HEEHAW
JIGSAW
MCGRAW
OLDSAW
OUTLAW
OUTSAW
PAWPAW
PITSAW
PRELAW
QUAPAW
REDRAW
RETHAW
RIPSAW
RUBRAW
SEESAW
TAXLAW
THELAW
UNDRAW
UNTHAW
UPSHAW
WARSAW
YEEHAW

AX••••
AXEMAN
AXEMEN
AXENIC
AXHEAD
AXILLA
AXIOMS
AXIONS
AXISES
AXLIKE
AXONAL
AXONES
AXSEED

A••X••
ALEXAS
ALEXEI
ALEXEY
ALEXIA
ALEXIS
ANOXIA
ANOXIC
APEXES
ATAXIA
ATAXIC
ATOXIC

A••••X
ADIEUX
AGESIX
APPROX
AUSPEX

•AX•••
BAXTER
FAXERS
FAXING
LAXALT
LAXEST
LAXITY
MAXELL
MAXENE
MAXIMA
MAXIMS
MAXINE
MAXING
MAXIXE
MAXOUT
MAXSON
OAXACA
PAXTON
RAXING
SAXONS
SAXONY
TAXCUT
TAXERS
TAXIED
TAXIES
TAXING
TAXLAW
TAXMAN
TAXMEN
TAXOLS
WAXERS
WAXIER
WAXILY
WAXING

•A•X••
CALXES
MARXES

•A••X•
GALAXY
MAXIXE

•A•••X
BAYEUX
CALMEX
CARWAX
EARWAX
GASTAX
HADDIX
HALLUX
HANDAX
HATBOX
LARYNX
LASTEX
MAALOX
MADDOX
MADDUX
MADMAX
MANNIX
MARCIX
MARKIX
MATRIX
RATEDX
WACOTX

••AX••
ATAXIA
ATAXIC
COAXAL
COAXED
COAXER
COAXES
FLAXEN
FLAXES
HOAXED
HOAXER
HOAXES
IMAXES
KLAXON
PRAXES
PRAXIS
UNAXED

••A••X
BRANDX
INABOX
INAFIX
MAALOX
MEATAX
SEAFOX
SMALLX

•••AX•
BORAXO
BYTAXI
EUTAXY
GALAXY
ICEAXE
THEAXE
TJMAXX

•••A•X
TJMAXX

••••AX
CARWAX
CLIMAX
COLFAX
EARWAX
FORNAX
GASTAX
HANDAX
KOUFAX
MADMAX
MEATAX
NONTAX
PENTAX
PICKAX
POLEAX
PRETAX
PROTAX
SINTAX
SKIWAX
SURTAX
SYNTAX
THORAX
USETAX

AY••••
AYEAYE
AYESHA
AYESIR
AYRTON

A•Y•••
ABYSMS
ADYTUM
ALYDAR
ALYSSA
AMYTAN
ANYDAY
ANYHOW
ANYMAN
ANYOLD
ANYONE
ANYONS
ANYWAY
ARYANS
ASYLUM
ATYALE
ATYPIC

A••Y••
ALIYAH
ALIYOT
ALKYDS
ALKYLS
ALLYCE
ALLYLS
ANDYET
ARGYLE
ARGYLL

A•••Y•
ABBEYS
ACETYL
AJFOYT
ALLAYS
ALLEYN
ALLEYS
ALLOYS
ALWAYS
ANNOYS
ANONYM
ARRAYS
ARROYO
ASSAYS
AYEAYE
AZODYE

A••••Y
ABBACY
ACIDLY
ACUITY
AERIFY
AERILY
AFFRAY
AGEDLY
AGENCY
AIRDRY
AIRILY
AIRWAY
ALBANY
ALECKY
ALEXEY
ALLDAY

ALMATY ALTKEY AMBERY ANDREY ANERGY ANTONY ANYDAY ANYWAY APATHY APIARY ARCHLY ARGOSY ARGUFY ARIARY ARIDLY ARMORY ARTERY ARTILY ASBURY ASEASY ASHLEY ASKAMY ASMANY ASTLEY ASTRAY ATPLAY AUBREY AUDREY AUGURY AURIFY AVIARY AVIDLY AWEARY AWEDLY

•AY•••

BAYARD BAYERN BAYEUX BAYING BAYLOR BAYMAN BAYMEN BAYOUS BAYRUM BAYSAT CAYMAN CAYUGA CAYUSE DAYBED DAYGLO DAYHOP DAYJOB DAYLIT DAYOFF DAYOLD DAYONE DAYSPA DAYTON FAYARD FAYLEN GAYEST GAYNES GAYNOR HAYDEN HAYERS HAYING HAYLEY HAYMES HAYMOW HAYNES HAYNIE JAYCEE JAYMES JAYVEE KAYAKS KAYOED KAYYOW LAYBYS LAYERS LAYFOR LAYING LAYINS LAYLOW LAYMAN LAYMEN LAYOFF LAYOUT LAYSBY LAYSIN LAYSON LAYSTO LAYSUP LAYUPS MAYANS MAYBES MAYDAY MAYEST MAYFLY MAYHAP MAYHEM MAYIGO MAYING MAYORS MAYRON MAYTAG NAYSAY PAYCUT PAYDAY PAYEES PAYERS PAYFOR PAYING PAYNOW PAYOFF PAYOLA PAYOUT PAYPAL PAYSIN PAYSON PAYSUP PAYTON RAYBAN RAYGUN RAYING RAYONS SAYAAH SAYAYE SAYBOO SAYDIE SAYERS SAYEST SAYHEY SAYIDO SAYING SAYLES SAYNAY SAYSAH SAYSHI SAYSNO SAYSOK SAYSOS SAYSSO SAYYES TAYLOR WAYANS WAYLAY WAYLON WAYNES WAYOFF WAYOUT WAYSIN ZAYINS

•A•Y••

BAEYER BANYAN BARYON BATYAM CANYON EASYAS EASYGO GARYIN KAYYOW LADYDI LARYNX LAWYER MAGYAR MARYAM MARYII MARYJO PAPYRI SALYUT SANYOS SATYRS SAWYER SAYYES

•A••Y•

BALLYS CAMRYN CAMRYS CATHYS DACTYL DADDYO DADDYS DANDYL DANNYS DARRYL GAMAYS HARRYO HARRYS JACLYN LATOYA LAURYL LAURYN LAYBYS MADLYN MALAYA MALAYS MARTYR MASSYS MATEYS NAGOYA PAPAYA PARTYS RALLYE SATAYS SAYAYE TAMAYO VANRYN VATDYE

•A•••Y

BABBLY BADBOY BADDAY BADGUY BAGBOY BAILEY BAKERY BALDLY BARANY BARELY BARFLY BARLEY BARNEY BARONY BASELY BASIFY BASSEY BASSLY BATBOY BATDAY BATLEY CAGILY CAGNEY CALMLY CALORY CAMBOY CAMEBY CANARY CANOPY CARBOY CARKEY CARNEY CARREY CARSEY CARVEY CASEFY CATCHY CATHAY CATTOY CAUCHY CAVAFY CAVITY DABNEY DAFTLY DAILEY DAINTY DAMPLY DANGLY DANKLY DANNAY DARKLY DARNAY DATARY EARTHY EASEBY EASILY EASLEY EATERY FABRAY FAIRLY FAKERY FAMILY FARACY FARCRY FARLEY FAULTY FAWLTY GADFLY GAIETY GAINLY GALAXY GALLEY GALWAY GAMELY GAMILY GANGLY GANTRY GARVEY GASIFY GATSBY HACKLY HAILEY HALEVY HALLEY HALSEY HANGBY HANLEY HARDBY HARDLY HARLEY HARNEY HARVEY HAYLEY HAZILY JACOBY JALOPY JANGLY JANNEY JAPERY JAUNTY KANALY LACHEY LACHOY LACILY LACKEY LAIDBY LAMELY LANDRY LANKLY LANSKY LASTLY LATELY LAUREY LAXITY LAYSBY LAZBOY LAZILY MABLEY MAINLY MAIRZY MALADY MALORY MALTBY MANDAY MANLEY MANRAY MARBLY MARKEY MARLEY MARSHY MASSEY MAUNDY MAYDAY MAYFLY MAZILY NAJIMY NAMELY NAPERY NASEBY NAYSAY OAKLEY PACIFY PAINTY PALELY PALTRY PANFRY PANTRY PAPACY PAPERY PARITY PARKAY PARLAY PARLEY PARODY PARTLY PASSBY PASTRY PATCHY PATDAY PATDRY PAULEY PAYDAY RACEBY RACILY RADLEY RAHWAY RAINEY RAMIFY RAMSAY RAMSEY RANDRY RANKLY RAPTLY RAREFY RARELY RARITY RASHLY RATIFY RATTLY SACFLY SADDAY SAFELY SAFETY SAGELY SALARY SALIFY SANELY SANITY SASHAY SATINY SAVORY SAXONY SAYHEY SAYNAY TABKEY TAGDAY TAMELY TANGLY TANGUY TARTLY TAUTLY TAWDRY VAGARY VAINLY VALERY VALLEY VANITY VAPORY VARNEY VASILY VASTLY VAULTY VAUNTY WADDLY WAFERY WAFFLY WAGGLY WALKBY WAMBLY WARCRY WARILY WARMLY WATERY WATNEY WAVERY WAVILY WAXILY WAYLAY YARELY YAWKEY ZANILY

••AY••

BRAYED BRAYER CLAYEY CRAYON DLAYER DRAYED DWAYNE EBAYER ELAYER ELAYNE FLAYED FLAYER FRAYED GRAYED GRAYER GRAYLY ISAYNO OKAYED PLAYAS PLAYAT PLAYBY PLAYED PLAYER PLAYIT PLAYON PLAYTO PLAYUP PRAYED PRAYER PRAYTO QUAYLE SHAYNE SLAYED SLAYER SPAYED SPAYER STAYAT STAYED STAYER STAYIN STAYON STAYUP SWAYED SWAYER SWAYZE THAYER XRAYED

••A•Y•

GLADYS HEARYE PLATYS SEALYS SHARYN

••A••Y

APATHY BEACHY BEATTY BEAUTY BLABBY BLAKEY BLATTY BRAINY BRANDY BRANNY BRASHY BRASSY BRATTY BRAWNY CHAFFY CHALKY CHAMMY CHANCY CHANEY CHANTY CHARLY CHATTY CIASPY CLAMMY CLANCY CLANKY CLASSY CLAYEY CRABBY CRAFTY CRAGGY CRAMPY CRANKY CRANNY CRAWLY DEADLY DEAFLY DEARLY DRABLY DRAFTY DRAGGY DRANCY DRAWLY DUALLY FEALTY FLABBY FLAGGY FLAPPY FLASHY FLATLY FRAIDY FRANNY GLADLY GLASSY GNARLY GNATTY GOALBY GOAWAY GOAWRY GRABBY GRAINY GRAMMY GRANBY GRANDY GRANNY GRAPEY GRAPHY GRASSY GRAYLY HEALEY HEANEY HEARTY HEATHY ICALLY INADAY INARAY INAWAY KEARNY KNARRY LEACHY LEAKEY LEALTY LEANLY MCAVOY MEANEY MEANLY MEASLY MTAIRY NEARBY NEARLY NEATLY NIAMEY OCASEY ORALLY ORANGY OVALLY PEACHY PEARLY PLASHY PLAYBY POACHY QUACKY QUAGGY QUARRY REALLY REALTY SCANTY SCARRY SEAWAY SHABBY SHAGGY SHALEY SHALLY SHAMMY SHANDY SHANTY SHARPY SKANKY SLANGY SLAPPY SMALLY SMARMY SMARTY SNAGGY SNAPPY SNARKY SNARLY SNAZZY SPACEY SPANKY SPARKY STABLY STACEY STAGEY STALKY STARRY SWABBY SWAMPY SWANKY TEAPOY TOASTY TRACEY TRAMPY TRANNY TRAPPY TRASHY TWANGY UNABLY USABLY USARMY VIABLY WEAKLY WHALEY WHAMMY YEARLY YEASTY

•••AY•

ALLAYS ALWAYS ARRAYS ASSAYS AYEAYE BELAYS BYWAYS COPAYS DECAYS DELAYS EMBAYS ESSAYS FORAYS GAMAYS INLAYS MALAYA MALAYS MORAYS NOMAYO NOWAYS ONLAYS PAPAYA PITAYA RELAYS REPAYS RESAYS SATAYS SAYAYE SPLAYS SPRAYS STRAYS TAMAYO TODAYS TOKAYS UNLAYS UNSAYS UVRAYS

•••A•Y

ABBACY ALBANY ALMATY APIARY ARIARY ASEASY ASKAMY ASMANY AVIARY AWEARY BARANY BEWARY BIGAMY BINARY BLEARY BOTANY BOVARY BRIARY CANARY CAVAFY CEDARY CLEARY CREAKY CREAMY CREASY CROAKY CUDAHY CURACY DATARY DELANY DENARY DIGAMY DREAMY DREARY EUTAXY FARACY FLOATY FREAKY FRIARY GALAXY GLEAMY GOEASY GREASY HILARY IMEASY INFAMY KANALY KODALY LEGACY LITANY LUNACY MALADY MILADY MYBABY MYLADY NONARY NOTANY NOTARY OFFALY OGRADY OHBABY OLEARY PAPACY PIRACY QUEASY ROMANY ROSARY ROTARY SALARY SENARY SHOALY SLEAZY SMEARY SNEAKY SOMANY STEADY STEAMY STMARY SUGARY SWEATY TREATY TWEAKY UNEASY UNGAMY UNHAZY UNWARY USNAVY VAGARY VOTARY

••••AY

AFFRAY AIRWAY ALLDAY ANYDAY ANYWAY ASTRAY ATPLAY BADDAY BATDAY BELLAY BENDAY BENGAY BETRAY BIGDAY BISCAY BOMBAY BUFFAY BUNGAY BYPLAY CATHAY CONWAY CORDAY DANNAY DARNAY DEBRAY DEEJAY DEFRAY DELRAY DISMAY DOGDAY DORSAY ESTRAY FABRAY FENWAY FLYWAY FRIDAY GALWAY GOAWAY HEYDAY HOORAY HOTDAY HURRAY IFIMAY ILLSAY IMOKAY INADAY INARAY INAWAY INGRAY INPLAY INTRAY JETWAY KEYWAY LEEMAY LEEWAY MANDAY MANRAY MAYDAY MIDDAY MIDMAY MIDWAY MILLAY MISLAY MISSAY MONDAY MORNAY MURRAY NAYSAY NETPAY NEWDAY NEWWAY NORGAY NORWAY OFFDAY OLDWAY ONEDAY ONEWAY OUTLAY OUTPAY OUTSAY PARKAY PARLAY PATDAY PAYDAY PEDWAY PERDAY PINCAY PREDAY PREPAY RAHWAY RAMSAY REDBAY REPLAY RUNWAY SADDAY SASHAY SAYNAY SEAWAY SEGWAY SIRKAY SIXDAY SIXWAY SKYWAY SUBWAY SUNDAY SUNRAY TAGDAY TENDAY THEBAY THEWAY TORBAY TWODAY TWOWAY UNCLAY VEEJAY WAYLAY

AZ••••

AZALEA AZANIA AZARIA AZELMA AZERAS AZERIS AZIDES AZODYE AZOLES AZONAL AZONIC AZORES AZORIN AZRAEL AZTECA AZTECS AZTEKS AZUELA AZUKIS AZURED AZURES

A•Z•••

ADZING ADZUKI ALZADO ALZIRA ANZACS

A••Z••

AMAZED AMAZES AMAZIN AMAZON AREZZO

A•••Z•

ABLAZE ALONZO AREZZO ASSIZE

A••••Z

ALMAAZ ALRITZ AMOSOZ

•AZ•••

BAZAAR BAZOOS CAZALE DAZERS DAZING DAZZLE FAZING FAZOOL GAZEAT GAZEBO GAZEON GAZERS GAZING HAZANS HAZARD HAZELS HAZERS HAZIER HAZILY HAZING HAZMAT JAZZBO JAZZED JAZZER JAZZES JAZZUP KAZOOS LAZBOY LAZIER LAZILY LAZING LAZULI MAZDAS MAZIER MAZILY MAZING MAZOLA MAZUMA RAZERS RAZING RAZORS RAZZED RAZZES RAZZIE RAZZLE ZAZENS

•A•Z••

BAIZAS BAIZES BALZAC BANZAI BARZUN DANZIG DAZZLE GAUZES JANZEN JAZZBO JAZZED JAZZER JAZZES JAZZUP

KATZEN LASZLO MAAZEL MAHZOR MAIZES MANZON MATZOH MATZOS PANZER PATZER RAZZED RAZZES RAZZIE RAZZLE TARZAN

•A••Z•

CABEZA LAMAZE LAONZA LAOTZU LARAZA MAIRZY YAKUZA ZABRZE

•A•••Z

PARLEZ TABRIZ TAMMUZ VALDEZ

••AZ••

AMAZED AMAZES AMAZIN AMAZON BLAZED BLAZER BLAZES BLAZON BRAZEN BRAZIL BRAZOS BRAZZA BRAZZI CHAZAN CRAZED CRAZES FRAZER GHAZIS GLAZED GLAZER GLAZES GRAZED GRAZER GRAZES GRAZIE MAAZEL PIAZZA PIAZZI PLAZAS SHAZAM SMAZES SNAZZY ZSAZSA

••A•Z•

BRAZZA BRAZZI KWANZA PIAZZA PIAZZI SNAZZY STANZA STARZZ SWAYZE

••A••Z

CHAVEZ FRANTZ IBANEZ JUAREZ KRANTZ QUARTZ SMALLZ STARZZ XYANDZ

•••AZ•

ABLAZE BEDAZE LAMAZE LARAZA PIZAZZ SLEAZE SLEAZY UNHAZY UPGAZE

•••A•Z

ALMAAZ ERSATZ IGNATZ KUVASZ MESAAZ PIZAZZ YUMAAZ

••••AZ

ALMAAZ MESAAZ SHIRAZ YUMAAZ

BA••••

BAABAA BAAING BAALIM BABALU BABBLE BABBLY BABELS BABIED BABIER BABIES BABKAS BABOON BABOOS BABSON BACALL BACHED BACHES BACHIT BACKED BACKER BACKIN BACKUP BACKUS BACONS BADBOY BADCOP BADDAY BADDER BADDIE BADDOG BADEGG BADEMS BADEND BADFIT BADGER BADGES BADGUY BADHAM BADHAT BADLIE BADLOT BADMAN BADMEN BADOFF BADRAP BADUNS BAERGA BAEYER BAFFED BAFFER BAFFIN BAFFLE BAGBOY BAGDAD BAGELS BAGEND BAGFUL BAGGED BAGGER BAGGIE BAGJOB BAGMAN BAGMEN BAGNIO BAGSIT BAGWIG BAHAMA BAHIAN BAHNEN BAIKAL BAILED BAILEE BAILER BAILEY BAILON BAILOR BAINES BAIRNS BAISAS BAITED BAITER BAIZAS BAIZES BAKERS BAKERY BAKING BAKKER BAKSHI BAKULA BALAAM BALATA BALBOA BALDED BALDER BALDIE BALDLY BALDUR BALEEN BALERS BALINE BALING BALKAN BALKAT BALKED BALKER BALLAD BALLET BALLIN BALLON BALLOT BALLOU BALLST BALLUP BALLYS BALMER BALSAM BALSAS BALTIC BALZAC BAMAKO BAMBIS BAMBOO BANANA BANANE BANCOS BANDED BANDER BANDIT BANGED BANGER BANGLE BANGON BANGOR BANGUI BANGUP BANISH BANJOS BANJUL BANKED BANKER BANKIT BANKON BANKUP BANLON BANNED BANNEN BANNER BANONS BANQUE BANQUO BANTAM BANTER BANTUS BANYAN BANZAI BAOBAB BARACK BARADA BARAKA BARANY BARATA BARATO BARBAN BARBED BARBER BARBET BARBIE BARBRA BARCAR BARCOS BARDIC BARDOT BAREGE BARELY BAREST BARFLY BARGED BARGER BARGES BARHOP BARING BARITE BARIUM BARKAT BARKED BARKER BARKIN BARKLA BARLEY BARLOW BARMAN BARMEN BARNED BARNES BARNET BARNEY BARNUM BAROJA BAROLO BARONE BARONI BARONS BARONY BARQUE BARRED BARREL BARREN BARRES BARRET BARRIE BARRIO BARRIS BARRON BARROW BARTAB BARTEL BARTER BARTLE BARTOK BARTON BARUCH BARYON BARZUN BASALT BASELY BASEST BASHED BASHER BASHES BASHIN BASIAL BASICS BASIFY BASILS BASING BASINS BASKED BASKER BASKET BASKIN BASQUE BASRAH BASSES BASSET BASSEY BASSLY BASSOS BASTED BASTER BASTES BASTIA BATAAN BATBOY BATDAY BATEAU BATFOR BATHED BATHER BATHES BATHOS BATIKS BATING BATLEY BATMAN BATMEN BATONS BATSIN BATSON BATTED BATTEN BATTER BATTLE BATYAM BAUBLE BAULKS BAUMAN BAUMER BAUSCH BAVIER BAWLED BAWLER BAXTER BAYARD BAYERN BAYEUX BAYING BAYLOR BAYMAN BAYMEN BAYOUS BAYRUM BAYSAT BAZAAR BAZOOS

B•A•••

BAABAA BAAING BAALIM BEACHY BEACON BEADED BEADER BEADLE BEADUP BEAGLE BEAKED BEAKER BEALLS BEAMAN BEAMED BEAMER BEAMON BEAMUP BEANED BEANIE BEANOS BEAPAL BEARDS BEARER BEARON BEARSE BEARUP BEASTS BEATAT BEATEN BEATER BEATIT BEATLE BEATON BEATTY BEATUP BEAUTS BEAUTY BEAVER BEAVIS BHANGS BIAFRA BIALIK BIANCA BIANCO BIASED BIASES BLABBY BLACKS BLADED BLADER BLADES BLAFFS BLAINE BLAISE BLAKEY BLAMED BLAMER BLAMES BLANCA BLANCH BLANCO BLANDA BLANKS BLARED BLARES BLASTS BLATTY BLAZED BLAZER BLAZES BLAZON BMAJOR BOARDS BOASTS BOATED BOATEL BOATER BRACCO BRACED BRACER BRACES BRACHS BRACTS BRAHMA BRAHMS BRAIDS BRAINS BRAINY BRAISE BRAKED BRAKES BRAMAH BRANCA BRANCH BRANDI BRANDO BRANDS BRANDT BRANDX BRANDY BRANNY BRANTS BRAQUE BRASCO BRASHY BRASIL BRASOV BRASSY BRATSK BRATTY BRAVAS BRAVED BRAVER BRAVES BRAVOS BRAWLS BRAWNY BRAYED BRAYER BRAZEN BRAZIL BRAZOS BRAZZA BRAZZI BWANAS

B••A••

BABALU BACALL BAHAMA BALAAM BALATA BAMAKO BANANA BANANE BARACK BARADA BARAKA BARANY BARATA BARATO BASALT BATAAN BAYARD BAZAAR BECALM BECAME BEDAUB BEDAZE BEFAIR BEFALL BEHAIM BEHALF BEHAVE BEJART BELAIR BELATE BELAYS BEMATA BERATE BESAME BESANT BETAKE BEVANS BEWAIL BEWARE BEWARY BFLATS BICARB BIGAIR BIGAMY BIGAPE BINACA BINARY BINATE BLEACH BLEAKS BLEARS BLEARY BLEATS BLOATS BOGART BONACI BONAMI BORATE BORAXO BOTANY BOVARY BOYARS BREACH BREADS BREAKS BREAMS BREAST BREATH BRIANA BRIAND BRIARD BRIARS BRIARY BROACH BROADA BROAST BRYANT BSCALE BSHARP BSTARS BTEAMS BUGAKU BUKAVU BURANA BUTANE BYDATE BYHALF BYHAND BYLAND BYLAWS BYMAIL BYNAME BYPASS BYPAST BYPATH BYTALK BYTAXI BYWAYS

B•••A•

BAABAA BABKAS BADDAY BADHAM BADHAT BADMAN BADRAP BAGDAD BAGMAN BAHIAN BAIKAL BAISAS BAIZAS BALAAM BALKAN BALKAT BALLAD BALSAM BALSAS BALZAC BANTAM BANYAN BANZAI BAOBAB BARBAN BARCAR BARKAT BARMAN BARTAB BASIAL BASRAH BATAAN BATDAY BATEAU BATMAN BATYAM BAUMAN BAYMAN BAYSAT BAZAAR BEAMAN BEAPAL BEATAT BEDLAM BEEPAT BEGGAR BEHEAD BELDAM BELGAE BELIAL BELLAY BEMOAN BENDAY BENGAL BENGAY BERMAN BETRAY BETTAS BEULAH BHOPAL BHUTAN BIGBAD BIGCAR BIGCAT BIGDAY BIGEAR BIGFAN BIGMAC BIGMAN BILBAO BILDAD BIOGAS BIOLAB BIOTAS BIRMAN BISCAY BISSAU BITMAP BOBCAT BOLLAS BOLYAI BOMBAL BOMBAY BONHAM BONSAI BOOSAT BOREAL BOREAS BORMAN BOWMAN BOWOAR BOWSAW BOXCAR BRAMAH BRAVAS BRIDAL BROCAS BROGAN BROKAW BRUMAL BRUTAL BUBBAS BUCCAL BUCHAN BUENAS BUFFAY BULGAR BULLAE BUMRAP BUNGAY BUNYAN BUREAU BURIAL BURKAS BURLAP BURMAN BUROAK BURSAE BURSAL BURSAR BURSAS BUSMAN BUYSAT BWANAS BYPLAY BYROAD

B••••A

BAABAA BAERGA BAHAMA BAKULA BALATA BALBOA BANANA BARADA BARAKA BARATA BARBRA BARKLA BAROJA BASTIA BELUGA BEMATA BERTHA BETCHA BIAFRA BIANCA BIKILA BINACA BLANCA BLANDA BOCHSA BODEGA BOGOTA BOLENA BONITA BORGIA BOSNIA BRAHMA BRANCA BRAZZA BRENDA BRIANA BROADA BRYNZA BUDDHA BULOVA BUQSHA BURANA BUSHWA

•BA•••

ABACAB ABACAS ABACUS ABASED ABASER ABASES ABATED ABATER ABATES ABATIS ABATOR DBACKS EBANKS EBATES EBAYER IBADAN IBANEZ IBARRA NBAERS PBANDJ SBARRO UBANGI

•B•A••

ABBACY ABBADO ABLARE ABLATE ABLAZE ABOARD ABRADE ABRAMS EBOATS HBEAMS IBEAMS LBEAMS OBEAHS OBLADI OBLAST OBLATE OBTAIN UBOATS

•B••A•

ABACAB ABACAS ABOMAS ABORAL ABROAD ABSCAM FBIMAN IBADAN IBIZAN OBIWAN OBRIAN RBIMAN

•B•••A

ABOLLA IBARRA IBERIA

••BA••

ABBACY ABBADO ALBANO ALBANS ALBANY AMBAND ATBATS AUBADE BABALU CABALA CABALS CABANA COBAIN COBALT CUBAGE CUBANS DEBAGS DEBARK DEBARS DEBASE DEBATE EMBALM EMBANK EMBARK EMBARS EMBAYS ENBANC ESBATS EWBANK FMBAND GOBACK GOBANG HABANA HOBART IMBACK INBACK JSBACH KEBABS LABATT LOBATE MCBAIN MYBABY NOBAKE NOBALL OHBABY ONBAIL ONBASE ORBACH QABALA REBAGS REBAIT REBAKE REBALE REBANK REBARS REBATE RIBALD RIBAND RUBATI RUBATO SABADO SABALS SABATO SUBARU TABARD TOBAGO TUBAGE TUBATE TYBALT UNBAGS UNBAIT UNBALE UNBARE UNBARS URBANA URBANE URBANI URBANV USBANK WABASH WEBADS

••B•A•

BABKAS BOBCAT BUBBAS CABMAN CABRAL COBHAM COBRAS CUBFAN DABRAT DABSAT DEBRAH DEBRAY FABIAN FABRAY GIBEAT GIBRAN HABEAS HABLAR HUBCAP IMBEAT JABBAR JIBEAT JOBJAR KUBLAI LABIAL LABRAT LEBEAU LIBRAE LIBRAN LIBRAS LIBYAN LLBEAN MCBEAL MRBEAN NUBIAN PTBOAT RIBPAD RUBRAW SABRAS SUBPAR SUBWAR SUBWAY TABLAS TIBIAE TIBIAL TIBIAS TOBIAS TUBMAN UMBRAE UMBRAL UMBRAS UPBEAR UPBEAT VIBRAM WEBCAM ZEBRAS

••B••A

ARBELA CABALA

CABANA
CABEZA
CIBOLA
EUBOEA
FIBULA
HABANA
JOBYNA
LABREA
NEBULA
NUBIRA
QABALA
RIBERA
ROBBIA
RUBBIA
SABENA
SABINA
SUBSEA
TABULA
UMBRIA
URBANA

•••BA•

AIRBAG
ALABAM
AMEBAE
AMEBAS
ARUBAN
BAABAA
BAOBAB
BARBAN
BIGBAD
BILBAO
BOMBAL
BOMBAY
BUBBAS
CASBAH
CEIBAS
COMBAT
CYMBAL
DIDBAD
DISBAR
DJEBAR
DUNBAR
DURBAN
FIGBAR
FORBAD
GASBAG
GIGBAG
GIMBAL
GLOBAL
GRABAT
GROBAN
GYMBAG
HERBAL
ICEBAG
ISOBAR
JABBAR
KASBAH
KITBAG
KLIBAN
KOMBAT
LUMBAR
MAMBAS
MUMBAI
NOTBAD
NUMBAT
OLDBAT
OUTBAN
OUTBAT
RAGBAG
RAWBAR
RAYBAN
REDBAT
REDBAY
RUMBAS
SAMBAS
SCUBAS
SEABAG
SHEBAT
SINBAD
STABAT
TEABAG
THEBAN
THEBAR
THEBAY
TIEBAR
TIMBAL
TOOBAD
TORBAY
TOWBAR
TRIBAL
TURBAN
VERBAL
WETBAR
WOMBAT

•••B•A

ARABIA
BAABAA
BALBOA
BARBRA
CARBRA
CUMBIA
GAMBIA
JERBOA
JOGBRA
LAMBDA
LISBOA
OJIBWA
PETBOA
PHOBIA
PUEBLA
ROBBIA
RUBBIA
SERBIA
ZAMBIA

••••BA

AMOEBA
ARRIBA
CASABA
HECUBA
JOJOBA
MAKEBA
RHUMBA
ROOMBA
SCOOBA
THENBA

BB••••

BBGUNS
BBKING
BBQPIT
BBSHOT

B•B•••

BABALU
BABBLE
BABBLY
BABELS
BABIED
BABIER
BABIES
BABKAS
BABOON
BABOOS
BABSON
BEBOPS
BIBBED
BIBBER
BIBLES
BIBLIO
BOBBED
BOBBER
BOBBIE
BOBBIN
BOBBLE
BOBBLY
BOBBYS
BOBCAT
BOBSUP
BUBBAS
BUBBLE
BUBBLY
BUBKES

B••B••

BAABAA
BABBLE
BABBLY
BADBOY
BAGBOY
BALBOA
BAMBIS
BAMBOO
BAOBAB
BARBAN
BARBED
BARBER
BARBET
BARBIE
BARBRA
BATBOY
BAUBLE
BEDBUG
BEEBEE
BENBEN
BENBOW
BERBER
BIBBED
BIBBER
BIEBER
BIGBAD
BIGBEN
BIGBET
BIGBOI
BIGBOX
BIGBOY
BIGBUX
BILBAO
BIMBOS
BISBEE
BLABBY
BLOBBY
BLOBEL
BOBBED
BOBBER
BOBBIE
BOBBIN
BOBBLE
BOBBLY
BOBBYS
BOMBAL
BOMBAY
BOMBED
BOMBER
BOMBES
BONBON
BOOBOO
BOXBED
BOXBOY
BRIBED
BRIBEE
BRIBER
BRIBES
BUBBAS
BUBBLE
BUBBLY
BUGBOY
BUMBLE
BUMBRY
BURBLE
BURBLY
BURBOT
BUSBOY
BYEBYE

B•••B•

BLABBY
BLOBBY
BLURBS

B••••B

BAGJOB
BAOBAB
BARTAB
BEDAUB
BENUMB
BICARB
BIOLAB

•BB•••

ABBACY
ABBADO
ABBESS
ABBEYS
ABBOTS
ABBOTT
ABBREV
EBBETS
EBBING

•B••B•

ABOMBS
HBOMBS
NBOMBS

•B•••B

ABACAB
ABSORB

••BB••

BABBLE
BABBLY
BIBBED
BIBBER
BOBBED
BOBBER
BOBBIE
BOBBIN
BOBBLE
BOBBLY
BOBBYS
BUBBAS
BUBBLE
BUBBLY
CABBED
CABBIE
CIBBER
COBBLE
CUBBED
DABBED
DABBER
DABBLE
DEBBIE
DIBBLE
DOBBIN
DUBBED
DUBBER
DYBBUK
FABBER
FIBBED
FIBBER
FOBBED
GABBED
GABBER
GABBLE
GABBRO
GIBBER
GIBBON
GOBBLE
HEBBEL
HOBBES
HOBBIT
HOBBLE
HUBBLE
HUBBUB
JABBAR
JABBED
JABBER
JOBBED
JOBBER
KIBBEE
KIBBLE
LIBBED
LIBBER
LIBBYS
LOBBED
LOBBER
LUBBER
MOBBED
MOBBER
NABBED
NABBER
NIBBLE
NUBBED
NUBBER
NUBBIN
NUBBLE
NUBBLY
PEBBLE
PEBBLY
RABBET
RABBIS
RABBIT
RABBLE
REBBES
REBBIE
RIBBED
RIBBER
RIBBIT
RIBBON
ROBBED
ROBBER
ROBBIA
ROBBIE
RUBBED
RUBBER
RUBBIA
RUBBLE
RUBBLY
SOBBED
SOBBER
SUBBED
TABBED
TUBBED
WABBIT
WEBBED
WEBBER
WOBBLE
WOBBLY

••B•B•

CUBEBS
IMBIBE
KABOBS
KEBABS
MYBABY
NABOBS
OHBABY

••B••B

COBWEB
HOBNOB
HUBBUB
SUBDEB
SUBURB

•••BB•

BLABBY
BLOBBY
CHUBBY
CLUBBY
CRABBE
CRABBY
FLABBY
GLOBBY
GRABBY
GRUBBY
KNOBBY
SHABBY
SLOBBY
SNOBBY
SNUBBY
STUBBY
SWABBY
THEBBC

•••B•B

BAOBAB
HUBBUB
JIMBOB
SKIBIB
SKIBOB

••••BB

LOWEBB
MCNABB
MRPIBB
SQUIBB
TYCOBB

BC••••

BCCING
BCDEFG
BCELLS
BCLION

B•C•••

BACALL
BACHED
BACHES
BACHIT
BACKED
BACKER
BACKIN
BACKUP
BACKUS
BACONS
BCCING
BECALM
BECAME
BECHET
BECKER
BECKET
BECKON
BECOME
BECOOL
BICARB
BICEPS
BICHON
BICKER
BICORN
BOCCES
BOCCIE
BOCCIS
BOCHCO
BOCHSA
BSCALE
BUCCAL
BUCHAN
BUCKED
BUCKER
BUCKET
BUCKLE
BUCKUP

B••C••

BADCOP
BANCOS
BARCAR
BARCOS
BEACHY
BEACON
BERCEO
BETCHA
BIGCAR
BIGCAT
BINCHY
BISCAY
BLACKS
BLOCKS
BLOCKY
BOBCAT
BOCCES
BOCCIE
BOCCIS
BOLCOM
BOOCOO
BOTCHY
BOUCHE
BOXCAR
BRACCO
BRACED
BRACER
BRACES
BRACHS
BRACTS
BRECHT
BRICKS
BRICKY
BROCAS
BUCCAL
BUICKS
BUNCHE
BUNCHY
BUNCOS

B•••C•

BARACK
BARUCH
BASICS
BAUSCH
BEDECK
BENICE
BIANCA
BIANCO
BIERCE
BINACA
BISECT
BLANCA
BLANCH
BLANCO
BLEACH
BLENCH
BLOTCH
BOCHCO
BODICE
BONACI
BORSCH
BOUNCE
BOUNCY
BRACCO
BRANCA
BRANCH
BRASCO
BREACH
BREECH
BROACH
BRONCO
BRONCS
BROOCH
BRUNCH

B••••C

BALTIC
BALZAC
BARDIC
BELGIC
BELLOC
BIGMAC
BIONIC
BIOPIC
BIOTIC

•BC•••

ABCDEF
NBCRED

•B•C••

ABACAB
ABACAS
ABACUS
ABSCAM
DBACKS
IBICES

•B••C•

ABBACY
ABDUCE
ABDUCT
ABJECT
IBMPCS
OBJECT

••BC••

BOBCAT
DUBCEK
HUBCAP
JOBCUT
RIBCUT
WEBCAM

••B•C•

ABBACY
CUBICS
GOBACK
IMBACK
INBACK
JSBACH
LUBECK
ORBACH
REBECS
XEBECS

••B••C

ENBANC
ENBLOC
FABRIC
PUBLIC
RUBRIC

•••B•C

AMEBIC
ARABIC
IAMBIC
LIMBIC
NIOBIC
PHOBIC
QUEBEC
SORBIC
TERBIC
THEBBC

••••BC

FIVEBC
FOURBC
NINEBC
THEBBC

B•D•••

BADBOY
BADCOP
BADDAY
BADDER
BADDIE
BADDOG
BADEGG
BADEMS
BADEND
BADFIT
BADGER
BADGES
BADGUY
BADHAM
BADHAT
BADLIE
BADLOT
BADMAN
BADMEN
BADOFF
BADRAP
BADUNS
BCDEFG
BEDAUB
BEDAZE
BEDBUG
BEDDED
BEDECK
BEDEWS
BEDIMS
BEDLAM
BEDOGS
BEDSIT
BEDWIN
BIDDEN
BIDDER
BIDERS
BIDETS
BIDFOR
BIDING
BIDSIN
BIDSON
BIDSUP
BODEGA
BODETT
BODICE
BODIED
BODIES
BODILY
BODINE
BODING
BODKIN
BODLEY
BODUKE
BUDDED
BUDDER
BUDDHA
BUDGED
BUDGER
BUDGES
BUDGET
BUDGIE
BYDATE

B••D••

BADDAY
BADDER
BADDIE
BADDOG
BAGDAD
BALDED
BALDER
BALDIE
BALDLY
BALDUR
BANDED
BANDER
BANDIT
BARDIC
BARDOT
BATDAY
BEADED
BEADER
BEADLE
BEADUP
BEDDED
BELDAM
BENDAY
BENDED
BENDER
BENDIX
BIDDEN
BIDDER
BIGDAY
BIGDIG
BIGDOG
BIGDOS
BILDAD
BINDER
BINDLE
BINDTO
BINDUP
BIRDED
BIRDER
BIRDIE
BLADED
BLADER
BLADES
BLUDGE
BLYDEN
BOLDED
BOLDEN
BOLDER
BOLDLY
BONDED
BONDER
BOODLE
BORDEN
BORDER
BORDET
BOUDIN
BREDES
BRIDAL
BRIDES
BRIDGE
BRIDLE
BRODIE
BRUDER
BSIDES
BUDDED
BUDDER
BUDDHA
BULDEO
BUNDLE
BUNDTS
BURDEN

B•••D•

BARADA
BEARDS
BESIDE
BETIDE
BIONDI
BIPEDS
BIPODS
BLANDA
BLEEDS
BLENDE
BLENDS
BLINDS
BLONDE
BLONDS
BLOODS
BLOODY
BOARDS
BOLIDE
BORIDE
BOUNDS
BOVIDS
BRAIDS
BRANDI
BRANDO
BRANDS
BRANDT
BRANDX
BRANDY
BREADS
BREEDS
BREEDY
BRENDA
BROADA
BROODS
BROODY
BUILDS

B••••D

BABIED
BACHED
BACKED
BADEND
BAFFED
BAGDAD
BAGEND
BAGGED
BAILED
BAITED
BALDED
BALKED
BALLAD
BANDED
BANGED
BANKED
BANNED
BARBED
BARGED
BARKED
BARNED
BARRED
BASHED
BASKED
BASTED
BATHED
BATTED
BAWLED
BAYARD
BEADED
BEAKED
BEAMED
BEANED
BEDDED
BEEFED
BEEPED
BEGGED
BEGIRD
BEGOOD
BEHEAD
BEHELD
BEHIND
BEHOLD
BEKIND
BELIED
BELLED
BELTED
BENDED
BERMED
BESTED
BETTED
BEYOND
BIASED
BIBBED
BIFFED
BIFOLD
BIGBAD
BIGEND
BIGKID
BIGRED
BILDAD
BILGED
BILKED
BILLED
BINGED
BINNED
BIRDED
BIRLED
BIRRED
BITTED
BLADED
BLAMED
BLARED
BLAZED
BOATED
BOBBED
BODIED
BOFFED
BOGGED
BOILED
BOLDED
BOLTED
BOMBED
BONDED
BONGED
BONKED
BOOKED
BOOMED
BOOTED
BOOZED
BOPPED
BORKED
BOSSED
BOWLED
BOXBED
BRACED
BRAKED
BRAVED
BRAYED
BREWED
BRIAND
BRIARD
BRIBED
BRIGID
BRINED
BROWED
BRUXED
BUCKED
BUDDED
BUDGED
BUFFED
BUGGED
BUGLED
BUJOLD
BULGED
BULKED
BULLED
BUMMED
BUMPED
BUNGED
BUNKED
BUNTED
BUOYED
BURIED
BURLED
BURNED
BURPED
BURRED
BUSHED
BUSIED
BUSKED
BUSSED
BUSTED
BUTTED
BUZZED
BYHAND
BYLAND
BYROAD
BYWORD

•BD•••

ABDIEL
ABDUCE
ABDUCT

•B•D••

ABCDEF
ABIDED
ABIDER
ABIDES
ABODES
IBADAN
IBIDEM

•B••D•

ABBADO
ABRADE
EBONDS
OBLADI
PBANDJ
TBIRDS
TBONDS

•B•••D

ABASED
ABATED
ABIDED
ABOARD
ABOUND
ABROAD
ABSURD
ABUSED
NBCRED
OBEYED
OBTUND

••BD••

SUBDEB
SUBDUE

••B•D•

ABBADO
ALBEDO
AUBADE
EMBEDS
EMBODY
IMBEDS
LIBIDO
NOBODY
REBIDS
SABADO
STBEDE
UNBUDS
WEBADS

••B••D

AMBAND
AMBLED
BABIED
BIBBED
BOBBED
CABBED
CABLED
CUBBED
CUBOID
DABBED
DUBBED
FABLED
FIBBED
FMBAND
FOBBED
GABBED
GABLED
HOBOED
HYBRID
IMBUED
INBRED
JABBED
JOBBED
KOBOLD
LIBBED
LOBBED

MOBBED
MRBOND
NABBED
NUBBED
REBEND
REBIND
REBRED
RIBALD
RIBAND
RIBBED
RIBPAD
ROBBED
RUBBED
RUBIED
SOBBED
SUBBED
SUBGOD
SUBLID
TABARD
TABBED
TABLED
TABUED
TUBBED
UNBEND
UNBIND
UNBLED
UNBOLD
UPBIND
WEBBED
WEBFED

•••BD•

LAMBDA

•••B•D

AIRBUD
BARBED
BIBBED
BIGBAD
BOBBED
BOMBED
BOXBED
BRIBED
CABBED
CATBED
COMBED
CUBBED
CUEBID
CURBED
DABBED
DAUBED
DAYBED
DIDBAD
DISBUD
DOGBED
DUBBED
EARBUD
FIBBED
FOBBED
FORBAD
FORBID
GABBED
GARBED
GLOBED
HERBED
HOTBED
JABBED
JOBBED
LAMBED
LIBBED
LIMBED
LOBBED
LOWBID
MOBBED
MORBID
NABBED
NOTBAD
NUBBED
NUMBED
OUTBID
OUTBUD
PREBID
PROBED
REDBUD
RIBBED
ROBBED
RUBBED
SEABED
SINBAD
SOBBED
SUBBED
TABBED
TOOBAD
TOPBID
TUBBED
TURBID
VERBID
WEBBED

BE••••

BEACHY
BEACON
BEADED
BEADER
BEADLE
BEADUP
BEAGLE
BEAKED
BEAKER
BEALLS
BEAMAN
BEAMED
BEAMER
BEAMON
BEAMUP
BEANED
BEANIE
BEANOS
BEAPAL
BEARDS
BEARER
BEARON
BEARSE
BEARUP
BEASTS
BEATAT
BEATEN
BEATER
BEATIT
BEATLE
BEATON
BEATTY
BEATUP
BEAUTS
BEAUTY
BEAVER
BEAVIS
BEBOPS
BECALM
BECAME
BECHET
BECKER
BECKET
BECKON
BECOME
BECOOL
BEDAUB
BEDAZE
BEDBUG
BEDDED
BEDECK
BEDEWS
BEDIMS
BEDLAM
BEDOGS
BEDSIT
BEDWIN
BEEBEE
BEEFED
BEEFUP
BEEGEE
BEEMER
BEEPAT
BEEPED
BEEPER
BEETLE
BEEVES
BEEZER
BEFAIR
BEFALL
BEFELL
BEFIRM
BEFITS
BEFOGS
BEFOOL
BEFORE
BEFOUL
BEGEMS
BEGETS
BEGFOR
BEGGAR
BEGGED
BEGINS
BEGIRD
BEGIRT
BEGLEY
BEGOFF
BEGONE
BEGOOD
BEGUMS
BEHAIM
BEHALF
BEHAVE
BEHEAD
BEHELD
BEHEST
BEHIND
BEHOLD
BEHOME
BEHOOF
BEIGES
BEIGHT
BEIGNE
BEINGS
BEINON
BEIRUT
BEJART
BEKIND
BELAIR
BELATE
BELAYS
BELDAM
BELFRY
BELGAE
BELGIC
BELIAL
BELIED
BELIEF
BELIER
BELIES
BELIKE
BELIZE
BELLAY
BELLED
BELLES
BELLOC
BELLOW
BELLUM
BELOIT
BELONG
BELONS
BELTED
BELTER
BELTON
BELTUP
BELUGA
BELZER
BEMATA
BEMINE
BEMIRE
BEMOAN
BEMUSE
BENBEN
BENBOW
BENDAY
BENDED
BENDER
BENDIX
BENEKE
BENGAL
BENGAY
BENHUR
BENICE
BENIGN
BENING
BENITO
BENNIE
BENOIT
BENOTE
BENSEY
BENSON
BENTON
BENTOS
BENUMB
BENZOL
BERATE
BERBER
BERCEO
BEREFT
BERETS
BERGEN
BERGER
BERING
BERKOW
BERLIN
BERMAN
BERMED
BERNIE
BERTHA
BERTHE
BERTHS
BERTIE
BERWYN
BERYLS
BESAME
BESANT
BESETS
BESIDE
BESOMS
BESORE
BESOTS
BESSEL
BESSER
BESSIE
BESSON
BESTED
BESTER
BESTIR
BESTOW
BESURE
BETAKE
BETCHA
BETELS
BETHEL
BETIDE
BETONY
BETOOK
BETRAY
BETSEY
BETSON
BETSYS
BETTAS
BETTED
BETTER
BETTOR
BETTYE
BEULAH
BEURRE
BEVANS
BEVELS
BEVIES
BEWAIL
BEWARE
BEWARY
BEWELL
BEWIGS
BEYMER
BEYOND
BEZELS

B•E•••

BAERGA
BAEYER
BCELLS
BEEBEE
BEEFED
BEEFUP
BEEGEE
BEEMER
BEEPAT
BEEPED
BEEPER
BEETLE
BEEVES
BEEZER
BIEBER
BIERCE
BIERES
BLEACH
BLEAKS
BLEARS
BLEARY
BLEATS
BLEEDS
BLEEPS
BLEETH
BLENCH
BLENDE
BLENDS
BLEWIN
BLEWIT
BLEWON
BLEWUP
BOEING
BOESKY
BREACH
BREADS
BREAKS
BREAMS
BREAST
BREATH
BRECHT
BREDES
BREECH
BREEDS
BREEDY
BREEZE
BREEZY
BREMEN
BREMER
BRENDA
BRENLY
BRETON
BREUER
BREVES
BREVET
BREVIS
BREWED
BREWER
BREWUP
BREYER
BSEVEN
BTEAMS
BUENAS
BUENOS
BYEBYE
BYENOW

B••E••

BABELS
BADEGG
BADEMS
BADEND
BAGELS
BAGEND
BAKERS
BAKERY
BALEEN
BALERS
BAREGE
BARELY
BAREST
BASELY
BASEST
BATEAU
BAYERN
BAYEUX
BCDEFG
BEDECK
BEDEWS
BEFELL
BEGEMS
BEGETS
BEHEAD
BEHELD
BEHEST
BENEKE
BEREFT
BERETS
BESETS
BETELS
BEVELS
BEWELL
BEZELS
BICEPS
BIDERS
BIDETS
BIGEAR
BIGEND
BIGEYE
BIKERS
BIPEDS
BIREME
BISECT
BITEIN
BITEON
BITERS
BITEUP
BLEEDS
BLEEPS
BLEETH
BLUELY
BLUEOX
BLUEST
BLUESY
BLUETS
BODEGA
BODETT
BOGEYS
BOHEME
BOLENA
BOLERO
BOLEYN
BONERS
BONERZ
BONEUP
BOOERS
BOPEEP
BOREAL
BOREAS
BOREON
BORERS
BOREUP
BOTELS
BOWELS
BOWERS
BOWERY
BOXERS
BREECH
BREEDS
BREEDY
BREEZE
BREEZY
BRIEFS
BRIENZ
BRIERS
BRIERY
BUREAU
BURETS
BUTENE
BUTEOS
BUYERS
BYTENS

B•••E•

BABIED
BABIER
BABIES
BACHED
BACHES
BACKED
BACKER
BADDER
BADGER
BADGES
BADMEN
BAEYER
BAFFED
BAFFER
BAGGED
BAGGER
BAGMEN
BAHNEN
BAILED
BAILEE
BAILER
BAILEY
BAINES
BAITED
BAITER
BAIZES
BAKKER
BALDED
BALDER
BALEEN
BALKED
BALKER
BALLET
BALMER
BANDED
BANDER
BANGED
BANGER
BANKED
BANKER
BANNED
BANNEN
BANNER
BANTER
BARBED
BARBER
BARBET
BARGED
BARGER
BARGES
BARKED
BARKER
BARLEY
BARMEN
BARNED
BARNES
BARNET
BARNEY
BARRED
BARREL
BARREN
BARRES
BARRET
BARTEL
BARTER
BASHED
BASHER
BASHES
BASKED
BASKER
BASKET
BASSES
BASSET
BASSEY
BASTED
BASTER
BASTES
BATHED
BATHER
BATHES
BATLEY
BATMEN
BATTED
BATTEN
BATTER
BAUMER
BAVIER
BAWLED
BAWLER
BAXTER
BAYMEN
BEADED
BEADER
BEAKED
BEAKER
BEAMED
BEAMER
BEANED
BEARER
BEATEN
BEATER
BEAVER
BECHET
BECKER
BECKET
BEDDED
BEEBEE
BEEFED
BEEGEE
BEEMER
BEEPED
BEEPER
BEEVES
BEEZER
BEGGED
BEGLEY
BEIGES
BELIED
BELIEF
BELIER
BELIES
BELLED
BELLES
BELTED
BELTER
BELZER
BENBEN
BENDED
BENDER
BENSEY
BERBER
BERCEO
BERGEN
BERGER
BERMED
BESSEL
BESSER
BESTED
BESTER
BETHEL
BETSEY
BETTED
BETTER
BEVIES
BEYMER
BIASED
BIASES
BIBBED
BIBBER
BIBLES
BICKER
BIDDEN
BIDDER
BIEBER
BIERES
BIFFED
BIGBEN
BIGBET
BIGGER
BIGMEN
BIGRED
BIGTEN
BILGED
BILGES
BILKED
BILKER
BILLED
BILLER
BILLET
BINDER
BINGED
BINGER
BINGES
BINNED
BINNEY
BIOMES
BIRDED
BIRDER
BIRLED
BIRLER
BIRNEY
BIRRED
BISBEE
BISSET
BITNET
BITTED
BITTEN
BITTER
BLADED
BLADER
BLADES
BLAKEY
BLAMED
BLAMER
BLAMES
BLARED
BLARES
BLAZED
BLAZER
BLAZES
BLIMEY
BLIXEN
BLOBEL
BLOKES
BLOOEY
BLOWER
BLYDEN
BOATED
BOATEL
BOATER
BOBBED
BOBBER
BOCCES
BODIED
BODIES
BODLEY
BOFFED
BOGGED
BOGIES
BOGLES
BOHRER
BOILED
BOILER
BOITES
BOKKEN
BOLDED
BOLDEN
BOLDER
BOLGER
BOLTED
BOLTER
BOMBED
BOMBER
BOMBES
BONDED
BONDER
BONGED
BONIER
BONKED
BONNER
BONNES
BONNET
BONNEY
BONZES
BOOKED
BOOKEM
BOOKER
BOOMED
BOOMER
BOOTED
BOOTEE
BOOTER
BOOTES
BOOZED
BOOZER
BOOZES
BOPEEP
BOPPED
BOPPER
BORDEN
BORDER
BORDET
BORGES
BORKED
BORNEO
BOSLEY
BOSSED
BOSSES
BOTHER
BOTREE
BOULES
BOULEZ
BOWLED
BOWLER
BOWLES
BOWMEN
BOWYER
BOWZER
BOXBED
BOXIER
BOXSET
BOYLES
BRACED
BRACER
BRACES
BRAKED
BRAKES
BRAVED
BRAVER
BRAVES
BRAYED
BRAYER
BRAZEN
BREDES
BREMEN
BREMER
BREUER
BREVES
BREVET
BREWED
BREWER
BREYER
BRIBED
BRIBEE
BRIBER
BRIBES
BRIDES
BRINED
BRINER
BRINES
BRISES
BROKEN
BROKER
BROWED
BRUDER
BRUGES
BRULEE
BRUMEL
BRUMES
BRUNEI
BRUNET
BRUTES
BRUXED
BRUXES
BSEVEN
BSIDES
BTHREE
BTILES
BUBKES
BUCKED
BUCKER
BUCKET
BUDDED
BUDDER
BUDGED
BUDGER
BUDGES
BUDGET
BUFFED
BUFFER
BUFFET
BUGGED
BUGLED
BUGLER
BUGLES
BULDEO
BULGED
BULGES
BULKED
BULLED
BULLET
BULWER
BUMLEG
BUMMED
BUMMER
BUMPED
BUMPER
BUNGED
BUNGEE
BUNKED
BUNKER
BUNSEN
BUNTED
BUNTER
BUNUEL
BUOYED
BUPKES
BURDEN
BURGEE
BURGER
BURIED
BURIER
BURIES
BURLED
BURLER
BURLEY
BURNED
BURNER
BURNET
BURNEY
BURPED
BURPEE
BURRED
BUSHED
BUSHEL
BUSHER
BUSHES
BUSIED
BUSIER
BUSIES
BUSKED
BUSKER
BUSMEN
BUSSED
BUSSES
BUSTED
BUSTER
BUTLER
BUTTED
BUTTER
BUTTES
BUTYET
BUZZED
BUZZER
BUZZES
BYRNES
BYTHEN

B••••E

BABBLE
BADDIE
BADLIE
BAFFLE
BAGGIE
BAILEE
BALDIE
BALINE
BANANE
BANGLE
BANQUE
BARBIE
BAREGE
BARITE
BARONE
BARQUE
BARRIE
BARTLE
BASQUE
BATTLE
BAUBLE
BEADLE
BEAGLE
BEANIE
BEARSE
BEATLE
BECAME
BECOME
BEDAZE
BEEBEE
BEEGEE
BEETLE
BEFORE
BEGONE
BEHAVE
BEHOME
BEIGNE
BELATE
BELGAE
BELIKE
BELIZE
BEMINE
BEMIRE
BEMUSE
BENEKE
BENICE
BENNIE
BENOTE
BERATE
BERNIE
BERTHE
BERTIE
BESAME
BESIDE
BESORE
BESSIE
BESURE
BETAKE
BETIDE
BETTYE
BEURRE
BEWARE
BIERCE
BIGAPE
BIGEYE
BIGGIE
BIGJOE
BIGLIE
BIGONE
BIGTOE
BILLIE
BINATE
BINDLE
BINGLE
BINNIE
BIRDIE
BIREME
BISBEE
BISQUE
BLAINE
BLAISE
BLENDE
BLITHE
BLONDE
BLOOIE
BLOUSE
BLUDGE
BLYTHE
BMOVIE
BOBBIE
BOBBLE
BOCCIE
BODICE
BODINE
BODUKE
BOGGLE
BOHEME
BOLIDE
BONNIE
BOODLE
BOOGIE
BOOKIE
BOOTEE
BOOTHE
BOOTIE
BORATE
BORIDE
BOTREE
BOTTLE
BOUCHE
BOUFFE
BOUNCE
BOURKE
BOURNE
BOURSE
BOVINE

BOWTIE BRAISE BRAQUE BREEZE BRIBEE BRIDGE BRIDLE BRODIE BROGUE BRONTE BRONZE BROOKE BROSSE BROWNE BROWSE BRUISE BRULEE BSCALE BTHREE BUBBLE BUCKLE BUDGIE BULLAE BUMBLE BUNCHE BUNDLE BUNGEE BUNGLE BURBLE BURGEE BURGLE BURNIE BURPEE BURSAE BUSTLE BUTANE BUTENE BYDATE BYEBYE BYGONE BYJOVE BYLINE BYNAME BYROTE BYSSHE BYWIRE

•BE•••

ABELES EBERLE EBERLY HBEAMS IBEAMS IBERIA IBEXES LBEAMS OBEAHS OBELUS OBENTO OBERON OBERTO OBEYED OBEYER

•B•E••

ABBESS ABBEYS ABJECT ABLEST ABSENT EBBETS NBAERS OBJECT OBJETS OBSESS OBTEST OBVERT UBIETY

•B••E•

ABASED ABASER ABASES ABATED ABATER ABATES ABBREV ABCDEF ABDIEL ABELES ABIDED ABIDER ABIDES ABODES ABUSED ABUSER ABUSES EBATES EBAYER FBIMEN IBANEZ IBEXES IBICES IBIDEM IBISES NBCRED OBEYED OBEYER OBITER OBOLER OBRIEN RBIMEN TBONES XBOXES

•B•••E

ABDUCE ABJURE ABLARE ABLATE ABLAZE ABRADE EBERLE OBLATE OBLIGE OBTUSE TBOONE

••BE••

ABBESS ABBEYS ALBEDO ALBEIT ALBERS ALBERT AMBERS AMBERY ARBELA ATBEST BABELS CABELL CABERS CABEZA CUBEBS CUBERS EBBETS EDBERG EGBERT EKBERG ELBERT EMBEDS EMBERS ENBERG FIBERS GIBEAT GIBERS HABEAS HUBERT IMBEAT IMBEDS JIBEAT JOBETH LABELS LEBEAU LIBELS LIBERS LLBEAN LUBECK MABELL MCBEAL MOBERG MRBEAN NOBELS OSBERT REBECS REBELS REBEND REBENT REBETS RIBERA RIBEYE ROBERS ROBERT RUBELS RUBENS SABENA SABERS SEBERG SOBEIT SOBERS STBEDE TEBETS TUBERS UMBELS UMBERS UNBELT UNBEND UNBENT UPBEAR UPBEAT WEBERN WEBERS XEBECS

••B•E•

ABBREV AMBIEN AMBLED AMBLER AMBLES ARBRES AUBREY BABIED BABIER BABIES BIBBED BIBBER BIBLES BOBBED BOBBER BUBKES CABBED CABLED CABLER CABLES CABLET CABMEN CIBBER COBWEB CUBBED DABBED DABBER DABNEY DEBREU DEBTEE DOBLES DUBBED DUBBER DUBCEK EMBLEM EUBOEA FABBER FABLED FABLER FABLES FIBBED FIBBER FIBRES FOBBED GABBED GABBER GABLED GABLER GABLES GIBBER GIBLET GOBIES GOBLET GOBOES HEBBEL HEBREW HOBBES HOBOED HOBOES HUBLEY IMBUED IMBUES INBRED JABBED JABBER JOBBED JOBBER KIBBEE KUBLER LABFEE LABREA LEBRET LIBBED LIBBER LOBBED LOBBER LUBBER MABLEY MOBBED MOBBER MOBLEY NABBED NABBER NIBLET NOBLER NOBLES NUBBED NUBBER RABBET RABIES REBBES REBRED REBREW RIBBED RIBBER RIBLET ROBBED ROBBER ROBLES RUBBED RUBBER RUBIED RUBIES RUBLES RUBLEV SABLES SABRES SOBBED SOBBER SUBBED SUBDEB SUBLET SUBNET SUBSEA SUBSET TABBED TABKEY TABLED TABLES TABLET TABSET TABUED TOBIES TUBBED UNBLED VEBLEN WEBBED WEBBER WEBFED

••B••E

ALBINE AUBADE BABBLE BOBBIE BOBBLE BUBBLE CABBIE COBBLE CUBAGE DABBLE DEBASE DEBATE DEBBIE DEBONE DEBTEE DIBBLE DUBOSE EMBRUE GABBLE GOBBLE HABILE HOBBLE HUBBLE IMBIBE IMBRUE INBLUE JOBONE KIBBEE KIBBLE LABFEE LABILE LABINE LIBRAE LOBATE LOBULE MOBILE MRBLUE NIBBLE NOBAKE NOBILE NUBBLE NUBILE OKBYME ONBASE PEBBLE RABBLE REBAKE REBALE REBATE REBBIE REBORE REBOTE REBUKE RIBEYE RIBOSE ROBBIE RUBBLE SABINE STBEDE SUBDUE SUBTLE TIBIAE TUBAGE TUBATE TUBULE UMBRAE UNBALE UNBARE URBANE WOBBLE ZABRZE

•••BE•

ADOBES BARBED BARBER BARBET BEEBEE BENBEN BERBER BIBBED BIBBER BIEBER BIGBEN BIGBET BISBEE BLOBEL BOBBED BOBBER BOMBED BOMBER BOMBES BOXBED BRIBED BRIBEE BRIBER BRIBES CABBED CAMBER CATBED CIBBER COMBED COMBER CORBEL CUBBED CUMBER CURBED DABBED DABBER DAUBED DAUBER DAUBES DAWBER DAYBED DOGBED DOMBEY DRABEK DUBBED DUBBER DUMBER FABBER FERBER FIBBED FIBBER FOBBED FORBES GABBED GABBER GARBED GARBER GERBER GIBBER GIMBEL GLOBED GLOBES GOOBER GREBES GUMBEL HEBBEL HERBED HERBES HOBBES HOTBED HUMBER ILLBET ISABEL JABBED JABBER JAMBES JOBBED JOBBER KHYBER KIBBEE KNEBEL LAMBED LIBBED LIBBER LIEBER LIMBED LIMBER LOBBED LOBBER LUBBER LUMBER MAYBES MEEBER MEMBER MOBBED MOBBER NABBED NABBER NUBBED NUBBER NUMBED NUMBER OUTBEG PLEBES PROBED PROBER PROBES QUEBEC RABBET REBBES REUBEN RIBBED RIBBER ROBBED ROBBER RUBBED RUBBER SEABED SEABEE SIÉBEN SIRBEN SOBBED SOBBER SOMBER SORBET SUBBED TABBED THEBEE THEBES TIMBER TOMBES TREBEK TRIBES TUBBED UTUBES WEBBED WEBBER YOUBET

•••B•E

ALIBLE AMEBAE ARABLE BABBLE BARBIE BAUBLE BEEBEE BISBEE BOBBIE BOBBLE BRIBEE BUBBLE BUMBLE BURBLE BYEBYE CABBIE COBBLE CRABBE DABBLE DEBBIE DIABLE DIBBLE DOABLE DOUBLE EDIBLE ENABLE FEEBLE FOIBLE FUMBLE GABBLE GAMBLE GARBLE GOBBLE GRABLE HEEBIE HERBIE HOBBLE HOMBRE HUBBLE HUMBLE JUMBLE KEMBLE KIBBEE KIBBLE KIMBLE LIABLE MARBLE MUMBLE NEWBIE NIBBLE NIMBLE NOMBRE NUBBLE PEBBLE PROBIE RABBLE RAMBLE REBBIE ROBBIE RUBBLE RUMBLE SEABEE SOMBRE STABLE SUABLE THEBEE TIMBRE TREBLE TUMBLE UNABLE USABLE VIABLE WAMBLE WARBLE WOBBLE ZOMBIE

••••BE

ACHEBE AEROBE CANTBE CARIBE CRABBE DANUBE ENROBE FLAMBE IMBIBE IVTUBE JARABE JUJUBE LEFTBE LETSBE MCCABE MUGABE NEEDBE PHOEBE SCRIBE STROBE THISBE UNROBE WILLBE

BF••••

BFLATS

B•F•••

BAFFED BAFFER BAFFIN BAFFLE BEFAIR BEFALL BEFELL BEFIRM BEFITS BEFOGS BEFOOL BEFORE BEFOUL BIFFED BIFOLD BIFORM BOFFED BOFFIN BOFFOS BUFFAY BUFFED BUFFER BUFFET BUFFON BUFFOS BUFFUP BYFORM

B••F••

BADFIT BAFFED BAFFER BAFFIN BAFFLE BAGFUL BARFLY BATFOR BEEFED BEEFUP BEGFOR BELFRY BIAFRA BIDFOR BIFFED BIGFAN BIGFUN BLAFFS BLIFIL BLUFFO BLUFFS BOFFED BOFFIN BOFFOS BOTFLY BOUFFE BOWFIN BOXFUL BUFFAY BUFFED BUFFER BUFFET BUFFON BUFFOS BUFFUP

B•••F•

BADOFF BASIFY BCDEFG BEGOFF BEREFT BITOFF BLAFFS BLUFFO BLUFFS BOUFFE BRIEFS BUGOFF BUYOFF

B••••F

BADOFF BEGOFF BEHALF BEHOOF BELIEF BITOFF BUGOFF BUYOFF BYHALF

•B•••F

ABCDEF ABITOF

••BF••

CUBFAN LABFEE SOBFUL TUBFUL WEBFED

••B•F•

FOBOFF REBUFF RUBIFY RUBOFF

••B••F

FOBOFF GOBSOF REBUFF ROBSOF RUBOFF

BG••••

BGIRLS

B•G•••

BAGBOY BAGDAD BAGELS BAGEND BAGFUL BAGGED BAGGER BAGGIE BAGJOB BAGMAN BAGMEN BAGNIO BAGSIT BAGWIG BBGUNS BEGEMS BEGETS BEGFOR BEGGAR BEGGED BEGINS BEGIRD BEGIRT BEGLEY BEGOFF BEGONE BEGOOD BEGUMS BIGAIR BIGAMY BIGAPE BIGBAD BIGBEN BIGBET BIGBOI BIGBOX BIGBOY BIGBUX BIGCAR BIGCAT BIGDAY BIGDIG BIGDOG BIGDOS BIGEAR BIGEND BIGEYE BIGFAN BIGFUN BIGGER BIGGIE BIGGUN BIGGUY BIGHIT BIGHTS BIGHUG BIGJOE BIGKID BIGLIE BIGMAC BIGMAN BIGMEN BIGOIL BIGONE BIGOTS BIGRED BIGRIG BIGSKY BIGSUR BIGTEN BIGTOE BIGTOP BIGWIG BIGWIN BOGART BOGEYS BOGGED BOGGLE BOGIES BOGLES BOGOTA BUGAKU BUGBOY BUGGED BUGLED BUGLER BUGLES BUGOFF BUGOUT BYGONE BYGOSH

B••G••

BADGER BADGES BADGUY BAGGED BAGGER BAGGIE BANGED BANGER BANGLE BANGON BANGOR BANGUI BANGUP BARGED BARGER BARGES BEAGLE BEEGEE BEGGAR BEGGED BEIGES BEIGHT BEIGNE BELGAE BELGIC BENGAL BENGAY BERGEN BERGER BIGGER BIGGIE BIGGUN BIGGUY BILGED BILGES BINGED BINGER BINGES BINGLE BINGOS BIOGAS BIRGIT BLIGHT BOGGED BOGGLE BOLGER BONGED BONGOS BOOGIE BORGES BORGIA BOUGHS BOUGHT BRIGHT BRIGID BRIGIT BROGAN BROGUE BRUGES BUDGED BUDGER BUDGES BUDGET BUDGIE BUGGED BULGAR BULGED BULGES BULGUR BUNGAY BUNGED BUNGEE BUNGLE BURGEE BURGER BURGHS BURGLE BURGOO BURGOS

B•••G•

BADEGG BAERGA BAREGE BEDOGS BEFOGS BEINGS BELUGA BENIGN BEWIGS BHANGS BLUDGE BODEGA BOINGO BOINGS BOURGS BRIDGE BRINGS BROUGH

B••••G

BAAING BADDOG BADEGG BAGWIG BAKING BALING BARING BASING BATING BAYING BBKING BCCING BCDEFG BEDBUG BELONG BENING BERING BIDING BIGDIG BIGDOG BIGHUG BIGRIG BIGWIG BIKING BINNIG BITING BLUING BODING BOEING BONING BOOING BORING BOWING BOXING BUMLEG BUSING BUYING

•BG•••

BBGUNS OBGYNS

•B••G•

OBLIGE UBANGI

•B•••G

BBKING EBBING OBLONG

6 BE

••BG••
SUBGOD
SUBGUM

••B•G•
CUBAGE
DEBAGS
DEBUGS
EMBOGS
REBAGS
TOBAGO
TUBAGE
UNBAGS
VWBUGS

••B••G
ALBORG
COBURG
CUBING
CYBORG
EBBING
EDBERG
EKBERG
ENBERG
GIBING
GOBANG
JIBING
LUBING
MOBERG
ORBING
ROBING
SEBERG
TUBING
WEBLOG

•••B•G
AIRBAG
BEDBUG
FLUBUG
GASBAG
GIGBAG
GYMBAG
HOWBIG
HUMBUG
ICEBAG
KITBAG
LIEBIG
OUTBEG
RAGBAG
SEABAG
TEABAG
TOOBIG
WINBIG
WONBIG
YEABIG

BH••••
BHANGS
BHOPAL
BHUTAN
BHUTTO

B•H•••
BAHAMA
BAHIAN
BAHNEN
BEHAIM
BEHALF
BEHAVE
BEHEAD
BEHELD
BEHEST
BEHIND
BEHOLD
BEHOME
BEHOOF
BOHEME
BOHRER
BSHARP
BTHREE
BYHALF
BYHAND

B••H••
BACHED
BACHES
BACHIT
BADHAM
BADHAT
BARHOP
BASHED
BASHER
BASHES
BASHIN
BATHED
BATHER
BATHES
BATHOS
BBSHOT
BECHET
BENHUR
BETHEL
BICHON
BIGHIT
BIGHTS
BIGHUG
BISHOP
BOCHCO
BOCHSA
BONHAM
BOOHOO
BOTHER
BRAHMA
BRAHMS
BUCHAN
BUSHED
BUSHEL
BUSHER
BUSHES
BUSHWA
BUTHOW
BYTHEN

B•••H•
BAKSHI
BEACHY
BEIGHT
BERTHA
BERTHE
BERTHS
BETCHA
BINCHY
BIRTHS
BLIGHT
BLITHE
BLYTHE
BOLSHY
BOOTHE
BOOTHS
BOTCHY
BOUCHE
BOUGHS
BOUGHT
BRACHS
BRASHY
BRECHT
BRIGHT
BROPHY
BROTHS
BROTHY
BRUSHY
BUDDHA
BUNCHE
BUNCHY
BUQSHA
BURGHS
BUTWHO
BUTWHY
BYSSHE

B••••H
BANISH
BARUCH
BASRAH
BAUSCH
BEULAH
BLANCH
BLEACH
BLEETH
BLENCH
BLOTCH
BLUISH
BORSCH
BOYISH
BRAMAH
BRANCH
BREACH
BREATH
BREECH
BROACH
BROOCH
BROUGH
BRUNCH
BYGOSH
BYPATH

•BH•••
ABHORS

•B•H••
ABMHOS
ABOHMS
BBSHOT

•B••H•
OBEAHS

•B•••H
ABLUSH

••BH••
COBHAM
JOBHOP

••B••H
AMBUSH
DEBRAH
JOBETH
JSBACH
KIBOSH
ORBACH
WABASH

•••B•H
CASBAH
KASBAH

BI••••
BIAFRA
BIALIK
BIANCA
BIANCO
BIASED
BIASES
BIBBED
BIBBER
BIBLES
BIBLIO
BICARB
BICEPS
BICHON
BICKER
BICORN
BIDDEN
BIDDER
BIDERS
BIDETS
BIDFOR
BIDING
BIDSIN
BIDSON
BIDSUP
BIEBER
BIERCE
BIERES
BIFFED
BIFOLD
BIFORM
BIGAIR
BIGAMY
BIGAPE
BIGBAD
BIGBEN
BIGBET
BIGBOI
BIGBOX
BIGBOY
BIGBUX
BIGCAR
BIGCAT
BIGDAY
BIGDIG
BIGDOG
BIGDOS
BIGEAR
BIGEND
BIGEYE
BIGFAN
BIGFUN
BIGGER
BIGGIE
BIGGUN
BIGGUY
BIGHIT
BIGHTS
BIGHUG
BIGJOE
BIGKID
BIGLIE
BIGMAC
BIGMAN
BIGMEN
BIGOIL
BIGONE
BIGOTS
BIGRED
BIGRIG
BIGSKY
BIGSUR
BIGTEN
BIGTOE
BIGTOP
BIGWIG
BIGWIN
BIJOUS
BIJOUX
BIKERS
BIKILA
BIKING
BIKINI
BILBAO
BILDAD
BILGED
BILGES
BILKED
BILKER
BILLED
BILLER
BILLET
BILLIE
BILLIS
BILLOW
BILOXI
BIMBOS
BIMINI
BINACA
BINARY
BINATE
BINCHY
BINDER
BINDLE
BINDTO
BINDUP
BINGED
BINGER
BINGES
BINGLE
BINGOS
BINNED
BINNEY
BINNIE
BINNIG
BINYON
BIOGAS
BIOLAB
BIOMES
BIONDI
BIONIC
BIONTS
BIOPIC
BIOPSY
BIOTAS
BIOTIC
BIOTIN
BIPEDS
BIPODS
BIRDED
BIRDER
BIRDIE
BIREME
BIRGIT
BIRLED
BIRLER
BIRMAN
BIRNEY
BIRRED
BIRTHS
BISBEE
BISCAY
BISECT
BISHOP
BISONS
BISQUE
BISSAU
BISSET
BISTRO
BITEIN
BITEON
BITERS
BITEUP
BITING
BITMAP
BITNET
BITOFF
BITTED
BITTEN
BITTER
BIZKIT

B•I•••
BAIKAL
BAILED
BAILEE
BAILER
BAILEY
BAILON
BAILOR
BAINES
BAIRNS
BAISAS
BAITED
BAITER
BAIZAS
BAIZES
BEIGES
BEIGHT
BEIGNE
BEINGS
BEINON
BEIRUT
BGIRLS
BLIFIL
BLIGHT
BLIMEY
BLIMPS
BLINDS
BLINIS
BLINKS
BLINTZ
BLISTS
BLITHE
BLIXEN
BMINOR
BMINUS
BOILED
BOILER
BOILUP
BOINGO
BOINGS
BOITES
BRIANA
BRIAND
BRIARD
BRIARS
BRIARY
BRIBED
BRIBEE
BRIBER
BRIBES
BRICKS
BRICKY
BRIDAL
BRIDES
BRIDGE
BRIDLE
BRIEFS
BRIENZ
BRIERS
BRIERY
BRIGHT
BRIGID
BRIGIT
BRILLO
BRINED
BRINER
BRINES
BRINGS
BRINKS
BRISES
BRISKS
BRITON
BSIDES
BTILES
BUICKS
BUILDS

B••I••
BAAING
BABIED
BABIER
BABIES
BAHIAN
BAKING
BALINE
BALING
BANISH
BARING
BARITE
BARIUM
BASIAL
BASICS
BASIFY
BASILS
BASING
BASINS
BATIKS
BATING
BAVIER
BAYING
BBKING
BCCING
BCLION
BEDIMS
BEFIRM
BEFITS
BEGINS
BEGIRD
BEGIRT
BEHIND
BEKIND
BELIAL
BELIED
BELIEF
BELIER
BELIES
BELIKE
BELIZE
BEMINE
BEMIRE
BENICE
BENIGN
BENING
BENITO
BERING
BESIDE
BETIDE
BEVIES
BEWIGS
BIDING
BIKILA
BIKING
BIKINI
BIMINI
BITING
BLAINE
BLAISE
BLUING
BLUISH
BODICE
BODIED
BODIES
BODILY
BODINE
BODING
BOEING
BOGIES
BOLIDE
BONIER
BONING
BONITA
BONITO
BOOING
BORIDE
BORING
BOVIDS
BOVINE
BOWING
BOXIER
BOXILY
BOXING
BOYISH
BRAIDS
BRAINS
BRAINY
BRAISE
BROILS
BRUINS
BRUISE
BRUITS
BUNION
BURIAL
BURIED
BURIER
BURIES
BURINS
BUSIED
BUSIER
BUSIES
BUSILY
BUSING
BUYING
BUYINS
BYLINE
BYWIRE

B•••I•
BAALIM
BACHIT
BACKIN
BADDIE
BADFIT
BADLIE
BAFFIN
BAGGIE
BAGNIO
BAGSIT
BAGWIG
BALDIE
BALLIN
BALTIC
BAMBIS
BANDIT
BANKIT
BARBIE
BARDIC
BARKIN
BARRIE
BARRIO
BARRIS
BASHIN
BASKIN
BASTIA
BATSIN
BBQPIT
BEANIE
BEATIT
BEAVIS
BEDSIT
BEDWIN
BEFAIR
BEHAIM
BELAIR
BELGIC
BELOIT
BENDIX
BENNIE
BENOIT
BERLIN
BERNIE
BERTIE
BESSIE
BESTIR
BEWAIL
BIALIK
BIBLIO
BIDSIN
BIGAIR
BIGDIG
BIGGIE
BIGHIT
BIGKID
BIGLIE
BIGOIL
BIGRIG
BIGWIG
BIGWIN
BILLIE
BILLIS
BINNIE
BINNIG
BIONIC
BIOPIC
BIOTIC
BIOTIN
BIRDIE
BIRGIT
BITEIN
BIZKIT
BLEWIN
BLEWIT
BLIFIL
BLINIS
BLOOIE
BLOWIN
BLOWIT
BMOVIE
BOBBIE
BOBBIN
BOCCIE
BOCCIS
BODKIN
BOFFIN
BOLLIX
BONNIE
BOOGIE
BOOKIE
BOOKII
BOOKIV
BOOKIX
BOOTIE
BOOTIT
BORGIA
BOSNIA
BOUDIN
BOWFIN
BOWTIE
BRASIL
BRAZIL
BREVIS
BRIGID
BRIGIT
BRODIE
BROLIN
BROVIK
BUDGIE
BUPKIS
BURNIE
BURNIN
BUSTIN
BUTTIN
BUYSIN
BUYSIT
BYMAIL

B••••I
BAKSHI
BANGUI
BANZAI
BARONI
BIGBOI
BIKINI
BILOXI
BIMINI
BIONDI
BOLYAI
BONACI
BONAMI
BONSAI
BOOKII
BOOKVI
BORZOI
BRANDI
BRAZZI
BRUNEI
BUSONI
BYTAXI

•BI•••
ABIDED
ABIDER
ABIDES
ABITOF
FBIMAN
FBIMEN
IBICES
IBIDEM
IBISES
IBIZAN
OBISPO
OBITER
OBIWAN
RBIMAN
RBIMEN
TBILLS
TBIRDS
UBIETY

•B•I••
ABDIEL
BBKING
EBBING
OBLIGE
OBOIST
OBRIAN
OBRIEN

•B••I•
ABATIS
BBQPIT
IBERIA
OBTAIN

•B•••I
OBLADI
UBANGI
UBUROI

••BI••
ALBINE
ALBINO
ALBION
AMBIEN
AMBITS
BABIED
BABIER
BABIES
CABINS
CUBICS
CUBING
CUBISM
CUBIST
CUBITI
CUBITS
CYBILL
DEBITS
EBBING
ERBIUM
FABIAN
GIBILL
GIBING
GOBIES
HABILE
HABITS
IMBIBE
JIBING
KIBITZ
LABIAL
LABILE
LABINE
LABIUM
LIBIDO
LUBING
MOBILE
MOBIUS
MRBILL
NOBILE
NUBIAN
NUBILE
NUBIRA
ORBING
ORBITS
RABIES
REBIDS
REBILL
REBIND
RIBISI
ROBING
ROBINS
RUBIED
RUBIES
RUBIFY
RUBIKS
SABINA
SABINE
SUBITO
TIBIAE
TIBIAL
TIBIAS
TOBIAS
TOBIES
TOBITS
TUBING
TUBIST
UNBIND
UNBITS
UPBIND
VIBIST

••B•I•
ALBEIT
AMBLIN
BIBLIO
BOBBIE
BOBBIN
CABBIE
CABRIO
COBAIN
CUBOID
DEBBIE
DEBRIS
DOBBIN
DOBLIN
DUBLIN
DUBOIS
FABRIC
FIBRIN
GOBLIN
HOBBIT
HUBRIS
HYBRID
LIBRIS
LUBLIN
MCBAIN
NUBBIN
ONBAIL
PUBLIC
PUBLIX
RABBIS
RABBIT
REBAIT
REBBIE
REBOIL
RIBBIT
ROBBIA
ROBBIE
RUBBIA
RUBRIC
RUBSIN
SOBEIT
SUBLID
SUBMIT
TABRIZ
UMBRIA
UNBAIT
WABBIT

••B••I
CUBITI
KABUKI
KUBLAI
RIBISI
RUBATI
URBANI

•••BI•
ALIBIS
AMEBIC
ANUBIS
ARABIA
ARABIC
ASHBIN
BAMBIS
BARBIE
BOBBIE
BOBBIN
CABBIE
CORBIN
CUEBID
CUMBIA
DEBBIE
DOBBIN
DREBIN
DURBIN
FORBID
GAMBIA
GAMBIT
GERBIL
GLOBIN
HARBIN
HEEBIE
HENBIT
HERBIE
HOBBIT
HOWBIG
IAMBIC
INABIT
LIEBIG
LIMBIC
LOWBID
MORBID
NESBIT
NEWBIE
NIOBIC
NUBBIN
ONEBIT
ORIBIS
OUTBID
PHOBIA
PHOBIC
PREBID
PROBIE
RABBIS
RABBIT
REBBIE
RIBBIT
ROBBIA
ROBBIE
RUBBIA
SERBIA
SKIBIB
SORBIC
TERBIC
TIDBIT
TOOBIG
TOPBID
TURBID
TWOBIT
VERBID
WABBIT
WEEBIT
WINBIG
WONBIG
XZIBIT
YEABIG
ZAMBIA
ZOMBIE

•••B•I
BIGBOI
MUMBAI

••••BI
GIAMBI
INCUBI
ITURBI
JACOBI
KENOBI
MESABI
RHOMBI
THEFBI
WASABI

B•J•••
BEJART
BIJOUS
BIJOUX
BUJOLD
BYJOVE

B••J••
BAGJOB
BANJOS
BANJUL
BIGJOE
BMAJOR
BOOJUM

B•••J•
BAROJA

•BJ•••
ABJECT
ABJURE
OBJECT
OBJETS

•B•••J
PBANDJ

••BJ••
JOBJAR

B•K•••
BAKERS
BAKERY
BAKING
BAKKER
BAKSHI
BAKULA
BBKING
BEKIND
BIKERS
BIKILA
BIKING
BIKINI
BOKKEN
BUKAVU

B••K••
BABKAS
BACKED
BACKER
BACKIN
BACKUP
BACKUS
BAIKAL
BAKKER
BALKAN
BALKAT

BALKED BALKER BANKED BANKER BANKIT BANKON BANKUP BARKAT BARKED BARKER BARKIN BARKLA BASKED BASKER BASKET BASKIN BEAKED BEAKER BECKER BECKET BECKON BERKOW BICKER BIGKID BILKED BILKER BIZKIT BLAKEY BLOKES BODKIN BOKKEN BONKED BOOKED BOOKEM BOOKER BOOKIE BOOKII BOOKIV BOOKIX BOOKVI BORKED BRAKED BRAKES BROKAW BROKEN BROKER BUBKES BUCKED BUCKER BUCKET BUCKLE BUCKUP BULKED BULKUP BUNKED BUNKER BUNKOS BUNKUM BUPKES BUPKIS BUPKUS BURKAS BUSKED BUSKER BUTKUS

B•••K•

BAMAKO BARAKA BATIKS BAULKS BELIKE BENEKE BETAKE BIGSKY BLACKS BLANKS BLEAKS BLINKS BLOCKS BLOCKY BODUKE BOESKY BOURKE BREAKS BRICKS BRICKY BRINKS BRISKS BRONKO BROOKE BROOKS BROOKY BUGAKU BUICKS

B••••K

BARACK BARTOK BEDECK BETOOK BIALIK BRATSK BROVIK BUROAK BYTALK

•BK•••

BBKING

•B••K•

DBACKS EBANKS EBOOKS IBOOKS PBOOKS

••BK••

BABKAS BUBKES TABKEY

••B•K•

KABUKI NOBAKE REBAKE REBUKE RUBIKS

••B••K

DEBARK DEBUNK DUBCEK DYBBUK EMBANK EMBARK EWBANK GOBACK IMBACK INBACK INBULK LUBECK REBANK REBOOK USBANK

•••B•K

DRABEK DYBBUK REEBOK RHEBOK TREBEK

BL••••

BLABBY BLACKS BLADED BLADER BLADES BLAFFS BLAINE BLAISE BLAKEY BLAMED BLAMER BLAMES BLANCA BLANCH BLANCO BLANDA BLANKS BLARED BLARES BLASTS BLATTY BLAZED BLAZER BLAZES BLAZON BLEACH BLEAKS BLEARS BLEARY BLEATS BLEEDS BLEEPS BLEETH BLENCH BLENDE BLENDS BLEWIN BLEWIT BLEWON BLEWUP BLIFIL BLIGHT BLIMEY BLIMPS BLINDS BLINIS BLINKS BLINTZ BLISTS BLITHE BLIXEN BLOATS BLOBBY BLOBEL BLOCKS BLOCKY BLOKES BLONDE BLONDS BLOODS BLOODY BLOOEY BLOOIE BLOOMS BLOOMY BLOOPS BLOTCH BLOTTO BLOTTY BLOTUP BLOUNT BLOUSE BLOWER BLOWIN BLOWIT BLOWON BLOWSY BLOWUP BLOWZY BLUDGE BLUELY BLUEOX BLUEST BLUESY BLUETS BLUFFO BLUFFS BLUING BLUISH BLUNTS BLURBS BLURRY BLURTS BLYDEN BLYTHE BLYTON

B•L•••

BALAAM BALATA BALBOA BALDED BALDER BALDIE BALDLY BALDUR BALEEN BALERS BALINE BALING BALKAN BALKAT BALKED BALKER BALLAD BALLET BALLIN BALLON BALLOT BALLOU BALLST BALLUP BALLYS BALMER BALSAM BALSAS BALTIC BALZAC BCLION BELAIR BELATE BELAYS BELDAM BELFRY BELGAE BELGIC BELIAL BELIED BELIEF BELIER BELIES BELIKE BELIZE BELLAY BELLED BELLES BELLOC BELLOW BELLUM BELOIT BELONG BELONS BELTED BELTER BELTON BELTUP BELUGA BELZER BFLATS BILBAO BILDAD BILGED BILGES BILKED BILKER BILLED BILLER BILLET BILLIE BILLIS BILLOW BILOXI BOLCOM BOLDED BOLDEN BOLDER BOLDLY BOLENA BOLERO BOLEYN BOLGER BOLIDE BOLLAS BOLLIX BOLSHY BOLTED BOLTER BOLTON BOLTUP BOLYAI BULDEO BULGAR BULGED BULGES BULGUR BULKED BULKUP BULLAE BULLED BULLET BULOVA BULWER BYLAND BYLAWS BYLINE BYLOTS

B••L••

BAALIM BADLIE BADLOT BAILED BAILEE BAILER BAILEY BAILON BAILOR BALLAD BALLET BALLIN BALLON BALLOT BALLOU BALLST BALLUP BALLYS BANLON BARLEY BARLOW BATLEY BAULKS BAWLED BAWLER BAYLOR BCELLS BEALLS BEDLAM BEGLEY BELLAY BELLED BELLES BELLOC BELLOW BELLUM BERLIN BEULAH BIALIK BIBLES BIBLIO BIGLIE BILLED BILLER BILLET BILLIE BILLIS BILLOW BIOLAB BIRLED BIRLER BODLEY BOGLES BOILED BOILER BOILUP BOLLAS BOLLIX BOSLEY BOULES BOULEZ BOWLED BOWLER BOWLES BOYLES BRILLO BROLIN BROLLY BRULEE BTILES BUGLED BUGLER BUGLES BUILDS BULLAE BULLED BULLET BUMLEG BURLAP BURLED BURLER BURLEY BUTLER BYPLAY

B•••L•

BABALU BABBLE BABBLY BABELS BACALL BAFFLE BAGELS BAKULA BALDLY BANGLE BARELY BARFLY BARKLA BAROLO BARTLE BASALT BASELY BASILS BASSLY BATTLE BAUBLE BCELLS BEADLE BEAGLE BEALLS BEATLE BECALM BEETLE BEFALL BEFELL BEHALF BEHELD BEHOLD BERYLS BETELS BEVELS BEWELL BEZELS BGIRLS BIFOLD BIKILA BINDLE BINGLE BLUELY BOBBLE BOBBLY BODILY BOGGLE BOLDLY BOODLE BOTELS BOTFLY BOTTLE BOWELS BOXILY BRAWLS BRENLY BRIDLE BRILLO BROILS BROLLY BSCALE BUBBLE BUBBLY BUCKLE BUJOLD BUMBLE BUNDLE BUNGLE BURBLE BURBLY BURGLE BUSILY BUSTLE BYHALF BYTALK

B••••L

BACALL BAGFUL BAIKAL BANJUL BARREL BARTEL BASIAL BEAPAL BECOOL BEFALL BEFELL BEFOOL BEFOUL BELIAL BENGAL BENZOL BESSEL BETHEL BEWAIL BEWELL BHOPAL BIGOIL BLIFIL BLOBEL BOATEL BOMBAL BOREAL BOXFUL BRASIL BRAZIL BRIDAL BRUMAL BRUMEL BRUTAL BUCCAL BUNUEL BURIAL BURSAL BUSHEL BYMAIL

•BL•••

ABLARE ABLATE ABLAZE ABLEST ABLOOM ABLUSH OBLADI OBLAST OBLATE OBLIGE OBLONG

•B•L••

ABELES ABOLLA OBELUS OBOLER OBOLUS TBILLS UBOLTS

•B••L•

ABOLLA EBERLE EBERLY TBILLS

•B•••L

ABDIEL ABORAL

••BL••

AMBLED AMBLER AMBLES AMBLIN BIBLES BIBLIO CABLED CABLER CABLES CABLET DEBLUR DOBLES DOBLIN DUBLIN EMBLEM ENBLOC FABLED FABLER FABLES GABLED GABLER GABLES GIBLET GOBLET GOBLIN HABLAR HUBLEY INBLUE JOBLOT KUBLAI KUBLER LUBLIN MABLEY MOBLEY MRBLUE NIBLET NOBLER NOBLES PABLUM PUBLIC PUBLIX RIBLET ROBLES RUBLES RUBLEV SABLES SUBLET SUBLID SUBLOT TABLAS TABLED TABLES TABLET UNBLED VEBLEN WEBLOG

••B•L•

ARBELA BABALU BABBLE BABBLY BABELS BOBBLE BOBBLY BUBBLE BUBBLY CABALA CABALS CABELL CIBOLA COBALT COBBLE CYBILL DABBLE DIBBLE EMBALM FIBULA GABBLE GIBILL GOBBLE HABILE HOBBLE HUBBLE INBULK KIBBLE KOBOLD LABELS LABILE LIBELS LOBULE MABELL MOBILE MRBILL NEBULA NIBBLE NOBALL NOBELS NOBILE NUBBLE NUBBLY NUBILE PEBBLE PEBBLY QABALA RABBLE REBALE REBELS REBILL REBOLT RIBALD RUBBLE RUBBLY RUBELS SABALS SIBYLS SUBTLE SUBTLY TABULA TUBULE TYBALT UMBELS UNBALE UNBELT UNBOLD UNBOLT WOBBLE WOBBLY

••B••L

CABELL CABRAL CYBILL GIBILL HEBBEL LABIAL MABELL MCBEAL MRBILL NOBALL ONBAIL REBILL REBOIL SOBFUL TIBIAL TUBFUL UMBRAL

•••BL•

ALIBLE ARABLE BABBLE BABBLY BAUBLE BOBBLE BOBBLY BUBBLE BUBBLY BUMBLE BURBLE BURBLY COBBLE DABBLE DIABLE DIABLO DIBBLE DOABLE DOUBLE DOUBLY DRABLY DUMBLY EDIBLE EDIBLY ENABLE FEEBLE FEEBLY FOIBLE FUMBLE GABBLE GAMBLE GARBLE GLIBLY GOBBLE GRABLE HOBBLE HUBBLE HUMBLE HUMBLY JUMBLE JUMBLY KEMBLE KIBBLE KIMBLE LIABLE MARBLE MARBLY MUMBLE MUMBLY NIBBLE NIMBLE NIMBLY NUBBLE NUBBLY NUMBLY PEBBLE PEBBLY PUEBLA PUEBLO RABBLE RAMBLE RUBBLE RUBBLY RUMBLE RUMBLY STABLE STABLY SUABLE TREBLE TREBLY TUMBLE UNABLE UNABLY USABLE USABLY VIABLE VIABLY WAMBLE WAMBLY WARBLE WOBBLE WOBBLY

•••B•L

BLOBEL BOMBAL CORBEL CYMBAL DIABOL GAMBOL GERBIL GIMBAL GIMBEL GLOBAL GUMBEL HEBBEL HERBAL ISABEL KNEBEL SNOBOL SYMBOL TIMBAL TRIBAL TYDBOL VERBAL

BM••••

BMAJOR BMINOR BMINUS BMOVIE

B•M•••

BAMAKO BAMBIS BAMBOO BEMATA BEMINE BEMIRE BEMOAN BEMUSE BIMBOS BIMINI BOMBAL BOMBAY BOMBED BOMBER BOMBES BUMBLE BUMBRY BUMLEG BUMMED BUMMER BUMOUT BUMPED BUMPER BUMPPO BUMPUP BUMRAP BYMAIL

B••M••

BADMAN BADMEN BAGMAN BAGMEN BALMER BARMAN BARMEN BATMAN BATMEN BAUMAN BAUMER BAYMAN BAYMEN BEAMAN BEAMED BEAMER BEAMON BEAMUP BEEMER BERMAN BERMED BEYMER BIGMAC BIGMAN BIGMEN BIOMES BIRMAN BITMAP BLAMED BLAMER BLAMES BLIMEY BLIMPS BONMOT BOOMED BOOMER BORMAN BOWMAN BOWMEN BRAMAH BREMEN BREMER BRUMAL BRUMEL BRUMES BUMMED BUMMER BURMAN BUSMAN BUSMEN

B•••M•

BADEMS BAHAMA BECAME BECOME BEDIMS BEGEMS BEGUMS BEHOME BENUMB BESAME BESOMS BIGAMY BIREME BLOOMS BLOOMY BOHEME BONAMI BOSOMS BOSOMY BRAHMA BRAHMS BREAMS BROOMS BROOMY BTEAMS BYNAME

B••••M

BAALIM BADHAM BALAAM BALSAM BANTAM BARIUM BARNUM BATYAM BAYRUM BECALM BEDLAM BEFIRM BEHAIM BELDAM BELLUM BIFORM BOLCOM BONHAM BOOJUM BOOKEM BOTTOM BUNKUM BYFORM

•BM•••

ABMHOS IBMPCS

•B•M••

ABOMAS ABOMBS FBIMAN FBIMEN HBOMBS NBOMBS RBIMAN RBIMEN

•B••M•

ABOHMS ABRAMS ABYSMS HBEAMS IBEAMS LBEAMS

•B•••M

ABLOOM ABSCAM

IBIDEM

••BM••
CABMAN
CABMEN
SUBMIT
TUBMAN

••B•M•
ALBUMS
OKBYME

••B••M
COBHAM
CUBISM
EMBALM
EMBLEM
ERBIUM
GOBOOM
KABOOM
LABIUM
PABLUM
SHBOOM
SUBGUM
VIBRAM
WEBCAM

•••B•M
ALABAM
SKIBUM

B•N•••
BANANA
BANANE
BANCOS
BANDED
BANDER
BANDIT
BANGED
BANGER
BANGLE
BANGON
BANGOR
BANGUI
BANGUP
BANISH
BANJOS
BANJUL
BANKED
BANKER
BANKIT
BANKON
BANKUP
BANLON
BANNED
BANNEN
BANNER
BANONS
BANQUE
BANQUO
BANTAM
BANTER
BANTUS
BANYAN
BANZAI
BENBEN
BENBOW
BENDAY
BENDED
BENDER
BENDIX
BENEKE
BENGAL
BENGAY
BENHUR
BENICE
BENIGN
BENING
BENITO
BENNIE
BENOIT
BENOTE
BENSEY
BENSON
BENTON
BENTOS
BENUMB
BENZOL
BINACA
BINARY
BINATE
BINCHY
BINDER
BINDLE
BINDTO
BINDUP
BINGED
BINGER
BINGES
BINGLE
BINGOS
BINNED
BINNEY
BINNIE
BINNIG
BINYON
BONACI
BONAMI
BONBON
BONDED
BONDER
BONERS
BONERZ
BONEUP
BONGED
BONGOS
BONHAM
BONIER
BONING
BONITA
BONITO
BONKED
BONMOT
BONNER
BONNES
BONNET
BONNEY
BONNIE
BONSAI
BONTON
BONZES
BUNCHE
BUNCHY
BUNCOS
BUNDLE
BUNDTS
BUNGAY
BUNGED
BUNGEE
BUNGLE
BUNION
BUNKED
BUNKER
BUNKOS
BUNKUM
BUNSEN
BUNTED
BUNTER
BUNTON
BUNUEL
BUNYAN
BYNAME

B••N••
BAGNIO
BAHNEN
BAINES
BANNED
BANNEN
BANNER
BARNED
BARNES
BARNET
BARNEY
BARNUM
BEANED
BEANIE
BEANOS
BEINGS
BEINON
BENNIE
BERNIE
BHANGS
BIANCA
BIANCO
BINNED
BINNEY
BINNIE
BINNIG
BIONDI
BIONIC
BIONTS
BIRNEY
BITNET
BLANCA
BLANCH
BLANCO
BLANDA
BLANKS
BLENCH
BLENDE
BLENDS
BLINDS
BLINIS
BLINKS
BLINTZ
BLONDE
BLONDS
BLUNTS
BMINOR
BMINUS
BOINGO
BOINGS
BONNER
BONNES
BONNET
BONNEY
BONNIE
BORNEO
BOSNIA
BOUNCE
BOUNCY
BOUNDS
BOUNTY
BRANCA
BRANCH
BRANDI
BRANDO
BRANDS
BRANDT
BRANDX
BRANDY
BRANNY
BRANTS
BRENDA
BRENLY
BRINED
BRINER
BRINES
BRINGS
BRINKS
BRONCO
BRONCS
BRONKO
BRONTE
BRONZE
BRONZY
BRUNCH
BRUNEI
BRUNET
BRUNOR
BRUNTS
BRYNZA
BUENAS
BUENOS
BURNED
BURNER
BURNET
BURNEY
BURNIE
BURNIN
BURNUP
BUYNOW
BWANAS
BYENOW
BYRNES

B•••N•
BAAING
BACONS
BADEND
BADUNS
BAGEND
BAIRNS
BAKING
BALINE
BALING
BANANA
BANANE
BANONS
BARANY
BARING
BARONE
BARONI
BARONS
BARONY
BASING
BASINS
BATING
BATONS
BAYING
BBGUNS
BBKING
BCCING
BEGINS
BEGONE
BEHIND
BEIGNE
BEKIND
BELONG
BELONS
BEMINE
BENING
BERING
BESANT
BETONY
BEVANS
BEYOND
BIDING
BIGEND
BIGONE
BIKING
BIKINI
BIMINI
BISONS
BITING
BLAINE
BLOUNT
BLUING
BODINE
BODING
BOEING
BOLENA
BONING
BOOING
BORING
BOSONS
BOSUNS
BOTANY
BOURNE
BOVINE
BOWING
BOXING
BRAINS
BRAINY
BRANNY
BRAWNY
BRIANA
BRIAND
BRIENZ
BROWNE
BROWNS
BROWNU
BROWNY
BRUINS
BRYANT
BURANA
BURINS
BUSING
BUSONI
BUTANE
BUTENE
BUYING
BUYINS
BYGONE
BYHAND
BYLAND
BYLINE
BYTENS

B••••N
BABOON
BABSON
BACKIN
BADMAN
BADMEN
BAFFIN
BAGMAN
BAGMEN
BAHIAN
BAHNEN
BAILON
BALEEN
BALKAN
BALLIN
BALLON
BANGON
BANKON
BANLON
BANNEN
BANYAN
BARBAN
BARKIN
BARMAN
BARMEN
BARREN
BARRON
BARTON
BARYON
BARZUN
BASHIN
BASKIN
BATAAN
BATMAN
BATMEN
BATSIN
BATSON
BATTEN
BAUMAN
BAYERN
BAYMAN
BAYMEN
BCLION
BEACON
BEAMAN
BEAMON
BEARON
BEATEN
BEATON
BECKON
BEDWIN
BEINON
BELTON
BEMOAN
BENBEN
BENIGN
BENSON
BENTON
BERGEN
BERLIN
BERMAN
BERWYN
BESSON
BETSON
BHUTAN
BICHON
BICORN
BIDDEN
BIDSIN
BIDSON
BIGBEN
BIGFAN
BIGFUN
BIGGUN
BIGMAN
BIGMEN
BIGTEN
BIGWIN
BINYON
BIOTIN
BIRMAN
BITEIN
BITEON
BITTEN
BLAZON
BLEWIN
BLEWON
BLIXEN
BLOWIN
BLOWON
BLYDEN
BLYTON
BOBBIN
BODKIN
BOFFIN
BOKKEN
BOLDEN
BOLEYN
BOLTON
BONBON
BONTON
BORDEN
BOREON
BORMAN
BOSSON
BOSTON
BOUDIN
BOUTON
BOWFIN
BOWMAN
BOWMEN
BRAZEN
BREMEN
BRETON
BRITON
BROGAN
BROKEN
BROLIN
BRYSON
BSEVEN
BUCHAN
BUFFON
BUNION
BUNSEN
BUNTON
BUNYAN
BURDEN
BURMAN
BURNIN
BURTON
BUSMAN
BUSMEN
BUSTIN
BUTTIN
BUTTON
BUYSIN
BUYSON
BYTHEN

•B•N••
EBANKS
EBONDS
IBANEZ
OBENTO
PBANDJ
TBONDS
TBONES
UBANGI

•B••N•
ABOUND
ABSENT
BBGUNS
BBKING
EBBING
OBGYNS
OBLONG
OBTUND
TBOONE

•B•••N
ABUTON
FBIMAN
FBIMEN
IBADAN
IBIZAN
OBERON
OBIWAN
OBRIAN
OBRIEN
OBTAIN
RBIMAN
RBIMEN

••BN••
COBNUT
DABNEY
HOBNOB
SUBNET

••B•N•
ALBANO
ALBANS
ALBANY
ALBINE
ALBINO
AMBAND
CABANA
CABINS
CUBANS
CUBING
DEBONE
DEBONT
DEBUNK
DOBYNS
EBBING
EMBANK
ENBANC
EWBANK
FMBAND
GIBING
GOBANG
HABANA
JIBING
JOBONE
JOBYNA
LABINE
LUBING
MRBOND
ORBING
REBANK
REBEND
REBENT
REBIND
RIBAND
ROBING
ROBINS
RUBENS
SABENA
SABINA
SABINE
TUBING
UNBEND
UNBENT
UNBIND
UPBIND
URBANA
URBANE
URBANI
URBANV
USBANK

••B••N
ALBION
AMBIEN
AMBLIN
AUBURN
BABOON
BABSON
BOBBIN
CABMAN
CABMEN
COBAIN
COBURN
CUBFAN
DOBBIN
DOBLIN
DUBLIN
FABIAN
FIBRIN
GIBBON
GIBRAN
GIBSON
GOBLIN
HEBRON
HOBSON
INBORN
JOBSON
LEBRON
LEBRUN
LIBRAN
LIBYAN
LLBEAN
LUBLIN
MCBAIN
MRBEAN
NUBBIN
NUBIAN
OSBORN
REBORN
RIBBON
ROBSON
RUBSIN
RUBSON
SUBORN
TOBURN
TUBMAN
UNBORN
VEBLEN
WEBERN
WOBURN

•••B•N
ARUBAN
ASHBIN
BARBAN
BENBEN
BIGBEN
BOBBIN
BONBON
CARBON
CORBIN
DOBBIN
DREBIN
DURBAN
DURBIN
GIBBON
GLOBIN
GROBAN
HARBIN
KLIBAN
LISBON
NUBBIN
ONABUN
OUTBAN
RAYBAN
REUBEN
RIBBON
SIEBEN
SIRBEN
THEBAN
TURBAN

BO••••
BOARDS
BOASTS
BOATED
BOATEL
BOATER
BOBBED
BOBBER
BOBBIE
BOBBIN
BOBBLE
BOBBLY
BOBBYS
BOBCAT
BOBSUP
BOCCES
BOCCIE
BOCCIS
BOCHCO
BOCHSA
BODEGA
BODETT
BODICE
BODIED
BODIES
BODILY
BODINE
BODING
BODKIN
BODLEY
BODUKE
BOEING
BOESKY
BOFFED
BOFFIN
BOFFOS
BOGART
BOGEYS
BOGGED
BOGGLE
BOGIES
BOGLES
BOGOTA
BOHEME
BOHRER
BOILED
BOILER
BOILUP
BOINGO
BOINGS
BOITES
BOKKEN
BOLCOM
BOLDED
BOLDEN
BOLDER
BOLDLY
BOLENA
BOLERO
BOLEYN
BOLGER
BOLIDE
BOLLAS
BOLLIX
BOLSHY
BOLTED
BOLTER
BOLTON
BOLTUP
BOLYAI
BOMBAL
BOMBAY
BOMBED
BOMBER
BOMBES
BONACI
BONAMI
BONBON
BONDED
BONDER
BONERS
BONERZ
BONEUP
BONGED
BONGOS
BONHAM
BONIER
BONING
BONITA
BONITO
BONKED
BONMOT
BONNER
BONNES
BONNET
BONNEY
BONNIE
BONSAI
BONTON
BONZES
BOOBOO
BOOCOO
BOODLE
BOOERS
BOOGIE
BOOHOO
BOOING
BOOJUM
BOOKED
BOOKEM
BOOKER
BOOKIE
BOOKII
BOOKIV
BOOKIX
BOOKVI
BOOMED
BOOMER
BOOSAT
BOOSTS
BOOTED
BOOTEE
BOOTER
BOOTES
BOOTHE
BOOTHS
BOOTIE
BOOTIT
BOOTUP
BOOZED
BOOZER
BOOZES
BOPEEP
BOPPED
BOPPER
BORATE
BORAXO
BORDEN
BORDER
BORDET
BOREAL
BOREAS
BOREON
BORERS
BOREUP
BORGES
BORGIA
BORIDE
BORING
BORKED
BORMAN
BORNEO
BORROW
BORSCH
BORZOI
BOSLEY
BOSNIA
BOSOMS
BOSOMY
BOSONS
BOSSED
BOSSES
BOSSON
BOSTON
BOSUNS
BOTANY
BOTCHY
BOTELS
BOTFLY
BOTHER
BOTREE
BOTTLE
BOTTOM
BOUCHE
BOUDIN
BOUFFE
BOUGHS
BOUGHT
BOULES
BOULEZ
BOUNCE
BOUNCY
BOUNDS
BOUNTY
BOURGS
BOURKE
BOURNE
BOURSE
BOUTON
BOVARY
BOVIDS
BOVINE
BOWELS
BOWERS
BOWERY
BOWFIN
BOWING
BOWLED
BOWLER
BOWLES
BOWMAN
BOWMEN
BOWOAR
BOWOUT
BOWSAW
BOWSTO
BOWTIE
BOWWOW
BOWYER
BOWZER
BOXBED
BOXBOY
BOXCAR
BOXERS
BOXFUL
BOXIER
BOXILY
BOXING
BOXSET
BOXTOP
BOYARS
BOYISH
BOYLES
BOYTOY

B•O•••
BAOBAB
BHOPAL
BIOGAS
BIOLAB
BIOMES
BIONDI
BIONIC
BIONTS
BIOPIC
BIOPSY
BIOTAS
BIOTIC
BIOTIN
BLOATS
BLOBBY
BLOBEL
BLOCKS
BLOCKY
BLOKES
BLONDE
BLONDS
BLOODS
BLOODY
BLOOEY
BLOOIE
BLOOMS
BLOOMY
BLOOPS
BLOTCH
BLOTTO
BLOTTY
BLOTUP
BLOUNT
BLOUSE
BLOWER
BLOWIN
BLOWIT
BLOWON
BLOWSY
BLOWUP
BLOWZY
BMOVIE
BOOBOO
BOOCOO
BOODLE
BOOERS
BOOGIE
BOOHOO
BOOING
BOOJUM
BOOKED
BOOKEM
BOOKER
BOOKIE
BOOKII
BOOKIV
BOOKIX
BOOKVI
BOOMED
BOOMER
BOOSAT
BOOSTS
BOOTED
BOOTEE
BOOTER
BOOTES
BOOTHE
BOOTHS
BOOTIE
BOOTIT
BOOTUP
BOOZED
BOOZER
BOOZES
BROACH
BROADA
BROAST
BROCAS
BRODIE
BROGAN
BROGUE
BROILS
BROKAW
BROKEN
BROKER
BROLIN
BROLLY
BRONCO
BRONCS
BRONKO
BRONTE
BRONZE
BRONZY
BROOCH
BROODS
BROODY
BROOKE
BROOKS
BROOKY
BROOMS
BROOMY
BROPHY
BROSSE
BROTHS
BROTHY
BROUGH
BROVIK
BROWED
BROWNE
BROWNS
BROWNU
BROWNY
BROWSE
BUOYED
BUOYUP

B••O••
BABOON
BABOOS
BACONS
BADOFF
BANONS
BAROJA
BAROLO
BARONE
BARONI
BARONS
BARONY
BATONS
BAYOUS
BAZOOS

BEBOPS BECOME BECOOL BEDOGS BEFOGS BEFOOL BEFORE BEFOUL BEGOFF BEGONE BEGOOD BEHOLD BEHOME BEHOOF BELOIT BELONG BELONS BEMOAN BENOIT BENOTE BESOMS BESORE BESOTS BETONY BETOOK BEYOND BICORN BIFOLD BIFORM BIGOIL BIGONE BIGOTS BIJOUS BIJOUX BILOXI BIPODS BISONS BITOFF BLOODS BLOODY BLOOEY BLOOIE BLOOMS BLOOMY BLOOPS BOGOTA BOSOMS BOSOMY BOSONS BOWOAR BOWOUT BROOCH BROODS BROODY BROOKE BROOKS BROOKY BROOMS BROOMY BUGOFF BUGOUT BUJOLD BULOVA BUMOUT BUROAK BUSONI BUYOFF BUYOUT BYFORM BYGONE BYGOSH BYJOVE BYLOTS BYROAD BYROTE BYWORD

B•••O•

BABOON BABOOS BABSON BADBOY BADCOP BADDOG BADLOT BAGBOY BAGJOB BAILON BAILOR BALBOA BALLON BALLOT BALLOU BAMBOO BANCOS BANGON BANGOR BANJOS BANKON BANLON BARCOS BARDOT BARHOP BARLOW BARRON BARROW BARTOK BARTON BARYON BASSOS BATBOY BATFOR BATHOS BATSON BAYLOR BAZOOS BBSHOT BCLION BEACON BEAMON BEANOS BEARON BEATON BECKON BECOOL BEFOOL BEGFOR BEGOOD BEHOOF BEINON BELLOC BELLOW BELTON BENBOW BENSON BENTON BENTOS BENZOL BERKOW BESSON BESTOW BETOOK BETSON BETTOR BICHON BIDFOR BIDSON BIGBOI BIGBOX BIGBOY BIGDOG BIGDOS BIGJOE BIGTOE BIGTOP BILLOW BIMBOS BINGOS BINYON BISHOP BITEON BLAZON BLEWON BLOWON BLUEOX BLYTON BMAJOR BMINOR BOFFOS BOLCOM BOLTON BONBON BONGOS BONMOT BONTON BOOBOO BOOCOO BOOHOO BOREON BORROW BORZOI BOSSON BOSTON BOTTOM BOUTON BOWWOW BOXBOY BOXTOP BOYTOY BRASOV BRAVOS BRAZOS BRETON BRITON BRUNOR BRYSON BUENOS BUFFON BUFFOS BUGBOY BUNCOS BUNION BUNKOS BUNTON BURBOT BURGOO BURGOS BURROS BURROW BURTON BUSBOY BUTEOS BUTHOW BUTTON BUYNOW BUYSON BYENOW BYTWOS

B••••O

BAGNIO BAMAKO BAMBOO BANQUO BARATO BAROLO BARRIO BENITO BERCEO BHUTTO BIANCO BIBLIO BILBAO BINDTO BISTRO BLANCO BLOTTO BLUFFO BOCHCO BOINGO BOLERO BONITO BOOBOO BOOCOO BOOHOO BORAXO BORNEO BOWSTO BRACCO BRANDO BRASCO BRILLO BRONCO BRONKO BULDEO BUMPPO BURGOO BUTWHO

•BO•••

ABOARD ABODES ABOHMS ABOLLA ABOMAS ABOMBS ABORAL ABORTS ABOUND EBOATS EBONDS EBOOKS HBOMBS IBOOKS NBOMBS OBOIST OBOLER OBOLUS PBOOKS TBONDS TBONES TBOONE UBOATS UBOLTS XBOXES

•B•O••

ABBOTS ABBOTT ABHORS ABLOOM ABROAD ABSORB EBOOKS IBOOKS OBLONG PBOOKS TBOONE

•B••O•

ABATOR ABITOF ABLOOM ABMHOS ABUTON BBSHOT OBERON UBUROI

•B•••O

ABBADO OBENTO OBERTO OBISPO SBARRO

••BO••

ABBOTS ABBOTT ALBORG ARBORS ARBOUR BABOON BABOOS BEBOPS CIBOLA CUBOID CYBORG DEBONE DEBONT DUBOIS DUBOSE ELBOWS EMBODY EMBOGS EMBOSS EMBOWS EUBOEA FOBOFF GOBOES GOBOOM GOBOTS HOBOED HOBOES INBORN JABOTS JOBONE KABOBS KABOOM KIBOSH KOBOLD LABORS LABOUR MRBOND NABOBS NABORS NOBODY OSBORN OXBOWS POBOYS PTBOAT REBOIL REBOLT REBOOK REBOOT REBOPS REBORE REBORN REBOTE REBOZO RIBOSE ROBOTS RUBOFF RUBOUT SABOTS SHBOOM SUBORN TABOOS TABORS TOBOOT UNBOLD UNBOLT UNBORN UPBOWS

••B•O•

ALBION BABOON BABOOS BABSON DEBTOR DOBROS ENBLOC GIBBON GIBSON GOBOOM GOBSOF HEBRON HOBNOB HOBSON JOBHOP JOBLOT JOBSON KABOOM LEBRON LIBROS REBOOK REBOOT RIBBON ROBROY ROBSOF ROBSON RUBSON SHBOOM SUBGOD SUBLOT TABOOS TOBOOT WEBLOG

••B••O

ABBADO ALBANO ALBEDO ALBINO BIBLIO CABRIO EMBRYO GABBRO LIBIDO REBOZO RUBATO SABADO SABATO SUBITO TOBAGO

•••BO•

ADOBOS BADBOY BAGBOY BALBOA BAMBOO BATBOY BENBOW BIGBOI BIGBOX BIGBOY BIMBOS BONBON BOOBOO BOXBOY BUGBOY BURBOT BUSBOY CAMBOY CARBON CARBOS CARBOY COMBOS COWBOY DIABOL DOCBOY DUMBOS FEMBOT FLYBOY FOGBOW GAMBOL GIBBON GUMBOS HARBOR HATBOX HOTBOT HOTBOX ICEBOX INABOX IROBOT JERBOA JIMBOB JUMBOS LAZBOY LESBOS LIMBOS LISBOA LISBON LOWBOY MAMBOS MMMBOP OLDBOY OUTBOW OUTBOX PEGBOX PEPBOY PETBOA PHOBOS PINBOY RAMBOS REEBOK RHEBOK RIBBON SAYBOO SHEBOP SKIBOB SKYBOX SNOBOL SPYBOT SUNBOW SYMBOL TAMBOR TEEBOX TOMBOY TURBOS TURBOT TYDBOL

•••B•O

BAMBOO BILBAO BOOBOO DIABLO GABBRO HASBRO PUEBLO SAYBOO

••••BO

AKIMBO CRAMBO GAZEBO JAZZBO LAVABO MALABO NINGBO PHLEBO PICABO PLUMBO SASEBO TRUMBO

B•P•••

BIPEDS BIPODS BOPEEP BOPPED BOPPER BUPKES BUPKIS BUPKUS BYPASS BYPAST BYPATH BYPLAY

B••P••

BBQPIT BEAPAL BEEPAT BEEPED BEEPER BHOPAL BIOPIC BIOPSY BOPPED BOPPER BROPHY BUMPED BUMPER BUMPPO BUMPUP BURPED BURPEE

B•••P•

BEBOPS BICEPS BIGAPE BLEEPS BLIMPS BLOOPS BUMPPO

B••••P

BACKUP BADCOP BADRAP BALLUP BANGUP BANKUP BARHOP BEADUP BEAMUP BEARUP BEATUP BEEFUP BELTUP BIDSUP BIGTOP BINDUP BISHOP BITEUP BITMAP BLEWUP BLOTUP BLOWUP BOBSUP BOILUP BOLTUP BONEUP BOOTUP BOPEEP BOREUP BOXTOP BREWUP BSHARP BUCKUP BUFFUP BULKUP BUMPUP BUMRAP BUOYUP BURLAP BURNUP BUSTUP BUYSUP

•B•P••

BBQPIT IBMPCS

•B••P•

ABRUPT OBISPO

••BP••

RIBPAD SUBPAR

••B•P•

BEBOPS KGBSPY REBOPS

••B••P

BOBSUP HUBCAP JOBHOP RUBSUP

•••B•P

CLUBUP MMMBOP SHEBOP

B•Q•••

BBQPIT BUQSHA

B••Q••

BANQUE BANQUO BARQUE BASQUE BISQUE BRAQUE

•BQ•••

BBQPIT

BR••••

BRACCO BRACED BRACER BRACES BRACHS BRACTS BRAHMA BRAHMS BRAIDS BRAINS BRAINY BRAISE BRAKED BRAKES BRAMAH BRANCA BRANCH BRANDI BRANDO BRANDS BRANDT BRANDX BRANDY BRANNY BRANTS BRAQUE BRASCO BRASHY BRASIL BRASOV BRASSY BRATSK BRATTY BRAVAS BRAVED BRAVER BRAVES BRAVOS BRAWLS BRAWNY BRAYED BRAYER BRAZEN BRAZIL BRAZOS BRAZZA BRAZZI BREACH BREADS BREAKS BREAMS BREAST BREATH BRECHT BREDES BREECH BREEDS BREEDY BREEZE BREEZY BREMEN BREMER BRENDA BRENLY BRETON BREUER BREVES BREVET BREVIS BREWED BREWER BREWUP BREYER BRIANA BRIAND BRIARD BRIARS BRIARY BRIBED BRIBEE BRIBER BRIBES BRICKS BRICKY BRIDAL BRIDES BRIDGE BRIDLE BRIEFS BRIENZ BRIERS BRIERY BRIGHT BRIGID BRIGIT BRILLO BRINED BRINER BRINES BRINGS BRINKS BRISES BRISKS BRITON BROACH BROADA BROAST BROCAS BRODIE BROGAN BROGUE BROILS BROKAW BROKEN BROKER BROLIN BROLLY BRONCO BRONCS BRONKO BRONTE BRONZE BRONZY BROOCH BROODS BROODY BROOKE BROOKS BROOKY BROOMS BROOMY BROPHY BROSSE BROTHS BROTHY BROUGH BROVIK BROWED BROWNE BROWNS BROWNU BROWNY BROWSE BRUDER BRUGES BRUINS BRUISE BRUITS BRULEE BRUMAL BRUMEL BRUMES BRUNCH BRUNEI BRUNET BRUNOR BRUNTS BRUSHY BRUTAL BRUTES BRUTUS BRUXED BRUXES BRYANT BRYNZA BRYSON

B•R•••

BARACK BARADA BARAKA BARANY BARATA BARATO BARBAN BARBED BARBER BARBET BARBIE BARBRA BARCAR BARCOS BARDIC BARDOT BAREGE BARELY BAREST BARFLY BARGED BARGER BARGES BARHOP BARING BARITE BARIUM BARKAT BARKED BARKER BARKIN BARKLA BARLEY BARLOW BARMAN BARMEN BARNED BARNES BARNET BARNEY BARNUM BAROJA BAROLO BARONE BARONI BARONS BARONY BARQUE BARRED BARREL BARREN BARRES BARRET BARRIE BARRIO BARRIS BARRON BARROW BARTAB BARTEL BARTER BARTLE BARTOK BARTON BARUCH BARYON BARZUN BERATE BERBER BERCEO BEREFT BERETS BERGEN BERGER BERING BERKOW BERLIN BERMAN BERMED BERNIE BERTHA BERTHE BERTHS BERTIE BERWYN BERYLS BIRDED BIRDER BIRDIE BIREME BIRGIT BIRLED BIRLER BIRMAN BIRNEY BIRRED BIRTHS BORATE BORAXO BORDEN BORDER BORDET BOREAL BOREAS BOREON BORERS BOREUP BORGES BORGIA BORIDE BORING BORKED BORMAN BORNEO BORROW BORSCH BORZOI BURANA BURBLE BURBLY BURBOT BURDEN BUREAU BURETS BURGEE BURGER BURGHS BURGLE BURGOO BURGOS BURIAL BURIED BURIER BURIES BURINS BURKAS BURLAP BURLED BURLER BURLEY BURMAN BURNED BURNER BURNET BURNEY BURNIE BURNIN BURNUP BUROAK BURPED BURPEE BURRED BURROS BURROW BURSAE BURSAL BURSAR BURSAS BURSTS BURTON BYRNES BYROAD BYROTE

B••R••

BADRAP BAERGA BAIRNS BARRED BARREL BARREN BARRES BARRET BARRIE BARRIO BARRIS BARRON BARROW BASRAH BAYRUM BEARDS BEARER BEARON

BEARSE
BEARUP
BEIRUT
BETRAY
BEURRE
BGIRLS
BIERCE
BIERES
BIGRED
BIGRIG
BIRRED
BLARED
BLARES
BLURBS
BLURRY
BLURTS
BOARDS
BOHRER
BORROW
BOTREE
BOURGS
BOURKE
BOURNE
BOURSE
BTHREE
BUMRAP
BURRED
BURROS
BURROW

B•••R•
BAKERS
BAKERY
BALERS
BARBRA
BAYARD
BAYERN
BEFIRM
BEFORE
BEGIRD
BEGIRT
BEJART
BELFRY
BEMIRE
BESORE
BESURE
BEURRE
BEWARE
BEWARY
BIAFRA
BICARB
BICORN
BIDERS
BIFORM
BIKERS
BINARY
BISTRO
BITERS
BLEARS
BLEARY
BLURRY
BOGART
BOLERO
BONERS
BONERZ
BOOERS
BORERS
BOVARY
BOWERS
BOWERY
BOXERS
BOYARS
BRIARD
BRIARS
BRIARY
BRIERS
BRIERY
BSHARP
BSTARS
BUMBRY
BUYERS
BYFORM
BYWIRE
BYWORD

B••••R
BABIER
BACKER
BADDER
BADGER
BAEYER
BAFFER
BAGGER
BAILER
BAILOR
BAITER
BAKKER
BALDER
BALDUR
BALKER
BALMER
BANDER
BANGER
BANGOR
BANKER
BANNER
BANTER
BARBER
BARCAR
BARGER
BARKER
BARTER
BASHER
BASKER
BASTER
BATFOR
BATHER
BATTER
BAUMER
BAVIER
BAWLER
BAXTER
BAYLOR
BAZAAR
BEADER
BEAKER
BEAMER
BEARER
BEATER
BEAVER
BECKER
BEEMER
BEEPER
BEEZER
BEFAIR
BEGFOR
BEGGAR
BELAIR
BELIER
BELTER
BELZER
BENDER
BENHUR
BERBER
BERGER
BESSER
BESTER
BESTIR
BETTER
BETTOR
BEYMER
BIBBER
BICKER
BIDDER
BIDFOR
BIEBER
BIGAIR
BIGCAR
BIGEAR
BIGGER
BIGSUR
BILKER
BILLER
BINDER
BINGER
BIRDER
BIRLER
BITTER
BLADER
BLAMER
BLAZER
BLOWER
BMAJOR
BMINOR
BOATER
BOBBER
BOHRER
BOILER
BOLDER
BOLGER
BOLTER
BOMBER
BONDER
BONIER
BONNER
BOOKER
BOOMER
BOOTER
BOOZER
BOPPER
BORDER
BOTHER
BOWLER
BOWOAR
BOWYER
BOWZER
BOXCAR
BOXIER
BRACER
BRAVER
BRAYER
BREMER
BREUER
BREWER
BREYER
BRIBER
BRINER
BROKER
BRUDER
BRUNOR
BUCKER
BUDDER
BUDGER
BUFFER
BUGLER
BULGAR
BULGUR
BULWER
BUMMER
BUMPER
BUNKER
BUNTER
BURGER
BURIER
BURLER
BURNER
BURSAR
BUSHER
BUSIER
BUSKER
BUSTER
BUTLER
BUTTER
BUZZER

•BR•••
ABRADE
ABRAMS
ABROAD
ABRUPT
OBRIAN
OBRIEN

•B•R••
ABBREV
ABORAL
ABORTS
EBERLE
EBERLY
IBARRA
IBERIA
NBCRED
OBERON
OBERTO
SBARRO
TBIRDS
UBUROI

•B••R•
ABHORS
ABJURE
ABLARE
ABOARD
ABSORB
ABSURD
IBARRA
NBAERS
OBVERT
SBARRO

•B•••R
ABASER
ABATER
ABATOR
ABIDER
ABUSER
EBAYER
OBEYER
OBITER
OBOLER

••BR••
ABBREV
ARBRES
AUBREY
CABRAL
CABRIO
COBRAS
DABRAT
DEBRAH
DEBRAY
DEBREU
DEBRIS
DOBROS
ELBRUS
EMBRUE
EMBRYO
FABRAY
FABRIC
FIBRES
FIBRIN
GIBRAN
HEBREW
HEBRON
HUBRIS
HYBRID
IMBRUE
INBRED
LABRAT
LABREA
LEBRET
LEBRON
LEBRUN
LIBRAE
LIBRAN
LIBRAS
LIBRIS
LIBROS
REBRED
REBREW
ROBROY
RUBRAW
RUBRIC
SABRAS
SABRES
TABRIZ
UMBRAE
UMBRAL
UMBRAS
UMBRIA
VIBRAM
ZABRZE
ZEBRAS

••B•R•
ALBERS
ALBERT
ALBORG
AMBERS
AMBERY
ARBORS
ASBURY
AUBURN
CABERS
COBURG
COBURN
CUBERS
CYBORG
DEBARK
DEBARS
DEBURR
EDBERG
EGBERT
EKBERG
ELBERT
ELBURZ
EMBARK
EMBARS
EMBERS
ENBERG
FIBERS
GABBRO
GIBERS
HOBART
HUBERT
INBORN
LABORS
LIBERS
MOBERG
NABORS
NUBIRA
OSBERT
OSBORN
REBARS
REBORE
REBORN
REBURY
RIBERA
ROBERS
ROBERT
SABERS
SEBERG
SOBERS
SUBARU
SUBORN
SUBURB
TABARD
TABORS
TOBURN
TUBERS
UMBERS
UNBARE
UNBARS
UNBORN
UNBURY
WEBERN
WEBERS
WOBURN

••B••R
AMBLER
ARBOUR
BABIER
BIBBER
BOBBER
CABLER
CIBBER
DABBER
DEBLUR
DEBTOR
DEBURR
DUBBER
FABBER
FABLER
FIBBER
GABBER
GABLER
GIBBER
HABLAR
JABBAR
JABBER
JOBBER
JOBJAR
KUBLER
LABOUR
LIBBER
LOBBER
LUBBER
MOBBER
NABBER
NOBLER
NUBBER
RIBBER
ROBBER
RUBBER
SOBBER
SUBPAR
SUBWAR
UPBEAR
WEBBER

•••BR•
BARBRA
BUMBRY
CARBRA
GABBRO
HASBRO
HOMBRE
JOGBRA
NOMBRE
SOMBRE
TIMBRE

•••B•R
BARBER
BERBER
BIBBER
BIEBER
BOBBER
BOMBER
BRIBER
CAMBER
CIBBER
COMBER
CUMBER
DABBER
DAUBER
DAWBER
DISBAR
DJEBAR
DUBBER
DUMBER
DUNBAR
FABBER
FERBER
FIBBER
FIGBAR
GABBER
GARBER
GERBER
GIBBER
GOOBER
HARBOR
HUMBER
ISOBAR
JABBAR
JABBER
JOBBER
KHYBER
LIBBER
LIEBER
LIMBER
LOBBER
LUBBER
LUMBAR
LUMBER
MEEBER
MEMBER
MOBBER
NABBER
NUBBER
NUMBER
PROBER
RAWBAR
RIBBER
ROBBER
RUBBER
SOBBER
SOMBER
TAMBOR
THEBAR
TIEBAR
TIMBER
TOWBAR
WEBBER
WETBAR
WILBUR

••••BR
CEREBR

BS••••
BSCALE
BSEVEN
BSHARP
BSIDES
BSTARS

B•S•••
BASALT
BASELY
BASEST
BASHED
BASHER
BASHES
BASHIN
BASIAL
BASICS
BASIFY
BASILS
BASING
BASINS
BASKED
BASKER
BASKET
BASKIN
BASQUE
BASRAH
BASSES
BASSET
BASSEY
BASSLY
BASSOS
BASTED
BASTER
BASTES
BASTIA
BBSHOT
BESAME
BESANT
BESETS
BESIDE
BESOMS
BESORE
BESOTS
BESSEL
BESSER
BESSIE
BESSON
BESTED
BESTER
BESTIR
BESTOW
BESURE
BISBEE
BISCAY
BISECT
BISHOP
BISONS
BISQUE
BISSAU
BISSET
BISTRO
BOSLEY
BOSNIA
BOSOMS
BOSOMY
BOSONS
BOSSED
BOSSES
BOSSON
BOSTON
BOSUNS
BUSBOY
BUSHED
BUSHEL
BUSHER
BUSHES
BUSHWA
BUSIED
BUSIER
BUSIES
BUSILY
BUSING
BUSKED
BUSKER
BUSMAN
BUSMEN
BUSONI
BUSSED
BUSSES
BUSTED
BUSTER
BUSTIN
BUSTLE
BUSTUP
BYSSHE

B••S••
BABSON
BAGSIT
BAISAS
BAKSHI
BALSAM
BALSAS
BASSES
BASSET
BASSEY
BASSLY
BASSOS
BATSIN
BATSON
BAUSCH
BAYSAT
BEASTS
BEDSIT
BENSEY
BENSON
BESSEL
BESSER
BESSIE
BESSON
BETSEY
BETSON
BETSYS
BIASED
BIASES
BIDSIN
BIDSON
BIDSUP
BIGSKY
BIGSUR
BISSAU
BISSET
BLASTS
BLISTS
BOASTS
BOBSUP
BOESKY
BOLSHY
BONSAI
BOOSAT
BOOSTS
BORSCH
BOSSED
BOSSES
BOSSON
BOWSAW
BOWSTO
BOXSET
BRASCO
BRASHY
BRASIL
BRASOV
BRASSY
BRISES
BRISKS
BROSSE
BRUSHY
BRYSON
BUNSEN
BUQSHA
BURSAE
BURSAL
BURSAR
BURSAS
BURSTS
BUSSED
BUSSES
BUYSAT
BUYSIN
BUYSIT
BUYSON
BUYSUP
BYSSHE

B•••S•
BALLST
BANISH
BAREST
BASEST
BEARSE
BEHEST
BEMUSE
BIOPSY
BLAISE
BLOUSE
BLOWSY
BLUEST
BLUESY
BLUISH
BOCHSA
BOURSE
BOYISH
BRAISE
BRASSY
BRATSK
BREAST
BROAST
BROSSE
BROWSE
BRUISE
BYGOSH
BYPASS
BYPAST

B••••S
BABELS
BABIES
BABKAS
BABOOS
BACHES
BACKUS
BACONS
BADEMS
BADGES
BADUNS
BAGELS
BAINES
BAIRNS
BAISAS
BAIZAS
BAIZES
BAKERS
BALERS
BALLYS
BALSAS
BAMBIS
BANCOS
BANJOS
BANONS
BANTUS
BARCOS
BARGES
BARNES
BARONS
BARRES
BARRIS
BASHES
BASICS
BASILS
BASINS
BASSES
BASSOS
BASTES
BATHES
BATHOS
BATIKS
BATONS
BAULKS
BAYOUS
BAZOOS
BBGUNS
BCELLS
BEALLS
BEANOS
BEARDS
BEASTS
BEAUTS
BEAVIS
BEBOPS
BEDEWS
BEDIMS
BEDOGS
BEEVES
BEFITS
BEFOGS
BEGEMS
BEGETS
BEGINS
BEGUMS
BEIGES
BEINGS
BELAYS
BELIES
BELLES
BELONS
BENTOS
BERETS
BERTHS
BERYLS
BESETS
BESOMS
BESOTS
BETELS
BETSYS
BETTAS
BEVANS
BEVELS
BEVIES
BEWIGS
BEZELS
BFLATS
BGIRLS
BHANGS
BIASES
BIBLES
BICEPS
BIDERS
BIDETS
BIERES
BIGDOS
BIGHTS
BIGOTS
BIJOUS
BIKERS
BILGES
BILLIS
BIMBOS
BINGES
BINGOS
BIOGAS
BIOMES
BIONTS
BIOTAS
BIPEDS
BIPODS
BIRTHS
BISONS
BITERS
BLACKS
BLADES
BLAFFS
BLAMES
BLANKS
BLARES
BLASTS
BLAZES
BLEAKS
BLEARS
BLEATS
BLEEDS
BLEEPS
BLENDS
BLIMPS
BLINDS
BLINIS
BLINKS
BLISTS
BLOATS
BLOCKS
BLOKES
BLONDS
BLOODS
BLOOMS
BLOOPS
BLUETS
BLUFFS
BLUNTS
BLURBS
BLURTS
BMINUS
BOARDS
BOASTS
BOBBYS
BOCCES
BOCCIS
BODIES
BOFFOS
BOGEYS
BOGIES
BOGLES
BOINGS
BOITES
BOLLAS
BOMBES
BONERS
BONGOS
BONNES
BONZES
BOOERS
BOOSTS
BOOTES
BOOTHS
BOOZES
BOREAS
BORERS
BORGES
BOSOMS
BOSONS
BOSSES
BOSUNS
BOTELS
BOUGHS
BOULES
BOUNDS
BOURGS
BOVIDS
BOWELS
BOWERS
BOWLES
BOXERS
BOYARS
BOYLES
BRACES
BRACHS
BRACTS
BRAHMS
BRAIDS
BRAINS
BRAKES
BRANDS
BRANTS
BRAVAS
BRAVES
BRAVOS
BRAWLS
BRAZOS
BREADS
BREAKS
BREAMS
BREDES
BREEDS
BREVES
BREVIS
BRIARS
BRIBES
BRICKS
BRIDES
BRIEFS
BRIERS
BRINES
BRINGS
BRINKS
BRISES
BRISKS
BROCAS
BROILS
BRONCS
BROODS
BROOKS
BROOMS
BROTHS
BROWNS
BRUGES
BRUINS
BRUITS
BRUMES
BRUNTS
BRUTES
BRUTUS
BRUXES
BSIDES
BSTARS
BTEAMS
BTILES
BUBBAS
BUBKES
BUDGES
BUENAS
BUENOS
BUFFOS
BUGLES
BUICKS
BUILDS
BULGES
BUNCOS
BUNDTS
BUNKOS
BUPKES
BUPKIS
BUPKUS
BURETS
BURGHS
BURGOS
BURIES
BURINS
BURKAS
BURROS
BURSAS
BURSTS
BUSHES
BUSIES
BUSSES
BUTEOS
BUTKUS
BUTTES
BUTUTS
BUYERS
BUYINS
BUZZES
BWANAS
BYLAWS
BYLOTS
BYPASS
BYRNES
BYTENS
BYTWOS
BYWAYS

•BS•••
ABSCAM
ABSENT
ABSORB
ABSURD
BBSHOT
OBSESS

•B•S••
ABASED

6 BS

ABASER
ABASES
ABUSED
ABUSER
ABUSES
ABYSMS
IBISES
OBISPO

•B••S•

ABBESS
ABLEST
ABLUSH
OBLAST
OBOIST
OBSESS
OBTEST
OBTUSE

•B•••S

ABACAS
ABACUS
ABASES
ABATES
ABATIS
ABBESS
ABBEYS
ABBOTS
ABELES
ABHORS
ABIDES
ABMHOS
ABODES
ABOHMS
ABOMAS
ABOMBS
ABORTS
ABRAMS
ABUSES
ABYSMS
BBGUNS
DBACKS
EBANKS
EBATES
EBBETS
EBOATS
EBONDS
EBOOKS
HBEAMS
HBOMBS
IBEAMS
IBEXES
IBICES
IBISES
IBMPCS
IBOOKS
LBEAMS
NBAERS
NBOMBS
OBEAHS
OBELUS
OBGYNS
OBJETS
OBOLUS
OBSESS
PBOOKS
TBILLS
TBIRDS
TBONDS
TBONES
UBOATS
UBOLTS
XBOXES

••BS••

BABSON
BOBSUP
DABSAT
GIBSON
GOBSOF
HOBSON
JOBSON
KGBSPY
PABSTS
ROBSOF
ROBSON
RUBSIN
RUBSON
RUBSUP
SUBSEA
SUBSET
TABSET

••B•S•

ABBESS
AMBUSH
ATBEST
CUBISM
CUBIST
DEBASE
DUBOSE
EMBOSS
GOBUST
IMBUSY
KIBOSH
ONBASE
RIBISI
RIBOSE
ROBUST
TUBIST
UNBUSY
VIBIST
WABASH

••B••S

ABBESS
ABBEYS
ABBOTS
ALBANS
ALBERS
ALBUMS
AMBERS
AMBITS
AMBLES
ARBORS
ARBRES
ATBATS
BABELS
BABIES
BABKAS
BABOOS
BEBOPS
BIBLES
BOBBYS
BUBBAS
BUBKES
CABALS
CABERS
CABINS
CABLES
COBRAS
CUBANS
CUBEBS
CUBERS
CUBICS
CUBITS
DEBAGS
DEBARS
DEBITS
DEBRIS
DEBUGS
DEBUTS
DOBLES
DOBROS
DOBYNS
DUBOIS
EBBETS
ELBOWS
ELBRUS
EMBARS
EMBAYS
EMBEDS
EMBERS
EMBOGS
EMBOSS
EMBOWS
ESBATS
FABLES
FIBERS
FIBRES
GABLES
GIBERS
GOBIES
GOBOES
GOBOTS
HABEAS
HABITS
HOBBES
HOBOES
HUBRIS
IMBEDS
IMBUES
JABOTS
KABOBS
KEBABS
LABELS
LABORS
LIBBYS
LIBELS
LIBERS
LIBRAS
LIBRIS
LIBROS
MOBIUS
NABOBS
NABORS
NOBELS
NOBLES
NOBUTS
ORBITS
OXBOWS
PABSTS
POBOYS
RABBIS
RABIES
REBAGS
REBARS
REBBES
REBECS
REBELS
REBETS
REBIDS
REBOPS
REBUTS
REBUYS
ROBERS
ROBINS
ROBLES
ROBOTS
RUBELS
RUBENS
RUBIES
RUBIKS
RUBLES
SABALS
SABERS
SABLES
SABOTS
SABRAS
SABRES
SIBYLS
SOBERS
TABLAS
TABLES
TABOOS
TABORS
TEBETS
TIBIAS
TOBIAS
TOBIES
TOBITS
TUBERS
UMBELS
UMBERS
UMBRAS
UNBAGS
UNBARS
UNBITS
UNBUDS
UPBOWS
VWBUGS
WEBADS
WEBERS
XEBECS
ZEBRAS

•••BS•

PROBST

•••B•S

ADOBES
ADOBOS
AIRBUS
ALIBIS
AMEBAS
ANUBIS
BAMBIS
BIMBOS
BOBBYS
BOMBES
BRIBES
BUBBAS
CARBOS
CEIBAS
COLBYS
COMBOS
DAUBES
DOUBTS
DUMBOS
EREBUS
FLYBYS
FORBES
FURBYS
GLOBES
GREBES
GUMBOS
HERBES
HOBBES
IAMBUS
JAMBES
JUMBOS
KOMBUS
LAYBYS
LESBOS
LIBBYS
LIEBYS
LIMBOS
MAMBAS
MAMBOS
MAYBES
NIMBUS
ORIBIS
PHOBOS
PLEBES
PROBES
RABBIS
RAMBOS
REBBES
RUMBAS
SAMBAS
SCUBAS
THEBES
TOMBES
TRIBES
TURBOS
UTUBES

••••BS

ABOMBS
ADLIBS
BLURBS
CARIBS
CAROBS
CELEBS
CLIMBS
COHABS
CRUMBS
CUBEBS
DEMOBS
DWEEBS
EXCUBS
EXURBS
HBOMBS
KABOBS
KEBABS
MCJOBS
MCRIBS
NABOBS
NBOMBS
PCLABS
PLANBS
PLUMBS
RAJABS
REDUBS
REHABS
REPUBS
RHOMBS
RHUMBS
SAHIBS
SCRUBS
SHRUBS
SQUABS
SQUIBS
TENLBS
THROBS
THUMBS
TYPEBS
VOCABS
ZHLOBS
ZHLUBS

BT••••

BTEAMS
BTHREE
BTILES

B•T•••

BATAAN
BATBOY
BATDAY
BATEAU
BATFOR
BATHED
BATHER
BATHES
BATHOS
BATIKS
BATING
BATLEY
BATMAN
BATMEN
BATONS
BATSIN
BATSON
BATTED
BATTEN
BATTER
BATTLE
BATYAM
BETAKE
BETCHA
BETELS
BETHEL
BETIDE
BETONY
BETOOK
BETRAY
BETSEY
BETSON
BETSYS
BETTAS
BETTED
BETTER
BETTOR
BETTYE
BITEIN
BITEON
BITERS
BITEUP
BITING
BITMAP
BITNET
BITOFF
BITTED
BITTEN
BITTER
BOTANY
BOTCHY
BOTELS
BOTFLY
BOTHER
BOTREE
BOTTLE
BOTTOM
BSTARS
BUTANE
BUTENE
BUTEOS
BUTHOW
BUTKUS
BUTLER
BUTTED
BUTTER
BUTTES
BUTTIN
BUTTON
BUTUTS
BUTWHO
BUTWHY
BUTYET
BYTALK
BYTAXI
BYTENS
BYTHEN
BYTWOS

B••T••

BAITED
BAITER
BALTIC
BANTAM
BANTER
BANTUS
BARTAB
BARTEL
BARTER
BARTLE
BARTOK
BARTON
BASTED
BASTER
BASTES
BASTIA
BATTED
BATTEN
BATTER
BATTLE
BAXTER
BEATAT
BEATEN
BEATER
BEATIT
BEATLE
BEATON
BEATTY
BEATUP
BEETLE
BELTED
BELTER
BELTON
BELTUP
BENTON
BENTOS
BERTHA
BERTHE
BERTHS
BERTIE
BESTED
BESTER
BESTIR
BESTOW
BETTAS
BETTED
BETTER
BETTOR
BETTYE
BHUTAN
BHUTTO
BIGTEN
BIGTOE
BIGTOP
BIOTAS
BIOTIC
BIOTIN
BIRTHS
BISTRO
BITTED
BITTEN
BITTER
BLATTY
BLITHE
BLOTCH
BLOTTO
BLOTTY
BLOTUP
BLYTHE
BLYTON
BOATED
BOATEL
BOATER
BOITES
BOLTED
BOLTER
BOLTON
BOLTUP
BONTON
BOOTED
BOOTEE
BOOTER
BOOTES
BOOTHE
BOOTHS
BOOTIE
BOOTIT
BOOTUP
BOSTON
BOTTLE
BOTTOM
BOUTON
BOWTIE
BOXTOP
BOYTOY
BRATSK
BRATTY
BRETON
BRITON
BROTHS
BROTHY
BRUTAL
BRUTES
BRUTUS
BUNTED
BUNTER
BUNTON
BURTON
BUSTED
BUSTER
BUSTIN
BUSTLE
BUSTUP
BUTTED
BUTTER
BUTTES
BUTTIN
BUTTON

B•••T•

BALATA
BARATA
BARATO
BARITE
BEASTS
BEATTY
BEAUTS
BEAUTY
BEFITS
BEGETS
BELATE
BEMATA
BENITO
BENOTE
BERATE
BERETS
BESETS
BESOTS
BFLATS
BHUTTO
BIDETS
BIGHTS
BIGOTS
BINATE
BINDTO
BIONTS
BLASTS
BLATTY
BLEATS
BLEETH
BLINTZ
BLISTS
BLOATS
BLOTTO
BLOTTY
BLUETS
BLUNTS
BLURTS
BOASTS
BODETT
BOGOTA
BONITA
BONITO
BOOSTS
BORATE
BOUNTY
BOWSTO
BRACTS
BRANTS
BRATTY
BREATH
BRONTE
BRUITS
BRUNTS
BUNDTS
BURETS
BURSTS
BUTUTS
BYDATE
BYLOTS
BYPATH
BYROTE

B••••T

BACHIT
BADFIT
BADHAT
BADLOT
BAGSIT
BALKAT
BALLET
BALLOT
BALLST
BANDIT
BANKIT
BARBET
BARDOT
BAREST
BARKAT
BARNET
BARRET
BASALT
BASEST
BASKET
BASSET
BAYSAT
BBQPIT
BBSHOT
BEATAT
BEATIT
BECHET
BECKET
BEDSIT
BEEPAT
BEGIRT
BEHEST
BEIGHT
BEIRUT
BEJART
BELOIT
BENOIT
BEREFT
BESANT
BIGBET
BIGCAT
BIGHIT
BILLET
BIRGIT
BISECT
BISSET
BITNET
BIZKIT
BLEWIT
BLIGHT
BLOUNT
BLOWIT
BLUEST
BOBCAT
BODETT
BOGART
BONMOT
BONNET
BOOSAT
BOOTIT
BORDET
BOUGHT
BOWOUT
BOXSET
BRANDT
BREAST
BRECHT
BREVET
BRIGHT
BRIGIT
BROAST
BRUNET
BRYANT
BUCKET
BUDGET
BUFFET
BUGOUT
BULLET
BUMOUT
BURBOT
BURNET
BUTYET
BUYOUT
BUYSAT
BUYSIT
BYPAST

•BT•••

OBTAIN
OBTEST
OBTUND
OBTUSE

•B•T••

ABATED
ABATER
ABATES
ABATIS
ABATOR
ABITOF
ABUTON
EBATES
OBITER

•B••T•

ABBOTS
ABBOTT
ABLATE
ABORTS
EBBETS
EBOATS
OBENTO
OBERTO
OBJETS
OBLATE
UBIETY
UBOATS
UBOLTS

•B•••T

ABBOTT
ABDUCT
ABJECT
ABLEST
ABRUPT
ABSENT
BBQPIT
BBSHOT
OBJECT
OBLAST
OBOIST
OBTEST
OBVERT

••BT••

DEBTEE
DEBTOR
SUBTLE
SUBTLY

••B•T•

ABBOTS
ABBOTT
AMBITS
ATBATS
CUBITI
CUBITS
DEBATE
DEBITS
DEBUTS
EBBETS
ESBATS
GOBOTS
HABITS
JABOTS
JOBETH
KIBITZ
LABATT
LOBATE
MOBUTU
NOBUTS
ORBITS
PABSTS
REBATE
REBETS
REBOTE
REBUTS
ROBOTS
RUBATI
RUBATO
SABATO
SABOTS
SUBITO
TEBETS
TOBITS
TUBATE
UNBITS

••B••T

ABBOTT
ALBEIT
ALBERT
ATBEST
BOBCAT
CABLET
COBALT
COBNUT
CUBIST
DABRAT
DABSAT
DEBONT
EGBERT
ELBERT
GIBEAT
GIBLET
GOBLET
GOBUST
HOBART
HOBBIT
HUBERT
IMBEAT
JIBEAT
JOBCUT
JOBLOT
LABATT
LABRAT
LEBRET
NIBLET
OSBERT
PTBOAT
RABBET
RABBIT
REBAIT
REBENT
REBOLT
REBOOT
RIBBIT
RIBCUT
RIBLET
ROBERT
ROBUST
RUBOUT
SOBEIT
SUBLET
SUBLOT
SUBMIT
SUBNET
SUBSET
TABLET
TABSET
TOBOOT
TUBIST
TYBALT
UNBAIT
UNBELT
UNBENT
UNBOLT
UPBEAT
VIBIST
WABBIT

•••BT•

DOUBTS

•••B•T

ALLBUT
BARBET
BIGBET
BURBOT
COMBAT
FEMBOT
GAMBIT
GRABAT
HENBIT
HOBBIT
HOTBOT
ILLBET
INABIT
IROBOT
KOMBAT
KORBUT
NESBIT
NUMBAT
OLDBAT
ONEBIT
OUTBAT
PROBST
RABBET
RABBIT
REDBAT
RIBBIT
SHEBAT
SORBET
SPYBOT
STABAT
TIDBIT
TURBOT
TWOBIT
WABBIT
WEEBIT
WOMBAT
XZIBIT
YESBUT
YOUBET

••••BT

INDEBT

BU••••

BUBBAS
BUBBLE
BUBBLY
BUBKES
BUCCAL
BUCHAN
BUCKED
BUCKER
BUCKET
BUCKLE
BUCKUP
BUDDED
BUDDER
BUDDHA
BUDGED
BUDGER
BUDGES
BUDGET
BUDGIE
BUENAS
BUENOS
BUFFAY
BUFFED
BUFFER
BUFFET
BUFFON
BUFFOS
BUFFUP
BUGAKU
BUGBOY
BUGGED
BUGLED
BUGLER
BUGLES
BUGOFF
BUGOUT
BUICKS
BUILDS
BUJOLD
BUKAVU
BULDEO
BULGAR
BULGED
BULGES
BULGUR
BULKED
BULKUP
BULLAE
BULLED
BULLET
BULOVA
BULWER
BUMBLE
BUMBRY
BUMLEG
BUMMED
BUMMER
BUMOUT
BUMPED
BUMPER
BUMPPO
BUMPUP
BUMRAP
BUNCHE
BUNCHY
BUNCOS
BUNDLE
BUNDTS
BUNGAY
BUNGED
BUNGEE
BUNGLE
BUNION
BUNKED
BUNKER
BUNKOS
BUNKUM
BUNSEN
BUNTED
BUNTER
BUNTON
BUNUEL
BUNYAN
BUOYED
BUOYUP
BUPKES
BUPKIS
BUPKUS
BUQSHA
BURANA
BURBLE
BURBLY
BURBOT
BURDEN
BUREAU
BURETS
BURGEE
BURGER
BURGHS
BURGLE

BURGOO
BURGOS
BURIAL
BURIED
BURIER
BURIES
BURINS
BURKAS
BURLAP
BURLED
BURLER
BURLEY
BURMAN
BURNED
BURNER
BURNET
BURNEY
BURNIE
BURNIN
BURNUP
BUROAK
BURPED
BURPEE
BURRED
BURROS
BURROW
BURSAE
BURSAL
BURSAR
BURSAS
BURSTS
BURTON
BUSBOY
BUSHED
BUSHEL
BUSHER
BUSHES
BUSHWA
BUSIED
BUSIER
BUSIES
BUSILY
BUSING
BUSKED
BUSKER
BUSMAN
BUSMEN
BUSONI
BUSSED
BUSSES
BUSTED
BUSTER
BUSTIN
BUSTLE
BUSTUP
BUTANE
BUTENE
BUTEOS
BUTHOW
BUTKUS
BUTLER
BUTTED
BUTTER
BUTTES
BUTTIN
BUTTON
BUTUTS
BUTWHO
BUTWHY
BUTYET
BUYERS
BUYING
BUYINS
BUYNOW
BUYOFF
BUYOUT
BUYSAT
BUYSIN
BUYSIT
BUYSON
BUYSUP
BUZZED
BUZZER
BUZZES

B•U•••
BAUBLE
BAULKS
BAUMAN
BAUMER
BAUSCH
BEULAH
BEURRE
BHUTAN
BHUTTO
BLUDGE
BLUELY
BLUEOX
BLUEST
BLUESY
BLUETS
BLUFFO
BLUFFS
BLUING
BLUISH
BLUNTS
BLURBS
BLURRY
BLURTS
BOUCHE
BOUDIN
BOUFFE
BOUGHS
BOUGHT
BOULES
BOULEZ
BOUNCE
BOUNCY
BOUNDS
BOUNTY
BOURGS
BOURKE
BOURNE
BOURSE
BOUTON
BRUDER
BRUGES
BRUINS
BRUISE
BRUITS
BRULEE
BRUMAL
BRUMEL
BRUMES
BRUNCH
BRUNEI
BRUNET
BRUNOR
BRUNTS
BRUSHY
BRUTAL
BRUTES
BRUTUS
BRUXED
BRUXES

B••U••
BADUNS
BAKULA
BARUCH
BBGUNS
BEAUTS
BEAUTY
BEGUMS
BELUGA
BEMUSE
BENUMB
BESURE
BLOUNT
BLOUSE
BODUKE
BOSUNS
BREUER
BROUGH
BUNUEL
BUTUTS

B•••U•
BACKUP
BACKUS
BADGUY
BAGFUL
BALDUR
BALLUP
BANGUI
BANGUP
BANJUL
BANKUP
BANQUE
BANQUO
BANTUS
BARIUM
BARNUM
BARQUE
BARZUN
BASQUE
BAYEUX
BAYOUS
BAYRUM
BEADUP
BEAMUP
BEARUP
BEATUP
BEDAUB
BEDBUG
BEEFUP
BEFOUL
BEIRUT
BELLUM
BELTUP
BENHUR
BIDSUP
BIGBUX
BIGFUN
BIGGUN
BIGGUY
BIGHUG
BIGSUR
BIJOUS
BIJOUX
BINDUP
BISQUE
BITEUP
BLEWUP
BLOTUP
BLOWUP
BMINUS
BOBSUP
BOILUP
BOLTUP
BONEUP
BOOJUM
BOOTUP
BOREUP
BOWOUT
BOXFUL
BRAQUE
BREWUP
BROGUE
BRUTUS
BUCKUP
BUFFUP
BUGOUT
BULGUR
BULKUP
BUMOUT
BUMPUP
BUNKUM
BUOYUP
BUPKUS
BURNUP
BUSTUP
BUTKUS
BUYOUT
BUYSUP

B••••U
BABALU
BALLOU
BATEAU
BISSAU
BROWNU
BUGAKU
BUKAVU
BUREAU

•BU•••
ABUSED
ABUSER
ABUSES
ABUTON
UBUROI

•B•U••
ABDUCE
ABDUCT
ABJURE
ABLUSH
ABOUND
ABRUPT
ABSURD
BBGUNS
OBTUND
OBTUSE

•B••U•
ABACUS
OBELUS
OBOLUS

••BU••
ALBUMS
AMBUSH
ASBURY
AUBURN
COBURG
COBURN
DEBUGS
DEBUNK
DEBURR
DEBUTS
ELBURZ
FIBULA
GOBUST
IMBUED
IMBUES
IMBUSY
INBULK
KABUKI
LOBULE
MOBUTU
NEBULA
NOBUTS
REBUFF
REBUKE
REBURY
REBUTS
REBUYS
ROBUST
SUBURB
TABUED
TABULA
TOBURN
TUBULE
UNBUDS
UNBURY
UNBUSY
VWBUGS
WOBURN

••B•U•
ARBOUR
BOBSUP
COBNUT
DEBLUR
DYBBUK
ELBRUS
EMBRUE
ERBIUM
HUBBUB
IMBRUE
INBLUE
JOBCUT
LABIUM
LABOUR
LEBRUN
MOBIUS
MRBLUE
PABLUM
RIBCUT
RUBOUT
RUBSUP
SOBFUL
SUBDUE
SUBGUM
TUBFUL

••B••U
BABALU
DEBREU
LEBEAU
MOBUTU
SUBARU

•••BU•
AIRBUD
AIRBUS
ALLBUT
BEDBUG
BIGBUX
CLUBUP
DISBUD
DYBBUK
EARBUD
EREBUS
FLUBUG
HUBBUB
HUMBUG
IAMBUS
KOMBUS
KORBUT
NIMBUS
ONABUN
OUTBUD
OUTBUY
PREBUY
REDBUD
SKIBUM
WILBUR
YESBUT

••••BU
MALIBU

B•V•••
BAVIER
BEVANS
BEVELS
BEVIES
BOVARY
BOVIDS
BOVINE

B••V••
BEAVER
BEAVIS
BEEVES
BMOVIE
BRAVAS
BRAVED
BRAVER
BRAVES
BRAVOS
BREVES
BREVET
BREVIS
BROVIK
BSEVEN

B•••V•
BEHAVE
BOOKVI
BUKAVU
BULOVA
BYJOVE

B••••V
BOOKIV
BRASOV

•BV•••
OBVERT

•B•••V
ABBREV

••B••V
ABBREV
RUBLEV
URBANV

BW••••
BWANAS

B•W•••
BAWLED
BAWLER
BEWAIL
BEWARE
BEWARY
BEWELL
BEWIGS
BOWELS
BOWERS
BOWERY
BOWFIN
BOWING
BOWLED
BOWLER
BOWLES
BOWMAN
BOWMEN
BOWOAR
BOWOUT
BOWSAW
BOWSTO
BOWTIE
BOWWOW
BOWYER
BOWZER
BYWAYS
BYWIRE
BYWORD

B••W••
BAGWIG
BEDWIN
BERWYN
BIGWIG
BIGWIN
BLEWIN
BLEWIT
BLEWON
BLEWUP
BLOWER
BLOWIN
BLOWIT
BLOWON
BLOWSY
BLOWUP
BLOWZY
BOWWOW
BRAWLS
BRAWNY
BREWED
BREWER
BREWUP
BROWED
BROWNE
BROWNS
BROWNU
BROWNY
BROWSE
BULWER
BUTWHO
BUTWHY
BYTWOS

B•••W•
BEDEWS
BUSHWA
BYLAWS

B••••W
BARLOW
BARROW
BELLOW
BENBOW
BERKOW
BESTOW
BILLOW
BORROW
BOWSAW
BOWWOW
BROKAW
BURROW
BUTHOW
BUYNOW
BYENOW

•B•W••
OBIWAN

••BW••
COBWEB
SUBWAR
SUBWAY

••B•W•
ELBOWS
EMBOWS
OXBOWS
UPBOWS

••B••W
HEBREW
REBREW
RUBRAW

•••BW•
OJIBWA

•••B•W
BENBOW
FOGBOW
OUTBOW
SUNBOW

B•X•••
BAXTER
BOXBED
BOXBOY
BOXCAR
BOXERS
BOXFUL
BOXIER
BOXILY
BOXING
BOXSET
BOXTOP

B••X••
BLIXEN
BRUXED
BRUXES

B•••X•
BILOXI
BORAXO
BYTAXI

B••••X
BAYEUX
BENDIX
BIGBOX
BIGBUX
BIJOUX
BLUEOX
BOLLIX
BOOKIX
BRANDX

•B•X••
IBEXES
XBOXES

••B••X
PUBLIX

•••B•X
BIGBOX
BIGBUX
HATBOX
HOTBOX
ICEBOX
INABOX
OUTBOX
PEGBOX
SKYBOX
TEEBOX

BY••••
BYDATE
BYEBYE
BYENOW
BYFORM
BYGONE
BYGOSH
BYHALF
BYHAND
BYJOVE
BYLAND
BYLAWS
BYLINE
BYLOTS
BYMAIL
BYNAME
BYPASS
BYPAST
BYPATH
BYPLAY
BYRNES
BYROAD
BYROTE
BYSSHE
BYTALK
BYTAXI
BYTENS
BYTHEN
BYTWOS
BYWAYS
BYWIRE
BYWORD

B•Y•••
BAYARD
BAYERN
BAYEUX
BAYING
BAYLOR
BAYMAN
BAYMEN
BAYOUS
BAYRUM
BAYSAT
BEYMER
BEYOND
BLYDEN
BLYTHE
BLYTON
BOYARS
BOYISH
BOYLES
BOYTOY
BRYANT
BRYNZA
BRYSON
BUYERS
BUYING
BUYINS
BUYNOW
BUYOFF
BUYOUT
BUYSAT
BUYSIN
BUYSIT
BUYSON
BUYSUP

B••Y••
BAEYER
BANYAN
BARYON
BATYAM
BERYLS
BINYON
BOLYAI
BOWYER
BRAYED
BRAYER
BREYER
BUNYAN
BUOYED
BUOYUP
BUTYET

B•••Y•
BALLYS
BELAYS
BERWYN
BETSYS
BETTYE
BIGEYE
BOBBYS
BOGEYS
BOLEYN
BYEBYE
BYWAYS

B••••Y
BABBLY
BADBOY
BADDAY
BADGUY
BAGBOY
BAILEY
BAKERY
BALDLY
BARANY
BARELY
BARFLY
BARLEY
BARNEY
BARONY
BASELY
BASIFY
BASSEY
BASSLY
BATBOY
BATDAY
BATLEY
BEACHY
BEATTY
BEAUTY
BEGLEY
BELFRY
BELLAY
BENDAY
BENGAY
BENSEY
BETONY
BETRAY
BETSEY
BEWARY
BIGAMY
BIGBOY
BIGDAY
BIGGUY
BIGSKY
BINARY
BINCHY
BINNEY
BIOPSY
BIRNEY
BISCAY
BLABBY
BLAKEY
BLATTY
BLEARY
BLIMEY
BLOBBY
BLOCKY
BLOODY
BLOOEY
BLOOMY
BLOTTY
BLOWSY
BLOWZY
BLUELY
BLUESY
BLURRY
BOBBLY
BODILY
BODLEY
BOESKY
BOLDLY
BOLSHY
BOMBAY
BONNEY
BOSLEY
BOSOMY
BOTANY
BOTCHY
BOTFLY
BOUNCY
BOUNTY
BOVARY
BOWERY
BOXBOY
BOXILY
BOYTOY
BRAINY
BRANDY
BRANNY
BRASHY
BRASSY
BRATTY
BRAWNY
BREEDY
BREEZY
BRENLY
BRIARY
BRICKY
BRIERY
BROLLY
BRONZY
BROODY
BROOKY
BROOMY
BROPHY
BROTHY
BROWNY
BRUSHY
BUBBLY
BUFFAY
BUGBOY
BUMBRY
BUNCHY
BUNGAY
BURBLY
BURLEY
BURNEY
BUSBOY
BUSILY
BUTWHY
BYPLAY

•BY•••
ABYSMS

•B•Y••
EBAYER
OBEYED
OBEYER
OBGYNS

•B••Y•
ABBEYS

•B•••Y
ABBACY
EBERLY
UBIETY

••BY••
DOBYNS
JOBYNA
LIBYAN
OKBYME
SIBYLS

••B•Y•
ABBEYS
BOBBYS
EMBAYS
EMBRYO
LIBBYS
POBOYS
REBUYS
RIBEYE

••B••Y
ABBACY
ALBANY
AMBERY
ASBURY
AUBREY
BABBLY
BOBBLY
BUBBLY
DABNEY
DEBRAY
EMBODY
FABRAY
HUBLEY
IMBUSY
KGBSPY
MABLEY
MOBLEY
MYBABY
NOBODY
NUBBLY
OHBABY
PEBBLY
REBURY
ROBROY
RUBBLY
RUBIFY
SUBTLY
SUBWAY
TABKEY
UNBURY
UNBUSY
WOBBLY

•••BY•
BOBBYS
BYEBYE
COLBYS
FLYBYS
FURBYS
LAYBYS
LIBBYS
LIEBYS

•••B•Y
BABBLY
BADBOY
BAGBOY
BATBOY
BIGBOY
BLABBY
BLOBBY
BOBBLY
BOMBAY
BOXBOY
BUBBLY
BUGBOY
BUMBRY
BURBLY
BUSBOY
CAMBOY
CARBOY
CHUBBY
CLUBBY
COWBOY
CRABBY
DOCBOY
DOMBEY
DOUBLY
DRABLY
DUMBLY
EDIBLY
FEEBLY
FLABBY
FLYBOY
GLIBLY
GLOBBY
GRABBY
GRUBBY
HUMBLY
JUMBLY
KNOBBY
LAZBOY
LOWBOY
MARBLY
MUMBLY
NIMBLY
NUBBLY
NUMBLY
OLDBOY
OUTBUY
PEBBLY
PEPBOY
PINBOY
PREBUY
REDBAY
RUBBLY
RUMBLY
SHABBY
SLOBBY
SNOBBY
SNUBBY
STABLY
STUBBY
SWABBY
THEBAY
TOMBOY
TORBAY
TREBLY
UNABLY
USABLY
VIABLY
WAMBLY
WOBBLY

••••BY
BLABBY
BLOBBY
CAMEBY
CHUBBY
CLUBBY
COMEBY
CRABBY
CROSBY
CRUMBY
DOESBY
DONEBY
DROPBY
DWEEBY
EASEBY
EKEDBY
EKESBY
FILEBY
FLABBY
FLEWBY
FLITBY
GATSBY
GETSBY
GLOBBY
GOALBY
GOESBY
GONEBY
GOODBY
GRABBY
GRANBY
GRUBBY
HANGBY
HARDBY
HEREBY
HORNBY
HUNGBY
JACOBY
KNOBBY
LAIDBY
LAYSBY
LETSBY
MALTBY
MYBABY
NASEBY
NEARBY
OHBABY
PASSBY
PHILBY
PLAYBY
PUTSBY
RACEBY
RIDEBY
RODEBY
ROLLBY
RUNSBY

RUSHBY SCOOBY SELLBY SENDBY SENTBY SETSBY SHABBY SHELBY SHOTBY SITSBY SKIPBY SLIPBY SLOBBY SNOBBY SNUBBY STOPBY STUBBY SWABBY TICKBY TRILBY WALKBY WENTBY WHITBY WINSBY ZIPSBY

B•Z•••

BAZAAR BAZOOS BEZELS BIZKIT BUZZED BUZZER BUZZES

B••Z••

BAIZAS BAIZES BALZAC BANZAI BARZUN BEEZER BELZER BENZOL BLAZED BLAZER BLAZES BLAZON BONZES BOOZED BOOZER BOOZES BORZOI BOWZER BRAZEN BRAZIL BRAZOS BRAZZA BRAZZI BUZZED BUZZER BUZZES

B•••Z•

BEDAZE BELIZE BLOWZY BRAZZA BRAZZI BREEZE BREEZY BRONZE BRONZY BRYNZA

B••••Z

BLINTZ BONERZ BOULEZ BRIENZ

•B•Z••

IBIZAN

•B••Z•

ABLAZE

•B•••Z

IBANEZ

••B•Z•

CABEZA REBOZO ZABRZE

••B••Z

ELBURZ KIBITZ TABRIZ

CA••••

CABALA CABALS CABANA CABBED CABBIE CABELL CABERS CABEZA CABINS CABLED CABLER CABLES CABLET CABMAN CABMEN CABRAL CABRIO CACAOS CACHED CACHES CACHET CACKLE CACTUS CADDIE CADEAU CADENT CADETS CADGED CADGER CADGES CADMIC CADMUS CADRES CAESAR CAFTAN CAGEIN CAGERS CAGEUP CAGIER CAGILY CAGING CAGNEY CAGUAS CAHIER CAHILL CAHOOT CAICOS CAIMAN CAIRNS CAJOLE CAJUNS CAKEUP CAKIER CAKING CALAIS CALASH CALDER CALGON CALICO CALIFS CALIPH CALKED CALKER CALLAN CALLAO CALLAS CALLED CALLEE CALLER CALLES CALLIN CALLIT CALLME CALLON CALLOW CALLTO CALLUP CALLUS CALMED CALMER CALMEX CALMLY CALORY CALVED CALVES CALVET CALVIN CALXES CAMARO CAMBER CAMBOY CAMDEN CAMEAS CAMEAT CAMEBY CAMEIN CAMELS CAMEON CAMEOS CAMERA CAMETO CAMEUP CAMINO CAMION CAMISE CAMMIE CAMOES CAMPED CAMPER CAMPOS CAMPUP CAMPUS CAMRYN CAMRYS CANAAN CANADA CANALS CANAPE CANARD CANARY CANCAN CANCEL CANCER CANCHA CANCUN CANDIA CANDID CANDLE CANDOR CANERS CANFUL CANIDS CANIER CANIFF CANINE CANING CANKER CANLIT CANNAS CANNED CANNEL CANNER CANNES CANNON CANNOT CANOED CANOER CANOES CANOLA CANONS CANOPY CANOVA CANTAB CANTAL CANTBE CANTED CANTER CANTLE CANTON CANTOO CANTOR CANTOS CANUCK CANULA CANUTE CANVAS CANYON CAPERS CAPFUL CAPGUN CAPITA CAPLET CAPNUT CAPONE CAPONI CAPONS CAPOTE CAPPED CAPPER CAPRID CAPRIS CAPTOR CARAFE CARATS CARBON CARBOS CARBOY CARBRA CARDED CARDER CARDIA CARDIN CARDIO CAREEN CAREER CAREOF CARERS CARESS CARETO CARETS CARFUL CARGOS CARHOP CARIBE CARIBS CARIES CARINA CARING CARIOU CARKEY CARLIN CARLOS CARLOT CARLOW CARMAN CARMEL CARMEN CARNAC CARNAL CARNAP CARNER CARNES CARNET CARNEY CAROBS CAROLE CAROLI CAROLL CAROLS CAROMS CARONI CARPAL CARPAT CARPED CARPEL CARPER CARPET CARPUS CARREL CARREY CARRIE CARROL CARROT CARSEY CARSON CARTED CARTEL CARTER CARTES CARTIN CARTON CARTOP CARUSO CARVED CARVEL CARVER CARVES CARVEY CARWAX CASABA CASALS CASAVA CASBAH CASEFY CASEIN CASERN CASERS CASHED CASHES CASHEW CASHIN CASING CASINO CASIOS CASITA CASKED CASKET CASPAR CASPER CASQUE CASSIA CASSIE CASSIM CASSIN CASSIO CASSIS CASTED CASTEL CASTER CASTES CASTLE CASTON CASTOR CASTRO CASTUP CASUAL CATALO CATANO CATBED CATCHY CATDOM CATENA CATERA CATERS CATFIT CATGUT CATHAY CATHER CATHYS CATION CATKIN CATLIN CATMAN CATMEN CATNAP CATNIP CATRIG CATSAT CATSIT CATSUP CATTLE CATTON CATTOY CAUCHY CAUCUS CAUDAD CAUDAL CAUGHT CAULKS CAUSAL CAUSED CAUSER CAUSES CAVAFY CAVEAT CAVEIN CAVELL CAVERN CAVERS CAVETT CAVIAR CAVIES CAVILS CAVING CAVITY CAVORT CAWCAW CAWDOR CAWING CAYMAN CAYUGA CAYUSE CAZALE

C•A•••

CEASED CEASES CHACEL CHACHA CHACHI CHACUN CHAFED CHAFER CHAFES CHAFFS CHAFFY CHAINE CHAINS CHAIRS CHAISE CHAKRA CHALET CHALKS CHALKY CHAMMY CHAMPS CHANCE CHANCY CHANDU CHANEL CHANEY CHANGE CHANGO CHANTE CHANTS CHANTY CHAPEL CHAPIN CHARDS CHARGE CHARLY CHARMS CHARON CHARRO CHARTA CHARTS CHASED CHASER CHASES CHASMS CHASSE CHASTE CHATTY CHATUP CHAVEZ CHAWED CHAZAN CIARDI CIASPY CLACKS CLADIN CLAIMS CLAIRE CLAIRS CLAMMA CLAMMY CLAMOR CLAMPS CLAMUP CLANCY CLANGS CLANKS CLANKY CLAQUE CLARET CLARKE CLAROS CLASPS CLASSA CLASSE CLASSY CLAUDE CLAUSE CLAVES CLAVIN CLAWAT CLAWED CLAWER CLAYEY CMAJOR COACTS COALED COALER COAPTS COARSE COASTS COATED COATEE COATER COATES COATIS COAXAL COAXED COAXER COAXES CRABBE CRABBY CRACKD CRACKS CRACOW CRADLE CRAFTS CRAFTY CRAGGY CRAIGT CRAINS CRAKES CRAMBO CRAMER CRAMIN CRAMPS CRAMPY CRANED CRANES CRANIA CRANIO CRANKS CRANKY CRANNY CRAPED CRAPES CRATED CRATER CRATES CRAVAT CRAVED CRAVEN CRAVER CRAVES CRAWLS CRAWLY CRAYON CRAZED CRAZES CUANDO CUANTO CUATRO CYANIC CYANID

C••A••

CABALA CABALS CABANA CACAOS CALAIS CALASH CAMARO CANAAN CANADA CANALS CANAPE CANARD CANARY CARAFE CARATS CASABA CASALS CASAVA CATALO CATANO CAVAFY CAZALE CCLAMP CDCASE CDRACK CDRATE CEDARN CEDARS CEDARY CERATE CERATO CESARE CESARS CETANE CFLATS CHEAPO CHEATS CHIANG CHOATE CICADA CIGARS CLEANS CLEARS CLEARY CLEATS CLEAVE CLOAKS COBAIN COBALT COHABS COLADA COMATE CONAIR CONANT COPALS COPAYS CORACI CORALS COTANS COWARD CREAKS CREAKY CREAMS CREAMY CREASE CREASY CREATE CROAKS CROAKY CROATS CSCALE CSHARP CSTARS CUBAGE CUBANS CUDAHY CUNARD CURACY CURADS CURARE CURATE CUSACK CYCADS CYRANO

C•••A•

CABMAN CABRAL CADEAU CAESAR CAFTAN CAGUAS CAIMAN CALLAN CALLAO CALLAS CAMEAS CAMEAT CANAAN CANCAN CANNAS CANTAB CANTAL CANVAS CARMAN CARNAC CARNAL CARNAP CARPAL CARPAT CARWAX CASBAH CASPAR CASUAL CATHAY CATMAN CATNAP CATSAT CAUDAD CAUDAL CAUSAL CAVEAT CAVIAR CAWCAW CAYMAN CEIBAS CELLAE CELLAR CENTAI CENTAL CENTAS CEPHAL CEREAL CERNAN CESTAS CHAZAN CHELAE CHEVAL CHICAS CHINAS CHIRAC CHIVAS CHORAL CIERAS CIUDAD CLAWAT CLIMAT CLIMAX CLONAL COAXAL COBHAM COBRAS COCOAS COEVAL COGNAC COLFAX COLLAR COLLAT COLMAN COLMAR COMBAT COMEAS COMEAT COMMAS COMPAQ COMPAS COMSAT CONFAB CONGAS CONLAN CONMAN CONRAD CONTAC CONWAY COOGAN COPCAR COPRAS CORDAY CORFAM CORMAN CORRAL CORSAS COSMAS COSTAE COSTAL COSTAR COSTAS COTTAE COTTAS COUGAR COWMAN CRAVAT CRETAN CRURAL CRUZAN CTSCAN CUBFAN CUICAS CUNEAL CUPPAS CURIAE CUSHAW CUSPAL CYMBAL

C••••A

CABALA CABANA CABEZA CAMERA CANADA CANCHA CANDIA CANOLA CANOVA CANULA CAPITA CARBRA CARDIA CARINA CASABA CASAVA CASITA CASSIA CATENA CATERA CAYUGA CELICA CEPEDA CESSNA CETERA CHACHA CHAKRA CHARTA CHEETA CHICHA CHINUA CHITRA CHOLLA CHOPRA CHROMA CHUPPA CHYNNA CIBOLA CICADA CINEMA CLAMMA CLASSA COELIA COLADA COLIMA COMIDA CONCHA CONTRA COPULA CORDIA CORNEA CORONA CORYZA COULDA COVINA COWPEA CRANIA CRENNA CREUSA CRIMEA CSONKA CUESTA CUMBIA CUPOLA

•CA•••

ACACIA ACADIA ACARID DCAREA ECARDS ECARTE ICALLY ICANSO ICARIA ICARUS MCADOO MCAFEE MCAVOY OCASEK OCASEY SCAASI SCAGGS SCALAR SCALDS SCALED SCALER SCALES SCALIA SCALPS SCAMPI SCAMPS SCANTS SCANTY SCARAB SCARCE SCARED SCARER SCARES SCARFS SCARNE SCARPS SCARRY SCARUM SCATHE

•C•A••

ACKACK ACUATE CCLAMP ECKART ECLAIR ECLASS ECLATS ICEAGE ICEAXE LCHAIM MCBAIN MCCABE MCCAIN MCCANN MCHALE MCHARG MCLAIN MCNABB MCNAIR OCCAMS OCEANS OCTADS OCTANE OCTANS OCTANT OCTAVE OCTAVO PCLABS SCAASI SCHAAP SCHAVS SCLAFF SCRAGS SCRAMS SCRAPE SCRAPS SCRAWL UCLANS

•C••A•

ACELAS ACETAL ACTSAS ACTUAL ACURAS ECOLAB ECOLAW ICEBAG ICECAP ICEDAM ICEMAN KCSTAR MCBEAL MCCRAE MCEWAN MCGRAW MCKEAN MCLEAN OCEDAR OCICAT OCULAR SCALAR SCARAB SCENAS SCHAAP SCHWAB SCHWAS SCREAK SCREAM SCUBAS

•C•••A

ACACIA ACADIA ACEDIA ACTIVA DCAREA ECZEMA ICARIA ICETEA MCCREA RCCOLA SCALIA SCHEMA SCLERA SCOOBA SCORIA SCOTIA SCYLLA

••CA••

ALCAPP ARCADE ARCANA ARCANE ARCARO ASCALE BACALL BECALM BECAME BICARB BSCALE CACAOS CDCASE CICADA

CSCALE
CYCADS
DACAPO
DECADE
DECADS
DECAFS
DECALS
DECAMP
DECANT
DECAPS
DECARE
DECAYS
DSCALE
DUCATS
ENCAGE
ENCAMP
ENCASE
ESCALE
ESCAPE
ESCARP
ESCAUT
FACADE
FSCALE
GOCART
GSCALE
HECATE
IDCARD
INCAIC
INCANS
INCANT
INCAPS
INCASE
INCASH
JACALS
JICAMA
LACAGE
LACASA
LACAVA
LECAIN
LOCALE
LOCALS
LOCANE
LOCATE
MACACO
MACAPA
MACAWS
MCCABE
MCCAIN
MCCANN
NICADS
OCCAMS
ONCALL
OSCANS
OSCARS
OXCART
PECANS
PICABO
PICARA
PICARD
PICARO
RECAGE
RECALL
RECANE
RECANS
RECANT
RECAPS
RECASE
RECAST
RICANS
SECADA
SECANT
SOCANI
TECATE
TICALS
TUCANA
UNCAGE
UNCAKE
UNCALM
UNCAPS
UNCASE
UNCASK
UNCAST
UPCARD
UPCAST
VACANT
VACATE
VICARS
VOCABS
VOCALS
WECARE
ZOCALO

••C•A•

ARCTAN
BUCCAL
BUCHAN
COCOAS
DACHAS
DECLAW
DRCLAW
DUCTAL
FACIAE
FACIAL
FACIAS
HICKAM
JACKAL
LUCIAN
LYCRAS
MACRAE
MCCRAE
MECCAN
MECCAS
MICMAC
MOCHAS
MUCHAS
NACHAS
NECTAR
NICIAS
NUCHAE
NUCHAL
PACMAN
PECKAT
PICKAT
PICKAX
RACIAL
RECLAD
RECOAL
RECOAT
RICRAC
RICTAL
ROCHAT
SOCIAL
SUCHAS
TICTAC
UNCIAL
UNCLAD
UNCLAY
VACLAV
WICCAN
YUCCAS

••C••A

ALCINA
ARCANA
BOCHSA
CICADA
ENCINA
EXCUSA
FACULA
HECUBA
ISCHIA
JICAMA
LACASA
LACAVA
LACTEA
LACUNA
LUCIDA
MACAPA
MACULA
MCCREA
NICOLA
PACULA
PICARA
RCCOLA
RICOLA
SECADA
TACOMA
TUCANA
UNCOLA
VECTRA
VICUNA

•••CA•

ABACAB
ABACAS
ABSCAM
AMICAL
APICAL
ARECAS
ARTCAR
ASHCAN
BARCAR
BIGCAR
BIGCAT
BISCAY
BOBCAT
BOXCAR
BROCAS
BUCCAL
CANCAN
CAWCAW
CHICAS
COPCAR
CTSCAN
CUICAS
DORCAS
DUNCAN
EPICAL
ERICAS
FATCAT
FINCAS
FISCAL
FRACAS
GASCAN
GASCAP
GELCAP
HEPCAT
HOTCAP
HOTCAR
HUBCAP
ICECAP
IFICAN
IPECAC
JAMCAM
LAICAL
LAPCAT
LASCAR
LEICAS
LOWCAL
MADCAP
MECCAN
MECCAS
MESCAL
MIDCAP
MUDCAT
MUSCAT
NASCAR
NEWCAR
OCICAT
OILCAN
OLDCAR
ONECAR
PARCAE
PASCAL
PETCAT
PINCAY
PONCAS
RASCAL
REDCAP
RESCAN
REXCAT
SEACAT
SKICAP
SKYCAM
SKYCAP
SNOCAT
SPYCAM
THECAN
THECAR
TINCAN
TOECAP
TOMCAT
TOPCAT
TOUCAN
TOWCAR
TOYCAR
TUSCAN
TWOCAR
UNOCAL
UTICAN
VULCAN
WEBCAM
WICCAN
YUCCAS

•••C•A

ACACIA
ALICIA
BETCHA
CANCHA
CHACHA
CHICHA
CONCHA
EJECTA
EXACTA
FASCIA
FLICKA
FRICKA
FULCRA
GARCIA
GOTCHA
JASCHA
KWACHA
LANCIA
MANCHA
MARCIA
MISCHA
MURCIA
PASCUA
PERCHA
SANCTA
THECIA
TRICIA

••••CA

AFRICA
ALPACA
ARNICA
ATTICA
AZTECA
BIANCA
BINACA
BLANCA
BRANCA
CELICA
DESICA
DODECA
EROICA
FRANCA
FRESCA
ITASCA
ITHACA
JAMOCA
KONICA
MARACA
MEDICA
MONICA
NAPACA
OAXACA
OJAICA
PATACA
SENECA
SILICA
SIRICA
VIVECA
VIVICA
WASECA

C•B•••

CABALA
CABALS
CABANA
CABBED
CABBIE
CABELL
CABERS
CABEZA
CABINS
CABLED
CABLER
CABLES
CABLET
CABMAN
CABMEN
CABRAL
CABRIO
CIBBER
CIBOLA
COBAIN
COBALT
COBBLE
COBHAM
COBNUT
COBRAS
COBURG
COBURN
COBWEB
CUBAGE
CUBANS
CUBBED
CUBEBS
CUBERS
CUBFAN
CUBICS
CUBING
CUBISM
CUBIST
CUBITI
CUBITS
CUBOID
CYBILL
CYBORG

C••B••

CABBED
CABBIE
CAMBER
CAMBOY
CARBON
CARBOS
CARBOY
CARBRA
CASBAH
CATBED
CEIBAS
CHUBBY
CIBBER
CLUBBY
CLUBUP
COBBLE
COLBYS
COMBAT
COMBED
COMBER
COMBOS
CORBEL
CORBIN
COWBOY
CRABBE
CRABBY
CUBBED
CUEBID
CUMBER
CUMBIA
CURBED
CYMBAL

C•••B•

CAMEBY
CANTBE
CARIBE
CARIBS
CAROBS
CASABA
CELEBS
CEREBR
CHUBBY
CLIMBS
CLUBBY
COHABS
COMEBY
CRABBE
CRABBY
CRAMBO
CROSBY
CRUMBS
CRUMBY
CUBEBS

C••••B

CANTAB
CECILB
CHERUB
COBWEB
CONFAB
CONJOB

•CB•••

MCBAIN
MCBEAL

•C•B••

ICEBAG
ICEBOX
SCUBAS

•C••B•

ACHEBE
MCCABE
MCJOBS
MCNABB
MCRIBS
PCLABS
SCOOBA
SCOOBY
SCRIBE
SCRUBS

•C•••B

ECOLAB
MCNABB
RCRUMB
SCARAB
SCHEIB
SCHLUB
SCHWAB

••CB••

DOCBOY

••C•B•

EXCUBS
HECUBA
INCUBI
JACOBI
JACOBY
MCCABE
PICABO
RACEBY
TICKBY
TYCOBB
VOCABS

••C••B

BICARB
CECILB
MACOMB
RECOMB
TYCOBB
UNCURB

•••C•B

ABACAB
ALICEB

CC••••

CCLAMP
CCLEFS

C•C•••

CACAOS
CACHED
CACHES
CACHET
CACKLE
CACTUS
CDCASE
CECILB
CECILE
CICADA
CICELY
CICERO
COCCUS
COCCYX
COCKED
COCKER
COCKLE
COCOAS
COCOON
CSCALE
CUCKOO
CYCADS
CYCLED
CYCLER
CYCLES
CYCLIC
CYCLOS

C••C••

CAICOS
CANCAN
CANCEL
CANCER
CANCHA
CANCUN
CATCHY
CAUCHY
CAUCUS
CAWCAW
CHACEL
CHACHA
CHACHI
CHACUN
CHECKS
CHICAS
CHICER
CHICHA
CHICHI
CHICKS
CHICLE
CHICLY
CHICOS
CHOCKS
CHUCKS
CHUCKY
CIRCLE
CIRCUM
CIRCUS
CISCOS
CLACKS
CLICHE
CLICHY
CLICKS
CLOCHE
CLOCKS
CLUCKS
COACTS
COCCUS
COCCYX
CONCHA
CONCHO
CONCHS
CONCUR
COPCAR
CRACKD
CRACKS
CRACOW
CRECHE
CRICKS
CROCKS
CROCUS
CRUCES
CTSCAN
CUICAS
CZECHS

C•••C•

CALICO
CANUCK
CDRACK
CELICA
CHANCE
CHANCY
CHEECH
CHINCH
CHOICE
CHURCH
CIVICS
CLANCY
CLENCH
CLINCH
CLUTCH
COERCE
COLECO
COLICS
COMICE
COMICS
CONICS
CONOCO
CORACI
COSECS
COSTCO
CRISCO
CROTCH
CROUCH
CRUNCH
CRUTCH
CUBICS
CULTCH
CURACY
CUSACK
CUSECS
CYNICS

C••••C

CADMIC
CARNAC
CEDRIC
CELTIC
CHEMIC
CHIRAC
CHORIC
CITRIC
CLERIC
CLINIC
COGNAC
CONTAC
COPTIC
COSMIC
COURIC
CRITIC
CULTIC
CUPRIC
CYANIC
CYCLIC
CYMRIC
CYSTIC

•CC•••

ACCEDE
ACCENT
ACCEPT
ACCESS
ACCORD
ACCOST
ACCRUE
ACCTNO
ACCUSE
BCCING
ECCLES
MCCABE
MCCAIN
MCCANN
MCCORD
MCCRAE
MCCREA
OCCAMS
OCCULT
OCCUPY
OCCURS
RCCOLA

•C•C••

ACACIA
ICECAP
ICICLE
OCICAT

•C••C•

ACKACK
MCDUCK
OCLOCK
SCARCE
SCHICK
SCONCE
SCORCH
SCOTCH

•C•••C

ACETIC
ACIDIC
ECESIC
ECHOIC
ICONIC
SCENIC

••CC••

ARCCOS
BOCCES
BOCCIE
BOCCIS
BUCCAL
COCCUS
COCCYX
HICCUP
LOCCIT
MECCAN
MECCAS
PICCHU
PUCCIS
SICCED
SOCCER
SUCCOR
TICCED
WICCAN
YUCCAS

••C•C•

BOCHCO
DECOCT
ENCYCL
MACACO
RECOCK
ROCOCO

••C••C

ARCSEC
ARCTIC
CYCLIC
ETCETC
HECTIC
INCAIC
LACTIC
MICMAC
PICNIC
PICRIC
RICRAC
TACTIC
TICTAC
UNCHIC

•••CC•

BRACCO
GRUCCI
STUCCO

•••C•C

IPECAC
ZINCIC

CD••••

CDCASE
CDEFGH
CDRACK
CDRATE
CDROMS

C•D•••

CADDIE
CADEAU
CADENT
CADETS
CADGED
CADGER
CADGES
CADMIC
CADMUS
CADRES
CEDARN
CEDARS
CEDARY
CEDERS
CEDING
CEDRIC
CIDERS
CIDERY
CODDLE
CODERS
CODGER
CODIFY
CODING
CODONS
CODYWY
CUDAHY
CUDDLE
CUDDLY
CUDGEL
CYDERS

C••D••

CADDIE
CALDER
CAMDEN
CANDIA
CANDID
CANDLE
CANDOR
CARDED
CARDER
CARDIA
CARDIN
CARDIO
CATDOM
CAUDAD
CAUDAL
CAWDOR
CHEDER
CHIDED
CHIDER
CHIDES
CINDER
CIUDAD
CLADIN
CLODDY
CLYDES
CODDLE
COEDIT
COLDER
COLDLY
COMDEN
COMDEX
COMDRS
CONDOR
CONDOS
COODER
CORDAY
CORDED
CORDER
CORDIA
CORDON
COYDOG
CRADLE
CREDIT
CREDOS
CRUDDY
CRUDER
CRUDES
CRUDUP
CUDDLE
CUDDLY
CUEDIN
CURDED
CURDLE

C•••D•

CANADA
CANIDS
CEPEDA
CHANDU
CHARDS
CHILDE
CHORDS
CIARDI
CICADA
CLAUDE
CLODDY
CLOUDS
CLOUDY
COLADA
COMEDY
COMIDA
COULDA
COULDI
CREEDS
CROWDS
CRUDDY
CUANDO
CUPIDS
CURADS
CYCADS

C••••D

CABBED
CABLED
CACHED
CADGED
CALKED
CALLED
CALMED
CALVED
CAMPED
CANARD
CANDID
CANNED
CANOED
CANTED
CAPPED
CAPRID
CARDED
CARPED
CARTED
CARVED
CASHED
CASKED
CASTED
CATBED
CAUDAD
CAUSED
CEASED
CEILED
CELLED
CENSED
CERVID
CESSED
CHAFED
CHASED
CHAWED
CHEFED
CHEWED
CHIDED
CHIMED
CHOKED
CHOWED
CHUTED
CITIED
CIUDAD
CLAWED
CLEWED
CLONED
CLOSED
CLOYED
COALED
COATED
COAXED
COCKED
COGGED
COIFED
COILED
COINED
COMBED
COMPED
CONFED
CONKED
CONNED
CONOID
CONRAD
COOEED
COOKED
COOLED
COOPED
COPIED
COPPED
CORDED
CORKED
CORNED
CORVID
COSHED
COSIED
COSTED
COWARD
COWLED
COZIED
CRACKD
CRANED
CRAPED
CRATED
CRAVED
CRAZED
CREPED
CREWED
CROWED
CUBBED
CUBOID
CUEBID
CUFFED
CULLED
CUNARD
CUPPED
CURBED
CURDED
CURLED
CURRED
CURSED
CURVED
CUSPED
CUSPID
CUSSED
CYANID
CYCLED

•CD•••

BCDEFG
MCDUCK

•C•D••

ACADIA
ACEDIA
ACEDIT
ACIDIC
ACIDLY
ICEDAM
ICEDIN
ICEDIT
ICEDUP
MCADOO
OCEDAR

•C••D•

ACCEDE
ECARDS
OCTADS
SCALDS
SCOLDS
SCRODS

•C•••D

ACARID
ACCORD
ECHOED
ECKERD
ICOULD
MCCORD
OCHRED
SCALED
SCARED
SCOPED
SCORED
SCREED

••CD••
ABCDEF

••C•D•
ACCEDE
ARCADE
CICADA
CYCADS
DECADE
DECADS
DECIDE
DECODE
ENCODE
ESCUDO
EXCIDE
FACADE
INCODE
LUCIDA
NICADS
RECEDE
RECODE
SECADA
SECEDE

••C••D
ACCORD
ARCHED
ASCEND
ASCOLD
BACHED
BACKED
BUCKED
CACHED
COCKED
CYCLED
DECKED
DOCKED
DUCKED
DUCTED
EMCEED
ETCHED
EUCLID
EXCEED
FECUND
GOCOED
GOCOLD
HACKED
HOCKED
IDCARD
IMCOLD
INCHED
ITCHED
JACKED
JOCUND
KICKED
LACKED
LICKED
LOCKED
LUCKED
MCCORD
MOCKED
MUCKED
NACRED
NBCRED
NECKED
NICHED
NICKED
NOCKED
OHCRUD
ORCHID
PACKED
PECKED
PICARD
PICKED
RACKED
RECKED
RECLAD
RECORD
RECUED
ROCKED
RUCKED
SACKED
SACRED
SECOND
SICCED
SOCKED
SUCKED
TACKED
TICCED
TICKED
TUCKED
UNCLAD
UPCARD
WICKED

•••C•D
BRACED
CRACKD
DANCED
DEICED
DEUCED
EDUCED
FARCED
FENCED
FORCED
GRACED
JUICED
LANCED
MERCED
MINCED
PEPCID
PIECED
PLACED
PLACID
PRICED
RANCID
REDCOD
REICED
SAUCED
SICCED
SLICED
SPACED
SPICED
SYNCED
TALCED
THECID
TICCED
TRACED
UNICED
VISCID
VOICED
WINCED
ZINCED

••••CD
USEDCD

CE••••
CEASED
CEASES
CECILB
CECILE
CEDARN
CEDARS
CEDARY
CEDERS
CEDING
CEDRIC
CEIBAS
CEILED
CELEBS
CELERY
CELICA
CELINE
CELLAE
CELLAR
CELLED
CELLOS
CELTIC
CEMENT
CENSED
CENSER
CENSES
CENSOR
CENSUS
CENTAI
CENTAL
CENTAS
CENTER
CENTOS
CENTRE
CENTRI
CENTRO
CENTUM
CEORLS
CEPEDA
CEPHAL
CERATE
CERATO
CEREAL
CEREBR
CEREUS
CERISE
CERIUM
CERNAN
CERROS
CERTIF
CERVID
CESARE
CESARS
CESIUM
CESSED
CESSES
CESSNA
CESTAS
CESTUS
CETANE
CETERA
CEYLON

C•E•••
CAESAR
CDEFGH
CHEAPO
CHEATS
CHECKS
CHEDER
CHEECH
CHEEKS
CHEEKY
CHEEPS
CHEERS
CHEERY
CHEESE
CHEESY
CHEETA
CHEFED
CHEKOV
CHELAE
CHEMIC
CHEMIN
CHENEY
CHENIN
CHEOPS
CHEQUE
CHERIE
CHERRY
CHERTS
CHERTY
CHERUB
CHERYL
CHESTS
CHESTY
CHEVAL
CHEVET
CHEVON
CHEVRE
CHEVYS
CHEWED
CHEWER
CHEWON
CHEWUP
CIELOS
CIERAS
CLEANS
CLEARS
CLEARY
CLEATS
CLEAVE
CLEEKS
CLEESE
CLEFTS
CLENCH
CLERGY
CLERIC
CLERKS
CLEVER
CLEVES
CLEWED
COEDIT
COELIA
COERCE
COEURS
COEVAL
CREAKS
CREAKY
CREAMS
CREAMY
CREASE
CREASY
CREATE
CRECHE
CREDIT
CREDOS
CREEDS
CREEKS
CREELS
CREEPO
CREEPS
CREEPY
CREMER
CREMES
CRENEL
CRENNA
CREOLE
CREPED
CREPES
CRESOL
CRESSY
CRESTS
CRETAN
CRETIN
CREUSA
CREUSE
CREWED
CREWEL
CUEBID
CUEDIN
CUEING
CUESIN
CUESTA
CUESUP
CUETIP
CZECHS
CZERNY

C••E••
CABELL
CABERS
CABEZA
CADEAU
CADENT
CADETS
CAGEIN
CAGERS
CAGEUP
CAKEUP
CAMEAS
CAMEAT
CAMEBY
CAMEIN
CAMELS
CAMEON
CAMEOS
CAMERA
CAMETO
CAMEUP
CANERS
CAPERS
CAREEN
CAREER
CAREOF
CARERS
CARESS
CARETO
CARETS
CASEFY
CASEIN
CASERN
CASERS
CATENA
CATERA
CATERS
CAVEAT
CAVEIN
CAVELL
CAVERN
CAVERS
CAVETT
CCLEFS
CEDERS
CELEBS
CELERY
CEMENT
CEPEDA
CEREAL
CEREBR
CEREUS
CETERA
CHEECH
CHEEKS
CHEEKY
CHEEPS
CHEERS
CHEERY
CHEESE
CHEESY
CHEETA
CHIEFS
CHIENS
CICELY
CICERO
CIDERS
CIDERY
CINEMA
CINEOL
CITEES
CITERS
CIVETS
CLEEKS
CLEESE
CLIENT
CLOETE
CLUEIN
CLUERS
CODERS
COGENT
COHEIR
COHERE
COLECO
COLEUS
COMEAS
COMEAT
COMEBY
COMEDY
COMEIN
COMELY
COMEOF
COMEON
COMERS
COMETH
COMETO
COMETS
COMEUP
CONERS
CONEYS
COOEED
COOEES
COOERS
COPERS
CORERS
COSECS
COSELL
COSETS
COVENS
COVENT
COVERS
COVERT
COVETS
COVEYS
COWENS
COWERS
COYEST
COZENS
CREEDS
CREEKS
CREELS
CREEPO
CREEPS
CREEPY
CRIERS
CRUETS
CRYERS
CUBEBS
CUBERS
CULETS
CUNEAL
CUPELS
CURERS
CURETS
CUSECS
CUTELY
CUTEST
CUTESY
CUTEYS
CUVEES
CYDERS

C•••E•
CABBED
CABLED
CABLER
CABLES
CABLET
CABMEN
CACHED
CACHES
CACHET
CADGED
CADGER
CADGES
CADRES
CAGIER
CAGNEY
CAHIER
CAKIER
CALDER
CALKED
CALKER
CALLED
CALLEE
CALLER
CALLES
CALMED
CALMER
CALMEX
CALVED
CALVES
CALVET
CALXES
CAMBER
CAMDEN
CAMOES
CAMPED
CAMPER
CANCEL
CANCER
CANIER
CANKER
CANNED
CANNEL
CANNER
CANNES
CANOED
CANOER
CANOES
CANTED
CANTER
CAPLET
CAPPED
CAPPER
CARDED
CARDER
CAREEN
CAREER
CARIES
CARKEY
CARMEL
CARMEN
CARNER
CARNES
CARNET
CARNEY
CARPED
CARPEL
CARPER
CARPET
CARREL
CARREY
CARSEY
CARTED
CARTEL
CARTER
CARTES
CARVED
CARVEL
CARVER
CARVES
CARVEY
CASHED
CASHES
CASHEW
CASKED
CASKET
CASPER
CASTED
CASTEL
CASTER
CASTES
CATBED
CATHER
CATMEN
CAUSED
CAUSER
CAUSES
CAVIES
CEASED
CEASES
CEILED
CELLED
CENSED
CENSER
CENSES
CENTER
CESSED
CESSES
CHACEL
CHAFED
CHAFER
CHAFES
CHALET
CHANEL
CHANEY
CHAPEL
CHASED
CHASER
CHASES
CHAVEZ
CHAWED
CHEDER
CHEFED
CHENEY
CHEVET
CHEWED
CHEWER
CHICER
CHIDED
CHIDER
CHIDES
CHILES
CHIMED
CHIMER
CHIMES
CHINES
CHISEL
CHIVES
CHOKED
CHOKER
CHOKES
CHOLER
CHOREO
CHORES
CHOSEN
CHOWED
CHUTED
CHUTES
CIBBER
CINDER
CIPHER
CISKEI
CITEES
CITIED
CITIES
CLARET
CLAVES
CLAWED
CLAWER
CLAYEY
CLEVER
CLEVES
CLEWED
CLIMES
CLONED
CLONER
CLONES
CLOSED
CLOSER
CLOSES
CLOSET
CLOVEN
CLOVER
CLOVES
CLOYED
CLYDES
CNOTES
COALED
COALER
COATED
COATEE
COATER
COATES
COAXED
COAXER
COAXES
COBWEB
COCKED
COCKER
CODGER
COFFEE
COFFER
COGGED
COHOES
COIFED
COILED
COILER
COINED
COINER
COKIER
COKIES
COLDER
COLLET
COLTER
COMBED
COMBER
COMDEN
COMDEX
COMPED
COMPEL
COMTES
CONFED
CONFER
CONGER
CONGES
CONIES
CONKED
CONKER
CONMEN
CONNED
CONNEE
CONVEX
CONVEY
COODER
COOEED
COOEES
COOKED
COOKER
COOLED
COOLER
COOLEY
COONEY
COOPED
COOPER
COOTER
COPIED
COPIER
COPIES
COPLEY
COPPED
COPPER
COPSES
COPTER
CORBEL
CORDED
CORDER
CORKED
CORKER
CORNEA
CORNED
CORNEL
CORNER
CORNET
CORREO
CORSET
CORTES
CORTEX
CORTEZ
CORVEE
COSHED
COSHER
COSHES
COSIED
COSIER
COSIES
COSSET
COSTED
COTLER
COTTEN
COTTER
COULEE
COUPES
COUTER
COWIER
COWLED
COWLEY
COWMEN
COWPEA
COWPER
COZIED
COZIER
COZIES
CRAKES
CRAMER
CRANED
CRANES
CRAPED
CRAPES
CRATED
CRATER
CRATES
CRAVED
CRAVEN
CRAVER
CRAVES
CRAZED
CRAZES
CREMER
CREMES
CRENEL
CREPED
CREPES
CREWED
CREWEL
CRIKEY
CRIMEA
CRIMES
CRIPES
CRISES
CRONES
CRORES
CROWED
CROWER
CRUCES
CRUDER
CRUDES
CRUSES
CRUXES
CTILES
CUBBED
CUDGEL
CUFFED
CULLED
CULLEN
CULLER
CULLET
CUMBER
CUORES
CUPPED
CURBED
CURDED
CURFEW
CURIES
CURLED
CURLER
CURLEW
CURLEY
CURRED
CURSED
CURSER
CURSES
CURTER
CURVED
CURVES
CURVET
CUSPED
CUSSED
CUSSER
CUSSES
CUSTER
CUTIES
CUTLER
CUTLET
CUTTER
CUVEES
CUVIER
CUYLER
CYCLED
CYCLER
CYCLES
CYGNET
CYPHER

C••••E
CABBIE
CACKLE
CADDIE
CAJOLE
CALLEE
CALLME
CAMISE
CAMMIE
CANAPE
CANDLE
CANINE
CANTBE
CANTLE
CANUTE
CAPONE
CAPOTE
CARAFE
CARIBE
CAROLE
CARRIE
CASQUE
CASSIE
CASTLE
CATTLE
CAYUSE
CAZALE
CDCASE
CDRATE
CECILE
CELINE
CELLAE
CENTRE
CERATE
CERISE
CESARE
CETANE
CHAINE
CHAISE
CHANCE
CHANGE
CHANTE
CHARGE
CHASSE
CHASTE
CHEESE
CHELAE
CHEQUE
CHERIE
CHEVRE
CHICLE
CHIGOE
CHILDE
CHOATE
CHOICE
CHOOSE
CHROME
CIGGIE
CINQUE
CIRCLE
CIRQUE
CLAIRE
CLAQUE
CLARKE
CLASSE
CLAUDE
CLAUSE
CLEAVE
CLEESE
CLICHE
CLIQUE
CLOCHE
CLOETE
CLOTHE
COARSE
COATEE
COBBLE
COCKLE
CODDLE
COERCE
COFFEE
COGGLE
COHERE
COIGNE
COLLIE
COMATE
COMICE
CONNEE
CONNIE
CONTRE
CONURE
COOKIE
COOLIE
COOTIE
CORPSE
CORVEE
COSINE
COSTAE
COTTAE
COULEE
COUPLE
COURSE
COWRIE
COYOTE
CRABBE
CRADLE
CREASE
CREATE
CRECHE
CREOLE
CREUSE
CRINGE
CROIRE
CROSSE
CROUSE
CROUTE
CROWNE
CRUISE
CRUSOE
CSCALE
CUBAGE
CUDDLE
CUPULE
CURARE
CURATE
CURDLE
CURIAE
CURITE

•CE•••
ACEDIA
ACEDIT
ACELAS
ACEOUT
ACESIT
ACESUP
ACETAL
ACETIC
ACETYL
BCELLS
DCELLS
ECESIC
ECESIS
ICEAGE
ICEAXE
ICEBAG
ICEBOX
ICECAP
ICEDAM
ICEDIN
ICEDIT
ICEDUP
ICEFOG
ICEMAN
ICEMEN
ICEOUT
ICEPOP
ICERUN
ICESIN
ICESIT
ICESUP
ICETEA
ICEUPS
MCEWAN
MCEWEN
OCEANS
OCEDAR
OCELLI
OCELOT
SCENAS
SCENEI
SCENES
SCENEV
SCENIC
SCENTS
TCELLS

•C•E••
ACCEDE
ACCENT
ACCEPT
ACCESS
ACHEBE
ACHENE
ACHERS
BCDEFG
CCLEFS
ECKERD
ECZEMA
GCLEFS
ICIEST
MCBEAL
MCKEAN
MCKEON
MCKERN
MCLEAN
MCNEIL
OCHERS
OCHERY
OCTETS
SCHEIB
SCHELL
SCHEMA
SCHEME
SCLERA
SCREAK
SCREAM
SCREED
SCREEN
SCREES

SCREWS
SCREWY
YCLEPT

•C••E•
ACHIER
ACUMEN
ACUTER
ACUTES
DCAREA
ECCLES
ECHOED
ECHOER
ECHOES
ECOLES
ICEMEN
ICETEA
ICKIER
MCAFEE
MCCREA
MCEWEN
MCGREW
MCKUEN
MCPHEE
OCASEK
OCASEY
OCHRED
OCHRES
OCONEE
PCUSER
SCALED
SCALER
SCALES
SCARED
SCARER
SCARES
SCENEI
SCENES
SCENEV
SCHLEP
SCONES
SCOPED
SCOPES
SCORED
SCORER
SCORES
SCOTER
SCREED
SCREEN
SCREES

•C•••E
ACCEDE
ACCRUE
ACCUSE
ACHEBE
ACHENE
ACTIVE
ACTONE
ACUATE
ECARTE
ECORSE
ECTYPE
ICEAGE
ICEAXE
ICICLE
MCAFEE
MCCABE
MCCRAE
MCHALE
MCPHEE
OCONEE
OCTANE
OCTAVE
SCARCE
SCARNE
SCATHE
SCHEME
SCONCE
SCOUPE
SCRAPE
SCRIBE
SCURVE
SCYTHE

••CE••
AACELL
ACCEDE
ACCENT
ACCEPT
ACCESS
ASCEND
ASCENT
BICEPS
CICELY
CICERO
DECEIT
DECENT
DICERS
DOCENT
EMCEED
EMCEES
EOCENE
ESCENT
ETCETC
EXCEED
EXCELS
EXCEPT
EXCESS
FACEIT
FACEON
FACERS
FACETS
FACEUP
HACEKS
INCENT
INCEPT
LACEON
LACERS
LACEUP
LUCENT
LYCEES
LYCEUM
MACERS
NICELY
NICENE
NICEST
NICETY
NOCENT
PACERS
RACEBY
RACEIN
RACEME
RACERS
RACETO
RACEUP
RECEDE
RECENT
RECESS
RICERS
SECEDE
ULCERS

••C•E•
AACHEN
ABCDEF
ANCIEN
ARCHED
ARCHER
ARCHES
ARCSEC
BACHED
BACHES
BACKED
BACKER
BECHET
BECKER
BECKET
BICKER
BOCCES
BUCKED
BUCKER
BUCKET
CACHED
CACHES
CACHET
COCKED
COCKER
CYCLED
CYCLER
CYCLES
DECKED
DECKER
DECREE
DICIER
DICKER
DICKEY
DOCKED
DOCKER
DOCKET
DUCKED
DUCKER
DUCTED
ECCLES
EMCEED
EMCEES
ENCRES
ESCHER
ESCHEW
ETCHED
ETCHER
ETCHES
EUCKEN
EXCEED
FACIES
FICHES
GOCOED
HACKED
HACKER
HICKEY
HOCKED
HOCKER
HOCKEY
INCHED
INCHER
INCHES
ITCHED
ITCHES
JACKED
JACKET
JOCKEY
KICKED
KICKER
KOCHEL
KOCHER
KUCHEN
LACHEY
LACIER
LACKED
LACKEY
LACTEA
LECHER
LECTER
LICHEE
LICHEN
LICKED
LICKER
LOCHER
LOCKED
LOCKER
LOCKET
LUCIEN
LUCKED
LYCEES
MACLEN
MACLES
MACNEE
MCCREA
MICHEL
MICKEY
MOCKED
MOCKER
MUCKED
MUCKER
NACRED
NACRES
NBCRED
NECKED
NECKER
NICHED
NICHES
NICKED
NICKEL
NICKER
NOCHES
NOCKED
NUCLEI
NUCLEO
ONCLES
OUCHES
PACIER
PACKED
PACKER
PACKET
PACTEN
PECHES
PECKED
PICHEL
PICKED
PICKER
PICKET
POCKET
PUCKER
RACHEL
RACIER
RACKED
RACKER
RACKET
RECHEW
RECKED
RECUED
RECUES
RICHEN
RICHER
RICHES
RICHET
RICKEY
ROCHET
ROCKED
ROCKER
ROCKET
RUCHES
RUCKED
RUCKER
SACHEM
SACHER
SACHET
SACKED
SACKER
SACRED
SECKEL
SECRET
SICCED
SICKEN
SICKER
SOCCER
SOCKED
SOCKET
SOCLES
SUCKED
SUCKER
SUCRES
TACKED
TACKER
TACTEL
TICCED
TICKED
TICKER
TICKET
TUCKED
TUCKER
TVCREW
UECKER
UNCLES
VACHEL
VACHES
WACKER
WICKED
WICKER
WICKET
ZUCKER

••C••E
ACCEDE
ACCRUE
ACCUSE
ALCOVE
ARCADE
ARCANE
ARCHIE
ASCALE
BECAME
BECOME
BOCCIE
BSCALE
BUCKLE
CACKLE
CDCASE
CECILE
COCKLE
CSCALE
DECADE
DECARE
DECIDE
DECILE
DECKLE
DECODE
DECREE
DICKIE
DOCILE
DSCALE
DUCKIE
ENCAGE
ENCASE
ENCODE
ENCORE
EOCENE
ESCALE
ESCAPE
EUCHRE
EXCIDE
EXCISE
EXCITE
EXCUSE
FACADE
FACIAE
FACILE
FICHTE
FICKLE
FOCSLE
FSCALE
GSCALE
HACKIE
HACKLE
HECATE
HECKLE
INCASE
INCISE
INCITE
INCODE
INCOME
INCUSE
JACKIE
JECKLE
JOCOSE
LACAGE
LICHEE
LOCALE
LOCANE
LOCATE
LUCILE
LUCINE
LUCITE
MACKIE
MACNEE
MACRAE
MCCABE
MCCRAE
NICENE
NICOLE
NUCHAE
OOCYTE
OSCINE
OSCULE
PICKLE
PICONE
RACEME
RACINE
RECAGE
RECANE
RECASE
RECEDE
RECIFE
RECIPE
RECITE
RECODE
RECURE
RECUSE
RICHIE
RICKIE
ROCKIE
ROCKNE
SACQUE
SECEDE
SECURE
SICKLE
TACKLE
TECATE
TECHIE
TICKLE
TOCOME
UNCAGE
UNCAKE
UNCASE
UNCORE
UNCUTE
VACATE
WECARE

•••CE•
ALICEB
ALICES
AMICES
APICES
AVOCET
BERCEO
BOCCES
BRACED
BRACER
BRACES
CANCEL
CANCER
CHACEL
CHICER
CRUCES
DANCED
DANCER
DANCES
DARCEL
DEICED
DEICER
DEICES
DEUCED
DEUCES
DUBCEK
DULCET
DUNCES
EDUCED
EDUCES
EXOCET
FARCED
FARCES
FASCES
FAUCET
FENCED
FENCER
FENCES
FORCED
FORCER
FORCES
GLACES
GORCEY
GRACED
GRACES
GROCER
IBICES
JAYCEE
JUICED
JUICER
JUICES
LANCED
LANCER
LANCES
LANCET
MARCEL
MERCED
MERCER
MINCED
MINCER
MINCES
NIECES
NUECES
OUNCES
PARCEL
PIECED
PIECER
PIECES
PINCER
PISCES
PLACED
PLACER
PLACES
PLOCES
PRICED
PRICER
PRICES
PRICEY
REICED
REICES
RONCEY
ROYCES
SAUCED
SAUCER
SAUCES
SICCED
SLICED
SLICER
SLICES
SOCCER
SPACED
SPACEK
SPACER
SPACES
SPACEY
SPICED
SPICER
SPICES
STACEY
SYNCED
TALCED
TERCEL
TERCES
TICCED
TRACED
TRACER
TRACES
TRACEY
TRECES
TRICEP
TRICES
TRUCES
UNICED
UNICEF
UNICES
VOICED
VOICER
VOICES
WENCES
WINCED
WINCER
WINCES
ZINCED

•••C•E
AMECHE
APACHE
BOCCIE
BOUCHE
BUNCHE
CHICLE
CIRCLE
CLICHE
CLOCHE
CRECHE
FESCUE
FIACRE
FLECHE
FORCHE
FRICKE
GAUCHE
GRACIE
ICICLE
JAYCEE
LANCIE
LOUCHE
MANCHE
MARCHE
MARCIE
MISCUE
MUNCIE
MUSCLE
ORACLE
PARCAE
PENCHE
PSYCHE
QUICHE
RASCHE
RESCUE
ROSCOE
RUNCIE
SIECLE
SPECIE
THICKE
TOUCHE
TRACHE
TROCHE

••••CE
ABDUCE
ADDUCE
ADVICE
AGENCE
AIRACE
ALLYCE
ALSACE
AMERCE
APIECE
ATONCE
BENICE
BIERCE
BODICE
BOUNCE
CHANCE
CHOICE
COERCE
COMICE
DEDUCE
DEFACE
DEVICE
DRRICE
DRYICE
EFFACE
ELANCE
ELLICE
ENFACE
ENLACE
ENTICE
EUNICE
EVINCE
FELICE
FIANCE
FIERCE
FLEECE
FRANCE
GFORCE
GLANCE
GREECE
HORACE
IGNACE
INDUCE
JANICE
JOUNCE
LUTECE
MALICE
MENACE
NODICE
NOTICE
NOVICE
NUANCE
OFFICE
ONRICE
PALACE
PEARCE
PEERCE
PEIRCE
PIERCE
PLAICE
POLICE
POUNCE
PRANCE
PRINCE
PUMICE
QUINCE
REDACE
REDUCE
REFACE
RELACE
RYENCE
SCARCE
SCONCE
SEAICE
SEANCE
SEDUCE
SLUICE
SOLACE
SOURCE
SPENCE
SPLICE
SPRUCE
STANCE
TENACE
THENCE
THRACE
THRICE
TIERCE
TRANCE
UNLACE
UNNICE
USANCE
VELOCE
VENICE
VIVACE
WHENCE

CF••••
CFLATS

C•F•••
CAFTAN
COFFEE
COFFER
COFFIN
CUFFED

C••F••
CANFUL
CAPFUL
CARFUL
CATFIT
CDEFGH
CHAFED
CHAFER
CHAFES
CHAFFS
CHAFFY
CHEFED
CHUFFS
CHUFFY
CLEFTS
CLIFFS
CLIFFY
COFFEE
COFFER
COFFIN
COIFED
COLFAX
COMFIT
CONFAB
CONFED
CONFER
CONFIT
CORFAM
CRAFTS
CRAFTY
CROFTS
CRYFOR
CUBFAN
CUFFED
CUPFUL
CURFEW

C•••F•
CALIFS
CANIFF
CARAFE
CASEFY
CAVAFY
CCLEFS
CHAFFS
CHAFFY
CHIEFS
CHUFFS
CHUFFY
CITIFY
CLIFFS
CLIFFY
CODIFY
CRYOFF
CUTOFF

C••••F
CANIFF
CAREOF
CERTIF
COMEOF
CRYOFF
CUTOFF

•C•F••
ACTFOR
ICEFOG
MCAFEE
SCOFFS
SCUFFS

•C••F•
BCDEFG
CCLEFS
GCLEFS
SCARFS
SCLAFF
SCOFFS
SCRUFF
SCUFFS
SCURFY

•C•••F
SCLAFF
SCRUFF

••CF••
SACFLY

••C•F•
DECAFS
PACIFY
RECIFE
UNCUFF

••C••F
ABCDEF
MUCHOF
SICKOF
UNCUFF

•••C•F
UNICEF

C•G•••
CAGEIN
CAGERS
CAGEUP
CAGIER
CAGILY
CAGING
CAGNEY
CAGUAS
CIGARS
CIGGIE
COGENT
COGGED
COGGLE
COGITO
COGNAC
CYGNET
CYGNUS

C••G••
CADGED
CADGER
CADGES
CALGON
CAPGUN
CARGOS
CATGUT
CAUGHT
CHIGOE
CIGGIE
CLOGGY
CLOGUP
CODGER
COGGED
COGGLE
COIGNE
COIGNS
CONGAS
CONGER
CONGES
CONGOU
COOGAN
CORGIS
COUGAR
COUGHS
CRAGGY
CUDGEL

C•••G•
CAYUGA
CDEFGH
CHANGE
CHANGO
CHARGE
CHOUGH
CLANGS
CLERGY
CLINGS
CLINGY
CLOGGY
CLOUGH
COSIGN
CRAGGY
CRAIGT
CRINGE
CUBAGE

C••••G
CAGING
CAKING
CANING
CARING
CASING
CATRIG
CAVING
CAWING
CEDING
CHIANG
CITING
CLUING
COBURG
CODING
COKING
COMING
CONING
COOING
COPING
CORING
COVING
COWING
COXING
COYDOG
CRYING
CUBING
CUEING
CURING
CYBORG

•CG•••
MCGILL
MCGRAW
MCGREW

•C•G••
SCAGGS

•C••G•
ICEAGE
ICINGS
MCHUGH
SCAGGS
SCRAGS

•C•••G
ACHING
ACTING
BCCING
BCDEFG
ICEBAG
ICEFOG
ICHING
MCHARG

••C•G•
ENCAGE
LACAGE
RECAGE
UNCAGE

••C••G
ARCING
BCCING
DICING
FACING
LACING
PACING
RACING
RICING
UNCLOG

CH••••
CHACEL
CHACHA
CHACHI
CHACUN
CHAFED
CHAFER
CHAFES
CHAFFS
CHAFFY
CHAINE
CHAINS
CHAIRS
CHAISE
CHAKRA
CHALET
CHALKS
CHALKY
CHAMMY
CHAMPS
CHANCE
CHANCY
CHANDU
CHANEL
CHANEY
CHANGE
CHANGO
CHANTE
CHANTS
CHANTY
CHAPEL
CHAPIN
CHARDS
CHARGE
CHARLY
CHARMS
CHARON
CHARRO
CHARTA
CHARTS
CHASED
CHASER
CHASES
CHASMS
CHASSE
CHASTE
CHATTY
CHATUP
CHAVEZ
CHAWED
CHAZAN

CHEAPO
CHEATS
CHECKS
CHEDER
CHEECH
CHEEKS
CHEEKY
CHEEPS
CHEERS
CHEERY
CHEESE
CHEESY
CHEETA
CHEFED
CHEKOV
CHELAE
CHEMIC
CHEMIN
CHENEY
CHENIN
CHEOPS
CHEQUE
CHERIE
CHERRY
CHERTS
CHERTY
CHERUB
CHERYL
CHESTS
CHESTY
CHEVAL
CHEVET
CHEVON
CHEVRE
CHEVYS
CHEWED
CHEWER
CHEWON
CHEWUP
CHIANG
CHICAS
CHICER
CHICHA
CHICHI
CHICKS
CHICLE
CHICLY
CHICOS
CHIDED
CHIDER
CHIDES
CHIEFS
CHIENS
CHIGOE
CHILDE
CHILES
CHILIS
CHILLI
CHILLS
CHILLY
CHIMED
CHIMER
CHIMES
CHIMPS
CHINAS
CHINCH
CHINES
CHINKS
CHINKY
CHINOS
CHINTZ
CHINUA
CHINUP
CHIPIN
CHIPUP
CHIRAC
CHIRHO
CHIRON
CHIRPS
CHIRPY
CHIRRS
CHISEL
CHISOX
CHISUM
CHITON
CHITRA
CHITTY
CHIVAS
CHIVES
CHLORO
CHOATE
CHOCKS
CHOICE
CHOIRS
CHOKED
CHOKER
CHOKES
CHOLER
CHOLLA
CHOLOS
CHOMPS
CHOOSE
CHOOSY
CHOPIN
CHOPPY
CHOPRA
CHOPUP
CHORAL
CHORDS
CHOREO
CHORES
CHORIC
CHORIO
CHOROS
CHORUS
CHOSEN
CHOUGH
CHOWED
CHRISM
CHRIST
CHROMA
CHROME
CHROMO
CHROMY
CHRONO
CHUBBY
CHUCKS
CHUCKY
CHUFFS
CHUFFY
CHUHSI
CHUMMY
CHUMPS
CHUNKS
CHUNKY
CHUPPA
CHURCH
CHURLS
CHURNS
CHURRO
CHUTED
CHUTES
CHYNNA
CHYRON

C•H•••

CAHIER
CAHILL
CAHOOT
COHABS
COHEIR
COHERE
COHOES
COHORT
COHOST
CSHARP

C••H••

CACHED
CACHES
CACHET
CARHOP
CASHED
CASHES
CASHEW
CASHIN
CATHAY
CATHER
CATHYS
CEPHAL
CHUHSI
CIPHER
COBHAM
COSHED
COSHER
COSHES
CUSHAW
CYPHER

C•••H•

CANCHA
CATCHY
CAUCHY
CAUGHT
CHACHA
CHACHI
CHICHA
CHICHI
CHIRHO
CLICHE
CLICHY
CLOCHE
CLOTHE
CLOTHO
CLOTHS
CONCHA
CONCHO
CONCHS
COUGHS
CRECHE
CRWTHS
CUDAHY
CZECHS

C••••H

CALASH
CALIPH
CASBAH
CDEFGH
CHEECH
CHINCH
CHOUGH
CHURCH
CLENCH
CLINCH
CLOUGH
CLUTCH
COMETH
COOLTH
COWISH
COYISH
CROTCH
CROUCH
CRUNCH
CRUTCH
CULTCH

•CH•••

ACHEBE
ACHENE
ACHERS
ACHIER
ACHING
ECHOED
ECHOER
ECHOES
ECHOIC
ICHING
ICHIRO
ICHORS
ICHTHY
LCHAIM
MCHALE
MCHARG
MCHUGH
OCHERS
OCHERY
OCHRED
OCHRES
SCHAAP
SCHAVS
SCHEIB
SCHELL
SCHEMA
SCHEME
SCHICK
SCHISM
SCHIST
SCHLEP
SCHLUB
SCHMOS
SCHNOZ
SCHOLL
SCHOOL
SCHORR
SCHULZ
SCHUSS
SCHWAB
SCHWAS
VCHIPS

•C•H••

MCPHEE

•C••H•

ICHTHY
SCATHE
SCYTHE

•C•••H

JCLOTH
MCHUGH
SCORCH
SCOTCH

••CH••

AACHEN
AHCHOO
ANCHOR
ANCHOS
ARCHED
ARCHER
ARCHES
ARCHIE
ARCHLY
ARCHON
BACHED
BACHES
BACHIT
BECHET
BICHON
BOCHCO
BOCHSA
BUCHAN
CACHED
CACHES
CACHET
DACHAS
DUCHIN
ESCHER
ESCHEW
ETCHED
ETCHER
ETCHES
EUCHRE
FICHES
FICHTE
FICHUS
HACHOO
INCHED
INCHER
INCHES
INCHON
ISCHIA
ITCHED
ITCHES
KOCHEL
KOCHER
KUCHEN
LACHEY
LACHOY
LECHER
LICHEE
LICHEN
LOCHER
MACHOS
MICHEL
MOCHAS
MUCHAS
MUCHOF
NACHAS
NACHOS
NICHED
NICHES
NOCHES
NUCHAE
NUCHAL
ORCHID
OUCHES
PACHIN
PECHES
PICHEL
RACHEL
RECHEW
RICHEN
RICHER
RICHES
RICHET
RICHIE
RICHIN
RICHLY
ROCHAT
ROCHET
ROCHON
RUCHES
SACHEM
SACHER
SACHET
SUCHAS
TECHIE
TECHNO
TECHTV
UNCHIC
URCHIN
VACHEL
VACHES
YACHTS

••C•H•

PICCHU
RICOHS

••C••H

INCASH

•••CH•

AMECHE
APACHE
BEACHY
BETCHA
BINCHY
BOTCHY
BOUCHE
BRACHS
BRECHT
BUNCHE
BUNCHY
CANCHA
CATCHY
CAUCHY
CHACHA
CHACHI
CHICHA
CHICHI
CLICHE
CLICHY
CLOCHE
CONCHA
CONCHO
CONCHS
CRECHE
CZECHS
EPOCHS
FLECHE
FORCHE
GAUCHE
GAUCHO
GOTCHA
HONCHO
JASCHA
KIMCHI
KWACHA
LEACHY
LITCHI
LOUCHE
LUNCHY
MANCHA
MANCHE
MANCHU
MARCHE
MISCHA
MUNCHY
NOTCHY
ORACHS
PANCHO
PASCHS
PATCHY
PEACHY
PENCHE
PERCHA
PICCHU
PITCHY
POACHY
PONCHO
POUCHY
PSYCHE
PSYCHO
PSYCHS
PUNCHY
QUICHE
RANCHO
RASCHE
REECHO
SANCHO
SYNCHS
TAICHI
TETCHY
TORCHY
TOUCHE
TOUCHY
TRACHE
TROCHE
WELCHS
WITCHY

••••CH

ALMACH
ANARCH
ASMUCH
ASSUCH
ATTACH
AVOUCH
BARUCH
BAUSCH
BLANCH
BLEACH
BLENCH
BLOTCH
BORSCH
BRANCH
BREACH
BREECH
BROACH
BROOCH
BRUNCH
CHEECH
CHINCH
CHURCH
CLENCH
CLINCH
CLUTCH
CROTCH
CROUCH
CRUNCH
CRUTCH
CULTCH
DETACH
DEUTCH
DRENCH
EDKOCH
ENRICH
EPARCH
EXARCH
FLETCH
FLINCH
FRENCH
FRISCH
GLITCH
GRINCH
GROUCH
HAUNCH
HIRSCH
HITECH
HOOTCH
INARCH
JSBACH
KIRSCH
KITSCH
KLATCH
KVETCH
LAUNCH
LOLICH
LUKICH
MENSCH
MUNICH
ORBACH
PAUNCH
PESACH
POVICH
PREACH
PUTSCH
QUENCH
RAUNCH
SCORCH
SCOTCH
SEARCH
SKETCH
SKITCH
SLOUCH
SMIRCH
SMOOCH
SNATCH
SNITCH
SOMUCH
SPEECH
SPRACH
STANCH
STARCH
STENCH
STITCH
STORCH
SWATCH
SWITCH
THATCH
TRENCH
TWITCH
ULRICH
VOTECH
WRENCH
WRETCH
ZURICH

CI••••

CIARDI
CIASPY
CIBBER
CIBOLA
CICADA
CICELY
CICERO
CIDERS
CIDERY
CIELOS
CIERAS
CIGARS
CIGGIE
CILIUM
CIMINO
CINDER
CINEMA
CINEOL
CINQUE
CIPHER
CIRCLE
CIRCUM
CIRCUS
CIRQUE
CIRRUS
CISCOS
CISKEI
CITEES
CITERS
CITIED
CITIES
CITIFY
CITING
CITIUS
CITRIC
CITRIN
CITRON
CITRUS
CIUDAD
CIVETS
CIVICS
CIXOUS

C•I•••

CAICOS
CAIMAN
CAIRNS
CEIBAS
CEILED
CHIANG
CHICAS
CHICER
CHICHA
CHICHI
CHICKS
CHICLE
CHICLY
CHICOS
CHIDED
CHIDER
CHIDES
CHIEFS
CHIENS
CHIGOE
CHILDE
CHILES
CHILIS
CHILLI
CHILLS
CHILLY
CHIMED
CHIMER
CHIMES
CHIMPS
CHINAS
CHINCH
CHINES
CHINKS
CHINKY
CHINOS
CHINTZ
CHINUA
CHINUP
CHIPIN
CHIPUP
CHIRAC
CHIRHO
CHIRON
CHIRPS
CHIRPY
CHIRRS
CHISEL
CHISOX
CHISUM
CHITON
CHITRA
CHITTY
CHIVAS
CHIVES
CLICHE
CLICHY
CLICKS
CLIENT
CLIFFS
CLIFFY
CLIMAT
CLIMAX
CLIMBS
CLIMES
CLINCH
CLINGS
CLINGY
CLINIC
CLINKS
CLIPON
CLIQUE
CLIQUY
CMINOR
CMINUS
COIFED
COIGNE
COIGNS
COILED
COILER
COILUP
COINED
COINER
COINOP
CRICKS
CRIERS
CRIKEY
CRIMEA
CRIMES
CRIMPS
CRIMPY
CRINGE
CRIPES
CRISCO
CRISES
CRISIS
CRISPS
CRISPY
CRISTO
CRITIC
CTILES
CUICAS

C••I••

CABINS
CAGIER
CAGILY
CAGING
CAHIER
CAHILL
CAKIER
CAKING
CALICO
CALIFS
CALIPH
CAMINO
CAMION
CAMISE
CANIDS
CANIER
CANIFF
CANINE
CANING
CAPITA
CARIBE
CARIBS
CARIES
CARINA
CARING
CARIOU
CASING
CASINO
CASIOS
CASITA
CATION
CAVIAR
CAVIES
CAVILS
CAVING
CAVITY
CAWING
CECILB
CECILE
CEDING
CELICA
CELINE
CERISE
CERIUM
CESIUM
CHAINE
CHAINS
CHAIRS
CHAISE
CHOICE
CHOIRS
CHRISM
CHRIST
CILIUM
CIMINO
CITIED
CITIES
CITIFY
CITING
CITIUS
CIVICS
CLAIMS
CLAIRE
CLAIRS
CLUING
CODIFY
CODING
COGITO
COKIER
COKIES
COKING
COLICS
COLIMA
COMICE
COMICS
COMIDA
COMING
COMITY
CONICS
CONIES
CONING
COOING
COPIED
COPIER
COPIES
COPING
CORING
CORIUM
COSIED
COSIER
COSIES
COSIGN
COSILY
COSINE
COVINA
COVING
COWIER
COWING
COWISH
COXING
COYISH
COZIED
COZIER
COZIES
COZILY
CRAIGT
CRAINS
CROIRE
CRUISE
CRYING
CUBICS
CUBING
CUBISM
CUBIST
CUBITI
CUBITS
CUEING
CUMINS
CUPIDS
CURIAE
CURIES
CURING
CURIOS
CURITE
CURIUM
CUTIES
CUTINS
CUVIER
CYBILL
CYNICS

C•••I•

CABBIE
CABRIO
CADDIE
CADMIC
CAGEIN
CALAIS
CALLIN
CALLIT
CALVIN
CAMEIN
CAMMIE
CANDIA
CANDID
CANLIT
CAPRID
CAPRIS
CARDIA
CARDIN
CARDIO
CARLIN
CARRIE
CARTIN
CASEIN
CASHIN
CASSIA
CASSIE
CASSIM
CASSIN
CASSIO
CASSIS
CATFIT
CATKIN
CATLIN
CATNIP
CATRIG
CATSIT
CAVEIN
CEDRIC
CELTIC
CERTIF
CERVID
CHAPIN
CHEMIC
CHEMIN
CHENIN
CHERIE
CHILIS
CHIPIN
CHOPIN
CHORIC
CHORIO
CIGGIE
CITRIC
CITRIN
CLADIN
CLAVIN
CLERIC
CLINIC
CLORIS
CLOVIS
CLUEIN
COATIS
COBAIN
COEDIT
COELIA
COFFIN
COHEIR
COLLIE
COMEIN
COMFIT
COMMIT
COMMIX
CONAIR
CONFIT
CONNIE
CONOID
COOKIE
COOLIE
COOLIO
COOLIT
COOTIE
COPSIT
COPTIC
COQUIS
CORBIN
CORDIA
CORGIS
CORVID
CORWIN
COSMIC
COURIC
COUSIN
COWRIE
CRAMIN
CRANIA
CRANIO
CREDIT
CRETIN
CRISIS
CRITIC
CRONIN
CUBOID
CUEBID
CUEDIN
CUESIN
CUETIP
CULKIN
CULLIS
CULTIC
CUMBIA
CUPRIC
CURLIN
CURTIN
CURTIS
CURTIZ
CUSPID
CUSTIS
CUTSIN
CUTSIT
CYANIC
CYANID
CYCLIC
CYMRIC
CYSTIC

C••••I

CAPONI
CAROLI
CARONI
CENTAI
CENTRI
CHACHI
CHICHI
CHILLI
CHUHSI
CIARDI
CISKEI
COLONI
CORACI
COULDI
CUBITI
CUMULI

•CI•••

ACIDIC
ACIDLY
ICICLE
ICIEST
ICINGS
OCICAT
SCIONS
SCIPIO

•C•I••

ACHIER
ACHING
ACTIII
ACTING
ACTION
ACTIUM
ACTIVA
ACTIVE
ACUITY
BCCING
BCLION
ICHING
ICHIRO
ICKIER
MCGILL
MCRIBS
SCHICK
SCHISM
SCHIST
SCRIBE
SCRIMP
SCRIMS

SCRIPS
SCRIPT
VCHIPS

•C••I•
ACACIA
ACADIA
ACARID
ACEDIA
ACEDIT
ACESIT
ACETIC
ACIDIC
ACQUIT
ACTIII
ACTSIN
ECESIC
ECESIS
ECHOIC
ECLAIR
ICARIA
ICEDIN
ICEDIT
ICESIN
ICESIT
ICONIC
LCHAIM
MCBAIN
MCCAIN
MCLAIN
MCNAIR
MCNEIL
SCALIA
SCENIC
SCHEIB
SCIPIO
SCORIA
SCOTIA

•C•••I
ACTIII
OCELLI
OCTOPI
OCTROI
SCAASI
SCAMPI
SCENEI

••CI••
AECIUM
ALCINA
ANCIEN
ARCING
BCCING
CECILB
CECILE
DECIDE
DECILE
DECIUS
DICIER
DICING
DOCILE
ENCINA
ENCINO
EXCIDE
EXCISE
EXCITE
FACIAE
FACIAL
FACIAS
FACIES
FACILE
FACING
INCISE
INCITE
LACIER
LACILY
LACING
LUCIAN
LUCIDA
LUCIEN
LUCILE
LUCINE
LUCITE
LUCIUS
NACION
NICIAS
OPCITS
OSCINE
PACIER
PACIFY
PACING
PACINO
RACIAL
RACIER
RACILY
RACINE
RACING
RACINO
RACISM
RACIST
RECIFE
RECIPE
RECITE
RICING
SICILY
SOCIAL
TICINO
UNCIAL

••C•I•
ARCHIE
ARCSIN
ARCTIC
BACHIT
BACKIN
BOCCIE
BOCCIS
CYCLIC
DECEIT
DICKIE
DUCHIN
DUCKIE
EUCLID
FACEIT
HACKIE
HACKIT
HECTIC
INCAIC
ISCHIA
JACKIE
KICKIN
LACTIC
LECAIN
LOCCIT
LOCKIN
MACKIE
MCCAIN
ORCHID
PACHIN
PACKIN
PECTIN
PICNIC
PICRIC
PUCCIS
RACEIN
RECOIL
RECOIN
RICHIE
RICHIN
RICKIE
ROCKIE
ROCKIN
ROCKIT
SOCKIN
SUCKIN
TACTIC
TECHIE
TOCSIN
TUCKIN
UNCHIC
UNCLIP
UNCOIL
UPCOIL
URCHIN
VICTIM

••C••I
INCUBI
JACOBI
NUCLEI
SOCANI

•••CI•
ACACIA
AFLCIO
ALICIA
ANACIN
BOCCIE
BOCCIS
DANCIN
ELICIT
FASCIA
GARCIA
GLACIS
GRACIE
LANCIA
LANCIE
LOCCIT
MARCIA
MARCIE
MARCIL
MARCIX
MUNCIE
MURCIA
NIACIN
NUNCIO
PENCIL
PEPCID
PLACID
PRECIP
PRECIS
PUCCIS
RANCID
RUNCIE
SPECIE
THECIA
THECID
TRACII
TRICIA
URACIL
VINCIT
VISCID
ZINCIC

•••C•I
CHACHI
CHICHI
FRUCTI
GRUCCI
KIMCHI
LITCHI
TAICHI
TRACII

••••CI
BONACI
CORACI
DODICI
GRUCCI
MEDICI
SEDICI
UNDICI

C•J•••
CAJOLE
CAJUNS

C••J••
CMAJOR
CONJOB

•CJ•••
MCJOBS

••C•J•
NICKJR

C•K•••
CAKEUP
CAKIER
CAKING
COKIER
COKIES
COKING

C••K••
CACKLE
CALKED
CALKER
CANKER
CARKEY
CASKED
CASKET
CATKIN
CHAKRA
CHEKOV
CHOKED
CHOKER
CHOKES
CISKEI
COCKED
COCKER
COCKLE
CONKED
CONKER
COOKED
COOKER
COOKIE
COOKUP
CORKED
CORKER
CORKUP
CRAKES
CRIKEY
CUCKOO
CULKIN

C•••K•
CAULKS
CHALKS
CHALKY
CHECKS
CHEEKS
CHEEKY
CHICKS
CHINKS
CHINKY
CHOCKS
CHUCKS
CHUCKY
CHUNKS
CHUNKY
CLACKS
CLANKS
CLANKY
CLARKE
CLEEKS
CLERKS
CLICKS
CLINKS
CLOAKS
CLOCKS
CLONKS
CLUCKS
CLUNKS
CLUNKY
CRACKD
CRACKS
CRANKS
CRANKY
CREAKS
CREAKY
CREEKS
CRICKS
CROAKS
CROAKY
CROCKS
CROOKS
CSONKA

C••••K
CANUCK
CDRACK
CUSACK

•CK•••
ACKACK
ECKART
ECKERD
ICKIER
MCKEAN
MCKEON
MCKERN
MCKUEN

•C•••K
ACKACK
MCDUCK
OCASEK
OCLOCK
SCHICK
SCREAK

••CK••
BACKED
BACKER
BACKIN
BACKUP
BACKUS
BECKER
BECKET
BECKON
BICKER
BUCKED
BUCKER
BUCKET
BUCKLE
BUCKUP
CACKLE
COCKED
COCKER
COCKLE
CUCKOO
DECKED
DECKER
DECKLE
DICKER
DICKEY
DICKIE
DOCKED
DOCKER
DOCKET
DUCKED
DUCKER
DUCKIE
EUCKEN
FICKLE
GECKOS
HACKED
HACKER
HACKIE
HACKIT
HACKLE
HACKLY
HACKUP
HECKLE
HECKNO
HICKAM
HICKEY
HICKOK
HOCKED
HOCKER
HOCKEY
JACKAL
JACKED
JACKET
JACKIE
JACKUP
JECKLE
JOCKEY
JOCKOS
KICKED
KICKER
KICKIN
KICKUP
LACKED
LACKEY
LICKED
LICKER
LICKUP
LOCKED
LOCKER
LOCKET
LOCKIN
LOCKON
LOCKUP
LUCKED
MACKIE
MICKEY
MOCKED
MOCKER
MOCKUP
MUCKED
MUCKER
MUCKUP
NECKED
NECKER
NICKED
NICKEL
NICKER
NICKJR
NOCKED
PACKED
PACKER
PACKET
PACKIN
PACKON
PACKUP
PECKAT
PECKED
PICKAT
PICKAX
PICKED
PICKER
PICKET
PICKLE
PICKON
PICKUP
POCKET
PUCKER
RACKED
RACKER
RACKET
RACKUP
RECKED
RECKON
RICKEY
RICKIE
ROCKED
ROCKER
ROCKET
ROCKIE
ROCKIN
ROCKIT
ROCKNE
ROCKYV
RUCKED
RUCKER
RUCKUP
RUCKUS
SACKED
SACKER
SACKUP
SECKEL
SICKEN
SICKER
SICKLE
SICKLY
SICKOF
SICKOS
SOCKED
SOCKET
SOCKIN
SUCKED
SUCKER
SUCKIN
SUCKUP
TACKED
TACKER
TACKLE
TACKON
TACKUP
TICKBY
TICKED
TICKER
TICKET
TICKLE
TICKLY
TUCKED
TUCKER
TUCKIN
UECKER
WACKER
WACKOS
WICKED
WICKER
WICKET
ZUCKER

••C•K•
HACEKS
UNCAKE

••C••K
HICKOK
MTCOOK
RECOCK
RECOOK
RECORK
UNCASK
UNCORK

•••CK•
ALECKS
ALECKY
BLACKS
BLOCKS
BLOCKY
BRICKS
BRICKY
BUICKS
CHECKS
CHICKS
CHOCKS
CHUCKS
CHUCKY
CLACKS
CLICKS
CLOCKS
CLUCKS
CRACKD
CRACKS
CRICKS
CROCKS
DBACKS
DRECKS
DRECKY
FLACKS
FLECKS
FLECKY
FLICKA
FLICKS
FLOCKS
FRICKA
FRICKE
FROCKS
GLOCKS
KLICKS
KNACKS
KNICKS
KNOCKS
MERCKX
ORECKS
PANCKS
PLUCKS
PLUCKY
PRICKS
QUACKS
QUACKY
SHACKS
SHECKY
SHOCKS
SHUCKS
SLACKS
SLICKS
SMACKS
SMOCKS
SNACKS
SNICKS
SPECKS
STACKS
STICKS
STICKY
STOCKS
STOCKY
THICKE
TRACKS
TRICKS
TRICKY
TRUCKS
VNECKS
WHACKS
WRACKS
WRECKS
YOICKS
ZINCKY

•••C•K
DUBCEK
SPACEK

••••CK
ACKACK
ARRACK
ATTACK
AWHECK
BARACK
BEDECK
CANUCK
CDRACK
CUSACK
FRANCK
GOBACK
HIJACK
IMBACK
INBACK
INHOCK
INLUCK
KOPECK
LUBECK
MALICK
MCDUCK
MRDICK
MUSICK
NATICK
NOLUCK
OCLOCK
ONDECK
PENICK
PLANCK
RECOCK
REDOCK
REKICK
RELOCK
REMICK
REPACK
REPICK
RERACK
RETACK
SCHICK
SHLOCK
SHTICK
STNICK
STRUCK
THWACK
UNDOCK
UNLOCK
UNPACK
UNPICK
UNRACK
UNSICK
UNTACK
UNTUCK
UPTICK
WOMACK
YORICK
ZANUCK

CL••••
CLACKS
CLADIN
CLAIMS
CLAIRE
CLAIRS
CLAMMA
CLAMMY
CLAMOR
CLAMPS
CLAMUP
CLANCY
CLANGS
CLANKS
CLANKY
CLAQUE
CLARET
CLARKE
CLAROS
CLASPS
CLASSA
CLASSE
CLASSY
CLAUDE
CLAUSE
CLAVES
CLAVIN
CLAWAT
CLAWED
CLAWER
CLAYEY
CLEANS
CLEARS
CLEARY
CLEATS
CLEAVE
CLEEKS
CLEESE
CLEFTS
CLENCH
CLERGY
CLERIC
CLERKS
CLEVER
CLEVES
CLEWED
CLICHE
CLICHY
CLICKS
CLIENT
CLIFFS
CLIFFY
CLIMAT
CLIMAX
CLIMBS
CLIMES
CLINCH
CLINGS
CLINGY
CLINIC
CLINKS
CLIPON
CLIQUE
CLIQUY
CLOAKS
CLOCHE
CLOCKS
CLODDY
CLOETE
CLOGGY
CLOGUP
CLOMPS
CLONAL
CLONED
CLONER
CLONES
CLONKS
CLORIS
CLOROX
CLOSED
CLOSER
CLOSES
CLOSET
CLOTHE
CLOTHO
CLOTHS
CLOTTY
CLOTUP
CLOUDS
CLOUDY
CLOUGH
CLOUTS
CLOVEN
CLOVER
CLOVES
CLOVIS
CLOWNS
CLOYED
CLUBBY
CLUBUP
CLUCKS
CLUEIN
CLUERS
CLUING
CLUMPS
CLUMPY
CLUMSY
CLUNKS
CLUNKY
CLUTCH
CLYDES

C•L•••
CALAIS
CALASH
CALDER
CALGON
CALICO
CALIFS
CALIPH
CALKED
CALKER
CALLAN
CALLAO
CALLAS
CALLED
CALLEE
CALLER
CALLES
CALLIN
CALLIT
CALLME
CALLON
CALLOW
CALLTO
CALLUP
CALLUS
CALMED
CALMER
CALMEX
CALMLY
CALORY
CALVED
CALVES
CALVET
CALVIN
CALXES
CCLAMP
CCLEFS
CELEBS
CELERY
CELICA
CELINE
CELLAE
CELLAR
CELLED
CELLOS
CELTIC
CFLATS
CHLORO
CILIUM
COLADA
COLBYS
COLDER
COLDLY
COLECO
COLEUS
COLFAX
COLICS
COLIMA
COLLAR
COLLAT
COLLET
COLLIE
COLLOP
COLLOQ
COLMAN
COLMAR
COLONI
COLONS
COLONY
COLORS
COLOUR
COLSON
COLTER
COLTON
COLUMN
CULETS
CULKIN
CULLED
CULLEN
CULLER
CULLET
CULLIS
CULLUM
CULTCH
CULTIC
CULTUS

C••L••
CABLED
CABLER
CABLES
CABLET
CALLAN
CALLAO
CALLAS
CALLED
CALLEE
CALLER
CALLES
CALLIN
CALLIT
CALLME
CALLON
CALLOW
CALLTO
CALLUP
CALLUS
CANLIT
CAPLET
CARLIN
CARLOS
CARLOT
CARLOW
CATLIN
CAULKS
CEILED
CELLAE
CELLAR
CELLED
CELLOS
CEYLON
CHALET
CHALKS
CHALKY
CHELAE
CHILDE
CHILES
CHILIS
CHILLI
CHILLS
CHILLY
CHOLER
CHOLLA
CHOLOS
CIELOS
COALED
COALER
COELIA
COILED
COILER
COILUP
COLLAR
COLLAT
COLLET
COLLIE
COLLOP
COLLOQ
CONLAN
COOLED
COOLER
COOLEY
COOLIE
COOLIO
COOLIT
COOLLY
COOLTH
COOLTO
COPLEY
COTLER
COULDA
COULDI
COULEE
COWLED
COWLEY
CTILES
CULLED
CULLEN
CULLER
CULLET
CULLIS
CULLUM
CURLED
CURLER
CURLEW
CURLEY
CURLIN
CURLUP
CUTLER
CUTLET
CUYLER
CYCLED
CYCLER
CYCLES
CYCLIC
CYCLOS

C•••L•
CABALA
CABALS
CABELL
CACKLE
CAGILY
CAHILL
CAJOLE
CALMLY
CAMELS
CANALS
CANDLE
CANOLA
CANTLE
CANULA
CAROLE
CAROLI
CAROLL
CAROLS
CASALS
CASTLE
CATALO
CATTLE
CAVELL
CAVILS
CAZALE
CECILB
CECILE
CEORLS
CHARLY
CHICLE
CHICLY
CHILLI
CHILLS
CHILLY
CHOLLA
CHURLS
CIBOLA
CICELY
CIRCLE
COBALT
COBBLE
COCKLE
CODDLE
COGGLE
COLDLY
COMELY
COMPLY
COOLLY
COPALS
COPULA
CORALS
COSELL

COSILY
COSTLY
COUPLE
COZILY
CRADLE
CRAWLS
CRAWLY
CREELS
CREOLE
CSCALE
CUDDLE
CUDDLY
CUMULI
CUMULO
CUPELS
CUPOLA
CUPULE
CURDLE
CURTLY
CUTELY
CYBILL

C••••L

CABELL
CABRAL
CAHILL
CANCEL
CANFUL
CANNEL
CANTAL
CAPFUL
CARFUL
CARMEL
CARNAL
CAROLL
CARPAL
CARPEL
CARREL
CARROL
CARTEL
CARVEL
CASTEL
CASUAL
CAUDAL
CAUSAL
CAVELL
CENTAL
CEPHAL
CEREAL
CHACEL
CHANEL
CHAPEL
CHERYL
CHEVAL
CHISEL
CHORAL
CINEOL
CLONAL
COAXAL
COEVAL
COMPEL
CONSUL
CORBEL
CORNEL
CORRAL
COSELL
COSTAL
CRENEL
CRESOL
CREWEL
CRURAL
CUDGEL
CUNEAL
CUPFUL
CUSPAL
CYBILL
CYMBAL

•CL•••

BCLION
CCLAMP
CCLEFS
ECLAIR
ECLASS
ECLATS
GCLEFS
JCLOTH
MCLAIN
MCLEAN
OCLOCK
PCLABS
SCLAFF
SCLERA
UCLANS
YCLEPT

•C•L••

ACELAS
BCELLS
DCELLS
ECCLES
ECOLAB
ECOLAW
ECOLES
ICALLY
OCELLI
OCELOT
OCULAR
OCULUS
SCALAR
SCALDS
SCALED
SCALER
SCALES
SCALIA
SCALPS
SCHLEP
SCHLUB
SCOLDS
SCULLS
SCULLY
SCULPT
SCYLLA
TCELLS

•C••L•

ACIDLY
BCELLS
DCELLS
ICALLY
ICICLE
ICOULD
MCGILL
MCHALE
OCCULT
OCELLI
RCCOLA
SCHELL
SCHOLL
SCHULZ
SCOWLS
SCROLL
SCULLS
SCULLY
SCYLLA
TCELLS

•C•••L

ACETAL
ACETYL
ACTUAL
MCBEAL
MCGILL
MCNEIL
SCHELL
SCHOLL
SCHOOL
SCRAWL
SCROLL

••CL••

CYCLED
CYCLER
CYCLES
CYCLIC
CYCLOS
DECLAW
DECLOT
DRCLAW
ECCLES
EUCLID
JACLYN
LACLOS
MACLEN
MACLES
NUCLEI
NUCLEO
ONCLES
RECLAD
SOCLES
UNCLAD
UNCLAY
UNCLES
UNCLIP
UNCLOG
VACLAV

••C•L•

AACELL
ARCHLY
ASCALE
ASCOLD
BACALL
BECALM
BSCALE
BUCKLE
CACKLE
CECILB
CECILE
CICELY
COCKLE
CSCALE
DECALS
DECILE
DECKLE
DOCILE
DSCALE
ESCALE
EXCELS
FACILE
FACULA
FICKLE
FOCSLE
FSCALE
GOCOLD
GSCALE
HACKLE
HACKLY
HECKLE
IMCOLD
INCULT
JACALS
JECKLE
LACILY
LOCALE
LOCALS
LUCILE
MACULA
NICELY
NICOLA
NICOLE
NICOLO
OCCULT
ONCALL
OSCULE
PACULA
PICKLE
RACILY
RCCOLA
RECALL
RICHLY
RICOLA
SACFLY
SICILY
SICKLE
SICKLY
TACKLE
TICALS
TICKLE
TICKLY
UNCALM
UNCOLA
VOCALS
ZOCALO

••C••L

AACELL
ASCOOL
BACALL
BECOOL
BUCCAL
DACTYL
DUCTAL
ENCYCL
FACIAL
IMCOOL
JACKAL
KOCHEL
MICHEL
MRCOOL
NICKEL
NUCHAL
ONCALL
PICHEL
RACHEL
RACIAL
RECALL
RECOAL
RECOIL
RECOOL
RECURL
RICTAL
SECKEL
SOCIAL
TACTEL
UNCIAL
UNCOIL
UNCOOL
UNCURL
UPCOIL
UPCURL
VACHEL

•••CL•

CHICLE
CHICLY
CIRCLE
ICICLE
MUSCLE
MUSCLY
ORACLE
SIECLE

•••C•L

AMICAL
APICAL
BUCCAL
CANCEL
CHACEL
DARCEL
EPICAL
FISCAL
GLYCOL
LAICAL
LOWCAL
MARCEL
MARCIL
MESCAL
PARCEL
PASCAL
PENCIL
PROCOL
RASCAL
TERCEL
UNOCAL
URACIL

••••CL

ENCYCL

CM••••

CMAJOR
CMINOR
CMINUS

C•M•••

CAMARO
CAMBER
CAMBOY
CAMDEN
CAMEAS
CAMEAT
CAMEBY
CAMEIN
CAMELS
CAMEON
CAMEOS
CAMERA
CAMETO
CAMEUP
CAMINO
CAMION
CAMISE
CAMMIE
CAMOES
CAMPED
CAMPER
CAMPOS
CAMPUP
CAMPUS
CAMRYN
CAMRYS
CEMENT
CIMINO
COMATE
COMBAT
COMBED
COMBER
COMBOS
COMDEN
COMDEX
COMDRS
COMEAS
COMEAT
COMEBY
COMEDY
COMEIN
COMELY
COMEOF
COMEON
COMERS
COMETH
COMETO
COMETS
COMEUP
COMFIT
COMICE
COMICS
COMIDA
COMING
COMITY
COMMAS
COMMIT
COMMIX
COMMON
COMORO
COMPAQ
COMPAS
COMPED
COMPEL
COMPLY
COMPOS
COMPOZ
COMSAT
COMTES
CUMBER
CUMBIA
CUMINS
CUMULI
CUMULO
CYMBAL
CYMRIC

C••M••

CABMAN
CABMEN
CADMIC
CADMUS
CAIMAN
CALMED
CALMER
CALMEX
CALMLY
CAMMIE
CARMAN
CARMEL
CARMEN
CATMAN
CATMEN
CAYMAN
CHAMMY
CHAMPS
CHEMIC
CHEMIN
CHIMED
CHIMER
CHIMES
CHIMPS
CHOMPS
CHUMMY
CHUMPS
CLAMMA
CLAMMY
CLAMOR
CLAMPS
CLAMUP
CLIMAT
CLIMAX
CLIMBS
CLIMES
CLOMPS
CLUMPS
CLUMPY
CLUMSY
COLMAN
COLMAR
COMMAS
COMMIT
COMMIX
COMMON
CONMAN
CONMEN
CORMAN
COSMAS
COSMIC
COSMOS
COWMAN
COWMEN
CRAMBO
CRAMER
CRAMIN
CRAMPS
CRAMPY
CREMER
CREMES
CRIMEA
CRIMES
CRIMPS
CRIMPY
CRUMBS
CRUMBY
CRUMMY
CRUMPS

C•••M•

CALLME
CAROMS
CCLAMP
CDROMS
CHAMMY
CHARMS
CHASMS
CHROMA
CHROME
CHROMO
CHROMY
CHUMMY
CINEMA
CLAIMS
CLAMMA
CLAMMY
COLIMA
COLUMN
CREAMS
CREAMY
CRUMMY

C••••M

CASSIM
CATDOM
CENTUM
CERIUM
CESIUM
CHISUM
CHRISM
CILIUM
CIRCUM
COBHAM
CORFAM
CORIUM
CUBISM
CULLUM
CURIUM
CUSTOM

•C•M••

ACUMEN
ICEMAN
ICEMEN
SCAMPI
SCAMPS
SCHMOS
SCUMMY

•C••M•

CCLAMP
ECTOMY
ECZEMA
OCCAMS
RCRUMB
SCHEMA
SCHEME
SCRAMS
SCRIMP
SCRIMS
SCRUMS
SCUMMY

•C•••M

ACTIUM
ICEDAM
LCHAIM
SCARUM
SCHISM
SCREAM

••CM••

AWCMON
MICMAC
PACMAN

••C•M•

BECAME
BECOME
DECAMP
DOCOMO
ENCAMP
INCOME
JICAMA
MACOMB
MECUMS
OCCAMS
RACEME
RECOMB
TACOMA
TOCOME

••C••M

AECIUM
BECALM
DICTUM
FACTUM
HICKAM
LYCEUM
RACISM
SACHEM
SACRUM
UNCALM
VACUUM
VICTIM

•••C•M

ABSCAM
BOLCOM
CIRCUM
DOTCOM
JAMCAM
KIDCOM
NONCOM
ROMCOM
SATCOM
SITCOM
SKYCAM
SPYCAM
TALCUM
VIACOM
WEBCAM
ZITCOM

CN••••

CNOTES

C•N•••

CANAAN
CANADA
CANALS
CANAPE
CANARD
CANARY
CANCAN
CANCEL
CANCER
CANCHA
CANCUN
CANDIA
CANDID
CANDLE
CANDOR
CANERS
CANFUL
CANIDS
CANIER
CANIFF
CANINE
CANING
CANKER
CANLIT
CANNAS
CANNED
CANNEL
CANNER
CANNES
CANNON
CANNOT
CANOED
CANOER
CANOES
CANOLA
CANONS
CANOPY
CANOVA
CANTAB
CANTAL
CANTBE
CANTED
CANTER
CANTLE
CANTON
CANTOO
CANTOR
CANTOS
CANUCK
CANULA
CANUTE
CANVAS
CANYON
CENSED
CENSER
CENSES
CENSOR
CENSUS
CENTAI
CENTAL
CENTAS
CENTER
CENTOS
CENTRE
CENTRI
CENTRO
CENTUM
CINDER
CINEMA
CINEOL
CINQUE
CONAIR
CONANT
CONCHA
CONCHO
CONCHS
CONCUR
CONDOR
CONDOS
CONERS
CONEYS
CONFAB
CONFED
CONFER
CONFIT
CONGAS
CONGER
CONGES
CONGOU
CONICS
CONIES
CONING
CONJOB
CONKED
CONKER
CONLAN
CONMAN
CONMEN
CONNED
CONNEE
CONNIE
CONNOR
CONOCO
CONOID
CONRAD
CONROY
CONSUL
CONTAC
CONTRA
CONTRE
CONURE
CONVEX
CONVEY
CONVOY
CONWAY
CUNARD
CUNEAL
CYNICS

C••N••

CAGNEY
CANNAS
CANNED
CANNEL
CANNER
CANNES
CANNON
CANNOT
CAPNUT
CARNAC
CARNAL
CARNAP
CARNER
CARNES
CARNET
CARNEY
CATNAP
CATNIP
CERNAN
CHANCE
CHANCY
CHANDU
CHANEL
CHANEY
CHANGE
CHANGO
CHANTE
CHANTS
CHANTY
CHENEY
CHENIN
CHINAS
CHINCH
CHINES
CHINKS
CHINKY
CHINOS
CHINTZ
CHINUA
CHINUP
CHUNKS
CHUNKY
CHYNNA
CLANCY
CLANGS
CLANKS
CLANKY
CLENCH
CLINCH
CLINGS
CLINGY
CLINIC
CLINKS
CLONAL
CLONED
CLONER
CLONES
CLONKS
CLUNKS
CLUNKY
CMINOR
CMINUS
COBNUT
COGNAC
COINED
COINER
COINOP
CONNED
CONNEE
CONNIE
CONNOR
COONEY
CORNEA
CORNED
CORNEL
CORNER
CORNET
COUNTS
COUNTY
CPSNOW
CRANED
CRANES
CRANIA
CRANIO
CRANKS
CRANKY
CRANNY
CRENEL
CRENNA
CRINGE
CRONES
CRONIN
CRONUS
CRONYN
CRUNCH
CSONKA
CUANDO
CUANTO
CURNOW
CYANIC
CYANID
CYGNET
CYGNUS

C•••N•

CABANA
CABINS
CADENT
CAGING
CAIRNS
CAJUNS
CAKING
CAMINO
CANINE
CANING
CANONS
CAPONE
CAPONI
CAPONS
CARINA
CARING
CARONI
CASING
CASINO
CATANO
CATENA
CAVING
CAWING
CEDING
CELINE
CEMENT
CESSNA
CETANE
CHAINE
CHAINS
CHIANG
CHIENS
CHRONO
CHURNS
CHYNNA
CIMINO
CITING
CLEANS
CLIENT
CLOWNS
CLUING
CODING
CODONS
COGENT
COIGNE
COIGNS
COKING
COLONI
COLONS
COLONY
COMING
CONANT
CONING
COOING
COOWNS
COPING
CORING
CORONA
COSINE
COTANS
COVENS
COVENT
COVINA
COVING
COWENS
COWING
COXING
COZENS
CRAINS
CRANNY
CRENNA
CROONS
CROWNE
CROWNS
CRYING
CUBANS
CUBING
CUEING
CUMINS
CURING
CUTINS
CYRANO
CZERNY

C••••N

CABMAN
CABMEN
CAFTAN
CAGEIN
CAIMAN
CALGON
CALLAN
CALLIN
CALLON
CALVIN
CAMDEN
CAMEIN
CAMEON
CAMION
CAMRYN
CANAAN
CANCAN
CANCUN
CANNON
CANTON
CANYON
CAPGUN
CARBON
CARDIN
CAREEN
CARLIN
CARMAN
CARMEN
CARSON
CARTIN
CARTON
CASEIN
CASERN
CASHIN
CASSIN
CASTON
CATION
CATKIN
CATLIN
CATMAN
CATMEN
CATTON
CAVEIN
CAVERN
CAYMAN
CEDARN
CERNAN
CEYLON
CHACUN
CHAPIN
CHARON
CHAZAN
CHEMIN
CHENIN
CHEVON
CHEWON
CHIPIN
CHIRON
CHITON
CHOPIN
CHOSEN
CHYRON
CITRIN
CITRON
CLADIN
CLAVIN
CLIPON
CLOVEN
CLUEIN
COBAIN
COBURN
COCOON
COFFIN
COLMAN
COLSON
COLTON
COLUMN
COMDEN
COMEIN
COMEON
COMMON
CONLAN
CONMAN
CONMEN
COOGAN
CORBIN
CORDON
CORMAN
CORWIN
COSIGN
COTTEN
COTTON
COUPON
COUSIN
COWMAN
COWMEN
CRAMIN

CRAVEN
CRAYON
CRETAN
CRETIN
CRONIN
CRONYN
CROTON
CRUZAN
CTSCAN
CUBFAN
CUEDIN
CUESIN
CULKIN
CULLEN
CURLIN
CURTIN
CURZON
CUTSIN

•CN•••
MCNABB
MCNAIR
MCNEIL

•C•N••
ACTNOW
ICANSO
ICINGS
ICONIC
OCONEE
SCANTS
SCANTY
SCENAS
SCENEI
SCENES
SCENEV
SCENIC
SCENTS
SCHNOZ
SCONCE
SCONES

•C••N•
ACCENT
ACCTNO
ACHENE
ACHING
ACORNS
ACTING
ACTONE
BCCING
ICHING
MCCANN
OCEANS
OCTANE
OCTANS
OCTANT
SCARNE
SCIONS
SCORNS
UCLANS

•C•••N
ACTION
ACTSIN
ACTSON
ACUMEN
BCLION
ICEDIN
ICEMAN
ICEMEN
ICERUN
ICESIN
MCBAIN
MCCAIN
MCCANN
MCEWAN
MCEWEN
MCKEAN
MCKEON
MCKERN
MCKUEN
MCLAIN
MCLEAN
SCREEN

••CN••
MACNEE
PICNIC

••C•N•
ACCENT
ACCTNO
ALCINA
ARCANA
ARCANE
ARCING
ASCEND
ASCENT
BACONS
BCCING
DECANT
DECENT
DICING
DOCENT
ENCINA
ENCINO
EOCENE
ESCENT
EXCONS
FACING
FECUND
HECKNO
INCANS
INCANT
INCENT
JOCUND
LACING
LACUNA
LOCANE
LUCENT
LUCINE
MCCANN
NICENE
NOCENT
OSCANS
OSCINE
PACING
PACINO
PECANS
PICONE
POCONO
RACINE
RACING
RACINO
RECANE
RECANS
RECANT
RECENT
RECONS
RICANS
RICING
ROCKNE
SECANT
SECOND
SOCANI
TECHNO
TICINO
TUCANA
VACANT
VICUNA

••C••N
AACHEN
ANCIEN
ARCHON
ARCSIN
ARCTAN
AWCMON
BACKIN
BECKON
BICHON
BICORN
BUCHAN
COCOON
DACRON
DUCHIN
EUCKEN
FACEON
INCHON
JACLYN
KICKIN
KUCHEN
LACEON
LECAIN
LICHEN
LOCKIN
LOCKON
LUCIAN
LUCIEN
MACLEN
MACOUN
MACRON
MCCAIN
MCCANN
MECCAN
MICRON
NACION
PACHIN
PACKIN
PACKON
PACMAN
PACTEN
PECTIN
PICKON
RACEIN
RECKON
RECOIN
RICHEN
RICHIN
ROCHON
ROCKIN
SICKEN
SOCKIN
SUCKIN
TACKON
TOCSIN
TUCKIN
TUCSON
TYCOON
URCHIN
WICCAN

•••C•N
ANACIN
ASHCAN
BEACON
CANCAN
CANCUN
CHACUN
CTSCAN
DANCIN
DEACON
DEFCON
DUNCAN
FALCON
FLACON
GARCON
GASCAN
GASCON
IFICAN
MECCAN
NEOCON
NIACIN
OILCAN
RESCAN
THECAN
TINCAN
TOUCAN
TUSCAN
UTICAN
VULCAN
WICCAN
ZIRCON

CO••••
COACTS
COALED
COALER
COAPTS
COARSE
COASTS
COATED
COATEE
COATER
COATES
COATIS
COAXAL
COAXED
COAXER
COAXES
COBAIN
COBALT
COBBLE
COBHAM
COBNUT
COBRAS
COBURG
COBURN
COBWEB
COCCUS
COCCYX
COCKED
COCKER
COCKLE
COCOAS
COCOON
CODDLE
CODERS
CODGER
CODIFY
CODING
CODONS
CODYWY
COEDIT
COELIA
COERCE
COEURS
COEVAL
COFFEE
COFFER
COFFIN
COGENT
COGGED
COGGLE
COGITO
COGNAC
COHABS
COHEIR
COHERE
COHOES
COHORT
COHOST
COIFED
COIGNE
COIGNS
COILED
COILER
COILUP
COINED
COINER
COINOP
COKIER
COKIES
COKING
COLADA
COLBYS
COLDER
COLDLY
COLECO
COLEUS
COLFAX
COLICS
COLIMA
COLLAR
COLLAT
COLLET
COLLIE
COLLOP
COLLOQ
COLMAN
COLMAR
COLONI
COLONS
COLONY
COLORS
COLOUR
COLSON
COLTER
COLTON
COLUMN
COMATE
COMBAT
COMBED
COMBER
COMBOS
COMDEN
COMDEX
COMDRS
COMEAS
COMEAT
COMEBY
COMEDY
COMEIN
COMELY
COMEOF
COMEON
COMERS
COMETH
COMETO
COMETS
COMEUP
COMFIT
COMICE
COMICS
COMIDA
COMING
COMITY
COMMAS
COMMIT
COMMIX
COMMON
COMORO
COMPAQ
COMPAS
COMPED
COMPEL
COMPLY
COMPOS
COMPOZ
COMSAT
COMTES
CONAIR
CONANT
CONCHA
CONCHO
CONCHS
CONCUR
CONDOR
CONDOS
CONERS
CONEYS
CONFAB
CONFED
CONFER
CONFIT
CONGAS
CONGER
CONGES
CONGOU
CONICS
CONIES
CONING
CONJOB
CONKED
CONKER
CONLAN
CONMAN
CONMEN
CONNED
CONNEE
CONNIE
CONNOR
CONOCO
CONOID
CONRAD
CONROY
CONSUL
CONTAC
CONTRA
CONTRE
CONURE
CONVEX
CONVEY
CONVOY
CONWAY
COODER
COOEED
COOEES
COOERS
COOGAN
COOING
COOKED
COOKER
COOKIE
COOKUP
COOLED
COOLER
COOLEY
COOLIE
COOLIO
COOLIT
COOLLY
COOLTH
COOLTO
COONEY
COOPED
COOPER
COOPTS
COOPUP
COOTER
COOTIE
COOWNS
COPALS
COPAYS
COPCAR
COPERS
COPIED
COPIER
COPIES
COPING
COPLEY
COPOUT
COPPED
COPPER
COPRAS
COPSES
COPSIT
COPSTO
COPTER
COPTIC
COPULA
COQUIS
CORACI
CORALS
CORBEL
CORBIN
CORDAY
CORDED
CORDER
CORDIA
CORDON
CORERS
CORFAM
CORGIS
CORING
CORIUM
CORKED
CORKER
CORKUP
CORMAN
CORNEA
CORNED
CORNEL
CORNER
CORNET
CORONA
COROTS
CORPSE
CORPUS
CORRAL
CORREO
CORSAS
CORSET
CORTES
CORTEX
CORTEZ
CORTOT
CORVEE
CORVID
CORVUS
CORWIN
CORYZA
COSECS
COSELL
COSETS
COSHED
COSHER
COSHES
COSIED
COSIER
COSIES
COSIGN
COSILY
COSINE
COSMAS
COSMIC
COSMOS
COSSET
COSTAE
COSTAL
COSTAR
COSTAS
COSTCO
COSTED
COSTLY
COSYUP
COTANS
COTLER
COTTAE
COTTAS
COTTEN
COTTER
COTTON
COUGAR
COUGHS
COULDA
COULDI
COULEE
COUNTS
COUNTY
COUPES
COUPLE
COUPON
COURIC
COURSE
COURTS
COUSIN
COUTER
COVENS
COVENT
COVERS
COVERT
COVETS
COVEYS
COVINA
COVING
COWARD
COWBOY
COWENS
COWERS
COWIER
COWING
COWISH
COWLED
COWLEY
COWMAN
COWMEN
COWPEA
COWPER
COWPOX
COWRIE
COXING
COYDOG
COYEST
COYISH
COYOTE
COYPUS
COZENS
COZIED
COZIER
COZIES
COZILY
COZYUP

C•O•••
CEORLS
CHOATE
CHOCKS
CHOICE
CHOIRS
CHOKED
CHOKER
CHOKES
CHOLER
CHOLLA
CHOLOS
CHOMPS
CHOOSE
CHOOSY
CHOPIN
CHOPPY
CHOPRA
CHOPUP
CHORAL
CHORDS
CHOREO
CHORES
CHORIC
CHORIO
CHOROS
CHORUS
CHOSEN
CHOUGH
CHOWED
CLOAKS
CLOCHE
CLOCKS
CLODDY
CLOETE
CLOGGY
CLOGUP
CLOMPS
CLONAL
CLONED
CLONER
CLONES
CLONKS
CLORIS
CLOROX
CLOSED
CLOSER
CLOSES
CLOSET
CLOTHE
CLOTHO
CLOTHS
CLOTTY
CLOTUP
CLOUDS
CLOUDY
CLOUGH
CLOUTS
CLOVEN
CLOVER
CLOVES
CLOVIS
CLOWNS
CLOYED
CNOTES
COODER
COOEED
COOEES
COOERS
COOGAN
COOING
COOKED
COOKER
COOKIE
COOKUP
COOLED
COOLER
COOLEY
COOLIE
COOLIO
COOLIT
COOLLY
COOLTH
COOLTO
COONEY
COOPED
COOPER
COOPTS
COOPUP
COOTER
COOTIE
COOWNS
CROAKS
CROAKY
CROATS
CROCKS
CROCUS
CROFTS
CROIRE
CRONES
CRONIN
CRONUS
CRONYN
CROOKS
CROONS
CROPUP
CRORES
CROSBY
CROSSE
CROTCH
CROTON
CROUCH
CROUPS
CROUPY
CROUSE
CROUTE
CROWDS
CROWED
CROWER
CROWNE
CROWNS
CSONKA
CUORES

C••O••
CAHOOT
CAJOLE
CALORY
CAMOES
CANOED
CANOER
CANOES
CANOLA
CANONS
CANOPY
CANOVA
CAPONE
CAPONI
CAPONS
CAPOTE
CAROBS
CAROLE
CAROLI
CAROLL
CAROLS
CAROMS
CARONI
CAVORT
CDROMS
CHEOPS
CHLORO
CHOOSE
CHOOSY
CHROMA
CHROME
CHROMO
CHROMY
CHRONO
CIBOLA
CIXOUS
COCOAS
COCOON
CODONS
COHOES
COHORT
COHOST
COLONI
COLONS
COLONY
COLORS
COLOUR
COMORO
CONOCO
CONOID
COPOUT
CORONA
COROTS
COYOTE
CREOLE
CROOKS
CROONS
CRUORS
CRYOFF
CRYOUT
CSPOTS
CUBOID
CUPOLA
CUTOFF
CUTOUT
CWPOST
CYBORG

C•••O•
CACAOS
CAHOOT
CAICOS
CALGON
CALLON
CALLOW
CAMBOY
CAMEON
CAMEOS
CAMION
CAMPOS
CANDOR
CANNON
CANNOT
CANTON
CANTOO
CANTOR
CANTOS
CANYON
CAPTOR
CARBON
CARBOS
CARBOY
CAREOF
CARGOS
CARHOP
CARIOU
CARLOS
CARLOT
CARLOW
CARROL
CARROT
CARSON
CARTON
CARTOP
CASIOS
CASTON
CASTOR
CATDOM
CATION
CATTON
CATTOY
CAWDOR
CELLOS
CENSOR
CENTOS
CERROS
CEYLON
CHARON
CHEKOV
CHEVON
CHEWON
CHICOS
CHIGOE
CHINOS
CHIRON
CHISOX
CHITON
CHOLOS
CHOROS
CHYRON
CIELOS
CINEOL
CISCOS
CITRON
CLAMOR
CLAROS
CLIPON
CLOROX
CMAJOR
CMINOR
COCOON
COINOP
COLLOP
COLLOQ
COLSON
COLTON
COMBOS
COMEOF
COMEON
COMMON
COMPOS
COMPOZ
CONDOR
CONDOS
CONGOU
CONJOB
CONNOR
CONROY
CONVOY
CORDON
CORTOT
COSMOS
COTTON
COUPON
COWBOY
COWPOX
COYDOG
CPSNOW
CRACOW
CRAYON
CREDOS
CRESOL
CROTON
CRUSOE
CRYFOR
CUCKOO
CURIOS
CURNOW
CURSOR
CURZON
CUSTOM
CYCLOS

C••••O
CABRIO
CALICO
CALLAO
CALLTO
CAMARO
CAMETO
CAMINO
CANTOO
CARDIO
CARETO
CARUSO
CASINO
CASSIO
CASTRO
CATALO
CATANO
CENTRO
CERATO
CHANGO
CHARRO
CHEAPO
CHIRHO
CHLORO
CHOREO
CHORIO
CHROMO
CHRONO
CHURRO
CICERO
CIMINO
CLOTHO
COGITO
COLECO
COMETO
COMORO
CONCHO
CONOCO
COOLIO
COOLTO
COPSTO
CORREO
COSTCO
CRAMBO
CRANIO
CREEPO
CRISCO
CRISTO
CRYPTO
CUANDO
CUANTO
CUATRO
CUCKOO
CUMULO
CYRANO

•CO•••
ACORNS
ECOLAB
ECOLAW
ECOLES
ECORSE
ICONIC
ICOULD
OCONEE
SCOFFS
SCOLDS
SCONCE
SCONES
SCOOBA
SCOOBY
SCOOPS
SCOOTS
SCOPED
SCOPES
SCORCH
SCORED
SCORER
SCORES
SCORIA
SCORNS
SCOTCH
SCOTER
SCOTIA
SCOTTO
SCOTTS
SCOTTY
SCOUPE
SCOURS
SCOUTS
SCOWLS

•C•O••
ACCORD
ACCOST
ACEOUT
ACROSS
ACTONE
ACTORS
ACTOUT
ECHOED
ECHOER
ECHOES
ECHOIC
ECTOMY
ICEOUT
ICHORS
JCLOTH
MCCORD
MCJOBS
OCLOCK
OCTOOT
OCTOPI
RCCOLA
SCHOLL
SCHOOL
SCHORR
SCIONS

6 CO

SCOOBA SCOOBY SCOOPS SCOOTS SCRODS SCROLL

•C••O•

ACTFOR ACTION ACTNOW ACTSON BCLION ICEBOX ICEFOG ICEPOP MCADOO MCAVOY MCKEON OCELOT OCTOOT OCTROI SCHMOS SCHNOZ SCHOOL

•C•••O

ACCTNO ACTTWO ICANSO ICHIRO MCADOO OCTAVO SCIPIO SCOTTO

••CO••

ACCORD ACCOST ALCOTT ALCOVE ASCOLD ASCOOL ASCOTS ATCOST BACONS BECOME BECOOL BICORN COCOAS COCOON DECOCT DECODE DECORS DECOYS DICOTS DOCOMO ENCODE ENCORE ESCORT EXCONS FSCOTT GOCOED GOCOLD IMCOLD IMCOOL INCODE INCOME JACOBI JACOBY JOCOSE MACOMB MACOUN MCCORD MRCOOL MTCOOK NICOLA NICOLE NICOLO NOCOST PICONE PICOTS POCONO RCCOLA RECOAL RECOAT RECOCK RECODE RECOIL RECOIN RECOMB RECONS RECOOK RECOOL RECOPY RECORD RECORK RECOST RECOUP RICOHS RICOLA ROCOCO SECOND TACOMA TOCOME TYCOBB TYCOON UNCOIL UNCOLA UNCOOL UNCOOP UNCORE UNCORK UPCOIL WACOTX

••C•O•

AHCHOO ANCHOR ANCHOS ARCCOS ARCHON ASCOOL AWCMON BECKON BECOOL BICHON CACAOS COCOON CUCKOO CYCLOS DACRON DECLOT DOCBOY DOCTOR ESCROW FACEON FACTOR GECKOS HACHOO HECTOR HICKOK IMCOOL INCHON JOCKOS LACEON LACHOY LACLOS LECTOR LOCKON MACHOS MACRON MACROS MICRON MICROS MRCOOL MTCOOK MUCHOF NACHOS NACION PACKON PICKON PICTOR RECKON RECOOK RECOOL RECTOR RECTOS ROCHON SECTOR SICKOF SICKOS SUCCOR TACKON TUCSON TYCOON UNCLOG UNCOOL UNCOOP VECTOR VICTOR WACKOS

••C••O

ACCTNO AHCHOO ARCARO BOCHCO CICERO CUCKOO DACAPO DOCOMO ENCINO ESCUDO HACHOO HECKNO MACACO NICOLO NUCLEO PACINO PICABO PICARO POCONO RACETO RACINO ROCOCO TECHNO TICINO ZOCALO

•••CO•

ANTCOW ARCCOS BADCOP BANCOS BARCOS BEACON BOLCOM BOOCOO BUNCOS CAICOS CHICOS CISCOS CRACOW DEACON DEFCON DELCOS DISCOS DOTCOM FALCON FLACON GARCON GASCON GLYCOL IMACOP JUNCOS KIDCOM MARCOS MASCOT MOOCOW MOSCOW NARCOS NEOCON NONCOM PESCOW PETCOW PROCOL RANCOR REDCOD ROMCOM ROSCOE SATCOM SEACOW SITCOM SUCCOR TELCOS TRICOT VIACOM WILCOX ZIRCON ZITCOM

•••C•O

AFLCIO ALECTO BERCEO BOOCOO BRACCO CONCHO FRACTO GAUCHO HONCHO NUNCIO PANCHO PONCHO PSYCHO RANCHO REECHO SANCHO STUCCO VELCRO

••••CO

ALNICO ASARCO BIANCO BLANCO BOCHCO BRACCO BRASCO BRONCO CALICO COLECO CONOCO COSTCO CRISCO ENESCO ENRICO FIASCO FRANCO FRESCO FRISCO GRAECO GRIECO GYNECO HELICO MACACO MEDICO MEJICO MEXICO MONACO OROSCO OROZCO PHILCO ROCOCO SAFECO STUCCO SUNOCO TEXACO UNESCO VAILCO ZYDECO

CP••••

CPSNOW

C•P•••

CAPERS CAPFUL CAPGUN CAPITA CAPLET CAPNUT CAPONE CAPONI CAPONS CAPOTE CAPPED CAPPER CAPRID CAPRIS CAPTOR CEPEDA CEPHAL CIPHER COPALS COPAYS COPCAR COPERS COPIED COPIER COPIES COPING COPLEY COPOUT COPPED COPPER COPRAS COPSES COPSIT COPSTO COPTER COPTIC COPULA CSPOTS CUPELS CUPFUL CUPIDS CUPOLA CUPPAS CUPPED CUPRIC CUPULE CWPOST CYPHER CYPRUS

C••P••

CAMPED CAMPER CAMPOS CAMPUP CAMPUS CAPPED CAPPER CARPAL CARPAT CARPED CARPEL CARPER CARPET CARPUS CASPAR CASPER CHAPEL CHAPIN CHIPIN CHIPUP CHOPIN CHOPPY CHOPRA CHOPUP CHUPPA CLIPON COAPTS COMPAQ COMPAS COMPED COMPEL COMPLY COMPOS COMPOZ COOPED COOPER COOPTS COOPUP COPPED COPPER CORPSE CORPUS COUPES COUPLE COUPON COWPEA COWPER COWPOX COYPUS CRAPED CRAPES CREPED CREPES CRIPES CROPUP CRYPTO CRYPTS CUPPAS CUPPED CUSPAL CUSPED CUSPID

C•••P•

CALIPH CANAPE CANOPY CHAMPS CHEAPO CHEEPS CHEOPS CHIMPS CHIRPS CHIRPY CHOMPS CHOPPY CHUMPS CHUPPA CIASPY CLAMPS CLASPS CLOMPS CLUMPS CLUMPY CRAMPS CRAMPY CREEPO CREEPS CREEPY CRIMPS CRIMPY CRISPS CRISPY CROUPS CROUPY CRUMPS CUTUPS

C••••P

CAGEUP CAKEUP CALLUP CAMEUP CAMPUP CARHOP CARNAP CARTOP CASTUP CATNAP CATNIP CATSUP CCLAMP CHATUP CHEWUP CHINUP CHIPUP CHOPUP CLAMUP CLOGUP CLOTUP CLUBUP COILUP COINOP COLLOP COMEUP COOKUP COOPUP CORKUP COSYUP COZYUP CROPUP CRUDUP CSHARP CUESUP CUETIP CURLUP CUTSUP

•CP•••

MCPHEE

•C•P••

ICEPOP SCIPIO SCOPED SCOPES

•C••P•

ACCEPT ECTYPE ICEUPS OCCUPY OCTOPI SCALPS SCAMPI SCAMPS SCARPS SCOOPS SCOUPE SCRAPE SCRAPS SCRIPS SCRIPT SCULPT VCHIPS YCLEPT

•C•••P

ACESUP ACTSUP CCLAMP ICECAP ICEDUP ICEPOP ICESUP SCHAAP SCHLEP SCRIMP

••C•P•

ACCEPT ALCAPP BICEPS DACAPO DECAPS ESCAPE EXCEPT INCAPS INCEPT MACAPA OCCUPY RECAPS RECIPE RECOPY UNCAPS

••C••P

ALCAPP BACKUP BUCKUP DECAMP ENCAMP ESCARP FACEUP HACKUP HICCUP JACKUP KICKUP LACEUP LICKUP LOCKUP MOCKUP MUCKUP PACKUP PICKUP RACEUP RACKUP RECOUP RUCKUP SACKUP SUCKUP TACKUP UNCLIP UNCOOP

•••C•P

BADCOP EGGCUP EYECUP GASCAP GELCAP HICCUP HOTCAP HOTCUP HUBCAP ICECAP IMACOP MADCAP MIDCAP OILCUP PRECIP REDCAP SKICAP SKYCAP TEACUP TINCUP TOECAP TRICEP

C•Q•••

COQUIS

C••Q••

CASQUE CHEQUE CINQUE CIRQUE CLAQUE CLIQUE CLIQUY

C••••Q

COLLOQ COMPAQ

•CQ•••

ACQUIT

••CQ••

SACQUE

••••CQ

DEVICQ

CR••••

CRABBE CRABBY CRACKD CRACKS CRACOW CRADLE CRAFTS CRAFTY CRAGGY CRAIGT CRAINS CRAKES CRAMBO CRAMER CRAMIN CRAMPS CRAMPY CRANED CRANES CRANIA CRANIO CRANKS CRANKY CRANNY CRAPED CRAPES CRATED CRATER CRATES CRAVAT CRAVED CRAVEN CRAVER CRAVES CRAWLS CRAWLY CRAYON CRAZED CRAZES CREAKS CREAKY CREAMS CREAMY CREASE CREASY CREATE CRECHE CREDIT CREDOS CREEDS CREEKS CREELS CREEPO CREEPS CREEPY CREMER CREMES CRENEL CRENNA CREOLE CREPED CREPES CRESOL CRESSY CRESTS CRETAN CRETIN CREUSA CREUSE CREWED CREWEL CRICKS CRIERS CRIKEY CRIMEA CRIMES CRIMPS CRIMPY CRINGE CRIPES CRISCO CRISES CRISIS CRISPS CRISPY CRISTO CRITIC CROAKS CROAKY CROATS CROCKS CROCUS CROFTS CROIRE CRONES CRONIN CRONUS CRONYN CROOKS CROONS CROPUP CRORES CROSBY CROSSE CROTCH CROTON CROUCH CROUPS CROUPY CROUSE CROUTE CROWDS CROWED CROWER CROWNE CROWNS CRUCES CRUDDY CRUDER CRUDES CRUDUP CRUETS CRUISE CRUMBS CRUMBY CRUMMY CRUMPS CRUNCH CRUORS CRURAL CRUSES CRUSOE CRUSTS CRUSTY CRUTCH CRUXES CRUZAN CRWTHS CRYERS CRYFOR CRYING CRYOFF CRYOUT CRYPTO CRYPTS

C•R•••

CARAFE CARATS CARBON CARBOS CARBOY CARBRA CARDED CARDER CARDIA CARDIN CARDIO CAREEN CAREER CAREOF CARERS CARESS CARETO CARETS CARFUL CARGOS CARHOP CARIBE CARIBS CARIES CARINA CARING CARIOU CARKEY CARLIN CARLOS CARLOT CARLOW CARMAN CARMEL CARMEN CARNAC CARNAL CARNAP CARNER CARNES CARNET CARNEY CAROBS CAROLE CAROLI CAROLL CAROLS CAROMS CARONI CARPAL CARPAT CARPED CARPEL CARPER CARPET CARPUS CARREL CARREY CARRIE CARROL CARROT CARSEY CARSON CARTED CARTEL CARTER CARTES CARTIN CARTON CARTOP CARUSO CARVED CARVEL CARVER CARVES CARVEY CARWAX CDRACK CDRATE CDROMS CERATE CERATO CEREAL CEREBR CEREUS CERISE CERIUM CERNAN CERROS CERTIF CERVID CHRISM CHRIST CHROMA CHROME CHROMO CHROMY CHRONO CIRCLE CIRCUM CIRCUS CIRQUE CIRRUS CORACI CORALS CORBEL CORBIN CORDAY CORDED CORDER CORDIA CORDON CORERS CORFAM CORGIS CORING CORIUM CORKED CORKER CORKUP CORMAN CORNEA CORNED CORNEL CORNER CORNET CORONA COROTS CORPSE CORPUS CORRAL CORREO CORSAS CORSET CORTES CORTEX CORTEZ CORTOT CORVEE CORVID CORVUS CORWIN CORYZA CURACY CURADS CURARE CURATE CURBED CURDED CURDLE CURERS CURETS CURFEW CURIAE CURIES CURING CURIOS CURITE CURIUM CURLED CURLER CURLEW CURLEY CURLIN CURLUP CURNOW CURRED CURSED CURSER CURSES CURSOR CURTER CURTIN CURTIS CURTIZ CURTLY CURTSY CURVED CURVES CURVET CURZON CYRANO

C••R••

CABRAL CABRIO CADRES CAIRNS CAMRYN CAMRYS CAPRID CAPRIS CARREL CARREY CARRIE CARROL CARROT CATRIG CEDRIC CEORLS CERROS CHARDS CHARGE CHARLY CHARMS CHARON CHARRO CHARTA CHARTS CHERIE CHERRY CHERTS CHERTY CHERUB CHERYL CHIRAC CHIRHO CHIRON CHIRPS CHIRPY CHIRRS

CHORAL
CHORDS
CHOREO
CHORES
CHORIC
CHORIO
CHOROS
CHORUS
CHURCH
CHURLS
CHURNS
CHURRO
CHYRON
CIARDI
CIERAS
CIRRUS
CITRIC
CITRIN
CITRON
CITRUS
CLARET
CLARKE
CLAROS
CLERGY
CLERIC
CLERKS
CLORIS
CLOROX
COARSE
COBRAS
COERCE
CONRAD
CONROY
COPRAS
CORRAL
CORREO
COURIC
COURSE
COURTS
COWRIE
CRORES
CRURAL
CUORES
CUPRIC
CURRED
CYMRIC
CYPRUS
CZERNY

C•••R•

CABERS
CAGERS
CALORY
CAMARO
CAMERA
CANARD
CANARY
CANERS
CAPERS
CARBRA
CARERS
CASERN
CASERS
CASTRO
CATERA
CATERS
CAVERN
CAVERS
CAVORT
CEDARN
CEDARS
CEDARY
CEDERS
CELERY
CENTRE
CENTRI
CENTRO
CESARE
CESARS
CETERA
CHAIRS
CHAKRA
CHARRO
CHEERS
CHEERY
CHERRY
CHEVRE
CHIRRS
CHITRA
CHLORO
CHOIRS
CHOPRA
CHURRO
CICERO
CIDERS
CIDERY
CIGARS
CITERS
CLAIRE
CLAIRS
CLEARS
CLEARY
CLUERS
COBURG
COBURN
CODERS
COEURS
COHERE
COHORT
COLORS
COMDRS
COMERS
COMORO
CONERS
CONTRA
CONTRE
CONURE
COOERS
COPERS
CORERS
COVERS
COVERT
COWARD
COWERS
CRIERS
CROIRE
CRUORS
CRYERS
CSHARP
CSTARS
CUATRO
CUBERS
CUNARD
CURARE
CURERS
CYBORG
CYDERS

C••••R

CABLER
CADGER
CAESAR
CAGIER
CAHIER
CAKIER
CALDER
CALKER
CALLER
CALMER
CAMBER
CAMPER
CANCER
CANDOR
CANIER
CANKER
CANNER
CANOER
CANTER
CANTOR
CAPPER
CAPTOR
CARDER
CAREER
CARNER
CARPER
CARTER
CARVER
CASPAR
CASPER
CASTER
CASTOR
CATHER
CAUSER
CAVIAR
CAWDOR
CELLAR
CENSER
CENSOR
CENTER
CEREBR
CHAFER
CHASER
CHEDER
CHEWER
CHICER
CHIDER
CHIMER
CHOKER
CHOLER
CIBBER
CINDER
CIPHER
CLAMOR
CLAWER
CLEVER
CLONER
CLOSER
CLOVER
CMAJOR
CMINOR
COALER
COATER
COAXER
COCKER
CODGER
COFFER
COHEIR
COILER
COINER
COKIER
COLDER
COLLAR
COLMAR
COLOUR
COLTER
COMBER
CONAIR
CONCUR
CONDOR
CONFER
CONGER
CONKER
CONNOR
COODER
COOKER
COOLER
COOPER
COOTER
COPCAR
COPIER
COPPER
COPTER
CORDER
CORKER
CORNER
COSHER
COSIER
COSTAR
COTLER
COTTER
COUGAR
COUTER
COWIER
COWPER
COZIER
CRAMER
CRATER
CRAVER
CREMER
CROWER
CRUDER
CRYFOR
CULLER
CUMBER
CURLER
CURSER
CURSOR
CURTER
CUSSER
CUSTER
CUTLER
CUTTER
CUVIER
CUYLER
CYCLER
CYPHER

•CR•••

ACROSS
MCRIBS
RCRUMB
SCRAGS
SCRAMS
SCRAPE
SCRAPS
SCRAWL
SCREAK
SCREAM
SCREED
SCREEN
SCREES
SCREWS
SCREWY
SCRIBE
SCRIMP
SCRIMS
SCRIPS
SCRIPT
SCRODS
SCROLL
SCRUBS
SCRUFF
SCRUMS

•C•R••

ACARID
ACCRUE
ACORNS
ACURAS
DCAREA
ECARDS
ECARTE
ECORSE
ICARIA
ICARUS
ICERUN
MCCRAE
MCCREA
MCGRAW
MCGREW
OCHRED
OCHRES
OCTROI
SCARAB
SCARCE
SCARED
SCARER
SCARES
SCARFS
SCARNE
SCARPS
SCARRY
SCARUM
SCORCH
SCORED
SCORER
SCORES
SCORIA
SCORNS
SCURFY
SCURRY
SCURVE
SCURVY

•C••R•

ACCORD
ACHERS
ACTORS
ECKART
ECKERD
ICHIRO
ICHORS
MCCORD
MCHARG
MCKERN
OCCURS
OCHERS
OCHERY
SCARRY
SCHORR
SCLERA
SCOURS
SCURRY

•C•••R

ACHIER
ACTFOR
ACUTER
ECHOER
ECLAIR
ICKIER
KCSTAR
MCNAIR
OCEDAR
OCULAR
PCUSER
SCALAR
SCALER
SCARER
SCHORR
SCORER
SCOTER

••CR••

ACCRUE
DACRON
DECREE
ENCRES
ESCROW
LYCRAS
MACRAE
MACRON
MACROS
MCCRAE
MCCREA
MICRON
MICROS
NACRED
NACRES
NBCRED
OHCRUD
PICRIC
RICRAC
SACRED
SACRUM
SECRET
SUCRES
TVCREW

••C•R•

ACCORD
ARCARO
BICARB
BICORN
CICERO
DECARE
DECORS
DICERS
ENCORE
ESCARP
ESCORT
EUCHRE
FACERS
GOCART
IDCARD
INCURS
LACERS
MACERS
MCCORD
OCCURS
OSCARS
OXCART
PACERS
PICARA
PICARD
PICARO
RACERS
RECORD
RECORK
RECURE
RECURL
RECURS
RICERS
SECURE
ULCERS
UNCORE
UNCORK
UNCURB
UNCURL
UPCARD
UPCURL
VECTRA
VICARS
WECARE

••C••R

ANCHOR
ARCHER
BACKER
BECKER
BICKER
BUCKER
COCKER
CYCLER
DECKER
DICIER
DICKER
DOCKER
DOCTOR
DUCKER
ESCHER
ETCHER
FACTOR
HACKER
HECTOR
HOCKER
INCHER
KICKER
KOCHER
LACIER
LECHER
LECTER
LECTOR
LICKER
LOCHER
LOCKER
MOCKER
MUCKER
NECKER
NECTAR
NICKER
NICKJR
PACIER
PACKER
PICKER
PICTOR
PUCKER
RACIER
RACKER
RECTOR
RICHER
ROCKER
RUCKER
SACHER
SACKER
SECTOR
SICKER
SOCCER
SUCCOR
SUCKER
TACKER
TICKER
TUCKER
UECKER
VECTOR
VICTOR
WACKER
WICKER
ZUCKER

•••CR•

DESCRY
FARCRY
FIACRE
FULCRA
OUTCRY
TVVCRS
VELCRO
WARCRY

•••C•R

ARTCAR
BARCAR
BIGCAR
BOXCAR
BRACER
CANCER
CHICER
CONCUR
COPCAR
DANCER
DEICER
FENCER
FORCER
GROCER
HOTCAR
JUICER
LANCER
LASCAR
MERCER
MINCER
NASCAR
NEWCAR
OLDCAR
ONECAR
PIECER
PINCER
PLACER
PRICER
RANCOR
SAUCER
SLICER
SOCCER
SPACER
SPICER
SUCCOR
THECAR
TOWCAR
TOYCAR
TRACER
TWOCAR
VOICER
WINCER

CS••••

CSCALE
CSHARP
CSONKA
CSPOTS
CSTARS

C•S•••

CASABA
CASALS
CASAVA
CASBAH
CASEFY
CASEIN
CASERN
CASERS
CASHED
CASHES
CASHEW
CASHIN
CASING
CASINO
CASIOS
CASITA
CASKED
CASKET
CASPAR
CASPER
CASQUE
CASSIA
CASSIE
CASSIM
CASSIN
CASSIO
CASSIS
CASTED
CASTEL
CASTER
CASTES
CASTLE
CASTON
CASTOR
CASTRO
CASTUP
CASUAL
CESARE
CESARS
CESIUM
CESSED
CESSES
CESSNA
CESTAS
CESTUS
CISCOS
CISKEI
COSECS
COSELL
COSETS
COSHED
COSHER
COSHES
COSIED
COSIER
COSIES
COSIGN
COSILY
COSINE
COSMAS
COSMIC
COSMOS
COSSET
COSTAE
COSTAL
COSTAR
COSTAS
COSTCO
COSTED
COSTLY
COSYUP
CPSNOW
CTSCAN
CUSACK
CUSECS
CUSHAW
CUSPAL
CUSPED
CUSPID
CUSSED
CUSSER
CUSSES
CUSTER
CUSTIS
CUSTOM
CYSTIC

C••S••

CAESAR
CARSEY
CARSON
CASSIA
CASSIE
CASSIM
CASSIN
CASSIO
CASSIS
CATSAT
CATSIT
CATSUP
CAUSAL
CAUSED
CAUSER
CAUSES
CEASED
CEASES
CENSED
CENSER
CENSES
CENSOR
CENSUS
CESSED
CESSES
CESSNA
CHASED
CHASER
CHASES
CHASMS
CHASSE
CHASTE
CHESTS
CHESTY
CHISEL
CHISOX
CHISUM
CHOSEN
CIASPY
CLASPS
CLASSA
CLASSE
CLASSY
CLOSED
CLOSER
CLOSES
CLOSET
COASTS
COLSON
COMSAT
CONSUL
COPSES
COPSIT
COPSTO
CORSAS
CORSET
COSSET
COUSIN
CRESOL
CRESSY
CRESTS
CRISCO
CRISES
CRISIS
CRISPS
CRISPY
CRISTO
CROSBY
CROSSE
CRUSES
CRUSOE
CRUSTS
CRUSTY
CUESIN
CUESTA
CUESUP
CURSED
CURSER
CURSES
CURSOR
CUSSED
CUSSER
CUSSES
CUTSIN
CUTSIT
CUTSUP

C•••S•

CALASH
CAMISE
CARESS
CARUSO
CAYUSE
CDCASE
CERISE
CHAISE
CHASSE
CHEESE
CHEESY
CHOOSE
CHOOSY
CHRISM
CHRIST
CHUHSI
CLASSA
CLASSE
CLASSY
CLAUSE
CLEESE
CLUMSY
COARSE
COHOST
CORPSE
COURSE
COWISH
COYEST
COYISH
CREASE
CREASY
CRESSY
CREUSA
CREUSE
CROSSE
CROUSE
CRUISE
CUBISM
CUBIST
CURTSY
CUTEST
CUTESY
CWPOST

C••••S

CABALS
CABERS
CABINS
CABLES
CACAOS
CACHES
CACTUS
CADETS
CADGES
CADMUS
CADRES
CAGERS
CAGUAS
CAICOS
CAIRNS
CAJUNS
CALAIS
CALIFS
CALLAS
CALLES
CALLUS
CALVES
CALXES
CAMEAS
CAMELS
CAMEOS
CAMOES
CAMPOS
CAMPUS
CAMRYS
CANALS
CANERS
CANIDS
CANNAS
CANNES
CANOES
CANONS
CANTOS
CANVAS
CAPERS
CAPONS
CAPRIS
CARATS
CARBOS
CARERS
CARESS
CARETS
CARGOS
CARIBS
CARIES
CARLOS
CARNES
CAROBS
CAROLS
CAROMS
CARPUS
CARTES
CARVES
CASALS
CASERS
CASHES
CASIOS
CASSIS
CASTES
CATERS
CATHYS
CAUCUS
CAULKS
CAUSES
CAVERS
CAVIES
CAVILS
CCLEFS
CDROMS
CEASES
CEDARS
CEDERS
CEIBAS
CELEBS
CELLOS
CENSES
CENSUS
CENTAS
CENTOS
CEORLS
CEREUS
CERROS
CESARS
CESSES
CESTAS
CESTUS
CFLATS
CHAFES
CHAFFS
CHAINS
CHAIRS
CHALKS
CHAMPS
CHANTS
CHARDS
CHARMS
CHARTS
CHASES
CHASMS
CHEATS
CHECKS
CHEEKS
CHEEPS
CHEERS
CHEOPS
CHERTS
CHESTS
CHEVYS
CHICAS
CHICKS
CHICOS
CHIDES
CHIEFS
CHIENS
CHILES
CHILIS
CHILLS
CHIMES
CHIMPS
CHINAS
CHINES
CHINKS
CHINOS
CHIRPS
CHIRRS
CHIVAS
CHIVES
CHOCKS
CHOIRS
CHOKES
CHOLOS
CHOMPS
CHORDS
CHORES
CHOROS
CHORUS
CHUCKS
CHUFFS
CHUMPS
CHUNKS
CHURLS
CHURNS
CHUTES
CIDERS
CIELOS
CIERAS
CIGARS
CIRCUS
CIRRUS
CISCOS
CITEES
CITERS
CITIES
CITIUS
CITRUS
CIVETS
CIVICS
CIXOUS
CLACKS
CLAIMS
CLAIRS
CLAMPS
CLANGS
CLANKS
CLAROS
CLASPS
CLAVES
CLEANS
CLEARS
CLEATS
CLEEKS
CLEFTS
CLERKS
CLEVES
CLICKS
CLIFFS
CLIMBS
CLIMES
CLINGS
CLINKS
CLOAKS
CLOCKS
CLOMPS
CLONES
CLONKS
CLORIS
CLOSES
CLOTHS
CLOUDS
CLOUTS
CLOVES
CLOVIS
CLOWNS
CLUCKS
CLUERS
CLUMPS
CLUNKS
CLYDES
CMINUS
CNOTES
COACTS
COAPTS
COASTS
COATES
COATIS
COAXES
COBRAS
COCCUS
COCOAS
CODERS
CODONS
COEURS
COHABS
COHOES
COIGNS
COKIES
COLBYS
COLEUS
COLICS
COLONS
COLORS

COMBOS
COMDRS
COMEAS
COMERS
COMETS
COMICS
COMMAS
COMPAS
COMPOS
COMTES
CONCHS
CONDOS
CONERS
CONEYS
CONGAS
CONGES
CONICS
CONIES
COOEES
COOERS
COOPTS
COOWNS
COPALS
COPAYS
COPERS
COPIES
COPRAS
COPSES
COQUIS
CORALS
CORERS
CORGIS
COROTS
CORPUS
CORSAS
CORTES
CORVUS
COSECS
COSETS
COSHES
COSIES
COSMAS
COSMOS
COSTAS
COTANS
COTTAS
COUGHS
COUNTS
COUPES
COURTS
COVENS
COVERS
COVETS
COVEYS
COWENS
COWERS
COYPUS
COZENS
COZIES
CRACKS
CRAFTS
CRAINS
CRAKES
CRAMPS
CRANES
CRANKS
CRAPES
CRATES
CRAVES
CRAWLS
CRAZES
CREAKS
CREAMS
CREDOS
CREEDS
CREEKS
CREELS
CREEPS
CREMES
CREPES
CRESTS
CRICKS
CRIERS
CRIMES
CRIMPS
CRIPES
CRISES
CRISIS
CRISPS
CROAKS
CROATS
CROCKS
CROCUS
CROFTS
CRONES
CRONUS
CROOKS
CROONS
CRORES
CROUPS
CROWDS
CROWNS
CRUCES
CRUDES
CRUETS
CRUMBS
CRUMPS
CRUORS
CRUSES
CRUSTS
CRUXES
CRWTHS
CRYERS
CRYPTS
CSPOTS
CSTARS
CTILES
CUBANS
CUBEBS
CUBERS
CUBICS
CUBITS
CUICAS
CULETS
CULLIS
CULTUS
CUMINS
CUORES
CUPELS
CUPIDS
CUPPAS
CURADS
CURERS
CURETS
CURIES
CURIOS
CURSES
CURTIS
CURVES
CUSECS
CUSSES
CUSTIS
CUTEYS
CUTIES
CUTINS
CUTUPS
CUVEES
CYCADS
CYCLES
CYCLOS
CYDERS
CYGNUS
CYNICS
CYPRUS
CZECHS

•CS•••

KCSTAR

•C•S••

ACESIT
ACESUP
ACTSAS
ACTSIN
ACTSON
ACTSUP
ECESIC
ECESIS
ICESIN
ICESIT
ICESUP
OCASEK
OCASEY
PCUSER

•C••S•

ACCESS
ACCOST
ACCUSE
ACROSS
ECLASS
ECORSE
ICANSO
ICIEST
SCAASI
SCHISM
SCHIST
SCHUSS

•C•••S

ACCESS
ACELAS
ACHERS
ACORNS
ACROSS
ACTORS
ACTSAS
ACURAS
ACUTES
BCELLS
CCLEFS
DCELLS
ECARDS
ECCLES
ECESIS
ECHOES
ECLASS
ECLATS
ECOLES
GCLEFS
ICARUS
ICEUPS
ICHORS
ICINGS
MCJOBS
MCRIBS
OCCAMS
OCCURS
OCEANS
OCHERS
OCHRES
OCTADS
OCTANS
OCTETS
OCULUS
PCLABS
SCAGGS
SCALDS
SCALES
SCALPS
SCAMPS
SCANTS
SCARES
SCARFS
SCARPS
SCENAS
SCENES
SCENTS
SCHAVS
SCHMOS
SCHUSS
SCHWAS
SCIONS
SCOFFS
SCOLDS
SCONES
SCOOPS
SCOOTS
SCOPES
SCORES
SCORNS
SCOTTS
SCOURS
SCOUTS
SCOWLS
SCRAGS
SCRAMS
SCRAPS
SCREES
SCREWS
SCRIMS
SCRIPS
SCRODS
SCRUBS
SCRUMS
SCUBAS
SCUFFS
SCULLS
TCELLS
UCLANS
VCHIPS

••CS••

ARCSEC
ARCSIN
FOCSLE
TOCSIN
TUCSON

••C•S•

ACCESS
ACCOST
ACCUSE
ATCOST
BOCHSA
CDCASE
ENCASE
EXCESS
EXCISE
EXCUSA
EXCUSE
INCASE
INCASH
INCISE
INCUSE
JOCOSE
LACASA
LOCUST
NICEST
NOCOST
RACISM
RACIST
RECASE
RECAST
RECESS
RECOST
RECUSE
UNCASE
UNCASK
UNCAST
UPCAST

••C••S

ACCESS
ANCHOS
ARCCOS
ARCHES
ASCOTS
BACHES
BACKUS
BACONS
BICEPS
BOCCES
BOCCIS
CACAOS
CACHES
CACTUS
COCCUS
COCOAS
CYCADS
CYCLES
CYCLOS
DACHAS
DECADS
DECAFS
DECALS
DECAPS
DECAYS
DECIUS
DECORS
DECOYS
DICERS
DICOTS
DUCATS
ECCLES
EMCEES
ENCRES
ETCHES
EXCELS
EXCESS
EXCONS
EXCUBS
FACERS
FACETS
FACIAS
FACIES
FICHES
FICHUS
GECKOS
HACEKS
INCANS
INCAPS
INCHES
INCURS
ITCHES
JACALS
JOCKOS
LACERS
LACLOS
LOCALS
LUCIUS
LYCEES
LYCRAS
MACAWS
MACERS
MACHOS
MACLES
MACROS
MECCAS
MECUMS
MICROS
MOCHAS
MUCHAS
NACHAS
NACHOS
NACRES
NICADS
NICHES
NICIAS
NOCHES
OCCAMS
OCCURS
ONCLES
OPCITS
OSCANS
OSCARS
OUCHES
PACERS
PECANS
PECHES
PICOTS
PUCCIS
RACERS
RECANS
RECAPS
RECESS
RECONS
RECTOS
RECTUS
RECUES
RECURS
RECUTS
RICANS
RICERS
RICHES
RICOHS
RUCHES
RUCKUS
SICKOS
SOCLES
SUCHAS
SUCRES
TICALS
ULCERS
UNCAPS
UNCLES
VACHES
VICARS
VOCABS
VOCALS
WACKOS
YACHTS
YUCCAS

•••C•S

ABACAS
ABACUS
ALECKS
ALICES
AMICES
AMICUS
APICES
ARCCOS
ARECAS
BANCOS
BARCOS
BLACKS
BLOCKS
BOCCES
BOCCIS
BRACES
BRACHS
BRACTS
BRICKS
BROCAS
BUICKS
BUNCOS
CAICOS
CAUCUS
CHECKS
CHICAS
CHICKS
CHICOS
CHOCKS
CHUCKS
CIRCUS
CISCOS
CLACKS
CLICKS
CLOCKS
CLUCKS
COACTS
COCCUS
CONCHS
CRACKS
CRICKS
CROCKS
CROCUS
CRUCES
CUICAS
CZECHS
DANCES
DBACKS
DEICES
DELCOS
DEUCES
DISCOS
DISCUS
DORCAS
DRECKS
DUNCES
EDICTS
EDUCES
EDUCTS
EJECTS
ELECTS
ENACTS
EPACTS
EPOCHS
ERECTS
ERICAS
ERUCTS
EVICTS
EXACTS
FARCES
FASCES
FENCES
FINCAS
FLACKS
FLECKS
FLICKS
FLOCKS
FORCES
FRACAS
FROCKS
GLACES
GLACIS
GLOCKS
GRACES
IBICES
JUICES
JUNCOS
KLICKS
KNACKS
KNICKS
KNOCKS
LANCES
LEICAS
MARCOS
MARCUS
MECCAS
MINCES
MULCTS
NARCOS
NIECES
NUECES
ORACHS
ORECKS
OUNCES
PANCKS
PASCHS
PIECES
PISCES
PLACES
PLOCES
PLUCKS
PONCAS
PRECIS
PRICES
PRICKS
PSYCHS
PUCCIS
QUACKS
REACTS
REICES
ROYCES
SAUCES
SHACKS
SHOCKS
SHUCKS
SLACKS
SLICES
SLICKS
SMACKS
SMOCKS
SNACKS
SNICKS
SPACES
SPECKS
SPICES
STACKS
STICKS
STOCKS
SYNCHS
TELCOS
TERCES
TINCTS
TRACES
TRACKS
TRACTS
TRECES
TRICES
TRICKS
TRUCES
TRUCKS
TVVCRS
UNICES
VNECKS
VOICES
WELCHS
WENCES
WHACKS
WINCES
WRACKS
WRECKS
YOICKS
YUCCAS

••••CS

ANTICS
ANZACS
ASDICS
ASPICS
ATTICS
AZTECS
BASICS
BRONCS
CIVICS
COLICS
COMICS
CONICS
COSECS
CUBICS
CUSECS
CYNICS
DUROCS
ENIACS
ESTOCS
ETHICS
FRANCS
GLOUCS
HAVOCS
IBMPCS
IONICS
ISAACS
KOVACS
LILACS
LOGICS
LYRICS
MAGICS
MEDICS
MEDOCS
MIMICS
MUSICS
OLMECS
OPTICS
OSMICS
PANICS
REBECS
RELICS
SERACS
SONICS
STOICS
SUMACS
TONICS
TOPICS
TOXICS
TUNICS
XEBECS

CT••••

CTILES
CTSCAN

C•T•••

CATALO
CATANO
CATBED
CATCHY
CATDOM
CATENA
CATERA
CATERS
CATFIT
CATGUT
CATHAY
CATHER
CATHYS
CATION
CATKIN
CATLIN
CATMAN
CATMEN
CATNAP
CATNIP
CATRIG
CATSAT
CATSIT
CATSUP
CATTLE
CATTON
CATTOY
CETANE
CETERA
CITEES
CITERS
CITIED
CITIES
CITIFY
CITING
CITIUS
CITRIC
CITRIN
CITRON
CITRUS
COTANS
COTLER
COTTAE
COTTAS
COTTEN
COTTER
COTTON
CSTARS
CUTELY
CUTEST
CUTESY
CUTEYS
CUTIES
CUTINS
CUTLER
CUTLET
CUTOFF
CUTOUT
CUTSIN
CUTSIT
CUTSUP
CUTTER
CUTUPS

C••T••

CACTUS
CAFTAN
CANTAB
CANTAL
CANTBE
CANTED
CANTER
CANTLE
CANTON
CANTOO
CANTOR
CANTOS
CAPTOR
CARTED
CARTEL
CARTER
CARTES
CARTIN
CARTON
CARTOP
CASTED
CASTEL
CASTER
CASTES
CASTLE
CASTON
CASTOR
CASTRO
CASTUP
CATTLE
CATTON
CATTOY
CELTIC
CENTAI
CENTAL
CENTAS
CENTER
CENTOS
CENTRE
CENTRI
CENTRO
CENTUM
CERTIF
CESTAS
CESTUS
CHATTY
CHATUP
CHITON
CHITRA
CHITTY
CHUTED
CHUTES
CLOTHE
CLOTHO
CLOTHS
CLOTTY
CLOTUP
CLUTCH
CNOTES
COATED
COATEE
COATER
COATES
COATIS
COLTER
COLTON
COMTES
CONTAC
CONTRA
CONTRE
COOTER
COOTIE
COPTER
COPTIC
CORTES
CORTEX
CORTEZ
CORTOT
COSTAE
COSTAL
COSTAR
COSTAS
COSTCO
COSTED
COSTLY
COTTAE
COTTAS
COTTEN
COTTER
COTTON
COUTER
CRATED
CRATER
CRATES
CRETAN
CRETIN
CRITIC
CROTCH
CROTON
CRUTCH
CRWTHS
CUATRO
CUETIP
CULTCH
CULTIC
CULTUS
CURTER
CURTIN
CURTIS
CURTIZ
CURTLY
CURTSY
CUSTER
CUSTIS
CUSTOM
CUTTER
CYSTIC

C•••T•

CADETS
CALLTO
CAMETO
CANUTE
CAPITA
CAPOTE
CARATS
CARETO
CARETS
CASITA
CAVETT
CAVITY
CDRATE
CERATE
CERATO
CFLATS
CHANTE
CHANTS
CHANTY
CHARTA
CHARTS
CHASTE
CHATTY
CHEATS
CHEETA
CHERTS
CHERTY
CHESTS
CHESTY
CHINTZ
CHITTY
CHOATE
CIVETS
CLEATS
CLEFTS
CLOETE
CLOTTY
CLOUTS
COACTS
COAPTS
COASTS
COGITO
COMATE
COMETH
COMETO
COMETS
COMITY
COOLTH
COOLTO
COOPTS
COPSTO
COROTS
COSETS
COUNTS
COUNTY
COURTS
COVETS
COYOTE
CRAFTS
CRAFTY
CREATE
CRESTS
CRISTO
CROATS
CROFTS
CROUTE
CRUETS
CRUSTS
CRUSTY
CRYPTO
CRYPTS
CSPOTS
CUANTO
CUBITI
CUBITS
CUESTA
CULETS
CURATE
CURETS
CURITE

C••••T

CABLET
CACHET
CADENT
CAHOOT
CALLIT
CALVET
CAMEAT
CANLIT
CANNOT
CAPLET
CAPNUT
CARLOT
CARNET
CARPAT
CARPET
CARROT
CASKET
CATFIT
CATGUT
CATSAT
CATSIT
CAUGHT
CAVEAT
CAVETT
CAVORT
CEMENT
CHALET
CHEVET
CHRIST
CLARET
CLAWAT
CLIENT
CLIMAT
CLOSET
COBALT
COBNUT
COEDIT
COGENT
COHORT
COHOST
COLLAT
COLLET
COMBAT
COMEAT
COMFIT
COMMIT
COMSAT
CONANT
CONFIT
COOLIT
COPOUT
COPSIT
CORNET
CORSET
CORTOT
COSSET
COVENT
COVERT
COYEST
CRAIGT
CRAVAT
CREDIT
CRYOUT
CUBIST
CULLET
CURVET
CUTEST
CUTLET
CUTOUT
CUTSIT
CWPOST
CYGNET

•CT•••

ACTFOR
ACTIII
ACTING
ACTION
ACTIUM
ACTIVA
ACTIVE
ACTNOW
ACTONE
ACTORS
ACTOUT
ACTSAS
ACTSIN
ACTSON
ACTSUP
ACTTWO
ACTUAL
ECTOMY
ECTYPE
OCTADS
OCTANE
OCTANS
OCTANT
OCTAVE
OCTAVO

OCTETS
OCTOOT
OCTOPI
OCTROI

•C•T••
ACCTNO
ACETAL
ACETIC
ACETYL
ACTTWO
ACUTER
ACUTES
ICETEA
ICHTHY
KCSTAR
SCATHE
SCOTCH
SCOTER
SCOTIA
SCOTTO
SCOTTS
SCOTTY
SCYTHE

•C••T•
ACUATE
ACUITY
ECARTE
ECLATS
JCLOTH
OCTETS
SCANTS
SCANTY
SCENTS
SCOOTS
SCOTTO
SCOTTS
SCOTTY
SCOUTS

•C•••T
ACCENT
ACCEPT
ACCOST
ACEDIT
ACEOUT
ACESIT
ACQUIT
ACTOUT
ECKART
ICEDIT
ICEOUT
ICESIT
ICIEST
OCCULT
OCELOT
OCICAT
OCTANT
OCTOOT
SCHIST
SCRIPT
SCULPT
YCLEPT

••CT••
ACCTNO
ARCTAN
ARCTIC
CACTUS
DACTYL
DICTUM
DOCTOR
DUCTAL
DUCTED
FACTOR
FACTUM
HECTIC
HECTOR
LACTEA
LACTIC
LECTER
LECTOR
NECTAR
PACTEN
PECTIN
PICTOR
RECTOR
RECTOS
RECTUS
RICTAL
SECTOR
TACTEL
TACTIC
TICTAC
VECTOR
VECTRA
VICTIM
VICTOR

••C•T•
ALCOTT
ASCOTS
DICOTS
DUCATS
ETCETC
EXCITE
FACETS
FICHTE
FSCOTT
HECATE
INCITE
LOCATE
LUCITE
NICETY
OOCYTE
OPCITS
PICOTS
RACETO
RECITE
RECUTS
TECATE
TECHTV
UNCUTE
VACATE
WACOTX
YACHTS

••C••T
ACCENT
ACCEPT
ACCOST
ALCOTT
ASCENT
ATCOST
BACHIT
BECHET
BECKET
BUCKET
CACHET
DECANT
DECEIT
DECENT
DECLOT
DECOCT
DOCENT
DOCKET
ESCAUT
ESCENT
ESCORT
EXCEPT
FACEIT
FSCOTT
GOCART
HACKIT
INCANT
INCENT
INCEPT
INCULT
JACKET
LOCCIT
LOCKET
LOCUST
LUCENT
NICEST
NOCENT
NOCOST
OCCULT
OXCART
PACKET
PECKAT
PICKAT
PICKET
POCKET
RACIST
RACKET
RECANT
RECAST
RECENT
RECOAT
RECOST
RICHET
ROCHAT
ROCHET
ROCKET
ROCKIT
SACHET
SECANT
SECRET
SOCKET
TICKET
UNCAST
UPCAST
VACANT
WICKET

•••CT•
ALECTO
BRACTS
COACTS
EDICTS
EDUCTS
EJECTA
EJECTS
ELECTS
ENACTS
EPACTS
ERECTS
ERUCTS
EVICTS
EXACTA
EXACTS
FRACTO
FRUCTI
MULCTS
REACTS
SANCTA
TINCTS
TRACTS

•••C•T
AVOCET
BIGCAT
BOBCAT
BRECHT
DIECUT
DULCET
ELICIT
ENDCUT
EXOCET
FATCAT
FAUCET
HEPCAT
JOBCUT
LANCET
LAPCAT
LOCCIT
LOWCUT
MASCOT
MISCUT
MUDCAT
MUSCAT
OCICAT
OUTCUT
PAYCUT
PETCAT
PRECUT
REXCAT
RIBCUT
SEACAT
SNOCAT
TAXCUT
TOMCAT
TOPCAT
TRICOT
VINCIT

••••CT
ABDUCT
ABJECT
ADDICT
ADDUCT
AFFECT
ASPECT
BISECT
DECOCT
DEDUCT
DEFECT
DEJECT
DELICT
DEPICT
DETECT
DIDACT
DIRECT
EFFECT
EXPECT
EXSECT
IMPACT
INDICT
INDUCT
INFACT
INFECT
INJECT
INSECT
INTACT
MISACT
OBJECT
ONEACT
OUTACT
PREACT
REDACT
REJECT
RELICT
RELUCT
RESECT
SELECT
STRICT
TEAACT
THEACT
TWOACT
UNFACT

CU••••
CUANDO
CUANTO
CUATRO
CUBAGE
CUBANS
CUBBED
CUBEBS
CUBERS
CUBFAN
CUBICS
CUBING
CUBISM
CUBIST
CUBITI
CUBITS
CUBOID
CUCKOO
CUDAHY
CUDDLE
CUDDLY
CUDGEL
CUEBID
CUEDIN
CUEING
CUESIN
CUESTA
CUESUP
CUETIP
CUFFED
CUICAS
CULETS
CULKIN
CULLED
CULLEN
CULLER
CULLET
CULLIS
CULLUM
CULTCH
CULTIC
CULTUS
CUMBER
CUMBIA
CUMINS
CUMULI
CUMULO
CUNARD
CUNEAL
CUORES
CUPELS
CUPFUL
CUPIDS
CUPOLA
CUPPAS
CUPPED
CUPRIC
CUPULE
CURACY
CURADS
CURARE
CURATE
CURBED
CURDED
CURDLE
CURERS
CURETS
CURFEW
CURIAE
CURIES
CURING
CURIOS
CURITE
CURIUM
CURLED
CURLER
CURLEW
CURLEY
CURLIN
CURLUP
CURNOW
CURRED
CURSED
CURSER
CURSES
CURSOR
CURTER
CURTIN
CURTIS
CURTIZ
CURTLY
CURTSY
CURVED
CURVES
CURVET
CURZON
CUSACK
CUSECS
CUSHAW
CUSPAL
CUSPED
CUSPID
CUSSED
CUSSER
CUSSES
CUSTER
CUSTIS
CUSTOM
CUTELY
CUTEST
CUTESY
CUTEYS
CUTIES
CUTINS
CUTLER
CUTLET
CUTOFF
CUTOUT
CUTSIN
CUTSIT
CUTSUP
CUTTER
CUTUPS
CUVEES
CUVIER
CUYLER

C•U•••
CAUCHY
CAUCUS
CAUDAD
CAUDAL
CAUGHT
CAULKS
CAUSAL
CAUSED
CAUSER
CAUSES
CHUBBY
CHUCKS
CHUCKY
CHUFFS
CHUFFY
CHUHSI
CHUMMY
CHUMPS
CHUNKS
CHUNKY
CHUPPA
CHURCH
CHURLS
CHURNS
CHURRO
CHUTED
CHUTES
CIUDAD
CLUBBY
CLUBUP
CLUCKS
CLUEIN
CLUERS
CLUING
CLUMPS
CLUMPY
CLUMSY
CLUNKS
CLUNKY
CLUTCH
COUGAR
COUGHS
COULDA
COULDI
COULEE
COUNTS
COUNTY
COUPES
COUPLE
COUPON
COURIC
COURSE
COURTS
COUSIN
COUTER
CRUCES
CRUDDY
CRUDER
CRUDES
CRUDUP
CRUETS
CRUISE
CRUMBS
CRUMBY
CRUMMY
CRUMPS
CRUNCH
CRUORS
CRURAL
CRUSES
CRUSOE
CRUSTS
CRUSTY
CRUTCH
CRUXES
CRUZAN

C••U••
CAGUAS
CAJUNS
CANUCK
CANULA
CANUTE
CARUSO
CASUAL
CAYUGA
CAYUSE
CHOUGH
CLAUDE
CLAUSE
CLOUDS
CLOUDY
CLOUGH
CLOUTS
COBURG
COBURN
COEURS
COLUMN
CONURE
COPULA
COQUIS
CREUSA
CREUSE
CROUCH
CROUPS
CROUPY
CROUSE
CROUTE
CUMULI
CUMULO
CUPULE
CUTUPS

C•••U•
CACTUS
CADMUS
CAGEUP
CAKEUP
CALLUP
CALLUS
CAMEUP
CAMPUP
CAMPUS
CANCUN
CANFUL
CAPFUL
CAPGUN
CAPNUT
CARFUL
CARPUS
CASQUE
CASTUP
CATGUT
CATSUP
CAUCUS
CENSUS
CENTUM
CEREUS
CERIUM
CESIUM
CESTUS
CHACUN
CHATUP
CHEQUE
CHERUB
CHEWUP
CHINUA
CHINUP
CHIPUP
CHISUM
CHOPUP
CHORUS
CILIUM
CINQUE
CIRCUM
CIRCUS
CIRQUE
CIRRUS
CITIUS
CITRUS
CIXOUS
CLAMUP
CLAQUE
CLIQUE
CLIQUY
CLOGUP
CLOTUP
CLUBUP
CMINUS
COBNUT
COCCUS
COILUP
COLEUS
COLOUR
COMEUP
CONCUR
CONSUL
COOKUP
COOPUP
COPOUT
CORIUM
CORKUP
CORPUS
CORVUS
COSYUP
COYPUS
COZYUP
CROCUS
CRONUS
CROPUP
CRUDUP
CRYOUT
CUESUP
CULLUM
CULTUS
CUPFUL
CURIUM
CURLUP
CUTOUT
CUTSUP
CYGNUS
CYPRUS

C••••U
CADEAU
CARIOU
CHANDU
CONGOU

•CU•••
ACUATE
ACUITY
ACUMEN
ACURAS
ACUTER
ACUTES
OCULAR
OCULUS
PCUSER
SCUBAS
SCUFFS
SCULLS
SCULLY
SCULPT
SCUMMY
SCURFY
SCURRY
SCURVE
SCURVY
SCUZZY

•C•U••
ACCUSE
ACQUIT
ACTUAL
ICEUPS
ICOULD
MCDUCK
MCHUGH
MCKUEN
OCCULT
OCCUPY
OCCURS
RCRUMB
SCHULZ
SCHUSS
SCOUPE
SCOURS
SCOUTS
SCRUBS
SCRUFF
SCRUMS

•C••U•
ACCRUE
ACEOUT
ACESUP
ACTIUM
ACTOUT
ACTSUP
ICARUS
ICEDUP
ICEOUT
ICERUN
ICESUP
OCULUS
SCARUM
SCHLUB

••CU••
ACCUSE
ESCUDO
EXCUBS
EXCUSA
EXCUSE
FACULA
FECUND
HECUBA
INCUBI
INCULT
INCURS
INCUSE
JOCUND
LACUNA
LOCUST
MACULA
MECUMS
OCCULT
OCCUPY
OCCURS
OSCULE
PACULA
RECUED
RECUES
RECURE
RECURL
RECURS
RECUSE
RECUTS
SECURE
UNCUFF
UNCURB
UNCURL
UNCUTE
UPCURL
VACUUM
VICUNA

••C•U•
ACCRUE
AECIUM
BACKUP
BACKUS
BUCKUP
CACTUS
COCCUS
DECIUS
DICTUM
ESCAUT
FACEUP
FACTUM
FICHUS
HACKUP
HICCUP
JACKUP
KICKUP
LACEUP
LICKUP
LOCKUP
LUCIUS
LYCEUM
MACOUN
MOCKUP
MUCKUP
OHCRUD
PACKUP
PICKUP
RACEUP
RACKUP
RECOUP
RECTUS
RUCKUP
RUCKUS
SACKUP
SACQUE
SACRUM
SUCKUP
TACKUP
VACUUM

••C••U
PICCHU

•••CU•
ABACUS
AMICUS
CANCUN
CAUCUS
CHACUN
CIRCUM
CIRCUS
COCCUS
CONCUR
CROCUS
DIECUT
DISCUS
EGGCUP
ENDCUT
EYECUP
FESCUE
HICCUP
HOTCUP
JOBCUT
LOWCUT
MARCUS
MISCUE
MISCUT
OILCUP
OUTCUT
PASCUA
PAYCUT
PRECUT
RESCUE
RIBCUT
TALCUM
TAXCUT
TEACUP
TINCUP

•••C•U
MANCHU
PICCHU

••••CU
APERCU

C•V•••
CAVAFY
CAVEAT
CAVEIN
CAVELL
CAVERN
CAVERS
CAVETT
CAVIAR
CAVIES
CAVILS
CAVING
CAVITY
CAVORT
CIVETS
CIVICS
COVENS
COVENT
COVERS
COVERT
COVETS
COVEYS
COVINA
COVING
CUVEES
CUVIER

C••V••
CALVED
CALVES
CALVET
CALVIN
CANVAS
CARVED
CARVEL
CARVER
CARVES
CARVEY
CERVID
CHAVEZ
CHEVAL
CHEVET
CHEVON
CHEVRE
CHEVYS
CHIVAS
CHIVES
CLAVES
CLAVIN
CLEVER
CLEVES
CLOVEN
CLOVER
CLOVES
CLOVIS
COEVAL
CONVEX
CONVEY
CONVOY
CORVEE
CORVID
CORVUS
CRAVAT
CRAVED
CRAVEN
CRAVER
CRAVES
CURVED
CURVES
CURVET

C•••V•
CANOVA
CASAVA
CLEAVE

C••••V
CHEKOV

•C•V••
MCAVOY

•C••V•
ACTIVA
ACTIVE
OCTAVE
OCTAVO
SCHAVS
SCURVE
SCURVY

•C•••V
SCENEV

••C•V•
ALCOVE
LACAVA

••C••V
ROCKYV
TECHTV
VACLAV

CW••••
CWPOST

C•W•••
CAWCAW
CAWDOR
CAWING
COWARD
COWBOY
COWENS
COWERS
COWIER
COWING
COWISH
COWLED
COWLEY
COWMAN
COWMEN
COWPEA
COWPER
COWPOX
COWRIE
CRWTHS

C••W••
CARWAX
CHAWED
CHEWED
CHEWER
CHEWON
CHEWUP
CHOWED
CLAWAT
CLAWED
CLAWER
CLEWED
CLOWNS
COBWEB
CONWAY
COOWNS
CORWIN
CRAWLS
CRAWLY
CREWED
CREWEL
CROWDS
CROWED
CROWER
CROWNE
CROWNS

C•••W•
CODYWY

C••••W
CALLOW
CARLOW
CASHEW
CAWCAW
CPSNOW
CRACOW
CURFEW
CURLEW
CURNOW
CUSHAW

•C•W••
MCEWAN
MCEWEN
SCHWAB
SCHWAS
SCOWLS

•C••W•
ACTTWO
SCRAWL
SCREWS
SCREWY

•C•••W
ACTNOW
ECOLAW
MCGRAW
MCGREW

••C•W•
MACAWS

••C••W
DECLAW

DRCLAW
ESCHEW
ESCROW
RECHEW
TVCREW

•••C•W
ANTCOW
CAWCAW
CRACOW
MOOCOW
MOSCOW
PESCOW
PETCOW
SEACOW

C•X•••
CIXOUS
COXING

C••X••
CALXES
COAXAL
COAXED
COAXER
COAXES
CRUXES

C••••X
CALMEX
CARWAX
CHISOX
CLIMAX
CLOROX
COCCYX
COLFAX
COMDEX
COMMIX
CONVEX
CORTEX
COWPOX

•C••X•
ICEAXE

•C•••X
ICEBOX

••C••X
COCCYX
PICKAX
WACOTX

•••C•X
COCCYX
MARCIX
MERCKX
WILCOX

CY••••
CYANIC
CYANID
CYBILL
CYBORG
CYCADS
CYCLED
CYCLER
CYCLES
CYCLIC
CYCLOS
CYDERS
CYGNET
CYGNUS
CYMBAL
CYMRIC
CYNICS
CYPHER
CYPRUS
CYRANO
CYSTIC

C•Y•••
CAYMAN
CAYUGA
CAYUSE
CEYLON
CHYNNA
CHYRON
CLYDES
COYDOG
COYEST
COYISH
COYOTE
COYPUS
CRYERS
CRYFOR
CRYING
CRYOFF
CRYOUT
CRYPTO
CRYPTS
CUYLER

C••Y••
CANYON
CLAYEY
CLOYED
CODYWY
CORYZA
COSYUP
COZYUP
CRAYON

C•••Y•
CAMRYN
CAMRYS
CATHYS
CHERYL
CHEVYS
COCCYX
COLBYS
CONEYS
COPAYS
COVEYS
CRONYN
CUTEYS

C••••Y
CAGILY
CAGNEY
CALMLY
CALORY
CAMBOY
CAMEBY
CANARY
CANOPY
CARBOY
CARKEY
CARNEY
CARREY
CARSEY
CARVEY
CASEFY
CATCHY
CATHAY
CATTOY
CAUCHY
CAVAFY
CAVITY
CEDARY
CELERY
CHAFFY
CHALKY
CHAMMY
CHANCY
CHANEY
CHANTY
CHARLY
CHATTY
CHEEKY
CHEERY
CHEESY
CHENEY
CHERRY
CHERTY
CHESTY
CHICLY
CHILLY
CHINKY
CHIRPY
CHITTY
CHOOSY
CHOPPY
CHROMY
CHUBBY
CHUCKY
CHUFFY
CHUMMY
CHUNKY
CIASPY
CICELY
CIDERY
CITIFY
CLAMMY
CLANCY
CLANKY
CLASSY
CLAYEY
CLEARY
CLERGY
CLICHY
CLIFFY
CLINGY
CLIQUY
CLODDY
CLOGGY
CLOTTY
CLOUDY
CLUBBY
CLUMPY
CLUMSY
CLUNKY
CODIFY
CODYWY
COLDLY
COLONY
COMEBY
COMEDY
COMELY
COMITY
COMPLY
CONROY
CONVEY
CONVOY
CONWAY
COOLEY
COOLLY
COONEY
COPLEY
CORDAY
COSILY
COSTLY
COUNTY
COWBOY
COWLEY
COZILY
CRABBY
CRAFTY
CRAGGY
CRAMPY
CRANKY
CRANNY
CRAWLY
CREAKY
CREAMY
CREASY
CREEPY
CRESSY
CRIKEY
CRIMPY
CRISPY
CROAKY
CROSBY
CROUPY
CRUDDY
CRUMBY
CRUMMY
CRUSTY
CUDAHY
CUDDLY
CURACY
CURLEY
CURTLY
CURTSY
CUTELY
CUTESY
CZERNY

•CY•••
SCYLLA
SCYTHE

•C•Y••
ECTYPE

•C••Y•
ACETYL

•C•••Y
ACIDLY
ACUITY
ECTOMY
ICALLY
ICHTHY
MCAVOY
OCASEY
OCCUPY
OCHERY
SCANTY
SCARRY
SCOOBY
SCOTTY
SCREWY
SCULLY
SCUMMY
SCURFY
SCURRY
SCURVY
SCUZZY

••CY••
ENCYCL
OOCYTE

••C•Y•
COCCYX
DACTYL
DECAYS
DECOYS
JACLYN
ROCKYV

••C••Y
ARCHLY
CICELY
DICKEY
DOCBOY
HACKLY
HICKEY
HOCKEY
JACOBY
JOCKEY
LACHEY
LACHOY
LACILY
LACKEY
MICKEY
NICELY
NICETY
OCCUPY
PACIFY
RACEBY
RACILY
RECOPY
RICHLY
RICKEY
SACFLY
SICILY
SICKLY
TICKBY
TICKLY
UNCLAY

•••CY•
COCCYX

•••C•Y
ALECKY
BEACHY
BINCHY
BISCAY
BLOCKY
BOTCHY
BRICKY
BUNCHY
CATCHY
CAUCHY
CHICLY
CHUCKY
CLICHY
DESCRY
DRECKY
FARCRY
FLECKY
GORCEY
LEACHY
LUNCHY
MUNCHY
MUSCLY
NOTCHY
OUTCRY
PATCHY
PEACHY
PINCAY
PITCHY
PLUCKY
POACHY
POUCHY
PRICEY
PUNCHY
QUACKY
RONCEY
SHECKY
SPACEY
STACEY
STICKY
STOCKY
TETCHY
TORCHY
TOUCHY
TRACEY
TRICKY
WARCRY
WITCHY
ZINCKY

••••CY
ABBACY
AGENCY
BOUNCY
CHANCY
CLANCY
CURACY
DRANCY
FARACY
FLEECY
IDIOCY
JOUNCY
LEGACY
LUNACY
PAPACY
PIRACY
POLICY
QUINCY

CZ••••
CZECHS
CZERNY

C•Z•••
CAZALE
COZENS
COZIED
COZIER
COZIES
COZILY
COZYUP

C••Z••
CHAZAN
CRAZED
CRAZES
CRUZAN
CURZON

C•••Z•
CABEZA
CORYZA

C••••Z
CHAVEZ
CHINTZ
COMPOZ
CORTEZ
CURTIZ

•CZ•••
ECZEMA

•C•Z••
SCUZZY

•C••Z•
SCUZZY

•C•••Z
SCHNOZ
SCHULZ

DA••••
DABBED
DABBER
DABBLE
DABNEY
DABRAT
DABSAT
DACAPO
DACHAS
DACRON
DACTYL
DADDYO
DADDYS
DADGUM
DADOED
DADOES
DAEDAL
DAEMON
DAEWOO
DAFTER
DAFTLY
DAGAMA
DAGGER
DAGGOO
DAGMAR
DAHLIA
DAILEY
DAINTY
DAISES
DAKOTA
DALAND
DALASI
DALENE
DALETH
DALETS
DALLAS
DALLES
DALTON
DAMAGE
DAMASK
DAMATO
DAMIEN
DAMITA
DAMMED
DAMMER
DAMNED
DAMNER
DAMONE
DAMORE
DAMOUR
DAMPED
DAMPEN
DAMPER
DAMPLY
DAMSEL
DAMSON
DAMSUP
DANANG
DANCED
DANCER
DANCES
DANCIN
DANDER
DANDIE
DANDLE
DANDYL
DANGED
DANGER
DANGIT
DANGLE
DANGLY
DANGME
DANIEL
DANILO
DANIOS
DANISH
DANITE
DANKER
DANKLY
DANNAY
DANNER
DANNON
DANNYS
DANOVA
DANSES
DANSON
DANTEI
DANTES
DANTON
DANUBE
DANZIG
DAOSTA
DAPHNE
DAPPED
DAPPER
DAPPLE
DARCEL
DAREME
DARENT
DARERS
DAREST
DARETO
DARIEN
DARING
DARIUS
DARKEN
DARKER
DARKLE
DARKLY
DARLIN
DARNAY
DARNED
DARNER
DARNIT
DARREN
DARRIN
DARROW
DARRYL
DARTED
DARTER
DARTLE
DARWIN
DASHED
DASHER
DASHES
DASHIS
DASHIT
DASSIN
DATARY
DATERS
DATHAN
DATING
DATIVE
DATRIL
DATSUN
DAUBED
DAUBER
DAUBES
DAUDET
DAUNTS
DAVENS
DAVIDE
DAVIDI
DAVIDL
DAVIDO
DAVIES
DAVITS
DAWBER
DAWDLE
DAWNED
DAWNON
DAWSON
DAYBED
DAYGLO
DAYHOP
DAYJOB
DAYLIT
DAYOFF
DAYOLD
DAYONE
DAYSPA
DAYTON
DAZERS
DAZING
DAZZLE

D•A•••
DBACKS
DCAREA
DEACON
DEADEN
DEADER
DEADLY
DEADON
DEAFEN
DEAFER
DEAFLY
DEAFTO
DEAIRS
DEALER
DEALIN
DEALTO
DEALUP
DEANNA
DEARER
DEARIE
DEARLY
DEARME
DEARTH
DEARTO
DEASIL
DEATHS
DHARMA
DIABLE
DIABLO
DIABOL
DIADEM
DIALED
DIALER
DIALIN
DIALOG
DIALSO
DIALUP
DIANNE
DIAPER
DIARIO
DIATOM
DLAYER
DMAJOR
DMARKS
DNAASE
DNALAB
DNASES
DOABLE
DOAKES
DOALLS
DOASET
DRABEK
DRABLY
DRAFTS
DRAFTY
DRAGEE
DRAGGY
DRAGIN
DRAGON
DRAGUP
DRAINS
DRAKES
DRAKEU
DRAMAS
DRANCY
DRAPED
DRAPER
DRAPES
DRATIT
DRAWEE
DRAWER
DRAWIN
DRAWLS
DRAWLY
DRAWON
DRAWTO
DRAWUP
DRAYED
DUALLY
DUARTE
DWARFS
DWAYNE
DYADIC

D••A••
DACAPO
DAGAMA
DALAND
DALASI
DAMAGE
DAMASK
DAMATO
DANANG
DATARY
DEBAGS
DEBARK
DEBARS
DEBASE
DEBATE
DECADE
DECADS
DECAFS
DECALS
DECAMP
DECANT
DECAPS
DECARE
DECAYS
DEDANS
DEFACE
DEFAME
DEFANG
DEFATS
DEGAGE
DEHAIR
DEJAVU
DEKALB
DELAND
DELANO
DELANY
DELAYS
DEMAIN
DEMAND
DEMARK
DEMAST
DENADA
DENALI
DENARI
DENARS
DENARY
DEPART
DEPAUL
DEPAUW
DERAIL
DERAIN
DERATE
DERATS
DESADE
DESALT
DETACH
DETAIL
DETAIN
DETARS
DEVANE
DEWARS
DFLATS
DIDACT
DIGAMY
DILATE
DIMAGE
DINARS
DIRAMS
DISANT
DISARM
DITALI
DIVANS
DIZAIN
DNAASE
DOGAPE
DOLAPS
DOMAIN
DOMANI
DONALD
DONATE
DONATH
DORADO
DORAGS
DORATI
DOSADO
DOSAGE
DOTAGE
DOTARD
DOUANE
DREADS
DREAMS
DREAMT
DREAMY
DREARY
DRYADS
DSCALE
DSHARP
DUCATS
DUGALD
DUGARD
DUNANT
DURANT
DUVALL
DYNAMO
DYNAST
DYSART

D•••A•
DABRAT
DABSAT
DACHAS
DAEDAL
DAGMAR
DALLAS
DANNAY
DARNAY
DATHAN
DEBRAH
DEBRAY
DECLAW
DEDHAM
DEEJAY
DEEPAK
DEFEAT
DEFJAM
DEFOAM
DEFRAG
DEFRAY
DELEAD
DELIAN
DELMAR
DELRAY
DELTAS
DEMEAN
DENHAM
DENIAL
DENTAL
DEODAR
DERMAL
DERMAS
DERMAT
DESSAU
DEWLAP
DIDBAD
DIGRAM
DIGSAT
DIKTAT
DILLAR
DINEAT
DINKAS
DIRHAM
DISBAR
DISMAL
DISMAS
DISMAY
DISTAL
DJEBAR
DJILAS
DNALAB
DOGDAY
DOGEAR
DOGMAS
DOGNAP
DOGSAT
DOGTAG
DOLLAR
DOLMAN
DOLMAS
DOODAD
DOODAH
DOOHAN
DORCAS
DORIAN
DORSAD
DORSAL
DORSAY
DOSSAL
DOTHAN
DOTOAT
DOUGAL
DOULAS
DRAMAS
DRCLAW
DUCTAL
DUENAS
DUNBAR
DUNCAN
DUNDAS
DUNHAM
DUNLAP
DURBAN
DURHAM
DURRAS
DVORAK
DYEVAT

D••••A
DAGAMA
DAHLIA
DAKOTA
DAMITA
DANOVA
DAOSTA
DAYSPA
DCAREA
DEANNA
DEFLEA
DENADA
DENDRA
DERITA
DESETA
DESICA
DEVEGA
DHARMA
DODECA
DODOMA
DONORA
DUENNA
DUESSA
DULLEA
DURYEA

•DA•••
ADAGES
ADAGIO
ADAPTS
EDAMES
GDANSK
IDAHOS
IDARED
ODAMAE

•D•A••
ADDAMS
ADJANI
ADNATE
ADRATE
ADWARE
ADWARS
CDCASE
CDRACK
CDRATE
EDDAIC
EDGARD
EDGARS
EDUARD
EDVARD
EDWARD
IDCARD
IDEALS
IDEATE
IDTAGS
KDLANG

•D••A•
ADIDAS
ADONAI
ADRIAN
EDEMAS
ODAMAE
ODDMAN

•D•••A
EDESSA
EDWINA
ODESSA
ODETTA

••DA••
ADDAMS
ATDAWN
BEDAUB
BEDAZE
BYDATE
CEDARN
CEDARS
CEDARY
CUDAHY
DEDANS
DIDACT
EDDAIC
EMDASH
ENDALL
ENDASH
GODARD
GODARK
HADAGO
HODADS
INDASH
IODATE
JUDAEA
JUDAIC
KODAKS
KODALY
MADAMA
MADAME
MADAMS
MEDAKA
MEDALS
MIDAIR
MODALS
OHDARN
OLDAGE
ORDAIN
PEDALS
PEDANT
PEDATE
RADARS
REDACE
REDACT
REDANS
REDANT
REDARE
REDARN
REDATE
RODALE
SEDAKA
SEDANS
SEDATE
TODATE
TODAYS
UNDAMS

UPDART
UPDATE
VEDAIC

••D•A•
AIDMAN
ANDEAN
ANDRAE
AUDIAL
BADDAY
BADHAM
BADHAT
BADMAN
BADRAP
BEDLAM
CADEAU
DEDHAM
DIDBAD
ENDEAR
ENDMAN
ENDRAN
ENDSAT
ERDMAN
ESDRAS
GIDDAP
GODEAD
HADEAN
HEDRAL
HODIAK
HODMAN
HYDRAE
HYDRAS
INDIAN
JEDGAR
JUDEAN
KIDMAN
KIDNAP
KODIAK
LYDIAN
MADCAP
MADMAN
MADMAX
MADRAS
MEDGAR
MEDIAL
MEDIAN
MEDIAS
MIDCAP
MIDDAY
MIDIAN
MIDMAY
MIDWAY
MUDCAT
MYDEAR
NADSAT
NODEAL
NODEAR
NODSAT
ODDMAN
OGDOAD
OHDEAR
OHDRAT
OLDBAT
OLDCAR
OLDGAG
OLDHAM
OLDHAT
OLDMAN
OLDPAL
OLDSAW
OLDWAY
ORDEAL
PADUAN
PEDWAY
RADIAL
RADIAN
REDBAT
REDBAY
REDCAP
REDEAL
REDHAT
REDIAL
REDOAK
REDRAG
REDRAW
REDTAB
REDTAG
RODHAM
RODMAN
RUDMAN
SADDAM
SADDAY
TODDAO
TODMAN
UNDEAD
UNDRAW
VODKAS
ZODIAC

••D••A
ANDREA
BODEGA
BUDDHA
DODECA
DODOMA
EIDOLA
ENDORA
EUDORA
FEDORA
GODIVA
INDIRA
JUDAEA
JUDOKA
LADIDA
LADOGA
MADAMA
MADERA
MEDAKA
MEDICA
MEDINA
MEDUSA
MODELA
MODENA
PADOVA
REDSEA
SEDAKA
SEDONA
WADENA
ZADORA

•••DA•
ADIDAS
AIRDAM
ALLDAY
ALYDAR
AMIDAS
ANODAL
ANYDAY
AOUDAD
APODAL
BADDAY
BAGDAD
BATDAY
BELDAM
BENDAY
BIGDAY
BILDAD
BRIDAL
CAUDAD
CAUDAL
CIUDAD
CORDAY
DAEDAL
DEODAR
DOGDAY
DOODAD
DOODAH
DUNDAS
FEUDAL
FONDAS
FRIDAY
GIDDAP
GOODAT
GOUDAS
HAIDAS
HANDAX
HEYDAY
HONDAS
HOTDAY
HOWDAH
IBADAN
ICEDAM
INADAY
JORDAN
KASDAN
LANDAT
LANDAU
MANDAN
MANDAY
MAYDAY
MAZDAS
MIDDAY
MOLDAU
MONDAY
MYRDAL
NASDAQ
NEWDAY
OCEDAR
OFFDAY
ONEDAY
PAIDAD
PANDAS
PASDAR
PATDAY
PAYDAY
PERDAY
PINDAR
PRADAS
PREDAY
RANDAL
SADDAM
SADDAY
SAIDAH
SANDAL
SENDAK
SIXDAY
SUNDAE
SUNDAS
SUNDAY
TAGDAY
TENDAY
TODDAO
TWODAY
VANDAL
VEADAR
WHODAT

•••D•A
ACADIA
ACEDIA
ALUDRA
BUDDHA
CANDIA
CARDIA
CORDIA
DENDRA
ELODEA
EXEDRA
GRADEA
NOIDEA
SANDIA
SANDRA
SONDRA
STADIA
SVEDKA
TOLDYA
TREDIA
TUNDRA

••••DA
AGENDA
AMANDA
ARMADA
ARVADA
ASSTDA
BARADA
BLANDA
BRENDA
BROADA
CANADA
CEPEDA
CICADA
COLADA
COMIDA
COULDA
DENADA
FRIEDA
GLENDA
GLINDA
IMELDA
ISOLDA
JUMADA
KAUNDA
LADIDA
LAMBDA
LAVIDA
LERIDA
LUANDA
LUCIDA
MARIDA
MASADA
MERIDA
MIRADA
NARADA
NERUDA
NEVADA
OLINDA
ONEIDA
OREIDA
PAGODA
PANADA
POSADA
PRAVDA
RAMADA
RATEDA
RESEDA
RHONDA
RUANDA
RWANDA
SALADA
SECADA
STRADA
TIENDA
UGANDA
VIGODA
WOULDA

DB••••
DBACKS

D•B•••
DABBED
DABBER
DABBLE
DABNEY
DABRAT
DABSAT
DEBAGS
DEBARK
DEBARS
DEBASE
DEBATE
DEBBIE
DEBITS
DEBLUR
DEBONE
DEBONT
DEBRAH
DEBRAY
DEBREU
DEBRIS
DEBTEE
DEBTOR
DEBUGS
DEBUNK
DEBURR
DEBUTS
DIBBLE
DOBBIN
DOBLES
DOBLIN
DOBROS
DOBYNS
DUBBED
DUBBER
DUBCEK
DUBLIN
DUBOIS
DUBOSE
DYBBUK

D••B••
DABBED
DABBER
DABBLE
DAUBED
DAUBER
DAUBES
DAWBER
DAYBED
DEBBIE
DIABLE
DIABLO
DIABOL
DIBBLE
DIDBAD
DISBAR
DISBUD
DJEBAR
DOABLE
DOBBIN
DOCBOY
DOGBED
DOMBEY
DOUBLE
DOUBLY
DOUBTS
DRABEK
DRABLY
DREBIN
DUBBED
DUBBER
DUMBER
DUMBLY
DUMBOS
DUNBAR
DURBAN
DURBIN
DYBBUK

D•••B•
DANUBE
DEMOBS
DOESBY
DONEBY
DROPBY
DWEEBS
DWEEBY

D••••B
DAYJOB
DEKALB
DNALAB
DYEJOB

•DB•••
EDBERG

•D•B••
ADOBES
ADOBOS
EDIBLE
EDIBLY

•D••B•
ADLIBS

•D•••B
ADSORB
ADVERB
ODDJOB

••DB••
BADBOY
BEDBUG
DIDBAD
OLDBAT
OLDBOY
REDBAT
REDBAY
REDBUD
TIDBIT
TYDBOL

••D•B•
INDEBT
REDUBS
RIDEBY
RODEBY

••D••B
BEDAUB
MIDRIB
MODELB
ODDJOB
REDTAB

•••DB•
EKEDBY
GOODBY
HARDBY
LAIDBY
NEEDBE
SENDBY

•••D•B
GRADEB
SUBDEB

DC••••
DCAREA
DCELLS

D•C•••
DACAPO
DACHAS
DACRON
DACTYL
DECADE
DECADS
DECAFS
DECALS
DECAMP
DECANT
DECAPS
DECARE
DECAYS
DECEIT
DECENT
DECIDE
DECILE
DECIUS
DECKED
DECKER
DECKLE
DECLAW
DECLOT
DECOCT
DECODE
DECORS
DECOYS
DECREE
DICERS
DICIER
DICING
DICKER
DICKEY
DICKIE
DICOTS
DICTUM
DOCBOY
DOCENT
DOCILE
DOCKED
DOCKER
DOCKET
DOCOMO
DOCTOR
DRCLAW
DSCALE
DUCATS
DUCHIN
DUCKED
DUCKER
DUCKIE
DUCTAL
DUCTED

D••C••
DANCED
DANCER
DANCES
DANCIN
DARCEL
DBACKS
DEACON
DEFCON
DEICED
DEICER
DEICES
DELCOS
DESCRY
DEUCED
DEUCES
DIECUT
DISCOS
DISCUS
DORCAS
DOTCOM
DRECKS
DRECKY
DUBCEK
DULCET
DUNCAN
DUNCES

D•••C•
DECOCT
DEDUCE
DEDUCT
DEFACE
DEFECT
DEJECT
DELICT
DEPICT
DESICA
DETACH
DETECT
DEUTCH
DEVICE
DEVICQ
DIDACT
DIRECT
DODECA
DODICI
DRANCY
DRENCH
DRRICE
DRYICE
DUROCS

D••••C
DEIFIC
DELTIC
DERMIC
DYADIC

•DC•••
CDCASE
IDCARD

•D•C••
EDICTS
EDUCED
EDUCES
EDUCTS

•D••C•
ADDICT
ADDUCE
ADDUCT
ADVICE
CDRACK
EDKOCH
IDIOCY

•D•••C
ADONIC
EDDAIC
EDENIC
ODINIC

••DC••
BADCOP
ENDCUT
KIDCOM
MADCAP
MIDCAP
MUDCAT
OLDCAR
REDCAP
REDCOD

••D•C•
ABDUCE
ABDUCT
ADDICT
ADDUCE
ADDUCT
ASDICS
BEDECK
BODICE
DEDUCE
DEDUCT
DIDACT
DODECA
DODICI
INDICT
INDUCE
INDUCT
MCDUCK
MEDICA
MEDICI
MEDICO
MEDICS
MEDOCS
MRDICK
NODICE
ONDECK
REDACE
REDACT
REDOCK
REDUCE
SEDICI
SEDUCE
UNDICI
UNDOCK
ZYDECO

••D••C
ANDRIC
CADMIC
CEDRIC
EDDAIC
HYDRIC
JUDAIC
OLDVIC
VEDAIC
ZODIAC

•••DC•
USEDCD

•••D•C
ACIDIC
ANODIC
BARDIC
DYADIC
EPODIC
GEODIC
HENDEC
IRIDIC
NORDIC
OXIDIC
RUNDMC
SYNDIC

DD••••
DDMMYY

D•D•••
DADDYO
DADDYS
DADGUM
DADOED
DADOES
DEDANS
DEDHAM
DEDINI
DEDUCE
DEDUCT
DEDUVE
DIDACT
DIDBAD
DIDDLE
DIDDLY
DIDFOR
DIDIES
DIDION
DIDNOT
DIDOES
DODDER
DODECA
DODGED
DODGEM
DODGER
DODGES
DODICI
DODODO
DODOES
DODOMA
DRDOOM
DUDDLE
DUDEUP
DUDING
DUDISH
DUDLEY

D••D••
DADDYO
DADDYS
DAEDAL
DANDER
DANDIE
DANDLE
DANDYL
DAUDET
DAWDLE
DEADEN
DEADER
DEADLY
DEADON
DEEDED
DEEDEE
DEIDRE
DENDRA
DENDRI
DENDRO
DEODAR
DIADEM
DIDDLE
DIDDLY
DIKDIK
DINDIN
DIODES
DODDER
DOGDAY
DOGDOM
DONDER
DOODAD
DOODAH
DOODLE
DOTDOT
DREDGE
DRUDGE
DRYDEN
DUDDLE
DUMDUM
DUNDAS
DUNDEE
DYADIC

D•••D•
DAVIDE
DAVIDI
DAVIDL
DAVIDO
DECADE
DECADS
DECIDE
DECODE
DELUDE
DEMODE
DENADA
DENUDE
DERIDE
DESADE
DESODS
DIPODY
DIRNDL
DIVIDE
DODODO
DORADO
DOSADO
DOSIDO
DOTODO
DREADS
DROIDS
DRUIDS
DRYADS
DYNODE

D••••D
DABBED
DADOED
DALAND
DAMMED
DAMNED
DAMPED
DANCED
DANGED
DAPPED
DARNED
DARTED
DASHED
DAUBED
DAWNED
DAYBED
DAYOLD
DECKED
DEEDED
DEEMED
DEFEND
DEFIED
DEFORD
DEFUND
DEICED
DELAND
DELEAD
DELVED
DEMAND
DEMOED
DEMOND
DENIED
DENNED
DENTED
DEPEND
DESEED
DEUCED
DEVOID
DIALED
DIDBAD
DIETED
DIMMED
DINGED
DINNED
DINTED
DIOMED
DIPPED
DIRKED
DISBUD
DISHED
DISKED
DISSED
DOCKED
DODGED
DOFFED
DOGBED
DOGGED
DOGOOD
DOLLED
DONALD
DONNED
DOODAD
DOOMED
DOORED
DORSAD
DOSSED
DOTARD
DOTTED
DOUSED
DOWNED
DOWSED
DRAPED
DRAYED
DRONED
DUBBED
DUCKED
DUCTED
DUELED
DUETED
DUGALD
DUGARD
DULLED
DUMPED
DUNKED
DUNNED
DURNED
DUSKED
DUSTED

•DD•••
ADDAMS
ADDEND
ADDERS
ADDICT
ADDING
ADDINS
ADDLED
ADDLES
ADDONS
ADDSIN
ADDSON
ADDSTO
ADDSUP
ADDUCE
ADDUCT
EDDAIC
EDDIED
EDDIES
EDDOES
ODDEST
ODDISH
ODDITY
ODDJOB
ODDLOT
ODDMAN
ODDMEN
ODDSON
UDDERS

•D•D••
ADIDAS
IDIDIT
ODEDON
PDIDDY

•D••D•
IDOIDO
PDIDDY

•D•••D
ADDEND
ADDLED
ADORED
EDDIED
EDGARD
EDITED
EDMOND
EDMUND
EDUARD
EDUCED
EDVARD
EDWARD
EDWOOD
IDARED
IDCARD
ODORED

••DD••
BADDAY
BADDER
BADDIE
BADDOG
BEDDED
BIDDEN
BIDDER
BUDDED
BUDDER
BUDDHA
CADDIE
CODDLE
CUDDLE
CUDDLY
DADDYO
DADDYS
DIDDLE
DIDDLY
DODDER
DUDDLE
FADDLE
FIDDLE
FODDER
FUDDLE
GADDED
GADDER
GADDIS
GEDDES
GIDDAP
HADDEN
HADDIE
HADDIX
HIDDEN
HUDDIE
HUDDLE
KIDDED
KIDDER
KIDDIE
KIDDOS
LADDER
LADDIE
LIDDED
LUDDEN
MADDED
MADDEN
MADDER
MADDIE
MADDOG
MADDOX
MADDUX
MEDDLE
MIDDAY
MIDDIE
MIDDLE
MMDDYY
MUDDED
MUDDER
MUDDLE
NODDED
NODDER
OLDDOG
PADDED
PADDER
PADDLE
PEDDLE
PIDDLE
PODDED
PUDDLE
PUDDLY
REDDEN
REDDER
REDDIN
REDDOG
REDDOT
RIDDED
RIDDEN
RIDDER
RIDDLE
RODDED
RODDER
RUDDER
SADDAM
SADDAY
SADDEN
SADDER
SADDLE
SIDDUR
SODDED
SODDEN
SUDDEN
TODDAO

TODDLE
VEDDER
WADDED
WADDER
WADDLE
WADDLY
WEDDED
WEDDER
WIDDER
ZADDIK

••D•D•

DODODO
HODADS
IODIDE
LADIDA
LADYDI
MADEDO
SODIDI
TVDVDS
YODUDE

••D••D

ADDEND
ADDLED
BADEND
BEDDED
BODIED
BUDDED
BUDGED
CADGED
DADOED
DIDBAD
DODGED
EDDIED
ENDUED
FUDGED
GADDED
GODARD
GODEAD
HEDGED
INDEED
INDUED
JUDGED
KEDGED
KIDDED
KIDVID
LADLED
LIDDED
LODGED
MADDED
MADRID
MODRED
MUDDED
NODDED
NUDGED
OGDOAD
OLDSOD
PADDED
PODDED
REDBUD
REDCOD
REDEED
REDYED
RIDDED
RIDGED
RODDED
SEDGED
SIDLED
SODDED
SUDSED
TIDIED
UNDEAD
UNDYED
WADDED
WEDDED
WEDGED

•••DD•

ATODDS
CLODDY
CRUDDY
FREDDY
PDIDDY
QUIDDE
READDS
SHEDDS
SHODDY
SKIDDY

•••D•D

ABIDED
AOUDAD
ASHDOD
BAGDAD
BALDED
BANDED
BEADED
BEDDED
BENDED
BILDAD
BIRDED
BLADED
BOLDED
BONDED
BUDDED
CANDID
CARDED
CAUDAD
CHIDED
CIUDAD
CORDED
CURDED
DEEDED
DOODAD
ELIDED
ELUDED
ERODED
EVADED
EXUDED
FENDED
FEUDED
FOLDED
FORDED
FORDID
FUNDED
GADDED
GELDED
GILDED
GIRDED
GLIDED
GOADED
GRADED
GUIDED
HANDED
HEADED
HEEDED
HERDED
HOODED
HORDED
KIDDED
LANDED
LARDED
LAUDED
LEADED
LIDDED
LOADED
LOIDED
LORDED
MADDED
MELDED
MENDED
MINDED
MISDID
MOLDED
MUDDED
NEEDED
NODDED
OUTDID
PADDED
PAIDAD
PENDED
PODDED
PONDED
PRIDED
RAIDED
REEDED
RENDED
RIDDED
RODDED
SANDED
SEEDED
SHADED
SODDED
SORDID
SPADED
SUEDED
TENDED
TRADED
USEDCD
VENDED
VOIDED
WADDED
WARDED
WEDDED
WEEDED
WELDED
WENDED
WINDED
WOODED
WORDED
YARDED

••••DD

HOWODD
MISADD
OUTADD

DE••••

DEACON
DEADEN
DEADER
DEADLY
DEADON
DEAFEN
DEAFER
DEAFLY
DEAFTO
DEAIRS
DEALER
DEALIN
DEALTO
DEALUP
DEANNA
DEARER
DEARIE
DEARLY
DEARME
DEARTH
DEARTO
DEASIL
DEATHS
DEBAGS
DEBARK
DEBARS
DEBASE
DEBATE
DEBBIE
DEBITS
DEBLUR
DEBONE
DEBONT
DEBRAH
DEBRAY
DEBREU
DEBRIS
DEBTEE
DEBTOR
DEBUGS
DEBUNK
DEBURR
DEBUTS
DECADE
DECADS
DECAFS
DECALS
DECAMP
DECANT
DECAPS
DECARE
DECAYS
DECEIT
DECENT
DECIDE
DECILE
DECIUS
DECKED
DECKER
DECKLE
DECLAW
DECLOT
DECOCT
DECODE
DECORS
DECOYS
DECREE
DEDANS
DEDHAM
DEDINI
DEDUCE
DEDUCT
DEDUVE
DEEDED
DEEDEE
DEEJAY
DEEMED
DEENIE
DEEPAK
DEEPEN
DEEPER
DEEPLY
DEERES
DEEVER
DEFACE
DEFAME
DEFANG
DEFATS
DEFCON
DEFEAT
DEFECT
DEFEND
DEFERS
DEFFER
DEFGHI
DEFIED
DEFIER
DEFIES
DEFILE
DEFINE
DEFJAM
DEFLEA
DEFOAM
DEFOGS
DEFORD
DEFORE
DEFORM
DEFRAG
DEFRAY
DEFTER
DEFTLY
DEFUEL
DEFUND
DEFUSE
DEGAGE
DEGELS
DEGERM
DEGREE
DEGUMS
DEGUST
DEHAIR
DEHIRE
DEHMEL
DEHORN
DEICED
DEICER
DEICES
DEIDRE
DEIFIC
DEIGNS
DEIMOS
DEISTS
DEJAVU
DEJECT
DEJUNK
DEJURE
DEKALB
DEKING
DEKKER
DEKKOS
DELAND
DELANO
DELANY
DELAYS
DELCOS
DELEAD
DELETE
DELFTS
DELIAN
DELICT
DELINT
DELISH
DELIST
DELIUS
DELKEY
DELMAR
DELPHI
DELRAY
DELREY
DELRIO
DELROY
DELSOL
DELTAS
DELTIC
DELUDE
DELUGE
DELUGG
DELUXE
DELVED
DELVER
DELVES
DEMAIN
DEMAND
DEMARK
DEMAST
DEMEAN
DEMIES
DEMILO
DEMISE
DEMIST
DEMITS
DEMOBS
DEMODE
DEMOED
DEMOND
DEMONS
DEMOTE
DEMOTH
DEMURE
DEMURS
DENADA
DENALI
DENARI
DENARS
DENARY
DENDRA
DENDRI
DENDRO
DENHAM
DENIAL
DENIED
DENIER
DENIES
DENIMS
DENIRO
DENISE
DENMOM
DENNED
DENNIS
DENNYS
DENOTE
DENOVO
DENSER
DENTAL
DENTED
DENTIN
DENTON
DENUDE
DENVER
DENZEL
DEODAR
DEPART
DEPAUL
DEPAUW
DEPEND
DEPERE
DEPEST
DEPICT
DEPLOY
DEPONE
DEPORT
DEPOSE
DEPOTS
DEPTHS
DEPULP
DEPUTE
DEPUTY
DERAIL
DERAIN
DERATE
DERATS
DERIDE
DERITA
DERIVE
DERMAL
DERMAS
DERMAT
DERMIC
DERMIS
DERMOT
DEROSE
DERREK
DERUST
DESADE
DESALT
DESCRY
DESEED
DESERT
DESETA
DESICA
DESIGN
DESILT
DESILU
DESIRE
DESIST
DESLUM
DESMOG
DESNOS
DESODS
DESOTO
DESPOT
DESREE
DESSAU
DESTEM
DESTRY
DETACH
DETAIL
DETAIN
DETARS
DETECT
DETENT
DETERS
DETEST
DETMER
DETOTH
DETOUR
DETROP
DETTES
DETUNE
DEUCED
DEUCES
DEUTCH
DEUTER
DEVANE
DEVEGA
DEVEIN
DEVERE
DEVERS
DEVEST
DEVICE
DEVICQ
DEVILS
DEVINE
DEVISE
DEVITO
DEVOID
DEVOIR
DEVORE
DEVOTE
DEVOTO
DEVOUR
DEVOUT
DEWARS
DEWIER
DEWILY
DEWING
DEWIRE
DEWITT
DEWLAP
DEWOLF
DEWORM
DEXTER
DEXTRO

D•E•••

DAEDAL
DAEMON
DAEWOO
DCELLS
DEEDED
DEEDEE
DEEJAY
DEEMED
DEENIE
DEEPAK
DEEPEN
DEEPER
DEEPLY
DEERES
DEEVER
DHEIGH
DIECUT
DIEFOR
DIENES
DIEOFF
DIEOUT
DIEPPE
DIESEL
DIESES
DIESIS
DIETED
DIETER
DIETES
DIEZES
DJEBAR
DOESBY
DOESIN
DOESIT
DOESNT
DOESOK
DOESSO
DOESTO
DOESUP
DREADS
DREAMS
DREAMT
DREAMY
DREARY
DREBIN
DRECKS
DRECKY
DREDGE
DRENCH
DRESSY
DREVIL
DREWIN
DREWON
DREWTO
DREWUP
DREXEL
DREYER
DUELED
DUELER
DUELLO
DUENAS
DUENNA
DUENOS
DUESSA
DUETED
DUETTI
DUETTO
DWEEBS
DWEEBY
DWELLS
DYEING
DYEJOB
DYELOT
DYEVAT

D••E••

DALENE
DALETH
DALETS
DAREME
DARENT
DARERS
DAREST
DARETO
DATERS
DAVENS
DAZERS
DECEIT
DECENT
DEFEAT
DEFECT
DEFEND
DEFERS
DEGELS
DEGERM
DEJECT
DELEAD
DELETE
DEMEAN
DEPEND
DEPERE
DEPEST
DESEED
DESERT
DESETA
DETECT
DETENT
DETERS
DETEST
DEVEGA
DEVEIN
DEVERE
DEVERS
DEVEST
DICERS
DIGEST
DIKERS
DINEAT
DINEIN
DINEON
DINERO
DINERS
DIRECT
DIRELY
DIREST
DISERE
DISEUR
DIVEIN
DIVERS
DIVERT
DIVEST
DIYERS
DOCENT
DODECA
DOGEAR
DOLENZ
DONEBY
DONEES
DONEIN
DONEIT
DONEOK
DONESO
DONETO
DONETS
DONEUP
DOPERS
DOREEN
DOREMI
DOSERS
DOTELL
DOTEON
DOTERS
DOVEIN
DOWELL
DOWELS
DOWERS
DOWERY
DOYENS
DOZENS
DOZERS
DRIERS
DRIEST
DRYERS
DRYEST
DRYEYE
DUDEUP
DUPERS
DUPERY
DURESS
DUVETS
DWEEBS
DWEEBY
DYNELS

D•••E•

DABBED
DABBER
DABNEY
DADOED
DADOES
DAFTER
DAGGER
DAILEY
DAISES
DALLES
DAMIEN
DAMMED
DAMMER
DAMNED
DAMNER
DAMPED
DAMPEN
DAMPER
DAMSEL
DANCED
DANCER
DANCES
DANDER
DANGED
DANGER
DANIEL
DANKER
DANNER
DANSES
DANTEI
DANTES
DAPPED
DAPPER
DARCEL
DARIEN
DARKEN
DARKER
DARNED
DARNER
DARREN
DARTED
DARTER
DASHED
DASHER
DASHES
DAUBED
DAUBER
DAUBES
DAUDET
DAVIES
DAWBER
DAWNED
DAYBED
DCAREA
DEADEN
DEADER
DEAFEN
DEAFER
DEALER
DEARER
DEBREU
DEBTEE
DECKED
DECKER
DECREE
DEEDED
DEEDEE
DEEMED
DEEPEN
DEEPER
DEERES
DEEVER
DEFFER
DEFIED
DEFIER
DEFIES
DEFLEA
DEFTER
DEFUEL
DEGREE
DEHMEL
DEICED
DEICER
DEICES
DEKKER
DELKEY
DELREY
DELVED
DELVER
DELVES
DEMIES
DEMOED
DENIED
DENIER
DENIES
DENNED
DENSER
DENTED
DENVER
DENZEL
DERREK
DESEED
DESREE
DESTEM
DETMER
DETTES
DEUCED
DEUCES
DEUTER
DEWIER
DEXTER
DHOLES
DHOTEL
DIADEM
DIALED
DIALER
DIAPER
DICIER
DICKER
DICKEY
DIDIES
DIDOES
DIENES
DIESEL
DIESES
DIETED
DIETER
DIETES
DIEZES
DIFFER
DIGGER
DILLER
DILSEY
DIMMED
DIMMER
DINGED
DINGER
DINNED
DINNER
DINTED
DIODES
DIOMED
DIPLEX
DIPNET
DIPPED
DIPPER
DIRGES
DIRKED
DISHED
DISHES
DISKED
DISMES
DISNEY
DISPEL
DISSED
DISSES
DITHER
DITZES
DLAYER
DNASES
DOAKES
DOASET
DOBLES
DOCKED
DOCKER
DOCKET
DODDER
DODGED
DODGEM
DODGER
DODGES
DODOES
DOFFED
DOFFER
DOGBED
DOGGED
DOGIES
DOGLEG
DOKKEN
DOLLED
DOLLEY
DOMBEY
DOMREP
DONDER
DONEES
DONKEY
DONNED
DONNER
DOOLEY
DOOMED
DOORED
DOOVER
DOOZER
DOPIER
DOREEN
DORIES
DORMER
DORSET
DORSEY
DOSSED
DOSSES
DOTTED
DOTTER
DOURER
DOUSED
DOUSER
DOUSES
DOUZES
DOWNED
DOWNER
DOWNES
DOWNEY
DOWSED
DOWSER
DOWSES
DOXIES
DOZIER
DRABEK
DRAGEE
DRAKES
DRAKEU
DRAPED
DRAPER
DRAPES
DRAWEE
DRAWER
DRAYED
DREXEL
DREYER
DRIVEL
DRIVEN
DRIVER
DRIVES
DRONED
DRONER
DRONES
DROUET
DROVER
DROVES
DRUPES
DRUSES
DRUZES
DRYDEN
DTILES
DUBBED
DUBBER
DUBCEK
DUCKED
DUCKER
DUCTED
DUDLEY
DUELED
DUELER
DUETED
DUFFEL
DUFFER
DULCET
DULLEA
DULLED
DULLER
DULLES
DUMBER
DUMPED
DUMPER
DUNCES
DUNDEE
DUNKED
DUNKER
DUNNED
DUNNER
DUPLEX
DURFEY
DURNED
DURYEA
DUSKED
DUSTED
DUSTER
DUTIES

D••••E

DABBLE
DALENE
DAMAGE
DAMONE
DAMORE
DANDIE
DANDLE
DANGLE
DANGME
DANITE
DANUBE
DAPHNE
DAPPLE
DAREME
DARKLE
DARTLE
DATIVE
DAVIDE
DAWDLE
DAYONE
DAZZLE
DEARIE
DEARME
DEBASE
DEBATE
DEBBIE
DEBONE
DEBTEE
DECADE
DECARE
DECIDE
DECILE
DECKLE
DECODE
DECREE
DEDUCE
DEDUVE
DEEDEE
DEENIE
DEFACE
DEFAME
DEFILE

DEFINE
DEFORE
DEFUSE
DEGAGE
DEGREE
DEHIRE
DEIDRE
DEJURE
DELETE
DELUDE
DELUGE
DELUXE
DEMISE
DEMODE
DEMOTE
DEMURE
DENISE
DENOTE
DENUDE
DEPERE
DEPONE
DEPOSE
DEPUTE
DERATE
DERIDE
DERIVE
DEROSE
DESADE
DESIRE
DESREE
DETUNE
DEVANE
DEVERE
DEVICE
DEVINE
DEVISE
DEVORE
DEVOTE
DEWIRE
DIABLE
DIANNE
DIBBLE
DICKIE
DIDDLE
DIEPPE
DILATE
DILUTE
DIMAGE
DIMPLE
DINGLE
DIONNE
DIPOLE
DIRIGE
DISERE
DISUSE
DIVIDE
DIVINE
DNAASE
DOABLE
DOCILE
DOFINE
DOGAPE
DOGGIE
DOLIKE
DOLORE
DOMINE
DONATE
DONGLE
DONNIE
DOODLE
DOOGIE
DOOLIE
DOOZIE
DORINE
DORMIE
DOSAGE
DOTAGE
DOTIME
DOTTIE
DOTTLE
DOUANE
DOUBLE
DRAGEE
DRAWEE
DREDGE
DROGUE
DROWSE
DROXIE
DRRICE
DRUDGE
DRYEYE
DRYICE
DSCALE
DUARTE
DUBOSE
DUCKIE
DUDDLE
DUFFLE
DUNDEE
DWAYNE
DYNODE

•DE•••

ADEEMS
ADELEH
ADELIE
ADELLE
ADENIS
ADEPTS
ADESTE
CDEFGH
EDEMAS
EDENIC
EDERLE
EDESSA
IDEALS
IDEATE
IDENTI
IDENTS
ODEDON
ODELET
ODENSE
ODEONS
ODESSA
ODETTA
ODETTE

•D•E••

ADDEND
ADDERS
ADEEMS
ADFEES
ADHERE
ADIEUS
ADIEUX
ADRENO
ADREPS
ADVENT
ADVERB
ADVERT
ADWEEK
EDBERG
EDGEIN
EDGERS
EDSELS
IDLERS
IDLEST
ODDEST
UDDERS

•D••E•

ADAGES
ADDLED
ADDLES
ADELEH
ADFEES
ADOBES
ADORED
ADOREE
ADORER
ADORES
ADRIEN
ADWEEK
EDAMES
EDDIED
EDDIES
EDDOES
EDGIER
EDILES
EDITED
EDUCED
EDUCES
IDARED
ODDMEN
ODELET
ODORED

•D•••E

ADDUCE
ADELIE
ADELLE
ADESTE
ADHERE
ADJURE
ADMIRE
ADNATE
ADOREE
ADRATE
ADRIVE
ADVICE
ADVISE
ADWARE
CDCASE
CDRATE
EDERLE
EDIBLE
EDIRNE
IDEATE
ODAMAE
ODENSE
ODETTE

••DE••

ADDEND
ADDERS
AIDERS
ALDERS
ANDEAN
ANDERS
ARDENT
ASDEEP
BADEGG
BADEMS
BADEND
BCDEFG
BEDECK
BEDEWS
BIDERS
BIDETS
BODEGA
BODETT
CADEAU
CADENT
CADETS
CEDERS
CIDERS
CIDERY
CODERS
CYDERS
DODECA
DUDEUP
EIDERS
ELDERS
ELDEST
ENDEAR
ENDERS
FADEIN
FADERS
GIDEON
GODEAD
GODEEP
GODETS
GODEYS
HADEAN
HIDEHO
HIDEKI
HIDERS
INDEBT
INDEED
INDEEP
INDENT
JUDEAN
KADEEM
KADETT
KIDEOS
LADERS
LODENS
LUDENS
MADEDO
MADEGO
MADEIT
MADEOF
MADERA
MADERO
MADEUP
MODELA
MODELB
MODELS
MODELT
MODEMS
MODENA
MODERN
MODEST
MUDEEL
MYDEAR
NODEAL
NODEAR
NUDELY
NUDEST
ODDEST
OHDEAR
OLDELI
OLDEST
ONDECK
ORDEAL
ORDERS
REDEAL
REDEED
REDEEM
REDEFY
REDENY
REDEYE
RIDEBY
RIDEIN
RIDENT
RIDERS
RIDETO
RIDEUP
RODEBY
RODEIN
RODENT
RODEOS
RODETO
RODEUP
RUDELY
RUDERY
RUDEST
RYDELL
SEDERS
TEDEUM
UDDERS
UNDEAD
UNDEEP
UNDEFT
UNDERS
UNDEWY
VIDEOS
VIDERI
WADEIN
WADENA
WADERS
WEDELN
WEDELS
WIDELY
WIDENS
WIDEOF
WIDEST
YODELS
ZYDECO

••D•E•

ABDIEL
ADDLED
ADDLES
AIDMEN
ANDREA
ANDREI
ANDRES
ANDREW
ANDREY
ANDYET
ASDEEP
AUDREY
BADDER
BADGER
BADGES
BADMEN
BEDDED
BIDDEN
BIDDER
BODIED
BODIES
BODLEY
BUDDED
BUDDER
BUDGED
BUDGER
BUDGES
BUDGET
CADGED
CADGER
CADGES
CADRES
CODGER
CUDGEL
DADOED
DADOES
DIDIES
DIDOES
DODDER
DODGED
DODGEM
DODGER
DODGES
DODOES
DUDLEY
EDDIED
EDDIES
EDDOES
ENDMEN
ENDUED
ENDUES
FIDGET
FIDLER
FODDER
FUDGED
FUDGER
FUDGES
GADDED
GADDER
GADGET
GEDDES
GIDGET
GODEEP
HADDEN
HADJES
HEDGED
HEDGER
HEDGES
HEDLEY
HEDREN
HIDDEN
HODGES
HODMEN
INDEED
INDEEP
INDIES
INDUED
INDUES
JUDAEA
JUDGED
JUDGES
KADEEM
KEDGED
KEDGER
KEDGES
KIDDED
KIDDER
KIDNEY
LADDER
LADIES
LADLED
LADLER
LADLES
LEDGER
LEDGES
LIDDED
LODGED
LODGER
LODGES
LUDDEN
MADDED
MADDEN
MADDER
MADMEN
MADRES
MADSEN
MEDLEY
MIDGES
MIDGET
MIDLEG
MIDLER
MODRED
MUDDED
MUDDER
MUDEEL
MUDHEN
NODDED
NODDER
NUDGED
NUDGER
NUDGES
ODDMEN
OLDIES
OLDMEN
OODLES
PADDED
PADDER
PADRES
PODDED
RADLEY
RADNER
REDDEN
REDDER
REDEED
REDEEM
REDHEN
REDLEG
REDOER
REDOES
REDREW
REDSEA
REDTEN
REDYED
REDYES
RIDDED
RIDDEN
RIDDER
RIDGED
RIDGES
RIDLEY
RODDED
RODDER
RODMEN
RODNEY
RUDDER
RUDNER
SADDEN
SADDER
SADHES
SADLER
SEDGED
SEDGES
SEDLEY
SIDLED
SIDLES
SIDNEY
SODDED
SODDEN
SUDDEN
SUDSED
SUDSER
SUDSES
SYDNEY
TEDKEY
TIDIED
TIDIER
TIDIES
TODIES
UNDEEP
UNDIES
UNDOER
UNDOES
UNDREW
UNDSET
UNDYED
VEDDER
WADDED
WADDER
WEDDED
WEDDER
WEDGED
WEDGES
WIDDER
WIDGET

••D••E

ABDUCE
ADDUCE
AEDILE
ALDINE
ANDRAE
AUDILE
BADDIE
BADLIE
BEDAZE
BODICE
BODINE
BODUKE
BUDGIE
BYDATE
CADDIE
CODDLE
CUDDLE
DEDUCE
DEDUVE
DIDDLE
DUDDLE
ENDIVE
ENDURE
ENDUSE
FADDLE
FIDDLE
FUDDLE
HADDIE
HADONE
HUDDIE
HUDDLE
HYDRAE
IMDONE
INDITE
INDUCE
IODATE
IODIDE
IODINE
IODISE
IODIZE
KIDDIE
LADDIE
LADUKE
MADAME
MADDIE
MEDDLE
MIDDIE
MIDDLE
MODINE
MODULE
MUDDLE
MUDPIE
NADINE
NODICE
NODOSE
NODULE
OLDAGE
PADDLE
PEDATE
PEDDLE
PIDDLE
PUDDLE
RADOME
REDACE
REDARE
REDATE
REDEYE
REDONE
REDOSE
REDTIE
REDUCE
RIDDLE
RODALE
SADDLE
SEDATE
SEDUCE
SODOWE
TODATE
TODDLE
UNDINE
UNDONE
UPDATE
UPDIKE
UPDIVE
UPDOVE
WADDLE
WEDGIE
YODUDE

•••DE•

ABCDEF
ABIDED
ABIDER
ABIDES
ABODES
ALUDEL
AMADEO
AMEDEE
AMEDEO
AMIDES
ANADEM
ANODES
ARIDER
ASIDES
AVIDER
AZIDES
BADDER
BALDED
BALDER
BANDED
BANDER
BEADED
BEADER
BEDDED
BENDED
BENDER
BIDDEN
BIDDER
BINDER
BIRDED
BIRDER
BLADED
BLADER
BLADES
BLYDEN
BOLDED
BOLDEN
BOLDER
BONDED
BONDER
BORDEN
BORDER
BORDET
BREDES
BRIDES
BRUDER
BSIDES
BUDDED
BUDDER
BULDEO
BURDEN
CALDER
CAMDEN
CARDED
CARDER
CHEDER
CHIDED
CHIDER
CHIDES
CINDER
CLYDES
COLDER
COMDEN
COMDEX
COODER
CORDED
CORDER
CRUDER
CRUDES
CURDED
DANDER
DAUDET
DEADEN
DEADER
DEEDED
DEEDEE
DIADEM
DIODES
DODDER
DONDER
DRYDEN
DUNDEE
ELIDED
ELIDER
ELIDES
ELODEA
ELUDED
ELUDER
ELUDES
EPODES
ERODED
ERODER
ERODES
ETUDES
EUSDEN
EVADED
EVADER
EVADES
EXUDED
EXUDES
FEEDER
FENDED
FENDER
FEUDED
FINDER
FODDER
FOLDED
FOLDER
FONDER
FORDED
FUNDED
FUNDER
GADDED
GADDER
GANDER
GARDEN
GEDDES
GELDED
GENDER
GEODES
GILDED
GILDER
GIRDED
GIRDER
GLADES
GLIDED
GLIDER
GLIDES
GOADED
GOLDEN
GOODEN
GOODER
GOSDEN
GRADEA
GRADEB
GRADED
GRADER
GRADES
GRIDES
GUIDED
GUIDER
GUIDES
GULDEN
HADDEN
HAIDEE
HAMDEN
HANDED
HANDEL
HANDER
HARDEN
HARDER
HAYDEN
HEADED
HEADER
HEEDED
HEEDER
HEIDEN
HENDEC
HERDED
HERDER
HIDDEN
HINDER
HOLDEM
HOLDEN
HOLDER
HOODED
HORDED
HORDES
HOYDEN
HRIDER
HYADES
IBIDEM
IMIDES
IRIDES
KANDEL
KANDER
KEYDET
KIDDED
KIDDER
KINDER
LADDER
LANDED
LANDER
LARDED
LARDER
LAUDED
LAUDER
LEADED
LEADEN
LEADER
LEIDEN
LENDEE
LENDER
LEWDER
LEYDEN
LIDDED
LIEDER
LINDEN
LINDER
LOADED
LOADER
LOIDED
LORDED
LOUDEN
LOUDER
LUDDEN
LUNDEN
MADDED
MADDEN
MADDER
MAIDEN
MALDEN
MANDEL
MARDEN
MEADER
MELDED
MELDER
MENDED
MENDEL
MENDER
MENDES
MILDER
MILDEW
MINDED
MINDEN
MINDER
MOLDED
MOLDER
MONDES
MOSDEF
MUDDED
MUDDER
MULDER
MURDER
NEEDED
NEEDER
NODDED
NODDER
NOIDEA
OXIDES
PADDED
PADDER
PANDER
PEEDEE
PENDED
PODDED
PONDED
PONDER
POWDER
PRIDED
PRIDES
PRUDES
RAIDED
RAIDER
READER
REDDEN
REDDER
REEDED
REEDER
RENDED
RENDER
RHODES
RIDDED
RIDDEN
RIDDER
ROADEO
ROADER
RODDED
RODDER
RONDEL
RUDDER
SADDEN
SADDER
SANDED
SANDER
SEEDED
SEEDER
SENDEE
SENDER
SHADED
SHADER
SHADES
SLIDER
SLIDES
SNIDER
SNYDER
SODDED
SODDEN
SOLDER
SONDES
SPADED
SPADER
SPADES
SPIDER
SPIDEY
SPODES
SPYDER
STIDES
SUBDEB
SUDDEN
SUEDED
SUEDES
SUNDER
SWEDEN
SWEDES
TANDEM
TARDES
TENDED
TENDER
TILDEN
TILDES
TINDER
TRADED
TRADER
TRADES
TSADES
VALDEZ
VARDEN
VEDDER
VENDED
VENDEE
VENDER
VERDES
VOIDED
VOIDER
WADDED
WADDER
WALDEN
WANDER
WARDED
WARDEN
WARDER
WEDDED
WEDDER
WEEDED
WEEDER
WEIDER
WELDED
WELDER
WENDED
WIDDER
WILDER
WINDED
WINDER
WINDEX
WONDER
WOODED
WOODEN
WORDED
YARDED
YARDER
YONDER

•••D•E

AMEDEE
AZODYE
BADDIE
BALDIE
BEADLE
BINDLE
BIRDIE
BLUDGE
BOODLE
BRIDGE
BRIDLE
BRODIE
BUNDLE
CADDIE
CANDLE
CODDLE
CRADLE
CUDDLE
CURDLE
DANDIE
DANDLE
DAWDLE
DEEDEE
DEIDRE
DIDDLE
DOODLE
DREDGE
DRUDGE
DUDDLE
DUNDEE
FADDLE
FEEDME
FERDIE
FIDDLE
FLEDGE
FONDLE
FONDUE
FOODIE
FOUDRE
FRIDGE
FUDDLE
GIRDLE
GOLDIE
GOODIE
GORDIE
GRUDGE
HADDIE
HAIDEE
HANDKE

HANDLE
HOLDME
HOODIE
HUDDIE
HUDDLE
HURDLE
KIDDIE
KINDLE
KLUDGE
LADDIE
LENDEE
MADDIE
MEDDLE
MERDLE
MIDDIE
MIDDLE
MUDDLE
NEEDBE
NEEDLE
NOODGE
NOODLE
ONEDGE
PADDLE
PEDDLE
PEEDEE
PERDUE
PHEDRE
PIDDLE
PLEDGE
POODLE
POUDRE
PUDDLE
PURDUE
QUIDDE
README
RIDDLE
RITDYE
ROADIE
RUNDLE
SADDLE
SAYDIE
SENDEE
SLEDGE
SLUDGE
SMIDGE
SMUDGE
STODGE
SUBDUE
SUNDAE
TIEDYE
TODDLE
TOODLE
TRUDGE
UNEDGE
UNIDLE
VATDYE
VENDEE
VENDUE
WADDLE
WENDIE
WOODIE

••••DE
ABRADE
ACCEDE
ALLUDE
ARCADE
ASHADE
AUBADE
BESIDE
BETIDE
BLENDE
BLONDE
BOLIDE
BORIDE
CHILDE
CLAUDE
DAVIDE
DECADE
DECIDE
DECODE
DELUDE
DEMODE
DENUDE
DERIDE
DESADE
DIVIDE
DYNODE
ENCODE
ETRADE
EXCIDE
FACADE
GOURDE
GRANDE
HALIDE
ILLUDE
IMPEDE
INCODE
INSIDE
INVADE
IODIDE
ISOLDE
LEVADE
MRHYDE
ONSIDE
OXHIDE
PALADE
PARADE
PESADE
POMADE
QUIDDE
RECEDE
RECODE
REHIDE
REMADE
RERIDE
RERODE
RESIDE
SALADE
SECEDE
STBEDE
STJUDE
STRIDE
STRODE
TIRADE
TRIODE
UNLADE
UNMADE
UNRUDE
UPSIDE
UVALDE
YEOLDE
YODUDE

DF••••
DFLATS

D•F•••
DAFTER
DAFTLY
DEFACE
DEFAME
DEFANG
DEFATS
DEFCON
DEFEAT
DEFECT
DEFEND
DEFERS
DEFFER
DEFGHI
DEFIED
DEFIER
DEFIES
DEFILE
DEFINE
DEFJAM
DEFLEA
DEFOAM
DEFOGS
DEFORD
DEFORE
DEFORM
DEFRAG
DEFRAY
DEFTER
DEFTLY
DEFUEL
DEFUND
DEFUSE
DIFFER
DOFFED
DOFFER
DOFINE
DUFFEL
DUFFER
DUFFLE
DUFFYS

D••F••
DEAFEN
DEAFER
DEAFLY
DEAFTO
DEFFER
DEIFIC
DELFTS
DIDFOR
DIEFOR
DIFFER
DIGFOR
DOFFED
DOFFER
DOOFUS
DRAFTS
DRAFTY
DRIFTS
DRIFTY
DRYFLY
DRYFOG
DUFFEL
DUFFER
DUFFLE
DUFFYS
DUGFOR
DURFEY

D•••F•
DAYOFF
DECAFS
DIEOFF
DRYOFF
DWARFS

D••••F
DAYOFF
DEWOLF
DIEOFF
DOURIF
DRYOFF

•DF•••
ADFEES

•D•F••
CDEFGH

•D••F•
ADOLFO
ADRIFT

••DF••
AIDFUL
BADFIT
BIDFOR
DIDFOR
GADFLY
HADFUN
JUDFRY
MADFOR
MEDFLY
REDFIN
REDFIR
REDFOX

••D•F•
BADOFF
BCDEFG
CODIFY
LEDOFF
MIDOFF
MODIFY
NIDIFY
NODOFF
REDEFY
UNDEFT

••D••F
BADOFF
LEDOFF
MADEOF
MIDOFF
NODOFF
RIDSOF
RUDOLF
WIDEOF

•••D•F
ABCDEF
FONDOF
GELDOF
KINDOF
MOSDEF
TOLDOF
VOIDOF

D•G•••
DAGAMA
DAGGER
DAGGOO
DAGMAR
DEGAGE
DEGELS
DEGERM
DEGREE
DEGUMS
DEGUST
DIGAMY
DIGEST
DIGFOR
DIGGER
DIGITS
DIGLOT
DIGOUT
DIGRAM
DIGSAT
DIGSIN
DIGSIT
DIGSUP
DOGAPE
DOGBED
DOGDAY
DOGDOM
DOGEAR
DOGGED
DOGGIE
DOGIES
DOGLEG
DOGMAS
DOGNAP
DOGONS
DOGOOD
DOGRUN
DOGSAT
DOGSIT
DOGTAG
DOGTOY
DUGALD
DUGARD
DUGFOR
DUGONG
DUGOUT

D••G••
DADGUM
DAGGER
DAGGOO
DANGED
DANGER
DANGIT
DANGLE
DANGLY
DANGME
DAYGLO
DEFGHI
DEIGNS
DIGGER
DINGED
DINGER
DINGHY
DINGLE
DINGUS
DIRGES
DODGED
DODGEM
DODGER
DODGES
DOGGED
DOGGIE
DONGLE
DOOGIE
DOTGOV
DOUGAL
DOUGHS
DOUGHY
DRAGEE
DRAGGY
DRAGIN
DRAGON
DRAGUP
DROGUE
DWIGHT

D•••G•
DAMAGE
DEBAGS
DEBUGS
DEFOGS
DEGAGE
DELUGE
DELUGG
DESIGN
DEVEGA
DHEIGH
DIMAGE
DIRIGE
DIRIGO
DOINGS
DONTGO
DORAGS
DOSAGE
DOTAGE
DRAGGY
DREDGE
DRINGS
DRUDGE

D••••G
DANANG
DANZIG
DARING
DATING
DAZING
DEFANG
DEFRAG
DEKING
DELUGG
DESMOG
DEWING
DIALOG
DICING
DIKING
DIMING
DINING
DIVING
DOGLEG
DOGTAG
DOLING
DOMING
DOPING
DOSING
DOTING
DOTORG
DOZING
DRJUNG
DRKING
DRYFOG
DRYING
DUDING
DUGONG
DUKING
DUPING
DURING
DYEING

•DG•••
EDGARD
EDGARS
EDGEIN
EDGERS
EDGIER
EDGILY
EDGING

•D•G••
ADAGES
ADAGIO

•D••G•
CDEFGH
IDTAGS

•D•••G
ADDING
ADZING
EDBERG
EDGING
IDLING
KDLANG

••DG••
BADGER
BADGES
BADGUY
BUDGED
BUDGER
BUDGES
BUDGET
BUDGIE
CADGED
CADGER
CADGES
CODGER
CUDGEL
DADGUM
DODGED
DODGEM
DODGER
DODGES
FIDGET
FUDGED
FUDGER
FUDGES
GADGET
GIDGET
HEDGED
HEDGER
HEDGES
HODGES
JEDGAR
JUDGED
JUDGES
KEDGED
KEDGER
KEDGES
LEDGER
LEDGES
LODGED
LODGER
LODGES
MEDGAR
MIDGES
MIDGET
NUDGED
NUDGER
NUDGES
OLDGAG
PIDGIN
RIDGED
RIDGES
SEDGED
SEDGES
WEDGED
WEDGES
WEDGIE
WIDGET

••D•G•
BADEGG
BEDOGS
BODEGA
HADAGO
INDIGO
LADOGA
MADEGO
OLDAGE
REDIGS

••D••G
ADDING
AIDING
BADDOG
BADEGG
BCDEFG
BEDBUG
BIDING
BODING
CEDING
CODING
DUDING
ENDING
FADING
HIDING
JADING
LADING
LUDWIG
MADDOG
MADVIG
MIDLEG
OLDDOG
OLDGAG
REDDOG
REDING
REDLEG
REDRAG
REDTAG
RIDING
SIDING
TIDING
WADING
ZEDONG

•••DG•
BLUDGE
BRIDGE
DREDGE
DRUDGE
FLEDGE
FLEDGY
FORDGT
FRIDGE
GRUDGE
KLUDGE
KLUDGY
NOODGE
ONEDGE
PLEDGE
SLEDGE
SLUDGE
SLUDGY
SMIDGE
SMUDGE
SMUDGY
STODGE
STODGY
TRUDGE
UNEDGE

•••D•G
BADDOG
BIGDIG
BIGDOG
COYDOG
FOGDOG
GUNDOG
HOTDOG
LAPDOG
MADDOG
OLDDOG
PETDOG
PYEDOG
REDDOG
SEADOG
SUNDOG
TOPDOG
TOYDOG
YOUDIG

••••DG
RATEDG

DH••••
DHARMA
DHEIGH
DHOLES
DHOTEL
DHOTIS

D•H•••
DAHLIA
DEHAIR
DEHIRE
DEHMEL
DEHORN
DRHOOK
DSHARP

D••H••
DACHAS
DAPHNE
DASHED
DASHER
DASHES
DASHIS
DASHIT
DATHAN
DAYHOP
DEDHAM
DENHAM
DIRHAM
DISHED
DISHES
DISHUP
DITHER
DOOHAN
DOTHAN
DRPHIL
DUCHIN
DUNHAM
DURHAM

D•••H•
DEATHS
DEFGHI
DELPHI
DEPTHS
DINGHY
DOUGHS
DOUGHY
DWIGHT

D••••H
DALETH
DANISH
DEARTH
DEBRAH
DELISH
DEMOTH
DETACH
DETOTH
DEUTCH
DHEIGH
DONATH
DOODAH
DOVISH
DOWITH
DRENCH
DRRUTH
DRYISH
DUDISH
DULUTH

•DH•••
ADHERE

•D•H••
IDAHOS

•D•••H
ADELEH
ADOLPH
CDEFGH
EDKOCH
ODDISH

••DH••
ANDHOW
BADHAM
BADHAT
DEDHAM
MUDHEN
OLDHAM
OLDHAT
REDHAT
REDHEN
REDHOT
RODHAM
SADHES
SADHUS

••D•H•
BUDDHA
CUDAHY
HIDEHO
WIDTHS

••D••H
DUDISH
EMDASH
ENDASH
INDASH
JADISH
JUDITH
MODISH
ODDISH
OLDISH
RADISH
WIDISH

•••DH•
BUDDHA
GANDHI
LANDHO
SAIDHI

•••D•H
DOODAH
GOODOH
HOWDAH
SAIDAH

••••DH
RIYADH

DI••••
DIABLE
DIABLO
DIABOL
DIADEM
DIALED
DIALER
DIALIN
DIALOG
DIALSO
DIALUP
DIANNE
DIAPER
DIARIO
DIATOM
DIBBLE
DICERS
DICIER
DICING
DICKER
DICKEY
DICKIE
DICOTS
DICTUM
DIDACT
DIDBAD
DIDDLE
DIDDLY
DIDFOR
DIDIES
DIDION
DIDNOT
DIDOES
DIECUT
DIEFOR
DIENES
DIEOFF
DIEOUT
DIEPPE
DIESEL
DIESES
DIESIS
DIETED
DIETER
DIETES
DIEZES
DIFFER
DIGAMY
DIGEST
DIGFOR
DIGGER
DIGITS
DIGLOT
DIGOUT
DIGRAM
DIGSAT
DIGSIN
DIGSIT
DIGSUP
DIKDIK
DIKERS
DIKING
DIKTAT
DILATE
DILLAR
DILLER
DILLON
DILSEY
DILUTE
DIMAGE
DIMING
DIMITY
DIMMED
DIMMER
DIMOUT
DIMPLE
DIMPLY
DIMSUM
DIMWIT
DINARS
DINDIN
DINEAT
DINEIN
DINEON
DINERO
DINERS
DINGED
DINGER
DINGHY
DINGLE
DINGUS
DINING
DINKAS
DINKUM
DINNED
DINNER
DINTED
DIODES
DIOMED
DIONNE
DIOXIN
DIPLEX
DIPNET
DIPODY
DIPOLE
DIPPED
DIPPER
DIPSIN
DIPSOS
DIRAMS
DIRECT
DIRELY
DIREST
DIRGES
DIRHAM
DIRIGE
DIRIGO
DIRKED
DIRNDL
DISANT
DISARM
DISBAR
DISBUD
DISCOS
DISCUS
DISERE
DISEUR
DISHED
DISHES
DISHUP
DISKED
DISMAL
DISMAS
DISMAY
DISMES
DISNEY
DISOWN
DISPEL
DISSED
DISSES
DISTAL
DISTIL
DISTRO
DISUSE
DITALI
DITHER
DITTOS
DITZES
DIVANS
DIVEIN
DIVERS
DIVERT
DIVEST
DIVIDE
DIVINE
DIVING
DIVOTS
DIXITS
DIYERS
DIZAIN

D•I•••
DAILEY
DAINTY
DAISES
DEICED
DEICER
DEICES
DEIDRE
DEIFIC
DEIGNS
DEIMOS
DEISTS
DJILAS
DJINNI
DJINNS
DMINOR
DMINUS
DMITRI
DMITRY
DOINGS
DOITUP
DRIERS
DRIEST
DRIFTS
DRIFTY
DRILLS
DRINGS
DRINKS
DRIPON
DRIPPY
DRIQJR
DRIVEL
DRIVEN
DRIVER
DRIVES
DRIVIN
DTILES
DWIGHT

D••I••
DAMIEN
DAMITA
DANIEL
DANILO
DANIOS
DANISH
DANITE
DARIEN
DARING
DARIUS
DATING
DATIVE
DAVIDE
DAVIDI
DAVIDL
DAVIDO
DAVIES
DAVITS
DAZING
DEAIRS
DEBITS
DECIDE
DECILE
DECIUS
DEDINI
DEFIED
DEFIER
DEFIES
DEFILE
DEFINE
DEHIRE
DEKING
DELIAN
DELICT
DELINT
DELISH
DELIST
DELIUS
DEMIES
DEMILO
DEMISE
DEMIST
DEMITS
DENIAL
DENIED
DENIER
DENIES
DENIMS
DENIRO
DENISE
DEPICT
DERIDE
DERITA
DERIVE
DESICA
DESIGN
DESILT
DESILU
DESIRE
DESIST
DEVICE
DEVICQ
DEVILS
DEVINE
DEVISE
DEVITO
DEWIER
DEWILY
DEWING
DEWIRE
DEWITT
DHEIGH
DICIER
DICING
DIDIES
DIDION
DIGITS
DIKING
DIMING
DIMITY
DINING
DIRIGE
DIRIGO
DIVIDE
DIVINE
DIVING

DIXITS
DOCILE
DODICI
DOFINE
DOGIES
DOLIKE
DOLING
DOMINE
DOMING
DOMINI
DOMINO
DONITZ
DOPIER
DOPILY
DOPING
DORIAN
DORIES
DORINE
DORITO
DOSIDO
DOSING
DOTIME
DOTING
DOVISH
DOWITH
DOXIES
DOZIER
DOZILY
DOZING
DRAINS
DRKING
DROIDS
DROITS
DRRICE
DRUIDS
DRYICE
DRYING
DRYINK
DRYISH
DUDING
DUDISH
DUKING
DUPING
DURING
DUTIES
DYEING

D•••I•
DAHLIA
DANCIN
DANDIE
DANGIT
DANZIG
DARLIN
DARNIT
DARRIN
DARWIN
DASHIS
DASHIT
DASSIN
DATRIL
DAYLIT
DEALIN
DEARIE
DEASIL
DEBBIE
DEBRIS
DECEIT
DEENIE
DEHAIR
DEIFIC
DELRIO
DELTIC
DEMAIN
DENNIS
DENTIN
DERAIL
DERAIN
DERMIC
DERMIS
DETAIL
DETAIN
DEVEIN
DEVOID
DEVOIR
DHOTIS
DIALIN
DIARIO
DICKIE
DIESIS
DIGSIN
DIGSIT
DIKDIK
DIMWIT
DINDIN
DINEIN
DIOXIN
DIPSIN
DISTIL
DIVEIN
DIZAIN
DOBBIN
DOBLIN
DOESIN
DOESIT
DOGGIE
DOGSIT
DOMAIN
DONEIN
DONEIT
DONNIE
DOOGIE
DOOLIE
DOOZIE
DORMIE
DORRIT
DOTTIE
DOURIF
DOVEIN
DRAGIN
DRATIT
DRAWIN
DREBIN
DREVIL
DREWIN
DRIVIN
DROMIO
DROPIN
DROPIT
DROXIE
DRPHIL
DUBLIN
DUBOIS
DUCHIN
DUCKIE
DUNKIN
DUNLIN
DURBIN
DURNIT
DUSTIN
DYADIC

D••••I
DALASI
DANTEI
DAVIDI
DEDINI
DEFGHI
DELPHI
DENALI
DENARI
DENDRI
DITALI
DJINNI
DMITRI
DODICI
DOMANI
DOMINI
DORATI
DOREMI
DUETTI

•DI•••
ADIDAS
ADIEUS
ADIEUX
EDIBLE
EDIBLY
EDICTS
EDILES
EDIRNE
EDISON
EDITED
EDITIO
EDITOR
IDIDIT
IDIOCY
IDIOMS
IDIOTS
ODINIC
ODIOUS
ODISTS
ODIUMS
PDIDDY

•D•I••
ADDICT
ADDING
ADDINS
ADLIBS
ADMINS
ADMIRE
ADMITS
ADRIAN
ADRIEN
ADRIFT
ADRIVE
ADVICE
ADVILS
ADVISE
ADZING
EDDIED
EDDIES
EDGIER
EDGILY
EDGING
EDWINA
IDLING
IDOIDO
ODDISH
ODDITY

•D••I•
ADAGIO
ADDSIN
ADELIE
ADENIS
ADJOIN
ADONIC
ADONIS
ADROIT
EDDAIC
EDENIC
EDGEIN
EDITIO
IDIDIT
ODINIC

•D•••I
ADJANI
ADONAI
ADZUKI
IDENTI

••DI••
ABDIEL
ADDICT
ADDING
ADDINS
AEDILE
AIDING
ALDINE
ALDISS
ASDICS
AUDIAL
AUDILE
AUDIOS
AUDITS
BEDIMS
BIDING
BODICE
BODIED
BODIES
BODILY
BODINE
BODING
CEDING
CODIFY
CODING
DEDINI
DIDIES
DIDION
DODICI
DUDING
DUDISH
EDDIED
EDDIES
ENDING
ENDIVE
FADING
GODIVA
HIDING
HODIAK
INDIAN
INDICT
INDIES
INDIGO
INDIRA
INDITE
INDIUM
IODIDE
IODINE
IODISE
IODIZE
JADING
JADISH
JUDITH
KODIAK
LADIDA
LADIES
LADING
LADINO
LODINJ
LYDIAN
MEDIAL
MEDIAN
MEDIAS
MEDICA
MEDICI
MEDICO
MEDICS
MEDINA
MEDIUM
MEDIUS
MIDIAN
MODIFY
MODINE
MODISH
MRDICK
NADINE
NADIRS
NIDIFY
NODICE
NUDISM
NUDIST
NUDITY
ODDISH
ODDITY
OLDIES
OLDISH
ONDISK
ONDITS
PODIUM
RADIAL
RADIAN
RADIOS
RADISH
RADIUM
RADIUS
REDIAL
REDIGS
REDING
REDINK
REDIPS
RIDING
RODINO
RODION
SADISM
SADIST
SEDICI
SIDING
SODIDI
SODIUM
TEDIUM
TIDIED
TIDIER
TIDIES
TIDILY
TIDING
TODIES
UNDICI
UNDIES
UNDIMS
UNDINE
UPDIKE
UPDIVE
VEDIST
VIDIOT
WADING
WIDISH
ZODIAC

••D•I•
ADDSIN
ALDRIN
ANDRIC
BADDIE
BADFIT
BADLIE
BEDSIT
BEDWIN
BIDSIN
BODKIN
BUDGIE
CADDIE
CADMIC
CEDRIC
EDDAIC
ENDPIN
ENDSIN
ENDSIT
FADEIN
GADDIS
GODWIN
GODWIT
HADDIE
HADDIX
HADJIS
HUDDIE
HYDRIC
JUDAIC
KIDDIE
KIDLIT
KIDVID
LADDIE
LUDWIG
MADDIE
MADEIT
MADRID
MADVIG
MEDNIS
MIDAIR
MIDDIE
MIDRIB
MUDPIE
NUDNIK
OLDVIC
ORDAIN
PIDGIN
REDDIN
REDFIN
REDFIR
REDSIX
REDTIE
RIDEIN
RODEIN
RUDKIN
TIDBIT
VEDAIC
WADEIN
WEDGIE
ZADDIK

••D••I
ANDREI
DEDINI
DODICI
HIDEKI
LADYDI
MEDICI
MIDORI
MODULI
OLDELI
SEDICI
SODIDI
UNDICI
VIDERI

•••DI•
ACADIA
ACEDIA
ACEDIT
ACIDIC
AGADIR
AMADIS
ANODIC
BADDIE
BALDIE
BANDIT
BARDIC
BENDIX
BIGDIG
BIRDIE
BOUDIN
BRODIE
CADDIE
CANDIA
CANDID
CARDIA
CARDIN
CARDIO
CLADIN
COEDIT
CORDIA
CREDIT
CUEDIN
DANDIE
DIKDIK
DINDIN
DYADIC
ELADIO
EPODIC
FEEDIN
FERDIE
FOLDIN
FOODIE
FORDID
GADDIS
GEODIC
GOLDIE
GOODIE
GORDIE
GRODIN
HADDIE
HADDIX
HANDIN
HARDIN
HEADIN
HELDIN
HELDIT
HOLDIN
HOLDIT
HOODIE
HUDDIE
ICEDIN
ICEDIT
IDIDIT
IRIDIC
JARDIN
KIDDIE
LADDIE
LAIDIN
LANDIS
LEADIN
LOADIN
LORDIT
LUNDIS
MADDIE
MAHDIS
MARDIS
MIDDIE
MISDID
NORDIC
OUTDID
OXIDIC
PAIDIN
PANDIT
PUNDIT
READIN
REDDIN
REEDIT
ROADIE
SANDIA
SARDIS
SAUDIS
SAYDIE
SENDIN
SLIDIN
SOLDIT
SORDID
STADIA
STUDIO
SYNDIC
TIEDIN
TOEDIN
TOLDIT
TREDIA
TSADIS
USEDIN
VERDIN
WENDIE
WOODIE
YOUDIG
ZADDIK

•••D•I
DENDRI
GANDHI
NORDOI
QUADRI
SAIDHI

••••DI
ALGEDI
BIONDI
BRANDI
CIARDI
COULDI
DAVIDI
FALUDI
GEORDI
LADYDI
LUNEDI
OBLADI
SAMEDI
SODIDI
YEHUDI

DJ••••
DJEBAR
DJILAS
DJINNI
DJINNS

D•J•••
DEJAVU
DEJECT
DEJUNK
DEJURE
DRJUNG

D••J••
DAYJOB
DEEJAY
DEFJAM
DMAJOR
DONJON
DYEJOB

D•••J•
DRIQJR

•DJ•••
ADJANI
ADJOIN
ADJURE
ADJUST

•D•J••
ODDJOB

••DJ••
HADJES
HADJIS
ODDJOB

••D••J
LODINJ

••••DJ
PBANDJ

D•K•••
DAKOTA
DEKALB
DEKING
DEKKER
DEKKOS
DIKDIK
DIKERS
DIKING
DIKTAT
DOKKEN
DOKTOR
DRKING
DRKOOP
DUKING

D••K••
DANKER
DANKLY
DARKEN
DARKER
DARKLE
DARKLY
DECKED
DECKER
DECKLE
DEKKER
DEKKOS
DELKEY
DICKER
DICKEY
DICKIE
DINKAS
DINKUM
DIRKED
DISKED
DOAKES
DOCKED
DOCKER
DOCKET
DOKKEN
DONKEY
DRAKES
DRAKEU
DUCKED
DUCKER
DUCKIE
DUNKED
DUNKER
DUNKIN
DUSKED

D•••K•
DBACKS
DMARKS
DOLIKE
DRECKS
DRECKY
DRINKS

D••••K
DAMASK
DEBARK
DEBUNK
DEEPAK
DEJUNK
DEMARK
DERREK
DIKDIK
DOESOK
DONEOK
DRABEK
DRHOOK
DRYINK
DUBCEK
DVORAK
DYBBUK

•DK•••
EDKOCH

•D••K•
ADZUKI

•D•••K
ADWEEK
CDRACK
GDANSK

••DK••
BODKIN
RUDKIN
RUDKUS
TEDKEY
VODKAS

••D•K•
BODUKE
HIDEKI
JUDOKA
KODAKS
LADUKE
MEDAKA
REDSKY
SEDAKA
SUDOKU
UPDIKE

••D••K
ATDUSK
BEDECK
GODARK
HODIAK
KODIAK
MCDUCK
MRDICK
NUDNIK
ONDECK
ONDISK
PODUNK
REDINK
REDOAK
REDOCK
UNDOCK
ZADDIK
ZEDONK

•••DK•
HANDKE
SVEDKA

•••D•K
DIKDIK
ENIDOK
SAIDOK
SENDAK
ZADDIK

DL••••
DLAYER

D•L•••
DALAND
DALASI
DALENE
DALETH
DALETS
DALLAS
DALLES
DALTON
DELAND
DELANO
DELANY
DELAYS
DELCOS
DELEAD
DELETE
DELFTS
DELIAN
DELICT
DELINT
DELISH
DELIST
DELIUS
DELKEY
DELMAR
DELPHI
DELRAY
DELREY
DELRIO
DELROY
DELSOL
DELTAS
DELTIC
DELUDE
DELUGE
DELUGG
DELUXE
DELVED
DELVER
DELVES
DFLATS
DILATE
DILLAR
DILLER
DILLON
DILSEY
DILUTE
DOLAPS
DOLENZ
DOLIKE
DOLING
DOLLAR
DOLLED
DOLLEY
DOLLOP
DOLLUP
DOLMAN
DOLMAS
DOLORE
DOLORS
DOLOUR
DOLTON
DULCET
DULLEA
DULLED
DULLER
DULLES
DULUTH

D••L••
DAHLIA
DAILEY
DALLAS
DALLES
DARLIN
DAYLIT
DCELLS
DEALER
DEALIN
DEALTO
DEALUP
DEBLUR
DECLAW
DECLOT
DEFLEA
DEPLOY
DESLUM
DEWLAP
DHOLES
DIALED
DIALER
DIALIN
DIALOG
DIALSO
DIALUP
DIGLOT
DILLAR
DILLER
DILLON
DIPLEX
DJILAS
DNALAB
DOALLS
DOBLES
DOBLIN
DOGLEG
DOLLAR
DOLLED
DOLLEY
DOLLOP
DOLLUP
DOOLEY
DOOLIE
DOULAS
DRCLAW
DRILLS
DROLLS
DROLLY
DTILES
DUALLY
DUBLIN
DUDLEY
DUELED
DUELER
DUELLO
DULLEA
DULLED
DULLER
DULLES
DUNLAP
DUNLIN
DUNLOP
DUPLEX
DUPLOS
DWELLS
DYELOT

D•••L•
DABBLE
DAFTLY
DAMPLY
DANDLE
DANGLE
DANGLY
DANILO
DANKLY
DAPPLE
DARKLE
DARKLY
DARTLE
DAWDLE
DAYGLO
DAYOLD
DAZZLE
DCELLS
DEADLY
DEAFLY
DEARLY
DECALS
DECILE
DECKLE
DEEPLY
DEFILE
DEFTLY
DEGELS
DEKALB
DEMILO
DENALI
DEPULP
DESALT
DESILT
DESILU
DEVILS
DEWILY
DEWOLF
DIABLE
DIABLO
DIBBLE
DIDDLE
DIDDLY
DIMPLE
DIMPLY
DINGLE
DIPOLE
DIRELY
DITALI
DOABLE
DOALLS
DOCILE
DONALD
DONGLE
DOODLE
DOPILY
DOTELL
DOTTLE
DOUBLE
DOUBLY
DOURLY
DOWELL
DOWELS
DOZILY
DRABLY
DRAWLS
DRAWLY
DRILLS
DROLLS
DROLLY
DROOLS
DROOLY
DRYFLY
DSCALE
DUALLY
DUDDLE
DUELLO
DUFFLE
DUGALD
DUMBLY
DUVALL
DWELLS
DYNELS

D••••L
DACTYL
DAEDAL
DAMSEL
DANDYL
DANIEL
DARCEL
DARRYL
DATRIL
DAVIDL
DEASIL
DEFUEL
DEHMEL
DELSOL
DENIAL
DENTAL
DENZEL
DEPAUL
DERAIL
DERMAL
DETAIL
DHOTEL
DIABOL
DIESEL
DIRNDL
DISMAL
DISPEL
DISTAL
DISTIL
DORSAL
DOSSAL
DOTELL
DOUGAL
DOWELL
DREVIL
DREXEL
DRIVEL
DRPHIL
DUCTAL
DUFFEL
DUVALL

•DL•••
ADLIBS
IDLERS
IDLEST

IDLING
KDLANG

•D•L••
ADDLED
ADDLES
ADELEH
ADELIE
ADELLE
ADOLFO
ADOLPH
ADULTS
EDILES
IDOLUM
IDYLLS
ODDLOT
ODELET

•D••L•
ADELLE
ADVILS
EDERLE
EDGILY
EDIBLE
EDIBLY
EDSELS
IDEALS
IDYLLS
ODOULS

••DL••
ADDLED
ADDLES
BADLIE
BADLOT
BEDLAM
BODLEY
DUDLEY
FIDLER
HEDLEY
KIDLIT
LADLED
LADLER
LADLES
LUDLOW
LUDLUM
MADLYN
MEDLEY
MIDLEG
MIDLER
ODDLOT
OODLES
RADLEY
REDLEG
RIDLEY
SADLER
SEDLEY
SIDLED
SIDLES

••D•L•
AEDILE
ASDULL
AUDILE
BODILY
CODDLE
CUDDLE
CUDDLY
DIDDLE
DIDDLY
DUDDLE
EIDOLA
ENDALL
FADDLE
FIDDLE
FUDDLE
GADFLY
HUDDLE
KIDULT
KODALY
MEDALS
MEDDLE
MEDFLY
MIDDLE
MODALS
MODELA
MODELB
MODELS
MODELT
MODULE
MODULI
MODULO
MUDDLE
NODULE
NUDELY
OLDELI
PADDLE
PEDALS
PEDDLE
PIDDLE
PUDDLE
PUDDLY
RIDDLE
RODALE
RUDELY
RUDOLF
RYDELL
SADDLE
TIDILY
TODDLE
UNDULY
WADDLE
WADDLY
WEDELN
WEDELS
WIDELY
YODELS

••D••L
ABDIEL
AIDFUL
ASDULL
AUDIAL
CUDGEL
ENDALL
HEDRAL
MEDIAL
MUDEEL
NODEAL
OLDPAL
ORDEAL
RADIAL
REDEAL
REDIAL
RYDELL
TYDBOL

•••DL•
ACIDLY
AGEDLY
ARIDLY
AVIDLY
AWEDLY
BALDLY
BEADLE
BINDLE
BOLDLY
BOODLE
BRIDLE
BUNDLE
CANDLE
CODDLE
COLDLY
CRADLE
CUDDLE
CUDDLY
CURDLE
DANDLE
DAWDLE
DEADLY
DIDDLE
DIDDLY
DOODLE
DUDDLE
FADDLE
FIDDLE
FONDLE
FONDLY
FUDDLE
GIRDLE
GLADLY
GOODLY
HANDLE
HARDLY
HUDDLE
HURDLE
KINDLE
KINDLY
LEWDLY
LORDLY
LOUDLY
MEDDLE
MERDLE
MIDDLE
MILDLY
MUDDLE
NEEDLE
NOODLE
PADDLE
PANDLS
PEDDLE
PIDDLE
POODLE
PUDDLE
PUDDLY
RIDDLE
RUNDLE
SADDLE
STUDLY
TODDLE
TOODLE
UNIDLE
UNIDLY
WADDLE
WADDLY
WILDLY

•••D•L
ALUDEL
AMIDOL
ANODAL
APODAL
BRIDAL
CAUDAL
DAEDAL
DANDYL
FEUDAL
HANDEL
KANDEL
MANDEL
MENDEL
MYRDAL
OXYDOL
RANDAL
RONDEL
SANDAL
TVIDOL
VANDAL

••••DL
DAVIDL
DIRNDL
GRINDL

DM••••
DMAJOR
DMARKS
DMINOR
DMINUS
DMITRI
DMITRY

D•M•••
DAMAGE
DAMASK
DAMATO
DAMIEN
DAMITA
DAMMED
DAMMER
DAMNED
DAMNER
DAMONE
DAMORE
DAMOUR
DAMPED
DAMPEN
DAMPER
DAMPLY
DAMSEL
DAMSON
DAMSUP
DDMMYY
DEMAIN
DEMAND
DEMARK
DEMAST
DEMEAN
DEMIES
DEMILO
DEMISE
DEMIST
DEMITS
DEMOBS
DEMODE
DEMOED
DEMOND
DEMONS
DEMOTE
DEMOTH
DEMURE
DEMURS
DIMAGE
DIMING
DIMITY
DIMMED
DIMMER
DIMOUT
DIMPLE
DIMPLY
DIMSUM
DIMWIT
DOMAIN
DOMANI
DOMBEY
DOMINE
DOMING
DOMINI
DOMINO
DOMREP
DUMBER
DUMBLY
DUMBOS
DUMDUM
DUMONT
DUMPED
DUMPER
DUMPON
DUMPTY

D••M••
DAEMON
DAGMAR
DAMMED
DAMMER
DDMMYY
DEEMED
DEHMEL
DEIMOS
DELMAR
DENMOM
DERMAL
DERMAS
DERMAT
DERMIC
DERMIS
DERMOT
DESMOG
DETMER
DIMMED
DIMMER
DIOMED
DISMAL
DISMAS
DISMAY
DISMES
DOGMAS
DOLMAN
DOLMAS
DOOMED
DOOMTO
DORMER
DORMIE
DRAMAS
DROMIO
DRUMUP
DRYMOP
DUOMOS

D•••M•
DAGAMA
DANGME
DAREME
DEARME
DECAMP
DEFAME
DEGUMS
DENIMS
DHARMA
DIGAMY
DIRAMS
DOCOMO
DODOMA
DOREMI
DOSUMS
DOTIME
DREAMS
DREAMT
DREAMY
DURUMS
DYNAMO

D••••M
DADGUM
DEDHAM
DEFJAM
DEFOAM
DEFORM
DEGERM
DENHAM
DENMOM
DESLUM
DESTEM
DEWORM
DIADEM
DIATOM
DICTUM
DIGRAM
DIMSUM
DINKUM
DIRHAM
DISARM
DODGEM
DOGDOM
DORSUM
DOTCOM
DRDOOM
DUMDUM
DUNHAM
DURHAM

•DM•••
ADMINS
ADMIRE
ADMITS
DDMMYY
EDMOND
EDMUND

•D•M••
DDMMYY
EDAMES
EDEMAS
ODAMAE
ODDMAN
ODDMEN

•D••M•
ADDAMS
ADEEMS
CDROMS
IDIOMS
ODIUMS

•D•••M
ADYTUM
IDOLUM

••DM••
AIDMAN
AIDMEN
BADMAN
BADMEN
CADMIC
CADMUS
ENDMAN
ENDMEN
ERDMAN
HODMAN
HODMEN
KIDMAN
MADMAN
MADMAX
MADMEN
MIDMAY
ODDMAN
ODDMEN
OLDMAN
OLDMEN
RODMAN
RODMEN
RUDMAN
TODMAN

••D•M•
ADDAMS
BADEMS
BEDIMS
DODOMA
MADAMA
MADAME
MADAMS
MODEMS
RADOME
SEDUMS
UNDAMS
UNDIMS

••D••M
BADHAM
BEDLAM
DADGUM
DEDHAM
DODGEM
DRDOOM
INDIUM
KADEEM
KIDCOM
LUDLUM
MEDIUM
NUDISM
OLDHAM
PODIUM
RADIUM
REDEEM
REDRUM
RODHAM
SADDAM
SADISM
SODIUM
TEDEUM
TEDIUM

•••DM•
FEEDME
HOLDME
MANDMS
README
RUNDMC

•••D•M
AIRDAM
ANADEM
BELDAM
CATDOM
DIADEM
DOGDOM
DUMDUM
FANDOM
HOLDEM
IBIDEM
ICEDAM
RANDOM
SADDAM
SELDOM
TANDEM
WINDOM
WISDOM

DN••••
DNAASE
DNALAB
DNASES

D•N•••
DANANG
DANCED
DANCER
DANCES
DANCIN
DANDER
DANDIE
DANDLE
DANDYL
DANGED
DANGER
DANGIT
DANGLE
DANGLY
DANGME
DANIEL
DANILO
DANIOS
DANISH
DANITE
DANKER
DANKLY
DANNAY
DANNER
DANNON
DANNYS
DANOVA
DANSES
DANSON
DANTEI
DANTES
DANTON
DANUBE
DANZIG
DENADA
DENALI
DENARI
DENARS
DENARY
DENDRA
DENDRI
DENDRO
DENHAM
DENIAL
DENIED
DENIER
DENIES
DENIMS
DENIRO
DENISE
DENMOM
DENNED
DENNIS
DENNYS
DENOTE
DENOVO
DENSER
DENTAL
DENTED
DENTIN
DENTON
DENUDE
DENVER
DENZEL
DINARS
DINDIN
DINEAT
DINEIN
DINEON
DINERO
DINERS
DINGED
DINGER
DINGHY
DINGLE
DINGUS
DINING
DINKAS
DINKUM
DINNED
DINNER
DINTED
DONALD
DONATE
DONATH
DONDER
DONEBY
DONEES
DONEIN
DONEIT
DONEOK
DONESO
DONETO
DONETS
DONEUP
DONGLE
DONITZ
DONJON
DONKEY
DONNED
DONNER
DONNIE
DONORA
DONORS
DONOSO
DONTGO
DONUTS
DUNANT
DUNBAR
DUNCAN
DUNCES
DUNDAS
DUNDEE
DUNHAM
DUNKED
DUNKER
DUNKIN
DUNLAP
DUNLIN
DUNLOP
DUNNED
DUNNER
DYNAMO
DYNAST
DYNELS
DYNODE

D••N••
DABNEY
DAINTY
DAMNED
DAMNER
DANNAY
DANNER
DANNON
DANNYS
DARNAY
DARNED
DARNER
DARNIT
DAUNTS
DAWNED
DAWNON
DEANNA
DEENIE
DENNED
DENNIS
DENNYS
DESNOS
DIANNE
DIDNOT
DIENES
DINNED
DINNER
DIONNE
DIPNET
DIRNDL
DISNEY
DJINNI
DJINNS
DMINOR
DMINUS
DOGNAP
DOINGS
DONNED
DONNER
DONNIE
DOWNED
DOWNER
DOWNES
DOWNEY
DOWNON
DRANCY
DRENCH
DRINGS
DRINKS
DRONED
DRONER
DRONES
DUENAS
DUENNA
DUENOS
DUNNED
DUNNER
DURNED
DURNIT

D•••N•
DALAND
DALENE
DAMONE
DANANG
DAPHNE
DARENT
DARING
DATING
DAVENS
DAYONE
DAZING
DEANNA
DEBONE
DEBONT
DEBUNK
DECANT
DECENT
DEDANS
DEDINI
DEFANG
DEFEND
DEFINE
DEFUND
DEIGNS
DEJUNK
DEKING
DELAND
DELANO
DELANY
DELINT
DEMAND
DEMOND
DEMONS
DEPEND
DEPONE
DETENT
DETUNE
DEVANE
DEVINE
DEWING
DIANNE
DICING
DIKING
DIMING
DINING
DIONNE
DISANT
DIVANS
DIVINE
DIVING
DJINNI
DJINNS
DOBYNS
DOCENT
DOESNT
DOFINE
DOGONS
DOLENZ
DOLING
DOMANI
DOMINE
DOMING
DOMINI
DOMINO
DOPING
DORINE
DOSING
DOTING
DOUANE
DOYENS
DOZENS
DOZING
DRAINS
DRJUNG
DRKING
DROWNS
DRYING
DRYINK
DUDING
DUENNA
DUGONG
DUKING
DUMONT
DUNANT
DUPING
DUPONT
DURANT
DURING
DWAYNE
DYEING

D••••N
DACRON
DAEMON
DALTON
DAMIEN
DAMPEN
DAMSON
DANCIN
DANNON
DANSON
DANTON
DARIEN
DARKEN
DARLIN
DARREN
DARRIN
DARWIN
DASSIN
DATHAN
DATSUN
DAWNON
DAWSON
DAYTON
DEACON
DEADEN
DEADON
DEAFEN
DEALIN
DEEPEN
DEFCON
DEHORN
DELIAN
DEMAIN
DEMEAN
DENTIN
DENTON
DERAIN
DESIGN
DETAIN
DEVEIN
DIALIN
DIDION
DIGSIN
DILLON
DINDIN
DINEIN
DINEON
DIOXIN
DIPSIN
DISOWN
DIVEIN
DIZAIN
DOBBIN
DOBLIN
DOESIN
DOGRUN
DOKKEN
DOLMAN
DOLTON
DOMAIN
DONEIN
DONJON
DOOHAN
DOREEN
DORIAN
DOTEON
DOTHAN
DOVEIN
DOWNON
DOWSON
DRAGIN
DRAGON
DRAWIN
DRAWON
DREBIN
DREWIN
DREWON
DRIPON
DRIVEN
DRIVIN
DROPIN
DRYDEN
DRYRUN
DUBLIN
DUCHIN
DUMPON
DUNCAN
DUNKIN
DUNLIN
DURBAN
DURBIN
DUSTIN
DUTTON

•DN•••
ADNATE
ADNOUN

•D•N••
ADENIS
ADONAI
ADONIC
ADONIS
EDENIC
GDANSK
IDENTI
IDENTS
IDONOT
IDUNNO
ODENSE
ODINIC
ODONTO

•D••N•
ADDEND
ADDING
ADDINS
ADDONS
ADJANI
ADMINS
ADORNS
ADRENO
ADVENT
ADZING
EDGING
EDIRNE
EDMOND
EDMUND
EDWINA
EDWYNN
IDLING
IDUNNO
KDLANG
ODEONS

•D•••N
ADDSIN
ADDSON
ADJOIN
ADNOUN
ADRIAN
ADRIEN
EDGEIN
EDISON
EDWYNN
ODDMAN
ODDMEN
ODDSON
ODEDON

••DN••
DIDNOT
KIDNAP
KIDNEY
MEDNIS
NUDNIK
RADNER
RADNOR
RODNEY
RUDNER
SIDNEY
SYDNEY

••D•N•
ADDEND
ADDING
ADDINS
ADDONS
AIDING
ALDINE
ARDENT
BADEND
BADUNS
BIDING
BODINE
BODING
CADENT
CEDING
CODING
CODONS
DEDANS
DEDINI
DUDING
ENDING
FADING
HADONE
HIDING
IMDONE
INDENT
IODINE
JADING
LADING
LADINO
LODENS
LODINJ
LUDENS
MEDINA
MIDONS
MODENA
MODINE
NADINE
PEDANT
PODUNK
REDANS
REDANT
REDENY
REDING
REDINK
REDONE
RIDENT
RIDING
RODENT
RODINO
SEDANS
SEDONA
SIDING
TIDING
UNDINE

UNDONE
WADENA
WADING
WIDENS
ZEDONG
ZEDONK

••D••N
ADDSIN
ADDSON
AIDMAN
AIDMEN
ALDRIN
ANDEAN
ATDAWN
BADMAN
BADMEN
BEDWIN
BIDDEN
BIDSIN
BIDSON
BODKIN
CEDARN
DIDION
ENDMAN
ENDMEN
ENDPIN
ENDRAN
ENDRUN
ENDSIN
ENDSON
ERDMAN
FADEIN
GIDEON
GODOWN
GODSON
GODWIN
HADDEN
HADEAN
HADFUN
HADRON
HEDREN
HEDRON
HIDDEN
HODMAN
HODMEN
HUDSON
INDIAN
JUDEAN
JUDSON
KIDMAN
LUDDEN
LYDIAN
MADDEN
MADLYN
MADMAN
MADMEN
MADSEN
MEDIAN
MIDIAN
MODERN
MUDHEN
ODDMAN
ODDMEN
ODDSON
OHDARN
OLDMAN
OLDMEN
ORDAIN
PADUAN
PIDGIN
RADIAN
REDARN
REDDEN
REDDIN
REDFIN
REDHEN
REDSUN
REDTEN
RIDDEN
RIDEIN
RODEIN
RODION
RODMAN
RODMEN
RUDKIN
RUDMAN
SADDEN
SODDEN
SUDDEN
TODMAN
WADEIN
WEDELN

•••DN•
NEEDNT
SAIDNO

•••D•N
AVEDON
BIDDEN
BLYDEN
BOLDEN
BORDEN
BOUDIN
BURDEN
CAMDEN
CARDIN
CLADIN
COMDEN
CORDON
CUEDIN
DEADEN
DEADON
DINDIN
DRYDEN
EUSDEN
FEEDIN
FEEDON
FELDON
FOLDIN
GARDEN
GOLDEN
GOODEN
GORDON
GOSDEN
GRODIN
GULDEN
HADDEN
HAMDEN
HANDIN
HANDON
HARDEN
HARDIN
HAYDEN
HEADIN
HEADON
HEIDEN
HELDIN
HELDON
HIDDEN
HOLDEN
HOLDIN
HOLDON
HOUDON
HOYDEN
IBADAN
ICEDIN
JARDIN
JOEDON
JORDAN
KASDAN
LAIDIN
LAIDON
LANDON
LARDON
LEADEN
LEADIN
LEADON
LEIDEN
LEYDEN
LIEDON
LINDEN
LOADIN
LONDON
LOUDEN
LOUDON
LUDDEN
LUNDEN
LYNDON
MADDEN
MAIDEN
MALDEN
MANDAN
MARDEN
MINDEN
ODEDON
OWEDON
PAIDIN
PARDON
PRODON
RAWDON
READIN
READON
REDDEN
REDDIN
RIDDEN
SADDEN
SENDIN
SENDON
SHEDON
SLIDIN
SODDEN
SOLDON
SUDDEN
SWEDEN
TENDON
TIEDIN
TIEDON
TILDEN
TOEDIN
TOLDON
TRODON
USEDIN
USEDON
VARDEN
VERDIN
VERDON
VERDUN
VIRDON
WALDEN
WARDEN
WELDON
WOODEN

DO••••
DOABLE
DOAKES
DOALLS
DOASET
DOBBIN
DOBLES
DOBLIN
DOBROS
DOBYNS
DOCBOY
DOCENT
DOCILE
DOCKED
DOCKER
DOCKET
DOCOMO
DOCTOR
DODDER
DODECA
DODGED
DODGEM
DODGER
DODGES
DODICI
DODODO
DODOES
DODOMA
DOESBY
DOESIN
DOESIT
DOESNT
DOESOK
DOESSO
DOESTO
DOESUP
DOFFED
DOFFER
DOFINE
DOGAPE
DOGBED
DOGDAY
DOGDOM
DOGEAR
DOGGED
DOGGIE
DOGIES
DOGLEG
DOGMAS
DOGNAP
DOGONS
DOGOOD
DOGRUN
DOGSAT
DOGSIT
DOGTAG
DOGTOY
DOINGS
DOITUP
DOKKEN
DOKTOR
DOLAPS
DOLENZ
DOLIKE
DOLING
DOLLAR
DOLLED
DOLLEY
DOLLOP
DOLLUP
DOLMAN
DOLMAS
DOLORE
DOLORS
DOLOUR
DOLTON
DOMAIN
DOMANI
DOMBEY
DOMINE
DOMING
DOMINI
DOMINO
DOMREP
DONALD
DONATE
DONATH
DONDER
DONEBY
DONEES
DONEIN
DONEIT
DONEOK
DONESO
DONETO
DONETS
DONEUP
DONGLE
DONITZ
DONJON
DONKEY
DONNED
DONNER
DONNIE
DONORA
DONORS
DONOSO
DONTGO
DONUTS
DOODAD
DOODAH
DOODLE
DOOFUS
DOOGIE
DOOHAN
DOOLEY
DOOLIE
DOOMED
DOOMTO
DOORED
DOOVER
DOOWOP
DOOZER
DOOZIE
DOPERS
DOPIER
DOPILY
DOPING
DORADO
DORAGS
DORATI
DORCAS
DOREEN
DOREMI
DORIAN
DORIES
DORINE
DORITO
DORMER
DORMIE
DORRIT
DORSAD
DORSAL
DORSAY
DORSET
DORSEY
DORSUM
DOSADO
DOSAGE
DOSERS
DOSIDO
DOSING
DOSSAL
DOSSED
DOSSES
DOSUMS
DOTAGE
DOTARD
DOTCOM
DOTDOT
DOTELL
DOTEON
DOTERS
DOTGOV
DOTHAN
DOTIME
DOTING
DOTOAT
DOTODO
DOTORG
DOTTED
DOTTER
DOTTIE
DOTTLE
DOUANE
DOUBLE
DOUBLY
DOUBTS
DOUGAL
DOUGHS
DOUGHY
DOULAS
DOURER
DOURIF
DOURLY
DOUSED
DOUSER
DOUSES
DOUZES
DOVEIN
DOVISH
DOWELL
DOWELS
DOWERS
DOWERY
DOWITH
DOWNED
DOWNER
DOWNES
DOWNEY
DOWNON
DOWSED
DOWSER
DOWSES
DOWSON
DOXIES
DOYENS
DOZENS
DOZERS
DOZIER
DOZILY
DOZING

D•O•••
DAOSTA
DEODAR
DHOLES
DHOTEL
DHOTIS
DIODES
DIOMED
DIONNE
DIOXIN
DOODAD
DOODAH
DOODLE
DOOFUS
DOOGIE
DOOHAN
DOOLEY
DOOLIE
DOOMED
DOOMTO
DOORED
DOOVER
DOOWOP
DOOZER
DOOZIE
DROGUE
DROIDS
DROITS
DROLLS
DROLLY
DROMIO
DRONED
DRONER
DRONES
DROOLS
DROOLY
DROOPS
DROOPY
DROPBY
DROPIN
DROPIT
DROPSY
DROSSY
DROUET
DROVER
DROVES
DROWNS
DROWSE
DROWSY
DROXIE
DUOMOS
DVORAK

D••O••
DADOED
DADOES
DAKOTA
DAMONE
DAMORE
DAMOUR
DANOVA
DAYOFF
DAYOLD
DAYONE
DEBONE
DEBONT
DECOCT
DECODE
DECORS
DECOYS
DEFOAM
DEFOGS
DEFORD
DEFORE
DEFORM
DEHORN
DEMOBS
DEMODE
DEMOED
DEMOND
DEMONS
DEMOTE
DEMOTH
DENOTE
DENOVO
DEPONE
DEPORT
DEPOSE
DEPOTS
DEROSE
DESODS
DESOTO
DETOTH
DETOUR
DEVOID
DEVOIR
DEVORE
DEVOTE
DEVOTO
DEVOUR
DEVOUT
DEWOLF
DEWORM
DICOTS
DIDOES
DIEOFF
DIEOUT
DIGOUT
DIMOUT
DIPODY
DIPOLE
DISOWN
DIVOTS
DOCOMO
DODODO
DODOES
DODOMA
DOGONS
DOGOOD
DOLORE
DOLORS
DOLOUR
DONORA
DONORS
DONOSO
DOTOAT
DOTODO
DOTORG
DRDOOM
DRHOOK
DRKOOP
DROOLS
DROOLY
DROOPS
DROOPY
DRYOFF
DRYOUT
DUBOIS
DUBOSE
DUGONG
DUGOUT
DUMONT
DUPONT
DUROCS
DYNODE

D•••O•
DACRON
DAEMON
DAEWOO
DAGGOO
DALTON
DAMSON
DANIOS
DANNON
DANSON
DANTON
DARROW
DAWNON
DAWSON
DAYHOP
DAYJOB
DAYTON
DEACON
DEADON
DEBTOR
DECLOT
DEFCON
DEIMOS
DEKKOS
DELCOS
DELROY
DELSOL
DENMOM
DENTON
DEPLOY
DERMOT
DESMOG
DESNOS
DESPOT
DETROP
DIABOL
DIALOG
DIATOM
DIDFOR
DIDION
DIDNOT
DIEFOR
DIGFOR
DIGLOT
DILLON
DINEON
DIPSOS
DISCOS
DITTOS
DMAJOR
DMINOR
DOBROS
DOCBOY
DOCTOR
DOESOK
DOGDOM
DOGOOD
DOGTOY
DOKTOR
DOLLOP
DOLTON
DONEOK
DONJON
DOOWOP
DOTCOM
DOTDOT
DOTEON
DOTGOV
DOWNON
DOWSON
DRAGON
DRAWON
DRDOOM
DREWON
DRHOOK
DRIPON
DRKOOP
DRYFOG
DRYMOP
DRYROT
DUENOS
DUGFOR
DUMBOS
DUMPON
DUNLOP
DUOMOS
DUPLOS
DUTTON
DYEJOB
DYELOT

D••••O
DACAPO
DADDYO
DAEWOO
DAGGOO
DAMATO
DANILO
DARETO
DAVIDO
DAYGLO
DEAFTO
DEALTO
DEARTO
DELANO
DELRIO
DEMILO
DENDRO
DENIRO
DENOVO
DESOTO
DEVITO
DEVOTO
DEXTRO
DIABLO
DIALSO
DIARIO
DINERO
DIRIGO
DISTRO
DOCOMO
DODODO
DOESSO
DOESTO
DOMINO
DONESO
DONETO
DONOSO
DONTGO
DOOMTO
DORADO
DORITO
DOSADO
DOSIDO
DOTODO
DRAWTO
DREWTO
DROMIO
DUELLO
DUETTO
DYNAMO

•DO•••
ADOBES
ADOBOS
ADOLFO
ADOLPH
ADONAI
ADONIC
ADONIS
ADOPTS
ADORED
ADOREE
ADORER
ADORES
ADORNS
ADOUTS
IDOIDO
IDOLUM
IDONOT
IDOTOO
ODONTO
ODORED
ODOULS
ODOURS

•D•O••
ADDONS
ADJOIN
ADNOUN
ADROIT
ADSORB
CDROMS
EDDOES
EDKOCH
EDMOND
EDWOOD
IDIOCY
IDIOMS
IDIOTS
ODEONS
ODIOUS

•D••O•
ADDSON
ADOBOS
EDISON
EDITOR
EDWOOD
IDAHOS
IDONOT
IDOTOO
ODDJOB
ODDLOT
ODDSON
ODEDON

•D•••O
ADAGIO
ADDSTO
ADOLFO
ADRENO
EDITIO
IDOIDO
IDOTOO
IDUNNO
ODONTO

••DO••
ADDONS
ALDOUS
ARDORS
ARDOUR
BADOFF
BEDOGS
CODONS
DADOED
DADOES
DIDOES
DODODO
DODOES
DODOMA
DRDOOM
EDDOES
EIDOLA
ENDORA
ENDOWS
EUDORA
FEDORA
FODORS
GODOWN
HADONE
HADOUT
HIDOUT
IMDONE
INDOOR
JUDOKA
KIDORY
LADOGA
LEDOFF
LEDOUT
LEDOUX
MEDOCS
MIDOFF
MIDONS
MIDORI
NODOFF
NODOSE
NODOUS
OGDOAD
PADOVA
PODOUS
RADOME
REDOAK
REDOCK
REDOER
REDOES
REDONE
REDOSE
REDOUT
RUDOLF
SEDONA
SODOWE
SUDOKU
TUDORS
UNDOCK
UNDOER
UNDOES
UNDONE
UPDOVE
WIDOWS
XEDOUT
ZADORA
ZEDONG
ZEDONK

••D•O•
ADDSON
ANDHOW
ANDROS
AUDIOS
BADBOY
BADCOP
BADDOG
BADLOT
BIDFOR
BIDSON
DIDFOR
DIDION
DIDNOT
DRDOOM
ENDSON
GIDEON
GODSON
HADRON
HEDRON
HUDSON
HYDROS
HYDROX
INDOOR
JUDSON
KIDCOM
KIDDOS
KIDEOS
KUDROW
LUDLOW
MADDOG
MADDOX
MADEOF
MADFOR
ODDJOB
ODDLOT
ODDSON
OLDBOY
OLDDOG
OLDSOD
RADIOS
RADNOR
REDCOD
REDDOG
REDDOT
REDFOX
REDHOT
REDSOX
REDTOP
RIDSOF
RODEOS
RODION
TYDBOL
VIDEOS
VIDIOT
WIDEOF

••D••O
ADDSTO
DADDYO
DODODO
ENDURO
HADAGO
HIDEHO
INDIGO
LADINO
MADEDO
MADEGO
MADERO
MADURO
MEDICO
MODULO
NODSTO
OLDPRO
REDTWO
RIDETO
RODETO
RODINO
TODDAO
ZYDECO

•••DO•
AMIDOL
ARADOS
ASHDOD
AVEDON
BADDOG
BARDOT
BIGDOG
BIGDOS
CANDOR
CATDOM
CAWDOR
CONDOR
CONDOS
CORDON
COYDOG
CREDOS
DEADON
DOGDOM
DOTDOT
EJIDOS
ENIDOK
FANDOM
FEEDON
FELDON
FEODOR
FOGDOG
FONDOF
FYODOR
GELDOF
GOODOH
GORDON
GUNDOG
HANDON
HEADON
HELDON
HOLDON
HOODOO
HOTDOG
HOUDON
ISIDOR
JOEDON
KENDOS
KIDDOS
KINDOF
LAIDON
LANDON
LANDOR
LAPDOG
LARDON
LEADON
LIEDON
LONDON
LOSDOS
LOUDON
LYNDON
MADDOG
MADDOX
MCADOO
MEADOW
MONDOS
NORDOI
ODEDON
OLDDOG
OWEDON
OXYDOL
PARDON
PETDOG
PRODON
PYEDOG
RANDOM
RAWDON
READON
REDDOG
REDDOT
RONDOS
SAIDOK
SARDOU
SEADOG
SELDOM
SENDON
SHADOW
SHEDON
SKIDOO
SOLDON
SUNDOG
TENDON
THEDOW
TIEDON

TOLDOF
TOLDON
TONDOS
TOPDOG
TOYDOG
TRODON
TVIDOL
USEDON
VENDOR
VERDON
VIRDON
VOIDOF
VOODOO
WELDON
WINDOM
WINDOW
WISDOM
ZENDOS

•••D•O

AMADEO
AMEDEO
BINDTO
BULDEO
CARDIO
DADDYO
DENDRO
ELADIO
FEEDTO
FREDRO
GLADTO
HEADTO
HELDTO
HOLDTO
HOODOO
ISIDRO
LAIDTO
LANDHO
LEADTO
LENDTO
LIEDTO
LLADRO
MCADOO
NEEDTO
OWEDTO
PLEDTO
READTO
ROADEO
SAIDNO
SAIDSO
SAIDTO
SANDRO
SENDTO
SKIDOO
SOLDTO
STUDIO
TENDTO
TIEDTO
TODDAO
USEDTO
VOODOO
YSIDRO

••••DO

ABBADO
AIKIDO
ALBEDO
ALZADO
BRANDO
CUANDO
DAVIDO
DODODO
DORADO
DOSADO
DOSIDO
DOTODO
ESCUDO
ESTADO
HAIRDO
IDOIDO
ITLLDO
JURADO
KOMODO
LAREDO
LIBIDO
MADEDO
MAKEDO
MARIDO
MENUDO
MIKADO
MOVADO
MUSTDO
OVERDO
OVIEDO
PSEUDO
RAPIDO
SABADO
SAYIDO
SPEEDO
SUREDO
TOLEDO
TUXEDO
WEIRDO
WILLDO
WONTDO
YESIDO

D•P•••

DAPHNE
DAPPED
DAPPER
DAPPLE
DEPART
DEPAUL
DEPAUW
DEPEND
DEPERE
DEPEST
DEPICT
DEPLOY
DEPONE
DEPORT
DEPOSE
DEPOTS
DEPTHS
DEPULP
DEPUTE
DEPUTY
DIPLEX
DIPNET
DIPODY
DIPOLE
DIPPED
DIPPER
DIPSIN
DIPSOS
DOPERS
DOPIER
DOPILY
DOPING
DRPHIL
DUPERS
DUPERY
DUPING
DUPLEX
DUPLOS
DUPONT

D••P••

DAMPED
DAMPEN
DAMPER
DAMPLY
DAPPED
DAPPER
DAPPLE
DEEPAK
DEEPEN
DEEPER
DEEPLY
DELPHI
DESPOT
DIAPER
DIEPPE
DIMPLE
DIMPLY
DIPPED
DIPPER
DISPEL
DRAPED
DRAPER
DRAPES
DRIPON
DRIPPY
DROPBY
DROPIN
DROPIT
DROPSY
DRUPES
DUMPED
DUMPER
DUMPON
DUMPTY

D•••P•

DACAPO
DAYSPA
DECAPS
DIEPPE
DOGAPE
DOLAPS
DRIPPY
DROOPS
DROOPY

D••••P

DAMSUP
DAYHOP
DEALUP
DECAMP
DEPULP
DETROP
DEWLAP
DIALUP
DIGSUP
DISHUP
DOESUP
DOGNAP
DOITUP
DOLLOP
DOLLUP
DOMREP
DONEUP
DOOWOP
DRAGUP
DRAWUP
DREWUP
DRKOOP
DRUMUP
DRYMOP
DSHARP
DUDEUP
DUNLAP
DUNLOP
DUSTUP

•D•P••

ADAPTS
ADEPTS
ADOPTS

•D••P•

ADOLPH
ADREPS

•D•••P

ADDSUP

••DP••

ENDPIN
MUDPIE
OLDPAL
OLDPRO

••D•P•

REDIPS

••D••P

ADDSUP
ASDEEP
BADCOP
BADRAP
BIDSUP
DUDEUP
ENDSUP
GIDDAP
GODEEP
INDEEP
KIDNAP
MADCAP
MADEUP
MIDCAP
REDCAP
REDTOP
RIDEUP
RODEUP
TIDYUP
UNDEEP
WADSUP

•••D•P

BEADUP
BINDUP
CRUDUP
EYEDUP
FOLDUP
GIDDAP
HANDUP
HARDUP
HEADUP
HELDUP
HOLDUP
ICEDUP
LAIDUP
LANDUP
LEADUP
LOADUP
PAIDUP
READUP
SENDUP
SPEDUP
TEEDUP
TIEDUP
USEDUP
WINDUP

D••Q••

DRIQJR

D••••Q

DEVICQ

•••D•Q

NASDAQ

DR••••

DRABEK
DRABLY
DRAFTS
DRAFTY
DRAGEE
DRAGGY
DRAGIN
DRAGON
DRAGUP
DRAINS
DRAKES
DRAKEU
DRAMAS
DRANCY
DRAPED
DRAPER
DRAPES
DRATIT
DRAWEE
DRAWER
DRAWIN
DRAWLS
DRAWLY
DRAWON
DRAWTO
DRAWUP
DRAYED
DRCLAW
DRDOOM
DREADS
DREAMS
DREAMT
DREAMY
DREARY
DREBIN
DRECKS
DRECKY
DREDGE
DRENCH
DRESSY
DREVIL
DREWIN
DREWON
DREWTO
DREWUP
DREXEL
DREYER
DRHOOK
DRIERS
DRIEST
DRIFTS
DRIFTY
DRILLS
DRINGS
DRINKS
DRIPON
DRIPPY
DRIQJR
DRIVEL
DRIVEN
DRIVER
DRIVES
DRIVIN
DRJUNG
DRKING
DRKOOP
DROGUE
DROIDS
DROITS
DROLLS
DROLLY
DROMIO
DRONED
DRONER
DRONES
DROOLS
DROOLY
DROOPS
DROOPY
DROPBY
DROPIN
DROPIT
DROPSY
DROSSY
DROUET
DROVER
DROVES
DROWNS
DROWSE
DROWSY
DROXIE
DRPHIL
DRRICE
DRRUTH
DRUDGE
DRUIDS
DRUMUP
DRUPES
DRUSES
DRUZES
DRYADS
DRYDEN
DRYERS
DRYEST
DRYEYE
DRYFLY
DRYFOG
DRYICE
DRYING
DRYINK
DRYISH
DRYMOP
DRYOFF
DRYOUT
DRYROT
DRYRUN

D•R•••

DARCEL
DAREME
DARENT
DARERS
DAREST
DARETO
DARIEN
DARING
DARIUS
DARKEN
DARKER
DARKLE
DARKLY
DARLIN
DARNAY
DARNED
DARNER
DARNIT
DARREN
DARRIN
DARROW
DARRYL
DARTED
DARTER
DARTLE
DARWIN
DERAIL
DERAIN
DERATE
DERATS
DERIDE
DERITA
DERIVE
DERMAL
DERMAS
DERMAT
DERMIC
DERMIS
DERMOT
DEROSE
DERREK
DERUST
DIRAMS
DIRECT
DIRELY
DIREST
DIRGES
DIRHAM
DIRIGE
DIRIGO
DIRKED
DIRNDL
DORADO
DORAGS
DORATI
DORCAS
DOREEN
DOREMI
DORIAN
DORIES
DORINE
DORITO
DORMER
DORMIE
DORRIT
DORSAD
DORSAL
DORSAY
DORSET
DORSEY
DORSUM
DRRICE
DRRUTH
DURANT
DURBAN
DURBIN
DURESS
DURFEY
DURHAM
DURING
DURNED
DURNIT
DUROCS
DURRAS
DURUMS
DURYEA

D••R••

DABRAT
DACRON
DARREN
DARRIN
DARROW
DARRYL
DATRIL
DCAREA
DEARER
DEARIE
DEARLY
DEARME
DEARTH
DEARTO
DEBRAH
DEBRAY
DEBREU
DEBRIS
DECREE
DEERES
DEFRAG
DEFRAY
DEGREE
DELRAY
DELREY
DELRIO
DELROY
DERREK
DESREE
DETROP
DHARMA
DIARIO
DIGRAM
DMARKS
DOBROS
DOGRUN
DOMREP
DOORED
DORRIT
DOURER
DOURIF
DOURLY
DRYROT
DRYRUN
DUARTE
DURRAS
DVORAK
DWARFS

D•••R•

DAMORE
DARERS
DATARY
DATERS
DAZERS
DEAIRS
DEBARK
DEBARS
DEBURR
DECARE
DECORS
DEFERS
DEFORD
DEFORE
DEFORM
DEGERM
DEHIRE
DEHORN
DEIDRE
DEJURE
DEMARK
DEMURE
DEMURS
DENARI
DENARS
DENARY
DENDRA
DENDRI
DENDRO
DENIRO
DEPART
DEPERE
DEPORT
DESCRY
DESERT
DESIRE
DESTRY
DETARS
DETERS
DEVERE
DEVERS
DEVORE
DEWARS
DEWIRE
DEWORM
DEXTRO
DICERS
DIKERS
DINARS
DINERO
DINERS
DISARM
DISERE
DISTRO
DIVERS
DIVERT
DIYERS
DMITRI
DMITRY
DOLORE
DOLORS
DONORA
DONORS
DOPERS
DOSERS
DOTARD
DOTERS
DOTORG
DOWERS
DOWERY
DOZERS
DREARY
DRIERS
DRYERS
DSHARP
DUGARD
DUPERS
DUPERY
DYSART

D••••R

DABBER
DAFTER
DAGGER
DAGMAR
DAMMER
DAMNER
DAMOUR
DAMPER
DANCER
DANDER
DANGER
DANKER
DANNER
DAPPER
DARKER
DARNER
DARTER
DASHER
DAUBER
DAWBER
DEADER
DEAFER
DEALER
DEARER
DEBLUR
DEBTOR
DEBURR
DECKER
DEEPER
DEEVER
DEFFER
DEFIER
DEFTER
DEHAIR
DEICER
DEKKER
DELMAR
DELVER
DENIER
DENSER
DENVER
DEODAR
DETMER
DETOUR
DEUTER
DEVOIR
DEVOUR
DEWIER
DEXTER
DIALER
DIAPER
DICIER
DICKER
DIDFOR
DIEFOR
DIETER
DIFFER
DIGFOR
DIGGER
DILLAR
DILLER
DIMMER
DINGER
DINNER
DIPPER
DISBAR
DISEUR
DITHER
DJEBAR
DLAYER
DMAJOR
DMINOR
DOCKER
DOCTOR
DODDER
DODGER
DOFFER
DOGEAR
DOKTOR
DOLLAR
DOLOUR
DONDER
DONNER
DOOVER
DOOZER
DOPIER
DORMER
DOTTER
DOURER
DOUSER
DOWNER
DOWSER
DOZIER
DRAPER
DRAWER
DREYER
DRIQJR
DRIVER
DRONER
DROVER
DUBBER
DUCKER
DUELER
DUFFER
DUGFOR
DULLER
DUMBER
DUMPER
DUNBAR
DUNKER
DUNNER
DUSTER

•DR•••

ADRATE
ADRENO
ADREPS
ADRIAN
ADRIEN
ADRIFT
ADRIVE
ADROIT
CDRACK
CDRATE
CDROMS

•D•R••

ADORED
ADOREE
ADORER
ADORES
ADORNS
EDERLE
EDIRNE
IDARED
ODORED

•D••R•

ADDERS
ADHERE
ADJURE
ADMIRE
ADSORB
ADVERB
ADVERT
ADWARE
ADWARS
EDBERG
EDGARD
EDGARS
EDGERS
EDUARD
EDVARD
EDWARD
IDCARD
IDLERS
ODOURS
UDDERS

•D•••R

ADORER
EDGIER
EDITOR

••DR••

ALDRIN
ANDRAE
ANDREA
ANDREI
ANDRES
ANDREW
ANDREY
ANDRIC
ANDROS
AUDREY
BADRAP
CADRES
CEDRIC
ENDRAN
ENDRUN
ESDRAS
HADRON
HEDRAL
HEDREN
HEDRON
HYDRAE
HYDRAS
HYDRIC
HYDROS
HYDROX
HYDRUS
KUDROW
MADRAS
MADRES
MADRID
MIDRIB
MODRED
OHDRAT
PADRES
REDRAG
REDRAW
REDREW
REDRUM
UNDRAW
UNDREW

••D•R•

ADDERS
AIDERS
ALDERS
ANDERS
ARDORS
BIDERS
CEDARN
CEDARS
CEDARY
CEDERS
CIDERS
CIDERY
CODERS
CYDERS
EIDERS
ELDERS
ENDERS
ENDORA
ENDURE
ENDURO
EUDORA
FADERS
FEDORA
FODORS
GODARD
GODARK
HIDERS
INDIRA
JUDFRY
KIDORY
LADERS
MADERA
MADERO
MADURO
MIDORI
MODERN
NADIRS
OHDARN
OLDPRO
ORDERS
RADARS
REDARE
REDARN
RIDERS
RUDERY
SEDERS
TUDORS
UDDERS
UNDERS
UPDART
VIDERI
WADERS
ZADORA

••D••R

ARDOUR
BADDER
BADGER
BIDDER
BIDFOR
BUDDER
BUDGER
CADGER
CODGER
DIDFOR
DODDER
DODGER
ENDEAR
FIDLER
FODDER
FUDGER
GADDER
HEDGER
INDOOR
JEDGAR
KEDGER
KIDDER
LADDER
LADLER
LEDGER
LODGER
MADDER
MADFOR
MEDGAR
MIDAIR
MIDLER
MUDDER
MYDEAR
NODDER
NODEAR
NUDGER
OHDEAR
OLDCAR
PADDER
RADNER
RADNOR
REDDER
REDFIR
REDOER
RIDDER
RODDER
RUDDER
RUDNER
SADDER
SADLER
SIDDUR
SUDSER
TIDIER
UNDOER
VEDDER
WADDER
WEDDER
WIDDER

•••DR•

AIRDRY
ALUDRA
COMDRS
DEIDRE
DENDRA
DENDRI
DENDRO
EXEDRA
FOUDRE
FREDRO
GUIDRY
HENDRY
ILLDRY
ISIDRO
KUNDRY
LANDRY
LLADRO
PATDRY
PHEDRE
POUDRE
PREDRY
QUADRI
RANDRY
RUNDRY
SANDRA
SANDRO
SONDRA
SUNDRY
TAWDRY
TUNDRA
YSIDRO

•••D•R

ABIDER
AGADIR
ALYDAR
ARIDER
AVIDER
BADDER
BALDER
BALDUR
BANDER
BEADER
BENDER
BIDDER
BINDER
BIRDER
BLADER
BOLDER
BONDER
BORDER
BRUDER
BUDDER
CALDER
CANDOR

CARDER
CAWDOR
CHEDER
CHIDER
CINDER
COLDER
CONDOR
COODER
CORDER
CRUDER
DANDER
DEADER
DEODAR
DODDER
DONDER
ELIDER
ELUDER
ERODER
EVADER
FEEDER
FENDER
FEODOR
FINDER
FODDER
FOLDER
FONDER
FUNDER
FYODOR
GADDER
GANDER
GENDER
GILDER
GIRDER
GLIDER
GOODER
GRADER
GUIDER
HANDER
HARDER
HEADER
HEEDER
HERDER
HINDER
HOLDER
HRIDER
ISIDOR
KANDER
KIDDER
KINDER
LADDER
LANDER
LANDOR
LARDER
LAUDER
LEADER
LENDER
LEWDER
LIEDER
LINDER
LOADER
LOUDER
MADDER
MEADER
MELDER
MENDER
MILDER
MINDER
MOLDER

MUDDER
MULDER
MURDER
NEEDER
NODDER
OCEDAR
PADDER
PANDER
PASDAR
PINDAR
PONDER
POWDER
RAIDER
READER
REDDER
REEDER
RENDER
RIDDER
ROADER
RODDER
RUDDER
SADDER
SANDER
SEEDER
SENDER
SHADER
SIDDUR
SLIDER
SNIDER
SNYDER
SOLDER
SPADER
SPIDER
SPYDER
SUNDER
TENDER
TINDER
TRADER
VEADAR
VEDDER
VENDER
VENDOR
VOIDER
WADDER
WANDER
WARDER
WEDDER
WEEDER
WEIDER
WELDER
WIDDER
WILDER
WINDER
WONDER
YARDER
YONDER

••••DR
RATEDR
THIRDR

DS••••
DSCALE
DSHARP

D•S•••
DASHED
DASHER

DASHES
DASHIS
DASHIT
DASSIN
DESADE
DESALT
DESCRY
DESEED
DESERT
DESETA
DESICA
DESIGN
DESILT
DESILU
DESIRE
DESIST
DESLUM
DESMOG
DESNOS
DESODS
DESOTO
DESPOT
DESREE
DESSAU
DESTEM
DESTRY
DISANT
DISARM
DISBAR
DISBUD
DISCOS
DISCUS
DISERE
DISEUR
DISHED
DISHES
DISHUP
DISKED
DISMAL
DISMAS
DISMAY
DISMES
DISNEY
DISOWN
DISPEL
DISSED
DISSES
DISTAL
DISTIL
DISTRO
DISUSE
DOSADO
DOSAGE
DOSERS
DOSIDO
DOSING
DOSSAL
DOSSED
DOSSES
DOSUMS
DUSKED
DUSTED
DUSTER
DUSTIN
DUSTUP
DYSART

D••S••
DABSAT
DAISES
DAMSEL
DAMSON
DAMSUP
DANSES
DANSON
DAOSTA
DASSIN
DATSUN
DAWSON
DAYSPA
DEASIL
DEISTS
DELSOL
DENSER
DESSAU
DIESEL
DIESES
DIESIS
DIGSAT
DIGSIN
DIGSIT
DIGSUP
DILSEY
DIMSUM
DIPSIN
DIPSOS
DISSED
DISSES
DNASES
DOASET
DOESBY
DOESIN
DOESIT
DOESNT
DOESOK
DOESSO
DOESTO
DOESUP
DOGSAT
DOGSIT
DORSAD
DORSAL
DORSAY
DORSET
DORSEY
DORSUM
DOSSAL
DOSSED
DOSSES
DOUSED
DOUSER
DOUSES
DOWSED
DOWSER
DOWSES
DOWSON
DRESSY
DROSSY
DRUSES
DUESSA

D•••S•
DALASI
DAMASK
DANISH

DAREST
DEBASE
DEFUSE
DEGUST
DELISH
DELIST
DEMAST
DEMISE
DEMIST
DENISE
DEPEST
DEPOSE
DEROSE
DERUST
DESIST
DETEST
DEVEST
DEVISE
DIALSO
DIGEST
DIREST
DISUSE
DIVEST
DNAASE
DOESSO
DONESO
DONOSO
DOVISH
DRESSY
DRIEST
DROPSY
DROSSY
DROWSE
DROWSY
DRYEST
DRYISH
DUBOSE
DUDISH
DUESSA
DURESS
DYNAST

D••••S
DACHAS
DADDYS
DADOES
DAISES
DALETS
DALLAS
DALLES
DANCES
DANIOS
DANNYS
DANSES
DANTES
DARERS
DARIUS
DASHES
DASHIS
DATERS
DAUBES
DAUNTS
DAVENS
DAVIES
DAVITS
DAZERS
DBACKS
DCELLS

DEAIRS
DEATHS
DEBAGS
DEBARS
DEBITS
DEBRIS
DEBUGS
DEBUTS
DECADS
DECAFS
DECALS
DECAPS
DECAYS
DECIUS
DECORS
DECOYS
DEDANS
DEERES
DEFATS
DEFERS
DEFIES
DEFOGS
DEGELS
DEGUMS
DEICES
DEIGNS
DEIMOS
DEISTS
DEKKOS
DELAYS
DELCOS
DELFTS
DELIUS
DELTAS
DELVES
DEMIES
DEMITS
DEMOBS
DEMONS
DEMURS
DENARS
DENIES
DENIMS
DENNIS
DENNYS
DEPOTS
DEPTHS
DERATS
DERMAS
DERMIS
DESNOS
DESODS
DETARS
DETERS
DETTES
DEUCES
DEVERS
DEVILS
DEWARS
DFLATS
DHOLES
DHOTIS
DICERS
DICOTS
DIDIES
DIDOES
DIENES
DIESES

DIESIS
DIETES
DIEZES
DIGITS
DIKERS
DINARS
DINERS
DINGUS
DINKAS
DIODES
DIPSOS
DIRAMS
DIRGES
DISCOS
DISCUS
DISHES
DISMAS
DISMES
DISSES
DITTOS
DITZES
DIVANS
DIVERS
DIVOTS
DIXITS
DIYERS
DJILAS
DJINNS
DMARKS
DMINUS
DNASES
DOAKES
DOALLS
DOBLES
DOBROS
DOBYNS
DODGES
DODOES
DOGIES
DOGMAS
DOGONS
DOINGS
DOLAPS
DOLMAS
DOLORS
DONEES
DONETS
DONORS
DONUTS
DOOFUS
DOPERS
DORAGS
DORCAS
DORIES
DOSERS
DOSSES
DOSUMS
DOTERS
DOUBTS
DOUGHS
DOULAS
DOUSES
DOUZES
DOWELS
DOWERS
DOWNES
DOWSES
DOXIES

DOYENS
DOZENS
DOZERS
DRAFTS
DRAINS
DRAKES
DRAMAS
DRAPES
DRAWLS
DREADS
DREAMS
DRECKS
DRIERS
DRIFTS
DRILLS
DRINGS
DRINKS
DRIVES
DROIDS
DROITS
DROLLS
DRONES
DROOLS
DROOPS
DROVES
DROWNS
DRUIDS
DRUPES
DRUSES
DRUZES
DRYADS
DRYERS
DTILES
DUBOIS
DUCATS
DUENAS
DUENOS
DUFFYS
DULLES
DUMBOS
DUNCES
DUNDAS
DUOMOS
DUPERS
DUPLOS
DURESS
DUROCS
DURRAS
DURUMS
DUTIES
DUVETS
DWARFS
DWEEBS
DWELLS
DYNELS

•DS•••
ADSORB
EDSELS

•D•S••
ADDSIN
ADDSON
ADDSTO
ADDSUP
ADESTE
EDESSA
EDISON

ODDSON
ODESSA
ODISTS

•D••S•
ADJUST
ADVISE
CDCASE
EDESSA
GDANSK
IDLEST
ODDEST
ODDISH
ODENSE
ODESSA

•D•••S
ADAGES
ADAPTS
ADDAMS
ADDERS
ADDINS
ADDLES
ADDONS
ADEEMS
ADENIS
ADEPTS
ADFEES
ADIDAS
ADIEUS
ADLIBS
ADMINS
ADMITS
ADOBES
ADOBOS
ADONIS
ADOPTS
ADORES
ADORNS
ADOUTS
ADREPS
ADULTS
ADVILS
ADWARS
CDROMS
EDAMES
EDDIES
EDDOES
EDEMAS
EDGARS
EDGERS
EDICTS
EDILES
EDSELS
EDUCES
EDUCTS
IDAHOS
IDEALS
IDENTS
IDIOMS
IDIOTS
IDLERS
IDTAGS
IDYLLS
ODEONS
ODIOUS
ODISTS
ODIUMS

ODOULS
ODOURS
UDDERS

••DS••
ADDSIN
ADDSON
ADDSTO
ADDSUP
BEDSIT
BIDSIN
BIDSON
BIDSUP
ENDSAT
ENDSIN
ENDSIT
ENDSON
ENDSUP
GODSON
HUDSON
JUDSON
MADSEN
MIDSTS
NADSAT
NODSAT
NODSTO
ODDSON
OLDSAW
OLDSOD
REDSEA
REDSIX
REDSKY
REDSOX
REDSUN
RIDSOF
SUDSED
SUDSER
SUDSES
UNDSET
WADSUP

••D•S•
ALDISS
ATDUSK
DUDISH
ELDEST
EMDASH
ENDASH
ENDUSE
INDASH
IODISE
JADISH
MEDUSA
MODEST
MODISH
NODOSE
NUDEST
NUDISM
NUDIST
ODDEST
ODDISH
OLDEST
OLDISH
ONDISK
RADISH
REDOSE
REDUST
RUDEST

SADISM
SADIST
VEDIST
WIDEST
WIDISH

••D••S
ADDAMS
ADDERS
ADDINS
ADDLES
ADDONS
AIDERS
ALDERS
ALDISS
ALDOUS
ANDERS
ANDRES
ANDROS
ARDORS
ASDICS
AUDIOS
AUDITS
BADEMS
BADGES
BADUNS
BEDEWS
BEDIMS
BEDOGS
BIDERS
BIDETS
BODIES
BUDGES
CADETS
CADGES
CADMUS
CADRES
CEDARS
CEDERS
CIDERS
CODERS
CODONS
CYDERS
DADDYS
DADOES
DEDANS
DIDIES
DIDOES
DODGES
DODOES
EDDIES
EDDOES
EIDERS
ELDERS
ENDERS
ENDOWS
ENDUES
ESDRAS
FADERS
FODORS
FUDGES
GADDIS
GEDDES
GODETS
GODEYS
HADJES
HADJIS
HEDGES

HIDERS
HODADS
HODGES
HYDRAS
HYDROS
HYDRUS
INDIES
INDUES
JUDGES
KEDGES
KIDDOS
KIDEOS
KODAKS
KUDZUS
LADERS
LADIES
LADLES
LEDGES
LODENS
LODGES
LUDENS
MADAMS
MADRAS
MADRES
MEDALS
MEDIAS
MEDICS
MEDIUS
MEDNIS
MEDOCS
MIDGES
MIDONS
MIDSTS
MODALS
MODELS
MODEMS
NADIRS
NODOUS
NUDGES
OLDIES
ONDITS
OODLES
ORDERS
PADRES
PEDALS
PODOUS
RADARS
RADIOS
RADIUS
REDANS
REDIGS
REDIPS
REDOES
REDUBS
REDYES
RIDERS
RIDGES
RODEOS
RUDKUS
SADHES
SADHUS
SEDANS
SEDERS
SEDGES
SEDUMS
SIDLES
SUDSES
TIDIES

TODAYS
TODIES
TUDORS
TVDVDS
UDDERS
UNDAMS
UNDERS
UNDIES
UNDIMS
UNDOES
VIDEOS
VODKAS
WADERS
WEDELS
WEDGES
WIDENS
WIDOWS
WIDTHS
YODELS

•••DS•
AMIDST
SAIDSO
WOODSY

•••D•S
ABIDES
ABODES
ADIDAS
AMADIS
AMIDAS
AMIDES
ANODES
ARADOS
ASIDES
ATODDS
AZIDES
BIGDOS
BLADES
BREDES
BRIDES
BSIDES
BUNDTS
CHIDES
CLYDES
COMDRS
CONDOS
CREDOS
CRUDES
DADDYS
DIODES
DUNDAS
EJIDOS
ELIDES
ELUDES
EPODES
ERODES
ETUDES
EVADES
EXODUS
EXUDES
FONDAS
FONDUS
GADDIS
GEDDES
GEODES
GLADES
GLADYS

GLIDES
GOUDAS
GRADES
GRIDES
GUIDES
HAIDAS
HINDUS
HONDAS
HORDES
HYADES
IMIDES
IRIDES
KENDOS
KIDDOS
LANDIS
LANDUS
LOSDOS
LUNDIS
MAHDIS
MANDMS
MARDIS
MAZDAS
MENDES
MONDES
MONDOS
MOODYS
OXIDES
PANDAS
PANDLS
PINDUS
PRADAS
PRIDES
PRUDES
READDS
RHODES
RONDOS
SARDIS
SAUDIS
SHADES
SHEDDS
SLIDES
SONDES
SPADES
SPODES
STIDES
SUEDES
SUNDAS
SWEDES
TARDES
TILDES
TONDOS
TRADES
TSADES
TSADIS
VELDTS
VERDES
WENDYS
ZENDOS

••••DS
ALKYDS
AMENDS
APHIDS
AROIDS
ATODDS
AVOIDS
AWARDS
BEARDS

BIPEDS
BIPODS
BLEEDS
BLENDS
BLINDS
BLONDS
BLOODS
BOARDS
BOUNDS
BOVIDS
BRAIDS
BRANDS
BREADS
BREEDS
BROODS
BUILDS
CANIDS
CHARDS
CHORDS
CLOUDS
CREEDS
CROWDS
CUPIDS
CURADS
CYCADS
DECADS
DESODS
DREADS
DROIDS
DRUIDS
DRYADS
EBONDS
ECARDS
ELANDS
EMBEDS
EMENDS
EPHODS
FARADS
FELIDS
FIELDS
FIENDS
FIORDS
FJORDS
FLOODS
FLUIDS
FOUNDS
FRAUDS
FRONDS
GLANDS
GOURDS
GRANDS
GREEDS
GRINDS
GUARDS
GUILDS
HEXADS
HOARDS
HODADS
HOUNDS
HYOIDS
ILIADS
IMBEDS
JIHADS
KNEADS
LAIRDS
LAMEDS
LIPIDS
LLOYDS

LYRIDS
MONADS
MOPEDS
MOULDS
MOUNDS
NAIADS
NICADS
NOKIDS
NOMADS
OCTADS
OOPODS
OOTIDS
OREADS
OVOIDS
PLAIDS
PLEADS
POUNDS
PSEUDS
RANIDS
RAPIDS
READDS
REBIDS
REPADS
RESODS
REWEDS
ROUNDS
SALADS
SCALDS
SCOLDS
SCRODS
SHARDS
SHEDDS
SHREDS
SKALDS
SNOODS
SOLIDS
SOUNDS
SPEEDS
SPENDS
SQUADS
SQUIDS
STANDS
STEADS
STEEDS
STRADS
SWARDS
SWORDS
SYNODS
TBIRDS
TBONDS
THIRDS
TREADS
TRENDS
TRIADS
TVDVDS
TWEEDS
UNBUDS
UPENDS
URSIDS
VIANDS
WEALDS
WEBADS
WIELDS
WORLDS
WOUNDS
YEGODS
YIELDS
ZOOIDS
ZOUNDS

DT••••

DTILES

D•T•••

DATARY
DATERS
DATHAN
DATING
DATIVE
DATRIL
DATSUN
DETACH
DETAIL
DETAIN
DETARS
DETECT
DETENT
DETERS
DETEST
DETMER
DETOTH
DETOUR
DETROP
DETTES
DETUNE
DITALI
DITHER
DITTOS
DITZES
DOTAGE
DOTARD
DOTCOM
DOTDOT
DOTELL
DOTEON
DOTERS
DOTGOV
DOTHAN
DOTIME
DOTING
DOTOAT
DOTODO
DOTORG
DOTTED
DOTTER
DOTTIE
DOTTLE
DUTIES
DUTTON

D••T••

DACTYL
DAFTER
DAFTLY
DALTON
DANTEI
DANTES
DANTON
DARTED
DARTER
DARTLE
DAYTON
DEATHS
DEBTEE
DEBTOR
DEFTER
DEFTLY
DELTAS
DELTIC
DENTAL
DENTED
DENTIN
DENTON
DEPTHS
DESTEM
DESTRY
DETTES
DEUTCH
DEUTER
DEXTER
DEXTRO
DHOTEL
DHOTIS
DIATOM
DICTUM
DIETED
DIETER
DIETES
DIKTAT
DINTED
DISTAL
DISTIL
DISTRO
DITTOS
DMITRI
DMITRY
DOCTOR
DOGTAG
DOGTOY
DOITUP
DOKTOR
DOLTON
DONTGO
DOTTED
DOTTER
DOTTIE
DOTTLE
DRATIT
DUCTAL
DUCTED
DUETED
DUETTI
DUETTO
DUSTED
DUSTER
DUSTIN
DUSTUP
DUTTON

D•••T•

DAINTY
DAKOTA
DALETH
DALETS
DAMATO
DAMITA
DANITE
DAOSTA
DARETO
DAUNTS
DAVITS
DEAFTO
DEALTO
DEARTH
DEARTO
DEBATE
DEBITS
DEBUTS
DEFATS
DEISTS
DELETE
DELFTS
DEMITS
DEMOTE
DEMOTH
DENOTE
DEPOTS
DEPUTE
DEPUTY
DERATE
DERATS
DERITA
DESETA
DESOTO
DETOTH
DEVITO
DEVOTE
DEVOTO
DEWITT
DFLATS
DICOTS
DIGITS
DILATE
DILUTE
DIMITY
DIVOTS
DIXITS
DOESTO
DONATE
DONATH
DONETO
DONETS
DONITZ
DONUTS
DOOMTO
DORATI
DORITO
DOUBTS
DOWITH
DRAFTS
DRAFTY
DRAWTO
DREWTO
DRIFTS
DRIFTY
DROITS
DRRUTH
DUARTE
DUCATS
DUETTI
DUETTO
DULUTH
DUMPTY
DUVETS

D••••T

DABRAT
DABSAT
DANGIT
DARENT
DAREST
DARNIT
DASHIT
DAUDET
DAYLIT
DEBONT
DECANT
DECEIT
DECENT
DECLOT
DECOCT
DEDUCT
DEFEAT
DEFECT
DEGUST
DEJECT
DELICT
DELINT
DELIST
DEMAST
DEMIST
DEPART
DEPEST
DEPICT
DEPORT
DERMAT
DERMOT
DERUST
DESALT
DESERT
DESILT
DESIST
DESPOT
DETECT
DETENT
DETEST
DEVEST
DEVOUT
DEWITT
DIDACT
DIDNOT
DIECUT
DIEOUT
DIGEST
DIGLOT
DIGOUT
DIGSAT
DIGSIT
DIKTAT
DIMOUT
DIMWIT
DINEAT
DIPNET
DIRECT
DIREST
DISANT
DIVERT
DIVEST
DOASET
DOCENT
DOCKET
DOESIT
DOESNT
DOGSAT
DOGSIT
DONEIT
DORRIT
DORSET
DOTDOT
DOTOAT
DRATIT
DREAMT
DRIEST
DROPIT
DROUET
DRYEST
DRYOUT
DRYROT
DUGOUT
DULCET
DUMONT
DUNANT
DUPONT
DURANT
DURNIT
DWIGHT
DYELOT
DYEVAT
DYNAST
DYSART

•DT•••

IDTAGS

•D•T••

ADYTUM
EDITED
EDITIO
EDITOR
IDOTOO
ODETTA
ODETTE

•D••T•

ADAPTS
ADDSTO
ADEPTS
ADESTE
ADMITS
ADNATE
ADOPTS
ADOUTS
ADRATE
ADULTS
CDRATE
EDICTS
EDUCTS
IDEATE
IDENTI
IDENTS
IDIOTS
ODDITY
ODETTA
ODETTE
ODISTS
ODONTO

•D•••T

ADDICT
ADDUCT
ADJUST
ADRIFT
ADROIT
ADVENT
ADVERT
IDIDIT
IDLEST
IDONOT
ODDEST
ODDLOT
ODELET

••DT••

REDTAB
REDTAG
REDTEN
REDTIE
REDTOP
REDTWO
WIDTHS

••D•T•

ADDSTO
AUDITS
BIDETS
BODETT
BYDATE
CADETS
GODETS
INDITE
IODATE
JUDITH
KADETT
KPDUTY
MIDSTS
NODSTO
NUDITY
ODDITY
ONDITS
ONDUTY
PEDATE
REDATE
RIDETO
RODETO
SEDATE
TODATE
UPDATE

••D••T

ABDUCT
ADDICT
ADDUCT
ANDYET
ARDENT
BADFIT
BADHAT
BADLOT
BEDSIT
BODETT
BUDGET
CADENT
DEDUCT
DIDACT
DIDNOT
ELDEST
ENDCUT
ENDSAT
ENDSIT
FIDGET
GADGET
GIDGET
GODWIT
HADOUT
HIDOUT
INDEBT
INDENT
INDICT
INDUCT
KADETT
KIDLIT
KIDULT
LEDOUT
MADEIT
MIDGET
MODELT
MODEST
MUDCAT
NADSAT
NODSAT
NUDEST
NUDIST
ODDEST
ODDLOT
OHDRAT
OLDBAT
OLDEST
OLDHAT
PEDANT
REDACT
REDANT
REDBAT
REDDOT
REDHAT
REDHOT
REDOUT
REDUST
RIDENT
RODENT
RUDEST
SADIST
TIDBIT
UNDEFT
UNDSET
UPDART
VEDIST
VIDIOT
WIDEST
WIDGET
XEDOUT

•••DT•

BINDTO
BUNDTS
FEEDTO
GLADTO
HEADTO
HELDTO
HOLDTO
LAIDTO
LEADTO
LENDTO
LIEDTO
NEEDTO
OWEDTO
PLEDTO
READTO
SAIDTO
SENDTO
SOLDTO
TENDTO
TIEDTO
USEDTO
VELDTS

•••D•T

ACEDIT
AMIDST
BANDIT
BARDOT
BORDET
COEDIT
CREDIT
DAUDET
DOTDOT
FORDGT
GOODAT
HELDIT
HOLDIT
ICEDIT
IDIDIT
KEYDET
LANDAT
LORDIT
NEEDNT
PANDIT
PUNDIT
REDDOT
REEDIT
SOLDIT
TOLDIT
WHODAT

••••DT

ARENDT
BRANDT

DU••••

DUALLY
DUARTE
DUBBED
DUBBER
DUBCEK
DUBLIN
DUBOIS
DUBOSE
DUCATS
DUCHIN
DUCKED
DUCKER
DUCKIE
DUCTAL
DUCTED
DUDDLE
DUDEUP
DUDING
DUDISH
DUDLEY
DUELED
DUELER
DUELLO
DUENAS
DUENNA
DUENOS
DUESSA
DUETED
DUETTI
DUETTO
DUFFEL
DUFFER
DUFFLE
DUFFYS
DUGALD
DUGARD
DUGFOR
DUGONG
DUGOUT
DUKING
DULCET
DULLEA
DULLED
DULLER
DULLES
DULUTH
DUMBER
DUMBLY
DUMBOS
DUMDUM
DUMONT
DUMPED
DUMPER
DUMPON
DUMPTY
DUNANT
DUNBAR
DUNCAN
DUNCES
DUNDAS
DUNDEE
DUNHAM
DUNKED
DUNKER
DUNKIN
DUNLAP
DUNLIN
DUNLOP
DUNNED
DUNNER
DUOMOS
DUPERS
DUPERY
DUPING
DUPLEX
DUPLOS
DUPONT
DURANT
DURBAN
DURBIN
DURESS
DURFEY
DURHAM
DURING
DURNED
DURNIT
DUROCS
DURRAS
DURUMS
DURYEA
DUSKED
DUSTED
DUSTER
DUSTIN
DUSTUP
DUTIES
DUTTON
DUVALL
DUVETS

D•U•••

DAUBED
DAUBER
DAUBES
DAUDET
DAUNTS
DEUCED
DEUCES
DEUTCH
DEUTER
DOUANE
DOUBLE
DOUBLY
DOUBTS
DOUGAL
DOUGHS
DOUGHY
DOULAS
DOURER
DOURIF
DOURLY
DOUSED
DOUSER
DOUSES
DOUZES
DRUDGE
DRUIDS
DRUMUP
DRUPES
DRUSES
DRUZES

D••U••

DANUBE
DEBUGS
DEBUNK
DEBURR
DEBUTS
DEDUCE
DEDUCT
DEDUVE
DEFUEL
DEFUND
DEFUSE
DEGUMS
DEGUST
DEJUNK
DEJURE
DELUDE
DELUGE
DELUGG
DELUXE
DEMURE
DEMURS
DENUDE
DEPULP
DEPUTE
DEPUTY
DERUST
DETUNE
DILUTE
DISUSE
DONUTS
DOSUMS
DRJUNG
DROUET
DRRUTH
DULUTH
DURUMS

D•••U•

DADGUM
DAMOUR
DAMSUP
DARIUS
DATSUN
DEALUP
DEBLUR
DECIUS
DELIUS
DEPAUL
DEPAUW
DESLUM
DETOUR
DEVOUR
DEVOUT
DIALUP
DICTUM
DIECUT
DIEOUT
DIGOUT
DIGSUP
DIMOUT
DIMSUM
DINGUS
DINKUM
DISBUD
DISCUS
DISEUR
DISHUP
DMINUS
DOESUP
DOGRUN
DOITUP
DOLLUP
DOLOUR
DONEUP
DOOFUS
DORSUM
DRAGUP
DRAWUP
DREWUP
DROGUE
DRUMUP
DRYOUT
DRYRUN
DUDEUP
DUGOUT
DUMDUM
DUSTUP
DYBBUK

D••••U

DEBREU
DEJAVU
DESILU
DESSAU
DRAKEU

•DU•••

ADULTS
EDUARD
EDUCED
EDUCES
EDUCTS
IDUNNO

•D•U••

ADDUCE
ADDUCT
ADJURE
ADJUST
ADOUTS
ADZUKI
EDMUND
ODIUMS
ODOULS
ODOURS

•D••U•

ADDSUP
ADIEUS
ADIEUX
ADNOUN
ADYTUM
IDOLUM
ODIOUS

••DU••

ABDUCE
ABDUCT
ADDUCE
ADDUCT
ASDULL
ATDUSK
BADUNS
BODUKE
DEDUCE
DEDUCT
DEDUVE
ENDUED
ENDUES
ENDURE
ENDURO
ENDUSE
INDUCE
INDUCT
INDUED
INDUES
KIDULT
KPDUTY
LADUKE
MADURO
MCDUCK
MEDUSA
MODULE
MODULI
MODULO
NODULE
ONDUTY
PADUAN
PODUNK
REDUBS
REDUCE
REDUST
SEDUCE
SEDUMS
UNDULY
YODUDE

••D•U•

ADDSUP
AIDFUL
ALDOUS
ARDOUR
BADGUY
BEDAUB
BEDBUG
BIDSUP
CADMUS
DADGUM
DUDEUP
ENDCUT
ENDRUN
ENDSUP
HADFUN
HADOUT
HIDOUT
HYDRUS
INDIUM
KUDZUS
LEDOUT
LEDOUX
LUDLUM
MADDUX
MADEUP
MEDIUM
MEDIUS
NODOUS
PODIUM
PODOUS
RADIUM
RADIUS
REDBUD
REDOUT
REDRUM
REDSUN
RIDEUP
RODEUP
RUDKUS
SADHUS
SIDDUR
SODIUM
TEDEUM
TEDIUM
TIDYUP
WADSUP
XEDOUT

••D••U

CADEAU
SUDOKU

•••DU•

BALDUR
BEADUP
BINDUP
CRUDUP
DUMDUM
EXODUS
EYEDUP
FOLDUP
FONDUE
FONDUS
HANDUP
HARDUP
HEADUP
HELDUP
HINDUS
HOLDUP
ICEDUP
LAIDUP
LANDUP
LANDUS
LEADUP
LOADUP
MADDUX
PAIDUP
PERDUE
PINDUS
PURDUE
READUP
SENDUP
SIDDUR
SPEDUP
SUBDUE
TEEDUP
TIEDUP
USEDUP
VENDUE
VERDUN
WINDUP

•••D•U

LANDAU
MOLDAU
SARDOU

••••DU

CHANDU
XANADU

DV••••

DVORAK

D•V•••

DAVENS
DAVIDE
DAVIDI
DAVIDL
DAVIDO
DAVIES
DAVITS
DEVANE
DEVEGA
DEVEIN
DEVERE
DEVERS
DEVEST
DEVICE
DEVICQ
DEVILS
DEVINE
DEVISE
DEVITO
DEVOID
DEVOIR
DEVORE
DEVOTE
DEVOTO
DEVOUR
DEVOUT
DIVANS
DIVEIN
DIVERS
DIVERT
DIVEST
DIVIDE
DIVINE
DIVING
DIVOTS

DOVEIN
DOVISH
DUVALL
DUVETS

D••V••
DEEVER
DELVED
DELVER
DELVES
DENVER
DOOVER
DREVIL
DRIVEL
DRIVEN
DRIVER
DRIVES
DRIVIN
DROVER
DROVES
DYEVAT

D•••V•
DANOVA
DATIVE
DEDUVE
DEJAVU
DENOVO
DERIVE

D••••V
DOTGOV

•DV•••
ADVENT
ADVERB
ADVERT
ADVICE
ADVILS
ADVISE
EDVARD

•D••V•
ADRIVE

••DV••
KIDVID
MADVIG
OLDVIC
TVDVDS

••D•V•
DEDUVE
ENDIVE
GODIVA
PADOVA
UPDIVE
UPDOVE

DW••••
DWARFS
DWAYNE
DWEEBS
DWEEBY
DWELLS
DWIGHT

D•W•••
DAWBER
DAWDLE
DAWNED
DAWNON
DAWSON
DEWARS
DEWIER
DEWILY
DEWING
DEWIRE
DEWITT
DEWLAP
DEWOLF
DEWORM
DOWELL
DOWELS
DOWERS
DOWERY
DOWITH
DOWNED
DOWNER
DOWNES
DOWNEY
DOWNON
DOWSED
DOWSER
DOWSES
DOWSON

D••W••
DAEWOO
DARWIN
DIMWIT
DOOWOP
DRAWEE
DRAWER
DRAWIN
DRAWLS
DRAWLY
DRAWON
DRAWTO
DRAWUP
DREWIN
DREWON
DREWTO
DREWUP
DROWNS
DROWSE
DROWSY

D•••W•
DISOWN

D••••W
DARROW
DECLAW
DEPAUW
DRCLAW

•DW•••
ADWARE
ADWARS
ADWEEK
EDWARD
EDWINA
EDWOOD
EDWYNN

••DW••
BEDWIN
GODWIN
GODWIT
LUDWIG
MIDWAY
OLDWAY
PEDWAY

••D•W•
ATDAWN
BEDEWS
CODYWY
ENDOWS
GODOWN
REDTWO
SODOWE
UNDEWY
WIDOWS

••D••W
ANDHOW
ANDREW
KUDROW
LUDLOW
OLDSAW
REDRAW
REDREW
UNDRAW
UNDREW

•••D•W
MEADOW
MILDEW
SHADOW
THEDOW
WINDOW

D•X•••
DEXTER
DEXTRO
DIXITS
DOXIES

D••X••
DIOXIN
DREXEL
DROXIE

D•••X•
DELUXE

D••••X
DIPLEX
DUPLEX

•D•••X
ADIEUX

••D••X
HADDIX
HYDROX
LEDOUX
MADDOX
MADDUX
MADMAX
REDFOX
REDSIX
REDSOX

•••D•X
BENDIX
COMDEX
HADDIX
HANDAX
MADDOX
MADDUX
WINDEX

••••DX
BRANDX
RATEDX

DY••••
DYADIC
DYBBUK
DYEING
DYEJOB
DYELOT
DYEVAT
DYNAMO
DYNAST
DYNELS
DYNODE
DYSART

D•Y•••
DAYBED
DAYGLO
DAYHOP
DAYJOB
DAYLIT
DAYOFF
DAYOLD
DAYONE
DAYSPA
DAYTON
DIYERS
DOYENS
DRYADS
DRYDEN
DRYERS
DRYEST
DRYEYE
DRYFLY
DRYFOG
DRYICE
DRYING
DRYINK
DRYISH
DRYMOP
DRYOFF
DRYOUT
DRYROT
DRYRUN

D••Y••
DLAYER
DOBYNS
DRAYED
DREYER
DURYEA
DWAYNE

D•••Y•
DACTYL
DADDYO
DADDYS
DANDYL
DANNYS
DARRYL
DDMMYY
DECAYS
DECOYS
DELAYS
DENNYS
DRYEYE
DUFFYS

D••••Y
DABNEY
DAFTLY
DAILEY
DAINTY
DAMPLY
DANGLY
DANKLY
DANNAY
DARKLY
DARNAY
DATARY
DDMMYY
DEADLY
DEAFLY
DEARLY
DEBRAY
DEEJAY
DEEPLY
DEFRAY
DEFTLY
DELANY
DELKEY
DELRAY
DELREY
DELROY
DENARY
DEPLOY
DEPUTY
DESCRY
DESTRY
DEWILY
DICKEY
DIDDLY
DIGAMY
DILSEY
DIMITY
DIMPLY
DINGHY
DIPODY
DIRELY
DISMAY
DISNEY
DMITRY
DOCBOY
DOESBY
DOGDAY
DOGTOY
DOLLEY
DOMBEY
DONEBY
DONKEY
DOOLEY
DOPILY
DORSAY
DORSEY
DOUBLY
DOUGHY
DOURLY
DOWERY
DOWNEY
DOZILY
DRABLY
DRAFTY
DRAGGY
DRANCY
DRAWLY
DREAMY
DREARY
DRECKY
DRESSY
DRIFTY
DRIPPY
DROLLY
DROOLY
DROOPY
DROPBY
DROPSY
DROSSY
DROWSY
DRYFLY
DUALLY
DUDLEY
DUMBLY
DUMPTY
DUPERY
DURFEY
DWEEBY

•DY•••
ADYTUM
IDYLLS

•D•Y••
EDWYNN

•D••Y•
DDMMYY

•D•••Y
DDMMYY
EDGILY
EDIBLY
IDIOCY
ODDITY
PDIDDY

••DY••
ANDYET
CODYWY
LADYDI
REDYED
REDYES
TIDYUP
UNDYED

••D•Y•
DADDYO
DADDYS
GODEYS
MADLYN
MMDDYY
REDEYE
TODAYS

••D••Y
ANDREY
AUDREY
BADBOY
BADDAY
BADGUY
BODILY
BODLEY
CEDARY
CIDERY
CODIFY
CODYWY
CUDAHY
CUDDLY
DIDDLY
DUDLEY
GADFLY
HEDLEY
JUDFRY
KIDNEY
KIDORY
KODALY
KPDUTY
MEDFLY
MEDLEY
MIDDAY
MIDMAY
MIDWAY
MMDDYY
MODIFY
NIDIFY
NUDELY
NUDITY
ODDITY
OLDBOY
OLDWAY
ONDUTY
PEDWAY
PUDDLY
RADLEY
REDBAY
REDEFY
REDENY
REDSKY
RIDEBY
RIDLEY
RODEBY
RODNEY
RUDELY
RUDERY
SADDAY
SEDLEY
SIDNEY
SYDNEY
TEDKEY
TIDILY
UNDEWY
UNDULY
WADDLY
WIDELY

•••DY•
AZODYE
DADDYO
DADDYS
DANDYL
GLADYS
MMDDYY
MOODYS
RITDYE
TIEDYE
TOLDYA
VATDYE
WENDYS

•••D•Y
ACIDLY
AGEDLY
AIRDRY
ALLDAY
ANYDAY
ARIDLY
AVIDLY
AWEDLY
BADDAY
BALDLY
BATDAY
BENDAY
BIGDAY
BOLDLY
CLODDY
COLDLY
CORDAY
CRUDDY
CUDDLY
DEADLY
DIDDLY
DOGDAY
EKEDBY
FLEDGY
FONDLY
FREDDY
FRIDAY
GLADLY
GOODBY
GOODLY
GUIDRY
HARDBY
HARDLY
HENDRY
HEYDAY
HOTDAY
ILLDRY
INADAY
KINDLY
KLUDGY
KUNDRY
LAIDBY
LANDRY
LEWDLY
LORDLY
LOUDLY
MANDAY
MAYDAY
MIDDAY
MILDLY
MMDDYY
MONDAY
NEWDAY
OFFDAY
ONEDAY
PATDAY
PATDRY
PAYDAY
PDIDDY
PERDAY
PREDAY
PREDRY
PUDDLY
RANDRY
RUNDRY
SADDAY
SENDBY
SHODDY
SIXDAY
SKIDDY
SLUDGY
SMUDGY
SPIDEY
STODGY
STUDLY
SUNDAY
SUNDRY
TAGDAY
TAWDRY
TENDAY
TWODAY
UNIDLY
WADDLY
WILDLY
WOODSY

••••DY
BLOODY
BRANDY
BREEDY
BROODY
CLODDY
CLOUDY
COMEDY
CRUDDY
DIPODY
EMBODY
FRAIDY
FREDDY
GRANDY
GREEDY
GRUNDY
HOUNDY
MALADY
MAUNDY
MELODY
MILADY
MONODY
MOULDY
MYLADY
NOBODY
OGRADY
PARODY
PDIDDY
REMEDY
SHANDY
SHEEDY
SHINDY
SHODDY
SKIDDY
SPEEDY
SPENDY
STEADY
STURDY
TRENDY
TWEEDY
UNTIDY
WEIRDY
WIELDY

D•Z•••
DAZERS
DAZING
DAZZLE
DIZAIN
DOZENS
DOZERS
DOZIER
DOZILY
DOZING

D••Z••
DANZIG
DAZZLE
DENZEL
DIEZES
DITZES
DOOZER
DOOZIE
DOUZES
DRUZES

D••••Z
DOLENZ
DONITZ

•DZ•••
ADZING
ADZUKI

••DZ••
KUDZUS

••D•Z•
BEDAZE
IODIZE

•••D•Z
VALDEZ

••••DZ
XYANDZ

EA••••
EAGLED
EAGLES
EAGLET
EAGRES
EAKINS
EALING
EAMONN
EANNIE
EARBUD
EARFUL
EARING
EARLAP
EARLET
EARNED
EARNER
EARNIE
EARNIT
EARTAB
EARTAG
EARTHA
EARTHS
EARTHY
EARVIN
EARWAX
EARWIG
EASEBY
EASEIN
EASELS
EASEON
EASERS
EASEUP
EASIER
EASILY
EASING
EASLEY
EASTER
EASTLA
EASTON
EASYAS
EASYGO
EATERS
EATERY
EATING
EATOUT
EATSAT
EATSIN
EATSIT
EATSOF
EATSUP

E•A•••
EBANKS
EBATES
EBAYER
ECARDS
ECARTE
EDAMES
EGALES
ELADIO
ELAINE
ELANCE
ELANDS
ELANET
ELAPID
ELAPSE
ELATED
ELATER
ELATES
ELAYER
ELAYNE
EMAILS
EMAJOR
EMALLS
ENABLE
ENACTS
ENAMEL
ENAMOR
ENARMS
ENATES
EPACTS
EPARCH
ERASED
ERASER
ERASES
ESALEN
ETAGES
ETAILS
ETALIA
ETALII
ETAOIN
ETAPES
EVADED
EVADER
EVADES
EWAINE
EXACTA
EXACTS
EXALTS
EXARCH

E••A••
EBOATS
ECKART
ECLAIR
ECLASS
ECLATS
EDDAIC
EDGARD
EDGARS
EDUARD
EDVARD
EDWARD
EFFACE
EFLATS
EKLAND
ELGART
ELNATH
ELPAIS
ELPASO
ELUANT
ELUARD
ELUATE
EMBALM
EMBANK
EMBARK
EMBARS
EMBAYS
EMDASH
EMMAUS
EMPALE
EMPATH
ENBANC
ENCAGE
ENCAMP
ENCASE
ENDALL
ENDASH
ENFACE
ENFAIT
ENFANT
ENGAGE
ENHALO
ENHAUT
ENIACS
ENLACE
ENRAGE
ENRANK
ENRAPT
ENSATE
ENTAIL
EPHAHS
EQUALS
EQUATE
ERHARD
ERLANG
ERNANI
ERRAND
ERRANT
ERRARE
ERRATA
ERSATZ
ESBATS
ESCALE
ESCAPE
ESCARP
ESCAUT
ESHARP
ESPANA
ESSAIS
ESSAYS
ESTADO
ESTATE
ETHANE
ETRADE
EURAIL
EUTAXY
EWBANK
EXHALE
EXMATE
EXPAND
EXPATS
EXTANT
EXYANK
EZPASS
EZZARD

E•••A•
EARLAP
EARTAB
EARTAG
EARWAX
EASYAS
EATSAT
ECOLAB
ECOLAW
EDEMAS
EGGSAC
EGOYAN
ELFMAN
ELIJAH
EMQUAD
ENDEAR
ENDMAN
ENDRAN
ENDSAT
ENGRAM
ENNEAD
ENQUAD
ENSEAL
ENSEAT
ENTIAL
ENTRAP
ENWRAP
EOLIAN
EONIAN
EPICAL
EPINAL
ERDMAN
EREVAN
ERICAS
ERIVAN
ERSTAD
ERYKAH
ESDRAS
ESPIAL
ESTRAY
EVENAS
EXTRAS

E••••A
EARTHA
EASTLA
ECZEMA
EDESSA
EDWINA
EGERIA
EGESTA
EIDOLA
EIGHTA
EJECTA
ELISHA
ELISSA
ELLORA
ELMIRA
ELNORA
ELODEA
ELOISA
ELVIRA
ELYRIA
EMILIA
ENCINA
ENDORA
ENIGMA
ERIEPA
ERINNA
EROICA
ERRATA
ESPANA
ESPOSA
ETALIA
EUBOEA
EUDORA
EUPNEA
EUREKA
EUROPA
EXACTA
EXCUSA
EXEDRA

•EA•••
BEACHY
BEACON
BEADED
BEADER
BEADLE
BEADUP
BEAGLE
BEAKED
BEAKER
BEALLS
BEAMAN
BEAMED
BEAMER
BEAMON
BEAMUP
BEANED
BEANIE
BEANOS
BEAPAL
BEARDS
BEARER
BEARON
BEARSE
BEARUP
BEASTS
BEATAT
BEATEN
BEATER
BEATIT
BEATLE
BEATON
BEATTY
BEATUP
BEAUTS
BEAUTY
BEAVER
BEAVIS
CEASED
CEASES
DEACON
DEADEN
DEADER
DEADLY
DEADON
DEAFEN
DEAFER
DEAFLY
DEAFTO
DEAIRS
DEALER
DEALIN
DEALTO
DEALUP
DEANNA
DEARER
DEARIE
DEARLY
DEARME
DEARTH
DEARTO
DEASIL
DEATHS
FEALTY
FEARED
FEARER
FEASTS
GEARED
GEARTO
GEARUP
HEADED
HEADER
HEADIN
HEADON
HEADTO
HEADUP
HEALED
HEALER
HEALEY
HEALTH
HEALUP
HEANEY
HEAPED
HEAPER
HEAPON
HEAPUP
HEARER
HEARNS
HEAROF
HEARSE
HEARST

HEARTH
HEARTS
HEARTY
HEARYE
HEATED
HEATER
HEATHS
HEATHY
HEATON
HEATUP
HEAVED
HEAVEN
HEAVER
HEAVES
JEANED
JEANIE
JEANNE
KEARNS
KEARNY
KEATON
LEACHY
LEADED
LEADEN
LEADER
LEADIN
LEADON
LEADTO
LEADUP
LEAFED
LEAGUE
LEAKED
LEAKER
LEAKEY
LEAKIN
LEALTY
LEANED
LEANER
LEANIN
LEANLY
LEANNE
LEANON
LEANTO
LEAPAT
LEAPED
LEAPER
LEAPIN
LEAPON
LEAPUP
LEARNS
LEARNT
LEASED
LEASER
LEASES
LEASTS
LEAVED
LEAVEN
LEAVER
LEAVES
MEADER
MEADOW
MEAGER
MEAGRE
MEALIE
MEANER
MEANEY
MEANIE
MEANIT
MEANLY

MEANTO
MEASLE
MEASLY
MEATAX
MEATUS
NEALON
NEARBY
NEARED
NEARER
NEARLY
NEARTO
NEATEN
NEATER
NEATLY
PEACHY
PEAHEN
PEAKED
PEALED
PEALER
PEALES
PEANUT
PEAPOD
PEARCE
PEARLE
PEARLS
PEARLY
REACTS
READDS
READER
READIN
README
READON
READTO
READUP
REAGAN
REAIMS
REAIRS
REALER
REALES
REALIA
REALLY
REALMS
REALTY
REAMED
REAMER
REAPED
REAPER
REARED
REARER
REARMS
REARUP
REASKS
REASON
REATAS
REATTA
REAVED
REAVER
REAVES
REAVOW
SEAAIR
SEAARM
SEABAG
SEABED
SEABEE
SEACAT
SEACOW
SEADOG
SEAEEL

SEAFOX
SEAGAL
SEAGOD
SEAHAG
SEAICE
SEALAB
SEALED
SEALER
SEALIN
SEALUP
SEALYS
SEAMAN
SEAMAP
SEAMED
SEAMEN
SEAMER
SEAMUS
SEANCE
SEARCH
SEARED
SEARER
SEARLE
SEASON
SEATAC
SEATED
SEATER
SEATON
SEAVER
SEAWAY
TEAACT
TEABAG
TEACUP
TEAMED
TEAMUP
TEAPOT
TEAPOY
TEARAT
TEARED
TEARER
TEARIT
TEARUP
TEASED
TEASEL
TEASER
TEASES
TEASET
TEATRO
TEAURN
VEADAR
WEAKEN
WEAKER
WEAKLY
WEAKON
WEALDS
WEALTH
WEANED
WEANER
WEAPON
WEARER
WEARON
WEASEL
WEAVED
WEAVER
WEAVES
YEABIG
YEAGER
YEANED
YEARLY

YEARNS
YEASTS
YEASTY
ZEALOT

•E•A••

AERATE
BECALM
BECAME
BEDAUB
BEDAZE
BEFAIR
BEFALL
BEHAIM
BEHALF
BEHAVE
BEJART
BELAIR
BELATE
BELAYS
BEMATA
BERATE
BESAME
BESANT
BETAKE
BEVANS
BEWAIL
BEWARE
BEWARY
CEDARN
CEDARS
CEDARY
CERATE
CERATO
CESARE
CESARS
CETANE
DEBAGS
DEBARK
DEBARS
DEBASE
DEBATE
DECADE
DECADS
DECAFS
DECALS
DECAMP
DECANT
DECAPS
DECARE
DECAYS
DEDANS
DEFACE
DEFAME
DEFANG
DEFATS
DEGAGE
DEHAIR
DEJAVU
DEKALB
DELAND
DELANO
DELANY
DELAYS
DEMAIN
DEMAND
DEMARK
DEMAST

DENADA
DENALI
DENARI
DENARS
DENARY
DEPART
DEPAUL
DEPAUW
DERAIL
DERAIN
DERATE
DERATS
DESADE
DESALT
DETACH
DETAIL
DETAIN
DETARS
DEVANE
DEWARS
FEMALE
FERALS
GELATE
GELATI
GELATO
GEMARA
GERALD
GERARD
GETANA
GETANF
HECATE
HEMATO
HEPATO
HERALD
HEXADS
HEXANE
KEBABS
KERALA
LECAIN
LEEANN
LEGACY
LEGALS
LEGART
LEGATE
LEGATO
LELAND
LEMANS
LENAIN
LENAPE
LENARD
LESAGE
LEVADE
LEVANT
MEDAKA
MEDALS
MEGALO
MEGANE
MENACE
MENAGE
MESAAZ
MESABI
METALS
METATE
NEGATE
NEPALI
NEVADA
NEWAGE
NEWARK

PECANS
PEDALS
PEDANT
PEDATE
PELAGE
PESACH
PESADE
PETAIN
PETALE
PETALS
PETARD
REBAGS
REBAIT
REBAKE
REBALE
REBANK
REBARS
REBATE
RECAGE
RECALL
RECANE
RECANS
RECANT
RECAPS
RECASE
RECAST
REDACE
REDACT
REDANS
REDANT
REDARE
REDARN
REDATE
REEARN
REFACE
REFALL
REGAIN
REGALE
REGARD
REGAVE
REHABS
REHANG
REHASH
REHAUL
REJAIL
RELACE
RELAID
RELAND
RELAPS
RELATE
RELAYS
REMADE
REMAIL
REMAIN
REMAKE
REMAND
REMANS
REMAPS
REMARK
REMATE
REMATS
RENAIL
RENAME
RENARD
RENATA
RENATO
REPACK
REPADS

REPAGE
REPAID
REPAIR
REPANE
REPARK
REPASS
REPAST
REPAVE
REPAYS
RERACK
RERAKE
RERANK
RERATE
RESAID
RESALE
RESALT
RESAND
RESANG
RESAVE
RESAWN
RESAWS
RESAYS
RETACK
RETAGS
RETAIL
RETAIN
RETAKE
RETAME
RETANS
RETAPE
RETAPS
RETARD
RETARS
REVAMP
REWAKE
REWARD
REWARM
REWARN
REWASH
REXALL
SEAAIR
SEAARM
SECADA
SECANT
SEDAKA
SEDANS
SEDATE
SEEALL
SEMANA
SENARY
SENATE
SENATS
SEPALS
SERACS
SERAIS
SERAPE
SERAPH
SESAME
SEWAGE
SEWARD
TEAACT
TECATE
TEJANA
TEJANO
TENACE
TENANT
TERATO
TEXACO

TEXANS
VEDAIC
VEGANS
VELARS
WEBADS
WECARE
YEMANA
ZENANA

•E••A•

AEGEAN
AENEAS
AERIAL
BEAMAN
BEAPAL
BEATAT
BEDLAM
BEEPAT
BEGGAR
BEHEAD
BELDAM
BELGAE
BELIAL
BELLAY
BEMOAN
BENDAY
BENGAL
BENGAY
BERMAN
BETRAY
BETTAS
BEULAH
CEIBAS
CELLAE
CELLAR
CENTAI
CENTAL
CENTAS
CEPHAL
CEREAL
CERNAN
CESTAS
DEBRAH
DEBRAY
DECLAW
DEDHAM
DEEJAY
DEEPAK
DEFEAT
DEFJAM
DEFOAM
DEFRAG
DEFRAY
DELEAD
DELIAN
DELMAR
DELRAY
DELTAS
DEMEAN
DENHAM
DENIAL
DENTAL
DEODAR
DERMAL
DERMAS
DERMAT
DESSAU
DEWLAP

FELLAH
FELLAS
FENWAY
FERIAS
FERMAT
FERNAO
FESTAL
FESTAS
FEUDAL
GEEGAW
GELCAP
GELLAR
GEMMAE
GENIAL
GENOAN
GENOAS
GENUAL
GERMAN
GESTAE
GETFAR
GETMAD
GETSAB
GETSAC
GETSAD
GETSAT
GEWGAW
HEDRAL
HEEHAW
HEGOAT
HELLAS
HENNAS
HEPCAT
HEPTAD
HERBAL
HEREAT
HERMAN
HERNAN
HEYDAY
HEYMAN
JEDGAR
JEERAT
JETFAN
JETLAG
JETSAM
JETTAS
JETWAY
KEENAN
KEEPAT
KENNAN
KENYAN
KEPTAT
KEVLAR
KEYMAN
KEYPAD
KEYPAL
KEYWAY
LEAPAT
LEBEAU
LEEMAY
LEERAT
LEEWAY
LEGMAN
LEHMAN
LEHUAS
LEICAS
LEMMAS
LESHAN
LESTAT

LETHAL
LETSAT
MEATAX
MECCAN
MECCAS
MEDGAR
MEDIAL
MEDIAN
MEDIAS
MELMAC
MENIAL
MENSAL
MENSAN
MENTAL
MERMAN
MESAAZ
MESCAL
MESIAL
METFAN
NECTAR
NEENAH
NEIMAN
NEMEAN
NEPEAN
NERMAL
NERVAL
NETMAN
NETPAY
NEUMAN
NEURAL
NEWCAR
NEWDAY
NEWHAT
NEWMAN
NEWMAR
NEWWAY
NEXRAD
PECKAT
PEDWAY
PEEKAT
PEEPAT
PEERAT
PELHAM
PELLAM
PENMAN
PENPAL
PENTAD
PENTAX
PERDAY
PETCAT
PETNAP
PETRAT
PETSAT
REAGAN
REATAS
RECLAD
RECOAL
RECOAT
REDBAT
REDBAY
REDCAP
REDEAL
REDHAT
REDIAL
REDOAK
REDRAG
REDRAW
REDTAB

REDTAG
REFLAG
REGEAR
REGGAE
REGNAL
REGNAT
REGRAB
REHEAL
REHEAR
REHEAT
REINAS
RELEAD
RELEAP
RELOAD
RELOAN
RENGAS
RENTAL
REPEAL
REPEAT
REPLAN
REPLAY
REREAD
RESCAN
RESEAL
RESEAM
RESEAT
RESEAU
RESNAP
RESOAK
RESOAP
RESPAN
RESTAB
RESWAM
RETEAR
RETHAW
RETIAL
RETRAL
RETRAP
REVEAL
REWEAR
REWRAP
REXCAT
SEABAG
SEACAT
SEAGAL
SEAHAG
SEALAB
SEAMAN
SEAMAP
SEATAC
SEAWAY
SEENAS
SEESAS
SEESAW
SEGWAY
SENDAK
SENNAS
SEPIAS
SEPTAL
SERIAL
SERTAS
SETSAT
SEURAT
TEABAG
TEARAT
TEHRAN
TEKWAR
TENDAY

TERRAE
TERRAN
TESLAS
TESTAE
TETRAD
TETRAS
VEADAR
VEEJAY
VEINAL
VENIAL
VENTAS
VERBAL
VERNAL
VESPAS
VESTAL
VESTAS
WEBCAM
WEIMAR
WENTAT
WETBAR
WETNAP
WETRAG
YEEHAW
YELLAT
YENTAS
YEOMAN
YESIAM
YESMAN
ZEBRAS
ZEEMAN
ZESTAS

•E•••A

AEOLIA
BELUGA
BEMATA
BERTHA
BETCHA
CELICA
CEPEDA
CESSNA
CETERA
DEANNA
DEFLEA
DENADA
DENDRA
DERITA
DESETA
DESICA
DEVEGA
FEDORA
FEMORA
GEISHA
GEMARA
GENERA
GENEVA
GENOVA
GETANA
HECUBA
HEGIRA
HELENA
HERNIA
HESTIA
JEMIMA
JERBOA
KERALA
KESHIA
KEYOFA

LENGUA
LENINA
LEONIA
LERIDA
MEDAKA
MEDICA
MEDINA
MEDUSA
MELINA
MERIDA
NEBULA
NERUDA
NESTEA
NEVADA
NEWERA
PELOTA
PENNIA
PEORIA
PEPITA
PERCHA
PERLEA
PERSIA
PESETA
PESEWA
PETBOA
PETIPA
PETULA
REALIA
REATTA
REDSEA
REGINA
REMORA
RENATA
RESEDA
RETINA
SECADA
SEDAKA
SEDONA
SEGURA
SELENA
SEMANA
SENECA
SENORA
SENTRA
SEPHIA
SEPIRA
SERBIA
SERENA
SEVENA
TEJANA
TENUTA
TERESA
VECTRA
VENERA
VENORA
VERONA
VEZINA
YELENA
YEMANA
ZENANA

••EA••

AFEARD
ALEAST
ASEASY
ATEAMS
ATEASE
AWEARY

AYEAYE
BLEACH
BLEAKS
BLEARS
BLEARY
BLEATS
BREACH
BREADS
BREAKS
BREAMS
BREAST
BREATH
BTEAMS
CHEAPO
CHEATS
CLEANS
CLEARS
CLEARY
CLEATS
CLEAVE
CREAKS
CREAKY
CREAMS
CREAMY
CREASE
CREASY
CREATE
DREADS
DREAMS
DREAMT
DREAMY
DREARY
FREAKS
FREAKY
GLEAMS
GLEAMY
GLEANS
GOEASY
GREASE
GREASY
GREATS
GREAVE
HBEAMS
IBEAMS
ICEAGE
ICEAXE
IDEALS
IDEATE
ILEANA
IMEANT
IMEASY
KNEADS
LBEAMS
LEEANN
NLEAST
OBEAHS
OCEANS
OLEARY
OLEATE
OMEARA
ONEACT
ONEALL
ONEARM
OREADS
PAEANS
PLEADS
PLEASE
PLEATS

POEANA
PREACH
PREACT
PREAGE
PREAMP
PREARM
QUEASY
REEARN
SEEALL
SHEARS
SHEATH
SHEAVE
SLEAZE
SLEAZY
SMEARS
SMEARY
SNEAKS
SNEAKY
SPEAKS
SPEARE
SPEARS
STEADS
STEADY
STEAKS
STEALS
STEAMS
STEAMY
SUEANE
SUEANN
SWEARS
SWEATS
SWEATY
THEACT
THEAGE
THEAPE
THEASP
THEAXE
TREADS
TREATS
TREATY
TWEAKS
TWEAKY
UNEASE
UNEASY
WHEATS
WREAKS
WREATH

••E•A•

ACELAS
ACETAL
AGENAS
AKELAS
ALEGAR
ALEMAN
ALETAP
ALEXAS
AMEBAE
AMEBAS
APEMAN
ARECAS
ARENAS
AXEMAN
AZERAS
BEEPAT
BUENAS
CAESAR
CHELAE

CHEVAL
CIERAS
COEVAL
CRETAN
DAEDAL
DEEJAY
DEEPAK
DJEBAR
DUENAS
DYEVAT
EDEMAS
EREVAN
EVENAS
FAENAS
FLEWAT
FOEMAN
FRETAT
GEEGAW
GOESAT
HEEHAW
HIEMAL
HYENAS
HYETAL
ICEBAG
ICECAP
ICEDAM
ICEMAN
IPECAC
JEERAT
KEENAN
KEEPAT
KIERAN
LEEMAY
LEERAT
LEEWAY
MAENAD
MCEWAN
MOERAE
NEENAH
NIETAS
OCEDAR
OMEGAS
ONECAR
ONEDAY
ONELAP
ONEMAN
ONEWAY
OPERAS
PEEKAT
PEEPAT
PEERAT
PIEMAN
PIEPAN
PIETAS
PLEIAD
PLEXAL
PREDAY
PREFAB
PRELAW
PREPAY
PRETAX
PREWAR
SCENAS
SEENAS
SEESAS
SEESAW
SHEBAT
SHEVAT

SLEZAK
STEFAN
STELAR
STELAS
THEBAN
THEBAR
THEBAY
THECAN
THECAR
THEFAN
THEGAP
THEHAJ
THELAW
THEMAN
THERAM
THERAP
THERAT
THETAS
THEWAY
TIEBAR
TIETAC
TOECAP
TOETAP
TREPAN
USETAX
VEEJAY
WHELAN
WIEMAN
YEEHAW
ZEEMAN

••E••A

ACEDIA
AGENDA
ALEXIA
AMELIA
AMENRA
AMESIA
ANEMIA
AREOLA
ARETHA
AVESTA
AYESHA
AZELMA
BAERGA
BRENDA
CHEETA
COELIA
CRENNA
CREUSA
CUESTA
DUENNA
DUESSA
EDESSA
EGERIA
EGESTA
EJECTA
EXEDRA
FIESTA
FRESCA
GLENDA
GRETNA
IBERIA
ICETEA
ILEANA
IMELDA
LUELLA
MOESHA

MTETNA
ODESSA
ODETTA
OLESHA
OMEARA
OMERTA
ONEIDA
OREIDA
OREXIA
OSETRA
PAELLA
PIERIA
PLEURA
PNEUMA
POEANA
PREVIA
PUEBLA
SHEENA
SHEILA
SHERPA
SIENNA
SIERRA
SIESTA
STELLA
STERNA
SVEDKA
THECIA
THEEPA
THELMA
THENBA
THENRA
THESEA
THEUSA
TIENDA
TIERRA
TREDIA
TRENTA
VIEIRA
VIENNA
XTERRA

•••EA•

AEGEAN
AENEAS
AGLEAM
ANDEAN
ANNEAL
APNEAS
APPEAL
APPEAR
ARREAR
ASNEAR
ASNEAT
ASTEAL
AUGEAN
AUGEAS
AXHEAD
BATEAU
BEHEAD
BIGEAR
BOREAL
BOREAS
BUREAU
CADEAU
CAMEAS
CAMEAT
CAVEAT
CEREAL

COMEAS
COMEAT
CUNEAL
DEFEAT
DELEAD
DEMEAN
DINEAT
DOGEAR
ENDEAR
ENNEAD
ENSEAL
ENSEAT
FIREAT
FIVEAA
FIVEAD
FIVEAM
FUMEAT
GALEAE
GALEAO
GAPEAT
GATEAU
GAZEAT
GIBEAT
GILEAD
GODEAD
GONEAR
GONEAT
GOTEAM
HABEAS
HADEAN
HAVEAT
HEREAT
IMBEAT
INFEAR
INGEAR
INLEAF
INSEAM
IRREAL
ISWEAR
JIBEAT
JUDEAN
JUNEAU
KOREAN
LAGEAR
LEBEAU
LINEAL
LINEAR
LIVEAT
LLBEAN
LOREAL
MCBEAL
MCKEAN
MCLEAN
MOREAU
MRBEAN
MYDEAR
NEMEAN
NEPEAN
NIKEAD
NINEAD
NINEAM
NODEAL
NODEAR
NOLEAD
NOMEAK
NOMEAT
OHDEAR
OHYEAH

OISEAU
ORDEAL
ORGEAT
OSTEAL
OUTEAT
PALEAE
PINEAL
POKEAT
POLEAX
POSEAS
RAMEAU
RAVEAT
REDEAL
REGEAR
REHEAL
REHEAR
REHEAT
RELEAD
RELEAP
REPEAL
REPEAT
REREAD
RESEAL
RESEAM
RESEAT
RESEAU
RETEAR
REVEAL
REWEAR
ROSEAU
SAMEAS
SAVEAS
SCREAK
SCREAM
SINEAD
SOLEAS
SOREAT
SPREAD
SQUEAK
SQUEAL
STREAK
STREAM
SUREAM
THREAD
THREAT
TINEAL
TINEAR
TOREAT
TYPEAB
TYPEAS
UNDEAD
UNLEAD
UNLEAF
UNLEAN
UNNEAT
UNREAD
UNREAL
UNSEAL
UNSEAM
UNSEAT
UPBEAR
UPBEAT
UPHEAP
UPLEAP
UPREAR
UPTEAR
WAVEAT

•••E•A

ALHENA
AMOEBA
ANGELA
ARBELA
ASPERA
ATHENA
AZTECA
AZUELA
BODEGA
BOLENA
CABEZA
CAMERA
CATENA
CATERA
CEPEDA
CETERA
CHEETA
CINEMA
DESETA
DEVEGA
DODECA
ECZEMA
ERIEPA
EUREKA
FIVEAA
FRIEDA
GALENA
GENERA
GENEVA
GOLETA
HELENA
IOMEGA
JAMESA
LAMESA
LIGEIA
LOVEYA
MADERA
MAKEBA
MINETA
MODELA
MODENA
MONETA
MULETA
MUNERA
NEWERA
NOVELA
NOVENA
ORTEGA
PAMELA
PESETA
PESEWA
RATEDA
RESEDA
RIBERA
RIJEKA
RIVERA
ROWENA
SABENA
SCHEMA
SCLERA
SELENA
SENECA
SERENA
SEVENA
SHEENA
TERESA
THEEPA

THREEA
TOPEKA
VALERA
VENERA
VIVECA
WADENA
WALESA
WASECA
YELENA

••••EA

AIRSEA
ALTHEA
ANDREA
AZALEA
CORNEA
COWPEA
CRIMEA
DCAREA
DEFLEA
DULLEA
DURYEA
ELODEA
EUBOEA
EUPNEA
GRADEA
GUINEA
HOTTEA
ICETEA
INAREA
JUDAEA
LABREA
LACTEA
MATTEA
MCCREA
NAUSEA
NESTEA
NOIDEA
NOUMEA
PERLEA
PROTEA
REDSEA
SPIREA
SUBSEA
THESEA
THREEA

EB••••

EBANKS
EBATES
EBAYER
EBBETS
EBBING
EBERLE
EBERLY
EBOATS
EBONDS
EBOOKS

E•B•••

EBBETS
EBBING
EDBERG
EGBERT
EKBERG
ELBERT
ELBOWS
ELBRUS

ELBURZ
EMBALM
EMBANK
EMBARK
EMBARS
EMBAYS
EMBEDS
EMBERS
EMBLEM
EMBODY
EMBOGS
EMBOSS
EMBOWS
EMBRUE
EMBRYO
ENBANC
ENBERG
ENBLOC
ERBIUM
ESBATS
EUBOEA
EWBANK

E••B••

EARBUD
EDIBLE
EDIBLY
ENABLE
EREBUS

E•••B•

EASEBY
EKEDBY
EKESBY
ENROBE
EXCUBS
EXURBS

E••••B

EARTAB
ECOLAB
EIGHTB
ENTOMB

•EB•••

BEBOPS
DEBAGS
DEBARK
DEBARS
DEBASE
DEBATE
DEBBIE
DEBITS
DEBLUR
DEBONE
DEBONT
DEBRAH
DEBRAY
DEBREU
DEBRIS
DEBTEE
DEBTOR
DEBUGS
DEBUNK
DEBURR
DEBUTS
HEBBEL
HEBREW

HEBRON
KEBABS
LEBEAU
LEBRET
LEBRON
LEBRUN
NEBULA
PEBBLE
PEBBLY
REBAGS
REBAIT
REBAKE
REBALE
REBANK
REBARS
REBATE
REBBES
REBBIE
REBECS
REBELS
REBEND
REBENT
REBETS
REBIDS
REBILL
REBIND
REBOIL
REBOLT
REBOOK
REBOOT
REBOPS
REBORE
REBORN
REBOTE
REBOZO
REBRED
REBREW
REBUFF
REBUKE
REBURY
REBUTS
REBUYS
SEBERG
TEBETS
VEBLEN
WEBADS
WEBBED
WEBBER
WEBCAM
WEBERN
WEBERS
WEBFED
WEBLOG
XEBECS
ZEBRAS

•E•B••

BEDBUG
BEEBEE
BENBEN
BENBOW
BERBER
CEIBAS
DEBBIE
FEEBLE
FEEBLY
FEMBOT
FERBER

GERBER
GERBIL
HEBBEL
HEEBIE
HENBIT
HERBAL
HERBED
HERBES
HERBIE
JERBOA
KEMBLE
LESBOS
MEEBER
MEMBER
NESBIT
NEWBIE
PEBBLE
PEBBLY
PEGBOX
PEPBOY
PETBOA
REBBES
REBBIE
REDBAT
REDBAY
REDBUD
REEBOK
REUBEN
SEABAG
SEABED
SEABEE
SERBIA
TEABAG
TEEBOX
TERBIC
VERBAL
VERBID
WEBBED
WEBBER
WEEBIT
WETBAR
YEABIG
YESBUT

•E••B•

AEROBE
CELEBS
CEREBR
DEMOBS
GETSBY
HECUBA
HEREBY
KEBABS
KENOBI
LEFTBE
LETSBE
LETSBY
MESABI
NEARBY
NEEDBE
REDUBS
REHABS
REPUBS
SELLBY
SENDBY
SENTBY
SETSBY
TENLBS

WENTBY

•E•••B

BEDAUB
BENUMB
CECILB
DEKALB
GETSAB
KEYOFB
NEWJOB
RECOMB
REDTAB
REGRAB
RESORB
RESTAB
REVERB
SEALAB
SEVENB

••EB••

AMEBAE
AMEBAS
AMEBIC
BEEBEE
BIEBER
BYEBYE
CUEBID
DJEBAR
DREBIN
EREBUS
FEEBLE
FEEBLY
GREBES
HEEBIE
ICEBAG
ICEBOX
KNEBEL
LIEBER
LIEBIG
LIEBYS
MEEBER
ONEBIT
PLEBES
PREBID
PREBUY
PUEBLA
PUEBLO
QUEBEC
REEBOK
RHEBOK
SHEBAT
SHEBOP
SIEBEN
TEEBOX
THEBAN
THEBAR
THEBAY
THEBBC
THEBEE
THEBES
TIEBAR
TREBEK
TREBLE
TREBLY
WEEBIT

••E•B•

DOESBY

DWEEBS
DWEEBY
EKEDBY
EKESBY
FLEWBY
GOESBY
NEEDBE
SHELBY
THEBBC
THEFBI
THENBA

••E••B

CHERUB
DYEJOB
PREFAB
THEHUB
THEMOB
THEWEB

•••EB•

ACHEBE
AMOEBA
CAMEBY
CELEBS
CEREBR
COMEBY
CUBEBS
DONEBY
DWEEBS
DWEEBY
EASEBY
FILEBY
FIVEBC
GAZEBO
GONEBY
HEREBY
INDEBT
LOWEBB
MAKEBA
NASEBY
NINEBC
PHLEBO
PHOEBE
RACEBY
RIDEBY
RODEBY
SASEBO
TYPEBS

•••E•B

ADVERB
LOWEBB
MODELB
REVERB
SCHEIB
SEVENB
SUPERB
THREEB
TYPEAB

••••EB

ALICEB
COBWEB
GRADEB
SUBDEB
THEWEB
THREEB

ZAGREB

EC••••

ECARDS
ECARTE
ECCLES
ECESIC
ECESIS
ECHOED
ECHOER
ECHOES
ECHOIC
ECKART
ECKERD
ECLAIR
ECLASS
ECLATS
ECOLAB
ECOLAW
ECOLES
ECORSE
ECTOMY
ECTYPE
ECZEMA

E•C•••

ECCLES
EMCEED
EMCEES
ENCAGE
ENCAMP
ENCASE
ENCINA
ENCINO
ENCODE
ENCORE
ENCRES
ENCYCL
EOCENE
ESCALE
ESCAPE
ESCARP
ESCAUT
ESCENT
ESCHER
ESCHEW
ESCORT
ESCROW
ESCUDO
ETCETC
ETCHED
ETCHER
ETCHES
EUCHRE
EUCKEN
EUCLID
EXCEED
EXCELS
EXCEPT
EXCESS
EXCIDE
EXCISE
EXCITE
EXCONS
EXCUBS
EXCUSA
EXCUSE

E••C••

EDICTS
EDUCED
EDUCES
EDUCTS
EGGCUP
EJECTA
EJECTS
ELECTS
ELICIT
ENACTS
ENDCUT
EPACTS
EPICAL
EPOCHS
ERECTS
ERICAS
ERUCTS
EVICTS
EXACTA
EXACTS
EXOCET
EYECUP

E•••C•

EDKOCH
EFFACE
EFFECT
ELANCE
ELLICE
ENCYCL
ENESCO
ENFACE
ENIACS
ENLACE
ENRICH
ENRICO
ENTICE
EPARCH
EROICA
ESTOCS
ETHICS
EUNICE
EVINCE
EXARCH
EXPECT
EXSECT

E••••C

ECESIC
ECHOIC
EDDAIC
EDENIC
EGGSAC
EIGHTC
EMERIC
EMETIC
ENBANC
ENBLOC
EPODIC
EROTIC
ETCETC
ETHNIC
ETONIC
EXILIC
EXOTIC

•EC•••

AECIUM
BECALM
BECAME
BECHET
BECKER
BECKET
BECKON
BECOME
BECOOL
CECILB
CECILE
DECADE
DECADS
DECAFS
DECALS
DECAMP
DECANT
DECAPS
DECARE
DECAYS
DECEIT
DECENT
DECIDE
DECILE
DECIUS
DECKED
DECKER
DECKLE
DECLAW
DECLOT
DECOCT
DECODE
DECORS
DECOYS
DECREE
FECUND
GECKOS
HECATE
HECKLE
HECKNO
HECTIC
HECTOR
HECUBA
JECKLE
LECAIN
LECHER
LECTER
LECTOR
MECCAN
MECCAS
MECUMS
NECKED
NECKER
NECTAR
PECANS
PECHES
PECKAT
PECKED
PECTIN
RECAGE
RECALL
RECANE
RECANS
RECANT
RECAPS
RECASE
RECAST

RECEDE
RECENT
RECESS
RECHEW
RECIFE
RECIPE
RECITE
RECKED
RECKON
RECLAD
RECOAL
RECOAT
RECOCK
RECODE
RECOIL
RECOIN
RECOMB
RECONS
RECOOK
RECOOL
RECOPY
RECORD
RECORK
RECOST
RECOUP
RECTOR
RECTOS
RECTUS
RECUED
RECUES
RECURE
RECURL
RECURS
RECUSE
RECUTS
SECADA
SECANT
SECEDE
SECKEL
SECOND
SECRET
SECTOR
SECURE
TECATE
TECHIE
TECHNO
TECHTV
UECKER
VECTOR
VECTRA
WECARE

•E•C••

BEACHY
BEACON
BERCEO
BETCHA
DEACON
DEFCON
DEICED
DEICER
DEICES
DELCOS
DESCRY
DEUCED
DEUCES
FENCED
FENCER
FENCES
FESCUE
GELCAP
HEPCAT
LEACHY
LEICAS
MECCAN
MECCAS
MERCED
MERCER
MERCKX
MESCAL
NEOCON
NEWCAR
PEACHY
PENCHE
PENCIL
PEPCID
PERCHA
PESCOW
PETCAT
PETCOW
REACTS
REDCAP
REDCOD
REECHO
REICED
REICES
RESCAN
RESCUE
REXCAT
SEACAT
SEACOW
TEACUP
TELCOS
TERCEL
TERCES
TETCHY
VELCRO
WEBCAM
WELCHS
WENCES

•E••C•

BEDECK
BENICE
CELICA
DECOCT
DEDUCE
DEDUCT
DEFACE
DEFECT
DEJECT
DELICT
DEPICT
DESICA
DETACH
DETECT
DEUTCH
DEVICE
DEVICQ
FELICE
HELICO
LEGACY
MEDICA
MEDICI
MEDICO
MEDICS
MEDOCS
MEJICO
MENACE
MENSCH
MEXICO
PEARCE
PEERCE
PEIRCE
PENICK
PESACH
REBECS
RECOCK
REDACE
REDACT
REDOCK
REDUCE
REFACE
REJECT
REKICK
RELACE
RELICS
RELICT
RELOCK
RELUCT
REMICK
REPACK
REPICK
RERACK
RESECT
RETACK
SEAICE
SEANCE
SEARCH
SEDICI
SEDUCE
SELECT
SENECA
SERACS
TEAACT
TENACE
TEXACO
VELOCE
VENICE
XEBECS

•E•••C

BELGIC
BELLOC
CEDRIC
CELTIC
DEIFIC
DELTIC
DERMIC
FERENC
FERRIC
GEODIC
GESTIC
GETSAC
HECTIC
HENDEC
HEROIC
KEYOFC
MELMAC
METRIC
PELVIC
PEPTIC
SEATAC
SEPTIC
SEVENC
TERBIC
VEDAIC

••EC••

ALECKS
ALECKY
ALECTO
AMECHE
ARECAS
BRECHT
CHECKS
CRECHE
CZECHS
DIECUT
DRECKS
DRECKY
EJECTA
EJECTS
ELECTS
ERECTS
EYECUP
FLECHE
FLECKS
FLECKY
ICECAP
IPECAC
NIECES
NUECES
ONECAR
ORECKS
PIECED
PIECER
PIECES
PRECIP
PRECIS
PRECUT
REECHO
SHECKY
SIECLE
SPECIE
SPECKS
THECAN
THECAR
THECIA
THECID
TOECAP
TRECES
VNECKS
WRECKS

••E•C•

AGENCE
AGENCY
AMERCE
APERCU
BIERCE
BLEACH
BLENCH
BREACH
BREECH
CHEECH
CLENCH
COERCE
DRENCH
ENESCO
FIERCE
FLEECE
FLEECY
FLETCH
FRENCH
FRESCA
FRESCO
GREECE
KVETCH
ONEACT
PEERCE
PIERCE
PREACH
PREACT
QUENCH
RYENCE
SKETCH
SPEECH
SPENCE
STENCH
THEACT
THENCE
TIERCE
TRENCH
UNESCO
USEDCD
WHENCE
WRENCH
WRETCH

••E••C

ACETIC
AMEBIC
ANEMIC
AXENIC
CHEMIC
CLERIC
ECESIC
EDENIC
EMERIC
EMETIC
GAELIC
IPECAC
IRENIC
NOETIC
ONESEC
POETIC
QUEBEC
SCENIC
STERIC
THEBBC
TIETAC
UNEPIC

•••EC•

ABJECT
AFFECT
APIECE
ASPECT
AWHECK
AZTECA
AZTECS
BEDECK
BISECT
BREECH
CHEECH
COLECO
COSECS
CUSECS
DEFECT
DEJECT
DETECT
DIRECT
DODECA
EFFECT
EXPECT
EXSECT
FLEECE
FLEECY
GRAECO
GREECE
GRIECO
GYNECO
HITECH
INFECT
INJECT
INSECT
KOPECK
LUBECK
LUTECE
OBJECT
OLMECS
ONDECK
REBECS
REJECT
RESECT
SAFECO
SELECT
SENECA
SPEECH
VIVECA
VOTECH
WASECA
XEBECS
ZYDECO

•••E•C

ETCETC
FERENC
FIVEBC
HOMEEC
MALEIC
NINEBC
SEVENC
THREEC

••••EC

ARCSEC
HENDEC
HOMEEC
INASEC
MIXTEC
ONESEC
ONSPEC
PARSEC
QUEBEC
THREEC
TOLTEC

ED••••

EDAMES
EDBERG
EDDAIC
EDDIED
EDDIES
EDDOES
EDEMAS
EDENIC
EDERLE
EDESSA
EDGARD
EDGARS
EDGEIN
EDGERS
EDGIER
EDGILY
EDGING
EDIBLE
EDIBLY
EDICTS
EDILES
EDIRNE
EDISON
EDITED
EDITIO
EDITOR
EDKOCH
EDMOND
EDMUND
EDSELS
EDUARD
EDUCED
EDUCES
EDUCTS
EDVARD
EDWARD
EDWINA
EDWOOD
EDWYNN

E•D•••

EDDAIC
EDDIED
EDDIES
EDDOES
EIDERS
EIDOLA
ELDERS
ELDEST
EMDASH
ENDALL
ENDASH
ENDCUT
ENDEAR
ENDERS
ENDING
ENDIVE
ENDMAN
ENDMEN
ENDORA
ENDOWS
ENDPIN
ENDRAN
ENDRUN
ENDSAT
ENDSIN
ENDSIT
ENDSON
ENDSUP
ENDUED
ENDUES
ENDURE
ENDURO
ENDUSE
ERDMAN
ESDRAS
EUDORA

E••D••

EJIDOS
EKEDBY
ELADIO
ELIDED
ELIDER
ELIDES
ELODEA
ELUDED
ELUDER
ELUDES
ENIDOK
EPODES
EPODIC
ERODED
ERODER
ERODES
ETUDES
EUSDEN
EVADED
EVADER
EVADES
EXEDRA
EXODUS
EXUDED
EXUDES
EYEDUP

E•••D•

EBONDS
ECARDS
ELANDS
EMBEDS
EMBODY
EMENDS
ENCODE
EPHODS
ESCUDO
ESTADO
ETRADE
EXCIDE

E••••D

EAGLED
EARBUD
EARNED
ECHOED
ECKERD
EDDIED
EDGARD
EDITED
EDMOND
EDMUND
EDUARD
EDUCED
EDVARD
EDWARD
EDWOOD
EFILED
EIGHTD
EKLAND
ELAPID
ELATED
ELIDED
ELOPED
ELUARD
ELUDED
ELUTED
ELWOOD
EMCEED
EMOTED
EMQUAD
ENDUED
ENFOLD
ENGILD
ENGIRD
ENNEAD
ENQUAD
ENSUED
ENURED
ENVIED
ENWIND
EQUOID
ERASED
ERHARD
ERODED
ERRAND
ERSTAD
ESPIED
ETCHED
EUCLID
EVADED
EVENED
EVOKED
EXCEED
EXILED
EXITED
EXPAND
EXPEND
EXTEND
EXUDED
EYELID
EYVIND
EZZARD

•ED•••

AEDILE
BEDAUB
BEDAZE
BEDBUG
BEDDED
BEDECK
BEDEWS
BEDIMS
BEDLAM
BEDOGS
BEDSIT
BEDWIN
CEDARN
CEDARS
CEDARY
CEDERS
CEDING
CEDRIC
DEDANS
DEDHAM
DEDINI
DEDUCE
DEDUCT
DEDUVE
FEDORA
GEDDES
HEDGED
HEDGER
HEDGES
HEDLEY
HEDRAL
HEDREN
HEDRON
JEDGAR
KEDGED
KEDGER
KEDGES
LEDGER
LEDGES
LEDOFF
LEDOUT
LEDOUX
MEDAKA
MEDALS
MEDDLE
MEDFLY
MEDGAR
MEDIAL
MEDIAN
MEDIAS
MEDICA
MEDICI
MEDICO
MEDICS
MEDINA
MEDIUM
MEDIUS
MEDLEY
MEDNIS
MEDOCS
MEDUSA
PEDALS
PEDANT
PEDATE
PEDDLE
PEDWAY
REDACE
REDACT
REDANS
REDANT
REDARE
REDARN
REDATE
REDBAT
REDBAY
REDBUD
REDCAP
REDCOD
REDDEN
REDDER
REDDIN
REDDOG
REDDOT
REDEAL
REDEED
REDEEM
REDEFY
REDENY
REDEYE
REDFIN
REDFIR
REDFOX
REDHAT
REDHEN
REDHOT
REDIAL
REDIGS
REDING
REDINK
REDIPS
REDLEG
REDOAK
REDOCK
REDOER
REDOES
REDONE
REDOSE
REDOUT
REDRAG
REDRAW
REDREW
REDRUM
REDSEA
REDSIX
REDSKY
REDSOX
REDSUN
REDTAB
REDTAG
REDTEN
REDTIE
REDTOP
REDTWO
REDUBS
REDUCE
REDUST
REDYED
REDYES
SEDAKA
SEDANS
SEDATE
SEDERS
SEDGED
SEDGES
SEDICI
SEDLEY
SEDONA
SEDUCE
SEDUMS
TEDEUM
TEDIUM
TEDKEY
VEDAIC
VEDDER
VEDIST
WEDDED
WEDDER
WEDELN
WEDELS
WEDGED
WEDGES
WEDGIE
XEDOUT
ZEDONG
ZEDONK

•E•D••

BEADED
BEADER
BEADLE
BEADUP
BEDDED
BELDAM
BENDAY
BENDED
BENDER
BENDIX
DEADEN
DEADER
DEADLY
DEADON
DEEDED
DEEDEE
DEIDRE
DENDRA
DENDRI
DENDRO
DEODAR
FEEDER
FEEDIN
FEEDME
FEEDON
FEEDTO
FELDON
FENDED
FENDER
FEODOR
FERDIE
FEUDAL
FEUDED
GEDDES
GELDED
GELDOF
GENDER
GEODES
GEODIC
HEADED
HEADER
HEADIN
HEADON
HEADTO
HEADUP
HEEDED
HEEDER
HEIDEN
HELDIN
HELDIT
HELDON
HELDTO
HELDUP
HENDEC
HENDRY
HERDED
HERDER
HEYDAY
KENDOS
KEYDET
LEADED
LEADEN
LEADER
LEADIN
LEADON
LEADTO
LEADUP
LEIDEN
LENDEE
LENDER
LENDTO
LEWDER
LEWDLY
LEYDEN
MEADER
MEADOW
MEDDLE
MELDED
MELDER
MENDED
MENDEL
MENDER
MENDES
MERDLE
NEEDBE
NEEDED
NEEDER
NEEDLE
NEEDNT
NEEDTO
NEWDAY
PEDDLE
PEEDEE
PENDED
PERDAY
PERDUE
PETDOG
READDS
READER
READIN
README
READON
READTO
READUP
REDDEN
REDDER
REDDIN
REDDOG
REDDOT
REEDED
REEDER
REEDIT
RENDED
RENDER
SEADOG
SEEDED
SEEDER
SELDOM
SENDAK
SENDBY
SENDEE
SENDER
SENDIN
SENDON
SENDTO
SENDUP
TEEDUP
TENDAY
TENDED
TENDER
TENDON
TENDTO
VEADAR
VEDDER
VELDTS
VENDED
VENDEE
VENDER
VENDOR
VENDUE
VERDES
VERDIN
VERDON
VERDUN
WEDDED
WEDDER
WEEDED
WEEDER
WEIDER
WELDED
WELDER
WELDON
WENDED
WENDIE
WENDYS
ZENDOS

•E••D•

BEARDS
BESIDE
BETIDE
CEPEDA
DECADE
DECADS
DECIDE
DECODE
DELUDE
DEMODE
DENADA
DENUDE
DERIDE
DESADE
DESODS
FELIDS
GEORDI
HEXADS
LERIDA
LEVADE
MELODY
MENUDO
MERIDA
NERUDA
NEVADA
PESADE
READDS
REBIDS
RECEDE
RECODE
REHIDE
REMADE
REMEDY
REPADS
RERIDE
RERODE
RESEDA
RESIDE
RESODS
REWEDS
SECADA
SECEDE
WEALDS
WEBADS
WEIRDO
WEIRDY
YEGODS
YEHUDI
YEOLDE
YESIDO

•E•••D

AENEID
BEADED
BEAKED
BEAMED
BEANED
BEDDED
BEEFED
BEEPED
BEGGED
BEGIRD
BEGOOD
BEHEAD
BEHELD
BEHIND
BEHOLD
BEKIND
BELIED
BELLED
BELTED
BENDED
BERMED
BESTED
BETTED
BEYOND
CEASED
CEILED
CELLED
CENSED
CERVID
CESSED
DECKED
DEEDED
DEEMED
DEFEND
DEFIED
DEFORD
DEFUND
DEICED
DELAND
DELEAD
DELVED
DEMAND
DEMOED
DEMOND
DENIED
DENNED
DENTED
DEPEND
DESEED
DEUCED
DEVOID
FEARED
FECUND
FELLED
FELTED
FENCED
FENDED
FERVID
FESSED
FEUDED
FEZZED
GEARED
GEEKED
GELDED
GELLED
GEMMED
GERALD
GERARD
GERUND

GETMAD
GETOLD
GETRID
GETSAD
HEADED
HEALED
HEAPED
HEATED
HEAVED
HEDGED
HEEDED
HEELED
HEFTED
HELMED
HELPED
HEMMED
HEPTAD
HERALD
HERBED
HERDED
HESIOD
JEANED
JEERED
JELLED
JERKED
JESTED
JETTED
KEDGED
KEELED
KEENED
KEGGED
KENNED
KERNED
KEYOFD
KEYPAD
LEADED
LEAFED
LEAKED
LEANED
LEAPED
LEASED
LEAVED
LEERED
LEGEND
LEGGED
LELAND
LEMOND
LENARD
LENSED
LEONID
LETTED
LEVEED
LEVIED
MELDED
MELTED
MENDED
MEOWED
MERCED
MERGED
MESHED
MESSED
METHOD
METRED
MEWLED
NEARED
NECKED
NEEDED
NEREID

NERVED
NESTED
NETTED
NEWKID
NEXRAD
PEAKED
PEALED
PEAPOD
PECKED
PEEKED
PEELED
PEENED
PEEPED
PEERED
PEEVED
PEGGED
PELTED
PENDED
PENNED
PENROD
PENTAD
PEPCID
PEPPED
PEQUOD
PERIOD
PERKED
PERMED
PERNOD
PETARD
PETTED
REAMED
REAPED
REARED
REAVED
REBEND
REBIND
REBRED
RECKED
RECLAD
RECORD
RECUED
REDBUD
REDCOD
REDEED
REDYED
REEDED
REEFED
REEKED
REELED
REEVED
REFEED
REFFED
REFIED
REFIND
REFOLD
REFUND
REGARD
REGILD
REGIRD
REHELD
REHOED
REHOLD
REICED
REINED
RELAID
RELAND
RELEAD
RELEND

RELIED
RELOAD
REMAND
REMEND
REMIND
REMOLD
RENARD
RENDED
RENTED
REPAID
REPLED
REPPED
REREAD
RESAID
RESAND
RESEED
RESEND
RESHOD
RESOLD
RESTED
RETARD
RETIED
RETOLD
RETROD
RETTED
REUNED
REUSED
REVEND
REVVED
REWARD
REWELD
REWIND
REWORD
SEABED
SEAGOD
SEALED
SEAMED
SEARED
SEATED
SECOND
SEDGED
SEEDED
SEEMED
SEEPED
SEERED
SEGUED
SEINED
SEIZED
SENSED
SERVED
SEVEND
SEWARD
TEAMED
TEARED
TEASED
TEEMED
TEHEED
TEMPED
TENDED
TENSED
TENTED
TERMED
TESTED
TETRAD
TEXTED
VEERED
VEGGED
VEILED

VEINED
VENDED
VENTED
VERBID
VERGED
VERSED
VESPID
VESTED
VETOED
VETTED
WEANED
WEAVED
WEBBED
WEBFED
WEDDED
WEDGED
WEEDED
WEENED
WELDED
WELLED
WELTED
WENDED
WETTED
YEANED
YELLED
YELPED
YENNED
YENSID
YESSED
ZEROED
ZESTED

••ED••

ACEDIA
ACEDIT
AGEDLY
AMEDEE
AMEDEO
AVEDON
AWEDLY
BREDES
CHEDER
COEDIT
CREDIT
CREDOS
CUEDIN
DAEDAL
DEEDED
DEEDEE
DREDGE
EKEDBY
EXEDRA
EYEDUP
FEEDER
FEEDIN
FEEDME
FEEDON
FEEDTO
FLEDGE
FLEDGY
FREDDY
FREDRO
HEEDED
HEEDER
ICEDAM
ICEDIN
ICEDIT
ICEDUP
JOEDON
LIEDER
LIEDON
LIEDTO
NEEDBE
NEEDED
NEEDER
NEEDLE
NEEDNT
NEEDTO
OCEDAR
ODEDON
ONEDAY
ONEDGE
OWEDON
OWEDTO
PEEDEE
PHEDRE
PLEDGE
PLEDTO
PREDAY
PREDRY
PYEDOG
REEDED
REEDER
REEDIT
SEEDED
SEEDER
SHEDDS
SHEDON
SLEDGE
SPEDUP
SUEDED
SUEDES
SVEDKA
SWEDEN
SWEDES
TEEDUP
THEDOW
TIEDIN
TIEDON
TIEDTO
TIEDUP
TIEDYE
TOEDIN
TREDIA
UNEDGE
USEDCD
USEDIN
USEDON
USEDTO
USEDUP
WEEDED
WEEDER

••E•D•

AGENDA
AMENDS
ARENDT
BLEEDS
BLENDE
BLENDS
BREADS
BREEDS
BREEDY
BRENDA
CREEDS
DREADS
EMENDS
FIELDS
FIENDS
FREDDY
GLENDA
GREEDS
GREEDY
IMELDA
KNEADS
ONEIDA
OREADS
OREIDA
OVERDO
PLEADS
PSEUDO
PSEUDS
SHEDDS
SHEEDY
SPEEDO
SPEEDS
SPEEDY
SPENDS
SPENDY
STEADS
STEADY
STEEDS
TIENDA
TREADS
TRENDS
TRENDY
TWEEDS
TWEEDY
UPENDS
WIELDS
WIELDY
YIELDS

••E••D

AFEARD
AGEOLD
ANELED
BEEFED
BEEPED
BREWED
CHEFED
CHEWED
CLEWED
CREPED
CREWED
CUEBID
DEEDED
DEEMED
DIETED
DUELED
DUETED
EVENED
EYELID
FLEXED
FOETID
FREUND
FUELED
GEEKED
GREYED
HEEDED
HEELED
ITEMED
JEERED
KEELED
KEENED
LEERED
MAENAD
NEEDED
OBEYED
OLERUD
OMENED
OPENED
PEEKED
PEELED
PEENED
PEEPED
PEERED
PEEVED
PIECED
PLEIAD
PREBID
PREMED
PREYED
QUEUED
REEDED
REEFED
REEKED
REELED
REEVED
SEEDED
SEEMED
SEEPED
SEERED
SIEGED
SIEVED
SKEWED
SLEWED
SPEWED
STEWED
SUEDED
TEEMED
THECID
THEEND
THEFED
THEKID
THEMED
THERED
THEROD
THETED
TIERED
TIEROD
TREPID
USEDCD
USERID
VEERED
VIEWED
WEEDED
WEENED
WHERED

•••ED•

ACCEDE
ALBEDO
ALGEDI
BIPEDS
BLEEDS
BREEDS
BREEDY
CEPEDA
COMEDY
CREEDS
EMBEDS
FRIEDA
GREEDS
GREEDY
IMBEDS
IMPEDE
LAMEDS
LAREDO
LUNEDI
MADEDO
MAKEDO
MOPEDS
OVIEDO
RATEDA
RATEDG
RATEDR
RATEDX
RECEDE
REMEDY
RESEDA
REWEDS
SAMEDI
SECEDE
SHEEDY
SHREDS
SPEEDO
SPEEDS
SPEEDY
STBEDE
STEEDS
SUREDO
TOLEDO
TUXEDO
TWEEDS
TWEEDY

•••E•D

ADDEND
AENEID
AFIELD
AGREED
ANTEED
APPEND
ASCEND
ATTEND
AUGEND
AXHEAD
AXSEED
BADEND
BAGEND
BEHEAD
BEHELD
BIGEND
COOEED
DEFEND
DELEAD
DEPEND
DESEED
ECKERD
EMCEED
ENNEAD
EXCEED
EXPEND
EXTEND
FAGEND
FAKEID
FIVEAD
FRIEND
GILEAD
GODEAD
IMPEND
INDEED
INNEED
INTEND
LEGEND
LEVEED
LOWEND
NEREID
NIKEAD
NINEAD
NOLEAD
NONEED
OFFEND
OSTEND
PUREED
REBEND
REDEED
REFEED
REHELD
RELEAD
RELEND
REMEND
REREAD
RESEED
RESEND
REVEND
REWELD
SCREED
SEVEND
SHIELD
SHREWD
SINEAD
SPREAD
TAGEND
TEHEED
THEEND
THREAD
THREED
UNBEND
UNDEAD
UNHEED
UNHELD
UNLEAD
UNREAD
UNSELD
UPHELD
UPSEND

••••ED

ABASED
ABATED
ABIDED
ABUSED
ADDLED
ADORED
AGREED
AISLED
ALATED
ALFRED
ALINED
ALIPED
ALLIED
AMAZED
AMBLED
AMUSED
ANELED
ANGLED
ANKLED
ANTEED
ARCHED
ARGUED
ATONED
AUTOED
AVOWED
AWAKED
AXSEED
AZURED
BABIED
BACHED
BACKED
BAFFED
BAGGED
BAILED
BAITED
BALDED
BALKED
BANDED
BANGED
BANKED
BANNED
BARBED
BARGED
BARKED
BARNED
BARRED
BASHED
BASKED
BASTED
BATHED
BATTED
BAWLED
BEADED
BEAKED
BEAMED
BEANED
BEDDED
BEEFED
BEEPED
BEGGED
BELIED
BELLED
BELTED
BENDED
BERMED
BESTED
BETTED
BIASED
BIBBED
BIFFED
BIGRED
BILGED
BILKED
BILLED
BINGED
BINNED
BIRDED
BIRLED
BIRRED
BITTED
BLADED
BLAMED
BLARED
BLAZED
BOATED
BOBBED
BODIED
BOFFED
BOGGED
BOILED
BOLDED
BOLTED
BOMBED
BONDED
BONGED
BONKED
BOOKED
BOOMED
BOOTED
BOOZED
BOPPED
BORKED
BOSSED
BOWLED
BOXBED
BRACED
BRAKED
BRAVED
BRAYED
BREWED
BRIBED
BRINED
BROWED
BRUXED
BUCKED
BUDDED
BUDGED
BUFFED
BUGGED
BUGLED
BULGED
BULKED
BULLED
BUMMED
BUMPED
BUNGED
BUNKED
BUNTED
BUOYED
BURIED
BURLED
BURNED
BURPED
BURRED
BUSHED
BUSIED
BUSKED
BUSSED
BUSTED
BUTTED
BUZZED
CABBED
CABLED
CACHED
CADGED
CALKED
CALLED
CALMED
CALVED
CAMPED
CANNED
CANOED
CANTED
CAPPED
CARDED
CARPED
CARTED
CARVED
CASHED
CASKED
CASTED
CATBED
CAUSED
CEASED
CEILED
CELLED
CENSED
CESSED
CHAFED
CHASED
CHAWED
CHEFED
CHEWED
CHIDED
CHIMED
CHOKED
CHOWED
CHUTED
CITIED
CLAWED
CLEWED
CLONED
CLOSED
CLOYED
COALED
COATED
COAXED
COCKED
COGGED
COIFED
COILED
COINED
COMBED
COMPED
CONFED
CONKED
CONNED
COOEED
COOKED
COOLED
COOPED
COPIED
COPPED
CORDED
CORKED
CORNED
COSHED
COSIED
COSTED
COWLED
COZIED
CRANED
CRAPED
CRATED
CRAVED
CRAZED
CREPED
CREWED
CROWED
CUBBED
CUFFED
CULLED
CUPPED
CURBED
CURDED
CURLED
CURRED
CURSED
CURVED
CUSPED
CUSSED
CYCLED
DABBED
DADOED
DAMMED
DAMNED
DAMPED
DANCED
DANGED
DAPPED
DARNED
DARTED
DASHED
DAUBED
DAWNED
DAYBED
DECKED
DEEDED
DEEMED
DEFIED
DEICED
DELVED
DEMOED
DENIED
DENNED
DENTED
DESEED
DEUCED
DIALED
DIETED
DIMMED
DINGED
DINNED
DINTED
DIOMED
DIPPED
DIRKED
DISHED
DISKED
DISSED
DOCKED
DODGED
DOFFED
DOGBED
DOGGED
DOLLED
DONNED
DOOMED
DOORED
DOSSED
DOTTED
DOUSED
DOWNED
DOWSED
DRAPED
DRAYED
DRONED
DUBBED
DUCKED
DUCTED
DUELED
DUETED
DULLED
DUMPED
DUNKED
DUNNED
DURNED
DUSKED
DUSTED
EAGLED
EARNED
ECHOED
EDDIED
EDITED
EDUCED
EFILED
ELATED
ELIDED
ELOPED
ELUDED
ELUTED
EMCEED
EMOTED
ENDUED
ENSUED
ENURED
ENVIED
ERASED
ERODED
ESPIED
ETCHED
EVADED
EVENED
EVOKED
EXCEED
EXILED
EXITED
EXUDED
FABLED
FAILED
FAIRED
FANGED
FANNED
FARCED
FARMED
FASTED
FATTED
FAWNED
FEARED
FELLED
FELTED
FENCED
FENDED
FESSED
FEUDED
FEZZED
FIBBED
FILLED
FILMED
FINKED
FINNED
FIRMED
FISHED
FISTED
FITTED
FIZZED
FLAKED
FLAMED
FLARED
FLAWED
FLAYED
FLEXED
FLOWED
FLUTED
FLUXED
FOALED
FOAMED
FOBBED
FOGGED
FOILED
FOLDED
FOOLED
FOOTED
FORCED
FORDED
FORGED
FORKED
FORMED
FOULED
FOWLED
FRAMED
FRAYED
FUDGED
FUELED
FUNDED
FUNKED
FUNNED
FURLED
FURRED
FUSSED
FUTZED
FUZZED
GABBED
GABLED
GADDED
GAFFED
GAGGED
GAINED
GAITED
GALLED
GAMMED
GANGED
GAOLED
GAPPED
GARBED
GASHED
GASPED
GASSED
GAUGED
GAWKED
GAWPED
GEARED
GEEKED
GELDED
GELLED
GEMMED
GIFTED
GIGGED
GILDED
GILLED
GIMPED
GINNED
GIRDED
GIRTED
GITTED
GLARED

GLAZED
GLIDED
GLOBED
GLOVED
GLOWED
GNAWED
GOADED
GOCOED
GOLFED
GONGED
GOOFED
GOOSED
GORGED
GORMED
GOUGED
GOWNED
GRACED
GRADED
GRATED
GRAVED
GRAYED
GRAZED
GREYED
GRIMED
GRIPED
GROPED
GROVED
GUIDED
GUILED
GULFED
GULLED
GULPED
GUMMED
GUNNED
GUSHED
GUSTED
GUTTED
GYPPED
HACKED
HAFTED
HAILED
HAIRED
HALOED
HALTED
HALVED
HAMMED
HANDED
HANGED
HARKED
HARMED
HARPED
HASHED
HASPED
HASTED
HATRED
HATTED
HAULED
HAWKED
HEADED
HEALED
HEAPED
HEATED
HEAVED
HEDGED
HEEDED
HEELED
HEFTED
HELMED

HELPED
HEMMED
HERBED
HERDED
HILLED
HILTED
HINGED
HINTED
HIPPED
HISSED
HOAXED
HOBOED
HOCKED
HOGGED
HONIED
HONKED
HOODED
HOOFED
HOOKED
HOOPED
HOOTED
HOPPED
HORDED
HORNED
HORSED
HOSTED
HOTBED
HOUSED
HOWLED
HUFFED
HUGGED
HULKED
HULLED
HUMMED
HUMPED
HUNTED
HURLED
HUSHED
HUSKED
HUTTED
HYMNED
HYPOED
IDARED
ILLFED
IMAGED
IMBUED
IMPLED
INBRED
INCHED
INDEED
INDUED
INNEED
INURED
IRISED
IRONED
ISSUED
ITCHED
ITEMED
ITRIED
JABBED
JACKED
JAGGED
JAILED
JAMMED
JARRED
JAZZED
JEANED
JEERED

JELLED
JERKED
JESTED
JETTED
JIGGED
JILTED
JINXED
JOBBED
JOGGED
JOINED
JOLTED
JOSHED
JOTTED
JOWLED
JUDGED
JUGGED
JUICED
JUMPED
JUNKED
JURIED
JUTTED
KAYOED
KEDGED
KEELED
KEENED
KEGGED
KENNED
KERNED
KICKED
KIDDED
KILLED
KILNED
KILTED
KINGED
KINKED
KIPPED
KISSED
KITTED
KNIFED
LACKED
LADLED
LAGGED
LAIRED
LALLED
LAMBED
LAMMED
LANCED
LANDED
LAPPED
LAPSED
LARDED
LARKED
LASHED
LASTED
LATHED
LAUDED
LEADED
LEAFED
LEAKED
LEANED
LEAPED
LEASED
LEAVED
LEERED
LEGGED
LENSED
LETTED
LEVEED

LEVIED
LIBBED
LICKED
LIDDED
LIFTED
LILIED
LILTED
LIMBED
LIMNED
LIMPED
LINKED
LINTED
LIPPED
LISPED
LISTED
LOADED
LOAFED
LOAMED
LOANED
LOBBED
LOCKED
LODGED
LOFTED
LOGGED
LOIDED
LOLLED
LONGED
LOOKED
LOOMED
LOOPED
LOOSED
LOOTED
LOPPED
LORDED
LOTTED
LOUSED
LUCKED
LUFFED
LUGGED
LULLED
LUMPED
LUNGED
LURKED
LUSTED
MADDED
MAILED
MAIMED
MALTED
MANNED
MAPPED
MARKED
MARLED
MARRED
MASHED
MASKED
MASSED
MASTED
MATTED
MAULED
MELDED
MELTED
MENDED
MEOWED
MERCED
MERGED
MESHED
MESSED
METRED

MEWLED
MIFFED
MILKED
MILLED
MINCED
MINDED
MINTED
MISFED
MISLED
MISSED
MISTED
MITRED
MOANED
MOATED
MOBBED
MOCKED
MODRED
MOILED
MOLDED
MOLTED
MONIED
MOONED
MOORED
MOOTED
MOPPED
MOSHED
MOSSED
MOUSED
MUCKED
MUDDED
MUFFED
MUGGED
MULLED
MUMMED
MUSHED
MUSSED
NABBED
NACRED
NAGGED
NAILED
NAPPED
NBCRED
NEARED
NECKED
NEEDED
NERVED
NESTED
NETTED
NICHED
NICKED
NIPPED
NOCKED
NODDED
NOISED
NONEED
NONFED
NOOSED
NOSHED
NUBBED
NUDGED
NULLED
NUMBED
NURSED
NUTTED
OBEYED
OCHRED
ODORED
OINKED

OKAYED
OMENED
OPENED
OPINED
ORATED
OUSTED
OUTLED
PACKED
PADDED
PAINED
PAIRED
PALLED
PALMED
PANNED
PANTED
PARGED
PARKED
PARRED
PARSED
PARTED
PASSED
PASTED
PATTED
PAUSED
PAWNED
PEAKED
PEALED
PECKED
PEEKED
PEELED
PEENED
PEEPED
PEERED
PEEVED
PEGGED
PELTED
PENDED
PENNED
PEPPED
PERKED
PERMED
PETTED
PHASED
PHONED
PHYSED
PICKED
PIECED
PIGGED
PILLED
PINGED
PINKED
PINNED
PIQUED
PISHED
PITHED
PITIED
PITTED
PLACED
PLANED
PLATED
PLAYED
PLOWED
PLUMED
PODDED
POISED
POLLED
PONDED
PONIED

POOHED
POOLED
POOPED
POPPED
PORKED
PORTED
POSTED
POTTED
POUFED
POURED
POUTED
PRATED
PRAYED
PREMED
PREYED
PRICED
PRIDED
PRIMED
PRISED
PRIZED
PROBED
PROSED
PROVED
PRUNED
PUFFED
PULLED
PULPED
PULSED
PUMPED
PUNNED
PUNTED
PUPPED
PUREED
PURGED
PURLED
PURRED
PURSED
PUSHED
PUTTED
QUAKED
QUEUED
QUIRED
QUOTED
RACKED
RAFTED
RAGGED
RAIDED
RAILED
RAINED
RAISED
RAMMED
RAMPED
RANGED
RANKED
RANTED
RAPPED
RASPED
RATTED
RAZZED
REAMED
REAPED
REARED
REAVED
REBRED
RECKED
RECUED
REDEED
REDYED

REEDED
REEFED
REEKED
REELED
REEVED
REFEED
REFFED
REFIED
REHOED
REICED
REINED
RELIED
RENDED
RENTED
REPLED
REPPED
RESEED
RESTED
RETIED
RETTED
REUNED
REUSED
REVVED
RHYMED
RIBBED
RIDDED
RIDGED
RIFFED
RIFLED
RIFTED
RIGGED
RIMMED
RINGED
RINSED
RIOTED
RIPPED
RISKED
ROAMED
ROARED
ROBBED
ROCKED
RODDED
ROGUED
ROILED
ROLFED
ROLLED
ROMPED
ROOFED
ROOKED
ROOMED
ROOTED
ROTTED
ROUGED
ROUSED
ROUTED
RRATED
RSVPED
RUBBED
RUBIED
RUCKED
RUFFED
RUGGED
RUINED
RUSHED
RUSTED
RUTTED
SACKED
SACRED

SAGGED
SAILED
SALTED
SALVED
SANDED
SAPPED
SASHED
SASSED
SAUCED
SAWRED
SCALED
SCARED
SCOPED
SCORED
SCREED
SEABED
SEALED
SEAMED
SEARED
SEATED
SEDGED
SEEDED
SEEMED
SEEPED
SEERED
SEGUED
SEINED
SEIZED
SENSED
SERVED
SHADED
SHAMED
SHAPED
SHARED
SHAVED
SHINED
SHOOED
SHOVED
SHOWED
SICCED
SIDLED
SIEGED
SIEVED
SIFTED
SIGHED
SIGNED
SILOED
SILTED
SINGED
SINNED
SIPPED
SKATED
SKEWED
SLAKED
SLATED
SLAVED
SLAYED
SLEWED
SLICED
SLIMED
SLOPED
SLOWED
SMILED
SMOKED
SNAKED
SNARED
SNIPED
SNORED

SNOWED
SOAKED
SOAPED
SOARED
SOBBED
SOCKED
SODDED
SOILED
SOLOED
SOLVED
SOPPED
SORTED
SOTTED
SOURED
SOUSED
SPACED
SPADED
SPARED
SPAYED
SPEWED
SPICED
SPIKED
SPINED
SPIRED
SPITED
SPOKED
SPUMED
STAGED
STAKED
STALED
STARED
STATED
STAVED
STAYED
STEWED
STOKED
STONED
STORED
STOWED
STYLED
SUBBED
SUCKED
SUDSED
SUEDED
SUITED
SULKED
SUMMED
SUNNED
SUPPED
SURFED
SURGED
SUSSED
SWAYED
SWIPED
SYNCED
TABBED
TABLED
TABUED
TACKED
TAGGED
TAILED
TALCED
TALKED
TAMPED
TANGED
TANKED
TANNED
TAPPED

TARRED
TARTED
TASKED
TASTED
TATTED
TAXIED
TEAMED
TEARED
TEASED
TEEMED
TEHEED
TEMPED
TENDED
TENSED
TENTED
TERMED
TESTED
TEXTED
THAWED
THEFED
THEMED
THERED
THETED
THREED
TICCED
TICKED
TIDIED
TIERED
TIFFED
TILLED
TILTED
TINGED
TINNED
TINTED
TIPPED
TITHED
TITLED
TITRED
TOGAED
TOGGED
TOILED
TOLLED
TONGED
TOOLED
TOOTED
TOPPED
TOSSED
TOTTED
TOURED
TOUTED
TRACED
TRADED
TROWED
TUBBED
TUCKED
TUFTED
TUGGED
TURFED
TURNED
TUSKED
TUTTED
TUTUED
TWINED
UNAGED
UNAWED
UNAXED
UNBLED
UNDYED

UNHEED
UNHOED
UNHUED
UNICED
UNIPED
UNITED
UNOWED
UNRUED
UNSHED
UNSUED
UNTIED
UNUSED
VALUED
VALVED
VAMPED
VANNED
VARIED
VATTED
VEERED
VEGGED
VEILED
VEINED
VENDED
VENTED
VERGED
VERSED
VESTED
VETOED
VETTED
VIALED
VIEWED
VISAED
VOGUED
VOICED
VOIDED
WADDED
WAFTED
WAGGED
WAILED
WAITED
WAIVED
WALKED
WALLED
WANNED
WANTED
WARDED
WARMED
WARNED
WARPED
WARRED
WARTED
WASHED
WASLED
WASTED
WEANED
WEAVED
WEBBED
WEBFED
WEDDED
WEDGED
WEEDED
WEENED
WELDED
WELLED
WELTED
WENDED
WETTED
WHALED

WHERED
WHILED
WHINED
WHITED
WICKED
WIFIED
WIGGED
WILLED
WILTED
WIMPED
WINCED
WINDED
WINGED
WINKED
WISHED
WISPED
WITTED
WOLFED
WONTED
WOODED
WOOFED
WORDED
WORKED
WORMED
XRATED
XRAYED
YAKKED
YANKED
YAPPED
YARDED
YARNED
YAWNED
YAWPED
YEANED
YELLED
YELPED
YENNED
YESSED
YIPPED
YOLKED
YOWLED
YOYOED
YUKKED
ZAGGED
ZAPPED
ZEROED
ZESTED
ZIGGED
ZINCED
ZINGED
ZIPPED
ZIZZED
ZONKED
ZOOMED

EE••••

EELERS
EELERY
EELIER
EELING
EELPOT
EENSIE
EERIER
EERILY
EEYORE

E•E•••

EBERLE
EBERLY
ECESIC
ECESIS
EDEMAS
EDENIC
EDERLE
EDESSA
EGERIA
EGESTA
EGESTS
EJECTA
EJECTS
EKEDBY
EKELOF
EKEOUT
EKESBY
ELECTS
ELEGIT
ELEMIS
ELEVEN
ELEVES
ELEVON
EMEERS
EMENDS
EMERGE
EMERIC
EMERIL
EMETIC
EMEUTE
ENERGY
ENEROS
ENESCO
EREBUS
ERECTS
ERENOW
ERESTU
EREVAN
ESENIN
ETERNE
EVELYN
EVENAS
EVENED
EVENER
EVENIF
EVENLY
EVENSO
EVENTS
EVENUP
EVERLY
EVERSO
EVERTS
EXEDRA
EXEMPT
EXERTS
EXETER
EXEUNT
EYECUP
EYEDUP
EYEFUL
EYEING
EYELET
EYELID
EYEPIT
EYESUP

E••E••

EASEBY
EASEIN
EASELS
EASEON
EASERS
EASEUP
EATERS
EATERY
EBBETS
ECKERD
ECZEMA
EDBERG
EDGEIN
EDGERS
EDSELS
EELERS
EELERY
EFFECT
EFFETE
EGBERT
EGGERS
EGGERT
EGRESS
EGRETS
EIDERS
EILEEN
EILERS
EILERT
EIRENE
EISELE
EKBERG
EKUELE
ELBERT
ELDERS
ELDEST
ELIELI
ELLERY
ELMERS
ELRENO
ELVERS
EMBEDS
EMBERS
EMCEED
EMCEES
EMEERS
EMMETS
EMMETT
EMPERY
ENBERG
ENDEAR
ENDERS
ENGELS
ENMESH
ENNEAD
ENSEAL
ENSEAT
ENTERO
ENTERS
ENVEIL
EOCENE
ERIEPA
ERNEST
ESCENT
ESKERS
ESSENE
ESTEEM
ESTERS
ETCETC
ETHENE
ETHERS

ETSEQQ
EUGENE
EULESS
EUREKA
EXCEED
EXCELS
EXCEPT
EXCESS
EXMETS
EXPECT
EXPELS
EXPEND
EXPERT
EXSECT
EXSERT
EXTEND
EXTENT
EXTERN

E•••E•

EAGLED
EAGLES
EAGLET
EAGRES
EARLET
EARNED
EARNER
EASIER
EASLEY
EASTER
EBATES
EBAYER
ECCLES
ECHOED
ECHOER
ECHOES
ECOLES
EDAMES
EDDIED
EDDIES
EDDOES
EDGIER
EDILES
EDITED
EDUCED
EDUCES
EELIER
EERIER
EFILED
EFILES
EGALES
EGGIER
EGGLER
EGISES
EGUREN
EIFFEL
EILEEN
EISLEY
EISNER
EITHER
ELANET
ELATED
ELATER
ELATES
ELAYER
ELEVEN
ELEVES
ELIDED
ELIDER
ELIDES
ELISEO
ELITER
ELITES
ELMIER
ELODEA
ELOGES
ELOPED
ELOPER
ELOPES
ELUDED
ELUDER
ELUDES
ELUTED
ELUTES
ELYSEE
EMBLEM
EMCEED
EMCEES
EMINEM
EMOTED
EMOTER
EMOTES
ENAMEL
ENATES
ENCRES
ENDMEN
ENDUED
ENDUES
ENOTES
ENSLER
ENSUED
ENSUES
ENTREE
ENTREZ
ENURED
ENURES
ENVIED
ENVIER
ENVIES
EPODES
EPOPEE
EPOSES
EPOWER
ERASED
ERASER
ERASES
ERODED
ERODER
ERODES
ESALEN
ESCHER
ESCHEW
ESPIED
ESPIER
ESPIES
ESTEEM
ESTHER
ETAGES
ETAPES
ETCHED
ETCHER
ETCHES
ETILES
ETUDES
EUBOEA
EUCKEN
EUPNEA
EUSDEN
EVADED
EVADER
EVADES
EVENED
EVENER
EVILER
EVITES
EVOKED
EVOKER
EVOKES
EXCEED
EXETER
EXILED
EXILER
EXILES
EXITED
EXOCET
EXUDED
EXUDES
EYELET
EYRIES
EZINES

E••••E

EANNIE
EARNIE
EBERLE
ECARTE
ECORSE
ECTYPE
EDERLE
EDIBLE
EDIRNE
EENSIE
EEYORE
EFFACE
EFFETE
EFFUSE
EGLISE
EIGHTE
EIRENE
EISELE
EKUELE
ELAINE
ELANCE
ELAPSE
ELAYNE
ELLICE
ELMIRE
ELMORE
ELOISE
ELUATE
ELYSEE
EMBRUE
EMERGE
EMEUTE
EMIGRE
EMILIE
EMPALE
EMPIRE
ENABLE
ENCAGE
ENCASE
ENCODE
ENCORE
ENDIVE
ENDURE
ENDUSE
ENFACE
ENGAGE
ENGINE
ENISLE
ENLACE
ENORME
ENRAGE
ENROBE
ENSATE
ENSILE
ENSURE
ENTICE
ENTIRE
ENTREE
ENZYME
EOCENE
EPOPEE
EPOQUE
EQUATE
EQUINE
ERMINE
ERRARE
ESCALE
ESCAPE
ESSENE
ESTATE
ESTIME
ETERNE
ETHANE
ETHENE
ETOILE
ETRADE
ETTORE
EUCHRE
EUGENE
EUNICE
EUROPE
EVINCE
EVOLVE
EVONNE
EVULSE
EWAINE
EXCIDE
EXCISE
EXCITE
EXCUSE
EXHALE
EXHUME
EXMATE
EXMORE
EXPIRE
EXPOSE
EXWIFE

•EE•••

BEEBEE
BEEFED
BEEFUP
BEEGEE
BEEMER
BEEPAT
BEEPED
BEEPER
BEETLE
BEEVES
BEEZER
DEEDED
DEEDEE
DEEJAY
DEEMED
DEENIE
DEEPAK
DEEPEN
DEEPER
DEEPLY
DEERES
DEEVER
FEEBLE
FEEBLY
FEEDER
FEEDIN
FEEDME
FEEDON
FEEDTO
FEEING
FEEJEE
FEELER
FEELOK
GEEGAW
GEEING
GEEKED
GEESON
GEEZER
HEEBIE
HEEDED
HEEDER
HEEGER
HEEHAW
HEEHEE
HEELED
HEELER
JEERAT
JEERED
JEERER
JEETER
JEEVES
KEELED
KEELER
KEENAN
KEENED
KEENEN
KEENER
KEENLY
KEENON
KEEPAT
KEEPER
KEEPIN
KEEPIT
KEEPON
KEEPTO
KEEPUP
LEEANN
LEEKIE
LEELEE
LEEMAY
LEERAT
LEERED
LEERER
LEEVES
LEEWAY
MEEBER
MEEKER
MEEKLY
MEETER
MEETLY
MEETUP
NEEDBE
NEEDED
NEEDER
NEEDLE
NEEDNT
NEEDTO
NEELIX
NEENAH
NEESON
PEEDEE
PEEKAT
PEEKED
PEEKER
PEEKIN
PEELED
PEELER
PEENED
PEEPAT
PEEPED
PEEPER
PEERAT
PEERCE
PEERED
PEERIN
PEEVED
PEEVES
PEEWEE
REEARN
REEBOK
REECHO
REEDED
REEDER
REEDIT
REEFED
REEFER
REEKED
REEKER
REEKOF
REELED
REELER
REELIN
REELUP
REEMIT
REENIE
REESES
REEVED
REEVES
SEEALL
SEEDED
SEEDER
SEEFIT
SEEGER
SEEING
SEEKER
SEEMED
SEEMLY
SEEMTO
SEENAS
SEENIN
SEENTO
SEENUP
SEEOFF
SEEOUT
SEEPED
SEEPIN
SEERED
SEESAS
SEESAW
SEESIN
SEESTO
SEESUP
SEETHE
SEEYOU
TEEBOX
TEEDUP
TEEHEE
TEEING
TEEMED
TEENER
TEENIE
TEENSY
TEEOFF
TEEPEE
TEESUP
TEETER
TEETHE
TEEVEE
VEEJAY
VEERED
WEEBIT
WEEDED
WEEDER
WEEKLY
WEENED
WEENIE
WEENSY
WEEONE
WEEPER
WEEUNS
WEEVIL
WEEZER
YEEHAW
ZEEMAN

•E•E••

AEGEAN
AENEAS
AENEID
BEDECK
BEDEWS
BEFELL
BEGEMS
BEGETS
BEHEAD
BEHELD
BEHEST
BENEKE
BEREFT
BERETS
BESETS
BETELS
BEVELS
BEWELL
BEZELS
CEDERS
CELEBS
CELERY
CEMENT
CEPEDA
CEREAL
CEREBR
CEREUS
CETERA
DECEIT
DECENT
DEFEAT
DEFECT
DEFEND
DEFERS
DEGELS
DEGERM
DEJECT
DELEAD
DELETE
DEMEAN
DEPEND
DEPERE
DEPEST
DESEED
DESERT
DESETA
DETECT
DETENT
DETERS
DETEST
DEVEGA
DEVEIN
DEVERE
DEVERS
DEVEST
EELERS
EELERY
FERENC
FEVERS
FEWEST
FEYEST
GELEES
GELETT
GENERA
GENETS
GENEVA
GENEVE
GERENT
HELENA
HELENE
HELENS
HEREAT
HEREBY
HEREIN
HEREOF
HEREON
HERESY
HERETO
HETERO
HEWERS
HEXERS
JEREMY
JEWELS
JEWETT
LEBEAU
LEGEND
LEPERS
LEVEED
LEVEES
LEVELS
LEVENE
LEVERS
LEVERT
MELEES
MELETE
MERELY
MEREST
METEOR
METERS
MEWERS
MEYERS
NEMEAN
NEPEAN
NEREID
NEVERS
NEWELL
NEWELS
NEWERA
NEWEST
PEGEEN
PELEUS
PESETA
PESEWA
PETERI
PETERS
PEWEES
REBECS
REBELS
REBEND
REBENT
REBETS
RECEDE
RECENT
RECESS
REDEAL
REDEED
REDEEM
REDEFY
REDENY
REDEYE
REFEED
REFELL
REFERS
REGEAR
REGELS
REGENT
REHEAL
REHEAR
REHEAT
REHEEL
REHELD
REHEMS
REJECT
REKEYS
RELEAD
RELEAP
RELEND
RELENT
RELETS
RELEVE
RELEVY
REMEDY
REMEET
REMELT
REMEND
RENEGE
RENEST
RENEWS
REPEAL
REPEAT
REPEGS
REPELS
REPENS
REPENT
REPERK
REREAD
REREEL
RERENT
RESEAL
RESEAM
RESEAT
RESEAU
RESECT
RESEDA
RESEED
RESEEK
RESEEN
RESEES
RESELL
RESEND
RESENT
RESETS
RESEWN
RESEWS
RETEAR
RETELL
RETEST
REVEAL
REVELS
REVEND
REVERB
REVERE
REVERS
REVERT
REVEST
REVETS
REWEAR
REWEDS
REWELD
REWETS
REZERO
SEAEEL
SEBERG
SECEDE
SEDERS
SELECT
SELENA
SELENE
SEMELE
SENECA
SERENA
SERENE
SEVENA
SEVENB
SEVENC
SEVEND
SEVENE
SEVENS
SEVERE
SEVERN
SEVERS
SEWELL
SEWERS
SEXERS
TEBETS
TEDEUM
TEHEED
TEHEES
TENEEE
TENETS
TEPEES
TERESA
TERETE
TEVERE
TEVETS
VENEER
VENERA
VENETO
VEREEN
VEREIN
VEXERS
WEBERN
WEBERS
WEDELN
WEDELS
WERENT
XEBECS
YELENA
YEMENI

•E••E•

AERIER
AERIES
AETHER
BEADED
BEADER
BEAKED
BEAKER
BEAMED
BEAMER
BEANED
BEARER
BEATEN
BEATER
BEAVER
BECHET
BECKER
BECKET
BEDDED
BEEBEE
BEEFED
BEEGEE
BEEMER
BEEPED
BEEPER
BEEVES
BEEZER
BEGGED
BEGLEY
BEIGES
BELIED
BELIEF
BELIER
BELIES
BELLED
BELLES
BELTED
BELTER
BELZER
BENBEN
BENDED
BENDER
BENSEY
BERBER
BERCEO
BERGEN
BERGER
BERMED
BESSEL
BESSER
BESTED
BESTER
BETHEL
BETSEY
BETTED
BETTER
BEVIES
BEYMER
CEASED
CEASES
CEILED
CELLED
CENSED
CENSER
CENSES
CENTER
CESSED
CESSES
DEADEN
DEADER
DEAFEN
DEAFER
DEALER
DEARER
DEBREU
DEBTEE
DECKED
DECKER
DECREE
DEEDED
DEEDEE
DEEMED
DEEPEN
DEEPER
DEERES
DEEVER
DEFFER
DEFIED
DEFIER
DEFIES
DEFLEA
DEFTER
DEFUEL
DEGREE
DEHMEL
DEICED
DEICER
DEICES
DEKKER
DELKEY
DELREY
DELVED
DELVER
DELVES
DEMIES
DEMOED
DENIED
DENIER
DENIES
DENNED
DENSER
DENTED
DENVER
DENZEL
DERREK
DESEED
DESREE
DESTEM
DETMER
DETTES
DEUCED
DEUCES
DEUTER
DEWIER
DEXTER
EELIER
EERIER
FEARED
FEARER
FEEDER
FEEJEE
FEELER
FELLED
FELLER
FELTED
FEMMES
FENCED
FENCER
FENCES
FENDED
FENDER
FENNEL
FENNER
FERBER
FERRER
FERRET
FESSED
FESSES
FESTER
FETTER
FEUDED
FEZZED
FEZZES
GEARED
GEDDES
GEEKED
GEEZER
GEFFEN
GEIGER
GEISEL
GELDED
GELEES
GELLED
GELLER
GELPEN
GELSEY
GEMMED
GENDER
GENIES
GENRES
GENTES
GENXER
GEODES
GERBER
GESTES
GETHEP
GETSET
GETTER
GETWET
GEYSER
HEADED
HEADER
HEALED
HEALER
HEALEY
HEANEY
HEAPED
HEAPER
HEARER
HEATED
HEATER
HEAVED
HEAVEN
HEAVER
HEAVES
HEBBEL
HEBREW
HEDGED
HEDGER
HEDGES
HEDLEY
HEDREN
HEEDED
HEEDER
HEEGER
HEEHEE
HEELED
HEELER
HEFNER
HEFTED
HEFTER
HEGGEN
HEGYES
HEHHEH
HEIDEN
HEIFER
HELLER
HELMED
HELMER
HELMET
HELPED
HELPER
HELTER
HEMMED
HEMMER
HEMPEN
HENDEC
HENGES
HENLEY
HENNER
HEPPER
HERBED
HERBES
HERDED
HERDER
HERMES
HEROES
HERPET
HERREN
HERSEY
HERVEY
HESTER
HEURES
HEUSEN
JEANED
JEERED
JEERER
JEETER
JEEVES
JELLED
JENNER
JENNET
JENNEY
JENSEN
JERKED
JERKER
JERSEY
JESSEL
JESTED
JESTER
JETSET
JETTED
KEDGED
KEDGER
KEDGES
KEELED
KEELER
KEENED
KEENEN
KEENER
KEEPER
KEGGED
KEGGER
KEGLER
KEITEL
KELLER
KELLEY
KELSEY
KENNED
KENNEL
KENNER
KEPLER
KERNED
KERNEL
KERNES
KERSEE
KEYDET
KEYMEN
KEYNES
KEYSER
LEADED
LEADEN
LEADER
LEAFED
LEAKED
LEAKER
LEAKEY
LEANED
LEANER
LEAPED
LEAPER
LEASED
LEASER
LEASES
LEAVED
LEAVEN
LEAVER
LEAVES
LEBRET
LECHER
LECTER
LEDGER
LEDGES
LEELEE
LEERED
LEERER
LEEVES
LEGGED
LEGMEN
LEGREE
LEHNEN
LEHRER
LEIDEN

LEISEN LEITER LEMUEL LENDEE LENDER LENSED LENSES LENTEN LERNER LESLEY LESSEE LESSEN LESSER LESTER LETTED LETTER LEVEED LEVEES LEVIED LEVIER LEVIES LEWDER LEYDEN MEADER MEAGER MEANER MEANEY MEDLEY MEEBER MEEKER MEETER MEGREZ MELDED MELDER MELEES MELTED MELTER MEMBER MENDED MENDEL MENDER MENDES MENKEN MENNEN MENTEE MEOWED MEOWER MERCED MERCER MERGED MERGEE MERGER MERGES MERKEL MERMEN MERSEY MESHED MESHES MESMER MESNES MESSED MESSES METIER METRED METRES MEWLED MEWLER NEARED

NEARER NEATEN NEATER NECKED NECKER NEEDED NEEDER NEPHEW NERVED NERVES NESSEN NESSES NESTEA NESTED NESTER NETHER NETMEN NETTED NETTER NEUTER NEWIES NEWLEY NEXTEL OERTER PEAHEN PEAKED PEALED PEALER PEALES PECHES PECKED PEEDEE PEEKED PEEKER PEELED PEELER PEENED PEEPED PEEPER PEERED PEEVED PEEVES PEEWEE PEGEEN PEGGED PEGLEG PEGLER PEKOES PELLET PELTED PELTER PENDED PENMEN PENNED PENNER PENNEY PENSEE PENTEL PEPPED PEPPER PERKED PERLEA PERMED PERTER PESTER PETREL PETTED PETTER

PETTET PEVNEY PEWEES PEWTER READER REALER REALES REAMED REAMER REAPED REAPER REARED REARER REAVED REAVER REAVES REBBES REBRED REBREW RECHEW RECKED RECUED RECUES REDDEN REDDER REDEED REDEEM REDHEN REDLEG REDOER REDOES REDREW REDSEA REDTEN REDYED REDYES REEDED REEDER REEFED REEFER REEKED REEKER REELED REELER REESES REEVED REEVES REFEED REFFED REFIED REFIES REFLEW REFLEX REFUEL REGLES REGRET REGREW REHEEL REHOED REHOES REICED REICES REIGER REINED REINER REINES REISER REITER

RELIED RELIEF RELIER RELIES REMEET REMSEN RENDED RENDER RENNES RENNET RENTED RENTEE RENTER RENTES REOPEN REPLED REPPED REREEL RESEED RESEEK RESEEN RESEES RESHES RESTED RESTER RESTES RETIED RETIEF RETIES RETTED REUBEN REUNED REUNER REUNES REUSED REUSER REUSES REUTER REVIEW REVUES REVVED REYLES SEABED SEABEE SEAEEL SEALED SEALER SEAMED SEAMEN SEAMER SEARED SEARER SEATED SEATER SEAVER SECKEL SECRET SEDGED SEDGES SEDLEY SEEDED SEEDER SEEGER SEEKER SEEMED SEEPED SEERED SEGUED

SEGUES SEINED SEINER SEINES SEIZED SEIZER SEIZES SELLER SELTEN SELVES SEMPER SENDEE SENDER SENSED SENSEI SENSEN SENSES SEPTET SEQUEL SERGEI SERGES SERIES SERVED SERVER SERVES SESTET SETFEE SETTEE SETTER SETZER SEVRES SEXIER SEXTET TEAMED TEARED TEARER TEASED TEASEL TEASER TEASES TEASET TEDKEY TEEHEE TEEMED TEENER TEEPEE TEETER TEEVEE TEHEED TEHEES TELLER TELNET TEMPED TEMPEH TEMPER TENDED TENDER TENEEE TENLEY TENNER TENSED TENSER TENSES TENTED TENTER TEPEES TERCEL TERCES

TERKEL TERMED TERMES TERNES TERRES TERRET TERSER TESTED TESTEE TESTER TETHER TETLEY TETZEL TEXMEX TEXTED UECKER VEBLEN VEDDER VEERED VEGGED VEGGES VEILED VEILER VEINED VELSEN VELVET VENDED VENDEE VENDER VENEER VENNER VENTED VENTER VENUES VERDES VEREEN VERGED VERGER VERGES VERJEE VERNET VERSED VERSES VERSET VERTEX VERVES VESPER VESSEL VESTED VESTEE VETOED VETOER VETOES VETTED VETTER VETTES WEAKEN WEAKER WEANED WEANER WEARER WEASEL WEAVED WEAVER WEAVES WEBBED WEBBER WEBFED

WEDDED WEDDER WEDGED WEDGES WEEDED WEEDER WEENED WEEPER WEEZER WEIDER WELDED WELDER WELLED WELLER WELLES WELTED WELTER WENCES WENDED WENNER WERFEL WERKER WERNER WESKER WESLEY WESSEX WESTER WETTED WETTER XERXES YEAGER YEANED YELLED YELLER YELPED YELPER YENNED YEOMEN YERKES YESMEN YESSED YESSES YESTER YESYES ZENGER ZEROED ZEROES ZESTED ZESTER

•E•••E

AEDILE AERATE AEROBE BEADLE BEAGLE BEANIE BEARSE BEATLE BECAME BECOME BEDAZE BEEBEE BEEGEE BEETLE BEFORE BEGONE BEHAVE

BEHOME BEIGNE BELATE BELGAE BELIKE BELIZE BEMINE BEMIRE BEMUSE BENEKE BENICE BENNIE BENOTE BERATE BERNIE BERTHE BERTIE BESAME BESIDE BESORE BESSIE BESURE BETAKE BETIDE BETTYE BEURRE BEWARE CECILE CELINE CELLAE CENTRE CERATE CERISE CESARE CETANE DEARIE DEARME DEBASE DEBATE DEBBIE DEBONE DEBTEE DECADE DECARE DECIDE DECILE DECKLE DECODE DECREE DEDUCE DEDUVE DEEDEE DEENIE DEFACE DEFAME DEFILE DEFINE DEFORE DEFUSE DEGAGE DEGREE DEHIRE DEIDRE DEJURE DELETE DELUDE DELUGE DELUXE

DEMISE DEMODE DEMOTE DEMURE DENISE DENOTE DENUDE DEPERE DEPONE DEPOSE DEPUTE DERATE DERIDE DERIVE DEROSE DESADE DESIRE DESREE DETUNE DEVANE DEVERE DEVICE DEVINE DEVISE DEVORE DEVOTE DEWIRE EENSIE EEYORE FEEBLE FEEDME FEEJEE FELICE FELINE FELIPE FEMALE FERDIE FERGIE FERULE FESCUE FETTLE GELATE GEMMAE GENEVE GENOME GENTLE GEORGE GERTIE GESTAE HEARSE HEARYE HECATE HECKLE HEEBIE HEEHEE HEINIE HEINSE HELENE HELPME HERBIE HEXANE HEXOSE JEANIE JEANNE JECKLE JEJUNE JENNIE JEROME

JESSYE KELLIE KELPIE KEMBLE KERSEE KETONE KETTLE KEWPIE LEAGUE LEANNE LEEKIE LEELEE LEFTBE LEGATE LEGREE LEGUME LENAPE LENDEE LENGLE LENNIE LENORE LESAGE LESLIE LESSEE LETSBE LETTRE LETUSE LEUTZE LEVADE LEVENE LEVINE LEVITE MEAGRE MEALIE MEANIE MEASLE MEDDLE MEGANE MELETE MENACE MENAGE MENTEE MENTHE MERDLE MERGEE MEROPE MERRIE METATE METTLE NEEDBE NEEDLE NEGATE NEISSE NELLIE NERONE NESSIE NESTLE NETTLE NEWAGE NEWBIE NEWSIE OENONE OEUVRE PEARCE PEARLE PEBBLE PEDATE PEDDLE

PEEDEE PEERCE PEEWEE PEIRCE PELAGE PENCHE PENSEE PEOPLE PERDUE PERINE PERUKE PERUSE PESADE PESTLE PETALE PETITE PETRIE PEYOTE README REBAKE REBALE REBATE REBBIE REBORE REBOTE REBUKE RECAGE RECANE RECASE RECEDE RECIFE RECIPE RECITE RECODE RECURE RECUSE REDACE REDARE REDATE REDEYE REDONE REDOSE REDTIE REDUCE REENIE REFACE REFILE REFINE REFIRE REFUGE REFUSE REFUTE REGALE REGAVE REGGAE REGGIE REGIME REGIVE REGLUE REHIDE REHIRE REHONE RELACE RELATE RELEVE RELINE RELIVE RELOSE

RELUME REMADE REMAKE REMATE REMINE REMISE REMOTE REMOVE RENAME RENEGE RENNIE RENOTE RENTEE REPAGE REPANE REPAVE REPINE REPOSE REPUTE RERAKE RERATE RERIDE RERISE RERODE REROSE RESALE RESAVE RESCUE RESHOE RESIDE RESILE RESITE RESIZE RESOLE RESUME RETAKE RETAME RETAPE RETILE RETIME RETIRE RETONE RETORE RETUNE RETYPE REURGE REVERE REVILE REVISE REVIVE REVOKE REVOTE REWAKE REWIPE REWIRE REWOKE REWORE REWOVE REYOKE REZONE SEABEE SEAICE SEANCE SEARLE SECEDE SECURE SEDATE SEDUCE

SEETHE SELENE SEMELE SEMITE SEMPLE SEMPRE SENATE SENDEE SENILE SERAPE SERENE SESAME SESSUE SETFEE SETOSE SETTEE SETTLE SEVENE SEVERE SEWAGE TECATE TECHIE TEEHEE TEENIE TEEPEE TEETHE TEEVEE TEKKIE TELLME TEMPLE TENACE TENEEE TENONE TENURE TERETE TERRAE TESSIE TESTAE TESTEE TEVERE VEGGIE VEINTE VELOCE VELURE VENDEE VENDUE VENICE VENIRE VENITE VENOSE VENULE VERITE VERJEE VESTEE WECARE WEDGIE WEENIE WEEONE WENDIE WESTIE WETONE YEOLDE YERTLE YETTIE

••EE••

ADEEMS AMEERS AVEENO BLEEDS BLEEPS BLEETH BREECH BREEDS BREEDY BREEZE BREEZY CHEECH CHEEKS CHEEKY CHEEPS CHEERS CHEERY CHEESE CHEESY CHEETA CLEEKS CLEESE CREEDS CREEKS CREELS CREEPO CREEPS CREEPY DWEEBS DWEEBY EMEERS FLEECE FLEECY FLEERS FLEETS FREELY FREEOF FREERS FREEST FREETO FREEUP FREEZE GREECE GREEDS GREEDY GREEKS GREENE GREENS GREENY GREETS ISEEIT KNEELS OKEEFE ONEEEE ONEEGG ONEEYE PREENS QUEENE QUEENS QUEERS RHEEMS SHEEDY SHEEHY SHEENA SHEENS SHEENY SHEERS SHEESH SHEETS SKEETS

SLEEKS SLEEKY SLEEPS SLEEPY SLEETS SLEETY SLEEVE SNEERS SNEERY SNEEZE SNEEZY SPEECH SPEEDO SPEEDS SPEEDY STEEDS STEELE STEELS STEELY STEEPS STEERS STEEVE SWEEPS SWEETS THEEND THEEPA THEEYE TWEEDS TWEEDY TWEENS TWEENY TWEETS TWEETY TWEEZE WHEELS WHEEZE WHEEZY

••E•E•

ABELES ADELEH AGETEN AKENES ALEKEG ALEVEL ALEVES ALEXEI ALEXEY AMEDEE AMEDEO ANELED ANELES APELET APEMEN APEXES ARETES ASEVER AXEMEN BAEYER BEEBEE BEEFED BEEGEE BEEMER BEEPED BEEPER BEEVES BEEZER BIEBER

BIERES
BREDES
BREMEN
BREMER
BREUER
BREVES
BREVET
BREWED
BREWER
BREYER
BSEVEN
CHEDER
CHEFED
CHENEY
CHEVET
CHEWED
CHEWER
CLEVER
CLEVES
CLEWED
CREMER
CREMES
CRENEL
CREPED
CREPES
CREWED
CREWEL
DEEDED
DEEDEE
DEEMED
DEEPEN
DEEPER
DEERES
DEEVER
DIENES
DIESEL
DIESES
DIETED
DIETER
DIETES
DIEZES
DREXEL
DREYER
DUELED
DUELER
DUETED
ELEVEN
ELEVES
EVENED
EVENER
EXETER
EYELET
FEEDER
FEEJEE
FEELER
FIEVEL
FLEXED
FLEXES
FOEMEN
FRERES
FREWER
FUELED
FUELER
GEEKED
GEEZER
GREBES
GRETEL
GREYED

GREYER
GSEVEN
HEEDED
HEEDER
HEEGER
HEEHEE
HEELED
HEELER
IBEXES
ICEMEN
ICETEA
ILEXES
INEVER
IPETER
ITEMED
JAEGER
JEERED
JEERER
JEETER
JEEVES
JOETEX
JUEVES
KEELED
KEELER
KEENED
KEENEN
KEENER
KEEPER
KIEFER
KNEBEL
KRENEK
KREWES
LEELEE
LEERED
LEERER
LEEVES
LIEBER
LIEDER
LIEFER
LIEGES
LIENEE
MCEWEN
MEEBER
MEEKER
MEETER
MIELES
NEEDED
NEEDER
NIECES
NIEVES
NUECES
NUEVES
OBEYED
OBEYER
ODELET
OLEVEL
OMELET
OMENED
ONEEEE
ONELEG
ONEMEG
ONESEC
ONESET
ONETEN
OPENED
OPENER
OXEYES
OYEZES

PEEDEE
PEEKED
PEEKER
PEELED
PEELER
PEENED
PEEPED
PEEPER
PEERED
PEEVED
PEEVES
PEEWEE
PIECED
PIECER
PIECES
PIELET
PIEMEN
PIETER
PLEBES
PLEXES
POEMES
POETES
PREFER
PREMED
PREMET
PRESET
PRETER
PREXES
PREYED
PREYER
QUEBEC
QUELER
QUEUED
QUEUER
QUEUES
REEDED
REEDER
REEFED
REEFER
REEKED
REEKER
REELED
REELER
REESES
REEVED
REEVES
RHEMES
RIESEN
ROEPER
SCENEI
SCENES
SCENEV
SEEDED
SEEDER
SEEGER
SEEKER
SEEMED
SEEPED
SEERED
SHEKEL
SHEREE
SIEBEN
SIEGED
SIEGEL
SIEGES
SIETES
SIEVED
SIEVES

SKEWED
SKEWER
SLEWED
SPEWED
SPEWER
STELES
STEREO
STERES
STEVEN
STEWED
STEWER
SUEDED
SUEDES
SWEDEN
SWEDES
TEEHEE
TEEMED
TEENER
TEEPEE
TEETER
TEEVEE
THEBEE
THEBES
THEFED
THEMED
THEMES
THEMET
THENET
THERED
THEREF
THERES
THESEA
THESES
THETED
THEVET
THEWEB
TIERED
TMESES
TREBEK
TRECES
TREXES
UNEVEN
USENET
VEERED
VIEWED
VIEWER
WEEDED
WEEDER
WEENED
WEEPER
WEEZER
WHERED
WHERES
WHEYEY
WIENER
WIESEL

••E••E

ADELIE
ADELLE
ADESTE
AGENCE
AGEONE
AHERNE
ALEGRE
ALETTE
AMEBAE
AMECHE
AMEDEE
AMELIE
AMERCE
AREOLE
ATEASE
ATERRE
AVENGE
AVENUE
AVERSE
AYEAYE
BEEBEE
BEEGEE
BEETLE
BIERCE
BLENDE
BREEZE
BYEBYE
CHEESE
CHELAE
CHEQUE
CHERIE
CHEVRE
CLEAVE
CLEESE
COERCE
CREASE
CREATE
CRECHE
CREOLE
CREUSE
DEEDEE
DEENIE
DIEPPE
DREDGE
EBERLE
EDERLE
EMERGE
EMEUTE
ETERNE
FAERIE
FAEROE
FEEBLE
FEEDME
FEEJEE
FIERCE
FLECHE
FLEDGE
FLEECE
FLENSE
FREEZE
GLENNE
GOETHE
GREASE
GREAVE
GREECE
GREENE
GUERRE
HEEBIE
HEEHEE
ICEAGE
ICEAXE
IDEATE
INESSE
ISERVE
KAETHE
KLEINE
KRESGE
LEEKIE
LEELEE
LIENEE
MOERAE
NEEDBE
NEEDLE
NIENTE
ODENSE
ODETTE
OKEEFE
OLEATE
OLEOLE
ONEDGE
ONEEEE
ONEEYE
ONEONE
ORELSE
ORENSE
PEEDEE
PEERCE
PEEWEE
PHEDRE
PIERCE
PIERRE
PLEASE
PLEDGE
PREAGE
PREMIE
PREVUE
PUENTE
QUEENE
REENIE
RYENCE
SEETHE
SHEAVE
SHELVE
SHEREE
SIECLE
SLEAZE
SLEDGE
SLEEVE
SNEEZE
SPEARE
SPECIE
SPENCE
STEELE
STEEVE
STEPPE
STERNE
STEVIE
STEWIE
SUEANE
SVELTE
SWERVE
TEEHEE
TEENIE
TEEPEE
TEETHE
TEEVEE
THEAGE
THEAPE
THEAXE
THEBEE
THEEYE
THENCE
THEONE
THEYRE
THEYVE
TIEDYE
TIERCE
TREBLE
TREIZE
TRENTE
TSETSE
TWEEZE
TWELVE
UNEASE
UNEDGE
VIELLE
VIENNE
WEENIE
WEEONE
WHEEZE
WHENCE
WIENIE
YVETTE

•••EE•

ADFEES
ADWEEK
AGREED
AGREER
AGREES
AILEEN
ALLEES
ANNEES
ANTEED
ASDEEP
ASLEEP
ASTEEP
ATHEEL
AXSEED
BALEEN
BOPEEP
CAREEN
CAREER
CITEES
COOEED
COOEES
CUVEES
DESEED
DONEES
DOREEN
EILEEN
EMCEED
EMCEES
ESTEEM
EXCEED
FIVEEE
FUSEES
GELEES
GODEEP
HAKEEM
HIREES
HOMEEC
INDEED
INDEEP
INNEED
KADEEM
KAREEM
LAREES
LATEEN
LEVEED
LEVEES
LYCEES
MELEES
MOREEN
MUDEEL
MUSEES
NINEEE
NOFEES
NONEED
NOREEN
ONEEEE
PAYEES
PEGEEN
PEWEES
POTEEN
PUREED
PUREES
RANEES
RAREES
REDEED
REDEEM
REFEED
REHEEL
REMEET
REREEL
RESEED
RESEEK
RESEEN
RESEES
RUPEES
SAREES
SATEEN
SCREED
SCREEN
SCREES
SEAEEL
SIXEEE
SPLEEN
SPREES
STREEP
STREET
TEHEED
TEHEES
TENEEE
TEPEES
THREEA
THREEB
THREEC
THREED
THREEE
THREES
TOHEEL
TOPEES
TUREEN
TUTEES
TWOEEE
UNDEEP
UNHEED
UNMEET
UNPEEL
UNREEL
UNSEEN
UPKEEP
VENEER
VEREEN

•••E•E

ACCEDE
ACHEBE
ACHENE
ADHERE
ALKENE
ALLEGE
ALLELE
AMPERE
APIECE
ARIEGE
ARLENE
ARPEGE
ARRETE
ARSENE
ATHENE
BAREGE
BENEKE
BIGEYE
BIREME
BOHEME
BREEZE
BUTENE
CHEESE
CLEESE
CLOETE
COHERE
DALENE
DAREME
DELETE
DEPERE
DEVERE
DISERE
DRYEYE
EFFETE
EIRENE
EISELE
EKUELE
EOCENE
ESSENE
ETHENE
EUGENE
FILENE
FIVEEE
FLEECE
FREEZE
FRIEZE
GALEAE
GAMETE
GENEVE
GISELE
GLIERE
GREECE
GREENE
GRIESE
GRIEVE
GYRENE
HELENE
IMHERE
IMPEDE
INHERE
IRLENE
ISMENE
JOLENE
LATENE
LEVENE
LORENE
LURENE
LUTECE
MAKEME
MANEGE
MAXENE
MELETE
NICENE
NINEEE
OKEEFE
ONEEEE
ONEEYE
PALEAE
PAREVE
PAVESE
PHOEBE
POPEYE
QUEENE
RACEME
RECEDE
REDEYE
RELEVE
RENEGE
REVERE
RIBEYE
ROGERE
SAVEME
SCHEME
SECEDE
SELENE
SEMELE
SERENE
SEVENE
SEVERE
SHREVE
SIXEEE
SLEEVE
SNEEZE
SPHERE
STBEDE
STEELE
STEEVE
STPETE
SURETE
TALESE
TENEEE
TERETE
TEVERE
THEEYE
THIEVE
THREEE
TONEME
TWEEZE
TWOEEE
UNSERE
UPHERE
VALENE
VALERE
VARESE
WHEEZE

••••EE

ADOREE
AMEDEE
ANGLEE
ANNLEE
APOGEE
ASFREE
ASHLEE
ATMFEE
ATTLEE
BAILEE
BEEBEE
BEEGEE
BISBEE
BOOTEE
BOTREE
BRIBEE
BRULEE
BTHREE
BUNGEE
BURGEE
BURPEE
CALLEE
COATEE
COFFEE
CONNEE
CORVEE
COULEE
DEBTEE
DECREE
DEEDEE
DEGREE
DESREE
DRAGEE
DRAWEE
DUNDEE
ELYSEE
ENTREE
EPOPEE
FEEJEE
FIVEEE
FOUREE
FRISEE
GAMGEE
GIFTEE
GOATEE
GOFREE
GURNEE
HAIDEE
HEEHEE
HUMVEE
IAGREE
ILLSEE
IMFREE
JAFFEE
JAYCEE
JAYVEE
KERSEE
KIBBEE
LABFEE
LEELEE
LEGREE
LENDEE
LESSEE
LICHEE
LIENEE
LISTEE
LOOKEE
MACNEE
MANTEE
MARLEE
MARMEE
MAUMEE
MCAFEE
MCPHEE
MENTEE
MERGEE
MONKEE
NINEEE
OCONEE
ONEEEE
OUTSEE
PARSEE
PAWNEE
PEEDEE
PEEWEE
PENSEE
POLLEE
PONGEE
PUTTEE
QUOTEE
RENTEE
RUSHEE
SANTEE
SEABEE
SENDEE
SETFEE
SETTEE
SHEREE
SIGNEE
SIRREE
SIXEEE
SOIREE
SOISEE
SWANEE
TAHNEE
TASTEE
TEEHEE
TEEPEE
TEEVEE
TENEEE
TESTEE
THEBEE
THREEE
TIPPEE
TOATEE
TOFFEE
TOUPEE
TOWHEE
TRALEE
TWOEEE
UNFREE
VALLEE
VENDEE
VERJEE
VESTEE
YANKEE
YIPPEE
YOUSEE

EF••••

EFFACE
EFFECT
EFFETE
EFFIGY
EFFLUX
EFFORT
EFFUSE
EFGHIJ
EFILED
EFILES
EFLATS

E•F•••

EFFACE
EFFECT
EFFETE
EFFIGY
EFFLUX
EFFORT
EFFUSE
EIFFEL
ELFISH
ELFMAN
ELFOWL
ENFACE
ENFAIT
ENFANT
ENFOLD
ERFURT

E••F••

EARFUL
EIFFEL
EYEFUL

E•••F•

EXWIFE

E••••F

EATSOF
EKELOF
ENGULF
EVENIF

•EF•••

BEFAIR
BEFALL
BEFELL
BEFIRM
BEFITS
BEFOGS
BEFOOL
BEFORE
BEFOUL
DEFACE
DEFAME
DEFANG
DEFATS
DEFCON
DEFEAT
DEFECT
DEFEND
DEFERS
DEFFER
DEFGHI
DEFIED
DEFIER
DEFIES
DEFILE
DEFINE
DEFJAM
DEFLEA
DEFOAM
DEFOGS
DEFORD
DEFORE
DEFORM
DEFRAG
DEFRAY
DEFTER
DEFTLY
DEFUEL
DEFUND
DEFUSE
GEFFEN
HEFLIN
HEFNER
HEFTED
HEFTER
KEFIRS
LEFTBE
LEFTIN
LEFTIT
LEFTOF
LEFTON
REFACE
REFALL
REFEED
REFELL
REFERS
REFFED
REFIED
REFIES
REFILE
REFILL
REFILM
REFIND
REFINE
REFIRE
REFITS
REFLAG
REFLEW
REFLEX
REFLOW
REFLUX
REFOLD
REFORM
REFUEL
REFUGE
REFUND
REFUSE
REFUTE
TEFLON

•E•F••

BEEFED
BEEFUP
BEGFOR
BELFRY
DEAFEN
DEAFER
DEAFLY
DEAFTO
DEFFER
DEIFIC
DELFTS
FEOFFS
GEFFEN
GETFAR
GETFIT
HEIFER
JETFAN
LEAFED
LETFLY
MEDFLY
MEIFUN
METFAN
NETFUL
PEPFUL
REDFIN
REDFIR
REDFOX
REEFED
REEFER
REFFED
RENFRO
REPFOR
SEAFOX
SEEFIT
SETFEE
SETFOR
WEBFED
WERFEL
WETFLY
YENFOR

•E••F•

AERIFY
BEGOFF
BEREFT
DECAFS
FEOFFS
GETOFF
KEYOFA
KEYOFB
KEYOFC
KEYOFD
KEYOFF
KEYOFG
LEDOFF
LETOFF
REBUFF
RECIFE
REDEFY
REGIFT
RESIFT
SEEOFF
SERIFS
SETOFF
TEEOFF
VERIFY

•E•••F

BEGOFF
BEHALF
BEHOOF
BELIEF
CERTIF
DEWOLF
GELDOF
GETANF
GETOFF
HEAROF
HEREOF
KEYOFF
LEDOFF
LEFTOF
LETOFF
REBUFF
REEKOF
RELIEF
REROOF
RETIEF
RETURF
SEEOFF
SETOFF
TEEOFF
TELLOF
TERRIF

••EF••

BEEFED
BEEFUP
CDEFGH

CHEFED CLEFTS DIEFOR EYEFUL ICEFOG IREFUL KIEFER LIEFER LIEFLY LIEFOR OLEFIN PREFAB PREFER PREFIX REEFED REEFER RUEFUL SEEFIT STEFAN STEFFI STEFOY SUEFOR THEFAN THEFBI THEFED THEFLY THEFOG THEFOX THEFTS USEFOR USEFUL VIEFOR WOEFUL

••E•F•

DIEOFF OKEEFE ONEOFF SEEOFF STEFFI TEEOFF THENFL TIEOFF

••E••F

DIEOFF EKELOF EVENIF FREEOF KNEWOF ONEOFF REEKOF SEEOFF TEEOFF THEREF TIEOFF

•••EF•

BCDEFG BEREFT BRIEFS CASEFY CCLEFS CHIEFS GANEFS GCLEFS GOLEFT GRIEFS ISLEFT OKEEFE RAREFY REDEFY TUMEFY UNDEFT UNLEFT

•••E•F

CAREOF COMEOF FIVEOF FREEOF GAVEOF GIVEOF HEREOF IMPERF INLEAF ITSELF LATEOF MADEOF MAKEOF MYSELF SUREOF TIREOF UNLEAF WIDEOF

••••EF

ABCDEF BELIEF JOZSEF MOSDEF RELIEF RETIEF THEREF UNICEF

EG••••

EGALES EGBERT EGERIA EGESTA EGESTS EGGCUP EGGERS EGGERT EGGIER EGGING EGGLER EGGNOG EGGSAC EGGSON EGISES EGLISE EGMONT EGOISM EGOIST EGOYAN EGRESS EGRETS EGUREN

E•G•••

EAGLED EAGLES EAGLET EAGRES EDGARD EDGARS EDGEIN EDGERS EDGIER EDGILY EDGING EFGHIJ EGGCUP EGGERS EGGERT EGGIER EGGING EGGLER EGGNOG EGGSAC EGGSON EIGHTA EIGHTB EIGHTC EIGHTD EIGHTE EIGHTH EIGHTS EIGHTY ELGART ENGAGE ENGELS ENGILD ENGINE ENGIRD ENGIRT ENGLIT ENGLUT ENGRAM ENGULF ERGOTS EUGENE EXGOVS

E••G••

ELEGIT ELOGES EMIGRE ENIGMA ETAGES

E•••G•

EASYGO EFFIGY EMBOGS EMERGE ENCAGE ENERGY ENGAGE ENOUGH ENRAGE ENSIGN ERYNGO EULOGY EWINGS

E••••G

EALING EARING EARTAG EARWIG EASING EATING EBBING EDBERG EDGING EELING EGGING EGGNOG EKBERG ENBERG ENDING EPILOG EPPING ERLANG ERRING ERVING ETTING EYEING

•EG•••

AEGEAN BEGEMS BEGETS BEGFOR BEGGAR BEGGED BEGINS BEGIRD BEGIRT BEGLEY BEGOFF BEGONE BEGOOD BEGUMS DEGAGE DEGELS DEGERM DEGREE DEGUMS DEGUST HEGGEN HEGIRA HEGOAT HEGYES KEGGED KEGGER KEGLER LEGACY LEGALS LEGART LEGATE LEGATO LEGEND LEGGED LEGION LEGIST LEGMAN LEGMEN LEGREE LEGROS LEGSIT LEGUIN LEGUME MEGALO MEGANE MEGOHM MEGREZ MEGRIM NEGATE PEGBOX PEGEEN PEGGED PEGLEG PEGLER PEGTOP REGAIN REGALE REGARD REGAVE REGEAR REGELS REGENT REGGAE REGGIE REGIFT REGILD REGIME REGINA REGION REGIRD REGIUS REGIVE REGLES REGLOW REGLUE REGNAL REGNAT REGNUM REGRAB REGRET REGREW REGRIP REGROW SEGUED SEGUES SEGURA SEGWAY TEGRIN VEGANS VEGGED VEGGES VEGGIE VEGOUT YEGODS

•E•G••

BEAGLE BEEGEE BEGGAR BEGGED BEIGES BEIGHT BEIGNE BELGAE BELGIC BENGAL BENGAY BERGEN BERGER DEFGHI DEIGNS FEIGNS FERGIE GEEGAW GEIGER GEIGHT GEWGAW HEDGED HEDGER HEDGES HEEGER HEGGEN HEIGHT HENGES IEIGHT JEDGAR JETGUN KEDGED KEDGER KEDGES KEGGED KEGGER LEAGUE LEDGER LEDGES LEGGED LENGLE LENGTH LENGUA MEAGER MEAGRE MEDGAR MERGED MERGEE MERGER MERGES NEIGHS PEGGED PENGPU REAGAN REGGAE REGGIE REIGER REIGNS RENGAS SEAGAL SEAGOD SEDGED SEDGES SEEGER SERGEI SERGES SERGIO VEGGED VEGGES VEGGIE VEIGHT VERGED VERGER VERGES VERGIL WEDGED WEDGES WEDGIE WEIGHS WEIGHT YEAGER ZENGER

•E••G•

BEDOGS BEFOGS BEINGS BELUGA BENIGN BEWIGS DEBAGS DEBUGS DEFOGS DEGAGE DELUGE DELUGG DESIGN DEVEGA GEORGE GEORGI GEORGY LEHIGH LESAGE LETSGO MENAGE NEWAGE PELAGE REBAGS RECAGE REDIGS REFUGE REJIGS RELOGS RENEGE REPAGE REPEGS REPUGN RERIGS RESIGN RETAGS REURGE SEWAGE

•E•••G

BEDBUG BELONG BENING BERING CEDING DEFANG DEFRAG DEKING DELUGG DESMOG DEWING EELING FEEING FETING GEEING GEHRIG HERZOG HEWING HEXING JETLAG KENNYG KEYING KEYOFG MEKONG METING MEWING PEGLEG PEKING PETDOG PETPIG REDDOG REDING REDLEG REDRAG REDTAG REFLAG REHANG REHUNG RESANG RESING RETTIG SEABAG SEADOG SEAHAG SEBERG SEEING SEWING TEABAG TEEING VEXING WEBLOG WETRAG WETTIG YEABIG ZEDONG

••EG••

ALEGAR ALEGRE ALEGUP BEEGEE ELEGIT FUEGOS GEEGAW GREGOR HEEGER JAEGER JUEGOS LIEGES OMEGAS ONEGIN OREGON SEEGER SIEGED SIEGEL SIEGES THEGAP

••E•G•

ANERGY AVENGE AWEIGH BAERGA CDEFGH CLERGY DHEIGH DREDGE EMERGE ENERGY FLEDGE FLEDGY ICEAGE KRESGE ONEDGE ONEEGG PLEDGE PREAGE SLEDGE SLEIGH THEAGE UNEDGE

••E••G

AGEING ALEKEG BOEING CUEING DYEING EYEING FEEING GEEING GIEING HIEING HOEING ICEBAG ICEFOG KOENIG LIEBIG ONEEGG ONELEG ONEMEG PRELOG PYEDOG SEEING STENOG TEEING THEFOG TOEING

•••EG•

ALLEGE ARIEGE ARPEGE BADEGG BAREGE BODEGA DEVEGA FOREGO IOMEGA MADEGO MAKEGO MANEGE NONEGO ONEEGG ORTEGA OSWEGO OTSEGO OWLEGG PHLEGM RAWEGG RENEGE REPEGS UNPEGS

•••E•G

BADEGG BCDEFG EDBERG EKBERG ENBERG LIPENG MOBERG ONEEGG OWLEGG RATEDG RAWEGG SEBERG SUPERG

••••EG

ALEKEG BUMLEG DOGLEG MIDLEG NUTMEG ONELEG ONEMEG OUTBEG PEGLEG REDLEG

E•H•••

ECHOED ECHOER ECHOES ECHOIC ENHALO ENHAUT EPHAHS EPHODS EPHORS EPHRON ERHARD ESHARP ESHKOL ETHANE ETHENE ETHERS ETHICS ETHIOP ETHNIC ETHNOS ETHYLS EXHALE EXHORT EXHUME

E••H••

EFGHIJ EIGHTA EIGHTB EIGHTC EIGHTD EIGHTE EIGHTH EIGHTS EIGHTY EITHER ESCHER ESCHEW ESTHER ETCHED ETCHER ETCHES EUCHRE

E•••H•

EARTHA EARTHS EARTHY ELISHA EPHAHS EPOCHS

E••••H

EDKOCH EIGHTH ELFISH ELIJAH ELNATH ELVISH EMDASH EMPATH ENDASH ENMESH ENOUGH ENRICH EOLITH EPARCH ERYKAH EXARCH

•EH•••

BEHAIM BEHALF BEHAVE BEHEAD BEHELD BEHEST BEHIND BEHOLD BEHOME BEHOOF DEHAIR DEHIRE DEHMEL DEHORN GEHRIG HEHHEH LEHIGH LEHMAN LEHNEN LEHRER LEHUAS NEHRUS REHABS REHANG REHASH REHAUL REHEAL REHEAR REHEAT REHEEL REHELD REHEMS REHIDE REHIRE REHITS REHOED REHOES REHOLD REHONE REHOOK REHUNG TEHEED TEHEES TEHRAN YEHUDI

•E•H••

AETHER BECHET BENHUR BETHEL CEPHAL DEDHAM DENHAM GETHEP GETHIP GETHOT HEEHAW HEEHEE HEHHEH JETHRO KESHIA LECHER LESHAN LETHAL MEOHMY MESHED MESHES METHOD METHYL NEPHEW NEPHRO NETHER NETHOU NEWHAT PEAHEN PECHES PELHAM RECHEW REDHAT REDHEN REDHOT RESHES RESHIP RESHOD RESHOE RESHOT RESHOW RESHUT RETHAW SEAHAG SENHOR SEPHIA TECHIE TECHNO TECHTV TEEHEE TENHUT TETHER TETHYS YEEHAW ZEPHYR

•E••H•

BEACHY BEIGHT BERTHA BERTHE BERTHS BETCHA DEATHS DEFGHI DELPHI DEPTHS GEIGHT GEISHA HEATHS HEATHY HEIGHT IEIGHT LEACHY MEGOHM MENTHE NEIGHS NEOSHO PEACHY PENCHE PERCHA REECHO SEETHE SEZWHO TEETHE TENTHS TETCHY VEIGHT WEIGHS WEIGHT WELCHS

•E•••H

BEULAH DEARTH DEBRAH DELISH DEMOTH DETACH DETOTH DEUTCH FELLAH FETISH HEALTH HEARTH HEHHEH HEWISH JEWISH LEHIGH LENGTH MENSCH NEENAH NEWISH PERISH PESACH REHASH RELISH REWASH SEARCH SERAPH TEMPEH WEALTH ZENITH

••EH••

HEEHAW HEEHEE ONEHIT TEEHEE THEHAJ THEHUB YEEHAW

••E•H•

ALEPHS AMECHE ARETHA AYESHA BRECHT CRECHE CZECHS FLECHE FLESHY GOETHE KAETHE MOESHA OBEAHS OLESHA REECHO SEETHE SHEEHY STETHO TEETHE THENHL THEWHO

••E••H

ADELEH ATENTH AWEIGH BLEACH BLEETH BLENCH BREACH BREATH BREECH CDEFGH CHEECH CLENCH DHEIGH DRENCH FLETCH FRENCH GUELPH KVETCH NEENAH ONEISH PREACH QUENCH SHEATH SHEESH SHEIKH SKETCH SLEIGH SLEUTH SMERSH SPEECH STENCH TRENCH WREATH WRENCH WRETCH

•••EH•

HIDEHO SHEEHY

•••E•H

AFRESH BLEETH BREECH CHEECH COMETH DALETH ENMESH GARETH GIVETH HITECH JOBETH JOSEPH LIVETH OHYEAH RULETH SAMEKH SHEESH SPEECH TAKETH THRESH UNMESH VOTECH

••••EH

ADELEH HEHHEH TEMPEH

EI••••

EIDERS EIDOLA EIFFEL EIGHTA EIGHTB EIGHTC EIGHTD EIGHTE EIGHTH EIGHTS EIGHTY EILEEN EILERS EILERT EIRENE EISELE EISLEY EISNER EITHER

E•I•••

EDIBLE EDIBLY EDICTS EDILES EDIRNE EDISON EDITED EDITIO EDITOR EFILED EFILES EGISES EJIDOS ELICIT ELIDED ELIDER ELIDES ELIELI ELIJAH ELINOR ELISEO ELISHA ELISSA ELISTS ELITER ELITES ELIXIR EMIGRE EMILIA

EMILIE
EMILIO
EMILYS
EMINEM
EMINOR
ENIACS
ENIDOK
ENIGMA
ENISLE
EPICAL
EPILOG
EPINAL
ERICAS
ERIEPA
ERINNA
ERINYS
ERIVAN
ETILES
EVICTS
EVILER
EVILLY
EVINCE
EVITES
EWINGS
EXILED
EXILER
EXILES
EXILIC
EXISTS
EXITED
EXITUS
EZINES

E••I••

EAKINS
EALING
EARING
EASIER
EASILY
EASING
EATING
EBBING
EDDIED
EDDIES
EDGIER
EDGILY
EDGING
EDWINA
EELIER
EELING
EERIER
EERILY
EFFIGY
EGGIER
EGGING
EGLISE
EGOISM
EGOIST
ELAINE
ELFISH
ELLICE
ELLIOS
ELLIOT
ELMIER
ELMIRA
ELMIRE
ELNINO
ELOISA
ELOISE
ELVIRA
ELVISH
EMAILS
EMMITT
EMPIRE
ENCINA
ENCINO
ENDING
ENDIVE
ENGILD
ENGINE
ENGIRD
ENGIRT
ENLINK
ENLIST
ENMITY
ENNIUS
ENOILS
ENRICH
ENRICO
ENSIGN
ENSILE
ENTIAL
ENTICE
ENTIRE
ENTITY
ENVIED
ENVIER
ENVIES
ENVIRO
ENWIND
EOLIAN
EOLITH
EONIAN
EOSINS
EPPING
EQUINE
EQUIPS
EQUITY
ERBIUM
ERMINE
EROICA
ERRING
ERVING
ESKIMO
ESPIAL
ESPIED
ESPIER
ESPIES
ESPIOS
ESTIME
ETAILS
ETHICS
ETHIOP
ETOILE
ETTING
EUNICE
EWAINE
EXCIDE
EXCISE
EXCITE
EXPIRE
EXPIRY
EXWIFE
EYEING
EYRIES
EYVIND

E•••I•

EANNIE
EARNIE
EARNIT
EARVIN
EARWIG
EASEIN
EATSIN
EATSIT
ECESIC
ECESIS
ECHOIC
ECLAIR
EDDAIC
EDENIC
EDGEIN
EDITIO
EENSIE
EFGHIJ
EGERIA
ELADIO
ELAPID
ELEGIT
ELEMIS
ELICIT
ELIXIR
ELPAIS
ELYRIA
ELYTIS
EMERIC
EMERIL
EMETIC
EMILIA
EMILIE
EMILIO
ENDPIN
ENDSIN
ENDSIT
ENFAIT
ENGLIT
ENJOIN
ENNUIS
ENOKIS
ENTAIL
ENVEIL
ENVOIS
EPODIC
EQUOID
EROTIC
ESENIN
ESPRIT
ESSAIS
ESTLIN
ETALIA
ETALII
ETAOIN
ETHNIC
ETONIC
EUCLID
EURAIL
EUSTIS
EVENIF
EXILIC
EXOTIC
EYELID
EYEPIT

E••••I

ELIELI
ERNANI
ETALII

•EI•••

BEIGES
BEIGHT
BEIGNE
BEINGS
BEINON
BEIRUT
CEIBAS
CEILED
DEICED
DEICER
DEICES
DEIDRE
DEIFIC
DEIGNS
DEIMOS
DEISTS
FEIGNS
FEINTS
FEISTY
GEIGER
GEIGHT
GEISEL
GEISHA
HEIDEN
HEIFER
HEIGHT
HEINIE
HEINSE
HEISTS
IEIGHT
KEITEL
LEICAS
LEIDEN
LEISEN
LEITER
MEIFUN
NEIGHS
NEIMAN
NEISSE
PEIRCE
REICED
REICES
REIGER
REIGNS
REILLY
REINAS
REINED
REINER
REINES
REININ
REINKS
REISER
REITER
SEIKOS
SEINED
SEINER
SEINES
SEISMO
SEISMS
SEIZED
SEIZER
SEIZES
SEIZOR
VEIGHT
VEILED
VEILER
VEINAL
VEINED
VEINTE
WEIDER
WEIGHS
WEIGHT
WEIMAR
WEIRDO
WEIRDY

•E•I••

AECIUM
AEDILE
AERIAL
AERIER
AERIES
AERIFY
AERILY
AERIOS
BEDIMS
BEFIRM
BEFITS
BEGINS
BEGIRD
BEGIRT
BEHIND
BEKIND
BELIAL
BELIED
BELIEF
BELIER
BELIES
BELIKE
BELIZE
BEMINE
BEMIRE
BENICE
BENIGN
BENING
BENITO
BERING
BESIDE
BETIDE
BEVIES
BEWIGS
CECILB
CECILE
CEDING
CELICA
CELINE
CERISE
CERIUM
CESIUM
DEAIRS
DEBITS
DECIDE
DECILE
DECIUS
DEDINI
DEFIED
DEFIER
DEFIES
DEFILE
DEFINE
DEHIRE
DEKING
DELIAN
DELICT
DELINT
DELISH
DELIST
DELIUS
DEMIES
DEMILO
DEMISE
DEMIST
DEMITS
DENIAL
DENIED
DENIER
DENIES
DENIMS
DENIRO
DENISE
DEPICT
DERIDE
DERITA
DERIVE
DESICA
DESIGN
DESILT
DESILU
DESIRE
DESIST
DEVICE
DEVICQ
DEVILS
DEVINE
DEVISE
DEVITO
DEWIER
DEWILY
DEWING
DEWIRE
DEWITT
EELIER
EELING
EERIER
EERILY
FEEING
FELICE
FELIDS
FELINE
FELIPE
FELIXI
FELIXV
FERIAS
FERITY
FETING
FETISH
GEEING
GEMINI
GENIAL
GENIES
GENIUS
HEGIRA
HELICO
HELIOS
HELIUM
HESIOD
HEWING
HEWISH
HEWITT
HEXING
JEMIMA
JEWISH
KEFIRS
KEYING
LEGION
LEGIST
LEHIGH
LENINA
LENITY
LEOIII
LERIDA
LESION
LEVIED
LEVIER
LEVIES
LEVINE
LEVITE
LEVITT
LEVITY
MEDIAL
MEDIAN
MEDIAS
MEDICA
MEDICI
MEDICO
MEDICS
MEDINA
MEDIUM
MEDIUS
MEJICO
MELINA
MENIAL
MERIDA
MERINO
MERITS
MESIAL
METIER
METING
MEWING
MEXICO
NEVILL
NEVINS
NEWIES
NEWISH
PEKING
PELION
PENICK
PEPINO
PEPITA
PERILS
PERINE
PERIOD
PERISH
PERITI
PETIPA
PETITE
PEWITS
REAIMS
REAIRS
REBIDS
REBILL
REBIND
RECIFE
RECIPE
RECITE
REDIAL
REDIGS
REDING
REDINK
REDIPS
REFIED
REFIES
REFILE
REFILL
REFILM
REFIND
REFINE
REFIRE
REFITS
REGIFT
REGILD
REGIME
REGINA
REGION
REGIRD
REGIUS
REGIVE
REHIDE
REHIRE
REHITS
REJIGS
REKICK
RELICS
RELICT
RELIED
RELIEF
RELIER
RELIES
RELINE
RELINK
RELISH
RELIST
RELIVE
REMICK
REMILL
REMIND
REMINE
REMINI
REMINT
REMISE
REMISS
REMITS
RENINS
REOILS
REPICK
REPINE
REPINS
RERIDE
RERIGS
RERISE
RESIDE
RESIFT
RESIGN
RESILE
RESING
RESINK
RESINS
RESINY
RESIST
RESITE
RESITS
RESIZE
RETIAL
RETIED
RETIEF
RETIES
RETILE
RETILL
RETIME
RETINA
RETINS
RETINT
RETIPS
RETIRE
REVIEW
REVILE
REVISE
REVIVE
REWIND
REWINS
REWIPE
REWIRE
REZIPS
SEAICE
SEDICI
SEEING
SEMITE
SENILE
SENIOR
SENITI
SEPIAS
SEPIRA
SERIAL
SERIES
SERIFS
SERINS
SEWING
SEWIST
SEXIER
SEXILY
SEXISM
SEXIST
TEDIUM
TEEING
VEDIST
VENIAL
VENICE
VENINS
VENIRE
VENITE
VERIFY
VERILY
VERISM
VERIST
VERITE
VERITY
VEXING
VEZINA
YESIAM
YESIDO
ZENIST
ZENITH

•E••I•

AENEID
AEOLIA
BEANIE
BEATIT
BEAVIS
BEDSIT
BEDWIN
BEFAIR
BEHAIM
BELAIR
BELGIC
BELOIT
BENDIX
BENNIE
BENOIT
BERLIN
BERNIE
BERTIE
BESSIE
BESTIR
BEWAIL
CEDRIC
CELTIC
CERTIF
CERVID
DEALIN
DEARIE
DEASIL
DEBBIE
DEBRIS
DECEIT
DEENIE
DEHAIR
DEIFIC
DELRIO
DELTIC
DEMAIN
DENNIS
DENTIN
DERAIL
DERAIN
DERMIC
DERMIS
DETAIL
DETAIN
DEVEIN
DEVOID
DEVOIR
EENSIE
FEEDIN
FELLIN
FERDIE
FERGIE
FERMIS
FERRIC
FERRIS
FERVID
GEHRIG
GEODIC
GERBIL
GERTIE
GERVIN
GESTIC
GETFIT
GETHIP
GETRID
GETSIN
GETSIT
GETTIN
HEADIN
HECTIC
HEEBIE
HEFLIN
HEINIE
HELDIN
HELDIT
HELPIN
HEMSIN
HENBIT
HENRIK
HERBIE
HEREIN
HERMIT
HERNIA
HEROIC
HEROIN
HESTIA
JEANIE
JENNIE
JERKIN
JESUIT
KEEPIN
KEEPIT
KELLIE
KELPIE
KELVIN
KEMPIS
KENSIT
KEPTIN
KERMIT
KERWIN
KESHIA
KEWPIE
KEYSIN
LEADIN
LEAKIN
LEANIN
LEAPIN
LECAIN
LEEKIE
LEFTIN
LEFTIT
LEGSIT
LEGUIN
LELOIR
LENAIN
LENNIE
LENTIL
LEOIII
LEONIA
LEONID
LEOVII
LEOXII
LESLIE
LESMIZ
LETRIP
LETSIN
MEALIE
MEANIE
MEANIT
MEDNIS
MEGRIM
MELVIL
MELVIN
MEMOIR
MENNIN
MENTIS
MERLIN
MERRIE
MESSIN
METRIC
NEELIX
NELLIE
NELLIS
NEREID
NESBIT
NESSIE
NESTIN
NEWBIE
NEWKID
NEWSIE
PECTIN
PEEKIN
PEERIN
PELVIC
PELVIS
PENCIL
PENNIA
PENNIS
PENSIN
PEORIA
PEPCID
PEPSIN
PEPTIC
PERKIN
PERMIT
PERRIN
PERSIA
PERSIS
PETAIN
PETPIG
PETRIE
PETSIT
PETTIS
PETTIT
READIN
REALIA
REBAIT
REBBIE
REBOIL
RECOIL
RECOIN
REDDIN
REDFIN
REDFIR
REDSIX
REDTIE
REEDIT
REELIN
REEMIT
REENIE
REGAIN
REGGIE
REGRIP
REININ
REJAIL
REJOIN
REKNIT
RELAID
REMAIL
REMAIN
RENAIL
RENNIE
RENNIN
RENOIR
REPAID
REPAIR
RESAID
RESHIP
RESNIK
RESOIL
RESPIN
RESTIR
RESUIT
RESWIM
RETAIL
RETAIN
RETRIM
RETTIG
REVOIR
SEAAIR
SEALIN
SEEFIT
SEENIN
SEEPIN
SEESIN
SELLIT
SENDIN
SENTIN
SEPHIA
SEPTIC
SEQUIN
SERAIS
SERBIA
SERGIO
SERKIN
SERKIS
SETSIN
SEWNIN
SEWSIN
TEARIT
TECHIE
TEENIE
TEGRIN
TEKKIE
TELLIT
TENNIS
TENPIN
TERBIC
TERRIF
TERRIS
TESSIE
TESSIO
TETRIS
VEDAIC
VEGGIE
VERBID
VERDIN
VEREIN
VERGIL
VERMIN
VESPID
WEDGIE
WEEBIT
WEENIE
WEEVIL
WENDIE
WENTIN
WESKIT
WESTIE
WESTIN
WETTIG
YEABIG
YENSID
YESSIR
YETTIE
ZEROIN
ZEUXIS

•E•••I

CENTAI
CENTRI
DEDINI
DEFGHI
DELPHI
DENALI
DENARI
DENDRI
FELIXI
GELATI
GEMINI
GEORDI
GEORGI
HENRYI
JETSKI
KENOBI
LEOIII
LEOVII
LEOXII
MEDICI
MESABI
NEPALI
NEROLI
NEVSKI
PELOSI
PERITI
PETERI
REMINI
RENVOI
SEDICI
SENITI
SENSEI
SERGEI
SESQUI
VENUTI
YEHUDI
YEMENI

••EI••

AGEING
AGEISM
AGEIST
AWEIGH
BOEING
CUEING
DHEIGH
DYEING
EYEING
FEEING
GEEING
GIEING
GNEISS
GREIST
HIEING
HOEING
KLEINE
KLEIST
KWEISI
OLEINS
ONEIDA
ONEILL
ONEIRO
ONEISH
OREIDA
PLEIAD
RHEIMS
SEEING
SHEIKH
SHEIKS
SHEILA
SKEINS
SLEIGH
STEINS
TEEING
THEIRS
THEISM
THEIST
TIEINS
TOEING
TOEINS
TREIZE
VIEIRA

••E•I•

ACEDIA
ACEDIT
ACESIT
ACETIC
ADELIE
ADENIS
AGESIX
ALEXIA
ALEXIS
AMEBIC
AMELIA
AMELIE
AMESIA
ANEMIA
ANEMIC
AXENIC
AYESIR
AZERIS
BLEWIN
BLEWIT
BREVIS
CHEMIC
CHEMIN
CHENIN
CHERIE
CLERIC
COEDIT
COELIA
CREDIT
CRETIN
CUEBID
CUEDIN
CUESIN
CUETIP
DEENIE
DIESIS
DOESIN
DOESIT
DREBIN
DREVIL
DREWIN
ECESIC
ECESIS
EDENIC
EGERIA
ELEGIT
ELEMIS
EMERIC
EMERIL
EMETIC
ESENIN

EVENIF EYELID EYEPIT FAERIE FEEDIN FLEWIN FOETID GAELIC GOESIN HEEBIE IBERIA ICEDIN ICEDIT ICESIN ICESIT IGETIT IRENIC ISEEIT ISELIN KEEPIN KEEPIT KNEWIT KOENIG LEEKIE LIEBIG LIESIN LIEVIO NEELIX NOESIS NOETIC NOEXIT OLEFIN ONEBIT ONEGIN ONEHIT ONEPIN OPENIT OREXIA OREXIS OVERIT PEEKIN PEERIN PIERIA PIETIN POETIC PREBID PRECIP PRECIS PREFIX PRELIM PREMIE PREMIX PREVIA PREVIN REEDIT REELIN REEMIT REENIE SCENIC SEEFIT SEENIN SEEPIN SEESIN SPECIE STEPIN STERIC STEVIE STEWIE TEENIE THECIA THECID THEKID THELIP THEPIT THESIS THETIS THEWIZ TIEDIN TIEPIN TIESIN TMESIS TOEDIN TOESIN TREDIA TREPID UNEPIC UNEVIL USEDIN USERID USESIN WEEBIT WEENIE WEEVIL WIENIE

••E•I

ALEXEI DUETTI IDENTI KWEISI MUESLI NIELLI OCELLI RIENZI SCENEI SHERRI STEFFI THEFBI

•••EI•

AENEID ALBEIT ANSEIS ARNEIS BITEIN CAGEIN CAMEIN CASEIN CAVEIN CLUEIN COHEIR COMEIN DECEIT DEVEIN DINEIN DIVEIN DONEIN DONEIT DOVEIN EASEIN EDGEIN ENVEIL FACEIT FADEIN FAKEID FAKEIT FILEIN GAVEIN GIVEIN GONEIN HATEIT HAVEIN HAVEIT HEREIN HOMEIN HONEIN ISEEIT ISSEIS LIFEIS LIGEIA LIVEIN LOMEIN LOSEIT LOVEIN LOVEIT LUREIN MADEIT MAKEIT MALEIC MCNEIL MOVEIN MOVEIT NAMEIT NEREID NISEIS NOSEIN PILEIN PIPEIN POPEIL RACEIN RAKEIN RIDEIN RODEIN ROPEIN SAVEIT SCHEIB SOBEIT SOLEIL SUREIS TAKEIN TAKEIT TOREIT TUNEIN TYPEIN UNVEIL VEREIN VOTEIN WADEIN WAVEIN WIREIN

•••E•I

ALGEDI ANGELI DOREMI ELIELI HIDEKI HUMERI JAMESI LAPERI LATERI LIGETI LUNEDI OLDELI PETERI SAMEDI VIDERI YEMENI

••••EI

ALEXEI ANDREI BRUNEI CISKEI DANTEI GLUTEI MALLEI NIKKEI NUCLEI ROLLEI SANSEI SCENEI SENSEI SERGEI TAIPEI

EJ••••

EJECTA EJECTS EJIDOS

E•J•••

ENJOIN ENJOYS

E••J••

ELIJAH EMAJOR

E••••J

EFGHIJ

•EJ•••

BEJART DEJAVU DEJECT DEJUNK DEJURE JEJUNE MEJICO REJAIL REJECT REJIGS REJOIN TEJANA TEJANO

•E•J••

DEEJAY DEFJAM FEEJEE MENJOU NEWJOB VEEJAY VERJEE

••EJ••

DEEJAY DYEJOB FEEJEE VEEJAY

••E••J

AGENTJ THEHAJ

•••E•J

INTERJ JAMESJ

EK••••

EKBERG EKEDBY EKELOF EKEOUT EKESBY EKLAND EKUELE

E•K•••

EAKINS ECKART ECKERD EDKOCH ELKONV ELKTON ESKERS ESKIMO

E••K••

ENOKIS ERYKAH ESHKOL EUCKEN EVOKED EVOKER EVOKES

E•••K•

EBANKS EBOOKS EUREKA

E••••K

EMBANK EMBARK ENIDOK ENLINK ENRANK EWBANK EXYANK

•EK•••

BEKIND DEKALB DEKING DEKKER DEKKOS JEKYLL MEKONG PEKING PEKOES REKEYS REKICK REKNIT REKNOT TEKKIE TEKWAR

•E•K••

BEAKED BEAKER BECKER BECKET BECKON BERKOW DECKED DECKER DECKLE DEKKER DEKKOS DELKEY GECKOS GEEKED HECKLE HECKNO JECKLE JERKED JERKER JERKIN JERKUP KEOKUK LEAKED LEAKER LEAKEY LEAKIN LEEKIE MEEKER MEEKLY MENKEN MERKEL NECKED NECKER NEWKID PEAKED PECKAT PECKED PEEKAT PEEKED PEEKER PEEKIN PERKED PERKIN PERKUP RECKED RECKON REEKED REEKER REEKOF SECKEL SEEKER SEIKOS SERKIN SERKIS TEDKEY TEKKIE TERKEL UECKER WEAKEN WEAKER WEAKLY WEAKON WEEKLY WERKER WESKER WESKIT YERKES

•E••K•

BELIKE BENEKE BETAKE JETSKI LEMOKO MEDAKA MERCKX NEVSKI NEVSKY PERUKE REASKS REBAKE REBUKE REDSKY REINKS REMAKE RERAKE RETAKE REVOKE REWAKE REWOKE REYOKE SEDAKA

•E•••K

BEDECK BETOOK DEBARK DEBUNK DEEPAK DEJUNK DEMARK DERREK FEELOK FELTOK HENRIK HENRYK KEOKUK NEWARK PENICK REBANK REBOOK RECOCK RECOOK RECORK REDINK REDOAK REDOCK REEBOK REHOOK REKICK RELINK RELOCK RELOOK REMARK REMICK REPACK REPARK REPERK REPICK RERACK RERANK RESEEK RESINK RESNIK RESOAK RETACK RETOOK REWORK SENDAK ZEDONK

••EK••

ALEKEG CHEKOV GEEKED LEEKIE MEEKER MEEKLY NIEKRO PEEKAT PEEKED PEEKER PEEKIN REEKED REEKER REEKOF SEEKER SHEKEL THEKID WEEKLY

••E•K•

ALECKS ALECKY BLEAKS BOESKY BREAKS CHECKS CHEEKS CHEEKY CLEEKS CLERKS CREAKS CREAKY CREEKS DRECKS DRECKY FLECKS FLECKY FREAKS FREAKY GREEKS ORECKS SHECKY SHEIKH SHEIKS SLEEKS SLEEKY SNEAKS SNEAKY SPEAKS SPECKS STEAKS SVEDKA TWEAKS TWEAKY VNECKS WHELKS WREAKS WRECKS

••E••K

AGENTK DEEPAK DOESOK FEELOK KRENEK REEBOK RHEBOK SLEZAK TREBEK

•••EK•

AZTEKS BENEKE CHEEKS CHEEKY CLEEKS CREEKS EUREKA GREEKS HACEKS HIDEKI KOPEKS RIJEKA SAMEKH SLEEKS SLEEKY TOPEKA

•••E•K

ADWEEK AWHECK BEDECK DONEOK JAMESK KOPECK LUBECK NOMEAK ONDECK REPERK RESEEK SCREAK SQUEAK STREAK

••••EK

ADWEEK DERREK DRABEK DUBCEK FLOREK KRENEK OCASEK RESEEK SAITEK SHRIEK SPACEK TARLEK TREBEK

EL••••

ELADIO ELAINE ELANCE ELANDS ELANET ELAPID ELAPSE ELATED ELATER ELATES ELAYER ELAYNE ELBERT ELBOWS ELBRUS ELBURZ ELDERS ELDEST ELECTS ELEGIT ELEMIS ELEVEN ELEVES ELEVON ELFISH ELFMAN ELFOWL ELGART ELICIT ELIDED ELIDER ELIDES ELIELI ELIJAH ELINOR ELISEO ELISHA ELISSA ELISTS ELITER ELITES ELIXIR ELKONV ELKTON ELLERY ELLICE ELLIOS ELLIOT ELLORA ELMERS ELMIER ELMIRA ELMIRE ELMONT ELMORE ELNATH ELNINO ELNORA ELODEA ELOGES ELOISA ELOISE ELOPED ELOPER ELOPES ELPAIS ELPASO ELRENO ELSTON ELTORO ELUANT ELUARD ELUATE ELUDED ELUDER ELUDES ELUTED ELUTES ELVERS ELVIRA ELVISH ELWOOD ELYRIA ELYSEE ELYTIS

E•L•••

EALING ECLAIR ECLASS ECLATS EELERS EELERY EELIER EELING EELPOT EFLATS EGLISE EILEEN EILERS EILERT EKLAND ELLERY ELLICE ELLIOS ELLIOT ELLORA ENLACE ENLINK ENLIST EOLIAN EOLITH ERLANG EULESS EULOGY

E••L••

EAGLED EAGLES EAGLET EARLAP EARLET EASLEY ECCLES ECOLAB ECOLAW ECOLES EDILES EFFLUX EFILED EFILES EGALES EGGLER EISLEY EKELOF EMALLS EMBLEM EMILIA EMILIE EMILIO EMILYS EMPLOY ENBLOC ENGLIT ENGLUT ENSLER EPILOG ESALEN ESTLIN ETALIA ETALII ETILES EUCLID EVELYN EVILER EVILLY EVOLVE EVULSE EXALTS EXILED EXILER EXILES EXILIC EXULTS EYELET EYELID

E•••L•

EASELS EASILY EASTLA EBERLE EBERLY EDERLE EDGILY EDIBLE EDIBLY EDSELS EERILY EIDOLA EISELE EKUELE ELIELI EMAILS EMALLS EMBALM EMPALE ENABLE ENDALL ENFOLD ENGELS ENGILD ENGULF ENHALO ENISLE ENOILS ENROLL ENROLS ENSILE EQUALS ERROLL ESCALE ETAILS ETHYLS ETOILE EVENLY EVERLY EVILLY EXCELS EXHALE EXPELS EXTOLL EXTOLS

E••••L

EARFUL EIFFEL ELFOWL EMERIL ENAMEL ENCYCL ENDALL ENROLL ENSEAL ENSOUL ENTAIL ENTIAL ENVEIL EPICAL EPINAL ERROLL ESHKOL ESPIAL ETYMOL EURAIL EXTOLL EYEFUL

•EL•••

BELAIR BELATE BELAYS BELDAM BELFRY BELGAE BELGIC BELIAL BELIED BELIEF BELIER BELIES BELIKE BELIZE BELLAY BELLED BELLES BELLOC BELLOW BELLUM BELOIT BELONG BELONS BELTED BELTER BELTON BELTUP BELUGA BELZER CELEBS CELERY CELICA CELINE CELLAE CELLAR CELLED CELLOS CELTIC DELAND DELANO DELANY DELAYS DELCOS DELEAD DELETE DELFTS DELIAN DELICT DELINT DELISH DELIST DELIUS DELKEY DELMAR DELPHI DELRAY DELREY DELRIO DELROY DELSOL DELTAS DELTIC DELUDE DELUGE DELUGG DELUXE DELVED DELVER DELVES EELERS EELERY EELIER EELING EELPOT FELDON FELICE FELIDS FELINE FELIPE FELIXI FELIXV FELLAH FELLAS FELLED FELLER FELLIN FELLON FELLOW FELLTO FELONS FELONY FELSON FELTED FELTOK GELATE GELATI GELATO GELCAP GELDED GELDOF GELEES GELETT GELLAR GELLED GELLER GELPEN GELSEY HELDIN HELDIT HELDON HELDTO HELDUP HELENA HELENE HELENS HELICO HELIOS HELIUM HELLAS HELLER HELLNO HELLON HELLOS HELMED HELMER HELMET HELMUT HELOTS HELPED HELPER HELPIN HELPME HELPON HELPUP HELTER JELLED JELLOS KELLER KELLEY KELLIE KELLYS KELPIE KELSEY KELTON KELVIN LELAND LELOIR MELDED MELDER MELEES MELETE MELINA MELLON MELLOW MELMAC MELODY MELONS MELOTT MELTED MELTER MELTON MELVIL MELVIN MELVYN NELLIE NELLIS NELSON PELAGE PELEUS PELHAM PELION PELLAM PELLET PELOSI PELOTA PELTED PELTER PELTRY PELVIC

PELVIS
RELACE
RELAID
RELAND
RELAPS
RELATE
RELAYS
RELEAD
RELEAP
RELEND
RELENT
RELETS
RELEVE
RELEVY
RELICS
RELICT
RELIED
RELIEF
RELIER
RELIES
RELINE
RELINK
RELISH
RELIST
RELIVE
RELOAD
RELOAN
RELOCK
RELOGS
RELOOK
RELOSE
RELOST
RELUCT
RELUME
RELYON
SELDOM
SELECT
SELENA
SELENE
SELLBY
SELLER
SELLIT
SELLON
SELLTO
SELTEN
SELVES
TELCOS
TELLER
TELLIT
TELLME
TELLOF
TELLON
TELNET
VELARS
VELCRO
VELDTS
VELLUM
VELOCE
VELOUR
VELSEN
VELURE
VELVET
WELCHS
WELDED
WELDER
WELDON
WELLED
WELLER
WELLES
WELLUP
WELTED
WELTER
YELENA
YELLAT
YELLED
YELLER
YELLOW
YELPED
YELPER

•E•L••

AEOLIA
AEOLUS
BEALLS
BEDLAM
BEGLEY
BELLAY
BELLED
BELLES
BELLOC
BELLOW
BELLUM
BERLIN
BEULAH
CEILED
CELLAE
CELLAR
CELLED
CELLOS
CEYLON
DEALER
DEALIN
DEALTO
DEALUP
DEBLUR
DECLAW
DECLOT
DEFLEA
DEPLOY
DESLUM
DEWLAP
FEALTY
FEELER
FEELOK
FELLAH
FELLAS
FELLED
FELLER
FELLIN
FELLON
FELLOW
FELLTO
GELLAR
GELLED
GELLER
HEALED
HEALER
HEALEY
HEALTH
HEALUP
HEDLEY
HEELED
HEELER
HEFLIN
HELLAS
HELLER
HELLNO
HELLON
HELLOS
HENLEY
JELLED
JELLOS
JETLAG
KEELED
KEELER
KEGLER
KELLER
KELLEY
KELLIE
KELLYS
KEPLER
KEVLAR
LEALTY
LEELEE
LESLEY
LESLIE
MEALIE
MEDLEY
MELLON
MELLOW
MERLIN
MERLOT
MEWLED
MEWLER
NEALON
NEELIX
NELLIE
NELLIS
NEWLEY
PEALED
PEALER
PEALES
PEELED
PEELER
PEGLEG
PEGLER
PELLAM
PELLET
PEPLUM
PERLEA
REALER
REALES
REALIA
REALLY
REALMS
REALTY
RECLAD
REDLEG
REELED
REELER
REELIN
REELUP
REFLAG
REFLEW
REFLEX
REFLOW
REFLUX
REGLES
REGLOW
REGLUE
REILLY
REPLAN
REPLAY
REPLED
REPLOT
REPLOW
REVLON
REYLES
SEALAB
SEALED
SEALER
SEALIN
SEALUP
SEALYS
SEDLEY
SELLBY
SELLER
SELLIT
SELLON
SELLTO
TEFLON
TELLER
TELLIT
TELLME
TELLOF
TELLON
TENLBS
TENLEY
TESLAS
TETLEY
VEBLEN
VEILED
VEILER
VELLUM
WEALDS
WEALTH
WEBLOG
WELLED
WELLER
WELLES
WELLUP
WESLEY
YELLAT
YELLED
YELLER
YELLOW
YEOLDE
ZEALOT

•E••L•

AEDILE
AERILY
BEADLE
BEAGLE
BEALLS
BEATLE
BECALM
BEETLE
BEFALL
BEFELL
BEHALF
BEHELD
BEHOLD
BERYLS
BETELS
BEVELS
BEWELL
BEZELS
CECILB
CECILE
CEORLS
DEADLY
DEAFLY
DEARLY
DECALS
DECILE
DECKLE
DEEPLY
DEFILE
DEFTLY
DEGELS
DEKALB
DEMILO
DENALI
DEPULP
DESALT
DESILT
DESILU
DEVILS
DEWILY
DEWOLF
EERILY
FEEBLE
FEEBLY
FEMALE
FERALS
FERULE
FETTLE
GENTLE
GENTLY
GERALD
GETOLD
HECKLE
HERALD
JECKLE
JEKYLL
JEWELS
KEENLY
KEMBLE
KERALA
KETTLE
LEANLY
LEGALS
LENGLE
LETFLY
LEVELS
LEWDLY
MEANLY
MEASLE
MEASLY
MEDALS
MEDDLE
MEDFLY
MEEKLY
MEETLY
MEGALO
MERDLE
MERELY
MERYLL
METALS
METTLE
NEARLY
NEATLY
NEBULA
NEEDLE
NEPALI
NEROLI
NESTLE
NETTLE
NETTLY
NEVILL
NEWELL
NEWELS
NEWULM
PEARLE
PEARLS
PEARLY
PEBBLE
PEBBLY
PEDALS
PEDDLE
PENULT
PEOPLE
PERILS
PERTLY
PESTLE
PETALE
PETALS
PETULA
REALLY
REBALE
REBELS
REBILL
REBOLT
RECALL
REFALL
REFELL
REFILE
REFILL
REFILM
REFOLD
REGALE
REGELS
REGILD
REHELD
REHOLD
REILLY
REMELT
REMILL
REMOLD
REOILS
REPELS
REPOLL
REROLL
RESALE
RESALT
RESELL
RESILE
RESOLD
RESOLE
RESULT
RETELL
RETILE
RETILL
RETOLD
REVELS
REVILE
REVOLT
REWELD
REXALL
SEARLE
SEEALL
SEEMLY
SEMELE
SEMPLE
SENILE
SEPALS
SETTLE
SEWELL
SEXILY
TEMPLE
VENULE
VERILY
WEAKLY
WEDELN
WEDELS
WEEKLY
WETFLY
YEARLY
YERTLE

•E•••L

AERIAL
BEAPAL
BECOOL
BEFALL
BEFELL
BEFOOL
BEFOUL
BELIAL
BENGAL
BENZOL
BESSEL
BETHEL
BEWAIL
BEWELL
CENTAL
CEPHAL
CEREAL
DEASIL
DEFUEL
DEHMEL
DELSOL
DENIAL
DENTAL
DENZEL
DEPAUL
DERAIL
DERMAL
DETAIL
FENNEL
FESTAL
FEUDAL
GEISEL
GENIAL
GENUAL
GERBIL
HEBBEL
HEDRAL
HERBAL
JEKYLL
JESSEL
KEITEL
KENNEL
KERNEL
KEYPAL
LEMUEL
LENTIL
LETHAL
MEDIAL
MELVIL
MENDEL
MENIAL
MENSAL
MENTAL
MERKEL
MERYLL
MESCAL
MESIAL
METHYL
NERMAL
NERVAL
NETFUL
NEURAL
NEUROL
NEVILL
NEWELL
NEXTEL
PENCIL
PENPAL
PENTEL
PEPFUL
PETREL
PETROL
REBILL
REBOIL
RECALL
RECOAL
RECOIL
RECOOL
RECURL
REDEAL
REDIAL
REFALL
REFELL
REFILL
REFUEL
REGNAL
REHAUL
REHEAL
REHEEL
REJAIL
REMAIL
REMILL
RENAIL
RENTAL
REPEAL
REPOLL
REREEL
REROLL
RESEAL
RESELL
RESOIL
RETAIL
RETELL
RETIAL
RETILL
RETOOL
RETRAL
REVEAL
REXALL
SEAEEL
SEAGAL
SECKEL
SEEALL
SEPTAL
SEQUEL
SERIAL
SEWELL
TEASEL
TERCEL
TERKEL
TETZEL
VEINAL
VENIAL
VERBAL
VERGIL
VERNAL
VESSEL
VESTAL
WEASEL
WEEVIL
WERFEL

••EL••

ABELES
ACELAS
ADELEH
ADELIE
ADELLE
AIELLO
AKELAS
AMELIA
AMELIE
ANELED
ANELES
APELET
AZELMA
BCELLS
CHELAE
CIELOS
COELIA
DCELLS
DUELED
DUELER
DUELLO
DWELLS
DYELOT
EKELOF
EVELYN
EYELET
EYELID
FEELER
FEELOK
FIELDS
FUELED
FUELER
FUELUP
GAELIC
GUELPH
HEELED
HEELER
IMELDA
ISELIN
KEELED
KEELER
KNELLS
KVELLS
LEELEE
LIELOW
LUELLA
MIELES
NEELIX
NIELLI
NIELLO
OBELUS
OCELLI
OCELOT
ODELET
OMELET
ONELAP
ONELEG
ORELSE
OTELLO
PAELLA
PEELED
PEELER
PHELPS
PIELET
PRELAW
PRELIM
PRELOG
QUELER
QUELLS
REELED
REELER
REELIN
REELUP
RKELLY
SHELBY
SHELLS
SHELTY
SHELVE
SMELLS
SMELLY
SMELTS
SNELLS
SPELLS
STELAR
STELAS
STELES
STELLA
STELMO
SVELTE
SWELLS
TCELLS
THELAW
THELIP
THELMA
THELOT
TWELVE
VIELLE
WHELAN
WHELKS
WHELMS
WHELPS
WIELDS
WIELDY
YIELDS

••E•L•

ADELLE
AGEDLY
AGEOLD
AIELLO
AREOLA
AREOLE
AWEDLY
BCELLS
BEETLE
BRENLY
CREELS
CREOLE
DCELLS
DEEPLY
DUELLO
DWELLS
EBERLE
EBERLY
EDERLE
EVENLY
EVERLY
FEEBLE
FEEBLY
FREELY
GREYLY
IDEALS
ISEULT
KEENLY
KNEELS
KNELLS
KVELLS
LIEFLY
LUELLA
MEEKLY
MEETLY
MUESLI
NEEDLE
NIELLI
NIELLO
OCELLI
OLEOLE
ONEALL
ONEILL
OPENLY
OTELLO
OVERLY
PAELLA
PUEBLA
PUEBLO
QUELLS
RKELLY
SEEALL
SEEMLY
SHEILA
SHELLS
SIECLE
SMELLS
SMELLY
SNELLS
SPELLS
STEALS
STEELE
STEELS
STEELY
STELLA
SWELLS
TCELLS
THEFLY
THEYLL
TREBLE
TREBLY
VIELLE
WEEKLY
WHEELS
WHENLL

••E••L

ACETAL
ACETYL
ALEVEL
CHERYL
CHEVAL
COEVAL
CRENEL
CRESOL
CREWEL
DAEDAL
DIESEL
DREVIL
DREXEL
EMERIL
EYEFUL
FIEVEL
GRETEL
HIEMAL
HYETAL
IREFUL
KNEBEL
OLEVEL
ONEALL
ONEILL
PHENOL
PLEXAL
RUEFUL
SEEALL
SHEKEL
SHERYL
SIEGEL
STEROL
THENFL
THENHL
THEYLL
UNEVIL
USEFUL
WEEVIL
WHENLL
WIESEL
WOEFUL

•••EL•

AACELL
AFIELD
ALLELE
ANGELA
ANGELI
ANGELL
ANGELO
ANGELS
ANSELM
APPELS
ARBELA
ARPELS
ARTELS
ASWELL
AZUELA
BABELS
BAGELS
BARELY
BASELY
BEFELL
BEHELD
BETELS
BEVELS
BEWELL
BEZELS
BLUELY
BOTELS
BOWELS
CABELL
CAMELS
CAVELL
CICELY
COMELY
COSELL
CREELS
CUPELS
CUTELY
DEGELS
DIRELY
DOTELL
DOWELL
DOWELS
DYNELS
EASELS
EDSELS
EISELE
EKUELE
ELIELI
ENGELS
EXCELS
EXPELS
FINELY
FREELY
FRIELS
GAMELY
GAVELS
GILELS
GIMELS
GISELE
GOWELL
GRUELS
HAMELN
HAZELS
HOMELY
HOSELS
HOTELS
HOVELS
HOWELL
HUGELY
IMPELS
INGELS
ITSELF
JEWELS
KAPELL
KNEELS
KOPELL
LABELS
LAMELY
LAPELS
LATELY
LEVELS
LIBELS
LIKELY
LIVELY
LONELY
LOVELL
LOVELY
LOWELL
MABELL
MAXELL
MERELY
MODELA
MODELB
MODELS
MODELT
MORELS
MOTELS
MUTELY
MYSELF
NAMELY
NAVELS
NEWELL
NEWELS
NICELY
NOBELS
NOHELP
NORELL
NOVELA
NOVELS
NUDELY
OFHELP
OHWELL
OLDELI
ORIELS
ORWELL
OUSELS
OUZELS
PALELY
PAMELA
PANELS
PIXELS
POMELO
POWELL
PURELY
RARELY
RATELS
RAVELS
REBELS
REFELL
REGELS
REHELD
REMELT
REPELS
RESELL
RETELL
REVELS
REWELD
RIFELY
RIPELY
RONELY
ROWELS
RUBELS
RUDELY
RYDELL
SAFELY
SAGELY
SANELY
SCHELL
SEMELE
SEWELL
SHIELD
SOLELY
SORELY
SPIELS
STEELE
STEELS
STEELY
SURELY
TAMELY
TAVELS
TIMELY
TOWELS
TUPELO
UMBELS
UNBELT
UNFELT
UNHELD
UNHELM
UNSELD
UNSELL
UNWELL
UPHELD
UPWELL
VILELY
VOWELS
VOWELY
WEDELN
WEDELS
WHEELS
WIDELY
WIFELY
WISELY
YARELY
YODELS
YOKELS

•••E•L

AACELL
ANGELL
ANNEAL
APPEAL
ASTEAL
ASWELL
ATHEEL
BEFELL
BEWELL
BOREAL
CABELL
CAVELL
CEREAL
CINEOL
COSELL
CUNEAL
DOTELL
DOWELL
ENSEAL
ENVEIL
GOWELL
HOWELL
IRREAL
KAPELL
KOPELL
LINEAL
LOREAL
LOVELL
LOWELL
MABELL
MAXELL
MCBEAL
MCNEIL
MUDEEL
NEWELL
NODEAL
NORELL
OHWELL
ORDEAL
ORWELL
OSTEAL
PINEAL
POPEIL
POWELL
REDEAL
REFELL
REHEAL
REHEEL
REPEAL
REREEL
RESEAL
RESELL

RETELL
REVEAL
RYDELL
SCHELL
SEAEEL
SEWELL
SHTETL
SOLEIL
SQUEAL
TINEAL
TOHEEL
UNPEEL
UNREAL
UNREEL
UNSEAL
UNSELL
UNVEIL
UNWELL
UPWELL

••••EL

ABDIEL
ALEVEL
ALUDEL
AMSTEL
ATHEEL
AZRAEL
BARREL
BARTEL
BESSEL
BETHEL
BLOBEL
BOATEL
BRUMEL
BUNUEL
BUSHEL
CANCEL
CANNEL
CARMEL
CARPEL
CARREL
CARTEL
CARVEL
CASTEL
CHACEL
CHANEL
CHAPEL
CHISEL
COMPEL
CORBEL
CORNEL
CRENEL
CREWEL
CUDGEL
DAMSEL
DANIEL
DARCEL
DEFUEL
DEHMEL
DENZEL
DHOTEL
DIESEL
DISPEL
DREXEL
DRIVEL
DUFFEL
EIFFEL
ENAMEL
FARFEL
FENNEL
FIEVEL
FINKEL
FUNNEL
GEISEL
GIMBEL
GOSPEL
GRAVEL
GRETEL
GROVEL
GUMBEL
GUNSEL
HALLEL
HANDEL
HANSEL
HASSEL
HEBBEL
HILLEL
HIMMEL
HORMEL
HOSTEL
HUMMEL
IJSSEL
ISABEL
ISOHEL
ISRAEL
JESSEL
KANDEL
KEITEL
KENNEL
KERNEL
KISSEL
KNEBEL
KOCHEL
KOPPEL
KOSSEL
KUMMEL
KUNZEL
LAUREL
LEMUEL
LINTEL
LIONEL
MAAZEL
MANDEL
MANTEL
MANUEL
MARCEL
MARIEL
MARTEL
MARVEL
MATTEL
MENDEL
MERKEL
MICHEL
MIGUEL
MONTEL
MORREL
MORSEL
MOSTEL
MUDEEL
MURIEL
MUSSEL
MUTUEL
NEXTEL
NICKEL
OLEVEL
ORAJEL
PARCEL
PASSEL
PASTEL
PENTEL
PETREL
PICHEL
POMMEL
PROPEL
PUMMEL
RACHEL
RAFAEL
RANGEL
RAPPEL
RAQUEL
REFUEL
REHEEL
REREEL
ROMMEL
RONDEL
RUNNEL
RUSSEL
SAMUEL
SEAEEL
SECKEL
SEQUEL
SHEKEL
SHOVEL
SIEGEL
SISKEL
SKYTEL
SNIVEL
SORREL
SPINEL
SWIVEL
TACTEL
TASSEL
TEASEL
TERCEL
TERKEL
TETZEL
TINSEL
TOHEEL
TRAVEL
TROWEL
TUNNEL
UNPEEL
UNREEL
VACHEL
VESSEL
WANKEL
WEASEL
WERFEL
WIESEL
ZIFFEL

EM••••

EMAILS
EMAJOR
EMALLS
EMBALM
EMBANK
EMBARK
EMBARS
EMBAYS
EMBEDS
EMBERS
EMBLEM
EMBODY
EMBOGS
EMBOSS
EMBOWS
EMBRUE
EMBRYO
EMCEED
EMCEES
EMDASH
EMEERS
EMENDS
EMERGE
EMERIC
EMERIL
EMETIC
EMEUTE
EMIGRE
EMILIA
EMILIE
EMILIO
EMILYS
EMINEM
EMINOR
EMMAUS
EMMETS
EMMETT
EMMITT
EMORYU
EMOTED
EMOTER
EMOTES
EMPALE
EMPATH
EMPERY
EMPIRE
EMPLOY
EMPSON
EMPTOR
EMQUAD

E•M•••

EAMONN
EDMOND
EDMUND
EGMONT
ELMERS
ELMIER
ELMIRA
ELMIRE
ELMONT
ELMORE
EMMAUS
EMMETS
EMMETT
EMMITT
ENMESH
ENMITY
ERMINE
EXMATE
EXMETS
EXMOOR
EXMORE

E••M••

EDAMES
EDEMAS
ELEMIS
ELFMAN
ENAMEL
ENAMOR
ENDMAN
ENDMEN
ERDMAN
ETYMOL
ETYMON
EXEMPT

E•••M•

ECTOMY
ECZEMA
ENARMS
ENCAMP
ENIGMA
ENORME
ENTOMB
ENTOMO
ENZYME
ESKIMO
ESTIME
EXHUME

E••••M

EGOISM
EMBALM
EMBLEM
EMINEM
ENGRAM
EPONYM
ERBIUM
ESTEEM
EUONYM
EXONYM

•EM•••

BEMATA
BEMINE
BEMIRE
BEMOAN
BEMUSE
CEMENT
DEMAIN
DEMAND
DEMARK
DEMAST
DEMEAN
DEMIES
DEMILO
DEMISE
DEMIST
DEMITS
DEMOBS
DEMODE
DEMOED
DEMOND
DEMONS
DEMOTE
DEMOTH
DEMURE
DEMURS
FEMALE
FEMBOT
FEMMES
FEMORA
FEMURS
GEMARA
GEMINI
GEMMAE
GEMMED
HEMATO
HEMMED
HEMMER
HEMPEN
HEMSIN
JEMIMA
KEMBLE
KEMPIS
LEMANS
LEMMAS
LEMMON
LEMNOS
LEMOKO
LEMOND
LEMONS
LEMONY
LEMUEL
LEMURS
MEMBER
MEMOIR
MEMORY
NEMEAN
REMADE
REMAIL
REMAIN
REMAKE
REMAND
REMANS
REMAPS
REMARK
REMATE
REMATS
REMEDY
REMEET
REMELT
REMEND
REMICK
REMILL
REMIND
REMINE
REMINI
REMINT
REMISE
REMISS
REMITS
REMOLD
REMOPS
REMORA
REMOTE
REMOVE
REMOWN
REMOWS
REMSEN
SEMANA
SEMELE
SEMITE
SEMPER
SEMPLE
SEMPRE
TEMPED
TEMPEH
TEMPER
TEMPLE
TEMPOS
TEMPTS
TEMPUS
YEMANA
YEMENI

•E•M••

BEAMAN
BEAMED
BEAMER
BEAMON
BEAMUP
BEEMER
BERMAN
BERMED
BEYMER
DEEMED
DEHMEL
DEIMOS
DELMAR
DENMOM
DERMAL
DERMAS
DERMAT
DERMIC
DERMIS
DERMOT
DESMOG
DETMER
FEMMES
FERMAT
FERMIS
GEMMAE
GEMMED
GERMAN
GETMAD
HELMED
HELMER
HELMET
HELMUT
HEMMED
HEMMER
HERMAN
HERMES
HERMIT
HERMON
HEYMAN
KERMIT
KEYMAN
KEYMEN
LEEMAY
LEGMAN
LEGMEN
LEHMAN
LEMMAS
LEMMON
LESMIZ
MELMAC
MERMAN
MERMEN
MESMER
NEIMAN
NERMAL
NETMAN
NETMEN
NEUMAN
NEWMAN
NEWMAR
PENMAN
PENMEN
PERMED
PERMIT
REAMED
REAMER
REEMIT
SEAMAN
SEAMAP
SEAMED
SEAMEN
SEAMER
SEAMUS
SEEMED
SEEMLY
SEEMTO
SERMON
TEAMED
TEAMUP
TEEMED
TERMED
TERMES
TEXMEX
VERMIN
WEIMAR
WETMOP
YEOMAN
YEOMEN
YESMAN
YESMEN
ZEEMAN

•E••M•

BECAME
BECOME
BEDIMS
BEGEMS
BEGUMS
BEHOME
BENUMB
BESAME
BESOMS
DEARME
DECAMP
DEFAME
DEGUMS
DENIMS
FEEDME
GENOME
HELPME
JEMIMA
JEREMY
JEROME
LEGUME
MECUMS
MEOHMY
README
REAIMS
REALMS
REARMS
RECOMB
REGIME
REHEMS
RELUME
RENAME
REPUMP
RESUME
RETAME
RETIME
REVAMP
SEDUMS
SEISMO
SEISMS
SERUMS
SESAME
TELLME
VENOMS

•E•••M

AECIUM
BECALM
BEDLAM
BEFIRM
BEHAIM
BELDAM
BELLUM
CENTUM
CERIUM
CESIUM
DEDHAM
DEFJAM
DEFOAM
DEFORM
DEGERM
DENHAM
DENMOM
DESLUM
DESTEM
DEWORM
HELIUM
JETSAM
MEDIUM
MEGOHM
MEGRIM
NEWSOM
NEWULM
PELHAM
PELLAM
PEPLUM
REDEEM
REDRUM
REFILM
REFORM
REGNUM
RESEAM
RESWAM
RESWIM
RETRIM
REWARM
SEAARM
SELDOM
SEPTUM
SEXISM
TEDEUM
TEDIUM
VELLUM
VERISM
WEBCAM
YESIAM

••EM••

ALEMAN
ANEMIA
ANEMIC
APEMAN
APEMEN
ATEMPO
AXEMAN
AXEMEN
BEEMER
BREMEN
BREMER
CHEMIC
CHEMIN
CREMER
CREMES
DAEMON
DEEMED
EDEMAS
ELEMIS
EXEMPT
FOEMAN
FOEMEN
HIEMAL
ICEMAN
ICEMEN
ITEMED
LEEMAY
NOEMON
ONEMAN
ONEMEG
PIEMAN
PIEMEN
POEMES
PREMED
PREMET
PREMIE
PREMIX
QUEMOY
REEMIT
RHEMES
SEEMED
SEEMLY
SEEMTO
STEMMY
TEEMED
THEMAN
THEMED
THEMES
THEMET
THEMOB
THEMRS
TIEMPO
TREMOR
WIEMAN
ZEEMAN

••E•M•

ADEEMS
ATEAMS
AZELMA
BREAMS
BTEAMS
CREAMS
CREAMY
DREAMS
DREAMT
DREAMY
FEEDME
GLEAMS
GLEAMY
HBEAMS
IBEAMS
LBEAMS
OLEUMS
PNEUMA
PNEUMO
PREAMP
RHEEMS
RHEIMS
RHEUMS
RHEUMY
STEAMS
STEAMY
STELMO
STEMMY
THELMA
THERMO
THERMS
WHELMS

••E••M

AGEISM
FRENUM
ICEDAM
ONEARM
PHENOM
PLENUM
PREARM
PRELIM
THEISM
THERAM

•••EM•

ADEEMS
BADEMS
BEGEMS
BIREME
BOHEME
CINEMA
DAREME
DOREMI
ECZEMA
GOLEMS
HAREMS
JEREMY
MAKEME
MODEMS
PROEMS
RACEME
REHEMS
RHEEMS
SAVEME
SCHEMA
SCHEME
SOLEMN
TONEME
TOTEMS
XYLEMS

•••E•M

AGLEAM
ANSELM
DEGERM
ESTEEM
FIVEAM
FIVEPM
GOTEAM
HAKEEM
INSEAM
JAMESM
KADEEM
KAREEM
LAPERM
LYCEUM
MUSEUM
NINEAM
NINEPM
PHLEGM
PILEUM
REDEEM
RESEAM
SCREAM
STREAM
SUREAM
TEDEUM
TOTERM
UNHELM
UNSEAM

••••EM

ANADEM
ANTHEM
ARNHEM
AUNTEM
BOOKEM
DESTEM
DIADEM
DODGEM
EMBLEM
EMINEM
ESTEEM
HAKEEM
HARLEM
HOLDEM
IBIDEM
KADEEM
KAREEM
MAYHEM
MOSLEM
PHLOEM
PROTEM
REDEEM
SACHEM
SHOLEM
SYSTEM
TANDEM
WILLEM

EN••••

ENABLE
ENACTS
ENAMEL
ENAMOR
ENARMS
ENATES
ENBANC
ENBERG
ENBLOC
ENCAGE
ENCAMP
ENCASE
ENCINA
ENCINO
ENCODE
ENCORE
ENCRES
ENCYCL
ENDALL
ENDASH
ENDCUT
ENDEAR
ENDERS
ENDING
ENDIVE
ENDMAN
ENDMEN
ENDORA
ENDOWS
ENDPIN
ENDRAN
ENDRUN
ENDSAT
ENDSIN
ENDSIT
ENDSON
ENDSUP
ENDUED
ENDUES
ENDURE
ENDURO
ENDUSE
ENERGY
ENEROS
ENESCO
ENFACE
ENFAIT
ENFANT
ENFOLD
ENGAGE
ENGELS
ENGILD
ENGINE
ENGIRD
ENGIRT
ENGLIT
ENGLUT
ENGRAM
ENGULF
ENHALO
ENHAUT
ENIACS
ENIDOK
ENIGMA
ENISLE
ENJOIN
ENJOYS
ENLACE
ENLINK
ENLIST
ENMESH
ENMITY
ENNEAD
ENNIUS
ENNUIS
ENOILS
ENOKIS
ENORME
ENOTES
ENOUGH
ENQUAD
ENRAGE
ENRANK
ENRAPT
ENRICH
ENRICO
ENROBE
ENROLL
ENROLS
ENROOT
ENSATE
ENSEAL
ENSEAT
ENSIGN
ENSILE
ENSLER
ENSOUL
ENSUED
ENSUES
ENSURE
ENTAIL
ENTERO
ENTERS
ENTIAL
ENTICE
ENTIRE
ENTITY
ENTOMB
ENTOMO
ENTRAP
ENTREE
ENTREZ
ENURED
ENURES
ENVEIL
ENVIED
ENVIER
ENVIES
ENVIRO
ENVOIS
ENVOYS
ENWIND
ENWRAP
ENZYME

E•N•••

EANNIE
EENSIE
ELNATH
ELNINO
ELNORA
ENNEAD
ENNIUS
ENNUIS
EONIAN
ERNANI
ERNEST
EUNICE

E••N••

EANNIE
EARNED
EARNER
EARNIE
EARNIT
EBANKS
EBONDS
EDENIC
EGGNOG
EISNER
ELANCE
ELANDS
ELANET
ELINOR
EMENDS
EMINEM
EMINOR
EPINAL
EPONYM
ERENOW
ERINNA
ERINYS
ERYNGO
ESENIN
ETHNIC
ETHNOS
ETONIC
EUONYM
EUPNEA
EVENAS
EVENED
EVENER
EVENIF
EVENLY
EVENSO
EVENTS
EVENUP
EVINCE
EVONNE
EWINGS
EXONYM
EZINES

E•••N•

EAKINS
EALING
EAMONN
EARING
EASING
EATING
EBBING
EDGING
EDIRNE
EDMOND
EDMUND
EDWINA
EDWYNN
EELING
EGGING
EGMONT
EIRENE
EKLAND
ELAINE
ELAYNE
ELKONV
ELMONT
ELNINO
ELRENO
ELUANT
EMBANK
ENBANC
ENCINA
ENCINO
ENDING
ENFANT
ENGINE
ENLINK
ENRANK
ENWIND
EOCENE
EOSINS
EPPING
EPSONS
EQUINE
ERINNA
ERLANG
ERMINE
ERNANI

ERRAND
ERRANT
ERRING
ERVING
ESCENT
ESPANA
ESSENE
ETERNE
ETHANE
ETHENE
ETTING
EUGENE
EVONNE
EWAINE
EWBANK
EXCONS
EXEUNT
EXPAND
EXPEND
EXTANT
EXTEND
EXTENT
EXYANK
EYEING
EYVIND

E••••N

EAMONN
EARVIN
EASEIN
EASEON
EASTON
EATSIN
EDGEIN
EDISON
EDWYNN
EGGSON
EGOYAN
EGUREN
EILEEN
ELEVEN
ELEVON
ELFMAN
ELKTON
ELSTON
EMPSON
ENDMAN
ENDMEN
ENDPIN
ENDRAN
ENDRUN
ENDSIN
ENDSON
ENJOIN
ENSIGN
EOLIAN
EONIAN
EPHRON
ERDMAN
EREVAN
ERIVAN
ESALEN
ESENIN
ESTLIN
ETAOIN
ETYMON
EUCKEN
EUSDEN
EVELYN
EXTERN

•EN•••

AENEAS
AENEID
BENBEN
BENBOW
BENDAY
BENDED
BENDER
BENDIX
BENEKE
BENGAL
BENGAY
BENHUR
BENICE
BENIGN
BENING
BENITO
BENNIE
BENOIT
BENOTE
BENSEY
BENSON
BENTON
BENTOS
BENUMB
BENZOL
CENSED
CENSER
CENSES
CENSOR
CENSUS
CENTAI
CENTAL
CENTAS
CENTER
CENTOS
CENTRE
CENTRI
CENTRO
CENTUM
DENADA
DENALI
DENARI
DENARS
DENARY
DENDRA
DENDRI
DENDRO
DENHAM
DENIAL
DENIED
DENIER
DENIES
DENIMS
DENIRO
DENISE
DENMOM
DENNED
DENNIS
DENNYS
DENOTE
DENOVO
DENSER
DENTAL
DENTED
DENTIN
DENTON
DENUDE
DENVER
DENZEL
EENSIE
FENCED
FENCER
FENCES
FENDED
FENDER
FENNEL
FENNER
FENWAY
GENDER
GENERA
GENETS
GENEVA
GENEVE
GENIAL
GENIES
GENIUS
GENOAN
GENOAS
GENOME
GENOVA
GENRES
GENTES
GENTLE
GENTLY
GENTRY
GENUAL
GENXER
HENBIT
HENDEC
HENDRY
HENGES
HENLEY
HENNAS
HENNER
HENRIK
HENRYI
HENRYK
HENRYV
HENSON
JENNER
JENNET
JENNEY
JENNIE
JENSEN
KENDOS
KENNAN
KENNED
KENNEL
KENNER
KENNYG
KENOBI
KENSIT
KENTON
KENYAN
KENYON
LENAIN
LENAPE
LENARD
LENDEE
LENDER
LENDTO
LENGLE
LENGTH
LENGUA
LENINA
LENITY
LENNIE
LENNON
LENNOX
LENORE
LENOVO
LENSED
LENSES
LENTEN
LENTIL
LENTOS
LENTTO
MENACE
MENAGE
MENDED
MENDEL
MENDER
MENDES
MENIAL
MENJOU
MENKEN
MENNEN
MENNIN
MENSAL
MENSAN
MENSCH
MENTAL
MENTEE
MENTHE
MENTIS
MENTOR
MENTOS
MENUDO
OENONE
PENCHE
PENCIL
PENDED
PENGPU
PENICK
PENMAN
PENMEN
PENNED
PENNER
PENNEY
PENNIA
PENNIS
PENNON
PENPAL
PENROD
PENSEE
PENSIN
PENSUP
PENTAD
PENTAX
PENTEL
PENTUP
PENULT
PENURY
RENAIL
RENAME
RENARD
RENATA
RENATO
RENDED
RENDER
RENEGE
RENEST
RENEWS
RENFRO
RENGAS
RENINS
RENNES
RENNET
RENNIE
RENNIN
RENOIR
RENONV
RENOTE
RENOWN
RENTAL
RENTED
RENTEE
RENTER
RENTES
RENTON
RENTTO
RENVOI
SENARY
SENATE
SENATS
SENDAK
SENDBY
SENDEE
SENDER
SENDIN
SENDON
SENDTO
SENDUP
SENECA
SENHOR
SENILE
SENIOR
SENITI
SENNAS
SENORA
SENORS
SENSED
SENSEI
SENSEN
SENSES
SENSOR
SENTBY
SENTIN
SENTON
SENTRA
SENTRY
SENTTO
SENTUP
TENACE
TENANT
TENDAY
TENDED
TENDER
TENDON
TENDTO
TENEEE
TENETS
TENHUT
TENLBS
TENLEY
TENNER
TENNIS
TENONE
TENONS
TENORS
TENPIN
TENSED
TENSER
TENSES
TENSOR
TENTED
TENTER
TENTHS
TENTON
TENTWO
TENURE
TENUTA
TENUTO
VENDED
VENDEE
VENDER
VENDOR
VENDUE
VENEER
VENERA
VENETO
VENIAL
VENICE
VENINS
VENIRE
VENITE
VENNER
VENOMS
VENORA
VENOSE
VENOUS
VENTAS
VENTED
VENTER
VENUES
VENULE
VENUTI
WENCES
WENDED
WENDIE
WENDYS
WENNER
WENTAT
WENTBY
WENTIN
WENTON
WENTTO
WENTUP
YENFOR
YENNED
YENSID
YENTAS
ZENANA
ZENDOS
ZENGER
ZENIST
ZENITH

•E•N••

BEANED
BEANIE
BEANOS
BEINGS
BEINON
BENNIE
BERNIE
CERNAN
DEANNA
DEENIE
DENNED
DENNIS
DENNYS
DESNOS
FEINTS
FENNEL
FENNER
FERNAO
HEANEY
HEFNER
HEINIE
HEINSE
HENNAS
HENNER
HERNAN
HERNIA
HEXNUT
JEANED
JEANIE
JEANNE
JENNER
JENNET
JENNEY
JENNIE
KEENAN
KEENED
KEENEN
KEENER
KEENLY
KEENON
KENNAN
KENNED
KENNEL
KENNER
KENNYG
KERNED
KERNEL
KERNES
KEYNES
LEANED
LEANER
LEANIN
LEANLY
LEANNE
LEANON
LEANTO
LEHNEN
LEMNOS
LENNIE
LENNON
LENNOX
LEONIA
LEONID
LERNER
MEANER
MEANEY
MEANIE
MEANIT
MEANLY
MEANTO
MEDNIS
MENNEN
MENNIN
MESNES
NEENAH
NERNST
PEANUT
PEENED
PENNED
PENNER
PENNEY
PENNIA
PENNIS
PENNON
PERNOD
PETNAP
PEVNEY
REENIE
REGNAL
REGNAT
REGNUM
REINAS
REINED
REINER
REINES
REININ
REINKS
REKNIT
REKNOT
RENNES
RENNET
RENNIE
RENNIN
RESNAP
RESNIK
REUNED
REUNER
REUNES
SEANCE
SEENAS
SEENIN
SEENTO
SEENUP
SEINED
SEINER
SEINES
SENNAS
SEWNIN
SEWNON
SEWNUP
TEENER
TEENIE
TEENSY
TELNET
TENNER
TENNIS
TERNES
VEINAL
VEINED
VEINTE
VENNER
VERNAL
VERNET
VERNON
WEANED
WEANER
WEENED
WEENIE
WEENSY
WENNER
WERNER
WETNAP
YEANED
YENNED

•E••N•

BEGINS
BEGONE
BEHIND
BEIGNE
BEKIND
BELONG
BELONS
BEMINE
BENING
BERING
BESANT
BETONY
BEVANS
BEYOND
CEDING
CELINE
CEMENT
CESSNA
CETANE
DEANNA
DEBONE
DEBONT
DEBUNK
DECANT
DECENT
DEDANS
DEDINI
DEFANG
DEFEND
DEFINE
DEFUND
DEIGNS
DEJUNK
DEKING
DELAND
DELANO
DELANY
DELINT
DEMAND
DEMOND
DEMONS
DEPEND
DEPONE
DETENT
DETUNE
DEVANE
DEVINE
DEWING
EELING
FECUND
FEEING
FEIGNS
FELINE
FELONS
FELONY
FERENC
FETING
GEEING
GEMINI
GERENT
GERUND
GETANA
GETANF
HEARNS
HECKNO
HELENA
HELENE
HELENS
HELLNO
HERONS
HEWING
HEXANE
HEXING
JEANNE
JEJUNE
JEVONS
KEARNS
KEARNY
KETONE
KEYING
LEANNE
LEARNS
LEARNT
LEEANN
LEGEND
LELAND
LEMANS
LEMOND
LEMONS
LEMONY
LENINA
LEVANT
LEVENE
LEVINE
MEDINA
MEGANE
MEKONG
MELINA
MELONS
MERINO
MESONS
METING
MEWING
NEEDNT
NERONE
NEVINS
OENONE
PECANS
PEDANT
PEKING
PEPINO
PERINE
REBANK
REBEND
REBENT
REBIND
RECANE
RECANS
RECANT
RECENT
RECONS
REDANS
REDANT
REDENY
REDING
REDINK
REDONE
REFIND
REFINE
REFUND
REGENT
REGINA
REHANG
REHONE
REHUNG
REIGNS
RELAND
RELEND
RELENT
RELINE
RELINK
REMAND
REMANS
REMEND
REMIND
REMINE
REMINI
REMINT
RENINS
RENONV
REOWNS
REPANE
REPENS
REPENT
REPINE
REPINS
RERANK
RERENT
RERUNS
RESAND
RESANG
RESEND
RESENT
RESING
RESINK
RESINS
RESINY
RETANS
RETINA
RETINS
RETINT
RETONE
RETUNE
REVEND
REWIND
REWINS
REZONE
SECANT
SECOND
SEDANS
SEDONA
SEEING
SELENA
SELENE
SEMANA
SERENA
SERENE
SERINS
SEVENA
SEVENB
SEVENC
SEVEND
SEVENE
SEVENS
SEWING
SEWONS
TECHNO
TEEING
TEJANA
TEJANO
TENANT
TENONE
TENONS
TETONS
TEXANS
VEGANS
VENINS
VERONA
VEXING
VEZINA
WEEONE
WEEUNS
WERENT
WETONE
YEARNS
YELENA
YEMANA
YEMENI
ZEDONG
ZEDONK
ZENANA

•E•••N

AEGEAN
BEACON
BEAMAN
BEAMON
BEARON
BEATEN
BEATON
BECKON
BEDWIN
BEINON
BELTON
BEMOAN
BENBEN
BENIGN
BENSON
BENTON
BERGEN
BERLIN
BERMAN
BERWYN
BESSON
BETSON
CEDARN
CERNAN
CEYLON
DEACON
DEADEN
DEADON
DEAFEN
DEALIN
DEEPEN
DEFCON
DEHORN
DELIAN
DEMAIN
DEMEAN
DENTIN
DENTON
DERAIN
DESIGN
DETAIN
DEVEIN
FEEDIN
FEEDON
FELDON
FELLIN
FELLON
FELSON
GEESON
GEFFEN
GELPEN
GENOAN
GERMAN
GERVIN
GETSIN
GETSON
GETTIN
HEADIN
HEADON
HEAPON
HEATON
HEAVEN
HEBRON
HEDREN
HEDRON
HEFLIN
HEGGEN
HEIDEN
HELDIN
HELDON
HELLON
HELPIN
HELPON
HEMPEN
HEMSIN
HENSON
HEREIN
HEREON
HERMAN
HERMON
HERNAN
HEROIN
HERREN
HESTON
HEUSEN
HEYMAN
JENSEN
JERKIN
JETFAN
JETGUN
JETSON
KEATON
KEENAN
KEENEN
KEENON
KEEPIN
KEEPON
KELTON
KELVIN
KENNAN
KENTON
KENYAN
KENYON
KEPTIN
KEPTON
KERWIN
KEYMAN
KEYMEN
KEYSIN
KEYSON
LEADEN
LEADIN
LEADON
LEAKIN
LEANIN
LEANON
LEAPIN
LEAPON
LEAVEN
LEBRON
LEBRUN
LECAIN
LEEANN
LEFTIN
LEFTON
LEGION
LEGMAN
LEGMEN
LEGUIN
LEHMAN
LEHNEN
LEIDEN
LEISEN
LEMMON
LENAIN
LENNON
LENTEN
LEPTON
LESHAN
LESION
LESSEN
LESSON
LETSIN
LETSON
LEYDEN
MECCAN
MEDIAN
MEIFUN
MELLON
MELTON
MELVIN
MELVYN
MENKEN
MENNEN
MENNIN
MENSAN
MERLIN
MERMAN
MERMEN
MERTON
MERVYN
MESSIN
METFAN
NEALON
NEATEN
NEESON
NEIMAN
NELSON
NEMEAN
NEOCON
NEPEAN
NESSEN
NESTIN
NETMAN
NETMEN
NETTON
NEUMAN
NEURON
NEWMAN
NEWTON
PEAHEN
PECTIN
PEEKIN
PEERIN
PEGEEN
PELION
PENMAN
PENMEN
PENNON
PENSIN
PEPSIN
PERKIN
PERRIN
PERSON
PETAIN
PEYTON
READIN
READON
REAGAN
REASON
REBORN
RECKON
RECOIN
REDARN
REDDEN
REDDIN
REDFIN
REDHEN
REDSUN
REDTEN
REEARN
REELIN
REGAIN
REGION
REININ
REJOIN
RELOAN
RELYON
REMAIN
REMOWN
REMSEN
RENNIN
RENOWN
RENTON
REOPEN
REPLAN
REPUGN
RESAWN
RESCAN
RESEEN
RESEWN
RESIGN
RESOWN
RESPAN
RESPIN
RESTON
RETAIN
RETORN
RETTON
RETURN
REUBEN
REVLON
REVSON
REWARN
REWORN
SEALIN
SEAMAN
SEAMEN
SEASON
SEATON

SEENIN
SEEPIN
SEESIN
SELLON
SELTEN
SENDIN
SENDON
SENSEN
SENTIN
SENTON
SEQUIN
SERKIN
SERMON
SETSIN
SETSON
SEVERN
SEWNIN
SEWNON
SEWSIN
SEWSON
SEXTON
TEAURN
TEFLON
TEGRIN
TEHRAN
TELLON
TENDON
TENPIN
TENTON
TERRAN
TEUTON
VEBLEN
VELSEN
VERDIN
VERDON
VERDUN
VEREEN
VEREIN
VERMIN
VERNON
WEAKEN
WEAKON
WEAPON
WEARON
WEBERN
WEDELN
WELDON
WENTIN
WENTON
WESSON
WESTIN
WESTON
YEOMAN
YEOMEN
YESMAN
YESMEN
ZEEMAN
ZEROIN

••EN••

ADENIS
AGENAS
AGENCE
AGENCY
AGENDA
AGENTJ
AGENTK
AGENTS
AKENES
AMENDS
AMENRA
AMENTS
ARENAS
ARENDT
ATENTH
AVENGE
AVENUE
AXENIC
BLENCH
BLENDE
BLENDS
BRENDA
BRENLY
BUENAS
BUENOS
BYENOW
CHENEY
CHENIN
CLENCH
CRENEL
CRENNA
DEENIE
DIENES
DRENCH
DUENAS
DUENNA
DUENOS
EDENIC
EMENDS
ERENOW
ESENIN
EVENAS
EVENED
EVENER
EVENIF
EVENLY
EVENSO
EVENTS
EVENUP
FAENAS
FIENDS
FLENSE
FRENCH
FRENUM
FRENZY
GLENDA
GLENNE
HYENAS
IDENTI
IDENTS
IRENIC
KEENAN
KEENED
KEENEN
KEENER
KEENLY
KEENON
KOENIG
KRENEK
LIENEE
LIENOR
MAENAD
NEENAH
NIENTE
OBENTO
ODENSE
OHENRY
OMENED
OPENED
OPENER
OPENIT
OPENLY
OPENON
OPENTO
OPENUP
ORENSE
PEENED
PHENOL
PHENOM
PLENTY
PLENUM
PRENUP
PUENTE
PUENZO
QUENCH
REENIE
RIENZI
RYENCE
SCENAS
SCENEI
SCENES
SCENEV
SCENIC
SCENTS
SEENAS
SEENIN
SEENTO
SEENUP
SIENNA
SPENCE
SPENDS
SPENDY
STENCH
STENOG
STENOS
STENTS
SUENOS
TEENER
TEENIE
TEENSY
THENBA
THENCE
THENET
THENFL
THENHL
THENRA
TIENDA
TRENCH
TRENDS
TRENDY
TRENTA
TRENTE
TRENTO
TWENTY
UPENDS
USENET
VIENNA
VIENNE
WEENED
WEENIE
WEENSY
WHENCE
WHENLL
WIENER
WIENIE
WRENCH

••E•N•

AGEING
AGEONE
AHERNE
AVEENO
BOEING
CLEANS
CRENNA
CUEING
CZERNY
DOESNT
DUENNA
DYEING
ETERNE
EXEUNT
EYEING
FEEING
FREONS
FRESNO
FREUND
GEEING
GIEING
GLEANS
GLENNE
GREENE
GREENS
GREENY
GRETNA
HIEING
HOEING
ILEANA
IMEANT
KLEINE
LEEANN
MTETNA
NEEDNT
OCEANS
ODEONS
OLEINS
ONEONE
PAEANS
POEANA
PREENS
QUEENE
QUEENS
SEEING
SHEENA
SHEENS
SHEENY
SIENNA
SKEINS
STEINS
STERNA
STERNE
STERNO
STERNS
SUEANE
SUEANN
TEEING
THEEND
THEONE
TIEINS
TOEING
TOEINS
TWEENS
TWEENY
VIENNA
VIENNE
WEEONE
WEEUNS

••E••N

AGETEN
ALEMAN
APEMAN
APEMEN
AVEDON
AXEMAN
AXEMEN
BLEWIN
BLEWON
BREMEN
BRETON
BSEVEN
CHEMIN
CHENIN
CHEVON
CHEWON
CRETAN
CRETIN
CUEDIN
CUESIN
DAEMON
DEEPEN
DOESIN
DREBIN
DREWIN
DREWON
ELEVEN
ELEVON
EREVAN
ESENIN
EVELYN
FEEDIN
FEEDON
FLEWIN
FLEWON
FOEMAN
FOEMEN
GEESON
GOESIN
GOESON
GREWON
GSEVEN
ICEDIN
ICEMAN
ICEMEN
ICERUN
ICESIN
ISELIN
JOEDON
KEENAN
KEENEN
KEENON
KEEPIN
KEEPON
KIERAN
KIERON
KMESON
LEEANN
LIEDON
LIESIN
LIESON
MCEWAN
MCEWEN
NEESON
NOEMON
OBERON
ODEDON
OLEFIN
OLESON
ONEGIN
ONEMAN
ONEPIN
ONERUN
ONETEN
ONETON
OPENON
OREGON
OWEDON
OWESON
PEEKIN
PEERIN
PIEMAN
PIEMEN
PIEPAN
PIETIN
PREVIN
PREYON
QUEZON
REEARN
REELIN
RIESEN
SEENIN
SEEPIN
SEESIN
SHEDON
SIEBEN
STEFAN
STEPIN
STEPON
STEVEN
SUEANN
SWEDEN
THEBAN
THECAN
THEFAN
THEMAN
THERON
THESON
THESUN
TIEDIN
TIEDON
TIEPIN
TIESIN
TIESON
TOEDIN
TOESIN
TREPAN
UNEVEN
USEDIN
USEDON
USESIN
USESON
WHELAN
WIEMAN
ZEEMAN

•••EN•

ABSENT
ACCENT
ACHENE
ADDEND
ADRENO
ADVENT
ALHENA
ALIENS
ALKENE
AMIENS
APPEND
ARDENT
ARGENT
ARLENE
ARSENE
ARSENO
ASCEND
ASCENT
ASPENS
ASSENT
ATHENA
ATHENE
ATHENS
ATTEND
AUGEND
AVEENO
BADEND
BAGEND
BIGEND
BOLENA
BRIENZ
BUTENE
BYTENS
CADENT
CATENA
CEMENT
CHIENS
CLIENT
COGENT
COVENS
COVENT
COWENS
COZENS
DALENE
DARENT
DAVENS
DECENT
DEFEND
DEPEND
DETENT
DOCENT
DOLENZ
DOYENS
DOZENS
EIRENE
ELRENO
EOCENE
ESCENT
ESSENE
ETHENE
EUGENE
EXPEND
EXTEND
EXTENT
FAGEND
FERENC
FILENE
FIVENO
FLUENT
FOMENT
FRIEND
GALENA
GERENT
GIVENS
GREENE
GREENS
GREENY
GYRENE
HAVENO
HAVENS
HAVENT
HELENA
HELENE
HELENS
IMPEND
INCENT
INDENT
INTEND
INTENS
INTENT
INVENT
IRLENE
ISMENE
JOLENE
LAMENT
LATENE
LATENS
LATENT
LEGEND
LEVENE
LIKENS
LINENS
LINENY
LIPENG
LIVENS
LODENS
LORENE
LORENZ
LOWEND
LUCENT
LUDENS
LUMENS
LURENE
MAVENS
MAXENE
MODENA
MOMENT
MORENO
NICENE
NOCENT
NORENT
NOVENA
NUGENT
OFFEND
ORIENT
OSTEND
PARENS
PARENT
PATENS
PATENT
POTENT
PREENS
QUEENE
QUEENS
RAMENS
RAVENS
REBEND
REBENT
RECENT
REDENY
REGENT
RELEND
RELENT
REMEND
REPENS
REPENT
RERENT
RESEND
RESENT
REVEND
RIDENT
RIPENS
RODENT
ROWENA
ROWENS
RUBENS
SABENA
SELENA
SELENE
SERENA
SERENE
SEVENA
SEVENB
SEVENC
SEVEND
SEVENE
SEVENS
SHEENA
SHEENS
SHEENY
SILENT
SIRENS
TAGEND
TALENT
THEEND
TOKENS
TORENT
TWEENS
TWEENY
UNBEND
UNBENT
UNLENT
UNPENS
UNPENT
UNRENT
UNSENT
UPSEND
UPSENT
URGENT
VALENE
VALENS
VALENT
VIXENS
VOTENO
WADENA
WAKENS
WERENT
WIDENS
WIZENS
WOMENS
YELENA
YEMENI
ZAZENS

•••E•N

AEGEAN
AILEEN
ALLEYN
ANDEAN
ASTERN
AUGEAN
BALEEN
BAYERN
BITEIN
BITEON
BOLEYN
BOREON
CAGEIN
CAMEIN
CAMEON
CAREEN
CASEIN
CASERN
CAVEIN
CAVERN
CLUEIN
COMEIN
COMEON
DEMEAN
DEVEIN
DINEIN
DINEON
DIVEIN
DONEIN
DOREEN
DOTEON
DOVEIN
EASEIN
EASEON
EDGEIN
EILEEN
EXTERN
FACEON
FADEIN
FILEIN
FIREON
GAVEIN
GAVEON
GAZEON
GIDEON
GIVEIN
GIVEON
GLUEON
GONEIN
GONEON
GOVERN
HADEAN
HAMELN
HAVEIN
HAVEON
HEREIN
HEREON
HIREON
HOMEIN
HONEIN
INTERN
JUDEAN
KOREAN
LACEON
LATEEN
LATEON
LAVERN
LIVEIN
LIVEON
LLBEAN
LOMEIN
LOVEIN
LUREIN
MCKEAN
MCKEON
MCKERN
MCLEAN
MODERN
MOREEN
MOVEIN
MOVEON
MRBEAN
MUSEON
NEMEAN
NEPEAN
NOREEN
NOSEIN
PEGEEN
PIGEON
PILEIN
PILEON
PIPEIN
POTEEN
RACEIN
RAKEIN
RAVEON
RESEEN
RESEWN
RIDEIN
RODEIN
ROPEIN
RULEON
SATEEN
SAVEON
SCREEN
SEVERN
SIMEON
SOLEMN
SPLEEN
STREWN
TAKEIN
TAKEON
TAPEON
TAVERN
TUNEIN
TUREEN
TYPEIN
UNHEWN
UNLEAN
UNSEEN
UNSEWN
URGEON
VEREEN
VEREIN
VOTEIN
VOTEON
WADEIN
WAVEIN
WEBERN
WEDELN
WIREIN
WOREON
WYVERN

••••EN

AACHEN
ACUMEN
ADRIEN
AGETEN
AIDMEN
AILEEN
AIRMEN
ALFVEN
ALGREN
ALLMEN
AMBIEN
ANCIEN
APEMEN
ARISEN
ASHMEN
AUSTEN
AWAKEN
AWOKEN
AXEMEN
BADMEN
BAGMEN
BAHNEN
BALEEN
BANNEN
BARMEN
BARREN
BATMEN
BATTEN
BAYMEN
BEATEN
BENBEN
BERGEN
BIDDEN
BIGBEN
BIGMEN
BIGTEN
BITTEN
BLIXEN
BLYDEN
BOKKEN
BOLDEN
BORDEN
BOWMEN
BRAZEN
BREMEN
BROKEN
BSEVEN
BUNSEN
BURDEN
BUSMEN
BYTHEN
CABMEN
CAMDEN
CAREEN
CARMEN
CATMEN
CHOSEN
CLOVEN
COMDEN
CONMEN
COTTEN
COWMEN
CRAVEN
CULLEN
DAMIEN
DAMPEN
DARIEN
DARKEN
DARREN
DEADEN
DEAFEN
DEEPEN
DOKKEN
DOREEN
DRIVEN
DRYDEN
EGUREN
EILEEN
ELEVEN
ENDMEN
ESALEN
EUCKEN
EUSDEN
FALLEN
FASTEN
FATTEN
FAYLEN
FBIMEN
FINSEN
FLAXEN
FLYMEN
FOEMEN
FRAUEN
FROZEN
GAGMEN
GARDEN
GASMEN
GEFFEN
GELPEN
GLUTEN
GOLDEN
GOODEN
GOOSEN
GOSDEN
GOSHEN
GOTTEN
GRAVEN
GSEVEN
GULDEN
GUNMEN
HAAGEN
HADDEN
HAMDEN
HAPPEN
HARDEN
HARKEN
HASTEN
HAYDEN
HEAVEN
HEDREN
HEGGEN
HEIDEN
HEMPEN
HERREN
HEUSEN
HIDDEN
HITMEN
HODMEN
HOLDEN
HOYDEN
HYPHEN
ICEMEN
IFTHEN
IMOGEN
JANSEN
JANZEN
JENSEN
JULIEN
KALLEN
KARLEN
KATZEN
KEENEN
KEYMEN
KITAEN
KITTEN
KRAKEN
KUCHEN
LARMEN
LARSEN
LASSEN
LATEEN
LATHEN
LAUREN
LAWMEN
LAYMEN
LEADEN
LEAVEN
LEGMEN
LEHNEN
LEIDEN
LEISEN
LENTEN
LESSEN
LEYDEN
LICHEN
LINDEN
LISTEN
LOOSEN
LOUDEN
LOWMEN
LUCIEN
LUDDEN
LUMPEN
LUNDEN
MACLEN
MADDEN
MADMEN
MADSEN
MAIDEN
MAJGEN
MALDEN
MARDEN
MARTEN
MATMEN
MCEWEN
MCKUEN
MENKEN
MENNEN
MERMEN
MINDEN
MIRREN
MITTEN
MIZZEN
MOLTEN
MOREEN
MORGEN
MORTEN
MUDHEN
NANSEN
NEATEN
NESSEN
NETMEN
NGUYEN
NISSEN
NONMEN
NOREEN
NUNGEN
OARMEN
OBRIEN
ODDMEN
OILMEN
OLDMEN
ONETEN
ORIGEN
ORTHEN
OXYGEN
PACTEN
PATTEN
PEAHEN
PEGEEN
PENMEN
PIEMEN
PIGMEN
PIGPEN
PINKEN
PITMEN
PLATEN
POLLEN
POTEEN
PROVEN
RAGMEN
RBIMEN
REDDEN
REDHEN
REDTEN
REMSEN
REOPEN
RESEEN
REUBEN
RICHEN
RIDDEN
RIESEN
RIPKEN
RODMEN
ROSSEN
ROSTEN
ROTTEN
SADDEN
SALTEN
SATEEN
SCREEN
SEAMEN
SELTEN
SENSEN
SHAKEN
SHAVEN
SICKEN
SIEBEN
SILKEN
SIRBEN
SIXTEN
SKYMEN
SLOVEN
SODDEN
SOFTEN
SOTHEN
SPLEEN
SPOKEN
STAMEN
STATEN
STEVEN
STOLEN
SUDDEN
SULLEN

SUNKEN
SWEDEN
TAUTEN
TAXMEN
TILDEN
TINMEN
TOPMEN
TOPTEN
TRAVEN
TUREEN
UNEVEN
UNOPEN
UNSEEN
USOPEN
VARDEN
VEBLEN
VELSEN
VEREEN
VIVIEN
WALDEN
WALKEN
WARDEN
WARREN
WEAKEN
WHITEN
WOODEN
WOOLEN
WORSEN
WYNKEN
YATSEN
YEOMEN
YESMEN

EO••••

EOCENE
EOLIAN
EOLITH
EONIAN
EOSINS

E•O•••

EBOATS
EBONDS
EBOOKS
ECOLAB
ECOLAW
ECOLES
ECORSE
EGOISM
EGOIST
EGOYAN
ELODEA
ELOGES
ELOISA
ELOISE
ELOPED
ELOPER
ELOPES
EMORYU
EMOTED
EMOTER
EMOTES
ENOILS
ENOKIS
ENORME
ENOTES
ENOUGH
EPOCHS
EPODES
EPODIC
EPONYM
EPOPEE
EPOQUE
EPOSES
EPOWER
ERODED
ERODER
ERODES
EROICA
EROTIC
ETOILE
ETONIC
EUONYM
EVOKED
EVOKER
EVOKES
EVOLVE
EVONNE
EXOCET
EXODUS
EXONYM
EXOTIC

E••O••

EAMONN
EATOUT
EBOOKS
ECHOED
ECHOER
ECHOES
ECHOIC
ECTOMY
EDDOES
EDKOCH
EDMOND
EDWOOD
EEYORE
EFFORT
EGMONT
EIDOLA
EKEOUT
ELBOWS
ELFOWL
ELKONV
ELLORA
ELMONT
ELMORE
ELNORA
ELTORO
ELWOOD
EMBODY
EMBOGS
EMBOSS
EMBOWS
ENCODE
ENCORE
ENDORA
ENDOWS
ENFOLD
ENJOIN
ENJOYS
ENROBE
ENROLL
ENROLS
ENROOT
ENSOUL
ENTOMB
ENTOMO
ENVOIS
ENVOYS
EPHODS
EPHORS
EPSONS
EQUOID
ERGOTS
ERROLL
ERRORS
ESCORT
ESPOSA
ESPOSO
ESTOCS
ESTOPS
ETAOIN
ETTORE
EUBOEA
EUDORA
EULOGY
EUROPA
EUROPE
EXCONS
EXGOVS
EXHORT
EXMOOR
EXMORE
EXPORT
EXPOSE
EXPOST
EXTOLL
EXTOLS
EXTORT

E•••O•

EASEON
EASTON
EATSOF
EDISON
EDITOR
EDWOOD
EELPOT
EGGNOG
EGGSON
EJIDOS
EKELOF
ELEVON
ELINOR
ELKTON
ELLIOS
ELLIOT
ELSTON
ELWOOD
EMAJOR
EMINOR
EMPLOY
EMPSON
EMPTOR
ENAMOR
ENBLOC
ENDSON
ENEROS
ENIDOK
ENROOT
EPHRON
EPILOG
ERENOW
ESCROW
ESHKOL
ESPIOS
ETHIOP
ETHNOS
ETYMOL
ETYMON
EXMOOR

E••••O

EASYGO
EDITIO
ELADIO
ELISEO
ELNINO
ELPASO
ELRENO
ELTORO
EMBRYO
EMILIO
ENCINO
ENDURO
ENESCO
ENHALO
ENRICO
ENTERO
ENTOMO
ENVIRO
ERYNGO
ESCUDO
ESKIMO
ESPOSO
ESTADO
EVENSO
EVERSO

•EO•••

AEOLIA
AEOLUS
CEORLS
DEODAR
FEODOR
FEOFFS
GEODES
GEODIC
GEORDI
GEORGE
GEORGI
GEORGY
KEOKUK
LEOIII
LEONIA
LEONID
LEOVII
LEOXII
MEOHMY
MEOWED
MEOWER
NEOCON
NEOSHO
PEOPLE
PEORIA
REOILS
REOPEN
REOWNS
YEOLDE
YEOMAN
YEOMEN

•E•O••

AEROBE
AESOPS
BEBOPS
BECOME
BECOOL
BEDOGS
BEFOGS
BEFOOL
BEFORE
BEFOUL
BEGOFF
BEGONE
BEGOOD
BEHOLD
BEHOME
BEHOOF
BELOIT
BELONG
BELONS
BEMOAN
BENOIT
BENOTE
BESOMS
BESORE
BESOTS
BETONY
BETOOK
BEYOND
DEBONE
DEBONT
DECOCT
DECODE
DECORS
DECOYS
DEFOAM
DEFOGS
DEFORD
DEFORE
DEFORM
DEHORN
DEMOBS
DEMODE
DEMOED
DEMOND
DEMONS
DEMOTE
DEMOTH
DENOTE
DENOVO
DEPONE
DEPORT
DEPOSE
DEPOTS
DEROSE
DESODS
DESOTO
DETOTH
DETOUR
DEVOID
DEVOIR
DEVORE
DEVOTE
DEVOTO
DEVOUR
DEVOUT
DEWOLF
DEWORM
EEYORE
FEDORA
FELONS
FELONY
FEMORA
FEROUS
FETORS
GENOAN
GENOAS
GENOME
GENOVA
GETOFF
GETOLD
GETOUT
HEGOAT
HELOTS
HEROES
HEROIC
HEROIN
HERONS
HESOUT
HEXOSE
JEROME
JEVONS
KENOBI
KETONE
KEYOFA
KEYOFB
KEYOFC
KEYOFD
KEYOFF
KEYOFG
LEDOFF
LEDOUT
LEDOUX
LELOIR
LEMOKO
LEMOND
LEMONS
LEMONY
LENORE
LENOVO
LEROUX
LETOFF
LETOUR
LETOUT
MEDOCS
MEGOHM
MEKONG
MELODY
MELONS
MELOTT
MEMOIR
MEMORY
MEROPE
MEROPS
MESONS
NEROLI
NERONE
OENONE
PEKOES
PELOSI
PELOTA
PEYOTE
REBOIL
REBOLT
REBOOK
REBOOT
REBOPS
REBORE
REBORN
REBOTE
REBOZO
RECOAL
RECOAT
RECOCK
RECODE
RECOIL
RECOIN
RECOMB
RECONS
RECOOK
RECOOL
RECOPY
RECORD
RECORK
RECOST
RECOUP
REDOAK
REDOCK
REDOER
REDOES
REDONE
REDOSE
REDOUT
REFOLD
REFORM
REHOED
REHOES
REHOLD
REHONE
REHOOK
REJOIN
RELOAD
RELOAN
RELOCK
RELOGS
RELOOK
RELOSE
RELOST
REMOLD
REMOPS
REMORA
REMOTE
REMOVE
REMOWN
REMOWS
RENOIR
RENONV
RENOTE
RENOWN
REPOLL
REPORT
REPOSE
REPOST
REPOTS
REPOUR
RERODE
REROLL
REROOF
REROOT
REROSE
RESOAK
RESOAP
RESODS
RESOIL
RESOLD
RESOLE
RESORB
RESORT
RESOWN
RESOWS
RETOLD
RETONE
RETOOK
RETOOL
RETOPS
RETORE
RETORN
RETORT
RETOSS
RETOUR
RETOWS
REVOIR
REVOKE
REVOLT
REVOTE
REWOKE
REWORD
REWORE
REWORK
REWORN
REWOVE
REYOKE
REZONE
SECOND
SEDONA
SEEOFF
SEEOUT
SENORA
SENORS
SEPOYS
SEROUS
SETOFF
SETOSE
SETOUT
SEWONS
TEEOFF
TENONE
TENONS
TENORS
TETONS
VEGOUT
VELOCE
VELOUR
VENOMS
VENORA
VENOSE
VENOUS
VERONA
VETOED
VETOER
VETOES
WEEONE
WETONE
XEDOUT
XESOUT
YEGODS
ZEDONG
ZEDONK
ZEROED
ZEROES
ZEROIN

•E••O•

AERIOS
BEACON
BEAMON
BEANOS
BEARON
BEATON
BECKON
BECOOL
BEFOOL
BEGFOR
BEGOOD
BEHOOF
BEINON
BELLOC
BELLOW
BELTON
BENBOW
BENSON
BENTON
BENTOS
BENZOL
BERKOW
BESSON
BESTOW
BETOOK
BETSON
BETTOR
CELLOS
CENSOR
CENTOS
CERROS
CEYLON
DEACON
DEADON
DEBTOR
DECLOT
DEFCON
DEIMOS
DEKKOS
DELCOS
DELROY
DELSOL
DENMOM
DENTON
DEPLOY
DERMOT
DESMOG
DESNOS
DESPOT
DETROP
EELPOT
FEEDON
FEELOK
FELDON
FELLON
FELLOW
FELSON
FELTOK
FEMBOT
FEODOR
FERVOR
GECKOS
GEESON
GELDOF
GETHOT
GETSON
HEADON
HEAPON
HEAROF
HEATON
HEBRON
HECTOR
HEDRON
HELDON
HELIOS
HELLON
HELLOS
HELPON
HENSON
HEREOF
HEREON
HERMON
HERZOG
HESIOD
HESTON
HEYYOU
JELLOS
JERBOA
JETSON
KEATON
KEENON
KEEPON
KELTON
KENDOS
KENTON
KENYON
KEPTON
KEYSON
LEADON
LEANON
LEAPON
LEBRON
LECTOR
LEFTOF
LEFTON
LEGION
LEGROS
LEMMON
LEMNOS
LENNON
LENNOX
LENTOS
LEPTON
LESBOS
LESION
LESSON
LESSOR
LETSON
MEADOW
MELLON
MELLOW
MELTON
MENJOU
MENTOR
MENTOS
MERLOT
MERTON
METEOR
METHOD
METROS
MEZZOS
NEALON
NEESON
NELSON
NEOCON
NESTOR
NETHOU
NETTON
NEUROL
NEURON
NEWJOB
NEWSOM
NEWTON
NEWTOY
PEAPOD
PEGBOX
PEGTOP
PELION
PENNON
PENROD
PEPBOY
PEQUOD
PEQUOT
PERIOD
PERNOD
PERROS
PERSON
PESCOW
PESTOS
PETBOA
PETCOW
PETDOG
PETROL
PETTOY
PEYTON
READON
REASON
REAVOW
REBOOK
REBOOT
RECKON
RECOOK
RECOOL
RECTOR
RECTOS
REDCOD
REDDOG
REDDOT
REDFOX
REDHOT
REDSOX
REDTOP
REEBOK
REEKOF
REFLOW
REGION
REGLOW
REGROW
REHOOK
REKNOT
RELOOK
RELYON
RENTON
RENVOI
REPFOR
REPLOT
REPLOW
REPROS
REROOF
REROOT
RESHOD
RESHOE
RESHOT
RESHOW
RESPOT
RESTON
RESTOW
RETOOK
RETOOL
RETROD
RETROS
RETTON
REVLON
REVSON
SEACOW
SEADOG
SEAFOX
SEAGOD
SEASON
SEATON
SECTOR
SEEYOU
SEIKOS
SEIZOR
SELDOM
SELLON
SENDON
SENHOR
SENIOR
SENSOR
SENTON
SERMON
SERVOS
SETFOR
SETSON
SETTOS
SEWNON
SEWSON
SEXPOT
SEXTON
SEZYOU
TEAPOT
TEAPOY
TEEBOX
TEFLON
TELCOS
TELLOF
TELLON
TEMPOS
TENDON
TENSOR
TENTON
TERROR
TEUTON
VECTOR
VENDOR
VERDON
VERNON
VERSOS
WEAKON
WEAPON
WEARON
WEBLOG
WELDON
WENTON
WESSON
WESTON
WETMOP
YELLOW
YENFOR
YESYOU
ZEALOT
ZENDOS

•E•••O

BENITO
BERCEO
CENTRO
CERATO
DEAFTO
DEALTO
DEARTO
DELANO
DELRIO
DEMILO
DENDRO
DENIRO
DENOVO
DESOTO
DEVITO
DEVOTO
DEXTRO
FEEDTO
FELLTO
FERNAO
GEARTO
GELATO
GETSTO
HEADTO
HECKNO
HELDTO
HELICO
HELLNO
HEMATO
HEPATO
HERETO
HETERO
HEWSTO
JETHRO
KEEPTO
KEPTTO
LEADTO
LEANTO
LEGATO
LEMOKO
LENDTO
LENOVO
LENTTO
LETSGO
MEANTO
MEDICO
MEGALO
MEJICO
MENUDO
MERINO
MEXICO
NEARTO
NEEDTO
NEOSHO
NEPHRO
NEXTTO
PEPINO
READTO
REBOZO
REDTWO
REECHO
RENATO
RENFRO
RENTTO
REZERO
SEEMTO
SEENTO
SEESTO
SEISMO
SELLTO
SENDTO
SENTTO
SERGIO
SETSTO
SEZWHO
TEATRO
TECHNO
TEJANO
TENDTO
TENTWO
TENUTO
TERATO
TESSIO
TEXACO
VELCRO
VENETO
WEIRDO
WENTTO
YESIDO

••EO••

ACEOUT
AGEOLD
AGEONE
AGEOUT
AREOLA
AREOLE
ATEOUT
CHEOPS
CREOLE
DIEOFF
DIEOUT
EKEOUT
FREONS
ICEOUT
ODEONS
OLEOLE
ONEOFF
ONEONE
ONEOUT
OREOOS
PREOPS
SEEOFF
SEEOUT
TEEOFF
THEONE
THEORY
TIEOFF
UVEOUS
WEEONE

••E•O•

ALEROS
ARETOO
AVEDON
BLEWON
BRETON
BUENOS
BYENOW
CHEKOV
CHEVON
CHEWON
CIELOS
CREDOS
CRESOL
DAEMON
DAEWOO
DIEFOR
DOESOK
DREWON
DUENOS
DYEJOB
DYELOT
EKELOF
ELEVON
ENEROS
ERENOW
FAEROE
FEEDON
FEELOK
FIEROS
FLEWON
FLEXOR
FREEOF
FUEGOS
GEESON
GOESON
GREGOR
GREWON
HUEVOS
ICEBOX
ICEFOG
ICEPOP
JOEDON
JUEGOS
KEENON
KEEPON
KIERON
KMESON
KNEWOF
LIEDON
LIEFOR
LIELOW
LIENOR
LIESON
NEESON
NIETOS
NOEMON
OBERON
OCELOT
ODEDON
OLESON
ONETON
OPENON
OREGON
OREOOS
OWEDON
OWESON
PHENOL
PHENOM
PLEXOR
PRELOG
PRETOR
PREYON
PYEDOG
QUEMOY
QUESOS
QUEZON
REEBOK
REEKOF

RHEBOK
RHETOR
SEEYOU
SHEBOP
SHEDON
STEFOY
STENOG
STENOS
STEPON
STEROL
SUEFOR
SUENOS
TEEBOX
THEDOW
THEFOG
THEFOX
THELOT
THEMOB
THEROD
THERON
THESON
THESOX
THETOP
THETOY
TIEDON
TIEROD
TIESON
TREMOR
TREVOR
USEDON
USEFOR
USESON
VIEFOR

••E••O

AGETWO
AIELLO
ALECTO
ALEPPO
AMEDEO
ARETOO
AREZZO
ATEMPO
AVEENO
CHEAPO
CREEPO
DAEWOO
DOESSO
DOESTO
DREWTO
DUELLO
DUETTO
ENESCO
EVENSO
EVERSO
FEEDTO
FLEWTO
FREDRO
FREETO
FRESCO
FRESNO
GHETTO
GOESTO
KEEPTO
KLEPTO
LIEDTO
LIESTO
LIEVIO
NEEDTO
NIEKRO
NIELLO
OBENTO
OBERTO
ONEIRO
ONETWO
OPENTO
OTELLO
OVERDO
OWEDTO
PIETRO
PLEDTO
PNEUMO
PRESTO
PSEUDO
PUEBLO
PUENZO
PUERTO
REECHO
SEEMTO
SEENTO
SEESTO
SPEEDO
STELMO
STEREO
STERNO
STETHO
THERMO
THEWHO
TIEDTO
TIEMPO
TIESTO
TRENTO
UNESCO
USEDTO

•••EO•

BITEON
BLUEOX
BOREON
BUTEOS
CAMEON
CAMEOS
CAREOF
CINEOL
COMEOF
COMEON
DINEON
DONEOK
DOTEON
EASEON
FACEON
FIREON
FIVEOF
FREEOF
GAVEOF
GAVEON
GAZEON
GIDEON
GIVEOF
GIVEON
GLUEON
GONEON
HAVEON
HEREOF
HEREON
HIREON
KIDEOS
LACEON
LATEOF
LATEON
LIVEON
MADEOF
MAKEOF
MCKEON
METEOR
MIMEOS
MOVEON
MUSEON
MUSEOS
PASEOS
PIGEON
PILEON
RAVEON
RODEOS
ROLEOS
ROMEOS
RULEON
SAVEON
SIMEON
SUREOF
TAKEON
TAPEON
TIREOF
TYPEOS
URGEON
VIDEOS
VIREOS
VOTEON
WIDEOF
WOREON

•••E•O

ADRENO
ALBEDO
ANGELO
ANTERO
ARSENO
ASTERO
AVEENO
BOLERO
CAMETO
CARETO
CICERO
COLECO
COMETO
CREEPO
DARETO
DINERO
DONESO
DONETO
ELRENO
ENTERO
FIVENO
FIVETO
FOREGO
FREETO
GALEAO
GAVETO
GAZEBO
GIVETO
GLUETO
GONETO
GRAECO
GRIECO
GYNECO
HATETO
HAVENO
HAVETO
HERETO
HETERO
HIDEHO
HOPESO
HOPETO
HOVETO
LAREDO
LATERO
LATETO
LIKESO
LIKETO
LOSETO
LOVETO
MADEDO
MADEGO
MADERO
MAKEDO
MAKEGO
MANERO
MORENO
MORESO
MOVETO
MYHERO
NONEGO
NUMERO
OSWEGO
OTSEGO
OVIEDO
PARETO
PHLEBO
PINERO
POMELO
RACETO
REZERO
RIDETO
RISETO
RODETO
ROMERO
ROSETO
SAFECO
SASEBO
SOWETO
SPEEDO
SUREDO
TAKETO
TOLEDO
TORERO
TRUETO
TUNETO
TUPELO
TUXEDO
UNHERO
VALERO
VENETO
VOTENO
WAVETO
WISETO
ZYDECO

••••EO

ALIVEO
AMADEO
AMEDEO
BERCEO
BORNEO
BULDEO
CHOREO
CORREO
ELISEO
NUCLEO
OROMEO
POMPEO
ROADEO
STEREO

EP••••

EPACTS
EPARCH
EPHAHS
EPHODS
EPHORS
EPHRON
EPICAL
EPILOG
EPINAL
EPOCHS
EPODES
EPODIC
EPONYM
EPOPEE
EPOQUE
EPOSES
EPOWER
EPPING
EPSONS

E•P•••

ELPAIS
ELPASO
EMPALE
EMPATH
EMPERY
EMPIRE
EMPLOY
EMPSON
EMPTOR
EPPING
ESPANA
ESPIAL
ESPIED
ESPIER
ESPIES
ESPIOS
ESPOSA
ESPOSO
ESPRIT
EUPNEA
EXPAND
EXPATS
EXPECT
EXPELS
EXPEND
EXPERT
EXPIRE
EXPIRY
EXPORT
EXPOSE
EXPOST
EZPASS

E••P••

EELPOT
ELAPID
ELAPSE
ELOPED
ELOPER
ELOPES
ENDPIN
EPOPEE
ERUPTS
ETAPES
EYEPIT

E•••P•

ECTYPE
ENRAPT
EQUIPS
ERIEPA
ESCAPE
ESTOPS
EUROPA
EUROPE
EXCEPT
EXEMPT

E••••P

EARLAP
EASEUP
EATSUP
EGGCUP
ENCAMP
ENDSUP
ENTRAP
ENWRAP
ESCARP
ESHARP
ETHIOP
EVENUP
EYECUP
EYEDUP
EYESUP

•EP•••

CEPEDA
CEPHAL
DEPART
DEPAUL
DEPAUW
DEPEND
DEPERE
DEPEST
DEPICT
DEPLOY
DEPONE
DEPORT
DEPOSE
DEPOTS
DEPTHS
DEPULP
DEPUTE
DEPUTY
HEPATO
HEPCAT
HEPPER
HEPTAD
KEPLER
KEPTAT
KEPTIN
KEPTON
KEPTTO
KEPTUP
LEPERS
LEPTON
NEPALI
NEPEAN
NEPHEW
NEPHRO
PEPBOY
PEPCID
PEPFUL
PEPINO
PEPITA
PEPLUM
PEPPED
PEPPER
PEPSIN
PEPSUP
PEPTIC
REPACK
REPADS
REPAGE
REPAID
REPAIR
REPANE
REPARK
REPASS
REPAST
REPAVE
REPAYS
REPEAL
REPEAT
REPEGS
REPELS
REPENS
REPENT
REPERK
REPFOR
REPICK
REPINE
REPINS
REPLAN
REPLAY
REPLED
REPLOT
REPLOW
REPOLL
REPORT
REPOSE
REPOST
REPOTS
REPOUR
REPPED
REPROS
REPUBS
REPUGN
REPUMP
REPUTE
SEPALS
SEPHIA
SEPIAS
SEPIRA
SEPOYS
SEPTAL
SEPTET
SEPTIC
SEPTUM
TEPEES
ZEPHYR

•E•P••

BEAPAL
BEEPAT
BEEPED
BEEPER
DEEPAK
DEEPEN
DEEPER
DEEPLY
DELPHI
DESPOT
EELPOT
GELPEN
HEAPED
HEAPER
HEAPON
HEAPUP
HELPED
HELPER
HELPIN
HELPME
HELPON
HELPUP
HEMPEN
HEPPER
HERPET
KEEPAT
KEEPER
KEEPIN
KEEPIT
KEEPON
KEEPTO
KEEPUP
KELPIE
KEMPIS
KEWPIE
KEYPAD
KEYPAL
LEAPAT
LEAPED
LEAPER
LEAPIN
LEAPON
LEAPUP
NETPAY
PEAPOD
PEEPAT
PEEPED
PEEPER
PENPAL
PEOPLE
PEPPED
PEPPER
PETPIG
PETPUP
REAPED
REAPER
REOPEN
REPPED
RESPAN
RESPIN
RESPOT
SEEPED
SEEPIN
SEMPER
SEMPLE
SEMPRE
SEXPOT
TEAPOT
TEAPOY
TEEPEE
TEMPED
TEMPEH
TEMPER
TEMPLE
TEMPOS
TEMPTS
TEMPUS
TENPIN
VESPAS
VESPER
VESPID
WEAPON
WEEPER
YELPED
YELPER

•E••P•

AESOPS
BEBOPS
DECAPS
FELIPE
GETUPS
LENAPE
LETUPS
MEROPE
MEROPS
PENGPU
PETIPA
REBOPS
RECAPS
RECIPE
RECOPY
REDIPS
RELAPS
REMAPS
REMOPS
RETAPE
RETAPS
RETIPS
RETOPS
RETYPE
REWIPE
REZIPS
SERAPE
SERAPH
SETUPS

•E•••P

BEADUP
BEAMUP
BEARUP
BEATUP
BEEFUP
BELTUP
DEALUP
DECAMP
DEPULP
DETROP
DEWLAP
FESSUP
GEARUP
GELCAP
GETHEP
GETHIP
GETSUP
HEADUP
HEALUP
HEAPUP
HEATUP
HELDUP
HELPUP
JERKUP
KEEPUP
KEPTUP
KEYSUP
LEADUP
LEAPUP
LETRIP
LETSUP
MEETUP
MESSUP
NEXTUP
PEGTOP
PENSUP
PENTUP
PEPSUP
PERKUP
PETNAP
PETPUP
READUP
REARUP
RECOUP
REDCAP
REDTOP
REELUP
REGRIP
RELEAP
REPUMP
RESHIP
RESNAP
RESOAP
RESTUP
RETRAP
REVAMP
REVSUP
REWRAP
SEALUP
SEAMAP
SEENUP
SEESUP
SENDUP
SENTUP
SETSUP
SEWNUP
SEWSUP
TEACUP
TEAMUP
TEARUP
TEEDUP
TEESUP
WELLUP
WENTUP
WETMOP
WETNAP

••EP••

ADEPTS
ALEPHS
ALEPPO
BEEPAT
BEEPED
BEEPER
CREPED
CREPES
DEEPAK
DEEPEN
DEEPER
DEEPLY
DIEPPE
EYEPIT
ICEPOP
KEEPAT
KEEPER
KEEPIN
KEEPIT
KEEPON
KEEPTO
KEEPUP
KLEPTO
ONEPIN
PEEPAT
PEEPED
PEEPER
PIEPAN
PREPAY
PREPPY
ROEPER
SEEPED
SEEPIN
STEPIN
STEPON
STEPPE
STEPUP
TEEPEE
THEPIT
THEPRU
TIEPIN
TREPAN
TREPID
UNEPIC
WEEPER

••E•P•

ALEPPO
ATEMPO
BLEEPS
CHEAPO
CHEEPS
CHEOPS
CREEPO
CREEPS
CREEPY
DIEPPE
EXEMPT
GUELPH
ICEUPS
ONEUPS
PHELPS
PREOPS
PREPPY
SHERPA
SLEEPS
SLEEPY
STEEPS
STEPPE
SWEEPS
THEAPE
THEEPA
THESPS
THESPY
TIEMPO
TIEUPS
TWERPS
WHELPS

••E••P

ACESUP
ALEGUP
ALETAP
BEEFUP
BLEWUP
BREWUP
CHEWUP
CUESUP
CUETIP
DOESUP
DREWUP
EVENUP
EYECUP
EYEDUP
EYESUP
FLEWUP
FREEUP
FUELUP
GOESUP
GREWUP
ICECAP
ICEDUP
ICEPOP
ICESUP
KEEPUP
MEETUP
ONELAP
OPENUP
PREAMP
PRECIP
PRENUP
REELUP
SEENUP
SEESUP
SHEBOP
SPEDUP
STEPUP
TEEDUP
TEESUP
THEASP
THEGAP
THELIP
THERAP
THETOP
TIEDUP
TIESUP
TOECAP
TOETAP
USEDUP
USESUP

•••EP•

ACCEPT
ADREPS
BICEPS
BLEEPS
CHEEPS
CREEPO
CREEPS
CREEPY
ERIEPA
EXCEPT
FIVEPM
INCEPT
JOSEPH
JULEPS
NINEPM
SALEPS
SLEEPS
SLEEPY
STEEPS
STREPS
SWEEPS
THEEPA
UNKEPT
UNWEPT
YCLEPT

•••E•P

ANTEUP
ASDEEP
ASLEEP
ASTEEP
BITEUP
BONEUP
BOPEEP
BOREUP
CAGEUP
CAKEUP
CAMEUP
COMEUP
DONEUP
DUDEUP
EASEUP
FACEUP
FIREUP
FIVEUP
FREEUP
GAVEUP
GIVEUP
GODEEP
GONEUP
HAVEUP
HIKEUP
HOLEUP
HYPEUP
INDEEP
LACEUP
LINEUP
MADEUP
MAKEUP
MOVEUP
NINEUP
NOHELP
NOSEUP
OFHELP
PAGEUP
PILEUP
PIPEUP
RACEUP
RAKEUP
RAVEUP
RELEAP
RIDEUP
RILEUP
RISEUP
RODEUP
ROPEUP
ROSEUP
SAVEUP
SIZEUP
STREEP
TAKEUP
TAPEUP
TONEUP
TOREUP
TOTEUP
TRUEUP
TUNEUP
TYPEUP
UNDEEP
UPHEAP
UPKEEP
UPLEAP
WAKEUP
WIPEUP
WIREUP
WISEUP
WOKEUP

••••EP

ASDEEP
ASLEEP
ASTEEP
BOPEEP
DOMREP
GETHEP
GODEEP
GOTHEP
INDEEP
INSTEP
NOSTEP
SCHLEP
STREEP
TRICEP
UNDEEP
UNSTEP
UPKEEP
UPSTEP

EQ••••

EQUALS
EQUATE
EQUINE
EQUIPS
EQUITY
EQUOID

E•Q•••

EMQUAD
ENQUAD

E••Q••

EPOQUE

E•••Q•

ETSEQQ

E••••Q

ETSEQQ

•EQ•••

PEQUOD
PEQUOT
SEQUEL
SEQUIN

•E•Q••

SESQUI

•E•••Q

DEVICQ

••EQ••

CHEQUE

•••EQ•

ETSEQQ

•••E•Q

ETSEQQ

••••EQ

SUZIEQ

ER••••

ERASED
ERASER
ERASES
ERBIUM
ERDMAN
EREBUS
ERECTS
ERENOW
ERESTU
EREVAN
ERFURT
ERGOTS
ERHARD
ERICAS
ERIEPA
ERINNA
ERINYS
ERIVAN
ERLANG
ERMINE
ERNANI
ERNEST
ERODED
ERODER
ERODES
EROICA
EROTIC
ERRAND
ERRANT
ERRARE
ERRATA
ERRING
ERROLL
ERRORS
ERSATZ
ERSTAD
ERUCTS
ERUPTS
ERVING
ERYKAH
ERYNGO

E•R•••

EARBUD
EARFUL
EARING
EARLAP
EARLET
EARNED
EARNER
EARNIE
EARNIT

EARTAB
EARTAG
EARTHA
EARTHS
EARTHY
EARVIN
EARWAX
EARWIG
EERIER
EERILY
EGRESS
EGRETS
EIRENE
ELRENO
ENRAGE
ENRANK
ENRAPT
ENRICH
ENRICO
ENROBE
ENROLL
ENROLS
ENROOT
ERRAND
ERRANT
ERRARE
ERRATA
ERRING
ERROLL
ERRORS
ETRADE
EURAIL
EUREKA
EUROPA
EUROPE
EYRIES

E••R••

EAGRES
EBERLE
EBERLY
ECARDS
ECARTE
ECORSE
EDERLE
EDIRNE
EGERIA
EGUREN
ELBRUS
ELYRIA
EMBRUE
EMBRYO
EMERGE
EMERIC
EMERIL
EMORYU
ENARMS
ENCRES
ENDRAN
ENDRUN
ENERGY
ENEROS
ENGRAM
ENORME
ENTRAP
ENTREE
ENTREZ
ENURED
ENURES
ENWRAP
EPARCH
EPHRON
ESCROW
ESDRAS
ESPRIT
ESTRAY
ETERNE
EVERLY
EVERSO
EVERTS
EXARCH
EXERTS
EXTRAS
EXURBS

E•••R•

EASERS
EATERS
EATERY
ECKART
ECKERD
EDBERG
EDGARD
EDGARS
EDGERS
EDUARD
EDVARD
EDWARD
EELERS
EELERY
EEYORE
EFFORT
EGBERT
EGGERS
EGGERT
EIDERS
EILERS
EILERT
EKBERG
ELBERT
ELBURZ
ELDERS
ELGART
ELLERY
ELLORA
ELMERS
ELMIRA
ELMIRE
ELMORE
ELNORA
ELTORO
ELUARD
ELVERS
ELVIRA
EMBARK
EMBARS
EMBERS
EMEERS
EMIGRE
EMPERY
EMPIRE
ENBERG
ENCORE
ENDERS
ENDORA
ENDURE
ENDURO
ENGIRD
ENGIRT
ENSURE
ENTERO
ENTERS
ENTIRE
ENVIRO
EPHORS
ERFURT
ERHARD
ERRARE
ERRORS
ESCARP
ESCORT
ESHARP
ESKERS
ESTERS
ETHERS
ETTORE
EUCHRE
EUDORA
EXEDRA
EXHORT
EXMORE
EXPERT
EXPIRE
EXPIRY
EXPORT
EXSERT
EXTERN
EXTORT
EZZARD

E••••R

EARNER
EASIER
EASTER
EBAYER
ECHOER
ECLAIR
EDGIER
EDITOR
EELIER
EERIER
EGGIER
EGGLER
EISNER
EITHER
ELATER
ELAYER
ELIDER
ELINOR
ELITER
ELIXIR
ELMIER
ELOPER
ELUDER
EMAJOR
EMINOR
EMOTER
EMPTOR
ENAMOR
ENDEAR
ENSLER
ENVIER
EPOWER
ERASER
ERODER
ESCHER
ESPIER
ESTHER
ETCHER
EVADER
EVENER
EVILER
EVOKER
EXETER
EXILER
EXMOOR

•ER•••

AERATE
AERIAL
AERIER
AERIES
AERIFY
AERILY
AERIOS
AEROBE
BERATE
BERBER
BERCEO
BEREFT
BERETS
BERGEN
BERGER
BERING
BERKOW
BERLIN
BERMAN
BERMED
BERNIE
BERTHA
BERTHE
BERTHS
BERTIE
BERWYN
BERYLS
CERATE
CERATO
CEREAL
CEREBR
CEREUS
CERISE
CERIUM
CERNAN
CERROS
CERTIF
CERVID
DERAIL
DERAIN
DERATE
DERATS
DERIDE
DERITA
DERIVE
DERMAL
DERMAS
DERMAT
DERMIC
DERMIS
DERMOT
DEROSE
DERREK
DERUST
EERIER
EERILY
FERALS
FERBER
FERDIE
FERENC
FERGIE
FERIAS
FERITY
FERMAT
FERMIS
FERNAO
FEROUS
FERRER
FERRET
FERRIC
FERRIS
FERULE
FERVID
FERVOR
GERALD
GERARD
GERBER
GERBIL
GERENT
GERMAN
GERTIE
GERUND
GERVIN
HERALD
HERBAL
HERBED
HERBES
HERBIE
HERDED
HERDER
HEREAT
HEREBY
HEREIN
HEREOF
HEREON
HERESY
HERETO
HERMAN
HERMES
HERMIT
HERMON
HERNAN
HERNIA
HEROES
HEROIC
HEROIN
HERONS
HERPET
HERREN
HERSEY
HERVEY
HERZOG
JERBOA
JEREMY
JERKED
JERKER
JERKIN
JERKUP
JEROME
JERSEY
KERALA
KERMIT
KERNED
KERNEL
KERNES
KERSEE
KERWIN
LERIDA
LERNER
LEROUX
MERCED
MERCER
MERCKX
MERDLE
MERELY
MEREST
MERGED
MERGEE
MERGER
MERGES
MERIDA
MERINO
MERITS
MERKEL
MERLIN
MERLOT
MERMAN
MERMEN
MEROPE
MEROPS
MERRIE
MERSEY
MERTON
MERVYN
MERYLL
NEREID
NERMAL
NERNST
NEROLI
NERONE
NERUDA
NERVAL
NERVED
NERVES
OERTER
PERCHA
PERDAY
PERDUE
PERILS
PERINE
PERIOD
PERISH
PERITI
PERKED
PERKIN
PERKUP
PERLEA
PERMED
PERMIT
PERNOD
PERRIN
PERROS
PERSIA
PERSIS
PERSON
PERTER
PERTLY
PERUKE
PERUSE
PERUTZ
RERACK
RERAKE
RERANK
RERATE
REREAD
REREEL
RERENT
RERIDE
RERIGS
RERISE
RERODE
REROLL
REROOF
REROOT
REROSE
RERUNS
SERACS
SERAIS
SERAPE
SERAPH
SERBIA
SERENA
SERENE
SERGEI
SERGES
SERGIO
SERIAL
SERIES
SERIFS
SERINS
SERKIN
SERKIS
SERMON
SEROUS
SERTAS
SERUMS
SERVED
SERVER
SERVES
SERVOS
TERATO
TERBIC
TERCEL
TERCES
TERESA
TERETE
TERKEL
TERMED
TERMES
TERNES
TERRAE
TERRAN
TERRES
TERRET
TERRIF
TERRIS
TERROR
TERSER
VERBAL
VERBID
VERDES
VERDIN
VERDON
VERDUN
VEREEN
VEREIN
VERGED
VERGER
VERGES
VERGIL
VERIFY
VERILY
VERISM
VERIST
VERITE
VERITY
VERJEE
VERMIN
VERNAL
VERNET
VERNON
VERONA
VERSED
VERSES
VERSET
VERSOS
VERSTS
VERSUS
VERTEX
VERVES
WERENT
WERFEL
WERKER
WERNER
XERXES
YERKES
YERTLE
ZEROED
ZEROES
ZEROIN

•E•R••

BEARDS
BEARER
BEARON
BEARSE
BEARUP
BEIRUT
BETRAY
BEURRE
CEDRIC
CEORLS
CERROS
DEARER
DEARIE
DEARLY
DEARME
DEARTH
DEARTO
DEBRAH
DEBRAY
DEBREU
DEBRIS
DECREE
DEERES
DEFRAG
DEFRAY
DEGREE
DELRAY
DELREY
DELRIO
DELROY
DERREK
DESREE
DETROP
FEARED
FEARER
FERRER
FERRET
FERRIC
FERRIS
GEARED
GEARTO
GEARUP
GEHRIG
GENRES
GEORDI
GEORGE
GEORGI
GEORGY
GETRID
HEARER
HEARNS
HEAROF
HEARSE
HEARST
HEARTH
HEARTS
HEARTY
HEARYE
HEBREW
HEBRON
HEDRAL
HEDREN
HEDRON
HENRIK
HENRYI
HENRYK
HENRYV
HERREN
HEURES
JEERAT
JEERED
JEERER
KEARNS
KEARNY
LEARNS
LEARNT
LEBRET
LEBRON
LEBRUN
LEERAT
LEERED
LEERER
LEGREE
LEGROS
LEHRER
LETRIP
MEGREZ
MEGRIM
MERRIE
METRED
METRES
METRIC
METROS
NEARBY
NEARED
NEARER
NEARLY
NEARTO
NEHRUS
NEURAL
NEUROL
NEURON
NEXRAD
PEARCE
PEARLE
PEARLS
PEARLY
PEERAT
PEERCE
PEERED
PEERIN
PEIRCE
PENROD
PEORIA
PERRIN
PERROS
PETRAT
PETREL
PETRIE
PETROL
REARED
REARER
REARMS
REARUP
REBRED
REBREW
REDRAG
REDRAW
REDREW
REDRUM
REGRAB
REGRET
REGREW
REGRIP
REGROW
REPROS
RETRAL
RETRAP
RETRIM
RETROD
RETROS
REURGE
REWRAP
SEARCH
SEARED
SEARER
SEARLE
SECRET
SEERED
SEURAT
SEVRES
TEARAT
TEARED
TEARER
TEARIT
TEARUP
TEGRIN
TEHRAN
TERRAE
TERRAN
TERRES
TERRET
TERRIF
TERRIS
TERROR
TETRAD
TETRAS
TETRIS
VEERED
WEARER
WEARON
WEIRDO
WEIRDY
WETRAG
YEARLY
YEARNS
ZEBRAS

•E••R•

BEFIRM
BEFORE
BEGIRD
BEGIRT
BEJART
BELFRY
BEMIRE
BESORE
BESURE
BEURRE
BEWARE
BEWARY
CEDARN
CEDARS
CEDARY
CEDERS
CELERY
CENTRE
CENTRI
CENTRO
CESARE
CESARS
CETERA
DEAIRS
DEBARK
DEBARS
DEBURR
DECARE
DECORS
DEFERS
DEFORD
DEFORE
DEFORM
DEGERM
DEHIRE
DEHORN
DEIDRE
DEJURE
DEMARK
DEMURE
DEMURS
DENARI
DENARS
DENARY
DENDRA
DENDRI
DENDRO
DENIRO
DEPART
DEPERE
DEPORT
DESCRY
DESERT
DESIRE
DESTRY
DETARS
DETERS
DEVERE
DEVERS
DEVORE
DEWARS
DEWIRE
DEWORM
DEXTRO
EELERS
EELERY
EEYORE
FEDORA
FEMORA
FEMURS
FETORS
FEVERS
GEMARA
GENERA
GENTRY
GERARD
HEGIRA
HENDRY
HETERO
HEWERS
HEXERS
JETHRO
KEFIRS
LEGART
LEMURS
LENARD
LENORE
LEPERS
LETTRE
LEVERS
LEVERT
MEAGRE
MEMORY
MESSRS
METERS
MEWERS
MEYERS
NEPHRO
NEVERS
NEWARK
NEWERA
OEUVRE
PELTRY
PENURY
PETARD
PETERI
PETERS
REAIRS
REBARS
REBORE
REBORN
REBURY
RECORD
RECORK
RECURE
RECURL
RECURS
REDARE
REDARN
REEARN
REFERS
REFIRE
REFORM
REGARD
REGIRD
REHIRE
REMARK
REMORA
RENARD
RENFRO
REPARK
REPERK
REPORT
RESORB
RESORT
RETARD
RETARS
RETIRE
RETORE
RETORN
RETORT
RETURF
RETURN
REVERB
REVERE
REVERS
REVERT
REWARD
REWARM
REWARN
REWIRE
REWORD
REWORE
REWORK
REWORN
REZERO
SEAARM
SEBERG
SECURE
SEDERS
SEGURA
SEMPRE
SENARY
SENORA
SENORS
SENTRA
SENTRY
SEPIRA
SEVERE
SEVERN
SEVERS
SEWARD
SEWERS
SEXERS
TEATRO
TEAURN
TENORS
TENURE
TEVERE
VECTRA
VELARS
VELCRO
VELURE
VENERA
VENIRE
VENORA
VESTRY
VEXERS
WEBERN
WEBERS
WECARE

•E•••R

AERIER
AETHER
BEADER
BEAKER
BEAMER
BEARER
BEATER
BEAVER
BECKER
BEEMER
BEEPER
BEEZER
BEFAIR
BEGFOR
BEGGAR
BELAIR
BELIER
BELTER
BELZER
BENDER
BENHUR
BERBER
BERGER
BESSER
BESTER
BESTIR
BETTER
BETTOR
BEYMER
CELLAR
CENSER
CENSOR
CENTER
CEREBR
DEADER
DEAFER
DEALER
DEARER
DEBLUR
DEBTOR
DEBURR
DECKER
DEEPER
DEEVER
DEFFER
DEFIER
DEFTER
DEHAIR
DEICER
DEKKER
DELMAR
DELVER
DENIER
DENSER
DENVER
DEODAR
DETMER
DETOUR
DEUTER
DEVOIR
DEVOUR
DEWIER
DEXTER
EELIER
EERIER
FEARER
FEEDER
FEELER
FELLER
FENCER
FENDER
FENNER
FEODOR
FERBER
FERRER
FERVOR
FESTER
FETTER
GEEZER
GEIGER
GELLAR
GELLER
GENDER
GENXER
GERBER
GETFAR
GETTER
GEYSER
HEADER
HEALER
HEAPER
HEARER
HEATER
HEAVER
HECTOR
HEDGER
HEEDER
HEEGER
HEELER
HEFNER
HEFTER
HEIFER
HELLER
HELMER
HELPER
HELTER
HEMMER
HENNER
HEPPER
HERDER
HESTER
JEDGAR
JEERER
JEETER
JENNER
JERKER
JESTER
KEDGER
KEELER
KEENER
KEEPER
KEGGER
KEGLER
KELLER
KENNER
KEPLER
KEVLAR
KEYSER
LEADER
LEAKER
LEANER
LEAPER
LEASER
LEAVER
LECHER
LECTER
LECTOR
LEDGER

LEERER
LEHRER
LEITER
LELOIR
LENDER
LERNER
LESSER
LESSOR
LESTER
LETOUR
LETTER
LEVIER
LEWDER
MEADER
MEAGER
MEANER
MEDGAR
MEEBER
MEEKER
MEETER
MELDER
MELTER
MEMBER
MEMOIR
MENDER
MENTOR
MEOWER
MERCER
MERGER
MESMER
METEOR
METIER
MEWLER
NEARER
NEATER
NECKER
NECTAR
NEEDER
NESTER
NESTOR
NETHER
NETTER
NEUTER
NEWCAR
NEWMAR
OERTER
PEALER
PEEKER
PEELER
PEEPER
PEGLER
PELTER
PENNER
PEPPER
PERTER
PESTER
PETTER
PEWTER
READER
REALER
REAMER
REAPER
REARER
REAVER
RECTOR
REDDER
REDFIR
REDOER
REEDER
REEFER
REEKER
REELER
REGEAR
REHEAR
REIGER
REINER
REISER
REITER
RELIER
RENDER
RENOIR
RENTER
REPAIR
REPFOR
REPOUR
RESTER
RESTIR
RETEAR
RETOUR
REUNER
REUSER
REUTER
REVOIR
REWEAR
SEAAIR
SEALER
SEAMER
SEARER
SEATER
SEAVER
SECTOR
SEEDER
SEEGER
SEEKER
SEINER
SEIZER
SEIZOR
SELLER
SEMPER
SENDER
SENHOR
SENIOR
SENSOR
SERVER
SETFOR
SETTER
SETZER
SEXIER
TEARER
TEASER
TEENER
TEETER
TEKWAR
TELLER
TEMPER
TENDER
TENNER
TENSER
TENSOR
TENTER
TERROR
TERSER
TESTER
TETHER
UECKER
VEADAR
VECTOR
VEDDER
VEILER
VELOUR
VENDER
VENDOR
VENEER
VENNER
VENTER
VERGER
VESPER
VETOER
VETTER
WEAKER
WEANER
WEARER
WEAVER
WEBBER
WEDDER
WEEDER
WEEPER
WEEZER
WEIDER
WEIMAR
WELDER
WELLER
WELTER
WENNER
WERKER
WERNER
WESKER
WESTER
WETBAR
WETTER
YEAGER
YELLER
YELPER
YENFOR
YESSIR
YESTER
ZENGER
ZEPHYR
ZESTER

••ER••

AHERNE
ALEROS
ALERTS
AMERCE
ANERGY
APERCU
ATERRE
AVERSE
AVERTS
AZERAS
AZERIS
BAERGA
BIERCE
BIERES
CHERIE
CHERRY
CHERTS
CHERTY
CHERUB
CHERYL
CIERAS
CLERGY
CLERIC
CLERKS
COERCE
CZERNY
DEERES
EBERLE
EBERLY
EDERLE
EGERIA
EMERGE
EMERIC
EMERIL
ENERGY
ENEROS
ETERNE
EVERLY
EVERSO
EVERTS
EXERTS
FAERIE
FAEROE
FIERCE
FIEROS
FRERES
GUERRE
IBERIA
ICERUN
ISERVE
JEERAT
JEERED
JEERER
KIERAN
KIERON
LEERAT
LEERED
LEERER
MOERAE
OBERON
OBERTO
OLERUD
OMERTA
ONERUN
OPERAS
OVERDO
OVERIT
OVERLY
PEERAT
PEERCE
PEERED
PEERIN
PIERCE
PIERIA
PIERRE
PUERTO
QWERTY
SEERED
SHEREE
SHERPA
SHERRI
SHERRY
SHERYL
SIERRA
SMERSH
SPERRY
STEREO
STERES
STERIC
STERNA
STERNE
STERNO
STERNS
STEROL
SWERVE
THERAM
THERAP
THERAT
THERED
THEREF
THERES
THERMO
THERMS
THEROD
THERON
TIERCE
TIERED
TIEROD
TIERRA
TWERPS
USERID
VEERED
WHERED
WHERES
WHERRY
XTERRA

••E•R•

AFEARD
ALEGRE
AMEERS
AMENRA
ATERRE
AWEARY
BLEARS
BLEARY
CHEERS
CHEERY
CHERRY
CHEVRE
CLEARS
CLEARY
COEURS
DREARY
EMEERS
EXEDRA
FLEERS
FLEURS
FREDRO
FREERS
GUERRE
NIEKRO
OHENRY
OLEARY
OMEARA
ONEARM
ONEIRO
OSETRA
PHEDRE
PIERRE
PIETRO
PLEURA
POETRY
PREARM
PREDRY
QUEERS
REEARN
SHEARS
SHEERS
SHERRI
SHERRY
SIERRA
SMEARS
SMEARY
SNEERS
SNEERY
SOEURS
SPEARE
SPEARS
SPERRY
STEERS
SWEARS
THEIRS
THEMRS
THENRA
THEORY
THEPRU
THEYRE
TIERRA
VIEIRA
WHERRY
XTERRA

••E••R

ALEGAR
ASEVER
AYESIR
BAEYER
BEEMER
BEEPER
BEEZER
BIEBER
BREMER
BREUER
BREWER
BREYER
CAESAR
CHEDER
CHEWER
CLEVER
CREMER
DEEPER
DEEVER
DIEFOR
DIETER
DJEBAR
DREYER
DUELER
EVENER
EXETER
FEEDER
FEELER
FLEXOR
FREWER
FUELER
GEEZER
GREGOR
GREYER
HEEDER
HEEGER
HEELER
INEVER
IPETER
JAEGER
JEERER
JEETER
KEELER
KEENER
KEEPER
KIEFER
LEERER
LIEBER
LIEDER
LIEFER
LIEFOR
LIENOR
MEEBER
MEEKER
MEETER
NEEDER
OBEYER
OCEDAR
ONECAR
OPENER
PEEKER
PEELER
PEEPER
PIECER
PIETER
PLEXOR
PREFER
PRETER
PRETOR
PREWAR
PREYER
QUELER
QUEUER
REEDER
REEFER
REEKER
REELER
RHETOR
ROEPER
SEEDER
SEEGER
SEEKER
SKEWER
SPEWER
STELAR
STEWER
SUEFOR
TEENER
TEETER
THEBAR
THECAR
TIEBAR
TREMOR
TREVOR
USEFOR
VIEFOR
VIEWER
WEEDER
WEEPER
WEEZER
WIENER

•••ER•

ACHERS
ADDERS
ADHERE
ADVERB
ADVERT
AFTERS
AIDERS
AIMERS
AIRERS
ALBERS
ALBERT
ALDERS
ALPERT
ALTERS
AMBERS
AMBERY
AMEERS
AMPERE
ANDERS
ANGERS
ANTERO
AOLERS
APPERT
ARMERS
ARTERY
ASKERS
ASPERA
ASSERT
ASTERN
ASTERO
ASTERS
AUGERS
BAKERS
BAKERY
BALERS
BAYERN
BIDERS
BIKERS
BITERS
BOLERO
BONERS
BONERZ
BOOERS
BORERS
BOWERS
BOWERY
BOXERS
BRIERS
BRIERY
BUYERS
CABERS
CAGERS
CAMERA
CANERS
CAPERS
CARERS
CASERN
CASERS
CATERA
CATERS
CAVERN
CAVERS
CEDERS
CELERY
CETERA
CHEERS
CHEERY
CICERO
CIDERS
CIDERY
CITERS
CLUERS
CODERS
COHERE
COMERS
CONERS
COOERS
COPERS
CORERS
COVERS
COVERT
COWERS
CRIERS
CRYERS
CUBERS
CURERS
CYDERS
DARERS
DATERS
DAZERS
DEFERS
DEGERM
DEPERE
DESERT
DETERS
DEVERE
DEVERS
DICERS
DIKERS
DINERO
DINERS
DISERE
DIVERS
DIVERT
DIYERS
DOPERS
DOSERS
DOTERS
DOWERS
DOWERY
DOZERS
DRIERS
DRYERS
DUPERS
DUPERY
EASERS
EATERS
EATERY
ECKERD
EDBERG
EDGERS
EELERS
EELERY
EGBERT
EGGERS
EGGERT
EIDERS
EILERS
EILERT
EKBERG
ELBERT
ELDERS
ELLERY
ELMERS
ELVERS
EMBERS
EMEERS
EMPERY
ENBERG
ENDERS
ENTERO
ENTERS
ESKERS
ESTERS
ETHERS
EXPERT
EXSERT
EXTERN
FACERS
FADERS
FAKERS
FAKERY
FARERS
FAXERS
FEVERS
FIBERS
FIFERS
FILERS
FINERY
FIRERS
FIVERS
FIXERS
FLEERS
FLIERS
FLYERS
FOYERS
FREERS
FRIERS
FRYERS
FUMERS
GAMERS
GAPERS
GATERS
GAZERS
GENERA
GIBERS
GIVERS
GLIERE
GLUERS
GOFERS
GOMERS
GONERS
GORERS
GOVERN
HATERS
HAYERS
HAZERS
HETERO
HEWERS
HEXERS
HIDERS
HIKERS
HIRERS
HIVERS
HOLERS
HOMERS
HONERS
HOPERS
HOSERS
HOVERS
HUBERT
HUMERI
HYPERS
IDLERS
IMHERE
IMPERF
INFERS
INHERE
INKERS
INNERS
INSERT
INTERJ
INTERN
INTERS
INVERT
IRKERS
JAPERS
JAPERY
JAVERT
JIVERS
JOKERS
KHMERS
KITERS
LACERS
LADERS
LAGERS
LAKERS
LAPERI
LAPERM
LASERS
LATERI
LATERO
LAVERN
LAVERS
LAYERS
LEPERS
LEVERS
LEVERT
LIBERS
LIFERS
LIGERS
LIKERS
LINERS
LITERS
LIVERS
LIVERY
LONERS
LOPERS
LOSERS
LOVERS
LOWERS
LOWERY
LUGERS
LURERS
MACERS
MADERA
MADERO
MAKERS
MANERO
MASERS
MASERU
MATERS
MCKERN
METERS
MEWERS
MEYERS
MILERS
MIMERS
MINERS
MISERS
MISERY
MITERS
MIXERS
MOBERG
MODERN
MOOERS
MOPERS
MOPERY
MOVERS
MOWERS
MOYERS
MUNERA
MUSERS
MYHERO
NAMERS
NAPERY
NBAERS
NEVERS
NEWERA
NFLERS
NHLERS
NINERS
NITERS
NITERY
NIXERS
NOSERS
NOTERS
NUMERO
OARERS
OATERS
OBVERT
OCHERS
OCHERY
OFFERS
OGLERS
OILERS
OLMERT
ORDERS
ORNERY
ORRERY
OSBERT
OSIERS
OSTERS
OTHERS
OTTERS
OWLERY
OWNERS
PACERS
PAGERS
PAPERS
PAPERY
PARERS
PATERS
PAVERS
PAWERS
PAYERS
PETERI
PETERS
PIKERS
PILERS
PINERO
PINERS
PINERY
PIPERS
PLIERS
POKERS
POKERY
POLERS
PORERS
POSERS
POWERS
PRIERS
PRYERS
PULERS
QUEERS
RACERS
RAGERS
RAKERS
RASERS
RATERS
RAVERS
RAZERS
REFERS
REPERK
REVERB
REVERE
REVERS
REVERT
REZERO
RIBERA
RICERS
RIDERS
RIKERS
RILERS
RIMERS
RISERS
RIVERA
RIVERS
ROBERS
ROBERT
ROGERE
ROGERS
ROMERO
ROPERS
ROPERY
ROSERY
ROVERS
ROWERS
RUDERY
RULERS
RUPERT
SABERS
SAVERS
SAWERS
SAYERS
SCLERA
SEBERG
SEDERS
SEVERE
SEVERN
SEVERS
SEWERS
SEXERS
SHEERS
SHOERS
SIXERS
SIZERS
SKIERS
SNEERS
SNEERY
SOBERS
SOLERS
SOMERS
SOWERS
SPHERE
SPIERS
STEERS
STIERS
SUPERB
SUPERG
SUPERS
TAKERS
TALERS
TAMERS
TAPERS
TASERS
TATERS
TAVERN
TAXERS
TEVERE
TIGERS
TILERS
TILERY
TIMERS
TITERS
TONERS
TOPERS
TORERO
TOTERM
TOTERS
TOWERS
TOWERY
TOYERS
TRIERS
TRYERS
TUBERS
TUNERS
TYLERS
TYPERS
UDDERS
ULCERS
UMBERS
UNDERS
UNHERO
UNSERE
UPHERE
UPPERS
URGERS
USHERS
UTTERS
VALERA
VALERE
VALERO
VALERY
VENERA
VEXERS
VIDERI
VINERS
VINERY
VIPERS
VOMERS
VOTERS
VOWERS
WADERS
WAFERS
WAFERY
WAGERS
WAKERS
WATERS
WATERY
WAVERS
WAVERY
WAXERS
WEBERN
WEBERS
WINERY
WIPERS
WIRERS
WOOERS
WYLERS
WYVERN
ZONERS

•••E•R

AGREER
APPEAR
ARREAR
ASNEAR
AUTEUR
BIGEAR
CAREER
CEREBR
COHEIR
DISEUR
DOGEAR
ENDEAR
GONEAR
INFEAR
INGEAR
ISWEAR
LAGEAR
LINEAR
METEOR
MSIEUR
MYDEAR
NODEAR
OHDEAR
POSEUR
RATEDR
REGEAR
REHEAR
RETEAR
REWEAR
TINEAR
UPBEAR
UPREAR
UPTEAR
VENEER

••••ER

ABASER
ABATER
ABIDER
ABUSER
ACHIER
ACUTER
ADORER
AERIER
AETHER
AGILER
AGREER
AIRIER
ALINER
AMBLER
AMPLER
AMUSER
ANGLER
ANSWER
ANTHER
ANTLER
ARCHER
ARGUER
ARIDER
ARTIER
ASEVER
ASHIER
ASTHER
ATONER
AUSTER
AVIDER
AVOWER

AWAKER	BLOWER	CANKER	CRAMER	DIPPER	EXETER	FUMIER	GUNNER	HOOVER	KEEPER	LENDER	MARKER	NATTER	PEGLER	PUNKER
AWARER	BOATER	CANNER	CRATER	DITHER	EXILER	FUNDER	GUNTER	HOPPER	KEGGER	LERNER	MARNER	NEARER	PELTER	PUNNER
BABIER	BOBBER	CANOER	CRAVER	DLAYER	FABBER	FUSSER	GUSHER	HORNER	KEGLER	LESSER	MARRER	NEATER	PENNER	PUNTER
BACKER	BOHRER	CANTER	CREMER	DOCKER	FABLER	GABBER	GUTTER	HOSIER	KELLER	LESTER	MASHER	NECKER	PEPPER	PURRER
BADDER	BOILER	CAPPER	CROWER	DODDER	FAFNER	GABLER	GYPPER	HOTTER	KENNER	LETTER	MASKER	NEEDER	PERTER	PURSER
BADGER	BOLDER	CARDER	CRUDER	DODGER	FAINER	GADDER	HACKER	HOWLER	KEPLER	LEVIER	MASTER	NESTER	PESTER	PUSHER
BAEYER	BOLGER	CAREER	CULLER	DOFFER	FAIRER	GAFFER	HAGLER	HOWSER	KEYSER	LEWDER	MATHER	NETHER	PETTER	PUTTER
BAFFER	BOLTER	CARNER	CUMBER	DONDER	FALLER	GAGGER	HAILER	HRIDER	KHYBER	LIBBER	MATTER	NETTER	PEWTER	QUAKER
BAGGER	BOMBER	CARPER	CURLER	DONNER	FALSER	GAINER	HALTER	HUGGER	KICKER	LICKER	MAULER	NEUTER	PFIZER	QUAVER
BAILER	BONDER	CARTER	CURSER	DOOVER	FALTER	GAITER	HALVER	HULLER	KIDDER	LIEBER	MAUSER	NICKER	PHASER	QUELER
BAITER	BONIER	CARVER	CURTER	DOOZER	FANNER	GAMIER	HAMMER	HUMBER	KIEFER	LIEDER	MAZIER	NIGHER	PHONER	QUEUER
BAKKER	BONNER	CASPER	CUSSER	DOPIER	FARMER	GAMMER	HAMPER	HUMMER	KILLER	LIEFER	MEADER	NIPPER	PICKER	QUIVER
BALDER	BOOKER	CASTER	CUSTER	DORMER	FASTER	GANDER	HANDER	HUNGER	KILMER	LIFTER	MEAGER	NOBLER	PIECER	QUOTER
BALKER	BOOMER	CATHER	CUTLER	DOTTER	FATHER	GANGER	HANGER	HUNKER	KILTER	LIMBER	MEANER	NODDER	PIETER	RACIER
BALMER	BOOTER	CAUSER	CUTTER	DOURER	FATTER	GAOLER	HANKER	HUNTER	KINDER	LIMIER	MEEBER	NOONER	PILFER	RACKER
BANDER	BOOZER	CENSER	CUVIER	DOUSER	FAWNER	GARBER	HARDER	HURLER	KIPPER	LIMNER	MEEKER	NOOSER	PINCER	RADNER
BANGER	BOPPER	CENTER	CUYLER	DOWNER	FEARER	GARNER	HARKER	HURTER	KISSER	LIMPER	MEETER	NOSHER	PINGER	RAFTER
BANKER	BORDER	CHAFER	CYCLER	DOWSER	FEEDER	GARTER	HARMER	HUSKER	KNIFER	LINDER	MELDER	NOSIER	PINIER	RAIDER
BANNER	BOTHER	CHASER	CYPHER	DOZIER	FEELER	GASPER	HARPER	ICKIER	KNOWER	LINGER	MELTER	NOSTER	PINKER	RAILER
BANTER	BOWLER	CHEDER	DABBER	DRAPER	FELLER	GASSER	HATTER	IFFIER	KOCHER	LINIER	MEMBER	NUBBER	PINNER	RAINER
BARBER	BOWYER	CHEWER	DAFTER	DRAWER	FENCER	GASTER	HAULER	IMAGER	KOHLER	LINKER	MENDER	NUDGER	PINTER	RAISER
BARGER	BOWZER	CHICER	DAGGER	DREYER	FENDER	GATHER	HAWKER	INANER	KOSHER	LINTER	MEOWER	NUMBER	PIPIER	RAMMER
BARKER	BOXIER	CHIDER	DAMMER	DRIVER	FENNER	GAUGER	HAWSER	INCHER	KOSTER	LINZER	MERCER	NURSER	PITIER	RANGER
BARTER	BRACER	CHIMER	DAMNER	DRONER	FERBER	GAWKER	HAZIER	INEVER	KOTTER	LIPPER	MERGER	NUTTER	PLACER	RANKER
BASHER	BRAVER	CHOKER	DAMPER	DROVER	FERRER	GAWPER	HEADER	INKIER	KRAMER	LISPER	MESMER	OAKIER	PLANER	RANTER
BASKER	BRAYER	CHOLER	DANCER	DUBBER	FESTER	GEEZER	HEALER	IPETER	KROGER	LISTER	METIER	OATIER	PLATER	RAPIER
BASTER	BREMER	CIBBER	DANDER	DUCKER	FETTER	GEIGER	HEAPER	IRATER	KRONER	LITHER	MEWLER	OBEYER	PLAYER	RAPPER
BATHER	BREUER	CINDER	DANGER	DUELER	FIBBER	GELLER	HEARER	IRONER	KRUGER	LITTER	MIDLER	OBITER	PLOMER	RAPTER
BATTER	BREWER	CIPHER	DANKER	DUFFER	FIDLER	GENDER	HEATER	ISOMER	KUBLER	LOADER	MILDER	OBOLER	PLOVER	RASHER
BAUMER	BREYER	CLAWER	DANNER	DULLER	FILLER	GENXER	HEAVER	ISSUER	LACIER	LOAFER	MILKER	OERTER	PLOWER	RASPER
BAVIER	BRIBER	CLEVER	DAPPER	DUMBER	FILTER	GERBER	HEDGER	JABBER	LADDER	LOANER	MILLER	OILIER	POGNER	RASTER
BAWLER	BRINER	CLONER	DARKER	DUMPER	FINDER	GETTER	HEEDER	JAEGER	LADLER	LOBBER	MILNER	OINKER	POISER	RATHER
BAXTER	BROKER	CLOSER	DARNER	DUNKER	FINGER	GEYSER	HEEGER	JAGGER	LAFFER	LOCHER	MINCER	OLIVER	POKIER	RATNER
BEADER	BRUDER	CLOVER	DARTER	DUNNER	FIRMER	GIBBER	HEELER	JAILER	LAGGER	LOCKER	MINDER	ONAGER	POLLER	RATTER
BEAKER	BUCKER	COALER	DASHER	DUSTER	FISHER	GILDER	HEFNER	JAMMER	LAKIER	LODGER	MINTER	OOZIER	PONDER	READER
BEAMER	BUDDER	COATER	DAUBER	EARNER	FITTER	GINGER	HEFTER	JASPER	LANCER	LOFTER	MIRIER	OPENER	POOLER	REALER
BEARER	BUDGER	COAXER	DAWBER	EASIER	FIZZER	GIPPER	HEIFER	JAVIER	LANDER	LOGGER	MISTER	OPINER	POORER	REAMER
BEATER	BUFFER	COCKER	DEADER	EASTER	FLAKER	GIRDER	HELLER	JAZZER	LANGER	LOGIER	MOANER	OSTLER	POPPER	REAPER
BEAVER	BUGLER	CODGER	DEAFER	EBAYER	FLAMER	GLASER	HELMER	JEERER	LANIER	LOITER	MOBBER	OUSTER	PORKER	REARER
BECKER	BULWER	COFFER	DEALER	ECHOER	FLAYER	GLAZER	HELPER	JEETER	LANKER	LOLLER	MOCKER	OWLIER	PORTER	REAVER
BEEMER	BUMMER	COILER	DEARER	EDGIER	FLOWER	GLIDER	HELTER	JENNER	LAPPER	LONGER	MOILER	OYSTER	POSHER	REDDER
BEEPER	BUMPER	COINER	DECKER	EELIER	FLUTER	GLOVER	HEMMER	JERKER	LAPSER	LOOKER	MOLDER	PACIER	POSTER	REDOER
BEEZER	BUNKER	COKIER	DEEPER	EERIER	FOAMER	GLOWER	HENNER	JESTER	LARDER	LOOPER	MOLTER	PACKER	POTHER	REEDER
BELIER	BUNTER	COLDER	DEEVER	EGGIER	FODDER	GLUIER	HEPPER	JIGGER	LARGER	LOOSER	MONGER	PADDER	POTTER	REEFER
BELTER	BURGER	COLTER	DEFFER	EGGLER	FOGGER	GNAWER	HERDER	JILTER	LARKER	LOOTER	MOONER	PALMER	POURER	REEKER
BELZER	BURIER	COMBER	DEFIER	EISNER	FOKKER	GOITER	HESTER	JINXER	LARTER	LOPPER	MOOTER	PALTER	POUTER	REELER
BENDER	BURLER	CONFER	DEFTER	EITHER	FOLDER	GOLFER	HIGHER	JITTER	LASHER	LOTTER	MOPIER	PAMPER	POWDER	REIGER
BERBER	BURNER	CONGER	DEICER	ELATER	FOLGER	GOOBER	HILLER	JIVIER	LASKER	LOUDER	MOPPER	PANDER	POYSER	REINER
BERGER	BUSHER	CONKER	DEKKER	ELAYER	FONDER	GOODER	HINDER	JOBBER	LASSER	LOUVER	MOSHER	PANIER	PRATER	REISER
BESSER	BUSIER	COODER	DELVER	ELIDER	FOOLER	GOOIER	HINTER	JOGGER	LATHER	LUBBER	MOTHER	PANNER	PRAWER	REITER
BESTER	BUSKER	COOKER	DENIER	ELITER	FOOTER	GOOVER	HIPPER	JOINER	LATTER	LUGGER	MOUSER	PANTER	PRAYER	RELIER
BETTER	BUSTER	COOLER	DENSER	ELMIER	FORCER	GOPHER	HISSER	JOKIER	LAUDER	LULLER	MUCKER	PANZER	PREFER	RENDER
BEYMER	BUTLER	COOPER	DENVER	ELOPER	FORGER	GORGER	HITHER	JOLTER	LAUPER	LUMBER	MUDDER	PAPIER	PRETER	RENTER
BIBBER	BUTTER	COOTER	DETMER	ELUDER	FORKER	GORIER	HITTER	JOSHER	LAUTER	LUMPER	MUGGER	PARGER	PREYER	RESTER
BICKER	BUZZER	COPIER	DEUTER	EMOTER	FORMER	GOUGER	HOAXER	JOTTER	LAWYER	LUNGER	MULDER	PARKER	PRICER	REUNER
BIDDER	CABLER	COPPER	DEWIER	ENSLER	FOSTER	GRADER	HOCKER	JOYNER	LAZIER	LUNKER	MULLER	PARSER	PRIMER	REUSER
BIEBER	CADGER	COPTER	DEXTER	ENVIER	FOULER	GRATER	HOFFER	JUICER	LEADER	LURKER	MUMMER	PASSER	PROBER	REUTER
BIGGER	CAGIER	CORDER	DIALER	EPOWER	FOWLER	GRAVER	HOHNER	JUMPER	LEAKER	LUSHER	MURDER	PASTER	PROPER	RHYMER
BILKER	CAHIER	CORKER	DIAPER	ERASER	FOXIER	GRAYER	HOKIER	JUNGER	LEANER	LUSTER	MUSHER	PATTER	PROSER	RIBBER
BILLER	CAKIER	CORNER	DICIER	ERODER	FRAMER	GRAZER	HOLDER	JUNKER	LEAPER	LUTHER	MUSTER	PATZER	PROVER	RICHER
BINDER	CALDER	COSHER	DICKER	ESCHER	FRASER	GREYER	HOLIER	JUSTER	LEASER	MADDER	MUTTER	PAUPER	PRUNER	RIDDER
BINGER	CALKER	COSIER	DIETER	ESPIER	FRATER	GRIPER	HOLLER	KAISER	LEAVER	MAHLER	NABBER	PAUSER	PUCKER	RIFLER
BIRDER	CALLER	COTLER	DIFFER	ESTHER	FRAZER	GROCER	HOMIER	KANDER	LECHER	MAILER	NAGGER	PAWNER	PUFFER	RIGGER
BIRLER	CALMER	COTTER	DIGGER	ETCHER	FREWER	GROPER	HONKER	KARRER	LECTER	MAIMER	NAILER	PCUSER	PULLER	RIMIER
BITTER	CAMBER	COUTER	DILLER	EVADER	FUDGER	GROVER	HOOFER	KAVNER	LEDGER	MAINER	NAIVER	PEALER	PULPER	RINGER
BLADER	CAMPER	COWIER	DIMMER	EVENER	FUELER	GROWER	HOOKER	KEDGER	LEERER	MANGER	NAPIER	PEEKER	PULVER	RINSER
BLAMER	CANCER	COWPER	DINGER	EVILER	FUHRER	GUIDER	HOOPER	KEELER	LEHRER	MANNER	NAPPER	PEELER	PUMPER	RIOTER
BLAZER	CANIER	COZIER	DINNER	EVOKER	FULLER	GULPER	HOOTER	KEENER	LEITER	MAPPER	NASSER	PEEPER	PUNIER	RIPPER

RISKER
RITTER
ROADER
ROAMER
ROARER
ROBBER
ROCKER
RODDER
ROEPER
ROHMER
ROHRER
ROLFER
ROLLER
ROMPER
ROOFER
ROOKER
ROOMER
ROOTER
ROPIER
ROSIER
ROSTER
ROTTER
ROUSER
ROUTER
RUBBER
RUCKER
RUDDER
RUDNER
RUINER
RULIER
RUMMER
RUNNER
RUSHER
RUTGER
RUTTER
SACHER
SACKER
SADDER
SADLER
SAGIER
SAILER
SALTER
SALVER
SANDER
SANGER
SAPPER
SASSER
SAUCER
SAWYER
SCALER
SCARER
SCORER
SCOTER
SEALER
SEAMER
SEARER
SEATER
SEAVER
SEEDER
SEEGER
SEEKER
SEINER
SEIZER
SELLER
SEMPER
SENDER
SERVER
SETTER
SETZER
SEXIER
SHADER
SHAKER
SHAPER
SHARER
SHAVER
SHINER
SHIRER
SHIVER
SHOVER
SHOWER
SICKER
SIFTER
SIGHER
SIGLER
SIGNER
SILVER
SIMMER
SIMPER
SINGER
SINKER
SINNER
SIPPER
SISLER
SISTER
SITTER
SKATER
SKEWER
SLAKER
SLATER
SLAVER
SLAYER
SLICER
SLIDER
SLIVER
SLOPER
SLOWER
SMILER
SMITER
SMOKER
SNAKER
SNARER
SNIDER
SNIPER
SNORER
SNYDER
SOAKER
SOAPER
SOARER
SOBBER
SOCCER
SOFTER
SOLDER
SOLVER
SOMBER
SOMMER
SOONER
SORTER
SOUPER
SOURER
SOUTER
SPACER
SPADER
SPARER
SPAYER
SPEWER
SPICER
SPIDER
SPIKER
SPINER
SPRIER
SPRYER
SPYDER
STAGER
STALER
STARER
STATER
STAYER
STEWER
STOKER
STONER
STORER
STOVER
STOWER
STYLER
SUAVER
SUCKER
SUDSER
SUFFER
SULKER
SUMMER
SUMNER
SUMTER
SUNDER
SUPPER
SURFER
SUTTER
SWAYER
SWIPER
TACKER
TAGGER
TAILER
TALKER
TALLER
TAMPER
TANKER
TANNER
TAPPER
TARTER
TASTER
TATLER
TATTER
TAUTER
TEARER
TEASER
TEENER
TEETER
TELLER
TEMPER
TENDER
TENNER
TENSER
TENTER
TERSER
TESTER
TETHER
THALER
THAWER
THAYER
TICKER
TIDIER
TIGGER
TILLER
TILTER
TIMBER
TINDER
TINIER
TINKER
TINNER
TINTER
TIPPER
TITHER
TITTER
TOILER
TOLLER
TONIER
TOOLER
TOOTER
TOPPER
TOSSER
TOTTER
TOURER
TOUTER
TOWNER
TRACER
TRADER
TRITER
TROYER
TUCKER
TUGGER
TUPPER
TURNER
TUSKER
TWINER
TWOFER
UECKER
UGLIER
ULSTER
UNDOER
UNITER
UNTIER
UPOVER
USURER
VAGUER
VAINER
VALUER
VAMPER
VANIER
VARIER
VASTER
VEDDER
VEILER
VENDER
VENEER
VENNER
VENTER
VERGER
VESPER
VETOER
VETTER
VIEWER
VINIER
VIZIER
VOGUER
VOICER
VOIDER
WACKER
WADDER
WAFTER
WAGGER
WAGNER
WAILER
WAITER
WAIVER
WALKER
WALLER
WALTER
WANDER
WANIER
WANNER
WANTER
WAPNER
WARDER
WARIER
WARMER
WARNER
WARPER
WASHER
WASSER
WASTER
WAVIER
WAXIER
WEAKER
WEANER
WEARER
WEAVER
WEBBER
WEDDER
WEEDER
WEEPER
WEEZER
WEIDER
WELDER
WELLER
WELTER
WENNER
WERKER
WERNER
WESKER
WESTER
WETTER
WHALER
WHINER
WHITER
WICKER
WIDDER
WIENER
WIGNER
WILDER
WILIER
WILLER
WIMMER
WINCER
WINDER
WINGER
WINIER
WINKER
WINNER
WINTER
WIRIER
WISHER
WISTER
WITHER
WITTER
WOHLER
WOLPER
WONDER
WOOFER
WORKER
WORMER
WRITER
WYNTER
XAVIER
XYSTER
YAKKER
YAMMER
YANKER
YAPPER
YARDER
YASSER
YATTER
YAWNER
YAWPER
YEAGER
YELLER
YELPER
YESTER
YONDER
YORKER
YOWLER
ZANIER
ZAPPER
ZENGER
ZESTER
ZIMMER
ZINGER
ZIPPER
ZITHER
ZONKER
ZOOIER
ZUCKER

ES••••

ESALEN
ESBATS
ESCALE
ESCAPE
ESCARP
ESCAUT
ESCENT
ESCHER
ESCHEW
ESCORT
ESCROW
ESCUDO
ESDRAS
ESENIN
ESHARP
ESHKOL
ESKERS
ESKIMO
ESPANA
ESPIAL
ESPIED
ESPIER
ESPIES
ESPIOS
ESPOSA
ESPOSO
ESPRIT
ESSAIS
ESSAYS
ESSENE
ESTADO
ESTATE
ESTEEM
ESTERS
ESTHER
ESTIME
ESTLIN
ESTOCS
ESTOPS
ESTRAY

E•S•••

EASEBY
EASEIN
EASELS
EASEON
EASERS
EASEUP
EASIER
EASILY
EASING
EASLEY
EASTER
EASTLA
EASTON
EASYAS
EASYGO
EDSELS
EISELE
EISLEY
EISNER
ELSTON
ENSATE
ENSEAL
ENSEAT
ENSIGN
ENSILE
ENSLER
ENSOUL
ENSUED
ENSUES
ENSURE
EOSINS
EPSONS
ERSATZ
ERSTAD
ESSAIS
ESSAYS
ESSENE
ETSEQQ
EUSDEN
EUSTIS
EXSECT
EXSERT

E••S••

EATSAT
EATSIN
EATSIT
EATSOF
EATSUP
ECESIC
ECESIS
EDESSA
EDISON
EENSIE
EGESTA
EGESTS
EGGSAC
EGGSON
EGISES
EKESBY
ELISEO
EL1SHA
ELISSA
ELISTS
ELYSEE
EMPSON
ENDSAT
ENDSIN
ENDSIT
ENDSON
ENDSUP
ENESCO
ENISLE
EPOSES
ERASED
ERASER
ERASES
ERESTU
EXISTS
EYESUP

E•••S•

ECLASS
ECORSE
EDESSA
EFFUSE
EGLISE
EGOISM
EGOIST
EGRESS
ELAPSE
ELDEST
ELFISH
ELISSA
ELOISA
ELOISE
ELPASO
ELVISH
EMBOSS
EMDASH
ENCASE
ENDASH
ENDUSE
ENLIST
ENMESH
ERNEST
ESPOSA
ESPOSO
EULESS
EVENSO
EVERSO
EVULSE
EXCESS
EXCISE
EXCUSA
EXCUSE
EXPOSE
EXPOST
EZPASS

E••••S

EAGLES
EAGRES
EAKINS
EARTHS
EASELS
EASERS
EASYAS
EATERS
EBANKS
EBATES
EBBETS
EBOATS
EBONDS
EBOOKS
ECARDS
ECCLES
ECESIS
ECHOES
ECLASS
ECLATS
ECOLES
EDAMES
EDDIES
EDDOES
EDEMAS
EDGARS
EDGERS
EDICTS
EDILES
EDSELS
EDUCES
EDUCTS
EELERS
EFILES
EFLATS
EGALES
EGESTS
EGGERS
EGISES
EGRESS
EGRETS
EIDERS
EIGHTS
EILERS
EJECTS
EJIDOS
ELANDS
ELATES
ELBOWS
ELBRUS
ELDERS
ELECTS
ELEMIS
ELEVES
ELIDES
ELISTS
ELITES
ELLIOS
ELMERS
ELOGES
ELOPES
ELPAIS
ELUDES
ELUTES
ELVERS
ELYTIS
EMAILS
EMALLS
EMBARS
EMBAYS
EMBEDS
EMBERS
EMBOGS
EMBOSS
EMBOWS
EMCEES
EMEERS
EMENDS
EMILYS
EMMAUS
EMMETS
EMOTES
ENACTS
ENARMS
ENATES
ENCRES
ENDERS
ENDOWS
ENDUES
ENEROS
ENGELS
ENIACS
ENJOYS
ENNIUS
ENNUIS
ENOILS
ENOKIS
ENOTES
ENROLS
ENSUES
ENTERS
ENURES
ENVIES
ENVOIS
ENVOYS
EOSINS
EPACTS
EPHAHS
EPHODS
EPHORS
EPOCHS
EPODES
EPOSES
EPSONS
EQUALS
EQUIPS
ERASES
EREBUS
ERECTS
ERGOTS
ERICAS
ERINYS
ERODES
ERRORS
ERUCTS
ERUPTS
ESBATS
ESDRAS
ESKERS
ESPIES
ESPIOS
ESSAIS
ESSAYS
ESTERS
ESTOCS
ESTOPS
ETAGES
ETAILS
ETAPES
ETCHES
ETHERS
ETHICS
ETHNOS
ETHYLS
ETILES
ETUDES
EULESS
EUSTIS
EVADES
EVENAS
EVENTS
EVERTS
EVICTS
EVITES
EVOKES
EWINGS
EXACTS
EXALTS
EXCELS
EXCESS
EXCONS
EXCUBS
EXERTS
EXGOVS
EXILES
EXISTS
EXITUS
EXMETS
EXODUS
EXPATS
EXPELS
EXTOLS
EXTRAS
EXUDES
EXULTS
EXURBS
EYRIES
EZINES
EZPASS

•ES•••

AESOPS
BESAME
BESANT
BESETS
BESIDE
BESOMS
BESORE
BESOTS
BESSEL
BESSER
BESSIE
BESSON
BESTED
BESTER
BESTIR
BESTOW
BESURE
CESARE
CESARS
CESIUM
CESSED
CESSES
CESSNA
CESTAS
CESTUS
DESADE
DESALT
DESCRY
DESEED
DESERT
DESETA
DESICA
DESIGN
DESILT
DESILU
DESIRE
DESIST
DESLUM
DESMOG
DESNOS
DESODS
DESOTO
DESPOT
DESREE
DESSAU
DESTEM
DESTRY
FESCUE
FESSED
FESSES
FESSUP
FESTAL
FESTAS
FESTER
FESTUS
GESTAE
GESTES
GESTIC
HESIOD
HESOUT
HESTER
HESTIA
HESTON
JESSEL
JESSYE
JESTED
JESTER
JESUIT
KESHIA
LESAGE
LESBOS
LESHAN
LESION
LESLEY
LESLIE
LESMIZ
LESSEE
LESSEN
LESSER
LESSON
LESSOR
LESTAT
LESTER
MESAAZ
MESABI
MESCAL
MESHED
MESHES
MESIAL
MESMER
MESNES
MESONS
MESSED
MESSES
MESSIN
MESSRS
MESSUP
NESBIT
NESSEN
NESSES
NESSIE
NESSUS
NESTEA
NESTED
NESTER
NESTIN
NESTLE
NESTOR
PESACH
PESADE
PESCOW
PESETA
PESEWA
PESTER
PESTLE
PESTOS
RESAID
RESALE
RESALT
RESAND
RESANG
RESAVE
RESAWN
RESAWS
RESAYS
RESCAN
RESCUE
RESEAL
RESEAM
RESEAT
RESEAU
RESECT
RESEDA
RESEED
RESEEK
RESEEN
RESEES
RESELL
RESEND
RESENT
RESETS
RESEWN
RESEWS
RESHES
RESHIP
RESHOD
RESHOE
RESHOT
RESHOW
RESHUT
RESIDE
RESIFT
RESIGN
RESILE
RESING
RESINK
RESINS
RESINY
RESIST
RESITE
RESITS
RESIZE
RESNAP
RESNIK
RESOAK
RESOAP
RESODS
RESOIL
RESOLD
RESOLE
RESORB
RESORT
RESOWN
RESOWS
RESPAN
RESPIN
RESPOT
RESTAB
RESTED
RESTER
RESTES
RESTIR
RESTON
RESTOW
RESTUP
RESUIT
RESULT
RESUME
RESWAM
RESWIM
SESAME
SESQUI
SESSUE
SESTET
TESLAS
TESSIE
TESSIO
TESTAE
TESTED
TESTEE
TESTER
VESPAS
VESPER
VESPID
VESSEL
VESTAL
VESTAS
VESTED
VESTEE
VESTRY
WESKER
WESKIT
WESLEY
WESSEX
WESSON
WESTER
WESTIE
WESTIN
WESTON
XESOUT
YESBUT
YESIAM
YESIDO
YESMAN
YESMEN
YESSED
YESSES
YESSIR
YESTER
YESYES
YESYOU
ZESTAS
ZESTED
ZESTER

•E•S••

BEASTS
BEDSIT
BENSEY
BENSON
BESSEL
BESSER
BESSIE
BESSON
BETSEY
BETSON
BETSYS
CEASED
CEASES
CENSED
CENSER
CENSES
CENSOR
CENSUS
CESSED
CESSES
CESSNA
DEASIL
DEISTS
DELSOL
DENSER
DESSAU
EENSIE
FEASTS
FEISTY
FELSON
FESSED
FESSES
FESSUP
GEESON
GEISEL
GEISHA
GELSEY
GETSAB
GETSAC
GETSAD
GETSAT
GETSBY
GETSET
GETSIN
GETSIT
GETSON
GETSTO
GETSUP
GEYSER
HEISTS
HEMSIN
HENSON
HERSEY
HEUSEN
HEWSTO
JENSEN
JERSEY
JESSEL
JESSYE
JETSAM
JETSET
JETSKI
JETSON
KELSEY
KENSIT
KERSEE
KEYSER

KEYSIN KEYSON KEYSUP LEASED LEASER LEASES LEASTS LEGSIT LEISEN LENSED LENSES LESSEE LESSEN LESSER LESSON LESSOR LETSAT LETSBE LETSBY LETSGO LETSIN LETSON LETSUP MEASLE MEASLY MENSAL MENSAN MENSCH MERSEY MESSED MESSES MESSIN MESSRS MESSUP NEESON NEISSE NELSON NEOSHO NESSEN NESSES NESSIE NESSUS NEVSKI NEVSKY NEWSIE NEWSOM PENSEE PENSIN PENSUP PEPSIN PEPSUP PERSIA PERSIS PERSON PETSAT PETSIT REASKS REASON REDSEA REDSIX REDSKY REDSOX REDSUN REESES REISER REMSEN REUSED REUSER

REUSES REVSON REVSUP SEASON SEESAS SEESAW SEESIN SEESTO SEESUP SEISMO SEISMS SENSED SENSEI SENSEN SENSES SENSOR SESSUE SETSAT SETSBY SETSIN SETSON SETSTO SETSUP SEWSIN SEWSON SEWSUP TEASED TEASEL TEASER TEASES TEASET TEESUP TENSED TENSER TENSES TENSOR TERSER TESSIE TESSIO VELSEN VERSED VERSES VERSET VERSOS VERSTS VERSUS VESSEL WEASEL WESSEX WESSON YEASTS YEASTY YENSID YESSED YESSES YESSIR

•E••S•

BEARSE BEHEST BEMUSE CERISE DEBASE DEFUSE DEGUST DELISH DELIST DEMAST DEMISE DEMIST DENISE DEPEST DEPOSE DEROSE DERUST DESIST DETEST DEVEST DEVISE FETISH FEWEST FEYEST HEARSE HEARST HEINSE HERESY HEWISH HEXOSE JEWISH LEGIST LETUSE MEDUSA MEREST NEISSE NERNST NEWEST NEWISH PELOSI PERISH PERUSE RECASE RECAST RECESS RECOST RECUSE REDOSE REDUST REFUSE REHASH RELISH RELIST RELOSE RELOST REMISE REMISS RENEST REPASS REPAST REPOSE REPOST RERISE REROSE RESIST RETEST RETOSS REVEST REVISE REWASH SETOSE SEWIST SEXISM SEXIST TEENSY TERESA VEDIST VENOSE VERISM VERIST WEENSY ZENIST

•E•••S

AENEAS AEOLUS AERIES AERIOS AESOPS BEALLS BEANOS BEARDS BEASTS BEAUTS BEAVIS BEBOPS BEDEWS BEDIMS BEDOGS BEEVES BEFITS BEFOGS BEGEMS BEGETS BEGINS BEGUMS BEIGES BEINGS BELAYS BELIES BELLES BELONS BENTOS BERETS BERTHS BERYLS BESETS BESOMS BESOTS BETELS BETSYS BETTAS BEVANS BEVELS BEVIES BEWIGS BEZELS CEASES CEDARS CEDERS CEIBAS CELEBS CELLOS CENSES CENSUS CENTAS CENTOS CEORLS CEREUS CERROS CESARS CESSES CESTAS CESTUS DEAIRS DEATHS

DEBAGS DEBARS DEBITS DEBRIS DEBUGS DEBUTS DECADS DECAFS DECALS DECAPS DECAYS DECIUS DECORS DECOYS DEDANS DEERES DEFATS DEFERS DEFIES DEFOGS DEGELS DEGUMS DEICES DEIGNS DEIMOS DEISTS DEKKOS DELAYS DELCOS DELFTS DELIUS DELTAS DELVES DEMIES DEMITS DEMOBS DEMONS DEMURS DENARS DENIES DENIMS DENNIS DENNYS DEPOTS DEPTHS DERATS DERMAS DERMIS DESNOS DESODS DETARS DETERS DETTES DEUCES DEVERS DEVILS DEWARS EELERS FEASTS FEIGNS FEINTS FELIDS FELLAS FELONS FEMMES FEMURS FENCES FEOFFS

FERALS FERIAS FERMIS FEROUS FERRIS FESSES FESTAS FESTUS FETORS FEVERS FEZZES GECKOS GEDDES GELEES GENETS GENIES GENIUS GENOAS GENRES GENTES GEODES GESTES GETUPS HEARNS HEARTS HEATHS HEAVES HEDGES HEGYES HEISTS HELENS HELIOS HELLAS HELLOS HELOTS HENGES HENNAS HERBES HERMES HEROES HERONS HEURES HEWERS HEXADS HEXERS JEEVES JELLOS JETTAS JEVONS JEWELS KEARNS KEBABS KEDGES KEFIRS KELLYS KEMPIS KENDOS KERNES KEYNES LEARNS LEASES LEASTS LEAVES LEDGES LEEVES LEGALS LEGROS LEHUAS

LEICAS LEMANS LEMMAS LEMNOS LEMONS LEMURS LENSES LENTOS LEPERS LESBOS LETUPS LEVEES LEVELS LEVERS LEVIES MEATUS MECCAS MECUMS MEDALS MEDIAS MEDICS MEDIUS MEDNIS MEDOCS MELEES MELONS MENDES MENTIS MENTOS MERGES MERITS MEROPS MESHES MESNES MESONS MESSES MESSRS METALS METERS METRES METROS MEWERS MEYERS MEZZOS NEHRUS NEIGHS NELLIS NERVES NESSES NESSUS NEVERS NEVINS NEWELS NEWIES PEALES PEARLS PECANS PECHES PEDALS PEEVES PEKOES PELEUS PELVIS PENNIS PERILS PERROS PERSIS PESTOS

PETALS PETERS PETTIS PEWEES PEWITS REACTS READDS REAIMS REAIRS REALES REALMS REARMS REASKS REATAS REAVES REBAGS REBARS REBBES REBECS REBELS REBETS REBIDS REBOPS REBUTS REBUYS RECANS RECAPS RECESS RECONS RECTOS RECTUS RECUES RECURS RECUTS REDANS REDIGS REDIPS REDOES REDUBS REDYES REESES REEVES REFERS REFIES REFITS REGELS REGIUS REGLES REHABS REHEMS REHITS REHOES REICES REIGNS REINAS REINES REINKS REJIGS REKEYS RELAPS RELAYS RELETS RELICS RELIES RELOGS REMANS REMAPS REMATS

REMISS REMITS REMOPS REMOWS RENEWS RENGAS RENINS RENNES RENTES REOILS REOWNS REPADS REPASS REPAYS REPEGS REPELS REPENS REPINS REPOTS REPROS REPUBS RERIGS RERUNS RESAWS RESAYS RESEES RESETS RESEWS RESHES RESINS RESITS RESODS RESOWS RESTES RETAGS RETANS RETAPS RETARS RETIES RETINS RETIPS RETOPS RETOSS RETOWS RETROS REUNES REUSES REVELS REVERS REVETS REVUES REWEDS REWETS REWINS REYLES REZIPS SEALYS SEAMUS SEDANS SEDERS SEDGES SEDUMS SEENAS SEESAS SEGUES SEIKOS SEINES SEISMS

SEIZES SELVES SENATS SENNAS SENORS SENSES SEPALS SEPIAS SEPOYS SERACS SERAIS SERGES SERIES SERIFS SERINS SERKIS SEROUS SERTAS SERUMS SERVES SERVOS SETTOS SETUPS SEVENS SEVERS SEVRES SEWERS SEWONS SEXERS TEASES TEBETS TEHEES TELCOS TEMPOS TEMPTS TEMPUS TENETS TENLBS TENNIS TENONS TENORS TENSES TENTHS TEPEES TERCES TERMES TERNES TERRES TERRIS TESLAS TETHYS TETONS TETRAS TETRIS TEVETS TEXANS VEGANS VEGGES VELARS VELDTS VENINS VENOMS VENOUS VENTAS VENUES VERDES VERGES VERSES

VERSOS VERSTS VERSUS VERVES VESPAS VESTAS VETOES VETTES VEXERS WEALDS WEAVES WEBADS WEBERS WEDELS WEDGES WEEUNS WEIGHS WELCHS WELLES WENCES WENDYS XEBECS XERXES YEARNS YEASTS YEGODS YENTAS YERKES YESSES YESYES ZEBRAS ZENDOS ZEROES ZESTAS ZEUXIS

••ES••

ACESIT ACESUP ADESTE AGESIX AMESIA ATESTS AVESTA AYESHA AYESIR BOESKY CAESAR CHESTS CHESTY CRESOL CRESSY CRESTS CUESIN CUESTA CUESUP DIESEL DIESES DIESIS DOESBY DOESIN DOESIT DOESNT DOESOK DOESSO DOESTO DOESUP DRESSY DUESSA ECESIC ECESIS EDESSA EGESTA EGESTS EKESBY ENESCO ERESTU EYESUP FIESTA FLESHY FRESCA FRESCO FRESNO GEESON GOESAT GOESBY GOESIN GOESON GOESTO GOESUP GUESTS HTESTS ICESIN ICESIT ICESUP INESSE KMESON KRESGE LIESIN LIESON LIESTO MOESHA MUESLI NEESON NOESIS NTESTS ODESSA OLESHA OLESON ONESEC ONESET OWESON PRESET PRESTO QUESOS QUESTS REESES RHESUS RIESEN SEESAS SEESAW SEESIN SEESTO SEESUP SIESTA TEESUP THESEA THESES THESIS THESON THESOX THESPS THESPY THESUN TIESIN TIESON TIESTO TIESUP TMESES TMESIS TOESIN TRESSY UNESCO USESIN USESON USESUP WIESEL WRESTS

••E•S•

AGEISM AGEIST ALEAST ASEASY ATEASE AVERSE BREAST CHEESE CHEESY CLEESE CREASE CREASY CRESSY CREUSA CREUSE DOESSO DRESSY DUESSA EDESSA EVENSO EVERSO FLENSE FREEST GNEISS GOEASY GREASE GREASY GREIST IMEASY INESSE KLEIST KWEISI NLEAST ODENSE ODESSA ONEISH ORELSE ORENSE PLEASE QUEASY SHEESH SMERSH TEENSY THEASP THEISM THEIST THEUSA TRESSY TSETSE UNEASE UNEASY WEENSY

••E••S

ABELES ACELAS ADEEMS ADENIS ADEPTS AGENAS AGENTS AKELAS AKENES ALECKS ALEPHS ALEROS ALERTS ALEUTS ALEVES ALEXAS ALEXIS AMEBAS AMEERS AMENDS AMENTS ANELES APEXES ARECAS ARENAS ARETES ATEAMS ATESTS AVERTS AZERAS AZERIS BCELLS BEEVES BIERES BLEAKS BLEARS BLEATS BLEEDS BLEEPS BLENDS BREADS BREAKS BREAMS BREDES BREEDS BREVES BREVIS BTEAMS BUENAS BUENOS CHEATS CHECKS CHEEKS CHEEPS CHEERS CHEOPS CHERTS CHESTS CHEVYS CIELOS CIERAS CLEANS CLEARS CLEATS CLEEKS CLEFTS CLERKS

CLEVES COEURS CREAKS CREAMS CREDOS CREEDS CREEKS CREELS CREEPS CREMES CREPES CRESTS CZECHS DCELLS DEERES DIENES DIESES DIESIS DIETES DIEZES DREADS DREAMS DRECKS DUENAS DUENOS DWEEBS DWELLS ECESIS EDEMAS EGESTS EJECTS ELECTS ELEMIS ELEVES EMEERS EMENDS ENEROS EREBUS ERECTS EVENAS EVENTS EVERTS EXERTS FAENAS FIELDS FIENDS FIEROS FLECKS FLEERS FLEETS FLEURS FLEXES FREAKS FREERS FREONS FRERES FUEGOS GLEAMS GLEANS GNEISS GREATS GREBES GREEDS GREEKS GREENS GREETS GUESTS HBEAMS

HTESTS
HUEVOS
HYENAS
IBEAMS
IBEXES
ICEUPS
IDEALS
IDENTS
ILEXES
JEEVES
JUEGOS
JUEVES
KNEADS
KNEELS
KNELLS
KREWES
KVELLS
LBEAMS
LEEVES
LIEBYS
LIEGES
LIEUTS
MIELES
NIECES
NIETAS
NIETOS
NIEVES
NOESIS
NTESTS
NUECES
NUEVES
OBEAHS
OBELUS
OCEANS
ODEONS
OLEINS
OLEUMS
OMEGAS
ONEUPS
OPERAS
OREADS
ORECKS
OREOOS
OREXIS
OXEYES
OYEZES
PAEANS
PEEVES
PHELPS
PIECES
PIETAS
PLEADS
PLEATS
PLEBES
PLEXES
PLEXUS
POEMES
POETES
PRECIS
PREENS
PREOPS
PREXES
PSEUDS
QUEENS
QUEERS
QUELLS
QUESOS
QUESTS
QUEUES
REESES
REEVES
RHEEMS
RHEIMS
RHEMES
RHESUS
RHEUMS
SCENAS
SCENES
SCENTS
SEENAS
SEESAS
SHEARS
SHEDDS
SHEENS
SHEERS
SHEETS
SHEIKS
SHELLS
SIEGES
SIETES
SIEVES
SKEETS
SKEINS
SLEEKS
SLEEPS
SLEETS
SMEARS
SMELLS
SMELTS
SNEAKS
SNEERS
SNELLS
SOEURS
SPEAKS
SPEARS
SPECKS
SPEEDS
SPELLS
SPENDS
STEADS
STEAKS
STEALS
STEAMS
STEEDS
STEELS
STEEPS
STEERS
STEINS
STELAS
STELES
STENOS
STENTS
STERES
STERNS
SUEDES
SUENOS
SWEARS
SWEATS
SWEDES
SWEEPS
SWEETS
SWELLS
TCELLS
THEBES
THEFTS
THEIRS
THEMES
THEMRS
THERES
THERMS
THESES
THESIS
THESPS
THETAS
THETIS
TIEINS
TIEUPS
TMESES
TMESIS
TOEINS
TREADS
TREATS
TRECES
TRENDS
TREXES
TWEAKS
TWEEDS
TWEENS
TWEETS
TWERPS
UPENDS
UVEOUS
VNECKS
WEEUNS
WHEATS
WHEELS
WHELKS
WHELMS
WHELPS
WHERES
WIELDS
WREAKS
WRECKS
WRESTS
YIELDS

•••ES•

ABBESS
ABLEST
ACCESS
AFRESH
ALWEST
APTEST
ARNESS
ARREST
ARTEST
ASSESS
ATBEST
ATREST
ATTEST
AWLESS
BAREST
BASEST
BEHEST
BLUEST
BLUESY
CARESS
CHEESE
CHEESY
CLEESE
COYEST
CUTEST
CUTESY
DAREST
DEPEST
DETEST
DEVEST
DIGEST
DIREST
DIVEST
DONESO
DRIEST
DRYEST
DURESS
EGRESS
ELDEST
ENMESH
ERNEST
EULESS
EXCESS
FEWEST
FEYEST
FINEST
FOREST
FREEST
GAMEST
GAYEST
GOWEST
GRIESE
HALEST
HERESY
HITEST
HONEST
HOPESO
HUGEST
ICIEST
IDLEST
IGUESS
ILLEST
INFEST
INGEST
INJEST
INNESS
INVEST
IQTEST
JAMESA
JAMESI
JAMESJ
JAMESK
JAMESM
JAMESS
JAMEST
JAMESV
JONESS
JONESY
LAMESA
LAMEST
LATEST
LAXEST
LIKESO
LIVEST
LOWEST
MAYEST
MEREST
MODEST
MOLEST
MORESO
MUTEST
NEWEST
NICEST
NLWEST
NOLESS
NUDEST
OBSESS
OBTEST
ODDEST
OGRESS
OLDEST
PALEST
PAVESE
PRIEST
PUREST
RAREST
RAWEST
RECESS
RENEST
RETEST
REVEST
RIFEST
RIPEST
RUDEST
SAFEST
SAGEST
SANEST
SAYEST
SHEESH
SHIEST
SHYEST
SLIEST
SLYEST
SOREST
STRESS
SUREST
TALESE
TAMEST
TERESA
THRESH
TRUEST
UNLESS
UNMESH
UNREST
VARESE
VILEST
WALESA
WIDEST
WISEST
WRIEST
WRYEST
YAREST

•••E•S

ABBESS
ABBEYS
ACCESS
ACHERS
ADDERS
ADEEMS
ADFEES
ADIEUS
ADREPS
AENEAS
AFTERS
AGLETS
AGREES
AIDERS
AIMERS
AIRERS
ALBERS
ALDERS
ALIENS
ALLEES
ALLEYS
ALTERS
AMBERS
AMEERS
AMIENS
AMVETS
ANDERS
ANGELS
ANGERS
ANNEES
ANSEIS
AOLERS
APNEAS
APPELS
ARMERS
ARMETS
ARNEIS
ARNESS
ARPELS
ARTELS
ASKERS
ASPENS
ASSESS
ASSETS
ASTERS
ATHENS
ATREUS
AUGEAS
AUGERS
AWLESS
AZTECS
AZTEKS
BABELS
BADEMS
BAGELS
BAKERS
BALERS
BEDEWS
BEGEMS
BEGETS
BERETS
BESETS
BETELS
BEVELS
BEZELS
BICEPS
BIDERS
BIDETS
BIKERS
BIPEDS
BITERS
BLEEDS
BLEEPS
BLUETS
BOGEYS
BONERS
BOOERS
BOREAS
BORERS
BOTELS
BOWELS
BOWERS
BOXERS
BREEDS
BRIEFS
BRIERS
BURETS
BUTEOS
BUYERS
BYTENS
CABERS
CADETS
CAGERS
CAMEAS
CAMELS
CAMEOS
CANERS
CAPERS
CARERS
CARESS
CARETS
CASERS
CATERS
CAVERS
CCLEFS
CEDERS
CELEBS
CEREUS
CHEEKS
CHEEPS
CHEERS
CHIEFS
CHIENS
CIDERS
CITEES
CITERS
CIVETS
CLEEKS
CLUERS
CODERS
COLEUS
COMEAS
COMERS
COMETS
CONERS
CONEYS
COOEES
COOERS
COPERS
CORERS
COSECS
COSETS
COVENS
COVERS
COVETS
COVEYS
COWENS
COWERS
COZENS
CREEDS
CREEKS
CREELS
CREEPS
CRIERS
CRUETS
CRYERS
CUBEBS
CUBERS
CULETS
CUPELS
CURERS
CURETS
CUSECS
CUTEYS
CUVEES
CYDERS
DALETS
DARERS
DATERS
DAVENS
DAZERS
DEFERS
DEGELS
DETERS
DEVERS
DICERS
DIKERS
DINERS
DIVERS
DIYERS
DONEES
DONETS
DOPERS
DOSERS
DOTERS
DOWELS
DOWERS
DOYENS
DOZENS
DOZERS
DRIERS
DRYERS
DUPERS
DURESS
DUVETS
DWEEBS
DYNELS
EASELS
EASERS
EATERS
EBBETS
EDGERS
EDSELS
EELERS
EGGERS
EGRESS
EGRETS
EIDERS
EILERS
ELDERS
ELMERS
ELVERS
EMBEDS
EMBERS
EMCEES
EMEERS
EMMETS
ENDERS
ENGELS
ENTERS
ESKERS
ESTERS
ETHERS
EULESS
EXCELS
EXCESS
EXMETS
EXPELS
FACERS
FACETS
FADERS
FAKERS
FARERS
FAXERS
FEVERS
FIBERS
FIFERS
FILERS
FILETS
FIRERS
FIVERS
FIVEWS
FIXERS
FLEERS
FLEETS
FLIERS
FLYERS
FOGEYS
FOLEYS
FOYERS
FREERS
FRIELS
FRIERS
FRYERS
FUMERS
FUSEES
GAMERS
GANEFS
GAPERS
GATERS
GAVELS
GAZERS
GCLEFS
GELEES
GENETS
GIBERS
GILELS
GIMELS
GIVENS
GIVERS
GLUERS
GODETS
GODEYS
GOFERS
GOLEMS
GOMERS
GONERS
GORERS
GREEDS
GREEKS
GREENS
GREETS
GRIEFS
GRUELS
HABEAS
HACEKS
HAREMS
HATERS
HAVENS
HAYERS
HAZELS
HAZERS
HELENS
HEWERS
HEXERS
HIDERS
HIKERS
HIREES
HIRERS
HIVERS
HOLERS
HOMERS
HOMEYS
HONERS
HONEYS
HOPERS
HOSELS
HOSERS
HOTELS
HOVELS
HOVERS
HYPERS
IDLERS
IGUESS
IMBEDS
IMPELS
INFERS
INGELS
INKERS
INLETS
INNERS
INNESS
INSETS
INTENS
INTERS
IRKERS
ISLETS
ISLEYS
ISSEIS
JAMESS
JAPERS
JEWELS
JIVERS
JOKERS
JONESS
JULEPS
KHMERS
KIDEOS
KITERS
KNEELS
KOPEKS
LABELS
LACERS
LADERS
LAGERS
LAKERS
LAMEDS
LAPELS
LAREES
LASERS
LATENS
LAVERS
LAYERS
LEPERS
LEVEES
LEVELS
LEVERS
LIBELS
LIBERS
LIFEIS
LIFERS
LIGERS
LIKENS
LIKERS
LINENS
LINERS
LITERS
LIVENS
LIVERS
LODENS
LONERS
LOOEYS
LOPERS
LOSERS
LOVERS
LOVEYS
LOWERS
LUDENS
LUGERS
LUMENS
LURERS
LYCEES
MACERS
MAKERS
MANETS
MASERS
MATERS
MATEYS
MAVENS
MELEES
METERS
MEWERS
MEYERS
MILERS
MIMEOS
MIMERS
MINERS
MISERS
MITERS
MIXERS
MODELS
MODEMS
MONETS
MONEYS
MOOERS
MOPEDS
MOPERS
MORELS
MOSEYS
MOTELS
MOTETS
MOVERS
MOWERS
MOYERS
MULEYS
MUSEES
MUSEOS
MUSERS
NAMERS
NAVELS
NBAERS
NEVERS
NEWELS
NFLERS
NHLERS
NINERS
NISEIS
NITERS
NIXERS
NOBELS
NOFEES
NOLESS
NONETS
NONEWS
NOPETS
NOSERS
NOTERS
NOVELS
NYJETS
NYMETS
OARERS
OATERS
OBJETS
OBSESS
OCHERS
OCTETS
OFFERS
OGLERS
OGRESS
OILERS
OLMECS
ONSETS
ORDERS
ORIELS
OSIERS
OSSETS
OSTERS
OTHERS
OTTERS
OUSELS
OUZELS
OWLETS
OWNERS
PACERS
PAGERS
PANELS
PAPERS
PARENS
PARERS
PAREUS
PASEOS
PATENS
PATERS
PAVERS
PAWERS
PAYEES
PAYERS
PELEUS
PETERS
PEWEES
PIKERS
PILERS
PILEUS
PINERS
PIPERS
PIPETS
PIXELS
PLIERS
POKERS
POKEYS
POLERS
PORERS
POSEAS
POSERS
POWERS
PREENS
PRIERS
PROEMS
PRYERS
PULERS
PUREES
QUEENS
QUEERS
QUIETS
RACERS
RAGERS
RAKERS
RAMENS
RAMETS
RANEES
RAREES
RASERS
RATELS
RATERS
RAVELS
RAVENS
RAVERS
RAZERS
REBECS
REBELS
REBETS
RECESS
REFERS
REGELS
REHEMS
REKEYS
RELETS
RENEWS
REPEGS
REPELS
REPENS
RESEES
RESETS
RESEWS
REVELS
REVERS
REVETS
REWEDS
REWETS
RHEEMS
RICERS
RIDERS
RIKERS
RILERS
RIMERS
RIPENS
RISERS
RIVERS
RIVETS
ROBERS
RODEOS
ROGERS
ROGETS
ROLEOS
ROMEOS
ROPERS
ROVERS
ROWELS
ROWENS
ROWERS
RUBELS
RUBENS
RULERS
RUPEES
SABERS
SALEPS
SAMEAS
SAREES
SAVEAS
SAVERS
SAWERS
SAYERS
SCREES
SCREWS
SEDERS
SEVENS
SEVERS
SEWERS
SEXERS
SHEENS
SHEERS
SHEETS
SHOERS
SHREDS
SHREWS
SINEWS
SIRENS
SIXERS
SIZERS
SKEETS
SKIERS
SLEEKS
SLEEPS
SLEETS
SNEERS
SOBERS
SOLEAS
SOLERS
SOLEUS
SOMERS
SOWERS
SPEEDS
SPIELS
SPIERS
SPREES
STEEDS
STEELS
STEEPS
STEERS
STIERS
STREPS
STRESS
STREWS
SUPERS
SUREIS
SWEEPS
SWEETS
TAKERS
TALERS
TAMERS
TAPERS
TASERS
TATERS
TAVELS
TAXERS
TEBETS
TEHEES
TENETS
TEPEES
TEVETS
THREES
TIGERS
TILERS
TIMERS
TITERS
TOKENS
TONERS
TOPEES
TOPERS
TOTEMS
TOTERS
TOWELS
TOWERS
TOYERS
TRIERS
TRYERS
TUBERS
TUNERS
TUTEES
TVSETS
TWEEDS
TWEENS
TWEETS
TYLERS
TYPEAS
TYPEBS
TYPEOS
TYPERS
UDDERS
ULCERS
UMBELS
UMBERS
UNDERS
UNLESS
UNMEWS
UNPEGS
UNPENS
UNSEWS
UPPERS
UPSETS
URAEUS
URGERS
USHERS
USNEWS
UTTERS
VALENS
VALETS
VEXERS
VIDEOS
VINERS
VIPERS
VIREOS
VIXENS
VOMERS
VOTERS
VOWELS
VOWERS
WADERS
WAFERS
WAGERS
WAKENS
WAKERS
WATERS
WAVERS
WAXERS
WEBERS
WEDELS
WHEELS
WIDENS
WIPERS
WIRERS
WIZENS
WOMENS
WOOERS
WYLERS
XEBECS
XYLEMS
YODELS
YOKELS

ZAZENS
ZONERS

••••ES

ABASES
ABATES
ABELES
ABIDES
ABODES
ABUSES
ACUTES
ADAGES
ADDLES
ADFEES
ADOBES
ADORES
AERIES
AGAMES
AGATES
AGAVES
AGGIES
AGONES
AGREES
AISLES
AKENES
ALEVES
ALICES
ALIKES
ALINES
ALKIES
ALLEES
ALLIES
AMAZES
AMBLES
AMICES
AMIDES
AMINES
AMOLES
AMORES
AMUSES
ANDRES
ANELES
ANGLES
ANIMES
ANISES
ANKLES
ANNEES
ANNIES
ANODES
ANOLES
ANTRES
APEXES
APICES
APPLES
ARAMES
ARBRES
ARCHES
ARETES
ARGUES
ARISES
ARMIES
ARNIES
ASIDES
ASTRES
ATILES
ATISES
ATONES
AWAKES

AXISES
AXONES
AZIDES
AZOLES
AZORES
AZURES
BABIES
BACHES
BADGES
BAINES
BAIZES
BARGES
BARNES
BARRES
BASHES
BASSES
BASTES
BATHES
BEEVES
BEIGES
BELIES
BELLES
BEVIES
BIASES
BIBLES
BIERES
BILGES
BINGES
BIOMES
BLADES
BLAMES
BLARES
BLAZES
BLOKES
BOCCES
BODIES
BOGIES
BOGLES
BOITES
BOMBES
BONNES
BONZES
BOOTES
BOOZES
BORGES
BOSSES
BOULES
BOWLES
BOYLES
BRACES
BRAKES
BRAVES
BREDES
BREVES
BRIBES
BRIDES
BRINES
BRISES
BRUGES
BRUMES
BRUTES
BRUXES
BSIDES
BTILES
BUBKES
BUDGES
BUGLES
BULGES

BUPKES
BURIES
BUSHES
BUSIES
BUSSES
BUTTES
BUZZES
BYRNES
CABLES
CACHES
CADGES
CADRES
CALLES
CALVES
CALXES
CAMOES
CANNES
CANOES
CARIES
CARNES
CARTES
CARVES
CASHES
CASTES
CAUSES
CAVIES
CEASES
CENSES
CESSES
CHAFES
CHASES
CHIDES
CHILES
CHIMES
CHINES
CHIVES
CHOKES
CHORES
CHUTES
CITEES
CITIES
CLAVES
CLEVES
CLIMES
CLONES
CLOSES
CLOVES
CLYDES
CNOTES
COATES
COAXES
COHOES
COKIES
COMTES
CONGES
CONIES
COOEES
COPIES
COPSES
CORTES
COSHES
COSIES
COUPES
COZIES
CRAKES
CRANES
CRAPES
CRATES

CRAVES
CRAZES
CREMES
CREPES
CRIMES
CRIPES
CRISES
CRONES
CRORES
CRUCES
CRUDES
CRUSES
CRUXES
CTILES
CUORES
CURIES
CURSES
CURVES
CUSSES
CUTIES
CUVEES
CYCLES
DADOES
DAISES
DALLES
DANCES
DANSES
DANTES
DASHES
DAUBES
DAVIES
DEERES
DEFIES
DEICES
DELVES
DEMIES
DENIES
DETTES
DEUCES
DHOLES
DIDIES
DIDOES
DIENES
DIESES
DIETES
DIEZES
DIODES
DIRGES
DISHES
DISMES
DISSES
DITZES
DNASES
DOAKES
DOBLES
DODGES
DODOES
DOGIES
DONEES
DORIES
DOSSES
DOUSES
DOUZES
DOWNES
DOWSES
DOXIES
DRAKES
DRAPES

DRIVES
DRONES
DROVES
DRUPES
DRUSES
DRUZES
DTILES
DULLES
DUNCES
DUTIES
EAGLES
EAGRES
EBATES
ECCLES
ECHOES
ECOLES
EDAMES
EDDIES
EDDOES
EDILES
EDUCES
EFILES
EGALES
EGISES
ELATES
ELEVES
ELIDES
ELITES
ELOGES
ELOPES
ELUDES
ELUTES
EMCEES
EMOTES
ENATES
ENCRES
ENDUES
ENOTES
ENSUES
ENURES
ENVIES
EPODES
EPOSES
ERASES
ERODES
ESPIES
ETAGES
ETAPES
ETCHES
ETILES
ETUDES
EVADES
EVITES
EVOKES
EXILES
EXUDES
EYRIES
EZINES
FABLES
FACIES
FAITES
FARCES
FAROES
FASCES
FAUTES
FAUVES
FAWKES
FEMMES

FENCES
FESSES
FEZZES
FHOLES
FIBRES
FICHES
FILLES
FISHES
FIZZES
FLAKES
FLAMES
FLARES
FLAXES
FLEXES
FLORES
FLUKES
FLUMES
FLUTES
FLUXES
FOGIES
FOLIES
FORBES
FORCES
FORGES
FORTES
FOSSES
FOWLES
FRAKES
FRAMES
FRERES
FRIGES
FRISES
FRITES
FTILES
FUDGES
FUGUES
FURIES
FURZES
FUSEES
FUSSES
FUTZES
FUZZES
GABLES
GAFFES
GAINES
GANGES
GASHES
GASSES
GAUGES
GAUZES
GAYNES
GEDDES
GELEES
GENIES
GENRES
GENTES
GEODES
GESTES
GIGUES
GIJOES
GIMMES
GLACES
GLADES
GLARES
GLAZES
GLIDES
GLOBES
GLOVES

GLUTES
GNOMES
GNOSES
GNOTES
GOBIES
GOBOES
GOOSES
GORGES
GORSES
GOUGES
GRACES
GRADES
GRAPES
GRATES
GRAVES
GRAZES
GREBES
GRIDES
GRIMES
GRIPES
GROPES
GROVES
GTILES
GUIDES
GUILES
GUISES
GUSHES
HADJES
HAINES
HAJJES
HALOES
HALVES
HANSES
HAOLES
HASHES
HASTES
HAWSES
HAYMES
HAYNES
HEAVES
HEDGES
HEGYES
HENGES
HERBES
HERMES
HEROES
HEURES
HINGES
HIREES
HISSES
HOAXES
HOBBES
HOBOES
HODGES
HOKIES
HOLIES
HOLMES
HOMIES
HOMMES
HOOVES
HORDES
HORSES
HOSSES
HOUSES
HOYLES
HTILES
HUGHES
HUSHES

HYADES
IBEXES
IBICES
IBISES
ILEXES
IMAGES
IMAXES
IMBUES
IMIDES
IMINES
IMMIES
INAGES
INCHES
INDIES
INDUES
INGLES
INGRES
INKLES
INNIES
INONES
INURES
IRIDES
IRISES
ISSUES
ISTLES
ISTRES
ITCHES
ITILES
JAMBES
JAUNES
JAURES
JAYMES
JAZZES
JEEVES
JINXES
JOSHES
JOSSES
JOULES
JTILES
JUDGES
JUEVES
JUICES
JURIES
KEDGES
KERNES
KEYNES
KISSES
KNAVES
KNIFES
KNIVES
KOPJES
KREWES
KTILES
LADIES
LADLES
LANCES
LAPSES
LAREES
LARGES
LASHES
LASSES
LATHES
LATKES
LATTES
LEASES
LEAVES
LEDGES
LEEVES

LENSES
LEVEES
LEVIES
LIANES
LIEGES
LIGNES
LILIES
LISLES
LISSES
LITRES
LIVRES
LOAVES
LODGES
LONGES
LOOIES
LOOSES
LORIES
LOSSES
LOUIES
LOUPES
LOUSES
LOWRES
LTILES
LUNGES
LUSHES
LUTZES
LWAVES
LYCEES
LYNXES
MACLES
MADRES
MAIRES
MAIZES
MANSES
MAPLES
MARTES
MARXES
MASHES
MASSES
MATJES
MATTES
MAUVES
MAYBES
MELEES
MENDES
MERGES
MESHES
MESNES
MESSES
METRES
MIDGES
MIELES
MILLES
MILNES
MINCES
MINXES
MISSES
MITRES
MOINES
MOIRES
MOISES
MOJOES
MONDES
MONIES
MOSHES
MOSSES
MOUSES
MOVIES

MTILES
MURRES
MUSEES
MUSHES
MUSSES
MYOPES
NACRES
NANTES
NAPLES
NAPPES
NASHES
NAUTES
NAVIES
NERVES
NESSES
NEWIES
NICHES
NIECES
NIEVES
NITRES
NIXIES
NOBLES
NOCHES
NOFEES
NOIRES
NOISES
NOONES
NOOSES
NOSHES
NTILES
NUDGES
NUECES
NUEVES
NURSES
OCHRES
OGIVES
OLAKES
OLDIES
OLIVES
OLORES
ONCLES
ONUSES
ONYXES
OODLES
OPINES
OPUSES
ORALES
ORATES
ORGIES
ORYXES
OSAGES
OTILES
OTOSES
OUCHES
OUNCES
OUTIES
OVINES
OVULES
OXEYES
OXIDES
OYEZES
PADRES
PAISES
PANNES
PARGES
PARKES
PARSES
PASSES

PASTES
PAUSES
PAYEES
PEALES
PECHES
PEEVES
PEKOES
PEWEES
PHASES
PHONES
PIECES
PIQUES
PISCES
PISHES
PISTES
PITIES
PIUTES
PIXIES
PLACES
PLAGES
PLANES
PLATES
PLEBES
PLEXES
PLOCES
PLUIES
PLUMES
PLUSES
POEMES
POETES
POIRES
POISES
POKIES
POMMES
PONIES
PORTES
POSIES
POSSES
POULES
PRATES
PRAXES
PREXES
PRICES
PRIDES
PRIMES
PRIZES
PROBES
PROLES
PROSES
PROVES
PRUDES
PRUNES
PTILES
PULSES
PUREES
PURGES
PURSES
PUSHES
PUSSES
QTILES
QUAKES
QUALES
QUEUES
QUIRES
QUOTES
RABIES
RAINES
RAISES

RAMIES
RAMSES
RANEES
RANGES
RAREES
RASHES
RASSES
RAZZES
REALES
REAVES
REBBES
RECUES
REDOES
REDYES
REESES
REEVES
REFIES
REGLES
REHOES
REICES
REINES
RELIES
RENNES
RENTES
RESEES
RESHES
RESTES
RETIES
REUNES
REUSES
REVUES
REYLES
RHAMES
RHEMES
RHODES
RHYMES
RICHES
RIDGES
RIFLES
RILLES
RINSES
RITZES
ROBLES
ROGUES
ROSIES
ROUGES
ROUSES
ROUTES
ROYCES
RTILES
RUBIES
RUBLES
RUCHES
RUPEES
RUSHES
RUSSES
SABLES
SABRES
SADHES
SALLES
SALVES
SAREES
SARGES
SASHES
SASSES
SAUCES
SAUTES
SAYLES

SAYYES
SCALES
SCARES
SCENES
SCONES
SCOPES
SCORES
SCREES
SEDGES
SEGUES
SEINES
SEIZES
SELVES
SENSES
SERGES
SERIES
SERVES
SEVRES
SHADES
SHAKES
SHALES
SHAMES
SHAPES
SHARES
SHAVES
SHINES
SHIRES
SHORES
SHOVES
SIDLES
SIEGES
SIETES
SIEVES
SINGES
SKATES
SLAKES
SLATES
SLAVES
SLICES
SLIDES
SLIMES
SLOPES
SMAZES
SMILES
SMITES
SMOKES
SMORES
SNAKES
SNARES
SNIPES
SNOPES
SNORES
SOAVES
SOCLES
SOLVES
SONDES
SOUSES
SPACES
SPADES
SPARES
SPATES
SPICES
SPIKES
SPILES
SPINES
SPIRES
SPITES
SPODES

SPOKES
SPORES
SPREES
SPUMES
STAGES
STAKES
STALES
STAPES
STARES
STASES
STATES
STAVES
STELES
STERES
STIDES
STILES
STIPES
STOKES
STOLES
STONES
STORES
STOVES
STUPES
STYLES
SUCRES
SUDSES
SUEDES
SUITES
SURGES
SUSSES
SWALES
SWEDES
SWIPES
TABLES
TAHOES
TANTES
TARDES
TARTES
TASSES
TASTES
TAUPES
TAXIES
TBONES
TEASES
TEHEES
TENSES
TEPEES
TERCES
TERMES
TERNES
TERRES
THALES
THAMES
THANES
THEBES
THEMES
THERES
THESES
THOLES
THREES
THROES
THYMES
TIDIES
TIGRES
TILDES
TINGES
TITHES
TITLES

TITRES
TMESES
TNOTES
TOBIES
TODIES
TOGUES
TOILES
TOMBES
TONNES
TOPEES
TOQUES
TORIES
TORRES
TORTES
TOSSES
TRACES
TRADES
TRANES
TRAVES
TRECES
TREXES
TRIBES
TRICES
TRIKES
TRINES
TRIPES
TROPES
TROVES
TRUCES
TSADES
TTILES
TULLES
TUQUES
TUSHES
TUSSES
TUTEES
TWINES
UGLIES
UKASES
UNCLES
UNDIES
UNDOES
UNGUES
UNICES
UNITES
UNTIES
USAGES
UTUBES
VACHES
VALSES
VALUES
VALVES
VANNES
VARIES
VEGGES
VENUES
VERDES
VERGES
VERSES
VERVES
VETOES
VETTES
VOGUES
VOICES
VOILES
VOSGES
VSIXES
VTILES

WAIVES	ETSEQQ	ELATED	ERRATA	ESPRIT	GETRID	NETTED	RETOSS	BELTED	GETTIN	NEATLY	RESTOW	WESTER	GEARTO	REHITS
WARNES	ETTING	ELATER	ERSATZ	EXCEPT	GETSAB	NETTER	RETOUR	BELTER	HEATED	NECTAR	RESTUP	WESTIE	GELATE	RELATE
WASHES	ETTORE	ELATES	ERUCTS	EXEMPT	GETSAC	NETTLE	RETOWS	BELTON	HEATER	NESTEA	RETTED	WESTIN	GELATI	RELETS
WASTES	ETUDES	ELITER	ERUPTS	EXEUNT	GETSAD	NETTLY	RETRAL	BELTUP	HEATHS	NESTED	RETTIG	WESTON	GELATO	REMATE
WAYNES	ETYMOL	ELITES	ESBATS	EXHORT	GETSAT	NETTON	RETRAP	BENTON	HEATHY	NESTER	RETTON	WETTED	GELETT	REMATS
WEAVES	ETYMON	ELKTON	ESTATE	EXOCET	GETSBY	PETAIN	RETRIM	BENTOS	HEATON	NESTIN	REUTER	WETTER	GENETS	REMITS
WEDGES		ELSTON	ETCETC	EXPECT	GETSET	PETALE	RETROD	BERTHA	HEATUP	NESTLE	SEATAC	WETTIG	GETSTO	REMOTE
WELLES	**E•T•••**	ELUTED	EVENTS	EXPERT	GETSIN	PETALS	RETROS	BERTHE	HECTIC	NESTOR	SEATED	YENTAS	HEADTO	RENATA
WENCES	EATERS	ELUTES	EVERTS	EXPORT	GETSIT	PETARD	RETTED	BERTHS	HECTOR	NETTED	SEATER	YERTLE	HEALTH	RENATO
WHALES	EATERY	ELYTIS	EVICTS	EXPOST	GETSON	PETBOA	RETTIG	BERTIE	HEFTED	NETTER	SEATON	YESTER	HEARTH	RENOTE
WHERES	EATING	EMETIC	EXACTA	EXSECT	GETSTO	PETCAT	RETTON	BESTED	HEFTER	NETTLE	SECTOR	YETTIE	HEARTS	RENTTO
WHILES	EATOUT	EMOTED	EXACTS	EXSERT	GETSUP	PETCOW	RETUNE	BESTER	HELTER	NETTLY	SEETHE	ZESTAS	HEARTY	REPOTS
WHINES	EATSAT	EMOTER	EXALTS	EXTANT	GETTER	PETDOG	RETURF	BESTIR	HEPTAD	NETTON	SELTEN	ZESTED	HECATE	REPUTE
WHITES	EATSIN	EMOTES	EXCITE	EXTENT	GETTIN	PETERI	RETURN	BESTOW	HESTER	NEUTER	SENTBY	ZESTER	HEISTS	RERATE
WHOLES	EATSIT	EMPTOR	EXERTS	EXTORT	GETUPS	PETERS	RETYPE	BETTAS	HESTIA	NEWTON	SENTIN		HELDTO	RESETS
WHYYES	EATSOF	ENATES	EXISTS	EYELET	GETWET	PETIPA	SETFEE	BETTED	HESTON	NEWTOY	SENTON	**•E••T•**	HELOTS	RESITE
WIFIES	EATSUP	ENOTES	EXMATE	EYEPIT	HETERO	PETITE	SETFOR	BETTER	JEETER	NEXTEL	SENTRA	AERATE	HEMATO	RESITS
WILKES	ECTOMY	EROTIC	EXMETS		JETFAN	PETNAP	SETOFF	BETTOR	JESTED	NEXTTO	SENTRY	BEASTS	HEPATO	REVETS
WINCES	ECTYPE	ERSTAD	EXPATS	**•ET•••**	JETGUN	PETPIG	SETOSE	BETTYE	JESTER	NEXTUP	SENTTO	BEATTY	HERETO	REVOTE
WISHES	EITHER	EUSTIS	EXULTS	AETHER	JETHRO	PETPUP	SETOUT	CELTIC	JETTAS	OERTER	SENTUP	BEAUTS	HEWITT	REWETS
WIZZES	ELTORO	EVITES		BETAKE	JETLAG	PETRAT	SETSAT	CENTAI	JETTED	PECTIN	SEPTAL	BEAUTY	HEWSTO	SEDATE
WOLVES	ENTAIL	EXETER	**E••••T**	BETCHA	JETSAM	PETREL	SETSBY	CENTAL	KEATON	PEGTOP	SEPTET	BEFITS	JEWETT	SEEMTO
WRITES	ENTERO	EXITED	EAGLET	BETELS	JETSET	PETRIE	SETSIN	CENTAS	KEITEL	PELTED	SEPTIC	BEGETS	KEEPTO	SEENTO
WTILES	ENTERS	EXITUS	EARLET	BETHEL	JETSKI	PETROL	SETSON	CENTER	KELTON	PELTER	SEPTUM	BELATE	KEPTTO	SEESTO
WUSSES	ENTIAL	EXOTIC	EARNIT	BETIDE	JETSON	PETSAT	SETSTO	CENTOS	KENTON	PELTRY	SERTAS	BEMATA	LEADTO	SELLTO
XBOXES	ENTICE		EATOUT	BETONY	JETTAS	PETSIT	SETSUP	CENTRE	KEPTAT	PENTAD	SESTET	BENITO	LEALTY	SEMITE
XERXES	ENTIRE	**E•••T•**	EATSAT	BETOOK	JETTED	PETTED	SETTEE	CENTRI	KEPTIN	PENTAX	SETTEE	BENOTE	LEANTO	SENATE
XFILES	ENTITY	EBBETS	EATSIT	BETRAY	JETWAY	PETTER	SETTER	CENTRO	KEPTON	PENTEL	SETTER	BERATE	LEASTS	SENATS
XGAMES	ENTOMB	EBOATS	ECKART	BETSEY	KETONE	PETTET	SETTLE	CENTUM	KEPTTO	PENTUP	SETTLE	BERETS	LEGATE	SENDTO
XMASES	ENTOMO	ECARTE	EELPOT	BETSON	KETTLE	PETTIS	SETTOS	CERTIF	KEPTUP	PEPTIC	SETTOS	BESETS	LEGATO	SENITI
XTILES	ENTRAP	ECLATS	EFFECT	BETSYS	LETFLY	PETTIT	SETUPS	CESTAS	KETTLE	PERTER	SEXTET	BESOTS	LENDTO	SENTTO
XTYPES	ENTREE	EDICTS	EFFORT	BETTAS	LETHAL	PETTOY	SETZER	CESTUS	LECTER	PERTLY	SEXTON	CERATE	LENGTH	SETSTO
YALIES	ENTREZ	EDUCTS	EGBERT	BETTED	LETOFF	PETULA	TETCHY	DEATHS	LECTOR	PESTER	TEATRO	CERATO	LENITY	TEBETS
YERKES	ESTADO	EFFETE	EGGERT	BETTER	LETOUR	RETACK	TETHER	DEBTEE	LEFTBE	PESTLE	TEETER	DEAFTO	LENTTO	TECATE
YESSES	ESTATE	EFLATS	EGMONT	BETTOR	LETOUT	RETAGS	TETHYS	DEBTOR	LEFTIN	PESTOS	TEETHE	DEALTO	LEVITE	TECHTV
YESYES	ESTEEM	EGESTA	EGOIST	BETTYE	LETRIP	RETAIL	TETLEY	DEFTER	LEFTIT	PETTED	TENTED	DEARTH	LEVITT	TEMPTS
YTILES	ESTERS	EGESTS	EILERT	CETANE	LETSAT	RETAIN	TETONS	DEFTLY	LEFTOF	PETTER	TENTER	DEARTO	LEVITY	TENDTO
YUTZES	ESTHER	EGRETS	EKEOUT	CETERA	LETSBE	RETAKE	TETRAD	DELTAS	LEFTON	PETTET	TENTHS	DEBATE	MEANTO	TENETS
ZAIRES	ESTIME	EIGHTA	ELANET	DETACH	LETSBY	RETAME	TETRAS	DELTIC	LEITER	PETTIS	TENTON	DEBITS	MELETE	TENUTA
ZANIES	ESTLIN	EIGHTB	ELBERT	DETAIL	LETSGO	RETANS	TETRIS	DENTAL	LENTEN	PETTIT	TENTWO	DEBUTS	MELOTT	TENUTO
ZEROES	ESTOCS	EIGHTC	ELDEST	DETAIN	LETSIN	RETAPE	TETZEL	DENTED	LENTIL	PETTOY	TESTAE	DEFATS	MERITS	TERATO
ZIZZES	ESTOPS	EIGHTD	ELEGIT	DETARS	LETSON	RETAPS	VETOED	DENTIN	LENTOS	PEWTER	TESTED	DEISTS	METATE	TERETE
ZTILES	ESTRAY	EIGHTE	ELGART	DETECT	LETSUP	RETARD	VETOER	DENTON	LENTTO	PEYTON	TESTEE	DELETE	NEARTO	TEVETS
	ETTING	EIGHTH	ELICIT	DETENT	LETTED	RETARS	VETOES	DEPTHS	LEPTON	REATAS	TESTER	DELFTS	NEEDTO	VEINTE
ET••••	ETTORE	EIGHTS	ELLIOT	DETERS	LETTER	RETEAR	VETTED	DESTEM	LESTAT	REATTA	TEUTON	DEMITS	NEGATE	VELDTS
ETAGES	EUTAXY	EIGHTY	ELMONT	DETEST	LETTRE	RETELL	VETTER	DESTRY	LESTER	RECTOR	TEXTED	DEMOTE	NEXTTO	VENETO
ETAILS	EXTANT	EJECTA	ELUANT	DETMER	LETUPS	RETEST	VETTES	DETTES	LETTED	RECTOS	VECTOR	DEMOTH	PEDATE	VENITE
ETALIA	EXTEND	EJECTS	EMMETT	DETOTH	LETUSE	RETHAW	WETBAR	DEUTCH	LETTER	RECTUS	VECTRA	DENOTE	PELOTA	VENUTI
ETALII	EXTENT	ELECTS	EMMITT	DETOUR	METALS	RETIAL	WETFLY	DEUTER	LETTRE	REDTAB	VENTAS	DEPOTS	PEPITA	VERITE
ETAOIN	EXTERN	ELISTS	ENDCUT	DETROP	METATE	RETIED	WETMOP	DEXTER	LEUTZE	REDTAG	VENTED	DEPUTE	PERITI	VERITY
ETAPES	EXTOLL	ELNATH	ENDSAT	DETTES	METEOR	RETIEF	WETNAP	DEXTRO	MEATAX	REDTEN	VENTER	DEPUTY	PERUTZ	VERSTS
ETCETC	EXTOLS	ELUATE	ENDSIT	DETUNE	METERS	RETIES	WETONE	FELTED	MEATUS	REDTIE	VERTEX	DERATE	PESETA	WEALTH
ETCHED	EXTORT	EMEUTE	ENFAIT	FETING	METFAN	RETILE	WETRAG	FELTOK	MEETER	REDTOP	VESTAL	DERATS	PETITE	WENTTO
ETCHER	EXTRAS	EMMETS	ENFANT	FETISH	METHOD	RETILL	WETTED	FESTAL	MEETLY	REDTWO	VESTAS	DERITA	PEWITS	YEASTS
ETCHES		EMMETT	ENGIRT	FETORS	METHYL	RETIME	WETTER	FESTAS	MEETUP	REITER	VESTED	DESETA	PEYOTE	YEASTY
ETERNE	**E••T••**	EMMITT	ENGLIT	FETTER	METIER	RETINA	WETTIG	FESTER	MELTED	RENTAL	VESTEE	DESOTO	REACTS	ZENITH
ETHANE	EARTAB	EMPATH	ENGLUT	FETTLE	METING	RETINS	YETTIE	FESTUS	MELTER	RENTED	VESTRY	DETOTH	READTO	
ETHENE	EARTAG	ENACTS	ENHAUT	GETANA	METRED	RETINT		FETTER	MELTON	RENTEE	VETTED	DEVITO	REALTY	**•E•••T**
ETHERS	EARTHA	ENMITY	ENLIST	GETANF	METRES	RETIPS	**•E•T••**	FETTLE	MENTAL	RENTER	VETTER	DEVOTE	REATTA	BEATAT
ETHICS	EARTHS	ENSATE	ENRAPT	GETFAR	METRIC	RETIRE	BEATAT	GENTES	MENTEE	RENTES	VETTES	DEVOTO	REBATE	BEATIT
ETHIOP	EARTHY	ENTITY	ENROOT	GETFIT	METROS	RETOLD	BEATEN	GENTLE	MENTHE	RENTON	WELTED	DEWITT	REBETS	BECHET
ETHNIC	EASTER	EOLITH	ENSEAT	GETHEP	METTLE	RETONE	BEATER	GENTLY	MENTIS	RENTTO	WELTER	FEALTY	REBOTE	BECKET
ETHNOS	EASTLA	EPACTS	ERFURT	GETHIP	NETFUL	RETOOK	BEATIT	GENTRY	MENTOR	RESTAB	WENTAT	FEASTS	REBUTS	BEDSIT
ETHYLS	EASTON	EQUATE	ERNEST	GETHOT	NETHER	RETOOL	BEATLE	GERTIE	MENTOS	RESTED	WENTBY	FEEDTO	RECITE	BEEPAT
ETILES	EBATES	EQUITY	ERRANT	GETMAD	NETHOU	RETOPS	BEATON	GESTAE	MERTON	RESTER	WENTIN	FEINTS	RECUTS	BEGIRT
ETOILE	EDITED	ERECTS	ESCAUT	GETOFF	NETMAN	RETORE	BEATTY	GESTES	METTLE	RESTES	WENTON	FEISTY	REDATE	BEHEST
ETONIC	EDITIO	ERESTU	ESCENT	GETOLD	NETMEN	RETORN	BEATUP	GESTIC	NEATEN	RESTIR	WENTTO	FELLTO	REFITS	BEIGHT
ETRADE	EDITOR	ERGOTS	ESCORT	GETOUT	NETPAY	RETORT	BEETLE	GETTER	NEATER	RESTON	WENTUP	FERITY	REFUTE	BEIRUT

BEJART
BELOIT
BENOIT
BEREFT
BESANT
CEMENT
DEBONT
DECANT
DECEIT
DECENT
DECLOT
DECOCT
DEDUCT
DEFEAT
DEFECT
DEGUST
DEJECT
DELICT
DELINT
DELIST
DEMAST
DEMIST
DEPART
DEPEST
DEPICT
DEPORT
DERMAT
DERMOT
DERUST
DESALT
DESERT
DESILT
DESIST
DESPOT
DETECT
DETENT
DETEST
DEVEST
DEVOUT
DEWITT
EELPOT
FEMBOT
FERMAT
FERRET
FEWEST
FEYEST
GEIGHT
GELETT
GERENT
GETFIT
GETHOT
GETOUT
GETSAT
GETSET
GETSIT
GETWET
HEARST
HEGOAT
HEIGHT
HELDIT
HELMET
HELMUT
HENBIT
HEPCAT
HEREAT
HERMIT
HERPET
HESOUT
HEWITT
HEXNUT
IEIGHT
JEERAT
JENNET
JESUIT
JETSET
JEWETT
KEEPAT
KEEPIT
KENSIT
KEPTAT
KERMIT
KEYDET
LEAPAT
LEARNT
LEBRET
LEDOUT
LEERAT
LEFTIT
LEGART
LEGIST
LEGSIT
LESTAT
LETOUT
LETSAT
LEVANT
LEVERT
LEVITT
MEANIT
MELOTT
MEREST
MERLOT
NEEDNT
NERNST
NESBIT
NEWEST
NEWHAT
PEANUT
PECKAT
PEDANT
PEEKAT
PEEPAT
PEERAT
PELLET
PENULT
PEQUOT
PERMIT
PETCAT
PETRAT
PETSAT
PETSIT
PETTET
PETTIT
REBAIT
REBENT
REBOLT
REBOOT
RECANT
RECAST
RECENT
RECOAT
RECOST
REDACT
REDANT
REDBAT
REDDOT
REDHAT
REDHOT
REDOUT
REDUST
REEDIT
REEMIT
REGENT
REGIFT
REGNAT
REGRET
REHEAT
REJECT
REKNIT
REKNOT
RELENT
RELICT
RELIST
RELOST
RELUCT
REMEET
REMELT
REMINT
RENEST
RENNET
REPAST
REPEAT
REPENT
REPLOT
REPORT
REPOST
RERENT
REROOT
RESALT
RESEAT
RESECT
RESENT
RESHOT
RESHUT
RESIFT
RESIST
RESORT
RESPOT
RESUIT
RESULT
RETEST
RETINT
RETORT
REVERT
REVEST
REVOLT
REXCAT
SEACAT
SECANT
SECRET
SEEFIT
SEEOUT
SELECT
SELLIT
SEPTET
SESTET
SETOUT
SETSAT
SEURAT
SEWIST
SEXIST
SEXPOT
SEXTET
TEAACT
TEAPOT
TEARAT
TEARIT
TEASET
TELLIT
TELNET
TENANT
TENHUT
TERRET
VEDIST
VEGOUT
VEIGHT
VELVET
VERIST
VERNET
VERSET
WEEBIT
WEIGHT
WENTAT
WERENT
WESKIT
XEDOUT
XESOUT
YELLAT
YESBUT
ZEALOT
ZENIST

••ET••

ACETAL
ACETIC
ACETYL
AGETEN
AGETWO
ALETAP
ALETTE
ARETES
ARETHA
ARETOO
BEETLE
BRETON
CRETAN
CRETIN
CUETIP
DIETED
DIETER
DIETES
DUETED
DUETTI
DUETTO
EMETIC
EXETER
FLETCH
FOETID
FRETAT
FRETTY
GHETTO
GOETHE
GRETEL
GRETNA
HYETAL
ICETEA
IGETIT
IPETER
JEETER
JOETEX
KAETHE
KVETCH
MEETER
MEETLY
MEETUP
MTETNA
NIETAS
NIETOS
NOETIC
ODETTA
ODETTE
ONETEN
ONETON
ONETWO
OSETRA
PIETAS
PIETER
PIETIN
PIETRO
POETES
POETIC
POETRY
PRETAX
PRETER
PRETOR
PRETTY
RHETOR
SEETHE
SIETES
SKETCH
STETHO
TEETER
TEETHE
THETAS
THETED
THETIS
THETOP
THETOY
TIETAC
TOETAP
TSETSE
USETAX
WRETCH
YVETTE

••E•T•

ADEPTS
ADESTE
AGENTJ
AGENTK
AGENTS
ALECTO
ALERTS
ALETTE
ALEUTS
AMENTS
ATENTH
ATESTS
AVERTS
AVESTA
BLEATS
BLEETH
BREATH
CHEATS
CHEETA
CHERTS
CHERTY
CHESTS
CHESTY
CLEATS
CLEFTS
CREATE
CRESTS
CUESTA
DOESTO
DREWTO
DUETTI
DUETTO
EGESTA
EGESTS
EJECTA
EJECTS
ELECTS
EMEUTE
ERECTS
ERESTU
EVENTS
EVERTS
EXERTS
FEEDTO
FIESTA
FLEETS
FLEWTO
FREETO
FRETTY
GHETTO
GOESTO
GREATS
GREETS
GUESTS
HTESTS
IDEATE
IDENTI
IDENTS
KEEPTO
KLEPTO
LIEDTO
LIESTO
LIEUTS
NEEDTO
NIENTE
NTESTS
OBENTO
OBERTO
ODETTA
ODETTE
OLEATE
OMERTA
OPENTO
OWEDTO
PLEATS
PLEDTO
PLENTY
PRESTO
PRETTY
PUENTE
PUERTO
QUESTS
QWERTY
SCENTS
SEEMTO
SEENTO
SEESTO
SHEATH
SHEETS
SHELTY
SIESTA
SKEETS
SLEETS
SLEETY
SLEUTH
SMELTS
STENTS
SVELTE
SWEATS
SWEATY
SWEETS
THEFTS
TIEDTO
TIESTO
TREATS
TREATY
TRENTA
TRENTE
TRENTO
TWEETS
TWEETY
TWENTY
USEDTO
WHEATS
WREATH
WRESTS
YVETTE

••E••T

ACEDIT
ACEOUT
ACESIT
AGEIST
AGEOUT
ALEAST
APELET
ARENDT
ATEOUT
BEEPAT
BLEWIT
BREAST
BRECHT
BREVET
CHEVET
COEDIT
CREDIT
DIECUT
DIEOUT
DOESIT
DOESNT
DREAMT
DYELOT
DYEVAT
EKEOUT
ELEGIT
EXEMPT
EXEUNT
EYELET
EYEPIT
FLEWAT
FREEST
FRETAT
GOESAT
GREIST
ICEDIT
ICEOUT
ICESIT
IGETIT
IMEANT
ISEEIT
ISEULT
JEERAT
KEEPAT
KEEPIT
KLEIST
KNEWIT
LEERAT
NEEDNT
NLEAST
NOEXIT
OCELOT
ODELET
OMELET
ONEACT
ONEBIT
ONEHIT
ONEOUT
ONESET
OPENIT
OVERIT
PEEKAT
PEEPAT
PEERAT
PIELET
PREACT
PRECUT
PREMET
PRESET
REEDIT
REEMIT
SEEFIT
SEEOUT
SHEBAT
SHEVAT
THEACT
THEIST
THELOT
THEMET
THENET
THEPIT
THERAT
THEVET
USENET
WEEBIT

•••ET•

AGLETS
AMVETS
ARMETS
ARNETT
ARRETE
ASSETS
BEGETS
BERETS
BESETS
BIDETS
BLEETH
BLUETS
BODETT
BURETS
CADETS
CAMETO
CARETO
CARETS
CAVETT
CHEETA
CIVETS
CLOETE
COMETH
COMETO
COMETS
COSETS
COVETS
CRUETS
CULETS
CURETS
DALETH
DALETS
DARETO
DELETE
DESETA
DONETO
DONETS
DUVETS
EBBETS
EFFETE
EGRETS
EMMETS
EMMETT
ETCETC
EXMETS
FACETS
FILETS
FIVETO
FLEETS
FREETO
GAIETY
GAMETE
GARETH
GAVETO
GELETT
GENETS
GIVETH
GIVETO
GLUETO
GODETS
GOLETA
GONETO
GREETS
HATETO
HAVETO
HERETO
HOPETO
HOVETO
INLETS
INSETS
ISLETS
JEWETT
JOBETH
KADETT
LATETO
LIGETI
LIKETO
LIVETH
LIVETV
LOSETO
LOVETO
LOVETT
MANETS
MELETE
MINETA
MOIETY
MONETA
MONETS
MOTETS
MOVETO
MULETA
NICETY
NINETY
NONETS
NOPETS
NYJETS
NYMETS
OBJETS
OCTETS
ONSETS
OSSETS
OWLETS
PARETO
PESETA
PIPETS
PRUETT
QUIETS
RACETO
RAMETS
REBETS
RELETS
RESETS
REVETS
REWETS
RIDETO
RISETO
RIVETS
RODETO
ROGETS
ROSETO
RULETH
SAFETY
SHEETS
SHTETL
SKEETS
SLEETS
SLEETY
SOWETO
STPETE
SURETE
SURETY
SWEETS
TAKETH
TAKETO
TEBETS
TENETS
TERETE
TEVETS
TRUETO
TUNETO
TVSETS
TWEETS
TWEETY
UBIETY
UPSETS
VALETS
VENETO
WAVETO
WISETO

•••E•T

ABJECT
ABLEST
ABSENT
ACCENT
ACCEPT
ADVENT
ADVERT
AFFECT
ALBEIT
ALBERT
ALPERT
ALWEST
APPERT
APTEST
ARDENT
ARGENT
ARNETT
ARREST
ARTEST
ASCENT
ASNEAT
ASPECT
ASSENT
ASSERT
ATBEST
ATREST
ATTEST
BAREST
BASEST
BEHEST
BEREFT
BISECT
BLUEST
BODETT
CADENT
CAMEAT
CAVEAT
CAVETT
CEMENT
CLIENT
COGENT
COMEAT
COVENT
COVERT
COYEST
CUTEST
DARENT
DAREST
DECEIT
DECENT
DEFEAT
DEFECT
DEJECT
DEPEST
DESERT
DETECT
DETENT
DETEST
DEVEST
DIGEST
DINEAT
DIRECT
DIREST
DIVERT
DIVEST
DOCENT
DONEIT
DRIEST
DRYEST
EFFECT
EGBERT
EGGERT
EILERT
ELBERT
ELDEST
EMMETT
ENSEAT
ERNEST
ESCENT
EXCEPT
EXPECT
EXPERT
EXSECT
EXSERT
EXTENT
FACEIT
FAKEIT
FEWEST
FEYEST
FINEST
FIREAT
FLUENT
FOMENT
FOREST
FREEST
FUMEAT
GAMEST
GAPEAT
GAYEST
GAZEAT
GELETT
GERENT
GIBEAT
GOLEFT
GONEAT
GONEXT
GOWEST
HALEST
HATEIT
HAVEAT
HAVEIT
HAVENT
HEREAT
HITEST
HONEST
HUBERT
HUGEST
ICIEST
IDLEST
ILLEST
IMBEAT
IMNEXT
INCENT
INCEPT
INDEBT
INDENT
INFECT
INFEST
INGEST
INJECT
INJEST
INSECT
INSERT
INTENT
INVENT
INVERT
INVEST
IQTEST
ISEEIT
ISLEFT
JAMEST
JAVERT
JEWETT
JIBEAT
KADETT
LAMENT
LAMEST
LATENT
LATEST
LAXEST
LEVERT
LIVEAT
LIVEST
LOSEIT
LOVEIT
LOVETT
LOWEST
LUCENT
MADEIT
MAKEIT
MAYEST
MEREST
MODELT
MODEST
MOLEST
MOMENT
MOVEIT
MUTEST
NAMEIT
NEWEST
NICEST
NLWEST
NOCENT
NOMEAT
NORENT
NUDEST
NUGENT
OBJECT
OBTEST
OBVERT
ODDEST
OLDEST
OLMERT
ORGEAT
ORIENT
OSBERT
OUTEAT
PALEST
PARENT
PATENT
POKEAT
POTENT
PRIEST
PRUETT
PUREST
RAREST
RAVEAT
RAWEST
REBENT
RECENT
REGENT
REHEAT
REJECT
RELENT
REMEET
REMELT
RENEST
REPEAT
REPENT
RERENT
RESEAT
RESECT
RESENT
RETEST
REVERT
REVEST
RIDENT
RIFEST
RIPEST
ROBERT
RODENT
RUDEST
RUPERT
SAFEST
SAGEST
SANEST
SAVEIT
SAYEST
SELECT
SHIEST
SHYEST
SILENT
SLIEST
SLYEST
SOBEIT
SOREAT
SOREST
STREET
SUREST
TAKEIT
TALENT
TAMEST
THREAT
TOREAT
TOREIT
TORENT
TRUEST
UNBELT
UNBENT
UNDEFT
UNFELT
UNKEPT
UNLEFT
UNLENT
UNMEET
UNNEAT
UNPENT
UNRENT
UNREST
UNSEAT
UNSENT
UNWEPT
UPBEAT
UPNEXT
UPSENT
URGENT
URTEXT
VALENT
VILEST
WAVEAT
WERENT
WIDEST
WISEST
WRIEST
WRYEST
YAREST
YCLEPT

••••ET

AIGLET
AIGRET
ALLSET
ALLWET
AMORET
AMULET
ANDYET
ANKLET
APELET
APPLET
ARMLET
AROUET
AUKLET
AVOCET
BALLET
BARBET
BARNET
BARRET
BASKET
BASSET
BECHET
BECKET
BIGBET
BILLET
BISSET
BITNET
BONNET
BORDET
BOXSET
BREVET
BRUNET
BUCKET
BUDGET
BUFFET
BULLET
BURNET
BUTYET
CABLET
CACHET
CALVET
CAPLET
CARNET
CARPET
CASKET
CHALET
CHEVET
CLARET
CLOSET
COLLET
CORNET
CORSET
COSSET
CULLET
CURVET
CUTLET
CYGNET
DAUDET
DIPNET
DOASET
DOCKET
DORSET
DROUET
DULCET
EAGLET
EARLET
ELANET
EXOCET
EYELET
FANJET

FAUCET FERRET FIDGET FILLET FLORET FLYNET FORGET GADGET GANNET GARNET GARRET GASJET GASKET GETSET GETWET GIBLET GIDGET GIMLET GOBLET GOTSET GOTWET GOULET GULLET GUSSET HAMLET HELMET HERPET HORNET ILLBET ILLMET ILLSET IMARET INAPET INKJET JACKET JENNET JETSET JOLIET JULIET JUNKET KEYDET KISMET LANCET LAPPET LARTET LEBRET LIMPET LINNET LIONET LOCKET LOIRET LONGET LOWSET MAGNET MALLET MARKET MIDGET MILLET MINUET MISSET MONNET MOPPET MUFFET MULLET MUPPET MUSKET MUSSET NIBLET

NOIRET NONNET NOTYET NUGGET NUTLET ODELET OFFSET OMELET ONESET OUIMET OUTJET OUTLET OUTSET PACKET PALLET PELLET PETTET PIAGET PICKET PIELET PIGLET PIOLET PIPPET PIQUET PLANET POCKET POIRET PREMET PRESET PRIVET PROJET PULLET PUPPET RABBET RACKET RAMJET REGRET REMEET RENNET RIBLET RICHET RILLET ROCHET ROCKET ROSSET RUNLET RUSSET SACHET SAMLET SECRET SEPTET SESTET SEXTET SIGNET SOCKET SONNET SORBET SOVIET SPINET STREET STYLET SUBLET SUBNET SUBSET SUNSET SWIVET TABLET TABSET

TAPPET TARGET TASKET TEASET TELNET TERRET THEMET THENET THEVET TICKET TILLET TIPPET TISKET TOILET TRIJET TRIVET TUFFET TURRET UNDSET UNMEET USENET VARLET VELVET VERNET VERSET VIOLET WALLET WARVET WASMET WICKET WIDGET WIGLET YAPHET YOUBET

EU••••
EUBOEA EUCHRE EUCKEN EUCLID EUDORA EUGENE EULESS EULOGY EUNICE EUONYM EUPNEA EURAIL EUREKA EUROPA EUROPE EUSDEN EUSTIS EUTAXY

E•U•••
EDUARD EDUCED EDUCES EDUCTS EGUREN EKUELE ELUANT ELUARD ELUATE ELUDED ELUDER ELUDES ELUTED ELUTES ENURED ENURES EQUALS EQUATE EQUINE EQUIPS EQUITY EQUOID ERUCTS ERUPTS ETUDES EVULSE EXUDED EXUDES EXULTS EXURBS

E••U••
EDMUND EFFUSE ELBURZ EMEUTE EMQUAD ENDUED ENDUES ENDURE ENDURO ENDUSE ENGULF ENNUIS ENOUGH ENQUAD ENSUED ENSUES ENSURE ERFURT ESCUDO EXCUBS EXCUSA EXCUSE EXEUNT EXHUME

E•••U•
EARBUD EARFUL EASEUP EATOUT EATSUP EFFLUX EGGCUP EKEOUT ELBRUS EMBRUE EMMAUS ENDCUT ENDRUN ENDSUP ENGLUT ENHAUT ENNIUS ENSOUL EPOQUE ERBIUM EREBUS ESCAUT EVENUP EXITUS EXODUS EYECUP EYEDUP EYEFUL EYESUP

E••••U
EMORYU ERESTU

•EU•••
BEULAH BEURRE DEUCED DEUCES DEUTCH DEUTER FEUDAL FEUDED HEURES HEUSEN LEUTZE NEUMAN NEURAL NEUROL NEURON NEUTER OEUVRE REUBEN REUNED REUNER REUNES REURGE REUSED REUSER REUSES REUTER SEURAT TEUTON ZEUXIS

•E•U••
BEAUTS BEAUTY BEGUMS BELUGA BEMUSE BENUMB BESURE DEBUGS DEBUNK DEBURR DEBUTS DEDUCE DEDUCT DEDUVE DEFUEL DEFUND DEFUSE DEGUMS DEGUST DEJUNK DEJURE DELUDE DELUGE DELUGG DELUXE DEMURE DEMURS DENUDE DEPULP DEPUTE DEPUTY DERUST DETUNE FECUND FEMURS FERULE GENUAL GERUND GETUPS HECUBA JEJUNE JESUIT LEGUIN LEGUME LEHUAS LEMUEL LEMURS LETUPS LETUSE MECUMS MEDUSA MENUDO NEBULA NERUDA NEWULM PENULT PENURY PEQUOD PEQUOT PERUKE PERUSE PERUTZ PETULA REBUFF REBUKE REBURY REBUTS REBUYS RECUED RECUES RECURE RECURL RECURS RECUSE RECUTS REDUBS REDUCE REDUST REFUEL REFUGE REFUND REFUSE REFUTE REHUNG RELUCT RELUME REPUBS REPUGN REPUMP REPUTE RERUNS RESUIT RESULT RESUME RETUNE RETURF RETURN REVUES SECURE SEDUCE SEDUMS SEGUED SEGUES SEGURA SEQUEL SEQUIN SERUMS SETUPS TEAURN TENURE TENUTA TENUTO VELURE VENUES VENULE VENUTI WEEUNS YEHUDI

•E••U•
AECIUM AEOLUS BEADUP BEAMUP BEARUP BEATUP BEDAUB BEDBUG BEEFUP BEFOUL BEIRUT BELLUM BELTUP BENHUR CENSUS CENTUM CEREUS CERIUM CESIUM CESTUS DEALUP DEBLUR DECIUS DELIUS DEPAUL DEPAUW DESLUM DETOUR DEVOUR DEVOUT FEROUS FESCUE FESSUP FESTUS GEARUP GENIUS GETOUT GETSUP HEADUP HEALUP HEAPUP HEATUP HELDUP HELIUM HELMUT HELPUP HESOUT HEXNUT JERKUP JETGUN KEEPUP KEOKUK KEPTUP KEYSUP LEADUP LEAGUE LEAPUP LEBRUN LEDOUT LEDOUX LENGUA LEROUX LETOUR LETOUT LETSUP MEATUS MEDIUM MEDIUS MEETUP MEIFUN MESSUP NEHRUS NESSUS NETFUL NEXTUP PEANUT PELEUS PENSUP PENTUP PEPFUL PEPLUM PEPSUP PERDUE PERKUP PETPUP READUP REARUP RECOUP RECTUS REDBUD REDOUT REDRUM REDSUN REELUP REFLUX REGIUS REGLUE REGNUM REHAUL REPOUR RESCUE RESHUT RESTUP RETOUR REVSUP SEALUP SEAMUS SEENUP SEEOUT SEESUP SENDUP SENTUP SEPTUM SEROUS SESQUI SESSUE SETOUT SETSUP SEWNUP SEWSUP TEACUP TEAMUP TEARUP TEDEUM TEDIUM TEEDUP TEESUP TEMPUS TENHUT VEGOUT VELLUM VELOUR VENDUE VENOUS VERDUN VERSUS WELLUP WENTUP XEDOUT XESOUT YESBUT

•E•••U
DEBREU DEJAVU DESILU DESSAU HEYYOU LEBEAU MENJOU NETHOU PENGPU RESEAU SEEYOU SEZYOU YESYOU

••EU••
ALEUTS BREUER COEURS CREUSA CREUSE EMEUTE EXEUNT FLEURS FREUND ICEUPS ISEULT LIEUTS OLEUMS ONEUPS PLEURA PNEUMA PNEUMO PSEUDO PSEUDS QUEUED QUEUER QUEUES RHEUMS RHEUMY SLEUTH SOEURS THEUSA TIEUPS WEEUNS

••E•U•
ACEOUT ACESUP AGEOUT ALEGUP ATEOUT AVENUE BEEFUP BLEWUP BREWUP CHEQUE CHERUB CHEWUP CUESUP DIECUT DIEOUT DOESUP DREWUP EKEOUT EREBUS EVENUP EYECUP EYEDUP EYEFUL EYESUP FLEWUP FREEUP FRENUM FUELUP GOESUP GREWUP ICEDUP ICEOUT ICERUN ICESUP IREFUL KEEPUP MEETUP OBELUS OLERUD ONEOUT ONERUN OPENUP PLENUM PLEXUS PREBUY PRECUT PRENUP PREVUE REELUP RHESUS RUEFUL SEENUP SEEOUT SEESUP SPEDUP STEPUP TEEDUP TEESUP THEHUB THESUN TIEDUP TIESUP USEDUP USEFUL USESUP UVEOUS WOEFUL

••E••U
APERCU ERESTU SEEYOU THEPRU

•••EU•
ADIEUS ADIEUX ANTEUP ATREUS AUTEUR BAYEUX BITEUP BONEUP BOREUP CAGEUP CAKEUP CAMEUP CEREUS COLEUS COMEUP DISEUR DONEUP DUDEUP EASEUP FACEUP FIREUP FIVEUP FREEUP GAVEUP GIVEUP GONEUP HAVEUP HIKEUP HOLEUP HYPEUP LACEUP LINEUP LYCEUM MADEUP MAKEUP MOVEUP MSIEUR MUSEUM NINEUP NOSEUP PAGEUP PAREUS PELEUS PILEUM PILEUP PILEUS PIPEUP POSEUR RACEUP RAKEUP RAVEUP RIDEUP RILEUP RISEUP RODEUP ROPEUP ROSEUP SAVEUP SIZEUP SOLEUS TAKEUP TAPEUP TEDEUM TONEUP TOREUP TOTEUP TRUEUP TUNEUP TYPEUP URAEUS WAKEUP WIPEUP WIREUP WISEUP WOKEUP

•••E•U
BATEAU BUREAU CADEAU GATEAU JUNEAU LEBEAU MASERU MOREAU OISEAU RAMEAU RESEAU ROSEAU

••••EU
DEBREU DRAKEU INLIEU MILIEU

EV••••
EVADED EVADER EVADES EVELYN EVENAS EVENED EVENER EVENIF EVENLY EVENSO EVENTS EVENUP EVERLY EVERSO EVERTS EVICTS EVILER EVILLY EVINCE EVITES EVOKED EVOKER EVOKES EVOLVE EVONNE EVULSE

E•V•••
EDVARD ELVERS ELVIRA ELVISH ENVEIL ENVIED ENVIER ENVIES ENVIRO ENVOIS ENVOYS ERVING EYVIND

E••V••
EARVIN ELEVEN ELEVES ELEVON EREVAN ERIVAN

E•••V•
ENDIVE EVOLVE EXGOVS

E••••V
ELKONV

•EV•••
BEVANS BEVELS BEVIES DEVANE DEVEGA DEVEIN DEVERE DEVERS DEVEST DEVICE DEVICQ DEVILS DEVINE DEVISE DEVITO DEVOID DEVOIR DEVORE DEVOTE DEVOTO DEVOUR DEVOUT FEVERS JEVONS KEVLAR LEVADE LEVANT LEVEED LEVEES LEVELS LEVENE LEVERS LEVERT LEVIED LEVIER LEVIES LEVINE LEVITE LEVITT LEVITY NEVADA NEVERS NEVILL NEVINS NEVSKI NEVSKY PEVNEY REVAMP REVEAL REVELS REVEND REVERB REVERE REVERS REVERT REVEST REVETS REVIEW REVILE REVISE REVIVE REVLON REVOIR REVOKE REVOLT REVOTE REVSON REVSUP REVUES REVVED SEVENA SEVENB SEVENC SEVEND SEVENE SEVENS SEVERE SEVERN SEVERS SEVRES TEVERE TEVETS

•E•V••
BEAVER BEAVIS BEEVES CERVID DEEVER DELVED DELVER DELVES DENVER FERVID FERVOR GERVIN HEAVED HEAVEN HEAVER HEAVES HERVEY JEEVES KELVIN LEAVED LEAVEN LEAVER LEAVES LEEVES LEOVII MELVIL MELVIN MELVYN MERVYN NERVAL NERVED NERVES OEUVRE PEEVED PEEVES PELVIC PELVIS REAVED REAVER REAVES REAVOW REEVED REEVES RENVOI REVVED SEAVER SELVES SERVED SERVER SERVES SERVOS TEEVEE VELVET VERVES WEAVED WEAVER WEAVES WEEVIL

•E••V•
BEHAVE DEDUVE DEJAVU DENOVO DERIVE GENEVA GENEVE GENOVA LENOVO REGAVE REGIVE RELEVE RELEVY RELIVE REMOVE REPAVE RESAVE REVIVE REWOVE

•E•••V
FELIXV
HENRYV
RENONV
TECHTV

••EV••
ALEVEL
ALEVES
ASEVER
BEEVES
BREVES
BREVET
BREVIS
BSEVEN
CHEVAL
CHEVET
CHEVON
CHEVRE
CHEVYS
CLEVER
CLEVES
COEVAL
DEEVER
DREVIL
DYEVAT
ELEVEN
ELEVES
ELEVON
EREVAN
FIEVEL
GSEVEN
HUEVOS
INEVER
JEEVES
JUEVES
LEEVES
LIEVIO
NIEVES
NUEVES
OLEVEL
PEEVED
PEEVES
PREVIA
PREVIN
PREVUE
REEVED
REEVES
SHEVAT
SIEVED
SIEVES
STEVEN
STEVIE
TEEVEE
THEVET
TREVOR
UNEVEN
UNEVIL
WEEVIL

••E•V•
CLEAVE
GREAVE
ISERVE
SHEAVE
SHELVE
SLEEVE
STEEVE
SWERVE
THEYVE
TWELVE

••E••V
CHEKOV
SCENEV

•••EV•
GENEVA
GENEVE
GRIEVE
HALEVY
PAREVE
RELEVE
RELEVY
SHREVE
SLEEVE
STEEVE
THIEVE

•••E•V
JAMESV
LIVETV

••••EV
ABBREV
KISLEV
LAPTEV
MAGLEV
RUBLEV
SCENEV

EW••••
EWAINE
EWBANK
EWINGS

E•W•••
EDWARD
EDWINA
EDWOOD
EDWYNN
ELWOOD
ENWIND
ENWRAP
EXWIFE

E••W••
EARWAX
EARWIG
EPOWER

E•••W•
ELBOWS
ELFOWL
EMBOWS
ENDOWS

E••••W
ECOLAW
ERENOW
ESCHEW
ESCROW

•EW•••
BEWAIL
BEWARE
BEWARY
BEWELL
BEWIGS
DEWARS
DEWIER
DEWILY
DEWING
DEWIRE
DEWITT
DEWLAP
DEWOLF
DEWORM
FEWEST
GEWGAW
HEWERS
HEWING
HEWISH
HEWITT
HEWSTO
JEWELS
JEWETT
JEWISH
KEWPIE
LEWDER
LEWDLY
MEWERS
MEWING
MEWLED
MEWLER
NEWAGE
NEWARK
NEWBIE
NEWCAR
NEWDAY
NEWELL
NEWELS
NEWERA
NEWEST
NEWHAT
NEWIES
NEWISH
NEWJOB
NEWKID
NEWLEY
NEWMAN
NEWMAR
NEWSIE
NEWSOM
NEWTON
NEWTOY
NEWULM
NEWWAY
PEWEES
PEWITS
PEWTER
REWAKE
REWARD
REWARM
REWARN
REWASH
REWEAR
REWEDS
REWELD
REWETS
REWIND
REWINS
REWIPE
REWIRE
REWOKE
REWORD
REWORE
REWORK
REWORN
REWOVE
REWRAP
SEWAGE
SEWARD
SEWELL
SEWERS
SEWING
SEWIST
SEWNIN
SEWNON
SEWNUP
SEWONS
SEWSIN
SEWSON
SEWSUP

•E•W••
BEDWIN
BERWYN
FENWAY
GETWET
JETWAY
KERWIN
KEYWAY
LEEWAY
MEOWED
MEOWER
NEWWAY
PEDWAY
PEEWEE
REOWNS
RESWAM
RESWIM
SEAWAY
SEGWAY
SEZWHO
TEKWAR

•E••W•
BEDEWS
PESEWA
REDTWO
REMOWN
REMOWS
RENEWS
RENOWN
RESAWN
RESAWS
RESEWN
RESEWS
RESOWN
RESOWS
RETOWS
TENTWO

•E•••W
BELLOW
BENBOW
BERKOW
BESTOW
DECLAW
DEPAUW
FELLOW
GEEGAW
GEWGAW
HEBREW
HEEHAW
MEADOW
MELLOW
NEPHEW
PESCOW
PETCOW
REAVOW
REBREW
RECHEW
REDRAW
REDREW
REFLEW
REFLOW
REGLOW
REGREW
REGROW
REPLOW
RESHOW
RESTOW
RETHAW
REVIEW
SEACOW
SEESAW
YEEHAW
YELLOW

••EW••
BLEWIN
BLEWIT
BLEWON
BLEWUP
BREWED
BREWER
BREWUP
CHEWED
CHEWER
CHEWON
CHEWUP
CLEWED
CREWED
CREWEL
DAEWOO
DREWIN
DREWON
DREWTO
DREWUP
FLEWAT
FLEWBY
FLEWIN
FLEWON
FLEWTO
FLEWUP
FREWER
GREWON
GREWUP
KNEWIT
KNEWOF
KREWES
LEEWAY
MCEWAN
MCEWEN
ONEWAY
PEEWEE
PREWAR
SKEWED
SKEWER
SLEWED
SPEWED
SPEWER
STEWED
STEWER
STEWIE
THEWAY
THEWEB
THEWHO
THEWIZ
VIEWED
VIEWER

••E•W•
AGETWO
ONETWO

••E••W
BYENOW
ERENOW
GEEGAW
HEEHAW
LIELOW
PRELAW
SEESAW
THEDOW
THELAW
YEEHAW

•••EW•
BEDEWS
FIVEWS
NONEWS
PESEWA
RENEWS
RESEWN
RESEWS
SCREWS
SCREWY
SHREWD
SHREWS
SINEWS
SINEWY
STREWN
STREWS
UNDEWY
UNHEWN
UNMEWS
UNSEWN
UNSEWS
USNEWS

••••EW
ALLNEW
ANDREW
CASHEW
CURFEW
CURLEW
ESCHEW
HEBREW
INAFEW
INVIEW
MATHEW
MCGREW
MILDEW
NEPHEW
NONJEW
NOTNEW
ONVIEW
REBREW
RECHEW
REDREW
REFLEW
REGREW
REVIEW
TVCREW
UNDREW
UNSKEW
UPGREW

EX••••
EXACTA
EXACTS
EXALTS
EXARCH
EXCEED
EXCELS
EXCEPT
EXCESS
EXCIDE
EXCISE
EXCITE
EXCONS
EXCUBS
EXCUSA
EXCUSE
EXEDRA
EXEMPT
EXERTS
EXETER
EXEUNT
EXGOVS
EXHALE
EXHORT
EXHUME
EXILED
EXILER
EXILES
EXILIC
EXISTS
EXITED
EXITUS
EXMATE
EXMETS
EXMOOR
EXMORE
EXOCET
EXODUS
EXONYM
EXOTIC
EXPAND
EXPATS
EXPECT
EXPELS
EXPEND
EXPERT
EXPIRE
EXPIRY
EXPORT
EXPOSE
EXPOST
EXSECT
EXSERT
EXTANT
EXTEND
EXTENT
EXTERN
EXTOLL
EXTOLS
EXTORT
EXTRAS
EXUDED
EXUDES
EXULTS
EXURBS
EXWIFE
EXYANK

E••X••
ELIXIR

E•••X•
EUTAXY

E••••X
EARWAX
EFFLUX

•EX•••
DEXTER
DEXTRO
HEXADS
HEXANE
HEXERS
HEXING
HEXNUT
HEXOSE
MEXICO
NEXRAD
NEXTEL
NEXTTO
NEXTUP
REXALL
REXCAT
SEXERS
SEXIER
SEXILY
SEXISM
SEXIST
SEXPOT
SEXTET
SEXTON
TEXACO
TEXANS
TEXMEX
TEXTED
VEXERS
VEXING

•E•X••
GENXER
LEOXII
XERXES
ZEUXIS

•E••X•
DELUXE
FELIXI
FELIXV

•E•••X
BENDIX
LEDOUX
LENNOX
LEROUX
MEATAX
MERCKX
NEELIX
PEGBOX
PENTAX
REDFOX
REDSIX
REDSOX
REFLEX
REFLUX
SEAFOX
TEEBOX
TEXMEX
VERTEX
WESSEX

••EX••
ALEXAS
ALEXEI
ALEXEY
ALEXIA
ALEXIS
APEXES
DREXEL
FLEXED
FLEXES
FLEXOR
IBEXES
ILEXES
NOEXIT
OREXIA
OREXIS
PLEXAL
PLEXES
PLEXOR
PLEXUS
PREXES
TREXES

••E•X•
ICEAXE
THEAXE

••E••X
AGESIX
ICEBOX
JOETEX
NEELIX
PREFIX
PREMIX
PRETAX
TEEBOX
THEFOX
THESOX
USETAX

•••EX•
GONEXT
IMNEXT
UNSEXY
UPNEXT
URTEXT

•••E•X
ADIEUX
BAYEUX
BLUEOX
POLEAX
RATEDX

••••EX
AUSPEX
CALMEX
COMDEX
CONVEX
CORTEX
DIPLEX
DUPLEX
JOETEX
LASTEX
POLLEX
REFLEX
SUSSEX
TEXMEX
UNISEX
VERTEX
VORTEX
WESSEX
WINDEX

EY••••
EYECUP
EYEDUP
EYEFUL
EYEING
EYELET
EYELID
EYEPIT
EYESUP
EYRIES
EYVIND

E•Y•••
EEYORE
ELYRIA
ELYSEE
ELYTIS
ERYKAH
ERYNGO
ETYMOL
ETYMON
EXYANK

E••Y••
EASYAS
EASYGO
EBAYER
ECTYPE
EDWYNN
EGOYAN
ELAYER
ELAYNE
ENCYCL
ENZYME
ETHYLS

E•••Y•
EMBAYS
EMBRYO
EMILYS
EMORYU
ENJOYS
ENVOYS
EPONYM
ERINYS
ESSAYS
EUONYM
EVELYN
EXONYM

E••••Y
EARTHY
EASEBY
EASILY
EASLEY
EATERY
EBERLY
ECTOMY
EDGILY
EDIBLY
EELERY
EERILY
EFFIGY
EIGHTY
EISLEY
EKEDBY
EKESBY
ELLERY
EMBODY
EMPERY
EMPLOY
ENERGY
ENMITY
ENTITY
EQUITY
ESTRAY
EULOGY
EUTAXY
EVENLY
EVERLY
EVILLY
EXPIRY

•EY•••
BEYMER
BEYOND
CEYLON
EEYORE
FEYEST
GEYSER
HEYDAY
HEYMAN
HEYYOU
KEYDET
KEYING
KEYMAN
KEYMEN
KEYNES
KEYOFA
KEYOFB
KEYOFC
KEYOFD
KEYOFF
KEYOFG
KEYPAD
KEYPAL
KEYSER
KEYSIN
KEYSON
KEYSUP
KEYWAY
LEYDEN
MEYERS
PEYOTE
PEYTON
REYLES
REYOKE

•E•Y••
BERYLS
HEGYES
HEYYOU
JEKYLL
KENYAN
KENYON
MERYLL
REDYED
REDYES
RELYON
RETYPE
SEEYOU
SEZYOU
YESYES
YESYOU

•E••Y•
BELAYS
BERWYN
BETSYS
BETTYE
DECAYS
DECOYS
DELAYS
DENNYS
HEARYE
HENRYI
HENRYK
HENRYV
JESSYE
KELLYS
KENNYG
MELVYN
MERVYN
METHYL
REBUYS
REDEYE
REKEYS
RELAYS
REPAYS
RESAYS
SEALYS
SEPOYS
TETHYS
WENDYS
ZEPHYR

•E•••Y
AERIFY
AERILY
BEACHY
BEATTY
BEAUTY
BEGLEY
BELFRY
BELLAY
BENDAY
BENGAY
BENSEY
BETONY
BETRAY
BETSEY
BEWARY
CEDARY
CELERY
DEADLY
DEAFLY
DEARLY
DEBRAY
DEEJAY
DEEPLY
DEFRAY
DEFTLY
DELANY
DELKEY
DELRAY
DELREY
DELROY
DENARY
DEPLOY
DEPUTY
DESCRY
DESTRY
DEWILY
EELERY
EERILY
FEALTY
FEEBLY
FEISTY
FELONY
FENWAY
FERITY
GELSEY
GENTLY
GENTRY
GEORGY
GETSBY
HEALEY
HEANEY
HEARTY
HEATHY
HEDLEY
HENDRY
HENLEY
HEREBY
HERESY
HERSEY
HERVEY
HEYDAY
JENNEY
JEREMY
JERSEY
JETWAY
KEARNY
KEENLY
KELLEY
KELSEY
KEYWAY
LEACHY
LEAKEY
LEALTY
LEANLY
LEEMAY
LEEWAY
LEGACY
LEMONY
LENITY
LESLEY
LETFLY
LETSBY
LEVITY
LEWDLY
MEANEY
MEANLY
MEASLY
MEDFLY
MEDLEY
MEEKLY
MEETLY
MELODY
MEMORY
MEOHMY
MERELY
MERSEY
NEARBY
NEARLY
NEATLY
NETPAY
NETTLY
NEVSKY
NEWDAY
NEWLEY
NEWTOY
NEWWAY
PEACHY
PEARLY
PEBBLY
PEDWAY
PELTRY
PENNEY
PENURY
PEPBOY
PERDAY
PERTLY
PETTOY
PEVNEY
REALLY
REALTY
REBURY
RECOPY
REDBAY
REDEFY
REDENY
REDSKY
REILLY
RELEVY
REMEDY
REPLAY
RESINY
SEAWAY
SEDLEY
SEEMLY
SEGWAY
SELLBY
SENARY
SENDBY
SENTBY
SENTRY
SETSBY
SEXILY
TEAPOY
TEDKEY
TEENSY
TENDAY
TENLEY
TETCHY
TETLEY
VEEJAY
VERIFY
VERILY
VERITY
VESTRY
WEAKLY
WEEKLY
WEENSY
WEIRDY
WENTBY
WESLEY
WETFLY
YEARLY
YEASTY

••EY••
BAEYER
BREYER
DREYER
GREYED
GREYER
GREYLY
OBEYED
OBEYER
OXEYES
PREYED
PREYER
PREYON
SEEYOU
THEYLL
THEYRE
THEYVE
WHEYEY

••E•Y•
ACETYL
AYEAYE
BYEBYE
CHERYL
CHEVYS
EVELYN
LIEBYS
ONEEYE
SHERYL
THEEYE
TIEDYE

••E••Y
AGEDLY
AGENCY
ALECKY
ALEXEY
ANERGY
ASEASY
AWEARY
AWEDLY
BLEARY
BOESKY
BREEDY
BREEZY
BRENLY
CHEEKY
CHEERY
CHEESY
CHENEY
CHERRY
CHERTY
CHESTY

CLEARY
CLERGY
CREAKY
CREAMY
CREASY
CREEPY
CRESSY
CZERNY
DEEJAY
DEEPLY
DOESBY
DREAMY
DREARY
DRECKY
DRESSY
DWEEBY
EBERLY
EKEDBY
EKESBY
ENERGY
EVENLY
EVERLY
FEEBLY
FLECKY
FLEDGY
FLEECY
FLESHY
FLEWBY
FREAKY
FREDDY
FREELY
FRENZY
FRETTY
GLEAMY
GOEASY
GOESBY
GREASY
GREEDY
GREENY
GREYLY
IMEASY
KEENLY
LEEMAY
LEEWAY
LIEFLY
MEEKLY
MEETLY
OHENRY
OLEARY
ONEDAY
ONEWAY
OPENLY
OVERLY
PLENTY
POETRY
PREBUY
PREDAY
PREDRY
PREPAY
PREPPY
PRETTY
QUEASY
QUEMOY
QWERTY
RHEUMY
RKELLY
SEEMLY
SHECKY
SHEEDY
SHEEHY
SHEENY
SHELBY
SHELTY
SHERRY
SLEAZY
SLEEKY
SLEEPY
SLEETY
SMEARY
SMELLY
SNEAKY
SNEERY
SNEEZY
SPEEDY
SPENDY
SPERRY
STEADY
STEAMY
STEELY
STEFOY
STEMMY
SWEATY
TEENSY
THEBAY
THEFLY
THEORY
THESPY
THETOY
THEWAY
TREATY
TREBLY
TRENDY
TRESSY
TWEAKY
TWEEDY
TWEENY
TWEETY
TWENTY
UNEASY
VEEJAY
WEEKLY
WEENSY
WHEEZY
WHERRY
WHEYEY
WIELDY

•••EY•
ABBEYS
ALLEYN
ALLEYS
BIGEYE
BOGEYS
BOLEYN
CONEYS
COVEYS
CUTEYS
DRYEYE
FOGEYS
FOLEYS
GODEYS
HOMEYS
HONEYS
ISLEYS
LOOEYS
LOVEYA
LOVEYS
MATEYS
MONEYS
MOSEYS
MULEYS
ONEEYE
POKEYS
POPEYE
REDEYE
REKEYS
RIBEYE
THEEYE

•••E•Y
AMBERY
ARTERY
BAKERY
BARELY
BASELY
BLUELY
BLUESY
BOWERY
BREEDY
BREEZY
BRIERY
CAMEBY
CASEFY
CELERY
CHEEKY
CHEERY
CHEESY
CICELY
CIDERY
COMEBY
COMEDY
COMELY
CREEPY
CUTELY
CUTESY
DIRELY
DONEBY
DOWERY
DUPERY
DWEEBY
EASEBY
EATERY
EELERY
ELLERY
EMPERY
FAKERY
FILEBY
FINELY
FINERY
FLEECY
FREELY
GAIETY
GAMELY
GONEBY
GREEDY
GREENY
HALEVY
HEREBY
HERESY
HOMELY
HUGELY
JAPERY
JEREMY
JONESY
LAMELY
LATELY
LIKELY
LINENY
LIVELY
LIVERY
LONELY
LOVELY
LOWERY
MERELY
MISERY
MOIETY
MOPERY
MUTELY
NAMELY
NAPERY
NASEBY
NICELY
NICETY
NINETY
NITERY
NUDELY
OCHERY
ORNERY
ORRERY
OWLERY
PALELY
PAPERY
PINERY
POKERY
PURELY
RACEBY
RAREFY
RARELY
REDEFY
REDENY
RELEVY
REMEDY
RIDEBY
RIFELY
RIPELY
RODEBY
RONELY
ROPERY
ROSERY
RUDELY
RUDERY
SAFELY
SAFETY
SAGELY
SANELY
SCREWY
SHEEDY
SHEEHY
SHEENY
SINEWY
SLEEKY
SLEEPY
SLEETY
SNEERY
SNEEZY
SOLELY
SORELY
SPEEDY
STEELY
SURELY
SURETY
TAMELY
TILERY
TIMELY
TOWERY
TUMEFY
TWEEDY
TWEENY
TWEETY
UBIETY
UNDEWY
UNSEXY
VALERY
VILELY
VINERY
VOWELY
WAFERY
WATERY
WAVERY
WHEEZY
WIDELY
WIFELY
WINERY
WISELY
YARELY

••••EY
ALEXEY
ALTKEY
ANDREY
ASHLEY
ASTLEY
AUBREY
AUDREY
BAILEY
BARLEY
BARNEY
BASSEY
BATLEY
BEGLEY
BENSEY
BETSEY
BINNEY
BIRNEY
BLAKEY
BLIMEY
BLOOEY
BODLEY
BONNEY
BOSLEY
BURLEY
BURNEY
CAGNEY
CARKEY
CARNEY
CARREY
CARSEY
CARVEY
CHANEY
CHENEY
CLAYEY
CONVEY
COOLEY
COONEY
COPLEY
COWLEY
CRIKEY
CURLEY
DABNEY
DAILEY
DELKEY
DELREY
DICKEY
DILSEY
DISNEY
DOLLEY
DOMBEY
DONKEY
DOOLEY
DORSEY
DOWNEY
DUDLEY
DURFEY
EASLEY
EISLEY
FARLEY
FINLEY
FINNEY
FLOOEY
FLOREY
FLUKEY
FOSSEY
GALLEY
GARVEY
GELSEY
GILLEY
GOONEY
GOOSEY
GORCEY
GRAPEY
GURLEY
GURNEY
HAILEY
HALLEY
HALSEY
HANLEY
HARLEY
HARNEY
HARVEY
HAYLEY
HEALEY
HEANEY
HEDLEY
HENLEY
HERSEY
HERVEY
HICKEY
HOCKEY
HOLLEY
HOOKEY
HORSEY
HOTKEY
HUBLEY
HUNLEY
HURLEY
HUSSEY
HUXLEY
INGREY
JANNEY
JENNEY
JERSEY
JITNEY
JOCKEY
JOLLEY
KELLEY
KELSEY
KIDNEY
KINSEY
LACHEY
LACKEY
LAUREY
LEAKEY
LESLEY
LINNEY
LOONEY
LOOSEY
LOWKEY
LUMLEY
LURKEY
LYNLEY
MABLEY
MANLEY
MARKEY
MARLEY
MASSEY
MEANEY
MEDLEY
MERSEY
MICKEY
MISKEY
MOBLEY
MONKEY
MOONEY
MORLEY
MOSLEY
MOTLEY
MOUSEY
NEWLEY
NIAMEY
NIPSEY
OAKLEY
OCASEY
OFFKEY
ORKNEY
OSPREY
PARLEY
PAULEY
PENNEY
PEVNEY
PHONEY
PHOOEY
PITNEY
POMPEY
PRICEY
PTOOEY
PULLEY
PURVEY
PUTNEY
RADLEY
RAINEY
RAMSEY
RICKEY
RIDLEY
RIPLEY
RODNEY
ROMNEY
RONCEY
ROONEY
ROWLEY
SAYHEY
SEDLEY
SHALEY
SIDNEY
SISLEY
SMILEY
SMOKEY
SPACEY
SPIDEY
STACEY
STAGEY
STONEY
SURREY
SURVEY
SYDNEY
TABKEY
TEDKEY
TENLEY
TETLEY
TILLEY
TOOMEY
TORREY
TRACEY
TUNNEY
TURKEY
VALLEY
VARNEY
VOLLEY
WATNEY
WESLEY
WHALEY
WHEYEY
WHITEY
WIMSEY
WOLSEY
WOOLEY
WORLEY
YAWKEY

EZ••••
EZINES
EZPASS
EZZARD

E•Z•••
ECZEMA
ENZYME
EZZARD

E••••Z
ELBURZ
ENTREZ
ERSATZ

•EZ•••
BEZELS
FEZZED
FEZZES
MEZZOS
REZERO
REZIPS
REZONE
SEZWHO
SEZYOU
VEZINA

•E•Z••
BEEZER
BELZER
BENZOL
DENZEL
FEZZED
FEZZES
GEEZER
HERZOG
MEZZOS
SEIZED
SEIZER
SEIZES
SEIZOR
SETZER
TETZEL
WEEZER

•E••Z•
BEDAZE
BELIZE
LEUTZE
REBOZO
RESIZE

•E•••Z
LESMIZ
MEGREZ
MESAAZ
PERUTZ

••EZ••
AREZZO
BEEZER
DIEZES
GEEZER
OYEZES
QUEZON
SLEZAK
WEEZER

••E•Z•
AREZZO
BREEZE
BREEZY
FREEZE
FRENZY
PUENZO
RIENZI
SLEAZE
SLEAZY
SNEEZE
SNEEZY
TREIZE
TWEEZE
WHEEZE
WHEEZY

••E••Z
THEWIZ

•••EZ•
BREEZE
BREEZY
CABEZA
FREEZE
FRIEZE
SNEEZE
SNEEZY
TWEEZE
WHEEZE
WHEEZY

•••E•Z
BONERZ
BRIENZ
DOLENZ
LORENZ

••••EZ
BOULEZ
CHAVEZ
CORTEZ
ENTREZ
IBANEZ
JUAREZ
MEGREZ
MONTEZ
PARLEZ
TROPEZ
VALDEZ

FA••••
FABBER
FABIAN
FABLED
FABLER
FABLES
FABRAY
FABRIC
FACADE
FACEIT
FACEON
FACERS
FACETS
FACEUP
FACIAE
FACIAL
FACIAS
FACIES
FACILE
FACING
FACTOR
FACTUM
FACULA
FADDLE
FADEIN
FADERS
FADING
FAENAS
FAERIE
FAEROE
FAFNER
FAFNIR
FAGEND
FAGINS
FAGOTS
FAILED
FAILLE
FAILTO
FAIMAN
FAINER
FAINTS
FAIRED
FAIRER
FAIRLY
FAIRUP
FAISAL
FAITES
FAITHS
FAJITA
FAKEID
FAKEIT
FAKERS
FAKERY
FAKING
FAKIRS
FALALA
FALANA
FALCON
FALINE
FALLAL
FALLEN
FALLER
FALLIN
FALLON
FALLOW
FALLTO
FALSER
FALTER
FALUDI
FAMILY
FAMINE
FAMING
FAMISH
FAMOUS
FAMULI
FANDOM
FANFIC
FANGED
FANGIO
FANION
FANJET
FANNED
FANNER
FANNIE
FANONS
FANOUT
FANTAN
FANTAS
FAQIRS
FARACY
FARADS
FARAHS
FARCED
FARCES
FARCRY
FARERS
FARFEL
FARINA
FARING
FARLEY
FARLOW
FARMED
FARMER
FARNUM
FAROES
FAROFF
FAROUK
FAROUT
FARRAH
FARRAR
FARRIS
FARROW
FARUKI
FASCES
FASCIA
FASTED
FASTEN
FASTER
FATALE
FATCAT
FATHER
FATHOM
FATIMA
FATLIP
FATMAN
FATONE
FATSIS
FATTED
FATTEN
FATTER
FATWAS
FAUCET
FAULTS
FAULTY
FAUNAE
FAUNAL
FAUNAS
FAUNUS
FAUTES
FAUVES
FAVORS
FAVOUR
FAWKES
FAWLTY
FAWNED
FAWNER
FAWNON
FAXERS
FAXING
FAYARD
FAYLEN
FAZING
FAZOOL

F•A•••
FEALTY
FEARED
FEARER
FEASTS
FIACRE
FIANCE
FIASCO
FLABBY
FLACKS
FLACON
FLAGGY
FLAGON
FLAILS
FLAIRS
FLAKED
FLAKER
FLAKES
FLAMBE
FLAMED
FLAMER
FLAMES
FLANGE
FLANKS
FLAPPY
FLARED
FLARES
FLASHY
FLASKS
FLATLY
FLATTV
FLAUNT
FLAUTA
FLAVIA
FLAVOR
FLAWED
FLAXEN
FLAXES
FLAYED
FLAYER
FMAJOR
FOALED
FOAMED
FOAMER
FRACAS
FRACTO
FRAIDY
FRAISE
FRAKES
FRAMED
FRAMER
FRAMES
FRANCA
FRANCE
FRANCK
FRANCO
FRANCS
FRANKS
FRANNY
FRANTZ
FRAPPE
FRASER
FRATER
FRAUDS
FRAUEN
FRAYED
FRAZER

F••A••
FACADE
FALALA
FALANA
FARACY
FARADS
FARAHS
FATALE
FAYARD
FEMALE
FERALS
FFLATS
FIGARO
FINALE
FINALS
FIXATE
FLOATS
FLOATY
FLYASH
FMBAND
FOLATE
FORAGE
FORAYS
FREAKS
FREAKY
FRIARS
FRIARY
FSCALE
FSHARP
FSTARS
FUGARD
FUGATO

F•••A•
FABIAN
FABRAY
FACIAE
FACIAL
FACIAS
FAENAS
FAIMAN
FAISAL
FALLAL
FANTAN
FANTAS
FARRAH
FARRAR
FATCAT
FATMAN
FATWAS
FAUNAE
FAUNAL
FAUNAS
FBIMAN
FELLAH
FELLAS
FENWAY
FERIAS
FERMAT
FERNAO
FESTAL
FESTAS
FEUDAL
FIGBAR
FIJIAN
FILIAL
FINCAS
FINIAL
FINIAN
FINNAN
FIREAT
FISCAL
FIVEAA
FIVEAD
FIVEAM
FLEWAT
FLORAE
FLORAL
FLORAS
FLYMAN
FLYWAY
FOEMAN
FOLIAR
FONDAS
FONTAL
FORBAD
FORMAL
FORMAN
FORMAT
FORNAX
FORTAS
FOSSAE
FOURAA
FOURAD
FOURAM
FRACAS
FRETAT
FRIDAY
FRITAS
FRUGAL
FRYPAN
FULMAR
FUMEAT
FUNGAL
FURMAN
FUSSAT

F••••A
FACULA
FAJITA
FALALA
FALANA
FARINA
FASCIA
FATIMA
FEDORA
FEMORA
FIBULA
FIESTA
FIVEAA
FLAUTA
FLAVIA
FLICKA
FOURAA
FRANCA
FRESCA
FRICKA
FRIEDA
FRITTA
FRUSTA
FULCRA
FUSUMA
FUTUNA
FUTURA

•F•A••
AFEARD
AFFAIR
AFLAME
AFLARE
AFLATS
AFRAID
AFRAME
BFLATS
CFLATS
DFLATS
EFFACE
EFLATS
FFLATS
GFLATS
LFRANK
OFFALS
OFFALY
OFLATE

•F••A•
AFFRAY
AFGHAN
AFLOAT
IFICAN
IFIMAY
OFFDAY

•F•••A
AFRICA
SFORZA

••FA••
AAFAIR
AFFAIR
ARFARF

ASFAST
AUFAIT
BEFAIR
BEFALL
DEFACE
DEFAME
DEFANG
DEFATS
EFFACE
ENFACE
ENFAIT
ENFANT
GOFAST
INFACT
INFALL
INFAMY
INFANT
MUFASA
NOFAIR
OFFALS
OFFALY
RAFAEL
REFACE
REFALL
SAFARI
UNFACT
UNFAIR

••F•A•
AFFRAY
ASFLAT
BUFFAY
CAFTAN
DEFEAT
DEFJAM
DEFOAM
DEFRAG
DEFRAY
ELFMAN
GOFLAT
GUFFAW
INFEAR
MAFIAS
OFFDAY
REFLAG
UNFLAT
USFLAG

••F••A
DEFLEA
MUFASA
RAFFIA

•••FA•
ARAFAT
BIGFAN
BUFFAY
COLFAX
CONFAB
CORFAM
CUBFAN
GETFAR
GOTFAR
GUFFAW
HOWFAR
JETFAN
KOUFAX
LOOFAH
LOOFAS
LOWFAT
METFAN
NAKFAS
NONFAN
NONFAT
NOTFAR
PREFAB
RAMFAN
SHOFAR
SOXFAN
STEFAN
SULFAS
SUNFAN
THEFAN
TOOFAR

•••F•A
BIAFRA
RAFFIA

••••FA
KEYOFA

FB••••
FBIMAN
FBIMEN

F•B•••
FABBER
FABIAN
FABLED
FABLER
FABLES
FABRAY
FABRIC
FIBBED
FIBBER
FIBERS
FIBRES
FIBRIN
FIBULA
FMBAND
FOBBED
FOBOFF

F••B••
FABBER
FEEBLE
FEEBLY
FEMBOT
FERBER
FIBBED
FIBBER
FIGBAR
FLABBY
FLUBUG
FLYBOY
FLYBYS
FOBBED
FOGBOW
FOIBLE
FORBAD
FORBES
FORBID
FUMBLE
FURBYS

F•••B•
FILEBY
FIVEBC
FLABBY
FLAMBE
FLEWBY
FLITBY
FOURBC

••F•B•
LEFTBE

•••FB•
THEFBI

•••F•B
CONFAB
PREFAB

••••FB
KEYOFB

F•C•••
FACADE
FACEIT
FACEON
FACERS
FACETS
FACEUP
FACIAE
FACIAL
FACIAS
FACIES
FACILE
FACING
FACTOR
FACTUM
FACULA
FECUND
FICHES
FICHTE
FICHUS
FICKLE
FOCSLE
FSCALE
FSCOTT

F••C••
FALCON
FARCED
FARCES
FARCRY
FASCES
FASCIA
FATCAT
FAUCET
FENCED
FENCER
FENCES
FESCUE
FIACRE
FINCAS
FISCAL
FLACKS
FLACON
FLECHE
FLECKS
FLECKY
FLICKA
FLICKS
FLOCKS
FORCED
FORCER
FORCES
FORCHE
FRACAS
FRACTO
FRICKA
FRICKE
FROCKS
FRUCTI
FULCRA

F•••C•
FARACY
FELICE
FIANCE
FIASCO
FIERCE
FLEECE
FLEECY
FLETCH
FLINCH
FRANCA
FRANCE
FRANCK
FRANCO
FRANCS
FRENCH
FRESCA
FRESCO
FRISCH
FRISCO

F••••C
FABRIC
FANFIC
FERENC
FERRIC
FILMIC
FINNIC
FISTIC
FIVEBC
FORMIC
FOURBC
FROLIC

•F•C••
AFLCIO
IFICAN

•F••C•
AFFECT
AFRICA
EFFACE
EFFECT
GFORCE
OFFICE

••FC••
DEFCON

••F•C•
AFFECT
DEFACE
DEFECT
EFFACE
EFFECT
ENFACE
INFACT
INFECT
OFFICE
REFACE
SAFECO
UNFACT

•••F•C
DEIFIC
FANFIC
UNIFIC

••••FC
KEYOFC

F•D•••
FADDLE
FADEIN
FADERS
FADING
FEDORA
FIDDLE
FIDGET
FIDLER
FODDER
FODORS
FUDDLE
FUDGED
FUDGER
FUDGES

F••D••
FADDLE
FANDOM
FEEDER
FEEDIN
FEEDME
FEEDON
FEEDTO
FELDON
FENDED
FENDER
FEODOR
FERDIE
FEUDAL
FEUDED
FIDDLE
FINDER
FLEDGE
FLEDGY
FODDER
FOGDOG
FOLDED
FOLDER
FOLDIN
FOLDUP
FONDAS
FONDER
FONDLE
FONDLY
FONDOF
FONDUE
FONDUS
FOODIE
FORDED
FORDGT
FORDID
FOUDRE
FREDDY
FREDRO
FRIDAY
FRIDGE
FUDDLE
FUNDED
FUNDER
FYODOR

F•••D•
FACADE
FALUDI
FARADS
FELIDS
FIELDS
FIENDS
FIORDS
FJORDS
FLOODS
FLUIDS
FOUNDS
FRAIDY
FRAUDS
FREDDY
FRIEDA
FRONDS

F••••D
FABLED
FAGEND
FAILED
FAIRED
FAKEID
FANGED
FANNED
FARCED
FARMED
FASTED
FATTED
FAWNED
FAYARD
FEARED
FECUND
FELLED
FELTED
FENCED
FENDED
FERVID
FESSED
FEUDED
FEZZED
FIBBED
FILLED
FILMED
FINKED
FINNED
FIRMED
FISHED
FISTED
FITTED
FIVEAD
FIZZED
FLAKED
FLAMED
FLARED
FLAWED
FLAYED
FLEXED
FLORID
FLOWED
FLUTED
FLUXED
FLYROD
FMBAND
FOALED
FOAMED
FOBBED
FOETID
FOGGED
FOILED
FOLDED
FOOLED
FOOTED
FORBAD
FORBID
FORCED
FORDED
FORDID
FORGED
FORKED
FORMED
FOULED
FOURAD
FOWLED
FRAMED
FRAYED
FREUND
FRIEND
FRIGID
FUDGED
FUELED
FUGARD
FUNDED
FUNKED
FUNNED
FURLED
FURRED
FUSSED
FUTZED
FUZZED

•F•D••
OFFDAY

•F•••D
AFEARD
AFFORD
AFIELD
AFRAID
EFILED
OFFEND

••FD••
OFFDAY

••F••D
AFFORD
ALFRED
AUFOND
BAFFED
BIFFED
BIFOLD
BOFFED
BUFFED
CUFFED
DEFEND
DEFIED
DEFORD
DEFUND
DOFFED
ENFOLD
GAFFED
GIFTED
HAFTED
HEFTED
HUFFED
INFOLD
LIFTED
LOFTED
LUFFED
MIFFED
MUFFED
OFFEND
OXFORD
PUFFED
RAFTED
REFEED
REFFED
REFIED
REFIND
REFOLD
REFUND
RIFFED
RIFLED
RIFTED
RUFFED
SIFTED
TIFFED
TUFTED
UNFOLD
UNFOND
UPFOLD
WAFTED
WIFIED

•••F•D
BAFFED
BEEFED
BIFFED
BOFFED
BUFFED
CHAFED
CHEFED
COIFED
CONFED
CUFFED
DOFFED
GAFFED
GOLFED
GOOFED
GULFED
HOOFED
HUFFED
ILLFED
KNIFED
LEAFED
LOAFED
LUFFED
MIFFED
MISFED
MUFFED
NONFED
POUFED
PUFFED
REEFED
REFFED
RIFFED
ROLFED
ROOFED
RUFFED
SURFED
THEFED
TIFFED
TURFED
WEBFED
WOLFED
WOOFED

••••FD
KEYOFD

FE••••
FEALTY
FEARED
FEARER
FEASTS
FECUND
FEDORA
FEEBLE
FEEBLY
FEEDER
FEEDIN
FEEDME
FEEDON
FEEDTO
FEEING
FEEJEE
FEELER
FEELOK
FEIGNS
FEINTS
FEISTY
FELDON
FELICE
FELIDS
FELINE
FELIPE
FELIXI
FELIXV
FELLAH
FELLAS
FELLED
FELLER
FELLIN
FELLON
FELLOW
FELLTO
FELONS
FELONY
FELSON
FELTED
FELTOK
FEMALE
FEMBOT
FEMMES
FEMORA
FEMURS
FENCED
FENCER
FENCES
FENDED
FENDER
FENNEL
FENNER
FENWAY
FEODOR
FEOFFS
FERALS
FERBER
FERDIE
FERENC
FERGIE
FERIAS
FERITY
FERMAT
FERMIS
FERNAO
FEROUS
FERRER
FERRET
FERRIC
FERRIS
FERULE
FERVID
FERVOR
FESCUE
FESSED
FESSES
FESSUP
FESTAL
FESTAS
FESTER
FESTUS
FETING
FETISH
FETORS
FETTER
FETTLE
FEUDAL
FEUDED
FEVERS
FEWEST
FEYEST
FEZZED
FEZZES

F•E•••
FAENAS
FAERIE
FAEROE
FEEBLE
FEEBLY
FEEDER
FEEDIN
FEEDME
FEEDON
FEEDTO
FEEING
FEEJEE
FEELER
FEELOK
FIELDS
FIENDS
FIERCE
FIEROS
FIESTA
FIEVEL
FLECHE
FLECKS
FLECKY
FLEDGE
FLEDGY
FLEECE
FLEECY
FLEERS
FLEETS
FLENSE
FLESHY
FLETCH
FLEURS
FLEWAT
FLEWBY
FLEWIN
FLEWON
FLEWTO
FLEWUP
FLEXED
FLEXES
FLEXOR
FOEMAN
FOEMEN
FOETID
FREAKS
FREAKY
FREDDY
FREDRO
FREELY
FREEOF
FREERS
FREEST
FREETO
FREEUP
FREEZE
FRENCH
FRENUM
FRENZY
FREONS
FRERES
FRESCA
FRESCO
FRESNO
FRETAT
FRETTY
FREUND
FREWER
FUEGOS
FUELED
FUELER
FUELUP

F••E••
FACEIT
FACEON
FACERS
FACETS
FACEUP
FADEIN
FADERS
FAGEND
FAKEID
FAKEIT
FAKERS
FAKERY
FARERS
FAXERS
FERENC
FEVERS
FEWEST
FEYEST
FIBERS
FIFERS
FILEBY
FILEIN
FILENE
FILERS
FILETS
FINELY
FINERY
FINEST
FIREAT
FIREON
FIRERS
FIREUP
FIVEAA
FIVEAD
FIVEAM
FIVEBC
FIVEEE
FIVENO
FIVEOF
FIVEPM
FIVERS
FIVETO
FIVEUP
FIVEWS
FIXERS
FLEECE
FLEECY
FLEERS
FLEETS
FLIERS
FLUENT
FLYERS
FOGEYS
FOLEYS
FOMENT
FOREGO
FOREST
FOYERS
FREELY
FREEOF
FREERS
FREEST
FREETO
FREEUP
FREEZE
FRIEDA
FRIELS
FRIEND
FRIERS
FRIEZE
FRYERS
FUMEAT
FUMERS
FUSEES

F•••E•
FABBER
FABLED
FABLER
FABLES
FACIES
FAFNER
FAILED
FAINER
FAIRED
FAIRER
FAITES
FALLEN
FALLER
FALSER
FALTER
FANGED
FANJET
FANNED
FANNER
FARCED
FARCES
FARFEL
FARLEY
FARMED
FARMER
FAROES
FASCES
FASTED
FASTEN
FASTER
FATHER
FATTED
FATTEN
FATTER
FAUCET
FAUTES
FAUVES
FAWKES
FAWNED
FAWNER
FAYLEN
FBIMEN
FEARED
FEARER
FEEDER
FEEJEE
FEELER
FELLED
FELLER
FELTED
FEMMES
FENCED
FENCER
FENCES
FENDED
FENDER
FENNEL
FENNER
FERBER
FERRER
FERRET
FESSED
FESSES
FESTER
FETTER
FEUDED
FEZZED
FEZZES
FHOLES
FIBBED
FIBBER
FIBRES
FICHES
FIDGET
FIDLER
FIEVEL
FILLED
FILLER
FILLES
FILLET
FILMED
FILTER
FINDER
FINGER
FINKED
FINKEL
FINLEY
FINNED
FINNEY
FINSEN
FIRMED
FIRMER
FISHED
FISHER
FISHES
FISTED
FITTED
FITTER
FIVEEE
FIZZED
FIZZER
FIZZES
FLAKED
FLAKER
FLAKES
FLAMED
FLAMER
FLAMES
FLARED
FLARES
FLAWED
FLAXEN
FLAXES
FLAYED
FLAYER
FLEXED
FLEXES
FLOOEY
FLOREK
FLORES
FLORET
FLOREY
FLOWED
FLOWER
FLUKES
FLUKEY
FLUMES
FLUTED
FLUTER
FLUTES
FLUXED
FLUXES
FLYMEN
FLYNET
FOALED
FOAMED
FOAMER
FOBBED
FODDER
FOEMEN
FOGGED
FOGGER
FOGIES
FOILED
FOKKER
FOLDED
FOLDER
FOLGER
FOLIES
FONDER
FOOLED
FOOLER
FOOTED
FOOTER
FORBES
FORCED
FORCER
FORCES
FORDED
FORGED
FORGER
FORGES
FORGET
FORKED
FORKER
FORMED
FORMER
FORTES
FOSSES
FOSSEY
FOSTER
FOULED
FOULER
FOUREE
FOWLED
FOWLER
FOWLES
FOXIER
FRAKES
FRAMED
FRAMER
FRAMES
FRASER
FRATER
FRAUEN
FRAYED
FRAZER
FRERES
FREWER
FRIGES
FRISEE
FRISES
FRITES
FROZEN
FTILES
FUDGED
FUDGER
FUDGES
FUELED
FUELER
FUGUES
FUHRER
FULLER
FUMIER
FUNDED
FUNDER
FUNKED
FUNNED
FUNNEL
FURIES

FURLED
FURRED
FURZES
FUSEES
FUSSED
FUSSER
FUSSES
FUTZED
FUTZES
FUZZED
FUZZES

F••••E
FACADE
FACIAE
FACILE
FADDLE
FAERIE
FAEROE
FAILLE
FALINE
FAMINE
FANNIE
FATALE
FATONE
FAUNAE
FEEBLE
FEEDME
FEEJEE
FELICE
FELINE
FELIPE
FEMALE
FERDIE
FERGIE
FERULE
FESCUE
FETTLE
FIACRE
FIANCE
FICHTE
FICKLE
FIDDLE
FIERCE
FIGURE
FILENE
FILOSE
FINALE
FINITE
FIPPLE
FIVEEE
FIXATE
FIZZLE
FLAMBE
FLANGE
FLECHE
FLEDGE
FLEECE
FLENSE
FLORAE
FLUTIE
FOCSLE
FOIBLE
FOKINE
FOLATE
FOLKIE
FONDLE
FONDUE
FONZIE
FOODIE
FOOTLE
FOOZLE
FORAGE
FORCHE
FORONE
FOSSAE
FOUDRE
FOUREE
FOZZIE
FRAISE
FRANCE
FRAPPE
FREEZE
FRICKE
FRIDGE
FRIEZE
FRINGE
FRISEE
FRUNZE
FSCALE
FUDDLE
FUISSE
FUMBLE
FURORE
FUSILE
FUTILE
FUTURE

•FE•••
AFEARD

•F•E••
AFFECT
AFIELD
AFRESH
AFTERS
EFFECT
EFFETE
NFLERS
OFFEND
OFFERS
OFHELP

•F••E•
EFILED
EFILES
IFFIER
IFTHEN
OFFKEY
OFFSET
PFIZER
XFILES

•F•••E
AFFINE
AFLAME
AFLARE
AFRAME
EFFACE
EFFETE
EFFUSE
GFORCE
OFFICE
OFLATE
OFNOTE
OFYORE

••FE••
ADFEES
AFFECT
BEFELL
DEFEAT
DEFECT
DEFEND
DEFERS
EFFECT
EFFETE
FIFERS
GOFERS
INFEAR
INFECT
INFERS
INFEST
LIFEIS
LIFERS
NOFEES
OFFEND
OFFERS
REFEED
REFELL
REFERS
RIFELY
RIFEST
SAFECO
SAFELY
SAFEST
SAFETY
UNFELT
WAFERS
WAFERY
WIFELY

••F•E•
ADFEES
ALFRED
ALFVEN
ASFREE
BAFFED
BAFFER
BIFFED
BOFFED
BUFFED
BUFFER
BUFFET
COFFEE
COFFER
CUFFED
DAFTER
DEFFER
DEFIED
DEFIER
DEFIES
DEFLEA
DEFTER
DEFUEL
DIFFER
DOFFED
DOFFER
DUFFEL
DUFFER
EIFFEL
FAFNER
GAFFED
GAFFER
GAFFES
GEFFEN
GIFTED
GIFTEE
GOFREE
HAFTED
HEFNER
HEFTED
HEFTER
HOFFER
HUFFED
IFFIER
IMFREE
JAFFEE
LAFFER
LIFTED
LIFTER
LOFTED
LOFTER
LUFFED
MIFFED
MUFFED
MUFFET
NOFEES
OFFKEY
OFFSET
PUFFED
PUFFER
RAFAEL
RAFTED
RAFTER
REFEED
REFFED
REFIED
REFIES
REFLEW
REFLEX
REFUEL
RIFFED
RIFLED
RIFLER
RIFLES
RIFTED
RUFFED
SIFTED
SIFTER
SOFTEN
SOFTER
SUFFER
TIFFED
TOFFEE
TUFFET
TUFTED
UNFREE
WAFTED
WAFTER
WIFIED
WIFIES
ZIFFEL

••F••E
AFFINE
ALFINE
ASFREE
ATFIVE
BAFFLE
BEFORE
COFFEE
DEFACE
DEFAME
DEFILE
DEFINE
DEFORE
DEFUSE
DOFINE
DUFFLE
EFFACE
EFFETE
EFFUSE
ENFACE
GIFTEE
GOFREE
IMFINE
IMFREE
INFUSE
JAFFEE
JOFFRE
LEFTBE
MIFUNE
MUFFLE
OFFICE
ONFILE
ONFIRE
PIFFLE
RAFFLE
REFACE
REFILE
REFINE
REFIRE
REFUGE
REFUSE
REFUTE
RIFFLE
RUFFLE
SAFIRE
SOFINE
SOFTIE
TOFFEE
UNFILE
UNFINE
UNFREE
WAFFLE
WIFFLE

•••FE•
ATMFEE
BAFFED
BAFFER
BEEFED
BIFFED
BOFFED
BUFFED
BUFFER
BUFFET
CHAFED
CHAFER
CHAFES
CHEFED
COFFEE
COFFER
COIFED
CONFED
CONFER
CUFFED
CURFEW
DEAFEN
DEAFER
DEFFER
DIFFER
DOFFED
DOFFER
DUFFEL
DUFFER
DURFEY
EIFFEL
FARFEL
GAFFED
GAFFER
GAFFES
GEFFEN
GOLFED
GOLFER
GOOFED
GULFED
HEIFER
HOFFER
HOOFED
HOOFER
HUFFED
ILLFED
INAFEW
JAFFEE
KIEFER
KNIFED
KNIFER
KNIFES
LABFEE
LAFFER
LEAFED
LIEFER
LOAFED
LOAFER
LUFFED
MCAFEE
MIFFED
MISFED
MUFFED
MUFFET
NONFED
PILFER
POUFED
PREFER
PUFFED
PUFFER
REEFED
REEFER
REFFED
RIFFED
ROLFED
ROLFER
ROOFED
ROOFER
RUFFED
SETFEE
SUFFER
SURFED
SURFER
THEFED
TIFFED
TOFFEE
TUFFET
TURFED
TWOFER
WEBFED
WERFEL
WOLFED
WOOFED
WOOFER
ZIFFEL

•••F•E
ATMFEE
BAFFLE
BOUFFE
COFFEE
DUFFLE
JAFFEE
JOFFRE
LABFEE
MCAFEE
MUFFLE
PIAFFE
PIFFLE
PURFLE
RAFFLE
RIFFLE
RUFFLE
SETFEE
STIFLE
TOFFEE
TRIFLE
WAFFLE
WIFFLE

••••FE
BOUFFE
CARAFE
EXWIFE
MYLIFE
OKEEFE
PIAFFE
RECIFE
STRAFE
STRIFE
TOLIFE
UNRIFE
UNSAFE

FF••••
FFLATS

F•F•••
FAFNER
FAFNIR
FIFERS
FIFING
FIFTHS

F••F••
FANFIC
FARFEL
FEOFFS
FITFOR
FITFUL
FLUFFS
FLUFFY
FORFUN
FULFIL
FUNFUR

F•••F•
FAROFF
FEOFFS
FLUFFS
FLUFFY
FOBOFF

F••••F
FAROFF
FIVEOF
FOBOFF
FONDOF
FREEOF
FULLOF

•FF•••
AFFAIR
AFFECT
AFFINE
AFFIRM
AFFORD
AFFRAY
EFFACE
EFFECT
EFFETE
EFFIGY
EFFLUX
EFFORT
EFFUSE
IFFIER
OFFALS
OFFALY
OFFDAY
OFFEND
OFFERS
OFFICE
OFFING
OFFISH
OFFKEY
OFFSET
OFFUTT

•F•F••
AFIFTH
GFIFTY

••FF••
BAFFED
BAFFER
BAFFIN
BAFFLE
BIFFED
BOFFED
BOFFIN
BOFFOS
BUFFAY
BUFFED
BUFFER
BUFFET
BUFFON
BUFFOS
BUFFUP
COFFEE
COFFER
COFFIN
CUFFED
DEFFER
DIFFER
DOFFED
DOFFER
DUFFEL
DUFFER
DUFFLE
DUFFYS
EIFFEL
GAFFED
GAFFER
GAFFES
GEFFEN
GOFFIN
GUFFAW
HOFFER
HUFFED
JAFFEE
JOFFRE
LAFFER
LUFFED
MIFFED
MUFFED
MUFFET
MUFFIN
MUFFLE
PHFFFT
PIFFLE
PUFFED
PUFFER
PUFFIN
PUFFUP
RAFFIA
RAFFIN
RAFFLE
REFFED
RIFFED
RIFFLE
RUFFED
RUFFLE
RUFFLY
SOFFIT
SUFFER
SUFFIX
TIFFED
TIFFIN
TOFFEE
TUFFET
WAFFLE
WAFFLY
WIFFLE
ZIFFEL

••F•F•
PHFFFT

••F••F
ARFARF
LEFTOF

•••FF•
BLAFFS
BLUFFO
BLUFFS
BOUFFE
CHAFFS
CHAFFY
CHUFFS
CHUFFY
CLIFFS
CLIFFY
FEOFFS
FLUFFS
FLUFFY
KROFFT
PHFFFT
PIAFFE
POUFFY
QUAFFS
SCOFFS
SCUFFS
SKIFFS
SNIFFS
SNIFFY
SNUFFS
SNUFFY
SPIFFS
SPIFFY
STAFFS
STEFFI
STIFFS
STUFFS
STUFFY
WHIFFS

••••FF
BADOFF
BEGOFF
BITOFF
BUGOFF
BUYOFF
CANIFF
CRYOFF
CUTOFF
DAYOFF
DIEOFF
DRYOFF
FAROFF
FOBOFF
GETOFF
GOTOFF
GRAAFF
HITOFF
HOPOFF
ILLOFF
KEYOFF
LAYOFF
LEDOFF
LETOFF
LIPOFF
LOGOFF
LOPOFF
MANOFF
MIDOFF
NODOFF
ONEOFF
PAYOFF
POPOFF
PRYOFF
PUTOFF
RANOFF
RATOFF
REBUFF
RIPOFF
RUBOFF
RUNOFF
SAWOFF
SCLAFF
SCRUFF
SEEOFF
SETOFF
TAPOFF
TARIFF
TEEOFF
TIEOFF
TIPOFF
TOPOFF
UNCUFF
WASOFF
WAYOFF
ZIPOFF

FG••••
FGHIJK

F•G•••
FAGEND
FAGINS
FAGOTS
FIGARO
FIGBAR
FIGHTS
FIGURE
FOGBOW
FOGDOG
FOGEYS
FOGGED
FOGGER
FOGIES
FOGSIN
FOGSUP
FUGARD
FUGATO
FUGUES

F••G••
FANGED
FANGIO
FEIGNS
FERGIE
FIDGET
FINGER
FIZGIG
FLAGGY
FLAGON
FLIGHT
FOGGED
FOGGER
FOLGER
FORGED
FORGER
FORGES
FORGET
FORGOT
FOUGHT
FRIGES
FRIGHT
FRIGID
FROGGY
FRUGAL
FUDGED
FUDGER
FUDGES
FUEGOS
FUNGAL
FUNGUS

F•••G•
FLAGGY
FLANGE
FLEDGE
FLEDGY
FLINGS
FORAGE
FORDGT
FOREGO
FRIDGE
FRINGE
FRINGY
FROGGY

F••••G
FACING
FADING
FAKING
FAMING
FARING
FAXING
FAZING
FEEING
FETING
FIFING
FILING
FINING
FIRING
FIXING
FIZGIG
FLUBUG
FLYING
FOGDOG
FOXING
FRYING
FUMING
FUSING

•FG•••
AFGHAN
EFGHIJ

•F••G•
EFFIGY

•F•••G
OFFING

••FG••
DEFGHI

••F•G•
BEFOGS
DEFOGS
EFFIGY
REFUGE

••F••G
DEFANG
DEFRAG
FIFING
OFFING
REFLAG
USFLAG
ZAFTIG

•••FG•
CDEFGH

•••F•G
DRYFOG
ICEFOG
INAFOG
THEFOG

••••FG
BCDEFG
KEYOFG

FH••••
FHOLES

F•H•••
FGHIJK
FSHARP
FUHRER

F••H••
FATHER
FATHOM
FICHES
FICHTE
FICHUS
FIGHTS
FISHED
FISHER
FISHES

F•••H•
FAITHS
FARAHS
FIFTHS
FILTHY
FIRTHS
FLASHY
FLECHE
FLESHY
FLIGHT
FORCHE
FORWHY
FOUGHT
FRIGHT
FROTHS
FROTHY

F••••H
FAMISH
FARRAH
FELLAH
FETISH
FINISH
FLETCH
FLINCH
FLUISH
FLYASH
FOURTH
FRENCH
FRISCH
FYVUSH

•FH•••
OFHELP

•F•H••
AFGHAN
EFGHIJ
IFTHEN

•F•••H
AFIFTH
AFRESH
OFFISH

••F•H•
DEFGHI
FIFTHS

••F••H
ELFISH
GOFISH
OAFISH
OFFISH

•••F•H
AFIFTH
CDEFGH
LOOFAH

FI••••
FIACRE
FIANCE
FIASCO
FIBBED
FIBBER
FIBERS
FIBRES
FIBRIN
FIBULA
FICHES
FICHTE
FICHUS
FICKLE
FIDDLE
FIDGET
FIDLER
FIELDS
FIENDS
FIERCE
FIEROS
FIESTA
FIEVEL
FIFERS
FIFING
FIFTHS
FIGARO
FIGBAR
FIGHTS
FIGURE
FIJIAN
FILEBY
FILEIN
FILENE
FILERS
FILETS
FILIAL
FILING
FILLED
FILLER
FILLES
FILLET
FILLIN
FILLIP
FILLUP
FILMED
FILMIC
FILOSE
FILTER
FILTHY
FINALE
FINALS
FINCAS
FINDER
FINELY
FINERY
FINEST
FINGER
FINIAL
FINIAN
FINING
FINISH
FINITE
FINITO
FINKED
FINKEL
FINKON
FINLEY
FINNAN
FINNED
FINNEY
FINNIC
FINSEN
FIORDS
FIPPLE
FIREAT
FIREON
FIRERS
FIREUP
FIRING
FIRKIN
FIRMED
FIRMER
FIRMLY
FIRMUP
FIRSTR
FIRSTS
FIRTHS
FISCAL
FISHED
FISHER
FISHES
FISTED
FISTIC
FITFOR
FITFUL
FITOUT
FITSIN
FITSON
FITSUP
FITTED
FITTER
FIVEAA
FIVEAD
FIVEAM
FIVEBC
FIVEEE
FIVENO
FIVEOF
FIVEPM
FIVERS
FIVETO
FIVEUP
FIVEWS
FIXATE
FIXERS

FIXING FIXINS FIXITY FIXUPS FIZGIG FIZZED FIZZER FIZZES FIZZLE

F•I•••

FAILED FAILLE FAILTO FAIMAN FAINER FAINTS FAIRED FAIRER FAIRLY FAIRUP FAISAL FAITES FAITHS FBIMAN FBIMEN FEIGNS FEINTS FEISTY FLICKA FLICKS FLIERS FLIGHT FLIMSY FLINCH FLINGS FLINTS FLINTY FLIPUP FLIRTS FLIRTY FLITBY FLITIN FMINOR FOIBLE FOILED FOISTS FRIARS FRIARY FRICKA FRICKE FRIDAY FRIDGE FRIEDA FRIELS FRIEND FRIERS FRIEZE FRIGES FRIGHT FRIGID FRIJOL FRILLS FRILLY FRINGE FRINGY FRISCH FRISCO FRISEE FRISES FRISKS FRISKY FRITAS FRITES FRITOS FRITTA FRITTO FRITZI FRIVOL FRIZZY FTILES FUISSE

F••I••

FABIAN FACIAE FACIAL FACIAS FACIES FACILE FACING FADING FAGINS FAJITA FAKING FAKIRS FALINE FAMILY FAMINE FAMING FAMISH FANION FAQIRS FARINA FARING FATIMA FAXING FAZING FEEING FELICE FELIDS FELINE FELIPE FELIXI FELIXV FERIAS FERITY FETING FETISH FGHIJK FIFING FIJIAN FILIAL FILING FINIAL FINIAN FINING FINISH FINITE FINITO FIRING FIXING FIXINS FIXITY FLAILS FLAIRS FLUIDS FLUISH FLYING FLYINS FOGIES FOKINE FOLIAR FOLIES FOLIOS FOLIUM FORINT FOXIER FOXILY FOXING FRAIDY FRAISE FRUITS FRUITY FRYING FUMIER FUMING FURIES FUSILE FUSILS FUSING FUSION FUTILE

F•••I•

FABRIC FACEIT FADEIN FAERIE FAFNIR FAKEID FAKEIT FALLIN FANFIC FANGIO FANNIE FARRIS FASCIA FATLIP FATSIS FEEDIN FELLIN FERDIE FERGIE FERMIS FERRIC FERRIS FERVID FIBRIN FILEIN FILLIN FILLIP FILMIC FINNIC FIRKIN FISTIC FITSIN FIZGIG FLAVIA FLEWIN FLITIN FLOPIT FLORID FLORIN FLORIO FLOWIN FLUTIE FOETID FOGSIN FOLDIN FOLKIE FONZIE FOODIE FOOTIT FORBID FORDID FORMIC FORTIS FOSSIL FOZZIE FRIGID FROLIC FULFIL

F••••I

FALUDI FAMULI FARUKI FELIXI FRITZI FRUCTI FRUTTI

•FI•••

AFIELD AFIFTH EFILED EFILES GFIFTY IFICAN IFIMAY IFITIS PFIZER XFILES

•F•I••

AFFINE AFFIRM AFRICA EFFIGY IFFIER OFFICE OFFING OFFISH

•F••I•

AFFAIR AFLCIO AFRAID EFGHIJ IFITIS

••FI••

AFFINE AFFIRM ALFINE ATFIVE BEFIRM BEFITS DEFIED DEFIER DEFIES DEFILE DEFINE DOFINE EFFIGY ELFISH FIFING GOFISH IFFIER IMFINE INFIRM KEFIRS MAFIAS OAFISH OFFICE OFFING OFFISH ONFILE ONFILM ONFIRE PRFIRM REFIED REFIES REFILE REFILL REFILM REFIND REFINE REFIRE REFITS SAFIRE SOFINE SUFISM UNFILE UNFINE UNFIRM UNFITS WIFIED WIFIES

••F•I•

AAFAIR AFFAIR AUFAIT BAFFIN BEFAIR BOFFIN COFFIN ENFAIT FAFNIR GOFFIN HEFLIN LEFTIN LEFTIT LIFEIS MUFFIN MUFTIS NOFAIR PUFFIN RAFFIA RAFFIN RIFKIN SOFFIT SOFTIE SUFFIX TIFFIN UNFAIR ZAFTIG

••F••I

DEFGHI MTFUJI SAFARI

•••FI•

BADFIT BAFFIN BLIFIL BOFFIN BOWFIN CATFIT COFFIN COMFIT CONFIT DEIFIC FANFIC FULFIL GETFIT GOFFIN GOTFIT HOOFIT INAFIX MISFIT MUFFIN NOTFIT OLAFII OLAFIV OLEFIN OUTFIT PREFIX PROFIT PUFFIN RAFFIA RAFFIN RAMFIS REDFIN REDFIR SAWFIT SEEFIT SOFFIT SUFFIX SURFIN TIFFIN UNIFIC

•••F•I

OLAFII STEFFI THEFBI

••••FI

AMALFI STEFFI

FJ••••

FJORDS

F•J•••

FAJITA FIJIAN

F••J••

FANJET FEEJEE FMAJOR FORJOY FRIJOL

F•••J•

FGHIJK

•F•••J

EFGHIJ

••FJ••

DEFJAM

••F•J•

MTFUJI

F•K•••

FAKEID FAKEIT FAKERS FAKERY FAKING FAKIRS FOKINE FOKKER FTKNOX

F••K••

FAWKES FICKLE FINKED FINKEL FINKON FIRKIN FLAKED FLAKER FLAKES FLUKES FLUKEY FOKKER FOLKIE FOLKSY FORKED FORKER FORKUP FRAKES FUNKED

F•••K•

FARUKI FLACKS FLANKS FLASKS FLECKS FLECKY FLICKA FLICKS FLOCKS FLUNKS FLUNKY FRANKS FREAKS FREAKY FRICKA FRICKE FRISKS FRISKY FROCKS

F••••K

FAROUK FEELOK FELTOK FGHIJK FLOREK FRANCK

•F•K••

OFFKEY

•F•••K

LFRANK

••FK••

OFFKEY RIFKIN

••F••K

UNFORK

FL••••

FLABBY FLACKS FLACON FLAGGY FLAGON FLAILS FLAIRS FLAKED FLAKER FLAKES FLAMBE FLAMED FLAMER FLAMES FLANGE FLANKS FLAPPY FLARED FLARES FLASHY FLASKS FLATLY FLATTV FLAUNT FLAUTA FLAVIA FLAVOR FLAWED FLAXEN FLAXES FLAYED FLAYER FLECHE FLECKS FLECKY FLEDGE FLEDGY FLEECE FLEECY FLEERS FLEETS FLENSE FLESHY FLETCH FLEURS FLEWAT FLEWBY FLEWIN FLEWON FLEWTO FLEWUP FLEXED FLEXES FLEXOR FLICKA FLICKS FLIERS FLIGHT FLIMSY FLINCH FLINGS FLINTS FLINTY FLIPUP FLIRTS FLIRTY FLITBY FLITIN FLOATS FLOATY FLOCKS FLOODS FLOOEY FLOORS FLOPIT FLOPPY FLOPSY FLORAE FLORAL FLORAS FLOREK FLORES FLORET FLOREY FLORID FLORIN FLORIO FLOSSY FLOURS FLOURY FLOUTS FLOWED FLOWER FLOWIN FLUBUG FLUENT FLUFFS FLUFFY FLUIDS FLUISH FLUKES FLUKEY FLUMES FLUNKS FLUNKY FLUORO FLURRY FLUTED FLUTER FLUTES FLUTIE FLUXED FLUXES FLYASH FLYBOY FLYBYS FLYERS FLYING FLYINS FLYLOW FLYMAN FLYMEN FLYNET FLYOUT FLYROD FLYWAY

F•L•••

FALALA FALANA FALCON FALINE FALLAL FALLEN FALLER FALLIN FALLON FALLOW FALLTO FALSER FALTER FALUDI FELDON FELICE FELIDS FELINE FELIPE FELIXI FELIXV FELLAH FELLAS FELLED FELLER FELLIN FELLON FELLOW FELLTO FELONS FELONY FELSON FELTED FELTOK FFLATS FILEBY FILEIN FILENE FILERS FILETS FILIAL FILING FILLED FILLER FILLES FILLET FILLIN FILLIP FILLUP FILMED FILMIC FILOSE FILTER FILTHY FOLATE FOLDED FOLDER FOLDIN FOLDUP FOLEYS FOLGER FOLIAR FOLIES FOLIOS FOLIUM FOLKIE FOLKSY FOLLOW FOLSOM FULCRA FULFIL FULLER FULLOF FULLUP FULMAR FULTON

F••L••

FABLED FABLER FABLES FAILED FAILLE FAILTO FALLAL FALLEN FALLER FALLIN FALLON FALLOW FALLTO FARLEY FARLOW FATLIP FAULTS FAULTY FAWLTY FAYLEN FEALTY FEELER FEELOK FELLAH FELLAS FELLED FELLER FELLIN FELLON FELLOW FELLTO FHOLES FIDLER FIELDS FILLED FILLER FILLES FILLET FILLIN FILLIP FILLUP FINLEY FLYLOW FOALED FOILED FOLLOW FOOLED FOOLER FOULED FOULER FOULLY FOULUP FOWLED FOWLER FOWLES FRILLS FRILLY FROLIC FTILES FUELED FUELER FUELUP FULLER FULLOF FULLUP FURLED

F•••L•

FACILE FACULA FADDLE FAILLE FAIRLY FALALA FAMILY FAMULI FATALE FEEBLE FEEBLY FEMALE FERALS FERULE FETTLE FIBULA FICKLE FIDDLE FINALE FINALS FINELY FIPPLE FIRMLY FIZZLE FLAILS FLATLY FOCSLE FOIBLE FONDLE FONDLY FOOTLE FOOZLE FOULLY FOXILY FREELY FRIELS FRILLS FRILLY FSCALE FUDDLE FUMBLE FUSILE FUSILS FUTILE

F••••L

FACIAL FAISAL FALLAL FARFEL FAUNAL FAZOOL FENNEL FESTAL FEUDAL FIEVEL FILIAL FINIAL FINKEL FISCAL FITFUL FLORAL FONTAL FORMAL FOSSIL FRIJOL FRIVOL FRUGAL FULFIL FUNGAL FUNNEL

•FL•••

AFLAME AFLARE AFLATS AFLCIO AFLOAT BFLATS CFLATS DFLATS EFLATS FFLATS GFLATS NFLERS OFLATE

•F•L••

EFFLUX EFILED EFILES XFILES

•F••L•

AFIELD IFONLY OFFALS OFFALY OFHELP

••FL••

ASFLAT DEFLEA EFFLUX GOFLAT HEFLIN INFLOW INFLUX REFLAG REFLEW REFLEX REFLOW REFLUX RIFLED RIFLER RIFLES TEFLON UNFLAT UPFLOW USFLAG

••F•L•

BAFFLE BEFALL BEFELL BIFOLD DAFTLY DEFILE DEFTLY DUFFLE ENFOLD IMFULL INFALL INFOLD INFULL MUFFLE OFFALS OFFALY ONFILE ONFILM PIFFLE RAFFLE REFALL REFELL REFILE REFILL REFILM REFOLD RIFELY RIFFLE RUFFLE RUFFLY SAFELY SOFTLY UNFELT UNFILE UNFOLD UNFULL UPFOLD WAFFLE WAFFLY WIFELY WIFFLE

••F••L

BEFALL BEFELL BEFOOL BEFOUL DEFUEL DUFFEL EIFFEL ELFOWL IMFULL INFALL INFULL RAFAEL REFALL REFELL REFILL REFUEL UNFOUL UNFULL UNFURL ZIFFEL

•••FL•

BAFFLE BARFLY BOTFLY DEAFLY DRYFLY DUFFLE GADFLY LETFLY LIEFLY MAYFLY MEDFLY MUFFLE OUTFLY PIFFLE POPFLY PURFLE RAFFLE RIFFLE RUFFLE RUFFLY SACFLY STIFLE THEFLY TRIFLE WAFFLE WAFFLY WETFLY WIFFLE

•••F•L

AIDFUL AIMFUL ARMFUL ARTFUL BAGFUL BLIFIL BOXFUL CANFUL CAPFUL CARFUL CUPFUL DUFFEL EARFUL EIFFEL EYEFUL FARFEL FITFUL FULFIL HATFUL IREFUL JARFUL JOYFUL JUGFUL LAPFUL LAWFUL MANFUL MUGFUL NETFUL PANFUL PEPFUL POTFUL RUEFUL SINFUL SOBFUL

TUBFUL
URNFUL
USEFUL
VATFUL
WERFEL
WOEFUL
ZIFFEL

••••FL
THENFL

FM••••
FMAJOR
FMBAND
FMINOR

F•M•••
FAMILY
FAMINE
FAMING
FAMISH
FAMOUS
FAMULI
FEMALE
FEMBOT
FEMMES
FEMORA
FEMURS
FOMENT
FUMBLE
FUMEAT
FUMERS
FUMIER
FUMING

F••M••
FAIMAN
FARMED
FARMER
FATMAN
FBIMAN
FBIMEN
FEMMES
FERMAT
FERMIS
FILMED
FILMIC
FIRMED
FIRMER
FIRMLY
FIRMUP
FLAMBE
FLAMED
FLAMER
FLAMES
FLIMSY
FLUMES
FLYMAN
FLYMEN
FOAMED
FOAMER
FOEMAN
FOEMEN
FORMAL
FORMAN
FORMAT
FORMED
FORMER
FORMIC
FRAMED
FRAMER
FRAMES
FRUMPS
FRUMPY
FULMAR
FURMAN

F•••M•
FATIMA
FEEDME
FORUMS
FUSUMA

F••••M
FACTUM
FANDOM
FARNUM
FATHOM
FIVEAM
FIVEPM
FOLIUM
FOLSOM
FOURAM
FOURPM
FRENUM

•F•M••
IFIMAY

•F••M•
AFLAME
AFRAME

•F•••M
AFFIRM

••FM••
ELFMAN

••F•M•
DEFAME
INFAMY

••F••M
AFFIRM
BEFIRM
BIFORM
BYFORM
DEFJAM
DEFOAM
DEFORM
INFIRM
INFORM
ONFILM
PRFIRM
REFILM
REFORM
SUFISM
UNFIRM

•••F•M
CORFAM
PARFUM

F•N•••
FANDOM
FANFIC
FANGED
FANGIO
FANION
FANJET
FANNED
FANNER
FANNIE
FANONS
FANOUT
FANTAN
FANTAS
FENCED
FENCER
FENCES
FENDED
FENDER
FENNEL
FENNER
FENWAY
FINALE
FINALS
FINCAS
FINDER
FINELY
FINERY
FINEST
FINGER
FINIAL
FINIAN
FINING
FINISH
FINITE
FINITO
FINKED
FINKEL
FINKON
FINLEY
FINNAN
FINNED
FINNEY
FINNIC
FINSEN
FONDAS
FONDER
FONDLE
FONDLY
FONDOF
FONDUE
FONDUS
FONTAL
FONZIE
FUNDED
FUNDER
FUNFUR
FUNGAL
FUNGUS
FUNKED
FUNNED
FUNNEL
FUNRUN

F••N••
FAENAS
FAFNER
FAFNIR
FAINER
FAINTS
FANNED
FANNER
FANNIE
FARNUM
FAUNAE
FAUNAL
FAUNAS
FAUNUS
FAWNED
FAWNER
FAWNON
FEINTS
FENNEL
FENNER
FERNAO
FIANCE
FIENDS
FINNAN
FINNED
FINNEY
FINNIC
FLANGE
FLANKS
FLENSE
FLINCH
FLINGS
FLINTS
FLINTY
FLUNKS
FLUNKY
FLYNET
FMINOR
FORNAX
FORNOW
FOUNDS
FOUNTS
FRANCA
FRANCE
FRANCK
FRANCO
FRANCS
FRANKS
FRANNY
FRANTZ
FRENCH
FRENUM
FRENZY
FRINGE
FRINGY
FRONDS
FRONTS
FRUNZE
FTKNOX
FUNNED
FUNNEL

F•••N•
FACING
FADING
FAGEND
FAGINS
FAKING
FALANA
FALINE
FAMINE
FAMING
FANONS
FARINA
FARING
FATONE
FAXING
FAZING
FECUND
FEEING
FEIGNS
FELINE
FELONS
FELONY
FERENC
FETING
FIFING
FILENE
FILING
FINING
FIRING
FIVENO
FIXING
FIXINS
FLAUNT
FLUENT
FLYING
FLYINS
FMBAND
FOKINE
FOMENT
FORINT
FORONE
FOURNO
FOXING
FRANNY
FREONS
FRESNO
FREUND
FRIEND
FROWNS
FRYING
FUMING
FUSING
FUTONS
FUTUNA

F••••N
FABIAN
FACEON
FADEIN
FAIMAN
FALCON
FALLEN
FALLIN
FALLON
FANION
FANTAN
FASTEN
FATMAN
FATTEN
FAWNON
FAYLEN
FBIMAN
FBIMEN
FEEDIN
FEEDON
FELDON
FELLIN
FELLON
FELSON
FIBRIN
FIJIAN
FILEIN
FILLIN
FINIAN
FINKON
FINNAN
FINSEN
FIREON
FIRKIN
FITSIN
FITSON
FLACON
FLAGON
FLAXEN
FLEWIN
FLEWON
FLITIN
FLORIN
FLOWIN
FLYMAN
FLYMEN
FOEMAN
FOEMEN
FOGSIN
FOLDIN
FORFUN
FORMAN
FRAUEN
FROZEN
FRYPAN
FULTON
FUNRUN
FURMAN
FUSION

•FN•••
OFNOTE

•F•N••
IFONLY

•F••N•
AFFINE
LFRANK
OFFEND
OFFING

•F•••N
AFGHAN
IFICAN
IFTHEN

••FN••
FAFNER
FAFNIR
HEFNER

••F•N•
AFFINE
ALFINE
AUFOND
DEFANG
DEFEND
DEFINE
DEFUND
DOFINE
ENFANT
FIFING
IMFINE
INFANT
MIFUNE
OFFEND
OFFING
REFIND
REFINE
REFUND
SOFINE
UNFINE
UNFOND

••F••N
ALFVEN
BAFFIN
BOFFIN
BUFFON
CAFTAN
COFFIN
DEFCON
ELFMAN
GEFFEN
GOFFIN
HEFLIN
LEFTIN
LEFTON
LOFTON
MUFFIN
PUFFIN
RAFFIN
RIFKIN
SOFTEN
SOFTON
TEFLON
TIFFIN

•••F•N
BAFFIN
BIGFAN
BIGFUN
BOFFIN
BOWFIN
BUFFON
COFFIN
CUBFAN
DEAFEN
FORFUN
GEFFEN
GOFFIN
HADFUN
HASFUN
ITSFUN
JETFAN
MEIFUN
METFAN
MUFFIN
NONFAN
OLEFIN
PUFFIN
RAFFIN
RAMFAN
REDFIN
SOXFAN
STEFAN
SUNFAN
SURFIN
THEFAN
TIFFIN
WASFUN

FO••••
FOALED
FOAMED
FOAMER
FOBBED
FOBOFF
FOCSLE
FODDER
FODORS
FOEMAN
FOEMEN
FOETID
FOGBOW
FOGDOG
FOGEYS
FOGGED
FOGGER
FOGIES
FOGSIN
FOGSUP
FOIBLE
FOILED
FOISTS
FOKINE
FOKKER
FOLATE
FOLDED
FOLDER
FOLDIN
FOLDUP
FOLEYS
FOLGER
FOLIAR
FOLIES
FOLIOS
FOLIUM
FOLKIE
FOLKSY
FOLLOW
FOLSOM
FOMENT
FONDAS
FONDER
FONDLE
FONDLY
FONDOF
FONDUE
FONDUS
FONTAL
FONZIE
FOODIE
FOOLED
FOOLER
FOOTED
FOOTER
FOOTIT
FOOTLE
FOOTUP
FOOZLE
FORAGE
FORAYS
FORBAD
FORBES
FORBID
FORCED
FORCER
FORCES
FORCHE
FORDED
FORDGT
FORDID
FOREGO
FOREST
FORFUN
FORGED
FORGER
FORGES
FORGET
FORGOT
FORINT
FORJOY
FORKED
FORKER
FORKUP
FORMAL
FORMAN
FORMAT
FORMED
FORMER
FORMIC
FORNAX
FORNOW
FORONE
FORTAS
FORTES
FORTIS
FORUMS
FORWHY
FORYOU
FOSSAE
FOSSES
FOSSEY
FOSSIL
FOSTER
FOUDRE
FOUGHT
FOULED
FOULER
FOULLY
FOULUP
FOUNDS
FOUNTS
FOURAA
FOURAD
FOURAM
FOURBC
FOUREE
FOURNO
FOURPM
FOURTH
FOURUP
FOWLED
FOWLER
FOWLES
FOXIER
FOXILY
FOXING
FOYERS
FOZZIE

F•O•••
FEODOR
FEOFFS
FHOLES
FIORDS
FJORDS
FLOATS
FLOATY
FLOCKS
FLOODS
FLOOEY
FLOORS
FLOPIT
FLOPPY
FLOPSY
FLORAE
FLORAL
FLORAS
FLOREK
FLORES
FLORET
FLOREY
FLORID
FLORIN
FLORIO
FLOSSY
FLOURS
FLOURY
FLOUTS
FLOWED
FLOWER
FLOWIN
FOODIE
FOOLED
FOOLER
FOOTED
FOOTER
FOOTIT
FOOTLE
FOOTUP
FOOZLE
FROCKS
FROGGY
FROLIC
FRONDS
FRONTS
FROSTS
FROSTY
FROTHS
FROTHY
FROWNS
FROWZY
FROYOS
FROZEN
FYODOR

F••O••
FAGOTS
FAMOUS
FANONS
FANOUT
FAROES
FAROFF
FAROUK
FAROUT
FATONE
FAVORS
FAVOUR
FAZOOL
FEDORA
FELONS
FELONY
FEMORA
FEROUS
FETORS
FILOSE
FITOUT
FLOODS
FLOOEY
FLOORS
FLUORO
FLYOUT
FOBOFF
FODORS
FORONE
FREONS
FSCOTT
FSTOPS
FTROOP
FURORE
FURORS
FUTONS

F•••O•
FACEON
FACTOR
FAEROE
FALCON
FALLON
FALLOW
FANDOM
FANION
FARLOW
FARROW
FATHOM
FAWNON
FAZOOL
FEEDON
FEELOK
FELDON
FELLON
FELLOW
FELSON
FELTOK
FEMBOT
FEODOR
FERVOR
FIEROS
FINKON
FIREON
FITFOR
FITSON
FIVEOF
FLACON
FLAGON
FLAVOR
FLEWON
FLEXOR
FLYBOY
FLYLOW
FLYROD
FMAJOR
FMINOR
FOGBOW
FOGDOG
FOLIOS
FOLLOW
FOLSOM
FONDOF
FORGOT
FORJOY
FORNOW
FORYOU
FREEOF
FRIJOL
FRITOS
FRIVOL
FROYOS
FTKNOX
FTROOP
FUEGOS
FULLOF
FULTON
FURROW
FUSION
FYODOR

F••••O
FAILTO
FALLTO
FANGIO
FEEDTO
FELLTO
FERNAO
FIASCO
FIGARO
FINITO
FIVENO
FIVETO
FLEWTO
FLORIO
FLUORO
FOREGO
FOURNO
FRACTO
FRANCO
FREDRO
FREETO
FRESCO
FRESNO
FRISCO
FRITTO
FUGATO

•FO•••
GFORCE
IFONLY
IFORTY
NFORTY
SFORZA
VFOURS

•F•O••
AFFORD
AFLOAT
EFFORT
OFNOTE
OFYORE

•F•••O
AFLCIO

••FO••
AFFORD
AJFOYT
ATFOUR
AUFOND
BEFOGS
BEFOOL
BEFORE
BEFOUL
BIFOLD
BIFORM
BYFORM
DEFOAM
DEFOGS
DEFORD
DEFORE
DEFORM
EFFORT
ELFOWL
ENFOLD
INFOLD
INFORM
MYFOOT
ONFOOT
OXFORD
REFOLD
REFORM
RUFOUS
UNFOLD
UNFOND
UNFORK
UNFOUL
UNFOXY
UPFOLD

••F•O•
BEFOOL
BOFFOS
BUFFON
BUFFOS
DEFCON
INFLOW
LEFTOF
LEFTON
LOFTON
MYFOOT
ONFOOT
REFLOW
SOFTON
TEFLON
UPFLOW

••F••O
SAFECO

•••FO•
ACTFOR
AIMFOR
ALLFOR
ASKFOR
BATFOR
BEGFOR
BIDFOR
BOFFOS
BUFFON
BUFFOS
CRYFOR
DIDFOR
DIEFOR
DIGFOR
DRYFOG
DUGFOR
FITFOR
GUNFOR
HITFOR
ICEFOG
INAFOG
LAYFOR
LIEFOR
MADFOR
NOTFOR
OPTFOR
OUTFOR
OUTFOX
PAYFOR
RANFOR
REDFOX
REPFOR
RUNFOR
SATFOR
SEAFOX
SETFOR
SITFOR
SLYFOX
STEFOY
SUEFOR
THEFOG
THEFOX
TRYFOR
USEFOR
VIEFOR
WHYFOR
YENFOR

•••F•O
BLUFFO
DEAFTO
RENFRO

••••FO
ADOLFO
BLUFFO

F•P•••
FIPPLE

F••P••
FIPPLE
FLAPPY
FLIPUP
FLOPIT
FLOPPY
FLOPSY
FRAPPE
FRYPAN

F•••P•
FELIPE
FIVEPM
FIXUPS
FLAPPY
FLOPPY
FOURPM
FRAPPE
FRUMPS
FRUMPY
FSTOPS

F••••P
FACEUP
FAIRUP
FATLIP
FESSUP
FILLIP
FILLUP
FIREUP
FIRMUP
FITSUP
FIVEUP
FLEWUP
FLIPUP
FOGSUP
FOLDUP
FOOTUP
FORKUP
FOULUP
FOURUP
FREEUP
FSHARP
FTROOP
FUELUP
FULLUP
FUZZUP

•F•••P
OFHELP

••F••P
BUFFUP
LIFTUP
PUFFUP

•••F•P
BEEFUP
BUFFUP
GOOFUP
PUFFUP

F•Q•••
FAQIRS

FR••••
FRACAS
FRACTO
FRAIDY
FRAISE
FRAKES
FRAMED
FRAMER
FRAMES
FRANCA
FRANCE
FRANCK
FRANCO
FRANCS
FRANKS
FRANNY
FRANTZ
FRAPPE
FRASER
FRATER
FRAUDS
FRAUEN
FRAYED
FRAZER
FREAKS
FREAKY
FREDDY
FREDRO
FREELY

FREEOF
FREERS
FREEST
FREETO
FREEUP
FREEZE
FRENCH
FRENUM
FRENZY
FREONS
FRERES
FRESCA
FRESCO
FRESNO
FRETAT
FRETTY
FREUND
FREWER
FRIARS
FRIARY
FRICKA
FRICKE
FRIDAY
FRIDGE
FRIEDA
FRIELS
FRIEND
FRIERS
FRIEZE
FRIGES
FRIGHT
FRIGID
FRIJOL
FRILLS
FRILLY
FRINGE
FRINGY
FRISCH
FRISCO
FRISEE
FRISES
FRISKS
FRISKY
FRITAS
FRITES
FRITOS
FRITTA
FRITTO
FRITZI
FRIVOL
FRIZZY
FROCKS
FROGGY
FROLIC
FRONDS
FRONTS
FROSTS
FROSTY
FROTHS
FROTHY
FROWNS
FROWZY
FROYOS
FROZEN
FRUCTI
FRUGAL
FRUITS
FRUITY
FRUMPS
FRUMPY
FRUNZE
FRUSTA
FRUTTI
FRYERS
FRYING
FRYPAN

F•R•••

FARACY
FARADS
FARAHS
FARCED
FARCES
FARCRY
FARERS
FARFEL
FARINA
FARING
FARLEY
FARLOW
FARMED
FARMER
FARNUM
FAROES
FAROFF
FAROUK
FAROUT
FARRAH
FARRAR
FARRIS
FARROW
FARUKI
FERALS
FERBER
FERDIE
FERENC
FERGIE
FERIAS
FERITY
FERMAT
FERMIS
FERNAO
FEROUS
FERRER
FERRET
FERRIC
FERRIS
FERULE
FERVID
FERVOR
FIREAT
FIREON
FIRERS
FIREUP
FIRING
FIRKIN
FIRMED
FIRMER
FIRMLY
FIRMUP
FIRSTR
FIRSTS
FIRTHS
FORAGE
FORAYS
FORBAD
FORBES
FORBID
FORCED
FORCER
FORCES
FORCHE
FORDED
FORDGT
FORDID
FOREGO
FOREST
FORFUN
FORGED
FORGER
FORGES
FORGET
FORGOT
FORINT
FORJOY
FORKED
FORKER
FORKUP
FORMAL
FORMAN
FORMAT
FORMED
FORMER
FORMIC
FORNAX
FORNOW
FORONE
FORTAS
FORTES
FORTIS
FORUMS
FORWHY
FORYOU
FTROOP
FURBYS
FURIES
FURLED
FURMAN
FURORE
FURORS
FURRED
FURROW
FURZES

F••R••

FABRAY
FABRIC
FAERIE
FAEROE
FAIRED
FAIRER
FAIRLY
FAIRUP
FARRAH
FARRAR
FARRIS
FARROW
FEARED
FEARER
FERRER
FERRET
FERRIC
FERRIS
FIBRES
FIBRIN
FIERCE
FIEROS
FIORDS
FJORDS
FLARED
FLARES
FLIRTS
FLIRTY
FLORAE
FLORAL
FLORAS
FLOREK
FLORES
FLORET
FLOREY
FLORID
FLORIN
FLORIO
FLURRY
FLYROD
FOURAA
FOURAD
FOURAM
FOURBC
FOUREE
FOURNO
FOURPM
FOURTH
FOURUP
FRERES
FUHRER
FUNRUN
FURRED
FURROW

F•••R•

FACERS
FADERS
FAKERS
FAKERY
FAKIRS
FAQIRS
FARCRY
FARERS
FAVORS
FAXERS
FAYARD
FEDORA
FEMORA
FEMURS
FETORS
FEVERS
FIACRE
FIBERS
FIFERS
FIGARO
FIGURE
FILERS
FINERY
FIRERS
FIVERS
FIXERS
FLAIRS
FLEERS
FLEURS
FLIERS
FLOORS
FLOURS
FLOURY
FLUORO
FLURRY
FLYERS
FODORS
FOUDRE
FOYERS
FREDRO
FREERS
FRIARS
FRIARY
FRIERS
FRYERS
FSHARP
FSTARS
FUGARD
FULCRA
FUMERS
FURORE
FURORS
FUTURA
FUTURE

F••••R

FABBER
FABLER
FACTOR
FAFNER
FAFNIR
FAINER
FAIRER
FALLER
FALSER
FALTER
FANNER
FARMER
FARRAR
FASTER
FATHER
FATTER
FAVOUR
FAWNER
FEARER
FEEDER
FEELER
FELLER
FENCER
FENDER
FENNER
FEODOR
FERBER
FERRER
FERVOR
FESTER
FETTER
FIBBER
FIDLER
FIGBAR
FILLER
FILTER
FINDER
FINGER
FIRMER
FIRSTR
FISHER
FITFOR
FITTER
FIZZER
FLAKER
FLAMER
FLAVOR
FLAYER
FLEXOR
FLOWER
FLUTER
FMAJOR
FMINOR
FOAMER
FODDER
FOGGER
FOKKER
FOLDER
FOLGER
FOLIAR
FONDER
FOOLER
FOOTER
FORCER
FORGER
FORKER
FORMER
FOSTER
FOULER
FOWLER
FOXIER
FRAMER
FRASER
FRATER
FRAZER
FREWER
FUDGER
FUELER
FUHRER
FULLER
FULMAR
FUMIER
FUNDER
FUNFUR
FUSSER
FYODOR

•FR•••

AFRAID
AFRAME
AFRESH
AFRICA
LFRANK

•F•R••

AFFRAY
GFORCE
IFORTY
NFORTY
SFORZA

•F••R•

AFEARD
AFFIRM
AFFORD
AFLARE
AFTERS
EFFORT
NFLERS
OFFERS
OFYORE
VFOURS

•F•••R

AFFAIR
IFFIER
PFIZER

••FR••

AFFRAY
ALFRED
ASFREE
DEFRAG
DEFRAY
GOFREE
IMFREE
UNFREE

••F•R•

AFFIRM
AFFORD
ARFARF
BEFIRM
BEFORE
BIFORM
BYFORM
DEFERS
DEFORD
DEFORE
DEFORM
EFFORT
ERFURT
FIFERS
GOFERS
INFERS
INFIRM
INFORM
JOFFRE
KEFIRS
LIFERS
OFFERS
ONFIRE
OXFORD
PRFIRM
REFERS
REFIRE
REFORM
SAFARI
SAFIRE
UNFIRM
UNFORK
UNFURL
WAFERS
WAFERY

••F••R

AAFAIR
AFFAIR
ATFOUR
BAFFER
BEFAIR
BUFFER
COFFER
DAFTER
DEFFER
DEFIER
DEFTER
DIFFER
DOFFER
DUFFER
FAFNER
FAFNIR
GAFFER
HEFNER
HEFTER
HOFFER
IFFIER
INFEAR
LAFFER
LIFTER
LOFTER
NOFAIR
PUFFER
RAFTER
RIFLER
SIFTER
SOFTER
SUFFER
UNFAIR
WAFTER

•••FR•

BELFRY
BIAFRA
JOFFRE
JUDFRY
PANFRY
RENFRO

•••F•R

ACTFOR
AIMFOR
ALLFOR
ASKFOR
BAFFER
BATFOR
BEGFOR
BIDFOR
BUFFER
CHAFER
COFFER
CONFER
CRYFOR
DEAFER
DEFFER
DIDFOR
DIEFOR
DIFFER
DIGFOR
DOFFER
DUFFER
DUGFOR
FITFOR
FUNFUR
GAFFER
GETFAR
GOLFER
GOTFAR
GUNFOR
HEIFER
HITFOR
HOFFER
HOOFER
HOWFAR
KIEFER
KNIFER
LAFFER
LAYFOR
LIEFER
LIEFOR
LOAFER
MADFOR
NOTFAR
NOTFOR
OPTFOR
OUTFOR
PAYFOR
PILFER
PREFER
PUFFER
RANFOR
REDFIR
REEFER
REPFOR
ROLFER
ROOFER
RUNFOR
SATFOR
SETFOR
SHOFAR
SITFOR
SUEFOR
SUFFER
SULFUR
SURFER
TOOFAR
TRYFOR
TWOFER
USEFOR
VIEFOR
WHYFOR
WOOFER
YENFOR

FS••••

FSCALE
FSCOTT
FSHARP
FSTARS
FSTOPS

F•S•••

FASCES
FASCIA
FASTED
FASTEN
FASTER
FESCUE
FESSED
FESSES
FESSUP
FESTAL
FESTAS
FESTER
FESTUS
FISCAL
FISHED
FISHER
FISHES
FISTED
FISTIC
FOSSAE
FOSSES
FOSSEY
FOSSIL
FOSTER
FUSEES
FUSILE
FUSILS
FUSING
FUSION
FUSSAT
FUSSED
FUSSER
FUSSES
FUSUMA

F••S••

FAISAL
FALSER
FATSIS
FEASTS
FEISTY
FELSON
FESSED
FESSES
FESSUP
FIASCO
FIESTA
FINSEN
FIRSTR
FIRSTS
FITSIN
FITSON
FITSUP
FLASHY
FLASKS
FLESHY
FLOSSY
FOCSLE
FOGSIN
FOGSUP
FOISTS
FOLSOM
FOSSAE
FOSSES
FOSSEY
FOSSIL
FRASER
FRESCA
FRESCO
FRESNO
FRISCH
FRISCO
FRISEE
FRISES
FRISKS
FRISKY
FROSTS
FROSTY
FRUSTA
FUISSE
FUSSAT
FUSSED
FUSSER
FUSSES

F•••S•

FAMISH
FETISH
FEWEST
FEYEST
FILOSE
FINEST
FINISH
FLENSE
FLIMSY
FLOPSY
FLOSSY
FLUISH
FLYASH
FOLKSY
FOREST
FRAISE
FREEST
FUISSE
FYVUSH

F••••S

FABLES
FACERS
FACETS
FACIAS
FACIES
FADERS
FAENAS
FAGINS
FAGOTS
FAINTS
FAITES
FAITHS
FAKERS
FAKIRS
FAMOUS
FANONS
FANTAS
FAQIRS
FARADS
FARAHS
FARCES
FARERS
FAROES
FARRIS
FASCES
FATSIS
FATWAS
FAULTS
FAUNAS
FAUNUS
FAUTES
FAUVES
FAVORS
FAWKES
FAXERS
FEASTS
FEIGNS
FEINTS
FELIDS
FELLAS
FELONS
FEMMES
FEMURS
FENCES
FEOFFS
FERALS
FERIAS
FERMIS
FEROUS
FERRIS
FESSES
FESTAS
FESTUS
FETORS
FEVERS
FEZZES
FFLATS
FHOLES
FIBERS
FIBRES
FICHES
FICHUS
FIELDS
FIENDS
FIEROS
FIFERS
FIFTHS
FIGHTS
FILERS
FILETS
FILLES
FINALS
FINCAS
FIORDS
FIRERS
FIRSTS
FIRTHS
FISHES
FIVERS
FIVEWS
FIXERS
FIXINS
FIXUPS
FIZZES
FJORDS
FLACKS
FLAILS
FLAIRS
FLAKES
FLAMES
FLANKS
FLARES
FLASKS
FLAXES
FLECKS
FLEERS
FLEETS
FLEURS
FLEXES
FLICKS
FLIERS
FLINGS
FLINTS
FLIRTS
FLOATS
FLOCKS
FLOODS
FLOORS
FLORAS
FLORES
FLOURS
FLOUTS
FLUFFS
FLUIDS
FLUKES
FLUMES
FLUNKS
FLUTES
FLUXES
FLYBYS
FLYERS
FLYINS
FODORS
FOGEYS
FOGIES
FOISTS
FOLEYS
FOLIES
FOLIOS
FONDAS
FONDUS
FORAYS
FORBES
FORCES
FORGES
FORTAS
FORTES
FORTIS
FORUMS
FOSSES
FOUNDS
FOUNTS
FOWLES
FOYERS
FRACAS
FRAKES
FRAMES
FRANCS
FRANKS
FRAUDS
FREAKS
FREERS
FREONS
FRERES
FRIARS
FRIELS
FRIERS
FRIGES
FRILLS
FRISES
FRISKS
FRITAS
FRITES
FRITOS
FROCKS
FRONDS
FRONTS
FROSTS
FROTHS
FROWNS
FROYOS
FRUITS
FRUMPS
FRYERS
FSTARS
FSTOPS
FTILES
FUDGES
FUEGOS
FUGUES
FUMERS
FUNGUS
FURBYS
FURIES
FURORS
FURZES
FUSEES
FUSILS
FUSSES
FUTONS
FUTZES
FUZZES

•F•S••

OFFSET

•F••S•

AFRESH
EFFUSE
OFFISH

•F•••S

AFLATS
AFTERS
BFLATS
CFLATS
DFLATS
EFILES
EFLATS
FFLATS
GFLATS
IFITIS
NFLERS
OFFALS
OFFERS
VFOURS
XFILES

••FS••

OFFSET

••F•S•

ASFAST
DEFUSE
EFFUSE
ELFISH
GOFAST
GOFISH
INFEST
INFUSE
MUFASA
NOFUSS
OAFISH
OFFISH
REFUSE
RIFEST
SAFEST
SUFISM
TUFTSU

••F••S

ADFEES
BEFITS
BEFOGS
BOFFOS
BUFFOS
DEFATS
DEFERS
DEFIES
DEFOGS
DUFFYS
FIFERS
FIFTHS
GAFFES
GOFERS
INFERS
KEFIRS
LIFEIS
LIFERS
LOFTUS
MAFIAS
MUFTIS
NOFEES
NOFUSS
OFFALS
OFFERS
REFERS
REFIES
REFITS
RIFLES
RUFOUS
UNFITS
WAFERS
WIFIES

•••F•S

BLAFFS
BLUFFS
BOFFOS
BUFFOS
CHAFES
CHAFFS
CHUFFS
CLEFTS
CLIFFS
CRAFTS
CROFTS
DELFTS
DOOFUS
DRAFTS
DRIFTS
DUFFYS
FEOFFS
FLUFFS
GAFFES
GOOFUS
GRAFTS
GRIFTS
KNIFES
LOOFAS
NAKFAS
QUAFFS
RAMFIS
SCOFFS
SCUFFS
SHAFTS
SHIFTS
SKIFFS
SNAFUS
SNIFFS
SNUFFS
SPIFFS
STAFFS
STIFFS
STUFFS
SULFAS
SWIFTS
THEFTS
WHIFFS

••••FS

BLAFFS
BLUFFS
BRIEFS

CALIFS
CCLEFS
CHAFFS
CHIEFS
CHUFFS
CLIFFS
DECAFS
DWARFS
FEOFFS
FLUFFS
GANEFS
GCLEFS
GRIEFS
MOTIFS
PILAFS
PROOFS
QUAFFS
SCARFS
SCOFFS
SCUFFS
SERIFS
SKIFFS
SMURFS
SNARFS
SNIFFS
SNUFFS
SPIFFS
SPOOFS
STAFFS
STIFFS
STUFFS
WHARFS
WHIFFS

FT••••
FTILES
FTKNOX
FTROOP

F•T•••
FATALE
FATCAT
FATHER
FATHOM
FATIMA
FATLIP
FATMAN
FATONE
FATSIS
FATTED
FATTEN
FATTER
FATWAS
FETING
FETISH
FETORS
FETTER
FETTLE
FITFOR
FITFUL
FITOUT
FITSIN
FITSON
FITSUP
FITTED
FITTER
FSTARS
FSTOPS
FUTILE
FUTONS
FUTUNA
FUTURA
FUTURE
FUTZED
FUTZES

F••T••
FACTOR
FACTUM
FAITES
FAITHS
FALTER
FANTAN
FANTAS
FASTED
FASTEN
FASTER
FATTED
FATTEN
FATTER
FAUTES
FELTED
FELTOK
FESTAL
FESTAS
FESTER
FESTUS
FETTER
FETTLE
FIFTHS
FILTER
FILTHY
FIRTHS
FISTED
FISTIC
FITTED
FITTER
FLATLY
FLATTV
FLETCH
FLITBY
FLITIN
FLUTED
FLUTER
FLUTES
FLUTIE
FOETID
FONTAL
FOOTED
FOOTER
FOOTIT
FOOTLE
FOOTUP
FORTAS
FORTES
FORTIS
FOSTER
FRATER
FRETAT
FRETTY
FRITAS
FRITES
FRITOS
FRITTA
FRITTO
FRITZI
FROTHS
FROTHY
FRUTTI
FULTON

F•••T•
FACETS
FAGOTS
FAILTO
FAINTS
FAJITA
FALLTO
FAULTS
FAULTY
FAWLTY
FEALTY
FEASTS
FEEDTO
FEINTS
FEISTY
FELLTO
FERITY
FFLATS
FICHTE
FIESTA
FIGHTS
FILETS
FINITE
FINITO
FIRSTR
FIRSTS
FIVETO
FIXATE
FIXITY
FLATTV
FLAUTA
FLEETS
FLEWTO
FLINTS
FLINTY
FLIRTS
FLIRTY
FLOATS
FLOATY
FLOUTS
FOISTS
FOLATE
FOUNTS
FOURTH
FRACTO
FRANTZ
FREETO
FRETTY
FRITTA
FRITTO
FRONTS
FROSTS
FROSTY
FRUCTI
FRUITS
FRUITY
FRUSTA
FRUTTI
FSCOTT
FUGATO

F••••T
FACEIT
FAKEIT
FANJET
FANOUT
FAROUT
FATCAT
FAUCET
FEMBOT
FERMAT
FERRET
FEWEST
FEYEST
FIDGET
FILLET
FINEST
FIREAT
FITOUT
FLAUNT
FLEWAT
FLIGHT
FLOPIT
FLORET
FLUENT
FLYNET
FLYOUT
FOMENT
FOOTIT
FORDGT
FOREST
FORGET
FORGOT
FORINT
FORMAT
FOUGHT
FREEST
FRETAT
FRIGHT
FSCOTT
FUMEAT
FUSSAT

•FT•••
AFTERS
IFTHEN

•F•T••
IFITIS

•F••T•
AFIFTH
AFLATS
BFLATS
CFLATS
DFLATS
EFFETE
EFLATS
FFLATS
GFIFTY
GFLATS
IFORTY
NFORTY
OFFUTT
OFLATE
OFNOTE

•F•••T
AFFECT
AFLOAT
EFFECT
EFFORT
OFFSET
OFFUTT

••FT••
CAFTAN
DAFTER
DAFTLY
DEFTER
DEFTLY
FIFTHS
GIFTED
GIFTEE
HAFTED
HEFTED
HEFTER
LEFTBE
LEFTIN
LEFTIT
LEFTOF
LEFTON
LIFTED
LIFTER
LIFTUP
LOFTED
LOFTER
LOFTON
LOFTUS
MUFTIS
RAFTED
RAFTER
RIFTED
SIFTED
SIFTER
SOFTEN
SOFTER
SOFTIE
SOFTLY
SOFTON
TUFTED
TUFTSU
WAFTED
WAFTER
ZAFTIG

••F•T•
BEFITS
DEFATS
EFFETE
OFFUTT
REFITS
REFUTE
SAFETY
UNFITS

••F••T
AFFECT
AJFOYT
ASFAST
ASFLAT
AUFAIT
BUFFET
DEFEAT
DEFECT
EFFECT
EFFORT
ENFAIT
ENFANT
ERFURT
GOFAST
GOFLAT
INFACT
INFANT
INFECT
INFEST
LEFTIT
MUFFET
MYFOOT
OFFSET
OFFUTT
ONFOOT
PHFFFT
RIFEST
SAFEST
SOFFIT
TUFFET
UNFACT
UNFELT
UNFLAT

•••FT•
AFIFTH
CLEFTS
CRAFTS
CRAFTY
CROFTS
DEAFTO
DELFTS
DRAFTS
DRAFTY
DRIFTS
DRIFTY
GFIFTY
GRAFTS
GRIFTS
SHAFTS
SHIFTS
SHIFTY
SWIFTS
THEFTS

•••F•T
ARAFAT
BADFIT
BUFFET
CATFIT
COMFIT
CONFIT
GETFIT
GOTFIT
HOOFIT
KROFFT
LOWFAT
MISFIT
MUFFET
NONFAT
NOTFIT
OUTFIT
PHFFFT
PROFIT
SAWFIT
SEEFIT
SOFFIT
TUFFET

••••FT
ADRIFT
ASSOFT
BEREFT
GOLEFT
GOSOFT
ISLEFT
KROFFT
PHFFFT
REGIFT
RESIFT
SHRIFT
THRIFT
UNDEFT
UNHAFT
UNLEFT
UNSOFT
UPLIFT
UPWAFT

FU••••
FUDDLE
FUDGED
FUDGER
FUDGES
FUEGOS
FUELED
FUELER
FUELUP
FUGARD
FUGATO
FUGUES
FUHRER
FUISSE
FULCRA
FULFIL
FULLER
FULLOF
FULLUP
FULMAR
FULTON
FUMBLE
FUMEAT
FUMERS
FUMIER
FUMING
FUNDED
FUNDER
FUNFUR
FUNGAL
FUNGUS
FUNKED
FUNNED
FUNNEL
FUNRUN
FURBYS
FURIES
FURLED
FURMAN
FURORE
FURORS
FURRED
FURROW
FURZES
FUSEES
FUSILE
FUSILS
FUSING
FUSION
FUSSAT
FUSSED
FUSSER
FUSSES
FUSUMA
FUTILE
FUTONS
FUTUNA
FUTURA
FUTURE
FUTZED
FUTZES
FUZZED
FUZZES
FUZZUP

F•U•••
FAUCET
FAULTS
FAULTY
FAUNAE
FAUNAL
FAUNAS
FAUNUS
FAUTES
FAUVES
FEUDAL
FEUDED
FLUBUG
FLUENT
FLUFFS
FLUFFY
FLUIDS
FLUISH
FLUKES
FLUKEY
FLUMES
FLUNKS
FLUNKY
FLUORO
FLURRY
FLUTED
FLUTER
FLUTES
FLUTIE
FLUXED
FLUXES
FOUDRE
FOUGHT
FOULED
FOULER
FOULLY
FOULUP
FOUNDS
FOUNTS
FOURAA
FOURAD
FOURAM
FOURBC
FOUREE
FOURNO
FOURPM
FOURTH
FOURUP
FRUCTI
FRUGAL
FRUITS
FRUITY
FRUMPS
FRUMPY
FRUNZE
FRUSTA
FRUTTI

F••U••
FACULA
FALUDI
FAMULI
FARUKI
FECUND
FEMURS
FERULE
FIBULA
FIGURE
FIXUPS
FLAUNT
FLAUTA
FLEURS
FLOURS
FLOURY
FLOUTS
FORUMS
FRAUDS
FRAUEN
FREUND
FUGUES
FUSUMA
FUTUNA
FUTURA
FUTURE
FYVUSH

F•••U•
FACEUP
FACTUM
FAIRUP
FAMOUS
FANOUT
FARNUM
FAROUK
FAROUT
FAUNUS
FAVOUR
FEROUS
FESCUE
FESSUP
FESTUS
FICHUS
FILLUP
FIREUP
FIRMUP
FITFUL
FITOUT
FITSUP
FIVEUP
FLEWUP
FLIPUP
FLUBUG
FLYOUT
FOGSUP
FOLDUP
FOLIUM
FONDUE
FONDUS
FOOTUP
FORFUN
FORKUP
FOULUP
FOURUP
FREEUP
FRENUM
FUELUP
FULLUP
FUNFUR
FUNGUS
FUNRUN
FUZZUP

F••••U
FORYOU

•F•U••
EFFUSE
OFFUTT
VFOURS

•F••U•
EFFLUX

••FU••
DEFUEL
DEFUND
DEFUSE
EFFUSE
ERFURT
IMFULL
INFULL
INFUSE
MIFUNE
MTFUJI
NOFUSS
OFFUTT
REFUEL
REFUGE
REFUND
REFUSE
REFUTE
UNFULL
UNFURL

••F•U•
ATFOUR
BEFOUL
BUFFUP
EFFLUX
INFLUX
LIFTUP
LOFTUS
PUFFUP
REFLUX
RUFOUS
UNFOUL

••F••U
TUFTSU

•••FU•
AIDFUL
AIMFUL
ARMFUL
ARTFUL
BAGFUL
BEEFUP
BIGFUN
BOXFUL
BUFFUP
CANFUL
CAPFUL
CARFUL
CUPFUL
DOOFUS
EARFUL
EYEFUL
FITFUL
FORFUN
FUNFUR
GOOFUP
GOOFUS
HADFUN
HASFUN
HATFUL
IREFUL
ITSFUN
JARFUL
JOYFUL
JUGFUL
LAPFUL
LAWFUL
MANFUL
MEIFUN
MUGFUL
NETFUL
PANFUL
PARFUM
PEPFUL
POTFUL
PUFFUP
RUEFUL
SINFUL
SNAFUS
SOBFUL
SULFUR
TUBFUL
URNFUL
USEFUL
VATFUL
WASFUN
WOEFUL

••••FU
KUNGFU

F•V•••
FAVORS
FAVOUR
FEVERS
FIVEAA
FIVEAD
FIVEAM
FIVEBC
FIVEEE
FIVENO
FIVEOF
FIVEPM
FIVERS
FIVETO
FIVEUP
FIVEWS
FYVUSH

F••V••
FAUVES
FERVID
FERVOR
FIEVEL
FLAVIA
FLAVOR
FRIVOL

F••••V
FELIXV
FLATTV

••FV••
ALFVEN

••F•V•
ATFIVE

•••F•V
OLAFIV

F•W•••
FAWKES
FAWLTY
FAWNED
FAWNER
FAWNON
FEWEST
FOWLED
FOWLER
FOWLES

F••W••
FATWAS
FENWAY
FLAWED
FLEWAT
FLEWBY
FLEWIN
FLEWON
FLEWTO
FLEWUP
FLOWED
FLOWER
FLOWIN
FLYWAY
FORWHY
FREWER
FROWNS
FROWZY

F•••W•
FIVEWS

F••••W
FALLOW
FARLOW
FARROW
FELLOW
FLYLOW
FOGBOW
FOLLOW
FORNOW
FURROW

••F•W•
ELFOWL

••F••W
GUFFAW
INFLOW
REFLEW
REFLOW
UPFLOW

•••F•W
CURFEW
GUFFAW
INAFEW

F•X•••
FAXERS
FAXING
FIXATE
FIXERS
FIXING
FIXINS
FIXITY
FIXUPS
FOXIER
FOXILY
FOXING

F••X••
FLAXEN
FLAXES
FLEXED
FLEXES
FLEXOR
FLUXED
FLUXES

F•••X•
FELIXI
FELIXV

F••••X
FORNAX
FTKNOX

•F•••X
EFFLUX

••F•X•
UNFOXY

••F••X
EFFLUX
INFLUX
REFLEX
REFLUX
SUFFIX

•••F•X
COLFAX
INAFIX
KOUFAX
OUTFOX
PREFIX
REDFOX
SEAFOX
SLYFOX
SUFFIX
THEFOX

FY••••
FYODOR
FYVUSH

F•Y•••
FAYARD
FAYLEN
FEYEST
FLYASH
FLYBOY
FLYBYS
FLYERS
FLYING
FLYINS
FLYLOW
FLYMAN
FLYMEN
FLYNET
FLYOUT
FLYROD
FLYWAY
FOYERS
FRYERS
FRYING
FRYPAN

F••Y••
FLAYED
FLAYER
FORYOU
FRAYED
FROYOS

F•••Y•
FLYBYS
FOGEYS
FOLEYS
FORAYS
FURBYS

F••••Y
FABRAY
FAIRLY
FAKERY
FAMILY
FARACY
FARCRY
FARLEY
FAULTY
FAWLTY
FEALTY
FEEBLY
FEISTY
FELONY
FENWAY
FERITY
FILEBY
FILTHY
FINELY
FINERY
FINLEY
FINNEY
FIRMLY
FIXITY
FLABBY
FLAGGY
FLAPPY
FLASHY
FLATLY
FLECKY
FLEDGY
FLEECY
FLESHY
FLEWBY
FLIMSY
FLINTY
FLIRTY
FLITBY
FLOATY
FLOOEY
FLOPPY
FLOPSY
FLOREY
FLOSSY
FLOURY
FLUFFY
FLUKEY
FLUNKY
FLURRY
FLYBOY
FLYWAY
FOLKSY
FONDLY
FORJOY
FORWHY
FOSSEY
FOULLY
FOXILY
FRAIDY
FRANNY
FREAKY
FREDDY
FREELY
FRENZY
FRETTY
FRIARY
FRIDAY
FRILLY
FRINGY
FRISKY
FRIZZY
FROGGY
FROSTY
FROTHY
FROWZY
FRUITY
FRUMPY

•FY•••
OFYORE

•F•••Y
AFFRAY
EFFIGY
GFIFTY
IFIMAY
IFONLY
IFORTY
NFORTY
OFFALY
OFFDAY
OFFKEY

••F•Y•
AJFOYT
DUFFYS

••F••Y
AFFRAY
BUFFAY
DAFTLY
DEFRAY
DEFTLY
EFFIGY
INFAMY
OFFALY
OFFDAY
OFFKEY
RIFELY
RUFFLY
SAFELY
SAFETY
SOFTLY
UNFOXY
WAFERY
WAFFLY
WIFELY

•••FY•
DUFFYS

•••F•Y
BARFLY
BELFRY
BOTFLY
BUFFAY
CHAFFY
CHUFFY
CLIFFY
CRAFTY
DEAFLY
DRAFTY
DRIFTY
DRYFLY
DURFEY
FLUFFY
GADFLY
GFIFTY
JUDFRY
LETFLY
LIEFLY
MAYFLY
MEDFLY
OUTFLY
PANFRY
POPFLY
POUFFY
RUFFLY
SACFLY
SHIFTY
SNIFFY
SNUFFY
SPIFFY
STEFOY
STUFFY
THEFLY
WAFFLY
WETFLY

••••FY
AERIFY
ARGUFY
AURIFY
BASIFY
CASEFY
CAVAFY
CHAFFY
CHUFFY
CITIFY
CLIFFY
CODIFY
FLUFFY
GASIFY
MINIFY
MODIFY
NIDIFY
NOTIFY
OSSIFY
PACIFY
POUFFY
PURIFY
RAMIFY
RAREFY
RATIFY
REDEFY
RUBIFY
SALIFY
SCURFY
SNIFFY
SNUFFY
SPIFFY
STUFFY
TUMEFY
TYPIFY
UGLIFY
VERIFY
VILIFY
VINIFY
VIVIFY

F•Z•••
FAZING
FAZOOL
FEZZED
FEZZES
FIZGIG
FIZZED
FIZZER
FIZZES
FIZZLE
FOZZIE
FUZZED
FUZZES
FUZZUP

F••Z••
FEZZED
FEZZES
FIZZED
FIZZER
FIZZES
FIZZLE
FONZIE
FOOZLE
FOZZIE
FRAZER
FRIZZY
FROZEN
FURZES
FUTZED
FUTZES
FUZZED
FUZZES
FUZZUP

F•••Z•
FREEZE
FRENZY
FRIEZE
FRITZI
FRIZZY
FROWZY
FRUNZE

F••••Z
FRANTZ

•F•Z••
PFIZER

•F••Z•
SFORZA

GA••••
GABBED
GABBER
GABBLE
GABBRO
GABLED
GABLER
GABLES
GADDED
GADDER
GADDIS
GADFLY
GADGET
GAELIC
GAFFED
GAFFER
GAFFES
GAGGED
GAGGER
GAGGLE
GAGING
GAGLAW
GAGMAN
GAGMEN
GAIETY
GAIJIN
GAINED
GAINER
GAINES
GAINLY
GAINON
GAINST
GAITED
GAITER
GALANT
GALAXY
GALEAE
GALEAO
GALENA
GALLED
GALLEY
GALLIA
GALLIC
GALLON
GALLOP
GALLUP
GALOIS
GALOOT
GALOPS
GALORE
GALOSH
GALPAL
GALTON
GALWAY
GAMAYS
GAMBIA
GAMBIT
GAMBLE
GAMBOL
GAMELY
GAMERS
GAMEST
GAMETE
GAMGEE
GAMIER
GAMILY
GAMINE
GAMING
GAMINS
GAMMAS
GAMMED
GAMMER
GAMMON
GAMOUS
GAMUTS
GANDER
GANDHI
GANEFS
GANGED
GANGER
GANGES
GANGLY
GANGUP
GANNET
GANNON
GANTRY
GAOLED
GAOLER
GAPEAT
GAPERS
GAPING
GAPPED
GARAGE
GARBED
GARBER
GARBLE
GARCIA
GARCON
GARDEN
GARETH
GARGAN
GARGLE
GARISH
GARLIC
GARNER
GARNET
GARRET
GARSON
GARTER
GARVEY
GARYIN
GASBAG
GASCAN
GASCAP
GASCON
GASHED
GASHES
GASHOG
GASIFY
GASJET
GASKET
GASLIT
GASLOG
GASMAN
GASMEN
GASOIL
GASPAR
GASPED
GASPER
GASSED
GASSER
GASSES
GASTAX
GASTER
GASTON
GASTRO
GASWAR
GATEAU
GATERS
GATHER
GATING
GATLIN
GATORS
GATSBY
GAUCHE
GAUCHO
GAUGED
GAUGER
GAUGES
GAULLE
GAUZES
GAVEIN
GAVELS
GAVEOF
GAVEON
GAVETO
GAVEUP
GAVIAL
GAVOTS
GAVRAS
GAWAIN
GAWKAT
GAWKED
GAWKER
GAWPED
GAWPER
GAYEST
GAYNES
GAYNOR
GAZEAT
GAZEBO
GAZEON
GAZERS
GAZING

G•A•••
GDANSK
GEARED
GEARTO
GEARUP
GHAINS
GHAZIS
GIAMBI
GIANNI
GIANTS
GLACES
GLACIS
GLADES
GLADLY
GLADTO
GLADYS
GLAMOR
GLAMUP
GLANCE
GLANDS
GLARED
GLARES
GLARUS
GLASER
GLASSY
GLAZED
GLAZER
GLAZES
GMAJOR
GNARLS
GNARLY
GNARRS
GNATTY
GNAWAT
GNAWED
GNAWER
GNAWON
GOADED
GOALBY
GOALIE
GOATEE
GOATIT
GOAWAY
GOAWOL
GOAWRY
GRAAFF
GRABAT
GRABBY
GRABLE
GRACED
GRACES
GRACIE
GRADEA
GRADEB
GRADED
GRADER
GRADES
GRAECO
GRAFTS
GRAHAM
GRAILS
GRAINS
GRAINY
GRAMME
GRAMMY
GRAMPA
GRAMPS
GRANBY
GRANDE
GRANDS
GRANDY
GRANGE
GRANIT
GRANNY
GRANPA
GRANTS
GRAPES
GRAPEY
GRAPHO
GRAPHS
GRAPHY
GRAPPA
GRASPS
GRASSO
GRASSY
GRATAE
GRATED
GRATER
GRATES
GRATIA
GRATIN
GRATIS
GRAVAS
GRAVED
GRAVEL
GRAVEN
GRAVER
GRAVES
GRAVID
GRAYED
GRAYER
GRAYLY
GRAZED
GRAZER
GRAZES
GRAZIE
GUANOS
GUARDS
GUAVAS

G••A••
GALANT
GALAXY
GAMAYS
GARAGE
GAWAIN
GELATE
GELATI
GELATO
GEMARA
GERALD
GERARD
GETANA
GETANF
GFLATS
GIJANE
GITANO
GLEAMS
GLEAMY
GLEANS
GLOATS
GOBACK
GOBANG
GOCART
GODARD
GODARK
GOEASY
GOFAST
GOKART
GOLAME
GOLAST
GOPAST
GOTAMA
GOTANA
GOTANF
GRAAFF
GREASE
GREASY
GREATS
GREAVE
GROANS
GROATS
GSCALE
GSHARP
GSTAAD
GSTARS
GUIANA
GULAGS
GUYANA
GYRATE

G•••A•
GAGLAW
GAGMAN
GALEAE
GALEAO
GALPAL
GALWAY
GAMMAS
GAPEAT
GARGAN
GASBAG
GASCAN
GASCAP
GASMAN
GASPAR
GASTAX
GASWAR
GATEAU
GAVIAL
GAVRAS
GAWKAT
GAZEAT
GEEGAW
GELCAP
GELLAR
GEMMAE
GENIAL
GENOAN
GENOAS
GENUAL
GERMAN
GESTAE
GETFAR
GETMAD
GETSAB
GETSAC
GETSAD
GETSAT
GEWGAW
GIBEAT
GIBRAN
GIDDAP
GIGBAG
GILEAD
GILLAN
GILMAN
GIMBAL
GLOBAL
GNAWAT
GOAWAY
GODEAD
GOESAT
GOFLAT
GONEAR
GONEAT
GOODAT
GORHAM
GOSTAG
GOTEAM
GOTFAR
GOTHAM
GOTMAD
GOUDAS
GRABAT
GRAHAM
GRATAE
GRAVAS
GRINAT
GROBAN
GSTAAD
GUAVAS
GUFFAW
GUINAN
GUITAR
GULLAH
GUNLAP
GUNLAW
GUNMAN
GUNNAR
GUSTAV
GUTMAN
GUZMAN
GYMBAG
GYMRAT
GYOZAS

G••••A
GALENA
GALLIA
GAMBIA
GARCIA
GEISHA
GEMARA
GENERA
GENEVA
GENOVA
GETANA
GLENDA
GLINDA
GLINKA
GLORIA
GLOSSA
GODIVA
GOLETA
GOTAMA
GOTANA
GOTCHA
GRADEA
GRAMPA
GRANPA
GRAPPA
GRATIA
GRETNA
GRISHA
GUIANA
GUINEA
GURKHA
GUYANA

•GA•••
AGADIR
AGAMAS
AGAMES
AGARIC
AGASSI
AGATES
AGATHA
AGAVES
AGAWAM
EGALES
OGAUGE
PGAPRO
UGANDA
UGARTE
XGAMES

•G•A••
AGHAST
AGLAIA
AGLARE
AGNAIL
AGNATE
IGNACE
IGNATZ
IGUANA
OGHAMS
OGLALA
OGRADY
UGGAMS

•G••A•
AGAMAS
AGAWAM
AGENAS
AGITAS
AGLEAM
AGORAE
AGORAS
EGGSAC
EGOYAN
OGDOAD
OGIVAL
SGTMAJ

•G•••A
AGATHA
AGENDA
AGLAIA
EGERIA
EGESTA
IGOTTA
IGUANA
OGLALA
UGANDA

••GA••
ARGALI
ASGARD
BIGAIR
BIGAMY
BIGAPE
BOGART
BUGAKU
CIGARS
DAGAMA
DEGAGE
DIGAMY
DOGAPE
DUGALD
DUGARD
EDGARD
EDGARS
ELGART
ENGAGE
FIGARO
FUGARD
FUGATO
HOGANS
IMGAME
INGATE
KAGAWA
KIGALI
LEGACY
LEGALS
LEGART
LEGATE
LEGATO
LIGAND
LIGATE
LOGANS
MEGALO
MEGANE
MUGABE
NAGANO
NEGATE
ORGANA
ORGANS
PAGANS
REGAIN
REGALE
REGARD
REGAVE
RIGANS
RIGATI
SUGARS
SUGARY
TOGAED
TSGARP
TVGAME
UGGAMS
UNGAGS
UNGAMY
UNGAVA
UPGAZE
VAGARY
VEGANS
WIGAND

••G•A•
AEGEAN
AFGHAN
AUGEAN
AUGEAS
BAGDAD
BAGMAN
BEGGAR
BIGBAD
BIGCAR
BIGCAT
BIGDAY
BIGEAR
BIGFAN
BIGMAC
BIGMAN
CAGUAS
COGNAC
DAGMAR
DIGRAM
DIGSAT
DOGDAY
DOGEAR
DOGMAS
DOGNAP
DOGSAT
DOGTAG
EGGSAC
ENGRAM
FIGBAR
GAGLAW
GAGMAN
GIGBAG
HAGGAI
HAGMAN
HEGOAT
IMGLAD
INGEAR
INGMAR
INGOAL
INGRAM
INGRAY
JAGUAR
JIGSAW
LAGEAR
LEGMAN
LOGJAM
MAGIAN
MAGMAS
MAGYAR
MCGRAW
NAGNAG
NAGSAT
ORGEAT
PIGMAN
RAGBAG
RAGLAN
RAGMAN
RAGNAR
RAGTAG
REGEAR
REGGAE
REGNAL
REGNAT
REGRAB
RUGRAT
SEGWAY
SIGHAT
SIGMAS
SIGNAL
TAGDAY
TUGSAT
UNGLAD
UNGUAL
VIGIAS
WIGWAG
WIGWAM
ZIGZAG

••G••A
ANGELA
ANGLIA
ANGOLA
ANGORA
BOGOTA
DAGAMA
EIGHTA
HEGIRA
JOGBRA
KAGAWA
LAGUNA
LIGEIA
LOGGIA
NAGOYA
ORGANA
OUGHTA
PAGLIA
PAGODA
RAGUSA
REGINA
SEGURA
UNGAVA
UNGULA
VIGODA
ZYGOMA

•••GA•
AARGAU
ALEGAR
AMIGAS
BEGGAR
BELGAE
BENGAL
BENGAY
BIOGAS
BROGAN
BULGAR
BUNGAY
CONGAS
COOGAN
COUGAR
DOUGAL
FRUGAL
FUNGAL
GARGAN
GEEGAW
GEWGAW
HAGGAI
HANGAR
HORGAN
JEDGAR
MANGAS
MEDGAR
MORGAN
NONGAS
NORGAY
NOUGAT
OLDGAG
OMEGAS
OUTGAS
PISGAH
POLGAR
REAGAN
REGGAE
RENGAS
SEAGAL
SLOGAN
TAIGAS
TARGAS
THEGAP
TONGAN
VARGAS
VIRGAS
VULGAR

•••G•A
ALOGIA
BORGIA
ENIGMA
LENGUA
LINGUA
LOGGIA
PHAGIA
QUAGGA
STIGMA
VIAGRA

••••GA
AURIGA
BAERGA
BELUGA
BODEGA
CAYUGA
DEVEGA
IOMEGA
LADOGA
MALAGA
ORTEGA
PAANGA
QUAGGA
ZUNIGA

G•B•••
GABBED
GABBER
GABBLE
GABBRO
GABLED
GABLER
GABLES
GIBBER
GIBBON
GIBEAT
GIBERS
GIBILL
GIBING
GIBLET
GIBRAN
GIBSON
GOBACK
GOBANG
GOBBLE
GOBIES
GOBLET
GOBLIN
GOBOES
GOBOOM
GOBOTS
GOBSOF
GOBUST

G••B••
GABBED
GABBER
GABBLE
GABBRO
GAMBIA
GAMBIT
GAMBLE
GAMBOL
GARBED
GARBER
GARBLE
GASBAG
GERBER
GERBIL
GIBBER
GIBBON
GIGBAG
GIMBAL
GIMBEL
GLIBLY
GLOBAL
GLOBBY
GLOBED
GLOBES
GLOBIN
GOBBLE
GOOBER
GRABAT
GRABBY
GRABLE
GREBES
GROBAN
GRUBBY
GUMBEL
GUMBOS
GYMBAG

G•••B•
GATSBY
GAZEBO
GETSBY
GIAMBI
GLOBBY
GOALBY
GOESBY
GONEBY
GOODBY
GRABBY
GRANBY
GRUBBY

G••••B
GETSAB
GRADEB

•GB•••
EGBERT
KGBSPY

••GB••
BAGBOY
BIGBAD
BIGBEN
BIGBET
BIGBOI
BIGBOX
BIGBOY
BIGBUX
BUGBOY
DOGBED
FIGBAR
FOGBOW
GIGBAG
JOGBRA
PEGBOX
RAGBAG

••G•B•
MUGABE

••G••B
BAGJOB
EIGHTB
RAGHIB
REGRAB
UNGLIB
ZAGREB

•••GB•
HANGBY
HUNGBY
NINGBO

GC••••
GCLEFS

G•C•••
GECKOS
GOCART
GOCOED
GOCOLD
GSCALE

G••C••
GARCIA
GARCON
GASCAN
GASCAP
GASCON
GAUCHE
GAUCHO
GELCAP
GLACES
GLACIS
GLOCKS
GLYCOL
GORCEY
GOTCHA
GRACED
GRACES
GRACIE
GROCER
GRUCCI

G•••C•
GFORCE
GLANCE
GLITCH
GLOUCS
GOBACK
GRAECO
GREECE
GRIECO
GRINCH
GROUCH
GRUCCI
GYNECO

G••••C
GAELIC
GALLIC
GARLIC
GEODIC
GESTIC
GETSAC
GNOMIC
GOTHIC

•G•C••
EGGCUP

•G••C•
AGENCE
AGENCY
IGNACE

•G•••C
AGARIC
EGGSAC

••GC••
BIGCAR
BIGCAT
EGGCUP

••G•C•
LEGACY
LOGICS
MAGICS

••G••C
ANGLIC
BIGMAC
COGNAC
EGGSAC
EIGHTC
HYGRIC

•••G•C
BELGIC
TRAGIC

GD••••
GDANSK

G•D•••
GADDED
GADDER
GADDIS
GADFLY
GADGET
GEDDES
GIDDAP
GIDEON
GIDGET
GODARD
GODARK
GODEAD
GODEEP
GODETS
GODEYS
GODIVA
GODOWN
GODSON
GODWIN
GODWIT

G••D••
GADDED
GADDER
GADDIS
GANDER
GANDHI
GARDEN
GEDDES
GELDED
GELDOF
GENDER
GEODES
GEODIC
GIDDAP
GILDED
GILDER
GIRDED
GIRDER
GIRDLE
GLADES
GLADLY
GLADTO
GLADYS
GLIDED
GLIDER
GLIDES
GOADED
GOLDEN
GOLDIE
GOODAT
GOODBY
GOODEN
GOODER
GOODIE
GOODLY
GOODOH
GORDIE
GORDON
GOSDEN
GOUDAS
GRADEA
GRADEB
GRADED
GRADER
GRADES
GRIDES
GRODIN
GRUDGE
GUIDED
GUIDER
GUIDES
GUIDRY
GULDEN
GUNDOG

G•••D•
GEORDI
GLANDS
GLENDA
GLINDA
GOURDE
GOURDS
GRANDE
GRANDS
GRANDY
GREEDS
GREEDY
GRINDL
GRINDS
GRUNDY
GUARDS
GUILDS

G••••D
GABBED
GABLED
GADDED
GAFFED
GAGGED
GAINED
GAITED
GALLED
GAMMED
GANGED
GAOLED
GAPPED
GARBED
GASHED
GASPED
GASSED
GAUGED
GAWKED
GAWPED
GEARED
GEEKED
GELDED
GELLED
GEMMED
GERALD
GERARD
GERUND
GETMAD
GETOLD
GETRID
GETSAD
GIFTED
GIGGED
GILDED
GILEAD
GILLED
GIMPED
GINNED
GIRDED
GIRTED
GITTED
GLARED
GLAZED
GLIDED
GLOBED
GLOVED
GLOWED
GNAWED
GOADED
GOCOED
GOCOLD
GODARD
GODEAD
GOLFED
GONGED
GOOFED
GOOSED
GORGED
GORMED
GOTMAD
GOTOLD
GOTRID
GOUGED
GOUNOD
GOWILD
GOWNED
GRACED
GRADED
GRATED
GRAVED
GRAVID
GRAYED
GRAZED
GREYED
GRIMED
GRIPED
GROPED
GROUND
GROVED
GSTAAD
GUIDED
GUILED
GULFED
GULLED
GULPED
GUMMED
GUNNED
GUSHED
GUSTED
GUTTED
GYPPED

•GD•••
OGDOAD

•G•D••
AGADIR
AGEDLY

•G••D•
AGENDA
OGRADY
UGANDA

•G•••D
AGEOLD
AGREED
OGDOAD

••GD••
BAGDAD
BIGDAY
BIGDIG
BIGDOG
BIGDOS
DOGDAY
DOGDOM
FOGDOG
TAGDAY

••G•D•
ALGEDI
PAGODA
VIGODA
YEGODS

••G••D
ANGLED
ARGUED
ASGARD
ASGOOD
AUGEND
BAGDAD
BAGEND
BAGGED
BEGGED
BEGIRD
BEGOOD
BIGBAD
BIGEND
BIGKID
BIGRED
BOGGED
BUGGED
BUGLED
COGGED
DOGBED
DOGGED
DOGOOD
DUGALD
DUGARD
EAGLED
EDGARD
EIGHTD
ENGILD
ENGIRD
FAGEND
FOGGED
FUGARD
GAGGED
GIGGED
HOGGED
HUGGED
IMGLAD
IMGOOD
INGOLD
INGOOD
INGRID
JAGGED
JIGGED
JOGGED
JUGGED
KEGGED
LAGGED
LEGEND
LEGGED
LIGAND
LOGGED
LUGGED
MUGGED
NAGGED
NOGOOD
OSGOOD
PEGGED
PIGGED
RAGGED
REGARD
REGILD
REGIRD
RIGGED
ROGUED
RUGGED
SAGGED
SEGUED
SIGHED
SIGNED
SIGURD
TAGEND
TAGGED
TOGAED
TOGGED
TUGGED
UNGIRD
UNGLAD
UPGIRD
VEGGED
VOGUED
WAGGED
WIGAND
WIGGED
ZAGGED
ZIGGED

•••G•D
BAGGED
BANGED
BARGED
BEGGED
BILGED
BINGED
BOGGED
BONGED
BRIGID
BUDGED
BUGGED
BULGED
BUNGED
CADGED
COGGED
DANGED
DINGED
DODGED
DOGGED
FANGED
FOGGED
FORGED
FRIGID
FUDGED
GAGGED
GANGED
GAUGED
GIGGED
GONGED
GORGED
GOUGED
HANGED
HEDGED
HINGED
HOGGED
HUGGED
IMAGED
JAGGED
JIGGED
JOGGED
JUDGED
JUGGED
KEDGED
KEGGED
KINGED
LAGGED
LEGGED
LODGED
LOGGED
LONGED
LUGGED
LUNGED
MERGED
MUGGED
NAGGED
NONGOD
NUDGED
PARGED
PEGGED
PIGGED
PINGED
PONGID
PURGED
RAGGED
RANGED
RIDGED
RIGGED
RINGED
ROUGED
RUGGED
SAGGED
SEAGOD
SEDGED
SIEGED
SINGED
STAGED
SUBGOD
SUNGOD
SURGED
TAGGED
TANGED
TINGED
TINGOD
TOGGED
TONGED
TUGGED
TURGID
UNAGED
VEGGED
VERGED
WAGGED
WARGOD
WEDGED
WIGGED
WINGED
ZAGGED
ZIGGED
ZINGED

GE••••
GEARED
GEARTO
GEARUP
GECKOS
GEDDES
GEEGAW
GEEING
GEEKED
GEESON
GEEZER
GEFFEN
GEHRIG
GEIGER
GEIGHT
GEISEL
GEISHA
GELATE
GELATI
GELATO
GELCAP
GELDED
GELDOF
GELEES
GELETT
GELLAR
GELLED
GELLER
GELPEN
GELSEY
GEMARA
GEMINI
GEMMAE
GEMMED
GENDER
GENERA
GENETS
GENEVA
GENEVE
GENIAL
GENIES
GENIUS
GENOAN
GENOAS
GENOME
GENOVA
GENRES
GENTES
GENTLE
GENTLY
GENTRY
GENUAL
GENXER
GEODES
GEODIC
GEORDI
GEORGE
GEORGI
GEORGY
GERALD
GERARD
GERBER
GERBIL
GERENT
GERMAN
GERTIE
GERUND
GERVIN
GESTAE
GESTES
GESTIC
GETANA
GETANF
GETFAR
GETFIT
GETHEP
GETHIP
GETHOT
GETMAD
GETOFF
GETOLD
GETOUT
GETRID
GETSAB
GETSAC
GETSAD
GETSAT
GETSBY
GETSET
GETSIN
GETSIT
GETSON
GETSTO
GETSUP
GETTER
GETTIN
GETUPS
GETWET
GEWGAW
GEYSER

G•E•••
GAELIC
GEEGAW
GEEING
GEEKED
GEESON
GEEZER
GHETTO
GIEING
GLEAMS
GLEAMY
GLEANS
GLENDA
GLENNE
GNEISS
GOEASY
GOESAT
GOESBY
GOESIN
GOESON
GOESTO
GOESUP
GOETHE
GREASE
GREASY
GREATS
GREAVE
GREBES
GREECE
GREEDS
GREEDY
GREEKS
GREENE
GREENS
GREENY
GREETS
GREGOR
GREIST
GRETEL
GRETNA
GREWON
GREWUP
GREYED
GREYER
GREYLY
GSEVEN
GUELPH
GUERRE
GUESTS

G••E••
GAIETY
GALEAE
GALEAO
GALENA
GAMELY
GAMERS
GAMEST
GAMETE
GANEFS
GAPEAT
GAPERS
GARETH
GATEAU
GATERS
GAVEIN
GAVELS
GAVEOF
GAVEON
GAVETO
GAVEUP
GAYEST
GAZEAT
GAZEBO
GAZEON
GAZERS
GCLEFS
GELEES
GELETT
GENERA
GENETS
GENEVA
GENEVE
GERENT
GIBEAT
GIBERS
GIDEON
GILEAD
GILELS
GIMELS
GISELE
GIVEIN
GIVENS
GIVEOF
GIVEON
GIVERS
GIVETH
GIVETO
GIVEUP
GLIERE
GLUEON
GLUERS
GLUETO
GODEAD
GODEEP
GODETS
GODEYS
GOFERS
GOLEFT
GOLEMS
GOLETA
GOMERS
GONEAR
GONEAT
GONEBY
GONEIN
GONEON
GONERS
GONETO
GONEUP
GONEXT
GORERS
GOTEAM
GOVERN
GOWELL
GOWEST
GRAECO
GREECE
GREEDS
GREEDY
GREEKS
GREENE
GREENS
GREENY
GREETS
GRIECO
GRIEFS
GRIESE
GRIEVE
GRUELS
GYNECO
GYRENE

G•••E•
GABBED
GABBER
GABLED
GABLER
GABLES
GADDED
GADDER
GADGET
GAFFED
GAFFER
GAFFES
GAGGED
GAGGER
GAGMEN
GAINED
GAINER
GAINES
GAITED
GAITER
GALLED
GALLEY
GAMGEE
GAMIER
GAMMED
GAMMER
GANDER
GANGED
GANGER
GANGES
GANNET
GAOLED
GAOLER
GAPPED
GARBED
GARBER
GARDEN
GARNER
GARNET
GARRET
GARTER
GARVEY
GASHED
GASHES
GASJET
GASKET
GASMEN
GASPED
GASPER
GASSED
GASSER
GASSES
GASTER
GATHER
GAUGED
GAUGER
GAUGES
GAUZES
GAWKED
GAWKER
GAWPED
GAWPER
GAYNES
GEARED
GEDDES
GEEKED
GEEZER
GEFFEN
GEIGER
GEISEL
GELDED
GELEES
GELLED
GELLER
GELPEN
GELSEY
GEMMED
GENDER
GENIES
GENRES
GENTES
GENXER
GEODES
GERBER
GESTES
GETHEP
GETSET
GETTER
GETWET
GEYSER
GIBBER
GIBLET
GIDGET
GIFTED
GIFTEE
GIGGED
GIGUES
GIJOES
GILDED
GILDER
GILLED
GILLEY
GIMBEL
GIMLET
GIMMES
GIMPED
GINGER
GINNED
GIPPER
GIRDED
GIRDER
GIRTED
GITTED
GLACES
GLADES
GLARED
GLARES
GLASER
GLAZED
GLAZER
GLAZES
GLIDED
GLIDER
GLIDES
GLOBED
GLOBES
GLOVED
GLOVER
GLOVES
GLOWED
GLOWER
GLUIER
GLUTEI
GLUTEN
GLUTES
GNAWED
GNAWER
GNOMES
GNOSES
GNOTES
GOADED
GOATEE
GOBIES
GOBLET
GOBOES
GOCOED
GODEEP
GOFREE
GOITER
GOLDEN
GOLFED
GOLFER
GONGED
GOOBER
GOODEN
GOODER
GOOFED
GOOIER
GOONEY
GOOSED
GOOSEN
GOOSES
GOOSEY
GOOVER
GOPHER
GORCEY
GORGED
GORGER
GORGES
GORIER
GORMED
GORSES
GOSDEN
GOSHEN
GOSPEL
GOTHEP
GOTSET
GOTTEN
GOTWET
GOUGED
GOUGER
GOUGES
GOULET
GOWNED
GRACED
GRACES
GRADEA
GRADEB
GRADED
GRADER
GRADES
GRAPES
GRAPEY
GRATED
GRATER
GRATES
GRAVED
GRAVEL
GRAVEN
GRAVER
GRAVES
GRAYED
GRAYER
GRAZED
GRAZER
GRAZES
GREBES
GRETEL
GREYED
GREYER
GRIDES
GRIMED
GRIMES
GRIPED
GRIPER
GRIPES
GROCER
GROPED
GROPER
GROPES
GROVED
GROVEL
GROVER
GROVES
GROWER
GSEVEN
GTILES
GUIDED
GUIDER
GUIDES
GUILED
GUILES
GUINEA
GUISES
GULDEN
GULFED
GULLED
GULLET
GULPED
GULPER
GUMBEL
GUMMED
GUNMEN
GUNNED
GUNNER
GUNSEL
GUNTER
GURLEY
GURNEE
GURNEY
GUSHED
GUSHER
GUSHES
GUSSET
GUSTED
GUTTED
GUTTER
GYPPED

GYPPER

G••••E

GABBLE
GAGGLE
GALEAE
GALORE
GAMBLE
GAMETE
GAMGEE
GAMINE
GARAGE
GARBLE
GARGLE
GAUCHE
GAULLE
GELATE
GEMMAE
GENEVE
GENOME
GENTLE
GEORGE
GERTIE
GESTAE
GFORCE
GIFTEE
GIGGLE
GIJANE
GIMMIE
GINNIE
GIRDLE
GIRLIE
GISELE
GLANCE
GLENNE
GLIERE
GLURGE
GOALIE
GOATEE
GOBBLE
GOETHE
GOFREE
GOGGLE
GOHOME
GOLAME
GOLDIE
GOLIKE
GOLIVE
GOODIE
GOOGLE
GOONIE
GORDIE
GOURDE
GRABLE
GRACIE
GRAMME
GRANDE
GRANGE
GRATAE
GRAZIE
GREASE
GREAVE
GREECE
GREENE
GRIESE
GRIEVE
GRILLE
GRIMKE
GRIPPE
GROOVE
GROSSE
GROUSE
GRUDGE
GRUNGE
GSCALE
GUERRE
GUNITE
GURGLE
GURNEE
GUZZLE
GWYNNE
GYRATE
GYRENE

•GE•••

AGEDLY
AGEING
AGEISM
AGEIST
AGENAS
AGENCE
AGENCY
AGENDA
AGENTJ
AGENTK
AGENTS
AGEOLD
AGEONE
AGEOUT
AGESIX
AGETEN
AGETWO
EGERIA
EGESTA
EGESTS
IGETIT

•G•E••

AGLEAM
AGLETS
AGREED
AGREER
AGREES
EGBERT
EGGERS
EGGERT
EGRESS
EGRETS
IGUESS
OGLERS
OGRESS

•G••E•

AGAMES
AGATES
AGAVES
AGETEN
AGGIES
AGILER
AGONES
AGREED
AGREER
AGREES
EGALES
EGGIER
EGGLER
EGISES
EGUREN
NGUYEN
OGIVES
UGLIER
UGLIES
XGAMES

•G•••E

AGENCE
AGEONE
AGLARE
AGNATE
AGORAE
EGLISE
IGNACE
IGNITE
IGNORE
OGAUGE
UGARTE
UGSOME

••GE••

AEGEAN
ALGEDI
ANGELA
ANGELI
ANGELL
ANGELO
ANGELS
ANGERS
ARGENT
AUGEAN
AUGEAS
AUGEND
AUGERS
BAGELS
BAGEND
BEGEMS
BEGETS
BIGEAR
BIGEND
BIGEYE
BOGEYS
CAGEIN
CAGERS
CAGEUP
COGENT
DEGELS
DEGERM
DIGEST
DOGEAR
EDGEIN
EDGERS
EGGERS
EGGERT
ENGELS
EUGENE
FAGEND
FOGEYS
HUGELY
HUGEST
INGEAR
INGELS
INGEST
LAGEAR
LAGERS
LEGEND
LIGEIA
LIGERS
LIGETI
LUGERS
NUGENT
ORGEAT
PAGERS
PAGEUP
PEGEEN
PIGEON
RAGERS
REGEAR
REGELS
REGENT
ROGERE
ROGERS
ROGETS
SAGELY
SAGEST
TAGEND
TIGERS
URGENT
URGEON
URGERS
WAGERS

••G•E•

AGGIES
AIGLET
AIGRET
ALGREN
ANGLED
ANGLEE
ANGLER
ANGLES
ARGUED
ARGUER
ARGUES
BAGGED
BAGGER
BAGMEN
BEGGED
BEGLEY
BIGBEN
BIGBET
BIGGER
BIGMEN
BIGRED
BIGTEN
BOGGED
BOGIES
BOGLES
BUGGED
BUGLED
BUGLER
BUGLES
CAGIER
CAGNEY
COGGED
CYGNET
DAGGER
DEGREE
DIGGER
DOGBED
DOGGED
DOGIES
DOGLEG
EAGLED
EAGLES
EAGLET
EAGRES
EDGIER
EGGIER
EGGLER
FOGGED
FOGGER
FOGIES
FUGUES
GAGGED
GAGGER
GAGMEN
GIGGED
GIGUES
HAGLER
HEGGEN
HEGYES
HIGHER
HOGGED
HUGGED
HUGGER
HUGHES
IAGREE
INGLES
INGRES
INGREY
JAGGED
JAGGER
JIGGED
JIGGER
JOGGED
JOGGER
JUGGED
KEGGED
KEGGER
KEGLER
LAGGED
LAGGER
LEGGED
LEGMEN
LEGREE
LIGNES
LOGGED
LOGGER
LOGIER
LUGGED
LUGGER
MAGLEV
MAGNET
MCGREW
MEGREZ
MIGUEL
MUGGED
MUGGER
NAGGED
NAGGER
NIGHER
NUGGET
ORGIES
PEGEEN
PEGGED
PEGLEG
PEGLER
PIGGED
PIGLET
PIGMEN
PIGPEN
POGNER
RAGGED
RAGMEN
REGLES
REGRET
REGREW
RIGGED
RIGGER
ROGUED
ROGUES
RUGGED
SAGGED
SAGIER
SEGUED
SEGUES
SIGHED
SIGHER
SIGLER
SIGNED
SIGNEE
SIGNER
SIGNET
TAGGED
TAGGER
TIGGER
TIGRES
TOGAED
TOGGED
TOGUES
TUGGED
TUGGER
UNGUES
UPGREW
VAGUER
VEGGED
VEGGES
VOGUED
VOGUER
VOGUES
WAGGED
WAGGER
WAGNER
WIGGED
WIGLET
WIGNER
ZAGGED
ZAGREB
ZIGGED

••G••E

ALGORE
ANGLEE
ARGIVE
ARGYLE
AUGITE
BAGGIE
BEGONE
BIGAPE
BIGEYE
BIGGIE
BIGJOE
BIGLIE
BIGONE
BIGTOE
BOGGLE
BYGONE
CIGGIE
COGGLE
DEGAGE
DEGREE
DOGAPE
DOGGIE
EIGHTE
ENGAGE
ENGINE
EUGENE
FIGURE
GAGGLE
GIGGLE
GOGGLE
HAGGLE
HIGGLE
HOGTIE
HUGHIE
IAGREE
IMGAME
IMGONE
INGATE
JIGGLE
JOGGLE
JUGGLE
LEGATE
LEGREE
LEGUME
LIGATE
MAGGIE
MAGLIE
MAGPIE
MEGANE
MUGABE
MUGGLE
NEGATE
NIGGLE
PIGGIE
PUGGLE
REGALE
REGAVE
REGGAE
REGGIE
REGIME
REGIVE
REGLUE
ROGERE
SIGNEE
TAGORE
TOGGLE
TVGAME
UNGLUE
UPGAZE
VEGGIE
WAGGLE
WIGGLE
ZYGOTE

•••GE•

ADAGES
APOGEE
BADGER
BADGES
BAGGED
BAGGER
BANGED
BANGER
BARGED
BARGER
BARGES
BEEGEE
BEGGED
BEIGES
BERGEN
BERGER
BIGGER
BILGED
BILGES
BINGED
BINGER
BINGES
BOGGED
BOLGER
BONGED
BORGES
BRUGES
BUDGED
BUDGER
BUDGES
BUDGET
BUGGED
BULGED
BULGES
BUNGED
BUNGEE
BURGEE
BURGER
CADGED
CADGER
CADGES
CODGER
COGGED
CONGER
CONGES
CUDGEL
DAGGER
DANGED
DANGER
DIGGER
DINGED
DINGER
DIRGES
DODGED
DODGEM
DODGER
DODGES
DOGGED
DRAGEE
ELOGES
ETAGES
FANGED
FIDGET
FINGER
FOGGED
FOGGER
FOLGER
FORGED
FORGER
FORGES
FORGET
FRIGES
FUDGED
FUDGER
FUDGES
GADGET
GAGGED
GAGGER
GAMGEE
GANGED
GANGER
GANGES
GAUGED
GAUGER
GAUGES
GEIGER
GIDGET
GIGGED
GINGER
GONGED
GORGED
GORGER
GORGES
GOUGED
GOUGER
GOUGES
HAAGEN
HANGED
HANGER
HEDGED
HEDGER
HEDGES
HEEGER
HEGGEN
HENGES
HINGED
HINGES
HODGES
HOGGED
HUGGED
HUGGER
HUNGER
IMAGED
IMAGER
IMAGES
IMOGEN
INAGES
JAEGER
JAGGED
JAGGER
JIGGED
JIGGER
JOGGED
JOGGER
JUDGED
JUDGES
JUGGED
JUNGER
KEDGED
KEDGER
KEDGES
KEGGED
KEGGER
KINGED
KROGER
KRUGER
LAGGED
LAGGER
LANGER
LARGER
LARGES
LEDGER
LEDGES
LEGGED
LIEGES
LINGER
LODGED
LODGER
LODGES
LOGGED
LOGGER
LONGED
LONGER
LONGES
LONGET
LUGGED
LUGGER
LUNGED
LUNGER
LUNGES
MAJGEN
MANGER
MEAGER
MERGED
MERGEE
MERGER
MERGES
MIDGES
MIDGET
MONGER
MORGEN
MUGGED
MUGGER
NAGGED
NAGGER
NUDGED
NUDGER
NUDGES
NUGGET
NUNGEN
ONAGER
ORIGEN
OSAGES
OXYGEN
PARGED
PARGER
PARGES
PEGGED
PIAGET
PIGGED
PINGED
PINGER
PLAGES
PONGEE
PURGED
PURGES
RAGGED
RANGED
RANGEL
RANGER
RANGES
REIGER
RIDGED
RIDGES
RIGGED
RIGGER
RINGED
RINGER
ROUGED
ROUGES
RUGGED
RUTGER
SAGGED
SANGER
SARGES
SEDGED
SEDGES
SEEGER
SERGEI
SERGES
SIEGED
SIEGEL
SIEGES
SINGED
SINGER
SINGES
STAGED
STAGER
STAGES
STAGEY
SURGED
SURGES
TAGGED
TAGGER
TANGED
TARGET
TIGGER
TINGED
TINGES
TOGGED
TONGED
TUGGED
TUGGER
UNAGED
USAGES
VEGGED
VEGGES
VERGED
VERGER
VERGES
VOSGES
WAGGED
WAGGER
WEDGED
WEDGES
WIDGET
WIGGED
WINGED
WINGER
YEAGER
ZAGGED
ZENGER
ZIGGED
ZINGED
ZINGER

•••G•E

ALEGRE
APOGEE
BAGGIE
BANGLE
BEAGLE
BEEGEE
BEIGNE
BELGAE
BIGGIE
BINGLE
BOGGLE
BOOGIE
BROGUE
BUDGIE
BUNGEE
BUNGLE
BURGEE
BURGLE
CHIGOE
CIGGIE
COGGLE
COIGNE
DANGLE
DANGME
DINGLE
DOGGIE
DONGLE
DOOGIE
DRAGEE
DROGUE
EMIGRE
FERGIE
GAGGLE
GAMGEE
GARGLE
GIGGLE
GOGGLE
GOOGLE
GURGLE
HAGGLE
HIGGLE
HINGLE
HOAGIE
JANGLE
JIGGLE
JINGLE
JOGGLE
JUGGLE
JUNGLE
KINGME
LEAGUE
LENGLE
LINGLE
LONGUE
MAGGIE
MANGLE
MARGIE
MEAGRE
MERGEE
MINGLE
MORGUE
MUGGLE
NIGGLE
NOOGIE
PIGGIE
PLAGUE
PONGEE
PRAGUE
PUGGLE
REGGAE
REGGIE
SANGRE
SINGLE
SOIGNE
STOGIE
TANGLE
TINGLE
TOGGLE
TONGUE
TRYGVE
VEGGIE
WAGGLE
WANGLE
WEDGIE
WIGGLE
WOOGIE

••••GE

ALLEGE
ARIEGE
ARPEGE
AVENGE
BAREGE
BLUDGE
BRIDGE
CHANGE
CHARGE
CRINGE
CUBAGE
DAMAGE
DEGAGE
DELUGE
DIMAGE
DIRIGE
DOSAGE
DOTAGE
DREDGE
DRUDGE
EMERGE
ENCAGE
ENGAGE
ENRAGE
FLANGE
FLEDGE
FORAGE
FRIDGE
FRINGE
GARAGE
GEORGE
GLURGE
GRANGE
GRUDGE
GRUNGE
HOMAGE
ICEAGE
INNAGE
KLUDGE
KRESGE
LACAGE
LAVAGE
LESAGE
LINAGE
LOUNGE
LOVAGE
MANAGE
MANEGE
MENAGE
MIRAGE
NEWAGE
NONAGE
NOODGE
OARAGE
OBLIGE
OGAUGE
OHMAGE
OLDAGE
ONEDGE
ORANGE
OUTAGE
PELAGE
PIPAGE
PLEDGE
PLUNGE
POTAGE
PREAGE
RAVAGE
RECAGE
REFUGE
RENEGE
REPAGE
REURGE
SAVAGE
SEWAGE
SILAGE
SLEDGE
SLUDGE
SMIDGE
SMUDGE
SPONGE
STODGE
STOOGE
THEAGE
TOWAGE
TRIAGE
TRUDGE
TUBAGE
TWINGE
ULLAGE
UNCAGE
UNEDGE
UNSAGE
VISAGE
VOYAGE
XLARGE

GF••••

GFIFTY
GFLATS
GFORCE

G•F•••

GAFFED
GAFFER
GAFFES
GEFFEN
GIFTED
GIFTEE
GOFAST
GOFERS
GOFFIN
GOFISH
GOFLAT
GOFREE
GUFFAW

G••F••

GADFLY
GAFFED
GAFFER
GAFFES
GEFFEN
GETFAR
GETFIT
GFIFTY
GOFFIN
GOLFED
GOLFER
GOOFED
GOOFUP
GOOFUS
GOTFAR
GOTFIT
GRAFTS
GRIFTS
GUFFAW
GULFED
GUNFOR

G•••F•

GANEFS
GASIFY
GCLEFS
GETOFF
GOLEFT
GOSOFT
GOTOFF
GRAAFF
GRIEFS

G••••F

GAVEOF
GELDOF
GETANF
GETOFF
GIVEOF
GOBSOF
GOTANF
GOTOFF
GRAAFF

•G••F•

UGLIFY

••GF••

BAGFUL
BEGFOR
BIGFAN
BIGFUN
DIGFOR
DUGFOR
JUGFUL
MUGFUL

••G•F•

ARGUFY
BEGOFF
BUGOFF
LOGOFF
REGIFT

••G••F

BEGOFF
BUGOFF
ENGULF
INGULF
LOGOFF

•••GF•

KUNGFU

G•G•••

GAGGED
GAGGER
GAGGLE
GAGING
GAGLAW
GAGMAN
GAGMEN

GIGBAG
GIGGED
GIGGLE
GIGGLY
GIGOLO
GIGOTS
GIGUES
GOGGLE
GOGGLY
GOGIRL
GUGINO

G••G••
GADGET
GAGGED
GAGGER
GAGGLE
GAMGEE
GANGED
GANGER
GANGES
GANGLY
GANGUP
GARGAN
GARGLE
GAUGED
GAUGER
GAUGES
GEEGAW
GEIGER
GEIGHT
GEWGAW
GIDGET
GIGGED
GIGGLE
GIGGLY
GINGER
GINGKO
GIUGNO
GLOGGS
GOGGLE
GOGGLY
GONGED
GOOGLE
GOOGLY
GOOGOL
GOOGOO
GORGED
GORGER
GORGES
GORGON
GOUGED
GOUGER
GOUGES
GREGOR
GRIGRI
GROGGY
GUNGHO
GURGLE

G•••G•
GARAGE
GEORGE
GEORGI
GEORGY
GINKGO
GLOGGS
GLURGE
GOINGS
GONOGO
GRANGE
GRINGO
GROGGY
GRUDGE
GRUNGE
GRUNGY
GULAGS

G••••G
GAGING
GAMING
GAPING
GASBAG
GASHOG
GASLOG
GATING
GAZING
GEEING
GEHRIG
GIBING
GIEING
GIGBAG
GIVING
GLUING
GOBANG
GOLONG
GORING
GOSTAG
GRUING
GUNDOG
GUYING
GYMBAG
GYRING

•GG•••
AGGIES
EGGCUP
EGGERS
EGGERT
EGGIER
EGGING
EGGLER
EGGNOG
EGGSAC
EGGSON
IGGING
IGGINS
UGGAMS

•G••G•
OGAUGE

•G•••G
AGEING
EGGING
EGGNOG
IGGING
OGLING

••GG••
BAGGED
BAGGER
BAGGIE
BEGGAR
BEGGED
BIGGER
BIGGIE
BIGGUN
BIGGUY
BOGGED
BOGGLE
BUGGED
CIGGIE
COGGED
COGGLE
DAGGER
DAGGOO
DIGGER
DOGGED
DOGGIE
FOGGED
FOGGER
GAGGED
GAGGER
GAGGLE
GIGGED
GIGGLE
GIGGLY
GOGGLE
GOGGLY
HAGGAI
HAGGIS
HAGGLE
HEGGEN
HIGGLE
HOGGED
HUGGED
HUGGER
JAGGED
JAGGER
JIGGED
JIGGER
JIGGLE
JIGGLY
JOGGED
JOGGER
JOGGLE
JUGGED
JUGGLE
KEGGED
KEGGER
LAGGED
LAGGER
LEGGED
LOGGED
LOGGER
LOGGIA
LUGGED
LUGGER
MAGGIE
MAGGIO
MAGGOT
MUGGED
MUGGER
MUGGLE
NAGGED
NAGGER
NIGGLE
NOGGIN
NUGGET
PEGGED
PIGGED
PIGGIE
PUGGLE
RAGGED
REGGAE
REGGIE
RIGGED
RIGGER
RUGGED
SAGGED
TAGGED
TAGGER
TIGGER
TOGGED
TOGGLE
TUGGED
TUGGER
VEGGED
VEGGES
VEGGIE
WAGGED
WAGGER
WAGGLE
WAGGLY
WIGGED
WIGGIN
WIGGLE
WIGGLY
ZAGGED
ZIGGED

••G•G•
DEGAGE
ENGAGE
UNGAGS

••G••G
BAGWIG
BIGDIG
BIGDOG
BIGHUG
BIGRIG
BIGWIG
CAGING
DOGLEG
DOGTAG
DUGONG
EDGING
EGGING
EGGNOG
FOGDOG
GAGING
GIGBAG
IGGING
LUGING
NAGNAG
PAGING
PEGLEG
RAGBAG
RAGING
RAGRUG
RAGTAG
URGING
WAGING
WIGWAG
ZIGZAG

•••GG•
CLOGGY
CRAGGY
DRAGGY
FLAGGY
FROGGY
GLOGGS
GROGGY
QUAGGA
QUAGGY
SCAGGS
SHAGGY
SKAGGS
SLUGGO
SMOGGY
SNAGGY
TROGGS
TWIGGY

•••G•G
FIZGIG
OLDGAG

••••GG
BADEGG
DELUGG
ONEEGG
OWLEGG
RAWEGG

GH••••
GHAINS
GHAZIS
GHETTO
GHIJKL
GHIRSH
GHOSTS
GHOSTY
GHOULS

G•H•••
GEHRIG
GOHOME
GSHARP

G••H••
GASHED
GASHES
GASHOG
GATHER
GETHEP
GETHIP
GETHOT
GOPHER
GORHAM
GOSHEN
GOTHAM
GOTHEP
GOTHIC
GOTHIP
GOTHOT
GRAHAM
GUSHED
GUSHER
GUSHES

G•••H•
GANDHI
GAUCHE
GAUCHO
GEIGHT
GEISHA
GIRTHS
GLYPHS
GOETHE
GOTCHA
GRAPHO
GRAPHS
GRAPHY
GRISHA
GUNGHO
GUNSHY
GURKHA

G••••H
GALOSH
GARETH
GARISH
GHIRSH
GIVETH
GLITCH
GOFISH
GOODOH
GOWITH
GRINCH
GROUCH
GROWTH
GUELPH
GULLAH

•GH•••
AGHAST
FGHIJK
OGHAMS

•G••H•
AGATHA

•G•••H
AGUISH
OGRISH

••GH••
AFGHAN
AUGHTS
BIGHIT
BIGHTS
BIGHUG
EFGHIJ
EIGHTA
EIGHTB
EIGHTC
EIGHTD
EIGHTE
EIGHTH
EIGHTS
EIGHTY
FIGHTS
HIGHER
HIGHIQ
HIGHLY
HIGHON
HIGHUP
HUGHES
HUGHIE
LIGHTS
MIGHTS
MIGHTY
NIGHER
NIGHON
NIGHTS
NIGHTY
OUGHTA
OUGHTS
RAGHIB
RIGHTO
RIGHTS
RIGHTY
SIGHAT
SIGHED
SIGHER
SIGHTS
TIGHTS
WIGHTS

••G•H•
MEGOHM

••G••H
BYGOSH
EIGHTH
MYGOSH
OHGOSH

•••GH•
ALIGHT
ARIGHT
BEIGHT
BLIGHT
BOUGHS
BOUGHT
BRIGHT
BURGHS
CAUGHT
COUGHS
DEFGHI
DINGHY
DOUGHS
DOUGHY
DWIGHT
FLIGHT
FOUGHT
FRIGHT
GEIGHT
GUNGHO
HAIGHT
HEIGHT
IEIGHT
IMIGHT
KNIGHT
LAUGHS
NAUGHT
NEIGHS
NOUGHT
PLIGHT
ROUGHS
SLIGHT
SOUGHT
TAUGHT
THIGHS
TOUGHS
TOUGHY
VAUGHN
VEIGHT
VOIGHT
WEIGHS
WEIGHT
WRIGHT

•••G•H
LENGTH
PISGAH

••••GH
AAAUGH
ARMAGH
AWEIGH
BROUGH
CDEFGH
CHOUGH
CLOUGH
DHEIGH
ENOUGH
LEHIGH
MCHUGH
ONHIGH
PLOUGH
SLEIGH
SLOUGH
THOUGH
TROUGH
UNNIGH

GI••••
GIAMBI
GIANNI
GIANTS
GIBBER
GIBBON
GIBEAT
GIBERS
GIBILL
GIBING
GIBLET
GIBRAN
GIBSON
GIDDAP
GIDEON
GIDGET
GIEING
GIFTED
GIFTEE
GIGBAG
GIGGED
GIGGLE
GIGGLY
GIGOLO
GIGOTS
GIGUES
GIJANE
GIJOES
GILDED
GILDER
GILEAD
GILELS
GILLAN
GILLED
GILLEY
GILLIS
GILMAN
GILPIN
GILROY
GIMBAL
GIMBEL
GIMELS
GIMLET
GIMMES
GIMMIE
GIMPED
GINGER
GINGKO
GINKGO
GINNED
GINNIE
GINSUP
GIORNO
GIOTTO
GIPPER
GIRDED
GIRDER
GIRDLE
GIRLIE
GIRTED
GIRTHS
GISELE
GISMOS
GITANO
GITTED
GIUGNO
GIVEIN
GIVENS
GIVEOF
GIVEON
GIVERS
GIVETH
GIVETO
GIVEUP
GIVING
GIZMOS

G•I•••
GAIETY
GAIJIN
GAINED
GAINER
GAINES
GAINLY
GAINON
GAINST
GAITED
GAITER
GEIGER
GEIGHT
GEISEL
GEISHA
GFIFTY
GHIJKL
GHIRSH
GLIBLY
GLIDED
GLIDER
GLIDES
GLIERE
GLINDA
GLINKA
GLINTS
GLINTY
GLITCH
GLITZY
GMINOR
GOINGS
GOINTO
GOITER
GRIDES
GRIECO
GRIEFS
GRIESE
GRIEVE
GRIFTS
GRIGRI
GRILLE
GRILLS
GRIMED
GRIMES
GRIMKE
GRIMLY
GRIMMS
GRIMMY
GRINAT
GRINCH
GRINDL
GRINDS
GRINGO
GRIOTS
GRIPED
GRIPER
GRIPES
GRIPPE
GRIPPY
GRISHA
GRISLY
GRISTS
GRITTI
GRITTY
GSIXTY
GTILES
GUIANA
GUIDED
GUIDER
GUIDES
GUIDRY
GUILDS
GUILED
GUILES
GUILTY
GUINAN
GUINEA
GUISES
GUITAR
GUITRY

G••I••
GAGING
GAMIER
GAMILY
GAMINE
GAMING
GAMINS
GAPING
GARISH
GASIFY
GATING
GAVIAL
GAZING
GEEING
GEMINI
GENIAL
GENIES
GENIUS
GHAINS
GIBILL
GIBING
GIEING
GIVING
GLUIER
GLUING
GNEISS
GOBIES
GODIVA
GOFISH
GOGIRL
GOLIKE
GOLIMP
GOLINO
GOLIVE
GOOIER
GORIER
GORILY
GORING
GORIOT
GOWILD
GOWITH
GRAILS
GRAINS
GRAINY
GREIST
GROINS
GRUING
GSUITS
GUGINO
GUNITE
GURION
GUYING
GYRING

G•••I•
GADDIS
GAELIC
GAIJIN
GALLIA
GALLIC
GALOIS
GAMBIA
GAMBIT
GARCIA
GARLIC
GARYIN
GASLIT
GASOIL
GATLIN
GAVEIN
GAWAIN
GEHRIG
GEODIC
GERBIL
GERTIE
GERVIN
GESTIC
GETFIT
GETHIP
GETRID
GETSIN
GETSIT
GETTIN
GHAZIS
GILLIS
GILPIN
GIMMIE
GINNIE
GIRLIE
GIVEIN
GLACIS
GLOBIN
GLORIA
GLYNIS
GNOMIC
GNOSIS
GOALIE
GOATIT
GOBLIN
GODWIN
GODWIT
GOESIN
GOFFIN
GOLDIE
GONEIN
GOODIE
GOONIE
GOONIN
GORDIE
GOSLIN
GOSSIP
GOTFIT
GOTHIC
GOTHIP
GOTOIT
GOTRID
GRACIE
GRANIT
GRATIA
GRATIN
GRATIS
GRAVID
GRAZIE
GRODIN
GROMIT
GRUMIO
GUNSIT

G••••I
GANDHI
GELATI
GEMINI
GEORDI
GEORGI
GIAMBI
GIANNI
GLUTEI
GRIGRI
GRITTI
GRUCCI

•GI•••
AGILER
AGITAS
BGIRLS
EGISES
OGIVAL
OGIVES

•G•I••
AGEING
AGEISM
AGEIST
AGGIES
AGLINT
AGUISH
EGGIER
EGGING
EGLISE
EGOISM
EGOIST
FGHIJK
IGGING
IGGINS
IGNITE
OGLING
OGRISH
UGLIER
UGLIES
UGLIFY
UGLILY

•G••I•
AGADIR
AGARIC
AGESIX
AGLAIA
AGNAIL
EGERIA
IGETIT
IGOTIT

•G•••I
AGASSI
AGOUTI

••GI••
AGGIES
ARGIVE
AUGITE
BEGINS
BEGIRD
BEGIRT
BOGIES
CAGIER
CAGILY
CAGING
COGITO
DIGITS
DOGIES
EDGIER
EDGILY
EDGING
EGGIER
EGGING
ENGILD
ENGINE
ENGIRD
ENGIRT
FAGINS
FOGIES
GAGING
GOGIRL
GUGINO
HEGIRA
IGGING
IGGINS
ITGIRL
LEGION
LEGIST
LOGICS
LOGIER
LOGILY
LOGINS
LUGING
MAGIAN
MAGICS
MCGILL
MYGIRL
ORGIES
PAGING
RAGING
REGIFT
REGILD
REGIME
REGINA
REGION
REGIRD
REGIUS
REGIVE
SAGIER
SIGILS
UNGILT
UNGIRD
UNGIRT
UPGIRD
UPGIRT
URGING
VIGIAS
VIGILS
WAGING
YOGINI
YOGISM

••G•I•
ANGLIA
ANGLIC
BAGGIE
BAGNIO
BAGSIT
BAGWIG
BIGAIR
BIGDIG
BIGGIE
BIGHIT
BIGKID
BIGLIE
BIGOIL
BIGRIG
BIGWIG
BIGWIN
CAGEIN
CIGGIE
DIGSIN
DIGSIT
DOGGIE
DOGSIT
EDGEIN
EFGHIJ
ENGLIT
FOGSIN
HAGGIS
HIGHIQ
HOGTIE
HUGHIE
HYGRIC
INGRID
LEGSIT
LEGUIN
LIGEIA
LIGNIN
LOGGIA
LOGSIN
LUGLIO
MAGGIE
MAGGIO
MAGLIE
MAGPIE
MEGRIM
NOGGIN
PAGLIA
PIGGIE
PIGSIT
RAGHIB
REGAIN
REGGIE
REGRIP
SIGNIN
TEGRIN
TIGRIS
TUGRIK
UNGLIB
UNGRIP
UNGUIS
VEGGIE
WIGGIN

••G••I
ALGEDI
ANGELI
ARGALI
BIGBOI
HAGGAI
KIGALI
LIGETI
LUGOSI
RIGATI
YOGINI

•••GI•
ADAGIO
ALOGIA
BAGGIE
BELGIC
BIGGIE
BIRGIT
BOOGIE
BORGIA
BRIGID
BRIGIT
BUDGIE
CIGGIE
CORGIS
DANGIT
DOGGIE
DOOGIE
DRAGIN
ELEGIT
FANGIO
FERGIE
FIZGIG
FRIGID
HAGGIS
HANGIN
HINGIS
HOAGIE
HUNGIN
LOGGIA
MAGGIE
MAGGIO
MARGIE
MARGIN

NOGGIN
NOOGIE
ONEGIN
ORIGIN
PHAGIA
PIDGIN
PIGGIE
PLUGIN
PONGID
RANGIN
REGGIE
RINGIN
RUNGIN
SERGIO
SHOGIS
SINGIN
STOGIE
TRAGIC
TURGID
VEGGIE
VERGIL
VIRGIL
VIRGIN
WEDGIE
WIGGIN
WINGIT
WOOGIE
XINGIN

•••G•I
BANGUI
DEFGHI
GRIGRI
HAGGAI
MOWGLI
SERGEI
SNUGLI

••••GI
GEORGI
UBANGI

G•J•••
GIJANE
GIJOES

G••J••
GAIJIN
GASJET
GHIJKL
GMAJOR

•G••J•
FGHIJK

•G•••J
AGENTJ
SGTMAJ

••GJ••
BAGJOB
BIGJOE
LOGJAM

••G••J
EFGHIJ

G•K•••
GOKART

G••K••
GASKET
GAWKAT
GAWKED
GAWKER
GECKOS
GEEKED
GINKGO
GURKHA

G•••K•
GHIJKL
GINGKO
GLINKA
GLOCKS
GOLIKE
GREEKS
GRIMKE

G••••K
GDANSK
GOBACK
GODARK

•G•••K
AGENTK
FGHIJK

••GK••
ANGKOR
BIGKID

••G•K•
BIGSKY
BUGAKU

••G••K
TUGRIK

•••GK•
GINGKO

GL••••
GLACES
GLACIS
GLADES
GLADLY
GLADTO
GLADYS
GLAMOR
GLAMUP
GLANCE
GLANDS
GLARED
GLARES
GLARUS
GLASER
GLASSY
GLAZED
GLAZER
GLAZES
GLEAMS
GLEAMY
GLEANS
GLENDA
GLENNE
GLIBLY
GLIDED
GLIDER
GLIDES
GLIERE
GLINDA
GLINKA
GLINTS
GLINTY
GLITCH
GLITZY
GLOATS
GLOBAL
GLOBBY
GLOBED
GLOBES
GLOBIN
GLOCKS
GLOGGS
GLOOMS
GLOOMY
GLOPPY
GLORIA
GLOSSA
GLOSSO
GLOSSY
GLOTTO
GLOUCS
GLOVED
GLOVER
GLOVES
GLOWED
GLOWER
GLUEON
GLUERS
GLUETO
GLUIER
GLUING
GLUMLY
GLUONS
GLURGE
GLUTEI
GLUTEN
GLUTES
GLYCOL
GLYNIS
GLYPHS
GLYPTO

G•L•••
GALANT
GALAXY
GALEAE
GALEAO
GALENA
GALLED
GALLEY
GALLIA
GALLIC
GALLON
GALLOP
GALLUP
GALOIS
GALOOT
GALOPS
GALORE
GALOSH
GALPAL
GALTON
GALWAY
GCLEFS
GELATE
GELATI
GELATO
GELCAP
GELDED
GELDOF
GELEES
GELETT
GELLAR
GELLED
GELLER
GELPEN
GELSEY
GFLATS
GILDED
GILDER
GILEAD
GILELS
GILLAN
GILLED
GILLEY
GILLIS
GILMAN
GILPIN
GILROY
GOLAME
GOLAST
GOLDEN
GOLDIE
GOLEFT
GOLEMS
GOLETA
GOLFED
GOLFER
GOLIKE
GOLIMP
GOLINO
GOLIVE
GOLLUM
GOLONG
GULAGS
GULDEN
GULFED
GULLAH
GULLED
GULLET
GULPED
GULPER

G••L••
GABLED
GABLER
GABLES
GAELIC
GAGLAW
GALLED
GALLEY
GALLIA
GALLIC
GALLON
GALLOP
GALLUP
GAOLED
GAOLER
GARLIC
GASLIT
GASLOG
GATLIN
GAULLE
GELLAR
GELLED
GELLER
GIBLET
GILLAN
GILLED
GILLEY
GILLIS
GIMLET
GIRLIE
GOALBY
GOALIE
GOBLET
GOBLIN
GOFLAT
GOLLUM
GOSLIN
GOSLOW
GOULET
GRILLE
GRILLS
GTILES
GUELPH
GUILDS
GUILED
GUILES
GUILTY
GULLAH
GULLED
GULLET
GUNLAP
GUNLAW
GURLEY

G•••L•
GABBLE
GADFLY
GAGGLE
GAINLY
GAMBLE
GAMELY
GAMILY
GANGLY
GARBLE
GARGLE
GAULLE
GAVELS
GENTLE
GENTLY
GERALD
GETOLD
GHOULS
GIBILL
GIGGLE
GIGGLY
GIGOLO
GILELS
GIMELS
GIRDLE
GISELE
GLADLY
GLIBLY
GLUMLY
GNARLS
GNARLY
GOBBLE
GOCOLD
GOGGLE
GOGGLY
GOODLY
GOOGLE
GOOGLY
GORILY
GOSOLO
GOTOLD
GOWELL
GOWILD
GRABLE
GRAILS
GRAYLY
GREYLY
GRILLE
GRILLS
GRIMLY
GRISLY
GROWLS
GROWLY
GRRRLS
GRUELS
GSCALE
GURGLE
GUZZLE

G••••L
GALPAL
GAMBOL
GASOIL
GAVIAL
GEISEL
GENIAL
GENUAL
GERBIL
GHIJKL
GIBILL
GIMBAL
GIMBEL
GLOBAL
GLYCOL
GOAWOL
GOGIRL
GOOGOL
GOSPEL
GOWELL
GRAVEL
GRETEL
GRINDL
GROVEL
GUMBEL
GUNSEL

•GL•••
AGLAIA
AGLARE
AGLEAM
AGLETS
AGLINT
EGLISE
IGLOOS
OGLALA
OGLERS
OGLING
UGLIER
UGLIES
UGLIFY
UGLILY

•G•L••
AGILER
EGALES
EGGLER

•G••L•
AGEDLY
AGEOLD
BGIRLS
OGLALA
UGLILY

•G•••L
AGNAIL
OGIVAL

••GL••
AIGLET
ANGLED
ANGLEE
ANGLER
ANGLES
ANGLIA
ANGLIC
ANGLOS
BEGLEY
BIGLIE
BOGLES
BUGLED
BUGLER
BUGLES
DIGLOT
DOGLEG
EAGLED
EAGLES
EAGLET
EGGLER
ENGLIT
ENGLUT
GAGLAW
HAGLER
IMGLAD
INGLES
JAGLOM
KEGLER
LUGLIO
MAGLEV
MAGLIE
PAGLIA
PEGLEG
PEGLER
PIGLET
RAGLAN
REGLES
REGLOW
REGLUE
SIGLER
TIGLON
UNGLAD
UNGLIB
UNGLUE
WIGLET

••G•L•
ANGELA
ANGELI
ANGELL
ANGELO
ANGELS
ANGOLA
ARGALI
ARGYLE
ARGYLL
BAGELS
BOGGLE
CAGILY
COGGLE
DEGELS
DUGALD
EDGILY
ENGELS
ENGILD
ENGULF
GAGGLE
GIGGLE
GIGGLY
GIGOLO
GOGGLE
GOGGLY
HAGGLE
HIGGLE
HIGHLY
HUGELY
INGELS
INGOLD
INGULF
JIGGLE
JIGGLY
JOGGLE
JUGGLE
KIGALI
LEGALS
LOGILY
MCGILL
MEGALO
MOGULS
MUGGLE
NIGGLE
PUGGLE
REGALE
REGELS
REGILD
SAGELY
SIGILS
TOGGLE
UNGILT
UNGULA
VIGILS
WAGGLE
WAGGLY
WIGGLE
WIGGLY

••G••L
ANGELL
ARGYLL
BAGFUL
BIGOIL
GOGIRL
INGOAL
ITGIRL
JUGFUL
MAGNOL
MCGILL
MIGUEL
MUGFUL
MYGIRL
PAGNOL
REGNAL
SIGNAL
UNGUAL

•••GL•
BANGLE
BEAGLE
BINGLE
BOGGLE
BUNGLE
BURGLE
COGGLE
DANGLE
DANGLY
DAYGLO
DINGLE
DONGLE
GAGGLE
GANGLY
GARGLE
GIGGLE
GIGGLY
GOGGLE
GOGGLY
GOOGLE
GOOGLY
GURGLE
HAGGLE
HIGGLE
HINGLE
JANGLE
JANGLY
JIGGLE
JIGGLY
JINGLE
JINGLY
JOGGLE
JUGGLE
JUNGLE
JUNGLY
KINGLY
LENGLE
LINGLE
LONGLY
MANGLE
MINGLE
MOWGLI
MUGGLE
NIGGLE
PUGGLE
SINGLE
SINGLY
SMUGLY
SNUGLI
SNUGLY
TANGLE
TANGLY
TINGLE
TINGLY
TOGGLE
WAGGLE
WAGGLY
WANGLE
WIGGLE
WIGGLY

•••G•L
BENGAL
CUDGEL
DOUGAL
FRUGAL
FUNGAL
GOOGOL
HANGUL
MONGOL
RANGEL
SEAGAL
SIEGEL
VERGIL
VIRGIL

GM••••
GMAJOR
GMINOR

G•M•••
GAMAYS
GAMBIA
GAMBIT
GAMBLE
GAMBOL
GAMELY
GAMERS
GAMEST
GAMETE
GAMGEE
GAMIER
GAMILY
GAMINE
GAMING
GAMINS
GAMMAS
GAMMED
GAMMER
GAMMON
GAMOUS
GAMUTS
GEMARA
GEMINI
GEMMAE
GEMMED
GIMBAL
GIMBEL
GIMELS
GIMLET
GIMMES
GIMMIE
GIMPED
GOMERS
GUMBEL
GUMBOS
GUMMED
GUMSUP
GYMBAG
GYMRAT

G••M••
GAGMAN
GAGMEN
GAMMAS
GAMMED
GAMMER
GAMMON
GASMAN
GASMEN
GEMMAE
GEMMED
GERMAN
GETMAD
GIAMBI
GILMAN
GIMMES
GIMMIE
GISMOS
GIZMOS
GLAMOR
GLAMUP
GLUMLY
GNOMES
GNOMIC
GNOMON
GORMED
GOTMAD
GRAMME
GRAMMY
GRAMPA
GRAMPS
GRIMED
GRIMES
GRIMKE
GRIMLY
GRIMMS
GRIMMY
GROMIT
GRUMIO
GRUMPS
GRUMPY
GUMMED
GUNMAN
GUNMEN
GUTMAN
GUZMAN

G•••M•
GENOME
GLEAMS
GLEAMY
GLOOMS
GLOOMY
GOHOME
GOLAME
GOLEMS
GOLIMP
GOTAMA
GRAMME
GRAMMY
GRIMMS
GRIMMY
GROOMS

G••••M
GOBOOM
GOLLUM
GORHAM
GOTEAM
GOTHAM
GRAHAM
GYPSUM

•GM•••
EGMONT

•G•M••
AGAMAS
AGAMES
SGTMAJ
XGAMES

•G••M•
OGHAMS
UGGAMS
UGSOME

•G•••M
AGAWAM
AGEISM
AGLEAM
EGOISM

••GM••
BAGMAN
BAGMEN
BIGMAC
BIGMAN
BIGMEN
DAGMAR
DOGMAS
GAGMAN
GAGMEN
HAGMAN
INGMAR
LEGMAN
LEGMEN
MAGMAS
PIGMAN
PIGMEN
RAGMAN
RAGMEN
RAGMOP
SIGMAS

••G•M•
BEGEMS
BEGUMS
BIGAMY
DAGAMA
DEGUMS
DIGAMY
IMGAME
LEGUME
REGIME
TVGAME
UGGAMS
UNGAMY
ZYGOMA

••G••M
DEGERM
DIGRAM
DOGDOM
ENGRAM
INGRAM
JAGLOM
LIGNUM
LOGJAM
MAGNUM
MEGOHM
MEGRIM
REGNUM
WIGWAM
YOGISM

•••GM•
DANGME
ENIGMA
KINGME
STIGMA

•••G•M
ARTGUM
DADGUM
DODGEM
SUBGUM

••••GM
PHLEGM

GN••••
GNARLS
GNARLY
GNARRS
GNATTY
GNAWAT
GNAWED
GNAWER
GNAWON
GNEISS
GNOMES
GNOMIC
GNOMON
GNOSES
GNOSIS
GNOTES

G•N•••
GANDER
GANDHI
GANEFS
GANGED
GANGER
GANGES
GANGLY
GANGUP
GANNET
GANNON
GANTRY
GENDER
GENERA
GENETS
GENEVA
GENEVE
GENIAL
GENIES
GENIUS
GENOAN
GENOAS
GENOME
GENOVA
GENRES
GENTES
GENTLE
GENTLY
GENTRY
GENUAL
GENXER
GINGER
GINGKO
GINKGO
GINNED
GINNIE
GINSUP
GONEAR
GONEAT
GONEBY
GONEIN
GONEON
GONERS
GONETO
GONEUP
GONEXT
GONGED
GONOGO
GONUTS
GUNDOG
GUNFOR
GUNGHO
GUNITE
GUNLAP
GUNLAW
GUNMAN
GUNMEN
GUNNAR
GUNNED
GUNNER
GUNSEL
GUNSHY
GUNSIT
GUNTER
GYNECO
GYNOUS

G••N••
GAINED
GAINER
GAINES
GAINLY
GAINON
GAINST
GANNET
GANNON
GARNER
GARNET
GAYNES
GAYNOR
GDANSK
GIANNI
GIANTS
GINNED
GINNIE
GLANCE
GLANDS
GLENDA
GLENNE
GLINDA
GLINKA
GLINTS
GLINTY
GLYNIS
GMINOR
GOINGS
GOINTO
GOONEY
GOONIE
GOONIN
GOUNOD
GOWNED
GRANBY
GRANDE
GRANDS
GRANDY
GRANGE
GRANIT
GRANNY
GRANPA
GRANTS
GRINAT
GRINCH
GRINDL
GRINDS
GRINGO
GRUNDY
GRUNGE
GRUNGY
GRUNTS
GUANOS
GUINAN
GUINEA
GUNNAR
GUNNED
GUNNER
GURNEE
GURNEY
GUVNOR
GWYNNE

G•••N•
GAGING
GALANT
GALENA
GAMINE
GAMING
GAMINS
GAPING
GATING
GAZING
GEEING
GEMINI
GERENT
GERUND
GETANA
GETANF
GHAINS
GIANNI
GIBING
GIEING
GIJANE
GIORNO
GITANO
GIUGNO
GIVENS
GIVING
GLEANS
GLENNE
GLUING
GLUONS
GOBANG
GOLINO
GOLONG
GORING

GOTANA
GOTANF
GRAINS
GRAINY
GRANNY
GREENE
GREENS
GREENY
GRETNA
GROANS
GROINS
GROUND
GROZNY
GRUING
GUGINO
GUIANA
GUYANA
GUYING
GWYNNE
GYRENE
GYRING

G••••N
GAGMAN
GAGMEN
GAIJIN
GAINON
GALLON
GALTON
GAMMON
GANNON
GARCON
GARDEN
GARGAN
GARSON
GARYIN
GASCAN
GASCON
GASMAN
GASMEN
GASTON
GATLIN
GAVEIN
GAVEON
GAWAIN
GAZEON
GEESON
GEFFEN
GELPEN
GENOAN
GERMAN
GERVIN
GETSIN
GETSON
GETTIN
GIBBON
GIBRAN
GIBSON
GIDEON
GILLAN
GILMAN
GILPIN
GIVEIN
GIVEON
GLOBIN
GLUEON
GLUTEN
GNAWON

GNOMON
GOBLIN
GODOWN
GODSON
GODWIN
GOESIN
GOESON
GOFFIN
GOLDEN
GONEIN
GONEON
GOODEN
GOONIN
GOOSEN
GORDON
GORGON
GOSDEN
GOSHEN
GOSLIN
GOTTEN
GOVERN
GRATIN
GRAVEN
GREWON
GROBAN
GRODIN
GROTON
GROWON
GSEVEN
GUINAN
GULDEN
GUNMAN
GUNMEN
GURION
GUTMAN
GUTZON
GUZMAN

•GN•••
AGNAIL
AGNATE
IGNACE
IGNATZ
IGNITE
IGNORE

•G•N••
AGENAS
AGENCE
AGENCY
AGENDA
AGENTJ
AGENTK
AGENTS
AGONES
EGGNOG
UGANDA

•G••N•
AGEING
AGEONE
AGLINT
EGGING
EGMONT
IGGING
IGGINS
IGUANA
OGLING

•G•••N
AGETEN
EGGSON
EGOYAN
EGUREN
NGUYEN

••GN••
BAGNIO
CAGNEY
COGNAC
CYGNET
CYGNUS
DOGNAP
EGGNOG
HOGNUT
LIGNES
LIGNIN
LIGNUM
LUGNUT
MAGNET
MAGNOL
MAGNON
MAGNUM
MAGNUS
MIGNON
NAGNAG
PAGNOL
PIGNUT
POGNER
RAGNAR
REGNAL
REGNAT
REGNUM
SIGNAL
SIGNED
SIGNEE
SIGNER
SIGNET
SIGNIN
SIGNON
SIGNOR
SIGNUP
WAGNER
WIGNER
ZAGNUT

••G•N•
ARGENT
AUGEND
BAGEND
BBGUNS
BEGINS
BEGONE
BIGEND
BIGONE
BYGONE
CAGING
COGENT
DOGONS
DUGONG
EDGING
EGGING
ENGINE
EUGENE
FAGEND
FAGINS
GAGING
GUGINO
HOGANS
IGGING
IGGINS
IMGONE
LAGUNA
LEGEND
LIGAND
LOGANS
LOGINS
LOGONS
LUGING
MEGANE
NAGANO
NUGENT
OBGYNS
ORGANA
ORGANS
PAGANS
PAGING
RAGING
REGENT
REGINA
RIGANS
TAGEND
TIGONS
URGENT
URGING
VEGANS
WAGING
WAGONS
WIGAND
YOGINI

••G••N
AEGEAN
AFGHAN
ALGREN
AUGEAN
BAGMAN
BAGMEN
BIGBEN
BIGFAN
BIGFUN
BIGGUN
BIGMAN
BIGMEN
BIGTEN
BIGWIN
CAGEIN
DIGSIN
DOGRUN
EDGEIN
EGGSON
FOGSIN
GAGMAN
GAGMEN
HAGMAN
HEGGEN
HIGHON
LAGOON
LEGION
LEGMAN
LEGMEN
LEGUIN
LIGNIN
LOGSIN
LOGSON
MAGIAN
MAGNON
MIGNON
NIGHON
NOGGIN
PEGEEN
PIGEON
PIGMAN
PIGMEN
PIGPEN
RAGLAN
RAGMAN
RAGMEN
RAGSON
REGAIN
REGION
SIGNIN
SIGNON
TAGSON
TEGRIN
TIGLON
TUGSON
URGEON
WIGGIN

•••GN•
ALIGNS
BEIGNE
COIGNE
COIGNS
DEIGNS
FEIGNS
GIUGNO
REIGNS
SOIGNE
VSIGNS

•••G•N
AIRGUN
ARAGON
BANGON
BERGEN
BIGGUN
BROGAN
CALGON
CAPGUN
COOGAN
DRAGIN
DRAGON
FLAGON
GARGAN
GORGON
HAAGEN
HANGIN
HANGON
HEGGEN
HORGAN
HUNGIN
HUNGON
IMOGEN
ISOGON
JARGON
JETGUN
MAJGEN
MARGIN
MORGAN
MORGEN
NOGGIN
NUNGEN
ONEGIN
OREGON
ORIGEN
ORIGIN
OUTGUN
OXYGEN
PIDGIN
PLUGIN
POPGUN
PROGUN
RANGIN
RAYGUN
REAGAN
RINGIN
RUNGIN
SAIGON
SARGON
SHOGUN
SINGIN
SIXGUN
SLOGAN
TONGAN
TOPGUN
TOYGUN
TRIGON
VAUGHN
VIRGIN
WIGGIN
XINGIN
YANGON
ZIPGUN

••••GN
ASSIGN
ATSIGN
BENIGN
COSIGN
DESIGN
ENSIGN
IMPUGN
MALIGN
OKSIGN
OPPUGN
REPUGN
RESIGN

GO••••
GOADED
GOALBY
GOALIE
GOATEE
GOATIT
GOAWAY
GOAWOL
GOAWRY
GOBACK
GOBANG
GOBBLE
GOBIES
GOBLET
GOBLIN
GOBOES
GOBOOM
GOBOTS
GOBSOF
GOBUST
GOCART
GOCOED
GOCOLD
GODARD
GODARK
GODEAD
GODEEP
GODETS
GODEYS
GODIVA
GODOWN
GODSON
GODWIN
GODWIT
GOEASY
GOESAT
GOESBY
GOESIN
GOESON
GOESTO
GOESUP
GOETHE
GOFAST
GOFERS
GOFFIN
GOFISH
GOFLAT
GOFREE
GOGGLE
GOGGLY
GOGIRL
GOHOME
GOINGS
GOINTO
GOITER
GOKART
GOLAME
GOLAST
GOLDEN
GOLDIE
GOLEFT
GOLEMS
GOLETA
GOLFED
GOLFER
GOLIKE
GOLIMP
GOLINO
GOLIVE
GOLLUM
GOLONG
GOMERS
GONEAR
GONEAT
GONEBY
GONEIN
GONEON
GONERS
GONETO
GONEUP
GONEXT
GONGED
GONOGO
GONUTS
GOOBER
GOODAT
GOODBY
GOODEN
GOODER
GOODIE
GOODLY
GOODOH
GOOFED
GOOFUP
GOOFUS
GOOGLE
GOOGLY
GOOGOL
GOOGOO
GOOIER
GOONEY
GOONIE
GOONIN
GOOSED
GOOSEN
GOOSES
GOOSEY
GOOVER
GOPAST
GOPHER
GORCEY
GORDIE
GORDON
GORERS
GORGED
GORGER
GORGES
GORGON
GORHAM
GORIER
GORILY
GORING
GORIOT
GORMED
GORSES
GOSDEN
GOSHEN
GOSLIN
GOSLOW
GOSOFT
GOSOLO
GOSOUR
GOSPEL
GOSSIP
GOSTAG
GOTAMA
GOTANA
GOTANF
GOTCHA
GOTEAM
GOTFAR
GOTFIT
GOTHAM
GOTHEP
GOTHIC
GOTHIP
GOTHOT
GOTMAD
GOTOFF
GOTOIT
GOTOLD
GOTOUT
GOTRID
GOTSET
GOTTEN
GOTWET
GOTYOU
GOUDAS
GOUGED
GOUGER
GOUGES
GOULET
GOUNOD
GOUPTO
GOURDE
GOURDS
GOVERN
GOWELL
GOWEST
GOWILD
GOWITH
GOWNED

G•O•••
GAOLED
GAOLER
GEODES
GEODIC
GEORDI
GEORGE
GEORGI
GEORGY
GFORCE
GHOSTS
GHOSTY
GHOULS
GIORNO
GIOTTO
GLOATS
GLOBAL
GLOBBY
GLOBED
GLOBES
GLOBIN
GLOCKS
GLOGGS
GLOOMS
GLOOMY
GLOPPY
GLORIA
GLOSSA
GLOSSO
GLOSSY
GLOTTO
GLOUCS
GLOVED
GLOVER
GLOVES
GLOWED
GLOWER
GNOMES
GNOMIC
GNOMON
GNOSES
GNOSIS
GNOTES
GOOBER
GOODAT
GOODBY
GOODEN
GOODER
GOODIE
GOODLY
GOODOH
GOOFED
GOOFUP
GOOFUS
GOOGLE
GOOGLY
GOOGOL
GOOGOO
GOOIER
GOONEY
GOONIE
GOONIN
GOOSED
GOOSEN
GOOSES
GOOSEY
GOOVER
GROANS
GROATS
GROBAN
GROCER
GRODIN
GROGGY
GROINS
GROMIT
GROOMS
GROOVE
GROOVY
GROPED
GROPER
GROPES
GROSSE
GROSSO
GROSZY
GROTON
GROTTO
GROTTY
GROUCH
GROUND
GROUPS
GROUSE
GROUTS
GROUTY
GROVED
GROVEL
GROVER
GROVES
GROWER
GROWLS
GROWLY
GROWON
GROWTH
GROWUP
GROZNY
GYOZAS

G••O••
GALOIS
GALOOT
GALOPS
GALORE
GALOSH
GAMOUS
GASOIL
GATORS
GAVOTS
GENOAN
GENOAS
GENOME
GENOVA
GETOFF
GETOLD
GETOUT
GIGOLO
GIGOTS
GIJOES
GLOOMS
GLOOMY
GLUONS
GOBOES
GOBOOM
GOBOTS
GOCOED
GOCOLD
GODOWN
GOHOME
GOLONG
GONOGO
GOSOFT
GOSOLO
GOSOUR
GOTOFF
GOTOIT
GOTOLD
GOTOUT
GRIOTS
GROOMS
GROOVE
GROOVY
GYNOUS

G•••O•
GAINON
GALLON
GALLOP
GALOOT
GALTON
GAMBOL
GAMMON
GANNON
GARCON
GARSON
GASCON
GASHOG
GASLOG
GASTON
GAVEOF
GAVEON
GAYNOR
GAZEON
GECKOS
GEESON
GELDOF
GETHOT
GETSON
GIBBON
GIBSON
GIDEON
GILROY
GISMOS
GIVEOF
GIVEON
GIZMOS
GLAMOR
GLUEON
GLYCOL
GMAJOR
GMINOR
GNAWON
GNOMON
GOAWOL
GOBOOM
GOBSOF
GODSON
GOESON
GONEON
GOODOH
GOOGOL
GOOGOO
GORDON
GORGON
GORIOT
GOSLOW
GOTHOT
GOTYOU
GOUNOD
GREGOR
GREWON
GROTON
GROWON
GUANOS
GUMBOS
GUNDOG
GUNFOR
GURION
GUTZON
GUVNOR

G••••O
GABBRO
GALEAO
GASTRO
GAUCHO
GAVETO
GAZEBO
GEARTO
GELATO
GETSTO
GHETTO
GIGOLO
GINGKO
GINKGO
GIORNO
GIOTTO
GITANO
GIUGNO
GIVETO
GLADTO
GLOSSO
GLOTTO
GLUETO
GLYPTO
GOESTO
GOINTO
GOLINO
GONETO
GONOGO
GOOGOO
GOSOLO
GOUPTO
GRAECO
GRAPHO
GRASSO
GRIECO
GRINGO
GROSSO
GROTTO
GRUMIO
GUGINO
GUNGHO
GYNECO

•GO•••
AGONES
AGORAE
AGORAS
AGOROT
AGOSTO
AGOUTI
EGOISM
EGOIST
EGOYAN
IGOROT
IGOTIT
IGOTTA

•G•O••
AGEOLD
AGEONE
AGEOUT
EGMONT
IGLOOS
IGNORE
OGDOAD
UGSOME

•G••O•
AGOROT
EGGNOG
EGGSON
IGLOOS
IGOROT

•G•••O
AGETWO
AGOSTO
PGAPRO

••GO••
ALGORE
ANGOLA
ANGORA
ARGOSY
ARGOTS
ASGOOD
BEGOFF
BEGONE
BEGOOD
BIGOIL
BIGONE
BIGOTS
BOGOTA
BUGOFF
BUGOUT
BYGONE
BYGOSH
DIGOUT
DOGONS
DOGOOD
DUGONG
DUGOUT
ERGOTS
EXGOVS
FAGOTS
GIGOLO
GIGOTS
HEGOAT
IMGONE
IMGOOD
INGOAL
INGOLD
INGOOD
INGOTS
LAGOON
LOGOFF
LOGONS
LOGOUT
LTGOVS
LUGOSI
LUGOUT
MEGOHM
MYGOSH
NAGOYA
NOGOOD
OHGOSH
OSGOOD
PAGODA
PIGOUT
RAGOUT
RIGORS
RIGOUR
RIGOUT
TAGORE
TAGOUT
TIGONS
TOGOUT
VEGOUT
VIGODA
VIGORS
VIGOUR
WAGONS
WIGOUT
YEGODS
ZYGOMA
ZYGOTE

••G•O•
ANGKOR
ANGLOS
ASGOOD
BAGBOY
BAGJOB
BEGFOR
BEGOOD
BIGBOI
BIGBOX
BIGBOY
BIGDOG
BIGDOS
BIGJOE
BIGTOE
BIGTOP
BUGBOY
DAGGOO
DIGFOR
DIGLOT
DOGDOM
DOGOOD
DOGTOY
DUGFOR
EGGNOG
EGGSON
FOGBOW
FOGDOG
HIGHON
IMGOOD
INGOOD
JAGLOM
LAGOON
LEGION
LEGROS
LOGSON
MAGGOT
MAGNOL
MAGNON
MIGNON
NIGHON
NOGOOD
OSGOOD
PAGNOL
PEGBOX
PEGTOP
PIGEON
RAGMOP
RAGSON
RAGTOP
REGION
REGLOW
REGROW
SIGNON
SIGNOR
TAGSON
TIGLON
TUGSON
UPGROW
URGEON

••G••O
ANGELO
BAGNIO
COGITO
DAGGOO
FIGARO
FUGATO
GIGOLO
GUGINO
LEGATO
LUGLIO
MAGGIO
MEGALO
NAGANO
RIGHTO

•••GO•
AMIGOS
ARAGON
BANGON
BANGOR
BINGOS
BONGOS
BURGOO
BURGOS
CALGON
CARGOS
CHIGOE
CONGOU
DAGGOO
DOTGOV
DRAGON
FLAGON

FORGOT
FUEGOS
GOOGOL
GOOGOO
GORGON
GREGOR
HANGON
HUNGON
IMAGOS
ISOGON
JARGON
JUEGOS
LARGOS
MAGGOT
MANGOS
MARGOT
MONGOL
MONGOS
NONGOD
OREGON
SAIGON
SARGON
SEAGOD
SPIGOT
SUBGOD
SUNGOD
TANGOS
TINGOD
TRIGON
VIRGOS
WARGOD
YANGON

•••G•O
ADAGIO
BURGOO
DAGGOO
DAYGLO
FANGIO
GINGKO
GIUGNO
GOOGOO
GUNGHO
MAGGIO
NINGBO
SANGTO
SERGIO
SINGTO
SLUGGO
SUNGTO

••••GO
ANTIGO
ASIAGO
BOINGO
CHANGO
DIRIGO
DONTGO
EASYGO
ERYNGO
FOREGO
GINKGO
GONOGO
GRINGO
HADAGO
HASAGO
INDIGO
ITSAGO
LATIGO
LETSGO
MADEGO
MAKEGO
MAYIGO
NONEGO
OSWEGO
OTSEGO
PAPAGO
PASSGO
SLOWGO
SLUGGO
STOPGO
TOBAGO
VIRAGO
WONTGO

G•P•••
GAPEAT
GAPERS
GAPING
GAPPED
GIPPER
GOPAST
GOPHER
GYPPED
GYPPER
GYPSUM

G••P••
GALPAL
GAPPED
GASPAR
GASPED
GASPER
GAWPED
GAWPER
GELPEN
GILPIN
GIMPED
GIPPER
GLOPPY
GLYPHS
GLYPTO
GOSPEL
GOUPTO
GRAPES
GRAPEY
GRAPHO
GRAPHS
GRAPHY
GRAPPA
GRIPED
GRIPER
GRIPES
GRIPPE
GRIPPY
GROPED
GROPER
GROPES
GULPED
GULPER
GYPPED
GYPPER

G•••P•
GALOPS
GETUPS
GLOPPY
GRAMPA
GRAMPS
GRANPA
GRAPPA
GRASPS
GRIPPE
GRIPPY
GROUPS
GRUMPS
GRUMPY
GUELPH

G••••P
GALLOP
GALLUP
GANGUP
GASCAP
GAVEUP
GEARUP
GELCAP
GETHEP
GETHIP
GETSUP
GIDDAP
GINSUP
GIVEUP
GLAMUP
GODEEP
GOESUP
GOLIMP
GONEUP
GOOFUP
GOSSIP
GOTHEP
GOTHIP
GREWUP
GROWUP
GSHARP
GUMSUP
GUNLAP

•G•P••
PGAPRO

•G••P•
KGBSPY

•G•••P
EGGCUP

••GP••
MAGPIE
PIGPEN

••G•P•
BIGAPE
DOGAPE

••G••P
BIGTOP
CAGEUP
DIGSUP
DOGNAP
EGGCUP
FOGSUP
HIGHUP
PAGEUP
PEGTOP
RAGMOP
RAGTOP
REGRIP
RIGSUP
SIGNUP
TAGSUP
TOGSUP
TSGARP
UNGRIP

•••GP•
PENGPU

•••G•P
ALEGUP
BANGUP
CLOGUP
DRAGUP
GANGUP
HANGUP
HUNGUP
PLUGUP
RANGUP
RINGUP
RUNGUP
SNAGUP
THEGAP

••G••Q
HIGHIQ

GR••••
GRAAFF
GRABAT
GRABBY
GRABLE
GRACED
GRACES
GRACIE
GRADEA
GRADEB
GRADED
GRADER
GRADES
GRAECO
GRAFTS
GRAHAM
GRAILS
GRAINS
GRAINY
GRAMME
GRAMMY
GRAMPA
GRAMPS
GRANBY
GRANDE
GRANDS
GRANDY
GRANGE
GRANIT
GRANNY
GRANPA
GRANTS
GRAPES
GRAPEY
GRAPHO
GRAPHS
GRAPHY
GRAPPA
GRASPS
GRASSO
GRASSY
GRATAE
GRATED
GRATER
GRATES
GRATIA
GRATIN
GRATIS
GRAVAS
GRAVED
GRAVEL
GRAVEN
GRAVER
GRAVES
GRAVID
GRAYED
GRAYER
GRAYLY
GRAZED
GRAZER
GRAZES
GRAZIE
GREASE
GREASY
GREATS
GREAVE
GREBES
GREECE
GREEDS
GREEDY
GREEKS
GREENE
GREENS
GREENY
GREETS
GREGOR
GREIST
GRETEL
GRETNA
GREWON
GREWUP
GREYED
GREYER
GREYLY
GRIDES
GRIECO
GRIEFS
GRIESE
GRIEVE
GRIFTS
GRIGRI
GRILLE
GRILLS
GRIMED
GRIMES
GRIMKE
GRIMLY
GRIMMS
GRIMMY
GRINAT
GRINCH
GRINDL
GRINDS
GRINGO
GRIOTS
GRIPED
GRIPER
GRIPES
GRIPPE
GRIPPY
GRISHA
GRISLY
GRISTS
GRITTI
GRITTY
GROANS
GROATS
GROBAN
GROCER
GRODIN
GROGGY
GROINS
GROMIT
GROOMS
GROOVE
GROOVY
GROPED
GROPER
GROPES
GROSSE
GROSSO
GROSZY
GROTON
GROTTO
GROTTY
GROUCH
GROUND
GROUPS
GROUSE
GROUTS
GROUTY
GROVED
GROVEL
GROVER
GROVES
GROWER
GROWLS
GROWLY
GROWON
GROWTH
GROWUP
GROZNY
GRRRLS
GRUBBY
GRUCCI
GRUDGE
GRUELS
GRUING
GRUMIO
GRUMPS
GRUMPY
GRUNDY
GRUNGE
GRUNGY
GRUNTS

G•R•••
GARAGE
GARBED
GARBER
GARBLE
GARCIA
GARCON
GARDEN
GARETH
GARGAN
GARGLE
GARISH
GARLIC
GARNER
GARNET
GARRET
GARSON
GARTER
GARVEY
GARYIN
GERALD
GERARD
GERBER
GERBIL
GERENT
GERMAN
GERTIE
GERUND
GERVIN
GIRDED
GIRDER
GIRDLE
GIRLIE
GIRTED
GIRTHS
GORCEY
GORDIE
GORDON
GORERS
GORGED
GORGER
GORGES
GORGON
GORHAM
GORIER
GORILY
GORING
GORIOT
GORMED
GORSES
GRRRLS
GURGLE
GURION
GURKHA
GURLEY
GURNEE
GURNEY
GYRATE
GYRENE
GYRING

G••R••
GARRET
GAVRAS
GEARED
GEARTO
GEARUP
GEHRIG
GENRES
GEORDI
GEORGE
GEORGI
GEORGY
GETRID
GFORCE
GHIRSH
GIBRAN
GILROY
GIORNO
GLARED
GLARES
GLARUS
GLORIA
GLURGE
GNARLS
GNARLY
GNARRS
GOFREE
GOTRID
GOURDE
GOURDS
GRRRLS
GUARDS
GUERRE
GYMRAT

G•••R•
GABBRO
GALORE
GAMERS
GANTRY
GAPERS
GASTRO
GATERS
GATORS
GAZERS
GEMARA
GENERA
GENTRY
GERARD
GIBERS
GIVERS
GLIERE
GLUERS
GNARRS
GOAWRY
GOCART
GODARD
GODARK
GOFERS
GOGIRL
GOKART
GOMERS
GONERS
GORERS
GOVERN
GRIGRI
GSHARP
GSTARS
GUERRE
GUIDRY
GUITRY

G••••R
GABBER
GABLER
GADDER
GAFFER
GAGGER
GAINER
GAITER
GAMIER
GAMMER
GANDER
GANGER
GAOLER
GARBER
GARNER
GARTER
GASPAR
GASPER
GASSER
GASTER
GASWAR
GATHER
GAUGER
GAWKER
GAWPER
GAYNOR
GEEZER
GEIGER
GELLAR
GELLER
GENDER
GENXER
GERBER
GETFAR
GETTER
GEYSER
GIBBER
GILDER
GINGER
GIPPER
GIRDER
GLAMOR
GLASER
GLAZER
GLIDER
GLOVER
GLOWER
GLUIER
GMAJOR
GMINOR
GNAWER
GOITER
GOLFER
GONEAR
GOOBER
GOODER
GOOIER
GOOVER
GOPHER
GORGER
GORIER
GOSOUR
GOTFAR
GOUGER
GRADER
GRATER
GRAVER
GRAYER
GRAZER
GREGOR
GREYER
GRIPER
GROCER
GROPER
GROVER
GROWER
GUIDER
GUITAR
GULPER
GUNFOR
GUNNAR
GUNNER
GUNTER
GUSHER
GUTTER
GUVNOR
GYPPER

•GR•••
AGREED
AGREER
AGREES
EGRESS
EGRETS
OGRADY
OGRESS
OGRISH

•G•R••
AGARIC
AGORAE
AGORAS
AGOROT
BGIRLS
EGERIA
EGUREN
IGOROT
UGARTE

•G••R•
AGLARE
EGBERT
EGGERS
EGGERT
IGNORE
OGLERS
PGAPRO

•G•••R
AGADIR
AGILER
AGREER
EGGIER
EGGLER
UGLIER

••GR••
AIGRET
ALGREN
BIGRED
BIGRIG
DEGREE
DIGRAM
DOGRUN
EAGRES
ENGRAM
HYGRIC
IAGREE
INGRAM
INGRAY
INGRES
INGREY
INGRID
LEGREE
LEGROS
MCGRAW
MCGREW
MEGREZ
MEGRIM
RAGRUG
REGRAB
REGRET
REGREW
REGRIP
REGROW
RUGRAT
TEGRIN
TIGRES
TIGRIS
TUGRIK
UNGRIP
UPGREW
UPGROW
ZAGREB

••G•R•
ALGORE
ANGERS
ANGORA
ASGARD
AUGERS
AUGURS
AUGURY
BEGIRD
BEGIRT
BOGART
CAGERS
CIGARS
DEGERM
DUGARD
EDGARD
EDGARS
EDGERS
EGGERS
EGGERT
ELGART
ENGIRD
ENGIRT
FIGARO
FIGURE
FUGARD
GOGIRL
HEGIRA
ITGIRL
JOGBRA
LAGERS
LEGART
LIGERS
LUGERS
MYGIRL
PAGERS
RAGERS
REGARD
REGIRD
RIGORS
ROGERE
ROGERS
SEGURA
SIGURD
SUGARS
SUGARY
TAGORE
TIGERS
TSGARP
UNGIRD
UNGIRT
UPGIRD
UPGIRT
URGERS
VAGARY
VIGORS
WAGERS
YOGURT

••G••R
ANGKOR
ANGLER
ARGUER
BAGGER
BEGFOR
BEGGAR
BIGAIR
BIGCAR
BIGEAR
BIGGER
BIGSUR
BUGLER
CAGIER
DAGGER
DAGMAR
DIGFOR
DIGGER
DOGEAR
DUGFOR
EDGIER
EGGIER
EGGLER
FIGBAR
FOGGER
GAGGER
HAGLER
HIGHER
HUGGER
INGEAR
INGMAR
JAGGER
JAGUAR
JIGGER
JOGGER
KEGGER
KEGLER
LAGEAR
LAGGER
LOGGER
LOGIER
LUGGER
MAGYAR
MUGGER
NAGGER
NIGHER
PEGLER
POGNER
RAGNAR
REGEAR
RIGGER
RIGOUR
SAGIER
SIGHER
SIGLER
SIGNER
SIGNOR
TAGGER
TIGGER
TUGGER
VAGUER
VIGOUR
VOGUER
WAGGER
WAGNER
WIGNER

•••GR•
ALEGRE
EMIGRE
GRIGRI
HUNGRY
MEAGRE
SANGRE
VIAGRA

•••G•R
ALEGAR
BADGER
BAGGER
BANGER
BANGOR
BARGER
BEGGAR
BERGER
BIGGER
BINGER
BOLGER
BUDGER
BULGAR
BULGUR
BURGER
CADGER
CODGER
CONGER
COUGAR
DAGGER
DANGER
DIGGER
DINGER
DODGER
FINGER
FOGGER
FOLGER
FORGER
FUDGER
GAGGER
GANGER
GAUGER
GEIGER
GINGER
GORGER
GOUGER
GREGOR
HANGAR
HANGER
HEDGER
HEEGER
HUGGER
HUNGER
IMAGER
JAEGER
JAGGER
JEDGAR
JIGGER
JOGGER
JUNGER
KEDGER
KEGGER
KROGER
KRUGER
LAGGER
LANGER
LARGER
LEDGER
LINGER
LODGER
LOGGER
LONGER
LUGGER
LUNGER
MANGER
MEAGER
MEDGAR
MERGER
MONGER
MUGGER
NAGGER
NUDGER
ONAGER
PARGER
PINGER
POLGAR
RANGER
REIGER
RIGGER
RINGER
RUTGER
SANGER
SEEGER
SINGER
STAGER
TAGGER
TIGGER
TUGGER
VERGER
VULGAR
WAGGER
WINGER
YASGUR
YEAGER
ZENGER
ZINGER

GS••••
GSCALE
GSEVEN
GSHARP
GSIXTY
GSTAAD
GSTARS
GSUITS

G•S•••
GASBAG
GASCAN
GASCAP
GASCON
GASHED
GASHES
GASHOG
GASIFY
GASJET
GASKET
GASLIT
GASLOG
GASMAN
GASMEN
GASOIL
GASPAR
GASPED
GASPER
GASSED
GASSER
GASSES
GASTAX
GASTER
GASTON
GASTRO
GASWAR
GESTAE
GESTES
GESTIC
GISELE
GISMOS
GOSDEN
GOSHEN
GOSLIN
GOSLOW
GOSOFT
GOSOLO
GOSOUR
GOSPEL
GOSSIP
GOSTAG
GUSHED
GUSHER
GUSHES
GUSSET
GUSTAV
GUSTED

G••S••
GARSON
GASSED
GASSER
GASSES
GATSBY
GEESON
GEISEL
GEISHA
GELSEY
GETSAB
GETSAC
GETSAD
GETSAT
GETSBY
GETSET
GETSIN
GETSIT
GETSON
GETSTO
GETSUP
GEYSER
GHOSTS
GHOSTY
GIBSON
GINSUP
GLASER
GLASSY
GLOSSA

GLOSSO
GLOSSY
GNOSES
GNOSIS
GOBSOF
GODSON
GOESAT
GOESBY
GOESIN
GOESON
GOESTO
GOESUP
GOOSED
GOOSEN
GOOSES
GOOSEY
GORSES
GOSSIP
GOTSET
GRASPS
GRASSO
GRASSY
GRISHA
GRISLY
GRISTS
GROSSE
GROSSO
GROSZY
GUESTS
GUISES
GUMSUP
GUNSEL
GUNSHY
GUNSIT
GUSSET
GYPSUM

G•••S•

GAINST
GALOSH
GAMEST
GARISH
GAYEST
GDANSK
GHIRSH
GLASSY
GLOSSA
GLOSSO
GLOSSY
GNEISS
GOBUST
GOEASY
GOFAST
GOFISH
GOLAST
GOPAST
GOWEST
GRASSO
GRASSY
GREASE
GREASY
GREIST
GRIESE
GROSSE
GROSSO
GROUSE

G••••S

GABLES
GADDIS
GAFFES
GAINES
GALOIS
GALOPS
GAMAYS
GAMERS
GAMINS
GAMMAS
GAMOUS
GAMUTS
GANEFS
GANGES
GAPERS
GASHES
GASSES
GATERS
GATORS
GAUGES
GAUZES
GAVELS
GAVOTS
GAVRAS
GAYNES
GAZERS
GCLEFS
GECKOS
GEDDES
GELEES
GENETS
GENIES
GENIUS
GENOAS
GENRES
GENTES
GEODES
GESTES
GETUPS
GFLATS
GHAINS
GHAZIS
GHOSTS
GHOULS
GIANTS
GIBERS
GIGOTS
GIGUES
GIJOES
GILELS
GILLIS
GIMELS
GIMMES
GIRTHS
GISMOS
GIVENS
GIVERS
GIZMOS
GLACES
GLACIS
GLADES
GLADYS
GLANDS
GLARES
GLARUS
GLAZES
GLEAMS
GLEANS
GLIDES
GLINTS
GLOATS
GLOBES
GLOCKS
GLOGGS
GLOOMS
GLOUCS
GLOVES
GLUERS
GLUONS
GLUTES
GLYNIS
GLYPHS
GNARLS
GNARRS
GNEISS
GNOMES
GNOSES
GNOSIS
GNOTES
GOBIES
GOBOES
GOBOTS
GODETS
GODEYS
GOFERS
GOINGS
GOLEMS
GOMERS
GONERS
GONUTS
GOOFUS
GOOSES
GORERS
GORGES
GORSES
GOUDAS
GOUGES
GOURDS
GRACES
GRADES
GRAFTS
GRAILS
GRAINS
GRAMPS
GRANDS
GRANTS
GRAPES
GRAPHS
GRASPS
GRATES
GRATIS
GRAVAS
GRAVES
GRAZES
GREATS
GREBES
GREEDS
GREEKS
GREENS
GREETS
GRIDES
GRIEFS
GRIFTS
GRILLS
GRIMES
GRIMMS
GRINDS
GRIOTS
GRIPES
GRISTS
GROANS
GROATS
GROINS
GROOMS
GROPES
GROUPS
GROUTS
GROVES
GROWLS
GRRRLS
GRUELS
GRUMPS
GRUNTS
GSTARS
GSUITS
GTILES
GUANOS
GUARDS
GUAVAS
GUESTS
GUIDES
GUILDS
GUILES
GUISES
GULAGS
GUMBOS
GUSHES
GYNOUS
GYOZAS

•GS•••

UGSOME

•G•S••

AGASSI
AGESIX
AGOSTO
EGESTA
EGESTS
EGGSAC
EGGSON
EGISES
KGBSPY

•G••S•

AGASSI
AGEISM
AGEIST
AGHAST
AGUISH
EGLISE
EGOISM
EGOIST
EGRESS
IGUESS
OGRESS
OGRISH

•G•••S

AGAMAS
AGAMES
AGATES
AGAVES
AGENAS
AGENTS
AGGIES
AGITAS
AGLETS
AGONES
AGORAS
AGREES
BGIRLS
EGALES
EGESTS
EGGERS
EGISES
EGRESS
EGRETS
IGGINS
IGLOOS
IGUESS
OGHAMS
OGIVES
OGLERS
OGRESS
UGGAMS
UGLIES
XGAMES

••GS••

ANGSTS
BAGSIT
BIGSKY
BIGSUR
DIGSAT
DIGSIN
DIGSIT
DIGSUP
DOGSAT
DOGSIT
EGGSAC
EGGSON
FOGSIN
FOGSUP
JIGSAW
LEGSIT
LOGSIN
LOGSON
NAGSAT
PIGSIT
PIGSTY
RAGSON
RIGSUP
TAGSON
TAGSUP
TOGSUP
TUGSAT
TUGSON

••G•S•

ARGOSY
AUGUST
BYGOSH
DEGUST
DIGEST
HUGEST
INGEST
LEGIST
LUGOSI
MYGOSH
OHGOSH
RAGUSA
SAGEST
YOGISM

••G••S

AGGIES
ANGELS
ANGERS
ANGLES
ANGLOS
ANGSTS
ARGOTS
ARGUES
AUGEAS
AUGERS
AUGHTS
AUGURS
BAGELS
BBGUNS
BEGEMS
BEGETS
BEGINS
BEGUMS
BIGDOS
BIGHTS
BIGOTS
BOGEYS
BOGIES
BOGLES
BUGLES
CAGERS
CAGUAS
CIGARS
CYGNUS
DEGELS
DEGUMS
DIGITS
DOGIES
DOGMAS
DOGONS
EAGLES
EAGRES
EDGARS
EDGERS
EGGERS
EIGHTS
ENGELS
ERGOTS
EXGOVS
FAGINS
FAGOTS
FIGHTS
FOGEYS
FOGIES
FUGUES
GIGOTS
GIGUES
HAGGIS
HEGYES
HOGANS
HUGHES
IGGINS
INGELS
INGLES
INGOTS
INGRES
LAGERS
LEGALS
LEGROS
LIGERS
LIGHTS
LIGNES
LOGANS
LOGICS
LOGINS
LOGONS
LTGOVS
LUGERS
MAGICS
MAGMAS
MAGNUS
MIGHTS
MOGULS
NIGHTS
OBGYNS
ORGANS
ORGIES
OUGHTS
PAGANS
PAGERS
RAGERS
REGELS
REGIUS
REGLES
RIGANS
RIGHTS
RIGORS
ROGERS
ROGETS
ROGUES
SEGUES
SIGHTS
SIGILS
SIGMAS
SUGARS
TIGERS
TIGHTS
TIGONS
TIGRES
TIGRIS
TOGUES
UGGAMS
UNGAGS
UNGUES
UNGUIS
URGERS
VEGANS
VEGGES
VIGIAS
VIGILS
VIGORS
VOGUES
WAGERS
WAGONS
WIGHTS
YEGODS

•••GS•

MONGST

•••G•S

ADAGES
ALIGNS
AMIGAS
AMIGOS
BADGES
BARGES
BEIGES
BILGES
BINGES
BINGOS
BIOGAS
BONGOS
BORGES
BOUGHS
BRUGES
BUDGES
BULGES
BURGHS
BURGOS
CADGES
CARGOS
COIGNS
CONGAS
CONGES
CORGIS
COUGHS
DEIGNS
DINGUS
DIRGES
DODGES
DOUGHS
ELOGES
ETAGES
FEIGNS
FORGES
FRIGES
FUDGES
FUEGOS
FUNGUS
GANGES
GAUGES
GLOGGS
GORGES
GOUGES
HAGGIS
HEDGES
HENGES
HINGES
HINGIS
HODGES
IMAGES
IMAGOS
INAGES
JUDGES
JUEGOS
KEDGES
LARGES
LARGOS
LAUGHS
LEDGES
LIEGES
LINGUS
LODGES
LONGES
LUNGES
MANGAS
MANGOS
MERGES
MIDGES
MINGUS
MONGOS
NEIGHS
NONGAS
NUDGES
OMEGAS
OSAGES
OUTGAS
PARGES
PLAGES
PURGES
RANGES
REIGNS
RENGAS
RIDGES
ROUGES
ROUGHS
SARGES
SCAGGS
SEDGES
SERGES
SHOGIS
SIEGES
SINGES
SKAGGS
STAGES
SURGES
TAIGAS
TANGOS
TARGAS
THIGHS
TINGES
TOUGHS
TRAGUS
TROGGS
USAGES
VARGAS
VEGGES
VERGES
VIRGAS
VIRGOS
VOSGES
VSIGNS
VULGUS
WEDGES
WEIGHS

••••GS

ALONGS
BEDOGS
BEFOGS
BEINGS
BEWIGS
BHANGS
BOINGS
BOURGS
BRINGS
CLANGS
CLINGS
DEBAGS
DEBUGS
DEFOGS
DOINGS
DORAGS
DRINGS
EMBOGS
EWINGS
FLINGS
GLOGGS
GOINGS
GULAGS
HMONGS
ICINGS
IDTAGS
IKINGS
INRAGS
LIANGS
ORANGS
ORINGS
PRONGS
REBAGS
REDIGS
REJIGS
RELOGS
REPEGS
RERIGS
RETAGS
SCAGGS
SCRAGS
SHRUGS
SKAGGS
SLANGS
SLINGS
SPRIGS
STINGS
SWINGS
THINGS
THONGS
TROGGS
TWANGS
UNBAGS
UNGAGS
UNPEGS
UNRIGS
UNWIGS
VWBUGS
WHANGS
WRINGS
WRONGS

GT••••

GTILES

G•T•••

GATEAU
GATERS
GATHER
GATING
GATLIN
GATORS
GATSBY
GETANA
GETANF
GETFAR
GETFIT
GETHEP
GETHIP
GETHOT
GETMAD
GETOFF
GETOLD
GETOUT
GETRID
GETSAB
GETSAC
GETSAD
GETSAT
GETSBY
GETSET
GETSIN
GETSIT
GETSON
GETSTO
GETSUP
GETTER
GETTIN
GETUPS
GETWET
GITANO
GITTED
GOTAMA
GOTANA
GOTANF
GOTCHA
GOTEAM
GOTFAR
GOTFIT
GOTHAM
GOTHEP
GOTHIC
GOTHIP
GOTHOT
GOTMAD
GOTOFF
GOTOIT
GOTOLD
GOTOUT
GOTRID
GOTSET
GOTTEN
GOTWET
GOTYOU
GSTAAD
GSTARS
GUTMAN
GUTTED
GUTTER
GUTZON

G••T••

GAITED
GAITER
GALTON
GANTRY
GARTER
GASTAX
GASTER
GASTON
GASTRO
GENTES
GENTLE
GENTLY
GENTRY
GERTIE
GESTAE
GESTES
GESTIC
GETTER
GETTIN
GHETTO
GIFTED
GIFTEE
GIOTTO
GIRTED
GIRTHS
GITTED
GLITCH
GLITZY
GLOTTO
GLUTEI
GLUTEN
GLUTES
GNATTY
GNOTES
GOATEE
GOATIT
GOETHE
GOITER
GOSTAG
GOTTEN
GRATAE
GRATED
GRATER
GRATES
GRATIA
GRATIN
GRATIS
GRETEL
GRETNA
GRITTI
GRITTY
GROTON
GROTTO
GROTTY
GUITAR
GUITRY
GUNTER
GUSTAV
GUSTED
GUTTED
GUTTER

G•••T•

GAIETY
GAMETE
GAMUTS
GARETH
GAVETO
GAVOTS
GEARTO
GELATE
GELATI
GELATO
GELETT
GENETS
GETSTO
GFIFTY
GFLATS
GHETTO
GHOSTS
GHOSTY
GIANTS
GIGOTS
GIOTTO
GIVETH
GIVETO
GLADTO
GLINTS
GLINTY
GLOATS
GLOTTO
GLUETO
GLYPTO
GNATTY
GOBOTS
GODETS
GOESTO
GOINTO
GOLETA
GONETO
GONUTS
GOUPTO
GOWITH
GRAFTS
GRANTS
GREATS
GREETS
GRIFTS
GRIOTS
GRISTS
GRITTI
GRITTY
GROATS
GROTTO
GROTTY
GROUTS
GROUTY
GROWTH
GRUNTS
GSIXTY
GSUITS
GUESTS
GUILTY
GUNITE
GYRATE

G••••T

GADGET
GAINST
GALANT
GALOOT
GAMBIT
GAMEST
GANNET
GAPEAT
GARNET
GARRET
GASJET
GASKET
GASLIT
GAWKAT
GAYEST
GAZEAT
GEIGHT
GELETT
GERENT
GETFIT
GETHOT
GETOUT
GETSAT
GETSET
GETSIT
GETWET
GIBEAT
GIBLET
GIDGET
GIMLET
GNAWAT
GOATIT
GOBLET
GOBUST
GOCART
GODWIT
GOESAT
GOFAST
GOFLAT
GOKART
GOLAST
GOLEFT
GONEAT
GONEXT
GOODAT
GOPAST
GORIOT
GOSOFT
GOTFIT
GOTHOT
GOTOIT
GOTOUT
GOTSET
GOTWET
GOULET
GOWEST
GRABAT
GRANIT
GREIST
GRINAT
GROMIT
GULLET
GUNSIT
GUSSET
GYMRAT

•GT•••

SGTMAJ

•G•T••

AGATES
AGATHA
AGETEN
AGETWO
AGITAS
IGETIT
IGOTIT
IGOTTA

•G••T•

AGENTJ
AGENTK
AGENTS
AGLETS
AGNATE
AGOSTO
AGOUTI
EGESTA
EGESTS
EGRETS
IGNATZ
IGNITE
IGOTTA
UGARTE

•G•••T

AGEIST
AGEOUT
AGHAST
AGLINT
AGOROT
EGBERT
EGGERT
EGMONT
EGOIST
IGETIT
IGOROT
IGOTIT

••GT••

BIGTEN
BIGTOE
BIGTOP
DOGTAG
DOGTOY
HOGTIE
PEGTOP
RAGTAG
RAGTOP

••G•T•

ANGSTS
ARGOTS
AUGHTS
AUGITE
BEGETS
BIGHTS
BIGOTS
BOGOTA
COGITO
DIGITS
EIGHTA
EIGHTB
EIGHTC
EIGHTD
EIGHTE
EIGHTH
EIGHTS
EIGHTY
ERGOTS
FAGOTS
FIGHTS
FUGATO
GIGOTS
INGATE
INGOTS
LEGATE
LEGATO
LIGATE
LIGETI
LIGHTS
MIGHTS
MIGHTY
NEGATE
NIGHTS
NIGHTY
OUGHTA
OUGHTS
PIGSTY
RIGATI
RIGHTO
RIGHTS
RIGHTY
ROGETS
SIGHTS
TIGHTS
WIGHTS
ZYGOTE

••G••T

AIGLET
AIGRET
ARGENT

AUGUST BAGSIT BEGIRT BIGBET BIGCAT BIGHIT BOGART BUGOUT COGENT CYGNET DEGUST DIGEST DIGLOT DIGOUT DIGSAT DIGSIT DOGSAT DOGSIT DUGOUT EAGLET EGGERT ELGART ENGIRT ENGLIT ENGLUT HEGOAT HOGNUT HUGEST INGEST LEGART LEGIST LEGSIT LOGOUT LUGNUT LUGOUT MAGGOT MAGNET NAGSAT NUGENT NUGGET ORGEAT PIGLET PIGNUT PIGOUT PIGSIT RAGOUT REGENT REGIFT REGNAT REGRET RIGOUT RUGRAT SAGEST SIGHAT SIGNET TAGOUT TOGOUT TUGSAT UNGILT UNGIRT UPGIRT URGENT VEGOUT WIGLET WIGOUT YOGURT ZAGNUT

•••GT•
LENGTH SANGTO SINGTO SUNGTO

•••G•T
ALIGHT ARIGHT BEIGHT BIRGIT BLIGHT BOUGHT BRIGHT BRIGIT BUDGET CATGUT CAUGHT DANGIT DWIGHT ELEGIT FIDGET FLIGHT FORGET FORGOT FOUGHT FRIGHT GADGET GEIGHT GIDGET HAIGHT HEIGHT IEIGHT IMIGHT KNIGHT LONGET MAGGOT MARGOT MIDGET MONGST NAUGHT NOUGAT NOUGHT NUGGET PIAGET PLIGHT ROTGUT SLIGHT SOUGHT SPIGOT TARGET TAUGHT VEIGHT VOIGHT WEIGHT WIDGET WINGIT WRIGHT

••••GT
CRAIGT FORDGT

GU••••
GUANOS GUARDS GUAVAS GUELPH GUERRE GUESTS GUFFAW GUGINO GUIANA GUIDED GUIDER GUIDES GUIDRY GUILDS GUILED GUILES GUILTY GUINAN GUINEA GUISES GUITAR GUITRY GULAGS GULDEN GULFED GULLAH GULLED GULLET GULPED GULPER GUMBEL GUMBOS GUMMED GUMSUP GUNDOG GUNFOR GUNGHO GUNITE GUNLAP GUNLAW GUNMAN GUNMEN GUNNAR GUNNED GUNNER GUNSEL GUNSHY GUNSIT GUNTER GURGLE GURION GURKHA GURLEY GURNEE GURNEY GUSHED GUSHER GUSHES GUSSET GUSTAV GUSTED GUTMAN GUTTED GUTTER GUTZON GUVNOR GUYANA GUYING GUZMAN GUZZLE

G•U•••
GAUCHE GAUCHO GAUGED GAUGER GAUGES GAULLE GAUZES GIUGNO GLUEON GLUERS GLUETO GLUIER GLUING GLUMLY GLUONS GLURGE GLUTEI GLUTEN GLUTES GOUDAS GOUGED GOUGER GOUGES GOULET GOUNOD GOUPTO GOURDE GOURDS GRUBBY GRUCCI GRUDGE GRUELS GRUING GRUMIO GRUMPS GRUMPY GRUNDY GRUNGE GRUNGY GRUNTS GSUITS

G••U••
GAMUTS GENUAL GERUND GETUPS GHOULS GIGUES GLOUCS GOBUST GONUTS GROUCH GROUND GROUPS GROUSE GROUTS GROUTY

G•••U•
GALLUP GAMOUS GANGUP GAVEUP GEARUP GENIUS GETOUT GETSUP GINSUP GIVEUP GLAMUP GLARUS GOESUP GOLLUM GONEUP GOOFUP GOOFUS GOSOUR GOTOUT GREWUP GROWUP GUMSUP GYNOUS GYPSUM

G••••U
GATEAU GOTYOU

•GU•••
AGUISH EGUREN IGUANA IGUESS NGUYEN

•G•U••
AGOUTI OGAUGE

•G••U•
AGEOUT EGGCUP

••GU••
ARGUED ARGUER ARGUES ARGUFY AUGURS AUGURY AUGUST BBGUNS BEGUMS CAGUAS DEGUMS DEGUST ENGULF FIGURE FUGUES GIGUES INGULF JAGUAR LAGUNA LEGUIN LEGUME MIGUEL MOGULS RAGUSA ROGUED ROGUES SEGUED SEGUES SEGURA SIGURD TOGUES UNGUAL UNGUES UNGUIS UNGULA VAGUER VOGUED VOGUER VOGUES YOGURT

••G•U•
BAGFUL BIGBUX BIGFUN BIGGUN BIGGUY BIGHUG BIGSUR BUGOUT CAGEUP CYGNUS DIGOUT DIGSUP DOGRUN DUGOUT EGGCUP ENGLUT FOGSUP HIGHUP HOGNUT JUGFUL LIGNUM LOGOUT LUGNUT LUGOUT MAGNUM MAGNUS MUGFUL PAGEUP PIGNUT PIGOUT RAGOUT RAGRUG REGIUS REGLUE REGNUM RIGOUR RIGOUT RIGSUP SIGNUP TAGOUT TAGSUP TOGOUT TOGSUP UNGLUE VEGOUT VIGOUR WIGOUT ZAGNUT

••G••U
BUGAKU

•••GU•
AIRGUN ALEGUP ARTGUM BADGUY BANGUI BANGUP BIGGUN BIGGUY BROGUE BULGUR CAPGUN CATGUT CLOGUP DADGUM DINGUS DRAGUP DROGUE FUNGUS GANGUP HANGUL HANGUP HUNGUP JETGUN LEAGUE LENGUA LINGUA LINGUS LONGUE MINGUS MORGUE OUTGUN PLAGUE PLUGUP POPGUN PRAGUE PROGUN RANGUP RAYGUN RINGUP ROTGUT RUNGUP SHOGUN SIXGUN SNAGUP SUBGUM TANGUY TONGUE TOPGUN TOYGUN TRAGUS VULGUS YASGUR ZIPGUN

•••G•U
AARGAU CONGOU KUNGFU PENGPU

G•V•••
GAVEIN GAVELS GAVEOF GAVEON GAVETO GAVEUP GAVIAL GAVOTS GAVRAS GIVEIN GIVENS GIVEOF GIVEON GIVERS GIVETH GIVETO GIVEUP GIVING GOVERN GUVNOR

G••V••
GARVEY GERVIN GLOVED GLOVER GLOVES GOOVER GRAVAS GRAVED GRAVEL GRAVEN GRAVER GRAVES GRAVID GROVED GROVEL GROVER GROVES GSEVEN GUAVAS

G•••V•
GENEVA GENEVE GENOVA GODIVA GOLIVE GREAVE GRIEVE GROOVE GROOVY

G••••V
GUSTAV

•G•V••
AGAVES OGIVAL OGIVES

••G•V•
ARGIVE EXGOVS LTGOVS REGAVE REGIVE UNGAVA

••G••V
MAGLEV

•••GV•
TRYGVE

•••G•V
DOTGOV

GW••••
GWYNNE

G•W•••
GAWAIN GAWKAT GAWKED GAWKER GAWPED GAWPER GEWGAW GOWELL GOWEST GOWILD GOWITH GOWNED

G••W••
GALWAY GASWAR GETWET GLOWED GLOWER GNAWAT GNAWED GNAWER GNAWON GOAWAY GOAWOL GOAWRY GODWIN GODWIT GOTWET GREWON GREWUP GROWER GROWLS GROWLY GROWON GROWTH GROWUP

G•••W•
GODOWN

G••••W
GAGLAW GEEGAW GEWGAW GOSLOW GUFFAW GUNLAW

•G•W••
AGAWAM

•G••W•
AGETWO

••GW••
BAGWIG BIGWIG BIGWIN SEGWAY WIGWAG WIGWAM

••G•W•
KAGAWA

••G••W
FOGBOW GAGLAW JIGSAW MCGRAW MCGREW REGLOW REGREW REGROW UPGREW UPGROW

•••G•W
GEEGAW GEWGAW

G••X••
GENXER GSIXTY

G•••X•
GALAXY GONEXT

G••••X
GASTAX

•G•••X
AGESIX

••G••X
BIGBOX BIGBUX PEGBOX

GY••••
GYMBAG GYMRAT GYNECO GYNOUS GYOZAS GYPPED GYPPER GYPSUM GYRATE GYRENE GYRING

G•Y•••
GAYEST GAYNES GAYNOR GEYSER GLYCOL GLYNIS GLYPHS GLYPTO GUYANA GUYING GWYNNE

G••Y••
GARYIN GOTYOU GRAYED GRAYER GRAYLY GREYED GREYER GREYLY

G•••Y•
GAMAYS GLADYS GODEYS

G••••Y
GADFLY GAIETY GAINLY GALAXY GALLEY GALWAY GAMELY GAMILY GANGLY GANTRY GARVEY GASIFY GATSBY GELSEY GENTLY GENTRY GEORGY GETSBY GFIFTY GHOSTY GIGGLY GILLEY GILROY GLADLY GLASSY GLEAMY GLIBLY GLINTY GLITZY GLOBBY GLOOMY GLOPPY GLOSSY GLUMLY GNARLY GNATTY GOALBY GOAWAY GOAWRY GOEASY GOESBY GOGGLY GONEBY GOODBY GOODLY GOOGLY GOONEY GOOSEY GORCEY GORILY GRABBY GRAINY GRAMMY GRANBY GRANDY GRANNY GRAPEY GRAPHY GRASSY GRAYLY GREASY GREEDY GREENY GREYLY GRIMLY GRIMMY GRIPPY GRISLY GRITTY GROGGY GROOVY GROSZY GROTTY GROUTY GROWLY GROZNY GRUBBY GRUMPY GRUNDY GRUNGY GSIXTY GUIDRY GUILTY GUITRY GUNSHY GURLEY GURNEY

•G•Y••
EGOYAN NGUYEN

•G•••Y
AGEDLY AGENCY KGBSPY OGRADY UGLIFY UGLILY

••GY••
ARGYLE ARGYLL HEGYES MAGYAR OBGYNS

••G•Y•
BIGEYE BOGEYS FOGEYS NAGOYA

••G••Y
ARGOSY ARGUFY AUGURY BAGBOY BEGLEY BIGAMY BIGBOY BIGDAY BIGGUY BIGSKY BUGBOY CAGILY CAGNEY DIGAMY DOGDAY DOGTOY EDGILY EIGHTY GIGGLY GOGGLY HIGHLY HUGELY INGRAY INGREY JIGGLY LEGACY LOGILY MIGHTY NIGHTY PIGSTY RIGHTY SAGELY SEGWAY SUGARY TAGDAY UNGAMY VAGARY WAGGLY WIGGLY

•••G•Y
BADGUY BENGAY BIGGUY BUNGAY CLOGGY CRAGGY DANGLY DINGHY DOUGHY DRAGGY FLAGGY FROGGY GANGLY GIGGLY GOGGLY GOOGLY GROGGY HANGBY HUNGBY HUNGRY JANGLY JIGGLY JINGLY JUNGLY KINGLY LONGLY NORGAY QUAGGY SHAGGY SINGLY SMOGGY SMUGLY SNAGGY SNUGLY STAGEY TANGLY TANGUY TINGLY TOUGHY TWIGGY WAGGLY WIGGLY

••••GY
ANERGY CLERGY CLINGY CLOGGY CRAGGY DRAGGY EFFIGY ENERGY EULOGY FLAGGY FLEDGY FRINGY FROGGY GEORGY GROGGY GRUNGY KLUDGY OOLOGY ORANGY QUAGGY SHAGGY SLANGY SLUDGY SMOGGY SMUDGY SNAGGY SPONGY STINGY STODGY SWINGY SYZYGY THINGY TWANGY TWIGGY

G•Z•••
GAZEAT GAZEBO GAZEON GAZERS GAZING GIZMOS GUZMAN GUZZLE

G••Z••
GAUZES GEEZER GHAZIS GLAZED GLAZER GLAZES GRAZED GRAZER GRAZES GRAZIE GROZNY GUTZON GUZZLE GYOZAS

G•••Z•
GLITZY GROSZY

•G•••Z
IGNATZ

••GZ••
ZIGZAG

••G•Z•
UPGAZE

••G••Z
MEGREZ

HA••••
HAAGEN HAAKON HABANA HABEAS HABILE HABITS HABLAR HACEKS HACHOO HACKED HACKER HACKIE HACKIT HACKLE HACKLY HACKUP HADAGO HADDEN HADDIE HADDIX HADEAN HADFUN HADJES HADJIS HADONE HADOUT HADRON HAFTED HAGGAI HAGGIS HAGGLE HAGLER HAGMAN HAHAHA HAIDAS HAIDEE HAIGHT HAIKAI HAIKUS HAILED HAILER HAILEY HAINES HAIRDO HAIRED HAJJES HAJJIS HAKEEM HAKIMS HALALA HALEST

HALEVY
HALIDE
HALING
HALITE
HALLAM
HALLEL
HALLEY
HALLIE
HALLOO
HALLOS
HALLOW
HALLUX
HALOED
HALOES
HALOID
HALPIN
HALSEY
HALTED
HALTER
HALVAH
HALVAS
HALVED
HALVER
HALVES
HAMATE
HAMDEN
HAMELN
HAMILL
HAMITE
HAMLET
HAMLIN
HAMMED
HAMMER
HAMPER
HAMSUN
HAMSUP
HAMULI
HANDAX
HANDED
HANDEL
HANDER
HANDIN
HANDKE
HANDLE
HANDON
HANDUP
HANGAR
HANGBY
HANGED
HANGER
HANGIN
HANGON
HANGUL
HANGUP
HANKER
HANKIE
HANLEY
HANLON
HANNAH
HANSAS
HANSEL
HANSES
HANSOM
HANSON
HAOLES
HAPPEN
HARALD
HARARE
HARASS
HARBIN
HARBOR
HARDBY
HARDEN
HARDER
HARDIN
HARDLY
HARDUP
HAREMS
HARHAR
HARING
HARKED
HARKEN
HARKER
HARLAN
HARLEM
HARLEY
HARLIN
HARLOT
HARLOW
HARMED
HARMER
HARMON
HARNEY
HAROLD
HARPED
HARPER
HARPON
HARRAD
HARRAH
HARRIS
HARROW
HARRYO
HARRYS
HARVEY
HASAGO
HASBRO
HASFUN
HASHED
HASHES
HASONE
HASOUT
HASPED
HASSAM
HASSAN
HASSEL
HASSID
HASSLE
HASTED
HASTEN
HASTES
HATARI
HATBOX
HATEIT
HATERS
HATETO
HATFUL
HATHOR
HATING
HATPIN
HATRED
HATTED
HATTER
HATTIE
HAULED
HAULER
HAULIN
HAULUP
HAUNCH
HAUNTS
HAVANA
HAVASU
HAVEAT
HAVEIN
HAVEIT
HAVENO
HAVENS
HAVENT
HAVEON
HAVETO
HAVEUP
HAVING
HAVOCS
HAWAII
HAWHAW
HAWING
HAWKED
HAWKER
HAWSER
HAWSES
HAYDEN
HAYERS
HAYING
HAYLEY
HAYMES
HAYMOW
HAYNES
HAYNIE
HAZANS
HAZARD
HAZELS
HAZERS
HAZIER
HAZILY
HAZING
HAZMAT

H•A•••
HAAGEN
HAAKON
HEADED
HEADER
HEADIN
HEADON
HEADTO
HEADUP
HEALED
HEALER
HEALEY
HEALTH
HEALUP
HEANEY
HEAPED
HEAPER
HEAPON
HEAPUP
HEARER
HEARNS
HEAROF
HEARSE
HEARST
HEARTH
HEARTS
HEARTY
HEARYE
HEATED
HEATER
HEATHS
HEATHY
HEATON
HEATUP
HEAVED
HEAVEN
HEAVER
HEAVES
HIATAL
HIATUS
HOAGIE
HOARDS
HOARSE
HOAXED
HOAXER
HOAXES
HYADES
HYATTS

H••A••
HABANA
HADAGO
HAHAHA
HALALA
HAMATE
HARALD
HARARE
HARASS
HASAGO
HATARI
HAVANA
HAVASU
HAWAII
HAZANS
HAZARD
HBEAMS
HECATE
HEMATO
HEPATO
HERALD
HEXADS
HEXANE
HIHATS
HIJACK
HILARY
HIVAOA
HIYALL
HOBART
HODADS
HOGANS
HOMAGE
HORACE
HOTAIR
HOWARD
HUMANE
HUMANS

H•••A•
HABEAS
HABLAR
HADEAN
HAGGAI
HAGMAN
HAIDAS
HAIKAI
HALLAM
HALVAH
HALVAS
HANDAX
HANGAR
HANNAH
HANSAS
HARHAR
HARLAN
HARRAD
HARRAH
HASSAM
HASSAN
HAVEAT
HAWHAW
HAZMAT
HEDRAL
HEEHAW
HEGOAT
HELLAS
HENNAS
HEPCAT
HEPTAD
HERBAL
HEREAT
HERMAN
HERNAN
HEYDAY
HEYMAN
HIATAL
HICKAM
HIEMAL
HINTAT
HISSAT
HITMAN
HITSAT
HODIAK
HODMAN
HOLMAN
HONDAS
HONKAT
HOOHAH
HOOHAS
HOOKAH
HOORAH
HOORAY
HOOSAC
HOOTAT
HORGAN
HOSTAS
HOTCAP
HOTCAR
HOTDAY
HOTWAR
HOWDAH
HOWFAR
HOWLAT
HOWSAD
HUBCAP
HUPPAH
HURRAH
HURRAY
HUSSAR
HUZZAH
HYDRAE
HYDRAS
HYENAS
HYETAL
HYMNAL

H••••A
HABANA
HAHAHA
HALALA
HAVANA
HECUBA
HEGIRA
HELENA
HERNIA
HESTIA
HIVAOA
HOOPLA
HOTTEA
HRYVNA

•HA•••
BHANGS
CHACEL
CHACHA
CHACHI
CHACUN
CHAFED
CHAFER
CHAFES
CHAFFS
CHAFFY
CHAINE
CHAINS
CHAIRS
CHAISE
CHAKRA
CHALET
CHALKS
CHALKY
CHAMMY
CHAMPS
CHANCE
CHANCY
CHANDU
CHANEL
CHANEY
CHANGE
CHANGO
CHANTE
CHANTS
CHANTY
CHAPEL
CHAPIN
CHARDS
CHARGE
CHARLY
CHARMS
CHARON
CHARRO
CHARTA
CHARTS
CHASED
CHASER
CHASES
CHASMS
CHASSE
CHASTE
CHATTY
CHATUP
CHAVEZ
CHAWED
CHAZAN
DHARMA
GHAINS
GHAZIS
KHAKIS
KHALID
LHASAN
PHAGIA
PHAROS
PHASED
PHASER
PHASES
PHASIC
RHAMES
SHABBY
SHACKS
SHADED
SHADER
SHADES
SHADOW
SHAFTS
SHAGGY
SHAKEN
SHAKER
SHAKES
SHAKIN
SHAKOS
SHAKUR
SHALES
SHALEY
SHALIT
SHALLI
SHALLY
SHALOM
SHAMAN
SHAMED
SHAMES
SHAMIR
SHAMMY
SHAMUS
SHANDY
SHANIA
SHANKS
SHANTY
SHAPED
SHAPER
SHAPES
SHARDS
SHARED
SHARER
SHARES
SHARIF
SHARKS
SHARON
SHARPE
SHARPS
SHARPY
SHARYN
SHASTA
SHAVED
SHAVEN
SHAVER
SHAVES
SHAWLS
SHAYNE
SHAZAM
THALER
THALES
THALIA
THAMES
THANES
THANKS
THATCH
THATIS
THATLL
THAWED
THAWER
THAYER
UHAULS
WHACKS
WHALED
WHALER
WHALES
WHALEY
WHAMMO
WHAMMY
WHANGS
WHARFS
WHATIF
WHATLL
WHATVE

•H•A••
CHEAPO
CHEATS
CHIANG
CHOATE
OHBABY
OHDARN
OHMAGE
PHIALS
PHRASE
SHEARS
SHEATH
SHEAVE
SHOALS
SHOALY
SHOATS
SHRANK
THEACT
THEAGE
THEAPE
THEASP
THEAXE
THRACE
THRALL
THRASH
THWACK
THWART
UHLANS
WHEATS
WHOAMI

•H••A•
BHOPAL
BHUTAN
CHAZAN
CHELAE
CHEVAL
CHICAS
CHINAS
CHIRAC
CHIVAS
CHORAL
LHASAN
OHDEAR
OHDRAT
OHIOAN
OHYEAH
RHINAL
SHAMAN
SHAZAM
SHEBAT
SHEVAT
SHIRAZ
SHOFAR
SHOPAT
SHOTAT
SHUMAI
THEBAN
THEBAR
THEBAY
THECAN
THECAR
THEFAN
THEGAP
THEHAJ
THELAW
THEMAN
THERAM
THERAP
THERAT
THETAS
THEWAY
THOMAS
THORAX
THREAD
THREAT
THROAT
WHELAN
WHODAT
XHOSAS

•H•••A
AHIMSA
CHACHA
CHAKRA
CHARTA
CHEETA
CHICHA
CHINUA
CHITRA
CHOLLA
CHOPRA
CHROMA
CHUPPA
CHYNNA
DHARMA
PHAGIA
PHOBIA
RHONDA
RHUMBA
SHANIA
SHASTA
SHEENA
SHEILA
SHERPA
SHORTA
THALIA
THECIA
THEEPA
THELMA
THENBA
THENRA
THESEA
THEUSA
THREEA

••HA••
AGHAST
ALHAIG
ARHATS
ASHADE
ASHAME
ASHARP
ATHAND
BAHAMA
BEHAIM
BEHALF
BEHAVE
BSHARP
BYHALF
BYHAND
COHABS
CSHARP
DEHAIR
DSHARP
ENHALO
ENHAUT
EPHAHS
ERHARD
ESHARP
ETHANE
EXHALE
FSHARP
GSHARP
HAHAHA
HIHATS
INHALE
INHALF
INHAND
ITHACA
JIHADS
JOHANN
LCHAIM
MAHALO
MCHALE
MCHARG
MOHAIR
MOHAVE
MOHAWK
NOHANT
OGHAMS
ONHAND
OSHAWA
PSHAWS
REHABS
REHANG
REHASH
REHAUL
SAHARA
SCHAAP
SCHAVS
TSHAPE
UNHAFT
UNHAIR
UNHALE
UNHAND
UNHASP
UNHATS
UNHAZY
USHAPE
UTHANT
VIHARA
VSHAPE
YSHAPE

••H•A•
ASHCAN
ASHLAR
ASHMAN
ASHPAN
ASHRAM
AXHEAD
BAHIAN
BEHEAD
ISHTAR
LEHMAN
LEHUAS
OAHUAN
OTHMAR
RAHRAH
RAHWAY
REHEAL
REHEAR
REHEAT
SCHAAP
SCHWAB
SCHWAS
TEHRAN
UPHEAP
WAHWAH

••H••A
ALHENA
ATHENA
BAHAMA
DAHLIA
HAHAHA
ITHACA
KAHLUA
KAHUNA
OSHAWA
SAHARA
SCHEMA
VIHARA

•••HA•
AFGHAN
ALOHAS
ALPHAS
ATTHAT
BADHAM
BADHAT
BONHAM
BUCHAN
CATHAY
CEPHAL
COBHAM
CUSHAW
DACHAS
DATHAN
DEDHAM
DENHAM
DIRHAM
DOOHAN
DOTHAN
DUNHAM
DURHAM
GORHAM
GOTHAM
GRAHAM
HARHAR
HAWHAW
HEEHAW
HOOHAH
HOOHAS
INTHAT
ITZHAK
KASHAS
LAPHAM
LESHAN
LETHAL
LOTHAR
MAYHAP
MISHAP
MOCHAS
MOSHAV
MUCHAS
NACHAS
NATHAN
NEWHAT
NIIHAU
NUCHAE
NUCHAL
OLDHAM
OLDHAT
OMAHAN
OMAHAS
OMPHAL
ORPHAN
ORWHAT
PASHAS
PATHAN
PELHAM
RASHAD
REDHAT
RETHAW
ROCHAT
RODHAM
RUSHAT
SASHAY
SEAHAG
SIGHAT
SKIHAT
SOTHAT
SOWHAT
SUCHAS
SUNHAT
THEHAJ
TINHAT
TOPHAT
TOYHAT
TURHAN
UNTHAW
UPSHAW
UTAHAN
WASHAD
WITHAL
YEEHAW

•••H•A
ALTHEA
ASTHMA
BOCHSA
BRAHMA
BUSHWA
EIGHTA
ISCHIA
JOSHUA
KESHIA
KISHKA
MOTHRA
NAPHTA
NASHUA
OUGHTA
SEPHIA
SOPHIA
XINHUA

••••HA
AGATHA
ARETHA
AYESHA
BERTHA
BETCHA
BUDDHA
BUQSHA
CANCHA
CHACHA
CHICHA
CONCHA
EARTHA
ELISHA
GEISHA
GOTCHA
GRISHA
GURKHA
HAHAHA
JASCHA
KWACHA
LUNTHA
MANCHA
MARSHA
MARTHA
MISCHA
MOESHA
OLESHA
PERCHA
POISHA
SANTHA
TRISHA
YAMAHA

HB••••
HBEAMS
HBOMBS

H•B•••
HABANA
HABEAS
HABILE
HABITS
HABLAR
HEBBEL
HEBREW
HEBRON
HOBART
HOBBES
HOBBIT
HOBBLE
HOBNOB
HOBOED
HOBOES
HOBSON
HUBBLE
HUBBUB
HUBCAP
HUBERT
HUBLEY
HUBRIS
HYBRID

H••B••
HARBIN
HARBOR
HASBRO
HATBOX
HEBBEL
HEEBIE
HENBIT
HERBAL
HERBED
HERBES
HERBIE
HOBBES
HOBBIT
HOBBLE
HOMBRE
HOTBED
HOTBOT
HOTBOX
HOWBIG
HUBBLE
HUBBUB
HUMBER
HUMBLE
HUMBLY
HUMBUG

H•••B•
HANGBY
HARDBY
HBOMBS
HECUBA
HEREBY
HORNBY
HUNGBY

H••••B
HOBNOB
HOTTUB
HUBBUB

•HB•••
OHBABY
SHBOOM

•H•B••
CHUBBY
KHYBER
PHOBIA
PHOBIC
PHOBOS
RHEBOK
SHABBY
SHEBAT
SHEBOP
THEBAN
THEBAR
THEBAY
THEBBC
THEBEE
THEBES

•H••B•
CHUBBY
OHBABY
PHILBY
PHLEBO
PHOEBE
RHOMBI
RHOMBS
RHUMBA
RHUMBS
SHABBY
SHELBY
SHOTBY
SHRUBS
THEBBC
THEFBI
THENBA
THISBE
THROBS
THUMBS
WHITBY
ZHLOBS
ZHLUBS

•H•••B
CHERUB
THEHUB
THEMOB
THEWEB
THREEB

••HB••
ASHBIN

••H•B•
ACHEBE
COHABS
REHABS
SAHIBS

••H••B
ATHROB
SCHEIB
SCHLUB
SCHWAB

•••HB•
RUSHBY

•••H•B
EIGHTB
RAGHIB
THEHUB

H•C•••
HACEKS
HACHOO
HACKED
HACKER
HACKIE
HACKIT
HACKLE
HACKLY
HACKUP
HECATE
HECKLE
HECKNO
HECTIC

HECTOR
HECUBA
HICCUP
HICKAM
HICKEY
HICKOK
HOCKED
HOCKER
HOCKEY

H••C••

HEPCAT
HICCUP
HONCHO
HOTCAP
HOTCAR
HOTCUP
HUBCAP

H•••C•

HAUNCH
HAVOCS
HELICO
HIJACK
HIRSCH
HITECH
HOOTCH
HORACE

H••••C

HECTIC
HENDEC
HEROIC
HOMEEC
HOOSAC
HYDRIC
HYGRIC

•HC•••

AHCHOO
OHCRUD

•H•C••

CHACEL
CHACHA
CHACHI
CHACUN
CHECKS
CHICAS
CHICER
CHICHA
CHICHI
CHICKS
CHICLE
CHICLY
CHICOS
CHOCKS
CHUCKS
CHUCKY
SHACKS
SHECKY
SHOCKS
SHUCKS
THECAN
THECAR
THECIA
THECID
THICKE
WHACKS

•H••C•

CHANCE
CHANCY
CHEECH
CHINCH
CHOICE
CHURCH
PHILCO
SHLOCK
SHTICK
THATCH
THEACT
THENCE
THRACE
THRICE
THWACK
WHENCE

•H•••C

AHOLIC
CHEMIC
CHIRAC
CHORIC
PHASIC
PHILIC
PHOBIC
PHONIC
PHOTIC
PHYSIC
THEBBC
THORIC
THREEC
THYMIC

••HC••

ASHCAN

••H•C•

AWHECK
ETHICS
INHOCK
ITHACA
SCHICK

••H••C

ECHOIC
ETHNIC

•••HC•

BOCHCO

•••H•C

EIGHTC
GOTHIC
LITHIC
MYTHIC
ORPHIC
PATHIC
UNCHIC

H•D•••

HADAGO
HADDEN
HADDIE
HADDIX
HADEAN
HADFUN
HADJES
HADJIS
HADONE
HADOUT
HADRON
HEDGED
HEDGER
HEDGES
HEDLEY
HEDRAL
HEDREN
HEDRON
HIDDEN
HIDEHO
HIDEKI
HIDERS
HIDING
HIDOUT
HODADS
HODGES
HODIAK
HODMAN
HODMEN
HUDDIE
HUDDLE
HUDSON
HYDRAE
HYDRAS
HYDRIC
HYDROS
HYDROX
HYDRUS

H••D••

HADDEN
HADDIE
HADDIX
HAIDAS
HAIDEE
HAMDEN
HANDAX
HANDED
HANDEL
HANDER
HANDIN
HANDKE
HANDLE
HANDON
HANDUP
HARDBY
HARDEN
HARDER
HARDIN
HARDLY
HARDUP
HAYDEN
HEADED
HEADER
HEADIN
HEADON
HEADTO
HEADUP
HEEDED
HEEDER
HEIDEN
HELDIN
HELDIT
HELDON
HELDTO
HELDUP
HENDEC
HENDRY
HERDED
HERDER
HEYDAY
HIDDEN
HINDER
HINDUS
HOLDEM
HOLDEN
HOLDER
HOLDIN
HOLDIT
HOLDME
HOLDON
HOLDTO
HOLDUP
HONDAS
HOODED
HOODIE
HOODOO
HORDED
HORDES
HOTDAY
HOTDOG
HOUDON
HOWDAH
HOYDEN
HRIDER
HUDDIE
HUDDLE
HURDLE
HYADES

H•••D•

HAIRDO
HALIDE
HEXADS
HOARDS
HODADS
HOUNDS
HOUNDY
HOWODD
HYOIDS

H••••D

HACKED
HAFTED
HAILED
HAIRED
HALOED
HALOID
HALTED
HALVED
HAMMED
HANDED
HANGED
HARALD
HARKED
HARMED
HAROLD
HARPED
HARRAD
HASHED
HASPED
HASSID
HASTED
HATRED
HATTED
HAULED
HAWKED
HAZARD
HEADED
HEALED
HEAPED
HEATED
HEAVED
HEDGED
HEEDED
HEELED
HEFTED
HELMED
HELPED
HEMMED
HEPTAD
HERALD
HERBED
HERDED
HESIOD
HILLED
HILTED
HINGED
HINTED
HIPPED
HISSED
HOAXED
HOBOED
HOCKED
HOGGED
HONIED
HONKED
HOODED
HOOFED
HOOKED
HOOPED
HOOTED
HOPPED
HORDED
HORNED
HORRID
HORSED
HOSTED
HOTBED
HOTROD
HOUSED
HOWARD
HOWLED
HOWODD
HOWSAD
HUFFED
HUGGED
HULKED
HULLED
HUMMED
HUMPED
HUNTED
HURLED
HUSHED
HUSKED
HUTTED
HYBRID
HYMNED
HYPOED

•HD•••

OHDARN
OHDEAR
OHDRAT

•H•D••

CHEDER
CHIDED
CHIDER
CHIDES
PHEDRE
RHODES
SHADED
SHADER
SHADES
SHADOW
SHEDDS
SHEDON
SHODDY
THEDOW
WHODAT

•H••D•

CHANDU
CHARDS
CHILDE
CHORDS
RHONDA
SHANDY
SHARDS
SHEDDS
SHEEDY
SHINDY
SHODDY
SHREDS
THIRDR
THIRDS

•H•••D

CHAFED
CHASED
CHAWED
CHEFED
CHEWED
CHIDED
CHIMED
CHOKED
CHOWED
CHUTED
KHALID
OHCRUD
PHASED
PHONED
PHYSED
RHYMED
SHADED
SHAMED
SHAPED
SHARED
SHAVED
SHIELD
SHINED
SHOOED
SHOULD
SHOVED
SHOWED
SHREWD
SHROUD
THAWED
THECID
THEEND
THEFED
THEKID
THEMED
THERED
THEROD
THETED
THREAD
THREED
WHALED
WHERED
WHILED
WHINED
WHITED
WHWORD

••HD••

ASHDOD
MAHDIS

••H•D•

APHIDS
ASHADE
EPHODS
JIHADS
MRHYDE
OXHIDE
REHIDE
YEHUDI

••H••D

ASHDOD
ATHAND
AXHEAD
BEHEAD
BEHELD
BEHIND
BEHOLD
BYHAND
ECHOED
ERHARD
INHAND
MTHOOD
OCHRED
ONHAND
ONHOLD
REHELD
REHOED
REHOLD
TEHEED
UNHAND
UNHEED
UNHELD
UNHOED
UNHOOD
UNHUED
UPHELD
UPHOLD

•••H•D

ARCHED
BACHED
BASHED
BATHED
BUSHED
CACHED
CASHED
COSHED
DASHED
DISHED
EIGHTD
ETCHED
FISHED
GASHED
GUSHED
HASHED
HUSHED
INCHED
ITCHED
JOSHED
LASHED
LATHED
MASHED
MESHED
METHOD
MOSHED
MUSHED
NICHED
NOSHED
ORCHID
PISHED
PITHED
POOHED
PUSHED
RASHAD
RASHID
RESHOD
RUSHED
SASHED
SIGHED
TITHED
UNSHED
UNSHOD
WASHAD
WASHED
WISHED

HE••••

HEADED
HEADER
HEADIN
HEADON
HEADTO
HEADUP
HEALED
HEALER
HEALEY
HEALTH
HEALUP
HEANEY
HEAPED
HEAPER
HEAPON
HEAPUP
HEARER
HEARNS
HEAROF
HEARSE
HEARST
HEARTH
HEARTS
HEARTY
HEARYE
HEATED
HEATER
HEATHS
HEATHY
HEATON
HEATUP
HEAVED
HEAVEN
HEAVER
HEAVES
HEBBEL
HEBREW
HEBRON
HECATE
HECKLE
HECKNO
HECTIC
HECTOR
HECUBA
HEDGED
HEDGER
HEDGES
HEDLEY
HEDRAL
HEDREN
HEDRON
HEEBIE
HEEDED
HEEDER
HEEGER
HEEHAW
HEEHEE
HEELED
HEELER
HEFLIN
HEFNER
HEFTED
HEFTER
HEGGEN
HEGIRA
HEGOAT
HEGYES
HEHHEH
HEIDEN
HEIFER
HEIGHT
HEINIE
HEINSE
HEISTS
HELDIN
HELDIT
HELDON
HELDTO
HELDUP
HELENA
HELENE
HELENS
HELICO
HELIOS
HELIUM
HELLAS
HELLER
HELLNO
HELLON
HELLOS
HELMED
HELMER
HELMET
HELMUT
HELOTS
HELPED
HELPER
HELPIN
HELPME
HELPON
HELPUP
HELTER
HEMATO
HEMMED
HEMMER
HEMPEN
HEMSIN
HENBIT
HENDEC
HENDRY
HENGES
HENLEY
HENNAS
HENNER
HENRIK
HENRYI
HENRYK
HENRYV
HENSON
HEPATO
HEPCAT
HEPPER
HEPTAD
HERALD
HERBAL
HERBED
HERBES
HERBIE
HERDED
HERDER
HEREAT
HEREBY
HEREIN
HEREOF
HEREON
HERESY
HERETO
HERMAN
HERMES
HERMIT
HERMON
HERNAN
HERNIA
HEROES
HEROIC
HEROIN
HERONS
HERPET
HERREN
HERSEY
HERVEY
HERZOG
HESIOD
HESOUT
HESTER
HESTIA
HESTON
HETERO
HEURES
HEUSEN
HEWERS
HEWING
HEWISH
HEWITT
HEWSTO
HEXADS
HEXANE
HEXERS
HEXING
HEXNUT
HEXOSE
HEYDAY
HEYMAN
HEYYOU

H•E•••

HBEAMS
HEEBIE
HEEDED
HEEDER
HEEGER
HEEHAW
HEEHEE
HEELED
HEELER
HIEING
HIEMAL
HOEING
HTESTS
HUEVOS
HYENAS
HYETAL

H••E••

HABEAS
HACEKS
HADEAN
HAKEEM
HALEST
HALEVY
HAMELN
HAREMS
HATEIT
HATERS
HATETO
HAVEAT
HAVEIN
HAVEIT
HAVENO
HAVENS
HAVENT
HAVEON
HAVETO
HAVEUP
HAYERS
HAZELS
HAZERS
HELENA
HELENE
HELENS
HEREAT
HEREBY
HEREIN
HEREOF
HEREON
HERESY
HERETO
HETERO
HEWERS
HEXERS
HIDEHO
HIDEKI
HIDERS
HIKERS
HIKEUP
HIREES
HIREON
HIRERS
HITECH
HITEST
HIVERS
HOLERS
HOLEUP
HOMEEC
HOMEIN
HOMELY
HOMERS
HOMEYS
HONEIN
HONERS
HONEST
HONEYS
HOPERS
HOPESO
HOPETO
HOSELS
HOSERS
HOTELS
HOVELS
HOVERS
HOVETO
HOWELL
HUBERT
HUGELY
HUGEST
HUMERI
HYPERS
HYPEUP

H•••E•

HAAGEN
HACKED
HACKER
HADDEN
HADJES
HAFTED
HAGLER
HAIDEE
HAILED
HAILER
HAILEY
HAINES
HAIRED
HAJJES
HAKEEM
HALLEL
HALLEY
HALOED
HALOES
HALSEY
HALTED
HALTER
HALVED
HALVER
HALVES
HAMDEN
HAMLET
HAMMED
HAMMER
HAMPER
HANDED
HANDEL
HANDER
HANGED
HANGER
HANKER
HANLEY
HANSEL
HANSES
HAOLES
HAPPEN
HARDEN
HARDER
HARKED
HARKEN
HARKER
HARLEM
HARLEY
HARMED
HARMER
HARNEY
HARPED
HARPER
HARVEY
HASHED
HASHES
HASPED
HASSEL
HASTED
HASTEN
HASTES
HATRED
HATTED
HATTER
HAULED
HAULER
HAWKED
HAWKER
HAWSER
HAWSES
HAYDEN
HAYLEY
HAYMES
HAYNES
HAZIER
HEADED
HEADER
HEALED
HEALER
HEALEY
HEANEY
HEAPED
HEAPER
HEARER
HEATED
HEATER
HEAVED
HEAVEN
HEAVER
HEAVES
HEBBEL
HEBREW
HEDGED
HEDGER
HEDGES
HEDLEY
HEDREN
HEEDED
HEEDER
HEEGER
HEEHEE
HEELED
HEELER
HEFNER
HEFTED
HEFTER
HEGGEN
HEGYES
HEHHEH
HEIDEN
HEIFER
HELLER
HELMED
HELMER
HELMET
HELPED
HELPER
HELTER
HEMMED
HEMMER
HEMPEN
HENDEC
HENGES
HENLEY
HENNER
HEPPER
HERBED
HERBES
HERDED
HERDER
HERMES
HEROES
HERPET
HERREN
HERSEY
HERVEY
HESTER
HEURES
HEUSEN
HICKEY
HIDDEN
HIGHER
HILLED
HILLEL
HILLER
HILTED
HIMMEL
HINDER
HINGED
HINGES
HINTED
HINTER
HIPPED
HIPPER
HIREES
HISSED
HISSER
HISSES
HITHER
HITMEN
HITTER
HOAXED
HOAXER
HOAXES
HOBBES
HOBOED
HOBOES
HOCKED
HOCKER
HOCKEY
HODGES
HODMEN
HOFFER
HOGGED
HOHNER
HOKIER
HOKIES
HOLDEM
HOLDEN
HOLDER
HOLIER
HOLIES
HOLLER
HOLLEY
HOLMES
HOMEEC
HOMIER
HOMIES
HOMMES
HONIED
HONKED
HONKER
HOODED
HOOFED
HOOFER
HOOKED
HOOKER
HOOKEY
HOOPED
HOOPER
HOOTED
HOOTER
HOOVER
HOOVES
HOPPED
HOPPER
HORDED
HORDES
HORMEL
HORNED
HORNER
HORNET
HORSED
HORSES
HORSEY
HOSIER
HOSSES
HOSTED
HOSTEL
HOTBED
HOTKEY
HOTTEA
HOTTER
HOUSED
HOUSES
HOWLED
HOWLER
HOWSER
HOYDEN
HOYLES
HRIDER
HTILES

HUBLEY
HUFFED
HUGGED
HUGGER
HUGHES
HULKED
HULLED
HULLER
HUMBER
HUMMED
HUMMEL
HUMMER
HUMPED
HUMVEE
HUNGER
HUNKER
HUNLEY
HUNTED
HUNTER
HURLED
HURLER
HURLEY
HURTER
HUSHED
HUSHES
HUSKED
HUSKER
HUSSEY
HUTTED
HUXLEY
HYADES
HYMNED
HYPHEN
HYPOED

H••••E

HABILE
HACKIE
HACKLE
HADDIE
HADONE
HAGGLE
HAIDEE
HALIDE
HALITE
HALLIE
HAMATE
HAMITE
HANDKE
HANDLE
HANKIE
HARARE
HASONE
HASSLE
HATTIE
HAYNIE
HEARSE
HEARYE
HECATE
HECKLE
HEEBIE
HEEHEE
HEINIE
HEINSE
HELENE
HELPME
HERBIE
HEXANE
HEXOSE
HIGGLE
HINGLE
HINKLE
HIPPIE
HITONE
HOAGIE
HOARSE
HOBBLE
HOGTIE
HOLDME
HOMAGE
HOMBRE
HONORE
HOODIE
HOOPLE
HOOPOE
HOOTIE
HORACE
HOTONE
HOTTIE
HUBBLE
HUDDIE
HUDDLE
HUGHIE
HUMANE
HUMBLE
HUMVEE
HURDLE
HURTLE
HUSTLE
HUTONE
HYDRAE

•HE•••

AHERNE
CHEAPO
CHEATS
CHECKS
CHEDER
CHEECH
CHEEKS
CHEEKY
CHEEPS
CHEERS
CHEERY
CHEESE
CHEESY
CHEETA
CHEFED
CHEKOV
CHELAE
CHEMIC
CHEMIN
CHENEY
CHENIN
CHEOPS
CHEQUE
CHERIE
CHERRY
CHERTS
CHERTY
CHERUB
CHERYL
CHESTS
CHESTY
CHEVAL
CHEVET
CHEVON
CHEVRE
CHEVYS
CHEWED
CHEWER
CHEWON
CHEWUP
DHEIGH
GHETTO
OHENRY
PHEDRE
PHELPS
PHENOL
PHENOM
RHEBOK
RHEEMS
RHEIMS
RHEMES
RHESUS
RHETOR
RHEUMS
RHEUMY
SHEARS
SHEATH
SHEAVE
SHEBAT
SHEBOP
SHECKY
SHEDDS
SHEDON
SHEEDY
SHEEHY
SHEENA
SHEENS
SHEENY
SHEERS
SHEESH
SHEETS
SHEIKH
SHEIKS
SHEILA
SHEKEL
SHELBY
SHELLS
SHELTY
SHELVE
SHEREE
SHERPA
SHERRI
SHERRY
SHERYL
SHEVAT
THEACT
THEAGE
THEAPE
THEASP
THEAXE
THEBAN
THEBAR
THEBAY
THEBBC
THEBEE
THEBES
THECAN
THECAR
THECIA
THECID
THEDOW
THEEND
THEEPA
THEEYE
THEFAN
THEFBI
THEFED
THEFLY
THEFOG
THEFOX
THEFTS
THEGAP
THEHAJ
THEHUB
THEIRS
THEISM
THEIST
THEKID
THELAW
THELIP
THELMA
THELOT
THEMAN
THEMED
THEMES
THEMET
THEMOB
THEMRS
THENBA
THENCE
THENET
THENFL
THENHL
THENRA
THEONE
THEORY
THEPIT
THEPRU
THERAM
THERAP
THERAT
THERED
THEREF
THERES
THERMO
THERMS
THEROD
THERON
THESEA
THESES
THESIS
THESON
THESOX
THESPS
THESPY
THESUN
THETAS
THETED
THETIS
THETOP
THETOY
THEUSA
THEVET
THEWAY
THEWEB
THEWHO
THEWIZ
THEYLL
THEYRE
THEYVE
WHEATS
WHEELS
WHEEZE
WHEEZY
WHELAN
WHELKS
WHELMS
WHELPS
WHENCE
WHENLL
WHERED
WHERES
WHERRY
WHEYEY

•H•E••

CHEECH
CHEEKS
CHEEKY
CHEEPS
CHEERS
CHEERY
CHEESE
CHEESY
CHEETA
CHIEFS
CHIENS
KHMERS
NHLERS
OHDEAR
OHWELL
OHYEAH
PHLEBO
PHLEGM
PHOEBE
RHEEMS
SHEEDY
SHEEHY
SHEENA
SHEENS
SHEENY
SHEERS
SHEESH
SHEETS
SHIELD
SHIEST
SHOERS
SHREDS
SHREVE
SHREWD
SHREWS
SHTETL
SHYEST
THEEND
THEEPA
THEEYE
THIEVE
THREAD
THREAT
THREEA
THREEB
THREEC
THREED
THREEE
THREES
THRESH
WHEELS
WHEEZE
WHEEZY

•H••E•

CHACEL
CHAFED
CHAFER
CHAFES
CHALET
CHANEL
CHANEY
CHAPEL
CHASED
CHASER
CHASES
CHAVEZ
CHAWED
CHEDER
CHEFED
CHENEY
CHEVET
CHEWED
CHEWER
CHICER
CHIDED
CHIDER
CHIDES
CHILES
CHIMED
CHIMER
CHIMES
CHINES
CHISEL
CHIVES
CHOKED
CHOKER
CHOKES
CHOLER
CHOREO
CHORES
CHOSEN
CHOWED
CHUTED
CHUTES
DHOLES
DHOTEL
FHOLES
KHYBER
PHASED
PHASER
PHASES
PHLOEM
PHONED
PHONER
PHONES
PHONEY
PHOOEY
PHYSED
RHAMES
RHEMES
RHODES
RHYMED
RHYMER
RHYMES
SHADED
SHADER
SHADES
SHAKEN
SHAKER
SHAKES
SHALES
SHALEY
SHAMED
SHAMES
SHAPED
SHAPER
SHAPES
SHARED
SHARER
SHARES
SHAVED
SHAVEN
SHAVER
SHAVES
SHEKEL
SHEREE
SHINED
SHINER
SHINES
SHIRER
SHIRES
SHIVER
SHOLEM
SHOOED
SHORES
SHOVED
SHOVEL
SHOVER
SHOVES
SHOWED
SHOWER
SHRIEK
THALER
THALES
THAMES
THANES
THAWED
THAWER
THAYER
THEBEE
THEBES
THEFED
THEMED
THEMES
THEMET
THENET
THERED
THEREF
THERES
THESEA
THESES
THETED
THEVET
THEWEB
THOLES
THREEA
THREEB
THREEC
THREED
THREEE
THREES
THROES
THYMES
WHALED
WHALER
WHALES
WHALEY
WHERED
WHERES
WHEYEY
WHILED
WHILES
WHINED
WHINER
WHINES
WHITED
WHITEN
WHITER
WHITES
WHITEY
WHOLES
WHYYES

•H•••E

AHERNE
AHORSE
CHAINE
CHAISE
CHANCE
CHANGE
CHANTE
CHARGE
CHASSE
CHASTE
CHEESE
CHELAE
CHEQUE
CHERIE
CHEVRE
CHICLE
CHIGOE
CHILDE
CHOATE
CHOICE
CHOOSE
CHROME
LHOTSE
OHMAGE
OHSURE
PHEDRE
PHOEBE
PHRASE
SHARPE
SHAYNE
SHEAVE
SHELVE
SHEREE
SHIITE
SHOPPE
SHORTE
SHOWME
SHREVE
SHRIKE
SHRINE
SHRIVE
SHROVE
THEAGE
THEAPE
THEAXE
THEBEE
THEEYE
THENCE
THEONE
THEYRE
THEYVE
THICKE
THIEVE
THISBE
THORPE
THRACE
THREEE
THRICE
THRIVE
THRONE
THROVE
WHATVE
WHEEZE
WHENCE

••HE••

ACHEBE
ACHENE
ACHERS
ADHERE
ALHENA
ATHEEL
ATHENA
ATHENE
ATHENS
AWHECK
AXHEAD
BEHEAD
BEHELD
BEHEST
BOHEME
COHEIR
COHERE
ETHENE
ETHERS
IMHERE
INHERE
MYHERO
NOHELP
OCHERS
OCHERY
OFHELP
OTHERS
REHEAL
REHEAR
REHEAT
REHEEL
REHELD
REHEMS
SCHEIB
SCHELL
SCHEMA
SCHEME
SPHERE
TEHEED
TEHEES
TOHEEL
UNHEED
UNHELD
UNHELM
UNHERO
UNHEWN
UPHEAP
UPHELD
UPHERE
USHERS

••H•E•

ACHIER
ASHIER
ASHLEE
ASHLEY
ASHMEN
ATHEEL
BAHNEN
BOHRER
BTHREE
CAHIER
COHOES
DEHMEL
ECHOED
ECHOER
ECHOES
FUHRER
HEHHEH
HOHNER
KOHLER
LEHNEN
LEHRER
MAHLER
OCHRED
OCHRES
REHEEL
REHOED
REHOES
ROHMER
ROHRER
SCHLEP
TAHNEE
TAHOES
TEHEED
TEHEES
TOHEEL
UNHEED
UNHOED
UNHUED
WOHLER

••H••E

ACHEBE
ACHENE
ADHERE
ASHADE
ASHAME
ASHINE
ASHLEE
ASHORE
ATHENE
ATHOME
AWHILE
BEHAVE
BEHOME
BOHEME
BTHREE
COHERE
DEHIRE
ETHANE
ETHENE
EXHALE
EXHUME
GOHOME
IMHERE
IMHOME
INHALE
INHERE
INHOME
INHUME
LAHORE
MCHALE
MOHAVE
MRHYDE
NOHOPE
ONHIRE
OXHIDE
REHIDE
REHIRE
REHONE
SCHEME
SPHERE
TAHNEE
TSHAPE
UNHALE
UNHIRE
UPHERE
UPHOVE
USHAPE
VSHAPE
WAHINE
YSHAPE

•••HE•

AACHEN
AETHER
ALTHEA
ANTHEM
ANTHER
ARCHED
ARCHER
ARCHES
ARNHEM
ASTHER
BACHED
BACHES
BASHED
BASHER
BASHES
BATHED
BATHER
BATHES
BECHET
BETHEL
BOTHER
BUSHED
BUSHEL
BUSHER
BUSHES
BYTHEN
CACHED
CACHES
CACHET
CASHED
CASHES
CASHEW
CATHER
CIPHER
COSHED
COSHER
COSHES
CYPHER
DASHED
DASHER
DASHES
DISHED
DISHES
DITHER
EITHER
ESCHER
ESCHEW
ESTHER
ETCHED
ETCHER
ETCHES
FATHER
FICHES
FISHED
FISHER
FISHES
GASHED
GASHES
GATHER
GETHEP
GOPHER
GOSHEN
GOTHEP
GUSHED
GUSHER
GUSHES
HASHED
HASHES
HEEHEE
HEHHEH
HIGHER
HITHER
HUGHES
HUSHED
HUSHES
HYPHEN
IFTHEN
INCHED
INCHER
INCHES
ISOHEL
ITCHED
ITCHES
JOSHED
JOSHER
JOSHES
KOCHEL
KOCHER
KOSHER
KUCHEN
LACHEY
LASHED
LASHER
LASHES
LATHED
LATHEN
LATHER
LATHES
LECHER
LICHEE
LICHEN
LITHER
LOCHER
LUSHER
LUSHES
LUTHER
MASHED
MASHER
MASHES
MATHER
MATHEW
MAYHEM
MCPHEE
MESHED
MESHES
MICHEL
MOSHED
MOSHER
MOSHES
MOTHER
MUDHEN
MUSHED
MUSHER
MUSHES
NASHES
NEPHEW
NETHER
NICHED
NICHES
NIGHER
NOCHES
NOSHED
NOSHER
NOSHES
ORTHEN
OUCHES
PEAHEN
PECHES
PICHEL
PISHED
PISHES
PITHED
POOHED
POSHER
POTHER
PUSHED
PUSHER
PUSHES
RACHEL
RASHER
RASHES
RATHER
RECHEW
REDHEN
RESHES
RICHEN
RICHER
RICHES
RICHET
ROCHET
RUCHES
RUSHED
RUSHEE
RUSHER
RUSHES
SACHEM
SACHER
SACHET
SADHES
SASHED
SASHES
SAYHEY
SIGHED
SIGHER
SOTHEN
TEEHEE
TETHER
TITHED
TITHER
TITHES
TOWHEE
TUSHES
UNSHED
VACHEL
VACHES
WASHED
WASHER
WASHES
WISHED
WISHER
WISHES
WITHER
YAPHET
ZITHER

•••H•E

ARCHIE
DAPHNE
EIGHTE
EUCHRE
FICHTE
HEEHEE
HUGHIE
KATHIE
KISHKE
LICHEE
MASHIE
MCPHEE
NUCHAE
RESHOE
RICHIE
RUSHEE
RUTHIE
SOPHIE
TECHIE
TEEHEE
TOWHEE
TUSHIE
UNSHOE
WASHME
WASHOE

••••HE

AMECHE
APACHE
BERTHE
BLITHE
BLYTHE
BOOTHE
BOUCHE
BUNCHE
BYSSHE
CLICHE
CLOCHE
CLOTHE
CRECHE
FLECHE
FORCHE
GAUCHE
GOETHE
KAETHE
LOATHE
LOUCHE
MANCHE
MARCHE
MARTHE
MENTHE
OLATHE
PENCHE
PSYCHE
QUICHE
RASCHE
SCATHE
SCYTHE
SEETHE
SOOTHE
SPATHE
SWATHE
TEETHE
TOUCHE
TRACHE
TROCHE
WRITHE

H•F•••

HAFTED
HEFLIN
HEFNER
HEFTED
HEFTER
HOFFER
HUFFED

H••F••

HADFUN
HASFUN
HATFUL
HEIFER
HITFOR
HOFFER
HOOFED
HOOFER
HOOFIT
HOWFAR
HUFFED

H•••F•

HITOFF
HOPOFF

H••••F

HEAROF
HEREOF
HITOFF
HOPOFF

•HF•••

PHFFFT

•H•F••

CHAFED
CHAFER
CHAFES
CHAFFS
CHAFFY
CHEFED
CHUFFS
CHUFFY
PHFFFT
SHAFTS
SHIFTS
SHIFTY
SHOFAR
THEFAN

THEFBI
THEFED
THEFLY
THEFOG
THEFOX
THEFTS
WHIFFS
WHYFOR

•H••F•
CHAFFS
CHAFFY
CHIEFS
CHUFFS
CHUFFY
PHFFFT
SHRIFT
THENFL
THRIFT
WHARFS
WHIFFS

•H•••F
SHARIF
THEREF
WHATIF

••H•F•
UNHAFT

••H••F
BEHALF
BEHOOF
BYHALF
INHALF

•••H•F
MUCHOF

H•G•••
HAGGAI
HAGGIS
HAGGLE
HAGLER
HAGMAN
HEGGEN
HEGIRA
HEGOAT
HEGYES
HIGGLE
HIGHER
HIGHIQ
HIGHLY
HIGHON
HIGHUP
HOGANS
HOGGED
HOGNUT
HOGTIE
HUGELY
HUGEST
HUGGED
HUGGER
HUGHES
HUGHIE
HYGRIC

H••G••
HAAGEN
HAGGAI
HAGGIS
HAGGLE
HAIGHT
HANGAR
HANGBY
HANGED
HANGER
HANGIN
HANGON
HANGUL
HANGUP
HEDGED
HEDGER
HEDGES
HEEGER
HEGGEN
HEIGHT
HENGES
HIGGLE
HINGED
HINGES
HINGIS
HINGLE
HOAGIE
HODGES
HOGGED
HORGAN
HUGGED
HUGGER
HUNGBY
HUNGER
HUNGIN
HUNGON
HUNGRY
HUNGUP

H•••G•
HADAGO
HASAGO
HMONGS
HOMAGE

H••••G
HALING
HARING
HATING
HAVING
HAWING
HAYING
HAZING
HERZOG
HEWING
HEXING
HIDING
HIEING
HIKING
HIRING
HIVING
HOEING
HOKING
HOLING
HOMING
HONING
HOPING
HOSING
HOTDOG
HOWBIG
HUMBUG
HUSING
HYPING

•HG•••
OHGOSH

•H•G••
CHIGOE
PHAGIA
SHAGGY
SHOGIS
SHOGUN
THEGAP
THIGHS

•H••G•
BHANGS
CHANGE
CHANGO
CHARGE
CHOUGH
DHEIGH
OHMAGE
PHLEGM
SHAGGY
SHRUGS
THEAGE
THINGS
THINGY
THONGS
THOUGH
WHANGS

•H•••G
CHIANG
PHOTOG
SHYING
THEFOG
THRONG

••H•G•
LEHIGH
MCHUGH
ONHIGH

••H••G
AAHING
ACHING
ALHAIG
ASHING
ATHING
GEHRIG
ICHING
MCHARG
OOHING
REHANG
REHUNG
UNHUNG
USHING

•••H•G
BIGHUG
GASHOG
QUAHOG
SEAHAG

HH••••
HHOURS

H•H•••
HAHAHA
HEHHEH
HIHATS
HIHIHI
HLHUNT
HOHNER
HOHOHO
HOHUMS

H••H••
HACHOO
HARHAR
HASHED
HASHES
HATHOR
HAWHAW
HEEHAW
HEEHEE
HEHHEH
HIGHER
HIGHIQ
HIGHLY
HIGHON
HIGHUP
HIPHOP
HITHER
HOOHAH
HOOHAS
HUGHES
HUGHIE
HUSHED
HUSHES
HUSHUP
HYPHEN

H•••H•
HAHAHA
HAIGHT
HEATHS
HEATHY
HEIGHT
HIDEHO
HIHIHI
HOHOHO
HONCHO
HONSHU
HUMPHS

H••••H
HALVAH
HANNAH
HARRAH
HAUNCH
HEALTH
HEARTH
HEHHEH
HEWISH
HIRSCH
HITECH
HOOHAH
HOOKAH
HOORAH
HOOTCH
HOWDAH
HUPPAH
HURRAH
HUZZAH

•HH•••
SHHHHH

•H•H••
AHCHOO
CHUHSI
SHHHHH
THEHAJ
THEHUB

•H••H•
CHACHA
CHACHI
CHICHA
CHICHI
CHIRHO
RHYTHM
SHEEHY
SHHHHH
THENHL
THEWHO
THIGHS

•H•••H
CHEECH
CHINCH
CHOUGH
CHURCH
DHEIGH
GHIRSH
OHGOSH
OHYEAH
SHEATH
SHEESH
SHEIKH
SHHHHH
SHILOH
THATCH
THOUGH
THRASH
THRESH
THRUSH
WHOOSH

••HH••
HEHHEH
SHHHHH

••H•H•
EPHAHS
HAHAHA
HIHIHI
HOHOHO
ICHTHY
SHHHHH
YOHOHO

••H••H
HEHHEH
LEHIGH
MCHUGH
ONHIGH
RAHRAH
REHASH
SHHHHH
UNHUNH
WAHWAH

•••HH•
PYRHHO
SHHHHH

•••H•H
EIGHTH
HEHHEH
HOOHAH
SHHHHH

••••HH
SHHHHH

HI••••
HIATAL
HIATUS
HICCUP
HICKAM
HICKEY
HICKOK
HIDDEN
HIDEHO
HIDEKI
HIDERS
HIDING
HIDOUT
HIEING
HIEMAL
HIGGLE
HIGHER
HIGHIQ
HIGHLY
HIGHON
HIGHUP
HIHATS
HIHIHI
HIJACK
HIJKLM
HIKERS
HIKEUP
HIKING
HILARY
HILLED
HILLEL
HILLER
HILTED
HILTON
HIMMEL
HINDER
HINDUS
HINGED
HINGES
HINGIS
HINGLE
HINKLE
HINTAT
HINTED
HINTER
HINTON
HIPHOP
HIPPED
HIPPER
HIPPIE
HIPPOS
HIPPUS
HIREES
HIREON
HIRERS
HIRING
HIRSCH
HISSAT
HISSED
HISSER
HISSES
HITECH
HITEST
HITFOR
HITHER
HITINS
HITMAN
HITMEN
HITOFF
HITONE
HITOUT
HITSAT
HITSIT
HITSON
HITSUP
HITTER
HIVAOA
HIVERS
HIVING
HIYALL

H•I•••
HAIDAS
HAIDEE
HAIGHT
HAIKAI
HAIKUS
HAILED
HAILER
HAILEY
HAINES
HAIRDO
HAIRED
HEIDEN
HEIFER
HEIGHT
HEINIE
HEINSE
HEISTS
HOISIN
HOISTS
HRIDER
HTILES

H••I••
HABILE
HABITS
HAKIMS
HALIDE
HALING
HALITE
HAMILL
HAMITE
HARING
HATING
HAVING
HAWING
HAYING
HAZIER
HAZILY
HAZING
HEGIRA
HELICO
HELIOS
HELIUM
HESIOD
HEWING
HEWISH
HEWITT
HEXING
HIDING
HIEING
HIHIHI
HIKING
HIRING
HITINS
HIVING
HODIAK
HOEING
HOKIER
HOKIES
HOKILY
HOKING
HOLIER
HOLIES
HOLILY
HOLING
HOLISM
HOLIST
HOMIER
HOMIES
HOMILY
HOMING
HOMINY
HONIED
HONING
HOPING
HOSIER
HOSING
HUSING
HYOIDS
HYPING

H•••I•
HACKIE
HACKIT
HADDIE
HADDIX
HADJIS
HAGGIS
HAJJIS
HALLIE
HALOID
HALPIN
HAMLIN
HANDIN
HANGIN
HANKIE
HARBIN
HARDIN
HARLIN
HARRIS
HASSID
HATEIT
HATPIN
HATTIE
HAULIN
HAVEIN
HAVEIT
HAWAII
HAYNIE
HEADIN
HECTIC
HEEBIE
HEFLIN
HEINIE
HELDIN
HELDIT
HELPIN
HEMSIN
HENBIT
HENRIK
HERBIE
HEREIN
HERMIT
HERNIA
HEROIC
HEROIN
HESTIA
HIGHIQ
HINGIS
HIPPIE
HITSIT
HOAGIE
HOBBIT
HOGTIE
HOISIN
HOLDIN
HOLDIT
HOLLIS
HOMEIN
HONEIN
HOODIE
HOOFIT
HOOTIE
HOPKIN
HOPSIN
HORNIN
HORRID
HOTAIR
HOTOIL
HOTTIE
HOTTIP
HOURIS
HOWBIG
HOWLIN
HUBRIS
HUDDIE
HUGHIE
HUNGIN
HYBRID
HYDRIC
HYGRIC

H••••I
HAGGAI
HAIKAI
HAMULI
HATARI
HAWAII
HENRYI
HIDEKI
HIHIHI
HUMERI

•HI•••
AHIMSA
CHIANG
CHICAS
CHICER
CHICHA
CHICHI
CHICKS
CHICLE
CHICLY
CHICOS
CHIDED
CHIDER
CHIDES
CHIEFS
CHIENS
CHIGOE
CHILDE
CHILES
CHILIS
CHILLI
CHILLS
CHILLY
CHIMED
CHIMER
CHIMES
CHIMPS
CHINAS
CHINCH
CHINES
CHINKS
CHINKY
CHINOS
CHINTZ
CHINUA
CHINUP
CHIPIN
CHIPUP
CHIRAC
CHIRHO
CHIRON
CHIRPS
CHIRPY
CHIRRS
CHISEL
CHISOX
CHISUM
CHITON
CHITRA
CHITTY
CHIVAS
CHIVES
GHIJKL
GHIRSH
OHIOAN
PHIALS
PHILBY
PHILCO
PHILIC
PHILIP
PHILLY
RHINAL
RHINOS
SHIELD
SHIEST
SHIFTS
SHIFTY
SHIISM
SHIITE
SHILLS
SHILLY
SHILOH
SHIMMY
SHIMON
SHINDY
SHINED
SHINER
SHINES
SHINNY
SHINTO
SHIPTO
SHIRAZ
SHIRER
SHIRES
SHIRKS
SHIRRS
SHIRTS
SHIVER
THICKE
THIEVE
THIGHS
THILLS
THINGS
THINGY
THINKS
THINLY
THIRDR
THIRDS
THIRST
THIRTY
THISBE
WHIFFS
WHILED
WHILES
WHILST
WHIMSY
WHINED
WHINER
WHINES
WHINNY
WHIPIN
WHIPPY
WHIPUP
WHIRLS
WHIRLY
WHIRRS
WHISKS
WHISKY
WHITBY
WHITED
WHITEN
WHITER
WHITES
WHITEY
WHITTY
WHIZZY

•H•I••
CHAINE
CHAINS
CHAIRS
CHAISE
CHOICE
CHOIRS
CHRISM
CHRIST
DHEIGH
GHAINS
RHEIMS
SHEIKH
SHEIKS
SHEILA
SHIISM
SHIITE
SHRIEK
SHRIFT
SHRIKE
SHRILL
SHRIMP
SHRINE
SHRINK
SHRIVE
SHTICK
SHYING
THEIRS
THEISM
THEIST
THRICE
THRIFT
THRILL
THRIVE

•H••I•
AHOLIC
CHAPIN
CHEMIC
CHEMIN
CHENIN
CHERIE
CHILIS
CHIPIN
CHOPIN
CHORIC
CHORIO
DHOTIS
GHAZIS
KHAKIS
KHALID
PHAGIA
PHASIC
PHILIC
PHILIP
PHOBIA
PHOBIC
PHONIC
PHOTIC
PHYSIC
PHYSIO
SHAKIN
SHALIT
SHAMIR
SHANIA
SHARIF
SHOGIS
SHOJIS
SHOOIN
SHOWIN
SHUTIN
THALIA
THATIS
THECIA
THECID
THEKID
THELIP
THEPIT
THESIS
THETIS
THEWIZ
THORIC
THYMIC
WHATIF
WHIPIN
WHOSIN

•H•••I
CHACHI
CHICHI
CHILLI
CHUHSI
RHOMBI
SHALLI
SHERRI
SHORTI
SHUMAI
THEFBI
WHOAMI
WHOOPI

••HI••
AAHING
ACHIER
ACHING
ALHIRT
APHIDS
ASHIER
ASHINE
ASHING
ATHING
AWHILE
AWHIRL
BAHIAN
BEHIND
CAHIER
CAHILL
DEHIRE
ETHICS
ETHIOP
FGHIJK
HIHIHI
ICHING
ICHIRO
ITHINK
LEHIGH
NIHILO
NOHITS
ONHIGH
ONHIRE
OOHING
OXHIDE
REHIDE
REHIRE
REHITS
SAHIBS
SCHICK
SCHISM
SCHIST
SPHINX
TAHINI
TAHITI
TSHIRT
TVHITS
UNHIRE
UPHILL
USHING
VCHIPS
WAHINE

••H•I•
ALHAIG
ASHBIN
ASHPIT
BEHAIM
COHEIR
DAHLIA
DEHAIR
ECHOIC
ETHNIC
GEHRIG
JOHNII
JOHNIV
JOHNIX
KAHLIL
LCHAIM
MAHDIS
MOHAIR
SCHEIB
UNHAIR

••H••I
HIHIHI
JOHNII
JOHNVI
JOHNXI
TAHINI
TAHITI
YEHUDI

•••HI•
ARCHIE
BACHIT
BASHIN
BIGHIT
CASHIN
DASHIS
DASHIT
DRPHIL
DUCHIN
EFGHIJ
GETHIP
GOTHIC
GOTHIP
HIGHIQ
HUGHIE
ISCHIA
KATHIE
KESHIA
LITHIC
MASHIE
MATHIS
MISHIT
MYTHIC
NONHIT
NOTHIN
ONEHIT
ORCHID
ORPHIC
OUTHIT
PACHIN
PATHIC
PUSHIN
PUSHIT
RAGHIB
RASHID
RESHIP
RICHIE
RICHIN
RISHIS
ROSHIS
RUSHIN
RUTHIE
SEPHIA
SOPHIA
SOPHIE
SUSHIS
TECHIE
TILHIM
TOOHIP
TUSHIE
UNCHIC
UNSHIP
URCHIN
WISHIN
WITHIN
WITHIT
YASHIN

•••H•I
CHUHSI
ISTHMI
TISHRI
VASHTI

••••HI
BAKSHI
CHACHI
CHICHI
DEFGHI
DELPHI
GANDHI
HIHIHI
KIMCHI
LITCHI
SAIDHI
SAYSHI
TAICHI

H•J•••
HAJJES
HAJJIS
HIJACK
HIJKLM

H••J••
HADJES
HADJIS
HAJJES
HAJJIS

•H•J••
GHIJKL
SHOJIS

•H•••J
THEHAJ

••H•J•
FGHIJK

•••H•J
EFGHIJ
THEHAJ

••••HJ
RALPHJ

H•K•••
HAKEEM
HAKIMS
HIKERS
HIKEUP
HIKING
HOKIER
HOKIES
HOKILY
HOKING
HOKUMS
HYKSOS

H••K••
HAAKON
HACKED
HACKER
HACKIE
HACKIT
HACKLE
HACKLY
HACKUP
HAIKAI
HAIKUS
HANKER
HANKIE
HARKED
HARKEN
HARKER
HAWKED
HAWKER
HECKLE
HECKNO
HICKAM
HICKEY
HICKOK
HIJKLM
HINKLE
HOCKED
HOCKER
HOCKEY
HONKAT
HONKED
HONKER
HOOKAH
HOOKED
HOOKER
HOOKEY
HOOKON
HOOKUP
HOPKIN
HOTKEY
HULKED
HUNKER
HUSKED
HUSKER

H•••K•
HACEKS
HANDKE
HIDEKI

H••••K
HENRIK
HENRYK
HICKOK
HIJACK
HODIAK

•H•K••
CHAKRA
CHEKOV
CHOKED
CHOKER
CHOKES
KHAKIS
SHAKEN
SHAKER
SHAKES
SHAKIN
SHAKOS
SHAKUR
SHEKEL
THEKID
ZHUKOV

•H••K•
CHALKS
CHALKY
CHECKS
CHEEKS
CHEEKY
CHICKS
CHINKS
CHINKY
CHOCKS
CHUCKS
CHUCKY
CHUNKS
CHUNKY
GHIJKL
SHACKS
SHANKS
SHARKS
SHECKY
SHEIKH
SHEIKS
SHIRKS
SHOCKS
SHOPKO
SHRIKE
SHUCKS
THANKS
THICKE
THINKS
THUNKS
WHACKS
WHELKS
WHISKS
WHISKY

•H•••K
OHLOOK
RHEBOK
SHLOCK
SHNOOK
SHRANK
SHRIEK
SHRINK
SHRUNK
SHTICK
THWACK

••HK••
ESHKOL

••H••K
AWHECK
DRHOOK
FGHIJK
INHOCK
ITHINK
MOHAWK
REHOOK
SCHICK
UNHOOK
UNHUSK

•••HK•
KISHKA
KISHKE
ROTHKO

•••H•K
ITZHAK

HL••••
HLHUNT

H•L•••
HALALA
HALEST
HALEVY
HALIDE
HALING
HALITE
HALLAM
HALLEL
HALLEY
HALLIE
HALLOO
HALLOS
HALLOW
HALLUX
HALOED
HALOES
HALOID
HALPIN
HALSEY
HALTED
HALTER
HALVAH
HALVAS
HALVED
HALVER
HALVES
HELDIN
HELDIT
HELDON
HELDTO
HELDUP
HELENA
HELENE
HELENS
HELICO
HELIOS
HELIUM
HELLAS
HELLER
HELLNO
HELLON
HELLOS
HELMED
HELMER
HELMET
HELMUT
HELOTS
HELPED
HELPER
HELPIN
HELPME
HELPON
HELPUP
HELTER
HILARY
HILLED
HILLEL
HILLER
HILTED
HILTON
HOLDEM
HOLDEN
HOLDER
HOLDIN
HOLDIT
HOLDME
HOLDON
HOLDTO
HOLDUP
HOLERS
HOLEUP
HOLIER
HOLIES
HOLILY
HOLING
HOLISM
HOLIST
HOLLER
HOLLEY
HOLLIS
HOLLOW
HOLMAN
HOLMES
HULKED
HULLED
HULLER
HULLOS

H••L••
HABLAR
HAGLER
HAILED
HAILER
HAILEY
HALLAM
HALLEL
HALLEY
HALLIE
HALLOO
HALLOS
HALLOW
HALLUX
HAMLET
HAMLIN
HANLEY
HANLON
HAOLES
HARLAN
HARLEM
HARLEY
HARLIN
HARLOT
HARLOW
HAULED
HAULER
HAULIN
HAULUP
HAYLEY
HEALED
HEALER
HEALEY
HEALTH
HEALUP
HEDLEY
HEELED
HEELER
HEFLIN
HELLAS
HELLER
HELLNO
HELLON
HELLOS
HENLEY
HILLED
HILLEL
HILLER
HOLLER
HOLLEY
HOLLIS
HOLLOW
HOWLAT
HOWLED
HOWLER
HOWLIN
HOYLES
HTILES
HUBLEY
HULLED
HULLER
HULLOS
HUNLEY
HURLED
HURLER
HURLEY
HUXLEY

H•••L•
HABILE
HACKLE
HACKLY
HAGGLE
HALALA
HAMELN
HAMILL
HAMULI
HANDLE
HARALD
HARDLY
HAROLD
HASSLE
HAZELS
HAZILY
HECKLE
HERALD
HIGGLE
HIGHLY
HIJKLM
HINGLE
HINKLE
HIYALL
HOBBLE
HOKILY
HOLILY
HOMELY
HOMILY
HOOPLA
HOOPLE
HOSELS
HOSTLY
HOTELS
HOURLY
HOVELS
HOWELL
HUBBLE
HUDDLE
HUGELY
HUMBLE
HUMBLY
HURDLE
HURTLE
HUSTLE

H••••L
HALLEL
HAMILL
HANDEL
HANGUL
HANSEL
HASSEL
HATFUL
HEBBEL
HEDRAL
HERBAL
HIATAL
HIEMAL
HILLEL
HIMMEL
HIYALL
HORMEL
HOSTEL
HOTOIL
HOWELL
HUMMEL
HYETAL
HYMNAL

•HL•••
CHLORO
NHLERS
OHLOOK
PHLEBO
PHLEGM
PHLOEM
SHLOCK
UHLANS
ZHLOBS
ZHLUBS

•H•L••
AHOLIC
CHALET
CHALKS
CHALKY
CHELAE
CHILDE
CHILES
CHILIS
CHILLI
CHILLS
CHILLY
CHOLER
CHOLLA
CHOLOS
DHOLES
FHOLES
KHALID
PHELPS
PHILBY
PHILCO
PHILIC
PHILIP
PHILLY
PHYLLO
PHYLUM
SHALES
SHALEY
SHALIT
SHALLI
SHALLY
SHALOM
SHELBY
SHELLS
SHELTY
SHELVE
SHILLS
SHILLY
SHILOH
SHOLEM
SHOLOM
SHULTZ
THALER
THALES
THALIA
THELAW
THELIP
THELMA
THELOT
THILLS
THOLES
WHALED
WHALER
WHALES
WHALEY
WHELAN
WHELKS
WHELMS
WHELPS
WHILED
WHILES
WHILST
WHOLES
WHOLLY

•H••L•
CHARLY
CHICLE
CHICLY
CHILLI
CHILLS
CHILLY
CHOLLA
CHURLS
GHOULS
OHWELL
PHIALS
PHILLY
PHYLLO
SHALLI
SHALLY
SHAWLS
SHEILA
SHELLS
SHIELD
SHILLS
SHILLY
SHOALS
SHOALY
SHOULD
SHRILL
THATLL
THEFLY
THEYLL
THILLS
THINLY
THRALL
THRILL
THUSLY
UHAULS
WHATLL
WHEELS
WHENLL
WHIRLS
WHIRLY
WHOLLY
WHORLS

•H•••L
BHOPAL
CHACEL
CHANEL
CHAPEL
CHERYL
CHEVAL
CHISEL
CHORAL
DHOTEL
GHIJKL
OHWELL
PHENOL
RHINAL
SHEKEL
SHERYL
SHOVEL
SHRILL
SHTETL
THATLL
THENFL
THENHL
THEYLL
THRALL
THRILL
WHATLL
WHENLL

••HL••
ASHLAR
ASHLEE
ASHLEY
DAHLIA
KAHLIL
KAHLUA
KOHLER
MAHLER
SCHLEP
SCHLUB
WAHLOO
WOHLER

••H•L•
AWHILE
BEHALF
BEHELD
BEHOLD
BYHALF
CAHILL
ENHALO
ETHYLS
EXHALE
INHALE
INHALF
MAHALO
MCHALE
NIHILO
NOHELP
OFHELP
ONHOLD
OPHULS
REHELD
REHOLD
SCHELL
SCHOLL
SCHULZ
UNHALE
UNHELD
UNHELM
UNHOLY
UNHULL
UPHELD
UPHILL
UPHOLD

••H••L
ATHEEL
AWHIRL
CAHILL
DEHMEL
ESHKOL
KAHLIL
REHAUL
REHEAL
REHEEL
SCHELL
SCHOLL
SCHOOL
TOHEEL
UNHULL
UPHILL

•••HL•
ARCHLY
HIGHLY
LUSHLY
POSHLY
RASHLY
RICHLY

•••H•L
BETHEL
BUSHEL
CEPHAL
DRPHIL
ISOHEL
KOCHEL
LETHAL
METHYL
MICHEL
NUCHAL
OMPHAL
PICHEL
RACHEL
VACHEL
WARHOL
WITHAL

••••HL
JAWOHL
THENHL

HM••••
HMONGS

H•M•••
HAMATE
HAMDEN
HAMELN
HAMILL
HAMITE
HAMLET
HAMLIN
HAMMED
HAMMER
HAMPER
HAMSUN
HAMSUP
HAMULI
HEMATO
HEMMED
HEMMER
HEMPEN
HEMSIN
HIMMEL
HOMAGE
HOMBRE
HOMEEC
HOMEIN
HOMELY
HOMERS
HOMEYS
HOMIER
HOMIES
HOMILY
HOMING
HOMINY
HOMMES
HUMANE
HUMANS
HUMBER
HUMBLE
HUMBLY
HUMBUG
HUMERI
HUMMED
HUMMEL
HUMMER
HUMMUS
HUMORS
HUMOUR
HUMPED
HUMPHS
HUMPTY
HUMVEE
HYMNAL
HYMNED

H••M••
HAGMAN
HAMMED
HAMMER
HARMED
HARMER
HARMON
HAYMES
HAYMOW
HAZMAT
HBOMBS
HELMED
HELMER
HELMET
HELMUT
HEMMED
HEMMER
HERMAN
HERMES
HERMIT
HERMON
HEYMAN
HIEMAL
HIMMEL
HITMAN
HITMEN
HODMAN
HODMEN
HOLMAN
HOLMES
HOMMES
HORMEL
HORMUZ
HUMMED
HUMMEL
HUMMER
HUMMUS

H•••M•
HAKIMS
HAREMS
HBEAMS
HELPME
HOHUMS
HOKUMS
HOLDME

H••••M
HAKEEM
HALLAM
HANSOM
HARLEM
HASSAM
HELIUM
HICKAM
HIJKLM
HOLDEM
HOLISM

•HM•••
KHMERS
OHMAGE

•H•M••
AHIMSA
CHAMMY
CHAMPS
CHEMIC
CHEMIN
CHIMED
CHIMER
CHIMES
CHIMPS
CHOMPS
CHUMMY
CHUMPS
RHAMES
RHEMES
RHOMBI
RHOMBS
RHUMBA
RHUMBS
RHYMED
RHYMER
RHYMES
SHAMAN
SHAMED
SHAMES
SHAMIR
SHAMMY
SHAMUS
SHIMMY
SHIMON
SHUMAI
THAMES
THEMAN
THEMED
THEMES
THEMET
THEMOB
THEMRS
THOMAS
THUMBS
THUMPS
THYMES
THYMIC
THYMUS
WHAMMO
WHAMMY
WHIMSY
WHOMPS
WHOMSO

•H••M•
CHAMMY
CHARMS
CHASMS
CHROMA
CHROME
CHROMO
CHROMY
CHUMMY
DHARMA
KHOUMS
RHEEMS
RHEIMS
RHEUMS
RHEUMY
SHAMMY
SHIMMY
SHOWME
SHRIMP
THELMA
THERMO
THERMS
THRUMS
WHAMMO
WHAMMY
WHELMS
WHOAMI

•H•••M
CHISUM
CHRISM
PHENOM
PHLEGM
PHLOEM
PHYLUM
RHYTHM
SHALOM
SHAZAM
SHBOOM
SHIISM
SHOLEM
SHOLOM
THEISM
THERAM

••HM••
ASHMAN
ASHMEN
DEHMEL
LEHMAN
OTHMAR
ROHMER
SCHMOS

••H•M•
ASHAME
ATHOME
BAHAMA
BEHOME
BOHEME
EXHUME
GOHOME
HOHUMS
IMHOME
INHOME
INHUME
OGHAMS
REHEMS
SCHEMA
SCHEME

••H••M
ASHRAM
BEHAIM
LCHAIM
SCHISM
UNHELM

•••HM•
ABOHMS
ASTHMA
BRAHMA
BRAHMS
ISTHMI
MEOHMY
MYOHMY
WASHME

•••H•M
ANTHEM
ARNHEM
BADHAM
BONHAM
COBHAM
DEDHAM
DENHAM
DIRHAM
DUNHAM
DURHAM
FATHOM
GORHAM
GOTHAM
GRAHAM
LAPHAM
MAYHEM
OLDHAM
PELHAM
RODHAM
SACHEM
TILHIM

••••HM
MEGOHM
RHYTHM

H•N•••
HANDAX
HANDED
HANDEL
HANDER
HANDIN
HANDKE
HANDLE
HANDON
HANDUP
HANGAR
HANGBY
HANGED
HANGER
HANGIN
HANGON
HANGUL
HANGUP
HANKER
HANKIE
HANLEY
HANLON
HANNAH
HANSAS
HANSEL
HANSES
HANSOM
HANSON
HENBIT
HENDEC
HENDRY
HENGES
HENLEY
HENNAS
HENNER
HENRIK
HENRYI
HENRYK
HENRYV
HENSON
HINDER
HINDUS
HINGED
HINGES
HINGIS
HINGLE
HINKLE
HINTAT
HINTED
HINTER
HINTON
HONCHO
HONDAS
HONEIN
HONERS
HONEST
HONEYS
HONIED
HONING
HONKAT
HONKED
HONKER
HONORE
HONORS
HONOUR
HONSHU
HUNGBY
HUNGER
HUNGIN
HUNGON
HUNGRY
HUNGUP
HUNKER
HUNLEY
HUNTED
HUNTER
HUNTUP

H••N••
HAINES
HANNAH
HARNEY
HAUNCH
HAUNTS
HAYNES
HAYNIE
HEANEY
HEFNER
HEINIE
HEINSE
HENNAS
HENNER
HERNAN
HERNIA
HEXNUT
HMONGS
HOBNOB
HOGNUT
HOHNER
HORNBY
HORNED
HORNER
HORNET

HORNIN HOUNDS HOUNDY HOWNOW HYENAS HYMNAL HYMNED HYPNOS

H•••N•

HABANA HADONE HALING HARING HASONE HATING HAVANA HAVENO HAVENS HAVENT HAVING HAWING HAYING HAZANS HAZING HEARNS HECKNO HELENA HELENE HELENS HELLNO HERONS HEWING HEXANE HEXING HIDING HIEING HIKING HIRING HITINS HITONE HIVING HLHUNT HOEING HOGANS HOKING HOLING HOMING HOMINY HONING HOPING HOSING HOTONE HRYVNA HUMANE HUMANS HURONS HUSING HUTONE HYPING HYSONS

H••••N

HAAGEN HAAKON HADDEN HADEAN HADFUN HADRON HAGMAN HALPIN HAMDEN HAMELN HAMLIN HAMSUN HANDIN HANDON HANGIN HANGON HANLON HANSON HAPPEN HARBIN HARDEN HARDIN HARKEN HARLAN HARLIN HARMON HARPON HASFUN HASSAN HASTEN HATPIN HAULIN HAVEIN HAVEON HAYDEN HEADIN HEADON HEAPON HEATON HEAVEN HEBRON HEDREN HEDRON HEFLIN HEGGEN HEIDEN HELDIN HELDON HELLON HELPIN HELPON HEMPEN HEMSIN HENSON HEREIN HEREON HERMAN HERMON HERNAN HEROIN HERREN HESTON HEUSEN HEYMAN HIDDEN HIGHON HILTON HINTON HIREON HITMAN HITMEN HITSON HOBSON HODMAN HODMEN HOISIN HOLDEN HOLDIN HOLDON HOLMAN HOMEIN HONEIN HOOKON HOPKIN HOPSIN HOPSON HORGAN HORNIN HORTON HOUDON HOWLIN HOYDEN HUDSON HUNGIN HUNGON HUSTON HUTTON HYPHEN

•HN•••

OHNUTS SHNOOK

•H•N••

BHANGS CHANCE CHANCY CHANDU CHANEL CHANEY CHANGE CHANGO CHANTE CHANTS CHANTY CHENEY CHENIN CHINAS CHINCH CHINES CHINKS CHINKY CHINOS CHINTZ CHINUA CHINUP CHUNKS CHUNKY CHYNNA OHENRY PHENOL PHENOM PHONED PHONER PHONES PHONEY PHONIC PHONOS RHINAL RHINOS RHONDA SHANDY SHANIA SHANKS SHANTY SHINDY SHINED SHINER SHINES SHINNY SHINTO SHUNTS THANES THANKS THENBA THENCE THENET THENFL THENHL THENRA THINGS THINGY THINKS THINLY THONGS THUNKS WHANGS WHENCE WHENLL WHINED WHINER WHINES WHINNY WHYNOT WHYNOW

•H••N•

AHERNE CHAINE CHAINS CHIANG CHIENS CHRONO CHURNS CHYNNA GHAINS SHAYNE SHEENA SHEENS SHEENY SHINNY SHRANK SHRINE SHRINK SHRUNK SHYING THEEND THEONE THORNS THORNY THRONE THRONG UHLANS WHINNY

•H•••N

BHUTAN CHACUN CHAPIN CHARON CHAZAN CHEMIN CHENIN CHEVON CHEWON CHIPIN CHIRON CHITON CHOPIN CHOSEN CHYRON LHASAN OHDARN OHIOAN PHOTON SHAKEN SHAKIN SHAMAN SHARON SHARYN SHAVEN SHEDON SHIMON SHOGUN SHOOIN SHOWIN SHUTIN THEBAN THECAN THEFAN THEMAN THERON THESON THESUN THORON THROWN WHELAN WHIPIN WHITEN WHOSIN WHOWON

••HN••

BAHNEN ETHNIC ETHNOS HOHNER JOHNII JOHNIV JOHNIX JOHNNY JOHNVI JOHNXI JOHNXV JOHNXX LEHNEN SCHNOZ TAHNEE

••H•N•

AAHING ACHENE ACHING ALHENA ASHINE ASHING ATHAND ATHENA ATHENE ATHENS ATHING BEHIND BYHAND ETHANE ETHENE HLHUNT ICHING INHAND ITHINK JOHANN JOHNNY KAHUNA NOHANT ONHAND OOHING REHANG REHONE REHUNG SPHINX SPHYNX TAHINI UNHAND UNHUNG UNHUNH USHING UTHANT WAHINE

••H••N

ASHBIN ASHCAN ASHMAN ASHMEN ASHPAN ASHTON BAHIAN BAHNEN DEHORN EPHRON JOHANN LEHMAN LEHNEN OAHUAN TEHRAN UNHEWN

•••HN•

DAPHNE TECHNO UTAHNS VISHNU

•••H•N

AACHEN AFGHAN ARCHON BASHIN BICHON BUCHAN BYTHEN CASHIN DATHAN DOOHAN DOTHAN DUCHIN GOSHEN HIGHON HYPHEN IFTHEN INCHON KUCHEN LATHEN LESHAN LICHEN MUDHEN NATHAN NIGHON NOTHIN OMAHAN ORPHAN ORTHEN PACHIN PATHAN PEAHEN PUSHIN PUSHON PYTHON REDHEN RICHEN RICHIN ROCHON RUSHIN SIPHON SOTHEN TURHAN URCHIN UTAHAN WISHIN WISHON WITHIN YASHIN

••••HN

IIJOHN STJOHN UPJOHN VAUGHN

HO••••

HOAGIE HOARDS HOARSE HOAXED HOAXER HOAXES HOBART HOBBES HOBBIT HOBBLE HOBNOB HOBOED HOBOES HOBSON HOCKED HOCKER HOCKEY HODADS HODGES HODIAK HODMAN HODMEN HOEING HOFFER HOGANS HOGGED HOGNUT HOGTIE HOHNER HOHOHO HOHUMS HOISIN HOISTS HOKIER HOKIES HOKILY HOKING HOKUMS HOLDEM HOLDEN HOLDER HOLDIN HOLDIT HOLDME HOLDON HOLDTO HOLDUP HOLERS HOLEUP HOLIER HOLIES HOLILY HOLING HOLISM HOLIST HOLLER HOLLEY HOLLIS HOLLOW HOLMAN HOLMES HOMAGE HOMBRE HOMEEC HOMEIN HOMELY HOMERS HOMEYS HOMIER HOMIES HOMILY HOMING HOMINY HOMMES HONCHO HONDAS HONEIN HONERS HONEST HONEYS HONIED HONING HONKAT HONKED HONKER HONORE HONORS HONOUR HONSHU HOODED HOODIE HOODOO HOOFED HOOFER HOOFIT HOOHAH HOOHAS HOOKAH HOOKED HOOKER HOOKEY HOOKON HOOKUP HOOPED HOOPER HOOPLA HOOPLE HOOPOE HOORAH HOORAY HOOSAC HOOTAT HOOTCH HOOTED HOOTER HOOTIE HOOVER HOOVES HOPERS HOPESO HOPETO HOPING HOPKIN HOPOFF HOPOUT HOPPED HOPPER HOPSIN HOPSON HOPSTO HOPSUP HORACE HORDED HORDES HORGAN HORMEL HORMUZ HORNBY HORNED HORNER HORNET HORNIN HORRID HORROR HORSED HORSES HORSEY HORTON HOSELS HOSERS HOSIER HOSING HOSSES HOSTAS HOSTED HOSTEL HOSTLY HOTAIR HOTBED HOTBOT HOTBOX HOTCAP HOTCAR HOTCUP HOTDAY HOTDOG HOTELS HOTKEY HOTOIL HOTONE HOTPOT HOTROD HOTTEA HOTTER HOTTIE HOTTIP HOTTUB HOTWAR HOUDON HOUNDS HOUNDY HOURIS HOURLY HOUSED HOUSES HOVELS HOVERS HOVETO HOWARD HOWBIG HOWDAH HOWELL HOWFAR HOWLAT HOWLED HOWLER HOWLIN HOWNOW HOWODD HOWSAD HOWSER HOWTOS HOYDEN HOYLES

H•O•••

HAOLES HBOMBS HHOURS HMONGS HOODED HOODIE HOODOO HOOFED HOOFER HOOFIT HOOHAH HOOHAS HOOKAH HOOKED HOOKER HOOKEY HOOKON HOOKUP HOOPED HOOPER HOOPLA HOOPLE HOOPOE HOORAH HOORAY HOOSAC HOOTAT HOOTCH HOOTED HOOTER HOOTIE HOOVER HOOVES HYOIDS

H••O••

HADONE HADOUT HALOED HALOES HALOID HAROLD HASONE HASOUT HAVOCS HEGOAT HELOTS HEROES HEROIC HEROIN HERONS HESOUT HEXOSE HIDOUT HITOFF HITONE HITOUT HOBOED HOBOES HOHOHO HONORE HONORS HONOUR HOPOFF HOPOUT HOTOIL HOTONE HOWODD HUMORS HUMOUR HURONS HUTONE HYPOED HYSONS

H•••O•

HAAKON HACHOO HADRON HALLOO HALLOS HALLOW HANDON HANGON HANLON HANSOM HANSON HARBOR HARLOT HARLOW HARMON HARPON HARROW HATBOX HATHOR HAVEON HAYMOW HEADON HEAPON HEAROF HEATON HEBRON HECTOR HEDRON HELDON HELIOS HELLON HELLOS HELPON HENSON HEREOF HEREON HERMON HERZOG HESIOD HESTON HEYYOU HICKOK HIGHON HILTON HINTON HIPHOP HIPPOS HIREON HITFOR HITSON HIVAOA HOBNOB HOBSON HOLDON HOLLOW HOODOO HOOKON HOOPOE HOPSON HORROR HORTON HOTBOT HOTBOX HOTDOG HOTPOT HOTROD HOUDON HOWNOW HOWTOS HUDSON HUEVOS HULLOS HUNGON HUSTON HUTTON HYDROS HYDROX HYKSOS HYPNOS HYSSOP

H••••O

HACHOO HADAGO HAIRDO HALLOO HARRYO HASAGO HASBRO HATETO HAVENO HAVETO HEADTO HECKNO HELDTO HELICO HELLNO HEMATO HEPATO HERETO HETERO HEWSTO HIDEHO HOHOHO HOLDTO HONCHO HOODOO HOPESO HOPETO HOPSTO HOVETO HUTTWO

•HO•••

AHOLIC AHORSE BHOPAL CHOATE CHOCKS CHOICE CHOIRS CHOKED CHOKER CHOKES CHOLER CHOLLA CHOLOS CHOMPS CHOOSE CHOOSY CHOPIN CHOPPY CHOPRA CHOPUP CHORAL CHORDS CHOREO CHORES CHORIC CHORIO CHOROS CHORUS CHOSEN CHOUGH CHOWED DHOLES DHOTEL DHOTIS FHOLES GHOSTS GHOSTY GHOULS HHOURS KHOUMS LHOTSE PHOBIA PHOBIC PHOBOS PHOEBE PHONED PHONER PHONES PHONEY PHONIC PHONOS PHOOEY PHOTIC PHOTOG PHOTON PHOTOS RHODES RHOMBI RHOMBS RHONDA SHOALS SHOALY SHOATS SHOCKS SHODDY SHOERS SHOFAR SHOGIS SHOGUN SHOJIS SHOLEM SHOLOM SHOOED SHOOIN SHOOTS SHOPAT SHOPKO SHOPPE SHORES SHORTA SHORTE SHORTI SHORTO SHORTS SHORTU SHORTY SHORTZ SHOTAT SHOTBY SHOTUP SHOULD SHOUTS SHOVED SHOVEL SHOVER SHOVES SHOWED SHOWER SHOWIN SHOWME SHOWUP THOLES THOMAS THONGS THORAX THORIC THORNS THORNY THORON THORPE THOUGH WHOAMI WHODAT WHOLES WHOLLY WHOMPS WHOMSO WHOOPI WHOOPS WHOOSH WHORLS WHOSIN WHOWON XHOSAS

•H•O••

CHEOPS CHLORO CHOOSE CHOOSY CHROMA CHROME CHROMO CHROMY CHRONO OHGOSH OHIOAN OHLOOK PHLOEM PHOOEY SHBOOM SHLOCK SHNOOK SHOOED SHOOIN SHOOTS SHROUD SHROVE THEONE THEORY THROAT THROBS THROES THRONE THRONG THROVE THROWN THROWS WHOOPI WHOOPS WHOOSH WHWORD ZHLOBS

•H••O•

AHCHOO CHARON CHEKOV CHEVON CHEWON CHICOS

CHIGOE
CHINOS
CHIRON
CHISOX
CHITON
CHOLOS
CHOROS
CHYRON
OHLOOK
OHSTOP
PHAROS
PHENOL
PHENOM
PHOBOS
PHONOS
PHOTOG
PHOTON
PHOTOS
RHEBOK
RHETOR
RHINOS
SHADOW
SHAKOS
SHALOM
SHARON
SHBOOM
SHEBOP
SHEDON
SHILOH
SHIMON
SHNOOK
SHOLOM
THEDOW
THEFOG
THEFOX
THELOT
THEMOB
THEROD
THERON
THESON
THESOX
THETOP
THETOY
THORON
WHOWON
WHYFOR
WHYNOT
WHYNOW
WHYYOU
ZHUKOV

•H•••O

AHCHOO
BHUTTO
CHANGO
CHARRO
CHEAPO
CHIRHO
CHLORO
CHOREO
CHORIO
CHROMO
CHRONO
CHURRO
GHETTO
PHILCO
PHLEBO
PHYLLO
PHYSIO
SHINTO
SHIPTO
SHOPKO
SHORTO
THERMO
THEWHO
WHAMMO
WHOMSO

••HO••

ABHORS
ASHORE
ATHOME
BEHOLD
BEHOME
BEHOOF
CAHOOT
COHOES
COHORT
COHOST
DEHORN
DRHOOK
ECHOED
ECHOER
ECHOES
ECHOIC
EPHODS
EPHORS
EXHORT
GOHOME
HOHOHO
ICHORS
IMHOME
INHOCK
INHOME
LAHORE
MAHOUT
MTHOOD
NOHOPE
ONHOLD
REHOED
REHOES
REHOLD
REHONE
REHOOK
SCHOLL
SCHOOL
SCHORR
TAHOES
UNHOED
UNHOLY
UNHOOD
UNHOOK
UPHOLD
UPHOVE
WAHOOS
YAHOOS
YOHOHO

••H•O•

ASHDOD
ASHTON
ATHROB
ATHROW
BEHOOF
CAHOOT
DRHOOK
EPHRON
ESHKOL
ETHIOP
ETHNOS
MAHZOR
MTHOOD
REHOOK
SCHMOS
SCHNOZ
SCHOOL
UNHOOD
UNHOOK
WAHLOO
WAHOOS
YAHOOS

••H••O

ENHALO
HOHOHO
ICHIRO
MAHALO
MYHERO
NIHILO
UNHERO
WAHLOO
YOHOHO

•••HO•

ABMHOS
AHCHOO
ANCHOR
ANCHOS
ANDHOW
ANYHOW
ARCHON
AUTHOR
BARHOP
BATHOS
BBSHOT
BICHON
BISHOP
BOOHOO
BUTHOW
CARHOP
DAYHOP
FATHOM
GASHOG
GETHOT
GOTHOT
HACHOO
HATHOR
HIGHON
HIPHOP
IDAHOS
INCHON
ITSHOT
JOBHOP
LACHOY
LITHOS
LUTHOR
MACHOS
METHOD
MUCHOF
MYTHOS
NACHOS
NETHOU
NIGHON
NOSHOW
ONAHOP
ONSHOW
PATHOS
POTHOS
PUSHON
PYTHON
QUAHOG
REDHOT
RESHOD
RESHOE
RESHOT
RESHOW
ROCHON
SENHOR
SIPHON
TOOHOT
TVSHOW
UNSHOD
UNSHOE
UPSHOT
WARHOL
WASHOE
WASHOS
WISHON
YOOHOO

•••H•O

AHCHOO
ARTHRO
BOCHCO
BOOHOO
HACHOO
JETHRO
LASHTO
NEPHRO
PASHTO
PYRHHO
RIGHTO
ROTHKO
RUSHTO
TECHNO
WISHTO
YOOHOO

••••HO

BUTWHO
CHIRHO
CLOTHO
CONCHO
GAUCHO
GRAPHO
GUNGHO
HIDEHO
HOHOHO
HONCHO
LANDHO
MORPHO
NAVAHO
NEOSHO
PANCHO
PONCHO
PSYCHO
PYRHHO
RANCHO
REECHO
SANCHO
SAPPHO
SEZWHO
STETHO
THEWHO
YOHOHO

H•P•••

HAPPEN
HEPATO
HEPCAT
HEPPER
HEPTAD
HIPHOP
HIPPED
HIPPER
HIPPIE
HIPPOS
HIPPUS
HOPERS
HOPESO
HOPETO
HOPING
HOPKIN
HOPOFF
HOPOUT
HOPPED
HOPPER
HOPSIN
HOPSON
HOPSTO
HOPSUP
HUPPAH
HYPERS
HYPEUP
HYPHEN
HYPING
HYPNOS
HYPOED

H••P••

HALPIN
HAMPER
HAPPEN
HARPED
HARPER
HARPON
HASPED
HATPIN
HEAPED
HEAPER
HEAPON
HEAPUP
HELPED
HELPER
HELPIN
HELPME
HELPON
HELPUP
HEMPEN
HEPPER
HERPET
HIPPED
HIPPER
HIPPIE
HIPPOS
HIPPUS
HOOPED
HOOPER
HOOPLA
HOOPLE
HOOPOE
HOPPED
HOPPER
HOTPOT
HUMPED
HUMPHS
HUMPTY
HUPPAH

H••••P

HACKUP
HAMSUP
HANDUP
HANGUP
HARDUP
HAULUP
HAVEUP
HEADUP
HEALUP
HEAPUP
HEATUP
HELDUP
HELPUP
HICCUP
HIGHUP
HIKEUP
HIPHOP
HITSUP
HOLDUP
HOLEUP
HOOKUP
HOPSUP
HOTCAP
HOTCUP
HOTTIP
HUBCAP
HUNGUP
HUNTUP
HUSHUP
HYPEUP
HYSSOP

•H•P••

BHOPAL
CHAPEL
CHAPIN
CHIPIN
CHIPUP
CHOPIN
CHOPPY
CHOPRA
CHOPUP
CHUPPA
SHAPED
SHAPER
SHAPES
SHIPTO
SHOPAT
SHOPKO
SHOPPE
THEPIT
THEPRU
WHIPIN
WHIPPY
WHIPUP

•H••P•

CHAMPS
CHEAPO
CHEEPS
CHEOPS
CHIMPS
CHIRPS
CHIRPY
CHOMPS
CHOPPY
CHUMPS
CHUPPA
PHELPS
SHARPE
SHARPS
SHARPY
SHERPA
SHOPPE
THEAPE
THEEPA
THESPS
THESPY
THORPE
THUMPS
WHELPS
WHIPPY
WHOMPS
WHOOPI
WHOOPS

•H•••P

CHATUP
CHEWUP
CHINUP
CHIPUP
CHOPUP
OHSTOP
PHILIP
SHEBOP
SHOTUP
SHOWUP
SHRIMP
SHUTUP
THEASP
THEGAP
THELIP
THERAP
THETOP
WHIPUP

••HP••

ASHPAN
ASHPIT

••H•P•

NOHOPE
TSHAPE
USHAPE
VCHIPS
VSHAPE
YSHAPE

••H••P

ASHARP
BSHARP
CSHARP
DSHARP
ESHARP
ETHIOP
FSHARP
GSHARP
NOHELP
OFHELP
SCHAAP
SCHLEP
UNHASP
UPHEAP

•••H•P

BARHOP
BISHOP
CARHOP
DAYHOP
DISHUP
GETHEP
GETHIP
GOTHEP
GOTHIP
HIGHUP
HIPHOP
HUSHUP
JOBHOP
LASHUP
MASHUP
MAYHAP
MISHAP
ONAHOP
PUSHUP
RESHIP
TOOHIP
UNSHIP
WASHUP

H••••Q

HIGHIQ

•H•Q••

CHEQUE

•••H•Q

HIGHIQ

HR••••

HRIDER
HRYVNA

H•R•••

HARALD
HARARE
HARASS
HARBIN
HARBOR
HARDBY
HARDEN
HARDER
HARDIN
HARDLY
HARDUP
HAREMS
HARHAR
HARING
HARKED
HARKEN
HARKER
HARLAN
HARLEM
HARLEY
HARLIN
HARLOT
HARLOW
HARMED
HARMER
HARMON
HARNEY
HAROLD
HARPED
HARPER
HARPON
HARRAD
HARRAH
HARRIS
HARROW
HARRYO
HARRYS
HARVEY
HERALD
HERBAL
HERBED
HERBES
HERBIE
HERDED
HERDER
HEREAT
HEREBY
HEREIN
HEREOF
HEREON
HERESY
HERETO
HERMAN
HERMES
HERMIT
HERMON
HERNAN
HERNIA
HEROES
HEROIC
HEROIN
HERONS
HERPET
HERREN
HERSEY
HERVEY
HERZOG
HIREES
HIREON
HIRERS
HIRING
HIRSCH
HORACE
HORDED
HORDES
HORGAN
HORMEL
HORMUZ
HORNBY
HORNED
HORNER
HORNET
HORNIN
HORRID
HORROR
HORSED
HORSES
HORSEY
HORTON
HURDLE
HURLED
HURLER
HURLEY
HURONS
HURRAH
HURRAY
HURTER
HURTLE

H••R••

HADRON
HAIRDO
HAIRED
HARRAD
HARRAH
HARRIS
HARROW
HARRYO
HARRYS
HATRED
HEARER
HEARNS
HEAROF
HEARSE
HEARST
HEARTH
HEARTS
HEARTY
HEARYE
HEBREW
HEBRON
HEDRAL
HEDREN
HEDRON
HENRIK
HENRYI
HENRYK
HENRYV
HERREN
HEURES
HOARDS
HOARSE
HOORAH
HOORAY
HORRID
HORROR
HOTROD
HOURIS
HOURLY
HUBRIS
HURRAH
HURRAY
HYBRID
HYDRAE
HYDRAS
HYDRIC
HYDROS
HYDROX
HYDRUS
HYGRIC

H•••R•

HARARE
HASBRO
HATARI
HATERS
HAYERS
HAZARD
HAZERS
HEGIRA
HENDRY
HETERO
HEWERS
HEXERS
HHOURS
HIDERS
HIKERS
HILARY
HIRERS
HIVERS
HOBART
HOLERS
HOMBRE
HOMERS
HONERS
HONORE
HONORS
HOPERS
HOSERS
HOVERS
HOWARD
HUBERT
HUMERI
HUMORS
HUNGRY
HYPERS

H••••R

HABLAR
HACKER
HAGLER
HAILER
HALTER
HALVER
HAMMER
HAMPER
HANDER
HANGAR
HANGER
HANKER
HARBOR
HARDER
HARHAR
HARKER
HARMER
HARPER
HATHOR
HATTER
HAULER
HAWKER
HAWSER
HAZIER
HEADER
HEALER
HEAPER
HEARER
HEATER
HEAVER
HECTOR
HEDGER
HEEDER
HEEGER
HEELER
HEFNER
HEFTER
HEIFER
HELLER
HELMER
HELPER
HELTER
HEMMER
HENNER
HEPPER
HERDER
HESTER
HIGHER
HILLER
HINDER
HINTER
HIPPER
HISSER
HITFOR
HITHER
HITTER
HOAXER
HOCKER
HOFFER
HOHNER
HOKIER
HOLDER
HOLIER
HOLLER
HOMIER
HONKER
HONOUR
HOOFER
HOOKER
HOOPER
HOOTER
HOOVER
HOPPER
HORNER
HORROR
HOSIER
HOTAIR
HOTCAR
HOTTER
HOTWAR
HOWFAR
HOWLER
HOWSER
HRIDER
HUGGER
HULLER
HUMBER
HUMMER
HUMOUR
HUNGER
HUNKER
HUNTER
HURLER
HURTER
HUSKER
HUSSAR

•HR•••

CHRISM
CHRIST
CHROMA
CHROME
CHROMO
CHROMY
CHRONO
PHRASE
SHRANK
SHREDS
SHREVE
SHREWD
SHREWS
SHRIEK
SHRIFT
SHRIKE
SHRILL
SHRIMP
SHRINE
SHRINK
SHRIVE
SHROUD
SHROVE
SHRUBS
SHRUGS
SHRUNK
THRACE
THRALL
THRASH
THREAD
THREAT
THREEA
THREEB
THREEC
THREED
THREEE
THREES
THRESH
THRICE
THRIFT
THRILL
THRIVE
THROAT
THROBS
THROES
THRONE
THRONG
THROVE
THROWN
THROWS
THRUMS
THRUSH
THRUST

•H•R••

AHERNE
AHORSE
CHARDS
CHARGE
CHARLY
CHARMS
CHARON
CHARRO
CHARTA
CHARTS
CHERIE
CHERRY
CHERTS
CHERTY
CHERUB
CHERYL
CHIRAC
CHIRHO
CHIRON
CHIRPS
CHIRPY
CHIRRS
CHORAL
CHORDS
CHOREO
CHORES
CHORIC
CHORIO
CHOROS
CHORUS
CHURCH
CHURLS
CHURNS
CHURRO
CHYRON
DHARMA
GHIRSH
OHCRUD
OHDRAT
PHAROS
SHARDS
SHARED
SHARER
SHARES
SHARIF
SHARKS
SHARON
SHARPE
SHARPS
SHARPY
SHARYN
SHEREE
SHERPA
SHERRI
SHERRY
SHERYL
SHIRAZ
SHIRER
SHIRES
SHIRKS
SHIRRS
SHIRTS
SHORES
SHORTA
SHORTE
SHORTI
SHORTO
SHORTS
SHORTU
SHORTY
SHORTZ
THERAM
THERAP
THERAT
THERED
THEREF
THERES
THERMO
THERMS
THEROD
THERON
THIRDR
THIRDS
THIRST
THIRTY
THORAX
THORIC
THORNS
THORNY
THORON
THORPE
WHARFS
WHERED
WHERES
WHERRY
WHIRLS
WHIRLY
WHIRRS
WHORLS

•H••R•

CHAIRS
CHAKRA
CHARRO
CHEERS
CHEERY
CHERRY
CHEVRE
CHIRRS
CHITRA
CHLORO
CHOIRS
CHOPRA
CHURRO
HHOURS
KHMERS
NHLERS
OHDARN
OHENRY
OHSURE
PHEDRE
SHEARS
SHEERS
SHERRI
SHERRY
SHIRRS
SHOERS
THEIRS
THEMRS
THENRA
THEORY
THEPRU
THEYRE
THWART
WHERRY
WHIRRS
WHWORD

•H•••R

CHAFER
CHASER
CHEDER
CHEWER
CHICER
CHIDER
CHIMER
CHOKER
CHOLER
KHYBER
OHDEAR
PHASER
PHONER
RHETOR
RHYMER
SHADER
SHAKER

SHAKUR
SHAMIR
SHAPER
SHARER
SHAVER
SHINER
SHIRER
SHIVER
SHOFAR
SHOVER
SHOWER
THALER
THAWER
THAYER
THEBAR
THECAR
THIRDR
WHALER
WHINER
WHITER
WHYFOR

••HR••
ASHRAM
ATHROB
ATHROW
BOHRER
BTHREE
EPHRON
FUHRER
GEHRIG
LEHRER
NEHRUS
OCHRED
OCHRES
RAHRAH
ROHRER
TEHRAN

••H•R•
ABHORS
ACHERS
ADHERE
ALHIRT
ASHARP
ASHORE
AWHIRL
BSHARP
COHERE
COHORT
CSHARP
DEHIRE
DEHORN
DSHARP
EPHORS
ERHARD
ESHARP
ETHERS
EXHORT
FSHARP
GSHARP
ICHIRO
ICHORS
IMHERE
IMHURT
INHERE
LAHORE
MCHARG

MYHERO
OCHERS
OCHERY
ONHIRE
OTHERS
REHIRE
SAHARA
SCHORR
SPHERE
TSHIRT
UNHERO
UNHIRE
UNHURT
UPHERE
USHERS
VIHARA

••H••R
ACHIER
ASHIER
ASHLAR
BOHRER
CAHIER
COHEIR
DEHAIR
ECHOER
FUHRER
HOHNER
ISHTAR
KOHLER
LEHRER
MAHLER
MAHZOR
MOHAIR
OTHMAR
REHEAR
ROHMER
ROHRER
SCHORR
UNHAIR
WOHLER

•••HR•
ARTHRO
EUCHRE
JETHRO
MOTHRA
NEPHRO
TISHRI

•••H•R
AETHER
ANCHOR
ANTHER
ARCHER
ARTHUR
ASTHER
AUTHOR
BASHER
BATHER
BENHUR
BOTHER
BUSHER
CATHER
CIPHER
COSHER
CYPHER
DASHER

DITHER
EITHER
ESCHER
ESTHER
ETCHER
FATHER
FISHER
GATHER
GOPHER
GUSHER
HARHAR
HATHOR
HIGHER
HITHER
INCHER
JOSHER
KOCHER
KOSHER
LASHER
LATHER
LECHER
LITHER
LOCHER
LOTHAR
LUSHER
LUTHER
LUTHOR
MASHER
MATHER
MOSHER
MOTHER
MUSHER
NETHER
NIGHER
NOSHER
POSHER
POTHER
PUSHER
RASHER
RATHER
RICHER
RUSHER
SACHER
SENHOR
SIGHER
TETHER
TITHER
WASHER
WISHER
WITHER
ZEPHYR
ZITHER

H•S•••
HASAGO
HASBRO
HASFUN
HASHED
HASHES
HASONE
HASOUT
HASPED
HASSAM
HASSAN
HASSEL
HASSID
HASSLE
HASTED

HASTEN
HASTES
HESIOD
HESOUT
HESTER
HESTIA
HESTON
HISSAT
HISSED
HISSER
HISSES
HOSELS
HOSERS
HOSIER
HOSING
HOSSES
HOSTAS
HOSTED
HOSTEL
HOSTLY
HUSHED
HUSHES
HUSHUP
HUSING
HUSKED
HUSKER
HUSSAR
HUSSEY
HUSTLE
HUSTON
HYSONS
HYSSOP

H••S••
HALSEY
HAMSUN
HAMSUP
HANSAS
HANSEL
HANSES
HANSOM
HANSON
HASSAM
HASSAN
HASSEL
HASSID
HASSLE
HAWSER
HAWSES
HEISTS
HEMSIN
HENSON
HERSEY
HEUSEN
HEWSTO
HIRSCH
HISSAT
HISSED
HISSER
HISSES
HITSAT
HITSIT
HITSON
HITSUP
HOBSON
HOISIN
HOISTS
HONSHU

HOOSAC
HOPSIN
HOPSON
HOPSTO
HOPSUP
HORSED
HORSES
HORSEY
HOSSES
HOUSED
HOUSES
HOWSAD
HOWSER
HTESTS
HUDSON
HUSSAR
HUSSEY
HYKSOS
HYSSOP

H•••S•
HALEST
HARASS
HAVASU
HEARSE
HEARST
HEINSE
HERESY
HEWISH
HEXOSE
HITEST
HOARSE
HOLISM
HOLIST
HONEST
HOPESO
HUGEST

H••••S
HABEAS
HABITS
HACEKS
HADJES
HADJIS
HAGGIS
HAIDAS
HAIKUS
HAINES
HAJJES
HAJJIS
HAKIMS
HALLOS
HALOES
HALVAS
HALVES
HANSAS
HANSES
HAOLES
HARASS
HAREMS
HARRIS
HARRYS
HASHES
HASTES
HATERS
HAUNTS
HAVENS
HAVOCS

HAWSES
HAYERS
HAYMES
HAYNES
HAZANS
HAZELS
HAZERS
HBEAMS
HBOMBS
HEARNS
HEARTS
HEATHS
HEAVES
HEDGES
HEGYES
HEISTS
HELENS
HELIOS
HELLAS
HELLOS
HELOTS
HENGES
HENNAS
HERBES
HERMES
HEROES
HERONS
HEURES
HEWERS
HEXADS
HEXERS
HHOURS
HIATUS
HIDERS
HIHATS
HIKERS
HINDUS
HINGES
HINGIS
HIPPOS
HIPPUS
HIREES
HIRERS
HISSES
HITINS
HIVERS
HMONGS
HOARDS
HOAXES
HOBBES
HOBOES
HODADS
HODGES
HOGANS
HOHUMS
HOISTS
HOKIES
HOKUMS
HOLERS
HOLIES
HOLLIS
HOLMES
HOMERS
HOMEYS
HOMIES
HOMMES
HONDAS
HONERS

HONEYS
HONORS
HOOHAS
HOOVES
HOPERS
HORDES
HORSES
HOSELS
HOSERS
HOSSES
HOSTAS
HOTELS
HOUNDS
HOURIS
HOUSES
HOVELS
HOVERS
HOWTOS
HOYLES
HTESTS
HTILES
HUBRIS
HUEVOS
HUGHES
HULLOS
HUMANS
HUMMUS
HUMORS
HUMPHS
HURONS
HUSHES
HYADES
HYATTS
HYDRAS
HYDROS
HYDRUS
HYENAS
HYKSOS
HYOIDS
HYPERS
HYPNOS
HYSONS

•HS•••
OHSTOP
OHSURE

•H•S••
CHASED
CHASER
CHASES
CHASMS
CHASSE
CHASTE
CHESTS
CHESTY
CHISEL
CHISOX
CHISUM
CHOSEN
GHOSTS
GHOSTY
LHASAN
PHASED
PHASER
PHASES
PHASIC
PHYSED

PHYSIC
PHYSIO
RHESUS
SHASTA
THESEA
THESES
THESIS
THESON
THESOX
THESPS
THESPY
THESUN
THISBE
THUSLY
WHISKS
WHISKY
WHOSIN
XHOSAS

•H••S•
AHIMSA
AHORSE
CHAISE
CHASSE
CHEESE
CHEESY
CHOOSE
CHOOSY
CHRISM
CHRIST
CHUHSI
GHIRSH
LHOTSE
OHGOSH
PHRASE
SHEESH
SHIEST
SHIISM
SHYEST
THEASP
THEISM
THEIST
THEUSA
THIRST
THRASH
THRESH
THRUSH
THRUST
WHILST
WHIMSY
WHOMSO
WHOOSH

•H•••S
BHANGS
CHAFES
CHAFFS
CHAINS
CHAIRS
CHALKS
CHAMPS
CHANTS
CHARDS
CHARMS
CHARTS
CHASES
CHASMS
CHEATS

CHECKS
CHEEKS
CHEEPS
CHEERS
CHEOPS
CHERTS
CHESTS
CHEVYS
CHICAS
CHICKS
CHICOS
CHIDES
CHIEFS
CHIENS
CHILES
CHILIS
CHILLS
CHIMES
CHIMPS
CHINAS
CHINES
CHINKS
CHINOS
CHIRPS
CHIRRS
CHIVAS
CHIVES
CHOCKS
CHOIRS
CHOKES
CHOLOS
CHOMPS
CHORDS
CHORES
CHOROS
CHORUS
CHUCKS
CHUFFS
CHUMPS
CHUNKS
CHURLS
CHURNS
CHUTES
DHOLES
DHOTIS
FHOLES
GHAINS
GHAZIS
GHOSTS
GHOULS
HHOURS
KHAKIS
KHMERS
KHOUMS
NHLERS
OHNUTS
PHAROS
PHASES
PHELPS
PHIALS
PHOBOS
PHONES
PHONOS
PHOTOS
RHAMES
RHEEMS
RHEIMS
RHEMES

RHESUS
RHEUMS
RHINOS
RHODES
RHOMBS
RHUMBS
RHYMES
SHACKS
SHADES
SHAFTS
SHAKES
SHAKOS
SHALES
SHAMES
SHAMUS
SHANKS
SHAPES
SHARDS
SHARES
SHARKS
SHARPS
SHAVES
SHAWLS
SHEARS
SHEDDS
SHEENS
SHEERS
SHEETS
SHEIKS
SHELLS
SHIFTS
SHILLS
SHINES
SHIRES
SHIRKS
SHIRRS
SHIRTS
SHOALS
SHOATS
SHOCKS
SHOERS
SHOGIS
SHOJIS
SHOOTS
SHORES
SHORTS
SHOUTS
SHOVES
SHREDS
SHREWS
SHRUBS
SHRUGS
SHUCKS
SHUNTS
THALES
THAMES
THANES
THANKS
THATIS
THEBES
THEFTS
THEIRS
THEMES
THEMRS
THERES
THERMS
THESES
THESIS

THESPS
THETAS
THETIS
THIGHS
THILLS
THINGS
THINKS
THIRDS
THOLES
THOMAS
THONGS
THORNS
THREES
THROBS
THROES
THROWS
THRUMS
THUMBS
THUMPS
THUNKS
THYMES
THYMUS
UHAULS
UHLANS
WHACKS
WHALES
WHANGS
WHARFS
WHEATS
WHEELS
WHELKS
WHELMS
WHELPS
WHERES
WHIFFS
WHILES
WHINES
WHIRLS
WHIRRS
WHISKS
WHITES
WHOLES
WHOMPS
WHOOPS
WHORLS
WHYYES
XHOSAS
ZHLOBS
ZHLUBS

••H•S•
AGHAST
BEHEST
COHOST
REHASH
SCHISM
SCHIST
SCHUSS
UNHASP
UNHUSK

••H••S
ABHORS
ACHERS
APHIDS
ARHATS
ATHENS
COHABS

COHOES
ECHOES
EPHAHS
EPHODS
EPHORS
ETHERS
ETHICS
ETHNOS
ETHYLS
HIHATS
HOHUMS
ICHORS
JIHADS
LEHUAS
MAHDIS
NEHRUS
NOHITS
OCHERS
OCHRES
OGHAMS
OPHULS
OTHERS
PSHAWS
REHABS
REHEMS
REHITS
REHOES
SAHIBS
SCHAVS
SCHMOS
SCHUSS
SCHWAS
TAHOES
TEHEES
TVHITS
UNHATS
USHERS
VCHIPS
WAHOOS
YAHOOS

•••HS•
BOCHSA
CHUHSI

•••H•S
AARHUS
ABMHOS
ABOHMS
ALOHAS
ALPHAS
ANCHOS
ARCHES
AUGHTS
BACHES
BASHES
BATHES
BATHOS
BIGHTS
BRAHMS
BUSHES
CACHES
CASHES
CATHYS
COSHES
DACHAS
DASHES
DASHIS

DISHES
EIGHTS
ETCHES
FICHES
FICHUS
FIGHTS
FISHES
GASHES
GUSHES
HASHES
HOOHAS
HUGHES
HUSHES
IDAHOS
INCHES
ITCHES
JANHUS
JOSHES
KASHAS
LASHES
LATHES
LIGHTS
LITHOS
LUSHES
MACHOS
MASHES
MATHIS
MESHES
MIGHTS
MOCHAS
MOSHES
MUCHAS
MUSHES
MYTHOS
NACHAS
NACHOS
NASHES
NICHES
NIGHTS
NOCHES
NOSHES
OMAHAS
OUCHES
OUGHTS
PASHAS
PATHOS
PECHES
PISHES
POTHOS
PUSHES
RASHES
RESHES
RICHES
RIGHTS
RISHIS
ROSHIS
RUCHES
RUSHES
SADHES
SADHUS
SASHES
SIGHTS
SUCHAS
SUSHIS
TETHYS
TIGHTS
TITHES
TUSHES

TYPHUS
UTAHNS
VACHES
WASHES
WASHOS
WIGHTS
WISHES
WITHUS
YACHTS

••••HS
ALEPHS
BERTHS
BIRTHS
BOOTHS
BOUGHS
BRACHS
BROTHS
BURGHS
CLOTHS
CONCHS
COUGHS
CRWTHS
CZECHS
DEATHS
DEPTHS
DOUGHS
EARTHS
EPHAHS
EPOCHS
FAITHS
FARAHS
FIFTHS
FIRTHS
FROTHS
GIRTHS
GLYPHS
GRAPHS
HEATHS
HUMPHS
JONAHS
LAUGHS
LYMPHS
MIRTHS
MONTHS
MORPHS
MOUTHS
MYNAHS
MYRRHS
NEIGHS
NINTHS
NORTHS
NYMPHS
OBEAHS
OOMPHS
OPRAHS
ORACHS
PASCHS
PSYCHS
RAJAHS
RICOHS
ROUGHS
SIXTHS
SLOTHS
SMITHS
SNATHS
SOUTHS
STAPHS

STROHS
SURAHS
SWATHS
SYLPHS
SYNCHS
SYNTHS
TENTHS
THIGHS
TILTHS
TORAHS
TOUGHS
TROTHS
TRUTHS
WEIGHS
WELCHS
WIDTHS
WORTHS
WRATHS
YOUTHS

HT••••
HTESTS
HTILES

H•T•••
HATARI
HATBOX
HATEIT
HATERS
HATETO
HATFUL
HATHOR
HATING
HATPIN
HATRED
HATTED
HATTER
HATTIE
HETERO
HITECH
HITEST
HITFOR
HITHER
HITINS
HITMAN
HITMEN
HITOFF
HITONE
HITOUT
HITSAT
HITSIT
HITSON
HITSUP
HITTER
HOTAIR
HOTBED
HOTBOT
HOTBOX
HOTCAP
HOTCAR
HOTCUP
HOTDAY
HOTDOG
HOTELS
HOTKEY
HOTOIL
HOTONE
HOTPOT

HOTROD
HOTTEA
HOTTER
HOTTIE
HOTTIP
HOTTUB
HOTWAR
HUTONE
HUTTED
HUTTON
HUTTWO

H••T••
HAFTED
HALTED
HALTER
HASTED
HASTEN
HASTES
HATTED
HATTER
HATTIE
HEATED
HEATER
HEATHS
HEATHY
HEATON
HEATUP
HECTIC
HECTOR
HEFTED
HEFTER
HELTER
HEPTAD
HESTER
HESTIA
HESTON
HIATAL
HIATUS
HILTED
HILTON
HINTAT
HINTED
HINTER
HINTON
HITTER
HOGTIE
HOOTAT
HOOTCH
HOOTED
HOOTER
HOOTIE
HORTON
HOSTAS
HOSTED
HOSTEL
HOSTLY
HOTTEA
HOTTER
HOTTIE
HOTTIP
HOTTUB
HOWTOS
HUNTED
HUNTER
HUNTUP
HURTER
HURTLE
HUSTLE
HUSTON
HUTTED
HUTTON
HUTTWO
HYATTS
HYETAL

H•••T•
HABITS
HALITE
HAMATE
HAMITE
HATETO
HAUNTS
HAVETO
HEADTO
HEALTH
HEARTH
HEARTS
HEARTY
HECATE
HEISTS
HELDTO
HELOTS
HEMATO
HEPATO
HERETO
HEWITT
HEWSTO
HIHATS
HOISTS
HOLDTO
HOPETO
HOPSTO
HOVETO
HTESTS
HUMPTY
HYATTS

H••••T
HACKIT
HADOUT
HAIGHT
HALEST
HAMLET
HARLOT
HASOUT
HATEIT
HAVEAT
HAVEIT
HAVENT
HAZMAT
HEARST
HEGOAT
HEIGHT
HELDIT
HELMET
HELMUT
HENBIT
HEPCAT
HEREAT
HERMIT
HERPET
HESOUT
HEWITT
HEXNUT
HIDOUT
HINTAT
HISSAT
HITEST
HITOUT
HITSAT
HITSIT
HLHUNT
HOBART
HOBBIT
HOGNUT
HOLDIT
HOLIST
HONEST
HONKAT
HOOFIT
HOOTAT
HOPOUT
HORNET
HOTBOT
HOTPOT
HOWLAT
HUBERT
HUGEST

•HT•••
SHTETL
SHTICK

•H•T••
BHUTAN
BHUTTO
CHATTY
CHATUP
CHITON
CHITRA
CHITTY
CHUTED
CHUTES
DHOTEL
DHOTIS
GHETTO
LHOTSE
OHSTOP
PHOTIC
PHOTOG
PHOTON
PHOTOS
RHETOR
RHYTHM
SHOTAT
SHOTBY
SHOTUP
SHUTIN
SHUTUP
THATCH
THATIS
THATLL
THETAS
THETED
THETIS
THETOP
THETOY
WHATIF
WHATLL
WHATVE
WHITBY
WHITED
WHITEN
WHITER
WHITES
WHITEY
WHITTY

•H••T•
BHUTTO
CHANTE
CHANTS
CHANTY
CHARTA
CHARTS
CHASTE
CHATTY
CHEATS
CHEETA
CHERTS
CHERTY
CHESTS
CHESTY
CHINTZ
CHITTY
CHOATE
GHETTO
GHOSTS
GHOSTY
OHNUTS
SHAFTS
SHANTY
SHASTA
SHEATH
SHEETS
SHELTY
SHIFTS
SHIFTY
SHIITE
SHINTO
SHIPTO
SHIRTS
SHOATS
SHOOTS
SHORTA
SHORTE
SHORTI
SHORTO
SHORTS
SHORTU
SHORTY
SHORTZ
SHOUTS
SHTETL
SHULTZ
SHUNTS
THEFTS
THIRTY
WHEATS
WHITTY

•H•••T
CHALET
CHEVET
CHRIST
OHDRAT
PHFFFT
SHALIT
SHEBAT
SHEVAT
SHIEST
SHOPAT
SHOTAT
SHRIFT
SHYEST
THEACT
THEIST
THELOT
THEMET
THENET
THEPIT
THERAT
THEVET
THIRST
THREAT
THRIFT
THROAT
THRUST
THWART
WHILST
WHODAT
WHYNOT

••HT••
ASHTON
ICHTHY
ISHTAR

••H•T•
ARHATS
HIHATS
NOHITS
REHITS
TAHITI
TVHITS
UNHATS

••H••T
AGHAST
ALHIRT
ASHPIT
BEHEST
CAHOOT
COHORT
COHOST
ENHAUT
EXHORT
HLHUNT
IMHURT
MAHOUT
NOHANT
REHEAT
SCHIST
TSHIRT
UNHAFT
UNHURT
UTHANT

•••HT•
AUGHTS
BIGHTS
EIGHTA
EIGHTB
EIGHTC
EIGHTD
EIGHTE
EIGHTH
EIGHTS
EIGHTY
FICHTE
FIGHTS
LASHTO
LIGHTS
MIGHTS
MIGHTY
NAPHTA
NIGHTS
NIGHTY
OUGHTA
OUGHTS
PASHTO
RIGHTO
RIGHTS
RIGHTY
RUSHTO
SIGHTS
TECHTV
TIGHTS
VASHTI
WIGHTS
WISHTO
YACHTS

•••H•T
ATTHAT
BACHIT
BADHAT
BBSHOT
BECHET
BIGHIT
CACHET
DASHIT
GETHOT
GOTHOT
INTHAT
ITSHOT
MISHIT
NEWHAT
NONHIT
OLDHAT
ONEHIT
ORWHAT
OUTHIT
PUSHIT
REDHAT
REDHOT
RESHOT
RESHUT
RICHET
ROCHAT
ROCHET
RUSHAT
SACHET
SIGHAT
SKIHAT
SOTHAT
SOWHAT
SUNHAT
TENHUT
TINHAT
TOOHOT
TOPHAT
TOYHAT
UNSHUT
UPSHOT
WITHIT
YAPHET

••••HT
ALIGHT
ARIGHT
BEIGHT
BLIGHT
BOUGHT
BRECHT
BRIGHT
CAUGHT
DWIGHT
FLIGHT
FOUGHT
FRIGHT
GEIGHT
HAIGHT
HEIGHT
IEIGHT
IMIGHT
KNIGHT
NAUGHT
NOUGHT
PLIGHT
SLIGHT
SOUGHT
TAUGHT
VEIGHT
VOIGHT
WEIGHT
WRIGHT

HU••••
HUBBLE
HUBBUB
HUBCAP
HUBERT
HUBLEY
HUBRIS
HUDDIE
HUDDLE
HUDSON
HUEVOS
HUFFED
HUGELY
HUGEST
HUGGED
HUGGER
HUGHES
HUGHIE
HULKED
HULLED
HULLER
HULLOS
HUMANE
HUMANS
HUMBER
HUMBLE
HUMBLY
HUMBUG
HUMERI
HUMMED
HUMMEL
HUMMER
HUMMUS
HUMORS
HUMOUR
HUMPED
HUMPHS
HUMPTY
HUMVEE
HUNGBY
HUNGER
HUNGIN
HUNGON
HUNGRY
HUNGUP
HUNKER
HUNLEY
HUNTED
HUNTER
HUNTUP
HUPPAH
HURDLE
HURLED
HURLER
HURLEY
HURONS
HURRAH
HURRAY
HURTER
HURTLE
HUSHED
HUSHES
HUSHUP
HUSING
HUSKED
HUSKER
HUSSAR
HUSSEY
HUSTLE
HUSTON
HUTONE
HUTTED
HUTTON
HUTTWO
HUXLEY
HUZZAH

H•U•••
HAULED
HAULER
HAULIN
HAULUP
HAUNCH
HAUNTS
HEURES
HEUSEN
HOUDON
HOUNDS
HOUNDY
HOURIS
HOURLY
HOUSED
HOUSES

H••U••
HAMULI
HECUBA
HHOURS
HLHUNT
HOHUMS
HOKUMS

H•••U•
HACKUP
HADFUN
HADOUT
HAIKUS
HALLUX
HAMSUN
HAMSUP
HANDUP
HANGUL
HANGUP
HARDUP
HASFUN
HASOUT
HATFUL
HAULUP
HAVEUP
HEADUP
HEALUP
HEAPUP
HEATUP
HELDUP
HELIUM
HELMUT
HELPUP
HESOUT
HEXNUT
HIATUS
HICCUP
HIDOUT
HIGHUP
HIKEUP
HINDUS
HIPPUS
HITOUT
HITSUP
HOGNUT
HOLDUP
HOLEUP
HONOUR
HOOKUP
HOPOUT
HOPSUP
HORMUZ
HOTCUP
HOTTUB
HUBBUB
HUMBUG
HUMMUS
HUMOUR
HUNGUP
HUNTUP
HUSHUP
HYDRUS
HYPEUP

H••••U
HAVASU
HEYYOU
HONSHU

•HU•••
BHUTAN
BHUTTO
CHUBBY
CHUCKS
CHUCKY
CHUFFS
CHUFFY
CHUHSI
CHUMMY
CHUMPS
CHUNKS
CHUNKY
CHUPPA
CHURCH
CHURLS
CHURNS
CHURRO
CHUTED
CHUTES
RHUMBA
RHUMBS
SHUCKS
SHULTZ
SHUMAI
SHUNTS
SHUTIN
SHUTUP
THUMBS
THUMPS
THUNKS
THUSLY
ZHUKOV

•H•U••
CHOUGH
GHOULS
HHOURS
KHOUMS
OHNUTS
OHSURE
RHEUMS
RHEUMY
SHOULD
SHOUTS
SHRUBS
SHRUGS
SHRUNK
THEUSA
THOUGH
THRUMS
THRUSH
THRUST
UHAULS
ZHLUBS

•H••U•
CHACUN
CHATUP
CHEQUE
CHERUB
CHEWUP
CHINUA
CHINUP
CHIPUP
CHISUM
CHOPUP
CHORUS
OHCRUD
PHYLUM
RHESUS
SHAKUR
SHAMUS
SHOGUN
SHOTUP
SHOWUP
SHROUD
SHUTUP
THEHUB
THESUN
THYMUS
WHIPUP

•H•••U
CHANDU
SHORTU
THEPRU
WHYYOU

••HU••
EXHUME
HLHUNT
HOHUMS
IMHURT
INHUME
KAHUNA
LEHUAS
MCHUGH
OAHUAN
OPHULS
REHUNG
SCHULZ
SCHUSS
UNHUED
UNHULL
UNHUNG
UNHUNH
UNHURT
UNHUSK
YEHUDI

••H•U•
ENHAUT
KAHLUA
MAHOUT
NEHRUS
REHAUL
SCHLUB

•••HU•
AARHUS
ARTHUR
BENHUR
BIGHUG
DISHUP
FICHUS
HIGHUP
HUSHUP
JANHUS
JOSHUA
LASHUP
MASHUP
NASHUA
PUSHUP
RESHUT
SADHUS
TENHUT
THEHUB
TYPHUS
UNSHUT
WASHUP
WITHUS
XINHUA

•••H•U
NETHOU
NIIHAU
VISHNU

••••HU
HONSHU
KYUSHU
MANCHU
PICCHU

H•V•••
HAVANA
HAVASU
HAVEAT
HAVEIN
HAVEIT
HAVENO
HAVENS
HAVENT
HAVEON
HAVETO
HAVEUP
HAVING
HAVOCS
HIVAOA
HIVERS
HIVING
HOVELS
HOVERS
HOVETO

H••V••
HALVAH
HALVAS
HALVED
HALVER
HALVES
HARVEY
HEAVED
HEAVEN
HEAVER
HEAVES
HERVEY
HOOVER
HOOVES
HRYVNA
HUEVOS
HUMVEE

H•••V•
HALEVY

H••••V
HENRYV

•H•V••
CHAVEZ
CHEVAL
CHEVET
CHEVON
CHEVRE
CHEVYS
CHIVAS
CHIVES
SHAVED
SHAVEN
SHAVER
SHAVES
SHEVAT
SHIVER
SHOVED
SHOVEL
SHOVER
SHOVES
THEVET

•H••V•
SHEAVE
SHELVE
SHREVE
SHRIVE
SHROVE
THEYVE
THIEVE
THRIVE
THROVE
WHATVE

•H•••V
CHEKOV
ZHUKOV

••H•V•
BEHAVE
JOHNVI
MOHAVE
SCHAVS
UPHOVE

••H••V
JOHNIV
JOHNXV

•••H•V
MOSHAV
TECHTV

H•W•••
HAWAII
HAWHAW
HAWING
HAWKED
HAWKER
HAWSER
HAWSES
HEWERS
HEWING
HEWISH
HEWITT
HEWSTO
HOWARD
HOWBIG
HOWDAH
HOWELL
HOWFAR
HOWLAT
HOWLED
HOWLER
HOWLIN
HOWNOW
HOWODD
HOWSAD
HOWSER
HOWTOS

H••W••
HOTWAR

H•••W•
HUTTWO

H••••W
HALLOW
HARLOW
HARROW
HAWHAW
HAYMOW
HEBREW
HEEHAW
HOLLOW
HOWNOW

•HW•••
OHWELL
THWACK
THWART
WHWORD

•H•W••
CHAWED
CHEWED
CHEWER
CHEWON
CHEWUP
CHOWED
SHAWLS
SHOWED
SHOWER
SHOWIN
SHOWME
SHOWUP
THAWED
THAWER
THEWAY
THEWEB
THEWHO
THEWIZ
WHOWON

•H••W•
SHREWD
SHREWS
THROWN
THROWS

•H•••W
SHADOW
THEDOW
THELAW
WHYNOW

••HW••
RAHWAY
SCHWAB
SCHWAS
WAHWAH

••H•W•
MOHAWK
OSHAWA
PSHAWS
UNHEWN

••H••W
ATHROW

•••HW•
BUSHWA

•••H•W
ANDHOW
ANYHOW
BUTHOW
CASHEW
CUSHAW
ESCHEW
HAWHAW
HEEHAW
MATHEW
NEPHEW
NOSHOW
ONSHOW
RECHEW
RESHOW
RETHAW
TVSHOW
UNTHAW
UPSHAW
YEEHAW

H•X•••
HEXADS
HEXANE
HEXERS
HEXING
HEXNUT
HEXOSE
HUXLEY

H••X••
HOAXED
HOAXER
HOAXES

H••••X
HADDIX
HALLUX
HANDAX
HATBOX
HOTBOX
HYDROX

•H••X•
THEAXE

•H•••X
CHISOX
THEFOX
THESOX
THORAX

••H•X•
JOHNXI
JOHNXV
JOHNXX

••H••X
JOHNIX
JOHNXX
SPHINX
SPHYNX

HY••••
HYADES

HYATTS
HYBRID
HYDRAE
HYDRAS
HYDRIC
HYDROS
HYDROX
HYDRUS
HYENAS
HYETAL
HYGRIC
HYKSOS
HYMNAL
HYMNED
HYOIDS
HYPERS
HYPEUP
HYPHEN
HYPING
HYPNOS
HYPOED
HYSONS
HYSSOP

H•Y•••

HAYDEN
HAYERS
HAYING
HAYLEY
HAYMES
HAYMOW
HAYNES
HAYNIE
HEYDAY
HEYMAN
HEYYOU
HIYALL
HOYDEN
HOYLES
HRYVNA

H••Y••

HEGYES
HEYYOU

H•••Y•

HARRYO
HARRYS
HEARYE
HENRYI
HENRYK
HENRYV
HOMEYS
HONEYS

H••••Y

HACKLY
HAILEY
HALEVY
HALLEY
HALSEY
HANGBY
HANLEY
HARDBY
HARDLY
HARLEY
HARNEY
HARVEY
HAYLEY
HAZILY
HEALEY
HEANEY
HEARTY
HEATHY
HEDLEY
HENDRY
HENLEY
HEREBY
HERESY
HERSEY
HERVEY
HEYDAY
HICKEY
HIGHLY
HILARY
HOCKEY
HOKILY
HOLILY
HOLLEY
HOMELY
HOMILY
HOMINY
HOOKEY
HOORAY
HORNBY
HORSEY
HOSTLY
HOTDAY
HOTKEY
HOUNDY
HOURLY
HUBLEY
HUGELY
HUMBLY
HUMPTY
HUNGBY
HUNGRY
HUNLEY
HURLEY
HURRAY
HUSSEY
HUXLEY

•HY•••

CHYNNA
CHYRON
KHYBER
OHYEAH
PHYLLO
PHYLUM
PHYSED
PHYSIC
PHYSIO
RHYMED
RHYMER
RHYMES
RHYTHM
SHYEST
SHYING
THYMES
THYMIC
THYMUS
WHYFOR
WHYNOT
WHYNOW
WHYYES
WHYYOU

•H•Y••

SHAYNE
THAYER
THEYLL
THEYRE
THEYVE
WHEYEY
WHYYES
WHYYOU

•H••Y•

CHERYL
CHEVYS
SHARYN
SHERYL
THEEYE

•H•••Y

CHAFFY
CHALKY
CHAMMY
CHANCY
CHANEY
CHANTY
CHARLY
CHATTY
CHEEKY
CHEERY
CHEESY
CHENEY
CHERRY
CHERTY
CHESTY
CHICLY
CHILLY
CHINKY
CHIRPY
CHITTY
CHOOSY
CHOPPY
CHROMY
CHUBBY
CHUCKY
CHUFFY
CHUMMY
CHUNKY
GHOSTY
OHBABY
OHENRY
PHILBY
PHILLY
PHONEY
PHOOEY
RHEUMY
SHABBY
SHAGGY
SHALEY
SHALLY
SHAMMY
SHANDY
SHANTY
SHARPY
SHECKY
SHEEDY
SHEEHY
SHEENY
SHELBY
SHELTY
SHERRY
SHIFTY
SHILLY
SHIMMY
SHINDY
SHINNY
SHOALY
SHODDY
SHORTY
SHOTBY
THEBAY
THEFLY
THEORY
THESPY
THETOY
THEWAY
THINGY
THINLY
THIRTY
THORNY
THUSLY
WHALEY
WHAMMY
WHEEZY
WHERRY
WHEYEY
WHIMSY
WHINNY
WHIPPY
WHIRLY
WHISKY
WHITBY
WHITEY
WHITTY
WHIZZY
WHOLLY

••HY••

ETHYLS
MRHYDE
SPHYNX

••H••Y

ASHLEY
ICHTHY
JOHNNY
OCHERY
RAHWAY
UNHAZY
UNHOLY

•••HY•

CATHYS
METHYL
TETHYS
ZEPHYR

•••H•Y

ARCHLY
CATHAY
EIGHTY
HIGHLY
LACHEY
LACHOY
LUSHLY
MEOHMY
MIGHTY
MYOHMY
NIGHTY
POSHLY
RASHLY
RICHLY
RIGHTY
RUSHBY
SASHAY
SAYHEY

••••HY

APATHY
BEACHY
BINCHY
BOLSHY
BOTCHY
BRASHY
BROPHY
BROTHY
BRUSHY
BUNCHY
BUTWHY
CATCHY
CAUCHY
CLICHY
CUDAHY
DINGHY
DOUGHY
EARTHY
FILTHY
FLASHY
FLESHY
FORWHY
FROTHY
GRAPHY
GUNSHY
HEATHY
ICHTHY
LEACHY
LUNCHY
MARSHY
MOUTHY
MUNCHY
MURPHY
NOTCHY
PATCHY
PEACHY
PITCHY
PLASHY
PLUSHY
POACHY
POUCHY
PUNCHY
SHEEHY
SLITHY
SLOSHY
SLUSHY
SMITHY
SWISHY
TETCHY
TOOTHY
TORCHY
TOUCHY
TOUGHY
TRASHY
TROPHY
WITCHY
WORTHY

H•Z•••

HAZANS
HAZARD
HAZELS
HAZERS
HAZIER
HAZILY
HAZING
HAZMAT
HUZZAH

H••Z••

HERZOG
HUZZAH

H••••Z

HORMUZ

•H•Z••

CHAZAN
GHAZIS
SHAZAM
WHIZZY

•H••Z•

WHEEZE
WHEEZY
WHIZZY

•H•••Z

CHAVEZ
CHINTZ
SHIRAZ
SHORTZ
SHULTZ
THEWIZ

••HZ••

MAHZOR

••H•Z•

UNHAZY

••H••Z

SCHNOZ
SCHULZ

IA••••

IAGREE
IAMBIC
IAMBUS
IAMNOT
IAMSAM
IAMTOO
IATRIC

I•A•••

IBADAN
IBANEZ
IBARRA
ICALLY
ICANSO
ICARIA
ICARUS
IDAHOS
IDARED
IMACOP
IMAGED
IMAGER
IMAGES
IMAGOS
IMAMAN
IMARET
IMAXES
INABIT
INABOX
INADAY
INAFEW
INAFIX
INAFOG
INAGES
INAJAM
INANER
INAPET
INAPIE
INAPOD
INARAY
INARCH
INAREA
INAROW
INARUG
INARUT
INASEC
INATIE
INATUB
INAWAY
IRAISE
IRANIS
IRAQIS
IRATER
ISAACS
ISABEL
ISAIAH
ISAIAN
ISANTI
ISAYNO
ITALIA
ITALIC
ITASCA
IVANIV
IVANKA
IVANOV
IVANVI
IWANNA

I••A••

IBEAMS
ICEAGE
ICEAXE
IDCARD
IDEALS
IDEATE
IDTAGS
IGNACE
IGNATZ
IGUANA
ILEANA
ILIADS
IMBACK
IMEANT
IMEASY
IMGAME
IMLATE
IMPACT
IMPAIR
IMPALA
IMPALE
IMPART
INBACK
INCAIC
INCANS
INCANT
INCAPS
INCASE
INCASH
INDASH
INFACT
INFALL
INFAMY
INFANT
INGATE
INHALE
INHALF
INHAND
INJAIL
INLAID
INLAND
INLAWS
INLAYS
INMATE
INNAGE
INNATE
INPARK
INPART
INPAWN
INRAGS
INSANA
INSANE
INTACT
INTAKE
INVADE
INVAIN
INWANT
INWARD
IODATE
IOLANI
IOWANS
ISAACS
ISLAND
ISLATE
ISMAIL
ISRAEL
ISRAIR
ITHACA
ITSAGO

I•••A•

IAMSAM
IBADAN
IBIZAN
ICEBAG
ICECAP
ICEDAM
ICEMAN
IFICAN
IFIMAY
ILLSAY
IMAMAN
IMBEAT
IMGLAD
IMOKAY
INADAY
INAJAM
INARAY
INAWAY
INDIAN
INFEAR
INGEAR
INGMAR
INGOAL
INGRAM
INGRAY
INKPAD
INKSAC
INLEAF
INPLAY
INROAD
INSEAM
INSPAN
INSTAL
INTHAT
INTRAY
IONIAN
IPECAC
IRREAL
ISAIAH
ISAIAN
ISHTAR
ISOBAR
ISWEAR
ITSPAT
ITZHAK

I••••A

IBARRA
IBERIA
ICARIA
ICETEA
IGOTTA
IGUANA
ILEANA
IMELDA
IMPALA
INAREA
INDIRA
INSANA
IOMEGA
ISCHIA
ISOLDA
ISTRIA
ITALIA
ITASCA
ITHACA
IVANKA
IWANNA

•IA•••

BIAFRA
BIALIK
BIANCA
BIANCO
BIASED
BIASES
CIARDI
CIASPY
DIABLE
DIABLO
DIABOL
DIADEM
DIALED
DIALER
DIALIN
DIALOG
DIALSO
DIALUP
DIANNE
DIAPER
DIARIO
DIATOM
FIACRE
FIANCE
FIASCO
GIAMBI
GIANNI
GIANTS
HIATAL
HIATUS
KIARIO
LIABLE
LIAISE
LIANAS
LIANES
LIANGS
MIAMIS
MIAMIU
MIAOUS
MIAOWS
MIASMA
MIATAS
NIACIN
NIAMEY
PIAFFE
PIAGET
PIANOS
PIAZZA
PIAZZI
RIALTO
RIATAS
TIARAS
VIABLE
VIABLY
VIACOM
VIAGRA
VIALED
VIANDS
VIATOR

•I•A••

AIRACE
AIRARM
BICARB
BIGAIR
BIGAMY
BIGAPE
BINACA
BINARY
BINATE
CICADA
CIGARS
DIDACT
DIGAMY
DILATE
DIMAGE
DINARS
DIRAMS
DISANT
DISARM
DITALI
DIVANS
DIZAIN
FIGARO
FINALE
FINALS
FIXATE
GIJANE
GITANO
HIHATS
HIJACK
HILARY
HIVAOA
HIYALL
JICAMA
JIHADS
KIGALI
KITAEN
LIGAND
LIGATE
LILACS
LIMANS
LINAGE
LIPARI
LIPASE
LITANY
LIZALU
LIZARD
MIDAIR
MIKADO
MIKASA
MILADY
MILANO
MILANS
MIRADA
MIRAGE
MISACT
MISADD
MISAIM
NICADS
NISANS
PICABO
PICARA
PICARD
PICARO
PILAFS
PILATE
PILAUS
PINATA
PIPAGE
PIRACY
PIRANA
PIRATE
PISANO
PISANS
PITAYA
PIZAZZ
RIBALD
RIBAND
RICANS
RIGANS
RIGATI
RIMATE
RITARD
RIVALS
RIYADH
RIYALS
SILAGE
SISALS
SITARS
SIVANS
TICALS
TILAKS
TIRADE
TIRANA
TIRANE
TISANE
TITANS
VICARS
VIHARA
VIRAGO
VISAED
VISAGE
VITALE
VITALS
VITARA
VIVACE
VIVANT
WIGAND
WINANS
WIZARD

•I••A•

AIDMAN
AIKMAN
AIMSAT
AIRBAG
AIRDAM
AIRMAN
AIRSAC
AIRWAR
AIRWAY
BIGBAD
BIGCAR
BIGCAT
BIGDAY
BIGEAR
BIGFAN
BIGMAC
BIGMAN
BILBAO
BILDAD
BIOGAS
BIOLAB
BIOTAS
BIRMAN
BISCAY
BISSAU
BITMAP
CIERAS
CIUDAD
DIDBAD
DIGRAM
DIGSAT
DIKTAT
DILLAR
DINEAT
DINKAS
DIRHAM
DISBAR
DISMAL
DISMAS
DISMAY
DISTAL
FIGBAR
FIJIAN
FILIAL
FINCAS
FINIAL
FINIAN
FINNAN
FIREAT
FISCAL
FIVEAA
FIVEAD
FIVEAM
GIBEAT
GIBRAN
GIDDAP
GIGBAG
GILEAD
GILLAN
GILMAN
GIMBAL
HIATAL
HICKAM
HIEMAL
HINTAT
HISSAT
HITMAN
HITSAT
JIBEAT
JIGSAW
KIDMAN
KIDNAP
KIERAN
KINNAN
KIOWAN
KIOWAS
KIRMAN
KITBAG
KITKAT
LIANAS
LIBRAE
LIBRAN
LIBRAS
LIBYAN
LILIAN
LINEAL
LINEAR
LITVAK
LIVEAT
MIATAS
MICMAC
MIDCAP
MIDDAY
MIDIAN
MIDMAY
MIDWAY
MILLAY
MILSAP
MINOAN
MINYAN
MIRIAM
MISHAP
MISLAY
MISSAL
MISSAY
MITRAL
MITTAG
NICIAS
NIETAS
NIIHAU
NIKEAD
NINEAD
NINEAM
NINJAS
NIPSAT
NISSAN
OILCAN
OILMAN
OILPAN
OISEAU
PICKAT
PICKAX
PIEMAN
PIEPAN
PIETAS
PIGMAN
PILLAR
PINCAY
PINDAR
PINEAL
PINNAE
PINNAS
PINOAK
PISGAH
PITMAN
PITSAW
PIZZAS
QINTAR
RIATAS
RIBPAD
RICRAC
RICTAL
RIOJAS
RIOPAN
RIPRAP
RIPSAW
RITUAL
SIGHAT
SIGMAS
SIGNAL
SILVAS
SIMIAN
SINBAD
SINEAD
SINTAX
SIOUAN
SIRKAY
SIRRAH
SITPAT
SITSAT
SIXDAY
SIXWAY
TIARAS
TIBIAE
TIBIAL
TIBIAS
TICTAC
TIEBAR
TIETAC
TIKKAS
TILTAT
TIMBAL
TINCAN
TINEAL
TINEAR
TINHAT
TINIAN
TINMAN
TINPAN
TIPJAR
TIRIAC
TITIAN
UINTAS
VIBRAM
VIGIAS
VILLAS
VIOLAS
VIRGAS
VISTAS
VISUAL
VIVIAN
WICCAN
WIEMAN
WIGWAG
WIGWAM
WINKAT
WINSAT
WITHAL
ZIGZAG

•I•••A

AIRSEA
BIAFRA
BIANCA
BIKILA
BINACA
CIBOLA
CICADA
CINEMA
EIDOLA
EIGHTA
FIBULA
FIESTA
FIVEAA
HIVAOA
JICAMA
KISHKA
LIGEIA
LIKUTA
LINGUA
LIOTTA
LISBOA
MIASMA
MIKASA
MIKITA
MIMOSA
MINETA
MINIMA
MIRADA
MISCHA
MIZUNA
NICOLA
NIKITA
NIKOLA
PIAZZA
PICARA
PIERIA
PINATA
PIRANA
PITAYA
RIBERA
RICOLA
RIJEKA
RIVERA
SIENNA
SIERRA
SIESTA
SILICA

SIRICA
TIENDA
TIERRA
TIRANA
VIAGRA
VICUNA
VIEIRA
VIENNA
VIGODA
VIHARA
VITARA
VIVECA
VIVICA
VIZSLA
WINONA
XINHUA
ZINNIA

••IA••
APIARY
ARIANA
ARIANE
ARIARY
ASIAGO
ASIANS
AVIANS
AVIARY
AVIATE
BRIANA
BRIAND
BRIARD
BRIARS
BRIARY
CHIANG
ENIACS
FRIARS
FRIARY
GUIANA
ILIADS
NAIADS
OPIATE
ORIANA
ORIANI
PHIALS
PLIANT
TRIADS
TRIAGE
TRIALS
UMIAKS
UNIATE
UNIATS

••I•A•
ADIDAS
AGITAS
AKITAS
ALIYAH
AMICAL
AMIDAS
AMIGAS
ANIMAL
ANIMAS
APICAL
BAIKAL
BAISAS
BAIZAS
BRIDAL
CAIMAN
CEIBAS
CHICAS
CHINAS
CHIRAC
CHIVAS
CLIMAT
CLIMAX
CUICAS
DJILAS
ELIJAH
EPICAL
EPINAL
ERICAS
ERIVAN
FAIMAN
FAISAL
FBIMAN
FRIDAY
FRITAS
GRINAT
GUINAN
GUITAR
HAIDAS
HAIKAI
IBIZAN
IFICAN
IFIMAY
KLIBAN
LAICAL
LEICAS
MAITAI
NAIRAS
NEIMAN
NIIHAU
OBIWAN
OCICAT
OGIVAL
OHIOAN
OUIJAS
OVISAC
PAIDAD
PAISAN
PRIMAL
RAILAT
RAITAS
RBIMAN
REINAS
RHINAL
SAIDAH
SAIPAN
SHIRAZ
SKICAP
SKIHAT
SKIWAX
SPINAL
SPIRAL
SPIVAK
TAIGAS
TAIPAN
TAIWAN
TOILAT
TRIBAL
TRINAL
UNITAS
UNIVAC
UTICAN
VEINAL
WEIMAR

••I••A
AHIMSA
ALICIA
AMINTA
ANITRA
ARIANA
ARISTA
AXILLA
BRIANA
CHICHA
CHINUA
CHITRA
CRIMEA
ELISHA
ELISSA
EMILIA
ENIGMA
ERIEPA
ERINNA
FLICKA
FRICKA
FRIEDA
FRITTA
GEISHA
GLINDA
GLINKA
GRISHA
GUIANA
GUINEA
KAILUA
NOIDEA
OJIBWA
OLINDA
OLIVIA
ORIANA
ORISSA
POINTA
POISHA
QUINTA
SMILLA
SPIREA
STIGMA
TRICIA
TRISHA
TRIVIA

•••IA•
ADRIAN
AERIAL
APPIAN
ATRIAL
AUDIAL
BAHIAN
BASIAL
BELIAL
BURIAL
CAVIAR
CURIAE
DELIAN
DENIAL
DORIAN
ENTIAL
EOLIAN
EONIAN
ESPIAL
FABIAN
FACIAE
FACIAL
FACIAS
FERIAS
FIJIAN
FILIAL
FINIAL
FINIAN
FOLIAR
GAVIAL
GENIAL
HODIAK
INDIAN
IONIAN
ISAIAH
ISAIAN
JOSIAH
JOVIAL
JOVIAN
JULIAN
KODIAK
LABIAL
LAMIAE
LAMIAS
LARIAT
LILIAN
LUCIAN
LYDIAN
MAFIAS
MAGIAN
MALIAN
MANIAC
MANIAS
MARIAH
MARIAN
MARIAS
MEDIAL
MEDIAN
MEDIAS
MENIAL
MESIAL
MIDIAN
MIRIAM
MUSIAL
MYRIAD
NARIAL
NICIAS
NOKIAS
NOMIAL
NORIAS
NOVIAS
NUBIAN
OBRIAN
OSSIAN
PARIAH
PLEIAD
RACIAL
RADIAL
RADIAN
REDIAL
RETIAL
RUPIAH
SAMIAM
SEPIAS
SERIAL
SIMIAN
SOCIAL
STRIAE
SYRIAN
TIBIAE
TIBIAL
TIBIAS
TINIAN
TIRIAC
TITIAN
TOBIAS
UNCIAL
VARIAS
VENIAL
VIGIAS
VIVIAN
YESIAM
ZODIAC
ZONIAN
ZUNIAN

•••I•A
ACTIVA
AFRICA
ALAINA
ALCINA
ALTIMA
ALZIRA
AMRITA
ANNIKA
ANNINA
AQUILA
ARNICA
ARRIBA
ATTICA
ATTILA
AURIGA
BIKILA
BONITA
CAPITA
CARINA
CASITA
CELICA
COLIMA
COMIDA
COVINA
DAMITA
DERITA
DESICA
EDWINA
ELMIRA
ELOISA
ELVIRA
ENCINA
EROICA
FAJITA
FARINA
FATIMA
GODIVA
HEGIRA
INDIRA
JEMIMA
KARINA
KONICA
LADIDA
LAMINA
LANINA
LATINA
LAVIDA
LENINA
LERIDA
LOLITA
LOUISA
LUCIDA
LUMINA
MANILA
MARIDA
MARINA
MARISA
MAXIMA
MEDICA
MEDINA
MELINA
MERIDA
MIKITA
MINIMA
MOLINA
MONICA
MORITA
NARITA
NIKITA
NUBIRA
NUMINA
OJAICA
ONEIDA
OPTIMA
OREIDA
PAMINA
PATINA
PEPITA
PETIPA
PURINA
REGINA
RETINA
ROSINA
ROSITA
SABINA
SALINA
SALIVA
SEPIRA
SHEILA
SILICA
SIRICA
TALISA
TROIKA
ULTIMA
VEZINA
VIEIRA
VIVICA
YAKIMA
ZORINA
ZUNIGA

••••IA
ACACIA
ACADIA
ACEDIA
AEOLIA
AGLAIA
ALEXIA
ALICIA
ALOGIA
ALTRIA
AMALIA
AMELIA
AMESIA
ANEMIA
ANGLIA
ANOMIA
ANOXIA
ANTLIA
APULIA
ARABIA
ASONIA
ATAXIA
ATONIA
AZANIA
AZARIA
BASTIA
BORGIA
BOSNIA
CANDIA
CARDIA
CASSIA
COELIA
CORDIA
CRANIA
CUMBIA
DAHLIA
EGERIA
ELYRIA
EMILIA
ETALIA
FASCIA
FLAVIA
GALLIA
GAMBIA
GARCIA
GLORIA
GRATIA
HERNIA
HESTIA
IBERIA
ICARIA
ISCHIA
ISTRIA
ITALIA
KESHIA
LANCIA
LATRIA
LATVIA
LAURIA
LEONIA
LIGEIA
LOGGIA
MARCIA
MURCIA
MYOPIA
NARNIA
NUTRIA
OLIVIA
OREXIA
PAGLIA
PATRIA
PENNIA
PEORIA
PERSIA
PHAGIA
PHOBIA
PIERIA
PLUVIA
PORTIA
PREVIA
RAFFIA
REALIA
ROBBIA
RUBBIA
RUSSIA
SANDIA
SARNIA
SCALIA
SCORIA
SCOTIA
SEPHIA
SERBIA
SHANIA
SOPHIA
STADIA
SYLVIA
THALIA
THECIA
TREDIA
TRICIA
TRIVIA
UMBRIA
URANIA
UTOPIA
YTTRIA
ZAMBIA
ZINNIA
ZOYSIA

IB••••
IBADAN
IBANEZ
IBARRA
IBEAMS
IBERIA
IBEXES
IBICES
IBIDEM
IBISES
IBIZAN
IBMPCS
IBOOKS

I•B•••
IMBACK
IMBEAT
IMBEDS
IMBIBE
IMBRUE
IMBUED
IMBUES
IMBUSY
INBACK
INBLUE
INBORN
INBRED
INBULK

I••B••
IAMBIC
IAMBUS
ICEBAG
ICEBOX
ILLBET
INABIT
INABOX
IROBOT
ISABEL
ISOBAR

I•••B•
IMBIBE
INCUBI
INDEBT
ITURBI
IVTUBE

I••••B
INATUB

•IB•••
BIBBED
BIBBER
BIBLES
BIBLIO
CIBBER
CIBOLA
DIBBLE
FIBBED
FIBBER
FIBERS
FIBRES
FIBRIN
FIBULA
GIBBER
GIBBON
GIBEAT
GIBERS
GIBILL
GIBING
GIBLET
GIBRAN
GIBSON
JIBEAT
JIBING
KIBBEE
KIBBLE
KIBITZ
KIBOSH
LIBBED
LIBBER
LIBBYS
LIBELS
LIBERS
LIBIDO
LIBRAE
LIBRAN
LIBRAS
LIBRIS
LIBROS
LIBYAN
NIBBLE
NIBLET
RIBALD
RIBAND
RIBBED
RIBBER
RIBBIT
RIBBON
RIBCUT
RIBERA
RIBEYE
RIBISI
RIBLET
RIBOSE
RIBPAD
SIBYLS
TIBIAE
TIBIAL
TIBIAS
VIBIST
VIBRAM

•I•B••
AIRBAG
AIRBUD
AIRBUS
BIBBED
BIBBER
BIEBER
BIGBAD
BIGBEN
BIGBET
BIGBOI
BIGBOX
BIGBOY
BIGBUX
BILBAO
BIMBOS
BISBEE
CIBBER
DIABLE
DIABLO
DIABOL
DIBBLE
DIDBAD
DISBAR
DISBUD
FIBBED
FIBBER
FIGBAR
GIBBER
GIBBON
GIGBAG
GIMBAL
GIMBEL
JIMBOB
KIBBEE
KIBBLE
KIMBLE
KITBAG
LIABLE
LIBBED
LIBBER
LIBBYS
LIEBER
LIEBIG
LIEBYS
LIMBED
LIMBER
LIMBIC
LIMBOS
LISBOA
LISBON
NIBBLE
NIMBLE
NIMBLY
NIMBUS
NIOBIC
PINBOY
RIBBED
RIBBER
RIBBIT
RIBBON
SIEBEN
SINBAD
SIRBEN
TIDBIT
TIEBAR
TIMBAL
TIMBER
TIMBRE
VIABLE
VIABLY
WILBUR
WINBIG

•I••B•
FILEBY
FIVEBC
GIAMBI
NINEBC
NINGBO
PICABO
RIDEBY
SITSBY
TICKBY
WILLBE
WINSBY
ZIPSBY

•I•••B
BICARB
BIOLAB
EIGHTB
JIMBOB
MIDRIB
OILRUB

••IB••
ALIBIS
ALIBLE
BRIBED
BRIBEE
BRIBER
BRIBES
CEIBAS
EDIBLE
EDIBLY
FOIBLE
GLIBLY
KLIBAN
OJIBWA
ORIBIS
SKIBIB
SKIBOB
SKIBUM
TRIBAL
TRIBES
XZIBIT

••I•B•
AKIMBO
CLIMBS
FLITBY
LAIDBY
PHILBY
SKIPBY
SLIPBY
THISBE
TRILBY
WHITBY

••I••B
ALICEB
POINTB
SKIBIB
SKIBOB

•••IB•
ADLIBS
ARRIBA
CARIBE
CARIBS
IMBIBE
MALIBU
MCRIBS
MRPIBB
SAHIBS
SCRIBE
SQUIBB
SQUIBS

•••I•B
CECILB
LOUISB
MRPIBB
SQUIBB

••••IB
MIDRIB
OUTRIB
RAGHIB
SCHEIB
SKIBIB
UNGLIB

IC••••
ICALLY
ICANSO
ICARIA
ICARUS
ICEAGE
ICEAXE
ICEBAG
ICEBOX
ICECAP
ICEDAM
ICEDIN
ICEDIT
ICEDUP
ICEFOG
ICEMAN
ICEMEN
ICEOUT
ICEPOP
ICERUN
ICESIN
ICESIT
ICESUP
ICETEA
ICEUPS
ICHING
ICHIRO
ICHORS
ICHTHY
ICICLE
ICIEST
ICINGS
ICKIER
ICONIC
ICOULD

I•C•••
IDCARD
IMCOLD
IMCOOL
INCAIC
INCANS
INCANT
INCAPS
INCASE
INCASH
INCENT
INCEPT
INCHED
INCHER
INCHES
INCHON
INCISE
INCITE
INCODE
INCOME
INCUBI
INCULT
INCURS
INCUSE
ISCHIA
ITCHED
ITCHES

I••C••
IBICES
ICECAP
ICICLE
IFICAN
IMACOP
IPECAC

I•••C•
IBMPCS
IDIOCY
IGNACE
IMBACK
IMPACT
INARCH
INBACK
INDICT
INDUCE
INDUCT
INFACT
INFECT
INHOCK
INJECT
INLUCK
INSECT
INTACT
IONICS
ISAACS
ITASCA
ITHACA

I••••C
IAMBIC
IATRIC
ICONIC
INASEC
INCAIC
INKSAC
INSYNC
IPECAC
IRENIC
IRIDIC
IRITIC
IRONIC
ITALIC

•IC•••
BICARB
BICEPS
BICHON
BICKER
BICORN
CICADA
CICELY
CICERO
DICERS
DICIER
DICING
DICKER
DICKEY
DICKIE
DICOTS
DICTUM
FICHES
FICHTE
FICHUS
FICKLE
HICCUP
HICKAM
HICKEY
HICKOK
JICAMA
KICKED
KICKER
KICKIN
KICKUP
LICHEE
LICHEN
LICKED
LICKER
LICKUP
MICHEL
MICKEY
MICMAC
MICRON
MICROS
NICADS
NICELY
NICENE
NICEST
NICETY
NICHED
NICHES
NICIAS
NICKED
NICKEL
NICKER
NICKJR
NICOLA
NICOLE
NICOLO
PICABO
PICARA
PICARD
PICARO
PICCHU
PICHEL
PICKAT
PICKAX
PICKED
PICKER
PICKET
PICKLE
PICKON
PICKUP
PICNIC
PICONE
PICOTS
PICRIC
PICTOR
RICANS
RICERS
RICHEN
RICHER
RICHES
RICHET
RICHIE
RICHIN
RICHLY
RICING
RICKEY
RICKIE
RICOHS
RICOLA
RICRAC
RICTAL
SICCED
SICILY
SICKEN
SICKER
SICKLE
SICKLY
SICKOF
SICKOS
TICALS
TICCED
TICINO
TICKBY
TICKED
TICKER
TICKET
TICKLE
TICKLY
TICTAC
VICARS
VICTIM
VICTOR
VICUNA
WICCAN
WICKED
WICKER
WICKET

•I•C••
BIGCAR
BIGCAT
BINCHY
BISCAY
CIRCLE
CIRCUM
CIRCUS
CISCOS
DIECUT
DISCOS
DISCUS
FIACRE
FINCAS
FISCAL
HICCUP
KIDCOM

KIMCHI
LITCHI
MIDCAP
MINCED
MINCER
MINCES
MISCHA
MISCUE
MISCUT
NIACIN
NIECES
OILCAN
OILCUP
PICCHU
PIECED
PIECER
PIECES
PINCAY
PINCER
PISCES
PITCHY
RIBCUT
SICCED
SIECLE
SITCOM
TICCED
TINCAN
TINCTS
TINCUP
VIACOM
VINCIT
VISCID
WICCAN
WILCOX
WINCED
WINCER
WINCES
WITCHY
ZINCED
ZINCIC
ZINCKY
ZIRCON
ZITCOM

•I••C•

AIRACE
BIANCA
BIANCO
BIERCE
BINACA
BISECT
CIVICS
DIDACT
DIRECT
FIANCE
FIASCO
FIERCE
HIJACK
HIRSCH
HITECH
KIRSCH
KITSCH
LILACS
MIMICS
MISACT
PIERCE
PIRACY
SILICA
SIRICA
TIERCE
VIVACE
VIVECA
VIVICA

•I•••C

AIRSAC
BIGMAC
BIONIC
BIOPIC
BIOTIC
CITRIC
EIGHTC
FILMIC
FINNIC
FISTIC
FIVEBC
LIMBIC
LITHIC
MICMAC
MIXTEC
NINEBC
NIOBIC
NITRIC
PICNIC
PICRIC
RICRAC
TICTAC
TIETAC
TIRIAC
VITRIC
ZINCIC
ZIPLOC

••IC••

ALICEB
ALICES
ALICIA
AMICAL
AMICES
AMICUS
APICAL
APICES
BRICKS
BRICKY
BUICKS
CAICOS
CHICAS
CHICER
CHICHA
CHICHI
CHICKS
CHICLE
CHICLY
CHICOS
CLICHE
CLICHY
CLICKS
CRICKS
CUICAS
DEICED
DEICER
DEICES
EDICTS
ELICIT
EPICAL
ERICAS
EVICTS
FLICKA
FLICKS
FRICKA
FRICKE
IBICES
ICICLE
IFICAN
JUICED
JUICER
JUICES
KLICKS
KNICKS
LAICAL
LEICAS
OCICAT
PRICED
PRICER
PRICES
PRICEY
PRICKS
QUICHE
REICED
REICES
SKICAP
SLICED
SLICER
SLICES
SLICKS
SNICKS
SPICED
SPICER
SPICES
STICKS
STICKY
TAICHI
THICKE
TRICEP
TRICES
TRICIA
TRICKS
TRICKY
TRICOT
UNICED
UNICEF
UNICES
UTICAN
VOICED
VOICER
VOICES
YOICKS

••I•C•

APIECE
CHINCH
CLINCH
CRISCO
ENIACS
EVINCE
FLINCH
FRISCH
FRISCO
GLITCH
GRIECO
GRINCH
IDIOCY
PEIRCE
PHILCO
PRINCE
QUINCE
QUINCY
SKITCH
SMIRCH
SNITCH
STITCH
SWITCH
TWITCH
VAILCO

••I••C

ACIDIC
AJIJIC
CHIRAC
CLINIC
CRITIC
DEIFIC
EXILIC
IRIDIC
IRITIC
ODINIC
OTITIC
OVISAC
OXIDIC
PHILIC
STIVIC
UNIFIC
UNIVAC

•••IC•

ADDICT
ADVICE
AFRICA
ALNICO
ANTICS
ARNICA
ASDICS
ASPICS
ATTICA
ATTICS
BASICS
BENICE
BODICE
CALICO
CELICA
CHOICE
CIVICS
COLICS
COMICE
COMICS
CONICS
CUBICS
CYNICS
DELICT
DEPICT
DESICA
DEVICE
DEVICQ
DODICI
DRRICE
DRYICE
ELLICE
ENRICH
ENRICO
ENTICE
EROICA
ETHICS
EUNICE
FELICE
HELICO
INDICT
IONICS
JANICE
KONICA
LOGICS
LOLICH
LUKICH
LYRICS
MAGICS
MALICE
MALICK
MEDICA
MEDICI
MEDICO
MEDICS
MEJICO
MEXICO
MIMICS
MONICA
MRDICK
MUNICH
MUSICK
MUSICS
NATICK
NODICE
NOTICE
NOVICE
OFFICE
OJAICA
ONRICE
OPTICS
OSMICS
PANICS
PENICK
PLAICE
POLICE
POLICY
POVICH
PUMICE
REKICK
RELICS
RELICT
REMICK
REPICK
SCHICK
SEAICE
SEDICI
SHTICK
SILICA
SIRICA
SLUICE
SONICS
SPLICE
STNICK
STOICS
STRICT
THRICE
TONICS
TOPICS
TOXICS
TUNICS
ULRICH
UNDICI
UNNICE
UNPICK
UNSICK
UPTICK
VENICE
VIVICA
YORICK
ZURICH

•••I•C

MANIAC
TIRIAC
ZODIAC

••••IC

ACETIC
ACIDIC
ADONIC
AGARIC
AHOLIC
AJIJIC
ALARIC
ALTAIC
AMEBIC
ANDRIC
ANEMIC
ANGLIC
ANODIC
ANOMIC
ANOXIC
AORTIC
ARABIC
ARCTIC
ATAVIC
ATAXIC
ATOMIC
ATONIC
ATOXIC
ATYPIC
AXENIC
AZONIC
BALTIC
BARDIC
BELGIC
BIONIC
BIOPIC
BIOTIC
CADMIC
CEDRIC
CELTIC
CHEMIC
CHORIC
CITRIC
CLERIC
CLINIC
COPTIC
COSMIC
COURIC
CRITIC
CULTIC
CUPRIC
CYANIC
CYCLIC
CYMRIC
CYSTIC
DEIFIC
DELTIC
DERMIC
DYADIC
ECESIC
ECHOIC
EDDAIC
EDENIC
EMERIC
EMETIC
EPODIC
EROTIC
ETHNIC
ETONIC
EXILIC
EXOTIC
FABRIC
FANFIC
FERRIC
FILMIC
FINNIC
FISTIC
FORMIC
FROLIC
GAELIC
GALLIC
GARLIC
GEODIC
GESTIC
GNOMIC
GOTHIC
HECTIC
HEROIC
HYDRIC
HYGRIC
IAMBIC
IATRIC
ICONIC
INCAIC
IRENIC
IRIDIC
IRITIC
IRONIC
ITALIC
JUDAIC
KAONIC
KARMIC
LACTIC
LAURIC
LIMBIC
LITHIC
MALEIC
MANTIC
MASTIC
METRIC
MOSAIC
MYOPIC
MYSTIC
MYTHIC
NIOBIC
NITRIC
NOETIC
NORDIC
ODINIC
OLDVIC
ORPHIC
OTITIC
OXALIC
OXIDIC
OZONIC
PATHIC
PATRIC
PELVIC
PEPTIC
PHASIC
PHILIC
PHOBIC
PHONIC
PHOTIC
PHYSIC
PICNIC
PICRIC
POETIC
PUBLIC
ROMAIC
RUBRIC
RUSTIC
SCENIC
SEPTIC
SLAVIC
SORBIC
STATIC
STERIC
STIVIC
SYNDIC
TACTIC
TANNIC
TAURIC
TERBIC
THORIC
THYMIC
TRAGIC
TROPIC
TURKIC
UNCHIC
UNEPIC
UNIFIC
URALIC
URANIC
VEDAIC
VITRIC
VLASIC
YTTRIC
ZINCIC

ID••••

IDAHOS
IDARED
IDCARD
IDEALS
IDEATE
IDENTI
IDENTS
IDIDIT
IDIOCY
IDIOMS
IDIOTS
IDLERS
IDLEST
IDLING
IDOIDO
IDOLUM
IDONOT
IDOTOO
IDTAGS
IDUNNO
IDYLLS

I•D•••

IMDONE
INDASH
INDEBT
INDEED
INDEEP
INDENT
INDIAN
INDICT
INDIES
INDIGO
INDIRA
INDITE
INDIUM
INDOOR
INDUCE
INDUCT
INDUED
INDUES
IODATE
IODIDE
IODINE
IODISE
IODIZE

I••D••

IBADAN
IBIDEM
ICEDAM
ICEDIN
ICEDIT
ICEDUP
IDIDIT
ILLDRY
IMIDES
INADAY
IRIDES
IRIDIC
ISIDOR
ISIDRO

I•••D•

IDOIDO
ILIADS
ILLUDE
IMBEDS
IMELDA
IMPEDE
INCODE
INSIDE
INVADE
IODIDE
ISOLDA
ISOLDE
ITLLDO

I••••D

ICOULD
IDARED
IDCARD
IDOIDO
ILLFED
IMAGED
IMBUED
IMCOLD
IMGLAD
IMGOOD
IMPEND
IMPLED
IMSOLD
IMTOLD
INAPOD
INBRED
INCHED
INDEED
INDUED
INFOLD
INGOLD
INGOOD
INGRID
INHAND
INKIND
INKPAD
INLAID
INLAND
INMIND
INNEED
INROAD
INTEND
INURED
INWARD
IRISED
IRONED
ISLAND
ISOPOD
ISSUED
ITCHED
ITEMED
ITRIED
IWOULD

•ID•••

AIDERS
AIDFUL
AIDING
AIDMAN
AIDMEN
BIDDEN
BIDDER
BIDERS
BIDETS
BIDFOR
BIDING
BIDSIN
BIDSON
BIDSUP
CIDERS
CIDERY
DIDACT
DIDBAD
DIDDLE
DIDDLY
DIDFOR
DIDIES
DIDION
DIDNOT
DIDOES
EIDERS
EIDOLA
FIDDLE
FIDGET
FIDLER
GIDDAP
GIDEON
GIDGET
HIDDEN
HIDEHO
HIDEKI
HIDERS
HIDING
HIDOUT
KIDCOM
KIDDED
KIDDER
KIDDIE
KIDDOS
KIDEOS
KIDLIT
KIDMAN
KIDNAP
KIDNEY
KIDORY
KIDULT
KIDVID
LIDDED
MIDAIR
MIDCAP
MIDDAY
MIDDIE
MIDDLE
MIDGES
MIDGET
MIDIAN
MIDLEG
MIDLER
MIDMAY
MIDOFF
MIDONS
MIDORI
MIDRIB
MIDSTS
MIDWAY
NIDIFY
PIDDLE
PIDGIN
RIDDED
RIDDEN
RIDDER
RIDDLE
RIDEBY
RIDEIN
RIDENT
RIDERS
RIDETO
RIDEUP
RIDGED
RIDGES
RIDING
RIDLEY
RIDSOF
SIDDUR
SIDING
SIDLED
SIDLES
SIDNEY
TIDBIT
TIDIED
TIDIER
TIDIES
TIDILY
TIDING
TIDYUP
VIDEOS
VIDERI
VIDIOT
WIDDER
WIDELY
WIDENS
WIDEOF
WIDEST
WIDGET
WIDISH
WIDOWS
WIDTHS

•I•D••

AIRDAM
AIRDRY
BIDDEN
BIDDER
BIGDAY
BIGDIG
BIGDOG
BIGDOS
BILDAD
BINDER
BINDLE
BINDTO
BINDUP
BIRDED
BIRDER
BIRDIE
CINDER
CIUDAD
DIADEM
DIDDLE
DIDDLY
DIKDIK
DINDIN
DIODES
FIDDLE
FINDER
GIDDAP
GILDED
GILDER
GIRDED
GIRDER
GIRDLE
HIDDEN
HINDER
HINDUS
KIDDED
KIDDER
KIDDIE
KIDDOS
KINDER
KINDLE
KINDLY
KINDOF
LIDDED
LIEDER
LIEDON
LIEDTO
LINDEN
LINDER
MIDDAY
MIDDIE
MIDDLE
MILDER
MILDEW
MILDLY
MINDED
MINDEN
MINDER
MISDID
PIDDLE
PINDAR
PINDUS
RIDDED
RIDDEN
RIDDER
RIDDLE
RITDYE
SIDDUR
SIXDAY
TIEDIN
TIEDON
TIEDTO
TIEDUP
TIEDYE
TILDEN
TILDES
TINDER
VIRDON
WIDDER
WILDER
WILDLY
WINDED
WINDER
WINDEX
WINDOM
WINDOW
WINDUP
WISDOM

•I••D•

AIKIDO
BIONDI
BIPEDS
BIPODS
CIARDI
CICADA
DIPODY
DIRNDL
DIVIDE
FIELDS
FIENDS
FIORDS
JIHADS
LIBIDO
LIPIDS
MIKADO
MILADY
MIRADA
MISADD
NICADS
RIYADH
TIENDA
TIRADE
VIANDS
VIGODA
WIELDS
WIELDY
WILLDO
YIELDS

•I•••D

AIRBUD
AISLED
BIASED
BIBBED
BIFFED
BIFOLD
BIGBAD
BIGEND
BIGKID
BIGRED
BILDAD
BILGED
BILKED
BILLED
BINGED
BINNED
BIRDED
BIRLED
BIRRED
BITTED
CITIED
CIUDAD
DIALED
DIDBAD
DIETED
DIMMED
DINGED
DINNED
DINTED
DIOMED
DIPPED
DIRKED
DISBUD
DISHED
DISKED
DISSED
EIGHTD
FIBBED
FILLED
FILMED
FINKED
FINNED
FIRMED
FISHED
FISTED
FITTED
FIVEAD
FIZZED
GIFTED
GIGGED
GILDED
GILEAD
GILLED
GIMPED
GINNED
GIRDED
GIRTED
GITTED
HILLED
HILTED
HINGED
HINTED
HIPPED
HISSED
JIGGED
JILTED
JINXED
KICKED
KIDDED
KIDVID
KILLED
KILNED
KILTED
KINGED
KINKED
KIPPED
KISSED
KITTED
LIBBED
LICKED
LIDDED
LIFTED
LIGAND
LILIED
LILTED
LIMBED
LIMNED
LIMPED
LIMPID
LINKED
LINTED
LIPPED
LIQUID
LISPED
LISTED
LIZARD
MIFFED
MILKED
MILLED
MILORD
MINCED
MINDED
MINTED
MISADD
MISDID
MISFED
MISLED
MISSED
MISTED
MITRED
NICHED
NICKED
NIKEAD
NIMROD
NINEAD
NIPPED
OINKED
PICARD
PICKED
PIECED
PIGGED
PILLED
PINGED
PINKED
PINNED
PIQUED
PISHED
PITHED
PITIED
PITTED
RIBALD
RIBAND
RIBBED
RIBPAD
RIDDED
RIDGED
RIFFED
RIFLED
RIFTED
RIGGED
RIMMED
RINGED
RINSED

RIOTED
RIPPED
RISKED
RITARD
SICCED
SIDLED
SIEGED
SIEVED
SIFTED
SIGHED
SIGNED
SIGURD
SILOED
SILTED
SINBAD
SINEAD
SINGED
SINNED
SIPPED
TICCED
TICKED
TIDIED
TIERED
TIEROD
TIFFED
TILLED
TILTED
TINGED
TINGOD
TINNED
TINTED
TIPPED
TITHED
TITLED
TITRED
VIALED
VIEWED
VISAED
VISCID
WICKED
WIFIED
WIGAND
WIGGED
WILLED
WILTED
WIMPED
WINCED
WINDED
WINGED
WINKED
WISHED
WISPED
WITTED
WIZARD
YIPPED
ZIGGED
ZINCED
ZINGED
ZIPPED
ZIZZED

••ID••

ABIDED
ABIDER
ABIDES
ACIDIC
ACIDLY
ADIDAS
AMIDAS
AMIDES
AMIDOL
AMIDST
ARIDER
ARIDLY
ASIDES
AVIDER
AVIDLY
AZIDES
BRIDAL
BRIDES
BRIDGE
BRIDLE
BSIDES
CHIDED
CHIDER
CHIDES
DEIDRE
EJIDOS
ELIDED
ELIDER
ELIDES
ENIDOK
FRIDAY
FRIDGE
GLIDED
GLIDER
GLIDES
GRIDES
GUIDED
GUIDER
GUIDES
GUIDRY
HAIDAS
HAIDEE
HEIDEN
HRIDER
IBIDEM
IDIDIT
IMIDES
IRIDES
IRIDIC
ISIDOR
ISIDRO
LAIDBY
LAIDIN
LAIDON
LAIDTO
LAIDUP
LEIDEN
LOIDED
MAIDEN
NOIDEA
OXIDES
OXIDIC
PAIDAD
PAIDIN
PAIDUP
PDIDDY
PRIDED
PRIDES
QUIDDE
RAIDED
RAIDER
SAIDAH
SAIDHI
SAIDNO
SAIDOK
SAIDSO
SAIDTO
SKIDDY
SKIDOO
SLIDER
SLIDES
SLIDIN
SMIDGE
SNIDER
SPIDER
SPIDEY
STIDES
TVIDOL
UNIDLE
UNIDLY
VOIDED
VOIDER
VOIDOF
WEIDER
YSIDRO

••I•D•

BLINDS
BUILDS
CHILDE
FRIEDA
GLINDA
GRINDL
GRINDS
GUILDS
HAIRDO
ILIADS
LAIRDS
NAIADS
OLINDA
OVIEDO
PDIDDY
QUIDDE
SHINDY
SKIDDY
TBIRDS
THIRDR
THIRDS
TRIADS
TRIODE
WEIRDO
WEIRDY

••I••D

ABIDED
AFIELD
ALINED
ALIPED
BAILED
BAITED
BOILED
BRIAND
BRIARD
BRIBED
BRIGID
BRINED
CEILED
CHIDED
CHIMED
COIFED
COILED
COINED
DEICED
EDITED
EFILED
ELIDED
EXILED
EXITED
FAILED
FAIRED
FOILED
FRIEND
FRIGID
GAINED
GAITED
GLIDED
GRIMED
GRIPED
GUIDED
GUILED
HAILED
HAIRED
IRISED
JAILED
JOINED
JUICED
KNIFED
LAIRED
LOIDED
MAILED
MAIMED
MOILED
NAILED
NOISED
OPINED
PAIDAD
PAINED
PAIRED
POISED
PRICED
PRIDED
PRIMED
PRISED
PRIZED
QUIRED
RAIDED
RAILED
RAINED
RAISED
REICED
REINED
ROILED
RUINED
SAILED
SEINED
SEIZED
SHIELD
SHINED
SLICED
SLIMED
SMILED
SNIPED
SOILED
SPICED
SPIKED
SPINED
SPIRED
SPITED
SUITED
SWIPED
TAILED
TOILED
TRIPOD
TWINED
UNICED
UNIPED
UNIPOD
UNITED
VEILED
VEINED
VOICED
VOIDED
WAILED
WAITED
WAIVED
WHILED
WHINED
WHITED

•••ID•

AIKIDO
APHIDS
AROIDS
AVOIDS
BESIDE
BETIDE
BOLIDE
BORIDE
BOVIDS
BRAIDS
CANIDS
COMIDA
CUPIDS
DAVIDE
DAVIDI
DAVIDL
DAVIDO
DECIDE
DERIDE
DIVIDE
DOSIDO
DROIDS
DRUIDS
EXCIDE
FELIDS
FLUIDS
FRAIDY
HALIDE
HYOIDS
IDOIDO
INSIDE
IODIDE
LADIDA
LAVIDA
LERIDA
LIBIDO
LIPIDS
LUCIDA
LYRIDS
MARIDA
MARIDO
MERIDA
NOKIDS
ONEIDA
ONSIDE
OOTIDS
OREIDA
OVOIDS
OXHIDE
PLAIDS
RANIDS
RAPIDO
RAPIDS
REBIDS
REHIDE
RERIDE
RESIDE
SAYIDO
SODIDI
SOLIDS
SQUIDS
STRIDE
UNTIDY
UPSIDE
URSIDS
YESIDO
ZOOIDS

•••I•D

ALLIED
BABIED
BEGIRD
BEHIND
BEKIND
BELIED
BODIED
BURIED
BUSIED
CITIED
COPIED
COSIED
COZIED
DEFIED
DENIED
EDDIED
ENGILD
ENGIRD
ENVIED
ENWIND
ESPIED
EYVIND
GOWILD
HESIOD
HONIED
INKIND
INMIND
ITRIED
JURIED
LEVIED
LILIED
MONIED
MYRIAD
PERIOD
PITIED
PLEIAD
PONIED
REBIND
REFIED
REFIND
REGILD
REGIRD
RELIED
REMIND
RETIED
REWIND
RUBIED
TAXIED
TIDIED
UNBIND
UNGIRD
UNKIND
UNTIED
UNWILD
UNWIND
UPBIND
UPGIRD
UPWIND
VARIED
WIFIED

••••ID

ACARID
AENEID
AFRAID
ALKAID
ALTOID
ARAMID
ASTRID
BIGKID
BRIGID
CANDID
CAPRID
CERVID
CONOID
CORVID
CUBOID
CUEBID
CUSPID
CYANID
DEVOID
ELAPID
EQUOID
EUCLID
EYELID
FAKEID
FERVID
FLORID
FOETID
FORBID
FORDID
FRIGID
GETRID
GOTRID
GRAVID
HALOID
HASSID
HORRID
HYBRID
INGRID
INLAID
KHALID
KIDVID
LEONID
LIMPID
LIQUID
LOWBID
MADRID
MISDID
MORBID
NAVAID
NEREID
NEWKID
ONLAID
ORCHID
OUTBID
OUTDID
PALLID
PEPCID
PLACID
PONGID
POTLID
PREBID
PUTRID
RANCID
RASHID
RELAID
REPAID
RESAID
SORDID
STOLID
STUPID
SUBLID
THECID
THEKID
TOPBID
TOROID
TORPID
TORRID
TREPID
TURBID
TURGID
UNAVID
UNLAID
UNPAID
UNSAID
UNVOID
USERID
VERBID
VESPID
VISCID
XYLOID
YENSID

IE••••

IEIGHT

I•E•••

IBEAMS
IBERIA
IBEXES
ICEAGE
ICEAXE
ICEBAG
ICEBOX
ICECAP
ICEDAM
ICEDIN
ICEDIT
ICEDUP
ICEFOG
ICEMAN
ICEMEN
ICEOUT
ICEPOP
ICERUN
ICESIN
ICESIT
ICESUP
ICETEA
ICEUPS
IDEALS
IDEATE
IDENTI
IDENTS
IGETIT
ILEANA
ILEXES
IMEANT
IMEASY
IMELDA
INESSE
INEVER
IPECAC
IPETER
IREFUL
IRENIC
ISEEIT
ISELIN
ISERVE
ISEULT
ITEMED

I••E••

ICIEST
IDLERS
IDLEST
IGUESS
ILLEST
IMBEAT
IMBEDS
IMHERE
IMNEXT
IMPEDE
IMPELS
IMPEND
IMPERF
INCENT
INCEPT
INDEBT
INDEED
INDEEP
INDENT
INFEAR
INFECT
INFERS
INFEST
INGEAR
INGELS
INGEST
INHERE
INJECT
INJEST
INKERS
INLEAF
INLETS
INNEED
INNERS
INNESS
INSEAM
INSECT
INSERT
INSETS
INTEND
INTENS
INTENT
INTERJ
INTERN
INTERS
INVENT
INVERT
INVEST
IOMEGA
IQTEST
IRKERS
IRLENE
IRREAL
ISEEIT
ISLEFT
ISLETS
ISLEYS
ISMENE
ISSEIS
ISWEAR
ITSELF

I•••E•

IAGREE
IBANEZ
IBEXES
IBICES
IBIDEM
IBISES
ICEMEN
ICETEA
ICKIER
IDARED
IFFIER
IFTHEN
IJSSEL
ILEXES
ILLBET
ILLFED
ILLMET
ILLSEE
ILLSET
IMAGED
IMAGER
IMAGES
IMARET
IMAXES
IMBUED
IMBUES
IMFREE
IMIDES
IMINES
IMMIES
IMOGEN
IMPLED
INAFEW
INAGES
INANER
INAPET
INAREA
INASEC
INBRED
INCHED
INCHER
INCHES
INDEED
INDEEP
INDIES
INDUED
INDUES
INEVER
INGLES
INGRES
INGREY
INKIER
INKJET
INKLES
INLIEU
INNEED
INNIES
INONES
INSTEP
INURED
INURES
INVIEW
IPETER
IRATER
IRIDES
IRISED
IRISES
IRONED
IRONER
ISABEL
ISOHEL
ISOMER
ISRAEL
ISSUED
ISSUER
ISSUES
ISTLES
ISTRES
ITCHED
ITCHES
ITEMED
ITILES
ITRIED

I••••E

IAGREE
ICEAGE
ICEAXE
ICICLE
IDEATE
IGNACE
IGNITE
IGNORE
ILLSEE
ILLUDE
ILLUME
ILLUSE
IMBIBE
IMBRUE
IMDONE
IMFINE
IMFREE
IMGAME
IMGONE
IMHERE
IMHOME
IMLATE
IMLIKE
IMMUNE
IMMURE
IMPALE
IMPEDE
IMPOSE
IMPURE
IMPUTE
IMSURE
INAPIE
INATIE
INBLUE
INCASE
INCISE
INCITE
INCODE
INCOME
INCUSE
INDITE
INDUCE
INESSE
INFUSE
INGATE
INHALE
INHERE
INHOME
INHUME
INJOKE
INJUNE
INJURE
INLINE
INLOVE
INMATE
INNAGE
INNATE
INOUYE
INSANE
INSIDE
INSOLE
INSURE
INTAKE
INTIME
INTONE
INTUNE
INVADE
INVITE
INVOKE
INWOVE
IODATE
IODIDE
IODINE
IODISE
IODIZE
IONISE
IONIZE
IONONE
IRAISE
IRLENE
IRVINE
ISERVE
ISITME
ISLATE
ISLIKE
ISMENE
ISOLDE
IVTUBE

•IE•••

AIELLO
BIEBER
BIERCE
BIERES
CIELOS
CIERAS
DIECUT
DIEFOR
DIENES
DIEOFF
DIEOUT
DIEPPE
DIESEL
DIESES
DIESIS
DIETED
DIETER
DIETES
DIEZES
FIELDS
FIENDS
FIERCE
FIEROS
FIESTA
FIEVEL
GIEING
HIEING
HIEMAL
KIEFER
KIERAN
KIERON
LIEBER
LIEBIG
LIEBYS
LIEDER
LIEDON
LIEDTO
LIEFER
LIEFLY
LIEFOR
LIEGES
LIELOW
LIENEE
LIENOR
LIESIN
LIESON
LIESTO
LIEUTS
LIEVIO
MIELES
NIECES
NIEKRO
NIELLI
NIELLO
NIENTE
NIETAS
NIETOS
NIEVES
PIECED
PIECER
PIECES
PIELET
PIEMAN
PIEMEN
PIEPAN
PIERCE
PIERIA
PIERRE
PIETAS
PIETER
PIETIN
PIETRO
RIENZI
RIESEN
SIEBEN
SIECLE
SIEGED
SIEGEL
SIEGES
SIENNA
SIERRA
SIESTA
SIETES
SIEVED
SIEVES
TIEBAR
TIEDIN
TIEDON
TIEDTO
TIEDUP
TIEDYE
TIEINS
TIEMPO
TIENDA
TIEOFF
TIEPIN
TIERCE
TIERED
TIEROD
TIERRA
TIESIN
TIESON
TIESTO
TIESUP
TIETAC
TIEUPS
VIEFOR
VIEIRA
VIELLE
VIENNA
VIENNE
VIEWED
VIEWER
WIELDS
WIELDY
WIEMAN
WIENER
WIENIE
WIESEL
YIELDS

•I•E••

AIDERS
AILEEN
AIMERS
AIRERS
BICEPS
BIDERS
BIDETS
BIGEAR
BIGEND
BIGEYE
BIKERS
BIPEDS
BIREME
BISECT
BITEIN
BITEON
BITERS
BITEUP
CICELY
CICERO
CIDERS
CIDERY
CINEMA
CINEOL
CITEES
CITERS
CIVETS
DICERS
DIGEST
DIKERS
DINEAT
DINEIN
DINEON
DINERO
DINERS
DIRECT
DIRELY
DIREST
DISERE
DISEUR
DIVEIN
DIVERS
DIVERT
DIVEST
DIYERS
EIDERS
EILEEN
EILERS
EILERT
EIRENE
EISELE
FIBERS
FIFERS
FILEBY
FILEIN
FILENE
FILERS
FILETS
FINELY
FINERY
FINEST
FIREAT
FIREON
FIRERS
FIREUP
FIVEAA
FIVEAD
FIVEAM
FIVEBC
FIVEEE
FIVENO
FIVEOF
FIVEPM
FIVERS
FIVETO
FIVEUP
FIVEWS
FIXERS
GIBEAT
GIBERS
GIDEON
GILEAD
GILELS
GIMELS
GISELE
GIVEIN
GIVENS
GIVEOF
GIVEON
GIVERS
GIVETH
GIVETO
GIVEUP
HIDEHO
HIDEKI

HIDERS HIKERS HIKEUP HIREES HIREON HIRERS HITECH HITEST HIVERS JIBEAT JIVERS KIDEOS KITERS LIBELS LIBERS LIFEIS LIFERS LIGEIA LIGERS LIGETI LIKELY LIKENS LIKERS LIKESO LIKETO LINEAL LINEAR LINENS LINENY LINERS LINEUP LIPENG LITERS LIVEAT LIVEIN LIVELY LIVENS LIVEON LIVERS LIVERY LIVEST LIVETH LIVETV MILERS MIMEOS MIMERS MINERS MINETA MISERS MISERY MITERS MIXERS NICELY NICENE NICEST NICETY NIKEAD NINEAD NINEAM NINEBC NINEEE NINEPM NINERS NINETY NINEUP NISEIS NITERS NITERY

NIXERS OILERS OISEAU PIGEON PIKERS PILEIN PILEON PILERS PILEUM PILEUP PILEUS PINEAL PINERO PINERS PINERY PIPEIN PIPERS PIPETS PIPEUP PIXELS RIBERA RIBEYE RICERS RIDEBY RIDEIN RIDENT RIDERS RIDETO RIDEUP RIFELY RIFEST RIJEKA RIKERS RILERS RILEUP RIMERS RIPELY RIPENS RIPEST RISERS RISETO RISEUP RIVERA RIVERS RIVETS SILENT SIMEON SINEAD SINEWS SINEWY SIRENS SIXEEE SIXERS SIZERS SIZEUP TIGERS TILERS TILERY TIMELY TIMERS TINEAL TINEAR TIREOF TITERS VIDEOS VIDERI VILELY VILEST

VINERS VINERY VIPERS VIREOS VIVECA VIXENS WIDELY WIDENS WIDEOF WIDEST WIFELY WINERY WIPERS WIPEUP WIREIN WIRERS WIREUP WISELY WISEST WISETO WISEUP WIZENS

•I••E•

AIDMEN AIGLET AIGRET AILEEN AIRIER AIRMEN AIRSEA AISLED AISLES BIASED BIASES BIBBED BIBBER BIBLES BICKER BIDDEN BIDDER BIEBER BIERES BIFFED BIGBEN BIGBET BIGGER BIGMEN BIGRED BIGTEN BILGED BILGES BILKED BILKER BILLED BILLER BILLET BINDER BINGED BINGER BINGES BINNED BINNEY BIOMES BIRDED BIRDER BIRLED BIRLER

BIRNEY BIRRED BISBEE BISSET BITNET BITTED BITTEN BITTER CIBBER CINDER CIPHER CISKEI CITEES CITIED CITIES DIADEM DIALED DIALER DIAPER DICIER DICKER DICKEY DIDIES DIDOES DIENES DIESEL DIESES DIETED DIETER DIETES DIEZES DIFFER DIGGER DILLER DILSEY DIMMED DIMMER DINGED DINGER DINNED DINNER DINTED DIODES DIOMED DIPLEX DIPNET DIPPED DIPPER DIRGES DIRKED DISHED DISHES DISKED DISMES DISNEY DISPEL DISSED DISSES DITHER DITZES EIFFEL EILEEN EISLEY EISNER EITHER FIBBED FIBBER FIBRES

FICHES FIDGET FIDLER FIEVEL FILLED FILLER FILLES FILLET FILMED FILTER FINDER FINGER FINKED FINKEL FINLEY FINNED FINNEY FINSEN FIRMED FIRMER FISHED FISHER FISHES FISTED FITTED FITTER FIVEEE FIZZED FIZZER FIZZES GIBBER GIBLET GIDGET GIFTED GIFTEE GIGGED GIGUES GIJOES GILDED GILDER GILLED GILLEY GIMBEL GIMLET GIMMES GIMPED GINGER GINNED GIPPER GIRDED GIRDER GIRTED GITTED HICKEY HIDDEN HIGHER HILLED HILLEL HILLER HILTED HIMMEL HINDER HINGED HINGES HINTED HINTER HIPPED HIPPER

HIREES HISSED HISSER HISSES HITHER HITMEN HITTER JIGGED JIGGER JILTED JILTER JINXED JINXER JINXES JITNEY JITTER JIVIER KIBBEE KICKED KICKER KIDDED KIDDER KIDNEY KIEFER KILLED KILLER KILMER KILNED KILTED KILTER KINDER KINGED KINKED KINSEY KIPPED KIPPER KISLEV KISMET KISSED KISSEL KISSER KISSES KITAEN KITTED KITTEN LIANES LIBBED LIBBER LICHEE LICHEN LICKED LICKER LIDDED LIEBER LIEDER LIEFER LIEGES LIENEE LIFTED LIFTER LIGNES LILIED LILIES LILTED LIMBED LIMBER LIMIER LIMNED

LIMNER LIMPED LIMPER LIMPET LINDEN LINDER LINGER LINIER LINKED LINKER LINNET LINNEY LINTED LINTEL LINTER LINZER LIONEL LIONET LIPPED LIPPER LISLES LISPED LISPER LISSES LISTED LISTEE LISTEN LISTER LITHER LITRES LITTER LIVRES MICHEL MICKEY MIDGES MIDGET MIDLEG MIDLER MIELES MIFFED MIGUEL MILDER MILDEW MILIEU MILKED MILKER MILLED MILLER MILLES MILLET MILNER MILNES MINCED MINCER MINCES MINDED MINDEN MINDER MINTED MINTER MINUET MINXES MIR1ER MIRREN MISFED MISKEY MISLED MISSED

MISSES MISSET MISTED MISTER MITRED MITRES MITTEN MIXTEC MIZZEN NIAMEY NIBLET NICHED NICHES NICKED NICKEL NICKER NIECES NIEVES NIGHER NIKKEI NINEEE NIPPED NIPPER NIPSEY NISSEN NITRES NIXIES OILIER OILMEN OINKED OINKER PIAGET PICHEL PICKED PICKER PICKET PIECED PIECER PIECES PIELET PIEMEN PIETER PIGGED PIGLET PIGMEN PIGPEN PILFER PILLED PINCER PINGED PINGER PINIER PINKED PINKEN PINKER PINNED PINNER PINTER PIOLET PIPIER PIPPET PIQUED PIQUES PIQUET PISCES PISHED PISHES PISTES

PITHED PITIED PITIER PITIES PITMEN PITNEY PITTED PIUTES PIXIES RIBBED RIBBER RIBLET RICHEN RICHER RICHES RICHET RICKEY RIDDED RIDDEN RIDDER RIDGED RIDGES RIDLEY RIESEN RIFFED RIFLED RIFLER RIFLES RIFTED RIGGED RIGGER RILLES RILLET RIMIER RIMMED RINGED RINGER RINSED RINSER RINSES RIOTED RIOTER RIPKEN RIPLEY RIPPED RIPPER RISKED RISKER RITTER RITZES SICCED SICKEN SICKER SIDLED SIDLES SIDNEY SIEBEN SIEGED SIEGEL SIEGES SIETES SIEVED SIEVES SIFTED SIFTER SIGHED SIGHER SIGLER

SIGNED SIGNEE SIGNER SIGNET SILKEN SILOED SILTED SILVER SIMMER SIMPER SINGED SINGER SINGES SINKER SINNED SINNER SIPPED SIPPER SIRBEN SIRREE SISKEL SISLER SISLEY SISTER SITTER SIXEEE SIXTEN TICCED TICKED TICKER TICKET TIDIED TIDIER TIDIES TIERED TIFFED TIGGER TIGRES TILDEN TILDES TILLED TILLER TILLET TILLEY TILTED TILTER TIMBER TINDER TINGED TINGES TINIER TINKER TINMEN TINNED TINNER TINSEL TINTED TINTER TIPPED TIPPEE TIPPER TIPPET TISKET TITHED TITHER TITHES TITLED TITLES

TITRED TITRES TITTER VIALED VIEWED VIEWER VINIER VIOLET VISAED VIVIEN VIZIER WICKED WICKER WICKET WIDDER WIDGET WIENER WIESEL WIFIED WIFIES WIGGED WIGLET WIGNER WILDER WILIER WILKES WILLED WILLEM WILLER WILTED WIMMER WIMPED WIMSEY WINCED WINCER WINCES WINDED WINDER WINDEX WINGED WINGER WINIER WINKED WINKER WINNER WINTER WIRIER WISHED WISHER WISHES WISPED WISTER WITHER WITTED WITTER WIZZES YIPPED YIPPEE ZIFFEL ZIGGED ZIMMER ZINCED ZINGED ZINGER ZIPPED ZIPPER ZITHER ZIZZED

ZIZZES

•I•••E

AIRACE BIERCE BIGAPE BIGEYE BIGGIE BIGJOE BIGLIE BIGONE BIGTOE BILLIE BINATE BINDLE BINGLE BINNIE BIRDIE BIREME BISBEE BISQUE CIGGIE CINQUE CIRCLE CIRQUE DIABLE DIANNE DIBBLE DICKIE DIDDLE DIEPPE DILATE DILUTE DIMAGE DIMPLE DINGLE DIONNE DIPOLE DIRIGE DISERE DISUSE DIVIDE DIVINE EIGHTE EIRENE EISELE FIACRE FIANCE FICHTE FICKLE FIDDLE FIERCE FIGURE FILENE FILOSE FINALE FINITE FIPPLE FIVEEE FIXATE FIZZLE GIFTEE GIGGLE GIJANE GIMMIE GINNIE GIRDLE GIRLIE

GISELE HIGGLE HINGLE HINKLE HIPPIE HITONE JIGGLE JILLIE JIMMIE JINGLE KIBBEE KIBBLE KIDDIE KILTIE KIMBLE KINDLE KINGME KISHKE KISSME LIABLE LIAISE LIBRAE LICHEE LIENEE LIGATE LILLIE LINAGE LINGLE LIPASE LISTEE LITTLE LITTRE LIZZIE MIDDIE MIDDLE MIFUNE MILLIE MILTIE MINGLE MINIME MINNIE MINUTE MIRAGE MISCUE MISSME MISUSE MIZZLE NIBBLE NICENE NICOLE NIENTE NIGGLE NIMBLE NINEEE NIPPLE PIAFFE PICKLE PICONE PIDDLE PIERCE PIERRE PIFFLE PIGGIE PILATE PILOSE PIMPLE PINKIE PINNAE

PIPAGE PIRATE RIBEYE RIBOSE RICHIE RICKIE RIDDLE RIFFLE RIMATE RIMOSE RIMPLE RIPPLE RISQUE RITDYE SICKLE SIECLE SIGNEE SILAGE SIMILE SIMONE SIMPLE SINGLE SINISE SIRREE SISSLE SIXEEE SIXONE SIZZLE TIBIAE TICKLE TIEDYE TIERCE TILLIE TIMBRE TINGLE TINKLE TINORE TIPPEE TIPPLE TIPTOE TIRADE TIRANE TISANE TISSUE TITTLE VIABLE VIELLE VIENNE VINNIE VIRILE VIRTUE VISAGE VISINE VITALE VITTLE VIVACE WIENIE WIFFLE WIGGLE WILKIE WILLBE WILLIE WIMPLE WINKIE WINNIE YIPPEE YIPPIE

••IE••

ADIEUS ADIEUX AFIELD ALIENS AMIENS APIECE ARIEGE BRIEFS BRIENZ BRIERS BRIERY CHIEFS CHIENS CLIENT CRIERS DRIERS DRIEST ELIELI ERIEPA FLIERS FRIEDA FRIELS FRIEND FRIERS FRIEZE GAIETY GLIERE GRIECO GRIEFS GRIESE GRIEVE ICIEST MOIETY MSIEUR ORIELS ORIENT OSIERS OVIEDO PLIERS PRIERS PRIEST QUIETS SHIELD SHIEST SKIERS SLIEST SPIELS SPIERS STIERS THIEVE TRIERS UBIETY WRIEST

••I•E•

ABIDED ABIDER ABIDES AGILER ALICEB ALICES ALIKES ALINED ALINER ALINES ALIPED ALIVEO

AMICES
AMIDES
AMINES
ANIMES
ANISES
APICES
ARIDER
ARISEN
ARISES
ASIDES
ATILES
ATISES
AVIDER
AXISES
AZIDES
BAILED
BAILEE
BAILER
BAILEY
BAINES
BAITED
BAITER
BAIZES
BEIGES
BLIMEY
BLIXEN
BOILED
BOILER
BOITES
BRIBED
BRIBEE
BRIBER
BRIBES
BRIDES
BRINED
BRINER
BRINES
BRISES
BSIDES
BTILES
CEILED
CHICER
CHIDED
CHIDER
CHIDES
CHILES
CHIMED
CHIMER
CHIMES
CHINES
CHISEL
CHIVES
CLIMES
COIFED
COILED
COILER
COINED
COINER
CRIKEY
CRIMEA
CRIMES
CRIPES
CRISES
CTILES
DAILEY
DAISES
DEICED
DEICER

DEICES
DRIVEL
DRIVEN
DRIVER
DRIVES
DTILES
EDILES
EDITED
EFILED
EFILES
EGISES
ELIDED
ELIDER
ELIDES
ELISEO
ELITER
ELITES
EMINEM
ETILES
EVILER
EVITES
EXILED
EXILER
EXILES
EXITED
EZINES
FAILED
FAINER
FAIRED
FAIRER
FAITES
FBIMEN
FOILED
FRIGES
FRISEE
FRISES
FRITES
FTILES
GAINED
GAINER
GAINES
GAITED
GAITER
GEIGER
GEISEL
GLIDED
GLIDER
GLIDES
GOITER
GRIDES
GRIMED
GRIMES
GRIPED
GRIPER
GRIPES
GTILES
GUIDED
GUIDER
GUIDES
GUILED
GUILES
GUINEA
GUISES
HAIDEE
HAILED
HAILER
HAILEY
HAINES

HAIRED
HEIDEN
HEIFER
HRIDER
HTILES
IBICES
IBIDEM
IBISES
IMIDES
IMINES
IRIDES
IRISED
IRISES
ITILES
JAILED
JAILER
JOINED
JOINER
JTILES
JUICED
JUICER
JUICES
KAISER
KEITEL
KNIFED
KNIFER
KNIFES
KNIVES
KTILES
LAIRED
LEIDEN
LEISEN
LEITER
LOIDED
LOIRET
LOITER
LTILES
MAIDEN
MAILED
MAILER
MAIMED
MAIMER
MAINER
MAIRES
MAIZES
MOILED
MOILER
MOINES
MOIRES
MOISES
MTILES
NAILED
NAILER
NAIVER
NOIDEA
NOIRES
NOIRET
NOISED
NOISES
NTILES
OBITER
OGIVES
OLIVER
OLIVES
OPINED
OPINER
OPINES
ORIGEN

OTILES
OUIMET
OVINES
OXIDES
PAINED
PAIRED
PAISES
PFIZER
POIRES
POIRET
POISED
POISER
POISES
PRICED
PRICER
PRICES
PRICEY
PRIDED
PRIDES
PRIMED
PRIMER
PRIMES
PRISED
PRIVET
PRIZED
PRIZES
PTILES
QTILES
QUIRED
QUIRES
QUIVER
RAIDED
RAIDER
RAILED
RAILER
RAINED
RAINER
RAINES
RAINEY
RAISED
RAISER
RAISES
RBIMEN
REICED
REICES
REIGER
REINED
REINER
REINES
REISER
REITER
ROILED
RTILES
RUINED
RUINER
SAILED
SAILER
SAITEK
SEINED
SEINER
SEINES
SEIZED
SEIZER
SEIZES
SHINED
SHINER
SHINES
SHIRER

SHIRES
SHIVER
SLICED
SLICER
SLICES
SLIDER
SLIDES
SLIMED
SLIMES
SLIVER
SMILED
SMILER
SMILES
SMILEY
SMITER
SMITES
SNIDER
SNIPED
SNIPER
SNIPES
SNIVEL
SOILED
SOIREE
SOISEE
SPICED
SPICER
SPICES
SPIDER
SPIDEY
SPIKED
SPIKER
SPIKES
SPILES
SPINED
SPINEL
SPINER
SPINES
SPINET
SPIREA
SPIRED
SPIRES
SPITED
SPITES
STIDES
STILES
STIPES
SUITED
SUITES
SWIPED
SWIPER
SWIPES
SWIVEL
SWIVET
TAILED
TAILER
TAIPEI
TOILED
TOILER
TOILES
TOILET
TRIBES
TRICEP
TRICES
TRIJET
TRIKES
TRINES
TRIPES
TRITER

TRIVET
TTILES
TWINED
TWINER
TWINES
UNICED
UNICEF
UNICES
UNIPED
UNISEX
UNITED
UNITER
UNITES
VAINER
VEILED
VEILER
VEINED
VOICED
VOICER
VOICES
VOIDED
VOIDER
VOILES
VSIXES
VTILES
WAILED
WAILER
WAITED
WAITER
WAIVED
WAIVER
WAIVES
WEIDER
WHILED
WHILES
WHINED
WHINER
WHINES
WHITED
WHITEN
WHITER
WHITES
WHITEY
WRITER
WRITES
WTILES
XFILES
XTILES
YTILES
ZAIRES
ZTILES

••I••E

ALIBLE
AMITIE
APIECE
ARIANE
ARIEGE
ARIOSE
AVIATE
BAILEE
BEIGNE
BLITHE
BRIBEE
BRIDGE
BRIDLE
CHICLE
CHIGOE

CHILDE
CLICHE
CLIQUE
COIGNE
CRINGE
DEIDRE
EDIBLE
EDIRNE
EMIGRE
EMILIE
ENISLE
EVINCE
FAILLE
FOIBLE
FRICKE
FRIDGE
FRIEZE
FRINGE
FRISEE
FUISSE
GLIERE
GRIESE
GRIEVE
GRILLE
GRIMKE
GRIPPE
HAIDEE
HEINIE
HEINSE
ICICLE
ISITME
LAINIE
MAISIE
MAITRE
NEISSE
OPIATE
ORIOLE
OTIOSE
PAIUTE
PEIRCE
PLISSE
POINTE
POIVRE
PRINCE
PRINZE
QUICHE
QUIDDE
QUINCE
QUINTE
QUINZE
SAINTE
SHIITE
SMIDGE
SOIGNE
SOIREE
SOISEE
STIFLE
STILLE
SUISSE
THICKE
THIEVE
THISBE
TRIAGE
TRIFLE
TRIODE
TRIPLE
TRISTE
TRIUNE

TRIXIE
TUILLE
TWINGE
UNIATE
UNIDLE
UNIQUE
VEINTE
WRITHE

•••IE•

ABDIEL
ACHIER
ADRIEN
AERIER
AERIES
AGGIES
AIRIER
ALKIES
ALLIED
ALLIES
AMBIEN
ANCIEN
ANNIES
ARMIES
ARNIES
ARTIER
ASHIER
BABIED
BABIER
BABIES
BAVIER
BELIED
BELIEF
BELIER
BELIES
BEVIES
BODIED
BODIES
BOGIES
BONIER
BOXIER
BURIED
BURIER
BURIES
BUSIED
BUSIER
BUSIES
CAGIER
CAHIER
CAKIER
CANIER
CARIES
CAVIES
CITIED
CITIES
COKIER
COKIES
CONIES
COPIED
COPIER
COPIES
COSIED
COSIER
COSIES
COWIER
COZIED
COZIER
COZIES

CURIES
CUTIES
CUVIER
DAMIEN
DANIEL
DARIEN
DAVIES
DEFIED
DEFIER
DEFIES
DEMIES
DENIED
DENIER
DENIES
DEWIER
DICIER
DIDIES
DOGIES
DOPIER
DORIES
DOXIES
DOZIER
DUTIES
EASIER
EDDIED
EDDIES
EDGIER
EELIER
EERIER
EGGIER
ELMIER
ENVIED
ENVIER
ENVIES
ESPIED
ESPIER
ESPIES
EYRIES
FACIES
FOGIES
FOLIES
FOXIER
FUMIER
FURIES
GAMIER
GENIES
GLUIER
GOBIES
GOOIER
GORIER
HAZIER
HOKIER
HOKIES
HOLIER
HOLIES
HOMIER
HOMIES
HONIED
HOSIER
ICKIER
IFFIER
IMMIES
INDIES
INKIER
INLIEU
INNIES
INVIEW
ITRIED

JAVIER
JIVIER
JOKIER
JOLIET
JULIEN
JULIET
JURIED
JURIES
LACIER
LADIES
LAKIER
LANIER
LAZIER
LEVIED
LEVIER
LEVIES
LILIED
LILIES
LIMIER
LINIER
LOGIER
LOOIES
LORIES
LOUIES
LUCIEN
MARIEL
MAZIER
METIER
MILIEU
MIRIER
MONIED
MONIES
MOPIER
MOVIES
MURIEL
NAPIER
NAVIES
NEWIES
NIXIES
NOSIER
OAKIER
OATIER
OBRIEN
OILIER
OLDIES
ONVIEW
OOZIER
ORGIES
OUTIES
OWLIER
PACIER
PANIER
PAPIER
PINIER
PIPIER
PITIED
PITIER
PITIES
PIXIES
PLUIES
POKIER
POKIES
PONIED
PONIES
POSIES
PUNIER
RABIES
RACIER

RAMIES
RAPIER
REFIED
REFIES
RELIED
RELIEF
RELIER
RELIES
RETIED
RETIEF
RETIES
REVIEW
RIMIER
ROPIER
ROSIER
ROSIES
RUBIED
RUBIES
RULIER
SAGIER
SERIES
SEXIER
SHRIEK
SOVIET
SPRIER
SUZIEQ
TAXIED
TAXIES
TIDIED
TIDIER
TIDIES
TINIER
TOBIES
TODIES
TONIER
TORIES
UGLIER
UGLIES
UNDIES
UNTIED
UNTIER
UNTIES
VANIER
VARIED
VARIER
VARIES
VINIER
VIVIEN
VIZIER
WANIER
WARIER
WAVIER
WAXIER
WIFIED
WIFIES
WILIER
WINIER
WIRIER
XAVIER
YALIES
ZANIER
ZANIES
ZOOIER

•••I•E

ACTIVE
ADMIRE
ADRIVE

ADVICE
ADVISE
AEDILE
AFFINE
ALBINE
ALDINE
ALFINE
ALPINE
APLITE
APRILE
ARGIVE
ARRIVE
ASHINE
ASPIRE
ASSIZE
ATFIVE
ATNINE
ATTIRE
AUDILE
AUGITE
AWHILE
AXLIKE
BALINE
BARITE
BELIKE
BELIZE
BEMINE
BEMIRE
BENICE
BESIDE
BETIDE
BLAINE
BLAISE
BODICE
BODINE
BOLIDE
BORIDE
BOVINE
BRAISE
BRUISE
BYLINE
BYWIRE
CAMISE
CANINE
CARIBE
CECILE
CELINE
CERISE
CHAINE
CHAISE
CHOICE
CLAIRE
COMICE
COSINE
CROIRE
CRUISE
CURIAE
CURITE
DANITE
DATIVE
DAVIDE
DECIDE
DECILE
DEFILE
DEFINE
DEHIRE
DEMISE
DENISE

DERIDE
DERIVE
DESIRE
DEVICE
DEVINE
DEVISE
DEWIRE
DIRIGE
DIVIDE
DIVINE
DOCILE
DOFINE
DOLIKE
DOMINE
DORINE
DOTIME
DRRICE
DRYICE
EGLISE
ELAINE
ELLICE
ELMIRE
ELOISE
EMPIRE
ENDIVE
ENGINE
ENSILE
ENTICE
ENTIRE
EQUINE
ERMINE
ESTIME
ETOILE
EUNICE
EWAINE
EXCIDE
EXCISE
EXCITE
EXPIRE
EXWIFE
FACIAE
FACILE
FALINE
FAMINE
FELICE
FELINE
FELIPE
FINITE
FOKINE
FRAISE
FUSILE
FUTILE
GAMINE
GOLIKE
GOLIVE
GUNITE
HABILE
HALIDE
HALITE
HAMITE
IGNITE
IMBIBE
IMFINE
IMLIKE
INCISE
INCITE
INDITE
INLINE

INSIDE
INTIME
INVITE
IODIDE
IODINE
IODISE
IODIZE
IONISE
IONIZE
IRAISE
IRVINE
ISLIKE
JANICE
JANINE
KALINE
KLEINE
KURILE
LABILE
LABINE
LAMIAE
LARINE
LEVINE
LEVITE
LIAISE
LOUISE
LUCILE
LUCINE
LUCITE
LUPINE
LYSINE
MALICE
MARINE
MAXINE
MAXIXE
MINIME
MOBILE
MODINE
MOLINE
MOTILE
MOTIVE
MURINE
MYLIFE
NADINE
NANINE
NARINE
NATIVE
NOBILE
NODICE
NOJIVE
NORITE
NOTICE
NOTIME
NOVICE
NOWISE
NUBILE
OBLIGE
OFFICE
ONFILE
ONFIRE
ONHIRE
ONLINE
ONMIKE
ONRICE
ONSIDE
ONSITE
ONTIME
OOLITE
OSCINE

OXHIDE
OXLIKE
PATINE
PERINE
PETITE
PLAICE
POLICE
POLITE
PRAISE
PUMICE
PYRITE
RACINE
RANINE
RAPINE
RATINE
RATITE
RAVINE
RECIFE
RECIPE
RECITE
REFILE
REFINE
REFIRE
REGIME
REGIVE
REHIDE
REHIRE
RELINE
RELIVE
REMINE
REMISE
REPINE
RERIDE
RERISE
RESIDE
RESILE
RESITE
RESIZE
RETILE
RETIME
RETIRE
REVILE
REVISE
REVIVE
REWIPE
REWIRE
RUTILE
SABINE
SAFIRE
SALINE
SATIRE
SCRIBE
SEAICE
SEMITE
SENILE
SHIITE
SHRIKE
SHRINE
SHRIVE
SIMILE
SINISE
SLUICE
SOFINE
SPLICE
SPLINE
SPRITE
SQUIRE
STRIAE

STRIDE
STRIFE
STRIKE
STRIPE
STRIVE
SUPINE
THRICE
THRIVE
TIBIAE
TOLIFE
TONITE
TREIZE
TVTIME
UMPIRE
UNDINE
UNFILE
UNFINE
UNHIRE
UNLIKE
UNLIVE
UNNICE
UNPILE
UNRIFE
UNRIPE
UNWISE
UPDIKE
UPDIVE
UPPILE
UPRISE
UPSIDE
UPSIZE
UPTIME
URSINE
VALINE
VALISE
VENICE
VENIRE
VENITE
VERITE
VIRILE
VISINE
VOTIVE
WAHINE
XPRIZE

••••IE

ADELIE
AMALIE
AMELIE
AMITIE
ANOMIE
ARCHIE
AUNTIE
AUSSIE
BADDIE
BADLIE
BAGGIE
BALDIE
BARBIE
BARRIE
BEANIE
BENNIE
BERNIE
BERTIE
BESSIE
BIGGIE
BIGLIE
BILLIE
BINNIE
BIRDIE
BLOOIE
BMOVIE
BOBBIE
BOCCIE
BONNIE
BOOGIE
BOOKIE
BOOTIE
BOWTIE
BRODIE
BUDGIE
BURNIE
CABBIE
CADDIE
CAMMIE
CARRIE
CASSIE
CHERIE
CIGGIE
COLLIE
CONNIE
COOKIE
COOLIE
COOTIE
COWRIE
DANDIE
DEARIE
DEBBIE
DEENIE
DICKIE
DOGGIE
DONNIE
DOOGIE
DOOLIE
DOOZIE
DORMIE
DOTTIE
DROXIE
DUCKIE
EANNIE
EARNIE
EENSIE
EMILIE
FAERIE
FANNIE
FERDIE
FERGIE
FLUTIE
FOLKIE
FONZIE
FOODIE
FOZZIE
GERTIE
GIMMIE
GINNIE
GIRLIE
GOALIE
GOLDIE
GOODIE
GOONIE
GORDIE
GRACIE
GRAZIE
HACKIE
HADDIE
HALLIE
HANKIE
HATTIE
HAYNIE
HEEBIE
HEINIE
HERBIE
HIPPIE
HOAGIE
HOGTIE
HOODIE
HOOTIE
HOTTIE
HUDDIE
HUGHIE
INAPIE
INATIE
JACKIE
JEANIE
JENNIE
JILLIE
JIMMIE
JOANIE
JUNKIE
KARRIE
KATHIE
KELLIE
KELPIE
KEWPIE
KIDDIE
KILTIE
KOOKIE
LADDIE
LAINIE
LAJOIE
LANCIE
LASSIE
LAURIE
LEEKIE
LENNIE
LESLIE
LILLIE
LIZZIE
LONNIE
LOOKIE
LOONIE
LORRIE
MACKIE
MADDIE
MAGGIE
MAGLIE
MAGPIE
MAISIE
MARCIE
MARGIE
MARKIE
MARNIE
MASHIE
MATTIE
MEALIE
MEANIE
MERRIE
MIDDIE
MILLIE
MILTIE
MINNIE
MOLLIE
MOMMIE
MOOKIE
MOONIE
MORRIE
MUDPIE
MUNCIE
MUSKIE
NANNIE
NAPPIE
NELLIE
NESSIE
NEWBIE
NEWSIE
NOOGIE
OUTLIE
OUTVIE
PANTIE
PATRIE
PATTIE
PETRIE
PIGGIE
PINKIE
POSTIE
POTPIE
POTSIE
PREMIE
PROBIE
PUNKIE
PURLIE
QUAKIE
RAZZIE
REBBIE
REDTIE
REENIE
REGGIE
RENNIE
RICHIE
RICKIE
ROADIE
ROBBIE
ROCKIE
ROLLIE
RONNIE
ROOKIE
ROOMIE
ROOTIE
RUNCIE
RUTHIE
SALLIE
SAVOIE
SAYDIE
SKOKIE
SOFTIE
SOPHIE
SORTIE
SPECIE
STEVIE
STEWIE
STOGIE
STYMIE
TALKIE
TECHIE
TEENIE
TEKKIE
TESSIE
TILLIE
TOMMIE
TOONIE
TOOTIE
TOWNIE
TRIXIE
TUSHIE
VEGGIE
VINNIE
WALKIE
WEDGIE
WEENIE
WENDIE
WESTIE
WIENIE
WILKIE
WILLIE
WINKIE
WINNIE
WOODIE
WOOGIE
YETTIE
YIPPIE
YORKIE
YUPPIE
ZOMBIE

IF••••

IFFIER
IFICAN
IFIMAY
IFITIS
IFONLY
IFORTY
IFTHEN

I•F•••

IFFIER
IMFINE
IMFREE
IMFULL
INFACT
INFALL
INFAMY
INFANT
INFEAR
INFECT
INFERS
INFEST
INFIRM
INFLOW
INFLUX
INFOLD
INFORM
INFULL
INFUSE

I••F••

ICEFOG
ILLFED
INAFEW
INAFIX
INAFOG
IREFUL
ITSFUN

I•••F•

ILLOFF
ISLEFT

I••••F

ILLOFF
IMPERF
INGULF
INHALF
INLEAF
ITSELF

•IF•••

BIFFED
BIFOLD
BIFORM
DIFFER
EIFFEL
FIFERS
FIFING
FIFTHS
GIFTED
GIFTEE
LIFEIS
LIFERS
LIFTED
LIFTER
LIFTUP
MIFFED
MIFUNE
PIFFLE
RIFELY
RIFEST
RIFFED
RIFFLE
RIFKIN
RIFLED
RIFLER
RIFLES
RIFTED
SIFTED
SIFTER
TIFFED
TIFFIN
WIFELY
WIFFLE
WIFIED
WIFIES
ZIFFEL

•I•F••

AIDFUL
AIMFOR
AIMFUL
BIAFRA
BIDFOR
BIFFED
BIGFAN
BIGFUN
DIDFOR
DIEFOR
DIFFER
DIGFOR
EIFFEL
FITFOR
FITFUL
HITFOR
KIEFER
LIEFER
LIEFLY
LIEFOR
MIFFED
MISFED
MISFIT
PIAFFE
PIFFLE
PILFER
RIFFED
RIFFLE
SINFUL
SITFOR
TIFFED
TIFFIN
VIEFOR
WIFFLE
ZIFFEL

•I••F•

BITOFF
CITIFY
DIEOFF
HITOFF
LIPOFF
MIDOFF
MINIFY
NIDIFY
PIAFFE
PILAFS
RIPOFF
TIEOFF
TIPOFF
VILIFY
VINIFY
VIVIFY
ZIPOFF

•I•••F

BITOFF
DIEOFF
FIVEOF
GIVEOF
HITOFF
KINDOF
LIPOFF
MIDOFF
RIDSOF
RIPOFF
SICKOF
TIEOFF
TIPOFF
TIREOF
WIDEOF
ZIPOFF

••IF••

AFIFTH
BLIFIL
CLIFFS
CLIFFY
COIFED
DEIFIC
DRIFTS
DRIFTY
GFIFTY
GRIFTS
HEIFER
KNIFED
KNIFER
KNIFES
MEIFUN
SHIFTS
SHIFTY
SKIFFS
SNIFFS
SNIFFY
SPIFFS
SPIFFY
STIFFS
STIFLE
SWIFTS
TRIFLE
UNIFIC
WHIFFS

••I•F•

BRIEFS
CHIEFS
CLIFFS
CLIFFY
GRIEFS
SKIFFS
SNIFFS
SNIFFY
SPIFFS
SPIFFY
STIFFS
WHIFFS

••I••F

ABITOF
UNICEF
VOIDOF

•••IF•

ADRIFT
AERIFY
AURIFY
BASIFY
CALIFS
CANIFF
CITIFY
CODIFY
EXWIFE
GASIFY
MINIFY
MODIFY
MOTIFS
MYLIFE
NIDIFY
NOTIFY
OSSIFY
PACIFY
PURIFY
RAMIFY
RATIFY
RECIFE
REGIFT
RESIFT
RUBIFY
SALIFY
SERIFS
SHRIFT
STRIFE
TARIFF
THRIFT
TOLIFE
TYPIFY
UGLIFY
UNRIFE
UPLIFT
VERIFY
VILIFY
VINIFY
VIVIFY

•••I•F

BELIEF
CANIFF
RELIEF
RETIEF
TARIFF

••••IF

CERTIF
DOURIF
EVENIF
MASSIF
ONLYIF
SHARIF
TERRIF
WHATIF

IG••••

IGETIT
IGGING
IGGINS
IGLOOS
IGNACE
IGNATZ
IGNITE
IGNORE
IGOROT
IGOTIT
IGOTTA
IGUANA
IGUESS

I•G•••

IAGREE
IGGING
IGGINS
IMGAME
IMGLAD
IMGONE
IMGOOD
INGATE
INGEAR
INGELS
INGEST
INGLES
INGMAR
INGOAL
INGOLD
INGOOD
INGOTS
INGRAM
INGRAY
INGRES
INGREY
INGRID
INGULF
ITGIRL

I••G••

IEIGHT
IMAGED
IMAGER
IMAGES
IMAGOS
IMIGHT
IMOGEN
INAGES
ISOGON

I•••G•

ICEAGE
ICINGS
IDTAGS
IKINGS
IMPUGN
INDIGO
INNAGE
INRAGS
IOMEGA
ITSAGO

I••••G

ICEBAG
ICEFOG
ICHING
IDLING
IGGING
INAFOG
INARUG
INKING
INNING
IRKING
IRVING
ISLING

•IG•••

AIGLET
AIGRET
BIGAIR
BIGAMY
BIGAPE
BIGBAD
BIGBEN
BIGBET
BIGBOI
BIGBOX
BIGBOY
BIGBUX
BIGCAR
BIGCAT
BIGDAY
BIGDIG
BIGDOG
BIGDOS
BIGEAR
BIGEND
BIGEYE
BIGFAN
BIGFUN
BIGGER
BIGGIE
BIGGUN
BIGGUY
BIGHIT
BIGHTS
BIGHUG
BIGJOE
BIGKID
BIGLIE
BIGMAC
BIGMAN
BIGMEN
BIGOIL
BIGONE
BIGOTS
BIGRED
BIGRIG
BIGSKY
BIGSUR
BIGTEN
BIGTOE
BIGTOP
BIGWIG
BIGWIN
CIGARS
CIGGIE
DIGAMY
DIGEST
DIGFOR
DIGGER
DIGITS
DIGLOT
DIGOUT
DIGRAM
DIGSAT
DIGSIN
DIGSIT
DIGSUP
EIGHTA
EIGHTB
EIGHTC
EIGHTD
EIGHTE
EIGHTH
EIGHTS
EIGHTY
FIGARO
FIGBAR
FIGHTS
FIGURE
GIGBAG
GIGGED
GIGGLE
GIGGLY
GIGOLO
GIGOTS
GIGUES
HIGGLE
HIGHER
HIGHIQ
HIGHLY
HIGHON
HIGHUP
JIGGED
JIGGER
JIGGLE
JIGGLY
JIGSAW
KIGALI
LIGAND
LIGATE
LIGEIA
LIGERS
LIGETI
LIGHTS
LIGNES
LIGNIN
LIGNUM
MIGHTS
MIGHTY
MIGNON
MIGUEL
NIGGLE
NIGHER
NIGHON
NIGHTS
NIGHTY
PIGEON
PIGGED
PIGGIE
PIGLET
PIGMAN
PIGMEN
PIGNUT
PIGOUT
PIGPEN
PIGSIT
PIGSTY
RIGANS
RIGATI
RIGGED
RIGGER
RIGHTO
RIGHTS
RIGHTY
RIGORS
RIGOUR
RIGOUT
RIGSUP
SIGHAT
SIGHED
SIGHER
SIGHTS
SIGILS
SIGLER
SIGMAS
SIGNAL
SIGNED
SIGNEE
SIGNER
SIGNET
SIGNIN
SIGNON
SIGNOR
SIGNUP
SIGURD
TIGERS
TIGGER
TIGHTS
TIGLON
TIGONS
TIGRES
TIGRIS
VIGIAS
VIGILS
VIGODA
VIGORS
VIGOUR
WIGAND
WIGGED
WIGGIN
WIGGLE
WIGGLY
WIGHTS
WIGLET
WIGNER
WIGOUT
WIGWAG
WIGWAM
ZIGGED
ZIGZAG

•I•G••

AIRGUN
BIGGER
BIGGIE
BIGGUN
BIGGUY
BILGED
BILGES
BINGED
BINGER
BINGES
BINGLE
BINGOS
BIOGAS
BIRGIT
CIGGIE
DIGGER
DINGED
DINGER
DINGHY
DINGLE
DINGUS
DIRGES
FIDGET
FINGER
FIZGIG
GIDGET
GIGGED
GIGGLE
GIGGLY
GINGER
GINGKO
GIUGNO
HIGGLE
HINGED
HINGES
HINGIS
HINGLE
JIGGED
JIGGER
JIGGLE
JIGGLY
JINGLE
JINGLY
KINGED
KINGLY
KINGME
LIEGES
LINGER
LINGLE
LINGUA
LINGUS
MIDGES
MIDGET
MINGLE
MINGUS
NIGGLE
NINGBO
PIAGET
PIDGIN
PIGGED
PIGGIE
PINGED
PINGER
PISGAH
RIDGED
RIDGES
RIGGED
RIGGER
RINGED
RINGER
RINGIN
RINGUP
SIEGED
SIEGEL
SIEGES
SINGED
SINGER
SINGES
SINGIN
SINGLE
SINGLY
SINGTO
SIXGUN
TIGGER
TINGED
TINGES
TINGLE
TINGLY
TINGOD
VIAGRA
VIRGAS
VIRGIL
VIRGIN
VIRGOS
WIDGET
WIGGED
WIGGIN
WIGGLE
WIGGLY
WINGED
WINGER
WINGIT
XINGIN
ZIGGED
ZINGED
ZINGER
ZIPGUN

•I••G•

DIMAGE
DIRIGE
DIRIGO
GINKGO
LIANGS
LINAGE
MIRAGE
PIPAGE
SILAGE
VIRAGO
VISAGE

•I•••G

AIDING
AILING
AIMING
AIRBAG
AIRING
AIRLOG
BIDING
BIGDIG
BIGDOG
BIGHUG
BIGRIG
BIGWIG
BIKING
BINNIG
BITING
CITING
DIALOG
DICING
DIKING
DIMING
DINING
DIVING
FIFING
FILING
FINING
FIRING
FIXING
FIZGIG
GIBING
GIEING
GIGBAG
GIVING
HIDING
HIEING
HIKING
HIRING
HIVING
JIBING
JIVING
KITBAG
KITING
LIEBIG
LIKING
LIMING
LINING
LIPENG
LIVING
MIDLEG
MIKING
MIMING
MINING
MIRING
MITTAG
MIXING
NIXING
OILING
OILRIG
PIKING
PILING
PINING
PIPING
RICING
RIDING
RILING
RIMING
RISING
RIVING
SIDING
SIRING
SITING
SIZING
TIDING
TILING
TIMING
TIRING
VIKING
VINING

VISING
WIGWAG
WILING
WINBIG
WINING
WIPING
WIRING
WISING
WITTIG
WIVING
ZIGZAG

••IG••

ALIGHT
ALIGNS
AMIGAS
AMIGOS
ARIGHT
BEIGES
BEIGHT
BEIGNE
BLIGHT
BRIGHT
BRIGID
BRIGIT
CHIGOE
COIGNE
COIGNS
DEIGNS
DWIGHT
EMIGRE
ENIGMA
FEIGNS
FLIGHT
FRIGES
FRIGHT
FRIGID
GEIGER
GEIGHT
GRIGRI
HAIGHT
HEIGHT
IEIGHT
IMIGHT
KNIGHT
NEIGHS
ORIGEN
ORIGIN
PLIGHT
REIGER
REIGNS
SAIGON
SLIGHT
SOIGNE
SPIGOT
STIGMA
TAIGAS
THIGHS
TRIGON
TWIGGY
VEIGHT
VOIGHT
VSIGNS
WEIGHS
WEIGHT
WRIGHT

••I•G•

ARIEGE
ASIAGO
BEINGS
BOINGO
BOINGS
BRIDGE
BRINGS
CLINGS
CLINGY
CRINGE
DOINGS
DRINGS
EWINGS
FLINGS
FRIDGE
FRINGE
FRINGY
GOINGS
GRINGO
ICINGS
IKINGS
ORINGS
SLINGS
SMIDGE
STINGS
STINGY
SWINGS
SWINGY
THINGS
THINGY
TRIAGE
TWIGGY
TWINGE
WRINGS

••I••G

CHIANG
EPILOG
SKIING

•••IG•

ANTIGO
ASSIGN
ATSIGN
AURIGA
AWEIGH
BENIGN
BEWIGS
COSIGN
CRAIGT
DESIGN
DHEIGH
DIRIGE
DIRIGO
EFFIGY
ENSIGN
INDIGO
LATIGO
LEHIGH
MALIGN
MAYIGO
OBLIGE
OKSIGN
ONHIGH
REDIGS
REJIGS
RERIGS
RESIGN
SLEIGH
SPRIGS
UNNIGH
UNRIGS
UNWIGS
ZUNIGA

•••I•G

AAHING
ACHING
ACTING
ADDING
ADZING
AGEING
AIDING
AILING
AIMING
AIRING
ALVING
AMPING
ARCING
ARMING
ASHING
ASKING
ATHING
AWNING
BAAING
BAKING
BALING
BARING
BASING
BATING
BAYING
BBKING
BCCING
BENING
BERING
BIDING
BIKING
BITING
BLUING
BODING
BOEING
BONING
BOOING
BORING
BOWING
BOXING
BUSING
BUYING
CAGING
CAKING
CANING
CARING
CASING
CAVING
CAWING
CEDING
CITING
CLUING
CODING
COKING
COMING
CONING
COOING
COPING
CORING
COVING
COWING
COXING
CRYING
CUBING
CUEING
CURING
DARING
DATING
DAZING
DEKING
DEWING
DICING
DIKING
DIMING
DINING
DIVING
DOLING
DOMING
DOPING
DOSING
DOTING
DOZING
DRKING
DRYING
DUDING
DUKING
DUPING
DURING
DYEING
EALING
EARING
EASING
EATING
EBBING
EDGING
EELING
EGGING
ENDING
EPPING
ERRING
ERVING
ETTING
EYEING
FACING
FADING
FAKING
FAMING
FARING
FAXING
FAZING
FEEING
FETING
FIFING
FILING
FINING
FIRING
FIXING
FLYING
FOXING
FRYING
FUMING
FUSING
GAGING
GAMING
GAPING
GATING
GAZING
GEEING
GIBING
GIEING
GIVING
GLUING
GORING
GRUING
GUYING
GYRING
HALING
HARING
HATING
HAVING
HAWING
HAYING
HAZING
HEWING
HEXING
HIDING
HIEING
HIKING
HIRING
HIVING
HOEING
HOKING
HOLING
HOMING
HONING
HOPING
HOSING
HUSING
HYPING
ICHING
IDLING
IGGING
INKING
INNING
IRKING
IRVING
ISLING
JADING
JAPING
JAWING
JIBING
JIVING
JOKING
JOYING
JUKING
KEYING
KITING
LACING
LADING
LAMING
LASING
LAVING
LAWING
LAYING
LAZING
LIKING
LIMING
LINING
LIVING
LOPING
LORING
LOSING
LOVING
LOWING
LUBING
LUGING
LURING
MAKING
MATING
MAXING
MAYING
MAZING
METING
MEWING
MIKING
MIMING
MINING
MIRING
MIXING
MOOING
MOPING
MOVING
MOWING
MUSING
MUTING
NAMING
NIXING
NOSING
NOTING
NUKING
OARING
OFFING
OGLING
OILING
OOHING
OOZING
OPTING
ORBING
OUTING
OWNING
PACING
PAGING
PALING
PARING
PAVING
PAWING
PAYING
PEKING
PIKING
PILING
PINING
PIPING
PLYING
POKING
POLING
PORING
POSING
PRYING
PULING
RACING
RAGING
RAKING
RARING
RASING
RATING
RAVING
RAXING
RAYING
RAZING
REDING
RESING
RICING
RIDING
RILING
RIMING
RISING
RIVING
ROBING
ROPING
ROVING
ROWING
RULING
SATING
SAVING
SAWING
SAYING
SEEING
SEWING
SHYING
SIDING
SIRING
SITING
SIZING
SKIING
SKYING
SLUING
SOLING
SOWING
SPRING
SPYING
STRING
STYING
TAKING
TAMING
TAPING
TARING
TAXING
TEEING
TIDING
TILING
TIMING
TIRING
TOEING
TONING
TOPING
TOTING
TOWING
TOYING
TRUING
TRYING
TSKING
TUBING
TUNING
TURING
TYPING
UMPING
UPPING
URGING
USHING
VEXING
VIKING
VINING
VISING
VOTING
VOWING
WADING
WAGING
WAKING
WALING
WANING
WARING
WAVING
WAXING
WILING
WINING
WIPING
WIRING
WISING
WIVING
WOOING
WOWING
YAWING
YOKING
ZONING

••••IG

ALHAIG
BAGWIG
BIGDIG
BIGRIG
BIGWIG
BINNIG
CATRIG
DANZIG
EARWIG
FIZGIG
GEHRIG
HOWBIG
KOENIG
LIEBIG
LUDWIG
MADVIG
OILRIG
OUTRIG
PETPIG
RETTIG
TOOBIG
UNTRIG
WETTIG
WINBIG
WITTIG
WONBIG
YEABIG
YOUDIG
ZAFTIG

I•H•••

ICHING
ICHIRO
ICHORS
ICHTHY
IMHERE
IMHOME
IMHURT
INHALE
INHALF
INHAND
INHERE
INHOCK
INHOME
INHUME
ISHTAR
ITHACA
ITHINK

I••H••

IDAHOS
IFTHEN
INCHED
INCHER
INCHES
INCHON
INTHAT
ISCHIA
ISOHEL
ISTHMI
ITCHED
ITCHES
ITSHOT
ITZHAK

I•••H•

ICHTHY
IEIGHT
IIJOHN
IMIGHT

I••••H

IMPISH
INARCH
INCASH
INDASH
INRUSH
INWITH
IOMOTH
IRTYSH
ISAIAH

•IH•••

HIHATS
HIHIHI
JIHADS
NIHILO
VIHARA

•I•H••

BICHON
BIGHIT
BIGHTS
BIGHUG
BISHOP
CIPHER
DIRHAM
DISHED
DISHES
DISHUP
DITHER
EIGHTA
EIGHTB
EIGHTC
EIGHTD
EIGHTE
EIGHTH
EIGHTS
EIGHTY
EITHER
FICHES
FICHTE
FICHUS
FIGHTS
FISHED
FISHER
FISHES
HIGHER
HIGHIQ
HIGHLY
HIGHON
HIGHUP
HIPHOP
HITHER
KISHKA
KISHKE
LICHEE
LICHEN
LIGHTS
LITHER
LITHIC
LITHOS
MICHEL
MIGHTS
MIGHTY
MISHAP
MISHIT
NICHED
NICHES
NIGHER
NIGHON
NIGHTS
NIGHTY
NIIHAU
PICHEL
PISHED
PISHES
PITHED
RICHEN
RICHER
RICHES
RICHET
RICHIE
RICHIN
RICHLY
RIGHTO
RIGHTS
RIGHTY
RISHIS
SIGHAT
SIGHED
SIGHER
SIGHTS
SIPHON
TIGHTS
TILHIM
TINHAT
TISHRI
TITHED
TITHER
TITHES
VISHNU
WIGHTS
WISHED
WISHER
WISHES
WISHIN
WISHON
WISHTO
WITHAL
WITHER
WITHIN
WITHIT
WITHUS
XINHUA
ZITHER

•I••H•

BINCHY
BIRTHS
DINGHY
FIFTHS
FILTHY
FIRTHS
GIRTHS
HIDEHO
HIHIHI
IIJOHN
KIMCHI
LITCHI
MIRTHS
MISCHA
NINTHS
PICCHU
PITCHY
RICOHS
SIXTHS
TILTHS
WIDTHS
WITCHY

•I•••H

EIGHTH
FINISH
GIVETH
HIRSCH
HITECH
KIBOSH
KIRSCH
KITSCH
LILITH
LIVETH
PISGAH
RIYADH
SIRRAH
WIDISH
WINISH
ZIZITH

••IH••

NIIHAU
SKIHAT

••I•H•

ALIGHT
ARIGHT
BEIGHT
BLIGHT
BLITHE
BRIGHT
CHICHA
CHICHI
CHIRHO
CLICHE
CLICHY
DWIGHT
ELISHA
FAITHS
FLIGHT
FRIGHT
GEIGHT
GEISHA
GRISHA
HAIGHT
HEIGHT
IEIGHT
IMIGHT
KNIGHT
NEIGHS
PLIGHT
POISHA
QUICHE
SAIDHI
SLIGHT
SLITHY
SMITHS
SMITHY
SWISHY
TAICHI
THIGHS
TRISHA
VEIGHT
VOIGHT
WEIGHS
WEIGHT
WRIGHT
WRITHE

••I••H

AFIFTH
ALIOTH
ALIYAH
CHINCH
CLINCH
ELIJAH
FLINCH
FRISCH
GHIRSH
GLITCH
GRINCH
PLINTH
SAIDAH
SHILOH
SKITCH
SMIRCH
SNITCH
SPILTH
STITCH
SWITCH
TWITCH

•••IH•

HIHIHI

•••I•H

AGUISH
ASPISH
AWEIGH
BANISH
BLUISH
BOYISH
CALIPH
COWISH
COYISH
DANISH
DELISH
DHEIGH
DOVISH
DOWITH
DRYISH
DUDISH
ELFISH
ELVISH
ENRICH
EOLITH
FAMISH
FETISH
FINISH
FLUISH
GARISH
GOFISH
GOWITH
HEWISH
IMPISH
INWITH
ISAIAH
JADISH
JEWISH
JOSIAH
JUDITH
LATISH
LAVISH
LEHIGH
LILITH
LOLICH
LOWISH
LUKICH
MARIAH
MODISH
MOPISH
MULISH
MUNICH
NEWISH
OAFISH
ODDISH
OFFISH
OGRISH
OLDISH
ONEISH
ONHIGH
ORNITH
OWLISH
PALISH
PARIAH
PARISH
PERISH
POLISH
POPISH
POVICH
PUNISH
RADISH
RAKISH
RAVISH
RAWISH
RELISH
RUPIAH
SALISH
SHEIKH
SLEIGH
SQUISH
ULRICH
UNNIGH
UNWISH
UPPISH
VANISH
WIDISH
WINISH
WRAITH
ZENITH
ZIZITH
ZURICH

II••••

IIJOHN

I•I•••

IBICES
IBIDEM
IBISES
IBIZAN
ICICLE
ICIEST
ICINGS
IDIDIT
IDIOCY
IDIOMS
IDIOTS
IEIGHT
IFICAN
IFIMAY
IFITIS
IKINGS
ILIADS
IMIDES
IMIGHT
IMINES
INIONS
INITIO
IRIDES
IRIDIC
IRISED
IRISES
IRISIN
IRITIC
IRITIS
ISIDOR
ISIDRO
ISINTO
ISITME
ITILES
ITIOUS
ITISSO

I••I••

ICHING
ICHIRO
ICKIER
IDLING
IDOIDO
IFFIER
IGGING
IGGINS
IGNITE
IKOIKO
ILLINI
ILOILO
IMBIBE
IMFINE
IMLIKE
IMMIES
IMPISH
INCISE
INCITE
INDIAN
INDICT
INDIES
INDIGO
INDIRA
INDITE
INDIUM
INFIRM
INKIER
INKIND
INKING
INLIEU
INLINE
INMIND
INNIES
INNING
INPINK
INSIDE
INSIST
INSITU
INTIME
INUITS
INVIEW
INVITE
INVIVO
INWITH
IODIDE
IODINE
IODISE
IODIZE
IONIAN
IONICS
IONISE
IONIUM
IONIZE
IRAISE
IRKING
IRVINE
IRVING
ISAIAH
ISAIAN
ISLIKE
ISLING
ITGIRL
ITHINK
ITRIED

I•••I•

IAMBIC
IATRIC
IBERIA
ICARIA
ICEDIN
ICEDIT
ICESIN
ICESIT
ICONIC
IDIDIT
IFITIS
IGETIT
IGOTIT
ILLLIT
IMONIT
IMPAIR
INABIT
INAFIX
INAPIE
INATIE
INCAIC
INGRID
INITIO
INJAIL
INKSIN
INLAID
INSTIL

INSTIR
INTOIT
INTUIT
INUPIK
INVAIN
IRANIS
IRAQIS
IRENIC
IRIDIC
IRISIN
IRITIC
IRITIS
IRONIC
ISCHIA
ISEEIT
ISELIN
ISMAIL
ISRAIR
ISSEIS
ISTRIA
ITALIA
ITALIC
IVANIV

I••••I
IDENTI
ILLINI
INCUBI
IOLANI
ISANTI
ISTHMI
ITURBI
IVANVI

•II•••
NIIHAU

•I•I••
AIDING
AIKIDO
AILING
AIMING
AIRIER
AIRILY
AIRING
BIDING
BIKILA
BIKING
BIKINI
BIMINI
BITING
CILIUM
CIMINO
CITIED
CITIES
CITIFY
CITING
CITIUS
CIVICS
DICIER
DICING
DIDIES
DIDION
DIGITS
DIKING
DIMING
DIMITY
DINING
DIRIGE
DIRIGO
DIVIDE
DIVINE
DIVING
DIXITS
FIFING
FIJIAN
FILIAL
FILING
FINIAL
FINIAN
FINING
FINISH
FINITE
FINITO
FIRING
FIXING
FIXINS
FIXITY
GIBILL
GIBING
GIEING
GIVING
HIDING
HIEING
HIHIHI
HIKING
HIRING
HITINS
HIVING
JIBING
JIMINY
JIVIER
JIVING
KIBITZ
KILIMS
KITING
LIAISE
LIBIDO
LIKING
LILIAN
LILIED
LILIES
LILIOM
LILITH
LIMIER
LIMING
LIMITS
LINIER
LINING
LIPIDS
LIVING
MIDIAN
MIKING
MIKITA
MILIEU
MIMICS
MIMING
MINIFY
MINIMA
MINIME
MINIMI
MINIMS
MINING
MINION
MINITV
MIRIAM
MIRIER
MIRING
MIRINS
MIXING
NICIAS
NIDIFY
NIHILO
NIKITA
NIMINY
NIMITZ
NIXIES
NIXING
OILIER
OILILY
OILING
PIKING
PILING
PIMINY
PINIER
PINING
PINION
PIPIER
PIPING
PIPITS
PITIED
PITIER
PITIES
PIXIES
RIBISI
RICING
RIDING
RILING
RIMIER
RIMING
RIMINI
RISING
RIVING
SICILY
SIDING
SIGILS
SILICA
SIMIAN
SIMILE
SINISE
SIRICA
SIRING
SIRIUS
SISISI
SITING
SITINS
SIZING
TIBIAE
TIBIAL
TIBIAS
TICINO
TIDIED
TIDIER
TIDIES
TIDILY
TIDING
TIEINS
TILING
TIMING
TINIAN
TINIER
TINILY
TIPINS
TIRIAC
TIRING
TITIAN
VIBIST
VIDIOT
VIEIRA
VIGIAS
VIGILS
VIKING
VILIFY
VINIER
VINIFY
VINING
VIRILE
VISINE
VISING
VISION
VISITS
VIVIAN
VIVICA
VIVIEN
VIVIFY
VIZIER
VIZIRS
WIDISH
WIFIED
WIFIES
WILIER
WILILY
WILING
WINIER
WINING
WINISH
WIPING
WIRIER
WIRILY
WIRING
WISING
WIVING
ZIZITH

•I••I•
AIOLIS
BIALIK
BIBLIO
BIDSIN
BIGAIR
BIGDIG
BIGGIE
BIGHIT
BIGKID
BIGLIE
BIGOIL
BIGRIG
BIGWIG
BIGWIN
BILLIE
BILLIS
BINNIE
BINNIG
BIONIC
BIOPIC
BIOTIC
BIOTIN
BIRDIE
BIRGIT
BITEIN
BIZKIT
CIGGIE
CITRIC
CITRIN
DIALIN
DIARIO
DICKIE
DIESIS
DIGSIN
DIGSIT
DIKDIK
DIMWIT
DINDIN
DINEIN
DIOXIN
DIPSIN
DISTIL
DIVEIN
DIZAIN
FIBRIN
FILEIN
FILLIN
FILLIP
FILMIC
FINNIC
FIRKIN
FISTIC
FITSIN
FIZGIG
GILLIS
GILPIN
GIMMIE
GINNIE
GIRLIE
GIVEIN
HIGHIQ
HINGIS
HIPPIE
HITSIT
JILLIE
JIMMIE
JINNIS
KIARIO
KICKIN
KIDDIE
KIDLIT
KIDVID
KILTIE
KISSIN
LIBRIS
LIEBIG
LIESIN
LIEVIO
LIFEIS
LIGEIA
LIGNIN
LILKIM
LILLIE
LILLIS
LIMBIC
LIMPID
LIQUID
LITHIC
LIVEIN
LIZZIE
MIAMIS
MIAMIU
MIDAIR
MIDDIE
MIDRIB
MILLIE
MILTIE
MINNIE
MINUIT
MISAIM
MISDID
MISFIT
MISHIT
MISSIS
NIACIN
NIOBIC
NISEIS
NITRIC
NITWIT
OILLIT
OILRIG
PICNIC
PICRIC
PIDGIN
PIERIA
PIETIN
PIGGIE
PIGSIT
PILEIN
PINKIE
PINYIN
PIPEIN
PIPPIN
PIPPIP
PIRRIP
PISTIL
PITKIN
PIUSII
PIUSIV
PIUSIX
RIBBIT
RICHIE
RICHIN
RICKIE
RIDEIN
RIFKIN
RINGIN
RISHIS
RISKIT
SIGNIN
SIKKIM
SINGIN
SINKIN
SITSIN
SITTIN
SIXPIN
SIXSIX
TIDBIT
TIEDIN
TIEPIN
TIESIN
TIFFIN
TIGRIS
TIKRIT
TILHIM
TILLIE
TILLIS
TILSIT
TIPSIN
VICTIM
VINCIT
VINNIE
VIOLIN
VIRGIL
VIRGIN
VISCID
VITRIC
WIENIE
WIGGIN
WILKIE
WILLIE
WILLIS
WIMMIN
WINBIG
WINGIT
WINKIE
WINNIE
WINWIN
WIREIN
WISHIN
WITHIN
WITHIT
WITTIG
XINGIN
YIPPIE
ZINCIC
ZINNIA
ZIPSIN
ZIPSIT

•I•••I
BIGBOI
BIKINI
BILOXI
BIMINI
BIONDI
CIARDI
CISKEI
DITALI
GIAMBI
GIANNI
HIDEKI
HIHIHI
KIGALI
KIMCHI
KINSKI
LIGETI
LIPARI
LITCHI
MIDORI
MINIMI
NIELLI
NIKKEI
PIAZZI
PIUSII
PIUSVI
PIUSXI
RIBISI
RIENZI
RIGATI
RIMINI
RIVOLI
SISISI
TISHRI
TIVOLI
VIDERI

••II••
SHIISM
SHIITE
SKIING

••I•I•
ACIDIC
AJIJIC
ALIBIS
ALICIA
AMITIE
BLIFIL
BLINIS
BRIGID
BRIGIT
CHILIS
CHIPIN
CLINIC
CRISIS
CRITIC
DEIFIC
DRIVIN
EDITIO
ELICIT
ELIXIR
EMILIA
EMILIE
EMILIO
EXILIC
FLITIN
FRIGID
GAIJIN
HEINIE
HOISIN
IDIDIT
IFITIS
INITIO
IRIDIC
IRISIN
IRITIC
IRITIS
JOININ
LAIDIN
LAINIE
MAILIN
MAISIE
NAILIN
NAILIT
ODINIC
OLIVIA
ORIBIS
ORIGIN
OSIRIS
OTITIC
OTITIS
OXIDIC
PAIDIN
PHILIC
PHILIP
QUITIT
RAININ
RAISIN
REININ
SCIPIO
SKIBIB
SKIPIT
SLIDIN
SLIPIN
SOITIS
SPIRIT
STIRIN
STIVIC
TRICIA
TRIVIA
TRIXIE
TWILIT
UNIFIC
WHIPIN
XZIBIT

••I••I
ARIOSI
CHICHI
CHILLI
DJINNI
DMITRI
ELIELI
FRITZI
GRIGRI
GRITTI
HAIKAI
KRISTI
MAITAI
ORIANI
OUIOUI
PRIORI
PRIZZI
QUINTI
SAIDHI
TAICHI
TAIPEI

•••II•
ACTIII
LEOIII

•••I•I
ACTIII
ASSISI
BIKINI
BIMINI
CUBITI
DAVIDI
DEDINI
DODICI
DOMINI
FELIXI
GEMINI
HIHIHI
ILLINI
KWEISI
LATINI
LEOIII
LOUISI
MEDICI
MINIMI
ORSINI
PANINI
PARINI
PERITI
RAPINI
REMINI
RIBISI
RIMINI
ROTINI
SEDICI
SENITI
SISISI
SODIDI
SURIMI
TAHINI
TAHITI
UNDICI
WAPITI
YOGINI

••••II
ACTIII
BOOKII
ETALII
HAWAII
JOHNII
LEOIII
LEOVII
LEOXII
MARKII
MARYII
OLAFII
OLAVII
OTTOII
PARTII
PAULII
PIUSII
SALTII
SAVAII
TRACII

IJ••••
IJKLMN
IJSSEL

I•J•••
IIJOHN
INJAIL
INJECT
INJEST
INJOKE
INJULY
INJUNE
INJURE
INJURY

I••J••
INAJAM
INKJET

I••••J
INTERJ

•IJ•••
BIJOUS
BIJOUX
FIJIAN
GIJANE
GIJOES
HIJACK
HIJKLM
IIJOHN
RIJEKA

•I•J••
BIGJOE
NINJAS
RIOJAS
TIPJAR

•I••J•
NICKJR

••IJ••
AJIJIC
ELIJAH
FRIJOL
GAIJIN
GHIJKL
OUIJAS
TRIJET

••I•J•
DRIQJR

•••IJ•
FGHIJK
ROMIJN

•••I•J
LODINJ

••••IJ
EFGHIJ

IK••••
IKINGS
IKOIKO

I•K•••
ICKIER
IJKLMN
INKERS
INKIER
INKIND
INKING
INKJET
INKLES
INKPAD
INKPOT
INKSAC
INKSIN
IRKERS
IRKING

I••K••
IMOKAY

I•••K•
IBOOKS
IKOIKO
IMLIKE
INJOKE
INTAKE
INVOKE
ISLIKE
IVANKA

I••••K
IMBACK
INBACK
INBULK
INHOCK
INLUCK
INPARK
INPINK
INUPIK
ISNTOK
ITHINK
ITZHAK

•IK•••
AIKIDO
AIKMAN
BIKERS
BIKILA
BIKING
BIKINI
DIKDIK
DIKERS
DIKING
DIKTAT
HIKERS
HIKEUP
HIKING
KIKUYU
LIKELY
LIKENS
LIKERS
LIKESO
LIKETO
LIKING
LIKUTA
MIKADO
MIKASA
MIKING
MIKITA
NIKEAD
NIKITA
NIKKEI
NIKOLA
NIKONS
PIKERS
PIKING
RIKERS
SIKKIM
TIKKAS
TIKRIT
VIKING
VIKTOR

•I•K••
BICKER
BIGKID
BILKED
BILKER
BIZKIT
CISKEI
DICKER
DICKEY
DICKIE
DINKAS
DINKUM
DIRKED
DISKED
FICKLE
FINKED
FINKEL
FINKON
FIRKIN
GINKGO
HICKAM
HICKEY
HICKOK
HIJKLM
HINKLE
KICKED
KICKER
KICKIN
KICKUP
KINKED
KINKOS
KIRKUK
KITKAT
LICKED
LICKER
LICKUP
LILKIM
LINKED
LINKER
LINKUP
MICKEY
MILKED
MILKER
MISKEY
NICKED
NICKEL
NICKER
NICKJR
NIEKRO
NIKKEI
OINKED
OINKER
PICKAT
PICKAX
PICKED
PICKER
PICKET
PICKLE
PICKON
PICKUP
PINKED
PINKEN
PINKER
PINKIE
PINKOS
PITKIN
RICKEY
RICKIE
RIFKIN
RIPKEN
RISKED
RISKER
RISKIT
SICKEN
SICKER
SICKLE
SICKLY
SICKOF
SICKOS
SIKKIM
SILKEN
SINKER
SINKIN
SIRKAY
SISKEL
TICKBY
TICKED
TICKER
TICKET
TICKLE
TICKLY
TIKKAS
TINKER
TINKLE
TINKLY
TISKET
WICKED
WICKER
WICKET
WILKES
WILKIE
WINKAT
WINKED
WINKER
WINKIE

•I••K•
BIGSKY
GINGKO
HIDEKI
KINSKI
KIOSKS
KISHKA
KISHKE
RIJEKA
RIMSKY
TILAKS
ZINCKY

•I•••K
BIALIK
DIKDIK
HICKOK
HIJACK
KIRKUK
LITVAK
PINOAK

••IK••
ALIKES
BAIKAL
CRIKEY
HAIKAI
HAIKUS
SEIKOS
SPIKED
SPIKER
SPIKES
TRIKES

••I•K•
BLINKS
BRICKS
BRICKY
BRINKS
BRISKS
BUICKS
CHICKS
CHINKS
CHINKY
CLICKS
CLINKS
CRICKS
DRINKS
FLICKA
FLICKS
FRICKA
FRICKE
FRISKS
FRISKY
GHIJKL
GLINKA
GRIMKE
KLICKS
KNICKS
PLINKS
PRICKS
PRINKS
QUIRKS
QUIRKY
REINKS
SHIRKS
SKINKS
SLICKS
SLINKS
SLINKY
SMIRKS
SMIRKY
SNICKS
SPINKS
STICKS
STICKY
STINKO
STINKS
STINKY
THICKE
THINKS
TRICKS
TRICKY
UMIAKS
WHISKS
WHISKY
YOICKS

••I••K
ENIDOK
SAIDOK
SAITEK
SPIVAK

•••IK•
ANNIKA
AXLIKE
BATIKS
BELIKE
DOLIKE
GOLIKE
IKOIKO
IMLIKE
ISLIKE
LUNIKS
MARIKO
ONMIKE
OXLIKE
RUBIKS
SHEIKH
SHEIKS
SHRIKE
STRIKE
TROIKA
UNLIKE
UPDIKE

•••I•K
ATRISK
DRYINK
ENLINK
FGHIJK
HODIAK
INPINK
ITHINK
KODIAK

MALICK
MRDICK
MUSICK
NATICK
NORISK
ONDISK
PENICK
REDINK
REKICK
RELINK
REMICK
REPICK
RESINK
SCHICK
SHRIEK
SHRINK
SHTICK
SOYINK
STNICK
UNKINK
UNLINK
UNPICK
UNSICK
UPLINK
UPTICK
YORICK

••••IK
BIALIK
BROVIK
DIKDIK
HENRIK
INUPIK
JARVIK
NARVIK
NUDNIK
RESNIK
TUGRIK
ZADDIK

IL••••
ILEANA
ILEXES
ILIADS
ILLBET
ILLDRY
ILLEST
ILLFED
ILLINI
ILLLIT
ILLMET
ILLOFF
ILLSAY
ILLSEE
ILLSET
ILLUDE
ILLUME
ILLUSE
ILOILO

I•L•••
IDLERS
IDLEST
IDLING
IGLOOS
ILLBET
ILLDRY
ILLEST
ILLFED
ILLINI
ILLLIT
ILLMET
ILLOFF
ILLSAY
ILLSEE
ILLSET
ILLUDE
ILLUME
ILLUSE
IMLATE
IMLIKE
INLAID
INLAND
INLAWS
INLAYS
INLEAF
INLETS
INLIEU
INLINE
INLOVE
INLUCK
IOLANI
IRLENE
ISLAND
ISLATE
ISLEFT
ISLETS
ISLEYS
ISLIKE
ISLING
ITLLDO

I••L••
ICALLY
IDOLUM
IDYLLS
IJKLMN
ILLLIT
IMELDA
IMGLAD
IMPLED
INBLUE
INFLOW
INFLUX
INGLES
INKLES
INPLAY
ISELIN
ISOLDA
ISOLDE
ISTLES
ITALIA
ITALIC
ITILES
ITLLDO

I•••L•
ICALLY
ICICLE
ICOULD
IDEALS
IDYLLS
IFONLY
ILOILO
IMCOLD
IMFULL
IMPALA
IMPALE
IMPELS
IMSOLD
IMTOLD
INBULK
INCULT
INFALL
INFOLD
INFULL
INGELS
INGOLD
INGULF
INHALE
INHALF
INJULY
INSOLE
INSULT
ISEULT
ITSELF
IWOULD

I••••L
IJSSEL
IMCOOL
IMFULL
INFALL
INFULL
INGOAL
INJAIL
INSTAL
INSTIL
IREFUL
IRREAL
ISABEL
ISMAIL
ISOHEL
ISRAEL
ITGIRL

•IL•••
AILEEN
AILING
AILURO
BILBAO
BILDAD
BILGED
BILGES
BILKED
BILKER
BILLED
BILLER
BILLET
BILLIE
BILLIS
BILLOW
BILOXI
CILIUM
DILATE
DILLAR
DILLER
DILLON
DILSEY
DILUTE
EILEEN
EILERS
EILERT
FILEBY
FILEIN
FILENE
FILERS
FILETS
FILIAL
FILING
FILLED
FILLER
FILLES
FILLET
FILLIN
FILLIP
FILLUP
FILMED
FILMIC
FILOSE
FILTER
FILTHY
GILDED
GILDER
GILEAD
GILELS
GILLAN
GILLED
GILLEY
GILLIS
GILMAN
GILPIN
GILROY
HILARY
HILLED
HILLEL
HILLER
HILTED
HILTON
JILLIE
JILTED
JILTER
KILIMS
KILLED
KILLER
KILMER
KILNED
KILROY
KILTED
KILTER
KILTIE
LILACS
LILIAN
LILIED
LILIES
LILIOM
LILITH
LILKIM
LILLIE
LILLIS
LILTED
MILADY
MILANO
MILANS
MILDER
MILDEW
MILDLY
MILERS
MILIEU
MILKED
MILKER
MILLAY
MILLED
MILLER
MILLES
MILLET
MILLIE
MILNER
MILNES
MILORD
MILOSZ
MILSAP
MILTIE
MILTON
OILCAN
OILCUP
OILERS
OILIER
OILILY
OILING
OILLIT
OILMAN
OILMEN
OILPAN
OILRIG
OILRUB
PILAFS
PILATE
PILAUS
PILEIN
PILEON
PILERS
PILEUM
PILEUP
PILEUS
PILFER
PILING
PILLAR
PILLED
PILLOW
PILOSE
PILOTS
PILOUS
RILERS
RILEUP
RILING
RILLES
RILLET
SILAGE
SILENT
SILICA
SILKEN
SILOED
SILTED
SILVAS
SILVER
TILAKS
TILDEN
TILDES
TILERS
TILERY
TILHIM
TILING
TILLED
TILLER
TILLET
TILLEY
TILLIE
TILLIS
TILNOW
TILSIT
TILSON
TILTAT
TILTED
TILTER
TILTHS
TILTON
TILTUP
VILELY
VILEST
VILIFY
VILLAS
VILLON
WILBUR
WILCOX
WILDER
WILDLY
WILIER
WILILY
WILING
WILKES
WILKIE
WILLBE
WILLDO
WILLED
WILLEM
WILLER
WILLIE
WILLIS
WILLOW
WILLYS
WILMUT
WILSON
WILTED
WILTON

•I•L••
AIELLO
AIGLET
AIOLIS
AIRLOG
AISLED
AISLES
BIALIK
BIBLES
BIBLIO
BIGLIE
BILLED
BILLER
BILLET
BILLIE
BILLIS
BILLOW
BIOLAB
BIRLED
BIRLER
CIELOS
DIALED
DIALER
DIALIN
DIALOG
DIALSO
DIALUP
DIGLOT
DILLAR
DILLER
DILLON
DIPLEX
EISLEY
FIDLER
FIELDS
FILLED
FILLER
FILLES
FILLET
FILLIN
FILLIP
FILLUP
FINLEY
GIBLET
GILLAN
GILLED
GILLEY
GILLIS
GIMLET
GIRLIE
HILLED
HILLEL
HILLER
JILLIE
KIDLIT
KILLED
KILLER
KISLEV
LIELOW
LILLIE
LILLIS
LISLES
MIDLEG
MIDLER
MIELES
MILLAY
MILLED
MILLER
MILLES
MILLET
MILLIE
MISLAY
MISLED
NIBLET
NIELLI
NIELLO
OILLIT
PIELET
PIGLET
PILLAR
PILLED
PILLOW
PIOLET
RIALTO
RIBLET
RIDLEY
RIFLED
RIFLER
RIFLES
RILLES
RILLET
RIPLEY
SIDLED
SIDLES
SIGLER
SISLER
SISLEY
TIGLON
TILLED
TILLER
TILLET
TILLEY
TILLIE
TILLIS
TITLED
TITLES
VIALED
VIELLE
VILLAS
VILLON
VIOLAS
VIOLET
VIOLIN
WIELDS
WIELDY
WIGLET
WILLBE
WILLDO
WILLED
WILLEM
WILLER
WILLIE
WILLIS
WILLOW
WILLYS
YIELDS
ZIPLOC

•I••L•
AIELLO
AIRILY
BIFOLD
BIKILA
BINDLE
BINGLE
CIBOLA
CICELY
CIRCLE
DIABLE
DIABLO
DIBBLE
DIDDLE
DIDDLY
DIMPLE
DIMPLY
DINGLE
DIPOLE
DIRELY
DITALI
EIDOLA
EISELE
FIBULA
FICKLE
FIDDLE
FINALE
FINALS
FINELY
FIPPLE
FIRMLY
FIZZLE
GIBILL
GIGGLE
GIGGLY
GIGOLO
GILELS
GIMELS
GIRDLE
GISELE
HIGGLE
HIGHLY
HIJKLM
HINGLE
HINKLE
HIYALL
JIGGLE
JIGGLY
JINGLE
JINGLY
KIBBLE
KIDULT
KIGALI
KIMBLE
KINDLE
KINDLY
KINGLY
LIABLE
LIBELS
LIEFLY
LIKELY
LIMPLY
LINGLE
LIONLY
LITTLE
LIVELY
LIZALU
MIDDLE
MILDLY
MINGLE
MIZZLE
MIZZLY
NIBBLE
NICELY
NICOLA
NICOLE
NICOLO
NIELLI
NIELLO
NIGGLE
NIHILO
NIKOLA
NIMBLE
NIMBLY
NIPPLE
OILILY
PICKLE
PIDDLE
PIFFLE
PIMPLE
PIMPLY
PIXELS
RIBALD
RICHLY
RICOLA
RIDDLE
RIFELY
RIFFLE
RIMPLE
RIPELY
RIPPLE
RIPPLY
RIVALS
RIVOLI
RIYALS
SIBYLS
SICILY
SICKLE
SICKLY
SIECLE
SIGILS
SIMILE
SIMPLE
SIMPLY
SINGLE
SINGLY
SISALS
SISSLE
SIZZLE
TICALS
TICKLE
TICKLY
TIDILY
TIMELY
TINGLE
TINGLY
TINILY
TINKLE
TINKLY
TIPPLE
TITTLE
TIVOLI
VIABLE
VIABLY
VIELLE
VIGILS
VILELY
VINYLS
VIRILE
VITALE
VITALS
VITTLE
VIZSLA
WIDELY
WIFELY
WIFFLE
WIGGLE
WIGGLY
WILDLY
WILILY
WIMPLE
WIRILY
WISELY

•I•••L
AIDFUL
AIMFUL
BIGOIL
CINEOL
DIABOL
DIESEL
DIRNDL
DISMAL
DISPEL
DISTAL
DISTIL
EIFFEL
FIEVEL
FILIAL
FINIAL
FINKEL
FISCAL
FITFUL
GIBILL
GIMBAL
GIMBEL
HIATAL
HIEMAL
HILLEL
HIMMEL
HIYALL
KISSEL
LINEAL
LINTEL
LIONEL
MICHEL
MIGUEL
MISSAL
MITRAL
NICKEL
PICHEL
PINEAL
PISTIL
PISTOL
RICTAL
RITUAL
SIEGEL
SIGNAL
SINFUL
SISKEL
TIBIAL
TIMBAL
TINEAL
TINSEL
VIRGIL
VISUAL
WIESEL
WITHAL
ZIFFEL

••IL••
AGILER
ATILES
AXILLA
BAILED
BAILEE
BAILER
BAILEY
BAILON
BAILOR
BOILED
BOILER
BOILUP
BRILLO
BTILES
BUILDS
CEILED
CHILDE
CHILES
CHILIS
CHILLI
CHILLS
CHILLY
COILED
COILER
COILUP
CTILES
DAILEY
DJILAS
DRILLS
DTILES
EDILES
EFILED
EFILES
EMILIA
EMILIE
EMILIO
EMILYS
EPILOG
ETILES
EVILER
EVILLY
EXILED
EXILER
EXILES
EXILIC
FAILED
FAILLE
FAILTO
FOILED
FRILLS
FRILLY
FTILES
GRILLE
GRILLS
GTILES
GUILDS
GUILED
GUILES
GUILTY
HAILED
HAILER
HAILEY
HTILES
ITILES
JAILED
JAILER
JAILOR
JTILES
KAILUA
KTILES
LTILES
MAILED
MAILER
MAILIN
MAILTO
MOILED
MOILER
MTILES
NAILED
NAILER
NAILIN
NAILIT
NAILUP
NTILES
OTILES
PHILBY
PHILCO
PHILIC
PHILIP
PHILLY
POILUS
PTILES
QTILES
QUILLS
QUILTS
RAILAT
RAILED
RAILER
RAILON
REILLY
ROILED
ROILUP
RTILES
SAILED
SAILER
SAILON
SAILOR
SAILTO
SHILLS
SHILLY
SHILOH
SKILLS
SMILED
SMILER
SMILES
SMILEY
SMILLA
SOILED
SPILES
SPILLS
SPILTH
STILES
STILLE
STILLS
STILLY
STILTS
SWILLS
TAILED
TAILER
TAILOR
TBILLS
THILLS
TOILAT
TOILED
TOILER
TOILES
TOILET
TRILBY
TRILLO
TRILLS
TTILES
TUILLE
TWILIT
TWILLS
VAILCO
VEILED
VEILER
VOILES
VTILES
WAILED
WAILER
WHILED
WHILES
WHILST
WTILES
XFILES
XTILES
YTILES
ZTILES

••I•L•
ACIDLY
AFIELD
ALIBLE
ARIDLY
AVIDLY
AXILLA
BGIRLS
BRIDLE
BRILLO
CHICLE
CHICLY
CHILLI
CHILLS
CHILLY
DRILLS
EDIBLE
EDIBLY
ELIELI
ENISLE
EVILLY
FAILLE
FAIRLY
FOIBLE
FRIELS
FRILLS
FRILLY
GAINLY
GLIBLY
GRILLE
GRILLS
GRIMLY
GRISLY
ICICLE
MAINLY
ORIELS
ORIOLE
PHIALS
PHILLY
PRIMLY
QUILLS
REILLY
SHIELD
SHILLS
SHILLY
SKILLS
SKIRLS
SLIMLY
SMILLA
SPIELS
SPILLS
STIFLE
STILLE
STILLS
STILLY
SWILLS
SWIRLS
SWIRLY
SWIRLZ
TBILLS
THILLS
THINLY
TRIALS
TRIFLE
TRILLO
TRILLS
TRIMLY
TRIPLE
TRIPLY
TUILLE
TWILLS
TWIRLS
TWIRLY
UNIDLE
UNIDLY
VAINLY
WHIRLS
WHIRLY

••I••L
AMICAL
AMIDOL
ANIMAL
APICAL
BAIKAL
BLIFIL
BRIDAL
CHISEL
DRIVEL
EPICAL
EPINAL
FAISAL
FRIJOL
FRIVOL
GEISEL
GHIJKL
GRINDL
KEITEL
LAICAL
OGIVAL
PRIMAL
RHINAL
SNIVEL
SPINAL
SPINEL
SPIRAL
SWIVEL
TRIBAL
TRINAL
TVIDOL
VEINAL

•••IL•
ADVILS
AEDILE
AERILY
AIRILY
ANVILS
APRILE
APRILS
AQUILA
ARTILY
ATTILA
ATWILL
AUDILE
AVAILS
AVRILS
AWHILE
BASILS
BIKILA
BODILY
BOXILY
BROILS
BUSILY
CAGILY
CAHILL
CAVILS
CECILB
CECILE
COSILY
COZILY
CYBILL
DANILO
DECILE
DEFILE

DEMILO
DESILT
DESILU
DEVILS
DEWILY
DOCILE
DOPILY
DOZILY
EASILY
EDGILY
EERILY
EMAILS
ENGILD
ENOILS
ENSILE
ETAILS
ETOILE
FACILE
FAMILY
FLAILS
FOXILY
FUSILE
FUSILS
FUTILE
GAMILY
GIBILL
GORILY
GOWILD
GRAILS
HABILE
HAMILL
HAZILY
HOKILY
HOLILY
HOMILY
ILOILO
JOKILY
KURILE
LABILE
LACILY
LAZILY
LOGILY
LUCILE
MANILA
MARILU
MAZILY
MCGILL
MOBILE
MOTILE
MRBILL
NEVILL
NIHILO
NOBILE
NOSILY
NOTILL
NUBILE
OILILY
ONEILL
ONFILE
ONFILM
OOZILY
PERILS
POKILY
PUNILY
PUPILS
QUAILS
RACILY
REBILL
REFILE
REFILL
REFILM
REGILD
REMILL
REOILS
RESILE
RETILE
RETILL
REVILE
ROSILY
RUTILE
SENILE
SEXILY
SHEILA
SHRILL
SICILY
SIGILS
SIMILE
SNAILS
SPOILS
SPOILT
TAMILS
THRILL
TIDILY
TINILY
TRAILS
UGLILY
UNFILE
UNGILT
UNOILY
UNPILE
UNTILT
UNWILD
UNWILY
UPHILL
UPPILE
UPTILT
VASILY
VERILY
VIGILS
VIRILE
WARILY
WAVILY
WAXILY
WILILY
WIRILY
ZANILY

•••I•L

ABDIEL
AERIAL
ASWIRL
ATRIAL
ATWILL
AUDIAL
AWHIRL
BASIAL
BELIAL
BURIAL
CAHILL
CYBILL
DANIEL
DAVIDL
DENIAL
ENTIAL
ESPIAL
FACIAL
FILIAL
FINIAL
GAVIAL
GENIAL
GIBILL
GOGIRL
HAMILL
ITGIRL
JOVIAL
LABIAL
MARIEL
MCGILL
MEDIAL
MENIAL
MESIAL
MRBILL
MURIEL
MUSIAL
MYGIRL
NARIAL
NEVILL
NOMIAL
NOTILL
ONEILL
RACIAL
RADIAL
REBILL
REDIAL
REFILL
REMILL
RETIAL
RETILL
SERIAL
SHRILL
SOCIAL
THRILL
TIBIAL
UNCIAL
UPHILL
VENIAL

••••IL

AGNAIL
ASSAIL
BEWAIL
BIGOIL
BLIFIL
BRASIL
BRAZIL
BYMAIL
DATRIL
DEASIL
DERAIL
DETAIL
DISTIL
DREVIL
DRPHIL
EMERIL
ENTAIL
ENVEIL
EURAIL
FOSSIL
FULFIL
GASOIL
GERBIL
HOTOIL
INJAIL
INSTIL
ISMAIL
KAHLIL
LENTIL
MARCIL
MCNEIL
MELVIL
NOTAIL
NUTOIL
NYQUIL
ONBAIL
OXTAIL
PENCIL
PISTIL
POPEIL
REBOIL
RECOIL
REJAIL
REMAIL
RENAIL
RESOIL
RETAIL
SOLEIL
TAROIL
TONSIL
UNCOIL
UNEVIL
UNNAIL
UNVEIL
UPCOIL
URACIL
USMAIL
VERGIL
VIRGIL
WEEVIL

IM••••

IMACOP
IMAGED
IMAGER
IMAGES
IMAGOS
IMAMAN
IMARET
IMAXES
IMBACK
IMBEAT
IMBEDS
IMBIBE
IMBRUE
IMBUED
IMBUES
IMBUSY
IMCOLD
IMCOOL
IMDONE
IMEANT
IMEASY
IMELDA
IMFINE
IMFREE
IMFULL
IMGAME
IMGLAD
IMGONE
IMGOOD
IMHERE
IMHOME
IMHURT
IMIDES
IMIGHT
IMINES
IMLATE
IMLIKE
IMMIES
IMMUNE
IMMUNO
IMMURE
IMNEXT
IMOGEN
IMOKAY
IMONIT
IMPACT
IMPAIR
IMPALA
IMPALE
IMPART
IMPEDE
IMPELS
IMPEND
IMPERF
IMPISH
IMPLED
IMPORT
IMPOSE
IMPOST
IMPROV
IMPUGN
IMPURE
IMPUTE
IMSOLD
IMSURE
IMTOLD

I•M•••

IAMBIC
IAMBUS
IAMNOT
IAMSAM
IAMTOO
IBMPCS
IMMIES
IMMUNE
IMMUNO
IMMURE
INMATE
INMIND
INMOST
IOMEGA
IOMOTH
ISMAIL
ISMENE

I••M••

ICEMAN
ICEMEN
IFIMAY
ILLMET
IMAMAN
INGMAR
ISOMER
ITEMED

I•••M•

IBEAMS
IDIOMS
IJKLMN
ILLUME
IMGAME
IMHOME
INCOME
INFAMY
INHOME
INHUME
INTIME
ISITME
ISTHMI

I••••M

IAMSAM
IBIDEM
ICEDAM
IDOLUM
INAJAM
INDIUM
INFIRM
INFORM
INGRAM
INSEAM
IONIUM

•IM•••

AIMERS
AIMFOR
AIMFUL
AIMING
AIMSAT
BIMBOS
BIMINI
CIMINO
DIMAGE
DIMING
DIMITY
DIMMED
DIMMER
DIMOUT
DIMPLE
DIMPLY
DIMSUM
DIMWIT
GIMBAL
GIMBEL
GIMELS
GIMLET
GIMMES
GIMMIE
GIMPED
HIMMEL
JIMBOB
JIMINY
JIMMIE
JIMSON
KIMBLE
KIMCHI
KIMONO
LIMANS
LIMBED
LIMBER
LIMBIC
LIMBOS
LIMIER
LIMING
LIMITS
LIMNED
LIMNER
LIMPED
LIMPER
LIMPET
LIMPID
LIMPLY
MIMEOS
MIMERS
MIMICS
MIMING
MIMOSA
NIMBLE
NIMBLY
NIMBUS
NIMINY
NIMITZ
NIMROD
PIMINY
PIMPLE
PIMPLY
RIMATE
RIMERS
RIMIER
RIMING
RIMINI
RIMMED
RIMOSE
RIMOUS
RIMPLE
RIMSKY
SIMEON
SIMIAN
SIMILE
SIMMER
SIMONE
SIMPER
SIMPLE
SIMPLY
TIMBAL
TIMBER
TIMBRE
TIMELY
TIMERS
TIMING
WIMMER
WIMMIN
WIMPED
WIMPLE
WIMSEY
ZIMMER

•I•M••

AIDMAN
AIDMEN
AIKMAN
AIRMAN
AIRMEN
BIGMAC
BIGMAN
BIGMEN
BIOMES
BIRMAN
BITMAP
DIMMED
DIMMER
DIOMED
DISMAL
DISMAS
DISMAY
DISMES
FILMED
FILMIC
FIRMED
FIRMER
FIRMLY
FIRMUP
GIAMBI
GILMAN
GIMMES
GIMMIE
GISMOS
GIZMOS
HIEMAL
HIMMEL
HITMAN
HITMEN
JIMMIE
KIDMAN
KILMER
KIRMAN
KISMET
LITMUS
MIAMIS
MIAMIU
MICMAC
MIDMAY
NIAMEY
OILMAN
OILMEN
PIEMAN
PIEMEN
PIGMAN
PIGMEN
PITMAN
PITMEN
RIMMED
SIGMAS
SIMMER
TIEMPO
TINMAN
TINMEN
WIEMAN
WILMUT
WIMMER
WIMMIN
ZIMMER

•I••M•

BIGAMY
BIREME
CINEMA
DIGAMY
DIRAMS
JICAMA
KILIMS
KINGME
KISSME
MIASMA
MINIMA
MINIME
MINIMI
MINIMS
MISSME

•I•••M

AIRARM
AIRDAM
BIFORM
CILIUM
CIRCUM
DIADEM
DIATOM
DICTUM
DIGRAM
DIMSUM
DINKUM
DIRHAM
DISARM
FIVEAM
FIVEPM
HICKAM
HIJKLM
KIDCOM
LIGNUM
LILIOM
LILKIM
MIRIAM
MISAIM
NINEAM
NINEPM
PILEUM
SIKKIM
SITCOM
TILHIM
VIACOM
VIBRAM
VICTIM
WIGWAM
WILLEM
WINDOM
WISDOM
ZITCOM

••IM••

AHIMSA
AKIMBO
ANIMAL
ANIMAS
ANIMES
ANIMUS
ASIMOV
BLIMEY
BLIMPS
CAIMAN
CHIMED
CHIMER
CHIMES
CHIMPS
CLIMAT
CLIMAX
CLIMBS
CLIMES
CRIMEA
CRIMES
CRIMPS
CRIMPY
DEIMOS
FAIMAN
FBIMAN
FBIMEN
FLIMSY
GRIMED
GRIMES
GRIMKE
GRIMLY
GRIMMS
GRIMMY
IFIMAY
MAIMED
MAIMER
NEIMAN
OUIMET
PRIMAL
PRIMED
PRIMER
PRIMES
PRIMLY
PRIMOS
PRIMPS
PRIMUS
RBIMAN
RBIMEN
SHIMMY
SHIMON
SKIMPS
SKIMPY
SLIMED
SLIMES
SLIMLY
STIMPY
TRIMLY
WEIMAR
WHIMSY

••I•M•

AXIOMS
ENIGMA
GRIMMS
GRIMMY
IDIOMS
ISITME
ODIUMS
OPIUMS
PRISMS
PRIZMS
SEISMO
SEISMS
SHIMMY
STIGMA

••I••M

CHISUM
EMINEM
IBIDEM
SHIISM
SKIBUM
UNISOM

•••IM•

ALTIMA
BEDIMS
CLAIMS
COLIMA
DENIMS
DOTIME
ESKIMO
ESTIME
FATIMA
GOLIMP
HAKIMS
INTIME
JEMIMA
KILIMS
MAXIMA
MAXIMS
MINIMA
MINIME
MINIMI
MINIMS
NAJIMY
NOTIME
ONTIME
OPTIMA
OPTIMO
PURIMS
REAIMS
REGIME
RETIME
RHEIMS
SCRIMP
SCRIMS
SHRIMP
SURIMI
TVTIME
ULTIMA
ULTIMO
UNDIMS
UNLIMP
UPTIME
YAKIMA

•••I•M

ACTIUM
AECIUM
AFFIRM
AGEISM
ALLIUM
ATRIUM
AUTISM
BARIUM
BEFIRM
CERIUM
CESIUM
CHRISM
CILIUM
CORIUM
CUBISM
CURIUM
EGOISM
ERBIUM
FOLIUM
HELIUM
HOLISM
INDIUM
INFIRM
IONIUM
LABIUM
LILIOM
MAOISM
MEDIUM
MIRIAM
MOMISM
MONISM
NUDISM
OMNIUM
ONFILM
OSMIUM
PODIUM
PRFIRM
PURISM
RACISM
RADIUM
REFILM
SADISM
SAMIAM
SCHISM
SEXISM
SHIISM
SODIUM
SQUIRM
SUFISM
TAOISM
TEDIUM
THEISM
TRUISM
UNFIRM
VALIUM
VERISM
YESIAM
YOGISM

••••IM

ANTRIM
BAALIM
BEHAIM
CASSIM
LCHAIM
LILKIM
MAKSIM
MEGRIM
MISAIM
MUSLIM
PASSIM
PRELIM
RESWIM
RETRIM
SIKKIM
TILHIM
TUPTIM
UNPRIM
UNSLIM
VICTIM

IN••••

INABIT
INABOX
INADAY
INAFEW
INAFIX
INAFOG
INAGES
INAJAM
INANER
INAPET
INAPIE
INAPOD
INARAY
INARCH
INAREA
INAROW
INARUG
INARUT
INASEC
INATIE
INATUB
INAWAY
INBACK
INBLUE
INBORN
INBRED
INBULK
INCAIC
INCANS
INCANT
INCAPS
INCASE
INCASH
INCENT
INCEPT
INCHED
INCHER
INCHES
INCHON
INCISE
INCITE
INCODE
INCOME
INCUBI
INCULT
INCURS
INCUSE
INDASH
INDEBT
INDEED
INDEEP
INDENT
INDIAN
INDICT
INDIES
INDIGO
INDIRA
INDITE
INDIUM
INDOOR
INDUCE
INDUCT
INDUED
INDUES
INESSE
INEVER
INFACT
INFALL
INFAMY
INFANT
INFEAR
INFECT
INFERS
INFEST
INFIRM
INFLOW
INFLUX
INFOLD
INFORM
INFULL
INFUSE
INGATE
INGEAR
INGELS
INGEST
INGLES
INGMAR
INGOAL
INGOLD
INGOOD
INGOTS
INGRAM
INGRAY
INGRES
INGREY
INGRID
INGULF
INHALE
INHALF
INHAND
INHERE
INHOCK
INHOME
INHUME
INIONS
INITIO
INJAIL
INJECT
INJEST
INJOKE
INJULY
INJUNE
INJURE
INJURY
INKERS
INKIER
INKIND
INKING
INKJET
INKLES
INKPAD
INKPOT
INKSAC
INKSIN
INLAID
INLAND
INLAWS
INLAYS
INLEAF
INLETS
INLIEU
INLINE
INLOVE
INLUCK
INMATE
INMIND
INMOST
INNAGE
INNATE
INNEED
INNERS
INNESS
INNIES
INNING
INONES
INOUYE
INPARK
INPART
INPAWN
INPINK
INPLAY
INPORT
INPOUR
INPUTS
INRAGS
INROAD
INRUNS
INRUSH
INSANA
INSANE
INSEAM
INSECT
INSERT
INSETS
INSIDE
INSIST
INSITU
INSOLE
INSPAN
INSPOT
INSTAL
INSTEP
INSTIL
INSTIR
INSULT
INSURE
INSYNC
INTACT
INTAKE
INTEND
INTENS
INTENT
INTERJ
INTERN
INTERS
INTHAT
INTIME
INTOIT
INTONE
INTOTO
INTOWN
INTRAY
INTROS
INTUIT
INTUNE
INTURN
INTWOS
INUITS
INUPIK
INURED
INURES
INVADE
INVAIN
INVENT
INVERT
INVEST
INVIEW
INVITE
INVIVO
INVOKE
INWANT
INWARD
INWITH
INWOVE

I•N•••

IGNACE
IGNATZ
IGNITE
IGNORE
IMNEXT
INNAGE
INNATE
INNEED
INNERS
INNESS
INNIES
INNING
IONIAN

IONICS
IONISE
IONIUM
IONIZE
IONONE
ISNTOK

I••N••

IAMNOT
IBANEZ
ICANSO
ICINGS
ICONIC
IDENTI
IDENTS
IDONOT
IDUNNO
IFONLY
IKINGS
IMINES
IMONIT
INANER
INONES
IRANIS
IRENIC
IRONED
IRONER
IRONIC
IRONON
ISANTI
ISINTO
ITSNOT
IVANIV
IVANKA
IVANOV
IVANVI
IWANNA

I•••N•

ICHING
IDLING
IDUNNO
IGGING
IGGINS
IGUANA
ILEANA
ILLINI
IMDONE
IMEANT
IMFINE
IMGONE
IMMUNE
IMMUNO
IMPEND
INCANS
INCANT
INCENT
INDENT
INFANT
INHAND
INIONS
INJUNE
INKIND
INKING
INLAND
INLINE
INMIND
INNING
INPINK
INRUNS
INSANA
INSANE
INSYNC
INTEND
INTENS
INTENT
INTONE
INTUNE
INVENT
INWANT
IODINE
IOLANI
IONONE
IOWANS
IRKING
IRLENE
IRVINE
IRVING
ISAYNO
ISLAND
ISLING
ISMENE
ITHINK
IWANNA

I••••N

IBADAN
IBIZAN
ICEDIN
ICEMAN
ICEMEN
ICERUN
ICESIN
IFICAN
IFTHEN
IIJOHN
IJKLMN
IMAMAN
IMOGEN
IMPUGN
INBORN
INCHON
INDIAN
INKSIN
INPAWN
INSPAN
INTERN
INTOWN
INTURN
INVAIN
IONIAN
IRISIN
IRONON
ISAIAN
ISELIN
ISOGON
ITSFUN

•IN•••

AINTSO
BINACA
BINARY
BINATE
BINCHY
BINDER
BINDLE
BINDTO
BINDUP
BINGED
BINGER
BINGES
BINGLE
BINGOS
BINNED
BINNEY
BINNIE
BINNIG
BINYON
CINDER
CINEMA
CINEOL
CINQUE
DINARS
DINDIN
DINEAT
DINEIN
DINEON
DINERO
DINERS
DINGED
DINGER
DINGHY
DINGLE
DINGUS
DINING
DINKAS
DINKUM
DINNED
DINNER
DINTED
FINALE
FINALS
FINCAS
FINDER
FINELY
FINERY
FINEST
FINGER
FINIAL
FINIAN
FINING
FINISH
FINITE
FINITO
FINKED
FINKEL
FINKON
FINLEY
FINNAN
FINNED
FINNEY
FINNIC
FINSEN
GINGER
GINGKO
GINKGO
GINNED
GINNIE
GINSUP
HINDER
HINDUS
HINGED
HINGES
HINGIS
HINGLE
HINKLE
HINTAT
HINTED
HINTER
HINTON
JINGLE
JINGLY
JINNIS
JINXED
JINXER
JINXES
KINDER
KINDLE
KINDLY
KINDOF
KINGED
KINGLY
KINGME
KINKED
KINKOS
KINNAN
KINSEY
KINSKI
LINAGE
LINDEN
LINDER
LINEAL
LINEAR
LINENS
LINENY
LINERS
LINEUP
LINGER
LINGLE
LINGUA
LINGUS
LINIER
LINING
LINKED
LINKER
LINKUP
LINNET
LINNEY
LINTED
LINTEL
LINTER
LINTON
LINZER
MINCED
MINCER
MINCES
MINDED
MINDEN
MINDER
MINERS
MINETA
MINGLE
MINGUS
MINIFY
MINIMA
MINIME
MINIMI
MINIMS
MINING
MINION
MINITV
MINNIE
MINNOW
MINOAN
MINORS
MINOSO
MINTED
MINTER
MINUET
MINUIT
MINUTE
MINXES
MINYAN
NINEAD
NINEAM
NINEBC
NINEEE
NINEPM
NINERS
NINETY
NINEUP
NINGBO
NINJAS
NINONS
NINTHS
OINKED
OINKER
PINATA
PINBOY
PINCAY
PINCER
PINDAR
PINDUS
PINEAL
PINERO
PINERS
PINERY
PINGED
PINGER
PINIER
PINING
PINION
PINKED
PINKEN
PINKER
PINKIE
PINKOS
PINNAE
PINNAS
PINNED
PINNER
PINOAK
PINONS
PINOTS
PINSON
PINSUP
PINTER
PINTOS
PINUPS
PINYIN
PINZON
QINTAR
RINGED
RINGER
RINGIN
RINGUP
RINSED
RINSER
RINSES
SINBAD
SINEAD
SINEWS
SINEWY
SINFUL
SINGED
SINGER
SINGES
SINGIN
SINGLE
SINGLY
SINGTO
SINISE
SINKER
SINKIN
SINNED
SINNER
SINTAX
TINCAN
TINCTS
TINCUP
TINDER
TINEAL
TINEAR
TINGED
TINGES
TINGLE
TINGLY
TINGOD
TINHAT
TINIAN
TINIER
TINILY
TINKER
TINKLE
TINKLY
TINMAN
TINMEN
TINNED
TINNER
TINORE
TINPAN
TINPOT
TINSEL
TINTED
TINTER
UINTAS
VINCIT
VINERS
VINERY
VINIER
VINIFY
VINING
VINNIE
VINOUS
VINSON
VINTON
VINYLS
WINANS
WINBIG
WINCED
WINCER
WINCES
WINDED
WINDER
WINDEX
WINDOM
WINDOW
WINDUP
WINERY
WINGED
WINGER
WINGIT
WINIER
WINING
WINISH
WINKAT
WINKED
WINKER
WINKIE
WINNER
WINNIE
WINNOW
WINONA
WINOUT
WINSAT
WINSBY
WINSOR
WINTER
WINTRY
WINWIN
XINGIN
XINHUA
ZINCED
ZINCIC
ZINCKY
ZINGED
ZINGER
ZINNIA

•I•N••

BIANCA
BIANCO
BINNED
BINNEY
BINNIE
BINNIG
BIONDI
BIONIC
BIONTS
BIRNEY
BITNET
DIANNE
DIDNOT
DIENES
DINNED
DINNER
DIONNE
DIPNET
DIRNDL
DISNEY
EISNER
FIANCE
FIENDS
FINNAN
FINNED
FINNEY
FINNIC
GIANNI
GIANTS
GINNED
GINNIE
JINNIS
JITNEY
KIDNAP
KIDNEY
KILNED
KINNAN
LIANAS
LIANES
LIANGS
LIENEE
LIENOR
LIGNES
LIGNIN
LIGNUM
LIMNED
LIMNER
LINNET
LINNEY
LIONEL
LIONET
LIONLY
MIGNON
MILNER
MILNES
MINNIE
MINNOW
NIENTE
PIANOS
PICNIC
PIGNUT
PINNAE
PINNAS
PINNED
PINNER
PITNEY
RIENZI
SIDNEY
SIENNA
SIGNAL
SIGNED
SIGNEE
SIGNER
SIGNET
SIGNIN
SIGNON
SIGNOR
SIGNUP
SINNED
SINNER
TIENDA
TILNOW
TINNED
TINNER
VIANDS
VIENNA
VIENNE
VINNIE
WIENER
WIENIE
WIGNER
WINNER
WINNIE
WINNOW
ZINNIA

•I••N•

AIDING
AILING
AIMING
AIRING
BIDING
BIGEND
BIGONE
BIKING
BIKINI
BIMINI
BISONS
BITING
CIMINO
CITING
DIANNE
DICING
DIKING
DIMING
DINING
DIONNE
DISANT
DIVANS
DIVINE
DIVING
EIRENE
FIFING
FILENE
FILING
FINING
FIRING
FIVENO
FIXING
FIXINS
GIANNI
GIBING
GIEING
GIJANE
GIORNO
GITANO
GIUGNO
GIVENS
GIVING
HIDING
HIEING
HIKING
HIRING
HITINS
HITONE
HIVING
JIBING
JIMINY
JIVING
KIMONO
KITING
LIGAND
LIKENS
LIKING
LIMANS
LIMING
LINENS
LINENY
LINING
LIPENG
LITANY
LIVENS
LIVING
MIDONS
MIFUNE
MIKING
MILANO
MILANS
MIMING
MINING
MIRING
MIRINS
MIXING
MIZUNA
NICENE
NIKONS
NIMINY
NINONS
NISANS
NIXING
NIXONS
OILING
PICONE
PIKING
PILING
PIMINY
PINING
PINONS
PIPING
PIRANA
PISANO
PISANS
PITONS
RIBAND
RICANS
RICING
RIDENT
RIDING
RIGANS
RILING
RIMING
RIMINI
RIPENS
RISING
RIVING
SIDING
SIENNA
SILENT
SIMONE
SIRENS
SIRING
SITING
SITINS
SIVANS
SIXONE
SIZING
TICINO
TIDING
TIEINS
TIGONS
TILING
TIMING
TIPINS
TIRANA
TIRANE
TIRING
TISANE
TITANS
VICUNA
VIENNA
VIENNE
VIKING
VINING
VISHNU
VISINE
VISING
VIVANT
VIXENS
WIDENS
WIGAND
WILING
WINANS
WINING
WINONA
WIPING
WIRING
WISING
WIVING
WIZENS
ZIPONS

•I•••N

AIDMAN
AIDMEN
AIKMAN
AILEEN
AIRGUN
AIRMAN
AIRMEN
BICHON
BICORN
BIDDEN
BIDSIN
BIDSON
BIGBEN
BIGFAN
BIGFUN
BIGGUN
BIGMAN
BIGMEN
BIGTEN
BIGWIN
BINYON
BIOTIN
BIRMAN
BITEIN
BITEON
BITTEN
CITRIN
CITRON
DIALIN
DIDION
DIGSIN
DILLON
DINDIN
DINEIN
DINEON
DIOXIN
DIPSIN
DISOWN
DIVEIN
DIZAIN
EILEEN
FIBRIN
FIJIAN
FILEIN
FILLIN
FINIAN
FINKON
FINNAN
FINSEN
FIREON
FIRKIN
FITSIN
FITSON
GIBBON
GIBRAN
GIBSON
GIDEON
GILLAN
GILMAN
GILPIN
GIVEIN
GIVEON
HIDDEN
HIGHON
HILTON
HINTON
HIREON
HITMAN
HITMEN
HITSON
IIJOHN
JIMSON
KICKIN
KIDMAN
KIERAN
KIERON
KINNAN
KIOWAN
KIRMAN
KISSIN
KITAEN
KITTEN
LIBRAN
LIBYAN
LICHEN
LIEDON
LIESIN
LIESON
LIGNIN
LILIAN
LINDEN
LINTON
LIPTON
LISBON
LISTEN
LISTON
LIVEIN
LIVEON
MICRON
MIDIAN
MIGNON
MILTON
MINDEN
MINION
MINOAN
MINYAN
MIRREN
MITTEN
MIZZEN
NIACIN
NIGHON
NIPPON
NISSAN
NISSEN
OILCAN
OILMAN
OILMEN
OILPAN
PICKON
PIDGIN
PIEMAN
PIEMEN
PIEPAN
PIETIN
PIGEON
PIGMAN
PIGMEN
PIGPEN
PILEIN
PILEON
PINION
PINKEN
PINSON
PINYIN
PINZON
PIPEIN
PIPPIN
PISTON
PITKIN
PITMAN
PITMEN
RIBBON
RICHEN
RICHIN
RIDDEN
RIDEIN
RIESEN
RIFKIN
RINGIN
RIOPAN
RIPKEN
RIPSON
SICKEN
SIEBEN
SIGNIN
SIGNON
SILKEN
SIMEON
SIMIAN
SINGIN
SINKIN
SIOUAN
SIPHON
SIPSON
SIRBEN
SITSIN
SITSON
SITTIN
SIXGUN
SIXPIN
SIXTEN
TIEDIN
TIEDON
TIEPIN
TIESIN
TIESON
TIFFIN
TIGLON
TILDEN
TILSON
TILTON
TINCAN
TINIAN
TINMAN
TINMEN
TINPAN
TIPSIN
TITIAN
VILLON
VINSON
VINTON
VIOLIN
VIRDON
VIRGIN
VISION
VIVIAN
VIVIEN
WICCAN
WIEMAN
WIGGIN
WILSON
WILTON
WIMMIN
WINWIN
WIREIN
WISHIN
WISHON
WITHIN
XINGIN
ZIPGUN
ZIPSIN
ZIRCON

••IN••

AKINTO
ALINED
ALINER
ALINES
AMINES
AMINOR
AMINOS
AMINTA
AMINUS
BAINES
BEINGS
BEINON
BLINDS
BLINIS
BLINKS
BLINTZ
BMINOR
BMINUS
BOINGO
BOINGS
BRINED
BRINER
BRINES
BRINGS
BRINKS
CHINAS
CHINCH
CHINES
CHINKS
CHINKY
CHINOS
CHINTZ
CHINUA
CHINUP
CLINCH
CLINGS
CLINGY
CLINIC
CLINKS
CMINOR
CMINUS
COINED
COINER
COINOP
CRINGE
DAINTY
DJINNI
DJINNS
DMINOR
DMINUS
DOINGS
DRINGS
DRINKS
ELINOR
EMINEM
EMINOR
EPINAL
ERINNA
ERINYS
EVINCE
EWINGS
EZINES
FAINER
FAINTS
FEINTS
FLINCH
FLINGS
FLINTS
FLINTY
FMINOR
FRINGE
FRINGY
GAINED
GAINER
GAINES
GAINLY
GAINON
GAINST
GLINDA
GLINKA
GLINTS
GLINTY
GMINOR
GOINGS
GOINTO
GRINAT
GRINCH
GRINDL
GRINDS
GRINGO
GUINAN
GUINEA
HAINES
HEINIE
HEINSE
ICINGS
IKINGS
IMINES
ISINTO
JOINED
JOINER
JOININ
JOINTS
JOINUP
LAINIE
MAINER
MAINLY
MAINST
MOINES
ODINIC
OLINDA
OPINED
OPINER
OPINES

ORINGS
OVINES
PAINED
PAINTS
PAINTY
PLINKS
PLINTH
POINTA
POINTB
POINTE
POINTS
POINTY
PRINCE
PRINKS
PRINTS
PRINZE
QUINCE
QUINCY
QUINQU
QUINTA
QUINTE
QUINTI
QUINTS
QUINZE
RAINED
RAINER
RAINES
RAINEY
RAININ
RAINON
REINAS
REINED
REINER
REINES
REININ
REINKS
RHINAL
RHINOS
RUINED
RUINER
SAINTE
SAINTS
SEINED
SEINER
SEINES
SHINDY
SHINED
SHINER
SHINES
SHINNY
SHINTO
SKINKS
SKINNY
SLINGS
SLINKS
SLINKY
SPINAL
SPINED
SPINEL
SPINER
SPINES
SPINET
SPINKS
STINGS
STINGY
STINKO
STINKS
STINKY
STINTS
SWINGS
SWINGY
TAINTS
THINGS
THINGY
THINKS
THINLY
TMINUS
TRINAL
TRINES
TWINED
TWINER
TWINES
TWINGE
VAINER
VAINLY
VEINAL
VEINED
VEINTE
WHINED
WHINER
WHINES
WHINNY
WRINGS

••I•N•

ALIENS
ALIGNS
AMIENS
ANIONS
ARIANA
ARIANE
ASIANS
AVIANS
AXIONS
BAIRNS
BEIGNE
BRIANA
BRIAND
BRIENZ
CAIRNS
CHIANG
CHIENS
CLIENT
COIGNE
COIGNS
DEIGNS
DJINNI
DJINNS
EDIRNE
ERINNA
FEIGNS
FRIEND
GUIANA
INIONS
ONIONS
ONIONY
ORIANA
ORIANI
ORIENT
ORIONS
PLIANT
REIGNS
SAIDNO
SCIONS
SHINNY
SKIING
SKINNY
SOIGNE
TRIUNE
UNIONS
VSIGNS
WHINNY

••I••N

ALISON
ARISEN
AVISON
BAILON
BEINON
BLIXEN
BRITON
CAIMAN
CHIPIN
CHIRON
CHITON
CLIPON
DRIPON
DRIVEN
DRIVIN
EDISON
ERIVAN
FAIMAN
FBIMAN
FBIMEN
FLITIN
GAIJIN
GAINON
GUINAN
HEIDEN
HOISIN
IBIZAN
IFICAN
IRISIN
JOININ
KLIBAN
LAIDIN
LAIDON
LEIDEN
LEISEN
MAIDEN
MAILIN
MAISON
MEIFUN
NAILIN
NEIMAN
NOIRON
OBIWAN
OHIOAN
ORIGEN
ORIGIN
ORISON
PAIDIN
PAISAN
POISON
PRISON
RAILON
RAININ
RAINON
RAISIN
RAISON
RBIMAN
RBIMEN
REININ
SAIGON
SAILON
SAIPAN
SAISON
SHIMON
SKIRUN
SLIDIN
SLIPIN
SLIPON
SPITON
STIRIN
TAIPAN
TAIWAN
TRIGON
TRIPON
TRITON
UNISON
UTICAN
WAITON
WHIPIN
WHITEN

•••IN•

AAHING
ACHING
ACTING
ADDING
ADDINS
ADMINS
ADZING
AFFINE
AGEING
AGLINT
AIDING
AILING
AIMING
AIRING
ALAINA
ALBINE
ALBINO
ALCINA
ALDINE
ALFINE
ALPINE
ALVING
ALVINO
AMPING
ANNINA
ANOINT
AQUINO
ARCING
ARMING
AROINT
ASHINE
ASHING
ASKING
ATHING
ATKINS
ATNINE
AWNING
BAAING
BAKING
BALINE
BALING
BARING
BASING
BASINS
BATING
BAYING
BBKING
BCCING
BEGINS
BEHIND
BEKIND
BEMINE
BENING
BERING
BIDING
BIKING
BIKINI
BIMINI
BITING
BLAINE
BLUING
BODINE
BODING
BOEING
BONING
BOOING
BORING
BOVINE
BOWING
BOXING
BRAINS
BRAINY
BRUINS
BURINS
BUSING
BUYING
BUYINS
BYLINE
CABINS
CAGING
CAKING
CAMINO
CANINE
CANING
CARINA
CARING
CASING
CASINO
CAVING
CAWING
CEDING
CELINE
CHAINE
CHAINS
CIMINO
CITING
CLUING
CODING
COKING
COMING
CONING
COOING
COPING
CORING
COSINE
COVINA
COVING
COWING
COXING
CRAINS
CRYING
CUBING
CUEING
CUMINS
CURING
CUTINS
DARING
DATING
DAZING
DEDINI
DEFINE
DEKING
DELINT
DEVINE
DEWING
DICING
DIKING
DIMING
DINING
DIVINE
DIVING
DOFINE
DOLING
DOMINE
DOMING
DOMINI
DOMINO
DOPING
DORINE
DOSING
DOTING
DOZING
DRAINS
DRKING
DRYING
DRYINK
DUDING
DUKING
DUPING
DURING
DYEING
EAKINS
EALING
EARING
EASING
EATING
EBBING
EDGING
EDWINA
EELING
EGGING
ELAINE
ELNINO
ENCINA
ENCINO
ENDING
ENGINE
ENLINK
ENWIND
EOSINS
EPPING
EQUINE
ERMINE
ERRING
ERVING
ETTING
EWAINE
EYEING
EYVIND
FACING
FADING
FAGINS
FAKING
FALINE
FAMINE
FAMING
FARINA
FARING
FAXING
FAZING
FEEING
FELINE
FETING
FIFING
FILING
FINING
FIRING
FIXING
FIXINS
FLYING
FLYINS
FOKINE
FORINT
FOXING
FRYING
FUMING
FUSING
GAGING
GAMINE
GAMING
GAMINS
GAPING
GATING
GAZING
GEEING
GEMINI
GHAINS
GIBING
GIEING
GIVING
GLUING
GOLINO
GORING
GRAINS
GRAINY
GROINS
GRUING
GUGINO
GUYING
GYRING
HALING
HARING
HATING
HAVING
HAWING
HAYING
HAZING
HEWING
HEXING
HIDING
HIEING
HIKING
HIRING
HITINS
HIVING
HOEING
HOKING
HOLING
HOMING
HOMINY
HONING
HOPING
HOSING
HUSING
HYPING
ICHING
IDLING
IGGING
IGGINS
ILLINI
IMFINE
INKIND
INKING
INLINE
INMIND
INNING
INPINK
IODINE
IRKING
IRVINE
IRVING
ISLING
ITHINK
JADING
JANINE
JAPING
JAWING
JIBING
JIMINY
JIVING
JOKING
JOYING
JUKING
KALINE
KARINA
KEYING
KITING
KLEINE
LABINE
LACING
LADING
LADINO
LAMINA
LAMING
LANINA
LAPINS
LARINE
LASING
LATINA
LATINI
LATINO
LATINS
LAVING
LAWING
LAYING
LAYINS
LAZING
LENINA
LEVINE
LIKING
LIMING
LINING
LIVING
LODINJ
LOGINS
LOPING
LORING
LOSING
LOVING
LOWING
LUBING
LUCINE
LUGING
LUMINA
LUPINE
LUPINO
LURING
LYSINE
MAKING
MARINA
MARINE
MARINO
MATING
MATINS
MAVINS
MAXINE
MAXING
MAYING
MAZING
MEDINA
MELINA
MERINO
METING
MEWING
MIKING
MIMING
MINING
MIRING
MIRINS
MIXING
MODINE
MOLINA
MOLINE
MOOING
MOPING
MOVING
MOWING
MRJINX
MURINE
MUSING
MUTING
MUTINY
NADINE
NAMING
NANINE
NARINE
NEVINS
NIMINY
NIXING
NOSING
NOTING
NUKING
NUMINA
OARING
OFFING
OGLING
OILING
OLEINS
ONLINE
OOHING
OOZING
OPTING
ORBING
ORSINI
ORSINO
OSCINE
OUTING
OWNING
PACING
PACINO
PAGING
PALING
PAMINA
PANINI
PANINO
PARING
PARINI
PATINA
PATINE
PAVING
PAWING
PAYING
PEKING
PEPINO
PERINE
PIKING
PILING
PIMINY
PINING
PIPING
PLAINS
PLAINT
PLYING
POKING
POLING
PORING
POSING
PRYING
PULING
PURINA
QUAINT
QUOINS
RACINE
RACING
RACINO
RAGING
RAKING
RANINE
RAPINE
RAPINI
RARING
RASING
RATINE
RATING
RAVINE
RAVING
RAXING
RAYING
RAZING
REBIND
REDING
REDINK
REFIND
REFINE
REGINA
RELINE
RELINK
REMIND
REMINE
REMINI
REMINT
RENINS
REPINE
REPINS
RESING
RESINK
RESINS
RESINY
RETINA
RETINS
RETINT
REWIND
REWINS
RICING
RIDING
RILING
RIMING
RIMINI
RISING
RIVING
ROBING
ROBINS
RODINO
ROPING
ROSINA
ROSINS
ROSINY
ROTINI
ROVING
ROWING
RULING
RUNINS
RUTINS
SABINA
SABINE
SALINA
SALINE
SATING
SATINS
SATINY
SAVING
SAWING
SAYING
SEEING
SERINS
SEWING
SHRINE
SHRINK
SHYING
SIDING
SIRING
SITING
SITINS
SIZING
SKEINS
SKIING
SKYING
SLUING
SOFINE
SOLING
SOWING
SOYINK
SPHINX
SPLINE
SPLINT
SPRING
SPRINT
SPYING
SQUINT
STAINS
STEINS
STRING
STYING
SUPINE
SWAINS
TAHINI
TAKING
TAMING
TAPING
TAPINS
TARING
TAXING
TEEING
TICINO
TIDING
TIEINS
TILING
TIMING
TIPINS
TIRING
TOEING
TOEINS
TONING
TOPING
TORINO
TOTING
TOWING
TOXINS
TOYING
TRAINS
TRUING
TRYING
TSKING
TUBING
TUNING
TURING
TWAINS
TYPING
UMPING
UNBIND
UNDINE
UNFINE
UNKIND
UNKINK
UNLINK
UNPINS
UNWIND
UPBIND
UPLINK
UPPING
UPWIND
URGING
URSINE
USHING
USMINT
VALINE
VENINS
VEXING
VEZINA
VIKING
VINING
VISINE
VISING
VOTING
VOWING
WADING
WAGING
WAHINE
WAKING
WALING
WANING
WARING
WAVING
WAXING
WILING
WINING
WIPING
WIRING
WISING
WIVING
WOOING
WOWING
YAWING
YOGINI
YOKING
ZAYINS
ZONING
ZORINA

•••I•N

ACTION
ADRIAN
ADRIEN
ALBION
AMBIEN
AMNION
ANCIEN
APPIAN
ASSIGN
ATSIGN
BAHIAN
BCLION
BENIGN
BUNION
CAMION
CATION
COSIGN
DAMIEN
DARIEN
DELIAN
DESIGN
DIDION
DORIAN
ENSIGN
EOLIAN
EONIAN
FABIAN
FANION
FIJIAN
FINIAN
FUSION
GURION
INDIAN
IONIAN
ISAIAN
JOVIAN
JULIAN
JULIEN
LEGION
LESION
LILIAN
LOTION
LUCIAN
LUCIEN
LYDIAN
MAGIAN
MALIAN
MALIGN
MARIAN
MARION
MEDIAN
MIDIAN
MINION
MOTION
NACION
NATION
NOTION
NUBIAN
OBRIAN
OBRIEN
OKSIGN
OPTION
OSSIAN
PELION
PINION
POTION
RADIAN
RATION
REGION
RESIGN
RODION
ROMIJN
SIMIAN
SYRIAN
TINIAN
TITIAN
VISION
VIVIAN
VIVIEN
ZONIAN
ZUNIAN

••••IN

ACTSIN
ADDSIN
ADJOIN
ALDRIN
AMAZIN
AMBLIN
ANACIN
ANAKIN
ARCSIN
ASHBIN
ASKSIN
ATRAIN
ATTAIN
AUSTIN
AZORIN
BACKIN
BAFFIN
BALLIN
BARKIN
BASHIN
BASKIN
BATSIN
BEDWIN
BERLIN
BIDSIN
BIGWIN
BIOTIN
BITEIN
BLEWIN
BLOWIN
BOBBIN
BODKIN
BOFFIN
BOUDIN
BOWFIN
BROLIN
BURNIN
BUSTIN
BUTTIN
BUYSIN
CAGEIN
CALLIN
CALVIN
CAMEIN
CARDIN
CARLIN
CARTIN
CASEIN
CASHIN
CASSIN
CATKIN
CATLIN
CAVEIN
CHAPIN
CHEMIN
CHENIN
CHIPIN
CHOPIN
CITRIN
CLADIN
CLAVIN
CLUEIN
COBAIN
COFFIN
COMEIN
CORBIN
CORWIN
COUSIN
CRAMIN
CRETIN
CRONIN
CUEDIN
CUESIN
CULKIN
CURLIN
CURTIN
CUTSIN
DANCIN
DARLIN
DARRIN
DARWIN
DASSIN
DEALIN
DEMAIN
DENTIN
DERAIN
DETAIN
DEVEIN
DIALIN
DIGSIN
DINDIN
DINEIN
DIOXIN
DIPSIN
DIVEIN
DIZAIN
DOBBIN
DOBLIN
DOESIN
DOMAIN
DONEIN

DOVEIN
DRAGIN
DRAWIN
DREBIN
DREWIN
DRIVIN
DROPIN
DUBLIN
DUCHIN
DUNKIN
DUNLIN
DURBIN
DUSTIN
EARVIN
EASEIN
EATSIN
EDGEIN
ENDPIN
ENDSIN
ENJOIN
ESENIN
ESTLIN
ETAOIN
FADEIN
FALLIN
FEEDIN
FELLIN
FIBRIN
FILEIN
FILLIN
FIRKIN
FITSIN
FLEWIN
FLITIN
FLORIN
FLOWIN
FOGSIN
FOLDIN
GAIJIN
GARYIN
GATLIN
GAVEIN
GAWAIN
GERVIN
GETSIN
GETTIN
GILPIN
GIVEIN
GLOBIN
GOBLIN
GODWIN
GOESIN
GOFFIN
GONEIN
GOONIN
GOSLIN
GRATIN
GRODIN
HALPIN
HAMLIN
HANDIN
HANGIN
HARBIN
HARDIN
HARLIN
HATPIN
HAULIN
HAVEIN

HEADIN
HEFLIN
HELDIN
HELPIN
HEMSIN
HEREIN
HEROIN
HOISIN
HOLDIN
HOMEIN
HONEIN
HOPKIN
HOPSIN
HORNIN
HOWLIN
HUNGIN
ICEDIN
ICESIN
INKSIN
INVAIN
IRISIN
ISELIN
JAMSIN
JARDIN
JASMIN
JERKIN
JOININ
JOLTIN
JOPLIN
JUMPIN
JUSTIN
KAOLIN
KATRIN
KEEPIN
KELVIN
KEPTIN
KERWIN
KEYSIN
KICKIN
KISSIN
KUPRIN
LAIDIN
LANVIN
LARKIN
LAVAIN
LAYSIN
LEADIN
LEAKIN
LEANIN
LEAPIN
LECAIN
LEFTIN
LEGUIN
LENAIN
LETSIN
LIESIN
LIGNIN
LIVEIN
LOADIN
LOCKIN
LOGSIN
LOMEIN
LOOKIN
LORAIN
LOUVIN
LOVEIN
LUBLIN
LUMPIN

LUREIN
MAILIN
MALTIN
MARGIN
MARLIN
MARTIN
MARVIN
MASLIN
MATLIN
MCBAIN
MCCAIN
MCLAIN
MELVIN
MENNIN
MERLIN
MESSIN
MOTRIN
MOULIN
MOVEIN
MUFFIN
MULLIN
MUSLIN
MYOSIN
NAILIN
NAPKIN
NESTIN
NIACIN
NOGGIN
NORAIN
NOSEIN
NOTHIN
NUBBIN
NUTKIN
OBTAIN
OLEFIN
ONEGIN
ONEPIN
OPTSIN
ORDAIN
ORIGIN
OUTSIN
PACHIN
PACKIN
PAIDIN
PANSIN
PAQUIN
PAYSIN
PECTIN
PEEKIN
PEERIN
PENSIN
PEPSIN
PERKIN
PERRIN
PETAIN
PIDGIN
PIETIN
PILEIN
PINYIN
PIPEIN
PIPPIN
PITKIN
PLUGIN
POPLIN
POPSIN
POTVIN
POURIN
PREVIN

PUFFIN
PULLIN
PUPKIN
PUSHIN
PUTSIN
PUTTIN
RACEIN
RAFFIN
RAININ
RAISIN
RAKEIN
RAMSIN
RANGIN
RANKIN
RASKIN
RATLIN
READIN
RECOIN
REDDIN
REDFIN
REELIN
REGAIN
REININ
REJOIN
REMAIN
RENNIN
RESPIN
RETAIN
RICHIN
RIDEIN
RIFKIN
RINGIN
ROAMIN
ROCKIN
RODEIN
ROLLIN
ROMAIN
ROOTIN
ROPEIN
RUBSIN
RUDKIN
RUNGIN
RUNSIN
RUSHIN
RUSKIN
RUXPIN
SANKIN
SEALIN
SEENIN
SEEPIN
SEESIN
SENDIN
SENTIN
SEQUIN
SERKIN
SETSIN
SEWNIN
SEWSIN
SHAKIN
SHOOIN
SHOWIN
SHUTIN
SIGNIN
SINGIN
SINKIN
SITSIN
SITTIN
SIXPIN

SLIDIN
SLIPIN
SNOWIN
SOAKIN
SOCKIN
SPRAIN
STALIN
STARIN
STATIN
STAYIN
STEPIN
STIRIN
STOPIN
STOTIN
STRAIN
SUCKIN
SUNKIN
SURFIN
TAKEIN
TALKIN
TANNIN
TAPSIN
TAUPIN
TEGRIN
TENPIN
TIEDIN
TIEPIN
TIESIN
TIFFIN
TIPSIN
TOCSIN
TOEDIN
TOESIN
TOMLIN
TONKIN
TOOKIN
TOOTIN
TOSSIN
TOWSIN
TUCKIN
TUNEIN
TURNIN
TURPIN
TWOPIN
TYPEIN
UNAKIN
UNJOIN
UNVAIN
UPSPIN
URCHIN
USEDIN
USESIN
VERDIN
VEREIN
VERMIN
VIOLIN
VIRGIN
VOTEIN
WADEIN
WALKIN
WALLIN
WANTIN
WAVEIN
WAYSIN
WENTIN
WESTIN
WHIPIN
WHOSIN

WIGGIN
WIMMIN
WINWIN
WIREIN
WISHIN
WITHIN
WORKIN
XINGIN
YASHIN
YASMIN
YORKIN
YOUWIN
ZEROIN
ZIPSIN
ZOOMIN

IO••••

IODATE
IODIDE
IODINE
IODISE
IODIZE
IOLANI
IOMEGA
IOMOTH
IONIAN
IONICS
IONISE
IONIUM
IONIZE
IONONE
IOWANS

I•O•••

IBOOKS
ICONIC
ICOULD
IDOIDO
IDOLUM
IDONOT
IDOTOO
IFONLY
IFORTY
IGOROT
IGOTIT
IGOTTA
IKOIKO
ILOILO
IMOGEN
IMOKAY
IMONIT
INONES
INOUYE
IROBOT
IRONED
IRONER
IRONIC
IRONON
ISOBAR
ISOGON
ISOHEL
ISOLDA
ISOLDE
ISOMER
ISOPOD
IWOULD

I••O••

IBOOKS
ICEOUT
ICHORS
IDIOCY
IDIOMS
IDIOTS
IGLOOS
IGNORE
IIJOHN
ILLOFF
IMCOLD
IMCOOL
IMDONE
IMGONE
IMGOOD
IMHOME
IMPORT
IMPOSE
IMPOST
IMSOLD
IMTOLD
INBORN
INCODE
INCOME
INDOOR
INFOLD
INFORM
INGOAL
INGOLD
INGOOD
INGOTS
INHOCK
INHOME
INIONS
INJOKE
INLOVE
INMOST
INPORT
INPOUR
INROAD
INSOLE
INTOIT
INTONE
INTOTO
INTOWN
INVOKE
INWOVE
IOMOTH
IONONE
ITIOUS

I•••O•

IAMNOT
IAMTOO
ICEBOX
ICEFOG
ICEPOP
IDAHOS
IDONOT
IDOTOO
IGLOOS
IGOROT
IMACOP
IMAGOS
IMCOOL
IMGOOD
IMPROV

INABOX
INAFOG
INAPOD
INAROW
INCHON
INDOOR
INFLOW
INGOOD
INKPOT
INSPOT
INTROS
INTWOS
IROBOT
IRONON
ISIDOR
ISNTOK
ISOGON
ISOPOD
ITSHOT
ITSNOT
ITSYOU
IVANOV

I••••O

IAMTOO
ICANSO
ICHIRO
IDOIDO
IDOTOO
IDUNNO
IKOIKO
ILOILO
IMMUNO
INDIGO
INITIO
INTOTO
INVIVO
ISAYNO
ISIDRO
ISINTO
ITISSO
ITLLDO
ITSAGO

•IO•••

AIOLIS
BIOGAS
BIOLAB
BIOMES
BIONDI
BIONIC
BIONTS
BIOPIC
BIOPSY
BIOTAS
BIOTIC
BIOTIN
DIODES
DIOMED
DIONNE
DIOXIN
FIORDS
GIORNO
GIOTTO
KIOSKS
KIOWAN
KIOWAS
LIONEL

LIONET
LIONLY
LIOTTA
NIOBIC
PIOLET
RIOJAS
RIOPAN
RIOTED
RIOTER
SIOUAN
VIOLAS
VIOLET
VIOLIN
VIORST

•I•O••

AIROUT
BICORN
BIFOLD
BIFORM
BIGOIL
BIGONE
BIGOTS
BIJOUS
BIJOUX
BILOXI
BIPODS
BISONS
BITOFF
CIBOLA
CIXOUS
DICOTS
DIDOES
DIEOFF
DIEOUT
DIGOUT
DIMOUT
DIPODY
DIPOLE
DISOWN
DIVOTS
EIDOLA
FILOSE
FITOUT
GIGOLO
GIGOTS
GIJOES
HIDOUT
HITOFF
HITONE
HITOUT
IIJOHN
KIBOSH
KIDORY
KIMONO
LIPOFF
LIPOUT
LITOUT
MIAOUS
MIAOWS
MIDOFF
MIDONS
MIDORI
MILORD
MILOSZ
MIMOSA
MINOAN
MINORS

MINOSO
NICOLA
NICOLE
NICOLO
NIKOLA
NIKONS
NINONS
NIXONS
PICONE
PICOTS
PIGOUT
PILOSE
PILOTS
PILOUS
PINOAK
PINONS
PINOTS
PITONS
PITOTS
PIVOTS
RIBOSE
RICOHS
RICOLA
RIGORS
RIGOUR
RIGOUT
RIMOSE
RIMOUS
RIPOFF
RIPOST
RIPOUT
RIVOLI
SILOED
SIMONE
SITOUT
SIXONE
TIEOFF
TIGONS
TINORE
TIPOFF
TIVOLI
VIGODA
VIGORS
VIGOUR
VINOUS
VISORS
VIZORS
WIDOWS
WIGOUT
WINONA
WINOUT
ZIPOFF
ZIPONS
ZIPOUT

•I••O•

AIMFOR
AIRLOG
AIRPOP
AIRPOT
BICHON
BIDFOR
BIDSON
BIGBOI
BIGBOX
BIGBOY
BIGDOG
BIGDOS

BIGJOE
BIGTOE
BIGTOP
BILLOW
BIMBOS
BINGOS
BINYON
BISHOP
BITEON
CIELOS
CINEOL
CISCOS
CITRON
DIABOL
DIALOG
DIATOM
DIDFOR
DIDION
DIDNOT
DIEFOR
DIGFOR
DIGLOT
DILLON
DINEON
DIPSOS
DISCOS
DITTOS
FIEROS
FINKON
FIREON
FITFOR
FITSON
FIVEOF
GIBBON
GIBSON
GIDEON
GILROY
GISMOS
GIVEOF
GIVEON
GIZMOS
HICKOK
HIGHON
HILTON
HINTON
HIPHOP
HIPPOS
HIREON
HITFOR
HITSON
HIVAOA
JIMBOB
JIMSON
KIDCOM
KIDDOS
KIDEOS
KIERON
KILROY
KINDOF
KINKOS
LIBROS
LIEDON
LIEFOR
LIELOW
LIENOR
LIESON
LILIOM
LIMBOS

LINTON
LIPTON
LIQUOR
LISBOA
LISBON
LISTON
LITHOS
LIVEON
MICRON
MICROS
MIGNON
MILTON
MIMEOS
MINION
MINNOW
MIRROR
MIRROS
MITSOU
NIETOS
NIGHON
NIMROD
NIPPON
NITROS
PIANOS
PICKON
PICTOR
PIGEON
PILEON
PILLOW
PINBOY
PINION
PINKOS
PINSON
PINTOS
PINZON
PISTOL
PISTON
PISTOU
PITROW
RIBBON
RIDSOF
RIPSON
RITSOS
SICKOF
SICKOS
SIGNON
SIGNOR
SIMEON
SIPHON
SIPSON
SITCOM
SITFOR
SITSON
TIEDON
TIEROD
TIESON
TIGLON
TILNOW
TILSON
TILTON
TINGOD
TINPOT
TIPTOE
TIPTOP
TIREOF
TISSOT
VIACOM
VIATOR

VICTOR
VIDEOS
VIDIOT
VIEFOR
VIKTOR
VILLON
VINSON
VINTON
VIRDON
VIREOS
VIRGOS
VISION
WIDEOF
WILCOX
WILLOW
WILSON
WILTON
WINDOM
WINDOW
WINNOW
WINSOR
WISDOM
WISHON
ZIPLOC
ZIPPOS
ZIPTOP
ZIRCON
ZITCOM

•I•••O

AIELLO
AIKIDO
AILURO
AINTSO
BIANCO
BIBLIO
BILBAO
BINDTO
BISTRO
CICERO
CIMINO
DIABLO
DIALSO
DIARIO
DINERO
DIRIGO
DISTRO
FIASCO
FIGARO
FINITO
FIVENO
FIVETO
GIGOLO
GINGKO
GINKGO
GIORNO
GIOTTO
GITANO
GIUGNO
GIVETO
HIDEHO
KIARIO
KIMONO
LIBIDO
LIEDTO
LIESTO
LIEVIO
LIKESO

LIKETO
MIKADO
MILANO
MINOSO
NICOLO
NIEKRO
NIELLO
NIHILO
NINGBO
PICABO
PICARO
PIETRO
PINERO
PISANO
RIALTO
RIDETO
RIGHTO
RISETO
SINGTO
SIXTWO
TICINO
TIEDTO
TIEMPO
TIESTO
VIRAGO
WILLDO
WISETO
WISHTO

••IO••

ALIOTH
ALIOTO
ANIONS
ARIOSE
ARIOSI
ARIOSO
AXIOMS
AXIONS
GRIOTS
IDIOCY
IDIOMS
IDIOTS
INIONS
ITIOUS
ODIOUS
OHIOAN
ONIONS
ONIONY
ORIOLE
ORIONS
OTIOSE
OUIOUI
PRIORI
PRIORS
PRIORY
SCIONS
TRIODE
UNIONS

••I•O•

ABITOF
ALISON
ALIYOT
AMIDOL
AMIGOS
AMINOR
AMINOS
ASIMOV

AVISON
AVISOS
BAILON
BAILOR
BEINON
BMINOR
BRITON
CAICOS
CHICOS
CHIGOE
CHINOS
CHIRON
CHISOX
CHITON
CLIPON
CMINOR
COINOP
DEIMOS
DMINOR
DRIPON
EDISON
EDITOR
EJIDOS
ELINOR
EMINOR
ENIDOK
EPILOG
FMINOR
FRIJOL
FRITOS
FRIVOL
GAINON
GMINOR
ISIDOR
JAILOR
LAIDON
MAISON
NOIRON
ORISON
POIROT
POISON
POITOU
PRIMOS
PRISON
RAILON
RAINON
RAISON
RHINOS
SAIDOK
SAIGON
SAILON
SAILOR
SAISON
SEIKOS
SEIZOR
SHILOH
SHIMON
SKIBOB
SKIDOO
SKITOW
SLIPON
SPIGOT
SPITON
SUITOR
TAILOR
TRICOT
TRIGON
TRIPOD

TRIPON TRITON TVIDOL UNIPOD UNISOM UNISON VOIDOF WAITON

••I••O

AKIMBO AKINTO ALIOTO ALIVEO ARIOSO ARISTO ASIAGO BOINGO BRILLO CHIRHO CRISCO CRISTO EDITIO ELISEO EMILIO FAILTO FRISCO FRITTO GOINTO GRIECO GRINGO HAIRDO INITIO ISIDRO ISINTO ITISSO LAIDTO MAILTO OBISPO OVIEDO PHILCO SAIDNO SAIDSO SAIDTO SAILTO SCIPIO SEISMO SHINTO SHIPTO SKIDOO STINKO TRILLO VAILCO WEIRDO YSIDRO

•••IO•

ACTION AERIOS ALBION AMNION AMNIOS AUDIOS BCLION BUNION CAMION CARIOU CASIOS CATION CURIOS DANIOS DIDION ELLIOS ELLIOT ESPIOS ETHIOP FANION FOLIOS FUSION GORIOT GURION HELIOS HESIOD JOLIOT JUNIOR LEGION LESION LILIOM LOTION MARION MINION MOTION NACION NATION NOTION NOVIOS OPTION PATIOS PAVIOR PELION PERIOD PINION POLIOS POTION RADIOS RATION RATIOS REGION RODION SAVIOR SENIOR VIDIOT VISION

•••I•O

AIKIDO ALBINO ALNICO ALVINO ANTIGO AQUINO BENITO BONITO CALICO CAMINO CASINO CIMINO COGITO DANILO DAVIDO DEMILO DENIRO DEVITO DIRIGO DOMINO DORITO DOSIDO ELNINO ENCINO ENRICO ENVIRO ESKIMO FINITO GOLINO GUGINO HELICO ICHIRO IDOIDO IKOIKO ILOILO INDIGO INVIVO LADINO LATIGO LATINO LIBIDO LUPINO MARIDO MARIKO MARINO MAYIGO MEDICO MEJICO MERINO MEXICO MOJITO NIHILO ONEIRO OPTIMO ORSINO PACINO PANINO PEPINO RACINO RAPIDO RODINO SAYIDO SUBITO TICINO TORINO ULTIMO YESIDO

••••IO

ADAGIO AFLCIO BAGNIO BARRIO BIBLIO CABRIO CARDIO CASSIO CHORIO COOLIO CRANIO DELRIO DIARIO DROMIO EDITIO ELADIO EMILIO FANGIO FLORIO GRUMIO INITIO KIARIO LIEVIO LUGLIO MAGGIO NUNCIO NUNZIO PHYSIO PLUVIO QRATIO SCIPIO SERGIO STUDIO TESSIO

IP••••

IPECAC IPETER

I•P•••

IMPACT IMPAIR IMPALA IMPALE IMPART IMPEDE IMPELS IMPEND IMPERF IMPISH IMPLED IMPORT IMPOSE IMPOST IMPROV IMPUGN IMPURE IMPUTE INPARK INPART INPAWN INPINK INPLAY INPORT INPOUR INPUTS

I••P••

IBMPCS ICEPOP INAPET INAPIE INAPOD INKPAD INKPOT INSPAN INSPOT INUPIK ISOPOD ITSPAT

I•••P•

ICEUPS INCAPS INCEPT IRRUPT

I••••P

ICECAP ICEDUP ICEPOP ICESUP IMACOP INDEEP INSTEP

•IP•••

BIPEDS BIPODS CIPHER DIPLEX DIPNET DIPODY DIPOLE DIPPED DIPPER DIPSIN DIPSOS FIPPLE GIPPER HIPHOP HIPPED HIPPER HIPPIE HIPPOS HIPPUS KIPPED KIPPER KIPPUR LIPARI LIPASE LIPENG LIPIDS LIPOFF LIPOUT LIPPED LIPPER LIPTON NIPPED NIPPER NIPPLE NIPPON NIPSAT NIPSEY NIPUPS PIPAGE PIPEIN PIPERS PIPETS PIPEUP PIPIER PIPING PIPITS PIPPET PIPPIN PIPPIP RIPELY RIPENS RIPEST RIPKEN RIPLEY RIPOFF RIPOST RIPOUT RIPPED RIPPER RIPPLE RIPPLY RIPRAP RIPSAW RIPSON RIPSUP SIPHON SIPPED SIPPER SIPSON TIPINS TIPJAR TIPOFF TIPPED TIPPEE TIPPER TIPPET TIPPLE TIPSIN TIPSUP TIPTOE TIPTOP VIPERS WIPERS WIPEUP WIPING YIPPED YIPPEE YIPPIE ZIPGUN ZIPLOC ZIPOFF ZIPONS ZIPOUT ZIPPED ZIPPER ZIPPOS ZIPSBY ZIPSIN ZIPSIT ZIPSUP ZIPTOP

•I•P••

AIRPOP AIRPOT BIOPIC BIOPSY DIAPER DIEPPE DIMPLE DIMPLY DIPPED DIPPER DISPEL FIPPLE GILPIN GIMPED GIPPER HIPPED HIPPER HIPPIE HIPPOS HIPPUS KIPPED KIPPER KIPPUR LIMPED LIMPER LIMPET LIMPID LIMPLY LIPPED LIPPER LISPED LISPER NIPPED NIPPER NIPPLE NIPPON OILPAN PIEPAN PIGPEN PIMPLE PIMPLY PIPPET PIPPIN PIPPIP RIBPAD RIMPLE RIOPAN RIPPED RIPPER RIPPLE RIPPLY SIMPER SIMPLE SIMPLY SIPPED SIPPER SITPAT SIXPIN TIEPIN TINPAN TINPOT TIPPED TIPPEE TIPPER TIPPET TIPPLE WIMPED WIMPLE WISPED YIPPED YIPPEE YIPPIE ZIPPED ZIPPER ZIPPOS

•I••P•

BICEPS BIGAPE CIASPY DIEPPE FIVEPM FIXUPS MIXUPS NINEPM NIPUPS PINUPS SIRUPS SITUPS TIEMPO TIEUPS

•I•••P

AIRPOP AIRSUP BIDSUP BIGTOP BINDUP BISHOP BITEUP BITMAP DIALUP DIGSUP DISHUP FILLIP FILLUP FIREUP FIRMUP FITSUP FIVEUP GIDDAP GINSUP GIVEUP HICCUP HIGHUP HIKEUP HIPHOP HITSUP KICKUP KIDNAP KISSUP LICKUP LIFTUP LINEUP LINKUP MIDCAP MILSAP MISHAP MISTUP NINEUP OILCUP PICKUP PILEUP PINSUP PIPEUP PIPPIP PIRRIP RIDEUP RIGSUP RILEUP RINGUP RIPRAP RIPSUP RISEUP SIGNUP SITSUP SIZEUP TIDYUP TIEDUP TIESUP TILTUP TINCUP TIPSUP TIPTOP WINDUP WIPEUP WIREUP WISEUP ZIPSUP ZIPTOP

••IP••

ALIPED CHIPIN CHIPUP CLIPON CRIPES DRIPON DRIPPY FLIPUP GRIPED GRIPER GRIPES GRIPPE GRIPPY JAIPUR QUIPPY QUIPUS RAIPUR SAIPAN SCIPIO SHIPTO SKIPBY SKIPIT SKIPPY SLIPBY SLIPIN SLIPON SLIPPY SLIPUP SNIPED SNIPER SNIPES SNIPPY STIPES SWIPED SWIPER SWIPES TAIPAN TAIPEI TRIPES TRIPLE TRIPLY TRIPOD TRIPON TRIPUP UNIPED UNIPOD WHIPIN WHIPPY WHIPUP

••I•P•

BLIMPS CHIMPS CHIRPS CHIRPY CRIMPS CRIMPY CRISPS CRISPY DRIPPY ERIEPA GRIPPE GRIPPY KRISPY OBISPO PRIMPS QUIPPY SKIMPS SKIMPY SKIPPY SLIPPY SNIPPY STIMPY TWIRPS WHIPPY

••I••P

BOILUP CHINUP CHIPUP COILUP COINOP DOITUP FAIRUP FLIPUP JOINUP LAIDUP NAILUP PAIDUP PAIRUP PHILIP ROILUP SKICAP SLIPUP STIRUP SUITUP TRICEP TRIPUP WAITUP WHIPUP

•••IP•

CALIPH EQUIPS FELIPE NOTIPS OXLIPS PETIPA RECIPE REDIPS RETIPS REWIPE REZIPS SCRIPS SCRIPT STRIPE STRIPS STRIPY TULIPS UNRIPE UNRIPS UNZIPS VCHIPS

•••I•P

ETHIOP GOLIMP SCRIMP SHRIMP UNLIMP

••••IP

CATNIP CUETIP FATLIP FILLIP GETHIP GOSSIP GOTHIP HOTTIP LETRIP OUTLIP PHILIP PIPPIP PIRRIP PRECIP REGRIP RESHIP THELIP TOOHIP TURNIP UNCLIP UNGRIP UNSHIP

IQ••••

IQTEST

I••Q••

IRAQIS

•IQ•••

LIQUID LIQUOR PIQUED PIQUES PIQUET

•I•Q••

BISQUE CINQUE CIRQUE RISQUE

•I•••Q

HIGHIQ

••IQ••

CLIQUE CLIQUY DRIQJR UNIQUE

••I•Q•

QUINQU

•••IQ•

LOWIQS

•••I•Q

DEVICQ SUZIEQ

••••IQ

HIGHIQ

IR••••

IRAISE IRANIS IRAQIS IRATER IREFUL IRENIC IRIDES IRIDIC IRISED IRISES IRISIN IRITIC IRITIS IRKERS IRKING IRLENE IROBOT IRONED IRONER IRONIC IRONON IRREAL IRRUPT IRTYSH IRVINE IRVING

I•R•••

INRAGS INROAD INRUNS INRUSH IRREAL IRRUPT ISRAEL ISRAIR ITRIED

I••R••

IAGREE IATRIC IBARRA IBERIA ICARIA ICARUS ICERUN IDARED IFORTY IGOROT IMARET IMBRUE IMFREE IMPROV INARAY INARCH INAREA INAROW INARUG INARUT INBRED INGRAM INGRAY INGRES INGREY INGRID INTRAY INTROS INURED INURES ISERVE ISTRES ISTRIA ITURBI

I•••R•

IBARRA ICHIRO ICHORS IDCARD IDLERS IGNORE ILLDRY IMHERE IMHURT IMMURE IMPART IMPERF IMPORT IMPURE IMSURE INBORN INCURS INDIRA INFERS INFIRM INFORM INHERE INJURE INJURY INKERS INNERS INPARK INPART INPORT INSERT INSURE INTERJ INTERN INTERS INTURN INVERT INWARD IRKERS ISIDRO ITGIRL

I••••R

ICKIER IFFIER IMAGER IMPAIR INANER INCHER INDOOR INEVER INFEAR INGEAR INGMAR INKIER INPOUR INSTIR IPETER IRATER IRONER ISHTAR ISIDOR ISOBAR ISOMER ISRAIR ISSUER ISWEAR

•IR•••

AIRACE AIRARM AIRBAG AIRBUD AIRBUS AIRDAM AIRDRY AIRERS AIRGUN AIRIER AIRILY AIRING AIRLOG AIRMAN AIRMEN AIROUT AIRPOP AIRPOT AIRSAC AIRSEA AIRSUP AIRWAR AIRWAY BIRDED BIRDER BIRDIE BIREME BIRGIT BIRLED BIRLER BIRMAN BIRNEY BIRRED BIRTHS CIRCLE CIRCUM CIRCUS CIRQUE CIRRUS DIRAMS DIRECT DIRELY DIREST DIRGES DIRHAM DIRIGE DIRIGO DIRKED DIRNDL EIRENE FIREAT FIREON FIRERS FIREUP FIRING FIRKIN FIRMED FIRMER FIRMLY FIRMUP FIRSTR FIRSTS FIRTHS GIRDED GIRDER GIRDLE GIRLIE GIRTED GIRTHS HIREES HIREON HIRERS HIRING HIRSCH KIRKUK KIRMAN KIRSCH MIRADA MIRAGE MIRIAM MIRIER MIRING MIRINS MIRREN MIRROR MIRROS MIRTHS PIRACY PIRANA PIRATE PIRRIP SIRBEN SIRENS SIRICA SIRING SIRIUS SIRKAY SIRRAH SIRREE SIRUPS TIRADE TIRANA TIRANE TIREOF TIRIAC TIRING VIRAGO VIRDON VIREOS VIRGAS VIRGIL VIRGIN VIRGOS VIRILE VIRTUE VIRTUS WIREIN WIRERS WIREUP WIRIER WIRILY WIRING ZIRCON

•I•R••

AIGRET BIERCE BIERES BIGRED BIGRIG BIRRED CIARDI CIERAS CIRRUS CITRIC

CITRIN
CITRON
CITRUS
DIARIO
DIGRAM
FIBRES
FIBRIN
FIERCE
FIEROS
FIORDS
GIBRAN
GILROY
GIORNO
KIARIO
KIERAN
KIERON
KILROY
LIBRAE
LIBRAN
LIBRAS
LIBRIS
LIBROS
LITRES
LIVRES
MICRON
MICROS
MIDRIB
MIRREN
MIRROR
MIRROS
MITRAL
MITRED
MITRES
NIMROD
NITRES
NITRIC
NITROS
OILRIG
OILRUB
PICRIC
PIERCE
PIERIA
PIERRE
PIRRIP
PITROW
RICRAC
RIPRAP
SIERRA
SIRRAH
SIRREE
TIARAS
TIERCE
TIERED
TIEROD
TIERRA
TIGRES
TIGRIS
TIKRIT
TITRED
TITRES
VIBRAM
VIORST
VITRIC

•I••R•

AIDERS
AILURO
AIMERS
AIRARM
AIRDRY
AIRERS
BIAFRA
BICARB
BICORN
BIDERS
BIFORM
BIKERS
BINARY
BISTRO
BITERS
CICERO
CIDERS
CIDERY
CIGARS
CITERS
DICERS
DIKERS
DINARS
DINERO
DINERS
DISARM
DISERE
DISTRO
DIVERS
DIVERT
DIYERS
EIDERS
EILERS
EILERT
FIACRE
FIBERS
FIFERS
FIGARO
FIGURE
FILERS
FINERY
FIRERS
FIVERS
FIXERS
GIBERS
GIVERS
HIDERS
HIKERS
HILARY
HIRERS
HIVERS
JIVERS
KIDORY
KITERS
LIBERS
LIFERS
LIGERS
LIKERS
LINERS
LIPARI
LITERS
LITTRE
LIVERS
LIVERY
LIZARD
MIDORI
MILERS
MILORD
MIMERS
MINERS
MINORS
MISERS
MISERY
MITERS
MIXERS
NIEKRO
NINERS
NITERS
NITERY
NIXERS
OILERS
PICARA
PICARD
PICARO
PIERRE
PIETRO
PIKERS
PILERS
PINERO
PINERS
PINERY
PIPERS
RIBERA
RICERS
RIDERS
RIGORS
RIKERS
RILERS
RIMERS
RISERS
RITARD
RIVERA
RIVERS
SIERRA
SIGURD
SITARS
SIXERS
SIZERS
TIERRA
TIGERS
TILERS
TILERY
TIMBRE
TIMERS
TINORE
TISHRI
TITERS
VIAGRA
VICARS
VIDERI
VIEIRA
VIGORS
VIHARA
VINERS
VINERY
VIPERS
VISORS
VITARA
VIZIRS
VIZORS
WINERY
WINTRY
WIPERS
WIRERS
WIZARD

•I•••R

AIMFOR
AIRIER
AIRWAR
BIBBER
BICKER
BIDDER
BIDFOR
BIEBER
BIGAIR
BIGCAR
BIGEAR
BIGGER
BIGSUR
BILKER
BILLER
BINDER
BINGER
BIRDER
BIRLER
BITTER
CIBBER
CINDER
CIPHER
DIALER
DIAPER
DICIER
DICKER
DIDFOR
DIEFOR
DIETER
DIFFER
DIGFOR
DIGGER
DILLAR
DILLER
DIMMER
DINGER
DINNER
DIPPER
DISBAR
DISEUR
DITHER
EISNER
EITHER
FIBBER
FIDLER
FIGBAR
FILLER
FILTER
FINDER
FINGER
FIRMER
FIRSTR
FISHER
FITFOR
FITTER
FIZZER
GIBBER
GILDER
GINGER
GIPPER
GIRDER
HIGHER
HILLER
HINDER
HINTER
HIPPER
HISSER
HITFOR
HITHER
HITTER
JIGGER
JILTER
JINXER
JITTER
JIVIER
KICKER
KIDDER
KIEFER
KILLER
KILMER
KILTER
KINDER
KIPPER
KIPPUR
KISSER
LIBBER
LICKER
LIEBER
LIEDER
LIEFER
LIEFOR
LIENOR
LIFTER
LIMBER
LIMIER
LIMNER
LIMPER
LINDER
LINEAR
LINGER
LINIER
LINKER
LINTER
LINZER
LIPPER
LIQUOR
LISPER
LISTER
LITHER
LITTER
MIDAIR
MIDLER
MILDER
MILKER
MILLER
MILNER
MINCER
MINDER
MINTER
MIRIER
MIRROR
MISTER
NICKER
NICKJR
NIGHER
NIPPER
OILIER
OINKER
PICKER
PICTOR
PIECER
PIETER
PILFER
PILLAR
PINCER
PINDAR
PINGER
PINIER
PINKER
PINNER
PINTER
PIPIER
PITIER
QINTAR
RIBBER
RICHER
RIDDER
RIFLER
RIGGER
RIGOUR
RIMIER
RINGER
RINSER
RIOTER
RIPPER
RISKER
RITTER
SICKER
SIDDUR
SIFTER
SIGHER
SIGLER
SIGNER
SIGNOR
SILVER
SIMMER
SIMPER
SINGER
SINKER
SINNER
SIPPER
SISLER
SISTER
SITFOR
SITTER
TICKER
TIDIER
TIEBAR
TIGGER
TILLER
TILTER
TIMBER
TINDER
TINEAR
TINIER
TINKER
TINNER
TINTER
TIPJAR
TIPPER
TITHER
TITTER
VIATOR
VICTOR
VIEFOR
VIEWER
VIGOUR
VIKTOR
VINIER
VIZIER
WICKER
WIDDER
WIENER
WIGNER
WILBUR
WILDER
WILIER
WILLER
WIMMER
WINCER
WINDER
WINGER
WINIER
WINKER
WINNER
WINSOR
WINTER
WIRIER
WISHER
WISTER
WITHER
WITTER
ZIMMER
ZINGER
ZIPPER
ZITHER

••IR••

BAIRNS
BEIRUT
BGIRLS
CAIRNS
CHIRAC
CHIRHO
CHIRON
CHIRPS
CHIRPY
CHIRRS
EDIRNE
FAIRED
FAIRER
FAIRLY
FAIRUP
FLIRTS
FLIRTY
GHIRSH
HAIRDO
HAIRED
LAIRDS
LAIRED
LOIRET
MAIRES
MAIRZY
MOIRES
NAIRAS
NOIRES
NOIRET
NOIRON
OSIRIS
PAIRED
PAIRUP
PEIRCE
POIRES
POIRET
POIROT
QUIRED
QUIRES
QUIRKS
QUIRKY
QUIRTS
SHIRAZ
SHIRER
SHIRES
SHIRKS
SHIRRS
SHIRTS
SKIRLS
SKIRTS
SKIRUN
SMIRCH
SMIRKS
SMIRKY
SOIREE
SPIRAL
SPIREA
SPIRED
SPIRES
SPIRIT
STIRIN
STIRUP
SWIRLS
SWIRLY
SWIRLZ
TBIRDS
THIRDR
THIRDS
THIRST
THIRTY
TWIRLS
TWIRLY
TWIRPS
WEIRDO
WEIRDY
WHIRLS
WHIRLY
WHIRRS
ZAIRES

••I•R•

ANITRA
APIARY
ARIARY
AVIARY
BRIARD
BRIARS
BRIARY
BRIERS
BRIERY
CHIRRS
CHITRA
CRIERS
DEIDRE
DMITRI
DMITRY
DRIERS
EMIGRE
FLIERS
FRIARS
FRIARY
FRIERS
GLIERE
GRIGRI
GUIDRY
GUITRY
ISIDRO
MAITRE
OSIERS
PLIERS
POIVRE
PRIERS
PRIORI
PRIORS
PRIORY
SHIRRS
SKIERS
SPIERS
STIERS
TRIERS
WHIRRS
YSIDRO

••I••R

ABIDER
AGILER
ALINER
AMINOR
ARIDER
AVIDER
BAILER
BAILOR
BAITER
BMINOR
BOILER
BRIBER
BRINER
CHICER
CHIDER
CHIMER
CMINOR
COILER
COINER
DEICER
DMINOR
DRIQJR
DRIVER
EDITOR
ELIDER
ELINOR
ELITER
ELIXIR
EMINOR
EVILER
EXILER
FAINER
FAIRER
FMINOR
GAINER
GAITER
GEIGER
GLIDER
GMINOR
GOITER
GRIPER
GUIDER
GUITAR
HAILER
HEIFER
HRIDER
ISIDOR
JAILER
JAILOR
JAIPUR
JOINER
JUICER
KAISER
KNIFER
LEITER
LOITER
MAILER
MAIMER
MAINER
MOILER
MSIEUR
NAILER
NAIVER
OBITER
OLIVER
OPINER
PFIZER
POISER
PRICER
PRIMER
QUIVER
RAIDER
RAILER
RAINER
RAIPUR
RAISER
REIGER
REINER
REISER
REITER
RUINER
SAILER
SAILOR
SEINER
SEIZER
SEIZOR
SHINER
SHIRER
SHIVER
SLICER
SLIDER
SLIVER
SMILER
SMITER
SNIDER
SNIPER
SPICER
SPIDER
SPIKER
SPINER
SUITOR
SWIPER
TAILER
TAILOR
THIRDR
TOILER
TRITER
TWINER
UNITER
VAINER
VEILER
VOICER
VOIDER
WAILER
WAITER
WAIVER
WEIDER
WEIMAR
WHINER
WHITER
WRITER

•••IR•

ADMIRE
AFFIRM
ALHIRT
ALZIRA
ASPIRE
ASWIRL
ATTIRE
AWHIRL
BEFIRM
BEGIRD
BEGIRT
BEMIRE
BYWIRE
CHAIRS
CHOIRS
CLAIRE
CLAIRS
CROIRE
DEAIRS
DEHIRE
DENIRO
DESIRE
DEWIRE
ELMIRA
ELMIRE
ELVIRA
EMPIRE
ENGIRD
ENGIRT
ENTIRE
ENVIRO
EXPIRE
EXPIRY
FAKIRS
FAQIRS
FLAIRS
GOGIRL
HEGIRA
ICHIRO
INDIRA
INFIRM
ITGIRL
KEFIRS
MTAIRY
MYGIRL
NADIRS
NUBIRA
ONEIRO
ONFIRE
ONHIRE
PAMIRS
PRFIRM
REAIRS
REFIRE
REGIRD
REHIRE
RETIRE
REWIRE
SAFIRE
SATIRE
SEPIRA
SQUIRE
SQUIRM
SQUIRT
STAIRS
TAPIRS
THEIRS
TSHIRT
UMPIRE
UNFIRM
UNGIRD
UNGIRT
UNHIRE
UNMIRY
UPGIRD
UPGIRT
VENIRE
VIEIRA
VIZIRS

•••I•R

ACHIER
AERIER
AIRIER
ARTIER
ASHIER
BABIER
BAVIER
BELIER
BONIER
BOXIER
BURIER
BUSIER
CAGIER
CAHIER
CAKIER
CANIER
CAVIAR
COKIER
COPIER
COSIER
COWIER
COZIER
CUVIER
DEFIER
DENIER
DEWIER
DICIER
DOPIER
DOZIER
EASIER
EDGIER
EELIER
EERIER
EGGIER
ELMIER
ENVIER
ESPIER
FOLIAR
FOXIER
FUMIER
GAMIER
GLUIER
GOOIER
GORIER
HAZIER
HOKIER
HOLIER
HOMIER
HOSIER
ICKIER
IFFIER
INKIER
JAVIER
JIVIER
JOKIER
JUNIOR
LACIER
LAKIER
LANIER
LAZIER
LEVIER
LIMIER
LINIER
LOGIER
MAZIER
METIER
MIRIER
MOPIER
NAPIER
NOSIER
OAKIER
OATIER
OILIER
OOZIER
OWLIER
PACIER
PANIER
PAPIER
PAVIOR
PINIER
PIPIER
PITIER
POKIER
PUNIER
RACIER
RAPIER
RELIER
RIMIER
ROPIER
ROSIER
RULIER
SAGIER
SAVIOR
SENIOR
SEXIER
SPRIER
TIDIER
TINIER
TONIER
UGLIER
UNTIER
VANIER
VARIER
VINIER
VIZIER
WANIER
WARIER
WAVIER
WAXIER
WILIER
WINIER
WIRIER
XAVIER
ZANIER
ZOOIER

••••IR

AAFAIR
AFFAIR
AGADIR
ALTAIR
AUPAIR
AYESIR
BEFAIR
BELAIR
BESTIR
BIGAIR
COHEIR
CONAIR
DEHAIR
DEVOIR
ECLAIR
ELIXIR
FAFNIR
HOTAIR
IMPAIR
INSTIR
ISRAIR
LELOIR
MCNAIR
MEMOIR
MIDAIR
MOHAIR
NOFAIR
REDFIR
RENOIR
REPAIR
RESTIR
REVOIR
SAVOIR
SEAAIR
SHAMIR
UNFAIR
UNHAIR
UPSTIR
YESSIR

IS••••

ISAACS
ISABEL
ISAIAH
ISAIAN
ISANTI
ISAYNO
ISCHIA
ISEEIT
ISELIN
ISERVE
ISEULT
ISHTAR
ISIDOR
ISIDRO
ISINTO
ISITME
ISLAND
ISLATE
ISLEFT
ISLETS
ISLEYS
ISLIKE
ISLING
ISMAIL
ISMENE
ISNTOK
ISOBAR
ISOGON
ISOHEL
ISOLDA
ISOLDE
ISOMER
ISOPOD
ISRAEL
ISRAIR
ISSEIS
ISSUED
ISSUER
ISSUES
ISTHMI
ISTLES
ISTRES
ISTRIA
ISUZUS
ISWEAR

I•S•••

IJSSEL
IMSOLD
IMSURE
INSANA
INSANE
INSEAM
INSECT
INSERT
INSETS
INSIDE
INSIST
INSITU
INSOLE
INSPAN
INSPOT
INSTAL
INSTEP
INSTIL
INSTIR
INSULT
INSURE
INSYNC
ISSEIS
ISSUED
ISSUER
ISSUES
ITSAGO
ITSELF
ITSFUN
ITSHOT
ITSNOT
ITSPAT
ITSYOU

I••S••

IAMSAM
IBISES
ICESIN
ICESIT
ICESUP
IJSSEL
ILLSAY
ILLSEE
ILLSET
INASEC
INESSE
INKSAC
INKSIN
IRISED
IRISES
IRISIN
ITASCA
ITISSO

I•••S•

ICANSO

ICIEST
IDLEST
IGUESS
ILLEST
ILLUSE
IMBUSY
IMEASY
IMPISH
IMPOSE
IMPOST
INCASE
INCASH
INCISE
INCUSE
INDASH
INESSE
INFEST
INFUSE
INGEST
INJEST
INMOST
INNESS
INRUSH
INSIST
INVEST
IODISE
IONISE
IQTEST
IRAISE
IRTYSH
ITISSO

I••••S

IAMBUS
IBEAMS
IBEXES
IBICES
IBISES
IBMPCS
IBOOKS
ICARUS
ICEUPS
ICHORS
ICINGS
IDAHOS
IDEALS
IDENTS
IDIOMS
IDIOTS
IDLERS
IDTAGS
IDYLLS
IFITIS
IGGINS
IGLOOS
IGUESS
IKINGS
ILEXES
ILIADS
IMAGES
IMAGOS
IMAXES
IMBEDS
IMBUES
IMIDES
IMINES
IMMIES
IMPELS
INAGES
INCANS
INCAPS
INCHES
INCURS
INDIES
INDUES
INFERS
INGELS
INGLES
INGOTS
INGRES
INIONS
INKERS
INKLES
INLAWS
INLAYS
INLETS
INNERS
INNESS
INNIES
INONES
INPUTS
INRAGS
INRUNS
INSETS
INTENS
INTERS
INTROS
INTWOS
INUITS
INURES
IONICS
IOWANS
IRANIS
IRAQIS
IRIDES
IRISES
IRITIS
IRKERS
ISAACS
ISLETS
ISLEYS
ISSEIS
ISSUES
ISTLES
ISTRES
ISUZUS
ITCHES
ITILES
ITIOUS

•IS•••

AISLED
AISLES
BISBEE
BISCAY
BISECT
BISHOP
BISONS
BISQUE
BISSAU
BISSET
BISTRO
CISCOS
CISKEI
DISANT
DISARM
DISBAR
DISBUD
DISCOS
DISCUS
DISERE
DISEUR
DISHED
DISHES
DISHUP
DISKED
DISMAL
DISMAS
DISMAY
DISMES
DISNEY
DISOWN
DISPEL
DISSED
DISSES
DISTAL
DISTIL
DISTRO
DISUSE
EISELE
EISLEY
EISNER
FISCAL
FISHED
FISHER
FISHES
FISTED
FISTIC
GISELE
GISMOS
HISSAT
HISSED
HISSER
HISSES
KISHKA
KISHKE
KISLEV
KISMET
KISSED
KISSEL
KISSER
KISSES
KISSIN
KISSME
KISSUP
LISBOA
LISBON
LISLES
LISPED
LISPER
LISSES
LISTED
LISTEE
LISTEN
LISTER
LISTON
MISACT
MISADD
MISAIM
MISCHA
MISCUE
MISCUT
MISDID
MISERS
MISERY
MISFED
MISFIT
MISHAP
MISHIT
MISKEY
MISLAY
MISLED
MISSAL
MISSAY
MISSED
MISSES
MISSET
MISSIS
MISSME
MISSUS
MISTED
MISTER
MISTUP
MISUSE
NISANS
NISEIS
NISSAN
NISSEN
OISEAU
PISANO
PISANS
PISCES
PISGAH
PISHED
PISHES
PISTES
PISTIL
PISTOL
PISTON
PISTOU
RISERS
RISETO
RISEUP
RISHIS
RISING
RISKED
RISKER
RISKIT
RISQUE
SISALS
SISISI
SISKEL
SISLER
SISLEY
SISSLE
SISTER
TISANE
TISHRI
TISKET
TISSOT
TISSUE
VISAED
VISAGE
VISCID
VISHNU
VISINE
VISING
VISION
VISITS
VISORS
VISTAS
VISUAL
WISDOM
WISELY
WISEST
WISETO
WISEUP
WISHED
WISHER
WISHES
WISHIN
WISHON
WISHTO
WISING
WISPED
WISTER

•I•S••

AIMSAT
AIRSAC
AIRSEA
AIRSUP
BIASED
BIASES
BIDSIN
BIDSON
BIDSUP
BIGSKY
BIGSUR
BISSAU
BISSET
CIASPY
DIESEL
DIESES
DIESIS
DIGSAT
DIGSIN
DIGSIT
DIGSUP
DILSEY
DIMSUM
DIPSIN
DIPSOS
DISSED
DISSES
FIASCO
FIESTA
FINSEN
FIRSTR
FIRSTS
FITSIN
FITSON
FITSUP
GIBSON
GINSUP
HIRSCH
HISSAT
HISSED
HISSER
HISSES
HITSAT
HITSIT
HITSON
HITSUP
JIGSAW
JIMSON
KINSEY
KINSKI
KIOSKS
KIRSCH
KISSED
KISSEL
KISSER
KISSES
KISSIN
KISSME
KISSUP
KITSCH
LIESIN
LIESON
LIESTO
LISSES
MIASMA
MIDSTS
MILSAP
MISSAL
MISSAY
MISSED
MISSES
MISSET
MISSIS
MISSME
MISSUS
MITSOU
NIPSAT
NIPSEY
NISSAN
NISSEN
PIGSIT
PIGSTY
PINSON
PINSUP
PITSAW
PIUSII
PIUSIV
PIUSIX
PIUSVI
PIUSXI
RIDSOF
RIESEN
RIGSUP
RIMSKY
RINSED
RINSER
RINSES
RIPSAW
RIPSON
RIPSUP
RITSOS
SIESTA
SIPSON
SISSLE
SITSAT
SITSBY
SITSIN
SITSON
SITSUP
SIXSIX
TIESIN
TIESON
TIESTO
TIESUP
TILSIT
TILSON
TINSEL
TIPSIN
TIPSUP
TISSOT
TISSUE
VINSON
VIZSLA
WIESEL
WILSON
WIMSEY
WINSAT
WINSBY
WINSOR
ZIPSBY
ZIPSIN
ZIPSIT
ZIPSUP

•I••S•

AINTSO
BIOPSY
DIALSO
DIGEST
DIREST
DISUSE
DIVEST
FILOSE
FINEST
FINISH
HITEST
KIBOSH
LIAISE
LIKESO
LIPASE
LIVEST
MIKASA
MILOSZ
MIMOSA
MINOSO
MISUSE
NICEST
PILOSE
RIBISI
RIBOSE
RIFEST
RIMOSE
RIPEST
RIPOST
SINISE
SISISI
VIBIST
VILEST
VIORST
WIDEST
WIDISH
WINISH
WISEST

•I•••S

AIDERS
AIMERS
AIOLIS
AIRBUS
AIRERS
AISLES
BIASES
BIBLES
BICEPS
BIDERS
BIDETS
BIERES
BIGDOS
BIGHTS
BIGOTS
BIJOUS
BIKERS
BILGES
BILLIS
BIMBOS
BINGES
BINGOS
BIOGAS
BIOMES
BIONTS
BIOTAS
BIPEDS
BIPODS
BIRTHS
BISONS
BITERS
CIDERS
CIELOS
CIERAS
CIGARS
CIRCUS
CIRRUS
CISCOS
CITEES
CITERS
CITIES
CITIUS
CITRUS
CIVETS
CIVICS
CIXOUS
DICERS
DICOTS
DIDIES
DIDOES
DIENES
DIESES
DIESIS
DIETES
DIEZES
DIGITS
DIKERS
DINARS
DINERS
DINGUS
DINKAS
DIODES
DIPSOS
DIRAMS
DIRGES
DISCOS
DISCUS
DISHES
DISMAS
DISMES
DISSES
DITTOS
DITZES
DIVANS
DIVERS
DIVOTS
DIXITS
DIYERS
EIDERS
EIGHTS
EILERS
FIBERS
FIBRES
FICHES
FICHUS
FIELDS
FIENDS
FIEROS
FIFERS
FIFTHS
FIGHTS
FILERS
FILETS
FILLES
FINALS
FINCAS
FIORDS
FIRERS
FIRSTS
FIRTHS
FISHES
FIVERS
FIVEWS
FIXERS
FIXINS
FIXUPS
FIZZES
GIANTS
GIBERS
GIGOTS
GIGUES
GIJOES
GILELS
GILLIS
GIMELS
GIMMES
GIRTHS
GISMOS
GIVENS
GIVERS
GIZMOS
HIATUS
HIDERS
HIHATS
HIKERS
HINDUS
HINGES
HINGIS
HIPPOS
HIPPUS
HIREES
HIRERS
HISSES
HITINS
HIVERS
JIHADS
JINNIS
JINXES
JIVERS
KIDDOS
KIDEOS
KILIMS
KINKOS
KIOSKS
KIOWAS
KISSES
KITERS
LIANAS
LIANES
LIANGS
LIBBYS
LIBELS
LIBERS
LIBRAS
LIBRIS
LIBROS
LIEBYS
LIEGES
LIEUTS
LIFEIS
LIFERS
LIGERS
LIGHTS
LIGNES
LIKENS
LIKERS
LILACS
LILIES
LILLIS
LIMANS
LIMBOS
LIMITS
LINENS
LINERS
LINGUS
LIPIDS
LISLES
LISSES
LITERS
LITHOS
LITMUS
LITRES
LIVENS
LIVERS
LIVRES
MIAMIS
MIAOUS
MIAOWS
MIATAS
MICROS
MIDGES
MIDONS
MIDSTS
MIELES
MIGHTS
MILANS
MILERS
MILLES
MILNES
MIMEOS
MIMERS
MIMICS
MINCES
MINERS
MINGUS
MINIMS
MINORS
MINXES
MIRINS
MIRROS
MIRTHS
MISERS
MISSES
MISSIS
MISSUS
MITERS
MITRES
MIXERS
MIXUPS
NICADS
NICHES
NICIAS
NIECES
NIETAS
NIETOS
NIEVES
NIGHTS
NIKONS
NIMBUS
NINERS
NINJAS
NINONS
NINTHS
NIPUPS
NISANS
NISEIS
NITERS
NITRES
NITROS
NIXERS
NIXIES
NIXONS
OILERS
PIANOS
PICOTS
PIECES
PIETAS
PIKERS
PILAFS
PILAUS
PILERS
PILEUS
PILOTS
PILOUS
PINDUS
PINERS
PINKOS
PINNAS
PINONS
PINOTS
PINTOS
PINUPS
PIPERS
PIPETS
PIPITS
PIQUES
PISANS
PISCES
PISHES
PISTES
PITIES
PITONS
PITOTS
PIUTES
PIVOTS
PIXELS
PIXIES
PIZZAS
RIATAS
RICANS
RICERS
RICHES
RICOHS
RIDERS
RIDGES
RIFLES
RIGANS
RIGHTS
RIGORS
RIKERS
RILERS
RILLES
RIMERS
RIMOUS
RINSES
RIOJAS
RIPENS
RISERS
RISHIS
RITSOS
RITZES
RIVALS
RIVERS
RIVETS
RIYALS
SIBYLS
SICKOS
SIDLES
SIEGES
SIETES
SIEVES
SIGHTS
SIGILS
SIGMAS
SILVAS
SINEWS
SINGES
SIRENS
SIRIUS
SIRUPS
SISALS
SITARS
SITINS
SITUPS
SIVANS
SIXERS
SIXTHS
SIXTUS
SIZERS
TIARAS
TIBIAS
TICALS
TIDIES
TIEINS
TIEUPS
TIGERS
TIGHTS
TIGONS
TIGRES
TIGRIS
TIKKAS
TILAKS
TILDES
TILERS
TILLIS
TILTHS
TIMERS
TINCTS
TINGES
TIPINS
TITANS
TITERS
TITHES
TITLES
TITRES
UINTAS
VIANDS
VICARS
VIDEOS
VIGIAS
VIGILS
VIGORS
VILLAS
VINERS
VINOUS
VINYLS
VIOLAS
VIPERS
VIREOS
VIRGAS
VIRGOS
VIRTUS
VISITS
VISORS
VISTAS
VITALS
VIXENS
VIZIRS
VIZORS
WIDENS
WIDOWS
WIDTHS
WIELDS
WIFIES
WIGHTS
WILKES
WILLIS
WILLYS
WINANS
WINCES
WIPERS
WIRERS
WISHES
WITHUS
WIZENS
WIZZES
YIELDS
ZIPONS
ZIPPOS
ZIZZES

••IS••

ALISON
ALISTS
ANISES
ARISEN
ARISES
ARISTA
ARISTO
ATISES
AVISON
AVISOS
AXISES
BAISAS
BLISTS
BRISES
BRISKS
CHISEL
CHISOX
CHISUM
CRISCO
CRISES
CRISIS
CRISPS
CRISPY
CRISTO
DAISES
DEISTS
EDISON
EGISES
ELISEO
ELISHA
ELISSA
ELISTS
ENISLE
EXISTS
FAISAL
FEISTY
FOISTS
FRISCH
FRISCO
FRISEE
FRISES
FRISKS
FRISKY
FUISSE
GEISEL
GEISHA
GRISHA
GRISLY
GRISTS
GUISES
HEISTS
HOISIN
HOISTS
IBISES
IRISED
IRISES
IRISIN
ITISSO
JOISTS
KAISER
KRISPY
KRISTI
LEISEN
MAISIE
MAISON
MOISES
NEISSE
NOISED
NOISES
OBISPO
ODISTS
ORISON
ORISSA
OVISAC
PAISAN
PAISES
PLISSE
POISED
POISER
POISES
POISHA
POISON
PRISED
PRISMS
PRISON
PRISSY
RAISED
RAISER
RAISES
RAISIN
RAISON
REISER
SAISON
SEISMO
SEISMS
SOISEE
SUISSE
SWISHY
THISBE
TRISHA
TRISTE
TWISTS
TWISTY
UNISEX
UNISOM
UNISON
UNISYS
WAISTS
WHISKS
WHISKY
WRISTS

••I•S•

AHIMSA
AMIDST
ARIOSE
ARIOSI
ARIOSO
DRIEST
ELISSA
FLIMSY
FUISSE
GAINST
GHIRSH
GRIESE
HEINSE
ICIEST
ITISSO
MAINST
NEISSE
ORISSA
OTIOSE
PLISSE
PRIEST
PRISSY
SAIDSO
SHIEST
SHIISM
SLIEST
SUISSE
THIRST
WHILST
WHIMSY
WRIEST

••I••S

ABIDES
ADIDAS
ADIEUS
AGITAS
AKITAS
ALIBIS
ALICES
ALIENS
ALIGNS

ALIKES
ALINES
ALISTS
AMICES
AMICUS
AMIDAS
AMIDES
AMIENS
AMIGAS
AMIGOS
AMINES
AMINOS
AMINUS
ANIMAS
ANIMES
ANIMUS
ANIONS
ANISES
APICES
ARISES
ASIANS
ASIDES
ATILES
ATISES
AVIANS
AVISOS
AXIOMS
AXIONS
AXISES
AZIDES
BAINES
BAIRNS
BAISAS
BAIZAS
BAIZES
BEIGES
BEINGS
BGIRLS
BLIMPS
BLINDS
BLINIS
BLINKS
BLISTS
BMINUS
BOINGS
BOITES
BRIARS
BRIBES
BRICKS
BRIDES
BRIEFS
BRIERS
BRINES
BRINGS
BRINKS
BRISES
BRISKS
BSIDES
BTILES
BUICKS
BUILDS
CAICOS
CAIRNS
CEIBAS
CHICAS
CHICKS
CHICOS
CHIDES
CHIEFS
CHIENS
CHILES
CHILIS
CHILLS
CHIMES
CHIMPS
CHINAS
CHINES
CHINKS
CHINOS
CHIRPS
CHIRRS
CHIVAS
CHIVES
CLICKS
CLIFFS
CLIMBS
CLIMES
CLINGS
CLINKS
CMINUS
COIGNS
CRICKS
CRIERS
CRIMES
CRIMPS
CRIPES
CRISES
CRISIS
CRISPS
CTILES
CUICAS
DAISES
DEICES
DEIGNS
DEIMOS
DEISTS
DJILAS
DJINNS
DMINUS
DOINGS
DRIERS
DRIFTS
DRILLS
DRINGS
DRINKS
DRIVES
DTILES
EDICTS
EDILES
EFILES
EGISES
EJIDOS
ELIDES
ELISTS
ELITES
EMILYS
ENIACS
ERICAS
ERINYS
ETILES
EVICTS
EVITES
EWINGS
EXILES
EXISTS
EXITUS
EZINES
FAINTS
FAITES
FAITHS
FEIGNS
FEINTS
FLICKS
FLIERS
FLINGS
FLINTS
FLIRTS
FOISTS
FRIARS
FRIELS
FRIERS
FRIGES
FRILLS
FRISES
FRISKS
FRITAS
FRITES
FRITOS
FTILES
GAINES
GLIDES
GLINTS
GOINGS
GRIDES
GRIEFS
GRIFTS
GRILLS
GRIMES
GRIMMS
GRINDS
GRIOTS
GRIPES
GRISTS
GTILES
GUIDES
GUILDS
GUILES
GUISES
HAIDAS
HAIKUS
HAINES
HEISTS
HOISTS
HTILES
IBICES
IBISES
ICINGS
IDIOMS
IDIOTS
IFITIS
IKINGS
ILIADS
IMIDES
IMINES
INIONS
IRIDES
IRISES
IRITIS
ITILES
ITIOUS
JOINTS
JOISTS
JTILES
JUICES
KLICKS
KNICKS
KNIFES
KNIVES
KTILES
LAIRDS
LEICAS
LTILES
MAIRES
MAIZES
MOINES
MOIRES
MOISES
MTILES
NAIADS
NAIRAS
NEIGHS
NOIRES
NOISES
NTILES
ODIOUS
ODISTS
ODIUMS
OGIVES
OLIVES
ONIONS
OPINES
OPIUMS
ORIBIS
ORIELS
ORINGS
ORIONS
OSIERS
OSIRIS
OTILES
OTITIS
OUIJAS
OVINES
OXIDES
PAINTS
PAISES
PHIALS
PLIERS
PLINKS
POILUS
POINTS
POIRES
POISES
PRICES
PRICKS
PRIDES
PRIERS
PRIMES
PRIMOS
PRIMPS
PRIMUS
PRINKS
PRINTS
PRIORS
PRISMS
PRIZES
PRIZMS
PTILES
QTILES
QUIETS
QUILLS
QUILTS
QUINTS
QUIPUS
QUIRES
QUIRKS
QUIRTS
RAINES
RAISES
RAITAS
REICES
REIGNS
REINAS
REINES
REINKS
RHINOS
RTILES
SAINTS
SCIONS
SEIKOS
SEINES
SEISMS
SEIZES
SHIFTS
SHILLS
SHINES
SHIRES
SHIRKS
SHIRRS
SHIRTS
SKIERS
SKIFFS
SKILLS
SKIMPS
SKINKS
SKIRLS
SKIRTS
SLICES
SLICKS
SLIDES
SLIMES
SLINGS
SLINKS
SMILES
SMIRKS
SMITES
SMITHS
SNICKS
SNIFFS
SNIPES
SOITIS
SPICES
SPIELS
SPIERS
SPIFFS
SPIKES
SPILES
SPILLS
SPINES
SPINKS
SPIRES
SPITES
STICKS
STIDES
STIERS
STIFFS
STILES
STILLS
STILTS
STINGS
STINKS
STINTS
STIPES
SUITES
SWIFTS
SWILLS
SWINGS
SWIPES
SWIRLS
TAIGAS
TAINTS
TBILLS
TBIRDS
THIGHS
THILLS
THINGS
THINKS
THIRDS
TMINUS
TOILES
TRIADS
TRIALS
TRIBES
TRICES
TRICKS
TRIERS
TRIKES
TRILLS
TRINES
TRIPES
TTILES
TWILLS
TWINES
TWIRLS
TWIRPS
TWISTS
UMIAKS
UNIATS
UNICES
UNIONS
UNISYS
UNITAS
UNITES
VOICES
VOILES
VSIGNS
VSIXES
VTILES
WAISTS
WAIVES
WEIGHS
WHIFFS
WHILES
WHINES
WHIRLS
WHIRRS
WHISKS
WHITES
WRINGS
WRISTS
WRITES
WTILES
XFILES
XTILES
YOICKS
YTILES
ZAIRES
ZTILES

•••IS•

ADVISE
AGEISM
AGEIST
AGUISH
ALDISS
ARLISS
ARTIST
ASPISH
ASSISI
ASSIST
ATRISK
ATWIST
AURIST
AUTISM
AUTIST
BANISH
BLAISE
BLUISH
BOYISH
BRAISE
BRUISE
CAMISE
CERISE
CHAISE
CHRISM
CHRIST
COWISH
COYISH
CRUISE
CUBISM
CUBIST
DANISH
DELISH
DELIST
DEMISE
DEMIST
DENISE
DESIST
DEVISE
DOVISH
DRYISH
DUDISH
EGLISE
EGOISM
EGOIST
ELFISH
ELOISA
ELOISE
ELVISH
ENLIST
EXCISE
FAMISH
FETISH
FINISH
FLUISH
FRAISE
GARISH
GNEISS
GOFISH
GREIST
HEWISH
HOLISM
HOLIST
IMPISH
INCISE
INSIST
IODISE
IONISE
IRAISE
JADISH
JEWISH
JURIST
KLEIST
KSWISS
KWEISI
LAKIST
LATISH
LAVISH
LEGIST
LIAISE
LOUISA
LOUISB
LOUISE
LOUISI
LOUISV
LOUISX
LOWISH
LUTIST
LYRIST
MAOISM
MAOIST
MARISA
MARIST
MODISH
MOMISM
MONISM
MONIST
MOPISH
MULISH
NEWISH
NORISK
NOWISE
NUDISM
NUDIST
OAFISH
OBOIST
ODDISH
OFFISH
OGRISH
OLDISH
ONDISK
ONEISH
OWLISH
PALISH
PAPIST
PARISH
PERISH
POLISH
POPISH
PRAISE
PUNISH
PURISM
PURIST
RACISM
RACIST
RADISH
RAKISH
RAVISH
RAWISH
RAWIST
RELISH
RELIST
REMISE
REMISS
RERISE
RESIST
REVISE
RIBISI
SADISM
SADIST
SALISH
SCHISM
SCHIST
SEWIST
SEXISM
SEXIST
SHIISM
SINISE
SISISI
SQUISH
SUFISM
TALISA
TAOISM
TAOIST
TAVIST
THEISM
THEIST
TRUISM
TUBIST
TYPIST
UNWISE
UNWISH
UPPISH
UPRISE
VALISE
VANISH
VEDIST
VERISM
VERIST
VIBIST
WIDISH
WINISH
YOGISM
ZENIST

•••I•S

ADDINS
ADLIBS
ADMINS
ADMITS
ADVILS
AERIES
AERIOS
AGGIES
ALDISS
ALKIES
ALLIES
ALTIUS
AMBITS
AMNIOS
ANNIES
ANTICS
ANVILS
APHIDS
APRILS
ARLISS
ARMIES
ARNIES
AROIDS
ASDICS
ASPICS
ATKINS
ATTICS
AUDIOS
AUDITS
AVAILS
AVOIDS
AVRILS
AWAITS
BABIES
BASICS
BASILS
BASINS
BATIKS
BEDIMS
BEFITS
BEGINS
BELIES
BEVIES
BEWIGS
BODIES
BOGIES
BOVIDS
BRAIDS
BRAINS
BROILS
BRUINS
BRUITS
BURIES
BURINS
BUSIES
BUYINS
CABINS
CALIFS
CANIDS
CARIBS
CARIES
CASIOS
CAVIES
CAVILS
CHAINS
CHAIRS
CHOIRS
CITIES
CITIUS
CIVICS
CLAIMS
CLAIRS
COKIES
COLICS
COMICS
CONICS
CONIES
COPIES
COSIES
COZIES
CRAINS
CUBICS
CUBITS
CUMINS
CUPIDS
CURIES
CURIOS
CUTIES
CUTINS
CYNICS
DANIOS
DARIUS
DAVIES
DAVITS
DEAIRS
DEBITS
DECIUS
DEFIES
DELIUS
DEMIES
DEMITS
DENIES
DENIMS
DEVILS
DIDIES
DIGITS
DIXITS
DOGIES
DORIES
DOXIES
DRAINS
DROIDS
DROITS
DRUIDS
DUTIES
EAKINS
EDDIES
ELLIOS
EMAILS
ENNIUS
ENOILS
ENVIES
EOSINS
EQUIPS
ESPIES
ESPIOS
ETAILS
ETHICS
EYRIES
FACIAS
FACIES
FAGINS
FAKIRS
FAQIRS
FELIDS
FERIAS
FIXINS
FLAILS
FLAIRS
FLUIDS
FLYINS
FOGIES
FOLIES
FOLIOS
FRUITS
FURIES
FUSILS
GAMINS
GENIES
GENIUS
GHAINS
GNEISS
GOBIES
GRAILS
GRAINS
GROINS
GSUITS
HABITS
HAKIMS
HELIOS
HITINS
HOKIES
HOLIES
HOMIES
HYOIDS
IGGINS
IMMIES
INDIES
INNIES
INUITS
IONICS
JAVITS
JULIUS
JUNIUS
JURIES
KEFIRS
KILIMS
KRAITS
KSWISS
LADIES
LAMIAS
LAPINS
LATINS
LAYINS
LEVIES
LILIES
LIMITS
LIPIDS
LOGICS
LOGINS
LOOIES
LORIES
LOUIES
LOWIQS
LUCIUS
LUNIKS
LYRICS
LYRIDS
MAFIAS
MAGICS
MANIAS
MARIAS
MATINS
MAVINS
MAXIMS
MCRIBS
MEDIAS
MEDICS
MEDIUS
MERITS
MIMICS
MINIMS
MIRINS
MOBIUS
MONIES
MOTIFS
MOVIES
MUSICS
MUTIUS
NADIRS
NAVIES
NEVINS
NEWIES
NICIAS
NIXIES
NOHITS
NOKIAS
NOKIDS
NORIAS
NOTIPS
NOVIAS
NOVIOS
OLDIES
OLEINS
ONDITS
OOTIDS
OPCITS
OPTICS
ORBITS
ORGIES
OSMICS
OUTIES
OVOIDS
OXLIPS
PAMIRS
PANICS
PATIOS
PERILS
PEWITS
PIPITS
PITIES
PIXIES
PLAIDS
PLAINS
PLAITS
PLUIES
POKIES
POLIOS
PONIES
POSIES
POSITS
PUPILS
PURIMS
QUAILS
QUOINS
QUOITS
RABIES
RADIOS
RADIUS
RAMIES
RANIDS
RAPIDS
RATIOS
REAIMS
REAIRS
REBIDS
REDIGS
REDIPS
REFIES
REFITS
REGIUS
REHITS
REJIGS
RELICS
RELIES
REMISS
REMITS
RENINS
REOILS
REPINS
RERIGS
RESINS
RESITS
RETIES
RETINS
RETIPS
REWINS
REZIPS
RHEIMS
ROBINS
ROSIES
ROSINS
RUBIES
RUBIKS
RUNINS
RUTINS
SAHIBS
SATINS
SCRIMS
SCRIPS
SEPIAS
SERIES
SERIFS
SERINS
SHEIKS
SIGILS
SIRIUS
SITINS
SKEINS
SNAILS
SOLIDS
SONICS
SPLITS
SPOILS
SPRIGS
SPRITS
SQUIBS
SQUIDS
STAINS
STAIRS
STEINS
STOICS
STPIUS
STRIPS
SWAINS
TAMILS
TAPINS
TAPIRS
TAXIES
THEIRS
TIBIAS
TIDIES
TIEINS
TIPINS
TOBIAS
TOBIES
TOBITS
TODIES
TOEINS
TONICS
TOPICS
TORIES
TOXICS
TOXINS
TRAILS
TRAINS
TRAITS
TULIPS
TUNICS
TVHITS
TWAINS
UGLIES
UNBITS
UNDIES
UNDIMS
UNFITS
UNPINS
UNRIGS
UNRIPS
UNTIES
UNWIGS
UNZIPS
URSIDS
VARIAS
VARIES
VCHIPS
VENINS
VIGIAS
VIGILS
VISITS
VIZIRS
WIFIES
YALIES
ZANIES
ZAYINS
ZOOIDS

••••IS

ABATIS
ADENIS
ADONIS
AIOLIS
ALANIS
ALEXIS
ALIBIS
ALLAIS
AMADIS
AMATIS
ANSEIS
ANUBIS
ARAMIS
ARNEIS
ARTOIS
ATARIS
ATROIS
AZERIS
AZUKIS
BAMBIS
BARRIS
BEAVIS
BILLIS
BLINIS
BOCCIS
BREVIS
BUPKIS
CALAIS
CAPRIS
CASSIS
CHILIS
CLORIS
CLOVIS
COATIS
COQUIS
CORGIS
CRISIS
CULLIS
CURTIS
CUSTIS
DASHIS
DEBRIS
DENNIS
DERMIS
DHOTIS
DIESIS
DUBOIS

ECESIS
ELEMIS
ELPAIS
ELYTIS
ENNUIS
ENOKIS
ENVOIS
ESSAIS
EUSTIS
FARRIS
FATSIS
FERMIS
FERRIS
FORTIS
GADDIS
GALOIS
GHAZIS
GILLIS
GLACIS
GLYNIS
GNOSIS
GRATIS
HADJIS
HAGGIS
HAJJIS
HARRIS
HINGIS
HOLLIS
HOURIS
HUBRIS
IFITIS
IRANIS
IRAQIS
IRITIS
ISSEIS
JAMAIS
JINNIS
KANJIS
KEMPIS
KHAKIS
KRAVIS
LANAIS
LANDIS
LIBRIS
LIFEIS
LILLIS
LUNDIS
MAHDIS
MAJLIS
MANTIS
MAORIS
MAQUIS
MARDIS
MARVIS
MASAIS
MATHIS
MEDNIS
MENTIS
MIAMIS
MISSIS
MORRIS
MUFTIS
MULTIS
MYOSIS
NELLIS
NISEIS
NOESIS
NORRIS
OKAPIS
OMANIS
ORANIS
OREXIS
ORIBIS
OSIRIS
OTITIS
OTOMIS
OTOSIS
OXALIS
PALAIS
PARNIS
PARRIS
PASTIS
PATOIS
PELVIS
PENNIS
PERSIS
PETTIS
POORIS
PRAXIS
PRECIS
PUCCIS
RABBIS
RAMFIS
RISHIS
ROSHIS
SALMIS
SARDIS
SAUDIS
SERAIS
SERKIS
SHOGIS
SHOJIS
SOITIS
STASIS
SUNNIS
SUREIS
SUSHIS
SWAMIS
TENNIS
TERRIS
TETRIS
THATIS
THESIS
THETIS
TIGRIS
TILLIS
TMESIS
TRAVIS
TSADIS
TSURIS
TUTSIS
TUTTIS
UNAMIS
UNGUIS
VALAIS
VALOIS
WALLIS
WILLIS
YAQUIS
ZEUXIS

IT••••

ITALIA
ITALIC
ITASCA
ITCHED
ITCHES
ITEMED
ITGIRL
ITHACA
ITHINK
ITILES
ITIOUS
ITISSO
ITLLDO
ITRIED
ITSAGO
ITSELF
ITSFUN
ITSHOT
ITSNOT
ITSPAT
ITSYOU
ITURBI
ITZHAK

I•T•••

IATRIC
IDTAGS
IFTHEN
IMTOLD
INTACT
INTAKE
INTEND
INTENS
INTENT
INTERJ
INTERN
INTERS
INTHAT
INTIME
INTOIT
INTONE
INTOTO
INTOWN
INTRAY
INTROS
INTUIT
INTUNE
INTURN
INTWOS
IQTEST
IRTYSH
ISTHMI
ISTLES
ISTRES
ISTRIA
IVTUBE

I••T••

IAMTOO
ICETEA
ICHTHY
IDOTOO
IFITIS
IGETIT
IGOTIT
IGOTTA
INATIE
INATUB
INITIO
INSTAL
INSTEP
INSTIL
INSTIR
IPETER
IRATER
IRITIC
IRITIS
ISHTAR
ISITME
ISNTOK

I•••T•

IDEATE
IDENTI
IDENTS
IDIOTS
IFORTY
IGNATZ
IGNITE
IGOTTA
IMLATE
IMPUTE
INCITE
INDITE
INGATE
INGOTS
INLETS
INMATE
INNATE
INPUTS
INSETS
INSITU
INTOTO
INUITS
INVITE
INWITH
IODATE
IOMOTH
ISANTI
ISINTO
ISLATE
ISLETS

I••••T

IAMNOT
ICEDIT
ICEOUT
ICESIT
ICIEST
IDIDIT
IDLEST
IDONOT
IEIGHT
IGETIT
IGOROT
IGOTIT
ILLBET
ILLEST
ILLLIT
ILLMET
ILLSET
IMARET
IMBEAT
IMEANT
IMHURT
IMIGHT
IMNEXT
IMONIT
IMPACT
IMPART
IMPORT
IMPOST
INABIT
INAPET
INARUT
INCANT
INCENT
INCEPT
INCULT
INDEBT
INDENT
INDICT
INDUCT
INFACT
INFANT
INFECT
INFEST
INGEST
INJECT
INJEST
INKJET
INKPOT
INMOST
INPART
INPORT
INSECT
INSERT
INSIST
INSPOT
INSULT
INTACT
INTENT
INTHAT
INTOIT
INTUIT
INVENT
INVERT
INVEST
INWANT
IQTEST
IROBOT
IRRUPT
ISEEIT
ISEULT
ISLEFT
ITSHOT
ITSNOT
ITSPAT

•IT•••

BITEIN
BITEON
BITERS
BITEUP
BITING
BITMAP
BITNET
BITOFF
BITTED
BITTEN
BITTER
CITEES
CITERS
CITIED
CITIES
CITIFY
CITING
CITIUS
CITRIC
CITRIN
CITRON
CITRUS
DITALI
DITHER
DITTOS
DITZES
EITHER
FITFOR
FITFUL
FITOUT
FITSIN
FITSON
FITSUP
FITTED
FITTER
GITANO
GITTED
HITECH
HITEST
HITFOR
HITHER
HITINS
HITMAN
HITMEN
HITOFF
HITONE
HITOUT
HITSAT
HITSIT
HITSON
HITSUP
HITTER
JITNEY
JITTER
KITAEN
KITBAG
KITERS
KITING
KITKAT
KITSCH
KITTED
KITTEN
LITANY
LITCHI
LITERS
LITHER
LITHIC
LITHOS
LITMUS
LITOUT
LITRES
LITTER
LITTLE
LITTRE
LITVAK
MITERS
MITRAL
MITRED
MITRES
MITSOU
MITTAG
MITTEN
NITERS
NITERY
NITRES
NITRIC
NITROS
NITWIT
PITAYA
PITCHY
PITHED
PITIED
PITIER
PITIES
PITKIN
PITMAN
PITMEN
PITNEY
PITONS
PITOTS
PITROW
PITSAW
PITTED
RITARD
RITDYE
RITSOS
RITTER
RITUAL
RITZES
SITARS
SITCOM
SITFOR
SITING
SITINS
SITOUT
SITPAT
SITSAT
SITSBY
SITSIN
SITSON
SITSUP
SITTER
SITTIN
SITUPS
TITANS
TITERS
TITHED
TITHER
TITHES
TITIAN
TITLED
TITLES
TITRED
TITRES
TITTER
TITTLE
VITALE
VITALS
VITARA
VITRIC
VITTLE
WITCHY
WITHAL
WITHER
WITHIN
WITHIT
WITHUS
WITTED
WITTER
WITTIG
ZITCOM
ZITHER

•I•T••

AINTSO
BIGTEN
BIGTOE
BIGTOP
BIOTAS
BIOTIC
BIOTIN
BIRTHS
BISTRO
BITTED
BITTEN
BITTER
DIATOM
DICTUM
DIETED
DIETER
DIETES
DIKTAT
DINTED
DISTAL
DISTIL
DISTRO
DITTOS
FIFTHS
FILTER
FILTHY
FIRTHS
FISTED
FISTIC
FITTED
FITTER
GIFTED
GIFTEE
GIOTTO
GIRTED
GIRTHS
GITTED
HIATAL
HIATUS
HILTED
HILTON
HINTAT
HINTED
HINTER
HINTON
HITTER
JILTED
JILTER
JITTER
KILTED
KILTER
KILTIE
KITTED
KITTEN
LIFTED
LIFTER
LIFTUP
LILTED
LINTED
LINTEL
LINTER
LINTON
LIOTTA
LIPTON
LISTED
LISTEE
LISTEN
LISTER
LISTON
LITTER
LITTLE
LITTRE
MIATAS
MILTIE
MILTON
MINTED
MINTER
MIRTHS
MISTED
MISTER
MISTUP
MITTAG
MITTEN
MIXTEC
NIETAS
NIETOS
NINTHS
PICTOR
PIETAS
PIETER
PIETIN
PIETRO
PINTER
PINTOS
PISTES
PISTIL
PISTOL
PISTON
PISTOU
PITTED
PIUTES
QINTAR
RIATAS
RICTAL
RIFTED
RIOTED
RIOTER
RITTER
SIETES
SIFTED
SIFTER
SILTED
SINTAX
SISTER
SITTER
SITTIN
SIXTEN
SIXTHS
SIXTUS
SIXTWO
TICTAC
TIETAC
TILTAT
TILTED
TILTER
TILTHS
TILTON
TILTUP
TINTED
TINTER
TIPTOE
TIPTOP
TITTER
TITTLE
UINTAS
VIATOR
VICTIM
VICTOR
VIKTOR
VINTON
VIRTUE
VIRTUS
VISTAS
VITTLE
WIDTHS
WILTED
WILTON
WINTER
WINTRY
WISTER
WITTED
WITTER
WITTIG
ZIPTOP

•I••T•

BIDETS
BIGHTS
BIGOTS
BINATE
BINDTO
BIONTS
CIVETS
DICOTS
DIGITS
DILATE
DILUTE
DIMITY
DIVOTS
DIXITS
EIGHTA
EIGHTB
EIGHTC
EIGHTD
EIGHTE
EIGHTH
EIGHTS
EIGHTY
FICHTE
FIESTA
FIGHTS
FILETS
FINITE
FINITO
FIRSTR
FIRSTS
FIVETO
FIXATE
FIXITY
GIANTS
GIGOTS
GIOTTO
GIVETH
GIVETO
HIHATS
KIBITZ
LIEDTO
LIESTO
LIEUTS
LIGATE
LIGETI
LIGHTS
LIKETO
LIKUTA
LILITH
LIMITS
LIOTTA
LIVETH
LIVETV
MIDSTS
MIGHTS
MIGHTY
MIKITA
MINETA
MINITV
MINUTE
NICETY
NIENTE
NIGHTS
NIGHTY
NIKITA
NIMITZ
NINETY
PICOTS
PIGSTY
PILATE
PILOTS
PINATA
PINOTS
PIPETS
PIPITS
PIRATE
PITOTS
PIVOTS
RIALTO
RIDETO
RIGATI
RIGHTO
RIGHTS
RIGHTY
RIMATE
RISETO
RIVETS
SIESTA
SIGHTS
SINGTO
TIEDTO
TIESTO
TIGHTS
TINCTS
VISITS
WIGHTS
WISETO
WISHTO
ZIZITH

•I•••T

AIGLET
AIGRET
AIMSAT
AIROUT
AIRPOT
BIGBET
BIGCAT
BIGHIT
BILLET
BIRGIT
BISECT
BISSET
BITNET
BIZKIT
DIDACT
DIDNOT
DIECUT
DIEOUT
DIGEST
DIGLOT
DIGOUT
DIGSAT
DIGSIT
DIKTAT
DIMOUT
DIMWIT
DINEAT
DIPNET
DIRECT
DIREST
DISANT
DIVERT
DIVEST
EILERT
FIDGET
FILLET
FINEST
FIREAT
FITOUT
GIBEAT
GIBLET
GIDGET
GIMLET
HIDOUT
HINTAT
HISSAT
HITEST
HITOUT
HITSAT
HITSIT
JIBEAT
KIDLIT
KIDULT
KISMET
KITKAT
LIMPET
LINNET
LIONET
LIPOUT
LITOUT
LIVEAT
LIVEST
MIDGET
MILLET
MINUET
MINUIT
MISACT
MISCUT
MISFIT
MISHIT
MISSET
NIBLET
NICEST
NIPSAT
NITWIT
OILLIT
PIAGET
PICKAT
PICKET
PIELET
PIGLET
PIGNUT
PIGOUT
PIGSIT
PIOLET
PIPPET
PIQUET
RIBBIT
RIBCUT
RIBLET
RICHET
RIDENT
RIFEST
RIGOUT
RILLET
RIPEST
RIPOST
RIPOUT
RISKIT
SIGHAT
SIGNET
SILENT
SITOUT
SITPAT
SITSAT
TICKET
TIDBIT
TIKRIT
TILLET
TILSIT
TILTAT
TINHAT
TINPOT
TIPPET
TISKET
TISSOT
VIBIST
VIDIOT
VILEST
VINCIT
VIOLET
VIORST
VIVANT
WICKET
WIDEST
WIDGET
WIGLET
WIGOUT
WILMUT
WINGIT
WINKAT
WINOUT
WINSAT
WISEST
WITHIT
ZIPOUT
ZIPSIT

••IT••

ABITOF
AGITAS
AKITAS
AMITIE
ANITRA
BAITED
BAITER
BLITHE
BOITES
BRITON
CHITON
CHITRA
CHITTY
CRITIC
DMITRI
DMITRY
DOITUP
EDITED
EDITIO
EDITOR
ELITER
ELITES
EVITES
EXITED
EXITUS
FAITES
FAITHS
FLITBY
FLITIN
FRITAS
FRITES
FRITOS
FRITTA
FRITTO
FRITZI
GAITED
GAITER
GLITCH
GLITZY
GOITER
GRITTI
GRITTY
GUITAR
GUITRY
IFITIS
INITIO
IRITIC
IRITIS
ISITME
KEITEL
LEITER
LOITER
MAITAI
MAITRE
OBITER
OTITIC
OTITIS
POITOU
QUITIT
RAITAS
REITER
SAITEK
SKITCH
SKITOW
SLITHY
SMITER
SMITES
SMITHS
SMITHY
SMITTY
SNITCH
SOITIS
SPITED
SPITES
SPITON
STITCH
SUITED
SUITES
SUITOR
SUITUP
SWITCH
TRITER
TRITON
TWITCH
TWITTY
UNITAS
UNITED
UNITER
UNITES
WAITED
WAITER
WAITON
WAITUP
WHITBY
WHITED
WHITEN
WHITER
WHITES
WHITEY
WHITTY
WRITER
WRITES
WRITHE

••I•T•

AFIFTH
AKINTO
ALIOTH
ALIOTO
ALISTS
AMINTA
ARISTA
ARISTO
AVIATE
BLINTZ
BLISTS
CHINTZ
CHITTY
CRISTO
DAINTY
DEISTS
DRIFTS
DRIFTY
EDICTS
ELISTS
EVICTS
EXISTS
FAILTO
FAINTS
FEINTS
FEISTY
FLINTS
FLINTY
FLIRTS
FLIRTY
FOISTS
FRITTA
FRITTO
GAIETY
GFIFTY
GLINTS
GLINTY
GOINTO
GRIFTS
GRIOTS
GRISTS
GRITTI

GRITTY
GSIXTY
GUILTY
HEISTS
HOISTS
IDIOTS
ISINTO
JOINTS
JOISTS
KRISTI
LAIDTO
MAILTO
MOIETY
ODISTS
OPIATE
PAINTS
PAINTY
PAIUTE
PLINTH
POINTA
POINTB
POINTE
POINTS
POINTY
PRINTS
QUIETS
QUILTS
QUINTA
QUINTE
QUINTI
QUINTS
QUIRTS
SAIDTO
SAILTO
SAINTE
SAINTS
SHIFTS
SHIFTY
SHIITE
SHINTO
SHIPTO
SHIRTS
SKIRTS
SMITTY
SPILTH
STILTS
STINTS
SWIFTS
TAINTS
THIRTY
TRISTE
TWISTS
TWISTY
TWITTY
UBIETY
UNIATE
UNIATS
VEINTE
WAISTS
WHITTY
WRISTS

••I••T
ALIGHT
ALIYOT
AMIDST
ARIGHT
BEIGHT
BEIRUT
BLIGHT
BRIGHT
BRIGIT
CLIENT
CLIMAT
DRIEST
DWIGHT
ELICIT
FLIGHT
FRIGHT
GAINST
GEIGHT
GRINAT
HAIGHT
HEIGHT
ICIEST
IDIDIT
IEIGHT
IMIGHT
KNIGHT
LOIRET
MAINST
NAILIT
NOIRET
OCICAT
ORIENT
OUIMET
PLIANT
PLIGHT
POIRET
POIROT
PRIEST
PRIVET
QUITIT
RAILAT
SHIEST
SKIHAT
SKIPIT
SLIEST
SLIGHT
SPIGOT
SPINET
SPIRIT
SWIVET
THIRST
TOILAT
TOILET
TRICOT
TRIJET
TRIVET
TWILIT
VEIGHT
VOIGHT
WEIGHT
WHILST
WRIEST
WRIGHT
XZIBIT

•••IT•
ACUITY
ADMITS
ALRITZ
AMBITS
AMRITA
APLITE
AUDITS
AUGITE
AWAITS
BARITE
BEFITS
BENITO
BONITA
BONITO
BRUITS
CAPITA
CASITA
CAVITY
COGITO
COMITY
CUBITI
CUBITS
CURITE
DAMITA
DANITE
DAVITS
DEBITS
DEMITS
DERITA
DEVITO
DEWITT
DIGITS
DIMITY
DIXITS
DONITZ
DORITO
DOWITH
DROITS
EMMITT
ENMITY
ENTITY
EOLITH
EQUITY
EXCITE
FAJITA
FERITY
FINITE
FINITO
FIXITY
FRUITS
FRUITY
GOWITH
GSUITS
GUNITE
HABITS
HALITE
HAMITE
HEWITT
IGNITE
INCITE
INDITE
INSITU
INUITS
INVITE
INWITH
JAVITS
JUDITH
KIBITZ
KRAITS
KUNITZ
LAXITY
LENITY
LEVITE
LEVITT
LEVITY
LILITH
LIMITS
LOLITA
LUCITE
MERITS
MIKITA
MINITV
MOJITO
MORITA
MORITZ
NARITA
NIKITA
NIMITZ
NOHITS
NORITE
NUDITY
ODDITY
ONDITS
ONSITE
OOLITE
OPCITS
ORBITS
ORNITH
PARITY
PEPITA
PERITI
PETITE
PEWITS
PIPITS
PLAITS
POLITE
POLITY
POSITS
PURITY
PYRITE
QUOITS
RARITY
RATITE
RECITE
REFITS
REHITS
REMITS
RESITE
RESITS
ROSITA
SANITY
SEMITE
SENITI
SHIITE
SPLITS
SPRITE
SPRITS
SPRITZ
SUBITO
TAHITI
TOBITS
TONITE
TRAITS
TVHITS
UNBITS
UNFITS
UPPITY
VANITY
VENITE
VERITE
VERITY
VISITS
WAPITI
WRAITH
ZENITH
ZIZITH

•••I•T
ADDICT
ADRIFT
AGEIST
AGLINT
ALHIRT
ANOINT
AROINT
ARTIST
ASSIST
ATWIST
AURIST
AUTIST
BEGIRT
CHRIST
CRAIGT
CUBIST
DELICT
DELINT
DELIST
DEMIST
DEPICT
DESILT
DESIST
DEWITT
EGOIST
ELLIOT
EMMITT
ENGIRT
ENLIST
FORINT
GORIOT
GREIST
HEWITT
HOLIST
INDICT
INSIST
JOLIET
JOLIOT
JULIET
JURIST
KLEIST
LAKIST
LARIAT
LEGIST
LEVITT
LUTIST
LYRIST
MAOIST
MARIST
MONIST
NUDIST
OBOIST
PAPIST
PLAINT
PURIST
QUAINT
RACIST
RAWIST
REGIFT
RELICT
RELIST
REMINT
RESIFT
RESIST
RETINT
SADIST
SCHIST
SCRIPT
SEWIST
SEXIST
SHRIFT
SOVIET
SPLINT
SPOILT
SPRINT
SQUINT
SQUIRT
STRICT
TAOIST
TAVIST
THEIST
THRIFT
TSHIRT
TUBIST
TYPIST
UNGILT
UNGIRT
UNMIXT
UNTILT
UPGIRT
UPLIFT
UPTILT
USMINT
VEDIST
VERIST
VIBIST
VIDIOT
ZENIST

••••IT
ACEDIT
ACESIT
ACQUIT
ADROIT
ALBEIT
ANNUIT
ARMPIT
ASHPIT
ATTRIT
AUFAIT
AULAIT
BACHIT
BADFIT
BAGSIT
BANDIT
BANKIT
BBQPIT
BEATIT
BEDSIT
BELOIT
BENOIT
BIGHIT
BIRGIT
BIZKIT
BLEWIT
BLOWIT
BOOTIT
BRIGIT
BUYSIT
CALLIT
CANLIT
CATFIT
CATSIT
COEDIT
COMFIT
COMMIT
CONFIT
COOLIT
COPSIT
CREDIT
CUTSIT
DANGIT
DARNIT
DASHIT
DAYLIT
DECEIT
DIGSIT
DIMWIT
DOESIT
DOGSIT
DONEIT
DORRIT
DRATIT
DROPIT
DURNIT
EARNIT
EATSIT
ELEGIT
ELICIT
ENDSIT
ENFAIT
ENGLIT
ESPRIT
EYEPIT
FACEIT
FAKEIT
FLOPIT
FOOTIT
GAMBIT
GASLIT
GETFIT
GETSIT
GOATIT
GODWIT
GOTFIT
GOTOIT
GRANIT
GROMIT
GUNSIT
HACKIT
HATEIT
HAVEIT
HELDIT
HENBIT
HERMIT
HITSIT
HOBBIT
HOLDIT
HOOFIT
ICEDIT
ICESIT
IDIDIT
IGETIT
IGOTIT
ILLLIT
IMONIT
INABIT
INTOIT
INTUIT
ISEEIT
JESUIT
KEEPIT
KENSIT
KERMIT
KIDLIT
KNEWIT
KNOWIT
KUWAIT
LAMSIT
LEFTIT
LEGSIT
LOCCIT
LORDIT
LOSEIT
LOSTIT
LOVEIT
LUMPIT
MADEIT
MAKEIT
MEANIT
MINUIT
MISFIT
MISHIT
MOVEIT
NAILIT
NAMEIT
NESBIT
NITWIT
NOEXIT
NONHIT
NOTFIT
NOWAIT
OILLIT
ONEBIT
ONEHIT
OPENIT
OUTFIT
OUTHIT
OUTSIT
OUTWIT
OVERIT
PANDIT
PARKIT
PASTIT
PERMIT
PETSIT
PETTIT
PIGSIT
PLAYIT
POSTIT
PROFIT
PROSIT
PULPIT
PUNDIT
PUSHIT
QUITIT
RABBIT
REBAIT
REEDIT
REEMIT
REKNIT
RESUIT
RIBBIT
RISKIT
ROCKIT
SAVEIT
SAWFIT
SAWPIT
SEEFIT
SELLIT
SHALIT
SKIPIT
SKYLIT
SOBEIT
SOFFIT
SOLDIT
SPIRIT
STOPIT
STOWIT
STRAIT
SUBMIT
SUMMIT
SUNLIT
TAKEIT
TARPIT
TEARIT
TELLIT
THEPIT
TIDBIT
TIKRIT
TILSIT
TOLDIT
TOMTIT
TOOKIT
TOREIT
TWILIT
TWOBIT
UNBAIT
UNKNIT
UPTOIT
VINCIT
WABBIT
WEEBIT
WESKIT
WINGIT
WITHIT
XZIBIT
ZIPSIT

I•U•••
IDUNNO
IGUANA
IGUESS
INUITS
INUPIK
INURED
INURES
ISUZUS
ITURBI

I••U••
ICEUPS
ICOULD
ILLUDE
ILLUME
ILLUSE
IMBUED
IMBUES
IMBUSY
IMFULL
IMHURT
IMMUNE
IMMUNO
IMMURE
IMPUGN
IMPURE
IMPUTE
IMSURE
INBULK
INCUBI
INCULT
INCURS
INCUSE
INDUCE
INDUCT
INDUED
INDUES
INFULL
INFUSE
INGULF
INHUME
INJULY
INJUNE
INJURE
INJURY
INLUCK
INOUYE
INPUTS
INRUNS
INRUSH
INSULT
INSURE
INTUIT
INTUNE
INTURN
IRRUPT
ISEULT
ISSUED
ISSUER
ISSUES
IVTUBE
IWOULD

I•••U•
IAMBUS
ICARUS
ICEDUP
ICEOUT
ICERUN
ICESUP
IDOLUM
IMBRUE
INARUG
INARUT
INATUB
INBLUE
INDIUM
INFLUX
INPOUR
IONIUM
IREFUL
ISUZUS
ITIOUS
ITSFUN

I••••U
INLIEU
INSITU
ITSYOU

•IU•••
CIUDAD
GIUGNO
PIUSII
PIUSIV
PIUSIX
PIUSVI
PIUSXI
PIUTES

•I•U••
AILURO
DILUTE
DISUSE
FIBULA
FIGURE
FIXUPS
GIGUES
KIDULT
KIKUYU
LIEUTS
LIKUTA
LIQUID
LIQUOR
MIFUNE
MIGUEL
MINUET
MINUIT
MINUTE
MISUSE
MIXUPS
MIZUNA
NIPUPS
PINUPS
PIQUED
PIQUES
PIQUET
RITUAL
SIGURD
SIOUAN
SIRUPS
SITUPS
TIEUPS
VICUNA
VISUAL

•I••U•
AIDFUL
AIMFUL
AIRBUD
AIRBUS
AIRGUN
AIROUT
AIRSUP
BIDSUP
BIGBUX
BIGFUN
BIGGUN
BIGGUY
BIGHUG
BIGSUR
BIJOUS
BIJOUX
BINDUP
BISQUE
BITEUP
CILIUM
CINQUE
CIRCUM
CIRCUS
CIRQUE
CIRRUS
CITIUS
CITRUS
CIXOUS
DIALUP
DICTUM
DIECUT
DIEOUT
DIGOUT
DIGSUP
DIMOUT
DIMSUM
DINGUS
DINKUM
DISBUD
DISCUS
DISEUR
DISHUP
FICHUS
FILLUP
FIREUP
FIRMUP
FITFUL
FITOUT
FITSUP
FIVEUP
GINSUP
GIVEUP
HIATUS
HICCUP
HIDOUT
HIGHUP
HIKEUP
HINDUS
HIPPUS
HITOUT
HITSUP
KICKUP
KIPPUR
KIRKUK
KISSUP
LICKUP
LIFTUP
LIGNUM
LINEUP
LINGUA
LINGUS
LINKUP
LIPOUT
LITMUS
LITOUT
MIAOUS
MINGUS
MISCUE
MISCUT
MISSUS
MISTUP
NIMBUS
NINEUP
OILCUP
OILRUB
PICKUP
PIGNUT
PIGOUT
PILAUS
PILEUM
PILEUP
PILEUS
PILOUS
PINDUS
PINSUP
PIPEUP
RIBCUT
RIDEUP
RIGOUR
RIGOUT
RIGSUP
RILEUP
RIMOUS
RINGUP
RIPOUT
RIPSUP
RISEUP
RISQUE
SIDDUR
SIGNUP
SINFUL
SIRIUS
SITOUT
SITSUP
SIXGUN
SIXTUS
SIZEUP
TIDYUP
TIEDUP
TIESUP
TILTUP
TINCUP
TIPSUP
TISSUE
VIGOUR
VINOUS
VIRTUE
VIRTUS
WIGOUT
WILBUR
WILMUT
WINDUP
WINOUT
WIPEUP
WIREUP
WISEUP
WITHUS
XINHUA
ZIPGUN
ZIPOUT
ZIPSUP

•I•••U
BISSAU
KIKUYU
LIZALU
MIAMIU
MILIEU
MITSOU
NIIHAU
OISEAU
PICCHU
PISTOU
VISHNU

••IU••
ODIUMS
OPIUMS
PAIUTE
TRIUNE

••I•U•
ADIEUS
ADIEUX
AMICUS
AMINUS
ANIMUS
BEIRUT
BMINUS
BOILUP
CHINUA
CHINUP
CHIPUP
CHISUM
CLIQUE
CLIQUY
CMINUS
COILUP
DMINUS
DOITUP
EXITUS
FAIRUP
FLIPUP
HAIKUS
ITIOUS
JAIPUR
JOINUP
KAILUA
LAIDUP
MEIFUN
MSIEUR
NAILUP
ODIOUS
OUIOUI
PAIDUP
PAIRUP
POILUS
PRIMUS
QUIPUS
RAIPUR
ROILUP
SKIBUM
SKIRUN
SLIPUP
STIRUP
SUITUP
TMINUS
TRIPUP
UNIQUE
WAITUP
WHIPUP

••I••U
NIIHAU
POITOU
QUINQU

•••IU•
ACTIUM
AECIUM
ALLIUM
ALTIUS
ATRIUM
BARIUM
CERIUM
CESIUM
CILIUM
CITIUS
CORIUM
CURIUM
DARIUS
DECIUS
DELIUS
ENNIUS
ERBIUM
FOLIUM
GENIUS
HELIUM
INDIUM
IONIUM
JULIUS
JUNIUS
LABIUM
LUCIUS
MEDIUM
MEDIUS
MOBIUS
MUTIUS
OMNIUM
OSMIUM
PODIUM
RADIUM
RADIUS
REGIUS
SIRIUS
SODIUM
STPIUS
TEDIUM
VALIUM

•••I•U
CARIOU
DESILU
INLIEU
INSITU
MALIBU
MARILU
MILIEU

••••IU
MIAMIU

IV••••
IVANIV
IVANKA
IVANOV
IVANVI
IVTUBE

I•V•••
INVADE
INVAIN
INVENT
INVERT
INVEST
INVIEW
INVITE
INVIVO
INVOKE
IRVINE
IRVING

I••V••
INEVER

I•••V•
INLOVE

INVIVO
INWOVE
ISERVE
IVANVI

I••••V
IMPROV
IVANIV
IVANOV

•IV•••
CIVETS
CIVICS
DIVANS
DIVEIN
DIVERS
DIVERT
DIVEST
DIVIDE
DIVINE
DIVING
DIVOTS
FIVEAA
FIVEAD
FIVEAM
FIVEBC
FIVEEE
FIVENO
FIVEOF
FIVEPM
FIVERS
FIVETO
FIVEUP
FIVEWS
GIVEIN
GIVENS
GIVEOF
GIVEON
GIVERS
GIVETH
GIVETO
GIVEUP
GIVING
HIVAOA
HIVERS
HIVING
JIVERS
JIVIER
JIVING
LIVEAT
LIVEIN
LIVELY
LIVENS
LIVEON
LIVERS
LIVERY
LIVEST
LIVETH
LIVETV
LIVING
LIVRES
PIVOTS
RIVALS
RIVERA
RIVERS
RIVETS
RIVING
RIVOLI
SIVANS
TIVOLI
VIVACE
VIVANT
VIVECA
VIVIAN
VIVICA
VIVIEN
VIVIFY
WIVING

•I•V••
FIEVEL
KIDVID
LIEVIO
LITVAK
NIEVES
SIEVED
SIEVES
SILVAS
SILVER

•I••V•
PIUSVI

•I•••V
KISLEV
LIVETV
MINITV
PIUSIV

••IV••
ALIVEO
CHIVAS
CHIVES
DRIVEL
DRIVEN
DRIVER
DRIVES
DRIVIN
ERIVAN
FRIVOL
KNIVES
NAIVER
OGIVAL
OGIVES
OLIVER
OLIVES
OLIVIA
POIVRE
PRIVET
QUIVER
SHIVER
SLIVER
SNIVEL
SPIVAK
STIVIC
SWIVEL
SWIVET
TRIVET
TRIVIA
UNIVAC
WAIVED
WAIVER
WAIVES

••I•V•
GRIEVE
THIEVE

••I••V
ASIMOV

•••IV•
ACTIVA
ACTIVE
ADRIVE
ARGIVE
ARRIVE
ATFIVE
DATIVE
DERIVE
ENDIVE
GODIVA
GOLIVE
INVIVO
MOTIVE
NATIVE
NOJIVE
REGIVE
RELIVE
REVIVE
SALIVA
SHRIVE
STRIVE
THRIVE
UNLIVE
UPDIVE
VOTIVE

•••I•V
FELIXV
LOUISV
MINITV

••••IV
BOOKIV
IVANIV
JOHNIV
MARKIV
OLAFIV
OLAVIV
OTTOIV
PARTIV
PAULIV
PIUSIV

IW••••
IWANNA
IWOULD

I•W•••
INWANT
INWARD
INWITH
INWOVE
IOWANS
ISWEAR

I••W••
INAWAY
INTWOS

I•••W•
INLAWS
INPAWN
INTOWN

I••••W
INAFEW
INAROW
INFLOW
INVIEW

•I•W••
AIRWAR
AIRWAY
BIGWIG
BIGWIN
DIMWIT
KIOWAN
KIOWAS
MIDWAY
NITWIT
SIXWAY
VIEWED
VIEWER
WIGWAG
WIGWAM
WINWIN

•I••W•
DISOWN
FIVEWS
MIAOWS
SINEWS
SINEWY
SIXTWO
WIDOWS

•I•••W
BILLOW
JIGSAW
LIELOW
MILDEW
MINNOW
PILLOW
PITROW
PITSAW
RIPSAW
TILNOW
WILLOW
WINDOW
WINNOW

••IW••
OBIWAN
SKIWAX
TAIWAN

••I•W•
OJIBWA

••I••W
SKITOW

•••I•W
INVIEW
ONVIEW
REVIEW

I••X••
IBEXES
ILEXES
IMAXES

I•••X•
ICEAXE
IMNEXT

I••••X
ICEBOX
INABOX
INAFIX
INFLUX

•IX•••
CIXOUS
DIXITS
FIXATE
FIXERS
FIXING
FIXINS
FIXITY
FIXUPS
MIXERS
MIXING
MIXTEC
MIXUPS
NIXERS
NIXIES
NIXING
NIXONS
PIXELS
PIXIES
SIXDAY
SIXEEE
SIXERS
SIXGUN
SIXONE
SIXPIN
SIXSIX
SIXTEN
SIXTHS
SIXTUS
SIXTWO
SIXWAY
VIXENS

•I•X••
DIOXIN
JINXED
JINXER
JINXES
MINXES

•I••X•
BILOXI
PIUSXI

•I•••X
BIGBOX
BIGBUX
BIJOUX
DIPLEX
PICKAX
PIUSIX
SINTAX
SIXSIX
WILCOX
WINDEX

••IX••
BLIXEN
ELIXIR
GSIXTY
TRIXIE
VSIXES

••I••X
ADIEUX
CHISOX
CLIMAX
SKIWAX
UNISEX

•••IX•
FELIXI
FELIXV
MAXIXE
UNMIXT

•••I•X
LOUISX
MRJINX
SPHINX

••••IX
AGESIX
BENDIX
BOLLIX
BOOKIX
COMMIX
HADDIX
INAFIX
JOHNIX
MANNIX
MARCIX
MARKIX
MATRIX
NEELIX
PIUSIX
PREFIX
PREMIX
PROLIX
PUBLIX
REDSIX
RONMIX
SIXSIX
SUFFIX
TOMMIX

I•Y•••
IDYLLS

I••Y••
INSYNC
IRTYSH
ISAYNO
ITSYOU

I•••Y•
INLAYS
INOUYE
ISLEYS

I••••Y
ICALLY
ICHTHY
IDIOCY
IFIMAY
IFONLY
IFORTY
ILLDRY
ILLSAY
IMBUSY
IMEASY
IMOKAY
INADAY
INARAY
INAWAY
INFAMY
INGRAY
INGREY
INJULY
INJURY
INPLAY
INTRAY

•IY•••
DIYERS
HIYALL
RIYADH
RIYALS

•I•Y••
BINYON
LIBYAN
MINYAN
PINYIN
SIBYLS
TIDYUP
VINYLS

•I••Y•
BIGEYE
KIKUYU
LIBBYS
LIEBYS
PITAYA
RIBEYE
RITDYE
TIEDYE
WILLYS

•I•••Y
AIRDRY
AIRILY
AIRWAY
BIGAMY
BIGBOY
BIGDAY
BIGGUY
BIGSKY
BINARY
BINCHY
BINNEY
BIOPSY
BIRNEY
BISCAY
CIASPY
CICELY
CIDERY
CITIFY
DICKEY
DIDDLY
DIGAMY
DILSEY
DIMITY
DIMPLY
DINGHY
DIPODY
DIRELY
DISMAY
DISNEY
EIGHTY
EISLEY
FILEBY
FILTHY
FINELY
FINERY
FINLEY
FINNEY
FIRMLY
FIXITY
GIGGLY
GILLEY
GILROY
HICKEY
HIGHLY
HILARY
JIGGLY
JIMINY
JINGLY
JITNEY
KIDNEY
KIDORY
KILROY
KINDLY
KINGLY
KINSEY
LIEFLY
LIKELY
LIMPLY
LINENY
LINNEY
LIONLY
LITANY
LIVELY
LIVERY
MICKEY
MIDDAY
MIDMAY
MIDWAY
MIGHTY
MILADY
MILDLY
MILLAY
MINIFY
MISERY
MISKEY
MISLAY
MISSAY
MIZZLY
NIAMEY
NICELY
NICETY
NIDIFY
NIGHTY
NIMBLY
NIMINY
NINETY
NIPSEY
NITERY
OILILY
PIGSTY
PIMINY
PIMPLY
PINBOY
PINCAY
PINERY
PIRACY
PITCHY
PITNEY
RICHLY
RICKEY
RIDEBY
RIDLEY
RIFELY
RIGHTY
RIMSKY
RIPELY
RIPLEY
RIPPLY
SICILY
SICKLY
SIDNEY
SIMPLY
SINEWY
SINGLY
SIRKAY
SISLEY
SITSBY
SIXDAY
SIXWAY
TICKBY
TICKLY
TIDILY
TILERY
TILLEY
TIMELY
TINGLY
TINILY
TINKLY
VIABLY
VILELY
VILIFY
VINERY
VINIFY
VIVIFY
WIDELY
WIELDY
WIFELY
WIGGLY
WILDLY
WILILY
WIMSEY
WINERY
WINSBY
WINTRY
WIRILY
WISELY
WITCHY
ZINCKY
ZIPSBY

••IY••
ALIYAH
ALIYOT

••I•Y•
EMILYS
ERINYS
UNISYS

••I••Y
ACIDLY
APIARY
ARIARY
ARIDLY
AVIARY
AVIDLY
BAILEY
BLIMEY
BRIARY
BRICKY
BRIERY
CHICLY
CHILLY
CHINKY
CHIRPY
CHITTY
CLICHY
CLIFFY
CLINGY
CLIQUY
CRIKEY
CRIMPY
CRISPY
DAILEY
DAINTY
DMITRY
DRIFTY
DRIPPY
EDIBLY
EVILLY
FAIRLY
FEISTY
FLIMSY
FLINTY
FLIRTY
FLITBY
FRIARY
FRIDAY
FRILLY
FRINGY
FRISKY
FRIZZY
GAIETY
GAINLY
GFIFTY
GLIBLY
GLINTY
GLITZY
GRIMLY
GRIMMY
GRIPPY
GRISLY
GRITTY
GSIXTY
GUIDRY
GUILTY
GUITRY
HAILEY
IDIOCY
IFIMAY
KRISPY
LAIDBY
MAINLY
MAIRZY
MOIETY
ONIONY
PAINTY
PDIDDY
PHILBY
PHILLY
POINTY
PRICEY
PRIMLY
PRIORY
PRISSY
QUINCY
QUIPPY
QUIRKY
RAINEY
REILLY
SHIFTY
SHILLY
SHIMMY
SHINDY
SHINNY
SKIDDY
SKIMPY
SKINNY
SKIPBY
SKIPPY
SLIMLY
SLINKY
SLIPBY
SLIPPY
SLITHY
SMILEY
SMIRKY
SMITHY
SMITTY
SNIFFY
SNIPPY
SPIDEY
SPIFFY
STICKY
STILLY
STIMPY
STINGY
STINKY
SWINGY
SWIRLY
SWISHY
THINGY
THINLY
THIRTY
TRICKY
TRILBY
TRIMLY
TRIPLY
TWIGGY
TWIRLY
TWISTY
TWITTY
UBIETY
UNIDLY
VAINLY
WEIRDY
WHIMSY
WHINNY
WHIPPY
WHIRLY
WHISKY
WHITBY
WHITEY
WHITTY
WHIZZY

•••I•Y
ACUITY
AERIFY
AERILY
AIRILY
ARTILY
AURIFY
BASIFY
BODILY
BOXILY
BRAINY
BUSILY
CAGILY
CAVITY
CITIFY
CODIFY
COMITY
COSILY
COZILY
DEWILY
DIMITY
DOPILY
DOZILY
EASILY
EDGILY
EERILY
EFFIGY
ENMITY
ENTITY
EQUITY
EXPIRY
FAMILY
FERITY
FIXITY
FOXILY
FRAIDY
FRUITY
GAMILY
GASIFY
GORILY
GRAINY
HAZILY
HOKILY
HOLILY
HOMILY
HOMINY
JIMINY
JOKILY
LACILY
LAXITY
LAZILY
LENITY
LEVITY
LOGILY
MAZILY
MINIFY
MODIFY
MTAIRY
MUTINY
NAJIMY
NIDIFY
NIMINY
NOSILY
NOTIFY
NUDITY
ODDITY
OILILY
OOZILY
OSSIFY
PACIFY
PARITY
PIMINY
POKILY
POLICY
POLITY
PUNILY
PURIFY
PURITY
RACILY
RAMIFY
RARITY
RATIFY
RESINY
ROSILY
ROSINY
RUBIFY
SALIFY
SANITY
SATINY
SEXILY
SICILY
STRIPY
TIDILY
TINILY
TYPIFY
UGLIFY
UGLILY
UNMIRY
UNOILY
UNTIDY
UNWILY
UPPITY
VANITY
VASILY
VERIFY
VERILY
VERITY
VILIFY
VINIFY
VIVIFY
WARILY
WAVILY
WAXILY
WILILY
WIRILY
ZANILY

I•Z•••
ITZHAK

I••Z••
IBIZAN
ISUZUS

I•••Z•
IODIZE
IONIZE

I••••Z
IBANEZ
IGNATZ

•IZ•••
BIZKIT
DIZAIN
FIZGIG
FIZZED
FIZZER
FIZZES
FIZZLE
GIZMOS
LIZALU
LIZARD
LIZZIE
MIZUNA
MIZZEN
MIZZLE
MIZZLY
PIZAZZ
PIZZAS
SIZERS
SIZEUP
SIZING
SIZZLE
VIZIER
VIZIRS
VIZORS
VIZSLA
WIZARD
WIZENS
WIZZES
ZIZITH
ZIZZED
ZIZZES

•I•Z••
DIEZES
DITZES
FIZZED
FIZZER
FIZZES
FIZZLE
LINZER
LIZZIE
MIZZEN
MIZZLE
MIZZLY
PIAZZA
PIAZZI
PINZON
PIZZAS
RITZES
SIZZLE
WIZZES
ZIGZAG
ZIZZED
ZIZZES

•I••Z•
PIAZZA
PIAZZI
PIZAZZ
RIENZI

•I•••Z
KIBITZ
MILOSZ
NIMITZ
PIZAZZ

••IZ••
BAIZAS
BAIZES
FRIZZY
IBIZAN
MAIZES
PFIZER
PRIZED
PRIZES
PRIZMS
PRIZZI
SEIZED
SEIZER
SEIZES
SEIZOR
WHIZZY

••I•Z•
FRIEZE
FRITZI
FRIZZY
GLITZY
MAIRZY
PRINZE
PRIZZI
QUINZE
WHIZZY

••I••Z
BLINTZ
BRIENZ
CHINTZ
SHIRAZ
SWIRLZ

•••IZ•
ASSIZE
BELIZE
IODIZE
IONIZE
RESIZE
TREIZE
UPSIZE
XPRIZE

•••I•Z
ALRITZ
DONITZ
KIBITZ
KUNITZ
MORITZ
NIMITZ
SPRITZ

••••IZ
CURTIZ
LESMIZ
TABRIZ
THEWIZ

JA••••
JABBAR
JABBED
JABBER
JABOTS
JACALS
JACKAL
JACKED
JACKET
JACKIE
JACKUP
JACLYN

JACOBI
JACOBY
JADING
JADISH
JAEGER
JAFFEE
JAGGED
JAGGER
JAGLOM
JAGUAR
JAILED
JAILER
JAILOR
JAIPUR
JALAPA
JALOPY
JALPAS
JAMAAL
JAMAIS
JAMBES
JAMCAM
JAMESA
JAMESI
JAMESJ
JAMESK
JAMESM
JAMESS
JAMEST
JAMESV
JAMMED
JAMMER
JAMOCA
JAMOKE
JAMSIN
JAMSUP
JAMUPS
JANGLE
JANGLY
JANHUS
JANICE
JANINE
JANNEY
JANSEN
JANUAR
JANZEN
JAPANS
JAPERS
JAPERY
JAPING
JARABE
JARDIN
JARFUL
JARGON
JARJAR
JARRED
JARULE
JARVIK
JASCHA
JASMIN
JASPER
JAUNES
JAUNTS
JAUNTY
JAURES
JAVERT
JAVIER
JAVITS
JAWING
JAWOHL
JAWSAT
JAYCEE
JAYMES
JAYVEE
JAZZBO
JAZZED
JAZZER
JAZZES
JAZZUP

J•A•••
JEANED
JEANIE
JEANNE
JOANIE
JOANNA
JOANNE
JOANOU
JUAREZ

J••A••
JACALS
JALAPA
JAMAAL
JAMAIS
JAPANS
JARABE
JICAMA
JIHADS
JOHANN
JONAHS
JSBACH
JUDAEA
JUDAIC
JUMADA
JURADO

J•••A•
JABBAR
JACKAL
JAGUAR
JALPAS
JAMAAL
JAMCAM
JANUAR
JARJAR
JAWSAT
JEDGAR
JEERAT
JETFAN
JETLAG
JETSAM
JETTAS
JETWAY
JIBEAT
JIGSAW
JOBJAR
JORDAN
JOSIAH
JOVIAL
JOVIAN
JOYPAD
JUDEAN
JULIAN
JUMPAT
JUNEAU
JUNTAS
JUSTAS

J••••A
JALAPA
JAMESA
JAMOCA
JASCHA
JEMIMA
JERBOA
JICAMA
JOANNA
JOBYNA
JOGBRA
JOJOBA
JOSHUA
JUDAEA
JUDOKA
JUMADA

•JA•••
OJAICA

•J•A••
TJMAXX

•J••A•
AJOWAN
DJEBAR
DJILAS

•J•••A
EJECTA
OJAICA
OJIBWA

••JA••
ADJANI
BEJART
DEJAVU
GIJANE
HIJACK
INJAIL
MOJAVE
PAJAMA
RAJABS
RAJAHS
REJAIL
TEJANA
TEJANO
UNJAMS

••J•A•
FIJIAN
MAJOAD
PAJOAD
STJOAN

••J••A
ARJUNA
FAJITA
JOJOBA
PAJAMA
RIJEKA
TEJANA

•••JA•
DEEJAY
DEFJAM
ELIJAH
INAJAM
JARJAR
JOBJAR
LOGJAM
NINJAS
ONAJAG
OUIJAS
PUNJAB
RIOJAS
TIPJAR
TRAJAN
TROJAN
VEEJAY

••••JA
BAROJA

J•B•••
JABBAR
JABBED
JABBER
JABOTS
JIBEAT
JIBING
JOBBED
JOBBER
JOBCUT
JOBETH
JOBHOP
JOBJAR
JOBLOT
JOBONE
JOBSON
JOBYNA
JSBACH

J••B••
JABBAR
JABBED
JABBER
JAMBES
JERBOA
JIMBOB
JOBBED
JOBBER
JOGBRA
JUMBLE
JUMBLY
JUMBOS

J•••B•
JACOBI
JACOBY
JARABE
JAZZBO
JOJOBA
JUJUBE

J••••B
JIMBOB

•J•B••
DJEBAR
OJIBWA

••J•B•
JOJOBA
JUJUBE
MCJOBS
RAJABS

•••J•B
BAGJOB
CONJOB
DAYJOB
DYEJOB
NEWJOB
ODDJOB
PUNJAB
TOPJOB

JC••••
JCLOTH

J•C•••
JACALS
JACKAL
JACKED
JACKET
JACKIE
JACKUP
JACLYN
JACOBI
JACOBY
JECKLE
JICAMA
JOCKEY
JOCKOS
JOCOSE
JOCUND

J••C••
JAMCAM
JASCHA
JAYCEE
JOBCUT
JUICED
JUICER
JUICES
JUNCOS

J•••C•
JAMOCA
JANICE
JOUNCE
JOUNCY
JSBACH

J••••C
JUDAIC

•J•C••
EJECTA
EJECTS

•J••C•
OJAICA

•J•••C
AJIJIC

••J•C•
ABJECT
DEJECT
HIJACK
INJECT
MEJICO
OBJECT
REJECT

•••J•C
AJIJIC

J•D•••
JADING
JADISH
JEDGAR
JUDAEA
JUDAIC
JUDEAN
JUDFRY
JUDGED
JUDGES
JUDITH
JUDOKA
JUDSON

J••D••
JARDIN
JOEDON
JORDAN

J•••D•
JIHADS
JUMADA
JURADO

J••••D
JABBED
JACKED
JAGGED
JAILED
JAMMED
JARRED
JAZZED
JEANED
JEERED
JELLED
JERKED
JESTED
JETTED
JIGGED
JILTED
JINXED
JOBBED
JOCUND
JOGGED
JOINED
JOLTED
JOSHED
JOTTED
JOWLED
JOYPAD
JUDGED
JUGGED
JUICED
JUMPED
JUNKED
JURIED
JUTTED

•J•D••
EJIDOS

•J••D•
FJORDS

••J•D•
STJUDE

••J••D
BUJOLD
MAJOAD
PAJOAD

JE••••
JEANED
JEANIE
JEANNE
JECKLE
JEDGAR
JEERAT
JEERED
JEERER
JEETER
JEEVES
JEJUNE
JEKYLL
JELLED
JELLOS
JEMIMA
JENNER
JENNET
JENNEY
JENNIE
JENSEN
JERBOA
JEREMY
JERKED
JERKER
JERKIN
JERKUP
JEROME
JERSEY
JESSEL
JESSYE
JESTED
JESTER
JESUIT
JETFAN
JETGUN
JETHRO
JETLAG
JETSAM
JETSET
JETSKI
JETSON
JETTAS
JETTED
JETWAY
JEVONS
JEWELS
JEWETT
JEWISH

J•E•••
JAEGER
JEERAT
JEERED
JEERER
JEETER
JEEVES
JOEDON
JOETEX
JUEGOS
JUEVES

J••E••
JAMESA
JAMESI
JAMESJ
JAMESK
JAMESM
JAMESS
JAMEST
JAMESV
JAPERS
JAPERY
JAVERT
JEREMY
JEWELS
JEWETT
JIBEAT
JIVERS
JOBETH
JOKERS
JOLENE
JONESS
JONESY
JOSEPH
JUDEAN
JULEPS
JUNEAU

J•••E•
JABBED
JABBER
JACKED
JACKET
JAEGER
JAFFEE
JAGGED
JAGGER
JAILED
JAILER
JAMBES
JAMMED
JAMMER
JANNEY
JANSEN
JANZEN
JARRED
JASPER
JAUNES
JAURES
JAVIER
JAYCEE
JAYMES
JAYVEE
JAZZED
JAZZER
JAZZES
JEANED
JEERED
JEERER
JEETER
JEEVES
JELLED
JENNER
JENNET
JENNEY
JENSEN
JERKED
JERKER
JERSEY
JESSEL
JESTED
JESTER
JETSET
JETTED
JIGGED
JIGGER
JILTED
JILTER
JINXED
JINXER
JINXES
JITNEY
JITTER
JIVIER
JOBBED
JOBBER
JOCKEY
JOETEX
JOGGED
JOGGER
JOINED
JOINER
JOKIER
JOLIET
JOLLEY
JOLTED
JOLTER
JOSHED
JOSHER
JOSHES
JOSSES
JOTTED
JOTTER
JOULES
JOWLED
JOYNER
JOZSEF
JTILES
JUAREZ
JUDAEA
JUDGED
JUDGES
JUEVES
JUGGED
JUICED
JUICER
JUICES
JULIEN
JULIET
JUMPED
JUMPER
JUNGER
JUNKED
JUNKER
JUNKET
JURIED
JURIES
JUSTER
JUTTED

J••••E
JACKIE
JAFFEE
JAMOKE
JANGLE
JANICE
JANINE
JARABE
JARULE
JAYCEE
JAYVEE
JEANIE
JEANNE
JECKLE
JEJUNE
JENNIE
JEROME
JESSYE
JIGGLE
JILLIE
JIMMIE
JINGLE
JOANIE
JOANNE
JOBONE
JOCOSE
JOFFRE
JOGGLE
JOLENE
JOSTLE
JOUNCE
JUGGLE
JUJUBE
JUMBLE
JUNGLE
JUNKIE
JUSQUE
JUSTME

•JE•••
DJEBAR
EJECTA
EJECTS

•J••E•
IJSSEL

••JE••
ABJECT
DEJECT
INJECT
INJEST
NYJETS
OBJECT
OBJETS
REJECT
RIJEKA

••J•E•
GIJOES
HAJJES
MAJGEN
MOJOES

••J••E
ABJURE
ADJURE
BYJOVE
CAJOLE
DEJURE
GIJANE
INJOKE
INJUNE
INJURE
JEJUNE
JUJUBE
LAJOIE
MOJAVE
NOJIVE
NOJOKE
STJUDE

•••JE•
FANJET
FEEJEE
GASJET
HADJES
HAJJES
INKJET
KOPJES
MATJES
NONJEW
ORAJEL
OUTJET
PROJET
RAMJET
TRIJET
VERJEE

•••J•E
BIGJOE
FEEJEE
MARJOE
VERJEE

••••JE
SKOPJE

J•F•••
JAFFEE
JOFFRE

J••F••
JAFFEE
JARFUL
JETFAN
JOFFRE
JOYFUL
JUDFRY
JUGFUL

J••••F
JOZSEF

•JF•••
AJFOYT

J•G•••
JAGGED
JAGGER
JAGLOM
JAGUAR
JIGGED
JIGGER
JIGGLE
JIGGLY
JIGSAW
JOGBRA
JOGGED
JOGGER
JOGGLE
JUGFUL
JUGGED
JUGGLE

J••G••
JAEGER
JAGGED
JAGGER
JANGLE
JANGLY
JARGON
JEDGAR
JETGUN
JIGGED
JIGGER
JIGGLE
JIGGLY
JINGLE
JINGLY
JOGGED
JOGGER
JOGGLE
JUDGED
JUDGES
JUEGOS
JUGGED
JUGGLE
JUNGER
JUNGLE
JUNGLY

J••••G
JADING
JAPING
JAWING
JETLAG
JIBING
JIVING
JOKING
JOYING
JUKING

••JG••
MAJGEN

••J•G•
REJIGS

••J••G
DRJUNG

•••J•G
ONAJAG

J•H•••
JIHADS
JOHANN
JOHNII
JOHNIV
JOHNIX
JOHNNY
JOHNVI
JOHNXI
JOHNXV
JOHNXX

J••H••
JANHUS
JETHRO
JOBHOP
JOSHED
JOSHER
JOSHES
JOSHUA

J•••H•
JASCHA
JAWOHL
JONAHS

J••••H
JADISH
JCLOTH
JEWISH
JOBETH
JOSEPH
JOSIAH
JSBACH
JUDITH

••J•H•
IIJOHN
RAJAHS
STJOHN
UPJOHN

•••J•H
ELIJAH

JI••••
JIBEAT
JIBING
JICAMA
JIGGED
JIGGER
JIGGLE
JIGGLY
JIGSAW
JIHADS
JILLIE
JILTED
JILTER
JIMBOB
JIMINY
JIMMIE
JIMSON
JINGLE
JINGLY
JINNIS
JINXED
JINXER
JINXES
JITNEY
JITTER
JIVERS
JIVIER
JIVING

J•I•••
JAILED
JAILER
JAILOR
JAIPUR
JOINED
JOINER
JOININ
JOINTS
JOINUP
JOISTS
JTILES
JUICED
JUICER
JUICES

J••I••
JADING
JADISH
JANICE
JANINE
JAPING
JAVIER
JAVITS
JAWING
JEMIMA
JEWISH
JIBING
JIMINY
JIVIER
JIVING
JOKIER
JOKILY
JOKING
JOLIET
JOLIOT
JOSIAH
JOVIAL
JOVIAN
JOYING
JUDITH
JUKING
JULIAN
JULIEN
JULIET
JULIUS
JUNIOR
JUNIUS
JURIED
JURIES
JURIST

J•••I•
JACKIE
JAMAIS
JAMSIN
JARDIN
JARVIK
JASMIN
JEANIE
JENNIE
JERKIN
JESUIT
JILLIE
JIMMIE
JINNIS
JOANIE
JOHNII
JOHNIV
JOHNIX
JOININ
JOLTIN
JOPLIN
JUDAIC
JUMPIN
JUNKIE
JUSTIN

J••••I
JACOBI
JAMESI
JETSKI
JOHNII
JOHNVI
JOHNXI

•JI•••
AJIJIC
DJILAS
DJINNI
DJINNS
EJIDOS
OJIBWA

•J•I••
OJAICA

•J••I•
AJIJIC

•J•••I
DJINNI

••JI••
FAJITA
FIJIAN
MEJICO
MOJITO
MRJINX
NAJIMY
NOJIVE
REJIGS

••J•I•
ADJOIN
ENJOIN
HAJJIS
INJAIL
LAJOIE
MAJLIS
REJAIL
REJOIN
UNJOIN

••J••I
ADJANI

•••JI•
AJIJIC
GAIJIN
HADJIS
HAJJIS
KANJIS
SHOJIS

••••JI
MTFUJI
ROMAJI

J•J•••
JEJUNE
JOJOBA

JUJUBE

J••J••
JARJAR
JOBJAR

J••••J
JAMESJ

•J•J••
AJIJIC

••JJ••
HAJJES
HAJJIS

JK••••
JKLMNO

J•K•••
JEKYLL
JOKERS
JOKIER
JOKILY
JOKING
JUKING

J••K••
JACKAL
JACKED
JACKET
JACKIE
JACKUP
JECKLE
JERKED
JERKER
JERKIN
JERKUP
JOCKEY
JOCKOS
JUNKED
JUNKER
JUNKET
JUNKIE

J•••K•
JAMOKE
JETSKI
JUDOKA

J••••K
JAMESK
JARVIK

•JK•••
IJKLMN

••JK••
HIJKLM

••J•K•
INJOKE
NOJOKE
RIJEKA

••J••K
DEJUNK
HIJACK

•••JK•
GHIJKL
STOJKO

••••JK
FGHIJK

J•L•••
JALAPA
JALOPY
JALPAS
JCLOTH
JELLED
JELLOS
JILLIE
JILTED
JILTER
JKLMNO
JOLENE
JOLIET
JOLIOT
JOLLEY
JOLSON
JOLTED
JOLTER
JOLTIN
JULEPS
JULIAN
JULIEN
JULIET
JULIUS

J••L••
JACLYN
JAGLOM
JAILED
JAILER
JAILOR
JELLED
JELLOS
JETLAG
JILLIE
JOBLOT
JOLLEY
JOPLIN
JOULES
JOWLED
JTILES

J•••L•
JACALS
JANGLE
JANGLY
JARULE
JECKLE
JEKYLL
JEWELS
JIGGLE
JIGGLY
JINGLE
JINGLY
JOGGLE
JOKILY
JOSTLE
JUGGLE
JUMBLE
JUMBLY
JUNGLE
JUNGLY
JUSTLY

J••••L
JACKAL
JAMAAL
JARFUL
JAWOHL
JEKYLL
JESSEL
JOVIAL
JOYFUL
JUGFUL

•J•L••
DJILAS
IJKLMN

•J•••L
IJSSEL

••JL••
MAJLIS

••J•L•
BUJOLD
CAJOLE
HIJKLM
INJULY
PUJOLS

••J••L
INJAIL
REJAIL

•••J•L
BANJUL
FRIJOL
GHIJKL
ORAJEL

J•M•••
JAMAAL
JAMAIS
JAMBES
JAMCAM
JAMESA
JAMESI
JAMESJ
JAMESK
JAMESM
JAMESS
JAMEST
JAMESV
JAMMED
JAMMER
JAMOCA
JAMOKE
JAMSIN
JAMSUP
JAMUPS
JEMIMA
JIMBOB
JIMINY
JIMMIE
JIMSON
JUMADA
JUMBLE
JUMBLY
JUMBOS
JUMPAT
JUMPED
JUMPER
JUMPIN
JUMPON
JUMPUP

J••M••
JAMMED
JAMMER
JASMIN
JAYMES
JIMMIE
JKLMNO

J•••M•
JEMIMA
JEREMY
JEROME
JICAMA
JORUMS
JUSTME

J••••M
JAGLOM
JAMCAM
JAMESM
JETSAM

•JM•••
TJMAXX

•J••M•
IJKLMN

••J•M•
NAJIMY
PAJAMA
UNJAMS

••J••M
HIJKLM

•••J•M
BOOJUM
DEFJAM
INAJAM
LOGJAM

J•N•••
JANGLE
JANGLY
JANHUS
JANICE
JANINE
JANNEY
JANSEN
JANUAR
JANZEN
JENNER
JENNET
JENNEY
JENNIE
JENSEN
JINGLE
JINGLY
JINNIS
JINXED
JINXER
JINXES
JONAHS
JONESS
JONESY
JONSON
JUNCOS
JUNEAU
JUNGER
JUNGLE
JUNGLY
JUNIOR
JUNIUS
JUNKED
JUNKER
JUNKET
JUNKIE
JUNTAS
JUNTOS

J••N••
JANNEY
JAUNES
JAUNTS
JAUNTY
JEANED
JEANIE
JEANNE
JENNER
JENNET
JENNEY
JENNIE
JINNIS
JITNEY
JOANIE
JOANNA
JOANNE
JOANOU
JOHNII
JOHNIV
JOHNIX
JOHNNY
JOHNVI
JOHNXI
JOHNXV
JOHNXX
JOINED
JOINER
JOININ
JOINTS
JOINUP
JOUNCE
JOUNCY
JOYNER

J•••N•
JADING
JANINE
JAPANS
JAPING
JAWING
JEANNE
JEJUNE
JEVONS
JIBING
JIMINY
JIVING
JKLMNO
JOANNA
JOANNE
JOBONE
JOBYNA
JOCUND
JOHANN
JOHNNY
JOKING
JOLENE
JOURNO
JOYING
JUKING

J••••N
JACLYN
JAMSIN
JANSEN
JANZEN
JARDIN
JARGON
JASMIN
JENSEN
JERKIN
JETFAN
JETGUN
JETSON
JIMSON
JOBSON
JOEDON
JOHANN
JOININ
JOLSON
JOLTIN
JONSON
JOPLIN
JORDAN
JOVIAN
JUDEAN
JUDSON
JULIAN
JULIEN
JUMPIN
JUMPON
JUSTIN

•J•N••
DJINNI
DJINNS

•J••N•
DJINNI
DJINNS

•J•••N
AJOWAN
IJKLMN

••J•N•
ADJANI
ARJUNA
CAJUNS
DEJUNK
DRJUNG
GIJANE
INJUNE
JEJUNE
MRJINX
TEJANA
TEJANO

••J••N
ADJOIN
ENJOIN
FIJIAN
IIJOHN
MAJGEN
REJOIN
STJOAN
STJOHN
UNJOIN
UPJOHN

•••J•N
DONJON
GAIJIN
TRAJAN
TROJAN

••••JN
ROMIJN

JO••••
JOANIE
JOANNA
JOANNE
JOANOU
JOBBED
JOBBER
JOBCUT
JOBETH
JOBHOP
JOBJAR
JOBLOT
JOBONE
JOBSON
JOBYNA
JOCKEY
JOCKOS
JOCOSE
JOCUND
JOEDON
JOETEX
JOFFRE
JOGBRA
JOGGED
JOGGER
JOGGLE
JOHANN
JOHNII
JOHNIV
JOHNIX
JOHNNY
JOHNVI
JOHNXI
JOHNXV
JOHNXX
JOINED
JOINER
JOININ
JOINTS
JOINUP
JOISTS
JOJOBA
JOKERS
JOKIER
JOKILY
JOKING
JOLENE
JOLIET
JOLIOT
JOLLEY
JOLSON
JOLTED
JOLTER
JOLTIN
JONAHS
JONESS
JONESY
JONSON
JOPLIN
JORDAN
JORUMS
JOSEPH
JOSHED
JOSHER
JOSHES
JOSHUA
JOSIAH
JOSSES
JOSTLE
JOTTED
JOTTER
JOULES
JOUNCE
JOUNCY
JOURNO
JOUSTS
JOVIAL
JOVIAN
JOWLED
JOYFUL
JOYING
JOYNER
JOYOUS
JOYPAD
JOZSEF

J••O••
JABOTS
JACOBI
JACOBY
JALOPY
JAMOCA
JAMOKE
JAWOHL
JCLOTH
JEROME
JEVONS
JOBONE
JOCOSE
JOJOBA
JOYOUS
JUDOKA
JURORS

J•••O•
JAGLOM
JAILOR
JARGON
JELLOS
JERBOA
JETSON
JIMBOB
JIMSON
JOANOU
JOBHOP
JOBLOT
JOBSON
JOCKOS
JOEDON
JOLIOT
JOLSON
JONSON
JUDSON
JUEGOS
JUMBOS
JUMPON
JUNCOS
JUNIOR
JUNTOS

J••••O
JAZZBO
JETHRO
JKLMNO
JOURNO
JURADO
JUSTSO

•JO•••
AJOWAN
FJORDS

•J•O••
AJFOYT

•J••O•
EJIDOS

••JO••
ADJOIN
ANJOUS
BIJOUS
BIJOUX
BUJOLD
BYJOVE
CAJOLE
ENJOIN
ENJOYS
GIJOES
IIJOHN
INJOKE
JOJOBA
LAJOIE
MAJOAD
MAJORS
MCJOBS
MOJOES
NOJOKE
PAJOAD
PUJOLS
REJOIN
STJOAN
STJOHN
UNJOIN
UPJOHN

••J••O
MEJICO
MOJITO
TEJANO

•••JO•
AMAJOR
BAGJOB
BANJOS
BIGJOE
BMAJOR
CMAJOR
CONJOB
DAYJOB
DMAJOR
DONJON
DYEJOB
EMAJOR
FMAJOR
FORJOY
FRIJOL
GMAJOR
MARJOE
MENJOU
NEWJOB
ODDJOB
TOPJOB

•••J•O
STOJKO

••••JO
MARYJO
NAVAJO

J•P•••
JAPANS
JAPERS
JAPERY
JAPING
JOPLIN

J••P••
JAIPUR
JALPAS
JASPER
JOYPAD
JUMPAT
JUMPED
JUMPER
JUMPIN
JUMPON
JUMPUP

J•••P•
JALAPA
JALOPY
JAMUPS
JOSEPH
JULEPS

J••••P
JACKUP
JAMSUP
JAZZUP
JERKUP
JOBHOP
JOINUP
JUMPUP

J••Q••
JUSQUE

J•R•••
JARABE
JARDIN
JARFUL
JARGON
JARJAR
JARRED
JARULE
JARVIK
JERBOA
JEREMY
JERKED
JERKER
JERKIN
JERKUP
JEROME
JERSEY
JORDAN
JORUMS
JURADO
JURIED
JURIES
JURIST
JURORS

J••R••
JARRED
JAURES
JEERAT
JEERED
JEERER
JOURNO
JUAREZ

J•••R•
JAPERS
JAPERY
JAVERT
JETHRO
JIVERS
JOFFRE
JOGBRA
JOKERS
JUDFRY
JURORS

J••••R
JABBAR
JABBER
JAEGER
JAGGER
JAGUAR
JAILER
JAILOR
JAIPUR
JAMMER
JANUAR
JARJAR
JASPER
JAVIER
JAZZER
JEDGAR
JEERER
JEETER
JENNER
JERKER
JESTER
JIGGER
JILTER
JINXER
JITTER
JIVIER
JOBBER
JOBJAR
JOGGER
JOINER
JOKIER
JOLTER
JOSHER
JOTTER
JOYNER
JUICER
JUMPER
JUNGER
JUNIOR
JUNKER
JUSTER

•J•R••
FJORDS

•J•••R
DJEBAR

••J•R•
ABJURE
ADJURE
BEJART
DEJURE
INJURE
INJURY
MAJORS

•••J•R
AMAJOR
BMAJOR
CMAJOR
DMAJOR
EMAJOR
FMAJOR
GMAJOR
JARJAR
JOBJAR
TIPJAR

••••JR
DRIQJR
NICKJR

JS••••
JSBACH

J•S•••
JASCHA
JASMIN
JASPER
JESSEL
JESSYE
JESTED
JESTER
JESUIT
JOSEPH
JOSHED
JOSHER
JOSHES
JOSHUA
JOSIAH
JOSSES
JOSTLE
JUSQUE
JUSTAS
JUSTER
JUSTIN
JUSTLY
JUSTME
JUSTSO
JUSTUS
JUSTYS

J••S••
JAMSIN
JAMSUP
JANSEN
JAWSAT
JENSEN
JERSEY
JESSEL
JESSYE
JETSAM
JETSET
JETSKI
JETSON
JIGSAW
JIMSON
JOBSON
JOISTS
JOLSON
JONSON
JOSSES
JOUSTS
JOZSEF
JUDSON

J•••S•
JADISH
JAMESA
JAMESI
JAMESJ
JAMESK
JAMESM
JAMESS
JAMEST
JAMESV
JEWISH
JOCOSE
JONESS
JONESY
JURIST
JUSTSO

J••••S
JABOTS
JACALS
JALPAS
JAMAIS
JAMBES
JAMESS
JAMUPS
JANHUS
JAPANS
JAPERS
JAUNES
JAUNTS
JAURES
JAVITS
JAYMES
JAZZES
JEEVES
JELLOS
JETTAS
JEVONS
JEWELS
JIHADS
JINNIS
JINXES
JIVERS
JOCKOS
JOINTS
JOISTS
JOKERS
JONAHS
JONESS
JORUMS
JOSHES
JOSSES
JOULES
JOUSTS
JOYOUS
JTILES
JUDGES
JUEGOS
JUEVES
JUICES
JULEPS
JULIUS
JUMBOS
JUNCOS
JUNIUS
JUNTAS
JUNTOS
JURIES
JURORS
JUSTAS
JUSTUS
JUSTYS

•JS•••
IJSSEL

•J•S••
IJSSEL

•J•••S
DJILAS
DJINNS
EJECTS
EJIDOS
FJORDS

••J•S•
ADJUST
INJEST
UNJUST

••J••S
ANJOUS
BIJOUS
CAJUNS
ENJOYS
GIJOES
HAJJES
HAJJIS
MAJLIS
MAJORS
MCJOBS
MOJOES
NYJETS
OBJETS
PUJOLS
RAJABS
RAJAHS
REJIGS
UNJAMS

•••J•S
BANJOS
HADJES
HADJIS
HAJJES
HAJJIS
KANJIS
KOPJES
MATJES
NINJAS
OUIJAS
RIOJAS
SHOJIS

••••JS
MTVVJS

JT••••
JTILES

J•T•••
JETFAN
JETGUN
JETHRO
JETLAG
JETSAM
JETSET
JETSKI
JETSON
JETTAS
JETTED
JETWAY
JITNEY
JITTER
JOTTED
JOTTER
JUTTED

J••T••
JEETER
JESTED
JESTER
JETTAS
JETTED
JILTED
JILTER
JITTER
JOETEX
JOLTED
JOLTER
JOLTIN
JOSTLE
JOTTED

JOTTER
JUNTAS
JUNTOS
JUSTAS
JUSTER
JUSTIN
JUSTLY
JUSTME
JUSTSO
JUSTUS
JUSTYS
JUTTED

J•••T•
JABOTS
JAUNTS
JAUNTY
JAVITS
JCLOTH
JEWETT
JOBETH
JOINTS
JOISTS
JOUSTS
JUDITH

J••••T
JACKET
JAMEST
JAVERT
JAWSAT
JEERAT
JENNET
JESUIT
JETSET
JEWETT
JIBEAT
JOBCUT
JOBLOT
JOLIET
JOLIOT
JULIET
JUMPAT
JUNKET
JURIST

•J••T•
EJECTA
EJECTS

•J•••T
AJFOYT

••J•T•
FAJITA
MOJITO
NYJETS
OBJETS

••J••T
ABJECT
ADJUST
BEJART
DEJECT
INJECT
INJEST
OBJECT
REJECT
UNJUST

•••J•T
FANJET
GASJET
INKJET
OUTJET
OUTJUT
PROJET
RAMJET
TRIJET

JU••••
JUAREZ
JUDAEA
JUDAIC
JUDEAN
JUDFRY
JUDGED
JUDGES
JUDITH
JUDOKA
JUDSON
JUEGOS
JUEVES
JUGFUL
JUGGED
JUGGLE
JUICED
JUICER
JUICES
JUJUBE
JUKING
JULEPS
JULIAN
JULIEN
JULIET
JULIUS
JUMADA
JUMBLE
JUMBLY
JUMBOS
JUMPAT
JUMPED
JUMPER
JUMPIN
JUMPON
JUMPUP
JUNCOS
JUNEAU
JUNGER
JUNGLE
JUNGLY
JUNIOR
JUNIUS
JUNKED
JUNKER
JUNKET
JUNKIE
JUNTAS
JUNTOS
JURADO
JURIED
JURIES
JURIST
JURORS
JUSQUE
JUSTAS
JUSTER
JUSTIN
JUSTLY
JUSTME
JUSTSO
JUSTUS
JUSTYS
JUTTED

J•U•••
JAUNES
JAUNTS
JAUNTY
JAURES
JOULES
JOUNCE
JOUNCY
JOURNO
JOUSTS

J••U••
JAGUAR
JAMUPS
JANUAR
JARULE
JEJUNE
JESUIT
JOCUND
JORUMS
JUJUBE

J•••U•
JACKUP
JAIPUR
JAMSUP
JANHUS
JARFUL
JAZZUP
JERKUP
JETGUN
JOBCUT
JOINUP
JOSHUA
JOYFUL
JOYOUS
JUGFUL
JULIUS
JUMPUP
JUNIUS
JUSQUE
JUSTUS

J••••U
JOANOU
JUNEAU

••JU••
ABJURE
ADJURE
ADJUST
ARJUNA
CAJUNS
DEJUNK
DEJURE
DRJUNG
INJULY
INJUNE
INJURE
INJURY
JEJUNE
JUJUBE
STJUDE
UNJUST

••J•U•
ANJOUS
BIJOUS
BIJOUX

••J••U
DEJAVU

•••JU•
BANJUL
BOOJUM
OUTJUT

•••J•U
MENJOU

J•V•••
JAVERT
JAVIER
JAVITS
JEVONS
JIVERS
JIVIER
JIVING
JOVIAL
JOVIAN

J••V••
JARVIK
JAYVEE
JEEVES
JUEVES

J•••V•
JOHNVI

J••••V
JAMESV
JOHNIV
JOHNXV

••J•V•
BYJOVE
DEJAVU
MOJAVE
NOJIVE

J•W•••
JAWING
JAWOHL
JAWSAT
JEWELS
JEWETT
JEWISH
JOWLED

J••W••
JETWAY

J••••W
JIGSAW

•J•W••
AJOWAN

•J••W•
OJIBWA

•••J•W
NONJEW

J••X••
JINXED
JINXER
JINXES

J•••X•
JOHNXI
JOHNXV
JOHNXX

J••••X
JOETEX
JOHNIX
JOHNXX

•J••X•
TJMAXX

•J•••X
TJMAXX

••J••X
BIJOUX
MRJINX

J•Y•••
JAYCEE
JAYMES
JAYVEE
JOYFUL
JOYING
JOYNER
JOYOUS
JOYPAD

J••Y••
JEKYLL
JOBYNA

J•••Y•
JACLYN
JESSYE
JUSTYS

J••••Y
JACOBY
JALOPY
JANGLY
JANNEY
JAPERY
JAUNTY
JENNEY
JEREMY
JERSEY
JETWAY
JIGGLY
JIMINY
JINGLY
JITNEY
JOCKEY
JOHNNY
JOKILY
JOLLEY
JONESY
JOUNCY
JUDFRY
JUMBLY
JUNGLY
JUSTLY

•J••Y•
AJFOYT

••J•Y•
ENJOYS

••J••Y
INJULY
INJURY
NAJIMY

•••J•Y
DEEJAY
FORJOY
VEEJAY

J•Z•••
JAZZBO
JAZZED
JAZZER
JAZZES
JAZZUP
JOZSEF

J••Z••
JANZEN
JAZZBO
JAZZED
JAZZER
JAZZES
JAZZUP

J••••Z
JUAREZ

KA••••
KABOBS
KABOOM
KABUKI
KADEEM
KADETT
KAETHE
KAGAWA
KAHLIL
KAHLUA
KAHUNA
KAILUA
KAISER
KAKAPO
KAKURO
KALINE
KALKAN
KALLEN
KALMAR
KAMALI
KANAKA
KANALY
KANATA
KANAWA
KANDEL
KANDER
KANJIS
KANSAN
KANSAS
KANTOR
KAOLIN
KAONIC
KAPELL
KAPLAN
KAPOKS
KAPPAS
KAPUTT
KARATE
KARATS
KAREEM
KARINA
KARKOV
KARLEN
KARMAS
KARMIC
KARNAK
KARPOV
KARRAS
KARRER
KARRIE
KARSTS
KASBAH
KASDAN
KASHAS
KATHIE
KATMAI
KATRIN
KATZEN
KAUNAS
KAUNDA
KAVNER
KAYAKS
KAYOED
KAYYOW
KAZOOS

K•A•••
KEARNS
KEARNY
KEATON
KHAKIS
KHALID
KIARIO
KLAATU
KLATCH
KLAXON
KMARTS
KNACKS
KNARRS
KNARRY
KNAVES
KOALAS
KRAALS
KRAITS
KRAKEN
KRAKOW
KRAMER
KRANTZ
KRASNA
KRAUSS
KRAVIS
KWACHA
KWANZA

K••A••
KAGAWA
KAKAPO
KAMALI
KANAKA
KANALY
KANATA
KANAWA
KARATE
KARATS
KAYAKS
KDLANG
KEBABS
KERALA
KIGALI
KITAEN
KLAATU
KNEADS
KODAKS
KODALY
KORANS
KORATS
KOVACS
KRAALS
KSTARS
KULAKS
KURALT
KUVASZ
KUWAIT

K•••A•
KALKAN
KALMAR
KANSAN
KANSAS
KAPLAN
KAPPAS
KARMAS
KARNAK
KARRAS
KASBAH
KASDAN
KASHAS
KATMAI
KAUNAS
KCSTAR
KEENAN
KEEPAT
KENNAN
KENYAN
KEPTAT
KEVLAR
KEYMAN
KEYPAD
KEYPAL
KEYWAY
KIDMAN
KIDNAP
KIERAN
KINNAN
KIOWAN
KIOWAS
KIRMAN
KITBAG
KITKAT
KLIBAN
KOALAS
KODIAK
KOMBAT
KONRAD
KOREAN
KORMAN
KOUFAX
KUBLAI

K••••A
KAGAWA
KAHLUA
KAHUNA
KAILUA
KANAKA
KANATA
KANAWA
KARINA
KAUNDA
KERALA
KESHIA
KEYOFA
KISHKA
KONICA
KORUNA
KRASNA
KWACHA
KWANZA

•KA•••
OKAPIS
OKAYED
SKAGGS
SKALDS
SKANKS
SKANKY
SKATED
SKATER
SKATES
UKASES

•K•A••
AKUAKU
EKLAND
OKSANA
SKOALS

•K••A•
AKELAS
AKITAS
SKICAP
SKIHAT
SKIWAX
SKYCAM
SKYCAP
SKYLAB
SKYMAN
SKYMAP
SKYWAY

•K•••A
OKSANA

••KA••
ACKACK
ALKAID
ALKALI
ANKARA
ASKAMY
ASKANT
BUKAVU
DEKALB
ECKART
GOKART
KAKAPO
MIKADO
MIKASA
ORKANS
TOKAYS
WAKAME
YUKATA
YUKAWA

••K•A•
AIKMAN
DIKTAT
INKPAD
INKSAC
MCKEAN
NAKFAS
NIKEAD
NOKIAS
OAKTAG
POKEAT
TEKWAR
TIKKAS
TOKLAS

••K••A
ANKARA
BAKULA
BIKILA
DAKOTA
LAKOTA
LIKUTA
MAKEBA
MAKUTA
MIKASA
MIKITA
NIKITA
NIKOLA
PAKULA
YAKIMA
YAKUZA
YUKATA
YUKAWA

•••KA•
BABKAS
BAIKAL
BALKAN
BALKAT
BARKAT
BROKAW
BURKAS
DINKAS
ERYKAH
GAWKAT
HAIKAI
HICKAM
HONKAT
HOOKAH
IMOKAY
JACKAL
KALKAN
KITKAT
LOOKAT
MARKAS
OSAKAN
PARKAS
PARKAV
PARKAY
PECKAT
PEEKAT
PICKAT
PICKAX
PLAKAT
POLKAS
PUNKAS
RYOKAN
SANKAS
SIRKAY
STUKAS
TALKAT
TANKAS
TIKKAS
TONKAS
VODKAS
WINKAT
WORKAT
YANKAT
YOAKAM

•••K•A
BARKLA
CHAKRA
GURKHA
LOOKMA
MARKKA
MOSKVA
YORKPA

••••KA
ALASKA
ANNIKA
APOPKA
BARAKA
CSONKA
EUREKA
FLICKA
FRICKA
GLINKA
IVANKA
JUDOKA
KANAKA
KISHKA
LUSAKA
MARKKA
MEDAKA
NOOTKA
POLSKA
RIJEKA
SEDAKA
SVEDKA
TANAKA
TOPEKA
TROIKA

K•B•••
KABOBS
KABOOM
KABUKI
KEBABS
KGBSPY
KIBBEE
KIBBLE
KIBITZ
KIBOSH
KOBOLD
KUBLAI
KUBLER

K••B••
KASBAH
KEMBLE
KHYBER
KIBBEE
KIBBLE
KIMBLE
KITBAG
KLIBAN
KNEBEL
KNOBBY
KOMBAT
KOMBUS
KORBUT

K•••B•
KABOBS
KEBABS
KENOBI
KNOBBY

K••••B
KEYOFB

•KB•••
EKBERG
OKBYME

•K•B••
SKIBIB
SKIBOB
SKIBUM
SKYBOX

•K••B•
AKIMBO
EKEDBY
EKESBY
SKIPBY

•K•••B
SKIBIB
SKIBOB
SKYLAB

••K•B•
MAKEBA

••K••B
DEKALB

•••KB•
TICKBY
WALKBY

KC••••
KCSTAR

K•C•••
KICKED
KICKER
KICKIN
KICKUP
KOCHEL
KOCHER
KUCHEN

K••C••
KIDCOM
KIMCHI
KLICKS
KNACKS
KNICKS
KNOCKS
KWACHA

K•••C•
KIRSCH
KITSCH
KLATCH
KONICA
KOPECK
KOVACS
KVETCH

K••••C
KAONIC
KARMIC
KEYOFC

•K•C••
SKICAP
SKYCAM
SKYCAP

•K••C•
SKETCH
SKITCH

••K•C•
ACKACK
EDKOCH
LUKICH
REKICK

••K••C
INKSAC

•••K•C
TURKIC

KD••••
KDLANG

K•D•••
KADEEM
KADETT
KEDGED
KEDGER
KEDGES
KIDCOM
KIDDED
KIDDER
KIDDIE
KIDDOS
KIDEOS
KIDLIT
KIDMAN
KIDNAP
KIDNEY
KIDORY
KIDULT
KIDVID
KODAKS
KODALY
KODIAK
KPDUTY
KUDROW
KUDZUS

K••D••
KANDEL
KANDER
KASDAN
KENDOS
KEYDET
KIDDED
KIDDER
KIDDIE
KIDDOS
KINDER
KINDLE
KINDLY
KINDOF
KLUDGE
KLUDGY
KUNDRY

K•••D•
KAUNDA
KNEADS
KOMODO

K••••D
KAYOED
KEDGED
KEELED
KEENED
KEGGED
KENNED
KERNED
KEYOFD
KEYPAD
KHALID
KICKED
KIDDED
KIDVID
KILLED
KILNED
KILTED
KINGED
KINKED
KIPPED
KISSED
KITTED
KNIFED
KOBOLD
KONRAD

•K•D••
EKEDBY
SKIDDY
SKIDOO

•K••D•
SKALDS
SKIDDY

•K•••D
EKLAND
OKAYED
SKATED
SKEWED

••KD••
DIKDIK

••K•D•
AIKIDO
ALKYDS
MAKEDO
MIKADO
NOKIDS

••K••D
ALKAID
ANKLED
BEKIND
ECKERD
FAKEID
INKIND
INKPAD
NIKEAD
UNKIND
YAKKED
YUKKED

•••K•D
AWAKED
BACKED
BALKED
BANKED
BARKED
BASKED
BEAKED
BIGKID
BILKED
BONKED
BOOKED
BORKED
BRAKED
BUCKED
BULKED
BUNKED
BUSKED
CALKED
CASKED
CHOKED
COCKED
CONKED
COOKED
CORKED
DECKED
DIRKED
DISKED
DOCKED
DUCKED
DUNKED
DUSKED
EVOKED
FINKED
FLAKED

FORKED
FUNKED
GAWKED
GEEKED
HACKED
HARKED
HAWKED
HOCKED
HONKED
HOOKED
HULKED
HUSKED
JACKED
JERKED
JUNKED
KICKED
KINKED
LACKED
LARKED
LEAKED
LICKED
LINKED
LOCKED
LOOKED
LUCKED
LURKED
MARKED
MASKED
MILKED
MOCKED
MUCKED
NECKED
NEWKID
NICKED
NOCKED
OINKED
PACKED
PARKED
PEAKED
PECKED
PEEKED
PERKED
PICKED
PINKED
PORKED
QUAKED
RACKED
RANKED
RECKED
REEKED
RISKED
ROCKED
ROOKED
RUCKED
SACKED
SLAKED
SMOKED
SNAKED
SOAKED
SOCKED
SPIKED
SPOKED
STAKED
STOKED
SUCKED
SULKED
TACKED
TALKED
TANKED
TASKED
THEKID
TICKED
TUCKED
TUSKED
WALKED
WICKED
WINKED
WORKED
YAKKED
YANKED
YOLKED
YUKKED
ZONKED

••••KD
CRACKD

KE••••
KEARNS
KEARNY
KEATON
KEBABS
KEDGED
KEDGER
KEDGES
KEELED
KEELER
KEENAN
KEENED
KEENEN
KEENER
KEENLY
KEENON
KEEPAT
KEEPER
KEEPIN
KEEPIT
KEEPON
KEEPTO
KEEPUP
KEFIRS
KEGGED
KEGGER
KEGLER
KEITEL
KELLER
KELLEY
KELLIE
KELLYS
KELPIE
KELSEY
KELTON
KELVIN
KEMBLE
KEMPIS
KENDOS
KENNAN
KENNED
KENNEL
KENNER
KENNYG
KENOBI
KENSIT
KENTON
KENYAN
KENYON
KEOKUK
KEPLER
KEPTAT
KEPTIN
KEPTON
KEPTTO
KEPTUP
KERALA
KERMIT
KERNED
KERNEL
KERNES
KERSEE
KERWIN
KESHIA
KETONE
KETTLE
KEVLAR
KEWPIE
KEYDET
KEYING
KEYMAN
KEYMEN
KEYNES
KEYOFA
KEYOFB
KEYOFC
KEYOFD
KEYOFF
KEYOFG
KEYPAD
KEYPAL
KEYSER
KEYSIN
KEYSON
KEYSUP
KEYWAY

K•E•••
KAETHE
KEELED
KEELER
KEENAN
KEENED
KEENEN
KEENER
KEENLY
KEENON
KEEPAT
KEEPER
KEEPIN
KEEPIT
KEEPON
KEEPTO
KEEPUP
KIEFER
KIERAN
KIERON
KLEINE
KLEIST
KLEPTO
KMESON
KNEADS
KNEBEL
KNEELS
KNELLS
KNEWIT
KNEWOF
KOENIG
KRENEK
KRESGE
KREWES
KVELLS
KVETCH
KWEISI

K••E••
KADEEM
KADETT
KAPELL
KAREEM
KHMERS
KIDEOS
KITERS
KNEELS
KOPECK
KOPEKS
KOPELL
KOREAN

K•••E•
KADEEM
KAISER
KALLEN
KANDEL
KANDER
KAREEM
KARLEN
KARRER
KATZEN
KAVNER
KAYOED
KEDGED
KEDGER
KEDGES
KEELED
KEELER
KEENED
KEENEN
KEENER
KEEPER
KEGGED
KEGGER
KEGLER
KEITEL
KELLER
KELLEY
KELSEY
KENNED
KENNEL
KENNER
KEPLER
KERNED
KERNEL
KERNES
KERSEE
KEYDET
KEYMEN
KEYNES
KEYSER
KHYBER
KIBBEE
KICKED
KICKER
KIDDED
KIDDER
KIDNEY
KIEFER
KILLED
KILLER
KILMER
KILNED
KILTED
KILTER
KINDER
KINGED
KINKED
KINSEY
KIPPED
KIPPER
KISLEV
KISMET
KISSED
KISSEL
KISSER
KISSES
KITAEN
KITTED
KITTEN
KNAVES
KNEBEL
KNIFED
KNIFER
KNIFES
KNIVES
KNOWER
KOCHEL
KOCHER
KOHLER
KOPJES
KOPPEL
KOSHER
KOSSEL
KOSTER
KOTTER
KRAKEN
KRAMER
KRENEK
KREWES
KROGER
KRONER
KRUGER
KTILES
KUBLER
KUCHEN
KUMMEL
KUNZEL

K••••E
KAETHE
KALINE
KARATE
KARRIE
KATHIE
KELLIE
KELPIE
KEMBLE
KERSEE
KETONE
KETTLE
KEWPIE
KIBBEE
KIBBLE
KIDDIE
KILTIE
KIMBLE
KINDLE
KINGME
KISHKE
KISSME
KLEINE
KLUDGE
KOOKIE
KOTTKE
KRESGE
KURILE

•KE•••
AKELAS
AKENES
EKEDBY
EKELOF
EKEOUT
EKESBY
OKEEFE
RKELLY
SKEETS
SKEINS
SKETCH
SKEWED
SKEWER

•K•E••
EKBERG
EKUELE
OKEEFE
SKEETS
SKIERS

•K••E•
AKENES
OKAYED
SKATED
SKATER
SKATES
SKEWED
SKEWER
SKYMEN
SKYTEL
UKASES

•K•••E
EKUELE
OKBYME
OKEEFE
SKOKIE
SKOPJE

••KE••
ALKENE
ASKERS
BAKERS
BAKERY
BIKERS
CAKEUP
DIKERS
ECKERD
ESKERS
FAKEID
FAKEIT
FAKERS
FAKERY
HAKEEM
HIKERS
HIKEUP
INKERS
IRKERS
JOKERS
LAKERS
LIKELY
LIKENS
LIKERS
LIKESO
LIKETO
MAKEBA
MAKEDO
MAKEGO
MAKEIT
MAKEME
MAKEOF
MAKERS
MAKEUP
MCKEAN
MCKEON
MCKERN
NIKEAD
PIKERS
POKEAT
POKERS
POKERY
POKEYS
RAKEIN
RAKERS
RAKEUP
REKEYS
RIKERS
TAKEIN
TAKEIT
TAKEON
TAKERS
TAKETH
TAKETO
TAKEUP
TOKENS
UNKEPT
UPKEEP
WAKENS
WAKERS
WAKEUP
WOKEUP
YOKELS

••K•E•
ALKIES
ANKLED
ANKLES
ANKLET
AUKLET
BAKKER
BOKKEN
CAKIER
COKIER
COKIES
DEKKER
DOKKEN
FOKKER
HAKEEM
HOKIER
HOKIES
ICKIER
INKIER
INKJET
INKLES
JOKIER
LAKIER
MCKUEN
NIKKEI
OAKIER
OAKLEY
ORKNEY
PEKOES
POKIER
POKIES
UPKEEP
YAKKED
YAKKER
YUKKED

••K••E
ALKENE
FOKINE
MAKEME
TEKKIE
WAKAME

•••KE•
ALEKEG
ALIKES
ALTKEY
AWAKED
AWAKEN
AWAKER
AWAKES
AWOKEN
BACKED
BACKER
BAKKER
BALKED
BALKER
BANKED
BANKER
BARKED
BARKER
BASKED
BASKER
BASKET
BEAKED
BEAKER
BECKER
BECKET
BICKER
BILKED
BILKER
BLAKEY
BLOKES
BOKKEN
BONKED
BOOKED
BOOKEM
BOOKER
BORKED
BRAKED
BRAKES
BROKEN
BROKER
BUBKES
BUCKED
BUCKER
BUCKET
BULKED
BUNKED
BUNKER
BUPKES
BUSKED
BUSKER
CALKED
CALKER
CANKER
CARKEY
CASKED
CASKET
CHOKED
CHOKER
CHOKES
CISKEI
COCKED
COCKER
CONKED
CONKER
COOKED
COOKER
CORKED
CORKER
CRAKES
CRIKEY
DANKER
DARKEN
DARKER
DECKED
DECKER
DEKKER
DELKEY
DICKER
DICKEY
DIRKED
DISKED
DOAKES
DOCKED
DOCKER
DOCKET
DOKKEN
DONKEY
DRAKES
DRAKEU
DUCKED
DUCKER
DUNKED
DUNKER
DUSKED
EUCKEN
EVOKED
EVOKER
EVOKES
FAWKES
FINKED
FINKEL
FLAKED
FLAKER
FLAKES
FLUKES
FLUKEY
FOKKER
FORKED
FORKER
FRAKES
FUNKED
GASKET
GAWKED
GAWKER
GEEKED
HACKED
HACKER
HANKER
HARKED
HARKEN
HARKER
HAWKED
HAWKER
HICKEY
HOCKED
HOCKER
HOCKEY
HONKED
HONKER
HOOKED
HOOKER
HOOKEY
HOTKEY
HULKED
HUNKER
HUSKED
HUSKER
JACKED
JACKET
JERKED
JERKER
JOCKEY
JUNKED
JUNKER
JUNKET
KICKED
KICKER
KINKED
KRAKEN
LACKED
LACKEY
LANKER
LARKED
LARKER
LASKER
LATKES
LEAKED
LEAKER
LEAKEY
LICKED
LICKER
LINKED
LINKER
LOCKED
LOCKER
LOCKET
LOOKED
LOOKEE
LOOKER
LOWKEY
LUCKED
LUNKER
LURKED
LURKER
LURKEY
MARKED
MARKER
MARKET
MARKEY
MASKED
MASKER
MEEKER
MENKEN
MERKEL
MICKEY
MILKED
MILKER
MISKEY
MOCKED
MOCKER
MONKEE
MONKEY
MUCKED
MUCKER
MUSKET
NECKED
NECKER
NICKED
NICKEL
NICKER
NIKKEI
NOCKED
OFFKEY
OINKED
OINKER
OLAKES
PACKED
PACKER
PACKET
PARKED
PARKER
PARKES
PEAKED
PECKED
PEEKED
PEEKER
PERKED
PICKED
PICKER
PICKET
PINKED
PINKEN
PINKER
POCKET
PORKED
PORKER
PUCKER
PUNKER
QUAKED
QUAKER
QUAKES
RACKED
RACKER
RACKET
RANKED
RANKER
RECKED
REEKED
REEKER
RICKEY
RIPKEN
RISKED
RISKER
ROCKED
ROCKER
ROCKET
ROOKED
ROOKER
RUCKED
RUCKER
SACKED
SACKER
SECKEL
SEEKER
SHAKEN
SHAKER
SHAKES
SHEKEL
SICKEN
SICKER
SILKEN
SINKER
SISKEL
SLAKED
SLAKER
SLAKES
SMOKED
SMOKER
SMOKES
SMOKEY
SNAKED
SNAKER
SNAKES
SOAKED
SOAKER
SOCKED
SOCKET
SPIKED
SPIKER
SPIKES
SPOKED
SPOKEN
SPOKES
STAKED
STAKES
STOKED
STOKER
STOKES
SUCKED
SUCKER
SULKED
SULKER
SUNKEN
TABKEY
TACKED
TACKER
TALKED
TALKER
TANKED
TANKER
TASKED
TASKET
TEDKEY
TERKEL
TICKED
TICKER
TICKET
TINKER
TISKET
TRIKES
TUCKED
TUCKER
TURKEY
TUSKED
TUSKER
UECKER
UNSKEW
WACKER
WALKED
WALKEN
WALKER
WANKEL
WEAKEN
WEAKER
WERKER
WESKER
WICKED
WICKER
WICKET
WILKES
WINKED
WINKER
WORKED
WORKER
WYNKEN
YAKKED
YAKKER
YANKED
YANKEE
YANKER
YAWKEY
YERKES
YOLKED
YORKER
YUKKED
ZONKED
ZONKER
ZUCKER

•••K•E
BOOKIE
BUCKLE
CACKLE
COCKLE
COOKIE
DARKLE
DECKLE
DICKIE
DUCKIE
FICKLE
FOLKIE
HACKIE
HACKLE
HANKIE
HECKLE
HINKLE
JACKIE
JECKLE
JUNKIE
KOOKIE
LEEKIE
LOOKEE
LOOKIE
MACKIE
MARKIE
MONKEE
MOOKIE
MUSKIE
PICKLE
PINKIE
PUNKIE
QUAKIE
RANKLE
RICKIE
ROCKIE
ROCKNE
ROOKIE
SICKLE
SKOKIE
TACKLE
TALKIE
TEKKIE
TICKLE
TINKLE
WALKIE
WILKIE
WINKIE
YANKEE
YORKIE

••••KE
ANANKE
AQUAKE
AXLIKE
BELIKE
BENEKE
BETAKE
BODUKE
BOURKE
BROOKE
CLARKE
DOLIKE
FRICKE
GOLIKE
GRIMKE
HANDKE
IMLIKE
INJOKE
INTAKE
INVOKE
ISLIKE
JAMOKE
KISHKE
KOTTKE
LADUKE
MOLTKE
NOBAKE
NOJOKE
ONMIKE
OXLIKE
PERUKE
REBAKE
REBUKE
REMAKE
RERAKE
RETAKE
REVOKE
REWAKE
REWOKE
REYOKE
ROURKE
SHRIKE
STLUKE
STRIKE
STROKE
THICKE
UNCAKE
UNLIKE
UNMAKE
UNYOKE
UPDIKE
UPTAKE

K•F•••
KEFIRS

K••F••
KIEFER
KNIFED
KNIFER
KNIFES
KOUFAX
KROFFT

K•••F•
KEYOFA
KEYOFB
KEYOFC
KEYOFD
KEYOFF
KEYOFG
KROFFT
KUNGFU

K••••F
KEYOFF
KINDOF
KNEWOF
KNOWOF

•K•F••
SKIFFS

•K••F•
OKEEFE
SKIFFS

•K•••F
EKELOF

••KF••
ASKFOR
NAKFAS

••K••F
ASKSOF
MAKEOF

•••K•F
REEKOF
SICKOF
TALKOF

KG••••
KGBSPY

K•G•••
KAGAWA
KEGGED
KEGGER
KEGLER
KIGALI

K••G••
KEDGED
KEDGER
KEDGES
KEGGED
KEGGER

KINGED
KINGLY
KINGME
KNIGHT
KROGER
KRUGER
KUNGFU

K•••G•
KLUDGE
KLUDGY
KRESGE

K••••G
KDLANG
KENNYG
KEYING
KEYOFG
KITBAG
KITING
KOENIG

•K•G••
SKAGGS

•K••G•
IKINGS
OKSIGN
SKAGGS

•K•••G
EKBERG
SKIING
SKYING

••K•G•
MAKEGO

••K••G
ASKING
BAKING
BBKING
BIKING
CAKING
COKING
DEKING
DIKING
DRKING
DUKING
FAKING
HIKING
HOKING
INKING
IRKING
JOKING
JUKING
LIKING
MAKING
MEKONG
MIKING
NUKING
OAKTAG
PEKING
PIKING
POKING
RAKING
TAKING
TSKING
VIKING
WAKING
YOKING

•••KG•
GINKGO

•••K•G
ALEKEG

KH••••
KHAKIS
KHALID
KHMERS
KHOUMS
KHYBER

K•H•••
KAHLIL
KAHLUA
KAHUNA
KOHLER

K••H••
KASHAS
KATHIE
KESHIA
KISHKA
KISHKE
KOCHEL
KOCHER
KOSHER
KUCHEN

K•••H•
KAETHE
KIMCHI
KNIGHT
KWACHA
KYUSHU

K••••H
KASBAH
KIBOSH
KIRSCH
KITSCH
KLATCH
KVETCH

•K•H••
SKIHAT

•K•••H
SKETCH
SKITCH

••K•H•
BAKSHI

••K••H
EDKOCH
LUKICH
RAKISH
TAKETH

•••KH•
GURKHA

•••K•H
ERYKAH
HOOKAH

••••KH
SAMEKH
SHEIKH

KI••••
KIARIO
KIBBEE
KIBBLE
KIBITZ
KIBOSH
KICKED
KICKER
KICKIN
KICKUP
KIDCOM
KIDDED
KIDDER
KIDDIE
KIDDOS
KIDEOS
KIDLIT
KIDMAN
KIDNAP
KIDNEY
KIDORY
KIDULT
KIDVID
KIEFER
KIERAN
KIERON
KIGALI
KIKUYU
KILIMS
KILLED
KILLER
KILMER
KILNED
KILROY
KILTED
KILTER
KILTIE
KIMBLE
KIMCHI
KIMONO
KINDER
KINDLE
KINDLY
KINDOF
KINGED
KINGLY
KINGME
KINKED
KINKOS
KINNAN
KINSEY
KINSKI
KIOSKS
KIOWAN
KIOWAS
KIPPED
KIPPER
KIPPUR
KIRKUK
KIRMAN
KIRSCH
KISHKA
KISHKE
KISLEV
KISMET
KISSED
KISSEL
KISSER
KISSES
KISSIN
KISSME
KISSUP
KITAEN
KITBAG
KITERS
KITING
KITKAT
KITSCH
KITTED
KITTEN

K•I•••
KAILUA
KAISER
KEITEL
KLIBAN
KLICKS
KNICKS
KNIFED
KNIFER
KNIFES
KNIGHT
KNIVES
KRISPY
KRISTI
KTILES

K••I••
KALINE
KARINA
KEFIRS
KEYING
KIBITZ
KILIMS
KITING
KLEINE
KLEIST
KODIAK
KONICA
KRAITS
KSWISS
KUNITZ
KURILE
KWEISI

K•••I•
KAHLIL
KANJIS
KAOLIN
KAONIC
KARMIC
KARRIE
KATHIE
KATRIN
KEEPIN
KEEPIT
KELLIE
KELPIE
KELVIN
KEMPIS
KENSIT
KEPTIN
KERMIT
KERWIN
KESHIA
KEWPIE
KEYSIN
KHAKIS
KHALID
KIARIO
KICKIN
KIDDIE
KIDLIT
KIDVID
KILTIE
KISSIN
KNEWIT
KNOWIT
KOENIG
KOOKIE
KRAVIS
KUPRIN
KUWAIT

K••••I
KABUKI
KAMALI
KATMAI
KENOBI
KIGALI
KIMCHI
KINSKI
KRISTI
KUBLAI
KWEISI

•KI•••
AKIMBO
AKINTO
AKITAS
IKINGS
SKIBIB
SKIBOB
SKIBUM
SKICAP
SKIDDY
SKIDOO
SKIERS
SKIFFS
SKIHAT
SKIING
SKILLS
SKIMPS
SKIMPY
SKINKS
SKINNY
SKIPBY
SKIPIT
SKIPPY
SKIRLS
SKIRTS
SKIRUN
SKITCH
SKITOW
SKIWAX

•K•I••
IKOIKO
OKSIGN
SKEINS
SKIING
SKYING

•K••I•
OKAPIS
SKIBIB
SKIPIT
SKOKIE
SKYLIT

••KI••
AIKIDO
ALKIES
ASKING
ATKINS
BAKING
BBKING
BEKIND
BIKILA
BIKING
BIKINI
CAKIER
CAKING
COKIER
COKIES
COKING
DEKING
DIKING
DRKING
DUKING
EAKINS
ESKIMO
FAKING
FAKIRS
FOKINE
HAKIMS
HIKING
HOKIER
HOKIES
HOKILY
HOKING
ICKIER
INKIER
INKIND
INKING
IRKING
JOKIER
JOKILY
JOKING
JUKING
LAKIER
LAKIST
LIKING
LUKICH
MAKING
MIKING
MIKITA
NIKITA
NOKIAS
NOKIDS
NUKING
OAKIER
PEKING
PIKING
POKIER
POKIES
POKILY
POKING
RAKING
RAKISH
REKICK
TAKING
TSKING
UNKIND
UNKINK
VIKING
WAKING
YAKIMA
YOKING

••K•I•
ALKAID
ASKSIN
DIKDIK
FAKEID
FAKEIT
INKSIN
MAKEIT
MAKSIM
RAKEIN
REKNIT
SIKKIM
TAKEIN
TAKEIT
TEKKIE
TIKRIT
UNKNIT

••K••I
ALKALI
BAKSHI
BIKINI
NIKKEI
TOKORI

•••KI•
ANAKIN
AZUKIS
BACKIN
BANKIT
BARKIN
BASKIN
BIGKID
BIZKIT
BODKIN
BOOKIE
BOOKII
BOOKIV
BOOKIX
BUPKIS
CATKIN
COOKIE
CULKIN
DICKIE
DUCKIE
DUNKIN
ENOKIS
FIRKIN
FOLKIE
HACKIE
HACKIT
HANKIE
HOPKIN
JACKIE
JERKIN
JUNKIE
KHAKIS
KICKIN
KOOKIE
LARKIN
LEAKIN
LEEKIE
LILKIM
LOCKIN
LOOKIE
LOOKIN
MACKIE
MARKIE
MARKII
MARKIV
MARKIX
MOOKIE
MUSKIE
NAPKIN
NEWKID
NUTKIN
PACKIN
PARKIT
PEEKIN
PERKIN
PINKIE
PITKIN
PUNKIE
PUPKIN
QUAKIE
RANKIN
RASKIN
RICKIE
RIFKIN
RISKIT
ROCKIE
ROCKIN
ROCKIT
ROOKIE
RUDKIN
RUSKIN
SANKIN
SERKIN
SERKIS
SHAKIN
SIKKIM
SINKIN
SKOKIE
SOAKIN
SOCKIN
SUCKIN
SUNKIN
TALKIE
TALKIN
TEKKIE
THEKID
TONKIN
TOOKIN
TOOKIT
TUCKIN
TURKIC
UNAKIN
WALKIE
WALKIN
WESKIT
WILKIE
WINKIE
WORKIN
YORKIE
YORKIN

•••K•I
BOOKII
BOOKVI
CISKEI
HAIKAI
MARKII
MARKVI
NIKKEI
SUUKYI

••••KI
ADZUKI
FARUKI
HIDEKI
JETSKI
KABUKI
KINSKI
NEVSKI
PATAKI
RUMAKI
SALUKI
SUZUKI

K••J••
KANJIS
KOPJES

•K••J•
SKOPJE

••KJ••
INKJET

•••KJ•
NICKJR

K•K•••
KAKAPO
KAKURO
KIKUYU
KOKOMO

K••K••
KALKAN
KARKOV
KEOKUK
KHAKIS
KICKED
KICKER
KICKIN
KICKUP
KINKED
KINKOS
KIRKUK
KITKAT
KOOKIE
KRAKEN
KRAKOW

K•••K•
KABUKI
KANAKA
KAPOKS
KAYAKS
KINSKI
KIOSKS
KISHKA
KISHKE
KLICKS
KNACKS
KNICKS
KNOCKS
KODAKS
KOPEKS
KOTTKE
KULAKS

K••••K
KARNAK
KEOKUK
KIRKUK
KODIAK
KOPECK
KRENEK

•K•K••
SKOKIE

•K••K•
AKUAKU
IKOIKO
SKANKS
SKANKY
SKINKS
SKULKS
SKUNKS
SKUNKY

••KK••
BAKKER
BOKKEN
DEKKER
DEKKOS
DOKKEN
FOKKER
NIKKEI
SIKKIM
TEKKIE
TIKKAS
YAKKED
YAKKER
YUKKED

••K••K
ACKACK
DIKDIK
MUKLUK
REKICK
TSKTSK
UNKINK

•••KK•
MARKKA

•••K•K
HICKOK
KEOKUK
KIRKUK

KL••••
KLAATU
KLATCH
KLAXON
KLEINE
KLEIST
KLEPTO
KLIBAN
KLICKS
KLMNOP
KLUDGE
KLUDGY
KLUTZY

K•L•••
KALINE
KALKAN
KALLEN
KALMAR
KDLANG
KELLER
KELLEY
KELLIE
KELLYS
KELPIE
KELSEY
KELTON
KELVIN
KILIMS
KILLED
KILLER
KILMER
KILNED
KILROY
KILTED
KILTER
KILTIE
KULAKS

K••L••
KAHLIL
KAHLUA
KAILUA
KALLEN
KAOLIN
KAPLAN
KARLEN
KEELED
KEELER
KEGLER
KELLER
KELLEY
KELLIE
KELLYS
KEPLER
KEVLAR
KHALID
KIDLIT
KILLED
KILLER
KISLEV
KNELLS
KNOLLS
KNOLLY
KOALAS
KOHLER
KRYLON
KRYLOV
KTILES
KUBLAI
KUBLER
KVELLS

K•••L•
KAMALI
KANALY
KAPELL
KEENLY
KEMBLE
KERALA
KETTLE
KIBBLE
KIDULT
KIGALI
KIMBLE
KINDLE
KINDLY
KINGLY
KNEELS
KNELLS
KNOLLS
KNOLLY
KNURLS
KNURLY
KOBOLD
KODALY
KOPELL
KRAALS
KURALT
KURILE
KVELLS

K••••L
KAHLIL
KANDEL
KAPELL
KEITEL
KENNEL
KERNEL
KEYPAL
KISSEL
KNEBEL
KOCHEL
KOPELL
KOPPEL
KOSSEL
KUMMEL
KUNZEL

•KL•••
EKLAND
JKLMNO

•K•L••
AKELAS
EKELOF
RKELLY
SKALDS
SKILLS
SKULKS
SKULLS
SKYLAB
SKYLIT

•K••L•
EKUELE
RKELLY
SKILLS
SKIRLS
SKOALS
SKULLS

•K•••L
SKYTEL

••KL••
ANKLED
ANKLES
ANKLET
AUKLET
IJKLMN
INKLES
MUKLUK
OAKLEY
TOKLAS

••K•L•
ALKALI
ALKYLS
BAKULA
BIKILA
DEKALB
HOKILY
JEKYLL
JOKILY
LIKELY
NIKOLA
PAKULA
POKILY
YOKELS

••K••L
JEKYLL

•••KL•
BARKLA
BUCKLE
CACKLE
COCKLE
DANKLY
DARKLE
DARKLY
DECKLE
FICKLE
HACKLE
HACKLY
HECKLE
HIJKLM
HINKLE
JECKLE
LANKLY
MEEKLY
PICKLE
RANKLE
RANKLY
SICKLE
SICKLY
TACKLE
TICKLE
TICKLY
TINKLE
TINKLY
WEAKLY
WEEKLY

•••K•L
BAIKAL
ESHKOL
FINKEL
JACKAL
MERKEL
NICKEL
SECKEL
SHEKEL
SISKEL
TERKEL
WANKEL

••••KL
GHIJKL

KM••••
KMARTS
KMESON

K•M•••
KAMALI
KEMBLE
KEMPIS
KHMERS
KIMBLE
KIMCHI
KIMONO
KLMNOP
KOMBAT
KOMBUS
KOMODO
KUMMEL

K••M••
KALMAR
KARMAS
KARMIC
KATMAI
KERMIT
KEYMAN
KEYMEN
KIDMAN
KILMER
KIRMAN
KISMET
KORMAN
KRAMER
KUMMEL

K•••M•
KHOUMS
KILIMS
KINGME
KISSME
KOKOMO

K••••M
KABOOM
KADEEM
KAREEM
KIDCOM

•K•M••
AKIMBO
JKLMNO
SKIMPS
SKIMPY
SKYMAN
SKYMAP
SKYMEN

•K••M•
OKBYME

•K•••M
SKIBUM
SKYCAM

••KM••
AIKMAN

••K•M•
ASKAMY
ESKIMO
HAKIMS
HOKUMS
IJKLMN
KOKOMO
MAKEME
OAKUMS
WAKAME
YAKIMA

••K••M
HAKEEM
MAKSIM
SIKKIM

•••KM•
LOOKMA

•••K•M
BOOKEM
BUNKUM
DINKUM
HICKAM
HIJKLM
LILKIM
SIKKIM
YOAKAM

KN••••
KNACKS
KNARRS
KNARRY
KNAVES
KNEADS
KNEBEL
KNEELS
KNELLS
KNEWIT
KNEWOF
KNICKS
KNIFED
KNIFER
KNIFES
KNIGHT
KNIVES
KNOBBY
KNOCKS
KNOLLS
KNOLLY
KNOTTS
KNOTTY
KNOTUP

KNOUTS
KNOWER
KNOWIT
KNOWNS
KNOWOF
KNURLS
KNURLY

K•N•••
KANAKA
KANALY
KANATA
KANAWA
KANDEL
KANDER
KANJIS
KANSAN
KANSAS
KANTOR
KENDOS
KENNAN
KENNED
KENNEL
KENNER
KENNYG
KENOBI
KENSIT
KENTON
KENYAN
KENYON
KINDER
KINDLE
KINDLY
KINDOF
KINGED
KINGLY
KINGME
KINKED
KINKOS
KINNAN
KINSEY
KINSKI
KONICA
KONRAD
KUNDRY
KUNGFU
KUNITZ
KUNZEL

K••N••
KAONIC
KARNAK
KAUNAS
KAUNDA
KAVNER
KEENAN
KEENED
KEENEN
KEENER
KEENLY
KEENON
KENNAN
KENNED
KENNEL
KENNER
KENNYG
KERNED
KERNEL
KERNES
KEYNES
KIDNAP
KIDNEY
KILNED
KINNAN
KLMNOP
KOENIG
KOONTZ
KRANTZ
KRENEK
KRONER
KRONOR
KRONUR
KWANZA

K•••N•
KAHUNA
KALINE
KARINA
KDLANG
KEARNS
KEARNY
KETONE
KEYING
KIMONO
KITING
KLEINE
KNOWNS
KORANS
KORUNA
KRASNA
KROONS

K••••N
KALKAN
KALLEN
KANSAN
KAOLIN
KAPLAN
KARLEN
KASDAN
KATRIN
KATZEN
KEATON
KEENAN
KEENEN
KEENON
KEEPIN
KEEPON
KELTON
KELVIN
KENNAN
KENTON
KENYAN
KENYON
KEPTIN
KEPTON
KERWIN
KEYMAN
KEYMEN
KEYSIN
KEYSON
KICKIN
KIDMAN
KIERAN
KIERON
KINNAN
KIOWAN
KIRMAN
KISSIN
KITAEN
KITTEN
KLAXON
KLIBAN
KMESON
KOREAN
KORMAN
KRAKEN
KRYLON
KUCHEN
KUPRIN

•KN•••
SKNXXX

•K•N••
AKENES
AKINTO
IKINGS
SKANKS
SKANKY
SKINKS
SKINNY
SKUNKS
SKUNKY

•K••N•
EKLAND
JKLMNO
OKSANA
SKEINS
SKIING
SKINNY
SKYING

•K•••N
OKSIGN
SKIRUN
SKYMAN
SKYMEN

••KN••
FTKNOX
ORKNEY
REKNIT
REKNOT
UNKNIT
UNKNOT

••K•N•
ALKENE
ASKANT
ASKING
ATKINS
BAKING
BBKING
BEKIND
BIKING
BIKINI
CAKING
COKING
DEKING
DIKING
DRKING
DUKING
EAKINS
ELKONV
FAKING
FOKINE
HIKING
HOKING
INKIND
INKING
IRKING
JOKING
JUKING
LIKENS
LIKING
MAKING
MEKONG
MIKING
NIKONS
NUKING
ORKANS
PEKING
PIKING
POKING
RAKING
TAKING
TOKENS
TSKING
UNKIND
UNKINK
VIKING
WAKENS
WAKING
YOKING
YUKONS

••K••N
AIKMAN
ASKSIN
BOKKEN
DOKKEN
ELKTON
IJKLMN
INKSIN
MCKEAN
MCKEON
MCKERN
MCKUEN
RAKEIN
TAKEIN
TAKEON

•••KN•
HECKNO
ROCKNE

•••K•N
ANAKIN
AWAKEN
AWOKEN
BACKIN
BALKAN
BANKON
BARKIN
BASKIN
BECKON
BODKIN
BOKKEN
BROKEN
CATKIN
CULKIN
DARKEN
DOKKEN
DUNKIN
EUCKEN
FINKON
FIRKIN
HAAKON
HARKEN
HOOKON
HOPKIN
JERKIN
KALKAN
KICKIN
KRAKEN
LARKIN
LEAKIN
LOCKIN
LOCKON
LOOKIN
LOOKON
MENKEN
NAPKIN
NUTKIN
OSAKAN
PACKIN
PACKON
PEEKIN
PERKIN
PICKON
PINKEN
PITKIN
PUPKIN
RANKIN
RASKIN
RECKON
RIFKIN
RIPKEN
ROCKIN
RUDKIN
RUSKIN
RYOKAN
SANKIN
SERKIN
SHAKEN
SHAKIN
SICKEN
SILKEN
SINKIN
SOAKIN
SOCKIN
SPOKEN
SUCKIN
SUNKEN
SUNKIN
TACKON
TALKIN
TALKON
TONKIN
TOOKIN
TOOKON
TUCKIN
UNAKIN
WALKEN
WALKIN
WALKON
WEAKEN
WEAKON
WORKIN
WORKON
WYNKEN
YANKON
YORKIN

KO••••
KOALAS
KOBOLD
KOCHEL
KOCHER
KODAKS
KODALY
KODIAK
KOENIG
KOHLER
KOKOMO
KOMBAT
KOMBUS
KOMODO
KONICA
KONRAD
KOOKIE
KOONTZ
KOPECK
KOPEKS
KOPELL
KOPJES
KOPPEL
KORANS
KORATS
KORBUT
KOREAN
KORMAN
KORUNA
KOSHER
KOSOVO
KOSSEL
KOSTER
KOTTER
KOTTKE
KOUFAX
KOVACS
KOWTOW

K•O•••
KAOLIN
KAONIC
KEOKUK
KHOUMS
KIOSKS
KIOWAN
KIOWAS
KNOBBY
KNOCKS
KNOLLS
KNOLLY
KNOTTS
KNOTTY
KNOTUP
KNOUTS
KNOWER
KNOWIT
KNOWNS
KNOWOF
KOOKIE
KOONTZ
KROFFT
KROGER
KRONER
KRONOR
KRONUR
KROONS

K••O••
KABOBS
KABOOM
KAPOKS
KAYOED
KAZOOS
KENOBI
KETONE
KEYOFA
KEYOFB
KEYOFC
KEYOFD
KEYOFF
KEYOFG
KIBOSH
KIDORY
KIMONO
KOBOLD
KOKOMO
KOMODO
KOSOVO
KROONS

K•••O•
KABOOM
KANTOR
KARKOV
KARPOV
KAYYOW
KAZOOS
KEATON
KEENON
KEEPON
KELTON
KENDOS
KENTON
KENYON
KEPTON
KEYSON
KIDCOM
KIDDOS
KIDEOS
KIERON
KILROY
KINDOF
KINKOS
KLAXON
KLMNOP
KMESON
KNEWOF
KNOWOF
KOWTOW
KRAKOW
KRONOR
KRYLON
KRYLOV
KUDROW

K••••O
KAKAPO
KAKURO
KEEPTO
KEPTTO
KIARIO
KIMONO
KLEPTO
KOKOMO
KOMODO
KOSOVO
KRYPTO

•KO•••
IKOIKO
SKOALS
SKOKIE
SKOPJE
SKORTS

•K•O••
EKEOUT

•K••O•
EKELOF
SKIBOB
SKIDOO
SKITOW
SKYBOX

•K•••O
AKIMBO
AKINTO
IKOIKO
JKLMNO
SKIDOO

••KO••
ASKOUT
DAKOTA
DRKOOP
EDKOCH
ELKONV
KOKOMO
LAKOTA
MEKONG
NIKOLA
NIKONS
PEKOES
TOKORI
YUKONS

••K•O•
ASKFOR
ASKSOF
DEKKOS
DOKTOR
DRKOOP
ELKTON
FTKNOX
HYKSOS
INKPOT
MAKEOF
MCKEON
REKNOT
TAKEON
UNKNOT
VIKTOR

••K••O
AIKIDO
ESKIMO
KAKAPO
KAKURO
KOKOMO
LIKESO
LIKETO
MAKEDO
MAKEGO
MIKADO
TAKETO

•••KO•
ANGKOR
BANKON
BECKON
BERKOW
BUNKOS
CHEKOV
CUCKOO
DEKKOS
ESHKOL
FINKON
GECKOS
HAAKON
HICKOK
HOOKON
JOCKOS
KARKOV
KINKOS
KRAKOW
LOCKON
LOOKON
MARKOV
MUSKOX
PACKON
PICKON
PINKOS
RECKON
REEKOF
SEIKOS
SHAKOS
SICKOF
SICKOS
TACKON
TALKOF
TALKON
TOOKON
WACKOS
WALKON
WEAKON
WORKON
YANKON
ZARKOV
ZHUKOV

•••K•O
CUCKOO
GINKGO
HECKNO
LOOKTO
NIEKRO
TALKTO
TOOKTO
WALKTO

••••KO
BAMAKO
BRONKO
GINGKO
IKOIKO
LEMOKO
MARIKO
ROTHKO
SHOPKO
STINKO
STOJKO

KP••••
KPDUTY

K•P•••
KAPELL
KAPLAN
KAPOKS
KAPPAS
KAPUTT
KEPLER
KEPTAT
KEPTIN
KEPTON
KEPTTO
KEPTUP
KIPPED
KIPPER
KIPPUR
KOPECK
KOPEKS
KOPELL
KOPJES
KOPPEL
KUPRIN

K••P••
KAPPAS
KARPOV
KEEPAT
KEEPER
KEEPIN
KEEPIT
KEEPON
KEEPTO
KEEPUP
KELPIE
KEMPIS
KEWPIE
KEYPAD
KEYPAL
KIPPED
KIPPER
KIPPUR
KLEPTO
KOPPEL
KRYPTO

K•••P•
KAKAPO
KGBSPY
KRISPY

K••••P
KEEPUP
KEPTUP
KEYSUP
KICKUP
KIDNAP
KISSUP
KLMNOP
KNOTUP

•K•P••
OKAPIS
SKIPBY
SKIPIT
SKIPPY
SKOPJE

•K••P•
SKIMPS
SKIMPY
SKIPPY

•K•••P
SKICAP
SKYCAP
SKYMAP

••KP••
INKPAD
INKPOT

••K•P•
KAKAPO
UNKEPT

••K••P
ASKSUP
CAKEUP
DRKOOP
HIKEUP
MAKEUP
RAKEUP
TAKEUP
UPKEEP
WAKEUP
WOKEUP

•••KP•
YORKPA

•••K•P
BACKUP
BANKUP
BUCKUP
BULKUP
COOKUP
CORKUP
FORKUP
HACKUP
HOOKUP
JACKUP
JERKUP
KICKUP
LICKUP
LINKUP
LOCKUP
LOOKUP
MARKUP
MOCKUP
MUCKUP
PACKUP
PERKUP
PICKUP
RACKUP
RUCKUP
SACKUP
SOAKUP
SUCKUP
TACKUP
TALKUP
TANKUP
TOOKUP
WALKUP
WORKUP

KR••••
KRAALS
KRAITS
KRAKEN
KRAKOW
KRAMER
KRANTZ
KRASNA
KRAUSS
KRAVIS
KRENEK
KRESGE
KREWES
KRISPY
KRISTI
KROFFT
KROGER
KRONER
KRONOR
KRONUR
KROONS
KRUGER
KRUSTY
KRYLON
KRYLOV
KRYPTO

K•R•••
KARATE
KARATS
KAREEM
KARINA
KARKOV
KARLEN
KARMAS
KARMIC
KARNAK
KARPOV
KARRAS
KARRER
KARRIE
KARSTS
KERALA
KERMIT
KERNED
KERNEL
KERNES
KERSEE
KERWIN
KIRKUK
KIRMAN
KIRSCH
KORANS
KORATS
KORBUT
KOREAN
KORMAN
KORUNA
KURALT
KURILE

K••R••
KARRAS
KARRER
KARRIE
KATRIN
KEARNS
KEARNY
KIARIO
KIERAN
KIERON
KILROY
KMARTS
KNARRS
KNARRY
KNURLS
KNURLY
KONRAD
KUDROW
KUPRIN

K•••R•
KAKURO
KEFIRS
KHMERS
KIDORY
KITERS
KNARRS
KNARRY
KSTARS
KUNDRY

K••••R
KAISER
KALMAR
KANDER
KANTOR
KARRER
KAVNER
KCSTAR
KEDGER
KEELER
KEENER
KEEPER
KEGGER
KEGLER
KELLER
KENNER
KEPLER
KEVLAR
KEYSER
KHYBER
KICKER
KIDDER
KIEFER
KILLER
KILMER
KILTER
KINDER
KIPPER
KIPPUR
KISSER
KNIFER
KNOWER
KOCHER
KOHLER
KOSHER
KOSTER
KOTTER
KRAMER
KROGER
KRONER
KRONOR
KRONUR
KRUGER
KUBLER

•K•R••
SKIRLS
SKIRTS
SKIRUN
SKORTS

•K••R•
EKBERG
SKIERS

•K•••R
SKATER
SKEWER

••KR••
TIKRIT

••K•R•
ANKARA
ASKERS
BAKERS
BAKERY
BIKERS
DIKERS
ECKART
ECKERD
ESKERS
FAKERS
FAKERY
FAKIRS
GOKART
HIKERS
INKERS
IRKERS
JOKERS
KAKURO
LAKERS
LIKERS
MAKERS
MCKERN
PIKERS
POKERS
POKERY
RAKERS
RIKERS
TAKERS
TOKORI
WAKERS

••K••R
ASKFOR
BAKKER
CAKIER
COKIER
DEKKER
DOKTOR
FOKKER
HOKIER
ICKIER
INKIER
JOKIER
LAKIER
OAKIER
POKIER
TEKWAR
VIKTOR
YAKKER

•••KR•
CHAKRA
NIEKRO

•••K•R
ANGKOR
AWAKER
BACKER
BAKKER
BALKER
BANKER
BARKER
BASKER
BEAKER
BECKER
BICKER
BILKER
BOOKER
BROKER
BUCKER
BUNKER
BUSKER
CALKER
CANKER
CHOKER
COCKER
CONKER
COOKER
CORKER
DANKER
DARKER
DECKER
DEKKER
DICKER
DOCKER
DUCKER
DUNKER
EVOKER
FLAKER
FOKKER
FORKER
GAWKER
HACKER
HANKER
HARKER
HAWKER
HOCKER
HONKER
HOOKER
HUNKER
HUSKER
JERKER
JUNKER
KICKER
LANKER
LARKER
LASKER
LEAKER

LICKER
LINKER
LOCKER
LOOKER
LUNKER
LURKER
MARKER
MASKER
MEEKER
MILKER
MOCKER
MUCKER
NECKER
NICKER
NICKJR
OINKER
PACKER
PARKER
PEEKER
PICKER
PINKER
PORKER
PUCKER
PUNKER
QUAKER
RACKER
RANKER
REEKER
RISKER.
ROCKER
ROOKER
RUCKER
SACKER
SEEKER
SHAKER
SHAKUR
SICKER
SINKER
SLAKER
SMOKER
SNAKER
SOAKER
SPIKER
STOKER
SUCKER
SULKER
TACKER
TALKER
TANKER
TICKER
TINKER
TUCKER
TUSKER
UECKER
WACKER
WALKER
WEAKER
WERKER
WESKER
WICKER
WINKER
WORKER
YAKKER
YANKER
YORKER
ZONKER
ZUCKER

KS••••
KSTARS
KSWISS

K•S•••
KASBAH
KASDAN
KASHAS
KCSTAR
KESHIA
KISHKA
KISHKE
KISLEV
KISMET
KISSED
KISSEL
KISSER
KISSES
KISSIN
KISSME
KISSUP
KOSHER
KOSOVO
KOSSEL
KOSTER

K••S••
KAISER
KANSAN
KANSAS
KARSTS
KELSEY
KENSIT
KERSEE
KEYSER
KEYSIN
KEYSON
KEYSUP
KGBSPY
KINSEY
KINSKI
KIOSKS
KIRSCH
KISSED
KISSEL
KISSER
KISSES
KISSIN
KISSME
KISSUP
KITSCH
KMESON
KOSSEL
KRASNA
KRESGE
KRISPY
KRISTI
KRUSTY
KYUSHU

K•••S•
KIBOSH
KLEIST
KRAUSS
KSWISS
KUVASZ
KWEISI

K••••S
KABOBS
KANJIS
KANSAS
KAPOKS
KAPPAS
KARATS
KARMAS
KARRAS
KARSTS
KASHAS
KAUNAS
KAYAKS
KAZOOS
KEARNS
KEBABS
KEDGES
KEFIRS
KELLYS
KEMPIS
KENDOS
KERNES
KEYNES
KHAKIS
KHMERS
KHOUMS
KIDDOS
KIDEOS
KILIMS
KINKOS
KIOSKS
KIOWAS
KISSES
KITERS
KLICKS
KMARTS
KNACKS
KNARRS
KNAVES
KNEADS
KNEELS
KNELLS
KNICKS
KNIFES
KNIVES
KNOCKS
KNOLLS
KNOTTS
KNOUTS
KNOWNS
KNURLS
KOALAS
KODAKS
KOMBUS
KOPEKS
KOPJES
KORANS
KORATS
KOVACS
KRAALS
KRAITS
KRAUSS
KRAVIS
KREWES
KROONS
KSTARS
KSWISS
KTILES
KUDZUS
KULAKS
KVELLS

•KS•••
OKSANA
OKSIGN

•K•S••
EKESBY
UKASES

•K•••S
AKELAS
AKENES
AKITAS
IKINGS
OKAPIS
SKAGGS
SKALDS
SKANKS
SKATES
SKEETS
SKEINS
SKIERS
SKIFFS
SKILLS
SKIMPS
SKINKS
SKIRLS
SKIRTS
SKOALS
SKORTS
SKULKS
SKULLS
SKUNKS
UKASES

••KS••
ASKSIN
ASKSOF
ASKSUP
BAKSHI
HYKSOS
INKSAC
INKSIN
MAKSIM

••K•S•
LAKIST
LIKESO
MIKASA
RAKISH
TSKTSK

••K••S
ALKIES
ALKYDS
ALKYLS
ANKLES
ASKERS
ATKINS
BAKERS
BIKERS
COKIES
DEKKOS
DIKERS
EAKINS
ESKERS
FAKERS
FAKIRS
HAKIMS
HIKERS
HOKIES
HOKUMS
HYKSOS
INKERS
INKLES
IRKERS
JOKERS
LAKERS
LIKENS
LIKERS
MAKERS
NAKFAS
NIKONS
NOKIAS
NOKIDS
OAKUMS
ORKANS
PEKOES
PIKERS
POKERS
POKEYS
POKIES
RAKERS
REKEYS
RIKERS
TAKERS
TIKKAS
TOKAYS
TOKENS
TOKLAS
WAKENS
WAKERS
YAKUTS
YOKELS
YUKONS

•••KS•
FOLKSY

•••K•S
ALECKS
ALIKES
AWAKES
AZUKIS
BABKAS
BACKUS
BLOKES
BRAKES
BUBKES
BUNKOS
BUPKES
BUPKIS
BUPKUS
BURKAS
BUTKUS
CHOKES
CRAKES
DEKKOS
DINKAS
DOAKES
DRAKES
ENOKIS
EVOKES
FAWKES
FLAKES
FLUKES
FRAKES
GECKOS
HAIKUS
JOCKOS
KHAKIS
KINKOS
LATKES
MARKAS
OLAKES
PARKAS
PARKES
PINKOS
POLKAS
PORKYS
PUNKAS
QUAKES
RUCKUS
RUDKUS
SANKAS
SEIKOS
SERKIS
SHAKES
SHAKOS
SICKOS
SLAKES
SMOKES
SNAKES
SPIKES
SPOKES
STAKES
STOKES
STUKAS
TANKAS
TIKKAS
TONKAS
TRIKES
VODKAS
WACKOS
WILKES
YERKES

••••KS
AZTEKS
BATIKS
BAULKS
BLACKS
BLANKS
BLEAKS
BLINKS
BLOCKS
BREAKS
BRICKS
BRINKS
BRISKS
BROOKS
BUICKS
CAULKS
CHALKS
CHECKS
CHEEKS
CHICKS
CHINKS
CHOCKS
CHUCKS
CHUNKS
CLACKS
CLANKS
CLEEKS
CLERKS
CLICKS
CLINKS
CLOAKS
CLOCKS
CLONKS
CLUCKS
CLUNKS
CRACKS
CRANKS
CREAKS
CREEKS
CRICKS
CROAKS
CROCKS
CROOKS
DBACKS
DMARKS
DRECKS
DRINKS
EBANKS
EBOOKS
FLACKS
FLANKS
FLASKS
FLECKS
FLICKS
FLOCKS
FLUNKS
FRANKS
FREAKS
FRISKS
FROCKS
GLOCKS
GREEKS
HACEKS
IBOOKS
KAPOKS
KAYAKS
KIOSKS
KLICKS
KNACKS
KNICKS
KNOCKS
KODAKS
KOPEKS
KULAKS
LUNIKS
ORECKS
OZARKS
PANCKS
PBOOKS
PLANKS
PLINKS
PLONKS
PLUCKS
PLUNKS
PRANKS
PRICKS
PRINKS
QUACKS
QUARKS
QUIRKS
REASKS
REINKS
RUBIKS
SHACKS
SHANKS
SHARKS
SHEIKS
SHIRKS
SHOCKS
SHUCKS
SKANKS
SKINKS
SKULKS
SKUNKS
SLACKS
SLEEKS
SLICKS
SLINKS
SMACKS
SMIRKS
SMOCKS
SNACKS
SNARKS
SNEAKS
SNICKS
SNOOKS
SPANKS
SPARKS
SPEAKS
SPECKS
SPINKS
SPOOKS
SPORKS
STACKS
STALKS
STEAKS
STICKS
STINKS
STOCKS
STORKS
THANKS
THINKS
THUNKS
TILAKS
TRACKS
TRICKS
TRUCKS
TRUNKS
TWEAKS
UMIAKS
VNECKS
WHACKS
WHELKS
WHISKS
WRACKS
WREAKS
WRECKS
YOICKS

KT••••
KTILES

K•T•••
KATHIE
KATMAI
KATRIN
KATZEN
KETONE
KETTLE
KITAEN
KITBAG
KITERS
KITING
KITKAT
KITSCH
KITTED
KITTEN
KOTTER
KOTTKE
KSTARS

K••T••
KAETHE
KANTOR
KCSTAR
KEATON
KEITEL
KELTON
KENTON
KEPTAT
KEPTIN
KEPTON
KEPTTO
KEPTUP
KETTLE
KILTED
KILTER
KILTIE
KITTED
KITTEN
KLATCH
KLUTZY
KNOTTS
KNOTTY
KNOTUP
KOSTER
KOTTER
KOTTKE
KOWTOW
KVETCH

K•••T•
KADETT
KANATA
KAPUTT
KARATE
KARATS
KARSTS
KEEPTO
KEPTTO
KIBITZ
KLAATU
KLEPTO
KMARTS
KNOTTS
KNOTTY
KNOUTS
KOONTZ
KORATS
KPDUTY
KRAITS
KRANTZ
KRISTI
KRUSTY
KRYPTO
KUNITZ

K••••T
KADETT
KAPUTT
KEEPAT
KEEPIT
KENSIT
KEPTAT
KERMIT
KEYDET
KIDLIT
KIDULT
KISMET
KITKAT
KLEIST
KNEWIT
KNIGHT
KNOWIT
KOMBAT
KORBUT
KROFFT
KURALT
KUWAIT

•K•T••
AKITAS
SKATED
SKATER
SKATES
SKETCH
SKITCH
SKITOW
SKYTEL

•K••T•
AKINTO
SKEETS
SKIRTS
SKORTS

•K•••T
EKEOUT
SKIHAT
SKIPIT
SKYLIT

••KT••
DIKTAT
DOKTOR
ELKTON
OAKTAG
TSKTSK
VIKTOR

••K•T•
DAKOTA
LAKOTA
LIKETO
LIKUTA
MAKUTA
MIKITA
NIKITA
TAKETH
TAKETO
YAKUTS
YUKATA

••K••T
ANKLET
ASKANT
ASKOUT
AUKLET
DIKTAT
ECKART
FAKEIT
GOKART
INKJET
INKPOT
LAKIST
MAKEIT
POKEAT
REKNIT
REKNOT
TAKEIT
TIKRIT
UNKEPT
UNKNIT
UNKNOT

•••KT•
LOOKTO
TALKTO
TOOKTO
WALKTO

•••K•T
BALKAT
BANKIT
BARKAT
BASKET
BECKET
BIZKIT
BUCKET
CASKET
DOCKET
GASKET
GAWKAT
HACKIT
HONKAT
JACKET
JUNKET
KITKAT
LOCKET
LOOKAT
MARKET
MUSKET
PACKET
PARKIT
PECKAT
PEEKAT
PICKAT
PICKET
PLAKAT
POCKET
RACKET
RISKIT
ROCKET
ROCKIT
SOCKET
TALKAT
TASKET
TICKET
TISKET
TOOKIT
WESKIT
WICKET
WINKAT
WORKAT
YANKAT

KU••••
KUBLAI
KUBLER
KUCHEN
KUDROW
KUDZUS
KULAKS
KUMMEL
KUNDRY
KUNGFU
KUNITZ
KUNZEL
KUPRIN
KURALT
KURILE
KUVASZ
KUWAIT

K•U•••
KAUNAS
KAUNDA
KLUDGE
KLUDGY
KLUTZY
KNURLS
KNURLY
KOUFAX
KRUGER
KRUSTY
KYUSHU

K••U••
KABUKI
KAHUNA
KAKURO
KAPUTT
KHOUMS
KIDULT
KIKUYU
KNOUTS
KORUNA
KPDUTY
KRAUSS

K•••U•
KAHLUA
KAILUA
KEEPUP
KEOKUK
KEPTUP
KEYSUP
KICKUP
KIPPUR
KIRKUK
KISSUP
KNOTUP
KOMBUS
KORBUT
KRONUR
KUDZUS

K••••U
KIKUYU
KLAATU
KUNGFU
KYUSHU

•KU•••
AKUAKU
EKUELE
SKULKS
SKULLS
SKUNKS
SKUNKY

•K••U•
EKEOUT
SKIBUM
SKIRUN

•K•••U
AKUAKU

••KU••
BAKULA
HOKUMS
KAKURO
KIKUYU
LIKUTA
MAKUTA
MCKUEN
OAKUMS
PAKULA
YAKUTS
YAKUZA

••K•U•
ASKOUT
ASKSUP
CAKEUP
HIKEUP
MAKEUP
MUKLUK
RAKEUP
TAKEUP
WAKEUP
WOKEUP

••K••U
BUKAVU
KIKUYU

•••KU•
BACKUP
BACKUS
BANKUP
BUCKUP
BULKUP
BUNKUM
BUPKUS
BUTKUS
COOKUP
CORKUP
DINKUM
FORKUP
HACKUP
HAIKUS
HOOKUP
JACKUP
JERKUP
KEOKUK
KICKUP
KIRKUK
LICKUP
LINKUP
LOCKUP
LOOKUP
MARKUP
MOCKUP
MUCKUP
PACKUP
PERKUP
PICKUP
RACKUP
RUCKUP
RUCKUS
RUDKUS
SACKUP
SHAKUR
SOAKUP
SUCKUP
TACKUP
TALKUP
TANKUP
TOOKUP
WALKUP
WORKUP

•••K•U
DRAKEU
RYUKYU

••••KU
AKUAKU
BUGAKU
SUDOKU

KV••••
KVELLS
KVETCH

K•V•••
KAVNER
KEVLAR
KOVACS
KUVASZ

K••V••
KELVIN
KIDVID
KNAVES
KNIVES
KRAVIS

K•••V•
KOSOVO

K••••V
KARKOV
KARPOV
KISLEV
KRYLOV

••K•V•
BUKAVU

••K••V
ELKONV

•••KV•
BOOKVI
MARKVI
MOSKVA

•••K•V
BOOKIV
CHEKOV
KARKOV
MARKIV
MARKOV
PARKAV
ROCKYV
ZARKOV
ZHUKOV

KW••••
KWACHA
KWANZA
KWEISI

K•W•••
KEWPIE
KOWTOW
KSWISS
KUWAIT

K••W••
KERWIN
KEYWAY
KIOWAN
KIOWAS
KNEWIT
KNEWOF
KNOWER
KNOWIT
KNOWNS
KNOWOF
KREWES

K•••W•
KAGAWA
KANAWA

K••••W
KAYYOW
KOWTOW
KRAKOW
KUDROW

•K•W••
SKEWED
SKEWER
SKIWAX
SKYWAY

•K•••W
SKITOW

••KW••
TEKWAR

••K•W•
YUKAWA

•••K•W
BERKOW
BROKAW
KRAKOW
UNSKEW

K••X••
KLAXON

K••••X
KOUFAX

•K•X••
SKNXXX

•K••X•
SKNXXX

•K•••X
SKIWAX
SKNXXX
SKYBOX

••K••X
FTKNOX

•••K•X
BOOKIX
MARKIX
MUSKOX
PICKAX

••••KX
MERCKX

KY••••
KYUSHU

K•Y•••
KAYAKS
KAYOED
KAYYOW
KEYDET
KEYING
KEYMAN
KEYMEN
KEYNES
KEYOFA
KEYOFB
KEYOFC
KEYOFD
KEYOFF
KEYOFG
KEYPAD
KEYPAL
KEYSER
KEYSIN
KEYSON
KEYSUP
KEYWAY
KHYBER
KRYLON
KRYLOV
KRYPTO

K••Y••
KAYYOW
KENYAN
KENYON

K•••Y•
KELLYS
KENNYG
KIKUYU

K••••Y
KANALY
KEARNY
KEENLY
KELLEY
KELSEY
KEYWAY
KGBSPY
KIDNEY
KIDORY
KILROY
KINDLY
KINGLY
KINSEY
KLUDGY
KLUTZY
KNARRY
KNOBBY
KNOLLY
KNOTTY
KNURLY
KODALY
KPDUTY
KRISPY
KRUSTY
KUNDRY

•KY•••
SKYBOX
SKYCAM
SKYCAP
SKYING
SKYLAB
SKYLIT
SKYMAN
SKYMAP
SKYMEN
SKYTEL
SKYWAY

•K•Y••
OKAYED
OKBYME

•K•••Y
EKEDBY
EKESBY
RKELLY
SKANKY
SKIDDY
SKIMPY
SKINNY
SKIPBY
SKIPPY
SKUNKY
SKYWAY

••KY••
ALKYDS
ALKYLS
JEKYLL

••K•Y•
KIKUYU
POKEYS
REKEYS
TOKAYS

••K••Y
ASKAMY
BAKERY
FAKERY
HOKILY
JOKILY
LIKELY
OAKLEY
ORKNEY
POKERY
POKILY

•••KY•
PORKYS
ROCKYV
RYUKYU
SUUKYI

•••K•Y
ALTKEY
BLAKEY
CARKEY
CRIKEY
DANKLY
DARKLY
DELKEY
DICKEY
DONKEY
FLUKEY
FOLKSY
HACKLY
HICKEY
HOCKEY
HOOKEY
HOTKEY
IMOKAY
JOCKEY
LACKEY
LANKLY
LEAKEY
LOWKEY
LURKEY
MARKEY
MEEKLY
MICKEY
MISKEY
MONKEY
OFFKEY
PARKAY
RANKLY
RICKEY
SICKLY
SIRKAY
SMOKEY
TABKEY
TEDKEY
TICKBY
TICKLY
TINKLY
TURKEY
WALKBY
WEAKLY
WEEKLY
YAWKEY

••••KY
ALECKY
BIGSKY
BLOCKY
BOESKY
BRICKY
BROOKY
CHALKY
CHEEKY
CHINKY
CHUCKY
CHUNKY
CLANKY
CLUNKY
CRANKY
CREAKY
CROAKY
DRECKY
FLECKY
FLUNKY
FREAKY
FRISKY
LANSKY
NEVSKY
PLUCKY
PLUNKY
PROSKY
QUACKY
QUIRKY
REDSKY
RIMSKY
SHECKY
SKANKY
SKUNKY
SLEEKY
SLINKY
SMIRKY
SNARKY
SNEAKY
SPANKY
SPARKY
SPOOKY
SPUNKY
STALKY
STICKY
STINKY
STOCKY
SWANKY
TRICKY
TWEAKY
WHISKY
ZINCKY

K•Z•••
KAZOOS

K••Z••
KATZEN
KUDZUS
KUNZEL

K•••Z•
KLUTZY
KWANZA

K••••Z
KIBITZ
KOONTZ
KRANTZ
KUNITZ
KUVASZ

••K•Z•
YAKUZA

LA••••
LAALAA
LABATT
LABELS
LABFEE
LABIAL
LABILE
LABINE
LABIUM
LABORS
LABOUR
LABRAT
LABREA
LACAGE
LACASA
LACAVA
LACEON
LACERS
LACEUP
LACHEY
LACHOY
LACIER
LACILY
LACING
LACKED
LACKEY
LACLOS
LACTEA
LACTIC
LACUNA
LADDER
LADDIE
LADERS
LADIDA
LADIES
LADING
LADINO
LADLED
LADLER
LADLES
LADOGA
LADUKE
LADYDI
LAFFER
LAGEAR
LAGERS
LAGGED
LAGGER
LAGOON
LAGUNA
LAHORE
LAICAL
LAIDBY
LAIDIN
LAIDON
LAIDTO
LAIDUP
LAINIE
LAIRDS
LAIRED
LAJOIE
LAKERS
LAKIER
LAKIST
LAKOTA
LALALA
LALLED
LAMARR
LAMAZE
LAMBDA
LAMBED
LAMEDS
LAMELY
LAMENT
LAMESA
LAMEST
LAMIAE
LAMIAS
LAMINA
LAMING
LAMMED
LAMONT
LAMOUR
LAMSIT
LANAIS
LANARK
LANATE
LANCED
LANCER
LANCES
LANCET
LANCIA
LANCIE
LANDAT
LANDAU
LANDED
LANDER
LANDHO
LANDIS
LANDON
LANDOR
LANDRY
LANDUP
LANDUS
LANGER
LANIER
LANINA
LANKER
LANKLY
LANOSE
LANSKY
LANSON
LANTOS
LANVAL
LANVIN
LAONZA
LAOTSE
LAOTZU
LAPCAT
LAPDOG
LAPELS
LAPERI
LAPERM
LAPFUL
LAPHAM
LAPINS
LAPPED
LAPPER
LAPPET
LAPSAT
LAPSED
LAPSER
LAPSES
LAPSUP
LAPSUS
LAPTEV
LAPTOP
LAPUTA
LARAMS
LARAZA
LARDED
LARDER
LARDON
LAREDO
LAREES
LARGER
LARGES
LARGOS
LARIAT
LARINE
LARKED
LARKER
LARKIN
LARMEN
LARMOR
LAROSA
LARRUP
LARSEN
LARSON
LARTER
LARTET
LARVAE
LARVAL
LARVAS
LARYNX
LASCAR
LASERS
LASHED
LASHER
LASHES
LASHTO
LASHUP
LASING
LASKER
LASSEN
LASSER
LASSES
LASSIE
LASSOS
LASTED
LASTEX
LASTLY
LASTRA
LASTUP
LASZLO
LATEEN
LATELY
LATENE
LATENS
LATENT
LATEOF
LATEON
LATERI
LATERO
LATEST
LATETO
LATHED
LATHEN
LATHER
LATHES
LATIGO
LATINA
LATINI
LATINO
LATINS
LATISH
LATKES
LATOUR
LATOYA
LATRIA
LATTER
LATTES
LATVIA
LAUDED
LAUDER
LAUGHS
LAULAU
LAUNCH
LAUPER
LAUREL
LAUREN
LAUREY
LAURIA
LAURIC
LAURIE
LAURYL
LAURYN
LAUTER
LAVABO
LAVAGE
LAVAIN
LAVERN
LAVERS
LAVIDA
LAVING
LAVISH
LAWFUL
LAWING
LAWMAN
LAWMEN
LAWSON
LAWTON
LAWYER
LAXALT
LAXEST
LAXITY
LAYBYS
LAYERS
LAYFOR
LAYING
LAYINS
LAYLOW
LAYMAN
LAYMEN
LAYOFF
LAYOUT
LAYSBY
LAYSIN
LAYSON
LAYSTO
LAYSUP
LAYUPS
LAZBOY
LAZIER
LAZILY
LAZING
LAZULI

L•A•••
LAALAA
LEACHY
LEADED
LEADEN
LEADER
LEADIN
LEADON
LEADTO
LEADUP
LEAFED
LEAGUE
LEAKED
LEAKER
LEAKEY
LEAKIN
LEALTY
LEANED
LEANER
LEANIN
LEANLY
LEANNE
LEANON
LEANTO
LEAPAT
LEAPED
LEAPER
LEAPIN
LEAPON
LEAPUP
LEARNS
LEARNT
LEASED
LEASER
LEASES
LEASTS
LEAVED
LEAVEN
LEAVER
LEAVES
LHASAN
LIABLE
LIAISE
LIANAS
LIANES
LIANGS
LLADRO
LLAMAS
LLANOS
LOADED
LOADER
LOADIN
LOADUP
LOAFED
LOAFER
LOAMED
LOANED
LOANER
LOATHE
LOAVES
LUANDA
LWAVES

L••A••
LABATT
LACAGE
LACASA
LACAVA
LALALA
LAMARR
LAMAZE
LANAIS
LANARK
LANATE
LARAMS
LARAZA
LAVABO
LAVAGE
LAVAIN
LAXALT
LBEAMS
LCHAIM
LECAIN
LEEANN
LEGACY
LEGALS
LEGART
LEGATE
LEGATO
LELAND
LEMANS
LENAIN
LENAPE
LENARD
LESAGE
LEVADE
LEVANT
LFRANK
LIGAND
LIGATE
LILACS
LIMANS
LINAGE
LIPARI
LIPASE
LITANY
LIZALU
LIZARD
LOBATE
LOCALE
LOCALS
LOCANE
LOCATE
LOGANS
LORAIN
LORANS
LOUANN
LOVAGE
LOYALE
LUNACY
LUNATE
LUSAKA
LUXATE

L•••A•
LAALAA
LABIAL
LABRAT
LAGEAR
LAICAL
LAMIAE
LAMIAS
LANDAT
LANDAU
LANVAL
LAPCAT
LAPHAM
LAPSAT
LARIAT
LARVAE
LARVAL
LARVAS
LASCAR
LAULAU
LAWMAN
LAYMAN
LEAPAT
LEBEAU
LEEMAY
LEERAT
LEEWAY
LEGMAN
LEHMAN
LEHUAS
LEICAS
LEMMAS
LESHAN
LESTAT
LETHAL
LETSAT
LHASAN
LIANAS
LIBRAE
LIBRAN
LIBRAS
LIBYAN
LILIAN
LINEAL
LINEAR
LITVAK
LIVEAT
LLAMAS
LLBEAN
LOGJAM
LOOFAH
LOOFAS
LOOKAT
LOQUAT
LOREAL
LOTHAR
LOUMAS
LOWCAL
LOWFAT
LOWMAN
LOWTAR
LUCIAN
LUMBAR
LYCRAS
LYDIAN

L••••A
LAALAA
LABREA
LACASA
LACAVA
LACTEA
LACUNA
LADIDA
LADOGA
LAGUNA
LAKOTA
LALALA
LAMBDA
LAMESA
LAMINA
LANCIA
LANINA
LAONZA
LAPUTA
LARAZA
LAROSA
LASTRA
LATINA
LATOYA
LATRIA
LATVIA
LAURIA
LAVIDA
LENGUA
LENINA
LEONIA
LERIDA
LIGEIA
LIKUTA
LINGUA
LIOTTA
LISBOA
LOGGIA
LOLITA
LOOKMA
LOOMPA
LOUISA
LOVEYA
LOYOLA
LUANDA
LUCIDA
LUELLA
LUMINA
LUNTHA
LUNULA
LUSAKA
LUSTRA

•LA•••
ALABAM
ALAINA
ALALAS
ALAMOS
ALANIS
ALANON
ALARIC
ALARMS
ALARUM
ALASKA
ALATED
BLABBY
BLACKS
BLADED
BLADER
BLADES
BLAFFS
BLAINE
BLAISE
BLAKEY
BLAMED
BLAMER
BLAMES
BLANCA
BLANCH
BLANCO
BLANDA
BLANKS
BLARED
BLARES
BLASTS
BLATTY
BLAZED
BLAZER
BLAZES
BLAZON
CLACKS
CLADIN
CLAIMS
CLAIRE
CLAIRS
CLAMMA
CLAMMY
CLAMOR
CLAMPS
CLAMUP
CLANCY
CLANGS
CLANKS
CLANKY
CLAQUE
CLARET
CLARKE
CLAROS
CLASPS
CLASSA
CLASSE
CLASSY
CLAUDE
CLAUSE
CLAVES
CLAVIN
CLAWAT
CLAWED
CLAWER
CLAYEY
DLAYER
ELADIO
ELAINE
ELANCE
ELANDS
ELANET
ELAPID
ELAPSE
ELATED
ELATER
ELATES
ELAYER
ELAYNE
FLABBY
FLACKS
FLACON
FLAGGY
FLAGON
FLAILS
FLAIRS
FLAKED
FLAKER
FLAKES
FLAMBE
FLAMED
FLAMER
FLAMES
FLANGE
FLANKS
FLAPPY
FLARED
FLARES
FLASHY
FLASKS
FLATLY
FLATTV
FLAUNT
FLAUTA
FLAVIA
FLAVOR
FLAWED
FLAXEN
FLAXES
FLAYED
FLAYER
GLACES
GLACIS
GLADES
GLADLY
GLADTO
GLADYS
GLAMOR
GLAMUP
GLANCE
GLANDS
GLARED
GLARES
GLARUS
GLASER
GLASSY
GLAZED
GLAZER
GLAZES
KLAATU
KLATCH
KLAXON
LLADRO
LLAMAS
LLANOS
OLAFII
OLAFIV
OLAKES
OLATHE
OLAVII
OLAVIV
PLACED
PLACER
PLACES
PLACID
PLAGES
PLAGUE
PLAICE
PLAIDS
PLAINS
PLAINT
PLAITS
PLAKAT
PLANAR
PLANAS
PLANBS
PLANCK
PLANED
PLANER
PLANES
PLANET
PLANKS
PLANON
PLANTE
PLANTO
PLANTS
PLAQUE
PLASHY
PLASMA
PLASMO
PLATED
PLATEN
PLATER
PLATES
PLATOS
PLATTE
PLATYS
PLAYAS
PLAYAT
PLAYBY
PLAYED
PLAYER
PLAYIT
PLAYON
PLAYTO
PLAYUP
PLAZAS
SLACKS
SLAKED
SLAKER
SLAKES
SLALOM
SLAMON
SLANGS
SLANGY
SLANTS
SLAPON
SLAPPY
SLATED
SLATER
SLATES
SLAVED
SLAVER
SLAVES
SLAVIC
SLAYED
SLAYER
VLASIC
XLARGE

•L•A••
ALBANO
ALBANS
ALBANY
ALCAPP
ALEAST
ALHAIG
ALKAID
ALKALI
ALLAIS
ALLAYS
ALMAAZ
ALMACH
ALMATY
ALNASL
ALPACA
ALSACE
ALTAIC
ALTAIR
ALTARF
ALTARS
ALVARO

ALWAYS
ALZADO
BLEACH
BLEAKS
BLEARS
BLEARY
BLEATS
BLOATS
CLEANS
CLEARS
CLEARY
CLEATS
CLEAVE
CLOAKS
ELGART
ELNATH
ELPAIS
ELPASO
ELUANT
ELUARD
ELUATE
FLOATS
FLOATY
FLYASH
GLEAMS
GLEAMY
GLEANS
GLOATS
ILEANA
ILIADS
KLAATU
NLEAST
OLDAGE
OLEARY
OLEATE
PLEADS
PLEASE
PLEATS
PLIANT
SLEAZE
SLEAZY
SLOANE
ULLAGE

•L••A•

ALABAM
ALALAS
ALEGAR
ALEMAN
ALETAP
ALEXAS
ALIYAH
ALLDAY
ALLMAN
ALMAAZ
ALOHAS
ALOMAR
ALPHAS
ALTMAN
ALTTAB
ALULAE
ALULAR
ALYDAR
CLAWAT
CLIMAT
CLIMAX
CLONAL
ELFMAN
ELIJAH
FLEWAT
FLORAE
FLORAL
FLORAS
FLYMAN
FLYWAY
GLOBAL
ILLSAY
KLIBAN
LLAMAS
LLBEAN
OLDBAT
OLDCAR
OLDGAG
OLDHAM
OLDHAT
OLDMAN
OLDPAL
OLDSAW
OLDWAY
PLAKAT
PLANAR
PLANAS
PLAYAS
PLAYAT
PLAZAS
PLEIAD
PLEXAL
PLURAL
SLEZAK
SLOGAN
SLOVAK
ULLMAN
ULTRAS

•L•••A

ALAINA
ALASKA
ALCINA
ALEXIA
ALHENA
ALICIA
ALOGIA
ALPACA
ALTHEA
ALTIMA
ALTRIA
ALUDRA
ALUMNA
ALYSSA
ALZIRA
BLANCA
BLANDA
CLAMMA
CLASSA
ELISHA
ELISSA
ELLORA
ELMIRA
ELNORA
ELODEA
ELOISA
ELVIRA
ELYRIA
FLAUTA
FLAVIA
FLICKA
GLENDA
GLINDA
GLINKA
GLORIA
GLOSSA
ILEANA
OLESHA
OLINDA
OLIVIA
PLASMA
PLEURA
PLUVIA
ULTIMA

••LA••

ABLARE
ABLATE
ABLAZE
AFLAME
AFLARE
AFLATS
AGLAIA
AGLARE
ALLAIS
ALLAYS
ASLANT
ATLAST
AULAIT
BALAAM
BALATA
BELAIR
BELATE
BELAYS
BFLATS
BYLAND
BYLAWS
CALAIS
CALASH
CCLAMP
CFLATS
COLADA
DALAND
DALASI
DELAND
DELANO
DELANY
DELAYS
DFLATS
DILATE
DOLAPS
ECLAIR
ECLASS
ECLATS
EFLATS
EKLAND
ENLACE
ERLANG
FALALA
FALANA
FFLATS
FOLATE
GALANT
GALAXY
GELATE
GELATI
GELATO
GFLATS
GOLAME
GOLAST
GULAGS
HALALA
HILARY
IMLATE
INLAID
INLAND
INLAWS
INLAYS
IOLANI
ISLAND
ISLATE
JALAPA
KDLANG
KULAKS
LALALA
LELAND
LILACS
MALABO
MALADY
MALAGA
MALARS
MALAWI
MALAYA
MALAYS
MCLAIN
MILADY
MILANO
MILANS
MOLARS
MYLADY
MYLARS
OBLADI
OBLAST
OBLATE
OFLATE
OGLALA
ONLAID
ONLAND
ONLATE
ONLAYS
OOLALA
PALACE
PALADE
PALAIS
PALATE
PCLABS
PELAGE
PILAFS
PILATE
PILAUS
POLAND
POLARA
RELACE
RELAID
RELAND
RELAPS
RELATE
RELAYS
ROLAND
SALAAM
SALADA
SALADE
SALADS
SALAMI
SALARY
SCLAFF
SILAGE
SOLACE
SOLANO
SOLANS
SOLARA
SOLATI
SPLASH
SPLATS
SPLAYS
TILAKS
TOLARS
TOLAST
TULANE
TULARE
TVLAND
UCLANS
UHLANS
ULLAGE
UMLAUT
UNLACE
UNLADE
UNLAID
UNLASH
UNLAYS
UPLAND
UPLAST
UPLATE
VALAIS
VELARS
VOLANS
VOLANT
VOLARE

••L•A•

AFLOAT
AGLEAM
ALLDAY
ALLMAN
BALAAM
BALKAN
BALKAT
BALLAD
BALSAM
BALSAS
BALZAC
BELDAM
BELGAE
BELIAL
BELLAY
BILBAO
BILDAD
BOLLAS
BOLYAI
BULGAR
BULLAE
CALLAN
CALLAO
CALLAS
CELLAE
CELLAR
COLFAX
COLLAR
COLLAT
COLMAN
COLMAR
DALLAS
DELEAD
DELIAN
DELMAR
DELRAY
DELTAS
DILLAR
DOLLAR
DOLMAN
DOLMAS
EOLIAN
FALLAL
FELLAH
FELLAS
FILIAL
FOLIAR
FULMAR
GALEAE
GALEAO
GALPAL
GALWAY
GELCAP
GELLAR
GILEAD
GILLAN
GILMAN
GULLAH
HALLAM
HALVAH
HALVAS
HELLAS
HOLMAN
ILLSAY
INLEAF
JALPAS
JULIAN
KALKAN
KALMAR
LILIAN
MALIAN
MCLEAN
MELMAC
MILLAY
MILSAP
MOLDAU
MOLNAR
MULLAH
MULLAS
NOLEAD
NOLOAD
OILCAN
OILMAN
OILPAN
ONLOAD
ONLOAN
PALEAE
PALLAS
PALMAR
PALMAS
PELHAM
PELLAM
PILLAR
POLEAX
POLGAR
POLKAS
POLLAK
PULSAR
RELEAD
RELEAP
RELOAD
RELOAN
SALAAM
SALMAN
SALSAS
SILVAS
SOLEAS
SULFAS
SULTAN
SYLVAN
TALKAT
TILTAT
TULSAN
ULLMAN
UNLEAD
UNLEAF
UNLEAN
UNLOAD
UPLEAP
UPLOAD
VILLAS
VULCAN
VULGAR
YELLAT
ZOLTAN

••L••A

AGLAIA
ARLOVA
BALATA
BALBOA
BELUGA
BOLENA
BULOVA
CELICA
COLADA
COLIMA
DULLEA
ELLORA
FALALA
FALANA
FULCRA
GALENA
GALLIA
GOLETA
HALALA
HELENA
JALAPA
LALALA
LOLITA
MALAGA
MALAYA
MELINA
MOLINA
MULETA
OGLALA
OOLALA
PALOMA
PELOTA
POLARA
POLSKA
SALADA
SALINA
SALIVA
SCLERA
SELENA
SILICA
SOLARA
SYLVIA
TALISA
TOLDYA
VALERA
VALOVA
WALESA
YELENA

•••LA•

ACELAS
AKELAS
ALALAS
ALULAE
ALULAR
ASFLAT
ASHLAR
ATPLAY
BALLAD
BEDLAM
BELLAY
BEULAH
BIOLAB
BOLLAS
BULLAE
BURLAP
BYPLAY
CALLAN
CALLAO
CALLAS
CELLAE
CELLAR
CHELAE
COLLAR
COLLAT
CONLAN
DALLAS
DECLAW
DEWLAP
DILLAR
DJILAS
DNALAB
DOLLAR
DOULAS
DRCLAW
DUNLAP
EARLAP
ECOLAB
ECOLAW
FALLAL
FELLAH
FELLAS
GAGLAW
GELLAR
GILLAN
GOFLAT
GULLAH
GUNLAP
GUNLAW
HABLAR
HALLAM
HARLAN
HELLAS
HOWLAT
IMGLAD
INPLAY
JETLAG
KAPLAN
KEVLAR
KOALAS
KUBLAI
LAALAA
LAULAU
MILLAY
MISLAY
MOOLAH
MULLAH
MULLAS
NOWLAN
NYALAS
OCULAR
ONELAP
OUTLAW
OUTLAY
OVULAR
PALLAS
PARLAY
PELLAM
PILLAR
POLLAK
POPLAR
PRELAW
RAGLAN
RAILAT
RECLAD
REFLAG
REPLAN
REPLAY
SCALAR
SEALAB
SKYLAB
STALAG
STELAR
STELAS
STOLAE
STOLAF
STOLAS
TABLAS
TAXLAW
TESLAS
THELAW
TOILAT
TOKLAS
TRALAS
UNCLAD
UNCLAY
UNFLAT
UNGLAD
UNPLAN
USFLAG
UVULAE
UVULAR
UVULAS
VACLAV
VASLAV
VILLAS
VIOLAS
WAYLAY
WHELAN
YELLAT

•••L•A

ABOLLA
AEOLIA
AMALIA
AMELIA
ANGLIA
ANTLIA
APULIA
AXILLA
AZALEA
AZELMA
CHOLLA
COELIA
COULDA
DAHLIA
DEFLEA
DULLEA
EMILIA
ETALIA
GALLIA
IMELDA
ISOLDA
ITALIA
KAHLUA
KAILUA
LAALAA
LUELLA
PAELLA
PAGLIA
PERLEA
REALIA
SCALIA
SCYLLA
SMALLA
SMILLA
STELLA
THALIA
THELMA
WOULDA

••••LA

ABOLLA
ANGELA
ANGOLA
AQUILA
ARBELA
AREOLA
ATTILA
AXILLA
AZUELA
BAKULA
BARKLA
BIKILA
CABALA
CANOLA
CANULA
CHOLLA
CIBOLA
COPULA
CUPOLA
EASTLA
EIDOLA
FACULA
FALALA
FIBULA
HALALA
HOOPLA
IMPALA
KERALA
LALALA
LOYOLA
LUELLA
LUNULA
MACULA
MANILA
MASALA
MAZOLA
MODELA
NEBULA
NICOLA
NIKOLA
NOVELA
OGLALA
OOLALA
PACULA
PAELLA
PAKULA
PAMELA
PAYOLA
PETULA
PUEBLA
QABALA
RCCOLA
RICOLA
ROMOLA
SCYLLA
SHEILA
SMALLA
SMILLA
STELLA
TABULA
UNCOLA
UNGULA
UPSALA
URSULA
VIZSLA

LB••••

LBEAMS

L•B•••

LABATT
LABELS
LABFEE
LABIAL
LABILE
LABINE
LABIUM
LABORS
LABOUR
LABRAT
LABREA
LEBEAU
LEBRET
LEBRON
LEBRUN
LIBBED
LIBBER
LIBBYS
LIBELS
LIBERS
LIBIDO
LIBRAE
LIBRAN
LIBRAS
LIBRIS
LIBROS
LIBYAN
LLBEAN
LOBATE
LOBBED
LOBBER
LOBULE
LUBBER
LUBECK
LUBING
LUBLIN

L••B••

LAMBDA
LAMBED
LAYBYS
LAZBOY
LESBOS
LIABLE
LIBBED
LIBBER
LIBBYS
LIEBER
LIEBIG
LIEBYS
LIMBED
LIMBER
LIMBIC
LIMBOS
LISBOA
LISBON
LOBBED
LOBBER
LOWBID
LOWBOY
LUBBER
LUMBAR
LUMBER

L•••B•

LAIDBY
LAVABO
LAYSBY
LEFTBE
LETSBE
LETSBY
LOWEBB

L••••B

LOUISB
LOWEBB

•LB•••

ALBANO
ALBANS
ALBANY
ALBEDO
ALBEIT
ALBERS
ALBERT
ALBINE
ALBINO
ALBION
ALBORG
ALBUMS
ELBERT
ELBOWS
ELBRUS
ELBURZ
LLBEAN

•L•B••

ALABAM
ALIBIS
ALIBLE
ALLBUT
BLABBY
BLOBBY
BLOBEL
CLUBBY
CLUBUP
FLABBY
FLUBUG
FLYBOY
FLYBYS
GLIBLY
GLOBAL
GLOBBY
GLOBED
GLOBES
GLOBIN
ILLBET
KLIBAN
OLDBAT
OLDBOY
PLEBES
SLOBBY

•L••B•

BLABBY
BLOBBY
BLURBS
CLIMBS
CLUBBY
FLABBY
FLAMBE
FLEWBY
FLITBY
GLOBBY
PLANBS
PLAYBY
PLUMBO
PLUMBS
SLIPBY
SLOBBY

•L•••B

ALICEB
ALTTAB

••LB••

ALLBUT
BALBOA
BILBAO
COLBYS
ILLBET
WILBUR

••L•B•

ADLIBS
CELEBS
FILEBY
MALABO
MALIBU
MALTBY
PCLABS
PHLEBO
ROLLBY
SELLBY
WALKBY
WILLBE
ZHLOBS
ZHLUBS

••L••B

APLOMB
OILRUB

•••LB•

GOALBY
PHILBY
ROLLBY
SELLBY
SHELBY
TENLBS
TRILBY
WILLBE

•••L•B

BIOLAB
DNALAB
ECOLAB
SCHLUB
SEALAB
SKYLAB
SMALLB
UNGLIB

••••LB

CECILB
DEKALB
MODELB
SMALLB

LC••••

LCHAIM

L•C•••

LACAGE
LACASA
LACAVA
LACEON
LACERS
LACEUP
LACHEY
LACHOY
LACIER
LACILY
LACING
LACKED
LACKEY
LACLOS
LACTEA
LACTIC
LACUNA
LECAIN
LECHER
LECTER
LECTOR
LICHEE
LICHEN
LICKED
LICKER
LICKUP
LOCALE
LOCALS
LOCANE
LOCATE
LOCCIT
LOCHER
LOCKED
LOCKER
LOCKET
LOCKIN
LOCKON
LOCKUP
LOCUST
LUCENT
LUCIAN
LUCIDA
LUCIEN
LUCILE
LUCINE
LUCITE
LUCIUS
LUCKED
LYCEES
LYCEUM
LYCRAS

L••C••

LAICAL
LANCED
LANCER
LANCES
LANCET
LANCIA
LANCIE
LAPCAT
LASCAR
LEACHY
LEICAS
LITCHI
LOCCIT
LOUCHE
LOWCAL
LOWCUT
LUNCHY

L•••C•

LAUNCH
LEGACY
LILACS
LOGICS
LOLICH
LUBECK
LUKICH
LUNACY
LUTECE
LYRICS

L••••C

LACTIC
LAURIC
LIMBIC
LITHIC
LOMPOC

•LC•••

ALCAPP
ALCINA
ALCOTT
ALCOVE
ULCERS

•L•C••

ALECKS
ALECKY
ALECTO
ALICEB

ALICES
ALICIA
BLACKS
BLOCKS
BLOCKY
CLACKS
CLICHE
CLICHY
CLICKS
CLOCHE
CLOCKS
CLUCKS
ELECTS
ELICIT
FLACKS
FLACON
FLECHE
FLECKS
FLECKY
FLICKA
FLICKS
FLOCKS
GLACES
GLACIS
GLOCKS
GLYCOL
KLICKS
OLDCAR
PLACED
PLACER
PLACES
PLACID
PLOCES
PLUCKS
PLUCKY
SLACKS
SLICED
SLICER
SLICES
SLICKS

•L••C•
ALLYCE
ALMACH
ALNICO
ALPACA
ALSACE
BLANCA
BLANCH
BLANCO
BLEACH
BLENCH
BLOTCH
CLANCY
CLENCH
CLINCH
CLUTCH
ELANCE
ELLICE
FLEECE
FLEECY
FLETCH
FLINCH
GLANCE
GLITCH
GLOUCS
KLATCH
OLMECS
PLAICE
PLANCK
SLOUCH
SLUICE
ULRICH

•L•••C
ALARIC
ALTAIC
CLERIC
CLINIC
OLDVIC
SLAVIC
VLASIC

••LC••
AFLCIO
BOLCOM
DELCOS
DULCET
FALCON
FULCRA
GELCAP
MULCTS
OILCAN
OILCUP
TALCED
TALCUM
TELCOS
VELCRO
VULCAN
WELCHS
WILCOX

••L•C•
ALLYCE
CALICO
CELICA
COLECO
COLICS
CULTCH
DELICT
ELLICE
ENLACE
FELICE
HELICO
INLUCK
LILACS
LOLICH
MALICE
MALICK
NOLUCK
OCLOCK
PALACE
POLICE
POLICY
RELACE
RELICS
RELICT
RELOCK
RELUCT
SELECT
SHLOCK
SILICA
SOLACE
SPLICE
UNLACE
UNLOCK
VELOCE

••L••C
BALTIC
BALZAC
BELGIC
BELLOC
CELTIC
CULTIC
DELTIC
FILMIC
GALLIC
MALEIC
MELMAC
PELVIC
TOLTEC

•••LC•
PHILCO
VAILCO

•••L•C
AHOLIC
ANGLIC
BELLOC
CYCLIC
ENBLOC
EXILIC
FROLIC
GAELIC
GALLIC
GARLIC
ITALIC
OXALIC
PHILIC
PUBLIC
SMALLC
URALIC
ZIPLOC

••••LC
SMALLC

L•D•••
LADDER
LADDIE
LADERS
LADIDA
LADIES
LADING
LADINO
LADLED
LADLER
LADLES
LADOGA
LADUKE
LADYDI
LEDGER
LEDGES
LEDOFF
LEDOUT
LEDOUX
LIDDED
LODENS
LODGED
LODGER
LODGES
LODINJ
LUDDEN
LUDENS
LUDLOW
LUDLUM
LUDWIG
LYDIAN

L••D••
LADDER
LADDIE
LAIDBY
LAIDIN
LAIDON
LAIDTO
LAIDUP
LANDAT
LANDAU
LANDED
LANDER
LANDHO
LANDIS
LANDON
LANDOR
LANDRY
LANDUP
LANDUS
LAPDOG
LARDED
LARDER
LARDON
LAUDED
LAUDER
LEADED
LEADEN
LEADER
LEADIN
LEADON
LEADTO
LEADUP
LEIDEN
LENDEE
LENDER
LENDTO
LEWDER
LEWDLY
LEYDEN
LIDDED
LIEDER
LIEDON
LIEDTO
LINDEN
LINDER
LLADRO
LOADED
LOADER
LOADIN
LOADUP
LOIDED
LONDON
LORDED
LORDIT
LORDLY
LOSDOS
LOUDEN
LOUDER
LOUDLY
LOUDON
LUDDEN
LUNDEN
LUNDIS
LYNDON

L•••D•
LADIDA
LADYDI
LAIRDS
LAMBDA
LAMEDS
LAREDO
LAVIDA
LERIDA
LEVADE
LIBIDO
LIPIDS
LLOYDS
LUANDA
LUCIDA
LUNEDI
LYRIDS

L••••D
LACKED
LADLED
LAGGED
LAIRED
LALLED
LAMBED
LAMMED
LANCED
LANDED
LAPPED
LAPSED
LARDED
LARKED
LASHED
LASTED
LATHED
LAUDED
LEADED
LEAFED
LEAKED
LEANED
LEAPED
LEASED
LEAVED
LEERED
LEGEND
LEGGED
LELAND
LEMOND
LENARD
LENSED
LEONID
LETTED
LEVEED
LEVIED
LIBBED
LICKED
LIDDED
LIFTED
LIGAND
LILIED
LILTED
LIMBED
LIMNED
LIMPED
LIMPID
LINKED
LINTED
LIPPED
LIQUID
LISPED
LISTED
LIZARD
LOADED
LOAFED
LOAMED
LOANED
LOBBED
LOCKED
LODGED
LOFTED
LOGGED
LOIDED
LOLLED
LOMOND
LONGED
LOOKED
LOOMED
LOOPED
LOOSED
LOOTED
LOPPED
LORDED
LOTTED
LOUSED
LOWBID
LOWEND
LUCKED
LUFFED
LUGGED
LULLED
LUMPED
LUNGED
LURKED
LUSTED
LYNYRD

•LD•••
ALDERS
ALDINE
ALDISS
ALDOUS
ALDRIN
ELDERS
ELDEST
OLDAGE
OLDBAT
OLDBOY
OLDCAR
OLDDOG
OLDELI
OLDEST
OLDGAG
OLDHAM
OLDHAT
OLDIES
OLDISH
OLDMAN
OLDMEN
OLDPAL
OLDPRO
OLDSAW
OLDSOD
OLDVIC
OLDWAY

•L•D••
ALLDAY
ALUDEL
ALUDRA
ALYDAR
BLADED
BLADER
BLADES
BLUDGE
BLYDEN
CLADIN
CLODDY
CLYDES
ELADIO
ELIDED
ELIDER
ELIDES
ELODEA
ELUDED
ELUDER
ELUDES
FLEDGE
FLEDGY
GLADES
GLADLY
GLADTO
GLADYS
GLIDED
GLIDER
GLIDES
ILLDRY
KLUDGE
KLUDGY
LLADRO
OLDDOG
PLEDGE
PLEDTO
SLEDGE
SLIDER
SLIDES
SLIDIN
SLUDGE
SLUDGY

•L••D•
ALBEDO
ALGEDI
ALKYDS
ALLUDE
ALZADO
BLANDA
BLEEDS
BLENDE
BLENDS
BLINDS
BLONDE
BLONDS
BLOODS
BLOODY
CLAUDE
CLODDY
CLOUDS
CLOUDY
ELANDS
FLOODS
FLUIDS
GLANDS
GLENDA
GLINDA
ILIADS
ILLUDE
LLOYDS
OLINDA
PLAIDS
PLEADS

•L•••D
ALATED
ALFRED
ALINED
ALIPED
ALKAID
ALLIED
ALMOND
ALTOID
BLADED
BLAMED
BLARED
BLAZED
CLAWED
CLEWED
CLONED
CLOSED
CLOYED
ELAPID
ELATED
ELIDED
ELOPED
ELUARD
ELUDED
ELUTED
ELWOOD
FLAKED
FLAMED
FLARED
FLAWED
FLAYED
FLEXED
FLORID
FLOWED
FLUTED
FLUXED
FLYROD
GLARED
GLAZED
GLIDED
GLOBED
GLOVED
GLOWED
ILLFED
OLDSOD
OLERUD
PLACED
PLACID
PLANED
PLATED
PLAYED
PLEIAD
PLOWED
PLUMED
SLAKED
SLATED
SLAVED
SLAYED
SLEWED
SLICED
SLIMED
SLOPED
SLOWED

••LD••
ALLDAY
BALDED
BALDER
BALDIE
BALDLY
BALDUR
BELDAM
BILDAD
BOLDED
BOLDEN
BOLDER
BOLDLY
BULDEO
CALDER
COLDER
COLDLY
FELDON
FOLDED
FOLDER
FOLDIN
FOLDUP
GELDED
GELDOF
GILDED
GILDER
GOLDEN
GOLDIE
GULDEN
HELDIN
HELDIT
HELDON
HELDTO
HELDUP
HOLDEM
HOLDEN
HOLDER
HOLDIN
HOLDIT
HOLDME
HOLDON
HOLDTO
HOLDUP
ILLDRY
MALDEN
MELDED
MELDER
MILDER
MILDEW
MILDLY
MOLDAU
MOLDED
MOLDER
MULDER
SELDOM
SOLDER
SOLDIT
SOLDON
SOLDTO
TILDEN
TILDES
TOLDIT
TOLDOF
TOLDON
TOLDYA
VALDEZ
VELDTS
WALDEN
WELDED
WELDER
WELDON
WILDER
WILDLY

••L•D•
ALLUDE
BOLIDE
COLADA
DELUDE
FALUDI
FELIDS
HALIDE
ILLUDE
ITLLDO
MALADY
MELODY
MILADY
MYLADY
OBLADI
PALADE
SALADA
SALADE
SALADS
SOLIDS
TOLEDO
UNLADE
WILLDO

••L••D
ALLIED
BALDED
BALKED
BALLAD
BELIED
BELLED
BELTED
BILDAD
BILGED
BILKED
BILLED
BOLDED
BOLTED
BULGED
BULKED
BULLED
BYLAND
CALKED
CALLED
CALMED
CALVED
CELLED
CULLED
DALAND
DELAND
DELEAD
DELVED
DOLLED
DULLED
EKLAND
FELLED
FELTED
FILLED
FILMED
FOLDED
GALLED
GELDED
GELLED
GILDED
GILEAD
GILLED
GOLFED
GULFED
GULLED
GULPED
HALOED
HALOID
HALTED
HALVED
HELMED
HELPED
HILLED
HILTED
HULKED
HULLED
ILLFED
INLAID
INLAND
ISLAND
JELLED
JILTED
JOLTED
KILLED
KILNED
KILTED
LALLED
LELAND
LILIED
LILTED
LOLLED
LULLED
MALTED
MELDED
MELTED
MILKED
MILLED
MILORD
MOLDED
MOLTED
MULLED
MYLORD
NOLEAD
NOLOAD
NULLED
ONLAID
ONLAND
ONLOAD
PALLED
PALLID
PALMED
PELTED
PILLED
POLAND
POLLED
PULLED
PULPED
PULSED
RELAID
RELAND
RELEAD
RELEND
RELIED
RELOAD
ROLAND
ROLFED
ROLLED
SALTED
SALVED
SILOED
SILTED
SOLOED
SOLVED
SULKED
TALCED
TALKED
TALMUD
TILLED
TILTED
TOLLED
TVLAND
UNLAID
UNLEAD
UNLOAD
UPLAND
UPLOAD
VALUED
VALVED
WALKED
WALLED
WELDED
WELLED
WELTED
WILLED
WILTED
WOLFED
XYLOID
YELLED
YELPED
YOLKED

•••LD•
BUILDS
CHILDE
COULDA
COULDI
FIELDS
GUILDS
IMELDA
ISOLDA
ISOLDE
ITLLDO
MOULDS
MOULDY
SCALDS
SCOLDS
SKALDS
UVALDE
WEALDS
WIELDS
WIELDY
WILLDO
WORLDS
WOULDA
YEOLDE
YIELDS

•••L•D
ADDLED
AISLED
AMBLED
ANELED
ANGLED
ANKLED
BAILED
BALLAD
BAWLED
BELLED
BILLED
BIRLED
BOILED
BOWLED
BUGLED
BULLED
BURLED
CABLED
CALLED
CEILED
CELLED
COALED
COILED
COOLED
COWLED
CULLED
CURLED
CYCLED
DIALED
DOLLED
DUELED
DULLED
EAGLED
EFILED
EUCLID
EXILED
EYELID
FABLED
FAILED
FELLED
FILLED
FOALED
FOILED
FOOLED
FOULED
FOWLED
FUELED
FURLED
GABLED
GALLED
GAOLED
GELLED
GILLED
GUILED
GULLED
HAILED
HAULED
HEALED
HEELED
HILLED
HOWLED
HULLED
HURLED
IMGLAD
IMPLED
JAILED
JELLED
JOWLED
KEELED
KHALID
KILLED
LADLED
LALLED
LOLLED
LULLED
MAILED
MARLED
MAULED
MEWLED
MILLED
MISLED
MOILED
MULLED
NAILED
NULLED
OUTLED
PALLED
PALLID
PEALED
PEELED
PILLED
POLLED
POOLED
POTLID
PULLED
PURLED
RAILED
RECLAD
REELED
REPLED
RIFLED
ROILED
ROLLED
SAILED
SCALED
SEALED
SIDLED
SMALLD
SMILED
SOILED
STALED
STOLID
STYLED
SUBLID
TABLED
TAILED
TILLED
TITLED
TOILED
TOLLED
TOOLED
UNBLED
UNCLAD
UNGLAD
VEILED
VIALED
WAILED
WALLED
WASLED
WELLED
WHALED
WHILED
WILLED
YELLED
YOWLED

••••LD
AFIELD
AGEOLD
ANYOLD
ARNOLD
ASCOLD
BEHELD
BEHOLD
BIFOLD
BUJOLD
DAYOLD
DONALD
DUGALD
ENFOLD
ENGILD
GERALD
GETOLD
GOCOLD
GOTOLD
GOWILD
HARALD
HAROLD
HERALD
ICOULD
IMCOLD
IMSOLD
IMTOLD
INFOLD
INGOLD
IWOULD
KOBOLD
ONHOLD
OSWALD
REFOLD
REGILD
REHELD
REHOLD
REMOLD
RESOLD
RETOLD
REWELD
RIBALD
RONALD
SHIELD
SHOULD
SMALLD
UNBOLD
UNFOLD
UNHELD
UNMOLD
UNSELD
UNSOLD
UNTOLD
UNWILD
UPFOLD
UPHELD
UPHOLD
WASOLD

LE••••
LEACHY
LEADED
LEADEN
LEADER
LEADIN
LEADON
LEADTO
LEADUP

LEAFED LEAGUE LEAKED LEAKER LEAKEY LEAKIN LEALTY LEANED LEANER LEANIN LEANLY LEANNE LEANON LEANTO LEAPAT LEAPED LEAPER LEAPIN LEAPON LEAPUP LEARNS LEARNT LEASED LEASER LEASES LEASTS LEAVED LEAVEN LEAVER LEAVES LEBEAU LEBRET LEBRON LEBRUN LECAIN LECHER LECTER LECTOR LEDGER LEDGES LEDOFF LEDOUT LEDOUX LEEANN LEEKIE LEELEE LEEMAY LEERAT LEERED LEERER LEEVES LEEWAY LEFTBE LEFTIN LEFTIT LEFTOF LEFTON LEGACY LEGALS LEGART LEGATE LEGATO LEGEND LEGGED LEGION LEGIST LEGMAN LEGMEN

LEGREE LEGROS LEGSIT LEGUIN LEGUME LEHIGH LEHMAN LEHNEN LEHRER LEHUAS LEICAS LEIDEN LEISEN LEITER LELAND LELOIR LEMANS LEMMAS LEMMON LEMNOS LEMOKO LEMOND LEMONS LEMONY LEMUEL LEMURS LENAIN LENAPE LENARD LENDEE LENDER LENDTO LENGLE LENGTH LENGUA LENINA LENITY LENNIE LENNON LENNOX LENORE LENOVO LENSED LENSES LENTEN LENTIL LENTOS LENTTO LEOIII LEONIA LEONID LEOVII LEOXII LEPERS LEPTON LERIDA LERNER LEROUX LESAGE LESBOS LESHAN LESION LESLEY LESLIE LESMIZ LESSEE LESSEN LESSER

LESSON LESSOR LESTAT LESTER LETFLY LETHAL LETOFF LETOUR LETOUT LETRIP LETSAT LETSBE LETSBY LETSGO LETSIN LETSON LETSUP LETTED LETTER LETTRE LETUPS LETUSE LEUTZE LEVADE LEVANT LEVEED LEVEES LEVELS LEVENE LEVERS LEVERT LEVIED LEVIER LEVIES LEVINE LEVITE LEVITT LEVITY LEWDER LEWDLY LEYDEN

L•E•••

LBEAMS LEEANN LEEKIE LEELEE LEEMAY LEERAT LEERED LEERER LEEVES LEEWAY LIEBER LIEBIG LIEBYS LIEDER LIEDON LIEDTO LIEFER LIEFLY LIEFOR LIEGES LIELOW LIENEE LIENOR LIESIN LIESON LIESTO LIEUTS LIEVIO LUELLA

L••E••

LABELS LACEON LACERS LACEUP LADERS LAGEAR LAGERS LAKERS LAMEDS LAMELY LAMENT LAMESA LAMEST LAPELS LAPERI LAPERM LAREDO LAREES LASERS LATEEN LATELY LATENE LATENS LATENT LATEOF LATEON LATERI LATERO LATEST LATETO LAVERN LAVERS LAXEST LAYERS LEBEAU LEGEND LEPERS LEVEED LEVEES LEVELS LEVENE LEVERS LEVERT LIBELS LIBERS LIFEIS LIFERS LIGEIA LIGERS LIGETI LIKELY LIKENS LIKERS LIKESO LIKETO LINEAL LINEAR LINENS LINENY LINERS LINEUP LIPENG

LITERS LIVEAT LIVEIN LIVELY LIVENS LIVEON LIVERS LIVERY LIVEST LIVETH LIVETV LLBEAN LODENS LOMEIN LONELY LONERS LOOEYS LOPERS LOREAL LORENE LORENZ LOSEIT LOSERS LOSETO LOVEIN LOVEIT LOVELL LOVELY LOVERS LOVETO LOVETT LOVEYA LOVEYS LOWEBB LOWELL LOWEND LOWERS LOWERY LOWEST LUBECK LUCENT LUDENS LUGERS LUMENS LUNEDI LUREIN LURENE LURERS LUTECE LYCEES LYCEUM

L•••E•

LABFEE LABREA LACHEY LACIER LACKED LACKEY LACTEA LADDER LADIES LADLED LADLER LADLES LAFFER LAGGED LAGGER

LAIRED LAKIER LALLED LAMBED LAMMED LANCED LANCER LANCES LANCET LANDED LANDER LANGER LANIER LANKER LAPPED LAPPER LAPPET LAPSED LAPSER LAPSES LAPTEV LARDED LARDER LAREES LARGER LARGES LARKED LARKER LARMEN LARSEN LARTER LARTET LASHED LASHER LASHES LASKER LASSEN LASSER LASSES LASTED LASTEX LATEEN LATHED LATHEN LATHER LATHES LATKES LATTER LATTES LAUDED LAUDER LAUPER LAUREL LAUREN LAUREY LAUTER LAWMEN LAWYER LAYMEN LAZIER LEADED LEADEN LEADER LEAFED LEAKED LEAKER LEAKEY LEANED

LEANER LEAPED LEAPER LEASED LEASER LEASES LEAVED LEAVEN LEAVER LEAVES LEBRET LECHER LECTER LEDGER LEDGES LEELEE LEERED LEERER LEEVES LEGGED LEGMEN LEGREE LEHNEN LEHRER LEIDEN LEISEN LEITER LEMUEL LENDEE LENDER LENSED LENSES LENTEN LERNER LESLEY LESSEE LESSEN LESSER LESTER LETTED LETTER LEVEED LEVEES LEVIED LEVIER LEVIES LEWDER LEYDEN LIANES LIBBED LIBBER LICHEE LICHEN LICKED LICKER LIDDED LIEBER LIEDER LIEFER LIEGES LIENEE LIFTED LIFTER LIGNES LILIED LILIES LILTED LIMBED

LIMBER LIMIER LIMNED LIMNER LIMPED LIMPER LIMPET LINDEN LINDER LINGER LINIER LINKED LINKER LINNET LINNEY LINTED LINTEL LINTER LINZER LIONEL LIONET LIPPED LIPPER LISLES LISPED LISPER LISSES LISTED LISTEE LISTEN LISTER LITHER LITRES LITTER LIVRES LOADED LOADER LOAFED LOAFER LOAMED LOANED LOANER LOAVES LOBBED LOBBER LOCHER LOCKED LOCKER LOCKET LODGED LODGER LODGES LOFTED LOFTER LOGGED LOGGER LOGIER LOIDED LOIRET LOITER LOLLED LOLLER LONGED LONGER LONGES LONGET LOOIES LOOKED

LOOKEE LOOKER LOOMED LOONEY LOOPED LOOPER LOOSED LOOSEN LOOSER LOOSES LOOSEY LOOTED LOOTER LOPPED LOPPER LORDED LORIES LOSSES LOTTED LOTTER LOUDEN LOUDER LOUIES LOUPES LOUSED LOUSES LOUVER LOWKEY LOWMEN LOWRES LOWSET LTILES LUBBER LUCIEN LUCKED LUDDEN LUFFED LUGGED LUGGER LULLED LULLER LUMBER LUMLEY LUMPED LUMPEN LUMPER LUNDEN LUNGED LUNGER LUNGES LUNKER LURKED LURKER LURKEY LUSHER LUSHES LUSTED LUSTER LUTHER LUTZES LWAVES LYCEES LYNLEY LYNXES

L••••E

LABFEE LABILE LABINE LACAGE LADDIE LADUKE LAHORE LAINIE LAJOIE LAMAZE LAMIAE LANATE LANCIE LANOSE LAOTSE LARINE LARVAE LASSIE LATENE LAURIE LAVAGE LEAGUE LEANNE LEEKIE LEELEE LEFTBE LEGATE LEGREE LEGUME LENAPE LENDEE LENGLE LENNIE LENORE LESAGE LESLIE LESSEE LETSBE LETTRE LETUSE LEUTZE LEVADE LEVENE LEVINE LEVITE LHOTSE LIABLE LIAISE LIBRAE LICHEE LIENEE LIGATE LILLIE LINAGE LINGLE LIPASE LISTEE LITTLE LITTRE LIZZIE LOATHE LOBATE LOBULE LOCALE LOCANE LOCATE LONGUE LONNIE LOOKEE LOOKIE

LOONIE LORENE LORRIE LOUCHE LOUISE LOUNGE LOUVRE LOVAGE LOYALE LUCILE LUCINE LUCITE LUNATE LUPINE LUPONE LURENE LUSTRE LUTECE LUXATE LYONNE LYSINE

•LE•••

ALEAST ALECKS ALECKY ALECTO ALEGAR ALEGRE ALEGUP ALEKEG ALEMAN ALEPHS ALEPPO ALEROS ALERTS ALETAP ALETTE ALEUTS ALEVEL ALEVES ALEXAS ALEXEI ALEXEY ALEXIA ALEXIS BLEACH BLEAKS BLEARS BLEARY BLEATS BLEEDS BLEEPS BLEETH BLENCH BLENDE BLENDS BLEWIN BLEWIT BLEWON BLEWUP CLEANS CLEARS CLEARY CLEATS CLEAVE CLEEKS CLEESE

CLEFTS CLENCH CLERGY CLERIC CLERKS CLEVER CLEVES CLEWED ELECTS ELEGIT ELEMIS ELEVEN ELEVES ELEVON FLECHE FLECKS FLECKY FLEDGE FLEDGY FLEECE FLEECY FLEERS FLEETS FLENSE FLESHY FLETCH FLEURS FLEWAT FLEWBY FLEWIN FLEWON FLEWTO FLEWUP FLEXED FLEXES FLEXOR GLEAMS GLEAMY GLEANS GLENDA GLENNE ILEANA ILEXES KLEINE KLEIST KLEPTO NLEAST OLEARY OLEATE OLEFIN OLEINS OLEOLE OLERUD OLESHA OLESON OLEUMS OLEVEL PLEADS PLEASE PLEATS PLEBES PLEDGE PLEDTO PLEIAD PLENTY PLENUM PLEURA PLEXAL

PLEXES PLEXOR PLEXUS SLEAZE SLEAZY SLEDGE SLEEKS SLEEKY SLEEPS SLEEPY SLEETS SLEETY SLEEVE SLEIGH SLEUTH SLEWED SLEZAK

•L•E••

ALBEDO ALBEIT ALBERS ALBERT ALDERS ALGEDI ALHENA ALIENS ALKENE ALLEES ALLEGE ALLELE ALLEYN ALLEYS ALPERT ALTERS ALWEST BLEEDS BLEEPS BLEETH BLUELY BLUEOX BLUEST BLUESY BLUETS CLEEKS CLEESE CLIENT CLOETE CLUEIN CLUERS ELBERT ELDERS ELDEST ELIELI ELLERY ELMERS ELRENO ELVERS FLEECE FLEECY FLEERS FLEETS FLIERS FLUENT FLYERS GLIERE GLUEON GLUERS

GLUETO ILLEST LLBEAN NLWEST OLDELI OLDEST OLMECS OLMERT PLIERS SLEEKS SLEEKY SLEEPS SLEEPY SLEETS SLEETY SLEEVE SLIEST SLYEST ULCERS

•L••E•

ALATED ALEKEG ALEVEL ALEVES ALEXEI ALEXEY ALFRED ALFVEN ALGREN ALICEB ALICES ALIKES ALINED ALINER ALINES ALIPED ALIVEO ALKIES ALLEES ALLIED ALLIES ALLMEN ALLNEW ALLSET ALLWET ALTHEA ALTKEY ALUDEL BLADED BLADER BLADES BLAKEY BLAMED BLAMER BLAMES BLARED BLARES BLAZED BLAZER BLAZES BLIMEY BLIXEN BLOBEL BLOKES BLOOEY BLOWER BLYDEN

CLARET CLAVES CLAWED CLAWER CLAYEY CLEVER CLEVES CLEWED CLIMES CLONED CLONER CLONES CLOSED CLOSER CLOSES CLOSET CLOVEN CLOVER CLOVES CLOYED CLYDES DLAYER ELANET ELATED ELATER ELATES ELAYER ELEVEN ELEVES ELIDED ELIDER ELIDES ELISEO ELITER ELITES ELMIER ELODEA ELOGES ELOPED ELOPER ELOPES ELUDED ELUDER ELUDES ELUTED ELUTES ELYSEE FLAKED FLAKER FLAKES FLAMED FLAMER FLAMES FLARED FLARES FLAWED FLAXEN FLAXES FLAYED FLAYER FLEXED FLEXES FLOOEY FLOREK FLORES FLORET FLOREY FLOWED

FLOWER FLUKES FLUKEY FLUMES FLUTED FLUTER FLUTES FLUXED FLUXES FLYMEN FLYNET GLACES GLADES GLARED GLARES GLASER GLAZED GLAZER GLAZES GLIDED GLIDER GLIDES GLOBED GLOBES GLOVED GLOVER GLOVES GLOWED GLOWER GLUIER GLUTEI GLUTEN GLUTES ILEXES ILLBET ILLFED ILLMET ILLSEE ILLSET OLAKES OLDIES OLDMEN OLEVEL OLIVER OLIVES OLORES PLACED PLACER PLACES PLAGES PLANED PLANER PLANES PLANET PLATED PLATEN PLATER PLATES PLAYED PLAYER PLEBES PLEXES PLOCES PLOMER PLOVER PLOWED PLOWER PLUIES PLUMED PLUMES PLUSES SLAKED SLAKER SLAKES SLATED SLATER SLATES SLAVED SLAVER SLAVES SLAYED SLAYER SLEWED SLICED SLICER SLICES SLIDER SLIDES SLIMED SLIMES SLIVER SLOPED SLOPER SLOPES SLOVEN SLOWED SLOWER ULSTER

•L•••E

ALBINE ALCOVE ALDINE ALEGRE ALETTE ALFINE ALGORE ALIBLE ALKENE ALLEGE ALLELE ALLUDE ALLURE ALLYCE ALPINE ALSACE ALULAE BLAINE BLAISE BLENDE BLITHE BLONDE BLOOIE BLOUSE BLUDGE BLYTHE CLAIRE CLAQUE CLARKE CLASSE CLAUDE CLAUSE CLEAVE CLEESE CLICHE CLIQUE CLOCHE CLOETE CLOTHE ELAINE ELANCE ELAPSE ELAYNE ELLICE ELMIRE ELMORE ELOISE ELUATE ELYSEE FLAMBE FLANGE FLECHE FLEDGE FLEECE FLENSE FLORAE FLUTIE GLANCE GLENNE GLIERE GLURGE ILLSEE ILLUDE ILLUME ILLUSE KLEINE KLUDGE OLATHE OLDAGE OLEATE OLEOLE PLAGUE PLAICE PLANTE PLAQUE PLATTE PLEASE PLEDGE PLISSE PLUNGE SLEAZE SLEDGE SLEEVE SLOANE SLUDGE SLUICE ULLAGE XLARGE

••LE••

ABLEST AGLEAM AGLETS AILEEN ALLEES ALLEGE ALLELE ALLEYN ALLEYS AOLERS ARLENE ASLEEP AWLESS BALEEN BALERS BOLENA BOLERO BOLEYN CCLEFS CELEBS CELERY COLECO COLEUS CULETS DALENE DALETH DALETS DELEAD DELETE DOLENZ EELERS EELERY EILEEN EILERS EILERT ELLERY EULESS FILEBY FILEIN FILENE FILERS FILETS FOLEYS GALEAE GALEAO GALENA GCLEFS GELEES GELETT GILEAD GILELS GOLEFT GOLEMS GOLETA HALEST HALEVY HELENA HELENE HELENS HOLERS HOLEUP IDLERS IDLEST ILLEST INLEAF INLETS IRLENE ISLEFT ISLETS ISLEYS JOLENE JULEPS MALEIC MCLEAN MELEES MELETE MILERS MOLEST MULETA MULEYS NFLERS NHLERS NOLEAD NOLESS OGLERS OILERS OWLEGG OWLERY OWLETS PALEAE PALELY PALEST PELEUS PHLEBO PHLEGM PILEIN PILEON PILERS PILEUM PILEUP PILEUS POLEAX POLERS PULERS RELEAD RELEAP RELEND RELENT RELETS RELEVE RELEVY RILERS RILEUP ROLEOS RULEON RULERS RULETH SALEPS SCLERA SELECT SELENA SELENE SILENT SOLEAS SOLEIL SOLELY SOLEMN SOLERS SOLEUS SPLEEN TALENT TALERS TALESE TILERS TILERY TOLEDO TYLERS UNLEAD UNLEAF UNLEAN UNLEFT UNLENT UNLESS UPLEAP VALENE VALENS VALENT VALERA VALERE VALERO VALERY VALETS VILELY VILEST WALESA WYLERS XYLEMS YCLEPT YELENA

••L•E•

AILEEN ALLEES ALLIED ALLIES ALLMEN ALLNEW ALLSET ALLWET ASLEEP BALDED BALDER BALEEN BALKED BALKER BALLET BALMER BELIED BELIEF BELIER BELIES BELLED BELLES BELTED BELTER BELZER BILGED BILGES BILKED BILKER BILLED BILLER BILLET BOLDED BOLDEN BOLDER BOLGER BOLTED BOLTER BULDEO BULGED BULGES BULKED BULLED BULLET BULWER CALDER CALKED CALKER CALLED CALLEE CALLER CALLES CALMED CALMER CALMEX CALVED CALVES CALVET CALXES CELLED COLDER COLLET COLTER CULLED CULLEN CULLER CULLET DALLES DELKEY DELREY DELVED DELVER DELVES DILLER DILSEY DOLLED DOLLEY DULCET DULLEA DULLED DULLER DULLES EELIER EILEEN FALLEN FALLER FALSER FALTER FELLED FELLER FELTED FILLED FILLER FILLES FILLET FILMED FILTER FOLDED FOLDER FOLGER FOLIES FULLER GALLED GALLEY GELDED GELEES GELLED GELLER GELPEN GELSEY GILDED GILDER GILLED GILLEY GOLDEN GOLFED GOLFER GULDEN GULFED GULLED GULLET GULPED GULPER HALLEL HALLEY HALOED HALOES HALSEY HALTED HALTER HALVED HALVER HALVES HELLER HELMED HELMER HELMET HELPED HELPER HELTER HILLED HILLEL HILLER HILTED HOLDEM HOLDEN HOLDER HOLIER HOLIES HOLLER HOLLEY HOLMES HULKED HULLED HULLER ILLBET ILLFED ILLMET ILLSEE ILLSET INLIEU JELLED JILTED JILTER JOLIET JOLLEY JOLTED JOLTER JULIEN JULIET KALLEN KELLER KELLEY KELSEY KILLED KILLER KILMER KILNED KILTED KILTER LALLED LILIED LILIES LILTED LOLLED LOLLER LULLED LULLER MALDEN MALLEI MALLET MALTED MELDED MELDER MELEES MELTED MELTER MILDER MILDEW MILIEU MILKED MILKER MILLED MILLER MILLES MILLET MILNER MILNES MOLDED MOLDER MOLTED MOLTEN MOLTER MULDER MULLED MULLER MULLET NULLED OILIER OILMEN OWLIER PALLED PALLET PALMED PALMER PALTER PELLET PELTED PELTER PHLOEM PILFER PILLED POLLED POLLEE POLLEN POLLER POLLEX PULLED PULLER PULLET PULLEY PULPED PULPER PULSED PULSES PULVER RELIED RELIEF RELIER RELIES RILLES RILLET ROLFED ROLFER ROLLED ROLLEI ROLLER RULIER SALLES SALTED SALTEN SALTER SALVED SALVER SALVES SELLER SELTEN SELVES SILKEN SILOED SILTED SILVER SOLDER SOLOED SOLVED SOLVER SOLVES SPLEEN SULKED SULKER SULLEN TALCED TALKED TALKER TALLER TELLER TELNET TILDEN TILDES TILLED TILLER TILLET TILLEY TILTED TILTER TOLLED TOLLER TOLTEC TULLES UGLIER UGLIES VALDEZ VALLEE VALLEY VALSES VALUED VALUER VALUES VALVED VALVES VELSEN VELVET VOLLEY WALDEN WALKED WALKEN WALKER WALLED WALLER WALLET WALTER WELDED WELDER WELLED WELLER WELLES WELTED WELTER WILDER WILIER WILKES WILLED WILLEM WILLER WILTED WOLFED WOLPER WOLSEY WOLVES YALIES YELLED YELLER YELPED YELPER YOLKED

••L••E

ABLARE ABLATE ABLAZE AFLAME AFLARE AGLARE ALLEGE ALLELE ALLUDE ALLURE ALLYCE APLITE ARLENE ASLOPE AXLIKE BALDIE BALINE BELATE BELGAE BELIKE BELIZE BILLIE BOLIDE BULLAE BYLINE CALLEE CALLME CELINE CELLAE COLLIE DALENE DELETE DELUDE DELUGE DELUXE DILATE DILUTE DOLIKE DOLORE EGLISE ELLICE ENLACE FALINE FELICE FELINE FELIPE FILENE FILOSE FOLATE FOLKIE GALEAE GALORE GELATE GOLAME GOLDIE GOLIKE GOLIVE HALIDE HALITE HALLIE HELENE HELPME HOLDME ILLSEE ILLUDE ILLUME ILLUSE IMLATE IMLIKE INLINE INLOVE IRLENE ISLATE ISLIKE JILLIE JOLENE KALINE KELLIE KELPIE KILTIE LILLIE MALICE MALONE MELETE MILLIE MILTIE MOLINE MOLLIE MOLTKE MYLIFE MYLOVE NELLIE NOLOSE OBLATE OBLIGE OFLATE ONLATE ONLINE OOLITE OXLIKE PALACE PALADE PALATE PALEAE PELAGE PILATE PILOSE POLICE POLITE POLLEE RALLYE RELACE RELATE RELEVE RELINE RELIVE RELOSE RELUME ROLLIE SALADE SALINE SALLIE SALOME SALUTE SELENE SILAGE SOLACE SOLUTE SPLICE SPLINE STLUKE TALESE TALKIE TELLME TILLIE TOLIFE TULANE TULARE ULLAGE UNLACE UNLADE UNLIKE UNLIVE UPLATE VALENE VALERE VALINE VALISE VALLEE VELOCE VELURE VOLARE VOLUME VOLUTE WALKIE WILKIE WILLBE WILLIE XYLOSE

•••LE•

ABELES ADDLED ADDLES ADELEH AGILER AIGLET AISLED AISLES AMBLED AMBLER AMBLES AMOLES AMPLER AMULET ANELED ANELES ANGLED ANGLEE ANGLER ANGLES ANKLED ANKLES ANKLET ANNLEE ANOLES ANTLER APELET APPLES APPLET ARMLET ASHLEE ASHLEY ASTLEY ATILES ATTLEE AUKLET AZALEA AZOLES BAILED BAILEE BAILER BAILEY BALLET BARLEY BATLEY BAWLED BAWLER BEGLEY BELLED BELLES BIBLES BILLED BILLER BILLET BIRLED BIRLER BODLEY BOGLES BOILED BOILER BOSLEY BOULES BOULEZ BOWLED BOWLER BOWLES BOYLES BRULEE BTILES BUGLED BUGLER BUGLES BULLED BULLET BUMLEG BURLED BURLER BURLEY BUTLER CABLED CABLER CABLES CABLET CALLED CALLEE CALLER CALLES CAPLET CEILED CELLED CHALET CHILES CHOLER COALED COALER COILED COILER COLLET COOLED COOLER COOLEY COPLEY COTLER COULEE COWLED COWLEY CTILES CULLED CULLEN CULLER CULLET CURLED CURLER CURLEW CURLEY CUTLER CUTLET CUYLER CYCLED CYCLER CYCLES DAILEY DALLES DEALER DEFLEA DHOLES DIALED DIALER DILLER DIPLEX DOBLES DOGLEG DOLLED DOLLEY DOOLEY DTILES DUDLEY DUELED DUELER DULLEA DULLED DULLER DULLES DUPLEX EAGLED EAGLES EAGLET EARLET EASLEY ECCLES ECOLES EDILES EFILED EFILES EGALES EGGLER EISLEY EMBLEM ENSLER ESALEN ETILES

EVILER
EXILED
EXILER
EXILES
EYELET
FABLED
FABLER
FABLES
FAILED
FALLEN
FALLER
FARLEY
FAYLEN
FEELER
FELLED
FELLER
FHOLES
FIDLER
FILLED
FILLER
FILLES
FILLET
FINLEY
FOALED
FOILED
FOOLED
FOOLER
FOULED
FOULER
FOWLED
FOWLER
FOWLES
FTILES
FUELED
FUELER
FULLER
FURLED
GABLED
GABLER
GABLES
GALLED
GALLEY
GAOLED
GAOLER
GELLED
GELLER
GIBLET
GILLED
GILLEY
GIMLET
GOBLET
GOULET
GTILES
GUILED
GUILES
GULLED
GULLET
GURLEY
HAGLER
HAILED
HAILER
HAILEY
HALLEL
HALLEY
HAMLET
HANLEY
HAOLES
HARLEM
HARLEY
HAULED
HAULER
HAYLEY
HEALED
HEALER
HEALEY
HEDLEY
HEELED
HEELER
HELLER
HENLEY
HILLED
HILLEL
HILLER
HOLLER
HOLLEY
HOWLED
HOWLER
HOYLES
HTILES
HUBLEY
HULLED
HULLER
HUNLEY
HURLED
HURLER
HURLEY
HUXLEY
IMPLED
INGLES
INKLES
ISTLES
ITILES
JAILED
JAILER
JELLED
JOLLEY
JOULES
JOWLED
JTILES
KALLEN
KARLEN
KEELED
KEELER
KEGLER
KELLER
KELLEY
KEPLER
KILLED
KILLER
KISLEV
KOHLER
KTILES
KUBLER
LADLED
LADLER
LADLES
LALLED
LEELEE
LESLEY
LISLES
LOLLED
LOLLER
LTILES
LULLED
LULLER
LUMLEY
LYNLEY
MABLEY
MACLEN
MACLES
MAGLEV
MAHLER
MAILED
MAILER
MALLEI
MALLET
MANLEY
MAPLES
MARLED
MARLEE
MARLEY
MAULED
MAULER
MEDLEY
MEWLED
MEWLER
MIDLEG
MIDLER
MIELES
MILLED
MILLER
MILLES
MILLET
MISLED
MOBLEY
MOILED
MOILER
MORLEY
MOSLEM
MOSLEY
MOTLEY
MTILES
MULLED
MULLER
MULLET
NAILED
NAILER
NAPLES
NEWLEY
NIBLET
NOBLER
NOBLES
NTILES
NUCLEI
NUCLEO
NULLED
NUTLET
OAKLEY
OBOLER
ODELET
OMELET
ONCLES
ONELEG
OODLES
ORALES
OSTLER
OTILES
OUTLED
OUTLET
OVULES
PALLED
PALLET
PARLEY
PARLEZ
PAULEY
PEALED
PEALER
PEALES
PEELED
PEELER
PEGLEG
PEGLER
PELLET
PERLEA
PIELET
PIGLET
PILLED
PIOLET
POLLED
POLLEE
POLLEN
POLLER
POLLEX
POOLED
POOLER
POULES
PROLES
PTILES
PULLED
PULLER
PULLET
PULLEY
PURLED
QTILES
QUALES
QUELER
RADLEY
RAILED
RAILER
REALER
REALES
REDLEG
REELED
REELER
REFLEW
REFLEX
REGLES
REPLED
REYLES
RIBLET
RIDLEY
RIFLED
RIFLER
RIFLES
RILLES
RILLET
RIPLEY
ROBLES
ROILED
ROLLED
ROLLEI
ROLLER
ROWLEY
RTILES
RUBLES
RUBLEV
RUNLET
SABLES
SADLER
SAILED
SAILER
SALLES
SAMLET
SAYLES
SCALED
SCALER
SCALES
SCHLEP
SEALED
SEALER
SEDLEY
SELLER
SHALES
SHALEY
SHOLEM
SIDLED
SIDLES
SIGLER
SISLER
SISLEY
SMILED
SMILER
SMILES
SMILEY
SOCLES
SOILED
SPILES
STALED
STALER
STALES
STELES
STILES
STOLEN
STOLES
STYLED
STYLER
STYLES
STYLET
SUBLET
SULLEN
SWALES
TABLED
TABLES
TABLET
TAILED
TAILER
TALLER
TARLEK
TATLER
TELLER
TENLEY
TETLEY
THALER
THALES
THOLES
TILLED
TILLER
TILLET
TILLEY
TITLED
TITLES
TOILED
TOILER
TOILES
TOILET
TOLLED
TOLLER
TOOLED
TOOLER
TRALEE
TTILES
TULLES
UNBLED
UNCLES
VALLEE
VALLEY
VARLET
VEBLEN
VEILED
VEILER
VIALED
VIOLET
VOILES
VOLLEY
VTILES
WAILED
WAILER
WALLED
WALLER
WALLET
WASLED
WELLED
WELLER
WELLES
WESLEY
WHALED
WHALER
WHALES
WHALEY
WHILED
WHILES
WHOLES
WIGLET
WILLED
WILLEM
WILLER
WOHLER
WOOLEN
WOOLEY
WORLEY
WTILES
XFILES
XTILES
YELLED
YELLER
YOWLED
YOWLER
YTILES
ZTILES

•••L•E

ADELIE
ADELLE
ALULAE
AMALIE
AMELIE
ANGLEE
ANNLEE
ASHLEE
ATTLEE
AVULSE
BADLIE
BAILEE
BIGLIE
BILLIE
BRULEE
BULLAE
CALLEE
CALLME
CELLAE
CHELAE
CHILDE
COLLIE
COOLIE
COULEE
DOOLIE
EMILIE
EVOLVE
EVULSE
FAILLE
GAULLE
GIRLIE
GOALIE
GRILLE
HALLIE
INBLUE
ISOLDE
JILLIE
KELLIE
LEELEE
LESLIE
LILLIE
MAGLIE
MARLEE
MEALIE
MILLIE
MOLLIE
MRBLUE
NELLIE
ORELSE
OUTLIE
POLLEE
PURLIE
RALLYE
REGLUE
ROLLIE
RVALUE
SALLIE
SHELVE
SMALLE
STILLE
STOLAE
STOLLE
SVELTE
TELLME
TILLIE
TRALEE
TUILLE
TWELVE
UNGLUE
UVALDE
UVALUE
UVULAE
VALLEE
VIELLE
WILLBE
WILLIE
YEOLDE

••••LE

ADELLE
AEDILE
ALIBLE
ALLELE
AMPULE
APRILE
ARABLE
AREOLE
ARGYLE
ASCALE
ATYALE
AUDILE
AWHILE
BABBLE
BAFFLE
BANGLE
BARTLE
BATTLE
BAUBLE
BEADLE
BEAGLE
BEATLE
BEETLE
BINDLE
BINGLE
BOBBLE
BOGGLE
BOODLE
BOTTLE
BRIDLE
BSCALE
BUBBLE
BUCKLE
BUMBLE
BUNDLE
BUNGLE
BURBLE
BURGLE
BUSTLE
CACKLE
CAJOLE
CANDLE
CANTLE
CAROLE
CASTLE
CATTLE
CAZALE
CECILE
CHICLE
CIRCLE
COBBLE
COCKLE
CODDLE
COGGLE
COUPLE
CRADLE
CREOLE
CSCALE
CUDDLE
CUPULE
CURDLE
DABBLE
DANDLE
DANGLE
DAPPLE
DARKLE
DARTLE
DAWDLE
DAZZLE
DECILE
DECKLE
DEFILE
DIABLE
DIBBLE
DIDDLE
DIMPLE
DINGLE
DIPOLE
DOABLE
DOCILE
DONGLE
DOODLE
DOTTLE
DOUBLE
DSCALE
DUDDLE
DUFFLE
EBERLE
EDERLE
EDIBLE
EISELE
EKUELE
EMPALE
ENABLE
ENISLE
ENSILE
ESCALE
ETOILE
EXHALE
FACILE
FADDLE
FAILLE
FATALE
FEEBLE
FEMALE
FERULE
FETTLE
FICKLE
FIDDLE
FINALE
FIPPLE
FIZZLE
FOCSLE
FOIBLE
FONDLE
FOOTLE
FOOZLE
FSCALE
FUDDLE
FUMBLE
FUSILE
FUTILE
GABBLE
GAGGLE
GAMBLE
GARBLE
GARGLE
GAULLE
GENTLE
GIGGLE
GIRDLE
GISELE
GOBBLE
GOGGLE
GOOGLE
GRABLE
GRILLE
GSCALE
GURGLE
GUZZLE
HABILE
HACKLE
HAGGLE
HANDLE
HASSLE
HECKLE
HIGGLE
HINGLE
HINKLE
HOBBLE
HOOPLE
HUBBLE
HUDDLE
HUMBLE
HURDLE
HURTLE
HUSTLE
ICICLE
IMPALE
INHALE
INSOLE
JANGLE
JARULE
JECKLE
JIGGLE
JINGLE
JOGGLE
JOSTLE
JUGGLE
JUMBLE
JUNGLE
KEMBLE
KETTLE
KIBBLE
KIMBLE
KINDLE
KURILE
LABILE
LENGLE
LIABLE
LINGLE
LITTLE
LOBULE
LOCALE
LOYALE
LUCILE
MANGLE
MANTLE
MAPPLE
MARBLE
MARPLE
MCHALE
MEASLE
MEDDLE
MERDLE
METTLE
MIDDLE
MINGLE
MIZZLE
MOBILE
MODULE
MORALE
MOTILE
MOTTLE
MUDDLE
MUFFLE
MUGGLE
MUMBLE
MUSCLE
MUZZLE
MYRTLE
NATALE
NEEDLE
NESTLE
NETTLE
NIBBLE
NICOLE
NIGGLE
NIMBLE
NIPPLE
NOBILE
NODULE
NOODLE
NOSALE
NOZZLE
NTUPLE
NUBBLE
NUBILE
NUZZLE
OLEOLE
ONFILE
ONSALE
ORACLE
ORIOLE
OSCULE
OTOOLE
PADDLE
PAROLE
PEARLE
PEBBLE
PEDDLE
PEOPLE
PESTLE
PETALE
PICKLE
PIDDLE
PIFFLE
PIMPLE
POODLE
POPPLE
POSOLE
POZOLE
PUDDLE
PUGGLE
PURFLE
PURPLE
PUZZLE
QUAYLE
RABBLE
RAFFLE
RAMBLE
RANKLE
RASSLE
RATTLE
RAZZLE
REBALE
REFILE
REGALE
RESALE
RESILE
RESOLE
RETILE
REVILE
RIDDLE
RIFFLE
RIMPLE
RIPPLE
RODALE
ROOTLE
ROYALE
RUBBLE
RUFFLE
RUMBLE
RUMPLE
RUNDLE
RUSTLE
RUTILE
SADDLE
SAMPLE
SEARLE
SEMELE
SEMPLE
SENILE
SETTLE
SICKLE
SIECLE
SIMILE
SIMPLE
SINGLE
SISSLE
SIZZLE
SMALLE
STABLE
STAPLE
STEELE
STIFLE
STILLE
STOLLE
SUABLE
SUBTLE
SUPPLE
TACKLE
TAMALE
TANGLE
TATTLE
TEMPLE
TICKLE
TINGLE
TINKLE
TIPPLE
TITTLE
TODDLE
TOGGLE
TOODLE
TOOTLE
TOPPLE
TOUSLE
TREBLE
TRIFLE
TRIPLE
TUBULE
TUILLE
TUMBLE
TURTLE
TUSSLE
UNABLE
UNBALE
UNFILE
UNHALE
UNIDLE
UNPALE
UNPILE
UNSOLE
UPPILE
USABLE
VENULE
VIABLE
VIELLE
VIRILE
VITALE
VITTLE
WADDLE
WAFFLE
WAGGLE
WAMBLE
WANGLE
WARBLE
WATTLE
WIFFLE
WIGGLE
WIMPLE
WOBBLE
YERTLE
ZONULE

LF••••

LFRANK

L•F•••

LAFFER
LEFTBE
LEFTIN
LEFTIT
LEFTOF
LEFTON
LIFEIS
LIFERS
LIFTED
LIFTER
LIFTUP
LOFTED
LOFTER
LOFTON
LOFTUS
LUFFED

L••F••

LABFEE
LAFFER
LAPFUL
LAWFUL
LAYFOR
LEAFED
LETFLY
LIEFER
LIEFLY
LIEFOR
LOAFED
LOAFER
LOOFAH
LOOFAS
LOWFAT
LUFFED

L•••F•

LAYOFF
LEDOFF
LETOFF
LIPOFF
LOGOFF
LOPOFF

L••••F

LATEOF
LAYOFF
LEDOFF
LEFTOF
LETOFF
LIPOFF
LOGOFF
LOPOFF
LOTSOF

•LF•••

ALFINE
ALFRED
ALFVEN
ELFISH
ELFMAN
ELFOWL

•L•F••

ALLFOR
BLAFFS
BLIFIL
BLUFFO
BLUFFS
CLEFTS
CLIFFS
CLIFFY
FLUFFS
FLUFFY
ILLFED
OLAFII
OLAFIV
OLEFIN
SLYFOX

•L••F•

BLAFFS
BLUFFO
BLUFFS
CLIFFS
CLIFFY
FLUFFS
FLUFFY
ILLOFF

•L•••F

ALOTOF
ALTARF
ILLOFF

••LF••

ALLFOR
BELFRY
COLFAX
DELFTS
FULFIL
GOLFED
GOLFER
GULFED
ILLFED
PILFER
ROLFED
ROLFER
SULFAS
SULFUR
WOLFED

••L•F•

CALIFS
CCLEFS
GCLEFS
GOLEFT
ILLOFF
ISLEFT
MYLIFE
PILAFS
SALIFY
SCLAFF
TOLIFE
UGLIFY
UNLEFT
UPLIFT
VILIFY

••L••F

BELIEF
FULLOF
GELDOF
ILLOFF
INLEAF
ONLYIF
RELIEF
SCLAFF
TALKOF
TELLOF
TOLDOF
UNLEAF

•••LF•

ADOLFO
AMALFI

•••L•F

EKELOF
FULLOF
SMALLF
STOLAF
TELLOF

••••LF

BEHALF
BYHALF
DEWOLF
ENGULF
INGULF
INHALF
ITSELF
MYSELF
RUDOLF
SMALLF

L•G•••

LAGEAR
LAGERS
LAGGED
LAGGER
LAGOON
LAGUNA
LEGACY
LEGALS
LEGART
LEGATE
LEGATO
LEGEND
LEGGED
LEGION
LEGIST

LEGMAN LEGMEN LEGREE LEGROS LEGSIT LEGUIN LEGUME LIGAND LIGATE LIGEIA LIGERS LIGETI LIGHTS LIGNES LIGNIN LIGNUM LOGANS LOGGED LOGGER LOGGIA LOGICS LOGIER LOGILY LOGINS LOGJAM LOGOFF LOGONS LOGOUT LOGSIN LOGSON LTGOVS LUGERS LUGGED LUGGER LUGING LUGLIO LUGNUT LUGOSI LUGOUT

L••G••

LAGGED LAGGER LANGER LARGER LARGES LARGOS LAUGHS LEAGUE LEDGER LEDGES LEGGED LENGLE LENGTH LENGUA LIEGES LINGER LINGLE LINGUA LINGUS LODGED LODGER LODGES LOGGED LOGGER LOGGIA LONGED LONGER LONGES LONGET LONGLY LONGUE LUGGED LUGGER LUNGED LUNGER LUNGES

L•••G•

LACAGE LADOGA LATIGO LAVAGE LEHIGH LESAGE LETSGO LIANGS LINAGE LOUNGE LOVAGE

L••••G

LACING LADING LAMING LAPDOG LASING LAVING LAWING LAYING LAZING LIEBIG LIKING LIMING LINING LIPENG LIVING LOPING LORING LOSING LOVING LOWING LUBING LUDWIG LUGING LURING

•LG•••

ALGEDI ALGORE ALGREN ELGART

•L•G••

ALEGAR ALEGRE ALEGUP ALIGHT ALIGNS ALOGIA BLIGHT CLOGGY CLOGUP ELEGIT ELOGES FLAGGY FLAGON FLIGHT GLOGGS OLDGAG PLAGES PLAGUE PLIGHT PLUGIN PLUGUP SLIGHT SLOGAN SLUGGO

•L••G•

ALLEGE ALONGS BLUDGE CLANGS CLERGY CLINGS CLINGY CLOGGY CLOUGH FLAGGY FLANGE FLEDGE FLEDGY FLINGS GLOGGS GLURGE KLUDGE KLUDGY OLDAGE PLEDGE PLOUGH PLUNGE SLANGS SLANGY SLEDGE SLEIGH SLINGS SLOUGH SLOWGO SLUDGE SLUDGY SLUGGO ULLAGE XLARGE

•L•••G

ALBORG ALEKEG ALHAIG ALVING BLUING CLUING FLUBUG FLYING GLUING OLDDOG OLDGAG PLYING SLUING

••LG••

BELGAE BELGIC BILGED BILGES BOLGER BULGAR BULGED BULGES BULGUR CALGON FOLGER POLGAR VULGAR VULGUS

••L•G•

ALLEGE BELUGA DELUGE DELUGG EULOGY GULAGS MALAGA MALIGN OBLIGE OOLOGY OWLEGG PELAGE PHLEGM RELOGS SILAGE ULLAGE

••L••G

AILING BALING BELONG DELUGG DOLING EALING EELING ERLANG FILING GOLONG HALING HOLING IDLING ISLING KDLANG OBLONG OGLING OILING OILRIG OOLONG OWLEGG PALING PILING POLING PULING RILING RULING SOLING SOLONG TILING WALING WILING

•••L•G

AIRLOG ANALOG BUMLEG DIALOG DOGLEG EPILOG GASLOG JETLAG MIDLEG ONELEG PEGLEG PRELOG PROLOG REDLEG REFLAG SAWLOG SMALLG STALAG UNCLOG UNPLUG USFLAG WEBLOG

••••LG

SMALLG

LH••••

LHASAN LHOTSE

L•H•••

LAHORE LCHAIM LEHIGH LEHMAN LEHNEN LEHRER LEHUAS

L••H••

LACHEY LACHOY LAPHAM LASHED LASHER LASHES LASHTO LASHUP LATHED LATHEN LATHER LATHES LECHER LESHAN LETHAL LICHEE LICHEN LIGHTS LITHER LITHIC LITHOS LOCHER LOTHAR LUSHER LUSHES LUSHLY LUTHER LUTHOR

L•••H•

LANDHO LAUGHS LEACHY LITCHI LOATHE LOUCHE LUNCHY LUNTHA LYMPHS

L••••H

LATISH LAUNCH LAVISH LEHIGH LENGTH LILITH LIVETH LOLICH LOOFAH LOWISH LUKICH

•LH•••

ALHAIG ALHENA ALHIRT HLHUNT

•L•H••

ALOHAS ALPHAS ALTHEA OLDHAM OLDHAT

•L••H•

ALEPHS ALIGHT BLIGHT BLITHE BLYTHE CLICHE CLICHY CLOCHE CLOTHE CLOTHO CLOTHS ELISHA FLASHY FLECHE FLESHY FLIGHT GLYPHS OLATHE OLESHA PLASHY PLIGHT PLUSHY SLIGHT SLITHY SLOSHY SLOTHS SLUSHY

•L•••H

ALIOTH ALIYAH ALMACH BLANCH BLEACH BLEETH BLENCH BLOTCH BLUISH CLENCH CLINCH CLOUGH CLUTCH ELFISH ELIJAH ELNATH ELVISH FLETCH FLINCH FLUISH FLYASH GLITCH KLATCH OLDISH PLINTH PLOUGH SLEIGH SLEUTH SLOUGH SLOUGH ULRICH

••LH••

PELHAM TILHIM

••L•H•

BOLSHY DELPHI FILTHY RALPHJ SYLPHS TILTHS WELCHS

••L••H

ABLUSH ASLOSH CALASH CALIPH CULTCH DALETH DELISH DULUTH EOLITH FELLAH GALOSH GULLAH HALVAH JCLOTH LILITH LOLICH MULISH MULLAH OWLISH PALISH POLISH RELISH RULETH SALISH SPLASH SPLOSH UNLASH UNLUSH

•••L•H

ADELEH ADOLPH BEULAH COOLTH FELLAH GUELPH GULLAH HEALTH MOOLAH MULLAH SHILOH SMALLH SPILTH WEALTH

••••LH

SMALLH

LI••••

LIABLE LIAISE LIANAS LIANES LIANGS LIBBED LIBBER LIBBYS LIBELS LIBERS LIBIDO LIBRAE LIBRAN LIBRAS LIBRIS LIBROS LIBYAN LICHEE LICHEN LICKED LICKER LICKUP LIDDED LIEBER LIEBIG LIEBYS LIEDER LIEDON LIEDTO LIEFER LIEFLY LIEFOR LIEGES LIELOW LIENEE LIENOR LIESIN LIESON LIESTO LIEUTS LIEVIO LIFEIS LIFERS LIFTED LIFTER LIFTUP LIGAND LIGATE LIGEIA LIGERS LIGETI LIGHTS LIGNES LIGNIN LIGNUM LIKELY LIKENS LIKERS LIKESO LIKETO LIKING LIKUTA LILACS LILIAN LILIED LILIES LILIOM LILITH LILKIM LILLIE LILLIS LILTED LIMANS LIMBED LIMBER LIMBIC LIMBOS LIMIER LIMING LIMITS LIMNED LIMNER LIMPED LIMPER LIMPET LIMPID LIMPLY LINAGE LINDEN LINDER LINEAL LINEAR LINENS LINENY LINERS LINEUP LINGER LINGLE LINGUA LINGUS LINIER LINING LINKED LINKER LINKUP LINNET LINNEY LINTED LINTEL LINTER LINTON LINZER LIONEL LIONET LIONLY LIOTTA LIPARI LIPASE LIPENG LIPIDS LIPOFF LIPOUT LIPPED LIPPER LIPTON LIQUID LIQUOR LISBOA LISBON LISLES LISPED LISPER LISSES LISTED LISTEE LISTEN LISTER LISTON LITANY LITCHI LITERS LITHER LITHIC LITHOS LITMUS LITOUT LITRES LITTER LITTLE LITTRE LITVAK LIVEAT LIVEIN LIVELY LIVENS LIVEON LIVERS LIVERY LIVEST LIVETH LIVETV LIVING LIVRES LIZALU LIZARD LIZZIE

L•I•••

LAICAL LAIDBY LAIDIN LAIDON LAIDTO LAIDUP LAINIE LAIRDS LAIRED LEICAS LEIDEN LEISEN LEITER LOIDED LOIRET LOITER LTILES

L••I••

LABIAL LABILE LABINE LABIUM LACIER LACILY LACING LADIDA LADIES LADING LADINO LAKIER LAKIST LAMIAE LAMIAS LAMINA LAMING LANIER LANINA LAPINS LARIAT LARINE LASING LATIGO LATINA LATINI LATINO LATINS LATISH LAVIDA LAVING LAVISH LAWING LAXITY LAYING LAYINS LAZIER LAZILY LAZING LEGION LEGIST LEHIGH LENINA LENITY LEOIII LERIDA LESION LEVIED LEVIER LEVIES LEVINE LEVITE LEVITT LEVITY LIAISE LIBIDO LIKING LILIAN LILIED LILIES LILIOM LILITH LIMIER LIMING LIMITS LINIER LINING LIPIDS LIVING LODINJ LOGICS LOGIER LOGILY LOGINS LOLICH LOLITA LOOIES LOPING LORIES LORING LOSING LOTION LOUIES LOUISA LOUISB LOUISE LOUISI LOUISV LOUISX LOVING LOWING LOWIQS LOWISH LUBING LUCIAN LUCIDA LUCIEN LUCILE LUCINE LUCITE LUCIUS LUGING LUKICH LUMINA LUNIKS LUPINE LUPINO LURING LUTIST LYDIAN LYRICS LYRIDS LYRIST LYSINE

L•••I•

LACTIC LADDIE LAIDIN LAINIE LAJOIE LAMSIT LANAIS LANCIA LANCIE LANDIS LANVIN LARKIN LASSIE LATRIA LATVIA LAURIA LAURIC LAURIE LAVAIN LAYSIN LCHAIM LEADIN LEAKIN LEANIN LEAPIN LECAIN LEEKIE LEFTIN LEFTIT LEGSIT LEGUIN LELOIR LENAIN LENNIE LENTIL LEOIII LEONIA LEONID LEOVII LEOXII LESLIE LESMIZ LETRIP LETSIN LIBRIS LIEBIG LIESIN LIEVIO LIFEIS LIGEIA LIGNIN LILKIM LILLIE LILLIS LIMBIC LIMPID LIQUID LITHIC LIVEIN LIZZIE LOADIN LOCCIT LOCKIN LOGGIA LOGSIN LOMEIN LONNIE LOOKIE LOOKIN LOONIE LORAIN LORDIT LORRIE LOSEIT LOSTIT LOUVIN LOVEIN LOVEIT LOWBID LUBLIN LUDWIG LUGLIO LUMPIN LUMPIT LUNDIS LUREIN

L••••I

LADYDI LAPERI LATERI LATINI LAZULI LEOIII LEOVII LEOXII LIGETI LIPARI LITCHI LOUISI LUGOSI LUNEDI

•LI•••

ALIBIS ALIBLE ALICEB ALICES ALICIA ALIENS ALIGHT ALIGNS ALIKES ALINED ALINER ALINES ALIOTH ALIOTO ALIPED ALISON ALISTS ALIVEO ALIYAH ALIYOT BLIFIL BLIGHT BLIMEY BLIMPS BLINDS BLINIS BLINKS BLINTZ BLISTS BLITHE BLIXEN CLICHE CLICHY CLICKS CLIENT CLIFFS CLIFFY CLIMAT CLIMAX CLIMBS CLIMES CLINCH CLINGS CLINGY CLINIC CLINKS CLIPON CLIQUE CLIQUY ELICIT ELIDED ELIDER ELIDES ELIELI ELIJAH ELINOR ELISEO ELISHA ELISSA ELISTS ELITER ELITES ELIXIR FLICKA FLICKS FLIERS FLIGHT FLIMSY FLINCH FLINGS FLINTS FLINTY FLIPUP FLIRTS FLIRTY FLITBY FLITIN GLIBLY GLIDED GLIDER GLIDES GLIERE GLINDA GLINKA GLINTS GLINTY GLITCH GLITZY ILIADS KLIBAN KLICKS OLINDA OLIVER OLIVES OLIVIA PLIANT PLIERS PLIGHT PLINKS PLINTH PLISSE SLICED SLICER SLICES SLICKS SLIDER SLIDES SLIDIN SLIEST SLIGHT SLIMED SLIMES SLIMLY

SLINGS
SLINKS
SLINKY
SLIPBY
SLIPIN
SLIPON
SLIPPY
SLIPUP
SLITHY
SLIVER

•L•I••

ALAINA
ALBINE
ALBINO
ALBION
ALCINA
ALDINE
ALDISS
ALFINE
ALHIRT
ALKIES
ALLIED
ALLIES
ALLIUM
ALNICO
ALPINE
ALRITZ
ALTIMA
ALTIUS
ALVING
ALVINO
ALZIRA
BLAINE
BLAISE
BLUING
BLUISH
CLAIMS
CLAIRE
CLAIRS
CLUING
ELAINE
ELFISH
ELLICE
ELLIOS
ELLIOT
ELMIER
ELMIRA
ELMIRE
ELNINO
ELOISA
ELOISE
ELVIRA
ELVISH
FLAILS
FLAIRS
FLUIDS
FLUISH
FLYING
FLYINS
GLUIER
GLUING
ILLINI
ILOILO
KLEINE
KLEIST
OLDIES
OLDISH
OLEINS
PLAICE
PLAIDS
PLAINS
PLAINT
PLAITS
PLEIAD
PLUIES
PLYING
SLEIGH
SLUICE
SLUING
ULRICH
ULTIMA
ULTIMO

•L••I•

ALANIS
ALARIC
ALBEIT
ALDRIN
ALEXIA
ALEXIS
ALHAIG
ALIBIS
ALICIA
ALKAID
ALLAIS
ALOGIA
ALTAIC
ALTAIR
ALTOID
ALTRIA
BLEWIN
BLEWIT
BLIFIL
BLINIS
BLOOIE
BLOWIN
BLOWIT
CLADIN
CLAVIN
CLERIC
CLINIC
CLORIS
CLOVIS
CLUEIN
ELADIO
ELAPID
ELEGIT
ELEMIS
ELICIT
ELIXIR
ELPAIS
ELYRIA
ELYTIS
FLAVIA
FLEWIN
FLITIN
FLOPIT
FLORID
FLORIN
FLORIO
FLOWIN
FLUTIE
GLACIS
GLOBIN
GLORIA
GLYNIS
ILLLIT
OLAFII
OLAFIV
OLAVII
OLAVIV
OLDVIC
OLEFIN
OLIVIA
PLACID
PLAYIT
PLUGIN
PLUVIA
PLUVIO
SLAVIC
SLIDIN
SLIPIN
VLASIC

•L•••I

ALEXEI
ALGEDI
ALKALI
ALUMNI
ELIELI
GLUTEI
ILLINI
OLAFII
OLAVII
OLDELI

••LI••

ADLIBS
AGLINT
AILING
ALLIED
ALLIES
ALLIUM
APLITE
ARLISS
AXLIKE
BALINE
BALING
BCLION
BELIAL
BELIED
BELIEF
BELIER
BELIES
BELIKE
BELIZE
BOLIDE
BYLINE
CALICO
CALIFS
CALIPH
CELICA
CELINE
CILIUM
COLICS
COLIMA
DELIAN
DELICT
DELINT
DELISH
DELIST
DELIUS
DOLIKE
DOLING
EALING
EELIER
EELING
EGLISE
ELLICE
ELLIOS
ELLIOT
ENLINK
ENLIST
EOLIAN
EOLITH
FALINE
FELICE
FELIDS
FELINE
FELIPE
FELIXI
FELIXV
FILIAL
FILING
FOLIAR
FOLIES
FOLIOS
FOLIUM
GOLIKE
GOLIMP
GOLINO
GOLIVE
HALIDE
HALING
HALITE
HELICO
HELIOS
HELIUM
HOLIER
HOLIES
HOLILY
HOLING
HOLISM
HOLIST
IDLING
ILLINI
IMLIKE
INLIEU
INLINE
ISLIKE
ISLING
JOLIET
JOLIOT
JULIAN
JULIEN
JULIET
JULIUS
KALINE
KILIMS
LILIAN
LILIED
LILIES
LILIOM
LILITH
LOLICH
LOLITA
MALIAN
MALIBU
MALICE
MALICK
MALIGN
MELINA
M1LIEU
MOLINA
MOLINE
MULISH
MYLIFE
OBLIGE
OGLING
OILIER
OILILY
OILING
ONLINE
OOLITE
OWLIER
OWLISH
OXLIKE
OXLIPS
PALING
PALISH
PELION
PILING
POLICE
POLICY
POLING
POLIOS
POLISH
POLITE
POLITY
PULING
RELICS
RELICT
RELIED
RELIEF
RELIER
RELIES
RELINE
RELINK
RELISH
RELIST
RELIVE
RILING
RULIER
RULING
SALIFY
SALINA
SALINE
SALISH
SALIVA
SILICA
SOLIDS
SOLING
SPLICE
SPLINE
SPLINT
SPLITS
TALISA
TILING
TOLIFE
TULIPS
UGLIER
UGLIES
UGLIFY
UGLILY
UNLIKE
UNLIMP
UNLINK
UNLIVE
UPLIFT
UPLINK
VALINE
VALISE
VALIUM
VILIFY
WALING
WILIER
WILILY
WILING
YALIES

••L•I•

AFLCIO
AGLAIA
ALLAIS
AULAIT
BALDIE
BALLIN
BALTIC
BELAIR
BELGIC
BELOIT
BILLIE
BILLIS
BOLLIX
CALAIS
CALLIN
CALLIT
CALVIN
CELTIC
COLLIE
CULKIN
CULLIS
CULTIC
DELRIO
DELTIC
ECLAIR
FALLIN
FELLIN
FILEIN
FILLIN
FILLIP
FILMIC
FOLDIN
FOLKIE
FULFIL
GALLIA
GALLIC
GALOIS
GILLIS
GILPIN
GOLDIE
HALLIE
HALOID
HALPIN
HELDIN
HELDIT
HELPIN
HOLDIN
HOLDIT
HOLLIS
ILLLIT
INLAID
JILLIE
JOLTIN
KELLIE
KELPIE
KELVIN
KILTIE
LELOIR
LILKIM
LILLIE
LILLIS
MALEIC
MALTIN
MCLAIN
MELVIL
MELVIN
MILLIE
MILTIE
MOLLIE
MULLIN
MULTIS
NELLIE
NELLIS
OILLIT
OILRIG
ONLAID
ONLYIF
PALAIS
PALLID
PELVIC
PELVIS
PILEIN
PULLIN
PULPIT
RELAID
ROLLIE
ROLLIN
SALLIE
SALMIS
SALTII
SELLIT
SOLDIT
SOLEIL
SYLVIA
TALKIE
TALKIN
TELLIT
TILHIM
TILLIE
TILLIS
TILSIT
TOLDIT
UNLAID
VALAIS
VALOIS
WALKIE
WALKIN
WALLIN
WALLIS
WILKIE
WILLIE
WILLIS
XYLOID

••L••I

BILOXI
BOLYAI
COLONI
DALASI
DELPHI
FALUDI
FELIXI
GELATI
ILLINI
IOLANI
MALAWI
MALLEI
MALOTI
OBLADI
PELOSI
POLLOI
ROLLEI
SALAMI
SALTII
SALUKI
SOLATI

•••LI•

ADELIE
AEOLIA
AHOLIC
AIOLIS
AMALIA
AMALIE
AMBLIN
AMELIA
AMELIE
ANGLIA
ANGLIC
ANTLIA
APULIA
BAALIM
BADLIE
BALLIN
BERLIN
BIALIK
BIBLIO
BIGLIE
BILLIE
BILLIS
BOLLIX
BROLIN
CALLIN
CALLIT
CANLIT
CARLIN
CATLIN
CHILIS
COELIA
COLLIE
COOLIE
COOLIO
COOLIT
CULLIS
CURLIN
CYCLIC
DAHLIA
DARLIN
DAYLIT
DEALIN
DIALIN
DOBLIN
DOOLIE
DUBLIN
DUNLIN
EMILIA
EMILIE
EMILIO
ENGLIT
ESTLIN
ETALIA
ETALII
EUCLID
EXILIC
EYELID
FALLIN
FATLIP
FELLIN
FILLIN
FILLIP
FROLIC
GAELIC
GALLIA
GALLIC
GARLIC
GASLIT
GATLIN
GILLIS
GIRLIE
GOALIE
GOBLIN
GOSLIN
HALLIE
HAMLIN
HARLIN
HAULIN
HEFLIN
HOLLIS
HOWLIN
ILLLIT
ISELIN
ITALIA
ITALIC
JILLIE
JOPLIN
KAHLIL
KAOLIN
KELLIE
KHALID
KIDLIT
LESLIE
LILLIE
LILLIS
LUBLIN
LUGLIO
MAGLIE
MAILIN
MAJLIS
MARLIN
MASLIN
MATLIN
MEALIE
MERLIN
MILLIE
MOLLIE
MOULIN
MULLIN
MUSLIM
MUSLIN
NAILIN
NAILIT
NEELIX
NELLIE
NELLIS
OILLIT
OUTLIE
OUTLIP
OXALIC
OXALIS
PAGLIA
PALLID
PAULII
PAULIV
PHILIC
PHILIP
POPLIN
POTLID
PRELIM
PROLIX
PUBLIC
PUBLIX
PULLIN
PURLIE
RATLIN
REALIA
REELIN
ROLLIE
ROLLIN
SALLIE
SCALIA
SEALIN
SELLIT
SHALIT
SKYLIT
STALIN
STOLID
SUBLID
SUNLIT
TELLIT
THALIA
THELIP
TILLIE
TILLIS
TOMLIN
TWILIT
UNCLIP
UNGLIB
UNSLIM
URALIC
VIOLIN
WALLIN
WALLIS
WILLIE
WILLIS

•••L•I

AMALFI
CHILLI
COULDI
ETALII
KUBLAI
MALLEI
NIELLI
NUCLEI
OCELLI
PAULII
PAULVI
POLLOI
ROLLEI
SHALLI
SMALLI

••••LI

ALKALI
ANGELI
ANNULI
ARGALI
CAROLI
CHILLI
CUMULI
DENALI
DITALI
ELIELI
FAMULI
HAMULI
KAMALI
KIGALI
LAZULI
MODULI
MOWGLI
MUESLI
NAPOLI
NEPALI
NEROLI
NIELLI
OCELLI
OLDELI
POPULI
RIVOLI
SHALLI
SMALLI
SNUGLI
SOMALI
TIVOLI

L•J•••

LAJOIE

L••J••

LOGJAM

L••••J

LODINJ

•L•J••

ELIJAH

••L••J

RALPHJ

•••L•J

SMALLJ

••••LJ

SMALLJ

L•K•••

LAKERS
LAKIER
LAKIST
LAKOTA
LIKELY
LIKENS
LIKERS
LIKESO
LIKETO
LIKING
LIKUTA
LUKICH

L••K••

LACKED
LACKEY
LANKER
LANKLY
LARKED
LARKER
LARKIN
LASKER
LATKES
LEAKED
LEAKER
LEAKEY
LEAKIN
LEEKIE
LICKED
LICKER
LICKUP
LILKIM
LINKED
LINKER
LINKUP
LOCKED
LOCKER
LOCKET
LOCKIN
LOCKON
LOCKUP
LOOKAT
LOOKED
LOOKEE
LOOKER
LOOKIE
LOOKIN
LOOKMA
LOOKON
LOOKTO
LOOKUP
LOWKEY
LUCKED
LUNKER
LURKED
LURKER
LURKEY

L•••K•

LADUKE
LANSKY
LEMOKO
LUNIKS
LUSAKA

L••••K

LANARK
LFRANK
LITVAK
LUBECK

•LK•••

ALKAID
ALKALI
ALKENE
ALKIES
ALKYDS
ALKYLS
ELKONV
ELKTON

•L•K••

ALEKEG
ALIKES
ALTKEY
BLAKEY
BLOKES
FLAKED
FLAKER
FLAKES
FLUKES
FLUKEY
OLAKES
PLAKAT
SLAKED
SLAKER
SLAKES

•L••K•

ALASKA
ALECKS
ALECKY
BLACKS
BLANKS
BLEAKS
BLINKS
BLOCKS
BLOCKY
CLACKS
CLANKS
CLANKY
CLARKE
CLEEKS
CLERKS
CLICKS
CLINKS
CLOAKS
CLOCKS
CLONKS
CLUCKS
CLUNKS
CLUNKY
FLACKS
FLANKS
FLASKS
FLECKS
FLECKY
FLICKA
FLICKS
FLOCKS
FLUNKS
FLUNKY
GLINKA
GLOCKS
KLICKS
PLANKS
PLINKS
PLONKS
PLUCKS
PLUCKY
PLUNKS
PLUNKY
SLACKS
SLEEKS
SLEEKY
SLICKS
SLINKS
SLINKY

•L•••K

FLOREK
PLANCK
SLEZAK
SLOVAK

••LK••

BALKAN
BALKAT
BALKED
BALKER
BILKED
BILKER
BULKED
BULKUP
CALKED
CALKER
CULKIN
DELKEY
FOLKIE
FOLKSY
HULKED
KALKAN
LILKIM
MILKED
MILKER
POLKAS
SILKEN
SULKED
SULKER
TALKAT
TALKED
TALKER
TALKIE
TALKIN
TALKOF
TALKON
TALKTO
TALKUP
WALKBY
WALKED
WALKEN
WALKER
WALKIE
WALKIN
WALKON
WALKTO
WALKUP
WILKES
WILKIE
YOLKED

••L•K•

AXLIKE
BELIKE
DOLIKE
GOLIKE
IMLIKE
ISLIKE
KULAKS
MOLTKE
OXLIKE
POLSKA
SALUKI
STLUKE
TILAKS
UNLIKE

••L••K

ENLINK
FELTOK
INLUCK
MALICK
NOLUCK
OCLOCK
OHLOOK
POLLAK
RELINK
RELOCK
RELOOK
SHLOCK
UNLINK
UNLOCK
UPLINK

•••LK•

BAULKS
CAULKS
CHALKS
CHALKY
SKULKS
STALKS
STALKY
WHELKS

•••L•K

BIALIK
FEELOK
MUKLUK
POLLAK
SMALLK
TARLEK
URALSK

••••LK

BYTALK
INBULK
SMALLK
UPTALK

LL••••

LLADRO
LLAMAS
LLANOS
LLBEAN
LLOYDS

L•L•••

LALALA
LALLED
LELAND
LELOIR
LILACS
LILIAN
LILIED
LILIES
LILIOM
LILITH
LILKIM
LILLIE
LILLIS
LILTED
LOLICH
LOLITA
LOLLED
LOLLER
LULLED
LULLER

L••L••

LAALAA
LACLOS

LADLED
LADLER
LADLES
LALLED
LAULAU
LAYLOW
LEALTY
LEELEE
LESLEY
LESLIE
LIELOW
LILLIE
LILLIS
LISLES
LOLLED
LOLLER
LTILES
LUBLIN
LUDLOW
LUDLUM
LUELLA
LUGLIO
LULLED
LULLER
LUMLEY
LYNLEY

L•••L•

LABELS
LABILE
LACILY
LALALA
LAMELY
LANKLY
LAPELS
LASTLY
LASZLO
LATELY
LAXALT
LAZILY
LAZULI
LEANLY
LEGALS
LENGLE
LETFLY
LEVELS
LEWDLY
LIABLE
LIBELS
LIEFLY
LIKELY
LIMPLY
LINGLE
LIONLY
LITTLE
LIVELY
LIZALU
LOBULE
LOCALE
LOCALS
LOGILY
LONELY
LONGLY
LORDLY
LOUDLY
LOVELL
LOVELY
LOWELL
LOYALE
LOYOLA
LTSULU
LUCILE
LUELLA
LUNULA
LUSHLY

L••••L

LABIAL
LAICAL
LANVAL
LAPFUL
LARVAL
LAUREL
LAURYL
LAWFUL
LEMUEL
LENTIL
LETHAL
LINEAL
LINTEL
LIONEL
LONNOL
LOREAL
LOVELL
LOWCAL
LOWELL

•LL•••

ALLAIS
ALLAYS
ALLBUT
ALLDAY
ALLEES
ALLEGE
ALLELE
ALLEYN
ALLEYS
ALLFOR
ALLIED
ALLIES
ALLIUM
ALLMAN
ALLMEN
ALLNEW
ALLOTS
ALLOUT
ALLOWS
ALLOYS
ALLPRO
ALLSET
ALLUDE
ALLURE
ALLWET
ALLYCE
ALLYLS
ELLERY
ELLICE
ELLIOS
ELLIOT
ELLORA
ILLBET
ILLDRY
ILLEST
ILLFED
ILLINI
ILLLIT
ILLMET
ILLOFF
ILLSAY
ILLSEE
ILLSET
ILLUDE
ILLUME
ILLUSE
ULLAGE
ULLMAN

•L•L••

ALALAS
ALULAE
ALULAR
FLYLOW
ILLLIT
SLALOM

•L••L•

ALIBLE
ALKALI
ALKYLS
ALLELE
ALLYLS
BLUELY
ELIELI
FLAILS
FLATLY
GLADLY
GLIBLY
GLUMLY
ILOILO
OLDELI
OLEOLE
SLIMLY
SLOWLY

•L•••L

ALEVEL
ALNASL
ALUDEL
BLIFIL
BLOBEL
CLONAL
ELFOWL
FLORAL
GLOBAL
GLYCOL
OLDPAL
OLEVEL
PLEXAL
PLURAL

••LL••

BALLAD
BALLET
BALLIN
BALLON
BALLOT
BALLOU
BALLST
BALLUP
BALLYS
BELLAY
BELLED
BELLES
BELLOC
BELLOW
BELLUM
BILLED
BILLER
BILLET
BILLIE
BILLIS
BILLOW
BOLLAS
BOLLIX
BULLAE
BULLED
BULLET
CALLAN
CALLAO
CALLAS
CALLED
CALLEE
CALLER
CALLES
CALLIN
CALLIT
CALLME
CALLON
CALLOW
CALLTO
CALLUP
CALLUS
CELLAE
CELLAR
CELLED
CELLOS
COLLAR
COLLAT
COLLET
COLLIE
COLLOP
COLLOQ
CULLED
CULLEN
CULLER
CULLET
CULLIS
CULLUM
DALLAS
DALLES
DILLAR
DILLER
DILLON
DOLLAR
DOLLED
DOLLEY
DOLLOP
DOLLUP
DULLEA
DULLED
DULLER
DULLES
FALLAL
FALLEN
FALLER
FALLIN
FALLON
FALLOW
FALLTO
FELLAH
FELLAS
FELLED
FELLER
FELLIN
FELLON
FELLOW
FELLTO
FILLED
FILLER
FILLES
FILLET
FILLIN
FILLIP
FILLUP
FOLLOW
FULLER
FULLOF
FULLUP
GALLED
GALLEY
GALLIA
GALLIC
GALLON
GALLOP
GALLUP
GELLAR
GELLED
GELLER
GILLAN
GILLED
GILLEY
GILLIS
GOLLUM
GULLAH
GULLED
GULLET
HALLAM
HALLEL
HALLEY
HALLIE
HALLOO
HALLOS
HALLOW
HALLUX
HELLAS
HELLER
HELLNO
HELLON
HELLOS
HILLED
HILLEL
HILLER
HOLLER
HOLLEY
HOLLIS
HOLLOW
HULLED
HULLER
HULLOS
ILLLIT
ITLLDO
JELLED
JELLOS
JILLIE
JOLLEY
KALLEN
KELLER
KELLEY
KELLIE
KELLYS
KILLED
KILLER
LALLED
LILLIE
LILLIS
LOLLED
LOLLER
LULLED
LULLER
MALLEI
MALLET
MALLON
MALLOW
MELLON
MELLOW
MILLAY
MILLED
MILLER
MILLES
MILLET
MILLIE
MOLLIE
MOLLOY
MULLAH
MULLAS
MULLED
MULLER
MULLET
MULLIN
NELLIE
NELLIS
NULLED
NULLOS
OILLIT
PALLAS
PALLED
PALLET
PALLID
PALLOR
PELLAM
PELLET
PILLAR
PILLED
PILLOW
POLLAK
POLLED
POLLEE
POLLEN
POLLER
POLLEX
POLLOI
POLLOS
POLLUX
PULLED
PULLER
PULLET
PULLEY
PULLIN
PULLON
PULLUP
RALLYE
RILLES
RILLET
ROLLBY
ROLLED
ROLLEI
ROLLER
ROLLIE
ROLLIN
ROLLON
ROLLUP
SALLES
SALLIE
SALLOW
SELLBY
SELLER
SELLIT
SELLON
SELLTO
SULLEN
TALLER
TALLOW
TELLER
TELLIT
TELLME
TELLOF
TELLON
TILLED
TILLER
TILLET
TILLEY
TILLIE
TILLIS
TOLLED
TOLLER
TULLES
VALLEE
VALLEY
VELLUM
VILLAS
VILLON
VOLLEY
WALLED
WALLER
WALLET
WALLIN
WALLIS
WALLOP
WALLOW
WALLST
WALLUP
WELLED
WELLER
WELLES
WELLUP
WILLBE
WILLDO
WILLED
WILLEM
WILLER
WILLIE
WILLIS
WILLOW
WILLYS
YELLAT
YELLED
YELLER
YELLOW

••L•L•

ALLELE
ALLYLS
BALDLY
BOLDLY
CALMLY
COLDLY
FALALA
GILELS
HALALA
HOLILY
LALALA
MILDLY
OGLALA
OILILY
OOLALA
PALELY
SOLELY
UGLILY
VILELY
WILDLY
WILILY

••L••L

BELIAL
DELSOL
FALLAL
FILIAL
FULFIL
GALPAL
HALLEL
HILLEL
MELVIL
SOLEIL

•••LL•

ABOLLA
ADELLE
AIELLO
APOLLO
ATOLLS
AXILLA
BCELLS
BEALLS
BRILLO
BROLLY
CHILLI
CHILLS
CHILLY
CHOLLA
COOLLY
DCELLS
DOALLS
DRILLS
DROLLS
DROLLY
DUALLY
DUELLO
DWELLS
EMALLS
EVILLY
FAILLE
FOULLY
FRILLS
FRILLY
GAULLE
GRILLE
GRILLS
ICALLY
IDYLLS
KNELLS
KNOLLS
KNOLLY
KVELLS
LUELLA
NIELLI
NIELLO
OCELLI
ORALLY
OTELLO
OVALLY
PAELLA
PHILLY
PHYLLO
QUELLS
QUILLS
REALLY
REILLY
RKELLY
SCULLS
SCULLY
SCYLLA
SHALLI
SHALLY
SHELLS
SHILLS
SHILLY
SKILLS
SKULLS
SMALLA
SMALLB
SMALLC
SMALLD
SMALLE
SMALLF
SMALLG
SMALLH
SMALLI
SMALLJ
SMALLK
SMALLL
SMALLM
SMALLN
SMALLO
SMALLP
SMALLQ
SMALLR
SMALLS
SMALLT
SMALLU
SMALLV
SMALLW
SMALLX
SMALLY
SMALLZ
SMELLS
SMELLY
SMILLA
SNELLS
SPELLS
SPILLS
STALLS
STELLA
STILLE
STILLS
STILLY
STOLLE
SWELLS
SWILLS
TBILLS
TCELLS
THILLS
TRILLO
TRILLS
TROLLS
TUILLE
TWILLS
VIELLE
WHOLLY
WOOLLY

•••L•L

FALLAL
HALLEL
HILLEL
KAHLIL
SMALLL

••••LL

AACELL
ANGELL
APPALL
ARGYLL
ARNALL
ASDULL
ASTALL
ASWELL
ATWILL
BACALL
BEFALL
BEFELL
BEWELL
CABELL
CAHILL
CAROLL
CAVELL
COSELL
CYBILL
DOTELL
DOWELL
DUVALL
ENDALL
ENROLL
ERROLL
EXTOLL
GIBILL
GOWELL
HAMILL
HIYALL
HOWELL
IMFULL
INFALL
INFULL
JEKYLL
KAPELL
KOPELL
LOVELL
LOWELL
MABELL
MAXELL
MCGILL
MERYLL
MRBILL
NEVILL
NEWELL
NOBALL
NORELL
NOTALL
NOTILL
NOTOLL
OHWELL
ONCALL
ONEALL
ONEILL
ORWELL
POWELL
REBILL
RECALL
REFALL
REFELL
REFILL
REMILL
REPOLL
REROLL
RESELL
RETELL
RETILL
REXALL
RYDELL
SAWALL
SCHELL
SCHOLL
SCROLL
SEEALL
SEWELL
SHRILL
SMALLL
SQUALL
STROLL
THATLL
THEYLL
THRALL
THRILL
UNFULL
UNHULL
UNROLL
UNSELL
UNWALL
UNWELL
UPHILL
UPWELL
WHATLL
WHENLL
YOUALL

LM••••

LMNOPQ

L•M•••

LAMARR
LAMAZE
LAMBDA
LAMBED
LAMEDS
LAMELY
LAMENT
LAMESA
LAMEST
LAMIAE
LAMIAS
LAMINA
LAMING
LAMMED
LAMONT
LAMOUR
LAMSIT
LEMANS
LEMMAS
LEMMON
LEMNOS
LEMOKO
LEMOND
LEMONS
LEMONY
LEMUEL
LEMURS
LIMANS
LIMBED
LIMBER
LIMBIC
LIMBOS
LIMIER
LIMING
LIMITS
LIMNED
LIMNER
LIMPED
LIMPER
LIMPET
LIMPID
LIMPLY
LOMEIN
LOMOND
LOMPOC
LUMBAR
LUMBER
LUMENS
LUMINA
LUMLEY
LUMMOX
LUMPED
LUMPEN
LUMPER
LUMPIN
LUMPIT
LUMPUR
LYMPHS

L••M••

LAMMED
LARMEN
LARMOR
LAWMAN
LAWMEN
LAYMAN
LAYMEN
LEEMAY
LEGMAN
LEGMEN
LEHMAN
LEMMAS
LEMMON
LESMIZ
LITMUS
LLAMAS
LOAMED
LOOMED
LOOMPA
LOOMUP
LOUMAS
LOWMAN
LOWMEN
LUMMOX

L•••M•

LARAMS
LBEAMS
LEGUME
LOOKMA

L••••M

LABIUM
LAPERM
LAPHAM
LCHAIM
LIGNUM
LILIOM
LILKIM
LOGJAM
LUDLUM
LYCEUM

•LM•••

ALMAAZ
ALMACH
ALMATY
ALMOND
ALMOST
ALMVPS
ELMERS
ELMIER
ELMIRA
ELMIRE
ELMONT
ELMORE
KLMNOP
NLMVPS
OLMECS
OLMERT

•L•M••

ALAMOS
ALEMAN
ALLMAN
ALLMEN
ALOMAR
ALTMAN
ALUMNA
ALUMNI
BLAMED
BLAMER
BLAMES
BLIMEY
BLIMPS
CLAMMA
CLAMMY
CLAMOR
CLAMPS
CLAMUP
CLIMAT
CLIMAX
CLIMBS
CLIMES
CLOMPS
CLUMPS
CLUMPY
CLUMSY
ELEMIS
ELFMAN
FLAMBE
FLAMED
FLAMER
FLAMES
FLIMSY
FLUMES
FLYMAN
FLYMEN
GLAMOR
GLAMUP
GLUMLY
ILLMET
LLAMAS
OLDMAN
OLDMEN
PLOMER
PLUMBO
PLUMBS
PLUMED
PLUMES
PLUMMY
PLUMPS
SLAMON
SLIMED
SLIMES
SLIMLY
SLUMMY
SLUMPS
ULLMAN

•L••M•

ALARMS
ALBUMS
ALTIMA
BLOOMS
BLOOMY
CLAIMS
CLAMMA
CLAMMY
GLEAMS
GLEAMY
GLOOMS
GLOOMY
ILLUME
OLEUMS
PLASMA
PLASMO
PLUMMY
SLUMMY
ULTIMA
ULTIMO

•L•••M

ALABAM
ALARUM
ALLIUM
OLDHAM
PLENUM
SLALOM

••LM••

ALLMAN
ALLMEN
BALMER
CALMED
CALMER
CALMEX
CALMLY
COLMAN
COLMAR
DELMAR
DOLMAN
DOLMAS
FILMED
FILMIC
FULMAR
GILMAN
HELMED
HELMER
HELMET
HELMUT
HOLMAN
HOLMES
ILLMET
JKLMNO
KALMAR
KILMER
MELMAC
OILMAN
OILMEN
PALMAR
PALMAS
PALMED
PALMER
PULMON
SALMAN
SALMIS
SALMON
TALMUD
ULLMAN
WILMUT

••L•M•

AFLAME
APLOMB
CALLME
CCLAMP
COLIMA
COLUMN
GOLAME
GOLEMS
GOLIMP
HELPME
HOLDME
ILLUME
KILIMS
PALOMA
RELUME
SALAMI
SALOME
SOLEMN
TELLME
UNLIMP
VOLUME
XYLEMS

••L••M

ABLOOM
AGLEAM
ALLIUM
BALAAM
BALSAM
BELDAM
BELLUM
BOLCOM
CILIUM
CULLUM
FOLIUM
FOLSOM
GOLLUM
HALLAM
HELIUM

HOLDEM
HOLISM
LILIOM
LILKIM
PELHAM
PELLAM
PHLEGM
PHLOEM
PILEUM
SALAAM
SELDOM
TALCUM
TILHIM
VALIUM
VELLUM
WILLEM

•••LM•
AZELMA
CALLME
IJKLMN
PSALMS
QUALMS
REALMS
STELMO
TELLME
THELMA
WHELMS

•••L•M
ASYLUM
BAALIM
BEDLAM
BELLUM
CULLUM
DESLUM
EMBLEM
GOLLUM
HALLAM
HARLEM
IDOLUM
JAGLOM
LUDLUM
MOSLEM
MUSLIM
PABLUM
PELLAM
PEPLUM
PHYLUM
PRELIM
SHALOM
SHOLEM
SHOLOM
SLALOM
SMALLM
UNSLIM
VELLUM
WILLEM

••••LM
ANSELM
BECALM
EMBALM
HIJKLM
NAPALM
NEWULM
ONFILM
REFILM
SMALLM
UNCALM
UNHELM

L•N•••
LANAIS
LANARK
LANATE
LANCED
LANCER
LANCES
LANCET
LANCIA
LANCIE
LANDAT
LANDAU
LANDED
LANDER
LANDHO
LANDIS
LANDON
LANDOR
LANDRY
LANDUP
LANDUS
LANGER
LANIER
LANINA
LANKER
LANKLY
LANOSE
LANSKY
LANSON
LANTOS
LANVAL
LANVIN
LENAIN
LENAPE
LENARD
LENDEE
LENDER
LENDTO
LENGLE
LENGTH
LENGUA
LENINA
LENITY
LENNIE
LENNON
LENNOX
LENORE
LENOVO
LENSED
LENSES
LENTEN
LENTIL
LENTOS
LENTTO
LINAGE
LINDEN
LINDER
LINEAL
LINEAR
LINENS
LINENY
LINERS
LINEUP
LINGER
LINGLE
LINGUA
LINGUS
LINIER
LINING
LINKED
LINKER
LINKUP
LINNET
LINNEY
LINTED
LINTEL
LINTER
LINTON
LINZER
LMNOPQ
LONDON
LONELY
LONERS
LONGED
LONGER
LONGES
LONGET
LONGLY
LONGUE
LONNIE
LONNOL
LUNACY
LUNATE
LUNCHY
LUNDEN
LUNDIS
LUNEDI
LUNGED
LUNGER
LUNGES
LUNIKS
LUNKER
LUNTHA
LUNULA
LYNDON
LYNLEY
LYNXES
LYNYRD

L••N••
LAINIE
LAONZA
LAUNCH
LEANED
LEANER
LEANIN
LEANLY
LEANNE
LEANON
LEANTO
LEHNEN
LEMNOS
LENNIE
LENNON
LENNOX
LEONIA
LEONID
LERNER
LIANAS
LIANES
LIANGS
LIENEE
LIENOR
LIGNES
LIGNIN
LIGNUM
LIMNED
LIMNER
LINNET
LINNEY
LIONEL
LIONET
LIONLY
LLANOS
LOANED
LOANER
LONNIE
LONNOL
LOONEY
LOONIE
LOTNOS
LOUNGE
LUANDA
LUGNUT
LYONNE

L•••N•
LABINE
LACING
LACUNA
LADING
LADINO
LAGUNA
LAMENT
LAMINA
LAMING
LAMONT
LANINA
LAPINS
LARINE
LARYNX
LASING
LATENE
LATENS
LATENT
LATINA
LATINI
LATINO
LATINS
LAVING
LAWING
LAYING
LAYINS
LAZING
LEANNE
LEARNS
LEARNT
LEEANN
LEGEND
LELAND
LEMANS
LEMOND
LEMONS
LEMONY
LENINA
LEVANT
LEVENE
LEVINE
LFRANK
LIGAND
LIKENS
LIKING
LIMANS
LIMING
LINENS
LINENY
LINING
LIPENG
LITANY
LIVENS
LIVING
LOCANE
LODENS
LODINJ
LOGANS
LOGINS
LOGONS
LOMOND
LOPING
LORANS
LORENE
LORENZ
LORING
LOSING
LOUANN
LOVING
LOWEND
LOWING
LUBING
LUCENT
LUCINE
LUDENS
LUGING
LUMENS
LUMINA
LUPINE
LUPINO
LUPONE
LURENE
LURING
LYONNE
LYSINE

L••••N
LACEON
LAGOON
LAIDIN
LAIDON
LANDON
LANSON
LANVIN
LARDON
LARKIN
LARMEN
LARSEN
LARSON
LASSEN
LATEEN
LATEON
LATHEN
LAUREN
LAURYN
LAVAIN
LAVERN
LAWMAN
LAWMEN
LAWSON
LAWTON
LAYMAN
LAYMEN
LAYSIN
LAYSON
LEADEN
LEADIN
LEADON
LEAKIN
LEANIN
LEANON
LEAPIN
LEAPON
LEAVEN
LEBRON
LEBRUN
LECAIN
LEEANN
LEFTIN
LEFTON
LEGION
LEGMAN
LEGMEN
LEGUIN
LEHMAN
LEHNEN
LEIDEN
LEISEN
LEMMON
LENAIN
LENNON
LENTEN
LEPTON
LESHAN
LESION
LESSEN
LESSON
LETSIN
LETSON
LEYDEN
LHASAN
LIBRAN
LIBYAN
LICHEN
LIEDON
LIESIN
LIESON
LIGNIN
LILIAN
LINDEN
LINTON
LIPTON
LISBON
LISTEN
LISTON
LIVEIN
LIVEON
LLBEAN
LOADIN
LOCKIN
LOCKON
LOFTON
LOGSIN
LOGSON
LOMEIN
LONDON
LOOKIN
LOOKON
LOOSEN
LORAIN
LOTION
LOUANN
LOUDEN
LOUDON
LOUVIN
LOVEIN
LOWMAN
LOWMEN
LUBLIN
LUCIAN
LUCIEN
LUDDEN
LUMPEN
LUMPIN
LUNDEN
LUPTON
LUREIN
LYDIAN
LYNDON
LYTTON

•LN•••
ALNASL
ALNICO
ELNATH
ELNINO
ELNORA

•L•N••
ALANIS
ALANON
ALINED
ALINER
ALINES
ALLNEW
ALONGS
ALONSO
ALONZO
BLANCA
BLANCH
BLANCO
BLANDA
BLANKS
BLENCH
BLENDE
BLENDS
BLINDS
BLINIS
BLINKS
BLINTZ
BLONDE
BLONDS
BLUNTS
CLANCY
CLANGS
CLANKS
CLANKY
CLENCH
CLINCH
CLINGS
CLINGY
CLINIC
CLINKS
CLONAL
CLONED
CLONER
CLONES
CLONKS
CLUNKS
CLUNKY
ELANCE
ELANDS
ELANET
ELINOR
FLANGE
FLANKS
FLENSE
FLINCH
FLINGS
FLINTS
FLINTY
FLUNKS
FLUNKY
FLYNET
GLANCE
GLANDS
GLENDA
GLENNE
GLINDA
GLINKA
GLINTS
GLINTY
GLYNIS
KLMNOP
LLANOS
OLINDA
PLANAR
PLANAS
PLANBS
PLANCK
PLANED
PLANER
PLANES
PLANET
PLANKS
PLANON
PLANTE
PLANTO
PLANTS
PLENTY
PLENUM
PLINKS
PLINTH
PLONKS
PLUNGE
PLUNKS
PLUNKY
SLANGS
SLANGY
SLANTS
SLINGS
SLINKS
SLINKY

•L••N•
ALAINA
ALBANO
ALBANS
ALBANY
ALBINE
ALBINO
ALCINA
ALDINE
ALFINE
ALHENA
ALIENS
ALIGNS
ALKENE
ALMOND
ALPINE
ALUMNA
ALUMNI
ALVING
ALVINO
BLAINE
BLOUNT
BLUING
CLEANS
CLIENT
CLOWNS
CLUING
ELAINE
ELAYNE
ELKONV
ELMONT
ELNINO
ELRENO
ELUANT
FLAUNT
FLUENT
FLYING
FLYINS
GLEANS
GLENNE
GLUING
GLUONS
HLHUNT
ILEANA
ILLINI
KLEINE
OLEINS
PLAINS
PLAINT
PLIANT
PLYING
SLOANE
SLUING

•L•••N
ALANON
ALBION
ALDRIN
ALEMAN
ALFVEN
ALGREN
ALISON
ALLEYN
ALLMAN
ALLMEN
ALSTON
ALTMAN
BLAZON
BLEWIN
BLEWON
BLIXEN
BLOWIN
BLOWON
BLYDEN
BLYTON
CLADIN
CLAVIN
CLIPON
CLOVEN
CLUEIN
ELEVEN
ELEVON
ELFMAN
ELKTON
ELSTON
FLACON
FLAGON
FLAXEN
FLEWIN
FLEWON
FLITIN
FLORIN
FLOWIN
FLYMAN
FLYMEN
GLOBIN
GLUEON
GLUTEN
KLAXON
KLIBAN
LLBEAN
OLDMAN
OLDMEN
OLEFIN
OLESON
PLANON
PLATEN
PLAYON
PLOWON
PLUGIN
PLUTON
SLAMON
SLAPON
SLIDIN
SLIPIN
SLIPON
SLOGAN
SLOPON
SLOVEN
ULLMAN

••LN••
ALLNEW
KILNED
MILNER
MILNES
MOLNAR
TELNET
TILNOW
WALNUT

••L•N•
AGLINT
AILING
ARLENE
ASLANT
BALINE
BALING
BELONG
BELONS
BOLENA
BYLAND
BYLINE
CELINE
COLONI
COLONS
COLONY
DALAND
DALENE
DELAND
DELANO
DELANY
DELINT
DOLENZ
DOLING
EALING
EELING
EKLAND
ENLINK
ERLANG
FALANA
FALINE
FELINE
FELONS
FELONY
FILENE
FILING
GALANT
GALENA
GOLINO
GOLONG
HALING
HELENA
HELENE
HELENS
HELLNO
HOLING
IDLING
ILLINI
INLAND
INLINE
IOLANI
IRLENE
ISLAND
ISLING
JKLMNO
JOLENE
KALINE
KDLANG
LELAND
MALONE
MELINA
MELONS
MILANO
MILANS
MOLINA
MOLINE
NYLONS
OBLONG
OGLING
OILING
ONLAND
ONLINE
OOLONG
ORLONS
PALING
PILING
POLAND
POLING
PULING
PYLONS
RELAND
RELEND
RELENT
RELINE
RELINK
RILING
ROLAND
RULING
SALINA
SALINE
SALONS
SELENA
SELENE
SILENT
SOLANO
SOLANS
SOLING
SOLONG
SOLONS
SPLINE
SPLINT
TALENT
TALONS
TILING
TULANE
TVLAND
UCLANS
UHLANS
UNLENT
UNLINK
UPLAND
UPLINK
VALENE
VALENS
VALENT
VALINE
VOLANS
VOLANT
WALING
WILING
YELENA

••L••N
AILEEN
ALLEYN
ALLMAN
ALLMEN
BALEEN
BALKAN
BALLIN
BALLON
BCLION
BELTON
BOLDEN
BOLEYN
BOLTON
CALGON
CALLAN
CALLIN
CALLON
CALVIN
COLMAN
COLSON
COLTON
COLUMN
CULKIN
CULLEN
DALTON
DELIAN
DILLON
DOLMAN
DOLTON
EILEEN
EOLIAN
FALCON
FALLEN
FALLIN
FALLON
FELDON
FELLIN
FELLON
FELSON
FILEIN
FILLIN
FOLDIN
FULTON
GALLON
GALTON
GELPEN
GILLAN
GILMAN
GILPIN
GOLDEN
GULDEN
HALPIN
HELDIN
HELDON
HELLON
HELPIN
HELPON
HILTON
HOLDEN
HOLDIN
HOLDON
HOLMAN
JOLSON
JOLTIN
JULIAN
JULIEN
KALKAN
KALLEN
KELTON
KELVIN
LILIAN
MALDEN
MALIAN
MALIGN
MALLON
MALTIN
MCLAIN
MCLEAN
MELLON
MELTON
MELVIN
MELVYN
MILTON
MOLSON
MOLTEN
MULLIN
NELSON
OILCAN
OILMAN
OILMEN
OILPAN
ONLOAN
PELION
PILEIN
PILEON
POLLEN
PULLIN
PULLON
PULMON
RELOAN
RELYON
ROLLIN
ROLLON
RULEON
SALMAN
SALMON
SALOON
SALTEN
SALTON
SELLON
SELTEN
SILKEN
SOLDON
SOLEMN
SPLEEN
SULLEN
SULTAN
SYLVAN
TALKIN
TALKON
TELLON
TILDEN
TILSON
TILTON
TOLDON
TULSAN
ULLMAN
UNLEAN
VELSEN
VILLON
VULCAN
WALDEN
WALKEN
WALKIN
WALKON
WALLIN
WALTON
WELDON
WILSON
WILTON
ZOLTAN

•••LN•
HELLNO

•••L•N
AMBLIN
AVALON
BAILON
BALLIN
BALLON
BANLON
BERLIN
BROLIN
CALLAN
CALLIN
CALLON
CARLIN
CATLIN
CEYLON
CONLAN
CULLEN
CURLIN
DARLIN
DEALIN
DIALIN
DILLON
DOBLIN
DUBLIN
DUNLIN
ESALEN
ESTLIN
EVELYN
FALLEN
FALLIN
FALLON
FAYLEN
FELLIN
FELLON
FILLIN
GALLON
GATLIN
GILLAN
GOBLIN
GOSLIN
HAMLIN
HANLON
HARLAN
HARLIN
HAULIN
HEFLIN
HELLON
HOWLIN
IJKLMN
ISELIN
JACLYN
JOPLIN
KALLEN
KAOLIN
KAPLAN
KARLEN
KRYLON
LUBLIN
MACLEN
MADLYN
MAILIN
MALLON
MARLIN
MARLON
MASLIN
MATLIN
MELLON
MERLIN
MOULIN
MULLIN
MUSLIN
NAILIN
NEALON
NOWLAN
POLLEN
POPLIN
PULLIN
PULLON
RAGLAN
RAILON
RATLIN
REELIN
REPLAN
REVLON
ROLLIN
ROLLON
ROSLYN
SAILON

SEALIN
SELLON
SMALLN
STALIN
STOLEN
STOLON
SULLEN
TEFLON
TELLON
TIGLON
TOMLIN
TOULON
TRYLON
UNPLAN
VEBLEN
VILLON
VIOLIN
WALLIN
WAYLON
WHELAN
WOOLEN

••••LN
HAMELN
SMALLN
WEDELN

LO••••
LOADED
LOADER
LOADIN
LOADUP
LOAFED
LOAFER
LOAMED
LOANED
LOANER
LOATHE
LOAVES
LOBATE
LOBBED
LOBBER
LOBULE
LOCALE
LOCALS
LOCANE
LOCATE
LOCCIT
LOCHER
LOCKED
LOCKER
LOCKET
LOCKIN
LOCKON
LOCKUP
LOCUST
LODENS
LODGED
LODGER
LODGES
LODINJ
LOFTED
LOFTER
LOFTON
LOFTUS
LOGANS
LOGGED
LOGGER
LOGGIA
LOGICS
LOGIER
LOGILY
LOGINS
LOGJAM
LOGOFF
LOGONS
LOGOUT
LOGSIN
LOGSON
LOIDED
LOIRET
LOITER
LOLICH
LOLITA
LOLLED
LOLLER
LOMEIN
LOMOND
LOMPOC
LONDON
LONELY
LONERS
LONGED
LONGER
LONGES
LONGET
LONGLY
LONGUE
LONNIE
LONNOL
LOOEYS
LOOFAH
LOOFAS
LOOIES
LOOKAT
LOOKED
LOOKEE
LOOKER
LOOKIE
LOOKIN
LOOKMA
LOOKON
LOOKTO
LOOKUP
LOOMED
LOOMPA
LOOMUP
LOONEY
LOONIE
LOOPED
LOOPER
LOOSED
LOOSEN
LOOSER
LOOSES
LOOSEY
LOOTED
LOOTER
LOPERS
LOPING
LOPOFF
LOPPED
LOPPER
LOQUAT
LORAIN
LORANS
LORDED
LORDIT
LORDLY
LOREAL
LORENE
LORENZ
LORIES
LORING
LORRIE
LOSDOS
LOSEIT
LOSERS
LOSETO
LOSING
LOSSES
LOSTIT
LOSTTO
LOTHAR
LOTION
LOTNOS
LOTSOF
LOTTED
LOTTER
LOTTOS
LOUANN
LOUCHE
LOUDEN
LOUDER
LOUDLY
LOUDON
LOUIES
LOUISA
LOUISB
LOUISE
LOUISI
LOUISV
LOUISX
LOUMAS
LOUNGE
LOUPES
LOUSED
LOUSES
LOUVER
LOUVIN
LOUVRE
LOVAGE
LOVEIN
LOVEIT
LOVELL
LOVELY
LOVERS
LOVETO
LOVETT
LOVEYA
LOVEYS
LOVING
LOWBID
LOWBOY
LOWCAL
LOWCUT
LOWEBB
LOWELL
LOWEND
LOWERS
LOWERY
LOWEST
LOWFAT
LOWING
LOWIQS
LOWISH
LOWKEY
LOWMAN
LOWMEN
LOWRES
LOWSET
LOWTAR
LOWTOP
LOYALE
LOYOLA

L•O•••
LAONZA
LAOTSE
LAOTZU
LEOIII
LEONIA
LEONID
LEOVII
LEOXII
LHOTSE
LIONEL
LIONET
LIONLY
LIOTTA
LLOYDS
LOOEYS
LOOFAH
LOOFAS
LOOIES
LOOKAT
LOOKED
LOOKEE
LOOKER
LOOKIE
LOOKIN
LOOKMA
LOOKON
LOOKTO
LOOKUP
LOOMED
LOOMPA
LOOMUP
LOONEY
LOONIE
LOOPED
LOOPER
LOOSED
LOOSEN
LOOSER
LOOSES
LOOSEY
LOOTED
LOOTER
LYONNE

L••O••
LABORS
LABOUR
LADOGA
LAGOON
LAHORE
LAJOIE
LAKOTA
LAMONT
LAMOUR
LANOSE
LAROSA
LATOUR
LATOYA
LAYOFF
LAYOUT
LEDOFF
LEDOUT
LEDOUX
LELOIR
LEMOKO
LEMOND
LEMONS
LEMONY
LENORE
LENOVO
LEROUX
LETOFF
LETOUR
LETOUT
LIPOFF
LIPOUT
LITOUT
LMNOPQ
LOGOFF
LOGONS
LOGOUT
LOMOND
LOPOFF
LOYOLA
LTGOVS
LUGOSI
LUGOUT
LUPONE

L•••O•
LACEON
LACHOY
LACLOS
LAGOON
LAIDON
LANDON
LANDOR
LANSON
LANTOS
LAPDOG
LAPTOP
LARDON
LARGOS
LARMOR
LARSON
LASSOS
LATEOF
LATEON
LAWSON
LAWTON
LAYFOR
LAYLOW
LAYSON
LAZBOY
LEADON
LEANON
LEAPON
LEBRON
LECTOR
LEFTOF
LEFTON
LEGION
LEGROS
LEMMON
LEMNOS
LENNON
LENNOX
LENTOS
LEPTON
LESBOS
LESION
LESSON
LESSOR
LETSON
LIBROS
LIEDON
LIEFOR
LIELOW
LIENOR
LIESON
LILIOM
LIMBOS
LINTON
LIPTON
LIQUOR
LISBOA
LISBON
LISTON
LITHOS
LIVEON
LLANOS
LOCKON
LOFTON
LOGSON
LOMPOC
LONDON
LONNOL
LOOKON
LOSDOS
LOTION
LOTNOS
LOTSOF
LOTTOS
LOUDON
LOWBOY
LOWTOP
LUDLOW
LUMMOX
LUPTON
LUTHOR
LYNDON
LYTTON

L••••O
LADINO
LAIDTO
LANDHO
LAREDO
LASHTO
LASZLO
LATERO
LATETO
LATIGO
LATINO
LAVABO
LAYSTO
LEADTO
LEANTO
LEGATO
LEMOKO
LENDTO
LENOVO
LENTTO
LETSGO
LIBIDO
LIEDTO
LIESTO
LIEVIO
LIKESO
LIKETO
LLADRO
LOOKTO
LOSETO
LOSTTO
LOVETO
LUGLIO
LUPINO

•LO•••
ALOGIA
ALOHAS
ALOMAR
ALONGS
ALONSO
ALONZO
ALOTOF
BLOATS
BLOBBY
BLOBEL
BLOCKS
BLOCKY
BLOKES
BLONDE
BLONDS
BLOODS
BLOODY
BLOOEY
BLOOIE
BLOOMS
BLOOMY
BLOOPS
BLOTCH
BLOTTO
BLOTTY
BLOTUP
BLOUNT
BLOUSE
BLOWER
BLOWIN
BLOWIT
BLOWON
BLOWSY
BLOWUP
BLOWZY
CLOAKS
CLOCHE
CLOCKS
CLODDY
CLOETE
CLOGGY
CLOGUP
CLOMPS
CLONAL
CLONED
CLONER
CLONES
CLONKS
CLORIS
CLOROX
CLOSED
CLOSER
CLOSES
CLOSET
CLOTHE
CLOTHO
CLOTHS
CLOTTY
CLOTUP
CLOUDS
CLOUDY
CLOUGH
CLOUTS
CLOVEN
CLOVER
CLOVES
CLOVIS
CLOWNS
CLOYED
ELODEA
ELOGES
ELOISA
ELOISE
ELOPED
ELOPER
ELOPES
FLOATS
FLOATY
FLOCKS
FLOODS
FLOOEY
FLOORS
FLOPIT
FLOPPY
FLOPSY
FLORAE
FLORAL
FLORAS
FLOREK
FLORES
FLORET
FLOREY
FLORID
FLORIN
FLORIO
FLOSSY
FLOURS
FLOURY
FLOUTS
FLOWED
FLOWER
FLOWIN
GLOATS
GLOBAL
GLOBBY
GLOBED
GLOBES
GLOBIN
GLOCKS
GLOGGS
GLOOMS
GLOOMY
GLOPPY
GLORIA
GLOSSA
GLOSSO
GLOSSY
GLOTTO
GLOUCS
GLOVED
GLOVER
GLOVES
GLOWED
GLOWER
ILOILO
LLOYDS
OLORES
PLOCES
PLOMER
PLONKS
PLOTTY
PLOUGH
PLOVER
PLOWED
PLOWER
PLOWON
PLOWUP
SLOANE
SLOBBY
SLOGAN
SLOOPS
SLOOPY
SLOPED
SLOPER
SLOPES
SLOPON
SLOPPY
SLOSHY
SLOTHS
SLOUCH
SLOUGH
SLOVAK
SLOVEN
SLOWED
SLOWER
SLOWGO
SLOWLY
SLOWUP
ZLOTYS

•L•O••
ALBORG
ALCOTT
ALCOVE
ALDOUS
ALGORE
ALIOTH
ALIOTO
ALLOTS
ALLOUT
ALLOWS
ALLOYS
ALMOND
ALMOST
ALTOID
BLOODS
BLOODY
BLOOEY
BLOOIE
BLOOMS
BLOOMY
BLOOPS
ELBOWS
ELFOWL
ELKONV
ELLORA
ELMONT
ELMORE
ELNORA
ELTORO
ELWOOD
FLOODS
FLOOEY
FLOORS
FLUORO
FLYOUT
GLOOMS
GLOOMY
GLUONS
ILLOFF
OLEOLE
SLOOPS
SLOOPY

•L••O•
ALAMOS
ALANON
ALBION
ALEROS
ALISON
ALIYOT
ALLFOR
ALOTOF
ALSTON
BLAZON
BLEWON
BLOWON
BLUEOX
BLYTON
CLAMOR
CLAROS
CLIPON
CLOROX
ELEVON
ELINOR
ELKTON
ELLIOS
ELLIOT
ELSTON
ELWOOD
FLACON
FLAGON
FLAVOR
FLEWON
FLEXOR
FLYBOY
FLYLOW
FLYROD
GLAMOR
GLUEON
GLYCOL
KLAXON
KLMNOP
LLANOS
OLDBOY
OLDDOG
OLDSOD
OLESON
PLANON
PLATOS
PLAYON
PLEXOR
PLOWON
PLUTON
SLALOM
SLAMON
SLAPON
SLIPON
SLOPON
SLYFOX

•L•••O
ALBANO
ALBEDO
ALBINO
ALECTO
ALEPPO
ALIOTO
ALIVEO
ALLPRO
ALNICO
ALONSO
ALONZO
ALVARO
ALVINO
ALZADO
BLANCO
BLOTTO
BLUFFO
CLOTHO
ELADIO
ELISEO
ELNINO
ELPASO
ELRENO
ELTORO
FLEWTO
FLORIO
FLUORO
GLADTO
GLOSSO
GLOTTO
GLUETO
GLYPTO
ILOILO
KLEPTO
LLADRO
OLDPRO
PLANTO
PLASMO
PLAYTO
PLEDTO
PLUMBO
PLUVIO
SLOWGO
SLUGGO
ULTIMO

••LO••
ABLOOM
AFLOAT
ALLOTS
ALLOUT
ALLOWS
ALLOYS
APLOMB
ARLOVA
ASLOPE
ASLOSH
BELOIT
BELONG
BELONS
BILOXI
BULOVA
BYLOTS
CALORY
CHLORO
COLONI
COLONS
COLONY
COLORS
COLOUR
DOLORE
DOLORS
DOLOUR
ELLORA
EULOGY
FELONS
FELONY
FILOSE
GALOIS
GALOOT
GALOPS
GALORE
GALOSH
GOLONG
HALOED
HALOES
HALOID
HELOTS
IGLOOS
ILLOFF
INLOVE
JALOPY
JCLOTH
LELOIR
MALONE
MALORY
MALOTI
MELODY
MELONS
MELOTT
MILORD
MILOSZ
MYLORD
MYLOVE
NOLOAD
NOLOSE
NOLOSS
NYLONS
OBLONG
OCLOCK
OHLOOK
ONLOAD
ONLOAN
OOLOGY
OOLONG
ORLONS
ORLOPS
PALOMA
PELOSI
PELOTA
PHLOEM
PILOSE
PILOTS
PILOUS
PYLONS
RELOAD
RELOAN
RELOCK
RELOGS
RELOOK
RELOSE
RELOST
SALOME
SALONS
SALOON
SHLOCK
SILOED
SOLOED
SOLONG
SOLONS
SPLOSH
TALONS
UNLOAD
UNLOCK
UNLOOP
UNLOST
UPLOAD
VALOIS
VALORS
VALOUR
VALOVA
VELOCE
VELOUR
XYLOID
XYLOSE
ZHLOBS

••L•O•
ABLOOM
ALLFOR
BALBOA
BALLON
BALLOT
BALLOU
BCLION
BELLOC
BELLOW
BELTON
BILLOW
BOLCOM
BOLTON
CALGON
CALLON
CALLOW
CELLOS
COLLOP
COLLOQ
COLSON
COLTON
DALTON
DELCOS
DELROY
DELSOL
DILLON
DOLLOP
DOLTON
EELPOT
ELLIOS
ELLIOT
FALCON
FALLON
FALLOW
FELDON
FELLON
FELLOW
FELSON
FELTOK
FOLIOS
FOLLOW
FOLSOM
FULLOF
FULTON
GALLON
GALLOP
GALOOT
GALTON
GELDOF
GILROY
HALLOO
HALLOS
HALLOW
HELDON
HELIOS
HELLON
HELLOS
HELPON
HILTON
HOLDON
HOLLOW
HULLOS
IGLOOS
JELLOS
JOLIOT
JOLSON
KELTON
KILROY
LILIOM
MALLON
MALLOW
MELLON
MELLOW
MELTON
MILTON
MOLLOY
MOLSON
NELSON
NULLOS
OHLOOK
PALLOR
PELION
PILEON
PILLOW
POLIOS
POLLOI
POLLOS
POLPOT
PULLON
PULMON
RELOOK
RELYON
ROLEOS
ROLLON
RULEON
SALLOW
SALMON
SALOON
SALTON
SALVOR
SALVOS
SELDOM
SELLON
SOLDON
TALKOF
TALKON
TALLOW
TALTOS
TELCOS
TELLOF
TELLON
TILNOW
TILSON
TILTON
TOLDOF
TOLDON
UNLOOP
VILLON
VOLVOS
WALKON
WALLOP
WALLOW
WALTON
WELDON
WILCOX
WILLOW
WILSON
WILTON
YELLOW

••L••O
AFLCIO
AILURO
ALLPRO
BILBAO
BOLERO
BULDEO
CALICO
CALLAO
CALLTO
CHLORO
COLECO
DELANO
DELRIO
FALLTO
FELLTO
GALEAO
GELATO
GOLINO
HALLOO
HELDTO
HELICO
HELLNO
HOLDTO
ITLLDO
JKLMNO
MALABO
MILANO
PHLEBO
SALUTO
SELLTO
SOLANO
SOLDTO
TALKTO
TOLEDO
VALERO
VELCRO
WALKTO
WILLDO

•••LO•
AIRLOG
ANALOG
ANGLOS

ASSLOW
ATALOW
AVALON
BADLOT
BAILON
BAILOR
BALLON
BALLOT
BALLOU
BANLON
BARLOW
BAYLOR
BELLOC
BELLOW
BILLOW
CALLON
CALLOW
CARLOS
CARLOT
CARLOW
CELLOS
CEYLON
CHOLOS
CIELOS
COLLOP
COLLOQ
CYCLOS
DECLOT
DEPLOY
DIALOG
DIGLOT
DILLON
DOLLOP
DUNLOP
DUPLOS
DYELOT
EKELOF
EMPLOY
ENBLOC
EPILOG
FALLON
FALLOW
FARLOW
FEELOK
FELLON
FELLOW
FLYLOW
FOLLOW
FULLOF
GALLON
GALLOP
GASLOG
GOSLOW
HALLOO
HALLOS
HALLOW
HANLON
HARLOT
HARLOW
HELLON
HELLOS
HOLLOW
HULLOS
INFLOW
JAGLOM
JAILOR
JELLOS
JOBLOT
KRYLON
KRYLOV
LACLOS
LAYLOW
LIELOW
LUDLOW
MAALOX
MALLON
MALLOW
MARLON
MELLON
MELLOW
MERLOT
MOLLOY
NEALON
NULLOS
OCELOT
ODDLOT
PALLOR
PARLOR
PAVLOV
PILLOW
POLLOI
POLLOS
PRELOG
PROLOG
PULLON
RAILON
RANLOW
REFLOW
REGLOW
REPLOT
REPLOW
REVLON
ROLLON
RUNLOW
SAILON
SAILOR
SALLOW
SAWLOG
SELLON
SHALOM
SHILOH
SHOLOM
SLALOM
STOLON
SUBLOT
TAILOR
TALLOW
TAYLOR
TEFLON
TELLOF
TELLON
THELOT
TIGLON
TOOLOW
TOULON
TRYLON
UNCLOG
UNSLOW
UPFLOW
VILLON
WAHLOO
WALLOP
WALLOW
WAYLON
WEBLOG
WILLOW
YELLOW
ZEALOT
ZIPLOC

•••L•O

ADOLFO
AIELLO
APOLLO
BIBLIO
BRILLO
CALLAO
CALLTO
COOLIO
COOLTO
DEALTO
DIALSO
DUELLO
EMILIO
FAILTO
FALLTO
FELLTO
HALLOO
HELLNO
ITLLDO
LUGLIO
MAILTO
NIELLO
NUCLEO
OTELLO
PHILCO
PHYLLO
RIALTO
SAILTO
SELLTO
SMALLO
STELMO
TRILLO
VAILCO
WAHLOO
WILLDO

••••LO

AIELLO
ANGELO
APOLLO
BAROLO
BRILLO
CATALO
CUMULO
DANILO
DAYGLO
DEMILO
DIABLO
DUELLO
ENHALO
GIGOLO
GOSOLO
ILOILO
LASZLO
MAHALO
MEGALO
MODULO
NICOLO
NIELLO
NIHILO
OTELLO
PHYLLO
POMELO
PUEBLO
ROMULO
SMALLO
STMALO
TRILLO
TUPELO
ZOCALO

L•P•••

LAPCAT
LAPDOG
LAPELS
LAPERI
LAPERM
LAPFUL
LAPHAM
LAPINS
LAPPED
LAPPER
LAPPET
LAPSAT
LAPSED
LAPSER
LAPSES
LAPSUP
LAPSUS
LAPTEV
LAPTOP
LAPUTA
LEPERS
LEPTON
LIPARI
LIPASE
LIPENG
LIPIDS
LIPOFF
LIPOUT
LIPPED
LIPPER
LIPTON
LOPERS
LOPING
LOPOFF
LOPPED
LOPPER
LUPINE
LUPINO
LUPONE
LUPTON

L••P••

LAPPED
LAPPER
LAPPET
LAUPER
LEAPAT
LEAPED
LEAPER
LEAPIN
LEAPON
LEAPUP
LIMPED
LIMPER
LIMPET
LIMPID
LIMPLY
LIPPED
LIPPER
LISPED
LISPER
LOMPOC
LOOPED
LOOPER
LOPPED
LOPPER
LOUPES
LUMPED
LUMPEN
LUMPER
LUMPIN
LUMPIT
LUMPUR
LYMPHS

L•••P•

LAYUPS
LENAPE
LETUPS
LMNOPQ
LOOMPA

L••••P

LACEUP
LAIDUP
LANDUP
LAPSUP
LAPTOP
LARRUP
LASHUP
LASTUP
LAYSUP
LEADUP
LEAPUP
LETRIP
LETSUP
LICKUP
LIFTUP
LINEUP
LINKUP
LOADUP
LOCKUP
LOOKUP
LOOMUP
LOWTOP

•LP•••

ALPACA
ALPERT
ALPHAS
ALPINE
ELPAIS
ELPASO

•L•P••

ALEPHS
ALEPPO
ALIPED
ALLPRO
CLIPON
ELAPID
ELAPSE
ELOPED
ELOPER
ELOPES
FLAPPY
FLIPUP
FLOPIT
FLOPPY
FLOPSY
GLOPPY
GLYPHS
GLYPTO
KLEPTO
OLDPAL
OLDPRO
SLAPON
SLAPPY
SLIPBY
SLIPIN
SLIPON
SLIPPY
SLIPUP
SLOPED
SLOPER
SLOPES
SLOPON
SLOPPY

•L••P•

ALCAPP
ALEPPO
ALMVPS
BLEEPS
BLIMPS
BLOOPS
CLAMPS
CLASPS
CLOMPS
CLUMPS
CLUMPY
FLAPPY
FLOPPY
GLOPPY
NLMVPS
PLUMPS
SLAPPY
SLEEPS
SLEEPY
SLIPPY
SLOOPS
SLOOPY
SLOPPY
SLUMPS
SLURPS

•L•••P

ALCAPP
ALEGUP
ALETAP
BLEWUP
BLOTUP
BLOWUP
CLAMUP
CLOGUP
CLOTUP
CLUBUP
FLEWUP
FLIPUP
GLAMUP
KLMNOP
PLAYUP
PLOWUP
PLUGUP
SLIPUP
SLOWUP

••LP••

ALLPRO
DELPHI
EELPOT
GALPAL
GELPEN
GILPIN
GULPED
GULPER
HALPIN
HELPED
HELPER
HELPIN
HELPME
HELPON
HELPUP
JALPAS
KELPIE
OILPAN
POLPOT
PULPED
PULPER
PULPIT
RALPHJ
SYLPHS
WOLPER
YELPED
YELPER

••L•P•

ASLOPE
CALIPH
DOLAPS
FELIPE
GALOPS
JALAPA
JALOPY
JULEPS
ORLOPS
OXLIPS
POLYPS
RELAPS
SALEPS
TULIPS
YCLEPT

••L••P

ASLEEP
BALLUP
BELTUP
BOLTUP
BULKUP
CALLUP
CCLAMP
COLLOP
DOLLOP
DOLLUP
FILLIP
FILLUP
FOLDUP
FULLUP
GALLOP
GALLUP
GELCAP
GOLIMP
HELDUP
HELPUP
HOLDUP
HOLEUP
MILSAP
OILCUP
PILEUP
PULLUP
RELEAP
RILEUP
ROLLUP
TALKUP
TILTUP
UNLIMP
UNLOOP
UPLEAP
WALKUP
WALLOP
WALLUP
WELLUP

•••LP•

ADOLPH
GUELPH
PHELPS
SCALPS
SCULPT
WHELPS

•••L•P

BALLUP
BOILUP
BURLAP
CALLUP
COILUP
COLLOP
CURLUP
DEALUP
DEWLAP
DIALUP
DOLLOP
DOLLUP
DUNLAP
DUNLOP
EARLAP
FATLIP
FILLIP
FILLUP
FOULUP
FUELUP
FULLUP
GALLOP
GALLUP
GUNLAP
HAULUP
HEALUP
NAILUP
ONELAP
OUTLIP
PHILIP
PULLUP
REELUP
ROILUP
ROLLUP
SCHLEP
SEALUP
SMALLP
THELIP
TOOLUP
UNCLIP
WALLOP
WALLUP
WELLUP

••••LP

DEPULP
NOHELP
OFHELP
SMALLP

L•Q•••

LIQUID
LIQUOR
LOQUAT

L•••Q•

LOWIQS

L••••Q

LMNOPQ

•L•Q••

CLAQUE
CLIQUE
CLIQUY
PLAQUE

••L••Q

COLLOQ

•••L•Q

COLLOQ
SMALLQ

••••LQ

POSSLQ
SMALLQ

L•R•••

LARAMS
LARAZA
LARDED
LARDER
LARDON
LAREDO
LAREES
LARGER
LARGES
LARGOS
LARIAT
LARINE
LARKED
LARKER
LARKIN
LARMEN
LARMOR
LAROSA
LARRUP
LARSEN
LARSON
LARTER
LARTET
LARVAE
LARVAL
LARVAS
LARYNX
LERIDA
LERNER
LEROUX
LFRANK
LORAIN
LORANS
LORDED
LORDIT
LORDLY
LOREAL
LORENE
LORENZ
LORIES
LORING
LORRIE
LUREIN
LURENE
LURERS
LURING
LURKED
LURKER
LURKEY
LYRICS
LYRIDS
LYRIST

L••R••

LABRAT
LABREA
LAIRDS
LAIRED
LARRUP
LATRIA
LAUREL
LAUREN
LAUREY
LAURIA
LAURIC
LAURIE
LAURYL
LAURYN
LEARNS
LEARNT
LEBRET
LEBRON
LEBRUN
LEERAT
LEERED
LEERER
LEGREE
LEGROS
LEHRER
LETRIP
LIBRAE
LIBRAN
LIBRAS
LIBRIS
LIBROS
LITRES
LIVRES
LOIRET
LORRIE
LOWRES
LYCRAS

L•••R•

LABORS
LACERS
LADERS
LAGERS
LAHORE
LAKERS
LAMARR
LANARK
LANDRY
LAPERI
LAPERM
LASERS
LASTRA
LATERI
LATERO
LAVERN
LAVERS
LAYERS
LEGART
LEMURS
LENARD
LENORE
LEPERS
LETTRE
LEVERS
LEVERT
LIBERS
LIFERS
LIGERS
LIKERS
LINERS
LIPARI
LITERS
LITTRE
LIVERS
LIVERY
LIZARD
LLADRO
LONERS
LOPERS
LOSERS
LOUVRE
LOVERS
LOWERS
LOWERY
LUGERS
LURERS
LUSTRA
LUSTRE
LUXURY
LYNYRD

L••••R

LABOUR
LACIER
LADDER
LADLER
LAFFER
LAGEAR
LAGGER
LAKIER
LAMARR
LAMOUR
LANCER
LANDER
LANDOR
LANGER
LANIER
LANKER
LAPPER
LAPSER
LARDER
LARGER
LARKER
LARMOR
LARTER
LASCAR
LASHER
LASKER
LASSER
LATHER
LATOUR
LATTER
LAUDER
LAUPER
LAUTER
LAWYER
LAYFOR
LAZIER
LEADER
LEAKER
LEANER
LEAPER
LEASER
LEAVER
LECHER
LECTER
LECTOR
LEDGER
LEERER
LEHRER
LEITER
LELOIR
LENDER
LERNER
LESSER
LESSOR
LESTER
LETOUR
LETTER
LEVIER
LEWDER
LIBBER
LICKER
LIEBER
LIEDER
LIEFER
LIEFOR
LIENOR
LIFTER
LIMBER
LIMIER
LIMNER
LIMPER
LINDER
LINEAR
LINGER
LINIER
LINKER
LINTER
LINZER
LIPPER
LIQUOR
LISPER
LISTER
LITHER
LITTER
LOADER
LOAFER
LOANER
LOBBER
LOCHER
LOCKER
LODGER
LOFTER
LOGGER
LOGIER
LOITER
LOLLER
LONGER
LOOKER
LOOPER
LOOSER
LOOTER
LOPPER
LOTHAR
LOTTER
LOUDER
LOUVER
LOWTAR
LUBBER
LUGGER
LULLER
LUMBAR
LUMBER
LUMPER
LUMPUR
LUNGER
LUNKER
LURKER
LUSHER
LUSTER
LUTHER
LUTHOR

•LR•••

ALRITZ
ELRENO
ULRICH

•L•R••

ALARIC
ALARMS
ALARUM
ALDRIN
ALEROS
ALERTS
ALFRED
ALGREN
ALTRIA
BLARED
BLARES
BLURBS
BLURRY
BLURTS
CLARET
CLARKE
CLAROS
CLERGY
CLERIC
CLERKS
CLORIS
CLOROX
ELBRUS
ELYRIA
FLARED
FLARES
FLIRTS
FLIRTY
FLORAE
FLORAL
FLORAS
FLOREK
FLORES
FLORET
FLOREY
FLORID
FLORIN
FLORIO
FLURRY
FLYROD
GLARED
GLARES
GLARUS
GLORIA
GLURGE
OLERUD
OLORES
PLURAL
SLURPS
SLURRY
ULTRAS
XLARGE

•L••R•

ALBERS
ALBERT
ALBORG
ALDERS
ALEGRE
ALGORE
ALHIRT
ALLPRO
ALLURE
ALPERT
ALTARF
ALTARS
ALTERS
ALUDRA
ALVARO
ALZIRA
BLEARS
BLEARY
BLURRY
CLAIRE
CLAIRS
CLEARS
CLEARY
CLUERS
ELBERT
ELBURZ
ELDERS
ELGART
ELLERY
ELLORA
ELMERS
ELMIRA
ELMIRE
ELMORE
ELNORA
ELTORO
ELUARD
ELVERS
ELVIRA
FLAIRS
FLEERS
FLEURS
FLIERS
FLOORS
FLOURS
FLOURY
FLUORO
FLURRY
FLYERS
GLIERE
GLUERS
ILLDRY
LLADRO
OLDPRO
OLEARY
OLMERT
PLEURA
PLIERS
SLURRY
ULCERS

•L•••R

ALEGAR
ALINER
ALLFOR
ALOMAR
ALTAIR
ALULAR
ALYDAR
BLADER
BLAMER
BLAZER
BLOWER
CLAMOR
CLAWER
CLEVER
CLONER
CLOSER
CLOVER
DLAYER
ELATER
ELAYER
ELIDER
ELINOR
ELITER
ELIXIR
ELMIER
ELOPER
ELUDER
FLAKER
FLAMER
FLAVOR
FLAYER
FLEXOR
FLOWER
FLUTER
GLAMOR
GLASER
GLAZER
GLIDER
GLOVER
GLOWER
GLUIER
OLDCAR
OLIVER
PLACER
PLANAR
PLANER

PLATER
PLAYER
PLEXOR
PLOMER
PLOVER
PLOWER
SLAKER
SLATER
SLAVER
SLAYER
SLICER
SLIDER
SLIVER
SLOPER
SLOWER
ULSTER

••LR••

DELRAY
DELREY
DELRIO
DELROY
GILROY
KILROY
OILRIG
OILRUB
WALRUS

••L•R•

ABLARE
AFLARE
AGLARE
AILURO
ALLPRO
ALLURE
AOLERS
BALERS
BELFRY
BOLERO
CALORY
CELERY
CHLORO
COLORS
DOLORE
DOLORS
EELERS
EELERY
EILERS
EILERT
ELLERY
ELLORA
FILERS
FULCRA
GALORE
HILARY
HOLERS
IDLERS
ILLDRY
MALARS
MALORY
MILERS
MILORD
MOLARS
MYLARS
MYLORD
NFLERS
NHLERS
OGLERS
OILERS
OWLERY
PALTRY
PELTRY
PILERS
POLARA
POLERS
PULERS
RILERS
RULERS
SALARY
SCLERA
SOLARA
SOLERS
SULTRY
TALERS
TILERS
TILERY
TOLARS
TULARE
TYLERS
VALERA
VALERE
VALERO
VALERY
VALORS
VELARS
VELCRO
VELURE
VOLARE
WYLERS

••L••R

ALLFOR
BALDER
BALDUR
BALKER
BALMER
BELAIR
BELIER
BELTER
BELZER
BILKER
BILLER
BOLDER
BOLGER
BOLTER
BULGAR
BULGUR
BULWER
CALDER
CALKER
CALLER
CALMER
CELLAR
COLDER
COLLAR
COLMAR
COLOUR
COLTER
CULLER
DELMAR
DELVER
DILLAR
DILLER
DOLLAR
DOLOUR
DULLER
ECLAIR
EELIER
FALLER
FALSER
FALTER
FELLER
FILLER
FILTER
FOLDER
FOLGER
FOLIAR
FULLER
FULMAR
GELLAR
GELLER
GILDER
GOLFER
GULPER
HALTER
HALVER
HELLER
HELMER
HELPER
HELTER
HILLER
HOLDER
HOLIER
HOLLER
HULLER
JILTER
JOLTER
KALMAR
KELLER
KILLER
KILMER
KILTER
LELOIR
LOLLER
LULLER
MELDER
MELTER
MILDER
MILKER
MILLER
MILNER
MOLDER
MOLNAR
MOLTER
MULDER
MULLER
OILIER
OWLIER
PALLOR
PALMAR
PALMER
PALTER
PELTER
PILFER
PILLAR
POLGAR
POLLER
PULLER
PULPER
PULSAR
PULVER
RELIER
ROLFER
ROLLER
RULIER
SALTER
SALVER
SALVOR
SELLER
SILVER
SOLDER
SOLVER
SULFUR
SULKER
TALKER
TALLER
TELLER
TILLER
TILTER
TOLLER
UGLIER
VALOUR
VALUER
VELOUR
VULGAR
WALKER
WALLER
WALTER
WELDER
WELLER
WELTER
WILBUR
WILDER
WILIER
WILLER
WOLPER
YELLER
YELPER

•••L•R

AGILER
ALULAR
AMBLER
AMPLER
ANGLER
ANTLER
ASHLAR
BAILER
BAILOR
BAWLER
BAYLOR
BILLER
BIRLER
BOILER
BOWLER
BUGLER
BURLER
BUTLER
CABLER
CALLER
CELLAR
CHOLER
COALER
COILER
COLLAR
COOLER
COTLER
CULLER
CURLER
CUTLER
CUYLER
CYCLER
DEALER
DEBLUR
DIALER
DILLAR
DILLER
DOLLAR
DUELER
DULLER
EGGLER
ENSLER
EVILER
EXILER
FABLER
FALLER
FEELER
FELLER
FIDLER
FILLER
FOOLER
FOULER
FOWLER
FUELER
FULLER
GABLER
GAOLER
GELLAR
GELLER
HABLAR
HAGLER
HAILER
HAULER
HEALER
HEELER
HELLER
HILLER
HOLLER
HOWLER
HULLER
HURLER
JAILER
JAILOR
KEELER
KEGLER
KELLER
KEPLER
KEVLAR
KILLER
KOHLER
KUBLER
LADLER
LOLLER
LULLER
MAHLER
MAILER
MAULER
MEWLER
MIDLER
MILLER
MOILER
MULLER
NAILER
NOBLER
OBOLER
OCULAR
OSTLER
OVULAR
PALLOR
PARLOR
PEALER
PEELER
PEGLER
PILLAR
POLLER
POOLER
POPLAR
PULLER
QUELER
RAILER
REALER
REELER
RIFLER
ROLLER
SADLER
SAILER
SAILOR
SCALAR
SCALER
SEALER
SELLER
SIGLER
SISLER
SMALLR
SMILER
STALER
STELAR
STYLER
TAILER
TAILOR
TALLER
TATLER
TAYLOR
TELLER
THALER
TILLER
TOILER
TOLLER
TOOLER
UVULAR
VEILER
WAILER
WALLER
WELLER
WHALER
WILLER
WOHLER
YELLER
YOWLER

••••LR

SMALLR

L•S•••

LASCAR
LASERS
LASHED
LASHER
LASHES
LASHTO
LASHUP
LASING
LASKER
LASSEN
LASSER
LASSES
LASSIE
LASSOS
LASTED
LASTEX
LASTLY
LASTRA
LASTUP
LASZLO
LESAGE
LESBOS
LESHAN
LESION
LESLEY
LESLIE
LESMIZ
LESSEE
LESSEN
LESSER
LESSON
LESSOR
LESTAT
LESTER
LISBOA
LISBON
LISLES
LISPED
LISPER
LISSES
LISTED
LISTEE
LISTEN
LISTER
LISTON
LOSDOS
LOSEIT
LOSERS
LOSETO
LOSING
LOSSES
LOSTIT
LOSTTO
LTSULU
LUSAKA
LUSHER
LUSHES
LUSHLY
LUSTED
LUSTER
LUSTRA
LUSTRE
LYSINE

L••S••

LAMSIT
LANSKY
LANSON
LAPSAT
LAPSED
LAPSER
LAPSES
LAPSUP
LAPSUS
LARSEN
LARSON
LASSEN
LASSER
LASSES
LASSIE
LASSOS
LAWSON
LAYSBY
LAYSIN
LAYSON
LAYSTO
LAYSUP
LEASED
LEASER
LEASES
LEASTS
LEGSIT
LEISEN
LENSED
LENSES
LESSEE
LESSEN
LESSER
LESSON
LESSOR
LETSAT
LETSBE
LETSBY
LETSGO
LETSIN
LETSON
LETSUP
LHASAN
LIESIN
LIESON
LIESTO
LISSES
LOGSIN
LOGSON
LOOSED
LOOSEN
LOOSER
LOOSES
LOOSEY
LOSSES
LOTSOF
LOUSED
LOUSES
LOWSET

L•••S•

LACASA
LAKIST
LAMESA
LAMEST
LANOSE
LAOTSE
LAROSA
LATEST
LATISH
LAVISH
LAXEST
LEGIST
LETUSE
LHOTSE
LIAISE
LIKESO
LIPASE
LIVEST
LOCUST
LOUISA
LOUISB
LOUISE
LOUISI
LOUISV
LOUISX
LOWEST
LOWISH
LUGOSI
LUTIST
LYRIST

L••••S

LABELS
LABORS
LACERS
LACLOS
LADERS
LADIES
LADLES
LAGERS
LAIRDS
LAKERS
LAMEDS
LAMIAS
LANAIS
LANCES
LANDIS
LANDUS
LANTOS
LAPELS
LAPINS
LAPSES
LAPSUS
LARAMS
LAREES
LARGES
LARGOS
LARVAS
LASERS
LASHES
LASSES
LASSOS
LATENS
LATHES
LATINS
LATKES
LATTES
LAUGHS
LAVERS
LAYBYS
LAYERS
LAYINS
LAYUPS
LBEAMS
LEARNS
LEASES
LEASTS
LEAVES
LEDGES
LEEVES
LEGALS
LEGROS
LEHUAS
LEICAS
LEMANS
LEMMAS
LEMNOS
LEMONS
LEMURS
LENSES
LENTOS
LEPERS
LESBOS
LETUPS
LEVEES
LEVELS
LEVERS
LEVIES
LIANAS
LIANES
LIANGS
LIBBYS
LIBELS
LIBERS
LIBRAS
LIBRIS
LIBROS
LIEBYS
LIEGES
LIEUTS
LIFEIS
LIFERS
LIGERS
LIGHTS
LIGNES
LIKENS
LIKERS
LILACS
LILIES
LILLIS
LIMANS
LIMBOS
LIMITS
LINENS
LINERS
LINGUS
LIPIDS
LISLES
LISSES
LITERS
LITHOS
LITMUS
LITRES
LIVENS
LIVERS
LIVRES
LLAMAS
LLANOS
LLOYDS
LOAVES
LOCALS
LODENS
LODGES
LOFTUS
LOGANS
LOGICS
LOGINS
LOGONS
LONERS
LONGES
LOOEYS
LOOFAS
LOOIES
LOOSES
LOPERS
LORANS
LORIES
LOSDOS
LOSERS
LOSSES
LOTNOS
LOTTOS
LOUIES
LOUMAS
LOUPES
LOUSES
LOVERS
LOVEYS
LOWERS
LOWIQS
LOWRES
LTGOVS
LTILES
LUCIUS
LUDENS
LUGERS
LUMENS
LUNDIS
LUNGES
LUNIKS
LURERS
LUSHES
LUTZES
LWAVES
LYCEES
LYCRAS
LYMPHS
LYNXES
LYRICS
LYRIDS

•LS•••

ALSACE
ALSTON
ELSTON
ULSTER

•L•S••

ALASKA
ALISON
ALISTS
ALLSET
ALYSSA
BLASTS
BLISTS
CLASPS
CLASSA
CLASSE
CLASSY
CLOSED
CLOSER
CLOSES
CLOSET
ELISEO
ELISHA
ELISSA
ELISTS
ELYSEE
FLASHY
FLASKS
FLESHY
FLOSSY
GLASER
GLASSY
GLOSSA
GLOSSO
GLOSSY
ILLSAY
ILLSEE
ILLSET
OLDSAW
OLDSOD
OLESHA
OLESON
PLASHY
PLASMA
PLASMO
PLISSE
PLUSES
PLUSHY
SLOSHY
SLUSHY
VLASIC

•L••S•

ALDISS
ALEAST
ALMOST
ALNASL
ALONSO
ALWEST
ALYSSA
BLAISE
BLOUSE
BLOWSY
BLUEST
BLUESY
BLUISH
CLASSA
CLASSE
CLASSY
CLAUSE
CLEESE
CLUMSY
ELAPSE
ELDEST
ELFISH
ELISSA
ELOISA
ELOISE
ELPASO
ELVISH
FLENSE
FLIMSY
FLOPSY
FLOSSY
FLUISH
FLYASH
GLASSY
GLOSSA
GLOSSO
GLOSSY
ILLEST
ILLUSE
KLEIST
NLEAST
NLWEST
OLDEST
OLDISH
PLEASE
PLISSE
SLIEST
SLYEST

•L•••S

ALALAS
ALAMOS
ALANIS
ALARMS
ALBANS
ALBERS
ALBUMS
ALDERS
ALDISS
ALDOUS
ALECKS
ALEPHS
ALEROS
ALERTS
ALEUTS
ALEVES
ALEXAS
ALEXIS
ALIBIS
ALICES
ALIENS
ALIGNS
ALIKES
ALINES
ALISTS
ALKIES
ALKYDS
ALKYLS
ALLAIS
ALLAYS
ALLEES
ALLEYS
ALLIES
ALLOTS
ALLOWS
ALLOYS
ALLYLS
ALMVPS
ALOHAS
ALONGS
ALPHAS
ALTARS
ALTERS
ALTIUS
ALWAYS
BLACKS
BLADES
BLAFFS
BLAMES
BLANKS
BLARES
BLASTS
BLAZES
BLEAKS
BLEARS
BLEATS
BLEEDS
BLEEPS
BLENDS
BLIMPS
BLINDS
BLINIS
BLINKS
BLISTS
BLOATS
BLOCKS
BLOKES
BLONDS
BLOODS
BLOOMS
BLOOPS
BLUETS
BLUFFS
BLUNTS
BLURBS
BLURTS
CLACKS
CLAIMS
CLAIRS
CLAMPS
CLANGS
CLANKS
CLAROS
CLASPS
CLAVES
CLEANS
CLEARS
CLEATS
CLEEKS
CLEFTS
CLERKS
CLEVES
CLICKS
CLIFFS
CLIMBS
CLIMES
CLINGS
CLINKS
CLOAKS
CLOCKS
CLOMPS
CLONES
CLONKS
CLORIS
CLOSES
CLOTHS
CLOUDS
CLOUTS
CLOVES
CLOVIS
CLOWNS
CLUCKS
CLUERS
CLUMPS
CLUNKS
CLYDES
ELANDS
ELATES
ELBOWS
ELBRUS
ELDERS
ELECTS
ELEMIS
ELEVES
ELIDES
ELISTS
ELITES
ELLIOS
ELMERS
ELOGES
ELOPES
ELPAIS
ELUDES
ELUTES
ELVERS
ELYTIS
FLACKS
FLAILS
FLAIRS
FLAKES
FLAMES
FLANKS
FLARES
FLASKS
FLAXES
FLECKS
FLEERS
FLEETS
FLEURS
FLEXES
FLICKS
FLIERS
FLINGS
FLINTS
FLIRTS
FLOATS
FLOCKS
FLOODS
FLOORS
FLORAS
FLORES
FLOURS
FLOUTS
FLUFFS
FLUIDS
FLUKES
FLUMES
FLUNKS
FLUTES
FLUXES
FLYBYS
FLYERS
FLYINS
GLACES
GLACIS
GLADES
GLADYS
GLANDS
GLARES
GLARUS
GLAZES
GLEAMS
GLEANS
GLIDES
GLINTS
GLOATS
GLOBES
GLOCKS
GLOGGS
GLOOMS
GLOUCS
GLOVES
GLUERS
GLUONS
GLUTES
GLYNIS
GLYPHS
ILEXES
ILIADS
KLICKS
LLAMAS
LLANOS
LLOYDS
NLMVPS
OLAKES

OLDIES OLEINS OLEUMS OLIVES OLMECS OLORES PLACES PLAGES PLAIDS PLAINS PLAITS PLANAS PLANBS PLANES PLANKS PLANTS PLATES PLATOS PLATYS PLAYAS PLAZAS PLEADS PLEATS PLEBES PLEXES PLEXUS PLIERS PLINKS PLOCES PLONKS PLUCKS PLUIES PLUMBS PLUMES PLUMPS PLUNKS PLUSES PLUTUS SLACKS SLAKES SLANGS SLANTS SLATES SLAVES SLEEKS SLEEPS SLEETS SLICES SLICKS SLIDES SLIMES SLINGS SLINKS SLOOPS SLOPES SLOTHS SLUMPS SLURPS ULCERS ULTRAS ZLOTYS

••LS••

ALLSET BALSAM BALSAS BOLSHY COLSON DELSOL DILSEY FALSER FELSON FOLSOM GELSEY HALSEY ILLSAY ILLSEE ILLSET JOLSON KELSEY MILSAP MOLSON NELSON POLSKA PULSAR PULSED PULSES SALSAS TILSIT TILSON TULSAN VALSES VELSEN WILSON WOLSEY

••L•S•

ABLEST ABLUSH ARLISS ASLOSH ATLAST AWLESS BALLST CALASH DALASI DELISH DELIST ECLASS EGLISE ENLIST EULESS FILOSE FOLKSY GALOSH GOLAST HALEST HOLISM HOLIST IDLEST ILLEST ILLUSE MILOSZ MOLEST MULISH NOLESS NOLOSE NOLOSS OBLAST OWLISH PALEST PALISH PELOSI PILOSE POLISH RELISH RELIST RELOSE RELOST SALISH SPLASH SPLOSH TALESE TALISA TOLAST UNLASH UNLESS UNLOST UNLUSH UPLAST VALISE VILEST WALESA WALLST XYLOSE

••L••S

ADLIBS AFLATS AGLETS ALLAIS ALLAYS ALLEES ALLEYS ALLIES ALLOTS ALLOWS ALLOYS ALLYLS AOLERS ARLISS AWLESS BALERS BALLYS BALSAS BELAYS BELIES BELLES BELONS BFLATS BILGES BILLIS BOLLAS BULGES BYLAWS BYLOTS CALAIS CALIFS CALLAS CALLES CALLUS CALVES CALXES CCLEFS CELEBS CELLOS CFLATS COLBYS COLEUS COLICS COLONS COLORS CULETS CULLIS CULTUS DALETS DALLAS DALLES DELAYS DELCOS DELFTS DELIUS DELTAS DELVES DFLATS DOLAPS DOLMAS DOLORS DULLES ECLASS ECLATS EELERS EFLATS EILERS ELLIOS EULESS FELIDS FELLAS FELONS FFLATS FILERS FILETS FILLES FOLEYS FOLIES FOLIOS GALOIS GALOPS GCLEFS GELEES GFLATS GILELS GILLIS GOLEMS GULAGS HALLOS HALOES HALVAS HALVES HELENS HELIOS HELLAS HELLOS HELOTS HOLERS HOLIES HOLLIS HOLMES HULLOS IDLERS IGLOOS INLAWS INLAYS INLETS ISLETS ISLEYS JALPAS JELLOS JULEPS JULIUS KELLYS KILIMS KULAKS LILACS LILIES LILLIS MALARS MALAYS MELEES MELONS MILANS MILERS MILLES MILNES MOLARS MULCTS MULEYS MULLAS MULTIS MYLARS NELLIS NFLERS NHLERS NOLESS NOLOSS NULLOS NYLONS OGLERS OILERS ONLAYS ORLONS ORLOPS OWLETS OXLIPS PALAIS PALLAS PALMAS PCLABS PELEUS PELVIS PILAFS PILAUS PILERS PILEUS PILOTS PILOUS POLERS POLIOS POLKAS POLLOS POLYPS PULERS PULSES PYLONS RELAPS RELAYS RELETS RELICS RELIES RELOGS RILERS RILLES ROLEOS RULERS SALADS SALEPS SALLES SALMIS SALONS SALSAS SALVES SALVOS SELVES SILVAS SOLANS SOLEAS SOLERS SOLEUS SOLIDS SOLONS SOLVES SPLATS SPLAYS SPLITS SULFAS SYLPHS TALERS TALONS TALTOS TELCOS TILAKS TILDES TILERS TILLIS TILTHS TOLARS TULIPS TULLES TYLERS UCLANS UGLIES UHLANS UNLAYS UNLESS VALAIS VALENS VALETS VALOIS VALORS VALSES VALUES VALVES VELARS VÊLDTS VILLAS VOLANS VOLVOS VULGUS WALLIS WALRUS WELCHS WELLES WILKES WILLIS WILLYS WOLVES WYLERS XYLEMS YALIES ZHLOBS ZHLUBS

•••LS•

AVULSE BALLST DIALSO EVULSE ORELSE URALSK WALLST WHILST

•••L•S

ABELES ACELAS ADDLES ADULTS AEOLUS AIOLIS AISLES AKELAS ALALAS AMBLES AMOLES ANELES ANGLES ANGLOS ANKLES ANOLES APPLES ATILES ATOLLS AZOLES BALLYS BAULKS BCELLS BEALLS BELLES BIBLES BILLIS BOGLES BOLLAS BOULES BOWLES BOYLES BTILES BUGLES BUILDS CABLES CALLAS CALLES CALLUS CARLOS CAULKS CELLOS CHALKS CHILES CHILIS CHILLS CHOLOS CIELOS CTILES CULLIS CYCLES CYCLOS DALLAS DALLES DCELLS DHOLES DJILAS DOALLS DOBLES DOULAS DRILLS DROLLS DTILES DULLES DUPLOS DWELLS EAGLES ECCLES ECOLES EDILES EFILES EGALES EMALLS EMILYS ETILES EXALTS EXILES EXULTS FABLES FAULTS FELLAS FHOLES FIELDS FILLES FOWLES FRILLS FTILES GABLES GILLIS GRILLS GTILES GUILDS GUILES HALLOS HAOLES HELLAS HELLOS HOLLIS HOYLES HTILES HULLOS IDYLLS INGLES INKLES ISTLES ITILES JELLOS JOULES JTILES KELLYS KNELLS KNOLLS KOALAS KTILES KVELLS LACLOS LADLES LILLIS LISLES LTILES MACLES MAJLIS MAPLES MIELES MILLES MOULDS MOULTS MTILES MULLAS NAPLES NELLIS NOBLES NTILES NULLOS NYALAS OBELUS OBOLUS OCULUS ONCLES OODLES ORALES OTILES OVULES OXALIS PALLAS PEALES PHELPS POILUS POLLOS POULES POULTS PROLES PSALMS PTILES QTILES QUALES QUALMS QUELLS QUILLS QUILTS REALES REALMS REGLES REYLES RIFLES RILLES ROBLES RTILES RUBLES SABLES SALLES SAULTS SAYLES SCALDS SCALES SCALPS SCOLDS SCULLS SEALYS SHALES SHELLS SHILLS SIDLES SKALDS SKILLS SKULKS SKULLS SMALLS SMELLS SMELTS SMILES SMOLTS SNELLS SOCLES SPELLS SPILES SPILLS STALES STALKS STALLS STELAS STELES STILES STILLS STILTS STOLAS STOLES STYLES STYLUS SWALES SWELLS SWILLS TABLAS TABLES TBILLS TCELLS TENLBS TESLAS THALES THILLS THOLES TILLIS TITLES TOILES TOKLAS TRALAS TRILLS TROLLS TTILES TULLES TWILLS UBOLTS UNCLES UVULAS VAULTS VILLAS VIOLAS VOILES VTILES WALLIS WEALDS WELLES WHALES WHELKS WHELMS WHELPS WHILES WHOLES WIELDS WILLIS WILLYS WORLDS WTILES XFILES XTILES YIELDS YTILES ZTILES

••••LS

ADVILS ALKYLS ALLYLS ANGELS ANNALS ANNULS ANVILS APPALS APPELS APRILS ARPELS ARTELS ATOLLS AVAILS AVRILS BABELS BAGELS BASILS BCELLS BEALLS BERYLS BETELS BEVELS BEZELS BGIRLS BOTELS BOWELS BRAWLS BROILS CABALS CAMELS CANALS CAROLS CASALS CAVILS CEORLS CHILLS CHURLS COPALS CORALS CRAWLS CREELS CUPELS DCELLS DECALS DEGELS DEVILS DOALLS DOWELS DRAWLS DRILLS DROLLS DROOLS DWELLS DYNELS EASELS EDSELS EMAILS EMALLS ENGELS ENOILS ENROLS EQUALS ETAILS ETHYLS EXCELS EXPELS EXTOLS FERALS FINALS FLAILS FRIELS FRILLS FUSILS GAVELS GHOULS GILELS GIMELS GNARLS GRAILS GRILLS GROWLS GRRRLS GRUELS HAZELS HOSELS HOTELS HOVELS IDEALS IDYLLS IMPELS INGELS JACALS JEWELS KNEELS KNELLS KNOLLS KNURLS KRAALS KVELLS LABELS LAPELS LEGALS LEVELS LIBELS LOCALS MEDALS METALS MODALS MODELS MOGULS MORALS MORELS MOTELS MURALS NASALS NAVELS NEWELS NOBELS NOPALS NOVELS ODOULS OFFALS OPHULS ORIELS OUSELS OUZELS PANDLS PANELS PAROLS PEARLS PEDALS PERILS PETALS PHIALS PIXELS PROWLS PUJOLS PUPILS QUAILS QUELLS QUILLS RATELS RAVELS REBELS REGELS REOILS REPELS REVELS RIVALS RIYALS ROWELS ROYALS RUBELS SABALS SCOWLS SCULLS SEPALS SHAWLS SHELLS SHILLS SHOALS SIBYLS SIGILS SISALS SKILLS SKIRLS SKOALS SKULLS SMALLS SMELLS SNAILS SNARLS SNELLS SPELLS SPIELS SPILLS SPOILS SPOOLS STALLS STEALS STEELS STILLS STOOLS SWELLS SWILLS SWIRLS TAMILS TAVELS TAXOLS TBILLS TCELLS THILLS TICALS TOTALS TOWELS TRAILS TRAWLS TRIALS TRILLS TROLLS TWILLS TWIRLS UHAULS UMBELS USUALS VIGILS VINYLS VITALS VOCALS VOWELS WEDELS WHEELS WHIRLS WHORLS YODELS YOKELS

LT••••

LTGOVS LTILES LTSULU

L•T•••

LATEEN LATELY LATENE LATENS LATENT LATEOF LATEON LATERI LATERO LATEST LATETO LATHED LATHEN LATHER LATHES LATIGO LATINA LATINI LATINO LATINS LATISH LATKES LATOUR LATOYA LATRIA LATTER LATTES LATVIA LETFLY LETHAL LETOFF LETOUR LETOUT LETRIP LETSAT LETSBE LETSBY LETSGO LETSIN LETSON LETSUP LETTED LETTER LETTRE LETUPS LETUSE LITANY LITCHI LITERS LITHER LITHIC LITHOS LITMUS LITOUT LITRES LITTER LITTLE LITTRE LITVAK LOTHAR LOTION LOTNOS LOTSOF LOTTED LOTTER LOTTOS LUTECE LUTHER LUTHOR LUTIST LUTZES LYTTON

L••T••

LACTEA LACTIC LANTOS LAOTSE LAOTZU LAPTEV LAPTOP LARTER LARTET LASTED LASTEX LASTLY LASTRA LASTUP LATTER LATTES LAUTER LAWTON LECTER LECTOR LEFTBE LEFTIN LEFTIT LEFTOF LEFTON LEITER LENTEN LENTIL LENTOS LENTTO LEPTON LESTAT LESTER LETTED LETTER LETTRE LEUTZE LHOTSE LIFTED LIFTER LIFTUP LILTED LINTED LINTEL LINTER LINTON LIOTTA LIPTON LISTED

LISTEE
LISTEN
LISTER
LISTON
LITTER
LITTLE
LITTRE
LOATHE
LOFTED
LOFTER
LOFTON
LOFTUS
LOITER
LOOTED
LOOTER
LOSTIT
LOSTTO
LOTTED
LOTTER
LOTTOS
LOWTAR
LOWTOP
LUNTHA
LUPTON
LUSTED
LUSTER
LUSTRA
LUSTRE
LYTTON

L•••T•

LABATT
LAIDTO
LAKOTA
LANATE
LAPUTA
LASHTO
LATETO
LAXITY
LAYSTO
LEADTO
LEALTY
LEANTO
LEASTS
LEGATE
LEGATO
LENDTO
LENGTH
LENITY
LENTTO
LEVITE
LEVITT
LEVITY
LIEDTO
LIESTO
LIEUTS
LIGATE
LIGETI
LIGHTS
LIKETO
LIKUTA
LILITH
LIMITS
LIOTTA
LIVETH
LIVETV
LOBATE
LOCATE
LOLITA
LOOKTO
LOSETO
LOSTTO
LOVETO
LOVETT
LUCITE
LUNATE
LUXATE

L••••T

LABATT
LABRAT
LAKIST
LAMENT
LAMEST
LAMONT
LAMSIT
LANCET
LANDAT
LAPCAT
LAPPET
LAPSAT
LARIAT
LARTET
LATENT
LATEST
LAXALT
LAXEST
LAYOUT
LEAPAT
LEARNT
LEBRET
LEDOUT
LEERAT
LEFTIT
LEGART
LEGIST
LEGSIT
LESTAT
LETOUT
LETSAT
LEVANT
LEVERT
LEVITT
LIMPET
LINNET
LIONET
LIPOUT
LITOUT
LIVEAT
LIVEST
LOCCIT
LOCKET
LOCUST
LOGOUT
LOIRET
LONGET
LOOKAT
LOQUAT
LORDIT
LOSEIT
LOSTIT
LOVEIT
LOVETT
LOWCUT
LOWEST
LOWFAT
LOWSET
LUCENT
LUGNUT
LUGOUT
LUMPIT
LUTIST
LYRIST

•LT•••

ALTAIC
ALTAIR
ALTARF
ALTARS
ALTERS
ALTHEA
ALTIMA
ALTIUS
ALTKEY
ALTMAN
ALTOID
ALTRIA
ALTTAB
ELTORO
ULTIMA
ULTIMO
ULTRAS

•L•T••

ALATED
ALETAP
ALETTE
ALOTOF
ALSTON
ALTTAB
BLATTY
BLITHE
BLOTCH
BLOTTO
BLOTTY
BLOTUP
BLYTHE
BLYTON
CLOTHE
CLOTHO
CLOTHS
CLOTTY
CLOTUP
CLUTCH
ELATED
ELATER
ELATES
ELITER
ELITES
ELKTON
ELSTON
ELUTED
ELUTES
ELYTIS
FLATLY
FLATTV
FLETCH
FLITBY
FLITIN
FLUTED
FLUTER
FLUTES
FLUTIE
GLITCH
GLITZY
GLOTTO
GLUTEI
GLUTEN
GLUTES
KLATCH
KLUTZY
OLATHE
PLATED
PLATEN
PLATER
PLATES
PLATOS
PLATTE
PLATYS
PLOTTY
PLUTON
PLUTUS
SLATED
SLATER
SLATES
SLITHY
SLOTHS
ULSTER
ZLOTYS

•L••T•

ALCOTT
ALECTO
ALERTS
ALETTE
ALEUTS
ALIOTH
ALIOTO
ALISTS
ALLOTS
ALMATY
ALRITZ
BLASTS
BLATTY
BLEATS
BLEETH
BLINTZ
BLISTS
BLOATS
BLOTTO
BLOTTY
BLUETS
BLUNTS
BLURTS
CLEATS
CLEFTS
CLOETE
CLOTTY
CLOUTS
ELECTS
ELISTS
ELNATH
ELUATE
FLATTV
FLAUTA
FLEETS
FLEWTO
FLINTS
FLINTY
FLIRTS
FLIRTY
FLOATS
FLOATY
FLOUTS
GLADTO
GLINTS
GLINTY
GLOATS
GLOTTO
GLUETO
GLYPTO
KLAATU
KLEPTO
OLEATE
PLAITS
PLANTE
PLANTO
PLANTS
PLATTE
PLAYTO
PLEATS
PLEDTO
PLENTY
PLINTH
PLOTTY
SLANTS
SLEETS
SLEETY
SLEUTH

•L•••T

ALBEIT
ALBERT
ALCOTT
ALEAST
ALHIRT
ALIGHT
ALIYOT
ALLBUT
ALLOUT
ALLSET
ALLWET
ALMOST
ALPERT
ALWEST
BLEWIT
BLIGHT
BLOUNT
BLOWIT
BLUEST
CLARET
CLAWAT
CLIENT
CLIMAT
CLOSET
ELANET
ELBERT
ELDEST
ELEGIT
ELGART
ELICIT
ELLIOT
ELMONT
ELUANT
FLAUNT
FLEWAT
FLIGHT
FLOPIT
FLORET
FLUENT
FLYNET
FLYOUT
HLHUNT
ILLBET
ILLEST
ILLLIT
ILLMET
ILLSET
KLEIST
NLEAST
NLWEST
OLDBAT
OLDEST
OLDHAT
OLMERT
PLAINT
PLAKAT
PLANET
PLAYAT
PLAYIT
PLIANT
PLIGHT
SLIEST
SLIGHT
SLYEST

••LT••

BALTIC
BELTED
BELTER
BELTON
BELTUP
BOLTED
BOLTER
BOLTON
BOLTUP
CELTIC
COLTER
COLTON
CULTCH
CULTIC
CULTUS
DALTON
DELTAS
DELTIC
DOLTON
FALTER
FELTED
FELTOK
FILTER
FILTHY
FULTON
GALTON
HALTED
HALTER
HELTER
HILTED
HILTON
JILTED
JILTER
JOLTED
JOLTER
JOLTIN
KELTON
KILTED
KILTER
KILTIE
LILTED
MALTBY
MALTED
MALTIN
MELTED
MELTER
MELTON
MILTIE
MILTON
MOLTED
MOLTEN
MOLTER
MOLTKE
MULTIS
PALTER
PALTRY
PELTED
PELTER
PELTRY
SALTED
SALTEN
SALTER
SALTII
SALTON
SELTEN
SILTED
SULTAN
SULTRY
TALTOS
TILTAT
TILTED
TILTER
TILTHS
TILTON
TILTUP
TOLTEC
WALTER
WALTON
WELTED
WELTER
WILTED
WILTON
ZOLTAN

••L•T•

ABLATE
AFLATS
AGLETS
ALLOTS
APLITE
BALATA
BELATE
BFLATS
BYLOTS
CALLTO
CFLATS
CULETS
DALETH
DALETS
DELETE
DELFTS
DFLATS
DILATE
DILUTE
DULUTH
ECLATS
EFLATS
EOLITH
FALLTO
FELLTO
FFLATS
FILETS
FOLATE
GELATE
GELATI
GELATO
GELETT
GFLATS
GOLETA
HALITE
HELDTO
HELOTS
HOLDTO
IMLATE
INLETS
ISLATE
ISLETS
JCLOTH
LILITH
LOLITA
MALOTI
MELETE
MELOTT
MULCTS
MULETA
OBLATE
OFLATE
ONLATE
OOLITE
OWLETS
PALATE
PELOTA
PILATE
PILOTS
POLITE
POLITY
RELATE
RELETS
RULETH
SALUTE
SALUTO
SELLTO
SOLATI
SOLDTO
SOLUTE
SPLATS
SPLITS
TALKTO
UPLATE
VALETS
VELDTS
VOLUTE
WALKTO

••L••T

ABLEST
AFLOAT
AGLINT
ALLBUT
ALLOUT
ALLSET
ALLWET
ASLANT
ATLAST
AULAIT
BALKAT
BALLET
BALLOT
BALLST
BELOIT
BILLET
BULLET
CALLIT
CALVET
COLLAT
COLLET
CULLET
DELICT
DELINT
DELIST
DULCET
EELPOT
EILERT
ELLIOT
ENLIST
FILLET
GALANT
GALOOT
GELETT
GOLAST
GOLEFT
GULLET
HALEST
HELDIT
HELMET
HELMUT
HOLDIT
HOLIST
IDLEST
ILLBET
ILLEST
ILLLIT
ILLMET
ILLSET
ISLEFT
JOLIET
JOLIOT
JULIET
MALLET
MELOTT
MILLET
MOLEST
MULLET
OBLAST
OILLIT
PALEST
PALLET
PELLET
POLPOT
PULLET
PULPIT
RELENT
RELICT
RELIST
RELOST
RELUCT
RILLET
SALYUT
SELECT
SELLIT
SILENT
SOLDIT
SPLINT
TALENT
TALKAT
TELLIT
TELNET
TILLET
TILSIT
TILTAT
TOLAST
TOLDIT
UMLAUT
UNLEFT
UNLENT
UNLOST
UPLAST
UPLIFT
VALENT
VELVET
VILEST
VOLANT
WALLET
WALLST
WALNUT
WILMUT
YCLEPT
YELLAT

•••LT•

ADULTS
CALLTO
COOLTH
COOLTO
DEALTO
EXALTS
EXULTS
FAILTO
FALLTO
FAULTS
FAULTY
FAWLTY
FEALTY
FELLTO
GUILTY
HEALTH
LEALTY
MAILTO
MOULTS
POULTS
QUILTS
REALTY
RIALTO
SAILTO
SAULTS
SELLTO
SHELTY
SHULTZ
SMELTS
SMOLTS
SPILTH
STILTS
STOLTZ
SVELTE
UBOLTS
VAULTS
VAULTY
WEALTH

•••L•T

AIGLET
AMULET
ANKLET
APELET
APPLET
ARMLET
ASFLAT
AUKLET
BADLOT
BALLET
BALLOT
BALLST
BILLET
BULLET
CABLET
CALLIT
CANLIT
CAPLET
CARLOT
CHALET
COLLAT
COLLET
COOLIT
CULLET
CUTLET
DAYLIT
DECLOT
DIGLOT
DYELOT
EAGLET
EARLET
ENGLIT
ENGLUT
EYELET
FILLET
GASLIT
GIBLET
GIMLET
GOBLET
GOFLAT
GOULET
GULLET
HAMLET
HARLOT
HOWLAT
ILLLIT
JOBLOT
KIDLIT
MALLET
MERLOT
MILLET
MULLET
NAILIT
NIBLET
NUTLET
OCELOT
ODDLOT
ODELET
OILLIT
OMELET
OUTLET
PALLET
PELLET
PIELET
PIGLET
PIOLET
PULLET
RAILAT
REPLOT
RIBLET
RILLET
RUNLET
SAMLET
SCULPT
SELLIT
SHALIT
SKYLIT
SMALLT
STYLET
SUBLET
SUBLOT
SUNLIT
TABLET
TELLIT
THELOT
TILLET
TOILAT
TOILET
TWILIT
UNFLAT
VARLET
VIOLET
WALLET
WALLST
WHILST
WIGLET
YELLAT
ZEALOT

••••LT

BASALT
COBALT
DESALT
DESILT
INCULT
INSULT
ISEULT
KIDULT
KURALT
LAXALT
MODELT
MOROLT
NOSALT
OCCULT
PENULT
REBOLT
REMELT
RESALT
RESULT
REVOLT
SMALLT
SPOILT
TUMULT
TYBALT
UNBELT
UNBOLT
UNFELT
UNGILT
UNTILT
UPTILT

LU••••

LUANDA
LUBBER
LUBECK
LUBING
LUBLIN
LUCENT
LUCIAN
LUCIDA
LUCIEN
LUCILE
LUCINE
LUCITE
LUCIUS
LUCKED
LUDDEN
LUDENS
LUDLOW
LUDLUM
LUDWIG
LUELLA
LUFFED
LUGERS
LUGGED
LUGGER
LUGING
LUGLIO
LUGNUT
LUGOSI
LUGOUT
LUKICH
LULLED
LULLER
LUMBAR
LUMBER
LUMENS
LUMINA
LUMLEY
LUMMOX
LUMPED
LUMPEN
LUMPER
LUMPIN
LUMPIT
LUMPUR
LUNACY
LUNATE
LUNCHY
LUNDEN
LUNDIS
LUNEDI
LUNGED
LUNGER
LUNGES
LUNIKS
LUNKER
LUNTHA
LUNULA
LUPINE
LUPINO
LUPONE
LUPTON
LUREIN
LURENE
LURERS
LURING
LURKED
LURKER
LURKEY
LUSAKA
LUSHER
LUSHES
LUSHLY
LUSTED
LUSTER
LUSTRA
LUSTRE
LUTECE
LUTHER
LUTHOR
LUTIST
LUTZES
LUXATE
LUXURY

L•U•••

LAUDED
LAUDER
LAUGHS
LAULAU
LAUNCH
LAUPER
LAUREL
LAUREN
LAUREY
LAURIA
LAURIC
LAURIE
LAURYL
LAURYN
LAUTER
LEUTZE
LOUANN
LOUCHE
LOUDEN
LOUDER
LOUDLY
LOUDON
LOUIES
LOUISA
LOUISB
LOUISE
LOUISI
LOUISV
LOUISX
LOUMAS
LOUNGE
LOUPES
LOUSED
LOUSES
LOUVER
LOUVIN
LOUVRE

L••U••

LACUNA
LADUKE
LAGUNA
LAPUTA
LAYUPS
LAZULI
LEGUIN
LEGUME
LEHUAS
LEMUEL
LEMURS
LETUPS
LETUSE
LIEUTS
LIKUTA
LIQUID
LIQUOR
LOBULE
LOCUST
LOQUAT
LTSULU
LUNULA
LUXURY

L•••U•

LABIUM
LABOUR
LACEUP
LAIDUP
LAMOUR
LANDUP
LANDUS
LAPFUL
LAPSUP
LAPSUS
LARRUP
LASHUP
LASTUP
LATOUR
LAWFUL
LAYOUT
LAYSUP
LEADUP
LEAGUE
LEAPUP
LEBRUN
LEDOUT
LEDOUX
LENGUA
LEROUX
LETOUR
LETOUT
LETSUP
LICKUP
LIFTUP
LIGNUM
LINEUP
LINGUA
LINGUS
LINKUP
LIPOUT
LITMUS
LITOUT
LOADUP
LOCKUP
LOFTUS
LOGOUT
LONGUE
LOOKUP
LOOMUP
LOWCUT
LUCIUS
LUDLUM
LUGNUT
LUGOUT
LUMPUR
LYCEUM

L••••U

LANDAU
LAOTZU
LAULAU
LEBEAU
LIZALU
LTSULU

•LU•••
ALUDEL ALUDRA ALULAE ALULAR ALUMNA ALUMNI BLUDGE BLUELY BLUEOX BLUEST BLUESY BLUETS BLUFFO BLUFFS BLUING BLUISH BLUNTS BLURBS BLURRY BLURTS CLUBBY CLUBUP CLUCKS CLUEIN CLUERS CLUING CLUMPS CLUMPY CLUMSY CLUNKS CLUNKY CLUTCH ELUANT ELUARD ELUATE ELUDED ELUDER ELUDES ELUTED ELUTES FLUBUG FLUENT FLUFFS FLUFFY FLUIDS FLUISH FLUKES FLUKEY FLUMES FLUNKS FLUNKY FLUORO FLURRY FLUTED FLUTER FLUTES FLUTIE FLUXED FLUXES GLUEON GLUERS GLUETO GLUIER GLUING GLUMLY GLUONS GLURGE GLUTEI GLUTEN GLUTES KLUDGE KLUDGY KLUTZY PLUCKS PLUCKY PLUGIN PLUGUP PLUIES PLUMBO PLUMBS PLUMED PLUMES PLUMMY PLUMPS PLUNGE PLUNKS PLUNKY PLURAL PLUSES PLUSHY PLUTON PLUTUS PLUVIA PLUVIO SLUDGE SLUDGY SLUGGO SLUICE SLUING SLUMMY SLUMPS SLURPS SLURRY SLUSHY

•L•U••
ALBUMS ALEUTS ALLUDE ALLURE BLOUNT BLOUSE CLAUDE CLAUSE CLOUDS CLOUDY CLOUGH CLOUTS ELBURZ FLAUNT FLAUTA FLEURS FLOURS FLOURY FLOUTS GLOUCS HLHUNT ILLUDE ILLUME ILLUSE OLEUMS PLEURA PLOUGH SLEUTH SLOUCH SLOUGH

•L••U•
ALARUM ALDOUS ALEGUP ALLBUT ALLIUM ALLOUT ALTIUS BLEWUP BLOTUP BLOWUP CLAMUP CLAQUE CLIQUE CLIQUY CLOGUP CLOTUP CLUBUP ELBRUS FLEWUP FLIPUP FLUBUG FLYOUT GLAMUP GLARUS OLERUD PLAGUE PLAQUE PLAYUP PLENUM PLEXUS PLOWUP PLUGUP PLUTUS SLIPUP SLOWUP

•L•••U
KLAATU

••LU••
ABLUSH AILURO ALLUDE ALLURE BELUGA COLUMN DELUDE DELUGE DELUGG DELUXE DILUTE DULUTH FALUDI ILLUDE ILLUME ILLUSE INLUCK NOLUCK RELUCT RELUME SALUKI SALUTE SALUTO SOLUTE STLUKE UNLUSH VALUED VALUER VALUES VELURE VOLUME VOLUTE ZHLUBS

••L•U•
ALLBUT ALLIUM ALLOUT BALDUR BALLUP BELLUM BELTUP BOLTUP BULGUR BULKUP CALLUP CALLUS CILIUM COLEUS COLOUR CULLUM CULTUS DELIUS DOLLUP DOLOUR FILLUP FOLDUP FOLIUM FULLUP GALLUP GOLLUM HALLUX HELDUP HELIUM HELMUT HELPUP HOLDUP HOLEUP JULIUS OILCUP OILRUB PELEUS PILAUS PILEUM PILEUP PILEUS PILOUS POLLUX PULLUP RILEUP ROLLUP SALYUT SOLEUS SULFUR TALCUM TALKUP TALMUD TILTUP UMLAUT VALIUM VALOUR VELLUM VELOUR VULGUS WALKUP WALLUP WALNUT WALRUS WELLUP WILBUR WILMUT

••L••U
BALLOU INLIEU MALIBU MILIEU MOLDAU

•••LU•
AEOLUS ASYLUM BALLUP BELLUM BOILUP CALLUP CALLUS COILUP CULLUM CURLUP DEALUP DEBLUR DESLUM DIALUP DOLLUP EFFLUX ENGLUT FILLUP FOULUP FUELUP FULLUP GALLUP GOLLUM HALLUX HAULUP HEALUP IDOLUM INBLUE INFLUX KAHLUA KAILUA LUDLUM MRBLUE MUKLUK NAILUP OBELUS OBOLUS OCULUS PABLUM PEPLUM PHYLUM POILUS POLLUX PULLUP REELUP REFLUX REGLUE ROILUP ROLLUP RVALUE SCHLUB SEALUP STYLUS TOOLUP UNGLUE UNPLUG UVALUE VELLUM WALLUP WELLUP

•••L•U
BALLOU LAULAU SMALLU

••••LU
BABALU DESILU LIZALU LTSULU MARILU MRSULU ORMOLU SMALLU TUVALU

L•V•••
LAVABO LAVAGE LAVAIN LAVERN LAVERS LAVIDA LAVING LAVISH LEVADE LEVANT LEVEED LEVEES LEVELS LEVENE LEVERS LEVERT LEVIED LEVIER LEVIES LEVINE LEVITE LEVITT LEVITY LIVEAT LIVEIN LIVELY LIVENS LIVEON LIVERS LIVERY LIVEST LIVETH LIVETV LIVING LIVRES LOVAGE LOVEIN LOVEIT LOVELL LOVELY LOVERS LOVETO LOVETT LOVEYA LOVEYS LOVING

L••V••
LANVAL LANVIN LARVAE LARVAL LARVAS LATVIA LEAVED LEAVEN LEAVER LEAVES LEEVES LEOVII LIEVIO LITVAK LOAVES LOUVER LOUVIN LOUVRE LWAVES

L•••V•
LACAVA LENOVO LTGOVS

L••••V
LAPTEV LIVETV LOUISV

•LV•••
ALVARO ALVING ALVINO ELVERS ELVIRA ELVISH

•L•V••
ALEVEL ALEVES ALFVEN ALIVEO ALMVPS CLAVES CLAVIN CLEVER CLEVES CLOVEN CLOVER CLOVES CLOVIS ELEVEN ELEVES ELEVON FLAVIA FLAVOR GLOVED GLOVER GLOVES NLMVPS OLAVII OLAVIV OLDVIC OLEVEL OLIVER OLIVES OLIVIA PLOVER PLUVIA PLUVIO SLAVED SLAVER SLAVES SLAVIC SLIVER SLOVAK SLOVEN

•L••V•
ALCOVE CLEAVE SLEEVE

•L•••V
ELKONV FLATTV OLAFIV OLAVIV

••LV••
CALVED CALVES CALVET CALVIN DELVED DELVER DELVES HALVAH HALVAS HALVED HALVER HALVES KELVIN MELVIL MELVIN MELVYN PELVIC PELVIS PULVER SALVED SALVER SALVES SALVOR SALVOS SELVES SILVAS SILVER SOLVED SOLVER SOLVES SYLVAN SYLVIA VALVED VALVES VELVET VOLVOS WOLVES

••L•V•
ARLOVA BULOVA GOLIVE HALEVY INLOVE MYLOVE RELEVE RELEVY RELIVE SALIVA UNLIVE VALOVA

••L••V
FELIXV

•••LV•
EVOLVE PAULVI SHELVE TWELVE

•••L•V
KISLEV KRYLOV MAGLEV PAULIV PAVLOV RUBLEV SMALLV VACLAV VASLAV

••••LV
SMALLV

LW••••
LWAVES

L•W•••
LAWFUL LAWING LAWMAN LAWMEN LAWSON LAWTON LAWYER LEWDER LEWDLY LOWBID LOWBOY LOWCAL LOWCUT LOWEBB LOWELL LOWEND LOWERS LOWERY LOWEST LOWFAT LOWING LOWIQS LOWISH LOWKEY LOWMAN LOWMEN LOWRES LOWSET LOWTAR LOWTOP

L••W••
LEEWAY LUDWIG

L••••W
LAYLOW LIELOW LUDLOW

•LW•••
ALWAYS ALWEST ELWOOD NLWEST

•L•W••
ALLWET BLEWIN BLEWIT BLEWON BLEWUP BLOWER BLOWIN BLOWIT BLOWON BLOWSY BLOWUP BLOWZY CLAWAT CLAWED CLAWER CLEWED CLOWNS FLAWED FLEWAT FLEWBY FLEWIN FLEWON FLEWTO FLEWUP FLOWED FLOWER FLOWIN FLYWAY GLOWED GLOWER OLDWAY PLOWED PLOWER PLOWON PLOWUP SLEWED SLOWED SLOWER SLOWGO SLOWLY SLOWUP

•L••W•
ALLOWS ELBOWS ELFOWL

•L•••W
ALLNEW FLYLOW OLDSAW

••LW••
ALLWET BULWER GALWAY

••L•W•
ALLOWS BYLAWS INLAWS MALAWI

••L••W
ALLNEW BELLOW BILLOW CALLOW FALLOW FELLOW FOLLOW HALLOW HOLLOW MALLOW MELLOW MILDEW PILLOW SALLOW TALLOW TILNOW WALLOW WILLOW YELLOW

•••L•W
ASSLOW ATALOW BARLOW BELLOW BILLOW CALLOW CARLOW CURLEW DECLAW DRCLAW ECOLAW FALLOW FARLOW FELLOW FLYLOW FOLLOW GAGLAW GOSLOW GUNLAW HALLOW HARLOW HOLLOW INFLOW LAYLOW LIELOW LUDLOW MALLOW MELLOW OUTLAW PILLOW PRELAW RANLOW REFLEW REFLOW REGLOW REPLOW RUNLOW SALLOW SMALLW TALLOW TAXLAW THELAW TOOLOW UNSLOW UPFLOW WALLOW WILLOW YELLOW

••••LW
SMALLW

L•X•••
LAXALT LAXEST LAXITY LUXATE LUXURY

L••X••
LEOXII LYNXES

L••••X
LARYNX LASTEX LEDOUX LENNOX LEROUX LOUISX LUMMOX

•L•X••
ALEXAS ALEXEI ALEXEY ALEXIA ALEXIS BLIXEN ELIXIR FLAXEN FLAXES FLEXED FLEXES FLEXOR FLUXED FLUXES ILEXES KLAXON PLEXAL PLEXES PLEXOR PLEXUS

•L•••X
BLUEOX CLIMAX CLOROX SLYFOX

••LX••
CALXES

••L•X•
BILOXI DELUXE FELIXI FELIXV GALAXY

••L••X
BOLLIX CALMEX COLFAX HALLUX POLEAX POLLEX POLLUX WILCOX

•••L•X
BOLLIX DIPLEX DUPLEX EFFLUX HALLUX INFLUX MAALOX NEELIX POLLEX POLLUX PROLIX PUBLIX REFLEX REFLUX SMALLX

••••LX
PROULX SMALLX

LY••••
LYCEES LYCEUM LYCRAS LYDIAN LYMPHS LYNDON LYNLEY LYNXES LYNYRD LYONNE LYRICS LYRIDS LYRIST LYSINE LYTTON

L•Y•••
LAYBYS LAYERS LAYFOR LAYING LAYINS LAYLOW LAYMAN LAYMEN LAYOFF LAYOUT LAYSBY LAYSIN LAYSON LAYSTO LAYSUP LAYUPS LEYDEN LOYALE LOYOLA

L••Y••
LADYDI LARYNX LAWYER LIBYAN LLOYDS LYNYRD

L•••Y•
LATOYA LAURYL LAURYN LAYBYS LIBBYS LIEBYS LOOEYS LOVEYA LOVEYS

L••••Y
LACHEY LACHOY LACILY LACKEY LAIDBY LAMELY LANDRY LANKLY LANSKY LASTLY LATELY LAUREY LAXITY LAYSBY LAZBOY LAZILY LEACHY LEAKEY LEALTY LEANLY LEEMAY LEEWAY LEGACY LEMONY LENITY LESLEY LETFLY LETSBY LEVITY LEWDLY LIEFLY LIKELY LIMPLY LINENY LINNEY LIONLY LITANY LIVELY LIVERY LOGILY LONELY LONGLY LOONEY LOOSEY LORDLY LOUDLY LOVELY LOWBOY LOWERY LOWKEY LUMLEY LUNACY LUNCHY LURKEY LUSHLY LUXURY LYNLEY

•LY•••
ALYDAR ALYSSA BLYDEN BLYTHE BLYTON CLYDES ELYRIA ELYSEE ELYTIS FLYASH FLYBOY FLYBYS FLYERS FLYING FLYINS FLYLOW FLYMAN FLYMEN FLYNET FLYOUT FLYROD FLYWAY GLYCOL GLYNIS GLYPHS GLYPTO PLYING SLYEST SLYFOX

•L•Y••
ALIYAH ALIYOT ALKYDS ALKYLS ALLYCE ALLYLS CLAYEY CLOYED DLAYER ELAYER ELAYNE FLAYED FLAYER

LLOYDS
PLAYAS
PLAYAT
PLAYBY
PLAYED
PLAYER
PLAYIT
PLAYON
PLAYTO
PLAYUP
SLAYED
SLAYER

•L••Y•
ALLAYS
ALLEYN
ALLEYS
ALLOYS
ALWAYS
FLYBYS
GLADYS
PLATYS
ZLOTYS

•L•••Y
ALBANY
ALECKY
ALEXEY
ALLDAY
ALMATY
ALTKEY
BLABBY
BLAKEY
BLATTY
BLEARY
BLIMEY
BLOBBY
BLOCKY
BLOODY
BLOOEY
BLOOMY
BLOTTY
BLOWSY
BLOWZY
BLUELY
BLUESY
BLURRY
CLAMMY
CLANCY
CLANKY
CLASSY
CLAYEY
CLEARY
CLERGY
CLICHY
CLIFFY
CLINGY
CLIQUY
CLODDY
CLOGGY
CLOTTY
CLOUDY
CLUBBY
CLUMPY
CLUMSY
CLUNKY
ELLERY
FLABBY
FLAGGY
FLAPPY
FLASHY
FLATLY
FLECKY
FLEDGY
FLEECY
FLESHY
FLEWBY
FLIMSY
FLINTY
FLIRTY
FLITBY
FLOATY
FLOOEY
FLOPPY
FLOPSY
FLOREY
FLOSSY
FLOURY
FLUFFY
FLUKEY
FLUNKY
FLURRY
FLYBOY
FLYWAY
GLADLY
GLASSY
GLEAMY
GLIBLY
GLINTY
GLITZY
GLOBBY
GLOOMY
GLOPPY
GLOSSY
GLUMLY
ILLDRY
ILLSAY
KLUDGY
KLUTZY
OLDBOY
OLDWAY
OLEARY
PLASHY
PLAYBY
PLENTY
PLOTTY
PLUCKY
PLUMMY
PLUNKY
PLUSHY
SLANGY
SLAPPY
SLEAZY
SLEEKY
SLEEPY
SLEETY
SLIMLY
SLINKY
SLIPBY
SLIPPY
SLITHY
SLOBBY
SLOOPY
SLOPPY
SLOSHY
SLOWLY
SLUDGY
SLUMMY
SLURRY
SLUSHY

••LY••
ALLYCE
ALLYLS
BOLYAI
ONLYIF
POLYPS
RELYON
SALYUT

••L•Y•
ALLAYS
ALLEYN
ALLEYS
ALLOYS
BALLYS
BELAYS
BOLEYN
COLBYS
DELAYS
FOLEYS
INLAYS
ISLEYS
KELLYS
MALAYA
MALAYS
MELVYN
MULEYS
ONLAYS
RALLYE
RELAYS
SPLAYS
TOLDYA
UNLAYS
WILLYS

••L••Y
ALLDAY
BALDLY
BELFRY
BELLAY
BOLDLY
BOLSHY
CALMLY
CALORY
CELERY
COLDLY
COLONY
DELANY
DELKEY
DELRAY
DELREY
DELROY
DILSEY
DOLLEY
EELERY
ELLERY
EULOGY
FELONY
FILEBY
FILTHY
FOLKSY
GALAXY
GALLEY
GALWAY
GELSEY
GILLEY
GILROY
HALEVY
HALLEY
HALSEY
HILARY
HOLILY
HOLLEY
ILLDRY
ILLSAY
JALOPY
JOLLEY
KELLEY
KELSEY
KILROY
MALADY
MALORY
MALTBY
MELODY
MILADY
MILDLY
MILLAY
MOLLOY
MYLADY
OILILY
OOLOGY
OWLERY
PALELY
PALTRY
PELTRY
POLICY
POLITY
PULLEY
RELEVY
ROLLBY
SALARY
SALIFY
SELLBY
SOLELY
SULTRY
TILERY
TILLEY
UGLIFY
UGLILY
VALERY
VALLEY
VILELY
VILIFY
VOLLEY
WALKBY
WILDLY
WILILY
WOLSEY

•••LY•
BALLYS
EMILYS
EVELYN
JACLYN
KELLYS
MADLYN
RALLYE
ROSLYN
SEALYS
WILLYS

•••L•Y
ASHLEY
ASTLEY
ATPLAY
BAILEY
BARLEY
BATLEY
BEGLEY
BELLAY
BODLEY
BOSLEY
BROLLY
BURLEY
BYPLAY
CHALKY
CHILLY
COOLEY
COOLLY
COPLEY
COWLEY
CURLEY
DAILEY
DEPLOY
DOLLEY
DOOLEY
DROLLY
DUALLY
DUDLEY
EASLEY
EISLEY
EMPLOY
EVILLY
FARLEY
FAULTY
FAWLTY
FEALTY
FINLEY
FOULLY
FRILLY
GALLEY
GILLEY
GOALBY
GUILTY
GURLEY
HAILEY
HALLEY
HANLEY
HARLEY
HAYLEY
HEALEY
HEDLEY
HENLEY
HOLLEY
HUBLEY
HUNLEY
HURLEY
HUXLEY
ICALLY
INPLAY
JOLLEY
KELLEY
KNOLLY
LEALTY
LESLEY
LUMLEY
LYNLEY
MABLEY
MANLEY
MARLEY
MEDLEY
MILLAY
MISLAY
MOBLEY
MOLLOY
MORLEY
MOSLEY
MOTLEY
MOULDY
NEWLEY
OAKLEY
ORALLY
OUTLAY
OVALLY
PARLAY
PARLEY
PAULEY
PHILBY
PHILLY
PULLEY
RADLEY
REALLY
REALTY
REILLY
REPLAY
RIDLEY
RIPLEY
RKELLY
ROLLBY
ROWLEY
SCULLY
SEDLEY
SELLBY
SHALEY
SHALLY
SHELBY
SHELTY
SHILLY
SISLEY
SMALLY
SMELLY
SMILEY
STALKY
STILLY
TENLEY
TETLEY
TILLEY
TRILBY
UNCLAY
VALLEY
VAULTY
VOLLEY
WAYLAY
WESLEY
WHALEY
WHOLLY
WIELDY
WOOLEY
WOOLLY
WORLEY

••••LY
ACIDLY
AERILY
AGEDLY
AIRILY
ARCHLY
ARIDLY
ARTILY
AVIDLY
AWEDLY
BABBLY
BALDLY
BARELY
BARFLY
BASELY
BASSLY
BLUELY
BOBBLY
BODILY
BOLDLY
BOTFLY
BOXILY
BRENLY
BROLLY
BUBBLY
BURBLY
BUSILY
CAGILY
CALMLY
CHARLY
CHICLY
CHILLY
CICELY
COLDLY
COMELY
COMPLY
COOLLY
COSILY
COSTLY
COZILY
CRAWLY
CUDDLY
CURTLY
CUTELY
DAFTLY
DAMPLY
DANGLY
DANKLY
DARKLY
DEADLY
DEAFLY
DEARLY
DEEPLY
DEFTLY
DEWILY
DIDDLY
DIMPLY
DIRELY
DOPILY
DOUBLY
DOURLY
DOZILY
DRABLY
DRAWLY
DROLLY
DROOLY
DRYFLY
DUALLY
DUMBLY
EASILY
EBERLY
EDGILY
EDIBLY
EERILY
EVENLY
EVERLY
EVILLY
FAIRLY
FAMILY
FEEBLY
FINELY
FIRMLY
FLATLY
FONDLY
FOULLY
FOXILY
FREELY
FRILLY
GADFLY
GAINLY
GAMELY
GAMILY
GANGLY
GENTLY
GIGGLY
GLADLY
GLIBLY
GLUMLY
GNARLY
GOGGLY
GOODLY
GOOGLY
GORILY
GRAYLY
GREYLY
GRIMLY
GRISLY
GROWLY
HACKLY
HARDLY
HAZILY
HIGHLY
HOKILY
HOLILY
HOMELY
HOMILY
HOSTLY
HOURLY
HUGELY
HUMBLY
ICALLY
IFONLY
INJULY
JANGLY
JIGGLY
JINGLY
JOKILY
JUMBLY
JUNGLY
JUSTLY
KANALY
KEENLY
KINDLY
KINGLY
KNOLLY
KNURLY
KODALY
LACILY
LAMELY
LANKLY
LASTLY
LATELY
LAZILY
LEANLY
LETFLY
LEWDLY
LIEFLY
LIKELY
LIMPLY
LIONLY
LIVELY
LOGILY
LONELY
LONGLY
LORDLY
LOUDLY
LOVELY
LUSHLY
MAINLY
MARBLY
MAYFLY
MAZILY
MEANLY
MEASLY
MEDFLY
MEEKLY
MEETLY
MERELY
MILDLY
MIZZLY
MOSTLY
MUMBLY
MUSCLY
MUTELY
NAMELY
NEARLY
NEATLY
NETTLY
NICELY
NIMBLY
NOSILY
NUBBLY
NUDELY
NUMBLY
OFFALY
OILILY
OOZILY
OPENLY
ORALLY
OUTFLY
OVALLY
OVERLY
PALELY
PARTLY
PEARLY
PEBBLY
PERTLY
PHILLY
PIMPLY
POKILY
POORLY
POPFLY
PORTLY
POSHLY
PRIMLY
PUDDLY
PUNILY
PURELY
PURPLY
RACILY
RANKLY
RAPTLY
RARELY
RASHLY
RATTLY
REALLY
REILLY
RICHLY
RIFELY
RIPELY
RIPPLY
RKELLY
RONELY
ROSILY
RUBBLY
RUDELY
RUFFLY
RUMBLY
RUMPLY
SACFLY
SAFELY
SAGELY
SANELY
SCULLY
SEEMLY
SEXILY
SHALLY
SHILLY
SHOALY
SICILY
SICKLY
SIMPLY
SINGLY
SLIMLY
SLOWLY
SMALLY
SMELLY
SMUGLY
SNARLY
SNUGLY
SOFTLY
SOLELY
SORELY
SOURLY
SPRYLY
STABLY
STEELY
STILLY
STOOLY
STUDLY
SUBTLY
SUPPLY
SURELY
SWIRLY
TAMELY
TANGLY
TARTLY
TAUTLY
THEFLY
THINLY
THUSLY
TICKLY
TIDILY
TIMELY
TINGLY
TINILY
TINKLY
TREBLY
TRIMLY
TRIPLY
TWIRLY
TWOPLY
UGLILY
UNABLY
UNDULY
UNHOLY
UNIDLY
UNOILY
UNRULY
UNWILY
USABLY
VAINLY
VASILY
VASTLY
VERILY
VIABLY
VILELY
VOWELY
WADDLY
WAFFLY
WAGGLY
WAMBLY
WARILY
WARMLY
WAVILY
WAXILY
WEAKLY
WEEKLY
WETFLY
WHIRLY
WHOLLY
WIDELY
WIFELY
WIGGLY
WILDLY
WILILY
WIRILY
WISELY
WOBBLY
WOOLLY
YARELY
YEARLY
ZANILY

L•Z•••
LAZBOY
LAZIER
LAZILY
LAZING
LAZULI
LIZALU
LIZARD
LIZZIE

L••Z••
LASZLO
LINZER
LIZZIE
LUTZES

L•••Z•
LAMAZE
LAONZA
LAOTZU
LARAZA
LEUTZE

L••••Z
LESMIZ
LORENZ

•LZ•••
ALZADO
ALZIRA

•L•Z••
BLAZED
BLAZER
BLAZES
BLAZON
GLAZED
GLAZER
GLAZES
PLAZAS
SLEZAK

•L••Z•
ALONZO
BLOWZY
GLITZY
KLUTZY
SLEAZE
SLEAZY

•L•••Z
ALMAAZ
ALRITZ
BLINTZ
ELBURZ

••LZ••
BALZAC
BELZER

••L•Z•
ABLAZE
BELIZE

••L••Z
DOLENZ
MILOSZ
VALDEZ

•••L•Z
BOULEZ
PARLEZ
SHULTZ
SMALLZ
STOLTZ

••••LZ
SCHULZ
SMALLZ
SWIRLZ

MA••••
MAALOX
MAAZEL
MABELL
MABLEY
MACACO
MACAPA
MACAWS
MACERS
MACHOS
MACKIE
MACLEN
MACLES
MACNEE
MACOMB
MACOUN
MACRAE
MACRON
MACROS
MACULA
MADAMA
MADAME
MADAMS
MADCAP
MADDED
MADDEN
MADDER
MADDIE
MADDOG
MADDOX
MADDUX
MADEDO
MADEGO
MADEIT
MADEOF
MADERA
MADERO
MADEUP
MADFOR
MADLYN
MADMAN
MADMAX
MADMEN
MADRAS
MADRES
MADRID
MADSEN
MADURO
MADVIG
MAENAD
MAFIAS
MAGGIE
MAGGIO
MAGGOT
MAGIAN
MAGICS
MAGLEV
MAGLIE
MAGMAS
MAGNET
MAGNOL
MAGNON
MAGNUM
MAGNUS
MAGPIE
MAGYAR
MAHALO
MAHDIS
MAHLER
MAHOUT
MAHZOR
MAIDEN
MAILED
MAILER
MAILIN
MAILTO
MAIMED
MAIMER
MAINER
MAINLY
MAINST
MAIRES
MAIRZY
MAISIE
MAISON
MAITAI
MAITRE
MAIZES
MAJGEN
MAJLIS
MAJOAD
MAJORS
MAKEBA
MAKEDO
MAKEGO
MAKEIT
MAKEME
MAKEOF
MAKERS
MAKEUP
MAKING
MAKSIM
MAKUTA
MALABO
MALADY
MALAGA
MALARS
MALAWI
MALAYA
MALAYS
MALDEN
MALEIC
MALIAN
MALIBU
MALICE
MALICK
MALIGN
MALLEI
MALLET
MALLON
MALLOW
MALONE
MALORY
MALOTI
MALTBY
MALTED
MALTIN
MAMBAS
MAMBOS
MAMMAL
MAMMAS
MAMMON
MANAGE
MANAMA
MANANA
MANAOS
MANAPE
MANATS
MANCHA
MANCHE
MANCHU
MANDAN
MANDAY
MANDEL
MANDMS
MANEGE
MANERO
MANETS
MANFUL
MANGAS
MANGER
MANGLE
MANGOS
MANIAC
MANIAS
MANILA
MANLEY
MANNAS
MANNED
MANNER
MANNIX
MANNON
MANOFF
MANORS
MANQUE
MANRAY
MANSES
MANTAS
MANTEE
MANTEL
MANTIC
MANTIS
MANTLE
MANTRA
MANTUA
MANUAL
MANUEL
MANURE
MANUSH
MANUTE
MANZON
MAOISM
MAOIST
MAORIS
MAOTAI
MAPLES
MAPOUT
MAPPED
MAPPER
MAPPLE
MAPUTO
MAQUIS
MARACA
MARAUD
MARBLE
MARBLY
MARCEL
MARCHE
MARCIA
MARCIE
MARCIL
MARCIX
MARCOS
MARCUS
MARDEN
MARDIS
MARGIE
MARGIN
MARGOT
MARIAH
MARIAN
MARIAS
MARIDA
MARIDO

MARIEL
MARIKO
MARILU
MARINA
MARINE
MARINO
MARION
MARISA
MARIST
MARJOE
MARKAS
MARKED
MARKER
MARKET
MARKEY
MARKIE
MARKII
MARKIV
MARKIX
MARKKA
MARKOV
MARKUP
MARKVI
MARLED
MARLEE
MARLEY
MARLIN
MARLON
MARMEE
MARMOT
MARNER
MARNIE
MAROON
MARPLE
MARQUE
MARRED
MARRER
MARRON
MARROW
MARSHA
MARSHY
MARTEL
MARTEN
MARTES
MARTHA
MARTHE
MARTIN
MARTYR
MARVEL
MARVIN
MARVIS
MARXES
MARYAM
MARYII
MARYJO
MASADA
MASAIS
MASALA
MASCOT
MASERS
MASERU
MASHED
MASHER
MASHES
MASHIE
MASHUP
MASKED
MASKER
MASLIN
MASONS
MASQUE
MASSED
MASSES
MASSEY
MASSIF
MASSON
MASSYS
MASTED
MASTER
MASTIC
MATERS
MATEYS
MATHER
MATHEW
MATHIS
MATING
MATINS
MATJES
MATLIN
MATMAN
MATMEN
MATRIX
MATRON
MATSON
MATSUI
MATSUO
MATTEA
MATTED
MATTEL
MATTER
MATTES
MATTIE
MATURE
MATZOH
MATZOS
MAULED
MAULER
MAUMAU
MAUMEE
MAUNDY
MAUSER
MAUVES
MAVENS
MAVINS
MAWSON
MAXELL
MAXENE
MAXIMA
MAXIMS
MAXINE
MAXING
MAXIXE
MAXOUT
MAXSON
MAYANS
MAYBES
MAYDAY
MAYEST
MAYFLY
MAYHAP
MAYHEM
MAYIGO
MAYING
MAYORS
MAYRON
MAYTAG
MAZDAS
MAZIER
MAZILY
MAZING
MAZOLA
MAZUMA

M•A•••

MAALOX
MAAZEL
MCADOO
MCAFEE
MCAVOY
MEADER
MEADOW
MEAGER
MEAGRE
MEALIE
MEANER
MEANEY
MEANIE
MEANIT
MEANLY
MEANTO
MEASLE
MEASLY
MEATAX
MEATUS
MIAMIS
MIAMIU
MIAOUS
MIAOWS
MIASMA
MIATAS
MOANED
MOANER
MOATED
MTAIRY

M••A••

MACACO
MACAPA
MACAWS
MADAMA
MADAME
MADAMS
MAHALO
MALABO
MALADY
MALAGA
MALARS
MALAWI
MALAYA
MALAYS
MANAGE
MANAMA
MANANA
MANAOS
MANAPE
MANATS
MARACA
MARAUD
MASADA
MASAIS
MASALA
MAYANS
MCBAIN
MCCABE
MCCAIN
MCCANN
MCHALE
MCHARG
MCLAIN
MCNABB
MCNAIR
MEDAKA
MEDALS
MEGALO
MEGANE
MENACE
MENAGE
MESAAZ
MESABI
METALS
METATE
MIDAIR
MIKADO
MIKASA
MILADY
MILANO
MILANS
MIRADA
MIRAGE
MISACT
MISADD
MISAIM
MODALS
MOHAIR
MOHAVE
MOHAWK
MOJAVE
MOLARS
MONACO
MONADS
MONAMI
MORALE
MORALS
MORANT
MORASS
MORATH
MORAYS
MOSAIC
MOVADO
MOZART
MRPAWS
MSTARS
MUFASA
MUGABE
MURALS
MURANO
MUTANT
MUTATE
MYBABY
MYLADY
MYLARS
MYNAHS

M•••A•

MACRAE
MADCAP
MADMAN
MADMAX
MADRAS
MAENAD
MAFIAS
MAGIAN
MAGMAS
MAGYAR
MAITAI
MAJOAD
MALIAN
MAMBAS
MAMMAL
MAMMAS
MANDAN
MANDAY
MANGAS
MANIAC
MANIAS
MANNAS
MANRAY
MANTAS
MANUAL
MAOTAI
MARIAH
MARIAN
MARIAS
MARKAS
MARYAM
MATMAN
MAUMAU
MAYDAY
MAYHAP
MAYTAG
MAZDAS
MCBEAL
MCCRAE
MCEWAN
MCGRAW
MCKEAN
MCLEAN
MEATAX
MECCAN
MECCAS
MEDGAR
MEDIAL
MEDIAN
MEDIAS
MELMAC
MENIAL
MENSAL
MENSAN
MENTAL
MERMAN
MESAAZ
MESCAL
MESIAL
METFAN
MIATAS
MICMAC
MIDCAP
MIDDAY
MIDIAN
MIDMAY
MIDWAY
MILLAY
MILSAP
MINOAN
MINYAN
MIRIAM
MISHAP
MISLAY
MISSAL
MISSAY
MITRAL
MITTAG
MOCHAS
MOERAE
MOLDAU
MOLNAR
MOMMAS
MONDAY
MONTAG
MONZAS
MOOLAH
MOREAU
MORGAN
MORNAY
MORTAL
MORTAR
MOSHAV
MOSSAD
MRBEAN
MSQUAD
MUCHAS
MUDCAT
MULLAH
MULLAS
MUMBAI
MURRAY
MUSCAT
MUSIAL
MUTUAL
MYDEAR
MYRDAL
MYRIAD

M••••A

MACAPA
MACULA
MADAMA
MADERA
MAKEBA
MAKUTA
MALAGA
MALAYA
MANAMA
MANANA
MANCHA
MANILA
MANTRA
MANTUA
MARACA
MARCIA
MARIDA
MARINA
MARISA
MARKKA
MARSHA
MARTHA
MASADA
MASALA
MATTEA
MAXIMA
MAZOLA
MAZUMA
MCCREA
MEDAKA
MEDICA
MEDINA
MEDUSA
MELINA
MERIDA
MIASMA
MIKASA
MIKITA
MIMOSA
MINETA
MINIMA
MIRADA
MISCHA
MIZUNA
MODELA
MODENA
MOESHA
MOLINA
MONETA
MONICA
MORITA
MOSKVA
MOTHRA
MTETNA
MTOSSA
MUFASA
MULETA
MUNERA
MURCIA
MYOPIA

•MA•••

AMADEO
AMADIS
AMAJOR
AMALFI
AMALIA
AMALIE
AMANAS
AMANDA
AMANTI
AMANTS
AMARNA
AMATIS
AMATOL
AMAZED
AMAZES
AMAZIN
AMAZON
BMAJOR
CMAJOR
DMAJOR
DMARKS
EMAILS
EMAJOR
EMALLS
FMAJOR
GMAJOR
IMACOP
IMAGED
IMAGER
IMAGES
IMAGOS
IMAMAN
IMARET
IMAXES
KMARTS
OMAHAN
OMAHAS
OMANIS
OMASUM
SMACKS
SMALLA
SMALLB
SMALLC
SMALLD
SMALLE
SMALLF
SMALLG
SMALLH
SMALLI
SMALLJ
SMALLK
SMALLL
SMALLM
SMALLN
SMALLO
SMALLP
SMALLQ
SMALLR
SMALLS
SMALLT
SMALLU
SMALLV
SMALLW
SMALLX
SMALLY
SMALLZ
SMARMY
SMARTS
SMARTY
SMAZES
XMASES

•M•A••

AMBAND
EMBALM
EMBANK
EMBARK
EMBARS
EMBAYS
EMDASH
EMMAUS
EMPALE
EMPATH
FMBAND
IMBACK
IMEANT
IMEASY
IMGAME
IMLATE
IMPACT
IMPAIR
IMPALA
IMPALE
IMPART
OMEARA
SMEARS
SMEARY
UMIAKS
UMLAUT
UMTATA

•M••A•

AMANAS
AMEBAE
AMEBAS
AMICAL
AMIDAS
AMIGAS
AMORAL
AMTRAC
AMTRAK
AMYTAN
EMQUAD
IMAMAN
IMBEAT
IMGLAD
IMOKAY
OMAHAN
OMAHAS
OMEGAS
OMPHAL
UMBRAE
UMBRAL
UMBRAS

•M•••A

AMALIA
AMANDA
AMARNA
AMELIA
AMENRA
AMESIA
AMINTA
AMOEBA
AMONRA
AMRITA
EMILIA
IMELDA
IMPALA
OMEARA
OMERTA
SMALLA
SMILLA
SMYRNA
UMBRIA
UMTATA

••MA••

ALMAAZ
ALMACH
ALMATY
ARMADA
ARMAGH
ARMAND
ARMANI
ASMANY
ASMARA
ATMANS
BAMAKO
BEMATA
BYMAIL
CAMARO
COMATE
DAMAGE
DAMASK
DAMATO
DEMAIN
DEMAND
DEMARK
DEMAST
DIMAGE
DOMAIN
DOMANI
EMMAUS
EXMATE
FEMALE
GAMAYS
GEMARA
HAMATE
HEMATO
HOMAGE
HUMANE
HUMANS
INMATE
ISMAIL
JAMAAL
JAMAIS
JUMADA
KAMALI
LAMARR
LAMAZE
LEMANS
LIMANS
NAMATH
NOMAAM
NOMADS
NOMAYO
OHMAGE
POMADE
RAMADA
RAMAPO
RAMATE
REMADE
REMAIL
REMAIN
REMAKE
REMAND
REMANS
REMAPS
REMARK
REMATE
REMATS
RIMATE
ROMAIC
ROMAIN
ROMAJI
ROMANI
ROMANO
ROMANS
ROMANY
RUMAKI
SAMARA
SEMANA
SOMALI
SOMANY
SOMATA
STMALO
STMARK
STMARY
SUMACS
TAMALE
TAMARA
TAMAYO
TJMAXX
TOMATO
UNMADE
UNMAKE
UNMANS
UNMASK
UNMAST
UNMATE
USMAIL
WOMACK
WOMANS
YAMAHA
YAMANI
YEMANA
YUMAAZ
YUMANS
ZYMASE

••M•A•

AIMSAT
ALMAAZ
BEMOAN
BOMBAL
BOMBAY
BUMRAP
CAMEAS
CAMEAT
COMBAT
COMEAS
COMEAT
COMMAS
COMPAQ
COMPAS
COMSAT
CYMBAL
DEMEAN
FUMEAT
GAMMAS
GEMMAE
GIMBAL
GYMBAG
GYMRAT
HYMNAL
IAMSAM
JAMAAL
JAMCAM
JUMPAT
KOMBAT
LAMIAE
LAMIAS
LEMMAS
LUMBAR
MAMBAS
MAMMAL
MAMMAS
MOMMAS
MUMBAI
NEMEAN
NOMAAM
NOMEAK
NOMEAT
NOMIAL
NUMBAT
OOMPAH
PAMPAS
RAMEAU
RAMFAN
RAMPAL
RAMSAY
RUMBAS
SAMBAS
SAMEAS
SAMIAM
SAMOAN
SAMPAN
SIMIAN
TAMTAM
TIMBAL
TOMCAT
WOMBAT
YUMAAZ

••M••A

ARMADA
ASMARA
BEMATA
CAMERA
COMIDA
CUMBIA
DAMITA
ELMIRA
FEMORA
GAMBIA
GEMARA
IOMEGA
JAMESA
JAMOCA
JEMIMA
JUMADA
LAMBDA
LAMESA
LAMINA
LUMINA
MIMOSA
NUMINA
PAMELA
PAMINA
POMONA
RAMADA
RAMONA
REMORA
ROMOLA
SAMARA
SAMOSA
SEMANA
SOMATA
TAMARA
YAMAHA
YAMUNA
YEMANA
ZAMBIA
ZAMORA

•••MA•

AAAMAP
ABOMAS
AGAMAS
AIDMAN
AIKMAN
AIRMAN
ALEMAN
ALLMAN
ALOMAR
ALTMAN
ANIMAL
ANIMAS
ANYMAN
APEMAN
AROMAS
ASHMAN
ATAMAN
AXEMAN
BADMAN
BAGMAN
BARMAN
BATMAN
BAUMAN
BAYMAN
BEAMAN
BERMAN
BIGMAC
BIGMAN
BIRMAN
BITMAP
BORMAN
BOWMAN
BRAMAH
BRUMAL
BURMAN
BUSMAN
CABMAN
CAIMAN
CARMAN
CATMAN
CAYMAN
CLIMAT
CLIMAX
COLMAN
COLMAR
COMMAS
CONMAN
CORMAN
COSMAS
COWMAN
DAGMAR
DELMAR
DERMAL
DERMAS
DERMAT
DISMAL
DISMAS
DISMAY
DOGMAS
DOLMAN
DOLMAS
DRAMAS
EDEMAS
ELFMAN
ENDMAN
ERDMAN
FAIMAN
FATMAN
FBIMAN
FERMAT
FLYMAN
FOEMAN
FORMAL
FORMAN
FORMAT
FULMAR
FURMAN
GAGMAN
GAMMAS
GASMAN
GEMMAE
GERMAN
GETMAD
GILMAN
GOTMAD
GUNMAN
GUTMAN
GUZMAN
HAGMAN
HAZMAT
HERMAN
HEYMAN
HIEMAL
HITMAN
HODMAN
HOLMAN
ICEMAN
IFIMAY
IMAMAN
INGMAR
KALMAR
KARMAS
KATMAI
KEYMAN
KIDMAN
KIRMAN
KORMAN
LAWMAN
LAYMAN
LEEMAY
LEGMAN
LEHMAN
LEMMAS
LLAMAS
LOUMAS
LOWMAN
MADMAN
MADMAX
MAGMAS
MAMMAL
MAMMAS
MATMAN
MAUMAU
MELMAC
MERMAN
MICMAC
MIDMAY
MOMMAS
NEIMAN
NERMAL
NETMAN
NEUMAN
NEWMAN
NEWMAR
NONMAN
NORMAL
NORMAN
OARMAN
ODAMAE
ODDMAN
OILMAN
OLDMAN
ONEMAN
OTHMAR
OUTMAN
PACMAN
PALMAR
PALMAS
PENMAN
PIEMAN
PIGMAN
PITMAN
PRIMAL
RAGMAN
RBIMAN
RODMAN
RUDMAN
SALMAN
SEAMAN
SEAMAP
SGTMAJ
SHAMAN
SHUMAI
SIGMAS
SKYMAN
SKYMAP
STOMAS
TARMAC
TASMAN
TAXMAN
THEMAN
THOMAS
TINMAN
TOAMAN
TODMAN
TOPMAN
TRUMAN
TUBMAN
TWOMAN
TWYMAN
ULLMAN
WEIMAR
WIEMAN
YEOMAN
YESMAN
ZEEMAN

•••M•A

AHIMSA
ALUMNA
ANEMIA
ANOMIA
CLAMMA
CRIMEA
GRAMPA
LOOMPA
NOUMEA
RHUMBA
ROOMBA

••••MA

ALTIMA
ASTHMA
AZELMA
BAHAMA
BRAHMA
CHROMA
CINEMA
CLAMMA
COLIMA
DAGAMA
DHARMA
DODOMA
ECZEMA
ENIGMA
FATIMA
FUSUMA
GOTAMA
JEMIMA
JICAMA
LOOKMA
MADAMA
MANAMA
MAXIMA
MAZUMA
MIASMA
MINIMA

OPTIMA
PAJAMA
PALOMA
PANAMA
PLASMA
PNEUMA
SCHEMA
SONOMA
STIGMA
TACOMA
THELMA
TOYAMA
TRAUMA
ULTIMA
YAKIMA
YOYOMA
ZYGOMA

M•B•••
MABELL
MABLEY
MCBAIN
MCBEAL
MOBBED
MOBBER
MOBERG
MOBILE
MOBIUS
MOBLEY
MOBUTU
MRBEAN
MRBILL
MRBLUE
MRBOND
MYBABY

M••B••
MAMBAS
MAMBOS
MARBLE
MARBLY
MAYBES
MEEBER
MEMBER
MMMBOP
MOBBED
MOBBER
MORBID
MUMBAI
MUMBLE
MUMBLY

M•••B•
MAKEBA
MALABO
MALIBU
MALTBY
MCCABE
MCJOBS
MCNABB
MCRIBS
MESABI
MRPIBB
MUGABE
MYBABY

M••••B
MACOMB
MCNABB
MIDRIB
MODELB
MRPIBB

•MB•••
AMBAND
AMBERS
AMBERY
AMBIEN
AMBITS
AMBLED
AMBLER
AMBLES
AMBLIN
AMBUSH
EMBALM
EMBANK
EMBARK
EMBARS
EMBAYS
EMBEDS
EMBERS
EMBLEM
EMBODY
EMBOGS
EMBOSS
EMBOWS
EMBRUE
EMBRYO
FMBAND
IMBACK
IMBEAT
IMBEDS
IMBIBE
IMBRUE
IMBUED
IMBUES
IMBUSY
UMBELS
UMBERS
UMBRAE
UMBRAL
UMBRAS
UMBRIA

•M•B••
AMEBAE
AMEBAS
AMEBIC
MMMBOP

•M••B•
AMOEBA
IMBIBE

•M•••B
SMALLB

••MB••
BAMBIS
BAMBOO
BIMBOS
BOMBAL
BOMBAY
BOMBED
BOMBER
BOMBES
BUMBLE
BUMBRY
CAMBER
CAMBOY
COMBAT
COMBED
COMBER
COMBOS
CUMBER
CUMBIA
CYMBAL
DOMBEY
DUMBER
DUMBLY
DUMBOS
FEMBOT
FUMBLE
GAMBIA
GAMBIT
GAMBLE
GAMBOL
GIMBAL
GIMBEL
GUMBEL
GUMBOS
GYMBAG
HOMBRE
HUMBER
HUMBLE
HUMBLY
HUMBUG
IAMBIC
IAMBUS
JAMBES
JIMBOB
JUMBLE
JUMBLY
JUMBOS
KEMBLE
KIMBLE
KOMBAT
KOMBUS
LAMBDA
LAMBED
LIMBED
LIMBER
LIMBIC
LIMBOS
LUMBAR
LUMBER
MAMBAS
MAMBOS
MEMBER
MMMBOP
MUMBAI
MUMBLE
MUMBLY
NIMBLE
NIMBLY
NIMBUS
NOMBRE
NUMBAT
NUMBED
NUMBER
NUMBLY
RAMBLE
RAMBOS
RUMBAS
RUMBLE
RUMBLY
SAMBAS
SOMBER
SOMBRE
SYMBOL
TAMBOR
TIMBAL
TIMBER
TIMBRE
TOMBES
TOMBOY
TUMBLE
WAMBLE
WAMBLY
WOMBAT
ZAMBIA
ZOMBIE

••M•B•
CAMEBY
COMEBY
DEMOBS

••M••B
JIMBOB

•••MB•
ABOMBS
AKIMBO
CLIMBS
CRAMBO
CRUMBS
CRUMBY
FLAMBE
GIAMBI
HBOMBS
NBOMBS
PLUMBO
PLUMBS
RHOMBI
RHOMBS
RHUMBA
RHUMBS
ROOMBA
THUMBS
TRUMBO

•••M•B
THEMOB

••••MB
APLOMB
BENUMB
ENTOMB
MACOMB
RCRUMB
RECOMB

MC••••
MCADOO
MCAFEE
MCAVOY
MCBAIN
MCBEAL
MCCABE
MCCAIN
MCCANN
MCCORD
MCCRAE
MCCREA
MCDUCK
MCEWAN
MCEWEN
MCGILL
MCGRAW
MCGREW
MCHALE
MCHARG
MCHUGH
MCJOBS
MCKEAN
MCKEON
MCKERN
MCKUEN
MCLAIN
MCLEAN
MCNABB
MCNAIR
MCNEIL
MCPHEE
MCRIBS

M•C•••
MACACO
MACAPA
MACAWS
MACERS
MACHOS
MACKIE
MACLEN
MACLES
MACNEE
MACOMB
MACOUN
MACRAE
MACRON
MACROS
MACULA
MCCABE
MCCAIN
MCCANN
MCCORD
MCCRAE
MCCREA
MECCAN
MECCAS
MECUMS
MICHEL
MICKEY
MICMAC
MICRON
MICROS
MOCHAS
MOCKED
MOCKER
MOCKUP
MRCOOL
MTCOOK
MUCHAS
MUCHOF
MUCKED
MUCKER
MUCKUP

M••C••
MADCAP
MANCHA
MANCHE
MANCHU
MARCEL
MARCHE
MARCIA
MARCIE
MARCIL
MARCIX
MARCOS
MARCUS
MASCOT
MECCAN
MECCAS
MERCED
MERCER
MERCKX
MESCAL
MIDCAP
MINCED
MINCER
MINCES
MISCHA
MISCUE
MISCUT
MOOCOW
MOSCOW
MUDCAT
MULCTS
MUNCHY
MUNCIE
MURCIA
MUSCAT
MUSCLE
MUSCLY

M•••C•
MACACO
MAGICS
MALICE
MALICK
MARACA
MCDUCK
MEDICA
MEDICI
MEDICO
MEDICS
MEDOCS
MEJICO
MENACE
MENSCH
MEXICO
MIMICS
MISACT
MONACO
MONICA
MRDICK
MUNICH
MUSICK
MUSICS

M••••C
MALEIC
MANIAC
MANTIC
MASTIC
MELMAC
METRIC
MICMAC
MIXTEC
MOSAIC
MYOPIC
MYSTIC
MYTHIC

•MC•••
EMCEED
EMCEES
IMCOLD
IMCOOL

•M•C••
AMECHE
AMICAL
AMICES
AMICUS
IMACOP
SMACKS
SMOCKS

•M••C•
AMERCE
IMBACK
IMPACT
SMIRCH
SMOOCH

•M•••C
AMEBIC
AMTRAC
EMERIC
EMETIC
SMALLC

••MC••
JAMCAM
KIMCHI
ROMCOM
TOMCAT

••M•C•
ALMACH
ASMUCH
COMICE
COMICS
IBMPCS
JAMOCA
MIMICS
OLMECS
OSMICS
PUMICE
REMICK
SOMUCH
SUMACS
WOMACK

••M••C
CYMRIC
HOMEEC
IAMBIC
LIMBIC
LOMPOC
ROMAIC

•••M•C
ANEMIC
ANOMIC
ATOMIC
BIGMAC
CADMIC
CHEMIC
COSMIC
DERMIC
FILMIC
FORMIC
GNOMIC
KARMIC
MELMAC
MICMAC
TARMAC
THYMIC

••••MC
RUNDMC

M•D•••
MADAMA
MADAME
MADAMS
MADCAP
MADDED
MADDEN
MADDER
MADDIE
MADDOG
MADDOX
MADDUX
MADEDO
MADEGO
MADEIT
MADEOF
MADERA
MADERO
MADEUP
MADFOR
MADLYN
MADMAN
MADMAX
MADMEN
MADRAS
MADRES
MADRID
MADSEN
MADURO
MADVIG
MCDUCK
MEDAKA
MEDALS
MEDDLE
MEDFLY
MEDGAR
MEDIAL
MEDIAN
MEDIAS
MEDICA
MEDICI
MEDICO
MEDICS
MEDINA
MEDIUM
MEDIUS
MEDLEY
MEDNIS
MEDOCS
MEDUSA
MIDAIR
MIDCAP
MIDDAY
MIDDIE
MIDDLE
MIDGES
MIDGET
MIDIAN
MIDLEG
MIDLER
MIDMAY
MIDOFF
MIDONS
MIDORI
MIDRIB
MIDSTS
MIDWAY
MMDDYY
MODALS
MODELA
MODELB
MODELS
MODELT
MODEMS
MODENA
MODERN
MODEST
MODIFY
MODINE
MODISH
MODRED
MODULE
MODULI
MODULO
MRDICK
MUDCAT
MUDDED
MUDDER
MUDDLE
MUDEEL
MUDHEN
MUDPIE
MYDEAR

M••D••
MADDED
MADDEN
MADDER
MADDIE
MADDOG
MADDOX
MADDUX
MAHDIS
MAIDEN
MALDEN
MANDAN
MANDAY
MANDEL
MANDMS
MARDEN
MARDIS
MAYDAY
MAZDAS
MCADOO
MEADER
MEADOW
MEDDLE
MELDED
MELDER
MENDED
MENDEL
MENDER
MENDES
MERDLE
MIDDAY
MIDDIE
MIDDLE
MILDER
MILDEW
MILDLY
MINDED
MINDEN
MINDER
MISDID
MMDDYY
MOLDAU
MOLDED
MOLDER
MONDAY
MONDES
MONDOS
MOODYS
MOSDEF
MUDDED
MUDDER
MUDDLE
MULDER
MURDER
MYRDAL

M•••D•
MADEDO
MAKEDO
MALADY
MARIDA
MARIDO
MASADA
MAUNDY
MELODY
MENUDO
MERIDA
MIKADO
MILADY
MIRADA
MISADD
MONADS
MONODY
MOPEDS
MOULDS
MOULDY
MOUNDS
MOVADO
MRHYDE
MUSTDO
MYLADY

M••••D
MADDED
MADRID
MAENAD
MAILED
MAIMED
MAJOAD
MALTED
MANNED
MAPPED
MARAUD
MARKED
MARLED
MARRED
MASHED
MASKED
MASSED
MASTED
MATTED
MAULED
MCCORD
MELDED
MELTED
MENDED
MEOWED
MERCED
MERGED
MESHED
MESSED
METHOD
METRED
MEWLED
MIFFED
MILKED
MILLED
MILORD
MINCED
MINDED
MINTED
MISADD
MISDID
MISFED
MISLED
MISSED
MISTED
MITRED
MOANED
MOATED
MOBBED
MOCKED
MODRED
MOILED
MOLDED
MOLTED
MONIED
MOONED
MOORED
MOOTED
MOPPED
MORBID
MOSHED
MOSSAD
MOSSED
MOUSED
MRBOND
MSQUAD
MTHOOD
MUCKED
MUDDED
MUFFED
MUGGED
MULLED
MUMMED
MUSHED
MUSSED
MYLORD
MYRIAD
MYWORD

•MD•••
EMDASH
IMDONE
MMDDYY

•M•D••
AMADEO
AMADIS
AMEDEE
AMEDEO
AMIDAS
AMIDES
AMIDOL
AMIDST
IMIDES
MMDDYY
SMIDGE
SMUDGE
SMUDGY

•M••D•
AMANDA
AMENDS
EMBEDS
EMBODY
EMENDS
IMBEDS
IMELDA
IMPEDE

•M•••D
AMAZED
AMBAND
AMBLED
AMUSED
EMCEED
EMOTED
EMQUAD
FMBAND
IMAGED
IMBUED
IMCOLD
IMGLAD
IMGOOD
IMPEND
IMPLED
IMSOLD
IMTOLD
OMENED
SMALLD
SMILED
SMOKED

••MD••
CAMDEN
COMDEN
COMDEX
COMDRS
DUMDUM
HAMDEN

••M•D•
ARMADA
COMEDY
COMIDA
DEMODE
JUMADA
KOMODO
LAMBDA
LAMEDS
NOMADS
POMADE
RAMADA
REMADE
REMEDY
SAMEDI
UNMADE

••M••D
ALMOND
ARMAND
BOMBED
BUMMED
BUMPED
CAMPED
COMBED
COMPED
DAMMED
DAMNED
DAMPED
DEMAND
DEMOED
DEMOND
DIMMED
DUMPED
EDMOND
EDMUND
GAMMED
GEMMED
GIMPED
GUMMED
HAMMED
HEMMED
HUMMED
HUMPED
HYMNED
INMIND
JAMMED
JUMPED
LAMBED
LAMMED
LEMOND
LIMBED
LIMNED
LIMPED
LIMPID
LOMOND
LUMPED
MUMMED
NIMROD
NUMBED
ORMOND
OSMOND
OSMUND
PUMPED
RAMMED
RAMPED
RAMROD
REMAND
REMEND
REMIND
REMOLD
RIMMED
ROMPED
SUMMED
TAMPED
TEMPED
UNMOLD
VAMPED
WIMPED

•••M•D
ARAMID
BEAMED
BERMED
BLAMED
BOOMED
BUMMED
CALMED
CHIMED
DAMMED
DEEMED
DIMMED
DIOMED
DOOMED
FARMED
FILMED
FIRMED
FLAMED
FOAMED
FORMED
FRAMED
GAMMED
GEMMED
GETMAD
GORMED
GOTMAD
GRIMED
GUMMED
HAMMED
HARMED
HELMED
HEMMED
HUMMED
ITEMED
JAMMED
LAMMED
LOAMED
LOOMED
MAIMED
MUMMED
PALMED
PERMED
PLUMED
PREMED
PRIMED
RAMMED
REAMED
RHYMED
RIMMED
ROAMED
ROOMED
SEAMED
SEEMED
SHAMED
SLIMED
SPUMED
SUMMED
TALMUD
TEAMED
TEEMED
TERMED
THEMED
WARMED
WORMED
ZOOMED

ME••••
MEADER
MEADOW
MEAGER
MEAGRE
MEALIE
MEANER
MEANEY
MEANIE
MEANIT
MEANLY
MEANTO
MEASLE
MEASLY
MEATAX
MEATUS
MECCAN
MECCAS
MECUMS
MEDAKA
MEDALS
MEDDLE
MEDFLY
MEDGAR
MEDIAL
MEDIAN
MEDIAS
MEDICA
MEDICI
MEDICO
MEDICS
MEDINA
MEDIUM
MEDIUS
MEDLEY
MEDNIS
MEDOCS
MEDUSA
MEEBER
MEEKER
MEEKLY
MEETER
MEETLY
MEETUP
MEGALO
MEGANE
MEGOHM
MEGREZ
MEGRIM
MEIFUN
MEJICO
MEKONG
MELDED
MELDER
MELEES
MELETE
MELINA
MELLON
MELLOW
MELMAC
MELODY

MELONS MELOTT MELTED MELTER MELTON MELVIL MELVIN MELVYN MEMBER MEMOIR MEMORY MENACE MENAGE MENDED MENDEL MENDER MENDES MENIAL MENJOU MENKEN MENNEN MENNIN MENSAL MENSAN MENSCH MENTAL MENTEE MENTHE MENTIS MENTOR MENTOS MENUDO MEOHMY MEOWED MEOWER MERCED MERCER MERCKX MERDLE MERELY MEREST MERGED MERGEE MERGER MERGES MERIDA MERINO MERITS MERKEL MERLIN MERLOT MERMAN MERMEN MEROPE MEROPS MERRIE MERSEY MERTON MERVYN MERYLL MESAAZ MESABI MESCAL MESHED MESHES MESIAL MESMER MESNES MESONS MESSED MESSES MESSIN MESSRS MESSUP METALS METATE METEOR METERS METFAN METHOD METHYL METIER METING METRED METRES METRIC METROS METTLE MEWERS MEWING MEWLED MEWLER MEXICO MEYERS MEZZOS

M•E•••

MAENAD MCEWAN MCEWEN MEEBER MEEKER MEEKLY MEETER MEETLY MEETUP MIELES MOERAE MOESHA MTETNA MUESLI

M••E••

MABELL MACERS MADEDO MADEGO MADEIT MADEOF MADERA MADERO MADEUP MAKEBA MAKEDO MAKEGO MAKEIT MAKEME MAKEOF MAKERS MAKEUP MALEIC MANEGE MANERO MANETS MASERS MASERU MATERS MATEYS MAVENS MAXELL MAXENE MAYEST MCBEAL MCKEAN MCKEON MCKERN MCLEAN MCNEIL MELEES MELETE MERELY MEREST METEOR METERS MEWERS MEYERS MILERS MIMEOS MIMERS MINERS MINETA MISERS MISERY MITERS MIXERS MOBERG MODELA MODELB MODELS MODELT MODEMS MODENA MODERN MODEST MOIETY MOLEST MOMENT MONETA MONETS MONEYS MOOERS MOPEDS MOPERS MOPERY MOREAU MOREEN MORELS MORENO MORESO MOSEYS MOTELS MOTETS MOVEIN MOVEIT MOVEON MOVERS MOVETO MOVEUP MOWERS MOYERS MRBEAN MSIEUR MUDEEL MULETA MULEYS MUNERA MUSEES MUSEON MUSEOS MUSERS MUSEUM MUTELY MUTEST MYDEAR MYHERO MYSELF

M•••E•

MAAZEL MABLEY MACLEN MACLES MACNEE MADDED MADDEN MADDER MADMEN MADRES MADSEN MAGLEV MAGNET MAHLER MAIDEN MAILED MAILER MAIMED MAIMER MAINER MAIRES MAIZES MAJGEN MALDEN MALLEI MALLET MALTED MANDEL MANGER MANLEY MANNED MANNER MANSES MANTEE MANTEL MANUEL MAPLES MAPPED MAPPER MARCEL MARDEN MARIEL MARKED MARKER MARKET MARKEY MARLED MARLEE MARLEY MARMEE MARNER MARRED MARRER MARTEL MARTEN MARTES MARVEL MARXES MASHED MASHER MASHES MASKED MASKER MASSED MASSES MASSEY MASTED MASTER MATHER MATHEW MATJES MATMEN MATTEA MATTED MATTEL MATTER MATTES MAULED MAULER MAUMEE MAUSER MAUVES MAYBES MAYHEM MAZIER MCAFEE MCCREA MCEWEN MCGREW MCKUEN MCPHEE MEADER MEAGER MEANER MEANEY MEDLEY MEEBER MEEKER MEETER MEGREZ MELDED MELDER MELEES MELTED MELTER MEMBER MENDED MENDEL MENDER MENDES MENKEN MENNEN MENTEE MEOWED MEOWER MERCED MERCER MERGED MERGEE MERGER MERGES MERKEL MERMEN MERSEY MESHED MESHES MESMER MESNES MESSED MESSES METIER METRED METRES MEWLED MEWLER MICHEL MICKEY MIDGES MIDGET MIDLEG MIDLER MIELES MIFFED MIGUEL MILDER MILDEW MILIEU MILKED MILKER MILLED MILLER MILLES MILLET MILNER MILNES MINCED MINCER MINCES MINDED MINDEN MINDER MINTED MINTER MINUET MINXES MIRIER MIRREN MISFED MISKEY MISLED MISSED MISSES MISSET MISTED MISTER MITRED MITRES MITTEN MIXTEC MIZZEN MOANED MOANER MOATED MOBBED MOBBER MOBLEY MOCKED MOCKER MODRED MOILED MOILER MOINES MOIRES MOISES MOJOES MOLDED MOLDER MOLTED MOLTEN MOLTER MONDES MONGER MONIED MONIES MONKEE MONKEY MONNET MONTEL MONTEZ MOONED MOONER MOONEY MOORED MOOTED MOOTER MOPIER MOPPED MOPPER MOPPET MOREEN MORGEN MORLEY MORREL MORSEL MORTEN MOSDEF MOSHED MOSHER MOSHES MOSLEM MOSLEY MOSSED MOSSES MOSTEL MOTHER MOTLEY MOUSED MOUSER MOUSES MOUSEY MOVIES MTILES MUCKED MUCKER MUDDED MUDDER MUDEEL MUDHEN MUFFED MUFFET MUGGED MUGGER MULDER MULLED MULLER MULLET MUMMED MUMMER MUPPET MURDER MURIEL MURRES MUSEES MUSHED MUSHER MUSHES MUSKET MUSSED MUSSEL MUSSES MUSSET MUSTER MUTTER MUTUEL MYOPES

M••••E

MACKIE MACNEE MACRAE MADAME MADDIE MAGGIE MAGLIE MAGPIE MAISIE MAITRE MAKEME MALICE MALONE MANAGE MANAPE MANCHE MANEGE MANGLE MANQUE MANTEE MANTLE MANURE MANUTE MAPPLE MARBLE MARCHE MARCIE MARGIE MARINE MARJOE MARKIE MARLEE MARMEE MARNIE MARPLE MARQUE MARTHE MASHIE MASQUE MATTIE MATURE MAUMEE MAXENE MAXINE MAXIXE MCAFEE MCCABE MCCRAE MCHALE MCPHEE MEAGRE MEALIE MEANIE MEASLE MEDDLE MEGANE MELETE MENACE MENAGE MENTEE MENTHE MERDLE MERGEE MEROPE MERRIE METATE METTLE MIDDIE MIDDLE MIFUNE MILLIE MILTIE MINGLE MINIME MINNIE MINUTE MIRAGE MISCUE MISSME MISUSE MIZZLE MOBILE MODINE MODULE MOERAE MOHAVE MOJAVE MOLINE MOLLIE MOLTKE MOMMIE MONKEE MONROE MOOKIE MOONIE MORALE MORGUE MOROSE MORRIE MOSQUE MOTILE MOTIVE MOTTLE MOUSSE MRBLUE MRHYDE MUDDLE MUDPIE MUFFLE MUGABE MUGGLE MUMBLE MUNCIE MUNROE MURINE MUSCLE MUSKIE MUTATE MUZZLE MYLIFE MYLOVE MYRTLE MYSORE

•ME•••

AMEBAE AMEBAS AMEBIC AMECHE AMEDEE AMEDEO AMEERS AMELIA AMELIE AMENDS AMENRA AMENTS AMERCE AMESIA EMEERS EMENDS EMERGE EMERIC EMERIL EMETIC EMEUTE IMEANT IMEASY IMELDA KMESON OMEARA OMEGAS OMELET OMENED OMERTA SMEARS SMEARY SMELLS SMELLY SMELTS SMERSH TMESES TMESIS

•M•E••

AMBERS AMBERY AMEERS AMIENS AMOEBA AMPERE AMVETS EMBEDS EMBERS EMCEED EMCEES EMEERS EMMETS EMMETT EMPERY IMBEAT IMBEDS IMHERE IMNEXT IMPEDE IMPELS IMPEND IMPERF UMBELS UMBERS

•M••E•

AMADEO AMAZED AMAZES AMBIEN AMBLED AMBLER AMBLES AMEDEE AMEDEO AMICES AMIDES AMINES AMOLES AMORES AMORET AMPLER AMSTEL AMULET AMUSED AMUSER AMUSES EMBLEM EMCEED EMCEES EMINEM EMOTED EMOTER EMOTES IMAGED IMAGER IMAGES IMARET IMAXES IMBUED IMBUES IMFREE IMIDES IMINES IMMIES IMOGEN IMPLED OMELET OMENED SMAZES SMILED SMILER SMILES SMILEY SMITER SMITES SMOKED SMOKER SMOKES SMOKEY SMORES TMESES XMASES

•M•••E

AMALIE AMEBAE AMECHE AMEDEE AMELIE AMERCE AMITIE AMPERE AMPULE BMOVIE EMBRUE EMERGE EMEUTE EMIGRE EMILIE EMPALE EMPIRE IMBIBE IMBRUE IMDONE IMFINE IMFREE IMGAME IMGONE IMHERE IMHOME IMLATE IMLIKE IMMUNE IMMURE IMPALE IMPEDE IMPOSE IMPURE IMPUTE IMSURE SMALLE SMIDGE SMUDGE UMBRAE UMPIRE

••ME••

AIMERS ARMERS ARMETS CAMEAS CAMEAT CAMEBY CAMEIN CAMELS CAMEON CAMEOS CAMERA CAMETO CAMEUP CEMENT COMEAS COMEAT COMEBY COMEDY COMEIN COMELY COMEOF COMEON COMERS COMETH COMETO COMETS COMEUP DEMEAN ELMERS EMMETS EMMETT ENMESH EXMETS FOMENT FUMEAT FUMERS GAMELY GAMERS GAMEST GAMETE GIMELS GOMERS HAMELN HOMEEC HOMEIN HOMELY HOMERS HOMEYS HUMERI IOMEGA ISMENE JAMESA JAMESI JAMESJ JAMESK JAMESM JAMESS JAMEST JAMESV KHMERS LAMEDS LAMELY LAMENT LAMESA LAMEST LOMEIN LUMENS MIMEOS MIMERS MOMENT NAMEIT NAMELY NAMERS NEMEAN NOMEAK NOMEAT NUMERO NYMETS OLMECS OLMERT PAMELA POMELO RAMEAU RAMENS RAMETS REMEDY REMEET REMELT REMEND RIMERS ROMEOS ROMERO SAMEAS SAMEDI SAMEKH SEMELE SIMEON SOMERS TAMELY TAMERS TAMEST TIMELY TIMERS TUMEFY UNMEET UNMESH UNMEWS VOMERS WOMENS YEMENI

••M•E•

ARMIES ARMLET ATMFEE BOMBED BOMBER BOMBES BUMLEG BUMMED BUMMER BUMPED BUMPER CAMBER CAMDEN CAMOES CAMPED CAMPER COMBED COMBER COMDEN COMDEX COMPED COMPEL COMTES CUMBER DAMIEN DAMMED DAMMER DAMNED DAMNER DAMPED DAMPEN DAMPER DAMSEL DEMIES DEMOED DIMMED DIMMER DOMBEY DOMREP DUMBER DUMPED DUMPER ELMIER FEMMES FUMIER GAMGEE GAMIER GAMMED GAMMER GEMMED GIMBEL GIMLET GIMMES GIMPED GUMBEL GUMMED HAMDEN HAMLET HAMMED HAMMER HAMPER HEMMED HEMMER HEMPEN HIMMEL HOMEEC HOMIER HOMIES HOMMES HUMBER HUMMED HUMMEL HUMMER HUMPED HUMVEE HYMNED IMMIES JAMBES JAMMED JAMMER JUMPED JUMPER KUMMEL LAMBED LAMMED LEMUEL LIMBED LIMBER LIMIER LIMNED LIMNER LIMPED LIMPER LIMPET LUMBER LUMLEY LUMPED LUMPEN LUMPER MEMBER MUMMED MUMMER NUMBED NUMBER PAMPER POMMEL POMMES POMPEO POMPEY PUMMEL PUMPED PUMPER RAMIES RAMJET RAMMED RAMMER RAMPED RAMSES RAMSEY

REMEET
REMSEN
RIMIER
RIMMED
ROMMEL
ROMNEY
ROMPED
ROMPER
RUMMER
SAMLET
SAMUEL
SEMPER
SIMMER
SIMPER
SOMBER
SOMMER
SUMMED
SUMMER
SUMNER
SUMTER
TAMPED
TAMPER
TEMPED
TEMPEH
TEMPER
TIMBER
TOMBES
UNMEET
VAMPED
VAMPER
WIMMER
WIMPED
WIMSEY
YAMMER
ZIMMER

••M••E
ADMIRE
ATMFEE
BEMINE
BEMIRE
BEMUSE
BUMBLE
CAMISE
CAMMIE
COMATE
COMICE
DAMAGE
DAMONE
DAMORE
DEMISE
DEMODE
DEMOTE
DEMURE
DIMAGE
DIMPLE
DOMINE
ELMIRE
ELMORE
ERMINE
EXMATE
EXMORE
FAMINE
FEMALE
FUMBLE
GAMBLE
GAMETE
GAMGEE
GAMINE
GEMMAE
GIMMIE
HAMATE
HAMITE
HOMAGE
HOMBRE
HUMANE
HUMBLE
HUMVEE
IMMUNE
IMMURE
INMATE
ISMENE
JAMOKE
JIMMIE
JUMBLE
KEMBLE
KIMBLE
LAMAZE
LAMIAE
MOMMIE
MUMBLE
NIMBLE
NOMBRE
NOMORE
OHMAGE
ONMIKE
OSMOSE
PIMPLE
POMADE
PUMICE
RAMATE
RAMBLE
RAMONE
RAMOSE
REMADE
REMAKE
REMATE
REMINE
REMISE
REMOTE
REMOVE
RIMATE
RIMOSE
RIMPLE
RUMBLE
RUMPLE
SAMPLE
SEMELE
SEMITE
SEMPLE
SEMPRE
SIMILE
SIMONE
SIMPLE
SOMBRE
TAMALE
TEMPLE
TIMBRE
TOMMIE
TUMBLE
UNMADE
UNMAKE
UNMATE
WAMBLE
WIMPLE
ZOMBIE
ZYMASE

•••ME•
ACUMEN
AGAMES
AIDMEN
AIRMEN
ALLMEN
ANIMES
APEMEN
ARAMES
ASHMEN
AXEMEN
BADMEN
BAGMEN
BALMER
BARMEN
BATMEN
BAUMER
BAYMEN
BEAMED
BEAMER
BEEMER
BERMED
BEYMER
BIGMEN
BIOMES
BLAMED
BLAMER
BLAMES
BLIMEY
BOOMED
BOOMER
BOWMEN
BREMEN
BREMER
BRUMEL
BRUMES
BUMMED
BUMMER
BUSMEN
CABMEN
CALMED
CALMER
CALMEX
CARMEL
CARMEN
CATMEN
CHIMED
CHIMER
CHIMES
CLIMES
CONMEN
COWMEN
CRAMER
CREMER
CREMES
CRIMEA
CRIMES
DAMMED
DAMMER
DEEMED
DEHMEL
DETMER
DIMMED
DIMMER
DIOMED
DISMES
DOOMED
DORMER
EDAMES
ENAMEL
ENDMEN
FARMED
FARMER
FBIMEN
FEMMES
FILMED
FIRMED
FIRMER
FLAMED
FLAMER
FLAMES
FLUMES
FLYMEN
FOAMED
FOAMER
FOEMEN
FORMED
FORMER
FRAMED
FRAMER
FRAMES
GAGMEN
GAMMED
GAMMER
GASMEN
GEMMED
GIMMES
GNOMES
GORMED
GRIMED
GRIMES
GUMMED
GUNMEN
HAMMED
HAMMER
HARMED
HARMER
HAYMES
HELMED
HELMER
HELMET
HEMMED
HEMMER
HERMES
HIMMEL
HITMEN
HODMEN
HOLMES
HOMMES
HORMEL
HUMMED
HUMMEL
HUMMER
ICEMEN
ILLMET
ISOMER
ITEMED
JAMMED
JAMMER
JAYMES
KEYMEN
KILMER
KISMET
KRAMER
KUMMEL
LAMMED
LARMEN
LAWMEN
LAYMEN
LEGMEN
LOAMED
LOOMED
LOWMEN
MADMEN
MAIMED
MAIMER
MARMEE
MATMEN
MAUMEE
MERMEN
MESMER
MUMMED
MUMMER
NETMEN
NIAMEY
NONMEN
NOUMEA
NUTMEG
OARMEN
ODDMEN
OILMEN
OLDMEN
ONEMEG
OROMEO
OUIMET
PALMED
PALMER
PENMEN
PERMED
PIEMEN
PIGMEN
PITMEN
PLOMER
PLUMED
PLUMES
POEMES
POMMEL
POMMES
PREMED
PREMET
PRIMED
PRIMER
PRIMES
PUMMEL
RAGMEN
RAMMED
RAMMER
RBIMEN
REAMED
REAMER
RHAMES
RHEMES
RHYMED
RHYMER
RHYMES
RIMMED
ROAMED
ROAMER
RODMEN
ROHMER
ROMMEL
ROOMED
ROOMER
RUMMER
SEAMED
SEAMEN
SEAMER
SEEMED
SHAMED
SHAMES
SIMMER
SKYMEN
SLIMED
SLIMES
SOMMER
SPUMED
SPUMES
STAMEN
SUMMED
SUMMER
TAXMEN
TEAMED
TEEMED
TERMED
TERMES
TEXMEX
THAMES
THEMED
THEMES
THEMET
THYMES
TINMEN
TOOMEY
TOPMEN
WARMED
WARMER
WASMET
WIMMER
WORMED
WORMER
XGAMES
YAMMER
YEOMEN
YESMEN
ZIMMER
ZOOMED

•••M•E
ANOMIE
CAMMIE
DORMIE
FLAMBE
GEMMAE
GIMMIE
GRAMME
GRIMKE
JIMMIE
MARMEE
MAUMEE
MOMMIE
ODAMAE
PREMIE
ROOMIE
STYMIE
TOMMIE
TROMPE

••••ME
AFLAME
AFRAME
ASHAME
ASSUME
ATHOME
BECAME
BECOME
BEHOME
BESAME
BIREME
BOHEME
BYNAME
CALLME
CHROME
DANGME
DAREME
DEARME
DEFAME
DOTIME
ENORME
ENZYME
ESTIME
EXHUME
FEEDME
GENOME
GOHOME
GOLAME
GRAMME
HELPME
HOLDME
ILLUME
IMGAME
IMHOME
INCOME
INHOME
INHUME
INTIME
ISITME
JEROME
JUSTME
KINGME
KISSME
LEGUME
MADAME
MAKEME
MINIME
MISSME
NONAME
NOTIME
OKBYME
ONTIME
RACEME
RADOME
README
REGIME
RELUME
RENAME
RESUME
RETAME
RETIME
SALOME
SAVEME
SCHEME
SESAME
SHOWME
TELLME
TOCOME
TONEME
TVGAME
TVTIME
UGSOME
UNTAME
UPTIME
VOLUME
WAKAME
WASHME

M•F•••
MAFIAS
MIFFED
MIFUNE
MTFUJI
MUFASA
MUFFED
MUFFET
MUFFIN
MUFFLE
MUFTIS
MYFOOT

M••F••
MADFOR
MANFUL
MAYFLY
MCAFEE
MEDFLY
MEIFUN
METFAN
MIFFED
MISFED
MISFIT
MUFFED
MUFFET
MUFFIN
MUFFLE
MUGFUL

M•••F•
MANOFF
MIDOFF
MINIFY
MODIFY
MOTIFS
MYLIFE

M••••F
MADEOF
MAKEOF
MANOFF
MASSIF
MIDOFF
MOSDEF
MOSTOF
MUCHOF
MYSELF

•MF•••
IMFINE
IMFREE
IMFULL

•M••F•
AMALFI
SMURFS

•M•••F
IMPERF
SMALLF

••MF••
AIMFOR
AIMFUL
ARMFUL
ATMFEE
COMFIT
RAMFAN
RAMFIS

••M•F•
RAMIFY
TUMEFY

••M••F
COMEOF

M•G•••
MAGGIE
MAGGIO
MAGGOT
MAGIAN
MAGICS
MAGLEV
MAGLIE
MAGMAS
MAGNET
MAGNOL
MAGNON
MAGNUM
MAGNUS
MAGPIE
MAGYAR
MCGILL
MCGRAW
MCGREW
MEGALO
MEGANE
MEGOHM
MEGREZ
MEGRIM
MIGHTS
MIGHTY
MIGNON
MIGUEL
MOGULS
MUGABE
MUGFUL
MUGGED
MUGGER
MUGGLE
MYGIRL
MYGOSH

M••G••
MAGGIE
MAGGIO
MAGGOT
MAJGEN
MANGAS
MANGER
MANGLE
MANGOS
MARGIE
MARGIN
MARGOT
MEAGER
MEAGRE
MEDGAR
MERGED
MERGEE
MERGER
MERGES
MIDGES
MIDGET
MINGLE
MINGUS
MONGER
MONGOL
MONGOS
MONGST
MORGAN
MORGEN
MORGUE
MOWGLI
MUGGED
MUGGER
MUGGLE

M•••G•
MADEGO
MAKEGO
MALAGA
MALIGN
MANAGE
MANEGE
MAYIGO
MCHUGH
MENAGE
MIRAGE

M••••G
MADDOG
MADVIG
MAKING
MATING
MAXING
MAYING
MAYTAG
MAZING
MCHARG
MEKONG
METING
MEWING
MIDLEG
MIKING
MIMING
MINING
MIRING
MITTAG
MIXING
MOBERG
MONTAG
MOOING
MOPING
MOVING
MOWING
MRWONG
MUSING
MUTING

•MG•••
IMGAME
IMGLAD
IMGONE
IMGOOD

•M•G••
AMIGAS
AMIGOS
EMIGRE
IMAGED
IMAGER
IMAGES
IMAGOS
IMIGHT
IMOGEN
OMEGAS
SMOGGY
SMUGLY

•M••G•
EMBOGS
EMERGE
HMONGS
IMPUGN
SMIDGE
SMOGGY
SMUDGE
SMUDGY

•M•••G
AMPING
SMALLG
UMPING

••MG••
GAMGEE

••M•G•
ARMAGH
DAMAGE
DIMAGE
HOMAGE
IOMEGA
OHMAGE

••M••G
AIMING
ARMING
BUMLEG
COMING
DIMING
DOMING
FAMING
FUMING
GAMING
GYMBAG
HOMING
HUMBUG
LAMING
LIMING
MIMING
NAMING
RIMING
TAMING
TIMING

•••M•G
DESMOG
NUTMEG
ONEMEG
UNSMUG

M•H•••
MAHALO
MAHDIS
MAHLER
MAHOUT
MAHZOR
MCHALE
MCHARG
MCHUGH
MOHAIR
MOHAVE
MOHAWK
MRHYDE
MTHOOD
MYHERO

M••H••
MACHOS
MASHED
MASHER
MASHES
MASHIE
MASHUP
MATHER
MATHEW
MATHIS
MAYHAP
MAYHEM
MCPHEE
MEOHMY
MESHED
MESHES
METHOD
METHYL
MICHEL
MIGHTS
MIGHTY
MISHAP
MISHIT
MOCHAS
MOSHAV
MOSHED
MOSHER
MOSHES
MOTHER
MOTHRA
MUCHAS
MUCHOF
MUDHEN
MUSHED
MUSHER
MUSHES
MYOHMY
MYTHIC
MYTHOS

M•••H•
MANCHA
MANCHE
MANCHU
MARCHE
MARSHA
MARSHY
MARTHA
MARTHE
MEGOHM
MENTHE
MIRTHS
MISCHA
MOESHA
MONTHS
MORPHO
MORPHS
MOUTHS
MOUTHY
MUNCHY
MURPHY
MYNAHS
MYRRHS

M••••H
MANUSH
MARIAH
MATZOH
MCHUGH
MENSCH
MODISH
MOOLAH
MOPISH
MORATH
MULISH
MULLAH
MUNICH
MYGOSH

•MH•••
IMHERE
IMHOME
IMHURT

•M•H••
OMAHAN
OMAHAS
OMPHAL

•M••H•
AMECHE
IMIGHT
SMITHS
SMITHY

•M•••H
AMBUSH
AMONTH
EMDASH
EMPATH
IMPISH
SMALLH
SMERSH
SMIRCH
SMOOCH
SMOOSH
SMOOTH

••MH••
ABMHOS

••M•H•
HUMPHS
KIMCHI
LYMPHS
NYMPHS
OOMPHS
YAMAHA

••M••H
ALMACH
ARMAGH
ASMUCH
COMETH
DEMOTH
ENMESH
FAMISH
IOMOTH
NAMATH
OOMPAH
SAMEKH
SOMUCH
TEMPEH
UNMESH

•••M•H
BRAMAH
WARMTH

MI••••
MIAMIS
MIAMIU
MIAOUS
MIAOWS
MIASMA
MIATAS
MICHEL
MICKEY
MICMAC
MICRON
MICROS
MIDAIR
MIDCAP
MIDDAY
MIDDIE
MIDDLE
MIDGES
MIDGET
MIDIAN
MIDLEG
MIDLER
MIDMAY
MIDOFF
MIDONS
MIDORI
MIDRIB
MIDSTS
MIDWAY
MIELES
MIFFED
MIFUNE
MIGHTS
MIGHTY
MIGNON
MIGUEL
MIKADO
MIKASA
MIKING
MIKITA
MILADY
MILANO
MILANS
MILDER
MILDEW
MILDLY
MILERS
MILIEU
MILKED
MILKER
MILLAY
MILLED
MILLER
MILLES
MILLET
MILLIE
MILNER
MILNES
MILORD
MILOSZ
MILSAP
MILTIE
MILTON
MIMEOS
MIMERS
MIMICS
MIMING
MIMOSA
MINCED
MINCER
MINCES
MINDED
MINDEN
MINDER
MINERS
MINETA
MINGLE
MINGUS
MINIFY
MINIMA
MINIME
MINIMI
MINIMS
MINING
MINION
MINITV
MINNIE
MINNOW
MINOAN
MINORS
MINOSO
MINTED
MINTER
MINUET
MINUIT
MINUTE
MINXES
MINYAN
MIRADA
MIRAGE
MIRIAM
MIRIER
MIRING
MIRINS
MIRREN
MIRROR
MIRROS
MIRTHS
MISACT
MISADD
MISAIM
MISCHA
MISCUE
MISCUT
MISDID
MISERS

MISERY
MISFED
MISFIT
MISHAP
MISHIT
MISKEY
MISLAY
MISLED
MISSAL
MISSAY
MISSED
MISSES
MISSET
MISSIS
MISSME
MISSUS
MISTED
MISTER
MISTUP
MISUSE
MITERS
MITRAL
MITRED
MITRES
MITSOU
MITTAG
MITTEN
MIXERS
MIXING
MIXTEC
MIXUPS
MIZUNA
MIZZEN
MIZZLE
MIZZLY

M•I•••

MAIDEN
MAILED
MAILER
MAILIN
MAILTO
MAIMED
MAIMER
MAINER
MAINLY
MAINST
MAIRES
MAIRZY
MAISIE
MAISON
MAITAI
MAITRE
MAIZES
MEIFUN
MOIETY
MOILED
MOILER
MOINES
MOIRES
MOISES
MSIEUR
MTILES

M••I••

MAFIAS
MAGIAN
MAGICS
MAKING
MALIAN
MALIBU
MALICE
MALICK
MALIGN
MANIAC
MANIAS
MANILA
MAOISM
MAOIST
MARIAH
MARIAN
MARIAS
MARIDA
MARIDO
MARIEL
MARIKO
MARILU
MARINA
MARINE
MARINO
MARION
MARISA
MARIST
MATING
MATINS
MAVINS
MAXIMA
MAXIMS
MAXINE
MAXING
MAXIXE
MAYIGO
MAYING
MAZIER
MAZILY
MAZING
MCGILL
MCRIBS
MEDIAL
MEDIAN
MEDIAS
MEDICA
MEDICI
MEDICO
MEDICS
MEDINA
MEDIUM
MEDIUS
MEJICO
MELINA
MENIAL
MERIDA
MERINO
MERITS
MESIAL
METIER
METING
MEWING
MEXICO
MIDIAN
MIKING
MIKITA
MILIEU
MIMICS
MIMING
MINIFY
MINIMA
MINIME
MINIMI
MINIMS
MINING
MINION
MINITV
MIRIAM
MIRIER
MIRING
MIRINS
MIXING
MOBILE
MOBIUS
MODIFY
MODINE
MODISH
MOJITO
MOLINA
MOLINE
MOMISM
MONICA
MONIED
MONIES
MONISM
MONIST
MOOING
MOPIER
MOPING
MOPISH
MORITA
MORITZ
MOTIFS
MOTILE
MOTION
MOTIVE
MOVIES
MOVING
MOWING
MRBILL
MRDICK
MRJINX
MRPIBB
MTAIRY
MULISH
MUNICH
MURIEL
MURINE
MUSIAL
MUSICK
MUSICS
MUSING
MUTING
MUTINY
MUTIUS
MYGIRL
MYLIFE
MYRIAD

M•••I•

MACKIE
MADDIE
MADEIT
MADRID
MADVIG
MAGGIE
MAGGIO
MAGLIE
MAGPIE
MAHDIS
MAILIN
MAISIE
MAJLIS
MAKEIT
MAKSIM
MALEIC
MALTIN
MANNIX
MANTIC
MANTIS
MAORIS
MAQUIS
MARCIA
MARCIE
MARCIL
MARCIX
MARDIS
MARGIE
MARGIN
MARKIE
MARKII
MARKIV
MARKIX
MARLIN
MARNIE
MARTIN
MARVIN
MARVIS
MARYII
MASAIS
MASHIE
MASLIN
MASSIF
MASTIC
MATHIS
MATLIN
MATRIX
MATTIE
MCBAIN
MCCAIN
MCLAIN
MCNAIR
MCNEIL
MEALIE
MEANIE
MEANIT
MEDNIS
MEGRIM
MELVIL
MELVIN
MEMOIR
MENNIN
MENTIS
MERLIN
MERRIE
MESSIN
METRIC
MIAMIS
MIAMIU
MIDAIR
MIDDIE
MIDRIB
MILLIE
MILTIE
MINNIE
MINUIT
MISAIM
MISDID
MISFIT
MISHIT
MISSIS
MOHAIR
MOLLIE
MOMMIE
MOOKIE
MOONIE
MORBID
MORRIE
MORRIS
MOSAIC
MOTRIN
MOULIN
MOVEIN
MOVEIT
MUDPIE
MUFFIN
MUFTIS
MULLIN
MULTIS
MUNCIE
MURCIA
MUSKIE
MUSLIM
MUSLIN
MYOPIA
MYOPIC
MYOSIN
MYOSIS
MYSTIC
MYTHIC

M••••I

MAITAI
MALAWI
MALLEI
MALOTI
MAOTAI
MARKII
MARKVI
MARYII
MATSUI
MEDICI
MESABI
MIDORI
MINIMI
MODULI
MONAMI
MORONI
MOWGLI
MTFUJI
MUESLI
MUMBAI

•MI•••

AMICAL
AMICES
AMICUS
AMIDAS
AMIDES
AMIDOL
AMIDST
AMIENS
AMIGAS
AMIGOS
AMINES
AMINOR
AMINOS
AMINTA
AMINUS
AMITIE
BMINOR
BMINUS
CMINOR
CMINUS
DMINOR
DMINUS
DMITRI
DMITRY
EMIGRE
EMILIA
EMILIE
EMILIO
EMILYS
EMINEM
EMINOR
FMINOR
GMINOR
IMIDES
IMIGHT
IMINES
SMIDGE
SMILED
SMILER
SMILES
SMILEY
SMILLA
SMIRCH
SMIRKS
SMIRKY
SMITER
SMITES
SMITHS
SMITHY
SMITTY
TMINUS
UMIAKS

•M•I••

AMBIEN
AMBITS
AMNION
AMNIOS
AMPING
AMRITA
EMAILS
EMMITT
EMPIRE
IMBIBE
IMFINE
IMLIKE
IMMIES
IMPISH
OMNIUM
UMPING
UMPIRE

•M••I•

AMADIS
AMALIA
AMALIE
AMATIS
AMAZIN
AMBLIN
AMEBIC
AMELIA
AMELIE
AMESIA
AMITIE
BMOVIE
EMERIC
EMERIL
EMETIC
EMILIA
EMILIE
EMILIO
IMONIT
IMPAIR
OMANIS
TMESIS
UMBRIA

•M•••I

AMALFI
AMANTI
DMITRI
SMALLI

••MI••

ADMINS
ADMIRE
ADMITS
AIMING
ARMIES
ARMING
BEMINE
BEMIRE
BIMINI
CAMINO
CAMION
CAMISE
CIMINO
COMICE
COMICS
COMIDA
COMING
COMITY
CUMINS
DAMIEN
DAMITA
DEMIES
DEMILO
DEMISE
DEMIST
DEMITS
DIMING
DIMITY
DOMINE
DOMING
DOMINI
DOMINO
ELMIER
ELMIRA
ELMIRE
EMMITT
ENMITY
ERMINE
FAMILY
FAMINE
FAMING
FAMISH
FUMIER
FUMING
GAMIER
GAMILY
GAMINE
GAMING
GAMINS
GEMINI
HAMILL
HAMITE
HOMIER
HOMIES
HOMILY
HOMING
HOMINY
IMMIES
INMIND
JEMIMA
JIMINY
LAMIAE
LAMIAS
LAMINA
LAMING
LIMIER
LIMING
LIMITS
LUMINA
MIMICS
MIMING
MOMISM
NAMING
NIMINY
NIMITZ
NOMIAL
NUMINA
ONMIKE
OSMICS
OSMIUM
PAMINA
PAMIRS
PIMINY
PUMICE
RAMIES
RAMIFY
REMICK
REMILL
REMIND
REMINE
REMINI
REMINT
REMISE
REMISS
REMITS
RIMIER
RIMING
RIMINI
ROMIJN
SAMIAM
SEMITE
SIMIAN
SIMILE
TAMILS
TAMING
TIMING
UNMIRY
UNMIXT
USMINT

••M•I•

ARMPIT
BAMBIS
BYMAIL
CAMEIN
CAMMIE
COMEIN
COMFIT
COMMIT
COMMIX
CUMBIA
CYMRIC
DEMAIN
DIMWIT
DOMAIN
GAMBIA
GAMBIT
GIMMIE
HAMLIN
HEMSIN
HOMEIN
IAMBIC
ISMAIL
JAMAIS
JAMSIN
JIMMIE
JUMPIN
KEMPIS
LAMSIT
LIMBIC
LIMPID
LOMEIN
LUMPIN
LUMPIT
MEMOIR
MOMMIE
NAMEIT
RAMFIS
RAMSIN
REMAIL
REMAIN
ROMAIC
ROMAIN
SUMMIT
TOMLIN
TOMMIE
TOMMIX
TOMTIT
USMAIL
WIMMIN
ZAMBIA
ZOMBIE

••M••I

ARMANI
BIMINI
CUMULI
DOMANI
DOMINI
FAMULI
GEMINI
HAMULI
HUMERI
JAMESI
KAMALI
KIMCHI
MUMBAI
REMINI
RIMINI
ROMAJI
ROMANI
RUMAKI
SAMEDI
SOMALI
SOMONI
YAMANI
YEMENI

•••MI•

ANEMIA
ANEMIC
ANOMIA
ANOMIC
ANOMIE
ARAMID
ARAMIS
ATOMIC
CADMIC
CAMMIE
CHEMIC
CHEMIN
COMMIT
COMMIX
COSMIC
CRAMIN
DERMIC
DERMIS
DORMIE
DROMIO
ELEMIS
FERMIS
FILMIC
FORMIC
GIMMIE
GNOMIC
GROMIT
GRUMIO
HERMIT
JASMIN
JIMMIE
KARMIC
KERMIT
LESMIZ
MIAMIS
MIAMIU
MOMMIE
OTOMIS
PERMIT
PREMIE
PREMIX
REEMIT
ROAMIN
RONMIX
ROOMIE
SALMIS
SHAMIR
STYMIE
SUBMIT
SUMMIT
SWAMIS
THYMIC
TOMMIE
TOMMIX
UNAMIS
VERMIN
WIMMIN
YASMIN
ZOOMIN

•••M•I

ALUMNI
GIAMBI
KATMAI
PASMOI
RHOMBI
SCAMPI
SHUMAI

••••MI

BONAMI
DOREMI
ISTHMI
MINIMI
MONAMI
SALAMI
SURIMI
TATAMI
WHOAMI

M•J•••

MAJGEN
MAJLIS
MAJOAD
MAJORS
MCJOBS
MEJICO
MOJAVE
MOJITO
MOJOES
MRJINX

M••J••

MARJOE
MATJES
MENJOU

M•••J•

MARYJO
MTFUJI
MTVVJS

•M•J••

AMAJOR
BMAJOR
CMAJOR
DMAJOR
EMAJOR
FMAJOR
GMAJOR

•M•••J

SMALLJ

••MJ••

RAMJET

••M•J•

ROMAJI
ROMIJN

••M••J

JAMESJ

•••M•J

SGTMAJ

M•K•••

MAKEBA
MAKEDO
MAKEGO
MAKEIT
MAKEME
MAKEOF
MAKERS
MAKEUP
MAKING
MAKSIM
MAKUTA
MCKEAN
MCKEON
MCKERN
MCKUEN
MEKONG
MIKADO
MIKASA
MIKING
MIKITA
MUKLUK

M••K••

MACKIE
MARKAS
MARKED
MARKER
MARKET
MARKEY
MARKIE
MARKII
MARKIV
MARKIX
MARKKA
MARKOV
MARKUP
MARKVI
MASKED
MASKER
MEEKER
MEEKLY
MENKEN
MERKEL
MICKEY
MILKED
MILKER
MISKEY
MOCKED
MOCKER
MOCKUP
MONKEE
MONKEY
MOOKIE
MOSKVA
MUCKED
MUCKER
MUCKUP
MUSKET
MUSKIE
MUSKOX

M•••K•

MARIKO
MARKKA
MEDAKA
MERCKX
MOLTKE

M••••K

MALICK
MCDUCK
MOHAWK
MRDICK
MTCOOK
MUKLUK
MUSICK

•M•K••

IMOKAY
SMOKED
SMOKER
SMOKES
SMOKEY

•M••K•

DMARKS
IMLIKE
SMACKS
SMIRKS
SMIRKY
SMOCKS
UMIAKS

•M•••K

AMTRAK
EMBANK
EMBARK
IMBACK
SMALLK

••M•K•

BAMAKO
JAMOKE
LEMOKO
ONMIKE
REMAKE
RIMSKY
RUMAKI
SAMEKH
UNMAKE

••M••K

ARMONK
DAMASK
DEMARK
JAMESK
NOMEAK
REMARK
REMICK
STMARK
UNMASK
WOMACK

•••MK•

GRIMKE

M•L•••

MALABO
MALADY
MALAGA
MALARS
MALAWI
MALAYA
MALAYS
MALDEN
MALEIC
MALIAN
MALIBU
MALICE
MALICK
MALIGN
MALLEI
MALLET
MALLON
MALLOW
MALONE
MALORY
MALOTI
MALTBY
MALTED
MALTIN
MCLAIN
MCLEAN
MELDED
MELDER
MELEES
MELETE
MELINA
MELLON
MELLOW
MELMAC
MELODY
MELONS
MELOTT
MELTED
MELTER
MELTON
MELVIL
MELVIN
MELVYN
MILADY
MILANO
MILANS
MILDER
MILDEW
MILDLY
MILERS
MILIEU
MILKED
MILKER
MILLAY
MILLED
MILLER
MILLES
MILLET
MILLIE
MILNER
MILNES
MILORD
MILOSZ
MILSAP
MILTIE
MILTON
MOLARS
MOLDAU
MOLDED
MOLDER
MOLEST
MOLINA
MOLINE
MOLLIE
MOLLOY
MOLNAR
MOLSON
MOLTED
MOLTEN
MOLTER
MOLTKE
MULCTS
MULDER
MULETA
MULEYS
MULISH
MULLAH
MULLAS
MULLED
MULLER
MULLET
MULLIN
MULTIS
MYLADY
MYLARS
MYLIFE
MYLORD
MYLOVE

M••L••

MAALOX
MABLEY
MACLEN
MACLES
MADLYN
MAGLEV
MAGLIE
MAHLER
MAILED
MAILER
MAILIN
MAILTO
MAJLIS
MALLEI
MALLET
MALLON
MALLOW
MANLEY
MAPLES
MARLED
MARLEE
MARLEY
MARLIN
MARLON
MASLIN
MATLIN
MAULED
MAULER
MEALIE
MEDLEY
MELLON
MELLOW
MERLIN
MERLOT
MEWLED
MEWLER
MIDLEG
MIDLER
MIELES
MILLAY
MILLED

MILLER
MILLES
MILLET
MILLIE
MISLAY
MISLED
MOBLEY
MOILED
MOILER
MOLLIE
MOLLOY
MOOLAH
MORLEY
MOSLEM
MOSLEY
MOTLEY
MOULDS
MOULDY
MOULIN
MOULTS
MRBLUE
MTILES
MUKLUK
MULLAH
MULLAS
MULLED
MULLER
MULLET
MULLIN
MUSLIM
MUSLIN

M•••L•
MABELL
MACULA
MAHALO
MAINLY
MANGLE
MANILA
MANTLE
MAPPLE
MARBLE
MARBLY
MARILU
MARPLE
MASALA
MAXELL
MAYFLY
MAZILY
MAZOLA
MCGILL
MCHALE
MEANLY
MEASLE
MEASLY
MEDALS
MEDDLE
MEDFLY
MEEKLY
MEETLY
MEGALO
MERDLE
MERELY
MERYLL
METALS
METTLE
MIDDLE
MILDLY
MINGLE
MIZZLE
MIZZLY
MOBILE
MODALS
MODELA
MODELB
MODELS
MODELT
MODULE
MODULI
MODULO
MOGULS
MORALE
MORALS
MORELS
MOROLT
MOSTLY
MOTELS
MOTILE
MOTTLE
MOWGLI
MRBILL
MRSULU
MUDDLE
MUESLI
MUFFLE
MUGGLE
MUMBLE
MUMBLY
MURALS
MUSCLE
MUSCLY
MUTELY
MUZZLE
MYRTLE
MYSELF

M••••L
MAAZEL
MABELL
MAGNOL
MAMMAL
MANDEL
MANFUL
MANTEL
MANUAL
MANUEL
MARCEL
MARCIL
MARIEL
MARTEL
MARVEL
MATTEL
MAXELL
MCBEAL
MCGILL
MCNEIL
MEDIAL
MELVIL
MENDEL
MENIAL
MENSAL
MENTAL
MERKEL
MERYLL
MESCAL
MESIAL
METHYL
MICHEL
MIGUEL
MISSAL
MITRAL
MONGOL
MONTEL
MORREL
MORSEL
MORTAL
MOSTEL
MRBILL
MRCOOL
MUDEEL
MUGFUL
MURIEL
MUSIAL
MUSSEL
MUTUAL
MUTUEL
MYGIRL
MYRDAL

•ML•••
IMLATE
IMLIKE
UMLAUT

•M•L••
AMALFI
AMALIA
AMALIE
AMBLED
AMBLER
AMBLES
AMBLIN
AMELIA
AMELIE
AMOLES
AMPLER
AMULET
EMALLS
EMBLEM
EMILIA
EMILIE
EMILIO
EMILYS
EMPLOY
IMELDA
IMGLAD
IMPLED
OMELET
SMALLA
SMALLB
SMALLC
SMALLD
SMALLE
SMALLF
SMALLG
SMALLH
SMALLI
SMALLJ
SMALLK
SMALLL
SMALLM
SMALLN
SMALLO
SMALLP
SMALLQ
SMALLR
SMALLS
SMALLT
SMALLU
SMALLV
SMALLW
SMALLX
SMALLY
SMALLZ
SMELLS
SMELLY
SMELTS
SMILED
SMILER
SMILES
SMILEY
SMILLA
SMOLTS

•M••L•
AMPULE
EMAILS
EMALLS
EMBALM
EMPALE
IMCOLD
IMFULL
IMPALA
IMPALE
IMPELS
IMSOLD
IMTOLD
SMALLA
SMALLB
SMALLC
SMALLD
SMALLE
SMALLF
SMALLG
SMALLH
SMALLI
SMALLJ
SMALLK
SMALLL
SMALLM
SMALLN
SMALLO
SMALLP
SMALLQ
SMALLR
SMALLS
SMALLT
SMALLU
SMALLV
SMALLW
SMALLX
SMALLY
SMALLZ
SMELLS
SMELLY
SMILLA
SMUGLY
UMBELS

•M•••L
AMATOL
AMICAL
AMIDOL
AMORAL
AMSTEL
EMERIL
IMCOOL
IMFULL
OMPHAL
SMALLL
UMBRAL

••ML••
ARMLET
BUMLEG
GIMLET
HAMLET
HAMLIN
LUMLEY
SAMLET
TOMLIN

••M•L•
BUMBLE
CAMELS
COMELY
COMPLY
CUMULI
CUMULO
DAMPLY
DEMILO
DIMPLE
DIMPLY
DUMBLY
FAMILY
FAMULI
FEMALE
FUMBLE
GAMBLE
GAMELY
GAMILY
GIMELS
HAMELN
HAMILL
HAMULI
HOMELY
HOMILY
HUMBLE
HUMBLY
JUMBLE
JUMBLY
KAMALI
KEMBLE
KIMBLE
LAMELY
LIMPLY
MUMBLE
MUMBLY
NAMELY
NIMBLE
NIMBLY
NUMBLY
ORMOLU
PAMELA
PIMPLE
PIMPLY
POMELO
RAMBLE
REMELT
REMILL
REMOLD
RIMPLE
ROMOLA
ROMULO
RUMBLE
RUMBLY
RUMPLE
RUMPLY
SAMPLE
SEMELE
SEMPLE
SIMILE
SIMPLE
SIMPLY
SOMALI
STMALO
TAMALE
TAMELY
TAMILS
TEMPLE
TIMELY
TUMBLE
TUMULT
UNMOLD
WAMBLE
WAMBLY
WIMPLE

••M••L
AIMFUL
ARMFUL
BOMBAL
BYMAIL
COMPEL
CYMBAL
DAMSEL
GAMBOL
GIMBAL
GIMBEL
GUMBEL
HAMILL
HIMMEL
HUMMEL
HYMNAL
ISMAIL
JAMAAL
KUMMEL
LEMUEL
MAMMAL
NOMIAL
POMMEL
PUMMEL
RAMPAL
REMAIL
REMILL
ROMMEL
SAMUEL
SYMBOL
TIMBAL
USMAIL

•••ML•
CALMLY
FIRMLY
GLUMLY
GRIMLY
PRIMLY
SEEMLY
SLIMLY
TRIMLY
WARMLY

•••M•L
ANIMAL
BRUMAL
BRUMEL
CARMEL
DEHMEL
DERMAL
DISMAL
ENAMEL
ETYMOL
FORMAL
HIEMAL
HIMMEL
HORMEL
HUMMEL
KUMMEL
MAMMAL
NERMAL
NORMAL
POMMEL
PRIMAL
PUMMEL
ROMMEL

MM••••
MMDDYY
MMMBOP

M•M•••
MAMBAS
MAMBOS
MAMMAL
MAMMAS
MAMMON
MEMBER
MEMOIR
MEMORY
MIMEOS
MIMERS
MIMICS
MIMING
MIMOSA
MMMBOP
MOMENT
MOMISM
MOMMAS
MOMMIE
MRMOTO
MUMBAI
MUMBLE
MUMBLY
MUMMED
MUMMER
MUMMYS
MYMYMY

M••M••
MADMAN
MADMAX
MADMEN
MAGMAS
MAIMED
MAIMER
MAMMAL
MAMMAS
MAMMON
MARMEE
MARMOT
MATMAN
MATMEN
MAUMAU
MAUMEE
MELMAC
MERMAN
MERMEN
MESMER
MIAMIS
MIAMIU
MICMAC
MIDMAY
MOMMAS
MOMMIE
MORMON
MUMMED
MUMMER
MUMMYS
MURMUR
MUUMUU

M•••M•
MACOMB
MADAMA
MADAME
MADAMS
MAKEME
MANAMA
MANDMS
MAXIMA
MAXIMS
MAZUMA
MECUMS
MEOHMY
MIASMA
MINIMA
MINIME
MINIMI
MINIMS
MISSME
MODEMS
MONAMI
MYMYMY
MYOHMY

M••••M
MAGNUM
MAKSIM
MAOISM
MARYAM
MAYHEM
MEDIUM
MEGOHM
MEGRIM
MIRIAM
MISAIM
MOMISM
MONISM
MOSLEM
MUSEUM
MUSLIM

•MM•••
EMMAUS
EMMETS
EMMETT
EMMITT
IMMIES
IMMUNE
IMMUNO
IMMURE
MMMBOP

•M•M••
IMAMAN

•M••M•
IMGAME
IMHOME
SMARMY

•M•••M
EMBALM
EMBLEM
EMINEM
OMASUM
OMNIUM
SMALLM

••MM••
BUMMED
BUMMER
CAMMIE
COMMAS
COMMIT
COMMIX
COMMON
DAMMED
DAMMER
DDMMYY
DIMMED
DIMMER
FEMMES
GAMMAS
GAMMED
GAMMER
GAMMON
GEMMAE
GEMMED
GIMMES
GIMMIE
GUMMED
HAMMED
HAMMER
HEMMED
HEMMER
HIMMEL
HOMMES
HUMMED
HUMMEL
HUMMER
HUMMUS
JAMMED
JAMMER
JIMMIE
KUMMEL
LAMMED
LEMMAS
LEMMON
LUMMOX
MAMMAL
MAMMAS
MAMMON
MOMMAS
MOMMIE
MUMMED
MUMMER
MUMMYS
POMMEL
POMMES
PUMMEL
RAMMED
RAMMER
RIMMED
ROMMEL
RUMMER
SIMMER
SOMMER
SUMMED
SUMMER
SUMMIT
SUMMON
TAMMUZ
TOMMIE
TOMMIX
WIMMER
WIMMIN
YAMMER
ZIMMER

••M•M•
JEMIMA
MYMYMY

••M••M
DIMSUM
DUMDUM
IAMSAM
JAMCAM
JAMESM
MOMISM
NOMAAM
OSMIUM
POMPOM
ROMCOM
SAMIAM
TAMTAM
TOMTOM
WAMPUM
YUMYUM

•••MM•
CHAMMY
CHUMMY
CLAMMA
CLAMMY
CRUMMY
GRAMME
GRAMMY
GRIMMS
GRIMMY
PLUMMY
SCUMMY
SHAMMY
SHIMMY
SLUMMY
STEMMY
WHAMMO
WHAMMY

•••M•M
DENMOM

MN••••
MNOPQR

M•N•••
MANAGE
MANAMA
MANANA
MANAOS
MANAPE
MANATS
MANCHA
MANCHE
MANCHU
MANDAN
MANDAY
MANDEL
MANDMS
MANEGE
MANERO
MANETS
MANFUL
MANGAS
MANGER
MANGLE
MANGOS
MANIAC
MANIAS
MANILA
MANLEY
MANNAS
MANNED
MANNER
MANNIX
MANNON
MANOFF
MANORS
MANQUE
MANRAY
MANSES
MANTAS
MANTEE
MANTEL
MANTIC
MANTIS
MANTLE
MANTRA
MANTUA
MANUAL
MANUEL
MANURE
MANUSH
MANUTE
MANZON
MCNABB
MCNAIR
MCNEIL
MENACE
MENAGE
MENDED
MENDEL
MENDER
MENDES
MENIAL
MENJOU
MENKEN
MENNEN
MENNIN
MENSAL
MENSAN
MENSCH
MENTAL
MENTEE
MENTHE
MENTIS
MENTOR
MENTOS
MENUDO
MINCED
MINCER
MINCES
MINDED
MINDEN
MINDER
MINERS
MINETA
MINGLE
MINGUS
MINIFY
MINIMA
MINIME
MINIMI
MINIMS
MINING
MINION
MINITV
MINNIE
MINNOW
MINOAN
MINORS
MINOSO
MINTED
MINTER
MINUET
MINUIT
MINUTE
MINXES
MINYAN
MONACO
MONADS
MONAMI
MONDAY
MONDES
MONDOS
MONETA
MONETS
MONEYS
MONGER
MONGOL
MONGOS
MONGST
MONICA
MONIED
MONIES
MONISM
MONIST
MONKEE
MONKEY
MONNET
MONODY
MONROE
MONTAG
MONTEL
MONTEZ
MONTHS
MONZAS
MUNCHY
MUNCIE
MUNERA
MUNICH
MUNROE
MYNAHS

M••N••
MACNEE
MAENAD
MAGNET
MAGNOL
MAGNON
MAGNUM
MAGNUS
MAINER
MAINLY
MAINST
MANNAS
MANNED
MANNER
MANNIX
MANNON
MARNER
MARNIE
MAUNDY
MEANER
MEANEY
MEANIE
MEANIT
MEANLY
MEANTO
MEDNIS
MENNEN
MENNIN
MESNES
MIGNON
MILNER
MILNES
MINNIE
MINNOW
MOANED
MOANER
MOINES
MOLNAR
MONNET
MOONED
MOONER
MOONEY
MOONIE
MORNAY
MOUNDS
MOUNTS
MOUNTY

M•••N•
MAKING
MALONE
MANANA
MARINA
MARINE
MARINO
MASONS
MATING
MATINS
MAVENS
MAVINS
MAXENE
MAXINE
MAXING
MAYANS
MAYING
MAZING
MCCANN
MEDINA
MEGANE
MEKONG
MELINA
MELONS
MERINO
MESONS
METING
MEWING
MIDONS
MIFUNE
MIKING
MILANO
MILANS
MIMING
MINING
MIRING
MIRINS
MIXING
MIZUNA
MODENA
MODINE
MOLINA
MOLINE
MOMENT
MOOING
MOPING
MORANT
MORENO
MORONI
MORONS
MOURNS
MOVING
MOWING
MRBOND
MRJINX
MRWONG
MTETNA
MURANO
MURINE
MUSING
MUSTNT
MUTANT
MUTING
MUTINY
MUTONS

M••••N
MACLEN
MACOUN
MACRON
MADDEN
MADLYN
MADMAN
MADMEN
MADSEN
MAGIAN
MAGNON
MAIDEN
MAILIN
MAISON
MAJGEN
MALDEN
MALIAN
MALIGN
MALLON
MALTIN
MAMMON
MANDAN
MANNON
MANZON
MARDEN
MARGIN
MARIAN
MARION
MARLIN
MARLON
MAROON
MARRON
MARTEN
MARTIN
MARVIN
MASLIN
MASSON
MATLIN
MATMAN
MATMEN
MATRON
MATSON
MAWSON
MAXSON
MAYRON
MCBAIN
MCCAIN
MCCANN
MCEWAN
MCEWEN
MCKEAN
MCKEON
MCKERN
MCKUEN
MCLAIN
MCLEAN
MECCAN
MEDIAN
MEIFUN
MELLON
MELTON
MELVIN
MELVYN
MENKEN
MENNEN
MENNIN
MENSAN
MERLIN
MERMAN
MERMEN
MERTON
MERVYN
MESSIN
METFAN
MICRON
MIDIAN
MIGNON
MILTON
MINDEN
MINION
MINOAN

MINYAN
MIRREN
MITTEN
MIZZEN
MODERN
MOLSON
MOLTEN
MOREEN
MORGAN
MORGEN
MORMON
MORTEN
MORTON
MOTION
MOTOWN
MOTRIN
MOULIN
MOVEIN
MOVEON
MRBEAN
MUDHEN
MUFFIN
MULLIN
MUSEON
MUSLIN
MUTTON
MYOSIN
MYTURN

•MN•••

AMNION
AMNIOS
IMNEXT
LMNOPQ
OMNIUM

•M•N••

AMANAS
AMANDA
AMANTI
AMANTS
AMENDS
AMENRA
AMENTS
AMINES
AMINOR
AMINOS
AMINTA
AMINUS
AMONRA
AMONTH
BMINOR
BMINUS
CMINOR
CMINUS
DMINOR
DMINUS
EMENDS
EMINEM
EMINOR
FMINOR
GMINOR
HMONGS
IMINES
IMONIT
OMANIS
OMENED
TMINUS

•M••N•

AMARNA
AMBAND
AMIENS
AMOUNT
AMPING
EMBANK
FMBAND
IMDONE
IMEANT
IMFINE
IMGONE
IMMUNE
IMMUNO
IMPEND
SMYRNA
UMPING

•M•••N

AMAZIN
AMAZON
AMBIEN
AMBLIN
AMNION
AMYTAN
EMPSON
IMAMAN
IMOGEN
IMPUGN
KMESON
OMAHAN
SMALLN

••MN••

DAMNED
DAMNER
HYMNAL
HYMNED
IAMNOT
KLMNOP
LEMNOS
LIMNED
LIMNER
ROMNEY
SUMNER

••M•N•

ADMINS
AIMING
ALMOND
ARMAND
ARMANI
ARMING
ARMONK
ASMANY
ATMANS
AUMONT
BEMINE
BIMINI
CAMINO
CEMENT
CIMINO
COMING
CUMINS
DAMONE
DEMAND
DEMOND
DEMONS
DIMING
DOMANI
DOMINE
DOMING
DOMINI
DOMINO
DUMONT
EAMONN
EDMOND
EDMUND
EGMONT
ELMONT
ERMINE
FAMINE
FAMING
FOMENT
FUMING
GAMINE
GAMING
GAMINS
GEMINI
HOMING
HOMINY
HUMANE
HUMANS
IMMUNE
IMMUNO
INMIND
ISMENE
JIMINY
KIMONO
LAMENT
LAMINA
LAMING
LAMONT
LEMANS
LEMOND
LEMONS
LEMONY
LIMANS
LIMING
LOMOND
LUMENS
LUMINA
MIMING
MOMENT
NAMING
NIMINY
NUMINA
ORMOND
OSMOND
OSMUND
PAMINA
PIMINY
POMONA
RAMENS
RAMONA
RAMONE
REMAND
REMANS
REMEND
REMIND
REMINE
REMINI
REMINT
RIMING
RIMINI
ROMANI
ROMANO
ROMANS
ROMANY
SEMANA
SIMONE
SOMANY
SOMONI
TAMING
TIMING
UNMANS
USMINT
WOMANS
WOMENS
YAMANI
YAMUNA
YEMANA
YEMENI
YUMANS

••M••N

BEMOAN
CAMDEN
CAMEIN
CAMEON
CAMION
CAMRYN
COMDEN
COMEIN
COMEON
COMMON
DAMIEN
DAMPEN
DAMSON
DEMAIN
DEMEAN
DOMAIN
DUMPON
EAMONN
GAMMON
HAMDEN
HAMELN
HAMLIN
HAMSUN
HEMPEN
HEMSIN
HOMEIN
JAMSIN
JIMSON
JUMPIN
JUMPON
LEMMON
LOMEIN
LUMPEN
LUMPIN
MAMMON
NEMEAN
POMPON
RAMFAN
RAMSIN
RAMSON
REMAIN
REMOWN
REMSEN
ROMAIN
ROMIJN
SAMOAN
SAMPAN
SAMSON
SIMEON
SIMIAN
SUMMON
TOMLIN
UNMOWN
WIMMIN

•••MN•

ALUMNA
ALUMNI
JKLMNO

•••M•N

ACUMEN
AIDMAN
AIDMEN
AIKMAN
AIRMAN
AIRMEN
ALEMAN
ALLMAN
ALLMEN
ALTMAN
ANYMAN
APEMAN
APEMEN
ASHMAN
ASHMEN
ATAMAN
AWCMON
AXEMAN
AXEMEN
BADMAN
BADMEN
BAGMAN
BAGMEN
BARMAN
BARMEN
BATMAN
BATMEN
BAUMAN
BAYMAN
BAYMEN
BEAMAN
BEAMON
BERMAN
BIGMAN
BIGMEN
BIRMAN
BORMAN
BOWMAN
BOWMEN
BREMEN
BURMAN
BUSMAN
BUSMEN
CABMAN
CABMEN
CAIMAN
CARMAN
CARMEN
CATMAN
CATMEN
CAYMAN
CHEMIN
COLMAN
COMMON
CONMAN
CONMEN
CORMAN
COWMAN
COWMEN
CRAMIN
DAEMON
DOLMAN
ELFMAN
ENDMAN
ENDMEN
ERDMAN
ETYMON
FAIMAN
FATMAN
FBIMAN
FBIMEN
FLYMAN
FLYMEN
FOEMAN
FOEMEN
FORMAN
FURMAN
GAGMAN
GAGMEN
GAMMON
GASMAN
GASMEN
GERMAN
GILMAN
GNOMON
GUNMAN
GUNMEN
GUTMAN
GUZMAN
HAGMAN
HARMON
HERMAN
HERMON
HEYMAN
HITMAN
HITMEN
HODMAN
HODMEN
HOLMAN
ICEMAN
ICEMEN
IMAMAN
JASMIN
KEYMAN
KEYMEN
KIDMAN
KIRMAN
KORMAN
LARMEN
LAWMAN
LAWMEN
LAYMAN
LAYMEN
LEGMAN
LEGMEN
LEHMAN
LEMMON
LOWMAN
LOWMEN
MADMAN
MADMEN
MAMMON
MATMAN
MATMEN
MERMAN
MERMEN
MORMON
NEIMAN
NETMAN
NETMEN
NEUMAN
NEWMAN
NOEMON
NONMAN
NONMEN
NORMAN
OARMAN
OARMEN
ODDMAN
ODDMEN
OILMAN
OILMEN
OLDMAN
OLDMEN
ONEMAN
OUTMAN
PACMAN
PENMAN
PENMEN
PIEMAN
PIEMEN
PIGMAN
PIGMEN
PITMAN
PITMEN
PULMON
RAGMAN
RAGMEN
RBIMAN
RBIMEN
ROAMIN
RODMAN
RODMEN
RUDMAN
SALMAN
SALMON
SEAMAN
SEAMEN
SERMON
SHAMAN
SHIMON
SKYMAN
SKYMEN
SLAMON
STAMEN
SUMMON
TASMAN
TAXMAN
TAXMEN
THEMAN
TINMAN
TINMEN
TOAMAN
TODMAN
TOPMAN
TOPMEN
TRUMAN
TUBMAN
TWOMAN
TWYMAN
ULLMAN
VERMIN
WIEMAN
WIMMIN
YASMIN
YEOMAN
YEOMEN
YESMAN
YESMEN
ZEEMAN
ZOOMIN

••••MN

AUTUMN
COLUMN
IJKLMN
SOLEMN

MO••••

MOANED
MOANER
MOATED
MOBBED
MOBBER
MOBERG
MOBILE
MOBIUS
MOBLEY
MOBUTU
MOCHAS
MOCKED
MOCKER
MOCKUP
MODALS
MODELA
MODELB
MODELS
MODELT
MODEMS
MODENA
MODERN
MODEST
MODIFY
MODINE
MODISH
MODRED
MODULE
MODULI
MODULO
MOERAE
MOESHA
MOGULS
MOHAIR
MOHAVE
MOHAWK
MOIETY
MOILED
MOILER
MOINES
MOIRES
MOISES
MOJAVE
MOJITO
MOJOES
MOLARS
MOLDAU
MOLDED
MOLDER
MOLEST
MOLINA
MOLINE
MOLLIE
MOLLOY
MOLNAR
MOLSON
MOLTED
MOLTEN
MOLTER
MOLTKE
MOMENT
MOMISM
MOMMAS
MOMMIE
MONACO
MONADS
MONAMI
MONDAY
MONDES
MONDOS
MONETA
MONETS
MONEYS
MONGER
MONGOL
MONGOS
MONGST
MONICA
MONIED
MONIES
MONISM
MONIST
MONKEE
MONKEY
MONNET
MONODY
MONROE
MONTAG
MONTEL
MONTEZ
MONTHS
MONZAS
MOOCOW
MOODYS
MOOERS
MOOING
MOOKIE
MOOLAH
MOONED
MOONER
MOONEY
MOONIE
MOORED
MOOTED
MOOTER
MOPEDS
MOPERS
MOPERY
MOPIER
MOPING
MOPISH
MOPPED
MOPPER
MOPPET
MOPSUP
MOPTOP
MOPUPS
MORALE
MORALS
MORANT
MORASS
MORATH
MORAYS
MORBID
MOREAU
MOREEN
MORELS
MORENO
MORESO
MORGAN
MORGEN
MORGUE
MORITA
MORITZ
MORLEY
MORMON
MORNAY
MOROLT
MORONI
MORONS
MOROSE
MOROSS
MORPHO
MORPHS
MORREL
MORRIE
MORRIS
MORROW
MORSEL
MORTAL
MORTAR
MORTEN
MORTON
MOSAIC
MOSCOW
MOSDEF
MOSEYS
MOSHAV
MOSHED
MOSHER
MOSHES
MOSKVA
MOSLEM
MOSLEY
MOSQUE
MOSSAD
MOSSED
MOSSES
MOSTEL
MOSTLY
MOSTOF
MOTELS
MOTETS
MOTHER
MOTHRA
MOTIFS
MOTILE
MOTION
MOTIVE
MOTLEY
MOTORS
MOTOWN
MOTRIN
MOTTLE
MOTTOS
MOTTST
MOULDS
MOULDY
MOULIN
MOULTS
MOUNDS
MOUNTS
MOUNTY
MOURNS
MOUSED
MOUSER
MOUSES
MOUSEY
MOUSSE
MOUTHS
MOUTHY
MOVADO
MOVEIN
MOVEIT
MOVEON
MOVERS
MOVETO
MOVEUP
MOVIES
MOVING
MOWERS
MOWGLI
MOWING
MOYERS
MOZART

M•O•••

MAOISM
MAOIST
MAORIS
MAOTAI
MEOHMY
MEOWED
MEOWER
MNOPQR
MOOCOW
MOODYS
MOOERS
MOOING
MOOKIE
MOOLAH
MOONED
MOONER
MOONEY
MOONIE
MOORED
MOOTED
MOOTER
MTOSSA
MYOHMY
MYOPES
MYOPIA
MYOPIC
MYOSIN
MYOSIS

M••O••

MACOMB
MACOUN
MAHOUT
MAJOAD
MAJORS
MALONE
MALORY
MALOTI
MANOFF
MANORS
MAPOUT
MAROON
MASONS
MAXOUT
MAYORS
MAZOLA
MCCORD
MCJOBS
MEDOCS
MEGOHM
MEKONG
MELODY
MELONS
MELOTT
MEMOIR
MEMORY
MEROPE
MEROPS
MESONS
MIAOUS
MIAOWS
MIDOFF
MIDONS
MIDORI
MILORD
MILOSZ
MIMOSA
MINOAN
MINORS
MINOSO
MOJOES
MONODY
MOROLT
MORONI
MORONS
MOROSE
MOROSS
MOTORS
MOTOWN
MRBOND
MRCOOL
MRMOTO
MRWONG
MTCOOK
MTHOOD
MUTONS
MYFOOT
MYGOSH
MYLORD
MYLOVE
MYSORE
MYWORD

M•••O•

MAALOX
MACHOS
MACRON
MACROS
MADDOG
MADDOX
MADEOF
MADFOR
MAGGOT
MAGNOL
MAGNON
MAHZOR
MAISON
MAKEOF
MALLON
MALLOW
MAMBOS
MAMMON
MANAOS
MANGOS
MANNON
MANZON
MARCOS
MARGOT
MARION
MARJOE
MARKOV
MARLON
MARMOT
MAROON
MARRON
MARROW
MASCOT
MASSON
MATRON
MATSON
MATZOH
MATZOS
MAWSON
MAXSON
MAYRON
MCADOO
MCAVOY
MCKEON
MEADOW
MELLON
MELLOW
MELTON
MENJOU
MENTOR
MENTOS
MERLOT
MERTON
METEOR
METHOD
METROS
MEZZOS
MICRON
MICROS
MIGNON
MILTON
MIMEOS
MINION
MINNOW
MIRROR
MIRROS
MITSOU
MMMBOP
MOLLOY
MOLSON
MONDOS
MONGOL
MONGOS
MONROE
MOOCOW
MOPTOP
MORMON
MORROW
MORTON
MOSCOW
MOSTOF
MOTION
MOTTOS
MOVEON
MRCOOL
MTCOOK
MTHOOD
MUCHOF
MUNROE
MURROW
MUSEON
MUSEOS
MUSKOX
MUTTON
MYFOOT
MYTHOS

M••••O

MACACO
MADEDO
MADEGO
MADERO
MADURO
MAGGIO
MAHALO
MAILTO
MAKEDO
MAKEGO
MALABO
MANERO
MAPUTO
MARIDO
MARIKO
MARINO
MARYJO
MATSUO
MAYIGO
MCADOO
MEANTO
MEDICO
MEGALO
MEJICO
MENUDO
MERINO
MEXICO
MIKADO
MILANO
MINOSO
MODULO
MOJITO
MONACO
MORENO
MORESO
MORPHO
MOVADO
MOVETO
MRMOTO
MURANO
MUSTDO
MYHERO

•MO•••

AMOEBA
AMOLES
AMONRA
AMONTH
AMORAL
AMORES
AMORET
AMOSOZ
AMOUNT
AMOURS
BMOVIE
EMORYU
EMOTED
EMOTER
EMOTES
HMONGS
IMOGEN
IMOKAY
IMONIT
SMOCKS
SMOGGY
SMOKED
SMOKER
SMOKES
SMOKEY
SMOLTS
SMOOCH
SMOOSH
SMOOTH
SMORES

•M•O••

EMBODY
EMBOGS
EMBOSS
EMBOWS
IMCOLD
IMCOOL
IMDONE
IMGONE
IMGOOD
IMHOME
IMPORT
IMPOSE
IMPOST
IMSOLD
IMTOLD
LMNOPQ
SMOOCH
SMOOSH
SMOOTH

•M••O•

AMAJOR
AMATOL
AMAZON
AMIDOL
AMIGOS
AMINOR
AMINOS
AMNION
AMNIOS
AMOSOZ
BMAJOR
BMINOR
CMAJOR
CMINOR
DMAJOR
DMINOR
EMAJOR
EMINOR
EMPLOY
EMPSON

EMPTOR
FMAJOR
FMINOR
GMAJOR
GMINOR
IMACOP
IMAGOS
IMCOOL
IMGOOD
IMPROV
KMESON
MMMBOP

•M•••O

AMADEO
AMEDEO
EMBRYO
EMILIO
IMMUNO
SMALLO

••MO••

ALMOND
ALMOST
ARMONK
ARMORS
ARMORY
ARMOUR
ATMOST
AUMONT
BEMOAN
BUMOUT
CAMOES
COMORO
DAMONE
DAMORE
DAMOUR
DEMOBS
DEMODE
DEMOED
DEMOND
DEMONS
DEMOTE
DEMOTH
DIMOUT
DUMONT
EAMONN
EDMOND
EGMONT
ELMONT
ELMORE
EXMOOR
EXMORE
FAMOUS
FEMORA
GAMOUS
HUMORS
HUMOUR
INMOST
IOMOTH
JAMOCA
JAMOKE
KIMONO
KOMODO
LAMONT
LAMOUR
LEMOKO
LEMOND
LEMONS
LEMONY
LOMOND
MEMOIR
MEMORY
MIMOSA
MRMOTO
NOMORE
ORMOLU
ORMOND
OSMOND
OSMOSE
POMONA
RAMONA
RAMONE
RAMOSE
REMOLD
REMOPS
REMORA
REMOTE
REMOVE
REMOWN
REMOWS
RIMOSE
RIMOUS
ROMOLA
RUMORS
RUMOUR
SAMOAN
SAMOSA
SIMONE
SOMONI
UNMOLD
UNMOOR
UNMOWN
UPMOST
UTMOST
ZAMORA

••M•O•

ABMHOS
AIMFOR
BAMBOO
BIMBOS
CAMBOY
CAMEON
CAMEOS
CAMION
CAMPOS
COMBOS
COMEOF
COMEON
COMMON
COMPOS
COMPOZ
DAMSON
DUMBOS
DUMPON
EXMOOR
FEMBOT
GAMBOL
GAMMON
GUMBOS
IAMNOT
IAMTOO
JIMBOB
JIMSON
JUMBOS
JUMPON
KLMNOP
LEMMON
LEMNOS
LIMBOS
LOMPOC
LUMMOX
MAMBOS
MAMMON
MIMEOS
MMMBOP
NIMROD
POMPOM
POMPON
RAMBOS
RAMROD
RAMSON
ROMCOM
ROMEOS
SAMSON
SIMEON
SUMMON
SYMBOL
TAMBOR
TEMPOS
TOMBOY
TOMTOM
UNMOOR
YOMTOV

••M••O

BAMAKO
BAMBOO
BUMPPO
CAMARO
CAMETO
CAMINO
CIMINO
COMETO
COMORO
CUMULO
DAMATO
DEMILO
DOMINO
HEMATO
IAMTOO
IMMUNO
KIMONO
KOMODO
LEMOKO
MRMOTO
NOMAYO
NUMERO
POMELO
POMPEO
RAMAPO
ROMANO
ROMERO
ROMULO
STMALO
TAMAYO
TOMATO

•••MO•

ALAMOS
ASIMOV
AWCMON
BEAMON
BONMOT
CLAMOR
COMMON
COSMOS
DAEMON
DEIMOS
DENMOM
DERMOT
DESMOG
DRYMOP
DUOMOS
ENAMOR
ETYMOL
ETYMON
GAMMON
GISMOS
GIZMOS
GLAMOR
GNOMON
HARMON
HAYMOW
HERMON
LARMOR
LEMMON
LUMMOX
MAMMON
MARMOT
MORMON
NOEMON
PASMOI
PATMOS
PRIMOS
PROMOS
PULMON
QUEMOY
RAGMOP
SALMON
SCHMOS
SERMON
SHIMON
SLAMON
STAMOS
SUMMON
THEMOB
TREMOR
WETMOP

•••M•O

AKIMBO
ATEMPO
CRAMBO
DOOMTO
DROMIO
GRUMIO
JKLMNO
OROMEO
PLUMBO
SEEMTO
TIEMPO
TRUMBO
WARMTO
WHAMMO
WHOMSO

••••MO

CHROMO
DOCOMO
DYNAMO
ENTOMO
ESKIMO
KOKOMO
OPTIMO
PLASMO
PNEUMO
SEISMO
STELMO
THERMO
ULTIMO
WHAMMO

M•P•••

MAPLES
MAPOUT
MAPPED
MAPPER
MAPPLE
MAPUTO
MCPHEE
MOPEDS
MOPERS
MOPERY
MOPIER
MOPING
MOPISH
MOPPED
MOPPER
MOPPET
MOPSUP
MOPTOP
MOPUPS
MRPAWS
MRPIBB
MUPPET

M••P••

MAGPIE
MAPPED
MAPPER
MAPPLE
MARPLE
MNOPQR
MOPPED
MOPPER
MOPPET
MORPHO
MORPHS
MUDPIE
MUPPET
MURPHY
MYOPES
MYOPIA
MYOPIC

M•••P•

MACAPA
MANAPE
MEROPE
MEROPS
MIXUPS
MOPUPS

M••••P

MADCAP
MADEUP
MAKEUP
MARKUP
MASHUP
MAYHAP
MEETUP
MESSUP
MIDCAP
MILSAP
MISHAP
MISTUP
MMMBOP
MOCKUP
MOPSUP
MOPTOP
MOVEUP
MUCKUP
MUSSUP

•MP•••

AMPERE
AMPING
AMPLER
AMPSUP
AMPULE
EMPALE
EMPATH
EMPERY
EMPIRE
EMPLOY
EMPSON
EMPTOR
IMPACT
IMPAIR
IMPALA
IMPALE
IMPART
IMPEDE
IMPELS
IMPEND
IMPERF
IMPISH
IMPLED
IMPORT
IMPOSE
IMPOST
IMPROV
IMPUGN
IMPURE
IMPUTE
OMPHAL
UMPING
UMPIRE

•M••P•

LMNOPQ

•M•••P

AMPSUP
IMACOP
MMMBOP
SMALLP

••MP••

ARMPIT
BUMPED
BUMPER
BUMPPO
BUMPUP
CAMPED
CAMPER
CAMPOS
CAMPUP
CAMPUS
COMPAQ
COMPAS
COMPED
COMPEL
COMPLY
COMPOS
COMPOZ
DAMPED
DAMPEN
DAMPER
DAMPLY
DIMPLE
DIMPLY
DUMPED
DUMPER
DUMPON
DUMPTY
GIMPED
HAMPER
HEMPEN
HUMPED
HUMPHS
HUMPTY
IBMPCS
JUMPAT
JUMPED
JUMPER
JUMPIN
JUMPON
JUMPUP
KEMPIS
LIMPED
LIMPER
LIMPET
LIMPID
LIMPLY
LOMPOC
LUMPED
LUMPEN
LUMPER
LUMPIN
LUMPIT
LUMPUR
LYMPHS
NYMPHS
OOMPAH
OOMPHS
PAMPAS
PAMPER
PIMPLE
PIMPLY
POMPEO
POMPEY
POMPOM
POMPON
PUMPED
PUMPER
PUMPUP
RAMPAL
RAMPED
RAMPUP
RIMPLE
ROMPED
ROMPER
RUMPLE
RUMPLY
RUMPUS
SAMPAN
SAMPLE
SEMPER
SEMPLE
SEMPRE
SIMPER
SIMPLE
SIMPLY
TAMPED
TAMPER
TEMPED
TEMPEH
TEMPER
TEMPLE
TEMPOS
TEMPTS
TEMPUS
VAMPED
VAMPER
WAMPUM
WIMPED
WIMPLE

••M•P•

ALMVPS
BUMPPO
JAMUPS
NLMVPS
RAMAPO
REMAPS
REMOPS
SUMUPS

••M••P

BUMPUP
BUMRAP
CAMEUP
CAMPUP
COMEUP
DAMSUP
DOMREP
GUMSUP
HAMSUP
JAMSUP
JUMPUP
KLMNOP
MMMBOP
PUMPUP
RAMPUP
SUMSUP

•••MP•

ATEMPO
BLIMPS
CHAMPS
CHIMPS
CHOMPS
CHUMPS
CLAMPS
CLOMPS
CLUMPS
CLUMPY
CRAMPS
CRAMPY
CRIMPS
CRIMPY
CRUMPS
EXEMPT
FRUMPS
FRUMPY
GRAMPA
GRAMPS
GRUMPS
GRUMPY
LOOMPA
PLUMPS
PRIMPS
PROMPT
SCAMPI
SCAMPS
SKIMPS
SKIMPY
SLUMPS
STAMPS
STIMPY
STOMPS
STUMPS
STUMPY
SWAMPS
SWAMPY
THUMPS
TIEMPO
TRAMPS
TRAMPY
TROMPE
TROMPS
TRUMPS
WHOMPS

•••M•P

AAAMAP
BEAMUP
BITMAP
CLAMUP
DRUMUP
DRYMOP
FIRMUP
GLAMUP
LOOMUP
RAGMOP
SEAMAP
SKYMAP
SWAMUP
TEAMUP
WARMUP
WETMOP

••••MP

CCLAMP
DECAMP
ENCAMP
GOLIMP
ONRAMP
PREAMP
REPUMP
REVAMP
SCRIMP
SHRIMP
UNLIMP

M•Q•••

MAQUIS
MSQUAD

M••Q••

MANQUE
MARQUE
MASQUE
MOSQUE

M•••Q•

MNOPQR

•MQ•••

EMQUAD

•M•••Q

LMNOPQ
SMALLQ

••M••Q

COMPAQ

MR••••

MRBEAN
MRBILL
MRBLUE
MRBOND
MRCOOL
MRDICK
MRHYDE
MRJINX
MRMOTO
MRPAWS
MRPIBB
MRSULU
MRWONG

M•R•••

MARACA
MARAUD
MARBLE
MARBLY
MARCEL
MARCHE
MARCIA
MARCIE
MARCIL
MARCIX
MARCOS
MARCUS
MARDEN
MARDIS
MARGIE
MARGIN
MARGOT
MARIAH
MARIAN
MARIAS
MARIDA
MARIDO
MARIEL
MARIKO
MARILU
MARINA
MARINE
MARINO
MARION
MARISA
MARIST
MARJOE
MARKAS
MARKED
MARKER
MARKET
MARKEY
MARKIE
MARKII
MARKIV
MARKIX
MARKKA
MARKOV
MARKUP
MARKVI
MARLED
MARLEE
MARLEY
MARLIN
MARLON
MARMEE
MARMOT
MARNER
MARNIE
MAROON
MARPLE
MARQUE
MARRED
MARRER
MARRON
MARROW
MARSHA
MARSHY
MARTEL
MARTEN
MARTES
MARTHA
MARTHE
MARTIN
MARTYR
MARVEL
MARVIN
MARVIS
MARXES
MARYAM
MARYII
MARYJO
MCRIBS
MERCED
MERCER
MERCKX
MERDLE
MERELY
MEREST
MERGED
MERGEE
MERGER
MERGES
MERIDA
MERINO
MERITS
MERKEL
MERLIN
MERLOT
MERMAN
MERMEN
MEROPE
MEROPS
MERRIE
MERSEY
MERTON
MERVYN
MERYLL
MIRADA
MIRAGE
MIRIAM
MIRIER
MIRING
MIRINS
MIRREN
MIRROR
MIRROS
MIRTHS
MORALE
MORALS
MORANT
MORASS
MORATH
MORAYS
MORBID
MOREAU
MOREEN
MORELS
MORENO
MORESO
MORGAN
MORGEN
MORGUE
MORITA
MORITZ
MORLEY
MORMON
MORNAY
MOROLT
MORONI
MORONS
MOROSE
MOROSS
MORPHO
MORPHS
MORREL
MORRIE
MORRIS
MORROW
MORSEL
MORTAL
MORTAR
MORTEN
MORTON
MURALS
MURANO
MURCIA
MURDER
MURIEL
MURINE
MURMUR
MURPHY
MURRAY
MURRES
MURROW
MYRDAL
MYRIAD
MYRRHS
MYRTLE

M••R••

MACRAE
MACRON
MACROS
MADRAS
MADRES
MADRID
MAIRES
MAIRZY
MANRAY
MAORIS
MARRED
MARRER
MARRON
MARROW
MATRIX
MATRON
MAYRON
MCCRAE
MCCREA
MCGRAW
MCGREW
MEGREZ
MEGRIM
MERRIE
METRED
METRES
METRIC
METROS
MICRON
MICROS
MIDRIB
MIRREN
MIRROR
MIRROS
MITRAL
MITRED
MITRES
MODRED
MOERAE
MOIRES
MONROE
MOORED
MORREL
MORRIE
MORRIS
MORROW
MOTRIN
MOURNS
MUNROE
MURRAY
MURRES
MURROW
MYRRHS

M•••R•

MACERS
MADERA
MADERO
MADURO
MAITRE
MAJORS
MAKERS
MALARS
MALORY
MANERO
MANORS
MANTRA
MANURE
MASERS
MASERU
MATERS
MATURE
MAYORS
MCCORD
MCHARG
MCKERN
MEAGRE
MEMORY
MESSRS
METERS
MEWERS
MEYERS
MIDORI
MILERS
MILORD
MIMERS
MINERS
MINORS
MISERS
MISERY
MITERS
MIXERS
MOBERG
MODERN
MOLARS
MOOERS
MOPERS
MOPERY
MOTHRA
MOTORS
MOVERS
MOWERS
MOYERS
MOZART
MSTARS
MTAIRY
MUNERA
MUSERS
MYGIRL
MYHERO
MYLARS
MYLORD
MYSORE
MYTURN
MYWORD

M••••R

MADDER
MADFOR
MAGYAR
MAHLER
MAHZOR
MAILER
MAIMER
MAINER
MANGER
MANNER
MAPPER
MARKER
MARNER
MARRER
MARTYR
MASHER
MASKER
MASTER
MATHER
MATTER
MAULER
MAUSER
MAZIER
MCNAIR
MEADER
MEAGER
MEANER
MEDGAR
MEEBER
MEEKER
MEETER
MELDER
MELTER
MEMBER
MEMOIR
MENDER
MENTOR
MEOWER
MERCER
MERGER
MESMER
METEOR
METIER
MEWLER
MIDAIR
MIDLER
MILDER
MILKER
MILLER
MILNER
MINCER
MINDER
MINTER
MIRIER
MIRROR
MISTER
MNOPQR
MOANER
MOBBER
MOCKER
MOHAIR
MOILER
MOLDER
MOLNAR
MOLTER
MONGER
MOONER
MOOTER
MOPIER
MOPPER
MORTAR
MOSHER
MOTHER
MOUSER
MSIEUR
MUCKER
MUDDER
MUGGER
MULDER
MULLER
MUMMER
MURDER
MURMUR
MUSHER
MUSTER
MUTTER
MYDEAR

•MR•••

AMRITA

•M•R••
AMARNA
AMERCE
AMORAL
AMORES
AMORET
AMTRAC
AMTRAK
DMARKS
EMBRUE
EMBRYO
EMERGE
EMERIC
EMERIL
EMORYU
IMARET
IMBRUE
IMFREE
IMPROV
KMARTS
OMERTA
SMARMY
SMARTS
SMARTY
SMERSH
SMIRCH
SMIRKS
SMIRKY
SMORES
SMURFS
SMYRNA
UMBRAE
UMBRAL
UMBRAS
UMBRIA

•M••R•
AMBERS
AMBERY
AMEERS
AMENRA
AMONRA
AMOURS
AMPERE
DMITRI
DMITRY
EMBARK
EMBARS
EMBERS
EMEERS
EMIGRE
EMPERY
EMPIRE
IMHERE
IMHURT
IMMURE
IMPART
IMPERF
IMPORT
IMPURE
IMSURE
OMEARA
SMEARS
SMEARY
UMBERS
UMPIRE

•M•••R
AMAJOR
AMBLER
AMINOR
AMPLER
AMUSER
BMAJOR
BMINOR
CMAJOR
CMINOR
DMAJOR
DMINOR
EMAJOR
EMINOR
EMOTER
EMPTOR
FMAJOR
FMINOR
GMAJOR
GMINOR
IMAGER
IMPAIR
SMALLR
SMILER
SMITER
SMOKER

••MR••
BUMRAP
CAMRYN
CAMRYS
CYMRIC
DOMREP
GYMRAT
NIMROD
RAMROD

••M•R•
ADMIRE
AIMERS
ARMERS
ARMORS
ARMORY
ASMARA
BEMIRE
BUMBRY
CAMARO
CAMERA
COMDRS
COMERS
COMORO
DAMORE
DEMARK
DEMURE
DEMURS
ELMERS
ELMIRA
ELMIRE
ELMORE
EXMORE
FEMORA
FEMURS
FUMERS
GAMERS
GEMARA
GOMERS
HOMBRE
HOMERS
HUMERI
HUMORS
IMMURE
KHMERS
LAMARR
LEMURS
MEMORY
MIMERS
NAMERS
NOMBRE
NOMORE
NUMERO
OLMERT
PAMIRS
REMARK
REMORA
RIMERS
ROMERO
RUMORS
SAMARA
SEMPRE
SOMBRE
SOMERS
STMARK
STMARY
TAMARA
TAMERS
TIMBRE
TIMERS
UNMIRY
VOMERS
ZAMORA

••M••R
AIMFOR
ARMOUR
BOMBER
BUMMER
BUMPER
CAMBER
CAMPER
COMBER
CUMBER
DAMMER
DAMNER
DAMOUR
DAMPER
DIMMER
DUMBER
DUMPER
ELMIER
EXMOOR
FUMIER
GAMIER
GAMMER
HAMMER
HAMPER
HEMMER
HOMIER
HUMBER
HUMMER
HUMOUR
JAMMER
JUMPER
LAMARR
LAMOUR
LIMBER
LIMIER
LIMNER
LIMPER
LUMBAR
LUMBER
LUMPER
LUMPUR
MEMBER
MEMOIR
MUMMER
NUMBER
PAMPER
PUMPER
RAMMER
RIMIER
ROMPER
RUMMER
RUMOUR
SEMPER
SIMMER
SIMPER
SOMBER
SOMMER
SUMMER
SUMNER
SUMTER
TAMBOR
TAMPER
TEMPER
TIMBER
UNMOOR
VAMPER
WIMMER
YAMMER
ZIMMER

•••MR•
THEMRS

•••M•R
ALOMAR
BALMER
BAUMER
BEAMER
BEEMER
BEYMER
BLAMER
BOOMER
BREMER
BUMMER
CALMER
CHIMER
CLAMOR
COLMAR
CRAMER
CREMER
DAGMAR
DAMMER
DELMAR
DETMER
DIMMER
DORMER
ENAMOR
FARMER
FIRMER
FLAMER
FOAMER
FORMER
FRAMER
FULMAR
GAMMER
GLAMOR
HAMMER
HARMER
HELMER
HEMMER
HUMMER
INGMAR
ISOMER
JAMMER
KALMAR
KILMER
KRAMER
LARMOR
MAIMER
MESMER
MUMMER
MURMUR
NEWMAR
OTHMAR
PALMAR
PALMER
PLOMER
PRIMER
RAMMER
REAMER
RHYMER
ROAMER
ROHMER
ROOMER
RUMMER
SEAMER
SHAMIR
SIMMER
SOMMER
SUMMER
TREMOR
WARMER
WEIMAR
WIMMER
WORMER
YAMMER
ZIMMER

MS••••
MSIEUR
MSQUAD
MSTARS

M•S•••
MASADA
MASAIS
MASALA
MASCOT
MASERS
MASERU
MASHED
MASHER
MASHES
MASHIE
MASHUP
MASKED
MASKER
MASLIN
MASONS
MASQUE
MASSED
MASSES
MASSEY
MASSIF
MASSON
MASSYS
MASTED
MASTER
MASTIC
MESAAZ
MESABI
MESCAL
MESHED
MESHES
MESIAL
MESMER
MESNES
MESONS
MESSED
MESSES
MESSIN
MESSRS
MESSUP
MISACT
MISADD
MISAIM
MISCHA
MISCUE
MISCUT
MISDID
MISERS
MISERY
MISFED
MISFIT
MISHAP
MISHIT
MISKEY
MISLAY
MISLED
MISSAL
MISSAY
MISSED
MISSES
MISSET
MISSIS
MISSME
MISSUS
MISTED
MISTER
MISTUP
MISUSE
MOSAIC
MOSCOW
MOSDEF
MOSEYS
MOSHAV
MOSHED
MOSHER
MOSHES
MOSKVA
MOSLEM
MOSLEY
MOSQUE
MOSSAD
MOSSED
MOSSES
MOSTEL
MOSTLY
MOSTOF
MRSULU
MUSCAT
MUSCLE
MUSCLY
MUSEES
MUSEON
MUSEOS
MUSERS
MUSEUM
MUSHED
MUSHER
MUSHES
MUSIAL
MUSICK
MUSICS
MUSING
MUSKET
MUSKIE
MUSKOX
MUSLIM
MUSLIN
MUSSED
MUSSEL
MUSSES
MUSSET
MUSSUP
MUSTDO
MUSTER
MUSTNT
MYSELF
MYSORE
MYSTIC

M••S••
MADSEN
MAISIE
MAISON
MAKSIM
MANSES
MARSHA
MARSHY
MASSED
MASSES
MASSEY
MASSIF
MASSON
MASSYS
MATSON
MATSUI
MATSUO
MAUSER
MAWSON
MAXSON
MEASLE
MEASLY
MENSAL
MENSAN
MENSCH
MERSEY
MESSED
MESSES
MESSIN
MESSRS
MESSUP
MIASMA
MIDSTS
MILSAP
MISSAL
MISSAY
MISSED
MISSES
MISSET
MISSIS
MISSME
MISSUS
MITSOU
MOESHA
MOISES
MOLSON
MOPSUP
MORSEL
MOSSAD
MOSSED
MOSSES
MOUSED
MOUSER
MOUSES
MOUSEY
MOUSSE
MTOSSA
MUESLI
MUSSED
MUSSEL
MUSSES
MUSSET
MUSSUP
MYOSIN
MYOSIS

M•••S•
MAINST
MANUSH
MAOISM
MAOIST
MARISA
MARIST
MAYEST
MEDUSA
MEREST
MIKASA
MILOSZ
MIMOSA
MINOSO
MISUSE
MODEST
MODISH
MOLEST
MOMISM
MONGST
MONISM
MONIST
MOPISH
MORASS
MORESO
MOROSE
MOROSS
MOTTST
MOUSSE
MTOSSA
MUFASA
MULISH
MUTEST
MYGOSH

M••••S
MACAWS
MACERS
MACHOS
MACLES
MACROS
MADAMS
MADRAS
MADRES
MAFIAS
MAGICS
MAGMAS
MAGNUS
MAHDIS
MAIRES
MAIZES
MAJLIS
MAJORS
MAKERS
MALARS
MALAYS
MAMBAS
MAMBOS
MAMMAS
MANAOS
MANATS
MANDMS
MANETS
MANGAS
MANGOS
MANIAS
MANNAS
MANORS
MANSES
MANTAS
MANTIS
MAORIS
MAPLES
MAQUIS
MARCOS
MARCUS
MARDIS
MARIAS
MARKAS
MARTES
MARVIS
MARXES
MASAIS
MASERS
MASHES
MASONS
MASSES
MASSYS
MATERS
MATEYS
MATHIS
MATINS
MATJES
MATTES
MATZOS
MAUVES
MAVENS
MAVINS
MAXIMS
MAYANS
MAYBES
MAYORS
MAZDAS
MCJOBS
MCRIBS
MEATUS
MECCAS
MECUMS
MEDALS
MEDIAS
MEDICS
MEDIUS
MEDNIS
MEDOCS
MELEES
MELONS
MENDES
MENTIS
MENTOS
MERGES
MERITS
MEROPS
MESHES
MESNES
MESONS
MESSES
MESSRS
METALS
METERS
METRES
METROS
MEWERS
MEYERS
MEZZOS
MIAMIS
MIAOUS
MIAOWS
MIATAS
MICROS
MIDGES
MIDONS
MIDSTS
MIELES
MIGHTS
MILANS
MILERS
MILLES
MILNES
MIMEOS
MIMERS
MIMICS
MINCES
MINERS
MINGUS
MINIMS
MINORS
MINXES
MIRINS
MIRROS
MIRTHS
MISERS
MISSES
MISSIS
MISSUS
MITERS
MITRES
MIXERS
MIXUPS
MOBIUS
MOCHAS
MODALS
MODELS
MODEMS
MOGULS
MOINES
MOIRES
MOISES
MOJOES
MOLARS
MOMMAS
MONADS
MONDES
MONDOS
MONETS
MONEYS
MONGOS
MONIES
MONTHS
MONZAS
MOODYS
MOOERS
MOPEDS
MOPERS
MOPUPS
MORALS
MORASS
MORAYS
MORELS
MORONS
MOROSS
MORPHS
MORRIS
MOSEYS
MOSHES
MOSSES
MOTELS
MOTETS
MOTIFS
MOTORS
MOTTOS
MOULDS
MOULTS
MOUNDS
MOUNTS
MOURNS
MOUSES
MOUTHS
MOVERS
MOVIES
MOWERS
MOYERS
MRPAWS
MSTARS
MTILES
MTVVJS
MUCHAS
MUFTIS
MULCTS
MULEYS
MULLAS
MULTIS
MUMMYS
MURALS
MURRES
MUSEES
MUSEOS
MUSERS
MUSHES
MUSICS
MUSSES
MUTIUS
MUTONS
MYLARS
MYNAHS
MYOPES
MYOSIS
MYRRHS
MYTHOS

•MS•••
AMSTEL
IMSOLD
IMSURE

•M•S••
AMESIA
AMOSOZ
AMPSUP
AMUSED
AMUSER
AMUSES
EMPSON
KMESON
OMASUM
TMESES
TMESIS
XMASES

•M••S•
AMBUSH
AMIDST
EMBOSS
EMDASH
IMBUSY
IMEASY
IMPISH
IMPOSE
IMPOST
SMERSH
SMOOSH

•M•••S
AMADIS
AMANAS
AMANTS
AMATIS
AMAZES
AMBERS
AMBITS
AMBLES
AMEBAS
AMEERS
AMENDS
AMENTS
AMICES
AMICUS
AMIDAS
AMIDES
AMIENS
AMIGAS
AMIGOS
AMINES
AMINOS
AMINUS
AMNIOS
AMOLES
AMORES
AMOURS
AMUSES
AMVETS
BMINUS
CMINUS
DMARKS
DMINUS
EMAILS
EMALLS
EMBARS
EMBAYS
EMBEDS
EMBERS
EMBOGS
EMBOSS
EMBOWS
EMCEES
EMEERS
EMENDS
EMILYS
EMMAUS
EMMETS
EMOTES
HMONGS
IMAGES
IMAGOS
IMAXES
IMBEDS
IMBUES
IMIDES
IMINES
IMMIES
IMPELS
KMARTS
OMAHAS
OMANIS
OMEGAS
SMACKS
SMALLS
SMARTS
SMAZES
SMEARS
SMELLS
SMELTS
SMILES
SMIRKS
SMITES
SMITHS
SMOCKS
SMOKES
SMOLTS
SMORES
SMURFS
TMESES
TMESIS
TMINUS
UMBELS
UMBERS
UMBRAS
UMIAKS
XMASES

••MS••
AIMSAT
COMSAT
DAMSEL
DAMSON
DAMSUP
DIMSUM
GUMSUP
HAMSUN
HAMSUP
HEMSIN
IAMSAM
JAMSIN
JAMSUP
JIMSON
LAMSIT
RAMSAY
RAMSES
RAMSEY
RAMSIN
RAMSON
REMSEN
RIMSKY
SAMSON
SUMSUP
WIMSEY

••M•S•
ALMOST
ATMOST
BEMUSE
CAMISE
DAMASK
DEMAST
DEMISE
DEMIST
ENMESH
FAMISH
GAMEST
INMOST
JAMESA
JAMESI
JAMESJ
JAMESK
JAMESM
JAMESS
JAMEST
JAMESV
LAMESA
LAMEST
MIMOSA
MOMISM
OSMOSE
RAMOSE
REMISE
REMISS
RIMOSE
SAMOSA
TAMEST
UNMASK
UNMAST
UNMESH
UPMOST
UTMOST
ZYMASE

••M••S
ABMHOS
ADMINS
ADMITS
AIMERS
ALMVPS
ARMERS
ARMETS
ARMIES
ARMORS
ATMANS
BAMBIS
BIMBOS
BOMBES
CAMEAS
CAMELS
CAMEOS
CAMOES
CAMPOS
CAMPUS
CAMRYS
COMBOS
COMDRS
COMEAS
COMERS
COMETS
COMICS
COMMAS
COMPAS
COMPOS
COMTES
CUMINS
DEMIES
DEMITS
DEMOBS
DEMONS
DEMURS
DUMBOS
ELMERS
EMMAUS
EMMETS
EXMETS
FAMOUS
FEMMES
FEMURS
FUMERS
GAMAYS
GAMERS
GAMINS
GAMMAS
GAMOUS
GAMUTS
GIMELS
GIMMES
GOMERS
GUMBOS
HOMERS
HOMEYS
HOMIES
HOMMES
HUMANS
HUMMUS
HUMORS
HUMPHS
IAMBUS
IBMPCS
IMMIES
JAMAIS
JAMBES
JAMESS
JAMUPS
JUMBOS
KEMPIS
KHMERS
KOMBUS
LAMEDS
LAMIAS
LEMANS

LEMMAS
LEMNOS
LEMONS
LEMURS
LIMANS
LIMBOS
LIMITS
LUMENS
LYMPHS
MAMBAS
MAMBOS
MAMMAS
MIMEOS
MIMERS
MIMICS
MOMMAS
MUMMYS
NAMERS
NIMBUS
NLMVPS
NOMADS
NYMETS
NYMPHS
OLMECS
OOMPHS
OSMICS
PAMIRS
PAMPAS
POMMES
RAMBOS
RAMENS
RAMETS
RAMFIS
RAMIES
RAMSES
REMANS
REMAPS
REMATS
REMISS
REMITS
REMOPS
REMOWS
RIMERS
RIMOUS
ROMANS
ROMEOS
RUMBAS
RUMORS
RUMPUS
SAMBAS
SAMEAS
SOMERS
SUMACS
SUMUPS
TAMERS
TAMILS
TEMPOS
TEMPTS
TEMPUS
TIMERS
TOMBES
UNMANS
UNMEWS
VOMERS
WOMANS
WOMENS
YUMANS

•••MS•
AHIMSA
CLUMSY
FLIMSY
WHIMSY
WHOMSO

•••M•S
ABOMAS
ABOMBS
AGAMAS
AGAMES
ALAMOS
ANIMAS
ANIMES
ANIMUS
ARAMES
ARAMIS
AROMAS
BIOMES
BLAMES
BLIMPS
BRUMES
CADMUS
CHAMPS
CHIMES
CHIMPS
CHOMPS
CHUMPS
CLAMPS
CLIMBS
CLIMES
CLOMPS
CLUMPS
COMMAS
COSMAS
COSMOS
CRAMPS
CREMES
CRIMES
CRIMPS
CRUMBS
CRUMPS
DEIMOS
DERMAS
DERMIS
DISMAS
DISMES
DOGMAS
DOLMAS
DRAMAS
DUOMOS
EDAMES
EDEMAS
ELEMIS
FEMMES
FERMIS
FLAMES
FLUMES
FRAMES
FRUMPS
GAMMAS
GIMMES
GISMOS
GIZMOS
GNOMES
GRAMPS
GRIMES
GRIMMS
GRUMPS
HAYMES
HBOMBS
HERMES
HOLMES
HOMMES
HUMMUS
JAYMES
KARMAS
LEMMAS
LITMUS
LLAMAS
LOUMAS
MAGMAS
MAMMAS
MIAMIS
MOMMAS
MUMMYS
NBOMBS
OTOMIS
PALMAS
PATMOS
PLUMBS
PLUMES
PLUMPS
POEMES
POMMES
PRIMES
PRIMOS
PRIMPS
PRIMUS
PROMOS
RHAMES
RHEMES
RHOMBS
RHUMBS
RHYMES
SALMIS
SCAMPS
SCHMOS
SEAMUS
SHAMES
SHAMUS
SIGMAS
SKIMPS
SLIMES
SLUMPS
SPUMES
STAMOS
STAMPS
STOMAS
STOMPS
STUMPS
SWAMIS
SWAMPS
TERMES
THAMES
THEMES
THEMRS
THOMAS
THUMBS
THUMPS
THYMES
THYMUS
TRAMPS
TROMPS
TRUMPS
UNAMIS
VARMUS
WHOMPS
XGAMES

••••MS
ABOHMS
ABRAMS
ABYSMS
ADDAMS
ADEEMS
ALARMS
ALBUMS
ATEAMS
AXIOMS
BADEMS
BEDIMS
BEGEMS
BEGUMS
BESOMS
BLOOMS
BOSOMS
BRAHMS
BREAMS
BROOMS
BTEAMS
CAROMS
CDROMS
CHARMS
CHASMS
CLAIMS
CREAMS
DEGUMS
DENIMS
DIRAMS
DOSUMS
DREAMS
DURUMS
ENARMS
FORUMS
GLEAMS
GLOOMS
GOLEMS
GRIMMS
GROOMS
HAKIMS
HAREMS
HBEAMS
HOHUMS
HOKUMS
IBEAMS
IDIOMS
JORUMS
KHOUMS
KILIMS
LARAMS
LBEAMS
MADAMS
MANDMS
MAXIMS
MECUMS
MINIMS
MODEMS
OAKUMS
OCCAMS
ODIUMS
OGHAMS
OLEUMS
OPIUMS
PRISMS
PRIZMS
PROAMS
PROEMS
PSALMS
PURIMS
QUALMS
REAIMS
REALMS
REARMS
REHEMS
RHEEMS
RHEIMS
RHEUMS
SCRAMS
SCRIMS
SCRUMS
SEDUMS
SEISMS
SERUMS
SPASMS
STEAMS
STORMS
STRUMS
SWARMS
THERMS
THRUMS
TOTEMS
UGGAMS
UNARMS
UNDAMS
UNDIMS
UNJAMS
VENOMS
VROOMS
WHELMS
XYLEMS

MT••••
MTAIRY
MTCOOK
MTETNA
MTFUJI
MTHOOD
MTILES
MTOSSA
MTVVJS

M•T•••
MATERS
MATEYS
MATHER
MATHEW
MATHIS
MATING
MATINS
MATJES
MATLIN
MATMAN
MATMEN
MATRIX
MATRON
MATSON
MATSUI
MATSUO
MATTEA
MATTED
MATTEL
MATTER
MATTES
MATTIE
MATURE
MATZOH
MATZOS
METALS
METATE
METEOR
METERS
METFAN
METHOD
METHYL
METIER
METING
METRED
METRES
METRIC
METROS
METTLE
MITERS
MITRAL
MITRED
MITRES
MITSOU
MITTAG
MITTEN
MOTELS
MOTETS
MOTHER
MOTHRA
MOTIFS
MOTILE
MOTION
MOTIVE
MOTLEY
MOTORS
MOTOWN
MOTRIN
MOTTLE
MOTTOS
MOTTST
MSTARS
MUTANT
MUTATE
MUTELY
MUTEST
MUTING
MUTINY
MUTIUS
MUTONS
MUTTER
MUTTON
MUTUAL
MUTUEL
MYTHIC
MYTHOS
MYTURN

M••T••
MAITAI
MAITRE
MALTBY
MALTED
MALTIN
MANTAS
MANTEE
MANTEL
MANTIC
MANTIS
MANTLE
MANTRA
MANTUA
MAOTAI
MARTEL
MARTEN
MARTES
MARTHA
MARTHE
MARTIN
MARTYR
MASTED
MASTER
MASTIC
MATTEA
MATTED
MATTEL
MATTER
MATTES
MATTIE
MAYTAG
MEATAX
MEATUS
MEETER
MEETLY
MEETUP
MELTED
MELTER
MELTON
MENTAL
MENTEE
MENTHE
MENTIS
MENTOR
MENTOS
MERTON
METTLE
MIATAS
MILTIE
MILTON
MINTED
MINTER
MIRTHS
MISTED
MISTER
MISTUP
MITTAG
MITTEN
MIXTEC
MOATED
MOLTED
MOLTEN
MOLTER
MOLTKE
MONTAG
MONTEL
MONTEZ
MONTHS
MOOTED
MOOTER
MOPTOP
MORTAL
MORTAR
MORTEN
MORTON
MOSTEL
MOSTLY
MOSTOF
MOTTLE
MOTTOS
MOTTST
MOUTHS
MOUTHY
MTETNA
MUFTIS
MULTIS
MUSTDO
MUSTER
MUSTNT
MUTTER
MUTTON
MYRTLE
MYSTIC

M•••T•
MAILTO
MAKUTA
MALOTI
MANATS
MANETS
MANUTE
MAPUTO
MEANTO
MELETE
MELOTT
MERITS
METATE
MIDSTS
MIGHTS
MIGHTY
MIKITA
MINETA
MINITV
MINUTE
MOBUTU
MOIETY
MOJITO
MONETA
MONETS
MORATH
MORITA
MORITZ
MOTETS
MOULTS
MOUNTS
MOUNTY
MOVETO
MRMOTO
MULCTS
MULETA
MUTATE

M••••T
MADEIT
MAGGOT
MAGNET
MAHOUT
MAINST
MAKEIT
MALLET
MAOIST
MAPOUT
MARGOT
MARIST
MARKET
MARMOT
MASCOT
MAXOUT
MAYEST
MEANIT
MELOTT
MEREST
MERLOT
MIDGET
MILLET
MINUET
MINUIT
MISACT
MISCUT
MISFIT
MISHIT
MISSET
MODELT
MODEST
MOLEST
MOMENT
MONGST
MONIST
MONNET
MOPPET
MORANT
MOROLT
MOTTST
MOVEIT
MOZART
MUDCAT
MUFFET
MULLET
MUPPET
MUSCAT
MUSKET
MUSSET
MUSTNT
MUTANT
MUTEST
MYFOOT

•MT•••
AMTRAC
AMTRAK
IMTOLD
UMTATA

•M•T••
AMATIS
AMATOL
AMITIE
AMSTEL
AMYTAN
DMITRI
DMITRY
EMETIC
EMOTED
EMOTER
EMOTES
EMPTOR
SMITER
SMITES
SMITHS
SMITHY
SMITTY
SMUTTY

•M••T•
AMANTI
AMANTS
AMBITS
AMENTS
AMINTA
AMONTH
AMRITA
AMVETS
EMEUTE
EMMETS
EMMETT
EMMITT
EMPATH
IMLATE
IMPUTE
KMARTS
OMERTA
SMARTS
SMARTY
SMELTS
SMITTY
SMOLTS
SMOOTH
SMUTTY
UMTATA

•M•••T
AMIDST
AMORET
AMOUNT
AMULET
EMMETT
EMMITT
IMARET
IMBEAT
IMEANT
IMHURT
IMIGHT
IMNEXT
IMONIT
IMPACT
IMPART
IMPORT
IMPOST
OMELET
SMALLT
UMLAUT

••MT••
COMTES
IAMTOO
SUMTER
TAMTAM
TOMTIT
TOMTOM
YOMTOV

••M•T•
ADMITS
ALMATY
ARMETS
BEMATA
CAMETO
COMATE
COMETH
COMETO
COMETS
COMITY
DAMATO
DAMITA
DEMITS
DEMOTE
DEMOTH
DIMITY
DUMPTY
EMMETS
EMMETT
EMMITT
ENMITY
EXMATE
EXMETS
GAMETE
GAMUTS
HAMATE
HAMITE
HEMATO
HUMPTY
INMATE
IOMOTH
LIMITS
MRMOTO
NAMATH
NIMITZ
NYMETS
RAMATE
RAMETS
REMATE
REMATS
REMITS
REMOTE
RIMATE
SEMITE
SOMATA
TEMPTS
TOMATO
UNMATE

••M••T
AIMSAT
ALMOST
ARMLET
ARMPIT
ATMOST
AUMONT
BUMOUT
CAMEAT
CEMENT
COMBAT
COMEAT
COMFIT
COMMIT
COMSAT
DEMAST
DEMIST
DIMOUT
DIMWIT
DUMONT
EGMONT
ELMONT
EMMETT
EMMITT
FEMBOT
FOMENT
FUMEAT
GAMBIT
GAMEST
GIMLET
GYMRAT
HAMLET
IAMNOT
INMOST
JAMEST
JUMPAT
KOMBAT
LAMENT
LAMEST
LAMONT
LAMSIT
LIMPET
LUMPIT
MOMENT
NAMEIT
NOMEAT
NUMBAT
OLMERT
RAMJET
REMEET
REMELT
REMINT
SAMLET
SUMMIT
TAMEST
TOMCAT
TOMTIT
TUMULT
UNMAST
UNMEET
UNMIXT
UPMOST
USMINT
UTMOST
WOMBAT

•••MT•
DOOMTO
SEEMTO
WARMTH
WARMTO

•••M•T
BONMOT
CLIMAT
COMMIT
DERMAT
DERMOT
EXEMPT
FERMAT
FORMAT
GROMIT
HAZMAT
HELMET
HELMUT
HERMIT
ILLMET
KERMIT
KISMET
MARMOT
OUIMET
PERMIT
PREMET
PROMPT
REEMIT
SUBMIT
SUMMIT
THEMET
WASMET
WILMUT

••••MT
DREAMT

MU••••
MUCHAS
MUCHOF
MUCKED
MUCKER
MUCKUP
MUDCAT
MUDDED
MUDDER
MUDDLE
MUDEEL
MUDHEN
MUDPIE
MUESLI
MUFASA
MUFFED
MUFFET
MUFFIN
MUFFLE
MUFTIS
MUGABE
MUGFUL
MUGGED
MUGGER
MUGGLE
MUKLUK
MULCTS
MULDER
MULETA
MULEYS
MULISH
MULLAH
MULLAS
MULLED
MULLER
MULLET
MULLIN
MULTIS
MUMBAI
MUMBLE
MUMBLY
MUMMED
MUMMER
MUMMYS
MUNCHY
MUNCIE
MUNERA
MUNICH
MUNROE
MUPPET
MURALS
MURANO
MURCIA
MURDER
MURIEL
MURINE
MURMUR
MURPHY
MURRAY
MURRES
MURROW
MUSCAT
MUSCLE
MUSCLY
MUSEES
MUSEON
MUSEOS
MUSERS
MUSEUM
MUSHED
MUSHER
MUSHES
MUSIAL
MUSICK
MUSICS
MUSING
MUSKET
MUSKIE
MUSKOX
MUSLIM
MUSLIN
MUSSED
MUSSEL
MUSSES
MUSSET
MUSSUP
MUSTDO
MUSTER
MUSTNT
MUTANT
MUTATE
MUTELY
MUTEST
MUTING
MUTINY
MUTIUS
MUTONS
MUTTER
MUTTON
MUTUAL
MUTUEL
MUUMUU
MUZZLE

M•U•••
MAULED
MAULER
MAUMAU
MAUMEE
MAUNDY
MAUSER
MAUVES
MOULDS
MOULDY
MOULIN
MOULTS
MOUNDS
MOUNTS
MOUNTY
MOURNS
MOUSED
MOUSER
MOUSES
MOUSEY
MOUSSE
MOUTHS
MOUTHY
MUUMUU

M••U••
MACULA
MADURO
MAKUTA
MANUAL
MANUEL
MANURE
MANUSH
MANUTE
MAPUTO
MAQUIS
MATURE
MAZUMA
MCDUCK
MCHUGH
MCKUEN
MECUMS
MEDUSA
MENUDO
MIFUNE
MIGUEL
MINUET
MINUIT
MINUTE
MISUSE
MIXUPS
MIZUNA
MOBUTU
MODULE
MODULI
MODULO
MOGULS
MOPUPS
MRSULU
MSQUAD
MTFUJI
MUTUAL
MUTUEL
MYTURN

M•••U•
MACOUN
MADDUX
MADEUP
MAGNUM
MAGNUS
MAHOUT
MAKEUP
MANFUL
MANQUE
MANTUA
MAPOUT
MARAUD
MARCUS
MARKUP
MARQUE
MASHUP
MASQUE
MATSUI
MATSUO
MAXOUT
MEATUS
MEDIUM
MEDIUS
MEETUP

MEIFUN
MESSUP
MIAOUS
MINGUS
MISCUE
MISCUT
MISSUS
MISTUP
MOBIUS
MOCKUP
MOPSUP
MORGUE
MOSQUE
MOVEUP
MRBLUE
MSIEUR
MUCKUP
MUGFUL
MUKLUK
MURMUR
MUSEUM
MUSSUP
MUTIUS
MUUMUU

M••••U
MALIBU
MANCHU
MARILU
MASERU
MAUMAU
MENJOU
MIAMIU
MILIEU
MITSOU
MOBUTU
MOLDAU
MOREAU
MRSULU
MUUMUU

•MU•••
AMULET
AMUSED
AMUSER
AMUSES
SMUDGE
SMUDGY
SMUGLY
SMURFS
SMUTTY

•M•U••
AMBUSH
AMOUNT
AMOURS
AMPULE
EMEUTE
EMQUAD
IMBUED
IMBUES
IMBUSY
IMFULL
IMHURT
IMMUNE
IMMUNO
IMMURE
IMPUGN
IMPURE
IMPUTE
IMSURE

•M••U•
AMICUS
AMINUS
AMPSUP
BMINUS
CMINUS
DMINUS
EMBRUE
EMMAUS
IMBRUE
OMASUM
OMNIUM
TMINUS
UMLAUT

•M•••U
EMORYU
SMALLU

••MU••
ASMUCH
BEMUSE
CUMULI
CUMULO
DEMURE
DEMURS
EDMUND
FAMULI
FEMURS
GAMUTS
HAMULI
IMMUNE
IMMUNO
IMMURE
JAMUPS
LEMUEL
LEMURS
OSMUND
ROMULO
SAMUEL
SOMUCH
SUMUPS
TUMULT
YAMUNA

••M•U•
AIMFUL
ARMFUL
ARMOUR
BUMOUT
BUMPUP
CAMEUP
CAMPUP
CAMPUS
COMEUP
DAMOUR
DAMSUP
DIMOUT
DIMSUM
DUMDUM
EMMAUS
FAMOUS
GAMOUS
GUMSUP
HAMSUN
HAMSUP
HUMBUG
HUMMUS
HUMOUR
IAMBUS
JAMSUP
JUMPUP
KOMBUS
LAMOUR
LUMPUR
NIMBUS
OSMIUM
PUMPUP
RAMPUP
RIMOUS
RUMOUR
RUMPUS
SUMSUP
TAMMUZ
TEMPUS
WAMPUM
YUMYUM

••M••U
ORMOLU
RAMEAU

•••MU•
ANIMUS
BEAMUP
CADMUS
CLAMUP
DRUMUP
FIRMUP
GLAMUP
HELMUT
HORMUZ
HUMMUS
LITMUS
LOOMUP
MURMUR
MUUMUU
PRIMUS
SEAMUS
SHAMUS
SWAMUP
TALMUD
TAMMUZ
TEAMUP
THYMUS
UNSMUG
VARMUS
WARMUP
WILMUT

•••M•U
MAUMAU
MIAMIU
MUUMUU

M•V•••
MAVENS
MAVINS
MOVADO
MOVEIN
MOVEIT
MOVEON
MOVERS
MOVETO
MOVEUP
MOVIES
MOVING
MTVVJS

M••V••
MADVIG
MARVEL
MARVIN
MARVIS
MAUVES
MCAVOY
MELVIL
MELVIN
MELVYN
MERVYN
MTVVJS

M•••V•
MARKVI
MOHAVE
MOJAVE
MOSKVA
MOTIVE
MYLOVE

M••••V
MAGLEV
MARKIV
MARKOV
MINITV
MOSHAV

•MV•••
AMVETS

•M•V••
BMOVIE

•M•••V
IMPROV
SMALLV

••MV••
ALMVPS
HUMVEE
NLMVPS

••M•V•
REMOVE

••M••V
JAMESV
YOMTOV

•••M•V
ASIMOV

M•W•••
MAWSON
MEWERS
MEWING
MEWLED
MEWLER
MOWERS
MOWGLI
MOWING
MRWONG
MYWORD

M••W••
MCEWAN
MCEWEN
MEOWED
MEOWER
MIDWAY

M•••W•
MACAWS
MALAWI
MIAOWS
MOHAWK
MOTOWN
MRPAWS

M••••W
MALLOW
MARROW
MATHEW
MCGRAW
MCGREW
MEADOW
MELLOW
MILDEW
MINNOW
MOOCOW
MORROW
MOSCOW
MURROW

•M••W•
EMBOWS

•M•••W
SMALLW

••MW••
DIMWIT

••M•W•
REMOWN
REMOWS
UNMEWS
UNMOWN

•••M•W
HAYMOW

M•X•••
MAXELL
MAXENE
MAXIMA
MAXIMS
MAXINE
MAXING
MAXIXE
MAXOUT
MAXSON
MEXICO
MIXERS
MIXING
MIXTEC
MIXUPS

M••X••
MARXES
MINXES

M•••X•
MAXIXE

M••••X
MAALOX
MADDOX
MADDUX
MADMAX
MANNIX
MARCIX
MARKIX
MATRIX
MEATAX
MERCKX
MRJINX
MUSKOX

•M•X••
IMAXES

•M••X•
IMNEXT

•M•••X
SMALLX

••M•X•
TJMAXX
UNMIXT

••M••X
COMDEX
COMMIX
LUMMOX
TJMAXX
TOMMIX

•••M•X
CALMEX
CLIMAX
COMMIX
LUMMOX
MADMAX
PREMIX
RONMIX
TEXMEX
TOMMIX

MY••••
MYBABY
MYDEAR
MYFOOT
MYGIRL
MYGOSH
MYHERO
MYLADY
MYLARS
MYLIFE
MYLORD
MYLOVE
MYMYMY
MYNAHS
MYOHMY
MYOPES
MYOPIA
MYOPIC
MYOSIN
MYOSIS
MYRDAL
MYRIAD
MYRRHS
MYRTLE
MYSELF
MYSORE
MYSTIC
MYTHIC
MYTHOS
MYTURN
MYWORD

M•Y•••
MAYANS
MAYBES
MAYDAY
MAYEST
MAYFLY
MAYHAP
MAYHEM
MAYIGO
MAYING
MAYORS
MAYRON
MAYTAG
MEYERS
MOYERS

M••Y••
MAGYAR
MARYAM
MARYII
MARYJO
MERYLL
MINYAN
MRHYDE
MYMYMY

M•••Y•
MADLYN
MALAYA
MALAYS
MARTYR
MASSYS
MATEYS
MELVYN
MERVYN
METHYL
MMDDYY
MONEYS
MOODYS
MORAYS
MOSEYS
MULEYS
MUMMYS

M••••Y
MABLEY
MAINLY
MAIRZY
MALADY
MALORY
MALTBY
MANDAY
MANLEY
MANRAY
MARBLY
MARKEY
MARLEY
MARSHY
MASSEY
MAUNDY
MAYDAY
MAYFLY
MAZILY
MCAVOY
MEANEY
MEANLY
MEASLY
MEDFLY
MEDLEY
MEEKLY
MEETLY
MELODY
MEMORY
MEOHMY
MERELY
MERSEY
MICKEY
MIDDAY
MIDMAY
MIDWAY
MIGHTY
MILADY
MILDLY
MILLAY
MINIFY
MISERY
MISKEY
MISLAY
MISSAY
MIZZLY
MMDDYY
MOBLEY
MODIFY
MOIETY
MOLLOY
MONDAY
MONKEY
MONODY
MOONEY
MOPERY
MORLEY
MORNAY
MOSLEY
MOSTLY
MOTLEY
MOULDY
MOUNTY
MOUSEY
MOUTHY
MTAIRY
MUMBLY
MUNCHY
MURPHY
MURRAY
MUSCLY
MUTELY
MUTINY
MYBABY
MYLADY
MYMYMY
MYOHMY

•MY•••
AMYTAN
SMYRNA

•M••Y•
EMBAYS
EMBRYO
EMILYS
EMORYU
MMDDYY

•M•••Y
AMBERY
DMITRY
EMBODY
EMPERY
EMPLOY
IMBUSY
IMEASY
IMOKAY
MMDDYY
SMALLY
SMARMY
SMARTY
SMEARY
SMELLY
SMILEY
SMIRKY
SMITHY
SMITTY
SMOGGY
SMOKEY
SMUDGY
SMUGLY
SMUTTY

••MY••
MYMYMY
YUMYUM

••M•Y•
CAMRYN
CAMRYS
DDMMYY
GAMAYS
HOMEYS
MUMMYS
NOMAYO
TAMAYO

••M••Y
ALMATY
ARMORY
ASMANY
BOMBAY
BUMBRY
CAMBOY
CAMEBY
COMEBY
COMEDY
COMELY
COMITY
COMPLY
DAMPLY
DDMMYY
DIMITY
DIMPLY
DOMBEY
DUMBLY
DUMPTY
ENMITY
FAMILY
GAMELY
GAMILY
HOMELY
HOMILY
HOMINY
HUMBLY
HUMPTY
JIMINY
JUMBLY
LAMELY
LEMONY
LIMPLY
LUMLEY
MEMORY
MUMBLY
MYMYMY
NAMELY
NIMBLY
NIMINY
NUMBLY
PIMINY
PIMPLY
POMPEY
RAMIFY
RAMSAY
RAMSEY
REMEDY
RIMSKY
ROMANY
ROMNEY
RUMBLY
RUMPLY
SIMPLY
SOMANY
STMARY
TAMELY
TIMELY
TOMBOY
TUMEFY
UNMIRY
WAMBLY
WIMSEY

•••MY•
DDMMYY
MUMMYS

•••M•Y
BLIMEY
CALMLY
CHAMMY
CHUMMY
CLAMMY
CLUMPY
CLUMSY
CRAMPY
CRIMPY
CRUMBY
CRUMMY
DDMMYY
DDMMYY
DISMAY
FIRMLY
FLIMSY
FRUMPY
GLUMLY
GRAMMY
GRIMLY
GRIMMY
GRUMPY
IFIMAY
LEEMAY
MIDMAY
NIAMEY
PLUMMY
PRIMLY
QUEMOY
SCUMMY
SEEMLY
SHAMMY
SHIMMY
SKIMPY
SLIMLY
SLUMMY
STEMMY
STIMPY
STUMPY
SWAMPY
TOOMEY
TRAMPY
TRIMLY
WARMLY
WHAMMY
WHIMSY

••••MY
ASKAMY
BIGAMY
BLOOMY
BOSOMY
BROOMY
CHAMMY
CHROMY
CHUMMY
CLAMMY
CREAMY
CRUMMY
DIGAMY
DREAMY
ECTOMY
GLEAMY
GLOOMY
GRAMMY
GRIMMY
INFAMY
JEREMY
MEOHMY
MYMYMY
MYOHMY
NAJIMY
PLUMMY
RHEUMY
SCUMMY
SHAMMY
SHIMMY
SLUMMY
SMARMY
STEAMY
STEMMY
STORMY
UNGAMY
USARMY
WHAMMY

M•Z•••
MAZDAS
MAZIER
MAZILY
MAZING
MAZOLA
MAZUMA
MEZZOS
MIZUNA
MIZZEN
MIZZLE
MIZZLY
MOZART
MUZZLE

M••Z••
MAAZEL
MAHZOR
MAIZES
MANZON
MATZOH
MATZOS
MEZZOS
MIZZEN
MIZZLE
MIZZLY
MONZAS
MUZZLE

M•••Z•
MAIRZY

M••••Z
MEGREZ
MESAAZ
MILOSZ
MONTEZ
MORITZ

•M•Z••
AMAZED
AMAZES
AMAZIN
AMAZON
SMAZES

•M•••Z
AMOSOZ
SMALLZ

••M•Z•
LAMAZE

••M••Z
ALMAAZ
COMPOZ
NIMITZ
TAMMUZ
YUMAAZ

•••M•Z
HORMUZ
LESMIZ
TAMMUZ

NA••••
NABBED
NABBER
NABOBS
NABORS
NACHAS
NACHOS
NACION
NACRED
NACRES
NADINE
NADIRS
NADSAT
NAGANO
NAGGED
NAGGER
NAGNAG
NAGOYA
NAGSAT
NAIADS
NAILED
NAILER
NAILIN
NAILIT
NAILUP
NAIRAS
NAIVER
NAJIMY
NAKFAS
NAMATH
NAMEIT
NAMELY
NAMERS
NAMING
NANINE
NANNIE
NANOOK
NANSEN
NANTES
NAPACA
NAPALM
NAPERY
NAPHTA
NAPIER
NAPKIN
NAPLES
NAPOLI
NAPPED
NAPPER
NAPPES
NAPPIE
NARADA
NARCOS
NARIAL
NARINE
NARITA
NARNIA
NARROW
NARVIK
NASALS
NASCAR
NASDAQ
NASEBY
NASHES
NASHUA
NASSAU
NASSER
NATALE
NATANT
NATHAN
NATICK
NATION
NATIVE
NATRON
NATTER
NATURE
NAUGHT
NAUSEA
NAUTES
NAVAHO
NAVAID
NAVAJO
NAVELS
NAVIES
NAYSAY

N•A•••
NBAERS
NEALON
NEARBY
NEARED
NEARER
NEARLY
NEARTO
NEATEN
NEATER
NEATLY
NIACIN
NIAMEY
NUANCE
NYALAS

N••A••
NAGANO
NAIADS
NAMATH
NAPACA
NAPALM
NARADA
NASALS
NATALE
NATANT
NAVAHO
NAVAID
NAVAJO
NEGATE
NEPALI
NEVADA
NEWAGE
NEWARK
NICADS
NISANS
NLEAST
NOBAKE
NOBALL
NOFAIR
NOHANT
NOMAAM
NOMADS
NOMAYO
NONAGE
NONAME
NONART
NONARY
NOPALS
NORAIN
NOSALE
NOSALT
NOTAIL
NOTALL
NOTANY
NOTARY
NOTATE
NOVATO
NOWAIT
NOWAYS
NSTARS
NUTATE
NYYANK

N•••A•
NACHAS
NADSAT
NAGNAG
NAGSAT
NAIRAS
NAKFAS
NARIAL
NASCAR
NASDAQ
NASSAU
NATHAN
NAYSAY
NECTAR
NEENAH
NEIMAN
NEMEAN
NEPEAN
NERMAL
NERVAL
NETMAN
NETPAY
NEUMAN
NEURAL
NEWCAR
NEWDAY
NEWHAT
NEWMAN
NEWMAR
NEWWAY
NEXRAD
NICIAS
NIETAS
NIIHAU
NIKEAD
NINEAD
NINEAM
NINJAS
NIPSAT
NISSAN
NODEAL
NODEAR
NODSAT
NOKIAS
NOLEAD
NOLOAD
NOMAAM
NOMEAK
NOMEAT
NOMIAL
NONFAN
NONFAT
NONGAS
NONMAN

NONPAR
NONTAN
NONTAX
NONWAR
NOONAN
NORGAY
NORIAS
NORMAL
NORMAN
NORVAL
NORWAY
NOSOAP
NOTBAD
NOTFAR
NOUGAT
NOUNAL
NOVIAS
NOWLAN
NUBIAN
NUCHAE
NUCHAL
NUMBAT
NYALAS

N••••A

NAGOYA
NAPACA
NAPHTA
NARADA
NARITA
NARNIA
NASHUA
NAUSEA
NEBULA
NERUDA
NESTEA
NEVADA
NEWERA
NICOLA
NIKITA
NIKOLA
NOIDEA
NOOTKA
NOSTRA
NOUMEA
NOVELA
NOVENA
NUBIRA
NUMINA
NUTRIA

•NA•••

ANACIN
ANADEM
ANAKIN
ANALOG
ANANAS
ANANKE
ANARCH
ANATTO
DNAASE
DNALAB
DNASES
ENABLE
ENACTS
ENAMEL
ENAMOR
ENARMS
ENATES
GNARLS
GNARLY
GNARRS
GNATTY
GNAWAT
GNAWED
GNAWER
GNAWON
INABIT
INABOX
INADAY
INAFEW
INAFIX
INAFOG
INAGES
INAJAM
INANER
INAPET
INAPIE
INAPOD
INARAY
INARCH
INAREA
INAROW
INARUG
INARUT
INASEC
INATIE
INATUB
INAWAY
KNACKS
KNARRS
KNARRY
KNAVES
ONABUN
ONAGER
ONAHOP
ONAJAG
ONAPAR
ONAUTO
RNAASE
SNACKS
SNAFUS
SNAGGY
SNAGUP
SNAILS
SNAKED
SNAKER
SNAKES
SNAPAT
SNAPON
SNAPPY
SNAPTO
SNAPUP
SNARED
SNARER
SNARES
SNARFS
SNARKS
SNARKY
SNARLS
SNARLY
SNATCH
SNATHS
SNAZZY
UNABLE
UNABLY
UNAGED
UNAKIN
UNAMIS
UNARMS
UNAVID
UNAWED
UNAXED

•N•A••

ANKARA
ANNALS
ANSARA
ANSATE
ANTAWN
ANWANG
ANZACS
DNAASE
ENBANC
ENCAGE
ENCAMP
ENCASE
ENDALL
ENDASH
ENFACE
ENFAIT
ENFANT
ENGAGE
ENHALO
ENHAUT
ENIACS
ENLACE
ENRAGE
ENRANK
ENRAPT
ENSATE
ENTAIL
INBACK
INCAIC
INCANS
INCANT
INCAPS
INCASE
INCASH
INDASH
INFACT
INFALL
INFAMY
INFANT
INGATE
INHALE
INHALF
INHAND
INJAIL
INLAID
INLAND
INLAWS
INLAYS
INMATE
INNAGE
INNATE
INPARK
INPART
INPAWN
INRAGS
INSANA
INSANE
INTACT
INTAKE
INVADE
INVAIN
INWANT
INWARD
KNEADS
ONBAIL
ONBASE
ONCALL
ONEACT
ONEALL
ONEARM
ONHAND
ONLAID
ONLAND
ONLATE
ONLAYS
ONRAMP
ONSALE
ONTAPE
ONWARD
RNAASE
SNEAKS
SNEAKY
UNBAGS
UNBAIT
UNBALE
UNBARE
UNBARS
UNCAGE
UNCAKE
UNCALM
UNCAPS
UNCASE
UNCASK
UNCAST
UNDAMS
UNEASE
UNEASY
UNFACT
UNFAIR
UNGAGS
UNGAMY
UNGAVA
UNHAFT
UNHAIR
UNHALE
UNHAND
UNHASP
UNHATS
UNHAZY
UNIATE
UNIATS
UNJAMS
UNLACE
UNLADE
UNLAID
UNLASH
UNLAYS
UNMADE
UNMAKE
UNMANS
UNMASK
UNMAST
UNMATE
UNNAIL
UNPACK
UNPAID
UNPALE
UNPAWN
UNRACK
UNRASH
UNSAFE
UNSAGE
UNSAID
UNSAWN
UNSAYS
UNTACK
UNTAME
UNTAPE
UNTAUT
UNVAIN
UNWALL
UNWARY

•N••A•

ANANAS
ANDEAN
ANDRAE
ANIMAL
ANIMAS
ANNEAL
ANNUAL
ANODAL
ANORAK
ANTRAL
ANYDAY
ANYMAN
ANYWAY
DNALAB
ENDEAR
ENDMAN
ENDRAN
ENDSAT
ENGRAM
ENNEAD
ENQUAD
ENSEAL
ENSEAT
ENTIAL
ENTRAP
ENWRAP
GNAWAT
INADAY
INAJAM
INARAY
INAWAY
INDIAN
INFEAR
INGEAR
INGMAR
INGOAL
INGRAM
INGRAY
INKPAD
INKSAC
INLEAF
INPLAY
INROAD
INSEAM
INSPAN
INSTAL
INTHAT
INTRAY
ONAJAG
ONAPAR
ONECAR
ONEDAY
ONELAP
ONEMAN
ONEWAY
ONLOAD
ONLOAN
ONSTAR
SNAPAT
SNOCAT
UNCIAL
UNCLAD
UNCLAY
UNDEAD
UNDRAW
UNFLAT
UNGLAD
UNGUAL
UNITAS
UNIVAC
UNLEAD
UNLEAF
UNLEAN
UNLOAD
UNNEAT
UNOCAL
UNORAL
UNPLAN
UNREAD
UNREAL
UNSEAL
UNSEAM
UNSEAT
UNSNAG
UNSNAP
UNSPAN
UNTHAW
UNTRAP
UNWRAP

•N•••A

ANDREA
ANEMIA
ANGELA
ANGLIA
ANGOLA
ANGORA
ANITRA
ANKARA
ANNIKA
ANNINA
ANOMIA
ANOXIA
ANSARA
ANTLIA
ENCINA
ENDORA
ENIGMA
INAREA
INDIRA
INSANA
ONEIDA
PNEUMA
UNCOLA
UNGAVA
UNGULA

••NA••

ADNATE
AGNAIL
AGNATE
ALNASL
ANNALS
ARNALL
BANANA
BANANE
BINACA
BINARY
BINATE
BONACI
BONAMI
BYNAME
CANAAN
CANADA
CANALS
CANAPE
CANARD
CANARY
CONAIR
CONANT
CUNARD
DANANG
DENADA
DENALI
DENARI
DENARS
DENARY
DINARS
DONALD
DONATE
DONATH
DUNANT
DYNAMO
DYNAST
ELNATH
ERNANI
FINALE
FINALS
IGNACE
IGNATZ
INNAGE
INNATE
JONAHS
KANAKA
KANALY
KANATA
KANAWA
LANAIS
LANARK
LANATE
LENAIN
LENAPE
LENARD
LINAGE
LUNACY
LUNATE
MANAGE
MANAMA
MANANA
MANAOS
MANAPE
MANATS
MCNABB
MCNAIR
MENACE
MENAGE
MONACO
MONADS
MONAMI
MYNAHS
NONAGE
NONAME
NONART
NONARY
ORNATE
OXNARD
PANADA
PANAMA
PINATA
RENAIL
RENAME
RENARD
RENATA
RENATO
RONALD
SENARY
SENATE
SENATS
SONANT
SONARS
SONATA
TANAKA
TANANA
TENACE
TENANT
UNNAIL
USNAVY
VANARK
WINANS
XANADU
ZENANA

••N•A•

AENEAS
ANNEAL
ANNUAL
APNEAS
ASNEAR
ASNEAT
BANTAM
BANYAN
BANZAI
BENDAY
BENGAL
BENGAY
BONHAM
BONSAI
BUNGAY
BUNYAN
CANAAN
CANCAN
CANNAS
CANTAB
CANTAL
CANVAS
CENTAI
CENTAL
CENTAS
CONFAB
CONGAS
CONLAN
CONMAN
CONRAD
CONTAC
CONWAY
CUNEAL
DANNAY
DENHAM
DENIAL
DENTAL
DINEAT
DINKAS
DUNBAR
DUNCAN
DUNDAS
DUNHAM
DUNLAP
ENNEAD
EONIAN
FANTAN
FANTAS
FENWAY
FINCAS
FINIAL
FINIAN
FINNAN
FONDAS
FONTAL
FUNGAL
GENIAL
GENOAN
GENOAS
GENUAL
GONEAR
GONEAT
GUNLAP
GUNLAW
GUNMAN
GUNNAR
HANDAX
HANGAR
HANNAH
HANSAS
HENNAS
HINTAT
HONDAS
HONKAT
IONIAN
JANUAR
JUNEAU
JUNTAS
KANSAN
KANSAS
KENNAN
KENYAN
KINNAN
KONRAD
LANDAT
LANDAU
LANVAL
LINEAL
LINEAR
MANDAN
MANDAY
MANGAS
MANIAC
MANIAS
MANNAS
MANRAY
MANTAS
MANUAL
MENIAL
MENSAL
MENSAN
MENTAL
MINOAN
MINYAN
MONDAY
MONTAG
MONZAS
NINEAD
NINEAM
NINJAS
NONFAN
NONFAT
NONGAS
NONMAN
NONPAR
NONTAN
NONTAX
NONWAR
PANDAS
PENMAN
PENPAL
PENTAD
PENTAX
PINCAY
PINDAR
PINEAL
PINNAE
PINNAS
PINOAK
PONCAS
PUNJAB
PUNKAS
PUNTAS
QANTAS
QINTAR
RANDAL
RANTAT
RENGAS
RENTAL
RUNSAT
RUNWAY
SANDAL
SANKAS
SANTAS
SENDAK
SENNAS
SINBAD
SINEAD
SINTAX
SONTAG
SUNDAE
SUNDAS
SUNDAY
SUNFAN
SUNHAT
SUNRAY
SUNTAN
SYNTAX
TANKAS
TANOAK
TENDAY
TINCAN
TINEAL
TINEAR
TINHAT
TINIAN
TINMAN
TINPAN
TONGAN
TONKAS
UINTAS
UNNEAT
VANDAL
VENIAL
VENTAS
WANTAD
WENTAT
WINKAT
WINSAT
YANKAT
YENTAS
ZANTAC
ZONIAN
ZUNIAN

••N••A

ANNIKA
ANNINA
ARNICA
BANANA
BINACA
BONITA
CANADA
CANCHA
CANDIA
CANOLA
CANOVA
CANULA
CINEMA
CONCHA
CONTRA
DANOVA
DENADA
DENDRA
DONORA
ELNORA
GENERA
GENEVA
GENOVA
KANAKA
KANATA
KANAWA
KONICA
LANCIA
LANINA
LENGUA
LENINA
LINGUA
LUNTHA
LUNULA
MANAMA
MANANA
MANCHA
MANILA
MANTRA
MANTUA
MINETA
MINIMA
MONETA
MONICA
MUNERA
PANADA
PANAMA
PENNIA
PINATA
RENATA
SANCTA
SANDIA
SANDRA
SANTHA
SENECA
SENORA
SENTRA
SONATA
SONDRA
SONOMA
SONORA
TANAKA
TANANA
TANTRA
TENUTA
TUNDRA
VENERA
VENORA
WINONA
XINHUA
ZENANA
ZINNIA
ZUNIGA

•••NA•

ADONAI
AGENAS
AMANAS
ANANAS
ARENAS
ASANAS
ATONAL
AXONAL
AZONAL
BUENAS
BWANAS
CANNAS
CARNAC
CARNAL
CARNAP
CATNAP
CERNAN
CHINAS
CLONAL
COGNAC
DANNAY
DARNAY
DOGNAP
DUENAS
EPINAL
EVENAS
FAENAS
FAUNAE
FAUNAL
FAUNAS
FERNAO
FINNAN
FORNAX
GRINAT
GUINAN
GUNNAR
HANNAH
HENNAS
HERNAN
HYENAS
HYMNAL
KARNAK
KAUNAS
KEENAN
KENNAN
KIDNAP
KINNAN
LIANAS
MAENAD
MANNAS
MOLNAR
MORNAY
NAGNAG
NEENAH
NOONAN
NOUNAL
PETNAP
PINNAE
PINNAS
PLANAR
PLANAS
POZNAN
PRANAS
PUTNAM
RAGNAR
REGNAL
REGNAT
REINAS
RESNAP
RHINAL
SAUNAS
SAYNAY
SCENAS
SEENAS
SENNAS
SIGNAL
SOONAS
SPINAL
TRINAL
UNSNAG
UNSNAP
VARNAS
VEINAL
VERNAL
WETNAP

•••N•A

AGENDA
AMANDA
AMENRA
AMINTA
AMONRA
ASONIA
ATONIA
AZANIA
BIANCA
BLANCA
BLANDA
BOSNIA
BRANCA
BRENDA
BRYNZA
CHINUA
CHYNNA
CORNEA
CRANIA
CRENNA
CSONKA
DEANNA
DUENNA
ERINNA
EUPNEA
FRANCA
GLENDA
GLINDA
GLINKA
GRANPA
GUINEA
HERNIA
IVANKA
IWANNA
JOANNA
KAUNDA
KWANZA
LAONZA
LEONIA
LUANDA
NARNIA
OLINDA
PAANGA
PENNIA
POINTA
QUANTA
QUINTA
RHONDA
RUANDA
RWANDA
SARNIA
SHANIA
SIENNA
STANZA
THENBA
THENRA
TIENDA
TRENTA
UGANDA
URANIA
VIENNA
ZINNIA

••••NA

ALAINA
ALCINA
ALHENA
ALUMNA
AMARNA
ANNINA
ARCANA
ARIANA
ARJUNA
ASTANA
ATHENA
BANANA
BOLENA
BRIANA
BURANA
CABANA
CARINA
CATENA
CESSNA
CHYNNA
CORONA
COVINA
CRENNA
DEANNA
DUENNA
EDWINA
ENCINA
ERINNA
ESPANA
FALANA
FARINA
FUTUNA
GALENA
GETANA
GOTANA
GRETNA
GUIANA
GUYANA
HABANA
HAVANA
HELENA
HRYVNA
IGUANA
ILEANA
INSANA
IWANNA
JOANNA
JOBYNA
KAHUNA
KARINA
KORUNA
KRASNA
LACUNA
LAGUNA
LAMINA
LANINA
LATINA
LENINA
LUMINA
MANANA
MARINA
MEDINA
MELINA
MIZUNA
MODENA
MOLINA
MTETNA
NOVENA
NUMINA
OKSANA
ORGANA
ORIANA
PAMINA
PARANA
PATINA
PIRANA
POEANA
POMONA
PURINA
RAMONA
REGINA
RETINA
ROSINA
ROWENA
ROXANA
SABENA
SABINA
SALINA
SAVANA
SEDONA
SELENA
SEMANA
SERENA
SEVENA
SHEENA
SIENNA

SMYRNA
STERNA
TANANA
TEJANA
TIRANA
TUCANA
URBANA
VERONA
VEZINA
VICUNA
VIENNA
WADENA
WINONA
YAMUNA
YELENA
YEMANA
ZENANA
ZORINA

NB••••

NBAERS
NBCRED
NBOMBS

N•B•••

NABBED
NABBER
NABOBS
NABORS
NEBULA
NIBBLE
NIBLET
NOBAKE
NOBALL
NOBELS
NOBILE
NOBLER
NOBLES
NOBODY
NOBUTS
NUBBED
NUBBER
NUBBIN
NUBBLE
NUBBLY
NUBIAN
NUBILE
NUBIRA

N••B••

NABBED
NABBER
NESBIT
NEWBIE
NIBBLE
NIMBLE
NIMBLY
NIMBUS
NIOBIC
NOMBRE
NOTBAD
NUBBED
NUBBER
NUBBIN
NUBBLE
NUBBLY
NUMBAT
NUMBED
NUMBER
NUMBLY

N•••B•

NABOBS
NASEBY
NBOMBS
NEARBY
NEEDBE
NINEBC
NINGBO

N••••B

NEWJOB
NOPROB

•NB•••

ENBANC
ENBERG
ENBLOC
INBACK
INBLUE
INBORN
INBRED
INBULK
ONBAIL
ONBASE
UNBAGS
UNBAIT
UNBALE
UNBARE
UNBARS
UNBELT
UNBEND
UNBENT
UNBIND
UNBITS
UNBLED
UNBOLD
UNBOLT
UNBORN
UNBUDS
UNBURY
UNBUSY

•N•B••

ANUBIS
ENABLE
INABIT
INABOX
KNEBEL
KNOBBY
ONABUN
ONEBIT
SNOBBY
SNOBOL
SNUBBY
UNABLE
UNABLY

•N••B•

ENROBE
INCUBI
INDEBT
KNOBBY
SNOBBY
SNUBBY
UNROBE

•N•••B

DNALAB
ENTOMB
INATUB
UNCURB
UNGLIB

••NB••

BENBEN
BENBOW
BONBON
DUNBAR
HENBIT
PINBOY
SINBAD
SUNBOW
WINBIG
WONBIG

••N•B•

CANTBE
DANUBE
DONEBY
GONEBY
HANGBY
HUNGBY
KENOBI
MCNABB
NINEBC
NINGBO
RUNSBY
SENDBY
SENTBY
TENLBS
WENTBY
WINSBY

••N••B

BENUMB
CANTAB
CONFAB
CONJOB
MCNABB
PUNJAB

•••NB•

GRANBY
HORNBY
PLANBS
THENBA

•••N•B

HOBNOB
POINTB

••••NB

SEVENB
SUSANB

N•C•••

NACHAS
NACHOS
NACION
NACRED
NACRES
NBCRED
NECKED
NECKER
NECTAR
NICADS
NICELY
NICENE
NICEST
NICETY
NICHED
NICHES
NICIAS
NICKED
NICKEL
NICKER
NICKJR
NICOLA
NICOLE
NICOLO
NOCENT
NOCHES
NOCKED
NOCOST
NUCHAE
NUCHAL
NUCLEI
NUCLEO

N••C••

NARCOS
NASCAR
NEOCON
NEWCAR
NIACIN
NIECES
NONCOM
NOTCHY
NUECES
NUNCIO

N•••C•

NAPACA
NATICK
NODICE
NOLUCK
NOTICE
NOVICE
NUANCE

N••••C

NINEBC
NIOBIC
NITRIC
NOETIC
NORDIC

•NC•••

ANCHOR
ANCHOS
ANCIEN
ENCAGE
ENCAMP
ENCASE
ENCINA
ENCINO
ENCODE
ENCORE
ENCRES
ENCYCL
INCAIC
INCANS
INCANT
INCAPS
INCASE
INCASH
INCENT
INCEPT
INCHED
INCHER
INCHES
INCHON
INCISE
INCITE
INCODE
INCOME
INCUBI
INCULT
INCURS
INCUSE
ONCALL
ONCLES
UNCAGE
UNCAKE
UNCALM
UNCAPS
UNCASE
UNCASK
UNCAST
UNCHIC
UNCIAL
UNCLAD
UNCLAY
UNCLES
UNCLIP
UNCLOG
UNCOIL
UNCOLA
UNCOOL
UNCOOP
UNCORE
UNCORK
UNCUFF
UNCURB
UNCURL
UNCUTE

•N•C••

ANACIN
ANTCOW
ENACTS
ENDCUT
KNACKS
KNICKS
KNOCKS
ONECAR
SNACKS
SNICKS
SNOCAT
UNICED
UNICEF
UNICES
UNOCAL
VNECKS

•N••C•

ANARCH
ANTICS
ANZACS
ENCYCL
ENESCO
ENFACE
ENIACS
ENLACE
ENRICH
ENRICO
ENTICE
INARCH
INBACK
INDICT
INDUCE
INDUCT
INFACT
INFECT
INHOCK
INJECT
INLUCK
INSECT
INTACT
ONDECK
ONEACT
ONRICE
SNATCH
SNITCH
UNDICI
UNDOCK
UNESCO
UNFACT
UNLACE
UNLOCK
UNNICE
UNPACK
UNPICK
UNRACK
UNSICK
UNTACK
UNTUCK

•N•••C

ANDRIC
ANEMIC
ANGLIC
ANODIC
ANOMIC
ANOXIC
ENBANC
ENBLOC
GNOMIC
INASEC
INCAIC
INKSAC
INSYNC
ONESEC
ONSPEC
UNCHIC
UNEPIC
UNIFIC
UNIVAC

••NC••

BANCOS
BINCHY
BUNCHE
BUNCHY
BUNCOS
CANCAN
CANCEL
CANCER
CANCHA
CANCUN
CONCHA
CONCHO
CONCHS
CONCUR
DANCED
DANCER
DANCES
DANCIN
DUNCAN
DUNCES
FENCED
FENCER
FENCES
FINCAS
HONCHO
JUNCOS
LANCED
LANCER
LANCES
LANCET
LANCIA
LANCIE
LUNCHY
MANCHA
MANCHE
MANCHU
MINCED
MINCER
MINCES
MUNCHY
MUNCIE
NONCOM
NUNCIO
OUNCES
PANCHO
PANCKS
PENCHE
PENCIL
PINCAY
PINCER
PONCAS
PONCHO
PUNCHY
RANCHO
RANCID
RANCOR
RONCEY
RUNCIE
SANCHO
SANCTA
SYNCED
SYNCHS
TINCAN
TINCTS
TINCUP
VINCIT
WENCES
WINCED
WINCER
WINCES
ZINCED
ZINCIC
ZINCKY

••N•C•

ALNICO
ARNICA
BENICE
BINACA
BONACI
CANUCK
CONICS
CONOCO
CYNICS
EUNICE
GYNECO
IGNACE
IONICS
JANICE
KONICA
LUNACY
MENACE
MENSCH
MONACO
MONICA
MUNICH
PANICS
PENICK
SENECA
SONICS
STNICK
SUNOCO
TENACE
TONICS
TUNICS
UNNICE
VENICE
ZANUCK

••N••C

CONTAC
FANFIC
FINNIC
HENDEC
MANIAC
MANTIC
NINEBC
RUNDMC
SYNDIC
TANNIC
ZANTAC
ZINCIC

•••NC•

AGENCE
AGENCY
ATONCE
BIANCA
BIANCO
BLANCA
BLANCH
BLANCO
BLENCH
BOUNCE
BOUNCY
BRANCA
BRANCH
BRONCO
BRONCS
BRUNCH
CHANCE
CHANCY
CHINCH
CLANCY
CLENCH
CLINCH
CRUNCH
DRANCY
DRENCH
ELANCE
EVINCE
FIANCE
FLINCH
FRANCA
FRANCE
FRANCK
FRANCO
FRANCS
FRENCH
GLANCE
GRINCH
HAUNCH
JOUNCE
JOUNCY
LAUNCH
NUANCE
PAUNCH
PLANCK
POUNCE
PRANCE
PRINCE
QUENCH
QUINCE
QUINCY
RAUNCH
RYENCE
SCONCE
SEANCE
SPENCE
STANCE
STANCH
STENCH
THENCE
TRANCE
TRENCH
USANCE
WHENCE
WRENCH

•••N•C

ADONIC
ATONIC
AXENIC
AZONIC
BIONIC
CARNAC
CLINIC
COGNAC
CYANIC
EDENIC
ETHNIC
ETONIC
FINNIC
ICONIC
IRENIC
IRONIC
KAONIC
ODINIC
OZONIC
PHONIC
PICNIC
SCENIC
TANNIC
URANIC

••••NC

ENBANC
FERENC
INSYNC
SEVENC

N•D•••

NADINE
NADIRS
NADSAT
NIDIFY
NODDED
NODDER
NODEAL
NODEAR
NODICE
NODOFF
NODOSE
NODOUS
NODSAT
NODSTO
NODULE
NUDELY
NUDEST
NUDGED
NUDGER
NUDGES
NUDISM
NUDIST
NUDITY
NUDNIK

N••D••

NASDAQ
NEEDBE
NEEDED
NEEDER
NEEDLE
NEEDNT
NEEDTO
NEWDAY
NODDED
NODDER
NOIDEA
NOODGE
NOODLE
NORDIC
NORDOI

N•••D•

NAIADS
NARADA
NERUDA
NEVADA
NICADS
NOBODY
NOKIDS
NOMADS

N••••D

NABBED
NACRED
NAGGED
NAILED
NAPPED
NAVAID
NBCRED
NEARED
NECKED
NEEDED
NEREID
NERVED
NESTED
NETTED
NEWKID
NEXRAD
NICHED
NICKED
NIKEAD
NIMROD
NINEAD
NIPPED
NOCKED
NODDED
NOGOOD
NOISED
NOLEAD
NOLOAD
NONEED
NONFED
NONGOD
NOOSED
NOSHED
NOTBAD
NUBBED
NUDGED
NULLED
NUMBED
NURSED
NUTTED

•ND•••

ANDEAN
ANDERS
ANDHOW
ANDRAE
ANDREA
ANDREI
ANDRES
ANDREW
ANDREY
ANDRIC
ANDROS
ANDYET
ENDALL
ENDASH
ENDCUT
ENDEAR
ENDERS
ENDING
ENDIVE
ENDMAN
ENDMEN
ENDORA
ENDOWS
ENDPIN
ENDRAN
ENDRUN
ENDSAT
ENDSIN
ENDSIT
ENDSON
ENDSUP
ENDUED
ENDUES
ENDURE
ENDURO
ENDUSE
INDASH
INDEBT
INDEED
INDEEP
INDENT
INDIAN
INDICT
INDIES
INDIGO
INDIRA
INDITE
INDIUM
INDOOR
INDUCE
INDUCT
INDUED
INDUES
ONDECK
ONDISK
ONDITS
ONDUTY
UNDAMS
UNDEAD
UNDEEP
UNDEFT
UNDERS
UNDEWY
UNDICI
UNDIES
UNDIMS
UNDINE
UNDOCK
UNDOER
UNDOES
UNDONE
UNDRAW
UNDREW
UNDSET
UNDULY
UNDYED

•N•D••

ANADEM
ANODAL
ANODES
ANODIC
ANYDAY
ENIDOK
INADAY
ONEDAY
ONEDGE
SNIDER
SNYDER
UNEDGE
UNIDLE
UNIDLY

•N••D•

ENCODE
INCODE
INSIDE
INVADE
KNEADS
ONEIDA
ONSIDE
SNOODS
UNBUDS
UNLADE
UNMADE
UNRUDE
UNTIDY

•N•••D

ANELED
ANGLED
ANKLED
ANTEED
ANYOLD
ENDUED
ENFOLD
ENGILD
ENGIRD
ENNEAD
ENQUAD
ENSUED
ENURED
ENVIED
ENWIND
GNAWED
INAPOD
INBRED
INCHED
INDEED
INDUED
INFOLD
INGOLD
INGOOD
INGRID
INHAND
INKIND
INKPAD
INLAID
INLAND
INMIND
INNEED
INROAD
INTEND
INURED
INWARD
KNIFED
ONHAND
ONHOLD
ONLAID
ONLAND
ONLOAD
ONWARD
SNAKED
SNARED
SNIPED
SNORED
SNOWED
UNAGED
UNAVID
UNAWED
UNAXED
UNBEND
UNBIND
UNBLED
UNBOLD
UNCLAD
UNDEAD
UNDYED
UNFOLD
UNFOND
UNGIRD
UNGLAD
UNHAND
UNHEED
UNHELD
UNHOED
UNHOOD
UNHUED
UNICED
UNIPED
UNIPOD
UNITED
UNKIND
UNLAID
UNLEAD
UNLOAD
UNMOLD
UNOWED
UNPAID
UNREAD
UNRUED
UNSAID
UNSELD
UNSHED
UNSHOD
UNSOLD
UNSUED
UNTIED
UNTOLD
UNTROD
UNUSED
UNVOID
UNWILD
UNWIND

••ND••

BANDED
BANDER
BANDIT
BENDAY
BENDED
BENDER
BENDIX
BINDER
BINDLE
BINDTO
BINDUP
BONDED
BONDER
BUNDLE
BUNDTS
CANDIA
CANDID
CANDLE
CANDOR
CINDER
CONDOR
CONDOS
DANDER
DANDIE
DANDLE
DANDYL
DENDRA
DENDRI
DENDRO
DINDIN
DONDER
DUNDAS
DUNDEE
FANDOM
FENDED
FENDER
FINDER
FONDAS
FONDER
FONDLE
FONDLY
FONDOF
FONDUE
FONDUS
FUNDED
FUNDER
GANDER
GANDHI
GENDER
GUNDOG
HANDAX
HANDED
HANDEL
HANDER
HANDIN
HANDKE
HANDLE
HANDON
HANDUP
HENDEC
HENDRY
HINDER
HINDUS
HONDAS
KANDEL
KANDER
KENDOS
KINDER
KINDLE
KINDLY
KINDOF
KUNDRY
LANDAT
LANDAU
LANDED
LANDER
LANDHO
LANDIS
LANDON
LANDOR
LANDRY
LANDUP
LANDUS
LENDEE
LENDER
LENDTO
LINDEN
LINDER
LONDON
LUNDEN
LUNDIS
LYNDON
MANDAN
MANDAY
MANDEL
MANDMS
MENDED

MENDEL
MENDER
MENDES
MINDED
MINDEN
MINDER
MONDAY
MONDES
MONDOS
PANDAS
PANDER
PANDIT
PANDLS
PENDED
PINDAR
PINDUS
PONDED
PONDER
PUNDIT
RANDAL
RANDOM
RANDRY
RENDED
RENDER
RONDEL
RONDOS
RUNDLE
RUNDMC
RUNDRY
SANDAL
SANDED
SANDER
SANDIA
SANDRA
SANDRO
SENDAK
SENDBY
SENDEE
SENDER
SENDIN
SENDON
SENDTO
SENDUP
SONDES
SONDRA
SUNDAE
SUNDAS
SUNDAY
SUNDER
SUNDOG
SUNDRY
SYNDIC
TANDEM
TENDAY
TENDED
TENDER
TENDON
TENDTO
TINDER
TONDOS
TUNDRA
VANDAL
VENDED
VENDEE
VENDER
VENDOR
VENDUE
WANDER
WENDED
WENDIE
WENDYS
WINDED
WINDER
WINDEX
WINDOM
WINDOW
WINDUP
WONDER
YONDER
ZENDOS

••N•D•

CANADA
CANIDS
DENADA
DENUDE
DYNODE
LUNEDI
MENUDO
MONADS
MONODY
PANADA
RANIDS
SYNODS
WONTDO
XANADU

••N••D

AENEID
ARNOLD
BANDED
BANGED
BANKED
BANNED
BENDED
BINGED
BINNED
BONDED
BONGED
BONKED
BUNGED
BUNKED
BUNTED
CANARD
CANDID
CANNED
CANOED
CANTED
CENSED
CONFED
CONKED
CONNED
CONOID
CONRAD
CUNARD
DANCED
DANGED
DENIED
DENNED
DENTED
DINGED
DINNED
DINTED
DONALD
DONNED
DUNKED
DUNNED
ENNEAD
FANGED
FANNED
FENCED
FENDED
FINKED
FINNED
FUNDED
FUNKED
FUNNED
GANGED
GINNED
GONGED
GUNNED
HANDED
HANGED
HINGED
HINTED
HONIED
HONKED
HUNTED
INNEED
JINXED
JUNKED
KENNED
KINGED
KINKED
KONRAD
LANCED
LANDED
LENARD
LENSED
LINKED
LINTED
LONGED
LUNGED
LYNYRD
MANNED
MENDED
MINCED
MINDED
MINTED
MONIED
NINEAD
NONEED
NONFED
NONGOD
OINKED
OXNARD
PANNED
PANTED
PENDED
PENNED
PENROD
PENTAD
PINGED
PINKED
PINNED
PONDED
PONGID
PONIED
PUNNED
PUNTED
RANCID
RANGED
RANKED
RANTED
RENARD
RENDED
RENTED
RINGED
RINSED
RONALD
SANDED
SENSED
SINBAD
SINEAD
SINGED
SINNED
SUNGOD
SUNNED
SYNCED
TANGED
TANKED
TANNED
TENDED
TENSED
TENTED
TINGED
TINGOD
TINNED
TINTED
TONGED
VANNED
VENDED
VENTED
WANNED
WANTAD
WANTED
WENDED
WINCED
WINDED
WINGED
WINKED
WONTED
YANKED
YENNED
YENSID
ZINCED
ZINGED
ZONKED

•••ND•

AGENDA
AMANDA
AMENDS
ARENDT
BIONDI
BLANDA
BLENDE
BLENDS
BLINDS
BLONDE
BLONDS
BOUNDS
BRANDI
BRANDO
BRANDS
BRANDT
BRANDX
BRANDY
BRENDA
CHANDU
CUANDO
DIRNDL
EBONDS
ELANDS
EMENDS
FIENDS
FOUNDS
FRONDS
GLANDS
GLENDA
GLINDA
GRANDE
GRANDS
GRANDY
GRINDL
GRINDS
GRUNDY
HOUNDS
HOUNDY
KAUNDA
LUANDA
MAUNDY
MOUNDS
OLINDA
PBANDJ
POUNDS
RHONDA
ROUNDS
RUANDA
RWANDA
SHANDY
SHINDY
SOUNDS
SPENDS
SPENDY
STANDS
TBONDS
TIENDA
TRENDS
TRENDY
UGANDA
UPENDS
VIANDS
WOUNDS
XYANDZ
ZOUNDS

•••N•D

ALINED
ATONED
BANNED
BARNED
BEANED
BINNED
BRINED
BURNED
CANNED
CLONED
COINED
CONNED
CORNED
CRANED
CYANID
DAMNED
DARNED
DAWNED
DENNED
DINNED
DONNED
DOWNED
DRONED
DUNNED
DURNED
EARNED
EVENED
FANNED
FAWNED
FINNED
FUNNED
GAINED
GINNED
GOUNOD
GOWNED
GUNNED
HORNED
HYMNED
IRONED
JEANED
JOINED
KEENED
KENNED
KERNED
KILNED
LEANED
LEONID
LIMNED
LOANED
MAENAD
MANNED
MOANED
MOONED
OMENED
OPENED
OPINED
PAINED
PANNED
PAWNED
PEENED
PENNED
PERNOD
PHONED
PINNED
PLANED
PRUNED
PUNNED
RAINED
REINED
REUNED
RUINED
SEINED
SHINED
SIGNED
SINNED
SPINED
STONED
SUNNED
TANNED
TINNED
TURNED
TWINED
VANNED
VEINED
WANNED
WARNED
WEANED
WEENED
WHINED
YARNED
YAWNED
YEANED
YENNED

••••ND

ABOUND
ADDEND
ALMOND
AMBAND
APPEND
ARMAND
AROUND
ASCEND
ATHAND
ATTEND
AUFOND
AUGEND
BADEND
BAGEND
BEHIND
BEKIND
BEYOND
BIGEND
BRIAND
BYHAND
BYLAND
DALAND
DEFEND
DEFUND
DELAND
DEMAND
DEMOND
DEPEND
EDMOND
EDMUND
EKLAND
ENWIND
ERRAND
EXPAND
EXPEND
EXTEND
EYVIND
FAGEND
FECUND
FMBAND
FREUND
FRIEND
GERUND
GROUND
IMPEND
INHAND
INKIND
INLAND
INMIND
INTEND
ISLAND
JOCUND
LEGEND
LELAND
LEMOND
LIGAND
LOMOND
LOWEND
MRBOND
OBTUND
OFFEND
ONHAND
ONLAND
ORMOND
OSMOND
OSMUND
OSTEND
POLAND
REBEND
REBIND
REFIND
REFUND
RELAND
RELEND
REMAND
REMEND
REMIND
RESAND
RESEND
REVEND
REWIND
RIBAND
ROLAND
ROTUND
SECOND
SEVEND
STRAND
TAGEND
THEEND
TVLAND
UNBEND
UNBIND
UNFOND
UNHAND
UNKIND
UNWIND
UPBIND
UPLAND
UPSEND
UPWIND
WIGAND

NE••••

NEALON
NEARBY
NEARED
NEARER
NEARLY
NEARTO
NEATEN
NEATER
NEATLY
NEBULA
NECKED
NECKER
NECTAR
NEEDBE
NEEDED
NEEDER
NEEDLE
NEEDNT
NEEDTO
NEELIX
NEENAH
NEESON
NEGATE
NEHRUS
NEIGHS
NEIMAN
NEISSE
NELLIE
NELLIS
NELSON
NEMEAN
NEOCON
NEOSHO
NEPALI
NEPEAN
NEPHEW
NEPHRO
NEREID
NERMAL
NERNST
NEROLI
NERONE
NERUDA
NERVAL
NERVED
NERVES
NESBIT
NESSEN
NESSES
NESSIE
NESSUS
NESTEA
NESTED
NESTER
NESTIN
NESTLE
NESTOR
NETFUL
NETHER
NETHOU
NETMAN
NETMEN
NETPAY
NETTED
NETTER
NETTLE
NETTLY
NETTON
NEUMAN
NEURAL
NEUROL
NEURON
NEUTER
NEVADA
NEVERS
NEVILL
NEVINS
NEVSKI
NEVSKY
NEWAGE
NEWARK
NEWBIE
NEWCAR
NEWDAY
NEWELL
NEWELS
NEWERA
NEWEST
NEWHAT
NEWIES
NEWISH
NEWJOB
NEWKID
NEWLEY
NEWMAN
NEWMAR
NEWSIE
NEWSOM
NEWTON
NEWTOY
NEWULM
NEWWAY
NEXRAD
NEXTEL
NEXTTO
NEXTUP

N•E•••

NEEDBE
NEEDED
NEEDER
NEEDLE
NEEDNT
NEEDTO
NEELIX
NEENAH
NEESON
NIECES
NIEKRO
NIELLI
NIELLO
NIENTE
NIETAS
NIETOS
NIEVES
NLEAST
NOEMON
NOESIS
NOETIC
NOEXIT
NTESTS
NUECES
NUEVES

N••E••

NAMEIT
NAMELY
NAMERS
NAPERY
NASEBY
NAVELS
NBAERS
NEMEAN
NEPEAN
NEREID
NEVERS
NEWELL
NEWELS
NEWERA
NEWEST
NFLERS
NHLERS
NICELY
NICENE
NICEST
NICETY
NIKEAD
NINEAD
NINEAM
NINEBC
NINEEE
NINEPM
NINERS
NINETY
NINEUP
NISEIS
NITERS
NITERY
NIXERS
NLWEST
NOBELS
NOCENT
NODEAL
NODEAR
NOFEES
NOHELP
NOLEAD
NOLESS
NOMEAK
NOMEAT
NONEED
NONEGO
NONETS
NONEWS
NOPETS
NOREEN
NORELL
NORENT
NOSEIN
NOSERS
NOSEUP
NOTERS
NOVELA
NOVELS
NOVENA
NUDELY
NUDEST
NUGENT
NUMERO
NYJETS
NYMETS

N•••E•

NABBED
NABBER
NACRED
NACRES
NAGGED
NAGGER
NAILED
NAILER
NAIVER
NANSEN
NANTES
NAPIER
NAPLES
NAPPED
NAPPER
NAPPES
NASHES
NASSER
NATTER
NAUSEA
NAUTES
NAVIES
NBCRED
NEARED
NEARER
NEATEN
NEATER
NECKED
NECKER
NEEDED
NEEDER
NEPHEW
NERVED
NERVES
NESSEN
NESSES
NESTEA
NESTED
NESTER
NETHER
NETMEN
NETTED
NETTER
NEUTER
NEWIES
NEWLEY
NEXTEL
NGUYEN
NIAMEY
NIBLET
NICHED
NICHES
NICKED
NICKEL
NICKER
NIECES
NIEVES
NIGHER
NIKKEI
NINEEE
NIPPED
NIPPER
NIPSEY
NISSEN
NITRES
NIXIES
NOBLER
NOBLES
NOCHES
NOCKED
NODDED
NODDER
NOFEES
NOIDEA
NOIRES
NOIRET
NOISED
NOISES
NONEED
NONFED
NONJEW
NONMEN
NONNET
NOONER
NOONES
NOOSED
NOOSER
NOOSES
NOREEN
NOSHED
NOSHER
NOSHES
NOSIER
NOSTEP
NOSTER
NOTNEW
NOTYET
NOUMEA
NTILES
NUBBED
NUBBER
NUCLEI
NUCLEO
NUDGED
NUDGER
NUDGES
NUECES
NUEVES
NUGGET
NULLED
NUMBED
NUMBER
NUNGEN
NURSED
NURSER
NURSES
NUTLET
NUTMEG
NUTTED
NUTTER

N••••E

NADINE
NANINE
NANNIE
NAPPIE
NARINE
NATALE
NATIVE
NATURE
NEEDBE
NEEDLE
NEGATE
NEISSE
NELLIE
NERONE
NESSIE
NESTLE
NETTLE
NEWAGE
NEWBIE
NEWSIE
NIBBLE
NICENE
NICOLE
NIENTE
NIGGLE
NIMBLE
NINEEE
NIPPLE
NOBAKE
NOBILE
NODICE
NODOSE
NODULE
NOHOPE
NOJIVE
NOJOKE
NOLOSE
NOMBRE
NOMORE
NONAGE
NONAME
NONUSE
NOODGE
NOODLE
NOOGIE
NORITE
NOSALE
NOTATE
NOTICE
NOTIME
NOTONE
NOVICE
NOVOTE
NOWISE
NOZZLE
NTUPLE
NUANCE
NUBBLE
NUBILE
NUCHAE
NUTATE
NUZZLE

•NE•••

ANELED
ANELES
ANEMIA
ANEMIC
ANERGY
ENERGY
ENEROS
ENESCO
GNEISS
INESSE
INEVER
KNEADS
KNEBEL
KNEELS
KNELLS
KNEWIT
KNEWOF
ONEACT
ONEALL
ONEARM
ONEBIT
ONECAR
ONEDAY
ONEDGE
ONEEEE
ONEEGG
ONEEYE
ONEGIN
ONEHIT
ONEIDA
ONEILL
ONEIRO
ONEISH
ONELAP
ONELEG
ONEMAN
ONEMEG
ONEOFF
ONEONE
ONEOUT
ONEPIN
ONERUN
ONESEC
ONESET
ONETEN
ONETON
ONETWO
ONEUPS
ONEWAY
PNEUMA
PNEUMO
SNEAKS
SNEAKY
SNEERS
SNEERY
SNEEZE
SNEEZY
SNELLS
UNEASE
UNEASY
UNEDGE
UNEPIC
UNESCO
UNEVEN
UNEVIL
VNECKS

•N•E••

ANDEAN
ANDERS
ANGELA
ANGELI
ANGELL
ANGELO
ANGELS
ANGERS
ANNEAL
ANNEES
ANSEIS
ANSELM
ANTEED
ANTERO
ANTEUP
ENBERG
ENDEAR
ENDERS
ENGELS
ENMESH
ENNEAD
ENSEAL
ENSEAT
ENTERO
ENTERS
ENVEIL
INCENT
INCEPT
INDEBT
INDEED
INDEEP
INDENT
INFEAR
INFECT
INFERS
INFEST
INGEAR
INGELS
INGEST
INHERE
INJECT
INJEST
INKERS
INLEAF
INLETS
INNEED
INNERS

INNESS
INSEAM
INSECT
INSERT
INSETS
INTEND
INTENS
INTENT
INTERJ
INTERN
INTERS
INVENT
INVERT
INVEST
KNEELS
ONDECK
ONEEEE
ONEEGG
ONEEYE
ONSETS
SNEERS
SNEERY
SNEEZE
SNEEZY
UNBELT
UNBEND
UNBENT
UNDEAD
UNDEEP
UNDEFT
UNDERS
UNDEWY
UNFELT
UNHEED
UNHELD
UNHELM
UNHERO
UNHEWN
UNKEPT
UNLEAD
UNLEAF
UNLEAN
UNLEFT
UNLENT
UNLESS
UNMEET
UNMESH
UNMEWS
UNNEAT
UNPEEL
UNPEGS
UNPENS
UNPENT
UNREAD
UNREAL
UNREEL
UNRENT
UNREST
UNSEAL
UNSEAM
UNSEAT
UNSEEN
UNSELD
UNSELL
UNSENT
UNSERE
UNSEWN
UNSEWS
UNSEXY
UNVEIL
UNWELL
UNWEPT

•N••E•

ANADEM
ANCIEN
ANDREA
ANDREI
ANDRES
ANDREW
ANDREY
ANDYET
ANELED
ANELES
ANGLED
ANGLEE
ANGLER
ANGLES
ANIMES
ANISES
ANKLED
ANKLES
ANKLET
ANNEES
ANNIES
ANNLEE
ANODES
ANOLES
ANSWER
ANTEED
ANTHEM
ANTHER
ANTLER
ANTRES
CNOTES
DNASES
ENAMEL
ENATES
ENCRES
ENDMEN
ENDUED
ENDUES
ENOTES
ENSLER
ENSUED
ENSUES
ENTREE
ENTREZ
ENURED
ENURES
ENVIED
ENVIER
ENVIES
GNAWED
GNAWER
GNOMES
GNOSES
GNOTES
INAFEW
INAGES
INANER
INAPET
INAREA
INASEC
INBRED
INCHED
INCHER
INCHES
INDEED
INDEEP
INDIES
INDUED
INDUES
INEVER
INGLES
INGRES
INGREY
INKIER
INKJET
INKLES
INLIEU
INNEED
INNIES
INONES
INSTEP
INURED
INURES
INVIEW
KNAVES
KNEBEL
KNIFED
KNIFER
KNIFES
KNIVES
KNOWER
ONAGER
ONCLES
ONEEEE
ONELEG
ONEMEG
ONESEC
ONESET
ONETEN
ONSPEC
ONUSES
ONVIEW
ONYXES
SNAKED
SNAKER
SNAKES
SNARED
SNARER
SNARES
SNIDER
SNIPED
SNIPER
SNIPES
SNIVEL
SNOPES
SNORED
SNORER
SNORES
SNOWED
SNYDER
TNOTES
UNAGED
UNAWED
UNAXED
UNBLED
UNCLES
UNDEEP
UNDIES
UNDOER
UNDOES
UNDREW
UNDSET
UNDYED
UNEVEN
UNFREE
UNGUES
UNHEED
UNHOED
UNHUED
UNICED
UNICEF
UNICES
UNIPED
UNISEX
UNITED
UNITER
UNITES
UNMEET
UNOPEN
UNOWED
UNPEEL
UNREEL
UNRUED
UNSEEN
UNSHED
UNSKEW
UNSTEP
UNSUED
UNTIED
UNTIER
UNTIES
UNUSED

•N•••E

ANANKE
ANDRAE
ANGLEE
ANNLEE
ANOMIE
ANSATE
ANTONE
ANYONE
DNAASE
ENABLE
ENCAGE
ENCASE
ENCODE
ENCORE
ENDIVE
ENDURE
ENDUSE
ENFACE
ENGAGE
ENGINE
ENISLE
ENLACE
ENORME
ENRAGE
ENROBE
ENSATE
ENSILE
ENSURE
ENTICE
ENTIRE
ENTREE
ENZYME
INAPIE
INATIE
INBLUE
INCASE
INCISE
INCITE
INCODE
INCOME
INCUSE
INDITE
INDUCE
INESSE
INFUSE
INGATE
INHALE
INHERE
INHOME
INHUME
INJOKE
INJUNE
INJURE
INLINE
INLOVE
INMATE
INNAGE
INNATE
INOUYE
INSANE
INSIDE
INSOLE
INSURE
INTAKE
INTIME
INTONE
INTUNE
INVADE
INVITE
INVOKE
INWOVE
ONBASE
ONEDGE
ONEEEE
ONEEYE
ONEONE
ONFILE
ONFIRE
ONHIRE
ONLATE
ONLINE
ONMIKE
ONRICE
ONSALE
ONSIDE
ONSITE
ONTAPE
ONTIME
RNAASE
SNEEZE
SNOOZE
UNABLE
UNBALE
UNBARE
UNCAGE
UNCAKE
UNCASE
UNCORE
UNCUTE
UNDINE
UNDONE
UNEASE
UNEDGE
UNFILE
UNFINE
UNFREE
UNGLUE
UNHALE
UNHIRE
UNIATE
UNIDLE
UNIQUE
UNLACE
UNLADE
UNLIKE
UNLIVE
UNMADE
UNMAKE
UNMATE
UNNICE
UNPALE
UNPILE
UNPURE
UNRIFE
UNRIPE
UNROBE
UNROPE
UNROVE
UNRUDE
UNSAFE
UNSAGE
UNSERE
UNSHOE
UNSOLE
UNSORE
UNSURE
UNTAME
UNTAPE
UNTRUE
UNTUNE
UNWISE
UNWOVE
UNYOKE
UNZONE

••NE••

AENEAS
AENEID
ANNEAL
ANNEES
APNEAS
ARNEIS
ARNESS
ARNETT
ASNEAR
ASNEAT
BENEKE
BONERS
BONERZ
BONEUP
CANERS
CINEMA
CINEOL
CONERS
CONEYS
CUNEAL
DINEAT
DINEIN
DINEON
DINERO
DINERS
DONEBY
DONEES
DONEIN
DONEIT
DONEOK
DONESO
DONETO
DONETS
DONEUP
DYNELS
ENNEAD
ERNEST
FINELY
FINERY
FINEST
GANEFS
GENERA
GENETS
GENEVA
GENEVE
GONEAR
GONEAT
GONEBY
GONEIN
GONEON
GONERS
GONETO
GONEUP
GONEXT
GYNECO
HONEIN
HONERS
HONEST
HONEYS
IMNEXT
INNEED
INNERS
INNESS
JONESS
JONESY
JUNEAU
LINEAL
LINEAR
LINENS
LINENY
LINERS
LINEUP
LONELY
LONERS
LUNEDI
MANEGE
MANERO
MANETS
MCNEIL
MINERS
MINETA
MONETA
MONETS
MONEYS
MUNERA
NINEAD
NINEAM
NINEBC
NINEEE
NINEPM
NINERS
NINETY
NINEUP
NONEED
NONEGO
NONETS
NONEWS
ORNERY
OWNERS
PANELS
PINEAL
PINERO
PINERS
PINERY
RANEES
RENEGE
RENEST
RENEWS
RONELY
SANELY
SANEST
SENECA
SINEAD
SINEWS
SINEWY
TENEEE
TENETS
TINEAL
TINEAR
TONEME
TONERS
TONEUP
TUNEIN
TUNERS
TUNETO
TUNEUP
UNNEAT
UPNEXT
USNEWS
VENEER
VENERA
VENETO
VINERS
VINERY
WINERY
ZONERS

••N•E•

ANNEES
ANNIES
ANNLEE
ARNHEM
ARNIES
AUNTEM
BANDED
BANDER
BANGED
BANGER
BANKED
BANKER
BANNED
BANNEN
BANNER
BANTER
BENBEN
BENDED
BENDER
BENSEY
BINDER
BINGED
BINGER
BINGES
BINNED
BINNEY
BONDED
BONDER
BONGED
BONIER
BONKED
BONNER
BONNES
BONNET
BONNEY
BONZES
BUNGED
BUNGEE
BUNKED
BUNKER
BUNSEN
BUNTED
BUNTER
BUNUEL
CANCEL
CANCER
CANIER
CANKER
CANNED
CANNEL
CANNER
CANNES
CANOED
CANOER
CANOES
CANTED
CANTER
CENSED
CENSER
CENSES
CENTER
CINDER
CONFED
CONFER
CONGER
CONGES
CONIES
CONKED
CONKER
CONMEN
CONNED
CONNEE
CONVEX
CONVEY
DANCED
DANCER
DANCES
DANDER
DANGED
DANGER
DANIEL
DANKER
DANNER
DANSES
DANTEI
DANTES
DENIED
DENIER
DENIES
DENNED
DENSER
DENTED
DENVER
DENZEL
DINGED
DINGER
DINNED
DINNER
DINTED
DONDER
DONEES
DONKEY
DONNED
DONNER
DUNCES
DUNDEE
DUNKED
DUNKER
DUNNED
DUNNER
FANGED
FANJET
FANNED
FANNER
FENCED
FENCER
FENCES
FENDED
FENDER
FENNEL
FENNER
FINDER
FINGER
FINKED
FINKEL
FINLEY
FINNED
FINNEY
FINSEN
FONDER
FUNDED
FUNDER
FUNKED
FUNNED
FUNNEL
GANDER
GANGED
GANGER
GANGES
GANNET
GENDER
GENIES
GENRES
GENTES
GENXER
GINGER
GINNED
GONGED
GUNMEN
GUNNED
GUNNER
GUNSEL
GUNTER
HANDED
HANDEL
HANDER
HANGED
HANGER
HANKER
HANLEY
HANSEL
HANSES
HENDEC
HENGES
HENLEY
HENNER
HINDER
HINGED
HINGES
HINTED
HINTER
HONIED
HONKED
HONKER
HUNGER
HUNKER
HUNLEY
HUNTED
HUNTER
INNEED
INNIES
JANNEY
JANSEN
JANZEN
JENNER
JENNET
JENNEY
JENSEN
JINXED
JINXER
JINXES
JUNGER
JUNKED
JUNKER
JUNKET
KANDEL
KANDER
KENNED
KENNEL
KENNER
KINDER
KINGED
KINKED
KINSEY
KUNZEL
LANCED
LANCER
LANCES
LANCET
LANDED
LANDER
LANGER
LANIER
LANKER
LENDEE
LENDER
LENSED
LENSES
LENTEN
LINDEN
LINDER
LINGER
LINIER
LINKED
LINKER
LINNET
LINNEY
LINTED
LINTEL
LINTER
LINZER
LONGED
LONGER
LONGES
LONGET
LUNDEN
LUNGED
LUNGER
LUNGES
LUNKER
LYNLEY
LYNXES
MANDEL
MANGER
MANLEY
MANNED
MANNER
MANSES
MANTEE
MANTEL
MANUEL
MENDED
MENDEL
MENDER
MENDES
MENKEN
MENNEN
MENTEE
MINCED
MINCER
MINCES
MINDED
MINDEN
MINDER
MINTED
MINTER
MINUET
MINXES
MONDES
MONGER
MONIED
MONIES
MONKEE
MONKEY
MONNET
MONTEL
MONTEZ
NANSEN
NANTES
NINEEE
NONEED
NONFED
NONJEW
NONMEN
NONNET
NUNGEN
OINKED
OINKER
OUNCES
PANDER
PANIER
PANNED
PANNER
PANNES
PANTED
PANTER
PANZER
PENDED
PENMEN
PENNED
PENNER
PENNEY
PENSEE
PENTEL
PINCER
PINGED
PINGER
PINIER
PINKED
PINKEN
PINKER
PINNED
PINNER
PINTER
PONDED
PONDER
PONGEE
PONIED
PONIES
PUNIER
PUNKER
PUNNED
PUNNER
PUNTED
PUNTER
RANEES
RANGED
RANGEL
RANGER
RANGES
RANKED
RANKER
RANTED
RANTER
RENDED
RENDER
RENNES
RENNET
RENTED
RENTEE
RENTER
RENTES
RINGED
RINGER
RINSED
RINSER
RINSES
RONCEY
RONDEL
RUNLET
RUNNEL
RUNNER
SANDED
SANDER
SANGER
SANSEI
SANTEE
SENDEE
SENDER
SENSED
SENSEI
SENSEN
SENSES
SINGED
SINGER
SINGES
SINKER
SINNED
SINNER
SONDES
SONNET
SUNDER
SUNKEN
SUNNED
SUNSET
SYNCED
TANDEM
TANGED
TANKED
TANKER
TANNED
TANNER
TANTES
TENDED
TENDER
TENEEE
TENLEY
TENNER
TENSED
TENSER
TENSES
TENTED
TENTER
TINDER
TINGED
TINGES
TINIER
TINKER
TINMEN
TINNED
TINNER
TINSEL
TINTED
TINTER
TONGED
TONIER
TONNES
TUNNEL
TUNNEY
VANIER
VANNED
VANNES
VENDED
VENDEE
VENDER
VENEER
VENNER
VENTED
VENTER
VENUES
VINIER
WANDER
WANIER
WANKEL
WANNED
WANNER
WANTED
WANTER
WENCES
WENDED
WENNER
WINCED
WINCER
WINCES
WINDED
WINDER
WINDEX
WINGED
WINGER
WINIER
WINKED
WINKER
WINNER
WINTER
WONDER
WONTED
WYNKEN
WYNTER
YANKED
YANKEE
YANKER
YENNED
YONDER
ZANIER
ZANIES
ZENGER
ZINCED
ZINGED
ZINGER
ZONKED
ZONKER

••N••E

ADNATE
AGNATE
ANNLEE
ATNINE
AUNTIE
BANANE
BANGLE
BANQUE
BENEKE
BENICE
BENNIE
BENOTE
BINATE
BINDLE
BINGLE
BINNIE
BONNIE
BUNCHE
BUNDLE
BUNGEE
BUNGLE
BYNAME
CANAPE
CANDLE
CANINE
CANTBE
CANTLE
CANUTE
CENTRE
CINQUE
CONNEE
CONNIE
CONTRE
CONURE
DANDIE

DANDLE
DANGLE
DANGME
DANITE
DANUBE
DENISE
DENOTE
DENUDE
DINGLE
DONATE
DONGLE
DONNIE
DUNDEE
DYNODE
EANNIE
EENSIE
EUNICE
FANNIE
FINALE
FINITE
FONDLE
FONDUE
FONZIE
GENEVE
GENOME
GENTLE
GINNIE
GUNITE
HANDKE
HANDLE
HANKIE
HINGLE
HINKLE
HONORE
IGNACE
IGNITE
IGNORE
INNAGE
INNATE
IONISE
IONIZE
IONONE
JANGLE
JANICE
JANINE
JENNIE
JINGLE
JUNGLE
JUNKIE
KINDLE
KINGME
LANATE
LANCIE
LANOSE
LENAPE
LENDEE
LENGLE
LENNIE
LENORE
LINAGE
LINGLE
LONGUE
LONNIE
LUNATE
MANAGE
MANAPE
MANCHE
MANEGE
MANGLE
MANQUE
MANTEE
MANTLE
MANURE
MANUTE
MENACE
MENAGE
MENTEE
MENTHE
MINGLE
MINIME
MINNIE
MINUTE
MONKEE
MONROE
MUNCIE
MUNROE
NANINE
NANNIE
NINEEE
NONAGE
NONAME
NONUSE
OENONE
OFNOTE
ORNATE
PANOPE
PANTIE
PENCHE
PENSEE
PINKIE
PINNAE
PONGEE
PUNKIE
RANINE
RANKLE
RENAME
RENEGE
RENNIE
RENOTE
RENTEE
RONNIE
RUNCIE
RUNDLE
SANGRE
SANTEE
SENATE
SENDEE
SENILE
SINGLE
SINISE
SUNDAE
TANGLE
TENACE
TENEEE
TENONE
TENURE
TINGLE
TINKLE
TINORE
TONEME
TONGUE
TONITE
UNNICE
VENDEE
VENDUE
VENICE
VENIRE
VENITE
VENOSE
VENULE
VINNIE
WANGLE
WENDIE
WINKIE
WINNIE
YANKEE
ZONULE

•••NE•

AGONES
AKENES
ALINED
ALINER
ALINES
ALLNEW
AMINES
ATONED
ATONER
ATONES
AXONES
BAHNEN
BAINES
BANNED
BANNEN
BANNER
BARNED
BARNES
BARNET
BARNEY
BEANED
BINNED
BINNEY
BIRNEY
BITNET
BONNER
BONNES
BONNET
BONNEY
BORNEO
BRINED
BRINER
BRINES
BRUNEI
BRUNET
BURNED
BURNER
BURNET
BURNEY
BYRNES
CAGNEY
CANNED
CANNEL
CANNER
CANNES
CARNER
CARNES
CARNET
CARNEY
CHANEL
CHANEY
CHENEY
CHINES
CLONED
CLONER
CLONES
COINED
COINER
CONNED
CONNEE
COONEY
CORNEA
CORNED
CORNEL
CORNER
CORNET
CRANED
CRANES
CRENEL
CRONES
CYGNET
DABNEY
DAMNED
DAMNER
DANNER
DARNED
DARNER
DAWNED
DENNED
DIENES
DINNED
DINNER
DIPNET
DISNEY
DONNED
DONNER
DOWNED
DOWNER
DOWNES
DOWNEY
DRONED
DRONER
DRONES
DUNNED
DUNNER
DURNED
EARNED
EARNER
EISNER
ELANET
EMINEM
EUPNEA
EVENED
EVENER
EZINES
FAFNER
FAINER
FANNED
FANNER
FAWNED
FAWNER
FENNEL
FENNER
FINNED
FINNEY
FLYNET
FUNNED
FUNNEL
GAINED
GAINER
GAINES
GANNET
GARNER
GARNET
GAYNES
GINNED
GOONEY
GOWNED
GUINEA
GUNNED
GUNNER
GURNEE
GURNEY
HAINES
HARNEY
HAYNES
HEANEY
HEFNER
HENNER
HOHNER
HORNED
HORNER
HORNET
HYMNED
IBANEZ
IMINES
INANER
INONES
IRONED
IRONER
JANNEY
JAUNES
JEANED
JENNER
JENNET
JENNEY
JITNEY
JOINED
JOINER
JOYNER
KAVNER
KEENED
KEENEN
KEENER
KENNED
KENNEL
KENNER
KERNED
KERNEL
KERNES
KEYNES
KIDNEY
KILNED
KRENEK
KRONER
LEANED
LEANER
LEHNEN
LERNER
LIANES
LIENEE
LIGNES
LIMNED
LIMNER
LINNET
LINNEY
LIONEL
LIONET
LOANED
LOANER
LOONEY
MACNEE
MAGNET
MAINER
MANNED
MANNER
MARNER
MEANER
MEANEY
MENNEN
MESNES
MILNER
MILNES
MOANED
MOANER
MOINES
MONNET
MOONED
MOONER
MOONEY
NONNET
NOONER
NOONES
NOTNEW
OCONEE
OMENED
OPENED
OPENER
OPINED
OPINER
OPINES
ORKNEY
OVINES
PAINED
PANNED
PANNER
PANNES
PAWNED
PAWNEE
PAWNER
PEENED
PENNED
PENNER
PENNEY
PEVNEY
PHONED
PHONER
PHONES
PHONEY
PINNED
PINNER
PITNEY
PLANED
PLANER
PLANES
PLANET
POGNER
PRUNED
PRUNER
PRUNES
PUNNED
PUNNER
PUTNEY
RADNER
RAINED
RAINER
RAINES
RAINEY
RATNER
REINED
REINER
REINES
RENNES
RENNET
REUNED
REUNER
REUNES
RODNEY
ROMNEY
ROONEY
RUDNER
RUINED
RUINER
RUNNEL
RUNNER
SCENEI
SCENES
SCENEV
SCONES
SEINED
SEINER
SEINES
SHINED
SHINER
SHINES
SIDNEY
SIGNED
SIGNEE
SIGNER
SIGNET
SINNED
SINNER
SONNET
SOONER
SPINED
SPINEL
SPINER
SPINES
SPINET
STONED
STONER
STONES
STONEY
SUBNET
SUMNER
SUNNED
SWANEE
SYDNEY
TAHNEE
TANNED
TANNER
TBONES
TEENER
TELNET
TENNER
TERNES
THANES
THENET
TINNED
TINNER
TONNES
TOWNER
TRANES
TRINES
TUNNEL
TUNNEY
TURNED
TURNER
TWINED
TWINER
TWINES
USENET
VAINER
VANNED
VANNES
VARNEY
VEINED
VENNER
VERNET
WAGNER
WANNED
WANNER
WAPNER
WARNED
WARNER
WARNES
WATNEY
WAYNES
WEANED
WEANER
WEENED
WENNER
WERNER
WHINED
WHINER
WHINES
WIENER
WIGNER
WINNER
YARNED
YAWNED
YAWNER
YEANED
YENNED

•••N•E

AGENCE
ANANKE
ASANTE
ATONCE
AVENGE
AVENUE
BEANIE
BENNIE
BERNIE
BINNIE
BLENDE
BLONDE
BONNIE
BOUNCE
BRONTE
BRONZE
BURNIE
CHANCE
CHANGE
CHANTE
CONNEE
CONNIE
CRINGE
DEENIE
DIANNE
DIONNE
DONNIE
EANNIE
EARNIE
ELANCE
EVINCE
EVONNE
FANNIE
FAUNAE
FIANCE
FLANGE
FLENSE
FRANCE
FRINGE
FRUNZE
GINNIE
GLANCE
GLENNE
GOONIE
GRANDE
GRANGE
GRUNGE
GURNEE
GWYNNE
HAYNIE
HEINIE
HEINSE
JEANIE
JEANNE
JENNIE
JOANIE
JOANNE
JOUNCE
LAINIE
LEANNE
LENNIE
LIENEE
LONNIE
LOONIE
LOUNGE
LYONNE
MACNEE
MARNIE
MEANIE
MINNIE
MOONIE
NANNIE
NIENTE
NUANCE
OCONEE
ODENSE
ORANGE
ORENSE
PAWNEE
PINNAE
PLANTE
PLUNGE
POINTE
POUNCE
PRANCE
PRINCE
PRINZE
PRYNNE
PUENTE
QUINCE
QUINTE
QUINZE
REENIE
RENNIE
RONNIE
RYENCE
SAINTE
SCONCE
SEANCE
SIGNEE
SPENCE
SPONGE
STANCE
SWANEE
TAHNEE
TEENIE
THENCE
TOONIE
TOWNIE
TRANCE
TRENTE
TWINGE
USANCE
VEINTE
VIENNE
VINNIE
WEENIE
WHENCE
WIENIE
WINNIE
YVONNE

••••NE

ACHENE
ACTONE
AFFINE
AGEONE
AHERNE
ALBINE
ALDINE
ALFINE
ALKENE
ALPINE
ANTONE
ANYONE
ARCANE
ARIANE
ARLENE
ARSENE
ASHINE
ATHENE
ATNINE
ATTUNE
BALINE
BANANE
BARONE
BEGONE
BEIGNE
BEMINE
BIGONE
BLAINE
BODINE
BOURNE
BOVINE
BROWNE
BUTANE
BUTENE
BYGONE
BYLINE
CANINE
CAPONE
CELINE
CETANE
CHAINE
COIGNE
COSINE
CROWNE
DALENE
DAMONE
DAPHNE
DAYONE
DEBONE
DEFINE
DEPONE
DETUNE
DEVANE
DEVINE
DIANNE
DIONNE
DIVINE
DOFINE
DOMINE
DORINE
DOUANE
DWAYNE
EDIRNE
EIRENE
ELAINE
ELAYNE
ENGINE
EOCENE
EQUINE
ERMINE
ESSENE
ETERNE
ETHANE
ETHENE
EUGENE
EVONNE
EWAINE
FALINE
FAMINE
FATONE
FELINE
FILENE
FOKINE
FORONE
GAMINE
GIJANE
GLENNE
GREENE
GWYNNE
GYRENE
HADONE
HASONE
HELENE
HEXANE
HITONE
HOTONE
HUMANE
HUTONE
IMDONE
IMFINE
IMGONE
IMMUNE
INJUNE
INLINE
INSANE
INTONE
INTUNE
IODINE
IONONE
IRLENE
IRVINE
ISMENE
JANINE
JEANNE
JEJUNE
JOANNE
JOBONE
JOLENE
KALINE
KETONE
KLEINE
LABINE
LARINE
LATENE
LEANNE
LEVENE
LEVINE
LOCANE
LORENE
LUCINE
LUPINE
LUPONE
LURENE
LYONNE
LYSINE
MALONE
MARINE
MAXENE
MAXINE
MEGANE
MIFUNE
MODINE
MOLINE
MURINE
NADINE
NANINE
NARINE
NERONE
NICENE
NOTONE
OCTANE
OENONE
ONEONE
ONLINE
OSCINE
OTTONE
PATINE
PAVANE
PERINE
PICONE
PRYNNE
QUEENE
RACINE
RAMONE
RANINE
RAPINE
RATINE
RAVINE
RECANE
REDONE
REFINE
REHONE
RELINE
REMINE
REPANE
REPINE
RETONE
RETUNE
REZONE
ROCKNE
ROXANE
SABINE
SALINE
SCARNE
SELENE
SERENE
SEVENE
SHAYNE
SHRINE
SIMONE
SIXONE
SLOANE
SOFINE
SOIGNE
SPLINE
STERNE
SUEANE
SUPINE
TBOONE
TENONE
THEONE
THRONE
TIRANE
TISANE
TRIUNE
TRYONE
TULANE
TYRONE
UNDINE
UNDONE
UNFINE
UNTUNE
UNZONE
URBANE
URSINE
VALENE
VALINE
VIENNE
VISINE
WAHINE
WEEONE
WETONE
YVONNE

NF••••

NFLERS
NFORTY

N•F•••

NOFAIR
NOFEES
NOFUSS

N••F••

NAKFAS
NETFUL
NONFAN
NONFAT
NONFED
NOTFAR
NOTFIT
NOTFOR

N•••F•

NIDIFY
NODOFF
NOTIFY

N••••F

NODOFF

•NF•••

ENFACE
ENFAIT
ENFANT
ENFOLD
INFACT
INFALL
INFAMY
INFANT
INFEAR
INFECT
INFERS
INFEST
INFIRM
INFLOW
INFLUX
INFOLD
INFORM
INFULL
INFUSE
ONFILE
ONFILM
ONFIRE
ONFOOT
UNFACT
UNFAIR
UNFELT
UNFILE
UNFINE
UNFIRM
UNFITS
UNFLAT
UNFOLD
UNFOND
UNFORK
UNFOUL
UNFOXY
UNFREE
UNFULL
UNFURL

•N•F••

INAFEW
INAFIX
INAFOG
KNIFED
KNIFER
KNIFES
SNAFUS
SNIFFS
SNIFFY
SNUFFS
SNUFFY
UNIFIC

•N••F•

ONEOFF
SNARFS
SNIFFS
SNIFFY
SNUFFS
SNUFFY
UNCUFF
UNDEFT
UNHAFT
UNLEFT
UNRIFE
UNSAFE
UNSOFT

•N•••F

ENGULF
INGULF
INHALF
INLEAF
KNEWOF
KNOWOF
ONEOFF
ONLYIF
UNCUFF
UNICEF
UNLEAF
UNROOF

••NF••

CANFUL
CONFAB
CONFED
CONFER
CONFIT
FANFIC
FUNFUR
GUNFOR
MANFUL
NONFAN
NONFAT
NONFED
PANFRY
PANFUL
RANFOR
RENFRO
RUNFOR
SINFUL
SUNFAN
URNFUL
YENFOR

••N•F•

CANIFF
GANEFS
KUNGFU
MANOFF
MINIFY
RANOFF
RUNOFF
VINIFY

••N••F

CANIFF
FONDOF
KINDOF
MANOFF
RANOFF
RUNOFF
TONSOF

•••NF•

THENFL

•••N•F

ATONOF

EVENIF
WARNOF

••••NF
GETANF
GOTANF

NG••••
NGUYEN

N•G•••
NAGANO
NAGGED
NAGGER
NAGNAG
NAGOYA
NAGSAT
NEGATE
NIGGLE
NIGHER
NIGHON
NIGHTS
NIGHTY
NOGGIN
NOGOOD
NUGENT
NUGGET

N••G••
NAGGED
NAGGER
NAUGHT
NEIGHS
NIGGLE
NINGBO
NOGGIN
NONGAS
NONGOD
NOOGIE
NORGAY
NOUGAT
NOUGHT
NUDGED
NUDGER
NUDGES
NUGGET
NUNGEN

N•••G•
NEWAGE
NONAGE
NONEGO
NOODGE

N••••G
NAGNAG
NAMING
NIXING
NOSING
NOTING
NUKING
NUTMEG

•NG•••
ANGELA
ANGELI
ANGELL
ANGELO
ANGELS
ANGERS
ANGKOR
ANGLED
ANGLEE
ANGLER
ANGLES
ANGLIA
ANGLIC
ANGLOS
ANGOLA
ANGORA
ANGSTS
ENGAGE
ENGELS
ENGILD
ENGINE
ENGIRD
ENGIRT
ENGLIT
ENGLUT
ENGRAM
ENGULF
INGATE
INGEAR
INGELS
INGEST
INGLES
INGMAR
INGOAL
INGOLD
INGOOD
INGOTS
INGRAM
INGRAY
INGRES
INGREY
INGRID
INGULF
UNGAGS
UNGAMY
UNGAVA
UNGILT
UNGIRD
UNGIRT
UNGLAD
UNGLIB
UNGLUE
UNGRIP
UNGUAL
UNGUES
UNGUIS
UNGULA

•N•G••
ENIGMA
INAGES
KNIGHT
ONAGER
ONEGIN
SNAGGY
SNAGUP
SNUGLI
SNUGLY
UNAGED

•N••G•
ANERGY
ANTIGO
ENCAGE
ENERGY
ENGAGE
ENOUGH
ENRAGE
ENSIGN
INDIGO
INNAGE
INRAGS
ONEDGE
ONEEGG
ONHIGH
SNAGGY
UNBAGS
UNCAGE
UNEDGE
UNGAGS
UNNIGH
UNPEGS
UNRIGS
UNSAGE
UNWIGS

•N•••G
ANALOG
ANWANG
ENBERG
ENDING
INAFOG
INARUG
INKING
INNING
ONAJAG
ONEEGG
ONELEG
ONEMEG
UNCLOG
UNHUNG
UNPLUG
UNRUNG
UNSMUG
UNSNAG
UNSNUG
UNSUNG
UNTRIG

••NG••
BANGED
BANGER
BANGLE
BANGON
BANGOR
BANGUI
BANGUP
BENGAL
BENGAY
BINGED
BINGER
BINGES
BINGLE
BINGOS
BONGED
BONGOS
BUNGAY
BUNGED
BUNGEE
BUNGLE
CONGAS
CONGER
CONGES
CONGOU
DANGED
DANGER
DANGIT
DANGLE
DANGLY
DANGME
DINGED
DINGER
DINGHY
DINGLE
DINGUS
DONGLE
FANGED
FANGIO
FINGER
FUNGAL
FUNGUS
GANGED
GANGER
GANGES
GANGLY
GANGUP
GINGER
GINGKO
GONGED
GUNGHO
HANGAR
HANGBY
HANGED
HANGER
HANGIN
HANGON
HANGUL
HANGUP
HENGES
HINGED
HINGES
HINGIS
HINGLE
HUNGBY
HUNGER
HUNGIN
HUNGON
HUNGRY
HUNGUP
JANGLE
JANGLY
JINGLE
JINGLY
JUNGER
JUNGLE
JUNGLY
KINGED
KINGLY
KINGME
KUNGFU
LANGER
LENGLE
LENGTH
LENGUA
LINGER
LINGLE
LINGUA
LINGUS
LONGED
LONGER
LONGES
LONGET
LONGLY
LONGUE
LUNGED
LUNGER
LUNGES
MANGAS
MANGER
MANGLE
MANGOS
MINGLE
MINGUS
MONGER
MONGOL
MONGOS
MONGST
NINGBO
NONGAS
NONGOD
NUNGEN
PENGPU
PINGED
PINGER
PONGEE
PONGID
RANGED
RANGEL
RANGER
RANGES
RANGIN
RANGUP
RENGAS
RINGED
RINGER
RINGIN
RINGUP
RUNGIN
RUNGUP
SANGER
SANGRE
SANGTO
SINGED
SINGER
SINGES
SINGIN
SINGLE
SINGLY
SINGTO
SUNGOD
SUNGTO
TANGED
TANGLE
TANGLY
TANGOS
TANGUY
TINGED
TINGES
TINGLE
TINGLY
TINGOD
TONGAN
TONGED
TONGUE
WANGLE
WINGED
WINGER
WINGIT
XINGIN
YANGON
ZENGER
ZINGED
ZINGER

••N•G•
BENIGN
DONTGO
GINKGO
GONOGO
INNAGE
LINAGE
MANAGE
MANEGE
MENAGE
NONAGE
NONEGO
RENEGE
UNNIGH
WONTGO
ZUNIGA

••N••G
AWNING
BENING
BINNIG
BONING
CANING
CONING
DANANG
DANZIG
DINING
FINING
GUNDOG
HONING
INNING
KENNYG
LINING
MINING
MONTAG
OWNING
PINING
SONTAG
SUNDOG
TONING
TUNING
VINING
WANING
WINBIG
WINING
WONBIG
ZONING

•••NG•
ALONGS
AVENGE
BEINGS
BHANGS
BOINGO
BOINGS
BRINGS
CHANGE
CHANGO
CLANGS
CLINGS
CLINGY
CRINGE
DOINGS
DRINGS
ERYNGO
EWINGS
FLANGE
FLINGS
FRINGE
FRINGY
GOINGS
GRANGE
GRINGO
GRUNGE
GRUNGY
HMONGS
ICINGS
IKINGS
LIANGS
LOUNGE
ORANGE
ORANGS
ORANGY
ORINGS
PAANGA
PLUNGE
PRONGS
SLANGS
SLANGY
SLINGS
SPONGE
SPONGY
STINGS
STINGY
SWINGS
SWINGY
THINGS
THINGY
THONGS
TWANGS
TWANGY
TWINGE
UBANGI
WHANGS
WRINGS
WRONGS

•••N•G
BINNIG
EGGNOG
KENNYG
KOENIG
NAGNAG
STENOG
UNSNAG
UNSNUG

••••NG
AAHING
ACHING
ACTING
ADDING
ADZING
AGEING
AIDING
AILING
AIMING
AIRING
ALVING
AMPING
ANWANG
ARCING
ARMING
ASHING
ASKING
ATHING
AWNING
BAAING
BAKING
BALING
BARING
BASING
BATING
BAYING
BBKING
BCCING
BELONG
BENING
BERING
BIDING
BIKING
BITING
BLUING
BODING
BOEING
BONING
BOOING
BORING
BOWING
BOXING
BUSING
BUYING
CAGING
CAKING
CANING
CARING
CASING
CAVING
CAWING
CEDING
CHIANG
CITING
CLUING
CODING
COKING
COMING
CONING
COOING
COPING
CORING
COVING
COWING
COXING
CRYING
CUBING
CUEING
CURING
DANANG
DARING
DATING
DAZING
DEFANG
DEKING
DEWING
DICING
DIKING
DIMING
DINING
DIVING
DOLING
DOMING
DOPING
DOSING
DOTING
DOZING
DRJUNG
DRKING
DRYING
DUDING
DUGONG
DUKING
DUPING
DURING
DYEING
EALING
EARING
EASING
EATING
EBBING
EDGING
EELING
EGGING
ENDING
EPPING
ERLANG
ERRING
ERVING
ETTING
EYEING
FACING
FADING
FAKING
FAMING
FARING
FAXING
FAZING
FEEING
FETING
FIFING
FILING
FINING
FIRING
FIXING
FLYING
FOXING
FRYING
FUMING
FUSING
GAGING
GAMING
GAPING
GATING
GAZING
GEEING
GIBING
GIEING
GIVING
GLUING
GOBANG
GOLONG
GORING
GRUING
GUYING
GYRING
HALING
HARING
HATING
HAVING
HAWING
HAYING
HAZING
HEWING
HEXING
HIDING
HIEING
HIKING
HIRING
HIVING
HOEING
HOKING
HOLING
HOMING
HONING
HOPING
HOSING
HUSING
HYPING
ICHING
IDLING
IGGING
INKING
INNING
IRKING
IRVING
ISLING
JADING
JAPING
JAWING
JIBING
JIVING
JOKING
JOYING
JUKING
KDLANG
KEYING
KITING
LACING
LADING
LAMING
LASING
LAVING
LAWING
LAYING
LAZING
LIKING
LIMING
LINING
LIPENG
LIVING
LOPING
LORING
LOSING
LOVING
LOWING
LUBING
LUGING
LURING
MAKING
MATING
MAXING
MAYING
MAZING
MEKONG
METING
MEWING
MIKING
MIMING
MINING
MIRING
MIXING
MOOING
MOPING
MOVING
MOWING
MRWONG
MUSING
MUTING
NAMING
NIXING
NOSING
NOTING
NUKING
OARING
OBLONG
OFFING
OGLING
OILING
OOHING
OOLONG
OOZING
OPTING
ORBING
OUTING
OWNING
PACING
PAGING
PALING
PARING
PAVING
PAWING
PAYING
PEKING
PIKING
PILING
PINING
PIPING
PLYING
POKING
POLING
PORING
POSING
PRYING
PULING
RACING
RAGING
RAKING
RARING
RASING
RATING
RAVING
RAXING
RAYING
RAZING
REDING
REHANG
REHUNG
RESANG
RESING
RICING
RIDING
RILING
RIMING
RISING
RIVING
ROBING
ROPING
ROVING
ROWING
RULING
SARONG
SATING
SAVING
SAWING
SAYING
SEEING
SEWING
SHYING
SIDING
SIRING
SITING
SIZING
SKIING
SKYING
SLUING
SOLING
SOLONG
SOWING
SPRANG
SPRING
SPRUNG
SPYING
STRING
STRONG
STRUNG
STYING
TAKING
TAMING
TAPING
TARING
TAXING
TEEING
THRONG
TIDING
TILING
TIMING
TIRING
TOEING
TONING
TOPING
TOTING
TOWING
TOYING
TRUING
TRYING
TSKING
TUBING
TUNING
TURING
TYPING
UMPING
UNHUNG
UNRUNG
UNSUNG
UPPING
URGING
USHING
VEXING
VIKING
VINING
VISING
VOTING
VOWING
WADING
WAGING
WAKING
WALING
WANING
WARING
WAVING
WAXING
WILING
WINING
WIPING
WIRING
WISING
WIVING
WOOING
WOWING
YAWING
YOKING
YUTANG
ZEDONG
ZONING

NH••••
NHLERS

N•H•••
NEHRUS
NIHILO
NOHANT
NOHELP
NOHITS
NOHOPE

N••H••
NACHAS
NACHOS
NAPHTA
NASHES
NASHUA
NATHAN
NEPHEW
NEPHRO
NETHER
NETHOU
NEWHAT
NICHED
NICHES
NIGHER
NIGHON
NIGHTS
NIGHTY
NIIHAU
NOCHES
NONHIT
NOSHED
NOSHER
NOSHES
NOSHOW
NOTHIN
NUCHAE
NUCHAL

N•••H•
NAUGHT
NAVAHO
NEIGHS
NEOSHO
NINTHS
NORTHS
NOTCHY
NOUGHT
NYMPHS

N••••H
NAMATH
NEENAH
NEWISH
NORUSH

•NH•••
ENHALO
ENHAUT
INHALE
INHALF
INHAND
INHERE
INHOCK
INHOME
INHUME
ONHAND
ONHIGH
ONHIRE
ONHOLD
UNHAFT
UNHAIR
UNHALE
UNHAND
UNHASP
UNHATS
UNHAZY
UNHEED
UNHELD
UNHELM
UNHERO
UNHEWN
UNHIRE
UNHOED
UNHOLY
UNHOOD
UNHOOK
UNHUED
UNHULL
UNHUNG
UNHUNH
UNHURT
UNHUSK

•N•H••
ANCHOR
ANCHOS
ANDHOW
ANTHEM
ANTHER
ANYHOW
INCHED
INCHER
INCHES
INCHON
INTHAT
ONAHOP
ONEHIT
ONSHOW
UNCHIC
UNSHED
UNSHIP
UNSHOD
UNSHOE
UNSHUT
UNTHAW

•N••H•
KNIGHT
SNATHS

•N•••H
ANARCH
ENDASH
ENMESH
ENOUGH
ENRICH
INARCH
INCASH
INDASH
INRUSH
INWITH
ONEISH
ONHIGH
ONRUSH
SNATCH
SNITCH
UNHUNH
UNLASH
UNLUSH
UNMESH
UNNIGH
UNPOSH
UNRASH
UNWISH

••NH••
ARNHEM
BENHUR
BONHAM
DENHAM
DUNHAM
JANHUS
NONHIT
SENHOR
SUNHAT
TENHUT
TINHAT
XINHUA

••N•H•
BINCHY
BUNCHE
BUNCHY
CANCHA
CONCHA
CONCHO
CONCHS
DINGHY
GANDHI
GUNGHO
GUNSHY
HONCHO
HONSHU
JONAHS
LANDHO
LUNCHY

LUNTHA
MANCHA
MANCHE
MANCHU
MENTHE
MONTHS
MUNCHY
MYNAHS
NINTHS
PANCHO
PENCHE
PONCHO
PUNCHY
RANCHO
SANCHO
SANTHA
SYNCHS
SYNTHS
TENTHS

••N••H
BANISH
DANISH
DONATH
ELNATH
FINISH
HANNAH
LENGTH
MANUSH
MENSCH
MUNICH
ORNITH
PUNISH
UNNIGH
VANISH
WINISH
ZENITH

•••NH•
THENHL

•••N•H
AMONTH
ATENTH
BLANCH
BLENCH
BRANCH
BRUNCH
CHINCH
CLENCH
CLINCH
CRUNCH
DRENCH
FLINCH
FRENCH
GRINCH
HANNAH
HAUNCH
LAUNCH
NEENAH
PAUNCH
PLINTH
QUENCH
RAUNCH
STANCH
STENCH
TRENCH
WRENCH

••••NH
UNHUNH

NI••••
NIACIN
NIAMEY
NIBBLE
NIBLET
NICADS
NICELY
NICENE
NICEST
NICETY
NICHED
NICHES
NICIAS
NICKED
NICKEL
NICKER
NICKJR
NICOLA
NICOLE
NICOLO
NIDIFY
NIECES
NIEKRO
NIELLI
NIELLO
NIENTE
NIETAS
NIETOS
NIEVES
NIGGLE
NIGHER
NIGHON
NIGHTS
NIGHTY
NIHILO
NIIHAU
NIKEAD
NIKITA
NIKKEI
NIKOLA
NIKONS
NIMBLE
NIMBLY
NIMBUS
NIMINY
NIMITZ
NIMROD
NINEAD
NINEAM
NINEBC
NINEEE
NINEPM
NINERS
NINETY
NINEUP
NINGBO
NINJAS
NINONS
NINTHS
NIOBIC
NIPPED
NIPPER
NIPPLE
NIPPON
NIPSAT
NIPSEY
NIPUPS
NISANS
NISEIS
NISSAN
NISSEN
NITERS
NITERY
NITRES
NITRIC
NITROS
NITWIT
NIXERS
NIXIES
NIXING
NIXONS

N•I•••
NAIADS
NAILED
NAILER
NAILIN
NAILIT
NAILUP
NAIRAS
NAIVER
NEIGHS
NEIMAN
NEISSE
NIIHAU
NOIDEA
NOIRES
NOIRET
NOIRON
NOISED
NOISES
NTILES

N••I••
NACION
NADINE
NADIRS
NAJIMY
NAMING
NANINE
NAPIER
NARIAL
NARINE
NARITA
NATICK
NATION
NATIVE
NAVIES
NEVILL
NEVINS
NEWIES
NEWISH
NICIAS
NIDIFY
NIHILO
NIKITA
NIMINY
NIMITZ
NIXIES
NIXING
NOBILE
NODICE
NOHITS
NOJIVE
NOKIAS
NOKIDS
NOMIAL
NORIAS
NORISK
NORITE
NOSIER
NOSILY
NOSING
NOTICE
NOTIFY
NOTILL
NOTIME
NOTING
NOTION
NOTIPS
NOVIAS
NOVICE
NOVIOS
NOWISE
NUBIAN
NUBILE
NUBIRA
NUDISM
NUDIST
NUDITY
NUKING
NUMINA

N•••I•
NAILIN
NAILIT
NAMEIT
NANNIE
NAPKIN
NAPPIE
NARNIA
NARVIK
NAVAID
NEELIX
NELLIE
NELLIS
NEREID
NESBIT
NESSIE
NESTIN
NEWBIE
NEWKID
NEWSIE
NIACIN
NIOBIC
NISEIS
NITRIC
NITWIT
NOESIS
NOETIC
NOEXIT
NOFAIR
NOGGIN
NONHIT
NOOGIE
NORAIN
NORDIC
NORRIS
NOSEIN
NOTAIL
NOTFIT
NOTHIN
NOWAIT
NUBBIN
NUDNIK
NUNCIO
NUNZIO
NUTKIN
NUTOIL
NUTRIA
NYQUIL

N••••I
NAPOLI
NEPALI
NEROLI
NEVSKI
NIELLI
NIKKEI
NORDOI
NOYORI
NUCLEI

•NI•••
ANIMAL
ANIMAS
ANIMES
ANIMUS
ANIONS
ANISES
ANITRA
ENIACS
ENIDOK
ENIGMA
ENISLE
INIONS
INITIO
KNICKS
KNIFED
KNIFER
KNIFES
KNIGHT
KNIVES
ONIONS
ONIONY
SNICKS
SNIDER
SNIFFS
SNIFFY
SNIPED
SNIPER
SNIPES
SNIPPY
SNITCH
SNIVEL
UNIATE
UNIATS
UNICED
UNICEF
UNICES
UNIDLE
UNIDLY
UNIFIC
UNIONS
UNIPED
UNIPOD
UNIQUE
UNISEX
UNISOM
UNISON
UNISYS
UNITAS
UNITED
UNITER
UNITES
UNIVAC

•N•I••
ANCIEN
ANNIES
ANNIKA
ANNINA
ANOINT
ANTICS
ANTIGO
ANVILS
ENCINA
ENCINO
ENDING
ENDIVE
ENGILD
ENGINE
ENGIRD
ENGIRT
ENLINK
ENLIST
ENMITY
ENNIUS
ENOILS
ENRICH
ENRICO
ENSIGN
ENSILE
ENTIAL
ENTICE
ENTIRE
ENTITY
ENVIED
ENVIER
ENVIES
ENVIRO
ENWIND
GNEISS
INCISE
INCITE
INDIAN
INDICT
INDIES
INDIGO
INDIRA
INDITE
INDIUM
INFIRM
INKIER
INKIND
INKING
INLIEU
INLINE
INMIND
INNIES
INNING
INPINK
INSIDE
INSIST
INSITU
INTIME
INUITS
INVIEW
INVITE
INVIVO
INWITH
ONDISK
ONDITS
ONEIDA
ONEILL
ONEIRO
ONEISH
ONFILE
ONFILM
ONFIRE
ONHIGH
ONHIRE
ONLINE
ONMIKE
ONRICE
ONSIDE
ONSITE
ONTIME
ONVIEW
SNAILS
UNBIND
UNBITS
UNCIAL
UNDICI
UNDIES
UNDIMS
UNDINE
UNFILE
UNFINE
UNFIRM
UNFITS
UNGILT
UNGIRD
UNGIRT
UNHIRE
UNKIND
UNKINK
UNLIKE
UNLIMP
UNLINK
UNLIVE
UNMIRY
UNMIXT
UNNICE
UNNIGH
UNOILY
UNPICK
UNPILE
UNPINS
UNRIFE
UNRIGS
UNRIPE
UNRIPS
UNSICK
UNTIDY
UNTIED
UNTIER
UNTIES
UNTILT
UNWIGS
UNWILD
UNWILY
UNWIND
UNWISE
UNWISH
UNZIPS

•N••I•
ANACIN
ANAKIN
ANDRIC
ANEMIA
ANEMIC
ANGLIA
ANGLIC
ANNUIT
ANODIC
ANOMIA
ANOMIC
ANOMIE
ANOXIA
ANOXIC
ANSEIS
ANTLIA
ANTRIM
ANUBIS
ENDPIN
ENDSIN
ENDSIT
ENFAIT
ENGLIT
ENJOIN
ENNUIS
ENOKIS
ENTAIL
ENVEIL
ENVOIS
GNOMIC
GNOSIS
INABIT
INAFIX
INAPIE
INATIE
INCAIC
INGRID
INITIO
INJAIL
INKSIN
INLAID
INSTIL
INSTIR
INTOIT
INTUIT
INUPIK
INVAIN
KNEWIT
KNOWIT
ONBAIL
ONEBIT
ONEGIN
ONEHIT
ONEPIN
ONLAID
ONLYIF
SNOWIN
UNAKIN
UNAMIS
UNAVID
UNBAIT
UNCHIC
UNCLIP
UNCOIL
UNEPIC
UNEVIL
UNFAIR
UNGLIB
UNGRIP
UNGUIS
UNHAIR
UNIFIC
UNJOIN
UNKNIT
UNLAID
UNNAIL
UNPAID
UNPRIM
UNSAID
UNSHIP
UNSLIM
UNTRIG
UNVAIN
UNVEIL
UNVOID

•N•••I
ANDREI
ANGELI
ANNULI
INCUBI
SNORRI
SNUGLI
UNDICI

••NI••
ALNICO
AMNION
AMNIOS
ANNIES
ANNIKA
ANNINA
ARNICA
ARNIES
ATNINE
AWNING
BANISH
BENICE
BENIGN
BENING
BENITO
BONIER
BONING
BONITA
BONITO
BUNION
CANIDS
CANIER
CANIFF
CANINE
CANING
CONICS
CONIES
CONING
CYNICS
DANIEL
DANILO
DANIOS
DANISH
DANITE
DENIAL
DENIED
DENIER
DENIES
DENIMS
DENIRO
DENISE
DINING
DONITZ
ELNINO
ENNIUS
EONIAN
EUNICE
FANION
FINIAL
FINIAN
FINING
FINISH
FINITE
FINITO
GENIAL
GENIES
GENIUS
GUNITE
HONIED
HONING
IGNITE
INNIES
INNING
IONIAN
IONICS
IONISE
IONIUM
IONIZE
JANICE
JANINE
JUNIOR
JUNIUS
KONICA
KUNITZ
LANIER
LANINA
LENINA
LENITY
LINIER
LINING
LUNIKS
MANIAC
MANIAS
MANILA
MENIAL
MINIFY
MINIMA
MINIME
MINIMI
MINIMS
MINING
MINION
MINITV
MONICA
MONIED
MONIES
MONISM
MONIST
MUNICH
NANINE
OMNIUM
ORNITH
OWNING
PANICS
PANIER
PANINI
PANINO
PENICK
PINIER
PINING
PINION
PONIED
PONIES
PUNIER
PUNILY
PUNISH
RANIDS
RANINE
RENINS
RUNINS
SANITY
SENILE
SENIOR
SENITI
SINISE
SONICS
STNICK
TINIAN
TINIER
TINILY
TONICS
TONIER
TONING
TONITE
TUNICS
TUNING
UNNICE
UNNIGH
VANIER
VANISH
VANITY
VENIAL
VENICE
VENINS
VENIRE
VENITE
VINIER
VINIFY
VINING
WANIER
WANING
WINIER
WINING
WINISH
ZANIER
ZANIES
ZANILY
ZENIST
ZENITH
ZONIAN
ZONING
ZUNIAN
ZUNIGA

••N•I•
AENEID
AGNAIL
ANNUIT
ARNEIS
AUNTIE
BANDIT
BANKIT
BENDIX
BENNIE
BENOIT
BINNIE
BINNIG
BONNIE
CANDIA
CANDID
CANLIT
CONAIR
CONFIT
CONNIE
CONOID
DANCIN
DANDIE
DANGIT
DANZIG
DENNIS
DENTIN
DINDIN
DINEIN
DONEIN
DONEIT
DONNIE
DUNKIN
DUNLIN
EANNIE
EENSIE
ENNUIS
FANFIC
FANGIO
FANNIE
FINNIC
FONZIE
GINNIE
GONEIN
GUNSIT
HANDIN
HANGIN
HANKIE
HENBIT
HENRIK
HINGIS
HONEIN
HUNGIN
JENNIE
JINNIS
JUNKIE
KANJIS
KENSIT
LANAIS
LANCIA
LANCIE
LANDIS
LANVIN
LENAIN
LENNIE
LENTIL
LONNIE
LUNDIS
MANNIX
MANTIC
MANTIS
MCNAIR
MCNEIL
MENNIN
MENTIS
MINNIE
MINUIT
MUNCIE
NANNIE
NONHIT
NUNCIO
NUNZIO
PANDIT
PANSIN
PANTIE
PENCIL
PENNIA
PENNIS
PENSIN
PINKIE
PINYIN
PONGID
PUNDIT
PUNKIE
RANCID
RANGIN
RANKIN
RENAIL
RENNIE
RENNIN
RENOIR
RINGIN
RONMIX
RONNIE
RUNCIE
RUNGIN
RUNSIN
SANDIA
SANKIN
SENDIN
SENTIN
SINGIN
SINKIN
SUNKIN
SUNLIT
SUNNIS
SYNDIC
TANNIC
TANNIN
TENNIS
TENPIN
TONKIN
TONSIL
TUNEIN
UNNAIL
VINCIT
VINNIE
WANTIN
WENDIE
WENTIN
WINBIG
WINGIT
WINKIE
WINNIE
WINWIN
WONBIG
XINGIN
YENSID
ZINCIC
ZINNIA

••N••I
ANNULI
BANGUI
BANZAI
BONACI
BONAMI
BONSAI
CENTAI
CENTRI
DANTEI
DENALI
DENARI
DENDRI
ERNANI
GANDHI
HENRYI
KENOBI
KINSKI
LUNEDI
MINIMI
MONAMI
PANINI
RENVOI
SANSEI
SENITI
SENSEI
VENUTI
YANQUI
ZANONI

•••NI•
ADENIS
ADONIC
ADONIS
ALANIS
ASONIA
ATONIA
ATONIC
AXENIC
AZANIA
AZONIC
BAGNIO
BEANIE
BENNIE
BERNIE
BINNIE
BINNIG
BIONIC
BLINIS
BONNIE
BOSNIA
BURNIE
BURNIN
CATNIP
CHENIN
CLINIC
CONNIE
CRANIA
CRANIO
CRONIN
CYANIC
CYANID
DARNIT
DEENIE
DENNIS
DONNIE
DURNIT
EANNIE
EARNIE
EARNIT
EDENIC
ESENIN
ETHNIC
ETONIC
EVENIF
FAFNIR
FANNIE
FINNIC
GINNIE
GLYNIS
GOONIE
GOONIN
GRANIT
HAYNIE
HEINIE
HERNIA
HORNIN
ICONIC
IMONIT
IRANIS
IRENIC
IRONIC
IVANIV
JEANIE
JENNIE
JINNIS
JOANIE
JOHNII
JOHNIV
JOHNIX
JOININ
KAONIC
KOENIG
LAINIE
LEANIN
LENNIE
LEONIA
LEONID
LIGNIN
LONNIE
LOONIE
MANNIX
MARNIE
MEANIE
MEANIT
MEDNIS
MENNIN
MINNIE
MOONIE
NANNIE
NARNIA
NUDNIK
ODINIC
OMANIS
OPENIT
ORANIS
OZONIC
PARNIS
PENNIA
PENNIS
PHONIC
PICNIC
RAININ
REENIE
REININ
REKNIT
RENNIE
RENNIN
RESNIK
RONNIE

SARNIA SCENIC SEENIN SEWNIN SHANIA SIGNIN SUNNIS TANNIC TANNIN TEENIE TENNIS TOONIE TOWNIE TURNIN TURNIP UNKNIT URANIA URANIC VINNIE WEENIE WIENIE WINNIE ZINNIA

•••N•I

ADONAI AMANTI AVANTI BIONDI BRANDI BRUNEI DJINNI GIANNI IDENTI ISANTI IVANVI JOHNII JOHNVI JOHNXI QUINTI RIENZI SCENEI SOONYI UBANGI

••••NI

ADJANI ALUMNI ARMANI BARONI BIKINI BIMINI BUSONI CAPONI CARONI COLONI DEDINI DJINNI DOMANI DOMINI ERNANI GEMINI GIANNI ILLINI IOLANI LATINI MORONI ORIANI ORSINI PANINI PARINI RAPINI REMINI RIMINI ROMANI ROTINI SOCANI SOMONI TAHINI URBANI YAMANI YEMENI YOGINI ZANONI

N•J•••

NAJIMY NOJIVE NOJOKE NYJETS

N••J••

NEWJOB NINJAS NONJEW

N•••J•

NAVAJO NICKJR

•NJ•••

ANJOUS ENJOIN ENJOYS INJAIL INJECT INJEST INJOKE INJULY INJUNE INJURE INJURY UNJAMS UNJOIN UNJUST

•N•J••

INAJAM INKJET ONAJAG

•N•••J

INTERJ

••NJ••

BANJOS BANJUL CONJOB DONJON FANJET KANJIS MENJOU NINJAS NONJEW PUNJAB

•••N•J

AGENTJ PBANDJ

••••NJ

LODINJ

N•K•••

NAKFAS NIKEAD NIKITA NIKKEI NIKOLA NIKONS NOKIAS NOKIDS NUKING

N••K••

NAPKIN NECKED NECKER NEWKID NICKED NICKEL NICKER NICKJR NIEKRO NIKKEI NOCKED NUTKIN

N•••K•

NEVSKI NEVSKY NOBAKE NOJOKE NOOTKA

N••••K

NANOOK NARVIK NATICK NEWARK NOLUCK NOMEAK NORISK NUDNIK NYYANK

•NK•••

ANKARA ANKLED ANKLES ANKLET INKERS INKIER INKIND INKING INKJET INKLES INKPAD INKPOT INKSAC INKSIN UNKEPT UNKIND UNKINK UNKNIT UNKNOT

•N•K••

ANAKIN ANGKOR ENOKIS SNAKED SNAKER SNAKES UNAKIN UNSKEW

•N••K•

ANANKE ANNIKA INJOKE INTAKE INVOKE KNACKS KNICKS KNOCKS ONMIKE SNACKS SNARKS SNARKY SNEAKS SNEAKY SNICKS SNOOKS UNCAKE UNLIKE UNMAKE UNYOKE VNECKS

•N•••K

ANORAK ENIDOK ENLINK ENRANK INBACK INBULK INHOCK INLUCK INPARK INPINK INUPIK ONDECK ONDISK UNCASK UNCORK UNDOCK UNFORK UNHOOK UNHUSK UNKINK UNLINK UNLOCK UNMASK UNPACK UNPICK UNRACK UNSICK UNSUNK UNTACK UNTUCK

••NK••

BANKED BANKER BANKIT BANKON BANKUP BONKED BUNKED BUNKER BUNKOS BUNKUM CANKER CONKED CONKER DANKER DANKLY DINKAS DINKUM DONKEY DUNKED DUNKER DUNKIN FINKED FINKEL FINKON FUNKED GINKGO HANKER HANKIE HINKLE HONKAT HONKED HONKER HUNKER JUNKED JUNKER JUNKET JUNKIE KINKED KINKOS LANKER LANKLY LINKED LINKER LINKUP LUNKER MENKEN MONKEE MONKEY OINKED OINKER PINKED PINKEN PINKER PINKIE PINKOS PUNKAS PUNKER PUNKIE RANKED RANKER RANKIN RANKLE RANKLY SANKAS SANKIN SINKER SINKIN SUNKEN SUNKIN TANKAS TANKED TANKER TANKUP TINKER TINKLE TINKLY TONKAS TONKIN WANKEL WINKAT WINKED WINKER WINKIE WYNKEN YANKAT YANKED YANKEE YANKER YANKON ZONKED ZONKER

••N•K•

ANNIKA BENEKE GINGKO HANDKE KANAKA KINSKI LANSKY LUNIKS PANCKS TANAKA ZINCKY

••N••K

CANUCK DONEOK HENRIK HENRYK ISNTOK LANARK NANOOK PENICK PINOAK SENDAK SHNOOK STNICK TANOAK VANARK ZANUCK

•••NK•

ANANKE BLANKS BLINKS BRINKS BRONKO CHINKS CHINKY CHUNKS CHUNKY CLANKS CLANKY CLINKS CLONKS CLUNKS CLUNKY CRANKS CRANKY CSONKA DRINKS EBANKS FLANKS FLUNKS FLUNKY FRANKS GLINKA IVANKA PLANKS PLINKS PLONKS PLUNKS PLUNKY PRANKS PRINKS REINKS SHANKS SKANKS SKANKY SKINKS SKUNKS SKUNKY SLINKS SLINKY SPANKS SPANKY SPINKS SPUNKY STINKO STINKS STINKY SWANKY THANKS THINKS THUNKS TRUNKS

•••N•K

AGENTK FRANCK GDANSK KARNAK KRENEK NUDNIK PLANCK RESNIK

••••NK

ARMONK DEBUNK DEJUNK DRYINK EMBANK ENLINK ENRANK EWBANK EXYANK INPINK ITHINK LFRANK NYYANK PODUNK REBANK REDINK RELINK RERANK RESINK SHRANK SHRINK SHRUNK SOYINK STRUNK UNKINK UNLINK UNSUNK UPLINK USBANK ZEDONK

NL••••

NLEAST NLMVPS NLWEST

N•L•••

NELLIE NELLIS NELSON NFLERS NHLERS NOLEAD NOLESS NOLOAD NOLOSE NOLOSS NOLUCK NULLED NULLOS NYLONS

N••L••

NAILED NAILER NAILIN NAILIT NAILUP NAPLES NEALON NEELIX NELLIE NELLIS NEWLEY NIBLET NIELLI NIELLO NOBLER NOBLES NOWLAN NTILES NUCLEI NUCLEO NULLED NULLOS NUTLET NYALAS

N•••L•

NAMELY NAPALM NAPOLI NASALS NATALE NAVELS NEARLY NEATLY NEBULA NEEDLE NEPALI NEROLI NESTLE NETTLE NETTLY NEVILL NEWELL NEWELS NEWULM NIBBLE NICELY NICOLA NICOLE NICOLO NIELLI NIELLO NIGGLE NIHILO NIKOLA NIMBLE NIMBLY NIPPLE NOBALL NOBELS NOBILE NODULE NOHELP NOODLE NOPALS NORELL NOSALE NOSALT NOSILY NOTALL NOTILL NOTOLL NOVELA NOVELS NOZZLE NTUPLE NUBBLE NUBBLY NUBILE NUDELY NUMBLY NUZZLE

N••••L

NARIAL NERMAL NERVAL NETFUL NEURAL NEUROL NEVILL NEWELL NEXTEL NICKEL NOBALL NODEAL NOMIAL NORELL NORMAL NORVAL NOTAIL NOTALL NOTILL NOTOLL NOUNAL NUCHAL NUTOIL NYQUIL

•NL•••

ENLACE ENLINK ENLIST INLAID INLAND INLAWS INLAYS INLEAF INLETS INLIEU INLINE INLOVE INLUCK ONLAID ONLAND ONLATE ONLAYS ONLINE ONLOAD ONLOAN ONLYIF UNLACE UNLADE UNLAID UNLASH UNLAYS UNLEAD UNLEAF UNLEAN UNLEFT UNLENT UNLESS UNLIKE UNLIMP UNLINK UNLIVE UNLOAD UNLOCK UNLOOP UNLOST UNLUSH

•N•L••

ANALOG ANELED ANELES ANGLED ANGLEE ANGLER ANGLES ANGLIA ANGLIC ANGLOS ANKLED ANKLES ANKLET ANNLEE ANOLES ANTLER ANTLIA DNALAB ENBLOC ENGLIT ENGLUT ENSLER INBLUE INFLOW INFLUX INGLES INKLES INPLAY KNELLS KNOLLS KNOLLY ONCLES ONELAP ONELEG SNELLS UNBLED UNCLAD UNCLAY UNCLES UNCLIP UNCLOG UNFLAT UNGLAD UNGLIB UNGLUE UNPLAN UNPLUG UNSLIM UNSLOW

•N••L•

ANGELA ANGELI ANGELL ANGELO ANGELS ANGOLA ANNALS ANNULI ANNULS ANSELM ANVILS ANYOLD ENABLE ENDALL ENFOLD ENGELS ENGILD ENGULF ENHALO ENISLE ENOILS ENROLL ENROLS ENSILE GNARLS GNARLY INBULK INCULT INFALL INFOLD INFULL INGELS INGOLD INGULF INHALE INHALF INJULY INSOLE INSULT KNEELS KNELLS KNOLLS KNOLLY KNURLS KNURLY ONCALL ONEALL ONEILL ONFILE ONFILM ONHOLD ONSALE SNAILS SNARLS SNARLY SNELLS SNUGLI SNUGLY UNABLE UNABLY UNBALE UNBELT UNBOLD UNBOLT UNCALM UNCOLA UNDULY UNFELT UNFILE UNFOLD UNFULL UNGILT UNGULA UNHALE UNHELD UNHELM UNHOLY UNHULL UNIDLE UNIDLY UNMOLD UNOILY UNPALE UNPILE UNROLL UNRULY UNSELD UNSELL UNSOLD UNSOLE UNTILT UNTOLD UNWALL UNWELL UNWILD UNWILY

•N•••L

ANGELL ANIMAL ANNEAL ANNUAL ANODAL ANTRAL ENAMEL ENCYCL ENDALL ENROLL ENSEAL ENSOUL ENTAIL ENTIAL ENVEIL INFALL INFULL INGOAL INJAIL INSTAL INSTIL KNEBEL ONBAIL ONCALL ONEALL ONEILL SNIVEL SNOBOL UNCIAL UNCOIL UNCOOL UNCURL UNEVIL UNFOUL UNFULL UNFURL UNGUAL UNHULL UNNAIL UNOCAL UNORAL UNPEEL UNREAL UNREEL UNROLL UNSEAL UNSELL UNVEIL UNWALL UNWELL

••NL••

ANNLEE BANLON CANLIT CONLAN DUNLAP DUNLIN DUNLOP FINLEY GUNLAP GUNLAW HANLEY HANLON HENLEY HUNLEY LYNLEY MANLEY RANLOW RUNLET RUNLOW SUNLIT TENLBS TENLEY

••N•L•

ANNALS ANNULI ANNULS ARNALL ARNOLD BANGLE BINDLE BINGLE BUNDLE BUNGLE CANALS CANDLE CANOLA CANTLE CANULA DANDLE DANGLE DANGLY DANILO DANKLY DENALI DINGLE DONALD DONGLE DYNELS FINALE FINALS FINELY FONDLE FONDLY GANGLY GENTLE GENTLY HANDLE HINGLE HINKLE JANGLE JANGLY JINGLE JINGLY JUNGLE JUNGLY KANALY KINDLE KINDLY KINGLY LANKLY LENGLE LINGLE LONELY LONGLY LUNULA MANGLE MANILA MANTLE MINGLE PANDLS PANELS PENULT PUNILY RANKLE RANKLY RONALD RONELY RUNDLE SANELY SENILE SINGLE SINGLY TANGLE TANGLY TINGLE TINGLY TINILY TINKLE TINKLY VENULE VINYLS WANGLE ZANILY ZONULE

••N••L

AGNAIL ALNASL ANNEAL ANNUAL ARNALL BANJUL BENGAL BENZOL BUNUEL CANCEL CANFUL CANNEL CANTAL CENTAL CINEOL CONSUL CUNEAL DANDYL DANIEL DENIAL DENTAL DENZEL FENNEL FINIAL FINKEL FONTAL FUNGAL FUNNEL GENIAL GENUAL GUNSEL HANDEL HANGUL HANSEL KANDEL KENNEL KUNZEL LANVAL LENTIL LINEAL LINTEL LONNOL MANDEL MANFUL

MANTEL
MANUAL
MANUEL
MCNEIL
MENDEL
MENIAL
MENSAL
MENTAL
MONGOL
MONTEL
PANFUL
PENCIL
PENPAL
PENTEL
PINEAL
RANDAL
RANGEL
RENAIL
RENTAL
RONDEL
RUNNEL
SANDAL
SINFUL
TINEAL
TINSEL
TONSIL
TUNNEL
UNNAIL
URNFUL
VANDAL
VENIAL
WANKEL

•••NL•

BRENLY
EVENLY
GAINLY
IFONLY
KEENLY
LEANLY
LIONLY
MAINLY
MEANLY
OPENLY
THINLY
VAINLY
WHENLL

•••N•L

ATONAL
AXONAL
AZONAL
CANNEL
CARNAL
CHANEL
CLONAL
CORNEL
CRENEL
DIRNDL
EPINAL
FAUNAL
FENNEL
FUNNEL
GRINDL
HYMNAL
KENNEL
KERNEL
LIONEL
LONNOL
MAGNOL
NOUNAL
PAGNOL
PHENOL
REGNAL
RHINAL
RUNNEL
SIGNAL
SPINAL
SPINEL
THENFL
THENHL
TRINAL
TUNNEL
VEINAL
VERNAL
WHENLL

N•M•••

NAMATH
NAMEIT
NAMELY
NAMERS
NAMING
NEMEAN
NIMBLE
NIMBLY
NIMBUS
NIMINY
NIMITZ
NIMROD
NLMVPS
NOMAAM
NOMADS
NOMAYO
NOMBRE
NOMEAK
NOMEAT
NOMIAL
NOMORE
NUMBAT
NUMBED
NUMBER
NUMBLY
NUMERO
NUMINA
NYMETS
NYMPHS

N••M••

NBOMBS
NEIMAN
NERMAL
NETMAN
NETMEN
NEUMAN
NEWMAN
NEWMAR
NIAMEY
NOEMON
NONMAN
NONMEN
NORMAL
NORMAN
NOUMEA
NUTMEG

N•••M•

NAJIMY
NONAME
NOTIME

N••••M

NAPALM
NEWSOM
NEWULM
NINEAM
NINEPM
NOMAAM
NONCOM
NOROOM
NUDISM

•NM•••

ENMESH
ENMITY
INMATE
INMIND
INMOST
ONMIKE
UNMADE
UNMAKE
UNMANS
UNMASK
UNMAST
UNMATE
UNMEET
UNMESH
UNMEWS
UNMIRY
UNMIXT
UNMOLD
UNMOOR
UNMOWN

•N•M••

ANEMIA
ANEMIC
ANIMAL
ANIMAS
ANIMES
ANIMUS
ANOMIA
ANOMIC
ANOMIE
ANYMAN
ENAMEL
ENAMOR
ENDMAN
ENDMEN
GNOMES
GNOMIC
GNOMON
INGMAR
ONEMAN
ONEMEG
UNAMIS
UNSMUG

•N••M•

ENARMS
ENCAMP
ENIGMA
ENORME
ENTOMB
ENTOMO
ENZYME
INCOME
INFAMY
INHOME
INHUME
INTIME
ONRAMP
ONTIME
PNEUMA
PNEUMO
UNARMS
UNDAMS
UNDIMS
UNGAMY
UNJAMS
UNLIMP
UNTAME

•N•••M

ANADEM
ANONYM
ANSELM
ANTHEM
ANTRIM
ANTRUM
ENGRAM
INAJAM
INDIUM
INFIRM
INFORM
INGRAM
INSEAM
ONEARM
ONFILM
UNCALM
UNFIRM
UNHELM
UNISOM
UNPRIM
UNSEAM
UNSLIM

••NM••

BONMOT
CONMAN
CONMEN
DENMOM
GUNMAN
GUNMEN
NONMAN
NONMEN
PENMAN
PENMEN
RONMIX
TINMAN
TINMEN

••N•M•

BENUMB
BONAMI
BYNAME
CINEMA
DANGME
DENIMS
DYNAMO
GENOME
KINGME
MANAMA
MANDMS
MINIMA
MINIME
MINIMI
MINIMS
MONAMI
NONAME
PANAMA
RENAME
RUNDMC
SONOMA
TONEME
VENOMS

••N••M

ARNHEM
AUNTEM
BANTAM
BONHAM
BUNKUM
CENTUM
DENHAM
DENMOM
DINKUM
DUNHAM
FANDOM
HANSOM
IONIUM
MONISM
NINEAM
NINEPM
NONCOM
OMNIUM
RANDOM
RANSOM
TANDEM
WINDOM

•••N•M

ANONYM
BARNUM
EMINEM
EPONYM
EUONYM
EXONYM
FARNUM
FRENUM
LIGNUM
MAGNUM
PHENOM
PLENUM
PUTNAM
REGNUM

••••NM

TAOSNM

N•N•••

NANINE
NANNIE
NANOOK
NANSEN
NANTES
NINEAD
NINEAM
NINEBC
NINEEE
NINEPM
NINERS
NINETY
NINEUP
NINGBO
NINJAS
NINONS
NINTHS
NONAGE
NONAME
NONART
NONARY
NONCOM
NONEED
NONEGO
NONETS
NONEWS
NONFAN
NONFAT
NONFED
NONGAS
NONGOD
NONHIT
NONJEW
NONMAN
NONMEN
NONNET
NONONO
NONPAR
NONPRO
NONRUN
NONTAN
NONTAX
NONUSE
NONWAR
NUNCIO
NUNGEN
NUNZIO

N••N••

NAGNAG
NANNIE
NARNIA
NEENAH
NERNST
NIENTE
NONNET
NOONAN
NOONER
NOONES
NOTNEW
NOTNOW
NOUNAL
NOWNOW
NUANCE
NUDNIK

N•••N•

NADINE
NAGANO
NAMING
NANINE
NARINE
NATANT
NEEDNT
NERONE
NEVINS
NICENE
NIKONS
NIMINY
NINONS
NISANS
NIXING
NIXONS
NOCENT
NOHANT
NONONO
NORENT
NORUNS
NOSING
NOTANY
NOTING
NOTONE
NOVENA
NUGENT
NUKING
NUMINA
NYLONS
NYYANK

N••••N

NACION
NAILIN
NANSEN
NAPKIN
NATHAN
NATION
NATRON
NEALON
NEATEN
NEESON
NEIMAN
NELSON
NEMEAN
NEOCON
NEPEAN
NESSEN
NESTIN
NETMAN
NETMEN
NETTON
NEUMAN
NEURON
NEWMAN
NEWTON
NGUYEN
NIACIN
NIGHON
NIPPON
NISSAN
NISSEN
NOEMON
NOGGIN
NOIRON
NONFAN
NONMAN
NONMEN
NONRUN
NONTAN
NOONAN
NORAIN
NOREEN
NORMAN
NORTON
NOSEIN
NOTHIN
NOTION
NOWLAN
NUBBIN
NUBIAN
NUNGEN
NUTKIN

•NN•••

ANNALS
ANNEAL
ANNEES
ANNIES
ANNIKA
ANNINA
ANNLEE
ANNOYS
ANNUAL
ANNUIT
ANNULI
ANNULS
ENNEAD
ENNIUS
ENNUIS
INNAGE
INNATE
INNEED
INNERS
INNESS
INNIES
INNING
UNNAIL
UNNEAT
UNNICE
UNNIGH

•N•N••

ANANAS
ANANKE
ANONYM
INANER
INONES
UNKNIT
UNKNOT
UNSNAG
UNSNAP
UNSNUG

•N••N•

ANIONS
ANNINA
ANOINT
ANTONE
ANTONY
ANWANG
ANYONE
ANYONS
ENBANC
ENCINA
ENCINO
ENDING
ENFANT
ENGINE
ENLINK
ENRANK
ENWIND
INCANS
INCANT
INCENT
INDENT
INFANT
INHAND
INIONS
INJUNE
INKIND
INKING
INLAND
INLINE
INMIND
INNING
INPINK
INRUNS
INSANA
INSANE
INSYNC
INTEND
INTENS
INTENT
INTONE
INTUNE
INVENT
INWANT
KNOWNS
ONEONE
ONHAND
ONIONS
ONIONY
ONLAND
ONLINE
UNBEND
UNBENT
UNBIND
UNDINE
UNDONE
UNFINE
UNFOND
UNHAND
UNHUNG
UNHUNH
UNIONS
UNKIND
UNKINK
UNLENT
UNLINK
UNMANS
UNPENS
UNPENT
UNPINS
UNRENT
UNRUNG
UNSENT
UNSUNG
UNSUNK
UNTUNE
UNWIND
UNZONE

•N•••N

ANACIN
ANAKIN
ANCIEN
ANDEAN
ANTAWN
ANTRON
ANYMAN
ENDMAN
ENDMEN
ENDPIN
ENDRAN
ENDRUN
ENDSIN
ENDSON
ENJOIN
ENSIGN
GNAWON
GNOMON
INBORN
INCHON
INDIAN
INKSIN
INPAWN
INSPAN
INTERN
INTOWN
INTURN
INVAIN
ONABUN
ONEGIN
ONEMAN
ONEPIN
ONERUN
ONETEN
ONETON
ONLOAN
SNAPON
SNOWIN
UNAKIN
UNBORN
UNEVEN
UNHEWN
UNISON
UNJOIN
UNLEAN
UNMOWN
UNOPEN
UNPAWN
UNPLAN
UNSAWN
UNSEEN
UNSEWN
UNSOWN
UNSPAN
UNSPUN
UNTORN
UNVAIN
UNWORN

••NN••

BANNED
BANNEN
BANNER
BENNIE
BINNED
BINNEY
BINNIE
BINNIG
BONNER
BONNES
BONNET
BONNEY
BONNIE
CANNAS
CANNED
CANNEL
CANNER
CANNES
CANNON
CANNOT
CONNED
CONNEE
CONNIE
CONNOR
DANNAY
DANNER
DANNON
DANNYS
DENNED
DENNIS
DENNYS
DINNED
DINNER
DONNED
DONNER
DONNIE
DUNNED
DUNNER
EANNIE
FANNED
FANNER
FANNIE
FENNEL
FENNER
FINNAN
FINNED
FINNEY
FINNIC
FUNNED
FUNNEL
GANNET
GANNON
GINNED
GINNIE
GUNNAR
GUNNED
GUNNER
HANNAH
HENNAS
HENNER
JANNEY
JENNER
JENNET
JENNEY
JENNIE
JINNIS
KENNAN
KENNED
KENNEL
KENNER
KENNYG
KINNAN
LENNIE
LENNON
LENNOX
LINNET
LINNEY
LONNIE
LONNOL
MANNAS
MANNED
MANNER
MANNIX
MANNON
MENNEN
MENNIN
MINNIE
MINNOW
MONNET
NANNIE
NONNET
PANNED
PANNER
PANNES
PENNED
PENNER
PENNEY
PENNIA
PENNIS
PENNON
PINNAE
PINNAS
PINNED
PINNER
PUNNED
PUNNER
RENNES
RENNET
RENNIE
RENNIN
RONNIE
RUNNEL
RUNNER
SENNAS
SINNED
SINNER
SONNET
SUNNED
SUNNIS
TANNED
TANNER
TANNIC
TANNIN
TENNER
TENNIS
TINNED
TINNER
TONNES
TUNNEL
TUNNEY
VANNED
VANNES
VENNER
VINNIE
WANNED
WANNER
WENNER
WINNER
WINNIE
WINNOW
YENNED
ZINNIA

••N•N•

ANNINA
ATNINE
AWNING
BANANA
BANANE
BANONS
BENING
BONING
CANINE
CANING
CANONS
CONANT
CONING
DANANG
DINING
DUNANT
ELNINO
ERNANI
FANONS
FINING
HONING
INNING
IONONE
JANINE
LANINA
LENINA
LINENS
LINENY
LINING
MANANA
MINING
NANINE
NINONS
NONONO
OENONE
OWNING
PANINI
PANINO
PINING
PINONS
RANINE
RENINS
RENONV
RUNINS
RUNONS
SONANT
SUNUNU
TANANA
TENANT
TENONE
TENONS
TONING
TUNING
VENINS
VINING
WANING
WINANS
WINING
WINONA
ZANONI
ZENANA
ZONING

••N••N

ADNOUN
AMNION
ATNOON
BANGON
BANKON
BANLON
BANNEN
BANYAN
BENBEN
BENIGN
BENSON
BENTON
BINYON
BONBON
BONTON
BUNION
BUNSEN
BUNTON
BUNYAN
CANAAN
CANCAN
CANCUN
CANNON
CANTON
CANYON
CONLAN
CONMAN
CONMEN
DANCIN
DANNON
DANSON
DANTON
DENTIN
DENTON
DINDIN
DINEIN
DINEON
DONEIN
DONJON
DUNCAN
DUNKIN
DUNLIN
EONIAN
FANION
FANTAN
FINIAN
FINKON
FINNAN
FINSEN
FUNRUN
GANNON
GENOAN
GONEIN
GONEON
GUNMAN
GUNMEN
HANDIN
HANDON
HANGIN
HANGON
HANLON
HANSON
HENSON
HINTON
HONEIN
HUNGIN
HUNGON
IONIAN
JANSEN
JANZEN
JENSEN
JONSON
KANSAN
KENNAN
KENTON
KENYAN
KENYON
KINNAN
LANDON
LANSON
LANVIN
LENAIN
LENNON
LENTEN
LINDEN
LINTON
LONDON
LUNDEN
LYNDON
MANDAN
MANNON
MANZON
MENKEN
MENNEN
MENNIN
MENSAN
MINDEN
MINION
MINOAN
MINYAN
NANSEN
NONFAN
NONMAN
NONMEN
NONRUN
NONTAN
NUNGEN
PANSIN
PENMAN
PENMEN
PENNON
PENSIN
PINION
PINKEN
PINSON
PINYIN
PINZON
RANGIN
RANKIN
RENNIN
RENOWN
RENTON
RINGIN
RONSON
RUNGIN
RUNSIN
RUNSON
RUNYON
SANKIN
SENDIN
SENDON
SENSEN
SENTIN
SENTON
SINGIN
SINKIN
SUNFAN
SUNKEN
SUNKIN
SUNTAN
TANNIN
TENDON
TENPIN
TENTON
TINCAN
TINIAN
TINMAN
TINMEN
TINPAN

TONGAN
TONKIN
TUNEIN
VANRYN
VINSON
VINTON
WANTIN
WANTON
WENTIN
WENTON
WINWIN
WONTON
WYNKEN
WYNTON
XINGIN
YANGON
YANKON
ZONIAN
ZUNIAN

•••NN•

BRANNY
CHYNNA
CRANNY
CRENNA
DEANNA
DIANNE
DIONNE
DJINNI
DJINNS
DUENNA
ERINNA
EVONNE
FRANNY
GIANNI
GLENNE
GRANNY
GWYNNE
IDUNNO
IWANNA
JEANNE
JOANNA
JOANNE
JOHNNY
LEANNE
LYONNE
PRYNNE
SHINNY
SIENNA
SKINNY
SWANNS
TRANNY
VIENNA
VIENNE
WHINNY
YVONNE

•••N•N

ALANON
BAHNEN
BANNEN
BEINON
BURNIN
CANNON
CERNAN
CHENIN
CRONIN
CRONYN
DANNON
DAWNON
DOWNON
ESENIN
FAWNON
FINNAN
GAINON
GANNON
GOONIN
GUINAN
HERNAN
HORNIN
IRONON
JOININ
KEENAN
KEENEN
KEENON
KENNAN
KINNAN
LEANIN
LEANON
LEHNEN
LENNON
LIGNIN
MAGNON
MANNON
MENNEN
MENNIN
MIGNON
NOONAN
OPENON
PENNON
PLANON
POZNAN
RAININ
RAINON
REININ
RENNIN
SEENIN
SEWNIN
SEWNON
SIGNIN
SIGNON
TANNIN
TURNIN
TURNON
VERNON

••••NN

EAMONN
EDWYNN
JOHANN
LEEANN
LOUANN
MCCANN
SUEANN
SUSANN

NO••••

NOBAKE
NOBALL
NOBELS
NOBILE
NOBLER
NOBLES
NOBODY
NOBUTS
NOCENT
NOCHES
NOCKED
NOCOST
NODDED
NODDER
NODEAL
NODEAR
NODICE
NODOFF
NODOSE
NODOUS
NODSAT
NODSTO
NODULE
NOEMON
NOESIS
NOETIC
NOEXIT
NOFAIR
NOFEES
NOFUSS
NOGGIN
NOGOOD
NOHANT
NOHELP
NOHITS
NOHOPE
NOIDEA
NOIRES
NOIRET
NOIRON
NOISED
NOISES
NOJIVE
NOJOKE
NOKIAS
NOKIDS
NOLEAD
NOLESS
NOLOAD
NOLOSE
NOLOSS
NOLUCK
NOMAAM
NOMADS
NOMAYO
NOMBRE
NOMEAK
NOMEAT
NOMIAL
NOMORE
NONAGE
NONAME
NONART
NONARY
NONCOM
NONEED
NONEGO
NONETS
NONEWS
NONFAN
NONFAT
NONFED
NONGAS
NONGOD
NONHIT
NONJEW
NONMAN
NONMEN
NONNET
NONONO
NONPAR
NONPRO
NONRUN
NONTAN
NONTAX
NONUSE
NONWAR
NOODGE
NOODLE
NOOGIE
NOONAN
NOONER
NOONES
NOOSED
NOOSER
NOOSES
NOOTKA
NOPALS
NOPETS
NOPQRS
NOPROB
NORAIN
NORDIC
NORDOI
NOREEN
NORELL
NORENT
NORGAY
NORIAS
NORISK
NORITE
NORMAL
NORMAN
NOROOM
NORRIS
NORTHS
NORTON
NORUNS
NORUSH
NORVAL
NORWAY
NOSALE
NOSALT
NOSEIN
NOSERS
NOSEUP
NOSHED
NOSHER
NOSHES
NOSHOW
NOSIER
NOSILY
NOSING
NOSOAP
NOSTEP
NOSTER
NOSTRA
NOTAIL
NOTALL
NOTANY
NOTARY
NOTATE
NOTBAD
NOTCHY
NOTERS
NOTFAR
NOTFIT
NOTFOR
NOTHIN
NOTICE
NOTIFY
NOTILL
NOTIME
NOTING
NOTION
NOTIPS
NOTNEW
NOTNOW
NOTOLL
NOTONE
NOTOUT
NOTTOO
NOTYET
NOTYOU
NOUGAT
NOUGHT
NOUMEA
NOUNAL
NOVATO
NOVELA
NOVELS
NOVENA
NOVIAS
NOVICE
NOVIOS
NOVOTE
NOWAIT
NOWAYS
NOWISE
NOWLAN
NOWNOW
NOYORI
NOZZLE

N•O•••

NBOMBS
NEOCON
NEOSHO
NFORTY
NIOBIC
NOODGE
NOODLE
NOOGIE
NOONAN
NOONER
NOONES
NOOSED
NOOSER
NOOSES
NOOTKA

N••O••

NABOBS
NABORS
NAGOYA
NANOOK
NAPOLI
NEROLI
NERONE
NICOLA
NICOLE
NICOLO
NIKOLA
NIKONS
NINONS
NIXONS
NOBODY
NOCOST
NODOFF
NODOSE
NODOUS
NOGOOD
NOHOPE
NOJOKE
NOLOAD
NOLOSE
NOLOSS
NOMORE
NONONO
NOROOM
NOSOAP
NOTOLL
NOTONE
NOTOUT
NOVOTE
NOYORI
NUTOIL
NYLONS
NYPOST

N•••O•

NACHOS
NACION
NANOOK
NARCOS
NARROW
NATION
NATRON
NEALON
NEESON
NELSON
NEOCON
NESTOR
NETHOU
NETTON
NEUROL
NEURON
NEWJOB
NEWSOM
NEWTON
NEWTOY
NIETOS
NIGHON
NIMROD
NIPPON
NITROS
NOEMON
NOGOOD
NOIRON
NONCOM
NONGOD
NOPROB
NORDOI
NOROOM
NORTON
NOSHOW
NOTFOR
NOTION
NOTNOW
NOTTOO
NOTYOU
NOVIOS
NOWNOW
NULLOS

N••••O

NAGANO
NAVAHO
NAVAJO
NEARTO
NEEDTO
NEOSHO
NEPHRO
NEXTTO
NICOLO
NIEKRO
NIELLO
NIHILO
NINGBO
NODSTO
NOMAYO
NONEGO
NONONO
NONPRO
NOTTOO
NOVATO
NUCLEO
NUMERO
NUNCIO
NUNZIO

•NO•••

ANODAL
ANODES
ANODIC
ANOINT
ANOLES
ANOMIA
ANOMIC
ANOMIE
ANONYM
ANORAK
ANOXIA
ANOXIC
CNOTES
ENOILS
ENOKIS
ENORME
ENOTES
ENOUGH
GNOMES
GNOMIC
GNOMON
GNOSES
GNOSIS
GNOTES
INONES
INOUYE
KNOBBY
KNOCKS
KNOLLS
KNOLLY
KNOTTS
KNOTTY
KNOTUP
KNOUTS
KNOWER
KNOWIT
KNOWNS
KNOWOF
MNOPQR
SNOBBY
SNOBOL
SNOCAT
SNOODS
SNOOKS
SNOOPS
SNOOPY
SNOOTS
SNOOTY
SNOOZE
SNOOZY
SNOPES
SNORED
SNORER
SNORES
SNORRI
SNORTS
SNORTY
SNOUTS
SNOWED
SNOWIN
TNOTES
UNOCAL
UNOILY
UNOPEN
UNORAL
UNOWED

•N•O••

ANGOLA
ANGORA
ANIONS
ANJOUS
ANNOYS
ANTONE
ANTONY
ANYOLD
ANYONE
ANYONS
ENCODE
ENCORE
ENDORA
ENDOWS
ENFOLD
ENJOIN
ENJOYS
ENROBE
ENROLL
ENROLS
ENROOT
ENSOUL
ENTOMB
ENTOMO
ENVOIS
ENVOYS
INBORN
INCODE
INCOME
INDOOR
INFOLD
INFORM
INGOAL
INGOLD
INGOOD
INGOTS
INHOCK
INHOME
INIONS
INJOKE
INLOVE
INMOST
INPORT
INPOUR
INROAD
INSOLE
INTOIT
INTONE
INTOTO
INTOWN
INVOKE
INWOVE
ONEOFF
ONEONE
ONEOUT
ONFOOT
ONHOLD
ONIONS
ONIONY
ONLOAD
ONLOAN
ONPOST
ONTOUR
SNOODS
SNOOKS
SNOOPS
SNOOPY
SNOOTS
SNOOTY
SNOOZE
SNOOZY
UNBOLD
UNBOLT
UNBORN
UNCOIL
UNCOLA
UNCOOL
UNCOOP
UNCORE
UNCORK
UNDOCK
UNDOER
UNDOES
UNDONE
UNFOLD
UNFOND
UNFORK
UNFOUL
UNFOXY
UNHOED
UNHOLY
UNHOOD
UNHOOK
UNIONS
UNJOIN
UNLOAD
UNLOCK
UNLOOP
UNLOST
UNMOLD
UNMOOR
UNMOWN
UNPOSH
UNPOTS
UNROBE
UNROLL
UNROOF
UNROOT
UNROPE
UNROVE
UNSOFT
UNSOLD
UNSOLE
UNSORE
UNSORT
UNSOUR
UNSOWN
UNTOLD
UNTORN
UNVOID
UNWORN
UNWOVE
UNYOKE
UNZONE

•N••O•

ANALOG
ANCHOR
ANCHOS
ANDHOW
ANDROS
ANGKOR
ANGLOS
ANTCOW
ANTRON
ANYHOW
ENAMOR
ENBLOC
ENDSON
ENEROS
ENIDOK
ENROOT
GNAWON
GNOMON
INABOX
INAFOG
INAPOD
INAROW
INCHON
INDOOR
INFLOW
INGOOD
INKPOT
INSPOT
INTROS
INTWOS
KNEWOF
KNOWOF
ONAHOP
ONETON
ONFOOT
ONSHOW
SNAPON
SNOBOL
UNCLOG
UNCOOL
UNCOOP
UNHOOD
UNHOOK
UNIPOD
UNISOM
UNISON
UNKNOT
UNLOOP
UNMOOR
UNROOF
UNROOT
UNSHOD
UNSHOE
UNSLOW
UNSTOP
UNSTOW
UNTROD

•N•••O

ANATTO
ANGELO
ANTERO
ANTIGO
ENCINO
ENDURO
ENESCO
ENHALO
ENRICO
ENTERO
ENTOMO
ENVIRO
INDIGO
INITIO
INTOTO
INVIVO
ONAUTO
ONEIRO
ONETWO
PNEUMO
SNAPTO
UNESCO
UNHERO

••NO••

ADNOUN
ANNOYS
ARNOLD
ATNOON
BANONS
BENOIT
BENOTE
CANOED
CANOER
CANOES
CANOLA
CANONS
CANOPY
CANOVA
CONOCO
CONOID
DANOVA
DENOTE
DENOVO
DONORA
DONORS
DONOSO
DYNODE
ELNORA
FANONS
FANOUT
GENOAN
GENOAS
GENOME
GENOVA
GONOGO
GYNOUS
HONORE
HONORS
HONOUR
IGNORE
IONONE
KENOBI
LANOSE
LENORE
LENOVO
LMNOPQ
MANOFF
MANORS
MINOAN
MINORS
MINOSO
MONODY
NANOOK
NINONS
NONONO
OENONE
OFNOTE
PANOPE
PANOUT
PINOAK
PINONS
PINOTS
RANOFF
RANOUT
RENOIR
RENONV
RENOTE
RENOWN
RUNOFF
RUNONS
RUNOUT
SENORA
SENORS
SHNOOK
SONOMA
SONORA
SUNOCO
SYNODS
TANOAK
TENONE
TENONS
TENORS
TINORE
VENOMS
VENORA
VENOSE
VENOUS
VINOUS
WINONA
WINOUT
WONOUT
ZANONI

••N•O•

AMNION
AMNIOS
ATNOON
BANCOS
BANGON
BANGOR
BANJOS
BANKON
BANLON
BENBOW
BENSON
BENTON
BENTOS
BENZOL
BINGOS
BINYON
BONBON
BONGOS
BONMOT
BONTON
BUNCOS
BUNION
BUNKOS
BUNTON
CANDOR
CANNON
CANNOT
CANTON
CANTOO
CANTOR
CANTOS
CANYON
CENSOR
CENTOS
CINEOL
CONDOR
CONDOS
CONGOU
CONJOB
CONNOR
CONROY
CONVOY
DANIOS
DANNON
DANSON
DANTON
DENMOM
DENTON
DINEON
DONEOK
DONJON
DUNLOP
FANDOM
FANION
FINKON
FONDOF
GANNON
GONEON
GUNDOG
GUNFOR
HANDON
HANGON
HANLON
HANSOM
HANSON
HENSON
HINTON
HUNGON
ISNTOK
JONSON
JUNCOS
JUNIOR
JUNTOS
KANTOR
KENDOS
KENTON
KENYON
KINDOF
KINKOS
LANDON
LANDOR
LANSON
LANTOS
LENNON
LENNOX
LENTOS
LINTON
LONDON
LONNOL
LYNDON
MANAOS
MANGOS
MANNON
MANZON
MENJOU
MENTOR
MENTOS
MINION
MINNOW
MONDOS
MONGOL
MONGOS
MONROE
MUNROE
NANOOK
NONCOM
NONGOD
PANTOS
PENNON
PENROD
PINBOY
PINION
PINKOS
PINSON
PINTOS
PINZON
RANCOR
RANDOM
RANFOR
RANLOW
RANSOM
RENTON
RENVOI
RONDOS
RONSON
RUNFOR
RUNLOW
RUNSON
RUNYON
SANTOS
SANYOS
SENDON
SENHOR
SENIOR
SENSOR
SENTON
SHNOOK
SUNBOW
SUNDOG
SUNGOD
TANGOS
TENDON
TENSOR
TENTON
TINGOD
TINPOT
TONDOS
TONSOF
VENDOR
VINSON
VINTON
WANTON
WENTON
WINDOM
WINDOW
WINNOW
WINSOR
WONTON
WYNTON
YANGON
YANKON
YENFOR
ZENDOS

••N••O

AINTSO
ALNICO
BANQUO
BENITO
BINDTO
BONITO
CANTOO
CENTRO
CONCHO
CONOCO
DANILO
DENDRO
DENIRO
DENOVO
DINERO
DONESO
DONETO
DONOSO
DONTGO
DYNAMO
ELNINO
FANGIO
FINITO
GINGKO
GINKGO
GONETO
GONOGO
GUNGHO
GYNECO
HONCHO
LANDHO
LENDTO
LENOVO
LENTTO
MANERO
MENUDO
MINOSO
MONACO
NINGBO
NONEGO
NONONO
NONPRO
NUNCIO
NUNZIO
PANCHO
PANINO
PINERO
PONCHO

RANCHO
RENATO
RENFRO
RENTTO
RUNSTO
SANCHO
SANDRO
SANGTO
SENDTO
SENTTO
SINGTO
SUNGTO
SUNOCO
TENDTO
TENTWO
TENUTO
TUNETO
VENETO
WANTTO
WENTTO
WONTDO
WONTGO

•••NO•
ACTNOW
ALANON
AMINOR
AMINOS
ATONOF
BEANOS
BEINON
BMINOR
BRUNOR
BUENOS
BUYNOW
BYENOW
CANNON
CANNOT
CHINOS
CMINOR
COINOP
CONNOR
CPSNOW
CURNOW
DANNON
DAWNON
DESNOS
DIDNOT
DMINOR
DOWNON
DUENOS
EGGNOG
ELINOR
EMINOR
ERENOW
ETHNOS
FAWNON
FMINOR
FORNOW
FTKNOX
GAINON
GANNON
GAYNOR
GMINOR
GOUNOD
GUANOS
GUVNOR
HOBNOB
HOWNOW
HYPNOS
IAMNOT
IDONOT
IRONON
ITSNOT
IVANOV
JOANOU
KEENON
KLMNOP
KRONOR
LEANON
LEMNOS
LENNON
LENNOX
LIENOR
LLANOS
LONNOL
LOTNOS
MAGNOL
MAGNON
MANNON
MIGNON
MINNOW
NOTNOW
NOWNOW
OPENON
PAGNOL
PAYNOW
PENNON
PERNOD
PHENOL
PHENOM
PHONOS
PIANOS
PLANON
RADNOR
RAINON
REKNOT
RHINOS
SCHNOZ
SEWNON
SIGNON
SIGNOR
STENOG
STENOS
SUENOS
TILNOW
TURNON
UNKNOT
VERNON
WARNOF
WHYNOT
WHYNOW
WINNOW

•••N•O
AKINTO
ALONSO
ALONZO
BAGNIO
BIANCO
BLANCO
BOINGO
BORNEO
BRANDO
BRONCO
BRONKO
CHANGO
CRANIO
CUANDO
CUANTO
ERYNGO
EVENSO
FERNAO
FRANCO
GOINTO
GRINGO
ICANSO
IDUNNO
ISINTO
LEANTO
MEANTO
OBENTO
ODONTO
OPENTO
PLANTO
PRONTO
PUENZO
SEENTO
SHINTO
STINKO
TRENTO
TURNTO

••••NO
ACCTNO
ADRENO
ALBANO
ALBINO
ALVINO
AQUINO
ARSENO
AVEENO
CAMINO
CASINO
CATANO
CHRONO
CIMINO
CYRANO
DELANO
DOMINO
ELNINO
ELRENO
ENCINO
FIVENO
FOURNO
FRESNO
GIORNO
GITANO
GIUGNO
GOLINO
GUGINO
HAVENO
HECKNO
HELLNO
IDUNNO
IMMUNO
ISAYNO
JKLMNO
JOURNO
KIMONO
LADINO
LATINO
LUPINO
MARINO
MERINO
MILANO
MORENO
MURANO
NAGANO
NONONO
ORSINO
PACINO
PANINO
PEPINO
PISANO
POCONO
RACINO
RODINO
ROMANO
SAIDNO
SAYSNO
SOLANO
STERNO
TECHNO
TEJANO
TICINO
TORINO
VOTENO
YOSANO

N•P•••
NAPACA
NAPALM
NAPERY
NAPHTA
NAPIER
NAPKIN
NAPLES
NAPOLI
NAPPED
NAPPER
NAPPES
NAPPIE
NEPALI
NEPEAN
NEPHEW
NEPHRO
NIPPED
NIPPER
NIPPLE
NIPPON
NIPSAT
NIPSEY
NIPUPS
NOPALS
NOPETS
NOPQRS
NOPROB
NYPOST

N••P••
NAPPED
NAPPER
NAPPES
NAPPIE
NETPAY
NIPPED
NIPPER
NIPPLE
NIPPON
NONPAR
NONPRO
NTUPLE
NYMPHS

N•••P•
NINEPM
NIPUPS
NLMVPS
NOHOPE
NOTIPS

N••••P
NAILUP
NEXTUP
NINEUP
NOHELP
NOSEUP
NOSOAP
NOSTEP

•NP•••
INPARK
INPART
INPAWN
INPINK
INPLAY
INPORT
INPOUR
INPUTS
ONPOST
UNPACK
UNPAID
UNPALE
UNPAWN
UNPEEL
UNPEGS
UNPENS
UNPENT
UNPICK
UNPILE
UNPINS
UNPLAN
UNPLUG
UNPOSH
UNPOTS
UNPRIM
UNPURE

•N•P••
ENDPIN
INAPET
INAPIE
INAPOD
INKPAD
INKPOT
INSPAN
INSPOT
INUPIK
MNOPQR
ONAPAR
ONEPIN
ONSPEC
SNAPAT
SNAPON
SNAPPY
SNAPTO
SNAPUP
SNIPED
SNIPER
SNIPES
SNIPPY
SNOPES
UNEPIC
UNIPED
UNIPOD
UNOPEN
UNSPAN
UNSPUN

•N••P•
ENRAPT
INCAPS
INCEPT
ONEUPS
ONTAPE
SNAPPY
SNIPPY
SNOOPS
SNOOPY
UNCAPS
UNKEPT
UNRIPE
UNRIPS
UNROPE
UNTAPE
UNWEPT
UNZIPS

•N•••P
ANTEUP
ENCAMP
ENDSUP
ENTRAP
ENWRAP
INDEEP
INSTEP
KNOTUP
ONAHOP
ONELAP
ONRAMP
SNAGUP
SNAPUP
UNCLIP
UNCOOP
UNDEEP
UNGRIP
UNHASP
UNLIMP
UNLOOP
UNSHIP
UNSNAP
UNSTEP
UNSTOP
UNTRAP
UNWRAP

••NP••
NONPAR
NONPRO
PENPAL
TENPIN
TINPAN
TINPOT

••N•P•
CANAPE
CANOPY
LENAPE
LMNOPQ
MANAPE
NINEPM
PANOPE
PENGPU
PINUPS
RUNUPS
SUNUPS

••N••P
BANGUP
BANKUP
BINDUP
BONEUP
DONEUP
DUNLAP
DUNLOP
GANGUP
GINSUP
GONEUP
GUNLAP
HANDUP
HANGUP
HUNGUP
HUNTUP
LANDUP
LINEUP
LINKUP
NINEUP
OWNSUP
PENSUP
PENTUP
PINSUP
PONYUP
RANGUP
RINGUP
RUNGUP
RUNSUP
SENDUP
SENTUP
TANKUP
TINCUP
TONEUP
TUNEUP
WENTUP
WINDUP

•••NP•
GRANPA

•••N•P
BURNUP
CARNAP
CATNAP
CATNIP
CHINUP
COINOP
DOGNAP
EVENUP
JOINUP
KIDNAP
KLMNOP
OPENUP
PETNAP
PRENUP
RESNAP
SEENUP
SEWNUP
SIGNUP
TORNUP
TURNIP
TURNUP
UNSNAP
WETNAP

N•Q•••
NYQUIL

N••Q••
NOPQRS

N••••Q
NASDAQ

•NQ•••
ENQUAD

•N•Q••
UNIQUE

•N••Q•
MNOPQR

••NQ••
BANQUE
BANQUO
CINQUE
MANQUE
YANQUI

••N••Q
LMNOPQ

•••NQ•
QUINQU

N•R•••
NARADA
NARCOS
NARIAL
NARINE
NARITA
NARNIA
NARROW
NARVIK
NEREID
NERMAL
NERNST
NEROLI
NERONE
NERUDA
NERVAL
NERVED
NERVES
NORAIN
NORDIC
NORDOI
NOREEN
NORELL
NORENT
NORGAY
NORIAS
NORISK
NORITE
NORMAL
NORMAN
NOROOM
NORRIS
NORTHS
NORTON
NORUNS
NORUSH
NORVAL
NORWAY
NURSED
NURSER
NURSES

N••R••
NACRED
NACRES
NAIRAS
NARROW
NATRON
NBCRED
NEARBY
NEARED
NEARER
NEARLY
NEARTO
NEHRUS
NEURAL
NEUROL
NEURON
NEXRAD
NFORTY
NIMROD
NITRES
NITRIC
NITROS
NOIRES
NOIRET
NOIRON
NONRUN
NOPROB
NORRIS
NUTRIA

N•••R•
NABORS
NADIRS
NAMERS
NAPERY
NATURE
NBAERS
NEPHRO
NEVERS
NEWARK
NEWERA
NFLERS
NHLERS
NIEKRO
NINERS
NITERS
NITERY
NIXERS
NOMBRE
NOMORE
NONART
NONARY
NONPRO
NOPQRS
NOSERS
NOSTRA
NOTARY
NOTERS
NOYORI
NSTARS
NUBIRA
NUMERO

N••••R
NABBER
NAGGER
NAILER
NAIVER
NAPIER
NAPPER
NASCAR
NASSER
NATTER
NEARER
NEATER
NECKER
NECTAR
NEEDER
NESTER
NESTOR
NETHER
NETTER
NEUTER
NEWCAR
NEWMAR
NICKER
NICKJR
NIGHER
NIPPER
NOBLER
NODDER
NODEAR
NOFAIR
NONPAR
NONWAR
NOONER
NOOSER
NOSHER
NOSIER
NOSTER
NOTFAR
NOTFOR
NUBBER
NUDGER
NUMBER
NURSER
NUTTER

•NR•••
ENRAGE
ENRANK
ENRAPT
ENRICH
ENRICO
ENROBE
ENROLL
ENROLS
ENROOT
INRAGS
INROAD
INRUNS
INRUSH
ONRAMP
ONRICE
ONRUSH
UNRACK
UNRASH
UNREAD
UNREAL
UNREEL
UNRENT
UNREST
UNRIFE
UNRIGS
UNRIPE
UNRIPS
UNROBE
UNROLL
UNROOF
UNROOT
UNROPE
UNROVE
UNRUDE
UNRUED
UNRULY
UNRUNG
UNRUST

•N•R••
ANARCH
ANDRAE
ANDREA
ANDREI
ANDRES
ANDREW
ANDREY
ANDRIC
ANDROS
ANERGY
ANORAK
ANTRAL
ANTRES
ANTRIM
ANTRON
ANTRUM
ENARMS
ENCRES
ENDRAN
ENDRUN
ENERGY
ENEROS
ENGRAM
ENORME
ENTRAP
ENTREE
ENTREZ
ENURED
ENURES
ENWRAP
GNARLS
GNARLY
GNARRS
INARAY
INARCH
INAREA
INAROW
INARUG
INARUT
INBRED
INGRAM
INGRAY
INGRES
INGREY
INGRID
INTRAY
INTROS
INURED
INURES
KNARRS
KNARRY
KNURLS
KNURLY
ONERUN
SNARED
SNARER
SNARES
SNARFS
SNARKS
SNARKY
SNARLS
SNARLY
SNORED
SNORER
SNORES
SNORRI
SNORTS
SNORTY
UNARMS
UNDRAW
UNDREW
UNFREE
UNGRIP
UNORAL
UNPRIM
UNTRAP
UNTRIG
UNTROD
UNTRUE
UNWRAP

•N••R•
ANDERS
ANGERS
ANGORA
ANITRA
ANKARA
ANSARA
ANTERO
ENBERG
ENCORE
ENDERS
ENDORA
ENDURE
ENDURO
ENGIRD
ENGIRT
ENSURE
ENTERO
ENTERS
ENTIRE
ENVIRO
GNARRS
INBORN
INCURS
INDIRA
INFERS
INFIRM
INFORM
INHERE
INJURE
INJURY
INKERS
INNERS
INPARK
INPART
INPORT
INSERT
INSURE
INTERJ
INTERN
INTERS
INTURN
INVERT
INWARD
KNARRS
KNARRY
ONEARM
ONEIRO
ONFIRE
ONHIRE
ONWARD
SNEERS
SNEERY
SNORRI
UNBARE
UNBARS
UNBORN
UNBURY
UNCORE
UNCORK
UNCURB
UNCURL
UNDERS
UNFIRM
UNFORK
UNFURL
UNGIRD
UNGIRT
UNHERO
UNHIRE
UNHURT
UNMIRY
UNPURE
UNSERE
UNSORE
UNSORT
UNSURE
UNTORN
UNWARY
UNWORN

•N•••R
ANCHOR
ANGKOR
ANGLER
ANSWER
ANTHER
ANTLER
ENAMOR
ENDEAR
ENSLER
ENVIER
GNAWER
INANER
INCHER
INDOOR
INEVER
INFEAR
INGEAR
INGMAR
INKIER
INPOUR
INSTIR
KNIFER
KNOWER
MNOPQR
ONAGER
ONAPAR
ONECAR
ONSTAR
ONTOUR
SNAKER
SNARER
SNIDER
SNIPER
SNORER
SNYDER
UNDOER
UNFAIR
UNHAIR
UNITER
UNMOOR
UNSOUR
UNTIER

••NR••
CONRAD
CONROY
FUNRUN
GENRES
HENRIK
HENRYI
HENRYK
HENRYV
KONRAD
MANRAY
MONROE
MUNROE
NONRUN
PENROD
SUNRAY
VANRYN

••N•R•
BINARY
BONERS
BONERZ
CANARD
CANARY
CANERS
CENTRE
CENTRI
CENTRO
CONERS
CONTRA
CONTRE
CONURE
CUNARD
DENARI
DENARS
DENARY
DENDRA
DENDRI
DENDRO
DENIRO
DINARS
DINERO
DINERS
DONORA
DONORS
ELNORA
FINERY
GANTRY
GENERA
GENTRY
GONERS
HENDRY
HONERS
HONORE
HONORS
HUNGRY
IGNORE
INNERS
KUNDRY
LANARK
LANDRY
LENARD
LENORE
LINERS
LONERS
LYNYRD
MANERO
MANORS
MANTRA
MANURE
MINERS
MINORS
MUNERA
NINERS
NONART
NONARY
NONPRO
ORNERY
OWNERS
OXNARD
PANFRY
PANTRY
PENURY
PINERO
PINERS
PINERY
RANDRY
RENARD
RENFRO
RUNDRY
SANDRA
SANDRO
SANGRE
SENARY
SENORA
SENORS
SENTRA
SENTRY
SONARS
SONDRA
SONORA
SUNDRY
TANTRA
TENORS
TENURE
TINORE
TONERS
TUNDRA

TUNERS
VANARK
VENERA
VENIRE
VENORA
VINERS
VINERY
WINERY
WINTRY
ZONERS

••N••R
ASNEAR
BANDER
BANGER
BANGOR
BANKER
BANNER
BANTER
BENDER
BENHUR
BINDER
BINGER
BONDER
BONIER
BONNER
BUNKER
BUNTER
CANCER
CANDOR
CANIER
CANKER
CANNER
CANOER
CANTER
CANTOR
CENSER
CENSOR
CENTER
CINDER
CONAIR
CONCUR
CONDOR
CONFER
CONGER
CONKER
CONNOR
DANCER
DANDER
DANGER
DANKER
DANNER
DENIER
DENSER
DENVER
DINGER
DINNER
DONDER
DONNER
DUNBAR
DUNKER
DUNNER
FANNER
FENCER
FENDER
FENNER
FINDER
FINGER
FONDER
FUNDER
FUNFUR
GANDER
GANGER
GENDER
GENXER
GINGER
GONEAR
GUNFOR
GUNNAR
GUNNER
GUNTER
HANDER
HANGAR
HANGER
HANKER
HENNER
HINDER
HINTER
HONKER
HONOUR
HUNGER
HUNKER
HUNTER
JANUAR
JENNER
JINXER
JUNGER
JUNIOR
JUNKER
KANDER
KANTOR
KENNER
KINDER
LANCER
LANDER
LANDOR
LANGER
LANIER
LANKER
LENDER
LINDER
LINEAR
LINGER
LINIER
LINKER
LINTER
LINZER
LONGER
LUNGER
LUNKER
MANGER
MANNER
MCNAIR
MENDER
MENTOR
MINCER
MINDER
MINTER
MONGER
NONPAR
NONWAR
OINKER
PANDER
PANIER
PANNER
PANTER
PANZER
PENNER
PINCER
PINDAR
PINGER
PINIER
PINKER
PINNER
PINTER
PONDER
PUNIER
PUNKER
PUNNER
PUNTER
QINTAR
RANCOR
RANFOR
RANGER
RANKER
RANTER
RENDER
RENOIR
RENTER
RINGER
RINSER
RUNFOR
RUNNER
SANDER
SANGER
SENDER
SENHOR
SENIOR
SENSOR
SINGER
SINKER
SINNER
SUNDER
TANKER
TANNER
TENDER
TENNER
TENSER
TENSOR
TENTER
TINDER
TINEAR
TINIER
TINKER
TINNER
TINTER
TONIER
VANIER
VENDER
VENDOR
VENEER
VENNER
VENTER
VINIER
WANDER
WANIER
WANNER
WANTER
WENNER
WINCER
WINDER
WINGER
WINIER
WINKER
WINNER
WINSOR
WINTER
WONDER
WYNTER
YANKER
YENFOR
YONDER
ZANIER
ZENGER
ZINGER
ZONKER

•••NR•
AMENRA
AMONRA
OHENRY
THENRA

•••N•R
ALINER
AMINOR
ATONER
BANNER
BMINOR
BONNER
BRINER
BRUNOR
BURNER
CANNER
CARNER
CLONER
CMINOR
COINER
CONNOR
CORNER
DAMNER
DANNER
DARNER
DINNER
DMINOR
DONNER
DOWNER
DRONER
DUNNER
EARNER
EISNER
ELINOR
EMINOR
EVENER
FAFNER
FAFNIR
FAINER
FANNER
FAWNER
FENNER
FMINOR
GAINER
GARNER
GAYNOR
GMINOR
GUNNAR
GUNNER
GUVNOR
HEFNER
HENNER
HOHNER
HORNER
INANER
IRONER
JENNER
JOINER
JOYNER
KAVNER
KEENER
KENNER
KRONER
KRONOR
KRONUR
LEANER
LERNER
LIENOR
LIMNER
LOANER
MAINER
MANNER
MARNER
MEANER
MILNER
MOANER
MOLNAR
MOONER
NOONER
OPENER
OPINER
PANNER
PAWNER
PENNER
PHONER
PINNER
PLANAR
PLANER
POGNER
PRUNER
PUNNER
RADNER
RADNOR
RAGNAR
RAINER
RATNER
REINER
REUNER
RUDNER
RUINER
RUNNER
SEINER
SHINER
SIGNER
SIGNOR
SINNER
SOONER
SPINER
STONER
SUMNER
TANNER
TEENER
TENNER
TINNER
TOWNER
TURNER
TWINER
VAINER
VENNER
WAGNER
WANNER
WAPNER
WARNER
WEANER
WENNER
WERNER
WHINER
WIENER
WIGNER
WINNER
YAWNER

NS••••
NSTARS

N•S•••
NASALS
NASCAR
NASDAQ
NASEBY
NASHES
NASHUA
NASSAU
NASSER
NESBIT
NESSEN
NESSES
NESSIE
NESSUS
NESTEA
NESTED
NESTER
NESTIN
NESTLE
NESTOR
NISANS
NISEIS
NISSAN
NISSEN
NOSALE
NOSALT
NOSEIN
NOSERS
NOSEUP
NOSHED
NOSHER
NOSHES
NOSHOW
NOSIER
NOSILY
NOSING
NOSOAP
NOSTEP
NOSTER
NOSTRA

N••S••
NADSAT
NAGSAT
NANSEN
NASSAU
NASSER
NAUSEA
NAYSAY
NEESON
NEISSE
NELSON
NEOSHO
NESSEN
NESSES
NESSIE
NESSUS
NEVSKI
NEVSKY
NEWSIE
NEWSOM
NIPSAT
NIPSEY
NISSAN
NISSEN
NODSAT
NODSTO
NOESIS
NOISED
NOISES
NOOSED
NOOSER
NOOSES
NTESTS
NURSED
NURSER
NURSES

N•••S•
NEISSE
NERNST
NEWEST
NEWISH
NICEST
NLEAST
NLWEST
NOCOST
NODOSE
NOFUSS
NOLESS
NOLOSE
NOLOSS
NONUSE
NORISK
NORUSH
NOWISE
NUDEST
NUDISM
NUDIST
NYPOST

N••••S
NABOBS
NABORS
NACHAS
NACHOS
NACRES
NADIRS
NAIADS
NAIRAS
NAKFAS
NAMERS
NANTES
NAPLES
NAPPES
NARCOS
NASALS
NASHES
NAUTES
NAVELS
NAVIES
NBAERS
NBOMBS
NEHRUS
NEIGHS
NELLIS
NERVES
NESSES
NESSUS
NEVERS
NEVINS
NEWELS
NEWIES
NFLERS
NHLERS
NICADS
NICHES
NICIAS
NIECES
NIETAS
NIETOS
NIEVES
NIGHTS
NIKONS
NIMBUS
NINERS
NINJAS
NINONS
NINTHS
NIPUPS
NISANS
NISEIS
NITERS
NITRES
NITROS
NIXERS
NIXIES
NIXONS
NLMVPS
NOBELS
NOBLES
NOBUTS
NOCHES
NODOUS
NOESIS
NOFEES
NOFUSS
NOHITS
NOIRES
NOISES
NOKIAS
NOKIDS
NOLESS
NOLOSS
NOMADS
NONETS
NONEWS
NONGAS
NOONES
NOOSES
NOPALS
NOPETS
NOPQRS
NORIAS
NORRIS
NORTHS
NORUNS
NOSERS
NOSHES
NOTERS
NOTIPS
NOVELS
NOVIAS
NOVIOS
NOWAYS
NSTARS
NTESTS
NTILES
NUDGES
NUECES
NUEVES
NULLOS
NURSES
NYALAS
NYJETS
NYLONS
NYMETS
NYMPHS

•NS•••
ANSARA
ANSATE
ANSEIS
ANSELM
ANSWER
ENSATE
ENSEAL
ENSEAT
ENSIGN
ENSILE
ENSLER
ENSOUL
ENSUED
ENSUES
ENSURE
INSANA
INSANE
INSEAM
INSECT
INSERT
INSETS
INSIDE
INSIST
INSITU
INSOLE
INSPAN
INSPOT
INSTAL
INSTEP
INSTIL
INSTIR
INSULT
INSURE
INSYNC
ONSALE
ONSETS
ONSHOW
ONSIDE
ONSITE
ONSPEC
ONSTAR
UNSAFE
UNSAGE
UNSAID
UNSAWN
UNSAYS
UNSEAL
UNSEAM
UNSEAT
UNSEEN
UNSELD
UNSELL
UNSENT
UNSERE
UNSEWN
UNSEWS
UNSEXY
UNSHED
UNSHIP
UNSHOD
UNSHOE
UNSHUT
UNSICK
UNSKEW
UNSLIM
UNSLOW
UNSMUG
UNSNAG
UNSNAP
UNSNUG
UNSOFT
UNSOLD
UNSOLE
UNSORE
UNSORT
UNSOUR
UNSOWN
UNSPAN
UNSPUN
UNSTEP
UNSTOP
UNSTOW
UNSUED
UNSUNG
UNSUNK
UNSURE

•N•S••
ANGSTS
ANISES
DNASES
ENDSAT
ENDSIN
ENDSIT
ENDSON
ENDSUP
ENESCO
ENISLE
GNOSES
GNOSIS
INASEC
INESSE
INKSAC
INKSIN
ONESEC
ONESET
ONUSES
UNDSET
UNESCO
UNISEX
UNISOM
UNISON
UNISYS
UNUSED

•N••S•
DNAASE
ENCASE
ENDASH
ENDUSE
ENLIST
ENMESH
GNEISS
INCASE
INCASH
INCISE
INCUSE
INDASH
INESSE
INFEST
INFUSE
INGEST
INJEST
INMOST
INNESS
INRUSH
INSIST
INVEST
ONBASE
ONDISK
ONEISH
ONPOST
ONRUSH
RNAASE
UNBUSY
UNCASE
UNCASK
UNCAST
UNEASE
UNEASY
UNHASP
UNHUSK
UNJUST
UNLASH
UNLESS
UNLOST
UNLUSH
UNMASK
UNMAST
UNMESH
UNPOSH
UNRASH
UNREST
UNRUST
UNWISE
UNWISH

•N•••S
ANANAS
ANCHOS
ANDERS
ANDRES
ANDROS
ANELES
ANGELS
ANGERS
ANGLES
ANGLOS
ANGSTS
ANIMAS
ANIMES
ANIMUS
ANIONS
ANISES
ANJOUS
ANKLES
ANNALS
ANNEES
ANNIES
ANNOYS
ANNULS
ANODES
ANOLES
ANSEIS
ANTICS
ANTRES
ANUBIS
ANVILS
ANYONS
ANZACS
CNOTES
DNASES
ENACTS
ENARMS
ENATES
ENCRES
ENDERS
ENDOWS
ENDUES
ENEROS
ENGELS
ENIACS
ENJOYS
ENNIUS
ENNUIS
ENOILS
ENOKIS
ENOTES
ENROLS
ENSUES
ENTERS
ENURES
ENVIES
ENVOIS
ENVOYS
GNARLS
GNARRS
GNEISS
GNOMES
GNOSES
GNOSIS
GNOTES
INAGES
INCANS
INCAPS
INCHES
INCURS
INDIES
INDUES
INFERS
INGELS
INGLES
INGOTS
INGRES
INIONS
INKERS
INKLES
INLAWS
INLAYS
INLETS
INNERS
INNESS
INNIES
INONES
INPUTS
INRAGS
INRUNS
INSETS
INTENS
INTERS
INTROS
INTWOS
INUITS
INURES
KNACKS
KNARRS
KNAVES
KNEADS
KNEELS
KNELLS
KNICKS
KNIFES
KNIVES
KNOCKS
KNOLLS
KNOTTS
KNOUTS
KNOWNS
KNURLS
ONCLES
ONDITS
ONEUPS
ONIONS
ONLAYS
ONSETS
ONUSES
ONYXES
SNACKS
SNAFUS
SNAILS
SNAKES
SNARES
SNARFS
SNARKS
SNARLS
SNATHS
SNEAKS
SNEERS
SNELLS
SNICKS
SNIFFS
SNIPES
SNOODS
SNOOKS
SNOOPS
SNOOTS
SNOPES
SNORES
SNORTS
SNOUTS
SNUFFS
TNOTES
UNAMIS
UNARMS
UNBAGS
UNBARS
UNBITS
UNBUDS
UNCAPS
UNCLES
UNDAMS
UNDERS
UNDIES
UNDIMS
UNDOES
UNFITS
UNGAGS
UNGUES
UNGUIS
UNHATS
UNIATS
UNICES
UNIONS
UNISYS
UNITAS
UNITES
UNJAMS
UNLAYS
UNLESS
UNMANS
UNMEWS
UNPEGS
UNPENS
UNPINS
UNPOTS
UNRIGS
UNRIPS
UNSAYS
UNSEWS
UNTIES
UNWIGS
UNZIPS
VNECKS

••NS••
BENSEY
BENSON
BONSAI
BUNSEN
CENSED
CENSER
CENSES
CENSOR
CENSUS
CONSUL
DANSES
DANSON
DENSER
EENSIE
FINSEN
GINSUP
GUNSEL
GUNSHY
GUNSIT
HANSAS
HANSEL
HANSES
HANSOM
HANSON
HENSON
HONSHU
JANSEN
JENSEN
JONSON
KANSAN
KANSAS
KENSIT
KINSEY
KINSKI
LANSKY
LANSON
LENSED
LENSES
MANSES
MENSAL
MENSAN
MENSCH
NANSEN
OWNSUP
PANSIN
PENSEE
PENSIN
PENSUP
PINSON
PINSUP
RANSOM
RINSED
RINSER
RINSES
RONSON
RUNSAT
RUNSBY
RUNSIN
RUNSON
RUNSTO
RUNSUP
SANSEI
SENSED
SENSEI
SENSEN
SENSES
SENSOR
SUNSET
TENSED
TENSER
TENSES
TENSOR
TINSEL
TONSIL
TONSOF
VINSON
WINSAT
WINSBY
WINSOR
YENSID

••N•S•
AINTSO
ALNASL
ARNESS
BANISH
DANISH
DENISE
DONESO
DONOSO
DYNAST
ERNEST
FINEST
FINISH
HONEST
INNESS
IONISE
JONESS
JONESY
LANOSE
MANUSH
MINOSO

MONGST
MONISM
MONIST
NONUSE
PUNISH
RENEST
SANEST
SINISE
VANISH
VENOSE
WINISH
ZENIST

••N••S

AENEAS
AMNIOS
ANNALS
ANNEES
ANNIES
ANNOYS
ANNULS
APNEAS
ARNEIS
ARNESS
ARNIES
BANCOS
BANJOS
BANONS
BANTUS
BENTOS
BINGES
BINGOS
BONERS
BONGOS
BONNES
BONZES
BUNCOS
BUNDTS
BUNKOS
CANALS
CANERS
CANIDS
CANNAS
CANNES
CANOES
CANONS
CANTOS
CANVAS
CENSES
CENSUS
CENTAS
CENTOS
CONCHS
CONDOS
CONERS
CONEYS
CONGAS
CONGES
CONICS
CONIES
CYNICS
DANCES
DANIOS
DANNYS
DANSES
DANTES
DENARS
DENIES
DENIMS
DENNIS
DENNYS
DINARS
DINERS
DINGUS
DINKAS
DONEES
DONETS
DONORS
DONUTS
DUNCES
DUNDAS
DYNELS
ENNIUS
ENNUIS
FANONS
FANTAS
FENCES
FINALS
FINCAS
FONDAS
FONDUS
FUNGUS
GANEFS
GANGES
GENETS
GENIES
GENIUS
GENOAS
GENRES
GENTES
GONERS
GONUTS
GYNOUS
HANSAS
HANSES
HENGES
HENNAS
HINDUS
HINGES
HINGIS
HONDAS
HONERS
HONEYS
HONORS
INNERS
INNESS
INNIES
IONICS
JANHUS
JINNIS
JINXES
JONAHS
JONESS
JUNCOS
JUNIUS
JUNTAS
JUNTOS
KANJIS
KANSAS
KENDOS
KINKOS
LANAIS
LANCES
LANDIS
LANDUS
LANTOS
LENSES
LENTOS
LINENS
LINERS
LINGUS
LONERS
LONGES
LUNDIS
LUNGES
LUNIKS
LYNXES
MANAOS
MANATS
MANDMS
MANETS
MANGAS
MANGOS
MANIAS
MANNAS
MANORS
MANSES
MANTAS
MANTIS
MENDES
MENTIS
MENTOS
MINCES
MINERS
MINGUS
MINIMS
MINORS
MINXES
MONADS
MONDES
MONDOS
MONETS
MONEYS
MONGOS
MONIES
MONTHS
MONZAS
MYNAHS
NANTES
NINERS
NINJAS
NINONS
NINTHS
NONETS
NONEWS
NONGAS
OHNUTS
OUNCES
OWNERS
PANCKS
PANDAS
PANDLS
PANELS
PANICS
PANNES
PANTOS
PENNIS
PINDUS
PINERS
PINKOS
PINNAS
PINONS
PINOTS
PINTOS
PINUPS
PONCAS
PONIES
PONZUS
PUNKAS
PUNTAS
QANTAS
RANEES
RANGES
RANIDS
RENEWS
RENGAS
RENINS
RENNES
RENTES
RINSES
RONDOS
RUNINS
RUNONS
RUNUPS
SANKAS
SANTAS
SANTOS
SANYOS
SENATS
SENNAS
SENORS
SENSES
SINEWS
SINGES
SONARS
SONDES
SONICS
SUNDAS
SUNNIS
SUNUPS
SYNCHS
SYNODS
SYNTHS
TANGOS
TANKAS
TANTES
TENETS
TENLBS
TENNIS
TENONS
TENORS
TENSES
TENTHS
TINCTS
TINGES
TONDOS
TONERS
TONICS
TONKAS
TONNES
TUNERS
TUNICS
UINTAS
USNEWS
VANNES
VENINS
VENOMS
VENOUS
VENTAS
VENUES
VINERS
VINOUS
VINYLS
WENCES
WENDYS
WINANS
WINCES
YENTAS
ZANIES
ZENDOS
ZONERS

•••NS•

ALONSO
EVENSO
FLENSE
GAINST
GDANSK
HEINSE
ICANSO
MAINST
NERNST
ODENSE
ORENSE
TEENSY
WEENSY

•••N•S

ADENIS
ADONIS
AGENAS
AGENTS
AGONES
AKENES
ALANIS
ALINES
ALONGS
AMANAS
AMANTS
AMENDS
AMENTS
AMINES
AMINOS
AMINUS
ANANAS
ARENAS
ASANAS
ATONES
AXONES
BAINES
BARNES
BEANOS
BEINGS
BHANGS
BIONTS
BLANKS
BLENDS
BLINDS
BLINIS
BLINKS
BLONDS
BLUNTS
BMINUS
BOINGS
BONNES
BOUNDS
BRANDS
BRANTS
BRINES
BRINGS
BRINKS
BRONCS
BRUNTS
BUENAS
BUENOS
BWANAS
BYRNES
CANNAS
CANNES
CARNES
CHANTS
CHINAS
CHINES
CHINKS
CHINOS
CHUNKS
CLANGS
CLANKS
CLINGS
CLINKS
CLONES
CLONKS
CLUNKS
CMINUS
COUNTS
CRANES
CRANKS
CRONES
CRONUS
CYGNUS
DANNYS
DAUNTS
DENNIS
DENNYS
DESNOS
DIENES
DJINNS
DMINUS
DOINGS
DOWNES
DRINGS
DRINKS
DRONES
DUENAS
DUENOS
EBANKS
EBONDS
ELANDS
EMENDS
ERINYS
ETHNOS
EVENAS
EVENTS
EWINGS
EZINES
FAENAS
FAINTS
FAUNAS
FAUNUS
FEINTS
FIENDS
FLANKS
FLINGS
FLINTS
FLUNKS
FOUNDS
FOUNTS
FRANCS
FRANKS
FRONDS
FRONTS
GAINES
GAYNES
GIANTS
GLANDS
GLINTS
GLYNIS
GOINGS
GRANDS
GRANTS
GRINDS
GRUNTS
GUANOS
HAINES
HAUNTS
HAYNES
HENNAS
HMONGS
HOUNDS
HYENAS
HYPNOS
ICINGS
IDENTS
IKINGS
IMINES
INONES
IRANIS
JAUNES
JAUNTS
JINNIS
JOINTS
KAUNAS
KERNES
KEYNES
LEMNOS
LIANAS
LIANES
LIANGS
LIGNES
LLANOS
LOTNOS
MAGNUS
MANNAS
MEDNIS
MESNES
MILNES
MOINES
MOUNDS
MOUNTS
NOONES
OMANIS
OPINES
ORANGS
ORANIS
ORANTS
ORINGS
OVINES
PAINTS
PANNES
PARNIS
PENNIS
PHONES
PHONOS
PIANOS
PINNAS
PLANAS
PLANBS
PLANES
PLANKS
PLANTS
PLINKS
PLONKS
PLUNKS
POINTS
POUNDS
PRANAS
PRANKS
PRINKS
PRINTS
PRONGS
PRUNES
QUINTS
RAINES
REINAS
REINES
REINKS
RENNES
REUNES
RHINOS
ROUNDS
SAINTS
SAUNAS
SCANTS
SCENAS
SCENES
SCENTS
SCONES
SEENAS
SEINES
SENNAS
SHANKS
SHINES
SHUNTS
SKANKS
SKINKS
SKUNKS
SLANGS
SLANTS
SLINGS
SLINKS
SOONAS
SOUNDS
SPANKS
SPENDS
SPINES
SPINKS
STANDS
STENOS
STENTS
STINGS
STINKS
STINTS
STONES
STUNTS
SUENOS
SUNNIS
SWANNS
SWINGS
TAINTS
TAUNTS
TBONDS
TBONES
TENNIS
TERNES
THANES
THANKS
THINGS
THINKS
THONGS
THUNKS
TMINUS
TONNES
TRANES
TRENDS
TRINES
TRUNKS
TWANGS
TWINES
UPENDS
URANUS
VANNES
VARNAS
VAUNTS
VIANDS
WARNES
WAYNES
WHANGS
WHINES
WOUNDS
WRINGS
WRONGS
ZOUNDS

••••NS

ACORNS
ADDINS
ADDONS
ADMINS
ADORNS
ALBANS
ALIENS
ALIGNS
AMIENS
ANIONS
ANYONS
APRONS
ARSONS
ARYANS
ASIANS
ASPENS
ATHENS
ATKINS
ATMANS
AVIANS
AXIONS
BACONS
BADUNS
BAIRNS
BANONS
BARONS
BASINS
BATONS
BBGUNS
BEGINS
BELONS
BEVANS
BISONS
BOSONS
BOSUNS
BRAINS
BROWNS
BRUINS
BURINS
BUYINS
BYTENS
CABINS
CAIRNS
CAJUNS
CANONS
CAPONS
CHAINS
CHIENS
CHURNS
CLEANS
CLOWNS
CODONS
COIGNS
COLONS
COOWNS
COTANS
COVENS
COWENS
COZENS
CRAINS
CROONS
CROWNS
CUBANS
CUMINS
CUTINS
DAVENS
DEDANS
DEIGNS
DEMONS
DIVANS
DJINNS
DOBYNS
DOGONS
DOYENS
DOZENS
DRAINS
DROWNS
EAKINS
EOSINS
EPSONS
EXCONS
FAGINS
FANONS
FEIGNS
FELONS
FIXINS
FLYINS
FREONS
FROWNS
FUTONS
GAMINS
GHAINS
GIVENS
GLEANS
GLUONS
GRAINS
GREENS
GROANS
GROINS
HAVENS
HAZANS
HEARNS
HELENS
HERONS
HITINS
HOGANS
HUMANS
HURONS
HYSONS
IGGINS
INCANS
INIONS
INRUNS
INTENS
IOWANS
JAPANS
JEVONS
KEARNS
KNOWNS
KORANS
KROONS
LAPINS
LATENS
LATINS
LAYINS
LEARNS
LEMANS
LEMONS
LIKENS
LIMANS
LINENS
LIVENS
LODENS
LOGANS
LOGINS
LOGONS
LORANS
LUDENS
LUMENS
MASONS
MATINS
MAVENS
MAVINS
MAYANS
MELONS
MESONS
MIDONS
MILANS
MIRINS
MORONS
MOURNS
MUTONS
NEVINS
NIKONS
NINONS
NISANS
NIXONS
NORUNS
NYLONS
OBGYNS
OCEANS
OCTANS
ODEONS
OLEINS
ONIONS
ORGANS
ORIONS
ORKANS
ORLONS
OSCANS
PAEANS
PAGANS
PARENS
PATENS
PECANS
PINONS
PISANS
PITONS
PLAINS
PRAWNS
PREENS
PUTONS
PYLONS
QUEENS
QUOINS
RAMENS
RAVENS
RAYONS
RECANS
RECONS
REDANS
REIGNS
REMANS
RENINS
REOWNS
REPENS
REPINS
RERUNS
RESINS
RETANS
RETINS
REWINS
RICANS
RIGANS
RIPENS
ROBINS
ROMANS
ROSINS
ROWANS
ROWENS
RUBENS
RUNINS
RUNONS
RUTINS
SALONS
SARANS
SATINS
SAXONS
SCIONS
SCORNS
SEDANS
SERINS
SEVENS
SEWONS
SHEENS
SIRENS
SITINS
SIVANS
SKEINS
SOLANS
SOLONS
SPAWNS
SPOONS
SPURNS
STAINS
STEINS
STERNS
SWAINS
SWANNS
SWOONS
TALONS
TAPINS
TAUONS
TENONS
TETONS
TEXANS
THORNS
TIEINS
TIGONS
TIPINS
TITANS
TOEINS
TOKENS
TOXINS
TOYONS
TRAINS
TWAINS
TWEENS
TYSONS
UCLANS
UHLANS
UNIONS
UNMANS
UNPENS
UNPINS
UTAHNS
UTURNS
VALENS
VEGANS
VENINS
VIXENS
VOLANS
VSIGNS
WAGONS
WAKENS
WAYANS
WEEUNS
WIDENS
WINANS
WIZENS
WOMANS
WOMENS
YEARNS
YUKONS
YUMANS
ZAYINS
ZAZENS
ZIPONS

NT••••

NTESTS
NTILES
NTUPLE

N•T•••

NATALE
NATANT
NATHAN
NATICK
NATION
NATIVE
NATRON
NATTER
NATURE
NETFUL
NETHER
NETHOU
NETMAN
NETMEN
NETPAY
NETTED
NETTER
NETTLE
NETTLY
NETTON
NITERS
NITERY
NITRES
NITRIC
NITROS
NITWIT
NOTAIL
NOTALL
NOTANY
NOTARY
NOTATE
NOTBAD
NOTCHY
NOTERS
NOTFAR
NOTFIT
NOTFOR
NOTHIN
NOTICE
NOTIFY
NOTILL
NOTIME
NOTING
NOTION
NOTIPS
NOTNEW
NOTNOW
NOTOLL
NOTONE
NOTOUT
NOTTOO
NOTYET
NOTYOU
NSTARS
NUTATE
NUTKIN
NUTLET
NUTMEG
NUTOIL
NUTRIA
NUTTED
NUTTER

N••T••

NANTES
NATTER
NAUTES
NEATEN
NEATER
NEATLY
NECTAR
NESTEA
NESTED
NESTER
NESTIN
NESTLE
NESTOR
NETTED
NETTER
NETTLE
NETTLY
NETTON
NEUTER
NEWTON
NEWTOY
NEXTEL
NEXTTO
NEXTUP
NIETAS
NIETOS
NINTHS
NOETIC
NONTAN
NONTAX
NOOTKA
NORTHS
NORTON
NOSTEP
NOSTER
NOSTRA
NOTTOO
NUTTED
NUTTER

N•••T•

NAMATH
NAPHTA
NARITA
NEARTO
NEEDTO
NEGATE
NEXTTO
NFORTY
NICETY
NIENTE
NIGHTS
NIGHTY
NIKITA
NIMITZ
NINETY
NOBUTS
NODSTO
NOHITS
NONETS
NOPETS
NORITE
NOTATE
NOVATO
NOVOTE
NTESTS
NUDITY
NUTATE
NYJETS
NYMETS

N••••T

NADSAT
NAGSAT
NAILIT
NAMEIT
NATANT
NAUGHT
NEEDNT
NERNST
NESBIT
NEWEST
NEWHAT
NIBLET
NICEST
NIPSAT
NITWIT

NLEAST
NLWEST
NOCENT
NOCOST
NODSAT
NOEXIT
NOHANT
NOIRET
NOMEAT
NONART
NONFAT
NONHIT
NONNET
NORENT
NOSALT
NOTFIT
NOTOUT
NOTYET
NOUGAT
NOUGHT
NOWAIT
NUDEST
NUDIST
NUGENT
NUGGET
NUMBAT
NUTLET
NYPOST

•NT•••

ANTAWN
ANTCOW
ANTEED
ANTERO
ANTEUP
ANTHEM
ANTHER
ANTICS
ANTIGO
ANTLER
ANTLIA
ANTONE
ANTONY
ANTRAL
ANTRES
ANTRIM
ANTRON
ANTRUM
ENTAIL
ENTERO
ENTERS
ENTIAL
ENTICE
ENTIRE
ENTITY
ENTOMB
ENTOMO
ENTRAP
ENTREE
ENTREZ
INTACT
INTAKE
INTEND
INTENS
INTENT
INTERJ
INTERN
INTERS
INTHAT
INTIME
INTOIT
INTONE
INTOTO
INTOWN
INTRAY
INTROS
INTUIT
INTUNE
INTURN
INTWOS
ONTAPE
ONTIME
ONTOUR
UNTACK
UNTAME
UNTAPE
UNTAUT
UNTHAW
UNTIDY
UNTIED
UNTIER
UNTIES
UNTILT
UNTOLD
UNTORN
UNTRAP
UNTRIG
UNTROD
UNTRUE
UNTUCK
UNTUNE

•N•T••

ANATTO
ANITRA
CNOTES
ENATES
ENOTES
GNATTY
GNOTES
INATIE
INATUB
INITIO
INSTAL
INSTEP
INSTIL
INSTIR
KNOTTS
KNOTTY
KNOTUP
ONETEN
ONETON
ONETWO
ONSTAR
SNATCH
SNATHS
SNITCH
TNOTES
UNITAS
UNITED
UNITER
UNITES
UNSTEP
UNSTOP
UNSTOW

•N••T•

ANATTO
ANGSTS
ANSATE
ENACTS
ENMITY
ENSATE
ENTITY
GNATTY
INCITE
INDITE
INGATE
INGOTS
INLETS
INMATE
INNATE
INPUTS
INSETS
INSITU
INTOTO
INUITS
INVITE
INWITH
KNOTTS
KNOTTY
KNOUTS
ONAUTO
ONDITS
ONDUTY
ONLATE
ONSETS
ONSITE
SNAPTO
SNOOTS
SNOOTY
SNORTS
SNORTY
SNOUTS
UNBITS
UNCUTE
UNFITS
UNHATS
UNIATE
UNIATS
UNMATE
UNPOTS

•N•••T

ANDYET
ANKLET
ANNUIT
ANOINT
ENDCUT
ENDSAT
ENDSIT
ENFAIT
ENFANT
ENGIRT
ENGLIT
ENGLUT
ENHAUT
ENLIST
ENRAPT
ENROOT
ENSEAT
GNAWAT
INABIT
INAPET
INARUT
INCANT
INCENT
INCEPT
INCULT
INDEBT
INDENT
INDICT
INDUCT
INFACT
INFANT
INFECT
INFEST
INGEST
INJECT
INJEST
INKJET
INKPOT
INMOST
INPART
INPORT
INSECT
INSERT
INSIST
INSPOT
INSULT
INTACT
INTENT
INTHAT
INTOIT
INTUIT
INVENT
INVERT
INVEST
INWANT
KNEWIT
KNIGHT
KNOWIT
ONEACT
ONEBIT
ONEHIT
ONEOUT
ONESET
ONFOOT
ONPOST
SNAPAT
SNOCAT
UNBAIT
UNBELT
UNBENT
UNBOLT
UNCAST
UNDEFT
UNDSET
UNFACT
UNFELT
UNFLAT
UNGILT
UNGIRT
UNHAFT
UNHURT
UNJUST
UNKEPT
UNKNIT
UNKNOT
UNLEFT
UNLENT
UNLOST
UNMAST
UNMEET
UNMIXT
UNNEAT
UNPENT
UNRENT
UNREST
UNROOT
UNRUST
UNSEAT
UNSENT
UNSHUT
UNSOFT
UNSORT
UNTAUT
UNTILT
UNWEPT

••NT••

AINTSO
AUNTEM
AUNTIE
BANTAM
BANTER
BANTUS
BENTON
BENTOS
BONTON
BUNTED
BUNTER
BUNTON
CANTAB
CANTAL
CANTBE
CANTED
CANTER
CANTLE
CANTON
CANTOO
CANTOR
CANTOS
CENTAI
CENTAL
CENTAS
CENTER
CENTOS
CENTRE
CENTRI
CENTRO
CENTUM
CONTAC
CONTRA
CONTRE
DANTEI
DANTES
DANTON
DENTAL
DENTED
DENTIN
DENTON
DINTED
DONTGO
FANTAN
FANTAS
FONTAL
GANTRY
GENTES
GENTLE
GENTLY
GENTRY
GUNTER
HINTAT
HINTED
HINTER
HINTON
HUNTED
HUNTER
HUNTUP
ISNTOK
JUNTAS
JUNTOS
KANTOR
KENTON
LANTOS
LENTEN
LENTIL
LENTOS
LENTTO
LINTED
LINTEL
LINTER
LINTON
LUNTHA
MANTAS
MANTEE
MANTEL
MANTIC
MANTIS
MANTLE
MANTRA
MANTUA
MENTAL
MENTEE
MENTHE
MENTIS
MENTOR
MENTOS
MINTED
MINTER
MONTAG
MONTEL
MONTEZ
MONTHS
NANTES
NINTHS
NONTAN
NONTAX
PANTED
PANTER
PANTIE
PANTOS
PANTRY
PENTAD
PENTAX
PENTEL
PENTUP
PINTER
PINTOS
PUNTAS
PUNTED
PUNTER
QANTAS
QINTAR
RANTAT
RANTED
RANTER
RENTAL
RENTED
RENTEE
RENTER
RENTES
RENTON
RENTTO
SANTAS
SANTEE
SANTHA
SANTOS
SENTBY
SENTIN
SENTON
SENTRA
SENTRY
SENTTO
SENTUP
SINTAX
SONTAG
SUNTAN
SYNTAX
SYNTHS
TANTES
TANTRA
TENTED
TENTER
TENTHS
TENTON
TENTWO
TINTED
TINTER
UINTAS
VENTAS
VENTED
VENTER
VINTON
WANTAD
WANTED
WANTER
WANTIN
WANTON
WANTTO
WENTAT
WENTBY
WENTIN
WENTON
WENTTO
WENTUP
WINTER
WINTRY
WONTDO
WONTED
WONTGO
WONTON
WYNTER
WYNTON
YENTAS
ZANTAC

••N•T•

ADNATE
AGNATE
ARNETT
BENITO
BENOTE
BINATE
BINDTO
BONITA
BONITO
BUNDTS
CANUTE
DANITE
DENOTE
DONATE
DONATH
DONETO
DONETS
DONITZ
DONUTS
ELNATH
FINITE
FINITO
GENETS
GONETO
GONUTS
GUNITE
IGNATZ
IGNITE
INNATE
KANATA
KUNITZ
LANATE
LENDTO
LENGTH
LENITY
LENTTO
LUNATE
MANATS
MANETS
MANUTE
MINETA
MINITV
MINUTE
MONETA
MONETS
NINETY
NONETS
OFNOTE
OHNUTS
ORNATE
ORNITH
PINATA
PINOTS
RENATA
RENATO
RENOTE
RENTTO
RUNSTO
SANCTA
SANGTO
SANITY
SENATE
SENATS
SENDTO
SENITI
SENTTO
SINGTO
SONATA
SUNGTO
TENDTO
TENETS
TENUTA
TENUTO
TINCTS
TONITE
TUNETO
VANITY
VENETO
VENITE
VENUTI
WANTTO
WENTTO
ZENITH

••N••T

ANNUIT
ARNETT
ASNEAT
BANDIT
BANKIT
BENOIT
BONMOT
BONNET
CANLIT
CANNOT
CONANT
CONFIT
DANGIT
DINEAT
DONEIT
DUNANT
DYNAST
ERNEST
FANJET
FANOUT
FINEST
GANNET
GONEAT
GONEXT
GUNSIT
HENBIT
HINTAT
HONEST
HONKAT
IMNEXT
JENNET
JUNKET
KENSIT
LANCET
LANDAT
LINNET
LONGET
MINUET
MINUIT
MONGST
MONIST
MONNET
NONART
NONFAT
NONHIT
NONNET
PANDIT
PANOUT
PENULT
PUNDIT
RANOUT
RANTAT
RENEST
RENNET
RUNLET
RUNOUT
RUNSAT
SANEST
SONANT
SONNET
SUNHAT
SUNLIT
SUNSET
TENANT
TENHUT
TINHAT
TINPOT
UNNEAT
UPNEXT
VINCIT
WENTAT
WINGIT
WINKAT
WINOUT
WINSAT
WONOUT
YANKAT
ZENIST

•••NT•

AGENTJ
AGENTK
AGENTS
AKINTO
AMANTI
AMANTS
AMENTS
AMINTA
AMONTH
ASANTE
ATENTH
AVANTI
BIONTS
BLINTZ
BLUNTS
BOUNTY
BRANTS
BRONTE
BRUNTS
CHANTE
CHANTS
CHANTY
CHINTZ
COUNTS
COUNTY
CUANTO
DAINTY
DAUNTS
EVENTS
FAINTS
FEINTS
FLINTS
FLINTY
FOUNTS
FRANTZ
FRONTS
GIANTS
GLINTS
GLINTY
GOINTO
GRANTS
GRUNTS
HAUNTS
IDENTI
IDENTS
ISANTI
ISINTO
JAUNTS
JAUNTY
JOINTS
KOONTZ
KRANTZ
LEANTO
MEANTO
MOUNTS
MOUNTY
NIENTE
OBENTO
ODONTO
OPENTO
ORANTS
PAINTS
PAINTY
PLANTE
PLANTO
PLANTS
PLENTY
PLINTH
POINTA
POINTB
POINTE
POINTS
POINTY
PRINTS
PRONTO
PUENTE
QUANTA
QUINTA
QUINTE
QUINTI
QUINTS
SAINTE
SAINTS
SCANTS
SCANTY
SCENTS
SEENTO
SHANTY
SHINTO
SHUNTS
SLANTS
STENTS
STINTS
STUNTS
STUNTY
TAINTS
TAUNTS
TRENTA
TRENTE
TRENTO
TURNTO
TWENTY
VAUNTS
VAUNTY
VEINTE

•••N•T

ARENDT
BARNET
BITNET
BONNET
BRANDT
BRUNET
BURNET
CANNOT
CAPNUT
CARNET
COBNUT
CORNET
CYGNET
DARNIT
DIDNOT
DIPNET
DURNIT
EARNIT
ELANET
FLYNET
GAINST
GANNET
GARNET
GRANIT
GRINAT
HEXNUT
HOGNUT
HORNET
IAMNOT
IDONOT
IMONIT
ITSNOT
JENNET
LINNET
LIONET
LUGNUT
MAGNET
MAINST
MEANIT
MONNET
NERNST
NONNET
OPENIT
PEANUT
PIGNUT
PLANET
REGNAT
REKNIT
REKNOT
RENNET
SIGNET
SONNET
SPINET
SUBNET
TELNET
THENET
UNKNIT
UNKNOT
USENET
VERNET
WALNUT
WHYNOT
ZAGNUT

••••NT

ABSENT
ACCENT
ADVENT
AGLINT
AMOUNT
ANOINT
ARDENT
ARGENT
AROINT
ARRANT
ASCENT
ASKANT
ASLANT
ASSENT
AUMONT
AVAUNT
BESANT
BLOUNT
BRYANT
CADENT
CEMENT
CLIENT
COGENT
CONANT
COVENT
DARENT
DEBONT
DECANT
DECENT
DELINT
DETENT
DISANT
DOCENT
DOESNT
DUMONT
DUNANT
DUPONT
DURANT
EGMONT
ELMONT
ELUANT
ENFANT
ERRANT
ESCENT
EXEUNT
EXTANT
EXTENT
FLAUNT
FLUENT
FOMENT
FORINT
GALANT
GERENT
HAVENT
HLHUNT
IMEANT
INCANT
INCENT
INDENT
INFANT
INTENT
INVENT
INWANT
LAMENT
LAMONT
LATENT
LEARNT
LEVANT
LUCENT
MOMENT
MORANT
MUSTNT
MUTANT
NATANT
NEEDNT
NOCENT
NOHANT
NORENT
NUGENT
OCTANT
ORIENT
PARENT
PATENT
PEDANT
PLAINT
PLIANT
POTENT
QUAINT
REBENT
RECANT
RECENT
REDANT
REGENT
RELENT
REMINT
REPENT
RERENT
RESENT
RETINT
RIDENT
RODENT
SAVANT
SECANT
SILENT
SONANT
SPLINT
SPRINT
SQUINT
TALENT
TENANT
TORENT
TRUANT
TYRANT
UNBENT
UNLENT
UNPENT
UNRENT
UNSENT
UPSENT
URGENT
USMINT
UTHANT
VACANT
VALENT
VIVANT
VOLANT
WERENT

NU••••

NUANCE
NUBBED
NUBBER
NUBBIN
NUBBLE
NUBBLY
NUBIAN
NUBILE
NUBIRA
NUCHAE
NUCHAL
NUCLEI
NUCLEO
NUDELY
NUDEST
NUDGED
NUDGER
NUDGES
NUDISM
NUDIST
NUDITY
NUDNIK
NUECES
NUEVES
NUGENT
NUGGET
NUKING
NULLED
NULLOS
NUMBAT
NUMBED
NUMBER
NUMBLY
NUMERO
NUMINA
NUNCIO
NUNGEN
NUNZIO
NURSED
NURSER
NURSES
NUTATE
NUTKIN
NUTLET
NUTMEG
NUTOIL
NUTRIA
NUTTED
NUTTER
NUZZLE

N•U•••

NAUGHT
NAUSEA
NAUTES
NEUMAN
NEURAL
NEUROL
NEURON
NEUTER
NGUYEN
NOUGAT
NOUGHT
NOUMEA
NOUNAL
NTUPLE

N••U••

NATURE
NEBULA
NERUDA
NEWULM
NIPUPS
NOBUTS
NODULE
NOFUSS
NOLUCK
NONUSE
NORUNS
NORUSH
NYQUIL

N•••U•

NAILUP
NASHUA

NEHRUS
NESSUS
NETFUL
NEXTUP
NIMBUS
NINEUP
NODOUS
NONRUN
NOSEUP
NOTOUT

N••••U
NASSAU
NETHOU
NIIHAU
NOTYOU

•NU•••
ANUBIS
ENURED
ENURES
INUITS
INUPIK
INURED
INURES
KNURLS
KNURLY
ONUSES
SNUBBY
SNUFFS
SNUFFY
SNUGLI
SNUGLY
UNUSED

•N•U••
ANNUAL
ANNUIT
ANNULI
ANNULS
ENDUED
ENDUES
ENDURE
ENDURO
ENDUSE
ENGULF
ENNUIS
ENOUGH
ENQUAD
ENSUED
ENSUES
ENSURE
INBULK
INCUBI
INCULT
INCURS
INCUSE
INDUCE
INDUCT
INDUED
INDUES
INFULL
INFUSE
INGULF
INHUME
INJULY
INJUNE
INJURE
INJURY
INLUCK
INOUYE
INPUTS
INRUNS
INRUSH
INSULT
INSURE
INTUIT
INTUNE
INTURN
KNOUTS
ONAUTO
ONDUTY
ONEUPS
ONRUSH
PNEUMA
PNEUMO
SNOUTS
UNBUDS
UNBURY
UNBUSY
UNCUFF
UNCURB
UNCURL
UNCUTE
UNDULY
UNFULL
UNFURL
UNGUAL
UNGUES
UNGUIS
UNGULA
UNHUED
UNHULL
UNHUNG
UNHUNH
UNHURT
UNHUSK
UNJUST
UNLUSH
UNPURE
UNRUDE
UNRUED
UNRULY
UNRUNG
UNRUST
UNSUED
UNSUNG
UNSUNK
UNSURE
UNTUCK
UNTUNE

•N••U•
ANIMUS
ANJOUS
ANTEUP
ANTRUM
ENDCUT
ENDRUN
ENDSUP
ENGLUT
ENHAUT
ENNIUS
ENSOUL
INARUG
INARUT
INATUB
INBLUE
INDIUM
INFLUX
INPOUR
KNOTUP
ONABUN
ONEOUT
ONERUN
ONTOUR
SNAFUS
SNAGUP
SNAPUP
UNFOUL
UNGLUE
UNIQUE
UNPLUG
UNSHUT
UNSMUG
UNSNUG
UNSOUR
UNSPUN
UNTAUT
UNTRUE

•N•••U
INLIEU
INSITU

••NU••
ANNUAL
ANNUIT
ANNULI
ANNULS
BENUMB
BUNUEL
CANUCK
CANULA
CANUTE
CONURE
DANUBE
DENUDE
DONUTS
ENNUIS
GENUAL
GONUTS
JANUAR
LUNULA
MANUAL
MANUEL
MANURE
MANUSH
MANUTE
MENUDO
MINUET
MINUIT
MINUTE
NONUSE
OHNUTS
PENULT
PENURY
PINUPS
RUNUPS
SUNUNU
SUNUPS
TENURE
TENUTA
TENUTO
VENUES
VENULE
VENUTI
ZANUCK
ZONULE

••N•U•
ADNOUN
BANGUI
BANGUP
BANJUL
BANKUP
BANQUE
BANQUO
BANTUS
BENHUR
BINDUP
BONEUP
BUNKUM
CANCUN
CANFUL
CENSUS
CENTUM
CINQUE
CONCUR
CONSUL
DINGUS
DINKUM
DONEUP
ENNIUS
FANOUT
FONDUE
FONDUS
FUNFUR
FUNGUS
FUNRUN
GANGUP
GENIUS
GINSUP
GONEUP
GYNOUS
HANDUP
HANGUL
HANGUP
HINDUS
HONOUR
HUNGUP
HUNTUP
IONIUM
JANHUS
JUNIUS
LANDUP
LANDUS
LENGUA
LINEUP
LINGUA
LINGUS
LINKUP
LONGUE
MANFUL
MANQUE
MANTUA
MINGUS
NINEUP
NONRUN
OMNIUM
OWNSUP
PANFUL
PANOUT
PENSUP
PENTUP
PINDUS
PINSUP
PONYUP
PONZUS
RANGUP
RANOUT
RINGUP
RUNGUP
RUNOUT
RUNSUP
SENDUP
SENTUP
SINFUL
TANGUY
TANKUP
TENHUT
TINCUP
TONEUP
TONGUE
TUNEUP
URNFUL
VENDUE
VENOUS
VINOUS
WENTUP
WINDUP
WINOUT
WONOUT
XINHUA
YANQUI

••N••U
CONGOU
HONSHU
JUNEAU
KUNGFU
LANDAU
MANCHU
MENJOU
PENGPU
SUNUNU
XANADU

•••NU•
AMINUS
AVENUE
BARNUM
BMINUS
BURNUP
CAPNUT
CHINUA
CHINUP
CMINUS
COBNUT
CRONUS
CYGNUS
DMINUS
EVENUP
FARNUM
FAUNUS
FRENUM
HEXNUT
HOGNUT
JOINUP
KRONUR
LIGNUM
LUGNUT
MAGNUM
MAGNUS
OPENUP
PEANUT
PIGNUT
PLENUM
PRENUP
REGNUM
SEENUP
SEWNUP
SIGNUP
TMINUS
TORNUP
TURNUP
UNSNUG
URANUS
WALNUT
ZAGNUT

•••N•U
CHANDU
JOANOU
QUINQU

••••NU
BROWNU
SUNUNU
VISHNU

N•V•••
NAVAHO
NAVAID
NAVAJO
NAVELS
NAVIES
NEVADA
NEVERS
NEVILL
NEVINS
NEVSKI
NEVSKY
NOVATO
NOVELA
NOVELS
NOVENA
NOVIAS
NOVICE
NOVIOS
NOVOTE

N••V••
NAIVER
NARVIK
NERVAL
NERVED
NERVES
NIEVES
NLMVPS
NORVAL
NUEVES

N•••V•
NATIVE
NOJIVE

•NV•••
ANVILS
ENVEIL
ENVIED
ENVIER
ENVIES
ENVIRO
ENVOIS
ENVOYS
INVADE
INVAIN
INVENT
INVERT
INVEST
INVIEW
INVITE
INVIVO
INVOKE
ONVIEW
UNVAIN
UNVEIL
UNVOID

•N•V••
INEVER
KNAVES
KNIVES
SNIVEL
UNAVID
UNEVEN
UNEVIL
UNIVAC

•N••V•
ENDIVE
INLOVE
INVIVO
INWOVE
UNGAVA
UNLIVE
UNROVE
UNWOVE

••NV••
CANVAS
CONVEX
CONVEY
CONVOY
DENVER
LANVAL
LANVIN
RENVOI

••N•V•
CANOVA
DANOVA
DENOVO
GENEVA
GENEVE
GENOVA
LENOVO
USNAVY

••N••V
HENRYV
MINITV
RENONV

•••NV•
IVANVI
JOHNVI

•••N•V
IVANIV
IVANOV
JOHNIV
JOHNXV
SCENEV

••••NV
ELKONV
RENONV
URBANV

N•W•••
NEWAGE
NEWARK
NEWBIE
NEWCAR
NEWDAY
NEWELL
NEWELS
NEWERA
NEWEST
NEWHAT
NEWIES
NEWISH
NEWJOB
NEWKID
NEWLEY
NEWMAN
NEWMAR
NEWSIE
NEWSOM
NEWTON
NEWTOY
NEWULM
NEWWAY
NLWEST
NOWAIT
NOWAYS
NOWISE
NOWLAN
NOWNOW

N••W••
NEWWAY
NITWIT
NONWAR
NORWAY

N•••W•
NONEWS

N••••W
NARROW
NEPHEW
NONJEW
NOSHOW
NOTNEW
NOTNOW
NOWNOW

•NW•••
ANWANG
ENWIND
ENWRAP
INWANT
INWARD
INWITH
INWOVE
ONWARD
UNWALL
UNWARY
UNWELL
UNWEPT
UNWIGS
UNWILD
UNWILY
UNWIND
UNWISE
UNWISH
UNWORN
UNWOVE
UNWRAP

•N•W••
ANSWER
ANYWAY
GNAWAT
GNAWED
GNAWER
GNAWON
INAWAY
INTWOS
KNEWIT
KNEWOF
KNOWER
KNOWIT
KNOWNS
KNOWOF
ONEWAY
SNOWED
SNOWIN
UNAWED
UNOWED

•N••W•
ANTAWN
ENDOWS
INLAWS
INPAWN
INTOWN
ONETWO
UNDEWY
UNHEWN
UNMEWS
UNMOWN
UNPAWN
UNSAWN
UNSEWN
UNSEWS
UNSOWN

•N•••W
ANDHOW
ANDREW
ANTCOW
ANYHOW
INAFEW
INAROW
INFLOW
INVIEW
ONSHOW
ONVIEW
UNDRAW
UNDREW
UNSKEW
UNSLOW
UNSTOW
UNTHAW

••NW••
CONWAY
FENWAY
NONWAR
RUNWAY
WINWIN

••N•W•
KANAWA
NONEWS
RENEWS
RENOWN
SINEWS
SINEWY
TENTWO
USNEWS

••N••W
BENBOW
GUNLAW
MINNOW
NONJEW
RANLOW
RUNLOW
SUNBOW
WINDOW
WINNOW

•••N•W
ACTNOW
ALLNEW
BUYNOW
BYENOW
CPSNOW
CURNOW
ERENOW
FORNOW
HOWNOW
MINNOW
NOTNEW
NOTNOW
NOWNOW
PAYNOW
TILNOW
WHYNOW
WINNOW

N•X•••
NEXRAD
NEXTEL
NEXTTO
NEXTUP
NIXERS
NIXIES
NIXING
NIXONS

N••X••
NOEXIT

N••••X
NEELIX
NONTAX

•N•X••
ANOXIA
ANOXIC
ONYXES
UNAXED

•N••X•
UNFOXY
UNMIXT
UNSEXY

•N•••X
INABOX
INAFIX
INFLUX
UNISEX

••NX••
GENXER
JINXED
JINXER
JINXES
LYNXES
MINXES
SKNXXX

••N•X•
GONEXT
IMNEXT
SKNXXX
UPNEXT

••N••X
BENDIX
CONVEX
HANDAX
LENNOX
MANNIX
NONTAX
PENTAX
RONMIX
SINTAX
SKNXXX
SYNTAX
WINDEX

•••NX•
JOHNXI
JOHNXV
JOHNXX

•••N•X
BRANDX
FORNAX
FTKNOX
JOHNIX
JOHNXX
LENNOX
MANNIX

••••NX
LARYNX
MRJINX
SPHINX
SPHYNX

NY••••
NYALAS
NYJETS
NYLONS
NYMETS
NYMPHS
NYPOST
NYQUIL
NYYANK

N•Y•••
NAYSAY
NOYORI
NYYANK

N••Y••
NGUYEN
NOTYET
NOTYOU

N•••Y•
NAGOYA
NOMAYO
NOWAYS

N••••Y
NAJIMY
NAMELY
NAPERY
NASEBY
NAYSAY
NEARBY
NEARLY
NEATLY
NETPAY
NETTLY
NEVSKY
NEWDAY
NEWLEY
NEWTOY
NEWWAY
NFORTY
NIAMEY
NICELY
NICETY
NIDIFY
NIGHTY
NIMBLY
NIMINY
NINETY
NIPSEY
NITERY
NOBODY
NONARY
NORGAY
NORWAY
NOSILY
NOTANY
NOTARY
NOTCHY
NOTIFY
NUBBLY
NUDELY
NUDITY
NUMBLY

•NY•••
ANYDAY
ANYHOW
ANYMAN
ANYOLD
ANYONE
ANYONS
ANYWAY
ONYXES
SNYDER
UNYOKE

•N•Y••
ANDYET
ENCYCL
ENZYME
INSYNC
ONLYIF
UNDYED

•N••Y•
ANNOYS
ANONYM
ENJOYS
ENVOYS
INLAYS
INOUYE
ONEEYE
ONLAYS
UNISYS
UNLAYS
UNSAYS

•N•••Y
ANDREY
ANERGY
ANTONY
ANYDAY
ANYWAY
ENERGY
ENMITY
ENTITY
GNARLY
GNATTY
INADAY
INARAY
INAWAY
INFAMY
INGRAY
INGREY
INJULY
INJURY
INPLAY
INTRAY
KNARRY
KNOBBY
KNOLLY
KNOTTY
KNURLY
ONDUTY
ONEDAY
ONEWAY
ONIONY
SNAGGY
SNAPPY
SNARKY
SNARLY
SNAZZY
SNEAKY
SNEERY
SNEEZY
SNIFFY
SNIPPY
SNOBBY
SNOOPY
SNOOTY
SNOOZY
SNORTY
SNUBBY
SNUFFY
SNUGLY
UNABLY
UNBURY
UNBUSY
UNCLAY
UNDEWY
UNDULY
UNEASY
UNFOXY
UNGAMY
UNHAZY
UNHOLY
UNIDLY
UNMIRY
UNOILY
UNRULY
UNSEXY
UNTIDY
UNWARY
UNWILY

••NY••
BANYAN
BINYON
BUNYAN
CANYON
KENYAN
KENYON
LYNYRD
MINYAN
PINYIN
PONYUP
RUNYON
SANYOS
VINYLS

••N•Y•
ANNOYS
CONEYS
DANDYL
DANNYS
DENNYS
HENRYI
HENRYK
HENRYV
HONEYS
KENNYG
MONEYS
VANRYN
WENDYS

••N••Y
BENDAY
BENGAY
BENSEY
BINARY
BINCHY
BINNEY
BONNEY
BUNCHY
BUNGAY
CANARY
CANOPY
CONROY
CONVEY
CONVOY
CONWAY
DANGLY
DANKLY
DANNAY
DENARY
DINGHY
DONEBY
DONKEY
FENWAY
FINELY
FINERY
FINLEY
FINNEY
FONDLY
GANGLY
GANTRY
GENTLY
GENTRY
GONEBY
GUNSHY
HANGBY
HANLEY
HENDRY
HENLEY
HUNGBY
HUNGRY
HUNLEY
JANGLY
JANNEY
JENNEY
JINGLY
JONESY
JUNGLY
KANALY
KINDLY
KINGLY
KINSEY
KUNDRY
LANDRY
LANKLY
LANSKY
LENITY
LINENY
LINNEY
LONELY
LONGLY
LUNACY
LUNCHY
LYNLEY
MANDAY
MANLEY
MANRAY
MINIFY
MONDAY
MONKEY
MONODY
MUNCHY
NINETY

NONARY
ORNERY
PANFRY
PANTRY
PENNEY
PENURY
PINBOY
PINCAY
PINERY
PUNCHY
PUNILY
RANDRY
RANKLY
RONCEY
RONELY
RUNDRY
RUNSBY
RUNWAY
SANELY
SANITY
SENARY
SENDBY
SENTBY
SENTRY
SINEWY
SINGLY
SUNDAY
SUNDRY
SUNRAY
TANGLY
TANGUY
TENDAY
TENLEY
TINGLY
TINILY
TINKLY
TUNNEY
USNAVY
VANITY
VINERY
VINIFY
WENTBY
WINERY
WINSBY
WINTRY
ZANILY
ZINCKY

•••NY•

ANONYM
CRONYN
DANNYS
DENNYS
EPONYM
ERINYS
EUONYM
EXONYM
KENNYG
SOONYI

•••N•Y

AGENCY
BARNEY
BINNEY
BIRNEY
BONNEY
BOUNCY
BOUNTY
BRANDY
BRANNY
BRENLY
BRONZY
BURNEY
CAGNEY
CARNEY
CHANCY
CHANEY
CHANTY
CHENEY
CHINKY
CHUNKY
CLANCY
CLANKY
CLINGY
CLUNKY
COONEY
COUNTY
CRANKY
CRANNY
DABNEY
DAINTY
DANNAY
DARNAY
DISNEY
DOWNEY
DRANCY
EVENLY
FINNEY
FLINTY
FLUNKY
FRANNY
FRENZY
FRINGY
GAINLY
GLINTY
GOONEY
GRANBY
GRANDY
GRANNY
GRUNDY
GRUNGY
GURNEY
HARNEY
HEANEY
HORNBY
HOUNDY
IFONLY
JANNEY
JAUNTY
JENNEY
JITNEY
JOHNNY
JOUNCY
KEENLY
KIDNEY
LEANLY
LINNEY
LIONLY
LOONEY
MAINLY
MAUNDY
MEANEY
MEANLY
MOONEY
MORNAY
MOUNTY
OHENRY
OPENLY
ORANGY
ORKNEY
PAINTY
PENNEY
PEVNEY
PHONEY
PITNEY
PLENTY
PLUNKY
POINTY
PUTNEY
QUINCY
RAINEY
RODNEY
ROMNEY
ROONEY
SAYNAY
SCANTY
SHANDY
SHANTY
SHINDY
SHINNY
SIDNEY
SKANKY
SKINNY
SKUNKY
SLANGY
SLINKY
SPANKY
SPENDY
SPONGY
SPUNKY
STINGY
STINKY
STONEY
STUNTY
SWANKY
SWINGY
SYDNEY
TEENSY
THINGY
THINLY
TRANNY
TRENDY
TUNNEY
TWANGY
TWENTY
VAINLY
VARNEY
VAUNTY
WATNEY
WEENSY
WHINNY

••••NY

ALBANY
ANTONY
ASMANY
BARANY
BARONY
BETONY
BOTANY
BRAINY
BRANNY
BRAWNY
BROWNY
COLONY
CRANNY
CZERNY
DELANY
FELONY
FRANNY
GRAINY
GRANNY
GREENY
GROZNY
HOMINY
JIMINY
JOHNNY
KEARNY
LEMONY
LINENY
LITANY
MUTINY
NIMINY
NOTANY
ONIONY
PIMINY
REDENY
RESINY
ROMANY
ROSINY
SATINY
SAXONY
SHEENY
SHINNY
SKINNY
SOMANY
SPOONY
THORNY
TRANNY
TROYNY
TWEENY
WHINNY

N•Z•••

NOZZLE
NUZZLE

N••Z••

NOZZLE
NUNZIO
NUZZLE

N••••Z

NIMITZ

•NZ•••

ANZACS
ENZYME
UNZIPS
UNZONE

•N•Z••

SNAZZY

•N•Z•

SNAZZY
SNEEZE
SNEEZY
SNOOZE
SNOOZY
UNHAZY

•N•••Z

ENTREZ

••NZ••

BANZAI
BENZOL
BONZES
DANZIG
DENZEL
FONZIE
JANZEN
KUNZEL
LINZER
MANZON
MONZAS
NUNZIO
PANZER
PINZON
PONZUS

••N•Z•

IONIZE

••N••Z

BONERZ
DONITZ
IGNATZ
KUNITZ
MONTEZ

•••NZ•

ALONZO
BRONZE
BRONZY
BRYNZA
FRENZY
FRUNZE
KWANZA
LAONZA
PRINZE
PUENZO
QUINZE
RIENZI
STANZA

•••N•Z

BLINTZ
CHINTZ
FRANTZ
IBANEZ
KOONTZ
KRANTZ
SCHNOZ
XYANDZ

••••NZ

BRIENZ
DOLENZ
LORENZ

OA••••

OAFISH
OAHUAN
OAKIER
OAKLEY
OAKTAG
OAKUMS
OARAGE
OARERS
OARING
OARMAN
OARMEN
OATERS
OATIER
OAXACA

O•A•••

OCASEK
OCASEY
ODAMAE
OGAUGE
OJAICA
OKAPIS
OKAYED
OLAFII
OLAFIV
OLAKES
OLATHE
OLAVII
OLAVIV
OMAHAN
OMAHAS
OMANIS
OMASUM
ONABUN
ONAGER
ONAHOP
ONAJAG
ONAPAR
ONAUTO
OPAQUE
ORACHS
ORACLE
ORAJEL
ORALES
ORALLY
ORANGE
ORANGS
ORANGY
ORANIS
ORANTS
ORATED
ORATES
ORATOR
OSAGES
OSAKAN
OVALLY
OXALIC
OXALIS
OZARKS

O••A••

OARAGE
OAXACA
OBEAHS
OBLADI
OBLAST
OBLATE
OBTAIN
OCCAMS
OCEANS
OCTADS
OCTANE
OCTANS
OCTANT
OCTAVE
OCTAVO
OFFALS
OFFALY
OFLATE
OGHAMS
OGLALA
OGRADY
OHBABY
OHDARN
OHMAGE
OKSANA
OLDAGE
OLEARY
OLEATE
OMEARA
ONBAIL
ONBASE
ONCALL
ONEACT
ONEALL
ONEARM
ONHAND
ONLAID
ONLAND
ONLATE
ONLAYS
ONRAMP
ONSALE
ONTAPE
ONWARD
OOLALA
OPIATE
OPRAHS
ORBACH
ORDAIN
OREADS
ORGANA
ORGANS
ORIANA
ORIANI
ORKANS
ORNATE
OSCANS
OSCARS
OSHAWA
OSTARS
OSWALD
OTTAVA
OTTAWA
OUTACT
OUTADD
OUTAGE
OUTASK
OUTATE
OUTAWE
OXCART
OXNARD
OXTAIL

O•••A•

OAHUAN
OAKTAG
OARMAN
OBIWAN
OBRIAN
OCEDAR
OCICAT
OCULAR
ODAMAE
ODDMAN
OFFDAY
OGDOAD
OGIVAL
OHDEAR
OHDRAT
OHIOAN
OHYEAH
OILCAN
OILMAN
OILPAN
OISEAU
OLDBAT
OLDCAR
OLDGAG
OLDHAM
OLDHAT
OLDMAN
OLDPAL
OLDSAW
OLDWAY
OMAHAN
OMAHAS
OMEGAS
OMPHAL
ONAJAG
ONAPAR
ONECAR
ONEDAY
ONELAP
ONEMAN
ONEWAY
ONLOAD
ONLOAN
ONSTAR
OOMPAH
OPERAS
ORDEAL
ORGEAT
ORPHAN
ORWHAT
OSAKAN
OSSIAN
OSTEAL
OTHMAR
OUIJAS
OUTBAN
OUTBAT
OUTEAT
OUTGAS
OUTLAW
OUTLAY
OUTMAN
OUTPAY
OUTRAN
OUTRAP
OUTSAT
OUTSAW
OUTSAY
OUTWAR
OVISAC
OVULAR

O••••A

OAXACA
ODESSA
ODETTA
OGLALA
OJAICA
OJIBWA
OKSANA
OLESHA
OLINDA
OLIVIA
OMEARA
OMERTA
ONEIDA
OOLALA
OPTIMA
OREIDA
OREXIA
ORGANA
ORIANA
ORISSA
ORTEGA
OSETRA
OSHAWA
OTTAVA
OTTAWA
OUGHTA

•OA•••

BOARDS
BOASTS
BOATED
BOATEL
BOATER
COACTS
COALED
COALER
COAPTS
COARSE
COASTS
COATED
COATEE
COATER
COATES
COATIS
COAXAL
COAXED
COAXER
COAXES
DOABLE
DOAKES
DOALLS
DOASET
FOALED
FOAMED
FOAMER
GOADED
GOALBY
GOALIE
GOATEE
GOATIT
GOAWAY
GOAWOL
GOAWRY
HOAGIE
HOARDS
HOARSE
HOAXED
HOAXER
HOAXES
JOANIE
JOANNA
JOANNE
JOANOU
KOALAS
LOADED
LOADER
LOADIN
LOADUP
LOAFED
LOAFER
LOAMED
LOANED
LOANER
LOATHE
LOAVES
MOANED
MOANER
MOATED
POACHY
ROADEO
ROADER
ROADIE
ROAMED
ROAMER
ROAMIN
ROARAT
ROARED
ROARER
ROASTS
SOAKED
SOAKER
SOAKIN
SOAKUP
SOAPED
SOAPER
SOAPUP
SOARED
SOARER
SOASTO
SOAVES
TOAMAN
TOASTS
TOASTY
TOATEE
YOAKAM

•O•A••

BOGART
BONACI
BONAMI
BORATE
BORAXO
BOTANY
BOVARY
BOYARS
COBAIN
COBALT
COHABS
COLADA
COMATE
CONAIR
CONANT
COPALS
COPAYS
CORACI
CORALS
COTANS
COWARD
DOGAPE
DOLAPS
DOMAIN
DOMANI
DONALD
DONATE
DONATH
DORADO
DORAGS
DORATI
DOSADO
DOSAGE
DOTAGE
DOTARD
DOUANE
FOLATE
FORAGE
FORAYS
GOBACK
GOBANG
GOCART
GODARD
GODARK
GOEASY
GOFAST
GOKART
GOLAME
GOLAST
GOPAST
GOTAMA
GOTANA
GOTANF
HOBART
HODADS
HOGANS
HOMAGE
HORACE
HOTAIR
HOWARD
IODATE
IOLANI
IOWANS
JOHANN
JONAHS
KODAKS
KODALY
KORANS
KORATS
KOVACS
LOBATE
LOCALE
LOCALS
LOCANE
LOCATE
LOGANS
LORAIN
LORANS
LOUANN
LOVAGE
LOYALE
MODALS
MOHAIR
MOHAVE
MOHAWK
MOJAVE
MOLARS
MONACO
MONADS
MONAMI
MORALE
MORALS
MORANT
MORASS
MORATH
MORAYS
MOSAIC
MOVADO
MOZART
NOBAKE
NOBALL
NOFAIR
NOHANT
NOMAAM
NOMADS
NOMAYO
NONAGE
NONAME
NONART
NONARY
NOPALS
NORAIN
NOSALE
NOSALT
NOTAIL
NOTALL
NOTANY
NOTARY
NOTATE
NOVATO
NOWAIT
NOWAYS
OOLALA
POEANA
POLAND
POLARA
POMADE
POPART
POSADA
POTAGE
POTASH
POTATO
RODALE
ROLAND
ROMAIC
ROMAIN
ROMAJI
ROMANI
ROMANO
ROMANS
ROMANY
RONALD
ROSARY
ROTARY
ROTATE
ROWANS
ROXANA
ROXANE
ROYALE
ROYALS
SOCANI
SOLACE
SOLANO
SOLANS
SOLARA
SOLATI
SOMALI
SOMANY
SOMATA
SONANT
SONARS
SONATA
TOBAGO
TODATE
TODAYS
TOGAED
TOKAYS
TOLARS
TOLAST
TOMATO
TORAHS
TOTALS
TOWAGE
TOWARD
TOYAMA
VOCABS
VOCALS
VOLANS
VOLANT
VOLARE
VOTARY
VOYAGE
WOMACK
WOMANS
YOSANO
YOUALL
ZOCALO

•O••A•

AORTAE
AORTAL
AORTAS
AOUDAD
BOBCAT
BOLLAS
BOLYAI
BOMBAL
BOMBAY
BONHAM
BONSAI
BOOSAT
BOREAL
BOREAS
BORMAN
BOWMAN
BOWOAR
BOWSAW
BOXCAR
COAXAL
COBHAM
COBRAS
COCOAS
COEVAL
COGNAC
COLFAX
COLLAR
COLLAT
COLMAN
COLMAR
COMBAT
COMEAS
COMEAT
COMMAS
COMPAQ
COMPAS
COMSAT
CONFAB
CONGAS
CONLAN
CONMAN
CONRAD
CONTAC
CONWAY
COOGAN
COPCAR
COPRAS
CORDAY
CORFAM
CORMAN
CORRAL
CORSAS
COSMAS
COSTAE
COSTAL
COSTAR
COSTAS
COTTAE
COTTAS
COUGAR
COWMAN
DOGDAY
DOGEAR
DOGMAS
DOGNAP
DOGSAT
DOGTAG
DOLLAR
DOLMAN
DOLMAS
DOODAD
DOODAH
DOOHAN
DORCAS
DORIAN
DORSAD
DORSAL
DORSAY
DOSSAL
DOTHAN
DOTOAT
DOUGAL
DOULAS
EOLIAN
EONIAN
FOEMAN
FOLIAR
FONDAS
FONTAL
FORBAD
FORMAL
FORMAN
FORMAT
FORNAX
FORTAS
FOSSAE
FOURAA
FOURAD
FOURAM
GOAWAY
GODEAD
GOESAT
GOFLAT
GONEAR
GONEAT
GOODAT
GORHAM
GOSTAG
GOTEAM
GOTFAR
GOTHAM
GOTMAD
GOUDAS
HODIAK
HODMAN
HOLMAN
HONDAS
HONKAT
HOOHAH
HOOHAS
HOOKAH
HOORAH
HOORAY
HOOSAC
HOOTAT
HORGAN
HOSTAS
HOTCAP
HOTCAR
HOTDAY
HOTWAR
HOWDAH
HOWFAR
HOWLAT
HOWSAD
IONIAN
JOBJAR
JORDAN
JOSIAH
JOVIAL
JOVIAN
JOYPAD
KOALAS
KODIAK
KOMBAT
KONRAD
KOREAN
KORMAN
KOUFAX
LOGJAM
LOOFAH
LOOFAS
LOOKAT
LOQUAT
LOREAL
LOTHAR
LOUMAS
LOWCAL
LOWFAT
LOWMAN
LOWTAR
MOCHAS
MOERAE
MOLDAU
MOLNAR
MOMMAS
MONDAY
MONTAG
MONZAS
MOOLAH
MOREAU
MORGAN
MORNAY

MORTAL
MORTAR
MOSHAV
MOSSAD
NODEAL
NODEAR
NODSAT
NOKIAS
NOLEAD
NOLOAD
NOMAAM
NOMEAK
NOMEAT
NOMIAL
NONFAN
NONFAT
NONGAS
NONMAN
NONPAR
NONTAN
NONTAX
NONWAR
NOONAN
NORGAY
NORIAS
NORMAL
NORMAN
NORVAL
NORWAY
NOSOAP
NOTBAD
NOTFAR
NOUGAT
NOUNAL
NOVIAS
NOWLAN
OOMPAH
POKEAT
POLEAX
POLGAR
POLKAS
POLLAK
PONCAS
POORAT
POPLAR
POPPAS
PORTAL
POSEAS
POSTAL
POZNAN
ROARAT
ROCHAT
RODHAM
RODMAN
ROSEAU
SOCIAL
SOLEAS
SONTAG
SOONAS
SOREAT
SOSPAD
SOTHAT
SOWHAT
SOXFAN
TOAMAN
TOBIAS
TODDAO
TODMAN
TOECAP
TOETAP
TOILAT
TOKLAS
TOMCAT
TONGAN
TONKAS
TOOBAD
TOOFAR
TOOTAT
TOPCAT
TOPHAT
TOPMAN
TORBAY
TOREAT
TORTAS
TOUCAN
TOWBAR
TOWCAR
TOYCAR
TOYHAT
VODKAS
VORPAL
WOMBAT
WORKAT
YOAKAM
YOWZAH
ZODIAC
ZOLTAN
ZONIAN

•O•••A

BOCHSA
BODEGA
BOGOTA
BOLENA
BONITA
BORGIA
BOSNIA
COELIA
COLADA
COLIMA
COMIDA
CONCHA
CONTRA
COPULA
CORDIA
CORNEA
CORONA
CORYZA
COULDA
COVINA
COWPEA
DODECA
DODOMA
DONORA
FOURAA
GODIVA
GOLETA
GOTAMA
GOTANA
GOTCHA
HOOPLA
HOTTEA
IOMEGA
JOANNA
JOBYNA
JOGBRA
JOJOBA
JOSHUA
KONICA
KORUNA
LOGGIA
LOLITA
LOOKMA
LOOMPA
LOUISA
LOVEYA
LOYOLA
MODELA
MODENA
MOESHA
MOLINA
MONETA
MONICA
MORITA
MOSKVA
MOTHRA
NOIDEA
NOOTKA
NOSTRA
NOUMEA
NOVELA
NOVENA
OOLALA
POEANA
POINTA
POISHA
POLARA
POLSKA
POMONA
PORTIA
POSADA
ROBBIA
ROMOLA
ROOMBA
ROSINA
ROSITA
ROSTRA
ROWENA
ROXANA
SOLARA
SOMATA
SONATA
SONDRA
SONOMA
SONORA
SOPHIA
TOLDYA
TOPEKA
TOYAMA
TOYOTA
WOULDA
YORKPA
YOYOMA
ZORINA
ZOYSIA

••OA••

ABOARD
BLOATS
BROACH
BROADA
BROAST
CHOATE
CLOAKS
CROAKS
CROAKY
CROATS
EBOATS
FLOATS
FLOATY
GLOATS
GROANS
GROATS
PROAMS
PROART
SHOALS
SHOALY
SHOATS
SKOALS
SLOANE
STOATS
TWOACT
UBOATS
WHOAMI

••O•A•

ABOMAS
ABORAL
ADONAI
AGORAE
AGORAS
AJOWAN
ALOHAS
ALOMAR
AMORAL
ANODAL
ANORAK
APODAL
AROMAS
ASOSAN
ATONAL
AVOWAL
AXONAL
AZONAL
BAOBAB
BHOPAL
BIOGAS
BIOLAB
BIOTAS
BOOSAT
BROCAS
BROGAN
BROKAW
CHORAL
CLONAL
COOGAN
DEODAR
DOODAD
DOODAH
DOOHAN
DVORAK
ECOLAB
ECOLAW
EGOYAN
FLORAE
FLORAL
FLORAS
GLOBAL
GOODAT
GROBAN
GYOZAS
HOOHAH
HOOHAS
HOOKAH
HOORAH
HOORAY
HOOSAC
HOOTAT
IMOKAY
ISOBAR
KIOWAN
KIOWAS
LOOFAH
LOOFAS
LOOKAT
MAOTAI
MOOLAH
NOONAN
POORAT
PROTAX
PROWAR
PROYAS
PROZAC
QUOTAS
RIOJAS
RIOPAN
RYOKAN
SHOFAR
SHOPAT
SHOTAT
SIOUAN
SLOGAN
SLOVAK
SNOCAT
SOONAS
STOLAE
STOLAF
STOLAS
STOMAS
STOPAT
THOMAS
THORAX
TOOBAD
TOOFAR
TOOTAT
TROJAN
TWOCAR
TWODAY
TWOMAN
TWOWAY
UNOCAL
UNORAL
VIOLAS
WHODAT
XHOSAS
YEOMAN

••O••A

ABOLLA
AEOLIA
ALOGIA
AMOEBA
AMONRA
ANOMIA
ANOXIA
APOPKA
ASONIA
ATONIA
BROADA
CHOLLA
CHOPRA
CSONKA
DAOSTA
ELODEA
ELOISA
EROICA
GLORIA
GLOSSA
HOOPLA
IGOTTA
ISOLDA
LAONZA
LEONIA
LIOTTA
LOOKMA
LOOMPA
MTOSSA
MYOPIA
NOOTKA
PEORIA
PHOBIA
PROTEA
RHONDA
ROOMBA
SCOOBA
SCORIA
SCOTIA
SFORZA
SHORTA
TROIKA
UTOPIA

•••OA•

ABROAD
AFLOAT
BEMOAN
BOWOAR
BUROAK
BYROAD
COCOAS
DEFOAM
DOTOAT
GENOAN
GENOAS
HEGOAT
INGOAL
INROAD
MAJOAD
MINOAN
NOLOAD
NOSOAP
OGDOAD
OHIOAN
ONLOAD
ONLOAN
PAJOAD
PINOAK
PTBOAT
RECOAL
RECOAT
REDOAK
RELOAD
RELOAN
RESOAK
RESOAP
SAMOAN
STJOAN
TANOAK
THROAT
UNLOAD
UPLOAD
UPROAR
UPSOAR

•••O•A

ANGOLA
ANGORA
AREOLA
ARLOVA
AURORA
BAROJA
BOGOTA
BULOVA
CANOLA
CANOVA
CHROMA
CIBOLA
CORONA
CUPOLA
DAKOTA
DANOVA
DODOMA
DONORA
EIDOLA
ELLORA
ELNORA
ENDORA
ESPOSA
EUBOEA
EUDORA
EUROPA
FEDORA
FEMORA
GENOVA
JAMOCA
JOJOBA
JUDOKA
KEYOFA
LADOGA
LAKOTA
LAROSA
LATOYA
LOYOLA
MAZOLA
MIMOSA
NAGOYA
NICOLA
NIKOLA
PADOVA
PAGODA
PALOMA
PAYOLA
PELOTA
POMONA
RAMONA
RCCOLA
REMORA
RICOLA
ROMOLA
SAMOSA
SCOOBA
SEDONA
SENORA
SONOMA
SONORA
TACOMA
TOYOTA
UNCOLA
VALOVA
VENORA
VERONA
VIGODA
WINONA
YOYOMA
ZADORA
ZAMORA
ZYGOMA

••••OA

BALBOA
HIVAOA
JERBOA
LISBOA
PETBOA

OB••••

OBEAHS
OBELUS
OBENTO
OBERON
OBERTO
OBEYED
OBEYER
OBGYNS
OBISPO
OBITER
OBIWAN
OBJECT
OBJETS
OBLADI
OBLAST
OBLATE
OBLIGE
OBLONG
OBOIST
OBOLER
OBOLUS
OBRIAN
OBRIEN
OBSESS
OBTAIN
OBTEST
OBTUND
OBTUSE
OBVERT

O•B•••

OHBABY
OKBYME
ONBAIL
ONBASE
ORBACH
ORBING
ORBITS
OSBERT
OSBORN
OXBOWS

O••B••

OJIBWA
OLDBAT
OLDBOY
ONABUN
ONEBIT
ORIBIS
OUTBAN
OUTBAT
OUTBEG
OUTBID
OUTBOW
OUTBOX
OUTBUD
OUTBUY

O•••B•

OHBABY

O••••B

ODDJOB
OILRUB
OUTRIB

•OB•••

BOBBED
BOBBER
BOBBIE
BOBBIN
BOBBLE
BOBBLY
BOBBYS
BOBCAT
BOBSUP
COBAIN
COBALT
COBBLE
COBHAM
COBNUT
COBRAS
COBURG
COBURN
COBWEB
DOBBIN
DOBLES
DOBLIN
DOBROS
DOBYNS
FOBBED
FOBOFF
GOBACK
GOBANG
GOBBLE
GOBIES
GOBLET
GOBLIN
GOBOES
GOBOOM
GOBOTS
GOBSOF
GOBUST
HOBART
HOBBES
HOBBIT
HOBBLE
HOBNOB
HOBOED
HOBOES
HOBSON
JOBBED
JOBBER
JOBCUT
JOBETH
JOBHOP
JOBJAR
JOBLOT
JOBONE
JOBSON
JOBYNA
KOBOLD
LOBATE
LOBBED
LOBBER
LOBULE
MOBBED
MOBBER
MOBERG
MOBILE
MOBIUS
MOBLEY
MOBUTU
NOBAKE
NOBALL
NOBELS
NOBILE
NOBLER
NOBLES
NOBODY
NOBUTS
POBOYS
ROBBED
ROBBER
ROBBIA
ROBBIE
ROBERS
ROBERT
ROBING
ROBINS
ROBLES
ROBOTS
ROBROY
ROBSOF
ROBSON
ROBUST
SOBBED
SOBBER
SOBEIT
SOBERS
SOBFUL
TOBAGO
TOBIAS
TOBIES
TOBITS
TOBOOT
TOBURN
WOBBLE
WOBBLY
WOBURN

•O•B••

BOBBED
BOBBER
BOBBIE
BOBBIN
BOBBLE
BOBBLY
BOBBYS
BOMBAL
BOMBAY
BOMBED
BOMBER
BOMBES
BONBON
BOOBOO
BOXBED
BOXBOY
COBBLE
COLBYS
COMBAT
COMBED
COMBER
COMBOS
CORBEL
CORBIN
COWBOY
DOABLE
DOBBIN
DOCBOY
DOGBED
DOMBEY
DOUBLE
DOUBLY
DOUBTS
FOBBED
FOGBOW
FOIBLE
FORBAD
FORBES
FORBID
GOBBLE
GOOBER
HOBBES
HOBBIT
HOBBLE
HOMBRE
HOTBED
HOTBOT
HOTBOX
HOWBIG
JOBBED
JOBBER
JOGBRA
KOMBAT
KOMBUS
KORBUT
LOBBED
LOBBER
LOWBID
LOWBOY
MOBBED
MOBBER
MORBID
NOMBRE
NOTBAD
ROBBED
ROBBER
ROBBIA
ROBBIE
SOBBED
SOBBER
SOMBER
SOMBRE
SORBET
SORBIC
TOMBES
TOMBOY
TOOBAD
TOOBIG
TOPBID
TORBAY
TOWBAR
WOBBLE
WOBBLY
WOMBAT
WONBIG
YOUBET
ZOMBIE

•O••B•

COHABS
COMEBY
DOESBY
DONEBY
FOURBC
GOALBY
GOESBY
GONEBY
GOODBY
HORNBY
JOJOBA
LOWEBB
RODEBY
ROLLBY
ROOMBA
VOCABS

•O•••B

COBWEB
CONFAB
CONJOB
HOBNOB
HOTTUB
LOUISB
LOWEBB
MODELB
NOPROB
POINTB
TOPJOB

••OB••

ADOBES
ADOBOS
BAOBAB
BLOBBY
BLOBEL
BOOBOO
GLOBAL
GLOBBY
GLOBED
GLOBES
GLOBIN
GOOBER
GROBAN
IROBOT
ISOBAR
KNOBBY
NIOBIC
PHOBIA
PHOBIC
PHOBOS
PROBED
PROBER
PROBES
PROBIE
PROBST
SLOBBY
SNOBBY
SNOBOL
TOOBAD
TOOBIG
TWOBIT

••O•B•

ABOMBS
AMOEBA
BLOBBY
CROSBY
DROPBY
GLOBBY
GOODBY
HBOMBS
KNOBBY
NBOMBS
PHOEBE
RHOMBI
RHOMBS
ROOMBA
SCOOBA
SCOOBY
SHOTBY
SLOBBY
SNOBBY
STOPBY

••O••B

BAOBAB
BIOLAB
ECOLAB

•••OB•

AEROBE
CAROBS
DEMOBS
ENROBE
JACOBI
JACOBY
JOJOBA
KABOBS
KENOBI
MCJOBS
NABOBS
SCOOBA
SCOOBY
STROBE
THROBS
TYCOBB
UNROBE
ZHLOBS

•••O•B

ABSORB
ADSORB
APLOMB
ENTOMB
KEYOFB
MACOMB
RECOMB
RESORB
TYCOBB

••••OB

ATHROB
BAGJOB
CONJOB
DAYJOB
DYEJOB
HOBNOB
JIMBOB
NEWJOB
NOPROB
ODDJOB
SKIBOB
THEMOB
TOPJOB

OC••••

OCASEK
OCASEY
OCCAMS
OCCULT
OCCUPY
OCCURS
OCEANS
OCEDAR
OCELLI
OCELOT
OCHERS
OCHERY
OCHRED
OCHRES
OCICAT
OCLOCK
OCONEE
OCTADS
OCTANE
OCTANS
OCTANT
OCTAVE
OCTAVO
OCTETS
OCTOOT
OCTOPI
OCTROI
OCULAR
OCULUS

O•C•••

OCCAMS
OCCULT
OCCUPY
OCCURS
OHCRUD
ONCALL
ONCLES
OOCYTE
OPCITS
ORCHID
OSCANS
OSCARS
OSCINE
OSCULE
OUCHES
OXCART

O••C••

OCICAT
OILCAN
OILCUP
OLDCAR
ONECAR
ORACHS
ORACLE
ORECKS
OUNCES
OUTCRY
OUTCUT

O•••C•

OAXACA
OBJECT
OCLOCK
OFFICE
OJAICA
OLMECS
ONDECK
ONEACT
ONRICE
OPTICS
ORBACH
OROSCO
OROZCO
OSMICS
OUTACT

O••••C

ODINIC
OLDVIC
ONESEC
ONSPEC
ORPHIC
OTITIC
OVISAC
OXALIC
OXIDIC
OZONIC

•OC•••

BOCCES
BOCCIE
BOCCIS
BOCHCO
BOCHSA
COCCUS
COCCYX
COCKED
COCKER
COCKLE
COCOAS
COCOON
DOCBOY
DOCENT
DOCILE
DOCKED
DOCKER
DOCKET
DOCOMO
DOCTOR
EOCENE
FOCSLE
GOCART
GOCOED
GOCOLD
HOCKED
HOCKER
HOCKEY
JOCKEY
JOCKOS
JOCOSE
JOCUND
KOCHEL
KOCHER
LOCALE

LOCALS
LOCANE
LOCATE
LOCCIT
LOCHER
LOCKED
LOCKER
LOCKET
LOCKIN
LOCKON
LOCKUP
LOCUST
MOCHAS
MOCKED
MOCKER
MOCKUP
NOCENT
NOCHES
NOCKED
NOCOST
OOCYTE
POCKET
POCONO
ROCHAT
ROCHET
ROCHON
ROCKED
ROCKER
ROCKET
ROCKIE
ROCKIN
ROCKIT
ROCKNE
ROCKYV
ROCOCO
SOCANI
SOCCER
SOCIAL
SOCKED
SOCKET
SOCKIN
SOCLES
TOCOME
TOCSIN
VOCABS
VOCALS
ZOCALO

•O•C••

BOBCAT
BOCCES
BOCCIE
BOCCIS
BOLCOM
BOOCOO
BOTCHY
BOUCHE
BOXCAR
COACTS
COCCUS
COCCYX
CONCHA
CONCHO
CONCHS
CONCUR
COPCAR
DORCAS
DOTCOM
FORCED
FORCER
FORCES
FORCHE
GORCEY
GOTCHA
HONCHO
HOTCAP
HOTCAR
HOTCUP
JOBCUT
LOCCIT
LOUCHE
LOWCAL
LOWCUT
MOOCOW
MOSCOW
NONCOM
NOTCHY
POACHY
PONCAS
PONCHO
POUCHY
ROMCOM
RONCEY
ROSCOE
ROYCES
SOCCER
TOECAP
TOMCAT
TOPCAT
TORCHY
TOUCAN
TOUCHE
TOUCHY
TOWCAR
TOYCAR
VOICED
VOICER
VOICES
YOICKS

•O••C•

BOCHCO
BODICE
BONACI
BORSCH
BOUNCE
BOUNCY
COERCE
COLECO
COLICS
COMICE
COMICS
CONICS
CONOCO
CORACI
COSECS
COSTCO
DODECA
DODICI
GOBACK
HOOTCH
HORACE
IONICS
JOUNCE
JOUNCY
KONICA
KOPECK
KOVACS
LOGICS
LOLICH
MONACO
MONICA
NODICE
NOLUCK
NOTICE
NOVICE
POLICE
POLICY
POUNCE
POVIGH
ROCOCO
SOLACE
SOMUCH
SONICS
SOURCE
TONICS
TOPICS
TOXICS
VOTECH
WOMACK
YORICK

•O•••C

AORTIC
COGNAC
CONTAC
COPTIC
COSMIC
COURIC
FORMIC
FOURBC
GOTHIC
HOMEEC
HOOSAC
LOMPOC
MOSAIC
NOETIC
NORDIC
POETIC
ROMAIC
SORBIC
TOLTEC
ZODIAC

••OC••

AVOCET
BLOCKS
BLOCKY
BOOCOO
BROCAS
CHOCKS
CLOCHE
CLOCKS
CROCKS
CROCUS
EPOCHS
EXOCET
FLOCKS
FROCKS
GLOCKS
GROCER
KNOCKS
MOOCOW
NEOCON
PLOCES
PROCOL
SHOCKS
SMOCKS
SNOCAT
STOCKS
STOCKY
TROCHE
TWOCAR
UNOCAL

••O•C•

ATONCE
AVOUCH
BLOTCH
BROACH
BRONCO
BRONCS
BROOCH
CHOICE
CROTCH
CROUCH
EROICA
GFORCE
GLOUCS
GROUCH
HOOTCH
OROSCO
OROZCO
SCONCE
SCORCH
SCOTCH
SLOUCH
SMOOCH
STOICS
STORCH
TWOACT

••O••C

ADONIC
AHOLIC
ANODIC
ANOMIC
ANOXIC
ATOMIC
ATONIC
ATOXIC
AZONIC
BIONIC
BIOPIC
BIOTIC
CHORIC
EPODIC
EROTIC
ETONIC
EXOTIC
FROLIC
GEODIC
GNOMIC
HOOSAC
ICONIC
IRONIC
KAONIC
MYOPIC
NIOBIC
OZONIC
PHOBIC
PHONIC
PHOTIC
PROZAC
THORIC
TROPIC

•••OC•

BROOCH
CONOCO
DECOCT
DUROCS
EDKOCH
ESTOCS
HAVOCS
IDIOCY
INHOCK
JAMOCA
MEDOCS
OCLOCK
RECOCK
REDOCK
RELOCK
ROCOCO
SHLOCK
SMOOCH
SUNOCO
UNDOCK
UNLOCK
VELOCE

•••O•C

ECHOIC
HEROIC
KEYOFC

••••OC

BELLOC
ENBLOC
LOMPOC
ZIPLOC

OD••••

ODAMAE
ODDEST
ODDISH
ODDITY
ODDJOB
ODDLOT
ODDMAN
ODDMEN
ODDSON
ODEDON
ODELET
ODENSE
ODEONS
ODESSA
ODETTA
ODETTE
ODINIC
ODIOUS
ODISTS
ODIUMS
ODONTO
ODORED
ODOULS
ODOURS

O•D•••

ODDEST
ODDISH
ODDITY
ODDJOB
ODDLOT
ODDMAN
ODDMEN
ODDSON
OGDOAD
OHDARN
OHDEAR
OHDRAT
OLDAGE
OLDBAT
OLDBOY
OLDCAR
OLDDOG
OLDELI
OLDEST
OLDGAG
OLDHAM
OLDHAT
OLDIES
OLDISH
OLDMAN
OLDMEN
OLDPAL
OLDPRO
OLDSAW
OLDSOD
OLDVIC
OLDWAY
ONDECK
ONDISK
ONDITS
ONDUTY
OODLES
ORDAIN
ORDEAL
ORDERS

O••D••

OCEDAR
ODEDON
OFFDAY
OLDDOG
ONEDAY
ONEDGE
OUTDID
OWEDON
OWEDTO
OXIDES
OXIDIC
OXYDOL

O•••D•

OBLADI
OCTADS
OGRADY
OLINDA
ONEIDA
ONSIDE
OOPODS
OOTIDS
OREADS
OREIDA
OUTADD
OVERDO
OVIEDO
OVOIDS
OXHIDE

O••••D

OBEYED
OBTUND
OCHRED
ODORED
OFFEND
OGDOAD
OHCRUD
OINKED
OKAYED
OLDSOD
OLERUD
OMENED
ONHAND
ONHOLD
ONLAID
ONLAND
ONLOAD
ONWARD
OPENED
OPINED
ORATED
ORCHID
ORMOND
ORTRUD
OSGOOD
OSMOND
OSMUND
OSTEND
OSWALD
OUSTED
OUTADD
OUTBID
OUTBUD
OUTDID
OUTLED
OXFORD
OXNARD

•OD•••

BODEGA
BODETT
BODICE
BODIED
BODIES
BODILY
BODINE
BODING
BODKIN
BODLEY
BODUKE
CODDLE
CODERS
CODGER
CODIFY
CODING
CODONS
CODYWY
DODDER
DODECA
DODGED
DODGEM
DODGER
DODGES
DODICI
DODODO
DODOES
DODOMA
FODDER
FODORS
GODARD
GODARK
GODEAD
GODEEP
GODETS
GODEYS
GODIVA
GODOWN
GODSON
GODWIN
GODWIT
HODADS
HODGES
HODIAK
HODMAN
HODMEN
IODATE
IODIDE
IODINE
IODISE
IODIZE
KODAKS
KODALY
KODIAK
LODENS
LODGED
LODGER
LODGES
LODINJ
MODALS
MODELA
MODELB
MODELS
MODELT
MODEMS
MODENA
MODERN
MODEST
MODIFY
MODINE
MODISH
MODRED
MODULE
MODULI
MODULO
NODDED
NODDER
NODEAL
NODEAR
NODICE
NODOFF
NODOSE
NODOUS
NODSAT
NODSTO
NODULE
OODLES
PODDED
PODIUM
PODOUS
PODUNK
RODALE
RODDED
RODDER
RODEBY
RODEIN
RODENT
RODEOS
RODETO
RODEUP
RODHAM
RODINO
RODION
RODMAN
RODMEN
RODNEY
SODDED
SODDEN
SODIDI
SODIUM
SODOWE
TODATE
TODAYS
TODDAO
TODDLE
TODIES
TODMAN
VODKAS
YODELS
YODUDE
ZODIAC

•O•D••

AOUDAD
BOLDED
BOLDEN
BOLDER
BOLDLY
BONDED
BONDER
BOODLE
BORDEN
BORDER
BORDET
BOUDIN
CODDLE
COEDIT
COLDER
COLDLY
COMDEN
COMDEX
COMDRS
CONDOR
CONDOS
COODER
CORDAY
CORDED
CORDER
CORDIA
CORDON
COYDOG
DODDER
DOGDAY
DOGDOM
DONDER
DOODAD
DOODAH
DOODLE
DOTDOT
FODDER
FOGDOG
FOLDED
FOLDER
FOLDIN
FOLDUP
FONDAS
FONDER
FONDLE
FONDLY
FONDOF
FONDUE
FONDUS
FOODIE
FORDED
FORDGT
FORDID
FOUDRE
GOADED
GOLDEN
GOLDIE
GOODAT
GOODBY
GOODEN
GOODER
GOODIE
GOODLY
GOODOH
GORDIE
GORDON
GOSDEN
GOUDAS
HOLDEM
HOLDEN
HOLDER
HOLDIN
HOLDIT
HOLDME
HOLDON
HOLDTO
HOLDUP
HONDAS
HOODED
HOODIE
HOODOO
HORDED
HORDES
HOTDAY
HOTDOG
HOUDON
HOWDAH
HOYDEN
JOEDON
JORDAN
LOADED
LOADER
LOADIN
LOADUP
LOIDED
LONDON
LORDED
LORDIT
LORDLY
LOSDOS
LOUDEN
LOUDER
LOUDLY
LOUDON
MOLDAU
MOLDED
MOLDER
MONDAY
MONDES
MONDOS
MOODYS
MOSDEF
NODDED
NODDER
NOIDEA
NOODGE
NOODLE
NORDIC
NORDOI
PODDED
PONDED
PONDER
POODLE
POUDRE
POWDER
ROADEO
ROADER
ROADIE
RODDED
RODDER
RONDEL
RONDOS
SODDED
SODDEN
SOLDER
SOLDIT
SOLDON
SOLDTO
SONDES
SONDRA
SORDID
TODDAO
TODDLE
TOEDIN
TOLDIT
TOLDOF
TOLDON
TOLDYA
TONDOS
TOODLE
TOPDOG
TOYDOG
VOIDED
VOIDER
VOIDOF
VOODOO
WONDER
WOODED
WOODEN
WOODIE
WOODSY
WORDED
YONDER
YOUDIG

•O••D•

BOARDS
BOLIDE
BORIDE
BOUNDS
BOVIDS
COLADA
COMEDY
COMIDA
COULDA
COULDI
DODODO
DORADO
DOSADO
DOSIDO
DOTODO
FOUNDS
GOURDE
GOURDS
HOARDS
HODADS
HOUNDS
HOUNDY
HOWODD
IODIDE
KOMODO
MONADS
MONODY
MOPEDS
MOULDS
MOULDY
MOUNDS
MOVADO
NOBODY
NOKIDS
NOMADS
OOPODS
OOTIDS
POMADE
POSADA
POUNDS
ROUNDS
SODIDI
SOLIDS
SOUNDS
TOLEDO
WONTDO
WORLDS
WOULDA
WOUNDS
YODUDE
ZOOIDS
ZOUNDS

•O•••D

AOUDAD
BOATED
BOBBED
BODIED
BOFFED
BOGGED
BOILED
BOLDED
BOLTED
BOMBED
BONDED
BONGED
BONKED
BOOKED
BOOMED
BOOTED
BOOZED
BOPPED
BORKED
BOSSED
BOWLED
BOXBED
COALED
COATED
COAXED
COCKED
COGGED
COIFED
COILED
COINED
COMBED
COMPED
CONFED
CONKED
CONNED
CONOID
CONRAD
COOEED
COOKED
COOLED
COOPED
COPIED
COPPED
CORDED
CORKED
CORNED
CORVID
COSHED
COSIED
COSTED
COWARD
COWLED
COZIED
DOCKED
DODGED
DOFFED
DOGBED
DOGGED
DOGOOD
DOLLED
DONALD
DONNED
DOODAD
DOOMED
DOORED
DORSAD
DOSSED
DOTARD
DOTTED
DOUSED
DOWNED
DOWSED
FOALED
FOAMED
FOBBED
FOETID
FOGGED
FOILED
FOLDED
FOOLED
FOOTED
FORBAD
FORBID
FORCED
FORDED
FORDID
FORGED
FORKED
FORMED
FOULED
FOURAD
FOWLED
GOADED
GOCOED
GOCOLD
GODARD
GODEAD
GOLFED
GONGED
GOOFED
GOOSED
GORGED
GORMED
GOTMAD
GOTOLD
GOTRID
GOUGED
GOUNOD
GOWILD
GOWNED
HOAXED
HOBOED
HOCKED
HOGGED
HONIED
HONKED
HOODED
HOOFED
HOOKED
HOOPED
HOOTED
HOPPED
HORDED
HORNED
HORRID
HORSED
HOSTED
HOTBED
HOTROD
HOUSED
HOWARD
HOWLED
HOWODD
HOWSAD
JOBBED
JOCUND
JOGGED
JOINED
JOLTED
JOSHED
JOTTED
JOWLED
JOYPAD
KOBOLD
KONRAD
LOADED
LOAFED
LOAMED
LOANED
LOBBED
LOCKED
LODGED
LOFTED
LOGGED
LOIDED
LOLLED
LOMOND
LONGED
LOOKED
LOOMED
LOOPED
LOOSED
LOOTED
LOPPED
LORDED
LOTTED
LOUSED
LOWBID
LOWEND
MOANED
MOATED
MOBBED
MOCKED
MODRED
MOILED
MOLDED
MOLTED
MONIED
MOONED
MOORED
MOOTED
MOPPED
MORBID
MOSHED
MOSSAD
MOSSED
MOUSED
NOCKED
NODDED
NOGOOD
NOISED
NOLEAD
NOLOAD
NONEED
NONFED
NONGOD
NOOSED
NOSHED
NOTBAD
PODDED
POISED
POLAND
POLLED
PONDED
PONGID
PONIED
POOHED
POOLED
POOPED
POPPED
PORKED
PORTED
POSTED
POTLID
POTTED
POUFED
POURED
POUTED
ROAMED
ROARED
ROBBED
ROCKED
RODDED
ROGUED
ROILED
ROLAND

ROLFED
ROLLED
ROMPED
RONALD
ROOFED
ROOKED
ROOMED
ROOTED
ROTTED
ROTUND
ROUGED
ROUSED
ROUTED
SOAKED
SOAPED
SOARED
SOBBED
SOCKED
SODDED
SOILED
SOLOED
SOLVED
SOPPED
SORDID
SORTED
SOSPAD
SOTTED
SOURED
SOUSED
TOGAED
TOGGED
TOILED
TOLLED
TONGED
TOOBAD
TOOLED
TOOTED
TOPBID
TOPPED
TOROID
TORPID
TORRID
TOSSED
TOTTED
TOURED
TOUTED
TOWARD
VOGUED
VOICED
VOIDED
WOLFED
WONTED
WOODED
WOOFED
WORDED
WORKED
WORMED
YOLKED
YOWLED
YOYOED
ZONKED
ZOOMED

••OD••

ABODES
ANODAL
ANODES
ANODIC
APODAL
ATODDS
AZODYE
BOODLE
BRODIE
CLODDY
COODER
DEODAR
DIODES
DOODAD
DOODAH
DOODLE
ELODEA
EPODES
EPODIC
ERODED
ERODER
ERODES
EXODUS
FEODOR
FOODIE
FYODOR
GEODES
GEODIC
GOODAT
GOODBY
GOODEN
GOODER
GOODIE
GOODLY
GOODOH
GRODIN
HOODED
HOODIE
HOODOO
MOODYS
NOODGE
NOODLE
POODLE
PRODON
RHODES
SHODDY
SPODES
STODGE
STODGY
TOODLE
TRODON
TWODAY
VOODOO
WHODAT
WOODED
WOODEN
WOODIE
WOODSY

••O•D•

AROIDS
ATODDS
AVOIDS
BIONDI
BLONDE
BLONDS
BLOODS
BLOODY
BROADA
BROODS
BROODY
CHORDS
CLODDY
CLOUDS
CLOUDY
CROWDS
DROIDS
EBONDS
FIORDS
FJORDS
FLOODS
FRONDS
GEORDI
HYOIDS
IDOIDO
ISOLDA
ISOLDE
LLOYDS
OVOIDS
RHONDA
SCOLDS
SHODDY
SNOODS
SWORDS
TBONDS
YEOLDE
ZOOIDS

••O••D

ABOARD
ABOUND
ADORED
AROUND
ATONED
AVOWED
BOOKED
BOOMED
BOOTED
BOOZED
BROWED
BUOYED
CHOKED
CHOWED
CLONED
CLOSED
CLOYED
COOEED
COOKED
COOLED
COOPED
CROWED
DIOMED
DOODAD
DOOMED
DOORED
DRONED
ELOPED
EMOTED
ERODED
EVOKED
FLORID
FLOWED
FOOLED
FOOTED
GAOLED
GLOBED
GLOVED
GLOWED
GOOFED
GOOSED
GROPED
GROUND
GROVED
HOODED
HOOFED
HOOKED
HOOPED
HOOTED
ICOULD
IRONED
ISOPOD
IWOULD
LEONID
LOOKED
LOOMED
LOOPED
LOOSED
LOOTED
MEOWED
MOONED
MOORED
MOOTED
NOOSED
ODORED
PHONED
PLOWED
POOHED
POOLED
POOPED
PROBED
PROSED
PROVED
QUOTED
RIOTED
ROOFED
ROOKED
ROOMED
ROOTED
SCOPED
SCORED
SHOOED
SHOULD
SHOVED
SHOWED
SLOPED
SLOWED
SMOKED
SNORED
SNOWED
SPOKED
STOKED
STOLID
STONED
STORED
STOWED
TOOBAD
TOOLED
TOOTED
TROWED
UNOWED
WOODED
WOOFED
ZOOMED

•••OD•

BIPODS
BLOODS
BLOODY
BROODS
BROODY
DECODE
DEMODE
DESODS
DIPODY
DODODO
DOTODO
DYNODE
EMBODY
ENCODE
EPHODS
FLOODS
HOWODD
INCODE
KOMODO
MELODY
MONODY
NOBODY
OOPODS
PAGODA
PARODY
RECODE
RERODE
RESODS
SCRODS
SNOODS
STRODE
SYNODS
TRIODE
VIGODA
YEGODS

•••O•D

ABROAD
ACCORD
AFFORD
AGEOLD
ALMOND
ALTOID
ANYOLD
ARNOLD
ASCOLD
ASGOOD
ATWOOD
AUFOND
AUTOED
BEGOOD
BEHOLD
BEYOND
BIFOLD
BUJOLD
BYROAD
BYWORD
CANOED
CONOID
CUBOID
DADOED
DAYOLD
DEFORD
DEMOED
DEMOND
DEVOID
DOGOOD
ECHOED
EDMOND
EDWOOD
ELWOOD
ENFOLD
EQUOID
GETOLD
GOCOED
GOCOLD
GOTOLD
HALOED
HALOID
HAROLD
HOBOED
HOWODD
HYPOED
IMCOLD
IMGOOD
IMSOLD
IMTOLD
INFOLD
INGOLD
INGOOD
INROAD
KAYOED
KEYOFD
KOBOLD
LEMOND
LOMOND
MAJOAD
MCCORD
MILORD
MRBOND
MTHOOD
MYLORD
MYWORD
NOGOOD
NOLOAD
OGDOAD
ONHOLD
ONLOAD
ORMOND
OSGOOD
OSMOND
OXFORD
PAJOAD
RECORD
REFOLD
REHOED
REHOLD
RELOAD
REMOLD
RESOLD
RETOLD
REWORD
SECOND
SHOOED
SHROUD
SILOED
SOLOED
STROUD
TOROID
UNBOLD
UNFOLD
UNFOND
UNHOED
UNHOOD
UNLOAD
UNMOLD
UNSOLD
UNTOLD
UNVOID
UPFOLD
UPHOLD
UPLOAD
VETOED
WASOLD
WHWORD
XYLOID
YOYOED
ZEROED

••••OD

ASGOOD
ASHDOD
ATWOOD
BEGOOD
DOGOOD
EDWOOD
ELWOOD
FLYROD
GOUNOD
HESIOD
HOTROD
IMGOOD
INAPOD
INGOOD
ISOPOD
METHOD
MTHOOD
NIMROD
NOGOOD
NONGOD
OLDSOD
OSGOOD
PEAPOD
PENROD
PEQUOD
PERIOD
PERNOD
RAMROD
REDCOD
RESHOD
RETROD
SEAGOD
SUBGOD
SUNGOD
THEROD
TIEROD
TINGOD
TRIPOD
UNHOOD
UNIPOD
UNSHOD
UNTROD
WARGOD

OE••••

OENONE
OERTER
OEUVRE

O•E•••

OBEAHS
OBELUS
OBENTO
OBERON
OBERTO
OBEYED
OBEYER
OCEANS
OCEDAR
OCELLI
OCELOT
ODEDON
ODELET
ODENSE
ODEONS
ODESSA
ODETTA
ODETTE
OHENRY
OKEEFE
OLEARY
OLEATE
OLEFIN
OLEINS
OLEOLE
OLERUD
OLESHA
OLESON
OLEUMS
OLEVEL
OMEARA
OMEGAS
OMELET
OMENED
OMERTA
ONEACT
ONEALL
ONEARM
ONEBIT
ONECAR
ONEDAY
ONEDGE
ONEEEE
ONEEGG
ONEEYE
ONEGIN
ONEHIT
ONEIDA
ONEILL
ONEIRO
ONEISH
ONELAP
ONELEG
ONEMAN
ONEMEG
ONEOFF
ONEONE
ONEOUT
ONEPIN
ONERUN
ONESEC
ONESET
ONETEN
ONETON
ONETWO
ONEUPS
ONEWAY
OPENED
OPENER
OPENIT
OPENLY
OPENON
OPENTO
OPENUP
OPERAS
OREADS
ORECKS
OREGON
OREIDA
ORELSE
ORENSE
OREOOS
OREXIA
OREXIS
OSETRA
OTELLO
OVERDO
OVERIT
OVERLY
OWEDON
OWEDTO
OWESON
OXEYES
OYEZES

O••E••

OARERS
OATERS
OBJECT
OBJETS
OBSESS
OBTEST
OBVERT
OCHERS
OCHERY
OCTETS
ODDEST
OFFEND
OFFERS
OFHELP
OGLERS
OGRESS
OHDEAR
OHWELL
OHYEAH
OILERS
OISEAU
OKEEFE
OLDELI
OLDEST
OLMECS
OLMERT
ONDECK
ONEEEE
ONEEGG
ONEEYE
ONSETS
ORDEAL
ORDERS
ORGEAT
ORIELS
ORIENT
ORNERY
ORRERY
ORTEGA
ORWELL
OSBERT
OSIERS
OSSETS
OSTEAL
OSTEND
OSTERS
OSWEGO
OTHERS
OTSEGO
OTTERS
OUSELS
OUTEAT
OUZELS
OVIEDO
OWLEGG
OWLERY
OWLETS
OWNERS

O•••E•

OAKIER
OAKLEY
OARMEN
OATIER
OBEYED
OBEYER
OBITER
OBOLER
OBRIEN
OCASEK
OCASEY
OCHRED
OCHRES
OCONEE
ODDMEN
ODELET
ODORED
OERTER
OFFKEY
OFFSET
OGIVES
OILIER
OILMEN
OINKED
OINKER
OKAYED
OLAKES
OLDIES
OLDMEN
OLEVEL
OLIVER
OLIVES
OLORES
OMELET
OMENED
ONAGER
ONCLES
ONEEEE
ONELEG
ONEMEG
ONESEC
ONESET
ONETEN
ONSPEC
ONUSES
ONVIEW
ONYXES
OODLES
OOZIER
OPENED
OPENER
OPINED
OPINER
OPINES
OPUSES
ORAJEL
ORALES
ORATED
ORATES
ORGIES
ORIGEN
ORKNEY
OROMEO
ORTHEN
ORYXES
OSAGES
OSPREY
OSTLER
OTILES
OTOSES
OUCHES
OUIMET
OUNCES
OUSTED
OUSTER
OUTBEG
OUTIES
OUTJET
OUTLED
OUTLET
OUTSEE
OUTSET
OVINES
OVULES
OWLIER
OXEYES
OXIDES
OXYGEN
OYEZES
OYSTER

O••••E

OARAGE
OBLATE
OBLIGE
OBTUSE
OCONEE
OCTANE
OCTAVE
ODAMAE
ODENSE
ODETTE
OENONE
OEUVRE
OFFICE
OFLATE
OFNOTE
OFYORE
OGAUGE
OHMAGE
OHSURE
OKBYME
OKEEFE
OLATHE
OLDAGE
OLEATE
OLEOLE
ONBASE
ONEDGE
ONEEEE
ONEEYE
ONEONE
ONFILE
ONFIRE
ONHIRE
ONLATE
ONLINE
ONMIKE
ONRICE
ONSALE
ONSIDE
ONSITE
ONTAPE
ONTIME
OOCYTE
OOLITE
OPAQUE
OPIATE
OPPOSE
ORACLE
ORANGE
ORELSE
ORENSE
ORIOLE
ORNATE
OSCINE
OSCULE
OSMOSE
OTIOSE
OTOOLE
OTTONE
OUTAGE
OUTATE
OUTAWE
OUTLIE
OUTSEE
OUTVIE
OXHIDE
OXLIKE

•OE•••

BOEING
BOESKY
COEDIT
COELIA
COERCE
COEURS
COEVAL
DOESBY
DOESIN
DOESIT
DOESNT
DOESOK
DOESSO
DOESTO
DOESUP
FOEMAN
FOEMEN
FOETID
GOEASY
GOESAT
GOESBY
GOESIN
GOESON
GOESTO
GOESUP
GOETHE
HOEING
JOEDON
JOETEX
KOENIG
MOERAE
MOESHA
NOEMON
NOESIS
NOETIC
NOEXIT
POEANA
POEMES
POETES
POETIC
POETRY
ROEPER
SOEURS
TOECAP
TOEDIN
TOEING
TOEINS
TOESIN
TOETAP
WOEFUL

•O•E••

AOLERS
BODEGA
BODETT
BOGEYS
BOHEME
BOLENA
BOLERO
BOLEYN
BONERS
BONERZ
BONEUP
BOOERS
BOPEEP
BOREAL
BOREAS
BOREON
BORERS
BOREUP
BOTELS
BOWELS
BOWERS
BOWERY
BOXERS
CODERS
COGENT
COHEIR
COHERE
COLECO
COLEUS
COMEAS
COMEAT
COMEBY
COMEDY
COMEIN
COMELY
COMEOF
COMEON
COMERS
COMETH
COMETO
COMETS
COMEUP
CONERS
CONEYS
COOEED
COOEES
COOERS
COPERS
CORERS
COSECS
COSELL
COSETS
COVENS
COVENT
COVERS
COVERT
COVETS
COVEYS
COWENS
COWERS
COYEST
COZENS
DOCENT
DODECA
DOGEAR
DOLENZ
DONEBY
DONEES
DONEIN
DONEIT
DONEOK
DONESO
DONETO
DONETS
DONEUP
DOPERS
DOREEN
DOREMI
DOSERS
DOTELL
DOTEON
DOTERS
DOVEIN
DOWELL
DOWELS
DOWERS
DOWERY
DOYENS
DOZENS
DOZERS
EOCENE
FOGEYS
FOLEYS
FOMENT
FOREGO
FOREST
FOYERS
GODEAD
GODEEP
GODETS
GODEYS
GOFERS
GOLEFT
GOLEMS
GOLETA
GOMERS
GONEAR
GONEAT
GONEBY
GONEIN
GONEON
GONERS
GONETO
GONEUP
GONEXT
GORERS
GOTEAM
GOVERN
GOWELL
GOWEST
HOLERS
HOLEUP
HOMEEC
HOMEIN
HOMELY
HOMERS
HOMEYS
HONEIN
HONERS
HONEST
HONEYS
HOPERS
HOPESO
HOPETO
HOSELS
HOSERS
HOTELS
HOVELS
HOVERS
HOVETO
HOWELL
IOMEGA
JOBETH
JOKERS
JOLENE
JONESS
JONESY
JOSEPH
KOPECK
KOPEKS
KOPELL
KOREAN
LODENS
LOMEIN
LONELY
LONERS
LOOEYS
LOPERS
LOREAL
LORENE
LORENZ
LOSEIT
LOSERS
LOSETO
LOVEIN
LOVEIT
LOVELL
LOVELY
LOVERS
LOVETO
LOVETT
LOVEYA
LOVEYS
LOWEBB
LOWELL
LOWEND
LOWERS
LOWERY
LOWEST
MOBERG
MODELA
MODELB

MODELS
MODELT
MODEMS
MODENA
MODERN
MODEST
MOIETY
MOLEST
MOMENT
MONETA
MONETS
MONEYS
MOOERS
MOPEDS
MOPERS
MOPERY
MOREAU
MOREEN
MORELS
MORENO
MORESO
MOSEYS
MOTELS
MOTETS
MOVEIN
MOVEIT
MOVEON
MOVERS
MOVETO
MOVEUP
MOWERS
MOYERS
NOBELS
NOCENT
NODEAL
NODEAR
NOFEES
NOHELP
NOLEAD
NOLESS
NOMEAK
NOMEAT
NONEED
NONEGO
NONETS
NONEWS
NOPETS
NOREEN
NORELL
NORENT
NOSEIN
NOSERS
NOSEUP
NOTERS
NOVELA
NOVELS
NOVENA
POKEAT
POKERS
POKERY
POKEYS
POLEAX
POLERS
POMELO
POPEIL
POPEYE
PORERS
POSEAS
POSERS
POSEUR
POTEEN
POTENT
POWELL
POWERS
ROBERS
ROBERT
RODEBY
RODEIN
RODENT
RODEOS
RODETO
RODEUP
ROGERE
ROGERS
ROGETS
ROLEOS
ROMEOS
ROMERO
RONELY
ROPEIN
ROPERS
ROPERY
ROPEUP
ROSEAU
ROSERY
ROSETO
ROSEUP
ROVERS
ROWELS
ROWENA
ROWENS
ROWERS
SOBEIT
SOBERS
SOLEAS
SOLEIL
SOLELY
SOLEMN
SOLERS
SOLEUS
SOMERS
SOREAT
SORELY
SOREST
SOWERS
SOWETO
TOHEEL
TOKENS
TOLEDO
TONEME
TONERS
TONEUP
TOPEES
TOPEKA
TOPERS
TOREAT
TOREIT
TORENT
TORERO
TOREUP
TOTEMS
TOTERM
TOTERS
TOTEUP
TOWELS
TOWERS
TOWERY
TOYERS
VOMERS
VOTECH
VOTEIN
VOTENO
VOTEON
VOTERS
VOWELS
VOWELY
VOWERS
WOKEUP
WOMENS
WOOERS
WOREON
YODELS
YOKELS
ZONERS

•O••E•

BOATED
BOATEL
BOATER
BOBBED
BOBBER
BOCCES
BODIED
BODIES
BODLEY
BOFFED
BOGGED
BOGIES
BOGLES
BOHRER
BOILED
BOILER
BOITES
BOKKEN
BOLDED
BOLDEN
BOLDER
BOLGER
BOLTED
BOLTER
BOMBED
BOMBER
BOMBES
BONDED
BONDER
BONGED
BONIER
BONKED
BONNER
BONNES
BONNET
BONNEY
BONZES
BOOKED
BOOKEM
BOOKER
BOOMED
BOOMER
BOOTED
BOOTEE
BOOTER
BOOTES
BOOZED
BOOZER
BOOZES
BOPEEP
BOPPED
BOPPER
BORDEN
BORDER
BORDET
BORGES
BORKED
BORNEO
BOSLEY
BOSSED
BOSSES
BOTHER
BOTREE
BOULES
BOULEZ
BOWLED
BOWLER
BOWLES
BOWMEN
BOWYER
BOWZER
BOXBED
BOXIER
BOXSET
BOYLES
COALED
COALER
COATED
COATEE
COATER
COATES
COAXED
COAXER
COAXES
COBWEB
COCKED
COCKER
CODGER
COFFEE
COFFER
COGGED
COHOES
COIFED
COILED
COILER
COINED
COINER
COKIER
COKIES
COLDER
COLLET
COLTER
COMBED
COMBER
COMDEN
COMDEX
COMPED
COMPEL
COMTES
CONFED
CONFER
CONGER
CONGES
CONIES
CONKED
CONKER
CONMEN
CONNED
CONNEE
CONVEX
CONVEY
COODER
COOEED
COOEES
COOKED
COOKER
COOLED
COOLER
COOLEY
COONEY
COOPED
COOPER
COOTER
COPIED
COPIER
COPIES
COPLEY
COPPED
COPPER
COPSES
COPTER
CORBEL
CORDED
CORDER
CORKED
CORKER
CORNEA
CORNED
CORNEL
CORNER
CORNET
CORREO
CORSET
CORTES
CORTEX
CORTEZ
CORVEE
COSHED
COSHER
COSHES
COSIED
COSIER
COSIES
COSSET
COSTED
COTLER
COTTEN
COTTER
COULEE
COUPES
COUTER
COWIER
COWLED
COWLEY
COWMEN
COWPEA
COWPER
COZIED
COZIER
COZIES
DOAKES
DOASET
DOBLES
DOCKED
DOCKER
DOCKET
DODDER
DODGED
DODGEM
DODGER
DODGES
DODOES
DOFFED
DOFFER
DOGBED
DOGGED
DOGIES
DOGLEG
DOKKEN
DOLLED
DOLLEY
DOMBEY
DOMREP
DONDER
DONEES
DONKEY
DONNED
DONNER
DOOLEY
DOOMED
DOORED
DOOVER
DOOZER
DOPIER
DOREEN
DORIES
DORMER
DORSET
DORSEY
DOSSED
DOSSES
DOTTED
DOTTER
DOURER
DOUSED
DOUSER
DOUSES
DOUZES
DOWNED
DOWNER
DOWNES
DOWNEY
DOWSED
DOWSER
DOWSES
DOXIES
DOZIER
FOALED
FOAMED
FOAMER
FOBBED
FODDER
FOEMEN
FOGGED
FOGGER
FOGIES
FOILED
FOKKER
FOLDED
FOLDER
FOLGER
FOLIES
FONDER
FOOLED
FOOLER
FOOTED
FOOTER
FORBES
FORCED
FORCER
FORCES
FORDED
FORGED
FORGER
FORGES
FORGET
FORKED
FORKER
FORMED
FORMER
FORTES
FOSSES
FOSSEY
FOSTER
FOULED
FOULER
FOUREE
FOWLED
FOWLER
FOWLES
FOXIER
GOADED
GOATEE
GOBIES
GOBLET
GOBOES
GOCOED
GODEEP
GOFREE
GOITER
GOLDEN
GOLFED
GOLFER
GONGED
GOOBER
GOODEN
GOODER
GOOFED
GOOIER
GOONEY
GOOSED
GOOSEN
GOOSES
GOOSEY
GOOVER
GOPHER
GORCEY
GORGED
GORGER
GORGES
GORIER
GORMED
GORSES
GOSDEN
GOSHEN
GOSPEL
GOTHEP
GOTSET
GOTTEN
GOTWET
GOUGED
GOUGER
GOUGES
GOULET
GOWNED
HOAXED
HOAXER
HOAXES
HOBBES
HOBOED
HOBOES
HOCKED
HOCKER
HOCKEY
HODGES
HODMEN
HOFFER
HOGGED
HOHNER
HOKIER
HOKIES
HOLDEM
HOLDEN
HOLDER
HOLIER
HOLIES
HOLLER
HOLLEY
HOLMES
HOMEEC
HOMIER
HOMIES
HOMMES
HONIED
HONKED
HONKER
HOODED
HOOFED
HOOFER
HOOKED
HOOKER
HOOKEY
HOOPED
HOOPER
HOOTED
HOOTER
HOOVER
HOOVES
HOPPED
HOPPER
HORDED
HORDES
HORMEL
HORNED
HORNER
HORNET
HORSED
HORSES
HORSEY
HOSIER
HOSSES
HOSTED
HOSTEL
HOTBED
HOTKEY
HOTTEA
HOTTER
HOUSED
HOUSES
HOWLED
HOWLER
HOWSER
HOYDEN
HOYLES
JOBBED
JOBBER
JOCKEY
JOETEX
JOGGED
JOGGER
JOINED
JOINER
JOKIER
JOLIET
JOLLEY
JOLTED
JOLTER
JOSHED
JOSHER
JOSHES
JOSSES
JOTTED
JOTTER
JOULES
JOWLED
JOYNER
JOZSEF
KOCHEL
KOCHER
KOHLER
KOPJES
KOPPEL
KOSHER
KOSSEL
KOSTER
KOTTER
LOADED
LOADER
LOAFED
LOAFER
LOAMED
LOANED
LOANER
LOAVES
LOBBED
LOBBER
LOCHER
LOCKED
LOCKER
LOCKET
LODGED
LODGER
LODGES
LOFTED
LOFTER
LOGGED
LOGGER
LOGIER
LOIDED
LOIRET
LOITER
LOLLED
LOLLER
LONGED
LONGER
LONGES
LONGET
LOOIES
LOOKED
LOOKEE
LOOKER
LOOMED
LOONEY
LOOPED
LOOPER
LOOSED
LOOSEN
LOOSER
LOOSES
LOOSEY
LOOTED
LOOTER
LOPPED
LOPPER
LORDED
LORIES
LOSSES
LOTTED
LOTTER
LOUDEN
LOUDER
LOUIES
LOUPES
LOUSED
LOUSES
LOUVER
LOWKEY
LOWMEN
LOWRES
LOWSET
MOANED
MOANER
MOATED
MOBBED
MOBBER
MOBLEY
MOCKED
MOCKER
MODRED
MOILED
MOILER
MOINES
MOIRES
MOISES
MOJOES
MOLDED
MOLDER
MOLTED
MOLTEN
MOLTER
MONDES
MONGER
MONIED
MONIES
MONKEE
MONKEY
MONNET
MONTEL
MONTEZ
MOONED
MOONER
MOONEY
MOORED
MOOTED
MOOTER
MOPIER
MOPPED
MOPPER
MOPPET
MOREEN
MORGEN
MORLEY
MORREL
MORSEL
MORTEN
MOSDEF
MOSHED
MOSHER
MOSHES
MOSLEM
MOSLEY
MOSSED
MOSSES
MOSTEL
MOTHER
MOTLEY
MOUSED
MOUSER
MOUSES
MOUSEY
MOVIES
NOBLER
NOBLES
NOCHES
NOCKED
NODDED
NODDER
NOFEES
NOIDEA
NOIRES
NOIRET
NOISED
NOISES
NONEED
NONFED
NONJEW
NONMEN
NONNET
NOONER
NOONES
NOOSED
NOOSER
NOOSES
NOREEN
NOSHED
NOSHER
NOSHES
NOSIER
NOSTEP
NOSTER
NOTNEW
NOTYET
NOUMEA
OODLES
OOZIER
POCKET
PODDED
POEMES
POETES
POGNER
POIRES
POIRET
POISED
POISER
POISES
POKIER
POKIES
POLLED
POLLEE
POLLEN
POLLER
POLLEX
POMMEL
POMMES
POMPEO
POMPEY
PONDED
PONDER
PONGEE
PONIED
PONIES
POOHED
POOLED
POOLER
POOPED
POORER
POPPED
POPPER
PORKED
PORKER
PORTED
PORTER
PORTES
POSHER
POSIES
POSSES
POSTED
POSTER
POTEEN
POTHER
POTTED
POTTER
POUFED
POULES
POURED
POURER
POUTED
POUTER
POWDER
POYSER
ROADEO
ROADER
ROAMED
ROAMER
ROARED
ROARER
ROBBED
ROBBER
ROBLES
ROCHET
ROCKED
ROCKER
ROCKET
RODDED
RODDER
RODMEN
RODNEY
ROEPER
ROGUED
ROGUES
ROHMER
ROHRER
ROILED
ROLFED
ROLFER
ROLLED
ROLLEI
ROLLER
ROMMEL
ROMNEY
ROMPED
ROMPER
RONCEY
RONDEL
ROOFED
ROOFER
ROOKED
ROOKER
ROOMED
ROOMER
ROONEY
ROOTED
ROOTER
ROPIER
ROSIER
ROSIES
ROSSEN
ROSSET
ROSTEN
ROSTER
ROTTED
ROTTEN
ROTTER
ROUGED
ROUGES
ROUSED
ROUSER
ROUSES
ROUTED
ROUTER
ROUTES
ROWLEY
ROYCES
SOAKED
SOAKER
SOAPED
SOAPER
SOARED
SOARER
SOAVES
SOBBED
SOBBER
SOCCER
SOCKED
SOCKET
SOCLES
SODDED
SODDEN
SOFTEN
SOFTER
SOILED
SOIREE
SOISEE
SOLDER
SOLOED
SOLVED
SOLVER
SOLVES
SOMBER
SOMMER
SONDES
SONNET
SOONER
SOPPED
SORBET
SORREL
SORTED
SORTER
SOTHEN
SOTTED
SOUPER
SOURED
SOURER
SOUSED
SOUSES
SOUTER
SOVIET
TOATEE
TOBIES
TODIES
TOFFEE
TOGAED
TOGGED
TOGUES
TOHEEL
TOILED
TOILER
TOILES
TOILET
TOLLED
TOLLER
TOLTEC
TOMBES
TONGED
TONIER
TONNES
TOOLED
TOOLER
TOOMEY
TOOTED
TOOTER
TOPEES
TOPMEN
TOPPED
TOPPER
TOPTEN
TOQUES
TORIES
TORRES
TORREY
TORTES
TOSSED
TOSSER
TOSSES
TOTTED
TOTTER
TOUPEE
TOURED
TOURER
TOUTED
TOUTER
TOWHEE
TOWNER
VOGUED
VOGUER
VOGUES
VOICED
VOICER
VOICES
VOIDED
VOIDER
VOILES
VOLLEY
VORTEX
VOSGES
WOHLER
WOLFED
WOLPER
WOLSEY
WOLVES
WONDER
WONTED
WOODED
WOODEN
WOOFED
WOOFER
WOOLEN
WOOLEY
WORDED
WORKED
WORKER
WORLEY
WORMED
WORMER
WORSEN
YOLKED
YONDER
YORKER
YOUBET
YOUSEE
YOWLED
YOWLER
YOYOED
ZONKED
ZONKER
ZOOIER
ZOOMED

•O•••E

AORTAE
BOBBIE
BOBBLE
BOCCIE
BODICE
BODINE
BODUKE
BOGGLE
BOHEME
BOLIDE
BONNIE
BOODLE
BOOGIE
BOOKIE
BOOTEE
BOOTHE
BOOTIE
BORATE
BORIDE
BOTREE
BOTTLE
BOUCHE
BOUFFE
BOUNCE
BOURKE

BOURNE
BOURSE
BOVINE
BOWTIE
COARSE
COATEE
COBBLE
COCKLE
CODDLE
COERCE
COFFEE
COGGLE
COHERE
COIGNE
COLLIE
COMATE
COMICE
CONNEE
CONNIE
CONTRE
CONURE
COOKIE
COOLIE
COOTIE
CORPSE
CORVEE
COSINE
COSTAE
COTTAE
COULEE
COUPLE
COURSE
COWRIE
COYOTE
DOABLE
DOCILE
DOFINE
DOGAPE
DOGGIE
DOLIKE
DOLORE
DOMINE
DONATE
DONGLE
DONNIE
DOODLE
DOOGIE
DOOLIE
DOOZIE
DORINE
DORMIE
DOSAGE
DOTAGE
DOTIME
DOTTIE
DOTTLE
DOUANE
DOUBLE
EOCENE
FOCSLE
FOIBLE
FOKINE
FOLATE
FOLKIE
FONDLE
FONDUE
FONZIE
FOODIE
FOOTLE
FOOZLE
FORAGE
FORCHE
FORONE
FOSSAE
FOUDRE
FOUREE
FOZZIE
GOALIE
GOATEE
GOBBLE
GOETHE
GOFREE
GOGGLE
GOHOME
GOLAME
GOLDIE
GOLIKE
GOLIVE
GOODIE
GOOGLE
GOONIE
GORDIE
GOURDE
HOAGIE
HOARSE
HOBBLE
HOGTIE
HOLDME
HOMAGE
HOMBRE
HONORE
HOODIE
HOOPLE
HOOPOE
HOOTIE
HORACE
HOTONE
HOTTIE
IODATE
IODIDE
IODINE
IODISE
IODIZE
IONISE
IONIZE
IONONE
JOANIE
JOANNE
JOBONE
JOCOSE
JOFFRE
JOGGLE
JOLENE
JOSTLE
JOUNCE
KOOKIE
KOTTKE
LOATHE
LOBATE
LOBULE
LOCALE
LOCANE
LOCATE
LONGUE
LONNIE
LOOKEE
LOOKIE
LOONIE
LORENE
LORRIE
LOUCHE
LOUISE
LOUNGE
LOUVRE
LOVAGE
LOYALE
MOBILE
MODINE
MODULE
MOERAE
MOHAVE
MOJAVE
MOLINE
MOLLIE
MOLTKE
MOMMIE
MONKEE
MONROE
MOOKIE
MOONIE
MORALE
MORGUE
MOROSE
MORRIE
MOSQUE
MOTILE
MOTIVE
MOTTLE
MOUSSE
NOBAKE
NOBILE
NODICE
NODOSE
NODULE
NOHOPE
NOJIVE
NOJOKE
NOLOSE
NOMBRE
NOMORE
NONAGE
NONAME
NONUSE
NOODGE
NOODLE
NOOGIE
NORITE
NOSALE
NOTATE
NOTICE
NOTIME
NOTONE
NOVICE
NOVOTE
NOWISE
NOZZLE
OOCYTE
OOLITE
POINTE
POIVRE
POLICE
POLITE
POLLEE
POMADE
PONGEE
POODLE
POPEYE
POPPLE
POROSE
POSOLE
POSTIE
POTAGE
POTPIE
POTSIE
POUDRE
POUNCE
POUSSE
POZOLE
ROADIE
ROBBIE
ROCKIE
ROCKNE
RODALE
ROGERE
ROLLIE
RONNIE
ROOKIE
ROOMIE
ROOTIE
ROOTLE
ROSCOE
ROTATE
ROURKE
ROXANE
ROYALE
SODOWE
SOFINE
SOFTIE
SOIGNE
SOIREE
SOISEE
SOLACE
SOLUTE
SOMBRE
SOOTHE
SOPHIE
SORTIE
SOTRUE
SOURCE
TOATEE
TOCOME
TODATE
TODDLE
TOFFEE
TOGGLE
TOLIFE
TOMMIE
TONEME
TONGUE
TONITE
TOODLE
TOONIE
TOOTIE
TOOTLE
TOPPLE
TORQUE
TOUCHE
TOUPEE
TOUSLE
TOWAGE
TOWHEE
TOWNIE
VOLARE
VOLUME
VOLUTE
VOTIVE
VOYAGE
WOBBLE
WOODIE
WOOGIE
YODUDE
YORKIE
YOUSEE
ZOMBIE
ZONULE

••OE••

AMOEBA
BOOERS
CLOETE
COOEED
COOEES
COOERS
LOOEYS
MOOERS
PHOEBE
PROEMS
SHOERS
TWOEEE
WOOERS

••O•E•

ABODES
ADOBES
ADORED
ADOREE
ADORER
ADORES
AGONES
AMOLES
AMORES
AMORET
ANODES
ANOLES
APOGEE
AROUET
ATONED
ATONER
ATONES
AVOCET
AVOWED
AVOWER
AWOKEN
AXONES
AZOLES
AZORES
BIOMES
BLOBEL
BLOKES
BLOOEY
BLOWER
BOOKED
BOOKEM
BOOKER
BOOMED
BOOMER
BOOTED
BOOTEE
BOOTER
BOOTES
BOOZED
BOOZER
BOOZES
BROKEN
BROKER
BROWED
BUOYED
CHOKED
CHOKER
CHOKES
CHOLER
CHOREO
CHORES
CHOSEN
CHOWED
CLONED
CLONER
CLONES
CLOSED
CLOSER
CLOSES
CLOSET
CLOVEN
CLOVER
CLOVES
CLOYED
CNOTES
COODER
COOEED
COOEES
COOKED
COOKER
COOLED
COOLER
COOLEY
COONEY
COOPED
COOPER
COOTER
CRONES
CRORES
CROWED
CROWER
CUORES
DHOLES
DHOTEL
DIODES
DIOMED
DOOLEY
DOOMED
DOORED
DOOVER
DOOZER
DRONED
DRONER
DRONES
DROUET
DROVER
DROVES
ECOLES
ELODEA
ELOGES
ELOPED
ELOPER
ELOPES
EMOTED
EMOTER
EMOTES
ENOTES
EPODES
EPOPEE
EPOSES
EPOWER
ERODED
ERODER
ERODES
EVOKED
EVOKER
EVOKES
EXOCET
FHOLES
FLOOEY
FLOREK
FLORES
FLORET
FLOREY
FLOWED
FLOWER
FOOLED
FOOLER
FOOTED
FOOTER
FROZEN
GAOLED
GAOLER
GEODES
GLOBED
GLOBES
GLOVED
GLOVER
GLOVES
GLOWED
GLOWER
GNOMES
GNOSES
GNOTES
GOOBER
GOODEN
GOODER
GOOFED
GOOIER
GOONEY
GOOSED
GOOSEN
GOOSES
GOOSEY
GOOVER
GROCER
GROPED
GROPER
GROPES
GROVED
GROVEL
GROVER
GROVES
GROWER
HAOLES
HOODED
HOOFED
HOOFER
HOOKED
HOOKER
HOOKEY
HOOPED
HOOPER
HOOTED
HOOTER
HOOVER
HOOVES
IMOGEN
INONES
IRONED
IRONER
ISOHEL
ISOMER
KNOWER
KROGER
KRONER
LIONEL
LIONET
LOOIES
LOOKED
LOOKEE
LOOKER
LOOMED
LOONEY
LOOPED
LOOPER
LOOSED
LOOSEN
LOOSER
LOOSES
LOOSEY
LOOTED
LOOTER
MEOWED
MEOWER
MOONED
MOONER
MOONEY
MOORED
MOOTED
MOOTER
MYOPES
NOONER
NOONES
NOOSED
NOOSER
NOOSES
OBOLER
OCONEE
ODORED
OLORES
OROMEO
OTOSES
PHONED
PHONER
PHONES
PHONEY
PHOOEY
PIOLET
PLOCES
PLOMER
PLOVER
PLOWED
PLOWER
POOHED
POOLED
POOLER
POOPED
POORER
PROBED
PROBER
PROBES
PROJET
PROLES
PROPEL
PROPER
PROSED
PROSER
PROSES
PROTEA
PROTEM
PROVED
PROVEN
PROVER
PROVES
PTOOEY
QUOTED
QUOTEE
QUOTER
QUOTES
REOPEN
RHODES
RIOTED
RIOTER
ROOFED
ROOFER
ROOKED
ROOKER
ROOMED
ROOMER
ROONEY
ROOTED
ROOTER
SCONES
SCOPED
SCOPES
SCORED
SCORER
SCORES
SCOTER
SHOLEM
SHOOED
SHORES
SHOVED
SHOVEL
SHOVER
SHOVES
SHOWED
SHOWER
SLOPED
SLOPER
SLOPES
SLOVEN
SLOWED
SLOWER
SMOKED
SMOKER
SMOKES
SMOKEY
SMORES
SNOPES
SNORED
SNORER
SNORES
SNOWED
SOONER
SPODES
SPOKED
SPOKEN
SPOKES
SPORES
STOKED
STOKER
STOKES
STOLEN
STOLES
STONED
STONER
STONES
STONEY
STORED
STORER
STORES
STOVER
STOVES
STOWED
STOWER
TBONES
THOLES
TNOTES
TOOLED
TOOLER
TOOMEY
TOOTED
TOOTER
TROPES
TROPEZ
TROVES
TROWED
TROWEL
TROYER
TWOEEE
TWOFER
UNOPEN
UNOWED
UPOVER
USOPEN
VIOLET
WHOLES
WOODED
WOODEN
WOOFED
WOOFER
WOOLEN
WOOLEY
XBOXES
YEOMEN
ZOOIER
ZOOMED

••O••E

ADOREE
AGORAE
AHORSE
ANOMIE
APOGEE
AROUSE
ATONCE
AZODYE
BLONDE
BLOOIE
BLOUSE
BMOVIE
BOODLE
BOOGIE
BOOKIE
BOOTEE
BOOTHE
BOOTIE
BRODIE
BROGUE
BRONTE
BRONZE
BROOKE
BROSSE
BROWNE
BROWSE
CHOATE
CHOICE
CHOOSE
CLOCHE
CLOETE
CLOTHE
COOKIE
COOLIE
COOTIE
CROIRE
CROSSE
CROUSE
CROUTE
CROWNE
DIONNE
DOODLE
DOOGIE
DOOLIE
DOOZIE
DROGUE
DROWSE
DROXIE
ECORSE
ELOISE
ENORME
EPOPEE
EPOQUE
ETOILE
EVOLVE
EVONNE
FLORAE
FOODIE
FOOTLE
FOOZLE
GEORGE
GFORCE
GOODIE
GOOGLE
GOONIE
GROOVE
GROSSE
GROUSE
HOODIE
HOOPLE
HOOPOE
HOOTIE
INOUYE
ISOLDE
KOOKIE
LAOTSE
LHOTSE
LOOKEE
LOOKIE
LOONIE
LYONNE
MOOKIE
MOONIE
NOODGE
NOODLE
NOOGIE
OCONEE
OTOOLE
PEOPLE
PHOEBE
POODLE
PROBIE
PROPRE
PROWSE
QUOQUE
QUOTEE
ROOKIE
ROOMIE
ROOTIE
ROOTLE
SCONCE
SCOUPE
SHOPPE
SHORTE
SHOWME
SKOKIE
SKOPJE
SLOANE
SNOOZE
SOOTHE
SPONGE
SPOUSE
STODGE
STOGIE
STOLAE
STOLLE
STOOGE
TBOONE
THORPE
TOODLE
TOONIE
TOOTIE
TOOTLE
TROCHE
TROMPE
TROUPE
TWOEEE
WOODIE
WOOGIE
YEOLDE
YVONNE

•••OE•

AUTOED
BLOOEY
CAMOES
CANOED
CANOER
CANOES
COHOES
DADOED
DADOES
DEMOED
DIDOES
DODOES
ECHOED
ECHOER
ECHOES
EDDOES
EUBOEA
FAROES
FLOOEY
GIJOES
GOBOES
GOCOED
HALOED
HALOES
HEROES
HOBOED
HOBOES
HYPOED
KAYOED
MOJOES
PEKOES
PHLOEM
PHOOEY
PTOOEY
REDOER
REDOES
REHOED
REHOES
SHOOED
SILOED
SOLOED
TAHOES
THROES
UNDOER
UNDOES
UNHOED
VETOED
VETOER
VETOES
YOYOED
ZEROED
ZEROES

•••O•E

ACTONE
AEROBE
AGEONE
ALCOVE
ALGORE
ANTONE
ANYONE
APPOSE
AREOLE
ARIOSE
ASHORE
ASLOPE
ATHOME
BARONE
BECOME
BEFORE
BEGONE
BEHOME
BENOTE
BESORE
BIGONE
BLOOIE
BROOKE
BYGONE
BYJOVE
BYROTE
CAJOLE
CAPONE
CAPOTE
CAROLE
CHOOSE
CHROME
COYOTE
CREOLE
DAMONE
DAMORE
DAYONE
DEBONE
DECODE
DEFORE
DEMODE
DEMOTE
DENOTE
DEPONE
DEPOSE
DEROSE
DEVORE
DEVOTE
DIPOLE
DOLORE
DUBOSE
DYNODE
EEYORE
ELMORE
ENCODE
ENCORE
ENROBE
ETTORE
EUROPE
EXMORE
EXPOSE
FATONE
FILOSE
FORONE
FURORE
GALORE
GENOME
GOHOME
GROOVE
HADONE
HASONE
HEXOSE
HITONE
HONORE
HOTONE
HUTONE
IGNORE
IMDONE
IMGONE
IMHOME
IMPOSE
INCODE
INCOME
INHOME
INJOKE
INLOVE
INSOLE
INTONE
INVOKE
INWOVE
IONONE
JAMOKE
JEROME
JOBONE
JOCOSE
KETONE
LAHORE
LAJOIE
LANOSE
LENORE
LUPONE
MALONE
MEROPE
MOROSE
MYLOVE
MYSORE
NERONE
NICOLE
NODOSE
NOHOPE
NOJOKE
NOLOSE
NOMORE
NOTONE
NOVOTE
OENONE
OFNOTE
OFYORE
OLEOLE
ONEONE
OPPOSE
ORIOLE
OSMOSE
OTIOSE
OTOOLE
OTTONE
PANOPE
PAROLE
PEYOTE
PICONE
PILOSE
POROSE
POSOLE
POZOLE
RADOME
RAMONE
RAMOSE
REBORE
REBOTE
RECODE
REDONE
REDOSE
REHONE
RELOSE
REMOTE
REMOVE
RENOTE
REPOSE
RERODE
REROSE
RESOLE
RETONE
RETORE
REVOKE
REVOTE
REWOKE
REWORE
REWOVE
REYOKE
REZONE
RIBOSE
RIMOSE
SALOME
SAVOIE
SETOSE
SHROVE
SIMONE
SIXONE
SNOOZE
SODOWE

STOOGE STROBE STRODE STROKE STROVE TAGORE TBOONE TENONE THEONE THRONE THROVE TINORE TOCOME TRIODE TRYONE TYRONE UGSOME UNCORE UNDONE UNROBE UNROPE UNROVE UNSOLE UNSORE UNWOVE UNYOKE UNZONE UPDOVE UPHOVE UPROSE UPTORE VELOCE VENOSE WEEONE WETONE XYLOSE ZYGOTE

••••OE

BIGJOE BIGTOE CHIGOE CRUSOE FAEROE HOOPOE MARJOE MONROE MUNROE RESHOE ROSCOE TIPTOE UNSHOE WASHOE

OF••••

OFFALS OFFALY OFFDAY OFFEND OFFERS OFFICE OFFING OFFISH OFFKEY OFFSET OFFUTT OFHELP OFLATE OFNOTE OFYORE

O•F•••

OAFISH OFFALS OFFALY OFFDAY OFFEND OFFERS OFFICE OFFING OFFISH OFFKEY OFFSET OFFUTT ONFILE ONFILM ONFIRE ONFOOT OXFORD

O••F••

OLAFII OLAFIV OLEFIN OPTFOR OUTFIT OUTFLY OUTFOR OUTFOX

O•••F•

OKEEFE ONEOFF OSSIFY

O••••F

ONEOFF ONLYIF

•OF•••

BOFFED BOFFIN BOFFOS COFFEE COFFER COFFIN DOFFED DOFFER DOFINE GOFAST GOFERS GOFFIN GOFISH GOFLAT GOFREE HOFFER JOFFRE LOFTED LOFTER LOFTON LOFTUS NOFAIR NOFEES NOFUSS SOFFIT SOFINE SOFTEN SOFTER SOFTIE SOFTLY SOFTON TOFFEE

•O•F••

BOFFED BOFFIN BOFFOS BOTFLY BOUFFE BOWFIN BOXFUL COFFEE COFFER COFFIN COIFED COLFAX COMFIT CONFAB CONFED CONFER CONFIT CORFAM DOFFED DOFFER DOOFUS FORFUN GOFFIN GOLFED GOLFER GOOFED GOOFUP GOOFUS GOTFAR GOTFIT HOFFER HOOFED HOOFER HOOFIT HOWFAR JOFFRE JOYFUL KOUFAX LOAFED LOAFER LOOFAH LOOFAS LOWFAT NONFAN NONFAT NONFED NOTFAR NOTFIT NOTFOR POPFLY POTFUL POUFED POUFFY ROLFED ROLFER ROOFED ROOFER SOBFUL SOFFIT SOXFAN TOFFEE TOOFAR WOEFUL WOLFED WOOFED WOOFER

•O••F•

BOUFFE CODIFY FOBOFF GOLEFT GOSOFT GOTOFF HOPOFF LOGOFF LOPOFF MODIFY MOTIFS NODOFF NOTIFY POPOFF POUFFY TOLIFE TOPOFF

•O•••F

COMEOF DOURIF FOBOFF FONDOF GOBSOF GOTANF GOTOFF HOPOFF JOZSEF LOGOFF LOPOFF LOTSOF MOSDEF MOSTOF NODOFF POPOFF ROBSOF SORTOF TOLDOF TONSOF TOPOFF VOIDOF YOUSUF

••OF••

CROFTS DOOFUS FEOFFS GOOFED GOOFUP GOOFUS HOOFED HOOFER HOOFIT KROFFT LOOFAH LOOFAS PROFIT ROOFED ROOFER SCOFFS SHOFAR TOOFAR TWOFER WOOFED WOOFER

••O•F•

ADOLFO FEOFFS KROFFT PROOFS SCOFFS SPOOFS

••O••F

ALOTOF ATONOF KNOWOF STOLAF

•••OF•

ASSOFT BADOFF BEGOFF BITOFF BUGOFF BUYOFF CRYOFF CUTOFF DAYOFF DIEOFF DRYOFF FAROFF FOBOFF GETOFF GOSOFT GOTOFF HITOFF HOPOFF ILLOFF KEYOFA KEYOFB KEYOFC KEYOFD KEYOFF KEYOFG LAYOFF LEDOFF LETOFF LIPOFF LOGOFF LOPOFF MANOFF MIDOFF NODOFF ONEOFF PAYOFF POPOFF PROOFS PRYOFF PUTOFF RANOFF RATOFF RIPOFF RUBOFF RUNOFF SAWOFF SEEOFF SETOFF SPOOFS TAPOFF TEEOFF TIEOFF TIPOFF TOPOFF UNSOFT WASOFF WAYOFF ZIPOFF

•••O•F

BADOFF BEGOFF BEHOOF BITOFF BUGOFF BUYOFF CRYOFF CUTOFF DAYOFF DEWOLF DIEOFF DRYOFF FAROFF FOBOFF GETOFF GOTOFF HITOFF HOPOFF ILLOFF KEYOFF LAYOFF LEDOFF LETOFF LIPOFF LOGOFF LOPOFF MANOFF MIDOFF NODOFF ONEOFF PAYOFF POPOFF PRYOFF PUTOFF RANOFF RATOFF REROOF RIPOFF RUBOFF RUDOLF RUNOFF SAWOFF SEEOFF SETOFF TAPOFF TEEOFF TIEOFF TIPOFF TOPOFF UNROOF WASOFF WAYOFF ZIPOFF

••••OF

ABITOF ALOTOF ASKSOF ATONOF BEHOOF CAREOF COMEOF EATSOF EKELOF FIVEOF FONDOF FREEOF FULLOF GAVEOF GELDOF GIVEOF GOBSOF HEAROF HEREOF KINDOF KNEWOF KNOWOF LATEOF LEFTOF LOTSOF MADEOF MAKEOF MOSTOF MUCHOF PARTOF REEKOF REROOF RIDSOF ROBSOF SICKOF SORTOF SUREOF TALKOF TELLOF TIREOF TOLDOF TONSOF UNROOF VOIDOF WARNOF WIDEOF

OG••••

OGAUGE OGDOAD OGHAMS OGIVAL OGIVES OGLALA OGLERS OGLING OGRADY OGRESS OGRISH

O•G•••

OBGYNS OHGOSH ORGANA ORGANS ORGEAT ORGIES OSGOOD OUGHTA OUGHTS

O••G••

OLDGAG OMEGAS ONAGER ONEGIN OREGON ORIGEN ORIGIN OSAGES OUTGAS OUTGUN OXYGEN

O•••G•

OARAGE OBLIGE OGAUGE OHMAGE OKSIGN OLDAGE ONEDGE ONEEGG ONHIGH OOLOGY OPPUGN ORANGE ORANGS ORANGY ORINGS ORTEGA OSWEGO OTSEGO OUTAGE OWLEGG

O••••G

OAKTAG OARING OBLONG OFFING OGLING OILING OILRIG OLDDOG OLDGAG ONAJAG ONEEGG ONELEG ONEMEG OOHING OOLONG OOZING OPTING ORBING OUTBEG OUTING OUTRIG OWLEGG OWNING

•OG•••

BOGART BOGEYS BOGGED BOGGLE BOGIES BOGLES BOGOTA COGENT COGGED COGGLE COGITO COGNAC DOGAPE DOGBED DOGDAY DOGDOM DOGEAR DOGGED DOGGIE DOGIES DOGLEG DOGMAS DOGNAP DOGONS DOGOOD DOGRUN DOGSAT DOGSIT DOGTAG DOGTOY FOGBOW FOGDOG FOGEYS FOGGED FOGGER FOGIES FOGSIN FOGSUP GOGGLE GOGGLY GOGIRL HOGANS HOGGED HOGNUT HOGTIE JOGBRA JOGGED JOGGER JOGGLE LOGANS LOGGED LOGGER LOGGIA LOGICS LOGIER LOGILY LOGINS LOGJAM LOGOFF LOGONS LOGOUT LOGSIN LOGSON MOGULS NOGGIN NOGOOD POGNER ROGERE ROGERS ROGETS ROGUED ROGUES TOGAED TOGGED TOGGLE TOGOUT TOGSUP TOGUES VOGUED VOGUER VOGUES YOGINI YOGISM YOGURT

•O•G••

BOGGED BOGGLE BOLGER BONGED BONGOS BOOGIE BORGES BORGIA BOUGHS BOUGHT CODGER COGGED COGGLE COIGNE COIGNS CONGAS CONGER CONGES CONGOU COOGAN CORGIS COUGAR COUGHS DODGED DODGEM DODGER DODGES DOGGED DOGGIE DONGLE DOOGIE DOTGOV DOUGAL DOUGHS DOUGHY FOGGED FOGGER FOLGER FORGED FORGER FORGES FORGET FORGOT FOUGHT GOGGLE GOGGLY GONGED GOOGLE GOOGLY GOOGOL GOOGOO GORGED GORGER GORGES GORGON GOUGED GOUGER GOUGES HOAGIE HODGES HOGGED HORGAN JOGGED JOGGER JOGGLE LODGED LODGER LODGES LOGGED LOGGER LOGGIA LONGED LONGER LONGES LONGET LONGLY LONGUE MONGER MONGOL MONGOS MONGST MORGAN MORGEN MORGUE MOWGLI NOGGIN NONGAS NONGOD NOOGIE NORGAY NOUGAT NOUGHT POLGAR PONGEE PONGID POPGUN ROTGUT ROUGED ROUGES ROUGHS SOIGNE SOUGHT TOGGED TOGGLE TONGAN TONGED TONGUE TOPGUN TOUGHS TOUGHY TOYGUN VOIGHT VOSGES WOOGIE

•O••G•

BODEGA BOINGO BOINGS BOURGS COSIGN DOINGS DONTGO DORAGS DOSAGE DOTAGE FORAGE FORDGT FOREGO GOINGS GONOGO HOMAGE IOMEGA LOUNGE LOVAGE NONAGE NONEGO NOODGE OOLOGY POTAGE TOBAGO TOWAGE VOYAGE WONTGO

•O•••G

BODING BOEING BONING BOOING BORING BOWING BOXING COBURG CODING COKING COMING CONING COOING COPING CORING COVING COWING COXING COYDOG DOGLEG DOGTAG DOLING DOMING DOPING DOSING DOTING DOTORG DOZING FOGDOG FOXING GOBANG GOLONG GORING GOSTAG HOEING HOKING HOLING HOMING HONING HOPING HOSING HOTDOG HOWBIG JOKING JOYING KOENIG LOPING LORING LOSING LOVING LOWING MOBERG MONTAG MOOING MOPING MOVING MOWING NOSING NOTING OOHING OOLONG OOZING POKING POLING PORING POSING ROBING ROPING ROVING ROWING SOLING SOLONG SONTAG SOWING TOEING TONING TOOBIG TOPDOG TOPING TOTING TOWING TOYDOG TOYING VOTING VOWING WONBIG WOOING WOWING YOKING YOUDIG ZONING

••OG••

ALOGIA APOGEE BIOGAS BOOGIE BROGAN BROGUE CLOGGY CLOGUP COOGAN DOOGIE DROGUE ELOGES FROGGY GLOGGS GOOGLE GOOGLY GOOGOL GOOGOO GROGGY IMOGEN ISOGON KROGER NOOGIE PROGUN SHOGIS SHOGUN SLOGAN SMOGGY STOGIE TROGGS WOOGIE

••O•G•

ALONGS BROUGH CHOUGH CLOGGY CLOUGH ENOUGH FROGGY GEORGE GEORGI GEORGY GLOGGS GROGGY HMONGS NOODGE PLOUGH PRONGS SLOUGH SLOWGO SMOGGY SPONGE SPONGY STODGE STODGY STOOGE STOPGO THONGS THOUGH TROGGS TROUGH WRONGS

••O••G

BOOING COOING MOOING PHOTOG PROLOG TOOBIG WOOING

•••OG•

BEDOGS BEFOGS DEFOGS EMBOGS EULOGY GONOGO LADOGA OOLOGY RELOGS STOOGE

•••O•G

ALBORG BELONG CYBORG DOTORG DUGONG GOLONG KEYOFG MEKONG MRWONG OBLONG OOLONG SARONG SOLONG STRONG THRONG ZEDONG

••••OG

AIRLOG ANALOG BADDOG BIGDOG COYDOG DESMOG DIALOG DRYFOG EGGNOG EPILOG FOGDOG GASHOG GASLOG GUNDOG HERZOG HOTDOG ICEFOG INAFOG LAPDOG MADDOG OLDDOG PETDOG PHOTOG PRELOG PROLOG PYEDOG QUAHOG REDDOG SAWLOG SEADOG STENOG SUNDOG TAUROG THEFOG TOPDOG TOYDOG UNCLOG WEBLOG

OH••••

OHBABY OHCRUD OHDARN OHDEAR OHDRAT OHENRY OHGOSH OHIOAN OHLOOK

OHMAGE
OHNUTS
OHSTOP
OHSURE
OHWELL
OHYEAH

O•H•••
OAHUAN
OCHERS
OCHERY
OCHRED
OCHRES
OFHELP
OGHAMS
ONHAND
ONHIGH
ONHIRE
ONHOLD
OOHING
OPHULS
OSHAWA
OTHERS
OTHMAR
OXHIDE

O••H••
OLDHAM
OLDHAT
OMAHAN
OMAHAS
OMPHAL
ONAHOP
ONEHIT
ONSHOW
ORCHID
ORPHAN
ORPHIC
ORTHEN
ORWHAT
OUCHES
OUGHTA
OUGHTS
OUTHIT

O•••H•
OBEAHS
OLATHE
OLESHA
OOMPHS
OPRAHS
ORACHS

O••••H
OAFISH
ODDISH
OFFISH
OGRISH
OHGOSH
OHYEAH
OLDISH
ONEISH
ONHIGH
ONRUSH
OOMPAH
ORBACH
ORNITH
OWLISH

•OH•••
BOHEME
BOHRER
COHABS
COHEIR
COHERE
COHOES
COHORT
COHOST
GOHOME
HOHNER
HOHOHO
HOHUMS
JOHANN
JOHNII
JOHNIV
JOHNIX
JOHNNY
JOHNVI
JOHNXI
JOHNXV
JOHNXX
KOHLER
MOHAIR
MOHAVE
MOHAWK
NOHANT
NOHELP
NOHITS
NOHOPE
OOHING
ROHMER
ROHRER
TOHEEL
WOHLER
YOHOHO

•O•H••
BOCHCO
BOCHSA
BONHAM
BOOHOO
BOTHER
COBHAM
COSHED
COSHER
COSHES
DOOHAN
DOTHAN
GOPHER
GORHAM
GOSHEN
GOTHAM
GOTHEP
GOTHIC
GOTHIP
GOTHOT
HOOHAH
HOOHAS
JOBHOP
JOSHED
JOSHER
JOSHES
JOSHUA
KOCHEL
KOCHER
KOSHER
LOCHER
LOTHAR
MOCHAS
MOSHAV
MOSHED
MOSHER
MOSHES
MOTHER
MOTHRA
NOCHES
NONHIT
NOSHED
NOSHER
NOSHES
NOSHOW
NOTHIN
POOHED
POSHER
POSHLY
POTHER
POTHOS
ROCHAT
ROCHET
ROCHON
RODHAM
ROSHIS
ROTHKO
SOPHIA
SOPHIE
SOTHAT
SOTHEN
SOWHAT
TOOHIP
TOOHOT
TOPHAT
TOWHEE
TOYHAT
YOOHOO

•O••H•
BOLSHY
BOOTHE
BOOTHS
BOTCHY
BOUCHE
BOUGHS
BOUGHT
CONCHA
CONCHO
CONCHS
COUGHS
DOUGHS
DOUGHY
FORCHE
FORWHY
FOUGHT
GOETHE
GOTCHA
HOHOHO
HONCHO
HONSHU
JONAHS
LOATHE
LOUCHE
MOESHA
MONTHS
MORPHO
MORPHS
MOUTHS
MOUTHY
NORTHS
NOTCHY
NOUGHT
OOMPHS
POACHY
POISHA
PONCHO
POUCHY
ROUGHS
SOOTHE
SOUGHT
SOUTHS
TOOTHY
TORAHS
TORCHY
TOUCHE
TOUCHY
TOUGHS
TOUGHY
VOIGHT
WORTHS
WORTHY
YOHOHO
YOUTHS

•O•••H
BORSCH
BOYISH
COMETH
COOLTH
COWISH
COYISH
DONATH
DOODAH
DOVISH
DOWITH
EOLITH
FOURTH
GOFISH
GOODOH
GOWITH
HOOHAH
HOOKAH
HOORAH
HOOTCH
HOWDAH
IOMOTH
JOBETH
JOSEPH
JOSIAH
LOLICH
LOOFAH
LOWISH
MODISH
MOOLAH
MOPISH
MORATH
NORUSH
OOMPAH
POLISH
POPISH
POTASH
POVICH
SOMUCH
VOTECH
YOWZAH

••OH••
ABOHMS
ALOHAS
BOOHOO
DOOHAN
HOOHAH
HOOHAS
ISOHEL
MEOHMY
MYOHMY
POOHED
TOOHIP
TOOHOT
YOOHOO

••O•H•
BOOTHE
BOOTHS
BROPHY
BROTHS
BROTHY
CLOCHE
CLOTHE
CLOTHO
CLOTHS
EPOCHS
FROTHS
FROTHY
NEOSHO
SLOSHY
SLOTHS
SOOTHE
TOOTHY
TROCHE
TROPHY
TROTHS

••O••H
ADOLPH
AMONTH
AVOUCH
BLOTCH
BROACH
BROOCH
BROUGH
CHOUGH
CLOUGH
COOLTH
CROTCH
CROUCH
DOODAH
ENOUGH
GOODOH
GROUCH
GROWTH
HOOHAH
HOOKAH
HOORAH
HOOTCH
LOOFAH
MOOLAH
PLOUGH
SCORCH
SCOTCH
SLOUCH
SLOUGH
SMOOCH
SMOOSH
SMOOTH
STORCH
SWOOSH
THOUGH
TROUGH
WHOOSH

•••OH•
HOHOHO
IIJOHN
JAWOHL
MEGOHM
RICOHS
STJOHN
STROHS
UPJOHN
YOHOHO

•••O•H
ALIOTH
ASLOSH
BROOCH
BYGOSH
DEMOTH
DETOTH
EDKOCH
GALOSH
IOMOTH
JCLOTH
KIBOSH
MYGOSH
OHGOSH
SMOOCH
SMOOSH
SMOOTH
SPLOSH
SWOOSH
UNPOSH
WHOOSH

••••OH
GOODOH
MATZOH
SHILOH

OI••••
OILCAN
OILCUP
OILERS
OILIER
OILILY
OILING
OILLIT
OILMAN
OILMEN
OILPAN
OILRIG
OILRUB
OINKED
OINKER
OISEAU

O•I•••
OBISPO
OBITER
OBIWAN
OCICAT
ODINIC
ODIOUS
ODISTS
ODIUMS
OGIVAL
OGIVES
OHIOAN
OJIBWA
OLINDA
OLIVER
OLIVES
OLIVIA
ONIONS
ONIONY
OPIATE
OPINED
OPINER
OPINES
OPIUMS
ORIANA
ORIANI
ORIBIS
ORIELS
ORIENT
ORIGEN
ORIGIN
ORINGS
ORIOLE
ORIONS
ORISON
ORISSA
OSIERS
OSIRIS
OTILES
OTIOSE
OTITIC
OTITIS
OUIJAS
OUIMET
OUIOUI
OVIEDO
OVINES
OVISAC
OXIDES
OXIDIC

O••I••
OAFISH
OAKIER
OARING
OATIER
OBLIGE
OBOIST
OBRIAN
OBRIEN
ODDISH
ODDITY
OFFICE
OFFING
OFFISH
OGLING
OGRISH
OILIER
OILILY
OILING
OJAICA
OKSIGN
OLDIES
OLDISH
OLEINS
OMNIUM
ONDISK
ONDITS
ONEIDA
ONEILL
ONEIRO
ONEISH
ONFILE
ONFILM
ONFIRE
ONHIGH
ONHIRE
ONLINE
ONMIKE
ONRICE
ONSIDE
ONSITE
ONTIME
ONVIEW
OOHING
OOLITE
OOTIDS
OOZIER
OOZILY
OOZING
OPCITS
OPTICS
OPTIMA
OPTIMO
OPTING
OPTION
ORBING
ORBITS
OREIDA
ORGIES
ORNITH
ORSINI
ORSINO
OSCINE
OSMICS
OSMIUM
OSSIAN
OSSIFY
OUTIES
OUTING
OVOIDS
OWLIER
OWLISH
OWNING
OXHIDE
OXLIKE
OXLIPS

O•••I•
OBTAIN
ODINIC
OILLIT
OILRIG
OKAPIS
OLAFII
OLAFIV
OLAVII
OLAVIV
OLDVIC
OLEFIN
OLIVIA
OMANIS
ONBAIL
ONEBIT
ONEGIN
ONEHIT
ONEPIN
ONLAID
ONLYIF
OPENIT
OPTSIN
ORANIS
ORCHID
ORDAIN
OREXIA
OREXIS
ORIBIS
ORIGIN
ORPHIC
OSIRIS
OTITIC
OTITIS
OTOMIS
OTOSIS
OTTOII
OTTOIV
OUTBID
OUTDID
OUTFIT
OUTHIT
OUTLIE
OUTLIP
OUTRIB
OUTRIG
OUTSIN
OUTSIT
OUTVIE
OUTWIT
OVERIT
OXALIC
OXALIS
OXIDIC
OXTAIL
OZONIC

O••••I
OBLADI
OCELLI
OCTOPI
OCTROI
OLAFII
OLAVII
OLDELI
ORIANI
ORSINI
OTTOII
OUIOUI

•OI•••
BOILED
BOILER
BOILUP
BOINGO
BOINGS
BOITES
COIFED
COIGNE
COIGNS
COILED
COILER
COILUP
COINED
COINER
COINOP
DOINGS
DOITUP
FOIBLE
FOILED
FOISTS
GOINGS
GOINTO
GOITER
HOISIN
HOISTS
JOINED
JOINER
JOININ
JOINTS
JOINUP
JOISTS
LOIDED
LOIRET
LOITER
MOIETY
MOILED
MOILER
MOINES
MOIRES
MOISES
NOIDEA
NOIRES
NOIRET
NOIRON
NOISED
NOISES
POILUS
POINTA
POINTB
POINTE
POINTS
POINTY
POIRES
POIRET
POIROT
POISED
POISER
POISES
POISHA
POISON
POITOU
POIVRE
ROILED
ROILUP
SOIGNE
SOILED
SOIREE
SOISEE
SOITIS
TOILAT
TOILED
TOILER
TOILES
TOILET
VOICED
VOICER
VOICES
VOIDED
VOIDER
VOIDOF
VOIGHT
VOILES
YOICKS

•O•I••
BODICE
BODIED
BODIES
BODILY
BODINE
BODING
BOEING
BOGIES
BOLIDE
BONIER
BONING
BONITA
BONITO
BOOING
BORIDE
BORING
BOVIDS
BOVINE
BOWING
BOXIER
BOXILY
BOXING
BOYISH
CODIFY
CODING
COGITO
COKIER
COKIES
COKING
COLICS
COLIMA
COMICE
COMICS
COMIDA
COMING
COMITY
CONICS
CONIES
CONING
COOING
COPIED
COPIER
COPIES
COPING
CORING
CORIUM
COSIED
COSIER
COSIES
COSIGN
COSILY
COSINE
COVINA
COVING
COWIER
COWING
COWISH
COXING
COYISH
COZIED
COZIER
COZIES
COZILY
DOCILE
DODICI
DOFINE
DOGIES
DOLIKE
DOLING
DOMINE
DOMING
DOMINI
DOMINO
DONITZ
DOPIER
DOPILY
DOPING
DORIAN
DORIES
DORINE
DORITO
DOSIDO
DOSING
DOTIME
DOTING
DOVISH
DOWITH
DOXIES
DOZIER
DOZILY
DOZING
EOLIAN
EOLITH
EONIAN
EOSINS
FOGIES
FOKINE
FOLIAR
FOLIES
FOLIOS
FOLIUM
FORINT
FOXIER
FOXILY
FOXING
GOBIES
GODIVA
GOFISH
GOGIRL
GOLIKE
GOLIMP
GOLINO
GOLIVE
GOOIER
GORIER
GORILY
GORING
GORIOT
GOWILD
GOWITH
HODIAK
HOEING
HOKIER
HOKIES
HOKILY
HOKING
HOLIER
HOLIES
HOLILY
HOLING
HOLISM
HOLIST
HOMIER
HOMIES
HOMILY
HOMING
HOMINY
HONIED
HONING
HOPING
HOSIER
HOSING
IODIDE
IODINE
IODISE
IODIZE
IONIAN
IONICS
IONISE
IONIUM
IONIZE
JOKIER
JOKILY
JOKING
JOLIET
JOLIOT
JOSIAH
JOVIAL
JOVIAN
JOYING
KODIAK
KONICA
LODINJ
LOGICS
LOGIER
LOGILY
LOGINS
LOLICH
LOLITA
LOOIES
LOPING
LORIES
LORING
LOSING
LOTION
LOUIES
LOUISA
LOUISB
LOUISE
LOUISI
LOUISV
LOUISX
LOVING
LOWING
LOWIQS
LOWISH
MOBILE
MOBIUS
MODIFY
MODINE
MODISH
MOJITO
MOLINA
MOLINE
MOMISM
MONICA
MONIED
MONIES
MONISM
MONIST
MOOING
MOPIER
MOPING
MOPISH
MORITA
MORITZ
MOTIFS
MOTILE
MOTION
MOTIVE
MOVIES
MOVING
MOWING
NOBILE
NODICE
NOHITS
NOJIVE
NOKIAS
NOKIDS
NOMIAL
NORIAS
NORISK
NORITE
NOSIER
NOSILY
NOSING
NOTICE
NOTIFY
NOTILL
NOTIME
NOTING
NOTION
NOTIPS
NOVIAS
NOVICE
NOVIOS
NOWISE
OOHING
OOLITE
OOTIDS
OOZIER
OOZILY
OOZING
PODIUM
POKIER
POKIES
POKILY
POKING
POLICE
POLICY
POLING
POLIOS
POLISH
POLITE
POLITY
PONIED
PONIES
POPISH
PORING
POSIES
POSING
POSITS
POTION
POVICH
ROBING
ROBINS
RODINO
RODION
ROMIJN
ROPIER
ROPING
ROSIER
ROSIES
ROSILY
ROSINA
ROSINS
ROSINY
ROSITA
ROTINI
ROVING
ROWING
SOCIAL
SODIDI
SODIUM
SOFINE
SOLIDS
SOLING
SONICS
SOVIET
SOWING
SOYINK
TOBIAS
TOBIES
TOBITS
TODIES
TOEING
TOEINS
TOLIFE
TONICS
TONIER
TONING
TONITE
TOPICS
TOPING
TORIES
TORINO
TOTING
TOWING
TOXICS
TOXINS
TOYING
VOTING
VOTIVE
VOWING
WOOING
WOWING
YOGINI
YOGISM
YOKING
YORICK
ZODIAC
ZONIAN
ZONING
ZOOIDS
ZOOIER
ZORINA

•O••I•
AORTIC
BOBBIE
BOBBIN
BOCCIE
BOCCIS
BODKIN

BOFFIN
BOLLIX
BONNIE
BOOGIE
BOOKIE
BOOKII
BOOKIV
BOOKIX
BOOTIE
BOOTIT
BORGIA
BOSNIA
BOUDIN
BOWFIN
BOWTIE
COATIS
COBAIN
COEDIT
COELIA
COFFIN
COHEIR
COLLIE
COMEIN
COMFIT
COMMIT
COMMIX
CONAIR
CONFIT
CONNIE
CONOID
COOKIE
COOLIE
COOLIO
COOLIT
COOTIE
COPSIT
COPTIC
COQUIS
CORBIN
CORDIA
CORGIS
CORVID
CORWIN
COSMIC
COURIC
COUSIN
COWRIE
DOBBIN
DOBLIN
DOESIN
DOESIT
DOGGIE
DOGSIT
DOMAIN
DONEIN
DONEIT
DONNIE
DOOGIE
DOOLIE
DOOZIE
DORMIE
DORRIT
DOTTIE
DOURIF
DOVEIN
FOETID
FOGSIN
FOLDIN

FOLKIE
FONZIE
FOODIE
FOOTIT
FORBID
FORDID
FORMIC
FORTIS
FOSSIL
FOZZIE
GOALIE
GOATIT
GOBLIN
GODWIN
GODWIT
GOESIN
GOFFIN
GOLDIE
GONEIN
GOODIE
GOONIE
GOONIN
GORDIE
GOSLIN
GOSSIP
GOTFIT
GOTHIC
GOTHIP
GOTOIT
GOTRID
HOAGIE
HOBBIT
HOGTIE
HOISIN
HOLDIN
HOLDIT
HOLLIS
HOMEIN
HONEIN
HOODIE
HOOFIT
HOOTIE
HOPKIN
HOPSIN
HORNIN
HORRID
HOTAIR
HOTOIL
HOTTIE
HOTTIP
HOURIS
HOWBIG
HOWLIN
JOANIE
JOHNII
JOHNIV
JOHNIX
JOININ
JOLTIN
JOPLIN
KOENIG
KOOKIE
LOADIN
LOCCIT
LOCKIN
LOGGIA
LOGSIN
LOMEIN

LONNIE
LOOKIE
LOOKIN
LOONIE
LORAIN
LORDIT
LORRIE
LOSEIT
LOSTIT
LOUVIN
LOVEIN
LOVEIT
LOWBID
MOHAIR
MOLLIE
MOMMIE
MOOKIE
MOONIE
MORBID
MORRIE
MORRIS
MOSAIC
MOTRIN
MOULIN
MOVEIN
MOVEIT
NOESIS
NOETIC
NOEXIT
NOFAIR
NOGGIN
NONHIT
NOOGIE
NORAIN
NORDIC
NORRIS
NOSEIN
NOTAIL
NOTFIT
NOTHIN
NOWAIT
POETIC
PONGID
POORIS
POPEIL
POPLIN
POPSIN
PORTIA
POSTIE
POSTIT
POTLID
POTPIE
POTSIE
POTVIN
POURIN
ROADIE
ROAMIN
ROBBIA
ROBBIE
ROCKIE
ROCKIN
ROCKIT
RODEIN
ROLLIE
ROLLIN
ROMAIC
ROMAIN
RONMIX

RONNIE
ROOKIE
ROOMIE
ROOTIE
ROOTIN
ROPEIN
ROSHIS
SOAKIN
SOBEIT
SOCKIN
SOFFIT
SOFTIE
SOITIS
SOLDIT
SOLEIL
SOPHIA
SOPHIE
SORBIC
SORDID
SORTIE
TOCSIN
TOEDIN
TOESIN
TOLDIT
TOMLIN
TOMMIE
TOMMIX
TOMTIT
TONKIN
TONSIL
TOOBIG
TOOHIP
TOOKIN
TOOKIT
TOONIE
TOOTIE
TOOTIN
TOPBID
TOREIT
TOROID
TORPID
TORRID
TOSSIN
TOWNIE
TOWSIN
VOTEIN
WONBIG
WOODIE
WOOGIE
WORKIN
YORKIE
YORKIN
YOUDIG
YOUWIN
ZOMBIE
ZOOMIN
ZOYSIA

•O•••I
BOLYAI
BONACI
BONAMI
BONSAI
BOOKII
BOOKVI
BORZOI
COLONI
CORACI

COULDI
DODICI
DOMANI
DOMINI
DORATI
DOREMI
IOLANI
JOHNII
JOHNVI
JOHNXI
LOUISI
MODULI
MONAMI
MORONI
MOWGLI
NORDOI
NOYORI
POLLOI
POPULI
POTOSI
ROLLEI
ROMAJI
ROMANI
ROTINI
SOCANI
SODIDI
SOLATI
SOMALI
SOMONI
SOONYI
TOKORI
YOGINI

••OI••
ANOINT
AROIDS
AROINT
AVOIDS
BOOING
BROILS
CHOICE
CHOIRS
COOING
CROIRE
DROIDS
DROITS
EGOISM
EGOIST
ELOISA
ELOISE
ENOILS
EROICA
ETOILE
GOOIER
GROINS
HYOIDS
IDOIDO
IKOIKO
ILOILO
LEOIII
LOOIES
MAOISM
MAOIST
MOOING
OBOIST
OVOIDS
QUOINS
QUOITS

REOILS
SPOILS
SPOILT
STOICS
TAOISM
TAOIST
TROIKA
UNOILY
WOOING
ZOOIDS
ZOOIER

••O•I•
ADONIC
ADONIS
AEOLIA
AHOLIC
AIOLIS
ALOGIA
ANODIC
ANOMIA
ANOMIC
ANOMIE
ANOXIA
ANOXIC
ASONIA
ATOMIC
ATONIA
ATONIC
ATOXIC
AZONIC
AZORIN
BIONIC
BIOPIC
BIOTIC
BIOTIN
BLOOIE
BLOWIN
BLOWIT
BMOVIE
BOOGIE
BOOKIE
BOOKII
BOOKIV
BOOKIX
BOOTIE
BOOTIT
BRODIE
BROLIN
BROVIK
CHOPIN
CHORIC
CHORIO
CLORIS
CLOVIS
COOKIE
COOLIE
COOLIO
COOLIT
COOTIE
CRONIN
DHOTIS
DIOXIN
DOOGIE
DOOLIE
DOOZIE
DROMIO
DROPIN

DROPIT
DROXIE
ENOKIS
EPODIC
EROTIC
ETONIC
EXOTIC
FLOPIT
FLORID
FLORIN
FLORIO
FLOWIN
FOODIE
FOOTIT
FROLIC
GEODIC
GLOBIN
GLORIA
GNOMIC
GNOSIS
GOODIE
GOONIE
GOONIN
GRODIN
GROMIT
HOODIE
HOOFIT
HOOTIE
ICONIC
IGOTIT
IMONIT
IRONIC
KAOLIN
KAONIC
KNOWIT
KOOKIE
LEOIII
LEONIA
LEONID
LEOVII
LEOXII
LOOKIE
LOOKIN
LOONIE
MAORIS
MOOKIE
MOONIE
MYOPIA
MYOPIC
MYOSIN
MYOSIS
NIOBIC
NOOGIE
OTOMIS
OTOSIS
OZONIC
PEORIA
PHOBIA
PHOBIC
PHONIC
PHOTIC
POORIS
PROBIE
PROFIT
PROLIX
PROSIT
ROOKIE
ROOMIE

ROOTIE
ROOTIN
SCORIA
SCOTIA
SHOGIS
SHOJIS
SHOOIN
SHOWIN
SKOKIE
SNOWIN
STOGIE
STOLID
STOPIN
STOPIT
STOTIN
STOWIT
THORIC
TOOBIG
TOOHIP
TOOKIN
TOOKIT
TOONIE
TOOTIE
TOOTIN
TROPIC
TWOBIT
TWOPIN
UTOPIA
VIOLIN
WHOSIN
WOODIE
WOOGIE
ZOOMIN

••O••I
ADONAI
AGOUTI
BIONDI
BOOKII
BOOKVI
GEORDI
GEORGI
LEOIII
LEOVII
LEOXII
MAOTAI
RHOMBI
SHORTI
SNORRI
SOONYI
TSOTSI
WHOAMI
WHOOPI

•••OI•
ADJOIN
ADROIT
ALTOID
ARTOIS
ATROIS
BELOIT
BENOIT
BIGOIL
BLOOIE
CONOID
CUBOID
DEVOID
DEVOIR

DUBOIS
ECHOIC
ENJOIN
ENVOIS
EQUOID
ETAOIN
GALOIS
GASOIL
GOTOIT
HALOID
HEROIC
HEROIN
HOTOIL
INTOIT
LAJOIE
LELOIR
MEMOIR
NUTOIL
OTTOII
OTTOIV
PATOIS
REBOIL
RECOIL
RECOIN
REJOIN
RENOIR
RESOIL
REVOIR
SAVOIE
SAVOIR
SHOOIN
TAROIL
TOROID
UNCOIL
UNJOIN
UNVOID
UPCOIL
UPTOIT
VALOIS
XYLOID
ZEROIN

•••O•I
ARIOSI
BARONI
BILOXI
BUSONI
CAPONI
CAROLI
CARONI
COLONI
JACOBI
KENOBI
LUGOSI
MALOTI
MIDORI
MORONI
NAPOLI
NEROLI
NOYORI
OCTOPI
OTTOII
OUIOUI
PELOSI
POTOSI
PRIORI
RIVOLI
SATORI

SOMONI
TIVOLI
TOKORI
WHOOPI
ZANONI

••••OI
BIGBOI
BORZOI
NORDOI
OCTROI
PASMOI
POLLOI
RENVOI
UBUROI

OJ••••
OJAICA
OJIBWA

O•J•••
OBJECT
OBJETS

O••J••
ODDJOB
ONAJAG
ORAJEL
OUIJAS
OUTJET
OUTJUT

•OJ•••
JOJOBA
MOJAVE
MOJITO
MOJOES
NOJIVE
NOJOKE

•O•J••
BOOJUM
CONJOB
DONJON
FORJOY
JOBJAR
KOPJES
LOGJAM
NONJEW
TOPJOB

•O••J•
ROMAJI
ROMIJN

•O•••J
LODINJ

••OJ••
BOOJUM
PROJET
RIOJAS
SHOJIS
STOJKO
TROJAN

••O•J•
SKOPJE

•••OJ•
BAROJA

OK••••
OKAPIS
OKAYED
OKBYME
OKEEFE
OKSANA
OKSIGN

O•K•••
OAKIER
OAKLEY
OAKTAG
OAKUMS
ORKANS
ORKNEY

O••K••
OFFKEY
OINKED
OINKER
OLAKES
OSAKAN

O•••K•
ONMIKE
ORECKS
OXLIKE
OZARKS

O••••K
OCASEK
OCLOCK
OHLOOK
ONDECK
ONDISK
OUTASK

•OK•••
BOKKEN
COKIER
COKIES
COKING
DOKKEN
DOKTOR
FOKINE
FOKKER
GOKART
HOKIER
HOKIES
HOKILY
HOKING
HOKUMS
JOKERS
JOKIER
JOKILY
JOKING
KOKOMO
NOKIAS
NOKIDS
POKEAT
POKERS
POKERY
POKEYS
POKIER
POKIES

POKILY
POKING
TOKAYS
TOKENS
TOKLAS
TOKORI
WOKEUP
YOKELS
YOKING

•O•K••
BODKIN
BOKKEN
BONKED
BOOKED
BOOKEM
BOOKER
BOOKIE
BOOKII
BOOKIV
BOOKIX
BOOKVI
BORKED
COCKED
COCKER
COCKLE
CONKED
CONKER
COOKED
COOKER
COOKIE
COOKUP
CORKED
CORKER
CORKUP
DOAKES
DOCKED
DOCKER
DOCKET
DOKKEN
DONKEY
FOKKER
FOLKIE
FOLKSY
FORKED
FORKER
FORKUP
HOCKED
HOCKER
HOCKEY
HONKAT
HONKED
HONKER
HOOKAH
HOOKED
HOOKER
HOOKEY
HOOKON
HOOKUP
HOPKIN
HOTKEY
JOCKEY
JOCKOS
KOOKIE
LOCKED
LOCKER
LOCKET
LOCKIN

LOCKON
LOCKUP
LOOKAT
LOOKED
LOOKEE
LOOKER
LOOKIE
LOOKIN
LOOKMA
LOOKON
LOOKTO
LOOKUP
LOWKEY
MOCKED
MOCKER
MOCKUP
MONKEE
MONKEY
MOOKIE
MOSKVA
NOCKED
POCKET
POLKAS
PORKED
PORKER
PORKYS
ROCKED
ROCKER
ROCKET
ROCKIE
ROCKIN
ROCKIT
ROCKNE
ROCKYV
ROOKED
ROOKER
ROOKIE
SOAKED
SOAKER
SOAKIN
SOAKUP
SOCKED
SOCKET
SOCKIN
TONKAS
TONKIN
TOOKIN
TOOKIT
TOOKON
TOOKTO
TOOKUP
VODKAS
WORKAT
WORKED
WORKER
WORKIN
WORKON
WORKUP
YOAKAM
YOLKED
YORKER
YORKIE
YORKIN
YORKPA
ZONKED
ZONKER

•O••K•
BODUKE
BOESKY
BOURKE
DOLIKE
GOLIKE
KODAKS
KOPEKS
KOTTKE
MOLTKE
NOBAKE
NOJOKE
NOOTKA
POLSKA
ROTHKO
ROURKE
TOPEKA
YOICKS

•O•••K
DOESOK
DONEOK
GOBACK
GODARK
HODIAK
KODIAK
KOPECK
MOHAWK
NOLUCK
NOMEAK
NORISK
PODUNK
POLLAK
SOYINK
VOSTOK
WOMACK
YORICK

••OK••
AWOKEN
BLOKES
BOOKED
BOOKEM
BOOKER
BOOKIE
BOOKII
BOOKIV
BOOKIX
BOOKVI
BROKAW
BROKEN
BROKER
CHOKED
CHOKER
CHOKES
COOKED
COOKER
COOKIE
COOKUP
ENOKIS
EVOKED
EVOKER
EVOKES
HOOKAH
HOOKED
HOOKER
HOOKEY
HOOKON

HOOKUP
IMOKAY
KEOKUK
KOOKIE
LOOKAT
LOOKED
LOOKEE
LOOKER
LOOKIE
LOOKIN
LOOKMA
LOOKON
LOOKTO
LOOKUP
MOOKIE
ROOKED
ROOKER
ROOKIE
RYOKAN
SKOKIE
SMOKED
SMOKER
SMOKES
SMOKEY
SPOKED
SPOKEN
SPOKES
STOKED
STOKER
STOKES
TOOKIN
TOOKIT
TOOKON
TOOKTO
TOOKUP

••O•K•
APOPKA
BLOCKS
BLOCKY
BRONKO
BROOKE
BROOKS
BROOKY
CHOCKS
CLOAKS
CLOCKS
CLONKS
CROAKS
CROAKY
CROCKS
CROOKS
CSONKA
EBOOKS
FLOCKS
FROCKS
GLOCKS
IBOOKS
IKOIKO
KIOSKS
KNOCKS
NOOTKA
PBOOKS
PLONKS
PROSKY
SHOCKS
SHOPKO
SMOCKS

SNOOKS
SPOOKS
SPOOKY
SPORKS
STOCKS
STOCKY
STOJKO
STORKS
TROIKA

••O••K
ANORAK
BROVIK
DVORAK
FLOREK
KEOKUK
SLOVAK

•••OK•
BROOKE
BROOKS
BROOKY
CROOKS
EBOOKS
IBOOKS
INJOKE
INVOKE
JAMOKE
JUDOKA
KAPOKS
LEMOKO
NOJOKE
PBOOKS
REVOKE
REWOKE
REYOKE
SNOOKS
SPOOKS
SPOOKY
STROKE
SUDOKU
UNYOKE

•••O•K
ARMONK
ATWORK
BETOOK
BUROAK
DRHOOK
FAROUK
INHOCK
MTCOOK
NANOOK
OCLOCK
OHLOOK
PINOAK
REBOOK
RECOCK
RECOOK
RECORK
REDOAK
REDOCK
REHOOK
RELOCK
RELOOK
RESOAK
RETOOK
REWORK

SHLOCK
SHNOOK
TANOAK
UNCORK
UNDOCK
UNFORK
UNHOOK
UNLOCK
ZEDONK

••••OK
BARTOK
BETOOK
DOESOK
DONEOK
DRHOOK
ENIDOK
FEELOK
FELTOK
HICKOK
ISNTOK
MTCOOK
NANOOK
OHLOOK
REBOOK
RECOOK
REEBOK
REHOOK
RELOOK
RETOOK
RHEBOK
SAIDOK
SAYSOK
SHNOOK
UNHOOK
VOSTOK

OL••••
OLAFII
OLAFIV
OLAKES
OLATHE
OLAVII
OLAVIV
OLDAGE
OLDBAT
OLDBOY
OLDCAR
OLDDOG
OLDELI
OLDEST
OLDGAG
OLDHAM
OLDHAT
OLDIES
OLDISH
OLDMAN
OLDMEN
OLDPAL
OLDPRO
OLDSAW
OLDSOD
OLDVIC
OLDWAY
OLEARY
OLEATE
OLEFIN
OLEINS

OLEOLE
OLERUD
OLESHA
OLESON
OLEUMS
OLEVEL
OLINDA
OLIVER
OLIVES
OLIVIA
OLMECS
OLMERT
OLORES

O•L•••
OBLADI
OBLAST
OBLATE
OBLIGE
OBLONG
OCLOCK
OFLATE
OGLALA
OGLERS
OGLING
OHLOOK
OILCAN
OILCUP
OILERS
OILIER
OILILY
OILING
OILLIT
OILMAN
OILMEN
OILPAN
OILRIG
OILRUB
ONLAID
ONLAND
ONLATE
ONLAYS
ONLINE
ONLOAD
ONLOAN
ONLYIF
OOLALA
OOLITE
OOLOGY
OOLONG
ORLONS
ORLOPS
OWLEGG
OWLERY
OWLETS
OWLIER
OWLISH
OXLIKE
OXLIPS

O••L••
OAKLEY
OBELUS
OBOLER
OBOLUS
OCELLI
OCELOT
OCULAR

OCULUS
ODDLOT
ODELET
OILLIT
OMELET
ONCLES
ONELAP
ONELEG
OODLES
ORALES
ORALLY
ORELSE
OSTLER
OTELLO
OTILES
OUTLAW
OUTLAY
OUTLED
OUTLET
OUTLIE
OUTLIP
OVALLY
OVULAR
OVULES
OXALIC
OXALIS

O•••L•
OCCULT
OCELLI
ODOULS
OFFALS
OFFALY
OFHELP
OGLALA
OHWELL
OILILY
OLDELI
OLEOLE
ONCALL
ONEALL
ONEILL
ONFILE
ONFILM
ONHOLD
ONSALE
OOLALA
OOZILY
OPENLY
OPHULS
ORACLE
ORALLY
ORIELS
ORIOLE
ORMOLU
ORWELL
OSCULE
OSWALD
OTELLO
OTOOLE
OUSELS
OUTFLY
OUZELS
OVALLY
OVERLY

O••••L
OGIVAL

OHWELL
OLDPAL
OLEVEL
OMPHAL
ONBAIL
ONCALL
ONEALL
ONEILL
ORAJEL
ORDEAL
ORWELL
OSTEAL
OXTAIL
OXYDOL

•OL•••
AOLERS
BOLCOM
BOLDED
BOLDEN
BOLDER
BOLDLY
BOLENA
BOLERO
BOLEYN
BOLGER
BOLIDE
BOLLAS
BOLLIX
BOLSHY
BOLTED
BOLTER
BOLTON
BOLTUP
BOLYAI
COLADA
COLBYS
COLDER
COLDLY
COLECO
COLEUS
COLFAX
COLICS
COLIMA
COLLAR
COLLAT
COLLET
COLLIE
COLLOP
COLLOQ
COLMAN
COLMAR
COLONI
COLONS
COLONY
COLORS
COLOUR
COLSON
COLTER
COLTON
COLUMN
DOLAPS
DOLENZ
DOLIKE
DOLING
DOLLAR
DOLLED
DOLLEY

DOLLOP
DOLLUP
DOLMAN
DOLMAS
DOLORE
DOLORS
DOLOUR
DOLTON
EOLIAN
EOLITH
FOLATE
FOLDED
FOLDER
FOLDIN
FOLDUP
FOLEYS
FOLGER
FOLIAR
FOLIES
FOLIOS
FOLIUM
FOLKIE
FOLKSY
FOLLOW
FOLSOM
GOLAME
GOLAST
GOLDEN
GOLDIE
GOLEFT
GOLEMS
GOLETA
GOLFED
GOLFER
GOLIKE
GOLIMP
GOLINO
GOLIVE
GOLLUM
GOLONG
HOLDEM
HOLDEN
HOLDER
HOLDIN
HOLDIT
HOLDME
HOLDON
HOLDTO
HOLDUP
HOLERS
HOLEUP
HOLIER
HOLIES
HOLILY
HOLING
HOLISM
HOLIST
HOLLER
HOLLEY
HOLLIS
HOLLOW
HOLMAN
HOLMES
IOLANI
JOLENE
JOLIET
JOLIOT
JOLLEY

JOLSON
JOLTED
JOLTER
JOLTIN
LOLICH
LOLITA
LOLLED
LOLLER
MOLARS
MOLDAU
MOLDED
MOLDER
MOLEST
MOLINA
MOLINE
MOLLIE
MOLLOY
MOLNAR
MOLSON
MOLTED
MOLTEN
MOLTER
MOLTKE
NOLEAD
NOLESS
NOLOAD
NOLOSE
NOLOSS
NOLUCK
OOLALA
OOLITE
OOLOGY
OOLONG
POLAND
POLARA
POLEAX
POLERS
POLGAR
POLICE
POLICY
POLING
POLIOS
POLISH
POLITE
POLITY
POLKAS
POLLAK
POLLED
POLLEE
POLLEN
POLLER
POLLEX
POLLOI
POLLOS
POLLUX
POLPOT
POLSKA
POLYPS
ROLAND
ROLEOS
ROLFED
ROLFER
ROLLBY
ROLLED
ROLLEI
ROLLER
ROLLIE
ROLLIN

ROLLON
ROLLUP
SOLACE
SOLANO
SOLANS
SOLARA
SOLATI
SOLDER
SOLDIT
SOLDON
SOLDTO
SOLEAS
SOLEIL
SOLELY
SOLEMN
SOLERS
SOLEUS
SOLIDS
SOLING
SOLOED
SOLONG
SOLONS
SOLUTE
SOLVED
SOLVER
SOLVES
TOLARS
TOLAST
TOLDIT
TOLDOF
TOLDON
TOLDYA
TOLEDO
TOLIFE
TOLLED
TOLLER
TOLTEC
VOLANS
VOLANT
VOLARE
VOLLEY
VOLUME
VOLUTE
VOLVOS
WOLFED
WOLPER
WOLSEY
WOLVES
YOLKED
ZOLTAN

•O•L••
BODLEY
BOGLES
BOILED
BOILER
BOILUP
BOLLAS
BOLLIX
BOSLEY
BOULES
BOULEZ
BOWLED
BOWLER
BOWLES
BOYLES
COALED
COALER

COELIA
COILED
COILER
COILUP
COLLAR
COLLAT
COLLET
COLLIE
COLLOP
COLLOQ
CONLAN
COOLED
COOLER
COOLEY
COOLIE
COOLIO
COOLIT
COOLLY
COOLTH
COOLTO
COPLEY
COTLER
COULDA
COULDI
COULEE
COWLED
COWLEY
DOALLS
DOBLES
DOBLIN
DOGLEG
DOLLAR
DOLLED
DOLLEY
DOLLOP
DOLLUP
DOOLEY
DOOLIE
DOULAS
FOALED
FOILED
FOLLOW
FOOLED
FOOLER
FOULED
FOULER
FOULLY
FOULUP
FOWLED
FOWLER
FOWLES
GOALBY
GOALIE
GOBLET
GOBLIN
GOFLAT
GOLLUM
GOSLIN
GOSLOW
GOULET
HOLLER
HOLLEY
HOLLIS
HOLLOW
HOWLAT
HOWLED
HOWLER
HOWLIN

HOYLES
JOBLOT
JOLLEY
JOPLIN
JOULES
JOWLED
KOALAS
KOHLER
LOLLED
LOLLER
MOBLEY
MOILED
MOILER
MOLLIE
MOLLOY
MOOLAH
MORLEY
MOSLEM
MOSLEY
MOTLEY
MOULDS
MOULDY
MOULIN
MOULTS
NOBLER
NOBLES
NOWLAN
OODLES
POILUS
POLLAK
POLLED
POLLEE
POLLEN
POLLER
POLLEX
POLLOI
POLLOS
POLLUX
POOLED
POOLER
POPLAR
POPLIN
POTLID
POULES
POULTS
ROBLES
ROILED
ROILUP
ROLLBY
ROLLED
ROLLEI
ROLLER
ROLLIE
ROLLIN
ROLLON
ROLLUP
ROSLYN
ROWLEY
SOCLES
SOILED
TOILAT
TOILED
TOILER
TOILES
TOILET
TOKLAS
TOLLED
TOLLER

TOMLIN
TOOLED
TOOLER
TOOLOW
TOOLUP
TOULON
VOILES
VOLLEY
WOHLER
WOOLEN
WOOLEY
WOOLLY
WORLDS
WORLEY
WOULDA
YOWLED
YOWLER

•O••L•
BOBBLE
BOBBLY
BODILY
BOGGLE
BOLDLY
BOODLE
BOTELS
BOTFLY
BOTTLE
BOWELS
BOXILY
COBALT
COBBLE
COCKLE
CODDLE
COGGLE
COLDLY
COMELY
COMPLY
COOLLY
COPALS
COPULA
CORALS
COSELL
COSILY
COSTLY
COUPLE
COZILY
DOABLE
DOALLS
DOCILE
DONALD
DONGLE
DOODLE
DOPILY
DOTELL
DOTTLE
DOUBLE
DOUBLY
DOURLY
DOWELL
DOWELS
DOZILY
FOCSLE
FOIBLE
FONDLE
FONDLY
FOOTLE
FOOZLE

FOULLY
FOXILY
GOBBLE
GOCOLD
GOGGLE
GOGGLY
GOODLY
GOOGLE
GOOGLY
GORILY
GOSOLO
GOTOLD
GOWELL
GOWILD
HOBBLE
HOKILY
HOLILY
HOMELY
HOMILY
HOOPLA
HOOPLE
HOSELS
HOSTLY
HOTELS
HOURLY
HOVELS
HOWELL
JOGGLE
JOKILY
JOSTLE
KOBOLD
KODALY
KOPELL
LOBULE
LOCALE
LOCALS
LOGILY
LONELY
LONGLY
LORDLY
LOUDLY
LOVELL
LOVELY
LOWELL
LOYALE
LOYOLA
MOBILE
MODALS
MODELA
MODELB
MODELS
MODELT
MODULE
MODULI
MODULO
MOGULS
MORALE
MORALS
MORELS
MOROLT
MOSTLY
MOTELS
MOTILE
MOTTLE
MOWGLI
NOBALL
NOBELS
NOBILE

NODULE
NOHELP
NOODLE
NOPALS
NORELL
NOSALE
NOSALT
NOSILY
NOTALL
NOTILL
NOTOLL
NOVELA
NOVELS
NOZZLE
OOLALA
OOZILY
POKILY
POMELO
POODLE
POORLY
POPFLY
POPPLE
POPULI
PORTLY
POSHLY
POSOLE
POSSLQ
POWELL
POZOLE
RODALE
ROMOLA
ROMULO
RONALD
RONELY
ROOTLE
ROSILY
ROWELS
ROYALE
ROYALS
SOFTLY
SOLELY
SOMALI
SORELY
SOURLY
TODDLE
TOGGLE
TOODLE
TOOTLE
TOPPLE
TOTALS
TOUSLE
TOWELS
VOCALS
VOWELS
VOWELY
WOBBLE
WOBBLY
WOOLLY
YODELS
YOKELS
YOUALL
ZOCALO
ZONULE

•O•••L
AORTAL
BOATEL
BOMBAL

BOREAL
BOXFUL
COAXAL
COEVAL
COMPEL
CONSUL
CORBEL
CORNEL
CORRAL
COSELL
COSTAL
DORSAL
DOSSAL
DOTELL
DOUGAL
DOWELL
FONTAL
FORMAL
FOSSIL
GOAWOL
GOGIRL
GOOGOL
GOSPEL
GOWELL
HORMEL
HOSTEL
HOTOIL
HOWELL
JOVIAL
JOYFUL
KOCHEL
KOPELL
KOPPEL
KOSSEL
LONNOL
LOREAL
LOVELL
LOWCAL
LOWELL
MONGOL
MONTEL
MORREL
MORSEL
MORTAL
MOSTEL
NOBALL
NODEAL
NOMIAL
NORELL
NORMAL
NORVAL
NOTAIL
NOTALL
NOTILL
NOTOLL
NOUNAL
POMMEL
POPEIL
PORTAL
POSTAL
POTFUL
POWELL
ROMMEL
RONDEL
SOBFUL
SOCIAL
SOLEIL
SORREL

TOHEEL
TONSIL
VORPAL
WOEFUL
YOUALL

••OL••
ABOLLA
ADOLFO
ADOLPH
AEOLIA
AEOLUS
AHOLIC
AIOLIS
AMOLES
ANOLES
APOLLO
ATOLLS
AZOLES
BIOLAB
BROLIN
BROLLY
CHOLER
CHOLLA
CHOLOS
COOLED
COOLER
COOLEY
COOLIE
COOLIO
COOLIT
COOLLY
COOLTH
COOLTO
DHOLES
DOOLEY
DOOLIE
DROLLS
DROLLY
ECOLAB
ECOLAW
ECOLES
EVOLVE
FHOLES
FOOLED
FOOLER
FROLIC
GAOLED
GAOLER
HAOLES
IDOLUM
ISOLDA
ISOLDE
KAOLIN
KNOLLS
KNOLLY
MOOLAH
OBOLER
OBOLUS
PIOLET
POOLED
POOLER
PROLES
PROLIX
PROLOG
SCOLDS
SHOLEM
SHOLOM

SMOLTS STOLAE STOLAF STOLAS STOLEN STOLES STOLID STOLLE STOLON STOLTZ THOLES TOOLED TOOLER TOOLOW TOOLUP TROLLS UBOLTS VIOLAS VIOLET VIOLIN WHOLES WHOLLY WOOLEN WOOLEY WOOLLY YEOLDE

••O•L•

ABOLLA APOLLO ATOLLS BOODLE BROILS BROLLY CEORLS CHOLLA COOLLY DOODLE DROLLS DROLLY DROOLS DROOLY ENOILS ETOILE FOOTLE FOOZLE GHOULS GOODLY GOOGLE GOOGLY GROWLS GROWLY HOOPLA HOOPLE ICOULD IFONLY ILOILO IWOULD KNOLLS KNOLLY LIONLY NOODLE ODOULS OTOOLE PEOPLE POODLE POORLY PROULX PROWLS REOILS ROOTLE SCOWLS SHOALS SHOALY SHOULD SKOALS SLOWLY SPOILS SPOILT SPOOLS STOLLE STOOLS STOOLY TOODLE TOOTLE TROLLS TWOPLY UNOILY WHOLLY WHORLS WOOLLY

••O••L

ABORAL AMORAL ANODAL APODAL ATONAL AVOWAL AXONAL AZONAL BHOPAL BLOBEL CHORAL CLONAL DHOTEL FLORAL GLOBAL GOOGOL GROVEL ISOHEL LIONEL PROCOL PROPEL PROPYL SHOVEL SNOBOL TROWEL UNOCAL UNORAL

•••OL•

AGEOLD ANGOLA ANYOLD AREOLA AREOLE ARNOLD ASCOLD BAROLO BEHOLD BIFOLD BUJOLD CAJOLE CANOLA CAROLE CAROLI CAROLL CAROLS CIBOLA CREOLE CUPOLA DAYOLD DEWOLF DIPOLE DROOLS DROOLY EIDOLA ENFOLD ENROLL ENROLS ERROLL EXTOLL EXTOLS GETOLD GIGOLO GOCOLD GOSOLO GOTOLD HAROLD IMCOLD IMSOLD IMTOLD INFOLD INGOLD INSOLE KOBOLD LOYOLA MAZOLA MOROLT NAPOLI NEROLI NICOLA NICOLE NICOLO NIKOLA NOTOLL OLEOLE ONHOLD ORIOLE ORMOLU OTOOLE PAROLE PAROLS PAYOLA POSOLE POZOLE PUJOLS RCCOLA REBOLT REFOLD REHOLD REMOLD REPOLL REROLL RESOLD RESOLE RETOLD REVOLT RICOLA RIVOLI ROMOLA RUDOLF SCHOLL SCROLL SPOOLS STOOLS STOOLY STROLL TAXOLS TIVOLI UNBOLD UNBOLT UNCOLA UNFOLD UNHOLY UNMOLD UNROLL UNSOLD UNSOLE UNTOLD UPFOLD UPHOLD WASOLD

•••O•L

ASCOOL BECOOL BEFOOL BEFOUL BIGOIL CAROLL ELFOWL ENROLL ENSOUL ERROLL EXTOLL FAZOOL GASOIL HOTOIL IMCOOL INGOAL JAWOHL MRCOOL NOTOLL NUTOIL REBOIL RECOAL RECOIL RECOOL REPOLL REROLL RESOIL RETOOL SCHOLL SCHOOL SCROLL STROLL TAROIL UNCOIL UNCOOL UNFOUL UNROLL UPCOIL

••••OL

AMATOL AMIDOL ASCOOL BECOOL BEFOOL BENZOL CARROL CINEOL CRESOL DELSOL DIABOL ESHKOL ETYMOL FAZOOL FRIJOL FRIVOL GAMBOL GLYCOL GOAWOL GOOGOL IMCOOL LONNOL MAGNOL MONGOL MRCOOL NEUROL OXYDOL PAGNOL PATROL PETROL PHENOL PISTOL PROCOL RECOOL RETOOL SCHOOL SNOBOL STEROL SYMBOL TVIDOL TYDBOL UNCOOL WARHOL

OM••••

OMAHAN OMAHAS OMANIS OMASUM OMEARA OMEGAS OMELET OMENED OMERTA OMNIUM OMPHAL

O•M•••

OHMAGE OLMECS OLMERT ONMIKE OOMPAH OOMPHS ORMOLU ORMOND OSMICS OSMIUM OSMOND OSMOSE OSMUND

O••M••

OARMAN OARMEN ODAMAE ODDMAN ODDMEN OILMAN OILMEN OLDMAN OLDMEN ONEMAN ONEMEG OROMEO OTHMAR OTOMIS OUIMET OUTMAN

O•••M•

OAKUMS OCCAMS ODIUMS OGHAMS OKBYME OLEUMS ONRAMP ONTIME OPIUMS OPTIMA OPTIMO

O••••M

OLDHAM OMASUM OMNIUM ONEARM ONFILM OSMIUM OUTSUM

•OM•••

BOMBAL BOMBAY BOMBED BOMBER BOMBES COMATE COMBAT COMBED COMBER COMBOS COMDEN COMDEX COMDRS COMEAS COMEAT COMEBY COMEDY COMEIN COMELY COMEOF COMEON COMERS COMETH COMETO COMETS COMEUP COMFIT COMICE COMICS COMIDA COMING COMITY COMMAS COMMIT COMMIX COMMON COMORO COMPAQ COMPAS COMPED COMPEL COMPLY COMPOS COMPOZ COMSAT COMTES DOMAIN DOMANI DOMBEY DOMINE DOMING DOMINI DOMINO DOMREP FOMENT GOMERS HOMAGE HOMBRE HOMEEC HOMEIN HOMELY HOMERS HOMEYS HOMIER HOMIES HOMILY HOMING HOMINY HOMMES IOMEGA IOMOTH KOMBAT KOMBUS KOMODO LOMEIN LOMOND LOMPOC MOMENT MOMISM MOMMAS MOMMIE NOMAAM NOMADS NOMAYO NOMBRE NOMEAK NOMEAT NOMIAL NOMORE OOMPAH OOMPHS POMADE POMELO POMMEL POMMES POMONA POMPEO POMPEY POMPOM POMPON ROMAIC ROMAIN ROMAJI ROMANI ROMANO ROMANS ROMANY ROMCOM ROMEOS ROMERO ROMIJN ROMMEL ROMNEY ROMOLA ROMPED ROMPER ROMULO SOMALI SOMANY SOMATA SOMBER SOMBRE SOMERS SOMMER SOMONI SOMUCH TOMATO TOMBES TOMBOY TOMCAT TOMLIN TOMMIE TOMMIX TOMTIT TOMTOM VOMERS WOMACK WOMANS WOMBAT WOMENS YOMTOV ZOMBIE

•O•M••

BONMOT BOOMED BOOMER BORMAN BOWMAN BOWMEN COLMAN COLMAR COMMAS COMMIT COMMIX COMMON CONMAN CONMEN CORMAN COSMAS COSMIC COSMOS COWMAN COWMEN DOGMAS DOLMAN DOLMAS DOOMED DOOMTO DORMER DORMIE FOAMED FOAMER FOEMAN FOEMEN FORMAL FORMAN FORMAT FORMED FORMER FORMIC GORMED GOTMAD HODMAN HODMEN HOLMAN HOLMES HOMMES HORMEL HORMUZ KORMAN LOAMED LOOMED LOOMPA LOOMUP LOUMAS LOWMAN LOWMEN MOMMAS MOMMIE MORMON NOEMON NONMAN NONMEN NORMAL NORMAN NOUMEA POEMES POMMEL POMMES ROAMED ROAMER ROAMIN RODMAN RODMEN ROHMER ROMMEL RONMIX ROOMBA ROOMED ROOMER ROOMIE SOMMER TOAMAN TODMAN TOMMIE TOMMIX TOOMEY TOPMAN TOPMEN WORMED WORMER ZOOMED ZOOMIN

•O••M•

BOHEME BONAMI BOSOMS BOSOMY COLIMA COLUMN DOCOMO DODOMA DOREMI DOSUMS DOTIME FORUMS GOHOME GOLAME GOLEMS GOLIMP GOTAMA HOHUMS HOKUMS HOLDME JORUMS KOKOMO LOOKMA MODEMS MONAMI NONAME NOTIME SOLEMN SONOMA TOCOME TONEME TOTEMS TOYAMA VOLUME YOYOMA

•O•••M

BOLCOM BONHAM BOOJUM BOOKEM BOTTOM COBHAM CORFAM CORIUM DODGEM DOGDOM DORSUM DOTCOM FOLIUM FOLSOM FOURAM FOURPM GOBOOM GOLLUM GORHAM GOTEAM GOTHAM HOLDEM HOLISM IONIUM LOGJAM MOMISM MONISM MOSLEM NOMAAM NONCOM NOROOM PODIUM POMPOM POSSUM POSTUM RODHAM ROMCOM ROSSUM SODIUM TOMTOM TOTERM YOAKAM YOGISM

••OM••

ABOMAS ABOMBS ALOMAR ANOMIA ANOMIC ANOMIE AROMAS ATOMIC BIOMES BOOMED BOOMER CHOMPS CLOMPS DIOMED DOOMED DOOMTO DROMIO DUOMOS GNOMES GNOMIC GNOMON GROMIT HBOMBS ISOMER LOOMED LOOMPA LOOMUP NBOMBS OROMEO OTOMIS PLOMER PROMOS PROMPT RHOMBI RHOMBS ROOMBA ROOMED ROOMER ROOMIE STOMAS STOMPS THOMAS TOOMEY TROMPE TROMPS TWOMAN WHOMPS WHOMSO YEOMAN YEOMEN ZOOMED ZOOMIN

••O•M•

ABOHMS BLOOMS BLOOMY BROOMS BROOMY ENORME GLOOMS GLOOMY GROOMS KHOUMS LOOKMA MEOHMY MYOHMY PROAMS PROEMS SHOWME STORMS STORMY VROOMS WHOAMI

••O••M

ANONYM BOOJUM BOOKEM EGOISM EPONYM EUONYM EXONYM IDOLUM MAOISM PROTEM QUORUM SHOLEM SHOLOM TAOISM TAOSNM

•••OM•

APLOMB ATHOME AXIOMS BECOME BEHOME BESOMS BLOOMS BLOOMY BOSOMS BOSOMY BROOMS BROOMY CAROMS CDROMS CHROMA CHROME CHROMO CHROMY DOCOMO DODOMA ECTOMY ENTOMB ENTOMO GENOME GLOOMS GLOOMY GOHOME GROOMS IDIOMS IMHOME INCOME INHOME JEROME KOKOMO MACOMB PALOMA RADOME RECOMB SALOME SONOMA TACOMA TOCOME UGSOME VENOMS VROOMS YOYOMA ZYGOMA

•••O•M

ABLOOM BIFORM BYFORM DEFOAM DEFORM DEWORM DRDOOM GOBOOM INFORM KABOOM MEGOHM NOROOM PHLOEM REFORM SHBOOM TVROOM

••••OM

ABLOOM BOLCOM BOTTOM CATDOM CUSTOM DENMOM DIATOM DOGDOM DOTCOM DRDOOM FANDOM FATHOM FOLSOM GOBOOM HANSOM JAGLOM KABOOM KIDCOM LILIOM NEWSOM NONCOM NOROOM PHENOM POMPOM RANDOM RANSOM ROMCOM SATCOM SELDOM SHALOM SHBOOM SHOLOM SITCOM SLALOM TOMTOM TVROOM UNISOM VIACOM WINDOM WISDOM ZITCOM

ON••••

ONABUN ONAGER ONAHOP ONAJAG ONAPAR ONAUTO ONBAIL ONBASE ONCALL ONCLES ONDECK ONDISK ONDITS ONDUTY ONEACT ONEALL ONEARM ONEBIT ONECAR ONEDAY ONEDGE ONEEEE ONEEGG ONEEYE ONEGIN ONEHIT ONEIDA ONEILL ONEIRO ONEISH ONELAP ONELEG ONEMAN ONEMEG ONEOFF ONEONE ONEOUT ONEPIN ONERUN ONESEC ONESET ONETEN ONETON ONETWO ONEUPS ONEWAY ONFILE ONFILM ONFIRE ONFOOT ONHAND ONHIGH ONHIRE ONHOLD ONIONS ONIONY ONLAID ONLAND ONLATE ONLAYS ONLINE ONLOAD ONLOAN ONLYIF ONMIKE ONPOST ONRAMP ONRICE ONRUSH ONSALE ONSETS ONSHOW ONSIDE ONSITE ONSPEC ONSTAR ONTAPE ONTIME ONTOUR ONUSES ONVIEW ONWARD ONYXES

O•N•••

OENONE OFNOTE OHNUTS OINKED OINKER OMNIUM ORNATE ORNERY ORNITH OUNCES OWNERS OWNING OWNSUP OXNARD

O••N••

OBENTO OCONEE ODENSE ODINIC ODONTO OHENRY OLINDA OMANIS OMENED OPENED OPENER OPENIT OPENLY OPENON OPENTO OPENUP OPINED OPINER OPINES

ORANGE
ORANGS
ORANGY
ORANIS
ORANTS
ORENSE
ORINGS
ORKNEY
OVINES
OZONIC

O•••N•

OARING
OBGYNS
OBLONG
OBTUND
OCEANS
OCTANE
OCTANS
OCTANT
ODEONS
OENONE
OFFEND
OFFING
OGLING
OILING
OKSANA
OLEINS
ONEONE
ONHAND
ONIONS
ONIONY
ONLAND
ONLINE
OOHING
OOLONG
OOZING
OPTING
ORBING
ORGANA
ORGANS
ORIANA
ORIANI
ORIENT
ORIONS
ORKANS
ORLONS
ORMOND
ORSINI
ORSINO
OSCANS
OSCINE
OSMOND
OSMUND
OSTEND
OTTONE
OUTING
OWNING

O••••N

OAHUAN
OARMAN
OARMEN
OBERON
OBIWAN
OBRIAN
OBRIEN
OBTAIN
ODDMAN
ODDMEN
ODDSON
ODEDON
OHDARN
OHIOAN
OILCAN
OILMAN
OILMEN
OILPAN
OKSIGN
OLDMAN
OLDMEN
OLEFIN
OLESON
OMAHAN
ONABUN
ONEGIN
ONEMAN
ONEPIN
ONERUN
ONETEN
ONETON
ONLOAN
OPENON
OPPUGN
OPTION
OPTSIN
ORDAIN
OREGON
ORIGEN
ORIGIN
ORISON
ORPHAN
ORTHEN
OSAKAN
OSBORN
OSSIAN
OUTBAN
OUTGUN
OUTMAN
OUTRAN
OUTRUN
OUTSIN
OWEDON
OWESON
OXYGEN

•ON•••

BONACI
BONAMI
BONBON
BONDED
BONDER
BONERS
BONERZ
BONEUP
BONGED
BONGOS
BONHAM
BONIER
BONING
BONITA
BONITO
BONKED
BONMOT
BONNER
BONNES
BONNET
BONNEY
BONNIE
BONSAI
BONTON
BONZES
CONAIR
CONANT
CONCHA
CONCHO
CONCHS
CONCUR
CONDOR
CONDOS
CONERS
CONEYS
CONFAB
CONFED
CONFER
CONFIT
CONGAS
CONGER
CONGES
CONGOU
CONICS
CONIES
CONING
CONJOB
CONKED
CONKER
CONLAN
CONMAN
CONMEN
CONNED
CONNEE
CONNIE
CONNOR
CONOCO
CONOID
CONRAD
CONROY
CONSUL
CONTAC
CONTRA
CONTRE
CONURE
CONVEX
CONVEY
CONVOY
CONWAY
DONALD
DONATE
DONATH
DONDER
DONEBY
DONEES
DONEIN
DONEIT
DONEOK
DONESO
DONETO
DONETS
DONEUP
DONGLE
DONITZ
DONJON
DONKEY
DONNED
DONNER
DONNIE
DONORA
DONORS
DONOSO
DONTGO
DONUTS
EONIAN
FONDAS
FONDER
FONDLE
FONDLY
FONDOF
FONDUE
FONDUS
FONTAL
FONZIE
GONEAR
GONEAT
GONEBY
GONEIN
GONEON
GONERS
GONETO
GONEUP
GONEXT
GONGED
GONOGO
GONUTS
HONCHO
HONDAS
HONEIN
HONERS
HONEST
HONEYS
HONIED
HONING
HONKAT
HONKED
HONKER
HONORE
HONORS
HONOUR
HONSHU
IONIAN
IONICS
IONISE
IONIUM
IONIZE
IONONE
JONAHS
JONESS
JONESY
JONSON
KONICA
KONRAD
LONDON
LONELY
LONERS
LONGED
LONGER
LONGES
LONGET
LONGLY
LONGUE
LONNIE
LONNOL
MONACO
MONADS
MONAMI
MONDAY
MONDES
MONDOS
MONETA
MONETS
MONEYS
MONGER
MONGOL
MONGOS
MONGST
MONICA
MONIED
MONIES
MONISM
MONIST
MONKEE
MONKEY
MONNET
MONODY
MONROE
MONTAG
MONTEL
MONTEZ
MONTHS
MONZAS
NONAGE
NONAME
NONART
NONARY
NONCOM
NONEED
NONEGO
NONETS
NONEWS
NONFAN
NONFAT
NONFED
NONGAS
NONGOD
NONHIT
NONJEW
NONMAN
NONMEN
NONNET
NONONO
NONPAR
NONPRO
NONRUN
NONTAN
NONTAX
NONUSE
NONWAR
PONCAS
PONCHO
PONDED
PONDER
PONGEE
PONGID
PONIED
PONIES
PONYUP
PONZUS
RONALD
RONCEY
RONDEL
RONDOS
RONELY
RONMIX
RONNIE
RONSON
SONANT
SONARS
SONATA
SONDES
SONDRA
SONICS
SONNET
SONOMA
SONORA
SONTAG
TONDOS
TONEME
TONERS
TONEUP
TONGAN
TONGED
TONGUE
TONICS
TONIER
TONING
TONITE
TONKAS
TONKIN
TONNES
TONSIL
TONSOF
WONBIG
WONDER
WONOUT
WONTDO
WONTED
WONTGO
WONTON
YONDER
ZONERS
ZONIAN
ZONING
ZONKED
ZONKER
ZONULE

•O•N••

BOINGO
BOINGS
BONNER
BONNES
BONNET
BONNEY
BONNIE
BORNEO
BOSNIA
BOUNCE
BOUNCY
BOUNDS
BOUNTY
COBNUT
COGNAC
COINED
COINER
COINOP
CONNED
CONNEE
CONNIE
CONNOR
COONEY
CORNEA
CORNED
CORNEL
CORNER
CORNET
COUNTS
COUNTY
DOGNAP
DOINGS
DONNED
DONNER
DONNIE
DOWNED
DOWNER
DOWNES
DOWNEY
DOWNON
FORNAX
FORNOW
FOUNDS
FOUNTS
GOINGS
GOINTO
GOONEY
GOONIE
GOONIN
GOUNOD
GOWNED
HOBNOB
HOGNUT
HOHNER
HORNBY
HORNED
HORNER
HORNET
HORNIN
HOUNDS
HOUNDY
HOWNOW
JOANIE
JOANNA
JOANNE
JOANOU
JOHNII
JOHNIV
JOHNIX
JOHNNY
JOHNVI
JOHNXI
JOHNXV
JOHNXX
JOINED
JOINER
JOININ
JOINTS
JOINUP
JOUNCE
JOUNCY
JOYNER
KOENIG
KOONTZ
LOANED
LOANER
LONNIE
LONNOL
LOONEY
LOONIE
LOTNOS
LOUNGE
MOANED
MOANER
MOINES
MOLNAR
MONNET
MOONED
MOONER
MOONEY
MOONIE
MORNAY
MOUNDS
MOUNTS
MOUNTY
NONNET
NOONAN
NOONER
NOONES
NOTNEW
NOTNOW
NOUNAL
NOWNOW
POGNER
POINTA
POINTB
POINTE
POINTS
POINTY
POUNCE
POUNDS
POZNAN
RODNEY
ROMNEY
RONNIE
ROONEY
ROUNDS
SONNET
SOONAS
SOONER
SOONYI
SOUNDS
TONNES
TOONIE
TORNUP
TOWNER
TOWNIE
WOUNDS
ZOUNDS

•O••N•

BODINE
BODING
BOEING
BOLENA
BONING
BOOING
BORING
BOSONS
BOSUNS
BOTANY
BOURNE
BOVINE
BOWING
BOXING
CODING
CODONS
COGENT
COIGNE
COIGNS
COKING
COLONI
COLONS
COLONY
COMING
CONANT
CONING
COOING
COOWNS
COPING
CORING
CORONA
COSINE
COTANS
COVENS
COVENT
COVINA
COVING
COWENS
COWING
COXING
COZENS
DOBYNS
DOCENT
DOESNT
DOFINE
DOGONS
DOLENZ
DOLING
DOMANI
DOMINE
DOMING
DOMINI
DOMINO
DOPING
DORINE
DOSING
DOTING
DOUANE
DOYENS
DOZENS
DOZING
EOCENE
EOSINS
FOKINE
FOMENT
FORINT
FORONE
FOURNO
FOXING
GOBANG
GOLINO
GOLONG
GORING
GOTANA
GOTANF
HOEING
HOGANS
HOKING
HOLING
HOMING
HOMINY
HONING
HOPING
HOSING
HOTONE
IODINE
IOLANI
IONONE
IOWANS
JOANNA
JOANNE
JOBONE
JOBYNA
JOCUND
JOHANN
JOHNNY
JOKING
JOLENE
JOURNO
JOYING
KORANS
KORUNA
LOCANE
LODENS
LODINJ
LOGANS
LOGINS
LOGONS
LOMOND
LOPING
LORANS
LORENE
LORENZ
LORING
LOSING
LOUANN
LOVING
LOWEND
LOWING
MODENA
MODINE
MOLINA
MOLINE
MOMENT
MOOING
MOPING
MORANT
MORENO
MORONI
MORONS
MOURNS
MOVING
MOWING
NOCENT
NOHANT
NONONO
NORENT
NORUNS
NOSING
NOTANY
NOTING
NOTONE
NOVENA
OOHING
OOLONG
OOZING
POCONO
PODUNK
POEANA
POKING
POLAND
POLING
POMONA
PORING
POSING
POTENT
ROBING
ROBINS
ROCKNE
RODENT
RODINO
ROLAND
ROMANI
ROMANO
ROMANS
ROMANY
ROPING
ROSINA
ROSINS
ROSINY
ROTINI
ROTUND
ROVING
ROWANS
ROWENA
ROWENS
ROWING
ROXANA
ROXANE
SOCANI
SOFINE
SOIGNE
SOLANO
SOLANS
SOLING
SOLONG
SOLONS
SOMANY
SOMONI
SONANT
SOWING
SOYINK
TOEING
TOEINS
TOKENS
TONING
TOPING
TORENT
TORINO
TOTING
TOWING
TOXINS
TOYING
TOYONS
VOLANS
VOLANT
VOTENO
VOTING
VOWING
WOMANS
WOMENS
WOOING
WOWING
YOGINI
YOKING
YOSANO
ZONING
ZORINA

•O•••N

BOBBIN
BODKIN
BOFFIN
BOKKEN
BOLDEN
BOLEYN
BOLTON
BONBON
BONTON
BORDEN
BOREON
BORMAN
BOSSON
BOSTON
BOUDIN
BOUTON
BOWFIN
BOWMAN
BOWMEN
COBAIN
COBURN
COCOON
COFFIN
COLMAN
COLSON
COLTON
COLUMN
COMDEN
COMEIN
COMEON
COMMON
CONLAN
CONMAN
CONMEN
COOGAN
CORBIN
CORDON
CORMAN
CORWIN
COSIGN
COTTEN
COTTON
COUPON
COUSIN
COWMAN
COWMEN
DOBBIN
DOBLIN
DOESIN
DOGRUN
DOKKEN
DOLMAN
DOLTON
DOMAIN
DONEIN
DONJON
DOOHAN
DOREEN
DORIAN
DOTEON
DOTHAN
DOVEIN
DOWNON
DOWSON
EOLIAN
EONIAN
FOEMAN
FOEMEN
FOGSIN
FOLDIN
FORFUN
FORMAN
GOBLIN
GODOWN
GODSON
GODWIN
GOESIN
GOESON
GOFFIN
GOLDEN
GONEIN
GONEON
GOODEN
GOONIN
GOOSEN
GORDON
GORGON
GOSDEN
GOSHEN
GOSLIN
GOTTEN
GOVERN
HOBSON
HODMAN
HODMEN
HOISIN
HOLDEN
HOLDIN
HOLDON
HOLMAN
HOMEIN
HONEIN
HOOKON
HOPKIN
HOPSIN
HOPSON
HORGAN
HORNIN
HORTON
HOUDON
HOWLIN
HOYDEN
IONIAN
JOBSON
JOEDON
JOHANN
JOININ
JOLSON
JOLTIN
JONSON
JOPLIN
JORDAN
JOVIAN
KOREAN
KORMAN
LOADIN
LOCKIN
LOCKON
LOFTON
LOGSIN
LOGSON
LOMEIN
LONDON
LOOKIN
LOOKON
LOOSEN
LORAIN
LOTION
LOUANN
LOUDEN
LOUDON
LOUVIN
LOVEIN
LOWMAN
LOWMEN
MODERN
MOLSON
MOLTEN
MOREEN
MORGAN
MORGEN
MORMON
MORTEN
MORTON
MOTION
MOTOWN
MOTRIN
MOULIN
MOVEIN
MOVEON
NOEMON
NOGGIN
NOIRON
NONFAN
NONMAN
NONMEN
NONRUN
NONTAN
NOONAN
NORAIN
NOREEN
NORMAN
NORTON
NOSEIN
NOTHIN
NOTION
NOWLAN
POISON
POLLEN
POMPON
POPGUN
POPLIN
POPSIN
POSTON
POTEEN
POTION
POTVIN
POUPON
POURIN
POZNAN
ROAMIN
ROBSON
ROCHON
ROCKIN
RODEIN
RODION
RODMAN
RODMEN
ROLLIN
ROLLON
ROMAIN
ROMIJN
RONSON
ROOTIN
ROPEIN
ROSLYN
ROSSEN
ROSTEN
ROTTEN
SOAKIN
SOCKIN
SODDEN
SOFTEN
SOFTON
SOLDON
SOLEMN
SOSOON
SOTHEN
SOURON
SOXFAN
TOAMAN
TOBURN
TOCSIN
TODMAN
TOEDIN
TOESIN
TOLDON
TOMLIN
TONGAN
TONKIN
TOOKIN
TOOKON
TOOTIN
TOPGUN
TOPMAN
TOPMEN
TOPTEN
TOSSIN
TOUCAN
TOULON
TOWSIN
TOYGUN
VOTEIN
VOTEON
WOBURN
WONTON
WOODEN
WOOLEN
WOREON
WORKIN
WORKON
WORSEN
YORKIN
YOUWIN
ZOLTAN
ZONIAN
ZOOMIN

••ON••

ADONAI
ADONIC
ADONIS
AGONES
ALONGS
ALONSO
ALONZO
AMONRA
AMONTH
ANONYM
ASONIA
ATONAL
ATONCE
ATONED

ATONER
ATONES
ATONIA
ATONIC
ATONOF
AXONAL
AXONES
AZONAL
AZONIC
BIONDI
BIONIC
BIONTS
BLONDE
BLONDS
BRONCO
BRONCS
BRONKO
BRONTE
BRONZE
BRONZY
CLONAL
CLONED
CLONER
CLONES
CLONKS
COONEY
CRONES
CRONIN
CRONUS
CRONYN
CSONKA
DIONNE
DRONED
DRONER
DRONES
EBONDS
EPONYM
ETONIC
EUONYM
EVONNE
EXONYM
FRONDS
FRONTS
GOONEY
GOONIE
GOONIN
HMONGS
ICONIC
IDONOT
IFONLY
IMONIT
INONES
IRONED
IRONER
IRONIC
IRONON
KAONIC
KOONTZ
KRONER
KRONOR
KRONUR
LAONZA
LEONIA
LEONID
LIONEL
LIONET
LIONLY
LOONEY
LOONIE
LYONNE
MOONED
MOONER
MOONEY
MOONIE
NOONAN
NOONER
NOONES
OCONEE
ODONTO
OZONIC
PHONED
PHONER
PHONES
PHONEY
PHONIC
PHONOS
PLONKS
PRONGS
PRONTO
RHONDA
ROONEY
SCONCE
SCONES
SOONAS
SOONER
SOONYI
SPONGE
SPONGY
STONED
STONER
STONES
STONEY
TBONDS
TBONES
THONGS
TOONIE
WRONGS
YVONNE

••O•N•

ABOUND
ACORNS
ADORNS
AMOUNT
ANOINT
AROINT
AROUND
BLOUNT
BOOING
BROWNE
BROWNS
BROWNU
BROWNY
CLOWNS
COOING
COOWNS
CROONS
CROWNE
CROWNS
DIONNE
DROWNS
EVONNE
FROWNS
GIORNO
GROANS
GROINS
GROUND
GROZNY
KNOWNS
KROONS
LYONNE
MOOING
QUOINS
REOWNS
SCORNS
SLOANE
SPOONS
SPOONY
SWOONS
TAOSNM
TBOONE
THORNS
THORNY
TROYNY
WOOING
YVONNE

••O••N

AJOWAN
ASOSAN
AWOKEN
AZORIN
BIOTIN
BLOWIN
BLOWON
BROGAN
BROKEN
BROLIN
CHOPIN
CHOSEN
CLOVEN
COOGAN
CRONIN
CRONYN
CROTON
DIOXIN
DOOHAN
DROPIN
EGOYAN
FLORIN
FLOWIN
FROZEN
GLOBIN
GNOMON
GOODEN
GOONIN
GOOSEN
GROBAN
GRODIN
GROTON
GROWON
HOOKON
IMOGEN
IRONON
ISOGON
KAOLIN
KIOWAN
LOOKIN
LOOKON
LOOSEN
MYOSIN
NEOCON
NOONAN
PHOTON
PLOWON
PRODON
PROGUN
PROTON
PROVEN
REOPEN
RIOPAN
ROOTIN
RYOKAN
SHOGUN
SHOOIN
SHOWIN
SIOUAN
SLOGAN
SLOPON
SLOVEN
SNOWIN
SPOKEN
SPOTON
STOLEN
STOLON
STOPIN
STOTIN
THORON
TOOKIN
TOOKON
TOOTIN
TRODON
TROJAN
TWOMAN
TWOPIN
UNOPEN
USOPEN
VIOLIN
WHOSIN
WHOWON
WOODEN
WOOLEN
YEOMAN
YEOMEN
ZOOMIN

•••ON•

ACTONE
ADDONS
AGEONE
ALMOND
ANIONS
ANTONE
ANTONY
ANYONE
ANYONS
APRONS
ARMONK
ARSONS
AUFOND
AUMONT
AXIONS
BACONS
BANONS
BARONE
BARONI
BARONS
BARONY
BATONS
BEGONE
BELONG
BELONS
BETONY
BEYOND
BIGONE
BISONS
BOSONS
BUSONI
BYGONE
CANONS
CAPONE
CAPONI
CAPONS
CARONI
CHRONO
CODONS
COLONI
COLONS
COLONY
CORONA
CROONS
DAMONE
DAYONE
DEBONE
DEBONT
DEMOND
DEMONS
DEPONE
DOGONS
DUGONG
DUMONT
DUPONT
EAMONN
EDMOND
EGMONT
ELKONV
ELMONT
EPSONS
EXCONS
FANONS
FATONE
FELONS
FELONY
FORONE
FREONS
FUTONS
GLUONS
GOLONG
HADONE
HASONE
HERONS
HITONE
HOTONE
HURONS
HUTONE
HYSONS
IMDONE
IMGONE
INIONS
INTONE
IONONE
JEVONS
JOBONE
KETONE
KIMONO
KROONS
LAMONT
LEMOND
LEMONS
LEMONY
LOGONS
LOMOND
LUPONE
MALONE
MASONS
MEKONG
MELONS
MESONS
MIDONS
MORONI
MORONS
MRBOND
MRWONG
MUTONS
NERONE
NIKONS
NINONS
NIXONS
NONONO
NOTONE
NYLONS
OBLONG
ODEONS
OENONE
ONEONE
ONIONS
ONIONY
OOLONG
ORIONS
ORLONS
ORMOND
OSMOND
OTTONE
PICONE
PINONS
PITONS
POCONO
POMONA
PUTONS
PYLONS
RAMONA
RAMONE
RAYONS
RECONS
REDONE
REHONE
RENONV
RETONE
REZONE
RUNONS
SALONS
SARONG
SAXONS
SAXONY
SCIONS
SECOND
SEDONA
SEWONS
SIMONE
SIXONE
SOLONG
SOLONS
SOMONI
SPOONS
SPOONY
STRONG
SWOONS
TALONS
TAUONS
TBOONE
TENONE
TENONS
TETONS
THEONE
THRONE
THRONG
TIGONS
TOYONS
TRYONE
TYRONE
TYSONS
UNDONE
UNFOND
UNIONS
UNZONE
VERONA
WAGONS
WEEONE
WETONE
WINONA
YUKONS
ZANONI
ZEDONG
ZEDONK
ZIPONS

•••O•N

ADJOIN
ADNOUN
ASWOON
ATNOON
BABOON
BEMOAN
BICORN
COCOON
DEHORN
DISOWN
EAMONN
ENJOIN
ETAOIN
GENOAN
GODOWN
HEROIN
IIJOHN
INBORN
INTOWN
LAGOON
MACOUN
MAROON
MINOAN
MOTOWN
OHIOAN
ONLOAN
OSBORN
REBORN
RECOIN
REJOIN
RELOAN
REMOWN
RENOWN
RESOWN
RETORN
REWORN
SALOON
SAMOAN
SHOOIN
SOSOON
STJOAN
STJOHN
SUBORN
THROWN
TYCOON
UNBORN
UNJOIN
UNMOWN
UNSOWN
UNTORN
UNWORN
UPJOHN
UPTORN
UPTOWN
ZEROIN

••••ON

ABUTON
ACTION
ACTSON
ADDSON
ALANON
ALBION
ALISON
ALSTON
AMAZON
AMNION
ANTRON
ARAGON
ARCHON
ASHTON
ASWOON
ATNOON
AVALON
AVEDON
AVISON
AWCMON
AYRTON
BABOON
BABSON
BAILON
BALLON
BANGON
BANKON
BANLON
BARRON
BARTON
BARYON
BATSON
BCLION
BEACON
BEAMON
BEARON
BEATON
BECKON
BEINON
BELTON
BENSON
BENTON
BESSON
BETSON
BICHON
BIDSON
BINYON
BITEON
BLAZON
BLEWON
BLOWON
BLYTON
BOLTON
BONBON
BONTON
BOREON
BOSSON
BOSTON
BOUTON
BRETON
BRITON
BRYSON
BUFFON
BUNION
BUNTON
BURTON
BUTTON
BUYSON
CALGON
CALLON
CAMEON
CAMION
CANNON
CANTON
CANYON
CARBON
CARSON
CARTON
CASTON
CATION
CATTON
CEYLON
CHARON
CHEVON
CHEWON
CHIRON
CHITON
CHYRON
CITRON
CLIPON
COCOON
COLSON
COLTON
COMEON
COMMON
CORDON
COTTON
COUPON
CRAYON
CROTON
CURZON
DACRON
DAEMON
DALTON
DAMSON
DANNON
DANSON
DANTON
DAWNON
DAWSON
DAYTON
DEACON
DEADON
DEFCON
DENTON
DIDION
DILLON
DINEON
DOLTON
DONJON
DOTEON
DOWNON
DOWSON
DRAGON
DRAWON
DREWON
DRIPON
DUMPON
DUTTON
EASEON
EASTON
EDISON
EGGSON
ELEVON
ELKTON
ELSTON
EMPSON
ENDSON
EPHRON
ETYMON
FACEON
FALCON
FALLON
FANION
FAWNON
FEEDON
FELDON
FELLON
FELSON
FINKON
FIREON
FITSON
FLACON
FLAGON
FLEWON
FULTON
FUSION
GAINON
GALLON
GALTON
GAMMON
GANNON
GARCON
GARSON
GASCON
GASTON
GAVEON
GAZEON
GEESON
GETSON
GIBBON
GIBSON
GIDEON
GIVEON
GLUEON
GNAWON
GNOMON
GODSON
GOESON
GONEON
GORDON
GORGON
GREWON
GROTON
GROWON
GURION
GUTZON
HAAKON
HADRON
HANDON
HANGON
HANLON
HANSON
HARMON
HARPON
HAVEON
HEADON
HEAPON
HEATON
HEBRON
HEDRON
HELDON
HELLON
HELPON
HENSON
HEREON
HERMON
HESTON
HIGHON
HILTON
HINTON
HIREON
HITSON
HOBSON
HOLDON
HOOKON
HOPSON
HORTON
HOUDON
HUDSON
HUNGON
HUSTON
HUTTON
INCHON
IRONON
ISOGON
JARGON
JETSON
JIMSON
JOBSON
JOEDON
JOLSON
JONSON
JUDSON
JUMPON
KEATON
KEENON
KEEPON
KELTON
KENTON
KENYON
KEPTON
KEYSON
KIERON
KLAXON
KMESON
KRYLON
LACEON
LAGOON
LAIDON
LANDON
LANSON
LARDON
LARSON
LATEON
LAWSON
LAWTON
LAYSON
LEADON
LEANON
LEAPON
LEBRON
LEFTON
LEGION
LEMMON
LENNON
LEPTON
LESION
LESSON
LETSON
LIEDON
LIESON
LINTON
LIPTON
LISBON
LISTON
LIVEON
LOCKON
LOFTON
LOGSON
LONDON
LOOKON
LOTION
LOUDON
LUPTON
LYNDON
LYTTON
MACRON
MAGNON
MAISON
MALLON
MAMMON
MANNON
MANZON
MARION
MARLON
MAROON
MARRON
MASSON
MATRON
MATSON
MAWSON
MAXSON
MAYRON
MCKEON
MELLON
MELTON
MERTON
MICRON
MIGNON
MILTON
MINION
MOLSON
MORMON
MORTON
MOTION
MOVEON
MUSEON
MUTTON
NACION
NATION
NATRON
NEALON
NEESON
NELSON
NEOCON
NETTON
NEURON
NEWTON
NIGHON
NIPPON
NOEMON
NOIRON
NORTON
NOTION
OBERON
ODDSON
ODEDON
OLESON
ONETON
OPENON
OPTION
OREGON
ORISON
OWEDON
OWESON
PACKON
PARDON
PARSON
PARTON
PASSON
PATRON
PATTON
PAXTON
PAYSON
PAYTON
PELION
PENNON
PERSON
PEYTON
PHOTON
PICKON
PIGEON
PILEON
PINION
PINSON
PINZON
PISTON
PLANON
PLAYON
PLOWON
PLUTON
POISON
POMPON
POSTON
POTION
POUPON
PREYON
PRISON
PRODON
PROTON
PULLON
PULMON
PUSHON
PUTSON
PYTHON
QUEZON
RAGSON
RAILON
RAINON
RAISON
RAMSON
RAPSON
RATION
RATSON
RAVEON
RAWDON
READON
REASON
RECKON
REGION
RELYON
RENTON
RESTON
RETTON
REVLON
REVSON
RIBBON
RIPSON
ROBSON
ROCHON
RODION
ROLLON
RONSON
RUBSON
RULEON
RUNSON
RUNYON
SAIGON
SAILON
SAISON
SALMON
SALOON
SALTON
SAMSON
SARGON
SARTON
SASSON
SAURON
SAVEON
SEASON
SEATON
SELLON
SENDON
SENTON
SERMON
SETSON
SEWNON
SEWSON
SEXTON
SHARON
SHEDON
SHIMON
SIGNON
SIMEON
SIPHON
SIPSON
SITSON
SLAMON
SLAPON
SLIPON
SLOPON
SNAPON
SOFTON
SOLDON
SOSOON
SOURON
SPITON
SPOTON
SPURON
STAYON
STEPON
STOLON
STYRON
SUMMON
SUTTON
TACKON
TAGSON
TAKEON
TALKON
TAPEON
TAPSON
TARPON
TEFLON
TELLON
TENDON
TENTON
TEUTON
THERON
THESON
THORON
TIEDON
TIESON
TIGLON
TILSON
TILTON
TOLDON
TOOKON
TOULON
TRIGON
TRIPON
TRITON
TRODON
TRYLON
TUCSON
TUGSON
TURNON
TYCOON
UNISON
URGEON
USEDON
USESON
VERDON
VERNON
VILLON
VINSON
VINTON
VIRDON
VISION
VOTEON
WAITON
WALKON
WALTON
WANTON
WATSON
WAYLON
WEAKON
WEAPON
WEARON
WELDON
WENTON
WESSON
WESTON
WHOWON
WILSON
WILTON

WISHON
WONTON
WOREON
WORKON
WYNTON
YANGON
YANKON
ZIRCON

OO••••

OOCYTE
OODLES
OOHING
OOLALA
OOLITE
OOLOGY
OOLONG
OOMPAH
OOMPHS
OOPODS
OOTIDS
OOZIER
OOZILY
OOZING

O•O•••

OBOIST
OBOLER
OBOLUS
OCONEE
ODONTO
ODORED
ODOULS
ODOURS
OLORES
OPORTO
OROMEO
OROSCO
OROZCO
OTOMIS
OTOOLE
OTOSES
OTOSIS
OVOIDS
OWOSSO
OZONIC

O••O••

OBLONG
OCLOCK
OCTOOT
OCTOPI
ODEONS
ODIOUS
OENONE
OFNOTE
OFYORE
OGDOAD
OHGOSH
OHIOAN
OHLOOK
OLEOLE
ONEOFF
ONEONE
ONEOUT
ONFOOT
ONHOLD
ONIONS
ONIONY
ONLOAD
ONLOAN
ONPOST
ONTOUR
OOLOGY
OOLONG
OOPODS
OPPOSE
OPTOUT
OREOOS
ORIOLE
ORIONS
ORLONS
ORLOPS
ORMOLU
ORMOND
OSBORN
OSGOOD
OSMOND
OSMOSE
OTIOSE
OTOOLE
OTTOII
OTTOIV
OTTONE
OUIOUI
OXBOWS
OXFORD

O•••O•

OBERON
OCELOT
OCTOOT
OCTROI
ODDJOB
ODDLOT
ODDSON
ODEDON
OHLOOK
OHSTOP
OLDBOY
OLDDOG
OLDSOD
OLESON
ONAHOP
ONETON
ONFOOT
ONSHOW
OPENON
OPTFOR
OPTION
ORATOR
OREGON
OREOOS
ORISON
OSGOOD
OUTBOW
OUTBOX
OUTFOR
OUTFOX
OUTPOP
OUTROW
OWEDON
OWESON
OXYDOL

O••••O

OBENTO
OBERTO
OBISPO
OCTAVO
ODONTO
OLDPRO
ONAUTO
ONEIRO
ONETWO
OPENTO
OPORTO
OPTIMO
OPTSTO
OROMEO
OROSCO
OROZCO
ORSINO
OSWEGO
OTELLO
OTSEGO
OVERDO
OVIEDO
OWEDTO
OWOSSO

•OO•••

BOOBOO
BOOCOO
BOODLE
BOOERS
BOOGIE
BOOHOO
BOOING
BOOJUM
BOOKED
BOOKEM
BOOKER
BOOKIE
BOOKII
BOOKIV
BOOKIX
BOOKVI
BOOMED
BOOMER
BOOSAT
BOOSTS
BOOTED
BOOTEE
BOOTER
BOOTES
BOOTHE
BOOTHS
BOOTIE
BOOTIT
BOOTUP
BOOZED
BOOZER
BOOZES
COODER
COOEED
COOEES
COOERS
COOGAN
COOING
COOKED
COOKER
COOKIE
COOKUP
COOLED
COOLER
COOLEY
COOLIE
COOLIO
COOLIT
COOLLY
COOLTH
COOLTO
COONEY
COOPED
COOPER
COOPTS
COOPUP
COOTER
COOTIE
COOWNS
DOODAD
DOODAH
DOODLE
DOOFUS
DOOGIE
DOOHAN
DOOLEY
DOOLIE
DOOMED
DOOMTO
DOORED
DOOVER
DOOWOP
DOOZER
DOOZIE
FOODIE
FOOLED
FOOLER
FOOTED
FOOTER
FOOTIT
FOOTLE
FOOTUP
FOOZLE
GOOBER
GOODAT
GOODBY
GOODEN
GOODER
GOODIE
GOODLY
GOODOH
GOOFED
GOOFUP
GOOFUS
GOOGLE
GOOGLY
GOOGOL
GOOGOO
GOOIER
GOONEY
GOONIE
GOONIN
GOOSED
GOOSEN
GOOSES
GOOSEY
GOOVER
HOODED
HOODIE
HOODOO
HOOFED
HOOFER
HOOFIT
HOOHAH
HOOHAS
HOOKAH
HOOKED
HOOKER
HOOKEY
HOOKON
HOOKUP
HOOPED
HOOPER
HOOPLA
HOOPLE
HOOPOE
HOORAH
HOORAY
HOOSAC
HOOTAT
HOOTCH
HOOTED
HOOTER
HOOTIE
HOOVER
HOOVES
KOOKIE
KOONTZ
LOOEYS
LOOFAH
LOOFAS
LOOIES
LOOKAT
LOOKED
LOOKEE
LOOKER
LOOKIE
LOOKIN
LOOKMA
LOOKON
LOOKTO
LOOKUP
LOOMED
LOOMPA
LOOMUP
LOONEY
LOONIE
LOOPED
LOOPER
LOOSED
LOOSEN
LOOSER
LOOSES
LOOSEY
LOOTED
LOOTER
MOOCOW
MOODYS
MOOERS
MOOING
MOOKIE
MOOLAH
MOONED
MOONER
MOONEY
MOONIE
MOORED
MOOTED
MOOTER
NOODGE
NOODLE
NOOGIE
NOONAN
NOONER
NOONES
NOOSED
NOOSER
NOOSES
NOOTKA
POODLE
POOHED
POOLED
POOLER
POOPED
POORAT
POORER
POORIS
POORLY
ROOFED
ROOFER
ROOKED
ROOKER
ROOKIE
ROOMBA
ROOMED
ROOMER
ROOMIE
ROONEY
ROOSTS
ROOTED
ROOTER
ROOTIE
ROOTIN
ROOTLE
ROOTSY
ROOTUP
SOONAS
SOONER
SOONYI
SOOTHE
TOOBAD
TOOBIG
TOODLE
TOOFAR
TOOHIP
TOOHOT
TOOKIN
TOOKIT
TOOKON
TOOKTO
TOOKUP
TOOLED
TOOLER
TOOLOW
TOOLUP
TOOMEY
TOONIE
TOOTAT
TOOTED
TOOTER
TOOTHY
TOOTIE
TOOTIN
TOOTLE
TOOTOO
TOOTSY
VOODOO
WOODED
WOODEN
WOODIE
WOODSY
WOOERS
WOOFED
WOOFER
WOOGIE
WOOING
WOOLEN
WOOLEY
WOOLLY
WOOTSY
YOOHOO
ZOOIDS
ZOOIER
ZOOMED
ZOOMIN

•O•O••

BOGOTA
BOSOMS
BOSOMY
BOSONS
BOWOAR
BOWOUT
COCOAS
COCOON
CODONS
COHOES
COHORT
COHOST
COLONI
COLONS
COLONY
COLORS
COLOUR
COMORO
CONOCO
CONOID
COPOUT
CORONA
COROTS
COYOTE
DOCOMO
DODODO
DODOES
DODOMA
DOGONS
DOGOOD
DOLORE
DOLORS
DOLOUR
DONORA
DONORS
DONOSO
DOTOAT
DOTODO
DOTORG
FOBOFF
FODORS
FORONE
GOBOES
GOBOOM
GOBOTS
GOCOED
GOCOLD
GODOWN
GOHOME
GOLONG
GONOGO
GOSOFT
GOSOLO
GOSOUR
GOTOFF
GOTOIT
GOTOLD
GOTOUT
HOBOED
HOBOES
HOHOHO
HONORE
HONORS
HONOUR
HOPOFF
HOPOUT
HOTOIL
HOTONE
HOWODD
IOMOTH
IONONE
JOBONE
JOCOSE
JOJOBA
JOYOUS
KOBOLD
KOKOMO
KOMODO
KOSOVO
LOGOFF
LOGONS
LOGOUT
LOMOND
LOPOFF
LOYOLA
MOJOES
MONODY
MOROLT
MORONI
MORONS
MOROSE
MOROSS
MOTORS
MOTOWN
NOBODY
NOCOST
NODOFF
NODOSE
NODOUS
NOGOOD
NOHOPE
NOJOKE
NOLOAD
NOLOSE
NOLOSS
NOMORE
NONONO
NOROOM
NOSOAP
NOTOLL
NOTONE
NOTOUT
NOVOTE
NOYORI
OOLOGY
OOLONG
OOPODS
POBOYS
POCONO
PODOUS
POMONA
POPOFF
POPOUT
POROSE
POROUS
POSOLE
POTOSI
POZOLE
ROBOTS
ROCOCO
ROMOLA
ROTORS
SODOWE
SOLOED
SOLONG
SOLONS
SOMONI
SONOMA
SONORA
SOPORS
SOSOON
TOBOOT
TOCOME
TOGOUT
TOKORI
TOPOFF
TOPOUT
TOROID
TOYONS
TOYOTA
VOROUS
WONOUT
XOXOXO
YOHOHO
YOYOED
YOYOMA

•O••O•

BOFFOS
BOLCOM
BOLTON
BONBON
BONGOS
BONMOT
BONTON
BOOBOO
BOOCOO
BOOHOO
BOREON
BORROW
BORZOI
BOSSON
BOSTON
BOTTOM
BOUTON
BOWWOW
BOXBOY
BOXTOP
BOYTOY
COCOON
COINOP
COLLOP
COLLOQ
COLSON
COLTON
COMBOS
COMEOF
COMEON
COMMON
COMPOS
COMPOZ
CONDOR
CONDOS
CONGOU
CONJOB
CONNOR
CONROY
CONVOY
CORDON
CORTOT
COSMOS
COTTON
COUPON
COWBOY
COWPOX
COYDOG
DOBROS
DOCBOY
DOCTOR
DOESOK
DOGDOM
DOGOOD
DOGTOY
DOKTOR
DOLLOP
DOLTON
DONEOK
DONJON
DOOWOP
DOTCOM
DOTDOT
DOTEON
DOTGOV
DOWNON
DOWSON
FOGBOW
FOGDOG
FOLIOS
FOLLOW
FOLSOM
FONDOF
FORGOT
FORJOY
FORNOW
FORYOU
GOAWOL
GOBOOM
GOBSOF
GODSON
GOESON
GONEON
GOODOH
GOOGOL
GOOGOO
GORDON
GORGON
GORIOT
GOSLOW
GOTHOT
GOTYOU
GOUNOD
HOBNOB
HOBSON
HOLDON
HOLLOW
HOODOO
HOOKON
HOOPOE
HOPSON
HORROR
HORTON
HOTBOT
HOTBOX
HOTDOG
HOTPOT
HOTROD
HOUDON
HOWNOW
HOWTOS
JOANOU
JOBHOP
JOBLOT
JOBSON
JOCKOS
JOEDON
JOLIOT
JOLSON
JONSON
KOWTOW
LOCKON
LOFTON
LOGSON
LOMPOC
LONDON
LONNOL
LOOKON
LOSDOS
LOTION
LOTNOS
LOTSOF
LOTTOS
LOUDON
LOWBOY
LOWTOP
MOLLOY
MOLSON
MONDOS
MONGOL
MONGOS
MONROE
MOOCOW
MOPTOP
MORMON
MORROW
MORTON
MOSCOW
MOSTOF
MOTION
MOTTOS
MOVEON
NOEMON
NOGOOD
NOIRON
NONCOM
NONGOD
NOPROB
NORDOI
NOROOM
NORTON
NOSHOW
NOTFOR
NOTION
NOTNOW
NOTTOO
NOTYOU
NOVIOS
NOWNOW
POIROT
POISON
POITOU
POLIOS
POLLOI
POLLOS
POLPOT
POMPOM
POMPON
POPTOP
POSTON
POSTOP
POTHOS
POTION
POTTOS
POUPON
POWWOW
ROBROY
ROBSOF
ROBSON
ROCHON
RODEOS
RODION
ROLEOS
ROLLON
ROMCOM
ROMEOS
RONDOS
RONSON
ROSCOE
ROSTOV
SOFTON
SOLDON
SORROW
SORTOF
SOSOON
SOURON
TOBOOT
TOLDOF
TOLDON
TOMBOY
TOMTOM
TONDOS
TONSOF
TOOHOT
TOOKON
TOOLOW
TOOTOO
TOPDOG
TOPJOB
TOPROW
TORPOR
TORSOS
TOULON
TOYDOG
TOYTOP
VOIDOF
VOLVOS
VOODOO
VOSTOK
VOTEON
VOXPOP
WONTON
WOREON
WORKON
YOMTOV
YOOHOO

•O•••O

BOCHCO
BOINGO
BOLERO
BONITO
BOOBOO
BOOCOO
BOOHOO
BORAXO
BORNEO
BOWSTO
COGITO
COLECO
COMETO
COMORO
CONCHO
CONOCO
COOLIO
COOLTO
COPSTO
CORREO
COSTCO
DOCOMO
DODODO
DOESSO
DOESTO
DOMINO
DONESO
DONETO
DONOSO
DONTGO
DOOMTO
DORADO
DORITO
DOSADO
DOSIDO
DOTODO
FOREGO
FOURNO
GOESTO
GOINTO
GOLINO
GONETO
GONOGO
GOOGOO
GOSOLO
GOUPTO
HOHOHO
HOLDTO
HONCHO
HOODOO
HOPESO
HOPETO
HOPSTO
HOVETO
JOURNO
KOKOMO
KOMODO
KOSOVO
LOOKTO
LOSETO
LOSTTO
LOVETO
MODULO
MOJITO
MONACO
MORENO
MORESO
MORPHO
MOVADO
MOVETO
NODSTO
NOMAYO
NONEGO
NONONO
NONPRO
NOTTOO
NOVATO
POCONO
POMELO
POMPEO
PONCHO
POTATO
ROADEO
ROCOCO
RODETO
RODINO
ROMANO
ROMERO
ROMULO
ROSETO
ROTHKO
SOASTO
SOLANO
SOLDTO
SOWETO
TOBAGO
TODDAO
TOLEDO
TOMATO
TOOKTO
TOOTOO
TORERO
TORINO
VOODOO
VOTENO
WONTDO
WONTGO
XOXOXO
YOHOHO
YOOHOO
YOSANO
YOUTWO
ZOCALO

••OO••

BLOODS
BLOODY
BLOOEY
BLOOIE
BLOOMS
BLOOMY
BLOOPS
BROOCH
BROODS
BROODY
BROOKE
BROOKS
BROOKY
BROOMS
BROOMY
CHOOSE
CHOOSY
CROOKS
CROONS
DROOLS
DROOLY
DROOPS
DROOPY
EBOOKS
FLOODS
FLOOEY
FLOORS
GLOOMS
GLOOMY
GROOMS
GROOVE
GROOVY
IBOOKS
KROONS
OTOOLE
PBOOKS
PHOOEY
PROOFS
PTOOEY
SCOOBA
SCOOBY
SCOOPS
SCOOTS
SHOOED
SHOOIN
SHOOTS
SLOOPS
SLOOPY
SMOOCH
SMOOSH
SMOOTH
SNOODS
SNOOKS
SNOOPS
SNOOPY
SNOOTS
SNOOTY
SNOOZE
SNOOZY
SPOOFS
SPOOKS
SPOOKY
SPOOLS
SPOONS
SPOONY
SPOORS
STOOGE
STOOLS
STOOLY
STOOPS
SWOONS
SWOOPS
SWOOSH
TBOONE
TROOPS
VROOMS
WHOOPI
WHOOPS
WHOOSH

••O•O•

ADOBOS AGOROT ALOTOF AMOSOZ ATONOF BLOWON BOOBOO BOOCOO BOOHOO CHOLOS CHOROS CLOROX CROTON DOOWOP DUOMOS FEODOR FROYOS FYODOR GNOMON GOODOH GOOGOL GOOGOO GROTON GROWON HOODOO HOOKON HOOPOE IDONOT IDOTOO IGOROT IROBOT IRONON ISOGON ISOPOD KNOWOF KRONOR LOOKON MOOCOW NEOCON PHOBOS PHONOS PHOTOG PHOTON PHOTOS PLOWON PROCOL PRODON PROLOG PROMOS PROTON SHOLOM SLOPON SNOBOL SPOTON STOLON THORON TOOHOT TOOKON TOOLOW TOOTOO TRODON VOODOO WHOWON YOOHOO

••O••O

ADOLFO AGOSTO ALONSO ALONZO APOLLO BLOTTO BOOBOO BOOCOO BOOHOO BRONCO BRONKO CHOREO CHORIO CLOTHO COOLIO COOLTO DOOMTO DROMIO FLORIO GIORNO GIOTTO GLOSSO GLOTTO GOOGOO GROSSO GROTTO HOODOO IDOIDO IDOTOO IKOIKO ILOILO LOOKTO NEOSHO ODONTO OPORTO OROMEO OROSCO OROZCO OWOSSO PRONTO SCOTTO SHOPKO SHORTO SLOWGO STOJKO STOPGO TOOKTO TOOTOO TROPPO VOODOO WHOMSO YOOHOO

•••OO•

ABLOOM ASCOOL ASGOOD ASTOOP ASWOON ATNOON ATWOOD BABOON BABOOS BAZOOS BECOOL BEFOOL BEGOOD BEHOOF BETOOK CAHOOT COCOON DOGOOD DRDOOM DRHOOK DRKOOP EDWOOD ELWOOD ENROOT EXMOOR FAZOOL FTROOP GALOOT GOBOOM IGLOOS IMCOOL IMGOOD INDOOR INGOOD KABOOM KAZOOS LAGOON MAROON MRCOOL MTCOOK MTHOOD MYFOOT NANOOK NOGOOD NOROOM OCTOOT OHLOOK ONFOOT OREOOS OSGOOD REBOOK REBOOT RECOOK RECOOL REHOOK RELOOK REROOF REROOT RETOOK RETOOL SALOON SCHOOL SHBOOM SHNOOK SOSOON TABOOS TOBOOT TVROOM TYCOON UNCOOL UNCOOP UNHOOD UNHOOK UNLOOP UNMOOR UNROOF UNROOT UPROOT WAHOOS YAHOOS

•••O•O

ALIOTO ARIOSO ARROYO BAROLO CHLORO CHROMO CHRONO COMORO CONOCO DENOVO DESOTO DEVOTO DOCOMO DODODO DONOSO DOTODO ELTORO ENTOMO ESPOSO FLUORO GIGOLO GONOGO GOSOLO HOHOHO INTOTO KIMONO KOKOMO KOMODO KOSOVO LEMOKO LENOVO MINOSO MRMOTO NICOLO NONONO POCONO REBOZO ROCOCO SUNOCO XOXOXO YOHOHO

••••OO

AHCHOO ARETOO BAMBOO BOOBOO BOOCOO BOOHOO BURGOO CANTOO CUCKOO DAEWOO DAGGOO GOOGOO HACHOO HALLOO HOODOO IAMTOO IDOTOO MCADOO NOTTOO SAYBOO SKIDOO TATTOO TOOTOO VOODOO WAHLOO YOOHOO

OP••••

OPAQUE OPCITS OPENED OPENER OPENIT OPENLY OPENON OPENTO OPENUP OPERAS OPHULS OPIATE OPINED OPINER OPINES OPIUMS OPORTO OPPOSE OPPUGN OPQRST OPRAHS OPTFOR OPTICS OPTIMA OPTIMO OPTING OPTION OPTOUT OPTSIN OPTSTO OPUSES

O•P•••

OMPHAL ONPOST OOPODS OPPOSE OPPUGN ORPHAN ORPHIC OSPREY

O••P••

OILPAN OKAPIS OLDPAL OLDPRO ONAPAR ONEPIN ONSPEC OOMPAH OOMPHS OUTPAY OUTPOP OUTPRY OUTPUT

O•••P•

OBISPO OCCUPY OCTOPI ONEUPS ONTAPE ORLOPS OUTSPY OXLIPS

O••••P

OFHELP OHSTOP OILCUP ONAHOP ONELAP ONRAMP OPENUP OUTLIP OUTPOP OUTRAP OWNSUP

•OP•••

BOPEEP BOPPED BOPPER COPALS COPAYS COPCAR COPERS COPIED COPIER COPIES COPING COPLEY COPOUT COPPED COPPER COPRAS COPSES COPSIT COPSTO COPTER COPTIC COPULA DOPERS DOPIER DOPILY DOPING GOPAST GOPHER HOPERS HOPESO HOPETO HOPING HOPKIN HOPOFF HOPOUT HOPPED HOPPER HOPSIN HOPSON HOPSTO HOPSUP JOPLIN KOPECK KOPEKS KOPELL KOPJES KOPPEL LOPERS LOPING LOPOFF LOPPED LOPPER MOPEDS MOPERS MOPERY MOPIER MOPING MOPISH MOPPED MOPPER MOPPET MOPSUP MOPTOP MOPUPS NOPALS NOPETS NOPQRS NOPROB OOPODS POPART POPEIL POPEYE POPFLY POPGUN POPISH POPLAR POPLIN POPOFF POPOUT POPPAS POPPED POPPER POPPLE POPSIN POPSUP POPTOP POPULI POPUPS ROPEIN ROPERS ROPERY ROPEUP ROPIER ROPING SOPHIA SOPHIE SOPORS SOPPED SOPSUP TOPBID TOPCAT TOPDOG TOPEES TOPEKA TOPERS TOPGUN TOPHAT TOPICS TOPING TOPJOB TOPMAN TOPMEN TOPOFF TOPOUT TOPPED TOPPER TOPPLE TOPROW TOPSUP TOPTEN

•O•P••

BOPPED BOPPER COAPTS COMPAQ COMPAS COMPED COMPEL COMPLY COMPOS COMPOZ COOPED COOPER COOPTS COOPUP COPPED COPPER CORPSE CORPUS COUPES COUPLE COUPON COWPEA COWPER COWPOX COYPUS GOSPEL GOUPTO HOOPED HOOPER HOOPLA HOOPLE HOOPOE HOPPED HOPPER HOTPOT JOYPAD KOPPEL LOMPOC LOOPED LOOPER LOPPED LOPPER LOUPES MOPPED MOPPER MOPPET MORPHO MORPHS NONPAR NONPRO OOMPAH OOMPHS POLPOT POMPEO POMPEY POMPOM POMPON POOPED POPPAS POPPED POPPER POPPLE POTPIE POUPON ROEPER ROMPED ROMPER SOAPED SOAPER SOAPUP SOPPED SOSPAD SOUPER SOUPUP TOPPED TOPPER TOPPLE TORPID TORPOR TOUPEE VORPAL VOXPOP WOLPER

•O••P•

DOGAPE DOLAPS FOURPM JOSEPH LOOMPA MOPUPS NOHOPE NOTIPS POLYPS POPUPS YORKPA

•O•••P

BOBSUP BOILUP BOLTUP BONEUP BOOTUP BOPEEP BOREUP BOXTOP COILUP COINOP COLLOP COMEUP COOKUP COOPUP CORKUP COSYUP COZYUP DOESUP DOGNAP DOITUP DOLLOP DOLLUP DOMREP DONEUP DOOWOP FOGSUP FOLDUP FOOTUP FORKUP FOULUP FOURUP GODEEP GOESUP GOLIMP GONEUP GOOFUP GOSSIP GOTHEP GOTHIP HOLDUP HOLEUP HOOKUP HOPSUP HOTCAP HOTCUP HOTTIP JOBHOP JOINUP LOADUP LOCKUP LOOKUP LOOMUP LOWTOP MOCKUP MOPSUP MOPTOP MOVEUP NOHELP NOSEUP NOSOAP NOSTEP PONYUP POPSUP POPTOP POSTOP RODEUP ROILUP ROLLUP ROOTUP ROPEUP ROSEUP SOAKUP SOAPUP SOPSUP SOUPUP TOECAP TOETAP TOGSUP TONEUP TOOHIP TOOKUP TOOLUP TOPSUP TOREUP TORNUP TOSSUP TOTEUP TOTSUP TOYTOP VOXPOP WOKEUP WORKUP

••OP••

ADOPTS APOPKA BHOPAL BIOPIC BIOPSY BROPHY CHOPIN CHOPPY CHOPRA CHOPUP COOPED COOPER COOPTS COOPUP CROPUP DROPBY DROPIN DROPIT DROPSY ELOPED ELOPER ELOPES EPOPEE FLOPIT FLOPPY FLOPSY GLOPPY GROPED GROPER GROPES HOOPED HOOPER HOOPLA HOOPLE HOOPOE ISOPOD LOOPED LOOPER MNOPQR MYOPES MYOPIA MYOPIC PEOPLE POOPED PROPEL PROPER PROPRE PROPUP PROPYL REOPEN RIOPAN SCOPED SCOPES SHOPAT SHOPKO SHOPPE SKOPJE SLOPED SLOPER SLOPES SLOPON SLOPPY SNOPES STOPAT STOPBY STOPGO STOPIN STOPIT STOPUP TROPES TROPEZ TROPHY TROPIC TROPPO TWOPIN TWOPLY UNOPEN USOPEN UTOPIA

••O•P•

ADOLPH BLOOPS CHOMPS CHOPPY CLOMPS CROUPS CROUPY DROOPS DROOPY FLOPPY GLOPPY GROUPS LOOMPA PROMPT SCOOPS SCOUPE SHOPPE SLOOPS SLOOPY SLOPPY SNOOPS SNOOPY STOMPS STOOPS SWOOPS THORPE TROMPE TROMPS TROOPS TROPPO TROUPE WHOMPS WHOOPI WHOOPS

••O••P

BLOTUP BLOWUP BOOTUP BUOYUP CHOPUP CLOGUP CLOTUP COOKUP COOPUP CROPUP DOOWOP FOOTUP GOOFUP GROWUP HOOKUP KNOTUP LOOKUP LOOMUP PLOWUP PROPUP ROOTUP SHOTUP SHOWUP SLOWUP STOPUP TOOHIP TOOKUP TOOLUP TROTUP

•••OP•

AESOPS ASLOPE BEBOPS BLOOPS CANOPY CHEOPS DROOPS DROOPY ESTOPS EUROPA EUROPE FSTOPS GALOPS JALOPY LMNOPQ MEROPE MEROPS NOHOPE OCTOPI ORLOPS PANOPE PREOPS REBOPS RECOPY REMOPS RETOPS SCOOPS SLOOPS SLOOPY SNOOPS SNOOPY STOOPS STROPS SWOOPS SYSOPS TROOPS TSTOPS UNROPE WHOOPI WHOOPS

•••O•P

ASTOOP DRKOOP FTROOP NOSOAP RECOUP RESOAP UNCOOP UNLOOP

••••OP

AIRPOP ASTOOP BADCOP BARHOP BIGTOP BISHOP BOXTOP CARHOP CARTOP COINOP COLLOP DAYHOP DETROP DOLLOP DOOWOP DRKOOP DRYMOP DUNLOP ETHIOP FTROOP GALLOP HIPHOP HYSSOP ICEPOP IMACOP JOBHOP KLMNOP LAPTOP LOWTOP MMMBOP MOPTOP OHSTOP ONAHOP OUTPOP PEGTOP POPTOP POSTOP RAGMOP RAGTOP REDTOP SHEBOP THETOP TIPTOP TOYTOP UNCOOP UNLOOP UNSTOP UPPROP VOXPOP WALLOP WETMOP ZIPTOP

O•Q•••

OPQRST

O••Q••

OPAQUE

•OQ•••

COQUIS LOQUAT TOQUES

•O•Q••

MOSQUE NOPQRS TORQUE

•O••Q•

LOWIQS

•O•••Q

COLLOQ COMPAQ POSSLQ

••OQ••

EPOQUE QUOQUE

••O•Q•

MNOPQR

•••O•Q

LMNOPQ

••••OQ

COLLOQ

OR••••

ORACHS ORACLE ORAJEL ORALES ORALLY ORANGE ORANGS ORANGY ORANIS ORANTS ORATED ORATES ORATOR ORBACH ORBING ORBITS ORCHID ORDAIN ORDEAL ORDERS OREADS ORECKS OREGON OREIDA ORELSE ORENSE OREOOS OREXIA OREXIS ORGANA ORGANS ORGEAT ORGIES ORIANA ORIANI ORIBIS ORIELS ORIENT ORIGEN ORIGIN ORINGS ORIOLE ORIONS ORISON ORISSA ORKANS ORKNEY ORLONS ORLOPS ORMOLU ORMOND ORNATE ORNERY ORNITH OROMEO OROSCO OROZCO ORPHAN ORPHIC ORRERY ORSINI

ORSINO
ORTEGA
ORTHEN
ORTRUD
ORWELL
ORWHAT
ORYXES

O•R•••
OARAGE
OARERS
OARING
OARMAN
OARMEN
OBRIAN
OBRIEN
OERTER
OGRADY
OGRESS
OGRISH
ONRAMP
ONRICE
ONRUSH
OPRAHS
ORRERY

O••R••
OBERON
OBERTO
OCHRED
OCHRES
OCTROI
ODORED
OHCRUD
OHDRAT
OILRIG
OILRUB
OLERUD
OLORES
OMERTA
ONERUN
OPERAS
OPORTO
OPQRST
ORTRUD
OSIRIS
OSPREY
OUTRAN
OUTRAP
OUTRIB
OUTRIG
OUTROW
OUTRUN
OVERDO
OVERIT
OVERLY
OZARKS

O•••R•
OARERS
OATERS
OBVERT
OCCURS
OCHERS
OCHERY
ODOURS
OEUVRE
OFFERS
OFYORE
OGLERS
OHDARN
OHENRY
OHSURE
OILERS
OLDPRO
OLEARY
OLMERT
OMEARA
ONEARM
ONEIRO
ONFIRE
ONHIRE
ONWARD
ORDERS
ORNERY
ORRERY
OSBERT
OSBORN
OSCARS
OSETRA
OSIERS
OSTARS
OSTERS
OTHERS
OTTERS
OUTCRY
OUTPRY
OWLERY
OWNERS
OXCART
OXFORD
OXNARD

O••••R
OAKIER
OATIER
OBEYER
OBITER
OBOLER
OCEDAR
OCULAR
OERTER
OHDEAR
OILIER
OINKER
OLDCAR
OLIVER
ONAGER
ONAPAR
ONECAR
ONSTAR
ONTOUR
OOZIER
OPENER
OPINER
OPTFOR
ORATOR
OSTLER
OTHMAR
OUSTER
OUTFOR
OUTWAR
OVULAR
OWLIER
OYSTER

•OR•••
AORTAE
AORTAL
AORTAS
AORTIC
BORATE
BORAXO
BORDEN
BORDER
BORDET
BOREAL
BOREAS
BOREON
BORERS
BOREUP
BORGES
BORGIA
BORIDE
BORING
BORKED
BORMAN
BORNEO
BORROW
BORSCH
BORZOI
CORACI
CORALS
CORBEL
CORBIN
CORDAY
CORDED
CORDER
CORDIA
CORDON
CORERS
CORFAM
CORGIS
CORING
CORIUM
CORKED
CORKER
CORKUP
CORMAN
CORNEA
CORNED
CORNEL
CORNER
CORNET
CORONA
COROTS
CORPSE
CORPUS
CORRAL
CORREO
CORSAS
CORSET
CORTES
CORTEX
CORTEZ
CORTOT
CORVEE
CORVID
CORVUS
CORWIN
CORYZA
DORADO
DORAGS
DORATI
DORCAS
DOREEN
DOREMI
DORIAN
DORIES
DORINE
DORITO
DORMER
DORMIE
DORRIT
DORSAD
DORSAL
DORSAY
DORSET
DORSEY
DORSUM
FORAGE
FORAYS
FORBAD
FORBES
FORBID
FORCED
FORCER
FORCES
FORCHE
FORDED
FORDGT
FORDID
FOREGO
FOREST
FORFUN
FORGED
FORGER
FORGES
FORGET
FORGOT
FORINT
FORJOY
FORKED
FORKER
FORKUP
FORMAL
FORMAN
FORMAT
FORMED
FORMER
FORMIC
FORNAX
FORNOW
FORONE
FORTAS
FORTES
FORTIS
FORUMS
FORWHY
FORYOU
GORCEY
GORDIE
GORDON
GORERS
GORGED
GORGER
GORGES
GORGON
GORHAM
GORIER
GORILY
GORING
GORIOT
GORMED
GORSES
HORACE
HORDED
HORDES
HORGAN
HORMEL
HORMUZ
HORNBY
HORNED
HORNER
HORNET
HORNIN
HORRID
HORROR
HORSED
HORSES
HORSEY
HORTON
JORDAN
JORUMS
KORANS
KORATS
KORBUT
KOREAN
KORMAN
KORUNA
LORAIN
LORANS
LORDED
LORDIT
LORDLY
LOREAL
LORENE
LORENZ
LORIES
LORING
LORRIE
MORALE
MORALS
MORANT
MORASS
MORATH
MORAYS
MORBID
MOREAU
MOREEN
MORELS
MORENO
MORESO
MORGAN
MORGEN
MORGUE
MORITA
MORITZ
MORLEY
MORMON
MORNAY
MOROLT
MORONI
MORONS
MOROSE
MOROSS
MORPHO
MORPHS
MORREL
MORRIE
MORRIS
MORROW
MORSEL
MORTAL
MORTAR
MORTEN
MORTON
NORAIN
NORDIC
NORDOI
NOREEN
NORELL
NORENT
NORGAY
NORIAS
NORISK
NORITE
NORMAL
NORMAN
NOROOM
NORRIS
NORTHS
NORTON
NORUNS
NORUSH
NORVAL
NORWAY
PORERS
PORING
PORKED
PORKER
PORKYS
POROSE
POROUS
PORTAL
PORTED
PORTER
PORTES
PORTIA
PORTLY
SORBET
SORBIC
SORDID
SOREAT
SORELY
SOREST
SORREL
SORROW
SORTED
SORTER
SORTIE
SORTOF
TORAHS
TORBAY
TORCHY
TOREAT
TOREIT
TORENT
TORERO
TOREUP
TORIES
TORINO
TORNUP
TOROID
TORPID
TORPOR
TORQUE
TORRES
TORREY
TORRID
TORSOS
TORTAS
TORTES
VOROUS
VORPAL
VORTEX
WORDED
WOREON
WORKAT
WORKED
WORKER
WORKIN
WORKON
WORKUP
WORLDS
WORLEY
WORMED
WORMER
WORSEN
WORSTS
WORTHS
WORTHY
YORICK
YORKER
YORKIE
YORKIN
YORKPA
ZORINA

•O•R••
BOARDS
BOHRER
BORROW
BOTREE
BOURGS
BOURKE
BOURNE
BOURSE
COARSE
COBRAS
COERCE
CONRAD
CONROY
COPRAS
CORRAL
CORREO
COURIC
COURSE
COURTS
COWRIE
DOBROS
DOGRUN
DOMREP
DOORED
DORRIT
DOURER
DOURIF
DOURLY
FOURAA
FOURAD
FOURAM
FOURBC
FOUREE
FOURNO
FOURPM
FOURTH
FOURUP
GOFREE
GOTRID
GOURDE
GOURDS
HOARDS
HOARSE
HOORAH
HOORAY
HORRID
HORROR
HOTROD
HOURIS
HOURLY
JOURNO
KONRAD
LOIRET
LORRIE
LOWRES
MODRED
MOERAE
MOIRES
MONROE
MOORED
MORREL
MORRIE
MORRIS
MORROW
MOTRIN
MOURNS
NOIRES
NOIRET
NOIRON
NONRUN
NOPROB
NORRIS
POIRES
POIRET
POIROT
POORAT
POORER
POORIS
POORLY
POURED
POURER
POURIN
ROARAT
ROARED
ROARER
ROBROY
ROHRER
ROURKE
SOARED
SOARER
SOIREE
SORREL
SORROW
SOTRUE
SOURCE
SOURED
SOURER
SOURLY
SOURON
TOPROW
TORRES
TORREY
TORRID
TOURED
TOURER

•O••R•
AOLERS
BOGART
BOLERO
BONERS
BONERZ
BOOERS
BORERS
BOVARY
BOWERS
BOWERY
BOXERS
BOYARS
COBURG
COBURN
CODERS
COEURS
COHERE
COHORT
COLORS
COMDRS
COMERS
COMORO
CONERS
CONTRA
CONTRE
CONURE
COOERS
COPERS
CORERS
COVERS
COVERT
COWARD
COWERS
DOLORE
DOLORS
DONORA
DONORS
DOPERS
DOSERS
DOTARD
DOTERS
DOTORG
DOWERS
DOWERY
DOZERS
FODORS
FOUDRE
FOYERS
GOAWRY
GOCART
GODARD
GODARK
GOFERS
GOGIRL
GOKART
GOMERS
GONERS
GORERS
GOVERN
HOBART
HOLERS
HOMBRE
HOMERS
HONERS
HONORE
HONORS
HOPERS
HOSERS
HOVERS
HOWARD
JOFFRE
JOGBRA
JOKERS
LONERS
LOPERS
LOSERS
LOUVRE
LOVERS
LOWERS
LOWERY
MOBERG
MODERN
MOLARS
MOOERS
MOPERS
MOPERY
MOTHRA
MOTORS
MOVERS
MOWERS
MOYERS
MOZART
NOMBRE
NOMORE
NONART
NONARY
NONPRO
NOPQRS
NOSERS
NOSTRA
NOTARY
NOTERS
NOYORI
POETRY
POIVRE
POKERS
POKERY
POLARA
POLERS
POPART
PORERS
POSERS
POUDRE
POWERS
ROBERS
ROBERT
ROGERE
ROGERS
ROMERO
ROPERS
ROPERY
ROSARY
ROSERY
ROSTRA
ROTARY
ROTORS
ROVERS
ROWERS
SOBERS
SOEURS
SOLARA
SOLERS
SOMBRE
SOMERS
SONARS
SONDRA
SONORA
SOPORS
SOWERS
TOBURN
TOKORI
TOLARS
TONERS
TOPERS
TORERO
TOTERM
TOTERS
TOWARD
TOWERS
TOWERY
TOYERS
VOLARE
VOMERS
VOTARY
VOTERS
VOWERS
WOBURN
WOOERS
YOGURT
ZONERS

•O•••R
BOATER
BOBBER
BOHRER
BOILER
BOLDER
BOLGER
BOLTER
BOMBER
BONDER
BONIER
BONNER
BOOKER
BOOMER
BOOTER
BOOZER
BOPPER
BORDER
BOTHER
BOWLER
BOWOAR
BOWYER
BOWZER
BOXCAR
BOXIER
COALER
COATER
COAXER
COCKER
CODGER
COFFER
COHEIR
COILER
COINER
COKIER
COLDER
COLLAR
COLMAR
COLOUR
COLTER
COMBER
CONAIR
CONCUR
CONDOR
CONFER
CONGER
CONKER
CONNOR
COODER
COOKER
COOLER
COOPER
COOTER
COPCAR
COPIER
COPPER
COPTER
CORDER
CORKER
CORNER
COSHER
COSIER
COSTAR
COTLER
COTTER
COUGAR
COUTER
COWIER
COWPER
COZIER
DOCKER
DOCTOR
DODDER
DODGER
DOFFER
DOGEAR
DOKTOR
DOLLAR
DOLOUR
DONDER
DONNER
DOOVER
DOOZER
DOPIER
DORMER
DOTTER
DOURER
DOUSER
DOWNER
DOWSER
DOZIER
FOAMER
FODDER
FOGGER
FOKKER
FOLDER
FOLGER
FOLIAR
FONDER
FOOLER
FOOTER
FORCER
FORGER
FORKER
FORMER
FOSTER
FOULER
FOWLER
FOXIER
GOITER
GOLFER
GONEAR
GOOBER
GOODER
GOOIER
GOOVER
GOPHER
GORGER
GORIER
GOSOUR
GOTFAR
GOUGER
HOAXER
HOCKER
HOFFER
HOHNER
HOKIER
HOLDER
HOLIER
HOLLER
HOMIER
HONKER
HONOUR
HOOFER
HOOKER
HOOPER
HOOTER
HOOVER
HOPPER
HORNER
HORROR
HOSIER
HOTAIR
HOTCAR
HOTTER
HOTWAR
HOWFAR
HOWLER
HOWSER
JOBBER
JOBJAR
JOGGER
JOINER
JOKIER
JOLTER
JOSHER
JOTTER
JOYNER
KOCHER
KOHLER
KOSHER
KOSTER
KOTTER
LOADER
LOAFER
LOANER
LOBBER
LOCHER
LOCKER
LODGER
LOFTER
LOGGER
LOGIER
LOITER
LOLLER
LONGER
LOOKER
LOOPER
LOOSER
LOOTER
LOPPER
LOTHAR
LOTTER
LOUDER
LOUVER
LOWTAR
MOANER
MOBBER
MOCKER
MOHAIR
MOILER
MOLDER
MOLNAR
MOLTER
MONGER
MOONER
MOOTER
MOPIER
MOPPER
MORTAR
MOSHER
MOTHER
MOUSER
NOBLER
NODDER
NODEAR
NOFAIR
NONPAR
NONWAR
NOONER
NOOSER
NOSHER
NOSIER
NOSTER
NOTFAR
NOTFOR
OOZIER
POGNER
POISER
POKIER
POLGAR
POLLER
PONDER
POOLER
POORER
POPLAR
POPPER
PORKER
PORTER
POSEUR
POSHER
POSTER
POTHER
POTTER
POURER
POUTER
POWDER
POYSER
ROADER
ROAMER
ROARER
ROBBER
ROCKER
RODDER
ROEPER
ROHMER
ROHRER
ROLFER
ROLLER
ROMPER
ROOFER
ROOKER
ROOMER
ROOTER
ROPIER
ROSIER
ROSTER
ROTTER
ROUSER
ROUTER
SOAKER
SOAPER
SOARER
SOBBER
SOCCER
SOFTER
SOLDER
SOLVER
SOMBER
SOMMER
SOONER
SORTER
SOUPER
SOURER
SOUTER
TOILER
TOLLER
TONIER
TOOFAR
TOOLER
TOOTER
TOPPER
TORPOR
TOSSER
TOTTER
TOURER
TOUTER
TOWBAR
TOWCAR
TOWNER
TOYCAR
VOGUER
VOICER
VOIDER
WOHLER
WOLPER
WONDER
WOOFER
WORKER
WORMER
YONDER
YORKER
YOWLER
ZONKER
ZOOIER

••OR••
ABORAL
ABORTS
ACORNS
ADORED
ADOREE

ADORER ADORES ADORNS AGORAE AGORAS AGOROT AHORSE AMORAL AMORES AMORET ANORAK AZORES AZORIN CEORLS CHORAL CHORDS CHOREO CHORES CHORIC CHORIO CHOROS CHORUS CLORIS CLOROX CRORES CUORES DOORED DVORAK ECORSE EMORYU ENORME FIORDS FJORDS FLORAE FLORAL FLORAS FLOREK FLORES FLORET FLOREY FLORID FLORIN FLORIO GEORDI GEORGE GEORGI GEORGY GFORCE GIORNO GLORIA HOORAH HOORAY IFORTY IGOROT MAORIS MOORED NFORTY ODORED OLORES OPORTO PEORIA POORAT POORER POORIS POORLY QUORUM SCORCH SCORED

SCORER SCORES SCORIA SCORNS SFORZA SHORES SHORTA SHORTE SHORTI SHORTO SHORTS SHORTU SHORTY SHORTZ SKORTS SMORES SNORED SNORER SNORES SNORRI SNORTS SNORTY SPORES SPORKS SPORTS SPORTY STORCH STORED STORER STORES STORKS STORMS STORMY STORRS SWORDS THORAX THORIC THORNS THORNY THORON THORPE UNORAL VIORST WHORLS

••O•R•

ABOARD AMONRA AMOURS BOOERS CHOIRS CHOPRA COOERS CROIRE FLOORS FLOURS FLOURY HHOURS MOOERS ODOURS PROART PROPRE SCOURS SHOERS SNORRI SPOORS STORRS VFOURS

WOOERS

••O••R

ADORER ALOMAR ATONER AVOWER BLOWER BOOKER BOOMER BOOTER BOOZER BROKER CHOKER CHOLER CLONER CLOSER CLOVER COODER COOKER COOLER COOPER COOTER CROWER DEODAR DOOVER DOOZER DRONER DROVER ELOPER EMOTER EPOWER ERODER EVOKER FEODOR FLOWER FOOLER FOOTER FYODOR GAOLER GLOVER GLOWER GOOBER GOODER GOOIER GOOVER GROCER GROPER GROVER GROWER HOOFER HOOKER HOOPER HOOTER HOOVER IRONER ISOBAR ISOMER KNOWER KROGER KRONER KRONOR KRONUR LOOKER LOOPER LOOSER LOOTER MEOWER

MNOPQR MOONER MOOTER NOONER NOOSER OBOLER PHONER PLOMER PLOVER PLOWER POOLER POORER PROBER PROPER PROSER PROVER PROWAR QUOTER RIOTER ROOFER ROOKER ROOMER ROOTER SCORER SCOTER SHOFAR SHOVER SHOWER SLOPER SLOWER SMOKER SNORER SOONER STOKER STONER STORER STOVER STOWER TOOFAR TOOLER TOOTER TROYER TWOCAR TWOFER UPOVER WOOFER ZOOIER

•••OR•

ABHORS ABSORB ACCORD ACTORS ADSORB AFFORD ALBORG ALGORE ANGORA ARBORS ARDORS ARMORS ARMORY ASHORE ASSORT ATWORK AURORA BEFORE BESORE

BICORN BIFORM BYFORM BYWORD CALORY CAVORT CHLORO COHORT COLORS COMORO CRUORS CYBORG DAMORE DECORS DEFORD DEFORE DEFORM DEHORN DEPORT DEVORE DEWORM DOLORE DOLORS DONORA DONORS DOTORG EEYORE EFFORT ELLORA ELMORE ELNORA ELTORO ENCORE ENDORA EPHORS ERRORS ESCORT ETTORE EUDORA EXHORT EXMORE EXPORT EXTORT FAVORS FEDORA FEMORA FETORS FLOORS FLUORO FODORS FURORE FURORS GALORE GATORS HONORE HONORS HUMORS ICHORS IGNORE IMPORT INBORN INFORM INPORT JURORS KIDORY LABORS LAHORE LENORE

MAJORS MALORY MANORS MAYORS MCCORD MEMORY MIDORI MILORD MINORS MOTORS MYLORD MYSORE MYWORD NABORS NOMORE NOYORI OFYORE OSBORN OXFORD PRIORI PRIORS PRIORY RAZORS REBORE REBORN RECORD RECORK REFORM REMORA REPORT RESORB RESORT RETORE RETORN RETORT REWORD REWORE REWORK REWORN RIGORS ROTORS RUMORS SAPORS SATORI SAVORS SAVORY SCHORR SENORA SENORS SONORA SOPORS SPOORS SUBORN TABORS TAGORE TENORS THEORY TINORE TOKORI TUDORS TUTORS UNBORN UNCORE UNCORK UNFORK UNSORE UNSORT UNTORN

UNWORN UPTORE UPTORN VALORS VAPORS VAPORY VENORA VIGORS VISORS VIZORS WHWORD ZADORA ZAMORA

•••O•R

ARBOUR ARDOUR ARMOUR ATFOUR BOWOAR CANOER COLOUR DAMOUR DETOUR DEVOIR DEVOUR DOLOUR ECHOER EXMOOR FAVOUR GOSOUR HONOUR HUMOUR INDOOR INPOUR LABOUR LAMOUR LATOUR LELOIR LETOUR MEMOIR ONTOUR REDOER RENOIR REPOUR RETOUR REVOIR RIGOUR RUMOUR SAVOIR SAVOUR SCHORR UNDOER UNMOOR UNSOUR UPROAR UPSOAR USTOUR VALOUR VAPOUR VELOUR VETOER VIGOUR

••••OR

ABATOR ACTFOR AIMFOR

ALLFOR AMAJOR AMINOR ANCHOR ANGKOR ASKFOR AUTHOR BAILOR BANGOR BATFOR BAYLOR BEGFOR BETTOR BIDFOR BMAJOR BMINOR BRUNOR CANDOR CANTOR CAPTOR CASTOR CAWDOR CENSOR CLAMOR CMAJOR CMINOR CONDOR CONNOR CRYFOR CURSOR DEBTOR DIDFOR DIEFOR DIGFOR DMAJOR DMINOR DOCTOR DOKTOR DUGFOR EDITOR ELINOR EMAJOR EMINOR EMPTOR ENAMOR EXMOOR FACTOR FEODOR FERVOR FITFOR FLAVOR FLEXOR FMAJOR FMINOR FYODOR GAYNOR GLAMOR GMAJOR GMINOR GREGOR GUNFOR GUVNOR HARBOR HATHOR HECTOR HITFOR HORROR INDOOR

ISIDOR JAILOR JUNIOR KANTOR KRONOR LANDOR LARMOR LAYFOR LECTOR LESSOR LIEFOR LIENOR LIQUOR LUTHOR MADFOR MAHZOR MENTOR METEOR MIRROR NESTOR NOTFOR OPTFOR ORATOR OUTFOR PALLOR PARLOR PASTOR PAVIOR PAYFOR PICTOR PLEXOR PRETOR RADNOR RANCOR RANFOR RAPTOR RECTOR REPFOR RHETOR RUNFOR SAILOR SALVOR SARTOR SATFOR SAVIOR SECTOR SEIZOR SENHOR SENIOR SENSOR SETFOR SIGNOR SITFOR STATOR STUPOR SUCCOR SUEFOR SUITOR TAILOR TAMBOR TAYLOR TENSOR TERROR TORPOR TREMOR TREVOR TRYFOR UNMOOR

USEFOR VECTOR VENDOR VIATOR VICTOR VIEFOR VIKTOR WHYFOR WINSOR YENFOR

OS••••

OSAGES OSAKAN OSBERT OSBORN OSCANS OSCARS OSCINE OSCULE OSETRA OSGOOD OSHAWA OSIERS OSIRIS OSMICS OSMIUM OSMOND OSMOSE OSMUND OSPREY OSSETS OSSIAN OSSIFY OSTARS OSTEAL OSTEND OSTERS OSTLER OSWALD OSWEGO

O•S•••

OBSESS OHSTOP OHSURE OISEAU OKSANA OKSIGN ONSALE ONSETS ONSHOW ONSIDE ONSITE ONSPEC ONSTAR ORSINI ORSINO OSSETS OSSIAN OSSIFY OTSEGO OUSELS OUSTED OUSTER OYSTER

O••S••

OBISPO OCASEK OCASEY ODDSON ODESSA ODISTS OFFSET OLDSAW OLDSOD OLESHA OLESON OMASUM ONESEC ONESET ONUSES OPTSIN OPTSTO OPUSES ORISON ORISSA OROSCO OTOSES OTOSIS OUTSAT OUTSAW OUTSAY OUTSEE OUTSET OUTSIN OUTSIT OUTSPY OUTSUM OVISAC OWESON OWNSUP OWOSSO

O•••S•

OAFISH OBLAST OBOIST OBSESS OBTEST OBTUSE ODDEST ODDISH ODENSE ODESSA OFFISH OGRESS OGRISH OHGOSH OLDEST OLDISH ONBASE ONDISK ONEISH ONPOST ONRUSH OPPOSE OPQRST ORELSE ORENSE ORISSA OSMOSE OTIOSE OUTASK

OWLISH OWOSSO

O••••S

OAKUMS OARERS OATERS OBEAHS OBELUS OBGYNS OBJETS OBOLUS OBSESS OCCAMS OCCURS OCEANS OCHERS OCHRES OCTADS OCTANS OCTETS OCULUS ODEONS ODIOUS ODISTS ODIUMS ODOULS ODOURS OFFALS OFFERS OGHAMS OGIVES OGLERS OGRESS OHNUTS OILERS OKAPIS OLAKES OLDIES OLEINS OLEUMS OLIVES OLMECS OLORES OMAHAS OMANIS OMEGAS ONCLES ONDITS ONEUPS ONIONS ONLAYS ONSETS ONUSES ONYXES OODLES OOMPHS OOPODS OOTIDS OPCITS OPERAS OPHULS OPINES OPIUMS OPRAHS OPTICS OPUSES ORACHS

ORALES ORANGS ORANIS ORANTS ORATES ORBITS ORDERS OREADS ORECKS OREOOS OREXIS ORGANS ORGIES ORIBIS ORIELS ORINGS ORIONS ORKANS ORLONS ORLOPS ORYXES OSAGES OSCANS OSCARS OSIERS OSIRIS OSMICS OSSETS OSTARS OSTERS OTHERS OTILES OTITIS OTOMIS OTOSES OTOSIS OTTERS OUCHES OUGHTS OUIJAS OUNCES OUSELS OUTGAS OUTIES OUZELS OVINES OVOIDS OVULES OWLETS OWNERS OXALIS OXBOWS OXEYES OXIDES OXLIPS OYEZES OZARKS

•OS•••

BOSLEY BOSNIA BOSOMS BOSOMY BOSONS BOSSED BOSSES BOSSON BOSTON

BOSUNS COSECS COSELL COSETS COSHED COSHER COSHES COSIED COSIER COSIES COSIGN COSILY COSINE COSMAS COSMIC COSMOS COSSET COSTAE COSTAL COSTAR COSTAS COSTCO COSTED COSTLY COSYUP DOSADO DOSAGE DOSERS DOSIDO DOSING DOSSAL DOSSED DOSSES DOSUMS EOSINS FOSSAE FOSSES FOSSEY FOSSIL FOSTER GOSDEN GOSHEN GOSLIN GOSLOW GOSOFT GOSOLO GOSOUR GOSPEL GOSSIP GOSTAG HOSELS HOSERS HOSIER HOSING HOSSES HOSTAS HOSTED HOSTEL HOSTLY JOSEPH JOSHED JOSHER JOSHES JOSHUA JOSIAH JOSSES JOSTLE KOSHER

KOSOVO KOSSEL KOSTER LOSDOS LOSEIT LOSERS LOSETO LOSING LOSSES LOSTIT LOSTTO MOSAIC MOSCOW MOSDEF MOSEYS MOSHAV MOSHED MOSHER MOSHES MOSKVA MOSLEM MOSLEY MOSQUE MOSSAD MOSSED MOSSES MOSTEL MOSTLY MOSTOF NOSALE NOSALT NOSEIN NOSERS NOSEUP NOSHED NOSHER NOSHES NOSHOW NOSIER NOSILY NOSING NOSOAP NOSTEP NOSTER NOSTRA POSADA POSEAS POSERS POSEUR POSHER POSHLY POSIES POSING POSITS POSOLE POSSES POSSLQ POSSUM POSTAL POSTED POSTER POSTIE POSTIT POSTON POSTOP POSTUM ROSARY ROSCOE

ROSEAU
ROSERY
ROSETO
ROSEUP
ROSHIS
ROSIER
ROSIES
ROSILY
ROSINA
ROSINS
ROSINY
ROSITA
ROSLYN
ROSSEN
ROSSET
ROSSUM
ROSTEN
ROSTER
ROSTOV
ROSTRA
SOSOON
SOSPAD
TOSSED
TOSSER
TOSSES
TOSSIN
TOSSUP
VOSGES
VOSTOK
YOSANO

•O•S••

BOASTS
BOBSUP
BOESKY
BOLSHY
BONSAI
BOOSAT
BOOSTS
BORSCH
BOSSED
BOSSES
BOSSON
BOWSAW
BOWSTO
BOXSET
COASTS
COLSON
COMSAT
CONSUL
COPSES
COPSIT
COPSTO
CORSAS
CORSET
COSSET
COUSIN
DOASET
DOESBY
DOESIN
DOESIT
DOESNT
DOESOK
DOESSO
DOESTO
DOESUP
DOGSAT
DOGSIT
DORSAD
DORSAL
DORSAY
DORSET
DORSEY
DORSUM
DOSSAL
DOSSED
DOSSES
DOUSED
DOUSER
DOUSES
DOWSED
DOWSER
DOWSES
DOWSON
FOCSLE
FOGSIN
FOGSUP
FOISTS
FOLSOM
FOSSAE
FOSSES
FOSSEY
FOSSIL
GOBSOF
GODSON
GOESAT
GOESBY
GOESIN
GOESON
GOESTO
GOESUP
GOOSED
GOOSEN
GOOSES
GOOSEY
GORSES
GOSSIP
GOTSET
HOBSON
HOISIN
HOISTS
HONSHU
HOOSAC
HOPSIN
HOPSON
HOPSTO
HOPSUP
HORSED
HORSES
HORSEY
HOSSES
HOUSED
HOUSES
HOWSAD
HOWSER
JOBSON
JOISTS
JOLSON
JONSON
JOSSES
JOUSTS
JOZSEF
KOSSEL
LOGSIN
LOGSON
LOOSED
LOOSEN
LOOSER
LOOSES
LOOSEY
LOSSES
LOTSOF
LOUSED
LOUSES
LOWSET
MOESHA
MOISES
MOLSON
MOPSUP
MORSEL
MOSSAD
MOSSED
MOSSES
MOUSED
MOUSER
MOUSES
MOUSEY
MOUSSE
NODSAT
NODSTO
NOESIS
NOISED
NOISES
NOOSED
NOOSER
NOOSES
POISED
POISER
POISES
POISHA
POISON
POLSKA
POPSIN
POPSUP
POSSES
POSSLQ
POSSUM
POTSIE
POUSSE
POYSER
ROASTS
ROBSOF
ROBSON
RONSON
ROOSTS
ROSSEN
ROSSET
ROSSUM
ROUSED
ROUSER
ROUSES
ROUSTS
SOASTO
SOISEE
SOPSUP
SOUSED
SOUSES
TOASTS
TOASTY
TOCSIN
TOESIN
TOGSUP
TONSIL
TONSOF
TOPSUP
TORSOS
TOSSED
TOSSER
TOSSES
TOSSIN
TOSSUP
TOTSUP
TOUSLE
TOWSIN
WOLSEY
WORSEN
WORSTS
YOUSEE
YOUSUF
ZOYSIA

•O••S•

BOCHSA
BOURSE
BOYISH
COARSE
COHOST
CORPSE
COURSE
COWISH
COYEST
COYISH
DOESSO
DONESO
DONOSO
DOVISH
FOLKSY
FOREST
GOBUST
GOEASY
GOFAST
GOFISH
GOLAST
GOPAST
GOWEST
HOARSE
HOLISM
HOLIST
HONEST
HOPESO
IODISE
IONISE
JOCOSE
JONESS
JONESY
LOCUST
LOUISA
LOUISB
LOUISE
LOUISI
LOUISV
LOUISX
LOWEST
LOWISH
MODEST
MODISH
MOLEST
MOMISM
MONGST
MONISM
MONIST
MOPISH
MORASS
MORESO
MOROSE
MOROSS
MOTTST
MOUSSE
NOCOST
NODOSE
NOFUSS
NOLESS
NOLOSE
NOLOSS
NONUSE
NORISK
NORUSH
NOWISE
POLISH
POPISH
POROSE
POTASH
POTOSI
POUSSE
ROBUST
ROOTSY
SOREST
TOLAST
TOOTSY
WOODSY
WOOTSY
YOGISM

•O•••S

AOLERS
AORTAS
BOARDS
BOASTS
BOBBYS
BOCCES
BOCCIS
BODIES
BOFFOS
BOGEYS
BOGIES
BOGLES
BOINGS
BOITES
BOLLAS
BOMBES
BONERS
BONGOS
BONNES
BONZES
BOOERS
BOOSTS
BOOTES
BOOTHS
BOOZES
BOREAS
BORERS
BORGES
BOSOMS
BOSONS
BOSSES
BOSUNS
BOTELS
BOUGHS
BOULES
BOUNDS
BOURGS
BOVIDS
BOWELS
BOWERS
BOWLES
BOXERS
BOYARS
BOYLES
COACTS
COAPTS
COASTS
COATES
COATIS
COAXES
COBRAS
COCCUS
COCOAS
CODERS
CODONS
COEURS
COHABS
COHOES
COIGNS
COKIES
COLBYS
COLEUS
COLICS
COLONS
COLORS
COMBOS
COMDRS
COMEAS
COMERS
COMETS
COMICS
COMMAS
COMPAS
COMPOS
COMTES
CONCHS
CONDOS
CONERS
CONEYS
CONGAS
CONGES
CONICS
CONIES
COOEES
COOERS
COOPTS
COOWNS
COPALS
COPAYS
COPERS
COPIES
COPRAS
COPSES
COQUIS
CORALS
CORERS
CORGIS
COROTS
CORPUS
CORSAS
CORTES
CORVUS
COSECS
COSETS
COSHES
COSIES
COSMAS
COSMOS
COSTAS
COTANS
COTTAS
COUGHS
COUNTS
COUPES
COURTS
COVENS
COVERS
COVETS
COVEYS
COWENS
COWERS
COYPUS
COZENS
COZIES
DOAKES
DOALLS
DOBLES
DOBROS
DOBYNS
DODGES
DODOES
DOGIES
DOGMAS
DOGONS
DOINGS
DOLAPS
DOLMAS
DOLORS
DONEES
DONETS
DONORS
DONUTS
DOOFUS
DOPERS
DORAGS
DORCAS
DORIES
DOSERS
DOSSES
DOSUMS
DOTERS
DOUBTS
DOUGHS
DOULAS
DOUSES
DOUZES
DOWELS
DOWERS
DOWNES
DOWSES
DOXIES
DOYENS
DOZENS
DOZERS
EOSINS
FODORS
FOGEYS
FOGIES
FOISTS
FOLEYS
FOLIES
FOLIOS
FONDAS
FONDUS
FORAYS
FORBES
FORCES
FORGES
FORTAS
FORTES
FORTIS
FORUMS
FOSSES
FOUNDS
FOUNTS
FOWLES
FOYERS
GOBIES
GOBOES
GOBOTS
GODETS
GODEYS
GOFERS
GOINGS
GOLEMS
GOMERS
GONERS
GONUTS
GOOFUS
GOOSES
GORERS
GORGES
GORSES
GOUDAS
GOUGES
GOURDS
HOARDS
HOAXES
HOBBES
HOBOES
HODADS
HODGES
HOGANS
HOHUMS
HOISTS
HOKIES
HOKUMS
HOLERS
HOLIES
HOLLIS
HOLMES
HOMERS
HOMEYS
HOMIES
HOMMES
HONDAS
HONERS
HONEYS
HONORS
HOOHAS
HOOVES
HOPERS
HORDES
HORSES
HOSELS
HOSERS
HOSSES
HOSTAS
HOTELS
HOUNDS
HOURIS
HOUSES
HOVELS
HOVERS
HOWTOS
HOYLES
IONICS
IOWANS
JOCKOS
JOINTS
JOISTS
JOKERS
JONAHS
JONESS
JORUMS
JOSHES
JOSSES
JOULES
JOUSTS
JOYOUS
KOALAS
KODAKS
KOMBUS
KOPEKS
KOPJES
KORANS
KORATS
KOVACS
LOAVES
LOCALS
LODENS
LODGES
LOFTUS
LOGANS
LOGICS
LOGINS
LOGONS
LONERS
LONGES
LOOEYS
LOOFAS
LOOIES
LOOSES
LOPERS
LORANS
LORIES
LOSDOS
LOSERS
LOSSES
LOTNOS
LOTTOS
LOUIES
LOUMAS
LOUPES
LOUSES
LOVERS
LOVEYS
LOWERS
LOWIQS
LOWRES
MOBIUS
MOCHAS
MODALS
MODELS
MODEMS
MOGULS
MOINES
MOIRES
MOISES
MOJOES
MOLARS
MOMMAS
MONADS
MONDES
MONDOS
MONETS
MONEYS
MONGOS
MONIES
MONTHS
MONZAS
MOODYS
MOOERS
MOPEDS
MOPERS
MOPUPS
MORALS
MORASS
MORAYS
MORELS
MORONS
MOROSS
MORPHS
MORRIS
MOSEYS
MOSHES
MOSSES
MOTELS
MOTETS
MOTIFS
MOTORS
MOTTOS
MOULDS
MOULTS
MOUNDS
MOUNTS
MOURNS
MOUSES
MOUTHS
MOVERS
MOVIES
MOWERS
MOYERS
NOBELS
NOBLES
NOBUTS
NOCHES
NODOUS
NOESIS
NOFEES
NOFUSS
NOHITS
NOIRES
NOISES
NOKIAS
NOKIDS
NOLESS
NOLOSS
NOMADS
NONETS
NONEWS
NONGAS
NOONES
NOOSES
NOPALS
NOPETS
NOPQRS
NORIAS
NORRIS
NORTHS
NORUNS
NOSERS
NOSHES
NOTERS
NOTIPS
NOVELS
NOVIAS
NOVIOS
NOWAYS
OODLES
OOMPHS
OOPODS
OOTIDS
POBOYS
PODOUS
POEMES
POETES
POILUS
POINTS
POIRES
POISES
POKERS
POKEYS
POKIES
POLERS
POLIOS
POLKAS
POLLOS
POLYPS
POMMES
PONCAS
PONIES
PONZUS
POORIS
POPPAS
POPUPS
PORERS
PORKYS
POROUS
PORTES
POSEAS
POSERS
POSIES
POSITS
POSSES
POTHOS
POTTOS
POULES
POULTS
POUNDS
POWERS
ROASTS
ROBERS
ROBINS
ROBLES
ROBOTS
RODEOS
ROGERS
ROGETS
ROGUES
ROLEOS
ROMANS
ROMEOS
RONDOS
ROOSTS
ROPERS
ROSHIS
ROSIES
ROSINS
ROTORS
ROUGES
ROUGHS
ROUNDS
ROUSES
ROUSTS
ROUTES
ROVERS
ROWANS
ROWELS
ROWENS
ROWERS
ROYALS
ROYCES
SOAVES
SOBERS
SOCLES
SOEURS
SOITIS
SOLANS
SOLEAS
SOLERS
SOLEUS
SOLIDS
SOLONS
SOLVES
SOMERS
SONARS
SONDES
SONICS
SOONAS
SOPORS
SOUNDS
SOUSES
SOUTHS
SOWERS
TOASTS
TOBIAS
TOBIES
TOBITS
TODAYS
TODIES
TOEINS
TOGUES
TOILES
TOKAYS
TOKENS
TOKLAS
TOLARS
TOMBES
TONDOS
TONERS
TONICS
TONKAS
TONNES
TOPEES
TOPERS
TOPICS
TOQUES
TORAHS
TORIES
TORRES
TORSOS
TORTAS
TORTES
TOSSES
TOTALS
TOTEMS
TOTERS
TOUGHS
TOWELS
TOWERS
TOXICS
TOXINS
TOYERS
TOYONS
VOCABS
VOCALS
VODKAS
VOGUES
VOICES
VOILES
VOLANS
VOLVOS
VOMERS
VOROUS
VOSGES
VOTERS
VOWELS
VOWERS
WOLVES
WOMANS
WOMENS
WOOERS
WORLDS
WORSTS
WORTHS
WOUNDS
YODELS
YOICKS
YOKELS
YOUTHS
ZONERS
ZOOIDS
ZOUNDS

••OS••

AGOSTO
AMOSOZ
ASOSAN
BOOSAT
BOOSTS
BROSSE
CHOSEN
CLOSED
CLOSER
CLOSES
CLOSET
CROSBY
CROSSE
DAOSTA
DROSSY
EPOSES
FLOSSY
FROSTS
FROSTY
GHOSTS
GHOSTY
GLOSSA
GLOSSO
GLOSSY
GNOSES
GNOSIS
GOOSED
GOOSEN
GOOSES
GOOSEY
GROSSE
GROSSO
GROSZY
HOOSAC
KIOSKS
LOOSED
LOOSEN
LOOSER
LOOSES
LOOSEY
MTOSSA
MYOSIN
MYOSIS
NEOSHO
NOOSED
NOOSER
NOOSES
OROSCO
OTOSES
OTOSIS
OWOSSO
PROSED
PROSER
PROSES
PROSIT
PROSKY
ROOSTS
SLOSHY
TAOSNM
WHOSIN
XHOSAS

••O•S•

AHORSE
ALONSO
AROUSE
BIOPSY
BLOUSE
BLOWSY
BROAST
BROSSE
BROWSE
CHOOSE
CHOOSY
CROSSE
CROUSE
DROPSY
DROSSY
DROWSE
DROWSY
ECORSE
EGOISM
EGOIST
ELOISA
ELOISE
FLOPSY
FLOSSY
GLOSSA
GLOSSO
GLOSSY
GROSSE
GROSSO
GROUSE
LAOTSE
LHOTSE
MAOISM
MAOIST
MTOSSA
OBOIST
OWOSSO
PROBST
PROUST
PROWSE
ROOTSY
SMOOSH
SPOUSE
SWOOSH
TAOISM
TAOIST
TOOTSY
TSOTSI
VIORST
WHOMSO
WHOOSH
WOODSY
WOOTSY

••O••S

ABODES
ABOHMS
ABOMAS
ABOMBS
ABORTS
ACORNS
ADOBES
ADOBOS
ADONIS
ADOPTS
ADORES
ADORNS
ADOUTS
AEOLUS
AGONES
AGORAS
AIOLIS
ALOHAS
ALONGS
AMOLES
AMORES
AMOURS
ANODES
ANOLES
AROIDS
AROMAS
ATODDS
ATOLLS
ATONES
AVOIDS
AXONES
AZOLES
AZORES
BIOGAS
BIOMES
BIONTS
BIOTAS
BLOATS
BLOCKS
BLOKES
BLONDS
BLOODS

BLOOMS
BLOOPS
BOOERS
BOOSTS
BOOTES
BOOTHS
BOOZES
BROCAS
BROILS
BRONCS
BROODS
BROOKS
BROOMS
BROTHS
BROWNS
CEORLS
CHOCKS
CHOIRS
CHOKES
CHOLOS
CHOMPS
CHORDS
CHORES
CHOROS
CHORUS
CLOAKS
CLOCKS
CLOMPS
CLONES
CLONKS
CLORIS
CLOSES
CLOTHS
CLOUDS
CLOUTS
CLOVES
CLOVIS
CLOWNS
CNOTES
COOEES
COOERS
COOPTS
COOWNS
CROAKS
CROATS
CROCKS
CROCUS
CROFTS
CRONES
CRONUS
CROOKS
CROONS
CRORES
CROUPS
CROWDS
CROWNS
CUORES
DHOLES
DHOTIS
DIODES
DOOFUS
DROIDS
DROITS
DROLLS
DRONES
DROOLS
DROOPS
DROVES
DROWNS
DUOMOS
EBOATS
EBONDS
EBOOKS
ECOLES
ELOGES
ELOPES
EMOTES
ENOILS
ENOKIS
ENOTES
EPOCHS
EPODES
EPOSES
ERODES
EVOKES
EXODUS
FEOFFS
FHOLES
FIORDS
FJORDS
FLOATS
FLOCKS
FLOODS
FLOORS
FLORAS
FLORES
FLOURS
FLOUTS
FROCKS
FRONDS
FRONTS
FROSTS
FROTHS
FROWNS
FROYOS
GEODES
GHOSTS
GHOULS
GLOATS
GLOBES
GLOCKS
GLOGGS
GLOOMS
GLOUCS
GLOVES
GNOMES
GNOSES
GNOSIS
GNOTES
GOOFUS
GOOSES
GROANS
GROATS
GROINS
GROOMS
GROPES
GROUPS
GROUTS
GROVES
GROWLS
GYOZAS
HAOLES
HBOMBS
HHOURS
HMONGS
HOOHAS
HOOVES
HYOIDS
IBOOKS
INONES
KHOUMS
KIOSKS
KIOWAS
KNOCKS
KNOLLS
KNOTTS
KNOUTS
KNOWNS
KROONS
LLOYDS
LOOEYS
LOOFAS
LOOIES
LOOSES
MAORIS
MOODYS
MOOERS
MYOPES
MYOSIS
NBOMBS
NOONES
NOOSES
OBOLUS
ODOULS
ODOURS
OLORES
OTOMIS
OTOSES
OTOSIS
OVOIDS
PBOOKS
PHOBOS
PHONES
PHONOS
PHOTOS
PLOCES
PLONKS
POORIS
PROAMS
PROBES
PROEMS
PROLES
PROMOS
PRONGS
PROOFS
PROSES
PROVES
PROWLS
PROYAS
QUOINS
QUOITS
QUOTAS
QUOTES
REOILS
REOWNS
RHODES
RHOMBS
RIOJAS
ROOSTS
SCOFFS
SCOLDS
SCONES
SCOOPS
SCOOTS
SCOPES
SCORES
SCORNS
SCOTTS
SCOURS
SCOUTS
SCOWLS
SHOALS
SHOATS
SHOCKS
SHOERS
SHOGIS
SHOJIS
SHOOTS
SHORES
SHORTS
SHOUTS
SHOVES
SKOALS
SKORTS
SLOOPS
SLOPES
SLOTHS
SMOCKS
SMOKES
SMOLTS
SMORES
SNOODS
SNOOKS
SNOOPS
SNOOTS
SNOPES
SNORES
SNORTS
SNOUTS
SOONAS
SPODES
SPOILS
SPOKES
SPOOFS
SPOOKS
SPOOLS
SPOONS
SPOORS
SPORES
SPORKS
SPORTS
SPOUTS
STOATS
STOCKS
STOICS
STOKES
STOLAS
STOLES
STOMAS
STOMPS
STONES
STOOLS
STOOPS
STORES
STORKS
STORMS
STORRS
STOUTS
STOVES
SWOONS
SWOOPS
SWORDS
TBONDS
TBONES
THOLES
THOMAS
THONGS
THORNS
TNOTES
TROGGS
TROLLS
TROMPS
TROOPS
TROPES
TROTHS
TROUTS
TROVES
UBOATS
UBOLTS
VFOURS
VIOLAS
VROOMS
WHOLES
WHOMPS
WHOOPS
WHORLS
WOOERS
WRONGS
XBOXES
XHOSAS
ZLOTYS
ZOOIDS

•••OS•

ACCOST
ACROSS
ALMOST
APPOSE
ARGOSY
ARIOSE
ARIOSI
ARIOSO
ASLOSH
ATCOST
ATMOST
BYGOSH
CHOOSE
CHOOSY
COHOST
CWPOST
DEPOSE
DEROSE
DONOSO
DUBOSE
EMBOSS
ESPOSA
ESPOSO
EXPOSE
EXPOST
FILOSE
GALOSH
HEXOSE
IMPOSE
IMPOST
INMOST
JOCOSE
KIBOSH
LANOSE
LAROSA
LUGOSI
MILOSZ
MIMOSA
MINOSO
MOROSE
MOROSS
MYGOSH
NOCOST
NODOSE
NOLOSE
NOLOSS
NYPOST
OHGOSH
ONPOST
OPPOSE
OSMOSE
OTIOSE
PELOSI
PILOSE
POROSE
POTOSI
RAMOSE
RECOST
REDOSE
RELOSE
RELOST
REPOSE
REPOST
REROSE
RETOSS
RIBOSE
RIMOSE
RIPOST
SAMOSA
SETOSE
SMOOSH
SPLOSH
SWOOSH
UNLOST
UNPOSH
UPMOST
UPROSE
UPTOSS
UTMOST
VENOSE
WHOOSH
XYLOSE

•••O•S

ABBOTS
ABHORS
ACROSS
ACTORS
ADDONS
AESOPS
ALDOUS
ALLOTS
ALLOWS
ALLOYS
ANIONS
ANJOUS
ANNOYS
ANYONS
APRONS
ARBORS
ARDORS
ARGOTS
ARMORS
ARROWS
ARSONS
ARTOIS
ASCOTS
ATROIS
AUROUS
AXIOMS
AXIONS
BABOOS
BACONS
BANONS
BARONS
BATONS
BAYOUS
BAZOOS
BEBOPS
BEDOGS
BEFOGS
BELONS
BESOMS
BESOTS
BIGOTS
BIJOUS
BIPODS
BISONS
BLOODS
BLOOMS
BLOOPS
BOSOMS
BOSONS
BROODS
BROOKS
BROOMS
BYLOTS
CAMOES
CANOES
CANONS
CAPONS
CAROBS
CAROLS
CAROMS
CDROMS
CHEOPS
CIXOUS
COCOAS
CODONS
COHOES
COLONS
COLORS
COROTS
CROOKS
CROONS
CRUORS
CSPOTS
DADOES
DECORS
DECOYS
DEFOGS
DEMOBS
DEMONS
DEPOTS
DESODS
DICOTS
DIDOES
DIVOTS
DODOES
DOGONS
DOLORS
DONORS
DROOLS
DROOPS
DUBOIS
DUROCS
EBOOKS
ECHOES
EDDOES
ELBOWS
EMBOGS
EMBOSS
EMBOWS
ENDOWS
ENJOYS
ENROLS
ENVOIS
ENVOYS
EPHODS
EPHORS
EPSONS
ERGOTS
ERRORS
ESTOCS
ESTOPS
EXCONS
EXGOVS
EXTOLS
FAGOTS
FAMOUS
FANONS
FAROES
FAVORS
FELONS
FEROUS
FETORS
FLOODS
FLOORS
FODORS
FREONS
FSTOPS
FURORS
FUTONS
GALOIS
GALOPS
GAMOUS
GATORS
GAVOTS
GENOAS
GIGOTS
GIJOES
GLOOMS
GLUONS
GOBOES
GOBOTS
GRIOTS
GROOMS
GYNOUS
HALOES
HAVOCS
HELOTS
HEROES
HERONS
HOBOES
HONORS
HUMORS
HURONS
HYSONS
IBOOKS
ICHORS
IDIOMS
IDIOTS
IGLOOS
INGOTS
INIONS
ITIOUS
JABOTS
JEVONS
JOYOUS
JURORS
KABOBS
KAPOKS
KAZOOS
KROONS
LABORS
LEMONS
LOGONS
LTGOVS
MAJORS
MANORS
MASONS
MAYORS
MCJOBS
MEDOCS
MELONS
MEROPS
MESONS
MIAOUS
MIAOWS
MIDONS
MINORS
MOJOES
MORONS
MOROSS
MOTORS
MUTONS
NABOBS
NABORS
NIKONS
NINONS
NIXONS
NODOUS
NOLOSS
NYLONS
ODEONS
ODIOUS
ONIONS
OOPODS
OREOOS
ORIONS
ORLONS
ORLOPS
OXBOWS
PAROLS
PATOIS
PBOOKS
PEKOES
PICOTS
PILOTS
PILOUS
PINONS
PINOTS
PITONS
PITOTS
PIVOTS
POBOYS
PODOUS
POROUS
PREOPS
PRIORS
PROOFS
PUJOLS
PUTONS
PYLONS
RAYONS
RAZORS
REBOPS
RECONS
REDOES
REHOES
RELOGS
REMOPS
REMOWS
REPOTS
RESODS
RESOWS
RETOPS
RETOSS
RETOWS
RICOHS
RIGORS
RIMOUS
ROBOTS
ROTORS
RUFOUS
RUMORS
RUNONS
SABOTS
SALONS
SAPORS
SAVORS
SAXONS
SCIONS
SCOOPS
SCOOTS
SCRODS
SENORS
SEPOYS
SEROUS
SEWONS
SHOOTS
SLOOPS
SNOODS
SNOOKS
SNOOPS
SNOOTS
SOLONS
SOPORS
SPOOFS
SPOOKS
SPOOLS
SPOONS
SPOORS
STOOLS
STOOPS
STROHS
STROPS
SWOONS
SWOOPS
SYNODS
SYSOPS
TABOOS
TABORS
TAHOES
TALONS
TAROTS
TAUONS
TAXOLS
TENONS
TENORS
TETONS
THROBS
THROES
THROWS
TIGONS
TOYONS
TROOPS
TSTOPS
TUDORS
TUTORS
TYSONS
UNDOES
UNIONS
UNPOTS
UPBOWS
UPTOSS
UVEOUS
VALOIS
VALORS
VAPORS
VENOMS
VENOUS
VETOES
VIGORS
VINOUS
VISORS
VIZORS
VOROUS
VROOMS
WAGONS
WAHOOS
WHOOPS
WIDOWS
YAHOOS
YEGODS
YUKONS
ZEROES
ZHLOBS
ZIPONS

••••OS

ABMHOS
ADOBOS
AERIOS
ALAMOS
ALEROS
AMIGOS
AMINOS
AMNIOS
ANCHOS
ANDROS
ANGLOS
ARADOS
ARCCOS
ASTROS
AUDIOS
AVISOS
BABOOS
BANCOS
BANJOS
BARCOS
BASSOS
BATHOS
BAZOOS
BEANOS
BENTOS
BIGDOS
BIMBOS
BINGOS
BOFFOS
BONGOS
BRAVOS
BRAZOS
BUENOS
BUFFOS
BUNCOS
BUNKOS
BURGOS
BURROS
BUTEOS
BYTWOS
CACAOS
CAICOS
CAMEOS
CAMPOS
CANTOS
CARBOS
CARGOS
CARLOS
CASIOS
CELLOS
CENTOS
CERROS
CHICOS
CHINOS
CHOLOS
CHOROS
CIELOS
CISCOS
CLAROS
COMBOS
COMPOS
CONDOS
COSMOS
CREDOS
CURIOS
CYCLOS
DANIOS
DEIMOS
DEKKOS
DELCOS
DESNOS
DIPSOS
DISCOS
DITTOS
DOBROS
DUENOS
DUMBOS
DUOMOS
DUPLOS
EJIDOS
ELLIOS
ENEROS
ESPIOS
ETHNOS
FIEROS
FOLIOS
FRITOS
FROYOS
FUEGOS
GECKOS
GISMOS
GIZMOS
GUANOS
GUMBOS
HALLOS
HELIOS
HELLOS
HIPPOS
HOWTOS
HUEVOS
HULLOS
HYDROS
HYKSOS
HYPNOS
IDAHOS
IGLOOS
IMAGOS
INTROS
INTWOS
JELLOS
JOCKOS
JUEGOS
JUMBOS
JUNCOS
JUNTOS
KAZOOS
KENDOS
KIDDOS
KIDEOS
KINKOS
LACLOS
LANTOS
LARGOS
LASSOS
LEGROS
LEMNOS
LENTOS
LESBOS
LIBROS
LIMBOS
LITHOS
LLANOS
LOSDOS
LOTNOS
LOTTOS
MACHOS
MACROS
MAMBOS
MANAOS
MANGOS
MARCOS
MATZOS
MENTOS
METROS
MEZZOS
MICROS
MIMEOS
MIRROS
MONDOS
MONGOS
MOTTOS
MUSEOS
MYTHOS
NACHOS
NARCOS
NIETOS
NITROS
NOVIOS
NULLOS
OREOOS
PANTOS
PASEOS
PASSOS
PATHOS
PATIOS
PATMOS
PERROS
PESTOS
PHAROS
PHOBOS
PHONOS
PHOTOS
PIANOS
PINKOS
PINTOS
PLATOS
POLIOS
POLLOS
POTHOS
POTTOS
PRIMOS
PROMOS
QUESOS
RADIOS
RAMBOS
RATIOS
RECTOS
REPROS
RETROS
RHINOS
RITSOS
RODEOS
ROLEOS
ROMEOS
RONDOS
SALVOS
SANTOS
SANYOS
SAYSOS
SCHMOS
SEIKOS
SERVOS
SETTOS
SHAKOS
SICKOS
STAMOS
STENOS
SUENOS
TABOOS
TALTOS
TANGOS
TELCOS
TEMPOS
TONDOS
TORSOS
TURBOS
TYPEOS
VERSOS
VIDEOS
VIREOS
VIRGOS
VOLVOS
WACKOS
WAHOOS
WASHOS
YAHOOS
ZENDOS
ZIPPOS

OT••••

OTELLO
OTHERS
OTHMAR
OTILES
OTIOSE
OTITIC
OTITIS
OTOMIS
OTOOLE
OTOSES
OTOSIS
OTSEGO
OTTAVA
OTTAWA
OTTERS
OTTOII
OTTOIV
OTTONE

O•T•••

OATERS
OATIER
OBTAIN
OBTEST
OBTUND
OBTUSE
OCTADS
OCTANE
OCTANS
OCTANT
OCTAVE
OCTAVO
OCTETS
OCTOOT
OCTOPI
OCTROI
ONTAPE
ONTIME
ONTOUR
OOTIDS
OPTFOR
OPTICS
OPTIMA
OPTIMO
OPTING
OPTION
OPTOUT
OPTSIN
OPTSTO
ORTEGA
ORTHEN
ORTRUD
OSTARS
OSTEAL
OSTEND
OSTERS
OSTLER
OTTAVA
OTTAWA
OTTERS
OTTOII
OTTOIV
OTTONE
OUTACT
OUTADD

OUTAGE OUTASK OUTATE OUTAWE OUTBAN OUTBAT OUTBEG OUTBID OUTBOW OUTBOX OUTBUD OUTBUY OUTCRY OUTCUT OUTDID OUTEAT OUTFIT OUTFLY OUTFOR OUTFOX OUTGAS OUTGUN OUTHIT OUTIES OUTING OUTJET OUTJUT OUTLAW OUTLAY OUTLED OUTLET OUTLIE OUTLIP OUTMAN OUTPAY OUTPOP OUTPRY OUTPUT OUTRAN OUTRAP OUTRIB OUTRIG OUTROW OUTRUN OUTSAT OUTSAW OUTSAY OUTSEE OUTSET OUTSIN OUTSIT OUTSPY OUTSUM OUTVIE OUTWAR OUTWIT OXTAIL

O••T••

OAKTAG OBITER ODETTA ODETTE OERTER OHSTOP OLATHE ONETEN ONETON ONETWO ONSTAR ORATED ORATES ORATOR OSETRA OTITIC OTITIS OUSTED OUSTER OYSTER

O•••T•

OBENTO OBERTO OBJETS OBLATE OCTETS ODDITY ODETTA ODETTE ODISTS ODONTO OFFUTT OFLATE OFNOTE OHNUTS OLEATE OMERTA ONAUTO ONDITS ONDUTY ONLATE ONSETS ONSITE OOCYTE OOLITE OPCITS OPENTO OPIATE OPORTO OPTSTO ORANTS ORBITS ORNATE ORNITH OSSETS OUGHTA OUGHTS OUTATE OWEDTO OWLETS

O••••T

OBJECT OBLAST OBOIST OBTEST OBVERT OCCULT OCELOT OCICAT OCTANT OCTOOT ODDEST ODDLOT ODELET OFFSET OFFUTT OHDRAT OILLIT OLDBAT OLDEST OLDHAT OLMERT OMELET ONEACT ONEBIT ONEHIT ONEOUT ONESET ONFOOT ONPOST OPENIT OPQRST OPTOUT ORGEAT ORIENT ORWHAT OSBERT OUIMET OUTACT OUTBAT OUTCUT OUTEAT OUTFIT OUTHIT OUTJET OUTJUT OUTLET OUTPUT OUTSAT OUTSET OUTSIT OUTWIT OVERIT OXCART

•OT•••

BOTANY BOTCHY BOTELS BOTFLY BOTHER BOTREE BOTTLE BOTTOM COTANS COTLER COTTAE COTTAS COTTEN COTTER COTTON DOTAGE DOTARD DOTCOM DOTDOT DOTELL DOTEON DOTERS DOTGOV DOTHAN DOTIME DOTING DOTOAT DOTODO DOTORG DOTTED DOTTER DOTTIE DOTTLE GOTAMA GOTANA GOTANF GOTCHA GOTEAM GOTFAR GOTFIT GOTHAM GOTHEP GOTHIC GOTHIP GOTHOT GOTMAD GOTOFF GOTOIT GOTOLD GOTOUT GOTRID GOTSET GOTTEN GOTWET GOTYOU HOTAIR HOTBED HOTBOT HOTBOX HOTCAP HOTCAR HOTCUP HOTDAY HOTDOG HOTELS HOTKEY HOTOIL HOTONE HOTPOT HOTROD HOTTEA HOTTER HOTTIE HOTTIP HOTTUB HOTWAR JOTTED JOTTER KOTTER KOTTKE LOTHAR LOTION LOTNOS LOTSOF LOTTED LOTTER LOTTOS MOTELS MOTETS MOTHER MOTHRA MOTIFS MOTILE MOTION MOTIVE MOTLEY MOTORS MOTOWN MOTRIN MOTTLE MOTTOS MOTTST NOTAIL NOTALL NOTANY NOTARY NOTATE NOTBAD NOTCHY NOTERS NOTFAR NOTFIT NOTFOR NOTHIN NOTICE NOTIFY NOTILL NOTIME NOTING NOTION NOTIPS NOTNEW NOTNOW NOTOLL NOTONE NOTOUT NOTTOO NOTYET NOTYOU OOTIDS POTAGE POTASH POTATO POTEEN POTENT POTFUL POTHER POTHOS POTION POTLID POTOSI POTPIE POTSIE POTTED POTTER POTTOS POTVIN ROTARY ROTATE ROTGUT ROTHKO ROTINI ROTORS ROTTED ROTTEN ROTTER ROTUND SOTHAT SOTHEN SOTRUE SOTTED TOTALS TOTEMS TOTERM TOTERS TOTEUP TOTING TOTSUP TOTTED TOTTER VOTARY VOTECH VOTEIN VOTENO VOTEON VOTERS VOTING VOTIVE

•O•T••

AORTAE AORTAL AORTAS AORTIC BOATED BOATEL BOATER BOITES BOLTED BOLTER BOLTON BOLTUP BONTON BOOTED BOOTEE BOOTER BOOTES BOOTHE BOOTHS BOOTIE BOOTIT BOOTUP BOSTON BOTTLE BOTTOM BOUTON BOWTIE BOXTOP BOYTOY COATED COATEE COATER COATES COATIS COLTER COLTON COMTES CONTAC CONTRA CONTRE COOTER COOTIE COPTER COPTIC CORTES CORTEX CORTEZ CORTOT COSTAE COSTAL COSTAR COSTAS COSTCO COSTED COSTLY COTTAE COTTAS COTTEN COTTER COTTON COUTER DOCTOR DOGTAG DOGTOY DOITUP DOKTOR DOLTON DONTGO DOTTED DOTTER DOTTIE DOTTLE FOETID FONTAL FOOTED FOOTER FOOTIT FOOTLE FOOTUP FORTAS FORTES FORTIS FOSTER GOATEE GOATIT GOETHE GOITER GOSTAG GOTTEN HOGTIE HOOTAT HOOTCH HOOTED HOOTER HOOTIE HORTON HOSTAS HOSTED HOSTEL HOSTLY HOTTEA HOTTER HOTTIE HOTTIP HOTTUB HOWTOS JOETEX JOLTED JOLTER JOLTIN JOSTLE JOTTED JOTTER KOSTER KOTTER KOTTKE KOWTOW LOATHE LOFTED LOFTER LOFTON LOFTUS LOITER LOOTED LOOTER LOSTIT LOSTTO LOTTED LOTTER LOTTOS LOWTAR LOWTOP MOATED MOLTED MOLTEN MOLTER MOLTKE MONTAG MONTEL MONTEZ MONTHS MOOTED MOOTER MOPTOP MORTAL MORTAR MORTEN MORTON MOSTEL MOSTLY MOSTOF MOTTLE MOTTOS MOTTST MOUTHS MOUTHY NOETIC NONTAN NONTAX NOOTKA NORTHS NORTON NOSTEP NOSTER NOSTRA NOTTOO POETES POETIC POETRY POITOU POPTOP PORTAL PORTED PORTER PORTES PORTIA PORTLY POSTAL POSTED POSTER POSTIE POSTIT POSTON POSTOP POSTUM POTTED POTTER POTTOS POUTED POUTER ROOTED ROOTER ROOTIE ROOTIN ROOTLE ROOTSY ROOTUP ROSTEN ROSTER ROSTOV ROSTRA ROTTED ROTTEN ROTTER ROUTED ROUTER ROUTES SOFTEN SOFTER SOFTIE SOFTLY SOFTON SOITIS SONTAG SOOTHE SORTED SORTER SORTIE SORTOF SOTTED SOUTER SOUTHS TOATEE TOETAP TOLTEC TOMTIT TOMTOM TOOTAT TOOTED TOOTER TOOTHY TOOTIE TOOTIN TOOTLE TOOTOO TOOTSY TOPTEN TORTAS TORTES TOTTED TOTTER TOUTED TOUTER TOYTOP VORTEX VOSTOK WONTDO WONTED WONTGO WONTON WOOTSY WORTHS WORTHY YOMTOV YOUTHS YOUTWO ZOLTAN

•O••T•

BOASTS BODETT BOGOTA BONITA BONITO BOOSTS BORATE BOUNTY BOWSTO COACTS COAPTS COASTS COGITO COMATE COMETH COMETO COMETS COMITY COOLTH COOLTO COOPTS COPSTO COROTS COSETS COUNTS COUNTY COURTS COVETS COYOTE DOESTO DONATE DONATH DONETO DONETS DONITZ DONUTS DOOMTO DORATI DORITO DOUBTS DOWITH EOLITH FOISTS FOLATE FOUNTS FOURTH GOBOTS GODETS GOESTO GOINTO GOLETA GONETO GONUTS GOUPTO GOWITH HOISTS HOLDTO HOPETO HOPSTO HOVETO IODATE IOMOTH JOBETH JOINTS JOISTS JOUSTS KOONTZ KORATS LOBATE LOCATE LOLITA LOOKTO LOSETO LOSTTO LOVETO LOVETT MOBUTU MOIETY MOJITO MONETA MONETS MORATH MORITA MORITZ MOTETS MOULTS MOUNTS MOUNTY MOVETO NOBUTS NODSTO NOHITS NONETS NOPETS NORITE NOTATE NOVATO NOVOTE OOCYTE OOLITE POINTA POINTB POINTE POINTS POINTY POLITE POLITY POSITS POTATO POULTS ROASTS ROBOTS RODETO ROGETS ROOSTS ROSETO ROSITA ROTATE ROUSTS SOASTO SOLATI SOLDTO SOLUTE SOMATA SONATA SOWETO TOASTS TOASTY TOBITS TODATE TOMATO TONITE TOOKTO TOYOTA VOLUTE WORSTS

•O•••T

BOBCAT BODETT BOGART BONMOT BONNET BOOSAT BOOTIT BORDET BOUGHT BOWOUT BOXSET COBALT COBNUT COEDIT COGENT COHORT COHOST COLLAT COLLET COMBAT COMEAT COMFIT COMMIT COMSAT CONANT CONFIT COOLIT COPOUT COPSIT CORNET CORSET CORTOT COSSET COVENT COVERT COYEST DOASET DOCENT DOCKET DOESIT DOESNT DOGSAT DOGSIT DONEIT DORRIT DORSET DOTDOT DOTOAT FOMENT FOOTIT FORDGT FOREST FORGET FORGOT FORINT FORMAT FOUGHT GOATIT GOBLET GOBUST GOCART GODWIT GOESAT GOFAST GOFLAT GOKART GOLAST GOLEFT GONEAT GONEXT GOODAT GOPAST GORIOT GOSOFT GOTFIT GOTHOT GOTOIT GOTOUT GOTSET GOTWET GOULET GOWEST HOBART HOBBIT HOGNUT HOLDIT HOLIST HONEST HONKAT HOOFIT HOOTAT HOPOUT HORNET HOTBOT HOTPOT HOWLAT JOBCUT JOBLOT JOLIET JOLIOT KOMBAT KORBUT LOCCIT LOCKET LOCUST LOGOUT LOIRET LONGET LOOKAT LOQUAT LORDIT LOSEIT LOSTIT LOVEIT LOVETT LOWCUT LOWEST LOWFAT LOWSET MODELT MODEST MOLEST MOMENT MONGST MONIST MONNET MOPPET MORANT MOROLT MOTTST MOVEIT MOZART NOCENT NOCOST NODSAT NOEXIT NOHANT NOIRET NOMEAT NONART NONFAT NONHIT NONNET NORENT NOSALT NOTFIT NOTOUT NOTYET NOUGAT NOUGHT NOWAIT POCKET POIRET POIROT POKEAT POLPOT POORAT POPART POPOUT POSTIT POTENT ROARAT ROBERT ROBUST ROCHAT ROCHET ROCKET ROCKIT RODENT ROSSET ROTGUT SOBEIT SOCKET SOFFIT SOLDIT SONANT SONNET SORBET SOREAT SOREST SOTHAT SOUGHT SOVIET SOWHAT TOBOOT TOGOUT TOILAT TOILET TOLAST TOLDIT TOMCAT TOMTIT TOOHOT TOOKIT TOOTAT TOPCAT TOPHAT TOPOUT TOREAT TOREIT TORENT TOYHAT VOIGHT VOLANT WOMBAT WONOUT WORKAT YOGURT YOUBET

••OT••

ALOTOF BIOTAS BIOTIC BIOTIN BLOTCH BLOTTO BLOTTY BLOTUP BOOTED BOOTEE BOOTER BOOTES BOOTHE BOOTHS BOOTIE BOOTIT BOOTUP BROTHS BROTHY CLOTHE CLOTHO CLOTHS CLOTTY CLOTUP CNOTES COOTER COOTIE CROTCH CROTON DHOTEL DHOTIS EMOTED EMOTER EMOTES ENOTES EROTIC EXOTIC FOOTED FOOTER FOOTIT FOOTLE FOOTUP FROTHS FROTHY GIOTTO GLOTTO GNOTES GROTON GROTTO GROTTY HOOTAT HOOTCH HOOTED HOOTER HOOTIE

IDOTOO
IGOTIT
IGOTTA
KNOTTS
KNOTTY
KNOTUP
LAOTSE
LAOTZU
LHOTSE
LIOTTA
LOOTED
LOOTER
MAOTAI
MOOTED
MOOTER
NOOTKA
PHOTIC
PHOTOG
PHOTON
PHOTOS
PLOTTY
PROTAX
PROTEA
PROTEM
PROTON
QUOTAS
QUOTED
QUOTEE
QUOTER
QUOTES
RIOTED
RIOTER
ROOTED
ROOTER
ROOTIE
ROOTIN
ROOTLE
ROOTSY
ROOTUP
SCOTCH
SCOTER
SCOTIA
SCOTTO
SCOTTS
SCOTTY
SHOTAT
SHOTBY
SHOTUP
SLOTHS
SOOTHE
SPOTON
SPOTTV
SPOTTY
STOTIN
TNOTES
TOOTAT
TOOTED
TOOTER
TOOTHY
TOOTIE
TOOTIN
TOOTLE
TOOTOO
TOOTSY
TROTHS
TROTUP
TSOTSI
WOOTSY
ZLOTYS

••O•T•

ABORTS
ADOPTS
ADOUTS
AGOSTO
AGOUTI
AMONTH
BIONTS
BLOATS
BLOTTO
BLOTTY
BOOSTS
BRONTE
CHOATE
CLOETE
CLOTTY
CLOUTS
COOLTH
COOLTO
COOPTS
CROATS
CROFTS
CROUTE
DAOSTA
DOOMTO
DROITS
EBOATS
FLOATS
FLOATY
FLOUTS
FRONTS
FROSTS
FROSTY
GHOSTS
GHOSTY
GIOTTO
GLOATS
GLOTTO
GROATS
GROTTO
GROTTY
GROUTS
GROUTY
GROWTH
IFORTY
IGOTTA
KNOTTS
KNOTTY
KNOUTS
KOONTZ
LIOTTA
LOOKTO
NFORTY
ODONTO
OPORTO
PLOTTY
PRONTO
QUOITS
ROOSTS
SCOOTS
SCOTTO
SCOTTS
SCOTTY
SCOUTS
SHOATS
SHOOTS
SHORTA
SHORTE
SHORTI
SHORTO
SHORTS
SHORTU
SHORTY
SHORTZ
SHOUTS
SKORTS
SMOLTS
SMOOTH
SNOOTS
SNOOTY
SNORTS
SNORTY
SNOUTS
SPORTS
SPORTY
SPOTTV
SPOTTY
SPOUTS
STOATS
STOLTZ
STOUTS
TOOKTO
TROUTS
UBOATS
UBOLTS

••O••T

AGOROT
AMORET
AMOUNT
ANOINT
AROINT
AROUET
AVOCET
BLOUNT
BLOWIT
BOOSAT
BOOTIT
BROAST
CLOSET
COOLIT
DROPIT
DROUET
EGOIST
EXOCET
FLOPIT
FLORET
FOOTIT
GOODAT
GROMIT
HOOFIT
HOOTAT
IDONOT
IGOROT
IGOTIT
IMONIT
IROBOT
KNOWIT
KROFFT
LIONET
LOOKAT
MAOIST
OBOIST
PIOLET
POORAT
PROART
PROBST
PROFIT
PROJET
PROMPT
PROSIT
PROUST
SHOPAT
SHOTAT
SNOCAT
SPOILT
STOPAT
STOPIT
STOWIT
TAOIST
TOOHOT
TOOKIT
TOOTAT
TWOACT
TWOBIT
VIOLET
VIORST
WHODAT

•••OT•

ABBOTS
ABBOTT
ALCOTT
ALIOTH
ALIOTO
ALLOTS
ARGOTS
ASCOTS
BENOTE
BESOTS
BIGOTS
BOGOTA
BYLOTS
BYROTE
CAPOTE
COROTS
COYOTE
CSPOTS
DAKOTA
DEMOTE
DEMOTH
DENOTE
DEPOTS
DESOTO
DETOTH
DEVOTE
DEVOTO
DICOTS
DIVOTS
ERGOTS
FAGOTS
FSCOTT
GAVOTS
GIGOTS
GOBOTS
GRIOTS
HELOTS
IDIOTS
INGOTS
INTOTO
IOMOTH
JABOTS
JCLOTH
LAKOTA
MALOTI
MELOTT
MRMOTO
NOVOTE
OFNOTE
PELOTA
PEYOTE
PICOTS
PILOTS
PINOTS
PITOTS
PIVOTS
REBOTE
REMOTE
RENOTE
REPOTS
REVOTE
ROBOTS
SABOTS
SCOOTS
SHOOTS
SMOOTH
SNOOTS
SNOOTY
TAROTS
TOYOTA
UNPOTS
WACOTX
ZYGOTE

•••O•T

ABBOTT
ACCOST
ACEOUT
ACTOUT
ADROIT
AFLOAT
AGEOUT
AIROUT
AJFOYT
ALCOTT
ALLOUT
ALMOST
ASKOUT
ASSOFT
ASSORT
ATCOST
ATEOUT
ATMOST
AUMONT
BELOIT
BENOIT
BOWOUT
BUGOUT
BUMOUT
BUYOUT
CAHOOT
CAVORT
COHORT
COHOST
COPOUT
CRYOUT
CUTOUT
CWPOST
DEBONT
DECOCT
DEPORT
DEVOUT
DIEOUT
DIGOUT
DIMOUT
DOTOAT
DRYOUT
DUGOUT
DUMONT
DUPONT
EATOUT
EFFORT
EGMONT
EKEOUT
ELMONT
ENROOT
ESCORT
EXHORT
EXPORT
EXPOST
EXTORT
FANOUT
FAROUT
FITOUT
FLYOUT
FSCOTT
GALOOT
GETOUT
GOSOFT
GOTOIT
GOTOUT
HADOUT
HASOUT
HEGOAT
HESOUT
HIDOUT
HITOUT
HOPOUT
ICEOUT
IMPORT
IMPOST
INMOST
INPORT
INTOIT
LAMONT
LAYOUT
LEDOUT
LETOUT
LIPOUT
LITOUT
LOGOUT
LUGOUT
MAHOUT
MAPOUT
MAXOUT
MELOTT
MOROLT
MYFOOT
NOCOST
NOTOUT
NYPOST
OCTOOT
ONEOUT
ONFOOT
ONPOST
OPTOUT
PANOUT
PAYOUT
PIGOUT
POPOUT
PTBOAT
PUTOUT
RAGOUT
RANOUT
RATOUT
REBOLT
REBOOT
RECOAT
RECOST
REDOUT
RELOST
REPORT
REPOST
REROOT
RESORT
RETORT
REVOLT
RIGOUT
RIPOST
RIPOUT
RUBOUT
RUNOUT
SATOUT
SAWOUT
SEEOUT
SETOUT
SITOUT
SPROUT
SPYOUT
TAGOUT
TAPOUT
THROAT
TOBOOT
TOGOUT
TOPOUT
TRYOUT
UNBOLT
UNLOST
UNROOT
UNSOFT
UNSORT
UPMOST
UPROOT
UPTOIT
UTMOST
VEGOUT
WAYOUT
WIGOUT
WINOUT
WONOUT
XEDOUT
XESOUT
ZIPOUT

••••OT

AGOROT
AIRPOT
ALIYOT
BADLOT
BALLOT
BARDOT
BBSHOT
BONMOT
BURBOT
CAHOOT
CANNOT
CARLOT
CARROT
CORTOT
DECLOT
DERMOT
DESPOT
DIDNOT
DIGLOT
DOTDOT
DRYROT
DYELOT
EELPOT
ELLIOT
ENROOT
FEMBOT
FORGOT
GALOOT
GETHOT
GORIOT
GOTHOT
HARLOT
HOTBOT
HOTPOT
IAMNOT
IDONOT
IGOROT
INKPOT
INSPOT
IROBOT
ITSHOT
ITSNOT
JOBLOT
JOLIOT
MAGGOT
MARGOT
MARMOT
MASCOT
MERLOT
MYFOOT
OCELOT
OCTOOT
ODDLOT
ONFOOT
PARROT
PEQUOT
POIROT
POLPOT
REBOOT
REDDOT
REDHOT
REKNOT
REPLOT
REROOT
RESHOT
RESPOT
SEXPOT
SPIGOT
SPYBOT
SUBLOT
TEAPOT
THELOT
TINPOT
TISSOT
TOBOOT
TOOHOT
TRICOT
TURBOT
TVSPOT
UNKNOT
UNROOT
UPROOT
UPSHOT
VIDIOT
WHYNOT
ZEALOT

OU••••

OUCHES
OUGHTA
OUGHTS
OUIJAS
OUIMET
OUIOUI
OUNCES
OUSELS
OUSTED
OUSTER
OUTACT
OUTADD
OUTAGE
OUTASK
OUTATE
OUTAWE
OUTBAN
OUTBAT
OUTBEG
OUTBID
OUTBOW
OUTBOX
OUTBUD
OUTBUY
OUTCRY
OUTCUT
OUTDID
OUTEAT
OUTFIT
OUTFLY
OUTFOR
OUTFOX
OUTGAS
OUTGUN
OUTHIT
OUTIES
OUTING
OUTJET
OUTJUT
OUTLAW
OUTLAY
OUTLED
OUTLET
OUTLIE
OUTLIP
OUTMAN
OUTPAY
OUTPOP
OUTPRY
OUTPUT
OUTRAN
OUTRAP
OUTRIB
OUTRIG
OUTROW
OUTRUN
OUTSAT
OUTSAW
OUTSAY
OUTSEE
OUTSET
OUTSIN
OUTSIT
OUTSPY
OUTSUM
OUTVIE
OUTWAR
OUTWIT
OUZELS

O•U•••

OCULAR
OCULUS
OEUVRE
ONUSES
OPUSES
OVULAR
OVULES

O••U••

OAHUAN
OAKUMS
OBTUND
OBTUSE
OCCULT
OCCUPY
OCCURS
ODIUMS
ODOULS
ODOURS
OFFUTT
OGAUGE
OHNUTS
OHSURE
OLEUMS
ONAUTO
ONDUTY
ONEUPS
ONRUSH
OPHULS
OPIUMS
OPPUGN
OSCULE
OSMUND

O•••U•

OBELUS
OBOLUS
OCULUS
ODIOUS
OHCRUD
OILCUP
OILRUB
OLERUD
OMASUM
OMNIUM
ONABUN
ONEOUT
ONERUN
ONTOUR
OPAQUE
OPENUP
OPTOUT
ORTRUD
OSMIUM
OUIOUI
OUTBUD
OUTBUY
OUTCUT
OUTGUN
OUTJUT
OUTPUT
OUTRUN
OUTSUM
OWNSUP

O••••U

OISEAU
ORMOLU

•OU•••

AOUDAD
BOUCHE
BOUDIN
BOUFFE
BOUGHS
BOUGHT
BOULES
BOULEZ
BOUNCE
BOUNCY
BOUNDS
BOUNTY
BOURGS
BOURKE
BOURNE
BOURSE
BOUTON
COUGAR
COUGHS
COULDA
COULDI
COULEE
COUNTS
COUNTY
COUPES
COUPLE
COUPON
COURIC
COURSE
COURTS
COUSIN
COUTER
DOUANE
DOUBLE
DOUBLY
DOUBTS
DOUGAL
DOUGHS
DOUGHY
DOULAS
DOURER
DOURIF
DOURLY
DOUSED
DOUSER
DOUSES
DOUZES
FOUDRE
FOUGHT
FOULED
FOULER
FOULLY
FOULUP
FOUNDS
FOUNTS
FOURAA
FOURAD
FOURAM
FOURBC
FOUREE
FOURNO
FOURPM
FOURTH
FOURUP
GOUDAS
GOUGED
GOUGER
GOUGES
GOULET
GOUNOD
GOUPTO
GOURDE
GOURDS
HOUDON
HOUNDS
HOUNDY
HOURIS
HOURLY
HOUSED
HOUSES
JOULES
JOUNCE
JOUNCY
JOURNO
JOUSTS
KOUFAX
LOUANN
LOUCHE
LOUDEN
LOUDER
LOUDLY
LOUDON
LOUIES
LOUISA
LOUISB
LOUISE
LOUISI
LOUISV
LOUISX
LOUMAS
LOUNGE
LOUPES
LOUSED
LOUSES
LOUVER
LOUVIN
LOUVRE
MOULDS
MOULDY
MOULIN
MOULTS
MOUNDS
MOUNTS
MOUNTY
MOURNS
MOUSED
MOUSER
MOUSES
MOUSEY
MOUSSE
MOUTHS
MOUTHY
NOUGAT
NOUGHT
NOUMEA
NOUNAL
POUCHY
POUDRE
POUFED
POUFFY
POULES
POULTS
POUNCE
POUNDS
POUPON
POURED
POURER
POURIN
POUSSE
POUTED
POUTER
ROUGED
ROUGES
ROUGHS
ROUNDS
ROURKE
ROUSED
ROUSER
ROUSES
ROUSTS
ROUTED
ROUTER
ROUTES
SOUGHT
SOUNDS
SOUPER
SOUPUP
SOURCE
SOURED
SOURER
SOURLY
SOURON
SOUSED
SOUSES
SOUTER
SOUTHS
TOUCAN
TOUCHE
TOUCHY
TOUGHS
TOUGHY
TOULON
TOUPEE
TOURED
TOURER
TOUSLE
TOUTED
TOUTER
WOULDA
WOUNDS
YOUALL
YOUBET
YOUDIG
YOUSEE
YOUSUF
YOUTHS
YOUTWO
YOUWIN
ZOUNDS

•O•U••

BODUKE
BOSUNS
COBURG
COBURN
COEURS
COLUMN
CONURE
COPULA
COQUIS
DONUTS
DOSUMS
FORUMS
GOBUST
GONUTS
HOHUMS
HOKUMS
JOCUND
JORUMS
KORUNA
LOBULE
LOCUST
LOQUAT
MOBUTU
MODULE
MODULI
MODULO
MOGULS
MOPUPS
NOBUTS
NODULE
NOFUSS
NOLUCK
NONUSE
NORUNS
NORUSH
PODUNK
POPULI
POPUPS
ROBUST
ROGUED
ROGUES
ROMULO
ROTUND
SOEURS
SOLUTE
SOMUCH
TOBURN
TOGUES
TOQUES
VOGUED
VOGUER
VOGUES
VOLUME
VOLUTE
WOBURN
YODUDE
YOGURT
ZONULE

•O••U•

BOBSUP
BOILUP
BOLTUP
BONEUP
BOOJUM
BOOTUP
BOREUP
BOWOUT
BOXFUL
COBNUT
COCCUS
COILUP
COLEUS
COLOUR
COMEUP
CONCUR
CONSUL
COOKUP
COOPUP
COPOUT
CORIUM
CORKUP
CORPUS
CORVUS
COSYUP
COYPUS
COZYUP
DOESUP
DOGRUN
DOITUP
DOLLUP
DOLOUR
DONEUP
DOOFUS
DORSUM
FOGSUP
FOLDUP
FOLIUM
FONDUE
FONDUS
FOOTUP
FORFUN
FORKUP
FOULUP
FOURUP
GOESUP
GOLLUM
GONEUP
GOOFUP
GOOFUS
GOSOUR
GOTOUT
HOGNUT
HOLDUP
HOLEUP
HONOUR
HOOKUP
HOPOUT
HOPSUP
HORMUZ
HOTCUP
HOTTUB
IONIUM
JOBCUT
JOINUP
JOSHUA
JOYFUL
JOYOUS
KOMBUS
KORBUT
LOADUP
LOCKUP
LOFTUS
LOGOUT
LONGUE

LOOKUP
LOOMUP
LOWCUT
MOBIUS
MOCKUP
MOPSUP
MORGUE
MOSQUE
MOVEUP
NODOUS
NONRUN
NOSEUP
NOTOUT
PODIUM
PODOUS
POILUS
POLLUX
PONYUP
PONZUS
POPGUN
POPOUT
POPSUP
POROUS
POSEUR
POSSUM
POSTUM
POTFUL
RODEUP
ROILUP
ROLLUP
ROOTUP
ROPEUP
ROSEUP
ROSSUM
ROTGUT
SOAKUP
SOAPUP
SOBFUL
SODIUM
SOLEUS
SOPSUP
SOTRUE
SOUPUP
TOGOUT
TOGSUP
TONEUP
TONGUE
TOOKUP
TOOLUP
TOPGUN
TOPOUT
TOPSUP
TOREUP
TORNUP
TORQUE
TOSSUP
TOTEUP
TOTSUP
TOYGUN
VOROUS
WOEFUL
WOKEUP
WONOUT
WORKUP
YOUSUF

•O•••U
CONGOU
FORYOU
GOTYOU
HONSHU
JOANOU
MOBUTU
MOLDAU
MOREAU
NOTYOU
POITOU
ROSEAU

••OU••
ABOUND
ADOUTS
AGOUTI
AMOUNT
AMOURS
AROUET
AROUND
AROUSE
AVOUCH
BLOUNT
BLOUSE
BROUGH
CHOUGH
CLOUDS
CLOUDY
CLOUGH
CLOUTS
CROUCH
CROUPS
CROUPY
CROUSE
CROUTE
DROUET
ENOUGH
FLOURS
FLOURY
FLOUTS
GHOULS
GLOUCS
GROUCH
GROUND
GROUPS
GROUSE
GROUTS
GROUTY
HHOURS
ICOULD
INOUYE
IWOULD
KHOUMS
KNOUTS
ODOULS
ODOURS
PLOUGH
PROULX
PROUST
SCOUPE
SCOURS
SCOUTS
SHOULD
SHOUTS
SIOUAN
SLOUCH
SLOUGH
SNOUTS
SPOUSE
SPOUTS
STOUTS
THOUGH
TROUGH
TROUPE
TROUTS
VFOURS

••O•U•
AEOLUS
BLOTUP
BLOWUP
BOOJUM
BOOTUP
BROGUE
BUOYUP
CHOPUP
CHORUS
CLOGUP
CLOTUP
COOKUP
COOPUP
CROCUS
CRONUS
CROPUP
DOOFUS
DROGUE
EPOQUE
EXODUS
FOOTUP
GOOFUP
GOOFUS
GROWUP
HOOKUP
IDOLUM
KEOKUK
KNOTUP
KRONUR
LOOKUP
LOOMUP
OBOLUS
PLOWUP
PROGUN
PROPUP
QUOQUE
QUORUM
ROOTUP
SHOGUN
SHOTUP
SHOWUP
SLOWUP
STOPUP
TOOKUP
TOOLUP
TROTUP

••O••U
BROWNU
EMORYU
LAOTZU
SHORTU

•••OU•
ACEOUT
ACTOUT
ADNOUN
AGEOUT
AIROUT
ALDOUS
ALLOUT
ANJOUS
ARBOUR
ARDOUR
ARMOUR
ASKOUT
ATEOUT
ATFOUR
AUROUS
BAYOUS
BEFOUL
BIJOUS
BIJOUX
BOWOUT
BUGOUT
BUMOUT
BUYOUT
CIXOUS
COLOUR
COPOUT
CRYOUT
CUTOUT
DAMOUR
DETOUR
DEVOUR
DEVOUT
DIEOUT
DIGOUT
DIMOUT
DOLOUR
DRYOUT
DUGOUT
EATOUT
EKEOUT
ENSOUL
FAMOUS
FANOUT
FAROUK
FAROUT
FAVOUR
FEROUS
FITOUT
FLYOUT
GAMOUS
GETOUT
GOSOUR
GOTOUT
GYNOUS
HADOUT
HASOUT
HESOUT
HIDOUT
HITOUT
HONOUR
HOPOUT
HUMOUR
ICEOUT
INPOUR
ITIOUS
JOYOUS
LABOUR
LAMOUR
LATOUR
LAYOUT
LEDOUT
LEDOUX
LEROUX
LETOUR
LETOUT
LIPOUT
LITOUT
LOGOUT
LUGOUT
MACOUN
MAHOUT
MAPOUT
MAXOUT
MIAOUS
NODOUS
NOTOUT
ODIOUS
ONEOUT
ONTOUR
OPTOUT
OUIOUI
PANOUT
PAYOUT
PIGOUT
PILOUS
PODOUS
POPOUT
POROUS
PUTOUT
RAGOUT
RANOUT
RATOUT
RECOUP
REDOUT
REPOUR
RETOUR
RIGOUR
RIGOUT
RIMOUS
RIPOUT
RUBOUT
RUFOUS
RUMOUR
RUNOUT
SATOUT
SAVOUR
SAWOUT
SEEOUT
SEROUS
SETOUT
SHROUD
SITOUT
SPROUT
SPYOUT
STROUD
TAGOUT
TAPOUT
TOGOUT
TOPOUT
TRYOUT
UNFOUL
UNSOUR
USTOUR
UVEOUS
VALOUR
VAPOUR
VEGOUT
VELOUR
VENOUS
VIGOUR
VINOUS
VOROUS
WAYOUT
WIGOUT
WINOUT
WONOUT
XEDOUT
XESOUT
ZIPOUT

•••O•U
ORMOLU
SUDOKU

••••OU
BALLOU
CARIOU
CONGOU
FORYOU
GOTYOU
HEYYOU
ITSYOU
JOANOU
MENJOU
MITSOU
NETHOU
NOTYOU
PISTOU
POITOU
SARDOU
SEEYOU
SEZYOU
WHYYOU
YESYOU

OV••••
OVALLY
OVERDO
OVERIT
OVERLY
OVIEDO
OVINES
OVISAC
OVOIDS
OVULAR
OVULES

O•V•••
OBVERT
ONVIEW

O••V••
OEUVRE
OGIVAL
OGIVES
OLAVII
OLAVIV
OLDVIC
OLEVEL
OLIVER
OLIVES
OLIVIA
OUTVIE

O•••V•
OCTAVE
OCTAVO
OTTAVA

O••••V
OLAFIV
OLAVIV
OTTOIV

•OV•••
BOVARY
BOVIDS
BOVINE
COVENS
COVENT
COVERS
COVERT
COVETS
COVEYS
COVINA
COVING
DOVEIN
DOVISH
GOVERN
HOVELS
HOVERS
HOVETO
JOVIAL
JOVIAN
KOVACS
LOVAGE
LOVEIN
LOVEIT
LOVELL
LOVELY
LOVERS
LOVETO
LOVETT
LOVEYA
LOVEYS
LOVING
MOVADO
MOVEIN
MOVEIT
MOVEON
MOVERS
MOVETO
MOVEUP
MOVIES
MOVING
NOVATO
NOVELA
NOVELS
NOVENA
NOVIAS
NOVICE
NOVIOS
NOVOTE
POVICH
ROVERS
ROVING
SOVIET

•O•V••
COEVAL
CONVEX
CONVEY
CONVOY
CORVEE
CORVID
CORVUS
DOOVER
GOOVER
HOOVER
HOOVES
LOAVES
LOUVER
LOUVIN
LOUVRE
NORVAL
POIVRE
POTVIN
SOAVES
SOLVED
SOLVER
SOLVES
VOLVOS
WOLVES

•O••V•
BOOKVI
GODIVA
GOLIVE
JOHNVI
KOSOVO
MOHAVE
MOJAVE
MOSKVA
MOTIVE
NOJIVE
VOTIVE

•O•••V
BOOKIV
DOTGOV
JOHNIV
JOHNXV
LOUISV
MOSHAV
ROCKYV
ROSTOV
YOMTOV

••OV••
BMOVIE
BROVIK
CLOVEN
CLOVER
CLOVES
CLOVIS
DOOVER
DROVER
DROVES
GLOVED
GLOVER
GLOVES
GOOVER
GROVED
GROVEL
GROVER
GROVES
HOOVER
HOOVES
LEOVII
PLOVER
PROVED
PROVEN
PROVER
PROVES
SHOVED
SHOVEL
SHOVER
SHOVES
SLOVAK
SLOVEN
STOVER
STOVES
TROVES
UPOVER

••O•V•
BOOKVI
EVOLVE
GROOVE
GROOVY

••O••V
BOOKIV
SPOTTV

•••OV•
ALCOVE
ARLOVA
BULOVA
BYJOVE
CANOVA
DANOVA
DENOVO
EXGOVS
GENOVA
GROOVE
GROOVY
INLOVE
INWOVE
KOSOVO
LENOVO
LTGOVS
MYLOVE
PADOVA
REMOVE
REWOVE
SHROVE
STROVE
THROVE
UNROVE
UNWOVE
UPDOVE
UPHOVE
VALOVA

•••O•V
ELKONV
OTTOIV
RENONV

••••OV
ASIMOV
ASTROV
BRASOV
CHEKOV
DOTGOV
IMPROV
IVANOV
KARKOV
KARPOV
KRYLOV
MARKOV
PAVLOV
ROSTOV
YOMTOV
ZARKOV
ZHUKOV

OW••••
OWEDON
OWEDTO
OWESON
OWLEGG
OWLERY
OWLETS
OWLIER
OWLISH
OWNERS
OWNING
OWNSUP
OWOSSO

O•W•••
OHWELL
ONWARD
ORWELL
ORWHAT
OSWALD
OSWEGO

O••W••
OBIWAN
OLDWAY
ONEWAY
OUTWAR
OUTWIT

O•••W•
OJIBWA
ONETWO
OSHAWA
OTTAWA
OUTAWE
OXBOWS

O••••W
OLDSAW
ONSHOW
ONVIEW
OUTBOW
OUTLAW
OUTROW
OUTSAW

•OW•••
BOWELS
BOWERS
BOWERY
BOWFIN
BOWING
BOWLED
BOWLER
BOWLES
BOWMAN
BOWMEN
BOWOAR
BOWOUT
BOWSAW
BOWSTO
BOWTIE
BOWWOW
BOWYER
BOWZER
COWARD
COWBOY
COWENS
COWERS
COWIER
COWING
COWISH
COWLED
COWLEY
COWMAN
COWMEN
COWPEA
COWPER
COWPOX
COWRIE
DOWELL
DOWELS
DOWERS
DOWERY
DOWITH
DOWNED
DOWNER
DOWNES
DOWNEY
DOWNON
DOWSED
DOWSER
DOWSES
DOWSON
FOWLED
FOWLER
FOWLES
GOWELL
GOWEST
GOWILD
GOWITH
GOWNED
HOWARD
HOWBIG
HOWDAH
HOWELL
HOWFAR
HOWLAT
HOWLED
HOWLER
HOWLIN
HOWNOW
HOWODD
HOWSAD
HOWSER
HOWTOS
IOWANS
JOWLED
KOWTOW
LOWBID
LOWBOY
LOWCAL
LOWCUT
LOWEBB
LOWELL
LOWEND
LOWERS
LOWERY
LOWEST
LOWFAT
LOWING
LOWIQS
LOWISH
LOWKEY
LOWMAN
LOWMEN
LOWRES
LOWSET
LOWTAR
LOWTOP
MOWERS
MOWGLI
MOWING
NOWAIT
NOWAYS
NOWISE
NOWLAN
NOWNOW
POWDER
POWELL
POWERS
POWWOW
ROWANS
ROWELS
ROWENA
ROWENS
ROWERS
ROWING
ROWLEY
SOWERS
SOWETO
SOWHAT
SOWING
TOWAGE
TOWARD
TOWBAR
TOWCAR
TOWELS
TOWERS
TOWERY
TOWHEE
TOWING
TOWNER
TOWNIE
TOWSIN
VOWELS
VOWELY
VOWERS
VOWING
WOWING
YOWLED
YOWLER
YOWZAH

•O•W••
BOWWOW
COBWEB
CONWAY
COOWNS
CORWIN
DOOWOP
FORWHY
GOAWAY
GOAWOL
GOAWRY
GODWIN
GODWIT
GOTWET
HOTWAR
NONWAR
NORWAY
POWWOW
YOUWIN

•O••W•
CODYWY
GODOWN
MOHAWK
MOTOWN
NONEWS
SODOWE
YOUTWO

•O•••W
BORROW
BOWSAW
BOWWOW
FOGBOW
FOLLOW
FORNOW
GOSLOW
HOLLOW
HOWNOW
KOWTOW
MOOCOW
MORROW
MOSCOW
NONJEW
NOSHOW
NOTNEW
NOTNOW
NOWNOW
POWWOW
SORROW
TOOLOW
TOPROW

••OW••
AJOWAN
AVOWAL
AVOWED
AVOWER
BLOWER
BLOWIN
BLOWIT
BLOWON
BLOWSY
BLOWUP
BLOWZY
BROWED
BROWNE
BROWNS
BROWNU
BROWNY
BROWSE
CHOWED
CLOWNS
COOWNS
CROWDS
CROWED
CROWER
CROWNE
CROWNS
DOOWOP
DROWNS
DROWSE
DROWSY
EPOWER
FLOWED
FLOWER
FLOWIN
FROWNS
FROWZY
GLOWED
GLOWER
GROWER
GROWLS
GROWLY
GROWON
GROWTH
GROWUP
KIOWAN
KIOWAS
KNOWER
KNOWIT
KNOWNS
KNOWOF
MEOWED
MEOWER
PLOWED
PLOWER
PLOWON
PLOWUP
PROWAR
PROWLS
PROWSE
REOWNS
SCOWLS
SHOWED
SHOWER
SHOWIN
SHOWME
SHOWUP
SLOWED
SLOWER
SLOWGO
SLOWLY
SLOWUP
SNOWED
SNOWIN
STOWED
STOWER
STOWIT
TROWED
TROWEL
TWOWAY
UNOWED
WHOWON

••O••W
BROKAW
ECOLAW
MOOCOW
TOOLOW

•••OW•
ALLOWS
ARROWS
DISOWN
ELBOWS
ELFOWL
EMBOWS
ENDOWS
GODOWN
INTOWN
MIAOWS
MOTOWN
OXBOWS
REMOWN
REMOWS
RENOWN
RESOWN
RESOWS
RETOWS
SODOWE
THROWN
THROWS
UNMOWN
UNSOWN
UPBOWS
UPTOWN
WIDOWS

••••OW
ACTNOW
ANDHOW
ANTCOW
ANYHOW
ASSLOW
ATALOW
ATHROW
BARLOW
BARROW
BELLOW
BENBOW
BERKOW
BESTOW
BILLOW
BORROW
BOWWOW
BURROW
BUTHOW
BUYNOW
BYENOW
CALLOW
CARLOW
CPSNOW
CRACOW
CURNOW
DARROW
ERENOW
ESCROW
FALLOW
FARLOW
FARROW
FELLOW
FLYLOW
FOGBOW
FOLLOW
FORNOW
FURROW
GOSLOW
HALLOW
HARLOW
HARROW
HAYMOW
HOLLOW
HOWNOW
INAROW
INFLOW
KAYYOW
KOWTOW
KRAKOW

KUDROW
LAYLOW
LIELOW
LUDLOW
MALLOW
MARROW
MEADOW
MELLOW
MINNOW
MOOCOW
MORROW
MOSCOW
MURROW
NARROW
NOSHOW
NOTNOW
NOWNOW
ONSHOW
OUTBOW
OUTROW
PAYNOW
PESCOW
PETCOW
PILLOW
PITROW
POWWOW
RANLOW
REAVOW
REFLOW
REGLOW
REGROW
REPLOW
RESHOW
RESTOW
RUNLOW
SALLOW
SEACOW
SHADOW
SKITOW
SORROW
SUNBOW
TALLOW
THEDOW
TILNOW
TOOLOW
TOPROW
TVSHOW
UNSLOW
UNSTOW
UPFLOW
UPGROW
WALLOW
WHYNOW
WILLOW
WINDOW
WINNOW
YARROW
YELLOW

OX••••
OXALIC
OXALIS
OXBOWS
OXCART
OXEYES
OXFORD
OXHIDE
OXIDES
OXIDIC
OXLIKE
OXLIPS
OXNARD
OXTAIL
OXYDOL
OXYGEN

O•X•••
OAXACA

O••X••
ONYXES
OREXIA
OREXIS
ORYXES

O••••X
OUTBOX
OUTFOX

•OX•••
BOXBED
BOXBOY
BOXCAR
BOXERS
BOXFUL
BOXIER
BOXILY
BOXING
BOXSET
BOXTOP
COXING
DOXIES
FOXIER
FOXILY
FOXING
ROXANA
ROXANE
SOXFAN
TOXICS
TOXINS
VOXPOP
XOXOXO

•O•X••
COAXAL
COAXED
COAXER
COAXES
HOAXED
HOAXER
HOAXES
NOEXIT

•O••X•
BORAXO
GONEXT
JOHNXI
JOHNXV
JOHNXX
XOXOXO

•O•••X
BOLLIX
BOOKIX
COCCYX
COLFAX
COMDEX
COMMIX
CONVEX
CORTEX
COWPOX
FORNAX
HOTBOX
JOETEX
JOHNIX
JOHNXX
KOUFAX
LOUISX
NONTAX
POLEAX
POLLEX
POLLUX
RONMIX
TOMMIX
VORTEX

••OX••
ANOXIA
ANOXIC
ATOXIC
DIOXIN
DROXIE
LEOXII
XBOXES

••O••X
BOOKIX
CLOROX
PROLIX
PROTAX
PROULX
THORAX

•••OX•
BILOXI
UNFOXY
XOXOXO

•••O•X
BIJOUX
LEDOUX
LEROUX
WACOTX

••••OX
APPROX
BIGBOX
BLUEOX
CHISOX
CLOROX
COWPOX
FTKNOX
HATBOX
HOTBOX
HYDROX
ICEBOX
INABOX
LENNOX
LUMMOX
MAALOX
MADDOX
MUSKOX
OUTBOX
OUTFOX
PEGBOX
REDFOX
REDSOX
SEAFOX
SKYBOX
SLYFOX
TEEBOX
THEFOX
THESOX
WILCOX

OY••••
OYEZES
OYSTER

O•Y•••
OFYORE
OHYEAH
ONYXES
ORYXES
OXYDOL
OXYGEN

O••Y••
OBEYED
OBEYER
OBGYNS
OKAYED
OKBYME
ONLYIF
OOCYTE
OXEYES

O•••Y•
ONEEYE
ONLAYS

O••••Y
OAKLEY
OCASEY
OCCUPY
OCHERY
ODDITY
OFFALY
OFFDAY
OFFKEY
OGRADY
OHBABY
OHENRY
OILILY
OLDBOY
OLDWAY
OLEARY
ONDUTY
ONEDAY
ONEWAY
ONIONY
OOLOGY
OOZILY
OPENLY
ORALLY
ORANGY
ORKNEY
ORNERY
ORRERY
OSPREY
OSSIFY
OUTBUY
OUTCRY
OUTFLY
OUTLAY
OUTPAY
OUTPRY
OUTSAY
OUTSPY
OVALLY
OVERLY
OWLERY

•OY•••
BOYARS
BOYISH
BOYLES
BOYTOY
COYDOG
COYEST
COYISH
COYOTE
COYPUS
DOYENS
FOYERS
HOYDEN
HOYLES
JOYFUL
JOYING
JOYNER
JOYOUS
JOYPAD
LOYALE
LOYOLA
MOYERS
NOYORI
POYSER
ROYALE
ROYALS
ROYCES
SOYINK
TOYAMA
TOYCAR
TOYDOG
TOYERS
TOYGUN
TOYHAT
TOYING
TOYONS
TOYOTA
TOYTOP
VOYAGE
YOYOED
YOYOMA
ZOYSIA

•O•Y••
BOLYAI
BOWYER
CODYWY
CORYZA
COSYUP
COZYUP
DOBYNS
FORYOU
GOTYOU
JOBYNA
NOTYET
NOTYOU
OOCYTE
POLYPS
PONYUP

•O••Y•
BOBBYS
BOGEYS
BOLEYN
COCCYX
COLBYS
CONEYS
COPAYS
COVEYS
FOGEYS
FOLEYS
FORAYS
GODEYS
HOMEYS
HONEYS
LOOEYS
LOVEYA
LOVEYS
MONEYS
MOODYS
MORAYS
MOSEYS
NOMAYO
NOWAYS
POBOYS
POKEYS
POPEYE
PORKYS
ROCKYV
ROSLYN
SOONYI
TODAYS
TOKAYS
TOLDYA

•O•••Y
BOBBLY
BODILY
BODLEY
BOESKY
BOLDLY
BOLSHY
BOMBAY
BONNEY
BOSLEY
BOSOMY
BOTANY
BOTCHY
BOTFLY
BOUNCY
BOUNTY
BOVARY
BOWERY
BOXBOY
BOXILY
BOYTOY
CODIFY
CODYWY
COLDLY
COLONY
COMEBY
COMEDY
COMELY
COMITY
COMPLY
CONROY
CONVEY
CONVOY
CONWAY
COOLEY
COOLLY
COONEY
COPLEY
CORDAY
COSILY
COSTLY
COUNTY
COWBOY
COWLEY
COZILY
DOCBOY
DOESBY
DOGDAY
DOGTOY
DOLLEY
DOMBEY
DONEBY
DONKEY
DOOLEY
DOPILY
DORSAY
DORSEY
DOUBLY
DOUGHY
DOURLY
DOWERY
DOWNEY
DOZILY
FOLKSY
FONDLY
FORJOY
FORWHY
FOSSEY
FOULLY
FOXILY
GOALBY
GOAWAY
GOAWRY
GOEASY
GOESBY
GOGGLY
GONEBY
GOODBY
GOODLY
GOOGLY
GOONEY
GOOSEY
GORCEY
GORILY
HOCKEY
HOKILY
HOLILY
HOLLEY
HOMELY
HOMILY
HOMINY
HOOKEY
HOORAY
HORNBY
HORSEY
HOSTLY
HOTDAY
HOTKEY
HOUNDY
HOURLY
JOCKEY
JOHNNY
JOKILY
JOLLEY
JONESY
JOUNCY
KODALY
LOGILY
LONELY
LONGLY
LOONEY
LOOSEY
LORDLY
LOUDLY
LOVELY
LOWBOY
LOWERY
LOWKEY
MOBLEY
MODIFY
MOIETY
MOLLOY
MONDAY
MONKEY
MONODY
MOONEY
MOPERY
MORLEY
MORNAY
MOSLEY
MOSTLY
MOTLEY
MOULDY
MOUNTY
MOUSEY
MOUTHY
NOBODY
NONARY
NORGAY
NORWAY
NOSILY
NOTANY
NOTARY
NOTCHY
NOTIFY
OOLOGY
OOZILY
POACHY
POETRY
POINTY
POKERY
POKILY
POLICY
POLITY
POMPEY
POORLY
POPFLY
PORTLY
POSHLY
POUCHY
POUFFY
ROBROY
RODEBY
RODNEY
ROLLBY
ROMANY
ROMNEY
RONCEY
RONELY
ROONEY
ROOTSY
ROPERY
ROSARY
ROSERY
ROSILY
ROSINY
ROTARY
ROWLEY
SOFTLY
SOLELY
SOMANY
SORELY
SOURLY
TOASTY
TOMBOY
TOOMEY
TOOTHY
TOOTSY
TORBAY
TORCHY
TORREY
TOUCHY
TOUGHY
TOWERY
VOLLEY
VOTARY
VOWELY
WOBBLY
WOLSEY
WOODSY
WOOLEY
WOOLLY
WOOTSY
WORLEY
WORTHY

••OY••
BUOYED
BUOYUP
CLOYED
EGOYAN
FROYOS
LLOYDS
PROYAS
TROYER
TROYNY

••O•Y•
ANONYM
AZODYE
CRONYN
EMORYU
EPONYM
EUONYM
EXONYM
INOUYE
LOOEYS
MOODYS
PROPYL
SOONYI
ZLOTYS

••O••Y
BIOPSY
BLOBBY
BLOCKY
BLOODY
BLOOEY
BLOOMY
BLOTTY
BLOWSY
BLOWZY
BROLLY
BRONZY
BROODY
BROOKY
BROOMY
BROPHY
BROTHY
BROWNY
CHOOSY
CHOPPY
CLODDY
CLOGGY
CLOTTY
CLOUDY
COOLEY
COOLLY
COONEY
CROAKY
CROSBY
CROUPY
DOOLEY
DROLLY
DROOLY
DROOPY
DROPBY
DROPSY
DROSSY
DROWSY
FLOATY
FLOOEY
FLOPPY
FLOPSY
FLOREY
FLOSSY
FLOURY
FROGGY
FROSTY
FROTHY
FROWZY
GEORGY
GHOSTY
GLOBBY
GLOOMY
GLOPPY
GLOSSY
GOODBY
GOODLY
GOOGLY
GOONEY
GOOSEY
GROGGY
GROOVY
GROSZY
GROTTY
GROUTY
GROWLY
GROZNY
HOOKEY
HOORAY
IFONLY
IFORTY
IMOKAY
KNOBBY
KNOLLY
KNOTTY
LIONLY
LOONEY
LOOSEY
MEOHMY
MOONEY
MYOHMY
NFORTY
PHONEY
PHOOEY
PLOTTY
POORLY
PROSKY
PTOOEY
ROONEY
ROOTSY
SCOOBY
SCOTTY
SHOALY
SHODDY
SHORTY
SHOTBY
SLOBBY
SLOOPY
SLOPPY
SLOSHY
SLOWLY
SMOGGY
SMOKEY
SNOBBY
SNOOPY
SNOOTY
SNOOZY
SNORTY
SPONGY
SPOOKY
SPOONY
SPORTY
SPOTTY
STOCKY
STODGY
STONEY
STOOLY
STOPBY
STORMY
THORNY
TOOMEY
TOOTHY
TOOTSY
TROPHY
TROYNY
TWODAY
TWOPLY
TWOWAY
UNOILY
WHOLLY
WOODSY
WOOLEY
WOOLLY
WOOTSY

•••OY•
AJFOYT
ALLOYS
ANNOYS
ARROYO
DECOYS
ENJOYS
ENVOYS
LATOYA
NAGOYA
POBOYS
SEPOYS

•••O•Y
ANTONY
ARGOSY
ARMORY
BARONY
BETONY
BLOODY
BLOOEY
BLOOMY
BOSOMY
BROODY
BROOKY
BROOMY
CALORY
CANOPY
CHOOSY
CHROMY
COLONY
DIPODY
DROOLY
DROOPY
ECTOMY
EMBODY
EULOGY
FELONY
FLOOEY
GLOOMY
GROOVY
IDIOCY
JACOBY
JALOPY
KIDORY
LEMONY
MALORY
MELODY
MEMORY
MONODY
NOBODY
ONIONY
OOLOGY
PARODY
PHOOEY
PRIORY
PTOOEY
RECOPY
SAVORY
SAXONY
SCOOBY
SLOOPY
SNOOPY
SNOOTY
SNOOZY
SPOOKY
SPOONY
STOOLY
THEORY
UNFOXY
UNHOLY
VAPORY

••••OY
BADBOY
BAGBOY
BATBOY
BIGBOY
BOXBOY
BOYTOY
BUGBOY
BUSBOY
CAMBOY
CARBOY
CATTOY
CONROY
CONVOY
COWBOY
DELROY
DEPLOY
DOCBOY
DOGTOY
EMPLOY
FLYBOY
FORJOY
GILROY
KILROY
LACHOY
LAZBOY
LOWBOY
MCAVOY
MOLLOY
NEWTOY
OLDBOY
PEPBOY
PETTOY
PINBOY
QUEMOY
ROBROY
STEFOY
TEAPOY
THETOY
TOMBOY

OZ••••
OZARKS
OZONIC

O•Z•••
OOZIER
OOZILY
OOZING
OUZELS

O••Z••
OROZCO
OYEZES

•OZ•••
COZENS
COZIED
COZIER
COZIES
COZILY
COZYUP
DOZENS
DOZERS
DOZIER
DOZILY
DOZING
FOZZIE
JOZSEF
MOZART
NOZZLE
OOZIER
OOZILY
OOZING
POZNAN
POZOLE

•O•Z••
BONZES
BOOZED
BOOZER
BOOZES
BORZOI
BOWZER
DOOZER
DOOZIE
DOUZES
FONZIE
FOOZLE
FOZZIE
MONZAS
NOZZLE
PONZUS
YOWZAH

•O••Z•
CORYZA
IODIZE
IONIZE

•O•••Z
BONERZ
BOULEZ
COMPOZ
CORTEZ
DOLENZ
DONITZ
HORMUZ
KOONTZ
LORENZ
MONTEZ
MORITZ

••OZ••
BOOZED
BOOZER
BOOZES
DOOZER
DOOZIE
FOOZLE
FROZEN
GROZNY
GYOZAS
OROZCO
PROZAC

••O•Z•
ALONZO
BLOWZY
BRONZE
BRONZY
FROWZY
GROSZY
LAONZA
LAOTZU
SFORZA
SNOOZE
SNOOZY

••O••Z
AMOSOZ
KOONTZ
SHORTZ
STOLTZ
TROPEZ

•••OZ•
REBOZO
SNOOZE
SNOOZY

•••O•Z
MILOSZ

••••OZ
AMOSOZ
COMPOZ
SCHNOZ

PA••••
PAANGA
PABLUM
PABSTS
PACERS
PACHIN
PACIER
PACIFY
PACING
PACINO
PACKED
PACKER
PACKET
PACKIN
PACKON
PACKUP
PACMAN
PACTEN
PACULA
PADDED
PADDER
PADDLE
PADOVA
PADRES
PADUAN
PAEANS
PAELLA
PAGANS
PAGERS
PAGEUP
PAGING
PAGLIA
PAGNOL
PAGODA
PAIDAD
PAIDIN
PAIDUP
PAINED
PAINTS
PAINTY
PAIRED
PAIRUP
PAISAN

PAISES
PAIUTE
PAJAMA
PAJOAD
PAKULA
PALACE
PALADE
PALAIS
PALATE
PALEAE
PALELY
PALEST
PALING
PALISH
PALLAS
PALLED
PALLET
PALLID
PALLOR
PALMAR
PALMAS
PALMED
PALMER
PALOMA
PALTER
PALTRY
PAMELA
PAMINA
PAMIRS
PAMPAS
PAMPER
PANADA
PANAMA
PANCHO
PANCKS
PANDAS
PANDER
PANDIT
PANDLS
PANELS
PANFRY
PANFUL
PANICS
PANIER
PANINI
PANINO
PANNED
PANNER
PANNES
PANOPE
PANOUT
PANSIN
PANTED
PANTER
PANTIE
PANTOS
PANTRY
PANZER
PAPACY
PAPAGO
PAPAWS
PAPAYA
PAPERS
PAPERY
PAPIER
PAPIST
PAPPAS
PAPUAN
PAPYRI
PAQUIN
PARADE
PARANA
PARAPH
PARCAE
PARCEL
PARDON
PARENS
PARENT
PARERS
PARETO
PAREUS
PAREVE
PARFUM
PARGED
PARGER
PARGES
PARIAH
PARING
PARINI
PARISH
PARITY
PARKAS
PARKAV
PARKAY
PARKED
PARKER
PARKES
PARKIT
PARLAY
PARLEY
PARLEZ
PARLOR
PARNIS
PARODY
PAROLE
PAROLS
PARRED
PARRIS
PARROT
PARSEC
PARSED
PARSEE
PARSER
PARSES
PARSON
PARTED
PARTII
PARTIV
PARTLY
PARTOF
PARTON
PARTYS
PARURE
PASCAL
PASCHS
PASCUA
PASDAR
PASEOS
PASHAS
PASHTO
PASMOI
PASSAS
PASSAT
PASSBY
PASSED
PASSEL
PASSER
PASSES
PASSGO
PASSIM
PASSON
PASSOS
PASSTO
PASSUP
PASTAS
PASTED
PASTEL
PASTER
PASTES
PASTIS
PASTIT
PASTOR
PASTRY
PATACA
PATAKI
PATCHY
PATDAY
PATDRY
PATENS
PATENT
PATERS
PATHAN
PATHIC
PATHOS
PATINA
PATINE
PATIOS
PATMOS
PATOIS
PATRIA
PATRIC
PATRIE
PATROL
PATRON
PATTED
PATTEN
PATTER
PATTIE
PATTON
PATZER
PAULEY
PAULII
PAULIV
PAULVI
PAUNCH
PAUPER
PAUSAL
PAUSED
PAUSER
PAUSES
PAVANE
PAVERS
PAVESE
PAVING
PAVIOR
PAVLOV
PAWERS
PAWING
PAWNED
PAWNEE
PAWNER
PAWPAW
PAWSAT
PAXTON
PAYCUT
PAYDAY
PAYEES
PAYERS
PAYFOR
PAYING
PAYNOW
PAYOFF
PAYOLA
PAYOUT
PAYPAL
PAYSIN
PAYSON
PAYSUP
PAYTON

P•A•••

PAANGA
PBANDJ
PEACHY
PEAHEN
PEAKED
PEALED
PEALER
PEALES
PEANUT
PEAPOD
PEARCE
PEARLE
PEARLS
PEARLY
PGAPRO
PHAGIA
PHAROS
PHASED
PHASER
PHASES
PHASIC
PIAFFE
PIAGET
PIANOS
PIAZZA
PIAZZI
PLACED
PLACER
PLACES
PLACID
PLAGES
PLAGUE
PLAICE
PLAIDS
PLAINS
PLAINT
PLAITS
PLAKAT
PLANAR
PLANAS
PLANBS
PLANCK
PLANED
PLANER
PLANES
PLANET
PLANKS
PLANON
PLANTE
PLANTO
PLANTS
PLAQUE
PLASHY
PLASMA
PLASMO
PLATED
PLATEN
PLATER
PLATES
PLATOS
PLATTE
PLATYS
PLAYAS
PLAYAT
PLAYBY
PLAYED
PLAYER
PLAYIT
PLAYON
PLAYTO
PLAYUP
PLAZAS
POACHY
PRADAS
PRAGUE
PRAISE
PRANAS
PRANCE
PRANKS
PRATED
PRATER
PRATES
PRAVDA
PRAWER
PRAWNS
PRAXES
PRAXIS
PRAYED
PRAYER
PRAYTO
PSALMS

P••A••

PAEANS
PAGANS
PAJAMA
PALACE
PALADE
PALAIS
PALATE
PANADA
PANAMA
PAPACY
PAPAGO
PAPAWS
PAPAYA
PCLABS
PECANS
PEDALS
PEDANT
PEDATE
PELAGE
PESACH
PESADE
PETAIN
PETALE
PETALS
PETARD
PHIALS
PHRASE
PICABO
PICARA
PICARD
PICARO
PILAFS
PILATE
PILAUS
PINATA
PIPAGE
PIRACY
PIRANA
PIRATE
PISANO
PISANS
PITAYA
PIZAZZ
PLEADS
PLEASE
PLEATS
PLIANT
POEANA
POLAND
POLARA
POMADE
POPART
POSADA
POTAGE
POTASH
POTATO
PREACH
PREACT
PREAGE
PREAMP
PREARM
PROAMS
PROART
PSHAWS
PTRAPS
PUPATE

P•••A•

PACMAN
PADUAN
PAIDAD
PAISAN
PAJOAD
PALEAE
PALLAS
PALMAR
PALMAS
PAMPAS
PANDAS
PAPPAS
PAPUAN
PARCAE
PARIAH
PARKAS
PARKAV
PARKAY
PARLAY
PASCAL
PASDAR
PASHAS
PASSAS
PASSAT
PASTAS
PATDAY
PATHAN
PAUSAL
PAWPAW
PAWSAT
PAYDAY
PAYPAL
PECKAT
PEDWAY
PEEKAT
PEEPAT
PEERAT
PELHAM
PELLAM
PENMAN
PENPAL
PENTAD
PENTAX
PERDAY
PETCAT
PETNAP
PETRAT
PETSAT
PICKAT
PICKAX
PIEMAN
PIEPAN
PIETAS
PIGMAN
PILLAR
PINCAY
PINDAR
PINEAL
PINNAE
PINNAS
PINOAK
PISGAH
PITMAN
PITSAW
PIZZAS
PLAKAT
PLANAR
PLANAS
PLAYAS
PLAYAT
PLAZAS
PLEIAD
PLEXAL
PLURAL
POKEAT
POLEAX
POLGAR
POLKAS
POLLAK
PONCAS
POORAT
POPLAR
POPPAS
PORTAL
POSEAS
POSTAL
POZNAN
PRADAS
PRANAS
PREDAY
PREFAB
PRELAW
PREPAY
PRETAX
PREWAR
PRIMAL
PROTAX
PROWAR
PROYAS
PROZAC
PSYWAR
PTBOAT
PULSAR
PUNJAB
PUNKAS
PUNTAS
PUTNAM

P••••A

PAANGA
PACULA
PADOVA
PAELLA
PAGLIA
PAGODA
PAJAMA
PAKULA
PALOMA
PAMELA
PAMINA
PANADA
PANAMA
PAPAYA
PARANA
PASCUA
PATACA
PATINA
PATRIA
PAYOLA
PELOTA
PENNIA
PEORIA
PEPITA
PERCHA
PERLEA
PERSIA
PESETA
PESEWA
PETBOA
PETIPA
PETULA
PHAGIA
PHOBIA
PIAZZA
PICARA
PIERIA
PINATA
PIRANA
PITAYA
PLASMA
PLEURA
PLUVIA
PNEUMA
POEANA
POINTA
POISHA
POLARA
POLSKA
POMONA
PORTIA
POSADA
PRAVDA
PREVIA
PROTEA
PUEBLA
PURINA

•PA•••

APACHE
APATHY
EPACTS
EPARCH
OPAQUE
SPACED
SPACEK
SPACER
SPACES
SPACEY
SPADED
SPADER
SPADES
SPANKS
SPANKY
SPARED
SPARER
SPARES
SPARKS
SPARKY
SPARSE
SPARTA
SPASMS
SPATES
SPATHE
SPAWNS
SPAYED
SPAYER

•P•A••

APIARY
APPALL
APPALS
EPHAHS
OPIATE
OPRAHS
SPEAKS
SPEARE
SPEARS
SPLASH
SPLATS
SPLAYS
SPRACH
SPRAIN
SPRANG
SPRATS
SPRAWL
SPRAYS
UPCARD
UPCAST
UPDART
UPDATE
UPGAZE
UPLAND
UPLAST
UPLATE
UPRATE
UPSALA
UPTAKE
UPTALK
UPWAFT
UPWARD

•P••A•

APEMAN
APICAL
APNEAS
APODAL
APPEAL
APPEAR
APPIAN
EPICAL
EPINAL
IPECAC
OPERAS
SPINAL
SPIRAL
SPIVAK
SPREAD
SPYCAM
UPBEAR
UPBEAT
UPHEAP
UPLEAP
UPLOAD
UPREAR
UPROAR
UPSHAW
UPSOAR
UPTEAR

•P•••A

APOPKA
APULIA
OPTIMA
SPARTA
SPIREA
UPSALA

••PA••

ALPACA
APPALL
APPALS
AUPAIR
BYPASS
BYPAST
BYPATH
COPALS
COPAYS
DEPART
DEPAUL
DEPAUW
ELPAIS
ELPASO
EMPALE
EMPATH
ESPANA
EXPAND
EXPATS
EZPASS
GOPAST
HEPATO
IMPACT
IMPAIR
IMPALA
IMPALE
IMPART
INPARK
INPART
INPAWN
JAPANS
LIPARI
LIPASE
MRPAWS
NAPACA
NAPALM
NEPALI
NOPALS
PAPACY
PAPAGO
PAPAWS
PAPAYA
PIPAGE
POPART
PUPATE
REPACK
REPADS
REPAGE
REPAID
REPAIR
REPANE
REPARK
REPASS
REPAST
REPAVE
REPAYS
RVPARK
SEPALS
STPATS
STPAUL
UNPACK
UNPAID
UNPALE
UNPAWN
ZAPATA

••P•A•

ALPHAS
APPEAL
APPEAR
APPIAN
ATPLAY
BYPLAY
CEPHAL
COPCAR
COPRAS
CUPPAS
ESPIAL
GAPEAT
HEPCAT
HEPTAD
HUPPAH
INPLAY
KAPLAN
KAPPAS
KEPTAT
LAPCAT
LAPHAM
LAPSAT
NEPEAN
NIPSAT
OMPHAL
ORPHAN
PAPPAS
PAPUAN
POPLAR
POPPAS
REPEAL
REPEAT
REPLAN
REPLAY
RIPRAP
RIPSAW
RUPIAH
SEPIAS
SEPTAL
SUPRAS
TAPPAN
TIPJAR
TOPCAT
TOPHAT
TOPMAN
TYPEAB
TYPEAS
UNPLAN
YAPSAT

••P••A

ALPACA
ASPERA
CAPITA
CEPEDA
COPULA
CUPOLA
ESPANA
ESPOSA
EUPNEA
IMPALA
LAPUTA
NAPACA
NAPHTA
PAPAYA
PEPITA
SEPHIA
SEPIRA
SOPHIA
TOPEKA
ZAPATA

•••PA•

ASHPAN
BEAPAL
BEEPAT
BHOPAL
CARPAL
CARPAT
CASPAR
COMPAQ
COMPAS
CUPPAS
CUSPAL
DEEPAK
FRYPAN
GALPAL
GASPAR
HUPPAH
INKPAD
INSPAN
ITSPAT
JALPAS
JOYPAD
JUMPAT
KAPPAS
KEEPAT
KEYPAD
KEYPAL
LEAPAT
NETPAY
NONPAR
OILPAN
OLDPAL
ONAPAR
OOMPAH
OUTPAY
PAMPAS
PAPPAS
PAWPAW
PAYPAL
PEEPAT
PENPAL
PIEPAN
POPPAS
PREPAY
QUAPAW
RAMPAL
RASPAS
RESPAN
RIBPAD
RIOPAN
SAIPAN
SAMPAN
SATPAT
SHOPAT
SITPAT
SNAPAT
SOSPAD
STOPAT
STUPAS
SUBPAR
TAIPAN
TAPPAN
TINPAN
TREPAN
UNSPAN
VESPAS
VORPAL

•••P•A

APOPKA
CHOPRA
CHUPPA
COWPEA
GRAPPA
HOOPLA
MYOPIA
UTOPIA

••••PA

CHUPPA
DAYSPA
ERIEPA
EUROPA
GRAMPA
GRANPA
GRAPPA
JALAPA
LOOMPA
MACAPA
PETIPA
SHERPA
THEEPA
YORKPA

PB••••

PBANDJ
PBOOKS

P•B•••

PABLUM
PABSTS
PEBBLE
PEBBLY
POBOYS
PTBOAT
PUBLIC
PUBLIX

P••B••

PEBBLE
PEBBLY
PEGBOX
PEPBOY
PETBOA
PHOBIA
PHOBIC
PHOBOS
PINBOY
PLEBES
PREBID
PREBUY
PROBED
PROBER
PROBES
PROBIE
PROBST
PUEBLA
PUEBLO

P•••B•

PASSBY
PCLABS
PHILBY
PHLEBO
PHOEBE
PICABO
PLANBS
PLAYBY
PLUMBO
PLUMBS
PUTSBY

P••••B

POINTB
PREFAB
PUNJAB

•PB•••

UPBEAR
UPBEAT
UPBIND
UPBOWS

•P•B••

SPYBOT

•P•••B

APLOMB

••PB••

PEPBOY
TOPBID

••P•B•

MRPIBB
REPUBS
TYPEBS
ZIPSBY

••P••B

MRPIBB
NOPROB
SUPERB
TOPJOB
TYPEAB

•••PB•

DROPBY
SKIPBY
SLIPBY
STOPBY

PC••••

PCLABS
PCUSER

P•C•••

PACERS
PACHIN
PACIER
PACIFY
PACING
PACINO
PACKED
PACKER
PACKET
PACKIN
PACKON
PACKUP
PACMAN
PACTEN
PACULA
PECANS
PECHES
PECKAT
PECKED
PECTIN
PICABO
PICARA
PICARD
PICARO
PICCHU
PICHEL
PICKAT
PICKAX
PICKED
PICKER
PICKET
PICKLE
PICKON
PICKUP
PICNIC
PICONE
PICOTS

PICRIC
PICTOR
POCKET
POCONO
PUCCIS
PUCKER

P••C••

PANCHO
PANCKS
PARCAE
PARCEL
PASCAL
PASCHS
PASCUA
PATCHY
PAYCUT
PEACHY
PENCHE
PENCIL
PEPCID
PERCHA
PESCOW
PETCAT
PETCOW
PICCHU
PIECED
PIECER
PIECES
PINCAY
PINCER
PISCES
PITCHY
PLACED
PLACER
PLACES
PLACID
PLOCES
PLUCKS
PLUCKY
POACHY
PONCAS
PONCHO
POUCHY
PRECIP
PRECIS
PRECUT
PRICED
PRICER
PRICES
PRICEY
PRICKS
PROCOL
PSYCHE
PSYCHO
PSYCHS
PUCCIS
PUNCHY

P•••C•

PALACE
PANICS
PAPACY
PATACA
PAUNCH
PEARCE
PEERCE
PEIRCE
PENICK
PESACH
PHILCO
PIERCE
PIRACY
PLAICE
PLANCK
POLICE
POLICY
POUNCE
POVICH
PRANCE
PREACH
PREACT
PRINCE
PUMICE
PUTSCH

P••••C

PARSEC
PATHIC
PATRIC
PELVIC
PEPTIC
PHASIC
PHILIC
PHOBIC
PHONIC
PHOTIC
PHYSIC
PICNIC
PICRIC
POETIC
PROZAC
PUBLIC

•PC•••

OPCITS
UPCARD
UPCAST
UPCOIL
UPCURL

•P•C••

APACHE
APICAL
APICES
EPACTS
EPICAL
EPOCHS
IPECAC
SPACED
SPACEK
SPACER
SPACES
SPACEY
SPECIE
SPECKS
SPICED
SPICER
SPICES
SPYCAM

•P••C•

APERCU
APIECE
EPARCH
OPTICS
SPEECH
SPENCE
SPLICE
SPRACH
SPRUCE
UPTICK

•P•••C

EPODIC
IPECAC

••PC••

COPCAR
HEPCAT
LAPCAT
PEPCID
TOPCAT

••P•C•

ALPACA
ASPECT
ASPICS
DEPICT
EXPECT
IMPACT
KOPECK
NAPACA
PAPACY
REPACK
REPICK
TOPICS
UNPACK
UNPICK

••P••C

COPTIC
CUPRIC
ORPHIC
PEPTIC
SEPTIC
ZIPLOC

•••PC•

IBMPCS

•••P•C

ATYPIC
BIOPIC
LOMPOC
MYOPIC
ONSPEC
TROPIC
UNEPIC

PD••••

PDIDDY

P•D•••

PADDED
PADDER
PADDLE
PADOVA
PADRES
PADUAN
PEDALS
PEDANT
PEDATE
PEDDLE
PEDWAY
PIDDLE
PIDGIN
PODDED
PODIUM
PODOUS
PODUNK
PUDDLE
PUDDLY

P••D••

PADDED
PADDER
PADDLE
PAIDAD
PAIDIN
PAIDUP
PANDAS
PANDER
PANDIT
PANDLS
PARDON
PASDAR
PATDAY
PATDRY
PAYDAY
PDIDDY
PEDDLE
PEEDEE
PENDED
PERDAY
PERDUE
PETDOG
PHEDRE
PIDDLE
PINDAR
PINDUS
PLEDGE
PLEDTO
PODDED
PONDED
PONDER
POODLE
POUDRE
POWDER
PRADAS
PREDAY
PREDRY
PRIDED
PRIDES
PRODON
PRUDES
PUDDLE
PUDDLY
PUNDIT
PURDUE
PYEDOG

P•••D•

PAGODA
PALADE
PANADA
PARADE
PARODY
PBANDJ
PDIDDY
PESADE
PLAIDS
PLEADS
POMADE
POSADA
POUNDS
PRAVDA
PSEUDO
PSEUDS

P••••D

PACKED
PADDED
PAIDAD
PAINED
PAIRED
PAJOAD
PALLED
PALLID
PALMED
PANNED
PANTED
PARGED
PARKED
PARRED
PARSED
PARTED
PASSED
PASTED
PATTED
PAUSED
PAWNED
PEAKED
PEALED
PEAPOD
PECKED
PEEKED
PEELED
PEENED
PEEPED
PEERED
PEEVED
PEGGED
PELTED
PENDED
PENNED
PENROD
PENTAD
PEPCID
PEPPED
PEQUOD
PERIOD
PERKED
PERMED
PERNOD
PETARD
PETTED
PHASED
PHONED
PHYSED
PICARD
PICKED
PIECED
PIGGED
PILLED
PINGED
PINKED
PINNED
PIQUED
PISHED
PITHED
PITIED
PITTED
PLACED
PLACID
PLANED
PLATED
PLAYED
PLEIAD
PLOWED
PLUMED
PODDED
POISED
POLAND
POLLED
PONDED
PONGID
PONIED
POOHED
POOLED
POOPED
POPPED
PORKED
PORTED
POSTED
POTLID
POTTED
POUFED
POURED
POUTED
PRATED
PRAYED
PREBID
PREMED
PREYED
PRICED
PRIDED
PRIMED
PRISED
PRIZED
PROBED
PROSED
PROVED
PRUNED
PUFFED
PULLED
PULPED
PULSED
PUMPED
PUNNED
PUNTED
PUPPED
PUREED
PURGED
PURLED
PURRED
PURSED
PUSHED
PUTRID
PUTTED

•PD•••

KPDUTY
UPDART
UPDATE
UPDIKE
UPDIVE
UPDOVE

•P•D••

APODAL
EPODES
EPODIC
SPADED
SPADER
SPADES
SPEDUP
SPIDER
SPIDEY
SPODES
SPYDER

•P••D•

APHIDS
EPHODS
SPEEDO
SPEEDS
SPEEDY
SPENDS
SPENDY
UPENDS
UPSIDE

•P•••D

APPEND
OPENED
OPINED
SPACED
SPADED
SPARED
SPAYED
SPEWED
SPICED
SPIKED
SPINED
SPIRED
SPITED
SPOKED
SPREAD
SPUMED
UPBIND
UPCARD
UPFOLD
UPGIRD
UPHELD
UPHOLD
UPLAND
UPLOAD
UPSEND
UPWARD
UPWIND

••PD••

LAPDOG
TOPDOG

••P•D•

BIPEDS
BIPODS
CEPEDA
CUPIDS
DIPODY
IMPEDE
LIPIDS
MOPEDS
OOPODS
RAPIDO
RAPIDS
REPADS

••P••D

APPEND
BOPPED
CAPPED
CAPRID
COPIED
COPPED
CUPPED
DAPPED
DEPEND
DIPPED
ESPIED
EXPAND
EXPEND
GAPPED
GYPPED
HEPTAD
HIPPED
HOPPED
HYPOED
IMPEND
IMPLED
KIPPED
LAPPED
LAPSED
LIPPED
LOPPED
MAPPED
MOPPED
NAPPED
NIPPED
PEPCID
PEPPED
POPPED
PUPPED
RAPPED
REPAID
REPLED
REPPED
RIPPED
SAPPED
SIPPED
SOPPED
SUPPED
TAPPED
TIPPED
TOPBID
TOPPED
UNPAID
YAPPED
YIPPED
ZAPPED
ZIPPED

•••P•D

ALIPED
BEEPED
BOPPED
BUMPED
BURPED
CAMPED
CAPPED
CARPED
COMPED
COOPED
COPPED
CRAPED
CREPED
CUPPED
CUSPED
CUSPID
DAMPED
DAPPED
DIPPED
DRAPED
DUMPED
ELAPID
ELOPED
GAPPED
GASPED
GAWPED
GIMPED
GRIPED
GROPED
GULPED
GYPPED
HARPED
HASPED
HEAPED
HELPED
HIPPED
HOOPED
HOPPED
HUMPED
INAPOD
INKPAD
ISOPOD
JOYPAD
JUMPED
KEYPAD
KIPPED
LAPPED
LEAPED
LIMPED
LIMPID
LIPPED
LISPED
LOOPED
LOPPED
LUMPED
MAPPED
MOPPED
NAPPED
NIPPED
PEAPOD
PEEPED
PEPPED
POOPED
POPPED
PULPED
PUMPED
PUPPED
RAMPED
RAPPED
RASPED
REAPED
REPPED
RIBPAD
RIPPED
ROMPED
RSVPED
SAPPED
SCOPED
SEEPED
SHAPED
SIPPED
SLOPED
SNIPED
SOAPED
SOPPED
SOSPAD
STUPID
SUPPED
SWIPED
TAMPED
TAPPED
TEMPED
TIPPED
TOPPED
TORPID
TREPID
TRIPOD
UNIPED
UNIPOD
VAMPED
VESPID
WARPED
WIMPED
WISPED
YAPPED
YAWPED
YELPED
YIPPED
ZAPPED
ZIPPED

PE••••

PEACHY
PEAHEN
PEAKED
PEALED
PEALER
PEALES
PEANUT
PEAPOD
PEARCE
PEARLE
PEARLS
PEARLY
PEBBLE
PEBBLY
PECANS
PECHES
PECKAT
PECKED
PECTIN
PEDALS
PEDANT
PEDATE
PEDDLE
PEDWAY
PEEDEE
PEEKAT
PEEKED
PEEKER
PEEKIN
PEELED
PEELER
PEENED
PEEPAT
PEEPED
PEEPER
PEERAT
PEERCE
PEERED
PEERIN
PEEVED
PEEVES
PEEWEE
PEGBOX
PEGEEN
PEGGED
PEGLEG
PEGLER
PEGTOP
PEIRCE
PEKING
PEKOES
PELAGE
PELEUS
PELHAM
PELION
PELLAM
PELLET
PELOSI
PELOTA
PELTED
PELTER
PELTRY
PELVIC
PELVIS
PENCHE
PENCIL
PENDED
PENGPU
PENICK
PENMAN
PENMEN
PENNED
PENNER
PENNEY
PENNIA
PENNIS
PENNON
PENPAL
PENROD
PENSEE
PENSIN
PENSUP
PENTAD
PENTAX
PENTEL
PENTUP
PENULT
PENURY
PEOPLE
PEORIA
PEPBOY
PEPCID
PEPFUL
PEPINO
PEPITA
PEPLUM
PEPPED
PEPPER
PEPSIN
PEPSUP
PEPTIC
PEQUOD
PEQUOT
PERCHA
PERDAY
PERDUE
PERILS
PERINE
PERIOD
PERISH
PERITI
PERKED
PERKIN
PERKUP
PERLEA
PERMED
PERMIT
PERNOD
PERRIN
PERROS
PERSIA
PERSIS
PERSON
PERTER
PERTLY
PERUKE
PERUSE
PERUTZ
PESACH
PESADE
PESCOW
PESETA
PESEWA
PESTER
PESTLE
PESTOS
PETAIN
PETALE
PETALS
PETARD
PETBOA
PETCAT
PETCOW
PETDOG
PETERI
PETERS
PETIPA
PETITE
PETNAP
PETPIG
PETPUP
PETRAT
PETREL
PETRIE
PETROL
PETSAT
PETSIT
PETTED
PETTER
PETTET
PETTIS
PETTIT
PETTOY
PETULA
PEVNEY
PEWEES
PEWITS
PEWTER
PEYOTE
PEYTON

P•E•••

PAEANS
PAELLA
PEEDEE
PEEKAT
PEEKED
PEEKER
PEEKIN
PEELED
PEELER
PEENED
PEEPAT
PEEPED
PEEPER
PEERAT
PEERCE
PEERED
PEERIN
PEEVED
PEEVES
PEEWEE
PHEDRE
PHELPS
PHENOL
PHENOM
PIECED
PIECER
PIECES
PIELET
PIEMAN
PIEMEN
PIEPAN
PIERCE
PIERIA
PIERRE
PIETAS
PIETER
PIETIN
PIETRO
PLEADS
PLEASE
PLEATS
PLEBES
PLEDGE
PLEDTO
PLEIAD
PLENTY
PLENUM
PLEURA
PLEXAL
PLEXES
PLEXOR
PLEXUS
PNEUMA
PNEUMO
POEANA
POEMES
POETES
POETIC
POETRY
PREACH
PREACT
PREAGE
PREAMP
PREARM
PREBID
PREBUY
PRECIP
PRECIS
PRECUT
PREDAY
PREDRY
PREENS
PREFAB
PREFER
PREFIX
PRELAW
PRELIM
PRELOG
PREMED
PREMET
PREMIE
PREMIX
PRENUP
PREOPS
PREPAY
PREPPY
PRESET
PRESTO
PRETAX
PRETER
PRETOR
PRETTY
PREVIA
PREVIN
PREVUE
PREWAR
PREXES
PREYED
PREYER
PREYON
PSEUDO
PSEUDS
PUEBLA
PUEBLO
PUENTE
PUENZO
PUERTO
PYEDOG

P••E••

PACERS
PAGERS
PAGEUP
PALEAE
PALELY
PALEST
PAMELA
PANELS
PAPERS
PAPERY
PARENS
PARENT
PARERS
PARETO
PAREUS
PAREVE
PASEOS
PATENS
PATENT
PATERS
PAVERS
PAVESE
PAWERS
PAYEES
PAYERS
PEGEEN
PELEUS
PESETA
PESEWA
PETERI
PETERS
PEWEES
PHLEBO
PHLEGM
PHOEBE
PIGEON
PIKERS
PILEIN
PILEON
PILERS
PILEUM
PILEUP
PILEUS
PINEAL
PINERO
PINERS
PINERY
PIPEIN
PIPERS
PIPETS
PIPEUP
PIXELS
PLIERS
POKEAT
POKERS
POKERY
POKEYS
POLEAX
POLERS
POMELO
POPEIL
POPEYE
PORERS
POSEAS
POSERS
POSEUR
POTEEN
POTENT
POWELL
POWERS
PREENS
PRIERS
PRIEST
PROEMS
PRUETT
PRYERS
PULERS
PUREED
PUREES
PURELY
PUREST

P•••E•

PACIER
PACKED
PACKER
PACKET
PACTEN
PADDED
PADDER
PADRES
PAINED
PAIRED

PAISES PALLED PALLET PALMED PALMER PALTER PAMPER PANDER PANIER PANNED PANNER PANNES PANTED PANTER PANZER PAPIER PARCEL PARGED PARGER PARGES PARKED PARKER PARKES PARLEY PARLEZ PARRED PARSEC PARSED PARSEE PARSER PARSES PARTED PASSED PASSEL PASSER PASSES PASTED PASTEL PASTER PASTES PATTED PATTEN PATTER PATZER PAULEY PAUPER PAUSED PAUSER PAUSES PAWNED PAWNEE PAWNER PAYEES PCUSER PEAHEN PEAKED PEALED PEALER PEALES PECHES PECKED PEEDEE PEEKED PEEKER PEELED PEELER PEENED PEEPED

PEEPER PEERED PEEVED PEEVES PEEWEE PEGEEN PEGGED PEGLEG PEGLER PEKOES PELLET PELTED PELTER PENDED PENMEN PENNED PENNER PENNEY PENSEE PENTEL PEPPED PEPPER PERKED PERLEA PERMED PERTER PESTER PETREL PETTED PETTER PETTET PEVNEY PEWEES PEWTER PFIZER PHASED PHASER PHASES PHLOEM PHONED PHONER PHONES PHONEY PHOOEY PHYSED PIAGET PICHEL PICKED PICKER PICKET PIECED PIECER PIECES PIELET PIEMEN PIETER PIGGED PIGLET PIGMEN PIGPEN PILFER PILLED PINCER PINGED PINGER PINIER PINKED PINKEN

PINKER PINNED PINNER PINTER PIOLET PIPIER PIPPET PIQUED PIQUES PIQUET PISCES PISHED PISHES PISTES PITHED PITIED PITIER PITIES PITMEN PITNEY PITTED PIUTES PIXIES PLACED PLACER PLACES PLAGES PLANED PLANER PLANES PLANET PLATED PLATEN PLATER PLATES PLAYED PLAYER PLEBES PLEXES PLOCES PLOMER PLOVER PLOWED PLOWER PLUIES PLUMED PLUMES PLUSES POCKET PODDED POEMES POETES POGNER POIRES POIRET POISED POISER POISES POKIER POKIES POLLED POLLEE POLLEN POLLER POLLEX POMMEL POMMES POMPEO

POMPEY PONDED PONDER PONGEE PONIED PONIES POOHED POOLED POOLER POOPED POORER POPPED POPPER PORKED PORKER PORTED PORTER PORTES POSHER POSIES POSSES POSTED POSTER POTEEN POTHER POTTED POTTER POUFED POULES POURED POURER POUTED POUTER POWDER POYSER PRATED PRATER PRATES PRAWER PRAXES PRAYED PRAYER PREFER PREMED PREMET PRESET PRETER PREXES PREYED PREYER PRICED PRICER PRICES PRICEY PRIDED PRIDES PRIMED PRIMER PRIMES PRISED PRIVET PRIZED PRIZES PROBED PROBER PROBES PROJET PROLES

PROPEL PROPER PROSED PROSER PROSES PROTEA PROTEM PROVED PROVEN PROVER PROVES PRUDES PRUNED PRUNER PRUNES PTILES PTOOEY PUCKER PUFFED PUFFER PULLED PULLER PULLET PULLEY PULPED PULPER PULSED PULSES PULVER PUMMEL PUMPED PUMPER PUNIER PUNKER PUNNED PUNNER PUNTED PUNTER PUPPED PUPPET PUREED PUREES PURGED PURGES PURLED PURRED PURRER PURSED PURSER PURSES PURVEY PUSHED PUSHER PUSHES PUSSES PUTNEY PUTTED PUTTEE PUTTER

P••••E

PADDLE PAIUTE PALACE PALADE PALATE PALEAE PANOPE PANTIE PARADE PARCAE PAREVE PAROLE PARSEE PARURE PATINE PATRIE PATTIE PAVANE PAVESE PAWNEE PEARCE PEARLE PEBBLE PEDATE PEDDLE PEEDEE PEERCE PEEWEE PEIRCE PELAGE PENCHE PENSEE PEOPLE PERDUE PERINE PERUKE PERUSE PESADE PESTLE PETALE PETITE PETRIE PEYOTE PHEDRE PHOEBE PHRASE PIAFFE PICKLE PICONE PIDDLE PIERCE PIERRE PIFFLE PIGGIE PILATE PILOSE PIMPLE PINKIE PINNAE PIPAGE PIRATE PLAGUE PLAICE PLANTE PLAQUE PLATTE PLEASE PLEDGE PLISSE PLUNGE POINTE POIVRE POLICE POLITE POLLEE POMADE PONGEE POODLE POPEYE POPPLE POROSE POSOLE POSTIE POTAGE POTPIE POTSIE POUDRE POUNCE POUSSE POZOLE PRAGUE PRAISE PRANCE PREAGE PREMIE PREVUE PRINCE PRINZE PROBIE PROPRE PROWSE PRYNNE PSYCHE PUDDLE PUENTE PUGGLE PUMICE PUNKIE PUPATE PURDUE PURFLE PURLIE PURPLE PURSUE PUTTEE PUZZLE PYRITE

•PE•••

APELET APEMAN APEMEN APERCU APEXES IPECAC IPETER OPENED OPENER OPENIT OPENLY OPENON OPENTO OPENUP OPERAS SPEAKS SPEARE SPEARS SPECIE SPECKS SPEDUP SPEECH SPEEDO SPEEDS SPEEDY SPELLS SPENCE SPENDS SPENDY SPERRY SPEWED SPEWER UPENDS

•P•E••

APIECE APNEAS APPEAL APPEAR APPELS APPEND APPERT APTEST SPEECH SPEEDO SPEEDS SPEEDY SPHERE SPIELS SPIERS SPLEEN SPREAD SPREES UPBEAR UPBEAT UPHEAP UPHELD UPHERE UPKEEP UPLEAP UPNEXT UPPERS UPREAR UPSEND UPSENT UPSETS UPTEAR UPWELL

•P••E•

APELET APEMEN APEXES APICES APOGEE APPLES APPLET EPODES EPOPEE EPOSES EPOWER IPETER OPENED OPENER OPINED OPINER OPINES OPUSES SPACED SPACEK SPACER SPACES SPACEY SPADED SPADER SPADES SPARED SPARER SPARES SPATES SPAYED SPAYER SPEWED SPEWER SPICED SPICER SPICES SPIDER SPIDEY SPIKED SPIKER SPIKES SPILES SPINED SPINEL SPINER SPINES SPINET SPIREA SPIRED SPIRES SPITED SPITES SPLEEN SPODES SPOKED SPOKEN SPOKES SPORES SPREES SPRIER SPRYER SPUMED SPUMES SPYDER UPGREW UPKEEP UPOVER UPSTEP

•P•••E

APACHE APIECE APLITE APOGEE APPOSE APRILE EPOPEE EPOQUE OPAQUE OPIATE OPPOSE SPARSE SPATHE SPEARE SPECIE SPENCE SPHERE SPLICE SPLINE SPONGE SPOUSE SPRITE SPRUCE UPDATE UPDIKE UPDIVE UPDOVE UPGAZE UPHERE UPHOVE UPLATE UPPILE UPRATE UPRISE UPROSE UPSIDE UPSIZE UPTAKE UPTIME UPTORE XPRIZE

••PE••

ALPERT AMPERE APPEAL APPEAR APPELS APPEND APPERT ARPEGE ARPELS ASPECT ASPENS ASPERA BIPEDS BOPEEP CAPERS CEPEDA COPERS CUPELS DEPEND DEPERE DEPEST DOPERS DUPERS DUPERY EMPERY EXPECT EXPELS EXPEND EXPERT GAPEAT GAPERS HOPERS HOPESO HOPETO HYPERS HYPEUP IMPEDE IMPELS IMPEND IMPERF JAPERS JAPERY KAPELL KOPECK KOPEKS KOPELL LAPELS LAPERI LAPERM LEPERS LIPENG LOPERS MOPEDS MOPERS MOPERY NAPERY NEPEAN NOPETS PAPERS PAPERY PIPEIN PIPERS PIPETS PIPEUP POPEIL POPEYE REPEAL REPEAT REPEGS REPELS REPENS REPENT REPERK RIPELY RIPENS RIPEST ROPEIN ROPERS ROPERY ROPEUP RUPEES RUPERT STPETE SUPERB SUPERG SUPERS TAPEON TAPERS TAPEUP TEPEES TOPEES TOPEKA TOPERS TUPELO TYPEAB TYPEAS TYPEBS TYPEIN TYPEOS TYPERS TYPEUP UNPEEL UNPEGS UNPENS UNPENT UPPERS VIPERS WIPERS WIPEUP

••P•E•

AMPLER APPLES APPLET BOPEEP BOPPED BOPPER BUPKES CAPLET CAPPED CAPPER CIPHER COPIED COPIER COPIES COPLEY COPPED COPPER COPSES COPTER CUPPED CYPHER DAPPED DAPPER DIPLEX DIPNET DIPPED DIPPER DOPIER DUPLEX ESPIED ESPIER ESPIES EUPNEA GAPPED GIPPER GOPHER GYPPED GYPPER HAPPEN HEPPER HIPPED HIPPER HOPPED HOPPER HYPHEN HYPOED IMPLED KEPLER KIPPED KIPPER KOPJES KOPPEL LAPPED LAPPER LAPPET LAPSED LAPSER LAPSES LAPTEV LIPPED LIPPER LOPPED LOPPER MAPLES MAPPED MAPPER MCPHEE MOPIER MOPPED MOPPER MOPPET MUPPET NAPIER NAPLES NAPPED NAPPER NAPPES NEPHEW NIPPED NIPPER NIPSEY OSPREY PAPIER PEPPED PEPPER PIPIER PIPPET POPPED POPPER PUPPED PUPPET RAPIER RAPPED RAPPEL RAPPER RAPTER REPLED REPPED RIPKEN RIPLEY RIPPED RIPPER ROPIER RUPEES SAPPED SAPPER SEPTET SIPPED SIPPER SOPPED SUPPED SUPPER TAPPED TAPPER TAPPET TEPEES TIPPED TIPPEE TIPPER TIPPET TOPEES TOPMEN TOPPED TOPPER TOPTEN TUPPER UNPEEL WAPNER YAPHET YAPPED YAPPER YIPPED YIPPEE ZAPPED ZAPPER ZIPPED ZIPPER

••P••E

ALPINE AMPERE AMPULE APPOSE ARPEGE ASPIRE ASPURE CAPONE CAPOTE CUPULE DAPHNE DAPPLE DEPERE DEPONE DEPOSE DEPUTE DIPOLE EMPALE EMPIRE EXPIRE EXPOSE FIPPLE HIPPIE IMPALE IMPEDE IMPOSE IMPURE IMPUTE LIPASE LUPINE LUPONE MAPPLE MCPHEE NAPPIE NIPPLE OPPOSE PIPAGE POPEYE POPPLE PUPATE RAPINE REPAGE REPANE REPAVE REPINE REPOSE REPUTE RIPPLE SOPHIE STPETE SUPINE SUPPLE TIPPEE TIPPLE TIPTOE TOPPLE UMPIRE UNPALE UNPILE UNPURE UPPILE YIPPEE YIPPIE YUPPIE

•••PE•

ALIPED AUSPEX BEEPED BEEPER BOPPED BOPPER BUMPED BUMPER BURPED BURPEE CAMPED CAMPER CAPPED CAPPER CARPED CARPEL CARPER CARPET CASPER CHAPEL COMPED COMPEL COOPED COOPER COPPED COPPER COUPES COWPEA COWPER CRAPED CRAPES CREPED CREPES CRIPES CUPPED CUSPED DAMPED DAMPEN DAMPER DAPPED DAPPER DEEPEN DEEPER DIAPER DIPPED DIPPER DISPEL DRAPED DRAPER DRAPES DRUPES DUMPED DUMPER ELOPED ELOPER ELOPES EPOPEE ETAPES GAPPED GASPED GASPER GAWPED GAWPER GELPEN GIMPED GIPPER GOSPEL GRAPES GRAPEY

GRIPED
GRIPER
GRIPES
GROPED
GROPER
GROPES
GULPED
GULPER
GYPPED
GYPPER
HAMPER
HAPPEN
HARPED
HARPER
HASPED
HEAPED
HEAPER
HELPED
HELPER
HEMPEN
HEPPER
HERPET
HIPPED
HIPPER
HOOPED
HOOPER
HOPPED
HOPPER
HUMPED
INAPET
JASPER
JUMPED
JUMPER
KEEPER
KIPPED
KIPPER
KOPPEL
LAPPED
LAPPER
LAPPET
LAUPER
LEAPED
LEAPER
LIMPED
LIMPER
LIMPET
LIPPED
LIPPER
LISPED
LISPER
LOOPED
LOOPER
LOPPED
LOPPER
LOUPES
LUMPED
LUMPEN
LUMPER
MAPPED
MAPPER
MOPPED
MOPPER
MOPPET
MUPPET
MYOPES
NAPPED
NAPPER
NAPPES
NIPPED
NIPPER
ONSPEC
PAMPER
PAUPER
PEEPED
PEEPER
PEPPED
PEPPER
PIGPEN
PIPPET
POMPEO
POMPEY
POOPED
POPPED
POPPER
PROPEL
PROPER
PULPED
PULPER
PUMPED
PUMPER
PUPPED
PUPPET
RAMPED
RAPPED
RAPPEL
RAPPER
RASPED
RASPER
REAPED
REAPER
REOPEN
REPPED
RIPPED
RIPPER
ROEPER
ROMPED
ROMPER
RSVPED
SAPPED
SAPPER
SCOPED
SCOPES
SEEPED
SEMPER
SHAPED
SHAPER
SHAPES
SIMPER
SIPPED
SIPPER
SLOPED
SLOPER
SLOPES
SNIPED
SNIPER
SNIPES
SNOPES
SOAPED
SOAPER
SOPPED
SOUPER
STAPES
STIPES
STUPES
SUPPED
SUPPER
SWIPED
SWIPER
SWIPES
TAIPEI
TAMPED
TAMPER
TAPPED
TAPPER
TAPPET
TAUPES
TEEPEE
TEMPED
TEMPEH
TEMPER
TIPPED
TIPPEE
TIPPER
TIPPET
TOPPED
TOPPER
TOUPEE
TRIPES
TROPES
TROPEZ
TUPPER
UNIPED
UNOPEN
USOPEN
VAMPED
VAMPER
VESPER
WARPED
WARPER
WEEPER
WIMPED
WISPED
WOLPER
XTYPES
YAPPED
YAPPER
YAWPED
YAWPER
YELPED
YELPER
YIPPED
YIPPEE
ZAPPED
ZAPPER
ZIPPED
ZIPPER

•••P•E

BURPEE
CORPSE
COUPLE
DAPPLE
DIEPPE
DIMPLE
ELAPSE
EPOPEE
FIPPLE
FRAPPE
GRIPPE
HELPME
HIPPIE
HOOPLE
HOOPOE
INAPIE
KELPIE
KEWPIE
MAGPIE
MAPPLE
MARPLE
MUDPIE
NAPPIE
NIPPLE
NTUPLE
PEOPLE
PIMPLE
POPPLE
POTPIE
PROPRE
PURPLE
RIMPLE
RIPPLE
RUMPLE
SAMPLE
SEMPLE
SEMPRE
SHOPPE
SIMPLE
SKOPJE
STAPLE
STEPPE
SUPPLE
TEEPEE
TEMPLE
TIPPEE
TIPPLE
TOPPLE
TOUPEE
TRIPLE
WIMPLE
YIPPEE
YIPPIE
YUPPIE

••••PE

ASLOPE
BIGAPE
CANAPE
DIEPPE
DOGAPE
ECTYPE
ESCAPE
EUROPE
FELIPE
FRAPPE
GRIPPE
LENAPE
MANAPE
MEROPE
NOHOPE
ONTAPE
PANOPE
RECIPE
RETAPE
RETYPE
REWIPE
SCOUPE
SCRAPE
SERAPE
SHARPE
SHOPPE
STEPPE
STRIPE
THEAPE
THORPE
TROMPE
TROUPE
TSHAPE
TVTAPE
UNRIPE
UNROPE
UNTAPE
USHAPE
VSHAPE
YSHAPE

PF••••

PFIZER

P•F•••

PHFFFT
PIFFLE
PRFIRM
PUFFED
PUFFER
PUFFIN
PUFFUP

P••F••

PANFRY
PANFUL
PARFUM
PAYFOR
PEPFUL
PHFFFT
PIAFFE
PIFFLE
PILFER
POPFLY
POTFUL
POUFED
POUFFY
PREFAB
PREFER
PREFIX
PROFIT
PUFFED
PUFFER
PUFFIN
PUFFUP
PURFLE

P•••F•

PACIFY
PAYOFF
PHFFFT
PIAFFE
PILAFS
POPOFF
POUFFY
PROOFS
PRYOFF
PURIFY
PUTOFF

P••••F

PARTOF
PAYOFF
POPOFF
PRYOFF
PUTOFF

•PF•••

UPFLOW
UPFOLD

•P•F••

OPTFOR
SPIFFS
SPIFFY

•P••F•

SPIFFS
SPIFFY
SPOOFS
UPLIFT
UPWAFT

••PF••

CAPFUL
CUPFUL
LAPFUL
PEPFUL
POPFLY
REPFOR

••P•F•

HOPOFF
LIPOFF
LOPOFF
POPOFF
RIPOFF
TAPOFF
TIPOFF
TOPOFF
TYPIFY
ZIPOFF

••P••F

HOPOFF
IMPERF
LIPOFF
LOPOFF
POPOFF
RIPOFF
TAPOFF
TIPOFF
TOPOFF
ZIPOFF

•••P•F

STAPUF

PG••••

PGAPRO

P•G•••

PAGANS
PAGERS
PAGEUP
PAGING
PAGLIA
PAGNOL
PAGODA
PEGBOX
PEGEEN
PEGGED
PEGLEG
PEGLER
PEGTOP
PIGEON
PIGGED
PIGGIE
PIGLET
PIGMAN
PIGMEN
PIGNUT
PIGOUT
PIGPEN
PIGSIT
PIGSTY
POGNER
PUGGLE

P••G••

PARGED
PARGER
PARGES
PEGGED
PENGPU
PHAGIA
PIAGET
PIDGIN
PIGGED
PIGGIE
PINGED
PINGER
PISGAH
PLAGES
PLAGUE
PLIGHT
PLUGIN
PLUGUP
POLGAR
PONGEE
PONGID
POPGUN
PRAGUE
PROGUN
PUGGLE
PURGED
PURGES

P•••G•

PAANGA
PAPAGO
PASSGO
PELAGE
PHLEGM
PIPAGE
PLEDGE
PLOUGH
PLUNGE
POTAGE
PREAGE
PRONGS

P••••G

PACING
PAGING
PALING
PARING
PAVING
PAWING
PAYING
PEGLEG
PEKING
PETDOG
PETPIG
PHOTOG
PIKING
PILING
PINING
PIPING
PLYING
POKING
POLING
PORING
POSING
PRELOG
PROLOG
PRYING
PULING
PYEDOG

•PG•••

UPGAZE
UPGIRD
UPGIRT
UPGREW
UPGROW

•P•G••

APOGEE
SPIGOT

•P••G•

OPPUGN
SPONGE
SPONGY
SPRIGS

•P•••G

EPILOG
EPPING
OPTING
SPRANG
SPRING
SPRUNG
SPYING
UPPING

••PG••

CAPGUN
POPGUN
TOPGUN
ZIPGUN

••P•G•

ARPEGE
IMPUGN
OPPUGN
PAPAGO
PIPAGE
REPAGE
REPEGS
REPUGN
UNPEGS

••P••G

AMPING
COPING
DOPING
DUPING
EPPING
GAPING
HOPING
HYPING
JAPING
LAPDOG
LIPENG
LOPING
MOPING
PIPING
ROPING
SUPERG
TAPING
TOPDOG
TOPING
TYPING
UMPING
UNPLUG
UPPING
WIPING

•••PG•

STOPGO

•••P•G

PETPIG

PH••••

PHAGIA
PHAROS
PHASED
PHASER
PHASES
PHASIC
PHEDRE
PHELPS
PHENOL
PHENOM
PHFFFT
PHIALS
PHILBY
PHILCO
PHILIC
PHILIP
PHILLY
PHLEBO
PHLEGM
PHLOEM
PHOBIA
PHOBIC
PHOBOS
PHOEBE
PHONED
PHONER
PHONES
PHONEY
PHONIC
PHONOS
PHOOEY
PHOTIC
PHOTOG
PHOTON
PHOTOS
PHRASE
PHYLLO
PHYLUM
PHYSED
PHYSIC
PHYSIO

P•H•••

PSHAWS

P••H••

PACHIN
PASHAS
PASHTO
PATHAN
PATHIC
PATHOS
PEAHEN
PECHES
PELHAM
PICHEL
PISHED
PISHES
PITHED
POOHED
POSHER
POSHLY
POTHER
POTHOS
PUSHED
PUSHER
PUSHES
PUSHIN
PUSHIT
PUSHON
PUSHUP
PYRHHO
PYTHON

P•••H•

PANCHO
PASCHS
PATCHY
PEACHY
PENCHE
PERCHA
PICCHU
PITCHY
PLASHY
PLIGHT
PLUSHY
POACHY
POISHA
PONCHO
POUCHY
PSYCHE
PSYCHO
PSYCHS
PUNCHY
PYRHHO

P••••H

PALISH
PARAPH
PARIAH
PARISH
PAUNCH
PERISH
PESACH
PISGAH
PLINTH
PLOUGH
POLISH
POPISH
POTASH
POVICH
PREACH
PUNISH
PUTSCH

•PH•••

APHIDS
EPHAHS
EPHODS
EPHORS
EPHRON
OPHULS
SPHERE
SPHINX
SPHYNX
UPHEAP
UPHELD
UPHERE
UPHILL
UPHOLD
UPHOVE

•P•H••

UPSHAW
UPSHOT

•P••H•

APACHE
APATHY
EPHAHS
EPOCHS
OPRAHS
SPATHE
UPJOHN

•P•••H

EPARCH
SPEECH
SPILTH
SPLASH
SPLOSH
SPRACH
UPPISH
UPRUSH

••PH••

ALPHAS
CEPHAL
CIPHER
CYPHER
DAPHNE
DRPHIL
GOPHER
HIPHOP
HYPHEN
LAPHAM
MCPHEE
NAPHTA
NEPHEW
NEPHRO
OMPHAL
ORPHAN
ORPHIC
SEPHIA
SIPHON
SOPHIA
SOPHIE
TOPHAT
TYPHUS
YAPHET
ZEPHYR

••P•H•

DEPTHS
SAPPHO

••P••H

ASPISH
BYPATH
EMPATH
HUPPAH
IMPISH
MOPISH
POPISH
RUPIAH
UNPOSH
UPPISH

•••PH•

ALEPHS
BROPHY
DELPHI
GLYPHS
GRAPHO
GRAPHS
GRAPHY
HUMPHS
LYMPHS
MORPHO
MORPHS
MURPHY
NYMPHS
OOMPHS
RALPHJ
SAPPHO
STAPHS
SYLPHS
TROPHY

•••P•H

HUPPAH
OOMPAH
TEMPEH

••••PH

ADOLPH
CALIPH
GUELPH
JOSEPH
PARAPH
SERAPH

PI••••

PIAFFE
PIAGET
PIANOS
PIAZZA
PIAZZI
PICABO
PICARA
PICARD
PICARO
PICCHU
PICHEL
PICKAT
PICKAX
PICKED
PICKER
PICKET
PICKLE
PICKON
PICKUP
PICNIC
PICONE
PICOTS
PICRIC
PICTOR
PIDDLE
PIDGIN
PIECED
PIECER
PIECES
PIELET
PIEMAN
PIEMEN
PIEPAN
PIERCE
PIERIA
PIERRE
PIETAS
PIETER
PIETIN
PIETRO
PIFFLE
PIGEON
PIGGED
PIGGIE
PIGLET
PIGMAN
PIGMEN
PIGNUT
PIGOUT
PIGPEN
PIGSIT
PIGSTY
PIKERS
PIKING
PILAFS
PILATE
PILAUS
PILEIN
PILEON
PILERS
PILEUM
PILEUP
PILEUS
PILFER
PILING
PILLAR
PILLED
PILLOW
PILOSE
PILOTS
PILOUS
PIMINY
PIMPLE
PIMPLY
PINATA
PINBOY
PINCAY
PINCER
PINDAR
PINDUS
PINEAL
PINERO
PINERS
PINERY
PINGED
PINGER
PINIER
PINING
PINION
PINKED
PINKEN
PINKER
PINKIE
PINKOS
PINNAE
PINNAS
PINNED
PINNER
PINOAK
PINONS
PINOTS
PINSON
PINSUP
PINTER
PINTOS
PINUPS
PINYIN
PINZON
PIOLET
PIPAGE
PIPEIN
PIPERS
PIPETS
PIPEUP
PIPIER
PIPING
PIPITS
PIPPET
PIPPIN
PIPPIP
PIQUED
PIQUES
PIQUET
PIRACY
PIRANA
PIRATE
PIRRIP
PISANO
PISANS
PISCES
PISGAH
PISHED
PISHES
PISTES
PISTIL
PISTOL
PISTON
PISTOU
PITAYA
PITCHY
PITHED
PITIED
PITIER
PITIES
PITKIN
PITMAN
PITMEN
PITNEY
PITONS
PITOTS
PITROW
PITSAW
PITTED
PIUSII
PIUSIV
PIUSIX
PIUSVI
PIUSXI
PIUTES
PIVOTS
PIXELS
PIXIES
PIZAZZ
PIZZAS

P•I•••

PAIDAD
PAIDIN
PAIDUP
PAINED
PAINTS
PAINTY
PAIRED
PAIRUP
PAISAN
PAISES
PAIUTE
PDIDDY
PEIRCE
PFIZER
PHIALS
PHILBY
PHILCO
PHILIC
PHILIP
PHILLY
PLIANT
PLIERS
PLIGHT
PLINKS
PLINTH
PLISSE
POILUS
POINTA
POINTB
POINTE
POINTS
POINTY
POIRES
POIRET
POIROT
POISED
POISER
POISES
POISHA
POISON
POITOU
POIVRE
PRICED
PRICER
PRICES
PRICEY
PRICKS
PRIDED
PRIDES
PRIERS
PRIEST

PRIMAL PRIMED PRIMER PRIMES PRIMLY PRIMOS PRIMPS PRIMUS PRINCE PRINKS PRINTS PRINZE PRIORI PRIORS PRIORY PRISED PRISMS PRISON PRISSY PRIVET PRIZED PRIZES PRIZMS PRIZZI PTILES

P••I••

PACIER PACIFY PACING PACINO PAGING PALING PALISH PAMINA PAMIRS PANICS PANIER PANINI PANINO PAPIER PAPIST PARIAH PARING PARINI PARISH PARITY PATINA PATINE PATIOS PAVING PAVIOR PAWING PAYING PEKING PELION PENICK PEPINO PEPITA PERILS PERINE PERIOD PERISH PERITI PETIPA PETITE PEWITS PIKING PILING PIMINY PINIER PINING PINION PIPIER PIPING PIPITS PITIED PITIER PITIES PIXIES PLAICE PLAIDS PLAINS PLAINT PLAITS PLEIAD PLUIES PLYING PODIUM POKIER POKIES POKILY POKING POLICE POLICY POLING POLIOS POLISH POLITE POLITY PONIED PONIES POPISH PORING POSIES POSING POSITS POTION POVICH PRAISE PRFIRM PRYING PULING PUMICE PUNIER PUNILY PUNISH PUPILS PURIFY PURIMS PURINA PURISM PURIST PURITY PYRITE

P•••I•

PACHIN PACKIN PAGLIA PAIDIN PALAIS PALLID PANDIT PANSIN PANTIE PAQUIN PARKIT PARNIS PARRIS PARTII PARTIV PASSIM PASTIS PASTIT PATHIC PATOIS PATRIA PATRIC PATRIE PATTIE PAULII PAULIV PAYSIN PECTIN PEEKIN PEERIN PELVIC PELVIS PENCIL PENNIA PENNIS PENSIN PEORIA PEPCID PEPSIN PEPTIC PERKIN PERMIT PERRIN PERSIA PERSIS PETAIN PETPIG PETRIE PETSIT PETTIS PETTIT PHAGIA PHASIC PHILIC PHILIP PHOBIA PHOBIC PHONIC PHOTIC PHYSIC PHYSIO PICNIC PICRIC PIDGIN PIERIA PIETIN PIGGIE PIGSIT PILEIN PINKIE PINYIN PIPEIN PIPPIN PIPPIP PIRRIP PISTIL PITKIN PIUSII PIUSIV PIUSIX PLACID PLAYIT PLUGIN PLUVIA PLUVIO POETIC PONGID POORIS POPEIL POPLIN POPSIN PORTIA POSTIE POSTIT POTLID POTPIE POTSIE POTVIN POURIN PRAXIS PREBID PRECIP PRECIS PREFIX PRELIM PREMIE PREMIX PREVIA PREVIN PROBIE PROFIT PROLIX PROSIT PUBLIC PUBLIX PUCCIS PUFFIN PULLIN PULPIT PUNDIT PUNKIE PUPKIN PURLIE PUSHIN PUSHIT PUTRID PUTSIN PUTTIN

P••••I

PANINI PAPYRI PARINI PARTII PASMOI PATAKI PAULII PAULVI PELOSI PERITI PETERI PIAZZI PIUSII PIUSVI PIUSXI POLLOI POPULI POTOSI PRIORI PRIZZI

•PI•••

APIARY APICAL APICES APIECE EPICAL EPILOG EPINAL OPIATE OPINED OPINER OPINES OPIUMS SPICED SPICER SPICES SPIDER SPIDEY SPIELS SPIERS SPIFFS SPIFFY SPIGOT SPIKED SPIKER SPIKES SPILES SPILLS SPILTH SPINAL SPINED SPINEL SPINER SPINES SPINET SPINKS SPIRAL SPIREA SPIRED SPIRES SPIRIT SPITED SPITES SPITON SPIVAK

•P•I••

APHIDS APLITE APPIAN APRILE APRILS EPPING OPCITS OPTICS OPTIMA OPTIMO OPTING OPTION SPHINX SPLICE SPLINE SPLINT SPLITS SPOILS SPOILT SPRIER SPRIGS SPRING SPRINT SPRITE SPRITS SPRITZ SPYING UPBIND UPDIKE UPDIVE UPGIRD UPGIRT UPHILL UPLIFT UPLINK UPPILE UPPING UPPISH UPPITY UPRISE UPSIDE UPSIZE UPTICK UPTILT UPTIME UPWIND XPRIZE

•P••I•

APULIA EPODIC OPENIT OPTSIN SPECIE SPIRIT SPRAIN UPCOIL UPSPIN UPSTIR UPTOIT

••PI••

ALPINE AMPING APPIAN ASPICS ASPIRE ASPISH CAPITA COPIED COPIER COPIES COPING CUPIDS DEPICT DOPIER DOPILY DOPING DUPING EMPIRE EPPING ESPIAL ESPIED ESPIER ESPIES ESPIOS EXPIRE EXPIRY GAPING HOPING HYPING IMPISH INPINK JAPING LAPINS LIPIDS LOPING LUPINE LUPINO MOPIER MOPING MOPISH MRPIBB NAPIER PAPIER PAPIST PEPINO PEPITA PIPIER PIPING PIPITS POPISH PUPILS RAPIDO RAPIDS RAPIER RAPINE RAPINI REPICK REPINE REPINS ROPIER ROPING RUPIAH SEPIAS SEPIRA STPIUS SUPINE TAPING TAPINS TAPIRS TIPINS TOPICS TOPING TYPIFY TYPING TYPIST UMPING UMPIRE UNPICK UNPILE UNPINS UPPILE UPPING UPPISH UPPITY WAPITI WIPING

••P•I•

AUPAIR BUPKIS CAPRID CAPRIS COPSIT COPTIC CUPRIC DIPSIN DRPHIL ELPAIS ESPRIT HIPPIE HOPKIN HOPSIN IMPAIR JOPLIN KEPTIN KUPRIN NAPKIN NAPPIE ORPHIC PEPCID PEPSIN PEPTIC PIPEIN PIPPIN PIPPIP POPEIL POPLIN POPSIN PUPKIN REPAID REPAIR ROPEIN SEPHIA SEPTIC SOPHIA SOPHIE TAPSIN TIPSIN TOPBID TUPTIM TYPEIN UNPAID UNPRIM YIPPIE YUPPIE ZIPSIN ZIPSIT

••P••I

CAPONI LAPERI LIPARI NAPOLI NEPALI PAPYRI POPULI RAPINI WAPITI

•••PI•

ARMPIT ASHPIT ATYPIC BBQPIT BIOPIC CHAPIN CHIPIN CHOPIN CUSPID DROPIN DROPIT ELAPID ENDPIN EYEPIT FLOPIT GILPIN HALPIN HATPIN HELPIN HIPPIE INAPIE INUPIK JUMPIN KEEPIN KEEPIT KELPIE KEMPIS KEWPIE LEAPIN LIMPID LUMPIN LUMPIT MAGPIE MUDPIE MYOPIA MYOPIC NAPPIE OKAPIS ONEPIN PETPIG PIPPIN PIPPIP POTPIE PULPIT RESPIN RUXPIN SAWPIT SCIPIO SEEPIN SIXPIN SKIPIT SLIPIN STEPIN STOPIN STOPIT STUPID TARPIT TAUPIN TENPIN THEPIT TIEPIN TORPID TREPID TROPIC TURPIN TWOPIN UNEPIC UPSPIN UTOPIA VESPID WHIPIN YIPPIE YUPPIE

•••P•I

DELPHI TAIPEI

••••PI

OCTOPI SCAMPI WHOOPI

P•J•••

PAJAMA PAJOAD PUJOLS

P••J••

PROJET PUNJAB

P••••J

PBANDJ

•PJ•••

UPJOHN

••PJ••

KOPJES TIPJAR TOPJOB

•••PJ•

SKOPJE

•••P•J

RALPHJ

P•K•••

PAKULA PEKING PEKOES PIKERS PIKING POKEAT POKERS POKERY POKEYS POKIER POKIES POKILY POKING

P••K••

PACKED PACKER PACKET PACKIN PACKON PACKUP PARKAS PARKAV PARKAY PARKED PARKER PARKES PARKIT PEAKED PECKAT PECKED PEEKAT PEEKED PEEKER PEEKIN PERKED PERKIN PERKUP PICKAT PICKAX PICKED PICKER PICKET PICKLE PICKON PICKUP PINKED PINKEN PINKER PINKIE PINKOS PITKIN PLAKAT POCKET POLKAS PORKED PORKER PORKYS PUCKER PUNKAS PUNKER PUNKIE PUPKIN

P•••K•

PANCKS PATAKI PBOOKS PERUKE PLANKS PLINKS PLONKS PLUCKS PLUCKY PLUNKS PLUNKY POLSKA PRANKS PRICKS PRINKS PROSKY

P••••K

PENICK PINOAK PLANCK PODUNK POLLAK

•PK•••

UPKEEP

•P•K••

SPIKED SPIKER SPIKES SPOKED SPOKEN SPOKES

•P••K•

APOPKA SPANKS SPANKY SPARKS SPARKY SPEAKS SPECKS SPINKS SPOOKS SPOOKY SPORKS SPUNKY UPDIKE UPTAKE

•P•••K

SPACEK SPIVAK UPLINK UPTALK UPTICK

••PK••

BUPKES BUPKIS BUPKUS HOPKIN NAPKIN PUPKIN RIPKEN

••P•K•

KAPOKS KOPEKS TOPEKA

••P••K

INPARK INPINK KOPECK REPACK REPARK REPERK REPICK RVPARK UNPACK UNPICK

•••PK•

APOPKA SHOPKO

•••P•K

DEEPAK INUPIK

PL••••

PLACED PLACER PLACES PLACID PLAGES PLAGUE PLAICE PLAIDS PLAINS PLAINT PLAITS PLAKAT PLANAR PLANAS PLANBS PLANCK PLANED PLANER PLANES PLANET PLANKS PLANON PLANTE PLANTO PLANTS PLAQUE PLASHY PLASMA PLASMO PLATED PLATEN PLATER PLATES PLATOS PLATTE PLATYS PLAYAS PLAYAT PLAYBY PLAYED PLAYER PLAYIT PLAYON PLAYTO PLAYUP PLAZAS PLEADS PLEASE PLEATS PLEBES PLEDGE PLEDTO PLEIAD PLENTY PLENUM PLEURA PLEXAL PLEXES PLEXOR PLEXUS PLIANT PLIERS PLIGHT PLINKS PLINTH PLISSE PLOCES PLOMER PLONKS PLOTTY PLOUGH PLOVER PLOWED PLOWER PLOWON PLOWUP PLUCKS PLUCKY PLUGIN PLUGUP PLUIES PLUMBO PLUMBS PLUMED PLUMES PLUMMY PLUMPS PLUNGE PLUNKS PLUNKY PLURAL PLUSES PLUSHY PLUTON PLUTUS PLUVIA PLUVIO PLYING

P•L•••

PALACE PALADE PALAIS PALATE PALEAE PALELY PALEST PALING PALISH PALLAS PALLED PALLET PALLID PALLOR PALMAR PALMAS PALMED PALMER PALOMA PALTER PALTRY PCLABS PELAGE PELEUS PELHAM PELION PELLAM PELLET PELOSI PELOTA PELTED PELTER PELTRY PELVIC PELVIS PHLEBO PHLEGM PHLOEM PILAFS PILATE PILAUS PILEIN PILEON PILERS PILEUM PILEUP PILEUS PILFER PILING PILLAR PILLED PILLOW PILOSE PILOTS PILOUS POLAND POLARA POLEAX POLERS POLGAR POLICE POLICY POLING POLIOS POLISH POLITE POLITY POLKAS POLLAK POLLED POLLEE POLLEN POLLER POLLEX POLLOI POLLOS POLLUX POLPOT POLSKA POLYPS PULERS PULING PULLED PULLER PULLET PULLEY PULLIN PULLON PULLUP PULMON PULPED PULPER PULPIT PULSAR PULSED PULSES PULVER PYLONS

P••L••

PABLUM PAELLA PAGLIA PALLAS PALLED PALLET PALLID PALLOR PARLAY PARLEY PARLEZ PARLOR PAULEY PAULII

PAULIV
PAULVI
PAVLOV
PEALED
PEALER
PEALES
PEELED
PEELER
PEGLEG
PEGLER
PELLAM
PELLET
PEPLUM
PERLEA
PHELPS
PHILBY
PHILCO
PHILIC
PHILIP
PHILLY
PHYLLO
PHYLUM
PIELET
PIGLET
PILLAR
PILLED
PILLOW
PIOLET
POILUS
POLLAK
POLLED
POLLEE
POLLEN
POLLER
POLLEX
POLLOI
POLLOS
POLLUX
POOLED
POOLER
POPLAR
POPLIN
POTLID
POULES
POULTS
PRELAW
PRELIM
PRELOG
PROLES
PROLIX
PROLOG
PSALMS
PTILES
PUBLIC
PUBLIX
PULLED
PULLER
PULLET
PULLEY
PULLIN
PULLON
PULLUP
PURLED
PURLIE

P•••L•

PACULA
PADDLE
PAELLA
PAKULA
PALELY
PAMELA
PANDLS
PANELS
PAROLE
PAROLS
PARTLY
PAYOLA
PEARLE
PEARLS
PEARLY
PEBBLE
PEBBLY
PEDALS
PEDDLE
PENULT
PEOPLE
PERILS
PERTLY
PESTLE
PETALE
PETALS
PETULA
PHIALS
PHILLY
PHYLLO
PICKLE
PIDDLE
PIFFLE
PIMPLE
PIMPLY
PIXELS
POKILY
POMELO
POODLE
POORLY
POPFLY
POPPLE
POPULI
PORTLY
POSHLY
POSOLE
POSSLQ
POWELL
POZOLE
PRIMLY
PROULX
PROWLS
PUDDLE
PUDDLY
PUEBLA
PUEBLO
PUGGLE
PUJOLS
PUNILY
PUPILS
PURELY
PURFLE
PURPLE
PURPLY
PUZZLE

P••••L

PAGNOL
PANFUL
PARCEL
PASCAL
PASSEL
PASTEL
PATROL
PAUSAL
PAYPAL
PENCIL
PENPAL
PENTEL
PEPFUL
PETREL
PETROL
PHENOL
PICHEL
PINEAL
PISTIL
PISTOL
PLEXAL
PLURAL
POMMEL
POPEIL
PORTAL
POSTAL
POTFUL
POWELL
PRIMAL
PROCOL
PROPEL
PROPYL
PUMMEL

•PL•••

APLITE
APLOMB
SPLASH
SPLATS
SPLAYS
SPLEEN
SPLICE
SPLINE
SPL1NT
SPLITS
SPLOSH
UPLAND
UPLAST
UPLATE
UPLEAP
UPLIFT
UPLINK
UPLOAD

•P•L••

APELET
APOLLO
APPLES
APPLET
APULIA
EPILOG
SPELLS
SPILES
SPILLS
SPILTH
UPFLOW

•P••L•

APOLLO
APPALL
APPALS
APPELS
APRILE
APRILS
OPENLY
OPHULS
SPELLS
SPIELS
SPILLS
SPOILS
SPOILT
SPOOLS
SPRYLY
UPFOLD
UPHELD
UPHILL
UPHOLD
UPPILE
UPSALA
UPTALK
UPTILT
UPWELL

•P•••L

APICAL
APODAL
APPALL
APPEAL
EPICAL
EPINAL
SPINAL
SPINEL
SPIRAL
SPRAWL
UPCOIL
UPCURL
UPHILL
UPWELL

••PL••

AMPLER
APPLES
APPLET
ATPLAY
BYPLAY
CAPLET
COPLEY
DEPLOY
DIPLEX
DUPLEX
DUPLOS
EMPLOY
IMPLED
INPLAY
JOPLIN
KAPLAN
KEPLER
MAPLES
NAPLES
PEPLUM
POPLAR
POPLIN
REPLAN
REPLAY
REPLED
REPLOT
REPLOW
RIPLEY
UNPLAN
UNPLUG
ZIPLOC

••P•L•

AMPULE
APPALL
APPALS
APPELS
ARPELS
COPALS
COPULA
CUPELS
CUPOLA
CUPULE
DAPPLE
DEPULP
DIPOLE
DOPILY
EMPALE
EXPELS
FIPPLE
IMPALA
IMPALE
IMPELS
KAPELL
KOPELL
LAPELS
MAPPLE
NAPALM
NAPOLI
NEPALI
NIPPLE
NOPALS
POPFLY
POPPLE
POPULI
PUPILS
RAPTLY
REPELS
REPOLL
RIPELY
RIPPLE
RIPPLY
SEPALS
SUPPLE
SUPPLY
TIPPLE
TOPPLE
TUPELO
UNPALE
UNPILE
UPPILE

••P••L

APPALL
APPEAL
CAPFUL
CEPHAL
CUPFUL
DEPAUL
DRPHIL
ESPIAL
KAPELL
KOPELL
KOPPEL
LAPFUL
OMPHAL
PEPFUL
POPEIL
RAPPEL
REPEAL
REPOLL
SEPTAL
STPAUL
UNPEEL

•••PL•

COMPLY
COUPLE
DAMPLY
DAPPLE
DEEPLY
DIMPLE
DIMPLY
FIPPLE
HOOPLA
HOOPLE
LIMPLY
MAPPLE
MARPLE
NIPPLE
NTUPLE
PEOPLE
PIMPLE
PIMPLY
POPPLE
PURPLE
PURPLY
RIMPLE
RIPPLE
RIPPLY
RUMPLE
RUMPLY
SAMPLE
SEMPLE
SIMPLE
SIMPLY
STAPLE
SUPPLE
SUPPLY
TEMPLE
TIPPLE
TOPPLE
TRIPLE
TRIPLY
TWOPLY
WIMPLE

•••P•L

BEAPAL
BHOPAL
CARPAL
CARPEL
CHAPEL
COMPEL
CUSPAL
DISPEL
GALPAL
GOSPEL
KEYPAL
KOPPEL
OLDPAL
PAYPAL
PENPAL
PROPEL
PROPYL
RAMPAL
RAPPEL
VORPAL

P•M•••

PAMELA
PAMINA
PAMIRS
PAMPAS
PAMPER
PIMINY
PIMPLE
PIMPLY
POMADE
POMELO
POMMEL
POMMES
POMONA
POMPEO
POMPEY
POMPOM
POMPON
PUMICE
PUMMEL
PUMPED
PUMPER
PUMPUP

P••M••

PACMAN
PALMAR
PALMAS
PALMED
PALMER
PASMOI
PATMOS
PENMAN
PENMEN
PERMED
PERMIT
PIEMAN
PIEMEN
PIGMAN
PIGMEN
PITMAN
PITMEN
PLOMER
PLUMBO
PLUMBS
PLUMED
PLUMES
PLUMMY
PLUMPS
POEMES
POMMEL
POMMES
PREMED
PREMET
PREMIE
PREMIX
PRIMAL
PRIMED
PRIMER
PRIMES
PRIMLY
PRIMOS
PRIMPS
PRIMUS
PROMOS
PROMPT
PULMON
PUMMEL

P•••M•

PAJAMA
PALOMA
PANAMA
PLASMA
PLASMO
PLUMMY
PNEUMA
PNEUMO
PREAMP
PRISMS
PRIZMS
PROAMS
PROEMS
PSALMS
PURIMS

P••••M

PABLUM
PARFUM
PASSIM
PELHAM
PELLAM
PEPLUM
PHENOM
PHLEGM
PHLOEM
PHYLUM
PILEUM
PLENUM
PODIUM
POMPOM
POSSUM
POSTUM
PREARM
PRELIM
PRFIRM
PROTEM
PURISM
PUTNAM

•PM•••

UPMOST

•P•M••

APEMAN
APEMEN
SPUMED
SPUMES

•P••M•

APLOMB
OPIUMS
OPTIMA
OPTIMO
SPASMS
UPTIME

•P•••M

EPONYM
SPYCAM

••PM••

TOPMAN
TOPMEN

••P•M•

REPUMP

••P••M

GYPSUM
LAPERM
LAPHAM
NAPALM
PEPLUM
SEPTUM
TUPTIM
UNPRIM

•••PM•

HELPME

•••P•M

POMPOM
WAMPUM

••••PM

FIVEPM
FOURPM
NINEPM

PN••••

PNEUMA
PNEUMO

P•N•••

PANADA
PANAMA
PANCHO
PANCKS
PANDAS
PANDER
PANDIT
PANDLS
PANELS
PANFRY
PANFUL
PANICS
PANIER
PANINI
PANINO
PANNED
PANNER
PANNES
PANOPE
PANOUT
PANSIN
PANTED
PANTER
PANTIE
PANTOS
PANTRY
PANZER
PENCHE
PENCIL
PENDED
PENGPU
PENICK
PENMAN
PENMEN
PENNED
PENNER
PENNEY
PENNIA
PENNIS
PENNON
PENPAL
PENROD
PENSEE
PENSIN
PENSUP
PENTAD
PENTAX
PENTEL
PENTUP
PENULT
PENURY
PINATA
PINBOY
PINCAY
PINCER
PINDAR
PINDUS
PINEAL
PINERO
PINERS
PINERY
PINGED
PINGER
PINIER
PINING
PINION
PINKED
PINKEN
PINKER
PINKIE
PINKOS
PINNAE
PINNAS
PINNED
PINNER
PINOAK
PINONS
PINOTS
PINSON
PINSUP
PINTER
PINTOS
PINUPS
PINYIN
PINZON
PONCAS
PONCHO
PONDED
PONDER
PONGEE
PONGID
PONIED
PONIES
PONYUP
PONZUS
PUNCHY
PUNDIT
PUNIER
PUNILY
PUNISH
PUNJAB
PUNKAS
PUNKER
PUNKIE
PUNNED
PUNNER
PUNTAS
PUNTED
PUNTER

P••N••

PAANGA
PAGNOL
PAINED
PAINTS
PAINTY
PANNED
PANNER
PANNES
PARNIS
PAUNCH
PAWNED
PAWNEE
PAWNER
PAYNOW
PBANDJ
PEANUT
PEENED
PENNED
PENNER
PENNEY
PENNIA
PENNIS
PENNON
PERNOD
PETNAP
PEVNEY
PHENOL
PHENOM
PHONED
PHONER
PHONES
PHONEY
PHONIC
PHONOS
PIANOS
PICNIC
PIGNUT
PINNAE
PINNAS
PINNED
PINNER
PITNEY
PLANAR
PLANAS
PLANBS
PLANCK
PLANED
PLANER
PLANES
PLANET
PLANKS
PLANON
PLANTE
PLANTO
PLANTS
PLENTY
PLENUM
PLINKS
PLINTH
PLONKS
PLUNGE
PLUNKS
PLUNKY
POGNER
POINTA
POINTB
POINTE
POINTS
POINTY
POUNCE
POUNDS
POZNAN
PRANAS
PRANCE
PRANKS
PRENUP
PRINCE
PRINKS
PRINTS
PRINZE
PRONGS
PRONTO
PRUNED
PRUNER
PRUNES
PRYNNE
PUENTE
PUENZO
PUNNED
PUNNER
PUTNAM
PUTNEY

P•••N•

PACING
PACINO
PAEANS
PAGANS
PAGING
PALING
PAMINA
PANINI
PANINO
PARANA
PARENS
PARENT
PARING
PARINI
PATENS
PATENT
PATINA
PATINE
PAVANE
PAVING
PAWING
PAYING
PECANS
PEDANT
PEKING
PEPINO
PERINE
PICONE
PIKING
PILING
PIMINY
PINING
PINONS
PIPING
PIRANA
PISANO
PISANS
PITONS
PLAINS
PLAINT
PLIANT
PLYING
POCONO
PODUNK
POEANA
POKING
POLAND
POLING
POMONA
PORING
POSING
POTENT
PRAWNS
PREENS
PRYING
PRYNNE
PULING
PURINA
PUTONS
PYLONS

P••••N

PACHIN
PACKIN
PACKON
PACMAN
PACTEN
PADUAN
PAIDIN
PAISAN
PANSIN
PAPUAN
PAQUIN
PARDON
PARSON
PARTON
PASSON
PATHAN
PATRON
PATTEN
PATTON
PAXTON
PAYSIN
PAYSON
PAYTON
PEAHEN
PECTIN
PEEKIN
PEERIN
PEGEEN
PELION
PENMAN
PENMEN
PENNON
PENSIN
PEPSIN
PERKIN
PERRIN
PERSON
PETAIN
PEYTON
PHOTON
PICKON
PIDGIN
PIEMAN
PIEMEN
PIEPAN
PIETIN
PI'GEON
PIGMAN
PIGMEN
PIGPEN
PILEIN
PILEON
PINION
PINKEN
PINSON
PINYIN
PINZON
PIPEIN
PIPPIN
PISTON
PITKIN
PITMAN
PITMEN
PLANON
PLATEN
PLAYON
PLOWON
PLUGIN
PLUTON
POISON
POLLEN
POMPON
POPGUN
POPLIN
POPSIN
POSTON
POTEEN
POTION
POTVIN
POUPON
POURIN
POZNAN
PREVIN
PREYON
PRISON
PRODON
PROGUN
PROTON
PROVEN
PUFFIN
PULLIN
PULLON
PULMON
PUPKIN
PUSHIN
PUSHON
PUTSIN
PUTSON
PUTTIN
PYTHON

•PN•••

APNEAS
UPNEXT

•P•N••

CPSNOW
EPINAL
EPONYM
OPENED
OPENER
OPENIT
OPENLY
OPENON
OPENTO
OPENUP
OPINED
OPINER
OPINES
SPANKS
SPANKY
SPENCE
SPENDS
SPENDY
SPINAL
SPINED
SPINEL
SPINER
SPINES
SPINET
SPINKS
SPONGE
SPONGY
SPUNKY
UPENDS

•P••N•

APPEND
APRONS
EPPING
EPSONS
OPTING
SPAWNS
SPHINX
SPHYNX
SPLINE
SPLINT
SPOONS
SPOONY
SPRANG
SPRING
SPRINT
SPRUNG
SPURNS
SPYING
UPBIND
UPLAND
UPLINK
UPPING
UPSEND
UPSENT
UPWIND

•P•••N

APEMAN
APEMEN
APPIAN
EPHRON
OPENON
OPPUGN
OPTION
OPTSIN
SPITON
SPLEEN
SPOKEN

SPOTON SPRAIN SPURON UPJOHN UPSPIN UPTORN UPTOWN UPTURN

••PN••

CAPNUT DIPNET EUPNEA HYPNOS WAPNER

••P•N•

ALPINE AMPING APPEND ASPENS CAPONE CAPONI CAPONS COPING DAPHNE DEPEND DEPONE DOPING DUPING DUPONT EPPING ESPANA EXPAND EXPEND GAPING HOPING HYPING IMPEND INPINK JAPANS JAPING LAPINS LIPENG LOPING LUPINE LUPINO LUPONE MOPING PEPINO PIPING RAPINE RAPINI REPANE REPENS REPENT REPINE REPINS RIPENS ROPING SUPINE TAPING TAPINS TIPINS TOPING TYPING UMPING UNPENS UNPENT UNPINS UPPING WIPING ZIPONS

••P••N

APPIAN CAPGUN DIPSIN EMPSON HAPPEN HOPKIN HOPSIN HOPSON HYPHEN IMPUGN INPAWN JOPLIN KAPLAN KEPTIN KEPTON KUPRIN LEPTON LIPTON LUPTON NAPKIN NEPEAN NIPPON OPPUGN ORPHAN PAPUAN PEPSIN PIPEIN PIPPIN POPGUN POPLIN POPSIN PUPKIN RAPSON REPLAN REPUGN RIPKEN RIPSON ROPEIN SIPHON SIPSON TAPEON TAPPAN TAPSIN TAPSON TIPSIN TOPGUN TOPMAN TOPMEN TOPTEN TYPEIN UNPAWN UNPLAN ZIPGUN ZIPSIN

•••P•N

ASHPAN CHAPIN CHIPIN CHOPIN CLIPON COUPON DAMPEN DEEPEN DRIPON DROPIN DUMPON ENDPIN FRYPAN GELPEN GILPIN HALPIN HAPPEN HARPON HATPIN HEAPON HELPIN HELPON HEMPEN INSPAN JUMPIN JUMPON KEEPIN KEEPON LEAPIN LEAPON LUMPEN LUMPIN NIPPON OILPAN ONEPIN PIEPAN PIGPEN PIPPIN POMPON POUPON REOPEN RESPAN RESPIN RIOPAN RUXPIN SAIPAN SAMPAN SEEPIN SIXPIN SLAPON SLIPIN SLIPON SLOPON SNAPON STEPIN STEPON STOPIN TAIPAN TAPPAN TARPON TAUPIN TENPIN TIEPIN TINPAN TREPAN TRIPON TURPIN TWOPIN UNOPEN UNSPAN UNSPUN UPSPIN USOPEN WEAPON WHIPIN

PO••••

POACHY POBOYS POCKET POCONO PODDED PODIUM PODOUS PODUNK POEANA POEMES POETES POETIC POETRY POGNER POILUS POINTA POINTB POINTE POINTS POINTY POIRES POIRET POIROT POISED POISER POISES POISHA POISON POITOU POIVRE POKEAT POKERS POKERY POKEYS POKIER POKIES POKILY POKING POLAND POLARA POLEAX POLERS POLGAR POLICE POLICY POLING POLIOS POLISH POLITE POLITY POLKAS POLLAK POLLED POLLEE POLLEN POLLER POLLEX POLLOI POLLOS POLLUX POLPOT POLSKA POLYPS POMADE POMELO POMMEL POMMES POMONA POMPEO POMPEY POMPOM POMPON PONCAS PONCHO PONDED PONDER PONGEE PONGID PONIED PONIES PONYUP PONZUS POODLE POOHED POOLED POOLER POOPED POORAT POORER POORIS POORLY POPART POPEIL POPEYE POPFLY POPGUN POPISH POPLAR POPLIN POPOFF POPOUT POPPAS POPPED POPPER POPPLE POPSIN POPSUP POPTOP POPULI POPUPS PORERS PORING PORKED PORKER PORKYS POROSE POROUS PORTAL PORTED PORTER PORTES PORTIA PORTLY POSADA POSEAS POSERS POSEUR POSHER POSHLY POSIES POSING POSITS POSOLE POSSES POSSLQ POSSUM POSTAL POSTED POSTER POSTIE POSTIT POSTON POSTOP POSTUM POTAGE POTASH POTATO POTEEN POTENT POTFUL POTHER POTHOS POTION POTLID POTOSI POTPIE POTSIE POTTED POTTER POTTOS POTVIN POUCHY POUDRE POUFED POUFFY POULES POULTS POUNCE POUNDS POUPON POURED POURER POURIN POUSSE POUTED POUTER POVICH POWDER POWELL POWERS POWWOW POYSER POZNAN POZOLE

P•O•••

PBOOKS PEOPLE PEORIA PHOBIA PHOBIC PHOBOS PHOEBE PHONED PHONER PHONES PHONEY PHONIC PHONOS PHOOEY PHOTIC PHOTOG PHOTON PHOTOS PIOLET PLOCES PLOMER PLONKS PLOTTY PLOUGH PLOVER PLOWED PLOWER PLOWON PLOWUP POODLE POOHED POOLED POOLER POOPED POORAT POORER POORIS POORLY PROAMS PROART PROBED PROBER PROBES PROBIE PROBST PROCOL PRODON PROEMS PROFIT PROGUN PROJET PROLES PROLIX PROLOG PROMOS PROMPT PRONGS PRONTO PROOFS PROPEL PROPER PROPRE PROPUP PROPYL PROSED PROSER PROSES PROSIT PROSKY PROTAX PROTEA PROTEM PROTON PROULX PROUST PROVED PROVEN PROVER PROVES PROWAR PROWLS PROWSE PROYAS PROZAC PTOOEY

P••O••

PADOVA PAGODA PAJOAD PALOMA PANOPE PANOUT PARODY PAROLE PAROLS PATOIS PAYOFF PAYOLA PAYOUT PBOOKS PEKOES PELOSI PELOTA PEYOTE PHLOEM PHOOEY PICONE PICOTS PIGOUT PILOSE PILOTS PILOUS PINOAK PINONS PINOTS PITONS PITOTS PIVOTS POBOYS POCONO PODOUS POMONA POPOFF POPOUT POROSE POROUS POSOLE POTOSI POZOLE PREOPS PRIORI PRIORS PRIORY PROOFS PRYOFF PTBOAT PTOOEY PUJOLS PUTOFF PUTONS PUTOUT PYLONS

P•••O•

PACKON PAGNOL PALLOR PANTOS PARDON PARLOR PARROT PARSON PARTOF PARTON PASEOS PASMOI PASSON PASSOS PASTOR PATHOS PATIOS PATMOS PATROL PATRON PATTON PAVIOR PAVLOV PAXTON PAYFOR PAYNOW PAYSON PAYTON PEAPOD PEGBOX PEGTOP PELION PENNON PENROD PEPBOY PEQUOD PEQUOT PERIOD PERNOD PERROS PERSON PESCOW PESTOS PETBOA PETCOW PETDOG PETROL PETTOY PEYTON PHAROS PHENOL PHENOM PHOBOS PHONOS PHOTOG PHOTON PHOTOS PIANOS PICKON PICTOR PIGEON PILEON PILLOW PINBOY PINION PINKOS PINSON PINTOS PINZON PISTOL PISTON PISTOU PITROW PLANON PLATOS PLAYON PLEXOR PLOWON PLUTON POIROT POISON POITOU POLIOS POLLOI POLLOS POLPOT POMPOM POMPON POPTOP POSTON POSTOP POTHOS POTION POTTOS POUPON POWWOW PRELOG PRETOR PREYON PRIMOS PRISON PROCOL PRODON PROLOG PROMOS PROTON PULLON PULMON PUSHON PUTSON PYEDOG PYTHON

P••••O

PACINO PANCHO PANINO PAPAGO PARETO PASHTO PASSGO PASSTO PEPINO PGAPRO PHILCO PHLEBO PHYLLO PHYSIO PICABO PICARO PIETRO PINERO PISANO PLANTO PLASMO PLAYTO PLEDTO PLUMBO PLUVIO PNEUMO POCONO POMELO POMPEO PONCHO POTATO PRAYTO PRESTO PRONTO PSEUDO PSYCHO PUEBLO PUENZO PUERTO PUTSTO PYRHHO

•PO•••

APODAL APOGEE APOLLO APOPKA EPOCHS EPODES EPODIC EPONYM EPOPEE EPOQUE EPOSES EPOWER OPORTO SPODES SPOILS SPOILT SPOKED SPOKEN SPOKES SPONGE SPONGY SPOOFS SPOOKS SPOOKY SPOOLS SPOONS SPOONY SPOORS SPORES SPORKS SPORTS SPORTY SPOTON SPOTTV SPOTTY SPOUSE SPOUTS UPOVER

•P•O••

APLOMB APPOSE APRONS EPHODS EPHORS EPSONS OPPOSE OPTOUT SPLOSH SPOOFS SPOOKS SPOOKY SPOOLS SPOONS SPOONY SPOORS SPROUT SPYOUT UPBOWS UPCOIL UPDOVE UPFOLD UPHOLD UPHOVE UPJOHN UPLOAD UPMOST UPROAR UPROOT UPROSE UPSOAR UPTOIT UPTORE UPTORN UPTOSS UPTOWN

•P••O•

APPROX CPSNOW EPHRON EPILOG OPENON OPTFOR OPTION SPIGOT SPITON SPOTON SPURON SPYBOT UPFLOW UPGROW UPPROP UPROOT UPSHOT

•P•••O

APOLLO OPENTO OPORTO OPTIMO OPTSTO SPEEDO

••PO••

APPOSE BIPODS CAPONE CAPONI CAPONS CAPOTE COPOUT CSPOTS CUPOLA CWPOST DEPONE DEPORT DEPOSE DEPOTS DIPODY DIPOLE DUPONT ESPOSA ESPOSO EXPORT EXPOSE EXPOST HOPOFF HOPOUT HYPOED IMPORT IMPOSE IMPOST INPORT INPOUR KAPOKS LIPOFF LIPOUT LOPOFF LUPONE MAPOUT NAPOLI NYPOST ONPOST OOPODS OPPOSE POPOFF POPOUT REPOLL REPORT REPOSE REPOST REPOTS REPOUR RIPOFF RIPOST RIPOUT SAPORS SEPOYS SOPORS TAPOFF TAPOUT TIPOFF TOPOFF TOPOUT UNPOSH UNPOTS VAPORS VAPORY VAPOUR ZIPOFF ZIPONS ZIPOUT

••P•O•

APPROX CAPTOR DEPLOY DIPSOS DUPLOS EMPLOY EMPSON EMPTOR ESPIOS HIPHOP HIPPOS HOPSON HYPNOS IMPROV KEPTON LAPDOG LAPTOP LEPTON LIPTON LUPTON MOPTOP NIPPON NOPROB PEPBOY POPTOP RAPSON RAPTOR REPFOR REPLOT REPLOW REPROS RIPSON SIPHON SIPSON TAPEON TAPSON TIPTOE TIPTOP TOPDOG TOPJOB TOPROW TYPEOS UPPROP ZIPLOC ZIPPOS ZIPTOP

••P••O

COPSTO ELPASO ESPOSO HEPATO HOPESO HOPETO HOPSTO KEPTTO LUPINO MAPUTO NEPHRO PAPAGO PEPINO RAPIDO SAPPHO TUPELO

•••PO•

AIRPOP AIRPOT CAMPOS CLIPON COMPOS COMPOZ COUPON COWPOX DESPOT DRIPON DUMPON EELPOT HARPON HEAPON HELPON HIPPOS HOOPOE HOTPOT ICEPOP INAPOD INKPOT INSPOT ISOPOD JUMPON KARPOV KEEPON LEAPON LOMPOC NIPPON OUTPOP PEAPOD POLPOT POMPOM POMPON POUPON RESPOT SEXPOT SLAPON SLIPON SLOPON SNAPON STEPON STUPOR TARPON TEAPOT TEAPOY TEMPOS TINPOT TORPOR TRIPOD TRIPON TVSPOT UNIPOD VOXPOP WEAPON ZIPPOS

•••P•O

ALEPPO ALLPRO BUMPPO CRYPTO GLYPTO GOUPTO GRAPHO KEEPTO KLEPTO KRYPTO MORPHO NONPRO OLDPRO PGAPRO POMPEO SAPPHO SCIPIO SHIPTO SHOPKO SNAPTO STOPGO TROPPO

••••PO

ALEPPO

ATEMPO BUMPPO CHEAPO CREEPO DACAPO KAKAPO OBISPO RAMAPO TIEMPO TROPPO

P•P•••

PAPACY PAPAGO PAPAWS PAPAYA PAPERS PAPERY PAPIER PAPIST PAPPAS PAPUAN PAPYRI PEPBOY PEPCID PEPFUL PEPINO PEPITA PEPLUM PEPPED PEPPER PEPSIN PEPSUP PEPTIC PIPAGE PIPEIN PIPERS PIPETS PIPEUP PIPIER PIPING PIPITS PIPPET PIPPIN PIPPIP POPART POPEIL POPEYE POPFLY POPGUN POPISH POPLAR POPLIN POPOFF POPOUT POPPAS POPPED POPPER POPPLE POPSIN POPSUP POPTOP POPULI POPUPS PUPATE PUPILS PUPKIN PUPPED PUPPET

P••P••

PAMPAS PAMPER PAPPAS PAUPER PAWPAW PAYPAL PEAPOD PEEPAT PEEPED PEEPER PENPAL PEOPLE PEPPED PEPPER PETPIG PETPUP PGAPRO PIEPAN PIGPEN PIMPLE PIMPLY PIPPET PIPPIN PIPPIP POLPOT POMPEO POMPEY POMPOM POMPON POOPED POPPAS POPPED POPPER POPPLE POTPIE POUPON PREPAY PREPPY PROPEL PROPER PROPRE PROPUP PROPYL PULPED PULPER PULPIT PUMPED PUMPER PUMPUP PUPPED PUPPET PURPLE PURPLY PUTPUT

P•••P•

PANOPE PARAPH PENGPU PETIPA PHELPS PINUPS PLUMPS POLYPS POPUPS PREOPS PREPPY PRIMPS PROMPT PTRAPS

P••••P

PACKUP PAGEUP PAIDUP PAIRUP PASSUP PAYSUP PEGTOP PENSUP PENTUP PEPSUP PERKUP PETNAP PETPUP PHILIP PICKUP PILEUP PINSUP PIPEUP PIPPIP PIRRIP PLAYUP PLOWUP PLUGUP PONYUP POPSUP POPTOP POSTOP PREAMP PRECIP PRENUP PROPUP PUFFUP PULLUP PUMPUP PUSHUP PUTSUP

•PP•••

APPALL APPALS APPEAL APPEAR APPELS APPEND APPERT APPIAN APPLES APPLET APPOSE APPROX EPPING OPPOSE OPPUGN UPPERS UPPILE UPPING UPPISH UPPITY UPPROP

•P•P••

APOPKA EPOPEE UPSPIN

•P•••P

OPENUP SPEDUP UPHEAP UPKEEP UPLEAP UPPROP UPSTEP

••PP••

BOPPED BOPPER CAPPED CAPPER COPPED COPPER CUPPAS CUPPED DAPPED DAPPER DAPPLE DIPPED DIPPER FIPPLE GAPPED GIPPER GYPPED GYPPER HAPPEN HEPPER HIPPED HIPPER HIPPIE HIPPOS HIPPUS HOPPED HOPPER HUPPAH KAPPAS KIPPED KIPPER KIPPUR KOPPEL LAPPED LAPPER LAPPET LIPPED LIPPER LOPPED LOPPER MAPPED MAPPER MAPPLE MOPPED MOPPER MOPPET MUPPET NAPPED NAPPER NAPPES NAPPIE NIPPED NIPPER NIPPLE NIPPON PAPPAS PEPPED PEPPER PIPPET PIPPIN PIPPIP POPPAS POPPED POPPER POPPLE PUPPED PUPPET RAPPED RAPPEL RAPPER REPPED RIPPED RIPPER RIPPLE RIPPLY SAPPED SAPPER SAPPHO SIPPED SIPPER SOPPED SUPPED SUPPER SUPPLE SUPPLY TAPPAN TAPPED TAPPER TAPPET TIPPED TIPPEE TIPPER TIPPET TIPPLE TOPPED TOPPER TOPPLE TUPPER YAPPED YAPPER YIPPED YIPPEE YIPPIE YUPPIE ZAPPED ZAPPER ZIPPED ZIPPER ZIPPOS

••P•P•

MOPUPS NIPUPS POPUPS

••P••P

AMPSUP BOPEEP DEPULP HIPHOP HOPSUP HYPEUP KEPTUP LAPSUP LAPTOP MOPSUP MOPTOP PEPSUP PIPEUP PIPPIP POPSUP POPTOP REPUMP RIPRAP RIPSUP ROPEUP SOPSUP TAPEUP TIPSUP TIPTOP TOPSUP TYPEUP UPPROP WIPEUP ZIPSUP ZIPTOP

•••PP•

ALEPPO BUMPPO CHOPPY CHUPPA DIEPPE DRIPPY FLAPPY FLOPPY FRAPPE GLOPPY GRAPPA GRIPPE GRIPPY PREPPY QUIPPY SHOPPE SKIPPY SLAPPY SLIPPY SLOPPY SNAPPY SNIPPY STEPPE TRAPPY TROPPO WHIPPY

•••P•P

AIRPOP BUMPUP CAMPUP CHIPUP CHOPUP COOPUP CROPUP FLIPUP HEAPUP HELPUP ICEPOP JUMPUP KEEPUP LEAPUP OUTPOP PETPUP PIPPIP PROPUP PUMPUP RAMPUP SLIPUP SNAPUP SOAPUP SOUPUP STEPUP STOPUP TRIPUP VOXPOP WHIPUP WRAPUP

••••PP

ALCAPP

PQ••••

PQRSTU

P•Q•••

PAQUIN PEQUOD PEQUOT PIQUED PIQUES PIQUET

P••Q••

PLAQUE

P••••Q

POSSLQ

•PQ•••

OPQRST

•P•Q••

EPOQUE OPAQUE

••PQ••

NOPQRS

•••PQ•

MNOPQR

•••P•Q

COMPAQ

••••PQ

LMNOPQ

PR••••

PRADAS PRAGUE PRAISE PRANAS PRANCE PRANKS PRATED PRATER PRATES PRAVDA PRAWER PRAWNS PRAXES PRAXIS PRAYED PRAYER PRAYTO PREACH PREACT PREAGE PREAMP PREARM PREBID PREBUY PRECIP PRECIS PRECUT PREDAY PREDRY PREENS PREFAB PREFER PREFIX PRELAW PRELIM PRELOG PREMED PREMET PREMIE PREMIX PRENUP PREOPS PREPAY PREPPY PRESET PRESTO PRETAX PRETER PRETOR PRETTY PREVIA PREVIN PREVUE PREWAR PREXES PREYED PREYER PREYON PRFIRM PRICED PRICER PRICES PRICEY PRICKS PRIDED PRIDES PRIERS PRIEST PRIMAL PRIMED PRIMER PRIMES PRIMLY PRIMOS PRIMPS PRIMUS PRINCE PRINKS PRINTS PRINZE PRIORI PRIORS PRIORY PRISED PRISMS PRISON PRISSY PRIVET PRIZED PRIZES PRIZMS PRIZZI PROAMS PROART PROBED PROBER PROBES PROBIE PROBST PROCOL PRODON PROEMS PROFIT PROGUN PROJET PROLES PROLIX PROLOG PROMOS PROMPT PRONGS PRONTO PROOFS PROPEL PROPER PROPRE PROPUP PROPYL PROSED PROSER PROSES PROSIT PROSKY PROTAX PROTEA PROTEM PROTON PROULX PROUST PROVED PROVEN PROVER PROVES PROWAR PROWLS PROWSE PROYAS PROZAC PRUDES PRUETT PRUNED PRUNER PRUNES PRYERS PRYING PRYNNE PRYOFF

P•R•••

PARADE PARANA PARAPH PARCAE PARCEL PARDON PARENS PARENT PARERS PARETO PAREUS PAREVE PARFUM PARGED PARGER PARGES PARIAH PARING PARINI PARISH PARITY PARKAS PARKAV PARKAY PARKED PARKER PARKES PARKIT PARLAY PARLEY PARLEZ PARLOR PARNIS PARODY PAROLE PAROLS PARRED PARRIS PARROT PARSEC PARSED PARSEE PARSER PARSES PARSON PARTED PARTII PARTIV PARTLY PARTOF PARTON PARTYS PARURE PERCHA PERDAY PERDUE PERILS PERINE PERIOD PERISH PERITI PERKED PERKIN PERKUP PERLEA PERMED PERMIT PERNOD PERRIN PERROS PERSIA PERSIS PERSON PERTER PERTLY PERUKE PERUSE PERUTZ PHRASE PIRACY PIRANA PIRATE PIRRIP PORERS PORING PORKED PORKER PORKYS POROSE POROUS PORTAL PORTED PORTER PORTES PORTIA PORTLY PQRSTU PTRAPS PURDUE PUREED PUREES PURELY PUREST PURFLE PURGED PURGES PURIFY PURIMS PURINA PURISM PURIST PURITY PURLED PURLIE PURPLE PURPLY PURRED PURRER PURSED PURSER PURSES PURSUE PURVEY PYRHHO PYRITE

P••R••

PADRES PAIRED PAIRUP PARRED PARRIS PARROT PATRIA PATRIC PATRIE PATROL PATRON PEARCE PEARLE PEARLS PEARLY PEERAT PEERCE PEERED PEERIN PEIRCE PENROD PEORIA PERRIN PERROS PETRAT PETREL PETRIE PETROL PHAROS PICRIC PIERCE PIERIA PIERRE PIRRIP PITROW PLURAL POIRES POIRET POIROT POORAT POORER POORIS POORLY POURED POURER POURIN PUERTO PURRED PURRER PUTRID

P•••R•

PACERS PAGERS PALTRY PAMIRS PANFRY PANTRY PAPERS PAPERY PAPYRI PARERS PARURE PASTRY PATDRY PATERS PAVERS PAWERS PAYERS PELTRY PENURY PETARD PETERI PETERS PGAPRO PHEDRE PICARA PICARD PICARO PIERRE PIETRO PIKERS PILERS PINERO PINERS PINERY PIPERS PLEURA PLIERS POETRY POIVRE POKERS POKERY POLARA POLERS POPART PORERS POSERS POUDRE POWERS PREARM PREDRY PRFIRM PRIERS PRIORI PRIORS PRIORY PROART PROPRE PRYERS PULERS

P••••R

PACIER PACKER PADDER PALLOR PALMAR PALMER PALTER PAMPER PANDER PANIER PANNER PANTER PANZER PAPIER PARGER PARKER PARLOR PARSER PASDAR PASSER PASTER PASTOR PATTER PATZER PAUPER PAUSER PAVIOR PAWNER PAYFOR PCUSER PEALER PEEKER PEELER PEEPER PEGLER PELTER PENNER PEPPER PERTER PESTER PETTER PEWTER PFIZER PHASER PHONER PICKER PICTOR PIECER PIETER PILFER PILLAR PINCER PINDAR PINGER PINIER PINKER PINNER PINTER PIPIER PITIER PLACER PLANAR PLANER PLATER PLAYER PLEXOR PLOMER PLOVER PLOWER POGNER POISER POKIER POLGAR POLLER PONDER POOLER POORER POPLAR POPPER PORKER PORTER POSEUR POSHER POSTER POTHER POTTER POURER POUTER POWDER POYSER PRATER PRAWER PRAYER PREFER PRETER PRETOR PREWAR PREYER PRICER PRIMER PROBER PROPER PROSER PROVER PROWAR PRUNER PSYWAR PUCKER PUFFER PULLER PULPER PULSAR PULVER PUMPER PUNIER PUNKER PUNNER PUNTER PURRER PURSER PUSHER PUTTER

•PR•••

APRILE APRILS APRONS OPRAHS SPRACH SPRAIN SPRANG SPRATS SPRAWL SPRAYS SPREAD SPREES SPRIER SPRIGS SPRING SPRINT SPRITE SPRITS SPRITZ SPROUT SPRUCE SPRUNG SPRYER SPRYLY UPRATE UPREAR UPRISE UPROAR UPROOT UPROSE UPRUSH XPRIZE

•P•R••

APERCU APPROX EPARCH EPHRON OPERAS OPORTO OPQRST

SPARED
SPARER
SPARES
SPARKS
SPARKY
SPARSE
SPARTA
SPERRY
SPIRAL
SPIREA
SPIRED
SPIRES
SPIRIT
SPORES
SPORKS
SPORTS
SPORTY
SPURNS
SPURON
SPURTS
UPGREW
UPGROW
UPPROP

•P••R•

APIARY
APPERT
EPHORS
SPEARE
SPEARS
SPERRY
SPHERE
SPIERS
SPOORS
UPCARD
UPCURL
UPDART
UPGIRD
UPGIRT
UPHERE
UPPERS
UPTORE
UPTORN
UPTURN
UPWARD

•P•••R

APPEAR
EPOWER
IPETER
OPENER
OPINER
OPTFOR
SPACER
SPADER
SPARER
SPAYER
SPEWER
SPICER
SPIDER
SPIKER
SPINER
SPRIER
SPRYER
SPYDER
UPBEAR
UPOVER
UPREAR
UPROAR
UPSOAR
UPSTIR
UPTEAR

••PR••

APPROX
CAPRID
CAPRIS
COPRAS
CUPRIC
CYPRUS
ESPRIT
IMPROV
KUPRIN
NOPROB
OSPREY
REPROS
RIPRAP
SUPRAS
TOPROW
UNPRIM
UPPROP

••P•R•

ALPERT
AMPERE
APPERT
ASPERA
ASPIRE
ASPURE
CAPERS
COPERS
DEPART
DEPERE
DEPORT
DOPERS
DUPERS
DUPERY
EMPERY
EMPIRE
EXPERT
EXPIRE
EXPIRY
EXPORT
GAPERS
HOPERS
HYPERS
IMPART
IMPERF
IMPORT
IMPURE
INPARK
INPART
INPORT
JAPERS
JAPERY
LAPERI
LAPERM
LEPERS
LIPARI
LOPERS
MOPERS
MOPERY
NAPERY
NEPHRO
NOPQRS
PAPERS
PAPERY
PAPYRI
PIPERS
POPART
REPARK
REPERK
REPORT
ROPERS
ROPERY
RUPERT
RVPARK
SAPORS
SEPIRA
SOPORS
SUPERB
SUPERG
SUPERS
TAPERS
TAPIRS
TOPERS
TYPERS
UMPIRE
UNPURE
UPPERS
VAPORS
VAPORY
VIPERS
WIPERS

••P••R

AMPLER
APPEAR
AUPAIR
BOPPER
CAPPER
CAPTOR
CIPHER
COPCAR
COPIER
COPPER
COPTER
CYPHER
DAPPER
DIPPER
DOPIER
EMPTOR
ESPIER
GIPPER
GOPHER
GYPPER
HEPPER
HIPPER
HOPPER
IMPAIR
INPOUR
KEPLER
KIPPER
KIPPUR
LAPPER
LAPSER
LIPPER
LOPPER
MAPPER
MOPIER
MOPPER
NAPIER
NAPPER
NIPPER
PAPIER
PEPPER
PIPIER
POPLAR
POPPER
RAPIER
RAPPER
RAPTER
RAPTOR
REPAIR
REPFOR
REPOUR
RIPPER
ROPIER
SAPPER
SIPPER
SUPPER
TAPPER
TIPJAR
TIPPER
TOPPER
TUPPER
VAPOUR
WAPNER
YAPPER
ZAPPER
ZEPHYR
ZIPPER

•••PR•

ALLPRO
CHOPRA
NONPRO
OLDPRO
OUTPRY
PGAPRO
PROPRE
SEMPRE
THEPRU

•••P•R

BEEPER
BOPPER
BUMPER
CAMPER
CAPPER
CARPER
CASPAR
CASPER
COOPER
COPPER
COWPER
DAMPER
DAPPER
DEEPER
DIAPER
DIPPER
DRAPER
DUMPER
ELOPER
GASPAR
GASPER
GAWPER
GIPPER
GRIPER
GROPER
GULPER
GYPPER
HAMPER
HARPER
HEAPER
HELPER
HEPPER
HIPPER
HOOPER
HOPPER
JAIPUR
JASPER
JUMPER
KEEPER
KIPPER
KIPPUR
LAPPER
LAUPER
LEAPER
LIMPER
LIPPER
LISPER
LOOPER
LOPPER
LUMPER
LUMPUR
MAPPER
MNOPQR
MOPPER
NAPPER
NIPPER
NONPAR
ONAPAR
PAMPER
PAUPER
PEEPER
PEPPER
POPPER
PROPER
PULPER
PUMPER
RAIPUR
RAPPER
RASPER
REAPER
RIPPER
ROEPER
ROMPER
SAPPER
SEMPER
SHAPER
SIMPER
SIPPER
SLOPER
SNIPER
SOAPER
SOUPER
STUPOR
SUBPAR
SUPPER
SWIPER
TAMPER
TAPPER
TEMPER
TIPPER
TOPPER
TORPOR
TUPPER
VAMPER
VESPER
WARPER
WEEPER
WOLPER
YAPPER
YAWPER
YELPER
ZAPPER
ZIPPER

PS••••

PSALMS
PSEUDO
PSEUDS
PSHAWS
PSYCHE
PSYCHO
PSYCHS
PSYWAR

P•S•••

PASCAL
PASCHS
PASCUA
PASDAR
PASEOS
PASHAS
PASHTO
PASMOI
PASSAS
PASSAT
PASSBY
PASSED
PASSEL
PASSER
PASSES
PASSGO
PASSIM
PASSON
PASSOS
PASSTO
PASSUP
PASTAS
PASTED
PASTEL
PASTER
PASTES
PASTIS
PASTIT
PASTOR
PASTRY
PESACH
PESADE
PESCOW
PESETA
PESEWA
PESTER
PESTLE
PESTOS
PISANO
PISANS
PISCES
PISGAH
PISHED
PISHES
PISTES
PISTIL
PISTOL
PISTON
PISTOU
POSADA
POSEAS
POSERS
POSEUR
POSHER
POSHLY
POSIES
POSING
POSITS
POSOLE
POSSES
POSSLQ
POSSUM
POSTAL
POSTED
POSTER
POSTIE
POSTIT
POSTON
POSTOP
POSTUM
PUSHED
PUSHER
PUSHES
PUSHIN
PUSHIT
PUSHON
PUSHUP
PUSSES

P••S••

PABSTS
PAISAN
PAISES
PANSIN
PARSEC
PARSED
PARSEE
PARSER
PARSES
PARSON
PASSAS
PASSAT
PASSBY
PASSED
PASSEL
PASSER
PASSES
PASSGO
PASSIM
PASSON
PASSOS
PASSTO
PASSUP
PAUSAL
PAUSED
PAUSER
PAUSES
PAWSAT
PAYSIN
PAYSON
PAYSUP
PCUSER
PENSEE
PENSIN
PENSUP
PEPSIN
PEPSUP
PERSIA
PERSIS
PERSON
PETSAT
PETSIT
PHASED
PHASER
PHASES
PHASIC
PHYSED
PHYSIC
PHYSIO
PIGSIT
PIGSTY
PINSON
PINSUP
PITSAW
PIUSII
PIUSIV
PIUSIX
PIUSVI
PIUSXI
PLASHY
PLASMA
PLASMO
PLISSE
PLUSES
PLUSHY
POISED
POISER
POISES
POISHA
POISON
POLSKA
POPSIN
POPSUP
POSSES
POSSLQ
POSSUM
POTSIE
POUSSE
POYSER
PQRSTU
PRESET
PRESTO
PRISED
PRISMS
PRISON
PRISSY
PROSED
PROSER
PROSES
PROSIT
PROSKY
PULSAR
PULSED
PULSES
PURSED
PURSER
PURSES
PURSUE
PUSSES
PUTSBY
PUTSCH
PUTSIN
PUTSON
PUTSTO
PUTSUP

P•••S•

PALEST
PALISH
PAPIST
PARISH
PAVESE
PELOSI
PERISH
PERUSE
PHRASE
PILOSE
PLEASE
PLISSE
POLISH
POPISH
POROSE
POTASH
POTOSI
POUSSE
PRAISE
PRIEST
PRISSY
PROBST
PROUST
PROWSE
PUNISH
PUREST
PURISM
PURIST

P••••S

PABSTS
PACERS
PADRES
PAEANS
PAGANS
PAGERS
PAINTS
PAISES
PALAIS
PALLAS
PALMAS
PAMIRS
PAMPAS
PANCKS
PANDAS
PANDLS
PANELS
PANICS
PANNES
PANTOS
PAPAWS
PAPERS
PAPPAS
PARENS
PARERS
PAREUS
PARGES
PARKAS
PARKES
PARNIS
PAROLS
PARRIS
PARSES
PARTYS
PASCHS
PASEOS
PASHAS
PASSAS
PASSES
PASSOS
PASTAS
PASTES
PASTIS
PATENS
PATERS
PATHOS
PATIOS
PATMOS
PATOIS
PAUSES
PAVERS
PAWERS
PAYEES
PAYERS
PBOOKS
PCLABS
PEALES
PEARLS
PECANS
PECHES
PEDALS
PEEVES
PEKOES
PELEUS
PELVIS
PENNIS
PERILS
PERROS
PERSIS
PESTOS
PETALS
PETERS
PETTIS
PEWEES
PEWITS
PHAROS
PHASES
PHELPS
PHIALS
PHOBOS
PHONES
PHONOS
PHOTOS
PIANOS
PICOTS
PIECES
PIETAS
PIKERS
PILAFS
PILAUS
PILERS
PILEUS
PILOTS
PILOUS
PINDUS
PINERS
PINKOS
PINNAS
PINONS
PINOTS
PINTOS
PINUPS
PIPERS
PIPETS
PIPITS
PIQUES
PISANS
PISCES
PISHES
PISTES
PITIES
PITONS
PITOTS
PIUTES
PIVOTS
PIXELS
PIXIES
PIZZAS
PLACES
PLAGES
PLAIDS
PLAINS
PLAITS
PLANAS
PLANBS
PLANES
PLANKS
PLANTS
PLATES
PLATOS
PLATYS
PLAYAS
PLAZAS
PLEADS
PLEATS
PLEBES
PLEXES
PLEXUS
PLIERS
PLINKS
PLOCES
PLONKS
PLUCKS
PLUIES
PLUMBS
PLUMES
PLUMPS
PLUNKS
PLUSES
PLUTUS
POBOYS
PODOUS
POEMES
POETES
POILUS
POINTS
POIRES
POISES
POKERS
POKEYS
POKIES
POLERS
POLIOS
POLKAS
POLLOS
POLYPS
POMMES
PONCAS
PONIES
PONZUS
POORIS
POPPAS
POPUPS
PORERS
PORKYS
POROUS
PORTES
POSEAS
POSERS
POSIES
POSITS
POSSES
POTHOS
POTTOS
POULES
POULTS
POUNDS
POWERS
PRADAS
PRANAS
PRANKS
PRATES
PRAWNS
PRAXES
PRAXIS
PRECIS
PREENS
PREOPS
PREXES
PRICES
PRICKS
PRIDES
PRIERS
PRIMES
PRIMOS
PRIMPS
PRIMUS
PRINKS
PRINTS
PRIORS
PRISMS
PRIZES
PRIZMS
PROAMS
PROBES
PROEMS
PROLES
PROMOS
PRONGS
PROOFS
PROSES
PROVES
PROWLS
PROYAS
PRUDES
PRUNES
PRYERS
PSALMS
PSEUDS
PSHAWS
PSYCHS
PTILES
PTRAPS
PUCCIS
PUJOLS
PULERS
PULSES
PUNKAS
PUNTAS
PUPILS
PUREES
PURGES
PURIMS
PURSES
PUSHES
PUSSES
PUTONS
PYLONS

•PS•••

CPSNOW
EPSONS
UPSALA
UPSEND
UPSENT
UPSETS
UPSHAW
UPSHOT
UPSIDE
UPSIZE
UPSOAR
UPSPIN
UPSTEP
UPSTIR

•P•S••

EPOSES
OPTSIN
OPTSTO
OPUSES
SPASMS

•P••S•

APPOSE
APTEST
OPPOSE
OPQRST
SPARSE
SPLASH
SPLOSH
SPOUSE
UPCAST
UPLAST
UPMOST
UPPISH
UPRISE
UPROSE
UPRUSH
UPTOSS

•P•••S

APEXES
APHIDS
APICES
APNEAS
APPALS
APPELS
APPLES
APRILS
APRONS
EPACTS
EPHAHS
EPHODS
EPHORS
EPOCHS
EPODES
EPOSES
EPSONS
OPCITS
OPERAS
OPHULS
OPINES
OPIUMS
OPRAHS
OPTICS
OPUSES
SPACES
SPADES
SPANKS
SPARES
SPARKS
SPASMS
SPATES
SPAWNS
SPEAKS
SPEARS
SPECKS
SPEEDS
SPELLS
SPENDS
SPICES
SPIELS
SPIERS
SPIFFS
SPIKES
SPILES
SPILLS
SPINES
SPINKS
SPIRES
SPITES
SPLATS
SPLAYS
SPLITS
SPODES
SPOILS
SPOKES
SPOOFS
SPOOKS
SPOOLS
SPOONS
SPOORS
SPORES
SPORKS
SPORTS
SPOUTS
SPRATS
SPRAYS
SPREES
SPRIGS
SPRITS
SPUMES
SPURNS
SPURTS
UPBOWS
UPENDS
UPPERS
UPSETS
UPTOSS

••PS••

AMPSUP
COPSES
COPSIT
COPSTO
DIPSIN
DIPSOS
EMPSON
GYPSUM
HOPSIN
HOPSON
HOPSTO
HOPSUP
LAPSAT
LAPSED
LAPSER
LAPSES
LAPSUP
LAPSUS
MOPSUP
NIPSAT
NIPSEY
PEPSIN
PEPSUP
POPSIN
POPSUP
RAPSON
RIPSAW
RIPSON
RIPSUP
SIPSON
SOPSUP
TAPSIN
TAPSON
TIPSIN
TIPSUP
TOPSUP
YAPSAT
ZIPSBY
ZIPSIN
ZIPSIT
ZIPSUP

••P•S•

APPOSE
ASPISH
BYPASS
BYPAST
CWPOST
DEPEST
DEPOSE
ELPASO
ESPOSA
ESPOSO
EXPOSE
EXPOST
EZPASS
GOPAST
HOPESO
IMPISH
IMPOSE
IMPOST
LIPASE
MOPISH
NYPOST
ONPOST
OPPOSE
PAPIST
POPISH
REPASS
REPAST
REPOSE
REPOST

RIPEST
RIPOST
TYPIST
UNPOSH
UPPISH

••P••S

ALPHAS
APPALS
APPELS
APPLES
ARPELS
ASPENS
ASPICS
BIPEDS
BIPODS
BUPKES
BUPKIS
BUPKUS
BYPASS
CAPERS
CAPONS
CAPRIS
COPALS
COPAYS
COPERS
COPIES
COPRAS
COPSES
CSPOTS
CUPELS
CUPIDS
CUPPAS
CYPRUS
DEPOTS
DEPTHS
DIPSOS
DOPERS
DUPERS
DUPLOS
ELPAIS
ESPIES
ESPIOS
EXPATS
EXPELS
EZPASS
GAPERS
HIPPOS
HIPPUS
HOPERS
HYPERS
HYPNOS
IMPELS
INPUTS
JAPANS
JAPERS
KAPOKS
KAPPAS
KOPEKS
KOPJES
LAPELS
LAPINS
LAPSES
LAPSUS
LEPERS
LIPIDS
LOPERS
MAPLES
MOPEDS
MOPERS
MOPUPS
MRPAWS
NAPLES
NAPPES
NIPUPS
NOPALS
NOPETS
NOPQRS
OOPODS
PAPAWS
PAPERS
PAPPAS
PIPERS
PIPETS
PIPITS
POPPAS
POPUPS
PUPILS
RAPIDS
RAPTUS
REPADS
REPASS
REPAYS
REPEGS
REPELS
REPENS
REPINS
REPOTS
REPROS
REPUBS
RIPENS
ROPERS
RUPEES
SAPORS
SEPALS
SEPIAS
SEPOYS
SOPORS
STPATS
STPIUS
SUPERS
SUPRAS
TAPERS
TAPINS
TAPIRS
TEPEES
TIPINS
TOPEES
TOPERS
TOPICS
TYPEAS
TYPEBS
TYPEOS
TYPERS
TYPHUS
UNPEGS
UNPENS
UNPINS
UNPOTS
UPPERS
VAPORS
VIPERS
WIPERS
ZIPONS
ZIPPOS

•••PS•

BIOPSY
CORPSE
DROPSY
ELAPSE
FLOPSY

•••P•S

ADAPTS
ADEPTS
ADOPTS
ALEPHS
CAMPOS
CAMPUS
CARPUS
COAPTS
COMPAS
COMPOS
COOPTS
CORPUS
COUPES
COYPUS
CRAPES
CREPES
CRIPES
CRYPTS
CUPPAS
DRAPES
DRUPES
ELOPES
ERUPTS
ETAPES
GLYPHS
GRAPES
GRAPHS
GRIPES
GROPES
HIPPOS
HIPPUS
HUMPHS
IBMPCS
JALPAS
KAPPAS
KEMPIS
LOUPES
LYMPHS
MORPHS
MYOPES
NAPPES
NYMPHS
OKAPIS
OOMPHS
PAMPAS
PAPPAS
POPPAS
QUIPUS
RASPAS
RUMPUS
SCOPES
SHAPES
SLOPES
SNIPES
SNOPES
STAPES
STAPHS
STIPES
STUPAS
STUPES
SWIPES
SYLPHS
TAUPES
TEMPOS
TEMPTS
TEMPUS
TRIPES
TROPES
VESPAS
XTYPES
ZIPPOS

••••PS

ADREPS
AESOPS
ALMVPS
BEBOPS
BICEPS
BLEEPS
BLIMPS
BLOOPS
CHAMPS
CHEEPS
CHEOPS
CHIMPS
CHIRPS
CHOMPS
CHUMPS
CLAMPS
CLASPS
CLOMPS
CLUMPS
CRAMPS
CREEPS
CRIMPS
CRISPS
CROUPS
CRUMPS
CUTUPS
DECAPS
DOLAPS
DROOPS
EQUIPS
ESTOPS
FIXUPS
FRUMPS
FSTOPS
GALOPS
GETUPS
GRAMPS
GRASPS
GROUPS
GRUMPS
ICEUPS
INCAPS
JAMUPS
JULEPS
LAYUPS
LETUPS
MEROPS
MIXUPS
MOPUPS
NIPUPS
NLMVPS
NOTIPS
ONEUPS
ORLOPS
OXLIPS
PHELPS
PINUPS
PLUMPS
POLYPS
POPUPS
PREOPS
PRIMPS
PTRAPS
REBOPS
RECAPS
REDIPS
RELAPS
REMAPS
REMOPS
RETAPS
RETIPS
RETOPS
REZIPS
RUNUPS
SALEPS
SCALPS
SCAMPS
SCARPS
SCOOPS
SCRAPS
SCRIPS
SETUPS
SHARPS
SIRUPS
SITUPS
SKIMPS
SLEEPS
SLOOPS
SLUMPS
SLURPS
SNOOPS
STAMPS
STEEPS
STOMPS
STOOPS
STRAPS
STREPS
STRIPS
STROPS
STUMPS
SUMUPS
SUNUPS
SWAMPS
SWEEPS
SWOOPS
SYRUPS
SYSOPS
THESPS
THUMPS
TIEUPS
TRAMPS
TROMPS
TROOPS
TRUMPS
TSTOPS
TULIPS
TWERPS
TWIRPS
UNCAPS
UNRIPS
UNZIPS
USURPS
VCHIPS
WHELPS
WHOMPS
WHOOPS

PT••••

PTBOAT
PTILES
PTOOEY
PTRAPS

P•T•••

PATACA
PATAKI
PATCHY
PATDAY
PATDRY
PATENS
PATENT
PATERS
PATHAN
PATHIC
PATHOS
PATINA
PATINE
PATIOS
PATMOS
PATOIS
PATRIA
PATRIC
PATRIE
PATROL
PATRON
PATTED
PATTEN
PATTER
PATTIE
PATTON
PATZER
PETAIN
PETALE
PETALS
PETARD
PETBOA
PETCAT
PETCOW
PETDOG
PETERI
PETERS
PETIPA
PETITE
PETNAP
PETPIG
PETPUP
PETRAT
PETREL
PETRIE
PETROL
PETSAT
PETSIT
PETTED
PETTER
PETTET
PETTIS
PETTIT
PETTOY
PETULA
PITAYA
PITCHY
PITHED
PITIED
PITIER
PITIES
PITKIN
PITMAN
PITMEN
PITNEY
PITONS
PITOTS
PITROW
PITSAW
PITTED
POTAGE
POTASH
POTATO
POTEEN
POTENT
POTFUL
POTHER
POTHOS
POTION
POTLID
POTOSI
POTPIE
POTSIE
POTTED
POTTER
POTTOS
POTVIN
PUTNAM
PUTNEY
PUTOFF
PUTONS
PUTOUT
PUTPUT
PUTRID
PUTSBY
PUTSCH
PUTSIN
PUTSON
PUTSTO
PUTSUP
PUTTED
PUTTEE
PUTTER
PUTTIN
PYTHON

P••T••

PACTEN
PALTER
PALTRY
PANTED
PANTER
PANTIE
PANTOS
PANTRY
PARTED
PARTII
PARTIV
PARTLY
PARTOF
PARTON
PARTYS
PASTAS
PASTED
PASTEL
PASTER
PASTES
PASTIS
PASTIT
PASTOR
PASTRY
PATTED
PATTEN
PATTER
PATTIE
PATTON
PAXTON
PAYTON
PECTIN
PEGTOP
PELTED
PELTER
PELTRY
PENTAD
PENTAX
PENTEL
PENTUP
PEPTIC
PERTER
PERTLY
PESTER
PESTLE
PESTOS
PETTED
PETTER
PETTET
PETTIS
PETTIT
PETTOY
PEWTER
PEYTON
PHOTIC
PHOTOG
PHOTON
PHOTOS
PICTOR
PIETAS
PIETER
PIETIN
PIETRO
PINTER
PINTOS
PISTES
PISTIL
PISTOL
PISTON
PISTOU
PITTED
PIUTES
PLATED
PLATEN
PLATER
PLATES
PLATOS
PLATTE
PLATYS
PLOTTY
PLUTON
PLUTUS
POETES
POETIC
POETRY
POITOU
POPTOP
PORTAL
PORTED
PORTER
PORTES
PORTIA
PORTLY
POSTAL
POSTED
POSTER
POSTIE
POSTIT
POSTON
POSTOP
POSTUM
POTTED
POTTER
POTTOS
POUTED
POUTER
PRATED
PRATER
PRATES
PRETAX
PRETER
PRETOR
PRETTY
PROTAX
PROTEA
PROTEM
PROTON
PUNTAS
PUNTED
PUNTER
PUTTED
PUTTEE
PUTTER
PUTTIN

P•••T•

PABSTS
PAINTS
PAINTY
PAIUTE
PALATE
PARETO
PARITY
PASHTO
PASSTO
PEDATE
PELOTA
PEPITA
PERITI
PERUTZ
PESETA
PETITE
PEWITS
PEYOTE
PICOTS
PIGSTY
PILATE
PILOTS
PINATA
PINOTS
PIPETS
PIPITS
PIRATE
PITOTS
PIVOTS
PLAITS
PLANTE
PLANTO
PLANTS
PLATTE
PLAYTO
PLEATS
PLEDTO
PLENTY
PLINTH
PLOTTY
POINTA
POINTB
POINTE
POINTS
POINTY
POLITE
POLITY
POSITS
POTATO
POULTS
PQRSTU
PRAYTO
PRESTO
PRETTY
PRINTS
PRONTO
PRUETT
PUENTE
PUERTO
PUPATE
PURITY
PUTSTO
PYRITE

P••••T

PACKET
PALEST
PALLET
PANDIT
PANOUT
PAPIST
PARENT
PARKIT
PARROT
PASSAT
PASTIT
PATENT
PAWSAT
PAYCUT
PAYOUT
PEANUT
PECKAT
PEDANT
PEEKAT
PEEPAT
PEERAT
PELLET
PENULT
PEQUOT
PERMIT
PETCAT
PETRAT
PETSAT
PETSIT
PETTET
PETTIT
PHFFFT
PIAGET
PICKAT
PICKET
PIELET
PIGLET
PIGNUT
PIGOUT
PIGSIT
PIOLET
PIPPET
PIQUET
PLAINT
PLAKAT
PLANET
PLAYAT
PLAYIT
PLIANT
PLIGHT
POCKET
POIRET
POIROT
POKEAT
POLPOT
POORAT
POPART
POPOUT
POSTIT
POTENT
PREACT
PRECUT
PREMET
PRESET
PRIEST
PRIVET
PROART
PROBST
PROFIT
PROJET
PROMPT
PROSIT
PROUST
PRUETT
PTBOAT
PULLET
PULPIT
PUNDIT
PUPPET
PUREST
PURIST
PUSHIT
PUTOUT
PUTPUT

•PT•••

APTEST
OPTFOR
OPTICS
OPTIMA
OPTIMO
OPTING
OPTION
OPTOUT
OPTSIN
OPTSTO
UPTAKE
UPTALK
UPTEAR
UPTICK
UPTILT
UPTIME
UPTOIT
UPTORE
UPTORN
UPTOSS
UPTOWN
UPTURN

•P•T••

APATHY
IPETER
SPATES
SPATHE
SPITED
SPITES
SPITON
SPOTON
SPOTTV
SPOTTY
UPSTEP
UPSTIR

•P••T•

APLITE
EPACTS
KPDUTY
OPCITS
OPENTO
OPIATE
OPORTO
OPTSTO
SPARTA
SPILTH
SPLATS
SPLITS
SPORTS
SPORTY
SPOTTV
SPOTTY
SPOUTS
SPRATS
SPRITE
SPRITS
SPRITZ
SPURTS
UPDATE
UPLATE
UPPITY
UPRATE
UPSETS

•P•••T

APELET
APPERT
APPLET
APTEST
OPENIT
OPQRST
OPTOUT
SPIGOT
SPINET
SPIRIT
SPLINT
SPOILT
SPRINT
SPROUT
SPYBOT
SPYOUT
UPBEAT
UPCAST
UPDART
UPGIRT
UPLAST
UPLIFT
UPMOST
UPNEXT
UPROOT
UPSENT
UPSHOT
UPTILT
UPTOIT
UPWAFT

••PT••

CAPTOR
COPTER
COPTIC
DEPTHS
EMPTOR
HEPTAD
KEPTAT
KEPTIN
KEPTON
KEPTTO
KEPTUP
LAPTEV
LAPTOP
LEPTON
LIPTON
LUPTON
MOPTOP
PEPTIC
POPTOP
RAPTER
RAPTLY
RAPTOR
RAPTUS
SEPTAL
SEPTET
SEPTIC
SEPTUM
TIPTOE
TIPTOP
TOPTEN
TUPTIM
ZIPTOP

••P•T•

BYPATH
CAPITA
CAPOTE
COPSTO
CSPOTS
DEPOTS
DEPUTE
DEPUTY
EMPATH
EXPATS
HEPATO
HOPETO
HOPSTO
IMPUTE
INPUTS
KAPUTT
KEPTTO
LAPUTA
MAPUTO
NAPHTA
NOPETS
PEPITA
PIPETS
PIPITS
PUPATE
REPOTS
REPUTE
STPATS
STPETE
UNPOTS
UPPITY
WAPITI
ZAPATA

••P••T

ALPERT
APPERT
APPLET
ASPECT
BYPAST
CAPLET
CAPNUT
COPOUT
COPSIT
CWPOST
DEPART
DEPEST
DEPICT
DEPORT
DIPNET
DUPONT
ESPRIT
EXPECT
EXPERT
EXPORT
EXPOST
GAPEAT
GOPAST
HEPCAT
HOPOUT
IMPACT
IMPART
IMPORT
IMPOST
INPART
INPORT
KAPUTT
KEPTAT
LAPCAT
LAPPET
LAPSAT
LIPOUT
MAPOUT
MOPPET
MUPPET
NIPSAT
NYPOST
ONPOST
PAPIST
PIPPET
POPART
POPOUT
PUPPET
REPAST
REPEAT
REPENT
REPLOT
REPORT
REPOST
RIPEST
RIPOST
RIPOUT
RUPERT
SEPTET
TAPOUT
TAPPET
TIPPET
TOPCAT
TOPHAT
TOPOUT
TYPIST
UNPENT
YAPHET
YAPSAT
ZIPOUT
ZIPSIT

•••PT•

ADAPTS
ADEPTS
ADOPTS
COAPTS
COOPTS
CRYPTO
CRYPTS
DUMPTY
ERUPTS
GLYPTO
GOUPTO
HUMPTY
KEEPTO
KLEPTO
KRYPTO
SHIPTO
SNAPTO
TEMPTS

•••P•T

AIRPOT
ARMPIT
ASHPIT
BBQPIT
BEEPAT
CARPAT
CARPET
DESPOT
DROPIT
EELPOT
EYEPIT
FLOPIT
HERPET
HOTPOT
INAPET
INKPOT
INSPOT
ITSPAT
JUMPAT
KEEPAT
KEEPIT
LAPPET
LEAPAT
LIMPET

LUMPIT
MOPPET
MUPPET
OUTPUT
PEEPAT
PIPPET
POLPOT
PULPIT
PUPPET
PUTPUT
RESPOT
SATPAT
SAWPIT
SEXPOT
SHOPAT
SITPAT
SKIPIT
SNAPAT
STOPAT
STOPIT
TAPPET
TARPIT
TEAPOT
THEPIT
TINPOT
TIPPET
TVSPOT

••••PT
ABRUPT
ACCEPT
ENRAPT
EXCEPT
EXEMPT
INCEPT
IRRUPT
PROMPT
SCRIPT
SCULPT
UNKEPT
UNWEPT
YCLEPT

PU••••
PUBLIC
PUBLIX
PUCCIS
PUCKER
PUDDLE
PUDDLY
PUEBLA
PUEBLO
PUENTE
PUENZO
PUERTO
PUFFED
PUFFER
PUFFIN
PUFFUP
PUGGLE
PUJOLS
PULERS
PULING
PULLED
PULLER
PULLET
PULLEY
PULLIN
PULLON
PULLUP
PULMON
PULPED
PULPER
PULPIT
PULSAR
PULSED
PULSES
PULVER
PUMICE
PUMMEL
PUMPED
PUMPER
PUMPUP
PUNCHY
PUNDIT
PUNIER
PUNILY
PUNISH
PUNJAB
PUNKAS
PUNKER
PUNKIE
PUNNED
PUNNER
PUNTAS
PUNTED
PUNTER
PUPATE
PUPILS
PUPKIN
PUPPED
PUPPET
PURDUE
PUREED
PUREES
PURELY
PUREST
PURFLE
PURGED
PURGES
PURIFY
PURIMS
PURINA
PURISM
PURIST
PURITY
PURLED
PURLIE
PURPLE
PURPLY
PURRED
PURRER
PURSED
PURSER
PURSES
PURSUE
PURVEY
PUSHED
PUSHER
PUSHES
PUSHIN
PUSHIT
PUSHON
PUSHUP
PUSSES
PUTNAM
PUTNEY
PUTOFF
PUTONS
PUTOUT
PUTPUT
PUTRID
PUTSBY
PUTSCH
PUTSIN
PUTSON
PUTSTO
PUTSUP
PUTTED
PUTTEE
PUTTER
PUTTIN
PUZZLE

P•U•••
PAULEY
PAULII
PAULIV
PAULVI
PAUNCH
PAUPER
PAUSAL
PAUSED
PAUSER
PAUSES
PCUSER
PIUSII
PIUSIV
PIUSIX
PIUSVI
PIUSXI
PIUTES
PLUCKS
PLUCKY
PLUGIN
PLUGUP
PLUIES
PLUMBO
PLUMBS
PLUMED
PLUMES
PLUMMY
PLUMPS
PLUNGE
PLUNKS
PLUNKY
PLURAL
PLUSES
PLUSHY
PLUTON
PLUTUS
PLUVIA
PLUVIO
POUCHY
POUDRE
POUFED
POUFFY
POULES
POULTS
POUNCE
POUNDS
POUPON
POURED
POURER
POURIN
POUSSE
POUTED
POUTER
PRUDES
PRUETT
PRUNED
PRUNER
PRUNES

P••U••
PACULA
PADUAN
PAIUTE
PAKULA
PAPUAN
PAQUIN
PARURE
PENULT
PENURY
PEQUOD
PEQUOT
PERUKE
PERUSE
PERUTZ
PETULA
PINUPS
PIQUED
PIQUES
PIQUET
PLEURA
PLOUGH
PNEUMA
PNEUMO
PODUNK
POPULI
POPUPS
PROULX
PROUST
PSEUDO
PSEUDS

P•••U•
PABLUM
PACKUP
PAGEUP
PAIDUP
PAIRUP
PANFUL
PANOUT
PAREUS
PARFUM
PASCUA
PASSUP
PAYCUT
PAYOUT
PAYSUP
PEANUT
PELEUS
PENSUP
PENTUP
PEPFUL
PEPLUM
PEPSUP
PERDUE
PERKUP
PETPUP
PHYLUM
PICKUP
PIGNUT
PIGOUT
PILAUS
PILEUM
PILEUP
PILEUS
PILOUS
PINDUS
PINSUP
PIPEUP
PLAGUE
PLAQUE
PLAYUP
PLENUM
PLEXUS
PLOWUP
PLUGUP
PLUTUS
PODIUM
PODOUS
POILUS
POLLUX
PONYUP
PONZUS
POPGUN
POPOUT
POPSUP
POROUS
POSEUR
POSSUM
POSTUM
POTFUL
PRAGUE
PREBUY
PRECUT
PRENUP
PREVUE
PRIMUS
PROGUN
PROPUP
PUFFUP
PULLUP
PUMPUP
PURDUE
PURSUE
PUSHUP
PUTOUT
PUTPUT
PUTSUP

P••••U
PENGPU
PICCHU
PISTOU
POITOU
PQRSTU

•PU•••
APULIA
OPUSES
SPUMED
SPUMES
SPUNKY
SPURNS
SPURON
SPURTS

•P•U••
KPDUTY
OPHULS
OPIUMS
OPPUGN
SPOUSE
SPOUTS
SPRUCE
SPRUNG
UPCURL
UPRUSH
UPTURN

•P••U•
EPOQUE
OPAQUE
OPENUP
OPTOUT
SPEDUP
SPROUT
SPYOUT

•P•••U
APERCU

••PU••
AMPULE
ASPURE
COPULA
CUPULE
DEPULP
DEPUTE
DEPUTY
IMPUGN
IMPURE
IMPUTE
INPUTS
KAPUTT
LAPUTA
MAPUTO
MOPUPS
NIPUPS
OPPUGN
PAPUAN
POPULI
POPUPS
REPUBS
REPUGN
REPUMP
REPUTE
UNPURE

••P•U•
AMPSUP
BUPKUS
CAPFUL
CAPGUN
CAPNUT
COPOUT
CUPFUL
CYPRUS
DEPAUL
DEPAUW
GYPSUM
HIPPUS
HOPOUT
HOPSUP
HYPEUP
INPOUR
KEPTUP
KIPPUR
LAPFUL
LAPSUP
LAPSUS
LIPOUT
MAPOUT
MOPSUP
PEPFUL
PEPLUM
PEPSUP
PIPEUP
POPGUN
POPOUT
POPSUP
RAPTUS
REPOUR
RIPOUT
RIPSUP
ROPEUP
SEPTUM
SOPSUP
STPAUL
STPIUS
TAPEUP
TAPOUT
TIPSUP
TOPGUN
TOPOUT
TOPSUP
TYPEUP
TYPHUS
UNPLUG
VAPOUR
WIPEUP
ZIPGUN
ZIPOUT
ZIPSUP

•••PU•
BUMPUP
CAMPUP
CAMPUS
CARPUS
CHIPUP
CHOPUP
COOPUP
CORPUS
COYPUS
CROPUP
FLIPUP
HEAPUP
HELPUP
HIPPUS
JAIPUR
JUMPUP
KEEPUP
KIPPUR
LEAPUP
LUMPUR
OUTPUT
PETPUP
PROPUP
PUMPUP
PUTPUT
QUIPUS
RAIPUR
RAMPUP
RUMPUS
SLIPUP
SNAPUP
SOAPUP
SOUPUP
STAPUF
STEPUP
STOPUP
TEMPUS
TRIPUP
UNSPUN
WAMPUM
WHIPUP
WRAPUP

•••P•U
THEPRU

••••PU
PENGPU

P•V•••
PAVANE
PAVERS
PAVESE
PAVING
PAVIOR
PAVLOV
PEVNEY
PIVOTS
POVICH

P••V••
PEEVED
PEEVES
PELVIC
PELVIS
PLOVER
PLUVIA
PLUVIO
POIVRE
POTVIN
PRAVDA
PREVIA
PREVIN
PREVUE
PRIVET
PROVED
PROVEN
PROVER
PROVES
PULVER
PURVEY

P•••V•
PADOVA
PAREVE
PAULVI
PIUSVI

P••••V
PARKAV
PARTIV
PAULIV
PAVLOV
PIUSIV

•P•V••
SPIVAK
UPOVER

•P••V•
UPDIVE
UPDOVE
UPHOVE

•P•••V
SPOTTV

••P•V•
REPAVE

••P••V
IMPROV
LAPTEV

•••P•V
KARPOV

P•W•••
PAWERS
PAWING
PAWNED
PAWNEE
PAWNER
PAWPAW
PAWSAT
PEWEES
PEWITS
PEWTER
POWDER
POWELL
POWERS
POWWOW

P••W••
PEDWAY
PEEWEE
PLOWED
PLOWER
PLOWON
PLOWUP
POWWOW
PRAWER
PRAWNS
PREWAR
PROWAR
PROWLS
PROWSE
PSYWAR

P•••W•
PAPAWS
PESEWA
PSHAWS

P••••W
PAWPAW
PAYNOW
PESCOW
PETCOW
PILLOW
PITROW
PITSAW
POWWOW
PRELAW

•PW•••
UPWAFT
UPWARD
UPWELL
UPWIND

•P•W••
EPOWER
SPAWNS
SPEWED
SPEWER

•P••W•
SPRAWL
UPBOWS
UPTOWN

•P•••W
CPSNOW
UPFLOW
UPGREW
UPGROW
UPSHAW

••P•W•
INPAWN
MRPAWS
PAPAWS
UNPAWN

••P••W
DEPAUW
NEPHEW
REPLOW
RIPSAW
TOPROW

•••P•W
PAWPAW
QUAPAW

P•X•••
PAXTON
PIXELS
PIXIES

P••X••
PLEXAL
PLEXES
PLEXOR
PLEXUS
PRAXES
PRAXIS
PREXES

P•••X•
PIUSXI

P••••X
PEGBOX
PENTAX
PICKAX
PIUSIX
POLEAX
POLLEX
POLLUX
PREFIX
PREMIX
PRETAX
PROLIX
PROTAX
PROULX
PUBLIX

•P•X••
APEXES

•P••X•
UPNEXT

•P•••X
APPROX
SPHINX
SPHYNX

••P••X
APPROX
DIPLEX
DUPLEX

•••P•X
AUSPEX
COWPOX

PY••••
PYEDOG
PYLONS
PYRHHO
PYRITE
PYTHON

P•Y•••
PAYCUT
PAYDAY
PAYEES
PAYERS
PAYFOR
PAYING
PAYNOW
PAYOFF
PAYOLA
PAYOUT
PAYPAL
PAYSIN
PAYSON
PAYSUP
PAYTON
PEYOTE
PEYTON
PHYLLO
PHYLUM
PHYSED
PHYSIC
PHYSIO
PLYING
POYSER
PRYERS
PRYING
PRYNNE
PRYOFF
PSYCHE
PSYCHO
PSYCHS
PSYWAR

P••Y••
PAPYRI
PINYIN
PLAYAS
PLAYAT
PLAYBY
PLAYED
PLAYER
PLAYIT
PLAYON
PLAYTO
PLAYUP
POLYPS
PONYUP
PRAYED
PRAYER
PRAYTO
PREYED
PREYER
PREYON
PROYAS

P•••Y•
PAPAYA
PARTYS
PITAYA
PLATYS
POBOYS
POKEYS
POPEYE
PORKYS
PROPYL

P••••Y
PACIFY
PAINTY
PALELY
PALTRY
PANFRY
PANTRY
PAPACY
PAPERY
PARITY
PARKAY
PARLAY
PARLEY
PARODY
PARTLY
PASSBY
PASTRY
PATCHY
PATDAY
PATDRY
PAULEY
PAYDAY
PDIDDY
PEACHY
PEARLY
PEBBLY
PEDWAY
PELTRY
PENNEY
PENURY
PEPBOY
PERDAY
PERTLY
PETTOY
PEVNEY
PHILBY
PHILLY
PHONEY
PHOOEY
PIGSTY
PIMINY
PIMPLY
PINBOY
PINCAY
PINERY
PIRACY
PITCHY
PITNEY
PLASHY
PLAYBY
PLENTY
PLOTTY
PLUCKY
PLUMMY
PLUNKY
PLUSHY
POACHY
POETRY
POINTY
POKERY
POKILY
POLICY
POLITY
POMPEY
POORLY
POPFLY
PORTLY
POSHLY
POUCHY
POUFFY
PREBUY
PREDAY
PREDRY
PREPAY
PREPPY
PRETTY
PRICEY
PRIMLY
PRIORY
PRISSY
PROSKY
PTOOEY
PUDDLY
PULLEY
PUNCHY
PUNILY
PURELY
PURIFY
PURITY
PURPLY
PURVEY
PUTNEY
PUTSBY

•PY•••
SPYBOT
SPYCAM
SPYDER
SPYING
SPYOUT

•P•Y••
SPAYED
SPAYER
SPHYNX
SPRYER
SPRYLY

•P••Y•
EPONYM
SPLAYS
SPRAYS

•P•••Y
APATHY
APIARY
KPDUTY
OPENLY
SPACEY
SPANKY
SPARKY
SPEEDY
SPENDY
SPERRY
SPIDEY
SPIFFY
SPONGY
SPOOKY
SPOONY
SPORTY
SPOTTY
SPRYLY
SPUNKY
UPPITY

••PY••
PAPYRI

••P•Y•
COPAYS
PAPAYA
POPEYE
REPAYS
SEPOYS
ZEPHYR

••P••Y
ATPLAY
BYPLAY
COPLEY
DEPLOY
DEPUTY
DIPODY
DOPILY
DUPERY
EMPERY
EMPLOY
EXPIRY
INPLAY
JAPERY
MOPERY
NAPERY
NIPSEY
OSPREY
PAPACY
PAPERY
PEPBOY
POPFLY
RAPTLY
REPLAY
RIPELY
RIPLEY
RIPPLY
ROPERY
SUPPLY
TYPIFY
UPPITY
VAPORY
ZIPSBY

•••PY•
PROPYL

•••P•Y
BIOPSY
BROPHY
CHOPPY
COMPLY
DAMPLY
DEEPLY
DIMPLY
DRIPPY
DROPBY
DROPSY
DUMPTY
FLAPPY
FLOPPY
FLOPSY
GLOPPY
GRAPEY
GRAPHY
GRIPPY
HUMPTY
LIMPLY
MURPHY
NETPAY
OUTPAY
OUTPRY
PIMPLY
POMPEY
PREPAY
PREPPY
PURPLY
QUIPPY
RIPPLY
RUMPLY
SIMPLY
SKIPBY
SKIPPY
SLAPPY
SLIPBY
SLIPPY
SLOPPY
SNAPPY
SNIPPY
STOPBY
SUPPLY
TEAPOY
TRAPPY
TRIPLY
TROPHY
TWOPLY
WHIPPY

••••PY
CANOPY
CHIRPY
CHOPPY
CIASPY

CLUMPY
CRAMPY
CREEPY
CRIMPY
CRISPY
CROUPY
DRIPPY
DROOPY
FLAPPY
FLOPPY
FRUMPY
GLOPPY
GRIPPY
GRUMPY
JALOPY
KGBSPY
KRISPY
OCCUPY
OUTSPY
PREPPY
QUIPPY
RECOPY
SHARPY
SKIMPY
SKIPPY
SLAPPY
SLEEPY
SLIPPY
SLOOPY
SLOPPY
SNAPPY
SNIPPY
SNOOPY
STIMPY
STRIPY
STUMPY
SWAMPY
SYRUPY
THESPY
TRAMPY
TRAPPY
WHIPPY

P•Z•••
PIZAZZ
PIZZAS
POZNAN
POZOLE
PUZZLE

P••Z••
PANZER
PATZER
PFIZER
PIAZZA
PIAZZI
PINZON
PIZZAS
PLAZAS
PONZUS
PRIZED
PRIZES
PRIZMS
PRIZZI
PROZAC
PUZZLE

P•••Z•
PIAZZA
PIAZZI
PIZAZZ
PRINZE
PRIZZI
PUENZO

P••••Z
PARLEZ
PERUTZ
PIZAZZ

•P••Z•
UPGAZE
UPSIZE
XPRIZE

•P•••Z
SPRITZ

•••P•Z
COMPOZ
TROPEZ

QA••••
QABALA
QANTAS
QATARI

Q•A•••
QRATIO
QUACKS
QUACKY
QUADRI
QUAFFS
QUAGGA
QUAGGY
QUAHOG
QUAILS
QUAINT
QUAKED
QUAKER
QUAKES
QUAKIE
QUALES
QUALMS
QUANTA
QUAPAW
QUARKS
QUARRY
QUARTE
QUARTO
QUARTS
QUARTZ
QUASAR
QUATRE
QUAVER
QUAYLE

Q••A••
QABALA
QATARI
QUEASY

Q•••A•
QANTAS
QINTAR
QUAPAW
QUASAR
QUOTAS

Q••••A
QABALA
QUAGGA
QUANTA
QUINTA

•Q•A••
AQUAKE
EQUALS
EQUATE
SQUABS
SQUADS
SQUALL
SQUARE
SQUASH
SQUATS
SQUAWK
UQUARK

•Q••A•
SQUEAK
SQUEAL

•Q•••A
AQUILA

••Q•A•
EMQUAD
ENQUAD
LOQUAT
MSQUAD

••Q••A
BUQSHA

Q•B•••
QABALA

Q••B••
QUEBEC

•Q••B•
SQUABS
SQUIBB
SQUIBS

•Q•••B
SQUIBB

Q••C••
QUACKS
QUACKY
QUICHE

Q•••C•
QUENCH
QUINCE
QUINCY

Q••••C
QUEBEC

Q••D••
QUADRI
QUIDDE

Q•••D•
QUIDDE

Q••••D
QUAKED
QUEUED
QUIRED
QUOTED

•Q••D•
SQUADS
SQUIDS

•Q•••D
EQUOID

••Q••D
EMQUAD
ENQUAD
LIQUID
MSQUAD
PEQUOD
PIQUED

Q•E•••
QUEASY
QUEBEC
QUEENE
QUEENS
QUEERS
QUELER
QUELLS
QUEMOY
QUENCH
QUESOS
QUESTS
QUEUED
QUEUER
QUEUES
QUEZON
QWERTY

Q••E••
QUEENE
QUEENS
QUEERS
QUIETS

Q•••E•
QTILES
QUAKED
QUAKER
QUAKES
QUALES
QUAVER
QUEBEC
QUELER
QUEUED
QUEUER
QUEUES
QUIRED
QUIRES
QUIVER
QUOTED
QUOTEE
QUOTER
QUOTES

Q••••E
QUAKIE
QUARTE
QUATRE
QUAYLE
QUEENE
QUICHE
QUIDDE
QUINCE
QUINTE
QUINZE
QUOQUE
QUOTEE

•Q•E••
IQTEST
SQUEAK
SQUEAL

•Q•••E
AQUAKE
EQUATE
EQUINE
SQUARE
SQUIRE

••Q•E•
PIQUED
PIQUES
PIQUET
RAQUEL
SEQUEL
TOQUES
TUQUES

•••Q•E
BANQUE
BARQUE
BASQUE
BISQUE
BRAQUE
CASQUE
CHEQUE
CINQUE
CIRQUE
CLAQUE
CLIQUE
EPOQUE
JUSQUE
MANQUE
MARQUE
MASQUE
MOSQUE
OPAQUE
PLAQUE
QUOQUE
RISQUE
SACQUE
TORQUE
UNIQUE

Q••F••
QUAFFS

Q•••F•
QUAFFS

Q••G••
QUAGGA
QUAGGY

Q•••G•
QUAGGA
QUAGGY

Q••••G
QUAHOG

Q••H••
QUAHOG

Q•••H•
QUICHE

Q••••H
QUENCH

•Q•••H
SQUASH
SQUISH

••Q•H•
BUQSHA

QI••••
QINTAR

Q•I•••
QTILES
QUICHE
QUIDDE
QUIETS
QUILLS
QUILTS
QUINCE
QUINCY
QUINQU
QUINTA
QUINTE
QUINTI
QUINTS
QUINZE
QUIPPY
QUIPUS
QUIRED
QUIRES
QUIRKS
QUIRKY
QUIRTS
QUITIT
QUIVER

Q••I••
QUAILS
QUAINT
QUOINS
QUOITS

Q•••I•
QRATIO
QUAKIE
QUITIT

Q••••I
QATARI
QUADRI
QUINTI

•Q•I••
AQUILA
AQUINO
EQUINE
EQUIPS
EQUITY
SQUIBB
SQUIBS
SQUIDS
SQUINT
SQUIRE
SQUIRM
SQUIRT
SQUISH

•Q••I•
EQUOID

••QI••
FAQIRS

••Q•I•
ACQUIT
BBQPIT
COQUIS
LIQUID
MAQUIS
NYQUIL
PAQUIN
SEQUIN
YAQUIS

•••QI•
IRAQIS

•••Q•I
SESQUI
YANQUI

•••QJ•
DRIQJR

Q••K••
QUAKED
QUAKER
QUAKES
QUAKIE

Q•••K•
QUACKS
QUACKY
QUARKS
QUIRKS
QUIRKY

•Q••K•
AQUAKE

•Q•••K
SQUAWK
SQUEAK
UQUARK

Q•L•••
QTILES

Q••L••
QUALES
QUALMS
QUELER
QUELLS
QUILLS
QUILTS

Q•••L•
QABALA
QUAILS
QUAYLE
QUELLS
QUILLS

•Q••L•
AQUILA
EQUALS
SQUALL

•Q•••L
SQUALL
SQUEAL

••Q••L
NYQUIL
RAQUEL
SEQUEL

Q••M••
QUEMOY

Q•••M•
QUALMS

Q••••M
QUORUM

•Q•••M
SQUIRM

Q•N•••
QANTAS
QINTAR

Q••N••
QUANTA
QUENCH
QUINCE
QUINCY
QUINQU
QUINTA
QUINTE
QUINTI
QUINTS
QUINZE

Q•••N•
QUAINT
QUEENE
QUEENS
QUOINS

Q••••N
QUEZON

•Q••N•
AQUINO
EQUINE
SQUINT

••Q••N
PAQUIN
SEQUIN

Q•O•••
QUOINS
QUOITS
QUOQUE
QUORUM
QUOTAS
QUOTED
QUOTEE
QUOTER
QUOTES

Q•••O•
QUAHOG
QUEMOY
QUESOS
QUEZON

Q••••O
QRATIO
QUARTO

•Q•O••
EQUOID

•Q•••O
AQUINO

••Q•O•
LIQUOR
PEQUOD
PEQUOT

•••Q•O
BANQUO

Q••P••
QUAPAW
QUIPPY
QUIPUS

Q•••P•
QUIPPY

•Q••P•
EQUIPS

••QP••
BBQPIT

Q••Q••
QUOQUE

Q•••Q•
QUINQU

••••QQ
ETSEQQ

QR••••
QRATIO
QRSTUV

Q••R••
QUARKS
QUARRY
QUARTE
QUARTO
QUARTS
QUARTZ
QUIRED
QUIRES
QUIRKS
QUIRKY
QUIRTS
QUORUM
QWERTY

Q•••R•
QATARI
QUADRI
QUARRY
QUATRE
QUEERS

Q••••R
QINTAR
QUAKER
QUASAR
QUAVER
QUELER
QUEUER
QUIVER
QUOTER

•QR•••
PQRSTU

•Q••R•
SQUARE
SQUIRE
SQUIRM
SQUIRT
UQUARK

••QR••
OPQRST

••Q•R•
FAQIRS

••Q••R
LIQUOR

•••QR•
NOPQRS

•••Q•R
DRIQJR

••••QR
MNOPQR

Q•S•••
QRSTUV

Q••S••
QUASAR
QUESOS
QUESTS

Q•••S•
QUEASY

Q••••S
QANTAS
QTILES
QUACKS
QUAFFS
QUAILS
QUAKES
QUALES
QUALMS
QUARKS
QUARTS
QUEENS
QUEERS
QUELLS
QUESOS
QUESTS
QUEUES
QUIETS
QUILLS
QUILTS
QUINTS
QUIPUS
QUIRES
QUIRKS
QUIRTS
QUOINS
QUOITS
QUOTAS
QUOTES

•Q•S••
PQRSTU

•Q••S•
IQTEST
SQUASH
SQUISH

•Q•••S
EQUALS
EQUIPS
SQUABS
SQUADS
SQUATS
SQUIBS
SQUIDS

••QS••
BUQSHA

••Q•S•
OPQRST

••Q••S
COQUIS
FAQIRS
MAQUIS
PIQUES
TOQUES
TUQUES
YAQUIS

•••Q•S
IRAQIS
NOPQRS

••••QS
LOWIQS
SUZYQS

QT••••
QTILES

Q•T•••
QATARI

Q••T••
QANTAS
QINTAR
QRATIO
QRSTUV
QUATRE
QUITIT
QUOTAS
QUOTED
QUOTEE
QUOTER
QUOTES

Q•••T•
QUANTA
QUARTE
QUARTO
QUARTS
QUARTZ
QUESTS
QUIETS
QUILTS
QUINTA
QUINTE
QUINTI
QUINTS
QUIRTS
QUOITS
QWERTY

Q••••T
QUAINT
QUITIT

•QT•••
IQTEST

•Q••T•
EQUATE
EQUITY
PQRSTU
SQUATS

•Q•••T
IQTEST
SQUINT
SQUIRT

••Q••T
ACQUIT
BBQPIT
LOQUAT
OPQRST
PEQUOT
PIQUET

QU••••
QUACKS
QUACKY
QUADRI
QUAFFS
QUAGGA
QUAGGY
QUAHOG
QUAILS
QUAINT
QUAKED
QUAKER
QUAKES
QUAKIE
QUALES
QUALMS
QUANTA
QUAPAW
QUARKS
QUARRY
QUARTE
QUARTO
QUARTS
QUARTZ
QUASAR
QUATRE
QUAVER
QUAYLE
QUEASY
QUEBEC
QUEENE
QUEENS
QUEERS
QUELER
QUELLS
QUEMOY
QUENCH
QUESOS
QUESTS
QUEUED
QUEUER
QUEUES
QUEZON
QUICHE
QUIDDE
QUIETS
QUILLS
QUILTS
QUINCE
QUINCY
QUINQU
QUINTA
QUINTE
QUINTI
QUINTS
QUINZE
QUIPPY
QUIPUS
QUIRED
QUIRES
QUIRKS
QUIRKY
QUIRTS
QUITIT
QUIVER
QUOINS
QUOITS
QUOQUE
QUORUM
QUOTAS
QUOTED
QUOTEE
QUOTER
QUOTES

Q••U••
QUEUED
QUEUER
QUEUES

Q•••U•
QRSTUV
QUIPUS
QUOQUE
QUORUM

Q••••U
QUINQU

•QU•••
AQUAKE
AQUILA
AQUINO
EQUALS
EQUATE
EQUINE
EQUIPS
EQUITY
EQUOID
SQUABS
SQUADS
SQUALL
SQUARE
SQUASH
SQUATS
SQUAWK
SQUEAK
SQUEAL
SQUIBB
SQUIBS
SQUIDS
SQUINT
SQUIRE
SQUIRM
SQUIRT
SQUISH
UQUARK

•Q•••U
PQRSTU

••QU••
ACQUIT
COQUIS
EMQUAD
ENQUAD
LIQUID
LIQUOR
LOQUAT
MAQUIS
MSQUAD
NYQUIL
PAQUIN
PEQUOD
PEQUOT
PIQUED
PIQUES
PIQUET
RAQUEL
SEQUEL
SEQUIN
TOQUES
TUQUES
YAQUIS

•••QU•
BANQUE
BANQUO
BARQUE
BASQUE
BISQUE
BRAQUE
CASQUE
CHEQUE
CINQUE
CIRQUE
CLAQUE
CLIQUE
CLIQUY
EPOQUE
JUSQUE
MANQUE
MARQUE
MASQUE
MOSQUE
OPAQUE
PLAQUE
QUOQUE
RISQUE
SACQUE
SESQUI
TORQUE
UNIQUE
YANQUI

••••QU
QUINQU

Q••V••
QUAVER
QUIVER

Q••••V
QRSTUV

QW••••
QWERTY

Q••••W
QUAPAW

•Q••W•
SQUAWK

Q••Y••
QUAYLE

Q••••Y
QUACKY
QUAGGY
QUARRY
QUEASY
QUEMOY
QUINCY
QUIPPY
QUIRKY

6 PZ

QWERTY

•Q•••Y
EQUITY

•••Q•Y
CLIQUY

Q••Z••
QUEZON

Q•••Z•
QUINZE

Q••••Z
QUARTZ

RA••••
RABBET
RABBIS
RABBIT
RABBLE
RABIES
RACEBY
RACEIN
RACEME
RACERS
RACETO
RACEUP
RACHEL
RACIAL
RACIER
RACILY
RACINE
RACING
RACINO
RACISM
RACIST
RACKED
RACKER
RACKET
RACKUP
RADARS
RADIAL
RADIAN
RADIOS
RADISH
RADIUM
RADIUS
RADLEY
RADNER
RADNOR
RADOME
RAFAEL
RAFFIA
RAFFIN
RAFFLE
RAFTED
RAFTER
RAGBAG
RAGERS
RAGGED
RAGHIB
RAGING
RAGLAN
RAGMAN
RAGMEN
RAGMOP
RAGNAR
RAGOUT
RAGRUG
RAGSON
RAGTAG
RAGTOP
RAGUSA
RAHRAH
RAHWAY
RAIDED
RAIDER
RAILAT
RAILED
RAILER
RAILON
RAINED
RAINER
RAINES
RAINEY
RAININ
RAINON
RAIPUR
RAISED
RAISER
RAISES
RAISIN
RAISON
RAITAS
RAJABS
RAJAHS
RAKEIN
RAKERS
RAKEUP
RAKING
RAKISH
RALLYE
RALPHJ
RAMADA
RAMAPO
RAMATE
RAMBLE
RAMBOS
RAMEAU
RAMENS
RAMETS
RAMFAN
RAMFIS
RAMIES
RAMIFY
RAMJET
RAMMED
RAMMER
RAMONA
RAMONE
RAMOSE
RAMPAL
RAMPED
RAMPUP
RAMROD
RAMSAY
RAMSES
RAMSEY
RAMSIN
RAMSON
RANCHO
RANCID
RANCOR
RANDAL
RANDOM
RANDRY
RANEES
RANFOR
RANGED
RANGEL
RANGER
RANGES
RANGIN
RANGUP
RANIDS
RANINE
RANKED
RANKER
RANKIN
RANKLE
RANKLY
RANLOW
RANOFF
RANOUT
RANSOM
RANTAT
RANTED
RANTER
RAPIDO
RAPIDS
RAPIER
RAPINE
RAPINI
RAPPED
RAPPEL
RAPPER
RAPSON
RAPTER
RAPTLY
RAPTOR
RAPTUS
RAQUEL
RAREES
RAREFY
RARELY
RAREST
RARING
RARITY
RASCAL
RASCHE
RASERS
RASHAD
RASHER
RASHES
RASHID
RASHLY
RASING
RASKIN
RASPAS
RASPED
RASPER
RASSES
RASSLE
RASTAS
RASTER
RASURE
RATEDA
RATEDG
RATEDR
RATEDX
RATELS
RATERS
RATHER
RATIFY
RATINE
RATING
RATION
RATIOS
RATITE
RATLIN
RATNER
RATOFF
RATOUT
RATSON
RATTAN
RATTAT
RATTED
RATTER
RATTLE
RATTLY
RAUNCH
RAVAGE
RAVEAT
RAVELS
RAVENS
RAVEON
RAVERS
RAVEUP
RAVINE
RAVING
RAVISH
RAWBAR
RAWDON
RAWEGG
RAWEST
RAWISH
RAWIST
RAXING
RAYBAN
RAYGUN
RAYING
RAYONS
RAZERS
RAZING
RAZORS
RAZZED
RAZZES
RAZZIE
RAZZLE

R•A•••
REACTS
READDS
READER
READIN
README
READON
READTO
READUP
REAGAN
REAIMS
REAIRS
REALER
REALES
REALIA
REALLY
REALMS
REALTY
REAMED
REAMER
REAPED
REAPER
REARED
REARER
REARMS
REARUP
REASKS
REASON
REATAS
REATTA
REAVED
REAVER
REAVES
REAVOW
RHAMES
RIALTO
RIATAS
RNAASE
ROADEO
ROADER
ROADIE
ROAMED
ROAMER
ROAMIN
ROARAT
ROARED
ROARER
ROASTS
RRATED
RUANDA
RVALUE
RWANDA

R••A••
RADARS
RAFAEL
RAJABS
RAJAHS
RAMADA
RAMAPO
RAMATE
RAVAGE
REBAGS
REBAIT
REBAKE
REBALE
REBANK
REBARS
REBATE
RECAGE
RECALL
RECANE
RECANS
RECANT
RECAPS
RECASE
RECAST
REDACE
REDACT
REDANS
REDANT
REDARE
REDARN
REDATE
REEARN
REFACE
REFALL
REGAIN
REGALE
REGARD
REGAVE
REHABS
REHANG
REHASH
REHAUL
REJAIL
RELACE
RELAID
RELAND
RELAPS
RELATE
RELAYS
REMADE
REMAIL
REMAIN
REMAKE
REMAND
REMANS
REMAPS
REMARK
REMATE
REMATS
RENAIL
RENAME
RENARD
RENATA
RENATO
REPACK
REPADS
REPAGE
REPAID
REPAIR
REPANE
REPARK
REPASS
REPAST
REPAVE
REPAYS
RERACK
RERAKE
RERANK
RERATE
RESAID
RESALE
RESALT
RESAND
RESANG
RESAVE
RESAWN
RESAWS
RESAYS
RETACK
RETAGS
RETAIL
RETAIN
RETAKE
RETAME
RETANS
RETAPE
RETAPS
RETARD
RETARS
REVAMP
REWAKE
REWARD
REWARM
REWARN
REWASH
REXALL
RIBALD
RIBAND
RICANS
RIGANS
RIGATI
RIMATE
RITARD
RIVALS
RIYADH
RIYALS
RNAASE
RODALE
ROLAND
ROMAIC
ROMAIN
ROMAJI
ROMANI
ROMANO
ROMANS
ROMANY
RONALD
ROSARY
ROTARY
ROTATE
ROWANS
ROXANA
ROXANE
ROYALE
ROYALS
RUBATI
RUBATO
RUMAKI
RVPARK

R•••A•
RACIAL
RADIAL
RADIAN
RAGBAG
RAGLAN
RAGMAN
RAGNAR
RAGTAG
RAHRAH
RAHWAY
RAILAT
RAITAS
RAMEAU
RAMFAN
RAMPAL
RAMSAY
RANDAL
RANTAT
RASCAL
RASHAD
RASPAS
RASTAS
RATTAN
RATTAT
RAVEAT
RAWBAR
RAYBAN
RBIMAN
REAGAN
REATAS
RECLAD
RECOAL
RECOAT
REDBAT
REDBAY
REDCAP
REDEAL
REDHAT
REDIAL
REDOAK
REDRAG
REDRAW
REDTAB
REDTAG
REFLAG
REGEAR
REGGAE
REGNAL
REGNAT
REGRAB
REHEAL
REHEAR
REHEAT
REINAS
RELEAD
RELEAP
RELOAD
RELOAN
RENGAS
RENTAL
REPEAL
REPEAT
REPLAN
REPLAY
REREAD
RESCAN
RESEAL
RESEAM
RESEAT
RESEAU
RESNAP
RESOAK
RESOAP
RESPAN
RESTAB
RESWAM
RETEAR
RETHAW
RETIAL
RETRAL
RETRAP
REVEAL
REWEAR
REWRAP
REXCAT
RHINAL
RIATAS
RIBPAD
RICRAC
RICTAL
RIOJAS
RIOPAN
RIPRAP
RIPSAW
RITUAL
ROARAT
ROCHAT
RODHAM
RODMAN
ROSEAU
RUBRAW
RUDMAN
RUGRAT
RUMBAS
RUNSAT
RUNWAY
RUPIAH
RUSHAT
RUTTAN
RYOKAN

R••••A
RAFFIA
RAGUSA
RAMADA
RAMONA
RATEDA
RCCOLA
REALIA
REATTA
REDSEA
REGINA
REMORA
RENATA
RESEDA
RETINA
RHONDA
RHUMBA
RIBERA
RICOLA
RIJEKA
RIVERA
ROBBIA
ROMOLA
ROOMBA
ROSINA
ROSITA
ROSTRA
ROWENA
ROXANA
RUANDA
RUBBIA
RUSSIA
RWANDA

•RA•••
ARABIA
ARABIC
ARABLE
ARADOS
ARAFAT
ARAGON
ARAMES
ARAMID
ARAMIS
ARARAS
ARARAT
BRACCO
BRACED
BRACER
BRACES
BRACHS
BRACTS
BRAHMA
BRAHMS
BRAIDS
BRAINS
BRAINY
BRAISE
BRAKED
BRAKES
BRAMAH
BRANCA
BRANCH
BRANDI
BRANDO
BRANDS
BRANDT
BRANDX
BRANDY
BRANNY
BRANTS
BRAQUE
BRASCO
BRASHY
BRASIL
BRASOV
BRASSY
BRATSK
BRATTY
BRAVAS
BRAVED
BRAVER
BRAVES
BRAVOS
BRAWLS
BRAWNY
BRAYED
BRAYER
BRAZEN
BRAZIL
BRAZOS
BRAZZA
BRAZZI
CRABBE
CRABBY
CRACKD
CRACKS
CRACOW
CRADLE
CRAFTS
CRAFTY
CRAGGY
CRAIGT
CRAINS
CRAKES
CRAMBO
CRAMER
CRAMIN
CRAMPS
CRAMPY
CRANED
CRANES
CRANIA
CRANIO
CRANKS
CRANKY
CRANNY
CRAPED
CRAPES
CRATED
CRATER
CRATES
CRAVAT
CRAVED
CRAVEN
CRAVER
CRAVES
CRAWLS
CRAWLY
CRAYON
CRAZED
CRAZES
DRABEK
DRABLY
DRAFTS
DRAFTY
DRAGEE
DRAGGY
DRAGIN
DRAGON
DRAGUP
DRAINS
DRAKES
DRAKEU
DRAMAS
DRANCY
DRAPED
DRAPER
DRAPES
DRATIT
DRAWEE
DRAWER
DRAWIN
DRAWLS
DRAWLY
DRAWON
DRAWTO
DRAWUP
DRAYED
ERASED
ERASER
ERASES
FRACAS
FRACTO
FRAIDY
FRAISE
FRAKES
FRAMED
FRAMER
FRAMES
FRANCA
FRANCE
FRANCK
FRANCO
FRANCS
FRANKS
FRANNY
FRANTZ
FRAPPE
FRASER
FRATER
FRAUDS
FRAUEN
FRAYED
FRAZER
GRAAFF
GRABAT
GRABBY
GRABLE
GRACED
GRACES
GRACIE
GRADEA
GRADEB
GRADED
GRADER
GRADES
GRAECO
GRAFTS
GRAHAM
GRAILS
GRAINS
GRAINY
GRAMME
GRAMMY
GRAMPA
GRAMPS
GRANBY
GRANDE
GRANDS
GRANDY
GRANGE
GRANIT
GRANNY
GRANPA
GRANTS
GRAPES
GRAPEY
GRAPHO
GRAPHS
GRAPHY
GRAPPA
GRASPS
GRASSO
GRASSY
GRATAE
GRATED
GRATER
GRATES
GRATIA
GRATIN
GRATIS
GRAVAS
GRAVED
GRAVEL
GRAVEN
GRAVER
GRAVES
GRAVID
GRAYED
GRAYER
GRAYLY
GRAZED
GRAZER
GRAZES
GRAZIE
IRAISE
IRANIS
IRAQIS
IRATER
KRAALS
KRAITS
KRAKEN
KRAKOW
KRAMER
KRANTZ
KRASNA
KRAUSS
KRAVIS
ORACHS
ORACLE
ORAJEL
ORALES
ORALLY
ORANGE
ORANGS
ORANGY
ORANIS
ORANTS
ORATED
ORATES
ORATOR
PRADAS
PRAGUE
PRAISE
PRANAS
PRANCE
PRANKS
PRATED
PRATER
PRATES
PRAVDA
PRAWER
PRAWNS
PRAXES
PRAXIS
PRAYED
PRAYER
PRAYTO
QRATIO
RRATED
TRACED
TRACER
TRACES
TRACEY
TRACHE
TRACII
TRACKS
TRACTS
TRADED
TRADER
TRADES
TRAGIC
TRAGUS
TRAILS
TRAINS
TRAITS
TRAJAN
TRALAS
TRALEE
TRAMPS
TRAMPY
TRANCE
TRANES
TRANNY
TRAPPY
TRASHY
TRAUMA
TRAVEL
TRAVEN
TRAVES
TRAVIS
TRAWLS
URACIL
URAEUS
URALIC
URALSK
URANIA
URANIC
URANUS
WRACKS
WRAITH
WRAPUP
WRASSE
WRATHS
XRATED
XRAYED

•R•A••
ARCADE
ARCANA
ARCANE
ARCARO
ARFARF
ARGALI
ARHATS
ARIANA
ARIANE
ARIARY
ARMADA
ARMAGH
ARMAND
ARMANI
ARNALL
ARRACK
ARRANT
ARRAYS
ARTAUD
ARVADA
ARYANS
BREACH
BREADS
BREAKS
BREAMS
BREAST
BREATH
BRIANA
BRIAND
BRIARD
BRIARS
BRIARY
BROACH
BROADA
BROAST
BRYANT
CREAKS
CREAKY
CREAMS
CREAMY
CREASE
CREASY
CREATE
CROAKS
CROAKY
CROATS
DREADS
DREAMS
DREAMT
DREAMY
DREARY
DRYADS
ERHARD
ERLANG
ERNANI
ERRAND
ERRANT
ERRARE
ERRATA
ERSATZ
FREAKS
FREAKY
FRIARS
FRIARY
GRAAFF
GREASE
GREASY
GREATS
GREAVE
GROANS
GROATS
KRAALS
MRPAWS
ORBACH
ORDAIN
OREADS
ORGANA
ORGANS
ORIANA
ORIANI
ORKANS
ORNATE
PREACH
PREACT
PREAGE
PREAMP
PREARM
PROAMS
PROART
TREADS
TREATS
TREATY
TRIADS
TRIAGE
TRIALS
TRUANT
URBANA
URBANE
URBANI
URBANV
WREAKS
WREATH

•R••A•
ARAFAT
ARARAS
ARARAT
ARCTAN
ARECAS
ARENAS
AROMAS
ARREAR
ARTCAR
ARUBAN
BRAMAH
BRAVAS
BRIDAL
BROCAS
BROGAN
BROKAW
BRUMAL
BRUTAL
CRAVAT
CRETAN

CRURAL
CRUZAN
DRAMAS
DRCLAW
ERDMAN
EREVAN
ERICAS
ERIVAN
ERSTAD
ERYKAH
FRACAS
FRETAT
FRIDAY
FRITAS
FRUGAL
FRYPAN
GRABAT
GRAHAM
GRATAE
GRAVAS
GRINAT
GROBAN
IRREAL
MRBEAN
ORDEAL
ORGEAT
ORPHAN
ORWHAT
PRADAS
PRANAS
PREDAY
PREFAB
PRELAW
PREPAY
PRETAX
PREWAR
PRIMAL
PROTAX
PROWAR
PROYAS
PROZAC
TRAJAN
TRALAS
TREPAN
TRIBAL
TRINAL
TROJAN
TRUMAN

•R•••A

ARABIA
ARBELA
ARCANA
AREOLA
ARETHA
ARIANA
ARISTA
ARJUNA
ARLOVA
ARMADA
ARNICA
ARRIBA
ARVADA
BRAHMA
BRANCA
BRAZZA
BRENDA
BRIANA
BROADA
BRYNZA
CRANIA
CRENNA
CREUSA
CRIMEA
ERIEPA
ERINNA
EROICA
ERRATA
FRANCA
FRESCA
FRICKA
FRIEDA
FRITTA
FRUSTA
GRADEA
GRAMPA
GRANPA
GRAPPA
GRATIA
GRETNA
GRISHA
HRYVNA
KRASNA
OREIDA
OREXIA
ORGANA
ORIANA
ORISSA
ORTEGA
PRAVDA
PREVIA
PROTEA
TRAUMA
TREDIA
TRENTA
TRICIA
TRISHA
TRIVIA
TROIKA
URANIA
URBANA
URSULA

••RA••

ABRADE
ABRAMS
ADRATE
AERATE
AFRAID
AFRAME
AIRACE
AIRARM
ARRACK
ARRANT
ARRAYS
ASRARE
ATRAIN
AURATE
AZRAEL
BARACK
BARADA
BARAKA
BARANY
BARATA
BARATO
BERATE
BORATE
BORAXO
BURANA
CARAFE
CARATS
CDRACK
CDRATE
CERATE
CERATO
CORACI
CORALS
CURACY
CURADS
CURARE
CURATE
CYRANO
DERAIL
DERAIN
DERATE
DERATS
DIRAMS
DORADO
DORAGS
DORATI
DURANT
ENRAGE
ENRANK
ENRAPT
ERRAND
ERRANT
ERRARE
ERRATA
ETRADE
EURAIL
FARACY
FARADS
FARAHS
FERALS
FORAGE
FORAYS
GARAGE
GERALD
GERARD
GYRATE
HARALD
HARARE
HARASS
HERALD
HORACE
INRAGS
ISRAEL
ISRAIR
JARABE
JURADO
KARATE
KARATS
KERALA
KORANS
KORATS
KURALT
LARAMS
LARAZA
LFRANK
LORAIN
LORANS
MARACA
MARAUD
MIRADA
MIRAGE
MORALE
MORALS
MORANT
MORASS
MORATH
MORAYS
MURALS
MURANO
NARADA
NORAIN
OARAGE
OGRADY
ONRAMP
OPRAHS
PARADE
PARANA
PARAPH
PHRASE
PIRACY
PIRANA
PIRATE
PTRAPS
RERACK
RERAKE
RERANK
RERATE
SARANS
SCRAGS
SCRAMS
SCRAPE
SCRAPS
SCRAWL
SERACS
SERAIS
SERAPE
SERAPH
SHRANK
SPRACH
SPRAIN
SPRANG
SPRATS
SPRAWL
SPRAYS
STRADA
STRADS
STRAFE
STRAIN
STRAIT
STRAND
STRAPS
STRATA
STRATI
STRATO
STRATS
STRAUB
STRAWS
STRAYS
SURAHS
TARAWA
TERATO
THRACE
THRALL
THRASH
TIRADE
TIRANA
TIRANE
TORAHS
TYRANT
UNRACK
UNRASH
UPRATE
UVRAYS
VIRAGO

••R•A•

AARGAU
ABROAD
ADRIAN
AERIAL
AIRBAG
AIRDAM
AIRMAN
AIRSAC
AIRWAR
AIRWAY
AORTAE
AORTAL
AORTAS
ARREAR
ATRIAL
BARBAN
BARCAR
BARKAT
BARMAN
BARTAB
BERMAN
BIRMAN
BOREAL
BOREAS
BORMAN
BUREAU
BURIAL
BURKAS
BURLAP
BURMAN
BUROAK
BURSAE
BURSAL
BURSAR
BURSAS
BYROAD
CARMAN
CARNAC
CARNAL
CARNAP
CARPAL
CARPAT
CARWAX
CEREAL
CERNAN
CORDAY
CORFAM
CORMAN
CORRAL
CORSAS
CURIAE
DARNAY
DERMAL
DERMAS
DERMAT
DIRHAM
DORCAS
DORIAN
DORSAD
DORSAL
DORSAY
DURBAN
DURHAM
DURRAS
EARLAP
EARTAB
EARTAG
EARWAX
FARRAH
FARRAR
FERIAS
FERMAT
FERNAO
FIREAT
FORBAD
FORMAL
FORMAN
FORMAT
FORNAX
FORTAS
FURMAN
GARGAN
GERMAN
GORHAM
HARHAR
HARLAN
HARRAD
HARRAH
HERBAL
HEREAT
HERMAN
HERNAN
HORGAN
HURRAH
HURRAY
INROAD
IRREAL
JARJAR
JORDAN
KARMAS
KARNAK
KARRAS
KIRMAN
KOREAN
KORMAN
LARIAT
LARVAE
LARVAL
LARVAS
LOREAL
MARIAH
MARIAN
MARIAS
MARKAS
MARYAM
MERMAN
MIRIAM
MOREAU
MORGAN
MORNAY
MORTAL
MORTAR
MURRAY
MYRDAL
MYRIAD
NARIAL
NERMAL
NERVAL
NORGAY
NORIAS
NORMAL
NORMAN
NORVAL
NORWAY
OARMAN
OBRIAN
PARCAE
PARIAH
PARKAS
PARKAV
PARKAY
PARLAY
PERDAY
PORTAL
REREAD
SCREAK
SCREAM
SERIAL
SERTAS
SIRKAY
SIRRAH
SOREAT
SPREAD
STREAK
STREAM
STRIAE
SUREAM
SURTAX
SYRIAN
TARGAS
TARMAC
TARSAL
TARTAN
TARTAR
TARZAN
TERRAE
TERRAN
THREAD
THREAT
THROAT
TIRIAC
TORBAY
TOREAT
TORTAS
TURBAN
TURHAN
UNREAD
UNREAL
UPREAR
UPROAR
VARGAS
VARIAS
VARNAS
VERBAL
VERNAL
VIRGAS
VORPAL
WARSAW
WORKAT

••R••A

AFRICA
AIRSEA
AMRITA
ARRIBA
AURIGA
AURORA
BARADA
BARAKA
BARATA
BARBRA
BARKLA
BAROJA
BERTHA
BORGIA
BURANA
CARBRA
CARDIA
CARINA
CHROMA
CORDIA
CORNEA
CORONA
CORYZA
DERITA
DURYEA
EARTHA
ERRATA
EUREKA
EUROPA
FARINA
GARCIA
GURKHA
HERNIA
JERBOA
KARINA
KERALA
KORUNA
LARAZA
LAROSA
LERIDA
MARACA
MARCIA
MARIDA
MARINA
MARISA
MARKKA
MARSHA
MARTHA
MERIDA
MIRADA
MORITA
MURCIA
NARADA
NARITA
NARNIA
NERUDA
PARANA
PERCHA
PERLEA
PERSIA
PIRANA
PORTIA
PURINA
SARNIA
SERBIA
SERENA
SIRICA
STRADA
STRATA
TARAWA
TERESA
THREEA
TIRANA
VERONA
YORKPA
ZORINA

•••RA•

ABORAL
ACURAS
AFFRAY
AGORAE
AGORAS
AMORAL
AMTRAC
AMTRAK
ANDRAE
ANORAK
ANTRAL
ARARAS
ARARAT
ASHRAM
ASTRAL
ASTRAY
AZERAS
BADRAP
BASRAH
BETRAY
BUMRAP
CABRAL
CHIRAC
CHORAL
CIERAS
COBRAS
CONRAD
COPRAS
CORRAL
CRURAL
DABRAT
DEBRAH
DEBRAY
DEFRAG
DEFRAY
DELRAY
DIGRAM
DURRAS
DVORAK
ENDRAN
ENGRAM
ENTRAP
ENWRAP
ESDRAS
ESTRAY
EXTRAS
FABRAY
FARRAH
FARRAR
FLORAE
FLORAL
FLORAS
FOURAA
FOURAD
FOURAM
GAVRAS
GIBRAN
GYMRAT
HARRAD
HARRAH
HEDRAL
HOORAH
HOORAY
HURRAH
HURRAY
HYDRAE
HYDRAS
INARAY
INGRAM
INGRAY
INTRAY
JEERAT
KARRAS
KIERAN
KONRAD
LABRAT
LEERAT
LIBRAE
LIBRAN
LIBRAS
LYCRAS
MACRAE
MADRAS
MANRAY
MCCRAE
MCGRAW
MITRAL
MOERAE
MURRAY
NAIRAS
NEURAL
NEXRAD
OHDRAT
OPERAS
OUTRAN
OUTRAP
PEERAT
PETRAT
PLURAL
POORAT
RAHRAH
REDRAG
REDRAW
REGRAB
RETRAL
RETRAP
REWRAP
RICRAC
RIPRAP
ROARAT
RUBRAW
RUGRAT
SABRAS
SATRAP
SCARAB
SEURAT
SHIRAZ
SIRRAH
SPIRAL
SUNRAY
SUPRAS
SUTRAS
TATRAS
TEARAT
TEHRAN
TERRAE
TERRAN
TETRAD
TETRAS
THERAM
THERAP
THERAT
THORAX
TIARAS
TSTRAP
ULTRAS
UMBRAE
UMBRAL
UMBRAS
UNDRAW
UNORAL
UNTRAP
UNWRAP
VIBRAM
WETRAG
XSARAS
ZEBRAS

•••R•A

ALTRIA
AMARNA
ANDREA
AZARIA
BAERGA
CHARTA
DCAREA
DHARMA
EGERIA
ELYRIA
FOURAA
GLORIA
IBARRA
IBERIA
ICARIA
INAREA
ISTRIA
LABREA
LATRIA
LAURIA
MCCREA
NUTRIA
OMERTA
PATRIA
PEORIA
PIERIA
SCORIA
SFORZA
SHERPA
SHORTA
SIERRA
SMYRNA
SPARTA
SPIREA
STERNA
TIERRA
UMBRIA
XTERRA
YTTRIA

••••RA

ALUDRA
ALZIRA
AMENRA
AMONRA
ANGORA
ANITRA
ANKARA
ANSARA
ASMARA
ASPERA
AURORA
BARBRA
BIAFRA
CAMERA
CARBRA
CATERA
CETERA
CHAKRA
CHITRA
CHOPRA
CONTRA
DENDRA
DONORA
ELLORA
ELMIRA
ELNORA
ELVIRA
ENDORA
EUDORA
EXEDRA
FEDORA
FEMORA
FULCRA
FUTURA
GEMARA
GENERA
HEGIRA
IBARRA
INDIRA
JOGBRA
LASTRA
LUSTRA
MADERA
MANTRA
MOTHRA
MUNERA
NEWERA
NOSTRA
NUBIRA
OMEARA
OSETRA
PICARA
PLEURA
POLARA
REMORA
RIBERA
RIVERA
ROSTRA
SAHARA
SAMARA
SANDRA
SCLERA
SEGURA
SENORA
SENTRA
SEPIRA
SIERRA
SOLARA
SONDRA
SONORA
TAMARA
TANTRA
THENRA
TIERRA
TUNDRA
VALERA
VECTRA
VENERA
VENORA
VIAGRA
VIEIRA
VIHARA
VITARA
XTERRA
ZADORA
ZAMORA

RB••••

RBIMAN
RBIMEN

R•B•••

RABBET
RABBIS
RABBIT
RABBLE
RABIES
REBAGS
REBAIT
REBAKE
REBALE
REBANK
REBARS
REBATE
REBBES
REBBIE
REBECS
REBELS
REBEND
REBENT
REBETS
REBIDS
REBILL
REBIND
REBOIL
REBOLT
REBOOK
REBOOT
REBOPS
REBORE
REBORN
REBOTE
REBOZO
REBRED
REBREW
REBUFF
REBUKE
REBURY
REBUTS
REBUYS
RIBALD
RIBAND
RIBBED
RIBBER
RIBBIT
RIBBON
RIBCUT
RIBERA
RIBEYE
RIBISI
RIBLET
RIBOSE
RIBPAD
ROBBED
ROBBER
ROBBIA
ROBBIE
ROBERS
ROBERT
ROBING
ROBINS
ROBLES
ROBOTS
ROBROY
ROBSOF
ROBSON
ROBUST
RUBATI
RUBATO
RUBBED
RUBBER
RUBBIA
RUBBLE
RUBBLY
RUBELS
RUBENS
RUBIED
RUBIES
RUBIFY
RUBIKS
RUBLES
RUBLEV
RUBOFF
RUBOUT
RUBRAW
RUBRIC
RUBSIN
RUBSON
RUBSUP

R••B••

RABBET
RABBIS
RABBIT
RABBLE
RAGBAG
RAMBLE
RAMBOS
RAWBAR
RAYBAN
REBBES
REBBIE
REDBAT
REDBAY
REDBUD
REEBOK
REUBEN
RHEBOK
RIBBED
RIBBER
RIBBIT
RIBBON
ROBBED
ROBBER
ROBBIA
ROBBIE
RUBBED
RUBBER
RUBBIA
RUBBLE
RUBBLY
RUMBAS
RUMBLE
RUMBLY

R•••B•

RACEBY
RAJABS
REDUBS
REHABS
REPUBS
RHOMBI
RHOMBS
RHUMBA
RHUMBS
RIDEBY
RODEBY
ROLLBY
ROOMBA
RUNSBY
RUSHBY

R••••B

RAGHIB
RCRUMB
RECOMB
REDTAB
REGRAB
RESORB
RESTAB
REVERB

•RB•••

ARBELA
ARBORS
ARBOUR
ARBRES
ERBIUM
MRBEAN
MRBILL
MRBLUE
MRBOND
ORBACH
ORBING
ORBITS
URBANA
URBANE
URBANI
URBANV

•R•B••

ARABIA
ARABIC
ARABLE
ARUBAN
BRIBED
BRIBEE
BRIBER
BRIBES
CRABBE
CRABBY
DRABEK
DRABLY
DREBIN
EREBUS
GRABAT
GRABBY
GRABLE
GREBES
GROBAN
GRUBBY

IROBOT
ORIBIS
PREBID
PREBUY
PROBED
PROBER
PROBES
PROBIE
PROBST
TREBEK
TREBLE
TREBLY
TRIBAL
TRIBES

•R••B•

ARRIBA
CRABBE
CRABBY
CRAMBO
CROSBY
CRUMBS
CRUMBY
DROPBY
GRABBY
GRANBY
GRUBBY
MRPIBB
TRILBY
TRUMBO

•R•••B

GRADEB
MRPIBB
PREFAB

••RB••

AIRBAG
AIRBUD
AIRBUS
BARBAN
BARBED
BARBER
BARBET
BARBIE
BARBRA
BERBER
BURBLE
BURBLY
BURBOT
CARBON
CARBOS
CARBOY
CARBRA
CORBEL
CORBIN
CURBED
DURBAN
DURBIN
EARBUD
FERBER
FORBAD
FORBES
FORBID
FURBYS
GARBED
GARBER
GARBLE
GERBER
GERBIL
HARBIN
HARBOR
HERBAL
HERBED
HERBES
HERBIE
JERBOA
KORBUT
MARBLE
MARBLY
MORBID
SERBIA
SIRBEN
SORBET
SORBIC
TERBIC
TORBAY
TURBAN
TURBID
TURBOS
TURBOT
VERBAL
VERBID
WARBLE

••R•B•

AEROBE
ARRIBA
CARIBE
CARIBS
CAROBS
CEREBR
ENROBE
HARDBY
HEREBY
HORNBY
JARABE
MCRIBS
SCRIBE
SCRUBS
SHRUBS
STROBE
THROBS
UNROBE

••R••B

BARTAB
EARTAB
RCRUMB
STRAUB
THREEB

•••RB•

BLURBS
EXURBS
FOURBC
ITURBI
NEARBY

•••R•B

ATHROB
CHERUB
MIDRIB
NOPROB
OILRUB
OUTRIB
REGRAB
SCARAB
ZAGREB

••••RB

ABSORB
ADSORB
ADVERB
BICARB
RESORB
REVERB
SUBURB
SUPERB
UNCURB

RC••••

RCCOLA
RCRUMB

R•C•••

RACEBY
RACEIN
RACEME
RACERS
RACETO
RACEUP
RACHEL
RACIAL
RACIER
RACILY
RACINE
RACING
RACINO
RACISM
RACIST
RACKED
RACKER
RACKET
RACKUP
RCCOLA
RECAGE
RECALL
RECANE
RECANS
RECANT
RECAPS
RECASE
RECAST
RECEDE
RECENT
RECESS
RECHEW
RECIFE
RECIPE
RECITE
RECKED
RECKON
RECLAD
RECOAL
RECOAT
RECOCK
RECODE
RECOIL
RECOIN
RECOMB
RECONS
RECOOK
RECOOL
RECOPY
RECORD
RECORK
RECOST
RECOUP
RECTOR
RECTOS
RECTUS
RECUED
RECUES
RECURE
RECURL
RECURS
RECUSE
RECUTS
RICANS
RICERS
RICHEN
RICHER
RICHES
RICHET
RICHIE
RICHIN
RICHLY
RICING
RICKEY
RICKIE
RICOHS
RICOLA
RICRAC
RICTAL
ROCHAT
ROCHET
ROCHON
ROCKED
ROCKER
ROCKET
ROCKIE
ROCKIN
ROCKIT
ROCKNE
ROCKYV
ROCOCO
RUCHES
RUCKED
RUCKER
RUCKUP
RUCKUS

R••C••

RANCHO
RANCID
RANCOR
RASCAL
RASCHE
REACTS
REDCAP
REDCOD
REECHO
REICED
REICES
RESCAN
RESCUE
REXCAT
RIBCUT
ROMCOM
RONCEY
ROSCOE
ROYCES
RUNCIE

R•••C•

RAUNCH
REBECS
RECOCK
REDACE
REDACT
REDOCK
REDUCE
REFACE
REJECT
REKICK
RELACE
RELICS
RELICT
RELOCK
RELUCT
REMICK
REPACK
REPICK
RERACK
RESECT
RETACK
ROCOCO
RYENCE

R••••C

RICRAC
ROMAIC
RUBRIC
RUNDMC
RUSTIC

•RC•••

ARCADE
ARCANA
ARCANE
ARCARO
ARCCOS
ARCHED
ARCHER
ARCHES
ARCHIE
ARCHLY
ARCHON
ARCING
ARCSEC
ARCSIN
ARCTAN
ARCTIC
DRCLAW
MRCOOL
ORCHID
URCHIN

•R•C••

ARCCOS
ARECAS
ARTCAR
BRACCO
BRACED
BRACER
BRACES
BRACHS
BRACTS
BRECHT
BRICKS
BRICKY
BROCAS
CRACKD
CRACKS
CRACOW
CRECHE
CRICKS
CROCKS
CROCUS
CRUCES
DRECKS
DRECKY
ERECTS
ERICAS
ERUCTS
FRACAS
FRACTO
FRICKA
FRICKE
FROCKS
FRUCTI
GRACED
GRACES
GRACIE
GROCER
GRUCCI
ORACHS
ORACLE
ORECKS
PRECIP
PRECIS
PRECUT
PRICED
PRICER
PRICES
PRICEY
PRICKS
PROCOL
TRACED
TRACER
TRACES
TRACEY
TRACHE
TRACII
TRACKS
TRACTS
TRECES
TRICEP
TRICES
TRICIA
TRICKS
TRICKY
TRICOT
TROCHE
TRUCES
TRUCKS
URACIL
WRACKS
WRECKS

•R••C•

ARNICA
ARRACK
BRACCO
BRANCA
BRANCH
BRASCO
BREACH
BREECH
BROACH
BRONCO
BRONCS
BROOCH
BRUNCH
CRISCO
CROTCH
CROUCH
CRUNCH
CRUTCH
DRANCY
DRENCH
DRRICE
DRYICE
EROICA
FRANCA
FRANCE
FRANCK
FRANCO
FRANCS
FRENCH
FRESCA
FRESCO
FRISCH
FRISCO
GRAECO
GREECE
GRIECO
GRINCH
GROUCH
GRUCCI
MRDICK
ORBACH
OROSCO
OROZCO
PRANCE
PREACH
PREACT
PRINCE
TRANCE
TRENCH
WRENCH
WRETCH

•R•••C

ARABIC
ARCSEC
ARCTIC
CRITIC
EROTIC
FROLIC
IRENIC
IRIDIC
IRITIC
IRONIC
ORPHIC
PROZAC
TRAGIC
TROPIC
URALIC
URANIC

••RC••

BARCAR
BARCOS
BERCEO
CIRCLE
CIRCUM
CIRCUS
DARCEL
DORCAS
FARCED
FARCES
FARCRY
FORCED
FORCER
FORCES
FORCHE
GARCIA
GARCON
GORCEY
MARCEL
MARCHE
MARCIA
MARCIE
MARCIL
MARCIX
MARCOS
MARCUS
MERCED
MERCER
MERCKX
MURCIA
NARCOS
PARCAE
PARCEL
PERCHA
TERCEL
TERCES
TORCHY
WARCRY
ZIRCON

••R•C•

AFRICA
AIRACE
ARRACK
BARACK
BARUCH
BORSCH
CDRACK
CORACI
CURACY
DIRECT
DRRICE
DUROCS
ENRICH
ENRICO
FARACY
HIRSCH
HORACE
KIRSCH
LYRICS
MARACA
ONRICE
PIRACY
RERACK
SERACS
SIRICA
SPRACH
SPRUCE
STRICT
STRUCK
THRACE
THRICE
ULRICH
UNRACK
YORICK
ZURICH

••R••C

AIRSAC
AORTIC
BARDIC
CARNAC
DERMIC
FERENC
FERRIC
FORMIC
GARLIC
HEROIC
KARMIC
NORDIC
PARSEC
SORBIC
TARMAC
TERBIC
THREEC
TIRIAC
TURKIC

•••RC•

AMERCE
ANARCH
APERCU
ASARCO
BIERCE
CHURCH
COERCE
EPARCH
EXARCH
FIERCE
GFORCE
INARCH
PEARCE
PEERCE
PEIRCE
PIERCE
SCARCE
SCORCH
SEARCH
SMIRCH
SOURCE
STARCH
STORCH
TIERCE

•••R•C

AGARIC
ALARIC
AMTRAC
ANDRIC
CEDRIC
CHIRAC
CHORIC
CITRIC
CLERIC
COURIC
CUPRIC
CYMRIC
EMERIC
FABRIC
FERRIC
FOURBC
HYDRIC
HYGRIC
IATRIC
LAURIC
METRIC
NITRIC
PATRIC
PICRIC
RICRAC
RUBRIC
STERIC
TAURIC
THORIC
VITRIC
YTTRIC

R•D•••

RADARS
RADIAL
RADIAN
RADIOS
RADISH
RADIUM
RADIUS
RADLEY
RADNER
RADNOR
RADOME
REDACE
REDACT
REDANS
REDANT
REDARE
REDARN
REDATE
REDBAT
REDBAY
REDBUD
REDCAP
REDCOD
REDDEN
REDDER
REDDIN
REDDOG
REDDOT
REDEAL
REDEED
REDEEM
REDEFY
REDENY
REDEYE
REDFIN
REDFIR
REDFOX
REDHAT
REDHEN
REDHOT
REDIAL
REDIGS
REDING
REDINK
REDIPS
REDLEG
REDOAK
REDOCK
REDOER
REDOES
REDONE
REDOSE
REDOUT
REDRAG
REDRAW
REDREW
REDRUM
REDSEA
REDSIX
REDSKY
REDSOX
REDSUN
REDTAB
REDTAG
REDTEN
REDTIE
REDTOP
REDTWO
REDUBS
REDUCE
REDUST
REDYED
REDYES
RIDDED
RIDDEN
RIDDER
RIDDLE
RIDEBY
RIDEIN
RIDENT
RIDERS
RIDETO
RIDEUP
RIDGED
RIDGES
RIDING
RIDLEY
RIDSOF
RODALE
RODDED
RODDER
RODEBY
RODEIN
RODENT
RODEOS
RODETO
RODEUP
RODHAM
RODINO
RODION
RODMAN
RODMEN
RODNEY
RUDDER
RUDELY
RUDERY
RUDEST
RUDKIN
RUDKUS
RUDMAN
RUDNER
RUDOLF
RYDELL

R••D••

RAIDED
RAIDER
RANDAL
RANDOM
RANDRY
RAWDON
READDS
READER
READIN
README
READON
READTO
READUP
REDDEN
REDDER
REDDIN
REDDOG
REDDOT
REEDED
REEDER
REEDIT
RENDED
RENDER
RHODES
RIDDED
RIDDEN
RIDDER
RIDDLE
RITDYE
ROADEO
ROADER
ROADIE
RODDED
RODDER
RONDEL
RONDOS
RUDDER
RUNDLE
RUNDMC
RUNDRY

R•••D•

RAMADA
RANIDS
RAPIDO
RAPIDS
RATEDA
RATEDG
RATEDR
RATEDX
READDS
REBIDS
RECEDE
RECODE
REHIDE
REMADE
REMEDY
REPADS
RERIDE
RERODE
RESEDA
RESIDE
RESODS
REWEDS
RHONDA
RIYADH
ROUNDS
RUANDA
RWANDA

R••••D

RACKED
RAFTED
RAGGED
RAIDED
RAILED
RAINED
RAISED
RAMMED
RAMPED
RAMROD
RANCID
RANGED
RANKED
RANTED
RAPPED
RASHAD
RASHID
RASPED
RATTED
RAZZED
REAMED
REAPED
REARED
REAVED
REBEND
REBIND
REBRED
RECKED
RECLAD
RECORD
RECUED
REDBUD
REDCOD
REDEED
REDYED
REEDED
REEFED
REEKED
REELED
REEVED
REFEED
REFFED
REFIED
REFIND
REFOLD
REFUND
REGARD
REGILD
REGIRD
REHELD
REHOED
REHOLD
REICED
REINED
RELAID
RELAND
RELEAD
RELEND
RELIED
RELOAD
REMAND
REMEND
REMIND
REMOLD
RENARD
RENDED
RENTED
REPAID
REPLED
REPPED
REREAD
RESAID
RESAND
RESEED
RESEND
RESHOD
RESOLD
RESTED
RETARD
RETIED
RETOLD
RETROD
RETTED
REUNED
REUSED
REVEND
REVVED
REWARD
REWELD
REWIND
REWORD
RHYMED
RIBALD
RIBAND
RIBBED
RIBPAD
RIDDED
RIDGED
RIFFED
RIFLED
RIFTED
RIGGED
RIMMED
RINGED
RINSED
RIOTED
RIPPED
RISKED
RITARD
ROAMED
ROARED
ROBBED
ROCKED
RODDED
ROGUED
ROILED
ROLAND
ROLFED
ROLLED
ROMPED
RONALD
ROOFED
ROOKED
ROOMED
ROOTED
ROTTED
ROTUND
ROUGED
ROUSED
ROUTED
RRATED
RSVPED
RUBBED
RUBIED
RUCKED
RUFFED
RUGGED
RUINED
RUSHED
RUSTED
RUTTED

•RD•••

ARDENT
ARDORS
ARDOUR
DRDOOM
ERDMAN
MRDICK
ORDAIN
ORDEAL
ORDERS

•R•D••

ARADOS
ARIDER
ARIDLY
BREDES
BRIDAL
BRIDES
BRIDGE
BRIDLE
BRODIE
BRUDER
CRADLE
CREDIT
CREDOS
CRUDDY
CRUDER
CRUDES
CRUDUP
DREDGE
DRUDGE
DRYDEN
ERODED
ERODER
ERODES
FREDDY
FREDRO
FRIDAY
FRIDGE
GRADEA
GRADEB
GRADED
GRADER
GRADES
GRIDES
GRODIN
GRUDGE
HRIDER
IRIDES
IRIDIC
PRADAS
PREDAY
PREDRY
PRIDED
PRIDES
PRODON
PRUDES
TRADED
TRADER
TRADES
TREDIA

TRODON
TRUDGE

•R••D•
ARCADE
ARENDT
ARMADA
AROIDS
ARVADA
BRAIDS
BRANDI
BRANDO
BRANDS
BRANDT
BRANDX
BRANDY
BREADS
BREEDS
BREEDY
BRENDA
BROADA
BROODS
BROODY
CREEDS
CROWDS
CRUDDY
DREADS
DROIDS
DRUIDS
DRYADS
FRAIDY
FRAUDS
FREDDY
FRIEDA
FRONDS
GRANDE
GRANDS
GRANDY
GREEDS
GREEDY
GRINDL
GRINDS
GRUNDY
MRHYDE
OREADS
OREIDA
PRAVDA
TREADS
TRENDS
TRENDY
TRIADS
TRIODE
URSIDS

•R•••D
ARAMID
ARCHED
ARGUED
ARMAND
ARNOLD
AROUND
ARTAUD
BRACED
BRAKED
BRAVED
BRAYED
BREWED
BRIAND
BRIARD
BRIBED
BRIGID
BRINED
BROWED
BRUXED
CRACKD
CRANED
CRAPED
CRATED
CRAVED
CRAZED
CREPED
CREWED
CROWED
DRAPED
DRAYED
DRONED
ERASED
ERHARD
ERODED
ERRAND
ERSTAD
FRAMED
FRAYED
FREUND
FRIEND
FRIGID
GRACED
GRADED
GRATED
GRAVED
GRAVID
GRAYED
GRAZED
GREYED
GRIMED
GRIPED
GROPED
GROUND
GROVED
IRISED
IRONED
MRBOND
ORATED
ORCHID
ORMOND
ORTRUD
PRATED
PRAYED
PREBID
PREMED
PREYED
PRICED
PRIDED
PRIMED
PRISED
PRIZED
PROBED
PROSED
PROVED
PRUNED
RRATED
TRACED
TRADED
TREPID
TRIPOD
TROWED
XRATED
XRAYED

••RD••
AIRDAM
AIRDRY
BARDIC
BARDOT
BIRDED
BIRDER
BIRDIE
BORDEN
BORDER
BORDET
BURDEN
CARDED
CARDER
CARDIA
CARDIN
CARDIO
CORDAY
CORDED
CORDER
CORDIA
CORDON
CURDED
CURDLE
FERDIE
FORDED
FORDGT
FORDID
GARDEN
GIRDED
GIRDER
GIRDLE
GORDIE
GORDON
HARDBY
HARDEN
HARDER
HARDIN
HARDLY
HARDUP
HERDED
HERDER
HORDED
HORDES
HURDLE
JARDIN
JORDAN
LARDED
LARDER
LARDON
LORDED
LORDIT
LORDLY
MARDEN
MARDIS
MERDLE
MURDER
MYRDAL
NORDIC
NORDOI
PARDON
PERDAY
PERDUE
PURDUE
SARDIS
SARDOU
SORDID
TARDES
VARDEN
VERDES
VERDIN
VERDON
VERDUN
VIRDON
WARDED
WARDEN
WARDER
WORDED
YARDED
YARDER

••R•D•
ABRADE
BARADA
BORIDE
CURADS
DERIDE
DIRNDL
DORADO
ETRADE
FARADS
JURADO
LAREDO
LERIDA
LYRIDS
MARIDA
MARIDO
MERIDA
MIRADA
NARADA
NERUDA
OGRADY
PARADE
PARODY
RERIDE
RERODE
SCRODS
SHREDS
STRADA
STRADS
STRIDE
STRODE
SUREDO
TIRADE
UNRUDE
WORLDS

••R••D
ABROAD
AFRAID
AGREED
AIRBUD
BARBED
BARGED
BARKED
BARNED
BARRED
BERMED
BIRDED
BIRLED
BIRRED
BORKED
BURIED
BURLED
BURNED
BURPED
BURRED
BYROAD
CARDED
CARPED
CARTED
CARVED
CERVID
CORDED
CORKED
CORNED
CORVID
CURBED
CURDED
CURLED
CURRED
CURSED
CURVED
DARNED
DARTED
DIRKED
DORSAD
DURNED
EARBUD
EARNED
ERRAND
FARCED
FARMED
FERVID
FIRMED
FORBAD
FORBID
FORCED
FORDED
FORDID
FORGED
FORKED
FORMED
FURLED
FURRED
GARBED
GERALD
GERARD
GERUND
GIRDED
GIRTED
GORGED
GORMED
HARALD
HARKED
HARMED
HAROLD
HARPED
HARRAD
HERALD
HERBED
HERDED
HORDED
HORNED
HORRID
HORSED
HURLED
INROAD
ITRIED
JARRED
JERKED
JURIED
KERNED
LARDED
LARKED
LORDED
LURKED
MARAUD
MARKED
MARLED
MARRED
MERCED
MERGED
MORBID
MYRIAD
NEREID
NERVED
NURSED
PARGED
PARKED
PARRED
PARSED
PARTED
PERIOD
PERKED
PERMED
PERNOD
PORKED
PORTED
PUREED
PURGED
PURLED
PURRED
PURSED
REREAD
SCREED
SERVED
SHREWD
SHROUD
SORDID
SORTED
SPREAD
STRAND
STROUD
SURFED
SURGED
TARRED
TARTED
TERMED
THREAD
THREED
TOROID
TORPID
TORRID
TURBID
TURFED
TURGID
TURNED
UNREAD
UNRUED
VARIED
VERBID
VERGED
VERSED
WARDED
WARGOD
WARMED
WARNED
WARPED
WARRED
WARTED
WORDED
WORKED
WORMED
YARDED
YARNED
ZEROED

•••RD•
AWARDS
BEARDS
BOARDS
CHARDS
CHORDS
CIARDI
ECARDS
FIORDS
FJORDS
GEORDI
GOURDE
GOURDS
GUARDS
HAIRDO
HOARDS
LAIRDS
OVERDO
SHARDS
STURDY
SWARDS
SWORDS
TBIRDS
THIRDR
THIRDS
WEIRDO
WEIRDY

•••R•D
ACARID
ADORED
ALFRED
ASTRID
ASTRUD
AZURED
BARRED
BIGRED
BIRRED
BLARED
BURRED
CAPRID
CONRAD
CURRED
DOORED
ENURED
FAIRED
FEARED
FLARED
FLORID
FLYROD
FOURAD
FURRED
GEARED
GETRID
GLARED
GOTRID
HAIRED
HARRAD
HATRED
HORRID
HOTROD
HYBRID
IDARED
INBRED
INGRID
INURED
JARRED
JEERED
KONRAD
LAIRED
LEERED
MADRID
MARRED
METRED
MITRED
MODRED
MOORED
NACRED
NBCRED
NEARED
NEXRAD
NIMROD
OCHRED
ODORED
OHCRUD
OLERUD
ORTRUD
PAIRED
PARRED
PEERED
PENROD
POURED
PURRED
PUTRID
QUIRED
RAMROD
REARED
REBRED
RETROD
ROARED
SACRED
SAWRED
SCARED
SCORED
SEARED
SEERED
SHARED
SNARED
SNORED
SOARED
SOURED
SPARED
SPIRED
STARED
STORED
TARRED
TEARED
TETRAD
THERED
THEROD
TIERED
TIEROD
TITRED
TORRID
TOURED
UNTROD
USERID
VEERED
WARRED
WHERED

••••RD
ABOARD
ABSURD
ACCORD
AFEARD
AFFORD
ASGARD
BAYARD
BEGIRD
BRIARD
BYWORD
CANARD
COWARD
CUNARD
DEFORD
DOTARD
DUGARD
ECKERD
EDGARD
EDUARD
EDVARD
EDWARD
ELUARD
ENGIRD
ERHARD
EZZARD
FAYARD
FUGARD
GERARD
GODARD
HAZARD
HOWARD
IDCARD
INWARD
LENARD
LIZARD
LYNYRD
MCCORD
MILORD
MYLORD
MYWORD
ONWARD
OXFORD
OXNARD
PETARD
PICARD
RECORD
REGARD
REGIRD
RENARD
RETARD
REWARD
REWORD
RITARD
SEWARD
SIGURD
TABARD
TOWARD
UNGIRD
UPCARD
UPGIRD
UPWARD
WHWORD
WIZARD

RE••••
REACTS
READDS
READER
READIN
README
READON
READTO
READUP
REAGAN
REAIMS
REAIRS
REALER
REALES
REALIA
REALLY
REALMS
REALTY
REAMED
REAMER
REAPED
REAPER
REARED
REARER
REARMS
REARUP
REASKS
REASON
REATAS
REATTA
REAVED
REAVER
REAVES
REAVOW
REBAGS
REBAIT
REBAKE
REBALE
REBANK
REBARS
REBATE
REBBES
REBBIE
REBECS
REBELS
REBEND
REBENT
REBETS
REBIDS
REBILL
REBIND
REBOIL
REBOLT
REBOOK
REBOOT
REBOPS
REBORE
REBORN
REBOTE
REBOZO
REBRED
REBREW
REBUFF
REBUKE
REBURY
REBUTS
REBUYS
RECAGE
RECALL
RECANE
RECANS
RECANT
RECAPS
RECASE
RECAST
RECEDE
RECENT
RECESS
RECHEW
RECIFE
RECIPE
RECITE
RECKED
RECKON
RECLAD
RECOAL
RECOAT
RECOCK
RECODE
RECOIL
RECOIN
RECOMB
RECONS
RECOOK
RECOOL
RECOPY
RECORD
RECORK
RECOST
RECOUP
RECTOR
RECTOS
RECTUS
RECUED
RECUES
RECURE
RECURL
RECURS
RECUSE
RECUTS
REDACE
REDACT
REDANS
REDANT
REDARE
REDARN
REDATE
REDBAT
REDBAY
REDBUD
REDCAP
REDCOD
REDDEN
REDDER
REDDIN
REDDOG
REDDOT
REDEAL
REDEED
REDEEM
REDEFY
REDENY
REDEYE
REDFIN
REDFIR
REDFOX
REDHAT
REDHEN
REDHOT
REDIAL
REDIGS
REDING
REDINK
REDIPS
REDLEG
REDOAK
REDOCK
REDOER
REDOES
REDONE
REDOSE
REDOUT
REDRAG
REDRAW
REDREW
REDRUM
REDSEA
REDSIX
REDSKY
REDSOX
REDSUN
REDTAB
REDTAG
REDTEN
REDTIE
REDTOP
REDTWO
REDUBS
REDUCE
REDUST
REDYED
REDYES
REEARN
REEBOK
REECHO
REEDED
REEDER
REEDIT
REEFED
REEFER
REEKED
REEKER
REEKOF
REELED
REELER
REELIN
REELUP
REEMIT
REENIE
REESES
REEVED
REEVES
REFACE
REFALL
REFEED
REFELL
REFERS
REFFED
REFIED
REFIES
REFILE
REFILL
REFILM
REFIND
REFINE
REFIRE
REFITS
REFLAG
REFLEW
REFLEX
REFLOW
REFLUX
REFOLD
REFORM
REFUEL
REFUGE
REFUND
REFUSE
REFUTE
REGAIN
REGALE
REGARD
REGAVE
REGEAR
REGELS
REGENT
REGGAE
REGGIE
REGIFT
REGILD
REGIME
REGINA
REGION
REGIRD
REGIUS
REGIVE
REGLES
REGLOW
REGLUE
REGNAL
REGNAT
REGNUM
REGRAB
REGRET
REGREW
REGRIP
REGROW
REHABS
REHANG
REHASH
REHAUL
REHEAL
REHEAR
REHEAT
REHEEL
REHELD
REHEMS
REHIDE
REHIRE
REHITS
REHOED
REHOES
REHOLD
REHONE
REHOOK
REHUNG
REICED
REICES
REIGER
REIGNS
REILLY
REINAS
REINED
REINER
REINES
REININ
REINKS
REISER
REITER
REJAIL
REJECT
REJIGS
REJOIN
REKEYS
REKICK
REKNIT
REKNOT
RELACE
RELAID
RELAND
RELAPS
RELATE
RELAYS
RELEAD
RELEAP
RELEND
RELENT
RELETS
RELEVE
RELEVY
RELICS
RELICT
RELIED
RELIEF
RELIER
RELIES
RELINE
RELINK
RELISH
RELIST
RELIVE
RELOAD
RELOAN
RELOCK
RELOGS
RELOOK
RELOSE
RELOST
RELUCT
RELUME
RELYON
REMADE
REMAIL
REMAIN
REMAKE
REMAND
REMANS
REMAPS
REMARK
REMATE
REMATS
REMEDY
REMEET
REMELT
REMEND
REMICK
REMILL
REMIND
REMINE
REMINI
REMINT
REMISE
REMISS
REMITS
REMOLD
REMOPS
REMORA
REMOTE
REMOVE
REMOWN
REMOWS
REMSEN
RENAIL
RENAME
RENARD
RENATA
RENATO
RENDED
RENDER
RENEGE
RENEST
RENEWS
RENFRO
RENGAS
RENINS
RENNES
RENNET
RENNIE
RENNIN
RENOIR
RENONV
RENOTE
RENOWN
RENTAL
RENTED
RENTEE
RENTER
RENTES
RENTON
RENTTO
RENVOI
REOILS
REOPEN
REOWNS
REPACK
REPADS
REPAGE
REPAID
REPAIR
REPANE
REPARK
REPASS
REPAST
REPAVE
REPAYS
REPEAL
REPEAT
REPEGS
REPELS
REPENS
REPENT
REPERK
REPFOR
REPICK
REPINE
REPINS
REPLAN
REPLAY

REPLED
REPLOT
REPLOW
REPOLL
REPORT
REPOSE
REPOST
REPOTS
REPOUR
REPPED
REPROS
REPUBS
REPUGN
REPUMP
REPUTE
RERACK
RERAKE
RERANK
RERATE
REREAD
REREEL
RERENT
RERIDE
RERIGS
RERISE
RERODE
REROLL
REROOF
REROOT
REROSE
RERUNS
RESAID
RESALE
RESALT
RESAND
RESANG
RESAVE
RESAWN
RESAWS
RESAYS
RESCAN
RESCUE
RESEAL
RESEAM
RESEAT
RESEAU
RESECT
RESEDA
RESEED
RESEEK
RESEEN
RESEES
RESELL
RESEND
RESENT
RESETS
RESEWN
RESEWS
RESHES
RESHIP
RESHOD
RESHOE
RESHOT
RESHOW
RESHUT
RESIDE
RESIFT
RESIGN
RESILE
RESING
RESINK
RESINS
RESINY
RESIST
RESITE
RESITS
RESIZE
RESNAP
RESNIK
RESOAK
RESOAP
RESODS
RESOIL
RESOLD
RESOLE
RESORB
RESORT
RESOWN
RESOWS
RESPAN
RESPIN
RESPOT
RESTAB
RESTED
RESTER
RESTES
RESTIR
RESTON
RESTOW
RESTUP
RESUIT
RESULT
RESUME
RESWAM
RESWIM
RETACK
RETAGS
RETAIL
RETAIN
RETAKE
RETAME
RETANS
RETAPE
RETAPS
RETARD
RETARS
RETEAR
RETELL
RETEST
RETHAW
RETIAL
RETIED
RETIEF
RETIES
RETILE
RETILL
RETIME
RETINA
RETINS
RETINT
RETIPS
RETIRE
RETOLD
RETONE
RETOOK
RETOOL
RETOPS
RETORE
RETORN
RETORT
RETOSS
RETOUR
RETOWS
RETRAL
RETRAP
RETRIM
RETROD
RETROS
RETTED
RETTIG
RETTON
RETUNE
RETURF
RETURN
RETYPE
REUBEN
REUNED
REUNER
REUNES
REURGE
REUSED
REUSER
REUSES
REUTER
REVAMP
REVEAL
REVELS
REVEND
REVERB
REVERE
REVERS
REVERT
REVEST
REVETS
REVIEW
REVILE
REVISE
REVIVE
REVLON
REVOIR
REVOKE
REVOLT
REVOTE
REVSON
REVSUP
REVUES
REVVED
REWAKE
REWARD
REWARM
REWARN
REWASH
REWEAR
REWEDS
REWELD
REWETS
REWIND
REWINS
REWIPE
REWIRE
REWOKE
REWORD
REWORE
REWORK
REWORN
REWOVE
REWRAP
REXALL
REXCAT
REYLES
REYOKE
REZERO
REZIPS
REZONE

R•E•••

REEARN
REEBOK
REECHO
REEDED
REEDER
REEDIT
REEFED
REEFER
REEKED
REEKER
REEKOF
REELED
REELER
REELIN
REELUP
REEMIT
REENIE
REESES
REEVED
REEVES
RHEBOK
RHEEMS
RHEIMS
RHEMES
RHESUS
RHETOR
RHEUMS
RHEUMY
RIENZI
RIESEN
RKELLY
ROEPER
RUEFUL
RYENCE

R••E••

RACEBY
RACEIN
RACEME
RACERS
RACETO
RACEUP
RAGERS
RAKEIN
RAKERS
RAKEUP
RAMEAU
RAMENS
RAMETS
RANEES
RAREES
RAREFY
RARELY
RAREST
RASERS
RATEDA
RATEDG
RATEDR
RATEDX
RATELS
RATERS
RAVEAT
RAVELS
RAVENS
RAVEON
RAVERS
RAVEUP
RAWEGG
RAWEST
RAZERS
REBECS
REBELS
REBEND
REBENT
REBETS
RECEDE
RECENT
RECESS
REDEAL
REDEED
REDEEM
REDEFY
REDENY
REDEYE
REFEED
REFELL
REFERS
REGEAR
REGELS
REGENT
REHEAL
REHEAR
REHEAT
REHEEL
REHELD
REHEMS
REJECT
REKEYS
RELEAD
RELEAP
RELEND
RELENT
RELETS
RELEVE
RELEVY
REMEDY
REMEET
REMELT
REMEND
RENEGE
RENEST
RENEWS
REPEAL
REPEAT
REPEGS
REPELS
REPENS
REPENT
REPERK
REREAD
REREEL
RERENT
RESEAL
RESEAM
RESEAT
RESEAU
RESECT
RESEDA
RESEED
RESEEK
RESEEN
RESEES
RESELL
RESEND
RESENT
RESETS
RESEWN
RESEWS
RETEAR
RETELL
RETEST
REVEAL
REVELS
REVEND
REVERB
REVERE
REVERS
REVERT
REVEST
REVETS
REWEAR
REWEDS
REWELD
REWETS
REZERO
RHEEMS
RIBERA
RIBEYE
RICERS
RIDEBY
RIDEIN
RIDENT
RIDERS
RIDETO
RIDEUP
RIFELY
RIFEST
RIJEKA
RIKERS
RILERS
RILEUP
RIMERS
RIPELY
RIPENS
RIPEST
RISERS
RISETO
RISEUP
RIVERA
RIVERS
RIVETS
ROBERS
ROBERT
RODEBY
RODEIN
RODENT
RODEOS
RODETO
RODEUP
ROGERE
ROGERS
ROGETS
ROLEOS
ROMEOS
ROMERO
RONELY
ROPEIN
ROPERS
ROPERY
ROPEUP
ROSEAU
ROSERY
ROSETO
ROSEUP
ROVERS
ROWELS
ROWENA
ROWENS
ROWERS
RUBELS
RUBENS
RUDELY
RUDERY
RUDEST
RULEON
RULERS
RULETH
RUPEES
RUPERT
RYDELL

R•••E•

RABBET
RABIES
RACHEL
RACIER
RACKED
RACKER
RACKET
RADLEY
RADNER
RAFAEL
RAFTED
RAFTER
RAGGED
RAGMEN
RAIDED
RAIDER
RAILED
RAILER
RAINED
RAINER
RAINES
RAINEY
RAISED
RAISER
RAISES
RAMIES
RAMJET
RAMMED
RAMMER
RAMPED
RAMSES
RAMSEY
RANEES
RANGED
RANGEL
RANGER
RANGES
RANKED
RANKER
RANTED
RANTER
RAPIER
RAPPED
RAPPEL
RAPPER
RAPTER
RAQUEL
RAREES
RASHER
RASHES
RASPED
RASPER
RASSES
RASTER
RATHER
RATNER
RATTED
RATTER
RAZZED
RAZZES
RBIMEN
READER
REALER
REALES
REAMED
REAMER
REAPED
REAPER
REARED
REARER
REAVED
REAVER
REAVES
REBBES
REBRED
REBREW
RECHEW
RECKED
RECUED
RECUES
REDDEN
REDDER
REDEED
REDEEM
REDHEN
REDLEG
REDOER
REDOES
REDREW
REDSEA
REDTEN
REDYED
REDYES
REEDED
REEDER
REEFED
REEFER
REEKED
REEKER
REELED
REELER
REESES
REEVED
REEVES
REFEED
REFFED
REFIED
REFIES
REFLEW
REFLEX
REFUEL
REGLES
REGRET
REGREW
REHEEL
REHOED
REHOES
REICED
REICES
REIGER
REINED
REINER
REINES
REISER
REITER
RELIED
RELIEF
RELIER
RELIES
REMEET
REMSEN
RENDED
RENDER
RENNES
RENNET
RENTED
RENTEE
RENTER
RENTES
REOPEN
REPLED
REPPED
REREEL
RESEED
RESEEK
RESEEN
RESEES
RESHES
RESTED
RESTER
RESTES
RETIED
RETIEF
RETIES
RETTED
REUBEN
REUNED
REUNER
REUNES
REUSED
REUSER
REUSES
REUTER
REVIEW
REVUES
REVVED
REYLES
RHAMES
RHEMES
RHODES
RHYMED
RHYMER
RHYMES
RIBBED
RIBBER
RIBLET
RICHEN
RICHER
RICHES
RICHET
RICKEY
RIDDED
RIDDEN
RIDDER
RIDGED
RIDGES
RIDLEY
RIESEN
RIFFED
RIFLED
RIFLER
RIFLES
RIFTED
RIGGED
RIGGER
RILLES
RILLET
RIMIER
RIMMED
RINGED
RINGER
RINSED
RINSER
RINSES
RIOTED
RIOTER
RIPKEN
RIPLEY
RIPPED
RIPPER
RISKED
RISKER
RITTER
RITZES
ROADEO
ROADER
ROAMED
ROAMER
ROARED
ROARER
ROBBED
ROBBER
ROBLES
ROCHET
ROCKED
ROCKER
ROCKET
RODDED
RODDER
RODMEN
RODNEY
ROEPER
ROGUED
ROGUES
ROHMER
ROHRER
ROILED
ROLFED
ROLFER
ROLLED
ROLLEI
ROLLER
ROMMEL
ROMNEY
ROMPED
ROMPER
RONCEY
RONDEL
ROOFED
ROOFER
ROOKED
ROOKER
ROOMED
ROOMER
ROONEY
ROOTED
ROOTER
ROPIER
ROSIER
ROSIES
ROSSEN
ROSSET
ROSTEN
ROSTER
ROTTED
ROTTEN
ROTTER
ROUGED
ROUGES
ROUSED
ROUSER
ROUSES
ROUTED
ROUTER
ROUTES
ROWLEY
ROYCES
RRATED
RSVPED
RTILES
RUBBED
RUBBER
RUBIED
RUBIES
RUBLES
RUBLEV
RUCHES
RUCKED
RUCKER
RUDDER
RUDNER
RUFFED
RUGGED
RUINED
RUINER
RULIER
RUMMER
RUNLET
RUNNEL
RUNNER
RUPEES
RUSHED
RUSHEE
RUSHER
RUSHES
RUSSEL
RUSSES
RUSSET
RUSTED
RUTGER
RUTTED
RUTTER

R••••E

RABBLE
RACEME
RACINE
RADOME
RAFFLE
RALLYE
RAMATE
RAMBLE
RAMONE
RAMOSE
RANINE
RANKLE
RAPINE
RASCHE
RASSLE
RASURE
RATINE
RATITE
RATTLE
RAVAGE
RAVINE
RAZZIE
RAZZLE
README
REBAKE
REBALE
REBATE
REBBIE
REBORE
REBOTE
REBUKE
RECAGE
RECANE
RECASE
RECEDE
RECIFE
RECIPE
RECITE
RECODE
RECURE
RECUSE
REDACE
REDARE
REDATE
REDEYE
REDONE
REDOSE
REDTIE
REDUCE
REENIE
REFACE
REFILE
REFINE
REFIRE
REFUGE
REFUSE
REFUTE
REGALE
REGAVE
REGGAE
REGGIE
REGIME
REGIVE
REGLUE
REHIDE
REHIRE
REHONE
RELACE
RELATE
RELEVE
RELINE
RELIVE
RELOSE
RELUME
REMADE
REMAKE
REMATE
REMINE
REMISE
REMOTE
REMOVE
RENAME
RENEGE
RENNIE
RENOTE
RENTEE
REPAGE
REPANE
REPAVE
REPINE
REPOSE
REPUTE
RERAKE
RERATE
RERIDE
RERISE
RERODE
REROSE
RESALE
RESAVE
RESCUE
RESHOE
RESIDE
RESILE
RESITE
RESIZE
RESOLE
RESUME
RETAKE
RETAME
RETAPE
RETILE
RETIME
RETIRE
RETONE
RETORE
RETUNE
RETYPE
REURGE
REVERE
REVILE
REVISE
REVIVE
REVOKE
REVOTE
REWAKE
REWIPE
REWIRE
REWOKE
REWORE
REWOVE
REYOKE
REZONE
RIBEYE
RIBOSE
RICHIE
RICKIE
RIDDLE
RIFFLE
RIMATE
RIMOSE
RIMPLE
RIPPLE
RISQUE
RITDYE
RNAASE
ROADIE
ROBBIE
ROCKIE
ROCKNE
RODALE
ROGERE
ROLLIE
RONNIE
ROOKIE
ROOMIE
ROOTIE
ROOTLE
ROSCOE
ROTATE
ROURKE
ROXANE
ROYALE
RUBBLE
RUFFLE
RUMBLE
RUMPLE
RUNCIE
RUNDLE
RUSHEE
RUSTLE
RUTHIE
RUTILE
RVALUE
RYENCE

•RE•••

ARECAS
ARENAS
ARENDT
AREOLA
AREOLE
ARETES
ARETHA
ARETOO
AREZZO
BREACH
BREADS
BREAKS
BREAMS
BREAST
BREATH
BRECHT
BREDES
BREECH
BREEDS
BREEDY
BREEZE
BREEZY
BREMEN
BREMER
BRENDA
BRENLY
BRETON
BREUER
BREVES
BREVET
BREVIS
BREWED
BREWER
BREWUP
BREYER
CREAKS
CREAKY
CREAMS
CREAMY
CREASE
CREASY
CREATE
CRECHE
CREDIT
CREDOS
CREEDS
CREEKS
CREELS
CREEPO
CREEPS
CREEPY
CREMER
CREMES
CRENEL
CRENNA
CREOLE
CREPED
CREPES
CRESOL
CRESSY
CRESTS
CRETAN
CRETIN
CREUSA
CREUSE
CREWED
CREWEL
DREADS
DREAMS
DREAMT
DREAMY
DREARY
DREBIN
DRECKS
DRECKY
DREDGE
DRENCH
DRESSY
DREVIL
DREWIN
DREWON
DREWTO
DREWUP
DREXEL
DREYER
EREBUS
ERECTS
ERENOW
ERESTU
EREVAN
FREAKS

FREAKY FREDDY FREDRO FREELY FREEOF FREERS FREEST FREETO FREEUP FREEZE FRENCH FRENUM FRENZY FREONS FRERES FRESCA FRESCO FRESNO FRETAT FRETTY FREUND FREWER GREASE GREASY GREATS GREAVE GREBES GREECE GREEDS GREEDY GREEKS GREENE GREENS GREENY GREETS GREGOR GREIST GRETEL GRETNA GREWON GREWUP GREYED GREYER GREYLY IREFUL IRENIC KRENEK KRESGE KREWES OREADS ORECKS OREGON OREIDA ORELSE ORENSE OREOOS OREXIA OREXIS PREACH PREACT PREAGE PREAMP PREARM PREBID PREBUY PRECIP PRECIS PRECUT

PREDAY PREDRY PREENS PREFAB PREFER PREFIX PRELAW PRELIM PRELOG PREMED PREMET PREMIE PREMIX PRENUP PREOPS PREPAY PREPPY PRESET PRESTO PRETAX PRETER PRETOR PRETTY PREVIA PREVIN PREVUE PREWAR PREXES PREYED PREYER PREYON TREADS TREATS TREATY TREBEK TREBLE TREBLY TRECES TREDIA TREIZE TREMOR TRENCH TRENDS TRENDY TRENTA TRENTE TRENTO TREPAN TREPID TRESSY TREVOR TREXES WREAKS WREATH WRECKS WRENCH WRESTS WRETCH

•R•E••

ARBELA ARDENT ARGENT ARIEGE ARLENE ARMERS ARMETS ARNEIS ARNESS ARNETT ARPEGE ARPELS ARREAR ARREST ARRETE ARSENE ARSENO ARTELS ARTERY ARTEST BREECH BREEDS BREEDY BREEZE BREEZY BRIEFS BRIENZ BRIERS BRIERY CREEDS CREEKS CREELS CREEPO CREEPS CREEPY CRIERS CRUETS CRYERS DRIERS DRIEST DRYERS DRYEST DRYEYE ERIEPA ERNEST FREELY FREEOF FREERS FREEST FREETO FREEUP FREEZE FRIEDA FRIELS FRIEND FRIERS FRIEZE FRYERS GRAECO GREECE GREEDS GREEDY GREEKS GREENE GREENS GREENY GREETS GRIECO GRIEFS GRIESE GRIEVE GRUELS IRKERS IRLENE IRREAL MRBEAN

ORDEAL ORDERS ORGEAT ORIELS ORIENT ORNERY ORRERY ORTEGA ORWELL PREENS PRIERS PRIEST PROEMS PRUETT PRYERS TRIERS TRUEST TRUETO TRUEUP TRYERS URAEUS URGENT URGEON URGERS URTEXT WRIEST WRYEST

•R••E•

ARAMES ARBRES ARCHED ARCHER ARCHES ARCSEC ARETES ARGUED ARGUER ARGUES ARIDER ARISEN ARISES ARMIES ARMLET ARNHEM ARNIES AROUET ARTIER BRACED BRACER BRACES BRAKED BRAKES BRAVED BRAVER BRAVES BRAYED BRAYER BRAZEN BREDES BREMEN BREMER BREUER BREVES BREVET BREWED BREWER BREYER

BRIBED BRIBEE BRIBER BRIBES BRIDES BRINED BRINER BRINES BRISES BROKEN BROKER BROWED BRUDER BRUGES BRULEE BRUMEL BRUMES BRUNEI BRUNET BRUTES BRUXED BRUXES CRAKES CRAMER CRANED CRANES CRAPED CRAPES CRATED CRATER CRATES CRAVED CRAVEN CRAVER CRAVES CRAZED CRAZES CREMER CREMES CRENEL CREPED CREPES CREWED CREWEL CRIKEY CRIMEA CRIMES CRIPES CRISES CRONES CRORES CROWED CROWER CRUCES CRUDER CRUDES CRUSES CRUXES DRABEK DRAGEE DRAKES DRAKEU DRAPED DRAPER DRAPES DRAWEE DRAWER DRAYED

DREXEL DREYER DRIVEL DRIVEN DRIVER DRIVES DRONED DRONER DRONES DROUET DROVER DROVES DRUPES DRUSES DRUZES DRYDEN ERASED ERASER ERASES ERODED ERODER ERODES FRAKES FRAMED FRAMER FRAMES FRASER FRATER FRAUEN FRAYED FRAZER FRERES FREWER FRIGES FRISEE FRISES FRITES FROZEN GRACED GRACES GRADEA GRADEB GRADED GRADER GRADES GRAPES GRAPEY GRATED GRATER GRATES GRAVED GRAVEL GRAVEN GRAVER GRAVES GRAYED GRAYER GRAZED GRAZER GRAZES GREBES GRETEL GREYED GREYER GRIDES GRIMED GRIMES GRIPED

GRIPER GRIPES GROCER GROPED GROPER GROPES GROVED GROVEL GROVER GROVES GROWER HRIDER IRATER IRIDES IRISED IRISES IRONED IRONER KRAKEN KRAMER KRENEK KREWES KROGER KRONER KRUGER ORAJEL ORALES ORATED ORATES ORGIES ORIGEN ORKNEY OROMEO ORTHEN ORYXES PRATED PRATER PRATES PRAWER PRAXES PRAYED PRAYER PREFER PREMED PREMET PRESET PRETER PREXES PREYED PREYER PRICED PRICER PRICES PRICEY PRIDED PRIDES PRIMED PRIMER PRIMES PRISED PRIVET PRIZED PRIZES PROBED PROBER PROBES PROJET PROLES

PROPEL PROPER PROSED PROSER PROSES PROTEA PROTEM PROVED PROVEN PROVER PROVES PRUDES PRUNED PRUNER PRUNES RRATED TRACED TRACER TRACES TRACEY TRADED TRADER TRADES TRALEE TRANES TRAVEL TRAVEN TRAVES TREBEK TRECES TREXES TRIBES TRICEP TRICES TRIJET TRIKES TRINES TRIPES TRITER TRIVET TROPES TROPEZ TROVES TROWED TROWEL TROYER TRUCES WRITER WRITES XRATED XRAYED

•R•••E

ARABLE ARCADE ARCANE ARCHIE AREOLE ARGIVE ARGYLE ARIANE ARIEGE ARIOSE ARLENE AROUSE ARPEGE ARRETE ARRIVE ARSENE BRAISE BRAQUE BREEZE BRIBEE BRIDGE BRIDLE BRODIE BROGUE BRONTE BRONZE BROOKE BROSSE BROWNE BROWSE BRUISE BRULEE CRABBE CRADLE CREASE CREATE CRECHE CREOLE CREUSE CRINGE CROIRE CROSSE CROUSE CROUTE CROWNE CRUISE CRUSOE DRAGEE DRAWEE DREDGE DROGUE DROWSE DROXIE DRRICE DRUDGE DRYEYE DRYICE ERMINE ERRARE FRAISE FRANCE FRAPPE FREEZE FRICKE FRIDGE FRIEZE FRINGE FRISEE FRUNZE GRABLE GRACIE GRAMME GRANDE GRANGE GRATAE GRAZIE GREASE GREAVE GREECE GREENE GRIESE GRIEVE GRILLE

GRIMKE GRIPPE GROOVE GROSSE GROUSE GRUDGE GRUNGE IRAISE IRLENE IRVINE KRESGE MRBLUE MRHYDE ORACLE ORANGE ORELSE ORENSE ORIOLE ORNATE PRAGUE PRAISE PRANCE PREAGE PREMIE PREVUE PRINCE PRINZE PROBIE PROPRE PROWSE PRYNNE TRACHE TRALEE TRANCE TREBLE TREIZE TRENTE TRIAGE TRIFLE TRIODE TRIPLE TRISTE TRIUNE TRIXIE TROCHE TROMPE TROUPE TRUDGE TRYGVE TRYONE URBANE URSINE WRASSE WRITHE

••RE••

ADRENO ADREPS AFRESH AGREED AGREER AGREES AIRERS ARREAR ARREST ARRETE ATREST ATREUS BAREGE BARELY BAREST BEREFT BERETS BIREME BOREAL BOREAS BOREON BORERS BOREUP BUREAU BURETS CAREEN CAREER CAREOF CARERS CARESS CARETO CARETS CEREAL CEREBR CEREUS CORERS CURERS CURETS DAREME DARENT DARERS DAREST DARETO DIRECT DIRELY DIREST DOREEN DOREMI DURESS EGRESS EGRETS EIRENE ELRENO EUREKA FARERS FERENC FIREAT FIREON FIRERS FIREUP FOREGO FOREST GARETH GERENT GORERS GYRENE HAREMS HEREAT HEREBY HEREIN HEREOF HEREON HERESY HERETO HIREES HIREON HIRERS IRREAL JEREMY KAREEM

KOREAN LAREDO LAREES LOREAL LORENE LORENZ LUREIN LURENE LURERS MERELY MEREST MOREAU MOREEN MORELS MORENO MORESO NEREID NOREEN NORELL NORENT OARERS OGRESS ORRERY PARENS PARENT PARERS PARETO PAREUS PAREVE PORERS PUREED PUREES PURELY PUREST RAREES RAREFY RARELY RAREST REREAD REREEL RERENT SAREES SCREAK SCREAM SCREED SCREEN SCREES SCREWS SCREWY SERENA SERENE SHREDS SHREVE SHREWD SHREWS SIRENS SOREAT SORELY SOREST SPREAD SPREES STREAK STREAM STREEP STREET STREPS STRESS STREWN

STREWS SUREAM SUREDO SUREIS SURELY SUREOF SUREST SURETE SURETY TERESA TERETE THREAD THREAT THREEA THREEB THREEC THREED THREEE THREES THRESH TIREOF TOREAT TOREIT TORENT TORERO TOREUP TUREEN UNREAD UNREAL UNREEL UNRENT UNREST UPREAR VARESE VEREEN VEREIN VIREOS WERENT WIREIN WIRERS WIREUP WOREON YARELY YAREST

••R•E•

ADRIEN AERIER AERIES AGREED AGREER AGREES AIRIER AIRMEN AIRSEA AZRAEL BARBED BARBER BARBET BARGED BARGER BARGES BARKED BARKER BARLEY BARMEN BARNED BARNES BARNET BARNEY BARRED BARREL BARREN BARRES BARRET BARTEL BARTER BERBER BERCEO BERGEN BERGER BERMED BIRDED BIRDER BIRLED BIRLER BIRNEY BIRRED BORDEN BORDER BORDET BORGES BORKED BORNEO BURDEN BURGEE BURGER BURIED BURIER BURIES BURLED BURLER BURLEY BURNED BURNER BURNET BURNEY BURPED BURPEE BURRED BYRNES CARDED CARDER CAREEN CAREER CARIES CARKEY CARMEL CARMEN CARNER CARNES CARNET CARNEY CARPED CARPEL CARPER CARPET CARREL CARREY CARSEY CARTED CARTEL CARTER CARTES CARVED CARVEL

CARVER CARVES CARVEY CORBEL CORDED CORDER CORKED CORKER CORNEA CORNED CORNEL CORNER CORNET CORREO CORSET CORTES CORTEX CORTEZ CORVEE CURBED CURDED CURFEW CURIES CURLED CURLER CURLEW CURLEY CURRED CURSED CURSER CURSES CURTER CURVED CURVES CURVET DARCEL DARIEN DARKEN DARKER DARNED DARNER DARREN DARTED DARTER DERREK DIRGES DIRKED DOREEN DORIES DORMER DORSET DORSEY DURFEY DURNED DURYEA EARLET EARNED EARNER EERIER EYRIES FARCED FARCES FARFEL FARLEY FARMED FARMER FAROES FERBER

FERRER FERRET FIRMED FIRMER FORBES FORCED FORCER FORCES FORDED FORGED FORGER FORGES FORGET FORKED FORKER FORMED FORMER FORTES FURIES FURLED FURRED FURZES GARBED GARBER GARDEN GARNER GARNET GARRET GARTER GARVEY GERBER GIRDED GIRDER GIRTED GORCEY GORGED GORGER GORGES GORIER GORMED GORSES GURLEY GURNEE GURNEY HARDEN HARDER HARKED HARKEN HARKER HARLEM HARLEY HARMED HARMER HARNEY HARPED HARPER HARVEY HERBED HERBES HERDED HERDER HERMES HEROES HERPET HERREN HERSEY HERVEY HIREES

HORDED HORDES HORMEL HORNED HORNER HORNET HORSED HORSES HORSEY HURLED HURLER HURLEY HURTER ISRAEL ITRIED JARRED JERKED JERKER JERSEY JURIED JURIES KAREEM KARLEN KARRER KERNED KERNEL KERNES KERSEE LARDED LARDER LAREES LARGER LARGES LARKED LARKER LARMEN LARSEN LARTER LARTET LERNER LORDED LORIES LURKED LURKER LURKEY MARCEL MARDEN MARIEL MARKED MARKER MARKET MARKEY MARLED MARLEE MARLEY MARMEE MARNER MARRED MARRER MARTEL MARTEN MARTES MARVEL MARXES MERCED MERCER MERGED MERGEE

MERGER MERGES MERKEL MERMEN MERSEY MIRIER MIRREN MOREEN MORGEN MORLEY MORREL MORSEL MORTEN MURDER MURIEL MURRES NERVED NERVES NOREEN NURSED NURSER NURSES OARMEN OBRIEN OERTER PARCEL PARGED PARGER PARGES PARKED PARKER PARKES PARLEY PARLEZ PARRED PARSEC PARSED PARSEE PARSER PARSES PARTED PERKED PERLEA PERMED PERTER PORKED PORKER PORTED PORTER PORTES PUREED PUREES PURGED PURGES PURLED PURRED PURRER PURSED PURSER PURSES PURVEY RAREES REREEL SAREES SARGES SCREED SCREEN SCREES

SERGEI SERGES SERIES SERVED SERVER SERVES SHRIEK SIRBEN SIRREE SORBET SORREL SORTED SORTER SPREES SPRIER SPRYER STREEP STREET SURFED SURFER SURGED SURGES SURREY SURVEY TARDES TARGET TARLEK TARRED TARTED TARTER TARTES TERCEL TERCES TERKEL TERMED TERMES TERNES TERRES TERRET TERSER THREEA THREEB THREEC THREED THREEE THREES THROES TORIES TORRES TORREY TORTES TUREEN TURFED TURKEY TURNED TURNER TURRET UNREEL UNRUED VARDEN VARIED VARIER VARIES VARLET VARNEY VERDES VEREEN VERGED

VERGER VERGES VERJEE VERNET VERSED VERSES VERSET VERTEX VERVES VORTEX WARDED WARDEN WARDER WARIER WARMED WARMER WARNED WARNER WARNES WARPED WARPER WARRED WARREN WARTED WARVET WERFEL WERKER WERNER WIRIER WORDED WORKED WORKER WORLEY WORMED WORMER WORSEN XERXES YARDED YARDER YARNED YERKES YORKER ZEROED ZEROES

••R••E

ABRADE ADRATE ADRIVE AERATE AEROBE AFRAME AIRACE AORTAE APRILE ARRETE ARRIVE ASRARE AURATE BARBIE BAREGE BARITE BARONE BARQUE BARRIE BARTLE BERATE BERNIE

BERTHE BERTIE BIRDIE BIREME BORATE BORIDE BURBLE BURGEE BURGLE BURNIE BURPEE BURSAE BYROTE CARAFE CARIBE CAROLE CARRIE CDRATE CERATE CERISE CHROME CIRCLE CIRQUE CORPSE CORVEE CURARE CURATE CURDLE CURIAE CURITE DAREME DARKLE DARTLE DERATE DERIDE DERIVE DEROSE DIRIGE DORINE DORMIE DRRICE EARNIE EIRENE ENRAGE ENROBE ERRARE ETRADE EUROPE FERDIE FERGIE FERULE FORAGE FORCHE FORONE FURORE GARAGE GARBLE GARGLE GERTIE GIRDLE GIRLIE GORDIE GURGLE GURNEE GYRATE GYRENE HARARE HERBIE

HORACE HURDLE HURTLE JARABE JARULE JEROME KARATE KARRIE KERSEE KURILE LARINE LARVAE LORENE LORRIE LURENE MARBLE MARCHE MARCIE MARGIE MARINE MARJOE MARKIE MARLEE MARMEE MARNIE MARPLE MARQUE MARTHE MERDLE MERGEE MEROPE MERRIE MIRAGE MORALE MORGUE MOROSE MORRIE MURINE MYRTLE NARINE NERONE NORITE OARAGE ONRICE PARADE PARCAE PAREVE PAROLE PARSEE PARURE PERDUE PERINE PERUKE PERUSE PHRASE PIRATE POROSE PURDUE PURFLE PURLIE PURPLE PURSUE PYRITE RERAKE RERATE RERIDE RERISE RERODE

REROSE SARTRE SCRAPE SCRIBE SERAPE SERENE SHREVE SHRIKE SHRINE SHRIVE SHROVE SIRREE SORTIE SPRITE SPRUCE STRAFE STRIAE STRIDE STRIFE STRIKE STRIPE STRIVE STROBE STRODE STROKE STROVE SURETE TERETE TERRAE THRACE THREEE THRICE THRIVE THRONE THROVE TIRADE TIRANE TORQUE TURTLE TYRONE UNRIFE UNRIPE UNROBE UNROPE UNROVE UNRUDE UPRATE UPRISE UPROSE VARESE VERITE VERJEE VIRILE VIRTUE WARBLE XPRIZE YERTLE YORKIE

•••RE•

ABBREV ADORED ADOREE ADORER ADORES AIGRET ALFRED ALGREN

AMORES AMORET ANDREA ANDREI ANDRES ANDREW ANDREY ANTRES ARBRES ASFREE ASTRES AUBREY AUDREY AWARER AZORES AZURED AZURES BARRED BARREL BARREN BARRES BARRET BEARER BIERES BIGRED BIRRED BLARED BLARES BOHRER BOTREE BTHREE BURRED CADRES CARREL CARREY CHOREO CHORES CLARET CORREO CRORES CUORES CURRED DARREN DCAREA DEARER DEBREU DECREE DEERES DEGREE DELREY DERREK DESREE DOMREP DOORED DOURER EAGRES EGUREN ENCRES ENTREE ENTREZ ENURED ENURES FAIRED FAIRER FEARED FEARER FERRER FERRET

FIBRES FLARED FLARES FLOREK FLORES FLORET FLOREY FOUREE FRERES FUHRER FURRED GARRET GEARED GENRES GLARED GLARES GOFREE HAIRED HATRED HEARER HEBREW HEDREN HERREN HEURES IAGREE IDARED IMARET IMFREE INAREA INBRED INGRES INGREY INURED INURES ISTRES JARRED JAURES JEERED JEERER JUAREZ KARRER LABREA LAIRED LAUREL LAUREN LAUREY LEBRET LEERED LEERER LEGREE LEHRER LITRES LIVRES LOIRET LOWRES MADRES MAIRES MARRED MARRER MCCREA MCGREW MEGREZ METRED METRES MIRREN MITRED MITRES MODRED

MOIRES MOORED MORREL MURRES NACRED NACRES NBCRED NEARED NEARER NITRES NOIRES NOIRET OCHRED OCHRES ODORED OLORES OSPREY PADRES PAIRED PARRED PEERED PETREL POIRES POIRET POORER POURED POURER PURRED PURRER QUIRED QUIRES REARED REARER REBRED REBREW REDREW REGRET REGREW ROARED ROARER ROHRER SABRES SACRED SAWRED SCARED SCARER SCARES SCORED SCORER SCORES SEARED SEARER SECRET SEERED SEVRES SHARED SHARER SHARES SHEREE SHIRER SHIRES SHORES SIRREE SMORES SNARED SNARER SNARES SNORED

SNORER SNORES SOARED SOARER SOIREE SORREL SOURED SOURER SPARED SPARER SPARES SPIREA SPIRED SPIRES SPORES STARED STARER STARES STEREO STERES STORED STORER STORES SUCRES SURREY TARRED TEARED TEARER TERRES TERRET THERED THEREF THERES TIERED TIGRES TITRED TITRES TORRES TORREY TOURED TOURER TURRET TVCREW UNDREW UNFREE UPGREW USURER VEERED WARRED WARREN WEARER WHERED WHERES ZAGREB ZAIRES

•••R•E

ACCRUE ADOREE AGORAE AHERNE AHORSE AMERCE ANDRAE ASFREE ATERRE AVERSE BARRIE

BEARSE BEURRE BIERCE BOTREE BOURKE BOURNE BOURSE BTHREE CARRIE CHARGE CHERIE CLARKE COARSE COERCE COURSE COWRIE DEARIE DEARME DECREE DEGREE DESREE DUARTE EBERLE ECARTE ECORSE EDERLE EDIRNE EMBRUE EMERGE ENORME ENTREE ETERNE FAERIE FAEROE FIERCE FLORAE FOUREE GEORGE GFORCE GLURGE GOFREE GOURDE GUERRE HEARSE HEARYE HOARSE HYDRAE IAGREE IMBRUE IMFREE ISERVE KARRIE LAURIE LEGREE LIBRAE LORRIE MACRAE MCCRAE MERRIE MOERAE MONROE MORRIE MUNROE PATRIE PEARCE PEARLE PEERCE PEIRCE

PETRIE PIERCE PIERRE QUARTE REURGE ROURKE SCARCE SCARNE SCURVE SEARLE SHARPE SHEREE SHORTE SIRREE SOIREE SOTRUE SOURCE SPARSE STARVE STERNE SWERVE TERRAE THORPE TIERCE UGARTE UMBRAE UNFREE UNTRUE XLARGE ZABRZE

••••RE

ABJURE ABLARE ADHERE ADJURE ADMIRE ADWARE AFLARE AGLARE ALEGRE ALGORE ALLURE AMPERE ASHORE ASPIRE ASPURE ASRARE ASSURE ASTARE ATERRE ATTIRE BEFORE BEMIRE BESORE BESURE BEURRE BEWARE BYWIRE CENTRE CESARE CHEVRE CLAIRE COHERE CONTRE CONURE CROIRE CURARE

DAMORE DECARE DEFORE DEHIRE DEIDRE DEJURE DEMURE DEPERE DESIRE DEVERE DEVORE DEWIRE DISERE DOLORE EEYORE ELMIRE ELMORE EMIGRE EMPIRE ENCORE ENDURE ENSURE ENTIRE ERRARE ETTORE EUCHRE EXMORE EXPIRE FIACRE FIGURE FOUDRE FURORE FUTURE GALORE GLIERE GUERRE HARARE HOMBRE HONORE IGNORE IMHERE IMMURE IMPURE IMSURE INHERE INJURE INSURE JOFFRE LAHORE LENORE LETTRE LITTRE LOUVRE LUSTRE MAITRE MANURE MATURE MEAGRE MYSORE NATURE NOMBRE NOMORE OEUVRE OFYORE OHSURE ONFIRE ONHIRE PARURE

PHEDRE
PIERRE
POIVRE
POUDRE
PROPRE
QUATRE
RASURE
REBORE
RECURE
REDARE
REFIRE
REHIRE
RETIRE
RETORE
REVERE
REWIRE
REWORE
ROGERE
SAFIRE
SANGRE
SARTRE
SATIRE
SECURE
SEMPRE
SEVERE
SOMBRE
SPEARE
SPHERE
SQUARE
SQUIRE
SUTURE
TAGORE
TENURE
TEVERE
THEYRE
TIMBRE
TINORE
TULARE
UMPIRE
UNBARE
UNCORE
UNHIRE
UNPURE
UNSERE
UNSORE
UNSURE
UPHERE
UPTORE
VALERE
VELURE
VENIRE
VOLARE
WECARE

6 RF

R•F•••
RAFAEL
RAFFIA
RAFFIN
RAFFLE
RAFTED
RAFTER
REFACE
REFALL
REFEED
REFELL
REFERS
REFFED
REFIED
REFIES
REFILE
REFILL
REFILM
REFIND
REFINE
REFIRE
REFITS
REFLAG
REFLEW
REFLEX
REFLOW
REFLUX
REFOLD
REFORM
REFUEL
REFUGE
REFUND
REFUSE
REFUTE
RIFELY
RIFEST
RIFFED
RIFFLE
RIFKIN
RIFLED
RIFLER
RIFLES
RIFTED
RUFFED
RUFFLE
RUFFLY
RUFOUS

R••F••
RAFFIA
RAFFIN
RAFFLE
RAMFAN
RAMFIS
RANFOR
REDFIN
REDFIR
REDFOX
REEFED
REEFER
REFFED
RENFRO
REPFOR
RIFFED
RIFFLE
ROLFED
ROLFER
ROOFED
ROOFER
RUEFUL
RUFFED
RUFFLE
RUFFLY
RUNFOR

R•••F•
RAMIFY
RANOFF
RAREFY
RATIFY
RATOFF
REBUFF
RECIFE
REDEFY
REGIFT
RESIFT
RIPOFF
RUBIFY
RUBOFF
RUNOFF

R••••F
RANOFF
RATOFF
REBUFF
REEKOF
RELIEF
REROOF
RETIEF
RETURF
RIDSOF
RIPOFF
ROBSOF
RUBOFF
RUDOLF
RUNOFF

•RF•••
ARFARF
ERFURT
PRFIRM

•R•F••
ARAFAT
ARMFUL
ARTFUL
CRAFTS
CRAFTY
CROFTS
CRYFOR
DRAFTS
DRAFTY
DRIFTS
DRIFTY
DRYFLY
DRYFOG
GRAFTS
GRIFTS
IREFUL
KROFFT
PREFAB
PREFER
PREFIX
PROFIT
TRIFLE
TRYFOR
URNFUL

•R••F•
ARGUFY
BRIEFS
CRYOFF
DRYOFF
GRAAFF
GRIEFS
KROFFT
PROOFS
PRYOFF

•R•••F
ARFARF
CRYOFF
DRYOFF
FREEOF
GRAAFF
PRYOFF

••RF••
BARFLY
CARFUL
CORFAM
CURFEW
DURFEY
EARFUL
FARFEL
FORFUN
JARFUL
PARFUM
PURFLE
SURFED
SURFER
SURFIN
TURFED
WERFEL

••R•F•
ADRIFT
AERIFY
AURIFY
BEREFT
CARAFE
FAROFF
PURIFY
RAREFY
SCRUFF
SERIFS
SHRIFT
STRAFE
STRIFE
TARIFF
THRIFT
UNRIFE
VERIFY

••R••F
CAREOF
CERTIF
FAROFF
HEREOF
PARTOF
REROOF
SCRUFF
SORTOF
SUREOF
TARIFF
TERRIF
TIREOF
UNROOF
WARNOF

•••RF•
DWARFS
SCARFS
SCURFY
SMURFS
SNARFS
WHARFS

•••R•F
DOURIF
HEAROF
SHARIF
TERRIF
THEREF

••••RF
ALTARF
ARFARF
IMPERF
RETURF

R•G•••
RAGBAG
RAGERS
RAGGED
RAGHIB
RAGING
RAGLAN
RAGMAN
RAGMEN
RAGMOP
RAGNAR
RAGOUT
RAGRUG
RAGSON
RAGTAG
RAGTOP
RAGUSA
REGAIN
REGALE
REGARD
REGAVE
REGEAR
REGELS
REGENT
REGGAE
REGGIE
REGIFT
REGILD
REGIME
REGINA
REGION
REGIRD
REGIUS
REGIVE
REGLES
REGLOW
REGLUE
REGNAL
REGNAT
REGNUM
REGRAB
REGRET
REGREW
REGRIP
REGROW
RIGANS
RIGATI
RIGGED
RIGGER
RIGHTO
RIGHTS
RIGHTY
RIGORS
RIGOUR
RIGOUT
RIGSUP
ROGERE
ROGERS
ROGETS
ROGUED
ROGUES
RUGGED
RUGRAT

R••G••
RAGGED
RANGED
RANGEL
RANGER
RANGES
RANGIN
RANGUP
RAYGUN
REAGAN
REGGAE
REGGIE
REIGER
REIGNS
RENGAS
RIDGED
RIDGES
RIGGED
RIGGER
RINGED
RINGER
RINGIN
RINGUP
ROTGUT
ROUGED
ROUGES
ROUGHS
RUGGED
RUNGIN
RUNGUP
RUTGER

R•••G•
RAVAGE
RAWEGG
REBAGS
RECAGE
REDIGS
REFUGE
REJIGS
RELOGS
RENEGE
REPAGE
REPEGS
REPUGN
RERIGS
RESIGN
RETAGS
REURGE

R••••G
RACING
RAGBAG
RAGING
RAGRUG
RAGTAG
RAKING
RARING
RASING
RATEDG
RATING
RAVING
RAWEGG
RAXING
RAYING
RAZING
REDDOG
REDING
REDLEG
REDRAG
REDTAG
REFLAG
REHANG
REHUNG
RESANG
RESING
RETTIG
RICING
RIDING
RILING
RIMING
RISING
RIVING
ROBING
ROPING
ROVING
ROWING
RULING

•RG•••
ARGALI
ARGENT
ARGIVE
ARGOSY
ARGOTS
ARGUED
ARGUER
ARGUES
ARGUFY
ARGYLE
ARGYLL
ERGOTS
ORGANA
ORGANS
ORGEAT
ORGIES
URGENT
URGEON
URGERS
URGING

•R•G••
ARAGON
ARIGHT
ARTGUM
BRIGHT
BRIGID
BRIGIT
BROGAN
BROGUE
BRUGES
CRAGGY
DRAGEE
DRAGGY
DRAGIN
DRAGON
DRAGUP
DROGUE
FRIGES
FRIGHT
FRIGID
FROGGY
FRUGAL
GREGOR
GRIGRI
GROGGY
KROGER
KRUGER
OREGON
ORIGEN
ORIGIN
PRAGUE
PROGUN
TRAGIC
TRAGUS
TRIGON
TROGGS
TRYGVE
WRIGHT

•R••G•
ARIEGE
ARMAGH
ARPEGE
BRIDGE
BRINGS
BROUGH
CRAGGY
CRAIGT
CRINGE
DRAGGY
DREDGE
DRINGS
DRUDGE
ERYNGO
FRIDGE
FRINGE
FRINGY
FROGGY
GRANGE
GRINGO
GROGGY
GRUDGE
GRUNGE
GRUNGY
KRESGE
ORANGE
ORANGS
ORANGY
ORINGS
ORTEGA
PREAGE
PRONGS
TRIAGE
TROGGS
TROUGH
TRUDGE
WRINGS
WRONGS

•R•••G
ARCING
ARMING
CRYING
DRJUNG
DRKING
DRYFOG
DRYING
ERLANG
ERRING
ERVING
FRYING
GRUING
IRKING
IRVING
MRWONG
ORBING
PRELOG
PROLOG
PRYING
TRUING
TRYING
URGING

••RG••
AARGAU
AIRGUN
BARGED
BARGER
BARGES
BERGEN
BERGER
BIRGIT
BORGES
BORGIA
BURGEE
BURGER
BURGHS
BURGLE
BURGOO
BURGOS
CARGOS
CORGIS
DIRGES
FERGIE
FORGED
FORGER
FORGES
FORGET
FORGOT
GARGAN
GARGLE
GORGED
GORGER
GORGES
GORGON
GURGLE
HORGAN
JARGON
LARGER
LARGES
LARGOS
MARGIE
MARGIN
MARGOT
MERGED
MERGEE
MERGER
MERGES
MORGAN
MORGEN
MORGUE
NORGAY
PARGED
PARGER
PARGES
PURGED
PURGES
SARGES
SARGON
SERGEI
SERGES
SERGIO
SURGED
SURGES
TARGAS
TARGET
TURGID
VARGAS
VERGED
VERGER
VERGES
VERGIL
VIRGAS
VIRGIL
VIRGIN
VIRGOS
WARGOD

••R•G•
AURIGA
BAREGE
DIRIGE
DIRIGO
DORAGS
ENRAGE
FORAGE
FORDGT
FOREGO
GARAGE
INRAGS
MIRAGE
OARAGE
RERIGS
SCRAGS
SHRUGS
SPRIGS
UNRIGS
VIRAGO

••R••G
AIRBAG
AIRING
AIRLOG
BARING
BERING
BORING
CARING
CORING
CURING
DARING
DURING
EARING
EARTAG
EARWIG
ERRING
FARING
FIRING
GORING
GYRING
HARING
HERZOG
HIRING
LORING
LURING
MIRING
OARING
PARING
PORING
RARING
SARONG
SIRING
SPRANG
SPRING
SPRUNG
STRING
STRONG
STRUNG
TARING
THRONG
TIRING
TURING
UNRUNG
WARING
WIRING

•••RG•
ANERGY
BAERGA
BOURGS
CHARGE
CLERGY
EMERGE
ENERGY
GEORGE
GEORGI
GEORGY
GLURGE
REURGE
XLARGE

•••R•G
BIGRIG
CATRIG
DEFRAG
GEHRIG
INARUG
OILRIG
OUTRIG
RAGRUG
REDRAG
TAUROG
UNTRIG
WETRAG

••••RG
ALBORG
COBURG
CYBORG
DOTORG
EDBERG
EKBERG
ENBERG
MCHARG
MOBERG
SEBERG
SUPERG

RH••••
RHAMES
RHEBOK
RHEEMS
RHEIMS
RHEMES
RHESUS
RHETOR
RHEUMS
RHEUMY
RHINAL
RHINOS
RHODES
RHOMBI
RHOMBS
RHONDA
RHUMBA
RHUMBS
RHYMED
RHYMER
RHYMES
RHYTHM

R•H•••
RAHRAH
RAHWAY
REHABS
REHANG
REHASH
REHAUL
REHEAL
REHEAR
REHEAT
REHEEL
REHELD
REHEMS
REHIDE
REHIRE
REHITS
REHOED
REHOES
REHOLD
REHONE
REHOOK
REHUNG
ROHMER
ROHRER

R••H••
RACHEL
RAGHIB
RASHAD
RASHER
RASHES
RASHID
RASHLY
RATHER
RECHEW
REDHAT
REDHEN
REDHOT
RESHES
RESHIP
RESHOD
RESHOE
RESHOT
RESHOW
RESHUT
RETHAW
RICHEN
RICHER
RICHES
RICHET
RICHIE
RICHIN
RICHLY
RIGHTO
RIGHTS
RIGHTY
RISHIS
ROCHAT
ROCHET
ROCHON
RODHAM
ROSHIS
ROTHKO
RUCHES
RUSHAT
RUSHBY
RUSHED
RUSHEE
RUSHER
RUSHES
RUSHIN
RUSHTO
RUTHIE

R•••H•
RAJAHS
RALPHJ
RANCHO
RASCHE
REECHO
RHYTHM
RICOHS
ROUGHS

R••••H
RADISH
RAHRAH
RAKISH
RAUNCH
RAVISH
RAWISH
REHASH
RELISH
REWASH
RIYADH
RULETH
RUPIAH

•RH•••
ARHATS
DRHOOK
ERHARD
MRHYDE

•R•H••
ARCHED
ARCHER
ARCHES
ARCHIE
ARCHLY
ARCHON
ARNHEM
ARTHRO
ARTHUR
BRAHMA
BRAHMS
DRPHIL
GRAHAM
ORCHID
ORPHAN
ORPHIC
ORTHEN
ORWHAT
URCHIN

•R••H•
ARETHA
ARIGHT
BRACHS
BRASHY
BRECHT
BRIGHT
BROPHY
BROTHS
BROTHY
BRUSHY
CRECHE
CRWTHS
FRIGHT
FROTHS
FROTHY
GRAPHO
GRAPHS
GRAPHY
GRISHA
ORACHS
TRACHE
TRASHY
TRISHA
TROCHE
TROPHY
TROTHS
TRUTHS
WRATHS
WRIGHT
WRITHE

•R•••H
ARMAGH
BRAMAH
BRANCH
BREACH
BREATH
BREECH
BROACH
BROOCH
BROUGH
BRUNCH
CROTCH
CROUCH
CRUNCH
CRUTCH
DRENCH
DRRUTH
DRYISH
ERYKAH
FRENCH
FRISCH
GRINCH
GROUCH
GROWTH
IRTYSH
ORBACH
ORNITH
PREACH
TRENCH
TROUGH
WRAITH
WREATH
WRENCH
WRETCH

••RH••
AARHUS
BARHOP
CARHOP
DIRHAM
DURHAM
GORHAM
HARHAR
PYRHHO
TURHAN
WARHOL

••R•H•
BERTHA
BERTHE
BERTHS
BIRTHS
BURGHS
EARTHA
EARTHS
EARTHY
FARAHS
FIRTHS
FORCHE
FORWHY
GIRTHS
GURKHA
MARCHE
MARSHA
MARSHY
MARTHA
MARTHE
MIRTHS
MORPHO
MORPHS
MURPHY
MYRRHS
NORTHS
OPRAHS
PERCHA
PYRHHO
STROHS
SURAHS
TORAHS
TORCHY
WORTHS
WORTHY

••R••H
AFRESH
BARUCH
BORSCH
DRRUTH
ENRICH
FARRAH
GARETH
GARISH

HARRAH HIRSCH HURRAH INRUSH KIRSCH MARIAH MORATH NORUSH OGRISH ONRUSH PARAPH PARIAH PARISH PERISH SERAPH SIRRAH SPRACH THRASH THRESH THRUSH ULRICH UNRASH UPRUSH WARMTH ZURICH

•••RH•

CHIRHO MYRRHS

•••R•H

ANARCH BASRAH CHURCH DEARTH DEBRAH EPARCH EXARCH FARRAH FOURTH GHIRSH HARRAH HEARTH HOORAH HURRAH INARCH RAHRAH SCORCH SEARCH SIRRAH SMERSH SMIRCH STARCH STORCH

RI••••

RIALTO RIATAS RIBALD RIBAND RIBBED RIBBER RIBBIT RIBBON RIBCUT RIBERA RIBEYE RIBISI

RIBLET RIBOSE RIBPAD RICANS RICERS RICHEN RICHER RICHES RICHET RICHIE RICHIN RICHLY RICING RICKEY RICKIE RICOHS RICOLA RICRAC RICTAL RIDDED RIDDEN RIDDER RIDDLE RIDEBY RIDEIN RIDENT RIDERS RIDETO RIDEUP RIDGED RIDGES RIDING RIDLEY RIDSOF RIENZI RIESEN RIFELY RIFEST RIFFED RIFFLE RIFKIN RIFLED RIFLER RIFLES RIFTED RIGANS RIGATI RIGGED RIGGER RIGHTO RIGHTS RIGHTY RIGORS RIGOUR RIGOUT RIGSUP RIJEKA RIKERS RILERS RILEUP RILING RILLES RILLET RIMATE RIMERS RIMIER RIMING RIMINI

RIMMED RIMOSE RIMOUS RIMPLE RIMSKY RINGED RINGER RINGIN RINGUP RINSED RINSER RINSES RIOJAS RIOPAN RIOTED RIOTER RIPELY RIPENS RIPEST RIPKEN RIPLEY RIPOFF RIPOST RIPOUT RIPPED RIPPER RIPPLE RIPPLY RIPRAP RIPSAW RIPSON RIPSUP RISERS RISETO RISEUP RISHIS RISING RISKED RISKER RISKIT RISQUE RITARD RITDYE RITSOS RITTER RITUAL RITZES RIVALS RIVERA RIVERS RIVETS RIVING RIVOLI RIYADH RIYALS

R•I•••

RAIDED RAIDER RAILAT RAILED RAILER RAILON RAINED RAINER RAINES RAINEY RAININ

RAINON RAIPUR RAISED RAISER RAISES RAISIN RAISON RAITAS RBIMAN RBIMEN REICED REICES REIGER REIGNS REILLY REINAS REINED REINER REINES REININ REINKS REISER REITER RHINAL RHINOS ROILED ROILUP RTILES RUINED RUINER

R••I••

RABIES RACIAL RACIER RACILY RACINE RACING RACINO RACISM RACIST RADIAL RADIAN RADIOS RADISH RADIUM RADIUS RAGING RAKING RAKISH RAMIES RAMIFY RANIDS RANINE RAPIDO RAPIDS RAPIER RAPINE RAPINI RARING RARITY RASING RATIFY RATINE RATING RATION RATIOS RATITE

RAVINE RAVING RAVISH RAWISH RAWIST RAXING RAYING RAZING REAIMS REAIRS REBIDS REBILL REBIND RECIFE RECIPE RECITE REDIAL REDIGS REDING REDINK REDIPS REFIED REFIES REFILE REFILL REFILM REFIND REFINE REFIRE REFITS REGIFT REGILD REGIME REGINA REGION REGIRD REGIUS REGIVE REHIDE REHIRE REHITS REJIGS REKICK RELICS RELICT RELIED RELIEF RELIER RELIES RELINE RELINK RELISH RELIST RELIVE REMICK REMILL REMIND REMINE REMINI REMINT REMISE REMISS REMITS RENINS REOILS REPICK REPINE REPINS

RERIDE RERIGS RERISE RESIDE RESIFT RESIGN RESILE RESING RESINK RESINS RESINY RESIST RESITE RESITS RESIZE RETIAL RETIED RETIEF RETIES RETILE RETILL RETIME RETINA RETINS RETINT RETIPS RETIRE REVIEW REVILE REVISE REVIVE REWIND REWINS REWIPE REWIRE REZIPS RHEIMS RIBISI RICING RIDING RILING RIMIER RIMING RIMINI RISING RIVING ROBING ROBINS RODINO RODION ROMIJN ROPIER ROPING ROSIER ROSIES ROSILY ROSINA ROSINS ROSINY ROSITA ROTINI ROVING ROWING RUBIED RUBIES RUBIFY RUBIKS RULIER

RULING RUNINS RUPIAH RUTILE RUTINS

R•••I•

RABBIS RABBIT RACEIN RAFFIA RAFFIN RAGHIB RAININ RAISIN RAKEIN RAMFIS RAMSIN RANCID RANGIN RANKIN RASHID RASKIN RATLIN RAZZIE READIN REALIA REBAIT REBBIE REBOIL RECOIL RECOIN REDDIN REDFIN REDFIR REDSIX REDTIE REEDIT REELIN REEMIT REENIE REGAIN REGGIE REGRIP REININ REJAIL REJOIN REKNIT RELAID REMAIL REMAIN RENAIL RENNIE RENNIN RENOIR REPAID REPAIR RESAID RESHIP RESNIK RESOIL RESPIN RESTIR RESUIT RESWIM RETAIL RETAIN RETRIM

RETTIG REVOIR RIBBIT RICHIE RICHIN RICKIE RIDEIN RIFKIN RINGIN RISHIS RISKIT ROADIE ROAMIN ROBBIA ROBBIE ROCKIE ROCKIN ROCKIT RODEIN ROLLIE ROLLIN ROMAIC ROMAIN RONMIX RONNIE ROOKIE ROOMIE ROOTIE ROOTIN ROPEIN ROSHIS RUBBIA RUBRIC RUBSIN RUDKIN RUNCIE RUNGIN RUNSIN RUSHIN RUSKIN RUSSIA RUSTIC RUTHIE RUXPIN

R••••I

RAPINI REMINI RENVOI RHOMBI RIBISI RIENZI RIGATI RIMINI RIVOLI ROLLEI ROMAJI ROMANI ROTINI RUBATI RUMAKI

•RI•••

ARIANA ARIANE ARIARY ARIDER ARIDLY

ARIEGE ARIGHT ARIOSE ARIOSI ARIOSO ARISEN ARISES ARISTA ARISTO BRIANA BRIAND BRIARD BRIARS BRIARY BRIBED BRIBEE BRIBER BRIBES BRICKS BRICKY BRIDAL BRIDES BRIDGE BRIDLE BRIEFS BRIENZ BRIERS BRIERY BRIGHT BRIGID BRIGIT BRILLO BRINED BRINER BRINES BRINGS BRINKS BRISES BRISKS BRITON CRICKS CRIERS CRIKEY CRIMEA CRIMES CRIMPS CRIMPY CRINGE CRIPES CRISCO CRISES CRISIS CRISPS CRISPY CRISTO CRITIC DRIERS DRIEST DRIFTS DRIFTY DRILLS DRINGS DRINKS DRIPON DRIPPY DRIQJR DRIVEL DRIVEN

DRIVER DRIVES DRIVIN ERICAS ERIEPA ERINNA ERINYS ERIVAN FRIARS FRIARY FRICKA FRICKE FRIDAY FRIDGE FRIEDA FRIELS FRIEND FRIERS FRIEZE FRIGES FRIGHT FRIGID FRIJOL FRILLS FRILLY FRINGE FRINGY FRISCH FRISCO FRISEE FRISES FRISKS FRISKY FRITAS FRITES FRITOS FRITTA FRITTO FRITZI FRIVOL FRIZZY GRIDES GRIECO GRIEFS GRIESE GRIEVE GRIFTS GRIGRI GRILLE GRILLS GRIMED GRIMES GRIMKE GRIMLY GRIMMS GRIMMY GRINAT GRINCH GRINDL GRINDS GRINGO GRIOTS GRIPED GRIPER GRIPES GRIPPE GRIPPY GRISHA

GRISLY GRISTS GRITTI GRITTY HRIDER IRIDES IRIDIC IRISED IRISES IRISIN IRITIC IRITIS KRISPY KRISTI ORIANA ORIANI ORIBIS ORIELS ORIENT ORIGEN ORIGIN ORINGS ORIOLE ORIONS ORISON ORISSA PRICED PRICER PRICES PRICEY PRICKS PRIDED PRIDES PRIERS PRIEST PRIMAL PRIMED PRIMER PRIMES PRIMLY PRIMOS PRIMPS PRIMUS PRINCE PRINKS PRINTS PRINZE PRIORI PRIORS PRIORY PRISED PRISMS PRISON PRISSY PRIVET PRIZED PRIZES PRIZMS PRIZZI TRIADS TRIAGE TRIALS TRIBAL TRIBES TRICEP TRICES TRICIA TRICKS

TRICKY TRICOT TRIERS TRIFLE TRIGON TRIJET TRIKES TRILBY TRILLO TRILLS TRIMLY TRINAL TRINES TRIODE TRIPES TRIPLE TRIPLY TRIPOD TRIPON TRIPUP TRISHA TRISTE TRITER TRITON TRIUNE TRIVET TRIVIA TRIXIE WRIEST WRIGHT WRINGS WRISTS WRITER WRITES WRITHE

•R•I••

ARCING ARGIVE ARLISS ARMIES ARMING ARNICA ARNIES AROIDS AROINT ARRIBA ARRIVE ARTIER ARTILY ARTIST BRAIDS BRAINS BRAINY BRAISE BROILS BRUINS BRUISE BRUITS CRAIGT CRAINS CROIRE CRUISE CRYING DRAINS DRKING DROIDS DROITS

DRRICE DRUIDS DRYICE DRYING DRYINK DRYISH ERBIUM ERMINE EROICA ERRING ERVING FRAIDY FRAISE FRUITS FRUITY FRYING GRAILS GRAINS GRAINY GREIST GROINS GRUING IRAISE IRKING IRVINE IRVING KRAITS MRBILL MRDICK MRJINX MRPIBB ORBING ORBITS OREIDA ORGIES ORNITH ORSINI ORSINO PRAISE PRFIRM PRYING TRAILS TRAINS TRAITS TREIZE TROIKA TRUING TRUISM TRYING URGING URSIDS URSINE WRAITH

•R••I•

ARABIA ARABIC ARAMID ARAMIS ARCHIE ARCSIN ARCTIC ARMPIT ARNEIS ARTOIS BRASIL BRAZIL BREVIS

BRIGID BRIGIT BRODIE BROLIN BROVIK CRAMIN CRANIA CRANIO CREDIT CRETIN CRISIS CRITIC CRONIN DRAGIN DRATIT DRAWIN DREBIN DREVIL DREWIN DRIVIN DROMIO DROPIN DROPIT DROXIE DRPHIL EROTIC FRIGID FROLIC GRACIE GRANIT GRATIA GRATIN GRATIS GRAVID GRAZIE GRODIN GROMIT GRUMIO IRANIS IRAQIS IRENIC IRIDIC IRISIN IRITIC IRITIS IRONIC KRAVIS ORANIS ORCHID ORDAIN OREXIA OREXIS ORIBIS ORIGIN ORPHIC PRAXIS PREBID PRECIP PRECIS PREFIX PRELIM PREMIE PREMIX PREVIA PREVIN PROBIE PROFIT PROLIX

PROSIT QRATIO TRACII TRAGIC TRAVIS TREDIA TREPID TRICIA TRIVIA TRIXIE TROPIC URACIL URALIC URANIA URANIC URCHIN

•R•••I

ARGALI ARIOSI ARMANI BRANDI BRAZZI BRUNEI ERNANI FRITZI FRUCTI FRUTTI GRIGRI GRITTI GRUCCI KRISTI ORIANI ORSINI PRIORI PRIZZI TRACII URBANI

••RI••

ADRIAN ADRIEN ADRIFT ADRIVE AERIAL AERIER AERIES AERIFY AERILY AERIOS AFRICA AIRIER AIRILY AIRING ALRITZ AMRITA APRILE APRILS ARRIBA ARRIVE ATRIAL ATRISK ATRIUM AURIFY AURIGA AURIST AVRILS BARING

BARITE
BARIUM
BERING
BORIDE
BORING
BURIAL
BURIED
BURIER
BURIES
BURINS
CARIBE
CARIBS
CARIES
CARINA
CARING
CARIOU
CERISE
CERIUM
CHRISM
CHRIST
CORING
CORIUM
CURIAE
CURIES
CURING
CURIOS
CURITE
CURIUM
DARIEN
DARING
DARIUS
DERIDE
DERITA
DERIVE
DIRIGE
DIRIGO
DORIAN
DORIES
DORINE
DORITO
DRRICE
DURING
EARING
EERIER
EERILY
ENRICH
ENRICO
ERRING
EYRIES
FARINA
FARING
FERIAS
FERITY
FIRING
FORINT
FURIES
GARISH
GORIER
GORILY
GORING
GORIOT
GURION
GYRING
HARING
HIRING
ITRIED
JURIED
JURIES
JURIST
KARINA
KURILE
LARIAT
LARINE
LERIDA
LORIES
LORING
LURING
LYRICS
LYRIDS
LYRIST
MARIAH
MARIAN
MARIAS
MARIDA
MARIDO
MARIEL
MARIKO
MARILU
MARINA
MARINE
MARINO
MARION
MARISA
MARIST
MCRIBS
MERIDA
MERINO
MERITS
MIRIAM
MIRIER
MIRING
MIRINS
MORITA
MORITZ
MURIEL
MURINE
MYRIAD
NARIAL
NARINE
NARITA
NORIAS
NORISK
NORITE
OARING
OBRIAN
OBRIEN
OGRISH
ONRICE
PARIAH
PARING
PARINI
PARISH
PARITY
PERILS
PERINE
PERIOD
PERISH
PERITI
PORING
PURIFY
PURIMS
PURINA
PURISM
PURIST
PURITY
PYRITE
RARING
RARITY
RERIDE
RERIGS
RERISE
SCRIBE
SCRIMP
SCRIMS
SCRIPS
SCRIPT
SERIAL
SERIES
SERIFS
SERINS
SHRIEK
SHRIFT
SHRIKE
SHRILL
SHRIMP
SHRINE
SHRINK
SHRIVE
SIRICA
SIRING
SIRIUS
SPRIER
SPRIGS
SPRING
SPRINT
SPRITE
SPRITS
SPRITZ
STRIAE
STRICT
STRIDE
STRIFE
STRIKE
STRING
STRIPE
STRIPS
STRIPY
STRIVE
SURIMI
SYRIAN
TARIFF
TARING
THRICE
THRIFT
THRILL
THRIVE
TIRIAC
TIRING
TORIES
TORINO
TURING
ULRICH
UNRIFE
UNRIGS
UNRIPE
UNRIPS
UPRISE
VARIAS
VARIED
VARIER
VARIES
VERIFY
VERILY
VERISM
VERIST
VERITE
VERITY
VIRILE
WARIER
WARILY
WARING
WIRIER
WIRILY
WIRING
XPRIZE
YORICK
ZORINA
ZURICH

••R•I•

ADROIT
AFRAID
AORTIC
ATRAIN
ATROIS
BARBIE
BARDIC
BARKIN
BARRIE
BARRIO
BARRIS
BERLIN
BERNIE
BERTIE
BIRDIE
BIRGIT
BORGIA
BURNIE
BURNIN
CARDIA
CARDIN
CARDIO
CARLIN
CARRIE
CARTIN
CERTIF
CERVID
CORBIN
CORDIA
CORGIS
CORVID
CORWIN
CURLIN
CURTIN
CURTIS
CURTIZ
DARLIN
DARNIT
DARRIN
DARWIN
DERAIL
DERAIN
DERMIC
DERMIS
DORMIE
DORRIT
DURBIN
DURNIT
EARNIE
EARNIT
EARVIN
EARWIG
EURAIL
FARRIS
FERDIE
FERGIE
FERMIS
FERRIC
FERRIS
FERVID
FIRKIN
FORBID
FORDID
FORMIC
FORTIS
GARCIA
GARLIC
GARYIN
GERBIL
GERTIE
GERVIN
GIRLIE
GORDIE
HARBIN
HARDIN
HARLIN
HARRIS
HERBIE
HEREIN
HERMIT
HERNIA
HEROIC
HEROIN
HORNIN
HORRID
ISRAIR
JARDIN
JARVIK
JERKIN
KARMIC
KARRIE
KERMIT
KERWIN
LARKIN
LORAIN
LORDIT
LORRIE
LUREIN
MARCIA
MARCIE
MARCIL
MARCIX
MARDIS
MARGIE
MARGIN
MARKIE
MARKII
MARKIV
MARKIX
MARLIN
MARNIE
MARTIN
MARVIN
MARVIS
MARYII
MERLIN
MERRIE
MORBID
MORRIE
MORRIS
MURCIA
NARNIA
NARVIK
NEREID
NORAIN
NORDIC
NORRIS
PARKIT
PARNIS
PARRIS
PARTII
PARTIV
PERKIN
PERMIT
PERRIN
PERSIA
PERSIS
PIRRIP
PORTIA
PURLIE
SARDIS
SARNIA
SERAIS
SERBIA
SERGIO
SERKIN
SERKIS
SORBIC
SORDID
SORTIE
SPRAIN
STRAIN
STRAIT
SUREIS
SURFIN
TAROIL
TARPIT
TERBIC
TERRIF
TERRIS
TOREIT
TOROID
TORPID
TORRID
TURBID
TURGID
TURKIC
TURNIN
TURNIP
TURPIN
VERBID
VERDIN
VEREIN
VERGIL
VERMIN
VIRGIL
VIRGIN
WIREIN
WORKIN
YORKIE
YORKIN
ZEROIN

••R••I

BARONI
BORZOI
CAROLI
CARONI
CORACI
DORATI
DOREMI
FARUKI
MARKII
MARKVI
MARYII
MORONI
NEROLI
NORDOI
PARINI
PARTII
PERITI
SERGEI
STRATI
SURIMI

•••RI•

ACARID
AGARIC
ALARIC
ALDRIN
ALTRIA
ANDRIC
ANTRIM
ASTRID
ATARIS
ATTRIT
AZARIA
AZERIS
AZORIN
BARRIE
BARRIO
BARRIS
BIGRIG
CABRIO
CAPRID
CAPRIS
CARRIE
CATRIG
CEDRIC
CHERIE
CHORIC
CHORIO
CITRIC
CITRIN
CLERIC
CLORIS
COURIC
COWRIE
CUPRIC
CYMRIC
DARRIN
DATRIL
DEARIE
DEBRIS
DELRIO
DIARIO
DORRIT
DOURIF
EGERIA
ELYRIA
EMERIC
EMERIL
ESPRIT
FABRIC
FAERIE
FARRIS
FERRIC
FERRIS
FIBRIN
FLORID
FLORIN
FLORIO
GEHRIG
GETRID
GLORIA
GOTRID
HARRIS
HENRIK
HORRID
HOURIS
HUBRIS
HYBRID
HYDRIC
HYGRIC
IATRIC
IBERIA
ICARIA
INGRID
ISTRIA
KARRIE
KATRIN
KIARIO
KUPRIN
LATRIA
LAURIA
LAURIC
LAURIE
LETRIP
LIBRIS
LORRIE
MADRID
MAORIS
MATRIX
MEGRIM
MERRIE
METRIC
MIDRIB
MORRIE
MORRIS
MOTRIN
NITRIC
NORRIS
NUTRIA
OILRIG
OSIRIS
OUTRIB
OUTRIG
OVERIT
PARRIS
PATRIA
PATRIC
PATRIE
PEERIN
PEORIA
PERRIN
PETRIE
PICRIC
PIERIA
PIRRIP
POORIS
POURIN
PUTRID
REGRIP
RETRIM
RUBRIC
SCORIA
SHARIF
SPIRIT
STARIN
STERIC
STIRIN
TABRIZ
TAURIC
TEARIT
TEGRIN
TERRIF
TERRIS
TETRIS
THORIC
TIGRIS
TIKRIT
TORRID
TSURIS
TUGRIK
UMBRIA
UNGRIP
UNPRIM
UNTRIG
USERID
VITRIC
YTTRIA
YTTRIC

•••R•I

ANDREI
CIARDI
GEORDI
GEORGI
HENRYI
ITURBI
OCTROI
SHERRI
SHORTI
SNORRI
UBUROI

••••RI

CENTRI
DENARI
DENDRI
DMITRI
GRIGRI
HATARI
HUMERI
LAPERI
LATERI
LIPARI
MIDORI
NOYORI
PAPYRI
PETERI
PRIORI
QATARI
QUADRI
SAFARI
SATORI
SHERRI
SNORRI
SUVARI
TISHRI
TOKORI
VIDERI

R•J•••

RAJABS
RAJAHS
REJAIL
REJECT
REJIGS
REJOIN
RIJEKA

R••J••

RAMJET
RIOJAS

R•••J•

ROMAJI
ROMIJN

R••••J

RALPHJ

•RJ•••

ARJUNA
DRJUNG
MRJINX

•R•J••

FRIJOL
ORAJEL
PROJET
TRAJAN
TRIJET
TROJAN

•R••J•

DRIQJR

••RJ••

FORJOY
JARJAR
MARJOE
VERJEE

••R•J•

BAROJA
MARYJO

••••RJ

INTERJ

RK••••

RKELLY

R•K•••

RAKEIN
RAKERS
RAKEUP
RAKING
RAKISH
REKEYS
REKICK
REKNIT
REKNOT
RIKERS

R••K••

RACKED
RACKER
RACKET
RACKUP
RANKED
RANKER
RANKIN
RANKLE
RANKLY
RASKIN
RECKED
RECKON
REEKED
REEKER
REEKOF
RICKEY
RICKIE
RIFKIN
RIPKEN
RISKED
RISKER
RISKIT
ROCKED
ROCKER
ROCKET
ROCKIE
ROCKIN
ROCKIT
ROCKNE
ROCKYV
ROOKED
ROOKER
ROOKIE
RUCKED
RUCKER
RUCKUP
RUCKUS
RUDKIN
RUDKUS
RUSKIN
RYOKAN
RYUKYU

R•••K•

REASKS
REBAKE
REBUKE
REDSKY
REINKS
REMAKE
RERAKE
RETAKE
REVOKE
REWAKE
REWOKE
REYOKE
RIJEKA
RIMSKY
ROTHKO
ROURKE
RUBIKS
RUMAKI

R••••K

REBANK
REBOOK
RECOCK
RECOOK
RECORK
REDINK
REDOAK
REDOCK
REEBOK
REHOOK
REKICK
RELINK
RELOCK
RELOOK
REMARK
REMICK
REPACK
REPARK
REPERK
REPICK
RERACK
RERANK
RESEEK
RESINK
RESNIK
RESOAK
RETACK
RETOOK
REWORK
RHEBOK
RVPARK

•RK•••

DRKING
DRKOOP
IRKERS
IRKING
ORKANS
ORKNEY

•R•K••

BRAKED
BRAKES
BROKAW
BROKEN
BROKER
CRAKES
CRIKEY
DRAKES
DRAKEU
ERYKAH
FRAKES
KRAKEN
KRAKOW
TRIKES

•R••K•

BREAKS
BRICKS
BRICKY
BRINKS
BRISKS
BRONKO
BROOKE
BROOKS
BROOKY
CRACKD
CRACKS
CRANKS
CRANKY
CREAKS
CREAKY
CREEKS
CRICKS
CROAKS
CROAKY
CROCKS
CROOKS
DRECKS
DRECKY
DRINKS
FRANKS
FREAKS
FREAKY
FRICKA
FRICKE
FRISKS
FRISKY
FROCKS
GREEKS
GRIMKE
ORECKS
PRANKS
PRICKS
PRINKS
PROSKY
TRACKS
TRICKS
TRICKY
TROIKA
TRUCKS
TRUNKS
WRACKS
WREAKS
WRECKS

•R•••K

ARMONK
ARRACK
BRATSK
BROVIK
DRABEK
DRHOOK
DRYINK
FRANCK
KRENEK
MRDICK
TREBEK
URALSK

••RK••

BARKAT
BARKED
BARKER
BARKIN
BARKLA
BERKOW
BORKED
BURKAS
CARKEY
CORKED
CORKER
CORKUP
DARKEN
DARKER
DARKLE
DARKLY
DIRKED
FIRKIN
FORKED
FORKER
FORKUP
GURKHA
HARKED
HARKEN
HARKER
JERKED
JERKER
JERKIN
JERKUP
KARKOV
KIRKUK
LARKED
LARKER
LARKIN
LURKED
LURKER
LURKEY
MARKAS
MARKED
MARKER
MARKET
MARKEY
MARKIE
MARKII
MARKIV
MARKIX
MARKKA
MARKOV
MARKUP
MARKVI
MERKEL
PARKAS
PARKAV
PARKAY
PARKED
PARKER
PARKES
PARKIT
PERKED
PERKIN
PERKUP
PORKED
PORKER
PORKYS
SERKIN
SERKIS
SIRKAY
TERKEL
TURKEY
TURKIC
WERKER
WORKAT
WORKED
WORKER
WORKIN
WORKON
WORKUP
YERKES
YORKER
YORKIE
YORKIN
YORKPA
ZARKOV

••R•K•

BARAKA
EUREKA
FARUKI
MARIKO
MARKKA
MERCKX
PERUKE
RERAKE
SHRIKE
STRIKE
STROKE

••R••K

ARRACK
ATRISK
BARACK
BARTOK
BUROAK
CDRACK
DERREK
ENRANK
FAROUK
JARVIK
KARNAK
KIRKUK
LFRANK
NARVIK
NORISK
RERACK
RERANK
SCREAK
SHRANK
SHRIEK
SHRINK
SHRUNK
STREAK
STRUCK
STRUNK
TARLEK
UNRACK
YORICK

•••RK•

BOURKE
CLARKE
CLERKS
DMARKS
OZARKS
QUARKS
QUIRKS
QUIRKY
ROURKE
SHARKS
SHIRKS
SMIRKS
SMIRKY
SNARKS
SNARKY
SPARKS
SPARKY
SPORKS
STORKS

•••R•K

AMTRAK
ANORAK
DERREK
DVORAK
FLOREK
HENRIK
HENRYK
TUGRIK

••••RK
ATWORK
DEBARK
DEMARK
EMBARK
GODARK
INPARK
LANARK
NEWARK
RECORK
REMARK
REPARK
REPERK
REWORK
RVPARK
STMARK
UNCORK
UNFORK
UQUARK
VANARK

R•L•••
RALLYE
RALPHJ
RELACE
RELAID
RELAND
RELAPS
RELATE
RELAYS
RELEAD
RELEAP
RELEND
RELENT
RELETS
RELEVE
RELEVY
RELICS
RELICT
RELIED
RELIEF
RELIER
RELIES
RELINE
RELINK
RELISH
RELIST
RELIVE
RELOAD
RELOAN
RELOCK
RELOGS
RELOOK
RELOSE
RELOST
RELUCT
RELUME
RELYON
RILERS
RILEUP
RILING
RILLES
RILLET
ROLAND
ROLEOS
ROLFED
ROLFER
ROLLBY
ROLLED
ROLLEI
ROLLER
ROLLIE
ROLLIN
ROLLON
ROLLUP
RULEON
RULERS
RULETH
RULIER
RULING

R••L••
RADLEY
RAGLAN
RAILAT
RAILED
RAILER
RAILON
RALLYE
RANLOW
RATLIN
REALER
REALES
REALIA
REALLY
REALMS
REALTY
RECLAD
REDLEG
REELED
REELER
REELIN
REELUP
REFLAG
REFLEW
REFLEX
REFLOW
REFLUX
REGLES
REGLOW
REGLUE
REILLY
REPLAN
REPLAY
REPLED
REPLOT
REPLOW
REVLON
REYLES
RIALTO
RIBLET
RIDLEY
RIFLED
RIFLER
RIFLES
RILLES
RILLET
RIPLEY
RKELLY
ROBLES
ROILED
ROILUP
ROLLBY
ROLLED
ROLLEI
ROLLER
ROLLIE
ROLLIN
ROLLON
ROLLUP
ROSLYN
ROWLEY
RTILES
RUBLES
RUBLEV
RUNLET
RUNLOW
RVALUE

R•••L•
RABBLE
RACILY
RAFFLE
RAMBLE
RANKLE
RANKLY
RAPTLY
RARELY
RASHLY
RASSLE
RATELS
RATTLE
RATTLY
RAVELS
RAZZLE
RCCOLA
REALLY
REBALE
REBELS
REBILL
REBOLT
RECALL
REFALL
REFELL
REFILE
REFILL
REFILM
REFOLD
REGALE
REGELS
REGILD
REHELD
REHOLD
REILLY
REMELT
REMILL
REMOLD
REOILS
REPELS
REPOLL
REROLL
RESALE
RESALT
RESELL
RESILE
RESOLD
RESOLE
RESULT
RETELL
RETILE
RETILL
RETOLD
REVELS
REVILE
REVOLT
REWELD
REXALL
RIBALD
RICHLY
RICOLA
RIDDLE
RIFELY
RIFFLE
RIMPLE
RIPELY
RIPPLE
RIPPLY
RIVALS
RIVOLI
RIYALS
RKELLY
RODALE
ROMOLA
ROMULO
RONALD
RONELY
ROOTLE
ROSILY
ROWELS
ROYALE
ROYALS
RUBBLE
RUBBLY
RUBELS
RUDELY
RUDOLF
RUFFLE
RUFFLY
RUMBLE
RUMBLY
RUMPLE
RUMPLY
RUNDLE
RUSTLE
RUTILE
RYDELL

R••••L
RACHEL
RACIAL
RADIAL
RAFAEL
RAMPAL
RANDAL
RANGEL
RAPPEL
RAQUEL
RASCAL
REBILL
REBOIL
RECALL
RECOAL
RECOIL
RECOOL
RECURL
REDEAL
REDIAL
REFALL
REFELL
REFILL
REFUEL
REGNAL
REHAUL
REHEAL
REHEEL
REJAIL
REMAIL
REMILL
RENAIL
RENTAL
REPEAL
REPOLL
REREEL
REROLL
RESEAL
RESELL
RESOIL
RETAIL
RETELL
RETIAL
RETILL
RETOOL
RETRAL
REVEAL
REXALL
RHINAL
RICTAL
RITUAL
ROMMEL
RONDEL
RUEFUL
RUNNEL
RUSSEL
RYDELL

•RL•••
ARLENE
ARLISS
ARLOVA
ERLANG
IRLENE
ORLONS
ORLOPS

•R•L••
ARMLET
BRILLO
BROLIN
BROLLY
BRULEE
DRCLAW
DRILLS
DROLLS
DROLLY
FRILLS
FRILLY
FROLIC
GRILLE
GRILLS
KRYLON
KRYLOV
MRBLUE
ORALES
ORALLY
ORELSE
PRELAW
PRELIM
PRELOG
PROLES
PROLIX
PROLOG
TRALAS
TRALEE
TRILBY
TRILLO
TRILLS
TROLLS
TRYLON
URALIC
URALSK

•R••L•
ARABLE
ARBELA
ARCHLY
AREOLA
AREOLE
ARGALI
ARGYLE
ARGYLL
ARIDLY
ARNALL
ARNOLD
ARPELS
ARTELS
ARTILY
BRAWLS
BRENLY
BRIDLE
BRILLO
BROILS
BROLLY
CRADLE
CRAWLS
CRAWLY
CREELS
CREOLE
DRABLY
DRAWLS
DRAWLY
DRILLS
DROLLS
DROLLY
DROOLS
DROOLY
DRYFLY
ERROLL
FREELY
FRIELS
FRILLS
FRILLY
GRABLE
GRAILS
GRAYLY
GREYLY
GRILLE
GRILLS
GRIMLY
GRISLY
GROWLS
GROWLY
GRRRLS
GRUELS
KRAALS
MRBILL
MRSULU
ORACLE
ORALLY
ORIELS
ORIOLE
ORMOLU
ORWELL
PRIMLY
PROULX
PROWLS
TRAILS
TRAWLS
TREBLE
TREBLY
TRIALS
TRIFLE
TRILLO
TRILLS
TRIMLY
TRIPLE
TRIPLY
TROLLS
URSULA

•R•••L
ARGYLL
ARMFUL
ARNALL
ARTFUL
BRASIL
BRAZIL
BRIDAL
BRUMAL
BRUMEL
BRUTAL
CRENEL
CRESOL
CREWEL
CRURAL
DREVIL
DREXEL
DRIVEL
DRPHIL
ERROLL
FRIJOL
FRIVOL
FRUGAL
GRAVEL
GRETEL
GRINDL
GROVEL
IREFUL
IRREAL
MRBILL
MRCOOL
ORAJEL
ORDEAL
ORWELL
PRIMAL
PROCOL
PROPEL
PROPYL
TRAVEL
TRIBAL
TRINAL
TROWEL
URACIL
URNFUL

••RL••
AIRLOG
BARLEY
BARLOW
BERLIN
BIRLED
BIRLER
BURLAP
BURLED
BURLER
BURLEY
CARLIN
CARLOS
CARLOT
CARLOW
CURLED
CURLER
CURLEW
CURLEY
CURLIN
CURLUP
DARLIN
EARLAP
EARLET
FARLEY
FARLOW
FURLED
GARLIC
GIRLIE
GURLEY
HARLAN
HARLEM
HARLEY
HARLIN
HARLOT
HARLOW
HURLED
HURLER
HURLEY
KARLEN
MARLED
MARLEE
MARLEY
MARLIN
MARLON
MERLIN
MERLOT
MORLEY
PARLAY
PARLEY
PARLEZ
PARLOR
PERLEA
PURLED
PURLIE
TARLEK
VARLET
WORLDS
WORLEY

••R•L•
AERILY
AIRILY
APRILE
APRILS
AVRILS
BARELY
BARFLY
BARKLA
BAROLO
BARTLE
BERYLS
BURBLE
BURBLY
BURGLE
CAROLE
CAROLI
CAROLL
CAROLS
CIRCLE
CORALS
CURDLE
CURTLY
DARKLE
DARKLY
DARTLE
DIRELY
EERILY
ENROLL
ENROLS
ERROLL
FERALS
FERULE
FIRMLY
GARBLE
GARGLE
GERALD
GIRDLE
GORILY
GRRRLS
GURGLE
HARALD
HARDLY
HAROLD
HERALD
HURDLE
HURTLE
JARULE
KERALA
KURALT
KURILE
LORDLY
MARBLE
MARBLY
MARILU
MARPLE
MERDLE
MERELY
MERYLL
MORALE
MORALS
MORELS
MOROLT
MURALS
MYRTLE
NEROLI
NORELL
PAROLE
PAROLS
PARTLY
PERILS
PERTLY
PORTLY
PURELY
PURFLE
PURPLE
PURPLY
RARELY
REROLL
SCROLL
SHRILL
SORELY
SPRYLY
STROLL
SURELY
TARTLY
THRALL
THRILL
TURTLE
UNROLL
UNRULY
VERILY
VIRILE
WARBLE
WARILY
WARMLY
WIRILY
YARELY
YERTLE

••R••L
AERIAL
AORTAL
ATRIAL
AZRAEL
BARREL
BARTEL
BOREAL
BURIAL
BURSAL
CARFUL
CARMEL
CARNAL
CAROLL
CARPAL
CARPEL
CARREL
CARROL
CARTEL
CARVEL
CEREAL
CORBEL
CORNEL
CORRAL
DARCEL
DARRYL
DERAIL
DERMAL
DIRNDL
DORSAL
EARFUL
ENROLL
ERROLL
EURAIL
FARFEL
FORMAL
GERBIL
HERBAL
HORMEL
IRREAL
ISRAEL
JARFUL
KERNEL
LARVAL
LOREAL
MARCEL
MARCIL
MARIEL
MARTEL
MARVEL
MERKEL
MERYLL
MORREL
MORSEL
MORTAL
MURIEL
MYRDAL
NARIAL
NERMAL
NERVAL
NORELL
NORMAL
NORVAL
PARCEL
PORTAL
REREEL
REROLL
SCRAWL
SCROLL
SERIAL
SHRILL
SORREL
SPRAWL
STROLL
TAROIL
TARSAL
TERCEL
TERKEL
THRALL
THRILL
UNREAL
UNREEL
UNROLL
VERBAL
VERGIL
VERNAL
VIRGIL
VORPAL
WARHOL
WERFEL

•••RL•
BGIRLS
CEORLS
CHARLY
CHURLS
DEARLY
DOURLY
EBERLE
EBERLY
EDERLE
EVERLY
FAIRLY
GNARLS
GNARLY
GRRRLS
HOURLY
KNURLS
KNURLY
NEARLY
OVERLY
PEARLE
PEARLS
PEARLY
POORLY
SEARLE
SKIRLS
SNARLS
SNARLY
SOURLY
SWIRLS
SWIRLY
SWIRLZ
TWIRLS
TWIRLY
WHIRLS
WHIRLY
WHORLS
YEARLY

•••R•L
ABORAL
AMORAL
ANTRAL
ASTRAL
BARREL
CABRAL
CARREL
CARROL
CHERYL
CHORAL
CORRAL
CRURAL
DARRYL
DATRIL
EMERIL
FLORAL
HEDRAL
LAUREL
LAURYL
MITRAL
MORREL
NEURAL
NEUROL
PATROL
PETREL
PETROL
PLURAL
RETRAL
SHERYL
SORREL
SPIRAL
STEROL
UMBRAL
UNORAL

••••RL
ASWIRL
AWHIRL
GOGIRL
ITGIRL
MYGIRL
RECURL
UNCURL
UNFURL
UPCURL

R•M•••
RAMADA
RAMAPO
RAMATE
RAMBLE
RAMBOS
RAMEAU
RAMENS
RAMETS
RAMFAN
RAMFIS
RAMIES
RAMIFY
RAMJET
RAMMED
RAMMER
RAMONA
RAMONE
RAMOSE
RAMPAL
RAMPED
RAMPUP
RAMROD
RAMSAY
RAMSES
RAMSEY
RAMSIN
RAMSON
REMADE
REMAIL
REMAIN
REMAKE
REMAND
REMANS
REMAPS
REMARK
REMATE
REMATS
REMEDY
REMEET
REMELT
REMEND
REMICK
REMILL
REMIND
REMINE
REMINI
REMINT
REMISE
REMISS
REMITS
REMOLD
REMOPS
REMORA
REMOTE
REMOVE
REMOWN
REMOWS
REMSEN
RIMATE
RIMERS
RIMIER
RIMING
RIMINI
RIMMED
RIMOSE
RIMOUS
RIMPLE
RIMSKY
ROMAIC
ROMAIN
ROMAJI
ROMANI
ROMANO
ROMANS
ROMANY
ROMCOM
ROMEOS
ROMERO
ROMIJN
ROMMEL
ROMNEY
ROMOLA
ROMPED
ROMPER
ROMULO
RUMAKI
RUMBAS
RUMBLE
RUMBLY
RUMMER
RUMORS
RUMOUR
RUMPLE
RUMPLY
RUMPUS

R••M••
RAGMAN
RAGMEN
RAGMOP
RAMMED
RAMMER
RBIMAN
RBIMEN
REAMED
REAMER
REEMIT
RHAMES
RHEMES
RHOMBI
RHOMBS
RHUMBA
RHUMBS
RHYMED
RHYMER
RHYMES
RIMMED
ROAMED
ROAMER
ROAMIN
RODMAN
RODMEN
ROHMER
ROMMEL
RONMIX
ROOMBA
ROOMED
ROOMER
ROOMIE
RUDMAN
RUMMER

R•••M•
RACEME
RADOME
RCRUMB
README
REAIMS
REALMS
REARMS
RECOMB
REGIME
REHEMS
RELUME
RENAME
REPUMP
RESUME
RETAME
RETIME
REVAMP
RHEEMS
RHEIMS
RHEUMS
RHEUMY
RUNDMC

R••••M
RACISM
RADIUM
RANDOM
RANSOM
REDEEM
REDRUM
REFILM
REFORM
REGNUM
RESEAM
RESWAM
RESWIM
RETRIM
REWARM
RHYTHM
RODHAM
ROMCOM
ROSSUM

•RM•••
ARMADA
ARMAGH
ARMAND
ARMANI
ARMERS
ARMETS
ARMFUL
ARMIES
ARMING
ARMLET
ARMONK
ARMORS
ARMORY
ARMOUR
ARMPIT
ERMINE
MRMOTO
ORMOLU
ORMOND

•R•M••
ARAMES
ARAMID
ARAMIS
AROMAS
BRAMAH
BREMEN
BREMER
BRUMAL
BRUMEL
BRUMES

CRAMBO
CRAMER
CRAMIN
CRAMPS
CRAMPY
CREMER
CREMES
CRIMEA
CRIMES
CRIMPS
CRIMPY
CRUMBS
CRUMBY
CRUMMY
CRUMPS
DRAMAS
DROMIO
DRUMUP
DRYMOP
ERDMAN
FRAMED
FRAMER
FRAMES
FRUMPS
FRUMPY
GRAMME
GRAMMY
GRAMPA
GRAMPS
GRIMED
GRIMES
GRIMKE
GRIMLY
GRIMMS
GRIMMY
GROMIT
GRUMIO
GRUMPS
GRUMPY
KRAMER
OROMEO
PREMED
PREMET
PREMIE
PREMIX
PRIMAL
PRIMED
PRIMER
PRIMES
PRIMLY
PRIMOS
PRIMPS
PRIMUS
PROMOS
PROMPT
TRAMPS
TRAMPY
TREMOR
TRIMLY
TROMPE
TROMPS
TRUMAN
TRUMBO
TRUMPS

•R••M•

BRAHMA
BRAHMS
BREAMS
BROOMS
BROOMY
CREAMS
CREAMY
CRUMMY
DREAMS
DREAMT
DREAMY
GRAMME
GRAMMY
GRIMMS
GRIMMY
GROOMS
PREAMP
PRISMS
PRIZMS
PROAMS
PROEMS
TRAUMA
VROOMS

•R•••M

ARNHEM
ARTGUM
DRDOOM
ERBIUM
FRENUM
GRAHAM
PREARM
PRELIM
PRFIRM
PROTEM
TRUISM

••RM••

AIRMAN
AIRMEN
BARMAN
BARMEN
BERMAN
BERMED
BIRMAN
BORMAN
BURMAN
CARMAN
CARMEL
CARMEN
CORMAN
DERMAL
DERMAS
DERMAT
DERMIC
DERMIS
DERMOT
DORMER
DORMIE
FARMED
FARMER
FERMAT
FERMIS
FIRMED
FIRMER
FIRMLY
FIRMUP
FORMAL
FORMAN
FORMAT
FORMED
FORMER
FORMIC
FURMAN
GERMAN
GORMED
HARMED
HARMER
HARMON
HERMAN
HERMES
HERMIT
HERMON
HORMEL
HORMUZ
KARMAS
KARMIC
KERMIT
KIRMAN
KORMAN
LARMEN
LARMOR
MARMEE
MARMOT
MERMAN
MERMEN
MORMON
MURMUR
NERMAL
NORMAL
NORMAN
OARMAN
OARMEN
PERMED
PERMIT
SERMON
TARMAC
TERMED
TERMES
VARMUS
VERMIN
WARMED
WARMER
WARMLY
WARMTH
WARMTO
WARMUP
WORMED
WORMER

••R•M•

ABRAMS
AFRAME
BIREME
CAROMS
CDROMS
CHROMA
CHROME
CHROMO
CHROMY
DAREME
DIRAMS
DOREMI
DURUMS
FORUMS
HAREMS
JEREMY
JEROME
JORUMS
LARAMS
ONRAMP
PURIMS
RCRUMB
SCRAMS
SCRIMP
SCRIMS
SCRUMS
SERUMS
SHRIMP
STRUMS
SURIMI
THRUMS

••R••M

AIRARM
AIRDAM
ATRIUM
BARIUM
BARNUM
CERIUM
CHRISM
CIRCUM
CORFAM
CORIUM
CURIUM
DIRHAM
DORSUM
DURHAM
FARNUM
GORHAM
HARLEM
KAREEM
MARYAM
MIRIAM
NOROOM
PARFUM
PURISM
SCREAM
STREAM
SUREAM
TVROOM
VERISM

•••RM•

ALARMS
CHARMS
DEARME
DHARMA
ENARMS
ENORME
REARMS
SMARMY
STORMS
STORMY
SWARMS
THERMO
THERMS
UNARMS
USARMY

•••R•M

ALARUM
ANTRIM
ANTRUM
ASHRAM
BAYRUM
DIGRAM
ENGRAM
FOURAM
FOURPM
INGRAM
MEGRIM
QUORUM
REDRUM
RETRIM
SACRUM
SCARUM
THERAM
UNPRIM
VIBRAM

••••RM

AFFIRM
AIRARM
ASWARM
BEFIRM
BIFORM
BYFORM
DEFORM
DEGERM
DEWORM
DISARM
INFIRM
INFORM
LAPERM
ONEARM
PREARM
PRFIRM
REFORM
REWARM
SEAARM
SQUIRM
TOTERM
UNFIRM

RN••••

RNAASE

R•N•••

RANCHO
RANCID
RANCOR
RANDAL
RANDOM
RANDRY
RANEES
RANFOR
RANGED
RANGEL
RANGER
RANGES
RANGIN
RANGUP
RANIDS
RANINE
RANKED
RANKER
RANKIN
RANKLE
RANKLY
RANLOW
RANOFF
RANOUT
RANSOM
RANTAT
RANTED
RANTER
RENAIL
RENAME
RENARD
RENATA
RENATO
RENDED
RENDER
RENEGE
RENEST
RENEWS
RENFRO
RENGAS
RENINS
RENNES
RENNET
RENNIE
RENNIN
RENOIR
RENONV
RENOTE
RENOWN
RENTAL
RENTED
RENTEE
RENTER
RENTES
RENTON
RENTTO
RENVOI
RINGED
RINGER
RINGIN
RINGUP
RINSED
RINSER
RINSES
RONALD
RONCEY
RONDEL
RONDOS
RONELY
RONMIX
RONNIE
RONSON
RUNCIE
RUNDLE
RUNDMC
RUNDRY
RUNFOR
RUNGIN
RUNGUP
RUNINS
RUNLET
RUNLOW
RUNNEL
RUNNER
RUNOFF
RUNONS
RUNOUT
RUNSAT
RUNSBY
RUNSIN
RUNSON
RUNSTO
RUNSUP
RUNUPS
RUNWAY
RUNYON

R••N••

RADNER
RADNOR
RAGNAR
RAINED
RAINER
RAINES
RAINEY
RAININ
RAINON
RATNER
RAUNCH
REENIE
REGNAL
REGNAT
REGNUM
REINAS
REINED
REINER
REINES
REININ
REINKS
REKNIT
REKNOT
RENNES
RENNET
RENNIE
RENNIN
RESNAP
RESNIK
REUNED
REUNER
REUNES
RHINAL
RHINOS
RHONDA
RIENZI
RODNEY
ROMNEY
RONNIE
ROONEY
ROUNDS
RUANDA
RUDNER
RUINED
RUINER
RUNNEL
RUNNER
RWANDA
RYENCE

R•••N•

RACINE
RACING
RACINO
RAGING
RAKING
RAMENS
RAMONA
RAMONE
RANINE
RAPINE
RAPINI
RARING
RASING
RATINE
RATING
RAVENS
RAVINE
RAVING
RAXING
RAYING
RAYONS
RAZING
REBANK
REBEND
REBENT
REBIND
RECANE
RECANS
RECANT
RECENT
RECONS
REDANS
REDANT
REDENY
REDING
REDINK
REDONE
REFIND
REFINE
REFUND
REGENT
REGINA
REHANG
REHONE
REHUNG
REIGNS
RELAND
RELEND
RELENT
RELINE
RELINK
REMAND
REMANS
REMEND
REMIND
REMINE
REMINI
REMINT
RENINS
RENONV
REOWNS
REPANE
REPENS
REPENT
REPINE
REPINS
RERANK
RERENT
RERUNS
RESAND
RESANG
RESEND
RESENT
RESING
RESINK
RESINS
RESINY
RETANS
RETINA
RETINS
RETINT
RETONE
RETUNE
REVEND
REWIND
REWINS
REZONE
RIBAND
RICANS
RICING
RIDENT
RIDING
RIGANS
RILING
RIMING
RIMINI
RIPENS
RISING
RIVING
ROBING
ROBINS
ROCKNE
RODENT
RODINO
ROLAND
ROMANI
ROMANO
ROMANS
ROMANY
ROPING
ROSINA
ROSINS
ROSINY
ROTINI
ROTUND
ROVING
ROWANS
ROWENA
ROWENS
ROWING
ROXANA
ROXANE
RUBENS
RULING
RUNINS
RUNONS
RUTINS

R••••N

RACEIN
RADIAN
RAFFIN
RAGLAN
RAGMAN
RAGMEN
RAGSON
RAILON
RAININ
RAINON
RAISIN
RAISON
RAKEIN
RAMFAN
RAMSIN
RAMSON
RANGIN
RANKIN
RAPSON
RASKIN
RATION
RATLIN
RATSON
RATTAN
RAVEON
RAWDON
RAYBAN
RAYGUN
RBIMAN
RBIMEN
READIN
READON
REAGAN
REASON
REBORN
RECKON
RECOIN
REDARN
REDDEN
REDDIN
REDFIN
REDHEN
REDSUN
REDTEN
REEARN
REELIN
REGAIN
REGION
REININ
REJOIN
RELOAN
RELYON
REMAIN
REMOWN
REMSEN
RENNIN
RENOWN
RENTON
REOPEN
REPLAN
REPUGN
RESAWN
RESCAN
RESEEN
RESEWN
RESIGN
RESOWN
RESPAN
RESPIN
RESTON
RETAIN
RETORN
RETTON
RETURN
REUBEN
REVLON
REVSON
REWARN
REWORN
RIBBON
RICHEN
RICHIN
RIDDEN
RIDEIN
RIESEN
RIFKIN
RINGIN
RIOPAN
RIPKEN
RIPSON
ROAMIN
ROBSON
ROCHON
ROCKIN
RODEIN
RODION
RODMAN
RODMEN
ROLLIN
ROLLON
ROMAIN
ROMIJN
RONSON
ROOTIN
ROPEIN
ROSLYN
ROSSEN
ROSTEN
ROTTEN
RUBSIN
RUBSON
RUDKIN
RUDMAN
RULEON
RUNGIN
RUNSIN
RUNSON
RUNYON
RUSHIN
RUSKIN
RUTTAN
RUXPIN
RYOKAN

•RN•••

ARNALL
ARNEIS
ARNESS
ARNETT
ARNHEM
ARNICA
ARNIES
ARNOLD
ERNANI
ERNEST
ORNATE
ORNERY
ORNITH
URNFUL

•R•N••

ARENAS
ARENDT
BRANCA
BRANCH
BRANDI
BRANDO
BRANDS
BRANDT
BRANDX
BRANDY
BRANNY
BRANTS
BRENDA
BRENLY
BRINED
BRINER
BRINES
BRINGS
BRINKS
BRONCO
BRONCS
BRONKO
BRONTE
BRONZE
BRONZY
BRUNCH
BRUNEI
BRUNET
BRUNOR
BRUNTS
BRYNZA
CRANED
CRANES
CRANIA
CRANIO
CRANKS
CRANKY
CRANNY
CRENEL
CRENNA
CRINGE
CRONES
CRONIN
CRONUS
CRONYN
CRUNCH
DRANCY
DRENCH
DRINGS
DRINKS
DRONED
DRONER
DRONES
ERENOW
ERINNA
ERINYS
ERYNGO
FRANCA
FRANCE
FRANCK
FRANCO
FRANCS
FRANKS
FRANNY
FRANTZ
FRENCH
FRENUM
FRENZY
FRINGE
FRINGY
FRONDS
FRONTS
FRUNZE
GRANBY
GRANDE
GRANDS
GRANDY
GRANGE
GRANIT
GRANNY
GRANPA
GRANTS
GRINAT
GRINCH
GRINDL
GRINDS
GRINGO
GRUNDY
GRUNGE
GRUNGY
GRUNTS
IRANIS
IRENIC
IRONED
IRONER
IRONIC
IRONON
KRANTZ
KRENEK
KRONER
KRONOR
KRONUR
ORANGE
ORANGS
ORANGY
ORANIS
ORANTS
ORENSE
ORINGS
ORKNEY
PRANAS
PRANCE
PRANKS
PRENUP
PRINCE
PRINKS
PRINTS
PRINZE
PRONGS
PRONTO
PRUNED
PRUNER
PRUNES
PRYNNE
TRANCE
TRANES
TRANNY
TRENCH
TRENDS
TRENDY
TRENTA
TRENTE
TRENTO
TRINAL
TRINES
TRUNKS
URANIA
URANIC
URANUS
WRENCH
WRINGS
WRONGS

•R••N•

ARCANA
ARCANE
ARCING
ARDENT
ARGENT
ARIANA
ARIANE
ARJUNA
ARLENE
ARMAND
ARMANI
ARMING
ARMONK
AROINT
AROUND
ARRANT
ARSENE
ARSENO
ARSONS
ARYANS
BRAINS
BRAINY
BRANNY
BRAWNY
BRIANA
BRIAND
BRIENZ
BROWNE
BROWNS
BROWNU
BROWNY
BRUINS
BRYANT
CRAINS
CRANNY
CRENNA
CROONS
CROWNE
CROWNS
CRYING
DRAINS
DRJUNG
DRKING
DROWNS
DRYING
DRYINK
ERINNA
ERLANG
ERMINE
ERNANI
ERRAND
ERRANT
ERRING
ERVING
FRANNY
FREONS
FRESNO
FREUND
FRIEND
FROWNS
FRYING
GRAINS
GRAINY
GRANNY
GREENE
GREENS
GREENY
GRETNA
GROANS
GROINS
GROUND
GROZNY
GRUING
HRYVNA
IRKING
IRLENE
IRVINE
IRVING
KRASNA
KROONS
MRBOND
MRJINX
MRWONG
ORBING
ORGANA
ORGANS
ORIANA
ORIANI
ORIENT
ORIONS
ORKANS
ORLONS
ORMOND
ORSINI
ORSINO
PRAWNS
PREENS
PRYING
PRYNNE
TRAINS
TRANNY
TRIUNE
TROYNY
TRUANT
TRUING
TRYING
TRYONE
URBANA
URBANE
URBANI
URBANV
URGENT
URGING
URSINE

•R•••N

ARAGON
ARCHON
ARCSIN
ARCTAN
ARISEN
ARUBAN
BRAZEN
BREMEN
BRETON
BRITON
BROGAN
BROKEN
BROLIN
BRYSON
CRAMIN
CRAVEN
CRAYON
CRETAN
CRETIN
CRONIN
CRONYN
CROTON
CRUZAN
DRAGIN
DRAGON
DRAWIN

DRAWON
DREBIN
DREWIN
DREWON
DRIPON
DRIVEN
DRIVIN
DROPIN
DRYDEN
DRYRUN
ERDMAN
EREVAN
ERIVAN
FRAUEN
FROZEN
FRYPAN
GRATIN
GRAVEN
GREWON
GROBAN
GRODIN
GROTON
GROWON
IRISIN
IRONON
KRAKEN
KRYLON
MRBEAN
ORDAIN
OREGON
ORIGEN
ORIGIN
ORISON
ORPHAN
ORTHEN
PREVIN
PREYON
PRISON
PRODON
PROGUN
PROTON
PROVEN
TRAJAN
TRAVEN
TREPAN
TRIGON
TRIPON
TRITON
TRODON
TROJAN
TRUMAN
TRYLON
URCHIN
URGEON

••RN••
BARNED
BARNES
BARNET
BARNEY
BARNUM
BERNIE
BIRNEY
BORNEO
BURNED
BURNER
BURNET
BURNEY
BURNIE
BURNIN
BURNUP
BYRNES
CARNAC
CARNAL
CARNAP
CARNER
CARNES
CARNET
CARNEY
CERNAN
CORNEA
CORNED
CORNEL
CORNER
CORNET
CURNOW
DARNAY
DARNED
DARNER
DARNIT
DIRNDL
DURNED
DURNIT
EARNED
EARNER
EARNIE
EARNIT
FARNUM
FERNAO
FORNAX
FORNOW
GARNER
GARNET
GURNEE
GURNEY
HARNEY
HERNAN
HERNIA
HORNBY
HORNED
HORNER
HORNET
HORNIN
KARNAK
KERNED
KERNEL
KERNES
LERNER
MARNER
MARNIE
MORNAY
NARNIA
NERNST
PARNIS
PERNOD
SARNIA
TERNES
TORNUP
TURNED
TURNER
TURNIN
TURNIP
TURNON
TURNTO
TURNUP
VARNAS
VARNEY
VERNAL
VERNET
VERNON
WARNED
WARNER
WARNES
WARNOF
WERNER
YARNED

••R•N•
ADRENO
AIRING
APRONS
ARRANT
BARANY
BARING
BARONE
BARONI
BARONS
BARONY
BERING
BORING
BURANA
BURINS
CARINA
CARING
CARONI
CHRONO
CORING
CORONA
CURING
CYRANO
DARENT
DARING
DORINE
DURANT
DURING
EARING
EIRENE
ELRENO
ENRANK
ERRAND
ERRANT
ERRING
FARINA
FARING
FERENC
FIRING
FORINT
FORONE
GERENT
GERUND
GORING
GYRENE
GYRING
HARING
HERONS
HIRING
HURONS
INRUNS
KARINA
KORANS
KORUNA
LARINE
LARYNX
LFRANK
LORANS
LORENE
LORENZ
LORING
LURENE
LURING
MARINA
MARINE
MARINO
MERINO
MIRING
MIRINS
MORANT
MORENO
MORONI
MORONS
MURANO
MURINE
NARINE
NERONE
NORENT
NORUNS
OARING
PARANA
PARENS
PARENT
PARING
PARINI
PERINE
PIRANA
PORING
PURINA
RARING
RERANK
RERENT
RERUNS
SARANS
SARONG
SERENA
SERENE
SERINS
SHRANK
SHRINE
SHRINK
SHRUNK
SIRENS
SIRING
SPRANG
SPRING
SPRINT
SPRUNG
STRAND
STRING
STRONG
STRUNG
STRUNK
TARING
THRONE
THRONG
TIRANA
TIRANE
TIRING
TORENT
TORINO
TURING
TYRANT
TYRONE
UNRENT
UNRUNG
VERONA
WARING
WERENT
WIRING
ZORINA

••R••N
ADRIAN
ADRIEN
AIRGUN
AIRMAN
AIRMEN
ATRAIN
AYRTON
BARBAN
BARKIN
BARMAN
BARMEN
BARREN
BARRON
BARTON
BARYON
BARZUN
BERGEN
BERLIN
BERMAN
BERWYN
BIRMAN
BORDEN
BOREON
BORMAN
BURDEN
BURMAN
BURNIN
BURTON
CARBON
CARDIN
CAREEN
CARLIN
CARMAN
CARMEN
CARSON
CARTIN
CARTON
CERNAN
CORBIN
CORDON
CORMAN
CORWIN
CURLIN
CURTIN
CURZON
DARIEN
DARKEN
DARLIN
DARREN
DARRIN
DARWIN
DERAIN
DOREEN
DORIAN
DURBAN
DURBIN
EARVIN
FIREON
FIRKIN
FORFUN
FORMAN
FURMAN
GARCON
GARDEN
GARGAN
GARSON
GARYIN
GERMAN
GERVIN
GORDON
GORGON
GURION
HARBIN
HARDEN
HARDIN
HARKEN
HARLAN
HARLIN
HARMON
HARPON
HEREIN
HEREON
HERMAN
HERMON
HERNAN
HEROIN
HERREN
HIREON
HORGAN
HORNIN
HORTON
JARDIN
JARGON
JERKIN
JORDAN
KARLEN
KERWIN
KIRMAN
KOREAN
KORMAN
LARDON
LARKIN
LARMEN
LARSEN
LARSON
LORAIN
LUREIN
MARDEN
MARGIN
MARIAN
MARION
MARLIN
MARLON
MAROON
MARRON
MARTEN
MARTIN
MARVIN
MERLIN
MERMAN
MERMEN
MERTON
MERVYN
MIRREN
MOREEN
MORGAN
MORGEN
MORMON
MORTEN
MORTON
NORAIN
NOREEN
NORMAN
NORTON
OARMAN
OARMEN
OBRIAN
OBRIEN
PARDON
PARSON
PARTON
PERKIN
PERRIN
PERSON
SARGON
SARTON
SCREEN
SERKIN
SERMON
SIRBEN
SPRAIN
STRAIN
STREWN
SURFIN
SYRIAN
TARPON
TARTAN
TARZAN
TERRAN
THROWN
TURBAN
TUREEN
TURHAN
TURNIN
TURNON
TURPIN
VARDEN
VERDIN
VERDON
VERDUN
VEREEN
VEREIN
VERMIN
VERNON
VIRDON
VIRGIN
WARDEN
WARREN
WIREIN
WOREON
WORKIN
WORKON
WORSEN
YORKIN
ZEROIN
ZIRCON

•••RN•
ACORNS
ADORNS
AHERNE
AMARNA
BAIRNS
BOURNE
CAIRNS
CHURNS
CZERNY
EDIRNE
ETERNE
FOURNO
GIORNO
HEARNS
JOURNO
KEARNS
KEARNY
LEARNS
LEARNT
MOURNS
SCARNE
SCORNS
SMYRNA
SPURNS
STERNA
STERNE
STERNO
STERNS
THORNS
THORNY
UTURNS
YEARNS

•••R•N
ALDRIN
ALGREN
ANTRON
AZORIN
BARREN
BARRON
BEARON
CAMRYN
CHARON
CHIRON
CHYRON
CITRIN
CITRON
DACRON
DARREN
DARRIN
DOGRUN
DRYRUN
EGUREN
ENDRAN
ENDRUN
EPHRON
FIBRIN
FLORIN
FUNRUN
GIBRAN
HADRON
HEBRON
HEDREN
HEDRON
HERREN
ICERUN
KATRIN
KIERAN
KIERON
KUPRIN
LAUREN
LAURYN
LEBRON
LEBRUN
LIBRAN
MACRON
MARRON
MATRON
MAYRON
MICRON
MIRREN
MOTRIN
NATRON
NEURON
NOIRON
NONRUN
OBERON
ONERUN
OUTRAN
OUTRUN
PATRON
PEERIN
PERRIN
POURIN
SAURON
SHARON
SHARYN
SKIRUN
SOURON
SPURON
STARIN
STIRIN
STYRON
TEGRIN
TEHRAN
TERRAN
THERON
THORON
VANRYN
WARREN
WEARON

••••RN
ASTERN
AUBURN
BAYERN
BICORN
CASERN
CAVERN
CEDARN
COBURN
DEHORN
EXTERN
GOVERN
INBORN
INTERN
INTURN
LAVERN
MCKERN
MODERN
MYTURN
OHDARN
OSBORN
REBORN
REDARN
REEARN
RETORN
RETURN
REWARN
REWORN
SATURN
SEVERN
SUBORN
TAVERN
TEAURN
TOBURN
UNBORN
UNTORN
UNWORN
UPTORN
UPTURN
WEBERN
WOBURN
WYVERN

RO••••
ROADEO
ROADER
ROADIE
ROAMED
ROAMER
ROAMIN
ROARAT
ROARED
ROARER
ROASTS
ROBBED
ROBBER
ROBBIA
ROBBIE
ROBERS
ROBERT
ROBING
ROBINS
ROBLES
ROBOTS
ROBROY
ROBSOF
ROBSON
ROBUST
ROCHAT
ROCHET
ROCHON
ROCKED
ROCKER
ROCKET
ROCKIE
ROCKIN
ROCKIT
ROCKNE
ROCKYV
ROCOCO
RODALE
RODDED
RODDER
RODEBY
RODEIN
RODENT
RODEOS
RODETO
RODEUP
RODHAM
RODINO
RODION
RODMAN
RODMEN
RODNEY
ROEPER
ROGERE
ROGERS
ROGETS
ROGUED
ROGUES
ROHMER
ROHRER
ROILED
ROILUP
ROLAND
ROLEOS
ROLFED
ROLFER
ROLLBY
ROLLED
ROLLEI
ROLLER
ROLLIE
ROLLIN
ROLLON
ROLLUP
ROMAIC
ROMAIN
ROMAJI
ROMANI
ROMANO
ROMANS
ROMANY
ROMCOM
ROMEOS
ROMERO
ROMIJN
ROMMEL
ROMNEY
ROMOLA
ROMPED
ROMPER
ROMULO
RONALD
RONCEY
RONDEL
RONDOS
RONELY
RONMIX
RONNIE
RONSON
ROOFED
ROOFER
ROOKED
ROOKER
ROOKIE
ROOMBA
ROOMED
ROOMER
ROOMIE
ROONEY
ROOSTS
ROOTED
ROOTER
ROOTIE
ROOTIN
ROOTLE
ROOTSY
ROOTUP
ROPEIN
ROPERS
ROPERY
ROPEUP
ROPIER
ROPING
ROSARY
ROSCOE
ROSEAU
ROSERY
ROSETO
ROSEUP
ROSHIS
ROSIER
ROSIES
ROSILY
ROSINA
ROSINS
ROSINY
ROSITA
ROSLYN
ROSSEN
ROSSET
ROSSUM
ROSTEN
ROSTER
ROSTOV
ROSTRA
ROTARY
ROTATE
ROTGUT
ROTHKO
ROTINI
ROTORS
ROTTED
ROTTEN
ROTTER
ROTUND
ROUGED
ROUGES
ROUGHS
ROUNDS
ROURKE
ROUSED
ROUSER
ROUSES
ROUSTS
ROUTED
ROUTER
ROUTES
ROVERS
ROVING
ROWANS
ROWELS
ROWENA
ROWENS
ROWERS
ROWING
ROWLEY
ROXANA
ROXANE
ROYALE
ROYALS
ROYCES

R•O•••
REOILS
REOPEN
REOWNS
RHODES
RHOMBI
RHOMBS
RHONDA
RIOJAS
RIOPAN
RIOTED
RIOTER
ROOFED
ROOFER
ROOKED
ROOKER
ROOKIE
ROOMBA
ROOMED
ROOMER
ROOMIE
ROONEY
ROOSTS
ROOTED
ROOTER
ROOTIE
ROOTIN
ROOTLE
ROOTSY
ROOTUP
RYOKAN

R••O••
RADOME
RAGOUT
RAMONA
RAMONE
RAMOSE
RANOFF
RANOUT
RATOFF
RATOUT
RAYONS
RAZORS
RCCOLA
REBOIL
REBOLT
REBOOK
REBOOT
REBOPS
REBORE
REBORN
REBOTE
REBOZO
RECOAL
RECOAT
RECOCK
RECODE
RECOIL
RECOIN
RECOMB
RECONS
RECOOK
RECOOL
RECOPY
RECORD
RECORK
RECOST
RECOUP
REDOAK
REDOCK
REDOER
REDOES
REDONE
REDOSE
REDOUT
REFOLD
REFORM
REHOED
REHOES
REHOLD
REHONE
REHOOK
REJOIN
RELOAD
RELOAN
RELOCK
RELOGS
RELOOK
RELOSE
RELOST
REMOLD
REMOPS
REMORA
REMOTE
REMOVE
REMOWN
REMOWS
RENOIR
RENONV
RENOTE
RENOWN
REPOLL
REPORT
REPOSE
REPOST
REPOTS
REPOUR
RERODE
REROLL
REROOF
REROOT
REROSE
RESOAK
RESOAP
RESODS
RESOIL
RESOLD
RESOLE
RESORB
RESORT
RESOWN
RESOWS
RETOLD
RETONE
RETOOK
RETOOL
RETOPS
RETORE
RETORN
RETORT
RETOSS
RETOUR
RETOWS
REVOIR
REVOKE
REVOLT
REVOTE
REWOKE
REWORD
REWORE
REWORK
REWORN
REWOVE
REYOKE
REZONE
RIBOSE
RICOHS
RICOLA
RIGORS
RIGOUR
RIGOUT
RIMOSE
RIMOUS
RIPOFF
RIPOST
RIPOUT
RIVOLI
ROBOTS
ROCOCO
ROMOLA
ROTORS
RUBOFF
RUBOUT
RUDOLF
RUFOUS
RUMORS
RUMOUR
RUNOFF
RUNONS
RUNOUT

R•••O•
RADIOS
RADNOR
RAGMOP
RAGSON
RAGTOP
RAILON
RAINON
RAISON
RAMBOS
RAMROD
RAMSON
RANCOR
RANDOM
RANFOR
RANLOW
RANSOM
RAPSON
RAPTOR
RATION
RATIOS
RATSON
RAVEON
RAWDON
READON
REASON
REAVOW
REBOOK
REBOOT
RECKON
RECOOK
RECOOL
RECTOR
RECTOS
REDCOD
REDDOG
REDDOT
REDFOX
REDHOT
REDSOX
REDTOP
REEBOK
REEKOF

REFLOW
REGION
REGLOW
REGROW
REHOOK
REKNOT
RELOOK
RELYON
RENTON
RENVOI
REPFOR
REPLOT
REPLOW
REPROS
REROOF
REROOT
RESHOD
RESHOE
RESHOT
RESHOW
RESPOT
RESTON
RESTOW
RETOOK
RETOOL
RETROD
RETROS
RETTON
REVLON
REVSON
RHEBOK
RHETOR
RHINOS
RIBBON
RIDSOF
RIPSON
RITSOS
ROBROY
ROBSOF
ROBSON
ROCHON
RODEOS
RODION
ROLEOS
ROLLON
ROMCOM
ROMEOS
RONDOS
RONSON
ROSCOE
ROSTOV
RUBSON
RULEON
RUNFOR
RUNLOW
RUNSON
RUNYON

R••••O

RACETO
RACINO
RAMAPO
RANCHO
RAPIDO
READTO
REBOZO
REDTWO
REECHO
RENATO
RENFRO
RENTTO
REZERO
RIALTO
RIDETO
RIGHTO
RISETO
ROADEO
ROCOCO
RODETO
RODINO
ROMANO
ROMERO
ROMULO
ROSETO
ROTHKO
RUBATO
RUNSTO
RUSHTO

•RO•••

AROIDS
AROINT
AROMAS
AROUET
AROUND
AROUSE
BROACH
BROADA
BROAST
BROCAS
BRODIE
BROGAN
BROGUE
BROILS
BROKAW
BROKEN
BROKER
BROLIN
BROLLY
BRONCO
BRONCS
BRONKO
BRONTE
BRONZE
BRONZY
BROOCH
BROODS
BROODY
BROOKE
BROOKS
BROOKY
BROOMS
BROOMY
BROPHY
BROSSE
BROTHS
BROTHY
BROUGH
BROVIK
BROWED
BROWNE
BROWNS
BROWNU
BROWNY
BROWSE
CROAKS
CROAKY
CROATS
CROCKS
CROCUS
CROFTS
CROIRE
CRONES
CRONIN
CRONUS
CRONYN
CROOKS
CROONS
CROPUP
CRORES
CROSBY
CROSSE
CROTCH
CROTON
CROUCH
CROUPS
CROUPY
CROUSE
CROUTE
CROWDS
CROWED
CROWER
CROWNE
CROWNS
DROGUE
DROIDS
DROITS
DROLLS
DROLLY
DROMIO
DRONED
DRONER
DRONES
DROOLS
DROOLY
DROOPS
DROOPY
DROPBY
DROPIN
DROPIT
DROPSY
DROSSY
DROUET
DROVER
DROVES
DROWNS
DROWSE
DROWSY
DROXIE
ERODED
ERODER
ERODES
EROICA
EROTIC
FROCKS
FROGGY
FROLIC
FRONDS
FRONTS
FROSTS
FROSTY
FROTHS
FROTHY
FROWNS
FROWZY
FROYOS
FROZEN
GROANS
GROATS
GROBAN
GROCER
GRODIN
GROGGY
GROINS
GROMIT
GROOMS
GROOVE
GROOVY
GROPED
GROPER
GROPES
GROSSE
GROSSO
GROSZY
GROTON
GROTTO
GROTTY
GROUCH
GROUND
GROUPS
GROUSE
GROUTS
GROUTY
GROVED
GROVEL
GROVER
GROVES
GROWER
GROWLS
GROWLY
GROWON
GROWTH
GROWUP
GROZNY
IROBOT
IRONED
IRONER
IRONIC
IRONON
KROFFT
KROGER
KRONER
KRONOR
KRONUR
KROONS
OROMEO
OROSCO
OROZCO
PROAMS
PROART
PROBED
PROBER
PROBES
PROBIE
PROBST
PROCOL
PRODON
PROEMS
PROFIT
PROGUN
PROJET
PROLES
PROLIX
PROLOG
PROMOS
PROMPT
PRONGS
PRONTO
PROOFS
PROPEL
PROPER
PROPRE
PROPUP
PROPYL
PROSED
PROSER
PROSES
PROSIT
PROSKY
PROTAX
PROTEA
PROTEM
PROTON
PROULX
PROUST
PROVED
PROVEN
PROVER
PROVES
PROWAR
PROWLS
PROWSE
PROYAS
PROZAC
TROCHE
TRODON
TROGGS
TROIKA
TROJAN
TROLLS
TROMPE
TROMPS
TROOPS
TROPES
TROPEZ
TROPHY
TROPIC
TROPPO
TROTHS
TROTUP
TROUGH
TROUPE
TROUTS
TROVES
TROWED
TROWEL
TROYER
TROYNY
VROOMS
WRONGS

•R•O••

ARBORS
ARBOUR
ARDORS
ARDOUR
AREOLA
AREOLE
ARGOSY
ARGOTS
ARIOSE
ARIOSI
ARIOSO
ARLOVA
ARMONK
ARMORS
ARMORY
ARMOUR
ARNOLD
ARROWS
ARROYO
ARSONS
ARTOIS
BROOCH
BROODS
BROODY
BROOKE
BROOKS
BROOKY
BROOMS
BROOMY
CREOLE
CROOKS
CROONS
CRUORS
CRYOFF
CRYOUT
DRDOOM
DRHOOK
DRKOOP
DROOLS
DROOLY
DROOPS
DROOPY
DRYOFF
DRYOUT
ERGOTS
ERROLL
ERRORS
FREONS
GRIOTS
GROOMS
GROOVE
GROOVY
KROONS
MRBOND
MRCOOL
MRMOTO
MRWONG
OREOOS
ORIOLE
ORIONS
ORLONS
ORLOPS
ORMOLU
ORMOND
PREOPS
PRIORI
PRIORS
PRIORY
PROOFS
PRYOFF
TRIODE
TROOPS
TRYONE
TRYOUT
VROOMS

•R••O•

ARADOS
ARAGON
ARCCOS
ARCHON
ARETOO
BRASOV
BRAVOS
BRAZOS
BRETON
BRITON
BRUNOR
BRYSON
CRACOW
CRAYON
CREDOS
CRESOL
CROTON
CRUSOE
CRYFOR
DRAGON
DRAWON
DRDOOM
DREWON
DRHOOK
DRIPON
DRKOOP
DRYFOG
DRYMOP
DRYROT
ERENOW
FREEOF
FRIJOL
FRITOS
FRIVOL
FROYOS
GREGOR
GREWON
GROTON
GROWON
IROBOT
IRONON
KRAKOW
KRONOR
KRYLON
KRYLOV
MRCOOL
ORATOR
OREGON
OREOOS
ORISON
PRELOG
PRETOR
PREYON
PRIMOS
PRISON
PROCOL
PRODON
PROLOG
PROMOS
PROTON
TREMOR
TREVOR
TRICOT
TRIGON
TRIPOD
TRIPON
TRITON
TRODON
TRYFOR
TRYLON
URGEON

•R•••O

ARCARO
ARETOO
AREZZO
ARIOSO
ARISTO
ARROYO
ARSENO
ARTHRO
ARTURO
BRACCO
BRANDO
BRASCO
BRILLO
BRONCO
BRONKO
CRAMBO
CRANIO
CREEPO
CRISCO
CRISTO
CRYPTO
DRAWTO
DREWTO
DROMIO
ERYNGO
FRACTO
FRANCO
FREDRO
FREETO
FRESCO
FRESNO
FRISCO
FRITTO
GRAECO
GRAPHO
GRASSO
GRIECO
GRINGO
GROSSO
GROTTO
GRUMIO
KRYPTO
MRMOTO
OROMEO
OROSCO
OROZCO
ORSINO
PRAYTO
PRESTO
PRONTO
QRATIO
TRENTO
TRILLO
TROPPO
TRUETO
TRUMBO

••RO••

ABROAD
ACROSS
ADROIT
AEROBE
AIROUT
APRONS
ARROWS
ARROYO
ATROIS
AURORA
AUROUS
BAROJA
BAROLO
BARONE
BARONI
BARONS
BARONY
BUROAK
BYROAD
BYROTE
CAROBS
CAROLE
CAROLI
CAROLL
CAROLS
CAROMS
CARONI
CDROMS
CHROMA
CHROME
CHROMO
CHROMY
CHRONO
CORONA
COROTS
DEROSE
DUROCS
ENROBE
ENROLL
ENROLS
ENROOT
ERROLL
ERRORS
EUROPA
EUROPE
FAROES
FAROFF
FAROUK
FAROUT
FEROUS
FORONE
FTROOP
FURORE
FURORS
HAROLD
HEROES
HEROIC
HEROIN
HERONS
HURONS
INROAD
JEROME
JURORS
LAROSA
LEROUX
MAROON
MEROPE
MEROPS
MOROLT
MORONI
MORONS
MOROSE
MOROSS
NEROLI
NERONE
NOROOM
PARODY
PAROLE
PAROLS
POROSE
POROUS
RERODE
REROLL
REROOF
REROOT
REROSE
SARONG
SCRODS
SCROLL
SEROUS
SHROUD
SHROVE
SPROUT
STROBE
STRODE
STROHS
STROKE
STROLL
STRONG
STROPS
STROUD
STROVE
TAROIL
TAROTS
THROAT
THROBS
THROES
THRONE
THRONG
THROVE
THROWN
THROWS
TOROID
TVROOM
TYRONE
UNROBE
UNROLL
UNROOF
UNROOT
UNROPE
UNROVE
UPROAR
UPROOT
UPROSE
VERONA
VOROUS
ZEROED
ZEROES
ZEROIN

••R•O•

AERIOS
AIRLOG
AIRPOP
AIRPOT
AYRTON
BARCOS
BARDOT
BARHOP
BARLOW
BARRON
BARROW
BARTOK
BARTON
BARYON
BERKOW
BOREON
BORROW
BORZOI
BURBOT
BURGOO
BURGOS
BURROS
BURROW
BURTON
CARBON
CARBOS
CARBOY
CAREOF
CARGOS
CARHOP
CARIOU
CARLOS
CARLOT
CARLOW
CARROL
CARROT
CARSON
CARTON
CARTOP
CERROS
CORDON
CORTOT
CURIOS
CURNOW
CURSOR
CURZON
DARROW
DERMOT
ENROOT
FARLOW
FARROW
FERVOR
FIREON
FORGOT
FORJOY
FORNOW
FORYOU
FTROOP
FURROW
GARCON
GARSON
GORDON
GORGON
GORIOT
GURION
HARBOR
HARLOT
HARLOW
HARMON
HARPON
HARROW
HEREOF
HEREON
HERMON
HERZOG
HIREON
HORROR
HORTON
JARGON
JERBOA
KARKOV
KARPOV
LARDON
LARGOS
LARMOR
LARSON
MARCOS
MARGOT
MARION
MARJOE
MARKOV
MARLON
MARMOT
MAROON
MARRON
MARROW
MERLOT
MERTON
MIRROR
MIRROS
MORMON
MORROW
MORTON
MURROW
NARCOS
NARROW
NORDOI
NOROOM
NORTON
PARDON
PARLOR
PARROT
PARSON
PARTOF
PARTON
PERIOD
PERNOD
PERROS
PERSON
REROOF
REROOT
SARDOU
SARGON
SARTON
SARTOR
SERMON
SERVOS
SORROW
SORTOF
SUREOF
TARPON
TERROR
TIREOF
TORPOR
TORSOS
TURBOS
TURBOT
TURNON
TVROOM
UNROOF
UNROOT
UPROOT
VERDON
VERNON
VERSOS
VIRDON
VIREOS
VIRGOS
WARGOD
WARHOL
WARNOF
WOREON
WORKON
YARROW
ZARKOV
ZIRCON

••R••O

ADRENO
ARROYO
BARATO
BAROLO
BARRIO
BERCEO
BORAXO
BORNEO
BURGOO
CARDIO
CARETO
CARUSO
CERATO
CHROMO
CHRONO
CORREO
CYRANO
DARETO
DIRIGO
DORADO
DORITO
ELRENO
ENRICO
FERNAO
FOREGO
HARRYO
HERETO
JURADO
LAREDO
MARIDO
MARIKO
MARINO
MARYJO
MERINO
MORENO
MORESO
MORPHO
MURANO
PARETO
PYRHHO
SERGIO
STRATO
SUREDO
TERATO
TORERO
TORINO
TURNTO
VIRAGO
WARMTO

•••RO•

AGOROT
ALEROS
ANDROS
ANTRON
APPROX
ASTROS
ASTROV
ATHROB
ATHROW
BARRON
BARROW
BEARON
BORROW
BURROS
BURROW
CARROL
CARROT
CERROS
CHARON
CHIRON
CHOROS
CHYRON
CITRON
CLAROS
CLOROX
CONROY
DACRON
DARROW
DELROY
DETROP
DOBROS
DRYROT
ENEROS
EPHRON
ESCROW
FAEROE
FARROW
FIEROS
FLYROD
FURROW
GILROY
HADRON
HARROW
HEAROF
HEBRON
HEDRON
HORROR
HOTROD
HYDROS
HYDROX
IGOROT
IMPROV
INAROW
INTROS
KIERON
KILROY
KUDROW
LEBRON
LEGROS
LIBROS
MACRON
MACROS
MARRON
MARROW
MATRON
MAYRON
METROS
MICRON
MICROS
MIRROR
MIRROS
MONROE
MORROW
MUNROE
MURROW
NARROW
NATRON
NEUROL
NEURON
NIMROD
NITROS
NOIRON
NOPROB
OBERON
OCTROI
OUTROW
PARROT
PATROL
PATRON
PENROD
PERROS
PETROL
PHAROS
PITROW
POIROT
RAMROD
REGROW
REPROS
RETROD
RETROS
ROBROY
SAURON
SHARON
SORROW
SOURON
SPURON
STEROL
STYRON
TAUROG
TERROR
THEROD
THERON
THORON
TIEROD
TOPROW
UBUROI
UNTROD
UPGROW
UPPROP
WEARON
YARROW

•••R•O

ASARCO
BARRIO
CABRIO
CHARRO
CHIRHO
CHOREO
CHORIO
CHURRO
CORREO
DEARTO
DELRIO
DIARIO
EMBRYO
EVERSO
FLORIO
FOURNO
GEARTO

GIORNO
HAIRDO
HARRYO
JOURNO
KIARIO
NEARTO
OBERTO
OPORTO
OVERDO
PUERTO
QUARTO
SBARRO
SHORTO
STEREO
STERNO
THERMO
WEIRDO

••••RO

AILURO
ALLPRO
ALVARO
ANTERO
ARCARO
ARTHRO
ARTURO
ASTERO
AUSTRO
BISTRO
BOLERO
CAMARO
CASTRO
CENTRO
CHARRO
CHLORO
CHURRO
CICERO
COMORO
CUATRO
DENDRO
DENIRO
DEXTRO
DINERO
DISTRO
ELTORO
ENDURO
ENTERO
ENVIRO
FIGARO
FLUORO
FREDRO
GABBRO
GASTRO
HASBRO
HETERO
ICHIRO
ISIDRO
JETHRO
KAKURO
LATERO
LLADRO
MADERO
MADURO
MANERO
MYHERO
NEPHRO
NIEKRO
NONPRO
NUMERO
OLDPRO
ONEIRO
PGAPRO
PICARO
PIETRO
PINERO
RENFRO
REZERO
ROMERO
SANDRO
SBARRO
TEATRO
TORERO
UNHERO
VALERO
VELCRO
YSIDRO

R•P•••

RAPIDO
RAPIDS
RAPIER
RAPINE
RAPINI
RAPPED
RAPPEL
RAPPER
RAPSON
RAPTER
RAPTLY
RAPTOR
RAPTUS
REPACK
REPADS
REPAGE
REPAID
REPAIR
REPANE
REPARK
REPASS
REPAST
REPAVE
REPAYS
REPEAL
REPEAT
REPEGS
REPELS
REPENS
REPENT
REPERK
REPFOR
REPICK
REPINE
REPINS
REPLAN
REPLAY
REPLED
REPLOT
REPLOW
REPOLL
REPORT
REPOSE
REPOST
REPOTS
REPOUR
REPPED
REPROS
REPUBS
REPUGN
REPUMP
REPUTE
RIPELY
RIPENS
RIPEST
RIPKEN
RIPLEY
RIPOFF
RIPOST
RIPOUT
RIPPED
RIPPER
RIPPLE
RIPPLY
RIPRAP
RIPSAW
RIPSON
RIPSUP
ROPEIN
ROPERS
ROPERY
ROPEUP
ROPIER
ROPING
RUPEES
RUPERT
RUPIAH
RVPARK

R••P••

RAIPUR
RALPHJ
RAMPAL
RAMPED
RAMPUP
RAPPED
RAPPEL
RAPPER
RASPAS
RASPED
RASPER
REAPED
REAPER
REOPEN
REPPED
RESPAN
RESPIN
RESPOT
RIBPAD
RIMPLE
RIOPAN
RIPPED
RIPPER
RIPPLE
RIPPLY
ROEPER
ROMPED
ROMPER
RSVPED
RUMPLE
RUMPLY
RUMPUS
RUXPIN

R•••P•

RAMAPO
REBOPS
RECAPS
RECIPE
RECOPY
REDIPS
RELAPS
REMAPS
REMOPS
RETAPE
RETAPS
RETIPS
RETOPS
RETYPE
REWIPE
REZIPS
RUNUPS

R••••P

RACEUP
RACKUP
RAGMOP
RAGTOP
RAKEUP
RAMPUP
RANGUP
RAVEUP
READUP
REARUP
RECOUP
REDCAP
REDTOP
REELUP
REGRIP
RELEAP
REPUMP
RESHIP
RESNAP
RESOAP
RESTUP
RETRAP
REVAMP
REVSUP
REWRAP
RIDEUP
RIGSUP
RILEUP
RINGUP
RIPRAP
RIPSUP
RISEUP
RODEUP
ROILUP
ROLLUP
ROOTUP
ROPEUP
ROSEUP
RUBSUP
RUCKUP
RUNGUP
RUNSUP

•RP•••

ARPEGE
ARPELS
DRPHIL
MRPAWS
MRPIBB
ORPHAN
ORPHIC

•R•P••

ARMPIT
BROPHY
CRAPED
CRAPES
CREPED
CREPES
CRIPES
CROPUP
CRYPTO
CRYPTS
DRAPED
DRAPER
DRAPES
DRIPON
DRIPPY
DROPBY
DROPIN
DROPIT
DROPSY
DRUPES
ERUPTS
FRAPPE
FRYPAN
GRAPES
GRAPEY
GRAPHO
GRAPHS
GRAPHY
GRAPPA
GRIPED
GRIPER
GRIPES
GRIPPE
GRIPPY
GROPED
GROPER
GROPES
KRYPTO
PREPAY
PREPPY
PROPEL
PROPER
PROPRE
PROPUP
PROPYL
TRAPPY
TREPAN
TREPID
TRIPES
TRIPLE
TRIPLY
TRIPOD
TRIPON
TRIPUP
TROPES
TROPEZ
TROPHY
TROPIC
TROPPO
WRAPUP

•R••P•

CRAMPS
CRAMPY
CREEPO
CREEPS
CREEPY
CRIMPS
CRIMPY
CRISPS
CRISPY
CROUPS
CROUPY
CRUMPS
DRIPPY
DROOPS
DROOPY
ERIEPA
FRAPPE
FRUMPS
FRUMPY
GRAMPA
GRAMPS
GRANPA
GRAPPA
GRASPS
GRIPPE
GRIPPY
GROUPS
GRUMPS
GRUMPY
IRRUPT
KRISPY
ORLOPS
PREOPS
PREPPY
PRIMPS
PROMPT
TRAMPS
TRAMPY
TRAPPY
TROMPE
TROMPS
TROOPS
TROPPO
TROUPE
TRUMPS

•R•••P

BREWUP
CROPUP
CRUDUP
DRAGUP
DRAWUP
DREWUP
DRKOOP
DRUMUP
DRYMOP
FREEUP
GREWUP
GROWUP
PREAMP
PRECIP
PRENUP
PROPUP
TRICEP
TRIPUP
TROTUP
TRUEUP
WRAPUP

••RP••

AIRPOP
AIRPOT
BURPED
BURPEE
CARPAL
CARPAT
CARPED
CARPEL
CARPER
CARPET
CARPUS
CORPSE
CORPUS
HARPED
HARPER
HARPON
HERPET
KARPOV
MARPLE
MORPHO
MORPHS
MURPHY
PURPLE
PURPLY
TARPIT
TARPON
TORPID
TORPOR
TURPIN
VORPAL
WARPED
WARPER

••R•P•

ABRUPT
ADREPS
ENRAPT
EUROPA
EUROPE
IRRUPT
MEROPE
MEROPS
PARAPH
PTRAPS
SCRAPE
SCRAPS
SCRIPS
SCRIPT
SERAPE
SERAPH
SIRUPS
STRAPS
STREPS
STRIPE
STRIPS
STRIPY
STROPS
SYRUPS
SYRUPY
UNRIPE
UNRIPS
UNROPE
YORKPA

••R••P

AIRPOP
AIRSUP
BARHOP
BOREUP
BURLAP
BURNUP
CARHOP
CARNAP
CARTOP
CORKUP
CURLUP
EARLAP
FIREUP
FIRMUP
FORKUP
FTROOP
HARDUP
JERKUP
LARRUP
MARKUP
ONRAMP
PERKUP
PIRRIP
SCRIMP
SHRIMP
STREEP
TARTUP
TOREUP
TORNUP
TURNIP
TURNUP
WARMUP
WIREUP
WORKUP

•••RP•

CHIRPS
CHIRPY
FOURPM
SCARPS
SHARPE
SHARPS
SHARPY
SHERPA
SLURPS
THORPE
TWERPS
TWIRPS
USURPS

•••R•P

BADRAP
BEARUP
BUMRAP
DETROP
DOMREP
ENTRAP
ENWRAP
FAIRUP
FOURUP
GEARUP
LARRUP
LETRIP
OUTRAP
PAIRUP
PIRRIP
REARUP
REGRIP
RETRAP
REWRAP
RIPRAP
SATRAP
STIRUP
TEARUP
THERAP
TSTRAP
UNGRIP
UNTRAP
UNWRAP
UPPROP

••••RP

ASHARP
BSHARP
CSHARP
DSHARP
ESCARP
ESHARP
FSHARP
GSHARP
TSGARP

R•Q•••

RAQUEL

R••Q••

RISQUE

•R•Q••

BRAQUE
DRIQJR
IRAQIS

••RQ••

BARQUE
CIRQUE
MARQUE
TORQUE

RR••••

RRATED

R•R•••

RAREES
RAREFY
RARELY
RAREST
RARING
RARITY
RCRUMB
RERACK
RERAKE
RERANK
RERATE
REREAD
REREEL
RERENT
RERIDE
RERIGS
RERISE
RERODE
REROLL
REROOF
REROOT
REROSE
RERUNS

R••R••

RAGRUG
RAHRAH
RAMROD
REARED
REARER
REARMS
REARUP
REBRED
REBREW
REDRAG
REDRAW
REDREW
REDRUM
REGRAB
REGRET
REGREW
REGRIP
REGROW
REPROS
RETRAL
RETRAP
RETRIM
RETROD
RETROS
REURGE
REWRAP
RICRAC
RIPRAP
ROARAT
ROARED
ROARER
ROBROY
ROHRER
ROURKE
RUBRAW
RUBRIC
RUGRAT

R•••R•

RACERS
RADARS
RAGERS
RAKERS
RANDRY
RASERS
RASURE
RATERS
RAVERS
RAZERS
RAZORS
REAIRS
REBARS
REBORE
REBORN
REBURY
RECORD
RECORK
RECURE
RECURL
RECURS
REDARE
REDARN
REEARN
REFERS
REFIRE
REFORM
REGARD
REGIRD
REHIRE
REMARK
REMORA
RENARD
RENFRO
REPARK
REPERK
REPORT
RESORB
RESORT
RETARD
RETARS
RETIRE
RETORE
RETORN
RETORT
RETURF
RETURN
REVERB
REVERE
REVERS
REVERT
REWARD
REWARM
REWARN
REWIRE
REWORD
REWORE
REWORK
REWORN
REZERO
RIBERA
RICERS
RIDERS
RIGORS
RIKERS
RILERS
RIMERS
RISERS
RITARD
RIVERA
RIVERS
ROBERS
ROBERT
ROGERE
ROGERS
ROMERO
ROPERS
ROPERY
ROSARY
ROSERY
ROSTRA
ROTARY
ROTORS
ROVERS
ROWERS
RUDERY
RULERS
RUMORS
RUNDRY
RUPERT
RVPARK

R••••R

RACIER
RACKER
RADNER
RADNOR
RAFTER
RAGNAR
RAIDER
RAILER
RAINER
RAIPUR
RAISER
RAMMER
RANCOR
RANFOR
RANGER
RANKER
RANTER
RAPIER
RAPPER
RAPTER
RAPTOR
RASHER
RASPER
RASTER
RATEDR
RATHER
RATNER
RATTER
RAWBAR
READER
REALER
REAMER
REAPER
REARER
REAVER
RECTOR
REDDER
REDFIR
REDOER
REEDER
REEFER
REEKER
REELER
REGEAR
REHEAR
REIGER
REINER
REISER
REITER
RELIER
RENDER
RENOIR
RENTER
REPAIR
REPFOR
REPOUR
RESTER
RESTIR
RETEAR
RETOUR
REUNER
REUSER
REUTER
REVOIR
REWEAR
RHETOR
RHYMER
RIBBER
RICHER
RIDDER
RIFLER
RIGGER
RIGOUR
RIMIER
RINGER
RINSER
RIOTER
RIPPER
RISKER
RITTER
ROADER
ROAMER
ROARER
ROBBER
ROCKER
RODDER
ROEPER
ROHMER
ROHRER
ROLFER
ROLLER
ROMPER
ROOFER
ROOKER
ROOMER
ROOTER
ROPIER
ROSIER
ROSTER
ROTTER
ROUSER
ROUTER
RUBBER
RUCKER
RUDDER
RUDNER
RUINER
RULIER
RUMMER
RUMOUR
RUNFOR
RUNNER
RUSHER
RUTGER
RUTTER

•RR•••

ARRACK
ARRANT
ARRAYS
ARREAR
ARREST
ARRETE
ARRIBA
ARRIVE
ARROWS
ARROYO
DRRICE
DRRUTH
ERRAND
ERRANT
ERRARE
ERRATA
ERRING
ERROLL
ERRORS
GRRRLS
IRREAL
IRRUPT
ORRERY

•R•R••

ARARAS
ARARAT
ARBRES
CRORES
CRURAL
DRYROT
DRYRUN
FRERES
GRRRLS
ORTRUD

•R••R•

ARBORS
ARCARO
ARDORS
ARFARF
ARIARY
ARMERS
ARMORS
ARMORY
ARTERY
ARTHRO
ARTURO
BRIARD
BRIARS
BRIARY
BRIERS
BRIERY
CRIERS
CROIRE
CRUORS
CRYERS
DREARY
DRIERS
DRYERS
ERFURT
ERHARD
ERRARE
ERRORS
FREDRO
FREERS
FRIARS
FRIARY
FRIERS
FRYERS
GRIGRI
IRKERS
ORDERS
ORNERY
ORRERY
PREARM
PREDRY
PRFIRM
PRIERS
PRIORI
PRIORS
PRIORY
PROART
PROPRE
PRYERS
TRIERS
TRYERS
URGERS

•R•••R

ARBOUR
ARCHER
ARDOUR
ARGUER
ARIDER
ARMOUR
ARREAR
ARTCAR
ARTHUR
ARTIER
BRACER
BRAVER
BRAYER
BREMER
BREUER
BREWER
BREYER
BRIBER
BRINER
BROKER
BRUDER
BRUNOR
CRAMER
CRATER
CRAVER
CREMER
CROWER
CRUDER
CRYFOR
DRAPER
DRAWER
DREYER
DRIQJR
DRIVER
DRONER
DROVER
ERASER
ERODER
FRAMER
FRASER
FRATER
FRAZER
FREWER
GRADER
GRATER
GRAVER
GRAYER
GRAZER
GREGOR
GREYER
GRIPER
GROCER
GROPER
GROVER
GROWER
HRIDER
IRATER
IRONER
KRAMER
KROGER
KRONER
KRONOR
KRONUR
KRUGER
ORATOR
PRATER
PRAWER
PRAYER
PREFER
PRETER

PRETOR
PREWAR
PREYER
PRICER
PRIMER
PROBER
PROPER
PROSER
PROVER
PROWAR
PRUNER
TRACER
TRADER
TREMOR
TREVOR
TRITER
TROYER
TRYFOR
WRITER

••RR••
BARRED
BARREL
BARREN
BARRES
BARRET
BARRIE
BARRIO
BARRIS
BARRON
BARROW
BIRRED
BORROW
BURRED
BURROS
BURROW
CARREL
CARREY
CARRIE
CARROL
CARROT
CERROS
CIRRUS
CORRAL
CORREO
CURRED
DARREN
DARRIN
DARROW
DARRYL
DERREK
DORRIT
DURRAS
FARRAH
FARRAR
FARRIS
FARROW
FERRER
FERRET
FERRIC
FERRIS
FURRED
FURROW
GARRET
GRRRLS
HARRAD
HARRAH
HARRIS
HARROW
HARRYO
HARRYS
HERREN
HORRID
HORROR
HURRAH
HURRAY
JARRED
KARRAS
KARRER
KARRIE
LARRUP
LORRIE
MARRED
MARRER
MARRON
MARROW
MERRIE
MIRREN
MIRROR
MIRROS
MORREL
MORRIE
MORRIS
MORROW
MURRAY
MURRES
MURROW
MYRRHS
NARROW
NORRIS
PARRED
PARRIS
PARROT
PERRIN
PERROS
PIRRIP
PURRED
PURRER
SIRRAH
SIRREE
SORREL
SORROW
SURREY
TARRED
TERRAE
TERRAN
TERRES
TERRET
TERRIF
TERRIS
TERROR
TORRES
TORREY
TORRID
TURRET
WARRED
WARREN
YARROW

••R•R•
AIRARM
AIRDRY
AIRERS
ASRARE
AURORA
BARBRA
BORERS
CARBRA
CARERS
CORERS
CURARE
CURERS
DARERS
ERRARE
ERRORS
FARCRY
FARERS
FIRERS
FURORE
FURORS
GERARD
GORERS
HARARE
HIRERS
JURORS
LURERS
OARERS
ORRERY
PARERS
PARURE
PORERS
SARTRE
TORERO
WARCRY
WIRERS

••R••R
AERIER
AGREER
AIRIER
AIRWAR
ARREAR
BARBER
BARCAR
BARGER
BARKER
BARTER
BERBER
BERGER
BIRDER
BIRLER
BORDER
BURGER
BURIER
BURLER
BURNER
BURSAR
CARDER
CAREER
CARNER
CARPER
CARTER
CARVER
CEREBR
CORDER
CORKER
CORNER
CURLER
CURSER
CURSOR
CURTER
DARKER
DARNER
DARTER
DORMER
EARNER
EERIER
FARMER
FARRAR
FERBER
FERRER
FERVOR
FIRMER
FIRSTR
FORCER
FORGER
FORKER
FORMER
GARBER
GARNER
GARTER
GERBER
GIRDER
GORGER
GORIER
HARBOR
HARDER
HARHAR
HARKER
HARMER
HARPER
HERDER
HORNER
HORROR
HURLER
HURTER
ISRAIR
JARJAR
JERKER
KARRER
LARDER
LARGER
LARKER
LARMOR
LARTER
LERNER
LURKER
MARKER
MARNER
MARRER
MARTYR
MERCER
MERGER
MIRIER
MIRROR
MORTAR
MURDER
MURMUR
NURSER
OERTER
PARGER
PARKER
PARLOR
PARSER
PERTER
PORKER
PORTER
PURRER
PURSER
SARTOR
SERVER
SORTER
SPRIER
SPRYER
SURFER
TARTAR
TARTER
TERROR
TERSER
TORPOR
TURNER
UPREAR
UPROAR
VARIER
VERGER
WARDER
WARIER
WARMER
WARNER
WARPER
WERKER
WERNER
WIRIER
WORKER
WORMER
YARDER
YORKER

•••RR•
ATERRE
BEURRE
BLURRY
CHARRO
CHERRY
CHIRRS
CHURRO
FLURRY
GNARRS
GUERRE
IBARRA
KNARRS
KNARRY
PIERRE
QUARRY
SBARRO
SCARRY
SCURRY
SHERRI
SHERRY
SHIRRS
SIERRA
SLURRY
SNORRI
SPERRY
STARRY
STORRS
TIERRA
WHERRY
WHIRRS
XTERRA

•••R•R
ADORER
AWARER
BEARER
BOHRER
DEARER
DOURER
FAIRER
FARRAR
FEARER
FERRER
FUHRER
HEARER
HORROR
JEERER
KARRER
LEERER
LEHRER
MARRER
MIRROR
NEARER
POORER
POURER
PURRER
REARER
ROARER
ROHRER
SCARER
SCORER
SEARER
SHARER
SHIRER
SNARER
SNORER
SOARER
SOURER
SPARER
STARER
STORER
TEARER
TERROR
THIRDR
TOURER
USURER
WEARER

••••RR
DEBURR
LAMARR
SCHORR

RS••••
RSTUVW
RSVPED

R•S•••
RASCAL
RASCHE
RASERS
RASHAD
RASHER
RASHES
RASHID
RASHLY
RASING
RASKIN
RASPAS
RASPED
RASPER
RASSES
RASSLE
RASTAS
RASTER
RASURE
RESAID
RESALE
RESALT
RESAND
RESANG
RESAVE
RESAWN
RESAWS
RESAYS
RESCAN
RESCUE
RESEAL
RESEAM
RESEAT
RESEAU
RESECT
RESEDA
RESEED
RESEEK
RESEEN
RESEES
RESELL
RESEND
RESENT
RESETS
RESEWN
RESEWS
RESHES
RESHIP
RESHOD
RESHOE
RESHOT
RESHOW
RESHUT
RESIDE
RESIFT
RESIGN
RESILE
RESING
RESINK
RESINS
RESINY
RESIST
RESITE
RESITS
RESIZE
RESNAP
RESNIK
RESOAK
RESOAP
RESODS
RESOIL
RESOLD
RESOLE
RESORB
RESORT
RESOWN
RESOWS
RESPAN
RESPIN
RESPOT
RESTAB
RESTED
RESTER
RESTES
RESTIR
RESTON
RESTOW
RESTUP
RESUIT
RESULT
RESUME
RESWAM
RESWIM
RISERS
RISETO
RISEUP
RISHIS
RISING
RISKED
RISKER
RISKIT
RISQUE
ROSARY
ROSCOE
ROSEAU
ROSERY
ROSETO
ROSEUP
ROSHIS
ROSIER
ROSIES
ROSILY
ROSINA
ROSINS
ROSINY
ROSITA
ROSLYN
ROSSEN
ROSSET
ROSSUM
ROSTEN
ROSTER
ROSTOV
ROSTRA
RUSHAT
RUSHBY
RUSHED
RUSHEE
RUSHER
RUSHES
RUSHIN
RUSHTO
RUSKIN
RUSSEL
RUSSES
RUSSET
RUSSIA
RUSTED
RUSTIC
RUSTLE

R••S••
RAGSON
RAISED
RAISER
RAISES
RAISIN
RAISON
RAMSAY
RAMSES
RAMSEY
RAMSIN
RAMSON
RANSOM
RAPSON
RASSES
RASSLE
RATSON
REASKS
REASON
REDSEA
REDSIX
REDSKY
REDSOX
REDSUN
REESES
REISER
REMSEN
REUSED
REUSER
REUSES
REVSON
REVSUP
RHESUS
RIDSOF
RIESEN
RIGSUP
RIMSKY
RINSED
RINSER
RINSES
RIPSAW
RIPSON
RIPSUP
RITSOS
ROASTS
ROBSOF
ROBSON
RONSON
ROOSTS
ROSSEN
ROSSET
ROSSUM
ROUSED
ROUSER
ROUSES
ROUSTS
RUBSIN
RUBSON
RUBSUP
RUNSAT
RUNSBY
RUNSIN
RUNSON
RUNSTO
RUNSUP
RUSSEL
RUSSES
RUSSET
RUSSIA

R•••S•
RACISM
RACIST
RADISH
RAGUSA
RAKISH
RAMOSE
RAREST
RAVISH
RAWEST
RAWISH
RAWIST
RECASE
RECAST
RECESS
RECOST
RECUSE
REDOSE
REDUST
REFUSE
REHASH
RELISH
RELIST
RELOSE
RELOST
REMISE
REMISS
RENEST
REPASS
REPAST
REPOSE
REPOST
RERISE
REROSE
RESIST
RETEST
RETOSS
REVEST
REVISE
REWASH
RIBISI
RIBOSE
RIFEST
RIMOSE
RIPEST
RIPOST
RNAASE
ROBUST
ROOTSY
RUDEST

R••••S
RABBIS
RABIES
RACERS
RADARS
RADIOS
RADIUS
RAGERS
RAINES
RAISES
RAITAS
RAJABS
RAJAHS
RAKERS
RAMBOS
RAMENS
RAMETS
RAMFIS
RAMIES
RAMSES
RANEES
RANGES
RANIDS
RAPIDS
RAPTUS
RAREES
RASERS
RASHES
RASPAS
RASSES
RASTAS
RATELS
RATERS
RATIOS
RAVELS
RAVENS
RAVERS
RAYONS
RAZERS
RAZORS
RAZZES
REACTS
READDS
REAIMS
REAIRS
REALES
REALMS
REARMS
REASKS
REATAS
REAVES
REBAGS
REBARS
REBBES
REBECS
REBELS
REBETS
REBIDS
REBOPS
REBUTS
REBUYS
RECANS
RECAPS
RECESS
RECONS
RECTOS
RECTUS
RECUES
RECURS
RECUTS
REDANS
REDIGS
REDIPS
REDOES
REDUBS
REDYES
REESES
REEVES
REFERS
REFIES
REFITS
REGELS
REGIUS
REGLES
REHABS
REHEMS
REHITS
REHOES
REICES
REIGNS
REINAS
REINES
REINKS
REJIGS
REKEYS
RELAPS
RELAYS
RELETS
RELICS
RELIES
RELOGS
REMANS
REMAPS
REMATS
REMISS
REMITS
REMOPS
REMOWS
RENEWS
RENGAS
RENINS
RENNES
RENTES
REOILS
REOWNS
REPADS
REPASS
REPAYS
REPEGS
REPELS
REPENS
REPINS
REPOTS
REPROS
REPUBS
RERIGS
RERUNS
RESAWS
RESAYS
RESEES
RESETS
RESEWS
RESHES
RESINS
RESITS
RESODS
RESOWS
RESTES
RETAGS
RETANS
RETAPS
RETARS
RETIES
RETINS
RETIPS
RETOPS
RETOSS
RETOWS
RETROS
REUNES
REUSES
REVELS
REVERS
REVETS
REVUES
REWEDS
REWETS
REWINS
REYLES
REZIPS
RHAMES
RHEEMS
RHEIMS
RHEMES
RHESUS
RHEUMS
RHINOS
RHODES
RHOMBS
RHUMBS
RHYMES
RIATAS
RICANS
RICERS
RICHES
RICOHS
RIDERS
RIDGES
RIFLES
RIGANS
RIGHTS
RIGORS
RIKERS
RILERS
RILLES
RIMERS
RIMOUS
RINSES
RIOJAS
RIPENS
RISERS
RISHIS
RITSOS
RITZES
RIVALS
RIVERS
RIVETS
RIYALS
ROASTS
ROBERS
ROBINS
ROBLES
ROBOTS
RODEOS
ROGERS
ROGETS
ROGUES
ROLEOS
ROMANS
ROMEOS
RONDOS
ROOSTS
ROPERS
ROSHIS
ROSIES
ROSINS
ROTORS
ROUGES
ROUGHS
ROUNDS
ROUSES
ROUSTS
ROUTES
ROVERS
ROWANS
ROWELS
ROWENS
ROWERS
ROYALS
ROYCES
RTILES
RUBELS
RUBENS
RUBIES
RUBIKS
RUBLES
RUCHES
RUCKUS
RUDKUS
RUFOUS
RULERS
RUMBAS
RUMORS
RUMPUS
RUNINS
RUNONS
RUNUPS
RUPEES
RUSHES
RUSSES
RUTINS

•RS•••
ARSENE
ARSENO
ARSONS
ERSATZ
ERSTAD
MRSULU
ORSINI
ORSINO
QRSTUV
URSIDS
URSINE
URSULA

•R•S••
ARCSEC
ARCSIN
ARISEN
ARISES
ARISTA
ARISTO
BRASCO
BRASHY
BRASIL
BRASOV
BRASSY
BRISES
BRISKS
BROSSE
BRUSHY
BRYSON
CRESOL
CRESSY
CRESTS
CRISCO
CRISES
CRISIS
CRISPS
CRISPY
CRISTO
CROSBY
CROSSE
CRUSES
CRUSOE
CRUSTS
CRUSTY
DRESSY
DROSSY
DRUSES
ERASED
ERASER
ERASES
ERESTU
FRASER
FRESCA
FRESCO
FRESNO
FRISCH
FRISCO
FRISEE
FRISES
FRISKS
FRISKY
FROSTS
FROSTY
FRUSTA
GRASPS
GRASSO
GRASSY
GRISHA
GRISLY
GRISTS
GROSSE
GROSSO
GROSZY
IRISED
IRISES
IRISIN
KRASNA
KRESGE
KRISPY
KRISTI
KRUSTY
ORISON
ORISSA
OROSCO
PRESET
PRESTO
PRISED
PRISMS
PRISON
PRISSY
PROSED
PROSER
PROSES
PROSIT
PROSKY
TRASHY
TRESSY
TRISHA
TRISTE
TRUSTS
TRUSTY
TRYSTS
WRASSE
WRESTS
WRISTS

•R••S•
ARGOSY
ARIOSE
ARIOSI
ARIOSO
ARLISS
ARNESS
AROUSE
ARREST
ARTEST
ARTIST
BRAISE

BRASSY BRATSK BREAST BROAST BROSSE BROWSE BRUISE CREASE CREASY CRESSY CREUSA CREUSE CROSSE CROUSE CRUISE DRESSY DRIEST DROPSY DROSSY DROWSE DROWSY DRYEST DRYISH ERNEST FRAISE FREEST GRASSO GRASSY GREASE GREASY GREIST GRIESE GROSSE GROSSO GROUSE IRAISE IRTYSH KRAUSS ORELSE ORENSE ORISSA PRAISE PRIEST PRISSY PROBST PROUST PROWSE TRESSY TRUEST TRUISM URALSK WRASSE WRIEST WRYEST

•R•••S

ARADOS ARAMES ARAMIS ARARAS ARBORS ARBRES ARCCOS ARCHES ARDORS ARECAS ARENAS ARETES ARGOTS ARGUES ARHATS ARISES ARLISS ARMERS ARMETS ARMIES ARMORS ARNEIS ARNESS ARNIES AROIDS AROMAS ARPELS ARRAYS ARROWS ARSONS ARTELS ARTOIS ARYANS BRACES BRACHS BRACTS BRAHMS BRAIDS BRAINS BRAKES BRANDS BRANTS BRAVAS BRAVES BRAVOS BRAWLS BRAZOS BREADS BREAKS BREAMS BREDES BREEDS BREVES BREVIS BRIARS BRIBES BRICKS BRIDES BRIEFS BRIERS BRINES BRINGS BRINKS BRISES BRISKS BROCAS BROILS BRONCS BROODS BROOKS BROOMS BROTHS BROWNS BRUGES BRUINS BRUITS BRUMES BRUNTS BRUTES BRUTUS BRUXES CRACKS CRAFTS CRAINS CRAKES CRAMPS CRANES CRANKS CRAPES CRATES CRAVES CRAWLS CRAZES CREAKS CREAMS CREDOS CREEDS CREEKS CREELS CREEPS CREMES CREPES CRESTS CRICKS CRIERS CRIMES CRIMPS CRIPES CRISES CRISIS CRISPS CROAKS CROATS CROCKS CROCUS CROFTS CRONES CRONUS CROOKS CROONS CRORES CROUPS CROWDS CROWNS CRUCES CRUDES CRUETS CRUMBS CRUMPS CRUORS CRUSES CRUSTS CRUXES CRWTHS CRYERS CRYPTS DRAFTS DRAINS DRAKES DRAMAS DRAPES DRAWLS DREADS DREAMS DRECKS DRIERS DRIFTS DRILLS DRINGS DRINKS DRIVES DROIDS DROITS DROLLS DRONES DROOLS DROOPS DROVES DROWNS DRUIDS DRUPES DRUSES DRUZES DRYADS DRYERS ERASES EREBUS ERECTS ERGOTS ERICAS ERINYS ERODES ERRORS ERUCTS ERUPTS FRACAS FRAKES FRAMES FRANCS FRANKS FRAUDS FREAKS FREERS FREONS FRERES FRIARS FRIELS FRIERS FRIGES FRILLS FRISES FRISKS FRITAS FRITES FRITOS FROCKS FRONDS FRONTS FROSTS FROTHS FROWNS FROYOS FRUITS FRUMPS FRYERS GRACES GRADES GRAFTS GRAILS GRAINS GRAMPS GRANDS GRANTS GRAPES GRAPHS GRASPS GRATES GRATIS GRAVAS GRAVES GRAZES GREATS GREBES GREEDS GREEKS GREENS GREETS GRIDES GRIEFS GRIFTS GRILLS GRIMES GRIMMS GRINDS GRIOTS GRIPES GRISTS GROANS GROATS GROINS GROOMS GROPES GROUPS GROUTS GROVES GROWLS GRRRLS GRUELS GRUMPS GRUNTS IRANIS IRAQIS IRIDES IRISES IRITIS IRKERS KRAALS KRAITS KRAUSS KRAVIS KREWES KROONS MRPAWS ORACHS ORALES ORANGS ORANIS ORANTS ORATES ORBITS ORDERS OREADS ORECKS OREOOS OREXIS ORGANS ORGIES ORIBIS ORIELS ORINGS ORIONS ORKANS ORLONS ORLOPS ORYXES PRADAS PRANAS PRANKS PRATES PRAWNS PRAXES PRAXIS PRECIS PREENS PREOPS PREXES PRICES PRICKS PRIDES PRIERS PRIMES PRIMOS PRIMPS PRIMUS PRINKS PRINTS PRIORS PRISMS PRIZES PRIZMS PROAMS PROBES PROEMS PROLES PROMOS PRONGS PROOFS PROSES PROVES PROWLS PROYAS PRUDES PRUNES PRYERS TRACES TRACKS TRACTS TRADES TRAGUS TRAILS TRAINS TRAITS TRALAS TRAMPS TRANES TRAVES TRAVIS TRAWLS TREADS TREATS TRECES TRENDS TREXES TRIADS TRIALS TRIBES TRICES TRICKS TRIERS TRIKES TRILLS TRINES TRIPES TROGGS TROLLS TROMPS TROOPS TROPES TROTHS TROUTS TROVES TRUCES TRUCKS TRUMPS TRUNKS TRUSTS TRUTHS TRYERS TRYSTS URAEUS URANUS URGERS URSIDS VROOMS WRACKS WRATHS WREAKS WRECKS WRESTS WRINGS WRISTS WRITES WRONGS

••RS••

AIRSAC AIRSEA AIRSUP BORSCH BURSAE BURSAL BURSAR BURSAS BURSTS CARSEY CARSON CORSAS CORSET CURSED CURSER CURSES CURSOR DORSAD DORSAL DORSAY DORSET DORSEY DORSUM FIRSTR FIRSTS GARSON GORSES HERSEY HIRSCH HORSED HORSES HORSEY JERSEY KARSTS KERSEE KIRSCH LARSEN LARSON MARSHA MARSHY MERSEY MORSEL NURSED NURSER NURSES PARSEC PARSED PARSEE PARSER PARSES PARSON PERSIA PERSIS PERSON PQRSTU PURSED PURSER PURSES PURSUE TARSAL TARSUS TERSER TORSOS VERSED VERSES VERSET VERSOS VERSTS VERSUS WARSAW WORSEN WORSTS WURSTS

••R•S•

ACROSS AFRESH ARREST ATREST ATRISK AURIST BAREST CARESS CARUSO CERISE CHRISM CHRIST CORPSE CURTSY DAREST DEROSE DERUST DIREST DURESS EGRESS FOREST GARISH HARASS HERESY INRUSH JURIST LAROSA LYRIST MARISA MARIST MEREST MORASS MORESO MOROSE MOROSS NERNST NORISK NORUSH OGRESS OGRISH ONRUSH PARISH PERISH PERUSE PHRASE POROSE PUREST PURISM PURIST RAREST RERISE REROSE SOREST STRESS SUREST TERESA THRASH THRESH THRUSH THRUST UNRASH UNREST UNRUST UPRISE UPROSE UPRUSH VARESE VERISM VERIST YAREST

••R••S

AARHUS ABRAMS ACROSS ADREPS AERIES AERIOS AGREES AIRBUS AIRERS AORTAS APRILS APRONS ARRAYS ARROWS ATREUS ATROIS AUROUS AVRILS BARCOS BARGES BARNES BARONS BARRES BARRIS BERETS BERTHS BERYLS BIRTHS BOREAS BORERS BORGES BURETS BURGHS BURGOS BURIES BURINS BURKAS BURROS BURSAS BURSTS BYRNES CARATS CARBOS CARERS CARESS CARETS CARGOS CARIBS CARIES CARLOS CARNES CAROBS CAROLS CAROMS CARPUS CARTES CARVES CDROMS CEREUS CERROS CIRCUS CIRRUS CORALS CORERS CORGIS COROTS CORPUS CORSAS CORTES CORVUS CURADS CURERS CURETS CURIES CURIOS CURSES CURTIS CURVES DARERS DARIUS DERATS DERMAS DERMIS DIRAMS DIRGES DORAGS DORCAS DORIES DURESS DUROCS DURRAS DURUMS EARTHS EGRESS EGRETS ENROLS ERRORS EYRIES FARADS FARAHS FARCES FARERS FAROES FARRIS FERALS FERIAS FERMIS FEROUS FERRIS FIRERS FIRSTS FIRTHS FORAYS FORBES FORCES FORGES FORTAS FORTES FORTIS FORUMS FURBYS FURIES FURORS FURZES GIRTHS GORERS GORGES GORSES GRRRLS HARASS HAREMS HARRIS HARRYS HERBES HERMES HEROES HERONS HIREES HIRERS HORDES HORSES HURONS INRAGS INRUNS JORUMS JURIES JURORS KARATS KARMAS KARRAS KARSTS KERNES KORANS KORATS LARAMS LAREES LARGES LARGOS LARVAS LORANS LORIES LURERS LYRICS LYRIDS MARCOS MARCUS MARDIS MARIAS MARKAS MARTES MARVIS MARXES MCRIBS MERGES MERITS MEROPS MIRINS MIRROS MIRTHS MORALS MORASS MORAYS MORELS MORONS MOROSS MORPHS MORRIS MURALS MURRES MYRRHS NARCOS NERVES NORIAS NORRIS NORTHS NORUNS NURSES OARERS OGRESS OPRAHS PARENS PARERS PAREUS PARGES PARKAS PARKES PARNIS PAROLS PARRIS PARSES PARTYS PERILS PERROS PERSIS PORERS PORKYS POROUS PORTES PTRAPS PUREES PURGES PURIMS PURSES RAREES RERIGS RERUNS SARANS SARDIS SAREES SARGES SCRAGS SCRAMS SCRAPS SCREES SCREWS SCRIMS SCRIPS SCRODS SCRUBS SCRUMS SERACS SERAIS SERGES SERIES SERIFS SERINS SERKIS SEROUS SERTAS SERUMS SERVES SERVOS SHREDS SHREWS SHRUBS SHRUGS SIRENS SIRIUS SIRUPS SPRATS SPRAYS SPREES SPRIGS SPRITS STRADS STRAPS STRATS STRAWS STRAYS STREPS STRESS STREWS STRIPS STROHS STROPS STRUMS STRUTS SURAHS SUREIS SURGES SYRUPS TARDES TARGAS TAROTS TARSUS TARTES TERCES TERMES TERNES TERRES TERRIS THREES THROBS THROES THROWS THRUMS TORAHS TORIES TORRES TORSOS TORTAS TORTES TURBOS UNRIGS UNRIPS UVRAYS VARGAS VARIAS VARIES VARMUS VARNAS VERDES VERGES VERSES VERSOS VERSTS VERSUS VERVES VIREOS VIRGAS VIRGOS VIRTUS VOROUS WARNES WIRERS WORLDS WORSTS WORTHS WURSTS XERXES YERKES ZEROES

•••RS•

AHORSE AVERSE BEARSE BOURSE COARSE COURSE ECORSE EVERSO GHIRSH HEARSE HEARST HOARSE OPQRST SMERSH SPARSE THIRST VIORST

•••R•S

ABORTS ACORNS ACURAS ADORES ADORNS AGORAS ALARMS ALEROS ALERTS AMORES ANDRES ANDROS ANTRES ARARAS ARBRES ASTRES ASTROS ATARIS AVERTS AWARDS AZERAS AZERIS AZORES AZURES BAIRNS BARRES BARRIS BEARDS BGIRLS BIERES BLARES BLURBS BLURTS BOARDS BOURGS BURROS CADRES CAIRNS CAMRYS CAPRIS CEORLS CERROS CHARDS CHARMS CHARTS CHERTS CHIRPS CHIRRS CHORDS CHORES CHOROS CHORUS CHURLS CHURNS CIERAS CIRRUS CITRUS CLAROS CLERKS CLORIS COBRAS COPRAS COURTS CRORES CUORES CYPRUS DEBRIS DEERES DMARKS DOBROS DURRAS DWARFS EAGRES ECARDS ELBRUS ENARMS ENCRES ENEROS ENURES

ESDRAS
EVERTS
EXERTS
EXTRAS
EXURBS
FARRIS
FERRIS
FIBRES
FIEROS
FIORDS
FJORDS
FLARES
FLIRTS
FLORAS
FLORES
FRERES
GAVRAS
GENRES
GLARES
GLARUS
GNARLS
GNARRS
GOURDS
GRRRLS
GUARDS
HARRIS
HARRYS
HEARNS
HEARTS
HEURES
HOARDS
HOURIS
HUBRIS
HYDRAS
HYDROS
HYDRUS
ICARUS
INGRES
INTROS
INURES
ISTRES
JAURES
KARRAS
KEARNS
KMARTS
KNARRS
KNURLS
LAIRDS
LEARNS
LEGROS
LIBRAS
LIBRIS
LIBROS
LITRES
LIVRES
LOWRES
LYCRAS
MACROS
MADRAS
MADRES
MAIRES
MAORIS
METRES
METROS
MICROS
MIRROS
MITRES
MOIRES
MORRIS
MOURNS
MURRES
MYRRHS
NACRES
NAIRAS
NEHRUS
NITRES
NITROS
NOIRES
NORRIS
OCHRES
OLORES
OPERAS
OSIRIS
OZARKS
PADRES
PARRIS
PEARLS
PERROS
PHAROS
POIRES
POORIS
QUARKS
QUARTS
QUIRES
QUIRKS
QUIRTS
REARMS
REPROS
RETROS
SABRAS
SABRES
SAURUS
SCARES
SCARFS
SCARPS
SCORES
SCORNS
SEVRES
SHARDS
SHARES
SHARKS
SHARPS
SHIRES
SHIRKS
SHIRRS
SHIRTS
SHORES
SHORTS
SKIRLS
SKIRTS
SKORTS
SLURPS
SMARTS
SMIRKS
SMORES
SMURFS
SNARES
SNARFS
SNARKS
SNARLS
SNORES
SNORTS
SPARES
SPARKS
SPIRES
SPORES
SPORKS
SPORTS
SPURNS
SPURTS
STARES
STARTS
STERES
STERNS
STORES
STORKS
STORMS
STORRS
SUCRES
SUPRAS
SUTRAS
SWARDS
SWARMS
SWIRLS
SWORDS
TATRAS
TAURUS
TBIRDS
TERRES
TERRIS
TETRAS
TETRIS
THERES
THERMS
THIRDS
THORNS
TIARAS
TIGRES
TIGRIS
TITRES
TORRES
TSURIS
TWERPS
TWIRLS
TWIRPS
ULTRAS
UMBRAS
UNARMS
USURPS
UTURNS
WALRUS
WHARFS
WHERES
WHIRLS
WHIRRS
WHORLS
XSARAS
YEARNS
ZAIRES
ZEBRAS

••••RS

ABHORS
ACHERS
ACTORS
ADDERS
ADWARS
AFTERS
AIDERS
AIMERS
AIRERS
ALBERS
ALDERS
ALTARS
ALTERS
AMBERS
AMEERS
AMOURS
ANDERS
ANGERS
AOLERS
ARBORS
ARDORS
ARMERS
ARMORS
ASKERS
ASTERS
ATTARS
AUGERS
AUGURS
BAKERS
BALERS
BIDERS
BIKERS
BITERS
BLEARS
BONERS
BOOERS
BORERS
BOWERS
BOXERS
BOYARS
BRIARS
BRIERS
BSTARS
BUYERS
CABERS
CAGERS
CANERS
CAPERS
CARERS
CASERS
CATERS
CAVERS
CEDARS
CEDERS
CESARS
CHAIRS
CHEERS
CHIRRS
CHOIRS
CIDERS
CIGARS
CITERS
CLAIRS
CLEARS
CLUERS
CODERS
COEURS
COLORS
COMDRS
COMERS
CONERS
COOERS
COPERS
CORERS
COVERS
COWERS
CRIERS
CRUORS
CRYERS
CSTARS
CUBERS
CURERS
CYDERS
DARERS
DATERS
DAZERS
DEAIRS
DEBARS
DECORS
DEFERS
DEMURS
DENARS
DETARS
DETERS
DEVERS
DEWARS
DICERS
DIKERS
DINARS
DINERS
DIVERS
DIYERS
DOLORS
DONORS
DOPERS
DOSERS
DOTERS
DOWERS
DOZERS
DRIERS
DRYERS
DUPERS
EASERS
EATERS
EDGARS
EDGERS
EELERS
EGGERS
EIDERS
EILERS
ELDERS
ELMERS
ELVERS
EMBARS
EMBERS
EMEERS
ENDERS
ENTERS
EPHORS
ERRORS
ESKERS
ESTERS
ETHERS
FACERS
FADERS
FAKERS
FAKIRS
FAQIRS
FARERS
FAVORS
FAXERS
FEMURS
FETORS
FEVERS
FIBERS
FIFERS
FILERS
FIRERS
FIVERS
FIXERS
FLAIRS
FLEERS
FLEURS
FLIERS
FLOORS
FLOURS
FLYERS
FODORS
FOYERS
FREERS
FRIARS
FRIERS
FRYERS
FSTARS
FUMERS
FURORS
GAMERS
GAPERS
GATERS
GATORS
GAZERS
GIBERS
GIVERS
GLUERS
GNARRS
GOFERS
GOMERS
GONERS
GORERS
GSTARS
HATERS
HAYERS
HAZERS
HEWERS
HEXERS
HHOURS
HIDERS
HIKERS
HIRERS
HIVERS
HOLERS
HOMERS
HONERS
HONORS
HOPERS
HOSERS
HOVERS
HUMORS
HYPERS
ICHORS
IDLERS
INCURS
INFERS
INKERS
INNERS
INTERS
IRKERS
JAPERS
JIVERS
JOKERS
JURORS
KEFIRS
KHMERS
KITERS
KNARRS
KSTARS
LABORS
LACERS
LADERS
LAGERS
LAKERS
LASERS
LAVERS
LAYERS
LEMURS
LEPERS
LEVERS
LIBERS
LIFERS
LIGERS
LIKERS
LINERS
LITERS
LIVERS
LONERS
LOPERS
LOSERS
LOVERS
LOWERS
LUGERS
LURERS
MACERS
MAJORS
MAKERS
MALARS
MANORS
MASERS
MATERS
MAYORS
MESSRS
METERS
MEWERS
MEYERS
MILERS
MIMERS
MINERS
MINORS
MISERS
MITERS
MIXERS
MOLARS
MOOERS
MOPERS
MOTORS
MOVERS
MOWERS
MOYERS
MSTARS
MUSERS
MYLARS
NABORS
NADIRS
NAMERS
NBAERS
NEVERS
NFLERS
NHLERS
NINERS
NITERS
NIXERS
NOPQRS
NOSERS
NOTERS
NSTARS
OARERS
OATERS
OCCURS
OCHERS
ODOURS
OFFERS
OGLERS
OILERS
ORDERS
OSCARS
OSIERS
OSTARS
OSTERS
OTHERS
OTTERS
OWNERS
PACERS
PAGERS
PAMIRS
PAPERS
PARERS
PATERS
PAVERS
PAWERS
PAYERS
PETERS
PIKERS
PILERS
PINERS
PIPERS
PLIERS
POKERS
POLERS
PORERS
POSERS
POWERS
PRIERS
PRIORS
PRYERS
PULERS
QUEERS
RACERS
RADARS
RAGERS
RAKERS
RASERS
RATERS
RAVERS
RAZERS
RAZORS
REAIRS
REBARS
RECURS
REFERS
RETARS
REVERS
RICERS
RIDERS
RIGORS
RIKERS
RILERS
RIMERS
RISERS
RIVERS
ROBERS
ROGERS
ROPERS
ROTORS
ROVERS
ROWERS
RULERS
RUMORS
SABERS
SAPORS
SATYRS
SAVERS
SAVORS
SAWERS
SAYERS
SCOURS
SEDERS
SENORS
SEVERS
SEWERS
SEXERS
SHEARS
SHEERS
SHIRRS
SHOERS
SITARS
SIXERS
SIZERS
SKIERS
SMEARS
SNEERS
SOBERS
SOEURS
SOLERS
SOMERS
SONARS
SOPORS
SOWERS
SPEARS
SPIERS
SPOORS
SSTARS
STAIRS
STEERS
STIERS
STORRS
SUGARS
SUPERS
SWEARS
TABORS
TAKERS
TALERS
TAMERS
TAPERS
TAPIRS
TASERS
TATARS
TATERS
TAXERS
TENORS
THEIRS
THEMRS
TIGERS
TILERS
TIMERS
TITERS
TOLARS
TONERS
TOPERS
TOTERS
TOWERS
TOYERS
TRIERS
TRYERS
TUBERS
TUDORS
TUNERS
TUTORS
TVVCRS
TYLERS
TYPERS
UDDERS
ULCERS
UMBERS
UNBARS
UNDERS
UPPERS
URGERS
USHERS
UTTERS
VALORS
VAPORS
VELARS
VEXERS
VFOURS
VICARS
VIGORS
VINERS
VIPERS
VISORS
VIZIRS
VIZORS
VOMERS
VOTERS
VOWERS
WADERS
WAFERS
WAGERS
WAKERS
WATERS
WAVERS
WAXERS
WEBERS
WHIRRS
WIPERS
WIRERS
WOOERS
WYLERS
ZONERS

RT••••

RTILES

R•T•••

RATEDA
RATEDG
RATEDR
RATEDX
RATELS
RATERS
RATHER
RATIFY
RATINE
RATING
RATION
RATIOS
RATITE
RATLIN
RATNER
RATOFF
RATOUT
RATSON
RATTAN
RATTAT
RATTED
RATTER
RATTLE
RATTLY
RETACK
RETAGS
RETAIL
RETAIN
RETAKE
RETAME
RETANS
RETAPE
RETAPS
RETARD
RETARS
RETEAR
RETELL
RETEST
RETHAW
RETIAL
RETIED
RETIEF
RETIES
RETILE
RETILL
RETIME
RETINA
RETINS
RETINT
RETIPS
RETIRE
RETOLD
RETONE
RETOOK
RETOOL
RETOPS
RETORE
RETORN
RETORT
RETOSS
RETOUR
RETOWS
RETRAL
RETRAP
RETRIM
RETROD
RETROS
RETTED
RETTIG
RETTON
RETUNE
RETURF
RETURN
RETYPE
RITARD
RITDYE
RITSOS
RITTER
RITUAL
RITZES
ROTARY
ROTATE
ROTGUT
ROTHKO
ROTINI
ROTORS
ROTTED
ROTTEN
ROTTER
ROTUND
RSTUVW
RUTGER
RUTHIE
RUTILE
RUTINS
RUTTAN
RUTTED
RUTTER

R••T••

RAFTED
RAFTER
RAGTAG
RAGTOP
RAITAS
RANTAT
RANTED
RANTER
RAPTER
RAPTLY
RAPTOR
RAPTUS
RASTAS
RASTER
RATTAN
RATTAT
RATTED
RATTER
RATTLE
RATTLY
REATAS
REATTA
RECTOR
RECTOS
RECTUS
REDTAB
REDTAG
REDTEN
REDTIE
REDTOP
REDTWO
REITER
RENTAL
RENTED
RENTEE
RENTER
RENTES
RENTON
RENTTO
RESTAB
RESTED
RESTER
RESTES
RESTIR
RESTON
RESTOW
RESTUP
RETTED
RETTIG
RETTON
REUTER
RHETOR
RHYTHM
RIATAS
RICTAL
RIFTED
RIOTED
RIOTER
RITTER
ROOTED
ROOTER
ROOTIE
ROOTIN
ROOTLE
ROOTSY
ROOTUP
ROSTEN
ROSTER
ROSTOV
ROSTRA
ROTTED
ROTTEN
ROTTER
ROUTED
ROUTER
ROUTES
RRATED
RUSTED
RUSTIC
RUSTLE
RUTTAN
RUTTED
RUTTER

R•••T•

RACETO
RAMATE
RAMETS
RARITY
RATITE
REACTS
READTO
REALTY
REATTA
REBATE
REBETS
REBOTE
REBUTS
RECITE
RECUTS
REDATE
REFITS
REFUTE
REHITS
RELATE
RELETS
REMATE
REMATS
REMITS
REMOTE
RENATA
RENATO
RENOTE
RENTTO
REPOTS
REPUTE
RERATE
RESETS
RESITE
RESITS
REVETS
REVOTE
REWETS
RIALTO
RIDETO
RIGATI
RIGHTO
RIGHTS
RIGHTY
RIMATE
RISETO
RIVETS
ROASTS
ROBOTS
RODETO
ROGETS
ROOSTS
ROSETO
ROSITA
ROTATE
ROUSTS
RUBATI
RUBATO
RULETH
RUNSTO
RUSHTO

R••••T

RABBET
RABBIT
RACIST
RACKET
RAGOUT
RAILAT
RAMJET
RANOUT
RANTAT
RAREST
RATOUT
RATTAT
RAVEAT
RAWEST
RAWIST
REBAIT
REBENT
REBOLT
REBOOT
RECANT
RECAST
RECENT
RECOAT
RECOST
REDACT
REDANT
REDBAT
REDDOT
REDHAT
REDHOT
REDOUT
REDUST
REEDIT
REEMIT
REGENT
REGIFT
REGNAT
REGRET
REHEAT
REJECT
REKNIT
REKNOT
RELENT
RELICT
RELIST
RELOST
RELUCT
REMEET
REMELT
REMINT
RENEST
RENNET
REPAST
REPEAT
REPENT
REPLOT
REPORT
REPOST
RERENT
REROOT
RESALT
RESEAT
RESECT
RESENT
RESHOT
RESHUT
RESIFT
RESIST
RESORT
RESPOT
RESUIT
RESULT
RETEST
RETINT
RETORT
REVERT
REVEST
REVOLT
REXCAT
RIBBIT
RIBCUT
RIBLET
RICHET
RIDENT
RIFEST
RIGOUT
RILLET
RIPEST
RIPOST
RIPOUT
RISKIT
ROARAT
ROBERT
ROBUST
ROCHAT
ROCHET
ROCKET
ROCKIT
RODENT
ROSSET
ROTGUT
RUBOUT
RUDEST
RUGRAT
RUNLET
RUNOUT
RUNSAT
RUPERT

RUSHAT
RUSSET

•RT•••
ARTAUD
ARTCAR
ARTELS
ARTERY
ARTEST
ARTFUL
ARTGUM
ARTHRO
ARTHUR
ARTIER
ARTILY
ARTIST
ARTOIS
ARTURO
IRTYSH
ORTEGA
ORTHEN
ORTRUD
URTEXT

•R•T••
ARCTAN
ARCTIC
ARETES
ARETHA
ARETOO
BRATSK
BRATTY
BRETON
BRITON
BROTHS
BROTHY
BRUTAL
BRUTES
BRUTUS
CRATED
CRATER
CRATES
CRETAN
CRETIN
CRITIC
CROTCH
CROTON
CRUTCH
CRWTHS
DRATIT
EROTIC
ERSTAD
FRATER
FRETAT
FRETTY
FRITAS
FRITES
FRITOS
FRITTA
FRITTO
FRITZI
FROTHS
FROTHY
FRUTTI
GRATAE
GRATED
GRATER
GRATES
GRATIA
GRATIN
GRATIS
GRETEL
GRETNA
GRITTI
GRITTY
GROTON
GROTTO
GROTTY
IRATER
IRITIC
IRITIS
ORATED
ORATES
ORATOR
PRATED
PRATER
PRATES
PRETAX
PRETER
PRETOR
PRETTY
PROTAX
PROTEA
PROTEM
PROTON
QRATIO
QRSTUV
RRATED
TRITER
TRITON
TROTHS
TROTUP
TRUTHS
WRATHS
WRETCH
WRITER
WRITES
WRITHE
XRATED

•R••T•
ARGOTS
ARHATS
ARISTA
ARISTO
ARMETS
ARNETT
ARRETE
BRACTS
BRANTS
BRATTY
BREATH
BRONTE
BRUITS
BRUNTS
CRAFTS
CRAFTY
CREATE
CRESTS
CRISTO
CROATS
CROFTS
CROUTE
CRUETS
CRUSTS
CRUSTY
CRYPTO
CRYPTS
DRAFTS
DRAFTY
DRAWTO
DREWTO
DRIFTS
DRIFTY
DROITS
DRRUTH
ERECTS
ERESTU
ERGOTS
ERRATA
ERSATZ
ERUCTS
ERUPTS
FRACTO
FRANTZ
FREETO
FRETTY
FRITTA
FRITTO
FRONTS
FROSTS
FROSTY
FRUCTI
FRUITS
FRUITY
FRUSTA
FRUTTI
GRAFTS
GRANTS
GREATS
GREETS
GRIFTS
GRIOTS
GRISTS
GRITTI
GRITTY
GROATS
GROTTO
GROTTY
GROUTS
GROUTY
GROWTH
GRUNTS
KRAITS
KRANTZ
KRISTI
KRUSTY
KRYPTO
MRMOTO
ORANTS
ORBITS
ORNATE
ORNITH
PRAYTO
PRESTO
PRETTY
PRINTS
PRONTO
PRUETT
TRACTS
TRAITS
TREATS
TREATY
TRENTA
TRENTE
TRENTO
TRISTE
TROUTS
TRUETO
TRUSTS
TRUSTY
TRYSTS
WRAITH
WREATH
WRESTS
WRISTS

•R•••T
ARAFAT
ARARAT
ARDENT
ARENDT
ARGENT
ARIGHT
ARMLET
ARMPIT
ARNETT
AROINT
AROUET
ARRANT
ARREST
ARTEST
ARTIST
BRANDT
BREAST
BRECHT
BREVET
BRIGHT
BRIGIT
BROAST
BRUNET
BRYANT
CRAIGT
CRAVAT
CREDIT
CRYOUT
DRATIT
DREAMT
DRIEST
DROPIT
DROUET
DRYEST
DRYOUT
DRYROT
ERFURT
ERNEST
ERRANT
FREEST
FRETAT
FRIGHT
GRABAT
GRANIT
GREIST
GRINAT
GROMIT
IROBOT
IRRUPT
KROFFT
ORGEAT
ORIENT
ORWHAT
PREACT
PRECUT
PREMET
PRESET
PRIEST
PRIVET
PROART
PROBST
PROFIT
PROJET
PROMPT
PROSIT
PROUST
PRUETT
TRICOT
TRIJET
TRIVET
TRUANT
TRUEST
TRYOUT
URGENT
URTEXT
WRIEST
WRIGHT
WRYEST

••RT••
AORTAE
AORTAL
AORTAS
AORTIC
AYRTON
BARTAB
BARTEL
BARTER
BARTLE
BARTOK
BARTON
BERTHA
BERTHE
BERTHS
BERTIE
BIRTHS
BURTON
CARTED
CARTEL
CARTER
CARTES
CARTIN
CARTON
CARTOP
CERTIF
CORTES
CORTEX
CORTEZ
CORTOT
CURTER
CURTIN
CURTIS
CURTIZ
CURTLY
CURTSY
DARTED
DARTER
DARTLE
EARTAB
EARTAG
EARTHA
EARTHS
EARTHY
FIRTHS
FORTAS
FORTES
FORTIS
GARTER
GERTIE
GIRTED
GIRTHS
HORTON
HURTER
HURTLE
LARTER
LARTET
MARTEL
MARTEN
MARTES
MARTHA
MARTHE
MARTIN
MARTYR
MERTON
MIRTHS
MORTAL
MORTAR
MORTEN
MORTON
MYRTLE
NORTHS
NORTON
OERTER
PARTED
PARTII
PARTIV
PARTLY
PARTOF
PARTON
PARTYS
PERTER
PERTLY
PORTAL
PORTED
PORTER
PORTES
PORTIA
PORTLY
SARTON
SARTOR
SARTRE
SERTAS
SORTED
SORTER
SORTIE
SORTOF
SURTAX
TARTAN
TARTAR
TARTED
TARTER
TARTES
TARTLY
TARTUP
TORTAS
TORTES
TURTLE
VERTEX
VIRTUE
VIRTUS
VORTEX
WARTED
WORTHS
WORTHY
YERTLE

••R•T•
ADRATE
AERATE
ALRITZ
AMRITA
ARRETE
AURATE
BARATA
BARATO
BARITE
BERATE
BERETS
BORATE
BURETS
BURSTS
BYROTE
CARATS
CARETO
CARETS
CDRATE
CERATE
CERATO
COROTS
CURATE
CURETS
CURITE
DARETO
DERATE
DERATS
DERITA
DORATI
DORITO
DRRUTH
EGRETS
ERRATA
FERITY
FIRSTR
FIRSTS
GARETH
GYRATE
HERETO
KARATE
KARATS
KARSTS
KORATS
MERITS
MORATH
MORITA
MORITZ
NARITA
NORITE
PARETO
PARITY
PERITI
PERUTZ
PIRATE
PQRSTU
PURITY
PYRITE
RARITY
RERATE
SPRATS
SPRITE
SPRITS
SPRITZ
STRATA
STRATI
STRATO
STRATS
STRUTS
SURETE
SURETY
TAROTS
TERATO
TERETE
TURNTO
UPRATE
VERITE
VERITY
VERSTS
WARMTH
WARMTO
WORSTS
WURSTS

••R••T
ABRUPT
ADRIFT
ADROIT
AIROUT
AIRPOT
ARRANT
ARREST
ATREST
AURIST
BARBET
BARDOT
BAREST
BARKAT
BARNET
BARRET
BEREFT
BIRGIT
BORDET
BURBOT
BURNET
CARLOT
CARNET
CARPAT
CARPET
CARROT
CHRIST
CORNET
CORSET
CORTOT
CURVET
DARENT
DAREST
DARNIT
DERMAT
DERMOT
DERUST
DIRECT
DIREST
DORRIT
DORSET
DURANT
DURNIT
EARLET
EARNIT
ENRAPT
ENROOT
ERRANT
FAROUT
FERMAT
FERRET
FIREAT
FORDGT
FOREST
FORGET
FORGOT
FORINT
FORMAT
GARNET
GARRET
GERENT
GORIOT
HARLOT
HEREAT
HERMIT
HERPET
HORNET
IRRUPT
JURIST
KERMIT
KORBUT
KURALT
LARIAT
LARTET
LORDIT
LYRIST
MARGOT
MARIST
MARKET
MARMOT
MEREST
MERLOT
MORANT
MOROLT
NERNST
NORENT
PARENT
PARKIT
PARROT
PERMIT
PUREST
PURIST
RAREST
RERENT
REROOT
SCRIPT
SHRIFT
SORBET
SOREAT
SOREST
SPRINT
SPROUT
STRAIT
STREET
STRICT
SUREST
TARGET
TARPIT
TERRET
THREAT
THRIFT
THROAT
THRUST
TOREAT
TOREIT
TORENT
TURBOT
TURRET
TYRANT
UNRENT
UNREST
UNROOT
UNRUST
UPROOT
VARLET
VERIST
VERNET
VERSET
WARVET
WERENT
WORKAT
YAREST

•••RT•
ABORTS
ALERTS
AVERTS
BLURTS
CHARTA
CHARTS
CHERTS
CHERTY
COURTS
DEARTH
DEARTO
DUARTE
ECARTE
EVERTS
EXERTS
FLIRTS
FLIRTY
FOURTH
GEARTO
HEARTH
HEARTS
HEARTY
IFORTY
KMARTS
NEARTO
NFORTY
OBERTO
OMERTA
OPORTO
PUERTO
QUARTE
QUARTO
QUARTS
QUARTZ
QUIRTS
QWERTY
SHIRTS
SHORTA
SHORTE
SHORTI
SHORTO
SHORTS
SHORTU
SHORTY
SHORTZ
SKIRTS
SKORTS
SMARTS
SMARTY
SNORTS
SNORTY
SPARTA
SPORTS
SPORTY
SPURTS
STARTS
THIRTY
UGARTE

•••R•T
AGOROT
AIGRET
AMORET
ARARAT
ATTRIT
BARRET
BEIRUT
CARROT
CLARET
DABRAT
DORRIT
DRYROT
ESPRIT
FERRET
FLORET
GARRET
GYMRAT
HEARST
IGOROT
IMARET
INARUT
JEERAT
LABRAT
LEARNT
LEBRET
LEERAT
LOIRET
NOIRET
OHDRAT
OPQRST
OVERIT
PARROT
PEERAT
PETRAT
POIRET
POIROT
POORAT
REGRET
ROARAT
RUGRAT
SECRET
SEURAT
SPIRIT
TEARAT
TEARIT
TERRET
THERAT
THIRST
TIKRIT
TURRET
VIORST

••••RT
ADVERT
ALBERT
ALHIRT
ALPERT
APPERT
ASSERT
ASSORT
ASTART
BEGIRT
BEJART
BOGART
CAVORT
COHORT
COVERT
DEPART
DEPORT
DESERT
DIVERT
DYSART
ECKART
EFFORT
EGBERT
EGGERT
EILERT
ELBERT
ELGART
ENGIRT
ERFURT
ESCORT
EXHORT
EXPERT
EXPORT
EXSERT
EXTORT
GOCART
GOKART
HOBART
HUBERT
IMHURT
IMPART
IMPORT
INPART
INPORT
INSERT
INVERT
JAVERT
LEGART
LEVERT
MOZART
NONART
OBVERT
OLMERT
OSBERT
OXCART
POPART
PROART
REPORT
RESORT
RETORT
REVERT
ROBERT
RUPERT
SQUIRT
STUART
THWART
TSHIRT
UNGIRT
UNHURT
UNSORT
UPDART
UPGIRT
YOGURT

RU••••
RUANDA
RUBATI
RUBATO
RUBBED
RUBBER
RUBBIA
RUBBLE
RUBBLY
RUBELS
RUBENS
RUBIED
RUBIES
RUBIFY
RUBIKS
RUBLES
RUBLEV
RUBOFF
RUBOUT
RUBRAW
RUBRIC
RUBSIN
RUBSON
RUBSUP
RUCHES
RUCKED
RUCKER
RUCKUP
RUCKUS
RUDDER
RUDELY
RUDERY
RUDEST
RUDKIN
RUDKUS
RUDMAN
RUDNER
RUDOLF
RUEFUL
RUFFED
RUFFLE
RUFFLY
RUFOUS
RUGGED
RUGRAT
RUINED
RUINER
RULEON
RULERS
RULETH
RULIER
RULING
RUMAKI
RUMBAS
RUMBLE
RUMBLY
RUMMER
RUMORS
RUMOUR
RUMPLE
RUMPLY
RUMPUS
RUNCIE
RUNDLE
RUNDMC
RUNDRY
RUNFOR
RUNGIN
RUNGUP
RUNINS
RUNLET
RUNLOW
RUNNEL
RUNNER
RUNOFF
RUNONS
RUNOUT
RUNSAT
RUNSBY
RUNSIN
RUNSON
RUNSTO
RUNSUP
RUNUPS
RUNWAY
RUNYON
RUPEES
RUPERT
RUPIAH
RUSHAT
RUSHBY
RUSHED
RUSHEE
RUSHER
RUSHES
RUSHIN
RUSHTO
RUSKIN
RUSSEL
RUSSES
RUSSET
RUSSIA
RUSTED
RUSTIC
RUSTLE
RUTGER
RUTHIE
RUTILE
RUTINS
RUTTAN
RUTTED
RUTTER
RUXPIN

R•U•••
RAUNCH
REUBEN
REUNED
REUNER
REUNES
REURGE
REUSED
REUSER
REUSES
REUTER
RHUMBA
RHUMBS
ROUGED
ROUGES
ROUGHS
ROUNDS
ROURKE
ROUSED
ROUSER
ROUSES
ROUSTS
ROUTED
ROUTER
ROUTES
RYUKYU

R••U••
RAGUSA
RAQUEL
RASURE
RCRUMB
REBUFF
REBUKE
REBURY
REBUTS
REBUYS
RECUED
RECUES
RECURE
RECURL
RECURS
RECUSE
RECUTS
REDUBS
REDUCE
REDUST
REFUEL
REFUGE
REFUND
REFUSE
REFUTE
REHUNG
RELUCT
RELUME
REPUBS
REPUGN
REPUMP
REPUTE
RERUNS
RESUIT
RESULT
RESUME
RETUNE
RETURF
RETURN
REVUES
RHEUMS
RHEUMY
RITUAL
ROBUST
ROGUED
ROGUES
ROMULO
ROTUND
RSTUVW
RUNUPS

R•••U•
RACEUP
RACKUP
RADIUM
RADIUS
RAGOUT
RAGRUG
RAIPUR
RAKEUP

RAMPUP
RANGUP
RANOUT
RAPTUS
RATOUT
RAVEUP
RAYGUN
READUP
REARUP
RECOUP
RECTUS
REDBUD
REDOUT
REDRUM
REDSUN
REELUP
REFLUX
REGIUS
REGLUE
REGNUM
REHAUL
REPOUR
RESCUE
RESHUT
RESTUP
RETOUR
REVSUP
RHESUS
RIBCUT
RIDEUP
RIGOUR
RIGOUT
RIGSUP
RILEUP
RIMOUS
RINGUP
RIPOUT
RIPSUP
RISEUP
RISQUE
RODEUP
ROILUP
ROLLUP
ROOTUP
ROPEUP
ROSEUP
ROSSUM
ROTGUT
RUBOUT
RUBSUP
RUCKUP
RUCKUS
RUDKUS
RUEFUL
RUFOUS
RUMOUR
RUMPUS
RUNGUP
RUNOUT
RUNSUP
RVALUE

R••••U
RAMEAU
RESEAU
ROSEAU
RYUKYU

•RU•••
ARUBAN
BRUDER
BRUGES
BRUINS
BRUISE
BRUITS
BRULEE
BRUMAL
BRUMEL
BRUMES
BRUNCH
BRUNEI
BRUNET
BRUNOR
BRUNTS
BRUSHY
BRUTAL
BRUTES
BRUTUS
BRUXED
BRUXES
CRUCES
CRUDDY
CRUDER
CRUDES
CRUDUP
CRUETS
CRUISE
CRUMBS
CRUMBY
CRUMMY
CRUMPS
CRUNCH
CRUORS
CRURAL
CRUSES
CRUSOE
CRUSTS
CRUSTY
CRUTCH
CRUXES
CRUZAN
DRUDGE
DRUIDS
DRUMUP
DRUPES
DRUSES
DRUZES
ERUCTS
ERUPTS
FRUCTI
FRUGAL
FRUITS
FRUITY
FRUMPS
FRUMPY
FRUNZE
FRUSTA
FRUTTI
GRUBBY
GRUCCI
GRUDGE
GRUELS
GRUING
GRUMIO
GRUMPS
GRUMPY
GRUNDY
GRUNGE
GRUNGY
GRUNTS
KRUGER
KRUSTY
PRUDES
PRUETT
PRUNED
PRUNER
PRUNES
TRUANT
TRUCES
TRUCKS
TRUDGE
TRUEST
TRUETO
TRUEUP
TRUING
TRUISM
TRUMAN
TRUMBO
TRUMPS
TRUNKS
TRUSTS
TRUSTY
TRUTHS

•R•U••
ARGUED
ARGUER
ARGUES
ARGUFY
ARJUNA
AROUET
AROUND
AROUSE
ARTURO
BREUER
BROUGH
CREUSA
CREUSE
CROUCH
CROUPS
CROUPY
CROUSE
CROUTE
DRJUNG
DROUET
DRRUTH
ERFURT
FRAUDS
FRAUEN
FREUND
GROUCH
GROUND
GROUPS
GROUSE
GROUTS
GROUTY
IRRUPT
KRAUSS
MRSULU
PROULX
PROUST
TRAUMA
TRIUNE
TROUGH
TROUPE
TROUTS
URSULA

•R••U•
ARBOUR
ARDOUR
ARMFUL
ARMOUR
ARTAUD
ARTFUL
ARTGUM
ARTHUR
BRAQUE
BREWUP
BROGUE
BRUTUS
CROCUS
CRONUS
CROPUP
CRUDUP
CRYOUT
DRAGUP
DRAWUP
DREWUP
DROGUE
DRUMUP
DRYOUT
DRYRUN
ERBIUM
EREBUS
FREEUP
FRENUM
GREWUP
GROWUP
IREFUL
KRONUR
MRBLUE
ORTRUD
PRAGUE
PREBUY
PRECUT
PRENUP
PREVUE
PRIMUS
PROGUN
PROPUP
QRSTUV
TRAGUS
TRIPUP
TROTUP
TRUEUP
TRYOUT
URAEUS
URANUS
URNFUL
WRAPUP

•R•••U
BROWNU
DRAKEU
ERESTU
MRSULU
ORMOLU

••RU••
ABRUPT
BARUCH
CARUSO
DERUST
DRRUTH
DURUMS
FARUKI
FERULE
FORUMS
GERUND
INRUNS
INRUSH
IRRUPT
JARULE
JORUMS
KORUNA
NERUDA
NORUNS
NORUSH
ONRUSH
PARURE
PERUKE
PERUSE
PERUTZ
RCRUMB
RERUNS
SCRUBS
SCRUFF
SCRUMS
SERUMS
SHRUBS
SHRUGS
SHRUNK
SIRUPS
SPRUCE
SPRUNG
STRUCK
STRUMS
STRUNG
STRUNK
STRUTS
SYRUPS
SYRUPY
THRUMS
THRUSH
THRUST
UNRUDE
UNRUED
UNRULY
UNRUNG
UNRUST
UPRUSH

••R•U•
AARHUS
AIRBUD
AIRBUS
AIRGUN
AIROUT
AIRSUP
ATREUS
ATRIUM
AUROUS
BARIUM
BARNUM
BARQUE
BARZUN
BOREUP
BURNUP
CARFUL
CARPUS
CEREUS
CERIUM
CIRCUM
CIRCUS
CIRQUE
CIRRUS
CORIUM
CORKUP
CORPUS
CORVUS
CURIUM
CURLUP
DARIUS
DORSUM
EARBUD
EARFUL
FARNUM
FAROUK
FAROUT
FEROUS
FIREUP
FIRMUP
FORFUN
FORKUP
HARDUP
HORMUZ
JARFUL
JERKUP
KIRKUK
KORBUT
LARRUP
LEROUX
MARAUD
MARCUS
MARKUP
MARQUE
MORGUE
MURMUR
PAREUS
PARFUM
PERDUE
PERKUP
POROUS
PURDUE
PURSUE
SEROUS
SHROUD
SIRIUS
SPROUT
STRAUB
STROUD
TARSUS
TARTUP
TOREUP
TORNUP
TORQUE
TURNUP
VARMUS
VERDUN
VERSUS
VIRTUE
VIRTUS
VOROUS
WARMUP
WIREUP
WORKUP

••R••U
AARGAU
BUREAU
CARIOU
FORYOU
MARILU
MOREAU
PQRSTU
SARDOU

•••RU•
ACCRUE
ALARUM
ANTRUM
ASTRUD
BAYRUM
BEARUP
BEIRUT
CHERUB
CHORUS
CIRRUS
CITRUS
CYPRUS
DOGRUN
DRYRUN
ELBRUS
EMBRUE
ENDRUN
FAIRUP
FOURUP
FUNRUN
GEARUP
GLARUS
HYDRUS
ICARUS
ICERUN
IMBRUE
INARUG
INARUT
LARRUP
LEBRUN
NEHRUS
NONRUN
OHCRUD
OILRUB
OLERUD
ONERUN
ORTRUD
OUTRUN
PAIRUP
QUORUM
RAGRUG
REARUP
REDRUM
SACRUM
SAURUS
SCARUM
SKIRUN
SOTRUE
STIRUP
TAURUS
TEARUP
UNTRUE
WALRUS

•••R•U
APERCU
DEBREU
EMORYU
SHORTU

••••RU
MASERU
SUBARU
THEPRU

RV••••
RVALUE
RVPARK

R•V•••
RAVAGE
RAVEAT
RAVELS
RAVENS
RAVEON
RAVERS
RAVEUP
RAVINE
RAVING
RAVISH
REVAMP
REVEAL
REVELS
REVEND
REVERB
REVERE
REVERS
REVERT
REVEST
REVETS
REVIEW
REVILE
REVISE
REVIVE
REVLON
REVOIR
REVOKE
REVOLT
REVOTE
REVSON
REVSUP
REVUES
REVVED
RIVALS
RIVERA
RIVERS
RIVETS
RIVING
RIVOLI
ROVERS
ROVING
RSVPED

R••V••
REAVED
REAVER
REAVES
REAVOW
REEVED
REEVES
RENVOI
REVVED

R•••V•
REGAVE
REGIVE
RELEVE
RELEVY
RELIVE
REMOVE
REPAVE
RESAVE
REVIVE
REWOVE
RSTUVW

R••••V
RENONV
ROCKYV
ROSTOV
RUBLEV

•RV•••
ARVADA
ERVING
IRVINE
IRVING

•R•V••
BRAVAS
BRAVED
BRAVER
BRAVES
BRAVOS
BREVES
BREVET
BREVIS
BROVIK
CRAVAT
CRAVED
CRAVEN
CRAVER
CRAVES
DREVIL
DRIVEL
DRIVEN
DRIVER
DRIVES
DRIVIN
DROVER
DROVES
EREVAN
ERIVAN
FRIVOL
GRAVAS
GRAVED
GRAVEL
GRAVEN
GRAVER
GRAVES
GRAVID
GROVED
GROVEL
GROVER
GROVES
HRYVNA
KRAVIS
PRAVDA
PREVIA
PREVIN
PREVUE
PRIVET
PROVED
PROVEN
PROVER
PROVES
TRAVEL
TRAVEN
TRAVES
TRAVIS
TREVOR
TRIVET
TRIVIA
TROVES

•R••V•
ARGIVE
ARLOVA
ARRIVE
GREAVE
GRIEVE
GROOVE
GROOVY
TRYGVE

•R•••V
BRASOV
KRYLOV
QRSTUV
URBANV

••RV••
CARVED
CARVEL
CARVER
CARVES
CARVEY
CERVID
CORVEE
CORVID
CORVUS
CURVED
CURVES
CURVET
EARVIN
FERVID
FERVOR
GARVEY
GERVIN
HARVEY
HERVEY
JARVIK
LARVAE
LARVAL
LARVAS
MARVEL
MARVIN
MARVIS
MERVYN
NARVIK
NERVAL
NERVED
NERVES
NORVAL
PURVEY
SERVED
SERVER
SERVES
SERVOS
SURVEY
VERVES
WARVET

••R•V•
ADRIVE
ARRIVE
DERIVE
MARKVI
PAREVE
SHREVE
SHRIVE
SHROVE
STRIVE
STROVE
THRIVE
THROVE
UNROVE

••R••V
KARKOV
KARPOV
MARKIV
MARKOV
PARKAV
PARTIV
ZARKOV

•••RV•
ISERVE
SCURVE
SCURVY
STARVE
SWERVE

•••R•V
ABBREV
ASTROV
HENRYV
IMPROV

RW••••
RWANDA

R•W•••
RAWBAR
RAWDON
RAWEGG
RAWEST
RAWISH
RAWIST
REWAKE
REWARD
REWARM
REWARN
REWASH
REWEAR
REWEDS
REWELD
REWETS
REWIND
REWINS
REWIPE
REWIRE
REWOKE
REWORD
REWORE
REWORK
REWORN
REWOVE
REWRAP
ROWANS
ROWELS
ROWENA
ROWENS
ROWERS
ROWING
ROWLEY

R••W••
RAHWAY
REOWNS
RESWAM
RESWIM
RUNWAY

R•••W•
REDTWO
REMOWN
REMOWS
RENEWS
RENOWN
RESAWN
RESAWS
RESEWN
RESEWS
RESOWN
RESOWS
RETOWS

R••••W
RANLOW
REAVOW
REBREW
RECHEW
REDRAW
REDREW
REFLEW
REFLOW
REGLOW
REGREW
REGROW
REPLOW
RESHOW
RESTOW
RETHAW
REVIEW
RIPSAW
RSTUVW
RUBRAW
RUNLOW

•RW•••
CRWTHS
MRWONG
ORWELL
ORWHAT

•R•W••
BRAWLS
BRAWNY
BREWED
BREWER
BREWUP
BROWED
BROWNE
BROWNS
BROWNU
BROWNY
BROWSE
CRAWLS
CRAWLY
CREWED
CREWEL
CROWDS
CROWED
CROWER
CROWNE
CROWNS
DRAWEE
DRAWER
DRAWIN
DRAWLS
DRAWLY
DRAWON
DRAWTO
DRAWUP
DREWIN
DREWON
DREWTO
DREWUP
DROWNS
DROWSE
DROWSY
FREWER
FROWNS
FROWZY
GREWON
GREWUP
GROWER
GROWLS
GROWLY
GROWON
GROWTH
GROWUP
KREWES
PRAWER
PRAWNS
PREWAR
PROWAR
PROWLS
PROWSE
TRAWLS
TROWED
TROWEL

•R••W•
ARROWS
MRPAWS

•R•••W
BROKAW
CRACOW
DRCLAW
ERENOW
KRAKOW
PRELAW

••RW••
AIRWAR
AIRWAY
BERWYN
CARWAX
CORWIN
DARWIN
EARWAX
EARWIG
FORWHY
KERWIN
NORWAY

••R•W•
ARROWS
SCRAWL
SCREWS
SCREWY
SHREWD
SHREWS
SPRAWL
STRAWS
STREWN
STREWS
TARAWA
THROWN
THROWS

••R••W
BARLOW
BARROW
BERKOW
BORROW
BURROW
CARLOW
CURFEW
CURLEW
CURNOW
DARROW
FARLOW
FARROW
FORNOW
FURROW
HARLOW
HARROW
MARROW
MORROW
MURROW
NARROW
SORROW
WARSAW
YARROW

•••R•W
ANDREW
ATHROW
BARROW
BORROW
BURROW
DARROW
ESCROW
FARROW
FURROW
HARROW
HEBREW
INAROW
KUDROW
MARROW
MCGRAW
MCGREW
MORROW
MURROW
NARROW
OUTROW
PITROW
REBREW
REDRAW
REDREW
REGREW
REGROW
RUBRAW
SORROW
TOPROW
TVCREW
UNDRAW
UNDREW
UPGREW
UPGROW
YARROW

R•X•••
RAXING
REXALL
REXCAT
ROXANA
ROXANE
RUXPIN

R••••X
RATEDX
REDFOX
REDSIX
REDSOX
REFLEX
REFLUX
RONMIX

•R•X••
BRUXED
BRUXES
CRUXES
DREXEL
DROXIE
OREXIA
OREXIS
ORYXES
PRAXES
PRAXIS
PREXES
TREXES
TRIXIE

•R••X•
URTEXT

•R•••X
BRANDX
MRJINX
PREFIX
PREMIX
PRETAX
PROLIX
PROTAX
PROULX

••RX••
MARXES
XERXES

••R•X•
BORAXO

••R••X
CARWAX

CORTEX EARWAX FORNAX LARYNX LEROUX MARCIX MARKIX MERCKX SURTAX VERTEX VORTEX

•••R•X
APPROX CLOROX HYDROX MATRIX THORAX

RY••••
RYDELL RYENCE RYOKAN RYUKYU

R•Y•••
RAYBAN RAYGUN RAYING RAYONS REYLES REYOKE RHYMED RHYMER RHYMES RHYTHM RIYADH RIYALS ROYALE ROYALS ROYCES

R••Y••
REDYED REDYES RELYON RETYPE RUNYON

R•••Y•
RALLYE REBUYS REDEYE REKEYS RELAYS REPAYS RESAYS RIBEYE RITDYE ROCKYV ROSLYN RYUKYU

R••••Y
RACEBY RACILY RADLEY RAHWAY RAINEY RAMIFY RAMSAY RAMSEY RANDRY RANKLY RAPTLY RAREFY RARELY RARITY RASHLY RATIFY RATTLY REALLY REALTY REBURY RECOPY REDBAY REDEFY REDENY REDSKY REILLY RELEVY REMEDY REPLAY RESINY RHEUMY RICHLY RICKEY RIDEBY RIDLEY RIFELY RIGHTY RIMSKY RIPELY RIPLEY RIPPLY RKELLY ROBROY RODEBY RODNEY ROLLBY ROMANY ROMNEY RONCEY RONELY ROONEY ROOTSY ROPERY ROSARY ROSERY ROSILY ROSINY ROTARY ROWLEY RUBBLY RUBIFY RUDELY RUDERY RUFFLY RUMBLY RUMPLY RUNDRY RUNSBY RUNWAY RUSHBY

•RY•••
ARYANS BRYANT BRYNZA BRYSON CRYERS CRYFOR CRYING CRYOFF CRYOUT CRYPTO CRYPTS DRYADS DRYDEN DRYERS DRYEST DRYEYE DRYFLY DRYFOG DRYICE DRYING DRYINK DRYISH DRYMOP DRYOFF DRYOUT DRYROT DRYRUN ERYKAH ERYNGO FRYERS FRYING FRYPAN HRYVNA KRYLON KRYLOV KRYPTO ORYXES PRYERS PRYING PRYNNE PRYOFF TRYERS TRYFOR TRYGVE TRYING TRYLON TRYONE TRYOUT TRYSTS WRYEST

•R•Y••
ARGYLE ARGYLL BRAYED BRAYER BREYER CRAYON DRAYED DREYER FRAYED FROYOS GRAYED GRAYER GRAYLY GREYED GREYER GREYLY IRTYSH MRHYDE PRAYED PRAYER PRAYTO PREYED PREYER PREYON PROYAS TROYER TROYNY XRAYED

•R••Y•
ARRAYS ARROYO CRONYN DRYEYE ERINYS PROPYL

•R•••Y
ARCHLY ARGOSY ARGUFY ARIARY ARIDLY ARMORY ARTERY ARTILY BRAINY BRANDY BRANNY BRASHY BRASSY BRATTY BRAWNY BREEDY BREEZY BRENLY BRIARY BRICKY BRIERY BROLLY BRONZY BROODY BROOKY BROOMY BROPHY BROTHY BROWNY BRUSHY CRABBY CRAFTY CRAGGY CRAMPY CRANKY CRANNY CRAWLY CREAKY CREAMY CREASY CREEPY CRESSY CRIKEY CRIMPY CRISPY CROAKY CROSBY CROUPY CRUDDY CRUMBY CRUMMY CRUSTY DRABLY DRAFTY DRAGGY DRANCY DRAWLY DREAMY DREARY DRECKY DRESSY DRIFTY DRIPPY DROLLY DROOLY DROOPY DROPBY DROPSY DROSSY DROWSY DRYFLY FRAIDY FRANNY FREAKY FREDDY FREELY FRENZY FRETTY FRIARY FRIDAY FRILLY FRINGY FRISKY FRIZZY FROGGY FROSTY FROTHY FROWZY FRUITY FRUMPY GRABBY GRAINY GRAMMY GRANBY GRANDY GRANNY GRAPEY GRAPHY GRASSY GRAYLY GREASY GREEDY GREENY GREYLY GRIMLY GRIMMY GRIPPY GRISLY GRITTY GROGGY GROOVY GROSZY GROTTY GROUTY GROWLY GROZNY GRUBBY GRUMPY GRUNDY GRUNGY KRISPY KRUSTY ORALLY ORANGY ORKNEY ORNERY ORRERY PREBUY PREDAY PREDRY PREPAY PREPPY PRETTY PRICEY PRIMLY PRIORY PRISSY PROSKY TRACEY TRAMPY TRANNY TRAPPY TRASHY TREATY TREBLY TRENDY TRESSY TRICKY TRILBY TRIMLY TRIPLY TROPHY TROYNY TRUSTY

••RY••
BARYON BERYLS CORYZA DURYEA FORYOU GARYIN LARYNX MARYAM MARYII MARYJO MERYLL SPRYER SPRYLY

••R•Y•
ARRAYS ARROYO BERWYN DARRYL FORAYS FURBYS HARRYO HARRYS MARTYR MERVYN MORAYS PARTYS PORKYS SPRAYS STRAYS UVRAYS

••R••Y
AERIFY AERILY AIRDRY AIRILY AIRWAY AURIFY BARANY BARELY BARFLY BARLEY BARNEY BARONY BIRNEY BURBLY BURLEY BURNEY CARBOY CARKEY CARNEY CARREY CARSEY CARVEY CHROMY CORDAY CURACY CURLEY CURTLY CURTSY DARKLY DARNAY DIRELY DORSAY DORSEY DURFEY EARTHY EERILY FARACY FARCRY FARLEY FERITY FIRMLY FORJOY FORWHY GARVEY GORCEY GORILY GURLEY GURNEY HARDBY HARDLY HARLEY HARNEY HARVEY HEREBY HERESY HERSEY HERVEY HORNBY HORSEY HURLEY HURRAY JEREMY JERSEY LORDLY LURKEY MARBLY MARKEY MARLEY MARSHY MERELY MERSEY MORLEY MORNAY MURPHY MURRAY NORGAY NORWAY OGRADY ORRERY PARITY PARKAY PARLAY PARLEY PARODY PARTLY PERDAY PERTLY PIRACY PORTLY PURELY PURIFY PURITY PURPLY PURVEY RAREFY RARELY RARITY SCREWY SIRKAY SORELY SPRYLY STRIPY SURELY SURETY SURREY SURVEY SYRUPY TARTLY TORBAY TORCHY TORREY TURKEY UNRULY VARNEY VERIFY VERILY VERITY WARCRY WARILY WARMLY WIRILY WORLEY WORTHY YARELY

•••RY•
CAMRYN CAMRYS CHERYL DARRYL EMBRYO EMORYU HARRYO HARRYS HEARYE HENRYI HENRYK HENRYV LAURYL LAURYN SHARYN SHERYL VANRYN

•••R•Y
AFFRAY ANDREY ANERGY ASTRAY AUBREY AUDREY BETRAY BLURRY CARREY CHARLY CHERRY CHERTY CHIRPY CLERGY CONROY CZERNY DEARLY DEBRAY DEFRAY DELRAY DELREY DELROY DOURLY EBERLY ENERGY ESTRAY EVERLY FABRAY FAIRLY FLIRTY FLOREY FLURRY GEORGY GILROY GNARLY HEARTY HOORAY HOURLY HURRAY IFORTY INARAY INGRAY INGREY INTRAY KEARNY KILROY KNARRY KNURLY LAUREY MAIRZY MANRAY MURRAY NEARBY NEARLY NFORTY OSPREY OVERLY PEARLY POORLY QUARRY QUIRKY QWERTY ROBROY SCARRY SCURFY SCURRY SCURVY SHARPY SHERRY SHORTY SLURRY SMARMY SMARTY SMIRKY SNARKY SNARLY SNORTY SOURLY SPARKY SPERRY SPORTY STARRY STORMY STURDY SUNRAY SURREY SWIRLY THIRTY THORNY TORREY TWIRLY USARMY WEIRDY WHERRY WHIRLY YEARLY

••••RY
AIRDRY AMBERY APIARY ARIARY ARMORY ARTERY ASBURY AUGURY AVIARY AWEARY BAKERY BELFRY BEWARY BINARY BLEARY BLURRY BOVARY BOWERY BRIARY BRIERY BUMBRY CALORY CANARY CEDARY CELERY CHEERY CHERRY CIDERY CLEARY DATARY DENARY DESCRY DESTRY DMITRY DOWERY DREARY DUPERY EATERY EELERY ELLERY EMPERY EXPIRY FAKERY FARCRY FINERY FLOURY FLURRY FRIARY GANTRY GENTRY GOAWRY GUIDRY GUITRY HENDRY HILARY HUNGRY ILLDRY INJURY JAPERY JUDFRY KIDORY KNARRY KUNDRY LANDRY LIVERY LOWERY LUXURY MALORY MEMORY MISERY MOPERY MTAIRY NAPERY NITERY NONARY NOTARY OCHERY OHENRY OLEARY ORNERY ORRERY OUTCRY OUTPRY OWLERY PALTRY PANFRY PANTRY PAPERY PASTRY PATDRY PELTRY PENURY PINERY POETRY POKERY PREDRY PRIORY QUARRY RANDRY REBURY ROPERY ROSARY ROSERY ROTARY RUDERY RUNDRY SALARY SAVORY SCARRY SCURRY SENARY SENTRY SHERRY SLURRY SMEARY SNEERY SPERRY STARRY STMARY SUGARY SULTRY SUNDRY TAWDRY THEORY TILERY TOWERY UNBURY UNMIRY UNWARY VAGARY VALERY VAPORY VESTRY VINERY VOTARY WAFERY WARCRY WATERY WAVERY WHERRY WINERY WINTRY

R•Z•••
RAZERS RAZING RAZORS RAZZED RAZZES RAZZIE RAZZLE REZERO REZIPS REZONE

R••Z••
RAZZED RAZZES RAZZIE RAZZLE RITZES

R•••Z•
REBOZO RESIZE RIENZI

•R•Z••
AREZZO BRAZEN BRAZIL BRAZOS BRAZZA BRAZZI CRAZED CRAZES CRUZAN DRUZES FRAZER FRIZZY FROZEN GRAZED GRAZER GRAZES GRAZIE GROZNY OROZCO PRIZED PRIZES PRIZMS PRIZZI PROZAC

•R••Z•
AREZZO BRAZZA BRAZZI BREEZE BREEZY BRONZE BRONZY BRYNZA FREEZE FRENZY FRIEZE FRITZI FRIZZY FROWZY FRUNZE GROSZY PRINZE PRIZZI TREIZE

•R•••Z
BRIENZ ERSATZ FRANTZ KRANTZ TROPEZ

••RZ••
BARZUN BORZOI CURZON FURZES HERZOG TARZAN

••R•Z•
CORYZA LARAZA XPRIZE

••R••Z
ALRITZ CORTEZ CURTIZ HORMUZ LORENZ MORITZ PARLEZ PERUTZ SPRITZ

•••RZ•
MAIRZY SFORZA STARZZ ZABRZE

•••R•Z
ENTREZ JUAREZ MEGREZ QUARTZ SHIRAZ SHORTZ STARZZ SWIRLZ TABRIZ

••••RZ
BONERZ ELBURZ

SA••••
SABADO SABALS SABATO SABENA SABERS SABINA SABINE SABLES SABOTS SABRAS SABRES SACFLY SACHEM SACHER SACHET SACKED SACKER SACKUP SACQUE SACRED SACRUM SADDAM SADDAY SADDEN SADDER SADDLE SADHES SADHUS SADISM SADIST SADLER SAFARI SAFECO SAFELY SAFEST SAFETY SAFIRE SAGELY SAGEST SAGGED SAGIER SAHARA SAHIBS SAIDAH SAIDHI SAIDNO SAIDOK SAIDSO SAIDTO SAIGON SAILED SAILER SAILON SAILOR SAILTO SAINTE SAINTS SAIPAN SAISON SAITEK SALAAM SALADA SALADE SALADS SALAMI SALARY SALEPS SALIFY SALINA SALINE SALISH SALIVA SALLES SALLIE SALLOW SALMAN SALMIS SALMON SALOME SALONS SALOON SALSAS SALTED SALTEN SALTER SALTII SALTON SALUKI SALUTE SALUTO SALVED SALVER SALVES SALVOR

SALVOS
SALYUT
SAMARA
SAMBAS
SAMEAS
SAMEDI
SAMEKH
SAMIAM
SAMLET
SAMOAN
SAMOSA
SAMPAN
SAMPLE
SAMSON
SAMUEL
SANCHO
SANCTA
SANDAL
SANDED
SANDER
SANDIA
SANDRA
SANDRO
SANELY
SANEST
SANGER
SANGRE
SANGTO
SANITY
SANKAS
SANKIN
SANSEI
SANTAS
SANTEE
SANTHA
SANTOS
SANYOS
SAPORS
SAPPED
SAPPER
SAPPHO
SARANS
SARDIS
SARDOU
SAREES
SARGES
SARGON
SARNIA
SARONG
SARTON
SARTOR
SARTRE
SASEBO
SASHAY
SASHED
SASHES
SASSED
SASSER
SASSES
SASSON
SATAYS
SATCOM
SATEEN
SATFOR
SATING
SATINS
SATINY
SATIRE
SATORI
SATOUT
SATPAT
SATRAP
SATURN
SATYRS
SAUCED
SAUCER
SAUCES
SAUDIS
SAULTS
SAUNAS
SAURON
SAURUS
SAUTES
SAVAGE
SAVAII
SAVANA
SAVANT
SAVATE
SAVEAS
SAVEIT
SAVEME
SAVEON
SAVERS
SAVEUP
SAVING
SAVIOR
SAVOIE
SAVOIR
SAVORS
SAVORY
SAVOUR
SAWALL
SAWERS
SAWFIT
SAWING
SAWLOG
SAWOFF
SAWOUT
SAWPIT
SAWRED
SAWSUP
SAWYER
SAXONS
SAXONY
SAYAAH
SAYAYE
SAYBOO
SAYDIE
SAYERS
SAYEST
SAYHEY
SAYIDO
SAYING
SAYLES
SAYNAY
SAYSAH
SAYSHI
SAYSNO
SAYSOK
SAYSOS
SAYSSO
SAYYES

S•A•••

SBARRO
SCAASI
SCAGGS
SCALAR
SCALDS
SCALED
SCALER
SCALES
SCALIA
SCALPS
SCAMPI
SCAMPS
SCANTS
SCANTY
SCARAB
SCARCE
SCARED
SCARER
SCARES
SCARFS
SCARNE
SCARPS
SCARRY
SCARUM
SCATHE
SEAAIR
SEAARM
SEABAG
SEABED
SEABEE
SEACAT
SEACOW
SEADOG
SEAEEL
SEAFOX
SEAGAL
SEAGOD
SEAHAG
SEAICE
SEALAB
SEALED
SEALER
SEALIN
SEALUP
SEALYS
SEAMAN
SEAMAP
SEAMED
SEAMEN
SEAMER
SEAMUS
SEANCE
SEARCH
SEARED
SEARER
SEARLE
SEASON
SEATAC
SEATED
SEATER
SEATON
SEAVER
SEAWAY
SHABBY
SHACKS
SHADED
SHADER
SHADES
SHADOW
SHAFTS
SHAGGY
SHAKEN
SHAKER
SHAKES
SHAKIN
SHAKOS
SHAKUR
SHALES
SHALEY
SHALIT
SHALLI
SHALLY
SHALOM
SHAMAN
SHAMED
SHAMES
SHAMIR
SHAMMY
SHAMUS
SHANDY
SHANIA
SHANKS
SHANTY
SHAPED
SHAPER
SHAPES
SHARDS
SHARED
SHARER
SHARES
SHARIF
SHARKS
SHARON
SHARPE
SHARPS
SHARPY
SHARYN
SHASTA
SHAVED
SHAVEN
SHAVER
SHAVES
SHAWLS
SHAYNE
SHAZAM
SKAGGS
SKALDS
SKANKS
SKANKY
SKATED
SKATER
SKATES
SLACKS
SLAKED
SLAKER
SLAKES
SLALOM
SLAMON
SLANGS
SLANGY
SLANTS
SLAPON
SLAPPY
SLATED
SLATER
SLATES
SLAVED
SLAVER
SLAVES
SLAVIC
SLAYED
SLAYER
SMACKS
SMALLA
SMALLB
SMALLC
SMALLD
SMALLE
SMALLF
SMALLG
SMALLH
SMALLI
SMALLJ
SMALLK
SMALLL
SMALLM
SMALLN
SMALLO
SMALLP
SMALLQ
SMALLR
SMALLS
SMALLT
SMALLU
SMALLV
SMALLW
SMALLX
SMALLY
SMALLZ
SMARMY
SMARTS
SMARTY
SMAZES
SNACKS
SNAFUS
SNAGGY
SNAGUP
SNAILS
SNAKED
SNAKER
SNAKES
SNAPAT
SNAPON
SNAPPY
SNAPTO
SNAPUP
SNARED
SNARER
SNARES
SNARFS
SNARKS
SNARKY
SNARLS
SNARLY
SNATCH
SNATHS
SNAZZY
SOAKED
SOAKER
SOAKIN
SOAKUP
SOAPED
SOAPER
SOAPUP
SOARED
SOARER
SOASTO
SOAVES
SPACED
SPACEK
SPACER
SPACES
SPACEY
SPADED
SPADER
SPADES
SPANKS
SPANKY
SPARED
SPARER
SPARES
SPARKS
SPARKY
SPARSE
SPARTA
SPASMS
SPATES
SPATHE
SPAWNS
SPAYED
SPAYER
STABAT
STABLE
STABLY
STACEY
STACKS
STADIA
STAFFS
STAGED
STAGER
STAGES
STAGEY
STAINS
STAIRS
STAKED
STAKES
STALAG
STALED
STALER
STALES
STALIN
STALKS
STALKY
STALLS
STAMEN
STAMOS
STAMPS
STANCE
STANCH
STANDS
STANZA
STAPES
STAPHS
STAPLE
STAPUF
STARCH
STARED
STARER
STARES
STARIN
STARRY
STARTS
STARVE
STARZZ
STASES
STASIS
STATED
STATEN
STATER
STATES
STATIC
STATIN
STATOR
STATUE
STATUS
STAVED
STAVES
STAYAT
STAYED
STAYER
STAYIN
STAYON
STAYUP
SUABLE
SUAVER
SWABBY
SWAINS
SWALES
SWAMIS
SWAMPS
SWAMPY
SWAMUP
SWANEE
SWANKY
SWANNS
SWARDS
SWARMS
SWATAT
SWATCH
SWATHE
SWATHS
SWAYED
SWAYER
SWAYZE

S••A••

SABADO
SABALS
SABATO
SAFARI
SAHARA
SALAAM
SALADA
SALADE
SALADS
SALAMI
SALARY
SAMARA
SARANS
SATAYS
SAVAGE
SAVAII
SAVANA
SAVANT
SAVATE
SAWALL
SAYAAH
SAYAYE
SCAASI
SCHAAP
SCHAVS
SCLAFF
SCRAGS
SCRAMS
SCRAPE
SCRAPS
SCRAWL
SEAAIR
SEAARM
SECADA
SECANT
SEDAKA
SEDANS
SEDATE
SEEALL
SEMANA
SENARY
SENATE
SENATS
SEPALS
SERACS
SERAIS
SERAPE
SERAPH
SESAME
SEWAGE
SEWARD
SHEARS
SHEATH
SHEAVE
SHOALS
SHOALY
SHOATS
SHRANK
SILAGE
SISALS
SITARS
SIVANS
SKOALS
SLEAZE
SLEAZY
SLOANE
SMEARS
SMEARY
SNEAKS
SNEAKY
SOCANI
SOLACE
SOLANO
SOLANS
SOLARA
SOLATI
SOMALI
SOMANY
SOMATA
SONANT
SONARS
SONATA
SPEAKS
SPEARE
SPEARS
SPLASH
SPLATS
SPLAYS
SPRACH
SPRAIN
SPRANG
SPRATS
SPRAWL
SPRAYS
SQUABS
SQUADS
SQUALL
SQUARE
SQUASH
SQUATS
SQUAWK
SSTARS
STEADS
STEADY
STEAKS
STEALS
STEAMS
STEAMY
STMALO
STMARK
STMARY
STOATS
STPATS
STPAUL
STRADA
STRADS
STRAFE
STRAIN
STRAIT
STRAND
STRAPS
STRATA
STRATI
STRATO
STRATS
STRAUB
STRAWS
STRAYS
STUART
SUBARU
SUEANE
SUEANN
SUGARS
SUGARY
SUMACS
SURAHS
SUSANB
SUSANN
SUVARI
SWEARS
SWEATS
SWEATY

S•••A•

SABRAS
SADDAM
SADDAY
SAIDAH
SAIPAN
SALAAM
SALMAN
SALSAS
SAMBAS
SAMEAS
SAMIAM
SAMOAN
SAMPAN
SANDAL
SANKAS
SANTAS
SASHAY
SATPAT
SATRAP
SAUNAS
SAVEAS
SAYAAH
SAYNAY
SAYSAH
SCALAR
SCARAB
SCENAS
SCHAAP
SCHWAB
SCHWAS
SCREAK
SCREAM
SCUBAS
SEABAG
SEACAT
SEAGAL
SEAHAG
SEALAB
SEAMAN
SEAMAP
SEATAC
SEAWAY
SEENAS
SEESAS
SEESAW
SEGWAY
SENDAK
SENNAS
SEPIAS
SEPTAL
SERIAL
SERTAS
SETSAT
SEURAT
SGTMAJ
SHAMAN
SHAZAM
SHEBAT
SHEVAT
SHIRAZ
SHOFAR
SHOPAT
SHOTAT
SHUMAI
SIGHAT
SIGMAS
SIGNAL
SILVAS
SIMIAN
SINBAD
SINEAD
SINTAX
SIOUAN
SIRKAY
SIRRAH
SITPAT
SITSAT
SIXDAY
SIXWAY
SKICAP
SKIHAT
SKIWAX
SKYCAM
SKYCAP
SKYLAB
SKYMAN
SKYMAP
SKYWAY
SLEZAK
SLOGAN
SLOVAK
SNAPAT
SNOCAT
SOCIAL
SOLEAS
SONTAG
SOONAS
SOREAT
SOSPAD
SOTHAT
SOWHAT
SOXFAN
SPINAL
SPIRAL
SPIVAK
SPREAD
SPYCAM
SQUEAK
SQUEAL
STABAT
STALAG
STAYAT
STEFAN
STELAR
STELAS
STJOAN
STOLAE
STOLAF
STOLAS
STOMAS
STOPAT
STREAK
STREAM
STRIAE
STUKAS
STUPAS
SUBPAR
SUBWAR
SUBWAY
SUCHAS
SULFAS
SULTAN
SUNDAE
SUNDAS
SUNDAY
SUNFAN
SUNHAT
SUNRAY
SUNTAN
SUPRAS
SUREAM
SURTAX
SUTRAS
SWATAT
SYLVAN
SYNTAX
SYRIAN

S••••A

SABENA
SABINA
SAHARA
SALADA
SALINA
SALIVA
SAMARA
SAMOSA
SANCTA
SANDIA
SANDRA
SANTHA
SARNIA
SAVANA
SCALIA
SCHEMA
SCLERA
SCOOBA
SCORIA
SCOTIA
SCYLLA
SECADA
SEDAKA
SEDONA
SEGURA
SELENA
SEMANA
SENECA
SENORA
SENTRA
SEPHIA
SEPIRA
SERBIA
SERENA
SEVENA
SFORZA
SHANIA
SHASTA
SHEENA
SHEILA
SHERPA
SHORTA
SIENNA
SIERRA
SIESTA
SILICA
SIRICA
SMALLA
SMILLA
SMYRNA
SOLARA
SOMATA
SONATA
SONDRA
SONOMA
SONORA
SOPHIA
SPARTA
SPIREA
STADIA
STANZA
STELLA
STERNA
STIGMA
STRADA
STRATA
SUBSEA
SVEDKA
SYLVIA

•SA•••

ASANAS
ASANTE
ASARCO
ESALEN
ISAACS
ISABEL
ISAIAH
ISAIAN
ISANTI
ISAYNO
OSAGES
OSAKAN
PSALMS
TSADES
TSADIS
USABLE
USABLY
USAGES
USANCE
USARMY
USAUSA
XSARAS
ZSAZSA

•S•A••

ASCALE
ASEASY
ASFAST
ASGARD
ASHADE
ASHAME
ASHARP
ASIAGO
ASIANS
ASKAMY
ASKANT
ASLANT
ASMANY
ASMARA
ASRARE
ASSAIL
ASSAYS
ASTALL
ASTANA
ASTARE
ASTART
ASWARM
BSCALE
BSHARP
BSTARS
CSCALE
CSHARP
CSTARS
DSCALE
DSHARP
ESBATS
ESCALE
ESCAPE
ESCARP
ESCAUT
ESHARP
ESPANA
ESSAIS
ESSAYS
ESTADO
ESTATE
FSCALE
FSHARP
FSTARS
GSCALE
GSHARP
GSTAAD
GSTARS
ISAACS
ISLAND
ISLATE
ISMAIL
ISRAEL
ISRAIR
JSBACH
KSTARS
MSTARS
NSTARS
OSCANS
OSCARS
OSHAWA
OSTARS
OSWALD
PSHAWS
SSTARS
TSGARP
TSHAPE
USBANK
USHAPE
USMAIL
USNAVY
USUALS
VSHAPE
YSHAPE

•S••A•

ASANAS
ASFLAT
ASHCAN
ASHLAR
ASHMAN
ASHPAN
ASHRAM
ASNEAR
ASNEAT
ASOSAN
ASTEAL
ASTRAL
ASTRAY
ESDRAS
ESPIAL
ESTRAY
GSTAAD
ISAIAH
ISAIAN
ISHTAR
ISOBAR
ISWEAR
MSQUAD
OSAKAN
OSSIAN
OSTEAL
PSYWAR
TSTRAP
USETAX
USFLAG
XSARAS

•S•••A

ASMARA
ASONIA
ASPERA
ASSTDA
ASTANA
ASTHMA
CSONKA
ESPANA
ESPOSA
ISCHIA
ISOLDA
ISTRIA
OSETRA
OSHAWA
USAUSA
ZSAZSA

••SA••

ALSACE
ANSARA
ANSATE
ASSAIL
ASSAYS
BASALT
BESAME
BESANT
CASABA
CASALS
CASAVA
CESARE
CESARS
CUSACK
DESADE
DESALT
DISANT
DISARM
DOSADO
DOSAGE
DYSART
ENSATE
ERSATZ
ESSAIS
ESSAYS
HASAGO
INSANA
INSANE
ITSAGO
LESAGE
LUSAKA
MASADA
MASAIS
MASALA
MESAAZ
MESABI
MISACT
MISADD
MISAIM
MOSAIC
NASALS
NISANS
NOSALE
NOSALT
OKSANA
ONSALE
PESACH
PESADE
PISANO
PISANS
POSADA
RESAID
RESALE
RESALT

RESAND
RESANG
RESAVE
RESAWN
RESAWS
RESAYS
ROSARY
SESAME
SISALS
SUSANB
SUSANN
TISANE
UNSAFE
UNSAGE
UNSAID
UNSAWN
UNSAYS
UPSALA
VISAED
VISAGE
WASABI
YOSANO

••S•A•

ABSCAM
BASIAL
BASRAH
BISCAY
BISSAU
BUSMAN
CASBAH
CASPAR
CASUAL
CESTAS
COSMAS
COSTAE
COSTAL
COSTAR
COSTAS
CTSCAN
CUSHAW
CUSPAL
DESSAU
DISBAR
DISMAL
DISMAS
DISMAY
DISTAL
DOSSAL
EASYAS
ENSEAL
ENSEAT
ERSTAD
FESTAL
FESTAS
FISCAL
FOSSAE
FUSSAT
GASBAG
GASCAN
GASCAP
GASMAN
GASPAR
GASTAX
GASWAR
GESTAE
GOSTAG
GUSTAV
HASSAM
HASSAN
HISSAT
HOSTAS
HUSSAR
INSEAM
INSPAN
INSTAL
ITSPAT
JOSIAH
JUSTAS
KASBAH
KASDAN
KASHAS
KCSTAR
LASCAR
LESHAN
LESTAT
MESAAZ
MESCAL
MESIAL
MISHAP
MISLAY
MISSAL
MISSAY
MOSHAV
MOSSAD
MUSCAT
MUSIAL
NASCAR
NASDAQ
NASSAU
NISSAN
NOSOAP
OISEAU
ONSTAR
OSSIAN
PASCAL
PASDAR
PASHAS
PASSAS
PASSAT
PASTAS
PISGAH
POSEAS
POSTAL
RASCAL
RASHAD
RASPAS
RASTAS
RESCAN
RESEAL
RESEAM
RESEAT
RESEAU
RESNAP
RESOAK
RESOAP
RESPAN
RESTAB
RESWAM
ROSEAU
RUSHAT
SASHAY
SOSPAD
TASMAN
TESLAS
TESTAE
TUSCAN
TUSSAL
TVSTAR
UNSEAL
UNSEAM
UNSEAT
UNSNAG
UNSNAP
UNSPAN
UPSHAW
UPSOAR
VASLAV
VASSAL
VASSAR
VESPAS
VESTAL
VESTAS
VISTAS
VISUAL
WASHAD
WYSTAN
YESIAM
YESMAN
ZESTAS

••S••A

ANSARA
ASSTDA
BASTIA
BOSNIA
BUSHWA
CASABA
CASAVA
CASITA
CASSIA
CESSNA
DESETA
DESICA
EASTLA
FASCIA
FUSUMA
HESTIA
INSANA
JASCHA
JOSHUA
KESHIA
KISHKA
LASTRA
LISBOA
LUSAKA
LUSTRA
MASADA
MASALA
MISCHA
MOSKVA
NASHUA
NESTEA
NOSTRA
OKSANA
PASCUA
PESETA
PESEWA
POSADA
RESEDA
ROSINA
ROSITA
ROSTRA
RUSSIA
UPSALA
URSULA
WASECA

•••SA•

ACTSAS
AIMSAT
AIRSAC
ASOSAN
BAISAS
BALSAM
BALSAS
BAYSAT
BISSAU
BONSAI
BOOSAT
BOWSAW
BURSAE
BURSAL
BURSAR
BURSAS
BUYSAT
CAESAR
CATSAT
CAUSAL
COMSAT
CORSAS
DABSAT
DESSAU
DIGSAT
DOGSAT
DORSAD
DORSAL
DORSAY
DOSSAL
EATSAT
EGGSAC
ENDSAT
FAISAL
FOSSAE
FUSSAT
GETSAB
GETSAC
GETSAD
GETSAT
GOESAT
HANSAS
HASSAM
HASSAN
HISSAT
HITSAT
HOOSAC
HOWSAD
HUSSAR
IAMSAM
ILLSAY
INKSAC
JAWSAT
JETSAM
JIGSAW
KANSAN
KANSAS
LAPSAT
LETSAT
LHASAN
MENSAL
MENSAN
MILSAP
MISSAL
MISSAY
MOSSAD
NADSAT
NAGSAT
NASSAU
NAYSAY
NIPSAT
NISSAN
NODSAT
OLDSAW
OUTSAT
OUTSAW
OUTSAY
OVISAC
PAISAN
PASSAS
PASSAT
PAUSAL
PAWSAT
PETSAT
PITSAW
PULSAR
QUASAR
RAMSAY
RIPSAW
RUNSAT
SALSAS
SAYSAH
SEESAS
SEESAW
SETSAT
SITSAT
TARSAL
TUGSAT
TULSAN
TUSSAL
VASSAL
VASSAR
WARSAW
WAUSAU
WINSAT
XHOSAS
YAPSAT

•••S•A

AIRSEA
ALASKA
ALYSSA
AMESIA
ARISTA
AVESTA
AYESHA
BUQSHA
CASSIA
CESSNA
CLASSA
CUESTA
DAOSTA
DAYSPA
DUESSA
EDESSA
EGESTA
ELISHA
ELISSA
FIESTA
FRESCA
FRUSTA
GEISHA
GLOSSA
GRISHA
ITASCA
KRASNA
MARSHA
MIASMA
MOESHA
MTOSSA
NAUSEA
ODESSA
OLESHA
ORISSA
PERSIA
PLASMA
POISHA
POLSKA
REDSEA
RUSSIA
SHASTA
SIESTA
SUBSEA
THESEA
TRISHA
VIZSLA
ZOYSIA

••••SA

AHIMSA
ALYSSA
BOCHSA
CLASSA
CREUSA
DUESSA
EDESSA
ELISSA
ELOISA
ESPOSA
EXCUSA
GLOSSA
JAMESA
LACASA
LAMESA
LAROSA
LOUISA
MARISA
MEDUSA
MIKASA
MIMOSA
MTOSSA
MUFASA
ODESSA
ORISSA
RAGUSA
SAMOSA
TALISA
TERESA
THEUSA
USAUSA
WALESA
ZSAZSA

SB••••

SBARRO

S•B•••

SABADO
SABALS
SABATO
SABENA
SABERS
SABINA
SABINE
SABLES
SABOTS
SABRAS
SABRES
SEBERG
SHBOOM
SIBYLS
SOBBED
SOBBER
SOBEIT
SOBERS
SOBFUL
STBEDE
SUBARU
SUBBED
SUBDEB
SUBDUE
SUBGOD
SUBGUM
SUBITO
SUBLET
SUBLID
SUBLOT
SUBMIT
SUBNET
SUBORN
SUBPAR
SUBSEA
SUBSET
SUBTLE
SUBTLY
SUBURB
SUBWAR
SUBWAY

S••B••

SAMBAS
SAYBOO
SCUBAS
SEABAG
SEABED
SEABEE
SERBIA
SHABBY
SHEBAT
SHEBOP
SIEBEN
SINBAD
SIRBEN
SKIBIB
SKIBOB
SKIBUM
SKYBOX
SLOBBY
SNOBBY
SNOBOL
SNUBBY
SOBBED
SOBBER
SOMBER
SOMBRE
SORBET
SORBIC
SPYBOT
STABAT
STABLE
STABLY
STUBBY
SUABLE
SUBBED
SUNBOW
SWABBY
SYMBOL

S•••B•

SAHIBS
SASEBO
SCOOBA
SCOOBY
SCRIBE
SCRUBS
SELLBY
SENDBY
SENTBY
SETSBY
SHABBY
SHELBY
SHOTBY
SHRUBS
SITSBY
SKIPBY
SLIPBY
SLOBBY
SNOBBY
SNUBBY
SQUABS
SQUIBB
SQUIBS
STOPBY
STROBE
STUBBY
SWABBY

S••••B

SCARAB
SCHEIB
SCHLUB
SCHWAB
SEALAB
SEVENB
SKIBIB
SKIBOB
SKYLAB
SMALLB
SQUIBB
STRAUB
SUBDEB
SUBURB
SUPERB
SUSANB

•SB•••

ASBURY
ESBATS
JSBACH
OSBERT
OSBORN
USBANK

•S•B••

ASHBIN
ISABEL
ISOBAR
USABLE
USABLY

••SB••

BISBEE
BUSBOY
CASBAH
DISBAR
DISBUD
GASBAG
HASBRO
KASBAH
LESBOS
LISBOA
LISBON
NESBIT
YESBUT

••S•B•

CASABA
EASEBY
MESABI
NASEBY
PASSBY
RUSHBY
SASEBO
WASABI

••S••B

ABSORB
ADSORB
RESORB
RESTAB
SUSANB

•••SB•

CROSBY
DOESBY
EKESBY
GATSBY
GETSBY
GOESBY
LAYSBY
LETSBE
LETSBY
PASSBY
PUTSBY
RUNSBY
SETSBY
SITSBY
THISBE
WINSBY
ZIPSBY

•••S•B

GETSAB

••••SB

LOUISB

SC••••

SCAASI
SCAGGS
SCALAR
SCALDS
SCALED
SCALER
SCALES
SCALIA
SCALPS
SCAMPI
SCAMPS
SCANTS
SCANTY
SCARAB
SCARCE
SCARED
SCARER
SCARES
SCARFS
SCARNE
SCARPS
SCARRY
SCARUM
SCATHE
SCENAS
SCENEI
SCENES
SCENEV
SCENIC
SCENTS
SCHAAP
SCHAVS
SCHEIB
SCHELL
SCHEMA
SCHEME
SCHICK
SCHISM
SCHIST
SCHLEP
SCHLUB
SCHMOS
SCHNOZ
SCHOLL
SCHOOL
SCHORR
SCHULZ
SCHUSS
SCHWAB
SCHWAS
SCIONS
SCIPIO
SCLAFF
SCLERA
SCOFFS
SCOLDS
SCONCE
SCONES
SCOOBA
SCOOBY
SCOOPS
SCOOTS
SCOPED
SCOPES
SCORCH
SCORED
SCORER
SCORES
SCORIA
SCORNS
SCOTCH
SCOTER
SCOTIA
SCOTTO
SCOTTS
SCOTTY
SCOUPE
SCOURS
SCOUTS
SCOWLS
SCRAGS
SCRAMS
SCRAPE
SCRAPS
SCRAWL
SCREAK
SCREAM
SCREED
SCREEN
SCREES
SCREWS
SCREWY
SCRIBE
SCRIMP
SCRIMS
SCRIPS
SCRIPT
SCRODS
SCROLL
SCRUBS
SCRUFF
SCRUMS
SCUBAS
SCUFFS
SCULLS
SCULLY
SCULPT
SCUMMY
SCURFY
SCURRY
SCURVE
SCURVY
SCUZZY
SCYLLA
SCYTHE

S•C•••

SACFLY
SACHEM
SACHER
SACHET
SACKED
SACKER
SACKUP
SACQUE
SACRED
SACRUM
SECADA
SECANT
SECEDE
SECKEL
SECOND
SECRET
SECTOR
SECURE
SICCED
SICILY
SICKEN
SICKER
SICKLE
SICKLY
SICKOF
SICKOS
SOCANI
SOCCER
SOCIAL
SOCKED
SOCKET
SOCKIN
SOCLES
SUCCOR
SUCHAS
SUCKED
SUCKER
SUCKIN
SUCKUP
SUCRES

S••C••

SANCHO
SANCTA
SATCOM
SAUCED
SAUCER
SAUCES
SEACAT
SEACOW
SHACKS
SHECKY
SHOCKS
SHUCKS
SICCED
SIECLE
SITCOM
SKICAP
SKYCAM
SKYCAP
SLACKS
SLICED
SLICER
SLICES
SLICKS
SMACKS
SMOCKS
SNACKS
SNICKS
SNOCAT
SOCCER
SPACED
SPACEK
SPACER
SPACES
SPACEY
SPECIE
SPECKS
SPICED
SPICER
SPICES
SPYCAM
STACEY
STACKS
STICKS
STICKY
STOCKS
STOCKY
STUCCO
SUCCOR
SYNCED
SYNCHS

S•••C•

SAFECO
SCARCE
SCHICK
SCONCE
SCORCH
SCOTCH
SEAICE
SEANCE
SEARCH
SEDICI
SEDUCE
SELECT
SENECA
SERACS
SHLOCK
SHTICK
SILICA
SIRICA
SKETCH
SKITCH
SLOUCH
SLUICE
SMIRCH
SMOOCH
SNATCH
SNITCH
SOLACE
SOMUCH
SONICS
SOURCE
SPEECH
SPENCE
SPLICE
SPRACH
SPRUCE
STANCE
STANCH
STARCH
STENCH
STITCH
STNICK
STOICS
STORCH
STRICT
STRUCK
STUCCO
SUMACS
SUNOCO
SWATCH
SWITCH

S••••C

SCENIC
SEATAC
SEPTIC
SEVENC
SLAVIC
SMALLC
SORBIC
STATIC
STERIC
STIVIC
SYNDIC

•SC•••

ASCALE
ASCEND
ASCENT
ASCOLD
ASCOOL
ASCOTS
BSCALE
CSCALE
DSCALE
ESCALE
ESCAPE
ESCARP
ESCAUT
ESCENT
ESCHER
ESCHEW
ESCORT
ESCROW
ESCUDO
FSCALE
FSCOTT
GSCALE
ISCHIA
OSCANS
OSCARS
OSCINE
OSCULE

•S•C••

ASHCAN
PSYCHE
PSYCHO
PSYCHS

•S••C•

ASARCO
ASDICS
ASMUCH
ASPECT
ASPICS
ASSUCH
ESTOCS
ISAACS
JSBACH
OSMICS
USANCE
USEDCD

••SC••

ABSCAM
BISCAY
CISCOS
CTSCAN
DESCRY
DISCOS
DISCUS
FASCES
FASCIA
FESCUE
FISCAL
GASCAN
GASCAP
GASCON
JASCHA
LASCAR
MASCOT
MESCAL
MISCHA
MISCUE
MISCUT
MOSCOW
MUSCAT
MUSCLE
MUSCLY
NASCAR
PASCAL
PASCHS
PASCUA
PESCOW
PISCES
RASCAL
RASCHE
RESCAN
RESCUE
ROSCOE
TUSCAN
VISCID

••S•C•

ALSACE
ASSUCH
BASICS
BISECT
COSECS
COSTCO
CUSACK
CUSECS
DESICA
EXSECT
INSECT
MISACT
MUSICK
MUSICS
PESACH
RESECT
UNSICK
WASECA

••S••C

COSMIC
CYSTIC
FISTIC
GESTIC
INSYNC
MASTIC
MOSAIC
MYSTIC
ONSPEC
RUSTIC

•••SC•

BAUSCH
BORSCH
BRASCO
CRISCO
ENESCO
FIASCO
FRESCA
FRESCO
FRISCH
FRISCO
HIRSCH
ITASCA
KIRSCH
KITSCH
MENSCH
OROSCO
PUTSCH

UNESCO

•••S•C

AIRSAC
ARCSEC
ECESIC
EGGSAC
GETSAC
HOOSAC
INASEC
INKSAC
ONESEC
OVISAC
PARSEC
PHASIC
PHYSIC
VLASIC

S•D•••

SADDAM
SADDAY
SADDEN
SADDER
SADDLE
SADHES
SADHUS
SADISM
SADIST
SADLER
SEDAKA
SEDANS
SEDATE
SEDERS
SEDGED
SEDGES
SEDICI
SEDLEY
SEDONA
SEDUCE
SEDUMS
SIDDUR
SIDING
SIDLED
SIDLES
SIDNEY
SODDED
SODDEN
SODIDI
SODIUM
SODOWE
SUDDEN
SUDOKU
SUDSED
SUDSER
SUDSES
SYDNEY

S••D••

SADDAM
SADDAY
SADDEN
SADDER
SADDLE
SAIDAH
SAIDHI
SAIDNO
SAIDOK
SAIDSO
SAIDTO
SANDAL
SANDED
SANDER
SANDIA
SANDRA
SANDRO
SARDIS
SARDOU
SAUDIS
SAYDIE
SEADOG
SEEDED
SEEDER
SELDOM
SENDAK
SENDBY
SENDEE
SENDER
SENDIN
SENDON
SENDTO
SENDUP
SHADED
SHADER
SHADES
SHADOW
SHEDDS
SHEDON
SHODDY
SIDDUR
SIXDAY
SKIDDY
SKIDOO
SLEDGE
SLIDER
SLIDES
SLIDIN
SLUDGE
SLUDGY
SMIDGE
SMUDGE
SMUDGY
SNIDER
SNYDER
SODDED
SODDEN
SOLDER
SOLDIT
SOLDON
SOLDTO
SONDES
SONDRA
SORDID
SPADED
SPADER
SPADES
SPEDUP
SPIDER
SPIDEY
SPODES
SPYDER
STADIA
STIDES
STODGE
STODGY
STUDIO
STUDLY
SUBDEB
SUBDUE
SUDDEN
SUEDED
SUEDES
SUNDAE
SUNDAS
SUNDAY
SUNDER
SUNDOG
SUNDRY
SVEDKA
SWEDEN
SWEDES
SYNDIC

S•••D•

SABADO
SALADA
SALADE
SALADS
SAMEDI
SAYIDO
SCALDS
SCOLDS
SCRODS
SECADA
SECEDE
SHANDY
SHARDS
SHEDDS
SHEEDY
SHINDY
SHODDY
SHREDS
SKALDS
SKIDDY
SNOODS
SODIDI
SOLIDS
SOUNDS
SPEEDO
SPEEDS
SPEEDY
SPENDS
SPENDY
SQUADS
SQUIDS
STANDS
STBEDE
STEADS
STEADY
STEEDS
STJUDE
STRADA
STRADS
STRIDE
STRODE
STURDY
SUREDO
SWARDS
SWORDS
SYNODS

S••••D

SACKED
SACRED
SAGGED
SAILED
SALTED
SALVED
SANDED
SAPPED
SASHED
SASSED
SAUCED
SAWRED
SCALED
SCARED
SCOPED
SCORED
SCREED
SEABED
SEAGOD
SEALED
SEAMED
SEARED
SEATED
SECOND
SEDGED
SEEDED
SEEMED
SEEPED
SEERED
SEGUED
SEINED
SEIZED
SENSED
SERVED
SEVEND
SEWARD
SHADED
SHAMED
SHAPED
SHARED
SHAVED
SHIELD
SHINED
SHOOED
SHOULD
SHOVED
SHOWED
SHREWD
SHROUD
SICCED
SIDLED
SIEGED
SIEVED
SIFTED
SIGHED
SIGNED
SIGURD
SILOED
SILTED
SINBAD
SINEAD
SINGED
SINNED
SIPPED
SKATED
SKEWED
SLAKED
SLATED
SLAVED
SLAYED
SLEWED
SLICED
SLIMED
SLOPED
SLOWED
SMALLD
SMILED
SMOKED
SNAKED
SNARED
SNIPED
SNORED
SNOWED
SOAKED
SOAPED
SOARED
SOBBED
SOCKED
SODDED
SOILED
SOLOED
SOLVED
SOPPED
SORDID
SORTED
SOSPAD
SOTTED
SOURED
SOUSED
SPACED
SPADED
SPARED
SPAYED
SPEWED
SPICED
SPIKED
SPINED
SPIRED
SPITED
SPOKED
SPREAD
SPUMED
STAGED
STAKED
STALED
STARED
STATED
STAVED
STAYED
STEWED
STOKED
STOLID
STONED
STORED
STOWED
STRAND
STROUD
STUPID
STYLED
SUBBED
SUBGOD
SUBLID
SUCKED
SUDSED
SUEDED
SUITED
SULKED
SUMMED
SUNGOD
SUNNED
SUPPED
SURFED
SURGED
SUSSED
SWAYED
SWIPED
SYNCED

•SD•••

ASDEEP
ASDICS
ASDULL
ESDRAS

•S•D••

ASHDOD
ASIDES
BSIDES
ISIDOR
ISIDRO
TSADES
TSADIS
USEDCD
USEDIN
USEDON
USEDTO
USEDUP
YSIDRO

•S••D•

ASHADE
ASSTDA
ESCUDO
ESTADO
ISOLDA
ISOLDE
PSEUDO
PSEUDS

•S•••D

ASCEND
ASCOLD
ASGARD
ASGOOD
ASHDOD
ASTRID
ASTRUD
ESPIED
GSTAAD
ISLAND
ISOPOD
ISSUED
MSQUAD
OSGOOD
OSMOND
OSMUND
OSTEND
OSWALD
RSVPED
USEDCD
USERID

••SD••

EUSDEN
GOSDEN
KASDAN
LOSDOS
MISDID
MOSDEF
NASDAQ
PASDAR
WISDOM

••S•D•

ASSTDA
BESIDE
DESADE
DESODS
DOSADO
DOSIDO
INSIDE
MASADA
MISADD
MUSTDO
ONSIDE
PESADE
POSADA
RESEDA
RESIDE
RESODS
UPSIDE
URSIDS
YESIDO

••S••D

ABSURD
AISLED
ATSTUD
AXSEED
BASHED
BASKED
BASTED
BESTED
BOSSED
BUSHED
BUSIED
BUSKED
BUSSED
BUSTED
CASHED
CASKED
CASTED
CESSED
COSHED
COSIED
COSTED
CUSPED
CUSPID
CUSSED
DASHED
DESEED
DISBUD
DISHED
DISKED
DISSED
DOSSED
DUSKED
DUSTED
ENSUED
ERSTAD
FASTED
FESSED
FISHED
FISTED
FUSSED
GASHED
GASPED
GASSED
GUSHED
GUSTED
HASHED
HASPED
HASSID
HASTED
HESIOD
HISSED
HOSTED
HUSHED
HUSKED
IMSOLD
ISSUED
JESTED
JOSHED
KISSED
LASHED
LASTED
LISPED
LISTED
LUSTED
MASHED
MASKED
MASSED
MASTED
MESHED
MESSED
MISADD
MISDID
MISFED
MISLED
MISSED
MISTED
MOSHED
MOSSAD
MOSSED
MUSHED
MUSSED
NESTED
NOSHED
OUSTED
PASSED
PASTED
PISHED
POSTED
PUSHED
RASHAD
RASHID
RASPED
RESAID
RESAND
RESEED
RESEND
RESHOD
RESOLD
RESTED
RISKED
RUSHED
RUSTED
SASHED
SASSED
SOSPAD
SUSSED
TASKED
TASTED
TESTED
TOSSED
TUSKED
UNSAID
UNSELD
UNSHED
UNSHOD
UNSOLD
UNSUED
UPSEND
VESPID
VESTED
VISAED
VISCID
WASHAD
WASHED
WASLED
WASOLD
WASTED
WISHED
WISPED
YESSED
ZESTED

•••S•D

ABASED
ABUSED
AMUSED
BIASED
BOSSED
BUSSED
CAUSED
CEASED
CENSED
CESSED
CHASED
CLOSED
CURSED
CUSSED
DISSED
DORSAD
DOSSED
DOUSED
DOWSED
ERASED
FESSED
FUSSED
GASSED
GETSAD
GOOSED
HASSID
HISSED
HORSED
HOUSED
HOWSAD
IRISED
KISSED
LAPSED
LEASED
LENSED
LOOSED
LOUSED
MASSED
MESSED
MISSED
MOSSAD
MOSSED
MOUSED
MUSSED
NOISED
NOOSED
NURSED
OLDSOD
PARSED
PASSED
PAUSED
PHASED
PHYSED
POISED
PRISED
PROSED
PULSED
PURSED
RAISED
REUSED
RINSED
ROUSED
SASSED
SENSED
SOUSED
SUDSED
SUSSED
TEASED
TENSED
TOSSED
UNUSED
VERSED
YENSID
YESSED

SE••••

SEAAIR
SEAARM
SEABAG
SEABED
SEABEE
SEACAT
SEACOW
SEADOG
SEAEEL
SEAFOX
SEAGAL
SEAGOD
SEAHAG
SEAICE
SEALAB
SEALED
SEALER
SEALIN
SEALUP
SEALYS
SEAMAN
SEAMAP
SEAMED
SEAMEN
SEAMER
SEAMUS
SEANCE
SEARCH
SEARED
SEARER
SEARLE
SEASON
SEATAC
SEATED
SEATER
SEATON
SEAVER
SEAWAY
SEBERG
SECADA
SECANT
SECEDE
SECKEL
SECOND
SECRET
SECTOR
SECURE
SEDAKA
SEDANS
SEDATE
SEDERS
SEDGED
SEDGES
SEDICI
SEDLEY
SEDONA
SEDUCE
SEDUMS
SEEALL
SEEDED
SEEDER
SEEFIT
SEEGER
SEEING
SEEKER
SEEMED
SEEMLY
SEEMTO
SEENAS
SEENIN
SEENTO
SEENUP
SEEOFF
SEEOUT
SEEPED
SEEPIN
SEERED
SEESAS
SEESAW
SEESIN
SEESTO
SEESUP
SEETHE
SEEYOU
SEGUED
SEGUES
SEGURA
SEGWAY
SEIKOS
SEINED
SEINER
SEINES
SEISMO
SEISMS
SEIZED
SEIZER
SEIZES
SEIZOR
SELDOM
SELECT
SELENA
SELENE
SELLBY
SELLER
SELLIT
SELLON
SELLTO
SELTEN
SELVES
SEMANA
SEMELE
SEMITE
SEMPER
SEMPLE
SEMPRE
SENARY
SENATE
SENATS
SENDAK
SENDBY
SENDEE
SENDER
SENDIN
SENDON
SENDTO
SENDUP
SENECA
SENHOR
SENILE
SENIOR
SENITI
SENNAS
SENORA
SENORS
SENSED
SENSEI
SENSEN
SENSES
SENSOR
SENTBY
SENTIN
SENTON
SENTRA
SENTRY
SENTTO
SENTUP
SEPALS
SEPHIA
SEPIAS
SEPIRA
SEPOYS
SEPTAL
SEPTET
SEPTIC
SEPTUM
SEQUEL
SEQUIN
SERACS
SERAIS
SERAPE
SERAPH
SERBIA
SERENA
SERENE
SERGEI
SERGES
SERGIO
SERIAL
SERIES
SERIFS
SERINS
SERKIN
SERKIS
SERMON
SEROUS
SERTAS
SERUMS
SERVED
SERVER
SERVES
SERVOS
SESAME
SESQUI
SESSUE
SESTET
SETFEE
SETFOR
SETOFF
SETOSE
SETOUT
SETSAT
SETSBY
SETSIN
SETSON
SETSTO
SETSUP
SETTEE
SETTER
SETTLE
SETTOS
SETUPS
SETZER
SEURAT
SEVENA
SEVENB
SEVENC
SEVEND
SEVENE
SEVENS
SEVERE
SEVERN
SEVERS
SEVRES
SEWAGE
SEWARD
SEWELL
SEWERS
SEWING
SEWIST
SEWNIN
SEWNON
SEWNUP
SEWONS
SEWSIN
SEWSON
SEWSUP
SEXERS
SEXIER
SEXILY
SEXISM
SEXIST
SEXPOT
SEXTET
SEXTON
SEZWHO
SEZYOU

S•E•••

SCENAS
SCENEI
SCENES
SCENEV
SCENIC
SCENTS
SEEALL
SEEDED
SEEDER
SEEFIT
SEEGER
SEEING
SEEKER
SEEMED
SEEMLY
SEEMTO
SEENAS
SEENIN
SEENTO
SEENUP
SEEOFF
SEEOUT
SEEPED
SEEPIN
SEERED
SEESAS
SEESAW
SEESIN
SEESTO
SEESUP
SEETHE
SEEYOU
SHEARS
SHEATH
SHEAVE
SHEBAT
SHEBOP
SHECKY
SHEDDS
SHEDON
SHEEDY
SHEEHY
SHEENA
SHEENS
SHEENY
SHEERS
SHEESH
SHEETS
SHEIKH
SHEIKS
SHEILA
SHEKEL
SHELBY
SHELLS
SHELTY
SHELVE
SHEREE
SHERPA
SHERRI
SHERRY
SHERYL
SHEVAT
SIEBEN
SIECLE
SIEGED
SIEGEL
SIEGES
SIENNA
SIERRA
SIESTA
SIETES
SIEVED
SIEVES
SKEETS
SKEINS
SKETCH
SKEWED
SKEWER
SLEAZE
SLEAZY
SLEDGE
SLEEKS
SLEEKY
SLEEPS
SLEEPY
SLEETS
SLEETY
SLEEVE
SLEIGH
SLEUTH
SLEWED
SLEZAK
SMEARS
SMEARY
SMELLS
SMELLY
SMELTS
SMERSH
SNEAKS
SNEAKY
SNEERS
SNEERY
SNEEZE
SNEEZY
SNELLS
SOEURS
SPEAKS
SPEARE
SPEARS
SPECIE
SPECKS
SPEDUP
SPEECH
SPEEDO
SPEEDS
SPEEDY
SPELLS
SPENCE
SPENDS
SPENDY
SPERRY
SPEWED
SPEWER
STEADS
STEADY
STEAKS
STEALS
STEAMS
STEAMY
STEEDS
STEELE
STEELS
STEELY
STEEPS
STEERS
STEEVE
STEFAN

STEFFI
STEFOY
STEINS
STELAR
STELAS
STELES
STELLA
STELMO
STEMMY
STENCH
STENOG
STENOS
STENTS
STEPIN
STEPON
STEPPE
STEPUP
STEREO
STERES
STERIC
STERNA
STERNE
STERNO
STERNS
STEROL
STETHO
STEVEN
STEVIE
STEWED
STEWER
STEWIE
SUEANE
SUEANN
SUEDED
SUEDES
SUEFOR
SUENOS
SVEDKA
SVELTE
SWEARS
SWEATS
SWEATY
SWEDEN
SWEDES
SWEEPS
SWEETS
SWELLS
SWERVE

S••E••

SABENA
SABERS
SAFECO
SAFELY
SAFEST
SAFETY
SAGELY
SAGEST
SALEPS
SAMEAS
SAMEDI
SAMEKH
SANELY
SANEST
SAREES
SASEBO
SATEEN
SAVEAS
SAVEIT
SAVEME
SAVEON
SAVERS
SAVEUP
SAWERS
SAYERS
SAYEST
SCHEIB
SCHELL
SCHEMA
SCHEME
SCLERA
SCREAK
SCREAM
SCREED
SCREEN
SCREES
SCREWS
SCREWY
SEAEEL
SEBERG
SECEDE
SEDERS
SELECT
SELENA
SELENE
SEMELE
SENECA
SERENA
SERENE
SEVENA
SEVENB
SEVENC
SEVEND
SEVENE
SEVENS
SEVERE
SEVERN
SEVERS
SEWELL
SEWERS
SEXERS
SHEEDY
SHEEHY
SHEENA
SHEENS
SHEENY
SHEERS
SHEESH
SHEETS
SHIELD
SHIEST
SHOERS
SHREDS
SHREVE
SHREWD
SHREWS
SHTETL
SHYEST
SILENT
SIMEON
SINEAD
SINEWS
SINEWY
SIRENS
SIXEEE
SIXERS
SIZERS
SIZEUP
SKEETS
SKIERS
SLEEKS
SLEEKY
SLEEPS
SLEEPY
SLEETS
SLEETY
SLEEVE
SLIEST
SLYEST
SNEERS
SNEERY
SNEEZE
SNEEZY
SOBEIT
SOBERS
SOLEAS
SOLEIL
SOLELY
SOLEMN
SOLERS
SOLEUS
SOMERS
SOREAT
SORELY
SOREST
SOWERS
SOWETO
SPEECH
SPEEDO
SPEEDS
SPEEDY
SPHERE
SPIELS
SPIERS
SPLEEN
SPREAD
SPREES
SQUEAK
SQUEAL
STBEDE
STEEDS
STEELE
STEELS
STEELY
STEEPS
STEERS
STEEVE
STIERS
STPETE
STREAK
STREAM
STREEP
STREET
STREPS
STRESS
STREWN
STREWS
SUPERB
SUPERG
SUPERS
SUREAM
SUREDO
SUREIS
SURELY
SUREOF
SUREST
SURETE
SURETY
SWEEPS
SWEETS

S•••E•

SABLES
SABRES
SACHEM
SACHER
SACHET
SACKED
SACKER
SACRED
SADDEN
SADDER
SADHES
SADLER
SAGGED
SAGIER
SAILED
SAILER
SAITEK
SALLES
SALTED
SALTEN
SALTER
SALVED
SALVER
SALVES
SAMLET
SAMUEL
SANDED
SANDER
SANGER
SANSEI
SANTEE
SAPPED
SAPPER
SAREES
SARGES
SASHED
SASHES
SASSED
SASSER
SASSES
SATEEN
SAUCED
SAUCER
SAUCES
SAUTES
SAWRED
SAWYER
SAYHEY
SAYLES
SAYYES
SCALED
SCALER
SCALES
SCARED
SCARER
SCARES
SCENEI
SCENES
SCENEV
SCHLEP
SCONES
SCOPED
SCOPES
SCORED
SCORER
SCORES
SCOTER
SCREED
SCREEN
SCREES
SEABED
SEABEE
SEAEEL
SEALED
SEALER
SEAMED
SEAMEN
SEAMER
SEARED
SEARER
SEATED
SEATER
SEAVER
SECKEL
SECRET
SEDGED
SEDGES
SEDLEY
SEEDED
SEEDER
SEEGER
SEEKER
SEEMED
SEEPED
SEERED
SEGUED
SEGUES
SEINED
SEINER
SEINES
SEIZED
SEIZER
SEIZES
SELLER
SELTEN
SELVES
SEMPER
SENDEE
SENDER
SENSED
SENSEI
SENSEN
SENSES
SEPTET
SEQUEL
SERGEI
SERGES
SERIES
SERVED
SERVER
SERVES
SESTET
SETFEE
SETTEE
SETTER
SETZER
SEVRES
SEXIER
SEXTET
SHADED
SHADER
SHADES
SHAKEN
SHAKER
SHAKES
SHALES
SHALEY
SHAMED
SHAMES
SHAPED
SHAPER
SHAPES
SHARED
SHARER
SHARES
SHAVED
SHAVEN
SHAVER
SHAVES
SHEKEL
SHEREE
SHINED
SHINER
SHINES
SHIRER
SHIRES
SHIVER
SHOLEM
SHOOED
SHORES
SHOVED
SHOVEL
SHOVER
SHOVES
SHOWED
SHOWER
SHRIEK
SICCED
SICKEN
SICKER
SIDLED
SIDLES
SIDNEY
SIEBEN
SIEGED
SIEGEL
SIEGES
SIETES
SIEVED
SIEVES
SIFTED
SIFTER
SIGHED
SIGHER
SIGLER
SIGNED
SIGNEE
SIGNER
SIGNET
SILKEN
SILOED
SILTED
SILVER
SIMMER
SIMPER
SINGED
SINGER
SINGES
SINKER
SINNED
SINNER
SIPPED
SIPPER
SIRBEN
SIRREE
SISKEL
SISLER
SISLEY
SISTER
SITTER
SIXEEE
SIXTEN
SKATED
SKATER
SKATES
SKEWED
SKEWER
SKYMEN
SKYTEL
SLAKED
SLAKER
SLAKES
SLATED
SLATER
SLATES
SLAVED
SLAVER
SLAVES
SLAYED
SLAYER
SLEWED
SLICED
SLICER
SLICES
SLIDER
SLIDES
SLIMED
SLIMES
SLIVER
SLOPED
SLOPER
SLOPES
SLOVEN
SLOWED
SLOWER
SMAZES
SMILED
SMILER
SMILES
SMILEY
SMITER
SMITES
SMOKED
SMOKER
SMOKES
SMOKEY
SMORES
SNAKED
SNAKER
SNAKES
SNARED
SNARER
SNARES
SNIDER
SNIPED
SNIPER
SNIPES
SNIVEL
SNOPES
SNORED
SNORER
SNORES
SNOWED
SNYDER
SOAKED
SOAKER
SOAPED
SOAPER
SOARED
SOARER
SOAVES
SOBBED
SOBBER
SOCCER
SOCKED
SOCKET
SOCLES
SODDED
SODDEN
SOFTEN
SOFTER
SOILED
SOIREE
SOISEE
SOLDER
SOLOED
SOLVED
SOLVER
SOLVES
SOMBER
SOMMER
SONDES
SONNET
SOONER
SOPPED
SORBET
SORREL
SORTED
SORTER
SOTHEN
SOTTED
SOUPER
SOURED
SOURER
SOUSED
SOUSES
SOUTER
SOVIET
SPACED
SPACEK
SPACER
SPACES
SPACEY
SPADED
SPADER
SPADES
SPARED
SPARER
SPARES
SPATES
SPAYED
SPAYER
SPEWED
SPEWER
SPICED
SPICER
SPICES
SPIDER
SPIDEY
SPIKED
SPIKER
SPIKES
SPILES
SPINED
SPINEL
SPINER
SPINES
SPINET
SPIREA
SPIRED
SPIRES
SPITED
SPITES
SPLEEN
SPODES
SPOKED
SPOKEN
SPOKES
SPORES
SPREES
SPRIER
SPRYER
SPUMED
SPUMES
SPYDER
STACEY
STAGED
STAGER
STAGES
STAGEY
STAKED
STAKES
STALED
STALER
STALES
STAMEN
STAPES
STARED
STARER
STARES
STASES
STATED
STATEN
STATER
STATES
STAVED
STAVES
STAYED
STAYER
STELES
STEREO
STERES
STEVEN
STEWED
STEWER
STIDES
STILES
STIPES
STOKED
STOKER
STOKES
STOLEN
STOLES
STONED
STONER
STONES
STONEY
STORED
STORER
STORES
STOVER
STOVES
STOWED
STOWER
STREEP
STREET
STUPES
STYLED
STYLER
STYLES
STYLET
SUAVER
SUBBED
SUBDEB
SUBLET
SUBNET
SUBSEA
SUBSET
SUCKED
SUCKER
SUCRES
SUDDEN
SUDSED
SUDSER
SUDSES
SUEDED
SUEDES
SUFFER
SUITED
SUITES
SULKED
SULKER
SULLEN
SUMMED
SUMMER
SUMNER
SUMTER
SUNDER
SUNKEN
SUNNED
SUNSET
SUPPED
SUPPER
SURFED
SURFER
SURGED
SURGES
SURREY
SURVEY
SUSSED
SUSSES
SUSSEX
SUTTER
SUZIEQ
SWALES
SWANEE
SWAYED
SWAYER
SWEDEN
SWEDES
SWIPED
SWIPER
SWIPES
SWIVEL
SWIVET
SYDNEY
SYNCED
SYSTEM

S••••E

SABINE
SACQUE
SADDLE
SAFIRE
SAINTE
SALADE
SALINE
SALLIE
SALOME
SALUTE
SAMPLE
SANGRE
SANTEE
SARTRE
SATIRE
SAVAGE
SAVATE
SAVEME
SAVOIE
SAYAYE
SAYDIE
SCARCE
SCARNE
SCATHE
SCHEME
SCONCE
SCOUPE
SCRAPE
SCRIBE
SCURVE
SCYTHE
SEABEE
SEAICE
SEANCE
SEARLE
SECEDE
SECURE
SEDATE
SEDUCE
SEETHE
SELENE
SEMELE
SEMITE
SEMPLE
SEMPRE
SENATE
SENDEE
SENILE
SERAPE
SERENE
SESAME
SESSUE
SETFEE
SETOSE
SETTEE
SETTLE
SEVENE
SEVERE
SEWAGE
SHARPE
SHAYNE
SHEAVE
SHELVE
SHEREE
SHIITE
SHOPPE
SHORTE
SHOWME
SHREVE
SHRIKE
SHRINE
SHRIVE
SHROVE
SICKLE
SIECLE
SIGNEE
SILAGE
SIMILE
SIMONE
SIMPLE
SINGLE
SINISE
SIRREE
SISSLE
SIXEEE
SIXONE
SIZZLE
SKOKIE
SKOPJE
SLEAZE
SLEDGE
SLEEVE
SLOANE
SLUDGE
SLUICE
SMALLE
SMIDGE
SMUDGE
SNEEZE
SNOOZE
SODOWE
SOFINE
SOFTIE
SOIGNE
SOIREE
SOISEE
SOLACE
SOLUTE
SOMBRE
SOOTHE
SOPHIE
SORTIE
SOTRUE
SOURCE
SPARSE
SPATHE
SPEARE
SPECIE
SPENCE
SPHERE
SPLICE
SPLINE
SPONGE
SPOUSE
SPRITE
SPRUCE
SQUARE
SQUIRE
STABLE
STANCE
STAPLE
STARVE
STATUE
STBEDE
STEELE
STEEVE
STEPPE
STERNE
STEVIE
STEWIE
STIFLE
STILLE
STJUDE
STLUKE
STODGE
STOGIE
STOLAE
STOLLE
STOOGE
STPETE
STRAFE
STRIAE
STRIDE
STRIFE
STRIKE
STRIPE
STRIVE
STROBE
STRODE
STROKE
STROVE
STYMIE
SUABLE
SUBDUE
SUBTLE
SUEANE
SUISSE
SUNDAE
SUPINE
SUPPLE
SURETE
SUTURE
SVELTE
SWANEE
SWATHE
SWAYZE
SWERVE

•SE•••

ASEASY
ASEVER
BSEVEN
ESENIN
GSEVEN
ISEEIT
ISELIN
ISERVE
ISEULT
OSETRA
PSEUDO
PSEUDS
TSETSE
USEDCD
USEDIN
USEDON
USEDTO
USEDUP
USEFOR
USEFUL
USENET
USERID
USESIN
USESON
USESUP
USETAX

•S•E••

ASCEND
ASCENT
ASDEEP
ASKERS
ASLEEP
ASNEAR
ASNEAT
ASPECT
ASPENS
ASPERA
ASSENT
ASSERT
ASSESS
ASSETS
ASTEAL
ASTEEP
ASTERN
ASTERO
ASTERS
ASWELL
ESCENT
ESKERS
ESSENE
ESTEEM
ESTERS
ISEEIT
ISLEFT
ISLETS
ISLEYS
ISMENE
ISSEIS
ISWEAR
MSIEUR
OSBERT
OSIERS
OSSETS
OSTEAL
OSTEND
OSTERS
OSWEGO
USHERS
USNEWS

•S••E•

ASDEEP
ASEVER
ASFREE
ASHIER
ASHLEE
ASHLEY
ASHMEN
ASIDES
ASLEEP
ASTEEP
ASTHER
ASTLEY
ASTRES
BSEVEN
BSIDES
ESALEN
ESCHER
ESCHEW
ESPIED
ESPIER
ESPIES
ESTEEM
ESTHER
GSEVEN
ISABEL
ISOHEL
ISOMER
ISRAEL
ISSUED
ISSUER
ISSUES
ISTLES
ISTRES
OSAGES
OSPREY
OSTLER
RSVPED
TSADES
USAGES
USENET
USOPEN
USURER
VSIXES

•S•••E

ASANTE
ASCALE
ASFREE
ASHADE
ASHAME
ASHINE
ASHLEE
ASHORE
ASLOPE
ASPIRE
ASPURE
ASRARE
ASSIZE
ASSUME
ASSURE
ASTARE
ASTUTE
BSCALE
CSCALE
DSCALE
ESCALE
ESCAPE
ESSENE
ESTATE
ESTIME
FSCALE
GSCALE
ISERVE
ISITME
ISLATE
ISLIKE
ISMENE

ISOLDE
OSCINE
OSCULE
OSMOSE
PSYCHE
TSETSE
TSHAPE
USABLE
USANCE
USHAPE
VSHAPE
YSHAPE

••SE••

ABSENT
ANSEIS
ANSELM
ARSENE
ARSENO
ASSENT
ASSERT
ASSESS
ASSETS
AXSEED
BASELY
BASEST
BESETS
BISECT
CASEFY
CASEIN
CASERN
CASERS
COSECS
COSELL
COSETS
CUSECS
DESEED
DESERT
DESETA
DISERE
DISEUR
DOSERS
EASEBY
EASEIN
EASELS
EASEON
EASERS
EASEUP
EDSELS
EISELE
ENSEAL
ENSEAT
ESSENE
ETSEQQ
EXSECT
EXSERT
FUSEES
GISELE
HOSELS
HOSERS
INSEAM
INSECT
INSERT
INSETS
ISSEIS
ITSELF
JOSEPH
LASERS

LOSEIT
LOSERS
LOSETO
MASERS
MASERU
MISERS
MISERY
MOSEYS
MUSEES
MUSEON
MUSEOS
MUSERS
MUSEUM
MYSELF
NASEBY
NISEIS
NOSEIN
NOSERS
NOSEUP
OBSESS
OISEAU
ONSETS
OSSETS
OTSEGO
OUSELS
PASEOS
PESETA
PESEWA
POSEAS
POSERS
POSEUR
RASERS
RESEAL
RESEAM
RESEAT
RESEAU
RESECT
RESEDA
RESEED
RESEEK
RESEEN
RESEES
RESELL
RESEND
RESENT
RESETS
RESEWN
RESEWS
RISERS
RISETO
RISEUP
ROSEAU
ROSERY
ROSETO
ROSEUP
SASEBO
TASERS
TVSETS
UNSEAL
UNSEAM
UNSEAT
UNSEEN
UNSELD
UNSELL
UNSENT
UNSERE
UNSEWN
UNSEWS

UNSEXY
UPSEND
UPSENT
UPSETS
WASECA
WISELY
WISEST
WISETO
WISEUP

••S•E•

AISLED
AISLES
AMSTEL
ANSWER
AUSPEX
AUSTEN
AUSTER
AXSEED
BASHED
BASHER
BASHES
BASKED
BASKER
BASKET
BASSES
BASSET
BASSEY
BASTED
BASTER
BASTES
BESSEL
BESSER
BESTED
BESTER
BISBEE
BISSET
BOSLEY
BOSSED
BOSSES
BUSHED
BUSHEL
BUSHER
BUSHES
BUSIED
BUSIER
BUSIES
BUSKED
BUSKER
BUSMEN
BUSSED
BUSSES
BUSTED
BUSTER
CASHED
CASHES
CASHEW
CASKED
CASKET
CASPER
CASTED
CASTEL
CASTER
CASTES
CESSED
CESSES
CISKEI
COSHED

COSHER
COSHES
COSIED
COSIER
COSIES
COSSET
COSTED
CUSPED
CUSSED
CUSSER
CUSSES
CUSTER
DASHED
DASHER
DASHES
DESEED
DESREE
DESTEM
DISHED
DISHES
DISKED
DISMES
DISNEY
DISPEL
DISSED
DISSES
DOSSED
DOSSES
DUSKED
DUSTED
DUSTER
EASIER
EASLEY
EASTER
EISLEY
EISNER
ENSLER
ENSUED
ENSUES
EUSDEN
FASCES
FASTED
FASTEN
FASTER
FESSED
FESSES
FESTER
FISHED
FISHER
FISHES
FISTED
FOSSES
FOSSEY
FOSTER
FUSEES
FUSSED
FUSSER
FUSSES
GASHED
GASHES
GASJET
GASKET
GASMEN
GASPED
GASPER
GASSED
GASSER
GASSES

GASTER
GESTES
GOSDEN
GOSHEN
GOSPEL
GUSHED
GUSHER
GUSHES
GUSSET
GUSTED
HASHED
HASHES
HASPED
HASSEL
HASTED
HASTEN
HASTES
HESTER
HISSED
HISSER
HISSES
HOSIER
HOSSES
HOSTED
HOSTEL
HUSHED
HUSHES
HUSKED
HUSKER
HUSSEY
IJSSEL
INSTEP
ISSUED
ISSUER
ISSUES
JASPER
JESSEL
JESTED
JESTER
JOSHED
JOSHER
JOSHES
JOSSES
JUSTER
KISLEV
KISMET
KISSED
KISSEL
KISSER
KISSES
KOSHER
KOSSEL
KOSTER
LASHED
LASHER
LASHES
LASKER
LASSEN
LASSER
LASSES
LASTED
LASTEX
LESLEY
LESSEE
LESSEN
LESSER
LESTER
LISLES

LISPED
LISPER
LISSES
LISTED
LISTEE
LISTEN
LISTER
LOSSES
LUSHER
LUSHES
LUSTED
LUSTER
MASHED
MASHER
MASHES
MASKED
MASKER
MASSED
MASSES
MASSEY
MASTED
MASTER
MESHED
MESHES
MESMER
MESNES
MESSED
MESSES
MISFED
MISKEY
MISLED
MISSED
MISSES
MISSET
MISTED
MISTER
MOSDEF
MOSHED
MOSHER
MOSHES
MOSLEM
MOSLEY
MOSSED
MOSSES
MOSTEL
MUSEES
MUSHED
MUSHER
MUSHES
MUSKET
MUSSED
MUSSEL
MUSSES
MUSSET
MUSTER
NASHES
NASSER
NESSEN
NESSES
NESTEA
NESTED
NESTER
NISSEN
NOSHED
NOSHER
NOSHES
NOSIER
NOSTEP

NOSTER
ONSPEC
OUSTED
OUSTER
OYSTER
PASSED
PASSEL
PASSER
PASSES
PASTED
PASTEL
PASTER
PASTES
PESTER
PISCES
PISHED
PISHES
PISTES
POSHER
POSIES
POSSES
POSTED
POSTER
PUSHED
PUSHER
PUSHES
PUSSES
RASHER
RASHES
RASPED
RASPER
RASSES
RASTER
RESEED
RESEEK
RESEEN
RESEES
RESHES
RESTED
RESTER
RESTES
RISKED
RISKER
ROSIER
ROSIES
ROSSEN
ROSSET
ROSTEN
ROSTER
RUSHED
RUSHEE
RUSHER
RUSHES
RUSSEL
RUSSES
RUSSET
RUSTED
SASHED
SASHES
SASSED
SASSER
SASSES
SESTET
SISKEL
SISLER
SISLEY
SISTER
SUSSED

SUSSES
SUSSEX
SYSTEM
TASKED
TASKET
TASSEL
TASSES
TASTED
TASTEE
TASTER
TASTES
TESTED
TESTEE
TESTER
TISKET
TOSSED
TOSSER
TOSSES
TUSHES
TUSKED
TUSKER
TUSSES
ULSTER
UNSEEN
UNSHED
UNSKEW
UNSTEP
UNSUED
UPSTEP
VASTER
VESPER
VESSEL
VESTED
VESTEE
VISAED
VOSGES
WASHED
WASHER
WASHES
WASLED
WASMET
WASSER
WASTED
WASTER
WASTES
WESKER
WESLEY
WESSEX
WESTER
WISHED
WISHER
WISHES
WISPED
WISTER
WUSSES
XYSTER
YASSER
YESMEN
YESSED
YESSES
YESTER
YESYES
ZESTED
ZESTER

••S••E

ALSACE
ANSATE

ARSENE
ASSIZE
ASSUME
ASSURE
AUSSIE
BASQUE
BESAME
BESIDE
BESORE
BESSIE
BESURE
BISBEE
BISQUE
BUSTLE
BYSSHE
CASQUE
CASSIE
CASTLE
CESARE
COSINE
COSTAE
DESADE
DESIRE
DESREE
DISERE
DISUSE
DOSAGE
EISELE
ENSATE
ENSILE
ENSURE
ESSENE
FESCUE
FOSSAE
FUSILE
GESTAE
GISELE
HASONE
HASSLE
HUSTLE
IMSURE
INSANE
INSIDE
INSOLE
INSURE
JESSYE
JOSTLE
JUSQUE
JUSTME
KISHKE
KISSME
LASSIE
LESAGE
LESLIE
LESSEE
LISTEE
LUSTRE
LYSINE
MASHIE
MASQUE
MISCUE
MISSME
MISUSE
MOSQUE
MUSCLE
MUSKIE
MYSORE
NESSIE

NESTLE
NOSALE
OHSURE
ONSALE
ONSIDE
ONSITE
PESADE
PESTLE
POSOLE
POSTIE
RASCHE
RASSLE
RASURE
RESALE
RESAVE
RESCUE
RESHOE
RESIDE
RESILE
RESITE
RESIZE
RESOLE
RESUME
RISQUE
ROSCOE
RUSHEE
RUSTLE
SESAME
SESSUE
SISSLE
TASTEE
TESSIE
TESTAE
TESTEE
TISANE
TISSUE
TUSHIE
TUSSLE
UGSOME
UNSAFE
UNSAGE
UNSERE
UNSHOE
UNSOLE
UNSORE
UNSURE
UPSIDE
UPSIZE
URSINE
VESTEE
VISAGE
VISINE
WASHME
WASHOE
WESTIE

•••SE•

ABASED
ABASER
ABASES
ABUSED
ABUSER
ABUSES
AIRSEA
ALLSET
AMUSED
AMUSER
AMUSES

ANISES
ARCSEC
ARISEN
ARISES
ATISES
AXISES
BASSES
BASSET
BASSEY
BENSEY
BESSEL
BESSER
BETSEY
BIASED
BIASES
BISSET
BOSSED
BOSSES
BOXSET
BRISES
BUNSEN
BUSSED
BUSSES
CARSEY
CAUSED
CAUSER
CAUSES
CEASED
CEASES
CENSED
CENSER
CENSES
CESSED
CESSES
CHASED
CHASER
CHASES
CHISEL
CHOSEN
CLOSED
CLOSER
CLOSES
CLOSET
COPSES
CORSET
COSSET
CRISES
CRUSES
CURSED
CURSER
CURSES
CUSSED
CUSSER
CUSSES
DAISES
DAMSEL
DANSES
DENSER
DIESEL
DIESES
DILSEY
DISSED
DISSES
DNASES
DOASET
DORSET
DORSEY
DOSSED

DOSSES
DOUSED
DOUSER
DOUSES
DOWSED
DOWSER
DOWSES
DRUSES
EGISES
ELISEO
ELYSEE
EPOSES
ERASED
ERASER
ERASES
FALSER
FESSED
FESSES
FINSEN
FOSSES
FOSSEY
FRASER
FRISEE
FRISES
FUSSED
FUSSER
FUSSES
GASSED
GASSER
GASSES
GEISEL
GELSEY
GETSET
GEYSER
GLASER
GNOSES
GOOSED
GOOSEN
GOOSES
GOOSEY
GORSES
GOTSET
GUISES
GUNSEL
GUSSET
HALSEY
HANSEL
HANSES
HASSEL
HAWSER
HAWSES
HERSEY
HEUSEN
HISSED
HISSER
HISSES
HORSED
HORSES
HORSEY
HOSSES
HOUSED
HOUSES
HOWSER
HUSSEY
IBISES
IJSSEL
ILLSEE
ILLSET

INASEC
IRISED
IRISES
JANSEN
JENSEN
JERSEY
JESSEL
JETSET
JOSSES
JOZSEF
KAISER
KELSEY
KERSEE
KEYSER
KINSEY
KISSED
KISSEL
KISSER
KISSES
KOSSEL
LAPSED
LAPSER
LAPSES
LARSEN
LASSEN
LASSER
LASSES
LEASED
LEASER
LEASES
LEISEN
LENSED
LENSES
LESSEE
LESSEN
LESSER
LISSES
LOOSED
LOOSEN
LOOSER
LOOSES
LOOSEY
LOSSES
LOUSED
LOUSES
LOWSET
MADSEN
MANSES
MASSED
MASSES
MASSEY
MAUSER
MERSEY
MESSED
MESSES
MISSED
MISSES
MISSET
MOISES
MORSEL
MOSSED
MOSSES
MOUSED
MOUSER
MOUSES
MOUSEY
MUSSED
MUSSEL

MUSSES
MUSSET
NANSEN
NASSER
NAUSEA
NESSEN
NESSES
NIPSEY
NISSEN
NOISED
NOISES
NOOSED
NOOSER
NOOSES
NURSED
NURSER
NURSES
OCASEK
OCASEY
OFFSET
ONESEC
ONESET
ONUSES
OPUSES
OTOSES
OUTSEE
OUTSET
PAISES
PARSEC
PARSED
PARSEE
PARSER
PARSES
PASSED
PASSEL
PASSER
PASSES
PAUSED
PAUSER
PAUSES
PCUSER
PENSEE
PHASED
PHASER
PHASES
PHYSED
PLUSES
POISED
POISER
POISES
POSSES
POYSER
PRESET
PRISED
PROSED
PROSER
PROSES
PULSED
PULSES
PURSED
PURSER
PURSES
PUSSES
RAISED
RAISER
RAISES
RAMSES
RAMSEY

RASSES
REDSEA
REESES
REISER
REMSEN
REUSED
REUSER
REUSES
RIESEN
RINSED
RINSER
RINSES
ROSSEN
ROSSET
ROUSED
ROUSER
ROUSES
RUSSEL
RUSSES
RUSSET
SANSEI
SASSED
SASSER
SASSES
SENSED
SENSEI
SENSEN
SENSES
SOISEE
SOUSED
SOUSES
STASES
SUBSEA
SUBSET
SUDSED
SUDSER
SUDSES
SUNSET
SUSSED
SUSSES
SUSSEX
TABSET
TASSEL
TASSES
TEASED
TEASEL
TEASER
TEASES
TEASET
TENSED
TENSER
TENSES
TERSER
THESEA
THESES
TINSEL
TMESES
TOSSED
TOSSER
TOSSES
TUSSES
UKASES
UNDSET
UNISEX
UNUSED
VALSES
VELSEN
VERSED

VERSES
VERSET
VESSEL
WASSER
WEASEL
WESSEX
WIESEL
WIMSEY
WOLSEY
WORSEN
WUSSES
XMASES
YASSER
YATSEN
YESSED
YESSES
YOUSEE

•••S•E
ADESTE
AUSSIE
BESSIE
BROSSE
BURSAE
BYSSHE
CASSIE
CHASSE
CHASTE
CLASSE
CROSSE
CRUSOE
EENSIE
ELYSEE
ENISLE
FOCSLE
FOSSAE
FRISEE
FUISSE
GROSSE
HASSLE
ILLSEE
INESSE
JESSYE
KERSEE
KISSME
KRESGE
LASSIE
LESSEE
LETSBE
MAISIE
MEASLE
MISSME
MOUSSE
NEISSE
NESSIE
NEWSIE
OUTSEE
PARSEE
PENSEE
PLISSE
POTSIE
POUSSE
PURSUE
RASSLE
SESSUE
SISSLE
SOISEE
SUISSE
TESSIE
THISBE
TISSUE
TOUSLE
TRISTE
TUSSLE
WRASSE
YOUSEE

••••SE
ACCUSE
ADVISE
AHORSE
APPOSE
ARIOSE
AROUSE
ATEASE
AVERSE
AVULSE
BEARSE
BEMUSE
BLAISE
BLOUSE
BOURSE
BRAISE
BROSSE
BROWSE
BRUISE
CAMISE
CAYUSE
CDCASE
CERISE
CHAISE
CHASSE
CHEESE
CHOOSE
CLASSE
CLAUSE
CLEESE
COARSE
CORPSE
COURSE
CREASE
CREUSE
CROSSE
CROUSE
CRUISE
DEBASE
DEFUSE
DEMISE
DENISE
DEPOSE
DEROSE
DEVISE
DISUSE
DNAASE
DROWSE
DUBOSE
ECORSE
EFFUSE
EGLISE
ELAPSE
ELOISE
ENCASE
ENDUSE
EVULSE
EXCISE
EXCUSE
EXPOSE
FILOSE
FLENSE
FRAISE
FUISSE
GREASE
GRIESE
GROSSE
GROUSE
HEARSE
HEINSE
HEXOSE
HOARSE
ILLUSE
IMPOSE
INCASE
INCISE
INCUSE
INESSE
INFUSE
IODISE
IONISE
IRAISE
JOCOSE
LANOSE
LAOTSE
LETUSE
LHOTSE
LIAISE
LIPASE
LOUISE
MISUSE
MOROSE
MOUSSE
NEISSE
NODOSE
NOLOSE
NONUSE
NOWISE
OBTUSE
ODENSE
ONBASE
OPPOSE
ORELSE
ORENSE
OSMOSE
OTIOSE
PAVESE
PERUSE
PHRASE
PILOSE
PLEASE
PLISSE
POROSE
POUSSE
PRAISE
PROWSE
RAMOSE
RECASE
RECUSE
REDOSE
REFUSE
RELOSE
REMISE
REPOSE
RERISE
REROSE
REVISE
RIBOSE
RIMOSE
RNAASE
SETOSE
SINISE
SPARSE
SPOUSE
SUISSE
TALESE
TSETSE
UNCASE
UNEASE
UNWISE
UPRISE
UPROSE
VALISE
VARESE
VENOSE
WRASSE
XYLOSE
ZYMASE

SF••••
SFORZA

S•F•••
SAFARI
SAFECO
SAFELY
SAFEST
SAFETY
SAFIRE
SIFTED
SIFTER
SOFFIT
SOFINE
SOFTEN
SOFTER
SOFTIE
SOFTLY
SOFTON
SUFFER
SUFFIX
SUFISM

S••F••
SACFLY
SATFOR
SAWFIT
SCOFFS
SCUFFS
SEAFOX
SEEFIT
SETFEE
SETFOR
SHAFTS
SHIFTS
SHIFTY
SHOFAR
SINFUL
SITFOR
SKIFFS
SLYFOX
SNAFUS
SNIFFS
SNIFFY
SNUFFS
SNUFFY
SOBFUL
SOFFIT
SOXFAN
SPIFFS
SPIFFY
STAFFS
STEFAN
STEFFI
STEFOY
STIFFS
STIFLE
STUFFS
STUFFY
SUEFOR
SUFFER
SUFFIX
SULFAS
SULFUR
SUNFAN
SURFED
SURFER
SURFIN
SWIFTS

S•••F•
SALIFY
SAWOFF
SCARFS
SCLAFF
SCOFFS
SCRUFF
SCUFFS
SCURFY
SEEOFF
SERIFS
SETOFF
SHRIFT
SKIFFS
SMURFS
SNARFS
SNIFFS
SNIFFY
SNUFFS
SNUFFY
SPIFFS
SPIFFY
SPOOFS
STAFFS
STEFFI
STIFFS
STRAFE
STRIFE
STUFFS
STUFFY

S••••F
SAWOFF
SCLAFF
SCRUFF
SEEOFF
SETOFF
SHARIF
SICKOF
SMALLF
SORTOF
STAPUF
STOLAF
SUREOF

•SF•••
ASFAST
ASFLAT
ASFREE
USFLAG

•S•F••
ASKFOR
USEFOR
USEFUL

•S••F•
ASSOFT
ISLEFT
OSSIFY

•S•••F
ASKSOF

••SF••
HASFUN
ITSFUN
MISFED
MISFIT
WASFUN

••S•F•
ASSOFT
BASIFY
CASEFY
GASIFY
GOSOFT
OSSIFY
RESIFT
UNSAFE
UNSOFT
WASOFF

••S••F
ITSELF
MASSIF
MOSDEF
MOSTOF
MYSELF
WASOFF

•••S•F
ASKSOF
EATSOF
GOBSOF
JOZSEF
LOTSOF
MASSIF
RIDSOF
ROBSOF
TONSOF
YOUSUF

SG••••
SGTMAJ

S•G•••
SAGELY
SAGEST
SAGGED
SAGIER
SEGUED
SEGUES
SEGURA
SEGWAY
SIGHAT
SIGHED
SIGHER
SIGHTS
SIGILS
SIGLER
SIGMAS
SIGNAL
SIGNED
SIGNEE
SIGNER
SIGNET
SIGNIN
SIGNON
SIGNOR
SIGNUP
SIGURD
SUGARS
SUGARY

S••G••
SAGGED
SAIGON
SANGER
SANGRE
SANGTO
SARGES
SARGON
SCAGGS
SEAGAL
SEAGOD
SEDGED
SEDGES
SEEGER
SERGEI
SERGES
SERGIO
SHAGGY
SHOGIS
SHOGUN
SIEGED
SIEGEL
SIEGES
SINGED
SINGER
SINGES
SINGIN
SINGLE
SINGLY
SINGTO
SIXGUN
SKAGGS
SLIGHT
SLOGAN
SLUGGO
SMOGGY
SMUGLY
SNAGGY
SNAGUP
SNUGLI
SNUGLY
SOIGNE
SOUGHT
SPIGOT
STAGED
STAGER
STAGES
STAGEY
STIGMA
STOGIE
SUBGOD
SUBGUM
SUNGOD
SUNGTO
SURGED
SURGES

S•••G•
SAVAGE
SCAGGS
SCRAGS
SEWAGE
SHAGGY
SHRUGS
SILAGE
SKAGGS
SLANGS
SLANGY
SLEDGE
SLEIGH
SLINGS
SLOUGH
SLOWGO
SLUDGE
SLUDGY
SLUGGO
SMIDGE
SMOGGY
SMUDGE
SMUDGY
SNAGGY
SPONGE
SPONGY
SPRIGS
STINGS
STINGY
STODGE
STODGY
STOOGE
STOPGO
SWINGS
SWINGY
SYZYGY

S••••G
SARONG
SATING
SAVING
SAWING
SAWLOG
SAYING
SEABAG
SEADOG
SEAHAG
SEBERG
SEEING
SEWING
SHYING
SIDING
SIRING
SITING
SIZING
SKIING
SKYING
SLUING
SMALLG
SOLING
SOLONG
SONTAG
SOWING
SPRANG
SPRING
SPRUNG
SPYING
STALAG
STENOG
STRING
STRONG
STRUNG
STYING
SUNDOG
SUPERG

•SG•••
ASGARD
ASGOOD
OSGOOD
TSGARP

•S•G••
ISOGON
OSAGES
USAGES
VSIGNS

•S••G•
ASIAGO
ASSIGN
OSWEGO

•S•••G
ASHING
ASKING
ISLING
TSKING
USFLAG
USHING

••SG••
PISGAH
VOSGES
YASGUR

••S•G•
ASSIGN
ATSIGN
COSIGN
DESIGN
DOSAGE
EASYGO
ENSIGN
HASAGO
ITSAGO
LESAGE
OKSIGN
OTSEGO
PASSGO
RESIGN
UNSAGE
VISAGE

••S••G
BASING
BUSING
CASING
DESMOG
DOSING
EASING
FUSING
GASBAG
GASHOG
GASLOG
GOSTAG
HOSING
HUSING
LASING
LOSING
MUSING
NOSING
POSING
RASING
RESANG
RESING
RISING
UNSMUG
UNSNAG
UNSNUG
UNSUNG
VISING
WISING

•••SG•
KRESGE
LETSGO
PASSGO

SH••••
SHABBY
SHACKS
SHADED
SHADER
SHADES
SHADOW
SHAFTS
SHAGGY
SHAKEN
SHAKER
SHAKES
SHAKIN
SHAKOS
SHAKUR
SHALES
SHALEY
SHALIT
SHALLI
SHALLY
SHALOM
SHAMAN
SHAMED
SHAMES
SHAMIR
SHAMMY
SHAMUS
SHANDY
SHANIA
SHANKS
SHANTY
SHAPED
SHAPER
SHAPES
SHARDS
SHARED
SHARER
SHARES
SHARIF
SHARKS
SHARON
SHARPE
SHARPS
SHARPY
SHARYN
SHASTA
SHAVED
SHAVEN
SHAVER
SHAVES
SHAWLS
SHAYNE
SHAZAM
SHBOOM
SHEARS
SHEATH
SHEAVE
SHEBAT
SHEBOP
SHECKY
SHEDDS
SHEDON
SHEEDY
SHEEHY
SHEENA
SHEENS
SHEENY
SHEERS
SHEESH
SHEETS
SHEIKH
SHEIKS
SHEILA
SHEKEL
SHELBY
SHELLS
SHELTY
SHELVE
SHEREE
SHERPA
SHERRI
SHERRY
SHERYL
SHEVAT
SHHHHH
SHIELD
SHIEST
SHIFTS
SHIFTY
SHIISM
SHIITE
SHILLS
SHILLY
SHILOH
SHIMMY
SHIMON
SHINDY
SHINED
SHINER
SHINES
SHINNY
SHINTO
SHIPTO
SHIRAZ
SHIRER
SHIRES
SHIRKS
SHIRRS
SHIRTS
SHIVER
SHLOCK
SHNOOK
SHOALS
SHOALY
SHOATS
SHOCKS
SHODDY
SHOERS
SHOFAR
SHOGIS
SHOGUN
SHOJIS
SHOLEM
SHOLOM
SHOOED
SHOOIN
SHOOTS
SHOPAT
SHOPKO
SHOPPE
SHORES
SHORTA
SHORTE
SHORTI
SHORTO
SHORTS
SHORTU
SHORTY
SHORTZ
SHOTAT
SHOTBY
SHOTUP
SHOULD
SHOUTS
SHOVED
SHOVEL
SHOVER
SHOVES
SHOWED
SHOWER
SHOWIN
SHOWME
SHOWUP
SHRANK
SHREDS
SHREVE
SHREWD
SHREWS
SHRIEK
SHRIFT
SHRIKE
SHRILL
SHRIMP
SHRINE
SHRINK
SHRIVE
SHROUD
SHROVE
SHRUBS
SHRUGS
SHRUNK
SHTETL
SHTICK
SHUCKS
SHULTZ
SHUMAI
SHUNTS
SHUTIN
SHUTUP
SHYEST
SHYING

S•H•••
SAHARA
SAHIBS
SCHAAP
SCHAVS
SCHEIB
SCHELL
SCHEMA
SCHEME
SCHICK
SCHISM
SCHIST
SCHLEP
SCHLUB
SCHMOS
SCHNOZ
SCHOLL
SCHOOL
SCHORR
SCHULZ
SCHUSS
SCHWAB
SCHWAS
SHHHHH
SPHERE
SPHINX
SPHYNX

S••H••
SACHEM
SACHER
SACHET
SADHES
SADHUS
SASHAY
SASHED
SASHES
SAYHEY
SEAHAG
SENHOR
SEPHIA
SHHHHH
SIGHAT
SIGHED
SIGHER
SIGHTS
SIPHON
SKIHAT
SOPHIA
SOPHIE
SOTHAT
SOTHEN
SOWHAT
SUCHAS
SUNHAT
SUSHIS

S•••H•
SAIDHI
SANCHO
SANTHA
SAPPHO
SAYSHI
SCATHE
SCYTHE
SEETHE
SEZWHO
SHEEHY
SHHHHH
SIXTHS
SLIGHT
SLITHY
SLOSHY
SLOTHS
SLUSHY
SMITHS
SMITHY
SNATHS
SOOTHE
SOUGHT
SOUTHS
SPATHE
STAPHS
STETHO
STJOHN
STROHS
SURAHS
SWATHE
SWATHS
SWISHY
SYLPHS
SYNCHS
SYNTHS

S••••H
SAIDAH
SALISH
SAMEKH
SAYAAH
SAYSAH
SCORCH
SCOTCH
SEARCH
SERAPH
SHEATH
SHEESH
SHEIKH
SHHHHH
SHILOH
SIRRAH
SKETCH
SKITCH
SLEIGH
SLEUTH
SLOUCH
SLOUGH
SMALLH
SMERSH
SMIRCH
SMOOCH
SMOOSH
SMOOTH
SNATCH
SNITCH
SOMUCH
SPEECH
SPILTH
SPLASH
SPLOSH
SPRACH
SQUASH
SQUISH
STANCH
STARCH
STENCH
STITCH
STORCH
SWATCH
SWITCH
SWOOSH

•SH•••
ASHADE
ASHAME
ASHARP
ASHBIN
ASHCAN
ASHDOD
ASHIER
ASHINE
ASHING
ASHLAR
ASHLEE
ASHLEY
ASHMAN
ASHMEN
ASHORE
ASHPAN
ASHPIT
ASHRAM
ASHTON
BSHARP
CSHARP
DSHARP
ESHARP
ESHKOL
FSHARP
GSHARP
ISHTAR
OSHAWA
PSHAWS
TSHAPE
TSHIRT
USHAPE
USHERS
USHING
VSHAPE
YSHAPE

•S•H••
ASTHER
ASTHMA
ESCHER
ESCHEW
ESTHER
ISCHIA
ISOHEL
ISTHMI

•S••H•
PSYCHE

PSYCHO PSYCHS

•S•••H

ASLOSH ASMUCH ASPISH ASSUCH ISAIAH JSBACH

••SH••

BASHED BASHER BASHES BASHIN BBSHOT BISHOP BUSHED BUSHEL BUSHER BUSHES BUSHWA CASHED CASHES CASHEW CASHIN COSHED COSHER COSHES CUSHAW DASHED DASHER DASHES DASHIS DASHIT DISHED DISHES DISHUP FISHED FISHER FISHES GASHED GASHES GASHOG GOSHEN GUSHED GUSHER GUSHES HASHED HASHES HUSHED HUSHES HUSHUP ITSHOT JOSHED JOSHER JOSHES JOSHUA KASHAS KESHIA KISHKA KISHKE KOSHER LASHED LASHER LASHES LASHTO LASHUP LESHAN LUSHER LUSHES LUSHLY MASHED MASHER MASHES MASHIE MASHUP MESHED MESHES MISHAP MISHIT MOSHAV MOSHED MOSHER MOSHES MUSHED MUSHER MUSHES NASHES NASHUA NOSHED NOSHER NOSHES NOSHOW ONSHOW PASHAS PASHTO PISHED PISHES POSHER POSHLY PUSHED PUSHER PUSHES PUSHIN PUSHIT PUSHON PUSHUP RASHAD RASHER RASHES RASHID RASHLY RESHES RESHIP RESHOD RESHOE RESHOT RESHOW RESHUT RISHIS ROSHIS RUSHAT RUSHBY RUSHED RUSHEE RUSHER RUSHES RUSHIN RUSHTO SASHAY SASHED SASHES SUSHIS TISHRI TUSHES TUSHIE TVSHOW UNSHED UNSHIP UNSHOD UNSHOE UNSHUT UPSHAW UPSHOT VASHTI VISHNU WASHAD WASHED WASHER WASHES WASHME WASHOE WASHOS WASHUP WISHED WISHER WISHES WISHIN WISHON WISHTO YASHIN

••S•H•

BYSSHE JASCHA MISCHA PASCHS RASCHE

••S••H

ASSUCH BASRAH CASBAH JOSEPH JOSIAH KASBAH PESACH PISGAH

•••SH•

AYESHA BAKSHI BOLSHY BRASHY BRUSHY BUQSHA BYSSHE ELISHA FLASHY FLESHY GEISHA GRISHA GUNSHY HONSHU KYUSHU MARSHA MARSHY MOESHA NEOSHO OLESHA PLASHY PLUSHY POISHA SAYSHI SLOSHY SLUSHY SWISHY TRASHY TRISHA

•••S•H

BAUSCH BORSCH FRISCH HIRSCH KIRSCH KITSCH MENSCH PUTSCH SAYSAH

••••SH

ABLUSH AFRESH AGUISH AMBUSH ASLOSH ASPISH BANISH BLUISH BOYISH BYGOSH CALASH COWISH COYISH DANISH DELISH DOVISH DRYISH DUDISH ELFISH ELVISH EMDASH ENDASH ENMESH FAMISH FETISH FINISH FLUISH FLYASH FYVUSH GALOSH GARISH GHIRSH GOFISH HEWISH IMPISH INCASH INDASH INRUSH IRTYSH JADISH JEWISH KIBOSH LATISH LAVISH LOWISH MANUSH MODISH MOPISH MULISH MYGOSH NEWISH NORUSH OAFISH ODDISH OFFISH OGRISH OHGOSH OLDISH ONEISH ONRUSH OWLISH PALISH PARISH PERISH POLISH POPISH POTASH PUNISH RADISH RAKISH RAVISH RAWISH REHASH RELISH REWASH SALISH SHEESH SMERSH SMOOSH SPLASH SPLOSH SQUASH SQUISH SWOOSH THRASH THRESH THRUSH UNLASH UNLUSH UNMESH UNPOSH UNRASH UNWISH UPPISH UPRUSH VANISH WABASH WHOOSH WIDISH WINISH

SI••••

SIBYLS SICCED SICILY SICKEN SICKER SICKLE SICKLY SICKOF SICKOS SIDDUR SIDING SIDLED SIDLES SIDNEY SIEBEN SIECLE SIEGED SIEGEL SIEGES SIENNA SIERRA SIESTA SIETES SIEVED SIEVES SIFTED SIFTER SIGHAT SIGHED SIGHER SIGHTS SIGILS SIGLER SIGMAS SIGNAL SIGNED SIGNEE SIGNER SIGNET SIGNIN SIGNON SIGNOR SIGNUP SIGURD SIKKIM SILAGE SILENT SILICA SILKEN SILOED SILTED SILVAS SILVER SIMEON SIMIAN SIMILE SIMMER SIMONE SIMPER SIMPLE SIMPLY SINBAD SINEAD SINEWS SINEWY SINFUL SINGED SINGER SINGES SINGIN SINGLE SINGLY SINGTO SINISE SINKER SINKIN SINNED SINNER SINTAX SIOUAN SIPHON SIPPED SIPPER SIPSON SIRBEN SIRENS SIRICA SIRING SIRIUS SIRKAY SIRRAH SIRREE SIRUPS SISALS SISISI SISKEL SISLER SISLEY SISSLE SISTER SITARS SITCOM SITFOR SITING SITINS SITOUT SITPAT SITSAT SITSBY SITSIN SITSON SITSUP SITTER SITTIN SITUPS SIVANS SIXDAY SIXEEE SIXERS SIXGUN SIXONE SIXPIN SIXSIX SIXTEN SIXTHS SIXTUS SIXTWO SIXWAY SIZERS SIZEUP SIZING SIZZLE

S•I•••

SAIDAH SAIDHI SAIDNO SAIDOK SAIDSO SAIDTO SAIGON SAILED SAILER SAILON SAILOR SAILTO SAINTE SAINTS SAIPAN SAISON SAITEK SCIONS SCIPIO SEIKOS SEINED SEINER SEINES SEISMO SEISMS SEIZED SEIZER SEIZES SEIZOR SHIELD SHIEST SHIFTS SHIFTY SHIISM SHIITE SHILLS SHILLY SHILOH SHIMMY SHIMON SHINDY SHINED SHINER SHINES SHINNY SHINTO SHIPTO SHIRAZ SHIRER SHIRES SHIRKS SHIRRS SHIRTS SHIVER SKIBIB SKIBOB SKIBUM SKICAP SKIDDY SKIDOO SKIERS SKIFFS SKIHAT SKIING SKILLS SKIMPS SKIMPY SKINKS SKINNY SKIPBY SKIPIT SKIPPY SKIRLS SKIRTS SKIRUN SKITCH SKITOW SKIWAX SLICED SLICER SLICES SLICKS SLIDER SLIDES SLIDIN SLIEST SLIGHT SLIMED SLIMES SLIMLY SLINGS SLINKS SLINKY SLIPBY SLIPIN SLIPON SLIPPY SLIPUP SLITHY SLIVER SMIDGE SMILED SMILER SMILES SMILEY SMILLA SMIRCH SMIRKS SMIRKY SMITER SMITES SMITHS SMITHY SMITTY SNICKS SNIDER SNIFFS SNIFFY SNIPED SNIPER SNIPES SNIPPY SNITCH SNIVEL SOIGNE SOILED SOIREE SOISEE SOITIS SPICED SPICER SPICES SPIDER SPIDEY SPIELS SPIERS SPIFFS SPIFFY SPIGOT SPIKED SPIKER SPIKES SPILES SPILLS SPILTH SPINAL SPINED SPINEL SPINER SPINES SPINET SPINKS SPIRAL SPIREA SPIRED SPIRES SPIRIT SPITED SPITES SPITON SPIVAK STICKS STICKY STIDES STIERS STIFFS STIFLE STIGMA STILES STILLE STILLS STILLY STILTS STIMPY STINGS STINGY STINKO STINKS STINKY STINTS STIPES STIRIN STIRUP STITCH STIVIC SUISSE SUITED SUITES SUITOR SUITUP SWIFTS SWILLS SWINGS SWINGY SWIPED SWIPER SWIPES SWIRLS SWIRLY SWIRLZ SWISHY SWITCH SWIVEL SWIVET

S••I••

SABINA SABINE SADISM SADIST SAFIRE SAGIER SAHIBS SALIFY SALINA SALINE SALISH SALIVA SAMIAM SANITY SATING SATINS SATINY SATIRE SAVING SAVIOR SAWING SAYIDO SAYING SCHICK SCHISM SCHIST SCRIBE SCRIMP SCRIMS SCRIPS SCRIPT SEAICE SEDICI SEEING SEMITE SENILE SENIOR SENITI SEPIAS SEPIRA SERIAL SERIES SERIFS SERINS SEWING SEWIST SEXIER SEXILY SEXISM SEXIST SHEIKH SHEIKS SHEILA SHIISM SHIITE SHRIEK SHRIFT SHRIKE SHRILL SHRIMP SHRINE SHRINK SHRIVE SHTICK SHYING SICILY SIDING SIGILS SILICA SIMIAN SIMILE SINISE SIRICA SIRING SIRIUS SISISI SITING SITINS SIZING SKEINS SKIING SKYING SLEIGH SLUICE SLUING SNAILS SOCIAL SODIDI SODIUM SOFINE SOLIDS SOLING SONICS SOVIET SOWING SOYINK SPHINX SPLICE SPLINE SPLINT SPLITS SPOILS SPOILT SPRIER SPRIGS SPRING SPRINT SPRITE SPRITS SPRITZ SPYING SQUIBB SQUIBS SQUIDS SQUINT SQUIRE SQUIRM SQUIRT SQUISH STAINS STAIRS STEINS STNICK STOICS STPIUS STRIAE STRICT STRIDE STRIFE STRIKE STRING STRIPE STRIPS STRIPY STRIVE STYING SUBITO SUFISM SUPINE SURIMI SUZIEQ SWAINS SYRIAN

S•••I•

SALLIE SALMIS SALTII SANDIA SANKIN SARDIS SARNIA SAUDIS SAVAII SAVEIT SAVOIE SAVOIR SAWFIT SAWPIT SAYDIE SCALIA SCENIC SCHEIB SCIPIO SCORIA SCOTIA SEAAIR SEALIN SEEFIT SEENIN SEEPIN SEESIN SELLIT SENDIN SENTIN SEPHIA SEPTIC SEQUIN SERAIS SERBIA SERGIO SERKIN SERKIS SETSIN SEWNIN SEWSIN SHAKIN SHALIT SHAMIR SHANIA SHARIF SHOGIS SHOJIS SHOOIN SHOWIN SHUTIN SIGNIN SIKKIM SINGIN SINKIN SITSIN SITTIN SIXPIN SIXSIX SKIBIB SKIPIT SKOKIE SKYLIT SLAVIC SLIDIN SLIPIN SNOWIN SOAKIN SOBEIT SOCKIN SOFFIT SOFTIE SOITIS SOLDIT SOLEIL SOPHIA SOPHIE SORBIC SORDID SORTIE SPECIE SPIRIT SPRAIN STADIA STALIN STARIN STASIS STATIC STATIN STAYIN STEPIN STERIC STEVIE STEWIE STIRIN STIVIC STOGIE STOLID STOPIN STOPIT STOTIN STOWIT STRAIN STRAIT STUDIO STUPID STYMIE SUBLID SUBMIT SUCKIN SUFFIX SUMMIT SUNKIN SUNLIT SUNNIS SUREIS SURFIN SUSHIS SWAMIS SYLVIA SYNDIC

S••••I

SAFARI SAIDHI SALAMI SALTII SALUKI SAMEDI SANSEI SATORI SAVAII SAYSHI SCAASI SCAMPI SCENEI SEDICI SENITI SENSEI SERGEI SESQUI SHALLI SHERRI SHORTI SHUMAI SISISI SMALLI SNORRI SNUGLI SOCANI SODIDI SOLATI SOMALI SOMONI SOONYI STEFFI STRATI SURIMI SUUKYI SUVARI SUZUKI

•SI•••

ASIAGO ASIANS ASIDES ASIMOV BSIDES GSIXTY ISIDOR ISIDRO ISINTO ISITME MSIEUR OSIERS OSIRIS VSIGNS VSIXES YSIDRO

•S•I••

ASDICS ASHIER ASHINE ASHING ASKING ASPICS ASPIRE ASPISH ASSIGN ASSISI ASSIST ASSIZE ASWIRL ESKIMO ESPIAL ESPIED ESPIER ESPIES ESPIOS ESTIME GSUITS ISAIAH ISAIAN ISLIKE ISLING KSWISS OSCINE OSMICS

OSMIUM
OSSIAN
OSSIFY
TSHIRT
TSKING
USHING
USMINT

•S••I•
ASHBIN
ASHPIT
ASKSIN
ASONIA
ASSAIL
ASTRID
ESENIN
ESPRIT
ESSAIS
ESTLIN
ISCHIA
ISEEIT
ISELIN
ISMAIL
ISRAIR
ISSEIS
ISTRIA
OSIRIS
TSADIS
TSURIS
USEDIN
USERID
USESIN
USMAIL

•S•••I
ASSISI
ISANTI
ISTHMI
TSOTSI

••SI••
ASSIGN
ASSISI
ASSIST
ASSIZE
ATSIGN
BASIAL
BASICS
BASIFY
BASILS
BASING
BASINS
BESIDE
BUSIED
BUSIER
BUSIES
BUSILY
BUSING
CASING
CASINO
CASIOS
CASITA
CESIUM
COSIED
COSIER
COSIES
COSIGN
COSILY
COSINE
DESICA
DESIGN
DESILT
DESILU
DESIRE
DESIST
DOSIDO
DOSING
EASIER
EASILY
EASING
ENSIGN
ENSILE
EOSINS
FUSILE
FUSILS
FUSING
FUSION
GASIFY
HESIOD
HOSIER
HOSING
HUSING
INSIDE
INSIST
INSITU
JOSIAH
LASING
LESION
LOSING
LYSINE
MESIAL
MUSIAL
MUSICK
MUSICS
MUSING
NOSIER
NOSILY
NOSING
OKSIGN
ONSIDE
ONSITE
ORSINI
ORSINO
OSSIAN
OSSIFY
POSIES
POSING
POSITS
RASING
RESIDE
RESIFT
RESIGN
RESILE
RESING
RESINK
RESINS
RESINY
RESIST
RESITE
RESITS
RESIZE
RISING
ROSIER
ROSIES
ROSILY
ROSINA
ROSINS
ROSINY
ROSITA
SISISI
UNSICK
UPSIDE
UPSIZE
URSIDS
URSINE
VASILY
VISINE
VISING
VISION
VISITS
WISING
YESIAM
YESIDO

••S•I•
ANSEIS
ASSAIL
AUSSIE
AUSTIN
BASHIN
BASKIN
BASTIA
BESSIE
BESTIR
BOSNIA
BUSTIN
CASEIN
CASHIN
CASSIA
CASSIE
CASSIM
CASSIN
CASSIO
CASSIS
COSMIC
CUSPID
CUSTIS
CYSTIC
DASHIS
DASHIT
DASSIN
DISTIL
DUSTIN
EASEIN
ESSAIS
EUSTIS
FASCIA
FISTIC
FOSSIL
GASLIT
GASOIL
GESTIC
GOSLIN
GOSSIP
HASSID
HESTIA
INSTIL
INSTIR
ISSEIS
JASMIN
JESUIT
JUSTIN
KESHIA
KISSIN
LASSIE
LESLIE
LESMIZ
LOSEIT
LOSTIT
MASAIS
MASHIE
MASLIN
MASSIF
MASTIC
MESSIN
MISAIM
MISDID
MISFIT
MISHIT
MISSIS
MOSAIC
MUSKIE
MUSLIM
MUSLIN
MYSTIC
NESBIT
NESSIE
NESTIN
NISEIS
NOSEIN
PASSIM
PASTIS
PASTIT
PISTIL
POSTIE
POSTIT
PUSHIN
PUSHIT
RASHID
RASKIN
RESAID
RESHIP
RESNIK
RESOIL
RESPIN
RESTIR
RESUIT
RESWIM
RISHIS
RISKIT
ROSHIS
RUSHIN
RUSKIN
RUSSIA
RUSTIC
SUSHIS
TESSIE
TESSIO
TOSSIN
TUSHIE
UNSAID
UNSHIP
UNSLIM
UPSPIN
UPSTIR
VESPID
VISCID
WESKIT
WESTIE
WESTIN
WISHIN
YASHIN
YASMIN
YESSIR

••S••I
ASSISI
BUSONI
CISKEI
MESABI
ORSINI
PASMOI
SESQUI
SISISI
TISHRI
VASHTI
WASABI

•••SI•
ACESIT
ACTSIN
ADDSIN
AGESIX
AMESIA
ARCSIN
ASKSIN
AUSSIE
AYESIR
BAGSIT
BATSIN
BEDSIT
BESSIE
BIDSIN
BRASIL
BUYSIN
BUYSIT
CASSIA
CASSIE
CASSIM
CASSIN
CASSIO
CASSIS
CATSIT
COPSIT
COUSIN
CRISIS
CUESIN
CUTSIN
CUTSIT
DASSIN
DEASIL
DIESIS
DIGSIN
DIGSIT
DIPSIN
DOESIN
DOESIT
DOGSIT
EATSIN
EATSIT
ECESIC
ECESIS
EENSIE
ENDSIN
ENDSIT
FATSIS
FITSIN
FOGSIN
FOSSIL
GETSIN
GETSIT
GNOSIS
GOESIN
GOSSIP
GUNSIT
HASSID
HEMSIN
HITSIT
HOISIN
HOPSIN
ICESIN
ICESIT
INKSIN
IRISIN
JAMSIN
KENSIT
KEYSIN
KISSIN
LAMSIT
LASSIE
LAYSIN
LEGSIT
LETSIN
LIESIN
LOGSIN
MAISIE
MAKSIM
MASSIF
MESSIN
MISSIS
MYOSIN
MYOSIS
NESSIE
NEWSIE
NOESIS
OPTSIN
OTOSIS
OUTSIN
OUTSIT
PANSIN
PASSIM
PAYSIN
PENSIN
PEPSIN
PERSIA
PERSIS
PETSIT
PHASIC
PHYSIC
PHYSIO
PIGSIT
PIUSII
PIUSIV
PIUSIX
POPSIN
POTSIE
PROSIT
PUTSIN
RAISIN
RAMSIN
REDSIX
RUBSIN
RUNSIN
RUSSIA
SEESIN
SETSIN
SEWSIN
SITSIN
SIXSIX
STASIS
TAPSIN
TESSIE
TESSIO
THESIS
TIESIN
TILSIT
TIPSIN
TMESIS
TOCSIN
TOESIN
TONSIL
TOSSIN
TOWSIN
TUTSIS
USESIN
VLASIC
WAYSIN
WHOSIN
YENSID
YESSIR
ZIPSIN
ZIPSIT
ZOYSIA

•••S•I
AGASSI
BAKSHI
BONSAI
JETSKI
KINSKI
KRISTI
MATSUI
MUESLI
NEVSKI
PIUSII
PIUSVI
PIUSXI
SANSEI
SAYSHI
SENSEI

••••SI
AGASSI
ARIOSI
ASSISI
CHUHSI
DALASI
JAMESI
KWEISI
LOUISI
LUGOSI
PELOSI
POTOSI
RIBISI
SCAASI
SISISI
TSOTSI
WATUSI

S•J•••
STJOAN
STJOHN
STJUDE

S••J••
SHOJIS
STOJKO

S•••J•
SKOPJE

S••••J
SGTMAJ
SMALLJ

••SJ••
GASJET

••••SJ
JAMESJ

SK••••
SKAGGS
SKALDS
SKANKS
SKANKY
SKATED
SKATER
SKATES
SKEETS
SKEINS
SKETCH
SKEWED
SKEWER
SKIBIB
SKIBOB
SKIBUM
SKICAP
SKIDDY
SKIDOO
SKIERS
SKIFFS
SKIHAT
SKIING
SKILLS
SKIMPS
SKIMPY
SKINKS
SKINNY
SKIPBY
SKIPIT
SKIPPY
SKIRLS
SKIRTS
SKIRUN
SKITCH
SKITOW
SKIWAX
SKNXXX
SKOALS
SKOKIE
SKOPJE
SKORTS
SKULKS
SKULLS
SKUNKS
SKUNKY
SKYBOX
SKYCAM
SKYCAP
SKYING
SKYLAB
SKYLIT
SKYMAN
SKYMAP
SKYMEN
SKYTEL
SKYWAY

S•K•••
SIKKIM

S••K••
SACKED
SACKER
SACKUP
SANKAS
SANKIN
SECKEL
SEEKER
SEIKOS
SERKIN
SERKIS
SHAKEN
SHAKER
SHAKES
SHAKIN
SHAKOS
SHAKUR
SHEKEL
SICKEN
SICKER
SICKLE
SICKLY
SICKOF
SICKOS
SIKKIM
SILKEN
SINKER
SINKIN
SIRKAY
SISKEL
SKOKIE
SLAKED
SLAKER
SLAKES
SMOKED
SMOKER
SMOKES
SMOKEY
SNAKED
SNAKER
SNAKES
SOAKED
SOAKER
SOAKIN
SOAKUP
SOCKED
SOCKET
SOCKIN
SPIKED
SPIKER
SPIKES
SPOKED
SPOKEN
SPOKES
STAKED
STAKES
STOKED
STOKER
STOKES
STUKAS
SUCKED
SUCKER
SUCKIN
SUCKUP
SULKED
SULKER
SUNKEN
SUNKIN
SUUKYI

S•••K•
SALUKI
SAMEKH
SEDAKA
SHACKS
SHANKS
SHARKS
SHECKY
SHEIKH
SHEIKS
SHIRKS
SHOCKS
SHOPKO
SHRIKE
SHUCKS
SKANKS
SKANKY
SKINKS
SKULKS
SKUNKS
SKUNKY
SLACKS
SLEEKS
SLEEKY
SLICKS
SLINKS
SLINKY
SMACKS
SMIRKS
SMIRKY
SMOCKS
SNACKS
SNARKS
SNARKY
SNEAKS
SNEAKY
SNICKS
SNOOKS
SPANKS
SPANKY
SPARKS
SPARKY
SPEAKS
SPECKS
SPINKS
SPOOKS
SPOOKY
SPORKS
SPUNKY
STACKS
STALKS
STALKY
STEAKS
STICKS
STICKY
STINKO
STINKS
STINKY
STLUKE
STOCKS
STOCKY
STOJKO
STORKS
STRIKE
STROKE
SUDOKU
SUZUKI
SVEDKA
SWANKY

S••••K
SAIDOK
SAITEK
SAYSOK
SCHICK
SCREAK
SENDAK
SHLOCK
SHNOOK
SHRANK
SHRIEK
SHRINK
SHRUNK
SHTICK
SLEZAK
SLOVAK
SMALLK
SOYINK
SPACEK
SPIVAK
SQUAWK
SQUEAK
STMARK
STNICK
STREAK
STRUCK
STRUNK

•SK•••
ASKAMY
ASKANT
ASKERS
ASKFOR
ASKING
ASKOUT
ASKSIN
ASKSOF
ASKSUP
ESKERS
ESKIMO
TSKING
TSKTSK

•S•K••
ESHKOL
OSAKAN

•S••K•
CSONKA
ISLIKE

•S•••K
ISNTOK
TSKTSK
USBANK

••SK••
BASKED
BASKER
BASKET
BASKIN
BUSKED
BUSKER
CASKED
CASKET
CISKEI
DISKED
DUSKED
GASKET
HUSKED
HUSKER
LASKER
MASKED
MASKER
MISKEY
MOSKVA
MUSKET
MUSKIE
MUSKOX
RASKIN
RISKED
RISKER
RISKIT
RUSKIN
SISKEL
TASKED
TASKET
TISKET
TUSKED
TUSKER
UNSKEW
WESKER
WESKIT

••S•K•
KISHKA
KISHKE
LUSAKA

••S••K
CUSACK
MUSICK
RESEEK
RESINK
RESNIK
RESOAK
UNSICK
UNSUNK
VOSTOK

•••SK•
ALASKA
BIGSKY
BOESKY
BRISKS
FLASKS
FRISKS
FRISKY
JETSKI
KINSKI
KIOSKS
LANSKY
NEVSKI
NEVSKY
POLSKA
PROSKY
REASKS
REDSKY
RIMSKY
WHISKS
WHISKY

•••S•K
DOESOK
OCASEK
SAYSOK

••••SK
ATDUSK
ATRISK
BRATSK
DAMASK
GDANSK
JAMESK
NORISK
ONDISK
OUTASK
TSKTSK
UNCASK
UNHUSK
UNMASK
URALSK

SL••••
SLACKS
SLAKED
SLAKER
SLAKES
SLALOM
SLAMON
SLANGS
SLANGY
SLANTS
SLAPON
SLAPPY
SLATED
SLATER
SLATES
SLAVED
SLAVER
SLAVES
SLAVIC
SLAYED
SLAYER
SLEAZE
SLEAZY
SLEDGE
SLEEKS
SLEEKY
SLEEPS
SLEEPY
SLEETS
SLEETY
SLEEVE
SLEIGH
SLEUTH
SLEWED
SLEZAK
SLICED
SLICER
SLICES
SLICKS
SLIDER
SLIDES
SLIDIN
SLIEST
SLIGHT
SLIMED
SLIMES
SLIMLY
SLINGS
SLINKS
SLINKY
SLIPBY
SLIPIN
SLIPON
SLIPPY
SLIPUP
SLITHY
SLIVER
SLOANE
SLOBBY
SLOGAN
SLOOPS
SLOOPY
SLOPED
SLOPER
SLOPES
SLOPON
SLOPPY
SLOSHY
SLOTHS
SLOUCH
SLOUGH
SLOVAK
SLOVEN
SLOWED
SLOWER
SLOWGO
SLOWLY
SLOWUP
SLUDGE
SLUDGY
SLUGGO
SLUICE
SLUING
SLUMMY
SLUMPS
SLURPS
SLURRY
SLUSHY
SLYEST
SLYFOX

S•L•••
SALAAM
SALADA
SALADE
SALADS
SALAMI
SALARY
SALEPS
SALIFY
SALINA
SALINE
SALISH
SALIVA
SALLES
SALLIE
SALLOW
SALMAN
SALMIS
SALMON
SALOME
SALONS
SALOON
SALSAS
SALTED
SALTEN
SALTER
SALTII
SALTON
SALUKI
SALUTE
SALUTO
SALVED
SALVER
SALVES
SALVOR
SALVOS
SALYUT
SCLAFF
SCLERA
SELDOM
SELECT
SELENA
SELENE
SELLBY
SELLER
SELLIT
SELLON
SELLTO
SELTEN
SELVES
SHLOCK
SILAGE
SILENT
SILICA
SILKEN
SILOED
SILTED
SILVAS
SILVER
SOLACE
SOLANO
SOLANS
SOLARA
SOLATI
SOLDER
SOLDIT
SOLDON
SOLDTO
SOLEAS
SOLEIL
SOLELY
SOLEMN
SOLERS
SOLEUS
SOLIDS
SOLING
SOLOED
SOLONG
SOLONS
SOLUTE
SOLVED
SOLVER
SOLVES
SPLASH

SPLATS
SPLAYS
SPLEEN
SPLICE
SPLINE
SPLINT
SPLITS
SPLOSH
STLUKE
SULFAS
SULFUR
SULKED
SULKER
SULLEN
SULTAN
SULTRY
SYLPHS
SYLVAN
SYLVIA

S••L••

SABLES
SADLER
SAILED
SAILER
SAILON
SAILOR
SAILTO
SALLES
SALLIE
SALLOW
SAMLET
SAULTS
SAWLOG
SAYLES
SCALAR
SCALDS
SCALED
SCALER
SCALES
SCALIA
SCALPS
SCHLEP
SCHLUB
SCOLDS
SCULLS
SCULLY
SCULPT
SCYLLA
SEALAB
SEALED
SEALER
SEALIN
SEALUP
SEALYS
SEDLEY
SELLBY
SELLER
SELLIT
SELLON
SELLTO
SHALES
SHALEY
SHALIT
SHALLI
SHALLY
SHALOM
SHELBY
SHELLS
SHELTY
SHELVE
SHILLS
SHILLY
SHILOH
SHOLEM
SHOLOM
SHULTZ
SIDLED
SIDLES
SIGLER
SISLER
SISLEY
SKALDS
SKILLS
SKULKS
SKULLS
SKYLAB
SKYLIT
SLALOM
SMALLA
SMALLB
SMALLC
SMALLD
SMALLE
SMALLF
SMALLG
SMALLH
SMALLI
SMALLJ
SMALLK
SMALLL
SMALLM
SMALLN
SMALLO
SMALLP
SMALLQ
SMALLR
SMALLS
SMALLT
SMALLU
SMALLV
SMALLW
SMALLX
SMALLY
SMALLZ
SMELLS
SMELLY
SMELTS
SMILED
SMILER
SMILES
SMILEY
SMILLA
SMOLTS
SNELLS
SOCLES
SOILED
SPELLS
SPILES
SPILLS
SPILTH
STALAG
STALED
STALER
STALES
STALIN
STALKS
STALKY
STALLS
STELAR
STELAS
STELES
STELLA
STELMO
STILES
STILLE
STILLS
STILLY
STILTS
STOLAE
STOLAF
STOLAS
STOLEN
STOLES
STOLID
STOLLE
STOLON
STOLTZ
STYLED
STYLER
STYLES
STYLET
STYLUS
SUBLET
SUBLID
SUBLOT
SULLEN
SUNLIT
SVELTE
SWALES
SWELLS
SWILLS

S•••L•

SABALS
SACFLY
SADDLE
SAFELY
SAGELY
SAMPLE
SANELY
SAWALL
SCHELL
SCHOLL
SCHULZ
SCOWLS
SCROLL
SCULLS
SCULLY
SCYLLA
SEARLE
SEEALL
SEEMLY
SEMELE
SEMPLE
SENILE
SEPALS
SETTLE
SEWELL
SEXILY
SHALLI
SHALLY
SHAWLS
SHEILA
SHELLS
SHIELD
SHILLS
SHILLY
SHOALS
SHOALY
SHOULD
SHRILL
SIBYLS
SICILY
SICKLE
SICKLY
SIECLE
SIGILS
SIMILE
SIMPLE
SIMPLY
SINGLE
SINGLY
SISALS
SISSLE
SIZZLE
SKILLS
SKIRLS
SKOALS
SKULLS
SLIMLY
SLOWLY
SMALLA
SMALLB
SMALLC
SMALLD
SMALLE
SMALLF
SMALLG
SMALLH
SMALLI
SMALLJ
SMALLK
SMALLL
SMALLM
SMALLN
SMALLO
SMALLP
SMALLQ
SMALLR
SMALLS
SMALLT
SMALLU
SMALLV
SMALLW
SMALLX
SMALLY
SMALLZ
SMELLS
SMELLY
SMILLA
SMUGLY
SNAILS
SNARLS
SNARLY
SNELLS
SNUGLI
SNUGLY
SOFTLY
SOLELY
SOMALI
SORELY
SOURLY
SPELLS
SPIELS
SPILLS
SPOILS
SPOILT
SPOOLS
SPRYLY
SQUALL
STABLE
STABLY
STALLS
STAPLE
STEALS
STEELE
STEELS
STEELY
STELLA
STIFLE
STILLE
STILLS
STILLY
STMALO
STOLLE
STOOLS
STOOLY
STROLL
STUDLY
SUABLE
SUBTLE
SUBTLY
SUPPLE
SUPPLY
SURELY
SWELLS
SWILLS
SWIRLS
SWIRLY
SWIRLZ

S••••L

SAMUEL
SANDAL
SAWALL
SCHELL
SCHOLL
SCHOOL
SCRAWL
SCROLL
SEAEEL
SEAGAL
SECKEL
SEEALL
SEPTAL
SEQUEL
SERIAL
SEWELL
SHEKEL
SHERYL
SHOVEL
SHRILL
SHTETL
SIEGEL
SIGNAL
SINFUL
SISKEL
SKYTEL
SMALLL
SNIVEL
SNOBOL
SOBFUL
SOCIAL
SOLEIL
SORREL
SPINAL
SPINEL
SPIRAL
SPRAWL
SQUALL
SQUEAL
STEROL
STPAUL
STROLL
SWIVEL
SYMBOL

•SL•••

ASLANT
ASLEEP
ASLOPE
ASLOSH
ISLAND
ISLATE
ISLEFT
ISLETS
ISLEYS
ISLIKE
ISLING

•S•L••

ASFLAT
ASHLAR
ASHLEE
ASHLEY
ASSLOW
ASTLEY
ASYLUM
ESALEN
ESTLIN
ISELIN
ISOLDA
ISOLDE
ISTLES
OSTLER
PSALMS
USFLAG

•S••L•

ASCALE
ASCOLD
ASDULL
ASTALL
ASWELL
BSCALE
CSCALE
DSCALE
ESCALE
FSCALE
GSCALE
ISEULT
OSCULE
OSWALD
USABLE
USABLY
USUALS

•S•••L

ASCOOL
ASDULL
ASSAIL
ASTALL
ASTEAL
ASTRAL
ASWELL
ASWIRL
ESHKOL
ESPIAL
ISABEL
ISMAIL
ISOHEL
ISRAEL
OSTEAL
USEFUL
USMAIL

••SL••

AISLED
AISLES
ASSLOW
BOSLEY
DESLUM
EASLEY
EISLEY
ENSLER
GASLIT
GASLOG
GOSLIN
GOSLOW
KISLEV
LESLEY
LESLIE
LISLES
MASLIN
MISLAY
MISLED
MOSLEM
MOSLEY
MUSLIM
MUSLIN
ROSLYN
SISLER
SISLEY
TESLAS
UNSLIM
UNSLOW
VASLAV
WASLED
WESLEY

••S•L•

ANSELM
BASALT
BASELY
BASILS
BASSLY
BUSILY
BUSTLE
CASALS
CASTLE
COSELL
COSILY
COSTLY
DESALT
DESILT
DESILU
EASELS
EASILY
EASTLA
EDSELS
EISELE
ENSILE
FUSILE
FUSILS
GISELE
GOSOLO
HASSLE
HOSELS
HOSTLY
HUSTLE
IMSOLD
INSOLE
INSULT
ITSELF
JOSTLE
JUSTLY
LASTLY
LASZLO
LTSULU
LUSHLY
MASALA
MOSTLY
MRSULU
MUSCLE
MUSCLY
MYSELF
NASALS
NESTLE
NOSALE
NOSALT
NOSILY
ONSALE
OUSELS
PESTLE
POSHLY
POSOLE
POSSLQ
RASHLY
RASSLE
RESALE
RESALT
RESELL
RESILE
RESOLD
RESOLE
RESULT
ROSILY
RUSTLE
SISALS
SISSLE
TUSSLE
UNSELD
UNSELL
UNSOLD
UNSOLE
UPSALA
URSULA
VASILY
VASTLY
WASOLD
WISELY

••S••L

AMSTEL
ASSAIL
BASIAL
BESSEL
BUSHEL
CASTEL
CASUAL
COSELL
COSTAL
CUSPAL
DISMAL
DISPEL
DISTAL
DISTIL
DOSSAL
ENSEAL
ENSOUL
FESTAL
FISCAL
FOSSIL
GASOIL
GOSPEL
HASSEL
HOSTEL
IJSSEL
INSTAL
INSTIL
JESSEL
KISSEL
KOSSEL
MESCAL
MESIAL
MISSAL
MOSTEL
MUSIAL
MUSSEL
PASCAL
PASSEL
PASTEL
PISTIL
PISTOL
POSTAL
RASCAL
RESEAL
RESELL
RESOIL
RUSSEL
SISKEL
TASSEL
TUSSAL
UNSEAL
UNSELL
VASSAL
VESSEL
VESTAL
VISUAL

•••SL•

BASSLY
ENISLE
FOCSLE
GRISLY
HASSLE
MEASLE
MEASLY
MUESLI
POSSLQ
RASSLE
SISSLE
THUSLY
TOUSLE
TUSSLE
VIZSLA

•••S•L

BESSEL
BRASIL
BURSAL
CAUSAL
CHISEL
CONSUL
CRESOL
DAMSEL
DEASIL
DELSOL
DIESEL
DORSAL
DOSSAL
FAISAL
FOSSIL
GEISEL
GUNSEL
HANSEL
HASSEL
IJSSEL
JESSEL
KISSEL
KOSSEL
MENSAL
MISSAL
MORSEL
MUSSEL
PASSEL
PAUSAL
RUSSEL
TARSAL
TASSEL
TEASEL
TINSEL
TONSIL
TUSSAL
VASSAL
VESSEL
WEASEL
WIESEL

••••SL

ALNASL

SM••••

SMACKS
SMALLA
SMALLB
SMALLC
SMALLD
SMALLE
SMALLF
SMALLG
SMALLH
SMALLI
SMALLJ
SMALLK
SMALLL
SMALLM
SMALLN
SMALLO
SMALLP
SMALLQ
SMALLR
SMALLS
SMALLT
SMALLU
SMALLV
SMALLW
SMALLX
SMALLY
SMALLZ
SMARMY
SMARTS
SMARTY
SMAZES
SMEARS
SMEARY
SMELLS
SMELLY
SMELTS
SMERSH
SMIDGE
SMILED
SMILER
SMILES
SMILEY
SMILLA
SMIRCH
SMIRKS
SMIRKY
SMITER
SMITES
SMITHS
SMITHY
SMITTY
SMOCKS
SMOGGY
SMOKED
SMOKER
SMOKES
SMOKEY
SMOLTS
SMOOCH
SMOOSH
SMOOTH
SMORES
SMUDGE
SMUDGY
SMUGLY
SMURFS
SMUTTY
SMYRNA

S•M•••

SAMARA
SAMBAS
SAMEAS
SAMEDI
SAMEKH
SAMIAM
SAMLET
SAMOAN
SAMOSA
SAMPAN
SAMPLE
SAMSON
SAMUEL
SEMANA
SEMELE
SEMITE
SEMPER
SEMPLE
SEMPRE
SIMEON
SIMIAN
SIMILE
SIMMER
SIMONE
SIMPER
SIMPLE
SIMPLY
SOMALI
SOMANY
SOMATA
SOMBER
SOMBRE
SOMERS
SOMMER
SOMONI
SOMUCH
STMALO
STMARK
STMARY
SUMACS
SUMMED
SUMMER
SUMMIT
SUMMON
SUMNER
SUMSUP
SUMTER
SUMUPS
SYMBOL

S••M••

SALMAN
SALMIS
SALMON
SCAMPI
SCAMPS
SCHMOS
SCUMMY
SEAMAN
SEAMAP
SEAMED
SEAMEN
SEAMER
SEAMUS
SEEMED
SEEMLY
SEEMTO
SERMON
SGTMAJ
SHAMAN
SHAMED
SHAMES
SHAMIR
SHAMMY
SHAMUS
SHIMMY
SHIMON
SHUMAI
SIGMAS
SIMMER
SKIMPS
SKIMPY
SKYMAN
SKYMAP
SKYMEN
SLAMON
SLIMED
SLIMES
SLIMLY
SLUMMY
SLUMPS
SOMMER
SPUMED
SPUMES
STAMEN
STAMOS
STAMPS
STEMMY
STIMPY
STOMAS
STOMPS
STUMPS
STUMPY
STYMIE
SUBMIT
SUMMED
SUMMER
SUMMIT
SUMMON
SWAMIS
SWAMPS
SWAMPY
SWAMUP

S•••M•

SALAMI
SALOME
SAVEME
SCHEMA
SCHEME
SCRAMS
SCRIMP
SCRIMS
SCRUMS
SCUMMY
SEDUMS
SEISMO
SEISMS
SERUMS
SESAME
SHAMMY
SHIMMY
SHOWME
SHRIMP
SLUMMY
SMARMY
SOLEMN
SONOMA
SPASMS
STEAMS
STEAMY
STELMO
STEMMY
STIGMA
STORMS
STORMY
STRUMS
SURIMI
SWARMS

S••••M

SACHEM
SACRUM
SADDAM
SADISM
SALAAM
SAMIAM
SATCOM
SCARUM
SCHISM
SCREAM
SEAARM
SELDOM
SEPTUM
SEXISM
SHALOM
SHAZAM
SHBOOM
SHIISM
SHOLEM
SHOLOM
SIKKIM
SITCOM
SKIBUM
SKYCAM
SLALOM
SMALLM
SODIUM
SPYCAM
SQUIRM
STREAM
SUBGUM
SUFISM
SUREAM
SYSTEM

•SM•••

ASMANY
ASMARA
ASMUCH
ISMAIL
ISMENE
OSMICS
OSMIUM
OSMOND
OSMOSE
OSMUND
USMAIL
USMINT

•S•M••

ASHMAN
ASHMEN
ASIMOV
ISOMER

•S••M•

ASHAME
ASKAMY
ASSUME
ASTHMA
ESKIMO
ESTIME
ISITME
ISTHMI
PSALMS
USARMY

•S•••M

ASHRAM
ASWARM
ASYLUM
ESTEEM
OSMIUM

••SM••

BUSMAN
BUSMEN
COSMAS
COSMIC
COSMOS
DESMOG
DISMAL
DISMAS
DISMAY
DISMES
GASMAN
GASMEN
GISMOS
JASMIN
KISMET
LESMIZ
MESMER
PASMOI
TASMAN
UNSMUG
WASMET
YASMIN
YESMAN
YESMEN

••S•M•

ASSUME
BESAME
BESOMS
BOSOMS
BOSOMY
DOSUMS
FUSUMA
JUSTME
KISSME
MISSME
RESUME
SESAME
UGSOME
WASHME

••S••M

ABSCAM
ANSELM
CASSIM
CESIUM
CUSTOM
DESLUM
DESTEM
DISARM
HASSAM
INSEAM
MISAIM
MOSLEM
MUSEUM
MUSLIM
PASSIM
POSSUM
POSTUM
RESEAM

RESWAM RESWIM ROSSUM SYSTEM UNSEAM UNSLIM WISDOM YESIAM

•••SM•

ABYSMS CHASMS KISSME MIASMA MISSME PLASMA PLASMO PRISMS SEISMO SEISMS SPASMS

•••S•M

BALSAM CASSIM CHISUM DIMSUM DORSUM FOLSOM GYPSUM HANSOM HASSAM IAMSAM JETSAM MAKSIM NEWSOM OMASUM OUTSUM PASSIM POSSUM RANSOM ROSSUM TAOSNM UNISOM

••••SM

AGEISM AUTISM CHRISM CUBISM EGOISM HOLISM JAMESM MAOISM MOMISM MONISM NUDISM PURISM RACISM SADISM SCHISM SEXISM SHIISM SUFISM TAOISM THEISM TRUISM VERISM YOGISM

SN••••

SNACKS SNAFUS SNAGGY SNAGUP SNAILS SNAKED SNAKER SNAKES SNAPAT SNAPON SNAPPY SNAPTO SNAPUP SNARED SNARER SNARES SNARFS SNARKS SNARKY SNARLS SNARLY SNATCH SNATHS SNAZZY SNEAKS SNEAKY SNEERS SNEERY SNEEZE SNEEZY SNELLS SNICKS SNIDER SNIFFS SNIFFY SNIPED SNIPER SNIPES SNIPPY SNITCH SNIVEL SNOBBY SNOBOL SNOCAT SNOODS SNOOKS SNOOPS SNOOPY SNOOTS SNOOTY SNOOZE SNOOZY SNOPES SNORED SNORER SNORES SNORRI SNORTS SNORTY SNOUTS SNOWED SNOWIN SNUBBY SNUFFS SNUFFY SNUGLI SNUGLY SNYDER

S•N•••

SANCHO SANCTA SANDAL SANDED SANDER SANDIA SANDRA SANDRO SANELY SANEST SANGER SANGRE SANGTO SANITY SANKAS SANKIN SANSEI SANTAS SANTEE SANTHA SANTOS SANYOS SENARY SENATE SENATS SENDAK SENDBY SENDEE SENDER SENDIN SENDON SENDTO SENDUP SENECA SENHOR SENILE SENIOR SENITI SENNAS SENORA SENORS SENSED SENSEI SENSEN SENSES SENSOR SENTBY SENTIN SENTON SENTRA SENTRY SENTTO SENTUP SHNOOK SINBAD SINEAD SINEWS SINEWY SINFUL SINGED SINGER SINGES SINGIN SINGLE SINGLY SINGTO SINISE SINKER SINKIN SINNED SINNER SINTAX SKNXXX SONANT SONARS SONATA SONDES SONDRA SONICS SONNET SONOMA SONORA SONTAG STNICK SUNBOW SUNDAE SUNDAS SUNDAY SUNDER SUNDOG SUNDRY SUNFAN SUNGOD SUNGTO SUNHAT SUNKEN SUNKIN SUNLIT SUNNED SUNNIS SUNOCO SUNRAY SUNSET SUNTAN SUNUNU SUNUPS SYNCED SYNCHS SYNDIC SYNODS SYNTAX SYNTHS

S••N••

SAINTE SAINTS SARNIA SAUNAS SAYNAY SCANTS SCANTY SCENAS SCENEI SCENES SCENEV SCENIC SCENTS SCHNOZ SCONCE SCONES SEANCE SEENAS SEENIN SEENTO SEENUP SEINED SEINER SEINES SENNAS SEWNIN SEWNON SEWNUP SHANDY SHANIA SHANKS SHANTY SHINDY SHINED SHINER SHINES SHINNY SHINTO SHUNTS SIDNEY SIENNA SIGNAL SIGNED SIGNEE SIGNER SIGNET SIGNIN SIGNON SIGNOR SIGNUP SINNED SINNER SKANKS SKANKY SKINKS SKINNY SKUNKS SKUNKY SLANGS SLANGY SLANTS SLINGS SLINKS SLINKY SONNET SOONAS SOONER SOONYI SOUNDS SPANKS SPANKY SPENCE SPENDS SPENDY SPINAL SPINED SPINEL SPINER SPINES SPINET SPINKS SPONGE SPONGY SPUNKY STANCE STANCH STANDS STANZA STENCH STENOG STENOS STENTS STINGS STINGY STINKO STINKS STINKY STINTS STONED STONER STONES STONEY STUNTS STUNTY SUBNET SUENOS SUMNER SUNNED SUNNIS SWANEE SWANKY SWANNS SWINGS SWINGY SYDNEY

S•••N•

SABENA SABINA SABINE SAIDNO SALINA SALINE SALONS SARANS SARONG SATING SATINS SATINY SAVANA SAVANT SAVING SAWING SAXONS SAXONY SAYING SAYSNO SCARNE SCIONS SCORNS SECANT SECOND SEDANS SEDONA SEEING SELENA SELENE SEMANA SERENA SERENE SERINS SEVENA SEVENB SEVENC SEVEND SEVENE SEVENS SEWING SEWONS SHAYNE SHEENA SHEENS SHEENY SHINNY SHRANK SHRINE SHRINK SHRUNK SHYING SIDING SIENNA SILENT SIMONE SIRENS SIRING SITING SITINS SIVANS SIXONE SIZING SKEINS SKIING SKINNY SKYING SLOANE SLUING SMYRNA SOCANI SOFINE SOIGNE SOLANO SOLANS SOLING SOLONG SOLONS SOMANY SOMONI SONANT SOWING SOYINK SPAWNS SPHINX SPHYNX SPLINE SPLINT SPOONS SPOONY SPRANG SPRING SPRINT SPRUNG SPURNS SPYING SQUINT STAINS STEINS STERNA STERNE STERNO STERNS STRAND STRING STRONG STRUNG STRUNK STYING SUEANE SUEANN SUNUNU SUPINE SUSANB SUSANN SWAINS SWANNS SWOONS

S••••N

SADDEN SAIGON SAILON SAIPAN SAISON SALMAN SALMON SALOON SALTEN SALTON SAMOAN SAMPAN SAMSON SANKIN SARGON SARTON SASSON SATEEN SATURN SAURON SAVEON SCREEN SEALIN SEAMAN SEAMEN SEASON SEATON SEENIN SEEPIN SEESIN SELLON SELTEN SENDIN SENDON SENSEN SENTIN SENTON SEQUIN SERKIN SERMON SETSIN SETSON SEVERN SEWNIN SEWNON SEWSIN SEWSON SEXTON SHAKEN SHAKIN SHAMAN SHARON SHARYN SHAVEN SHEDON SHIMON SHOGUN SHOOIN SHOWIN SHUTIN SICKEN SIEBEN SIGNIN SIGNON SILKEN SIMEON SIMIAN SINGIN SINKIN SIOUAN SIPHON SIPSON SIRBEN SITSIN SITSON SITTIN SIXGUN SIXPIN SIXTEN SKIRUN SKYMAN SKYMEN SLAMON SLAPON SLIDIN SLIPIN SLIPON SLOGAN SLOPON SLOVEN SMALLN SNAPON SNOWIN SOAKIN SOCKIN SODDEN SOFTEN SOFTON SOLDON SOLEMN SOSOON SOTHEN SOURON SOXFAN SPITON SPLEEN SPOKEN SPOTON SPRAIN SPURON STALIN STAMEN STARIN STATEN STATIN STAYIN STAYON STEFAN STEPIN STEPON STEVEN STIRIN STJOAN STJOHN STOLEN STOLON STOPIN STOTIN STRAIN STREWN STYRON SUBORN SUCKIN SUDDEN SUEANN SULLEN SULTAN SUMMON SUNFAN SUNKEN SUNKIN SUNTAN SURFIN SUSANN SUTTON SWEDEN SYLVAN SYRIAN

•SN•••

ASNEAR ASNEAT ISNTOK USNAVY USNEWS

•S•N••

ASANAS ASANTE ASONIA CSONKA ESENIN ISANTI ISINTO USANCE USENET

•S••N•

ASCEND ASCENT ASHINE ASHING ASIANS ASKANT ASKING ASLANT ASMANY ASPENS ASSENT ASTANA ESCENT ESPANA ESSENE ISAYNO ISLAND ISLING ISMENE OSCANS OSCINE OSMOND OSMUND OSTEND TSKING USBANK USHING USMINT VSIGNS

•S•••N

ASHBIN ASHCAN ASHMAN ASHMEN ASHPAN ASHTON ASKSIN ASOSAN ASSIGN ASTERN ASWOON BSEVEN ESALEN ESENIN ESTLIN GSEVEN ISAIAN ISELIN ISOGON OSAKAN OSBORN OSSIAN USEDIN USEDON USESIN USESON USOPEN

••SN••

BOSNIA CPSNOW DESNOS DISNEY EISNER ITSNOT MESNES RESNAP RESNIK UNSNAG UNSNAP UNSNUG

••S•N•

ABSENT ARSENE ARSENO ARSONS ASSENT BASING BASINS BESANT BISONS BOSONS BOSUNS BUSING BUSONI CASING CASINO CESSNA COSINE DISANT DOSING EASING EOSINS EPSONS ESSENE FUSING HASONE HOSING HUSING HYSONS INSANA INSANE INSYNC LASING LOSING LYSINE MASONS MESONS MUSING MUSTNT NISANS NOSING OKSANA ORSINI ORSINO PISANO PISANS POSING RASING RESAND RESANG RESEND RESENT RESING RESINK RESINS RESINY RISING ROSINA ROSINS ROSINY SUSANB SUSANN TISANE TYSONS UNSENT UNSUNG UNSUNK UPSEND UPSENT URSINE VISHNU VISINE VISING WISING YOSANO

••S••N

ALSTON ASSIGN ATSIGN AUSTEN AUSTIN BASHIN BASKIN BESSON BOSSON BOSTON BUSMAN BUSMEN BUSTIN CASEIN CASERN CASHIN CASSIN CASTON COSIGN CTSCAN DASSIN DESIGN DISOWN DUSTIN EASEIN EASEON EASTON ELSTON ENSIGN EUSDEN FASTEN FUSION GASCAN GASCON GASMAN GASMEN GASTON GOSDEN GOSHEN GOSLIN HASFUN HASSAN HASTEN HESTON HUSTON INSPAN ITSFUN JASMIN JUSTIN KASDAN KISSIN LASSEN LESHAN LESION LESSEN LESSON LISBON LISTEN LISTON MASLIN MASSON MESSIN MUSEON MUSLIN NESSEN NESTIN NISSAN NISSEN NOSEIN OKSIGN OSSIAN PASSON PISTON POSTON PUSHIN PUSHON RASKIN RESAWN RESCAN RESEEN RESEWN RESIGN RESOWN RESPAN RESPIN RESTON ROSLYN ROSSEN ROSTEN RUSHIN RUSKIN SASSON SOSOON SUSANN TASMAN TOSSIN TUSCAN UNSAWN UNSEEN UNSEWN UNSOWN UNSPAN UNSPUN UPSPIN VISION WASFUN WESSON WESTIN WESTON WISHIN WISHON WYSTAN YASHIN YASMIN YESMAN YESMEN

•••SN•

CESSNA DOESNT FRESNO KRASNA SAYSNO TAOSNM

•••S•N

ACTSIN ACTSON ADDSIN ADDSON ALISON ARCSIN ARISEN ASKSIN ASOSAN AVISON BABSON BATSIN BATSON BENSON BESSON BETSON BIDSIN BIDSON BOSSON BRYSON BUNSEN BUYSIN BUYSON CARSON CASSIN CHOSEN COLSON COUSIN CUESIN CUTSIN DAMSON DANSON DASSIN DATSUN DAWSON DIGSIN DIPSIN DOESIN DOWSON EATSIN EDISON EGGSON EMPSON ENDSIN ENDSON FELSON FINSEN FITSIN FITSON FOGSIN GARSON GEESON GETSIN GETSON GIBSON GODSON GOESIN GOESON GOOSEN HAMSUN HANSON HASSAN HEMSIN HENSON HEUSEN HITSON HOBSON HOISIN HOPSIN HOPSON HUDSON ICESIN INKSIN IRISIN JAMSIN JANSEN JENSEN JETSON JIMSON JOBSON JOLSON JONSON JUDSON KANSAN

KEYSIN KEYSON KISSIN KMESON LANSON LARSEN LARSON LASSEN LAWSON LAYSIN LAYSON LEISEN LESSEN LESSON LETSIN LETSON LHASAN LIESIN LIESON LOGSIN LOGSON LOOSEN MADSEN MAISON MASSON MATSON MAWSON MAXSON MENSAN MESSIN MOLSON MYOSIN NANSEN NEESON NELSON NESSEN NISSAN NISSEN ODDSON OLESON OPTSIN ORISON OUTSIN OWESON PAISAN PANSIN PARSON PASSON PAYSIN PAYSON PENSIN PEPSIN PERSON PINSON POISON POPSIN PRISON PUTSIN PUTSON RAGSON RAISIN RAISON RAMSIN RAMSON RAPSON RATSON REASON REDSUN

REMSEN REVSON RIESEN RIPSON ROBSON RONSON ROSSEN RUBSIN RUBSON RUNSIN RUNSON SAISON SAMSON SASSON SEASON SEESIN SENSEN SETSIN SETSON SEWSIN SEWSON SIPSON SITSIN SITSON TAGSON TAPSIN TAPSON THESON THESUN TIESIN TIESON TILSON TIPSIN TOCSIN TOESIN TOSSIN TOWSIN TUCSON TUGSON TULSAN UNISON USESIN USESON VELSEN VINSON WATSON WAYSIN WESSON WHOSIN WILSON WORSEN YATSEN ZIPSIN

SO••••

SOAKED SOAKER SOAKIN SOAKUP SOAPED SOAPER SOAPUP SOARED SOARER SOASTO SOAVES SOBBED SOBBER

SOBEIT SOBERS SOBFUL SOCANI SOCCER SOCIAL SOCKED SOCKET SOCKIN SOCLES SODDED SODDEN SODIDI SODIUM SODOWE SOEURS SOFFIT SOFINE SOFTEN SOFTER SOFTIE SOFTLY SOFTON SOIGNE SOILED SOIREE SOISEE SOITIS SOLACE SOLANO SOLANS SOLARA SOLATI SOLDER SOLDIT SOLDON SOLDTO SOLEAS SOLEIL SOLELY SOLEMN SOLERS SOLEUS SOLIDS SOLING SOLOED SOLONG SOLONS SOLUTE SOLVED SOLVER SOLVES SOMALI SOMANY SOMATA SOMBER SOMBRE SOMERS SOMMER SOMONI SOMUCH SONANT SONARS SONATA SONDES SONDRA SONICS SONNET

SONOMA SONORA SONTAG SOONAS SOONER SOONYI SOOTHE SOPHIA SOPHIE SOPORS SOPPED SOPSUP SORBET SORBIC SORDID SOREAT SORELY SOREST SORREL SORROW SORTED SORTER SORTIE SORTOF SOSOON SOSPAD SOTHAT SOTHEN SOTRUE SOTTED SOUGHT SOUNDS SOUPER SOUPUP SOURCE SOURED SOURER SOURLY SOURON SOUSED SOUSES SOUTER SOUTHS SOVIET SOWERS SOWETO SOWHAT SOWING SOXFAN SOYINK

S•O•••

SCOFFS SCOLDS SCONCE SCONES SCOOBA SCOOBY SCOOPS SCOOTS SCOPED SCOPES SCORCH SCORED SCORER SCORES SCORIA SCORNS

SCOTCH SCOTER SCOTIA SCOTTO SCOTTS SCOTTY SCOUPE SCOURS SCOUTS SCOWLS SFORZA SHOALS SHOALY SHOATS SHOCKS SHODDY SHOERS SHOFAR SHOGIS SHOGUN SHOJIS SHOLEM SHOLOM SHOOED SHOOIN SHOOTS SHOPAT SHOPKO SHOPPE SHORES SHORTA SHORTE SHORTI SHORTO SHORTS SHORTU SHORTY SHORTZ SHOTAT SHOTBY SHOTUP SHOULD SHOUTS SHOVED SHOVEL SHOVER SHOVES SHOWED SHOWER SHOWIN SHOWME SHOWUP SIOUAN SKOALS SKOKIE SKOPJE SKORTS SLOANE SLOBBY SLOGAN SLOOPS SLOOPY SLOPED SLOPER SLOPES SLOPON SLOPPY SLOSHY

SLOTHS SLOUCH SLOUGH SLOVAK SLOVEN SLOWED SLOWER SLOWGO SLOWLY SLOWUP SMOCKS SMOGGY SMOKED SMOKER SMOKES SMOKEY SMOLTS SMOOCH SMOOSH SMOOTH SMORES SNOBBY SNOBOL SNOCAT SNOODS SNOOKS SNOOPS SNOOPY SNOOTS SNOOTY SNOOZE SNOOZY SNOPES SNORED SNORER SNORES SNORRI SNORTS SNORTY SNOUTS SNOWED SNOWIN SOONAS SOONER SOONYI SOOTHE SPODES SPOILS SPOILT SPOKED SPOKEN SPOKES SPONGE SPONGY SPOOFS SPOOKS SPOOKY SPOOLS SPOONS SPOONY SPOORS SPORES SPORKS SPORTS SPORTY SPOTON SPOTTV SPOTTY

SPOUSE SPOUTS STOATS STOCKS STOCKY STODGE STODGY STOGIE STOICS STOJKO STOKED STOKER STOKES STOLAE STOLAF STOLAS STOLEN STOLES STOLID STOLLE STOLON STOLTZ STOMAS STOMPS STONED STONER STONES STONEY STOOGE STOOLS STOOLY STOOPS STOPAT STOPBY STOPGO STOPIN STOPIT STOPUP STORCH STORED STORER STORES STORKS STORMS STORMY STORRS STOTIN STOUTS STOVER STOVES STOWED STOWER STOWIT SWOONS SWOOPS SWOOSH SWORDS

S••O••

SABOTS SALOME SALONS SALOON SAMOAN SAMOSA SAPORS SARONG SATORI

SATOUT SAVOIE SAVOIR SAVORS SAVORY SAVOUR SAWOFF SAWOUT SAXONS SAXONY SCHOLL SCHOOL SCHORR SCIONS SCOOBA SCOOBY SCOOPS SCOOTS SCRODS SCROLL SECOND SEDONA SEEOFF SEEOUT SENORA SENORS SEPOYS SEROUS SETOFF SETOSE SETOUT SEWONS SHBOOM SHLOCK SHNOOK SHOOED SHOOIN SHOOTS SHROUD SHROVE SILOED SIMONE SITOUT SIXONE SLOOPS SLOOPY SMOOCH SMOOSH SMOOTH SNOODS SNOOKS SNOOPS SNOOPY SNOOTS SNOOTY SNOOZE SNOOZY SODOWE SOLOED SOLONG SOLONS SOMONI SONOMA SONORA SOPORS SOSOON SPLOSH SPOOFS

SPOOKS SPOOKY SPOOLS SPOONS SPOONY SPOORS SPROUT SPYOUT STJOAN STJOHN STOOGE STOOLS STOOLY STOOPS STROBE STRODE STROHS STROKE STROLL STRONG STROPS STROUD STROVE SUBORN SUDOKU SUNOCO SWOONS SWOOPS SWOOSH SYNODS SYSOPS

S•••O•

SAIDOK SAIGON SAILON SAILOR SAISON SALLOW SALMON SALOON SALTON SALVOR SALVOS SAMSON SANTOS SANYOS SARDOU SARGON SARTON SARTOR SASSON SATCOM SATFOR SAURON SAVEON SAVIOR SAWLOG SAYBOO SAYSOK SAYSOS SCHMOS SCHNOZ SCHOOL SEACOW SEADOG SEAFOX SEAGOD

SEASON SEATON SECTOR SEEYOU SEIKOS SEIZOR SELDOM SELLON SENDON SENHOR SENIOR SENSOR SENTON SERMON SERVOS SETFOR SETSON SETTOS SEWNON SEWSON SEXPOT SEXTON SEZYOU SHADOW SHAKOS SHALOM SHARON SHBOOM SHEBOP SHEDON SHILOH SHIMON SHNOOK SHOLOM SICKOF SICKOS SIGNON SIGNOR SIMEON SIPHON SIPSON SITCOM SITFOR SITSON SKIBOB SKIDOO SKITOW SKYBOX SLALOM SLAMON SLAPON SLIPON SLOPON SLYFOX SNAPON SNOBOL SOFTON SOLDON SORROW SORTOF SOSOON SOURON SPIGOT SPITON SPOTON SPURON SPYBOT STAMOS

STATOR STAYON STEFOY STENOG STENOS STEPON STEROL STOLON STUPOR STYRON SUBGOD SUBLOT SUCCOR SUEFOR SUENOS SUITOR SUMMON SUNBOW SUNDOG SUNGOD SUREOF SUTTON SYMBOL

S••••O

SABADO SABATO SAFECO SAIDNO SAIDSO SAIDTO SAILTO SALUTO SANCHO SANDRO SANGTO SAPPHO SASEBO SAYBOO SAYIDO SAYSNO SAYSSO SBARRO SCIPIO SCOTTO SEEMTO SEENTO SEESTO SEISMO SELLTO SENDTO SENTTO SERGIO SETSTO SEZWHO SHINTO SHIPTO SHOPKO SHORTO SINGTO SIXTWO SKIDOO SLOWGO SLUGGO SMALLO SNAPTO SOASTO SOLANO

SOLDTO SOWETO SPEEDO STELMO STEREO STERNO STETHO STINKO STMALO STOJKO STOPGO STRATO STUCCO STUDIO SUBITO SUNGTO SUNOCO SUREDO

•SO•••

ASONIA ASOSAN CSONKA ISOBAR ISOGON ISOHEL ISOLDA ISOLDE ISOMER ISOPOD TSOTSI USOPEN

•S•O••

ASCOLD ASCOOL ASCOTS ASGOOD ASHORE ASKOUT ASLOPE ASLOSH ASSOFT ASSORT ASTOOP ASWOON CSPOTS ESCORT ESPOSA ESPOSO ESTOCS ESTOPS FSCOTT FSTOPS OSBORN OSGOOD OSMOND OSMOSE TSTOPS USTOUR

•S••O•

ASCOOL ASGOOD ASHDOD ASHTON ASIMOV ASKFOR

ASKSOF ASSLOW ASTOOP ASTROS ASTROV ASWOON ESCROW ESHKOL ESPIOS ISIDOR ISNTOK ISOGON ISOPOD OSGOOD USEDON USEFOR USESON

•S•••O

ASARCO ASIAGO ASTERO ESCUDO ESKIMO ESPOSO ESTADO ISAYNO ISIDRO ISINTO OSWEGO PSEUDO PSYCHO USEDTO YSIDRO

••SO••

ABSORB ADSORB AESOPS ARSONS ASSOFT ASSORT BESOMS BESORE BESOTS BISONS BOSOMS BOSOMY BOSONS BUSONI DESODS DESOTO DISOWN ENSOUL EPSONS GASOIL GOSOFT GOSOLO GOSOUR HASONE HASOUT HESOUT HYSONS IMSOLD INSOLE KOSOVO MASONS MESONS

MYSORE NOSOAP POSOLE RESOAK RESOAP RESODS RESOIL RESOLD RESOLE RESORB RESORT RESOWN RESOWS SOSOON SYSOPS TYSONS UGSOME UNSOFT UNSOLD UNSOLE UNSORE UNSORT UNSOUR UNSOWN UPSOAR VISORS WASOFF WASOLD XESOUT

••S•O•

ALSTON ASSLOW BASSOS BBSHOT BESSON BESTOW BISHOP BOSSON BOSTON BUSBOY CASIOS CASTON CASTOR CISCOS COSMOS CPSNOW CUSTOM DESMOG DESNOS DESPOT DISCOS EASEON EASTON ELSTON FUSION GASCON GASHOG GASLOG GASTON GISMOS GOSLOW HESIOD HESTON HUSTON HYSSOP INSPOT ITSHOT

ITSNOT ITSYOU LASSOS LESBOS LESION LESSON LESSOR LISBOA LISBON LISTON LOSDOS MASCOT MASSON MOSCOW MOSTOF MUSEON MUSEOS MUSKOX NESTOR NOSHOW OHSTOP ONSHOW PASEOS PASMOI PASSON PASSOS PASTOR PESCOW PESTOS PISTOL PISTON PISTOU POSTON POSTOP PUSHON RESHOD RESHOE RESHOT RESHOW RESPOT RESTON RESTOW ROSCOE ROSTOV SASSON SOSOON TISSOT TVSHOW TVSPOT UNSHOD UNSHOE UNSLOW UNSTOP UNSTOW UPSHOT VISION VOSTOK WASHOE WASHOS WESSON WESTON WISDOM WISHON YESYOU

••S••O

ARSENO AUSTRO

BISTRO
CASINO
CASSIO
CASTRO
COSTCO
DESOTO
DISTRO
DOSADO
DOSIDO
EASYGO
GASTRO
GOSOLO
HASAGO
HASBRO
ITSAGO
JUSTSO
KOSOVO
LASHTO
LASZLO
LOSETO
LOSTTO
MUSTDO
ORSINO
OTSEGO
PASHTO
PASSGO
PASSTO
PISANO
RISETO
ROSETO
RUSHTO
SASEBO
TESSIO
WISETO
WISHTO
YESIDO
YOSANO

•••SO•

ACTSON
ADDSON
ALISON
AMOSOZ
ASKSOF
AVISON
AVISOS
BABSON
BASSOS
BATSON
BENSON
BESSON
BETSON
BIDSON
BOSSON
BRASOV
BRYSON
BUYSON
CARSON
CENSOR
CHISOX
COLSON
CRESOL
CRUSOE
CURSOR
DAMSON
DANSON
DAWSON
DELSOL
DIPSOS
DOESOK
DOWSON
EATSOF
EDISON
EGGSON
EMPSON
ENDSON
FELSON
FITSON
FOLSOM
GARSON
GEESON
GETSON
GIBSON
GOBSOF
GODSON
GOESON
HANSOM
HANSON
HENSON
HITSON
HOBSON
HOPSON
HUDSON
HYKSOS
HYSSOP
JETSON
JIMSON
JOBSON
JOLSON
JONSON
JUDSON
KEYSON
KMESON
LANSON
LARSON
LASSOS
LAWSON
LAYSON
LESSON
LESSOR
LETSON
LIESON
LOGSON
LOTSOF
MAISON
MASSON
MATSON
MAWSON
MAXSON
MITSOU
MOLSON
NEESON
NELSON
NEWSOM
ODDSON
OLDSOD
OLESON
ORISON
OWESON
PARSON
PASSON
PASSOS
PAYSON
PERSON
PINSON
POISON
PRISON
PUTSON
QUESOS
RAGSON
RAISON
RAMSON
RANSOM
RAPSON
RATSON
REASON
REDSOX
REVSON
RIDSOF
RIPSON
RITSOS
ROBSOF
ROBSON
RONSON
RUBSON
RUNSON
SAISON
SAMSON
SASSON
SAYSOK
SAYSOS
SEASON
SENSOR
SETSON
SEWSON
SIPSON
SITSON
TAGSON
TAPSON
TENSOR
THESON
THESOX
TIESON
TILSON
TISSOT
TONSOF
TORSOS
TUCSON
TUGSON
UNISOM
UNISON
USESON
VERSOS
VINSON
WATSON
WESSON
WILSON
WINSOR

•••S•O

ADDSTO
AGOSTO
ARISTO
BOWSTO
BRASCO
CASSIO
COPSTO
CRISCO
CRISTO
DOESSO
DOESTO
ELISEO
ENESCO
FIASCO
FRESCO
FRESNO
FRISCO
GETSTO
GLOSSO
GOESTO
GRASSO
GROSSO
HEWSTO
HOPSTO
ITISSO
LAYSTO
LETSGO
LIESTO
MATSUO
NEOSHO
NODSTO
OBISPO
OPTSTO
OROSCO
OWOSSO
PASSGO
PASSTO
PHYSIO
PLASMO
PRESTO
PUTSTO
RUNSTO
SAYSNO
SAYSSO
SEESTO
SEISMO
SETSTO
SOASTO
TESSIO
TIESTO
UNESCO

••••SO

AINTSO
ALONSO
ARIOSO
CARUSO
DIALSO
DOESSO
DONESO
DONOSO
ELPASO
ESPOSO
EVENSO
EVERSO
GLOSSO
GRASSO
GROSSO
HOPESO
ICANSO
ITISSO
JUSTSO
LIKESO
MINOSO
MORESO
OWOSSO
SAIDSO
SAYSSO
WHOMSO

SP••••

SPACED
SPACEK
SPACER
SPACES
SPACEY
SPADED
SPADER
SPADES
SPANKS
SPANKY
SPARED
SPARER
SPARES
SPARKS
SPARKY
SPARSE
SPARTA
SPASMS
SPATES
SPATHE
SPAWNS
SPAYED
SPAYER
SPEAKS
SPEARE
SPEARS
SPECIE
SPECKS
SPEDUP
SPEECH
SPEEDO
SPEEDS
SPEEDY
SPELLS
SPENCE
SPENDS
SPENDY
SPERRY
SPEWED
SPEWER
SPHERE
SPHINX
SPHYNX
SPICED
SPICER
SPICES
SPIDER
SPIDEY
SPIELS
SPIERS
SPIFFS
SPIFFY
SPIGOT
SPIKED
SPIKER
SPIKES
SPILES
SPILLS
SPILTH
SPINAL
SPINED
SPINEL
SPINER
SPINES
SPINET
SPINKS
SPIRAL
SPIREA
SPIRED
SPIRES
SPIRIT
SPITED
SPITES
SPITON
SPIVAK
SPLASH
SPLATS
SPLAYS
SPLEEN
SPLICE
SPLINE
SPLINT
SPLITS
SPLOSH
SPODES
SPOILS
SPOILT
SPOKED
SPOKEN
SPOKES
SPONGE
SPONGY
SPOOFS
SPOOKS
SPOOKY
SPOOLS
SPOONS
SPOONY
SPOORS
SPORES
SPORKS
SPORTS
SPORTY
SPOTON
SPOTTV
SPOTTY
SPOUSE
SPOUTS
SPRACH
SPRAIN
SPRANG
SPRATS
SPRAWL
SPRAYS
SPREAD
SPREES
SPRIER
SPRIGS
SPRING
SPRINT
SPRITE
SPRITS
SPRITZ
SPROUT
SPRUCE
SPRUNG
SPRYER
SPRYLY
SPUMED
SPUMES
SPUNKY
SPURNS
SPURON
SPURTS
SPYBOT
SPYCAM
SPYDER
SPYING
SPYOUT

S•P•••

SAPORS
SAPPED
SAPPER
SAPPHO
SEPALS
SEPHIA
SEPIAS
SEPIRA
SEPOYS
SEPTAL
SEPTET
SEPTIC
SEPTUM
SIPHON
SIPPED
SIPPER
SIPSON
SOPHIA
SOPHIE
SOPORS
SOPPED
SOPSUP
STPATS
STPAUL
STPETE
STPIUS
SUPERB
SUPERG
SUPERS
SUPINE
SUPPED
SUPPER
SUPPLE
SUPPLY
SUPRAS

S••P••

SAIPAN
SAMPAN
SAMPLE
SAPPED
SAPPER
SAPPHO
SATPAT
SAWPIT
SCIPIO
SCOPED
SCOPES
SEEPED
SEEPIN
SEMPER
SEMPLE
SEMPRE
SEXPOT
SHAPED
SHAPER
SHAPES
SHIPTO
SHOPAT
SHOPKO
SHOPPE
SIMPER
SIMPLE
SIMPLY
SIPPED
SIPPER
SITPAT
SIXPIN
SKIPBY
SKIPIT
SKIPPY
SKOPJE
SLAPON
SLAPPY
SLIPBY
SLIPIN
SLIPON
SLIPPY
SLIPUP
SLOPED
SLOPER
SLOPES
SLOPON
SLOPPY
SNAPAT
SNAPON
SNAPPY
SNAPTO
SNAPUP
SNIPED
SNIPER
SNIPES
SNIPPY
SNOPES
SOAPED
SOAPER
SOAPUP
SOPPED
SOSPAD
SOUPER
SOUPUP
STAPES
STAPHS
STAPLE
STAPUF
STEPIN
STEPON
STEPPE
STEPUP
STIPES
STOPAT
STOPBY
STOPGO
STOPIN
STOPIT
STOPUP
STUPAS
STUPES
STUPID
STUPOR
SUBPAR
SUPPED
SUPPER
SUPPLE
SUPPLY
SWIPED
SWIPER
SWIPES
SYLPHS

S•••P•

SALEPS
SCALPS
SCAMPI
SCAMPS
SCARPS
SCOOPS
SCOUPE
SCRAPE
SCRAPS
SCRIPS
SCRIPT
SCULPT
SERAPE
SERAPH
SETUPS
SHARPE
SHARPS
SHARPY
SHERPA
SHOPPE
SIRUPS
SITUPS
SKIMPS
SKIMPY
SKIPPY
SLAPPY
SLEEPS
SLEEPY
SLIPPY
SLOOPS
SLOOPY
SLOPPY
SLUMPS
SLURPS
SNAPPY
SNIPPY
SNOOPS
SNOOPY
STAMPS
STEEPS
STEPPE
STIMPY
STOMPS
STOOPS
STRAPS
STREPS
STRIPE
STRIPS
STRIPY
STROPS
STUMPS
STUMPY
SUMUPS
SUNUPS
SWAMPS
SWAMPY
SWEEPS
SWOOPS
SYRUPS
SYRUPY
SYSOPS

S••••P

SACKUP
SATRAP
SAVEUP
SAWSUP
SCHAAP
SCHLEP
SCRIMP
SEALUP
SEAMAP
SEENUP
SEESUP
SENDUP
SENTUP
SETSUP
SEWNUP
SEWSUP
SHEBOP
SHOTUP
SHOWUP
SHRIMP
SHUTUP
SIGNUP
SITSUP
SIZEUP
SKICAP
SKYCAP
SKYMAP
SLIPUP
SLOWUP
SMALLP
SNAGUP
SNAPUP
SOAKUP
SOAPUP
SOPSUP
SOUPUP
SPEDUP
STAYUP
STEPUP
STIRUP
STOPUP
STREEP
SUCKUP
SUITUP
SUMSUP
SWAMUP

•SP•••

ASPECT
ASPENS
ASPERA
ASPICS
ASPIRE
ASPISH
ASPURE
CSPOTS
ESPANA
ESPIAL
ESPIED
ESPIER
ESPIES
ESPIOS
ESPOSA
ESPOSO
ESPRIT
OSPREY

•S•P••

ASHPAN
ASHPIT
ISOPOD
RSVPED
USOPEN

•S••P•

ASLOPE
ESCAPE
ESTOPS
FSTOPS
TSHAPE
TSTOPS
USHAPE
USURPS
VSHAPE
YSHAPE

•S•••P

ASDEEP
ASHARP
ASKSUP
ASLEEP
ASTEEP
ASTOOP
BSHARP
CSHARP
DSHARP
ESCARP
ESHARP
FSHARP
GSHARP
TSGARP
TSTRAP
USEDUP
USESUP

••SP••

AUSPEX
CASPAR
CASPER
CUSPAL
CUSPED
CUSPID
DESPOT
DISPEL
GASPAR
GASPED
GASPER
GOSPEL
HASPED
INSPAN
INSPOT
ITSPAT
JASPER
LISPED
LISPER
ONSPEC
RASPAS
RASPED
RASPER
RESPAN
RESPIN
RESPOT
SOSPAD
TVSPOT
UNSPAN
UNSPUN
UPSPIN
VESPAS
VESPER
VESPID
WISPED

••S•P•

AESOPS
JOSEPH
SYSOPS

••S••P

BISHOP
BUSTUP
CASTUP
COSYUP
DISHUP
DUSTUP
EASEUP
FESSUP
GASCAP
GOSSIP
HUSHUP
HYSSOP
INSTEP
KISSUP
LASHUP
LASTUP
MASHUP
MESSUP
MISHAP
MISTUP
MUSSUP
NOSEUP
NOSOAP
NOSTEP
OHSTOP
PASSUP
POSTOP
PUSHUP
RESHIP
RESNAP
RESOAP
RESTUP
RISEUP
ROSEUP
TOSSUP
UNSHIP
UNSNAP
UNSTEP
UNSTOP
UPSTEP
WASHUP
WISEUP

•••SP•

CIASPY
CLASPS
CRISPS
CRISPY
DAYSPA
GRASPS
KGBSPY
KRISPY
OBISPO
OUTSPY
THESPS
THESPY

•••S•P

ACESUP
ACTSUP
ADDSUP
AIRSUP
AMPSUP
ASKSUP
BIDSUP
BOBSUP
BUYSUP
CATSUP
CUESUP
CUTSUP
DAMSUP
DIGSUP
DOESUP
EATSUP
ENDSUP
EYESUP
FESSUP
FITSUP
FOGSUP
GETSUP
GINSUP
GOESUP
GOSSIP
GUMSUP
HAMSUP
HITSUP
HOPSUP
HYSSOP
ICESUP
JAMSUP
KEYSUP
KISSUP
LAPSUP
LAYSUP
LETSUP
MESSUP
MILSAP
MOPSUP
MUSSUP
OWNSUP
PASSUP
PAYSUP
PENSUP
PEPSUP
PINSUP
POPSUP
PUTSUP
REVSUP
RIGSUP
RIPSUP
RUBSUP
RUNSUP
SAWSUP
SEESUP
SETSUP
SEWSUP
SITSUP
SOPSUP
SUMSUP
TAGSUP
TEESUP
TIESUP
TIPSUP
TOGSUP
TOPSUP
TOSSUP
TOTSUP
USESUP
WADSUP
ZIPSUP

••••SP

THEASP
UNHASP

SQ••••

SQUABS
SQUADS
SQUALL
SQUARE
SQUASH
SQUATS
SQUAWK
SQUEAK
SQUEAL
SQUIBB
SQUIBS
SQUIDS
SQUINT
SQUIRE
SQUIRM
SQUIRT
SQUISH

S•Q•••

SEQUEL
SEQUIN

S••Q••

SACQUE
SESQUI

S•••Q•

SUZYQS

S••••Q

SMALLQ
SUZIEQ

•SQ•••

MSQUAD

••SQ••

BASQUE
BISQUE
CASQUE
JUSQUE
MASQUE
MOSQUE
RISQUE
SESQUI

••S•Q•

ETSEQQ

••S••Q

ETSEQQ
NASDAQ
POSSLQ

•••S•Q

POSSLQ

S•R•••

SARANS
SARDIS
SARDOU
SAREES
SARGES
SARGON
SARNIA
SARONG
SARTON
SARTOR
SARTRE
SCRAGS
SCRAMS
SCRAPE
SCRAPS
SCRAWL
SCREAK
SCREAM
SCREED
SCREEN
SCREES
SCREWS
SCREWY
SCRIBE
SCRIMP
SCRIMS
SCRIPS
SCRIPT
SCRODS
SCROLL
SCRUBS
SCRUFF
SCRUMS
SERACS
SERAIS
SERAPE
SERAPH
SERBIA
SERENA
SERENE
SERGEI
SERGES
SERGIO
SERIAL
SERIES
SERIFS
SERINS
SERKIN
SERKIS
SERMON
SEROUS
SERTAS
SERUMS
SERVED
SERVER
SERVES
SERVOS
SHRANK
SHREDS
SHREVE
SHREWD
SHREWS
SHRIEK
SHRIFT
SHRIKE
SHRILL
SHRIMP
SHRINE
SHRINK
SHRIVE
SHROUD
SHROVE
SHRUBS

SHRUGS
SHRUNK
SIRBEN
SIRENS
SIRICA
SIRING
SIRIUS
SIRKAY
SIRRAH
SIRREE
SIRUPS
SORBET
SORBIC
SORDID
SOREAT
SORELY
SOREST
SORREL
SORROW
SORTED
SORTER
SORTIE
SORTOF
SPRACH
SPRAIN
SPRANG
SPRATS
SPRAWL
SPRAYS
SPREAD
SPREES
SPRIER
SPRIGS
SPRING
SPRINT
SPRITE
SPRITS
SPRITZ
SPROUT
SPRUCE
SPRUNG
SPRYER
SPRYLY
STRADA
STRADS
STRAFE
STRAIN
STRAIT
STRAND
STRAPS
STRATA
STRATI
STRATO
STRATS
STRAUB
STRAWS
STRAYS
STREAK
STREAM
STREEP
STREET
STREPS
STRESS
STREWN
STREWS
STRIAE
STRICT
STRIDE
STRIFE
STRIKE
STRING
STRIPE
STRIPS
STRIPY
STRIVE
STROBE
STRODE
STROHS
STROKE
STROLL
STRONG
STROPS
STROUD
STROVE
STRUCK
STRUMS
STRUNG
STRUNK
STRUTS
SURAHS
SUREAM
SUREDO
SUREIS
SURELY
SUREOF
SUREST
SURETE
SURETY
SURFED
SURFER
SURFIN
SURGED
SURGES
SURIMI
SURREY
SURTAX
SURVEY
SYRIAN
SYRUPS
SYRUPY

S••R••

SABRAS
SABRES
SACRED
SACRUM
SATRAP
SAURON
SAURUS
SAWRED
SBARRO
SCARAB
SCARCE
SCARED
SCARER
SCARES
SCARFS
SCARNE
SCARPS
SCARRY
SCARUM
SCORCH
SCORED
SCORER
SCORES
SCORIA
SCORNS
SCURFY
SCURRY
SCURVE
SCURVY
SEARCH
SEARED
SEARER
SEARLE
SECRET
SEERED
SEURAT
SEVRES
SFORZA
SHARDS
SHARED
SHARER
SHARES
SHARIF
SHARKS
SHARON
SHARPE
SHARPS
SHARPY
SHARYN
SHEREE
SHERPA
SHERRI
SHERRY
SHERYL
SHIRAZ
SHIRER
SHIRES
SHIRKS
SHIRRS
SHIRTS
SHORES
SHORTA
SHORTE
SHORTI
SHORTO
SHORTS
SHORTU
SHORTY
SHORTZ
SIERRA
SIRRAH
SIRREE
SKIRLS
SKIRTS
SKIRUN
SKORTS
SLURPS
SLURRY
SMARMY
SMARTS
SMARTY
SMERSH
SMIRCH
SMIRKS
SMIRKY
SMORES
SMURFS
SMYRNA
SNARED
SNARER
SNARES
SNARFS
SNARKS
SNARKY
SNARLS
SNARLY
SNORED
SNORER
SNORES
SNORRI
SNORTS
SNORTY
SOARED
SOARER
SOIREE
SORREL
SORROW
SOTRUE
SOURCE
SOURED
SOURER
SOURLY
SOURON
SPARED
SPARER
SPARES
SPARKS
SPARKY
SPARSE
SPARTA
SPERRY
SPIRAL
SPIREA
SPIRED
SPIRES
SPIRIT
SPORES
SPORKS
SPORTS
SPORTY
SPURNS
SPURON
SPURTS
STARCH
STARED
STARER
STARES
STARIN
STARRY
STARTS
STARVE
STARZZ
STEREO
STERES
STERIC
STERNA
STERNE
STERNO
STERNS
STEROL
STIRIN
STIRUP
STORCH
STORED
STORER
STORES
STORKS
STORMS
STORMY
STORRS
STURDY
STYRON
SUCRES
SUNRAY
SUPRAS
SURREY
SUTRAS
SWARDS
SWARMS
SWERVE
SWIRLS
SWIRLY
SWIRLZ
SWORDS

S•••R•

SABERS
SAFARI
SAFIRE
SAHARA
SALARY
SAMARA
SANDRA
SANDRO
SANGRE
SAPORS
SARTRE
SATIRE
SATORI
SATURN
SATYRS
SAVERS
SAVORS
SAVORY
SAWERS
SAYERS
SBARRO
SCARRY
SCHORR
SCLERA
SCOURS
SCURRY
SEAARM
SEBERG
SECURE
SEDERS
SEGURA
SEMPRE
SENARY
SENORA
SENORS
SENTRA
SENTRY
SEPIRA
SEVERE
SEVERN
SEVERS
SEWARD
SEWERS
SEXERS
SHEARS
SHEERS
SHERRI
SHERRY
SHIRRS
SHOERS
SIERRA
SIGURD
SITARS
SIXERS
SIZERS
SKIERS
SLURRY
SMEARS
SMEARY
SNEERS
SNEERY
SNORRI
SOBERS
SOEURS
SOLARA
SOLERS
SOMBRE
SOMERS
SONARS
SONDRA
SONORA
SOPORS
SOWERS
SPEARE
SPEARS
SPERRY
SPHERE
SPIERS
SPOORS
SQUARE
SQUIRE
SQUIRM
SQUIRT
SSTARS
STAIRS
STARRY
STEERS
STIERS
STMARK
STMARY
STORRS
STUART
SUBARU
SUBORN
SUBURB
SUGARS
SUGARY
SULTRY
SUNDRY
SUPERB
SUPERG
SUPERS
SUTURE
SUVARI
SWEARS

S••••R

SACHER
SACKER
SADDER
SADLER
SAGIER
SAILER
SAILOR
SALTER
SALVER
SALVOR
SANDER
SANGER
SAPPER
SARTOR
SASSER
SATFOR
SAUCER
SAVIOR
SAVOIR
SAVOUR
SAWYER
SCALAR
SCALER
SCARER
SCHORR
SCORER
SCOTER
SEAAIR
SEALER
SEAMER
SEARER
SEATER
SEAVER
SECTOR
SEEDER
SEEGER
SEEKER
SEINER
SEIZER
SEIZOR
SELLER
SEMPER
SENDER
SENHOR
SENIOR
SENSOR
SERVER
SETFOR
SETTER
SETZER
SEXIER
SHADER
SHAKER
SHAKUR
SHAMIR
SHAPER
SHARER
SHAVER
SHINER
SHIRER
SHIVER
SHOFAR
SHOVER
SHOWER
SICKER
SIDDUR
SIFTER
SIGHER
SIGLER
SIGNER
SIGNOR
SILVER
SIMMER
SIMPER
SINGER
SINKER
SINNER
SIPPER
SISLER
SISTER
SITFOR
SITTER
SKATER
SKEWER
SLAKER
SLATER
SLAVER
SLAYER
SLICER
SLIDER
SLIVER
SLOPER
SLOWER
SMALLR
SMILER
SMITER
SMOKER
SNAKER
SNARER
SNIDER
SNIPER
SNORER
SNYDER
SOAKER
SOAPER
SOARER
SOBBER
SOCCER
SOFTER
SOLDER
SOLVER
SOMBER
SOMMER
SOONER
SORTER
SOUPER
SOURER
SOUTER
SPACER
SPADER
SPARER
SPAYER
SPEWER
SPICER
SPIDER
SPIKER
SPINER
SPRIER
SPRYER
SPYDER
STAGER
STALER
STARER
STATER
STATOR
STAYER
STELAR
STEWER
STOKER
STONER
STORER
STOVER
STOWER
STUPOR
STYLER
SUAVER
SUBPAR
SUBWAR
SUCCOR
SUCKER
SUDSER
SUEFOR
SUFFER
SUITOR
SULFUR
SULKER
SUMMER
SUMNER
SUMTER
SUNDER
SUPPER
SURFER
SUTTER
SWAYER
SWIPER

•SR•••

ASRARE
ISRAEL
ISRAIR

•S•R••

ASARCO
ASFREE
ASHRAM
ASTRAL
ASTRAY
ASTRES
ASTRID
ASTROS
ASTROV
ASTRUD
ESCROW
ESDRAS
ESPRIT
ESTRAY
ISERVE
ISTRES
ISTRIA
OSIRIS
OSPREY
TSTRAP
TSURIS
USARMY
USERID
USURER
USURPS
XSARAS

•S••R•

ASBURY
ASGARD
ASHARP
ASHORE
ASKERS
ASMARA
ASPERA
ASPIRE
ASPURE
ASRARE
ASSERT
ASSORT
ASSURE
ASTARE
ASTART
ASTERN
ASTERO
ASTERS
ASWARM
ASWIRL
BSHARP
BSTARS
CSHARP
CSTARS
DSHARP
ESCARP
ESCORT
ESHARP
ESKERS
ESTERS
FSHARP
FSTARS
GSHARP
GSTARS
ISIDRO
KSTARS
MSTARS
NSTARS
OSBERT
OSBORN
OSCARS
OSETRA
OSIERS
OSTARS
OSTERS
SSTARS
TSGARP
TSHIRT
USHERS
YSIDRO

•S•••R

ASEVER
ASHIER
ASHLAR
ASKFOR
ASNEAR
ASTHER
ESCHER
ESPIER
ESTHER
ISHTAR
ISIDOR
ISOBAR
ISOMER
ISRAIR
ISSUER
ISWEAR
MSIEUR
OSTLER
PSYWAR
USEFOR
USTOUR
USURER

••SR••

BASRAH
DESREE

••S•R•

ABSORB
ABSURD
ADSORB
ANSARA
ASSERT
ASSORT
ASSURE
AUSTRO
BESORE
BESURE
BISTRO
CASERN
CASERS
CASTRO
CESARE
CESARS
DESCRY
DESERT
DESIRE
DESTRY
DISARM
DISERE
DISTRO
DOSERS
DYSART
EASERS
ENSURE
EXSERT
GASTRO
HASBRO
HOSERS
IMSURE
INSERT
INSURE
LASERS
LASTRA
LOSERS
LUSTRA
LUSTRE
MASERS
MASERU
MESSRS
MISERS
MISERY
MUSERS
MYSORE
NOSERS
NOSTRA
OHSURE
PASTRY
POSERS
RASERS
RASURE
RESORB
RESORT
RISERS
ROSARY
ROSERY
ROSTRA
TASERS
TISHRI
UNSERE
UNSORE
UNSORT
UNSURE
VESTRY
VISORS

••S••R

ANSWER
AUSTER
BASHER
BASKER
BASTER
BESSER
BESTER
BESTIR
BUSHER
BUSIER
BUSKER
BUSTER
CASPAR
CASPER
CASTER
CASTOR
COSHER
COSIER
COSTAR
CUSSER
CUSTER
DASHER
DISBAR
DISEUR
DUSTER
EASIER
EASTER
EISNER
ENSLER
FASTER
FESTER
FISHER
FOSTER
FUSSER
GASPAR
GASPER
GASSER
GASTER
GASWAR
GOSOUR
GUSHER
HESTER
HISSER
HOSIER
HUSKER
HUSSAR
INSTIR
ISSUER
JASPER
JESTER
JOSHER
JUSTER
KCSTAR
KISSER
KOSHER
KOSTER
LASCAR
LASHER
LASKER
LASSER
LESSER
LESSOR
LESTER
LISPER
LISTER
LUSHER
LUSTER
MASHER
MASKER
MASTER
MESMER
MISTER
MOSHER
MUSHER
MUSTER
NASCAR
NASSER
NESTER
NESTOR
NOSHER
NOSIER
NOSTER
ONSTAR
OUSTER
OYSTER
PASDAR
PASSER
PASTER
PASTOR
PESTER
POSEUR
POSHER
POSTER
PUSHER
RASHER
RASPER
RASTER
RESTER
RESTIR
RISKER
ROSIER
ROSTER
RUSHER
SASSER
SISLER
SISTER
TASTER
TESTER
TOSSER
TUSKER
TVSTAR
ULSTER
UNSOUR
UPSOAR
UPSTIR
VASSAR
VASTER
VESPER
WASHER
WASSER
WASTER
WESKER
WESTER
WISHER
WISTER
XYSTER
YASGUR
YASSER
YESSIR
YESTER
ZESTER

•••SR•

MESSRS

•••S•R

ABASER
ABUSER
AMUSER
AYESIR
BESSER
BIGSUR
BURSAR
CAESAR
CAUSER
CENSER
CENSOR
CHASER
CLOSER
CURSER
CURSOR
CUSSER
DENSER
DOUSER
DOWSER
ERASER
FALSER
FIRSTR
FRASER
FUSSER
GASSER
GEYSER
GLASER
HAWSER
HISSER
HOWSER
HUSSAR
KAISER
KEYSER
KISSER
LAPSER
LASSER
LEASER
LESSER
LESSOR
LOOSER
MAUSER
MOUSER
NASSER
NOOSER
NURSER
PARSER
PASSER
PAUSER
PCUSER
PHASER
POISER
POYSER
PROSER
PULSAR
PURSER
QUASAR
RAISER
REISER
REUSER
RINSER
ROUSER
SASSER
SENSOR
SUDSER
TEASER
TENSER
TENSOR
TERSER
TOSSER
VASSAR
WASSER
WINSOR
YASSER
YESSIR

SS••••

SSTARS

S•S•••

SASEBO
SASHAY
SASHED
SASHES
SASSED
SASSER
SASSES
SASSON
SESAME
SESQUI
SESSUE
SESTET
SISALS
SISISI
SISKEL
SISLER
SISLEY
SISSLE
SISTER
SOSOON
SOSPAD
SUSANB
SUSANN
SUSHIS
SUSSED
SUSSES
SUSSEX
SYSOPS
SYSTEM

S••S••

SAISON
SALSAS
SAMSON
SANSEI
SASSED
SASSER
SASSES
SASSON
SAWSUP
SAYSAH
SAYSHI
SAYSNO
SAYSOK
SAYSOS
SAYSSO
SEASON
SEESAS
SEESAW
SEESIN
SEESTO
SEESUP
SEISMO
SEISMS
SENSED
SENSEI
SENSEN
SENSES
SENSOR
SESSUE
SETSAT

SETSBY
SETSIN
SETSON
SETSTO
SETSUP
SEWSIN
SEWSON
SEWSUP
SHASTA
SIESTA
SIPSON
SISSLE
SITSAT
SITSBY
SITSIN
SITSON
SITSUP
SIXSIX
SLOSHY
SLUSHY
SOASTO
SOISEE
SOPSUP
SOUSED
SOUSES
SPASMS
STASES
STASIS
SUBSEA
SUBSET
SUDSED
SUDSER
SUDSES
SUISSE
SUMSUP
SUNSET
SUSSED
SUSSES
SUSSEX
SWISHY

S•••S•

SADISM
SADIST
SAFEST
SAGEST
SAIDSO
SALISH
SAMOSA
SANEST
SAYEST
SAYSSO
SCAASI
SCHISM
SCHIST
SCHUSS
SETOSE
SEWIST
SEXISM
SEXIST
SHEESH
SHIEST
SHIISM
SHYEST
SINISE
SISISI
SLIEST
SLYEST
SMERSH
SMOOSH
SOREST
SPARSE
SPLASH
SPLOSH
SPOUSE
SQUASH
SQUISH
STRESS
SUFISM
SUISSE
SUREST
SWOOSH

S••••S

SABALS
SABERS
SABLES
SABOTS
SABRAS
SABRES
SADHES
SADHUS
SAHIBS
SAINTS
SALADS
SALEPS
SALLES
SALMIS
SALONS
SALSAS
SALVES
SALVOS
SAMBAS
SAMEAS
SANKAS
SANTAS
SANTOS
SANYOS
SAPORS
SARANS
SARDIS
SAREES
SARGES
SASHES
SASSES
SATAYS
SATINS
SATYRS
SAUCES
SAUDIS
SAULTS
SAUNAS
SAURUS
SAUTES
SAVEAS
SAVERS
SAVORS
SAWERS
SAXONS
SAYERS
SAYLES
SAYSOS
SAYYES
SCAGGS
SCALDS
SCALES
SCALPS
SCAMPS
SCANTS
SCARES
SCARFS
SCARPS
SCENAS
SCENES
SCENTS
SCHAVS
SCHMOS
SCHUSS
SCHWAS
SCIONS
SCOFFS
SCOLDS
SCONES
SCOOPS
SCOOTS
SCOPES
SCORES
SCORNS
SCOTTS
SCOURS
SCOUTS
SCOWLS
SCRAGS
SCRAMS
SCRAPS
SCREES
SCREWS
SCRIMS
SCRIPS
SCRODS
SCRUBS
SCRUMS
SCUBAS
SCUFFS
SCULLS
SEALYS
SEAMUS
SEDANS
SEDERS
SEDGES
SEDUMS
SEENAS
SEESAS
SEGUES
SEIKOS
SEINES
SEISMS
SEIZES
SELVES
SENATS
SENNAS
SENORS
SENSES
SEPALS
SEPIAS
SEPOYS
SERACS
SERAIS
SERGES
SERIES
SERIFS
SERINS
SERKIS
SEROUS
SERTAS
SERUMS
SERVES
SERVOS
SETTOS
SETUPS
SEVENS
SEVERS
SEVRES
SEWERS
SEWONS
SEXERS
SHACKS
SHADES
SHAFTS
SHAKES
SHAKOS
SHALES
SHAMES
SHAMUS
SHANKS
SHAPES
SHARDS
SHARES
SHARKS
SHARPS
SHAVES
SHAWLS
SHEARS
SHEDDS
SHEENS
SHEERS
SHEETS
SHEIKS
SHELLS
SHIFTS
SHILLS
SHINES
SHIRES
SHIRKS
SHIRRS
SHIRTS
SHOALS
SHOATS
SHOCKS
SHOERS
SHOGIS
SHOJIS
SHOOTS
SHORES
SHORTS
SHOUTS
SHOVES
SHREDS
SHREWS
SHRUBS
SHRUGS
SHUCKS
SHUNTS
SIBYLS
SICKOS
SIDLES
SIEGES
SIETES
SIEVES
SIGHTS
SIGILS
SIGMAS
SILVAS
SINEWS
SINGES
SIRENS
SIRIUS
SIRUPS
SISALS
SITARS
SITINS
SITUPS
SIVANS
SIXERS
SIXTHS
SIXTUS
SIZERS
SKAGGS
SKALDS
SKANKS
SKATES
SKEETS
SKEINS
SKIERS
SKIFFS
SKILLS
SKIMPS
SKINKS
SKIRLS
SKIRTS
SKOALS
SKORTS
SKULKS
SKULLS
SKUNKS
SLACKS
SLAKES
SLANGS
SLANTS
SLATES
SLAVES
SLEEKS
SLEEPS
SLEETS
SLICES
SLICKS
SLIDES
SLIMES
SLINGS
SLINKS
SLOOPS
SLOPES
SLOTHS
SLUMPS
SLURPS
SMACKS
SMALLS
SMARTS
SMAZES
SMEARS
SMELLS
SMELTS
SMILES
SMIRKS
SMITES
SMITHS
SMOCKS
SMOKES
SMOLTS
SMORES
SMURFS
SNACKS
SNAFUS
SNAILS
SNAKES
SNARES
SNARFS
SNARKS
SNARLS
SNATHS
SNEAKS
SNEERS
SNELLS
SNICKS
SNIFFS
SNIPES
SNOODS
SNOOKS
SNOOPS
SNOOTS
SNOPES
SNORES
SNORTS
SNOUTS
SNUFFS
SOAVES
SOBERS
SOCLES
SOEURS
SOITIS
SOLANS
SOLEAS
SOLERS
SOLEUS
SOLIDS
SOLONS
SOLVES
SOMERS
SONARS
SONDES
SONICS
SOONAS
SOPORS
SOUNDS
SOUSES
SOUTHS
SOWERS
SPACES
SPADES
SPANKS
SPARES
SPARKS
SPASMS
SPATES
SPAWNS
SPEAKS
SPEARS
SPECKS
SPEEDS
SPELLS
SPENDS
SPICES
SPIELS
SPIERS
SPIFFS
SPIKES
SPILES
SPILLS
SPINES
SPINKS
SPIRES
SPITES
SPLATS
SPLAYS
SPLITS
SPODES
SPOILS
SPOKES
SPOOFS
SPOOKS
SPOOLS
SPOONS
SPOORS
SPORES
SPORKS
SPORTS
SPOUTS
SPRATS
SPRAYS
SPREES
SPRIGS
SPRITS
SPUMES
SPURNS
SPURTS
SQUABS
SQUADS
SQUATS
SQUIBS
SQUIDS
SSTARS
STACKS
STAFFS
STAGES
STAINS
STAIRS
STAKES
STALES
STALKS
STALLS
STAMOS
STAMPS
STANDS
STAPES
STAPHS
STARES
STARTS
STASES
STASIS
STATES
STATUS
STAVES
STEADS
STEAKS
STEALS
STEAMS
STEEDS
STEELS
STEEPS
STEERS
STEINS
STELAS
STELES
STENOS
STENTS
STERES
STERNS
STICKS
STIDES
STIERS
STIFFS
STILES
STILLS
STILTS
STINGS
STINKS
STINTS
STIPES
STOATS
STOCKS
STOICS
STOKES
STOLAS
STOLES
STOMAS
STOMPS
STONES
STOOLS
STOOPS
STORES
STORKS
STORMS
STORRS
STOUTS
STOVES
STPATS
STPIUS
STRADS
STRAPS
STRATS
STRAWS
STRAYS
STREPS
STRESS
STREWS
STRIPS
STROHS
STROPS
STRUMS
STRUTS
STUFFS
STUKAS
STUMPS
STUNTS
STUPAS
STUPES
STYLES
STYLUS
SUCHAS
SUCRES
SUDSES
SUEDES
SUENOS
SUGARS
SUITES
SULFAS
SUMACS
SUMUPS
SUNDAS
SUNNIS
SUNUPS
SUPERS
SUPRAS
SURAHS
SUREIS
SURGES
SUSHIS
SUSSES
SUTRAS
SUZYQS
SWAINS
SWALES
SWAMIS
SWAMPS
SWANNS
SWARDS
SWARMS
SWATHS
SWEARS
SWEATS
SWEDES
SWEEPS
SWEETS
SWELLS
SWIFTS
SWILLS
SWINGS
SWIPES
SWIRLS
SWOONS
SWOOPS
SWORDS
SYLPHS
SYNCHS
SYNODS
SYNTHS
SYRUPS
SYSOPS

•SS•••

ASSAIL
ASSAYS
ASSENT
ASSERT
ASSESS
ASSETS
ASSIGN
ASSISI
ASSIST
ASSIZE
ASSLOW
ASSOFT
ASSORT
ASSTDA
ASSUCH
ASSUME
ASSURE
ESSAIS
ESSAYS
ESSENE
ISSEIS
ISSUED
ISSUER
ISSUES
OSSETS
OSSIAN
OSSIFY

•S•S••

ASKSIN
ASKSOF
ASKSUP
ASOSAN
USESIN
USESON
USESUP

•S••S•

ASEASY
ASFAST
ASLOSH
ASPISH
ASSESS
ASSISI
ASSIST
ESPOSA
ESPOSO
KSWISS
OSMOSE
TSETSE
TSKTSK
TSOTSI
USAUSA
ZSAZSA

•S•••S

ASANAS
ASCOTS
ASDICS
ASIANS
ASIDES
ASKERS
ASPENS
ASPICS
ASSAYS
ASSESS
ASSETS
ASTERS
ASTRES
ASTROS
BSIDES
BSTARS
CSPOTS
CSTARS
ESBATS
ESDRAS
ESKERS
ESPIES
ESPIOS
ESSAIS
ESSAYS
ESTERS
ESTOCS
ESTOPS
FSTARS
FSTOPS
GSTARS
GSUITS
ISAACS
ISLETS
ISLEYS
ISSEIS
ISSUES
ISTLES
ISTRES
ISUZUS
KSTARS
KSWISS
MSTARS
NSTARS
OSAGES
OSCANS
OSCARS
OSIERS
OSIRIS
OSMICS
OSSETS
OSTARS
OSTERS
PSALMS
PSEUDS
PSHAWS
PSYCHS
SSTARS
TSADES
TSADIS
TSTOPS
TSURIS
USAGES
USHERS
USNEWS
USUALS
USURPS
VSIGNS
VSIXES
XSARAS

••SS••

AUSSIE
BASSES
BASSET
BASSEY
BASSLY
BASSOS
BESSEL
BESSER
BESSIE
BESSON
BISSAU
BISSET
BOSSED
BOSSES
BOSSON
BUSSED
BUSSES
BYSSHE
CASSIA
CASSIE
CASSIM
CASSIN
CASSIO
CASSIS
CESSED
CESSES
CESSNA
COSSET
CUSSED
CUSSER
CUSSES
DASSIN
DESSAU
DISSED
DISSES
DOSSAL
DOSSED
DOSSES
FESSED
FESSES
FESSUP
FOSSAE
FOSSES
FOSSEY
FOSSIL
FUSSAT
FUSSED
FUSSER
FUSSES
GASSED
GASSER
GASSES
GOSSIP
GUSSET
HASSAM
HASSAN
HASSEL
HASSID
HASSLE
HISSAT
HISSED
HISSER
HISSES
HOSSES
HUSSAR
HUSSEY
HYSSOP
IJSSEL
JESSEL
JESSYE
JOSSES
KISSED
KISSEL
KISSER
KISSES
KISSIN
KISSME
KISSUP
KOSSEL
LASSEN
LASSER
LASSES
LASSIE
LASSOS
LESSEE
LESSEN
LESSER
LESSON
LESSOR
LISSES
LOSSES
MASSED
MASSES
MASSEY
MASSIF
MASSON
MASSYS
MESSED
MESSES
MESSIN
MESSRS
MESSUP
MISSAL
MISSAY
MISSED
MISSES
MISSET
MISSIS
MISSME
MISSUS
MOSSAD
MOSSED
MOSSES
MUSSED
MUSSEL
MUSSES
MUSSET
MUSSUP
NASSAU
NASSER
NESSEN
NESSES
NESSIE
NESSUS
NISSAN
NISSEN
PASSAS
PASSAT
PASSBY
PASSED
PASSEL
PASSER
PASSES
PASSGO
PASSIM
PASSON
PASSOS
PASSTO
PASSUP
POSSES
POSSLQ
POSSUM
PUSSES
RASSES
RASSLE
ROSSEN
ROSSET
ROSSUM
RUSSEL
RUSSES
RUSSET
RUSSIA
SASSED
SASSER
SASSES
SASSON
SESSUE
SISSLE
SUSSED
SUSSES
SUSSEX
TASSEL
TASSES
TESSIE
TESSIO
TISSOT
TISSUE
TOSSED
TOSSER
TOSSES
TOSSIN
TOSSUP
TUSSAL
TUSSES
TUSSLE
VASSAL
VASSAR
VESSEL
WASSER
WESSEX
WESSON
WUSSES
YASSER
YESSED
YESSES
YESSIR

••S•S•

ASSESS
ASSISI
ASSIST
BASEST
DESIST
DISUSE
INSIST
JUSTSO
MISUSE
OBSESS
RESIST
SISISI
WISEST

••S••S

AESOPS
AISLES
ANSEIS
ARSONS
ASSAYS
ASSESS
ASSETS
BASHES
BASICS
BASILS
BASINS
BASSES
BASSOS
BASTES
BESETS
BESOMS
BESOTS
BISONS
BOSOMS
BOSONS
BOSSES
BOSUNS
BUSHES
BUSIES
BUSSES
CASALS
CASERS
CASHES
CASIOS
CASSIS
CASTES
CESARS
CESSES
CESTAS
CESTUS
CISCOS
COSECS
COSETS
COSHES
COSIES
COSMAS
COSMOS
COSTAS
CUSECS
CUSSES
CUSTIS
DASHES
DASHIS
DESNOS
DESODS
DISCOS
DISCUS
DISHES
DISMAS
DISMES
DISSES
DOSERS
DOSSES
DOSUMS
EASELS
EASERS
EASYAS
EDSELS
ENSUES
EOSINS
EPSONS
ESSAIS
ESSAYS
EUSTIS
FASCES
FESSES
FESTAS
FESTUS
FISHES
FOSSES
FUSEES
FUSILS
FUSSES
GASHES
GASSES
GESTES
GISMOS
GUSHES
HASHES
HASTES
HISSES
HOSELS
HOSERS
HOSSES
HOSTAS
HUSHES
HYSONS
INSETS
ISSEIS
ISSUES
JOSHES
JOSSES
JUSTAS
JUSTUS
JUSTYS
KASHAS
KISSES
LASERS
LASHES
LASSES
LASSOS
LESBOS
LISLES
LISSES

LOSDOS LOSERS LOSSES LUSHES MASAIS MASERS MASHES MASONS MASSES MASSYS MESHES MESNES MESONS MESSES MESSRS MISERS MISSES MISSIS MISSUS MOSEYS MOSHES MOSSES MUSEES MUSEOS MUSERS MUSHES MUSICS MUSSES NASALS NASHES NESSES NESSUS NISANS NISEIS NOSERS NOSHES OBSESS ONSETS OSSETS OUSELS PASCHS PASEOS PASHAS PASSAS PASSES PASSOS PASTAS PASTES PASTIS PESTOS PISANS PISCES PISHES PISTES POSEAS POSERS POSIES POSITS POSSES PUSHES PUSSES RASERS RASHES RASPAS RASSES RASTAS RESAWS RESAYS

RESEES RESETS RESEWS RESHES RESINS RESITS RESODS RESOWS RESTES RISERS RISHIS ROSHIS ROSIES ROSINS RUSHES RUSSES SASHES SASSES SISALS SUSHIS SUSSES SYSOPS TASERS TASSES TASTES TESLAS TOSSES TUSHES TUSSES TVSETS TYSONS UNSAYS UNSEWS UPSETS URSIDS VASTUS VESPAS VESTAS VISITS VISORS VISTAS VOSGES WASHES WASHOS WASTES WISHES WUSSES XYSTUS YESSES YESYES ZESTAS

•••SS•

AGASSI ALYSSA BRASSY BROSSE CHASSE CLASSA CLASSE CLASSY CRESSY CROSSE DOESSO DRESSY DROSSY DUESSA EDESSA ELISSA FLOSSY FUISSE GLASSY GLOSSA GLOSSO GLOSSY GRASSO GRASSY GROSSE GROSSO INESSE ITISSO MOUSSE MTOSSA NEISSE ODESSA ORISSA OWOSSO PLISSE POUSSE PRISSY SAYSSO SUISSE TRESSY WRASSE

•••S•S

ABASES ABUSES ABYSMS ACTSAS ALISTS AMUSES ANGSTS ANISES ARISES ATESTS ATISES AVISOS AXISES BAISAS BALSAS BASSES BASSOS BEASTS BETSYS BIASES BLASTS BLISTS BOASTS BOOSTS BOSSES BRISES BRISKS BURSAS BURSTS BUSSES CASSIS CAUSES CEASES CENSES CENSUS CESSES CHASES CHASMS CHESTS CLASPS CLOSES COASTS COPSES CORSAS CRESTS CRISES CRISIS CRISPS CRUSES CRUSTS CURSES CUSSES DAISES DANSES DEISTS DIESES DIESIS DIPSOS DISSES DNASES DOSSES DOUSES DOWSES DRUSES ECESIS EGESTS EGISES ELISTS EPOSES ERASES EXISTS FATSIS FEASTS FESSES FIRSTS FLASKS FOISTS FOSSES FRISES FRISKS FROSTS FUSSES GASSES GHOSTS GNOSES GNOSIS GOOSES GORSES GRASPS GRISTS GUESTS GUISES HANSAS HANSES HAWSES HEISTS HISSES HOISTS HORSES HOSSES HOUSES HTESTS HYKSOS IBISES IRISES JOISTS JOSSES JOUSTS KANSAS KARSTS KIOSKS KISSES LAPSES LAPSUS LASSES LASSOS LEASES LEASTS LENSES LISSES LOOSES LOSSES LOUSES MANSES MASSES MASSYS MESSES MESSRS MIDSTS MISSES MISSIS MISSUS MOISES MOSSES MOUSES MUSSES MYOSIS NESSES NESSUS NOESIS NOISES NOOSES NTESTS NURSES ODISTS ONUSES OPUSES OTOSES OTOSIS PABSTS PAISES PARSES PASSAS PASSES PASSOS PAUSES PERSIS PHASES PLUSES POISES POSSES PRISMS PROSES PULSES PURSES PUSSES QUESOS QUESTS RAISES RAMSES RASSES REASKS REESES REUSES RHESUS RINSES RITSOS ROASTS ROOSTS ROUSES ROUSTS RUSSES SALSAS SASSES SAYSOS SEESAS SEISMS SENSES SOUSES SPASMS STASES STASIS SUDSES SUSSES TARSUS TASSES TEASES TENSES THESES THESIS THESPS TMESES TMESIS TOASTS TORSOS TOSSES TRUSTS TRYSTS TUSSES TUTSIS TWISTS UKASES UNISYS VALSES VERSES VERSOS VERSTS VERSUS WAISTS WHISKS WORSTS WRESTS WRISTS WURSTS WUSSES XHOSAS XMASES YEASTS YESSES

••••SS

ABBESS ACCESS ACROSS ALDISS ARLISS ARNESS ASSESS AWLESS BYPASS CARESS DURESS ECLASS EGRESS EMBOSS EULESS EXCESS EZPASS GNEISS HARASS IGUESS INNESS JAMESS JONESS KRAUSS KSWISS MORASS MOROSS NOFUSS NOLESS NOLOSS OBSESS OGRESS RECESS REMISS REPASS RETOSS SCHUSS STRESS UNLESS UPTOSS

ST••••

STABAT STABLE STABLY STACEY STACKS STADIA STAFFS STAGED STAGER STAGES STAGEY STAINS STAIRS STAKED STAKES STALAG STALED STALER STALES STALIN STALKS STALKY STALLS STAMEN STAMOS STAMPS STANCE STANCH STANDS STANZA STAPES STAPHS STAPLE STAPUF STARCH STARED STARER STARES STARIN STARRY STARTS STARVE STARZZ STASES STASIS STATED STATEN STATER STATES STATIC STATIN STATOR STATUE STATUS STAVED STAVES STAYAT STAYED STAYER STAYIN STAYON STAYUP STBEDE STEADS STEADY STEAKS STEALS STEAMS STEAMY STEEDS STEELE STEELS STEELY STEEPS STEERS STEEVE STEFAN STEFFI STEFOY STEINS STELAR STELAS STELES STELLA STELMO STEMMY STENCH STENOG STENOS STENTS STEPIN STEPON STEPPE STEPUP STEREO STERES STERIC STERNA STERNE STERNO STERNS STEROL STETHO STEVEN STEVIE STEWED STEWER STEWIE STICKS STICKY STIDES STIERS STIFFS STIFLE STIGMA STILES STILLE STILLS STILLY STILTS STIMPY STINGS STINGY STINKO STINKS STINKY STINTS STIPES STIRIN STIRUP STITCH STIVIC STJOAN STJOHN STJUDE STLUKE STMALO STMARK STMARY STNICK STOATS STOCKS STOCKY STODGE STODGY STOGIE STOICS STOJKO STOKED STOKER STOKES STOLAE STOLAF STOLAS STOLEN STOLES STOLID STOLLE STOLON STOLTZ STOMAS STOMPS STONED STONER STONES STONEY STOOGE STOOLS STOOLY STOOPS STOPAT STOPBY STOPGO STOPIN STOPIT STOPUP STORCH STORED STORER STORES STORKS STORMS STORMY STORRS STOTIN STOUTS STOVER STOVES STOWED STOWER STOWIT STPATS STPAUL STPETE STPIUS STRADA STRADS STRAFE STRAIN STRAIT STRAND STRAPS STRATA STRATI STRATO STRATS STRAUB STRAWS STRAYS STREAK STREAM STREEP STREET STREPS STRESS STREWN STREWS STRIAE STRICT STRIDE STRIFE STRIKE STRING STRIPE STRIPS STRIPY STRIVE STROBE STRODE STROHS STROKE STROLL STRONG STROPS STROUD STROVE STRUCK STRUMS STRUNG STRUNK STRUTS STUART STUBBY STUCCO STUDIO STUDLY STUFFS STUFFY STUKAS STUMPS STUMPY STUNTS STUNTY STUPAS STUPES STUPID STUPOR STURDY STUVWX STYING STYLED STYLER STYLES STYLET STYLUS STYMIE STYRON

S•T•••

SATAYS SATCOM SATEEN SATFOR SATING SATINS SATINY SATIRE SATORI SATOUT SATPAT SATRAP SATURN SATYRS SETFEE SETFOR SETOFF SETOSE SETOUT SETSAT SETSBY SETSIN SETSON SETSTO SETSUP SETTEE SETTER SETTLE SETTOS SETUPS SETZER SGTMAJ SHTETL SHTICK SITARS SITCOM SITFOR SITING SITINS SITOUT SITPAT SITSAT SITSBY SITSIN SITSON SITSUP SITTER SITTIN SITUPS SOTHAT SOTHEN SOTRUE SOTTED SSTARS SUTRAS SUTTER SUTTON SUTURE

S••T••

SAITEK SALTED SALTEN SALTER SALTII SALTON SANTAS SANTEE SANTHA SANTOS SARTON SARTOR SARTRE SAUTES SCATHE SCOTCH SCOTER SCOTIA SCOTTO SCOTTS SCOTTY SCYTHE SEATAC SEATED SEATER SEATON SECTOR SEETHE SELTEN SENTBY SENTIN SENTON SENTRA SENTRY SENTTO SENTUP SEPTAL SEPTET SEPTIC SEPTUM SERTAS SESTET SETTEE SETTER SETTLE SETTOS SEXTET SEXTON SHOTAT SHOTBY SHOTUP SHUTIN SHUTUP SIETES SIFTED SIFTER SILTED SINTAX SISTER SITTER SITTIN SIXTEN SIXTHS SIXTUS SIXTWO SKATED SKATER SKATES SKETCH SKITCH SKITOW SKYTEL SLATED SLATER SLATES SLITHY SLOTHS SMITER SMITES SMITHS SMITHY SMITTY SMUTTY SNATCH SNATHS SNITCH SOFTEN SOFTER SOFTIE SOFTLY SOFTON SOITIS SONTAG SOOTHE SORTED SORTER SORTIE SORTOF SOTTED SOUTER SOUTHS SPATES SPATHE SPITED SPITES SPITON SPOTON SPOTTV SPOTTY STATED STATEN STATER STATES STATIC STATIN STATOR STATUE STATUS STETHO STITCH STOTIN SUBTLE SUBTLY SUITED SUITES SUITOR SUITUP SULTAN SULTRY SUMTER SUNTAN SURTAX SUTTER SUTTON SWATAT SWATCH SWATHE SWATHS SWITCH SYNTAX SYNTHS SYSTEM

S•••T•

SABATO SABOTS SAFETY SAIDTO SAILTO SAINTE SAINTS SALUTE SALUTO SANCTA SANGTO SANITY SAULTS SAVATE SCANTS SCANTY SCENTS SCOOTS SCOTTO SCOTTS SCOTTY SCOUTS SEDATE SEEMTO SEENTO SEESTO SELLTO SEMITE SENATE SENATS SENDTO SENITI SENTTO SETSTO SHAFTS SHANTY SHASTA SHEATH SHEETS SHELTY SHIFTS SHIFTY SHIITE SHINTO SHIPTO SHIRTS SHOATS SHOOTS SHORTA SHORTE SHORTI SHORTO SHORTS SHORTU SHORTY SHORTZ SHOUTS SHTETL SHULTZ SHUNTS SIESTA SIGHTS SINGTO SKEETS SKIRTS SKORTS SLANTS SLEETS SLEETY SLEUTH SMARTS SMARTY SMELTS SMITTY SMOLTS SMOOTH SMUTTY SNAPTO SNOOTS SNOOTY SNORTS SNORTY SNOUTS SOASTO SOLATI SOLDTO SOLUTE SOMATA SONATA SOWETO SPARTA SPILTH SPLATS SPLITS SPORTS SPORTY SPOTTV SPOTTY SPOUTS SPRATS SPRITE SPRITS SPRITZ SPURTS SQUATS STARTS STENTS STILTS STINTS STOATS

STOLTZ
STOUTS
STPATS
STPETE
STRATA
STRATI
STRATO
STRATS
STRUTS
STUNTS
STUNTY
SUBITO
SUNGTO
SURETE
SURETY
SVELTE
SWEATS
SWEATY
SWEETS
SWIFTS

S••••T

SACHET
SADIST
SAFEST
SAGEST
SALYUT
SAMLET
SANEST
SATOUT
SATPAT
SAVANT
SAVEIT
SAWFIT
SAWOUT
SAWPIT
SAYEST
SCHIST
SCRIPT
SCULPT
SEACAT
SECANT
SECRET
SEEFIT
SEEOUT
SELECT
SELLIT
SEPTET
SESTET
SETOUT
SETSAT
SEURAT
SEWIST
SEXIST
SEXPOT
SEXTET
SHALIT
SHEBAT
SHEVAT
SHIEST
SHOPAT
SHOTAT
SHRIFT
SHYEST
SIGHAT
SIGNET
SILENT
SITOUT
SITPAT
SITSAT
SKIHAT
SKIPIT
SKYLIT
SLIEST
SLIGHT
SLYEST
SMALLT
SNAPAT
SNOCAT
SOBEIT
SOCKET
SOFFIT
SOLDIT
SONANT
SONNET
SORBET
SOREAT
SOREST
SOTHAT
SOUGHT
SOVIET
SOWHAT
SPIGOT
SPINET
SPIRIT
SPLINT
SPOILT
SPRINT
SPROUT
SPYBOT
SPYOUT
SQUINT
SQUIRT
STABAT
STAYAT
STOPAT
STOPIT
STOWIT
STRAIT
STREET
STRICT
STUART
STYLET
SUBLET
SUBLOT
SUBMIT
SUBNET
SUBSET
SUMMIT
SUNHAT
SUNLIT
SUNSET
SUREST
SWATAT
SWIVET

•ST•••

ASTALL
ASTANA
ASTARE
ASTART
ASTEAL
ASTEEP
ASTERN
ASTERO
ASTERS
ASTHER
ASTHMA
ASTLEY
ASTOOP
ASTRAL
ASTRAY
ASTRES
ASTRID
ASTROS
ASTROV
ASTRUD
ASTUTE
BSTARS
CSTARS
ESTADO
ESTATE
ESTEEM
ESTERS
ESTHER
ESTIME
ESTLIN
ESTOCS
ESTOPS
ESTRAY
FSTARS
FSTOPS
GSTAAD
GSTARS
ISTHMI
ISTLES
ISTRES
ISTRIA
KSTARS
MSTARS
NSTARS
OSTARS
OSTEAL
OSTEND
OSTERS
OSTLER
RSTUVW
SSTARS
TSTOPS
TSTRAP
USTOUR

•S•T••

ASHTON
ASSTDA
ISHTAR
ISITME
ISNTOK
OSETRA
TSETSE
TSKTSK
TSOTSI
USETAX

•S••T•

ASANTE
ASCOTS
ASSETS
ASTUTE
CSPOTS
ESBATS
ESTATE
FSCOTT
GSIXTY
GSUITS
ISANTI
ISINTO
ISLATE
ISLETS
OSSETS
USEDTO

•S•••T

ASCENT
ASFAST
ASFLAT
ASHPIT
ASKANT
ASKOUT
ASLANT
ASNEAT
ASPECT
ASSENT
ASSERT
ASSIST
ASSOFT
ASSORT
ASTART
ESCAUT
ESCENT
ESCORT
ESPRIT
FSCOTT
ISEEIT
ISEULT
ISLEFT
OSBERT
TSHIRT
USENET
USMINT

••ST••

ALSTON
AMSTEL
ASSTDA
ATSTUD
AUSTEN
AUSTER
AUSTIN
AUSTRO
BASTED
BASTER
BASTES
BASTIA
BESTED
BESTER
BESTIR
BESTOW
BISTRO
BOSTON
BUSTED
BUSTER
BUSTIN
BUSTLE
BUSTUP
CASTED
CASTEL
CASTER
CASTES
CASTLE
CASTON
CASTOR
CASTRO
CASTUP
CESTAS
CESTUS
COSTAE
COSTAL
COSTAR
COSTAS
COSTCO
COSTED
COSTLY
CUSTER
CUSTIS
CUSTOM
CYSTIC
DESTEM
DESTRY
DISTAL
DISTIL
DISTRO
DUSTED
DUSTER
DUSTIN
DUSTUP
EASTER
EASTLA
EASTON
ELSTON
ERSTAD
EUSTIS
FASTED
FASTEN
FASTER
FESTAL
FESTAS
FESTER
FESTUS
FISTED
FISTIC
FOSTER
GASTAX
GASTER
GASTON
GASTRO
GESTAE
GESTES
GESTIC
GOSTAG
GUSTAV
GUSTED
HASTED
HASTEN
HASTES
HESTER
HESTIA
HESTON
HOSTAS
HOSTED
HOSTEL
HOSTLY
HUSTLE
HUSTON
INSTAL
INSTEP
INSTIL
INSTIR
JESTED
JESTER
JOSTLE
JUSTAS
JUSTER
JUSTIN
JUSTLY
JUSTME
JUSTSO
JUSTUS
JUSTYS
KCSTAR
KOSTER
LASTED
LASTEX
LASTLY
LASTRA
LASTUP
LESTAT
LESTER
LISTED
LISTEE
LISTEN
LISTER
LISTON
LOSTIT
LOSTTO
LUSTED
LUSTER
LUSTRA
LUSTRE
MASTED
MASTER
MASTIC
MISTED
MISTER
MISTUP
MOSTEL
MOSTLY
MOSTOF
MUSTDO
MUSTER
MUSTNT
MYSTIC
NESTEA
NESTED
NESTER
NESTIN
NESTLE
NESTOR
NOSTEP
NOSTER
NOSTRA
OHSTOP
ONSTAR
OUSTED
OUSTER
OYSTER
PASTAS
PASTED
PASTEL
PASTER
PASTES
PASTIS
PASTIT
PASTOR
PASTRY
PESTER
PESTLE
PESTOS
PISTES
PISTIL
PISTOL
PISTON
PISTOU
POSTAL
POSTED
POSTER
POSTIE
POSTIT
POSTON
POSTOP
POSTUM
QRSTUV
RASTAS
RASTER
RESTAB
RESTED
RESTER
RESTES
RESTIR
RESTON
RESTOW
RESTUP
ROSTEN
ROSTER
ROSTOV
ROSTRA
RUSTED
RUSTIC
RUSTLE
SESTET
SISTER
SYSTEM
TASTED
TASTEE
TASTER
TASTES
TESTAE
TESTED
TESTEE
TESTER
TVSTAR
ULSTER
UNSTEP
UNSTOP
UNSTOW
UPSTEP
UPSTIR
VASTER
VASTLY
VASTUS
VESTAL
VESTAS
VESTED
VESTEE
VESTRY
VISTAS
VOSTOK
WASTED
WASTER
WASTES
WESTER
WESTIE
WESTIN
WESTON
WISTER
WYSTAN
XYSTER
XYSTUS
YESTER
ZESTAS
ZESTED
ZESTER

••S•T•

ANSATE
ASSETS
BESETS
BESOTS
CASITA
COSETS
DESETA
DESOTO
ENSATE
ERSATZ
INSETS
INSITU
LASHTO
LOSETO
LOSTTO
ONSETS
ONSITE
OSSETS
PASHTO
PASSTO
PESETA
POSITS
RESETS
RESITE
RESITS
RISETO
ROSETO
ROSITA
RUSHTO
TVSETS
UPSETS
VASHTI
VISITS
WISETO
WISHTO

••S••T

ABSENT
ASSENT
ASSERT
ASSIST
ASSOFT
ASSORT
BASALT
BASEST
BASKET
BASSET
BBSHOT
BESANT
BISECT
BISSET
CASKET
COSSET
DASHIT
DESALT
DESERT
DESILT
DESIST
DESPOT
DISANT
DYSART
ENSEAT
EXSECT
EXSERT
FUSSAT
GASJET
GASKET
GASLIT
GOSOFT
GUSSET
HASOUT
HESOUT
HISSAT
INSECT
INSERT
INSIST
INSPOT
INSULT
ITSHOT
ITSNOT
ITSPAT
JESUIT
KISMET
LESTAT
LOSEIT
LOSTIT
MASCOT
MISACT
MISCUT
MISFIT
MISHIT
MISSET
MUSCAT
MUSKET
MUSSET
MUSTNT
NESBIT
NOSALT
PASSAT
PASTIT
POSTIT
PUSHIT
RESALT
RESEAT
RESECT
RESENT
RESHOT
RESHUT
RESIFT
RESIST
RESORT
RESPOT
RESUIT
RESULT
RISKIT
ROSSET
RUSHAT
RUSSET
SESTET
TASKET
TISKET
TISSOT
TVSPOT
UNSEAT
UNSENT
UNSHUT
UNSOFT
UNSORT
UPSENT
UPSHOT
WASMET
WESKIT
WISEST
XESOUT
YESBUT

•••ST•

ADDSTO
ADESTE
AGOSTO
ALISTS
ANGSTS
ARISTA
ARISTO
ATESTS
AVESTA
BEASTS
BLASTS
BLISTS
BOASTS
BOOSTS
BOWSTO
BURSTS
CHASTE
CHESTS
CHESTY
COASTS
COPSTO
CRESTS
CRISTO
CRUSTS
CRUSTY
CUESTA
DAOSTA
DEISTS
DOESTO
EGESTA
EGESTS
ELISTS
ERESTU
EXISTS
FEASTS
FEISTY
FIESTA
FIRSTR
FIRSTS
FOISTS
FROSTS
FROSTY
FRUSTA
GETSTO
GHOSTS
GHOSTY
GOESTO
GRISTS
GUESTS
HEISTS
HEWSTO
HOISTS
HOPSTO
HTESTS
JOISTS
JOUSTS
KARSTS
KRISTI
KRUSTY
LAYSTO
LEASTS
LIESTO
MIDSTS
NODSTO
NTESTS
ODISTS
OPTSTO
PABSTS
PASSTO
PIGSTY
PORSTU
PRESTO
PUTSTO
QUESTS
ROASTS
ROOSTS
ROUSTS
RUNSTO
SEESTO
SETSTO
SHASTA
SIESTA
SOASTO
TIESTO
TOASTS
TOASTY
TRISTE
TRUSTS
TRUSTY
TRYSTS
TWISTS
TWISTY
VERSTS
WAISTS
WORSTS
WRESTS
WRISTS
WURSTS
YEASTS
YEASTY

•••S•T

ACESIT
AIMSAT
ALLSET
BAGSIT
BASSET
BAYSAT
BEDSIT
BISSET
BOOSAT
BOXSET
BUYSAT
BUYSIT
CATSAT
CATSIT
CLOSET
COMSAT
COPSIT
CORSET
COSSET
CUTSIT
DABSAT
DIGSAT
DIGSIT
DOASET
DOESIT
DOESNT
DOGSAT
DOGSIT
DORSET
EATSAT
EATSIT
ENDSAT
ENDSIT
FUSSAT
GETSAT
GETSET
GETSIT
GOESAT
GOTSET
GUNSIT
GUSSET
HISSAT
HITSAT
HITSIT
ICESIT
ILLSET
JAWSAT
JETSET
KENSIT
LAMSIT
LAPSAT
LEGSIT
LETSAT
LOWSET
MISSET
MUSSET
NADSAT
NAGSAT
NIPSAT
NODSAT
OFFSET
ONESET
OUTSAT
OUTSET
OUTSIT
PASSAT
PAWSAT
PETSAT
PETSIT
PIGSIT
PRESET
PROSIT
ROSSET
RUNSAT
RUSSET
SETSAT
SITSAT
SUBSET
SUNSET
TABSET
TEASET
TILSIT
TISSOT
TUGSAT
UNDSET
VERSET
WINSAT
YAPSAT
ZIPSIT

••••ST

ABLEST
ACCOST
ADJUST
AGEIST
AGHAST
ALEAST
ALMOST
ALWEST
AMIDST
APTEST
ARREST
ARTEST
ARTIST
ASFAST
ASSIST
ATBEST
ATCOST
ATLAST
ATMOST
ATREST
ATTEST
ATWIST
AUGUST
AURIST
AUTIST
BALLST
BAREST
BASEST
BEHEST
BLUEST
BREAST
BROAST
BYPAST
CHRIST
COHOST
COYEST
CUBIST
CUTEST
CWPOST
DAREST
DEGUST
DELIST
DEMAST
DEMIST
DEPEST
DERUST
DESIST
DETEST
DEVEST
DIGEST
DIREST
DIVEST
DRIEST
DRYEST
DYNAST
EGOIST
ELDEST
ENLIST
ERNEST
EXPOST
FEWEST
FEYEST
FINEST
FOREST
FREEST
GAINST
GAMEST
GAYEST
GOBUST
GOFAST
GOLAST
GOPAST
GOWEST
GREIST
HALEST
HEARST
HITEST
HOLIST
HONEST
HUGEST
ICIEST
IDLEST
ILLEST
IMPOST
INFEST
INGEST
INJEST
INMOST
INSIST
INVEST
IQTEST
JAMEST
JURIST
KLEIST
LAKIST
LAMEST
LATEST
LAXEST
LEGIST
LIVEST
LOCUST
LOWEST
LUTIST
LYRIST
MAINST
MAOIST
MARIST
MAYEST
MEREST
MODEST
MOLEST
MONGST
MONIST
MOTTST
MUTEST
NERNST
NEWEST
NICEST
NLEAST
NLWEST
NOCOST
NUDEST
NUDIST
NYPOST
OBLAST
OBOIST
OBTEST
ODDEST
OLDEST
ONPOST
OPQRST
PALEST
PAPIST
PRIEST
PROBST
PROUST
PUREST
PURIST
RACIST
RAREST
RAWEST
RAWIST
RECAST
RECOST
REDUST
RELIST
RELOST
RENEST
REPAST
REPOST
RESIST
RETEST
REVEST
RIFEST
RIPEST
RIPOST
ROBUST
RUDEST
SADIST
SAFEST
SAGEST
SANEST
SAYEST
SCHIST
SEWIST
SEXIST
SHIEST
SHYEST
SLIEST
SLYEST
SOREST
SUREST
TAMEST
TAOIST
TAVIST
THEIST
THIRST
THRUST
TOLAST
TRUEST
TUBIST
TYPIST
UNCAST
UNJUST
UNLOST
UNMAST
UNREST
UNRUST
UPCAST
UPLAST
UPMOST
UTMOST
VEDIST
VERIST
VIBIST
VILEST
VIORST
WALLST
WHILST
WIDEST
WISEST
WRIEST
WRYEST
YAREST
ZENIST

SU••••
SUABLE
SUAVER
SUBARU
SUBBED
SUBDEB
SUBDUE
SUBGOD
SUBGUM
SUBITO
SUBLET
SUBLID
SUBLOT
SUBMIT
SUBNET
SUBORN
SUBPAR
SUBSEA
SUBSET
SUBTLE
SUBTLY
SUBURB
SUBWAR
SUBWAY
SUCCOR
SUCHAS
SUCKED
SUCKER
SUCKIN
SUCKUP
SUCRES
SUDDEN
SUDOKU
SUDSED
SUDSER
SUDSES
SUEANE
SUEANN
SUEDED
SUEDES
SUEFOR
SUENOS
SUFFER
SUFFIX
SUFISM
SUGARS
SUGARY
SUISSE
SUITED
SUITES
SUITOR
SUITUP
SULFAS
SULFUR
SULKED
SULKER
SULLEN
SULTAN
SULTRY
SUMACS
SUMMED
SUMMER
SUMMIT
SUMMON
SUMNER
SUMSUP
SUMTER
SUMUPS
SUNBOW
SUNDAE
SUNDAS
SUNDAY
SUNDER
SUNDOG
SUNDRY
SUNFAN
SUNGOD
SUNGTO
SUNHAT
SUNKEN
SUNKIN
SUNLIT
SUNNED
SUNNIS
SUNOCO
SUNRAY
SUNSET
SUNTAN
SUNUNU
SUNUPS
SUPERB
SUPERG
SUPERS
SUPINE
SUPPED
SUPPER
SUPPLE
SUPPLY
SUPRAS
SURAHS
SUREAM
SUREDO
SUREIS
SURELY
SUREOF
SUREST
SURETE
SURETY
SURFED
SURFER
SURFIN
SURGED
SURGES
SURIMI
SURREY
SURTAX
SURVEY
SUSANB
SUSANN
SUSHIS
SUSSED
SUSSES
SUSSEX
SUTRAS
SUTTER
SUTTON
SUTURE
SUUKYI
SUVARI
SUZIEQ
SUZUKI
SUZYQS

S•U•••
SAUCED
SAUCER
SAUCES
SAUDIS
SAULTS
SAUNAS
SAURON
SAURUS
SAUTES
SCUBAS
SCUFFS
SCULLS
SCULLY
SCULPT
SCUMMY
SCURFY
SCURRY
SCURVE
SCURVY
SCUZZY
SEURAT
SHUCKS
SHULTZ
SHUMAI
SHUNTS
SHUTIN
SHUTUP
SKULKS
SKULLS
SKUNKS
SKUNKY
SLUDGE
SLUDGY
SLUGGO
SLUICE
SLUING
SLUMMY
SLUMPS
SLURPS
SLURRY
SLUSHY
SMUDGE
SMUDGY
SMUGLY
SMURFS
SMUTTY
SNUBBY
SNUFFS
SNUFFY
SNUGLI
SNUGLY
SOUGHT
SOUNDS
SOUPER
SOUPUP
SOURCE
SOURED
SOURER
SOURLY
SOURON
SOUSED
SOUSES
SOUTER
SOUTHS
SPUMED
SPUMES
SPUNKY
SPURNS
SPURON
SPURTS
SQUABS
SQUADS
SQUALL
SQUARE
SQUASH
SQUATS
SQUAWK
SQUEAK
SQUEAL
SQUIBB
SQUIBS
SQUIDS
SQUINT
SQUIRE
SQUIRM
SQUIRT
SQUISH
STUART
STUBBY
STUCCO
STUDIO
STUDLY
STUFFS
STUFFY
STUKAS
STUMPS
STUMPY
STUNTS
STUNTY
STUPAS
STUPES
STUPID
STUPOR
STURDY
STUVWX
SUUKYI

S••U••
SALUKI
SALUTE
SALUTO
SAMUEL
SATURN
SCHULZ
SCHUSS
SCOUPE
SCOURS
SCOUTS
SCRUBS
SCRUFF
SCRUMS
SECURE
SEDUCE
SEDUMS
SEGUED
SEGUES
SEGURA
SEQUEL
SEQUIN
SERUMS
SETUPS
SHOULD
SHOUTS
SHRUBS
SHRUGS
SHRUNK
SIGURD
SIOUAN
SIRUPS
SITUPS
SLEUTH
SLOUCH
SLOUGH
SNOUTS
SOEURS
SOLUTE
SOMUCH
SPOUSE
SPOUTS
SPRUCE
SPRUNG
STJUDE
STLUKE
STOUTS
STRUCK
STRUMS
STRUNG
STRUNK
STRUTS
SUBURB
SUMUPS
SUNUNU
SUNUPS
SUTURE
SUZUKI
SYRUPS
SYRUPY

S•••U•
SACKUP
SACQUE
SACRUM
SADHUS
SALYUT
SATOUT
SAURUS
SAVEUP
SAVOUR
SAWOUT
SAWSUP
SCARUM
SCHLUB
SEALUP
SEAMUS
SEENUP
SEEOUT
SEESUP
SENDUP
SENTUP
SEPTUM
SEROUS
SESQUI
SESSUE
SETOUT
SETSUP
SEWNUP
SEWSUP
SHAKUR
SHAMUS
SHOGUN
SHOTUP
SHOWUP
SHROUD
SHUTUP
SIDDUR
SIGNUP
SINFUL
SIRIUS
SITOUT
SITSUP
SIXGUN
SIXTUS
SIZEUP
SKIBUM
SKIRUN
SLIPUP
SLOWUP
SNAFUS
SNAGUP
SNAPUP
SOAKUP
SOAPUP
SOBFUL
SODIUM
SOLEUS
SOPSUP
SOTRUE
SOUPUP
SPEDUP
SPROUT
SPYOUT
STAPUF
STATUE
STATUS
STAYUP
STEPUP
STIRUP
STOPUP
STPAUL
STPIUS
STRAUB
STROUD
STYLUS
SUBDUE
SUBGUM
SUCKUP
SUITUP
SULFUR
SUMSUP
SWAMUP

S••••U
SARDOU
SEEYOU
SEZYOU
SHORTU
SMALLU
SUBARU
SUDOKU
SUNUNU

•SU•••
GSUITS
ISUZUS
TSURIS
USUALS
USURER
USURPS

•S•U••
ASBURY
ASDULL
ASMUCH
ASPURE
ASSUCH
ASSUME
ASSURE
ASTUTE
ESCUDO
ISEULT
ISSUED
ISSUER
ISSUES
MSQUAD
OSCULE
OSMUND
PSEUDO
PSEUDS
RSTUVW
USAUSA

•S••U•
ASKOUT
ASKSUP
ASTRUD
ASYLUM
ESCAUT
ISUZUS
MSIEUR
OSMIUM
USEDUP
USEFUL
USESUP
USTOUR

••SU••
ABSURD
ASSUCH
ASSUME
ASSURE
BESURE
BOSUNS
CASUAL
DISUSE
DOSUMS
ENSUED
ENSUES
ENSURE
FUSUMA
IMSURE
INSULT
INSURE
ISSUED
ISSUER
ISSUES
JESUIT
LTSULU
MISUSE
MRSULU
OHSURE
RASURE
RESUIT
RESULT
RESUME
UNSUED
UNSUNG
UNSUNK
UNSURE
URSULA
VISUAL

••S•U•
ATSTUD
BASQUE
BISQUE
BUSTUP
CASQUE
CASTUP
CESIUM
CESTUS
COSYUP
DESLUM
DISBUD
DISCUS
DISEUR
DISHUP
DUSTUP
EASEUP
ENSOUL
FESCUE
FESSUP
FESTUS
GOSOUR
HASFUN
HASOUT
HESOUT
HUSHUP
ITSFUN
JOSHUA
JUSQUE
JUSTUS
KISSUP
LASHUP
LASTUP
MASHUP
MASQUE
MESSUP
MISCUE
MISCUT
MISSUS
MISTUP
MOSQUE
MUSEUM
MUSSUP
NASHUA
NESSUS
NOSEUP
PASCUA
PASSUP
POSEUR
POSSUM
POSTUM
PUSHUP
QRSTUV
RESCUE
RESHUT
RESTUP
RISEUP
RISQUE
ROSEUP
ROSSUM
SESQUI
SESSUE
TISSUE
TOSSUP
UNSHUT
UNSMUG
UNSNUG
UNSOUR
UNSPUN
VASTUS
WASFUN
WASHUP
WISEUP
XESOUT
XYSTUS
YASGUR
YESBUT

••S••U
BISSAU
DESILU
DESSAU
INSITU
ITSYOU
LTSULU
MASERU
MRSULU
NASSAU
OISEAU
PISTOU
RESEAU
ROSEAU
VISHNU
YESYOU

•••SU•
ACESUP
ACTSUP
ADDSUP
AIRSUP
AMPSUP
ASKSUP
BIDSUP
BIGSUR
BOBSUP
BUYSUP
CATSUP
CENSUS
CHISUM
CONSUL
CUESUP
CUTSUP
DAMSUP
DATSUN
DIGSUP
DIMSUM
DOESUP
DORSUM
EATSUP
ENDSUP
EYESUP
FESSUP
FITSUP
FOGSUP
GETSUP
GINSUP
GOESUP
GUMSUP
GYPSUM
HAMSUN
HAMSUP
HITSUP
HOPSUP
ICESUP
JAMSUP
KEYSUP
KISSUP
LAPSUP
LAPSUS
LAYSUP
LETSUP
MATSUI
MATSUO
MESSUP
MISSUS
MOPSUP
MUSSUP
NESSUS
OMASUM
OUTSUM
OWNSUP
PASSUP
PAYSUP
PENSUP
PEPSUP
PINSUP
POPSUP
POSSUM
PURSUE
PUTSUP
REDSUN
REVSUP
RHESUS
RIGSUP
RIPSUP
ROSSUM
RUBSUP
RUNSUP
SAWSUP
SEESUP
SESSUE
SETSUP
SEWSUP
SITSUP
SOPSUP
SUMSUP
TAGSUP
TARSUS
TEESUP
THESUN
TIESUP
TIPSUP
TISSUE
TOGSUP
TOPSUP
TOSSUP
TOTSUP
USESUP
VERSUS
WADSUP
YOUSUF
ZIPSUP

•••S•U
BISSAU
DESSAU
ERESTU
HONSHU
KYUSHU
MITSOU
NASSAU
PQRSTU
WAUSAU

••••SU
HAVASU
TUFTSU

SV••••
SVEDKA
SVELTE

S•V•••
SAVAGE
SAVAII
SAVANA
SAVANT
SAVATE
SAVEAS
SAVEIT
SAVEME
SAVEON
SAVERS
SAVEUP
SAVING
SAVIOR
SAVOIE
SAVOIR
SAVORS
SAVORY
SAVOUR
SEVENA
SEVENB
SEVENC
SEVEND
SEVENE
SEVENS
SEVERE
SEVERN
SEVERS
SEVRES
SIVANS
SOVIET
SUVARI

S••V••
SALVED
SALVER
SALVES
SALVOR
SALVOS
SEAVER
SELVES
SERVED
SERVER
SERVES
SERVOS
SHAVED
SHAVEN
SHAVER
SHAVES
SHEVAT
SHIVER
SHOVED
SHOVEL
SHOVER
SHOVES
SIEVED
SIEVES
SILVAS
SILVER
SLAVED
SLAVER
SLAVES
SLAVIC
SLIVER
SLOVAK
SLOVEN
SNIVEL
SOAVES
SOLVED
SOLVER
SOLVES
SPIVAK
STAVED
STAVES
STEVEN
STEVIE
STIVIC
STOVER
STOVES
STUVWX
SUAVER
SURVEY
SWIVEL
SWIVET
SYLVAN
SYLVIA

S•••V•
SALIVA
SCHAVS
SCURVE
SCURVY
SHEAVE
SHELVE
SHREVE
SHRIVE
SHROVE
SLEEVE
STARVE
STEEVE
STRIVE
STROVE
SWERVE

S••••V
SCENEV
SMALLV
SPOTTV

•SV•••
RSVPED

•S•V••
ASEVER
BSEVEN
GSEVEN

•S••V•
ISERVE
RSTUVW
USNAVY

•S•••V
ASIMOV
ASTROV

••S•V•
CASAVA
KOSOVO
MOSKVA
RESAVE

••S••V
GUSTAV
KISLEV
MOSHAV
QRSTUV
ROSTOV
VASLAV

•••SV•
PIUSVI

•••S•V
BRASOV
PIUSIV

••••SV
JAMESV
LOUISV

SW••••
SWABBY
SWAINS
SWALES
SWAMIS
SWAMPS
SWAMPY
SWAMUP
SWANEE
SWANKY
SWANNS
SWARDS
SWARMS
SWATAT
SWATCH
SWATHE
SWATHS
SWAYED
SWAYER
SWAYZE
SWEARS
SWEATS
SWEATY
SWEDEN
SWEDES
SWEEPS
SWEETS
SWELLS
SWERVE
SWIFTS
SWILLS
SWINGS
SWINGY
SWIPED
SWIPER
SWIPES
SWIRLS
SWIRLY
SWIRLZ
SWISHY
SWITCH
SWIVEL
SWIVET
SWOONS
SWOOPS
SWOOSH
SWORDS

S•W•••
SAWALL
SAWERS
SAWFIT
SAWING
SAWLOG
SAWOFF
SAWOUT
SAWPIT
SAWRED
SAWSUP
SAWYER
SEWAGE
SEWARD
SEWELL
SEWERS
SEWING
SEWIST
SEWNIN
SEWNON
SEWNUP
SEWONS
SEWSIN
SEWSON
SEWSUP
SOWERS
SOWETO
SOWHAT
SOWING

S••W••
SCHWAB
SCHWAS
SCOWLS
SEAWAY
SEGWAY
SEZWHO
SHAWLS
SHOWED
SHOWER
SHOWIN
SHOWME
SHOWUP
SIXWAY
SKEWED
SKEWER
SKIWAX
SKYWAY
SLEWED
SLOWED
SLOWER
SLOWGO
SLOWLY
SLOWUP
SNOWED
SNOWIN
SPAWNS
SPEWED
SPEWER
STEWED
STEWER
STEWIE
STOWED
STOWER
STOWIT
SUBWAR
SUBWAY

S•••W•
SCRAWL
SCREWS
SCREWY
SHREWD
SHREWS
SINEWS
SINEWY
SIXTWO
SODOWE
SPRAWL
SQUAWK
STRAWS
STREWN
STREWS
STUVWX

S••••W
SALLOW
SEACOW
SEESAW
SHADOW
SKITOW
SMALLW
SORROW
SUNBOW

•SW•••
ASWARM
ASWELL
ASWIRL
ASWOON
ISWEAR
KSWISS
OSWALD
OSWEGO

•S•W••
PSYWAR

•S••W•
OSHAWA
PSHAWS
USNEWS

•S•••W
ASSLOW
ESCHEW
ESCROW
RSTUVW

••SW••
ANSWER
GASWAR
RESWAM
RESWIM

••S•W•
BUSHWA
DISOWN
PESEWA
RESAWN
RESAWS
RESEWN
RESEWS

RESOWN
RESOWS
UNSAWN
UNSEWN
UNSEWS
UNSOWN

••S••W
ASSLOW
BESTOW
CASHEW
CPSNOW
CUSHAW
GOSLOW
MOSCOW
NOSHOW
ONSHOW
PESCOW
RESHOW
RESTOW
TVSHOW
UNSKEW
UNSLOW
UNSTOW
UPSHAW

•••S•W
BOWSAW
JIGSAW
OLDSAW
OUTSAW
PITSAW
RIPSAW
SEESAW
WARSAW

S•X•••
SAXONS
SAXONY
SEXERS
SEXIER
SEXILY
SEXISM
SEXIST
SEXPOT
SEXTET
SEXTON
SIXDAY
SIXEEE
SIXERS
SIXGUN
SIXONE
SIXPIN
SIXSIX
SIXTEN
SIXTHS
SIXTUS
SIXTWO
SIXWAY
SOXFAN

S••X••
SKNXXX

S•••X•
SKNXXX

S••••X
SEAFOX
SINTAX
SIXSIX
SKIWAX
SKNXXX
SKYBOX
SLYFOX
SMALLX
SPHINX
SPHYNX
STUVWX
SUFFIX
SURTAX
SUSSEX
SYNTAX

•S•X••
GSIXTY
VSIXES

•S•••X
USETAX

••S•X•
UNSEXY

••S••X
AUSPEX
GASTAX
LASTEX
MUSKOX
SUSSEX
WESSEX

•••SX•
PIUSXI

•••S•X
AGESIX
CHISOX
PIUSIX
REDSIX
REDSOX
SIXSIX
SUSSEX
THESOX
UNISEX
WESSEX

••••SX
LOUISX

SY••••
SYDNEY
SYLPHS
SYLVAN
SYLVIA
SYMBOL
SYNCED
SYNCHS
SYNDIC
SYNODS
SYNTAX
SYNTHS
SYRIAN
SYRUPS
SYRUPY
SYSOPS
SYSTEM
SYZYGY

S•Y•••
SAYAAH
SAYAYE
SAYBOO
SAYDIE
SAYERS
SAYEST
SAYHEY
SAYIDO
SAYING
SAYLES
SAYNAY
SAYSAH
SAYSHI
SAYSNO
SAYSOK
SAYSOS
SAYSSO
SAYYES
SCYLLA
SCYTHE
SHYEST
SHYING
SKYBOX
SKYCAM
SKYCAP
SKYING
SKYLAB
SKYLIT
SKYMAN
SKYMAP
SKYMEN
SKYTEL
SKYWAY
SLYEST
SLYFOX
SMYRNA
SNYDER
SOYINK
SPYBOT
SPYCAM
SPYDER
SPYING
SPYOUT
STYING
STYLED
STYLER
STYLES
STYLET
STYLUS
STYMIE
STYRON

S••Y••
SALYUT
SANYOS
SATYRS
SAWYER
SAYYES
SEEYOU
SEZYOU
SHAYNE
SIBYLS
SLAYED
SLAYER
SPAYED
SPAYER
SPHYNX
SPRYER
SPRYLY
STAYAT
STAYED
STAYER
STAYIN
STAYON
STAYUP
SUZYQS
SWAYED
SWAYER
SWAYZE
SYZYGY

S•••Y•
SATAYS
SAYAYE
SEALYS
SEPOYS
SHARYN
SHERYL
SOONYI
SPLAYS
SPRAYS
STRAYS
SUUKYI

S••••Y
SACFLY
SADDAY
SAFELY
SAFETY
SAGELY
SALARY
SALIFY
SANELY
SANITY
SASHAY
SATINY
SAVORY
SAXONY
SAYHEY
SAYNAY
SCANTY
SCARRY
SCOOBY
SCOTTY
SCREWY
SCULLY
SCUMMY
SCURFY
SCURRY
SCURVY
SCUZZY
SEAWAY
SEDLEY
SEEMLY
SEGWAY
SELLBY
SENARY
SENDBY
SENTBY
SENTRY
SETSBY
SEXILY
SHABBY
SHAGGY
SHALEY
SHALLY
SHAMMY
SHANDY
SHANTY
SHARPY
SHECKY
SHEEDY
SHEEHY
SHEENY
SHELBY
SHELTY
SHERRY
SHIFTY
SHILLY
SHIMMY
SHINDY
SHINNY
SHOALY
SHODDY
SHORTY
SHOTBY
SICILY
SICKLY
SIDNEY
SIMPLY
SINEWY
SINGLY
SIRKAY
SISLEY
SITSBY
SIXDAY
SIXWAY
SKANKY
SKIDDY
SKIMPY
SKINNY
SKIPBY
SKIPPY
SKUNKY
SKYWAY
SLANGY
SLAPPY
SLEAZY
SLEEKY
SLEEPY
SLEETY
SLIMLY
SLINKY
SLIPBY
SLIPPY
SLITHY
SLOBBY
SLOOPY
SLOPPY
SLOSHY
SLOWLY
SLUDGY
SLUMMY
SLURRY
SLUSHY
SMALLY
SMARMY
SMARTY
SMEARY
SMELLY
SMILEY
SMIRKY
SMITHY
SMITTY
SMOGGY
SMOKEY
SMUDGY
SMUGLY
SMUTTY
SNAGGY
SNAPPY
SNARKY
SNARLY
SNAZZY
SNEAKY
SNEERY
SNEEZY
SNIFFY
SNIPPY
SNOBBY
SNOOPY
SNOOTY
SNOOZY
SNORTY
SNUBBY
SNUFFY
SNUGLY
SOFTLY
SOLELY
SOMANY
SORELY
SOURLY
SPACEY
SPANKY
SPARKY
SPEEDY
SPENDY
SPERRY
SPIDEY
SPIFFY
SPONGY
SPOOKY
SPOONY
SPORTY
SPOTTY
SPRYLY
SPUNKY
STABLY
STACEY
STAGEY
STALKY
STARRY
STEADY
STEAMY
STEELY
STEFOY
STEMMY
STICKY
STILLY
STIMPY
STINGY
STINKY
STMARY
STOCKY
STODGY
STONEY
STOOLY
STOPBY
STORMY
STRIPY
STUBBY
STUDLY
STUFFY
STUMPY
STUNTY
STURDY
SUBTLY
SUBWAY
SUGARY
SULTRY
SUNDAY
SUNDRY
SUNRAY
SUPPLY
SURELY
SURETY
SURREY
SURVEY
SWABBY
SWAMPY
SWANKY
SWEATY
SWINGY
SWIRLY
SWISHY
SYDNEY
SYRUPY
SYZYGY

•SY•••
ASYLUM
PSYCHE
PSYCHO
PSYCHS
PSYWAR

•S•Y••
ISAYNO

•S••Y•
ASSAYS
ESSAYS
ISLEYS

•S•••Y
ASBURY
ASEASY
ASHLEY
ASKAMY
ASMANY
ASTLEY
ASTRAY
ESTRAY
GSIXTY
OSPREY
OSSIFY
USABLY
USARMY
USNAVY

••SY••
COSYUP
EASYAS
EASYGO
INSYNC
ITSYOU
YESYES
YESYOU

••S•Y•
ASSAYS
ESSAYS
JESSYE
JUSTYS
MASSYS
MOSEYS
RESAYS
ROSLYN
UNSAYS

••S••Y
BASELY
BASIFY
BASSEY
BASSLY
BISCAY
BOSLEY
BOSOMY
BUSBOY
BUSILY
CASEFY
COSILY
COSTLY
DESCRY
DESTRY
DISMAY
DISNEY
EASEBY
EASILY
EASLEY
EISLEY
FOSSEY
GASIFY
HOSTLY
HUSSEY
JUSTLY
LASTLY
LESLEY
LUSHLY
MASSEY
MISERY
MISKEY
MISLAY
MISSAY
MOSLEY
MOSTLY
MUSCLY
NASEBY
NOSILY
OSSIFY
PASSBY
PASTRY
POSHLY
RASHLY
RESINY
ROSARY
ROSERY
ROSILY
ROSINY
RUSHBY
SASHAY
SJSLEY
UNSEXY
VASILY
VASTLY
VESTRY
WESLEY
WISELY

•••SY•
BETSYS
JESSYE
MASSYS
UNISYS

•••S•Y
BASSEY
BASSLY
BENSEY
BETSEY
BIGSKY
BOESKY
BOLSHY
BRASHY
BRASSY
BRUSHY
CARSEY
CHESTY
CIASPY
CLASSY
CRESSY
CRISPY
CROSBY
CRUSTY
DILSEY
DOESBY
DORSAY
DORSEY
DRESSY
DROSSY
EKESBY
FEISTY
FLASHY
FLESHY
FLOSSY
FOSSEY
FRISKY
FROSTY
GATSBY
GELSEY
GETSBY
GHOSTY
GLASSY
GLOSSY
GOESBY
GOOSEY
GRASSY
GRISLY
GROSZY
GUNSHY
HALSEY
HERSEY
HORSEY
HUSSEY
ILLSAY
JERSEY
KELSEY
KGBSPY
KINSEY
KRISPY
KRUSTY
LANSKY
LAYSBY
LETSBY
LOOSEY
MARSHY
MASSEY
MEASLY
MERSEY
MISSAY
MOUSEY
NAYSAY
NEVSKY
NIPSEY
OCASEY
OUTSAY
OUTSPY
PASSBY
PIGSTY
PLASHY
PLUSHY
PRISSY
PROSKY
PUTSBY
RAMSAY
RAMSEY
REDSKY
RIMSKY
RUNSBY
SETSBY
SITSBY
SLOSHY
SLUSHY
SWISHY
THESPY
THUSLY
TOASTY
TRASHY
TRESSY
TRUSTY
TWISTY
WHISKY
WIMSEY
WINSBY
WOLSEY
YEASTY
ZIPSBY

••••SY
ARGOSY
ASEASY
BIOPSY
BLOWSY
BLUESY
BRASSY
CHEESY
CHOOSY
CLASSY
CLUMSY
CREASY
CRESSY
CURTSY
CUTESY
DRESSY
DROPSY
DROSSY
DROWSY
FLIMSY
FLOPSY
FLOSSY
FOLKSY
GLASSY
GLOSSY
GOEASY
GRASSY
GREASY
HERESY
IMBUSY
IMEASY
JONESY
PRISSY
QUEASY
ROOTSY
TEENSY
TOOTSY
TRESSY
UNBUSY
UNEASY
WEENSY
WHIMSY
WOODSY
WOOTSY

S•Z•••
SEZWHO
SEZYOU
SIZERS
SIZEUP
SIZING
SIZZLE
SUZIEQ
SUZUKI
SUZYQS
SYZYGY

S••Z••
SCUZZY
SEIZED
SEIZER
SEIZES
SEIZOR
SETZER
SHAZAM
SIZZLE
SLEZAK
SMAZES
SNAZZY

S•••Z•
SCUZZY
SFORZA
SLEAZE
SLEAZY
SNAZZY
SNEEZE
SNEEZY
SNOOZE
SNOOZY
STANZA
STARZZ
SWAYZE

S••••Z
SCHNOZ
SCHULZ
SHIRAZ
SHORTZ
SHULTZ
SMALLZ
SPRITZ
STARZZ
STOLTZ
SWIRLZ

•S•Z••
ISUZUS
ZSAZSA

•S••Z•
ASSIZE

••SZ••
LASZLO

••S•Z•
ASSIZE
RESIZE
UPSIZE

••S••Z
ERSATZ
LESMIZ
MESAAZ

•••SZ•
GROSZY

•••S•Z
AMOSOZ

••••SZ
KUVASZ
MILOSZ

TA••••
TABARD
TABBED
TABKEY
TABLAS
TABLED
TABLES
TABLET
TABOOS
TABORS
TABRIZ
TABSET
TABUED
TABULA
TACKED
TACKER
TACKLE
TACKON
TACKUP
TACOMA
TACTEL
TACTIC
TAGDAY
TAGEND
TAGGED
TAGGER
TAGORE
TAGOUT
TAGSON
TAGSUP
TAHINI
TAHITI
TAHNEE
TAHOES
TAICHI
TAIGAS
TAILED
TAILER
TAILOR
TAINTS
TAIPAN
TAIPEI
TAIWAN
TAKEIN
TAKEIT
TAKEON
TAKERS
TAKETH
TAKETO
TAKEUP
TAKING
TALCED
TALCUM
TALENT
TALERS
TALESE
TALISA
TALKAT
TALKED
TALKER
TALKIE
TALKIN
TALKOF
TALKON
TALKTO
TALKUP
TALLER
TALLOW
TALMUD
TALONS
TALTOS
TAMALE
TAMARA
TAMAYO
TAMBOR
TAMELY
TAMERS
TAMEST
TAMILS
TAMING
TAMMUZ
TAMPED
TAMPER
TAMTAM
TANAKA
TANANA
TANDEM
TANGED
TANGLE
TANGLY
TANGOS
TANGUY
TANKAS
TANKED
TANKER
TANKUP
TANNED
TANNER
TANNIC
TANNIN
TANOAK
TANTES
TANTRA
TAOISM
TAOIST
TAOSNM
TAPEON
TAPERS
TAPEUP
TAPING
TAPINS
TAPIRS
TAPOFF
TAPOUT
TAPPAN
TAPPED
TAPPER
TAPPET
TAPSIN
TAPSON
TARAWA
TARDES
TARGAS
TARGET
TARIFF
TARING
TARLEK
TARMAC
TAROIL
TAROTS
TARPIT
TARPON
TARRED
TARSAL
TARSUS
TARTAN
TARTAR
TARTED
TARTER
TARTES
TARTLY
TARTUP
TARZAN
TASERS
TASKED
TASKET
TASMAN
TASSEL
TASSES
TASTED
TASTEE
TASTER
TASTES
TATAMI
TATARS
TATERS
TATLER
TATRAS
TATTED
TATTER
TATTLE
TATTOO
TAUGHT
TAUNTS
TAUONS
TAUPES
TAUPIN
TAURIC
TAUROG
TAURUS
TAUTEN
TAUTER
TAUTLY
TAVELS
TAVERN
TAVIST
TAWDRY
TAXCUT
TAXERS
TAXIED
TAXIES
TAXING
TAXLAW
TAXMAN
TAXMEN
TAXOLS
TAYLOR

T•A•••
TEAACT
TEABAG
TEACUP
TEAMED
TEAMUP
TEAPOT
TEAPOY
TEARAT
TEARED
TEARER
TEARIT
TEARUP
TEASED
TEASEL
TEASER
TEASES
TEASET
TEATRO
TEAURN
THALER
THALES
THALIA
THAMES
THANES
THANKS
THATCH
THATIS
THATLL
THAWED
THAWER
THAYER
TIARAS
TOAMAN
TOASTS
TOASTY
TOATEE
TRACED
TRACER
TRACES
TRACEY
TRACHE
TRACII
TRACKS
TRACTS
TRADED
TRADER

TRADES
TRAGIC
TRAGUS
TRAILS
TRAINS
TRAITS
TRAJAN
TRALAS
TRALEE
TRAMPS
TRAMPY
TRANCE
TRANES
TRANNY
TRAPPY
TRASHY
TRAUMA
TRAVEL
TRAVEN
TRAVES
TRAVIS
TRAWLS
TSADES
TSADIS
TWAINS
TWANGS
TWANGY

T••A••

TABARD
TAMALE
TAMARA
TAMAYO
TANAKA
TANANA
TARAWA
TATAMI
TATARS
TEAACT
TECATE
TEJANA
TEJANO
TENACE
TENANT
TERATO
TEXACO
TEXANS
THEACT
THEAGE
THEAPE
THEASP
THEAXE
THRACE
THRALL
THRASH
THWACK
THWART
TICALS
TILAKS
TIRADE
TIRANA
TIRANE
TISANE
TITANS
TJMAXX
TOBAGO
TODATE
TODAYS
TOGAED
TOKAYS
TOLARS
TOLAST
TOMATO
TORAHS
TOTALS
TOWAGE
TOWARD
TOYAMA
TREADS
TREATS
TREATY
TRIADS
TRIAGE
TRIALS
TRUANT
TSGARP
TSHAPE
TUBAGE
TUBATE
TUCANA
TULANE
TULARE
TUVALU
TVGAME
TVLAND
TVTAPE
TWEAKS
TWEAKY
TWOACT
TYBALT
TYRANT

T•••A•

TABLAS
TAGDAY
TAIGAS
TAIPAN
TAIWAN
TALKAT
TAMTAM
TANKAS
TANOAK
TAPPAN
TARGAS
TARMAC
TARSAL
TARTAN
TARTAR
TARZAN
TASMAN
TATRAS
TAXLAW
TAXMAN
TEABAG
TEARAT
TEHRAN
TEKWAR
TENDAY
TERRAE
TERRAN
TESLAS
TESTAE
TETRAD
TETRAS
THEBAN
THEBAR
THEBAY
THECAN
THECAR
THEFAN
THEGAP
THEHAJ
THELAW
THEMAN
THERAM
THERAP
THERAT
THETAS
THEWAY
THOMAS
THORAX
THREAD
THREAT
THROAT
TIARAS
TIBIAE
TIBIAL
TIBIAS
TICTAC
TIEBAR
TIETAC
TIKKAS
TILTAT
TIMBAL
TINCAN
TINEAL
TINEAR
TINHAT
TINIAN
TINMAN
TINPAN
TIPJAR
TIRIAC
TITIAN
TOAMAN
TOBIAS
TODDAO
TODMAN
TOECAP
TOETAP
TOILAT
TOKLAS
TOMCAT
TONGAN
TONKAS
TOOBAD
TOOFAR
TOOTAT
TOPCAT
TOPHAT
TOPMAN
TORBAY
TOREAT
TORTAS
TOUCAN
TOWBAR
TOWCAR
TOYCAR
TOYHAT
TRAJAN
TRALAS
TREPAN
TRIBAL
TRINAL
TROJAN
TRUMAN
TSTRAP
TUBMAN
TUGSAT
TULSAN
TURBAN
TURHAN
TUSCAN
TUSSAL
TVSTAR
TWOCAR
TWODAY
TWOMAN
TWOWAY
TWYMAN
TYPEAB
TYPEAS

T••••A

TABULA
TACOMA
TALISA
TAMARA
TANAKA
TANANA
TANTRA
TARAWA
TEJANA
TENUTA
TERESA
THALIA
THECIA
THEEPA
THELMA
THENBA
THENRA
THESEA
THEUSA
THREEA
TIENDA
TIERRA
TIRANA
TOLDYA
TOPEKA
TOYAMA
TOYOTA
TRAUMA
TREDIA
TRENTA
TRICIA
TRISHA
TRIVIA
TROIKA
TUCANA
TUNDRA

•TA•••

ATALOW
ATAMAN
ATARIS
ATAVIC
ATAXIA
ATAXIC
ETAGES
ETAILS
ETALIA
ETALII
ETAOIN
ETAPES
ITALIA
ITALIC
ITASCA
MTAIRY
STABAT
STABLE
STABLY
STACEY
STACKS
STADIA
STAFFS
STAGED
STAGER
STAGES
STAGEY
STAINS
STAIRS
STAKED
STAKES
STALAG
STALED
STALER
STALES
STALIN
STALKS
STALKY
STALLS
STAMEN
STAMOS
STAMPS
STANCE
STANCH
STANDS
STANZA
STAPES
STAPHS
STAPLE
STAPUF
STARCH
STARED
STARER
STARES
STARIN
STARRY
STARTS
STARVE
STARZZ
STASES
STASIS
STATED
STATEN
STATER
STATES
STATIC
STATIN
STATOR
STATUE
STATUS
STAVED
STAVES
STAYAT
STAYED
STAYER
STAYIN
STAYON
STAYUP
UTAHAN
UTAHNS

•T•A••

ATBATS
ATDAWN
ATEAMS
ATEASE
ATHAND
ATLAST
ATMANS
ATRAIN
ATTACH
ATTACK
ATTAIN
ATTARS
ATYALE
BTEAMS
ETHANE
ETRADE
ITHACA
ITSAGO
OTTAVA
OTTAWA
PTRAPS
STEADS
STEADY
STEAKS
STEALS
STEAMS
STEAMY
STMALO
STMARK
STMARY
STOATS
STPATS
STPAUL
STRADA
STRADS
STRAFE
STRAIN
STRAIT
STRAND
STRAPS
STRATA
STRATI
STRATO
STRATS
STRAUB
STRAWS
STRAYS
STUART
UTHANT

•T••A•

ATAMAN
ATONAL
ATPLAY
ATRIAL
ATTHAT
CTSCAN
ITSPAT
ITZHAK
OTHMAR
PTBOAT
STABAT
STALAG
STAYAT
STEFAN
STELAR
STELAS
STJOAN
STOLAE
STOLAF
STOLAS
STOMAS
STOPAT
STREAK
STREAM
STRIAE
STUKAS
STUPAS
UTAHAN
UTICAN

•T•••A

ATAXIA
ATHENA
ATONIA
ATTICA
ATTILA
ETALIA
ITALIA
ITASCA
ITHACA
MTETNA
MTOSSA
OTTAVA
OTTAWA
STADIA
STANZA
STELLA
STERNA
STIGMA
STRADA
STRATA
UTOPIA
XTERRA
YTTRIA

••TA••

ALTAIC
ALTAIR
ALTARF
ALTARS
ANTAWN
ARTAUD
ASTALL
ASTANA
ASTARE
ASTART
ATTACH
ATTACK
ATTAIN
ATTARS
BATAAN
BETAKE
BOTANY
BSTARS
BUTANE
BYTALK
BYTAXI
CATALO
CATANO
CETANE
COTANS
CSTARS
DATARY
DETACH
DETAIL
DETAIN
DETARS
DITALI
DOTAGE
DOTARD
ENTAIL
ESTADO
ESTATE
EUTAXY
EXTANT
FATALE
FSTARS
GETANA
GETANF
GITANO
GOTAMA
GOTANA
GOTANF
GSTAAD
GSTARS
HATARI
HOTAIR
IDTAGS
INTACT
INTAKE
KITAEN
KSTARS
LITANY
METALS
METATE
MSTARS
MUTANT
MUTATE
NATALE
NATANT
NOTAIL
NOTALL
NOTANY
NOTARY
NOTATE
NSTARS
NUTATE
OBTAIN
OCTADS
OCTANE
OCTANS
OCTANT
OCTAVE
OCTAVO
ONTAPE
OSTARS
OTTAVA
OTTAWA
OUTACT
OUTADD
OUTAGE
OUTASK
OUTATE
OUTAWE
OXTAIL
PATACA
PATAKI
PETAIN
PETALE
PETALS
PETARD
PITAYA
POTAGE
POTASH
POTATO
QATARI
RETACK
RETAGS
RETAIL
RETAIN
RETAKE
RETAME
RETANS
RETAPE
RETAPS
RETARD
RETARS
RITARD
ROTARY
ROTATE
SATAYS
SITARS
SSTARS
TATAMI
TATARS
TITANS
TOTALS
TVTAPE
UMTATA
UNTACK
UNTAME
UNTAPE
UNTAUT
UPTAKE
UPTALK
VITALE
VITALS
VITARA
VOTARY
YATATA
YUTANG

••T•A•

ACTSAS
ACTUAL
ALTMAN
ALTTAB
AMTRAC
AMTRAK
ANTRAL
ARTCAR
ASTEAL
ASTRAL
ASTRAY
ATTHAT
BATAAN
BATDAY
BATEAU
BATMAN
BATYAM
BETRAY
BETTAS
BITMAP
CATHAY
CATMAN
CATNAP
CATSAT
COTTAE
COTTAS
DATHAN
DOTHAN
DOTOAT
EATSAT
ENTIAL
ENTRAP
ESTRAY
EXTRAS
FATCAT
FATMAN
FATWAS
GATEAU
GETFAR
GETMAD
GETSAB
GETSAC
GETSAD
GETSAT
GOTEAM
GOTFAR
GOTHAM
GOTMAD
GSTAAD
GUTMAN
HITMAN
HITSAT
HOTCAP
HOTCAR
HOTDAY
HOTWAR
INTHAT
INTRAY
JETFAN
JETLAG
JETSAM
JETTAS
JETWAY
KATMAI
KITBAG
KITKAT
LETHAL
LETSAT
LITVAK
LOTHAR
MATMAN
METFAN
MITRAL
MITTAG
MUTUAL
NATHAN
NETMAN
NETPAY
NOTBAD
NOTFAR
OSTEAL
OUTBAN
OUTBAT
OUTEAT
OUTGAS
OUTLAW
OUTLAY
OUTMAN
OUTPAY
OUTRAN
OUTRAP
OUTSAT
OUTSAW
OUTSAY
OUTWAR
PATDAY
PATHAN
PETCAT
PETNAP
PETRAT
PETSAT
PITMAN
PITSAW
PUTNAM
RATTAN
RATTAT
RETEAR
RETHAW
RETIAL
RETRAL
RETRAP
RITUAL
RUTTAN
SATPAT
SATRAP
SETSAT
SGTMAJ
SITPAT
SITSAT
SOTHAT
SUTRAS
TATRAS
TETRAD
TETRAS
TITIAN
TSTRAP
ULTRAS
UNTHAW
UNTRAP
UPTEAR
WETBAR
WETNAP
WETRAG
WITHAL

••T••A

ACTIVA
ALTHEA
ALTIMA
ALTRIA
ANTLIA
ASTANA
ASTHMA
ATTICA
ATTILA
AZTECA
BETCHA
CATENA
CATERA
CETERA
FATIMA
FUTUNA
FUTURA
GETANA
GOTAMA
GOTANA
GOTCHA
HOTTEA
ISTRIA
LATINA
LATOYA
LATRIA
LATVIA
MATTEA
MOTHRA
NUTRIA
OPTIMA
ORTEGA
OTTAVA
OTTAWA
PATACA
PATINA
PATRIA
PETBOA
PETIPA
PETULA
PITAYA
RATEDA
RETINA
ULTIMA
UMTATA
VITARA
YATATA
YTTRIA

•••TA•

ACETAL
AGITAS
AKITAS
ALETAP
ALTTAB
AMYTAN
AORTAE
AORTAL
AORTAS
ARCTAN
AVATAR
BANTAM
BARTAB
BEATAT
BETTAS
BHUTAN
BIOTAS
BRUTAL
CAFTAN
CANTAB
CANTAL
CENTAI
CENTAL
CENTAS
CESTAS
CONTAC
COSTAE
COSTAL
COSTAR
COSTAS
COTTAE
COTTAS
CRETAN
DELTAS
DENTAL
DIKTAT
DISTAL
DOGTAG
DUCTAL
EARTAB
EARTAG
ERSTAD
FANTAN
FANTAS
FESTAL
FESTAS
FONTAL
FORTAS
FRETAT
FRITAS
GASTAX
GESTAE
GOSTAG
GRATAE
GUITAR
GUSTAV
HEPTAD
HIATAL
HINTAT
HOOTAT
HOSTAS
HYETAL
INSTAL
ISHTAR
JETTAS
JUNTAS
JUSTAS
KCSTAR
KEPTAT
LESTAT
LOWTAR
MAITAI
MANTAS
MAOTAI
MAYTAG
MEATAX
MENTAL
MIATAS
MITTAG
MONTAG
MORTAL
MORTAR
NECTAR
NIETAS
NONTAN
NONTAX
OAKTAG
ONSTAR
PASTAS
PENTAD
PENTAX
PIETAS
PORTAL
POSTAL
PRETAX
PROTAX
PUNTAS
QANTAS
QINTAR
QUOTAS
RAGTAG
RAITAS
RANTAT
RASTAS
RATTAN
RATTAT
REATAS
REDTAB
REDTAG
RENTAL
RESTAB
RIATAS
RICTAL
RUTTAN
SANTAS
SEATAC
SEPTAL
SERTAS
SHOTAT
SINTAX
SONTAG
SULTAN
SUNTAN
SURTAX
SWATAT
SYNTAX
TAMTAM
TARTAN
TARTAR
TESTAE
THETAS
TICTAC
TIETAC
TILTAT
TOETAP
TOOTAT
TORTAS
TVSTAR
UINTAS
UNITAS
USETAX
VENTAS
VESTAL
VESTAS
VISTAS
WANTAD
WENTAT
WYSTAN
YENTAS
ZANTAC
ZESTAS
ZOLTAN

•••T•A

AGATHA
ANITRA
ARETHA
ASSTDA
BASTIA
BERTHA
CHITRA
CONTRA
EARTHA
EASTLA
FRITTA
GRATIA
GRETNA
HESTIA
HOTTEA
ICETEA
IGOTTA
LACTEA
LASTRA
LIOTTA
LUNTHA
LUSTRA
MANTRA
MANTUA
MARTHA
MATTEA
MTETNA
NESTEA
NOOTKA
NOSTRA
ODETTA
OSETRA
PORTIA
PROTEA
REATTA
ROSTRA
SANTHA
SCOTIA
SENTRA
TANTRA
VECTRA

••••TA

AMINTA
AMRITA
ARISTA
AVESTA
BALATA
BARATA
BEMATA
BOGOTA
BONITA
CAPITA
CASITA
CHARTA
CHEETA
CUESTA
DAKOTA
DAMITA
DAOSTA
DERITA
DESETA
EGESTA
EIGHTA
EJECTA
ERRATA
EXACTA
FAJITA
FIESTA
FLAUTA
FRITTA
FRUSTA
GOLETA
IGOTTA
KANATA
LAKOTA
LAPUTA
LIKUTA
LIOTTA
LOLITA
MAKUTA
MIKITA
MINETA
MONETA
MORITA
MULETA
NAPHTA
NARITA
NIKITA
ODETTA
OMERTA
OUGHTA

PELOTA
PEPITA
PESETA
PINATA
POINTA
QUANTA
QUINTA
REATTA
RENATA
ROSITA
SANCTA
SHASTA
SHORTA
SIESTA
SOMATA
SONATA
SPARTA
STRATA
TENUTA
TOYOTA
TRENTA
UMTATA
YATATA
YUKATA
ZAPATA

TB••••
TBILLS
TBIRDS
TBONDS
TBONES
TBOONE

T•B•••
TABARD
TABBED
TABKEY
TABLAS
TABLED
TABLES
TABLET
TABOOS
TABORS
TABRIZ
TABSET
TABUED
TABULA
TEBETS
TIBIAE
TIBIAL
TIBIAS
TOBAGO
TOBIAS
TOBIES
TOBITS
TOBOOT
TOBURN
TUBAGE
TUBATE
TUBBED
TUBERS
TUBFUL
TUBING
TUBIST
TUBMAN
TUBULE
TYBALT

T••B••
TABBED
TAMBOR
TEABAG
TEEBOX
TERBIC
THEBAN
THEBAR
THEBAY
THEBBC
THEBEE
THEBES
TIDBIT
TIEBAR
TIMBAL
TIMBER
TIMBRE
TOMBES
TOMBOY
TOOBAD
TOOBIG
TOPBID
TORBAY
TOWBAR
TREBEK
TREBLE
TREBLY
TRIBAL
TRIBES
TUBBED
TUMBLE
TURBAN
TURBID
TURBOS
TURBOT
TWOBIT
TYDBOL

T•••B•
TENLBS
THEBBC
THEFBI
THENBA
THISBE
THROBS
THUMBS
TICKBY
TRILBY
TRUMBO
TYCOBB
TYPEBS

T••••B
THEHUB
THEMOB
THEWEB
THREEB
TOPJOB
TYCOBB
TYPEAB

•TB•••
ATBATS
ATBEST
PTBOAT
STBEDE

•T•B••
STABAT
STABLE
STABLY
STUBBY
UTUBES

•T••B•
ITURBI
STOPBY
STROBE
STUBBY

•T•••B
ATHROB
STRAUB

••TB••
BATBOY
CATBED
HATBOX
HOTBED
HOTBOT
HOTBOX
KITBAG
NOTBAD
OUTBAN
OUTBAT
OUTBEG
OUTBID
OUTBOW
OUTBOX
OUTBUD
OUTBUY
PETBOA
WETBAR

••T•B•
GATSBY
GETSBY
IVTUBE
LETSBE
LETSBY
PUTSBY
SETSBY
SITSBY

••T••B
ALTTAB
ENTOMB
GETSAB
HOTTUB
OUTRIB

•••TB•
CANTBE
FLITBY
LEFTBE
MALTBY
SENTBY
SHOTBY
WENTBY
WHITBY

•••T•B
ALTTAB
BARTAB
CANTAB
EARTAB
HOTTUB
INATUB
REDTAB
RESTAB

••••TB
EIGHTB
POINTB

TC••••
TCELLS

T•C•••
TACKED
TACKER
TACKLE
TACKON
TACKUP
TACOMA
TACTEL
TACTIC
TECATE
TECHIE
TECHNO
TECHTV
TICALS
TICCED
TICINO
TICKBY
TICKED
TICKER
TICKET
TICKLE
TICKLY
TICTAC
TOCOME
TOCSIN
TUCANA
TUCKED
TUCKER
TUCKIN
TUCSON
TVCREW
TYCOBB
TYCOON

T••C••
TAICHI
TALCED
TALCUM
TAXCUT
TEACUP
TELCOS
TERCEL
TERCES
TETCHY
THECAN
THECAR
THECIA
THECID
THICKE
TICCED
TINCAN
TINCTS
TINCUP
TOECAP
TOMCAT
TOPCAT
TORCHY
TOUCAN
TOUCHE
TOUCHY
TOWCAR
TOYCAR
TRACED
TRACER
TRACES
TRACEY
TRACHE
TRACII
TRACKS
TRACTS
TRECES
TRICEP
TRICES
TRICIA
TRICKS
TRICKY
TRICOT
TROCHE
TRUCES
TRUCKS
TUSCAN
TVVCRS
TWOCAR

T•••C•
TEAACT
TENACE
TEXACO
THATCH
THEACT
THENCE
THRACE
THRICE
THWACK
TIERCE
TONICS
TOPICS
TOXICS
TRANCE
TRENCH
TUNICS
TWITCH
TWOACT

T••••C
TACTIC
TANNIC
TARMAC
TAURIC
TERBIC
THEBBC
THORIC
THREEC
THYMIC
TICTAC
TIETAC
TIRIAC
TOLTEC
TRAGIC
TROPIC
TURKIC

•TC•••
ATCOST
ETCETC
ETCHED
ETCHER
ETCHES
ITCHED
ITCHES
MTCOOK

•T•C••
CTSCAN
STACEY
STACKS
STICKS
STICKY
STOCKS
STOCKY
STUCCO
UTICAN

•T••C•
ATONCE
ATTACH
ATTACK
ATTICA
ATTICS
ETHICS
ITASCA
ITHACA
STANCE
STANCH
STARCH
STENCH
STITCH
STNICK
STOICS
STORCH
STRICT
STRUCK
STUCCO

•T•••C
ATAVIC
ATAXIC
ATOMIC
ATONIC
ATOXIC
ATYPIC
ETCETC
ETHNIC
ETONIC
ITALIC
OTITIC
STATIC
STERIC
STIVIC
YTTRIC

••TC••
ANTCOW
ARTCAR
BETCHA
BOTCHY
CATCHY
DOTCOM
FATCAT
GOTCHA
HOTCAP
HOTCAR
HOTCUP
LITCHI
NOTCHY
OUTCRY
OUTCUT
PATCHY
PETCAT
PETCOW
PITCHY
SATCOM
SITCOM
TETCHY
WITCHY
ZITCOM

••T•C•
ANTICS
ATTACH
ATTACK
ATTICA
ATTICS
AZTECA
AZTECS
DETACH
DETECT
ENTICE
ESTOCS
HITECH
INTACT
KITSCH
LUTECE
NATICK
NOTICE
OPTICS
OUTACT
PATACA
PUTSCH
RETACK
SHTICK
UNTACK
UNTUCK
UPTICK
VOTECH

••T••C
ALTAIC
AMTRAC
CITRIC
GETSAC
GOTHIC
IATRIC
LITHIC
METRIC
MYTHIC
NITRIC
PATHIC
PATRIC
VITRIC
YTTRIC

•••TC•
BLOTCH
CLUTCH
COSTCO
CROTCH
CRUTCH
CULTCH
DEUTCH
FLETCH
GLITCH
HOOTCH
KLATCH
KVETCH
SCOTCH
SKETCH
SKITCH
SNATCH
SNITCH
STITCH
SWATCH
SWITCH
THATCH
TWITCH
WRETCH

•••T•C
ACETIC
AORTIC
ARCTIC
BALTIC
BIOTIC
CELTIC
CONTAC
COPTIC
CRITIC
CULTIC
CYSTIC
DELTIC
EMETIC
EROTIC
EXOTIC
FISTIC
GESTIC
HECTIC
IRITIC
LACTIC
MANTIC
MASTIC
MIXTEC
MYSTIC
NOETIC
OTITIC
PEPTIC
PHOTIC
POETIC
RUSTIC
SEATAC
SEPTIC
STATIC
TACTIC
TICTAC
TIETAC
TOLTEC
ZANTAC

••••TC
EIGHTC
ETCETC

T•D•••
TEDEUM
TEDIUM
TEDKEY
TIDBIT
TIDIED
TIDIER
TIDIES
TIDILY
TIDING
TIDYUP
TODATE
TODAYS
TODDAO
TODDLE
TODIES
TODMAN
TUDORS
TVDVDS
TYDBOL

T••D••
TAGDAY
TANDEM
TARDES
TAWDRY
TEEDUP
TENDAY
TENDED
TENDER
TENDON
TENDTO
THEDOW
TIEDIN
TIEDON
TIEDTO
TIEDUP
TIEDYE
TILDEN
TILDES
TINDER
TODDAO
TODDLE
TOEDIN
TOLDIT
TOLDOF
TOLDON
TOLDYA
TONDOS
TOODLE
TOPDOG
TOYDOG
TRADED
TRADER
TRADES
TREDIA
TRODON
TRUDGE
TSADES
TSADIS
TUNDRA
TVIDOL
TWODAY

T•••D•
TBIRDS
TBONDS
THIRDR
THIRDS
TIENDA
TIRADE
TOLEDO
TREADS
TRENDS
TRENDY
TRIADS
TRIODE
TUXEDO
TVDVDS
TWEEDS
TWEEDY

T••••D
TABARD
TABBED
TABLED
TABUED
TACKED
TAGEND
TAGGED
TAILED
TALCED
TALKED
TALMUD
TAMPED
TANGED
TANKED
TANNED
TAPPED
TARRED
TARTED
TASKED
TASTED
TATTED
TAXIED
TEAMED
TEARED
TEASED
TEEMED
TEHEED
TEMPED
TENDED
TENSED
TENTED
TERMED
TESTED
TETRAD
TEXTED
THAWED
THECID
THEEND
THEFED
THEKID
THEMED
THERED
THEROD
THETED
THREAD
THREED
TICCED
TICKED
TIDIED
TIERED
TIEROD
TIFFED
TILLED
TILTED
TINGED
TINGOD
TINNED
TINTED
TIPPED
TITHED
TITLED
TITRED
TOGAED
TOGGED
TOILED
TOLLED
TONGED
TOOBAD
TOOLED
TOOTED
TOPBID
TOPPED
TOROID
TORPID
TORRID
TOSSED
TOTTED
TOURED
TOUTED
TOWARD
TRACED
TRADED
TREPID
TRIPOD
TROWED
TUBBED
TUCKED
TUFTED
TUGGED
TURBID
TURFED
TURGID
TURNED
TUSKED
TUTTED
TUTUED
TVLAND
TWINED

•TD•••
ATDAWN
ATDUSK

•T•D••
ATODDS
ETUDES
STADIA
STIDES
STODGE
STODGY
STUDIO
STUDLY

•T••D•
ATODDS
ETRADE
ITLLDO
STANDS
STBEDE
STEADS
STEADY
STEEDS
STJUDE
STRADA
STRADS
STRIDE
STRODE
STURDY

•T•••D
ATHAND
ATONED
ATSTUD
ATTEND
ATWOOD
ETCHED
ITCHED
ITEMED
ITRIED
MTHOOD
STAGED
STAKED
STALED
STARED
STATED
STAVED
STAYED
STEWED
STOKED
STOLID
STONED
STORED
STOWED
STRAND
STROUD
STUPID
STYLED

••TD••
BATDAY
CATDOM
DOTDOT
HOTDAY
HOTDOG
OUTDID
PATDAY
PATDRY
PETDOG
RITDYE
VATDYE

••T•D•
BETIDE
DOTODO
ESTADO
OCTADS
OOTIDS
OUTADD
RATEDA
RATEDG
RATEDR
RATEDX
UNTIDY

••T••D
ALTOID
ANTEED
ARTAUD
ASTRID
ASTRUD
ATTEND
AUTOED
BATHED
BATTED
BETTED
BITTED
BUTTED
CATBED
CITIED
DOTARD
DOTTED
EXTEND
FATTED
FITTED
FUTZED
GETMAD
GETOLD
GETRID
GETSAD
GITTED
GOTMAD
GOTOLD
GOTRID
GSTAAD
GUTTED
HATRED
HATTED
HOTBED
HOTROD
HUTTED
IMTOLD
INTEND
JETTED
JOTTED
JUTTED
KITTED
LATHED
LETTED
LOTTED
MATTED
METHOD
METRED
MITRED
NETTED
NOTBAD
NUTTED
OBTUND
ORTRUD
OSTEND
OUTADD
OUTBID
OUTBUD
OUTDID
OUTLED
PATTED
PETARD
PETTED
PITHED
PITIED
PITTED
POTLID
POTTED
PUTRID
PUTTED
RATTED
RETARD
RETIED
RETOLD
RETROD
RETTED
RITARD
ROTTED
ROTUND
RUTTED
SOTTED
TATTED
TETRAD
TITHED
TITLED
TITRED
TOTTED
TUTTED
TUTUED
UNTIED
UNTOLD
UNTROD
VATTED
VETOED
VETTED
WETTED
WITTED

•••TD•
ASSTDA
MUSTDO
WONTDO

•••T•D
ABATED
ALATED
ATSTUD
BAITED
BASTED
BATTED
BELTED
BESTED
BETTED
BITTED
BOATED
BOLTED
BOOTED
BUNTED
BUSTED
BUTTED
CANTED
CARTED
CASTED
CHUTED
COATED
COSTED
CRATED
DARTED
DENTED
DIETED
DINTED
DOTTED
DUCTED
DUETED
DUSTED
EDITED
ELATED
ELUTED
EMOTED
ERSTAD
EXITED
FASTED
FATTED
FELTED
FISTED
FITTED
FLUTED
FOETID
FOOTED
GAITED
GIFTED
GIRTED
GITTED
GRATED
GUSTED
GUTTED
HAFTED
HALTED
HASTED
HATTED
HEATED
HEFTED
HEPTAD
HILTED
HINTED
HOOTED
HOSTED
HUNTED
HUTTED
JESTED
JETTED
JILTED
JOLTED
JOTTED
JUTTED
KILTED
KITTED
LASTED
LETTED
LIFTED
LILTED
LINTED
LISTED
LOFTED
LOOTED
LOTTED
LUSTED
MALTED
MASTED
MATTED
MELTED
MINTED
MISTED
MOATED
MOLTED
MOOTED
NESTED
NETTED
NUTTED
ORATED
OUSTED
PANTED
PARTED
PASTED
PATTED
PELTED
PENTAD
PETTED
PITTED
PLATED
PORTED
POSTED
POTTED
POUTED

PRATED
PUNTED
PUTTED
QUOTED
RAFTED
RANTED
RATTED
RENTED
RESTED
RETTED
RIFTED
RIOTED
ROOTED
ROTTED
ROUTED
RRATED
RUSTED
RUTTED
SALTED
SEATED
SIFTED
SILTED
SKATED
SLATED
SORTED
SOTTED
SPITED
STATED
SUITED
TARTED
TASTED
TATTED
TENTED
TESTED
TEXTED
THETED
TILTED
TINTED
TOOTED
TOTTED
TOUTED
TUFTED
TUTTED
UNITED
VATTED
VENTED
VESTED
VETTED
WAFTED
WAITED
WANTAD
WANTED
WARTED
WASTED
WELTED
WETTED
WHITED
WILTED
WITTED
WONTED
XRATED
ZESTED

••••TD
EIGHTD

TE••••
TEAACT
TEABAG
TEACUP
TEAMED
TEAMUP
TEAPOT
TEAPOY
TEARAT
TEARED
TEARER
TEARIT
TEARUP
TEASED
TEASEL
TEASER
TEASES
TEASET
TEATRO
TEAURN
TEBETS
TECATE
TECHIE
TECHNO
TECHTV
TEDEUM
TEDIUM
TEDKEY
TEEBOX
TEEDUP
TEEHEE
TEEING
TEEMED
TEENER
TEENIE
TEENSY
TEEOFF
TEEPEE
TEESUP
TEETER
TEETHE
TEEVEE
TEFLON
TEGRIN
TEHEED
TEHEES
TEHRAN
TEJANA
TEJANO
TEKKIE
TEKWAR
TELCOS
TELLER
TELLIT
TELLME
TELLOF
TELLON
TELNET
TEMPED
TEMPEH
TEMPER
TEMPLE
TEMPOS
TEMPTS
TEMPUS
TENACE
TENANT
TENDAY
TENDED
TENDER
TENDON
TENDTO
TENEEE
TENETS
TENHUT
TENLBS
TENLEY
TENNER
TENNIS
TENONE
TENONS
TENORS
TENPIN
TENSED
TENSER
TENSES
TENSOR
TENTED
TENTER
TENTHS
TENTON
TENTWO
TENURE
TENUTA
TENUTO
TEPEES
TERATO
TERBIC
TERCEL
TERCES
TERESA
TERETE
TERKEL
TERMED
TERMES
TERNES
TERRAE
TERRAN
TERRES
TERRET
TERRIF
TERRIS
TERROR
TERSER
TESLAS
TESSIE
TESSIO
TESTAE
TESTED
TESTEE
TESTER
TETCHY
TETHER
TETHYS
TETLEY
TETONS
TETRAD
TETRAS
TETRIS
TETZEL
TEUTON
TEVERE
TEVETS
TEXACO
TEXANS
TEXMEX
TEXTED

T•E•••
TCELLS
TEEBOX
TEEDUP
TEEHEE
TEEING
TEEMED
TEENER
TEENIE
TEENSY
TEEOFF
TEEPEE
TEESUP
TEETER
TEETHE
TEEVEE
THEACT
THEAGE
THEAPE
THEASP
THEAXE
THEBAN
THEBAR
THEBAY
THEBBC
THEBEE
THEBES
THECAN
THECAR
THECIA
THECID
THEDOW
THEEND
THEEPA
THEEYE
THEFAN
THEFBI
THEFED
THEFLY
THEFOG
THEFOX
THEFTS
THEGAP
THEHAJ
THEHUB
THEIRS
THEISM
THEIST
THEKID
THELAW
THELIP
THELMA
THELOT
THEMAN
THEMED
THEMES
THEMET
THEMOB
THEMRS
THENBA
THENCE
THENET
THENFL
THENHL
THENRA
THEONE
THEORY
THEPIT
THEPRU
THERAM
THERAP
THERAT
THERED
THEREF
THERES
THERMO
THERMS
THEROD
THERON
THESEA
THESES
THESIS
THESON
THESOX
THESPS
THESPY
THESUN
THETAS
THETED
THETIS
THETOP
THETOY
THEUSA
THEVET
THEWAY
THEWEB
THEWHO
THEWIZ
THEYLL
THEYRE
THEYVE
TIEBAR
TIEDIN
TIEDON
TIEDTO
TIEDUP
TIEDYE
TIEINS
TIEMPO
TIENDA
TIEOFF
TIEPIN
TIERCE
TIERED
TIEROD
TIERRA
TIESIN
TIESON
TIESTO
TIESUP
TIETAC
TIEUPS
TMESES
TMESIS
TOECAP
TOEDIN
TOEING
TOEINS
TOESIN
TOETAP
TREADS
TREATS
TREATY
TREBEK
TREBLE
TREBLY
TRECES
TREDIA
TREIZE
TREMOR
TRENCH
TRENDS
TRENDY
TRENTA
TRENTE
TRENTO
TREPAN
TREPID
TRESSY
TREVOR
TREXES
TSETSE
TWEAKS
TWEAKY
TWEEDS
TWEEDY
TWEENS
TWEENY
TWEETS
TWEETY
TWEEZE
TWELVE
TWENTY
TWERPS

T••E••
TAGEND
TAKEIN
TAKEIT
TAKEON
TAKERS
TAKETH
TAKETO
TAKEUP
TALENT
TALERS
TALESE
TAMELY
TAMERS
TAMEST
TAPEON
TAPERS
TAPEUP
TASERS
TATERS
TAVELS
TAVERN
TAXERS
TEBETS
TEDEUM
TEHEED
TEHEES
TENEEE
TENETS
TEPEES
TERESA
TERETE
TEVERE
TEVETS
THEEND
THEEPA
THEEYE
THIEVE
THREAD
THREAT
THREEA
THREEB
THREEC
THREED
THREEE
THREES
THRESH
TIGERS
TILERS
TILERY
TIMELY
TIMERS
TINEAL
TINEAR
TIREOF
TITERS
TOHEEL
TOKENS
TOLEDO
TONEME
TONERS
TONEUP
TOPEES
TOPEKA
TOPERS
TOREAT
TOREIT
TORENT
TORERO
TOREUP
TOTEMS
TOTERM
TOTERS
TOTEUP
TOWELS
TOWERS
TOWERY
TOYERS
TRIERS
TRUEST
TRUETO
TRUEUP
TRYERS
TUBERS
TUMEFY
TUNEIN
TUNERS
TUNETO
TUNEUP
TUPELO
TUREEN
TUTEES
TUXEDO
TVSETS
TWEEDS
TWEEDY
TWEENS
TWEENY
TWEETS
TWEETY
TWEEZE
TWOEEE
TYLERS
TYPEAB
TYPEAS
TYPEBS
TYPEIN
TYPEOS
TYPERS
TYPEUP

T•••E•
TABBED
TABKEY
TABLED
TABLES
TABLET
TABSET
TABUED
TACKED
TACKER
TACTEL
TAGGED
TAGGER
TAHNEE
TAHOES
TAILED
TAILER
TAIPEI
TALCED
TALKED
TALKER
TALLER
TAMPED
TAMPER
TANDEM
TANGED
TANKED
TANKER
TANNED
TANNER
TANTES
TAPPED
TAPPER
TAPPET
TARDES
TARGET
TARLEK
TARRED
TARTED
TARTER
TARTES
TASKED
TASKET
TASSEL
TASSES
TASTED
TASTEE
TASTER
TASTES
TATLER
TATTED
TATTER
TAUPES
TAUTEN
TAUTER
TAXIED
TAXIES
TAXMEN
TBONES
TEAMED
TEARED
TEARER
TEASED
TEASEL
TEASER
TEASES
TEASET
TEDKEY
TEEHEE
TEEMED
TEENER
TEEPEE
TEETER
TEEVEE
TEHEED
TEHEES
TELLER
TELNET
TEMPED
TEMPEH
TEMPER
TENDED
TENDER
TENEEE
TENLEY
TENNER
TENSED
TENSER
TENSES
TENTED
TENTER
TEPEES
TERCEL
TERCES
TERKEL
TERMED
TERMES
TERNES
TERRES
TERRET
TERSER
TESTED
TESTEE
TESTER
TETHER
TETLEY
TETZEL
TEXMEX
TEXTED
THALER
THALES
THAMES
THANES
THAWED
THAWER
THAYER
THEBEE
THEBES
THEFED
THEMED
THEMES
THEMET
THENET
THERED
THEREF
THERES
THESEA
THESES
THETED
THEVET
THEWEB
THOLES
THREEA
THREEB
THREEC
THREED
THREEE
THREES
THROES
THYMES
TICCED
TICKED
TICKER
TICKET
TIDIED
TIDIER
TIDIES
TIERED
TIFFED
TIGGER
TIGRES
TILDEN
TILDES
TILLED
TILLER
TILLET
TILLEY
TILTED
TILTER
TIMBER
TINDER
TINGED
TINGES
TINIER
TINKER
TINMEN
TINNED
TINNER
TINSEL
TINTED
TINTER
TIPPED
TIPPEE
TIPPER
TIPPET
TISKET
TITHED
TITHER
TITHES
TITLED
TITLES
TITRED
TITRES
TITTER
TMESES
TNOTES
TOATEE
TOBIES
TODIES
TOFFEE
TOGAED
TOGGED
TOGUES
TOHEEL
TOILED
TOILER
TOILES
TOILET
TOLLED
TOLLER
TOLTEC
TOMBES
TONGED
TONIER
TONNES
TOOLED
TOOLER
TOOMEY
TOOTED
TOOTER
TOPEES
TOPMEN
TOPPED
TOPPER
TOPTEN
TOQUES
TORIES
TORRES
TORREY
TORTES
TOSSED
TOSSER
TOSSES
TOTTED
TOTTER
TOUPEE
TOURED
TOURER
TOUTED
TOUTER
TOWHEE
TOWNER
TRACED
TRACER
TRACES
TRACEY
TRADED
TRADER
TRADES
TRALEE
TRANES
TRAVEL
TRAVEN
TRAVES
TREBEK
TRECES
TREXES
TRIBES
TRICEP
TRICES
TRIJET
TRIKES
TRINES
TRIPES
TRITER
TRIVET
TROPES
TROPEZ
TROVES
TROWED
TROWEL
TROYER
TRUCES
TSADES
TTILES
TUBBED
TUCKED
TUCKER
TUFFET
TUFTED
TUGGED
TUGGER
TULLES
TUNNEL
TUNNEY
TUPPER
TUQUES
TUREEN
TURFED
TURKEY
TURNED
TURNER
TURRET
TUSHES
TUSKED
TUSKER
TUSSES
TUTEES
TUTTED
TUTUED
TVCREW
TWINED
TWINER
TWINES
TWOEEE
TWOFER

T••••E
TACKLE
TAGORE
TAHNEE
TALESE
TALKIE
TAMALE
TANGLE
TASTEE
TATTLE
TBOONE
TECATE
TECHIE
TEEHEE
TEENIE
TEEPEE
TEETHE
TEEVEE
TEKKIE
TELLME
TEMPLE
TENACE
TENEEE
TENONE
TENURE
TERETE
TERRAE
TESSIE
TESTAE
TESTEE
TEVERE
THEAGE
THEAPE
THEAXE
THEBEE
THEEYE
THENCE
THEONE
THEYRE
THEYVE
THICKE
THIEVE
THISBE
THORPE
THRACE
THREEE
THRICE
THRIVE
THRONE
THROVE
TIBIAE
TICKLE
TIEDYE
TIERCE
TILLIE
TIMBRE
TINGLE
TINKLE
TINORE
TIPPEE
TIPPLE
TIPTOE
TIRADE
TIRANE
TISANE
TISSUE
TITTLE
TOATEE
TOCOME
TODATE
TODDLE
TOFFEE
TOGGLE
TOLIFE
TOMMIE
TONEME
TONGUE
TONITE
TOODLE
TOONIE
TOOTIE
TOOTLE
TOPPLE
TORQUE
TOUCHE
TOUPEE
TOUSLE
TOWAGE
TOWHEE
TOWNIE
TRACHE
TRALEE
TRANCE
TREBLE
TREIZE
TRENTE
TRIAGE
TRIFLE
TRIODE
TRIPLE
TRISTE
TRIUNE
TRIXIE
TROCHE
TROMPE
TROUPE
TRUDGE
TRYGVE
TRYONE
TSETSE
TSHAPE
TUBAGE
TUBATE
TUBULE
TUILLE
TULANE
TULARE
TUMBLE
TURTLE
TUSHIE
TUSSLE
TVGAME
TVTAPE
TVTIME
TWEEZE
TWELVE
TWINGE
TWOEEE
TYRONE

•TE•••
ATEAMS
ATEASE
ATEMPO
ATENTH
ATEOUT
ATERRE
ATESTS
BTEAMS
ETERNE
HTESTS
ITEMED
MTETNA
NTESTS
OTELLO
STEADS
STEADY
STEAKS
STEALS
STEAMS
STEAMY
STEEDS
STEELE
STEELS
STEELY
STEEPS
STEERS
STEEVE
STEFAN
STEFFI
STEFOY
STEINS
STELAR
STELAS
STELES
STELLA
STELMO
STEMMY
STENCH
STENOG
STENOS
STENTS
STEPIN
STEPON
STEPPE
STEPUP
STEREO
STERES
STERIC
STERNA
STERNE
STERNO
STERNS
STEROL
STETHO
STEVEN
STEVIE
STEWED
STEWER
STEWIE
XTERRA

•T•E••
ATBEST
ATHEEL
ATHENA
ATHENE
ATHENS
ATREST
ATREUS
ATTEND
ATTEST
ETCETC
ETHENE
ETHERS
ETSEQQ
ITSELF
OTHERS
OTSEGO
OTTERS
STBEDE
STEEDS
STEELE
STEELS
STEELY
STEEPS
STEERS
STEEVE
STIERS
STPETE
STREAK
STREAM
STREEP
STREET
STREPS
STRESS
STREWN
STREWS
UTTERS

•T••E•
ATHEEL
ATILES
ATISES
ATMFEE
ATONED
ATONER
ATONES
ATTLEE
BTHREE
BTILES
CTILES
DTILES

ETAGES
ETAPES
ETCHED
ETCHER
ETCHES
ETILES
ETUDES
FTILES
GTILES
HTILES
ITCHED
ITCHES
ITEMED
ITILES
ITRIED
JTILES
KTILES
LTILES
MTILES
NTILES
OTILES
OTOSES
PTILES
PTOOEY
QTILES
RTILES
STACEY
STAGED
STAGER
STAGES
STAGEY
STAKED
STAKES
STALED
STALER
STALES
STAMEN
STAPES
STARED
STARER
STARES
STASES
STATED
STATEN
STATER
STATES
STAVED
STAVES
STAYED
STAYER
STELES
STEREO
STERES
STEVEN
STEWED
STEWER
STIDES
STILES
STIPES
STOKED
STOKER
STOKES
STOLEN
STOLES
STONED
STONER
STONES
STONEY
STORED
STORER
STORES
STOVER
STOVES
STOWED
STOWER
STREEP
STREET
STUPES
STYLED
STYLER
STYLES
STYLET
TTILES
UTUBES
VTILES
WTILES
XTILES
XTYPES
YTILES
ZTILES

•T•••E

ATEASE
ATERRE
ATFIVE
ATHENE
ATHOME
ATMFEE
ATNINE
ATONCE
ATTIRE
ATTLEE
ATTUNE
ATYALE
BTHREE
ETERNE
ETHANE
ETHENE
ETOILE
ETRADE
ETTORE
NTUPLE
OTIOSE
OTOOLE
OTTONE
STABLE
STANCE
STAPLE
STARVE
STATUE
STBEDE
STEELE
STEEVE
STEPPE
STERNE
STEVIE
STEWIE
STIFLE
STILLE
STJUDE
STLUKE
STODGE
STOGIE
STOLAE
STOLLE
STOOGE
STPETE
STRAFE
STRIAE
STRIDE
STRIFE
STRIKE
STRIPE
STRIVE
STROBE
STRODE
STROKE
STROVE
STYMIE

••TE••

AFTERS
ALTERS
ANTEED
ANTERO
ANTEUP
APTEST
ARTELS
ARTERY
ARTEST
ASTEAL
ASTEEP
ASTERN
ASTERO
ASTERS
ATTEND
ATTEST
AUTEUR
AZTECA
AZTECS
AZTEKS
BATEAU
BETELS
BITEIN
BITEON
BITERS
BITEUP
BOTELS
BUTENE
BUTEOS
BYTENS
CATENA
CATERA
CATERS
CETERA
CITEES
CITERS
CUTELY
CUTEST
CUTESY
CUTEYS
DATERS
DETECT
DETENT
DETERS
DETEST
DOTELL
DOTEON
DOTERS
EATERS
EATERY
ENTERO
ENTERS
ESTEEM
ESTERS
EXTEND
EXTENT
EXTERN
GATEAU
GATERS
GOTEAM
HATEIT
HATERS
HATETO
HETERO
HITECH
HITEST
HOTELS
INTEND
INTENS
INTENT
INTERJ
INTERN
INTERS
IQTEST
KITERS
LATEEN
LATELY
LATENE
LATENS
LATENT
LATEOF
LATEON
LATERI
LATERO
LATEST
LATETO
LITERS
LUTECE
MATERS
MATEYS
METEOR
METERS
MITERS
MOTELS
MOTETS
MUTELY
MUTEST
NITERS
NITERY
NOTERS
OATERS
OBTEST
OCTETS
ORTEGA
OSTEAL
OSTEND
OSTERS
OTTERS
OUTEAT
PATENS
PATENT
PATERS
PETERI
PETERS
POTEEN
POTENT
RATEDA
RATEDG
RATEDR
RATEDX
RATELS
RATERS
RETEAR
RETELL
RETEST
SATEEN
SHTETL
TATERS
TITERS
TOTEMS
TOTERM
TOTERS
TOTEUP
TUTEES
UPTEAR
URTEXT
UTTERS
VOTECH
VOTEIN
VOTENO
VOTEON
VOTERS
WATERS
WATERY

••T•E•

AETHER
ALTHEA
ALTKEY
ANTEED
ANTHEM
ANTHER
ANTLER
ANTRES
ARTIER
ASTEEP
ASTHER
ASTLEY
ASTRES
ATTLEE
AUTOED
BATHED
BATHER
BATHES
BATLEY
BATMEN
BATTED
BATTEN
BATTER
BETHEL
BETSEY
BETTED
BETTER
BITNET
BITTED
BITTEN
BITTER
BOTHER
BOTREE
BUTLER
BUTTED
BUTTER
BUTTES
BUTYET
BYTHEN
CATBED
CATHER
CATMEN
CITEES
CITIED
CITIES
COTLER
COTTEN
COTTER
CUTIES
CUTLER
CUTLET
CUTTER
DETMER
DETTES
DITHER
DITZES
DOTTED
DOTTER
DUTIES
EITHER
ENTREE
ENTREZ
ESTEEM
ESTHER
FATHER
FATTED
FATTEN
FATTER
FETTER
FITTED
FITTER
FUTZED
FUTZES
GATHER
GETHEP
GETSET
GETTER
GETWET
GITTED
GOTHEP
GOTSET
GOTTEN
GOTWET
GUTTED
GUTTER
HATRED
HATTED
HATTER
HITHER
HITMEN
HITTER
HOTBED
HOTKEY
HOTTEA
HOTTER
HUTTED
IFTHEN
ISTLES
ISTRES
JETSET
JETTED
JITNEY
JITTER
JOTTED
JOTTER
JUTTED
KATZEN
KITAEN
KITTED
KITTEN
KOTTER
LATEEN
LATHED
LATHEN
LATHER
LATHES
LATKES
LATTER
LATTES
LETTED
LETTER
LITHER
LITRES
LITTER
LOTTED
LOTTER
LUTHER
LUTZES
MATHER
MATHEW
MATJES
MATMEN
MATTEA
MATTED
MATTEL
MATTER
MATTES
METIER
METRED
METRES
MITRED
MITRES
MITTEN
MOTHER
MOTLEY
MUTTER
MUTUEL
NATTER
NETHER
NETMEN
NETTED
NETTER
NITRES
NOTNEW
NOTYET
NUTLET
NUTMEG
NUTTED
NUTTER
OATIER
ORTHEN
OSTLER
OUTBEG
OUTIES
OUTJET
OUTLED
OUTLET
OUTSEE
OUTSET
PATTED
PATTEN
PATTER
PATZER
PETREL
PETTED
PETTER
PETTET
PITHED
PITIED
PITIER
PITIES
PITMEN
PITNEY
PITTED
POTEEN
POTHER
POTTED
POTTER
PUTNEY
PUTTED
PUTTEE
PUTTER
RATHER
RATNER
RATTED
RATTER
RETIED
RETIEF
RETIES
RETTED
RITTER
RITZES
ROTTED
ROTTEN
ROTTER
RUTGER
RUTTED
RUTTER
SATEEN
SETFEE
SETTEE
SETTER
SETZER
SITTER
SOTHEN
SOTTED
SUTTER
TATLER
TATTED
TATTER
TETHER
TETLEY
TETZEL
TITHED
TITHER
TITHES
TITLED
TITLES
TITRED
TITRES
TITTER
TOTTED
TOTTER
TUTEES
TUTTED
TUTUED
UNTIED
UNTIER
UNTIES
VATTED
VETOED
VETOER
VETOES
VETTED
VETTER
VETTES
WATNEY
WETTED
WETTER
WITHER
WITTED
WITTER
YATSEN
YATTER
YUTZES
ZITHER

••T••E

ACTIVE
ACTONE
ANTONE
ASTARE
ASTUTE
ATTIRE
ATTLEE
ATTUNE
BATTLE
BETAKE
BETIDE
BETTYE
BOTREE
BOTTLE
BUTANE
BUTENE
CATTLE
CETANE
COTTAE
DATIVE
DETUNE
DOTAGE
DOTIME
DOTTIE
DOTTLE
ECTYPE
ENTICE
ENTIRE
ENTREE
ESTATE
ESTIME
ETTORE
FATALE
FATONE
FETTLE
FUTILE
FUTURE
HATTIE
HITONE
HOTONE
HOTTIE
HUTONE
INTAKE
INTIME
INTONE
INTUNE
IVTUBE
KATHIE
KETONE
KETTLE
KOTTKE
LATENE
LETSBE
LETTRE
LETUSE
LITTLE
LITTRE
LUTECE
MATTIE
MATURE
METATE
METTLE
MOTILE
MOTIVE
MOTTLE
MUTATE
NATALE
NATIVE
NATURE
NETTLE
NOTATE
NOTICE
NOTIME
NOTONE
NUTATE
OBTUSE
OCTANE
OCTAVE
ONTAPE
ONTIME
OTTONE
OUTAGE
OUTATE
OUTAWE
OUTLIE
OUTSEE
OUTVIE
PATINE
PATRIE
PATTIE
PETALE
PETITE
PETRIE
POTAGE
POTPIE
POTSIE
PUTTEE
RATINE
RATITE
RATTLE
RETAKE
RETAME
RETAPE
RETILE
RETIME
RETIRE
RETONE
RETORE
RETUNE
RETYPE
RITDYE
ROTATE
RUTHIE
RUTILE
SATIRE
SETFEE
SETOSE
SETTEE
SETTLE
SOTRUE
SUTURE
TATTLE
TITTLE
TVTAPE
TVTIME
UNTAME
UNTAPE
UNTRUE
UNTUNE
UPTAKE
UPTIME
UPTORE
VATDYE
VITALE
VITTLE
VOTIVE
WATTLE
WETONE
YETTIE

•••TE•

ABATED
ABATER
ABATES
ACUTER
ACUTES
AGATES
AGETEN
ALATED
AMSTEL
ARETES
AUNTEM
AUSTEN
AUSTER
BAITED
BAITER
BANTER
BARTEL
BARTER
BASTED
BASTER
BASTES
BATTED
BATTEN
BATTER
BAXTER
BEATEN
BEATER
BELTED
BELTER
BESTED
BESTER
BETTED
BETTER
BIGTEN
BITTED
BITTEN
BITTER
BOATED
BOATEL
BOATER
BOITES
BOLTED
BOLTER
BOOTED
BOOTEE
BOOTER
BOOTES
BRUTES
BUNTED
BUNTER
BUSTED
BUSTER
BUTTED
BUTTER
BUTTES
CANTED
CANTER
CARTED
CARTEL
CARTER
CARTES
CASTED
CASTEL
CASTER
CASTES
CENTER
CHUTED
CHUTES
CNOTES
COATED
COATEE
COATER
COATES
COLTER
COMTES
COOTER
COPTER
CORTES
CORTEX
CORTEZ
COSTED
COTTEN
COTTER
COUTER
CRATED
CRATER
CRATES
CURTER
CUSTER
CUTTER
DAFTER
DANTEI
DANTES
DARTED
DARTER
DEBTEE
DEFTER
DENTED
DESTEM
DETTES
DEUTER
DEXTER
DHOTEL
DIETED
DIETER
DIETES
DINTED
DOTTED
DOTTER
DUCTED
DUETED
DUSTED
DUSTER
EASTER
EBATES
EDITED
ELATED
ELATER
ELATES
ELITER
ELITES
ELUTED
ELUTES
EMOTED
EMOTER
EMOTES
ENATES
ENOTES
EVITES
EXETER
EXITED
FAITES
FALTER
FASTED
FASTEN
FASTER
FATTED
FATTEN
FATTER
FAUTES
FELTED
FESTER
FETTER
FILTER
FISTED
FITTED
FITTER
FLUTED
FLUTER
FLUTES
FOOTED
FOOTER
FORTES
FOSTER
FRATER
FRITES
GAITED
GAITER
GARTER
GASTER
GENTES
GESTES
GETTER
GIFTED
GIFTEE
GIRTED
GITTED
GLUTEI
GLUTEN
GLUTES
GNOTES
GOATEE
GOITER
GOTTEN
GRATED
GRATER
GRATES
GRETEL
GUNTER
GUSTED
GUTTED
GUTTER
HAFTED
HALTED
HALTER
HASTED
HASTEN
HASTES
HATTED
HATTER
HEATED
HEATER
HEFTED
HEFTER
HELTER
HESTER
HILTED
HINTED
HINTER
HITTER
HOOTED
HOOTER
HOSTED
HOSTEL
HOTTEA
HOTTER
HUNTED
HUNTER
HURTER
HUTTED
ICETEA
INSTEP
IPETER
IRATER
JEETER
JESTED
JESTER
JETTED
JILTED
JILTER
JITTER
JOETEX
JOLTED
JOLTER
JOTTED
JOTTER
JUSTER
JUTTED
KEITEL
KILTED
KILTER
KITTED
KITTEN
KOSTER
KOTTER
LACTEA
LAPTEV
LARTER
LARTET
LASTED
LASTEX
LATTER
LATTES
LAUTER
LECTER
LEITER
LENTEN
LESTER
LETTED
LETTER
LIFTED
LIFTER
LILTED
LINTED
LINTEL
LINTER
LISTED
LISTEE
LISTEN
LISTER
LITTER
LOFTED
LOFTER
LOITER
LOOTED
LOOTER
LOTTED
LOTTER
LUSTED
LUSTER
MALTED
MANTEE
MANTEL
MARTEL
MARTEN
MARTES
MASTED
MASTER
MATTEA
MATTED
MATTEL
MATTER
MATTES
MEETER
MELTED
MELTER
MENTEE
MINTED
MINTER
MISTED
MISTER
MITTEN
MIXTEC
MOATED
MOLTED
MOLTEN
MOLTER
MONTEL
MONTEZ
MOOTED
MOOTER
MORTEN
MOSTEL
MUSTER
MUTTER
NANTES
NATTER
NAUTES
NEATEN
NEATER
NESTEA
NESTED
NESTER
NETTED
NETTER
NEUTER
NEXTEL
NOSTEP
NOSTER
NUTTED
NUTTER
OBITER
OERTER
ONETEN

ORATED ORATES OUSTED OUSTER OYSTER PACTEN PALTER PANTED PANTER PARTED PASTED PASTEL PASTER PASTES PATTED PATTEN PATTER PELTED PELTER PENTEL PERTER PESTER PETTED PETTER PETTET PEWTER PIETER PINTER PISTES PITTED PIUTES PLATED PLATEN PLATER PLATES POETES PORTED PORTER PORTES POSTED POSTER POTTED POTTER POUTED POUTER PRATED PRATER PRATES PRETER PROTEA PROTEM PUNTED PUNTER PUTTED PUTTEE PUTTER QUOTED QUOTEE QUOTER QUOTES RAFTED RAFTER RANTED RANTER RAPTER RASTER RATTED RATTER

REDTEN REITER RENTED RENTEE RENTER RENTES RESTED RESTER RESTES RETTED REUTER RIFTED RIOTED RIOTER RITTER ROOTED ROOTER ROSTEN ROSTER ROTTED ROTTEN ROTTER ROUTED ROUTER ROUTES RRATED RUSTED RUTTED RUTTER SAITEK SALTED SALTEN SALTER SANTEE SAUTES SCOTER SEATED SEATER SELTEN SEPTET SESTET SETTEE SETTER SEXTET SIETES SIFTED SIFTER SILTED SISTER SITTER SIXTEN SKATED SKATER SKATES SKYTEL SLATED SLATER SLATES SMITER SMITES SOFTEN SOFTER SORTED SORTER SOTTED SOUTER SPATES SPITED

SPITES STATED STATEN STATER STATES SUITED SUITES SUMTER SUTTER SYSTEM TACTEL TANTES TARTED TARTER TARTES TASTED TASTEE TASTER TASTES TATTED TATTER TAUTEN TAUTER TEETER TENTED TENTER TESTED TESTEE TESTER TEXTED THETED TILTED TILTER TINTED TINTER TITTER TNOTES TOATEE TOLTEC TOOTED TOOTER TOPTEN TORTES TOTTED TOTTER TOUTED TOUTER TRITER TUFTED TUTTED ULSTER UNITED UNITER UNITES UNSTEP UPSTEP VASTER VATTED VENTED VENTER VERTEX VESTED VESTEE VETTED VETTER VETTES VORTEX WAFTED

WAFTER WAITED WAITER WALTER WANTED WANTER WARTED WASTED WASTER WASTES WELTED WELTER WESTER WETTED WETTER WHITED WHITEN WHITER WHITES WHITEY WILTED WINTER WISTER WITTED WITTER WONTED WRITER WRITES WYNTER XRATED XYSTER YATTER YESTER ZESTED ZESTER

•••T•E

ALETTE AMITIE AORTAE AUNTIE BARTLE BATTLE BEATLE BEETLE BERTHE BERTIE BETTYE BIGTOE BLITHE BLYTHE BOOTEE BOOTHE BOOTIE BOTTLE BOWTIE BUSTLE CANTBE CANTLE CASTLE CATTLE CENTRE CLOTHE COATEE CONTRE COOTIE COSTAE COTTAE

DARTLE DEBTEE DOTTIE DOTTLE FETTLE FLUTIE FOOTLE GENTLE GERTIE GESTAE GIFTEE GOATEE GOETHE GRATAE HATTIE HOGTIE HOOTIE HOTTIE HURTLE HUSTLE INATIE ISITME JOSTLE JUSTME KAETHE KETTLE KILTIE KOTTKE LAOTSE LEFTBE LETTRE LEUTZE LHOTSE LISTEE LITTLE LITTRE LOATHE LUSTRE MAITRE MANTEE MANTLE MARTHE MATTIE MENTEE MENTHE METTLE MILTIE MOLTKE MOTTLE MYRTLE NESTLE NETTLE ODETTE OLATHE PANTIE PATTIE PESTLE PLATTE POSTIE PUTTEE QUATRE QUOTEE RATTLE REDTIE RENTEE ROOTIE ROOTLE RUSTLE

SANTEE SARTRE SCATHE SCYTHE SEETHE SETTEE SETTLE SOFTIE SOOTHE SORTIE SPATHE STATUE SUBTLE SWATHE TASTEE TATTLE TEETHE TESTAE TESTEE TIPTOE TITTLE TOATEE TOOTIE TOOTLE TSETSE TURTLE VESTEE VIRTUE VITTLE WATTLE WESTIE WHATVE WRITHE YERTLE YETTIE YVETTE

••••TE

ABLATE ACUATE ADESTE ADNATE ADRATE AERATE AGNATE ALETTE ANSATE APLITE ARRETE ASANTE ASTUTE AUGITE AURATE AVIATE BARITE BELATE BENOTE BERATE BINATE BORATE BRONTE BYDATE BYROTE CANUTE CAPOTE CDRATE CERATE CHANTE

CHASTE CHOATE CLOETE COMATE COYOTE CREATE CROUTE CURATE CURITE DANITE DEBATE DELETE DEMOTE DENOTE DEPUTE DERATE DEVOTE DILATE DILUTE DONATE DUARTE ECARTE EFFETE EIGHTE ELUATE EMEUTE ENSATE EQUATE ESTATE EXCITE EXMATE FICHTE FINITE FIXATE FOLATE GAMETE GELATE GUNITE GYRATE HALITE HAMATE HAMITE HECATE IDEATE IGNITE IMLATE IMPUTE INCITE INDITE INGATE INMATE INNATE INVITE IODATE ISLATE KARATE LANATE LEGATE LEVITE LIGATE LOBATE LOCATE LUCITE LUNATE LUXATE MANUTE MELETE METATE

MINUTE MUTATE NEGATE NIENTE NORITE NOTATE NOVOTE NUTATE OBLATE ODETTE OFLATE OFNOTE OLEATE ONLATE ONSITE OOCYTE OOLITE OPIATE ORNATE OUTATE PAIUTE PALATE PEDATE PETITE PEYOTE PILATE PIRATE PLANTE PLATTE POINTE POLITE PUENTE PUPATE PYRITE QUARTE QUINTE RAMATE RATITE REBATE REBOTE RECITE REDATE REFUTE RELATE REMATE REMOTE RENOTE REPUTE RERATE RESITE REVOTE RIMATE ROTATE SAINTE SALUTE SAVATE SEDATE SEMITE SENATE SHIITE SHORTE SOLUTE SPRITE STPETE SURETE SVELTE TECATE TERETE

TODATE TONITE TRENTE TRISTE TUBATE UGARTE UNCUTE UNIATE UNMATE UPDATE UPLATE UPRATE VACATE VEINTE VENITE VERITE VOLUTE YVETTE ZYGOTE

T•F•••

TEFLON TIFFED TIFFIN TOFFEE TUFFET TUFTED TUFTSU

T••F••

THEFAN THEFBI THEFED THEFLY THEFOG THEFOX THEFTS TIFFED TIFFIN TOFFEE TOOFAR TRIFLE TRYFOR TUBFUL TUFFET TURFED TWOFER

T•••F•

TAPOFF TARIFF TEEOFF THENFL THRIFT TIEOFF TIPOFF TOLIFE TOPOFF TUMEFY TYPIFY

T••••F

TALKOF TAPOFF TARIFF TEEOFF TELLOF TERRIF

THEREF TIEOFF TIPOFF TIREOF TOLDOF TONSOF TOPOFF

•TF•••

ATFIVE ATFOUR MTFUJI

•T•F••

ATMFEE ITSFUN STAFFS STEFAN STEFFI STEFOY STIFFS STIFLE STUFFS STUFFY

•T••F•

STAFFS STEFFI STIFFS STRAFE STRIFE STUFFS STUFFY

•T•••F

ATONOF ITSELF STAPUF STOLAF

••TF••

ACTFOR ARTFUL BATFOR BOTFLY CATFIT FITFOR FITFUL GETFAR GETFIT GOTFAR GOTFIT HATFUL HITFOR JETFAN LETFLY METFAN NETFUL NOTFAR NOTFIT NOTFOR OPTFOR OUTFIT OUTFLY OUTFOR OUTFOX POTFUL SATFOR

SETFEE SETFOR SITFOR VATFUL WETFLY

••T•F•

BITOFF CITIFY CUTOFF GETOFF GOTOFF HITOFF LETOFF MOTIFS NOTIFY PUTOFF RATIFY RATOFF SETOFF

••T••F

ALTARF BITOFF CUTOFF EATSOF GETANF GETOFF GOTANF GOTOFF HITOFF LATEOF LETOFF LOTSOF PUTOFF RATOFF RETIEF RETURF SETOFF

•••T•F

ABITOF ALOTOF CERTIF LEFTOF MOSTOF PARTOF SORTOF WHATIF

T•G•••

TAGDAY TAGEND TAGGED TAGGER TAGORE TAGOUT TAGSON TAGSUP TEGRIN TIGERS TIGGER TIGHTS TIGLON TIGONS TIGRES TIGRIS TOGAED

TOGGED TOGGLE TOGOUT TOGSUP TOGUES TSGARP TUGGED TUGGER TUGRIK TUGSAT TUGSON TVGAME

T••G••

TAGGED TAGGER TAIGAS TANGED TANGLE TANGLY TANGOS TANGUY TARGAS TARGET TAUGHT THEGAP THIGHS TIGGER TINGED TINGES TINGLE TINGLY TINGOD TOGGED TOGGLE TONGAN TONGED TONGUE TOPGUN TOUGHS TOUGHY TOYGUN TRAGIC TRAGUS TRIGON TROGGS TRYGVE TUGGED TUGGER TURGID TWIGGY

T•••G•

THEAGE THINGS THINGY THONGS THOUGH TOBAGO TOWAGE TRIAGE TROGGS TROUGH TRUDGE TUBAGE TWANGS TWANGY TWIGGY

TWINGE

T••••G

TAKING TAMING TAPING TARING TAUROG TAXING TEABAG TEEING THEFOG THRONG TIDING TILING TIMING TIRING TOEING TONING TOOBIG TOPDOG TOPING TOTING TOWING TOYDOG TOYING TRUING TRYING TSKING TUBING TUNING TURING TYPING

•TG•••

ITGIRL LTGOVS

•T•G••

ETAGES STAGED STAGER STAGES STAGEY STIGMA STOGIE

•T••G•

ATSIGN ITSAGO OTSEGO STINGS STINGY STODGE STODGY STOOGE STOPGO

•T•••G

ATHING ETTING STALAG STENOG STRING STRONG STRUNG STYING

••TG••

ARTGUM CATGUT DOTGOV JETGUN OUTGAS OUTGUN ROTGUT RUTGER

••T•G•

ANTIGO DOTAGE IDTAGS LATIGO LETSGO ORTEGA OUTAGE POTAGE RETAGS

••T••G

ACTING BATING BITING CATRIG CITING DATING DOTING DOTORG EATING ETTING FETING GATING HATING HOTDOG JETLAG KITBAG KITING MATING METING MITTAG MUTING NOTING NUTMEG OPTING OUTBEG OUTING OUTRIG PETDOG PETPIG RATEDG RATING RETTIG SATING SITING TOTING UNTRIG VOTING WETRAG WETTIG WITTIG YUTANG

•••TG•

DONTGO WONTGO

•••T•G

DOGTAG EARTAG GOSTAG MAYTAG MITTAG MONTAG OAKTAG PHOTOG RAGTAG REDTAG RETTIG SONTAG WETTIG WITTIG ZAFTIG

TH••••

THALER THALES THALIA THAMES THANES THANKS THATCH THATIS THATLL THAWED THAWER THAYER THEACT THEAGE THEAPE THEASP THEAXE THEBAN THEBAR THEBAY THEBBC THEBEE THEBES THECAN THECAR THECIA THECID THEDOW THEEND THEEPA THEEYE THEFAN THEFBI THEFED THEFLY THEFOG THEFOX THEFTS THEGAP THEHAJ THEHUB THEIRS THEISM THEIST THEKID THELAW THELIP THELMA THELOT THEMAN

THEMED
THEMES
THEMET
THEMOB
THEMRS
THENBA
THENCE
THENET
THENFL
THENHL
THENRA
THEONE
THEORY
THEPIT
THEPRU
THERAM
THERAP
THERAT
THERED
THEREF
THERES
THERMO
THERMS
THEROD
THERON
THESEA
THESES
THESIS
THESON
THESOX
THESPS
THESPY
THESUN
THETAS
THETED
THETIS
THETOP
THETOY
THEUSA
THEVET
THEWAY
THEWEB
THEWHO
THEWIZ
THEYLL
THEYRE
THEYVE
THICKE
THIEVE
THIGHS
THILLS
THINGS
THINGY
THINKS
THINLY
THIRDR
THIRDS
THIRST
THIRTY
THISBE
THOLES
THOMAS
THONGS
THORAX
THORIC
THORNS
THORNY
THORON
THORPE
THOUGH
THRACE
THRALL
THRASH
THREAD
THREAT
THREEA
THREEB
THREEC
THREED
THREEE
THREES
THRESH
THRICE
THRIFT
THRILL
THRIVE
THROAT
THROBS
THROES
THRONE
THRONG
THROVE
THROWN
THROWS
THRUMS
THRUSH
THRUST
THUMBS
THUMPS
THUNKS
THUSLY
THWACK
THWART
THYMES
THYMIC
THYMUS

T•H•••

TAHINI
TAHITI
TAHNEE
TAHOES
TEHEED
TEHEES
TEHRAN
TOHEEL
TSHAPE
TSHIRT
TVHITS

T••H••

TECHIE
TECHNO
TECHTV
TEEHEE
TENHUT
TETHER
TETHYS
THEHAJ
THEHUB
TIGHTS
TILHIM
TINHAT
TISHRI
TITHED
TITHER
TITHES
TOOHIP
TOOHOT
TOPHAT
TOWHEE
TOYHAT
TURHAN
TUSHES
TUSHIE
TVSHOW
TYPHUS

T•••H•

TAICHI
TAUGHT
TEETHE
TENTHS
TETCHY
THENHL
THEWHO
THIGHS
TILTHS
TOOTHY
TORAHS
TORCHY
TOUCHE
TOUCHY
TOUGHS
TOUGHY
TRACHE
TRASHY
TRISHA
TROCHE
TROPHY
TROTHS
TRUTHS

T••••H

TAKETH
TEMPEH
THATCH
THOUGH
THRASH
THRESH
THRUSH
TRENCH
TROUGH
TWITCH

•TH•••

ATHAND
ATHEEL
ATHENA
ATHENE
ATHENS
ATHING
ATHOME
ATHROB
ATHROW
BTHREE
ETHANE
ETHENE
ETHERS
ETHICS
ETHIOP
ETHNIC
ETHNOS
ETHYLS
ITHACA
ITHINK
MTHOOD
OTHERS
OTHMAR
UTHANT

•T•H••

ATTHAT
ETCHED
ETCHER
ETCHES
ITCHED
ITCHES
ITSHOT
ITZHAK
UTAHAN
UTAHNS

•T••H•

STAPHS
STETHO
STJOHN
STROHS

•T•••H

ATENTH
ATTACH
STANCH
STARCH
STENCH
STITCH
STORCH

••TH••

AETHER
ALTHEA
ANTHEM
ANTHER
ARTHRO
ARTHUR
ASTHER
ASTHMA
ATTHAT
AUTHOR
BATHED
BATHER
BATHES
BATHOS
BETHEL
BOTHER
BUTHOW
BYTHEN
CATHAY
CATHER
CATHYS
DATHAN
DITHER
DOTHAN
EITHER
ESTHER
FATHER
FATHOM
GATHER
GETHEP
GETHIP
GETHOT
GOTHAM
GOTHEP
GOTHIC
GOTHIP
GOTHOT
HATHOR
HITHER
IFTHEN
INTHAT
ISTHMI
JETHRO
KATHIE
LATHED
LATHEN
LATHER
LATHES
LETHAL
LITHER
LITHIC
LITHOS
LOTHAR
LUTHER
LUTHOR
MATHER
MATHEW
MATHIS
METHOD
METHYL
MOTHER
MOTHRA
MYTHIC
MYTHOS
NATHAN
NETHER
NETHOU
NOTHIN
ORTHEN
OUTHIT
PATHAN
PATHIC
PATHOS
PITHED
POTHER
POTHOS
PYTHON
RATHER
RETHAW
ROTHKO
RUTHIE
SOTHAT
SOTHEN
TETHER
TETHYS
TITHED
TITHER
TITHES
UNTHAW
WITHAL
WITHER
WITHIN
WITHIT
WITHUS
ZITHER

••T•H•

BETCHA
BOTCHY
BUTWHO
BUTWHY
CATCHY
GOTCHA
LITCHI
NOTCHY
PATCHY
PITCHY
TETCHY
WITCHY

••T••H

ATTACH
DETACH
DETOTH
FETISH
HITECH
IRTYSH
KITSCH
LATISH
MATZOH
POTASH
PUTSCH
VOTECH

•••TH•

AGATHA
APATHY
ARETHA
BERTHA
BERTHE
BERTHS
BIRTHS
BLITHE
BLYTHE
BOOTHE
BOOTHS
BROTHS
BROTHY
CLOTHE
CLOTHO
CLOTHS
CRWTHS
DEATHS
DEPTHS
EARTHA
EARTHS
EARTHY
FAITHS
FIFTHS
FILTHY
FIRTHS
FROTHS
FROTHY
GIRTHS
GOETHE
HEATHS
HEATHY
ICHTHY
KAETHE
LOATHE
LUNTHA
MARTHA
MARTHE
MENTHE
MIRTHS
MONTHS
MOUTHS
MOUTHY
NINTHS
NORTHS
OLATHE
RHYTHM
SANTHA
SCATHE
SCYTHE
SEETHE
SIXTHS
SLITHY
SLOTHS
SMITHS
SMITHY
SNATHS
SOOTHE
SOUTHS
SPATHE
STETHO
SWATHE
SWATHS
SYNTHS
TEETHE
TENTHS
TILTHS
TOOTHY
TROTHS
TRUTHS
WIDTHS
WORTHS
WORTHY
WRATHS
WRITHE
YOUTHS

•••T•H

BLOTCH
CLUTCH
CROTCH
CRUTCH
CULTCH
DEUTCH
FLETCH
GLITCH
HOOTCH
KLATCH
KVETCH
SCOTCH
SKETCH
SKITCH
SNATCH
SNITCH
STITCH
SWATCH
SWITCH
THATCH
TWITCH
WRETCH

••••TH

AFIFTH
ALIOTH
AMONTH
ATENTH
BLEETH
BREATH
BYPATH
COMETH
COOLTH
DALETH
DEARTH
DEMOTH
DETOTH
DONATH
DOWITH
DRRUTH
DULUTH
EIGHTH
ELNATH
EMPATH
EOLITH
FOURTH
GARETH
GIVETH
GOWITH
GROWTH
HEALTH
HEARTH
INWITH
IOMOTH
JCLOTH
JOBETH
JUDITH
LENGTH
LILITH
LIVETH
MORATH
NAMATH
ORNITH
PLINTH
RULETH
SHEATH
SLEUTH
SMOOTH
SPILTH
TAKETH
WARMTH
WEALTH
WRAITH
WREATH
ZENITH
ZIZITH

TI••••

TIARAS
TIBIAE
TIBIAL
TIBIAS
TICALS
TICCED
TICINO
TICKBY
TICKED
TICKER
TICKET
TICKLE
TICKLY
TICTAC
TIDBIT
TIDIED
TIDIER
TIDIES
TIDILY
TIDING
TIDYUP
TIEBAR
TIEDIN
TIEDON
TIEDTO
TIEDUP
TIEDYE
TIEINS
TIEMPO
TIENDA
TIEOFF
TIEPIN
TIERCE
TIERED
TIEROD
TIERRA
TIESIN
TIESON
TIESTO
TIESUP
TIETAC
TIEUPS
TIFFED
TIFFIN
TIGERS
TIGGER
TIGHTS
TIGLON
TIGONS
TIGRES
TIGRIS
TIKKAS
TIKRIT
TILAKS
TILDEN
TILDES
TILERS
TILERY
TILHIM
TILING
TILLED
TILLER
TILLET
TILLEY
TILLIE
TILLIS
TILNOW
TILSIT
TILSON
TILTAT
TILTED
TILTER
TILTHS
TILTON
TILTUP
TIMBAL
TIMBER
TIMBRE
TIMELY
TIMERS
TIMING
TINCAN
TINCTS
TINCUP
TINDER
TINEAL
TINEAR
TINGED
TINGES
TINGLE
TINGLY
TINGOD
TINHAT
TINIAN
TINIER
TINILY
TINKER
TINKLE
TINKLY
TINMAN
TINMEN
TINNED
TINNER
TINORE
TINPAN
TINPOT
TINSEL
TINTED
TINTER
TIPINS
TIPJAR
TIPOFF
TIPPED
TIPPEE
TIPPER
TIPPET
TIPPLE
TIPSIN
TIPSUP
TIPTOE
TIPTOP
TIRADE
TIRANA
TIRANE
TIREOF
TIRIAC
TIRING
TISANE
TISHRI
TISKET
TISSOT
TISSUE
TITANS
TITERS
TITHED
TITHER
TITHES
TITIAN
TITLED
TITLES
TITRED
TITRES
TITTER
TITTLE
TIVOLI

T•I•••

TAICHI
TAIGAS
TAILED
TAILER
TAILOR
TAINTS
TAIPAN
TAIPEI
TAIWAN
TBILLS
TBIRDS
THICKE
THIEVE
THIGHS
THILLS
THINGS
THINGY
THINKS
THINLY
THIRDR
THIRDS
THIRST
THIRTY
THISBE
TMINUS
TOILAT
TOILED
TOILER
TOILES
TOILET
TRIADS
TRIAGE
TRIALS
TRIBAL
TRIBES
TRICEP
TRICES
TRICIA
TRICKS
TRICKY
TRICOT
TRIERS
TRIFLE
TRIGON
TRIJET
TRIKES
TRILBY
TRILLO
TRILLS
TRIMLY
TRINAL
TRINES
TRIODE
TRIPES
TRIPLE
TRIPLY
TRIPOD
TRIPON
TRIPUP
TRISHA
TRISTE
TRITER
TRITON
TRIUNE
TRIVET
TRIVIA
TRIXIE
TTILES
TUILLE
TVIDOL
TWIGGY
TWILIT
TWILLS
TWINED
TWINER
TWINES
TWINGE
TWIRLS
TWIRLY
TWIRPS
TWISTS
TWISTY
TWITCH
TWITTY

T••I••

TAHINI
TAHITI
TAKING
TALISA
TAMILS
TAMING
TAOISM
TAOIST
TAPING
TAPINS
TAPIRS
TARIFF
TARING
TAVIST
TAXIED
TAXIES
TAXING
TEDIUM
TEEING
THEIRS
THEISM
THEIST
THRICE
THRIFT
THRILL
THRIVE
TIBIAE
TIBIAL
TIBIAS
TICINO
TIDIED
TIDIER
TIDIES
TIDILY
TIDING
TIEINS
TILING
TIMING
TINIAN
TINIER
TINILY
TIPINS
TIRIAC
TIRING
TITIAN
TOBIAS
TOBIES
TOBITS
TODIES
TOEING
TOEINS
TOLIFE
TONICS
TONIER
TONING
TONITE
TOPICS
TOPING
TORIES
TORINO
TOTING
TOWING
TOXICS
TOXINS
TOYING
TRAILS
TRAINS
TRAITS
TREIZE
TROIKA
TRUING
TRUISM
TRYING
TSHIRT
TSKING
TUBING
TUBIST
TULIPS
TUNICS
TUNING
TURING
TVHITS
TVTIME
TWAINS
TYPIFY
TYPING
TYPIST

T•••I•

TABRIZ
TACTIC
TAKEIN
TAKEIT
TALKIE
TALKIN
TANNIC
TANNIN
TAPSIN
TAROIL
TARPIT
TAUPIN
TAURIC
TEARIT
TECHIE
TEENIE
TEGRIN
TEKKIE
TELLIT
TENNIS
TENPIN
TERBIC
TERRIF
TERRIS
TESSIE
TESSIO
TETRIS
THALIA
THATIS
THECIA
THECID
THEKID
THELIP
THEPIT
THESIS
THETIS
THEWIZ
THORIC
THYMIC
TIDBIT
TIEDIN
TIEPIN
TIESIN
TIFFIN
TIGRIS
TIKRIT
TILHIM
TILLIE
TILLIS
TILSIT
TIPSIN
TMESIS
TOCSIN
TOEDIN
TOESIN
TOLDIT
TOMLIN
TOMMIE
TOMMIX
TOMTIT
TONKIN
TONSIL
TOOBIG
TOOHIP
TOOKIN
TOOKIT
TOONIE
TOOTIE
TOOTIN
TOPBID
TOREIT
TOROID
TORPID
TORRID
TOSSIN
TOWNIE
TOWSIN
TRACII
TRAGIC
TRAVIS
TREDIA
TREPID
TRICIA
TRIVIA
TRIXIE
TROPIC
TSADIS
TSURIS
TUCKIN
TUGRIK
TUNEIN
TUPTIM
TURBID
TURGID
TURKIC
TURNIN
TURNIP
TURPIN
TUSHIE
TUTSIS
TUTTIS
TWILIT
TWOBIT
TWOPIN
TYPEIN

T••••I

TAHINI
TAHITI
TAICHI
TAIPEI
TATAMI
THEFBI
TISHRI
TIVOLI
TOKORI
TRACII
TSOTSI

•TI•••

ATILES
ATISES
BTILES
CTILES
DTILES
ETILES
FTILES
GTILES
HTILES
ITILES
ITIOUS
ITISSO
JTILES
KTILES
LTILES
MTILES
NTILES
OTILES
OTIOSE
OTITIC
OTITIS
PTILES
QTILES
RTILES
STICKS
STICKY
STIDES
STIERS
STIFFS
STIFLE
STIGMA
STILES
STILLE
STILLS
STILLY
STILTS
STIMPY
STINGS
STINGY
STINKO
STINKS
STINKY
STINTS
STIPES
STIRIN
STIRUP
STITCH
STIVIC
TTILES
UTICAN
VTILES
WTILES
XTILES
YTILES
ZTILES

•T•I••

ATFIVE

ATHING
ATKINS
ATNINE
ATRIAL
ATRISK
ATRIUM
ATSIGN
ATTICA
ATTICS
ATTILA
ATTIRE
ATWILL
ATWIST
ETAILS
ETHICS
ETHIOP
ETOILE
ETTING
ITGIRL
ITHINK
ITRIED
MTAIRY
STAINS
STAIRS
STEINS
STNICK
STOICS
STPIUS
STRIAE
STRICT
STRIDE
STRIFE
STRIKE
STRING
STRIPE
STRIPS
STRIPY
STRIVE
STYING

•T••I•

ATARIS
ATAVIC
ATAXIA
ATAXIC
ATOMIC
ATONIA
ATONIC
ATOXIC
ATRAIN
ATROIS
ATTAIN
ATTRIT
ATYPIC
ETALIA
ETALII
ETAOIN
ETHNIC
ETONIC
ITALIA
ITALIC
OTITIC
OTITIS
OTOMIS
OTOSIS
OTTOII
OTTOIV
STADIA
STALIN
STARIN
STASIS
STATIC
STATIN
STAYIN
STEPIN
STERIC
STEVIE
STEWIE
STIRIN
STIVIC
STOGIE
STOLID
STOPIN
STOPIT
STOTIN
STOWIT
STRAIN
STRAIT
STUDIO
STUPID
STYMIE
UTOPIA
YTTRIA
YTTRIC

•T•••I

ETALII
ITURBI
MTFUJI
OTTOII
STEFFI
STRATI

••TI••

ACTIII
ACTING
ACTION
ACTIUM
ACTIVA
ACTIVE
ALTIMA
ALTIUS
ANTICS
ANTIGO
ARTIER
ARTILY
ARTIST
ATTICA
ATTICS
ATTILA
ATTIRE
AUTISM
AUTIST
BATIKS
BATING
BETIDE
BITING
CATION
CITIED
CITIES
CITIFY
CITING
CITIUS
CUTIES
CUTINS
DATING
DATIVE
DOTIME
DOTING
DUTIES
EATING
ENTIAL
ENTICE
ENTIRE
ENTITY
ESTIME
ETTING
FATIMA
FETING
FETISH
FUTILE
GATING
HATING
HITINS
INTIME
KITING
LATIGO
LATINA
LATINI
LATINO
LATINS
LATISH
LOTION
LUTIST
MATING
MATINS
METIER
METING
MOTIFS
MOTILE
MOTION
MOTIVE
MUTING
MUTINY
MUTIUS
NATICK
NATION
NATIVE
NOTICE
NOTIFY
NOTILL
NOTIME
NOTING
NOTION
NOTIPS
OATIER
ONTIME
OOTIDS
OPTICS
OPTIMA
OPTIMO
OPTING
OPTION
OUTIES
OUTING
PATINA
PATINE
PATIOS
PETIPA
PETITE
PITIED
PITIER
PITIES
POTION
RATIFY
RATINE
RATING
RATION
RATIOS
RATITE
RETIAL
RETIED
RETIEF
RETIES
RETILE
RETILL
RETIME
RETINA
RETINS
RETINT
RETIPS
RETIRE
ROTINI
RUTILE
RUTINS
SATING
SATINS
SATINY
SATIRE
SHTICK
SITING
SITINS
TITIAN
TOTING
TVTIME
ULTIMA
ULTIMO
UNTIDY
UNTIED
UNTIER
UNTIES
UNTILT
UPTICK
UPTILT
UPTIME
VOTING
VOTIVE

••T•I•

ACTIII
ACTSIN
ALTAIC
ALTAIR
ALTOID
ALTRIA
ANTLIA
ANTRIM
ARTOIS
ASTRID
ATTAIN
ATTRIT
BATSIN
BITEIN
BUTTIN
CATFIT
CATKIN
CATLIN
CATNIP
CATRIG
CATSIT
CITRIC
CITRIN
CUTSIN
CUTSIT
DATRIL
DETAIL
DETAIN
DOTTIE
EATSIN
EATSIT
ENTAIL
ESTLIN
FATLIP
FATSIS
FITSIN
GATLIN
GETFIT
GETHIP
GETRID
GETSIN
GETSIT
GETTIN
GOTFIT
GOTHIC
GOTHIP
GOTOIT
GOTRID
HATEIT
HATPIN
HATTIE
HITSIT
HOTAIR
HOTOIL
HOTTIE
HOTTIP
IATRIC
INTOIT
INTUIT
ISTRIA
KATHIE
KATRIN
LATRIA
LATVIA
LETRIP
LETSIN
LITHIC
MATHIS
MATLIN
MATRIX
MATTIE
METRIC
MOTRIN
MYTHIC
NITRIC
NITWIT
NOTAIL
NOTFIT
NOTHIN
NUTKIN
NUTOIL
NUTRIA
OBTAIN
OPTSIN
OTTOII
OTTOIV
OUTBID
OUTDID
OUTFIT
OUTHIT
OUTLIE
OUTLIP
OUTRIB
OUTRIG
OUTSIN
OUTSIT
OUTVIE
OUTWIT
OXTAIL
PATHIC
PATOIS
PATRIA
PATRIC
PATRIE
PATTIE
PETAIN
PETPIG
PETRIE
PETSIT
PETTIS
PETTIT
PITKIN
POTLID
POTPIE
POTSIE
POTVIN
PUTRID
PUTSIN
PUTTIN
RATLIN
RETAIL
RETAIN
RETRIM
RETTIG
RUTHIE
SETSIN
SITSIN
SITTIN
TETRIS
TUTSIS
TUTTIS
UNTRIG
UPTOIT
VITRIC
VOTEIN
WETTIG
WITHIN
WITHIT
WITTIG
YETTIE
YTTRIA
YTTRIC

••T••I

ACTIII
BYTAXI
DITALI
HATARI
ISTHMI
JETSKI
KATMAI
LATERI
LATINI
LITCHI
MATSUI
OCTOPI
OCTROI
OTTOII
PATAKI
PETERI
POTOSI
QATARI
ROTINI
SATORI
TATAMI
WATUSI

•••TI•

ABATIS
ACETIC
AMATIS
AMITIE
AORTIC
ARCTIC
AUNTIE
AUSTIN
BALTIC
BASTIA
BEATIT
BERTIE
BESTIR
BIOTIC
BIOTIN
BOOTIE
BOOTIT
BOWTIE
BUSTIN
BUTTIN
CARTIN
CELTIC
CERTIF
COATIS
COOTIE
COPTIC
CRETIN
CRITIC
CUETIP
CULTIC
CURTIN
CURTIS
CURTIZ
CUSTIS
CYSTIC
DELTIC
DENTIN
DHOTIS
DISTIL
DOTTIE
DRATIT
DUSTIN
EDITIO
ELYTIS
EMETIC
EROTIC
EUSTIS
EXOTIC
FISTIC
FLITIN
FLUTIE
FOETID
FOOTIT
FORTIS
GERTIE
GESTIC
GETTIN
GOATIT
GRATIA
GRATIN
GRATIS
HATTIE
HECTIC
HESTIA
HOGTIE
HOOTIE
HOTTIE
HOTTIP
IFITIS
IGETIT
IGOTIT
INATIE
INITIO
INSTIL
INSTIR
IRITIC
IRITIS
JOLTIN
JUSTIN
KEPTIN
KILTIE
LACTIC
LEFTIN
LEFTIT
LENTIL
LOSTIT
MALTIN
MANTIC
MANTIS
MARTIN
MASTIC
MATTIE
MENTIS
MILTIE
MUFTIS
MULTIS
MYSTIC
NESTIN
NOETIC
OTITIC
OTITIS
PANTIE
PARTII
PARTIV
PASTIS
PASTIT
PATTIE
PECTIN
PEPTIC
PETTIS
PETTIT
PHOTIC
PIETIN
PISTIL
POETIC
PORTIA
POSTIE
POSTIT
PUTTIN
QRATIO
QUITIT
REDTIE
RESTIR
RETTIG
ROOTIE
ROOTIN
RUSTIC
SALTII
SCOTIA
SENTIN
SEPTIC
SHUTIN
SITTIN
SOFTIE
SOITIS
SORTIE
STATIC
STATIN
STOTIN
TACTIC
THATIS
THETIS
TOMTIT
TOOTIE
TOOTIN
TUPTIM
TUTTIS
UPSTIR
VICTIM
WANTIN
WENTIN
WESTIE
WESTIN
WETTIG
WHATIF
WITTIG
YETTIE
ZAFTIG

•••T•I

CENTAI
CENTRI
DANTEI
DMITRI
DUETTI
FRITZI
FRUTTI
GLUTEI
GRITTI
MAITAI
MAOTAI
PARTII
SALTII
TSOTSI

••••TI

AGOUTI
AMANTI
AVANTI
CUBITI
DORATI
DUETTI
FRUCTI
FRUTTI
GELATI
GRITTI
IDENTI
ISANTI
KRISTI
LIGETI
MALOTI
PERITI
QUINTI
RIGATI
RUBATI
SENITI
SHORTI
SOLATI
STRATI
TAHITI
VASHTI
VENUTI
WAPITI

TJ••••

TJMAXX

T•J•••

TEJANA
TEJANO

T••J••

TIPJAR
TOPJOB
TRAJAN
TRIJET
TROJAN

T••••J

THEHAJ

•TJ•••

STJOAN
STJOHN
STJUDE

•T•J••

STOJKO

•T••J•

MTFUJI
MTVVJS

••TJ••

MATJES
OUTJET
OUTJUT

••T••J

INTERJ
SGTMAJ

••••TJ

AGENTJ

T•K•••

TAKEIN
TAKEIT
TAKEON
TAKERS
TAKETH
TAKETO
TAKEUP
TAKING
TEKKIE
TEKWAR
TIKKAS
TIKRIT
TOKAYS
TOKENS
TOKLAS
TOKORI
TSKING
TSKTSK

T••K••

TABKEY
TACKED
TACKER
TACKLE
TACKON
TACKUP
TALKAT
TALKED
TALKER
TALKIE
TALKIN
TALKOF
TALKON
TALKTO
TALKUP
TANKAS
TANKED
TANKER
TANKUP
TASKED
TASKET
TEDKEY
TEKKIE
TERKEL
THEKID
TICKBY
TICKED
TICKER
TICKET
TICKLE
TICKLY
TIKKAS
TINKER
TINKLE
TINKLY
TISKET
TONKAS
TONKIN
TOOKIN
TOOKIT
TOOKON
TOOKTO
TOOKUP
TRIKES
TUCKED
TUCKER
TUCKIN
TURKEY
TURKIC
TUSKED
TUSKER

T•••K•

TANAKA
THANKS
THICKE
THINKS
THUNKS
TILAKS
TOPEKA
TRACKS
TRICKS
TRICKY
TROIKA
TRUCKS
TRUNKS
TWEAKS
TWEAKY

T••••K

TANOAK
TARLEK
THWACK
TREBEK
TSKTSK
TUGRIK

•TK•••

ATKINS
FTKNOX

•T•K••

STAKED
STAKES
STOKED
STOKER
STOKES
STUKAS

•T••K•

STACKS
STALKS
STALKY
STEAKS
STICKS
STICKY
STINKO
STINKS
STINKY
STLUKE
STOCKS
STOCKY
STOJKO
STORKS
STRIKE
STROKE

•T•••K

ATDUSK
ATRISK
ATTACK
ATWORK
ITHINK
ITZHAK
MTCOOK
STMARK
STNICK
STREAK
STRUCK
STRUNK

••TK••

ALTKEY
BUTKUS
CATKIN
HOTKEY
KITKAT
LATKES
NUTKIN
PITKIN

••T•K•

AZTEKS
BATIKS
BETAKE
INTAKE
JETSKI
KOTTKE
PATAKI
RETAKE
ROTHKO
UPTAKE

••T••K

AMTRAK
ATTACK
BETOOK
BYTALK
LITVAK
NATICK
OUTASK
RETACK
RETOOK
SHTICK
UNTACK
UNTUCK
UPTALK
UPTICK

•••TK•

KOTTKE
MOLTKE
NOOTKA

•••T•K

BARTOK
BRATSK
FELTOK
ISNTOK
SAITEK
TSKTSK
VOSTOK

••••TK

AGENTK

T•L•••

TALCED
TALCUM
TALENT
TALERS
TALESE
TALISA
TALKAT
TALKED
TALKER
TALKIE
TALKIN
TALKOF
TALKON
TALKTO
TALKUP
TALLER
TALLOW
TALMUD
TALONS
TALTOS
TELCOS
TELLER
TELLIT
TELLME
TELLOF
TELLON
TELNET
TILAKS
TILDEN
TILDES
TILERS
TILERY
TILHIM
TILING
TILLED
TILLER
TILLET
TILLEY
TILLIE
TILLIS
TILNOW
TILSIT
TILSON
TILTAT
TILTED
TILTER
TILTHS
TILTON
TILTUP
TOLARS
TOLAST
TOLDIT
TOLDOF
TOLDON
TOLDYA
TOLEDO
TOLIFE
TOLLED
TOLLER
TOLTEC
TULANE
TULARE
TULIPS
TULLES
TULSAN
TVLAND
TYLERS

T••L••

TABLAS
TABLED
TABLES
TABLET
TAILED
TAILER
TAILOR
TALLER
TALLOW
TARLEK
TATLER
TAXLAW
TAYLOR
TBILLS
TCELLS
TEFLON
TELLER
TELLIT
TELLME
TELLOF
TELLON
TENLBS
TENLEY
TESLAS
TETLEY
THALER
THALES
THALIA
THELAW
THELIP
THELMA
THELOT
THILLS
THOLES
TIGLON
TILLED
TILLER
TILLET
TILLEY
TILLIE
TILLIS
TITLED
TITLES
TOILAT
TOILED
TOILER
TOILES
TOILET
TOKLAS
TOLLED
TOLLER
TOMLIN
TOOLED
TOOLER
TOOLOW
TOOLUP
TOULON
TRALAS
TRALEE
TRILBY
TRILLO
TRILLS
TROLLS
TRYLON
TTILES
TUILLE
TULLES
TWELVE
TWILIT
TWILLS

T•••L•

TABULA
TACKLE
TAMALE
TAMELY
TAMILS
TANGLE
TANGLY
TARTLY
TATTLE
TAUTLY
TAVELS
TAXOLS
TBILLS
TCELLS
TEMPLE
THATLL
THEFLY
THEYLL
THILLS

THINLY
THRALL
THRILL
THUSLY
TICALS
TICKLE
TICKLY
TIDILY
TIMELY
TINGLE
TINGLY
TINILY
TINKLE
TINKLY
TIPPLE
TITTLE
TIVOLI
TODDLE
TOGGLE
TOODLE
TOOTLE
TOPPLE
TOTALS
TOUSLE
TOWELS
TRAILS
TRAWLS
TREBLE
TREBLY
TRIALS
TRIFLE
TRILLO
TRILLS
TRIMLY
TRIPLE
TRIPLY
TROLLS
TUBULE
TUILLE
TUMBLE
TUMULT
TUPELO
TURTLE
TUSSLE
TUVALU
TWILLS
TWIRLS
TWIRLY
TWOPLY
TYBALT

T••••L

TACTEL
TAROIL
TARSAL
TASSEL
TEASEL
TERCEL
TERKEL
TETZEL
THATLL
THENFL
THENHL
THEYLL
THRALL
THRILL
TIBIAL
TIMBAL
TINEAL
TINSEL
TOHEEL
TONSIL
TRAVEL
TRIBAL
TRINAL
TROWEL
TUBFUL
TUNNEL
TUSSAL
TVIDOL
TYDBOL

•TL•••

ATLAST
ITLLDO
STLUKE

•T•L••

ATALOW
ATILES
ATOLLS
ATPLAY
ATTLEE
BTILES
CTILES
DTILES
ETALIA
ETALII
ETILES
FTILES
GTILES
HTILES
ITALIA
ITALIC
ITILES
ITLLDO
JTILES
KTILES
LTILES
MTILES
NTILES
OTELLO
OTILES
PTILES
QTILES
RTILES
STALAG
STALED
STALER
STALES
STALIN
STALKS
STALKY
STALLS
STELAR
STELAS
STELES
STELLA
STELMO
STILES
STILLE
STILLS
STILLY
STILTS
STOLAE
STOLAF
STOLAS
STOLEN
STOLES
STOLID
STOLLE
STOLON
STOLTZ
STYLED
STYLER
STYLES
STYLET
STYLUS
TTILES
VTILES
WTILES
XTILES
YTILES
ZTILES

•T••L•

ATOLLS
ATTILA
ATWILL
ATYALE
ETAILS
ETHYLS
ETOILE
ITSELF
LTSULU
NTUPLE
OTELLO
OTOOLE
STABLE
STABLY
STALLS
STAPLE
STEALS
STEELE
STEELS
STEELY
STELLA
STIFLE
STILLE
STILLS
STILLY
STMALO
STOLLE
STOOLS
STOOLY
STROLL
STUDLY

•T•••L

ATHEEL
ATONAL
ATRIAL
ATWILL
ETYMOL
ITGIRL
STEROL
STPAUL
STROLL

••TL••

ANTLER
ANTLIA
ASTLEY
ATTLEE
BATLEY
BUTLER
CATLIN
COTLER
CUTLER
CUTLET
ESTLIN
FATLIP
GATLIN
ISTLES
JETLAG
MATLIN
MOTLEY
NUTLET
OSTLER
OUTLAW
OUTLAY
OUTLED
OUTLET
OUTLIE
OUTLIP
POTLID
RATLIN
TATLER
TETLEY
TITLED
TITLES

••T•L•

ARTELS
ARTILY
ASTALL
ATTILA
BATTLE
BETELS
BOTELS
BOTFLY
BOTTLE
BYTALK
CATALO
CATTLE
CUTELY
DITALI
DOTELL
DOTTLE
EXTOLL
EXTOLS
FATALE
FETTLE
FUTILE
GETOLD
GOTOLD
HOTELS
IMTOLD
KETTLE
LATELY
LETFLY
LITTLE
METALS
METTLE
MOTELS
MOTILE
MOTTLE
MUTELY
NATALE
NETTLE
NETTLY
NOTALL
NOTILL
NOTOLL
OUTFLY
PETALE
PETALS
PETULA
RATELS
RATTLE
RATTLY
RETELL
RETILE
RETILL
RETOLD
RUTILE
SETTLE
TATTLE
TITTLE
TOTALS
UNTILT
UNTOLD
UPTALK
UPTILT
VITALE
VITALS
VITTLE
WATTLE
WETFLY

••T••L

ACTUAL
ANTRAL
ARTFUL
ASTALL
ASTEAL
ASTRAL
BETHEL
DATRIL
DETAIL
DOTELL
ENTAIL
ENTIAL
EXTOLL
FITFUL
HATFUL
HOTOIL
LETHAL
MATTEL
METHYL
MITRAL
MUTUAL
MUTUEL
NETFUL
NOTAIL
NOTALL
NOTILL
NOTOLL
NUTOIL
OSTEAL
OXTAIL
PATROL
PETREL
PETROL
POTFUL
RETAIL
RETELL
RETIAL
RETILL
RETOOL
RETRAL
RITUAL
SHTETL
TETZEL
VATFUL
WITHAL

•••TL•

BARTLE
BATTLE
BEATLE
BEETLE
BOTTLE
BUSTLE
CANTLE
CASTLE
CATTLE
COSTLY
CURTLY
DAFTLY
DARTLE
DEFTLY
DOTTLE
EASTLA
FETTLE
FLATLY
FOOTLE
GENTLE
GENTLY
HOSTLY
HURTLE
HUSTLE
JOSTLE
JUSTLY
KETTLE
LASTLY
LITTLE
MANTLE
MEETLY
METTLE
MOSTLY
MOTTLE
MYRTLE
NEATLY
NESTLE
NETTLE
NETTLY
PARTLY
PERTLY
PESTLE
PORTLY
RAPTLY
RATTLE
RATTLY
ROOTLE
RUSTLE
SETTLE
SOFTLY
SUBTLE
SUBTLY
TARTLY
TATTLE
TAUTLY
THATLL
TITTLE
TOOTLE
TURTLE
VASTLY
VITTLE
WATTLE
WHATLL
YERTLE

•••T•L

ACETAL
ACETYL
AMATOL
AMSTEL
AORTAL
BARTEL
BOATEL
BRUTAL
CANTAL
CARTEL
CASTEL
CENTAL
COSTAL
DACTYL
DENTAL
DHOTEL
DISTAL
DISTIL
DUCTAL
FESTAL
FONTAL
GRETEL
HIATAL
HOSTEL
HYETAL
INSTAL
INSTIL
KEITEL
LENTIL
LINTEL
MANTEL
MARTEL
MATTEL
MENTAL
MONTEL
MORTAL
MOSTEL
NEXTEL
PASTEL
PENTEL
PISTIL
PISTOL
PORTAL
POSTAL
RENTAL
RICTAL
SEPTAL
SKYTEL
TACTEL
THATLL
VESTAL
WHATLL

••••TL

SHTETL

TM••••

TMESES
TMESIS
TMINUS

T•M•••

TAMALE
TAMARA
TAMAYO
TAMBOR
TAMELY
TAMERS
TAMEST
TAMILS
TAMING
TAMMUZ
TAMPED
TAMPER
TAMTAM
TEMPED
TEMPEH
TEMPER
TEMPLE
TEMPOS
TEMPTS
TEMPUS
TIMBAL
TIMBER
TIMBRE
TIMELY
TIMERS
TIMING
TJMAXX
TOMATO
TOMBES
TOMBOY
TOMCAT
TOMLIN
TOMMIE
TOMMIX
TOMTIT
TOMTOM
TUMBLE
TUMEFY
TUMULT

T••M••

TALMUD
TAMMUZ
TARMAC
TASMAN
TAXMAN
TAXMEN
TEAMED
TEAMUP
TEEMED
TERMED
TERMES
TEXMEX
THAMES
THEMAN
THEMED
THEMES
THEMET
THEMOB
THEMRS
THOMAS
THUMBS
THUMPS
THYMES
THYMIC
THYMUS
TIEMPO
TINMAN
TINMEN
TOAMAN
TODMAN
TOMMIE
TOMMIX
TOOMEY
TOPMAN
TOPMEN
TRAMPS
TRAMPY
TREMOR
TRIMLY
TROMPE
TROMPS
TRUMAN
TRUMBO
TRUMPS
TUBMAN
TWOMAN
TWYMAN

T•••M•

TACOMA
TATAMI
TELLME
THELMA
THERMO
THERMS
THRUMS
TOCOME
TONEME
TOTEMS
TOYAMA
TRAUMA
TVGAME
TVTIME

T••••M

TALCUM
TAMTAM
TANDEM
TAOISM
TAOSNM
TEDEUM
TEDIUM
THEISM
THERAM
TILHIM
TOMTOM
TOTERM
TRUISM
TUPTIM
TVROOM

•TM•••

ATMANS
ATMFEE
ATMOST
STMALO
STMARK
STMARY
UTMOST

•T•M••

ATAMAN
ATEMPO
ATOMIC
ETYMOL
ETYMON
ITEMED
OTHMAR
OTOMIS
STAMEN
STAMOS
STAMPS
STEMMY
STIMPY
STOMAS
STOMPS
STUMPS
STUMPY
STYMIE

•T••M•

ATEAMS
ATHOME
BTEAMS
STEAMS
STEAMY
STELMO
STEMMY
STIGMA
STORMS
STORMY
STRUMS

•T•••M

ATRIUM
STREAM

••TM••

ALTMAN
BATMAN
BATMEN
BITMAP
CATMAN
CATMEN
DETMER
FATMAN
GETMAD
GOTMAD
GUTMAN
HITMAN
HITMEN
KATMAI
LITMUS
MATMAN
MATMEN
NETMAN
NETMEN
NUTMEG
OUTMAN
PATMOS
PITMAN
PITMEN
SGTMAJ
WETMOP

••T•M•

ALTIMA
ASTHMA
AUTUMN
DOTIME
ECTOMY
ENTOMB
ENTOMO
ESTIME
FATIMA
GOTAMA
INTIME
ISTHMI
NOTIME
ONTIME
OPTIMA
OPTIMO
RETAME
RETIME
TATAMI
TOTEMS
TVTIME
ULTIMA
ULTIMO
UNTAME
UPTIME

••T••M

ACTIUM
ANTHEM
ANTRIM
ANTRUM
ARTGUM
AUTISM
BATYAM
BOTTOM
CATDOM
DOTCOM
ESTEEM
FATHOM
GOTEAM
GOTHAM
JETSAM
OUTSUM
PUTNAM
RETRIM
SATCOM
SITCOM
TOTERM
ZITCOM

•••TM•

ISITME
JUSTME

•••T•M

ADYTUM
AUNTEM
BANTAM
BOTTOM
CENTUM
CUSTOM
DESTEM
DIATOM
DICTUM
FACTUM
POSTUM
PROTEM
RHYTHM
SEPTUM
SYSTEM
TAMTAM
TOMTOM
TUPTIM
VICTIM

TN••••

TNOTES

T•N•••

TANAKA
TANANA
TANDEM
TANGED
TANGLE
TANGLY
TANGOS
TANGUY
TANKAS
TANKED
TANKER
TANKUP
TANNED
TANNER
TANNIC
TANNIN
TANOAK
TANTES
TANTRA
TENACE
TENANT
TENDAY
TENDED
TENDER
TENDON
TENDTO
TENEEE
TENETS
TENHUT
TENLBS
TENLEY
TENNER
TENNIS
TENONE
TENONS
TENORS
TENPIN
TENSED
TENSER
TENSES
TENSOR
TENTED
TENTER
TENTHS
TENTON
TENTWO
TENURE
TENUTA
TENUTO
TINCAN
TINCTS
TINCUP
TINDER
TINEAL
TINEAR
TINGED
TINGES
TINGLE
TINGLY
TINGOD
TINHAT
TINIAN
TINIER
TINILY
TINKER
TINKLE
TINKLY
TINMAN
TINMEN
TINNED
TINNER
TINORE
TINPAN
TINPOT
TINSEL
TINTED
TINTER
TONDOS
TONEME
TONERS
TONEUP
TONGAN
TONGED
TONGUE
TONICS
TONIER
TONING
TONITE
TONKAS
TONKIN
TONNES
TONSIL
TONSOF
TUNDRA
TUNEIN
TUNERS
TUNETO
TUNEUP
TUNICS
TUNING
TUNNEL
TUNNEY

T••N••

TAHNEE
TAINTS
TANNED
TANNER
TANNIC
TANNIN
TAUNTS
TBONDS
TBONES
TEENER
TEENIE
TEENSY
TELNET
TENNER
TENNIS
TERNES
THANES
THANKS
THENBA
THENCE
THENET
THENFL
THENHL
THENRA
THINGS
THINGY
THINKS
THINLY
THONGS
THUNKS
TIENDA
TILNOW
TINNED
TINNER
TMINUS
TONNES
TOONIE
TORNUP
TOWNER
TOWNIE
TRANCE
TRANES
TRANNY
TRENCH
TRENDS
TRENDY
TRENTA
TRENTE
TRENTO
TRINAL
TRINES
TRUNKS
TUNNEL
TUNNEY
TURNED
TURNER
TURNIN
TURNIP
TURNON
TURNTO
TURNUP
TWANGS
TWANGY
TWENTY
TWINED
TWINER
TWINES
TWINGE

T•••N•

TAGEND
TAHINI
TAKING
TALENT
TALONS
TAMING
TANANA
TAOSNM
TAPING
TAPINS
TARING
TAUONS
TAXING
TBOONE
TECHNO
TEEING
TEJANA
TEJANO
TENANT
TENONE
TENONS
TETONS
TEXANS
THEEND
THEONE
THORNS
THORNY
THRONE
THRONG
TICINO
TIDING
TIEINS
TIGONS
TILING
TIMING
TIPINS
TIRANA
TIRANE
TIRING
TISANE
TITANS
TOEING
TOEINS
TOKENS
TONING
TOPING
TORENT
TORINO
TOTING
TOWING
TOXINS
TOYING
TOYONS
TRAINS
TRANNY
TRIUNE
TROYNY
TRUANT
TRUING
TRYING
TRYONE
TSKING
TUBING
TUCANA
TULANE
TUNING
TURING
TVLAND
TWAINS
TWEENS
TWEENY
TYPING
TYRANT
TYRONE
TYSONS

T••••N

TACKON
TAGSON
TAIPAN
TAIWAN
TAKEIN
TAKEON
TALKIN
TALKON
TANNIN
TAPEON
TAPPAN
TAPSIN
TAPSON
TARPON
TARTAN
TARZAN
TASMAN

TAUPIN
TAUTEN
TAVERN
TAXMAN
TAXMEN
TEAURN
TEFLON
TEGRIN
TEHRAN
TELLON
TENDON
TENPIN
TENTON
TERRAN
TEUTON
THEBAN
THECAN
THEFAN
THEMAN
THERON
THESON
THESUN
THORON
THROWN
TIEDIN
TIEDON
TIEPIN
TIESIN
TIESON
TIFFIN
TIGLON
TILDEN
TILSON
TILTON
TINCAN
TINIAN
TINMAN
TINMEN
TINPAN
TIPSIN
TITIAN
TOAMAN
TOBURN
TOCSIN
TODMAN
TOEDIN
TOESIN
TOLDON
TOMLIN
TONGAN
TONKIN
TOOKIN
TOOKON
TOOTIN
TOPGUN
TOPMAN
TOPMEN
TOPTEN
TOSSIN
TOUCAN
TOULON
TOWSIN
TOYGUN
TRAJAN
TRAVEN
TREPAN
TRIGON
TRIPON
TRITON
TRODON
TROJAN
TRUMAN
TRYLON
TUBMAN
TUCKIN
TUCSON
TUGSON
TULSAN
TUNEIN
TURBAN
TUREEN
TURHAN
TURNIN
TURNON
TURPIN
TUSCAN
TWOMAN
TWOPIN
TWYMAN
TYCOON
TYPEIN

•TN•••

ATNINE
ATNOON
STNICK

•T•N••

ATENTH
ATONAL
ATONCE
ATONED
ATONER
ATONES
ATONIA
ATONIC
ATONOF
ETHNIC
ETHNOS
ETONIC
FTKNOX
ITSNOT
STANCE
STANCH
STANDS
STANZA
STENCH
STENOG
STENOS
STENTS
STINGS
STINGY
STINKO
STINKS
STINKY
STINTS
STONED
STONER
STONES
STONEY
STUNTS
STUNTY

•T••N•

ATHAND
ATHENA
ATHENE
ATHENS
ATHING
ATKINS
ATMANS
ATNINE
ATTEND
ATTUNE
ETERNE
ETHANE
ETHENE
ETTING
ITHINK
MTETNA
OTTONE
STAINS
STEINS
STERNA
STERNE
STERNO
STERNS
STRAND
STRING
STRONG
STRUNG
STRUNK
STYING
UTAHNS
UTHANT
UTURNS

•T•••N

ATAMAN
ATDAWN
ATNOON
ATRAIN
ATSIGN
ATTAIN
CTSCAN
ETAOIN
ETYMON
ITSFUN
STALIN
STAMEN
STARIN
STATEN
STATIN
STAYIN
STAYON
STEFAN
STEPIN
STEPON
STEVEN
STIRIN
STJOAN
STJOHN
STOLEN
STOLON
STOPIN
STOTIN
STRAIN
STREWN
STYRON
UTAHAN
UTICAN

••TN••

ACTNOW
BITNET
CATNAP
CATNIP
JITNEY
LOTNOS
NOTNEW
NOTNOW
PETNAP
PITNEY
PUTNAM
PUTNEY
RATNER
WATNEY
WETNAP

••T•N•

ACTING
ACTONE
ANTONE
ANTONY
ASTANA
ATTEND
ATTUNE
BATING
BATONS
BETONY
BITING
BOTANY
BUTANE
BUTENE
BYTENS
CATANO
CATENA
CETANE
CITING
COTANS
CUTINS
DATING
DETENT
DETUNE
DOTING
EATING
ETTING
EXTANT
EXTEND
EXTENT
FATONE
FETING
FUTONS
FUTUNA
GATING
GETANA
GETANF
GITANO
GOTANA
GOTANF
HATING
HITINS
HITONE
HOTONE
HUTONE
INTEND
INTENS
INTENT
INTONE
INTUNE
KETONE
KITING
LATENE
LATENS
LATENT
LATINA
LATINI
LATINO
LATINS
LITANY
MATING
MATINS
METING
MUTANT
MUTING
MUTINY
MUTONS
NATANT
NOTANY
NOTING
NOTONE
OBTUND
OCTANE
OCTANS
OCTANT
OPTING
OSTEND
OTTONE
OUTING
PATENS
PATENT
PATINA
PATINE
PITONS
POTENT
PUTONS
RATINE
RATING
RETANS
RETINA
RETINS
RETINT
RETONE
RETUNE
ROTINI
ROTUND
RUTINS
SATING
SATINS
SATINY
SITING
SITINS
TETONS
TITANS
TOTING
UNTUNE
VOTENO
VOTING
WETONE
YUTANG

••T••N

ACTION
ACTSIN
ACTSON
ALTMAN
ANTAWN
ANTRON
ASTERN
ATTAIN
AUTUMN
BATAAN
BATMAN
BATMEN
BATSIN
BATSON
BATTEN
BETSON
BITEIN
BITEON
BITTEN
BUTTIN
BUTTON
BYTHEN
CATION
CATKIN
CATLIN
CATMAN
CATMEN
CATTON
CITRIN
CITRON
COTTEN
COTTON
CUTSIN
DATHAN
DATSUN
DETAIN
DOTEON
DOTHAN
DUTTON
EATSIN
ESTLIN
EXTERN
FATMAN
FATTEN
FITSIN
FITSON
GATLIN
GETSIN
GETSON
GETTIN
GOTTEN
GUTMAN
GUTZON
HATPIN
HITMAN
HITMEN
HITSON
HUTTON
IFTHEN
INTERN
INTOWN
INTURN
JETFAN
JETGUN
JETSON
KATRIN
KATZEN
KITAEN
KITTEN
LATEEN
LATEON
LATHEN
LETSIN
LETSON
LOTION
LYTTON
MATLIN
MATMAN
MATMEN
MATRON
MATSON
METFAN
MITTEN
MOTION
MOTOWN
MOTRIN
MUTTON
MYTURN
NATHAN
NATION
NATRON
NETMAN
NETMEN
NETTON
NOTHIN
NOTION
NUTKIN
OBTAIN
OPTION
OPTSIN
ORTHEN
OUTBAN
OUTGUN
OUTMAN
OUTRAN
OUTRUN
OUTSIN
PATHAN
PATRON
PATTEN
PATTON
PETAIN
PITKIN
PITMAN
PITMEN
POTEEN
POTION
POTVIN
PUTSIN
PUTSON
PUTTIN
PYTHON
RATION
RATLIN
RATSON
RATTAN
RETAIN
RETORN
RETTON
RETURN
ROTTEN
RUTTAN
SATEEN
SATURN
SETSIN
SETSON
SITSIN
SITSON
SITTIN
SOTHEN
SUTTON
TITIAN
UNTORN
UPTORN
UPTOWN
UPTURN
VOTEIN
VOTEON
WATSON
WITHIN
YATSEN

•••TN•

ACCTNO
GRETNA
MTETNA
MUSTNT

•••T•N

ABUTON
AGETEN
ALSTON
AMYTAN
ARCTAN
ASHTON
AUSTEN
AUSTIN
AYRTON
BARTON
BATTEN
BEATEN
BEATON
BELTON
BENTON
BHUTAN
BIGTEN
BIOTIN
BITTEN
BLYTON
BOLTON
BONTON
BOSTON
BOUTON
BRETON
BRITON
BUNTON
BURTON
BUSTIN
BUTTIN
BUTTON
CAFTAN
CANTON
CARTIN
CARTON
CASTON
CATTON
CHITON
COLTON
COTTEN
COTTON
CRETAN
CRETIN
CROTON
CURTIN
DALTON
DANTON
DAYTON
DENTIN
DENTON
DOLTON
DUSTIN
DUTTON
EASTON
ELKTON
ELSTON
FANTAN
FASTEN
FATTEN
FLITIN
FULTON
GALTON
GASTON
GETTIN
GLUTEN
GOTTEN
GRATIN
GROTON
HASTEN
HEATON
HESTON
HILTON
HINTON
HORTON
HUSTON
HUTTON
JOLTIN
JUSTIN
KEATON
KELTON
KENTON
KEPTIN
KEPTON
KITTEN
LAWTON
LEFTIN
LEFTON
LENTEN
LEPTON
LINTON
LIPTON
LISTEN
LISTON
LOFTON
LUPTON
LYTTON
MALTIN
MARTEN
MARTIN
MELTON
MERTON
MILTON
MITTEN
MOLTEN
MORTEN
MORTON
MUTTON
NEATEN
NESTIN
NETTON
NEWTON
NONTAN
NORTON
ONETEN
ONETON
PACTEN
PARTON
PATTEN
PATTON
PAXTON
PAYTON
PECTIN
PEYTON
PHOTON
PIETIN
PISTON
PLATEN
PLUTON
POSTON
PROTON
PUTTIN
RATTAN
REDTEN
RENTON
RESTON
RETTON
ROOTIN
ROSTEN
ROTTEN
RUTTAN
SALTEN
SALTON
SARTON
SEATON
SELTEN
SENTIN
SENTON
SEXTON
SHUTIN
SITTIN
SIXTEN
SOFTEN
SOFTON
SPITON
SPOTON
STATEN
STATIN
STOTIN
SULTAN
SUNTAN
SUTTON
TARTAN
TAUTEN
TENTON
TEUTON
TILTON
TOOTIN
TOPTEN
TRITON
VINTON
WAITON
WALTON
WANTIN
WANTON
WENTIN
WENTON
WESTIN
WESTON
WHITEN
WILTON
WONTON
WYNTON
WYSTAN
ZOLTAN

TO••••

TOAMAN
TOASTS
TOASTY
TOATEE
TOBAGO
TOBIAS
TOBIES
TOBITS
TOBOOT
TOBURN
TOCOME
TOCSIN
TODATE
TODAYS
TODDAO
TODDLE
TODIES
TODMAN
TOECAP
TOEDIN
TOEING
TOEINS
TOESIN
TOETAP
TOFFEE
TOGAED
TOGGED
TOGGLE
TOGOUT
TOGSUP
TOGUES
TOHEEL
TOILAT
TOILED
TOILER
TOILES
TOILET
TOKAYS
TOKENS
TOKLAS
TOKORI
TOLARS
TOLAST
TOLDIT
TOLDOF
TOLDON
TOLDYA
TOLEDO
TOLIFE
TOLLED
TOLLER
TOLTEC
TOMATO
TOMBES
TOMBOY
TOMCAT
TOMLIN
TOMMIE
TOMMIX
TOMTIT
TOMTOM
TONDOS
TONEME
TONERS
TONEUP
TONGAN
TONGED
TONGUE
TONICS
TONIER
TONING
TONITE
TONKAS
TONKIN
TONNES
TONSIL
TONSOF
TOOBAD
TOOBIG
TOODLE
TOOFAR
TOOHIP
TOOHOT
TOOKIN
TOOKIT
TOOKON
TOOKTO
TOOKUP
TOOLED
TOOLER
TOOLOW
TOOLUP
TOOMEY
TOONIE
TOOTAT
TOOTED
TOOTER
TOOTHY
TOOTIE
TOOTIN
TOOTLE
TOOTOO
TOOTSY
TOPBID
TOPCAT
TOPDOG
TOPEES
TOPEKA
TOPERS
TOPGUN
TOPHAT
TOPICS
TOPING
TOPJOB
TOPMAN
TOPMEN
TOPOFF
TOPOUT
TOPPED
TOPPER
TOPPLE
TOPROW
TOPSUP
TOPTEN
TOQUES
TORAHS
TORBAY
TORCHY
TOREAT
TOREIT
TORENT
TORERO
TOREUP
TORIES
TORINO
TORNUP
TOROID
TORPID
TORPOR
TORQUE
TORRES
TORREY
TORRID
TORSOS
TORTAS
TORTES
TOSSED
TOSSER
TOSSES
TOSSIN
TOSSUP
TOTALS
TOTEMS
TOTERM
TOTERS
TOTEUP
TOTING
TOTSUP
TOTTED
TOTTER
TOUCAN
TOUCHE
TOUCHY
TOUGHS
TOUGHY
TOULON
TOUPEE
TOURED
TOURER
TOUSLE
TOUTED
TOUTER
TOWAGE
TOWARD
TOWBAR
TOWCAR
TOWELS
TOWERS
TOWERY
TOWHEE
TOWING
TOWNER
TOWNIE
TOWSIN
TOXICS
TOXINS
TOYAMA
TOYCAR
TOYDOG
TOYERS
TOYGUN
TOYHAT
TOYING
TOYONS
TOYOTA
TOYTOP

T•O•••

TAOISM
TAOIST
TAOSNM
TBONDS
TBONES
TBOONE
THOLES
THOMAS
THONGS
THORAX
THORIC
THORNS
THORNY
THORON
THORPE
THOUGH
TNOTES
TOOBAD
TOOBIG
TOODLE
TOOFAR
TOOHIP
TOOHOT
TOOKIN
TOOKIT
TOOKON
TOOKTO
TOOKUP
TOOLED
TOOLER
TOOLOW
TOOLUP
TOOMEY
TOONIE
TOOTAT
TOOTED
TOOTER
TOOTHY
TOOTIE
TOOTIN
TOOTLE
TOOTOO
TOOTSY
TROCHE
TRODON
TROGGS
TROIKA
TROJAN
TROLLS
TROMPE
TROMPS
TROOPS
TROPES
TROPEZ
TROPHY
TROPIC
TROPPO
TROTHS
TROTUP
TROUGH
TROUPE
TROUTS
TROVES
TROWED
TROWEL
TROYER
TROYNY
TSOTSI
TWOACT
TWOBIT
TWOCAR
TWODAY
TWOEEE
TWOFER
TWOMAN
TWOPIN
TWOPLY
TWOWAY

T••O••

TABOOS
TABORS
TACOMA
TAGORE
TAGOUT
TAHOES
TALONS
TANOAK
TAPOFF
TAPOUT
TAROIL
TAROTS
TAUONS
TAXOLS
TBOONE
TEEOFF
TENONE
TENONS
TENORS
TETONS
THEONE
THEORY
THROAT
THROBS
THROES
THRONE
THRONG
THROVE
THROWN
THROWS
TIEOFF
TIGONS
TINORE
TIPOFF
TIVOLI
TOBOOT
TOCOME
TOGOUT
TOKORI
TOPOFF
TOPOUT
TOROID
TOYONS
TOYOTA
TRIODE
TROOPS
TRYONE
TRYOUT
TSTOPS
TUDORS
TUTORS
TVROOM
TYCOBB
TYCOON
TYRONE
TYSONS

T•••O•

TABOOS
TACKON
TAGSON
TAILOR
TAKEON
TALKOF
TALKON

TALLOW
TALTOS
TAMBOR
TANGOS
TAPEON
TAPSON
TARPON
TATTOO
TAUROG
TAYLOR
TEAPOT
TEAPOY
TEEBOX
TEFLON
TELCOS
TELLOF
TELLON
TEMPOS
TENDON
TENSOR
TENTON
TERROR
TEUTON
THEDOW
THEFOG
THEFOX
THELOT
THEMOB
THEROD
THERON
THESON
THESOX
THETOP
THETOY
THORON
TIEDON
TIEROD
TIESON
TIGLON
TILNOW
TILSON
TILTON
TINGOD
TINPOT
TIPTOE
TIPTOP
TIREOF
TISSOT
TOBOOT
TOLDOF
TOLDON
TOMBOY
TOMTOM
TONDOS
TONSOF
TOOHOT
TOOKON
TOOLOW
TOOTOO
TOPDOG
TOPJOB
TOPROW
TORPOR
TORSOS
TOULON
TOYDOG
TOYTOP
TREMOR
TREVOR
TRICOT
TRIGON
TRIPOD
TRIPON
TRITON
TRODON
TRYFOR
TRYLON
TUCSON
TUGSON
TURBOS
TURBOT
TURNON
TVIDOL
TVROOM
TVSHOW
TVSPOT
TYCOON
TYDBOL
TYPEOS

T••••O

TAKETO
TALKTO
TAMAYO
TATTOO
TEATRO
TECHNO
TEJANO
TENDTO
TENTWO
TENUTO
TERATO
TESSIO
TEXACO
THERMO
THEWHO
TICINO
TIEDTO
TIEMPO
TIESTO
TOBAGO
TODDAO
TOLEDO
TOMATO
TOOKTO
TOOTOO
TORERO
TORINO
TRENTO
TRILLO
TROPPO
TRUETO
TRUMBO
TUNETO
TUPELO
TURNTO
TUXEDO

•TO•••

ATODDS
ATOLLS
ATOMIC
ATONAL
ATONCE
ATONED
ATONER
ATONES
ATONIA
ATONIC
ATONOF
ATOXIC
ETOILE
ETONIC
MTOSSA
OTOMIS
OTOOLE
OTOSES
OTOSIS
PTOOEY
STOATS
STOCKS
STOCKY
STODGE
STODGY
STOGIE
STOICS
STOJKO
STOKED
STOKER
STOKES
STOLAE
STOLAF
STOLAS
STOLEN
STOLES
STOLID
STOLLE
STOLON
STOLTZ
STOMAS
STOMPS
STONED
STONER
STONES
STONEY
STOOGE
STOOLS
STOOLY
STOOPS
STOPAT
STOPBY
STOPGO
STOPIN
STOPIT
STOPUP
STORCH
STORED
STORER
STORES
STORKS
STORMS
STORMY
STORRS
STOTIN
STOUTS
STOVER
STOVES
STOWED
STOWER
STOWIT
UTOPIA

•T•O••

ATCOST
ATEOUT
ATFOUR
ATHOME
ATMOST
ATNOON
ATROIS
ATWOOD
ATWORK
ETAOIN
ETTORE
FTROOP
ITIOUS
LTGOVS
MTCOOK
MTHOOD
OTIOSE
OTOOLE
OTTOII
OTTOIV
OTTONE
PTBOAT
PTOOEY
STJOAN
STJOHN
STOOGE
STOOLS
STOOLY
STOOPS
STROBE
STRODE
STROHS
STROKE
STROLL
STRONG
STROPS
STROUD
STROVE
UTMOST

•T••O•

ATALOW
ATHROB
ATHROW
ATNOON
ATONOF
ATWOOD
ETHIOP
ETHNOS
ETYMOL
ETYMON
FTKNOX
FTROOP
ITSHOT
ITSNOT
ITSYOU
MTCOOK
MTHOOD
STAMOS
STATOR
STAYON
STEFOY
STENOG
STENOS
STEPON
STEROL
STOLON
STUPOR
STYRON

•T•••O

ATEMPO
ITISSO
ITLLDO
ITSAGO
OTELLO
OTSEGO
STELMO
STEREO
STERNO
STETHO
STINKO
STMALO
STOJKO
STOPGO
STRATO
STUCCO
STUDIO

••TO••

ACTONE
ACTORS
ACTOUT
ALTOID
ANTONE
ANTONY
ARTOIS
ASTOOP
AUTOED
BATONS
BETONY
BETOOK
BITOFF
CUTOFF
CUTOUT
DETOTH
DETOUR
DOTOAT
DOTODO
DOTORG
EATOUT
ECTOMY
ELTORO
ENTOMB
ENTOMO
ESTOCS
ESTOPS
ETTORE
EXTOLL
EXTOLS
EXTORT
FATONE
FETORS
FITOUT
FSTOPS
FUTONS
GATORS
GETOFF
GETOLD
GETOUT
GOTOFF
GOTOIT
GOTOLD
GOTOUT
HITOFF
HITONE
HITOUT
HOTOIL
HOTONE
HUTONE
IMTOLD
INTOIT
INTONE
INTOTO
INTOWN
KETONE
LATOUR
LATOYA
LETOFF
LETOUR
LETOUT
LITOUT
MOTORS
MOTOWN
MUTONS
NOTOLL
NOTONE
NOTOUT
NUTOIL
OCTOOT
OCTOPI
ONTOUR
OPTOUT
OTTOII
OTTOIV
OTTONE
PATOIS
PITONS
PITOTS
POTOSI
PUTOFF
PUTONS
PUTOUT
RATOFF
RATOUT
RETOLD
RETONE
RETOOK
RETOOL
RETOPS
RETORE
RETORN
RETORT
RETOSS
RETOUR
RETOWS
ROTORS
SATORI
SATOUT
SETOFF
SETOSE
SETOUT
SITOUT
TETONS
TSTOPS
TUTORS
UNTOLD
UNTORN
UPTOIT
UPTORE
UPTORN
UPTOSS
UPTOWN
USTOUR
VETOED
VETOER
VETOES
WETONE

••T•O•

ACTFOR
ACTION
ACTNOW
ACTSON
ANTCOW
ANTRON
ASTOOP
ASTROS
ASTROV
AUTHOR
BATBOY
BATFOR
BATHOS
BATSON
BETOOK
BETSON
BETTOR
BITEON
BOTTOM
BUTEOS
BUTHOW
BUTTON
BYTWOS
CATDOM
CATION
CATTON
CATTOY
CITRON
COTTON
DETROP
DITTOS
DOTCOM
DOTDOT
DOTEON
DOTGOV
DUTTON
EATSOF
FATHOM
FITFOR
FITSON
GETHOT
GETSON
GOTHOT
GOTYOU
GUTZON
HATBOX
HATHOR
HITFOR
HITSON
HOTBOT
HOTBOX
HOTDOG
HOTPOT
HOTROD
HUTTON
INTROS
INTWOS
JETSON
LATEOF
LATEON
LETSON
LITHOS
LOTION
LOTNOS
LOTSOF
LOTTOS
LUTHOR
LYTTON
MATRON
MATSON
MATZOH
MATZOS
METEOR
METHOD
METROS
MITSOU
MOTION
MOTTOS
MUTTON
MYTHOS
NATION
NATRON
NETHOU
NETTON
NITROS
NOTFOR
NOTION
NOTNOW
NOTTOO
NOTYOU
OCTOOT
OCTROI
OPTFOR
OPTION
OUTBOW
OUTBOX
OUTFOR
OUTFOX
OUTPOP
OUTROW
PATHOS
PATIOS
PATMOS
PATROL
PATRON
PATTON
PETBOA
PETCOW
PETDOG
PETROL
PETTOY
PITROW
POTHOS
POTION
POTTOS
PUTSON
PYTHON
RATION
RATIOS
RATSON
RETOOK
RETOOL
RETROD
RETROS
RETTON
RITSOS
SATCOM
SATFOR
SETFOR
SETSON
SETTOS
SITCOM
SITFOR
SITSON
SUTTON
TATTOO
UNTROD
VOTEON
WATSON
WETMOP
ZITCOM

••T••O

ACTTWO
ANTERO
ANTIGO
ARTHRO
ARTURO
ASTERO
BUTWHO
CATALO
CATANO
DOTODO
ELTORO
ENTERO
ENTOMO
ESTADO
GETSTO
GITANO
HATETO
HETERO
HUTTWO
INTOTO
JETHRO
LATERO
LATETO
LATIGO
LATINO
LETSGO
MATSUO
NOTTOO
OCTAVO
OPTIMO
OPTSTO
POTATO
PUTSTO
ROTHKO
SETSTO
TATTOO
ULTIMO
VOTENO

•••TO•

ABATOR
ABITOF
ABUTON
ALOTOF
ALSTON
AMATOL
ARETOO
ASHTON
AYRTON
BARTOK
BARTON
BEATON
BELTON
BENTON
BENTOS
BESTOW
BETTOR
BIGTOE
BIGTOP
BLYTON
BOLTON
BONTON
BOSTON
BOTTOM
BOUTON
BOXTOP
BOYTOY
BRETON
BRITON
BUNTON
BURTON
BUTTON
CANTON
CANTOO
CANTOR
CANTOS
CAPTOR
CARTON
CARTOP
CASTON
CASTOR
CATTON
CATTOY
CENTOS
CHITON
COLTON
CORTOT
COTTON
CROTON
CUSTOM
DALTON
DANTON
DAYTON
DEBTOR
DENTON
DIATOM
DITTOS
DOCTOR
DOGTOY
DOKTOR
DOLTON
DUTTON
EASTON
EDITOR
ELKTON
ELSTON
EMPTOR
FACTOR
FELTOK
FRITOS
FULTON
GALTON
GASTON
GROTON
HEATON
HECTOR
HESTON
HILTON
HINTON
HORTON
HOWTOS
HUSTON
HUTTON
IAMTOO
IDOTOO
ISNTOK
JUNTOS
KANTOR
KEATON
KELTON
KENTON
KEPTON
KOWTOW
LANTOS
LAPTOP
LAWTON
LECTOR
LEFTOF
LEFTON
LENTOS
LEPTON
LINTON
LIPTON
LISTON
LOFTON
LOTTOS
LOWTOP
LUPTON
LYTTON
MELTON
MENTOR
MENTOS
MERTON
MILTON
MOPTOP
MORTON
MOSTOF
MOTTOS
MUTTON
NESTOR
NETTON
NEWTON
NEWTOY
NIETOS
NORTON
NOTTOO
OHSTOP
ONETON
ORATOR
PANTOS
PARTOF
PARTON
PASTOR
PATTON
PAXTON
PAYTON
PEGTOP
PESTOS
PETTOY
PEYTON
PHOTOG
PHOTON
PHOTOS
PICTOR
PINTOS
PISTOL
PISTON
PISTOU
PLATOS
PLUTON
POITOU
POPTOP
POSTON
POSTOP
POTTOS
PRETOR
PROTON
RAGTOP
RAPTOR
RECTOR
RECTOS
REDTOP
RENTON
RESTON
RESTOW
RETTON
RHETOR
ROSTOV
SALTON
SANTOS
SARTON
SARTOR
SEATON
SECTOR
SENTON
SETTOS
SEXTON
SKITOW
SOFTON
SORTOF
SPITON
SPOTON
STATOR
SUITOR
SUTTON
TALTOS
TATTOO
TENTON
TEUTON
THETOP
THETOY
TILTON
TIPTOE
TIPTOP
TOMTOM
TOOTOO
TOYTOP
TRITON
UNSTOP
UNSTOW
VECTOR
VIATOR
VICTOR
VIKTOR
VINTON
VOSTOK
WAITON
WALTON
WANTON
WENTON
WESTON
WILTON
WONTON
WYNTON
YOMTOV
ZIPTOP

•••T•O

ACCTNO
ACTTWO
AGETWO
AINTSO
ANATTO
ARETOO
AUSTRO
BHUTTO
BISTRO
BLOTTO
CANTOO
CASTRO
CENTRO
CLOTHO
COSTCO
CUATRO
DEXTRO
DISTRO
DONTGO
DUETTO
EDITIO
FRITTO
GASTRO
GHETTO
GIOTTO
GLOTTO
GROTTO
HUTTWO
IAMTOO
IDOTOO
INITIO
JUSTSO
KEPTTO
LENTTO
LOSTTO
MUSTDO
NEXTTO
NOTTOO
ONETWO
PIETRO
QRATIO
REDTWO
RENTTO
SCOTTO
SENTTO
SIXTWO
STETHO
TATTOO
TEATRO
TENTWO
TOOTOO
WANTTO
WENTTO
WONTDO
WONTGO
YOUTWO

••••TO

ADDSTO
AGOSTO
AKINTO
ALECTO
ALIOTO
ANATTO
ARISTO
BARATO
BENITO
BHUTTO
BINDTO
BLOTTO
BONITO
BOWSTO
CALLTO
CAMETO
CARETO
CERATO
COGITO
COMETO
COOLTO
COPSTO
CRISTO
CRYPTO
CUANTO
DAMATO
DARETO
DEAFTO
DEALTO
DEARTO
DESOTO
DEVITO
DEVOTO
DOESTO
DONETO
DOOMTO
DORITO
DRAWTO
DREWTO
DUETTO
FAILTO
FALLTO
FEEDTO
FELLTO
FINITO
FIVETO
FLEWTO
FRACTO
FREETO
FRITTO
FUGATO
GAVETO
GEARTO
GELATO
GETSTO
GHETTO
GIOTTO
GIVETO
GLADTO
GLOTTO
GLUETO
GLYPTO
GOESTO
GOINTO
GONETO
GOUPTO
GROTTO
HATETO
HAVETO
HEADTO
HELDTO
HEMATO
HEPATO
HERETO
HEWSTO
HOLDTO
HOPETO
HOPSTO
HOVETO
INTOTO
ISINTO
KEEPTO
KEPTTO
KLEPTO
KRYPTO
LAIDTO
LASHTO
LATETO
LAYSTO
LEADTO
LEANTO
LEGATO
LENDTO
LENTTO
LIEDTO
LIESTO
LIKETO
LOOKTO
LOSETO
LOSTTO
LOVETO
MAILTO
MAPUTO
MEANTO
MOJITO
MOVETO
MRMOTO
NEARTO
NEEDTO
NEXTTO
NODSTO
NOVATO
OBENTO
OBERTO
ODONTO
ONAUTO
OPENTO
OPORTO
OPTSTO
OWEDTO
PARETO
PASHTO
PASSTO
PLANTO
PLAYTO
PLEDTO
POTATO
PRAYTO
PRESTO
PRONTO
PUERTO
PUTSTO
QUARTO
RACETO
READTO
RENATO
RENTTO
RIALTO
RIDETO
RIGHTO
RISETO
RODETO
ROSETO
RUBATO
RUNSTO
RUSHTO
SABATO
SAIDTO
SAILTO

SALUTO
SANGTO
SCOTTO
SEEMTO
SEENTO
SEESTO
SELLTO
SENDTO
SENTTO
SETSTO
SHINTO
SHIPTO
SHORTO
SINGTO
SNAPTO
SOASTO
SOLDTO
SOWETO
STRATO
SUBITO
SUNGTO
TAKETO
TALKTO
TENDTO
TENUTO
TERATO
TIEDTO
TIESTO
TOMATO
TOOKTO
TRENTO
TRUETO
TUNETO
TURNTO
USEDTO
VENETO
WALKTO
WANTTO
WARMTO
WAVETO
WENTTO
WISETO
WISHTO

T•P•••

TAPEON
TAPERS
TAPEUP
TAPING
TAPINS
TAPIRS
TAPOFF
TAPOUT
TAPPAN
TAPPED
TAPPER
TAPPET
TAPSIN
TAPSON
TEPEES
TIPINS
TIPJAR
TIPOFF
TIPPED
TIPPEE
TIPPER
TIPPET
TIPPLE
TIPSIN
TIPSUP
TIPTOE
TIPTOP
TOPBID
TOPCAT
TOPDOG
TOPEES
TOPEKA
TOPERS
TOPGUN
TOPHAT
TOPICS
TOPING
TOPJOB
TOPMAN
TOPMEN
TOPOFF
TOPOUT
TOPPED
TOPPER
TOPPLE
TOPROW
TOPSUP
TOPTEN
TUPELO
TUPPER
TUPTIM
TYPEAB
TYPEAS
TYPEBS
TYPEIN
TYPEOS
TYPERS
TYPEUP
TYPHUS
TYPIFY
TYPING
TYPIST

T••P••

TAIPAN
TAIPEI
TAMPED
TAMPER
TAPPAN
TAPPED
TAPPER
TAPPET
TARPIT
TARPON
TAUPES
TAUPIN
TEAPOT
TEAPOY
TEEPEE
TEMPED
TEMPEH
TEMPER
TEMPLE
TEMPOS
TEMPTS
TEMPUS
TENPIN
THEPIT
THEPRU
TIEPIN
TINPAN
TINPOT
TIPPED
TIPPEE
TIPPER
TIPPET
TIPPLE
TOPPED
TOPPER
TOPPLE
TORPID
TORPOR
TOUPEE
TRAPPY
TREPAN
TREPID
TRIPES
TRIPLE
TRIPLY
TRIPOD
TRIPON
TRIPUP
TROPES
TROPEZ
TROPHY
TROPIC
TROPPO
TUPPER
TURPIN
TVSPOT
TWOPIN
TWOPLY

T•••P•

THEAPE
THEEPA
THESPS
THESPY
THORPE
THUMPS
TIEMPO
TIEUPS
TRAMPS
TRAMPY
TRAPPY
TROMPE
TROMPS
TROOPS
TROPPO
TROUPE
TRUMPS
TSHAPE
TSTOPS
TULIPS
TVTAPE
TWERPS
TWIRPS

T••••P

TACKUP
TAGSUP
TAKEUP
TALKUP
TANKUP
TAPEUP
TARTUP
TEACUP
TEAMUP
TEARUP
TEEDUP
TEESUP
THEASP
THEGAP
THELIP
THERAP
THETOP
TIDYUP
TIEDUP
TIESUP
TILTUP
TINCUP
TIPSUP
TIPTOP
TOECAP
TOETAP
TOGSUP
TONEUP
TOOHIP
TOOKUP
TOOLUP
TOPSUP
TOREUP
TORNUP
TOSSUP
TOTEUP
TOTSUP
TOYTOP
TRICEP
TRIPUP
TROTUP
TRUEUP
TSGARP
TSTRAP
TUNEUP
TURNIP
TURNUP
TYPEUP

•TP•••

ATPLAY
STPATS
STPAUL
STPETE
STPIUS

•T•P••

ATYPIC
ETAPES
ITSPAT
NTUPLE
STAPES
STAPHS
STAPLE
STAPUF
STEPIN
STEPON
STEPPE
STEPUP
STIPES
STOPAT
STOPBY
STOPGO
STOPIN
STOPIT
STOPUP
STUPAS
STUPES
STUPID
STUPOR
UTOPIA
XTYPES

•T••P•

ATEMPO
PTRAPS
STAMPS
STEEPS
STEPPE
STIMPY
STOMPS
STOOPS
STRAPS
STREPS
STRIPE
STRIPS
STRIPY
STROPS
STUMPS
STUMPY

•T•••P

ETHIOP
FTROOP
STAYUP
STEPUP
STIRUP
STOPUP
STREEP

••TP••

HATPIN
HOTPOT
NETPAY
OUTPAY
OUTPOP
OUTPRY
OUTPUT
PETPIG
PETPUP
POTPIE
PUTPUT
SATPAT
SITPAT

••T•P•

CUTUPS
ECTYPE
ESTOPS
FSTOPS
GETUPS
LETUPS
NOTIPS
OCTOPI
ONTAPE
OUTSPY
PETIPA
RETAPE
RETAPS
RETIPS
RETOPS
RETYPE
SETUPS
SITUPS
TSTOPS
TVTAPE
UNTAPE

••T••P

ACTSUP
ANTEUP
ASTEEP
ASTOOP
BITEUP
BITMAP
CATNAP
CATNIP
CATSUP
CUTSUP
DETROP
EATSUP
ENTRAP
FATLIP
FITSUP
GETHEP
GETHIP
GETSUP
GOTHEP
GOTHIP
HITSUP
HOTCAP
HOTCUP
HOTTIP
LETRIP
LETSUP
OUTLIP
OUTPOP
OUTRAP
PETNAP
PETPUP
PUTSUP
RETRAP
SATRAP
SETSUP
SITSUP
TOTEUP
TOTSUP
TSTRAP
UNTRAP
WETMOP
WETNAP

•••T•P

ALETAP
BEATUP
BELTUP
BIGTOP
BLOTUP
BOLTUP
BOOTUP
BOXTOP
BUSTUP
CARTOP
CASTUP
CHATUP
CLOTUP
CUETIP
DOITUP
DUSTUP
FOOTUP
HEATUP
HOTTIP
HUNTUP
INSTEP
KEPTUP
KNOTUP
LAPTOP
LASTUP
LIFTUP
LOWTOP
MEETUP
MISTUP
MOPTOP
NEXTUP
NOSTEP
OHSTOP
PEGTOP
PENTUP
POPTOP
POSTOP
RAGTOP
REDTOP
RESTUP
ROOTUP
SENTUP
SHOTUP
SHUTUP
SUITUP
TARTUP
THETOP
TILTUP
TIPTOP
TOETAP
TOYTOP
TROTUP
UNSTEP
UNSTOP
UPSTEP
WAITUP
WENTUP
ZIPTOP

T•Q•••

TOQUES
TUQUES

T••Q••

TORQUE

•T••Q•

ETSEQQ

•T•••Q

ETSEQQ

TR••••

TRACED
TRACER
TRACES
TRACEY
TRACHE
TRACII
TRACKS
TRACTS
TRADED
TRADER
TRADES
TRAGIC
TRAGUS
TRAILS
TRAINS
TRAITS
TRAJAN
TRALAS
TRALEE
TRAMPS
TRAMPY
TRANCE
TRANES
TRANNY
TRAPPY
TRASHY
TRAUMA
TRAVEL
TRAVEN
TRAVES
TRAVIS
TRAWLS
TREADS
TREATS
TREATY
TREBEK
TREBLE
TREBLY
TRECES
TREDIA
TREIZE
TREMOR
TRENCH
TRENDS
TRENDY
TRENTA
TRENTE
TRENTO
TREPAN
TREPID
TRESSY
TREVOR
TREXES
TRIADS
TRIAGE
TRIALS
TRIBAL
TRIBES
TRICEP
TRICES
TRICIA
TRICKS
TRICKY
TRICOT
TRIERS
TRIFLE
TRIGON
TRIJET
TRIKES
TRILBY
TRILLO
TRILLS
TRIMLY
TRINAL
TRINES
TRIODE
TRIPES
TRIPLE
TRIPLY
TRIPOD
TRIPON
TRIPUP
TRISHA
TRISTE
TRITER
TRITON
TRIUNE
TRIVET
TRIVIA
TRIXIE
TROCHE
TRODON
TROGGS
TROIKA
TROJAN
TROLLS
TROMPE
TROMPS
TROOPS
TROPES
TROPEZ
TROPHY
TROPIC
TROPPO
TROTHS
TROTUP
TROUGH
TROUPE
TROUTS
TROVES
TROWED
TROWEL
TROYER
TROYNY
TRUANT
TRUCES
TRUCKS
TRUDGE
TRUEST
TRUETO
TRUEUP
TRUING
TRUISM
TRUMAN
TRUMBO
TRUMPS
TRUNKS
TRUSTS
TRUSTY
TRUTHS
TRYERS
TRYFOR
TRYGVE
TRYING
TRYLON
TRYONE
TRYOUT
TRYSTS

T•R•••

TARAWA
TARDES
TARGAS
TARGET
TARIFF
TARING
TARLEK
TARMAC
TAROIL
TAROTS
TARPIT
TARPON
TARRED
TARSAL
TARSUS
TARTAN
TARTAR
TARTED
TARTER
TARTES
TARTLY
TARTUP
TARZAN
TERATO
TERBIC
TERCEL
TERCES
TERESA
TERETE
TERKEL
TERMED
TERMES
TERNES
TERRAE
TERRAN
TERRES
TERRET
TERRIF
TERRIS
TERROR
TERSER
THRACE
THRALL
THRASH
THREAD
THREAT
THREEA
THREEB
THREEC
THREED
THREEE
THREES
THRESH
THRICE
THRIFT
THRILL
THRIVE
THROAT
THROBS
THROES
THRONE
THRONG
THROVE
THROWN
THROWS
THRUMS
THRUSH
THRUST
TIRADE
TIRANA
TIRANE
TIREOF
TIRIAC
TIRING
TORAHS
TORBAY
TORCHY
TOREAT
TOREIT
TORENT
TORERO
TOREUP
TORIES
TORINO
TORNUP
TOROID
TORPID
TORPOR
TORQUE
TORRES
TORREY
TORRID
TORSOS
TORTAS
TORTES
TURBAN
TURBID
TURBOS
TURBOT
TUREEN
TURFED
TURGID
TURHAN
TURING
TURKEY
TURKIC
TURNED
TURNER
TURNIN
TURNIP
TURNON
TURNTO
TURNUP
TURPIN
TURRET
TURTLE
TVROOM
TYRANT
TYRONE

T••R••

TABRIZ
TARRED
TATRAS
TAURIC
TAUROG
TAURUS
TBIRDS
TEARAT
TEARED
TEARER
TEARIT
TEARUP
TEGRIN
TEHRAN
TERRAE
TERRAN
TERRES
TERRET
TERRIF
TERRIS
TERROR
TETRAD
TETRAS
TETRIS
THERAM
THERAP
THERAT
THERED
THEREF
THERES
THERMO
THERMS
THEROD
THERON
THIRDR
THIRDS
THIRST
THIRTY
THORAX
THORIC
THORNS
THORNY
THORON
THORPE
TIARAS
TIERCE
TIERED
TIEROD
TIERRA
TIGRES
TIGRIS
TIKRIT
TITRED
TITRES
TOPROW
TORRES
TORREY
TORRID
TOURED
TOURER
TSTRAP
TSURIS
TUGRIK
TURRET
TVCREW
TWERPS
TWIRLS
TWIRLY
TWIRPS

T•••R•

TABARD
TABORS
TAGORE
TAKERS
TALERS
TAMARA
TAMERS
TANTRA
TAPERS
TAPIRS
TASERS
TATARS
TATERS
TAVERN
TAWDRY
TAXERS
TEATRO
TEAURN
TENORS
TENURE
TEVERE
THEIRS
THEMRS
THENRA
THEORY
THEPRU
THEYRE
THWART
TIERRA
TIGERS
TILERS
TILERY
TIMBRE
TIMERS
TINORE
TISHRI
TITERS
TOBURN
TOKORI
TOLARS
TONERS
TOPERS
TORERO
TOTERM
TOTERS
TOWARD
TOWERS
TOWERY
TOYERS
TRIERS
TRYERS
TSGARP
TSHIRT
TUBERS
TUDORS
TULARE
TUNDRA
TUNERS
TUTORS
TVVCRS
TYLERS
TYPERS

T••••R

TACKER
TAGGER
TAILER
TAILOR
TALKER
TALLER
TAMBOR
TAMPER
TANKER
TANNER
TAPPER
TARTAR
TARTER
TASTER
TATLER
TATTER
TAUTER
TAYLOR
TEARER
TEASER
TEENER
TEETER
TEKWAR
TELLER
TEMPER
TENDER
TENNER
TENSER
TENSOR
TENTER
TERROR
TERSER
TESTER
TETHER
THALER
THAWER
THAYER
THEBAR
THECAR
THIRDR
TICKER
TIDIER
TIEBAR
TIGGER
TILLER
TILTER
TIMBER
TINDER
TINEAR
TINIER
TINKER
TINNER
TINTER
TIPJAR
TIPPER
TITHER
TITTER
TOILER
TOLLER
TONIER
TOOFAR
TOOLER
TOOTER
TOPPER
TORPOR
TOSSER
TOTTER
TOURER
TOUTER
TOWBAR
TOWCAR
TOWNER
TOYCAR
TRACER
TRADER
TREMOR
TREVOR
TRITER
TROYER
TRYFOR
TUCKER
TUGGER
TUPPER
TURNER
TUSKER
TVSTAR
TWINER
TWOCAR
TWOFER

•TR•••

ATRAIN
ATREST
ATREUS
ATRIAL
ATRISK
ATRIUM
ATROIS
ETRADE
FTROOP
ITRIED
PTRAPS
STRADA
STRADS
STRAFE
STRAIN
STRAIT
STRAND
STRAPS
STRATA
STRATI
STRATO
STRATS
STRAUB
STRAWS
STRAYS
STREAK
STREAM
STREEP
STREET
STREPS
STRESS
STREWN
STREWS
STRIAE
STRICT
STRIDE
STRIFE
STRIKE
STRING
STRIPE
STRIPS
STRIPY
STRIVE
STROBE
STRODE
STROHS
STROKE
STROLL
STRONG
STROPS
STROUD
STROVE
STRUCK
STRUMS
STRUNG
STRUNK
STRUTS

•T•R••

ATARIS
ATERRE
ATHROB
ATHROW
ATTRIT
BTHREE
ETERNE
ITURBI
STARCH
STARED
STARER
STARES
STARIN
STARRY

STARTS
STARVE
STARZZ
STEREO
STERES
STERIC
STERNA
STERNE
STERNO
STERNS
STEROL
STIRIN
STIRUP
STORCH
STORED
STORER
STORES
STORKS
STORMS
STORMY
STORRS
STURDY
STYRON
UTURNS
XTERRA
YTTRIA
YTTRIC

•T••R•

ATERRE
ATTARS
ATTIRE
ATWORK
ETHERS
ETTORE
ITGIRL
MTAIRY
OTHERS
OTTERS
STAIRS
STARRY
STEERS
STIERS
STMARK
STMARY
STORRS
STUART
UTTERS
XTERRA

•T•••R

ATFOUR
ATONER
ETCHER
OTHMAR
STAGER
STALER
STARER
STATER
STATOR
STAYER
STELAR
STEWER
STOKER
STONER
STORER
STOVER
STOWER
STUPOR
STYLER

••TR••

ALTRIA
AMTRAC
AMTRAK
ANTRAL
ANTRES
ANTRIM
ANTRON
ANTRUM
ASTRAL
ASTRAY
ASTRES
ASTRID
ASTROS
ASTROV
ASTRUD
ATTRIT
BETRAY
BOTREE
CATRIG
CITRIC
CITRIN
CITRON
CITRUS
DATRIL
DETROP
ENTRAP
ENTREE
ENTREZ
ESTRAY
EXTRAS
GETRID
GOTRID
HATRED
HOTROD
IATRIC
INTRAY
INTROS
ISTRES
ISTRIA
KATRIN
LATRIA
LETRIP
LITRES
MATRIX
MATRON
METRED
METRES
METRIC
METROS
MITRAL
MITRED
MITRES
MOTRIN
NATRON
NITRES
NITRIC
NITROS
NUTRIA
OCTROI
ORTRUD
OUTRAN
OUTRAP
OUTRIB
OUTRIG
OUTROW
OUTRUN
PATRIA
PATRIC
PATRIE
PATROL
PATRON
PETRAT
PETREL
PETRIE
PETROL
PITROW
PUTRID
RETRAL
RETRAP
RETRIM
RETROD
RETROS
SATRAP
SOTRUE
SUTRAS
TATRAS
TETRAD
TETRAS
TETRIS
TITRED
TITRES
TSTRAP
ULTRAS
UNTRAP
UNTRIG
UNTROD
UNTRUE
VITRIC
WETRAG
YTTRIA
YTTRIC

••T•R•

ACTORS
AFTERS
ALTARF
ALTARS
ALTERS
ANTERO
ARTERY
ARTHRO
ARTURO
ASTARE
ASTART
ASTERN
ASTERO
ASTERS
ATTARS
ATTIRE
BITERS
BSTARS
CATERA
CATERS
CETERA
CITERS
CSTARS
DATARY
DATERS
DETARS
DETERS
DOTARD
DOTERS
DOTORG
EATERS
EATERY
ELTORO
ENTERO
ENTERS
ENTIRE
ESTERS
ETTORE
EXTERN
EXTORT
FETORS
FSTARS
FUTURA
FUTURE
GATERS
GATORS
GSTARS
HATARI
HATERS
HETERO
INTERJ
INTERN
INTERS
INTURN
JETHRO
KITERS
KSTARS
LATERI
LATERO
LETTRE
LITERS
LITTRE
MATERS
MATURE
METERS
MITERS
MOTHRA
MOTORS
MSTARS
MYTURN
NATURE
NITERS
NITERY
NOTARY
NOTERS
NSTARS
OATERS
OSTARS
OSTERS
OTTERS
OUTCRY
OUTPRY
PATDRY
PATERS
PETARD
PETERI
PETERS
QATARI
RATERS
RETARD
RETARS
RETIRE
RETORE
RETORN
RETORT
RETURF
RETURN
RITARD
ROTARY
ROTORS
SATIRE
SATORI
SATURN
SATYRS
SITARS
SSTARS
SUTURE
TATARS
TATERS
TITERS
TOTERM
TOTERS
TUTORS
UNTORN
UPTORE
UPTORN
UPTURN
UTTERS
VITARA
VOTARY
VOTERS
WATERS
WATERY

••T••R

ACTFOR
AETHER
ALTAIR
ANTHER
ANTLER
ARTCAR
ARTHUR
ARTIER
ASTHER
AUTEUR
AUTHOR
BATFOR
BATHER
BATTER
BETTER
BETTOR
BITTER
BOTHER
BUTLER
BUTTER
CATHER
COTLER
COTTER
CUTLER
CUTTER
DETMER
DETOUR
DITHER
DOTTER
EITHER
ESTHER
FATHER
FATTER
FETTER
FITFOR
FITTER
GATHER
GETFAR
GETTER
GOTFAR
GUTTER
HATHOR
HATTER
HITFOR
HITHER
HITTER
HOTAIR
HOTCAR
HOTTER
HOTWAR
JITTER
JOTTER
KOTTER
LATHER
LATOUR
LATTER
LETOUR
LETTER
LITHER
LITTER
LOTHAR
LOTTER
LUTHER
LUTHOR
MATHER
MATTER
METEOR
METIER
MOTHER
MUTTER
NATTER
NETHER
NETTER
NOTFAR
NOTFOR
NUTTER
OATIER
ONTOUR
OPTFOR
OSTLER
OUTFOR
OUTWAR
PATTER
PATZER
PETTER
PITIER
POTHER
POTTER
PUTTER
RATEDR
RATHER
RATNER
RATTER
RETEAR
RETOUR
RITTER
ROTTER
RUTGER
RUTTER
SATFOR
SETFOR
SETTER
SETZER
SITFOR
SITTER
SUTTER
TATLER
TATTER
TETHER
TITHER
TITTER
TOTTER
UNTIER
UPTEAR
USTOUR
VETOER
VETTER
WETBAR
WETTER
WITHER
WITTER
YATTER
ZITHER

•••TR•

ANITRA
AUSTRO
BISTRO
CASTRO
CENTRE
CENTRI
CENTRO
CHITRA
CONTRA
CONTRE
CUATRO
DESTRY
DEXTRO
DISTRO
DMITRI
DMITRY
GANTRY
GASTRO
GENTRY
GUITRY
LASTRA
LETTRE
LITTRE
LUSTRA
LUSTRE
MAITRE
MANTRA
NOSTRA
OSETRA
PALTRY
PANTRY
PASTRY
PELTRY
PIETRO
POETRY
QUATRE
ROSTRA
SARTRE
SENTRA
SENTRY
SULTRY
TANTRA
TEATRO
VECTRA
VESTRY
WINTRY

•••T•R

ABATER
ABATOR
ACUTER
AUSTER
AVATAR
BAITER
BANTER
BARTER
BASTER
BATTER
BAXTER
BEATER
BELTER
BESTER
BESTIR
BETTER
BETTOR
BITTER
BOATER
BOLTER
BOOTER
BUNTER
BUSTER
BUTTER
CANTER
CANTOR
CAPTOR
CARTER
CASTER
CASTOR
CENTER
COATER
COLTER
COOTER
COPTER
COSTAR
COTTER
COUTER
CRATER
CURTER
CUSTER
CUTTER
DAFTER
DARTER
DEBTOR
DEFTER
DEUTER
DEXTER
DIETER
DOCTOR
DOKTOR
DOTTER
DUSTER
EASTER
EDITOR
ELATER
ELITER
EMOTER
EMPTOR
EXETER
FACTOR
FALTER
FASTER
FATTER
FESTER
FETTER
FILTER
FITTER
FLUTER
FOOTER
FOSTER
FRATER
GAITER
GARTER
GASTER
GETTER
GOITER
GRATER
GUITAR
GUNTER
GUTTER
HALTER
HATTER
HEATER
HECTOR
HEFTER
HELTER
HESTER
HINTER
HITTER
HOOTER
HOTTER
HUNTER
HURTER
INSTIR
IPETER
IRATER
ISHTAR
JEETER
JESTER
JILTER
JITTER
JOLTER
JOTTER
JUSTER
KANTOR
KCSTAR
KILTER
KOSTER
KOTTER
LARTER
LATTER
LAUTER
LECTER
LECTOR
LEITER
LESTER
LETTER
LIFTER
LINTER
LISTER
LITTER
LOFTER
LOITER
LOOTER
LOTTER
LOWTAR
LUSTER
MARTYR
MASTER
MATTER
MEETER
MELTER
MENTOR
MINTER
MISTER
MOLTER
MOOTER
MORTAR
MUSTER
MUTTER
NATTER
NEATER
NECTAR
NESTER
NESTOR
NETTER
NEUTER
NOSTER
NUTTER
OBITER
OERTER
ONSTAR
ORATOR
OUSTER
OYSTER
PALTER
PANTER
PASTER
PASTOR
PATTER
PELTER
PERTER
PESTER
PETTER
PEWTER
PICTOR
PIETER
PINTER
PLATER
PORTER
POSTER
POTTER
POUTER
PRATER
PRETER
PRETOR
PUNTER
PUTTER
QINTAR
QUOTER
RAFTER
RANTER
RAPTER
RAPTOR
RASTER
RATTER
RECTOR
REITER
RENTER
RESTER
RESTIR
REUTER
RHETOR
RIOTER
RITTER
ROOTER
ROSTER
ROTTER
ROUTER
RUTTER
SALTER
SARTOR
SCOTER
SEATER
SECTOR
SETTER
SIFTER
SISTER
SITTER
SKATER
SLATER
SMITER
SOFTER
SORTER
SOUTER
STATER
STATOR
SUITOR
SUMTER
SUTTER
TARTAR
TARTER
TASTER
TATTER
TAUTER
TEETER
TENTER
TESTER
TILTER
TINTER
TITTER
TOOTER
TOTTER
TOUTER
TRITER
TVSTAR
ULSTER
UNITER
UPSTIR
VASTER
VECTOR
VENTER
VETTER
VIATOR
VICTOR
VIKTOR
WAFTER
WAITER
WALTER
WANTER
WASTER
WELTER
WESTER
WETTER
WHITER
WINTER
WISTER
WITTER
WRITER
WYNTER
XYSTER
YATTER
YESTER
ZESTER

••••TR

FIRSTR

TS••••

TSADES
TSADIS
TSETSE
TSGARP
TSHAPE
TSHIRT
TSKING
TSKTSK
TSOTSI
TSTOPS
TSTRAP
TSURIS

T•S•••

TASERS
TASKED
TASKET
TASMAN
TASSEL
TASSES
TASTED
TASTEE
TASTER
TASTES
TESLAS
TESSIE
TESSIO
TESTAE
TESTED
TESTEE
TESTER
TISANE
TISHRI
TISKET
TISSOT
TISSUE
TOSSED
TOSSER
TOSSES
TOSSIN
TOSSUP
TUSCAN
TUSHES
TUSHIE
TUSKED
TUSKER
TUSSAL
TUSSES
TUSSLE
TVSETS
TVSHOW
TVSPOT
TVSTAR
TYSONS

T••S••

TABSET
TAGSON
TAGSUP
TAOSNM
TAPSIN
TAPSON
TARSAL
TARSUS
TASSEL
TASSES
TEASED
TEASEL
TEASER
TEASES
TEASET
TEESUP
TENSED
TENSER
TENSES
TENSOR
TERSER
TESSIE
TESSIO
THESEA
THESES
THESIS
THESON
THESOX
THESPS
THESPY
THESUN
THISBE
THUSLY
TIESIN
TIESON
TIESTO
TIESUP
TILSIT
TILSON
TINSEL
TIPSIN
TIPSUP
TISSOT
TISSUE
TMESES
TMESIS
TOASTS
TOASTY
TOCSIN
TOESIN
TOGSUP
TONSIL
TONSOF
TOPSUP
TORSOS
TOSSED
TOSSER
TOSSES
TOSSIN
TOSSUP
TOTSUP
TOUSLE
TOWSIN
TRASHY
TRESSY
TRISHA
TRISTE
TRUSTS
TRUSTY
TRYSTS
TUCSON
TUGSAT
TUGSON
TULSAN
TUSSAL
TUSSES
TUSSLE
TUTSIS
TWISTS
TWISTY

T•••S•

TALESE
TALISA
TAMEST
TAOISM
TAOIST
TAVIST
TEENSY
TERESA
THEASP
THEISM
THEIST
THEUSA
THIRST
THRASH
THRESH
THRUSH
THRUST
TOLAST
TOOTSY
TRESSY
TRUEST
TRUISM
TSETSE
TSKTSK
TSOTSI
TUBIST
TUFTSU
TYPIST

T••••S

TABLAS
TABLES
TABOOS
TABORS
TAHOES
TAIGAS
TAINTS
TAKERS
TALERS
TALONS
TALTOS
TAMERS
TAMILS
TANGOS
TANKAS
TANTES
TAPERS
TAPINS
TAPIRS
TARDES
TARGAS
TAROTS
TARSUS
TARTES
TASERS
TASSES
TASTES
TATARS
TATERS
TATRAS
TAUNTS
TAUONS
TAUPES
TAURUS
TAVELS
TAXERS
TAXIES
TAXOLS
TBILLS
TBIRDS
TBONDS
TBONES
TCELLS
TEASES
TEBETS
TEHEES
TELCOS
TEMPOS
TEMPTS
TEMPUS
TENETS
TENLBS
TENNIS
TENONS
TENORS
TENSES
TENTHS
TEPEES
TERCES
TERMES
TERNES
TERRES
TERRIS
TESLAS
TETHYS
TETONS
TETRAS
TETRIS
TEVETS
TEXANS
THALES
THAMES
THANES
THANKS
THATIS
THEBES
THEFTS
THEIRS
THEMES
THEMRS
THERES
THERMS
THESES
THESIS
THESPS
THETAS
THETIS
THIGHS
THILLS
THINGS
THINKS
THIRDS
THOLES
THOMAS
THONGS
THORNS
THREES
THROBS
THROES
THROWS
THRUMS
THUMBS
THUMPS
THUNKS
THYMES
THYMUS
TIARAS
TIBIAS
TICALS

TIDIES
TIEINS
TIEUPS
TIGERS
TIGHTS
TIGONS
TIGRES
TIGRIS
TIKKAS
TILAKS
TILDES
TILERS
TILLIS
TILTHS
TIMERS
TINCTS
TINGES
TIPINS
TITANS
TITERS
TITHES
TITLES
TITRES
TMESES
TMESIS
TMINUS
TNOTES
TOASTS
TOBIAS
TOBIES
TOBITS
TODAYS
TODIES
TOEINS
TOGUES
TOILES
TOKAYS
TOKENS
TOKLAS
TOLARS
TOMBES
TONDOS
TONERS
TONICS
TONKAS
TONNES
TOPEES
TOPERS
TOPICS
TOQUES
TORAHS
TORIES
TORRES
TORSOS
TORTAS
TORTES
TOSSES
TOTALS
TOTEMS
TOTERS
TOUGHS
TOWELS
TOWERS
TOXICS
TOXINS
TOYERS
TOYONS
TRACES
TRACKS
TRACTS
TRADES
TRAGUS
TRAILS
TRAINS
TRAITS
TRALAS
TRAMPS
TRANES
TRAVES
TRAVIS
TRAWLS
TREADS
TREATS
TRECES
TRENDS
TREXES
TRIADS
TRIALS
TRIBES
TRICES
TRICKS
TRIERS
TRIKES
TRILLS
TRINES
TRIPES
TROGGS
TROLLS
TROMPS
TROOPS
TROPES
TROTHS
TROUTS
TROVES
TRUCES
TRUCKS
TRUMPS
TRUNKS
TRUSTS
TRUTHS
TRYERS
TRYSTS
TSADES
TSADIS
TSTOPS
TSURIS
TTILES
TUBERS
TUDORS
TULIPS
TULLES
TUNERS
TUNICS
TUQUES
TURBOS
TUSHES
TUSSES
TUTEES
TUTORS
TUTSIS
TUTTIS
TVDVDS
TVHITS
TVSETS
TVVCRS
TWAINS
TWANGS
TWEAKS
TWEEDS
TWEENS
TWEETS
TWERPS
TWILLS
TWINES
TWIRLS
TWIRPS
TWISTS
TYLERS
TYPEAS
TYPEBS
TYPEOS
TYPERS
TYPHUS
TYSONS

•TS•••

ATSIGN
ATSTUD
CTSCAN
ETSEQQ
ITSAGO
ITSELF
ITSFUN
ITSHOT
ITSNOT
ITSPAT
ITSYOU
LTSULU
OTSEGO

•T•S••

ATESTS
ATISES
HTESTS
ITASCA
ITISSO
MTOSSA
NTESTS
OTOSES
OTOSIS
STASES
STASIS

•T••S•

ATBEST
ATCOST
ATDUSK
ATEASE
ATLAST
ATMOST
ATREST
ATRISK
ATTEST
ATWIST
ITISSO
MTOSSA
OTIOSE
STRESS
UTMOST

•T•••S

ATARIS
ATBATS
ATEAMS
ATESTS
ATHENS
ATILES
ATISES
ATKINS
ATMANS
ATODDS
ATOLLS
ATONES
ATREUS
ATROIS
ATTARS
ATTICS
BTEAMS
BTILES
CTILES
DTILES
ETAGES
ETAILS
ETAPES
ETCHES
ETHERS
ETHICS
ETHNOS
ETHYLS
ETILES
ETUDES
FTILES
GTILES
HTESTS
HTILES
ITCHES
ITILES
ITIOUS
JTILES
KTILES
LTGOVS
LTILES
MTILES
MTVVJS
NTESTS
NTILES
OTHERS
OTILES
OTITIS
OTOMIS
OTOSES
OTOSIS
OTTERS
PTILES
PTRAPS
QTILES
RTILES
STACKS
STAFFS
STAGES
STAINS
STAIRS
STAKES
STALES
STALKS
STALLS
STAMOS
STAMPS
STANDS
STAPES
STAPHS
STARES
STARTS
STASES
STASIS
STATES
STATUS
STAVES
STEADS
STEAKS
STEALS
STEAMS
STEEDS
STEELS
STEEPS
STEERS
STEINS
STELAS
STELES
STENOS
STENTS
STERES
STERNS
STICKS
STIDES
STIERS
STIFFS
STILES
STILLS
STILTS
STINGS
STINKS
STINTS
STIPES
STOATS
STOCKS
STOICS
STOKES
STOLAS
STOLES
STOMAS
STOMPS
STONES
STOOLS
STOOPS
STORES
STORKS
STORMS
STORRS
STOUTS
STOVES
STPATS
STPIUS
STRADS
STRAPS
STRATS
STRAWS
STRAYS
STREPS
STRESS
STREWS
STRIPS
STROHS
STROPS
STRUMS
STRUTS
STUFFS
STUKAS
STUMPS
STUNTS
STUPAS
STUPES
STYLES
STYLUS
TTILES
UTAHNS
UTTERS
UTUBES
UTURNS
VTILES
WTILES
XTILES
XTYPES
YTILES
ZTILES

••TS••

ACTSAS
ACTSIN
ACTSON
ACTSUP
BATSIN
BATSON
BETSEY
BETSON
BETSYS
CATSAT
CATSIT
CATSUP
CUTSIN
CUTSIT
CUTSUP
DATSUN
EATSAT
EATSIN
EATSIT
EATSOF
EATSUP
FATSIS
FITSIN
FITSON
FITSUP
GATSBY
GETSAB
GETSAC
GETSAD
GETSAT
GETSBY
GETSET
GETSIN
GETSIT
GETSON
GETSTO
GETSUP
GOTSET
HITSAT
HITSIT
HITSON
HITSUP
JETSAM
JETSET
JETSKI
JETSON
KITSCH
LETSAT
LETSBE
LETSBY
LETSGO
LETSIN
LETSON
LETSUP
LOTSOF
MATSON
MATSUI
MATSUO
MITSOU
OPTSIN
OPTSTO
OUTSAT
OUTSAW
OUTSAY
OUTSEE
OUTSET
OUTSIN
OUTSIT
OUTSPY
OUTSUM
PETSAT
PETSIT
PITSAW
POTSIE
PUTSBY
PUTSCH
PUTSIN
PUTSON
PUTSTO
PUTSUP
RATSON
RITSOS
SETSAT
SETSBY
SETSIN
SETSON
SETSTO
SETSUP
SITSAT
SITSBY
SITSIN
SITSON
SITSUP
TOTSUP
TUTSIS
WATSON
YATSEN

••T•S•

APTEST
ARTEST
ARTIST
ATTEST
AUTISM
AUTIST
CUTEST
CUTESY
DETEST
FETISH
HITEST
IQTEST
IRTYSH
LATEST
LATISH
LETUSE
LUTIST
MOTTST
MUTEST
OBTEST
OBTUSE
OUTASK
POTASH
POTOSI
RETEST
RETOSS
SETOSE
UPTOSS
WATUSI

••T••S

ACTORS
ACTSAS
AFTERS
ALTARS
ALTERS
ALTIUS
ANTICS
ANTRES
ARTELS
ARTOIS
ASTERS
ASTRES
ASTROS
ATTARS
ATTICS
AZTECS
AZTEKS
BATHES
BATHOS
BATIKS
BATONS
BETELS
BETSYS
BETTAS
BITERS
BOTELS
BSTARS
BUTEOS
BUTKUS
BUTTES
BUTUTS
BYTENS
BYTWOS
CATERS
CATHYS
CITEES
CITERS
CITIES
CITIUS
CITRUS
COTANS
COTTAS
CSTARS
CUTEYS
CUTIES
CUTINS
CUTUPS
DATERS
DETARS
DETERS
DETTES
DITTOS
DITZES
DOTERS
DUTIES
EATERS
ENTERS
ESTERS
ESTOCS
ESTOPS
EXTOLS
EXTRAS
FATSIS
FATWAS
FETORS
FSTARS
FSTOPS
FUTONS
FUTZES
GATERS
GATORS
GETUPS
GSTARS
HATERS
HITINS
HOTELS
IDTAGS
INTENS
INTERS
INTROS
INTWOS
ISTLES
ISTRES
JETTAS
KITERS
KSTARS
LATENS
LATHES
LATINS
LATKES
LATTES
LETUPS
LITERS
LITHOS
LITMUS
LITRES
LOTNOS
LOTTOS
LUTZES
MATERS
MATEYS
MATHIS
MATINS
MATJES
MATTES
MATZOS
METALS
METERS
METRES
METROS
MITERS
MITRES
MOTELS
MOTETS
MOTIFS
MOTORS
MOTTOS
MSTARS
MUTIUS
MUTONS
MYTHOS
NITERS
NITRES
NITROS
NOTERS
NOTIPS
NSTARS
OATERS
OCTADS
OCTANS
OCTETS
OOTIDS
OPTICS
OSTARS
OSTERS
OTTERS
OUTGAS
OUTIES
PATENS
PATERS
PATHOS
PATIOS
PATMOS
PATOIS
PETALS
PETERS
PETTIS
PITIES
PITONS
PITOTS
POTHOS
POTTOS
PUTONS
RATELS
RATERS
RATIOS
RETAGS
RETANS
RETAPS
RETARS
RETIES
RETINS
RETIPS
RETOPS
RETOSS
RETOWS
RETROS
RITSOS
RITZES
ROTORS
RUTINS
SATAYS
SATINS
SATYRS
SETTOS
SETUPS
SITARS
SITINS
SITUPS
SSTARS
SUTRAS
TATARS
TATERS
TATRAS
TETHYS
TETONS
TETRAS
TETRIS
TITANS
TITERS
TITHES
TITLES
TITRES
TOTALS
TOTEMS
TOTERS
TSTOPS
TUTEES
TUTORS
TUTSIS
TUTTIS
ULTRAS
UNTIES
UPTOSS
UTTERS
VETOES
VETTES
VITALS
VOTERS
WATERS
WITHUS
YUTZES

•••TS•

AINTSO
BRATSK
CURTSY
JUSTSO
LAOTSE
LHOTSE
MOTTST
ROOTSY
TOOTSY
TSETSE
TSKTSK
TSOTSI
TUFTSU
WOOTSY

•••T•S

ABATES
ABATIS
ACUTES
AGATES
AGITAS
AKITAS
AMATIS
AORTAS
ARETES
BANTUS
BASTES
BENTOS
BERTHS
BETTAS
BIOTAS
BIRTHS
BOITES
BOOTES
BOOTHS
BROTHS
BRUTES
BRUTUS
BUTTES
CACTUS
CANTOS
CARTES
CASTES
CENTAS
CENTOS
CESTAS
CESTUS
CHUTES
CLOTHS
CNOTES
COATES
COATIS
COMTES
CORTES
COSTAS
COTTAS
CRATES
CRWTHS
CULTUS
CURTIS
CUSTIS
DANTES
DEATHS
DELTAS
DEPTHS
DETTES
DHOTIS
DIETES
DITTOS
EARTHS
EBATES
ELATES
ELITES
ELUTES
ELYTIS
EMOTES
ENATES
ENOTES
EUSTIS
EVITES
EXITUS
FAITES
FAITHS
FANTAS
FAUTES
FESTAS
FESTUS
FIFTHS
FIRTHS
FLUTES
FORTAS
FORTES
FORTIS
FRITAS
FRITES
FRITOS
FROTHS
GENTES
GESTES
GIRTHS
GLUTES
GNOTES
GRATES
GRATIS
HASTES
HEATHS
HIATUS
HOSTAS
HOWTOS
HYATTS
IFITIS
IRITIS
JETTAS
JUNTAS
JUNTOS
JUSTAS
JUSTUS
JUSTYS
KNOTTS
LANTOS
LATTES
LENTOS
LOFTUS
LOTTOS
MANTAS
MANTIS
MARTES
MATTES
MEATUS
MENTIS
MENTOS
MIATAS
MIRTHS
MONTHS
MOTTOS
MOUTHS
MUFTIS
MULTIS
NANTES
NAUTES
NIETAS
NIETOS
NINTHS
NORTHS
ORATES
OTITIS
PANTOS
PARTYS
PASTAS
PASTES
PASTIS
PESTOS
PETTIS
PHOTOS
PIETAS
PINTOS
PISTES
PIUTES
PLATES
PLATOS
PLATYS
PLUTUS
POETES
PORTES
POTTOS
PRATES
PUNTAS
QANTAS
QUOTAS
QUOTES
RAITAS
RAPTUS
RASTAS
REATAS
RECTOS
RECTUS
RENTES
RESTES
RIATAS
ROUTES
SANTAS
SANTOS
SAUTES
SCOTTS
SERTAS
SETTOS
SIETES
SIXTHS
SIXTUS
SKATES
SLATES
SLOTHS
SMITES
SMITHS
SNATHS
SOITIS
SOUTHS
SPATES
SPITES
STATES
STATUS
SUITES
SWATHS
SYNTHS
TALTOS
TANTES
TARTES
TASTES
TENTHS
THATIS
THETAS
THETIS
TILTHS
TNOTES
TORTAS
TORTES
TROTHS
TRUTHS
TUTTIS
UINTAS
UNITAS
UNITES
VASTUS
VENTAS
VESTAS
VETTES
VIRTUS
VISTAS
WASTES
WHITES
WIDTHS
WORTHS
WRATHS
WRITES
XYSTUS
YENTAS
YOUTHS
ZESTAS
ZLOTYS

••••TS

ABBOTS
ABORTS
ADAPTS
ADEPTS
ADMITS
ADOPTS
ADOUTS
ADULTS
AFLATS
AGENTS
AGLETS
ALERTS
ALEUTS
ALISTS
ALLOTS
AMANTS
AMBITS
AMENTS
AMVETS
ANGSTS
ARGOTS
ARHATS
ARMETS
ASCOTS
ASSETS
ATBATS
ATESTS
AUDITS
AUGHTS
AVERTS
AWAITS
BEASTS
BEAUTS
BEFITS
BEGETS
BERETS
BESETS
BESOTS
BFLATS
BIDETS
BIGHTS
BIGOTS
BIONTS
BLASTS
BLEATS
BLISTS
BLOATS
BLUETS
BLUNTS
BLURTS
BOASTS
BOOSTS
BRACTS
BRANTS
BRUITS
BRUNTS
BUNDTS
BURETS
BURSTS
BUTUTS
BYLOTS
CADETS
CARATS
CARETS
CFLATS
CHANTS
CHARTS
CHEATS
CHERTS
CHESTS
CIVETS
CLEATS
CLEFTS
CLOUTS
COACTS
COAPTS
COASTS
COMETS

COOPTS COROTS COSETS COUNTS COURTS COVETS CRAFTS CRESTS CROATS CROFTS CRUETS CRUSTS CRYPTS CSPOTS CUBITS CULETS CURETS DALETS DAUNTS DAVITS DEBITS DEBUTS DEFATS DEISTS DELFTS DEMITS DEPOTS DERATS DFLATS DICOTS DIGITS DIVOTS DIXITS DONETS DONUTS DOUBTS DRAFTS DRIFTS DROITS DUCATS DUVETS EBBETS EBOATS ECLATS EDICTS EDUCTS EFLATS EGESTS EGRETS EIGHTS EJECTS ELECTS ELISTS EMMETS ENACTS EPACTS ERECTS ERGOTS ERUCTS ERUPTS ESBATS EVENTS EVERTS EVICTS EXACTS EXALTS EXERTS EXISTS

EXMETS EXPATS EXULTS FACETS FAGOTS FAINTS FAULTS FEASTS FEINTS FFLATS FIGHTS FILETS FIRSTS FLEETS FLINTS FLIRTS FLOATS FLOUTS FOISTS FOUNTS FRONTS FROSTS FRUITS GAMUTS GAVOTS GENETS GFLATS GHOSTS GIANTS GIGOTS GLINTS GLOATS GOBOTS GODETS GONUTS GRAFTS GRANTS GREATS GREETS GRIFTS GRIOTS GRISTS GROATS GROUTS GRUNTS GSUITS GUESTS HABITS HAUNTS HEARTS HEISTS HELOTS HIHATS HOISTS HTESTS HYATTS IDENTS IDIOTS INGOTS INLETS INPUTS INSETS INUITS ISLETS JABOTS JAUNTS JAVITS JOINTS

JOISTS JOUSTS KARATS KARSTS KMARTS KNOTTS KNOUTS KORATS KRAITS LEASTS LIEUTS LIGHTS LIMITS MANATS MANETS MERITS MIDSTS MIGHTS MONETS MOTETS MOULTS MOUNTS MULCTS NIGHTS NOBUTS NOHITS NONETS NOPETS NTESTS NYJETS NYMETS OBJETS OCTETS ODISTS OHNUTS ONDITS ONSETS OPCITS ORANTS ORBITS OSSETS OUGHTS OWLETS PABSTS PAINTS PEWITS PICOTS PILOTS PINOTS PIPETS PIPITS PITOTS PIVOTS PLAITS PLANTS PLEATS POINTS POSITS POULTS PRINTS QUARTS QUESTS QUIETS QUILTS QUINTS QUIRTS QUOITS RAMETS

REACTS REBETS REBUTS RECUTS REFITS REHITS RELETS REMATS REMITS REPOTS RESETS RESITS REVETS REWETS RIGHTS RIVETS ROASTS ROBOTS ROGETS ROOSTS ROUSTS SABOTS SAINTS SAULTS SCANTS SCENTS SCOOTS SCOTTS SCOUTS SENATS SHAFTS SHEETS SHIFTS SHIRTS SHOATS SHOOTS SHORTS SHOUTS SHUNTS SIGHTS SKEETS SKIRTS SKORTS SLANTS SLEETS SMARTS SMELTS SMOLTS SNOOTS SNORTS SNOUTS SPLATS SPLITS SPORTS SPOUTS SPRATS SPRITS SPURTS SQUATS STARTS STENTS STILTS STINTS STOATS STOUTS STPATS STRATS STRUTS

STUNTS SWEATS SWEETS SWIFTS TAINTS TAROTS TAUNTS TEBETS TEMPTS TENETS TEVETS THEFTS TIGHTS TINCTS TOASTS TOBITS TRACTS TRAITS TREATS TROUTS TRUSTS TRYSTS TVHITS TVSETS TWEETS TWISTS UBOATS UBOLTS UNBITS UNFITS UNHATS UNIATS UNPOTS UPSETS VALETS VAULTS VAUNTS VELDTS VERSTS VISITS WAISTS WHEATS WIGHTS WORSTS WRESTS WRISTS WURSTS YACHTS YAKUTS YEASTS

TT••••

TTILES

T•T•••

TATAMI TATARS TATERS TATLER TATRAS TATTED TATTER TATTLE TATTOO TETCHY TETHER TETHYS TETLEY TETONS TETRAD TETRAS TETRIS TETZEL TITANS TITERS TITHED TITHER TITHES TITIAN TITLED TITLES TITRED TITRES TITTER TITTLE TOTALS TOTEMS TOTERM TOTERS TOTEUP TOTING TOTSUP TOTTED TOTTER TSTOPS TSTRAP TUTEES TUTORS TUTSIS TUTTED TUTTIS TUTTUT TUTUED TVTAPE TVTIME

T••T••

TACTEL TACTIC TALTOS TAMTAM TANTES TANTRA TARTAN TARTAR TARTED TARTER TARTES TARTLY TARTUP TASTED TASTEE TASTER TASTES TATTED TATTER TATTLE TATTOO TAUTEN TAUTER TAUTLY TEATRO TEETER TEETHE TENTED TENTER TENTHS TENTON TENTWO TESTAE TESTED TESTEE TESTER TEUTON TEXTED THATCH THATIS THATLL THETAS THETED THETIS THETOP THETOY TICTAC TIETAC TILTAT TILTED TILTER TILTHS TILTON TILTUP TINTED TINTER TIPTOE TIPTOP TITTER TITTLE TNOTES TOATEE TOETAP TOLTEC TOMTIT TOMTOM TOOTAT TOOTED TOOTER TOOTHY TOOTIE TOOTIN TOOTLE TOOTOO TOOTSY TOPTEN TORTAS TORTES TOTTED TOTTER TOUTED TOUTER TOYTOP TRITER TRITON TROTHS TROTUP TRUTHS TSETSE TSKTSK TSOTSI TUFTED TUFTSU TUPTIM TURTLE TUTTED TUTTIS TUTTUT TVSTAR TWITCH TWITTY

T•••T•

TAHITI TAINTS TAKETH TAKETO TALKTO TAROTS TAUNTS TEBETS TECATE TECHTV TEMPTS TENDTO TENETS TENUTA TENUTO TERATO TERETE TEVETS THEFTS THIRTY TIEDTO TIESTO TIGHTS TINCTS TOASTS TOASTY TOBITS TODATE TOMATO TONITE TOOKTO TOYOTA TRACTS TRAITS TREATS TREATY TRENTA TRENTE TRENTO TRISTE TROUTS TRUETO TRUSTS TRUSTY TRYSTS TUBATE TUNETO TURNTO TVHITS TVSETS TWEETS TWEETY TWENTY TWISTS TWISTY TWITTY

T••••T

TABLET TABSET TAGOUT TAKEIT TALENT TALKAT TAMEST TAOIST TAPOUT TAPPET TARGET TARPIT TASKET TAUGHT TAVIST TAXCUT TEAACT TEAPOT TEARAT TEARIT TEASET TELLIT TELNET TENANT TENHUT TERRET THEACT THEIST THELOT THEMET THENET THEPIT THERAT THEVET THIRST THREAT THRIFT THROAT THRUST THWART TICKET TIDBIT TIKRIT TILLET TILSIT TILTAT TINHAT TINPOT TIPPET TISKET TISSOT TOBOOT TOGOUT TOILAT TOILET TOLAST TOLDIT TOMCAT TOMTIT TOOHOT TOOKIT TOOTAT TOPCAT TOPHAT TOPOUT TOREAT TOREIT TORENT TOYHAT TRICOT TRIJET TRIVET TRUANT TRUEST TRYOUT TSHIRT TUBIST TUFFET TUGSAT TUMULT TURBOT TURRET TUTTUT TVSPOT TWILIT TWOACT TWOBIT TYBALT TYPIST TYRANT

•TT•••

ATTACH ATTACK ATTAIN ATTARS ATTEND ATTEST ATTHAT ATTICA ATTICS ATTILA ATTIRE ATTLEE ATTRIT ATTUNE ETTING ETTORE OTTAVA OTTAWA OTTERS OTTOII OTTOIV OTTONE UTTERS YTTRIA YTTRIC

•T•T••

ATSTUD MTETNA OTITIC OTITIS STATED STATEN STATER STATES STATIC STATIN STATOR STATUE STATUS STETHO STITCH STOTIN

•T••T•

ATBATS ATENTH ATESTS ETCETC HTESTS NTESTS STARTS STENTS STILTS STINTS STOATS STOLTZ STOUTS STPATS STPETE STRATA STRATI STRATO STRATS STRUTS STUNTS STUNTY

•T•••T

ATBEST ATCOST ATEOUT ATLAST ATMOST ATREST ATTEST ATTHAT ATTRIT ATWIST ITSHOT ITSNOT ITSPAT PTBOAT STABAT STAYAT STOPAT STOPIT STOWIT STRAIT STREET STRICT STUART STYLET UTHANT UTMOST

••TT••

ACTTWO ALTTAB BATTED BATTEN BATTER BATTLE BETTAS BETTED BETTER BETTOR BETTYE BITTED BITTEN BITTER BOTTLE BOTTOM BUTTED BUTTER BUTTES BUTTIN BUTTON CATTLE CATTON CATTOY COTTAE COTTAS COTTEN COTTER COTTON CUTTER DETTES DITTOS DOTTED DOTTER DOTTIE DOTTLE DUTTON FATTED FATTEN FATTER FETTER FETTLE FITTED FITTER GETTER GETTIN GITTED GOTTEN GUTTED GUTTER HATTED HATTER HATTIE HITTER HOTTEA HOTTER HOTTIE HOTTIP HOTTUB HUTTED HUTTON HUTTWO JETTAS JETTED JITTER JOTTED JOTTER JUTTED KETTLE KITTED KITTEN KOTTER KOTTKE LATTER LATTES LETTED LETTER LETTRE LITTER LITTLE LITTRE LOTTED LOTTER LOTTOS LYTTON MATTEA MATTED MATTEL MATTER MATTES MATTIE METTLE MITTAG MITTEN MOTTLE MOTTOS MOTTST MUTTER MUTTON NATTER NETTED NETTER NETTLE NETTLY NETTON NOTTOO NUTTED NUTTER PATTED PATTEN PATTER PATTIE PATTON PETTED PETTER PETTET PETTIS PETTIT PETTOY PITTED POTTED POTTER POTTOS PUTTED PUTTEE PUTTER PUTTIN RATTAN RATTAT RATTED RATTER RATTLE RATTLY RETTED RETTIG RETTON RITTER ROTTED ROTTEN ROTTER RUTTAN RUTTED RUTTER SETTEE SETTER SETTLE SETTOS SITTER SITTIN SOTTED SUTTER SUTTON TATTED TATTER TATTLE TATTOO TITTER TITTLE TOTTED TOTTER TUTTED TUTTIS TUTTUT VATTED VETTED VETTER VETTES VITTLE WATTLE WETTED WETTER WETTIG WITTED WITTER WITTIG YATTER YETTIE

••T•T•

ASTUTE BUTUTS DETOTH ENTITY ESTATE GETSTO HATETO INTOTO LATETO METATE MOTETS MUTATE NOTATE NUTATE OCTETS OPTSTO OUTATE PETITE PITOTS POTATO PUTSTO RATITE ROTATE SETSTO SHTETL UMTATA YATATA

••T••T

ACTOUT APTEST ARTEST ARTIST ASTART ATTEST ATTHAT ATTRIT AUTIST BITNET BUTYET CATFIT CATGUT CATSAT CATSIT CUTEST CUTLET CUTOUT CUTSIT DETECT DETENT DETEST DOTDOT DOTOAT EATOUT EATSAT EATSIT EXTANT EXTENT EXTORT FATCAT FITOUT GETFIT GETHOT GETOUT GETSAT GETSET GETSIT GETWET GOTFIT GOTHOT GOTOIT GOTOUT GOTSET GOTWET HATEIT HITEST HITOUT HITSAT HITSIT HOTBOT HOTPOT INTACT INTENT INTHAT INTOIT INTUIT IQTEST JETSET KITKAT LATENT LATEST LETOUT LETSAT LITOUT LUTIST MOTTST MUTANT MUTEST NATANT NITWIT NOTFIT NOTOUT NOTYET NUTLET OBTEST OCTANT OCTOOT OPTOUT OUTACT OUTBAT OUTCUT OUTEAT

OUTFIT OUTHIT OUTJET OUTJUT OUTLET OUTPUT OUTSAT OUTSET OUTSIT OUTWIT PATENT PETCAT PETRAT PETSAT PETSIT PETTET PETTIT POTENT PUTOUT PUTPUT RATOUT RATTAT RETEST RETINT RETORT ROTGUT SATOUT SATPAT SETOUT SETSAT SITOUT SITPAT SITSAT SOTHAT TUTTUT UNTAUT UNTILT UPTILT UPTOIT URTEXT WITHIT

•••TT•

ALETTE ANATTO BEATTY BHUTTO BLATTY BLOTTO BLOTTY BRATTY CHATTY CHITTY CLOTTY DUETTI DUETTO FLATTV FRETTY FRITTA FRITTO FRUTTI GHETTO GIOTTO GLOTTO GNATTY GRITTI GRITTY GROTTO GROTTY HYATTS IGOTTA KEPTTO KNOTTS KNOTTY LENTTO LIOTTA LOSTTO NEXTTO ODETTA ODETTE PLATTE PLOTTY PRETTY REATTA RENTTO SCOTTO SCOTTS SCOTTY SENTTO SMITTY SMUTTY SPOTTV SPOTTY TWITTY WANTTO WENTTO WHITTY YVETTE

•••T•T

BEATAT BEATIT BOOTIT CORTOT DIKTAT DRATIT FOOTIT FRETAT GOATIT HINTAT HOOTAT IGETIT IGOTIT KEPTAT LARTET LEFTIT LESTAT LOSTIT MOTTST MUSTNT PASTIT PETTET PETTIT POSTIT QUITIT RANTAT RATTAT SEPTET SESTET SEXTET SHOTAT SWATAT TILTAT TOMTIT TOOTAT TUTTUT WENTAT

••••TT

ABBOTT ALCOTT ARNETT BODETT CAVETT DEWITT EMMETT EMMITT FSCOTT GELETT HEWITT JEWETT KADETT KAPUTT LABATT LEVITT LOVETT MELOTT OFFUTT PRUETT

TU••••

TUBAGE TUBATE TUBBED TUBERS TUBFUL TUBING TUBIST TUBMAN TUBULE TUCANA TUCKED TUCKER TUCKIN TUCSON TUDORS TUFFET TUFTED TUFTSU TUGGED TUGGER TUGRIK TUGSAT TUGSON TUILLE TULANE TULARE TULIPS TULLES TULSAN TUMBLE TUMEFY TUMULT TUNDRA TUNEIN TUNERS TUNETO TUNEUP TUNICS TUNING TUNNEL TUNNEY TUPELO TUPPER TUPTIM TUQUES TURBAN TURBID TURBOS TURBOT TUREEN TURFED TURGID TURHAN TURING TURKEY TURKIC TURNED TURNER TURNIN TURNIP TURNON TURNTO TURNUP TURPIN TURRET TURTLE TUSCAN TUSHES TUSHIE TUSKED TUSKER TUSSAL TUSSES TUSSLE TUTEES TUTORS TUTSIS TUTTED TUTTIS TUTTUT TUTUED TUVALU TUVWXY TUXEDO

T•U•••

TAUGHT TAUNTS TAUONS TAUPES TAUPIN TAURIC TAUROG TAURUS TAUTEN TAUTER TAUTLY TEUTON THUMBS THUMPS THUNKS THUSLY TOUCAN TOUCHE TOUCHY TOUGHS TOUGHY TOULON TOUPEE TOURED TOURER TOUSLE TOUTED TOUTER TRUANT TRUCES TRUCKS TRUDGE TRUEST TRUETO TRUEUP TRUING TRUISM TRUMAN TRUMBO TRUMPS TRUNKS TRUSTS TRUSTY TRUTHS TSURIS

T••U••

TABUED TABULA TEAURN TENURE TENUTA TENUTO THEUSA THOUGH THRUMS THRUSH THRUST TIEUPS TOBURN TOGUES TOQUES TRAUMA TRIUNE TROUGH TROUPE TROUTS TUBULE TUMULT TUQUES TUTUED

T•••U•

TACKUP TAGOUT TAGSUP TAKEUP TALCUM TALKUP TALMUD TAMMUZ TANGUY TANKUP TAPEUP TAPOUT TARSUS TARTUP TAURUS TAXCUT TEACUP TEAMUP TEARUP TEDEUM TEDIUM TEEDUP TEESUP TEMPUS TENHUT THEHUB THESUN THYMUS TIDYUP TIEDUP TIESUP TILTUP TINCUP TIPSUP TISSUE TMINUS TOGOUT TOGSUP TONEUP TONGUE TOOKUP TOOLUP TOPGUN TOPOUT TOPSUP TOREUP TORNUP TORQUE TOSSUP TOTEUP TOTSUP TOYGUN TRAGUS TRIPUP TROTUP TRUEUP TRYOUT TUBFUL TUNEUP TURNUP TUTTUT TYPEUP TYPHUS

T••••U

THEPRU TUFTSU TUVALU

•TU•••

ETUDES ITURBI NTUPLE STUART STUBBY STUCCO STUDIO STUDLY STUFFS STUFFY STUKAS STUMPS STUMPY STUNTS STUNTY STUPAS STUPES STUPID STUPOR STURDY STUVWX UTUBES UTURNS

•T•U••

ATDUSK ATTUNE LTSULU MTFUJI STJUDE STLUKE STOUTS STRUCK STRUMS STRUNG STRUNK STRUTS

•T••U•

ATEOUT ATFOUR ATREUS ATRIUM ATSTUD ITIOUS ITSFUN STAPUF STATUE STATUS STAYUP STEPUP STIRUP STOPUP STPAUL STPIUS STRAUB STROUD STYLUS

•T•••U

ITSYOU LTSULU

••TU••

ACTUAL ARTURO ASTUTE ATTUNE AUTUMN BUTUTS CUTUPS DETUNE FUTUNA FUTURA FUTURE GETUPS INTUIT INTUNE INTURN IVTUBE LETUPS LETUSE MATURE MUTUAL MUTUEL MYTURN NATURE OBTUND OBTUSE PETULA RETUNE RETURF RETURN RITUAL ROTUND RSTUVW SATURN SETUPS SITUPS SUTURE TUTUED UNTUCK UNTUNE UPTURN WATUSI

••T•U•

ACTIUM ACTOUT ACTSUP ALTIUS ANTEUP ANTRUM ARTAUD ARTFUL ARTGUM ARTHUR ASTRUD AUTEUR BITEUP BUTKUS CATGUT CATSUP CITIUS CITRUS CUTOUT CUTSUP DATSUN DETOUR EATOUT EATSUP FITFUL FITOUT FITSUP GETOUT GETSUP GOTOUT HATFUL HITOUT HITSUP HOTCUP HOTTUB JETGUN LATOUR LETOUR LETOUT LETSUP LITMUS LITOUT MATSUI MATSUO MUTIUS NETFUL NOTOUT ONTOUR OPTOUT ORTRUD OUTBUD OUTBUY OUTCUT OUTGUN OUTJUT OUTPUT OUTRUN OUTSUM PETPUP POTFUL PUTOUT PUTPUT PUTSUP RATOUT RETOUR ROTGUT SATOUT SETOUT SETSUP SITOUT SITSUP SOTRUE TOTEUP TOTSUP TUTTUT UNTAUT UNTRUE USTOUR VATFUL WITHUS

••T••U

BATEAU GATEAU GOTYOU MITSOU NETHOU NOTYOU

•••TU•

ADYTUM ATSTUD BANTUS BEATUP BELTUP BLOTUP BOLTUP BOOTUP BRUTUS BUSTUP CACTUS CASTUP CENTUM CESTUS CHATUP CLOTUP CULTUS DICTUM DOITUP DUSTUP EXITUS FACTUM FESTUS FOOTUP HEATUP HIATUS HOTTUB HUNTUP INATUB JUSTUS KEPTUP KNOTUP LASTUP LIFTUP LOFTUS MANTUA MEATUS MEETUP MISTUP NEXTUP PENTUP PLUTUS POSTUM QRSTUV RAPTUS RECTUS RESTUP ROOTUP SENTUP SEPTUM SHOTUP SHUTUP SIXTUS STATUE STATUS SUITUP TARTUP TILTUP TROTUP TUTTUT VASTUS VIRTUE VIRTUS WAITUP WENTUP XYSTUS

•••T•U

LAOTZU PISTOU POITOU TUFTSU

••••TU

ERESTU INSITU KLAATU MOBUTU PQRSTU SHORTU

TV••••

TVCREW TVDVDS TVGAME TVHITS TVIDOL TVLAND TVROOM TVSETS TVSHOW TVSPOT TVSTAR TVTAPE TVTIME TVVCRS

T•V•••

TAVELS TAVERN TAVIST TEVERE TEVETS TIVOLI TUVALU TUVWXY TVVCRS

T••V••

TEEVEE THEVET TRAVEL TRAVEN TRAVES TRAVIS TREVOR TRIVET TRIVIA TROVES TVDVDS

T•••V•

THEYVE THIEVE THRIVE THROVE TRYGVE TWELVE

T••••V

TECHTV

•TV•••

MTVVJS

•T•V••

ATAVIC MTVVJS STAVED STAVES STEVEN STEVIE STIVIC STOVER STOVES STUVWX

•T••V•

ATFIVE LTGOVS OTTAVA STARVE STEEVE STRIVE STROVE

•T•••V

OTTOIV

••TV••

LATVIA LITVAK OUTVIE POTVIN

••T•V•

ACTIVA ACTIVE DATIVE MOTIVE NATIVE OCTAVE OCTAVO OTTAVA RSTUVW VOTIVE

••T••V

ASTROV DOTGOV OTTOIV

•••TV•

WHATVE

•••T•V

FLATTV GUSTAV LAPTEV PARTIV QRSTUV ROSTOV SPOTTV YOMTOV

••••TV

FLATTV LIVETV MINITV SPOTTV TECHTV

TW••••

TWAINS TWANGS TWANGY TWEAKS TWEAKY TWEEDS TWEEDY TWEENS TWEENY TWEETS TWEETY TWEEZE TWELVE TWENTY TWERPS TWIGGY TWILIT TWILLS TWINED TWINER TWINES TWINGE TWIRLS TWIRLY TWIRPS TWISTS TWISTY TWITCH TWITTY TWOACT TWOBIT TWOCAR TWODAY TWOEEE TWOFER TWOMAN TWOPIN TWOPLY TWOWAY TWYMAN

T•W•••

TAWDRY THWACK THWART TOWAGE TOWARD TOWBAR TOWCAR TOWELS TOWERS TOWERY TOWHEE TOWING TOWNER TOWNIE TOWSIN

T••W••

TAIWAN TEKWAR THAWED THAWER THEWAY THEWEB THEWHO THEWIZ TRAWLS TROWED TROWEL TUVWXY TWOWAY

T•••W•

TARAWA TENTWO THROWN THROWS

T••••W

TALLOW TAXLAW THEDOW THELAW TILNOW TOOLOW TOPROW TVCREW TVSHOW

•TW•••

ATWILL ATWIST ATWOOD ATWORK

•T•W••

STEWED STEWER STEWIE STOWED STOWER STOWIT

•T••W•

ATDAWN OTTAWA STRAWS STREWN STREWS STUVWX

•T•••W

ATALOW ATHROW

••TW••

BUTWHO BUTWHY BYTWOS FATWAS GETWET GOTWET HOTWAR INTWOS JETWAY NITWIT OUTWAR OUTWIT

••T•W•

ACTTWO ANTAWN HUTTWO INTOWN MOTOWN OTTAWA OUTAWE RETOWS UPTOWN

••T••W

ACTNOW ANTCOW BUTHOW MATHEW NOTNEW NOTNOW OUTBOW OUTLAW OUTROW OUTSAW PETCOW PITROW PITSAW RETHAW RSTUVW UNTHAW

•••TW•

ACTTWO AGETWO HUTTWO ONETWO REDTWO SIXTWO TENTWO YOUTWO

•••T•W

BESTOW KOWTOW RESTOW SKITOW UNSTOW

T•X•••

TAXCUT TAXERS TAXIED TAXIES TAXING TAXLAW TAXMAN TAXMEN TAXOLS TEXACO TEXANS TEXMEX TEXTED TOXICS TOXINS TUXEDO

T••X••

TREXES TRIXIE

T•••X•

THEAXE TJMAXX TUVWXY

T••••X

TEEBOX TEXMEX THEFOX THESOX THORAX TJMAXX TOMMIX

•T•X••

ATAXIA ATAXIC ATOXIC

•T•••X

FTKNOX STUVWX

••T•X•

BYTAXI EUTAXY URTEXT

••T••X

HATBOX HOTBOX MATRIX

OUTBOX
OUTFOX
RATEDX

•••T•X
CORTEX
GASTAX
JOETEX
LASTEX
MEATAX
NONTAX
PENTAX
PRETAX
PROTAX
SINTAX
SURTAX
SYNTAX
USETAX
VERTEX
VORTEX

••••TX
WACOTX

TY••••
TYBALT
TYCOBB
TYCOON
TYDBOL
TYLERS
TYPEAB
TYPEAS
TYPEBS
TYPEIN
TYPEOS
TYPERS
TYPEUP
TYPHUS
TYPIFY
TYPING
TYPIST
TYRANT
TYRONE
TYSONS

T•Y•••
TAYLOR
THYMES
THYMIC
THYMUS
TOYAMA
TOYCAR
TOYDOG
TOYERS
TOYGUN
TOYHAT
TOYING
TOYONS
TOYOTA
TOYTOP
TRYERS
TRYFOR
TRYGVE
TRYING
TRYLON
TRYONE
TRYOUT
TRYSTS
TWYMAN

T••Y••
THAYER
THEYLL
THEYRE
THEYVE
TIDYUP
TROYER
TROYNY

T•••Y•
TAMAYO
TETHYS
THEEYE
TIEDYE
TODAYS
TOKAYS
TOLDYA

T••••Y
TABKEY
TAGDAY
TAMELY
TANGLY
TANGUY
TARTLY
TAUTLY
TAWDRY
TEAPOY
TEDKEY
TEENSY
TENDAY
TENLEY
TETCHY
TETLEY
THEBAY
THEFLY
THEORY
THESPY
THETOY
THEWAY
THINGY
THINLY
THIRTY
THORNY
THUSLY
TICKBY
TICKLY
TIDILY
TILERY
TILLEY
TIMELY
TINGLY
TINILY
TINKLY
TOASTY
TOMBOY
TOOMEY
TOOTHY
TOOTSY
TORBAY
TORCHY
TORREY
TOUCHY
TOUGHY
TOWERY
TRACEY
TRAMPY
TRANNY
TRAPPY
TRASHY
TREATY
TREBLY
TRENDY
TRESSY
TRICKY
TRILBY
TRIMLY
TRIPLY
TROPHY
TROYNY
TRUSTY
TUMEFY
TUNNEY
TURKEY
TUVWXY
TWANGY
TWEAKY
TWEEDY
TWEENY
TWEETY
TWENTY
TWIGGY
TWIRLY
TWISTY
TWITTY
TWODAY
TWOPLY
TWOWAY
TYPIFY

•TY•••
ATYALE
ATYPIC
ETYMOL
ETYMON
STYING
STYLED
STYLER
STYLES
STYLET
STYLUS
STYMIE
STYRON
XTYPES

•T•Y••
ETHYLS
ITSYOU
STAYAT
STAYED
STAYER
STAYIN
STAYON
STAYUP

•T••Y•
STRAYS

•T•••Y
ATPLAY
MTAIRY
PTOOEY
STABLY
STACEY
STAGEY
STALKY
STARRY
STEADY
STEAMY
STEELY
STEFOY
STEMMY
STICKY
STILLY
STIMPY
STINGY
STINKY
STMARY
STOCKY
STODGY
STONEY
STOOLY
STOPBY
STORMY
STRIPY
STUBBY
STUDLY
STUFFY
STUMPY
STUNTY
STURDY

••TY••
BATYAM
BUTYET
ECTYPE
GOTYOU
IRTYSH
NOTYET
NOTYOU
RETYPE
SATYRS

••T•Y•
BETSYS
BETTYE
CATHYS
CUTEYS
LATOYA
MATEYS
METHYL
PITAYA
RITDYE
SATAYS
TETHYS
VATDYE

••T••Y
ALTKEY
ANTONY
ARTERY
ARTILY
ASTLEY
ASTRAY
BATBOY
BATDAY
BATLEY
BETONY
BETRAY
BETSEY
BOTANY
BOTCHY
BOTFLY
BUTWHY
CATCHY
CATHAY
CATTOY
CITIFY
CUTELY
CUTESY
DATARY
EATERY
ECTOMY
ENTITY
ESTRAY
EUTAXY
GATSBY
GETSBY
HOTDAY
HOTKEY
INTRAY
JETWAY
JITNEY
LATELY
LETFLY
LETSBY
LITANY
MOTLEY
MUTELY
MUTINY
NETPAY
NETTLY
NITERY
NOTANY
NOTARY
NOTCHY
NOTIFY
OUTBUY
OUTCRY
OUTFLY
OUTLAY
OUTPAY
OUTPRY
OUTSAY
OUTSPY
PATCHY
PATDAY
PATDRY
PETTOY
PITCHY
PITNEY
PUTNEY
PUTSBY
RATIFY
RATTLY
ROTARY
SATINY
SETSBY
SITSBY
TETCHY
TETLEY
UNTIDY
VOTARY
WATERY
WATNEY
WETFLY
WITCHY

•••TY•
ACETYL
BETTYE
DACTYL
JUSTYS
MARTYR
PARTYS
PLATYS
ZLOTYS

•••T•Y
APATHY
BEATTY
BLATTY
BLOTTY
BOYTOY
BRATTY
BROTHY
CATTOY
CHATTY
CHITTY
CLOTTY
COSTLY
CURTLY
CURTSY
DAFTLY
DEFTLY
DESTRY
DMITRY
DOGTOY
EARTHY
FILTHY
FLATLY
FLITBY
FRETTY
FROTHY
GANTRY
GENTLY
GENTRY
GLITZY
GNATTY
GRITTY
GROTTY
GUITRY
HEATHY
HOSTLY
ICHTHY
JUSTLY
KLUTZY
KNOTTY
LASTLY
MALTBY
MEETLY
MOSTLY
MOUTHY
NEATLY
NETTLY
NEWTOY
PALTRY
PANTRY
PARTLY
PASTRY
PELTRY
PERTLY
PETTOY
PLOTTY
POETRY
PORTLY
PRETTY
RAPTLY
RATTLY
ROOTSY
SCOTTY
SENTBY
SENTRY
SHOTBY
SLITHY
SMITHY
SMITTY
SMUTTY
SOFTLY
SPOTTY
SUBTLY
SULTRY
TARTLY
TAUTLY
THETOY
TOOTHY
TOOTSY
TWITTY
VASTLY
VESTRY
WENTBY
WHITBY
WHITEY
WHITTY
WINTRY
WOOTSY
WORTHY

••••TY
ACUITY
ALMATY
BEATTY
BEAUTY
BLATTY
BLOTTY
BOUNTY
BRATTY
CAVITY
CHANTY
CHATTY
CHERTY
CHESTY
CHITTY
CLOTTY
COMITY
COUNTY
CRAFTY
CRUSTY
DAINTY
DEPUTY
DIMITY
DRAFTY
DRIFTY
DUMPTY
EIGHTY
ENMITY
ENTITY
EQUITY
FAULTY
FAWLTY
FEALTY
FEISTY
FERITY
FIXITY
FLINTY
FLIRTY
FLOATY
FRETTY
FROSTY
FRUITY
GAIETY
GFIFTY
GHOSTY
GLINTY
GNATTY
GRITTY
GROTTY
GROUTY
GSIXTY
GUILTY
HEARTY
HUMPTY
IFORTY
JAUNTY
KNOTTY
KPDUTY
KRUSTY
LAXITY
LEALTY
LENITY
LEVITY
MIGHTY
MOIETY
MOUNTY
NFORTY
NICETY
NIGHTY
NINETY
NUDITY
ODDITY
ONDUTY
PAINTY
PARITY
PIGSTY
PLENTY
PLOTTY
POINTY
POLITY
PRETTY
PURITY
QWERTY
RARITY
REALTY
RIGHTY
SAFETY
SANITY
SCANTY
SCOTTY
SHANTY
SHELTY
SHIFTY
SHORTY
SLEETY
SMARTY
SMITTY
SMUTTY
SNOOTY
SNORTY
SPORTY
SPOTTY
STUNTY
SURETY
SWEATY
THIRTY
TOASTY
TREATY
TRUSTY
TWEETY
TWENTY
TWISTY
TWITTY
UBIETY
UPPITY
VANITY
VAULTY
VAUNTY
VERITY
WHITTY
YEASTY

T••Z••
TARZAN
TETZEL

T•••Z•
TREIZE
TWEEZE

T••••Z
TABRIZ
TAMMUZ
THEWIZ
TROPEZ

•TZ•••
ITZHAK

•T••Z•
STANZA
STARZZ

•T•••Z
STARZZ
STOLTZ

••TZ••
DITZES
FUTZED
FUTZES
GUTZON
KATZEN
LUTZES
MATZOH
MATZOS
PATZER
RITZES
SETZER
TETZEL
YUTZES

••T••Z
ENTREZ

•••TZ•
FRITZI
GLITZY
KLUTZY
LAOTZU
LEUTZE

•••T•Z
CORTEZ
CURTIZ
MONTEZ

••••TZ
ALRITZ
BLINTZ
CHINTZ
DONITZ
ERSATZ
FRANTZ
IGNATZ
KIBITZ
KOONTZ
KRANTZ
KUNITZ
MORITZ
NIMITZ
PERUTZ
QUARTZ
SHORTZ
SHULTZ
SPRITZ
STOLTZ

U•A•••
UBANGI
UGANDA
UGARTE
UHAULS
UKASES
UNABLE
UNABLY
UNAGED
UNAKIN
UNAMIS
UNARMS
UNAVID
UNAWED
UNAXED
URACIL
URAEUS
URALIC
URALSK
URANIA
URANIC
URANUS
USABLE
USABLY
USAGES
USANCE
USARMY
USAUSA
UTAHAN
UTAHNS
UVALDE
UVALUE

U••A••
UBOATS
UCLANS
UGGAMS
UHLANS
ULLAGE
UMIAKS
UMLAUT
UMTATA
UNBAGS
UNBAIT
UNBALE
UNBARE
UNBARS
UNCAGE
UNCAKE
UNCALM
UNCAPS
UNCASE
UNCASK
UNCAST
UNDAMS
UNEASE
UNEASY
UNFACT
UNFAIR
UNGAGS
UNGAMY
UNGAVA
UNHAFT
UNHAIR
UNHALE
UNHAND
UNHASP
UNHATS
UNHAZY
UNIATE
UNIATS
UNJAMS
UNLACE
UNLADE
UNLAID
UNLASH
UNLAYS
UNMADE
UNMAKE
UNMANS
UNMASK
UNMAST
UNMATE
UNNAIL
UNPACK
UNPAID
UNPALE
UNPAWN
UNRACK
UNRASH
UNSAFE
UNSAGE
UNSAID
UNSAWN
UNSAYS
UNTACK
UNTAME
UNTAPE
UNTAUT
UNVAIN
UNWALL
UNWARY
UPCARD
UPCAST
UPDART
UPDATE
UPGAZE
UPLAND
UPLAST
UPLATE
UPRATE
UPSALA
UPTAKE
UPTALK
UPWAFT
UPWARD
UQUARK
URBANA
URBANE
URBANI
URBANV
USBANK
USHAPE
USMAIL
USNAVY
USUALS
UTHANT
UVRAYS

U•••A•
UINTAS
ULLMAN
ULTRAS
UMBRAE
UMBRAL
UMBRAS
UNCIAL
UNCLAD
UNCLAY
UNDEAD
UNDRAW
UNFLAT
UNGLAD
UNGUAL
UNITAS
UNIVAC
UNLEAD
UNLEAF
UNLEAN
UNLOAD
UNNEAT
UNOCAL
UNORAL
UNPLAN
UNREAD
UNREAL
UNSEAL
UNSEAM
UNSEAT
UNSNAG
UNSNAP
UNSPAN
UNTHAW
UNTRAP
UNWRAP
UPBEAR
UPBEAT
UPHEAP
UPLEAP
UPLOAD
UPREAR
UPROAR
UPSHAW
UPSOAR
UPTEAR
USETAX
USFLAG
UTAHAN
UTICAN
UVULAE
UVULAR
UVULAS

U••••A
UGANDA
ULTIMA
UMBRIA
UMTATA
UNCOLA
UNGAVA
UNGULA
UPSALA
URANIA
URBANA
URSULA
USAUSA
UTOPIA

•UA•••
CUANDO
CUANTO
CUATRO
DUALLY
DUARTE
GUANOS
GUARDS
GUAVAS
JUAREZ
LUANDA
NUANCE
QUACKS
QUACKY
QUADRI
QUAFFS
QUAGGA
QUAGGY
QUAHOG
QUAILS
QUAINT
QUAKED
QUAKER
QUAKES
QUAKIE
QUALES
QUALMS
QUANTA
QUAPAW
QUARKS
QUARRY
QUARTE
QUARTO
QUARTS
QUARTZ
QUASAR
QUATRE
QUAVER
QUAYLE
RUANDA
SUABLE
SUAVER

•U•A••
AUBADE
AUFAIT
AULAIT
AUPAIR
AURATE
BUGAKU
BUKAVU
BURANA
BUTANE
CUBAGE
CUBANS
CUDAHY
CUNARD
CURACY
CURADS
CURARE
CURATE
CUSACK
DUCATS
DUGALD
DUGARD
DUNANT
DURANT
DUVALL
EURAIL
EUTAXY
FUGARD
FUGATO
GUIANA
GULAGS
GUYANA
HUMANE
HUMANS
JUDAEA
JUDAIC
JUMADA
JURADO
KULAKS
KURALT
KUVASZ
KUWAIT
LUNACY
LUNATE
LUSAKA
LUXATE
MUFASA
MUGABE
MURALS
MURANO
MUTANT
MUTATE
NUTATE
OUTACT
OUTADD
OUTAGE
OUTASK
OUTATE
OUTAWE
PUPATE
QUEASY
RUBATI
RUBATO
RUMAKI
SUBARU
SUEANE
SUEANN
SUGARS
SUGARY
SUMACS
SURAHS
SUSANB
SUSANN
SUVARI
TUBAGE
TUBATE
TUCANA
TULANE
TULARE
TUVALU
YUKATA
YUKAWA
YUMAAZ
YUMANS
YUTANG

•U••A•
AUDIAL
AUGEAN
AUGEAS
BUBBAS
BUCCAL
BUCHAN
BUENAS
BUFFAY
BULGAR
BULLAE
BUMRAP
BUNGAY
BUNYAN
BUREAU
BURIAL
BURKAS
BURLAP
BURMAN
BUROAK
BURSAE
BURSAL
BURSAR
BURSAS
BUSMAN
BUYSAT
CUBFAN
CUICAS
CUNEAL
CUPPAS
CURIAE
CUSHAW
CUSPAL
DUCTAL
DUENAS
DUNBAR
DUNCAN
DUNDAS
DUNHAM
DUNLAP
DURBAN
DURHAM
DURRAS
FULMAR
FUMEAT
FUNGAL
FURMAN
FUSSAT
GUAVAS
GUFFAW
GUINAN
GUITAR
GULLAH
GUNLAP
GUNLAW
GUNMAN
GUNNAR

GUSTAV GUTMAN GUZMAN HUBCAP HUPPAH HURRAH HURRAY HUSSAR HUZZAH JUDEAN JULIAN JUMPAT JUNEAU JUNTAS JUSTAS KUBLAI LUCIAN LUMBAR MUCHAS MUDCAT MULLAH MULLAS MUMBAI MURRAY MUSCAT MUSIAL MUTUAL NUBIAN NUCHAE NUCHAL NUMBAT OUIJAS OUTBAN OUTBAT OUTEAT OUTGAS OUTLAW OUTLAY OUTMAN OUTPAY OUTRAN OUTRAP OUTSAT OUTSAW OUTSAY OUTWAR PULSAR PUNJAB PUNKAS PUNTAS PUTNAM QUAPAW QUASAR QUOTAS RUBRAW RUDMAN RUGRAT RUMBAS RUNSAT RUNWAY RUPIAH RUSHAT RUTTAN SUBPAR SUBWAR SUBWAY SUCHAS SULFAS SULTAN SUNDAE SUNDAS SUNDAY SUNFAN SUNHAT SUNRAY SUNTAN SUPRAS SUREAM SURTAX SUTRAS TUBMAN TUGSAT TULSAN TURBAN TURHAN TUSCAN TUSSAL VULCAN VULGAR YUCCAS YUMAAZ ZUNIAN

•U•••A

AURIGA AURORA BUDDHA BULOVA BUQSHA BURANA BUSHWA CUESTA CUMBIA CUPOLA DUENNA DUESSA DULLEA DURYEA EUBOEA EUDORA EUPNEA EUREKA EUROPA FULCRA FUSUMA FUTUNA FUTURA GUIANA GUINEA GURKHA GUYANA JUDAEA JUDOKA JUMADA LUANDA LUCIDA LUELLA LUMINA LUNTHA LUNULA LUSAKA LUSTRA MUFASA MULETA MUNERA MURCIA NUBIRA NUMINA NUTRIA OUGHTA PUEBLA PURINA QUAGGA QUANTA QUINTA RUANDA RUBBIA RUSSIA SUBSEA TUCANA TUNDRA YUKATA YUKAWA ZUNIGA

••UA••

ACUATE AKUAKU AQUAKE DOUANE EDUARD ELUANT ELUARD ELUATE EQUALS EQUATE IGUANA LOUANN SQUABS SQUADS SQUALL SQUARE SQUASH SQUATS SQUAWK STUART TRUANT UQUARK USUALS YOUALL

••U•A•

ACURAS ALULAE ALULAR AOUDAD ARUBAN BAUMAN BEULAH BHUTAN BRUMAL BRUTAL CAUDAD CAUDAL CAUSAL CIUDAD COUGAR CRURAL CRUZAN DOUGAL DOULAS FAUNAE FAUNAL FAUNAS FEUDAL FOURAA FOURAD FOURAM FRUGAL GOUDAS KAUNAS KOUFAX LAULAU LOUMAS MAUMAU NEUMAN NEURAL NOUGAT NOUNAL OCULAR OVULAR PAUSAL PLURAL SAUNAS SCUBAS SEURAT SHUMAI SQUEAK SQUEAL STUKAS STUPAS TOUCAN TRUMAN UVULAE UVULAR UVULAS WAUSAU

••U••A

ALUDRA ALUMNA APULIA AQUILA AZUELA CHUPPA COULDA FOURAA FRUSTA IGUANA KAUNDA LAURIA LOUISA NAUSEA NOUMEA PLUVIA RHUMBA WOULDA

•••UA•

ACTUAL ANNUAL CAGUAS CASUAL EMQUAD ENQUAD GENUAL JAGUAR JANUAR LEHUAS LOQUAT MANUAL MSQUAD MUTUAL OAHUAN PADUAN PAPUAN RITUAL SIOUAN UNGUAL VISUAL

•••U•A

ARJUNA BAKULA BELUGA CANULA CAYUGA COPULA CREUSA EXCUSA FACULA FIBULA FLAUTA FUSUMA FUTUNA FUTURA HECUBA KAHUNA KORUNA LACUNA LAGUNA LAPUTA LIKUTA LUNULA MACULA MAKUTA MAZUMA MEDUSA MIZUNA NEBULA NERUDA PACULA PAKULA PETULA PLEURA PNEUMA RAGUSA SEGURA TABULA TENUTA THEUSA TRAUMA UNGULA URSULA USAUSA VICUNA YAKUZA YAMUNA

••••UA

CHINUA JOSHUA KAHLUA KAILUA LENGUA LINGUA MANTUA NASHUA PASCUA XINHUA

UB••••

UBANGI UBIETY UBOATS UBOLTS UBUROI

U•B•••

UMBELS UMBERS UMBRAE UMBRAL UMBRAS UMBRIA UNBAGS UNBAIT UNBALE UNBARE UNBARS UNBELT UNBEND UNBENT UNBIND UNBITS UNBLED UNBOLD UNBOLT UNBORN UNBUDS UNBURY UNBUSY UPBEAR UPBEAT UPBIND UPBOWS URBANA URBANE URBANI URBANV USBANK

U••B••

UNABLE UNABLY USABLE USABLY UTUBES

U•••B•

UNROBE

U••••B

UNCURB UNGLIB

•UB•••

AUBADE AUBREY AUBURN BUBBAS BUBBLE BUBBLY BUBKES CUBAGE CUBANS CUBBED CUBEBS CUBERS CUBFAN CUBICS CUBING CUBISM CUBIST CUBITI CUBITS CUBOID DUBBED DUBBER DUBCEK DUBLIN DUBOIS DUBOSE EUBOEA HUBBLE HUBBUB HUBCAP HUBERT HUBLEY HUBRIS KUBLAI KUBLER LUBBER LUBECK LUBING LUBLIN NUBBED NUBBER NUBBIN NUBBLE NUBBLY NUBIAN NUBILE NUBIRA PUBLIC PUBLIX RUBATI RUBATO RUBBED RUBBER RUBBIA RUBBLE RUBBLY RUBELS RUBENS RUBIED RUBIES RUBIFY RUBIKS RUBLES RUBLEV RUBOFF RUBOUT RUBRAW RUBRIC RUBSIN RUBSON RUBSUP SUBARU SUBBED SUBDEB SUBDUE SUBGOD SUBGUM SUBITO SUBLET SUBLID SUBLOT SUBMIT SUBNET SUBORN SUBPAR SUBSEA SUBSET SUBTLE SUBTLY SUBURB SUBWAR SUBWAY TUBAGE TUBATE TUBBED TUBERS TUBFUL TUBING TUBIST TUBMAN TUBULE

•U•B••

BUBBAS BUBBLE BUBBLY BUGBOY BUMBLE BUMBRY BURBLE BURBLY BURBOT BUSBOY CUBBED CUEBID CUMBER CUMBIA CURBED DUBBED DUBBER DUMBER DUMBLY DUMBOS DUNBAR DURBAN DURBIN FUMBLE FURBYS GUMBEL GUMBOS HUBBLE HUBBUB HUMBER HUMBLE HUMBLY HUMBUG JUMBLE JUMBLY JUMBOS LUBBER LUMBAR LUMBER MUMBAI MUMBLE MUMBLY NUBBED NUBBER NUBBIN NUBBLE NUBBLY NUMBAT NUMBED NUMBER NUMBLY OUTBAN OUTBAT OUTBEG OUTBID OUTBOW OUTBOX OUTBUD OUTBUY PUEBLA PUEBLO QUEBEC RUBBED RUBBER RUBBIA RUBBLE RUBBLY RUMBAS RUMBLE RUMBLY SUABLE SUBBED SUNBOW TUBBED TUMBLE TURBAN TURBID TURBOS TURBOT

•U••B•

CUBEBS HUNGBY JUJUBE MUGABE PUTSBY RUNSBY RUSHBY

•U•••B

HUBBUB OUTRIB PUNJAB SUBDEB SUBURB SUPERB SUSANB

••UB••

ANUBIS ARUBAN BAUBLE CHUBBY CLUBBY CLUBUP DAUBED DAUBER DAUBES DOUBLE DOUBLY DOUBTS FLUBUG GRUBBY REUBEN SCUBAS SNUBBY STUBBY UTUBES YOUBET

••U•B•

BLURBS CHUBBY CLUBBY CRUMBS CRUMBY EXURBS FOURBC GRUBBY ITURBI PLUMBO PLUMBS RHUMBA RHUMBS SNUBBY SQUABS SQUIBB SQUIBS STUBBY THUMBS TRUMBO

••U••B

LOUISB SQUIBB

•••UB•

DANUBE EXCUBS HECUBA INCUBI IVTUBE JUJUBE REDUBS REPUBS SCRUBS SHRUBS ZHLUBS

•••U•B

BENUMB RCRUMB SUBURB UNCURB

••••UB

BEDAUB CHERUB HOTTUB HUBBUB INATUB OILRUB SCHLUB STRAUB THEHUB

UC••••

UCLANS

U•C•••

UECKER ULCERS UNCAGE UNCAKE UNCALM UNCAPS UNCASE UNCASK UNCAST UNCHIC UNCIAL UNCLAD UNCLAY UNCLES UNCLIP UNCLOG UNCOIL UNCOLA UNCOOL UNCOOP UNCORE UNCORK UNCUFF UNCURB UNCURL UNCUTE UPCARD UPCAST UPCOIL UPCURL URCHIN

U••C••

UNICED UNICEF UNICES UNOCAL URACIL UTICAN

U•••C•

ULRICH UNDICI UNDOCK UNESCO UNFACT UNLACE UNLOCK UNNICE UNPACK UNPICK UNRACK UNSICK UNTACK UNTUCK UPTICK USANCE USEDCD

U••••C

UNCHIC UNEPIC UNIFIC UNIVAC URALIC URANIC

•UC•••

BUCCAL BUCHAN BUCKED BUCKER BUCKET BUCKLE BUCKUP CUCKOO DUCATS DUCHIN DUCKED DUCKER DUCKIE DUCTAL DUCTED EUCHRE EUCKEN EUCLID KUCHEN LUCENT LUCIAN LUCIDA LUCIEN LUCILE LUCINE LUCITE LUCIUS LUCKED MUCHAS MUCHOF MUCKED MUCKER MUCKUP NUCHAE NUCHAL NUCLEI NUCLEO OUCHES PUCCIS PUCKER RUCHES RUCKED RUCKER RUCKUP RUCKUS SUCCOR SUCHAS SUCKED SUCKER SUCKIN SUCKUP SUCRES TUCANA TUCKED TUCKER TUCKIN TUCSON YUCCAS ZUCKER

•U•C••

BUCCAL BUICKS BUNCHE BUNCHY BUNCOS CUICAS DUBCEK DULCET DUNCAN DUNCES FULCRA HUBCAP JUICED JUICER JUICES JUNCOS LUNCHY MUDCAT MULCTS MUNCHY MUNCIE MURCIA MUSCAT MUSCLE MUSCLY NUECES NUNCIO OUNCES OUTCRY OUTCUT PUCCIS PUNCHY QUACKS QUACKY QUICHE RUNCIE SUCCOR TUSCAN VULCAN YUCCAS

•U••C•

CUBICS CULTCH CURACY CUSACK CUSECS DUROCS EUNICE LUBECK LUKICH LUNACY LUTECE MUNICH MUSICK MUSICS NUANCE OUTACT PUMICE PUTSCH QUENCH QUINCE QUINCY SUMACS SUNOCO TUNICS ZURICH

•U•••C

CULTIC CUPRIC JUDAIC PUBLIC QUEBEC RUBRIC RUNDMC RUSTIC TURKIC

••UC••

BOUCHE CAUCHY CAUCUS CHUCKS CHUCKY CLUCKS CRUCES DEUCED DEUCES EDUCED EDUCES EDUCTS ERUCTS FAUCET FRUCTI GAUCHE GAUCHO GRUCCI LOUCHE PLUCKS PLUCKY POUCHY SAUCED SAUCER SAUCES SHUCKS STUCCO TOUCAN TOUCHE TOUCHY TRUCES TRUCKS

••U•C•

BAUSCH BOUNCE BOUNCY BRUNCH CHURCH CLUTCH CRUNCH CRUTCH DEUTCH GRUCCI HAUNCH JOUNCE JOUNCY LAUNCH PAUNCH POUNCE RAUNCH SLUICE SOURCE STUCCO

••U••C

COURIC FOURBC LAURIC TAURIC

•••UC•

ABDUCE ABDUCT ADDUCE ADDUCT ASMUCH ASSUCH AVOUCH BARUCH CANUCK CROUCH DEDUCE DEDUCT GLOUCS GROUCH INDUCE INDUCT INLUCK MCDUCK NOLUCK REDUCE RELUCT SEDUCE SLOUCH SOMUCH SPRUCE STRUCK UNTUCK ZANUCK

UD••••

UDDERS

U•D•••

UDDERS UNDAMS UNDEAD UNDEEP UNDEFT UNDERS UNDEWY UNDICI UNDIES UNDIMS UNDINE UNDOCK UNDOER UNDOES UNDONE UNDRAW UNDREW UNDSET UNDULY UNDYED UPDART UPDATE UPDIKE UPDIVE UPDOVE

U••D••

UNEDGE UNIDLE UNIDLY USEDCD USEDIN USEDON USEDTO USEDUP

U•••D•
UGANDA
UNBUDS
UNLADE
UNMADE
UNRUDE
UNTIDY
UPENDS
UPSIDE
URSIDS
UVALDE

U••••D
UNAGED
UNAVID
UNAWED
UNAXED
UNBEND
UNBIND
UNBLED
UNBOLD
UNCLAD
UNDEAD
UNDYED
UNFOLD
UNFOND
UNGIRD
UNGLAD
UNHAND
UNHEED
UNHELD
UNHOED
UNHOOD
UNHUED
UNICED
UNIPED
UNIPOD
UNITED
UNKIND
UNLAID
UNLEAD
UNLOAD
UNMOLD
UNOWED
UNPAID
UNREAD
UNRUED
UNSAID
UNSELD
UNSHED
UNSHOD
UNSOLD
UNSUED
UNTIED
UNTOLD
UNTROD
UNUSED
UNVOID
UNWILD
UNWIND
UPBIND
UPCARD
UPFOLD
UPGIRD
UPHELD
UPHOLD
UPLAND
UPLOAD
UPSEND
UPWARD
UPWIND
USEDCD
USERID

•UD•••
AUDIAL
AUDILE
AUDIOS
AUDITS
AUDREY
BUDDED
BUDDER
BUDDHA
BUDGED
BUDGER
BUDGES
BUDGET
BUDGIE
CUDAHY
CUDDLE
CUDDLY
CUDGEL
DUDDLE
DUDEUP
DUDING
DUDISH
DUDLEY
EUDORA
FUDDLE
FUDGED
FUDGER
FUDGES
HUDDIE
HUDDLE
HUDSON
JUDAEA
JUDAIC
JUDEAN
JUDFRY
JUDGED
JUDGES
JUDITH
JUDOKA
JUDSON
KUDROW
KUDZUS
LUDDEN
LUDENS
LUDLOW
LUDLUM
LUDWIG
MUDCAT
MUDDED
MUDDER
MUDDLE
MUDEEL
MUDHEN
MUDPIE
NUDELY
NUDEST
NUDGED
NUDGER
NUDGES
NUDISM
NUDIST
NUDITY
NUDNIK
PUDDLE
PUDDLY
RUDDER
RUDELY
RUDERY
RUDEST
RUDKIN
RUDKUS
RUDMAN
RUDNER
RUDOLF
SUDDEN
SUDOKU
SUDSED
SUDSER
SUDSES
TUDORS

•U•D••
BUDDED
BUDDER
BUDDHA
BULDEO
BUNDLE
BUNDTS
BURDEN
CUDDLE
CUDDLY
CUEDIN
CURDED
CURDLE
DUDDLE
DUMDUM
DUNDAS
DUNDEE
EUSDEN
FUDDLE
FUNDED
FUNDER
GUIDED
GUIDER
GUIDES
GUIDRY
GULDEN
GUNDOG
HUDDIE
HUDDLE
HURDLE
KUNDRY
LUDDEN
LUNDEN
LUNDIS
MUDDED
MUDDER
MUDDLE
MULDER
MURDER
OUTDID
PUDDLE
PUDDLY
PUNDIT
PURDUE
QUADRI
QUIDDE
RUDDER
RUNDLE
RUNDMC
RUNDRY
SUBDEB
SUBDUE
SUDDEN
SUEDED
SUEDES
SUNDAE
SUNDAS
SUNDAY
SUNDER
SUNDOG
SUNDRY
TUNDRA

•U••D•
AUBADE
BUILDS
CUANDO
CUPIDS
CURADS
GUARDS
GUILDS
JUMADA
JURADO
LUANDA
LUCIDA
LUNEDI
MUSTDO
OUTADD
QUIDDE
RUANDA
SUREDO
TUXEDO

•U•••D
AUFOND
AUGEND
AUTOED
BUCKED
BUDDED
BUDGED
BUFFED
BUGGED
BUGLED
BUJOLD
BULGED
BULKED
BULLED
BUMMED
BUMPED
BUNGED
BUNKED
BUNTED
BUOYED
BURIED
BURLED
BURNED
BURPED
BURRED
BUSHED
BUSIED
BUSKED
BUSSED
BUSTED
BUTTED
BUZZED
CUBBED
CUBOID
CUEBID
CUFFED
CULLED
CUNARD
CUPPED
CURBED
CURDED
CURLED
CURRED
CURSED
CURVED
CUSPED
CUSPID
CUSSED
DUBBED
DUCKED
DUCTED
DUELED
DUETED
DUGALD
DUGARD
DULLED
DUMPED
DUNKED
DUNNED
DURNED
DUSKED
DUSTED
EUCLID
FUDGED
FUELED
FUGARD
FUNDED
FUNKED
FUNNED
FURLED
FURRED
FUSSED
FUTZED
FUZZED
GUIDED
GUILED
GULFED
GULLED
GULPED
GUMMED
GUNNED
GUSHED
GUSTED
GUTTED
HUFFED
HUGGED
HULKED
HULLED
HUMMED
HUMPED
HUNTED
HURLED
HUSHED
HUSKED
HUTTED
JUDGED
JUGGED
JUICED
JUMPED
JUNKED
JURIED
JUTTED
LUCKED
LUFFED
LUGGED
LULLED
LUMPED
LUNGED
LURKED
LUSTED
MUCKED
MUDDED
MUFFED
MUGGED
MULLED
MUMMED
MUSHED
MUSSED
NUBBED
NUDGED
NULLED
NUMBED
NURSED
NUTTED
OUSTED
OUTADD
OUTBID
OUTBUD
OUTDID
OUTLED
PUFFED
PULLED
PULPED
PULSED
PUMPED
PUNNED
PUNTED
PUPPED
PUREED
PURGED
PURLED
PURRED
PURSED
PUSHED
PUTRID
PUTTED
QUAKED
QUEUED
QUIRED
QUOTED
RUBBED
RUBIED
RUCKED
RUFFED
RUGGED
RUINED
RUSHED
RUSTED
RUTTED
SUBBED
SUBGOD
SUBLID
SUCKED
SUDSED
SUEDED
SUITED
SULKED
SUMMED
SUNGOD
SUNNED
SUPPED
SURFED
SURGED
SUSSED
TUBBED
TUCKED
TUFTED
TUGGED
TURBID
TURFED
TURGID
TURNED
TUSKED
TUTTED
TUTUED
YUKKED

••UD••
ALUDEL
ALUDRA
AOUDAD
BLUDGE
BOUDIN
BRUDER
CAUDAD
CAUDAL
CIUDAD
CRUDDY
CRUDER
CRUDES
CRUDUP
DAUDET
DRUDGE
ELUDED
ELUDER
ELUDES
ETUDES
EXUDED
EXUDES
FEUDAL
FEUDED
FOUDRE
GOUDAS
GRUDGE
HOUDON
KLUDGE
KLUDGY
LAUDED
LAUDER
LOUDEN
LOUDER
LOUDLY
LOUDON
POUDRE
PRUDES
SAUDIS
SLUDGE
SLUDGY
SMUDGE
SMUDGY
STUDIO
STUDLY
TRUDGE
YOUDIG

••U•D•
BOUNDS
COULDA
COULDI
CRUDDY
DRUIDS
FLUIDS
FOUNDS
GOURDE
GOURDS
GRUNDY
HOUNDS
HOUNDY
KAUNDA
MAUNDY
MOULDS
MOULDY
MOUNDS
POUNDS
ROUNDS
SOUNDS
SQUADS
SQUIDS
STURDY
WOULDA
WOUNDS
ZOUNDS

••U••D
ABUSED
AMUSED
AOUDAD
AZURED
BRUXED
CAUDAD
CAUSED
CHUTED
CIUDAD
DAUBED
DEUCED
DOUSED
EDUARD
EDUCED
ELUARD
ELUDED
ELUTED
ENURED
EQUOID
EXUDED
FEUDED
FLUTED
FLUXED
FOULED
FOURAD
GAUGED
GOUGED
GOUNOD
HAULED
HOUSED
INURED
LAUDED
LOUSED
MAULED
MOUSED
PAUSED
PLUMED
POUFED
POURED
POUTED
PRUNED
REUNED
REUSED
ROUGED
ROUSED
ROUTED
SAUCED
SOURED
SOUSED
SPUMED
STUPID
TOURED
TOUTED
UNUSED

•••UD•
ALLUDE
CLAUDE
CLOUDS
CLOUDY
DELUDE
DENUDE
ESCUDO
FALUDI
FRAUDS
ILLUDE
MENUDO
NERUDA
PSEUDO
PSEUDS
STJUDE
UNBUDS
UNRUDE
YEHUDI
YODUDE

•••U•D
ABOUND
ABSURD
ARGUED
AROUND
DEFUND
EDMUND
EMQUAD
ENDUED
ENQUAD
ENSUED
FECUND
FREUND
GERUND
GROUND
ICOULD
IMBUED
INDUED
ISSUED
IWOULD
JOCUND
LIQUID
MSQUAD
OBTUND
OSMUND
PEQUOD
PIQUED
QUEUED
RECUED
REFUND
ROGUED
ROTUND
SEGUED
SHOULD
SIGURD
TABUED
TUTUED
UNHUED
UNRUED
UNSUED
VALUED
VOGUED

••••UD
AIRBUD
ARTAUD
ASTRUD
ATSTUD
DISBUD
EARBUD
MARAUD
OHCRUD
OLERUD
ORTRUD
OUTBUD
REDBUD
SHROUD
STROUD
TALMUD

UE••••
UECKER

U•E•••
UNEASE
UNEASY
UNEDGE
UNEPIC
UNESCO
UNEVEN
UNEVIL
UPENDS
USEDCD
USEDIN
USEDON
USEDTO
USEDUP
USEFOR
USEFUL
USENET
USERID
USESIN
USESON
USESUP
USETAX
UVEOUS

U••E••
UBIETY
UDDERS
ULCERS
UMBELS
UMBERS
UNBELT
UNBEND
UNBENT
UNDEAD
UNDEEP
UNDEFT
UNDERS
UNDEWY
UNFELT
UNHEED
UNHELD
UNHELM
UNHERO
UNHEWN
UNKEPT
UNLEAD
UNLEAF
UNLEAN
UNLEFT
UNLENT
UNLESS
UNMEET
UNMESH
UNMEWS
UNNEAT
UNPEEL
UNPEGS
UNPENS
UNPENT
UNREAD
UNREAL
UNREEL
UNRENT
UNREST
UNSEAL
UNSEAM
UNSEAT
UNSEEN
UNSELD
UNSELL
UNSENT
UNSERE
UNSEWN
UNSEWS
UNSEXY
UNVEIL
UNWELL
UNWEPT
UPBEAR
UPBEAT
UPHEAP
UPHELD
UPHERE
UPKEEP
UPLEAP
UPNEXT
UPPERS
UPREAR
UPSEND
UPSENT
UPSETS
UPTEAR
UPWELL
URAEUS
URGENT
URGEON
URGERS
URTEXT
USHERS
USNEWS
UTTERS

U•••E•
UECKER
UGLIER
UGLIES
UKASES
ULSTER
UNAGED
UNAWED
UNAXED
UNBLED
UNCLES
UNDEEP
UNDIES
UNDOER
UNDOES
UNDREW
UNDSET
UNDYED
UNEVEN
UNFREE
UNGUES
UNHEED
UNHOED
UNHUED
UNICED
UNICEF
UNICES
UNIPED
UNISEX
UNITED
UNITER
UNITES
UNMEET
UNOPEN
UNOWED
UNPEEL
UNREEL
UNRUED
UNSEEN
UNSHED
UNSKEW
UNSTEP
UNSUED
UNTIED
UNTIER
UNTIES
UNUSED
UPGREW
UPKEEP
UPOVER
UPSTEP
USAGES
USENET
USOPEN
USURER
UTUBES

U••••E
UGARTE
UGSOME
ULLAGE
UMBRAE
UMPIRE
UNABLE
UNBALE
UNBARE
UNCAGE
UNCAKE
UNCASE
UNCORE
UNCUTE
UNDINE
UNDONE
UNEASE
UNEDGE
UNFILE
UNFINE
UNFREE
UNGLUE
UNHALE
UNHIRE
UNIATE
UNIDLE
UNIQUE
UNLACE
UNLADE
UNLIKE
UNLIVE
UNMADE
UNMAKE
UNMATE
UNNICE
UNPALE
UNPILE
UNPURE
UNRIFE
UNRIPE
UNROBE
UNROPE
UNROVE
UNRUDE
UNSAFE
UNSAGE
UNSERE
UNSHOE
UNSOLE
UNSORE
UNSURE
UNTAME
UNTAPE
UNTRUE
UNTUNE
UNWISE
UNWOVE
UNYOKE
UNZONE
UPDATE
UPDIKE
UPDIVE
UPDOVE
UPGAZE
UPHERE
UPHOVE
UPLATE
UPPILE
UPRATE
UPRISE
UPROSE
UPSIDE
UPSIZE
UPTAKE
UPTIME
UPTORE
URBANE
URSINE
USABLE
USANCE
USHAPE
UVALDE
UVALUE
UVULAE

•UE•••
BUENAS
BUENOS
CUEBID
CUEDIN
CUEING
CUESIN
CUESTA
CUESUP
CUETIP
DUELED
DUELER
DUELLO
DUENAS
DUENNA
DUENOS
DUESSA
DUETED
DUETTI
DUETTO
FUEGOS
FUELED
FUELER
FUELUP
GUELPH
GUERRE
GUESTS
HUEVOS
JUEGOS
JUEVES
LUELLA
MUESLI
NUECES
NUEVES
PUEBLA
PUEBLO
PUENTE
PUENZO
PUERTO
QUEASY
QUEBEC
QUEENE
QUEENS
QUEERS
QUELER
QUELLS
QUEMOY
QUENCH
QUESOS
QUESTS
QUEUED
QUEUER
QUEUES
QUEZON
RUEFUL
SUEANE
SUEANN
SUEDED
SUEDES
SUEFOR
SUENOS

•U•E••
AUGEAN
AUGEAS
AUGEND
AUGERS
AUTEUR
BUREAU
BURETS
BUTENE
BUTEOS
BUYERS
CUBEBS
CUBERS
CULETS
CUNEAL
CUPELS
CURERS
CURETS
CUSECS
CUTELY
CUTEST
CUTESY
CUTEYS
CUVEES
DUDEUP
DUPERS
DUPERY
DURESS
DUVETS
EUGENE
EULESS
EUREKA
FUMEAT
FUMERS
FUSEES
HUBERT
HUGELY
HUGEST
HUMERI
JUDEAN
JULEPS
JUNEAU
LUBECK
LUCENT
LUDENS
LUGERS
LUMENS
LUNEDI
LUREIN
LURENE
LURERS
LUTECE
MUDEEL
MULETA
MULEYS
MUNERA
MUSEES
MUSEON
MUSEOS
MUSERS
MUSEUM
MUTELY
MUTEST
NUDELY
NUDEST
NUGENT
NUMERO
OUSELS
OUTEAT
OUZELS
PULERS
PUREED
PUREES
PURELY

PUREST QUEENE QUEENS QUEERS QUIETS RUBELS RUBENS RUDELY RUDERY RUDEST RULEON RULERS RULETH RUPEES RUPERT SUPERB SUPERG SUPERS SUREAM SUREDO SUREIS SURELY SUREOF SUREST SURETE SURETY TUBERS TUMEFY TUNEIN TUNERS TUNETO TUNEUP TUPELO TUREEN TUTEES TUXEDO

•U••E•

AUBREY AUDREY AUKLET AUNTEM AUSPEX AUSTEN AUSTER AUTOED BUBKES BUCKED BUCKER BUCKET BUDDED BUDDER BUDGED BUDGER BUDGES BUDGET BUFFED BUFFER BUFFET BUGGED BUGLED BUGLER BUGLES BULDEO BULGED BULGES BULKED BULLED

BULLET BULWER BUMLEG BUMMED BUMMER BUMPED BUMPER BUNGED BUNGEE BUNKED BUNKER BUNSEN BUNTED BUNTER BUNUEL BUOYED BUPKES BURDEN BURGEE BURGER BURIED BURIER BURIES BURLED BURLER BURLEY BURNED BURNER BURNET BURNEY BURPED BURPEE BURRED BUSHED BUSHEL BUSHER BUSHES BUSIED BUSIER BUSIES BUSKED BUSKER BUSMEN BUSSED BUSSES BUSTED BUSTER BUTLER BUTTED BUTTER BUTTES BUTYET BUZZED BUZZER BUZZES CUBBED CUDGEL CUFFED CULLED CULLEN CULLER CULLET CUMBER CUORES CUPPED CURBED CURDED CURFEW

CURIES CURLED CURLER CURLEW CURLEY CURRED CURSED CURSER CURSES CURTER CURVED CURVES CURVET CUSPED CUSSED CUSSER CUSSES CUSTER CUTIES CUTLER CUTLET CUTTER CUVEES CUVIER CUYLER DUBBED DUBBER DUBCEK DUCKED DUCKER DUCTED DUDLEY DUELED DUELER DUETED DUFFEL DUFFER DULCET DULLEA DULLED DULLER DULLES DUMBER DUMPED DUMPER DUNCES DUNDEE DUNKED DUNKER DUNNED DUNNER DUPLEX DURFEY DURNED DURYEA DUSKED DUSTED DUSTER DUTIES EUBOEA EUCKEN EUPNEA EUSDEN FUDGED FUDGER FUDGES FUELED FUELER

FUGUES FUHRER FULLER FUMIER FUNDED FUNDER FUNKED FUNNED FUNNEL FURIES FURLED FURRED FURZES FUSEES FUSSED FUSSER FUSSES FUTZED FUTZES FUZZED FUZZES GUIDED GUIDER GUIDES GUILED GUILES GUINEA GUISES GULDEN GULFED GULLED GULLET GULPED GULPER GUMBEL GUMMED GUNMEN GUNNED GUNNER GUNSEL GUNTER GURLEY GURNEE GURNEY GUSHED GUSHER GUSHES GUSSET GUSTED GUTTED GUTTER HUBLEY HUFFED HUGGED HUGGER HUGHES HULKED HULLED HULLER HUMBER HUMMED HUMMEL HUMMER HUMPED HUMVEE HUNGER HUNKER HUNLEY

HUNTED HUNTER HURLED HURLER HURLEY HURTER HUSHED HUSHES HUSKED HUSKER HUSSEY HUTTED HUXLEY JUAREZ JUDAEA JUDGED JUDGES JUEVES JUGGED JUICED JUICER JUICES JULIEN JULIET JUMPED JUMPER JUNGER JUNKED JUNKER JUNKET JURIED JURIES JUSTER JUTTED KUBLER KUCHEN KUMMEL KUNZEL LUBBER LUCIEN LUCKED LUDDEN LUFFED LUGGED LUGGER LULLED LULLER LUMBER LUMLEY LUMPED LUMPEN LUMPER LUNDEN LUNGED LUNGER LUNGES LUNKER LURKED LURKER LURKEY LUSHER LUSHES LUSTED LUSTER LUTHER LUTZES MUCKED MUCKER

MUDDED MUDDER MUDEEL MUDHEN MUFFED MUFFET MUGGED MUGGER MULDER MULLED MULLER MULLET MUMMED MUMMER MUPPET MURDER MURIEL MURRES MUSEES MUSHED MUSHER MUSHES MUSKET MUSSED MUSSEL MUSSES MUSSET MUSTER MUTTER MUTUEL NUBBED NUBBER NUCLEI NUCLEO NUDGED NUDGER NUDGES NUECES NUEVES NUGGET NULLED NUMBED NUMBER NUNGEN NURSED NURSER NURSES NUTLET NUTMEG NUTTED NUTTER OUCHES OUIMET OUNCES OUSTED OUSTER OUTBEG OUTIES OUTJET OUTLED OUTLET OUTSEE OUTSET PUCKER PUFFED PUFFER PULLED PULLER

PULLET PULLEY PULPED PULPER PULSED PULSES PULVER PUMMEL PUMPED PUMPER PUNIER PUNKER PUNNED PUNNER PUNTED PUNTER PUPPED PUPPET PUREED PUREES PURGED PURGES PURLED PURRED PURRER PURSED PURSER PURSES PURVEY PUSHED PUSHER PUSHES PUSSES PUTNEY PUTTED PUTTEE PUTTER QUAKED QUAKER QUAKES QUALES QUAVER QUEBEC QUELER QUEUED QUEUER QUEUES QUIRED QUIRES QUIVER QUOTED QUOTEE QUOTER QUOTES RUBBED RUBBER RUBIED RUBIES RUBLES RUBLEV RUCHES RUCKED RUCKER RUDDER RUDNER RUFFED RUGGED RUINED

RUINER RULIER RUMMER RUNLET RUNNEL RUNNER RUPEES RUSHED RUSHEE RUSHER RUSHES RUSSEL RUSSES RUSSET RUSTED RUTGER RUTTED RUTTER SUAVER SUBBED SUBDEB SUBLET SUBNET SUBSEA SUBSET SUCKED SUCKER SUCRES SUDDEN SUDSED SUDSER SUDSES SUEDED SUEDES SUFFER SUITED SUITES SULKED SULKER SULLEN SUMMED SUMMER SUMNER SUMTER SUNDER SUNKEN SUNNED SUNSET SUPPED SUPPER SURFED SURFER SURGED SURGES SURREY SURVEY SUSSED SUSSES SUSSEX SUTTER SUZIEQ TUBBED TUCKED TUCKER TUFFET TUFTED TUGGED TUGGER

TULLES TUNNEL TUNNEY TUPPER TUQUES TUREEN TURFED TURKEY TURNED TURNER TURRET TUSHES TUSKED TUSKER TUSSES TUTEES TUTTED TUTUED WUSSES YUKKED YUTZES ZUCKER

•U•••E

AUBADE AUDILE AUGITE AUNTIE AURATE AUSSIE BUBBLE BUCKLE BUDGIE BULLAE BUMBLE BUNCHE BUNDLE BUNGEE BUNGLE BURBLE BURGEE BURGLE BURNIE BURPEE BURSAE BUSTLE BUTANE BUTENE CUBAGE CUDDLE CUPULE CURARE CURATE CURDLE CURIAE CURITE DUARTE DUBOSE DUCKIE DUDDLE DUFFLE DUNDEE EUCHRE EUGENE EUNICE EUROPE FUDDLE FUISSE

FUMBLE FURORE FUSILE FUTILE FUTURE GUERRE GUNITE GURGLE GURNEE GUZZLE HUBBLE HUDDIE HUDDLE HUGHIE HUMANE HUMBLE HUMVEE HURDLE HURTLE HUSTLE HUTONE JUGGLE JUJUBE JUMBLE JUNGLE JUNKIE JUSQUE JUSTME KURILE LUCILE LUCINE LUCITE LUNATE LUPINE LUPONE LURENE LUSTRE LUTECE LUXATE MUDDLE MUDPIE MUFFLE MUGABE MUGGLE MUMBLE MUNCIE MUNROE MURINE MUSCLE MUSKIE MUTATE MUZZLE NUANCE NUBBLE NUBILE NUCHAE NUTATE NUZZLE OUTAGE OUTATE OUTAWE OUTLIE OUTSEE OUTVIE PUDDLE PUENTE PUGGLE PUMICE

PUNKIE PUPATE PURDUE PURFLE PURLIE PURPLE PURSUE PUTTEE PUZZLE QUAKIE QUARTE QUATRE QUAYLE QUEENE QUICHE QUIDDE QUINCE QUINTE QUINZE QUOQUE QUOTEE RUBBLE RUFFLE RUMBLE RUMPLE RUNCIE RUNDLE RUSHEE RUSTLE RUTHIE RUTILE SUABLE SUBDUE SUBTLE SUEANE SUISSE SUNDAE SUPINE SUPPLE SURETE SUTURE TUBAGE TUBATE TUBULE TUILLE TULANE TULARE TUMBLE TURTLE TUSHIE TUSSLE YUPPIE

••UE••

AZUELA BLUELY BLUEOX BLUEST BLUESY BLUETS CLUEIN CLUERS CRUETS EKUELE FLUENT GLUEON GLUERS GLUETO GRUELS IGUESS PRUETT SQUEAK SQUEAL TRUEST TRUETO TRUEUP

••U•E•

ABUSED ABUSER ABUSES ACUMEN ACUTER ACUTES ALUDEL AMULET AMUSED AMUSER AMUSES AZURED AZURES BAUMER BOULES BOULEZ BRUDER BRUGES BRULEE BRUMEL BRUMES BRUNEI BRUNET BRUTES BRUXED BRUXES CAUSED CAUSER CAUSES CHUTED CHUTES COULEE COUPES COUTER CRUCES CRUDER CRUDES CRUSES CRUXES DAUBED DAUBER DAUBES DAUDET DEUCED DEUCES DEUTER DOURER DOUSED DOUSER DOUSES DOUZES DRUPES DRUSES DRUZES EDUCED EDUCES EGUREN ELUDED

ELUDER ELUDES ELUTED ELUTES ENURED ENURES ETUDES EXUDED EXUDES FAUCET FAUTES FAUVES FEUDED FLUKES FLUKEY FLUMES FLUTED FLUTER FLUTES FLUXED FLUXES FOULED FOULER FOUREE GAUGED GAUGER GAUGES GAUZES GLUIER GLUTEI GLUTEN GLUTES GOUGED GOUGER GOUGES GOULET HAULED HAULER HEURES HEUSEN HOUSED HOUSES INURED INURES JAUNES JAURES JOULES KRUGER LAUDED LAUDER LAUPER LAUREL LAUREN LAUREY LAUTER LOUDEN LOUDER LOUIES LOUPES LOUSED LOUSES LOUVER MAULED MAULER MAUMEE MAUSER MAUVES MOUSED

MOUSER MOUSES MOUSEY NAUSEA NAUTES NEUTER NGUYEN NOUMEA ONUSES OPUSES OVULES PAULEY PAUPER PAUSED PAUSER PAUSES PCUSER PIUTES PLUIES PLUMED PLUMES PLUSES POUFED POULES POURED POURER POUTED POUTER PRUDES PRUNED PRUNER PRUNES REUBEN REUNED REUNER REUNES REUSED REUSER REUSES REUTER ROUGED ROUGES ROUSED ROUSER ROUSES ROUTED ROUTER ROUTES SAUCED SAUCER SAUCES SAUTES SOUPER SOURED SOURER SOUSED SOUSES SOUTER SPUMED SPUMES STUPES TAUPES TAUTEN TAUTER TOUPEE TOURED TOURER TOUTED

TOUTER TRUCES UNUSED USURER UTUBES YOUBET YOUSEE

••U••E

ACUATE ALULAE AQUAKE AVULSE BAUBLE BEURRE BLUDGE BOUCHE BOUFFE BOUNCE BOURKE BOURNE BOURSE BRUISE BRULEE COULEE COUPLE COURSE CRUISE CRUSOE DOUANE DOUBLE DRUDGE EKUELE ELUATE EQUATE EQUINE EVULSE FAUNAE FLUTIE FOUDRE FOUREE FRUNZE GAUCHE GAULLE GLURGE GOURDE GRUDGE GRUNGE JOUNCE KLUDGE LAURIE LEUTZE LOUCHE LOUISE LOUNGE LOUVRE MAUMEE MOUSSE NTUPLE OEUVRE PLUNGE POUDRE POUNCE POUSSE REURGE ROURKE SCURVE SLUDGE

SLUICE
SMUDGE
SOURCE
SQUARE
SQUIRE
TOUCHE
TOUPEE
TOUSLE
TRUDGE
UVULAE
YOUSEE

•••UE•
ARGUED
ARGUER
ARGUES
AROUET
BREUER
BUNUEL
DEFUEL
DROUET
ENDUED
ENDUES
ENSUED
ENSUES
FRAUEN
FUGUES
GIGUES
IMBUED
IMBUES
INDUED
INDUES
ISSUED
ISSUER
ISSUES
LEMUEL
MANUEL
MCKUEN
MIGUEL
MINUET
MUTUEL
PIQUED
PIQUES
PIQUET
QUEUED
QUEUER
QUEUES
RAQUEL
RECUED
RECUES
REFUEL
REVUES
ROGUED
ROGUES
SAMUEL
SEGUED
SEGUES
SEQUEL
TABUED
TOGUES
TOQUES
TUQUES
TUTUED
UNGUES
UNHUED
UNRUED
UNSUED
VAGUER
VALUED
VALUER
VALUES
VENUES
VOGUED
VOGUER
VOGUES

•••U•E
ABDUCE
ABJURE
ACCUSE
ADDUCE
ADJURE
ALLUDE
ALLURE
AMPULE
AROUSE
ASPURE
ASSUME
ASSURE
ASTUTE
ATTUNE
BEMUSE
BESURE
BLOUSE
BODUKE
CANUTE
CAYUSE
CLAUDE
CLAUSE
CONURE
CREUSE
CROUSE
CROUTE
CUPULE
DANUBE
DEDUCE
DEDUVE
DEFUSE
DEJURE
DELUDE
DELUGE
DELUXE
DEMURE
DENUDE
DEPUTE
DETUNE
DILUTE
DISUSE
EFFUSE
EMEUTE
ENDURE
ENDUSE
ENSURE
EXCUSE
EXHUME
FERULE
FIGURE
FUTURE
GROUSE
ILLUDE
ILLUME
ILLUSE
IMMUNE
IMMURE
IMPURE
IMPUTE
IMSURE
INCUSE
INDUCE
INFUSE
INHUME
INJUNE
INJURE
INOUYE
INSURE
INTUNE
IVTUBE
JARULE
JEJUNE
JUJUBE
LADUKE
LEGUME
LETUSE
LOBULE
MANURE
MANUTE
MATURE
MIFUNE
MINUTE
MISUSE
MODULE
NATURE
NODULE
NONUSE
OBTUSE
OGAUGE
OHSURE
OSCULE
PAIUTE
PARURE
PERUKE
PERUSE
RASURE
REBUKE
RECURE
RECUSE
REDUCE
REFUGE
REFUSE
REFUTE
RELUME
REPUTE
RESUME
RETUNE
SALUTE
SCOUPE
SECURE
SEDUCE
SOLUTE
SPOUSE
SPRUCE
STJUDE
STLUKE
SUTURE
TENURE
TRIUNE
TROUPE
TUBULE
UNCUTE
UNPURE
UNRUDE
UNSURE
UNTUNE
VELURE
VENULE
VOLUME
VOLUTE
YODUDE
ZONULE

••••UE
ACCRUE
AVENUE
BANQUE
BARQUE
BASQUE
BISQUE
BRAQUE
BROGUE
CASQUE
CHEQUE
CINQUE
CIRQUE
CLAQUE
CLIQUE
DROGUE
EMBRUE
EPOQUE
FESCUE
FONDUE
IMBRUE
INBLUE
JUSQUE
LEAGUE
LONGUE
MANQUE
MARQUE
MASQUE
MISCUE
MORGUE
MOSQUE
MRBLUE
OPAQUE
PERDUE
PLAGUE
PLAQUE
PRAGUE
PREVUE
PURDUE
PURSUE
QUOQUE
REGLUE
RESCUE
RISQUE
RVALUE
SACQUE
SESSUE
SOTRUE
STATUE
SUBDUE
TISSUE
TONGUE
TORQUE
UNGLUE
UNIQUE
UNTRUE
UVALUE
VENDUE
VIRTUE

U•F•••
UNFACT
UNFAIR
UNFELT
UNFILE
UNFINE
UNFIRM
UNFITS
UNFLAT
UNFOLD
UNFOND
UNFORK
UNFOUL
UNFOXY
UNFREE
UNFULL
UNFURL
UPFLOW
UPFOLD
USFLAG

U••F••
UNIFIC
URNFUL
USEFOR
USEFUL

U•••F•
UGLIFY
UNCUFF
UNDEFT
UNHAFT
UNLEFT
UNRIFE
UNSAFE
UNSOFT
UPLIFT
UPWAFT

U••••F
UNCUFF
UNICEF
UNLEAF
UNROOF

•UF•••
AUFAIT
AUFOND
BUFFAY
BUFFED
BUFFER
BUFFET
BUFFON
BUFFOS
BUFFUP
CUFFED
DUFFEL
DUFFER
DUFFLE
DUFFYS
GUFFAW
HUFFED
LUFFED
MUFASA
MUFFED
MUFFET
MUFFIN
MUFFLE
MUFTIS
PUFFED
PUFFER
PUFFIN
PUFFUP
RUFFED
RUFFLE
RUFFLY
RUFOUS
SUFFER
SUFFIX
SUFISM
TUFFET
TUFTED
TUFTSU

•U•F••
BUFFAY
BUFFED
BUFFER
BUFFET
BUFFON
BUFFOS
BUFFUP
CUBFAN
CUFFED
CUPFUL
CURFEW
DUFFEL
DUFFER
DUFFLE
DUFFYS
DUGFOR
DURFEY
FULFIL
FUNFUR
GUFFAW
GULFED
GUNFOR
HUFFED
JUDFRY
JUGFUL
LUFFED
MUFFED
MUFFET
MUFFIN
MUFFLE
MUGFUL
OUTFIT
OUTFLY
OUTFOR
OUTFOX
PUFFED
PUFFER
PUFFIN
PUFFUP
PURFLE
QUAFFS
RUEFUL
RUFFED
RUFFLE
RUFFLY
RUNFOR
SUEFOR
SUFFER
SUFFIX
SULFAS
SULFUR
SUNFAN
SURFED
SURFER
SURFIN
TUBFUL
TUFFET
TURFED

•U••F•
AURIFY
BUGOFF
BUYOFF
CUTOFF
KUNGFU
PURIFY
PUTOFF
QUAFFS
RUBIFY
RUBOFF
RUNOFF
TUMEFY

•U•••F
BUGOFF
BUYOFF
CUTOFF
FULLOF
MUCHOF
PUTOFF
RUBOFF
RUDOLF
RUNOFF
SUREOF

••UF••
BLUFFO
BLUFFS
BOUFFE
CHUFFS
CHUFFY
FLUFFS
FLUFFY
KOUFAX
POUFED
POUFFY
SCUFFS
SNUFFS
SNUFFY
STUFFS
STUFFY

••U•F•
BLUFFO
BLUFFS
BOUFFE
CHUFFS
CHUFFY
FLUFFS
FLUFFY
POUFFY
SCUFFS
SCURFY
SMURFS
SNUFFS
SNUFFY
STUFFS
STUFFY

••U••F
DOURIF
YOUSUF

•••UF•
ARGUFY
REBUFF
SCRUFF
UNCUFF

•••U•F
ENGULF
INGULF
REBUFF
RETURF
SCRUFF
UNCUFF

••••UF
STAPUF
YOUSUF

UG••••
UGANDA
UGARTE
UGGAMS
UGLIER
UGLIES
UGLIFY
UGLILY
UGSOME

U•G•••
UGGAMS
UNGAGS
UNGAMY
UNGAVA
UNGILT
UNGIRD
UNGIRT
UNGLAD
UNGLIB
UNGLUE
UNGRIP
UNGUAL
UNGUES
UNGUIS
UNGULA
UPGAZE
UPGIRD
UPGIRT
UPGREW
UPGROW
URGENT
URGEON
URGERS
URGING

U••G••
UNAGED
USAGES

U•••G•
UBANGI
ULLAGE
UNBAGS
UNCAGE
UNEDGE
UNGAGS
UNNIGH
UNPEGS
UNRIGS
UNSAGE
UNWIGS

U••••G
UMPING
UNCLOG
UNHUNG
UNPLUG
UNRUNG
UNSMUG
UNSNAG
UNSNUG
UNSUNG
UNTRIG
UPPING
URGING
USFLAG
USHING

•UG•••
AUGEAN
AUGEAS
AUGEND
AUGERS
AUGHTS
AUGITE
AUGURS
AUGURY
AUGUST
BUGAKU
BUGBOY
BUGGED
BUGLED
BUGLER
BUGLES
BUGOFF
BUGOUT
DUGALD
DUGARD
DUGFOR
DUGONG
DUGOUT
EUGENE
FUGARD
FUGATO
FUGUES
GUGINO
HUGELY
HUGEST
HUGGED
HUGGER
HUGHES
HUGHIE
JUGFUL
JUGGED
JUGGLE
LUGERS
LUGGED
LUGGER
LUGING
LUGLIO
LUGNUT
LUGOSI
LUGOUT
MUGABE
MUGFUL
MUGGED
MUGGER
MUGGLE
NUGENT
NUGGET
OUGHTA
OUGHTS
PUGGLE
RUGGED
RUGRAT
SUGARS
SUGARY
TUGGED
TUGGER
TUGRIK
TUGSAT
TUGSON

•U•G••
BUDGED
BUDGER
BUDGES
BUDGET
BUDGIE
BUGGED
BULGAR
BULGED
BULGES
BULGUR
BUNGAY
BUNGED
BUNGEE
BUNGLE
BURGEE
BURGER
BURGHS
BURGLE
BURGOO
BURGOS
CUDGEL
FUDGED
FUDGER
FUDGES
FUEGOS
FUNGAL
FUNGUS
GUNGHO
GURGLE
HUGGED
HUGGER
HUNGBY
HUNGER
HUNGIN
HUNGON
HUNGRY
HUNGUP
JUDGED
JUDGES
JUEGOS
JUGGED
JUGGLE
JUNGER
JUNGLE
JUNGLY
KUNGFU
LUGGED
LUGGER
LUNGED
LUNGER
LUNGES
MUGGED
MUGGER
MUGGLE
NUDGED
NUDGER
NUDGES
NUGGET
NUNGEN
OUTGAS
OUTGUN
PUGGLE
PURGED
PURGES
QUAGGA
QUAGGY
RUGGED
RUNGIN
RUNGUP
RUTGER
SUBGOD
SUBGUM
SUNGOD
SUNGTO
SURGED
SURGES
TUGGED
TUGGER
TURGID
VULGAR
VULGUS

•U••G•
AURIGA
CUBAGE
EULOGY
GULAGS
OUTAGE
QUAGGA
QUAGGY
TUBAGE
ZUNIGA

•U•••G
BUMLEG
BUSING
BUYING
CUBING
CUEING
CURING
DUDING
DUGONG
DUKING
DUPING
DURING
FUMING
FUSING
GUNDOG
GUYING
HUMBUG
HUSING
JUKING
LUBING
LUDWIG
LUGING
LURING
MUSING
MUTING
NUKING
NUTMEG
OUTBEG
OUTING
OUTRIG
PULING
QUAHOG
RULING
SUNDOG
SUPERG
TUBING
TUNING
TURING
YUTANG

••UG••
BOUGHS
BOUGHT
BRUGES
CAUGHT
COUGAR
COUGHS
DOUGAL
DOUGHS
DOUGHY
FOUGHT
FRUGAL
GAUGED
GAUGER
GAUGES
GIUGNO
GOUGED
GOUGER
GOUGES
KRUGER
LAUGHS
NAUGHT
NOUGAT
NOUGHT
PLUGIN
PLUGUP
ROUGED
ROUGES
ROUGHS
SLUGGO
SMUGLY
SNUGLI
SNUGLY
SOUGHT
TAUGHT
TOUGHS
TOUGHY
VAUGHN

••U•G•
BLUDGE
BOURGS
DRUDGE
GLURGE
GRUDGE
GRUNGE
GRUNGY
KLUDGE
KLUDGY
LOUNGE
PLUNGE
REURGE
SLUDGE
SLUDGY
SLUGGO
SMUDGE
SMUDGY
TRUDGE

••U••G
BLUING
CLUING
FLUBUG
GLUING
GRUING
SLUING
TAUROG
TRUING
YOUDIG

•••UG•
AAAUGH
BELUGA
BROUGH
CAYUGA
CHOUGH
CLOUGH
DEBUGS
DELUGE
DELUGG
ENOUGH
IMPUGN
MCHUGH
OGAUGE
OPPUGN
PLOUGH
REFUGE
REPUGN
SHRUGS
SLOUGH
THOUGH
TROUGH
VWBUGS

•••U•G
COBURG
DELUGG
DRJUNG
REHUNG
SPRUNG
STRUNG
UNHUNG
UNRUNG
UNSUNG

••••UG
BEDBUG
BIGHUG
FLUBUG
HUMBUG
INARUG
RAGRUG
UNPLUG
UNSMUG
UNSNUG

UH••••
UHAULS
UHLANS

U•H•••
UNHAFT
UNHAIR
UNHALE
UNHAND
UNHASP
UNHATS
UNHAZY
UNHEED
UNHELD
UNHELM
UNHERO
UNHEWN
UNHIRE
UNHOED
UNHOLY
UNHOOD
UNHOOK
UNHUED
UNHULL
UNHUNG
UNHUNH
UNHURT
UNHUSK
UPHEAP
UPHELD
UPHERE
UPHILL
UPHOLD
UPHOVE
USHAPE
USHERS
USHING
UTHANT

U••H••
UNCHIC
UNSHED
UNSHIP
UNSHOD
UNSHOE
UNSHUT
UNTHAW
UPSHAW
UPSHOT
URCHIN
UTAHAN
UTAHNS

U•••H•
UPJOHN

U••••H
ULRICH
UNHUNH
UNLASH
UNLUSH
UNMESH
UNNIGH
UNPOSH
UNRASH
UNWISH
UPPISH
UPRUSH

•UH•••
FUHRER

•U•H••
AUGHTS
AUTHOR
BUCHAN
BUSHED
BUSHEL
BUSHER
BUSHES
BUSHWA
BUTHOW
CUSHAW
DUCHIN
DUNHAM
DURHAM
EUCHRE
GUSHED
GUSHER
GUSHES
HUGHES
HUGHIE
HUSHED
HUSHES
HUSHUP
KUCHEN
LUSHER
LUSHES
LUSHLY
LUTHER
LUTHOR
MUCHAS
MUCHOF
MUDHEN
MUSHED
MUSHER
MUSHES
NUCHAE
NUCHAL
OUCHES
OUGHTA
OUGHTS
OUTHIT
PUSHED
PUSHER
PUSHES
PUSHIN
PUSHIT
PUSHON
PUSHUP
QUAHOG
RUCHES
RUSHAT
RUSHBY
RUSHED
RUSHEE
RUSHER
RUSHES
RUSHIN
RUSHTO
RUTHIE
SUCHAS
SUNHAT
SUSHIS
TURHAN
TUSHES
TUSHIE

•U••H•
BUDDHA

BUNCHE
BUNCHY
BUQSHA
BURGHS
BUTWHO
BUTWHY
CUDAHY
GUNGHO
GUNSHY
GURKHA
HUMPHS
LUNCHY
LUNTHA
MUNCHY
MURPHY
PUNCHY
QUICHE
SURAHS

•U•••H

CULTCH
DUDISH
DULUTH
GUELPH
GULLAH
HUPPAH
HURRAH
HUZZAH
JUDITH
LUKICH
MULISH
MULLAH
MUNICH
PUNISH
PUTSCH
QUENCH
RULETH
RUPIAH
ZURICH

••UH••

CHUHSI

••U•H•

BOUCHE
BOUGHS
BOUGHT
BRUSHY
CAUCHY
CAUGHT
COUGHS
DOUGHS
DOUGHY
FOUGHT
GAUCHE
GAUCHO
KYUSHU
LAUGHS
LOUCHE
MOUTHS
MOUTHY
NAUGHT
NOUGHT
PLUSHY
POUCHY
ROUGHS
SLUSHY
SOUGHT
SOUTHS
TAUGHT
TOUCHE
TOUCHY
TOUGHS
TOUGHY
TRUTHS
VAUGHN
YOUTHS

••U••H

AGUISH
BAUSCH
BEULAH
BLUISH
BRUNCH
CHURCH
CLUTCH
CRUNCH
CRUTCH
DEUTCH
FLUISH
FOURTH
HAUNCH
LAUNCH
PAUNCH
RAUNCH
SQUASH
SQUISH

•••U•H

AAAUGH
ABLUSH
AMBUSH
ASMUCH
ASSUCH
AVOUCH
BARUCH
BROUGH
CHOUGH
CLOUGH
CROUCH
DRRUTH
DULUTH
ENOUGH
FYVUSH
GROUCH
INRUSH
MANUSH
MCHUGH
NORUSH
ONRUSH
PLOUGH
SLEUTH
SLOUCH
SLOUGH
SOMUCH
THOUGH
THRUSH
TROUGH
UNHUNH
UNLUSH
UPRUSH

UI••••

UINTAS

U•I•••

UBIETY
UMIAKS
UNIATE
UNIATS
UNICED
UNICEF
UNICES
UNIDLE
UNIDLY
UNIFIC
UNIONS
UNIPED
UNIPOD
UNIQUE
UNISEX
UNISOM
UNISON
UNISYS
UNITAS
UNITED
UNITER
UNITES
UNIVAC
UTICAN

U••I••

UGLIER
UGLIES
UGLIFY
UGLILY
ULRICH
ULTIMA
ULTIMO
UMPING
UMPIRE
UNBIND
UNBITS
UNCIAL
UNDICI
UNDIES
UNDIMS
UNDINE
UNFILE
UNFINE
UNFIRM
UNFITS
UNGILT
UNGIRD
UNGIRT
UNHIRE
UNKIND
UNKINK
UNLIKE
UNLIMP
UNLINK
UNLIVE
UNMIRY
UNMIXT
UNNICE
UNNIGH
UNOILY
UNPICK
UNPILE
UNPINS
UNRIFE
UNRIGS
UNRIPE
UNRIPS
UNSICK
UNTIDY
UNTIED
UNTIER
UNTIES
UNTILT
UNWIGS
UNWILD
UNWILY
UNWIND
UNWISE
UNWISH
UNZIPS
UPBIND
UPDIKE
UPDIVE
UPGIRD
UPGIRT
UPHILL
UPLIFT
UPLINK
UPPILE
UPPING
UPPISH
UPPITY
UPRISE
UPSIDE
UPSIZE
UPTICK
UPTILT
UPTIME
UPWIND
URGING
URSIDS
URSINE
USHING
USMINT

U•••I•

UMBRIA
UNAKIN
UNAMIS
UNAVID
UNBAIT
UNCHIC
UNCLIP
UNCOIL
UNEPIC
UNEVIL
UNFAIR
UNGLIB
UNGRIP
UNGUIS
UNHAIR
UNIFIC
UNJOIN
UNKNIT
UNLAID
UNNAIL
UNPAID
UNPRIM
UNSAID
UNSHIP
UNSLIM
UNTRIG
UNVAIN
UNVEIL
UNVOID
UPCOIL
UPSPIN
UPSTIR
UPTOIT
URACIL
URALIC
URANIA
URANIC
URCHIN
USEDIN
USERID
USESIN
USMAIL
UTOPIA

U••••I

UBANGI
UBUROI
UNDICI
URBANI

•UI•••

BUICKS
BUILDS
CUICAS
FUISSE
GUIANA
GUIDED
GUIDER
GUIDES
GUIDRY
GUILDS
GUILED
GUILES
GUILTY
GUINAN
GUINEA
GUISES
GUITAR
GUITRY
JUICED
JUICER
JUICES
OUIJAS
OUIMET
OUIOUI
QUICHE
QUIDDE
QUIETS
QUILLS
QUILTS
QUINCE
QUINCY
QUINOU
QUINTA
QUINTE
QUINTI
QUINTS
QUINZE
QUIPPY
QUIPUS
QUIRED
QUIRES
QUIRKS
QUIRKY
QUIRTS
QUITIT
QUIVER
RUINED
RUINER
SUISSE
SUITED
SUITES
SUITOR
SUITUP
TUILLE

•U•I••

AUDIAL
AUDILE
AUDIOS
AUDITS
AUGITE
AURIFY
AURIGA
AURIST
AUTISM
AUTIST
BUNION
BURIAL
BURIED
BURIER
BURIES
BURINS
BUSIED
BUSIER
BUSIES
BUSILY
BUSING
BUYING
BUYINS
CUBICS
CUBING
CUBISM
CUBIST
CUBITI
CUBITS
CUEING
CUMINS
CUPIDS
CURIAE
CURIES
CURING
CURIOS
CURITE
CURIUM
CUTIES
CUTINS
CUVIER
DUDING
DUDISH
DUKING
DUPING
DURING
DUTIES
EUNICE
FUMIER
FUMING
FURIES
FUSILE
FUSILS
FUSING
FUSION
FUTILE
GUGINO
GUNITE
GURION
GUYING
HUSING
JUDITH
JUKING
JULIAN
JULIEN
JULIET
JULIUS
JUNIOR
JUNIUS
JURIED
JURIES
JURIST
KUNITZ
KURILE
LUBING
LUCIAN
LUCIDA
LUCIEN
LUCILE
LUCINE
LUCITE
LUCIUS
LUGING
LUKICH
LUMINA
LUNIKS
LUPINE
LUPINO
LURING
LUTIST
MULISH
MUNICH
MURIEL
MURINE
MUSIAL
MUSICK
MUSICS
MUSING
MUTING
MUTINY
MUTIUS
NUBIAN
NUBILE
NUBIRA
NUDISM
NUDIST
NUDITY
NUKING
NUMINA
OUTIES
OUTING
PULING
PUMICE
PUNIER
PUNILY
PUNISH
PUPILS
PURIFY
PURIMS
PURINA
PURISM
PURIST
PURITY
QUAILS
QUAINT
QUOINS
QUOITS
RUBIED
RUBIES
RUBIFY
RUBIKS
RULIER
RULING
RUNINS
RUPIAH
RUTILE
RUTINS
SUBITO
SUFISM
SUPINE
SURIMI
SUZIEQ
TUBING
TUBIST
TULIPS
TUNICS
TUNING
TURING
ZUNIAN
ZUNIGA
ZURICH

•U••I•

AUFAIT
AULAIT
AUNTIE
AUPAIR
AUSSIE
AUSTIN
BUDGIE
BUPKIS
BURNIE
BURNIN
BUSTIN
BUTTIN
BUYSIN
BUYSIT
CUBOID
CUEBID
CUEDIN
CUESIN
CUETIP
CULKIN
CULLIS
CULTIC
CUMBIA
CUPRIC
CURLIN
CURTIN
CURTIS
CURTIZ
CUSPID
CUSTIS
CUTSIN
CUTSIT
DUBLIN
DUBOIS
DUCHIN
DUCKIE
DUNKIN
DUNLIN
DURBIN
DURNIT
DUSTIN
EUCLID
EURAIL
EUSTIS
FULFIL
GUNSIT
HUBRIS
HUDDIE
HUGHIE
HUNGIN
JUDAIC
JUMPIN
JUNKIE
JUSTIN
KUPRIN
KUWAIT
LUBLIN
LUDWIG
LUGLIO
LUMPIN
LUMPIT
LUNDIS
LUREIN
MUDPIE
MUFFIN
MUFTIS
MULLIN
MULTIS
MUNCIE
MURCIA
MUSKIE
MUSLIM
MUSLIN
NUBBIN
NUDNIK
NUNCIO
NUNZIO
NUTKIN
NUTOIL
NUTRIA
OUTBID
OUTDID
OUTFIT
OUTHIT
OUTLIE
OUTLIP
OUTRIB
OUTRIG
OUTSIN
OUTSIT
OUTVIE
OUTWIT
PUBLIC
PUBLIX
PUCCIS
PUFFIN
PULLIN
PULPIT
PUNDIT
PUNKIE
PUPKIN
PURLIE
PUSHIN
PUSHIT
PUTRID
PUTSIN
PUTTIN
QUAKIE
QUITIT
RUBBIA
RUBRIC
RUBSIN
RUDKIN
RUNCIE
RUNGIN
RUNSIN
RUSHIN
RUSKIN
RUSSIA
RUSTIC
RUTHIE
RUXPIN
SUBLID
SUBMIT
SUCKIN
SUFFIX
SUMMIT
SUNKIN
SUNLIT
SUNNIS
SUREIS
SURFIN
SUSHIS
TUCKIN
TUGRIK
TUNEIN
TUPTIM
TURBID
TURGID
TURKIC
TURNIN
TURNIP
TURPIN
TUSHIE
TUTSIS
TUTTIS
YUPPIE

•U•••I

BUSONI
CUBITI
CUMULI
DUETTI
HUMERI
KUBLAI
LUGOSI
LUNEDI
MUESLI
MUMBAI
NUCLEI
OUIOUI
QUADRI
QUINTI
RUBATI
RUMAKI
SURIMI
SUUKYI
SUVARI
SUZUKI

••UI••

ACUITY
AGUISH
AQUILA
AQUINO
BLUING
BLUISH
BRUINS
BRUISE
BRUITS
CLUING
CRUISE
DRUIDS
EQUINE
EQUIPS
EQUITY
FLUIDS
FLUISH
FRUITS
FRUITY
GLUIER
GLUING
GRUING
GSUITS
INUITS
LOUIES
LOUISA
LOUISB
LOUISE
LOUISI
LOUISV
LOUISX
PLUIES
SLUICE
SLUING
SQUIBB
SQUIBS
SQUIDS
SQUINT
SQUIRE
SQUIRM
SQUIRT
SQUISH
TRUING
TRUISM

••U•I•

ANUBIS
APULIA
AZUKIS
BOUDIN
CLUEIN
COURIC
COUSIN
DOURIF
EQUOID
FLUTIE
GRUMIO
HAULIN
HOURIS
INUPIK
LAURIA
LAURIC
LAURIE
LOUVIN
MOULIN
PAULII
PAULIV
PIUSII
PIUSIV
PIUSIX
PLUGIN
PLUVIA
PLUVIO
POURIN
SAUDIS
SHUTIN
STUDIO
STUPID
TAUPIN
TAURIC
TSURIS
YOUDIG
YOUWIN
ZEUXIS

••U••I

ALUMNI
BRUNEI
CHUHSI
COULDI
FRUCTI
FRUTTI
GLUTEI
GRUCCI
ITURBI
LOUISI
PAULII
PAULVI
PIUSII
PIUSVI
PIUSXI
SHUMAI
SNUGLI
SUUKYI
UBUROI

•••UI•

ACQUIT
ANNUIT
COQUIS
ENNUIS
INTUIT
JESUIT
LEGUIN
LIQUID
MAQUIS
MINUIT
NYQUIL
PAQUIN
RESUIT
SEQUIN
UNGUIS
YAQUIS

•••U•I

ADZUKI
AGOUTI
ANNULI
CUMULI
FALUDI
FAMULI
FARUKI
HAMULI
INCUBI
KABUKI
LAZULI
MODULI
MTFUJI
POPULI
SALUKI
SUZUKI
VENUTI
WATUSI
YEHUDI

••••UI

BANGUI
MATSUI
OUIOUI
SESQUI
YANQUI

U•J•••

UNJAMS
UNJOIN
UNJUST
UPJOHN

•UJ•••

BUJOLD
JUJUBE
PUJOLS

•U•J••

OUIJAS
OUTJET
OUTJUT
PUNJAB

•••UJ•

MTFUJI

UK••••

UKASES

U•K•••

UNKEPT
UNKIND
UNKINK
UNKNIT
UNKNOT
UPKEEP

U••K••

UECKER
UNAKIN
UNSKEW

U•••K•

UMIAKS
UNCAKE
UNLIKE
UNMAKE
UNYOKE
UPDIKE
UPTAKE

U••••K

UNCASK
UNCORK
UNDOCK
UNFORK
UNHOOK
UNHUSK
UNKINK
UNLINK
UNLOCK
UNMASK
UNPACK
UNPICK
UNRACK
UNSICK
UNSUNK
UNTACK
UNTUCK
UPLINK
UPTALK
UPTICK
UQUARK
URALSK
USBANK

•UK•••

AUKLET
BUKAVU
DUKING
JUKING
LUKICH
MUKLUK
NUKING
YUKATA
YUKAWA
YUKKED
YUKONS

•U•K••

BUBKES
BUCKED
BUCKER
BUCKET
BUCKLE
BUCKUP
BULKED
BULKUP
BUNKED
BUNKER
BUNKOS
BUNKUM
BUPKES
BUPKIS
BUPKUS
BURKAS
BUSKED
BUSKER
BUTKUS
CUCKOO
CULKIN
DUCKED
DUCKER
DUCKIE
DUNKED
DUNKER
DUNKIN
DUSKED
EUCKEN
FUNKED
GURKHA
HULKED
HUNKER
HUSKED
HUSKER
JUNKED
JUNKER
JUNKET
JUNKIE
LUCKED
LUNKER
LURKED
LURKER
LURKEY
MUCKED
MUCKER
MUCKUP
MUSKET
MUSKIE
MUSKOX
NUTKIN
PUCKER
PUNKAS
PUNKER
PUNKIE
PUPKIN
QUAKED
QUAKER
QUAKES
QUAKIE
RUCKED
RUCKER
RUCKUP
RUCKUS
RUDKIN
RUDKUS
RUSKIN
SUCKED
SUCKER
SUCKIN
SUCKUP
SULKED
SULKER
SUNKEN
SUNKIN
SUUKYI
TUCKED
TUCKER
TUCKIN
TURKEY
TURKIC
TUSKED
TUSKER
YUKKED
ZUCKER

•U••K•

BUGAKU
BUICKS
EUREKA
JUDOKA
KULAKS
LUNIKS
LUSAKA
QUACKS
QUACKY
QUARKS
QUIRKS
QUIRKY
RUBIKS
RUMAKI
SUDOKU
SUZUKI

•U•••K

BUROAK
CUSACK
DUBCEK
LUBECK

MUKLUK
MUSICK
NUDNIK
OUTASK
TUGRIK

••UK••
AZUKIS
FLUKES
FLUKEY
RYUKYU
STUKAS
SUUKYI
ZHUKOV

••U•K•
AKUAKU
AQUAKE
BAULKS
BOURKE
CAULKS
CHUCKS
CHUCKY
CHUNKS
CHUNKY
CLUCKS
CLUNKS
CLUNKY
FLUNKS
FLUNKY
PLUCKS
PLUCKY
PLUNKS
PLUNKY
ROURKE
SHUCKS
SKULKS
SKUNKS
SKUNKY
SPUNKY
THUNKS
TRUCKS
TRUNKS

••U••K
INUPIK
SQUAWK
SQUEAK
UQUARK

•••UK•
ADZUKI
BODUKE
FARUKI
KABUKI
LADUKE
PERUKE
REBUKE
SALUKI
STLUKE
SUZUKI

•••U•K
ATDUSK
CANUCK
DEBUNK
DEJUNK
INBULK
INLUCK
MCDUCK
NOLUCK
PODUNK
SHRUNK
STRUCK
STRUNK
UNHUSK
UNSUNK
UNTUCK
ZANUCK

••••UK
DYBBUK
FAROUK
KEOKUK
KIRKUK
MUKLUK

UL••••
ULCERS
ULLAGE
ULLMAN
ULRICH
ULSTER
ULTIMA
ULTIMO
ULTRAS

U•L•••
UCLANS
UGLIER
UGLIES
UGLIFY
UGLILY
UHLANS
ULLAGE
ULLMAN
UMLAUT
UNLACE
UNLADE
UNLAID
UNLASH
UNLAYS
UNLEAD
UNLEAF
UNLEAN
UNLEFT
UNLENT
UNLESS
UNLIKE
UNLIMP
UNLINK
UNLIVE
UNLOAD
UNLOCK
UNLOOP
UNLOST
UNLUSH
UPLAND
UPLAST
UPLATE
UPLEAP
UPLIFT
UPLINK
UPLOAD

U••L••
UBOLTS
UNBLED
UNCLAD
UNCLAY
UNCLES
UNCLIP
UNCLOG
UNFLAT
UNGLAD
UNGLIB
UNGLUE
UNPLAN
UNPLUG
UNSLIM
UNSLOW
UPFLOW
URALIC
URALSK
USFLAG
UVALDE
UVALUE
UVULAE
UVULAR
UVULAS

U•••L•
UGLILY
UHAULS
UMBELS
UNABLE
UNABLY
UNBALE
UNBELT
UNBOLD
UNBOLT
UNCALM
UNCOLA
UNDULY
UNFELT
UNFILE
UNFOLD
UNFULL
UNGILT
UNGULA
UNHALE
UNHELD
UNHELM
UNHOLY
UNHULL
UNIDLE
UNIDLY
UNMOLD
UNOILY
UNPALE
UNPILE
UNROLL
UNRULY
UNSELD
UNSELL
UNSOLD
UNSOLE
UNTILT
UNTOLD
UNWALL
UNWELL
UNWILD
UNWILY
UPFOLD
UPHELD
UPHILL
UPHOLD
UPPILE
UPSALA
UPTALK
UPTILT
UPWELL
URSULA
USABLE
USABLY
USUALS

U••••L
UMBRAL
UNCIAL
UNCOIL
UNCOOL
UNCURL
UNEVIL
UNFOUL
UNFULL
UNFURL
UNGUAL
UNHULL
UNNAIL
UNOCAL
UNORAL
UNPEEL
UNREAL
UNREEL
UNROLL
UNSEAL
UNSELL
UNVEIL
UNWALL
UNWELL
UPCOIL
UPCURL
UPHILL
UPWELL
URACIL
URNFUL
USEFUL
USMAIL

•UL•••
AULAIT
BULDEO
BULGAR
BULGED
BULGES
BULGUR
BULKED
BULKUP
BULLAE
BULLED
BULLET
BULOVA
BULWER
CULETS
CULKIN
CULLED
CULLEN
CULLER
CULLET
CULLIS
CULLUM
CULTCH
CULTIC
CULTUS
DULCET
DULLEA
DULLED
DULLER
DULLES
DULUTH
EULESS
EULOGY
FULCRA
FULFIL
FULLER
FULLOF
FULLUP
FULMAR
FULTON
GULAGS
GULDEN
GULFED
GULLAH
GULLED
GULLET
GULPED
GULPER
HULKED
HULLED
HULLER
HULLOS
JULEPS
JULIAN
JULIEN
JULIET
JULIUS
KULAKS
LULLED
LULLER
MULCTS
MULDER
MULETA
MULEYS
MULISH
MULLAH
MULLAS
MULLED
MULLER
MULLET
MULLIN
MULTIS
NULLED
NULLOS
PULERS
PULING
PULLED
PULLER
PULLET
PULLEY
PULLIN
PULLON
PULLUP
PULMON
PULPED
PULPER
PULPIT
PULSAR
PULSED
PULSES
PULVER
RULEON
RULERS
RULETH
RULIER
RULING
SULFAS
SULFUR
SULKED
SULKER
SULLEN
SULTAN
SULTRY
TULANE
TULARE
TULIPS
TULLES
TULSAN
VULCAN
VULGAR
VULGUS

•U•L••
AUKLET
BUGLED
BUGLER
BUGLES
BUILDS
BULLAE
BULLED
BULLET
BUMLEG
BURLAP
BURLED
BURLER
BURLEY
BUTLER
CULLED
CULLEN
CULLER
CULLET
CULLIS
CULLUM
CURLED
CURLER
CURLEW
CURLEY
CURLIN
CURLUP
CUTLER
CUTLET
CUYLER
DUALLY
DUBLIN
DUDLEY
DUELED
DUELER
DUELLO
DULLEA
DULLED
DULLER
DULLES
DUNLAP
DUNLIN
DUNLOP
DUPLEX
DUPLOS
EUCLID
FUELED
FUELER
FUELUP
FULLER
FULLOF
FULLUP
FURLED
GUELPH
GUILDS
GUILED
GUILES
GUILTY
GULLAH
GULLED
GULLET
GUNLAP
GUNLAW
GURLEY
HUBLEY
HULLED
HULLER
HULLOS
HUNLEY
HURLED
HURLER
HURLEY
HUXLEY
KUBLAI
KUBLER
LUBLIN
LUDLOW
LUDLUM
LUELLA
LUGLIO
LULLED
LULLER
LUMLEY
MUKLUK
MULLAH
MULLAS
MULLED
MULLER
MULLET
MULLIN
MUSLIM
MUSLIN
NUCLEI
NUCLEO
NULLED
NULLOS
NUTLET
OUTLAW
OUTLAY
OUTLED
OUTLET
OUTLIE
OUTLIP
PUBLIC
PUBLIX
PULLED
PULLER
PULLET
PULLEY
PULLIN
PULLON
PULLUP
PURLED
PURLIE
QUALES
QUALMS
QUELER
QUELLS
QUILLS
QUILTS
RUBLES
RUBLEV
RUNLET
RUNLOW
SUBLET
SUBLID
SUBLOT
SULLEN
SUNLIT
TUILLE
TULLES

•U••L•
AUDILE
BUBBLE
BUBBLY
BUCKLE
BUJOLD
BUMBLE
BUNDLE
BUNGLE
BURBLE
BURBLY
BURGLE
BUSILY
BUSTLE
CUDDLE
CUDDLY
CUMULI
CUMULO
CUPELS
CUPOLA
CUPULE
CURDLE
CURTLY
CUTELY
DUALLY
DUDDLE
DUELLO
DUFFLE
DUGALD
DUMBLY
DUVALL
FUDDLE
FUMBLE
FUSILE
FUSILS
FUTILE
GURGLE
GUZZLE
HUBBLE
HUDDLE
HUGELY
HUMBLE
HUMBLY
HURDLE
HURTLE
HUSTLE
JUGGLE
JUMBLE
JUMBLY
JUNGLE
JUNGLY
JUSTLY
KURALT
KURILE
LUCILE
LUELLA
LUNULA
LUSHLY
MUDDLE
MUESLI
MUFFLE
MUGGLE
MUMBLE
MUMBLY
MURALS
MUSCLE
MUSCLY
MUTELY
MUZZLE
NUBBLE
NUBBLY
NUBILE
NUDELY
NUMBLY
NUZZLE
OUSELS
OUTFLY
OUZELS
PUDDLE
PUDDLY
PUEBLA
PUEBLO
PUGGLE
PUJOLS
PUNILY
PUPILS
PURELY
PURFLE
PURPLE
PURPLY
PUZZLE
QUAILS
QUAYLE
QUELLS
QUILLS
RUBBLE
RUBBLY
RUBELS
RUDELY
RUDOLF
RUFFLE
RUFFLY
RUMBLE
RUMBLY
RUMPLE
RUMPLY
RUNDLE
RUSTLE
RUTILE
SUABLE
SUBTLE
SUBTLY
SUPPLE
SUPPLY
SURELY
TUBULE
TUILLE
TUMBLE
TUMULT
TUPELO
TURTLE
TUSSLE
TUVALU

•U•••L
AUDIAL
BUCCAL
BUNUEL
BURIAL
BURSAL
BUSHEL
CUDGEL
CUNEAL
CUPFUL
CUSPAL
DUCTAL
DUFFEL
DUVALL
EURAIL
FULFIL
FUNGAL
FUNNEL
GUMBEL
GUNSEL
HUMMEL
JUGFUL
KUMMEL
KUNZEL
MUDEEL
MUGFUL
MURIEL
MUSIAL
MUSSEL
MUTUAL
MUTUEL
NUCHAL
NUTOIL
PUMMEL
RUEFUL
RUNNEL
RUSSEL
TUBFUL
TUNNEL
TUSSAL

••UL••
ADULTS
ALULAE
ALULAR
AMULET
APULIA
AVULSE
BAULKS
BEULAH
BOULES
BOULEZ
BRULEE
CAULKS
COULDA
COULDI
COULEE
DOULAS
EVULSE
EXULTS
FAULTS
FAULTY
FOULED
FOULER
FOULLY
FOULUP
GAULLE
GOULET
HAULED
HAULER
HAULIN
HAULUP
JOULES
LAULAU
MAULED
MAULER
MOULDS
MOULDY
MOULIN
MOULTS
OCULAR
OCULUS
OVULAR
OVULES
PAULEY
PAULII
PAULIV
PAULVI
POULES
POULTS
SAULTS
SCULLS
SCULLY
SCULPT
SHULTZ
SKULKS
SKULLS
TOULON
UVULAE
UVULAR
UVULAS
VAULTS
VAULTY
WOULDA

••U•L•
AQUILA
AZUELA
BAUBLE
BLUELY
CHURLS
COUPLE
DOUBLE
DOUBLY
DOURLY
EKUELE
EQUALS
FOULLY
GAULLE
GLUMLY
GRUELS
HOURLY
KNURLS
KNURLY
LOUDLY
NTUPLE
SCULLS
SCULLY
SKULLS
SMUGLY
SNUGLI
SNUGLY
SOURLY
SQUALL
STUDLY
TAUTLY
THUSLY
TOUSLE
USUALS
YOUALL

••U••L
ALUDEL
BRUMAL
BRUMEL
BRUTAL
CAUDAL
CAUSAL
CRURAL
DOUGAL
FAUNAL
FEUDAL
FRUGAL
LAUREL
LAURYL
NEURAL
NEUROL
NOUNAL
PAUSAL
PLURAL
SQUALL
SQUEAL
YOUALL

•••UL•
AMPULE
ANNULI
ANNULS
ASDULL
BAKULA
CANULA
COPULA
CUMULI
CUMULO
CUPULE
DEPULP
ENGULF
FACULA
FAMULI
FERULE
FIBULA
GHOULS
HAMULI
ICOULD
IMFULL
INBULK
INCULT
INFULL
INGULF
INJULY
INSULT
ISEULT
IWOULD
JARULE
KIDULT
LAZULI
LOBULE
LTSULU
LUNULA
MACULA
MODULE
MODULI
MODULO
MOGULS
MRSULU
NEBULA
NEWULM
NODULE
OCCULT
ODOULS
OPHULS
OSCULE
PACULA
PAKULA
PENULT
PETULA
POPULI
PROULX
RESULT
ROMULO
SCHULZ
SHOULD
TABULA
TUBULE
TUMULT
UHAULS
UNDULY
UNFULL
UNGULA
UNHULL
UNRULY
URSULA
VENULE
ZONULE

•••U•L
ACTUAL
ANNUAL
ASDULL
BUNUEL
CASUAL
DEFUEL
GENUAL
IMFULL
INFULL
LEMUEL
MANUAL
MANUEL
MIGUEL
MUTUAL
MUTUEL
NYQUIL
RAQUEL
RECURL
REFUEL
RITUAL
SAMUEL
SEQUEL
UNCURL
UNFULL
UNFURL
UNGUAL
UNHULL
UPCURL
VISUAL

••••UL
AIDFUL
AIMFUL
ARMFUL
ARTFUL
BAGFUL
BANJUL
BEFOUL
BOXFUL
CANFUL
CAPFUL
CARFUL
CONSUL
CUPFUL
DEPAUL
EARFUL
ENSOUL
EYEFUL
FITFUL
HANGUL
HATFUL
IREFUL
JARFUL
JOYFUL
JUGFUL
LAPFUL
LAWFUL
MANFUL
MUGFUL
NETFUL
PANFUL
PEPFUL
POTFUL
REHAUL
RUEFUL
SINFUL
SOBFUL
STPAUL
TUBFUL
UNFOUL
URNFUL
USEFUL
VATFUL
WOEFUL

UM••••
UMBELS
UMBERS
UMBRAE
UMBRAL
UMBRAS
UMBRIA
UMIAKS
UMLAUT
UMPING
UMPIRE
UMTATA

U•M•••
UNMADE
UNMAKE
UNMANS
UNMASK
UNMAST
UNMATE
UNMEET
UNMESH
UNMEWS
UNMIRY
UNMIXT
UNMOLD
UNMOOR
UNMOWN
UPMOST
USMAIL
USMINT
UTMOST

U••M••
ULLMAN
UNAMIS
UNSMUG

U•••M•
UGGAMS
UGSOME
ULTIMA
ULTIMO
UNARMS
UNDAMS
UNDIMS
UNGAMY
UNJAMS
UNLIMP
UNTAME
UPTIME
USARMY

U••••M
UNCALM
UNFIRM
UNHELM
UNISOM
UNPRIM
UNSEAM
UNSLIM

•UM•••
AUMONT
BUMBLE
BUMBRY
BUMLEG
BUMMED
BUMMER
BUMOUT
BUMPED
BUMPER
BUMPPO
BUMPUP
BUMRAP
CUMBER
CUMBIA
CUMINS
CUMULI
CUMULO
DUMBER
DUMBLY
DUMBOS
DUMDUM
DUMONT
DUMPED
DUMPER
DUMPON
DUMPTY
FUMBLE
FUMEAT

FUMERS	RUMMER	QUALMS	RHUMBA	TRAUMA	POSSUM	UNCORK	UNHEED	UNMASK	UNSELD	UNWORN	UPSEND	BUNKER	JUNIUS	RUNUPS
FUMIER	RUMORS	RUNDMC	RHUMBS	VOLUME	POSTUM	UNCUFF	UNHELD	UNMAST	UNSELL	UNWOVE	UPSENT	BUNKOS	JUNKED	RUNWAY
FUMING	RUMOUR	SURIMI	SCUMMY		QUORUM	UNCURB	UNHELM	UNMATE	UNSENT	UNWRAP	UPWIND	BUNKUM	JUNKER	RUNYON
GUMBEL	RUMPLE		SHUMAI	•••U•M	RADIUM	UNCURL	UNHERO	UNMEET	UNSERE	UNYOKE	URBANA	BUNSEN	JUNKET	SUNBOW
GUMBOS	RUMPLY	•U•••M	SLUMMY	NEWULM	REDRUM	UNCUTE	UNHEWN	UNMESH	UNSEWN	UNZIPS	URBANE	BUNTED	JUNKIE	SUNDAE
GUMMED	RUMPUS	AUNTEM	SLUMPS	VACUUM	REGNUM	UNDAMS	UNHIRE	UNMEWS	UNSEWS	UNZONE	URBANI	BUNTER	JUNTAS	SUNDAS
GUMSUP	SUMACS	AUTISM	SPUMED		ROSSUM	UNDEAD	UNHOED	UNMIRY	UNSEXY		URBANV	BUNTON	JUNTOS	SUNDAY
HUMANE	SUMMED	BUNKUM	SPUMES	••••UM	SACRUM	UNDEEP	UNHOLY	UNMIXT	UNSHED	U•N•••	URGENT	BUNUEL	KUNDRY	SUNDER
HUMANS	SUMMER	CUBISM	STUMPS	ACTIUM	SCARUM	UNDEFT	UNHOOD	UNMOLD	UNSHIP	UINTAS	URGING	BUNYAN	KUNGFU	SUNDOG
HUMBER	SUMMIT	CULLUM	STUMPY	ADYTUM	SEPTUM	UNDERS	UNHOOK	UNMOOR	UNSHOD	UNNAIL	URSINE	CUNARD	KUNITZ	SUNDRY
HUMBLE	SUMMON	CURIUM	THUMBS	AECIUM	SKIBUM	UNDEWY	UNHUED	UNMOWN	UNSHOE	UNNEAT	USBANK	CUNEAL	KUNZEL	SUNFAN
HUMBLY	SUMNER	CUSTOM	THUMPS	ALARUM	SODIUM	UNDICI	UNHULL	UNNAIL	UNSHUT	UNNICE	USHING	DUNANT	LUNACY	SUNGOD
HUMBUG	SUMSUP	DUMDUM	TRUMAN	ALLIUM	SUBGUM	UNDIES	UNHUNG	UNNEAT	UNSICK	UNNIGH	USMINT	DUNBAR	LUNATE	SUNGTO
HUMERI	SUMTER	DUNHAM	TRUMBO	ANTRUM	TALCUM	UNDIMS	UNHUNH	UNNICE	UNSKEW	UPNEXT	UTAHNS	DUNCAN	LUNCHY	SUNHAT
HUMMED	SUMUPS	DURHAM	TRUMPS	ARTGUM	TEDEUM	UNDINE	UNHURT	UNNIGH	UNSLIM	URNFUL	UTHANT	DUNCES	LUNDEN	SUNKEN
HUMMEL	TUMBLE	EUONYM		ASYLUM	TEDIUM	UNDOCK	UNHUSK	UNOCAL	UNSLOW	USNAVY	UTURNS	DUNDAS	LUNDIS	SUNKIN
HUMMER	TUMEFY	LUDLUM	••U•M•	ATRIUM	VACUUM	UNDOER	UNIATE	UNOILY	UNSMUG	USNEWS		DUNDEE	LUNEDI	SUNLIT
HUMMUS	TUMULT	MUSEUM	CHUMMY	BARIUM	VALIUM	UNDOES	UNIATS	UNOPEN	UNSNAG		U••••N	DUNHAM	LUNGED	SUNNED
HUMORS	YUMAAZ	MUSLIM	CRUMMY	BARNUM	VELLUM	UNDONE	UNICED	UNORAL	UNSNAP	U••N••	ULLMAN	DUNKED	LUNGER	SUNNIS
HUMOUR	YUMANS	NUDISM	PLUMMY	BAYRUM	WAMPUM	UNDRAW	UNICEF	UNOWED	UNSNUG	UBANGI	UNAKIN	DUNKER	LUNGES	SUNOCO
HUMPED	YUMYUM	OUTSUM	SCUMMY	BELLUM	YUMYUM	UNDREW	UNICES	UNPACK	UNSOFT	UGANDA	UNBORN	DUNKIN	LUNIKS	SUNRAY
HUMPHS		PURISM	SLUMMY	BOOJUM		UNDSET	UNIDLE	UNPAID	UNSOLD	UNKNIT	UNEVEN	DUNLAP	LUNKER	SUNSET
HUMPTY	•U•M••	PUTNAM		BUNKUM	UN••••	UNDULY	UNIDLY	UNPALE	UNSOLE	UNKNOT	UNHEWN	DUNLIN	LUNTHA	SUNTAN
HUMVEE	BUMMED	QUORUM	••U••M	CENTUM	UNABLE	UNDYED	UNIFIC	UNPAWN	UNSORE	UNSNAG	UNISON	DUNLOP	LUNULA	SUNUNU
JUMADA	BUMMER	SUBGUM	FOURAM	CERIUM	UNABLY	UNEASE	UNIONS	UNPEEL	UNSORT	UNSNAP	UNJOIN	DUNNED	MUNCHY	SUNUPS
JUMBLE	BURMAN	SUFISM	FOURPM	CESIUM	UNAGED	UNEASY	UNIPED	UNPEGS	UNSOUR	UNSNUG	UNLEAN	DUNNER	MUNCIE	TUNDRA
JUMBLY	BUSMAN	SUREAM	SQUIRM	CHISUM	UNAKIN	UNEDGE	UNIPOD	UNPENS	UNSOWN	UPENDS	UNMOWN	EUNICE	MUNERA	TUNEIN
JUMBOS	BUSMEN	TUPTIM	TRUISM	CILIUM	UNAMIS	UNEPIC	UNIQUE	UNPENT	UNSPAN	URANIA	UNOPEN	FUNDED	MUNICH	TUNERS
JUMPAT	DUOMOS	YUMYUM		CIRCUM	UNARMS	UNESCO	UNISEX	UNPICK	UNSPUN	URANIC	UNPAWN	FUNDER	MUNROE	TUNETO
JUMPED	FULMAR		•••UM•	CORIUM	UNAVID	UNEVEN	UNISOM	UNPILE	UNSTEP	URANUS	UNPLAN	FUNFUR	NUNCIO	TUNEUP
JUMPER	FURMAN	••UM••	ALBUMS	CULLUM	UNAWED	UNEVIL	UNISON	UNPINS	UNSTOP	USANCE	UNSAWN	FUNGAL	NUNGEN	TUNICS
JUMPIN	GUMMED	ACUMEN	ASSUME	CURIUM	UNAXED	UNFACT	UNISYS	UNPLAN	UNSTOW	USENET	UNSEEN	FUNGUS	NUNZIO	TUNING
JUMPON	GUNMAN	ALUMNA	AUTUMN	DADGUM	UNBAGS	UNFAIR	UNITAS	UNPLUG	UNSUED		UNSEWN	FUNKED	OUNCES	TUNNEL
JUMPUP	GUNMEN	ALUMNI	BEGUMS	DESLUM	UNBAIT	UNFELT	UNITED	UNPOSH	UNSUNG	U•••N•	UNSOWN	FUNNED	PUNCHY	TUNNEY
KUMMEL	GUTMAN	BAUMAN	BENUMB	DICTUM	UNBALE	UNFILE	UNITER	UNPOTS	UNSUNK	UCLANS	UNSPAN	FUNNEL	PUNDIT	ZUNIAN
LUMBAR	GUZMAN	BAUMER	COLUMN	DIMSUM	UNBARE	UNFINE	UNITES	UNPRIM	UNSURE	UHLANS	UNSPUN	FUNRUN	PUNIER	ZUNIGA
LUMBER	HUMMED	BRUMAL	DEGUMS	DINKUM	UNBARS	UNFIRM	UNIVAC	UNPURE	UNTACK	UMPING	UNTORN	GUNDOG	PUNILY	
LUMENS	HUMMEL	BRUMEL	DOSUMS	DORSUM	UNBELT	UNFITS	UNJAMS	UNRACK	UNTAME	UNBEND	UNVAIN	GUNFOR	PUNISH	•U•N••
LUMINA	HUMMER	BRUMES	DURUMS	DUMDUM	UNBEND	UNFLAT	UNJOIN	UNRASH	UNTAPE	UNBENT	UNWORN	GUNGHO	PUNJAB	BUENAS
LUMLEY	HUMMUS	CHUMMY	EXHUME	ERBIUM	UNBENT	UNFOLD	UNJUST	UNREAD	UNTAUT	UNBIND	UPJOHN	GUNITE	PUNKAS	BUENOS
LUMMOX	KUMMEL	CHUMPS	FORUMS	FACTUM	UNBIND	UNFOND	UNKEPT	UNREAL	UNTHAW	UNDINE	UPSPIN	GUNLAP	PUNKER	BURNED
LUMPED	LUMMOX	CLUMPS	FUSUMA	FARNUM	UNBITS	UNFORK	UNKIND	UNREEL	UNTIDY	UNDONE	UPTORN	GUNLAW	PUNKIE	BURNER
LUMPEN	MUMMED	CLUMPY	HOHUMS	FOLIUM	UNBLED	UNFOUL	UNKINK	UNRENT	UNTIED	UNFINE	UPTOWN	GUNMAN	PUNNED	BURNET
LUMPER	MUMMER	CLUMSY	HOKUMS	FRENUM	UNBOLD	UNFOXY	UNKNIT	UNREST	UNTIER	UNFOND	UPTURN	GUNMEN	PUNNER	BURNEY
LUMPIN	MUMMYS	CRUMBS	ILLUME	GOLLUM	UNBOLT	UNFREE	UNKNOT	UNRIFE	UNTIES	UNHAND	URCHIN	GUNNAR	PUNTAS	BURNIE
LUMPIT	MURMUR	CRUMBY	INHUME	GYPSUM	UNBORN	UNFULL	UNLACE	UNRIGS	UNTILT	UNHUNG	URGEON	GUNNED	PUNTED	BURNIN
LUMPUR	MUUMUU	CRUMMY	JORUMS	HELIUM	UNBUDS	UNFURL	UNLADE	UNRIPE	UNTOLD	UNHUNH	USEDIN	GUNNER	PUNTER	BURNUP
MUMBAI	NUTMEG	CRUMPS	KHOUMS	IDOLUM	UNBURY	UNGAGS	UNLAID	UNRIPS	UNTORN	UNIONS	USEDON	GUNSEL	RUNCIE	BUYNOW
MUMBLE	OUIMET	DRUMUP	LEGUME	INDIUM	UNBUSY	UNGAMY	UNLASH	UNROBE	UNTRAP	UNKIND	USESIN	GUNSHY	RUNDLE	CUANDO
MUMBLY	OUTMAN	FLUMES	MAZUMA	IONIUM	UNCAGE	UNGAVA	UNLAYS	UNROLL	UNTRIG	UNKINK	USESON	GUNSIT	RUNDMC	CUANTO
MUMMED	PULMON	FRUMPS	MECUMS	LABIUM	UNCAKE	UNGILT	UNLEAD	UNROOF	UNTROD	UNLENT	USOPEN	GUNTER	RUNDRY	CURNOW
MUMMER	PUMMEL	FRUMPY	OAKUMS	LIGNUM	UNCALM	UNGIRD	UNLEAF	UNROOT	UNTRUE	UNLINK	UTAHAN	HUNGBY	RUNFOR	DUENAS
MUMMYS	QUEMOY	GLUMLY	ODIUMS	LUDLUM	UNCAPS	UNGIRT	UNLEAN	UNROPE	UNTUCK	UNMANS	UTICAN	HUNGER	RUNGIN	DUENNA
NUMBAT	RUDMAN	GRUMIO	OLEUMS	LYCEUM	UNCASE	UNGLAD	UNLEFT	UNROVE	UNTUNE	UNPENS		HUNGIN	RUNGUP	DUENOS
NUMBED	RUMMER	GRUMPS	OPIUMS	MAGNUM	UNCASK	UNGLIB	UNLENT	UNRUDE	UNUSED	UNPENT	•UN•••	HUNGON	RUNINS	DUNNED
NUMBER	SUBMIT	GRUMPY	PNEUMA	MEDIUM	UNCAST	UNGLUE	UNLESS	UNRUED	UNVAIN	UNPINS	AUNTEM	HUNGRY	RUNLET	DUNNER
NUMBLY	SUMMED	LOUMAS	PNEUMO	MUSEUM	UNCHIC	UNGRIP	UNLIKE	UNRULY	UNVEIL	UNRENT	AUNTIE	HUNGUP	RUNLOW	DURNED
NUMERO	SUMMER	MAUMAU	RCRUMB	OMASUM	UNCIAL	UNGUAL	UNLIMP	UNRUNG	UNVOID	UNRUNG	BUNCHE	HUNKER	RUNNEL	DURNIT
NUMINA	SUMMIT	MAUMEE	RELUME	OMNIUM	UNCLAD	UNGUES	UNLINK	UNRUST	UNWALL	UNSENT	BUNCHY	HUNLEY	RUNNER	EUONYM
PUMICE	SUMMON	MUUMUU	REPUMP	OSMIUM	UNCLAY	UNGUIS	UNLIVE	UNSAFE	UNWARY	UNSUNG	BUNCOS	HUNTED	RUNOFF	EUPNEA
PUMMEL	TUBMAN	NEUMAN	RESUME	OUTSUM	UNCLES	UNGULA	UNLOAD	UNSAGE	UNWELL	UNSUNK	BUNDLE	HUNTER	RUNONS	FUNNED
PUMPED		NOUMEA	RHEUMS	PABLUM	UNCLIP	UNHAFT	UNLOCK	UNSAID	UNWEPT	UNTUNE	BUNDTS	HUNTUP	RUNOUT	FUNNEL
PUMPER	•U••M•	PLUMBO	RHEUMY	PARFUM	UNCLOG	UNHAIR	UNLOOP	UNSAWN	UNWIGS	UNWIND	BUNGAY	JUNCOS	RUNSAT	GUANOS
PUMPUP	AUTUMN	PLUMBS	SCRUMS	PEPLUM	UNCOIL	UNHALE	UNLOST	UNSAYS	UNWILD	UNZONE	BUNGED	JUNEAU	RUNSBY	GUINAN
RUMAKI	DURUMS	PLUMED	SEDUMS	PHYLUM	UNCOLA	UNHAND	UNLUSH	UNSEAL	UNWILY	UPBIND	BUNGEE	JUNGER	RUNSIN	GUINEA
RUMBAS	FUSUMA	PLUMES	SERUMS	PILEUM	UNCOOL	UNHASP	UNMADE	UNSEAM	UNWIND	UPLAND	BUNGLE	JUNGLE	RUNSON	GUNNAR
RUMBLE	JUSTME	PLUMMY	STRUMS	PLENUM	UNCOOP	UNHATS	UNMAKE	UNSEAT	UNWISE	UPLINK	BUNION	JUNGLY	RUNSTO	GUNNED
RUMBLY	PURIMS	PLUMPS	THRUMS	PODIUM	UNCORE	UNHAZY	UNMANS	UNSEEN	UNWISH	UPPING	BUNKED	JUNIOR	RUNSUP	GUNNER

GURNEE
GURNEY
GUVNOR
LUANDA
LUGNUT
NUANCE
NUDNIK
PUENTE
PUENZO
PUNNED
PUNNER
PUTNAM
PUTNEY
QUANTA
QUENCH
QUINCE
QUINCY
QUINQU
QUINTA
QUINTE
QUINTI
QUINTS
QUINZE
RUANDA
RUDNER
RUINED
RUINER
RUNNEL
RUNNER
SUBNET
SUENOS
SUMNER
SUNNED
SUNNIS
TUNNEL
TUNNEY
TURNED
TURNER
TURNIN
TURNIP
TURNON
TURNTO
TURNUP

•U••N•

AUFOND
AUGEND
AUMONT
BURANA
BURINS
BUSING
BUSONI
BUTANE
BUTENE
BUYING
BUYINS
CUBANS
CUBING
CUEING
CUMINS
CURING
CUTINS
DUDING
DUENNA
DUGONG
DUKING
DUMONT
DUNANT
DUPING
DUPONT
DURANT
DURING
EUGENE
FUMING
FUSING
FUTONS
FUTUNA
GUGINO
GUIANA
GUYANA
GUYING
HUMANE
HUMANS
HURONS
HUSING
HUTONE
JUKING
LUBING
LUCENT
LUCINE
LUDENS
LUGING
LUMENS
LUMINA
LUPINE
LUPINO
LUPONE
LURENE
LURING
MURANO
MURINE
MUSING
MUSTNT
MUTANT
MUTING
MUTINY
MUTONS
NUGENT
NUKING
NUMINA
OUTING
PULING
PURINA
PUTONS
QUAINT
QUEENE
QUEENS
QUOINS
RUBENS
RULING
RUNINS
RUNONS
RUTINS
SUEANE
SUEANN
SUNUNU
SUPINE
SUSANB
SUSANN
TUBING
TUCANA
TULANE
TUNING
TURING
YUKONS
YUMANS
YUTANG

•U•••N

AUBURN
AUGEAN
AUSTEN
AUSTIN
AUTUMN
BUCHAN
BUFFON
BUNION
BUNSEN
BUNTON
BUNYAN
BURDEN
BURMAN
BURNIN
BURTON
BUSMAN
BUSMEN
BUSTIN
BUTTIN
BUTTON
BUYSIN
BUYSON
CUBFAN
CUEDIN
CUESIN
CULKIN
CULLEN
CURLIN
CURTIN
CURZON
CUTSIN
DUBLIN
DUCHIN
DUMPON
DUNCAN
DUNKIN
DUNLIN
DURBAN
DURBIN
DUSTIN
DUTTON
EUCKEN
EUSDEN
FULTON
FUNRUN
FURMAN
FUSION
GUINAN
GULDEN
GUNMAN
GUNMEN
GURION
GUTMAN
GUTZON
GUZMAN
HUDSON
HUNGIN
HUNGON
HUSTON
HUTTON
JUDEAN
JUDSON
JULIAN
JULIEN
JUMPIN
JUMPON
JUSTIN
KUCHEN
KUPRIN
LUBLIN
LUCIAN
LUCIEN
LUDDEN
LUMPEN
LUMPIN
LUNDEN
LUPTON
LUREIN
MUDHEN
MUFFIN
MULLIN
MUSEON
MUSLIN
MUTTON
NUBBIN
NUBIAN
NUNGEN
NUTKIN
OUTBAN
OUTGUN
OUTMAN
OUTRAN
OUTRUN
OUTSIN
PUFFIN
PULLIN
PULLON
PULMON
PUPKIN
PUSHIN
PUSHON
PUTSIN
PUTSON
PUTTIN
QUEZON
RUBSIN
RUBSON
RUDKIN
RUDMAN
RULEON
RUNGIN
RUNSIN
RUNSON
RUNYON
RUSHIN
RUSKIN
RUTTAN
RUXPIN
SUBORN
SUCKIN
SUDDEN
SUEANN
SULLEN
SULTAN
SUMMON
SUNFAN
SUNKEN
SUNKIN
SUNTAN
SURFIN
SUSANN
SUTTON
TUBMAN
TUCKIN
TUCSON
TUGSON
TULSAN
TUNEIN
TURBAN
TUREEN
TURHAN
TURNIN
TURNON
TURPIN
TUSCAN
VULCAN
ZUNIAN

••UN••

BLUNTS
BOUNCE
BOUNCY
BOUNDS
BOUNTY
BRUNCH
BRUNEI
BRUNET
BRUNOR
BRUNTS
CHUNKS
CHUNKY
CLUNKS
CLUNKY
COUNTS
COUNTY
CRUNCH
DAUNTS
FAUNAE
FAUNAL
FAUNAS
FAUNUS
FLUNKS
FLUNKY
FOUNDS
FOUNTS
FRUNZE
GOUNOD
GRUNDY
GRUNGE
GRUNGY
GRUNTS
HAUNCH
HAUNTS
HOUNDS
HOUNDY
IDUNNO
JAUNES
JAUNTS
JAUNTY
JOUNCE
JOUNCY
KAUNAS
KAUNDA
LAUNCH
LOUNGE
MAUNDY
MOUNDS
MOUNTS
MOUNTY
NOUNAL
PAUNCH
PLUNGE
PLUNKS
PLUNKY
POUNCE
POUNDS
PRUNED
PRUNER
PRUNES
RAUNCH
REUNED
REUNER
REUNES
ROUNDS
SAUNAS
SHUNTS
SKUNKS
SKUNKY
SOUNDS
SPUNKY
STUNTS
STUNTY
TAUNTS
THUNKS
TRUNKS
VAUNTS
VAUNTY
WOUNDS
ZOUNDS

••U•N•

ALUMNA
ALUMNI
AQUINO
BLUING
BOURNE
BRUINS
CHURNS
CLUING
DOUANE
ELUANT
EQUINE
FLUENT
FOURNO
GIUGNO
GLUING
GLUONS
GRUING
IDUNNO
IGUANA
JOURNO
LOUANN
MOURNS
SLUING
SPURNS
SQUINT
TAUONS
TRUANT
TRUING
UTURNS

••U••N

ABUTON
ACUMEN
ARUBAN
BAUMAN
BHUTAN
BOUDIN
BOUTON
CLUEIN
COUPON
COUSIN
CRUZAN
EGUREN
GLUEON
GLUTEN
HAULIN
HEUSEN
HOUDON
LAUREN
LAURYN
LOUANN
LOUDEN
LOUDON
LOUVIN
MOULIN
NEUMAN
NEURON
NGUYEN
PLUGIN
PLUTON
POUPON
POURIN
REUBEN
SAURON
SHUTIN
SOURON
SPURON
TAUPIN
TAUTEN
TEUTON
TOUCAN
TOULON
TRUMAN
VAUGHN
YOUWIN

•••UN•

ABOUND
AMOUNT
ARJUNA
AROUND
ATTUNE
AVAUNT
BADUNS
BBGUNS
BLOUNT
BOSUNS
CAJUNS
DEBUNK
DEFUND
DEJUNK
DETUNE
DRJUNG
EDMUND
EXEUNT
FECUND
FLAUNT
FREUND
FUTUNA
GERUND
GROUND
HLHUNT
IMMUNE
IMMUNO
INJUNE
INRUNS
INTUNE
JEJUNE
JOCUND
KAHUNA
KORUNA
LACUNA
LAGUNA
MIFUNE
MIZUNA
NORUNS
OBTUND
OSMUND
PODUNK
REFUND
REHUNG
RERUNS
RETUNE
ROTUND
SHRUNK
SPRUNG
STRUNG
STRUNK
SUNUNU
TRIUNE
UNHUNG
UNHUNH
UNRUNG
UNSUNG
UNSUNK
UNTUNE
VICUNA
WEEUNS
YAMUNA

•••U•N

AUBURN
AUTUMN
COBURN
COLUMN
FRAUEN
IMPUGN
INTURN
LEGUIN
MCKUEN
MYTURN
OAHUAN
OPPUGN
PADUAN
PAPUAN
PAQUIN
REPUGN
RETURN
SATURN
SEQUIN
SIOUAN
TEAURN
TOBURN
UPTURN
WOBURN

••••UN

ADNOUN
AIRGUN
BARZUN
BIGFUN
BIGGUN
CANCUN
CAPGUN
CHACUN
DATSUN
DOGRUN
DRYRUN
ENDRUN
FORFUN
FUNRUN
HADFUN
HAMSUN
HASFUN
ICERUN
ITSFUN
JETGUN
LEBRUN
MACOUN
MEIFUN
NONRUN
ONABUN
ONERUN
OUTGUN
OUTRUN
POPGUN
PROGUN
RAYGUN
REDSUN
SHOGUN
SIXGUN
SKIRUN
THESUN
TOPGUN
TOYGUN
UNSPUN
VERDUN
WASFUN
ZIPGUN

U•O•••

UBOATS
UBOLTS
UNOCAL
UNOILY
UNOPEN
UNORAL
UNOWED
UPOVER
USOPEN
UTOPIA

U••O••

UGSOME
UNBOLD
UNBOLT
UNBORN
UNCOIL
UNCOLA
UNCOOL
UNCOOP
UNCORE
UNCORK
UNDOCK
UNDOER
UNDOES
UNDONE
UNFOLD
UNFOND
UNFORK
UNFOUL
UNFOXY
UNHOED
UNHOLY
UNHOOD
UNHOOK
UNIONS
UNJOIN
UNLOAD
UNLOCK
UNLOOP
UNLOST
UNMOLD
UNMOOR
UNMOWN
UNPOSH
UNPOTS
UNROBE
UNROLL
UNROOF
UNROOT
UNROPE
UNROVE
UNSOFT
UNSOLD
UNSOLE
UNSORE
UNSORT
UNSOUR
UNSOWN
UNTOLD
UNTORN
UNVOID
UNWORN
UNWOVE
UNYOKE
UNZONE
UPBOWS
UPCOIL
UPDOVE
UPFOLD
UPHOLD
UPHOVE
UPJOHN
UPLOAD
UPMOST
UPROAR
UPROOT
UPROSE
UPSOAR
UPTOIT
UPTORE
UPTORN
UPTOSS
UPTOWN
USTOUR
UTMOST
UVEOUS

U•••O•

UBUROI
UNCLOG
UNCOOL
UNCOOP
UNHOOD
UNHOOK
UNIPOD
UNISOM
UNISON
UNKNOT
UNLOOP
UNMOOR
UNROOF
UNROOT
UNSHOD
UNSHOE
UNSLOW
UNSTOP
UNSTOW
UNTROD
UPFLOW
UPGROW
UPPROP
UPROOT
UPSHOT
URGEON
USEDON
USEFOR
USESON

U••••O

ULTIMO
UNESCO
UNHERO
USEDTO

•UO•••

BUOYED
BUOYUP
CUORES
DUOMOS
EUONYM
QUOINS
QUOITS
QUOQUE
QUORUM
QUOTAS
QUOTED
QUOTEE
QUOTER
QUOTES

•U•O••

AUFOND
AUMONT
AURORA
AUROUS
AUTOED
BUGOFF
BUGOUT
BUJOLD
BULOVA
BUMOUT
BUROAK
BUSONI
BUYOFF
BUYOUT
CUBOID
CUPOLA
CUTOFF
CUTOUT
DUBOIS
DUBOSE
DUGONG
DUGOUT
DUMONT
DUPONT
DUROCS
EUBOEA
EUDORA
EULOGY
EUROPA
EUROPE
FURORE
FURORS
FUTONS
HUMORS
HUMOUR
HURONS
HUTONE
JUDOKA
JURORS
LUGOSI
LUGOUT
LUPONE
MUTONS
NUTOIL
OUIOUI
PUJOLS
PUTOFF
PUTONS
PUTOUT
RUBOFF
RUBOUT
RUDOLF
RUFOUS
RUMORS
RUMOUR
RUNOFF
RUNONS
RUNOUT
SUBORN
SUDOKU
SUNOCO
TUDORS
TUTORS
YUKONS

•U••O•

AUDIOS
AUTHOR
BUENOS
BUFFON
BUFFOS
BUGBOY
BUNCOS
BUNION
BUNKOS
BUNTON
BURBOT
BURGOO
BURGOS
BURROS
BURROW
BURTON
BUSBOY
BUTEOS
BUTHOW
BUTTON
BUYNOW
BUYSON
CUCKOO
CURIOS
CURNOW
CURSOR
CURZON
CUSTOM
DUENOS
DUGFOR
DUMBOS
DUMPON
DUNLOP
DUOMOS
DUPLOS
DUTTON
FUEGOS
FULLOF
FULTON
FURROW
FUSION
GUANOS
GUMBOS
GUNDOG
GUNFOR
GURION
GUTZON
GUVNOR
HUDSON
HUEVOS
HULLOS
HUNGON
HUSTON
HUTTON
JUDSON
JUEGOS
JUMBOS
JUMPON
JUNCOS
JUNIOR
JUNTOS
KUDROW
LUDLOW
LUMMOX
LUPTON
LUTHOR
MUCHOF
MUNROE
MURROW
MUSEON
MUSEOS
MUSKOX
MUTTON
NULLOS
OUTBOW
OUTBOX
OUTFOR
OUTFOX
OUTPOP
OUTROW
PULLON
PULMON
PUSHON
PUTSON
QUAHOG
QUEMOY
QUESOS
QUEZON
RUBSON
RULEON
RUNFOR
RUNLOW
RUNSON
RUNYON
SUBGOD
SUBLOT
SUCCOR
SUEFOR
SUENOS
SUITOR
SUMMON
SUNBOW
SUNDOG
SUNGOD
SUREOF
SUTTON
TUCSON
TUGSON
TURBOS
TURBOT
TURNON

•U•••O

AUSTRO
BULDEO
BUMPPO
BURGOO
BUTWHO
CUANDO
CUANTO
CUATRO
CUCKOO
CUMULO
DUELLO
DUETTO
FUGATO
GUGINO
GUNGHO
HUTTWO
JURADO
JUSTSO
LUGLIO
LUPINO
MURANO
MUSTDO
NUCLEO
NUMERO
NUNCIO
NUNZIO
PUEBLO
PUENZO
PUERTO
PUTSTO
QUARTO
RUBATO
RUNSTO
RUSHTO
SUBITO
SUNGTO
SUNOCO
SUREDO
TUNETO
TUPELO
TURNTO
TUXEDO

••UO••

CRUORS
EQUOID
FLUORO
GLUONS
TAUONS

••U•O•

ABUTON
BLUEOX
BOUTON
BRUNOR
COUPON
CRUSOE
GLUEON
GOUNOD
HOUDON
LOUDON
NEUROL
NEURON
PLUTON
POUPON
SAURON
SOURON
SPURON
STUPOR
TAUROG
TEUTON
TOULON
UBUROI
ZHUKOV

••U••O

AQUINO
BHUTTO
BLUFFO
CHURRO
FLUORO
FOURNO
GAUCHO
GIUGNO
GLUETO
GOUPTO
GRUMIO
IDUNNO
JOURNO
PLUMBO
PLUVIO
SLUGGO
STUCCO
STUDIO
TRUETO
TRUMBO
YOUTWO

•••UO•

LIQUOR
PEQUOD
PEQUOT

•••U•O

AILURO
ARTURO
CARUSO
CUMULO
ENDURO
ESCUDO
IMMUNO
KAKURO
MADURO
MAPUTO
MENUDO
MODULO
ONAUTO
PNEUMO

PSEUDO
ROMULO
SALUTO
TENUTO

••••UO
BANQUO
MATSUO

UP••••
UPBEAR
UPBEAT
UPBIND
UPBOWS
UPCARD
UPCAST
UPCOIL
UPCURL
UPDART
UPDATE
UPDIKE
UPDIVE
UPDOVE
UPENDS
UPFLOW
UPFOLD
UPGAZE
UPGIRD
UPGIRT
UPGREW
UPGROW
UPHEAP
UPHELD
UPHERE
UPHILL
UPHOLD
UPHOVE
UPJOHN
UPKEEP
UPLAND
UPLAST
UPLATE
UPLEAP
UPLIFT
UPLINK
UPLOAD
UPMOST
UPNEXT
UPOVER
UPPERS
UPPILE
UPPING
UPPISH
UPPITY
UPPROP
UPRATE
UPREAR
UPRISE
UPROAR
UPROOT
UPROSE
UPRUSH
UPSALA
UPSEND
UPSENT
UPSETS
UPSHAW
UPSHOT
UPSIDE
UPSIZE
UPSOAR
UPSPIN
UPSTEP
UPSTIR
UPTAKE
UPTALK
UPTEAR
UPTICK
UPTILT
UPTIME
UPTOIT
UPTORE
UPTORN
UPTOSS
UPTOWN
UPTURN
UPWAFT
UPWARD
UPWELL
UPWIND

U•P•••
UMPING
UMPIRE
UNPACK
UNPAID
UNPALE
UNPAWN
UNPEEL
UNPEGS
UNPENS
UNPENT
UNPICK
UNPILE
UNPINS
UNPLAN
UNPLUG
UNPOSH
UNPOTS
UNPRIM
UNPURE
UPPERS
UPPILE
UPPING
UPPISH
UPPITY
UPPROP

U••P••
UNEPIC
UNIPED
UNIPOD
UNOPEN
UNSPAN
UNSPUN
UPSPIN
USOPEN
UTOPIA

U•••P•
UNCAPS
UNKEPT
UNRIPE
UNRIPS
UNROPE
UNTAPE
UNWEPT
UNZIPS
USHAPE
USURPS

U••••P
UNCLIP
UNCOOP
UNDEEP
UNGRIP
UNHASP
UNLIMP
UNLOOP
UNSHIP
UNSNAP
UNSTEP
UNSTOP
UNTRAP
UNWRAP
UPHEAP
UPKEEP
UPLEAP
UPPROP
UPSTEP
USEDUP
USESUP

•UP•••
AUPAIR
BUPKES
BUPKIS
BUPKUS
CUPELS
CUPFUL
CUPIDS
CUPOLA
CUPPAS
CUPPED
CUPRIC
CUPULE
DUPERS
DUPERY
DUPING
DUPLEX
DUPLOS
DUPONT
EUPNEA
HUPPAH
KUPRIN
LUPINE
LUPINO
LUPONE
LUPTON
MUPPET
PUPATE
PUPILS
PUPKIN
PUPPED
PUPPET
RUPEES
RUPERT
RUPIAH
SUPERB
SUPERG
SUPERS
SUPINE
SUPPED
SUPPER
SUPPLE
SUPPLY
SUPRAS
TUPELO
TUPPER
TUPTIM
YUPPIE

•U•P••
AUSPEX
BUMPED
BUMPER
BUMPPO
BUMPUP
BURPED
BURPEE
CUPPAS
CUPPED
CUSPAL
CUSPED
CUSPID
DUMPED
DUMPER
DUMPON
DUMPTY
GULPED
GULPER
HUMPED
HUMPHS
HUMPTY
HUPPAH
JUMPAT
JUMPED
JUMPER
JUMPIN
JUMPON
JUMPUP
LUMPED
LUMPEN
LUMPER
LUMPIN
LUMPIT
LUMPUR
MUDPIE
MUPPET
MURPHY
OUTPAY
OUTPOP
OUTPRY
OUTPUT
PULPED
PULPER
PULPIT
PUMPED
PUMPER
PUMPUP
PUPPED
PUPPET
PURPLE
PURPLY
PUTPUT
QUAPAW
QUIPPY
QUIPUS
RUMPLE
RUMPLY
RUMPUS
RUXPIN
SUBPAR
SUPPED
SUPPER
SUPPLE
SUPPLY
TUPPER
TURPIN
YUPPIE

•U••P•
BUMPPO
CUTUPS
EUROPA
EUROPE
GUELPH
JULEPS
OUTSPY
QUIPPY
RUNUPS
SUMUPS
SUNUPS
TULIPS

•U•••P
BUCKUP
BUFFUP
BULKUP
BUMPUP
BUMRAP
BUOYUP
BURLAP
BURNUP
BUSTUP
BUYSUP
CUESUP
CUETIP
CURLUP
CUTSUP
DUDEUP
DUNLAP
DUNLOP
DUSTUP
FUELUP
FULLUP
FUZZUP
GUMSUP
GUNLAP
HUBCAP
HUNGUP
HUNTUP
HUSHUP
JUMPUP
MUCKUP
MUSSUP
OUTLIP
OUTPOP
OUTRAP
PUFFUP
PULLUP
PUMPUP
PUSHUP
PUTSUP
RUBSUP
RUCKUP
RUNGUP
RUNSUP
SUCKUP
SUITUP
SUMSUP
TUNEUP
TURNIP
TURNUP

••UP••
CHUPPA
COUPES
COUPLE
COUPON
DRUPES
ERUPTS
GOUPTO
INUPIK
LAUPER
LOUPES
NTUPLE
PAUPER
POUPON
SOUPER
SOUPUP
STUPAS
STUPES
STUPID
STUPOR
TAUPES
TAUPIN
TOUPEE

••U•P•
CHUMPS
CHUPPA
CLUMPS
CLUMPY
CRUMPS
EQUIPS
FOURPM
FRUMPS
FRUMPY
GRUMPS
GRUMPY
PLUMPS
SCULPT
SLUMPS
SLURPS
STUMPS
STUMPY
THUMPS
TRUMPS
USURPS

••U••P
CLUBUP
CRUDUP
DRUMUP
FOULUP
FOURUP
HAULUP
PLUGUP
SHUTUP
SOUPUP
TRUEUP

•••UP•
ABRUPT
CROUPS
CROUPY
CUTUPS
FIXUPS
GETUPS
GROUPS
ICEUPS
IRRUPT
JAMUPS
LAYUPS
LETUPS
MIXUPS
MOPUPS
NIPUPS
OCCUPY
ONEUPS
PINUPS
POPUPS
RUNUPS
SCOUPE
SETUPS
SIRUPS
SITUPS
SUMUPS
SUNUPS
SYRUPS
SYRUPY
TIEUPS
TROUPE

•••U•P
DEPULP
REPUMP

••••UP
ACESUP
ACTSUP
ADDSUP
AIRSUP
ALEGUP
AMPSUP
ANTEUP
ASKSUP
BACKUP
BALLUP
BANGUP
BANKUP
BEADUP
BEAMUP
BEARUP
BEATUP
BEEFUP
BELTUP
BIDSUP
BINDUP
BITEUP
BLEWUP
BLOTUP
BLOWUP
BOBSUP
BOILUP
BOLTUP
BONEUP
BOOTUP
BOREUP
BREWUP
BUCKUP
BUFFUP
BULKUP
BUMPUP
BUOYUP
BURNUP
BUSTUP
BUYSUP
CAGEUP
CAKEUP
CALLUP
CAMEUP
CAMPUP
CASTUP
CATSUP
CHATUP
CHEWUP
CHINUP
CHIPUP
CHOPUP
CLAMUP
CLOGUP
CLOTUP
CLUBUP
COILUP
COMEUP
COOKUP
COOPUP
CORKUP
COSYUP
COZYUP
CROPUP
CRUDUP
CUESUP
CURLUP
CUTSUP
DAMSUP
DEALUP
DIALUP
DIGSUP
DISHUP
DOESUP
DOITUP
DOLLUP
DONEUP
DRAGUP
DRAWUP
DREWUP
DRUMUP
DUDEUP
DUSTUP
EASEUP
EATSUP
EGGCUP
ENDSUP
EVENUP
EYECUP
EYEDUP
EYESUP
FACEUP
FAIRUP
FESSUP
FILLUP
FIREUP
FIRMUP
FITSUP
FIVEUP
FLEWUP
FLIPUP
FOGSUP
FOLDUP
FOOTUP
FORKUP
FOULUP
FOURUP
FREEUP
FUELUP
FULLUP
FUZZUP
GALLUP
GANGUP
GAVEUP
GEARUP
GETSUP
GINSUP
GIVEUP
GLAMUP
GOESUP
GONEUP
GOOFUP
GREWUP
GROWUP
GUMSUP
HACKUP
HAMSUP
HANDUP
HANGUP
HARDUP
HAULUP
HAVEUP
HEADUP
HEALUP
HEAPUP
HEATUP
HELDUP
HELPUP
HICCUP
HIGHUP
HIKEUP
HITSUP
HOLDUP
HOLEUP
HOOKUP
HOPSUP
HOTCUP
HUNGUP
HUNTUP
HUSHUP
HYPEUP
ICEDUP
ICESUP
JACKUP
JAMSUP
JAZZUP
JERKUP
JOINUP
JUMPUP
KEEPUP
KEPTUP
KEYSUP
KICKUP
KISSUP
KNOTUP
LACEUP
LAIDUP
LANDUP
LAPSUP
LARRUP
LASHUP
LASTUP
LAYSUP
LEADUP
LEAPUP
LETSUP
LICKUP
LIFTUP
LINEUP
LINKUP
LOADUP
LOCKUP
LOOKUP
LOOMUP
MADEUP
MAKEUP
MARKUP
MASHUP
MEETUP
MESSUP
MISTUP
MOCKUP
MOPSUP
MOVEUP
MUCKUP
MUSSUP
NAILUP
NEXTUP
NINEUP
NOSEUP
OILCUP
OPENUP
OWNSUP
PACKUP
PAGEUP
PAIDUP
PAIRUP
PASSUP
PAYSUP
PENSUP
PENTUP
PEPSUP
PERKUP
PETPUP
PICKUP
PILEUP
PINSUP
PIPEUP
PLAYUP
PLOWUP
PLUGUP
PONYUP
POPSUP
PRENUP
PROPUP
PUFFUP
PULLUP
PUMPUP
PUSHUP
PUTSUP
RACEUP
RACKUP
RAKEUP
RAMPUP
RANGUP
RAVEUP
READUP
REARUP
RECOUP
REELUP
RESTUP
REVSUP
RIDEUP
RIGSUP
RILEUP
RINGUP
RIPSUP
RISEUP
RODEUP
ROILUP
ROLLUP
ROOTUP
ROPEUP
ROSEUP
RUBSUP
RUCKUP
RUNGUP
RUNSUP
SACKUP
SAVEUP
SAWSUP
SEALUP
SEENUP
SEESUP
SENDUP
SENTUP
SETSUP
SEWNUP
SEWSUP
SHOTUP
SHOWUP
SHUTUP
SIGNUP
SITSUP
SIZEUP
SLIPUP
SLOWUP
SNAGUP
SNAPUP
SOAKUP
SOAPUP
SOPSUP
SOUPUP
SPEDUP
STAYUP
STEPUP
STIRUP
STOPUP
SUCKUP
SUITUP
SUMSUP
SWAMUP
TACKUP
TAGSUP
TAKEUP
TALKUP
TANKUP
TAPEUP
TARTUP
TEACUP
TEAMUP
TEARUP
TEEDUP
TEESUP
TIDYUP
TIEDUP
TIESUP
TILTUP
TINCUP
TIPSUP
TOGSUP
TONEUP
TOOKUP
TOOLUP
TOPSUP
TOREUP
TORNUP
TOSSUP
TOTEUP
TOTSUP
TRIPUP
TROTUP
TRUEUP
TUNEUP
TURNUP
TYPEUP
USEDUP
USESUP
WADSUP
WAITUP
WAKEUP
WALKUP
WALLUP
WARMUP
WASHUP
WELLUP
WENTUP
WHIPUP
WINDUP
WIPEUP
WIREUP
WISEUP
WOKEUP
WORKUP
WRAPUP
ZIPSUP

UQ••••
UQUARK

U••Q••
UNIQUE

•UQ•••
BUQSHA
TUQUES

•U•Q••
JUSQUE
QUOQUE

•U••Q•
QUINQU
SUZYQS

•U•••Q
SUZIEQ

UR••••
URACIL
URAEUS
URALIC
URALSK
URANIA
URANIC
URANUS
URBANA
URBANE
URBANI
URBANV
URCHIN
URGENT
URGEON
URGERS
URGING
URNFUL
URSIDS
URSINE
URSULA
URTEXT

U•R•••
ULRICH
UNRACK
UNRASH
UNREAD
UNREAL
UNREEL
UNRENT
UNREST
UNRIFE
UNRIGS
UNRIPE
UNRIPS
UNROBE
UNROLL
UNROOF
UNROOT
UNROPE
UNROVE
UNRUDE
UNRUED
UNRULY
UNRUNG
UNRUST
UPRATE
UPREAR
UPRISE
UPROAR
UPROOT
UPROSE
UPRUSH
UVRAYS

U••R••
UBUROI
UGARTE
ULTRAS
UMBRAE
UMBRAL
UMBRAS
UMBRIA
UNARMS
UNDRAW
UNDREW
UNFREE
UNGRIP
UNORAL
UNPRIM
UNTRAP
UNTRIG
UNTROD
UNTRUE
UNWRAP
UPGREW
UPGROW
UPPROP
USARMY
USERID
USURER
USURPS
UTURNS

U•••R•
UDDERS
ULCERS
UMBERS
UMPIRE
UNBARE
UNBARS
UNBORN
UNBURY
UNCORE
UNCORK
UNCURB
UNCURL
UNDERS
UNFIRM
UNFORK
UNFURL
UNGIRD
UNGIRT
UNHERO
UNHIRE
UNHURT
UNMIRY
UNPURE
UNSERE
UNSORE
UNSORT
UNSURE
UNTORN
UNWARY
UNWORN
UPCARD
UPCURL
UPDART
UPGIRD
UPGIRT
UPHERE
UPPERS
UPTORE
UPTORN
UPTURN
UPWARD
UQUARK
URGERS
USHERS
UTTERS

U••••R
UECKER
UGLIER
ULSTER
UNDOER
UNFAIR
UNHAIR
UNITER
UNMOOR
UNSOUR
UNTIER
UPBEAR
UPOVER
UPREAR
UPROAR
UPSOAR
UPSTIR
UPTEAR
USEFOR
USTOUR
USURER
UVULAR

•UR•••
AURATE
AURIFY
AURIGA
AURIST
AURORA
AUROUS
BURANA
BURBLE
BURBLY
BURBOT
BURDEN
BUREAU
BURETS
BURGEE
BURGER
BURGHS
BURGLE
BURGOO
BURGOS
BURIAL
BURIED
BURIER
BURIES
BURINS
BURKAS
BURLAP
BURLED
BURLER
BURLEY
BURMAN
BURNED
BURNER
BURNET
BURNEY
BURNIE
BURNIN
BURNUP
BUROAK
BURPED
BURPEE
BURRED
BURROS
BURROW
BURSAE
BURSAL
BURSAR
BURSAS
BURSTS
BURTON
CURACY
CURADS
CURARE
CURATE
CURBED
CURDED
CURDLE
CURERS

CURETS
CURFEW
CURIAE
CURIES
CURING
CURIOS
CURITE
CURIUM
CURLED
CURLER
CURLEW
CURLEY
CURLIN
CURLUP
CURNOW
CURRED
CURSED
CURSER
CURSES
CURSOR
CURTER
CURTIN
CURTIS
CURTIZ
CURTLY
CURTSY
CURVED
CURVES
CURVET
CURZON
DURANT
DURBAN
DURBIN
DURESS
DURFEY
DURHAM
DURING
DURNED
DURNIT
DUROCS
DURRAS
DURUMS
DURYEA
EURAIL
EUREKA
EUROPA
EUROPE
FURBYS
FURIES
FURLED
FURMAN
FURORE
FURORS
FURRED
FURROW
FURZES
GURGLE
GURION
GURKHA
GURLEY
GURNEE
GURNEY
HURDLE
HURLED
HURLER
HURLEY
HURONS
HURRAH

HURRAY
HURTER
HURTLE
JURADO
JURIED
JURIES
JURIST
JURORS
KURALT
KURILE
LUREIN
LURENE
LURERS
LURING
LURKED
LURKER
LURKEY
MURALS
MURANO
MURCIA
MURDER
MURIEL
MURINE
MURMUR
MURPHY
MURRAY
MURRES
MURROW
NURSED
NURSER
NURSES
PURDUE
PUREED
PUREES
PURELY
PUREST
PURFLE
PURGED
PURGES
PURIFY
PURIMS
PURINA
PURISM
PURIST
PURITY
PURLED
PURLIE
PURPLE
PURPLY
PURRED
PURRER
PURSED
PURSER
PURSES
PURSUE
PURVEY
SURAHS
SUREAM
SUREDO
SUREIS
SURELY
SUREOF
SUREST
SURETE
SURETY
SURFED
SURFER
SURFIN

SURGED
SURGES
SURIMI
SURREY
SURTAX
SURVEY
TURBAN
TURBID
TURBOS
TURBOT
TUREEN
TURFED
TURGID
TURHAN
TURING
TURKEY
TURKIC
TURNED
TURNER
TURNIN
TURNIP
TURNON
TURNTO
TURNUP
TURPIN
TURRET
TURTLE
WURSTS
ZURICH

•U•R••
AUBREY
AUDREY
BUMRAP
BURRED
BURROS
BURROW
CUORES
CUPRIC
CURRED
DUARTE
DURRAS
FUHRER
FUNRUN
FURRED
FURROW
GUARDS
GUERRE
HUBRIS
HURRAH
HURRAY
JUAREZ
KUDROW
KUPRIN
MUNROE
MURRAY
MURRES
MURROW
NUTRIA
OUTRAN
OUTRAP
OUTRIB
OUTRIG
OUTROW
OUTRUN
PUERTO
PURRED
PURRER

PUTRID
QUARKS
QUARRY
QUARTE
QUARTO
QUARTS
QUARTZ
QUIRED
QUIRES
QUIRKS
QUIRKY
QUIRTS
QUORUM
RUBRAW
RUBRIC
RUGRAT
SUCRES
SUNRAY
SUPRAS
SURREY
SUTRAS
TUGRIK
TURRET

•U••R•
AUBURN
AUGERS
AUGURS
AUGURY
AURORA
AUSTRO
BUMBRY
BUYERS
CUATRO
CUBERS
CUNARD
CURARE
CURERS
DUGARD
DUPERS
DUPERY
EUCHRE
EUDORA
FUGARD
FULCRA
FUMERS
FURORE
FURORS
FUTURA
FUTURE
GUERRE
GUIDRY
GUITRY
HUBERT
HUMERI
HUMORS
HUNGRY
JUDFRY
JURORS
KUNDRY
LUGERS
LURERS
LUSTRA
LUSTRE
LUXURY
MUNERA
MUSERS
NUBIRA

NUMERO
OUTCRY
OUTPRY
PULERS
QUADRI
QUARRY
QUATRE
QUEERS
RUDERY
RULERS
RUMORS
RUNDRY
RUPERT
SUBARU
SUBORN
SUBURB
SUGARS
SUGARY
SULTRY
SUNDRY
SUPERB
SUPERG
SUPERS
SUTURE
SUVARI
TUBERS
TUDORS
TULARE
TUNDRA
TUNERS
TUTORS

•U•••R
AUPAIR
AUSTER
AUTEUR
AUTHOR
BUCKER
BUDDER
BUDGER
BUFFER
BUGLER
BULGAR
BULGUR
BULWER
BUMMER
BUMPER
BUNKER
BUNTER
BURGER
BURIER
BURLER
BURNER
BURSAR
BUSHER
BUSIER
BUSKER
BUSTER
BUTLER
BUTTER
BUZZER
CULLER
CUMBER
CURLER
CURSER
CURSOR
CURTER
CUSSER

CUSTER
CUTLER
CUTTER
CUVIER
CUYLER
DUBBER
DUCKER
DUELER
DUFFER
DUGFOR
DULLER
DUMBER
DUMPER
DUNBAR
DUNKER
DUNNER
DUSTER
FUDGER
FUELER
FUHRER
FULLER
FULMAR
FUMIER
FUNDER
FUNFUR
FUSSER
GUIDER
GUITAR
GULPER
GUNFOR
GUNNAR
GUNNER
GUNTER
GUSHER
GUTTER
GUVNOR
HUGGER
HULLER
HUMBER
HUMMER
HUMOUR
HUNGER
HUNKER
HUNTER
HURLER
HURTER
HUSKER
HUSSAR
JUICER
JUMPER
JUNGER
JUNIOR
JUNKER
JUSTER
KUBLER
LUBBER
LUGGER
LULLER
LUMBAR
LUMBER
LUMPER
LUMPUR
LUNGER
LUNKER
LURKER
LUSHER
LUSTER
LUTHER

LUTHOR
MUCKER
MUDDER
MUGGER
MULDER
MULLER
MUMMER
MURDER
MURMUR
MUSHER
MUSTER
MUTTER
NUBBER
NUDGER
NUMBER
NURSER
NUTTER
OUSTER
OUTFOR
OUTWAR
PUCKER
PUFFER
PULLER
PULPER
PULSAR
PULVER
PUMPER
PUNIER
PUNKER
PUNNER
PUNTER
PURRER
PURSER
PUSHER
PUTTER
QUAKER
QUASAR
QUAVER
QUELER
QUEUER
QUIVER
QUOTER
RUBBER
RUCKER
RUDDER
RUDNER
RUINER
RULIER
RUMMER
RUMOUR
RUNFOR
RUNNER
RUSHER
RUTGER
RUTTER
SUAVER
SUBPAR
SUBWAR
SUCCOR
SUCKER
SUDSER
SUEFOR
SUFFER
SUITOR
SULFUR
SULKER
SUMMER
SUMNER

SUMTER
SUNDER
SUPPER
SURFER
SUTTER
TUCKER
TUGGER
TUPPER
TURNER
TUSKER
VULGAR
ZUCKER

••UR••
ACURAS
AZURED
AZURES
BEURRE
BLURBS
BLURRY
BLURTS
BOURGS
BOURKE
BOURNE
BOURSE
CHURCH
CHURLS
CHURNS
CHURRO
COURIC
COURSE
COURTS
CRURAL
DOURER
DOURIF
DOURLY
EGUREN
ENURED
ENURES
EXURBS
FLURRY
FOURAA
FOURAD
FOURAM
FOURBC
FOUREE
FOURNO
FOURPM
FOURTH
FOURUP
GLURGE
GOURDE
GOURDS
HEURES
HOURIS
HOURLY
INURED
INURES
ITURBI
JAURES
JOURNO
KNURLS
KNURLY
LAUREL
LAUREN
LAUREY
LAURIA
LAURIC

LAURIE
LAURYL
LAURYN
MOURNS
NEURAL
NEUROL
NEURON
PLURAL
POURED
POURER
POURIN
REURGE
ROURKE
SAURON
SAURUS
SCURFY
SCURRY
SCURVE
SCURVY
SEURAT
SLURPS
SLURRY
SMURFS
SOURCE
SOURED
SOURER
SOURLY
SOURON
SPURNS
SPURON
SPURTS
STURDY
TAURIC
TAUROG
TAURUS
TOURED
TOURER
TSURIS
UBURQI
USURER
USURPS
UTURNS

••U•R•
ALUDRA
BEURRE
BLURRY
CHURRO
CLUERS
CRUORS
EDUARD
ELUARD
FLUORO
FLURRY
FOUDRE
GLUERS
LOUVRE
OEUVRE
POUDRE
SCURRY
SLURRY
SQUARE
SQUIRE
SQUIRM
SQUIRT
STUART
UQUARK

••U••R
ABUSER
ACUTER
ALULAR
AMUSER
BAUMER
BRUDER
BRUNOR
CAUSER
COUGAR
COUTER
CRUDER
DAUBER
DEUTER
DOURER
DOUSER
ELUDER
FLUTER
FOULER
GAUGER
GLUIER
GOUGER
HAULER
KRUGER
LAUDER
LAUPER
LAUTER
LOUDER
LOUVER
MAULER
MAUSER
MOUSER
NEUTER
OCULAR
OVULAR
PAUPER
PAUSER
PCUSER
POURER
POUTER
PRUNER
REUNER
REUSER
REUTER
ROUSER
ROUTER
SAUCER
SOUPER
SOURER
SOUTER
STUPOR
TAUTER
TOURER
TOUTER
USURER
UVULAR

•••UR•
ABJURE
ABSURD
ADJURE
AILURO
ALLURE
AMOURS
ARTURO
ASBURY
ASPURE
ASSURE

AUBURN
AUGURS
AUGURY
BESURE
COBURG
COBURN
COEURS
CONURE
DEBURR
DEJURE
DEMURE
DEMURS
ELBURZ
ENDURE
ENDURO
ENSURE
ERFURT
FEMURS
FIGURE
FLEURS
FLOURS
FLOURY
FUTURA
FUTURE
HHOURS
IMHURT
IMMURE
IMPURE
IMSURE
INCURS
INJURE
INJURY
INSURE
INTURN
KAKURO
LEMURS
LUXURY
MADURO
MANURE
MATURE
MYTURN
NATURE
OCCURS
ODOURS
OHSURE
PARURE
PENURY
PLEURA
RASURE
REBURY
RECURE
RECURL
RECURS
RETURF
RETURN
SATURN
SCOURS
SECURE
SEGURA
SIGURD
SOEURS
SUBURB
SUTURE
TEAURN
TENURE
TOBURN
UNBURY
UNCURB

UNCURL
UNFURL
UNHURT
UNPURE
UNSURE
UPCURL
UPTURN
VELURE
VFOURS
WOBURN
YOGURT

•••U•R
ARGUER
BREUER
DEBURR
ISSUER
JAGUAR
JANUAR
LIQUOR
QUEUER
VAGUER
VALUER
VOGUER

••••UR
ARBOUR
ARDOUR
ARMOUR
ARTHUR
ATFOUR
AUTEUR
BALDUR
BENHUR
BIGSUR
BULGUR
COLOUR
CONCUR
DAMOUR
DEBLUR
DETOUR
DEVOUR
DISEUR
DOLOUR
FAVOUR
FUNFUR
GOSOUR
HONOUR
HUMOUR
INPOUR
JAIPUR
KIPPUR
KRONUR
LABOUR
LAMOUR
LATOUR
LETOUR
LUMPUR
MSIEUR
MURMUR
ONTOUR
POSEUR
RAIPUR
REPOUR
RETOUR
RIGOUR
RUMOUR
SAVOUR

SHAKUR
SIDDUR
SULFUR
UNSOUR
USTOUR
VALOUR
VAPOUR
VELOUR
VIGOUR
WILBUR
YASGUR

US••••
USABLE
USABLY
USAGES
USANCE
USARMY
USAUSA
USBANK
USEDCD
USEDIN
USEDON
USEDTO
USEDUP
USEFOR
USEFUL
USENET
USERID
USESIN
USESON
USESUP
USETAX
USFLAG
USHAPE
USHERS
USHING
USMAIL
USMINT
USNAVY
USNEWS
USOPEN
USTOUR
USUALS
USURER
USURPS

U•S•••
UGSOME
ULSTER
UNSAFE
UNSAGE
UNSAID
UNSAWN
UNSAYS
UNSEAL
UNSEAM
UNSEAT
UNSEEN
UNSELD
UNSELL
UNSENT
UNSERE
UNSEWN
UNSEWS
UNSEXY
UNSHED
UNSHIP

UNSHOD
UNSHOE
UNSHUT
UNSICK
UNSKEW
UNSLIM
UNSLOW
UNSMUG
UNSNAG
UNSNAP
UNSNUG
UNSOFT
UNSOLD
UNSOLE
UNSORE
UNSORT
UNSOUR
UNSOWN
UNSPAN
UNSPUN
UNSTEP
UNSTOP
UNSTOW
UNSUED
UNSUNG
UNSUNK
UNSURE
UPSALA
UPSEND
UPSENT
UPSETS
UPSHAW
UPSHOT
UPSIDE
UPSIZE
UPSOAR
UPSPIN
UPSTEP
UPSTIR
URSIDS
URSINE
URSULA

U••S••
UKASES
UNDSET
UNESCO
UNISEX
UNISOM
UNISON
UNISYS
UNUSED
USESIN
USESON
USESUP

U•••S•
UNBUSY
UNCASE
UNCASK
UNCAST
UNEASE
UNEASY
UNHASP
UNHUSK
UNJUST
UNLASH
UNLESS

UNLOST
UNLUSH
UNMASK
UNMAST
UNMESH
UNPOSH
UNRASH
UNREST
UNRUST
UNWISE
UNWISH
UPCAST
UPLAST
UPMOST
UPPISH
UPRISE
UPROSE
UPRUSH
UPTOSS
URALSK
USAUSA
UTMOST

U••••S
UBOATS
UBOLTS
UCLANS
UDDERS
UGGAMS
UGLIES
UHAULS
UHLANS
UINTAS
UKASES
ULCERS
ULTRAS
UMBELS
UMBERS
UMBRAS
UMIAKS
UNAMIS
UNARMS
UNBAGS
UNBARS
UNBITS
UNBUDS
UNCAPS
UNCLES
UNDAMS
UNDERS
UNDIES
UNDIMS
UNDOES
UNFITS
UNGAGS
UNGUES
UNGUIS
UNHATS
UNIATS
UNICES
UNIONS
UNISYS
UNITAS
UNITES
UNJAMS
UNLAYS
UNLESS
UNMANS

UNMEWS
UNPEGS
UNPENS
UNPINS
UNPOTS
UNRIGS
UNRIPS
UNSAYS
UNSEWS
UNTIES
UNWIGS
UNZIPS
UPBOWS
UPENDS
UPPERS
UPSETS
UPTOSS
URAEUS
URANUS
URGERS
URSIDS
USAGES
USHERS
USNEWS
USUALS
USURPS
UTAHNS
UTTERS
UTUBES
UTURNS
UVEOUS
UVRAYS
UVULAS

•US•••

AUSPEX
AUSSIE
AUSTEN
AUSTER
AUSTIN
AUSTRO
BUSBOY
BUSHED
BUSHEL
BUSHER
BUSHES
BUSHWA
BUSIED
BUSIER
BUSIES
BUSILY
BUSING
BUSKED
BUSKER
BUSMAN
BUSMEN
BUSONI
BUSSED
BUSSES
BUSTED
BUSTER
BUSTIN
BUSTLE
BUSTUP
CUSACK
CUSECS
CUSHAW
CUSPAL
CUSPED
CUSPID
CUSSED
CUSSER
CUSSES
CUSTER
CUSTIS
CUSTOM
DUSKED
DUSTED
DUSTER
DUSTIN
DUSTUP
EUSDEN
EUSTIS
FUSEES
FUSILE
FUSILS
FUSING
FUSION
FUSSAT
FUSSED
FUSSER
FUSSES
FUSUMA
GUSHED
GUSHER
GUSHES
GUSSET
GUSTAV
GUSTED
HUSHED
HUSHES
HUSHUP
HUSING
HUSKED
HUSKER
HUSSAR
HUSSEY
HUSTLE
HUSTON
JUSQUE
JUSTAS
JUSTER
JUSTIN
JUSTLY
JUSTME
JUSTSO
JUSTUS
JUSTYS
LUSAKA
LUSHER
LUSHES
LUSHLY
LUSTED
LUSTER
LUSTRA
LUSTRE
MUSCAT
MUSCLE
MUSCLY
MUSEES
MUSEON
MUSEOS
MUSERS
MUSEUM
MUSHED
MUSHER
MUSHES
MUSIAL
MUSICK
MUSICS
MUSING
MUSKET
MUSKIE
MUSKOX
MUSLIM
MUSLIN
MUSSED
MUSSEL
MUSSES
MUSSET
MUSSUP
MUSTDO
MUSTER
MUSTNT
OUSELS
OUSTED
OUSTER
PUSHED
PUSHER
PUSHES
PUSHIN
PUSHIT
PUSHON
PUSHUP
PUSSES
RUSHAT
RUSHBY
RUSHED
RUSHEE
RUSHER
RUSHES
RUSHIN
RUSHTO
RUSKIN
RUSSEL
RUSSES
RUSSET
RUSSIA
RUSTED
RUSTIC
RUSTLE
SUSANB
SUSANN
SUSHIS
SUSSED
SUSSES
SUSSEX
TUSCAN
TUSHES
TUSHIE
TUSKED
TUSKER
TUSSAL
TUSSES
TUSSLE
WUSSES

•U•S••

AUSSIE
BUNSEN
BUQSHA
BURSAE
BURSAL
BURSAR
BURSAS
BURSTS
BUSSED
BUSSES
BUYSAT
BUYSIN
BUYSIT
BUYSON
BUYSUP
CUESIN
CUESTA
CUESUP
CURSED
CURSER
CURSES
CURSOR
CUSSED
CUSSER
CUSSES
CUTSIN
CUTSIT
CUTSUP
DUESSA
FUISSE
FUSSAT
FUSSED
FUSSER
FUSSES
GUESTS
GUISES
GUMSUP
GUNSEL
GUNSHY
GUNSIT
GUSSET
HUDSON
HUSSAR
HUSSEY
JUDSON
MUESLI
MUSSED
MUSSEL
MUSSES
MUSSET
MUSSUP
NURSED
NURSER
NURSES
OUTSAT
OUTSAW
OUTSAY
OUTSEE
OUTSET
OUTSIN
OUTSIT
OUTSPY
OUTSUM
PULSAR
PULSED
PULSES
PURSED
PURSER
PURSES
PURSUE
PUSSES
PUTSBY
PUTSCH
PUTSIN
PUTSON
PUTSTO
PUTSUP
QUASAR
QUESOS
QUESTS
RUBSIN
RUBSON
RUBSUP
RUNSAT
RUNSBY
RUNSIN
RUNSON
RUNSTO
RUNSUP
RUSSEL
RUSSES
RUSSET
RUSSIA
SUBSEA
SUBSET
SUDSED
SUDSER
SUDSES
SUISSE
SUMSUP
SUNSET
SUSSED
SUSSES
SUSSEX
TUCSON
TUGSAT
TUGSON
TULSAN
TUSSAL
TUSSES
TUSSLE
TUTSIS
WURSTS
WUSSES

•U••S•

AUGUST
AURIST
AUTISM
AUTIST
CUBISM
CUBIST
CURTSY
CUTEST
CUTESY
DUBOSE
DUDISH
DUESSA
DURESS
EULESS
FUISSE
HUGEST
JURIST
JUSTSO
KUVASZ
LUGOSI
LUTIST
MUFASA
MULISH
MUTEST
NUDEST
NUDISM
NUDIST
OUTASK
PUNISH
PUREST
PURISM
PURIST
QUEASY
RUDEST
SUFISM
SUISSE
SUREST
TUBIST
TUFTSU

•U•••S

AUDIOS
AUDITS
AUGEAS
AUGERS
AUGHTS
AUGURS
AUROUS
BUBBAS
BUBKES
BUDGES
BUENAS
BUENOS
BUFFOS
BUGLES
BUICKS
BUILDS
BULGES
BUNCOS
BUNDTS
BUNKOS
BUPKES
BUPKIS
BUPKUS
BURETS
BURGHS
BURGOS
BURIES
BURINS
BURKAS
BURROS
BURSAS
BURSTS
BUSHES
BUSIES
BUSSES
BUTEOS
BUTKUS
BUTTES
BUTUTS
BUYERS
BUYINS
BUZZES
CUBANS
CUBEBS
CUBERS
CUBICS
CUBITS
CUICAS
CULETS
CULLIS
CULTUS
CUMINS
CUORES
CUPELS
CUPIDS
CUPPAS
CURADS
CURERS
CURETS
CURIES
CURIOS
CURSES
CURTIS
CURVES
CUSECS
CUSSES
CUSTIS
CUTEYS
CUTIES
CUTINS
CUTUPS
CUVEES
DUBOIS
DUCATS
DUENAS
DUENOS
DUFFYS
DULLES
DUMBOS
DUNCES
DUNDAS
DUOMOS
DUPERS
DUPLOS
DURESS
DUROCS
DURRAS
DURUMS
DUTIES
DUVETS
EULESS
EUSTIS
FUDGES
FUEGOS
FUGUES
FUMERS
FUNGUS
FURBYS
FURIES
FURORS
FURZES
FUSEES
FUSILS
FUSSES
FUTONS
FUTZES
FUZZES
GUANOS
GUARDS
GUAVAS
GUESTS
GUIDES
GUILDS
GUILES
GUISES
GULAGS
GUMBOS
GUSHES
HUBRIS
HUEVOS
HUGHES
HULLOS
HUMANS
HUMMUS
HUMORS
HUMPHS
HURONS
HUSHES
JUDGES
JUEGOS
JUEVES
JUICES
JULEPS
JULIUS
JUMBOS
JUNCOS
JUNIUS
JUNTAS
JUNTOS
JURIES
JURORS
JUSTAS
JUSTUS
JUSTYS
KUDZUS
KULAKS
LUCIUS
LUDENS
LUGERS
LUMENS
LUNDIS
LUNGES
LUNIKS
LURERS
LUSHES
LUTZES
MUCHAS
MUFTIS
MULCTS
MULEYS
MULLAS
MULTIS
MUMMYS
MURALS
MURRES
MUSEES
MUSEOS
MUSERS
MUSHES
MUSICS
MUSSES
MUTIUS
MUTONS
NUDGES
NUECES
NUEVES
NULLOS
NURSES
OUCHES
OUGHTS
OUIJAS
OUNCES
OUSELS
OUTGAS
OUTIES
OUZELS
PUCCIS
PUJOLS
PULERS
PULSES
PUNKAS
PUNTAS
PUPILS
PUREES
PURGES
PURIMS
PURSES
PUSHES
PUSSES
PUTONS
QUACKS
QUAFFS
QUAILS
QUAKES
QUALES
QUALMS
QUARKS
QUARTS
QUEENS
QUEERS
QUELLS
QUESOS
QUESTS
QUEUES
QUIETS
QUILLS
QUILTS
QUINTS
QUIPUS
QUIRES
QUIRKS
QUIRTS
QUOINS
QUOITS
QUOTAS
QUOTES
RUBELS
RUBENS
RUBIES
RUBIKS
RUBLES
RUCHES
RUCKUS
RUDKUS
RUFOUS
RULERS
RUMBAS
RUMORS
RUMPUS
RUNINS
RUNONS
RUNUPS
RUPEES
RUSHES
RUSSES
RUTINS
SUCHAS
SUCRES
SUDSES
SUEDES
SUENOS
SUGARS
SUITES
SULFAS
SUMACS
SUMUPS
SUNDAS
SUNNIS
SUNUPS
SUPERS
SUPRAS
SURAHS
SUREIS
SURGES
SUSHIS
SUSSES
SUTRAS
SUZYQS
TUBERS
TUDORS
TULIPS
TULLES
TUNERS
TUNICS
TUQUES
TURBOS
TUSHES
TUSSES
TUTEES
TUTORS
TUTSIS
TUTTIS
VULGUS
WURSTS
WUSSES
YUCCAS
YUKONS
YUMANS
YUTZES

••US••

ABUSED
ABUSER
ABUSES
AMUSED
AMUSER
AMUSES
BAUSCH
BRUSHY
CAUSAL
CAUSED
CAUSER
CAUSES
COUSIN
CRUSES
CRUSOE
CRUSTS
CRUSTY
DOUSED
DOUSER
DOUSES
DRUSES
FRUSTA
HEUSEN
HOUSED
HOUSES
JOUSTS
KRUSTY
KYUSHU
LOUSED
LOUSES
MAUSER
MOUSED
MOUSER
MOUSES
MOUSEY
MOUSSE
NAUSEA
ONUSES
OPUSES
PAUSAL
PAUSED
PAUSER
PAUSES
PCUSER
PIUSII
PIUSIV
PIUSIX
PIUSVI
PIUSXI
PLUSES
PLUSHY
POUSSE
REUSED
REUSER
REUSES
ROUSED
ROUSER
ROUSES
ROUSTS
SLUSHY
SOUSED
SOUSES
THUSLY
TOUSLE
TRUSTS
TRUSTY
UNUSED
WAUSAU
YOUSEE
YOUSUF

••U•S•

AGUISH
AVULSE
BLUEST
BLUESY
BLUISH
BOURSE
BRUISE
CHUHSI
CLUMSY
COURSE
CRUISE
EVULSE
FLUISH
IGUESS
LOUISA
LOUISB
LOUISE
LOUISI
LOUISV
LOUISX
MOUSSE
POUSSE
SQUASH
SQUISH
TRUEST
TRUISM

••U••S

ABUSES
ACURAS
ACUTES
ADULTS
AMUSES
ANUBIS
AZUKIS
AZURES
BAULKS
BLUETS
BLUFFS
BLUNTS
BLURBS
BLURTS
BOUGHS
BOULES
BOUNDS
BOURGS
BRUGES
BRUINS
BRUITS
BRUMES
BRUNTS
BRUTES
BRUTUS
BRUXES
CAUCUS
CAULKS
CAUSES
CHUCKS
CHUFFS
CHUMPS
CHUNKS
CHURLS
CHURNS
CHUTES
CLUCKS
CLUERS
CLUMPS
CLUNKS
COUGHS
COUNTS
COUPES
COURTS
CRUCES
CRUDES
CRUETS
CRUMBS
CRUMPS
CRUORS
CRUSES
CRUSTS
CRUXES
DAUBES
DAUNTS
DEUCES
DOUBTS
DOUGHS
DOULAS
DOUSES
DOUZES
DRUIDS
DRUPES
DRUSES
DRUZES
EDUCES
EDUCTS
ELUDES
ELUTES
ENURES
EQUALS
EQUIPS
ERUCTS
ERUPTS
ETUDES
EXUDES
EXULTS
EXURBS
FAULTS
FAUNAS
FAUNUS
FAUTES
FAUVES
FLUFFS
FLUIDS
FLUKES
FLUMES
FLUNKS
FLUTES
FLUXES
FOUNDS
FOUNTS
FRUITS
FRUMPS
GAUGES
GAUZES
GLUERS
GLUONS
GLUTES
GOUDAS
GOUGES
GOURDS
GRUELS
GRUMPS
GRUNTS
GSUITS
HAUNTS
HEURES
HOUNDS
HOURIS
HOUSES
IGUESS
INUITS
INURES
ISUZUS
JAUNES
JAUNTS
JAURES
JOULES
JOUSTS
KAUNAS
KNURLS
LAUGHS
LOUIES
LOUMAS
LOUPES
LOUSES
MAUVES
MOULDS
MOULTS
MOUNDS
MOUNTS
MOURNS
MOUSES
MOUTHS
NAUTES
OCULUS
ONUSES
OPUSES
OVULES
PAUSES
PIUTES
PLUCKS
PLUIES
PLUMBS
PLUMES
PLUMPS
PLUNKS
PLUSES
PLUTUS
POULES
POULTS
POUNDS
PRUDES
PRUNES
REUNES
REUSES
RHUMBS
ROUGES
ROUGHS
ROUNDS
ROUSES
ROUSTS
ROUTES
SAUCES
SAUDIS
SAULTS
SAUNAS
SAURUS
SAUTES
SCUBAS
SCUFFS
SCULLS
SHUCKS
SHUNTS
SKULKS
SKULLS
SKUNKS
SLUMPS
SLURPS
SMURFS
SNUFFS
SOUNDS
SOUSES
SOUTHS
SPUMES
SPURNS
SPURTS
SQUABS
SQUADS
SQUATS
SQUIBS
SQUIDS
STUFFS
STUKAS
STUMPS
STUNTS
STUPAS
STUPES
TAUNTS
TAUONS
TAUPES
TAURUS
THUMBS
THUMPS
THUNKS
TOUGHS
TRUCES
TRUCKS
TRUMPS
TRUNKS
TRUSTS
TRUTHS
TSURIS
USUALS
USURPS
UTUBES
UTURNS
UVULAS
VAULTS
VAUNTS
WOUNDS
YOUTHS
ZEUXIS
ZOUNDS

•••US•

ABLUSH
ACCUSE
ADJUST
AMBUSH
AROUSE
ATDUSK
AUGUST
BEMUSE
BLOUSE
CARUSO
CAYUSE
CLAUSE
CREUSA
CREUSE
CROUSE
DEFUSE
DEGUST
DERUST
DISUSE
EFFUSE
ENDUSE
EXCUSA
EXCUSE
FYVUSH
GOBUST
GROUSE
ILLUSE
IMBUSY
INCUSE
INFUSE
INRUSH
KRAUSS
LETUSE
LOCUST
MANUSH
MEDUSA
MISUSE
NOFUSS
NONUSE
NORUSH
OBTUSE
ONRUSH
PERUSE
PROUST
RAGUSA
RECUSE
REDUST

REFUSE ROBUST SCHUSS SPOUSE THEUSA THRUSH THRUST UNBUSY UNHUSK UNJUST UNLUSH UNRUST UPRUSH USAUSA WATUSI

•••U•S

ADOUTS ALBUMS ALEUTS AMOURS ANNULS ARGUES AUGURS BADUNS BBGUNS BEAUTS BEGUMS BOSUNS BUTUTS CAGUAS CAJUNS CLOUDS CLOUTS COEURS COQUIS CROUPS CUTUPS DEBUGS DEBUTS DEGUMS DEMURS DONUTS DOSUMS DURUMS ENDUES ENNUIS ENSUES EXCUBS FEMURS FIXUPS FLEURS FLOURS FLOUTS FORUMS FRAUDS FUGUES GAMUTS GETUPS GHOULS GIGUES GLOUCS GONUTS GROUPS GROUTS HHOURS HOHUMS HOKUMS ICEUPS IMBUES INCURS INDUES INPUTS INRUNS ISSUES JAMUPS JORUMS KHOUMS KNOUTS KRAUSS LAYUPS LEHUAS LEMURS LETUPS LIEUTS MAQUIS MECUMS MIXUPS MOGULS MOPUPS NIPUPS NOBUTS NOFUSS NORUNS OAKUMS OCCURS ODIUMS ODOULS ODOURS OHNUTS OLEUMS ONEUPS OPHULS OPIUMS PINUPS PIQUES POPUPS PSEUDS QUEUES REBUTS REBUYS RECUES RECURS RECUTS REDUBS REPUBS RERUNS REVUES RHEUMS ROGUES RUNUPS SCHUSS SCOURS SCOUTS SCRUBS SCRUMS SEDUMS SEGUES SERUMS SETUPS SHOUTS SHRUBS SHRUGS SIRUPS SITUPS SNOUTS SOEURS SPOUTS STOUTS STRUMS STRUTS SUMUPS SUNUPS SYRUPS THRUMS TIEUPS TOGUES TOQUES TROUTS TUQUES UHAULS UNBUDS UNGUES UNGUIS VALUES VENUES VFOURS VOGUES VWBUGS WEEUNS YAKUTS YAQUIS ZHLUBS

••••US

AARHUS ABACUS ADIEUS AEOLUS AIRBUS ALDOUS ALTIUS AMICUS AMINUS ANIMUS ANJOUS ATREUS AUROUS BACKUS BANTUS BAYOUS BIJOUS BMINUS BRUTUS BUPKUS BUTKUS CACTUS CADMUS CALLUS CAMPUS CARPUS CAUCUS CENSUS CEREUS CESTUS CHORUS CIRCUS CIRRUS CITIUS CITRUS CIXOUS CMINUS COCCUS COLEUS CORPUS CORVUS COYPUS CROCUS CRONUS CULTUS CYGNUS CYPRUS DARIUS DECIUS DELIUS DINGUS DISCUS DMINUS DOOFUS ELBRUS EMMAUS ENNIUS EREBUS EXITUS EXODUS FAMOUS FAUNUS FEROUS FESTUS FICHUS FONDUS FUNGUS GAMOUS GENIUS GLARUS GOOFUS GYNOUS HAIKUS HIATUS HINDUS HIPPUS HUMMUS HYDRUS IAMBUS ICARUS ISUZUS ITIOUS JANHUS JOYOUS JULIUS JUNIUS JUSTUS KOMBUS KUDZUS LANDUS LAPSUS LINGUS LITMUS LOFTUS LUCIUS MAGNUS MARCUS MEATUS MEDIUS MIAOUS MINGUS MISSUS MOBIUS MUTIUS NEHRUS NESSUS NIMBUS NODOUS OBELUS OBOLUS OCULUS ODIOUS PAREUS PELEUS PILAUS PILEUS PILOUS PINDUS PLEXUS PLUTUS PODOUS POILUS PONZUS POROUS PRIMUS QUIPUS RADIUS RAPTUS RECTUS REGIUS RHESUS RIMOUS RUCKUS RUDKUS RUFOUS RUMPUS SADHUS SAURUS SEAMUS SEROUS SHAMUS SIRIUS SIXTUS SNAFUS SOLEUS STATUS STPIUS STYLUS TARSUS TAURUS TEMPUS THYMUS TMINUS TRAGUS TYPHUS URAEUS URANUS UVEOUS VARMUS VASTUS VENOUS VERSUS VINOUS VIRTUS VOROUS VULGUS WALRUS WITHUS XYSTUS

UT••••

UTAHAN UTAHNS UTHANT UTICAN UTMOST UTOPIA UTTERS UTUBES UTURNS

U•T•••

ULTIMA ULTIMO ULTRAS UMTATA UNTACK UNTAME UNTAPE UNTAUT UNTHAW UNTIDY UNTIED UNTIER UNTIES UNTILT UNTOLD UNTORN UNTRAP UNTRIG UNTROD UNTRUE UNTUCK UNTUNE UPTAKE UPTALK UPTEAR UPTICK UPTILT UPTIME UPTOIT UPTORE UPTORN UPTOSS UPTOWN UPTURN URTEXT USTOUR UTTERS

U••T••

UINTAS ULSTER UNITAS UNITED UNITER UNITES UNSTEP UNSTOP UNSTOW UPSTEP UPSTIR USETAX

U•••T•

UBIETY UBOATS UBOLTS UGARTE UMTATA UNBITS UNCUTE UNFITS UNHATS UNIATE UNIATS UNMATE UNPOTS UPDATE UPLATE UPPITY UPRATE UPSETS USEDTO

U••••T

UMLAUT UNBAIT UNBELT UNBENT UNBOLT UNCAST UNDEFT UNDSET UNFACT UNFELT UNFLAT UNGILT UNGIRT UNHAFT UNHURT UNJUST UNKEPT UNKNIT UNKNOT UNLEFT UNLENT UNLOST UNMAST UNMEET UNMIXT UNNEAT UNPENT UNRENT UNREST UNROOT UNRUST UNSEAT UNSENT UNSHUT UNSOFT UNSORT UNTAUT UNTILT UNWEPT UPBEAT UPCAST UPDART UPGIRT UPLAST UPLIFT UPMOST UPNEXT UPROOT UPSENT UPSHOT UPTILT UPTOIT UPWAFT URGENT URTEXT USENET USMINT UTHANT UTMOST

•UT•••

AUTEUR AUTHOR AUTISM AUTIST AUTOED AUTUMN BUTANE BUTENE BUTEOS BUTHOW BUTKUS BUTLER BUTTED BUTTER BUTTES BUTTIN BUTTON BUTUTS BUTWHO BUTWHY BUTYET CUTELY CUTEST CUTESY CUTEYS CUTIES CUTINS CUTLER CUTLET CUTOFF CUTOUT CUTSIN CUTSIT CUTSUP CUTTER CUTUPS DUTIES DUTTON EUTAXY FUTILE FUTONS FUTUNA FUTURA FUTURE FUTZED FUTZES GUTMAN GUTTED GUTTER GUTZON HUTONE HUTTED HUTTON HUTTWO JUTTED LUTECE LUTHER LUTHOR LUTIST LUTZES MUTANT MUTATE MUTELY MUTEST MUTING MUTINY MUTIUS MUTONS MUTTER MUTTON MUTUAL MUTUEL NUTATE NUTKIN NUTLET NUTMEG NUTOIL NUTRIA NUTTED NUTTER OUTACT OUTADD OUTAGE OUTASK OUTATE OUTAWE OUTBAN OUTBAT OUTBEG OUTBID OUTBOW OUTBOX OUTBUD OUTBUY OUTCRY OUTCUT OUTDID OUTEAT OUTFIT OUTFLY OUTFOR OUTFOX OUTGAS OUTGUN OUTHIT OUTIES OUTING OUTJET OUTJUT OUTLAW OUTLAY OUTLED OUTLET OUTLIE OUTLIP OUTMAN OUTPAY OUTPOP OUTPRY OUTPUT OUTRAN OUTRAP OUTRIB OUTRIG OUTROW OUTRUN OUTSAT OUTSAW OUTSAY OUTSEE OUTSET OUTSIN OUTSIT OUTSPY OUTSUM OUTVIE OUTWAR OUTWIT PUTNAM PUTNEY PUTOFF PUTONS PUTOUT PUTPUT PUTRID PUTSBY PUTSCH PUTSIN PUTSON PUTSTO PUTSUP PUTTED PUTTEE PUTTER PUTTIN RUTGER RUTHIE RUTILE RUTINS RUTTAN RUTTED RUTTER SUTRAS SUTTER SUTTON SUTURE TUTEES TUTORS TUTSIS TUTTED TUTTIS TUTTUT TUTUED YUTANG YUTZES

•U•T••

AUNTEM AUNTIE AUSTEN AUSTER AUSTIN AUSTRO BUNTED BUNTER BUNTON BURTON BUSTED BUSTER BUSTIN BUSTLE BUSTUP BUTTED BUTTER BUTTES BUTTIN BUTTON CUATRO CUETIP CULTCH CULTIC CULTUS CURTER CURTIN CURTIS CURTIZ CURTLY CURTSY CUSTER CUSTIS CUSTOM CUTTER DUCTAL DUCTED DUETED DUETTI DUETTO DUSTED DUSTER DUSTIN DUSTUP DUTTON EUSTIS FULTON GUITAR GUITRY GUNTER GUSTAV GUSTED GUTTED GUTTER HUNTED HUNTER HUNTUP HURTER HURTLE HUSTLE HUSTON HUTTED HUTTON HUTTWO JUNTAS JUNTOS JUSTAS JUSTER JUSTIN JUSTLY JUSTME JUSTSO JUSTUS JUSTYS JUTTED LUNTHA LUPTON LUSTED LUSTER LUSTRA LUSTRE MUFTIS MULTIS MUSTDO MUSTER MUSTNT MUTTER MUTTON NUTTED NUTTER OUSTED OUSTER PUNTAS PUNTED PUNTER PUTTED PUTTEE PUTTER PUTTIN QUATRE QUITIT QUOTAS QUOTED QUOTEE QUOTER QUOTES RUSTED RUSTIC RUSTLE RUTTAN RUTTED RUTTER SUBTLE SUBTLY SUITED SUITES SUITOR SUITUP SULTAN SULTRY SUMTER SUNTAN SURTAX SUTTER SUTTON TUFTED TUFTSU TUPTIM TURTLE TUTTED TUTTIS TUTTUT

•U••T•

AUDITS AUGHTS AUGITE AURATE BUNDTS BURETS BURSTS BUTUTS CUANTO CUBITI CUBITS CUESTA CULETS CURATE CURETS CURITE DUARTE DUCATS DUETTI DUETTO DULUTH DUMPTY DUVETS FUGATO GUESTS GUILTY GUNITE HUMPTY JUDITH KUNITZ LUCITE LUNATE LUXATE MULCTS MULETA MUTATE NUDITY NUTATE OUGHTA OUGHTS OUTATE PUENTE PUERTO PUPATE PURITY PUTSTO QUANTA QUARTE QUARTO QUARTS QUARTZ QUESTS QUIETS QUILTS QUINTA QUINTE QUINTI QUINTS QUIRTS QUOITS RUBATI RUBATO RULETH RUNSTO RUSHTO SUBITO SUNGTO SURETE SURETY TUBATE TUNETO TURNTO WURSTS YUKATA

•U•••T

AUFAIT AUGUST AUKLET AULAIT AUMONT AURIST AUTIST BUCKET BUDGET BUFFET BUGOUT BULLET BUMOUT BURBOT BURNET BUTYET BUYOUT BUYSAT BUYSIT CUBIST CULLET CURVET CUTEST CUTLET CUTOUT CUTSIT DUGOUT DULCET DUMONT DUNANT DUPONT DURANT DURNIT FUMEAT FUSSAT GULLET GUNSIT GUSSET HUBERT HUGEST JULIET JUMPAT JUNKET JURIST KURALT KUWAIT LUCENT LUGNUT LUGOUT LUMPIT LUTIST MUDCAT MUFFET MULLET MUPPET MUSCAT MUSKET MUSSET MUSTNT MUTANT MUTEST NUDEST NUDIST NUGENT NUGGET NUMBAT NUTLET OUIMET OUTACT OUTBAT OUTCUT OUTEAT OUTFIT OUTHIT OUTJET OUTJUT OUTLET OUTPUT OUTSAT OUTSET OUTSIT OUTWIT PULLET PULPIT PUNDIT PUPPET PUREST PURIST PUSHIT PUTOUT PUTPUT QUAINT QUITIT RUBOUT RUDEST RUGRAT RUNLET RUNOUT RUNSAT RUPERT RUSHAT RUSSET SUBLET SUBLOT SUBMIT SUBNET SUBSET SUMMIT SUNHAT SUNLIT SUNSET SUREST TUBIST TUFFET TUGSAT TUMULT TURBOT TURRET TUTTUT

••UT••

ABUTON ACUTER ACUTES BHUTAN BHUTTO BOUTON BRUTAL BRUTES BRUTUS CHUTED CHUTES CLUTCH COUTER CRUTCH DEUTCH

DEUTER
ELUTED
ELUTES
FAUTES
FLUTED
FLUTER
FLUTES
FLUTIE
FRUTTI
GLUTEI
GLUTEN
GLUTES
KLUTZY
LAUTER
LEUTZE
MOUTHS
MOUTHY
NAUTES
NEUTER
PIUTES
PLUTON
PLUTUS
POUTED
POUTER
REUTER
ROUTED
ROUTER
ROUTES
SAUTES
SHUTIN
SHUTUP
SMUTTY
SOUTER
SOUTHS
TAUTEN
TAUTER
TAUTLY
TEUTON
TOUTED
TOUTER
TRUTHS
YOUTHS
YOUTWO

••U•T•

ACUATE
ACUITY
ADULTS
BHUTTO
BLUETS
BLUNTS
BLURTS
BOUNTY
BRUITS
BRUNTS
COUNTS
COUNTY
COURTS
CRUETS
CRUSTS
CRUSTY
DAUNTS
DOUBTS
EDUCTS
ELUATE
EQUATE
EQUITY
ERUCTS
ERUPTS
EXULTS
FAULTS
FAULTY
FOUNTS
FOURTH
FRUCTI
FRUITS
FRUITY
FRUSTA
FRUTTI
GLUETO
GOUPTO
GRUNTS
GSUITS
HAUNTS
INUITS
JAUNTS
JAUNTY
JOUSTS
KRUSTY
MOULTS
MOUNTS
MOUNTY
POULTS
PRUETT
ROUSTS
SAULTS
SHULTZ
SHUNTS
SMUTTY
SPURTS
SQUATS
STUNTS
STUNTY
TAUNTS
TRUETO
TRUSTS
TRUSTY
VAULTS
VAULTY
VAUNTS
VAUNTY

••U••T

AMULET
BLUEST
BOUGHT
BRUNET
CAUGHT
DAUDET
ELUANT
FAUCET
FLUENT
FOUGHT
GOULET
NAUGHT
NOUGAT
NOUGHT
PRUETT
SCULPT
SEURAT
SOUGHT
SQUINT
SQUIRT
STUART
TAUGHT
TRUANT
TRUEST
YOUBET

•••UT•

ADOUTS
AGOUTI
ALEUTS
ASTUTE
BEAUTS
BEAUTY
BUTUTS
CANUTE
CLOUTS
CROUTE
DEBUTS
DEPUTE
DEPUTY
DILUTE
DONUTS
DRRUTH
DULUTH
EMEUTE
FLAUTA
FLOUTS
GAMUTS
GONUTS
GROUTS
GROUTY
IMPUTE
INPUTS
KAPUTT
KNOUTS
KPDUTY
LAPUTA
LIEUTS
LIKUTA
MAKUTA
MANUTE
MAPUTO
MINUTE
MOBUTU
NOBUTS
OFFUTT
OHNUTS
ONAUTO
ONDUTY
PAIUTE
PERUTZ
REBUTS
RECUTS
REFUTE
REPUTE
SALUTE
SALUTO
SCOUTS
SHOUTS
SLEUTH
SNOUTS
SOLUTE
SPOUTS
STOUTS
STRUTS
TENUTA
TENUTO
TROUTS
UNCUTE
VENUTI
VOLUTE
YAKUTS

•••U•T

ABDUCT
ABRUPT
ACQUIT
ADDUCT
ADJUST
AMOUNT
ANNUIT
AROUET
AUGUST
AVAUNT
BLOUNT
DEDUCT
DEGUST
DERUST
DROUET
ERFURT
EXEUNT
FLAUNT
GOBUST
HLHUNT
IMHURT
INCULT
INDUCT
INSULT
INTUIT
IRRUPT
ISEULT
JESUIT
KAPUTT
KIDULT
LOCUST
LOQUAT
MINUET
MINUIT
OCCULT
OFFUTT
PENULT
PEQUOT
PIQUET
PROUST
REDUST
RELUCT
RESUIT
RESULT
ROBUST
THRUST
TUMULT
UNHURT
UNJUST
UNRUST
YOGURT

••••UT

ACEOUT
ACTOUT
AGEOUT
AIROUT
ALLBUT
ALLOUT
ASKOUT
ATEOUT
BEIRUT
BOWOUT
BUGOUT
BUMOUT
BUYOUT
CAPNUT
CATGUT
COBNUT
COPOUT
CRYOUT
CUTOUT
DEVOUT
DIECUT
DIEOUT
DIGOUT
DIMOUT
DRYOUT
DUGOUT
EATOUT
EKEOUT
ENDCUT
ENGLUT
ENHAUT
ESCAUT
FANOUT
FAROUT
FITOUT
FLYOUT
GETOUT
GOTOUT
HADOUT
HASOUT
HELMUT
HESOUT
HEXNUT
HIDOUT
HITOUT
HOGNUT
HOPOUT
ICEOUT
INARUT
JOBCUT
KORBUT
LAYOUT
LEDOUT
LETOUT
LIPOUT
LITOUT
LOGOUT
LOWCUT
LUGNUT
LUGOUT
MAHOUT
MAPOUT
MAXOUT
MISCUT
NOTOUT
ONEOUT
OPTOUT
OUTCUT
OUTJUT
OUTPUT
PANOUT
PAYCUT
PAYOUT
PEANUT
PIGNUT
PIGOUT
POPOUT
PRECUT
PUTOUT
PUTPUT
RAGOUT
RANOUT
RATOUT
REDOUT
RESHUT
RIBCUT
RIGOUT
RIPOUT
ROTGUT
RUBOUT
RUNOUT
SALYUT
SATOUT
SAWOUT
SEEOUT
SETOUT
SITOUT
SPROUT
SPYOUT
TAGOUT
TAPOUT
TAXCUT
TENHUT
TOGOUT
TOPOUT
TRYOUT
TUTTUT
UMLAUT
UNSHUT
UNTAUT
VEGOUT
WALNUT
WAYOUT
WIGOUT
WILMUT
WINOUT
WONOUT
XEDOUT
XESOUT
YESBUT
ZAGNUT
ZIPOUT

U•U•••

UBUROI
UNUSED
UQUARK
USUALS
USURER
USURPS
UTUBES
UTURNS
UVULAE
UVULAR
UVULAS

U••U••

UHAULS
UNBUDS
UNBURY
UNBUSY
UNCUFF
UNCURB
UNCURL
UNCUTE
UNDULY
UNFULL
UNFURL
UNGUAL
UNGUES
UNGUIS
UNGULA
UNHUED
UNHULL
UNHUNG
UNHUNH
UNHURT
UNHUSK
UNJUST
UNLUSH
UNPURE
UNRUDE
UNRUED
UNRULY
UNRUNG
UNRUST
UNSUED
UNSUNG
UNSUNK
UNSURE
UNTUCK
UNTUNE
UPCURL
UPRUSH
UPTURN
URSULA
USAUSA

U•••U•

UMLAUT
UNFOUL
UNGLUE
UNIQUE
UNPLUG
UNSHUT
UNSMUG
UNSNUG
UNSOUR
UNSPUN
UNTAUT
UNTRUE
URAEUS
URANUS
URNFUL
USEDUP
USEFUL
USESUP
USTOUR
UVALUE
UVEOUS

•UU•••

MUUMUU
SUUKYI

•U•U••

AUBURN
AUGURS
AUGURY
AUGUST
AUTUMN
BUNUEL
BUTUTS
CUMULI
CUMULO
CUPULE
CUTUPS
DULUTH
DURUMS
FUGUES
FUSUMA
FUTUNA
FUTURA
FUTURE
JUJUBE
LUNULA
LUXURY
MUTUAL
MUTUEL
QUEUED
QUEUER
QUEUES
RUNUPS
SUBURB
SUMUPS
SUNUNU
SUNUPS
SUTURE
SUZUKI
TUBULE
TUMULT
TUQUES
TUTUED

•U••U•

AUROUS
AUTEUR
BUCKUP
BUFFUP
BUGOUT
BULGUR
BULKUP
BUMOUT
BUMPUP
BUNKUM
BUOYUP
BUPKUS
BURNUP
BUSTUP
BUTKUS
BUYOUT
BUYSUP
CUESUP
CULLUM
CULTUS
CUPFUL
CURIUM
CURLUP
CUTOUT
CUTSUP
DUDEUP
DUGOUT
DUMDUM
DUSTUP
FUELUP
FULLUP
FUNFUR
FUNGUS
FUNRUN
FUZZUP
GUMSUP
HUBBUB
HUMBUG
HUMMUS
HUMOUR
HUNGUP
HUNTUP
HUSHUP
JUGFUL
JULIUS
JUMPUP
JUNIUS
JUSQUE
JUSTUS
KUDZUS
LUCIUS
LUDLUM
LUGNUT
LUGOUT
LUMPUR
MUCKUP
MUGFUL
MUKLUK
MURMUR
MUSEUM
MUSSUP
MUTIUS
MUUMUU
OUIOUI
OUTBUD
OUTBUY
OUTCUT
OUTGUN
OUTJUT
OUTPUT
OUTRUN
OUTSUM
PUFFUP
PULLUP
PUMPUP
PURDUE
PURSUE
PUSHUP
PUTOUT
PUTPUT
PUTSUP
QUIPUS
QUOQUE
QUORUM
RUBOUT
RUBSUP
RUCKUP
RUCKUS
RUDKUS
RUEFUL
RUFOUS
RUMOUR
RUMPUS
RUNGUP
RUNOUT
RUNSUP
SUBDUE
SUBGUM
SUCKUP
SUITUP
SULFUR
SUMSUP
TUBFUL
TUNEUP
TURNUP
TUTTUT
VULGUS
YUMYUM

•U•••U

BUGAKU
BUKAVU
BUREAU
JUNEAU
KUNGFU
MUUMUU
QUINQU
SUBARU
SUDOKU
SUNUNU
TUFTSU
TUVALU

••U•U•

BRUTUS
CAUCUS
CLUBUP
CRUDUP
DRUMUP
FAUNUS
FLUBUG
FOULUP
FOURUP
HAULUP
ISUZUS
MUUMUU
OCULUS
PLUGUP
PLUTUS
SAURUS
SHUTUP
SOUPUP
TAURUS
TRUEUP
YOUSUF

••U••U

AKUAKU
KYUSHU
LAULAU
MAUMAU
MUUMUU
RYUKYU
WAUSAU

•••UU•

VACUUM

•••U•U

KIKUYU
LTSULU
MOBUTU
MRSULU
SUNUNU

••••UU

MUUMUU

UV••••

UVALDE
UVALUE
UVEOUS
UVRAYS
UVULAE
UVULAR
UVULAS
UVWXYZ

U•V•••

UNVAIN
UNVEIL
UNVOID

U••V••

UNAVID
UNEVEN
UNEVIL
UNIVAC
UPOVER

U•••V•

UNGAVA
UNLIVE
UNROVE
UNWOVE
UPDIVE
UPDOVE
UPHOVE
USNAVY

U••••V

URBANV

•UV•••

CUVEES
CUVIER
DUVALL
DUVETS
GUVNOR
KUVASZ
SUVARI
TUVALU
TUVWXY

•U•V••

CURVED
CURVES
CURVET
GUAVAS
HUEVOS
HUMVEE
JUEVES
NUEVES
OUTVIE
PULVER
PURVEY
QUAVER
QUIVER
SUAVER
SURVEY

•U••V•

BUKAVU
BULOVA

•U•••V

GUSTAV
RUBLEV

••UV••

FAUVES
LOUVER
LOUVIN
LOUVRE
MAUVES
OEUVRE
PLUVIA
PLUVIO
STUVWX

••U•V•

PAULVI
PIUSVI
SCURVE
SCURVY

••U••V

LOUISV
PAULIV
PIUSIV
ZHUKOV

•••UV•

DEDUVE
RSTUVW

••••UV

QRSTUV

U•W•••

UNWALL
UNWARY
UNWELL
UNWEPT
UNWIGS
UNWILD
UNWILY
UNWIND
UNWISE
UNWISH
UNWORN
UNWOVE
UNWRAP
UPWAFT
UPWARD
UPWELL
UPWIND
UVWXYZ

U••W••

UNAWED
UNOWED

U•••W•

UNDEWY
UNHEWN
UNMEWS
UNMOWN
UNPAWN
UNSAWN
UNSEWN
UNSEWS
UNSOWN
UPBOWS
UPTOWN
USNEWS

U••••W

UNDRAW
UNDREW
UNSKEW
UNSLOW
UNSTOW
UNTHAW
UPFLOW
UPGREW
UPGROW
UPSHAW

•UW•••

KUWAIT

•U•W••

BULWER
BUTWHO
BUTWHY
LUDWIG
OUTWAR
OUTWIT
RUNWAY
SUBWAR
SUBWAY
TUVWXY

•U••W•

BUSHWA
HUTTWO
OUTAWE
YUKAWA

•U•••W

BURROW
BUTHOW
BUYNOW
CURFEW
CURLEW
CURNOW
CUSHAW
FURROW
GUFFAW
GUNLAW
KUDROW
LUDLOW
MURROW
OUTBOW
OUTLAW
OUTROW
OUTSAW
QUAPAW
RUBRAW
RUNLOW
SUNBOW

••UW••

YOUWIN

••U•W•

SQUAWK
STUVWX
YOUTWO

•••U•W

RSTUVW

••••UW

DEPAUW

U••X••

UNAXED
UVWXYZ

U•••X•

UNFOXY
UNMIXT
UNSEXY
UPNEXT
URTEXT

U••••X

UNISEX
USETAX

•UX•••

HUXLEY
LUXATE
LUXURY
RUXPIN
TUXEDO

•U••X•

EUTAXY
TUVWXY

•U•••X

AUSPEX
DUPLEX
LUMMOX
MUSKOX
OUTBOX
OUTFOX
PUBLIX
SUFFIX
SURTAX
SUSSEX

••UX••

BRUXED
BRUXES
CRUXES
FLUXED
FLUXES
ZEUXIS

••U•X•

PIUSXI

••U••X

BLUEOX
KOUFAX
LOUISX
PIUSIX
STUVWX

•••UX•

DELUXE

•••U•X

PROULX

••••UX

ADIEUX
BAYEUX
BIGBUX
BIJOUX
EFFLUX
HALLUX
INFLUX
LEDOUX
LEROUX
MADDUX
POLLUX
REFLUX

U•Y•••

UNYOKE

U••Y••

UNDYED

U•••Y•

UNISYS
UNLAYS
UNSAYS
UVRAYS
UVWXYZ

U••••Y

UBIETY
UGLIFY
UGLILY
UNABLY
UNBURY
UNBUSY
UNCLAY
UNDEWY
UNDULY
UNEASY
UNFOXY
UNGAMY
UNHAZY
UNHOLY
UNIDLY
UNMIRY
UNOILY
UNRULY
UNSEXY
UNTIDY
UNWARY
UNWILY
UPPITY
USABLY
USARMY
USNAVY

•UY•••

BUYERS
BUYING
BUYINS
BUYNOW
BUYOFF

BUYOUT
BUYSAT
BUYSIN
BUYSIT
BUYSON
BUYSUP
CUYLER
GUYANA
GUYING

•U•Y••
BUNYAN
BUOYED
BUOYUP
BUTYET
DURYEA
QUAYLE
RUNYON
SUZYQS
YUMYUM

•U••Y•
CUTEYS
DUFFYS
EUONYM
FURBYS
JUSTYS
MULEYS
MUMMYS
SUUKYI

•U•••Y
AUBREY
AUDREY
AUGURY
AURIFY
BUBBLY
BUFFAY
BUGBOY
BUMBRY
BUNCHY
BUNGAY
BURBLY
BURLEY
BURNEY
BUSBOY
BUSILY
BUTWHY
CUDAHY
CUDDLY
CURACY
CURLEY
CURTLY
CURTSY
CUTELY
CUTESY
DUALLY
DUDLEY
DUMBLY
DUMPTY
DUPERY
DURFEY
EULOGY
EUTAXY
GUIDRY
GUILTY
GUITRY
GUNSHY
GURLEY
GURNEY
HUBLEY
HUGELY
HUMBLY
HUMPTY
HUNGBY
HUNGRY
HUNLEY
HURLEY
HURRAY
HUSSEY
HUXLEY
JUDFRY
JUMBLY
JUNGLY
JUSTLY
KUNDRY
LUMLEY
LUNACY
LUNCHY
LURKEY
LUSHLY
LUXURY
MUMBLY
MUNCHY
MURPHY
MURRAY
MUSCLY
MUTELY
MUTINY
NUBBLY
NUDELY
NUDITY
NUMBLY
OUTBUY
OUTCRY
OUTFLY
OUTLAY
OUTPAY
OUTPRY
OUTSAY
OUTSPY
PUDDLY
PULLEY
PUNCHY
PUNILY
PURELY
PURIFY
PURITY
PURPLY
PURVEY
PUTNEY
PUTSBY
QUACKY
QUAGGY
QUARRY
QUEASY
QUEMOY
QUINCY
QUIPPY
QUIRKY
RUBBLY
RUBIFY
RUDELY
RUDERY
RUFFLY
RUMBLY
RUMPLY
RUNDRY
RUNSBY
RUNWAY
RUSHBY
SUBTLY
SUBWAY
SUGARY
SULTRY
SUNDAY
SUNDRY
SUNRAY
SUPPLY
SURELY
SURETY
SURREY
SURVEY
TUMEFY
TUNNEY
TURKEY
TUVWXY

••UY••
NGUYEN

••U•Y•
LAURYL
LAURYN
RYUKYU
SUUKYI

••U••Y
ACUITY
BLUELY
BLUESY
BLURRY
BOUNCY
BOUNTY
BRUSHY
CAUCHY
CHUBBY
CHUCKY
CHUFFY
CHUMMY
CHUNKY
CLUBBY
CLUMPY
CLUMSY
CLUNKY
COUNTY
CRUDDY
CRUMBY
CRUMMY
CRUSTY
DOUBLY
DOUGHY
DOURLY
EQUITY
FAULTY
FLUFFY
FLUKEY
FLUNKY
FLURRY
FOULLY
FRUITY
FRUMPY
GLUMLY
GRUBBY
GRUMPY
GRUNDY
GRUNGY
HOUNDY
HOURLY
JAUNTY
JOUNCY
KLUDGY
KLUTZY
KNURLY
KRUSTY
LAUREY
LOUDLY
MAUNDY
MOULDY
MOUNTY
MOUSEY
MOUTHY
PAULEY
PLUCKY
PLUMMY
PLUNKY
PLUSHY
POUCHY
POUFFY
SCULLY
SCUMMY
SCURFY
SCURRY
SCURVY
SCUZZY
SKUNKY
SLUDGY
SLUMMY
SLURRY
SLUSHY
SMUDGY
SMUGLY
SMUTTY
SNUBBY
SNUFFY
SNUGLY
SOURLY
SPUNKY
STUBBY
STUDLY
STUFFY
STUMPY
STUNTY
STURDY
TAUTLY
THUSLY
TOUCHY
TOUGHY
TRUSTY
VAULTY
VAUNTY

•••UY•
INOUYE
KIKUYU
REBUYS

•••U•Y
ARGUFY
ASBURY
AUGURY
BEAUTY
CLOUDY
CROUPY
DEPUTY
FLOURY
GROUTY
IMBUSY
INJULY
INJURY
KPDUTY
LUXURY
OCCUPY
ONDUTY
PENURY
REBURY
RHEUMY
SYRUPY
UNBURY
UNBUSY
UNDULY
UNRULY

••••UY
BADGUY
BIGGUY
CLIQUY
OUTBUY
PREBUY
TANGUY

U•Z•••
UNZIPS
UNZONE

U•••Z•
UNHAZY
UPGAZE
UPSIZE

U••••Z
UVWXYZ

•UZ•••
BUZZED
BUZZER
BUZZES
FUZZED
FUZZES
FUZZUP
GUZMAN
GUZZLE
HUZZAH
MUZZLE
NUZZLE
OUZELS
PUZZLE
SUZIEQ
SUZUKI
SUZYQS

•U•Z••
BUZZED
BUZZER
BUZZES
CURZON
FURZES
FUTZED
FUTZES
FUZZED
FUZZES
FUZZUP
GUTZON
GUZZLE
HUZZAH
KUDZUS
KUNZEL
LUTZES
MUZZLE
NUNZIO
NUZZLE
PUZZLE
QUEZON
YUTZES

•U••Z•
PUENZO
QUINZE

•U•••Z
CURTIZ
JUAREZ
KUNITZ
KUVASZ
QUARTZ
YUMAAZ

••UZ••
CRUZAN
DOUZES
DRUZES
GAUZES
ISUZUS
SCUZZY

••U•Z•
FRUNZE
KLUTZY
LEUTZE
SCUZZY

••U••Z
BOULEZ
SHULTZ

•••UZ•
YAKUZA

•••U•Z
ELBURZ
PERUTZ
SCHULZ

••••UZ
HORMUZ
TAMMUZ

VA••••
VACANT
VACATE
VACHEL
VACHES
VACLAV
VACUUM
VAGARY
VAGUER
VAILCO
VAINER
VAINLY
VALAIS
VALDEZ
VALENE
VALENS
VALENT
VALERA
VALERE
VALERO
VALERY
VALETS
VALINE
VALISE
VALIUM
VALLEE
VALLEY
VALOIS
VALORS
VALOUR
VALOVA
VALSES
VALUED
VALUER
VALUES
VALVED
VALVES
VAMPED
VAMPER
VANARK
VANDAL
VANIER
VANISH
VANITY
VANNED
VANNES
VANRYN
VAPORS
VAPORY
VAPOUR
VARDEN
VARESE
VARGAS
VARIAS
VARIED
VARIER
VARIES
VARLET
VARMUS
VARNAS
VARNEY
VASHTI
VASILY
VASLAV
VASSAL
VASSAR
VASTER
VASTLY
VASTUS
VATDYE
VATFUL
VATTED
VAUGHN
VAULTS
VAULTY
VAUNTS
VAUNTY

V•A•••
VEADAR
VIABLE
VIABLY
VIACOM
VIAGRA
VIALED
VIANDS
VIATOR
VLASIC

V••A••
VACANT
VACATE
VAGARY
VALAIS
VANARK
VEDAIC
VEGANS
VELARS
VICARS
VIHARA
VIRAGO
VISAED
VISAGE
VITALE
VITALS
VITARA
VIVACE
VIVANT
VOCABS
VOCALS
VOLANS
VOLANT
VOLARE
VOTARY
VOYAGE
VSHAPE

V•••A•
VACLAV
VANDAL
VARGAS
VARIAS
VARNAS
VASLAV
VASSAL
VASSAR
VEADAR
VEEJAY
VEINAL
VENIAL
VENTAS
VERBAL
VERNAL
VESPAS
VESTAL
VESTAS
VIBRAM
VIGIAS
VILLAS
VIOLAS
VIRGAS
VISTAS
VISUAL
VIVIAN
VODKAS
VORPAL
VULCAN
VULGAR

V••••A
VALERA
VALOVA
VECTRA
VENERA
VENORA
VERONA
VEZINA
VIAGRA
VICUNA
VIEIRA
VIENNA
VIGODA
VIHARA
VITARA
VIVECA
VIVICA
VIZSLA

•VA•••
AVAILS
AVALON
AVANTI
AVATAR
AVAUNT
EVADED
EVADER
EVADES
IVANIV
IVANKA
IVANOV
IVANVI
OVALLY
RVALUE
UVALDE
UVALUE

•V•A••
AVIANS
AVIARY
AVIATE
RVPARK
TVGAME
TVLAND
TVTAPE
UVRAYS

•V••A•
AVATAR
AVOWAL
DVORAK
EVENAS
OVISAC
OVULAR
TVSTAR
UVULAE
UVULAR
UVULAS

•V•••A
AVESTA
IVANKA
SVEDKA

••VA••
ALVARO
ARVADA
BEVANS
BOVARY
CAVAFY
DEVANE
DIVANS
DUVALL
EDVARD
HAVANA
HAVASU
HIVAOA
INVADE
INVAIN
KOVACS
KUVASZ
LAVABO
LAVAGE
LAVAIN
LEVADE
LEVANT
LOVAGE
MOVADO
NAVAHO
NAVAID
NAVAJO
NEVADA
NOVATO
PAVANE
RAVAGE
REVAMP
RIVALS
SAVAGE
SAVAII
SAVANA
SAVANT
SAVATE
SIVANS
SUVARI
TUVALU
UNVAIN
VIVACE
VIVANT

••V•A•
CAVEAT
CAVIAR
FIVEAA
FIVEAD
FIVEAM
GAVIAL
GAVRAS
HAVEAT
JOVIAL
JOVIAN
KEVLAR
LIVEAT
NOVIAS
RAVEAT
REVEAL
SAVEAS
VIVIAN
WAVEAT

••V••A
ARVADA
COVINA
DEVEGA
ELVIRA
FIVEAA
HAVANA
HIVAOA
LAVIDA
LOVEYA
NEVADA
NOVELA
NOVENA
RIVERA
SAVANA
SEVENA
VIVECA
VIVICA

•••VA•
BRAVAS
CANVAS
CHEVAL
CHIVAS
COEVAL
CRAVAT
DYEVAT
EREVAN
ERIVAN
GRAVAS
GUAVAS
HALVAH
HALVAS
LANVAL
LARVAE
LARVAL
LARVAS
LITVAK
NERVAL
NORVAL
OGIVAL
SHEVAT
SILVAS
SLOVAK
SPIVAK
SYLVAN
UNIVAC

•••V•A
FLAVIA
HRYVNA
LATVIA
OLIVIA
PLUVIA
PRAVDA
PREVIA
SYLVIA
TRIVIA

••••VA
ACTIVA
ARLOVA
BULOVA
CANOVA
CASAVA
DANOVA
GENEVA
GENOVA
GODIVA
LACAVA
MOSKVA
OTTAVA
PADOVA
SALIVA
UNGAVA
VALOVA

V•B•••
VEBLEN
VIBIST
VIBRAM
VWBUGS

V••B••
VERBAL
VERBID
VIABLE
VIABLY

V•••B•
VOCABS

•V••B•
IVTUBE

••V•B•
FIVEBC
LAVABO

••V••B
ADVERB
REVERB
SEVENB

VC••••
VCHIPS

V•C•••
VACANT
VACATE
VACHEL
VACHES
VACLAV
VACUUM
VECTOR
VECTRA
VICARS
VICTIM
VICTOR
VICUNA
VOCABS
VOCALS

V••C••
VELCRO
VIACOM
VINCIT
VISCID
VNECKS
VOICED
VOICER
VOICES
VULCAN

V•••C•
VAILCO
VELOCE
VENICE
VIVACE
VIVECA
VIVICA
VOTECH

V••••C
VEDAIC
VITRIC
VLASIC

•VC•••
TVCREW

•V•C••
AVOCET
EVICTS
TVVCRS

•V••C•
AVOUCH
EVINCE
KVETCH

•V•••C
OVISAC

••VC••
TVVCRS

••V•C•
ADVICE
CIVICS
DEVICE
DEVICQ
HAVOCS
KOVACS
NOVICE
POVICH
VIVACE
VIVECA
VIVICA

••V••C
FIVEBC
SEVENC

•••V•C
ATAVIC
OLDVIC
PELVIC
SLAVIC
STIVIC
UNIVAC

V•D•••
VEDAIC
VEDDER
VEDIST
VIDEOS
VIDERI
VIDIOT
VODKAS

V••D••
VALDEZ
VANDAL
VARDEN
VATDYE
VEADAR
VEDDER
VELDTS
VENDED
VENDEE
VENDER
VENDOR
VENDUE
VERDES
VERDIN
VERDON
VERDUN
VIRDON
VOIDED
VOIDER
VOIDOF
VOODOO

V•••D•
VIANDS
VIGODA

V••••D
VALUED
VALVED
VAMPED
VANNED
VARIED
VATTED
VEERED
VEGGED
VEILED
VEINED
VENDED
VENTED
VERBID
VERGED
VERSED
VESPID
VESTED
VETOED
VETTED
VIALED
VIEWED
VISAED
VISCID
VOGÜED
VOICED
VOIDED

•VD•••
TVDVDS

•V•D••
AVEDON
AVIDER
AVIDLY
EVADED
EVADER
EVADES
SVEDKA
TVIDOL

•V••D•
AVOIDS
OVERDO
OVIEDO
OVOIDS
TVDVDS
UVALDE

•V•••D
AVOWED
EVADED
EVENED
EVOKED
TVLAND

••V•D•
ARVADA
BOVIDS
DAVIDE
DAVIDI
DAVIDL
DAVIDO
DIVIDE
INVADE
LAVIDA
LEVADE
MOVADO
NEVADA

••V••D
DEVOID
EDVARD
ENVIED
EYVIND
FIVEAD
LEVEED
LEVIED
NAVAID
REVEND
REVVED
RSVPED
SEVEND
UNVOID

•••VD•
PRAVDA
TVDVDS

•••V•D
BRAVED
CALVED
CARVED
CERVID
CORVID
CRAVED
CURVED
DELVED
FERVID
GLOVED
GRAVED

GRAVID GROVED HALVED HEAVED KIDVID LEAVED NERVED PEEVED PROVED REAVED REEVED REVVED SALVED SERVED SHAVED SHOVED SIEVED SLAVED SOLVED STAVED UNAVID VALVED WAIVED WEAVED

VE••••

VEADAR VEBLEN VECTOR VECTRA VEDAIC VEDDER VEDIST VEEJAY VEERED VEGANS VEGGED VEGGES VEGGIE VEGOUT VEIGHT VEILED VEILER VEINAL VEINED VEINTE VELARS VELCRO VELDTS VELLUM VELOCE VELOUR VELSEN VELURE VELVET VENDED VENDEE VENDER VENDOR VENDUE VENEER VENERA VENETO VENIAL VENICE VENINS VENIRE VENITE VENNER VENOMS VENORA VENOSE VENOUS VENTAS VENTED VENTER VENUES VENULE VENUTI VERBAL VERBID VERDES VERDIN VERDON VERDUN VEREEN VEREIN VERGED VERGER VERGES VERGIL VERIFY VERILY VERISM VERIST VERITE VERITY VERJEE VERMIN VERNAL VERNET VERNON VERONA VERSED VERSES VERSET VERSOS VERSTS VERSUS VERTEX VERVES VESPAS VESPER VESPID VESSEL VESTAL VESTAS VESTED VESTEE VESTRY VETOED VETOER VETOES VETTED VETTER VETTES VEXERS VEXING VEZINA

V•E•••

VEEJAY VEERED VIEFOR VIEIRA VIELLE VIENNA VIENNE VIEWED VIEWER VNECKS

V••E••

VALENE VALENS VALENT VALERA VALERE VALERO VALERY VALETS VARESE VENEER VENERA VENETO VEREEN VEREIN VEXERS VIDEOS VIDERI VILELY VILEST VINERS VINERY VIPERS VIREOS VIVECA VIXENS VOMERS VOTECH VOTEIN VOTENO VOTEON VOTERS VOWELS VOWELY VOWERS

V•••E•

VACHEL VACHES VAGUER VAINER VALDEZ VALLEE VALLEY VALSES VALUED VALUER VALUES VALVED VALVES VAMPED VAMPER VANIER VANNED VANNES VARDEN VARIED VARIER VARIES VARLET VARNEY VASTER VATTED VEBLEN VEDDER VEERED VEGGED VEGGES VEILED VEILER VEINED VELSEN VELVET VENDED VENDEE VENDER VENEER VENNER VENTED VENTER VENUES VERDES VEREEN VERGED VERGER VERGES VERJEE VERNET VERSED VERSES VERSET VERTEX VERVES VESPER VESSEL VESTED VESTEE VETOED VETOER VETOES VETTED VETTER VETTES VIALED VIEWED VIEWER VINIER VIOLET VISAED VIVIEN VIZIER VOGUED VOGUER VOGUES VOICED VOICER VOICES VOIDED VOIDER VOILES VOLLEY VORTEX VOSGES VSIXES VTILES

V••••E

VACATE VALENE VALERE VALINE VALISE VALLEE VARESE VATDYE VEGGIE VEINTE VELOCE VELURE VENDEE VENDUE VENICE VENIRE VENITE VENOSE VENULE VERITE VERJEE VESTEE VIABLE VIELLE VIENNE VINNIE VIRILE VIRTUE VISAGE VISINE VITALE VITTLE VIVACE VOLARE VOLUME VOLUTE VOTIVE VOYAGE VSHAPE

•VE•••

AVEDON AVEENO AVENGE AVENUE AVERSE AVERTS AVESTA EVELYN EVENAS EVENED EVENER EVENIF EVENLY EVENSO EVENTS EVENUP EVERLY EVERSO EVERTS KVELLS KVETCH OVERDO OVERIT OVERLY SVEDKA SVELTE UVEOUS YVETTE

•V•E••

AVEENO OVIEDO TVSETS

•V••E•

AVIDER AVOCET AVOWED AVOWER EVADED EVADER EVADES EVENED EVENER EVILER EVITES EVOKED EVOKER EVOKES OVINES OVULES TVCREW

•V•••E

AVENGE AVENUE AVERSE AVIATE AVULSE EVINCE EVOLVE EVONNE EVULSE IVTUBE RVALUE SVELTE TVGAME TVTAPE TVTIME UVALDE UVALUE UVULAE YVETTE YVONNE

••VE••

ADVENT ADVERB ADVERT AMVETS BEVELS CAVEAT CAVEIN CAVELL CAVERN CAVERS CAVETT CIVETS COVENS COVENT COVERS COVERT COVETS COVEYS CUVEES DAVENS DEVEGA DEVEIN DEVERE DEVERS DEVEST DIVEIN DIVERS DIVERT DIVEST DOVEIN DUVETS ELVERS ENVEIL FEVERS FIVEAA FIVEAD FIVEAM FIVEBC FIVEEE FIVENO FIVEOF FIVEPM FIVERS FIVETO FIVEUP FIVEWS GAVEIN GAVELS GAVEOF GAVEON GAVETO GAVEUP GIVEIN GIVENS GIVEOF GIVEON GIVERS GIVETH GIVETO GIVEUP GOVERN HAVEAT HAVEIN HAVEIT HAVENO HAVENS HAVENT HAVEON HAVETO HAVEUP HIVERS HOVELS HOVERS HOVETO INVENT INVERT INVEST JAVERT JIVERS LAVERN LAVERS LEVEED LEVEES LEVELS LEVENE LEVERS LEVERT LIVEAT LIVEIN LIVELY LIVENS LIVEON LIVERS LIVERY LIVEST LIVETH LIVETV LOVEIN LOVEIT LOVELL LOVELY LOVERS LOVETO LOVETT LOVEYA LOVEYS MAVENS MOVEIN MOVEIT MOVEON MOVERS MOVETO MOVEUP NAVELS NEVERS NOVELA NOVELS NOVENA OBVERT PAVERS PAVESE RAVEAT RAVELS RAVENS RAVEON RAVERS RAVEUP REVEAL REVELS REVEND REVERB REVERE REVERS REVERT REVEST REVETS RIVERA RIVERS RIVETS ROVERS SAVEAS SAVEIT SAVEME SAVEON SAVERS SAVEUP SEVENA SEVENB SEVENC SEVEND SEVENE SEVENS SEVERE SEVERN SEVERS TAVELS TAVERN TEVERE TEVETS UNVEIL VIVECA WAVEAT WAVEIN WAVERS WAVERY WAVETO WYVERN

••V•E•

BAVIER BEVIES CAVIES CUVEES CUVIER DAVIES ENVIED ENVIER ENVIES FIVEEE INVIEW JAVIER JIVIER KAVNER LEVEED LEVEES LEVIED LEVIER LEVIES LIVRES MOVIES NAVIES ONVIEW PEVNEY REVIEW REVUES REVVED RSVPED SEVRES SOVIET VIVIEN WAVIER XAVIER

••V••E

ADVICE ADVISE BOVINE DAVIDE DEVANE DEVERE DEVICE DEVINE DEVISE DEVORE DEVOTE DIVIDE DIVINE FIVEEE INVADE INVITE INVOKE IRVINE LAVAGE LEVADE LEVENE LEVINE LEVITE LOVAGE NOVICE NOVOTE PAVANE PAVESE RAVAGE RAVINE REVERE REVILE REVISE REVIVE REVOKE REVOTE SAVAGE SAVATE SAVEME SAVOIE SEVENE SEVERE TEVERE VIVACE

•••VE•

AGAVES ALEVEL ALEVES ALFVEN ALIVEO ASEVER BEAVER BEEVES BRAVED BRAVER BRAVES BREVES BREVET BSEVEN CALVED CALVES CALVET CARVED CARVEL CARVER CARVES CARVEY CHAVEZ CHEVET CHIVES CLAVES CLEVER CLEVES CLOVEN CLOVER CLOVES CONVEX CONVEY CORVEE CRAVED CRAVEN CRAVER CRAVES CURVED CURVES CURVET DEEVER DELVED DELVER DELVES DENVER DOOVER DRIVEL DRIVEN DRIVER DRIVES DROVER DROVES ELEVEN ELEVES FAUVES FIEVEL GARVEY GLOVED GLOVER GLOVES GOOVER GRAVED GRAVEL GRAVEN GRAVER GRAVES GROVED GROVEL GROVER GROVES GSEVEN HALVED HALVER HALVES HARVEY HEAVED HEAVEN HEAVER HEAVES HERVEY HOOVER HOOVES HUMVEE INEVER JAYVEE JEEVES JUEVES KNAVES KNIVES LEAVED LEAVEN LEAVER LEAVES LEEVES LOAVES LOUVER LWAVES MARVEL MAUVES NAIVER NERVED NERVES NIEVES NUEVES OGIVES OLEVEL OLIVER OLIVES PEEVED PEEVES PLOVER PRIVET PROVED PROVEN PROVER PROVES PULVER PURVEY QUAVER QUIVER REAVED REAVER REAVES REEVED REEVES REVVED SALVED SALVER SALVES SEAVER SELVES SERVED SERVER SERVES SHAVED SHAVEN SHAVER SHAVES SHIVER SHOVED SHOVEL SHOVER SHOVES SIEVED SIEVES SILVER SLAVED SLAVER SLAVES SLIVER SLOVEN SNIVEL SOAVES SOLVED SOLVER SOLVES STAVED STAVES STEVEN STOVER STOVES SUAVER SURVEY SWIVEL SWIVET TEEVEE THEVET TRAVEL TRAVEN TRAVES TRIVET TROVES UNEVEN UPOVER VALVED VALVES VELVET VERVES WAIVED WAIVER WAIVES WARVET WEAVED WEAVER WEAVES WOLVES

•••V•E

BMOVIE CHEVRE CORVEE HUMVEE JAYVEE LARVAE LOUVRE OEUVRE OUTVIE POIVRE PREVUE STEVIE TEEVEE

••••VE

ACTIVE ADRIVE ALCOVE ARGIVE ARRIVE ATFIVE BEHAVE BYJOVE CLEAVE DATIVE DEDUVE DERIVE ENDIVE EVOLVE GENEVE GOLIVE GREAVE GRIEVE GROOVE INLOVE INWOVE ISERVE MOHAVE MOJAVE MOTIVE MYLOVE NATIVE NOJIVE OCTAVE PAREVE REGAVE REGIVE RELEVE RELIVE REMOVE REPAVE RESAVE REVIVE REWOVE SCURVE SHEAVE SHELVE SHREVE SHRIVE SHROVE SLEEVE STARVE STEEVE STRIVE STROVE SWERVE THEYVE THIEVE THRIVE THROVE TRYGVE TWELVE UNLIVE UNROVE UNWOVE UPDIVE UPDOVE UPHOVE VOTIVE WHATVE

VF••••

VFOURS

V••F••

VATFUL VIEFOR

V•••F•

VERIFY VILIFY VINIFY VIVIFY

V••••F

VOIDOF

•V•••F

EVENIF

••V•F•

CAVAFY VIVIFY

••V••F

FIVEOF GAVEOF GIVEOF

V•G•••

VAGARY VAGUER VEGANS VEGGED VEGGES VEGGIE VEGOUT VIGIAS VIGILS VIGODA VIGORS VIGOUR VOGUED VOGUER VOGUES

V••G••

VARGAS VAUGHN VEGGED VEGGES VEGGIE VEIGHT VERGED VERGER VERGES VERGIL VIAGRA VIRGAS VIRGIL VIRGIN VIRGOS VOIGHT VOSGES VSIGNS VULGAR VULGUS

V•••G•

VIRAGO VISAGE VOYAGE VWBUGS

V••••G

VEXING VIKING VINING VISING VOTING VOWING

•VG•••

TVGAME

•V••G•

AVENGE

••V•G•

DEVEGA LAVAGE LOVAGE RAVAGE SAVAGE

••V••G

ALVING CAVING COVING DIVING

ERVING
GIVING
HAVING
HIVING
IRVING
JIVING
LAVING
LIVING
LOVING
MOVING
PAVING
RAVING
RIVING
ROVING
SAVING
WAVING
WIVING

•••V•G
MADVIG

V•H•••
VCHIPS
VIHARA
VSHAPE

V••H••
VACHEL
VACHES
VASHTI
VISHNU

V•••H•
VAUGHN
VEIGHT
VOIGHT

V••••H
VANISH
VOTECH

•VH•••
TVHITS

•V•H••
TVSHOW

•V•••H
AVOUCH
KVETCH

••V•H•
NAVAHO

••V••H
DOVISH
ELVISH
FYVUSH
GIVETH
LAVISH
LIVETH
POVICH
RAVISH

•••V•H
HALVAH

VI••••
VIABLE
VIABLY
VIACOM
VIAGRA
VIALED
VIANDS
VIATOR
VIBIST
VIBRAM
VICARS
VICTIM
VICTOR
VICUNA
VIDEOS
VIDERI
VIDIOT
VIEFOR
VIEIRA
VIELLE
VIENNA
VIENNE
VIEWED
VIEWER
VIGIAS
VIGILS
VIGODA
VIGORS
VIGOUR
VIHARA
VIKING
VIKTOR
VILELY
VILEST
VILIFY
VILLAS
VILLON
VINCIT
VINERS
VINERY
VINIER
VINIFY
VINING
VINNIE
VINOUS
VINSON
VINTON
VINYLS
VIOLAS
VIOLET
VIOLIN
VIORST
VIPERS
VIRAGO
VIRDON
VIREOS
VIRGAS
VIRGIL
VIRGIN
VIRGOS
VIRILE
VIRTUE
VIRTUS
VISAED
VISAGE
VISCID
VISHNU
VISINE
VISING
VISION
VISITS
VISORS
VISTAS
VISUAL
VITALE
VITALS
VITARA
VITRIC
VITTLE
VIVACE
VIVANT
VIVECA
VIVIAN
VIVICA
VIVIEN
VIVIFY
VIXENS
VIZIER
VIZIRS
VIZORS
VIZSLA

V•I•••
VAILCO
VAINER
VAINLY
VEIGHT
VEILED
VEILER
VEINAL
VEINED
VEINTE
VOICED
VOICER
VOICES
VOIDED
VOIDER
VOIDOF
VOIGHT
VOILES
VSIGNS
VSIXES
VTILES

V••I••
VALINE
VALISE
VALIUM
VANIER
VANISH
VANITY
VARIAS
VARIED
VARIER
VARIES
VASILY
VCHIPS
VEDIST
VENIAL
VENICE
VENINS
VENIRE
VENITE
VERIFY
VERILY
VERISM
VERIST
VERITE
VERITY
VEXING
VEZINA
VIBIST
VIDIOT
VIEIRA
VIGIAS
VIGILS
VIKING
VILIFY
VINIER
VINIFY
VINING
VIRILE
VISINE
VISING
VISION
VISITS
VIVIAN
VIVICA
VIVIEN
VIVIFY
VIZIER
VIZIRS
VOTING
VOTIVE
VOWING

V•••I•
VALAIS
VALOIS
VEDAIC
VEGGIE
VERBID
VERDIN
VEREIN
VERGIL
VERMIN
VESPID
VICTIM
VINCIT
VINNIE
VIOLIN
VIRGIL
VIRGIN
VISCID
VITRIC
VLASIC
VOTEIN

V••••I
VASHTI
VENUTI
VIDERI

•VI•••
AVIANS
AVIARY
AVIATE
AVIDER
AVIDLY
AVISON
AVISOS
EVICTS
EVILER
EVILLY
EVINCE
EVITES
OVIEDO
OVINES
OVISAC
TVIDOL

•V•I••
AVAILS
AVOIDS
AVRILS
OVOIDS
TVHITS
TVTIME

•V••I•
EVENIF
IVANIV
OVERIT

•V•••I
AVANTI
IVANVI

••VI••
ADVICE
ADVILS
ADVISE
ALVING
ALVINO
ANVILS
BAVIER
BEVIES
BOVIDS
BOVINE
CAVIAR
CAVIES
CAVILS
CAVING
CAVITY
CIVICS
COVINA
COVING
CUVIER
DAVIDE
DAVIDI
DAVIDL
DAVIDO
DAVIES
DAVITS
DEVICE
DEVICQ
DEVILS
DEVINE
DEVISE
DEVITO
DIVIDE
DIVINE
DIVING
DOVISH
ELVIRA
ELVISH
ENVIED
ENVIER
ENVIES
ENVIRO
ERVING
EYVIND
GAVIAL
GIVING
HAVING
HIVING
INVIEW
INVITE
INVIVO
IRVINE
IRVING
JAVIER
JAVITS
JIVIER
JIVING
JOVIAL
JOVIAN
LAVIDA
LAVING
LAVISH
LEVIED
LEVIER
LEVIES
LEVINE
LEVITE
LEVITT
LEVITY
LIVING
LOVING
MAVINS
MOVIES
MOVING
NAVIES
NEVILL
NEVINS
NOVIAS
NOVICE
NOVIOS
ONVIEW
PAVING
PAVIOR
POVICH
RAVINE
RAVING
RAVISH
REVIEW
REVILE
REVISE
REVIVE
RIVING
ROVING
SAVING
SAVIOR
SOVIET
TAVIST
VIVIAN
VIVICA
VIVIEN
VIVIFY
WAVIER
WAVILY
WAVING
WIVING
XAVIER

••V•I•
CAVEIN
DEVEIN
DEVOID
DEVOIR
DIVEIN
DOVEIN
ENVEIL
ENVOIS
GAVEIN
GIVEIN
HAVEIN
HAVEIT
INVAIN
LAVAIN
LIVEIN
LOVEIN
LOVEIT
MOVEIN
MOVEIT
NAVAID
REVOIR
SAVAII
SAVEIT
SAVOIE
SAVOIR
UNVAIN
UNVEIL
UNVOID
WAVEIN

••V••I
DAVIDI
NEVSKI
RIVOLI
SAVAII
SUVARI
TIVOLI

•••VI•
ATAVIC
BEAVIS
BMOVIE
BREVIS
BROVIK
CALVIN
CERVID
CLAVIN
CLOVIS
CORVID
DREVIL
DRIVIN
EARVIN
FERVID
FLAVIA
GERVIN
GRAVID
JARVIK
KELVIN
KIDVID
KRAVIS
LANVIN
LATVIA
LEOVII
LIEVIO
LOUVIN
MADVIG
MARVIN
MARVIS
MELVIL
MELVIN
NARVIK
OLAVII
OLAVIV
OLDVIC
OLIVIA
OUTVIE
PELVIC
PELVIS
PLUVIA
PLUVIO
POTVIN
PREVIA
PREVIN
SLAVIC
STEVIE
STIVIC
SYLVIA
TRAVIS
TRIVIA
UNAVID
UNEVIL
WEEVIL

•••V•I
LEOVII
OLAVII
RENVOI

••••VI
BOOKVI
IVANVI
JOHNVI
MARKVI
PAULVI
PIUSVI

V••J••
VEEJAY
VERJEE

••V•J•
MTVVJS
NAVAJO

•••VJ•
MTVVJS

V•K•••
VIKING
VIKTOR

V••K••
VODKAS

V•••K•
VNECKS

V••••K
VANARK
VOSTOK

•V•K••
EVOKED
EVOKER
EVOKES

•V••K•
IVANKA
SVEDKA

•V•••K
DVORAK
RVPARK

••V•K•
INVOKE
NEVSKI
NEVSKY
REVOKE

•••V•K
BROVIK
JARVIK
LITVAK
NARVIK
SLOVAK
SPIVAK

VL••••
VLASIC

V•L•••
VALAIS
VALDEZ
VALENE
VALENS
VALENT
VALERA
VALERE
VALERO
VALERY
VALETS
VALINE
VALISE
VALIUM
VALLEE
VALLEY
VALOIS
VALORS
VALOUR
VALOVA
VALSES
VALUED
VALUER
VALUES
VALVED
VALVES
VELARS
VELCRO
VELDTS
VELLUM
VELOCE
VELOUR
VELSEN
VELURE
VELVET
VILELY
VILEST
VILIFY
VILLAS
VILLON
VOLANS
VOLANT
VOLARE
VOLLEY
VOLUME
VOLUTE
VOLVOS
VULCAN
VULGAR
VULGUS

V••L••
VACLAV
VAILCO
VALLEE
VALLEY
VARLET
VASLAV
VAULTS
VAULTY
VEBLEN
VEILED
VEILER
VELLUM
VIALED
VIELLE
VILLAS
VILLON
VIOLAS
VIOLET
VIOLIN
VOILES
VOLLEY
VTILES

V•••L•
VAINLY
VASILY
VASTLY
VENULE
VERILY
VIABLE
VIABLY
VIELLE
VIGILS
VILELY
VINYLS
VIRILE
VITALE
VITALS
VITTLE
VIZSLA
VOCALS
VOWELS
VOWELY

V••••L
VACHEL
VANDAL
VASSAL
VATFUL
VEINAL
VENIAL
VERBAL
VERGIL
VERNAL
VESSEL
VESTAL
VIRGIL
VISUAL
VORPAL

•VL•••
TVLAND

•V•L••
AVALON
AVULSE
EVELYN
EVILER
EVILLY
EVOLVE
EVULSE
KVELLS
OVALLY
OVULAR
OVULES
RVALUE
SVELTE
UVALDE
UVALUE
UVULAE
UVULAR
UVULAS

•V••L•
AVAILS
AVIDLY
AVRILS
EVENLY
EVERLY
EVILLY
KVELLS
OVALLY
OVERLY

•V•••L
AVOWAL
TVIDOL

••VL••
KEVLAR
PAVLOV
REVLON

••V•L•
ADVILS
ANVILS
BEVELS
CAVELL
CAVILS
DEVILS
DUVALL
GAVELS
HOVELS
LEVELS
LIVELY
LOVELL
LOVELY
NAVELS
NEVILL
NOVELA
NOVELS
RAVELS
REVELS
REVILE
REVOLT
RIVALS
RIVOLI
TAVELS
TIVOLI
TUVALU
WAVILY

••V••L
CAVELL
DAVIDL
DUVALL
ENVEIL
GAVIAL
JOVIAL
LOVELL
NEVILL
REVEAL
UNVEIL

•••V•L
ALEVEL
CARVEL
CHEVAL
COEVAL
DREVIL
DRIVEL
FIEVEL
FRIVOL
GRAVEL
GROVEL
LANVAL
LARVAL
MARVEL
MELVIL
NERVAL
NORVAL
OGIVAL
OLEVEL
SHOVEL
SNIVEL
SWIVEL
TRAVEL
UNEVIL
WEEVIL

V•M•••
VAMPED
VAMPER
VOMERS

V••M••
VARMUS
VERMIN

V•••M•
VENOMS
VOLUME
VROOMS

V••••M
VACUUM
VALIUM
VELLUM
VERISM
VIACOM
VIBRAM
VICTIM

•V••M•
TVGAME
TVTIME

•V•••M
TVROOM

••V•M•
REVAMP
SAVEME

•••V•M
FIVEAM
FIVEPM

VN••••
VNECKS

V•N•••
VANARK
VANDAL
VANIER
VANISH
VANITY
VANNED
VANNES
VANRYN
VENDED
VENDEE
VENDER
VENDOR
VENDUE
VENEER
VENERA
VENETO
VENIAL
VENICE
VENINS
VENIRE
VENITE
VENNER
VENOMS
VENORA
VENOSE
VENOUS
VENTAS
VENTED
VENTER
VENUES
VENULE
VENUTI
VINCIT
VINERS
VINERY
VINIER
VINIFY
VINING
VINNIE
VINOUS
VINSON
VINTON
VINYLS

V••N••
VAINER
VAINLY
VANNED
VANNES
VARNAS
VARNEY
VAUNTS
VAUNTY
VEINAL
VEINED
VEINTE
VENNER
VERNAL
VERNET
VERNON
VIANDS
VIENNA
VIENNE
VINNIE

V•••N•
VACANT
VALENE
VALENS
VALENT
VALINE
VEGANS
VENINS
VERONA
VEXING
VEZINA
VICUNA
VIENNA
VIENNE
VIKING
VINING
VISHNU
VISINE
VISING
VIVANT
VIXENS
VOLANS
VOLANT
VOTENO
VOTING
VOWING
VSIGNS

V••••N
VANRYN
VARDEN
VAUGHN
VEBLEN
VELSEN
VERDIN
VERDON
VERDUN
VEREEN
VEREIN
VERMIN
VERNON
VILLON
VINSON
VINTON
VIOLIN
VIRDON
VIRGIN
VISION
VIVIAN
VIVIEN
VOTEIN
VOTEON
VULCAN

•V•N••
AVANTI
AVENGE
AVENUE
EVENAS
EVENED
EVENER
EVENIF
EVENLY
EVENSO
EVENTS
EVENUP
EVINCE
EVONNE
IVANIV
IVANKA
IVANOV
IVANVI
OVINES
YVONNE

•V••N•
AVAUNT
AVEENO
AVIANS
EVONNE
TVLAND
YVONNE

•V•••N
AVALON
AVEDON
AVISON
EVELYN

••VN••
GUVNOR
KAVNER
PEVNEY

••V•N•
ADVENT
ALVING
ALVINO
BEVANS
BOVINE
CAVING
COVENS
COVENT
COVINA
COVING
DAVENS
DEVANE
DEVINE
DIVANS
DIVINE
DIVING
ERVING
EYVIND

FIVENO GIVENS GIVING HAVANA HAVENO HAVENS HAVENT HAVING HIVING INVENT IRVINE IRVING JEVONS JIVING LAVING LEVANT LEVENE LEVINE LIVENS LIVING LOVING MAVENS MAVINS MOVING NEVINS NOVENA PAVANE PAVING RAVENS RAVINE RAVING REVEND RIVING ROVING SAVANA SAVANT SAVING SEVENA SEVENB SEVENC SEVEND SEVENE SEVENS SIVANS VIVANT WAVING WIVING

••V••N
CAVEIN CAVERN DEVEIN DIVEIN DOVEIN GAVEIN GAVEON GIVEIN GIVEON GOVERN HAVEIN HAVEON INVAIN JOVIAN LAVAIN LAVERN LIVEIN LIVEON LOVEIN MOVEIN MOVEON RAVEON REVLON REVSON SAVEON SEVERN TAVERN UNVAIN VIVIAN VIVIEN WAVEIN WYVERN

•••VN•
HRYVNA

•••V•N
ALFVEN BSEVEN CALVIN CHEVON CLAVIN CLOVEN CRAVEN DRIVEN DRIVIN EARVIN ELEVEN ELEVON EREVAN ERIVAN GERVIN GRAVEN GSEVEN HEAVEN KELVIN LANVIN LEAVEN LOUVIN MARVIN MELVIN MELVYN MERVYN POTVIN PREVIN PROVEN SHAVEN SLOVEN STEVEN SYLVAN TRAVEN UNEVEN

VO••••
VOCABS VOCALS VODKAS VOGUED VOGUER VOGUES VOICED VOICER VOICES VOIDED VOIDER VOIDOF VOIGHT VOILES VOLANS VOLANT VOLARE VOLLEY VOLUME VOLUTE VOLVOS VOMERS VOODOO VOROUS VORPAL VORTEX VOSGES VOSTOK VOTARY VOTECH VOTEIN VOTENO VOTEON VOTERS VOTING VOTIVE VOWELS VOWELY VOWERS VOWING VOXPOP VOYAGE

V•O•••
VFOURS VIOLAS VIOLET VIOLIN VIORST VOODOO VROOMS

V••O••
VALOIS VALORS VALOUR VALOVA VAPORS VAPORY VAPOUR VEGOUT VELOCE VELOUR VENOMS VENORA VENOSE VENOUS VERONA VETOED VETOER VETOES VIGODA VIGORS VIGOUR VINOUS VISORS VIZORS VOROUS VROOMS

V•••O•
VECTOR VENDOR VERDON VERNON VERSOS VIACOM VIATOR VICTOR VIDEOS VIDIOT VIEFOR VIKTOR VILLON VINSON VINTON VIRDON VIREOS VIRGOS VISION VOIDOF VOLVOS VOODOO VOSTOK VOTEON VOXPOP

V••••O
VAILCO VALERO VELCRO VENETO VIRAGO VOODOO VOTENO

•VO•••
AVOCET AVOIDS AVOUCH AVOWAL AVOWED AVOWER DVORAK EVOKED EVOKER EVOKES EVOLVE EVONNE OVOIDS YVONNE

•V•O••
TVROOM UVEOUS

•V••O•
AVALON AVEDON AVISON AVISOS IVANOV TVIDOL TVROOM TVSHOW TVSPOT

•V•••O
AVEENO EVENSO EVERSO OVERDO OVIEDO

••VO••
CAVORT DEVOID DEVOIR DEVORE DEVOTE DEVOTO DEVOUR DEVOUT DIVOTS ENVOIS ENVOYS FAVORS FAVOUR GAVOTS HAVOCS INVOKE JEVONS NOVOTE PIVOTS REVOIR REVOKE REVOLT REVOTE RIVOLI SAVOIE SAVOIR SAVORS SAVORY SAVOUR TIVOLI UNVOID

••V•O•
FIVEOF GAVEOF GAVEON GIVEOF GIVEON GUVNOR HAVEON HIVAOA LIVEON MOVEON NOVIOS PAVIOR PAVLOV RAVEON REVLON REVSON SAVEON SAVIOR

••V••O
ALVARO ALVINO DAVIDO DEVITO DEVOTO ENVIRO FIVENO FIVETO GAVETO GIVETO HAVENO HAVETO HOVETO INVIVO LAVABO LOVETO MOVADO MOVETO NAVAHO NAVAJO NOVATO WAVETO

•••VO•
BRAVOS CHEVON CONVOY ELEVON FERVOR FLAVOR FRIVOL HUEVOS MCAVOY REAVOW RENVOI SALVOR SALVOS SERVOS TREVOR VOLVOS

•••V•O
ALIVEO LIEVIO PLUVIO

••••VO
DENOVO INVIVO KOSOVO LENOVO OCTAVO

V•P•••
VAPORS VAPORY VAPOUR VIPERS

V••P••
VAMPED VAMPER VESPAS VESPER VESPID VORPAL VOXPOP

V•••P•
VCHIPS VSHAPE

V••••P
VOXPOP

•VP•••
RVPARK

•V•P••
TVSPOT

•V••P•
TVTAPE

•V•••P
EVENUP

••VP••
RSVPED

••V•P•
FIVEPM

••V••P
FIVEUP GAVEUP GIVEUP HAVEUP MOVEUP RAVEUP REVAMP REVSUP SAVEUP

•••VP•
ALMVPS NLMVPS

••V••Q
DEVICQ

VR••••
VROOMS

V•R•••
VARDEN VARESE VARGAS VARIAS VARIED VARIER VARIES VARLET VARMUS VARNAS VARNEY VERBAL VERBID VERDES VERDIN VERDON VERDUN VEREEN VEREIN VERGED VERGER VERGES VERGIL VERIFY VERILY VERISM VERIST VERITE VERITY VERJEE VERMIN VERNAL VERNET VERNON VERONA VERSED VERSES VERSET VERSOS VERSTS VERSUS VERTEX VERVES VIRAGO VIRDON VIREOS VIRGAS VIRGIL VIRGIN VIRGOS VIRILE VIRTUE VIRTUS VOROUS VORPAL VORTEX

V••R••
VANRYN VEERED VIBRAM VIORST VITRIC

V•••R•
VAGARY VALERA VALERE VALERO VALERY VALORS VANARK VAPORS VAPORY VECTRA VELARS VELCRO VELURE VENERA VENIRE VENORA VESTRY VEXERS VFOURS VIAGRA VICARS VIDERI VIEIRA VIGORS VIHARA VINERS VINERY VIPERS VISORS VITARA VIZIRS VIZORS VOLARE VOMERS VOTARY VOTERS VOWERS

V••••R
VAGUER VAINER VALOUR VALUER VAMPER VANIER VAPOUR VARIER VASSAR VASTER VEADAR VECTOR VEDDER VEILER VELOUR VENDER VENDOR VENEER VENNER VENTER VERGER VESPER VETOER VETTER VIATOR VICTOR VIEFOR VIEWER VIGOUR VIKTOR VINIER VIZIER VOGUER VOICER VOIDER VULGAR

•VR•••
AVRILS TVROOM UVRAYS

•V•R••
AVERSE AVERTS DVORAK EVERLY EVERSO EVERTS OVERDO OVERIT OVERLY TVCREW

•V••R•
AVIARY RVPARK TVVCRS

•V•••R
AVATAR AVIDER AVOWER EVADER EVENER EVILER EVOKER OVULAR TVSTAR UVULAR

••VR••
GAVRAS LIVRES SEVRES

••V•R•
ADVERB ADVERT ALVARO BOVARY CAVERN CAVERS CAVORT COVERS COVERT DEVERE DEVERS DEVORE DIVERS DIVERT EDVARD ELVERS ELVIRA ENVIRO FAVORS FEVERS FIVERS GIVERS GOVERN HIVERS HOVERS INVERT JAVERT JIVERS LAVERN LAVERS LEVERS LEVERT LIVERS LIVERY LOVERS MOVERS NEVERS OBVERT PAVERS RAVERS REVERB REVERE REVERS REVERT RIVERA RIVERS ROVERS SAVERS SAVORS SAVORY SEVERE SEVERN SEVERS SUVARI TAVERN TEVERE TVVCRS WAVERS WAVERY WYVERN

••V••R
BAVIER CAVIAR CUVIER DEVOIR DEVOUR ENVIER FAVOUR GUVNOR JAVIER JIVIER KAVNER KEVLAR LEVIER PAVIOR REVOIR SAVIOR SAVOIR SAVOUR WAVIER XAVIER

•••VR•
CHEVRE LOUVRE OEUVRE POIVRE

•••V•R
ASEVER BEAVER BRAVER CARVER CLEVER CLOVER CRAVER DEEVER DELVER DENVER DOOVER DRIVER DROVER FERVOR FLAVOR GLOVER GOOVER GRAVER GROVER HALVER HEAVER HOOVER INEVER LEAVER LOUVER NAIVER OLIVER PLOVER PROVER PULVER QUAVER QUIVER REAVER SALVER SALVOR SEAVER SERVER SHAVER SHIVER SHOVER SILVER SLAVER SLIVER SOLVER STOVER SUAVER TREVOR UPOVER WAIVER WEAVER

VS••••
VSHAPE VSIGNS VSIXES

V•S•••
VASHTI VASILY VASLAV VASSAL VASSAR VASTER VASTLY VASTUS VESPAS VESPER VESPID VESSEL VESTAL VESTAS VESTED VESTEE VESTRY VISAED VISAGE VISCID VISHNU VISINE VISING VISION VISITS VISORS VISTAS VISUAL VOSGES VOSTOK

V••S••
VALSES VASSAL VASSAR VELSEN VERSED VERSES VERSET VERSOS VERSTS VERSUS VESSEL VINSON VIZSLA VLASIC

V•••S•
VALISE VANISH VARESE VEDIST VENOSE VERISM VERIST VIBIST VILEST VIORST

V••••S
VACHES VALAIS VALENS VALETS VALOIS VALORS VALSES VALUES VALVES VANNES VAPORS VARGAS VARIAS VARIES VARMUS VARNAS VASTUS VAULTS VAUNTS VCHIPS VEGANS VEGGES VELARS VELDTS VENINS VENOMS VENOUS VENTAS VENUES VERDES VERGES VERSES VERSOS VERSTS VERSUS VERVES VESPAS VESTAS VETOES VETTES VEXERS VFOURS VIANDS VICARS VIDEOS VIGIAS VIGILS VIGORS VILLAS VINERS VINOUS VINYLS VIOLAS VIPERS VIREOS VIRGAS VIRGOS VIRTUS VISITS VISORS VISTAS VITALS VIXENS VIZIRS VIZORS VNECKS VOCABS VOCALS VODKAS VOGUES VOICES VOILES VOLANS VOLVOS VOMERS VOROUS VOSGES VOTERS VOWELS VOWERS VROOMS VSIGNS VSIXES VTILES VULGUS VWBUGS

•VS•••
TVSETS TVSHOW TVSPOT TVSTAR

•V•S••
AVESTA AVISON AVISOS OVISAC

•V••S•
AVERSE AVULSE EVENSO EVERSO EVULSE

•V•••S
AVAILS AVERTS AVIANS AVISOS AVOIDS AVRILS EVADES EVENAS EVENTS EVERTS EVICTS EVITES EVOKES KVELLS OVINES OVOIDS OVULES TVDVDS TVHITS TVSETS TVVCRS UVEOUS UVRAYS UVULAS

••VS••
NEVSKI NEVSKY REVSON REVSUP

••V•S•
ADVISE DEVEST DEVISE DIVEST DOVISH ELVISH FYVUSH HAVASU INVEST KUVASZ LAVISH LIVEST PAVESE RAVISH REVEST REVISE TAVIST

••V••S
ADVILS AMVETS ANVILS BEVANS BEVELS BEVIES BOVIDS CAVERS CAVIES CAVILS CIVETS CIVICS COVENS COVERS COVETS

COVEYS
CUVEES
DAVENS
DAVIES
DAVITS
DEVERS
DEVILS
DIVANS
DIVERS
DIVOTS
DUVETS
ELVERS
ENVIES
ENVOIS
ENVOYS
FAVORS
FEVERS
FIVERS
FIVEWS
GAVELS
GAVOTS
GAVRAS
GIVENS
GIVERS
HAVENS
HAVOCS
HIVERS
HOVELS
HOVERS
JAVITS
JEVONS
JIVERS
KOVACS
LAVERS
LEVEES
LEVELS
LEVERS
LEVIES
LIVENS
LIVERS
LIVRES
LOVERS
LOVEYS
MAVENS
MAVINS
MOVERS
MOVIES
MTVVJS
NAVELS
NAVIES
NEVERS
NEVINS
NOVELS
NOVIAS
NOVIOS
PAVERS
PIVOTS
RAVELS
RAVENS
RAVERS
REVELS
REVERS
REVETS
REVUES
RIVALS
RIVERS
RIVETS
ROVERS
SAVEAS
SAVERS
SAVORS
SEVENS
SEVERS
SEVRES
SIVANS
TAVELS
TEVETS
TVVCRS
WAVERS

•••V•S
AGAVES
ALEVES
ALMVPS
BEAVIS
BEEVES
BRAVAS
BRAVES
BRAVOS
BREVES
BREVIS
CALVES
CANVAS
CARVES
CHEVYS
CHIVAS
CHIVES
CLAVES
CLEVES
CLOVES
CLOVIS
CORVUS
CRAVES
CURVES
DELVES
DRIVES
DROVES
ELEVES
FAUVES
GLOVES
GRAVAS
GRAVES
GROVES
GUAVAS
HALVAS
HALVES
HEAVES
HOOVES
HUEVOS
JEEVES
JUEVES
KNAVES
KNIVES
KRAVIS
LARVAS
LEAVES
LEEVES
LOAVES
LWAVES
MARVIS
MAUVES
MTVVJS
NERVES
NIEVES
NLMVPS
NUEVES
OGIVES
OLIVES
PEEVES
PELVIS
PROVES
REAVES
REEVES
SALVES
SALVOS
SELVES
SERVES
SERVOS
SHAVES
SHOVES
SIEVES
SILVAS
SLAVES
SOAVES
SOLVES
STAVES
STOVES
TRAVES
TRAVIS
TROVES
TVDVDS
VALVES
VERVES
VOLVOS
WAIVES
WEAVES
WOLVES

••••VS
EXGOVS
LTGOVS
SCHAVS

VT••••
VTILES

V•T•••
VATDYE
VATFUL
VATTED
VETOED
VETOER
VETOES
VETTED
VETTER
VETTES
VITALE
VITALS
VITARA
VITRIC
VITTLE
VOTARY
VOTECH
VOTEIN
VOTENO
VOTEON
VOTERS
VOTING
VOTIVE

V••T••
VASTER
VASTLY
VASTUS
VATTED
VECTOR
VECTRA
VENTAS
VENTED
VENTER
VERTEX
VESTAL
VESTAS
VESTED
VESTEE
VESTRY
VETTED
VETTER
VETTES
VIATOR
VICTIM
VICTOR
VIKTOR
VINTON
VIRTUE
VIRTUS
VISTAS
VITTLE
VORTEX
VOSTOK

V•••T•
VACATE
VALETS
VANITY
VASHTI
VAULTS
VAULTY
VAUNTS
VAUNTY
VEINTE
VELDTS
VENETO
VENITE
VENUTI
VERITE
VERITY
VERSTS
VISITS
VOLUTE

V••••T
VACANT
VALENT
VARLET
VEDIST
VEGOUT
VEIGHT
VELVET
VERIST
VERNET
VERSET
VIBIST
VIDIOT
VILEST
VINCIT
VIOLET
VIORST
VIVANT
VOIGHT
VOLANT

•VT•••
IVTUBE
TVTAPE
TVTIME

•V•T••
AVATAR
EVITES
KVETCH
TVSTAR
YVETTE

•V••T•
AVANTI
AVERTS
AVESTA
AVIATE
EVENTS
EVERTS
EVICTS
SVELTE
TVHITS
TVSETS
YVETTE

•V•••T
AVAUNT
AVOCET
OVERIT
TVSPOT

••V•T•
AMVETS
CAVETT
CAVITY
CIVETS
COVETS
DAVITS
DEVITO
DEVOTE
DEVOTO
DIVOTS
DUVETS
FIVETO
GAVETO
GAVOTS
GIVETH
GIVETO
HAVETO
HOVETO
INVITE
JAVITS
LEVITE
LEVITT
LEVITY
LIVETH
LIVETV
LOVETO
LOVETT
MOVETO
NOVATO
NOVOTE
PIVOTS
REVETS
REVOTE
RIVETS
SAVATE
TEVETS
WAVETO

••V••T
ADVENT
ADVERT
CAVEAT
CAVETT
CAVORT
COVENT
COVERT
DEVEST
DEVOUT
DIVERT
DIVEST
HAVEAT
HAVEIT
HAVENT
INVENT
INVERT
INVEST
JAVERT
LEVANT
LEVERT
LEVITT
LIVEAT
LIVEST
LOVEIT
LOVETT
MOVEIT
OBVERT
RAVEAT
REVERT
REVEST
REVOLT
SAVANT
SAVEIT
SOVIET
TAVIST
VIVANT
WAVEAT

•••V•T
BREVET
CALVET
CHEVET
CRAVAT
CURVET
DYEVAT
PRIVET
SHEVAT
SWIVET
THEVET
TRIVET
VELVET
WARVET

VU••••
VULCAN
VULGAR
VULGUS

V•U•••
VAUGHN
VAULTS
VAULTY
VAUNTS
VAUNTY

V••U••
VACUUM
VAGUER
VALUED
VALUER
VALUES
VELURE
VENUES
VENULE
VENUTI
VFOURS
VICUNA
VISUAL
VOGUED
VOGUER
VOGUES
VOLUME
VOLUTE
VWBUGS

V•••U•
VACUUM
VALIUM
VALOUR
VAPOUR
VARMUS
VASTUS
VATFUL
VEGOUT
VELLUM
VELOUR
VENDUE
VENOUS
VERDUN
VERSUS
VIGOUR
VINOUS
VIRTUE
VIRTUS
VOROUS
VULGUS

V••••U
VISHNU

•VU•••
AVULSE
EVULSE
OVULAR
OVULES
UVULAE
UVULAR
UVULAS

•V•U••
AVAUNT
AVOUCH
IVTUBE

•V••U•
AVENUE
EVENUP
RVALUE
UVALUE
UVEOUS

••VU••
FYVUSH
REVUES

••V•U•
DEVOUR
DEVOUT
FAVOUR
FIVEUP
GAVEUP
GIVEUP
HAVEUP
MOVEUP
RAVEUP
REVSUP
SAVEUP
SAVOUR

••V••U
HAVASU
TUVALU

•••VU•
CORVUS
PREVUE

••••VU
BUKAVU
DEJAVU

V•V•••
VIVACE
VIVANT
VIVECA
VIVIAN
VIVICA
VIVIEN
VIVIFY

V••V••
VALVED
VALVES
VELVET
VERVES
VOLVOS

V•••V•
VALOVA
VOTIVE

V••••V
VACLAV
VASLAV

•VV•••
TVVCRS

•V•V••
TVDVDS

•V••V•
EVOLVE
IVANVI

•V•••V
IVANIV
IVANOV

••VV••
MTVVJS
REVVED

••V•V•
INVIVO
REVIVE

••V••V
LIVETV
PAVLOV

•••V•V
OLAVIV

VW••••
VWBUGS

V•W•••
VOWELS
VOWELY
VOWERS
VOWING

V••W••
VIEWED
VIEWER

•VW•••
UVWXYZ

•V•W••
AVOWAL
AVOWED
AVOWER

•V•••W
TVCREW
TVSHOW

••VW••
TUVWXY

••V•W•
FIVEWS

••V••W
INVIEW
ONVIEW
REVIEW

•••VW•
STUVWX

•••V•W
REAVOW

••••VW
RSTUVW

V•X•••
VEXERS
VEXING
VIXENS
VOXPOP

V••X••
VSIXES

V••••X
VERTEX
VORTEX

•V•X••
UVWXYZ

••V•X•
TUVWXY

•••V•X
CONVEX
STUVWX

V•Y•••
VOYAGE

V••Y••
VINYLS

V•••Y•
VANRYN
VATDYE

V••••Y
VAGARY
VAINLY
VALERY
VALLEY
VANITY
VAPORY
VARNEY
VASILY
VASTLY
VAULTY
VAUNTY
VEEJAY
VERIFY
VERILY
VERITY
VESTRY
VIABLY
VILELY
VILIFY
VINERY
VINIFY
VIVIFY
VOLLEY
VOTARY
VOWELY

•V••Y•
EVELYN
UVRAYS
UVWXYZ

•V•••Y
AVIARY
AVIDLY
EVENLY
EVERLY
EVILLY
OVALLY
OVERLY

••V•Y•
COVEYS
ENVOYS
LOVEYA
LOVEYS

••V••Y
BOVARY
CAVAFY
CAVITY
LEVITY
LIVELY
LIVERY
LOVELY
NEVSKY
PEVNEY
SAVORY
TUVWXY
VIVIFY
WAVERY
WAVILY

•••VY•
CHEVYS
MELVYN
MERVYN

•••V•Y
CARVEY
CONVEY
CONVOY
GARVEY
HARVEY
HERVEY
MCAVOY
PURVEY
SURVEY

••••VY
GROOVY
HALEVY
RELEVY
SCURVY
USNAVY

V•Z•••
VEZINA
VIZIER
VIZIRS
VIZORS
VIZSLA

V••••Z
VALDEZ

•V•••Z
UVWXYZ

••V••Z
KUVASZ

•••V•Z
CHAVEZ

WA••••
WABASH
WABBIT
WACKER
WACKOS
WACOTX
WADDED
WADDER
WADDLE
WADDLY
WADEIN
WADENA
WADERS
WADING
WADSUP
WAFERS
WAFERY
WAFFLE
WAFFLY
WAFTED
WAFTER
WAGERS
WAGGED
WAGGER
WAGGLE
WAGGLY
WAGING
WAGNER
WAGONS
WAHINE
WAHLOO
WAHOOS
WAHWAH
WAILED
WAILER
WAISTS
WAITED
WAITER
WAITON
WAITUP
WAIVED
WAIVER
WAIVES
WAKAME
WAKENS
WAKERS
WAKEUP
WAKING
WALDEN
WALESA
WALING
WALKBY
WALKED
WALKEN
WALKER
WALKIE
WALKIN
WALKON
WALKTO
WALKUP
WALLED
WALLER
WALLET
WALLIN
WALLIS
WALLOP
WALLOW
WALLST
WALLUP
WALNUT
WALRUS
WALTER
WALTON
WAMBLE
WAMBLY
WAMPUM
WANDER
WANGLE
WANIER
WANING
WANKEL
WANNED
WANNER
WANTAD
WANTED
WANTER
WANTIN
WANTON
WANTTO
WAPITI
WAPNER
WARBLE
WARCRY
WARDED
WARDEN
WARDER
WARGOD
WARHOL
WARIER
WARILY
WARING
WARMED
WARMER
WARMLY
WARMTH
WARMTO
WARMUP
WARNED
WARNER
WARNES
WARNOF
WARPED
WARPER
WARRED
WARREN
WARSAW
WARTED
WARVET
WASABI
WASECA
WASFUN
WASHAD
WASHED
WASHER
WASHES
WASHME
WASHOE
WASHOS
WASHUP
WASLED
WASMET
WASOFF
WASOLD
WASSER
WASTED
WASTER
WASTES
WATERS
WATERY
WATNEY
WATSON
WATTLE
WATUSI
WAUSAU
WAVEAT
WAVEIN
WAVERS
WAVERY
WAVETO
WAVIER
WAVILY
WAVING
WAXERS
WAXIER
WAXILY
WAXING
WAYANS
WAYLAY
WAYLON
WAYNES
WAYOFF
WAYOUT
WAYSIN

W•A•••
WEAKEN
WEAKER
WEAKLY
WEAKON
WEALDS
WEALTH
WEANED
WEANER
WEAPON
WEARER
WEARON
WEASEL
WEAVED
WEAVER
WEAVES
WHACKS
WHALED
WHALER
WHALES
WHALEY
WHAMMO
WHAMMY
WHANGS
WHARFS
WHATIF
WHATLL
WHATVE
WRACKS
WRAITH
WRAPUP
WRASSE
WRATHS

W••A••
WABASH
WAKAME
WASABI
WAYANS
WEBADS
WECARE
WHEATS
WHOAMI
WIGAND
WINANS
WIZARD
WOMACK
WOMANS
WREAKS
WREATH

W•••A•
WAHWAH
WANTAD
WARSAW
WASHAD
WAUSAU
WAVEAT
WAYLAY
WEBCAM
WEIMAR
WENTAT
WETBAR
WETNAP
WETRAG
WHELAN
WHODAT
WICCAN
WIEMAN
WIGWAG
WIGWAM
WINKAT
WINSAT
WITHAL
WOMBAT
WORKAT
WYSTAN

W••••A
WADENA
WALESA
WASECA
WINONA
WOULDA

•WA•••
AWAITS
AWAKED
AWAKEN
AWAKER
AWAKES
AWARDS
AWARER
BWANAS
DWARFS
DWAYNE
EWAINE
IWANNA
KWACHA
KWANZA
LWAVES

RWANDA SWABBY SWAINS SWALES SWAMIS SWAMPS SWAMPY SWAMUP SWANEE SWANKY SWANNS SWARDS SWARMS SWATAT SWATCH SWATHE SWATHS SWAYED SWAYER SWAYZE TWAINS TWANGS TWANGY

•W•A••

AWEARY EWBANK SWEARS SWEATS SWEATY TWEAKS TWEAKY TWOACT

•W••A•

BWANAS SWATAT TWOCAR TWODAY TWOMAN TWOWAY TWYMAN

•W•••A

IWANNA KWACHA KWANZA RWANDA

••WA••

ADWARE ADWARS ALWAYS ANWANG ASWARM BEWAIL BEWARE BEWARY BYWAYS COWARD DEWARS EDWARD GAWAIN HAWAII HOWARD INWANT INWARD IOWANS KUWAIT NEWAGE NEWARK NOWAIT NOWAYS ONWARD OSWALD REWAKE REWARD REWARM REWARN REWASH ROWANS SAWALL SEWAGE SEWARD THWACK THWART TOWAGE TOWARD UNWALL UNWARY UPWAFT UPWARD

••W•A•

BOWMAN BOWOAR BOWSAW CAWCAW COWMAN DEWLAP ENWRAP GAWKAT GEWGAW HAWHAW HOWDAH HOWFAR HOWLAT HOWSAD ISWEAR JAWSAT LAWMAN LOWCAL LOWFAT LOWMAN LOWTAR NEWCAR NEWDAY NEWHAT NEWMAN NEWMAR NEWWAY NOWLAN ORWHAT PAWPAW PAWSAT RAWBAR REWEAR REWRAP SOWHAT TOWBAR TOWCAR UNWRAP YOWZAH

••W••A

COWPEA EDWINA NEWERA ROWENA

•••WA•

AGAWAM AIRWAR AIRWAY AJOWAN ANYWAY AVOWAL CARWAX CLAWAT CONWAY EARWAX FATWAS FENWAY FLEWAT FLYWAY GALWAY GASWAR GNAWAT GOAWAY HOTWAR INAWAY JETWAY KEYWAY KIOWAN KIOWAS LEEWAY MCEWAN MIDWAY NEWWAY NONWAR NORWAY OBIWAN OLDWAY ONEWAY OUTWAR PEDWAY PREWAR PROWAR PSYWAR RAHWAY RESWAM RUNWAY SCHWAB SCHWAS SEAWAY SEGWAY SIXWAY SKIWAX SKYWAY SUBWAR SUBWAY TAIWAN TEKWAR THEWAY TWOWAY WAHWAH WIGWAG WIGWAM

••••WA

BUSHWA KAGAWA KANAWA OJIBWA OSHAWA OTTAWA PESEWA TARAWA YUKAWA

W•B•••

WABASH WABBIT WEBADS WEBBED WEBBER WEBCAM WEBERN WEBERS WEBFED WEBLOG WOBBLE WOBBLY WOBURN

W••B••

WABBIT WAMBLE WAMBLY WARBLE WEBBED WEBBER WEEBIT WETBAR WILBUR WINBIG WOBBLE WOBBLY WOMBAT WONBIG

W•••B•

WALKBY WASABI WENTBY WHITBY WILLBE WINSBY

•WB•••

EWBANK VWBUGS

•W•B••

SWABBY TWOBIT

•W••B•

DWEEBS DWEEBY SWABBY

••WB••

COWBOY DAWBER HOWBIG LOWBID LOWBOY NEWBIE RAWBAR TOWBAR

••W•B•

LOWEBB

••W••B

LOWEBB NEWJOB

•••WB•

FLEWBY

•••W•B

COBWEB SCHWAB THEWEB

W•C•••

WACKER WACKOS WACOTX WECARE WICCAN WICKED WICKER WICKET

W••C••

WARCRY WEBCAM WELCHS WENCES WHACKS WICCAN WILCOX WINCED WINCER WINCES WITCHY WRACKS WRECKS

W•••C•

WASECA WHENCE WOMACK WRENCH WRETCH

•WC•••

AWCMON

•W•C••

KWACHA TWOCAR

•W••C•

AWHECK SWATCH SWITCH TWITCH TWOACT

••WC••

CAWCAW LOWCAL LOWCUT NEWCAR TOWCAR

••W•C•

THWACK

W•D•••

WADDED WADDER WADDLE WADDLY WADEIN WADENA WADERS WADING WADSUP WEDDED WEDDER WEDELN WEDELS WEDGED WEDGES WEDGIE WIDDER WIDELY WIDENS WIDEOF WIDEST WIDGET WIDISH WIDOWS WIDTHS

W••D••

WADDED WADDER WADDLE WADDLY WALDEN WANDER WARDED WARDEN WARDER WEDDED WEDDER WEEDED WEEDER WEIDER WELDED WELDER WELDON WENDED WENDIE WENDYS WHODAT WIDDER WILDER WILDLY WINDED WINDER WINDEX WINDOM WINDOW WINDUP WISDOM WONDER WOODED WOODEN WOODIE WOODSY WORDED

W•••D•

WEALDS WEBADS WEIRDO WEIRDY WIELDS WIELDY WILLDO WONTDO WORLDS WOULDA WOUNDS

W••••D

WADDED WAFTED WAGGED WAILED WAITED WAIVED WALKED WALLED WANNED WANTAD WANTED WARDED WARGOD WARMED WARNED WARPED WARRED WARTED WASHAD WASHED WASLED WASOLD WASTED WEANED WEAVED WEBBED WEBFED WEDDED WEDGED WEEDED WEENED WELDED WELLED WELTED WENDED WETTED WHALED WHERED WHILED WHINED WHITED WHWORD WICKED WIFIED WIGAND WIGGED WILLED WILTED WIMPED WINCED WINDED WINGED WINKED WISHED WISPED WITTED WIZARD WOLFED WONTED WOODED WOOFED WORDED WORKED WORMED

•W•D••

AWEDLY OWEDON OWEDTO SWEDEN SWEDES TWODAY

•W••D•

AWARDS RWANDA SWARDS SWORDS TWEEDS TWEEDY

•W•••D

AWAKED IWOULD SWAYED SWIPED TWINED

••WD••

CAWDOR DAWDLE HOWDAH LEWDER LEWDLY NEWDAY POWDER RAWDON TAWDRY

••W•D•

HOWODD REWEDS

••W••D

ATWOOD BAWLED BOWLED BYWORD COWARD COWLED DAWNED DOWNED DOWSED EDWARD EDWOOD ELWOOD ENWIND FAWNED FOWLED GAWKED GAWPED GOWILD GOWNED HAWKED HOWARD HOWLED HOWODD HOWSAD INWARD JOWLED LOWBID LOWEND MEWLED MYWORD NEWKID ONWARD OSWALD PAWNED REWARD REWELD REWIND REWORD SAWRED SEWARD TOWARD UNWILD UNWIND UPWARD UPWIND WHWORD YAWNED YAWPED YOWLED

•••WD•

CROWDS

•••W•D

AVOWED BREWED BROWED CHAWED CHEWED CHOWED CLAWED CLEWED CREWED CROWED FLAWED FLOWED GLOWED GNAWED MEOWED PLOWED SHOWED SKEWED SLEWED SLOWED SNOWED SPEWED STEWED STOWED THAWED TROWED UNAWED UNOWED VIEWED

••••WD

SHREWD

WE••••

WEAKEN WEAKER WEAKLY WEAKON WEALDS WEALTH WEANED WEANER WEAPON WEARER WEARON WEASEL WEAVED WEAVER WEAVES WEBADS WEBBED WEBBER WEBCAM WEBERN WEBERS WEBFED WEBLOG WECARE WEDDED WEDDER WEDELN WEDELS WEDGED WEDGES WEDGIE WEEBIT WEEDED WEEDER WEEKLY WEENED WEENIE WEENSY WEEONE WEEPER WEEUNS WEEVIL WEEZER WEIDER WEIGHS WEIGHT WEIMAR WEIRDO WEIRDY WELCHS WELDED WELDER WELDON WELLED WELLER WELLES WELLUP WELTED WELTER WENCES WENDED WENDIE WENDYS WENNER WENTAT WENTBY WENTIN WENTON WENTTO WENTUP WERENT WERFEL WERKER WERNER WESKER WESKIT WESLEY WESSEX WESSON WESTER WESTIE WESTIN WESTON WETBAR WETFLY WETMOP WETNAP WETONE WETRAG WETTED WETTER WETTIG

W•E•••

WEEBIT WEEDED WEEDER WEEKLY WEENED WEENIE WEENSY WEEONE WEEPER WEEUNS WEEVIL WEEZER WHEATS WHEELS WHEEZE WHEEZY WHELAN WHELKS WHELMS WHELPS WHENCE WHENLL WHERED WHERES WHERRY WHEYEY WIELDS WIELDY WIEMAN WIENER WIENIE WIESEL WOEFUL WREAKS WREATH WRECKS WRENCH WRESTS WRETCH

W••E••

WADEIN WADENA WADERS WAFERS WAFERY WAGERS WAKENS WAKERS WAKEUP WALESA WASECA WATERS WATERY WAVEAT WAVEIN WAVERS WAVERY WAVETO WAXERS WEBERN WEBERS WEDELN WEDELS WERENT WHEELS WHEEZE WHEEZY WIDELY WIDENS WIDEOF WIDEST WIFELY WINERY WIPERS WIPEUP WIREIN WIRERS WIREUP WISELY WISEST WISETO WISEUP WIZENS WOKEUP WOMENS WOOERS WOREON WRIEST WRYEST WYLERS WYVERN

W•••E•

WACKER WADDED WADDER WAFTED WAFTER WAGGED WAGGER WAGNER WAILED WAILER WAITED WAITER WAIVED WAIVER WAIVES WALDEN WALKED WALKEN WALKER WALLED WALLER WALLET WALTER WANDER WANIER WANKEL WANNED WANNER WANTED WANTER WAPNER WARDED WARDEN WARDER WARIER WARMED WARMER WARNED WARNER WARNES WARPED WARPER WARRED WARREN WARTED WARVET WASHED WASHER WASHES WASLED WASMET WASSER WASTED WASTER WASTES WATNEY WAVIER WAXIER WAYNES WEAKEN WEAKER WEANED WEANER WEARER WEASEL WEAVED WEAVER WEAVES WEBBED WEBBER WEBFED WEDDED WEDDER WEDGED WEDGES WEEDED WEEDER WEENED WEEPER WEEZER WEIDER WELDED WELDER WELLED WELLER WELLES WELTED WELTER WENCES WENDED WENNER WERFEL WERKER WERNER WESKER WESLEY WESSEX WESTER WETTED WETTER WHALED WHALER WHALES WHALEY WHERED WHERES WHEYEY WHILED WHILES WHINED WHINER WHINES WHITED WHITEN WHITER WHITES WHITEY WHOLES WHYYES WICKED WICKER WICKET WIDDER WIDGET WIENER WIESEL WIFIED WIFIES WIGGED WIGLET WIGNER WILDER WILIER WILKES WILLED WILLEM WILLER WILTED WIMMER WIMPED WIMSEY WINCED WINCER WINCES WINDED WINDER WINDEX WINGED WINGER WINIER WINKED WINKER WINNER WINTER WIRIER WISHED WISHER WISHES WISPED WISTER WITHER WITTED WITTER WIZZES WOHLER WOLFED WOLPER WOLSEY WOLVES WONDER WONTED WOODED WOODEN WOOFED WOOFER WOOLEN WOOLEY WORDED WORKED WORKER WORLEY WORMED WORMER WORSEN WRITER WRITES WTILES WUSSES WYNKEN WYNTER

W••••E

WADDLE WAFFLE WAGGLE WAHINE WAKAME WALKIE WAMBLE WANGLE WARBLE WASHME

WASHOE
WATTLE
WECARE
WEDGIE
WEENIE
WEEONE
WENDIE
WESTIE
WETONE
WHATVE
WHEEZE
WHENCE
WIENIE
WIFFLE
WIGGLE
WILKIE
WILLBE
WILLIE
WIMPLE
WINKIE
WINNIE
WOBBLE
WOODIE
WOOGIE
WRASSE
WRITHE

•WE•••

AWEARY
AWEDLY
AWEIGH
DWEEBS
DWEEBY
DWELLS
KWEISI
OWEDON
OWEDTO
OWESON
QWERTY
SWEARS
SWEATS
SWEATY
SWEDEN
SWEDES
SWEEPS
SWEETS
SWELLS
SWERVE
TWEAKS
TWEAKY
TWEEDS
TWEEDY
TWEENS
TWEENY
TWEETS
TWEETY
TWEEZE
TWELVE
TWENTY
TWERPS

•W•E••

AWHECK
AWLESS
DWEEBS
DWEEBY
OWLEGG
OWLERY
OWLETS
OWNERS
SWEEPS
SWEETS
TWEEDS
TWEEDY
TWEENS
TWEENY
TWEETS
TWEETY
TWEEZE
TWOEEE

•W••E•

AWAKED
AWAKEN
AWAKER
AWAKES
AWARER
AWOKEN
LWAVES
OWLIER
SWALES
SWANEE
SWAYED
SWAYER
SWEDEN
SWEDES
SWIPED
SWIPER
SWIPES
SWIVEL
SWIVET
TWINED
TWINER
TWINES
TWOEEE
TWOFER

•W•••E

AWHILE
DWAYNE
EWAINE
GWYNNE
SWANEE
SWATHE
SWAYZE
SWERVE
TWEEZE
TWELVE
TWINGE
TWOEEE

••WE••

ADWEEK
ALWEST
ASWELL
BEWELL
BOWELS
BOWERS
BOWERY
COWENS
COWERS
DOWELL
DOWELS
DOWERS
DOWERY
FEWEST
GOWELL
GOWEST
HEWERS
HOWELL
ISWEAR
JEWELS
JEWETT
LOWEBB
LOWELL
LOWEND
LOWERS
LOWERY
LOWEST
MEWERS
MOWERS
NEWELL
NEWELS
NEWERA
NEWEST
NLWEST
OHWELL
ORWELL
OSWEGO
PAWERS
PEWEES
POWELL
POWERS
RAWEGG
RAWEST
REWEAR
REWEDS
REWELD
REWETS
ROWELS
ROWENA
ROWENS
ROWERS
SAWERS
SEWELL
SEWERS
SOWERS
SOWETO
TOWELS
TOWERS
TOWERY
UNWELL
UNWEPT
UPWELL
VOWELS
VOWELY
VOWERS

••W•E•

ADWEEK
BAWLED
BAWLER
BOWLED
BOWLER
BOWLES
BOWMEN
BOWYER
BOWZER
COWIER
COWLED
COWLEY
COWMEN
COWPEA
COWPER
DAWBER
DAWNED
DEWIER
DOWNED
DOWNER
DOWNES
DOWNEY
DOWSED
DOWSER
DOWSES
FAWKES
FAWNED
FAWNER
FOWLED
FOWLER
FOWLES
GAWKED
GAWKER
GAWPED
GAWPER
GOWNED
HAWKED
HAWKER
HAWSER
HAWSES
HOWLED
HOWLER
HOWSER
JOWLED
LAWMEN
LAWYER
LEWDER
LOWKEY
LOWMEN
LOWRES
LOWSET
MEWLED
MEWLER
NEWIES
NEWLEY
PAWNED
PAWNEE
PAWNER
PEWEES
PEWTER
POWDER
ROWLEY
SAWRED
SAWYER
TOWHEE
TOWNER
YAWKEY
YAWNED
YAWNER
YAWPED
YAWPER
YOWLED
YOWLER

••W••E

ADWARE
BEWARE
BOWTIE
BYWIRE
COWRIE
DAWDLE
DEWIRE
EXWIFE
INWOVE
KEWPIE
NEWAGE
NEWBIE
NEWSIE
NOWISE
PAWNEE
REWAKE
REWIPE
REWIRE
REWOKE
REWORE
REWOVE
SEWAGE
TOWAGE
TOWHEE
TOWNIE
UNWISE
UNWOVE

•••WE•

ALLWET
ANSWER
AVOWED
AVOWER
BLOWER
BREWED
BREWER
BROWED
BULWER
CHAWED
CHEWED
CHEWER
CHOWED
CLAWED
CLAWER
CLEWED
COBWEB
CREWED
CREWEL
CROWED
CROWER
DRAWEE
DRAWER
EPOWER
FLAWED
FLOWED
FLOWER
FREWER
GETWET
GLOWED
GLOWER
GNAWED
GNAWER
GOTWET
GROWER
KNOWER
KREWES
MCEWEN
MEOWED
MEOWER
PEEWEE
PLOWED
PLOWER
PRAWER
SHOWED
SHOWER
SKEWED
SKEWER
SLEWED
SLOWED
SLOWER
SNOWED
SPEWED
SPEWER
STEWED
STEWER
STOWED
STOWER
THAWED
THAWER
THEWEB
TROWED
TROWEL
UNAWED
UNOWED
VIEWED
VIEWER

•••W•E

BROWNE
BROWSE
CROWNE
DRAWEE
DROWSE
PEEWEE
PROWSE
SHOWME
STEWIE

••••WE

OUTAWE
SODOWE

W•F•••

WAFERS
WAFERY
WAFFLE
WAFFLY
WAFTED
WAFTER
WIFELY
WIFFLE
WIFIED
WIFIES

W••F••

WAFFLE
WAFFLY
WASFUN
WEBFED
WERFEL
WETFLY
WHIFFS
WHYFOR
WIFFLE
WOEFUL
WOLFED
WOOFED
WOOFER

W•••F•

WASOFF
WAYOFF
WHARFS
WHIFFS

W••••F

WARNOF
WASOFF
WAYOFF
WHATIF
WIDEOF

•W•F••

SWIFTS
TWOFER

•W••F•

DWARFS

••WF••

BOWFIN
HOWFAR
LAWFUL
LOWFAT
SAWFIT

••W•F•

EXWIFE
SAWOFF
UPWAFT

••W••F

DEWOLF
SAWOFF

•••W•F

KNEWOF
KNOWOF

W•G•••

WAGERS
WAGGED
WAGGER
WAGGLE
WAGGLY
WAGING
WAGNER
WAGONS
WIGAND
WIGGED
WIGGIN
WIGGLE
WIGGLY
WIGHTS
WIGLET
WIGNER
WIGOUT
WIGWAG
WIGWAM

W••G••

WAGGED
WAGGER
WAGGLE
WAGGLY
WANGLE
WARGOD
WEDGED
WEDGES
WEDGIE
WEIGHS
WEIGHT
WIDGET
WIGGED
WIGGIN
WIGGLE
WIGGLY
WINGED
WINGER
WINGIT
WOOGIE
WRIGHT

W•••G•

WHANGS
WONTGO
WRINGS
WRONGS

W••••G

WADING
WAGING
WAKING
WALING
WANING
WARING
WAVING
WAXING
WEBLOG
WETRAG
WETTIG
WIGWAG
WILING
WINBIG
WINING
WIPING
WIRING
WISING
WITTIG
WIVING
WONBIG
WOOING
WOWING

•W•G••

DWIGHT
TWIGGY

•W••G•

AWEIGH
EWINGS
OWLEGG
SWINGS
SWINGY
TWANGS
TWANGY
TWIGGY
TWINGE
VWBUGS

•W•••G

AWNING
OWLEGG
OWNING

••WG••

GEWGAW
MOWGLI

••W•G•

BEWIGS
NEWAGE
OSWEGO
RAWEGG
SEWAGE
TOWAGE
UNWIGS

••W••G

ANWANG
BOWING
CAWING
COWING
DEWING
HAWING
HEWING
HOWBIG
JAWING
LAWING
LOWING
MEWING
MOWING
MRWONG
PAWING
RAWEGG
ROWING
SAWING
SAWLOG
SEWING
SOWING
TOWING
VOWING
WOWING
YAWING

•••WG•

SLOWGO

•••W•G

BAGWIG
BIGWIG
EARWIG
LUDWIG
WIGWAG

WH••••

WHACKS
WHALED
WHALER
WHALES
WHALEY
WHAMMO
WHAMMY
WHANGS
WHARFS
WHATIF
WHATLL
WHATVE
WHEATS
WHEELS
WHEEZE
WHEEZY
WHELAN
WHELKS
WHELMS
WHELPS
WHENCE
WHENLL
WHERED
WHERES
WHERRY
WHEYEY
WHIFFS
WHILED
WHILES
WHILST
WHIMSY
WHINED
WHINER
WHINES
WHINNY
WHIPIN
WHIPPY
WHIPUP
WHIRLS
WHIRLY
WHIRRS
WHISKS
WHISKY
WHITBY
WHITED
WHITEN
WHITER
WHITES
WHITEY
WHITTY
WHIZZY
WHOAMI
WHODAT
WHOLES
WHOLLY
WHOMPS
WHOMSO
WHOOPI
WHOOPS
WHOOSH
WHORLS
WHOSIN
WHOWON
WHWORD
WHYFOR
WHYNOT
WHYNOW
WHYYES
WHYYOU

W•H•••

WAHINE
WAHLOO
WAHOOS
WAHWAH
WOHLER

W••H••

WARHOL
WASHAD
WASHED
WASHER
WASHES
WASHME
WASHOE
WASHOS
WASHUP
WIGHTS
WISHED
WISHER
WISHES
WISHIN
WISHON
WISHTO
WITHAL
WITHER
WITHIN
WITHIT
WITHUS

W•••H•

WEIGHS
WEIGHT
WELCHS
WIDTHS
WITCHY
WORTHS
WORTHY
WRATHS
WRIGHT
WRITHE

W••••H

WABASH
WAHWAH
WARMTH
WEALTH
WHOOSH
WIDISH
WINISH
WRAITH
WREATH
WRENCH
WRETCH

•WH•••

AWHECK
AWHILE
AWHIRL

•W••H•

DWIGHT
KWACHA
SWATHE
SWATHS
SWISHY

•W•••H

AWEIGH
OWLISH
SWATCH
SWITCH
SWOOSH
TWITCH

••WH••

HAWHAW
NEWHAT
ORWHAT
SOWHAT
TOWHEE

••W•H•

CRWTHS
JAWOHL

••W••H

COWISH
DOWITH
GOWITH
HEWISH
HOWDAH
INWITH
JEWISH
LOWISH
NEWISH
RAWISH
REWASH
UNWISH
YOWZAH

•••WH•

BUTWHO
BUTWHY
FORWHY
SEZWHO
THEWHO

•••W•H

GROWTH
WAHWAH

WI••••

WICCAN
WICKED
WICKER
WICKET
WIDDER
WIDELY
WIDENS
WIDEOF
WIDEST
WIDGET
WIDISH
WIDOWS
WIDTHS
WIELDS
WIELDY
WIEMAN
WIENER
WIENIE
WIESEL
WIFELY
WIFFLE
WIFIED
WIFIES
WIGAND
WIGGED
WIGGIN
WIGGLE
WIGGLY
WIGHTS
WIGLET
WIGNER
WIGOUT
WIGWAG
WIGWAM
WILBUR
WILCOX
WILDER
WILDLY
WILIER
WILILY
WILING
WILKES
WILKIE
WILLBE
WILLDO
WILLED
WILLEM
WILLER
WILLIE
WILLIS
WILLOW
WILLYS
WILMUT
WILSON
WILTED
WILTON
WIMMER
WIMMIN
WIMPED
WIMPLE
WIMSEY
WINANS
WINBIG
WINCED
WINCER
WINCES
WINDED
WINDER
WINDEX
WINDOM
WINDOW
WINDUP
WINERY
WINGED
WINGER
WINGIT
WINIER
WINING
WINISH
WINKAT
WINKED
WINKER
WINKIE
WINNER
WINNIE
WINNOW
WINONA
WINOUT
WINSAT
WINSBY
WINSOR
WINTER
WINTRY
WINWIN
WIPERS
WIPEUP
WIPING
WIREIN
WIRERS
WIREUP
WIRIER
WIRILY
WIRING
WISDOM
WISELY
WISEST
WISETO
WISEUP
WISHED
WISHER
WISHES
WISHIN
WISHON
WISHTO
WISING
WISPED
WISTER
WITCHY
WITHAL
WITHER
WITHIN
WITHIT
WITHUS
WITTED
WITTER
WITTIG
WIVING
WIZARD
WIZENS
WIZZES

W•I•••

WAILED
WAILER
WAISTS
WAITED
WAITER
WAITON
WAITUP
WAIVED
WAIVER
WAIVES
WEIDER
WEIGHS
WEIGHT
WEIMAR
WEIRDO
WEIRDY
WHIFFS
WHILED
WHILES
WHILST
WHIMSY
WHINED
WHINER
WHINES
WHINNY
WHIPIN
WHIPPY
WHIPUP
WHIRLS
WHIRLY
WHIRRS
WHISKS
WHISKY
WHITBY
WHITED
WHITEN
WHITER
WHITES
WHITEY
WHITTY
WHIZZY
WRIEST
WRIGHT
WRINGS
WRISTS
WRITER
WRITES
WRITHE
WTILES

W••I••

WADING
WAGING
WAHINE
WAKING
WALING
WANIER
WANING
WAPITI
WARIER
WARILY
WARING
WAVIER
WAVILY
WAVING
WAXIER
WAXILY
WAXING
WIDISH
WIFIED
WIFIES
WILIER
WILILY
WILING
WINIER
WINING
WINISH
WIPING
WIRIER
WIRILY
WIRING
WISING
WIVING
WOOING
WOWING
WRAITH

W•••I•

WABBIT
WADEIN
WALKIE
WALKIN
WALLIN
WALLIS
WANTIN
WAVEIN
WAYSIN
WEDGIE
WEEBIT
WEENIE
WEEVIL

WENDIE WENTIN WESKIT WESTIE WESTIN WETTIG WHATIF WHIPIN WHOSIN WIENIE WIGGIN WILKIE WILLIE WILLIS WIMMIN WINBIG WINGIT WINKIE WINNIE WINWIN WIREIN WISHIN WITHIN WITHIT WITTIG WONBIG WOODIE WOOGIE WORKIN

W••••I

WAPITI WASABI WATUSI WHOAMI WHOOPI

•WI•••

DWIGHT EWINGS SWIFTS SWILLS SWINGS SWINGY SWIPED SWIPER SWIPES SWIRLS SWIRLY SWIRLZ SWISHY SWITCH SWIVEL SWIVET TWIGGY TWILIT TWILLS TWINED TWINER TWINES TWINGE TWIRLS TWIRLY TWIRPS TWISTS TWISTY TWITCH TWITTY

•W•I••

AWAITS AWEIGH AWHILE AWHIRL AWNING EWAINE KWEISI OWLIER OWLISH OWNING SWAINS TWAINS

•W••I•

SWAMIS TWILIT TWOBIT TWOPIN

•W•••I

KWEISI

••WI••

ASWIRL ATWILL ATWIST BEWIGS BOWING BYWIRE CAWING COWIER COWING COWISH DEWIER DEWILY DEWING DEWIRE DEWITT DOWITH EDWINA ENWIND EXWIFE GOWILD GOWITH HAWING HEWING HEWISH HEWITT INWITH JAWING JEWISH KSWISS LAWING LOWING LOWIQS LOWISH MEWING MOWING NEWIES NEWISH NOWISE PAWING PEWITS RAWISH RAWIST REWIND REWINS REWIPE REWIRE ROWING SAWING SEWING SEWIST SOWING TOWING UNWIGS UNWILD UNWILY UNWIND UNWISE UNWISH UPWIND VOWING WOWING YAWING

••W•I•

BEWAIL BOWFIN BOWTIE COWRIE GAWAIN HAWAII HOWBIG HOWLIN KEWPIE KUWAIT LOWBID NEWBIE NEWKID NEWSIE NOWAIT SAWFIT SAWPIT SEWNIN SEWSIN TOWNIE TOWSIN

••W••I

HAWAII MOWGLI

•••WI•

BAGWIG BEDWIN BIGWIG BIGWIN BLEWIN BLEWIT BLOWIN BLOWIT CORWIN DARWIN DIMWIT DRAWIN DREWIN EARWIG FLEWIN FLOWIN GODWIN GODWIT KERWIN KNEWIT KNOWIT LUDWIG NITWIT OUTWIT RESWIM SHOWIN SNOWIN STEWIE STOWIT THEWIZ WINWIN YOUWIN

••••WI

MALAWI

••WJ••

NEWJOB

W•K•••

WAKAME WAKENS WAKERS WAKEUP WAKING WOKEUP

W••K••

WACKER WACKOS WALKBY WALKED WALKEN WALKER WALKIE WALKIN WALKON WALKTO WALKUP WANKEL WEAKEN WEAKER WEAKLY WEAKON WEEKLY WERKER WESKER WESKIT WICKED WICKER WICKET WILKES WILKIE WINKAT WINKED WINKER WINKIE WORKAT WORKED WORKER WORKIN WORKON WORKUP WYNKEN

W•••K•

WHACKS WHELKS WHISKS WHISKY WRACKS WREAKS WRECKS

W••••K

WOMACK

•W•K••

AWAKED AWAKEN AWAKER AWAKES AWOKEN

•W••K•

SWANKY TWEAKS TWEAKY

•W•••K

AWHECK EWBANK

••WK••

FAWKES GAWKAT GAWKED GAWKER HAWKED HAWKER LOWKEY NEWKID YAWKEY

••W•K•

REWAKE REWOKE

••W••K

ADWEEK ATWORK NEWARK REWORK THWACK

••••WK

MOHAWK SQUAWK

W•L•••

WALDEN WALESA WALING WALKBY WALKED WALKEN WALKER WALKIE WALKIN WALKON WALKTO WALKUP WALLED WALLER WALLET WALLIN WALLIS WALLOP WALLOW WALLST WALLUP WALNUT WALRUS WALTER WALTON WELCHS WELDED WELDER WELDON WELLED WELLER WELLES WELLUP WELTED WELTER WILBUR WILCOX WILDER WILDLY WILIER WILILY WILING WILKES WILKIE WILLBE WILLDO WILLED WILLEM WILLER WILLIE WILLIS WILLOW WILLYS WILMUT WILSON WILTED WILTON WOLFED WOLPER WOLSEY WOLVES WYLERS

W••L••

WAHLOO WAILED WAILER WALLED WALLER WALLET WALLIN WALLIS WALLOP WALLOW WALLST WALLUP WASLED WAYLAY WAYLON WEALDS WEALTH WEBLOG WELLED WELLER WELLES WELLUP WESLEY WHALED WHALER WHALES WHALEY WHELAN WHELKS WHELMS WHELPS WHILED WHILES WHILST WHOLES WHOLLY WIELDS WIELDY WIGLET WILLBE WILLDO WILLED WILLEM WILLER WILLIE WILLIS WILLOW WILLYS WOHLER WOOLEN WOOLEY WOOLLY WORLDS WORLEY WOULDA WTILES

W•••L•

WADDLE WADDLY WAFFLE WAFFLY WAGGLE WAGGLY WAMBLE WAMBLY WANGLE WARBLE WARILY WARMLY WASOLD WATTLE WAVILY WAXILY WEAKLY WEDELN WEDELS WEEKLY WETFLY WHATLL WHEELS WHENLL WHIRLS WHIRLY WHOLLY WHORLS WIDELY WIFELY WIFFLE WIGGLE WIGGLY WILDLY WILILY WIMPLE WIRILY WISELY WOBBLE WOBBLY WOOLLY

W••••L

WANKEL WARHOL WEASEL WEEVIL WERFEL WHATLL WHENLL WIESEL WITHAL WOEFUL

•WL•••

AWLESS OWLEGG OWLERY OWLETS OWLIER OWLISH

•W•L••

DWELLS SWALES SWELLS SWILLS TWELVE TWILIT TWILLS

•W••L•

AWEDLY AWHILE DWELLS IWOULD SWELLS SWILLS SWIRLS SWIRLY SWIRLZ TWILLS TWIRLS TWIRLY TWOPLY

•W•••L

AWHIRL SWIVEL

••WL••

BAWLED BAWLER BOWLED BOWLER BOWLES COWLED COWLEY DEWLAP FAWLTY FOWLED FOWLER FOWLES HOWLAT HOWLED HOWLER HOWLIN JOWLED MEWLED MEWLER NEWLEY NOWLAN ROWLEY SAWLOG YOWLED YOWLER

••W•L•

ASWELL ATWILL BEWELL BOWELS DAWDLE DEWILY DEWOLF DOWELL DOWELS GOWELL GOWILD HOWELL JEWELS LEWDLY LOWELL MOWGLI NEWELL NEWELS NEWULM OHWELL ORWELL OSWALD POWELL REWELD ROWELS SAWALL SEWELL TOWELS UNWALL UNWELL UNWILD UNWILY UPWELL VOWELS VOWELY

••W••L

ASWELL ASWIRL ATWILL BEWAIL BEWELL DOWELL GOWELL HOWELL JAWOHL LAWFUL LOWCAL LOWELL NEWELL OHWELL ORWELL POWELL SAWALL SEWELL UNWALL UNWELL UPWELL

•••WL•

BRAWLS CRAWLS CRAWLY DRAWLS DRAWLY GROWLS GROWLY PROWLS SCOWLS SHAWLS SLOWLY TRAWLS

•••W•L

AVOWAL CREWEL GOAWOL TROWEL

••••WL

ELFOWL SCRAWL SPRAWL

W•M•••

WAMBLE WAMBLY WAMPUM WIMMER WIMMIN WIMPED WIMPLE WIMSEY WOMACK WOMANS WOMBAT WOMENS

W••M••

WARMED WARMER WARMLY WARMTH WARMTO WARMUP WASMET WEIMAR WETMOP WHAMMO WHAMMY WHIMSY WHOMPS WHOMSO WIEMAN WILMUT WIMMER WIMMIN WORMED WORMER

W•••M•

WAKAME WASHME WHAMMO WHAMMY WHELMS WHOAMI

W••••M

WAMPUM WEBCAM WIGWAM WILLEM WINDOM WISDOM

•W•M••

AWCMON SWAMIS SWAMPS SWAMPY SWAMUP TWOMAN TWYMAN

•W••M•

SWARMS

••WM••

BOWMAN BOWMEN COWMAN COWMEN LAWMAN LAWMEN LOWMAN LOWMEN NEWMAN NEWMAR

••W••M

ASWARM DEWORM NEWSOM NEWULM REWARM

•••WM•

SHOWME

•••W•M

AGAWAM RESWAM RESWIM WIGWAM

W•N•••

WANDER WANGLE WANIER WANING WANKEL WANNED WANNER WANTAD WANTED WANTER WANTIN WANTON WANTTO WENCES WENDED WENDIE WENDYS WENNER WENTAT WENTBY WENTIN WENTON WENTTO WENTUP WINANS WINBIG WINCED WINCER WINCES WINDED WINDER WINDEX WINDOM WINDOW WINDUP WINERY WINGED WINGER WINGIT WINIER WINING WINISH WINKAT WINKED WINKER WINKIE WINNER WINNIE WINNOW WINONA WINOUT WINSAT WINSBY WINSOR WINTER WINTRY WINWIN WONBIG WONDER WONOUT WONTDO WONTED WONTGO WONTON WYNKEN WYNTER WYNTON

W••N••

WAGNER WALNUT WANNED WANNER WAPNER WARNED WARNER WARNES WARNOF WATNEY WAYNES WEANED WEANER WEENED WEENIE WEENSY WENNER WERNER WETNAP WHANGS WHENCE WHENLL WHINED WHINER WHINES WHINNY WHYNOT WHYNOW WIENER WIENIE WIGNER WINNER WINNIE WINNOW WOUNDS WRENCH WRINGS WRONGS

W•••N•

WADENA WADING WAGING WAGONS WAHINE WAKENS WAKING WALING WANING WARING WAVING WAXING WAYANS WEEONE WEEUNS WERENT WETONE WHINNY WIDENS WIGAND WILING WINANS WINING WINONA WIPING WIRING WISING WIVING WIZENS WOMANS WOMENS WOOING WOWING

W••••N

WADEIN WAITON WALDEN WALKEN WALKIN WALKON WALLIN WALTON WANTIN WANTON WARDEN WARREN WASFUN WATSON WAVEIN WAYLON WAYSIN WEAKEN WEAKON WEAPON WEARON WEBERN WEDELN WELDON WENTIN WENTON WESSON WESTIN WESTON WHELAN WHIPIN WHITEN WHOSIN WHOWON WICCAN WIEMAN WIGGIN WILSON WILTON WIMMIN WINWIN WIREIN WISHIN WISHON WITHIN WOBURN WONTON WOODEN WOOLEN WOREON WORKIN WORKON WORSEN WYNKEN WYNTON WYSTAN WYVERN

•WN•••

AWNING OWNERS OWNING OWNSUP

•W•N••

BWANAS EWINGS GWYNNE IWANNA KWANZA RWANDA SWANEE SWANKY SWANNS SWINGS SWINGY TWANGS TWANGY TWENTY TWINED TWINER TWINES TWINGE

•W••N•

AWNING DWAYNE EWAINE EWBANK GWYNNE IWANNA OWNING SWAINS SWANNS SWOONS TWAINS TWEENS TWEENY

•W•••N

AWAKEN AWCMON AWOKEN OWEDON OWESON SWEDEN TWOMAN TWOPIN TWYMAN

••WN••

DAWNED DAWNON DOWNED DOWNER DOWNES DOWNEY DOWNON FAWNED FAWNER

FAWNON
GOWNED
HOWNOW
NOWNOW
PAWNED
PAWNEE
PAWNER
SEWNIN
SEWNON
SEWNUP
TOWNER
TOWNIE
YAWNED
YAWNER

••W•N•
ANWANG
BOWING
CAWING
COWENS
COWING
DEWING
EDWINA
EDWYNN
ENWIND
HAWING
HEWING
INWANT
IOWANS
JAWING
LAWING
LOWEND
LOWING
MEWING
MOWING
MRWONG
PAWING
REWIND
REWINS
ROWANS
ROWENA
ROWENS
ROWING
SAWING
SEWING
SEWONS
SOWING
TOWING
UNWIND
UPWIND
VOWING
WOWING
YAWING

••W••N
ASWOON
BOWFIN
BOWMAN
BOWMEN
COWMAN
COWMEN
DAWNON
DAWSON
DOWNON
DOWSON
EDWYNN
FAWNON
GAWAIN
HOWLIN
LAWMAN
LAWMEN
LAWSON
LAWTON
LOWMAN
LOWMEN
MAWSON
NEWMAN
NEWTON
NOWLAN
RAWDON
REWARN
REWORN
SEWNIN
SEWNON
SEWSIN
SEWSON
TOWSIN
UNWORN

•••WN•
BRAWNY
BROWNE
BROWNS
BROWNU
BROWNY
CLOWNS
COOWNS
CROWNE
CROWNS
DROWNS
FROWNS
KNOWNS
PRAWNS
REOWNS
SPAWNS

•••W•N
AJOWAN
BEDWIN
BERWYN
BIGWIN
BLEWIN
BLEWON
BLOWIN
BLOWON
CHEWON
CORWIN
DARWIN
DRAWIN
DRAWON
DREWIN
DREWON
FLEWIN
FLEWON
FLOWIN
GNAWON
GODWIN
GREWON
GROWON
KERWIN
KIOWAN
MCEWAN
MCEWEN
OBIWAN
PLOWON
SHOWIN
SNOWIN
TAIWAN
WHOWON
WINWIN
YOUWIN

••••WN
ANTAWN
ATDAWN
DISOWN
GODOWN
INPAWN
INTOWN
MOTOWN
REMOWN
RENOWN
RESAWN
RESEWN
RESOWN
STREWN
THROWN
UNHEWN
UNMOWN
UNPAWN
UNSAWN
UNSEWN
UNSOWN
UPTOWN

WO••••
WOBBLE
WOBBLY
WOBURN
WOEFUL
WOHLER
WOKEUP
WOLFED
WOLPER
WOLSEY
WOLVES
WOMACK
WOMANS
WOMBAT
WOMENS
WONBIG
WONDER
WONOUT
WONTDO
WONTED
WONTGO
WONTON
WOODED
WOODEN
WOODIE
WOODSY
WOOERS
WOOFED
WOOFER
WOOGIE
WOOING
WOOLEN
WOOLEY
WOOLLY
WOOTSY
WORDED
WOREON
WORKAT
WORKED
WORKER
WORKIN
WORKON
WORKUP
WORLDS
WORLEY
WORMED
WORMER
WORSEN
WORSTS
WORTHS
WORTHY
WOULDA
WOUNDS
WOWING

W•O•••
WHOAMI
WHODAT
WHOLES
WHOLLY
WHOMPS
WHOMSO
WHOOPI
WHOOPS
WHOOSH
WHORLS
WHOSIN
WHOWON
WOODED
WOODEN
WOODIE
WOODSY
WOOERS
WOOFED
WOOFER
WOOGIE
WOOING
WOOLEN
WOOLEY
WOOLLY
WOOTSY
WRONGS

W••O••
WACOTX
WAGONS
WAHOOS
WASOFF
WASOLD
WAYOFF
WAYOUT
WEEONE
WETONE
WHOOPI
WHOOPS
WHOOSH
WHWORD
WIDOWS
WIGOUT
WINONA
WINOUT
WONOUT

W•••O•
WACKOS
WAHLOO
WAHOOS
WAITON
WALKON
WALLOP
WALLOW
WALTON
WANTON
WARGOD
WARHOL
WARNOF
WASHOE
WASHOS
WATSON
WAYLON
WEAKON
WEAPON
WEARON
WEBLOG
WELDON
WENTON
WESSON
WESTON
WETMOP
WHOWON
WHYFOR
WHYNOT
WHYNOW
WHYYOU
WIDEOF
WILCOX
WILLOW
WILSON
WILTON
WINDOM
WINDOW
WINNOW
WINSOR
WISDOM
WISHON
WONTON
WOREON
WORKON
WYNTON

W••••O
WAHLOO
WALKTO
WANTTO
WARMTO
WAVETO
WEIRDO
WENTTO
WHAMMO
WHOMSO
WILLDO
WISETO
WISHTO
WONTDO
WONTGO

•WO•••
AWOKEN
IWOULD
OWOSSO
SWOONS
SWOOPS
SWOOSH
SWORDS
TWOACT
TWOBIT
TWOCAR
TWODAY
TWOEEE
TWOFER
TWOMAN
TWOPIN
TWOPLY
TWOWAY

•W•O••
CWPOST
SWOONS
SWOOPS
SWOOSH

•W••O•
AWCMON
OWEDON
OWESON

•W•••O
OWEDTO
OWOSSO

••WO••
ASWOON
ATWOOD
ATWORK
BOWOAR
BOWOUT
BYWORD
DEWOLF
DEWORM
EDWOOD
ELWOOD
HOWODD
INWOVE
JAWOHL
MRWONG
MYWORD
REWOKE
REWORD
REWORE
REWORK
REWORN
REWOVE
SAWOFF
SAWOUT
SEWONS
UNWORN
UNWOVE
WHWORD

••W•O•
ASWOON
ATWOOD
BOWWOW
CAWDOR
COWBOY
COWPOX
DAWNON
DAWSON
DOWNON
DOWSON
EDWOOD
ELWOOD
FAWNON
HOWNOW
HOWTOS
KOWTOW
LAWSON
LAWTON
LOWBOY
LOWTOP
MAWSON
NEWJOB
NEWSOM
NEWTON
NEWTOY
NOWNOW
POWWOW
RAWDON
SAWLOG
SEWNON
SEWSON

••W••O
BOWSTO
HEWSTO
OSWEGO
SOWETO

•••WO•
BLEWON
BLOWON
BOWWOW
BYTWOS
CHEWON
DAEWOO
DOOWOP
DRAWON
DREWON
FLEWON
GNAWON
GOAWOL
GREWON
GROWON
INTWOS
KNEWOF
KNOWOF
PLOWON
POWWOW
WHOWON

•••W•O
BUTWHO
DAEWOO
DRAWTO
DREWTO
FLEWTO
SEZWHO
SLOWGO
THEWHO

••••WO
ACTTWO
AGETWO
HUTTWO
ONETWO
REDTWO
SIXTWO
TENTWO
YOUTWO

W•P•••
WAPITI
WAPNER
WIPERS
WIPEUP
WIPING

W••P••
WAMPUM
WARPED
WARPER
WEAPON
WEEPER
WHIPIN
WHIPPY
WHIPUP
WIMPED
WIMPLE
WISPED
WOLPER
WRAPUP

W•••P•
WHELPS
WHIPPY
WHOMPS
WHOOPI
WHOOPS

W••••P
WADSUP
WAITUP
WAKEUP
WALKUP
WALLOP
WALLUP
WARMUP
WASHUP
WELLUP
WENTUP
WETMOP
WETNAP
WHIPUP
WINDUP
WIPEUP
WIREUP
WISEUP
WOKEUP
WORKUP
WRAPUP

•WP•••
CWPOST

•W•P••
SWIPED
SWIPER
SWIPES
TWOPIN
TWOPLY

•W••P•
SWAMPS
SWAMPY
SWEEPS
SWOOPS
TWERPS
TWIRPS

•W•••P
OWNSUP
SWAMUP

••WP••
COWPEA
COWPER
COWPOX
GAWPED
GAWPER
KEWPIE
PAWPAW
SAWPIT
YAWPED
YAWPER

••W•P•
REWIPE
UNWEPT

••W••P
DEWLAP
ENWRAP
LOWTOP
REWRAP
SAWSUP
SEWNUP
SEWSUP
UNWRAP

•••W•P
BLEWUP
BLOWUP
BREWUP
CHEWUP
DOOWOP
DRAWUP
DREWUP
FLEWUP
GREWUP
GROWUP
PLOWUP
SHOWUP
SLOWUP

••W•Q•
LOWIQS

WR••••
WRACKS
WRAITH
WRAPUP
WRASSE
WRATHS
WREAKS
WREATH
WRECKS
WRENCH
WRESTS
WRETCH
WRIEST
WRIGHT
WRINGS
WRISTS
WRITER
WRITES
WRITHE
WRONGS
WRYEST

W•R•••
WARBLE
WARCRY
WARDED
WARDEN
WARDER
WARGOD
WARHOL
WARIER
WARILY
WARING
WARMED
WARMER
WARMLY
WARMTH
WARMTO
WARMUP
WARNED
WARNER
WARNES
WARNOF
WARPED
WARPER
WARRED
WARREN
WARSAW
WARTED
WARVET
WERENT
WERFEL
WERKER
WERNER
WIREIN
WIRERS
WIREUP
WIRIER
WIRILY
WIRING
WORDED
WOREON
WORKAT
WORKED
WORKER
WORKIN
WORKON
WORKUP
WORLDS
WORLEY
WORMED
WORMER
WORSEN
WORSTS
WORTHS
WORTHY
WURSTS

W••R••
WALRUS
WARRED
WARREN
WEARER
WEARON
WEIRDO
WEIRDY
WETRAG
WHARFS
WHERED
WHERES
WHERRY
WHIRLS
WHIRLY
WHIRRS
WHORLS

W•••R•
WADERS
WAFERS
WAFERY
WAGERS
WAKERS
WARCRY
WATERS
WATERY
WAVERS
WAVERY
WAXERS
WEBERN
WEBERS
WECARE
WHERRY
WHIRRS
WHWORD
WINERY
WINTRY
WIPERS
WIRERS
WIZARD
WOBURN
WOOERS
WYLERS
WYVERN

W••••R
WACKER
WADDER
WAFTER
WAGGER
WAGNER
WAILER
WAITER
WAIVER
WALKER
WALLER
WALTER
WANDER
WANIER
WANNER
WANTER
WAPNER
WARDER
WARIER
WARMER
WARNER
WARPER
WASHER
WASSER
WASTER
WAVIER
WAXIER
WEAKER
WEANER
WEARER
WEAVER
WEBBER
WEDDER
WEEDER
WEEPER
WEEZER
WEIDER
WEIMAR
WELDER
WELLER
WELTER
WENNER
WERKER
WERNER
WESKER
WESTER
WETBAR
WETTER
WHALER
WHINER
WHITER
WHYFOR
WICKER
WIDDER
WIENER
WIGNER
WILBUR
WILDER
WILIER
WILLER
WIMMER
WINCER
WINDER
WINGER
WINIER
WINKER
WINNER
WINSOR
WINTER
WIRIER
WISHER
WISTER
WITHER
WITTER
WOHLER
WOLPER
WONDER
WOOFER
WORKER
WORMER
WRITER
WYNTER

•W•R••
AWARDS
AWARER
DWARFS
QWERTY
SWARDS
SWARMS
SWERVE
SWIRLS
SWIRLY
SWIRLZ
SWORDS
TWERPS
TWIRLS
TWIRLY
TWIRPS

•W••R•
AWEARY
AWHIRL
OWLERY
OWNERS
SWEARS

•W•••R
AWAKER
AWARER
OWLIER
SWAYER
SWIPER
TWINER
TWOCAR
TWOFER

••WR••
COWRIE
ENWRAP
LOWRES
REWRAP
SAWRED
UNWRAP

••W•R•
ADWARE
ADWARS
ASWARM
ASWIRL
ATWORK
BEWARE
BEWARY
BOWERS
BOWERY
BYWIRE
BYWORD
COWARD
COWERS
DEWARS
DEWIRE
DEWORM
DOWERS
DOWERY
EDWARD
HEWERS
HOWARD
INWARD
LOWERS
LOWERY
MEWERS
MOWERS
MYWORD
NEWARK
NEWERA
ONWARD
PAWERS
POWERS
REWARD
REWARM
REWARN
REWIRE
REWORD
REWORE
REWORK
REWORN
ROWERS
SAWERS
SEWARD
SEWERS
SOWERS
TAWDRY
THWART
TOWARD
TOWERS
TOWERY
UNWARY
UNWORN
UPWARD
VOWERS
WHWORD

••W••R
BAWLER
BOWLER
BOWOAR
BOWYER
BOWZER
CAWDOR
COWIER
COWPER
DAWBER
DEWIER
DOWNER
DOWSER
FAWNER
FOWLER
GAWKER
GAWPER
HAWKER
HAWSER
HOWFAR
HOWLER
HOWSER
ISWEAR
LAWYER
LEWDER
LOWTAR
MEWLER
NEWCAR
NEWMAR
PAWNER
PEWTER
POWDER
RAWBAR
REWEAR
SAWYER
TOWBAR
TOWCAR
TOWNER
YAWNER
YAWPER
YOWLER

•••WR•
GOAWRY

•••W•R
AIRWAR
ANSWER
AVOWER
BLOWER
BREWER
BULWER
CHEWER
CLAWER
CROWER
DRAWER
EPOWER
FLOWER
FREWER
GASWAR
GLOWER
GNAWER
GROWER
HOTWAR
KNOWER
MEOWER
NONWAR
OUTWAR
PLOWER
PRAWER
PREWAR
PROWAR
PSYWAR
SHOWER
SKEWER
SLOWER
SPEWER
STEWER
STOWER
SUBWAR
TEKWAR
THAWER
VIEWER

W•S•••
WASABI
WASECA
WASFUN
WASHAD
WASHED
WASHER
WASHES
WASHME
WASHOE
WASHOS
WASHUP
WASLED
WASMET
WASOFF
WASOLD
WASSER
WASTED
WASTER
WASTES
WESKER
WESKIT
WESLEY

WESSEX
WESSON
WESTER
WESTIE
WESTIN
WESTON
WISDOM
WISELY
WISEST
WISETO
WISEUP
WISHED
WISHER
WISHES
WISHIN
WISHON
WISHTO
WISING
WISPED
WISTER
WUSSES
WYSTAN

W••S••
WADSUP
WAISTS
WARSAW
WASSER
WATSON
WAUSAU
WAYSIN
WEASEL
WESSEX
WESSON
WHISKS
WHISKY
WHOSIN
WIESEL
WILSON
WIMSEY
WINSAT
WINSBY
WINSOR
WOLSEY
WORSEN
WORSTS
WRASSE
WRESTS
WRISTS
WURSTS
WUSSES

W•••S•
WABASH
WALESA
WALLST
WATUSI
WEENSY
WHILST
WHIMSY
WHOMSO
WHOOSH
WIDEST
WIDISH
WINISH
WISEST
WOODSY
WOOTSY
WRASSE
WRIEST
WRYEST

W••••S
WACKOS
WADERS
WAFERS
WAGERS
WAGONS
WAHOOS
WAISTS
WAIVES
WAKENS
WAKERS
WALLIS
WALRUS
WARNES
WASHES
WASHOS
WASTES
WATERS
WAVERS
WAXERS
WAYANS
WAYNES
WEALDS
WEAVES
WEBADS
WEBERS
WEDELS
WEDGES
WEEUNS
WEIGHS
WELCHS
WELLES
WENCES
WENDYS
WHACKS
WHALES
WHANGS
WHARFS
WHEATS
WHEELS
WHELKS
WHELMS
WHELPS
WHERES
WHIFFS
WHILES
WHINES
WHIRLS
WHIRRS
WHISKS
WHITES
WHOLES
WHOMPS
WHOOPS
WHORLS
WHYYES
WIDENS
WIDOWS
WIDTHS
WIELDS
WIFIES
WIGHTS
WILKES
WILLIS
WILLYS
WINANS
WINCES
WIPERS
WIRERS
WISHES
WITHUS
WIZENS
WIZZES
WOLVES
WOMANS
WOMENS
WOOERS
WORLDS
WORSTS
WORTHS
WOUNDS
WRACKS
WRATHS
WREAKS
WRECKS
WRESTS
WRINGS
WRISTS
WRITES
WRONGS
WTILES
WURSTS
WUSSES
WYLERS

•W•S••
OWESON
OWNSUP
OWOSSO
SWISHY
TWISTS
TWISTY

•W••S•
AWLESS
CWPOST
KWEISI
OWLISH
OWOSSO
SWOOSH

•W•••S
AWAITS
AWAKES
AWARDS
AWLESS
BWANAS
DWARFS
DWEEBS
DWELLS
EWINGS
LWAVES
OWLETS
OWNERS
SWAINS
SWALES
SWAMIS
SWAMPS
SWANNS
SWARDS
SWARMS
SWATHS
SWEARS
SWEATS
SWEDES
SWEEPS
SWEETS
SWELLS
SWIFTS
SWILLS
SWINGS
SWIPES
SWIRLS
SWOONS
SWOOPS
SWORDS
TWAINS
TWANGS
TWEAKS
TWEEDS
TWEENS
TWEETS
TWERPS
TWILLS
TWINES
TWIRLS
TWIRPS
TWISTS
VWBUGS

••WS••
BOWSAW
BOWSTO
DAWSON
DOWSED
DOWSER
DOWSES
DOWSON
HAWSER
HAWSES
HEWSTO
HOWSAD
HOWSER
JAWSAT
LAWSON
LOWSET
MAWSON
NEWSIE
NEWSOM
PAWSAT
SAWSUP
SEWSIN
SEWSON
SEWSUP
TOWSIN

••W•S•
ALWEST
ATWIST
COWISH
FEWEST
GOWEST
HEWISH
JEWISH
KSWISS
LOWEST
LOWISH
NEWEST
NEWISH
NLWEST
NOWISE
RAWEST
RAWISH
RAWIST
REWASH
SEWIST
UNWISE
UNWISH

••W••S
ADWARS
ALWAYS
BEWIGS
BOWELS
BOWERS
BOWLES
BYWAYS
COWENS
COWERS
CRWTHS
DEWARS
DOWELS
DOWERS
DOWNES
DOWSES
FAWKES
FOWLES
HAWSES
HEWERS
HOWTOS
IOWANS
JEWELS
KSWISS
LOWERS
LOWIQS
LOWRES
MEWERS
MOWERS
NEWELS
NEWIES
NOWAYS
PAWERS
PEWEES
PEWITS
POWERS
REWEDS
REWETS
REWINS
ROWANS
ROWELS
ROWENS
ROWERS
SAWERS
SEWERS
SEWONS
SOWERS
TOWELS
TOWERS
UNWIGS
VOWELS
VOWERS

•••WS•
BLOWSY
BROWSE
DROWSE
DROWSY
PROWSE

•••W•S
BRAWLS
BROWNS
BYTWOS
CLOWNS
COOWNS
CRAWLS
CROWDS
CROWNS
DRAWLS
DROWNS
FATWAS
FROWNS
GROWLS
INTWOS
KIOWAS
KNOWNS
KREWES
PRAWNS
PROWLS
REOWNS
SCHWAS
SCOWLS
SHAWLS
SPAWNS
TRAWLS

••••WS
ALLOWS
ARROWS
BEDEWS
BYLAWS
ELBOWS
EMBOWS
ENDOWS
FIVEWS
INLAWS
MACAWS
MIAOWS
MRPAWS
NONEWS
OXBOWS
PAPAWS
PSHAWS
REMOWS
RENEWS
RESAWS
RESEWS
RESOWS
RETOWS
SCREWS
SHREWS
SINEWS
STRAWS
STREWS
THROWS
UNMEWS
UNSEWS
UPBOWS
USNEWS
WIDOWS

WT••••
WTILES

W•T•••
WATERS
WATERY
WATNEY
WATSON
WATTLE
WATUSI
WETBAR
WETFLY
WETMOP
WETNAP
WETONE
WETRAG
WETTED
WETTER
WETTIG
WITCHY
WITHAL
WITHER
WITHIN
WITHIT
WITHUS
WITTED
WITTER
WITTIG

W••T••
WAFTED
WAFTER
WAITED
WAITER
WAITON
WAITUP
WALTER
WALTON
WANTAD
WANTED
WANTER
WANTIN
WANTON
WANTTO
WARTED
WASTED
WASTER
WASTES
WATTLE
WELTED
WELTER
WENTAT
WENTBY
WENTIN
WENTON
WENTTO
WENTUP
WESTER
WESTIE
WESTIN
WESTON
WETTED
WETTER
WETTIG
WHATIF
WHATLL
WHATVE
WHITBY
WHITED
WHITEN
WHITER
WHITES
WHITEY
WHITTY
WIDTHS
WILTED
WILTON
WINTER
WINTRY
WISTER
WITTED
WITTER
WITTIG
WONTDO
WONTED
WONTGO
WONTON
WOOTSY
WORTHS
WORTHY
WRATHS
WRETCH
WRITER
WRITES
WRITHE
WYNTER
WYNTON
WYSTAN

W•••T•
WACOTX
WAISTS
WALKTO
WANTTO
WAPITI
WARMTH
WARMTO
WAVETO
WEALTH
WENTTO
WHEATS
WHITTY
WIGHTS
WISETO
WISHTO
WORSTS
WRAITH
WREATH
WRESTS
WRISTS
WURSTS

W••••T
WABBIT
WALLET
WALLST
WALNUT
WARVET
WASMET
WAVEAT
WAYOUT
WEEBIT
WEIGHT
WENTAT
WERENT
WESKIT
WHILST
WHODAT
WHYNOT
WICKET
WIDEST
WIDGET
WIGLET
WIGOUT
WILMUT
WINGIT
WINKAT
WINOUT
WINSAT
WISEST
WITHIT
WOMBAT
WONOUT
WORKAT
WRIEST
WRIGHT
WRYEST

•W•T••
SWATAT
SWATCH
SWATHE
SWATHS
SWITCH
TWITCH
TWITTY

•W••T•
AWAITS
OWEDTO
OWLETS
QWERTY
SWEATS
SWEATY
SWEETS
SWIFTS
TWEETS
TWEETY
TWENTY
TWISTS
TWISTY
TWITTY

•W•••T
CWPOST
DWIGHT
SWATAT
SWIVET
TWILIT
TWOACT
TWOBIT

••WT••
BOWTIE
CRWTHS
HOWTOS
KOWTOW
LAWTON
LOWTAR
LOWTOP
NEWTON
NEWTOY
PEWTER

••W•T•
BOWSTO
DEWITT
DOWITH
FAWLTY
GOWITH
HEWITT
HEWSTO
INWITH
JEWETT
PEWITS
REWETS
SOWETO

••W••T
ALWEST
ATWIST
BOWOUT
DEWITT
FEWEST
GAWKAT
GOWEST
HEWITT
HOWLAT
INWANT
JAWSAT
JEWETT
KUWAIT
LOWCUT
LOWEST
LOWFAT
LOWSET
NEWEST
NEWHAT
NLWEST
NOWAIT
ORWHAT
PAWSAT
RAWEST
RAWIST
SAWFIT
SAWOUT
SAWPIT
SEWIST
SOWHAT
THWART
UNWEPT
UPWAFT

•••WT•
DRAWTO
DREWTO
FLEWTO
GROWTH

•••W•T
ALLWET
BLEWIT
BLOWIT
CLAWAT
DIMWIT
FLEWAT
GETWET
GNAWAT
GODWIT
GOTWET
KNEWIT
KNOWIT
NITWIT
OUTWIT
STOWIT

WU••••
WURSTS
WUSSES

W•U•••
WAUSAU
WOULDA
WOUNDS

W••U••
WATUSI
WEEUNS
WOBURN

W•••U•
WADSUP
WAITUP
WAKEUP
WALKUP
WALLUP
WALNUT
WALRUS
WAMPUM
WARMUP
WASFUN
WASHUP
WAYOUT
WELLUP
WENTUP
WHIPUP
WIGOUT
WILBUR
WILMUT
WINDUP
WINOUT
WIPEUP
WIREUP
WISEUP
WITHUS
WOEFUL
WOKEUP
WONOUT
WORKUP
WRAPUP

W••••U
WAUSAU
WHYYOU

•W•U••
IWOULD
VWBUGS

•W••U•
OWNSUP
SWAMUP

••WU••
NEWULM

••W•U•
BOWOUT
LAWFUL
LOWCUT
SAWOUT
SAWSUP
SEWNUP
SEWSUP

•••WU•
BLEWUP
BLOWUP
BREWUP
CHEWUP
DRAWUP
DREWUP
FLEWUP
GREWUP
GROWUP
PLOWUP
SHOWUP
SLOWUP

•••W•U
BROWNU

W•V•••
WAVEAT
WAVEIN
WAVERS
WAVERY
WAVETO
WAVIER
WAVILY
WAVING
WIVING
WYVERN

W••V••
WAIVED
WAIVER
WAIVES
WARVET
WEAVED
WEAVER
WEAVES
WEEVIL
WOLVES

W•••V•
WHATVE

•W•V••
LWAVES
SWIVEL
SWIVET

•W••V•
SWERVE
TWELVE

••W•V•
INWOVE
REWOVE
UNWOVE

W•W•••
WHWORD
WOWING

W••W••
WAHWAH
WHOWON
WIGWAG
WIGWAM
WINWIN

W•••W•
WIDOWS

W••••W
WALLOW
WARSAW
WHYNOW
WILLOW
WINDOW
WINNOW

•W•W••
TWOWAY

••WW••
BOWWOW
NEWWAY
POWWOW

••W••W
BOWSAW
BOWWOW
CAWCAW
GEWGAW
HAWHAW
HOWNOW
KOWTOW
NOWNOW
PAWPAW
POWWOW

•••W•W
BOWWOW
POWWOW

W•X•••
WAXERS
WAXIER
WAXILY
WAXING

W••••X
WACOTX
WESSEX
WILCOX
WINDEX

••WX••
UVWXYZ

••W••X
COWPOX

•••WX•
TUVWXY

•••W•X
CARWAX
EARWAX
SKIWAX

••••WX
STUVWX

WY••••
WYLERS
WYNKEN
WYNTER
WYNTON
WYSTAN
WYVERN

W•Y•••
WAYANS
WAYLAY
WAYLON
WAYNES
WAYOFF
WAYOUT
WAYSIN
WHYFOR
WHYNOT
WHYNOW
WHYYES
WHYYOU
WRYEST

W••Y••
WHEYEY
WHYYES
WHYYOU

W•••Y•
WENDYS
WILLYS

W••••Y
WADDLY
WAFERY
WAFFLY
WAGGLY
WALKBY
WAMBLY
WARCRY
WARILY
WARMLY
WATERY
WATNEY
WAVERY
WAVILY
WAXILY
WAYLAY
WEAKLY
WEEKLY
WEENSY
WEIRDY
WENTBY
WESLEY
WETFLY
WHALEY
WHAMMY
WHEEZY
WHERRY
WHEYEY
WHIMSY
WHINNY
WHIPPY
WHIRLY
WHISKY
WHITBY
WHITEY
WHITTY
WHIZZY
WHOLLY
WIDELY
WIELDY
WIFELY
WIGGLY
WILDLY
WILILY
WIMSEY
WINERY
WINSBY
WINTRY
WIRILY
WISELY
WITCHY
WOBBLY
WOLSEY
WOODSY
WOOLEY
WOOLLY
WOOTSY
WORLEY
WORTHY

•WY•••
GWYNNE
TWYMAN

•W•Y••
DWAYNE
SWAYED
SWAYER
SWAYZE

•W•••Y
AWEARY
AWEDLY
DWEEBY
OWLERY
QWERTY
SWABBY
SWAMPY
SWANKY
SWEATY
SWINGY
SWIRLY
SWISHY
TWANGY
TWEAKY
TWEEDY
TWEENY
TWEETY
TWENTY
TWIGGY
TWIRLY

TWISTY
TWITTY
TWODAY
TWOPLY
TWOWAY

••WY••
BOWYER
EDWYNN
LAWYER
SAWYER

••W•Y•
ALWAYS
BYWAYS
NOWAYS
UVWXYZ

••W••Y
BEWARY
BOWERY
COWBOY
COWLEY
DEWILY
DOWERY
DOWNEY
FAWLTY
LEWDLY
LOWBOY
LOWERY
LOWKEY
NEWDAY
NEWLEY
NEWTOY
NEWWAY
ROWLEY
TAWDRY
TOWERY
UNWARY
UNWILY
VOWELY
YAWKEY

•••WY•
BERWYN

•••W•Y
AIRWAY
ANYWAY
BLOWSY
BLOWZY
BRAWNY
BROWNY
BUTWHY
CONWAY
CRAWLY
DRAWLY
DROWSY
FENWAY
FLEWBY
FLYWAY
FORWHY
FROWZY
GALWAY
GOAWAY
GOAWRY
GROWLY
INAWAY
JETWAY
KEYWAY
LEEWAY
MIDWAY
NEWWAY
NORWAY
OLDWAY
ONEWAY
PEDWAY
RAHWAY
RUNWAY
SEAWAY
SEGWAY
SIXWAY
SKYWAY
SLOWLY
SUBWAY
THEWAY
TUVWXY
TWOWAY

••••WY
CODYWY
SCREWY
SINEWY
UNDEWY

W•Z•••
WIZARD
WIZENS
WIZZES

W••Z••
WEEZER
WHIZZY
WIZZES

W•••Z•
WHEEZE
WHEEZY
WHIZZY

•W••Z•
KWANZA
SWAYZE
TWEEZE

•W•••Z
SWIRLZ

••WZ••
BOWZER
YOWZAH

••W••Z
UVWXYZ

•••WZ•
BLOWZY
FROWZY

•••W•Z
THEWIZ

XA••••
XANADU
XAVIER

X•A•••
XGAMES
XLARGE
XMASES
XRATED
XRAYED
XSARAS
XYANDZ

X••A••
XANADU

X•••A•
XHOSAS
XSARAS

X••••A
XINHUA
XTERRA

•XA•••
EXACTA
EXACTS
EXALTS
EXARCH
OXALIC
OXALIS

•X•A••
EXHALE
EXMATE
EXPAND
EXPATS
EXTANT
EXYANK
OXCART
OXNARD
OXTAIL

•X••A•
AXEMAN
AXHEAD
AXONAL
EXTRAS

•X•••A
AXILLA
EXACTA
EXCUSA
EXEDRA

••XA••
FIXATE
HEXADS
HEXANE
LAXALT
LUXATE
OAXACA
REXALL
ROXANA
ROXANE
TEXACO
TEXANS

••X•A•
BOXCAR
NEXRAD
REXCAT
SIXDAY
SIXWAY
SOXFAN
TAXLAW
TAXMAN

••X••A
MAXIMA
OAXACA
ROXANA

•••XA•
ALEXAS
COAXAL
PLEXAL

•••X•A
ALEXIA
ANOXIA
ATAXIA
OREXIA

XB••••
XBOXES

X•B•••
XEBECS

X••B••
XZIBIT

•XB•••
OXBOWS

•X••B•
EXCUBS
EXURBS

••XB••
BOXBED
BOXBOY

X•••C•
XEBECS

•XC•••
EXCEED
EXCELS
EXCEPT
EXCESS
EXCIDE
EXCISE
EXCITE
EXCONS
EXCUBS
EXCUSA
EXCUSE
OXCART

•X•C••
EXACTA
EXACTS
EXOCET

•X••C•
EXARCH
EXPECT
EXSECT

•X•••C
AXENIC
EXILIC
EXOTIC
OXALIC
OXIDIC

••XC••
BOXCAR
REXCAT
TAXCUT

••X•C•
MEXICO
OAXACA
TEXACO
TOXICS

••X••C
MIXTEC

•••X•C
ANOXIC
ATAXIC
ATOXIC

X•D•••
XEDOUT

X•••D•
XANADU
XYANDZ

X••••D
XRATED
XRAYED
XYLOID

•X•D••
EXEDRA
EXODUS
EXUDED
EXUDES
OXIDES
OXIDIC
OXYDOL

•X••D•
EXCIDE
OXHIDE

•X•••D
AXHEAD
AXSEED
EXCEED
EXILED
EXITED
EXPAND
EXPEND
EXTEND
EXUDED
OXFORD
OXNARD

••XD••
SIXDAY

••X•D•
HEXADS
TUXEDO

••X••D
BOXBED
NEXRAD
TAXIED
TEXTED

•••X•D
BRUXED
COAXED
FLEXED
FLUXED
HOAXED
JINXED
UNAXED

XE••••
XEBECS
XEDOUT
XERXES
XESOUT

X•E•••
XTERRA

X••E••
XEBECS
XYLEMS

X•••E•
XAVIER
XBOXES
XERXES
XFILES
XGAMES
XMASES
XRATED
XRAYED
XTILES
XTYPES
XYSTER

X••••E
XLARGE
XPRIZE
XYLOSE

•XE•••
AXEMAN
AXEMEN
AXENIC
EXEDRA
EXEMPT
EXERTS
EXETER
EXEUNT
OXEYES

•X•E••
AXHEAD
AXSEED
EXCEED
EXCELS
EXCEPT
EXCESS
EXMETS
EXPECT
EXPELS
EXPEND
EXPERT
EXSECT
EXSERT
EXTEND
EXTENT
EXTERN

•X••E•
AXEMEN
AXISES
AXONES
AXSEED
EXCEED
EXETER
EXILED
EXILER
EXILES
EXITED
EXOCET
EXUDED
EXUDES
OXEYES
OXIDES
OXYGEN

•X•••E
AXLIKE
EXCIDE
EXCISE
EXCITE
EXCUSE
EXHALE
EXHUME
EXMATE
EXMORE
EXPIRE
EXPOSE
EXWIFE
OXHIDE
OXLIKE

••XE••
BOXERS
FAXERS
FIXERS
HEXERS
LAXEST
MAXELL
MAXENE
MIXERS
NIXERS
PIXELS
SEXERS
SIXEEE
SIXERS
TAXERS
TUXEDO
VEXERS
VIXENS
WAXERS

••X•E•
BAXTER
BOXBED
BOXIER
BOXSET
DEXTER
DOXIES
FOXIER
HUXLEY
MIXTEC
NEXTEL
NIXIES
PIXIES
SEXIER
SEXTET
SIXEEE
SIXTEN
TAXIED
TAXIES
TAXMEN
TEXMEX
TEXTED
WAXIER

••X••E
FIXATE
HEXANE
HEXOSE
LUXATE
MAXENE
MAXINE
MAXIXE
ROXANE
SIXEEE
SIXONE

•••XE•
ALEXEI
ALEXEY
APEXES
BLIXEN
BRUXED
BRUXES
CALXES
COAXED
COAXER
COAXES
CRUXES
DREXEL
FLAXEN
FLAXES
FLEXED
FLEXES
FLUXED
FLUXES
GENXER
HOAXED
HOAXER
HOAXES
IBEXES
ILEXES
IMAXES
JINXED
JINXER
JINXES
LYNXES
MARXES
MINXES
ONYXES
ORYXES
PLEXES
PRAXES
PREXES
TREXES
UNAXED
VSIXES
XBOXES
XERXES

•••X•E
DROXIE
TRIXIE

••••XE
DELUXE
ICEAXE
MAXIXE
THEAXE

XF••••
XFILES

•XF•••
OXFORD

•X••F•
EXWIFE

••XF••
BOXFUL
SOXFAN

XG••••
XGAMES

X••G••
XINGIN

X•••G•
XLARGE

•XG•••
EXGOVS

•X•G••
OXYGEN

••XG••
SIXGUN

••X••G
BOXING
COXING
FAXING
FIXING
FOXING
HEXING
MAXING
MIXING
NIXING
RAXING
TAXING
VEXING
WAXING

XH••••
XHOSAS

X••H••
XINHUA

•XH•••
AXHEAD
EXHALE
EXHORT
EXHUME
OXHIDE

•X••H•
EXARCH

••X•H•
SIXTHS

XI••••
XINGIN
XINHUA

X•I•••
XFILES
XTILES
XZIBIT

X••I••
XAVIER
XPRIZE

X•••I•
XINGIN
XYLOID
XZIBIT

•XI•••
AXILLA
AXIOMS
AXIONS
AXISES
EXILED
EXILER
EXILES
EXILIC
EXISTS
EXITED
EXITUS
OXIDES
OXIDIC

•X•I••
AXLIKE
EXCIDE
EXCISE
EXCITE
EXPIRE
EXPIRY
EXWIFE
OXHIDE
OXLIKE
OXLIPS

•X••I•
AXENIC
EXILIC
EXOTIC
OXALIC
OXALIS
OXIDIC
OXTAIL

••XI••
BOXIER
BOXILY
BOXING
COXING
DIXITS
DOXIES
FAXING
FIXING
FIXINS
FIXITY
FOXIER
FOXILY
FOXING
HEXING
LAXITY
MAXIMA
MAXIMS
MAXINE
MAXING
MAXIXE
MEXICO
MIXING
NIXIES
NIXING
PIXIES
RAXING
SEXIER
SEXILY
SEXISM
SEXIST
TAXIED
TAXIES
TAXING
TOXICS
TOXINS
VEXING
WAXIER
WAXILY
WAXING

••X•I•
RUXPIN
SIXPIN
SIXSIX

•••XI•
ALEXIA
ALEXIS
ANOXIA
ANOXIC
ATAXIA
ATAXIC
ATOXIC
DIOXIN
DROXIE
ELIXIR
LEOXII
NOEXIT
OREXIA
OREXIS
PRAXIS
TRIXIE
ZEUXIS

•••X•I
ALEXEI
LEOXII

••••XI
BILOXI
BYTAXI
FELIXI
JOHNXI
PIUSXI

•X••K•
AXLIKE
OXLIKE

•X•••K
EXYANK

XL••••
XLARGE

X•L•••
XYLEMS
XYLOID
XYLOSE

X••L••
XFILES
XTILES

•XL•••
AXLIKE
OXLIKE
OXLIPS

•X•L••
AXILLA
EXALTS
EXILED
EXILER
EXILES
EXILIC
EXULTS
OXALIC
OXALIS

•X••L•
AXILLA
EXCELS
EXHALE
EXPELS
EXTOLL
EXTOLS

•X•••L
AXONAL
EXTOLL
OXTAIL
OXYDOL

••XL••
HUXLEY
TAXLAW

••X•L•
BOXILY
FOXILY
LAXALT
MAXELL
PIXELS
REXALL
SEXILY
TAXOLS
WAXILY

••X••L
BOXFUL
MAXELL
NEXTEL
REXALL

•••X•L
COAXAL
DREXEL
PLEXAL

XM••••
XMASES

X••M••
XGAMES

X•••M•
XYLEMS

•XM•••
EXMATE
EXMETS
EXMOOR
EXMORE

•X•M••
AXEMAN
AXEMEN
EXEMPT

•X••M•
AXIOMS
EXHUME

•X•••M
EXONYM

••XM••
TAXMAN
TAXMEN
TEXMEX

••X•M•
MAXIMA
MAXIMS

••X••M
SEXISM

X•N•••
XANADU
XINGIN
XINHUA

X••N••
XYANDZ

X••••N
XINGIN

•XN•••
OXNARD

•X•N••
AXENIC
AXONAL
AXONES
EXONYM

•X••N•
AXIONS
EXCONS
EXEUNT
EXPAND
EXPEND
EXTANT
EXTEND
EXTENT
EXYANK

•X•••N
AXEMAN
AXEMEN
EXTERN
OXYGEN

••XN••
HEXNUT

••X•N•
BOXING
COXING
FAXING
FIXING
FIXINS
FOXING
HEXANE
HEXING
MAXENE
MAXINE
MAXING
MIXING
NIXING
NIXONS
RAXING
ROXANA
ROXANE
SAXONS
SAXONY
SIXONE
TAXING
TEXANS
TOXINS
VEXING
VIXENS
WAXING

••X••N
MAXSON
PAXTON
RUXPIN
SEXTON
SIXGUN
SIXPIN
SIXTEN
SOXFAN
TAXMAN
TAXMEN

•••X•N
BLIXEN
DIOXIN
FLAXEN
KLAXON

XO••••
XOXOXO

X•O•••
XBOXES
XHOSAS

X••O••
XEDOUT
XESOUT
XOXOXO
XYLOID
XYLOSE

X••••O
XOXOXO

•XO•••
AXONAL
AXONES
EXOCET
EXODUS
EXONYM
EXOTIC

•X•O••
AXIOMS
AXIONS
EXCONS
EXGOVS
EXHORT
EXMOOR
EXMORE
EXPORT
EXPOSE
EXPOST
EXTOLL
EXTOLS
EXTORT
OXBOWS
OXFORD

•X••O•
EXMOOR
OXYDOL

••XO••
CIXOUS
HEXOSE

MAXOUT
NIXONS
SAXONS
SAXONY
SIXONE
TAXOLS
XOXOXO

••X•O•
BOXBOY
BOXTOP
MAXSON
PAXTON
SEXPOT
SEXTON
VOXPOP

••X••O
DEXTRO
MEXICO
NEXTTO
SIXTWO
TEXACO
TUXEDO
XOXOXO

•••XO•
FLEXOR
KLAXON
PLEXOR

••••XO
BORAXO
XOXOXO

XP••••
XPRIZE

X••P••
XTYPES

•XP•••
EXPAND
EXPATS
EXPECT
EXPELS
EXPEND
EXPERT
EXPIRE
EXPIRY
EXPORT
EXPOSE
EXPOST

•X••P•
EXCEPT
EXEMPT
OXLIPS

••XP••
RUXPIN
SEXPOT
SIXPIN
VOXPOP

••X•P•
FIXUPS
MIXUPS

••X••P
BOXTOP
NEXTUP
VOXPOP

XR••••
XRATED
XRAYED

X•R•••
XERXES
XPRIZE

X••R••
XLARGE
XSARAS
XTERRA

X•••R•
XTERRA

X••••R
XAVIER
XYSTER

•X•R••
EXARCH
EXERTS
EXTRAS
EXURBS

•X••R•
EXEDRA
EXHORT
EXMORE
EXPERT
EXPIRE
EXPIRY
EXPORT
EXSERT
EXTERN
EXTORT
OXCART
OXFORD
OXNARD

•X•••R
EXETER
EXILER
EXMOOR

••XR••
NEXRAD

••X•R•
BOXERS
DEXTRO
FAXERS
FIXERS
HEXERS
LUXURY
MIXERS
NIXERS
SEXERS
SIXERS
TAXERS
VEXERS
WAXERS

••X••R
BAXTER
BOXCAR
BOXIER
DEXTER
FOXIER
SEXIER
WAXIER

•••X•R
COAXER
ELIXIR
FLEXOR
GENXER
HOAXER
JINXER
PLEXOR

XS••••
XSARAS

X•S•••
XESOUT
XYSTER
XYSTUS

X••S••
XHOSAS
XMASES

X•••S•
XYLOSE

X••••S
XBOXES
XEBECS
XERXES
XFILES
XGAMES
XHOSAS
XMASES
XSARAS
XTILES
XTYPES
XYLEMS
XYSTUS

•XS•••
AXSEED
EXSECT
EXSERT

•X•S••
AXISES
EXISTS

•X••S•
EXCESS
EXCISE
EXCUSA
EXCUSE
EXPOSE
EXPOST

•X•••S
AXIOMS
AXIONS
AXISES
AXONES
EXACTS
EXALTS
EXCELS
EXCESS
EXCONS
EXCUBS
EXERTS
EXGOVS
EXILES
EXISTS
EXITUS
EXMETS
EXODUS
EXPATS
EXPELS
EXTOLS
EXTRAS
EXUDES
EXULTS
EXURBS
OXALIS
OXBOWS
OXEYES
OXIDES
OXLIPS

••XS••
BOXSET
MAXSON
SIXSIX

••X•S•
HEXOSE
LAXEST
SEXISM
SEXIST

••X••S
BOXERS
CIXOUS
DIXITS
DOXIES
FAXERS
FIXERS
FIXINS
FIXUPS
HEXADS
HEXERS
MAXIMS
MIXERS
MIXUPS
NIXERS
NIXIES
NIXONS
PIXELS
PIXIES
SAXONS
SEXERS
SIXERS
SIXTHS
SIXTUS
TAXERS
TAXIES
TAXOLS
TEXANS
TOXICS
TOXINS
VEXERS
VIXENS
WAXERS

•••X•S
ALEXAS
ALEXIS
APEXES
BRUXES
CALXES
COAXES
CRUXES
FLAXES
FLEXES
FLUXES
HOAXES
IBEXES
ILEXES
IMAXES
JINXES
LYNXES
MARXES
MINXES
ONYXES
OREXIS
ORYXES
PLEXES
PLEXUS
PRAXES
PRAXIS
PREXES
TREXES
VSIXES
XBOXES
XERXES
ZEUXIS

XT••••
XTERRA
XTILES
XTYPES

X••T••
XRATED
XYSTER
XYSTUS

X••••T
XEDOUT
XESOUT
XZIBIT

•XT•••
EXTANT
EXTEND
EXTENT
EXTERN
EXTOLL
EXTOLS
EXTORT
EXTRAS
OXTAIL

•X•T••
EXETER
EXITED
EXITUS
EXOTIC

•X••T•
EXACTA
EXACTS
EXALTS
EXCITE
EXERTS
EXISTS
EXMATE
EXMETS
EXPATS
EXULTS

•X•••T
EXCEPT
EXEMPT
EXEUNT
EXHORT
EXOCET
EXPECT
EXPERT
EXPORT
EXPOST
EXSECT
EXSERT
EXTANT
EXTENT
EXTORT
OXCART

••XT••
BAXTER
BOXTOP
DEXTER
DEXTRO
MIXTEC
NEXTEL
NEXTTO
NEXTUP
PAXTON
SEXTET
SEXTON
SIXTEN
SIXTHS
SIXTUS
SIXTWO
TEXTED

••X•T•
DIXITS
FIXATE
FIXITY
LAXITY
LUXATE
NEXTTO

••X••T
BOXSET
HEXNUT
LAXALT
LAXEST
MAXOUT
REXCAT
SEXIST
SEXPOT
SEXTET
TAXCUT

•••XT•
GSIXTY

•••X•T
NOEXIT

••••XT
GONEXT
IMNEXT
UNMIXT
UPNEXT
URTEXT

X•••U•
XEDOUT
XESOUT
XINHUA
XYSTUS

X••••U
XANADU

•XU•••
EXUDED
EXUDES
EXULTS
EXURBS

•X•U••
EXCUBS
EXCUSA
EXCUSE
EXEUNT
EXHUME

•X••U•
EXITUS
EXODUS

••XU••
FIXUPS
LUXURY
MIXUPS

••X•U•
BOXFUL
CIXOUS
HEXNUT
MAXOUT
NEXTUP
SIXGUN
SIXTUS
TAXCUT

•••XU•
PLEXUS

X•V•••
XAVIER

•X••V•
EXGOVS

••••XV
FELIXV
JOHNXV

•XW•••
EXWIFE

•X••W•
OXBOWS

••XW••
SIXWAY

••X•W•
SIXTWO

••X••W
TAXLAW

X•X•••
XOXOXO

X••X••
XBOXES
XERXES

X•••X•
XOXOXO

••X•X•
MAXIXE
XOXOXO

••X••X
SIXSIX
TEXMEX

•••XX•
SKNXXX

•••X•X
SKNXXX

••••XX
JOHNXX
SKNXXX
TJMAXX

XY••••
XYANDZ
XYLEMS
XYLOID
XYLOSE
XYSTER
XYSTUS

X•Y•••
XTYPES

X••Y••
XRAYED

•XY•••
EXYANK
OXYDOL
OXYGEN

•X•Y••
OXEYES

•X••Y•
EXONYM

•X•••Y
EXPIRY

••X••Y
BOXBOY
BOXILY
FIXITY
FOXILY
HUXLEY
LAXITY
LUXURY
SAXONY
SEXILY
SIXDAY
SIXWAY
WAXILY

•••XY•
UVWXYZ

•••X•Y
ALEXEY
GSIXTY

••••XY
EUTAXY
GALAXY
TUVWXY
UNFOXY
UNSEXY

XZ••••
XZIBIT

X•••Z•
XPRIZE

X••••Z
XYANDZ

•••X•Z
UVWXYZ

YA••••
YACHTS
YAHOOS
YAKIMA
YAKKED
YAKKER
YAKUTS
YAKUZA
YALIES
YAMAHA
YAMANI
YAMMER
YAMUNA
YANGON
YANKAT
YANKED
YANKEE
YANKER
YANKON
YANQUI
YAPHET
YAPPED
YAPPER
YAPSAT
YAQUIS
YARDED
YARDER
YARELY
YAREST
YARNED
YARROW
YASGUR
YASHIN
YASMIN
YASSER
YATATA
YATSEN
YATTER
YAWING
YAWKEY
YAWNED
YAWNER
YAWPED
YAWPER

Y•A•••
YEABIG
YEAGER
YEANED
YEARLY
YEARNS
YEASTS
YEASTY
YOAKAM

Y••A••
YAMAHA
YAMANI
YATATA
YEMANA
YOSANO
YOUALL
YSHAPE
YUKATA
YUKAWA
YUMAAZ
YUMANS
YUTANG

Y•••A•
YANKAT
YAPSAT
YEEHAW
YELLAT
YENTAS
YEOMAN
YESIAM
YESMAN
YOAKAM
YOWZAH
YUCCAS
YUMAAZ

Y••••A
YAKIMA
YAKUZA
YAMAHA
YAMUNA
YATATA
YELENA
YEMANA
YORKPA
YOYOMA
YTTRIA
YUKATA
YUKAWA

•YA•••
CYANIC
CYANID
DYADIC
HYADES
HYATTS
NYALAS
XYANDZ

•Y•A••
AYEAYE
BYDATE
BYHALF
BYHAND
BYLAND
BYLAWS
BYMAIL
BYNAME
BYPASS
BYPAST
BYPATH
BYTALK
BYTAXI
BYWAYS
CYCADS
CYRANO
DYNAMO
DYNAST
DYSART
GYRATE
MYBABY
MYLADY
MYLARS
MYNAHS
NYYANK
TYBALT
TYRANT
ZYMASE

•Y••A•
BYPLAY
BYROAD
CYMBAL
DYEVAT
GYMBAG
GYMRAT
GYOZAS
HYDRAE
HYDRAS
HYENAS
HYETAL
HYMNAL
LYCRAS
LYDIAN
MYDEAR
MYRDAL
MYRIAD
NYALAS
RYOKAN
SYLVAN
SYNTAX
SYRIAN
TYPEAB
TYPEAS
WYSTAN

•Y•••A
AYESHA
MYOPIA
SYLVIA
ZYGOMA

••YA••
ARYANS
ATYALE
BAYARD
BOYARS
BRYANT
DRYADS
EXYANK
FAYARD
FLYASH
GUYANA
HIYALL
KAYAKS
LOYALE
MAYANS
NYYANK
RIYADH
RIYALS
ROYALE
ROYALS
SAYAAH
SAYAYE
TOYAMA
VOYAGE
WAYANS

••Y•A•
ALYDAR
AMYTAN
ANYDAY
ANYMAN
ANYWAY
BAYMAN
BAYSAT
BUYSAT
CAYMAN
ERYKAH
FLYMAN
FLYWAY
FRYPAN
HEYDAY
HEYMAN
JOYPAD
KEYMAN
KEYPAD
KEYPAL
KEYWAY
LAYMAN
MAYDAY
MAYHAP
MAYTAG
NAYSAY
OHYEAH
PAYDAY
PAYPAL
PSYWAR
RAYBAN
SAYAAH
SAYNAY
SAYSAH
SKYCAM
SKYCAP
SKYLAB
SKYMAN
SKYMAP
SKYWAY
SPYCAM
TOYCAR
TOYHAT
TWYMAN
WAYLAY

••Y••A
ALYSSA
BRYNZA
CAYUGA
CHYNNA
DAYSPA
ELYRIA
GUYANA
HRYVNA
KEYOFA
LOYOLA
PAYOLA
SCYLLA
SMYRNA
TOYAMA
TOYOTA
YOYOMA
ZOYSIA

•••YA•
ALIYAH
BANYAN
BATYAM
BOLYAI
BUNYAN
EASYAS
EGOYAN
KENYAN
LIBYAN
MAGYAR
MARYAM
MINYAN
PLAYAS
PLAYAT
PROYAS
STAYAT

•••Y•A
CORYZA
DURYEA
JOBYNA

••••YA
LATOYA
LOVEYA
MALAYA
NAGOYA
PAPAYA
PITAYA
TOLDYA

Y••B••
YEABIG
YESBUT
YOUBET

•YB•••
CYBILL
CYBORG
DYBBUK
HYBRID
MYBABY
TYBALT

•Y•B••
BYEBYE
CYMBAL
DYBBUK
GYMBAG
SYMBOL
TYDBOL

•Y••B•
MYBABY
TYCOBB
TYPEBS

•Y•••B
DYEJOB
TYCOBB
TYPEAB

••YB••
DAYBED
FLYBOY
FLYBYS
KHYBER
LAYBYS
MAYBES
RAYBAN
SAYBOO
SKYBOX
SPYBOT

••Y•B•
LAYSBY

••Y••B
DAYJOB
KEYOFB
SKYLAB

•••YB•
PLAYBY

YC••••
YCLEPT

Y•C•••
YACHTS
YUCCAS

Y••C••
YOICKS
YUCCAS

Y•••C•
YORICK

Y••••C
YTTRIC

•YC•••
CYCADS
CYCLED
CYCLER
CYCLES
CYCLIC
CYCLOS
LYCEES
LYCEUM
LYCRAS
TYCOBB
TYCOON

•Y•C••
EYECUP
SYNCED
SYNCHS

•Y••C•
CYNICS
GYNECO
LYRICS
RYENCE
ZYDECO

•Y•••C
CYANIC
CYCLIC
CYMRIC
CYSTIC
DYADIC
HYDRIC
HYGRIC
MYOPIC
MYSTIC
MYTHIC
SYNDIC

••YC••
GLYCOL
JAYCEE
PAYCUT
PSYCHE
PSYCHO
PSYCHS
ROYCES
SKYCAM
SKYCAP
SPYCAM
TOYCAR

••Y•C•
DRYICE

••Y••C
ATYPIC
KEYOFC
PHYSIC
THYMIC

•••YC•
ALLYCE
ENCYCL

•••Y•C
INSYNC

Y•D•••
YODELS
YODUDE

Y••D••
YARDED
YARDER
YONDER
YOUDIG
YSIDRO

Y•••D•
YEGODS
YEHUDI
YEOLDE
YESIDO
YIELDS
YODUDE

Y••••D
YAKKED
YANKED
YAPPED
YARDED
YARNED
YAWNED
YAWPED
YEANED
YELLED
YELPED
YENNED
YENSID
YESSED
YIPPED
YOLKED
YOWLED
YOYOED
YUKKED

•YD•••
BYDATE
CYDERS
HYDRAE
HYDRAS
HYDRIC
HYDROS
HYDROX
HYDRUS
LYDIAN
MYDEAR
RYDELL
SYDNEY
TYDBOL
ZYDECO

•Y•D••
DYADIC
EYEDUP
FYODOR
HYADES
LYNDON
MYRDAL
PYEDOG
SYNDIC

•Y••D•
CYCADS
DYNODE
HYOIDS
LYRIDS
MYLADY
SYNODS
XYANDZ

•Y•••D
BYHAND
BYLAND
BYROAD
BYWORD
CYANID
CYCLED
EYELID
EYVIND
GYPPED
HYBRID
HYMNED
HYPOED
LYNYRD
MYLORD
MYRIAD
MYWORD
SYNCED
XYLOID

••YD••
ALYDAR
ANYDAY
BLYDEN
CLYDES
COYDOG
DRYDEN
HAYDEN
HEYDAY
HOYDEN
KEYDET
LEYDEN
MAYDAY
OXYDOL
PAYDAY
SAYDIE
SNYDER
SPYDER
TOYDOG

••Y•D•
DRYADS
RIYADH
SAYIDO

••Y••D
ANYOLD
BAYARD
BEYOND
DAYBED
DAYOLD
FAYARD
FLYROD
JOYPAD
KAYOED
KEYOFD
KEYPAD
PHYSED
RHYMED
STYLED
YOYOED

•••YD•
ALKYDS
LADYDI
LLOYDS
MRHYDE

•••Y•D
BRAYED
BUOYED
CLOYED
DRAYED
FLAYED
FRAYED
GRAYED
GREYED
LYNYRD
OBEYED
OKAYED
PLAYED
PRAYED
PREYED
REDYED
SLAYED
SPAYED
STAYED
SWAYED
UNDYED
XRAYED

YE••••
YEABIG
YEAGER
YEANED
YEARLY
YEARNS
YEASTS
YEASTY
YEEHAW
YEGODS
YEHUDI
YELENA
YELLAT
YELLED
YELLER
YELLOW
YELPED
YELPER
YEMANA
YEMENI
YENFOR
YENNED
YENSID
YENTAS
YEOLDE
YEOMAN
YEOMEN
YERKES
YERTLE
YESBUT
YESIAM
YESIDO
YESMAN
YESMEN
YESSED
YESSES
YESSIR
YESTER
YESYES
YESYOU
YETTIE

Y•E•••
YEEHAW
YIELDS
YVETTE

Y••E••
YARELY
YAREST
YCLEPT
YELENA
YEMENI
YODELS
YOKELS

Y•••E•
YAKKED
YAKKER
YALIES
YAMMER
YANKED
YANKEE
YANKER
YAPHET
YAPPED
YAPPER
YARDED
YARDER
YARNED
YASSER
YATSEN
YATTER
YAWKEY
YAWNED
YAWNER
YAWPED
YAWPER
YEAGER
YEANED
YELLED
YELLER
YELPED
YELPER
YENNED
YEOMEN
YERKES
YESMEN
YESSED
YESSES
YESTER
YESYES
YIPPED
YIPPEE
YOLKED
YONDER
YORKER
YOUBET
YOUSEE
YOWLED
YOWLER
YOYOED
YTILES
YUKKED
YUTZES

Y••••E
YANKEE
YEOLDE
YERTLE
YETTIE
YIPPEE
YIPPIE
YODUDE
YORKIE
YOUSEE
YSHAPE
YUPPIE
YVETTE
YVONNE

•YE•••
AYEAYE
AYESHA
AYESIR
BYEBYE
BYENOW
DYEING
DYEJOB
DYELOT
DYEVAT
EYECUP
EYEDUP
EYEFUL
EYEING
EYELET
EYELID
EYEPIT
EYESUP
HYENAS
HYETAL
OYEZES
PYEDOG
RYENCE

•Y•E••
BYTENS
CYDERS
DYNELS
GYNECO
GYRENE
HYPERS
HYPEUP
LYCEES
LYCEUM
MYDEAR
MYHERO
MYSELF
NYJETS
NYMETS
RYDELL
TYLERS
TYPEAB
TYPEAS
TYPEBS
TYPEIN
TYPEOS
TYPERS
TYPEUP
WYLERS
WYVERN
XYLEMS
ZYDECO

•Y••E•
BYRNES
BYTHEN
CYCLED
CYCLER
CYCLES
CYGNET
CYPHER
EYELET
EYRIES
GYPPED
GYPPER
HYADES
HYMNED
HYPHEN
HYPOED
LYCEES
LYNLEY
LYNXES
MYOPES
OYEZES
OYSTER
SYDNEY
SYNCED
SYSTEM
WYNKEN
WYNTER
XYSTER

•Y•••E
AYEAYE
BYDATE
BYEBYE
BYGONE
BYJOVE
BYLINE
BYNAME
BYROTE
BYSSHE
BYWIRE
DYNODE
GYRATE
GYRENE
HYDRAE
LYONNE
LYSINE
MYLIFE
MYLOVE
MYRTLE
MYSORE
PYRITE
RYENCE
TYRONE
XYLOSE
ZYGOTE
ZYMASE

••YE••
BAYERN
BAYEUX
BUYERS
COYEST
CRYERS
DIYERS
DOYENS
DRYERS
DRYEST
DRYEYE
FEYEST
FLYERS
FOYERS
FRYERS
GAYEST
HAYERS
LAYERS
MAYEST
MEYERS
MOYERS
OHYEAH
PAYEES
PAYERS
PRYERS
SAYERS
SAYEST
SHYEST
SLYEST
TOYERS
TRYERS
WRYEST

••Y•E•
BAYMEN
BEYMER
BLYDEN
BOYLES
CLYDES
CUYLER
DAYBED
DRYDEN
ELYSEE
FAYLEN
FLYMEN
FLYNET
GAYNES
GEYSER
HAYDEN
HAYLEY
HAYMES
HAYNES
HOYDEN
HOYLES
JAYCEE
JAYMES
JAYVEE
JOYNER
KAYOED
KEYDET
KEYMEN
KEYNES
KEYSER
KHYBER
LAYMEN
LEYDEN
MAYBES
MAYHEM
ONYXES
ORYXES
OXYGEN
PAYEES
PHYSED
POYSER
REYLES
RHYMED
RHYMER
RHYMES
ROYCES
SAYHEY
SAYLES
SAYYES
SKYMEN
SKYTEL
SNYDER
SPYDER
STYLED
STYLER
STYLES
STYLET
THYMES
WAYNES
WHYYES
XTYPES
YOYOED

••Y••E
ANYONE
ATYALE
BLYTHE
CAYUSE
COYOTE
DAYONE
DRYEYE
DRYICE
EEYORE
ELYSEE
GWYNNE
HAYNIE
JAYCEE
JAYVEE
LOYALE
OFYORE
PEYOTE
PRYNNE
PSYCHE
REYOKE
ROYALE
SAYAYE
SAYDIE
SCYTHE
STYMIE
TRYGVE
TRYONE
UNYOKE
VOYAGE

•••YE•
ANDYET
BAEYER
BOWYER
BRAYED
BRAYER
BREYER
BUOYED
BUTYET
CLAYEY
CLOYED
DLAYER
DRAYED
DREYER
DURYEA
EBAYER
ELAYER
FLAYED
FLAYER
FRAYED
GRAYED
GRAYER
GREYED
GREYER
HEGYES
LAWYER
NGUYEN
NOTYET
OBEYED
OBEYER
OKAYED
OXEYES
PLAYED
PLAYER
PRAYED
PRAYER
PREYED
PREYER
REDYED
REDYES
SAWYER
SAYYES
SLAYED
SLAYER
SPAYED
SPAYER
SPRYER
STAYED
STAYER
SWAYED
SWAYER
THAYER
TROYER
UNDYED
WHEYEY
WHYYES
XRAYED
YESYES

•••Y•E
ALLYCE
ARGYLE
DWAYNE
ECTYPE
ELAYNE
ENZYME
MRHYDE
OKBYME
OOCYTE
QUAYLE
RETYPE
SHAYNE
SWAYZE
THEYRE
THEYVE

••••YE
AYEAYE
AZODYE
BETTYE
BIGEYE
BYEBYE
DRYEYE
HEARYE
INOUYE
JESSYE
ONEEYE
POPEYE
RALLYE
REDEYE
RIBEYE
RITDYE
SAYAYE
THEEYE
TIEDYE
VATDYE

Y••F••
YENFOR

Y••••F
YOUSUF

•YF•••
BYFORM
MYFOOT

•Y•F••
EYEFUL

•Y••F•
MYLIFE
TYPIFY

•Y•••F
BYHALF
MYSELF

••YF••
CRYFOR
DRYFLY
DRYFOG
JOYFUL
LAYFOR
MAYFLY
PAYFOR
SLYFOX
TRYFOR
WHYFOR

••Y•F•
BUYOFF
CRYOFF
DAYOFF
DRYOFF
KEYOFA
KEYOFB
KEYOFC
KEYOFD
KEYOFF
KEYOFG
LAYOFF
PAYOFF
PRYOFF
WAYOFF

••Y••F
BUYOFF
CRYOFF
DAYOFF
DRYOFF
KEYOFF
LAYOFF
PAYOFF
PRYOFF
WAYOFF

•••Y•F
ONLYIF

Y•G•••
YEGODS
YOGINI
YOGISM
YOGURT

Y••G••
YANGON
YASGUR
YEAGER

Y••••G
YAWING
YEABIG
YOKING
YOUDIG
YUTANG

•YG•••
BYGONE
BYGOSH
CYGNET
CYGNUS
HYGRIC
MYGIRL
MYGOSH
ZYGOMA
ZYGOTE

•Y•G••
SYZYGY

•Y•••G
CYBORG
DYEING
EYEING
GYMBAG
GYRING
HYPING
PYEDOG
TYPING

••YG••
DAYGLO
OXYGEN
RAYGUN
TOYGUN
TRYGVE

••Y•G•
CAYUGA
ERYNGO
MAYIGO
VOYAGE

••Y••G
BAYING
BUYING
COYDOG
CRYING
DRYFOG
DRYING
FLYING
FRYING
GUYING
HAYING
JOYING
KEYING
KEYOFG
LAYING
MAYING
MAYTAG
PAYING
PLYING
PRYING
RAYING
SAYING
SHYING
SKYING
SPYING
STYING
TOYDOG
TOYING
TRYING

•••YG•
EASYGO
SYZYGY

••••YG
KENNYG

Y•H•••
YAHOOS
YEHUDI
YOHOHO
YSHAPE

Y••H••
YACHTS
YAPHET
YASHIN
YEEHAW
YOOHOO

Y•••H•
YAMAHA
YOHOHO
YOUTHS

Y••••H
YOWZAH

•YH•••
BYHALF
BYHAND
MYHERO

•Y•H••
BYTHEN
CYPHER
HYPHEN
MYOHMY
MYTHIC
MYTHOS
PYRHHO
PYTHON
TYPHUS

•Y••H•
AYESHA
BYSSHE
KYUSHU
LYMPHS
MYNAHS
MYRRHS
NYMPHS
PYRHHO
SYLPHS
SYNCHS
SYNTHS

•Y•••H
BYGOSH
BYPATH
FYVUSH
MYGOSH

••YH••
ANYHOW
DAYHOP
MAYHAP
MAYHEM
SAYHEY
TOYHAT

••Y•H•
BLYTHE
GLYPHS
PSYCHE
PSYCHO
PSYCHS
RHYTHM
SAYSHI
SCYTHE

••Y••H
BOYISH
COYISH
DRYISH
ERYKAH
FLYASH
OHYEAH
RIYADH
SAYAAH
SAYSAH

•••Y•H
ALIYAH
IRTYSH

YI••••
YIELDS
YIPPED
YIPPEE
YIPPIE

Y•I•••
YOICKS
YSIDRO
YTILES

Y••I••
YAKIMA
YALIES
YAWING
YESIAM
YESIDO
YOGINI
YOGISM
YOKING
YORICK

Y•••I•
YAQUIS
YASHIN
YASMIN
YEABIG
YENSID
YESSIR
YETTIE
YIPPIE
YORKIE
YORKIN
YOUDIG
YOUWIN
YTTRIA
YTTRIC
YUPPIE

Y••••I
YAMANI
YANQUI
YEHUDI
YEMENI
YOGINI

•Y•I••
BYLINE
BYWIRE
CYBILL
CYNICS
DYEING
EYEING
EYRIES
EYVIND
GYRING
HYOIDS
HYPING
LYDIAN
LYRICS
LYRIDS
LYRIST
LYSINE
MYGIRL
MYLIFE
MYRIAD
PYRITE
SYRIAN
TYPIFY
TYPING
TYPIST

•Y••I•
AYESIR
BYMAIL
CYANIC
CYANID
CYCLIC
CYMRIC
CYSTIC
DYADIC
EYELID
EYEPIT
HYBRID
HYDRIC
HYGRIC
MYOPIA
MYOPIC
MYOSIN
MYOSIS
MYSTIC
MYTHIC
NYQUIL
SYLVIA
SYNDIC
TYPEIN
XYLOID

•Y•••I
BYTAXI

••YI••
BAYING
BOYISH
BUYING
BUYINS
COYISH
CRYING
DRYICE
DRYING
DRYINK
DRYISH
FLYING
FLYINS
FRYING
GUYING
HAYING
JOYING
KEYING
LAYING
LAYINS
MAYIGO
MAYING
PAYING
PLYING
PRYING
RAYING
SAYIDO
SAYING
SHYING

SKYING SOYINK SPYING STYING TOYING TRYING ZAYINS

••Y•I•
ATYPIC BUYSIN BUYSIT DAYLIT ELYRIA ELYTIS GLYNIS HAYNIE KEYSIN LAYSIN PAYSIN PHYSIC PHYSIO SAYDIE SKYLIT STYMIE THYMIC WAYSIN ZOYSIA

••Y••I
NOYORI SAYSHI

•••YI•
GARYIN MARYII ONLYIF PINYIN PLAYIT STAYIN

•••Y•I
BOLYAI LADYDI MARYII PAPYRI

••••YI
HENRYI SOONYI SUUKYI

•YJ•••
BYJOVE NYJETS

•Y•J••
DYEJOB

••YJ••
DAYJOB

•••YJ•
MARYJO

Y•K•••
YAKIMA YAKKED YAKKER YAKUTS YAKUZA YOKELS YOKING YUKATA YUKAWA YUKKED YUKONS

Y••K••
YAKKED YAKKER YANKAT YANKED YANKEE YANKER YANKON YAWKEY YERKES YOAKAM YOLKED YORKER YORKIE YORKIN YORKPA YUKKED

Y•••K•
YOICKS

Y••••K
YORICK

•YK•••
HYKSOS

•Y•K••
RYOKAN RYUKYU WYNKEN

•Y•••K
BYTALK DYBBUK NYYANK

••YK••
ERYKAH

••Y•K•
KAYAKS REYOKE UNYOKE

••Y••K
DRYINK EXYANK NYYANK SAYSOK SOYINK

••••YK
HENRYK

Y•L•••
YALIES YCLEPT YELENA YELLAT YELLED YELLER YELLOW YELPED YELPER YOLKED

Y••L••
YELLAT YELLED YELLER YELLOW YEOLDE YIELDS YOWLED YOWLER YTILES

Y•••L•
YARELY YEARLY YERTLE YODELS YOKELS YOUALL

Y••••L
YOUALL

•YL•••
BYLAND BYLAWS BYLINE BYLOTS MYLADY MYLARS MYLIFE MYLORD MYLOVE NYLONS PYLONS SYLPHS SYLVAN SYLVIA TYLERS WYLERS XYLEMS XYLOID XYLOSE

•Y•L••
BYPLAY CYCLED CYCLER CYCLES CYCLIC CYCLOS DYELOT EYELET EYELID LYNLEY NYALAS

•Y••L•
BYHALF BYTALK CYBILL DYNELS MYRTLE MYSELF RYDELL TYBALT

•Y•••L
BYMAIL CYBILL CYMBAL EYEFUL HYETAL HYMNAL MYGIRL MYRDAL NYQUIL RYDELL SYMBOL TYDBOL

••YL••
ASYLUM BAYLOR BOYLES CEYLON CUYLER DAYLIT FAYLEN FLYLOW HAYLEY HOYLES IDYLLS KRYLON KRYLOV LAYLOW PHYLLO PHYLUM REYLES SAYLES SCYLLA SKYLAB SKYLIT STYLED STYLER STYLES STYLET STYLUS TAYLOR TRYLON WAYLAY WAYLON

••Y•L•
ANYOLD ATYALE DAYGLO DAYOLD DRYFLY HIYALL IDYLLS LOYALE LOYOLA MAYFLY PAYOLA PHYLLO RIYALS ROYALE ROYALS SCYLLA

••Y••L
ETYMOL GLYCOL HIYALL JOYFUL KEYPAL OXYDOL PAYPAL SKYTEL

•••YL•
ALKYLS ALLYLS ARGYLE ARGYLL BERYLS ETHYLS GRAYLY GREYLY JEKYLL MERYLL QUAYLE SIBYLS SPRYLY THEYLL VINYLS

•••Y•L
ARGYLL ENCYCL JEKYLL MERYLL THEYLL

••••YL
ACETYL CHERYL DACTYL DANDYL DARRYL LAURYL METHYL PROPYL SHERYL

Y•M•••
YAMAHA YAMANI YAMMER YAMUNA YEMANA YEMENI YOMTOV YUMAAZ YUMANS YUMYUM

Y••M••
YAMMER YASMIN YEOMAN YEOMEN YESMAN YESMEN

Y•••M•
YAKIMA YOYOMA

Y••••M
YESIAM YOAKAM YOGISM YUMYUM

•YM•••
BYMAIL CYMBAL CYMRIC GYMBAG GYMRAT HYMNAL HYMNED LYMPHS MYMYMY NYMETS NYMPHS SYMBOL ZYMASE

•Y••M•
BYNAME DYNAMO MYMYMY MYOHMY XYLEMS ZYGOMA

•Y•••M
BYFORM GYPSUM LYCEUM SYSTEM

••YM••
ANYMAN BAYMAN BAYMEN BEYMER CAYMAN DRYMOP ETYMOL ETYMON FLYMAN FLYMEN HAYMES HAYMOW HEYMAN JAYMES KEYMAN KEYMEN LAYMAN LAYMEN RHYMED RHYMER RHYMES SKYMAN SKYMAP SKYMEN STYMIE THYMES THYMIC THYMUS TWYMAN

••Y•M•
ABYSMS TOYAMA YOYOMA

••Y••M
ADYTUM ASYLUM BAYRUM MAYHEM PHYLUM RHYTHM SKYCAM SPYCAM

•••YM•
ENZYME MYMYMY OKBYME

•••Y•M
BATYAM MARYAM YUMYUM

••••YM
ANONYM EPONYM EUONYM EXONYM

Y•N•••
YANGON YANKAT YANKED YANKEE YANKER YANKON YANQUI YENFOR YENNED YENSID YENTAS YONDER

Y••N••
YARNED YAWNED YAWNER YEANED YENNED YVONNE

Y•••N•
YAMANI YAMUNA YAWING YEARNS YELENA YEMANA YEMENI YOGINI YOKING YOSANO YUKONS YUMANS YUTANG YVONNE

Y••••N
YANGON YANKON YASHIN YASMIN YATSEN YEOMAN YEOMEN YESMAN YESMEN YORKIN YOUWIN

•YN•••
BYNAME CYNICS DYNAMO DYNAST DYNELS DYNODE GYNECO GYNOUS LYNDON LYNLEY LYNXES LYNYRD MYNAHS SYNCED SYNCHS SYNDIC SYNODS SYNTAX SYNTHS WYNKEN WYNTER WYNTON

•Y•N••
BYENOW BYRNES CYANIC CYANID CYGNET CYGNUS HYENAS HYMNAL HYMNED HYPNOS LYONNE RYENCE SYDNEY XYANDZ

•Y••N•
BYGONE BYHAND BYLAND BYLINE BYTENS CYRANO DYEING EYEING EYVIND GYRENE GYRING HYPING HYSONS LYONNE LYSINE NYLONS NYYANK PYLONS TYPING TYRANT TYRONE TYSONS

•Y•••N
AYRTON BYTHEN HYPHEN LYDIAN LYNDON LYTTON MYOSIN MYTURN PYTHON RYOKAN SYLVAN SYRIAN TYCOON TYPEIN WYNKEN WYNTON WYSTAN WYVERN

••YN••
BRYNZA BUYNOW CHYNNA ERYNGO FLYNET GAYNES GAYNOR GLYNIS GWYNNE HAYNES HAYNIE JOYNER KEYNES PAYNOW PRYNNE SAYNAY WAYNES WHYNOT WHYNOW

••Y•N•
ANYONE ANYONS ARYANS BAYING BEYOND BRYANT BUYING BUYINS CHYNNA CRYING DAYONE DOYENS DRYING DRYINK EXYANK FLYING FLYINS FRYING GUYANA GUYING GWYNNE HAYING HRYVNA JOYING KEYING LAYING LAYINS MAYANS MAYING NYYANK PAYING PLYING PRYING PRYNNE RAYING RAYONS SAYING SAYSNO SHYING SKYING SMYRNA SOYINK SPYING STYING TOYING TOYONS TRYING TRYONE WAYANS ZAYINS

••Y••N
AMYTAN ANYMAN BAYERN BAYMAN BAYMEN BLYDEN BLYTON BRYSON BUYSIN BUYSON CAYMAN CEYLON CHYRON DAYTON DRYDEN DRYRUN ETYMON FAYLEN FLYMAN FLYMEN FRYPAN HAYDEN HEYMAN HOYDEN KEYMAN KEYMEN KEYSIN KEYSON KRYLON LAYMAN LAYMEN LAYSIN LAYSON LEYDEN MAYRON OXYGEN PAYSIN PAYSON PAYTON PEYTON RAYBAN RAYGUN SKYMAN SKYMEN STYRON TOYGUN TRYLON TWYMAN WAYLON WAYSIN

•••YN•
DOBYNS DWAYNE EDWYNN ELAYNE INSYNC ISAYNO JOBYNA LARYNX OBGYNS SHAYNE SPHYNX TROYNY

•••Y•N
BANYAN BARYON BINYON BUNYAN CANYON CRAYON EDWYNN EGOYAN GARYIN KENYAN KENYON LIBYAN MINYAN NGUYEN PINYIN PLAYON PREYON RELYON RUNYON STAYIN STAYON

••••YN
ALLEYN BERWYN BOLEYN CAMRYN CRONYN EVELYN JACLYN LAURYN MADLYN MELVYN MERVYN ROSLYN SHARYN VANRYN

YO••••
YOAKAM YODELS YODUDE YOGINI YOGISM YOGURT YOHOHO YOICKS YOKELS YOKING YOLKED YOMTOV YONDER YOOHOO YORICK YORKER YORKIE YORKIN YORKPA YOSANO YOUALL YOUBET YOUDIG YOUSEE YOUSUF YOUTHS YOUTWO YOUWIN YOWLED YOWLER YOWZAH YOYOED YOYOMA

Y•O•••
YEOLDE YEOMAN YEOMEN YOOHOO YVONNE

Y••O••
YAHOOS YEGODS YOHOHO YOYOED YOYOMA YUKONS

Y•••O•
YAHOOS YANGON YANKON YARROW YELLOW YENFOR YESYOU YOMTOV YOOHOO

Y••••O
YESIDO YOHOHO YOOHOO YOSANO YOUTWO YSIDRO

•YO•••
FYODOR GYOZAS HYOIDS LYONNE MYOHMY MYOPES MYOPIA MYOPIC MYOSIN MYOSIS RYOKAN

•Y•O••
BYFORM BYGONE BYGOSH BYJOVE BYLOTS BYROAD BYROTE BYWORD CYBORG DYNODE GYNOUS HYPOED HYSONS MYFOOT MYGOSH MYLORD MYLOVE MYSORE MYWORD NYLONS NYPOST PYLONS SYNODS SYSOPS TYCOBB TYCOON TYRONE TYSONS XYLOID XYLOSE ZYGOMA ZYGOTE

•Y••O•
AYRTON BYENOW BYTWOS CYCLOS DYEJOB DYELOT FYODOR HYDROS HYDROX HYKSOS HYPNOS HYSSOP LYNDON LYTTON MYFOOT MYTHOS PYEDOG PYTHON SYMBOL TYCOON TYDBOL TYPEOS WYNTON

•Y•••O
CYRANO DYNAMO GYNECO MYHERO PYRHHO ZYDECO

••YO••
ANYOLD ANYONE ANYONS BAYOUS BEYOND BUYOFF BUYOUT COYOTE CRYOFF CRYOUT DAYOFF DAYOLD DAYONE DRYOFF DRYOUT EEYORE FLYOUT JOYOUS KAYOED KEYOFA KEYOFB KEYOFC KEYOFD KEYOFF KEYOFG LAYOFF LAYOUT LOYOLA MAYORS NOYORI OFYORE PAYOFF PAYOLA PAYOUT PEYOTE PRYOFF RAYONS REYOKE SPYOUT TOYONS TOYOTA TRYONE TRYOUT UNYOKE WAYOFF WAYOUT YOYOED YOYOMA

••Y•O•
ANYHOW BAYLOR BLYTON BOYTOY BRYSON BUYNOW BUYSON CEYLON CHYRON COYDOG CRYFOR DAYHOP DAYJOB DAYTON DRYFOG DRYMOP DRYROT ETYMOL ETYMON FLYBOY FLYLOW FLYROD GAYNOR GLYCOL HAYMOW HEYYOU KAYYOW KEYSON KRYLON KRYLOV LAYFOR LAYLOW LAYSON MAYRON OXYDOL PAYFOR PAYNOW PAYSON PAYTON PEYTON SAYBOO SAYSOK SAYSOS SKYBOX SLYFOX SPYBOT STYRON TAYLOR TOYDOG TOYTOP

TRYFOR
TRYLON
WAYLON
WHYFOR
WHYNOT
WHYNOW
WHYYOU

••Y••O
CRYPTO
DAYGLO
ERYNGO
GLYPTO
KRYPTO
LAYSTO
MAYIGO
PHYLLO
PHYSIO
PSYCHO
SAYBOO
SAYIDO
SAYSNO
SAYSSO

•••YO•
ALIYOT
BARYON
BINYON
CANYON
CRAYON
FORYOU
FROYOS
GOTYOU
HEYYOU
ITSYOU
KAYYOW
KENYON
NOTYOU
PLAYON
PREYON
RELYON
RUNYON
SANYOS
SEEYOU
SEZYOU
STAYON
WHYYOU
YESYOU

•••Y•O
EASYGO
ISAYNO
MARYJO
PLAYTO
PRAYTO

••••YO
ARROYO
DADDYO
EMBRYO
HARRYO
NOMAYO
TAMAYO

Y•P•••
YAPHET
YAPPED
YAPPER
YAPSAT
YIPPED
YIPPEE
YIPPIE
YUPPIE

Y••P••
YAPPED
YAPPER
YAWPED
YAWPER
YELPED
YELPER
YIPPED
YIPPEE
YIPPIE
YUPPIE

Y•••P•
YCLEPT
YORKPA
YSHAPE

•YP•••
BYPASS
BYPAST
BYPATH
BYPLAY
CYPHER
CYPRUS
GYPPED
GYPPER
GYPSUM
HYPERS
HYPEUP
HYPHEN
HYPING
HYPNOS
HYPOED
NYPOST
TYPEAB
TYPEAS
TYPEBS
TYPEIN
TYPEOS
TYPERS
TYPEUP
TYPHUS
TYPIFY
TYPING
TYPIST

•Y•P••
EYEPIT
GYPPED
GYPPER
LYMPHS
MYOPES
MYOPIA
MYOPIC
NYMPHS
SYLPHS

•Y••P•
SYRUPS
SYRUPY
SYSOPS

•Y•••P
EYECUP
EYEDUP
EYESUP
HYPEUP
HYSSOP
TYPEUP

••YP••
ATYPIC
COYPUS
CRYPTO
CRYPTS
FRYPAN
GLYPHS
GLYPTO
JOYPAD
KEYPAD
KEYPAL
KRYPTO
PAYPAL
XTYPES

••Y•P•
DAYSPA
LAYUPS

••Y••P
BUYSUP
DAYHOP
DRYMOP
KEYSUP
LAYSUP
MAYHAP
PAYSUP
SKYCAP
SKYMAP
TOYTOP

•••YP•
ECTYPE
POLYPS
RETYPE

•••Y•P
BUOYUP
COSYUP
COZYUP
PLAYUP
PONYUP
STAYUP
TIDYUP

Y•Q•••
YAQUIS

Y••Q••
YANQUI

•YQ•••
NYQUIL

•••YQ•
SUZYQS

Y•R•••
YARDED
YARDER
YARELY
YAREST
YARNED
YARROW
YERKES
YERTLE
YORICK
YORKER
YORKIE
YORKIN
YORKPA

Y••R••
YARROW
YEARLY
YEARNS
YTTRIA
YTTRIC

Y•••R•
YOGURT
YSIDRO

Y••••R
YAKKER
YAMMER
YANKER
YAPPER
YARDER
YASGUR
YASSER
YATTER
YAWNER
YAWPER
YEAGER
YELLER
YELPER
YENFOR
YESSIR
YESTER
YONDER
YORKER
YOWLER

•YR•••
AYRTON
BYRNES
BYROAD
BYROTE
CYRANO
EYRIES
GYRATE
GYRENE
GYRING
LYRICS
LYRIDS
LYRIST
MYRDAL
MYRIAD
MYRRHS
MYRTLE
PYRHHO
PYRITE
SYRIAN
SYRUPS
SYRUPY
TYRANT
TYRONE

•Y•R••
CYMRIC
CYPRUS
GYMRAT
HYBRID
HYDRAE
HYDRAS
HYDRIC
HYDROS
HYDROX
HYDRUS
HYGRIC
LYCRAS
MYRRHS

•Y••R•
BYFORM
BYWIRE
BYWORD
CYBORG
CYDERS
DYSART
HYPERS
LYNYRD
MYGIRL
MYHERO
MYLARS
MYLORD
MYSORE
MYTURN
MYWORD
TYLERS
TYPERS
WYLERS
WYVERN

•Y•••R
AYESIR
CYCLER
CYPHER
FYODOR
GYPPER
MYDEAR
OYSTER
WYNTER
XYSTER

••YR••
BAYRUM
CHYRON
DRYROT
DRYRUN
ELYRIA
FLYROD
MAYRON
SMYRNA
STYRON

••Y•R•
BAYARD
BAYERN
BOYARS
BUYERS
CRYERS
DIYERS
DRYERS
EEYORE
FAYARD
FLYERS
FOYERS
FRYERS
HAYERS
LAYERS
MAYORS
MEYERS
MOYERS
NOYORI
OFYORE
PAYERS
PRYERS
SAYERS
TOYERS
TRYERS

••Y••R
ALYDAR
BAYLOR
BEYMER
CRYFOR
CUYLER
GAYNOR
GEYSER
JOYNER
KEYSER
KHYBER
LAYFOR
PAYFOR
POYSER
PSYWAR
RHYMER
SNYDER
SPYDER
STYLER
TAYLOR
TOYCAR
TRYFOR
WHYFOR

•••YR•
LYNYRD
PAPYRI
SATYRS
THEYRE

•••Y•R
BAEYER
BOWYER
BRAYER
BREYER
DLAYER
DREYER
EBAYER
ELAYER
FLAYER
GRAYER
GREYER
LAWYER
MAGYAR
OBEYER
PLAYER
PRAYER
PREYER
SAWYER
SLAYER
SPAYER
SPRYER
STAYER
SWAYER
THAYER
TROYER

••••YR
MARTYR
ZEPHYR

YS••••
YSHAPE
YSIDRO

Y•S•••
YASGUR
YASHIN
YASMIN
YASSER
YESBUT
YESIAM
YESIDO
YESMAN
YESMEN
YESSED
YESSES
YESSIR
YESTER
YESYES
YESYOU
YOSANO

Y••S••
YAPSAT
YASSER
YATSEN
YEASTS
YEASTY
YENSID
YESSED
YESSES
YESSIR
YOUSEE
YOUSUF

Y•••S•
YAREST
YOGISM

Y••••S
YACHTS
YAHOOS
YAKUTS
YALIES
YAQUIS
YEARNS
YEASTS
YEGODS
YENTAS
YERKES
YESSES
YESYES
YIELDS
YODELS
YOICKS
YOKELS
YOUTHS
YTILES
YUCCAS
YUKONS
YUMANS
YUTZES

•YS•••
BYSSHE
CYSTIC
DYSART
HYSONS
HYSSOP
LYSINE
MYSELF
MYSORE
MYSTIC
OYSTER
SYSOPS
SYSTEM
TYSONS
WYSTAN
XYSTER
XYSTUS

•Y•S••
AYESHA
AYESIR
BYSSHE
EYESUP
GYPSUM
HYKSOS
HYSSOP
KYUSHU
MYOSIN
MYOSIS

•Y••S•
BYGOSH
BYPASS
BYPAST
DYNAST
FYVUSH
LYRIST
MYGOSH
NYPOST
TYPIST
XYLOSE
ZYMASE

•Y•••S
BYLAWS
BYLOTS
BYPASS
BYRNES
BYTENS
BYTWOS
BYWAYS
CYCADS
CYCLES
CYCLOS
CYDERS
CYGNUS
CYNICS
CYPRUS
DYNELS
EYRIES
GYNOUS
GYOZAS
HYADES
HYATTS
HYDRAS
HYDROS
HYDRUS
HYENAS
HYKSOS
HYOIDS
HYPERS
HYPNOS
HYSONS
LYCEES
LYCRAS
LYMPHS
LYNXES
LYRICS
LYRIDS
MYLARS
MYNAHS
MYOPES
MYOSIS
MYRRHS
MYTHOS
NYALAS
NYJETS
NYLONS
NYMETS
NYMPHS
OYEZES
PYLONS
SYLPHS
SYNCHS
SYNODS
SYNTHS
SYRUPS
SYSOPS
TYLERS
TYPEAS
TYPEBS
TYPEOS
TYPERS
TYPHUS
TYSONS
WYLERS
XYLEMS
XYSTUS

••YS••
ABYSMS
ALYSSA
BAYSAT
BRYSON
BUYSAT
BUYSIN
BUYSIT
BUYSON
BUYSUP
DAYSPA
ELYSEE
GEYSER
KEYSER
KEYSIN
KEYSON
KEYSUP
LAYSBY
LAYSIN
LAYSON
LAYSTO
LAYSUP
NAYSAY
PAYSIN
PAYSON
PAYSUP
PHYSED
PHYSIC
PHYSIO
POYSER
SAYSAH
SAYSHI
SAYSNO
SAYSOK
SAYSOS
SAYSSO
TRYSTS
WAYSIN
ZOYSIA

••Y•S•
ALYSSA
BOYISH
CAYUSE
COYEST
COYISH
DRYEST
DRYISH
FEYEST
FLYASH
GAYEST
MAYEST
SAYEST
SAYSSO
SHYEST
SLYEST
WRYEST

••Y••S
ABYSMS
ANYONS
ARYANS
BAYOUS
BOYARS
BOYLES
BUYERS
BUYINS
CLYDES
COYPUS
CRYERS
CRYPTS
DIYERS
DOYENS
DRYADS
DRYERS
ELYTIS
FLYBYS
FLYERS
FLYINS
FOYERS
FRYERS
GAYNES
GLYNIS
GLYPHS
HAYERS
HAYMES
HAYNES
HOYLES
IDYLLS
JAYMES
JOYOUS
KAYAKS
KEYNES
LAYBYS
LAYERS
LAYINS
LAYUPS
MAYANS
MAYBES
MAYORS
MEYERS
MOYERS
ONYXES
ORYXES
PAYEES
PAYERS
PRYERS
PSYCHS
RAYONS
REYLES
RHYMES
RIYALS
ROYALS
ROYCES
SAYERS
SAYLES
SAYSOS
SAYYES
STYLES
STYLUS
THYMES
THYMUS
TOYERS
TOYONS
TRYERS
TRYSTS
WAYANS
WAYNES
WHYYES
XTYPES
ZAYINS

•••YS•
IRTYSH

•••Y•S
ALKYDS
ALKYLS
ALLYLS
BERYLS
DOBYNS
EASYAS
ETHYLS
FROYOS
HEGYES
LLOYDS
OBGYNS
OXEYES
PLAYAS
POLYPS
PROYAS
REDYES
SANYOS
SATYRS
SAYYES
SIBYLS
SUZYQS
VINYLS
WHYYES
YESYES

••••YS
ABBEYS
ALLAYS
ALLEYS
ALLOYS
ALWAYS
ANNOYS
ARRAYS
ASSAYS
BALLYS
BELAYS
BETSYS
BOBBYS
BOGEYS
BYWAYS
CAMRYS
CATHYS
CHEVYS
COLBYS
CONEYS
COPAYS
COVEYS
CUTEYS
DADDYS
DANNYS
DECAYS
DECOYS
DELAYS
DENNYS
DUFFYS
EMBAYS
EMILYS
ENJOYS
ENVOYS
ERINYS
ESSAYS
FLYBYS
FOGEYS
FOLEYS
FORAYS
FURBYS
GAMAYS
GLADYS
GODEYS
HARRYS
HOMEYS
HONEYS
INLAYS
ISLEYS
JUSTYS
KELLYS
LAYBYS
LIBBYS
LIEBYS
LOOEYS
LOVEYS
MALAYS
MASSYS
MATEYS
MONEYS
MOODYS
MORAYS
MOSEYS
MULEYS
MUMMYS
NOWAYS
ONLAYS
PARTYS
PLATYS
POBOYS
POKEYS
PORKYS
REBUYS
REKEYS
RELAYS
REPAYS
RESAYS
SATAYS
SEALYS
SEPOYS
SPLAYS
SPRAYS
STRAYS
TETHYS
TODAYS
TOKAYS
UNISYS
UNLAYS
UNSAYS
UVRAYS
WENDYS
WILLYS
ZLOTYS

YT••••
YTILES
YTTRIA
YTTRIC

Y•T•••
YATATA
YATSEN
YATTER
YETTIE
YTTRIA
YTTRIC
YUTANG
YUTZES

Y••T••
YATTER
YENTAS
YERTLE
YESTER
YETTIE
YOMTOV
YOUTHS
YOUTWO
YVETTE

Y•••T•
YACHTS
YAKUTS
YATATA
YEASTS
YEASTY
YUKATA
YVETTE

Y••••T
YANKAT
YAPHET
YAPSAT
YAREST
YCLEPT
YELLAT
YESBUT
YOGURT
YOUBET

•YT•••
BYTALK
BYTAXI
BYTENS
BYTHEN
BYTWOS
LYTTON
MYTHIC
MYTHOS
MYTURN
PYTHON

•Y•T••
AYRTON
CYSTIC
HYATTS
HYETAL
LYTTON
MYRTLE
MYSTIC
OYSTER
SYNTAX
SYNTHS
SYSTEM
WYNTER
WYNTON
WYSTAN
XYSTER
XYSTUS

•Y••T•
BYDATE
BYLOTS
BYPATH
BYROTE
GYRATE
HYATTS
NYJETS
NYMETS
PYRITE
ZYGOTE

•Y•••T
BYPAST
CYGNET
DYELOT
DYEVAT
DYNAST
DYSART
EYELET
EYEPIT
GYMRAT
LYRIST
MYFOOT
NYPOST
TYBALT
TYPIST
TYRANT

••YT••
ADYTUM
AMYTAN
BLYTHE
BLYTON
BOYTOY
DAYTON
ELYTIS
MAYTAG
PAYTON
PEYTON
RHYTHM
SCYTHE
SKYTEL
TOYTOP

••Y•T•
COYOTE
CRYPTO
CRYPTS
GLYPTO
KRYPTO
LAYSTO
PEYOTE
TOYOTA
TRYSTS

••Y••T
BAYSAT
BRYANT
BUYOUT
BUYSAT
BUYSIT
COYEST
CRYOUT
DAYLIT
DRYEST
DRYOUT
DRYROT
FEYEST
FLYNET
FLYOUT
GAYEST
KEYDET
LAYOUT
MAYEST
PAYCUT
PAYOUT
SAYEST
SHYEST
SKYLIT
SLYEST
SPYBOT
SPYOUT
STYLET

TOYHAT TRYOUT WAYOUT WHYNOT WRYEST

•••YT•
OOCYTE PLAYTO PRAYTO

•••Y•T
ALIYOT ANDYET BUTYET NOTYET PLAYAT PLAYIT SALYUT STAYAT

••••YT
AJFOYT

YU••••
YUCCAS YUKATA YUKAWA YUKKED YUKONS YUMAAZ YUMANS YUMYUM YUPPIE YUTANG YUTZES

Y•U•••
YOUALL YOUBET YOUDIG YOUSEE YOUSUF YOUTHS YOUTWO YOUWIN

Y••U••
YAKUTS YAKUZA YAMUNA YAQUIS YEHUDI YODUDE YOGURT

Y•••U•
YANQUI YASGUR YESBUT YOUSUF YUMYUM

Y••••U
YESYOU

•YU•••
KYUSHU RYUKYU

•Y•U••
FYVUSH MYTURN NYQUIL SYRUPS SYRUPY

•Y••U•
CYGNUS CYPRUS DYBBUK EYECUP EYEDUP EYEFUL EYESUP GYNOUS GYPSUM HYDRUS HYPEUP LYCEUM TYPEUP TYPHUS XYSTUS

•Y•••U
KYUSHU RYUKYU

••YU••
CAYUGA CAYUSE LAYUPS

••Y•U•
ADYTUM ASYLUM BAYEUX BAYOUS BAYRUM BUYOUT BUYSUP COYPUS CRYOUT DRYOUT DRYRUN FLYOUT JOYFUL JOYOUS KEYSUP LAYOUT LAYSUP PAYCUT PAYOUT PAYSUP PHYLUM RAYGUN SPYOUT STYLUS THYMUS TOYGUN TRYOUT WAYOUT

••Y••U
HEYYOU WHYYOU

•••YU•
BUOYUP COSYUP COZYUP PLAYUP PONYUP SALYUT STAYUP TIDYUP YUMYUM

•••Y•U
FORYOU GOTYOU HEYYOU ITSYOU NOTYOU SEEYOU SEZYOU WHYYOU YESYOU

••••YU
EMORYU KIKUYU RYUKYU

YV••••
YVETTE YVONNE

Y••••V
YOMTOV

•YV•••
EYVIND FYVUSH WYVERN

•Y•V••
DYEVAT SYLVAN SYLVIA

•Y••V•
BYJOVE MYLOVE

••YV••
HRYVNA JAYVEE

••Y•V•
TRYGVE

••Y••V
KRYLOV

•••YV•
THEYVE

••••YV
HENRYV ROCKYV

Y•W•••
YAWING YAWKEY YAWNED YAWNER YAWPED YAWPER YOWLED YOWLER YOWZAH

Y••W••
YOUWIN

Y•••W•
YOUTWO YUKAWA

Y••••W
YARROW YEEHAW YELLOW

•YW•••
BYWAYS BYWIRE BYWORD MYWORD

•Y•W••
BYTWOS

•Y••W•
BYLAWS

•Y•••W
BYENOW

••YW••
ANYWAY FLYWAY KEYWAY PSYWAR SKYWAY

••Y••W
ANYHOW BUYNOW FLYLOW HAYMOW KAYYOW LAYLOW PAYNOW WHYNOW

•••YW•
CODYWY

•••Y•W
KAYYOW

•Y•X••
LYNXES

•Y••X•
BYTAXI

•Y•••X
HYDROX SYNTAX

••YX••
ONYXES ORYXES

••Y••X
BAYEUX SKYBOX SLYFOX

•••Y•X
LARYNX SPHYNX

••••YX
COCCYX

Y•Y•••
YOYOED YOYOMA

Y••Y••
YESYES YESYOU YUMYUM

Y••••Y
YARELY YAWKEY YEARLY YEASTY

•YY•••
NYYANK

•Y•Y••
LYNYRD MYMYMY SYZYGY

•Y••Y•
AYEAYE BYEBYE BYWAYS RYUKYU

•Y•••Y
BYPLAY LYNLEY MYBABY MYLADY MYMYMY MYOHMY SYDNEY SYRUPY SYZYGY TYPIFY

••YY••
HEYYOU KAYYOW SAYYES WHYYES WHYYOU

••Y•Y•
DRYEYE FLYBYS LAYBYS SAYAYE

••Y••Y
ANYDAY ANYWAY BOYTOY DRYFLY FLYBOY FLYWAY HAYLEY HEYDAY KEYWAY LAYSBY MAYDAY MAYFLY NAYSAY PAYDAY SAYHEY SAYNAY SKYWAY WAYLAY

•••Y•Y
CLAYEY CODYWY GRAYLY GREYLY MYMYMY PLAYBY SPRYLY SYZYGY TROYNY WHEYEY

••••YY
DDMMYY MMDDYY

Y••Z••
YOWZAH YUTZES

Y•••Z•
YAKUZA

Y••••Z
YUMAAZ

•YZ•••
SYZYGY

•Y•Z••
GYOZAS OYEZES

•Y•••Z
XYANDZ

••Y•Z•
BRYNZA

•••YZ•
CORYZA SWAYZE

••••YZ
UVWXYZ

ZA••••
ZABRZE ZADDIK ZADORA ZAFTIG ZAGGED ZAGNUT ZAGREB ZAIRES ZAMBIA ZAMORA ZANIER ZANIES ZANILY ZANONI ZANTAC ZANUCK ZAPATA ZAPPED ZAPPER ZARKOV ZAYINS ZAZENS

Z•A•••
ZEALOT ZSAZSA

Z••A••
ZAPATA ZENANA ZOCALO ZYMASE

Z•••A•
ZANTAC ZEBRAS ZEEMAN ZESTAS ZIGZAG ZODIAC ZOLTAN ZONIAN ZUNIAN

Z••••A
ZADORA ZAMBIA ZAMORA ZAPATA ZENANA ZINNIA ZORINA ZOYSIA ZSAZSA ZUNIGA ZYGOMA

•ZA•••
AZALEA AZANIA AZARIA OZARKS

•Z•A••
AZRAEL EZPASS EZZARD

•Z••A•
AZERAS AZONAL

•Z•••A
AZALEA AZANIA AZARIA AZELMA AZTECA AZUELA

••ZA••
ALZADO ANZACS BAZAAR CAZALE DIZAIN EZZARD HAZANS HAZARD LIZALU LIZARD MOZART PIZAZZ WIZARD

••Z•A•
BAZAAR GAZEAT GUZMAN HAZMAT HUZZAH ITZHAK MAZDAS PIZZAS POZNAN

••Z••A
ALZIRA ECZEMA MAZOLA MAZUMA MIZUNA VEZINA VIZSLA

•••ZA•
BAIZAS BALZAC BANZAI CHAZAN CRUZAN GYOZAS HUZZAH IBIZAN MONZAS PIZZAS PLAZAS PROZAC SHAZAM SLEZAK TARZAN YOWZAH ZIGZAG

•••Z•A
BRAZZA PIAZZA ZSAZSA

••••ZA
BRAZZA BRYNZA CABEZA CORYZA KWANZA LAONZA LARAZA PIAZZA SFORZA STANZA YAKUZA

Z•B•••
ZABRZE ZEBRAS

Z••B••
ZAMBIA ZOMBIE

Z•••B•
ZHLOBS ZHLUBS ZIPSBY

Z••••B
ZAGREB

•Z•B••
XZIBIT

••ZB••
LAZBOY

••Z•B•
GAZEBO JAZZBO

•••ZB•
JAZZBO

Z•C•••
ZOCALO ZUCKER

Z••C••
ZINCED ZINCIC ZINCKY ZIRCON ZITCOM

Z•••C•
ZANUCK ZURICH ZYDECO

Z••••C
ZANTAC ZINCIC ZIPLOC ZODIAC

•Z•C••
CZECHS

•Z••C•
AZTECA AZTECS

•Z•••C
AZONIC OZONIC

••Z•C•
ANZACS

•••ZC•
OROZCO

•••Z•C
BALZAC PROZAC

Z•D•••
ZADDIK ZADORA ZEDONG ZEDONK ZODIAC ZYDECO

Z••D••
ZADDIK ZENDOS

Z•••D•
ZOOIDS ZOUNDS

Z••••D
ZAGGED ZAPPED ZEROED ZESTED ZIGGED ZINCED ZINGED ZIPPED ZIZZED ZONKED ZOOMED

•Z•D••
AZIDES AZODYE

•Z•••D
AZURED EZZARD

••ZD••
MAZDAS

••Z•D•
ALZADO

••Z••D
BUZZED COZIED EZZARD FEZZED FIZZED FUZZED HAZARD JAZZED LIZARD RAZZED WIZARD ZIZZED

•••Z•D
AMAZED BLAZED BOOZED BUZZED CRAZED FEZZED FIZZED FUTZED FUZZED GLAZED GRAZED JAZZED PRIZED RAZZED SEIZED ZIZZED

ZE••••
ZEALOT ZEBRAS ZEDONG ZEDONK ZEEMAN ZENANA ZENDOS ZENGER ZENIST ZENITH ZEPHYR ZEROED ZEROES ZEROIN ZESTAS ZESTED ZESTER ZEUXIS

Z•E•••
ZEEMAN

Z••E••
ZAZENS ZONERS ZYDECO

Z•••E•
ZAGGED ZAGREB ZAIRES ZANIER ZANIES ZAPPED ZAPPER ZENGER ZEROED ZEROES ZESTED ZESTER ZIFFEL ZIGGED ZIMMER ZINCED ZINGED ZINGER ZIPPED ZIPPER ZITHER ZIZZED ZIZZES ZONKED ZONKER ZOOIER ZOOMED ZTILES ZUCKER

Z••••E
ZABRZE ZOMBIE ZONULE ZYGOTE ZYMASE

•ZE•••
AZELMA AZERAS AZERIS CZECHS CZERNY

•Z•E••
AZTECA AZTECS AZTEKS AZUELA

•Z••E•
AZALEA AZIDES AZOLES AZORES AZRAEL AZURED AZURES EZINES

•Z•••E
AZODYE

••ZE••
BEZELS COZENS DAZERS DOZENS DOZERS ECZEMA GAZEAT GAZEBO GAZEON GAZERS HAZELS HAZERS OUZELS RAZERS REZERO SIZERS SIZEUP WIZENS ZAZENS

••Z•E•
BUZZED BUZZER BUZZES COZIED COZIER COZIES DOZIER FEZZED FEZZES FIZZED FIZZER FIZZES FUZZED FUZZES HAZIER JAZZED JAZZER JAZZES JOZSEF LAZIER MAZIER MIZZEN OOZIER RAZZED RAZZES SUZIEQ VIZIER WIZZES ZIZZED ZIZZES

••Z••E
CAZALE DAZZLE ENZYME FIZZLE FOZZIE GUZZLE LIZZIE MIZZLE MUZZLE NOZZLE NUZZLE POZOLE PUZZLE RAZZIE RAZZLE REZONE SIZZLE UNZONE

•••ZE•
AMAZED AMAZES BAIZES BEEZER BELZER BLAZED BLAZER BLAZES BONZES BOOZED BOOZER BOOZES BOWZER BRAZEN BUZZED BUZZER BUZZES CRAZED CRAZES DENZEL DIEZES DITZES DOOZER DOUZES DRUZES FEZZED FEZZES FIZZED FIZZER FIZZES FRAZER FROZEN FURZES FUTZED FUTZES FUZZED FUZZES GAUZES GEEZER GLAZED GLAZER GLAZES GRAZED GRAZER GRAZES JANZEN JAZZED JAZZER JAZZES KATZEN KUNZEL LINZER LUTZES MAAZEL MAIZES MIZZEN OYEZES PANZER PATZER PFIZER PRIZED PRIZES RAZZED RAZZES RITZES SEIZED SEIZER SEIZES SETZER SMAZES TETZEL WEEZER WIZZES YUTZES ZIZZED ZIZZES

•••Z•E
DAZZLE DOOZIE FIZZLE FONZIE FOOZLE FOZZIE GRAZIE GUZZLE LIZZIE MIZZLE MUZZLE NOZZLE NUZZLE PUZZLE RAZZIE RAZZLE SIZZLE

••••ZE
ABLAZE ASSIZE BEDAZE BELIZE BREEZE BRONZE FREEZE FRIEZE FRUNZE IODIZE IONIZE LAMAZE LEUTZE PRINZE QUINZE RESIZE SLEAZE SNEEZE SNOOZE SWAYZE TREIZE TWEEZE UPGAZE UPSIZE WHEEZE XPRIZE ZABRZE

Z•F•••
ZAFTIG ZIFFEL

Z••F••
ZIFFEL

Z•••F•
ZIPOFF

Z••••F
ZIPOFF

••Z••F
JOZSEF

Z•G•••
ZAGGED
ZAGNUT
ZAGREB
ZIGGED
ZIGZAG
ZYGOMA
ZYGOTE

Z••G••
ZAGGED
ZENGER
ZIGGED
ZINGED
ZINGER
ZIPGUN

Z•••G•
ZUNIGA

Z••••G
ZAFTIG
ZEDONG
ZIGZAG
ZONING

••ZG••
FIZGIG

••Z•G•
SYZYGY

••Z••G
ADZING
DAZING
DOZING
FAZING
FIZGIG
GAZING
HAZING
LAZING
MAZING
OOZING
RAZING
SIZING

•••Z•G
DANZIG
HERZOG
ZIGZAG

ZH••••
ZHLOBS
ZHLUBS
ZHUKOV

Z••H••
ZEPHYR
ZITHER

Z••••H
ZENITH
ZIZITH
ZURICH

•Z••H•
CZECHS

••ZH••
ITZHAK

••Z•H•
SEZWHO

••Z••H
HUZZAH
ZIZITH

•••Z•H
HUZZAH
MATZOH
YOWZAH

ZI••••
ZIFFEL
ZIGGED
ZIGZAG
ZIMMER
ZINCED
ZINCIC
ZINCKY
ZINGED
ZINGER
ZINNIA
ZIPGUN
ZIPLOC
ZIPOFF
ZIPONS
ZIPOUT
ZIPPED
ZIPPER
ZIPPOS
ZIPSBY
ZIPSIN
ZIPSIT
ZIPSUP
ZIPTOP
ZIRCON
ZITCOM
ZITHER
ZIZITH
ZIZZED
ZIZZES

Z•I•••
ZAIRES
ZTILES

Z••I••
ZANIER
ZANIES
ZANILY
ZAYINS
ZENIST
ZENITH
ZIZITH
ZODIAC
ZONIAN
ZONING
ZOOIDS
ZOOIER
ZORINA
ZUNIAN
ZUNIGA
ZURICH

Z•••I•
ZADDIK
ZAFTIG
ZAMBIA
ZEROIN
ZEUXIS
ZINCIC
ZINNIA
ZIPSIN
ZIPSIT
ZOMBIE
ZOOMIN
ZOYSIA

Z••••I
ZANONI

•ZI•••
AZIDES
EZINES
XZIBIT

•Z••I•
AZANIA
AZARIA
AZERIS
AZONIC
AZORIN
AZUKIS
OZONIC
XZIBIT

••ZI••
ADZING
ALZIRA
COZIED
COZIER
COZIES
COZILY
DAZING
DOZIER
DOZILY
DOZING
FAZING
GAZING
HAZIER
HAZILY
HAZING
LAZIER
LAZILY
LAZING
MAZIER
MAZILY
MAZING
OOZIER
OOZILY
OOZING
RAZING
REZIPS
SIZING
SUZIEQ
UNZIPS
VEZINA
VIZIER
VIZIRS
ZIZITH

••Z•I•
BIZKIT
DIZAIN
FIZGIG
FOZZIE
LIZZIE
RAZZIE

••Z••I
ADZUKI
LAZULI
SUZUKI

•••ZI•
AMAZIN
BRAZIL
DANZIG
DOOZIE
FONZIE
FOZZIE
GHAZIS
GRAZIE
LIZZIE
NUNZIO
RAZZIE

•••Z•I
BANZAI
BORZOI
BRAZZI
PIAZZI
PRIZZI

••••ZI
BRAZZI
FRITZI
PIAZZI
PRIZZI
RIENZI

Z••K••
ZARKOV
ZHUKOV
ZONKED
ZONKER
ZUCKER

Z•••K•
ZINCKY

Z••••K
ZADDIK
ZANUCK
ZEDONK

•Z•K••
AZUKIS

•Z••K•
AZTEKS
OZARKS

••ZK••
BIZKIT

••Z•K•
ADZUKI
SUZUKI

••Z••K
ITZHAK

•••Z•K
SLEZAK

ZL••••
ZLOTYS

Z•L•••
ZHLOBS
ZHLUBS
ZOLTAN

Z••L••
ZEALOT
ZIPLOC
ZTILES

Z•••L•
ZANILY
ZOCALO
ZONULE

Z••••L
ZIFFEL

•Z•L••
AZALEA
AZELMA
AZOLES

•Z••L•
AZUELA

•Z•••L
AZONAL
AZRAEL

••Z•L•
BEZELS
CAZALE
COZILY
DAZZLE
DOZILY
FIZZLE
GUZZLE
HAZELS
HAZILY
LAZILY
LAZULI
LIZALU
MAZILY
MAZOLA
MIZZLE
MIZZLY
MUZZLE
NOZZLE
NUZZLE
OOZILY
OUZELS
POZOLE
PUZZLE
RAZZLE
SIZZLE
VIZSLA

••Z••L
FAZOOL

•••ZL•
DAZZLE
FIZZLE
FOOZLE
GUZZLE
LASZLO
MIZZLE
MIZZLY
MUZZLE
NOZZLE
NUZZLE
PUZZLE
RAZZLE
SIZZLE

•••Z•L
BENZOL
BRAZIL
DENZEL
KUNZEL
MAAZEL
TETZEL

Z•M•••
ZAMBIA
ZAMORA
ZIMMER
ZOMBIE
ZYMASE

Z••M••
ZEEMAN
ZIMMER
ZOOMED
ZOOMIN

Z•••M•
ZYGOMA

Z••••M
ZITCOM

•Z••M•
AZELMA

••ZM••
GIZMOS
GUZMAN
HAZMAT

••Z•M•
ECZEMA
ENZYME
MAZUMA

•••ZM•
PRIZMS

•••Z•M
SHAZAM

Z•N•••
ZANIER
ZANIES
ZANILY
ZANONI
ZANTAC
ZANUCK
ZENANA
ZENDOS
ZENGER
ZENIST
ZENITH
ZINCED
ZINCIC
ZINCKY
ZINGED
ZINGER
ZINNIA
ZONERS
ZONIAN
ZONING
ZONKED
ZONKER
ZONULE
ZUNIAN
ZUNIGA

Z••N••
ZAGNUT
ZINNIA
ZOUNDS

Z•••N•
ZANONI
ZAYINS
ZAZENS
ZEDONG
ZEDONK
ZENANA
ZIPONS
ZONING
ZORINA

Z••••N
ZEEMAN
ZEROIN
ZIPGUN
ZIPSIN
ZIRCON
ZOLTAN
ZONIAN
ZOOMIN
ZUNIAN

•Z•N••
AZANIA
AZONAL
AZONIC
EZINES
OZONIC

•Z••N•
CZERNY

•Z•••N
AZORIN

••ZN••
POZNAN

••Z•N•
ADZING
COZENS
DAZING
DOZENS
DOZING
FAZING
GAZING
HAZANS
HAZING
LAZING
MAZING
MIZUNA
OOZING
RAZING
REZONE
SIZING
UNZONE
VEZINA
WIZENS
ZAZENS

••Z••N
DIZAIN
GAZEON
GUZMAN
MIZZEN
POZNAN

•••ZN•
GROZNY

•••Z•N
AMAZIN
AMAZON
BARZUN
BLAZON
BRAZEN
CHAZAN
CRUZAN
CURZON
FROZEN
GUTZON
IBIZAN
JANZEN
KATZEN
MANZON
MIZZEN
PINZON
QUEZON
TARZAN

ZO••••
ZOCALO
ZODIAC
ZOLTAN
ZOMBIE
ZONERS
ZONIAN
ZONING
ZONKED
ZONKER
ZONULE
ZOOIDS
ZOOIER
ZOOMED
ZOOMIN
ZORINA
ZOUNDS
ZOYSIA

Z•O•••
ZLOTYS
ZOOIDS
ZOOIER
ZOOMED
ZOOMIN

Z••O••
ZADORA
ZAMORA
ZANONI
ZEDONG
ZEDONK
ZEROED
ZEROES
ZEROIN
ZHLOBS
ZIPOFF
ZIPONS
ZIPOUT
ZYGOMA
ZYGOTE

Z•••O•
ZARKOV
ZEALOT
ZENDOS
ZHUKOV
ZIPLOC
ZIPPOS
ZIPTOP
ZIRCON
ZITCOM

Z••••O
ZOCALO
ZYDECO

•ZO•••
AZODYE
AZOLES
AZONAL
AZONIC
AZORES
AZORIN
OZONIC

••ZO••
BAZOOS
FAZOOL
KAZOOS
MAZOLA
POZOLE
RAZORS
REZONE
UNZONE
VIZORS

••Z•O•
BAZOOS
FAZOOL
GAZEON
GIZMOS
KAZOOS
LAZBOY
MEZZOS
SEZYOU

••Z••O
ALZADO
GAZEBO
JAZZBO
REZERO
SEZWHO

•••ZO•
AMAZON
BENZOL
BLAZON
BORZOI
BRAZOS
CURZON
GUTZON
HERZOG
MAHZOR
MANZON
MATZOH
MATZOS
MEZZOS
PINZON
QUEZON
SEIZOR

•••Z•O
AREZZO
JAZZBO
LASZLO
NUNZIO
OROZCO

••••ZO
ALONZO
AREZZO
PUENZO
REBOZO

Z•P•••
ZAPATA
ZAPPED
ZAPPER
ZEPHYR
ZIPGUN
ZIPLOC
ZIPOFF
ZIPONS
ZIPOUT
ZIPPED
ZIPPER
ZIPPOS
ZIPSBY
ZIPSIN
ZIPSIT
ZIPSUP
ZIPTOP

Z••P••
ZAPPED
ZAPPER
ZIPPED
ZIPPER
ZIPPOS

Z••••P
ZIPSUP
ZIPTOP

•ZP•••
EZPASS

••Z•P•
REZIPS
UNZIPS

••Z••P
COZYUP
FUZZUP
JAZZUP
SIZEUP

•••Z•P
FUZZUP
JAZZUP

••Z•Q•
SUZYQS

••Z••Q
SUZIEQ

Z•R•••
ZARKOV
ZEROED
ZEROES
ZEROIN
ZIRCON
ZORINA
ZURICH

Z••R••
ZABRZE
ZAGREB
ZAIRES
ZEBRAS

Z•••R•
ZADORA
ZAMORA
ZONERS

Z••••R
ZANIER
ZAPPER
ZENGER
ZEPHYR
ZESTER
ZIMMER
ZINGER
ZIPPER
ZITHER
ZONKER
ZOOIER
ZUCKER

•ZR•••
AZRAEL

•Z•R••
AZARIA
AZERAS
AZERIS
AZORES
AZORIN
AZURED
AZURES
CZERNY
OZARKS

•Z••R•
EZZARD

••Z•R•
ALZIRA
DAZERS
DOZERS
EZZARD
GAZERS
HAZARD
HAZERS
LIZARD
MOZART
RAZERS
RAZORS
REZERO
SIZERS
VIZIRS
VIZORS
WIZARD

••Z••R
BAZAAR
BUZZER
COZIER
DOZIER
FIZZER
HAZIER
JAZZER
LAZIER
MAZIER
OOZIER
VIZIER

•••Z•R
BEEZER
BELZER
BLAZER
BOOZER
BOWZER
BUZZER
DOOZER
FIZZER
FRAZER
GEEZER
GLAZER
GRAZER
JAZZER
LINZER
MAHZOR
PANZER
PATZER
PFIZER
SEIZER
SEIZOR
SETZER
WEEZER

ZS••••
ZSAZSA

Z•S•••
ZESTAS
ZESTED
ZESTER

Z••S••
ZIPSBY
ZIPSIN
ZIPSIT
ZIPSUP
ZOYSIA

Z•••S•
ZENIST
ZSAZSA
ZYMASE

Z••••S
ZAIRES
ZANIES
ZAYINS
ZAZENS
ZEBRAS
ZENDOS
ZEROES
ZESTAS
ZEUXIS
ZHLOBS
ZHLUBS
ZIPONS
ZIPPOS
ZIZZES
ZLOTYS
ZONERS
ZOOIDS
ZOUNDS
ZTILES

•Z••S•
EZPASS

•Z•••S
AZERAS
AZERIS
AZIDES
AZOLES
AZORES
AZTECS
AZTEKS
AZUKIS
AZURES
CZECHS
EZINES
EZPASS
OZARKS

••ZS••
JOZSEF
VIZSLA

••Z••S
ANZACS
BAZOOS
BEZELS
BUZZES
COZENS
COZIES
DAZERS
DOZENS
DOZERS
FEZZES
FIZZES
FUZZES
GAZERS
GIZMOS
HAZANS
HAZELS
HAZERS
JAZZES
KAZOOS
MAZDAS
MEZZOS
OUZELS
PIZZAS
RAZERS
RAZORS
RAZZES
REZIPS
SIZERS
SUZYQS
UNZIPS
VIZIRS
VIZORS
WIZENS
WIZZES
ZAZENS
ZIZZES

•••ZS•
ZSAZSA

•••Z•S
AMAZES
BAIZAS
BAIZES
BLAZES
BONZES
BOOZES
BRAZOS
BUZZES
CRAZES
DIEZES
DITZES
DOUZES
DRUZES
FEZZES
FIZZES
FURZES
FUTZES
FUZZES
GAUZES
GHAZIS
GLAZES
GRAZES
GYOZAS
ISUZUS
JAZZES
KUDZUS
LUTZES
MAIZES
MATZOS
MEZZOS
MONZAS
OYEZES
PIZZAS
PLAZAS
PONZUS
PRIZES
PRIZMS
RAZZES
RITZES
SEIZES
SMAZES
WIZZES
YUTZES
ZIZZES

ZT••••
ZTILES

Z•T•••
ZITCOM
ZITHER

Z••T••
ZAFTIG
ZANTAC
ZESTAS
ZESTED
ZESTER
ZIPTOP
ZLOTYS
ZOLTAN

Z•••T•
ZAPATA
ZENITH
ZIZITH
ZYGOTE

Z••••T
ZAGNUT
ZEALOT
ZENIST
ZIPOUT
ZIPSIT

•ZT•••
AZTECA
AZTECS
AZTEKS

•Z•••T	ZURICH	ZIPSUP	**••Z•U•**	PONZUS	**ZY••••**	ZINCKY	**••Z••Y**	SNAZZY	SNAZZY	ZIZZES	FIZZED	MEZZOS	ZIZZES	SCUZZY
XZIBIT			COZYUP		ZYDECO	ZIPSBY	COZILY	WHIZZY	SNEEZY	ZSAZSA	FIZZER	MIZZEN		SNAZZY
	Z•U•••	**•ZU•••**	FUZZUP	**••••ZU**	ZYGOMA		DOZILY		SNOOZY		FIZZES	MIZZLE	**••Z•Z•**	WHIZZY
••Z•T•	ZEUXIS	AZUELA	JAZZUP	LAOTZU	ZYGOTE	**•Z••Y•**	HAZILY	**••••ZY**	UNHAZY	**Z•••Z•**	FIZZLE	MIZZLY	PIZAZZ	
ZIZITH	ZHUKOV	AZUKIS	SIZEUP		ZYMASE	AZODYE	LAZBOY	BLOWZY	WHEEZY	ZABRZE	FOZZIE	MUZZLE		**••••ZZ**
	ZOUNDS	AZURED		**Z••••V**			LAZILY	BREEZY	WHIZZY		FUZZED	NOZZLE	**••Z••Z**	PIZAZZ
••Z••T		AZURES	**••Z••U**	ZARKOV	**Z•Y•••**	**•Z•••Y**	MAZILY	BRONZY		**•ZZ•••**	FUZZES	NUZZLE	PIZAZZ	STARZZ
BIZKIT	**Z••U••**		LIZALU	ZHUKOV	ZAYINS	CZERNY	MIZZLY	FRENZY	**Z•Z•••**	EZZARD	FUZZUP	PIZZAS		
GAZEAT	ZANUCK	**••ZU••**	SEZYOU		ZOYSIA		OOZILY	FRIZZY	ZAZENS		GUZZLE	PUZZLE	**•••ZZ•**	
HAZMAT	ZHLUBS	ADZUKI		**••ZW••**		**••ZY••**	SYZYGY	FROWZY	ZIZITH	**••ZZ••**	HUZZAH	RAZZED	AREZZO	
MOZART	ZONULE	LAZULI	**•••ZU•**	SEZWHO	**Z•••Y•**	COZYUP		GLITZY	ZIZZED	BUZZED	JAZZBO	RAZZES	BRAZZA	
		MAZUMA	BARZUN		ZEPHYR	ENZYME	**•••Z•Y**	GROSZY	ZIZZES	BUZZER	JAZZED	RAZZIE	BRAZZI	
ZU••••	**Z•••U•**	MIZUNA	FUZZUP	**Z••X••**	ZLOTYS	SEZYOU	FRIZZY	KLUTZY		BUZZES	JAZZER	RAZZLE	FRIZZY	
ZUCKER	ZAGNUT	SUZUKI	ISUZUS	ZEUXIS		SUZYQS	GROZNY	MAIRZY	**Z••Z••**	DAZZLE	JAZZES	SIZZLE	PIAZZA	
ZUNIAN	ZIPGUN		JAZZUP		**Z••••Y**	SYZYGY	MIZZLY	SCUZZY	ZIGZAG	FEZZED	JAZZUP	WIZZES	PIAZZI	
ZUNIGA	ZIPOUT		KUDZUS		ZANILY		SCUZZY	SLEAZY	ZIZZED	FEZZES	LIZZIE	ZIZZED	PRIZZI	

7

AA•••••
AAACELL
AAAMAPS
AACELLS
AAJUMBO
AALARGE
AALIYAH
AAMILNE
AARATED

A•A••••
AAACELL
AAAMAPS
ABALONE
ABANDON
ABASERS
ABASHED
ABASHES
ABASING
ABATERS
ABATING
ABATORS
ACACIAS
ACADEME
ACADEMY
ACADIAN
ACANTHI
ACARIDS
ACAUDAL
ADAGIOS
ADAMANT
ADAMITE
ADAMSES
ADAMSON
ADAPTED
ADAPTER
ADAPTOR
ADAPTTO
ADAWARE
ADAYAGO
AFARCRY
AFATLOT
AGAINST
AGAKHAN
AGALLOP
AGARICS
AGASSIZ
AGATINE
AHASSLE
AJACCIO
ALABAMA
ALABAMY
ALACKOF
ALADDIN
ALADINE
ALAKING
ALAMEDA
ALAMEIN
ALAMODE
ALAMOSA
ALANINE
ALANJAY
ALANNAH
ALARBUS
ALARCON
ALARMED
ALARMER
ALARUMS
ALASKAN
ALASKAS
ALASSAD
ALATEEN
ALAYING
AMADEUS
AMALGAM
AMANITA
AMANTIS
AMAPOLA
AMARONE
AMASSED
AMASSER
AMASSES
AMATEUR
AMATIVE
AMATOLS
AMATORY
AMAZING
AMAZONS
ANACINS
ANADEMS
ANAEMIA
ANAEMIC
ANAGRAM
ANAHEIM
ANALOGS
ANALOGY
ANALYSE
ANALYST
ANALYTE
ANALYZE
ANANIAS
ANAPEST
ANARCHS
ANARCHY
ANASAZI
ANATASE
ANATOLE
ANATOLY
ANATOMY
APACHES
APAIROF
APATITE
ARABIAN
ARABICA
ARABICS
ARABIST
ARABLES
ARACARI
ARACHNE
ARACHNO
ARAFTOF
ARAFURA
ARAGORN
ARALSEA
ARAMAIC
ARAMARK
ARAMEAN
ARAMIDS
ARANEID
ARANTXA
ARAPAHO
ASABODY
ASAGIFT
ASAGRAY
ASAJOKE
ASALARK
ASANTES
ASARULE
ASATEAM
ATABOIL
ATACAMA
ATACLIP
ATACOST
ATALOSS
ATAMANS
ATANEND
ATARAXY
ATATILT
ATATIME
ATATURK
ATAVISM
ATAVIST
AVAILED
AVALONS
AVANTIS
AVARICE
AVATARS
AWAITED
AWAITER
AWAKENS
AWAKERS
AWAKING
AWARDED
AWARDEE
AWARDER
AWAREOF
AWAREST
AWASHIN
AZALEAS
AZANIAN

A••A•••
AALARGE
AARATED
ABLATED
ABLATES
ABRADED
ABRADER
ABRADES
ABRAHAM
ABRAXAS
ABSALOM
ACKACKS
ACTABLE
ACTAEON
ADDABLE
ADDAXES
ADRATES
ADVANCE
AERATED
AERATES
AERATOR
AFEARED
AFFABLE
AFFABLY
AFFAIRE
AFFAIRS
AFRAMES
AGNAILS
AGNATES
AGNATIC
AHEADOF
AIRACES
AKSAKOV
ALBANIA
ALCAIDE
ALCALDE
ALCAZAR
ALDAVIS
ALEARDI
ALFALFA
ALGARVE
ALIASES
ALKALIS
ALLAGES
ALLANTE
ALLAYED
ALLAYER
ALMAATA
ALMADEN
ALMANAC
ALOADOF
ALPACAS
ALSATIA
ALVAREZ
AMHARIC
AMIABLE
AMIABLY
AMRADIO
ANDAMAN
ANDANTE
ANKARAN
ANNABEL
ANNAKIN
ANNALEE
ANNALES
ANNAMAY
ANNATTO
ANTACID
ANTARES
APHAGIA
APHAGIC
APHASIA
APHASIC
APPALLS
APPARAT
APPAREL
AQUAMAN
AQUARIA
AQUATIC
AQUAVIT
ARBACES
ARCADED
ARCADES
ARCADIA
ARCANUM
AREAMAP
AREARUG
AREAWAY
ARGALIS
ARGANTE
ARIADNE
ARIANES
ARMADAS
ARRABAL
ARRACKS
ARRAIGN
ARRANGE
ARRASES
ARRAYAL
ARRAYED
ARRAYER
ASCARED
ASFARAS
ASHAMED
ASHANTI
ASIAGOS
ASIATIC
ASKANCE
ASKAWAY
ASMARAN
ASSAILS
ASSANTE
ASSAULT
ASSAYED
ASSAYER
ASTAIRE
ASTARTE
ATEABIT
ATEALOT
ATEAWAY
ATFAULT
ATLANTA
ATLARGE
ATLASES
ATTABOY
ATTACHE
ATTACKS
ATTAINS
ATTAINT
ATWATER
AUBADES
AUPAIRS
AURALEE
AURALLY
AUSABLE
AUTARCH
AUTARKY
AVGASES
AVIANCA
AVIATED
AVIATES
AVIATIC
AVIATOR
AXIALLY
AYEAYES
AZKABAN

A•••A••
AAAMAPS
ABELARD
ABEYANT
ABIGAIL
ABREAST
ABROACH
ABSTAIN
ACCLAIM
ACERATE
ACETALS
ACETATE
ACREAGE
ACTUARY
ACTUATE
ADAMANT
ADAWARE
ADAYAGO
ADDSALT
ADONAIS
ADRIANA
ADSPACE
ADULATE
AERIALS
AFFIANT
AFFRAYS
AFGHANI
AFGHANS
AGEMATE
AGESAGO
AGITATE
AGITATO
AIRBAGS
AIRBALL
AIRBASE
AIRDAMS
AIRDATE
AIRFARE
AIRLANE
AIRMADA
AIRMAIL
AIRMASS
AIRPACK
AIRPARK
AIRRACE
AIRRAGE
AIRRAID
AIRSACS
AIRTANK
AIRTAXI
AIRWARS
AIRWAVE
AIRWAYS
AJOWANS
ALABAMA
ALABAMY
ALEGARS
ALETAPS
ALEYARD
ALIBABA
ALIDADE
ALIYAHS
ALLCAPS
ALLCASH
ALLEARS
ALLHAIL
ALLMALE
ALMAATA
ALOHAOE
ALPHARD
ALREADY
ALSHAIN
ALTTABS
AMERADA
AMIDALA
AMILATE
AMTRACK
AMTRACS
AMYLASE
ANASAZI
ANATASE
ANDEANS
ANDIAMO
ANDRADE
ANGLAIS
ANIMACY
ANIMALS
ANIMATE
ANIMATO
ANNEALS
ANNUALS
ANOMALY
ANORAKS
ANSPACH
ANTFARM
ANTIART
ANYWAYS
AOUDADS
APPEALS
APPEARS
APPEASE
APPLAUD
ARACARI
ARAMAIC
ARAMARK
ARAPAHO
ARCHAIC
ARCLAMP
ARCUATE
ARIGATO
ARIKARA
ARMBAND
ARMYANT
ARREARS
ARTCARS
ARTFAIR
ARTSALE
ARTWALL
ARTWARE
ARUBANS
ASALARK
ASBYATT
ASHCAKE
ASHCANS
ASHLAND
ASHLARS
ASHPANS
ASHRAMS
ASISAID
ASONANT
ASPHALT
ASPRAWL
ASSHARP
ASSUAGE
ATACAMA
ATAMANS
ATARAXY
ATELATE
ATGRADE
ATHEART
ATHWART
ATLEAST
ATMCARD
ATPEACE
ATSTAKE
ATTRACT
AUREATE
AVATARS
AVERAGE
AVOCADO
AVOWALS
AWKWARD
AXHEADS
AYNRAND
AZUSACA

A••••A•
AALIYAH
ABETTAL
ABIDJAN
ABOLLAE
ABRAHAM
ABRAXAS
ABUTTAL
ABYSMAL
ABYSSAL
ACACIAS
ACADIAN
ACAUDAL
ACCRUAL
ACCUSAL
ACROBAT
ACTEDAS
ACTIVAS
ADEPTAT
ADMIRAL
ADOLLAR
ADRENAL
ADWOMAN
AEOLIAN
AEROBAT
AFCTEAM
AFRICAN
AGAKHAN
AGENDAS
AGULHAS
AIMEDAT
AINTHAY
AIRBOAT
AIRHEAD
AIRPLAY
AIRTRAP
ALANJAY
ALANNAH
ALASKAN
ALASKAS
ALASSAD
ALBORAK
ALCAZAR
ALDORAY
ALLBRAN
ALLCLAD
ALLHEAL
ALLOWAY
ALLSTAR
ALLTHAT
ALMANAC
ALMSMAN
ALNILAM
ALNITAK
ALNIYAT
ALPACAS
ALSORAN
ALTIMAS
ALTOSAX
ALUMNAE
ALUMNAL
ALYKHAN
AMALGAM
AMESLAN
AMICHAI
AMISTAD
AMOEBAE
AMOEBAS
AMRITAS
AMSCRAY
ANAGRAM
ANANIAS
ANDAMAN
ANDREAS
ANEMIAS
ANGELAS
ANGOLAN
ANGORAS
ANGRYAT
ANGULAR
ANITRAS
ANKARAN
ANNAMAY
ANNULAR
ANTBEAR
ANTHRAX
ANTITAX
ANTIWAR
ANYROAD
APOGEAL
APOGEAN
APPARAT
APTERAL
APULIAN
AQUAMAN
AQUINAS
ARABIAN
ARAMEAN
ARCHWAY
AREAMAP
AREAWAY
AREOLAE
AREOLAR
AREOLAS
ARISTAE
ARISTAS
ARMADAS
ARMLOAD
ARNICAS
ARONNAX
AROUSAL
ARRABAL
ARRAYAL
ARRIVAL
ARSENAL
ARTISAN
ASAGRAY
ASATEAM
ASEXUAL
ASFARAS
ASHHEAP
ASHTRAY
ASKAWAY
ASMARAN
ASOCIAL
ASSTDAS
ASTHMAS
ASTOLAT
ASTREAM
ASUSUAL
ATEAWAY
AUGURAL
AURORAE
AURORAL
AURORAS
AUSTRAL
AUTOMAT
AVERNAL
AVESTAN
AVESTAS
AVIDFAN
AVIVIAN
AXEHEAD
AXILLAE
AXILLAR
AXILLAS
AZALEAS
AZANIAN
AZKABAN
AZOREAN
AZORIAN
AZTECAN

A•••••A
ABINTRA
ACEROLA
ACHIEVA
ADDENDA
ADELINA
ADRIANA
AGRIPPA
AIRMADA
ALABAMA
ALAMEDA
ALAMOSA
ALBANIA
ALBERTA
ALEGRIA
ALFALFA
ALFORJA
ALFREDA
ALGEBRA
ALGERIA
ALGIEBA
ALIBABA
ALLEGRA
ALLUVIA
ALMAATA
ALMERIA
ALSATIA
ALTOONA
ALUMINA
ALYOSHA
AMANITA
AMAPOLA
AMERADA
AMERICA
AMERIKA
AMIDALA
AMMONIA
AMNESIA
AMPHORA
AMREETA
ANAEMIA
ANDORRA
ANOSMIA
ANSONIA
ANTENNA
ANTIGUA
ANTONIA
APHAGIA
APHASIA
APHELIA
APHONIA
AQUARIA
ARABICA
ARAFURA
ARALSEA
ARANTXA
ARCADIA
ARIETTA
ARIKARA
ARIZONA
ARMENIA
ARUGULA
ASSUNTA
ASSYRIA
ASTORIA
ATACAMA
ATLANTA
AUGUSTA
AULETTA
AUREOLA
AUSTRIA
AUTOPIA
AVENIDA
AVIANCA
AVONLEA
AZUSACA

•AA••••
AAACELL
AAAMAPS
BAALISH
BAALISM
BAALIST
BAALITE
HAARLEM
MAANDPA
MAARTEN
PAANGAS
SAATCHI

•A•A•••
AALARGE
AARATED
BACARDI
BADAREA
BAHAISM
BAHAIST
BAHAMAS
BAHAMEN
BALABAN
BALANCE
BALASES
BALATAS
BALATON
BANACEK
BANALER
BANALLY
BANANAS
BANANES
BARACUS
BARANOF
BASALLY
BASALTS
BATAVIA
BAVARIA
BAYAREA
BAZAARS
CABALAS
CABALLE
CABANAS
CABARET
CADAVER
CALABRO
CALAMAR
CALANDO
CAMACHO
CAMAROS
CANALED
CANAPES
CANARDS
CANASTA
CAPABLE
CAPABLY
CAPADES
CAPAPIE
CARABOO
CARACAS
CARAFES
CARAMBA
CARAMEL
CARAMIA
CARAVAN
CARAVEL
CARAWAY
CASABAS
CASAVAS
CATALAN
CATALOG
CATALOS
CATALPA
CATANIA
CATAWBA
CAVALRY

DACAPOS	JAKARTA	MANANAS	RAJARAO	WASATCH	CADEAUX	FAISALI	HAZMATS	MANUALS	PAYCASH	TAGSALE	WAYLAYS	CARAWAY
DADAART	JAMAICA	MANATEE	RAKABLE	WAXABLE	CAESARS	FALCATE	JACKALS	MARCATO	PAYDAYS	TAKEAIM	WAYWARD	CARBRAS
DADAISM	JANACEK	MARACAS	RAMADAN	XANADUS	CAFTANS	FALLACY	JACKASS	MARGATE	PAYRATE	TAMBALA	YARDAGE	CARCOAT
DADAIST	JAVAMAN	MARANTZ	RAMADAS	YAMAHAS	CAIMANS	FALLALS	JAGUARS	MARGAUX	QADDAFI	TAMIAMI	YARDARM	CARDIAC
DALASIS	KAKAPOS	MARAUDS	RANAMOK	ZAGAZIG	CALGARY	FANBASE	JAMBAND	MARHAUS	RACHAEL	TAMMANY	ZACHARY	CARDIAL
DAMAGED	KANAKAS	MASARYK	RANATAB	ZAPATAS	CALVARY	FANFARE	JAMCAMS	MARIANA	RADIALS	TAMPAFL		CARINAE
DAMAGES	KARACHI	MATADOR	RANAWAY	ZAPATEO	CAMPARI	FANMAIL	JAMPACK	MARIANO	RADIANS	TAMTAMS	•A•••A•	CARINAS
DAMASKS	KARAJAN	MATALIN	RAPALLO		CANCANS	FANPALM	JANEANE	MARMARA	RADIANT	TANBARK	AALIYAH	CARLOAD
DAMASUS	KARAKUM	MAYALIN	RAPANUI	•A••A••	CANDACE	FANTAIL	JANUARY	MARSALA	RADIATE	TANKAGE	BABIYAR	CARLOAN
DANANAS	KARAOKE	MAZARIN	RATABLE	AAAMAPS	CANTABS	FANTANS	JAYWALK	MARYANN	RAEDAWN	TANKARD	BABYGAP	CARPSAT
DATABLE	KARASEA	NAIADES	RATAFIA	BABBAGE	CANTALS	FANTASM	JAYWARD	MASCARA	RAGBAGS	TANOAKS	BABYSAT	CARSEAT
DATABUS	KARATES	NAMABLE	RATATAT	BACHATA	CANTATA	FANTAST	JAZZAGE	MASSAGE	RAGLANS	TANTARA	BACCHAE	CASABAS
DATASET	KATAYEV	NAMABLY	RAVAGED	BADBACK	CANVASS	FANTASY	KABBALA	MAUMAUS	RAGMANS	TAPPANS	BACHMAN	CASAVAS
EARACHE	KAYAKED	NANAIMO	RAVAGER	BADCALL	CAPEANN	FAREAST	KAMPALA	MAUVAIS	RAILAGE	TARBABY	BACKBAR	CASELAW
EATABIT	KAYAKER	NAPALMS	RAVAGES	BADCASE	CAPTAIN	FARMAID	KANSANS	MAXBAER	RAMFANS	TARMACS	BACKBAY	CASHBAR
EATABLE	LABAMBA	NARAYAN	SABADOS	BADDAYS	CAPUANA	FARRAGO	LABIALS	MAYDAYS	RAMPAGE	TARSALS	BACKPAY	CASITAS
EATALOT	LABATTS	NASALLY	SAFARIS	BADHAIR	CARBARN	FATBACK	LABIATE	MAYFAIR	RAMPANT	TARTANS	BACKSAW	CASPIAN
EATAWAY	LADADOG	NATALIA	SAHARAN	BADHAND	CARCARE	FATCATS	LABRATS	MAYNARD	RAMPART	TARTARE	BACKWAY	CASSIAS
FABARES	LAFARGE	NATALIE	SALAAMS	BADHATS	CARCASS	FATFARM	LACTAID	MAYTAGS	RANBACK	TARTARS	BAGHDAD	CATALAN
FACADES	LAGASSE	NATASHA	SALABLE	BADLAND	CARFARE	GABBANA	LACTASE	NAHUATL	RANDALL	TARZANA	BAHAMAS	CATBOAT
FADAYEV	LAHAINA	NATATOR	SALADES	BADNAME	CARJACK	GAETANO	LACTATE	NAIPAUL	RANLAPS	TARZANS	BAITCAR	CATENAE
FALAFEL	LALAKER	NAVAHOS	SALADIN	BADPAST	CARNABY	GAGLAWS	LAGGARD	NARRATE	RANLATE	TATIANA	BAKEPAN	CATENAS
FANATIC	LALANNE	NAVAIDS	SALAMIS	BADRAPS	CARNAGE	GALEATE	LAMBADA	NARVAEZ	RANPAST	TAXBASE	BALABAN	CATERAS
FARADAY	LAMAISM	NAVAJOS	SALAZAR	BAGGAGE	CARPALS	GALLANT	LANDAUS	NASTASE	RANSACK	TAXLAWS	BALATAS	CATFLAP
FARAWAY	LAMAIST	NAVARRE	SAMARAS	BAGLADY	CARPARK	GALPALS	LANTANA	NATHANS	RAPHAEL	TAXPAID	BALBOAS	CATHEAD
FATALES	LAMARCK	NAYARIT	SAMARIA	BAHIANS	CARRARA	GALVANI	LANYARD	NAYSAID	RASCALS	TAXRATE	BALIHAI	CATSCAN
FATALLY	LAPALMA	OAXACAN	SARACEN	BAHRAIN	CARSALE	GALVANO	LAPCATS	NAYSAYS	RATPACK	TAXSALE	BALKSAT	CATSPAW
GAGARIN	LARAINE	PAJAMAS	SARALEE	BAKLAVA	CARTAGE	GAMBADO	LAPLACA	OAHUANS	RATRACE	TAYBACK	BANANAS	CAVEMAN
GAHAGAN	LARAMIE	PALABRA	SARANAC	BALKANS	CARTALK	GANDALF	LAPLACE	OAKCASK	RATTAIL	VACCARO	BANDEAU	CAVILAT
GALAHAD	LASAGNA	PALACES	SARAWAK	BALLADE	CARWASH	GARBAGE	LAPLAND	OAKLAND	RATTANS	VAGRANT	BANDSAW	CAYUGAS
GALANOS	LASAGNE	PALADIN	SARAZEN	BALLADS	CASCADE	GARBAGY	LAPLATA	OAKLAWN	RAWBARS	VALIANT	BARBEAU	DAHLIAS
GALANTS	LASALLE	PALAMAS	SATANIC	BALLARD	CASEATE	GARLAND	LAPSANG	OAKPARK	RAWDATA	VALUATE	BARCLAY	DAKOTAN
GALATEA	LAVABOS	PALANCE	SATATOP	BALLAST	CASPARY	GASBAGS	LAPWARE	OAKTAGS	RAYBANS	VALVATE	BAREXAM	DAKOTAS
GALATIA	LAVACHE	PALATAL	SAVABLE	BALMAIN	CASSABA	GASCANS	LARIATS	OATCAKE	SABBATH	VANCAMP	BARFBAG	DANANAS
GALAXES	LAVAGES	PALATES	SAVAGED	BALSAMS	CASSATT	GASCAPS	LASCALA	PACKAGE	SACCADE	VANDALS	BARKSAT	DANELAW
GALAXIE	LAVAINE	PALAVER	SAVAGER	BALSAMY	CASSAVA	GASLAMP	LASCARS	PACKARD	SADCAFE	VANSANT	BARSOAP	DANTEAN
GARAGED	LAVALSE	PALAZZI	SAVAGES	BANDAGE	CASUALS	GASMAIN	LASCAUX	PADRAIC	SADFATE	VANTAGE	BARTRAY	DARESAY
GARAGES	LAWANDA	PALAZZO	SAVALAS	BANDAID	CATCALL	GASMASK	LASTACT	PADUANS	SADSACK	VANUATU	BASEMAN	DARKMAN
HADACOW	LAYAWAY	PANACEA	SAVANAS	BANDANA	CATHAIR	GASPARD	LAULAUS	PAGEANT	SAGCARD	VANWARD	BASEPAY	DARKTAN
HADAFIT	LAZARUS	PANACHE	SAVANNA	BANTAMS	CATNAPS	GASTANK	LAWCASE	PAHLAVI	SAGUARO	VANZANT	BASINAL	DAYSPAS
HADAGAS	MACABRE	PANADAS	SAVANTS	BANYANS	CATTAIL	GASWARS	LAYBACK	PAIDADS	SAIDAAH	VARIANT	BASSSAX	DAYSTAR
HADAJOB	MACACOS	PANAMAS	SAVARIN	BANZAIS	CATTALO	GATEAUX	LAYBARE	PAISANO	SAIDAYE	VARIATE	BATEMAN	DAYWEAR
HADANIP	MACADAM	PANARAB	SAWATCH	BAOBABS	CATWALK	GATTACA	MACHAON	PAISANS	SALAAMS	VARLAAM	BATHMAT	EARFLAP
HADAROW	MACAQUE	PAPADOC	SAYABLE	BARBARA	CAUDATE	GAUTAMA	MACRAME	PALEALE	SALTANT	VASSALS	BATSMAN	EASTHAM
HADASAY	MADALYN	PAPAGOS	SAYAMEN	BARBARY	CAVEART	GAVIALS	MADCAPS	PALMARY	SALVAGE	WAHWAHS	BAYEDAT	EASTMAN
HADASET	MADAMES	PAPAYAS	TABARDS	BARBATE	CAVEATS	GAZZARA	MADDASH	PALMATE	SAMBAED	WAIKATO	BAYLEAF	EATAWAY
HADATIT	MADAMEX	PARABLE	TABARET	BARCARS	CAVIARE	HAGGARD	MAENADS	PALPATE	SAMBASS	WALLABY	CABALAS	EATENAT
HALALAS	MAGALOG	PARADED	TABASCO	BARGAIN	CAVIARS	HAIKAIS	MAGNANI	PANCAKE	SAMOANS	WALLACE	CABANAS	FACTUAL
HALAVAH	MAHALIA	PARADER	TAGALOG	BARMAID	CAYMANS	HALDANE	MAGNATE	PANGAEA	SAMPANS	WALLACH	CABEZAS	FACULAE
HAMACHI	MAHARIS	PARADES	TAGAMET	BARNABY	DABHAND	HALVAHS	MAGYARS	PAPUANS	SANDALS	WALMART	CAKEPAN	FADIMAN
HANAPER	MAHATMA	PARADOR	TAKABLE	BARNARD	DADAART	HALYARD	MAITAIS	PARBAKE	SANTAFE	WANNABE	CALAMAR	FAIRFAX
HASACOW	MAKABLE	PARADOX	TALARIA	BARRACK	DAKTARI	HANDAXE	MALEANT	PARFAIT	SANTANA	WANTADS	CALIBAN	FAIRWAY
HASAFIT	MALABAR	PARAGON	TAMABLE	BARRAGE	DARKAGE	HANGARS	MALIANS	PARIAHS	SAPSAGO	WANTAGH	CAMERAE	FAJITAS
HASAGAS	MALACCA	PARAIBA	TAMALES	BARTABS	DASTARD	HANSARP	MALLARD	PARKADE	SARCASM	WARBABY	CAMERAL	FARADAY
HASANIP	MALACHI	PARAMUS	TAMARAC	BARWARE	DAYCAMP	HARBACH	MALPASO	PARKAVE	SASHAYS	WARFARE	CAMERAS	FARAWAY
HASAROW	MALAGAN	PARAPET	TANAGER	BASMATI	DAYCARE	HARHARS	MALRAUX	PARLAYS	SATBACK	WARGAME	CANCHAS	FAREWAR
HASASAY	MALAGAS	PARAPHS	TARANTO	BASSALE	DAYGAME	HARLAND	MALTASE	PARTAKE	SATIATE	WARHAWK	CANIDAE	FARINAS
HASASET	MALAISE	PARASKI	TATAMIS	BASSANI	DAYMARE	HARRAHS	MALWARE	PASSADE	SATRAPS	WARPAGE	CANOLAS	FARMGAL
HASATIT	MALAMUD	PARASOL	TAXABLE	BASSANO	DAYPACK	HARTACK	MAMMALS	PASSADO	SATRAPY	WARPATH	CANTSAY	FASCIAE
HATABLE	MALARIA	PARATUS	VACANCY	BATDAYS	DAYSAIL	HARVARD	MANDALA	PASSAGE	SAUNAED	WARRANT	CANULAE	FASCIAL
HAVANAN	MALARKY	PASALLE	VACATED	BATEAUX	EARHART	HATBAND	MANDANS	PASSAIC	SAUSAGE	WASFAIR	CANULAS	FASCIAS
HAVANAS	MALAYAN	PATACAS	VACATES	BAUHAUS	EARLAPS	HATRACK	MANDATE	PASSANT	SAWPAST	WASLATE	CAPEMAY	FASTCAR
HAVARTI	MAMAMIA	PAVANES	VALADON	BAZAARS	EARMARK	HAULAGE	MANDAYS	PASSATS	SAYMASS	WASSAIL	CAPITAL	FATHEAD
HAZANIM	MANACLE	PAYABLE	VALANCE	CABBAGE	EARTABS	HAVEAGO	MANGANO	PATCASH	SAYSAAH	WASTAGE	CAPITAN	FAUXPAS
HAZARDS	MANAGED	QABALAH	VANADIC	CABBAGY	EARTAGS	HAWHAWS	MANIACS	PATHAND	SAYSAYE	WATTAGE	CAPSHAW	FAYWRAY
JACALES	MANAGER	QABALAS	WABASHA	CABBALA	EATCAKE	HAYBALE	MANKATO	PATHANS	SAYWAIT	WAYBACK	CAPSTAN	GAHAGAN
JACAMAR	MANAGES	QATARIS	WAKAMES	CABFARE	EATLATE	HAYRACK	MANMADE	PAWPAWS	TAGDAYS	WAYLAID	CARACAS	GAINSAY
JAIALAI	MANAGUA	RADAMES	WASABIS	CACHACA	FACIALS	HAYWARD	MANSARD	PAYBACK	TAGGANT	WAYLAND	CARAVAN	GALAHAD

GALENAS
GAMBIAN
GAMEBAG
GAMELAN
GAMELAW
GAMETAL
GANGSAW
GANGWAY
GAPEDAT
GAPESAT
GARNEAU
GASHEAT
GASLEAK
GASSMAN
GATEMAN
GATEWAY
GAVEEAR
GAVEWAY
GAVILAN
GAWKSAT
GAZEDAT
GAZESAT
HABITAT
HACKMAN
HACKSAW
HADAGAS
HADASAY
HADRIAN
HAITIAN
HALALAS
HALAVAH
HALFBAD
HALFDAY
HALFMAD
HALFRAW
HALFWAY
HALIFAX
HALLWAY
HANDBAG
HANDCAR
HANDSAW
HANGMAN
HANUKAH
HARDDAY
HARDHAT
HARDPAN
HARDWAY
HARTMAN
HASAGAS
HASASAY
HAVANAN
HAVANAS
HAWKMAN
JACAMAR
JACKDAW
JACKTAR
JAIALAI
JAMBEAU
JANEWAY
JAVAMAN
JAWEDAT
JAZZMAN
KAHUNAS
KAMERAD
KANAKAS
KANTIAN
KAPITAL
KARAJAN

KAUFMAN
LABCOAT
LABORAT
LACTEAL
LACUNAE
LACUNAL
LACUNAR
LACUNAS
LADIDAS
LADYDAY
LADYNAS
LAGUNAS
LAKOTAS
LAMBDAS
LAMBEAU
LAMINAE
LAMINAL
LAMINAR
LAMINAS
LANCIAS
LANDMAN
LANDSAT
LANDTAG
LANDTAX
LANGHAM
LANGWAY
LAOTIAN
LAPUTAN
LASTGAS
LASTLAP
LASTMAY
LATERAL
LATERAN
LATETAG
LATIFAH
LATINAS
LATVIAN
LAUGHAT
LAVERAN
LAYAWAY
MACADAM
MACGRAW
MACLEAN
MACULAE
MACULAR
MADEHAY
MADEMAD
MADEPAR
MADEWAR
MADEWAY
MADIGAN
MAGICAL
MAILBAG
MAILCAR
MAILMAN
MAINMAN
MAKEHAY
MAKEMAD
MAKEPAR
MAKEWAR
MAKEWAY
MALABAR
MALAGAN
MALAGAS
MALAYAN
MALECAT
MALLRAT
MANANAS

MANILAS
MANOWAR
MANSMAN
MANTRAP
MANTRAS
MANTUAN
MANXCAT
MANXMAN
MANYEAR
MARACAS
MARCEAU
MARDIAN
MARIDAS
MARINAS
MARITAL
MARKHAM
MARKKAA
MARRYAT
MARSBAR
MARSHAL
MARTIAL
MARTIAN
MARXIAN
MARYKAY
MATEWAN
MATHIAS
MATINAL
MATTHAU
MAUGHAM
MAUPRAT
MAURIAC
MAURIAT
MAXIMAL
MAXIMAS
MAYORAL
NAMEDAY
NAMETAG
NARAYAN
NARWHAL
NATURAL
NAUSEAM
NAVIDAD
NAVYMAN
OAKLEAF
OARSMAN
OATBRAN
OATMEAL
OAXACAN
PAANGAS
PACECAR
PACELAP
PACKRAT
PADUCAH
PAELLAS
PAGODAS
PAJAMAS
PALAMAS
PALATAL
PALOMAR
PALOMAS
PALUDAL
PANADAS
PANAMAS
PANARAB
PANCHAX
PANGRAM
PAPAYAS
PARKMAN

PARKWAY
PARTIAL
PARTWAY
PASCHAL
PATACAS
PATHWAY
PATINAS
PAWEDAT
PAYLOAD
PAYOLAS
QABALAH
QABALAS
RACECAR
RACEWAY
RADICAL
RADIOAD
RAFFIAS
RAILCAR
RAILMAN
RAILSAT
RAILWAY
RAINHAT
RAINMAN
RAJARAO
RAMADAN
RAMADAS
RAMSFAN
RANATAB
RANAWAY
RANTSAT
RAPIDAN
RAPSTAR
RAREGAS
RARITAN
RATATAT
RATECAP
RATTRAP
RAVENAL
RAWDEAL
RAWMEAT
RAYOVAC
SAFEWAY
SAGINAW
SAHARAN
SAIDAAH
SAIDNAY
SALAZAR
SALINAS
SALIVAS
SAMARAS
SAMEDAY
SAMOSAS
SAMOVAR
SAMPRAS
SAMURAI
SANBLAS
SANDBAG
SANDBAR
SANDDAB
SANDMAN
SANJUAN
SAPHEAD
SARANAC
SARAWAK
SAROYAN
SARUMAN
SAURIAN
SAVALAS

SAVANAS
SAYSAAH
SAYSNAY
SAYWHAT
TABLEAU
TABULAR
TACOMAS
TACTUAL
TAGTEAM
TAILWAG
TALIBAN
TALKSAT
TAMARAC
TANGRAM
TANKCAR
TAPEMAN
TASKBAR
TAUREAN
TAXICAB
TAXIMAN
TAXIWAY
TAXYEAR
VALJEAN
VANLOAD
VARLAAM
VATICAL
VATICAN
VAUGHAN
WAGEWAR
WAKSMAN
WALKMAN
WALKWAY
WALLMAP
WALTHAM
WARHEAD
WASHDAY
WASHRAG
WATTEAU
WAVEDAT
WAVESAT
WAXBEAN
XANTHAN
YAKIMAS
YALELAW
YALEMAN
YAMAHAS
YANKSAT
YARDMAN
YASHMAK
YAYTEAM
ZAIRIAN
ZAMBIAN
ZAPATAS

•A••••A

BACHATA
BACTRIA
BADAREA
BADIDEA
BAKLAVA
BAMBINA
BANDANA
BANDERA
BARBARA
BARBERA
BARBUDA
BARETTA
BARISTA

BATAVIA
BATISTA
BAVARIA
BAYAREA
BAZOOKA
CABBALA
CACHACA
CADENZA
CAESURA
CAHOKIA
CALDERA
CALISTA
CALMSEA
CAMBRIA
CAMILLA
CANASTA
CANDELA
CANDIDA
CANNULA
CANTATA
CANTINA
CANZONA
CAPELLA
CAPTIVA
CAPUANA
CARAMBA
CARAMIA
CARIOCA
CARLOTA
CARMELA
CARMINA
CARNERA
CARRARA
CARRERA
CASELLA
CASERTA
CASSABA
CASSAVA
CASSOLA
CATALPA
CATANIA
CATAWBA
CATFLEA
DACOSTA
DANIELA
DAPHNIA
DASILVA
DAYTONA
FAMILIA
GABBANA
GALATEA
GALATIA
GALICIA
GANGLIA
GANGSTA
GARDENA
GATTACA
GAUTAMA
GAZZARA
HANKIBA
IACOCCA
JAKARTA
JAMAICA
KABBALA
KACHINA
KAMPALA
KAPITSA
KARASEA

KATISHA
KATRINA
LABAMBA
LACERTA
LACONIA
LAHAINA
LAJOLLA
LAMBADA
LAMOTTA
LANTANA
LAPALMA
LAPLACA
LAPLATA
LARUSSA
LASAGNA
LASCALA
LASORDA
LATOSCA
LAVINIA
LAWANDA
LAZONGA
MAANDPA
MACHINA
MACONGA
MADEIRA
MADONNA
MAGENTA
MAGILLA
MAHALIA
MAHATMA
MAJORCA
MALACCA
MALARIA
MALLIKA
MALVINA
MAMAMIA
MANAGUA
MANDALA
MANDELA
MANTECA
MARIANA
MARILLA
MARIMBA
MARKKAA
MARKOVA
MARMARA
MARSALA
MARTINA
MARUSJA
MASCARA
MATILDA
MAXILLA
MAZEPPA
MAZURKA
NAMIBIA
NAPHTHA
NATALIA
NATASHA
NAUTICA
PALABRA
PALMYRA
PALOOKA
PANACEA
PANDORA
PANETTA
PANGAEA
PANTERA
PAPILLA

PAPRIKA
PARAIBA
PARTITA
PASTINA
PATELLA
PAULINA
PAVLOVA
RASBORA
RASHIDA
RATAFIA
RAVENNA
RAWDATA
SABRINA
SAGETEA
SALONGA
SALSODA
SALTSEA
SAMARIA
SAMBORA
SAMBUCA
SANGRIA
SANTANA
SATSUMA
SAVANNA
SAXTUBA
TABITHA
TAFFETA
TAKETEA
TALARIA
TAMBALA
TANTARA
TAPIOCA
TARZANA
TATIANA
TAVERNA
VALVULA
VAMPIRA
VANDURA
VANESSA
VANILLA
WABASHA
YASHICA
ZAKUSKA

••AA•••

DNAASES
ELAAIUN
SEAARMS

••A•A••

AAAMAPS
ADAMANT
ADAWARE
ADAYAGO
ALABAMA
ALABAMY
ANASAZI
ANATASE
ARACARI
ARAMAIC
ARAMARK
ARAPAHO
ASALARK
ATACAMA
ATAMANS
ATARAXY
AVATARS
BEATALL

BLATANT
BRANAGH
BRAVADA
BRAVADO
BYAHAIR
CHAGALL
CHAPALA
CHAPATI
CHARADE
CHAZANS
CLAMANT
CLAMATO
CLAVATE
CRAVATS
DEADAIR
DIAHANN
DNALABS
DOAGAIN
DRAMADY
DRAYAGE
EMANANT
EMANATE
GRADATE
GRAHAME
GRAHAMS
GRANADA
GRANARY
GUANACO
GUARANI
HEALALL
IMAMATE
INABALL
INACAST
INADAZE
INARAGE
INAVALE
JEANARP
KHANATE
KHATAMI
KLAMATH
LEAFAGE
LEAKAGE
LHASANS
MBABANE
MCADAMS
MEANAGE
MEATAXE
MIAHAMM
MIASARA
MTADAMS
NBAGAME
NIAGARA
OCALAFL
OCANADA
OFANAGE
OMAHANE
OMAHANS
ONADARE
ONADATE
ONALARK
OSAKANS
OXALATE
PEASANT
PHALANX
PHARAOH
PLACARD
PLACATE
PLAKATS

PLANATE
PLAYACT
QUAPAWS
QUASARS
QUAYAGE
READAPT
REAGANS
REAMASS
REAVAIL
REAWAKE
SCALAGE
SCALARS
SCARABS
SEABAGS
SEABASS
SEACALM
SEACATS
SEAFARE
SEAGATE
SEAHAWK
SEALABS
SEALANE
SEALANT
SEAMAPS
SEARACE
SEASALT
SEAWALL
SEAWARD
SEAWAYS
SHALALA
SHAMANS
SHANANA
SPANAIR
STALAGS
TEABAGS
TEABALL
TEACAKE
TEACART
TIARAED
TOAHAIR
TRALALA
TRAVAIL
UNAWAKE
UNAWARE
UTAHANS
VEADARS
WHATAMI
ZEALAND

••A••A•

ACACIAS
ACADIAN
ACAUDAL
AGAKHAN
ALANJAY
ALANNAH
ALASKAN
ALASKAS
ALASSAD
AMALGAM
ANAGRAM
ANANIAS
ARABIAN
ARAMEAN
ASAGRAY
ASATEAM
AZALEAS
AZANIAN

BEACHAM
BEANBAG
BEARCAT
BEARPAW
BEATSAT
BIAFRAN
BIAXIAL
BOATMAN
BRAHMAN
BRAHMAS
CHACHAS
CHAKRAS
CHALLAH
CHAPEAU
CHAPMAN
CHARMAN
CHARPAK
CHASMAL
CHATEAU
CHATHAM
CHAZZAN
CLAMBAR
CLAUSAL
CLAWSAT
COALCAR
COALGAS
COALTAR
COASTAL
COAXIAL
CPAEXAM
CRANIAL
CRASHAW
CRAWDAD
CSARDAS
CZARDAS
DEADPAN
DHARMAS
DIAGRAM
DIAPHAN
DOADEAL
DRAWBAR
DRAWMAN
DRAYMAN
EXACTAS
FHALOAN
FLAGDAY
FLAGMAN
FLAILAT
FLATCAR
FLATHAT
FLATTAX
FLAUTAS
FRACTAL
GHANIAN
GLACIAL
GLAREAT
GNAWSAT
GOAHEAD
GRABBAG
GRABBAR
GRABSAT
GRACIAS
GRADEAA
GRADUAL
GRAMMAR
GRAMPAS
GRANDAM
GRANPAS

GRAPPAS
GRASPAT
GRATIAS
GRAUMAN
GRAVLAX
GRAYJAY
GRAYLAG
HEADMAN
HEADSAW
HEADWAY
HEARSAY
HEATFAN
HEATRAY
HIALEAH
HJALMAR
IDAHOAN
INAHEAP
INASNAP
INATRAP
IRANIAN
ISABEAU
ISAHEAD
ITALIAN
KHAYYAM
KWACHAS
KWANZAA
KWANZAS
LEADMAN
LEAPDAY
LEAPSAT
LEAPTAT
LOAFPAN
MEATMAN
MIAMIAN
MIASMAL
MIASMAS
MUAMMAR
MYANMAR
NBATEAM
NEARPAR
OBADIAH
ONABIAS
ONALEAD
ONATEAR
PAANGAS
PEABEAN
PEACOAT
PHARLAP
PIAZZAS
PLANTAR
PLASMAS
PLATEAU
PLAYSAT
QUAGGAS
QUARTAN
REALMAN
REASSAY
REATTAS
ROADMAP
ROADTAR
ROADTAX
ROADWAY
ROARSAT
RUANDAS
RWANDAN
SCANDAL
SCATMAN
SEABOAT

SEAFOAM
SEAGRAM
SEASTAR
SHABBAT
SHANKAR
SHAVIAN
SKAGWAY
SMALLAD
SNAPSAT
SNARLAT
SOAPPAD
SPACIAL
SPARTAN
SPATIAL
STANZAS
STAREAT
STARMAN
STARMAP
STAYSAT
SWAGMAN
SWATSAT
SWAYBAR
TEALEAF
TEARGAS
TEARSAT
TEATRAY
THATWAY
TRAMCAR
TRAMPAS
TRAMWAY
TRANSAM
TRAUMAS
UGANDAN
UPAHEAD
WHATSAY
XRAYLAB
YEAHMAN
YEATEAM

••A•••A

ALABAMA
ALAMEDA
ALAMOSA
AMANITA
AMAPOLA
ANAEMIA
ARABICA
ARAFURA
ARALSEA
ARANTXA
ATACAMA
BLACULA
BRAVADA
BRAVURA
CHACHKA
CHALUPA
CHAPALA
CLAUDIA
CRAPOLA
CRAYOLA
CZARINA
DEADSEA
DRACHMA
DRACULA
ELANTRA
EVALUNA
GRADEAA
GRANADA

GRANDMA
GRANDPA
GRANITA
GRANOLA
IPANEMA
ISADORA
KWANZAA
MAANDPA
MIASARA
MYALGIA
NDAKOTA
NIAGARA
OCANADA
OCARINA
OTALGIA
PHAEDRA
PIANOLA
SCAPULA
SDAKOTA
SHAKIRA
SHALALA
SHANANA
SHARONA
SNAPPEA
SPATULA
STAMINA
SWANSEA
TEAMUSA
TRACHEA
TRALALA
TSARINA
TZARINA
ULANOVA
VIATICA

•••AA••

ALMAATA
BAZAARS
DADAART
DEWAART
SALAAMS

•••A•A•

ABRAHAM
ABRAXAS
ALCAZAR
ALMANAC
ALPACAS
ANDAMAN
ANKARAN
ANNAMAY
APPARAT
AQUAMAN
AREAMAP
AREAWAY
ARMADAS
ARRABAL
ARRAYAL
ASFARAS
ASKAWAY
ASMARAN
ATEAWAY
AZKABAN
BAHAMAS
BALABAN
BALATAS
BANANAS
BENATAR
BETAMAX
BETARAY
BROADAS
BROADAX
CABALAS
CABANAS
CALAMAR
CARACAS
CARAVAN
CARAWAY
CASABAS
CASAVAS
CATALAN
CHIAPAS
CICADAE
CICADAS
COLADAS
CURACAO
CUTAWAY
DANANAS
DIEAWAY
DINADAM
DUNAWAY
EATAWAY
EDNAMAY
ELEAZAR
ELLAMAE
FARADAY
FARAWAY
FLEABAG
FLYAWAY
FORADAY
GAHAGAN
GALAHAD
GETAWAY
GOTAWAY
GUJARAT
HADAGAS
HADASAY
HALALAS
HALAVAH
HASAGAS
HASASAY
HAVANAN
HAVANAS
HIDAWAY
HOPACAB
IDEAMAN
IGUANAS
IMPALAS
ISFAHAN
ITHACAN
JACAMAR
JAIALAI
JAVAMAN
JICAMAS
JUMADAS
KANAKAS
KARAJAN
LAYAWAY
LEDAWAY
LISAGAY
MACADAM
MALABAR
MALAGAN
MALAGAS
MALAYAN
MANANAS
MARACAS
MEDAKAS
MEDAWAR
MIKASAS
MIRADAS
MIRAMAR
MIRAMAX
MONACAN
MONADAL
MUBARAK
NARAYAN
NEVADAN
NONARAB
OAXACAN
OCTAVAL
OGLALAS
ONEACAT
ONEADAY
OTTAWAN
OTTAWAS
PAJAMAS
PALAMAS
PALATAL
PANADAS
PANAMAS
PANARAB
PAPAYAS
PATACAS
PEGAWAY
PHRASAL
PICARAS
PINATAS
PITAPAT
PITAYAS
POLARAS
POSADAS
PROARAB
PUTAWAY
QABALAH
QABALAS
RAJARAO
RAMADAN
RAMADAS
RANATAB
RANAWAY
RATATAT
RITAGAM
RITAMAE
ROTAWAY
RUNATAB
RUNAWAY
SAHARAN
SALAZAR
SAMARAS
SARANAC
SARAWAK
SAVALAS
SAVANAS
SEMANAS
SHYAWAY
SODACAN
SOFARAS
SOLARAS
SONATAS
STRATAS
SWEARAT
TAMARAC
TEJANAS
TITANAE
TOWAWAY
ULZANAS
UNNASAL
UNPAGAN
VIHARAS
VISAYAN
VITARAS
YAMAHAS
YOGAMAT
YUCATAN
YUKATAS
ZAPATAS
ZENANAS

•••A••A

ALBANIA
ALFALFA
ALMAATA
ALSATIA
APHAGIA
APHASIA
AQUARIA
ARCADIA
ATLANTA
AVIANCA
BADAREA
BATAVIA
BAVARIA
BAYAREA
BOBATEA
BONANZA
CANASTA
CARAMBA
CARAMIA
CATALPA
CATANIA
CATAWBA
CONAGRA
CROATIA
DEFALLA
DEPALMA
DRLAURA
ENCARTA
EURASIA
GALATEA
GALATIA
HIMALIA
HOSANNA
HYPATIA
IHEARYA
ILIAMNA
INFANTA
JAKARTA
JAMAICA
JOCASTA
JOHANNA
JUDAICA
KARASEA
KILAUEA
LABAMBA
LAHAINA
LAPALMA
LASAGNA
LAWANDA
LEGANZA
LUCANIA
MAHALIA
MAHATMA
MALACCA
MALARIA
MAMAMIA
MANAGUA
MEGAERA
MELANIA
MICAELA
MIRANDA
MORAVIA
MYLANTA
NATALIA
NATASHA
OCEANIA
OCTAVIA
OLEANNA
ORGANZA
PALABRA
PANACEA
PARAIBA
PERAHIA
PIRANHA
RATAFIA
REDALGA
REGALIA
REGATTA
ROMANIA
RORAIMA
ROSALIA
ROSANNA
RUMANIA
SAMARIA
SAVANNA
SEDALIA
SINATRA
SKIAREA
SOLARIA
SOMALIA
SUBAREA
SUMATRA
SUSANNA
TALARIA
TITANIA
VERANDA
VIDALIA
VISALIA
VIVARIA
WABASHA
YOLANDA
YUCAIPA
ZIMARRA

••••AA•

DENHAAG
FIVEAAA
FOURAAA
JIMKAAT
ROLVAAG
SAIDAAH
SAYSAAH
SELMAAL
VARLAAM
YESMAAM

••••A•A

ADRIANA
AIRMADA
ALABAMA
ALIBABA
ALMAATA
AMERADA
AMIDALA
ARIKARA
ATACAMA
AZUSACA
BACHATA
BAKLAVA
BANDANA
BARBARA
BIGMAMA
BIODATA
BOKHARA
BRAVADA
BUKHARA
CABBALA
CACHACA
CANTATA
CAPUANA
CARRARA
CASSABA
CASSAVA
CHAPALA
CHICANA
DIORAMA
DOGMATA
EDEMATA
ENTRADA
ESTRADA
FERMATA
FERRARA
FIVEAAA
FONTANA
FOURAAA
GABBANA
GATTACA
GAUTAMA
GAZZARA
GETSANA
GODMAMA
GODPAPA
GONZAGA
GRANADA
GRENADA
GUEVARA
HERMANA
HONIARA
IKEBANA
ILLEANA
INDIANA
JORDANA
JULIANA
KABBALA
KAMPALA
KITHARA
KOLKATA
LAMBADA
LANTANA
LAPLACA
LAPLATA
LASCALA
LEMMATA
LINEARA
LUCIANA
MANDALA
MARIANA
MARMARA
MARSALA
MASCARA
MESSALA
MIASARA
MOMBASA
MONTANA
MORGANA
MUSTAFA
NIAGARA
NIRVANA
OCANADA
OKINAWA
OOHLALA
OSTRAVA
OVIPARA
PANGAEA
PICCATA
POLTAVA
PREDATA
PRORATA
QUEPASA
RAWDATA
SANTANA
SHALALA
SHANANA
SMETANA
STOMATA
SULTANA
SYRIANA
TAMBALA
TANTARA
TARZANA
TATIANA
TIJUANA
TOCCATA
TOSTADA
TRALALA
TYMPANA
UPPSALA
VICDANA
WYOTANA

•••••AA

FIVEAAA
FOURAAA
GRADEAA
KWANZAA
MARKKAA
RUFIYAA
VIVICAA

AB•••••

ABALONE
ABANDON
ABASERS
ABASHED
ABASHES
ABASING
ABATERS
ABATING
ABATORS
ABBOTCY
ABCDEFG
ABCNEWS
ABDOMEN
ABDUCED
ABDUCES
ABDUCTS
ABELARD
ABETTAL
ABETTED
ABETTER
ABETTOR
ABEYANT
ABIDEBY
ABIDERS
ABIDING
ABIDJAN
ABIGAIL
ABILENE
ABILITY
ABINTRA
ABIOTIC
ABITIBI
ABJURED
ABJURER
ABJURES
ABLATED
ABLATES
ABOLISH
ABOLLAE
ABORTED
ABOUNDS
ABOUTIT
ABOUTTO
ABRADED
ABRADER
ABRADES
ABRAHAM
ABRAXAS
ABREAST
ABRIDGE
ABRILES
ABROACH
ABRUZZI
ABSALOM
ABSCISE
ABSCOND
ABSENCE
ABSENTS
ABSINTH
ABSOLUT
ABSOLVE
ABSORBS
ABSTAIN
ABUSERS
ABUSING
ABUSIVE
ABUTSON
ABUTTAL
ABUTTED
ABUTTER
ABYSMAL
ABYSSAL
ABYSSES

A•B••••

ABBOTCY
ALBANIA
ALBEDOS
ALBENIZ
ALBERTA
ALBERTI
ALBERTO
ALBINOS
ALBIREO
ALBORAK
ALBSURE
ALBUMEN
ALBUMIN
ALBUNDY
AMBIENS
AMBIENT
AMBLERS
AMBLING
AMBRIES
AMBROSE
ANBESOL
ARBACES
ARBITER
ARBOLES
ARBORED
ARBOURS
ARBUTUS
ASBYATT
AUBADES
AUBERGE
AUBURNS
AUBURNU

A••B•••

AIRBAGS
AIRBALL
AIRBASE
AIRBILL
AIRBOAT
AKEBONO
ALABAMA
ALABAMY
ALIBABA
ALIBIED
ALLBRAN
AMEBOID
AMIBLUE
ANTBEAR
ANTBIRD
ANYBODY
ARABIAN
ARABICA
ARABICS
ARABIST
ARABLES
ARLBERG
ARMBAND
ARMBONE
ARTBOOK
ARUBANS
ASABODY
ASHBERY
ASHBINS
ASHBURN
ASHBURY
ATABOIL

A•••B••

ACERBIC
ACROBAT
ACTABLE
ADDABLE
ADDIBLE
ADHIBIT
AEROBAT
AEROBES
AEROBIC
AFFABLE
AFFABLY
AGRIBIZ
ALARBUS
ALDUBIN
ALEMBIC
ALGEBRA
AMIABLE
AMIABLY
AMOEBAE
AMOEBAS
AMOEBIC
ANNABEL
ANTIBES
ARRABAL
ATEABIT
ATTABOY
AUDIBLE
AUDIBLY
AUDUBON
AUNTBEE
AUSABLE
AUTOBIO
AUTOBUS
AWEEBIT
AZKABAN

A••••B•

AAJUMBO
ABIDEBY
ABITIBI
ABSORBS
ADSORBS
ADVERBS
AIRTUBE
ALGIEBA
ALIBABA
ALLENBY
ALTTABS
ARECIBO
ASCRIBE

•AB••••

BABBAGE
BABBITT
BABBLED
BABBLER
BABBLES
BABCOCK
BABENCO
BABETTE
BABIEST
BABIYAR
BABOONS
BABYBOP
BABYGAP
BABYING
BABYISH
BABYLON
BABYOIL
BABYSAT
BABYSIT
CABALAS
CABALLE
CABANAS
CABARET
CABBAGE
CABBAGY
CABBALA
CABBIES
CABBING
CABEZAS
CABFARE
CABINET
CABLERS
CABLETS
CABLETV
CABLING
CABOOSE
CABRIDE
CABRINI
CABRIOS
DABBERS
DABBING
DABBLED
DABBLER
DABBLES
DABHAND
FABARES
FABBEST
FABERGE
FABFOUR
FABLERS
FABLING
FABRICS
FABRIZI
GABBANA
GABBERS
GABBIER
GABBING
GABBLED
GABBLES
GABBROS
GABFEST
GABRIEL
HABILIS
HABITAT
HABITED
HABITUE
JABBERS
JABBING
KABBALA
KABUKIS
LABAMBA
LABATTS
LABCOAT
LABELED
LABELER
LABELLE
LABFEES
LABIALS
LABIATE
LABMICE
LABORAT
LABORED
LABORER
LABOURS
LABRATS
LABTECH
LABTEST
LABTUBE
NABBERS
NABBING
NABISCO
NABOKOV
NABUCCO
PABLUMS
PABULUM
QABALAH
QABALAS
RABBETS
RABBITS
RABBITT
RABBITY
RABBLED
RABBLES
RABIDLY
SABADOS
SABBATH
SABERED
SABINES
SABRINA
TABARDS
TABARET
TABASCO
TABBIES
TABBING
TABITHA
TABKEYS
TABLEAU
TABLETS
TABLING
TABLOID
TABOOED
TABORET
TABOULI
TABSETS
TABUING
TABULAR
WABASHA
WABBITS
ZABUTON

•A•B•••

BABBAGE
BABBITT
BABBLED
BABBLER
BABBLES
BADBACK
BADBOYS
BAGBOYS
BALBOAS
BAMBIII
BAMBINA
BAMBINI
BAMBINO
BAMBOOS
BANBURY
BAOBABS
BARBARA
BARBARY
BARBATE
BARBEAU
BARBELL
BARBERA
BARBERS
BARBETS
BARBIES
BARBILL
BARBING
BARBUDA
BARBULE
BATBOYS
BAUBLES
CABBAGE
CABBAGY
CABBALA
CABBIES
CABBING
CADBURY
CAMBERS
CAMBOYS
CAMBRIA
CAMBRIC
CARBARN
CARBIDE
CARBINE
CARBONS
CARBOYS
CARBRAS
CATBEDS
CATBERT
CATBIRD
CATBOAT
CATBOWL
DABBERS
DABBING
DABBLED
DABBLER
DABBLES
DANBURY
DASBOOT
DAUBERS
DAUBING
DAYBEDS
DAYBOOK
EARBONE
EARBUDS
FABBEST
FANBASE
FANBELT
FATBACK
GABBANA
GABBERS
GABBIER
GABBING
GABBLED
GABBLES
GABBROS
GAMBADO
GAMBIAN
GAMBIER
GAMBITS
GAMBLED
GAMBLER
GAMBLES
GAMBOLS
GARBAGE
GARBAGY
GARBING
GARBLED
GARBLER
GARBLES
GASBAGS
HADBEEN
HADBEST
HAMBONE
HAMBURG
HARBACH
HARBORS
HARBOUR

HARBURG
HASBEEN
HATBAND
HATBRIM
HAYBALE
IAMBICS
IAMBIST
JABBERS
JABBING
JAMBAND
JAMBEAU
JAWBONE
JAYBIRD
KABBALA
LAMBADA
LAMBDAS
LAMBEAU
LAMBENT
LAMBERT
LAMBETH
LAMBING
LAMBKIN
LAPBELT
LAWBOOK
LAYBACK
LAYBARE
LAZBOYS
MACBETH
MAMBOED
MARBLED
MARBLER
MARBLES
MAXBAER
MAXBORN
MAYBESO
NABBERS
NABBING
OATBRAN
PACBELL
PARBAKE
PARBOIL
PAYBACK
RABBETS
RABBITS
RABBITT
RABBITY
RABBLED
RABBLES
RAEBURN
RAGBAGS
RAMBLED
RAMBLER
RAMBLES
RAMBLIN
RANBACK
RASBORA
RATBERT
RAWBARS
RAYBANS
RAYBURN
SABBATH
SAMBAED
SAMBASS
SAMBORA
SAMBUCA
SANBLAS
SANBORN
SATBACK
SAWBUCK
TABBIES
TABBING
TAMBALA
TAMBLYN
TANBARK
TARBABY
TARBELL
TAXBASE
TAYBACK
WABBITS
WAMBLED
WAMBLES
WARBABY
WARBLED
WARBLER
WARBLES
WARBOND
WARBURG
WAXBEAN
WAYBACK
WAYBILL
YASBECK
ZAMBEZI
ZAMBIAN
ZAMBONI

•A••B••

BABYBOP
BACKBAR
BACKBAY
BACKBIT
BALABAN
BALLBOY
BANDBOX
BARFBAG
CALABRO
CALIBAN
CALIBER
CALIBRE
CALLBOX
CALLBOY
CAMPBED
CAPABLE
CAPABLY
CARABOO
CARIBES
CARIBOO
CARIBOU
CASABAS
CASHBAR
CASHBOX
DATABLE
DATABUS
EATABIT
EATABLE
FAREBOX
FARMBOY
GAMEBAG
GAMEBOY
GAZEBOS
HALFBAD
HALIBUT
HANDBAG
HANGBYS
HATABLE
HAUTBOY
JACOBIN
JAZZBOS
LADYBUG
LAKEBED
LAVABOS
MACABRE
MAILBAG
MAILBIN
MAILBOX
MAKABLE
MALABAR
MALEBEE
MALTBIE
MARSBAR
NAMABLE
NAMABLY
NAMIBIA
PAGEBOY
PALABRA
PARABLE
PARIBUS
PAYABLE
RAILBUS
RAINBOW
RAKABLE
RAREBIT
RATABLE
SAFEBET
SAIDBOO
SALABLE
SALTBOX
SANDBAG
SANDBAR
SANDBOX
SANDBUR
SANIBEL
SAVABLE
SAYABLE
SAYSBOO
TAKABLE
TALIBAN
TALKBIG
TAMABLE
TASKBAR
TAXABLE
WASABIS
WAXABLE

•A•••B•

AAJUMBO
BADDEBT
BAGJOBS
BAOBABS
BARNABY
BARTABS
CANITBE
CANTABS
CARAMBA
CARNABY
CASSABA
CATAWBA
DAYJOBS
EARLOBE
EARTABS
EASEDBY
EASESBY
HADTOBE
HANGSBY
HANKIBA
HASTOBE
LABAMBA
LABTUBE
LAPROBE
LATROBE
LAZENBY
MADLIBS
MARIMBA
NAIROBI
PARAIBA
RACEDBY
RACESBY
SAXTUBA
TAKENBY
TARBABY
WALKSBY
WALLABY
WANNABE
WARBABY

•A••••B

BACKRUB
BANKJOB
BATHTUB
CARCLUB
CATCOMB
EASYJOB
FANCLUB
HADAJOB
PANARAB
PAYSTUB
RANATAB
SANDDAB
TAXICAB
VAPORUB
WARCLUB
WASHTUB

••AB•••

ALABAMA
ALABAMY
ARABIAN
ARABICA
ARABICS
ARABIST
ARABLES
ASABODY
ATABOIL
BLABBED
BLABBER
CHABLIS
CLABBER
CRABBED
CRABBER
CRABPOT
DIABLES
DIABLOS
DIABOLO
DRABBER
DRABBLE
ENABLED
ENABLER
ENABLES
EXABYTE
GOABOUT
GRABBAG
GRABBAR
GRABBED
GRABBER
GRABSAT
INABALL
INABIND
ISABEAU
MBABANE
MOABITE
ONABIAS
PEABEAN
PEABODY
SEABAGS
SEABASS
SEABEDS
SEABEES
SEABIRD
SEABLUE
SEABOAT
SEABORG
SHABBAT
SLABBED
STABBED
STABBER
STABILE
STABLED
STABLER
STABLES
SWABBED
SWABBER
TEABAGS
TEABALL
TRABERT
UPABOVE
USABLES

••A•B••

ALARBUS
BEANBAG
BEATBOX
BLABBED
BLABBER
BLAUBOK
BRAMBLE
BRAMBLY
CDALBUM
CHAMBER
CHAMBRE
CLABBER
CLAMBAR
CLAMBER
COALBIN
CRABBED
CRABBER
DRABBER
DRABBLE
DRAWBAR
ENARBOR
FLAMBED
FLAMBES
FLATBED
GEARBOX
GRABBAG
GRABBAR
GRABBED
GRABBER
PEATBOG
PLAYBOY
ROADBED
SHABBAT
SHAMBLE
SLABBED
SOAPBOX
SPAMBOT
STABBED
STABBER
SWABBED
SWABBER
SWAYBAR
TRAUBEL
YEAHBUT

••A••B•

BYANDBY
DNALABS
ETALIBI
LEAVEBE
PLACEBO
PLAYSBY
SCARABS
SEALABS
STANDBY

••A•••B

BEARCUB
XRAYLAB

•••AB••

ACTABLE
ADDABLE
AFFABLE
AFFABLY
AMIABLE
AMIABLY
ANNABEL
ARRABAL
ATEABIT
ATTABOY
AUSABLE
AZKABAN
BALABAN
BELABOR
BUGABOO
BUYABLE
CALABRO
CAPABLE
CAPABLY
CARABOO
CASABAS
CIMABUE
CITABLE
COHABIT
CURABLE
CURABLY
DATABLE
DATABUS
DISABLE
DRYABLE
DURABLE
DURABLY
EATABIT
EATABLE
EFFABLE
EFFABLY
ENDABLE
EQUABLE
EQUABLY
ERRABLE
EULABUS
FINABLE
FIXABLE
FLEABAG
FLYABLE
FORABIT
FRIABLE
FRYABLE
GETABLE
GIGABIT
HATABLE
HIDABLE
HIRABLE
ICHABOD
INHABIT
INLABOR
ITSABOY
LAVABOS
LESABRE
LIEABED
LIKABLE
LINABLE
LIVABLE
LOSABLE
LOVABLE
LOVABLY
MACABRE
MAKABLE
MALABAR
MEGABIT
MINABLE
MIRABEL
MIXABLE
MOVABLE
MOVABLY
MUTABLE
MUTABLY
NAMABLE
NAMABLY
NOTABIT
NOTABLE
NOTABLY
PALABRA
PARABLE
PAYABLE
PLIABLE
PLIABLY
POSABLE
POTABLE
RAKABLE
RATABLE
RECABLE
RELABEL
RETABLE
RIDABLE
ROSABUD
SALABLE
SAVABLE
SAYABLE
SEEABLE
SIZABLE
SIZABLY
SKIABLE
SOFABED
TAKABLE
TAMABLE
TAXABLE
TENABLE
TENABLY
THEABCS
TOTABLE
TOWABLE
TRIABLE
TUNABLE
TVTABLE
VENABLE
VOCABLE
VOCABLY
VOTABLE
WASABIS
WAXABLE
WIRABLE

•••A•B•

BEDAUBS
BICARBS
CARAMBA
CATAWBA
FLOATBY
ITMAYBE
LABAMBA
MOGAMBO
NOCARBS
PARAIBA
SNEAKBY
SWEARBY

•••A••B

GETAJOB
GOTAJOB
HADAJOB
HOPACAB
NONARAB
PANARAB
PROARAB
RANATAB
RUBADUB
RUNATAB
TUNASUB

••••AB•

ALIBABA
ALTTABS
BAOBABS
BARNABY
BARTABS
BIGBABY
BIOLABS
BURNABY
CANTABS
CARNABY
CASSABA
CONFABS
CRYBABY
DNALABS
EARTABS
HUSHABY
LULLABY
PREFABS
PUNJABI
REDTABS
REGRABS
RESTABS
ROCKABY
SCARABS
SEALABS
SYLLABI
TARBABY
THEBABE
THEBABY
TYPEABS
WALLABY
WANNABE
WARBABY

••••A•B

EWELAMB
LINEARB
LOWCARB
PETLAMB
POPEAFB
RHUBARB
THELAMB

•••••AB

CHEMLAB
GOBYCAB
GODTHAB
HOMELAB
HOPACAB
LEFTJAB
MINICAB
MINILAB
NONARAB
PANARAB
PEDICAB
PROARAB
PULLTAB
RANATAB
RUNATAB
SANDDAB
SHECRAB
SINUTAB
TAXICAB
TESTLAB
THECRAB
TRIMTAB
XRAYLAB

AC•••••

ACACIAS
ACADEME
ACADEMY
ACADIAN
ACANTHI
ACARIDS
ACAUDAL
ACCEDED
ACCEDER
ACCEDES
ACCENTS
ACCEPTS
ACCLAIM
ACCORDS
ACCOSTS
ACCOUNT
ACCRETE
ACCRUAL
ACCRUED
ACCRUES
ACCTNOS
ACCURST
ACCUSAL
ACCUSED
ACCUSER
ACCUSES
ACDELCO
ACEDOUT
ACEHIGH
ACERATE
ACERBIC
ACEROLA
ACEROSE
ACESOUT
ACETALS
ACETATE
ACETIFY
ACETONE
ACHEFOR
ACHENES
ACHERON
ACHESON
ACHIEST
ACHIEVA
ACHIEVE
ACHILLE
ACHTUNG
ACIDIFY
ACIDITY
ACINGIT
ACKACKS
ACOLYTE
ACONITE
ACORNED
ACOUPLE
ACQUIRE
ACQUITS
ACREAGE
ACRIDLY
ACROBAT
ACRONYM
ACRYLIC
ACTABLE
ACTAEON
ACTEDAS
ACTEDIN
ACTEDON
ACTEDUP
ACTFIVE
ACTFOUR
ACTIFED
ACTINON
ACTIONS
ACTIVAS
ACTIVES
ACTLIKE
ACTORLY
ACTRESS
ACTSFOR
ACTSOUT
ACTUARY
ACTUATE
ACTUPON
ACUMENS
ACUTELY
ACUTEST
ACYCLIC

A•C••••

AACELLS
ABCDEFG
ABCNEWS
ACCEDED
ACCEDER
ACCEDES
ACCENTS
ACCEPTS
ACCLAIM
ACCORDS
ACCOSTS
ACCOUNT
ACCRETE
ACCRUAL
ACCRUED
ACCRUES
ACCTNOS
ACCURST
ACCUSAL
ACCUSED
ACCUSER
ACCUSES
AFCTEAM
AHCHOOS
ALCAIDE
ALCALDE
ALCAZAR
ALCESTE
ALCHEMY
ALCOHOL
ALCOPOP
ALCOVES
ALCYONE
ANCHORS
ANCHOVY
ANCIENT
ARCADED
ARCADES
ARCADIA
ARCANUM
ARCHAIC
ARCHERS
ARCHERY
ARCHEST
ARCHFOE
ARCHIES
ARCHING
ARCHIVE
ARCHONS
ARCHSEE
ARCHWAY
ARCINGS
ARCLAMP
ARCSINE
ARCUATE
ARCWELD
ASCARED
ASCENDS
ASCENTS
ASCETIC
ASCRIBE
ATCROSS
AUCTION

A••C•••

AAACELL
ABSCISE
ABSCOND
ACACIAS
ACYCLIC
AIRCOOL
AIRCREW
AITCHES
AJACCIO
ALACKOF
ALLCAPS
ALLCASH
ALLCLAD
AMICHAI
AMSCRAY
ANACINS
ANTCOWS
APACHES
APECKOF
ARACARI
ARACHNE
ARACHNO
ARECIBO
ARTCARS
ASHCAKE
ASHCANS
ASOCIAL
ATACAMA
ATACLIP
ATACOST
ATECROW
ATMCARD
AVOCADO
AVOCETS

A•••C••

ABDUCED
ABDUCES
ABDUCTS
ACKACKS
ADDICTS
ADDUCED
ADDUCER
ADDUCES
ADDUCTS
ADVICES
AFARCRY
AFFECTS
AFRICAN
AGENCES
AIRACES
AJACCIO
ALARCON
ALENCON
ALNICOS
ALPACAS
AMERCED
AMERCER
AMERCES
ANARCHS
ANARCHY
ANTACID
APERCUS
APRICOT
ARBACES
ARDECHE
ARNICAS
ARRACKS
ARTICLE
ASPECTS
ATTACHE
ATTACKS
ATTICUS
ATTUCKS
AURICLE
AZTECAN

A••••C•

ABBOTCY
ABROACH
ABSENCE
ACDELCO
ADJUNCT
ADSPACE
ADVANCE
AFFLECK
AFFLICT
AGARICS
AIRDUCT
AIRLOCK
AIRPACK
AIRRACE
AIRSACS
AIRSICK
AIRSOCK
AIRWICK
ALDRICH
AMERICA
AMTRACK
AMTRACS
ANDSUCH
ANIMACY
ANSPACH
ANTIOCH
ANYLUCK
ARABICA
ARABICS
ARDENCY
ARMLOCK
ARTDECO
ARTROCK
ASKANCE
ASPENCO
ATDEUCE
ATLUNCH
ATOMICS
ATONICS
ATPEACE
ATTRACT
AUSPICE
AUTARCH
AVARICE
AVIANCA
AZUSACA

A•••••C

ABIOTIC
ACERBIC
ACRYLIC
ACYCLIC
AELFRIC
AEROBIC
AGNATIC
ALEMBIC
ALLELIC
ALMANAC
AMHARIC
AMMONIC
AMNESIC
AMOEBIC
ANAEMIC
ANGELIC

ANIONIC
ANOSMIC
APHAGIC
APHASIC
APHONIC
AQUATIC
ARAMAIC
ARCHAIC
ARSENIC
ARTHURC
ASCETIC
ASEPTIC
ASIATIC
AVIATIC
AVIONIC

•AC••••
AACELLS
BACARDI
BACCHAE
BACCHIC
BACCHUS
BACHATA
BACHING
BACHMAN
BACILLI
BACKBAR
BACKBAY
BACKBIT
BACKEND
BACKERS
BACKHOE
BACKING
BACKLIT
BACKLOG
BACKLOT
BACKOFF
BACKOUT
BACKPAY
BACKROW
BACKRUB
BACKSAW
BACKSIN
BACKSUP
BACKUPS
BACKWAY
BACTRIA
CACHACA
CACHETS
CACHING
CACIQUE
CACKLED
CACKLER
CACKLES
CACONYM
DACAPOS
DACOSTA
DACRONS
DACTYLS
FACADES
FACEDIT
FACEDON
FACEOFF
FACESIT
FACESON
FACETED
FACIALS
FACINGS
FACONNE
FACTFUL
FACTION
FACTOID
FACTORS
FACTORY
FACTUAL
FACULAE
FACULTY
HACKERS
HACKETT
HACKIES
HACKING
HACKLED
HACKLER
HACKLES
HACKMAN
HACKNEY
HACKOFF
HACKSAW
HACKSIT
HACKSUP
IACOCCA
JACALES
JACAMAR
JACCUSE
JACINTH
JACINTO
JACKALS
JACKASS
JACKDAW
JACKETS
JACKIEO
JACKING
JACKPOT
JACKSON
JACKSOO
JACKSUP
JACKTAR
JACOBIN
JACONET
JACQUES
JACUZZI
KACHINA
KACHING
LACEDUP
LACERTA
LACESON
LACESUP
LACEUPS
LACIEST
LACINGS
LACKEYS
LACKING
LACKWIT
LACONIA
LACONIC
LACOSTE
LACQUER
LACRIMO
LACTAID
LACTASE
LACTATE
LACTEAL
LACTOSE
LACUNAE
LACUNAL
LACUNAR
LACUNAS
LACUREE
MACABRE
MACACOS
MACADAM
MACAQUE
MACBETH
MACDUFF
MACEDON
MACGRAW
MACHAON
MACHETE
MACHINA
MACHINE
MACHONE
MACHREE
MACHSIX
MACHTWO
MACLEAN
MACLEOD
MACNEIL
MACONGA
MACOUNS
MACRAME
MACRONS
MACULAE
MACULAR
MACUSER
NACELLE
PACBELL
PACECAR
PACELAP
PACEOFF
PACHISI
PACIEST
PACIFIC
PACKAGE
PACKARD
PACKERS
PACKETS
PACKICE
PACKING
PACKOFF
PACKRAT
PACKSIN
PACKSON
PACKSUP
PACQUIN
RACCOON
RACECAR
RACEDBY
RACEDIN
RACEDTO
RACEDUP
RACEMES
RACESBY
RACESTO
RACESUP
RACEWAY
RACHAEL
RACIEST
RACINOS
RACISTS
RACKERS
RACKETS
RACKETY
RACKING
RACKOUT
RACKSUP
RACQUET
SACCADE
SACHEMS
SACHETS
SACKERS
SACKFUL
SACKING
SACKOUT
SACKSUP
SACLIKE
SACQUES
TACHYON
TACITLY
TACITUS
TACKERS
TACKIER
TACKILY
TACKING
TACKLED
TACKLER
TACKLES
TACKSON
TACKSUP
TACOMAS
TACONIC
TACTFUL
TACTICS
TACTILE
TACTUAL
VACANCY
VACATED
VACATES
VACCARO
VACCINE
VACUITY
VACUOLE
VACUOUS
VACUUMS
WACKEST
WACKIER
WACKILY
YACHTED
YACHTER
YACHTIE
ZACHARY

•A•C•••
AAACELL
BABCOCK
BACCHAE
BACCHIC
BACCHUS
BADCALL
BADCASE
BADCOLD
BALCONY
BARCARS
BARCLAY
BARCODE
BATCHED
BATCHES
BAYCITY
CALCIFY
CALCITE
CALCIUM
CALCULI
CANCANS
CANCELS
CANCERS
CANCHAS
CARCARE
CARCASS
CARCLUB
CARCOAT
CASCADE
CATCALL
CATCHER
CATCHES
CATCHON
CATCHOW
CATCHUP
CATCOMB
DANCERS
DANCING
DASCHLE
DAYCAMP
DAYCARE
EARCLIP
EATCAKE
EATCROW
FALCATE
FALCONS
FANCIED
FANCIER
FANCIES
FANCIFY
FANCILY
FANCLUB
FANCYUP
FARCEUR
FARCING
FASCIAE
FASCIAL
FASCIAS
FASCISM
FASCIST
FATCATS
FATCELL
FATCITY
FAUCETS
FAWCETT
GARCONS
GASCANS
GASCAPS
GASCONS
GASCONY
GAUCHER
GAUCHOS
HAECKEL
HALCYON
HANCOCK
HATCHED
HATCHER
HATCHES
HATCHET
JACCUSE
JAECKEL
JAMCAMS
JAYCEES
LABCOAT
LAICIZE
LANCERS
LANCETS
LANCIAS
LANCING
LANCOME
LAOCOON
LAPCATS
LARCENY
LARCHEN
LARCHES
LASCALA
LASCARS
LASCAUX
LATCHED
LATCHES
LATCHON
LAWCASE
MADCAPS
MADCHEN
MALCOLM
MANCINI
MANCUSO
MARCATO
MARCEAU
MARCELS
MARCHED
MARCHER
MARCHES
MARCHON
MARCONI
MARCUSE
MASCARA
MASCOTS
MATCHED
MATCHER
MATCHES
MATCHUP
NASCENT
NATCHEZ
OAKCASK
OATCAKE
PANCAKE
PANCHAX
PARCELS
PARCHED
PARCHES
PASCHAL
PASCOLI
PATCASH
PATCHED
PATCHEN
PATCHER
PATCHES
PATCHUP
PAUCITY
PAYCASH
PAYCUTS
RACCOON
RANCHED
RANCHER
RANCHES
RANCHOS
RANCORS
RANCOUR
RASCALS
RATCHET
RAUCOUS
SACCADE
SADCAFE
SAGCARD
SALCHOW
SANCTUM
SANCTUS
SARCASM
SATCHEL
SATCHMO
SATCOMS
SAUCERS
SAUCIER
SAUCILY
SAUCING
SAUCONY
SAWCHUK
TALCKED
TALCUMS
TAXCODE
TAXCUTS
VACCARO
VACCINE
VANCAMP
WALCOTT
WARCLUB
WATCHED
WATCHER
WATCHES
WATCHIT
WATCHTV
WAYCOOL

•A••C••
BAITCAR
BANACEK
BARACUS
CADUCEI
CALICES
CALICOS
CALYCES
CAMACHO
CANUCKS
CAPECOD
CAPUCHE
CARACAS
CASHCOW
CATSCAN
EARACHE
FAMICOM
FASTCAR
GALICIA
HADACOW
HAIRCUT
HALFCUT
HAMACHI
HANDCAR
HARICOT
HASACOW
IACOCCA
JANACEK
KARACHI
LAROCHE
LATICES
LAVACHE
MACACOS
MAGICAL
MAILCAR
MALACCA
MALACHI
MALECAT
MALICES
MANACLE
MANXCAT
MARACAS
NABUCCO
OAXACAN
PACECAR
PADUCAH
PALACES
PANACEA
PANACHE
PANICKY
PANICLE
PATACAS
PAUNCHY
RACECAR
RADICAL
RADICES
RADICLE
RAILCAR
RATECAP
RAUNCHY
SAATCHI
SARACEN
TANKCAR
TAXICAB
VANOCUR
VATICAL
VATICAN
WAVICLE

•A•••C•
BABCOCK
BABENCO
BADBACK
BADITCH
BADLUCK
BALANCE
BARLICK
BARRACK
CACHACA
CADENCE
CADENCY
CALTECH
CANDACE
CANDICE
CANNOCK
CANSECO
CAPRICE
CARIOCA
CARJACK
CASSOCK
CATORCE
DAVINCI
DAYPACK
EARLOCK
FABRICS
FAIENCE
FALLACY
FANFICS
FATBACK
GALLICO
GARLICS
GARRICK
GATTACA
GATWICK
HADDOCK
HAMHOCK
HAMMOCK
HANCOCK
HAPTICS
HARBACH
HARNICK
HARTACK
HASSOCK
HATRACK
HAYRACK
HAYRICK
IACOCCA
IAMBICS
IATRICS
JALISCO
JAMAICA
JAMPACK
LABMICE
LABTECH
LADOUCE
LAMARCK
LAPLACA
LAPLACE
LASTACT
LATENCY
LATOSCA
LATTICE
LAYBACK
MADLOCK
MAJORCA
MALACCA
MANIACS
MANRICO
MANTECA
MASTICS
MATLOCK
MATTOCK
MAURICE
NABISCO
NABUCCO
NATWICK
NAUTICA
OARLOCK
PACKICE
PADDOCK
PADLOCK
PALANCE
PAMLICO
PARSECS
PATENCY
PATRICE
PATRICK
PAYBACK
RANBACK
RANSACK
RATPACK
RATRACE
SADSACK
SAMBUCA
SATBACK
SAWATCH
SAWBUCK
TABASCO
TACTICS
TAMPICO
TAPIOCA
TARMACS
TAYBACK
VACANCY
VALANCE
VALENCE
VANDYCK
VANEYCK
VANWYCK
VARRICK
WALLACE
WALLACH
WARLOCK
WARWICK
WASATCH
WAYBACK
YANNICK
YASBECK
YASHICA

•A••••C
BACCHIC
BALDRIC
BASILIC
CALORIC
CAMBRIC
CANONIC
CARDIAC
CAUSTIC
FANATIC
FATIDIC
GASTRIC
HAMITIC
HASIDIC
LACONIC
LAENNEC
LAUTREC
MALEFIC
MANTRIC
MASONIC
MAURIAC
PACIFIC
PADRAIC
PAPADOC
PARODIC
PASSAIC
RAYKROC
RAYOVAC
SARANAC
SATANIC
SATIRIC
SATYRIC
TACONIC
TAMARAC
VANADIC
WAREPIC
XANTHIC
ZAPOTEC

••AC•••
AAACELL
ACACIAS
AJACCIO
ALACKOF
ANACINS
APACHES
ARACARI
ARACHNE
ARACHNO
ATACAMA
ATACLIP
ATACOST
BEACHAM
BEACHED
BEACHES
BEACONS
BLACKED
BLACKEN
BLACKER
BLACKIE
BLACKLY
BLACULA
BRACERO
BRACERS
BRACEUP
BRACING
BRACKEN
BRACKET
CHACHAS
CHACHKA
CLACKED
CLACKER
CLACTON
COACHED
COACHES
COACTED
CRACKED
CRACKER
CRACKLE
CRACKLY
CRACKUP
DEACONS
DNACODE
DRACHMA
DRACULA
EDACITY
ENACTED
ENACTOR
EVACUEE
EXACTAS
EXACTED
EXACTER
EXACTLY
EXACTOR
FIACRES
FLACCID
FLACKED
FLACONS
FRACTAL
GIACOMO
GLACEED
GLACIAL
GLACIER
GRACIAS
GRACILE
GRACING
GRACKLE
INACAST
JOACHIM
KRACKEL
KWACHAS
LEACHED
LEACHER
LEACHES
LEACOCK
OPACITY
ORACIES
ORACLES
PEACHED
PEACHES
PEACOAT
PEACOCK
PLACARD
PLACATE
PLACEBO
PLACERS
PLACIDO
PLACING
PLACKET
POACHED
POACHER
POACHES
PRACTIC
QUACKED
QUACKER
REACHED
REACHER
REACHES
REACHIN
REACHUP
REACTED
REACTOR
REACTTO
ROACHES
SCACCHI
SEACALM
SEACATS
SEACOWS
SHACKED
SHACKLE
SLACKED
SLACKEN
SLACKER
SLACKLY
SLACKUP
SMACKED
SMACKER
SMACKOF
SMACKUP
SNACKED
SNACKER
SNACKON
SPACELY
SPACERS
SPACIAL
SPACIER
SPACING
SPACKLE
STACKED
STACKER
STACKUP
TEACAKE
TEACART
TEACHER
TEACHES
TEACHIN
TEACOZY
TEACUPS
TRACERS
TRACERY
TRACHEA
TRACING
TRACKED
TRACKER
TRACTOR
UNACTED
URACILS
WHACKED
WHACKER
WRACKED
WRACKUP
XFACTOR

••A•C••
AFARCRY
AJACCIO
ALARCON
ANARCHS
ANARCHY
BEARCAT
BEARCUB
BEATCOP
BIANCHI
BLANCHE
BRANCHY
CHALCIS
CHANCED
CHANCEL
CHANCER
CHANCES
CHARCOT
CHAUCER
COALCAR
ELANCES
EPARCHS
EPARCHY
EXARCHS
FIANCEE
FIANCES
FIASCOS
FLACCID
FLATCAR
FRAICHE
FRANCES
FRANCHI
FRANCIS
GLANCED
GLANCES
LEANCUT
NUANCED
NUANCES
PLAICES
PRANCED
PRANCER
PRANCES
SAATCHI
SCACCHI
SCARCER
SEANCES
STANCES
STARCHY
THATCHY
TRAMCAR
TRANCED
TRANCES
USANCES

••A••C•
AGARICS
ARABICA
ARABICS
AVARICE
BLALOCK
BYANECK
CHALICE
CLARICE
DIALECT
GUANACO
ITALICS

KLATSCH
LEACOCK
ONAKICK
PEACOCK
PLAYACT
SEADUCK
SEARACE
SEASICK
STATICE
STATICS
STAUNCH
TEANECK
TRADUCE
VIADUCT
VIATICA

••A•••C

ANAEMIC
ARAMAIC
CHAOTIC
CHASMIC
CLASSIC
DHARMIC
DRASTIC
ELASTIC
FRANTIC
GRAPHIC
JEANLUC
MIASMIC
MYALGIC
NIANTIC
OTALGIC
PLASMIC
PLASTIC
PRACTIC
PSALMIC
QUADRIC
QUARTIC
STANNIC
TRAFFIC

•••AC••

ACKACKS
AIRACES
ALPACAS
ANTACID
ARBACES
ARRACKS
ATTACHE
ATTACKS
BANACEK
BARACUS
BONACIS
CAMACHO
CARACAS
CDRACKS
CENACLE
CORACLE
CURACAO
DEBACLE
DEFACED
DEFACER
DEFACES
DEFACTO
DIDACTS
EARACHE
EFFACED
EFFACER
EFFACES
ENFACED
ENFACES
ENLACED
ENLACES
EXFACTO
GOUACHE
HADACOW
HAMACHI
HASACOW
HIBACHI
HIJACKS
HITACHI
HOPACAB
HYRACES
IMPACTS
INVACUO
ITHACAN
JANACEK
KARACHI
LAVACHE
LIMACON
MACACOS
MALACCA
MALACHI
MANACLE
MARACAS
MENACED
MENACER
MENACES
MIRACLE
MISACTS
MONACAN
MRMACHO
NONACID
OAXACAN
ONEACAT
ONEACRE
ONEACTS
OUTACTS
PALACES
PANACEA
PANACHE
PATACAS
PREACHY
PREACID
PREACTS
REDACTS
REFACED
REFACES
RELACED
RELACES
REPACKS
RERACKS
RETACKS
SARACEN
SODACAN
SOLACED
SOLACER
SOLACES
TENACES
TENACRE
THWACKS
TOBACCO
TREACLE
TREACLY
TWOACRE
TWOACTS
UNFACED
UNFACTS
UNLACED
UNLACES
UNMACHO
UNPACED
UNPACKS
UNRACKS
UNTACKS

•••A•C•

ADVANCE
ASKANCE
AUTARCH
AVIANCA
BALANCE
BELASCO
BYCATCH
DEBAUCH
DEMARCO
DURANCE
ENHANCE
ERRANCY
FINANCE
FLEANCE
INFANCY
INMARCH
JAMAICA
JOMARCH
JUDAICA
LAMARCK
MALACCA
MONARCH
MOSAICS
MRDARCY
MRMARCH
MTMARCY
NOCATCH
PALANCE
PENANCE
PLIANCY
RELANCE
RELATCH
REMATCH
REPATCH
ROMANCE
SAWATCH
SCRATCH
SONANCE
TABASCO
TENANCY
THEABCS
TOBACCO
TRUANCY
UNFANCY
UNLATCH
VACANCY
VALANCE
WASATCH

•••A••C

AGNATIC
ALMANAC
AMHARIC
APHAGIC
APHASIC
AQUATIC
ASIATIC
AVIATIC
BOTANIC
CERAMIC
DINARIC
DRYADIC
DYNAMIC
ERRATIC
FANATIC
FORASEC
HEMATIC
HEPATIC
HEXADIC
ILIADIC
ISLAMIC
KORANIC
LUNATIC
MELANIC
MONADIC
NOMADIC
OCEANIC
OCTADIC
OGHAMIC
ORGANIC
OSMATIC
PAPADOC
PELAGIC
PIRATIC
ROMANIC
SARANAC
SATANIC
SCIATIC
SOMATIC
STEARIC
TAMARAC
TITANIC
TRIADIC
VANADIC
VENATIC
VOCALIC
YUCATEC

••••AC•

ABROACH
ADSPACE
AIRPACK
AIRRACE
AIRSACS
AMTRACK
AMTRACS
ANIMACY
ANSPACH
ATPEACE
ATTRACT
AZUSACA
BADBACK
BARRACK
BIGMACS
BUYBACK
CACHACA
CANDACE
CARJACK
COGNACS
COMPACT
CONRACK
CONTACS
CONTACT
CORMACK
COSSACK
COTEACH
CPEBACH
CUTBACK
DAYPACK
DETRACT
DOGFACE
DOGRACE
EGGSACS
EMBRACE
EMPLACE
EUSTACE
EXTRACT
FALLACY
FATBACK
FINBACK
FOREACH
FURNACE
GATTACA
GETBACK
GOTBACK
GRIMACE
GUANACO
HARBACH
HARTACK
HATRACK
HAYRACK
HITBACK
HOGBACK
HOTPACK
ICEPACK
IMPEACH
INBLACK
INEXACT
INFRACT
INKSACS
INPEACE
INPLACE
INREACH
INSPACE
JAMPACK
JETPACK
LAPLACA
LAPLACE
LASTACT
LAYBACK
LIEBACK
MANIACS
MESHACH
MICMACS
MUDPACK
MYSPACE
NEWFACE
NONFACT
NOPLACE
ONTRACK
OUTBACK
OUTFACE
OUTPACE
OUTRACE
OVERACT
OVISACS
PAYBACK
PDQBACH
PINNACE
PLAYACT
POLLACK
PREFACE
PRELACY
PREPACK
PRERACE
PRIMACY
PRIVACY
PUTBACK
RANBACK
RANSACK
RATPACK
RATRACE
REBRACE
REDFACE
REDJACK
REENACT
REFRACT
REPLACE
RESPACE
RESTACK
RETEACH
RETRACE
RETRACK
RETRACT
RICRACS
RIOTACT
RUNBACK
SADSACK
SATBACK
SEARACE
SETBACK
SITBACK
SIXPACK
SKIRACE
SKIRACK
SKYJACK
SOLOACT
SPINACH
STOMACH
SUBRACE
SURFACE
TARMACS
TAYBACK
TEDMACK
TERRACE
TESTACY
THESACK
TICTACS
TIEBACK
TIERACK
TIETACK
TIETACS
TWOFACE
UNBRACE
UNIVACS
UNSLACK
UNSTACK
UNTEACH
UNTRACK
UPREACH
VERSACE
WALLACE
WALLACH
WAYBACK
WINBACK
ZODIACS

••••A•C

ARAMAIC
ARCHAIC
DELTAIC
HEBRAIC
LEBLANC
MTBLANC
PADRAIC
PASSAIC
PROSAIC
VOLTAIC
ZEBRAIC

•••••AC

ALMANAC
BIVOUAC
CARDIAC
ELEGIAC
HYGELAC
KEROUAC
MAURIAC
MEDEVAC
MEDIVAC
MINIVAC
PONTIAC
POTOMAC
RAYOVAC
SARANAC
SHELLAC
SHOEPAC
SIMILAC
TAMARAC
THERIAC

AD•••••

ADAGIOS
ADAMANT
ADAMITE
ADAMSES
ADAMSON
ADAPTED
ADAPTER
ADAPTOR
ADAPTTO
ADAWARE
ADAYAGO
ADDABLE
ADDAXES
ADDEDIN
ADDEDLY
ADDEDON
ADDEDTO
ADDEDUP
ADDENDA
ADDENDS
ADDIBLE
ADDICTS
ADDISON
ADDLING
ADDONTO
ADDRESS
ADDSALT
ADDUCED
ADDUCER
ADDUCES
ADDUCTS
ADDUPTO
ADELIES
ADELINA
ADELINE
ADELPHI
ADENINE
ADENOID
ADEPTAT
ADEPTER
ADEPTLY
ADHERED
ADHERER
ADHERES
ADHIBIT
ADIPOSE
ADJOINS
ADJOURN
ADJUDGE
ADJUNCT
ADJURED
ADJURER
ADJURES
ADJUROR
ADJUSTS
ADMIRAL
ADMIRED
ADMIRER
ADMIRES
ADMITTO
ADMIXED
ADMIXES
ADNOUNS
ADOLLAR
ADOLPHE
ADONAIS
ADOPTED
ADOPTEE
ADOPTER
ADORERS
ADORING
ADORNED
ADORNER
ADRATES
ADRENAL
ADRIANA
ADSORBS
ADSPACE
ADULATE
ADULTLY
ADVANCE
ADVENTS
ADVERBS
ADVERSE
ADVERTS
ADVICES
ADVISED
ADVISEE
ADVISER
ADVISES
ADVISOR
ADWOMAN
ADWOMEN
ADZUKIS

A•D••••

ABDOMEN
ABDUCED
ABDUCES
ABDUCTS
ACDELCO
ADDABLE
ADDAXES
ADDEDIN
ADDEDLY
ADDEDON
ADDEDTO
ADDEDUP
ADDENDA
ADDENDS
ADDIBLE
ADDICTS
ADDISON
ADDLING
ADDONTO
ADDRESS
ADDSALT
ADDUCED
ADDUCER
ADDUCES
ADDUCTS
ADDUPTO
AEDILES
AIDLESS
ALDAVIS
ALDENTE
ALDORAY
ALDRICH
ALDUBIN
ANDAMAN
ANDANTE
ANDEANS
ANDIAMO
ANDIRON
ANDMORE
ANDORRA
ANDOVER
ANDRADE
ANDREAS
ANDRESS
ANDREWS
ANDROID
ANDROUS
ANDSOON
ANDSUCH
ANDTHEN
ARDECHE
ARDENCY
ARDMORE
ARDOURS
ARDUOUS
ATDEUCE
AUDIBLE
AUDIBLY
AUDILES
AUDITED
AUDITEE
AUDITOR
AUDUBON

A••D•••

ABCDEFG
ABIDEBY
ABIDERS
ABIDING
ABIDJAN
ACADEME
ACADEMY
ACADIAN
ACEDOUT
ACIDIFY
ACIDITY
AGEDOUT
AIRDAMS
AIRDATE
AIRDRIE
AIRDROP
AIRDUCT
ALADDIN
ALADINE
ALIDADE
ALLDONE
ALTDORF
ALUDELS
AMADEUS
AMIDALA
AMIDOLS
ANADEMS
ANODISE
ANODIZE
ANODYNE
AOUDADS
APEDIET
APODOUS
ARIDEST
ARIDITY
ARTDECO
ATEDIRT
AULDSOD
AVIDEST
AVIDFAN
AVIDITY
AZODYES

A•••D••

ABANDON
ABRADED
ABRADER
ABRADES
ABRIDGE
ACAUDAL
ACCEDED
ACCEDER
ACCEDES
ACRIDLY
ACTEDAS
ACTEDIN
ACTEDON
ACTEDUP
ADDEDIN
ADDEDLY
ADDEDON
ADDEDTO
ADDEDUP
ADJUDGE
AGENDAS
AGENDUM
AHEADOF
AIKIDOS
AIMEDAT
AIREDUP
ALADDIN
ALBEDOS
ALLUDED
ALLUDES
ALMADEN
ALOADOF
AMENDED
AMENDER
AMPEDUP
AMRADIO
ANTEDUP
APHIDES
APSIDES
ARCADED
ARCADES
ARCADIA
ARIADNE
ARLEDGE
ARMADAS
ARUNDEL
ASKEDIN
ASKEDOF
ASKEDUP
ASSTDAS
ASUNDER
AUBADES
AVOIDED
AVOIDER
AWARDED
AWARDEE
AWARDER

A••••D•

ABOUNDS
ACARIDS
ACCORDS
ADDENDA
ADDENDS
AFFORDS
AIRMADA
ALAMEDA
ALAMODE
ALBUNDY
ALCAIDE
ALCALDE
ALEARDI
ALFREDA
ALFREDE
ALFREDO
ALFREDU
ALIDADE
ALLENDE
ALMONDS
ALMONDY
ALREADY
ALTOIDS
AMERADA
ANDRADE
ANYBODY
AOUDADS
APPENDS
ARAMIDS
ARNOLDS
ASABODY
ASCENDS
ASTRIDE
ATGRADE
ATTENDS
AUGENDS
AVENIDA
AVOCADO
AXHEADS
AXSEEDS

A•••••D

AARATED
ABASHED
ABDUCED
ABELARD
ABETTED
ABJURED
ABLATED
ABORTED
ABRADED
ABSCOND
ABUTTED
ACCEDED
ACCRUED
ACCUSED
ACORNED
ACTIFED
ADAPTED
ADDUCED
ADENOID
ADHERED
ADJURED
ADMIRED
ADMIXED
ADOPTED
ADORNED
ADVISED
AERATED
AFEARED
AFFINED
AFFIXED
AGENTED
AGROUND
AIRHEAD
AIRRAID
ALARMED
ALASSAD
ALERTED
ALEYARD
ALIBIED
ALIGNED
ALLAYED
ALLCLAD
ALLEGED
ALLGOOD
ALLOWED
ALLOYED
ALLTIED
ALLTOLD
ALLUDED
ALLURED
ALPHARD
ALTERED
AMASSED
AMEBOID
AMENDED
AMERCED
AMERIND
AMISTAD
ANDROID
ANEROID
ANGERED
ANISEED
ANNELID
ANNEXED
ANNOYED
ANTACID
ANTBIRD
ANYKIND
ANYROAD
APPLAUD
APPLIED
APPOSED
APRONED
ARANEID
ARBORED
ARCADED
ARCWELD
ARMBAND
ARMLOAD
ARMORED
AROUSED
ARRAYED
ARRIVED
ASCARED
ASHAMED
ASHFORD
ASHLAND
ASISAID
ASPIRED
ASSAYED
ASSUMED
ASSURED
ASTOUND
ATANEND
ATMCARD
ATTHIRD
ATTIRED
ATTUNED
AUDITED
AUGURED
AULDSOD
AVAILED
AVENGED
AVERRED
AVERTED
AVIATED
AVOIDED
AVULSED
AWAITED
AWARDED
AWKWARD
AXEHEAD
AXELROD
AYKROYD
AYNRAND

•AD••••

BADAREA
BADBACK
BADBOYS
BADCALL
BADCASE
BADCOLD
BADDAYS
BADDEBT
BADDEED
BADDEST
BADDIES
BADDISH
BADDOGS
BADEGGS
BADENDS
BADENOV
BADFITS
BADFORM
BADGERS
BADGIRL
BADGUYS
BADHAIR

BADHAND
BADHATS
BADIDEA
BADITCH
BADJOKE
BADLAND
BADLIES
BADLOTS
BADLOVE
BADLUCK
BADMOOD
BADMOVE
BADNAME
BADNESS
BADNEWS
BADOMEN
BADPAST
BADRAPS
BADSHOT
BADSIGN
BADTIME
BADTRIP
BADWORD
CADAVER
CADBURY
CADDIED
CADDIES
CADDISH
CADEAUX
CADENCE
CADENCY
CADENZA
CADETTE
CADGERS
CADGING
CADMIUM
CADUCEI
DADAART
DADAISM
DADAIST
DADDIES
DADOING
EADGILS
FADAYEV
FADDIER
FADDIET
FADDISH
FADDISM
FADDIST
FADEDIN
FADEDLY
FADEINS
FADEOUT
FADESIN
FADIMAN
FADLIKE
GADDERS
GADDING
GADGETS
GADGETY
GADSDEN
HADACOW
HADAFIT
HADAGAS
HADAJOB
HADANIP
HADAROW
HADASAY
HADASET
HADATIT
HADBEEN
HADBEST
HADDOCK
HADDONE
HADFITS
HADOVER
HADPULL
HADRIAN
HADRONS
HADROOM
HADSOME
HADTIME
HADTOBE
JADEDLY
JADEITE
KADDISH
KADETTS
LADADOG
LADDERS
LADDIES
LADDISH
LADHOOD
LADIDAS
LADINGS
LADINOS
LADLERS
LADLING
LADOUCE
LADRONE
LADYBUG
LADYDAY
LADYISH
LADYKIN
LADYNAS
MADALYN
MADAMES
MADAMEX
MADCAPS
MADCHEN
MADDASH
MADDENS
MADDERS
MADDEST
MADDING
MADDISH
MADDOGS
MADEFIT
MADEFOR
MADEFUN
MADEHAY
MADEILL
MADEIRA
MADELON
MADEMAD
MADEOFF
MADEONE
MADEOUT
MADEPAR
MADERUN
MADEWAR
MADEWAY
MADIGAN
MADISON
MADLIBS
MADLOCK
MADNESS
MADONNA
MADRUSH
MADUROS
PADDERS
PADDIES
PADDING
PADDLED
PADDLER
PADDLES
PADDOCK
PADGETT
PADLOCK
PADRAIC
PADRONE
PADSITE
PADUANS
PADUCAH
QADDAFI
RADAMES
RADFORD
RADIALS
RADIANS
RADIANT
RADIATE
RADICAL
RADICES
RADICLE
RADIOAD
RADIODJ
RADIOED
RADIOER
RADIOIN
RADIXES
RADOMES
SADCAFE
SADDENS
SADDEST
SADDLED
SADDLER
SADDLES
SADEYED
SADEYES
SADFATE
SADISTS
SADNESS
SADSACK
SADSONG
TADPOLE
WADDELL
WADDERS
WADDING
WADDLED
WADDLER
WADDLES
WADEDIN
WADESIN
WADKINS
ZADKINE

•A•D•••

BADDAYS
BADDEBT
BADDEED
BADDEST
BADDIES
BADDISH
BADDOGS
BALDEST
BALDIES
BALDING
BALDISH
BALDRIC
BALDWIN
BANDAGE
BANDAID
BANDANA
BANDBOX
BANDEAU
BANDERA
BANDERS
BANDIDO
BANDIED
BANDIER
BANDIES
BANDING
BANDITO
BANDITS
BANDLET
BANDSAW
BARDEEN
BATDAYS
BAWDIER
BAWDILY
CADDIED
CADDIES
CADDISH
CALDERA
CALDERS
CALDRON
CANDACE
CANDELA
CANDENT
CANDICE
CANDIDA
CANDIDE
CANDIDS
CANDIED
CANDIES
CANDLED
CANDLER
CANDLES
CANDOUR
CARDERS
CARDIAC
CARDIAL
CARDIFF
CARDING
CARDIUM
CARDKEY
CARDOOR
CARDOZO
CATDOOR
CAUDATE
DADDIES
DANDERS
DANDIER
DANDIES
DANDIFY
DANDILY
DANDLED
DANDLER
DANDLES
DAWDLED
DAWDLER
DAWDLES
EARDROP
EARDRUM
EATDIRT
FADDIER
FADDIET
FADDISH
FADDISM
FADDIST
FANDOMS
GADDERS
GADDING
GANDALF
GANDERS
GARDENA
GARDENS
GARDNER
GAUDENS
GAUDERY
GAUDIER
GAUDIES
GAUDILY
HADDOCK
HADDONE
HALDANE
HANDAXE
HANDBAG
HANDCAR
HANDERS
HANDEYE
HANDFED
HANDFUL
HANDGUN
HANDIER
HANDILY
HANDING
HANDLED
HANDLER
HANDLES
HANDLIN
HANDOFF
HANDOUT
HANDSAW
HANDSEL
HANDSET
HANDSIN
HANDSON
HANDSUP
HANDYTO
HARDDAY
HARDEES
HARDENS
HARDEST
HARDHAT
HARDHIT
HARDIER
HARDILY
HARDING
HARDISH
HARDPAN
HARDPUT
HARDSET
HARDSIX
HARDTEN
HARDTOP
HARDWAY
HARDWON
HASDONE
JARDINE
JARDINS
KADDISH
LADDERS
LADDIES
LADDISH
LAIDFOR
LAIDLOW
LAIDOFF
LAIDOUT
LANDAUS
LANDERS
LANDING
LANDINI
LANDLER
LANDMAN
LANDMEN
LANDSAT
LANDSUP
LANDTAG
LANDTAX
LAPDOGS
LARDERS
LARDIER
LARDING
LARDNER
LARDONS
LAUDERS
LAUDING
LAYDOWN
MACDUFF
MADDASH
MADDENS
MADDERS
MADDEST
MADDING
MADDISH
MADDOGS
MAHDISM
MAHDIST
MAIDENS
MAIDISH
MALDIVE
MANDALA
MANDANS
MANDATE
MANDAYS
MANDELA
MANDOKI
MANDREL
MARDIAN
MAUDLIN
MAYDAYS
OAKDESK
PADDERS
PADDIES
PADDING
PADDLED
PADDLER
PADDLES
PADDOCK
PAIDADS
PAIDFOR
PAIDOFF
PAIDOUT
PANDERS
PANDITS
PANDORA
PARDNER
PARDONS
PATDOWN
PAYDAYS
PAYDIRT
QADDAFI
RAEDAWN
RAGDOLL
RAIDERS
RAIDING
RAMDOWN
RANDALL
RANDEEP
RANDIER
RANDOWN
RAWDATA
RAWDEAL
SADDENS
SADDEST
SADDLED
SADDLER
SADDLES
SAIDAAH
SAIDAYE
SAIDBOO
SAIDIDO
SAIDNAY
SANDALS
SANDBAG
SANDBAR
SANDBOX
SANDBUR
SANDDAB
SANDERS
SANDFLY
SANDHOG
SANDIER
SANDING
SANDLER
SANDLOT
SANDMAN
SANDMEN
SANDPIT
SARDINE
SATDOWN
SAWDUST
TAGDAYS
TANDEMS
TANDOOR
TARDIER
TARDILY
VANDALS
VANDIEN
VANDINE
VANDURA
VANDUYN
VANDYCK
VANDYKE
VATDYED
VATDYES
VAUDOIS
WADDELL
WADDERS
WADDING
WADDLED
WADDLER
WADDLES
WALDORF
WANDERS
WARDENS
WARDERS
WARDING
WARDOFF
YARDAGE
YARDARM
YARDERS
YARDING
YARDMAN
YARDMEN

•A••D••

BADIDEA
BAGHDAD
BASEDON
BAYEDAT
CAGEDIN
CAGEDUP
CAKEDUP
CAMEDUE
CANIDAE
CAPADES
CAREDTO
CAVEDIN
DAMPDRY
DASHDOT
DATEDLY
DAZEDLY
EARLDOM
EASEDBY
EASEDIN
EASEDON
EASEDUP
FACADES
FACEDIT
FACEDON
FADEDIN
FADEDLY
FAKEDIT
FALLDUE
FARADAY
FATIDIC
GADSDEN
GAPEDAT
GASEDUP
GAZEDAT
GAZEDON
HAIRDOS
HAIRDYE
HALFDAY
HALFDUG
HALIDES
HANGDOG
HARDDAY
HASIDIC
HASIDIM
HATEDIT
JACKDAW
JADEDLY
JANEDOE
JAWEDAT
KATYDID
LACEDUP
LADADOG
LADIDAS
LADYDAY
LAMBDAS
LANGDON
LAREDOS
LASTDON
LAUNDER
LAUNDRY
LAYODDS
MAANDPA
MACADAM
MACEDON
MAKEDOS
MALEDOG
MALODOR
MARIDAS
MARIDOS
MARSDEN
MATADOR
MAULDIN
MAUNDER
NAIADES
NAKEDLY
NAMEDAY
NAVIDAD
PAGODAS
PALADIN
PALEDRY
PALUDAL
PANADAS
PAPADOC
PARADED
PARADER
PARADES
PARADOR
PARADOX
PARODIC
PASTDUE
PATSDRY
PAVIDLY
PAWEDAT
RABIDLY
RACEDBY
RACEDIN
RACEDTO
RACEDUP
RAKEDIN
RAKEDUP
RAMADAN
RAMADAS
RAPIDAN
RAPIDER
RAPIDLY
RATEDPG
SABADOS
SALADES
SALADIN
SAMEDAY
SAMEDIS
SANDDAB
SAVEDON
SAVEDUP
TAPEDON
TAPEDUP
VALADON
VALIDID
VALIDLY
VANADIC
VAPIDLY
WADEDIN
WAKEDUP
WASHDAY
WAVEDAT
WAVEDIN
WAVEDTO
WAXEDUP
XANADUS

•A•••D•

BACARDI
BADENDS
BAGLADY
BALLADE
BALLADS
BANDIDO
BARBUDA
BARCODE
CABRIDE
CALANDO
CALENDS
CANARDS
CANDIDA
CANDIDE
CANDIDS
CARBIDE
CASCADE
CASSIDY
CATBEDS
CATHODE
DAYBEDS
DAYSIDE
EARBUDS
FAGENDS
FAKEIDS
FANTODS
FARSIDE
GAMBADO
GAPKIDS
HALOIDS
HAPKIDO
HAROLDI
HARRODS
HATREDS
HAYRIDE
HAZARDS
LAMBADA
LASORDA
LAWANDA
LAYODDS
MAENADS
MAKESDO
MALTEDS
MANMADE
MARAUDS
MATILDA
NAVAIDS
PAIDADS
PARKADE
PASSADE
PASSADO
RADIODJ
RAGGEDY
RAMRODS
RASHIDA
RAWHIDE
SACCADE
SAIDIDO
SALSODA
SAYSIDO
TABARDS
TAGENDS
TAXCODE
WANTADS
WARGODS
WAYSIDE
YAOUNDE

•A••••D

AARATED
BABBLED
BACKEND
BADCOLD
BADDEED
BADHAND
BADLAND
BADMOOD
BADWORD
BAFFLED
BAGHDAD
BAGNOLD
BALLARD
BANDAID
BANDIED
BANGLED
BARMAID
BARNARD
BARNRED
BARTEND
BATCHED
BATIKED
BATTLED
BAULKED
CACKLED
CADDIED
CAIRNED
CAJOLED
CAMELID
CAMEOED
CAMPBED
CANALED
CANDIED
CANDLED
CAPECOD
CAPERED
CARLOAD
CAROLED
CAROMED
CAROTID
CARRIED
CASQUED
CASTLED
CATBIRD
CATERED
CATEYED
CATFOOD
CATHEAD
CAULKED
CAVILED
DABBLED
DABHAND
DAGWOOD
DALLIED
DAMAGED
DANDLED
DANGLED
DAPPLED
DARKLED
DARKRED
DARTLED
DASTARD
DAUNTED
DAWDLED
DAYSEND
DAZZLED
EANMUND
EARTHED
EASELED
EASTEND
FACETED
FACTOID
FAGOTED
FAINTED
FANCIED
FANFOLD
FARGOND
FARMAID
FATHEAD
FAULTED
FAVORED
GABBLED
GALAHAD
GALOPED
GAMBLED
GARAGED
GARBLED
GARGLED
GARLAND
GASPARD
GAVELED
GAYLORD
HABITED
HACKLED
HAGGARD
HAGGLED
HALFBAD
HALFFED
HALFMAD
HALFROD
HALYARD
HAMMOND
HANDFED
HANDLED
HAPLOID
HARLAND
HARRIED
HARROLD
HARVARD
HASSLED
HATBAND
HATCHED
HAUNTED
HAYSEED
HAYWARD
JAMBAND
JANGLED
JAUNTED
JAYBIRD
JAYWARD
KAMERAD
KATYDID
KAYAKED
LABELED
LABORED
LACTAID
LADHOOD
LAGGARD
LAKEBED
LANFORD
LANGUID
LANYARD
LAPELED
LAPLAND
LASSOED
LATCHED
LATENED
LAUGHED
LAWFORD
LAYERED
MACLEOD
MADEMAD
MAITRED
MAJORED
MAKEMAD
MALAMUD
MALLARD
MAMBOED
MANAGED
MANFRED
MANGLED
MANHOOD
MANKIND
MANSARD
MANTLED
MANURED
MARBLED
MARCHED
MARRIED
MARSRED
MASONED
MASTOID
MATCHED
MATURED
MAYNARD
NANNIED
NATURED
NAVIDAD
NAYSAID
OAKLAND
OAKWOOD
PACKARD
PADDLED
PAINTED
PANELED
PAPERED
PARADED
PARCHED
PAROLED
PAROTID
PARRIED
PARTIED
PATCHED
PATHAND
PAYHEED
PAYLOAD
RABBLED
RADFORD
RADIOAD
RADIOED
RAFFLED
RAGWEED
RAINGOD
RALLIED
RAMBLED
RANCHED
RANKLED

RANWILD
RASSLED
RATTLED
RAVAGED
RAVELED
RAVENED
RAVINED
RAWFOOD
RAYMOND
RAZORED
SABERED
SADDLED
SADEYED
SAGCARD
SAINTED
SALLIED
SALUTED
SAMBAED
SAMEOLD
SAMLOYD
SAMOYED
SAMPLED
SANFORD
SAPHEAD
SAUNAED
SAUTEED
SAVAGED
SAVORED
SAVVIED
SAWWOOD
TABLOID
TABOOED
TACKLED
TAILEND
TAINTED
TALCKED
TALLIED
TALONED
TANGLED
TANGOED
TANKARD
TAPERED
TARRIED
TASERED
TATTLED
TAUNTED
TAXPAID
VACATED
VALETED
VALIDID
VANLOAD
VANWARD
VAPORED
VATDYED
VAULTED
VAUNTED
WADDLED
WAFERED
WAFFLED
WAGERED
WAGGLED
WAGONED
WAISTED
WAKENED
WALTZED
WAMBLED
WANGLED
WARBLED
WARBOND
WARHEAD
WARLORD
WATCHED
WATERED
WATFORD
WATTLED
WAVERED
WAYLAID
WAYLAND
WAYWARD
YACHTED

••AD•••

ACADEME
ACADEMY
ACADIAN
ALADDIN
ALADINE
AMADEUS
ANADEMS
BEADERS
BEADIER
BEADILY
BEADING
BEADLES
BEADSUP
BLADDER
BLADERS
BLADING
BRADLEE
BRADLEY
CLADDED
CRADLED
CRADLER
CRADLES
DEADAIR
DEADEND
DEADENS
DEADEST
DEADEYE
DEADPAN
DEADSEA
DEADSET
DIADEMS
DOADEAL
EVADERS
EVADING
GLADDEN
GLADDER
GLADEYE
GOADING
GRADATE
GRADEAA
GRADERS
GRADING
GRADUAL
HEADEND
HEADERS
HEADFOR
HEADFUL
HEADIER
HEADILY
HEADING
HEADMAN
HEADMEN
HEADOFF
HEADOUT
HEADPIN
HEADSAW
HEADSET
HEADSIN
HEADSTO
HEADSUP
HEADWAY
IMADEIT
INADAZE
ISADORA
ISADORE
LEADDOG
LEADENS
LEADERS
LEADETH
LEADIER
LEADING
LEADINS
LEADMAN
LEADMEN
LEADOFF
LEADORE
LEADOUT
LEADSIN
LEADSON
LEADSTO
LEADSUP
LEADUPS
LLADROS
LOADERS
LOADING
LOADSIN
LOADSOF
LOADSUP
MCADAMS
MEADOWS
MEADOWY
MTADAMS
OBADIAH
ONADARE
ONADATE
ONADIET
PRADESH
QUADRIC
RCADOME
READAPT
READDED
READERS
READFOR
READIED
READIER
READIES
READILY
READING
READMIT
READOFF
READOPT
READORN
READOUT
READSIN
READSON
READSTO
READSUP
ROADBED
ROADEOS
ROADERS
ROADHOG
ROADIES
ROADMAP
ROADTAR
ROADTAX
ROADWAY
SCADSOF
SEADOGS
SEADUCK
SEADUTY
SHADERS
SHADIER
SHADILY
SHADING
SHADOWS
SHADOWY
SHADROE
SPADERS
SPADING
STADIUM
STADLER
SWADDLE
TOADIED
TOADIES
TOADISH
TRADEIN
TRADEON
TRADERS
TRADEUP
TRADING
TRADUCE
TWADDLE
UNADDED
UNADEPT
UNADULT
VEADARS
VIADENT
VIADUCT

••A•D••

ABANDON
ACAUDAL
ALADDIN
AWARDED
AWARDEE
AWARDER
BEANDIP
BEARDED
BLADDER
BLANDER
BLANDLY
BOARDED
BOARDER
BOARDUP
BRAEDEN
BRAIDED
BRAIDER
BRANDED
BRANDER
BRANDON
BYANDBY
CLADDED
CLAMDIP
CLAUDEL
CLAUDIA
CLAUDIO
CRAWDAD
CSARDAS
CZARDAS
CZARDOM
DEARDEN
EVANDER
FLAGDAY
GLADDEN
GLADDER
GRANDAM
GRANDEE
GRANDER
GRANDLY
GRANDMA
GRANDPA
GUARDED
GUARDEE
GUARDER
HEARDOF
HOARDED
HOARDER
INAIDOF
ISAIDNO
KRAMDEN
LEADDOG
LEANDER
LEAPDAY
MAANDPA
MCARDLE
MEANDER
ONANDON
PBANDJS
PHAEDRA
PLAUDIT
PLAYDOH
PSANDQS
READDED
REARDON
REAUDIT
RUANDAS
RWANDAN
SCALDED
SCALDER
SCANDAL
SHAHDOM
SLANDER
SOANDSO
SPANDEX
STAIDER
STAIDLY
STANDBY
STANDEE
STANDER
STANDIN
STANDON
STANDTO
STANDUP
STARDOM
STAYDRY
SWADDLE
THANDIE
TSARDOM
TWADDLE
UGANDAN
UNADDED
UNAIDED
UPANDIN
WHAUDEN
XSANDOS

••A••D•

ACARIDS
ALAMEDA
ALAMODE
ARAMIDS
ASABODY
BRAVADA
BRAVADO
CHARADE
CYANIDE
CYANIDS
DIALEDO
DNACODE
DOASIDO
DRAMADY
DRAMEDY
ELAPIDS
GRANADA
IDAREDS
OCANADA
PEABODY
PEAPODS
PLACIDO
SCAREDY
SEABEDS
SEAGODS
SEASIDE
TRAGEDY
ULANUDE

••A•••D

ABASHED
ADAPTED
ALARMED
ALASSAD
AMASSED
ARANEID
ATANEND
AVAILED
AWAITED
AWARDED
BEACHED
BEARDED
BIASSED
BLABBED
BLACKED
BLANKED
BLASTED
BLATTED
BOARDED
BOASTED
BRAGGED
BRAIDED
BRAINED
BRAISED
BRANDED
BRAVOED
BRAWLED
CHAFFED
CHAINED
CHAIRED
CHALKED
CHAMPED
CHANCED
CHANGED
CHANTED
CHAPPED
CHARGED
CHARMED
CHARRED
CHARTED
CHASSED
CHATTED
CLACKED
CLADDED
CLAIMED
CLAMMED
CLAMPED
CLANGED
CLANKED
CLAPPED
CLASHED
CLASPED
CLASSED
COACHED
COACTED
COAPTED
COASTED
CRABBED
CRACKED
CRADLED
CRAFTED
CRAGGED
CRAMMED
CRAMPED
CRANKED
CRASHED
CRAWDAD
CRAWLED
DEADEND
DEAIRED
DEARGOD
DIALLED
DIAMOND
DRAFTED
DRAGGED
DRAINED
DRATTED
DRAWLED
DWARFED
EBANKED
ELAPSED
EMAILED
ENABLED
ENACTED
ENARMED
ETAILED
EXACTED
EXALTED
FEASTED
FLACCID
FLACKED
FLAGGED
FLAILED
FLAMBED
FLAMMED
FLANKED
FLAPPED
FLASHED
FLATBED
FLATTED
FRAGGED
FRANKED
GLACEED
GLANCED
GLASSED
GNARLED
GNARRED
GNASHED
GOAHEAD
GOATEED
GRABBED
GRAFTED
GRAINED
GRANTED
GRAPHED
GRASPED
GRASSED
GUARDED
HEADEND
HEARTED
HOARDED
HYALOID
INABIND
INAMOOD
INAWORD
ISAHEAD
KNARRED
LEACHED
LEAGUED
LEARNED
LEASHED
LEAWOOD
LIAISED
LOATHED
MIAOUED
MIAOWED
NUANCED
OFAKIND
OFAMIND
ONALEAD
PEACHED
PEARLED
PIAFFED
PLACARD
PLAGUED
PLAITED
PLANKED
PLANNED
PLANTED
PLASHED
PLATTED
POACHED
PRAISED
PRANCED
PRAWNED
QUACKED
QUAFFED
QUAILED
QUASHED
REACHED
REACTED
READDED
READIED
REAIMED
REAIRED
REAMEND
REAREND
REARMED
REASKED
ROADBED
ROASTED
SCALDED
SCALPED
SCAMMED
SCAMPED
SCANNED
SCANTED
SCARFED
SCARPED
SCARRED
SCARWID
SCATHED
SCATTED
SEABIRD
SEAFOOD
SEAWARD
SEAWEED
SHACKED
SHAFTED
SHAGGED
SHAMMED
SHANKED
SHARPED
SHAWLED
SLABBED
SLACKED
SLAMMED
SLANTED
SLAPPED
SLASHED
SLATTED
SMACKED
SMALLAD
SMARTED
SMASHED
SNACKED
SNAFUED
SNAGGED
SNAPPED
SNARFED
SNARLED
SOAPPAD
SPAMMED
SPANKED
SPANNED
SPARKED
SPARRED
SPATTED
SPAWNED
STABBED
STABLED
STACKED
STAFFED
STAGGED
STAINED
STAIRED
STALKED
STALLED
STAMPED
STAPLED
STARRED
STARTED
STARVED
STASHED
SWABBED
SWAMPED
SWANKED
SWAPPED
SWARMED
SWASHED
SWATHED
SWATTED
THANKED
TIARAED
TOADIED
TOASTED
TRACKED
TRAILED
TRAINED
TRAMMED
TRAMPED
TRANCED
TRAPPED
TRASHED
TRAWLED
TWANGED
UNACTED
UNADDED
UNAIDED
UNAIMED
UNAIRED
UNARMED
UNASKED
UNAXLED
UPAHEAD
VIALLED
WEARIED
WHACKED
WHAMMED
WHANGED
WHAPPED
WHARFED
WRACKED
WRAPPED
YEAREND
YEARNED
YEASTED
ZEALAND

•••AD••

ABRADED
ABRADER
ABRADES
AHEADOF
ALMADEN
ALOADOF
AMRADIO
ARCADED
ARCADES
ARCADIA
ARIADNE
ARMADAS
AUBADES
BREADED
BREADER
BREADTH
BROADAS
BROADAX
BROADEN
BROADER
BROADLY
CAPADES
CBRADIO
CELADON
CHEADLE
CICADAE
CICADAS
CITADEL
COLADAS
DECADES
DINADAM
DOSADOS
DREADED
DRYADES
DRYADIC
ECUADOR
ESTADOS
FACADES
FARADAY
FLEADIP
FMRADIO
FORADAY
HEXADIC
HODADDY
IDBADGE
ILIADIC
INVADED
INVADER
INVADES
JUMADAS
KNEADED
KNEADER
KOWADLO
LADADOG
LEVADES
MACADAM
MATADOR
MIKADOS
MIRADAS
MIRADOR
MISADDS
MOGADOR
MONADAL
MONADIC
MOVADOS
MRPADRE
NAIADES
NEVADAN
NOMADIC
OCTADIC
ONEADAY
OUTADDS
PALADIN
PANADAS
PAPADOC
PARADED
PARADER
PARADES
PARADOR
PARADOX
PESADES
PICADOR
PLEADED
PLEADER
PLEADTO
POMADED
POMADES
POSADAS
RAMADAN
RAMADAS
RUBADUB
SABADOS
SALADES
SALADIN
STEADED
TIRADES
TREADED
TREADER
TREADLE
TREADON
TRIADIC
UNFADED
UNJADED
UNLADED
UNLADEN
UNLADES
UNMADLY
UNSADLY
UNWADED
VALADON
VANADIC
XANADUS
XMRADIO

•••A•D•

ALCAIDE
ALCALDE
ALEARDI
BACARDI
BOGARDE
BOIARDO
BRIARDS
CALANDO
CANARDS
COWARDS
DEMANDS
DOTARDS
EDGARDO
EDUARDO
EDWARDG
EDWARDI
EDWARDR
EDWARDS
EDWARDV
ENGARDE
ERRANDS
EXPANDS
FMBANDS
GERALDO
HAZARDS
HERALDS
HODADDY
HOWARDK
HOWARDS
HOWARDU
IDCARDS
INLANDS
INNARDS
INWARDS
ISLANDS
LAWANDA
LIGANDS
LIZARDS
MARAUDS
MIRANDA
MISADDS
MTBALDY
NAVAIDS
NOCANDO
NOHANDS
ONWARDS
ORGANDY
ORLANDO
ORMANDY
OUTADDS
PETARDS
PICARDO
PICARDY
REGARDS
RELANDS
REMANDS
RENALDO
RESANDS
RETARDS
REWARDS
RIBALDS
RIBANDS
RICARDO
RINALDO
RITARDS
ROBARDS
ROLAIDS
SEWARDS
STRANDS
TABARDS
TEBALDI
TOWARDS
UNGAUDY
UNHANDS
UNHANDY
UNHARDY
UPCARDS
UPLANDS
UPWARDS
VERANDA
VIVALDI
WCHANDY
WIZARDS
YOLANDA
YOUANDI

•••A••D

AARATED
ABLATED
ABRADED
AERATED
AFEARED
ALLAYED
ANTACID
ARCADED
ARRAYED
ASCARED
ASHAMED
ASSAYED
AVIATED
BEDAZED
BEHAVED
BELATED
BELAYED
BERATED
BEWARED
BLEARED
BLEATED
BLOATED
BREADED
CANALED
CEDARED
CERATED
CHEATED
CLEANED
CLEARED
CLEATED
CLEAVED
CLOAKED
CREAKED

CREAMED
CREASED
CREATED
CROAKED
CURATED
DAMAGED
DEBASED
DEBATED
DECAPOD
DECAYED
DEFACED
DEFAMED
DELAYED
DERATED
DEWAXED
DILATED
DONATED
DREADED
DREAMED
EFFACED
EMBAYED
EMPALED
ENCAGED
ENCASED
ENFACED
ENGAGED
ENLACED
ENRAGED
EQUALED
EQUATED
ESCAPED
ESSAYED
ESTATED
EXHALED
FIXATED
FLOATED
FORAGED
FORAYED
FREAKED
GALAHAD
GARAGED
GELATED
GLEAMED
GLEANED
GLOATED
GREASED
GROANED
GYRATED
HEXAPOD
ICHABOD
IDEATED
IGUANID
IMPALED
IMPAVID
INCASED
INHALED
INVADED
INVALID
IODATED
KAYAKED
KNEADED
LIEABED
LIGATED
LOBATED
LOCATED
LSHAPED
LUNATED
LUXATED
MALAMUD
MANAGED
MEDALED
MELAMED
MENACED
METALED
MURALED
MUTATED
NEGATED
NONACID
NOTATED
NUTATED
OCEANID
OSHAPED
OUTAWED
PARADED
PEDALED
PETALED
PGRATED
PHRASED
PIRATED
PLEADED
PLEASED
PLEATED
POMADED
PREACID
PREAGED
PSHAWED
PUPATED
PYRAMID
RAVAGED
REBAKED
REBALED
REBATED
RECAGED
RECANED
RECASED
REDARED
REDATED
REFACED
REFAXED
REGALED
RELACED
RELATED
RELAXED
RELAYED
REMATED
RENAMED
REPAGED
REPAVED
RERAKED
RERATED
RESAVED
RESAWED
RETAMED
RETAPED
RETAXED
REWAKED
REWAXED
RIVALED
ROSABUD
ROTATED
SAVAGED
SCRAPED
SEDATED
SEPALED
SHEAFED
SHEARED
SHEAVED
SHOALED
SMEARED
SNEAKED
SOFABED
SOLACED
SPEARED
SPLAYED
SPRAYED
SQUALID
SQUARED
SSHAPED
STEADED
STEAMED
STRAFED
STRAYED
SUBARID
SUDAFED
SUGARED
SWEATED
TOTALED
TREADED
TREATED
TSHAPED
TWEAKED
UNBAKED
UNBALED
UNBARED
UNBASED
UNBATED
UNCAGED
UNCAKED
UNCANED
UNCAPED
UNCASED
UNDARED
UNDATED
UNDAZED
UNEAVED
UNFACED
UNFADED
UNFAKED
UNFAMED
UNFATED
UNFAZED
UNGATED
UNHATED
UNHAYED
UNHAZED
UNJADED
UNLACED
UNLADED
UNLAVED
UNLAXED
UNMANED
UNMATED
UNNAMED
UNPACED
UNPAGED
UNPALED
UNPARED
UNPAVED
UNPAWED
UNRAKED
UNRATED
UNRAYED
UNRAZED
UNSATED
UNSAVED
UNSAWED
UNTAMED
UNTAPED
UNTAXED
UNWADED
UNWAGED
UNWAKED
UNWANED
UNWAVED
UNWAXED
UPDATED
UPGAZED
UPRATED
USHAPED
VACATED
VISAGED
VOYAGED
VSHAPED
WREAKED
YSHAPED

••••AD•

AIRMADA
ALIDADE
ALREADY
AMERADA
ANDRADE
AOUDADS
ATGRADE
AVOCADO
AXHEADS
BAGLADY
BALLADE
BALLADS
BEHEADS
BRAVADA
BRAVADO
BRIGADE
BROCADE
BYROADS
CASCADE
CHARADE
COCKADE
COMRADE
CORRADE
CRUSADE
CRUZADO
DEGRADE
DELEADS
DOODADS
DRAMADY
ELPRADO
EMQUADS
ENNEADS
ENQUADS
ENTRADA
EPILADY
ESTRADA
FORBADE
FTMEADE
FURTADO
GAMBADO
GRANADA
GRENADA
GRENADE
HEPTADS
ILLMADE
IMREADY
INKPADS
INROADS
INTRADE
JOYPADS
KEYPADS
LAMBADA
LIMEADE
MAENADS
MANMADE
MERCADO
MYRIADS
NEWMADE
NEXRADS
NIKEADS
NOLOADS
NOTRADE
OCANADA
OGDOADS
OLDLADY
ONLOADS
PAIDADS
PARKADE
PASSADE
PASSADO
PENTADS
PERVADE
PREBADE
PREFADE
PREMADE
RECLADS
REGRADE
RELEADS
RELOADS
REREADS
RESPADE
RETRADE
RIBPADS
ROULADE
SACCADE
SOSPADS
SPREADS
TETRADS
THREADS
THREADY
TORNADO
TOSTADA
UNBLADE
UNHEADY
UNLEADS
UNLOADS
UNREADY
UNSHADE
UNSHADY
UPGRADE
UPLOADS
UPTRADE
WANTADS

••••A•D

ABELARD
AIRRAID
ALEYARD
ALPHARD
APPLAUD
ARMBAND
ASHLAND
ASISAID
ATMCARD
AWKWARD
AYNRAND
BADHAND
BADLAND
BALLARD
BANDAID
BARMAID
BARNARD
BEEYARD
BEHEARD
BERNARD
BIGBAND
BIGHAND
BOMBARD
BONNARD
BOYBAND
BRIGAND
BROWARD
BUSTARD
BUZZARD
COBRAND
COLLARD
COMMAND
CONGAED
COPLAND
COSTARD
COWHAND
CUECARD
CUSTARD
DABHAND
DASTARD
DEBEARD
DEFRAUD
DIEHARD
DILLARD
DISBAND
DISCARD
DULLARD
DURWARD
EDOUARD
EMERALD
ENGLAND
EYEHAND
FARMAID
FERNAND
FINLAND
FORWARD
FOULARD
FROWARD
GARLAND
GASPARD
GISCARD
GIZZARD
GODDARD
HAGGARD
HALYARD
HARLAND
HARVARD
HATBAND
HAYWARD
HENNAED
HEYWARD
HOLLAND
HOTHAND
HUBBARD
HUMBARD
HUSBAND
IBNSAUD
ICELAND
INBOARD
IRELAND
JAMBAND
JAYWARD
JUGBAND
JUTLAND
KEYCARD
KINCAID
KINKAID
KOOLAID
LACTAID
LAGGARD
LANYARD
LAPLAND
LEEWARD
LEGRAND
LEONARD
LEOPARD
LEOTARD
LEPPARD
LIVEAID
LOLLARD
LOMBARD
LOWCARD
LOWHAND
LOWLAND
LOWPAID
MALLARD
MANSARD
MAYNARD
MERMAID
MIDLAND
MILHAUD
MILLAND
MILLARD
MISLAID
MISSAID
MONTAND
MUSTARD
NAYSAID
NEDLAND
NEWHAND
NEWLAID
NONPAID
NORMAND
OAKLAND
OFFHAND
OILSAND
OLDHAND
OLDMAID
ONBOARD
ONEHAND
ONEYARD
ONGUARD
OPERAND
ORCHARD
OSTWALD
OUTLAID
OUTLAND
OUTPAID
OUTSAID
OUTWARD
PACKARD
PATHAND
PEPBAND
PEPPARD
PICCARD
PIEBALD
PIPCARD
PLACARD
POLKAED
POLLARD
POMMARD
PONIARD
PREPAID
REBOARD
REBRAND
REDCARD
REGNARD
REHEARD
REYNARD
REYNAUD
RICHARD
RIMBAUD
RITEAID
ROLLAND
RONSARD
ROSTAND
ROWLAND
RUDYARD
RUMBAED
RUTLAND
SAGCARD
SAMBAED
SAUNAED
SCUBAED
SEAWARD
SHEPARD
SKYWARD
STEWARD
SUBBAND
SUMMAND
SUNMAID
SUNWARD
SZILARD
TANKARD
TAXPAID
THEBAND
THEBARD
TIARAED
TOOHARD
TORVALD
TOYLAND
TRYHARD
TUSSAUD
UNBEARD
UNBRAID
UNGRAND
UNGUARD
UNHEARD
UNITARD
UNSTAID
UPBRAID
UPHOARD
UPSTAND
VANWARD
VILLARD
VINLAND
VISTAED
WAYLAID
WAYLAND
WAYWARD
WELLAND
WETLAND
WHOSAID
WIELAND
WILLARD
WOODARD
ZEALAND
ZEELAND

•••••AD

AIRHEAD
ALASSAD
ALLCLAD
AMISTAD
ANYROAD
ARMLOAD
AXEHEAD
BAGHDAD
BEOGRAD
BIGHEAD
BIGLEAD
BOWHEAD
BUSLOAD
CARLOAD
CATHEAD
CHILIAD
CRAWDAD
DOESBAD
DONEBAD
EGGHEAD
EIGHTAD
FATHEAD
FEELBAD
FELTBAD
FIFTYAD
FOOTPAD
FORTYAD
GALAHAD
GETSMAD
GOAHEAD
GODHEAD
GOESBAD
GOESMAD
GONEBAD
GONEMAD
HALFBAD
HALFMAD
HEELPAD
HELIPAD
HOTHEAD
HOTLEAD
ILLCLAD
IMPLEAD
INSTEAD
ISAHEAD
ISSUEAD
JUGHEAD
KAMERAD
KNEEPAD
LEWHOAD
LIKEMAD
LILYPAD
LIPREAD
LOOKSAD
LOWROAD
MADEMAD
MAKEMAD
MEMOPAD
MISLEAD
MISREAD
MOPHEAD
NAVIDAD
NOTEPAD
NOVISAD
OFFLOAD
OFFROAD
ONALEAD
OUTLEAD
OUTREAD
OVERSAD
PAYLOAD
PINHEAD
PITHEAD
POPUPAD
PRELOAD
PRINTAD
RADIOAD
REDHEAD
REKNEAD
REPLEAD
RETREAD
SAPHEAD
SEVENAD
SHINPAD
SINDBAD
SIXTYAD
SMALLAD
SOAPPAD
SOLEDAD
STEPDAD
SUBHEAD
THREEAD
TOBEHAD
TOMJOAD
TOWHEAD
TURNBAD
UNTREAD
UPAHEAD
VANLOAD
VENTRAD
VERYBAD
VERYMAD
VERYSAD
WARHEAD
WENTBAD
WENTMAD

AE•••••

AEDILES
AEGISES
AELFRIC
AEOLIAN
AERATED
AERATES
AERATOR
AERIALS
AERIEST
AEROBAT
AEROBES
AEROBIC
AEROSOL

A•E••••

ABELARD
ABETTAL
ABETTED
ABETTER
ABETTOR
ABEYANT
ACEDOUT
ACEHIGH
ACERATE
ACERBIC
ACEROLA
ACEROSE
ACESOUT
ACETALS
ACETATE
ACETIFY
ACETONE
ADELIES
ADELINA
ADELINE
ADELPHI
ADENINE
ADENOID
ADEPTAT
ADEPTER
ADEPTLY
AFEARED
AGEDOUT
AGEFIVE
AGEFOUR
AGEISTS
AGELESS
AGELONG
AGEMATE
AGENCES
AGENDAS
AGENDUM
AGENINE
AGENTED
AGENTRY
AGESAGO
AGESOUT
AHEADOF
AKEBONO
AKERLOF
ALEARDI
ALEGARS
ALEGRIA
ALEKEGS
ALEKSEI
ALEMBIC
ALENCON
ALERTED
ALERTER
ALERTLY
ALERTTO
ALETAPS
ALETTES
ALEVELS
ALEWIFE
ALEYARD
AMEBOID
AMENDED
AMENDER
AMENITY
AMERADA
AMERCED
AMERCER
AMERCES
AMERICA
AMERIGO
AMERIKA
AMERIND
AMESLAN
ANELING
ANEMIAS
ANEMONE
ANEROID
APECKOF
APEDIET
APELETS
APELIKE
APERCUS
APERIES
APERSON
APESUIT
AREAMAP
AREARUG
AREAWAY
ARECIBO
ARENOSE
ARENSKY
AREOLAE
AREOLAR
AREOLAS
AREOLES
ARETINO
ASEETHE
ASEPSIS
ASEPTIC
ASEXUAL
ATEABIT
ATEALOT
ATEAWAY
ATECROW
ATEDIRT
ATEIGHT
ATEINTO
ATEITUP
ATELATE
ATELESS
ATELIER
ATEMORE
ATEOVER
AVENGED
AVENGER
AVENGES
AVENIDA
AVENUEQ
AVENUES
AVERAGE
AVERELL
AVERILL
AVERNAL
AVERNUS
AVERRED
AVERTED
AVERTER
AVESTAN
AVESTAS
AVEYRON
AWEEBIT
AWELESS
AWESOME
AXEHEAD
AXELIKE
AXELROD
AYEAYES

A••E•••

AACELLS
ABREAST
ABSENCE
ABSENTS
ACCEDED
ACCEDER
ACCEDES
ACCENTS
ACCEPTS
ACDELCO
ACHEFOR
ACHENES
ACHERON
ACHESON
ACREAGE
ACTEDAS
ACTEDIN
ACTEDON
ACTEDUP
ADDEDIN
ADDEDLY
ADDEDON
ADDEDTO
ADDEDUP
ADDENDA
ADDENDS
ADHERED
ADHERER
ADHERES
ADRENAL
ADVENTS
ADVERBS
ADVERSE
ADVERTS
AFFECTS
AGREEON
AGREERS
AGREETO
AILERON
AIMEDAT
AIREDUP
ALBEDOS
ALBENIZ
ALBERTA
ALBERTI
ALBERTO
ALCESTE
ALDENTE
ALFEROV
ALGEBRA
ALGERIA
ALIENEE
ALIENOR
ALIENTO
ALKENES
ALLEARS
ALLEGED
ALLEGER
ALLEGES
ALLEGRA
ALLEGRO
ALLELES
ALLELIC
ALLELSE
ALLENBY
ALLENDE
ALLERGY
ALLEWIS
ALLEYES

ALMERIA
ALREADY
ALTERED
ALTERER
ALVEOLI
AMHERST
AMMETER
AMNERIS
AMNESIA
AMNESIC
AMNESTY
AMOEBAE
AMOEBAS
AMOEBIC
AMPEDUP
AMPERES
AMREETA
ANAEMIA
ANAEMIC
ANBESOL
ANDEANS
ANGELAS
ANGELES
ANGELIC
ANGELOU
ANGELUS
ANGERED
ANNEALS
ANNELID
ANNETTE
ANNEXED
ANNEXES
ANSELMO
ANTEDUP
ANTEING
ANTENNA
ANTERUS
ANTESUP
APHELIA
APLENTY
APPEALS
APPEARS
APPEASE
APPENDS
APPETIT
APTERAL
APTERYX
AQUEOUS
ARDECHE
ARDENCY
ARGENTI
ARGENTO
ARGENTS
ARIETTA
ARIETTE
ARLEDGE
ARMENIA
ARREARS
ARRESTS
ARSENAL
ARSENIC
ARSENIO
ARTEMIS
ARTEMUS
ARTERIO
ASCENDS
ASCENTS
ASCETIC
ASEETHE
ASKEDIN
ASKEDOF
ASKEDUP
ASLEWOF
ASPECTS
ASPENCO
ASPERSE
ASSENTS
ASSERTS
ASTERIX
ATDEUCE
ATHEART
ATHEISM
ATHEIST
ATLEAST
ATPEACE
ATSEVEN
ATTEMPT
ATTENDS
ATTESTS
AUBERGE
AUGENDS
AULETTA
AUREATE
AUREOLA
AUREOLE
AUTEURS
AWEEBIT
AXHEADS
AXSEEDS
AZTECAN

A•••E••

AAACELL
ABASERS
ABATERS
ABCDEFG
ABCNEWS
ABIDEBY
ABIDERS
ABILENE
ABUSERS
ACADEME
ACADEMY
ACCRETE
ACHIEST
ACHIEVA
ACHIEVE
ACTAEON
ACTRESS
ACUMENS
ACUTELY
ACUTEST
ADDRESS
ADORERS
AERIEST
AFCTEAM
AFFLECK
AGELESS
AGGRESS
AGILELY
AGILEST
AGREEON
AGREERS
AGREETO
AIDLESS
AIGLETS
AIGRETS
AILMENT
AIMLESS
AIRHEAD
AIRIEST
AIRLESS
AIRNESS
AIRVENT
ALAMEDA
ALAMEIN
ALATEEN
ALCHEMY
ALEKEGS
ALEVELS
ALFIERI
ALFREDA
ALFREDE
ALFREDO
ALFREDU
ALGIEBA
ALGIERS
ALGREEN
ALIMENT
ALINERS
ALIVETO
ALLHEAL
ALLHERE
ALLNESS
ALLNEWS
ALTKEYS
ALUDELS
AMADEUS
AMATEUR
AMBIENS
AMBIENT
AMBLERS
AMPLEST
AMREETA
AMSTELS
AMULETS
AMUSEME
AMUSERS
ANADEMS
ANAHEIM
ANAPEST
ANCIENT
ANDREAS
ANDRESS
ANDREWS
ANGLERS
ANISEED
ANKLERS
ANKLETS
ANSWERS
ANTBEAR
ANTHEIL
ANTHEMS
ANTHERS
ANTLERS
ANTWERP
ANXIETY
ANYNEWS
APELETS
APILEOF
APOGEAL
APOGEAN
APOGEES
APPLETS
APTNESS
ARAMEAN
ARANEID
ARCHERS
ARCHERY
ARCHEST
ARCWELD
ARGUERS
ARIDEST
ARLBERG
ARMLESS
ARMLETS
ARMREST
ARRIERE
ARTDECO
ARTFERN
ARTIEST
ARTLESS
ASATEAM
ASHBERY
ASHHEAP
ASHIEST
ASHLESS
ASSWEET
ASTREAM
ATANEND
ATELESS
ATHLETE
ATMFEES
ATONERS
AUGMENT
AUKLETS
AUSLESE
AUSTERE
AUSTERS
AVERELL
AVIDEST
AVOCETS
AVOWERS
AWAKENS
AWAKERS
AWAREOF
AWAREST
AWELESS
AWNLESS
AXEHEAD
AXSEEDS
AZALEAS
AZOREAN
AZULEJO

A••••E•

AARATED
ABASHED
ABASHES
ABDOMEN
ABDUCED
ABDUCES
ABETTED
ABETTER
ABJURED
ABJURER
ABJURES
ABLATED
ABLATES
ABORTED
ABRADED
ABRADER
ABRADES
ABRILES
ABUTTED
ABUTTER
ABYSSES
ACCEDED
ACCEDER
ACCEDES
ACCRUED
ACCRUES
ACCUSED
ACCUSER
ACCUSES
ACHENES
ACORNED
ACTIFED
ACTIVES
ADAMSES
ADAPTED
ADAPTER
ADDAXES
ADDUCED
ADDUCER
ADDUCES
ADELIES
ADEPTER
ADHERED
ADHERER
ADHERES
ADJURED
ADJURER
ADJURES
ADMIRED
ADMIRER
ADMIRES
ADMIXED
ADMIXES
ADOPTED
ADOPTEE
ADOPTER
ADORNED
ADORNER
ADRATES
ADVICES
ADVISED
ADVISEE
ADVISER
ADVISES
ADWOMEN
AEDILES
AEGISES
AERATED
AERATES
AEROBES
AFEARED
AFFINED
AFFINES
AFFIXED
AFFIXER
AFFIXES
AFRAMES
AGENCES
AGENTED
AGNATES
AGNOMEN
AGONIES
AGUTTER
AIRACES
AIRCREW
AITCHES
ALARMED
ALARMER
ALATEEN
ALBIREO
ALBUMEN
ALCOVES
ALEKSEI
ALERTED
ALERTER
ALETTES
ALGREEN
ALIASES
ALIBIED
ALIENEE
ALIGNED
ALIGNER
ALKENES
ALLAGES
ALLAYED
ALLAYER
ALLEGED
ALLEGER
ALLEGES
ALLELES
ALLEYES
ALLOPEZ
ALLOVER
ALLOWED
ALLOYED
ALLTIED
ALLUDED
ALLUDES
ALLURED
ALLURER
ALLURES
ALMADEN
ALMONER
ALMSMEN
ALPINER
ALPINES
ALROKER
ALROSEN
ALTERED
ALTERER
ALUNSER
ALVAREZ
AMASSED
AMASSER
AMASSES
AMBRIES
AMENDED
AMENDER
AMERCED
AMERCER
AMERCES
AMITIES
AMMETER
AMPERES
AMPULES
ANDOVER
ANDTHEN
ANGELES
ANGERED
ANGRIER
ANISEED
ANNABEL
ANNALEE
ANNALES
ANNEXED
ANNEXES
ANNOYED
ANNOYER
ANNULET
ANOMIES
ANOTHER
ANTARES
ANTIBES
ANTIGEN
ANTSIER
ANYONES
APACHES
APEDIET
APERIES
APHIDES
APLITES
APLUSES
APOGEES
APOTHEM
APPAREL
APPLIED
APPLIER
APPLIES
APPOSED
APPOSES
APRONED
APSIDES
AQUIFER
AQUIVER
ARABLES
ARALSEA
ARBACES
ARBITER
ARBOLES
ARBORED
ARCADED
ARCADES
ARCHIES
ARCHSEE
AREOLES
ARGUSES
ARGYLES
ARIANES
ARMORED
ARMORER
AROUSED
AROUSER
AROUSES
ARRASES
ARRAYED
ARRAYER
ARRISES
ARRIVED
ARRIVER
ARRIVES
ARTSIER
ARUNDEL
ARUSPEX
ASANTES
ASCARED
ASHAMED
ASHIVER
ASHTREE
ASIMMER
ASKOVER
ASPIRED
ASPIRER
ASPIRES
ASQUIET
ASSAYED
ASSAYER
ASSIZES
ASSUMED
ASSUMER
ASSUMES
ASSURED
ASSURER
ASSURES
ASSWEET
ASTUTER
ASUNDER
ATELIER
ATEOVER
ATHOMES
ATLASES
ATMFEES
ATOMIES
ATONIES
ATSEVEN
ATTHREE
ATTIMES
ATTIRED
ATTIRER
ATTIRES
ATTUNED
ATTUNES
ATTYGEN
ATWATER
AUBADES
AUDILES
AUDITED
AUDITEE
AUGITES
AUGURED
AUGURER
AUNTBEE
AUNTIES
AURALEE
AUSSIES
AUTOPEN
AVAILED
AVENGED
AVENGER
AVENGES
AVENUEQ
AVENUES
AVERRED
AVERTED
AVERTER
AVGASES
AVIATED
AVIATES
AVOIDED
AVOIDER
AVONLEA
AVULSED
AVULSES
AWAITED
AWAITER
AWARDED
AWARDEE
AWARDER
AYEAYES
AZINGER
AZODYES

A•••••E

AALARGE
AAMILNE
ABALONE
ABILENE
ABOLLAE
ABRIDGE
ABSCISE
ABSENCE
ABSOLVE
ABUSIVE
ACADEME
ACCRETE
ACERATE
ACEROSE
ACETATE
ACETONE
ACHIEVE
ACHILLE
ACOLYTE
ACONITE
ACOUPLE
ACQUIRE
ACREAGE
ACTABLE
ACTFIVE
ACTLIKE
ACTUATE
ADAMITE
ADAWARE
ADDABLE
ADDIBLE
ADELINE
ADENINE
ADIPOSE
ADJUDGE
ADOLPHE
ADOPTEE
ADSPACE
ADULATE
ADVANCE
ADVERSE
ADVISEE
AFFABLE
AFFAIRE
AGATINE
AGEFIVE
AGEMATE
AGENINE
AGITATE
AGONISE
AGONIZE
AHASSLE
AIRBASE
AIRDATE
AIRDRIE
AIRFARE
AIRFONE
AIRHOLE
AIRHOSE
AIRLANE
AIRLIKE
AIRLINE
AIRMILE
AIRRACE
AIRRAGE
AIRTIME
AIRTUBE
AIRWAVE
ALADINE
ALAMODE
ALANINE
ALBSURE
ALCAIDE
ALCALDE
ALCESTE
ALCYONE
ALDENTE
ALEWIFE
ALFONSE
ALFREDE
ALGARVE
ALIDADE
ALIENEE
ALIGOTE
ALITTLE
ALLANTE
ALLDONE
ALLELSE
ALLENDE
ALLGONE
ALLHERE
ALLMALE
ALLMINE
ALLOFME
ALLONGE
ALLOWME
ALLRISE
ALLTIME
ALLWISE
ALOHAOE
ALUMNAE
AMARONE
AMATIVE
AMBROSE
AMIABLE
AMIBLUE
AMILATE
AMINUTE
AMOEBAE
AMPOULE
AMUSEME
AMYLASE
ANALYSE
ANALYTE
ANALYZE
ANATASE
ANATOLE
ANDANTE
ANDMORE
ANDRADE
ANEMONE
ANILINE
ANIMATE
ANNALEE
ANNETTE
ANODISE
ANODIZE
ANODYNE
ANTIQUE
ANTLIKE
ANTOINE
ANYHOPE
ANYMORE
ANYTIME
ANYWISE
APATITE
APELIKE
APOSTLE
APPEASE
APPRISE
APPROVE
ARACHNE
ARCHFOE
ARCHIVE
ARCHSEE
ARCSINE
ARCUATE
ARDECHE
ARDMORE
ARENOSE
AREOLAE
ARGANTE
ARGONNE
ARIADNE
ARIETTE
ARISTAE
ARLEDGE
ARMBONE
ARMHOLE
ARMLIKE
ARMOIRE
ARRANGE
ARRIERE
ARSHILE
ARTICLE
ARTISTE
ARTSALE
ARTWARE
ASAJOKE
ASARULE
ASCRIBE
ASEETHE
ASHCAKE
ASHTREE
ASININE
ASKANCE
ASPERSE
ASSANTE
ASSLIKE
ASSUAGE
ASTAIRE
ASTARTE
ASTRIDE
ATATIME
ATDEUCE
ATELATE
ATEMORE
ATGRADE
ATHLETE
ATINGLE
ATIPTOE
ATISSUE
ATLARGE
ATOMISE
ATOMIZE
ATPEACE
ATSTAKE
ATTACHE
ATTHREE
ATTRITE
AUBERGE
AUDIBLE
AUDITEE
AUGUSTE
AUNTBEE
AURALEE
AUREATE
AUREOLE
AURICLE
AURORAE
AUSABLE
AUSLESE
AUSPICE
AUSTERE
AUTOMNE
AVARICE
AVERAGE
AWARDEE
AWESOME
AXELIKE
AXILLAE
AXLROSE
AZURITE

•AE••••

CAESARS
CAESURA
DAEMONS
DAEWOOS
FAERIES
FAEROES
GAETANO
HAECKEL
JAECKEL
JAEGERS
LAEMMLE
LAENNEC
LAERTES
MAENADS
MAESTRO
MAEWEST
PAELLAS
RAEBURN
RAEDAWN

•A•E•••

AACELLS
BABENCO
BABETTE
BADEGGS
BADENDS
BADENOV
BAGEHOT
BAKEOFF
BAKEPAN
BAKERST
BALEENS
BALEFUL
BANEFUL
BAREGES
BARENTS
BARETTA
BAREXAM
BASEDON
BASEHIT
BASEMAN
BASEMEN
BASENJI
BASEPAY
BASESIX
BASETEN
BASETWO
BATEAUX
BATEMAN
BAYEDAT
CABEZAS
CADEAUX
CADENCE
CADENCY
CADENZA
CADETTE
CAGEDIN
CAGEDUP
CAGEPET
CAGESUP
CAKEDUP
CAKEMIX
CAKEPAN
CAKESUP
CAKETIN
CALENDS
CAMEDUE
CAMELID
CAMELOT
CAMEOED
CAMEOFF
CAMEOUT
CAMERAE
CAMERAL
CAMERAS
CAMERON
CANETTI
CAPEANN
CAPECOD
CAPEESH
CAPELET
CAPELLA
CAPEMAY
CAPERED
CAREDTO
CAREENS
CAREERS
CAREFOR
CAREFUL
CARESTO
CASEATE
CASEINS
CASELAW
CASELLA
CASELOT
CASEOUS
CASEOUT
CASERNE
CASERNS
CASERTA
CATENAE
CATENAS
CATERAS
CATERED
CATERER
CATERTO
CATEYED
CAVEART
CAVEATS
CAVEDIN
CAVEINS

CAVEMAN	GAPEDAT	LATEENS	NAKEDLY	SALEMOR	WAVEDTO	BASTERS	CATBEDS	FARMERS	HACKETT	LADLERS	MANYEAR	PARCELS
CAVEMEN	GAPESAT	LATEFEE	NAMEDAY	SALERNO	WAVELET	BATHERS	CATBERT	FARMERY	HADBEEN	LAFLEUR	MAPPERS	PARGERS
CAVERNS	GASEDUP	LATENCY	NAMEONE	SAMEDAY	WAVEOFF	BATNEXT	CATFEET	FARNESS	HADBEST	LAGGERS	MARCEAU	PARKERS
CAVESIN	GASEITY	LATENED	NAMETAG	SAMEDIS	WAVERED	BATTENS	CATHEAD	FAROESE	HAILERS	LAKIEST	MARCELS	PARLEYS
CAYENNE	GASEOUS	LATENTS	NANETTE	SAMEKHS	WAVERER	BATTERS	CATSEYE	FARRELL	HALLEYS	LAMBEAU	MARGERY	PARSECS
DALETHS	GASESUP	LATERAL	PACECAR	SAMEOLD	WAVESAT	BATTERY	CAUSERS	FARSEER	HALTERS	LAMBENT	MARKERS	PARSEES
DANELAW	GATEAUX	LATERAN	PACELAP	SATEENS	WAVESIN	BAWLERS	DABBERS	FARWEST	HALVERS	LAMBERT	MARKETS	PARSERS
DANEYKO	GATELEG	LATERON	PACEOFF	SAVEDON	WAVESTO	BAYLEAF	DAFTEST	FASTENS	HAMLETS	LAMBETH	MARLENE	PARVENU
DAREFUL	GATEMAN	LATETAG	PAGEANT	SAVEDUP	WAXEDUP	CABLERS	DAGGERS	FASTEST	HAMMERS	LAMPERT	MARRERS	PASSELS
DARENOT	GATEMEN	LATEXES	PAGEBOY	SAVEFOR	WAXESUP	CABLETS	DAMMERS	FATCELL	HAMMETT	LANCERS	MARTENS	PASSERS
DARESAY	GATEWAY	LAVELLI	PAGEONE	SAVESON	YALELAW	CABLETV	DAMNERS	FATHEAD	HAMPERS	LANCETS	MARVELL	PASSEUL
DARESTO	GAVEEAR	LAVERAN	PAGESIX	SAVESUP	YALEMAN	CACHETS	DAMPENS	FATHERS	HANDERS	LANDERS	MARVELS	PASTEIN
DAREZZO	GAVELED	LAVERNE	PAGETWO	TAGENDS	YALEMEN	CADGERS	DAMPERS	FATLESS	HANDEYE	LANKEST	MASHERS	PASTELS
DATEDLY	GAVEOFF	LAYERED	PALEALE	TAKEAIM	ZANETTO	CAGIEST	DAMPEST	FATNESS	HANGERS	LANTERN	MASKERS	PASTERN
DAVEKOZ	GAVEOUT	LAYETTE	PALEDRY	TAKEFOR		CAHIERS	DAMSELS	FATTENS	HANKERS	LAPBELT	MASSEUR	PASTERS
DAZEDLY	GAVEWAY	LAZENBY	PALEMON	TAKEILL	•A••E••	CAIRENE	DANCERS	FATTEST	HAPLESS	LAPPERS	MASTERP	PASTEUP
EAGERER	GAZEBOS	MACEDON	PALERMO	TAKEINS	AAACELL	CAKIEST	DANDERS	FAUCETS	HAPPENS	LAPPETS	MASTERS	PASTEUR
EAGERLY	GAZEDAT	MADEFIT	PALETTE	TAKENBY	BABIEST	CALDERA	DANGELO	FAWCETT	HARDEES	LAPSERS	MASTERY	PATIENT
EASEDBY	GAZEDON	MADEFOR	PANELED	TAKENIN	BACKEND	CALDERS	DANGERS	FAWNERS	HARDENS	LARCENY	MATHERS	PATNESS
EASEDIN	GAZELLE	MADEFUN	PANETTA	TAKENON	BACKERS	CALKERS	DANIELA	GABBERS	HARDEST	LARDERS	MATHEWS	PATTERN
EASEDON	GAZESAT	MADEHAY	PAPEETE	TAKENTO	BADDEBT	CALLEES	DANIELJ	GABFEST	HARKENS	LARGELY	MATLESS	PATTERS
EASEDUP	GAZESON	MADEILL	PAPELES	TAKENUP	BADDEED	CALLERS	DANIELS	GADDERS	HARLEYS	LARGENT	MATTERS	PATZERS
EASEFUL	GAZETTE	MADEIRA	PAPERED	TAKEOFF	BADDEST	CALMEST	DANKEST	GADGETS	HARMERS	LARGEOJ	MAULERS	PAUPERS
EASELED	HAGERTY	MADELON	PAPERER	TAKEONE	BADGERS	CALTECH	DANSEUR	GADGETY	HARNESS	LARGESS	MAUREEN	PAUSERS
EASEOFF	HAMELIN	MADEMAD	PARENTS	TAKEOUT	BADNESS	CALVERT	DANTEAN	GAFFERS	HARPERS	LARGEST	MAUSERS	PAWNEES
EASEOUT	HAPENNY	MADEOFF	PATELLA	TAKESIN	BADNEWS	CAMBERS	DANTEII	GAGGERS	HARVEST	LARKERS	MAXWELL	PAWNERS
EASESBY	HATEDIT	MADEONE	PATENCY	TAKESIT	BAFFERS	CAMPERS	DANVERS	GAGREEL	HARWELL	LASHERS	MAYBESO	PAYHEED
EASESIN	HATEFUL	MADEOUT	PATENTS	TAKESON	BAGGERS	CANCELS	DARKENS	GAINERS	HASBEEN	LATEENS	MAYHEMS	PAYLESS
EASESON	HATESIT	MADEPAR	PATERNO	TAKESTO	BAGWELL	CANCERS	DARKEST	GAITERS	HASKELL	LATHERS	MAZIEST	PAYMENT
EASESUP	HAVEAGO	MADERUN	PAWEDAT	TAKESUP	BAHREIN	CANDELA	DARLEEN	GALLEON	HASTENS	LATHERY	NABBERS	PAYWELL
EATENAT	HAVEFUN	MADEWAR	RACECAR	TAKETEA	BAILEES	CANDENT	DARLENE	GALLERY	HASTERT	LATRELL	NAGGERS	RABBETS
EATENUP	HAVENER	MADEWAY	RACEDBY	TAKETEN	BAILERS	CANIEST	DARNELL	GALLEYS	HATLESS	LAUDERS	NAILERS	RACIEST
FABERGE	HAVENOT	MAGENTA	RACEDIN	TALENTS	BAITERS	CANKERS	DARNERS	GAMIEST	HATREDS	LAURELS	NAIVELY	RACKERS
FACEDIT	HAVEONE	MAJESTE	RACEDTO	TAPEDON	BALDEST	CANNELL	DARTERS	GAMMERS	HATTERS	LAURENT	NAIVEST	RACKETS
FACEDON	HAVEOUT	MAJESTY	RACEDUP	TAPEDUP	BALEENS	CANNELS	DARWELL	GANDERS	HAULERS	LAWLESS	NAIVETE	RACKETY
FACEOFF	HAYESES	MAJEURE	RACEMES	TAPEMAN	BALKERS	CANNERS	DASHERS	GANGERS	HAUTEUR	LAWYERS	NAIVETY	RAFTERS
FACESIT	IAPETUS	MAKEDOS	RACESBY	TAPEMEN	BALLETS	CANNERY	DAUBERS	GANNETS	HAWKERS	LAXNESS	NAPIERS	RAGGEDY
FACESON	JADEDLY	MAKEFIT	RACESTO	TAPERED	BANDEAU	CANOERS	DAYBEDS	GANNETT	HAWKEYE	LAZIEST	NAPLESS	RAGWEED
FACETED	JADEITE	MAKEFOR	RACESUP	TAPESON	BANDERA	CANSECO	DAYSEND	GAOLERS	HAWSERS	LAZZERI	NAPPERS	RAIDERS
FADEDIN	JAMESII	MAKEFUN	RACEWAY	TAPESUP	BANDERS	CANTEEN	DAYWEAR	GAPLESS	HAYSEED	MACBETH	NASCENT	RAILERS
FADEDLY	JAMESIV	MAKEHAY	RAGEFUL	TASERED	BANGERS	CANTERS	EAGLETS	GARDENA	HAZIEST	MACHETE	NATTERS	RAIMENT
FADEINS	JAMESON	MAKEILL	RAKEDIN	TAVERNA	BANKERS	CAPEESH	EARLESS	GARDENS	JABBERS	MACLEAN	NAUSEAM	RAISERS
FADEOUT	JAMESVI	MAKEMAD	RAKEDUP	TAVERNS	BANNERS	CAPLESS	EARLETS	GARMENT	JACKETS	MACLEOD	OAKDESK	RAISEUP
FADESIN	JANEANE	MAKEOFF	RAKEOFF	VALENCE	BANTERS	CAPLETS	EARNERS	GARNEAU	JAEGERS	MACNEIL	OAKFERN	RAMJETS
FAGENDS	JANEDOE	MAKEONE	RAKESIN	VALENTE	BARBEAU	CAPPERS	EARNEST	GARNERS	JAGLESS	MADDENS	OAKIEST	RAMMERS
FAIENCE	JANEIRO	MAKEOUT	RAKESUP	VALENTI	BARBELL	CARDERS	EASIEST	GARNETS	JAILERS	MADDERS	OAKLEAF	RAMSESI
FAKEDIT	JANEWAY	MAKEPAR	RALEIGH	VALERIE	BARBERA	CAREENS	EASTEGG	GARNETT	JAMBEAU	MADDEST	OARLESS	RANDEEP
FAKEFUR	JAVELIN	MAKERUN	RAMEKIN	VALETED	BARBERS	CAREERS	EASTEND	GARRETS	JAMMERS	MADNESS	OATMEAL	RANGERS
FAKEIDS	JAWEDAT	MAKESDO	RAMESES	VANESSA	BARBETS	CARKEYS	EASTERN	GARRETT	JAPHETH	MAEWEST	PACBELL	RANKERS
FAKEOUT	KADETTS	MAKESGO	RAREBIT	VANEXEL	BARDEEN	CARLENE	EASTERS	GARTERS	JARLESS	MAGLEVS	PACIEST	RANKEST
FAKESIT	KAMERAD	MAKESIT	RAREGAS	VANEYCK	BARGEIN	CARLESS	EATHERE	GASHEAT	JARRELL	MAGNETO	PACKERS	RANTERS
FANEUIL	KANEOHE	MAKESUP	RATECAP	WADEDIN	BARGERS	CARMELA	EATLESS	GASJETS	JARRETT	MAGNETS	PACKETS	RAPIERS
FAREAST	LABELED	MAKEUPS	RATEDPG	WADESIN	BARKEEP	CARNERA	FABBEST	GASKELL	JASPERS	MAIDENS	PADDERS	RAPPELS
FAREBOX	LABELER	MAKEWAR	RAVELED	WAFERED	BARKERS	CARNETS	FABLERS	GASKETS	JASPERY	MAILERS	PADGETT	RAPPERS
FAREWAR	LABELLE	MAKEWAY	RAVELLY	WAGERED	BARLESS	CARPELS	FAINEST	GASLEAK	JAWLESS	MAIMERS	PAIRERS	RASHERS
FATEFUL	LACEDUP	MALEANT	RAVELOE	WAGERER	BARLEYS	CARPERS	FAIREST	GASLESS	JAYCEES	MAINERS	PALLETS	RASHEST
FAYETTE	LACERTA	MALEBEE	RAVENAL	WAGEWAR	BARNEYS	CARPETS	FALLERS	GASPERS	JAYLENO	MAJGENS	PALMERS	RASPERS
GALEATE	LACESON	MALECAT	RAVENED	WAKEDUP	BARRELS	CARRELS	FALSELY	GASSERS	JAYVEES	MALLETS	PALTERS	RASTERS
GALENAS	LACESUP	MALEDOG	RAVENNA	WAKEFUL	BARRENS	CARRERA	FALSEST	GASTERO	JAZZERS	MALLEUS	PAMPERS	RATBERT
GALENTO	LACEUPS	MALEFIC	RAVEUPS	WAKENED	BARRETS	CARRERE	FALTERS	GATHERS	KAISERS	MALTEDS	PANDERS	RATTERS
GALETTE	LAFEMME	MALEHOG	RAWEGGS	WAKENER	BARRETT	CARSEAT	FALWELL	GAUDENS	KAYLENZ	MALTESE	PANIERS	RAWDEAL
GAMEBAG	LAKEBED	MALEPIG	SABERED	WAKESUP	BARTEND	CARTELS	FANBELT	GAUDERY	LABFEES	MANDELA	PANNERS	RAWMEAT
GAMEBOY	LAMENTS	MANEGES	SADEYED	WAKEUPS	BARTERS	CARTERS	FANFEST	GAUGERS	LABTECH	MANGERS	PANTENE	RAWNESS
GAMELAN	LANEONE	MANETTE	SADEYES	WAREPIC	BASHERS	CARVELS	FANJETS	GAVEEAR	LABTEST	MANHEIM	PANTERA	RAYLESS
GAMELAW	LANETWO	MARENGO	SAFEBET	WATERED	BASKETS	CARVERS	FANNERS	GAWKERS	LACIEST	MANLESS	PANTERS	RAYNELL
GAMELEG	LAPELED	MATEWAN	SAFEWAY	WATERER	BASKETT	CASHEWS	FARCEUR	GAWPERS	LACKEYS	MANNERS	PANZERS	SACHEMS
GAMETAL	LAPERMS	MAZEPPA	SAGEHEN	WAVEDAT	BASSETS	CASKETS	FARFELS	GAYNESS	LACTEAL	MANTECA	PAPEETE	SACHETS
GAMETES	LAREDOS	NACELLE	SAGETEA	WAVEDIN	BASSETT	CASTERS	FARLEFT	HACKERS	LADDERS	MANTELS	PAPIERS	SACKERS

SADDENS
SADDEST
SADNESS
SAGIEST
SAILERS
SALIENT
SALIERI
SALTERS
SALVERS
SAMLETS
SAMUELL
SANDERS
SANREMO
SANSEIS
SAPHEAD
SAPIENS
SAPIENT
SAPLESS
SAPPERS
SARGENT
SASSERS
SATEENS
SATIETY
SATWELL
SAUCERS
SAUTEED
SAWYERS
TABKEYS
TABLEAU
TABLETS
TABSETS
TACKERS
TAFFETA
TAGGERS
TAGTEAM
TAILEND
TAILERS
TALKERS
TALLEST
TAMPERS
TANDEMS
TANGELO
TANGENT
TANKERS
TANNERS
TANNERY
TANNEST
TAPPERS
TAPPETS
TARBELL
TARGETS
TARHEEL
TARTEST
TASSELS
TASTEIT
TASTERS
TATTERS
TATTERY
TAUREAN
TAUTENS
TAUTEST
TAXLESS
TAXLEVY
TAXYEAR
VAGUELY
VAGUEST
VAINEST
VALJEAN
VALLEJO
VALLEYS
VALUERS
VAMPERS
VANPELT
VAQUERO
VARIERS
VARIETY
VARLETS
VASTEST
WACKEST
WADDELL
WADDERS
WAFTERS
WAGGERS
WAGGERY
WAILERS
WAITERS
WAIVERS
WALKERS
WALLETS
WALLEYE
WALTERS
WANDERS
WANIEST
WANKELS
WANNESS
WANNEST
WANTERS
WARDENS
WARDERS
WARHEAD
WARHERO
WARIEST
WARLESS
WARMERS
WARMEST
WARPERS
WARRENG
WARRENS
WARVETS
WASHERS
WASTERS
WATTEAU
WAVIEST
WAXBEAN
WAXIEST
WAYLESS
XAVIERU
YAKKERS
YAMMERS
YANKEES
YANKERS
YAPPERS
YARDERS
YARNELL
YASBECK
YATTERS
YAWNERS
YAWPERS
YAYTEAM
ZAMBEZI
ZANIEST
ZAPPERS

•A•••E•

AARATED
BABBLED
BABBLER
BABBLES
BADAREA
BADDEED
BADDIES
BADIDEA
BADLIES
BADOMEN
BAFFIES
BAFFLED
BAFFLER
BAFFLES
BAGGIER
BAGGIES
BAHAMEN
BAILEES
BAINTER
BALASES
BALDIES
BALKIER
BALLMER
BALLUET
BALMIER
BALONEY
BAMMIES
BANACEK
BANALER
BANANES
BANDIED
BANDIER
BANDIES
BANDLET
BANGLED
BANGLES
BANJOES
BANKFEE
BANQUES
BANQUET
BANSHEE
BARBIES
BARDEEN
BAREGES
BARITES
BARKEEP
BARKIER
BARKLEY
BARMIER
BARNRED
BARONET
BARQUES
BARRIER
BARTLES
BARTLET
BASEMEN
BASETEN
BASQUES
BASSIER
BATCHED
BATCHES
BATIKED
BATSMEN
BATTIER
BATTLED
BATTLER
BATTLES
BAUBLES
BAULKED
BAULKER
BAWDIER
BAYAREA
BAYONET
BAYTREE
CABARET
CABBIES
CABINET
CACKLED
CACKLER
CACKLES
CADAVER
CADDIED
CADDIES
CADUCEI
CAGEPET
CAIRNED
CAJOLED
CAJOLER
CAJOLES
CALIBER
CALICES
CALIPER
CALLEES
CALMSEA
CALUMET
CALYCES
CALYXES
CAMEOED
CAMISES
CAMMIES
CAMPBED
CAMPIER
CANALED
CANAPES
CANDIED
CANDIES
CANDLED
CANDLER
CANDLES
CANINES
CANNIER
CANTEEN
CANTLES
CAPADES
CAPELET
CAPERED
CAPOTES
CAPULET
CARAFES
CARAMEL
CARAVEL
CARDKEY
CARFREE
CARGOES
CARIBES
CARNIES
CAROLED
CAROLER
CAROMED
CARRIED
CARRIER
CARRIES
CARTIER
CASHIER
CASQUED
CASQUES
CASTLED
CASTLES
CATCHER
CATCHES
CATERED
CATERER
CATEYED
CATFEET
CATFLEA
CATTIER
CAULKED
CAULKER
CAUTHEN
CAVEMEN
CAVILED
CAVILER
CAYUSES
DABBLED
DABBLER
DABBLES
DADDIES
DAFFIER
DAHOMEY
DAILIES
DAIMLER
DAIRIES
DAIRYER
DAISIES
DALLIED
DALLIER
DALLIES
DALTREY
DAMAGED
DAMAGES
DAMOSEL
DANDIER
DANDIES
DANDLED
DANDLER
DANDLES
DANGLED
DANGLER
DANGLES
DANIKEN
DANITES
DAPHNES
DAPPLED
DAPPLES
DARKLED
DARKLES
DARKRED
DARLEEN
DARTLED
DARTLES
DASHIER
DATASET
DATIVES
DAUMIER
DAUNTED
DAUNTER
DAUSSET
DAWDLED
DAWDLER
DAWDLES
DAZZLED
DAZZLER
DAZZLES
EAGERER
EARLIER
EARLIES
EARTHED
EARTHEN
EASELED
EATOVER
FABARES
FACADES
FACETED
FADAYEV
FADDIER
FADDIET
FAERIES
FAEROES
FAGOTED
FAILLES
FAINTED
FAINTER
FAIRIES
FAIRSEX
FALAFEL
FAMINES
FANCIED
FANCIER
FANCIES
FANSLER
FARRIER
FARSEER
FARTHER
FARTLEK
FASTNET
FATALES
FATFREE
FATONES
FATTIER
FAULTED
FAVORED
FAVORER
GABBIER
GABBLED
GABBLES
GABRIEL
GADSDEN
GAGGLES
GAGREEL
GAGSTER
GALATEA
GALAXES
GALILEE
GALILEI
GALILEO
GALOPED
GAMBIER
GAMBLED
GAMBLER
GAMBLES
GAMELEG
GAMETES
GAMINES
GANTLET
GARAGED
GARAGES
GARBLED
GARBLER
GARBLES
GARDNER
GARGLED
GARGLER
GARGLES
GASOVEN
GASSIER
GATELEG
GATEMEN
GAUCHER
GAUDIER
GAUDIES
GAUNTER
GAUSSES
GAUTIER
GAUZIER
GAVELED
GAWKIER
HAARLEM
HABITED
HACKIES
HACKLED
HACKLER
HACKLES
HACKNEY
HADASET
HADBEEN
HADOVER
HAECKEL
HAGGLED
HAGGLER
HAGGLES
HAIRGEL
HAIRIER
HAIRNET
HALFFED
HALFIES
HALIDES
HALITES
HALOGEN
HAMITES
HAMMIER
HAMSTER
HANAPER
HANDFED
HANDIER
HANDLED
HANDLER
HANDLES
HANDSEL
HANDSET
HANGMEN
HANGTEN
HANKIES
HANOVER
HAPPIER
HARDEES
HARDIER
HARDSET
HARDTEN
HARPIES
HARRIED
HARRIER
HARRIES
HARRIET
HARSHEN
HARSHER
HARTLEY
HASASET
HASBEEN
HASOVER
HASSLED
HASSLES
HASTIER
HATCHED
HATCHER
HATCHES
HATCHET
HAUNTED
HAUNTER
HAVENER
HAYESES
HAYSEED
JACALES
JACKIEO
JACONET
JACQUES
JAECKEL
JAGGIER
JAGGIES
JAMMIER
JAMMIES
JANACEK
JANGLED
JANGLER
JANGLES
JANSSEN
JANVIER
JAUNTED
JAYCEES
JAYVEES
JAZZIER
JAZZMEN
KAISHEK
KARASEA
KARATES
KASTLER
KATAYEV
KAYAKED
KAYAKER
LABELED
LABELER
LABFEES
LABORED
LABORER
LACQUER
LACUREE
LADDIES
LAENNEC
LAERTES
LAISSEZ
LAITIES
LAKEBED
LALAKER
LAMPREY
LANDLER
LANDMEN
LANGLEY
LANKIER
LAPELED
LARCHEN
LARCHES
LARDIER
LARDNER
LARKIER
LASSIES
LASSOED
LASSOER
LASSOES
LASTLEG
LATCHED
LATCHES
LATEFEE
LATENED
LATEXES
LATICES
LATIMES
LAUGHED
LAUGHER
LAUNDER
LAUTREC
LAVAGES
LAYERED
LAYOPEN
LAYOVER
MAARTEN
MACHREE
MACUSER
MADAMES
MADAMEX
MADCHEN
MAGPIES
MAHONEY
MAIGRET
MAILMEN
MAINMEN
MAITRED
MAITRES
MAJORED
MALEBEE
MALICES
MALMSEY
MALTIER
MAMBOED
MANAGED
MANAGER
MANAGES
MANATEE
MANDREL
MANEGES
MANFRED
MANGIER
MANGLED
MANGLER
MANGLES
MANGOES
MANLIER
MANNIES
MANTLED
MANTLES
MANTLET
MANURED
MANURES
MANXMEN
MARBLED
MARBLER
MARBLES
MARCHED
MARCHER
MARCHES
MARGRET
MARINER
MARINES
MARLIER
MARNIER
MARQUEE
MARQUES
MARQUEZ
MARRIED
MARRIES
MARSDEN
MARSHES
MARSRED
MARVIER
MASHIES
MASONED
MASQUER
MASQUES
MASSIER
MATCHED
MATCHER
MATCHES
MATHIEU
MATINEE
MATTHEW
MATURED
MATURER
MATURES
MAUNDER
MAUREEN
MAVISES
MAXBAER
MAXIXES
NAGGIER
NAIADES
NAILKEG
NAILSET
NANNIED
NANNIES
NAPPIER
NAPPIES
NAPSTER
NARTHEX
NARVAEZ
NASTIER
NASTIES
NATCHEZ
NATIVES
NATTIER
NATURED
NATUREL
NATURES
NAVYMEN
OAKTREE
OARSMEN
PADDIES
PADDLED
PADDLER
PADDLES
PAINTED
PAINTER
PAISLEY
PAIUTES
PALACES
PALATES
PALAVER
PALFREY
PALJOEY
PALLIER
PALMIER
PANACEA
PANELED
PANGAEA
PANNIER
PANSIES
PANTHER
PANTIES
PANTLEG
PAPELES
PAPERED
PAPERER
PAPPIES
PARADED
PARADER
PARADES
PARAPET
PARCHED
PARCHES
PARDNER
PAROLED
PAROLEE
PAROLES
PARQUET
PARRIED
PARRIER
PARRIES
PARSEES
PARSLEY
PARTIED
PARTIER
PARTIES
PARTNER
PARTYER
PARURES
PASSKEY
PASTIER
PASTIES
PATCHED
PATCHEN
PATCHER
PATCHES
PATRIES
PATSIES
PATTIES
PAULSEN
PAVANES
PAWNEES
PAYHEED
RABBLED
RABBLES
RACEMES
RACHAEL
RACQUET
RADAMES
RADICES
RADIOED
RADIOER
RADIXES
RADOMES
RAFFLED
RAFFLER
RAFFLES
RAGGIER
RAGGIES
RAGWEED
RAILMEN
RAINIER
RALLIED
RALLIER
RALLIES
RALLYES
RAMBLED
RAMBLER
RAMBLES
RAMESES
RAMIREZ
RAMONES
RANCHED
RANCHER
RANCHES
RANDEEP
RANDIER
RANFREE
RANGIER
RANKLED
RANKLES
RANOVER
RAPHAEL
RAPIDER
RAPINES
RASPIER
RASSLED
RASSLER
RASSLES
RASURES
RATCHET
RATINES
RATITES
RATTIER
RATTLED
RATTLER
RATTLES
RAVAGED
RAVAGER
RAVAGES
RAVELED
RAVENED
RAVINED
RAVINES
RAZORED
RAZZIES
SABERED
SABINES
SACQUES
SADDLED
SADDLER
SADDLES
SADEYED
SADEYES
SAFEBET
SAGEHEN
SAGETEA
SAGGIER
SAINTED
SAINTES
SALADES
SALINES
SALLIED
SALLIER
SALLIES
SALTIER
SALTSEA
SALUTED
SALUTER
SALUTES
SALVOES
SAMBAED
SAMISEN
SAMOSET
SAMOYED
SAMPLED
SAMPLER
SAMPLES
SANDIER
SANDLER
SANDMEN
SANIBEL
SAPPIER
SARACEN
SARALEE
SARAZEN
SASSIER
SATCHEL
SATINET
SATIRES
SAUCIER
SAUNAED
SAUNTER
SAUTEED
SAVAGED
SAVAGER
SAVAGES
SAVORED
SAVORER
SAVVIED
SAVVIER
SAVVIES
SAYAMEN
SAYOVER
SAYSYES
SAYWHEN
TABARET
TABBIES
TABOOED
TABORET
TACKIER
TACKLED
TACKLER
TACKLES
TAFFIES
TAGAMET
TAINTED
TAKETEA
TAKETEN
TALCKED
TALKIER
TALKIES
TALLIED
TALLIER
TALLIES
TALONED
TALUSES
TAMALES
TAMGLEN
TANAGER
TANGIER
TANGLED
TANGLER
TANGLES
TANGOED
TANGOER
TANSIES
TAPEMEN
TAPERED
TAPSTER
TARDIER
TARHEEL
TARRIED
TARRIER
TARRIES
TARTIER
TARTLET

TASERED
TASTIER
TATTIER
TATTLED
TATTLER
TATTLES
TAUNTED
TAUNTER
TAWNIER
TAXFREE
TAXIMEN
VACATED
VACATES
VALETED
VALINES
VALISES
VALOREM
VAMPIER
VANDIEN
VANEXEL
VANOWEN
VAPORED
VAPORER
VARITEK
VASQUEZ
VASTIER
VATDYED
VATDYES
VAULTED
VAULTER
VAUNTED
VAUNTER
WACKIER
WADDLED
WADDLER
WADDLES
WAFERED
WAFFLED
WAFFLER
WAFFLES
WAGERED
WAGERER
WAGGLED
WAGGLER
WAGGLES
WAGONED
WAGONER
WAHINES
WAISTED
WAKAMES
WAKENED
WAKENER
WALTHER
WALTZED
WALTZER
WALTZES
WAMBLED
WAMBLES
WANGLED
WANGLER
WANGLES
WARBLED
WARBLER
WARBLES
WARTIER
WASHIER
WASPIER
WASTREL
WATCHED
WATCHER
WATCHES
WATERED
WATERER
WATTLED
WATTLES
WAVELET
WAVERED
WAVERER
YACHTED
YACHTER
YAHTZEE
YALEMEN
YANKEES
YARDMEN
YAWNIER
ZAPATEO
ZAPOTEC
ZAPPIER
ZATOPEK

•A••••E

AALARGE
AAMILNE
BAALITE
BABBAGE
BABETTE
BACCHAE
BACKHOE
BADCASE
BADJOKE
BADLOVE
BADMOVE
BADNAME
BADTIME
BAGGAGE
BAGLIKE
BAGPIPE
BALANCE
BALLADE
BALLONE
BANDAGE
BANKFEE
BANKONE
BANSHEE
BAPTISE
BAPTIZE
BARBATE
BARBULE
BARCODE
BARNONE
BAROQUE
BARRAGE
BARWARE
BASSALE
BATISTE
BATLIKE
BAUXITE
BAYONNE
BAYTREE
CABALLE
CABBAGE
CABFARE
CABOOSE
CABRIDE
CACIQUE
CADENCE
CADETTE
CAIRENE
CALCITE
CALIBRE
CALORIE
CALOTTE
CALZONE
CAMEDUE
CAMERAE
CAMILLE
CAMRYLE
CANDACE
CANDICE
CANDIDE
CANIDAE
CANITBE
CANULAE
CANZONE
CAPABLE
CAPAPIE
CAPRICE
CAPRINE
CAPSIZE
CAPSULE
CAPTIVE
CAPTURE
CAPUCHE
CARBIDE
CARBINE
CARCARE
CARFARE
CARFREE
CARINAE
CARIOLE
CARLENE
CARLYLE
CARMINE
CARNAGE
CAROUSE
CARRERE
CARSALE
CARTAGE
CARTIRE
CASCADE
CASEATE
CASERNE
CASTILE
CATENAE
CATHODE
CATLIKE
CATORCE
CATSEYE
CAUDATE
CAVIARE
CAYENNE
DARKAGE
DARLENE
DASCHLE
DATABLE
DAYCARE
DAYGAME
DAYMARE
DAYSIDE
DAYTIME
EARACHE
EARBONE
EARHOLE
EARLIKE
EARLOBE
EASYONE
EATABLE
EATCAKE
EATHERE
EATLATE
EATMORE
FABERGE
FACONNE
FACULAE
FADLIKE
FAIENCE
FAILURE
FAIRUSE
FALCATE
FALLDUE
FAMILLE
FANBASE
FANFARE
FANLIKE
FANTINE
FANWISE
FANZINE
FARGONE
FARMORE
FAROESE
FARSIDE
FASCIAE
FASTONE
FATFREE
FATIGUE
FATLIKE
FAXLORE
FAYETTE
GAGLINE
GAGRULE
GALAXIE
GALEATE
GALETTE
GALILEE
GARBAGE
GARONNE
GAROTTE
GARPIKE
GARROTE
GASLINE
GASPIPE
GASTONE
GAVOTTE
GAZELLE
GAZETTE
HABITUE
HADDONE
HADSOME
HADTIME
HADTOBE
HAGLIKE
HAIRDYE
HALDANE
HAMBONE
HAMLINE
HANDAXE
HANDEYE
HARLINE
HASDONE
HASTIME
HASTOBE
HATABLE
HATLIKE
HATSIZE
HAULAGE
HAVEONE
HAWKEYE
HAYBALE
HAYRIDE
HAYWIRE
IAMLOVE
JACCUSE
JADEITE
JAMLIKE
JANEANE
JANEDOE
JARDINE
JASMINE
JAWBONE
JAWLIKE
JAWLINE
JAZZAGE
KANEOHE
KAPTURE
KARAOKE
KATRINE
LABELLE
LABIATE
LABMICE
LABTUBE
LACOSTE
LACTASE
LACTATE
LACTOSE
LACUNAE
LACUREE
LADOUCE
LADRONE
LAEMMLE
LAFARGE
LAFEMME
LAFITTE
LAGASSE
LAICIZE
LALANNE
LALIQUE
LAMINAE
LAMOTTE
LANCOME
LANEONE
LANOTTE
LAPLACE
LAPORTE
LAPROBE
LAPWARE
LARAINE
LARAMIE
LAROCHE
LASAGNE
LASALLE
LASTONE
LATEFEE
LATRINE
LATROBE
LATTICE
LAVACHE
LAVAINE
LAVALSE
LAVERNE
LAWCASE
LAWLIKE
LAYBARE
LAYETTE
MACABRE
MACAQUE
MACHETE
MACHINE
MACHONE
MACHREE
MACRAME
MACULAE
MADEONE
MAGNATE
MAGUIRE
MAJESTE
MAJEURE
MAKABLE
MAKEONE
MALAISE
MALDIVE
MALEBEE
MALTASE
MALTBIE
MALTESE
MALTOSE
MALWARE
MANACLE
MANATEE
MANDATE
MANETTE
MANHOLE
MANIPLE
MANLIKE
MANMADE
MANROPE
MANSIZE
MARCUSE
MARGATE
MARLENE
MARLOWE
MARQUEE
MARRYME
MARYURE
MASSAGE
MASSINE
MASSIVE
MATINEE
MATISSE
MAURICE
MAYPOLE
MAYTIME
MAYWINE
NACELLE
NAIVETE
NAMABLE
NAMEONE
NANETTE
NAPTIME
NARRATE
NASTASE
NATALIE
NATSUME
NAVARRE
OAKLIKE
OAKTREE
OARLIKE
OATCAKE
OATLIKE
PACKAGE
PACKICE
PADRONE
PADSITE
PAGEONE
PALANCE
PALEALE
PALETTE
PALMATE
PALPATE
PANACHE
PANCAKE
PANICLE
PANPIPE
PANTENE
PANTILE
PANTONE
PANURGE
PAPEETE
PAPOOSE
PARABLE
PARBAKE
PARFIVE
PARKADE
PARKAVE
PAROLEE
PARTAKE
PARTITE
PARTONE
PASALLE
PASSADE
PASSAGE
PASSIVE
PASTDUE
PASTIME
PASTURE
PATRICE
PAULINE
PAYABLE
PAYMORE
PAYRATE
RADIATE
RADICLE
RAGTIME
RAILAGE
RAKABLE
RALPHIE
RAMHOME
RAMLIKE
RAMPAGE
RANFREE
RANHOME
RANKINE
RANLATE
RAPTUNE
RAPTURE
RATABLE
RATHOLE
RATLIKE
RATLINE
RATRACE
RAVELOE
RAWHIDE
RAYLIKE
SACCADE
SACLIKE
SADCAFE
SADFATE
SAIDAYE
SALABLE
SALTINE
SALVAGE
SAMWISE
SANJOSE
SANTAFE
SAOTOME
SARALEE
SARDINE
SATHOME
SATIATE
SAUSAGE
SAVABLE
SAWLIKE
SAYABLE
SAYMORE
SAYSAYE
TACTILE
TADPOLE
TAGLIKE
TAGLINE
TAGSALE
TAKABLE
TAKEONE
TALLONE
TAMABLE
TANKAGE
TANLINE
TAPSHOE
TARTARE
TAURINE
TAXABLE
TAXBASE
TAXCODE
TAXFREE
TAXHIKE
TAXRATE
TAXSALE
VACCINE
VACUOLE
VALANCE
VALENCE
VALENTE
VALERIE
VALLONE
VALOTTE
VALUATE
VALVATE
VALVULE
VAMOOSE
VAMPIRE
VANDINE
VANDYKE
VANLINE
VANTAGE
VARIATE
WALKURE
WALLACE
WALLEYE
WALPOLE
WANNABE
WARFARE
WARGAME
WARLIKE
WARPAGE
WARTIME
WARZONE
WASLATE
WASSURE
WASTAGE
WATTAGE
WAVICLE
WAXABLE
WAXLIKE
WAYSIDE
YACHTIE
YAHTZEE
YANGTZE
YAOUNDE
YARDAGE
YASMINE
ZADKINE

••AE•••

ANAEMIA
ANAEMIC
BRAEDEN
CPAEXAM
PHAEDRA
PHAETON
PRAETOR
SEAEELS

••A•E••

AAACELL
ABASERS
ABATERS
ACADEME
ACADEMY
ALAMEDA
ALAMEIN
ALATEEN
AMADEUS
AMATEUR
ANADEMS
ANAHEIM
ANAPEST
ARAMEAN
ARANEID
ASATEAM
ATANEND
AWAKENS
AWAKERS
AWAREOF
AWAREST
AZALEAS
BEADERS
BEAHERO
BEAKERS
BEAMERS
BEANERY
BEARERS
BEATERS
BEAVERS
BLADERS
BLAKELY
BLAMEON
BLAMERS
BLAZERS
BLAZEUP
BOATELS
BOATERS
BRACERO
BRACERS
BRACEUP
BRALESS
BRAVELY
BRAVERY
BRAVEST
BRAYERS
BRAZENS
BYANECK
CHAFERS
CHALETS
CHANELS
CHAPEAU
CHAPELS
CHASERS
CHATEAU
CLARETS
CLAVELL
CLAWERS
COAGENT
COALERS
COATEES
COATERS
COAXERS
CRATERS
CRATEUP
CRAVENS
CRAVERS
DEADEND
DEADENS
DEADEST
DEADEYE
DEAFENS
DEAFEST
DEALERS
DEANERY
DEAREST
DIADEMS
DIALECT
DIALEDO
DIALERS
DIAPERS
DNATEST
DOADEAL
DRAGEES
DRAMEDY
DRAPERS
DRAPERY
DRAWEES
DRAWERS
EBAYERS
ELANETS
ELATERS
ENAMELS
ERASERS
ETAGERE
EVADERS
FEARERS
FLAKERS
FLAMERS
FLAMEUP
FLANEUR
FLAREUP
FLAYERS
FOAMERS
FRAMERS
FRAMEUP
FRATERS
GLACEED
GLADEYE
GLAREAT
GLAZERS
GNAWERS
GOAHEAD
GOATEED
GOATEES
GRADEAA
GRADERS
GRAPERY
GRATEON
GRATERS
GRATEUP
GRAVELS
GRAVELY
GRAVERS
GRAVEST
GRAYEST
GRAZERS
HEADEND
HEADERS
HEALERS
HEAPERS
HEARERS
HEATERS
HEAVEHO
HEAVENS
HEAVERS
HEAVETO
HIALEAH
HOAXERS
IDAREDS
IHATEIT
IHAVEIT
IMADEIT
IMAGERS
IMAGERY
IMAMESS
IMARETS
INAHEAP
INAMESS
INANELY
INANEST
INAWEOF
IPANEMA
IRATELY
IRATEST
ISABEAU
ISAHEAD
KNAVERY
KRAKENS
LEADENS
LEADERS
LEADETH
LEAKERS
LEAKEYS
LEANERS
LEANEST
LEAPERS
LEASERS
LEASETO
LEAVEBE
LEAVEIN
LEAVEIT
LEAVENS
LEAVEON
LLANERO
LOADERS
LOAFERS
LOANERS
MEANEST
MOANERS
NBATEAM
NEAREST
NEATENS
NEATEST
ONAGERS
ONALEAD
ONALERT
ONATEAR
PEABEAN
PEAHENS
PHASEIN
PHASERS
PLACEBO
PLACERS
PLANERS
PLANETS
PLATEAU
PLATENS
PLATERS
PLAYERS
PRADESH
PRATERS
PRAYERS
QUAKERS
QUAVERS
QUAVERY
READERS
REAGENT
REALEST
REAMEND
REAMERS
REAPERS
REAREND
REARERS
REAVERS
ROADEOS
ROADERS
ROAMERS
ROARERS
SCALENE
SCALERS
SCALEUP
SCAREDY
SCARERS
SCAREUP
SEABEDS
SEABEES
SEAEELS
SEAFERN
SEAHERO
SEALEGS
SEALERS
SEALERY
SEAMERS
SEARERS
SEATERS
SEAWEED
SHADERS
SHAKERS
SHAKEUP
SHAPELY
SHAPERS
SHAPEUP
SHAREIN
SHARERS
SHAVERS
SIAMESE
SKATERS
SLAKERS
SLATERS
SLAVERS
SLAVERY
SLAYERS
SNAKERS
SNARERS
SOAKERS
SOAPERS
SOARERS
SOAREWE
SPACELY
SPACERS
SPADERS
SPARELY
SPAREME
SPARERS
SPAREST
SPAYERS
STAGERS
STALELY
STALEST
STAMENS
STAREAT
STARERS
STATELY
STATERS
STAYERS
SUAVELY
SUAVEST
SWAYERS
TEALEAF
TEALESS
TEANECK
TEARERS
TEASELS
TEASERS
TEASETS
TEASEUP
THALERS
THAWERS
TRABERT
TRACERS
TRACERY
TRADEIN
TRADEON
TRADERS
TRADEUP
TRAGEDY
TRAPEZE
TRAVELS
TRAVERS
UNADEPT
UNALERT
UPAHEAD
VIADENT
WEAKENS
WEAKEST
WEANERS
WEARERS
WEASELS
WEAVERS
WHALERS
YEAREND
YEATEAM

••A••E•

ABASHED
ABASHES
ADAMSES
ADAPTED
ADAPTER
ALARMED
ALARMER
ALATEEN
AMASSED
AMASSER
AMASSES
APACHES
ARABLES
ARALSEA
ASANTES
AVAILED
AWAITED
AWAITER
AWARDED
AWARDEE
AWARDER
BEACHED
BEACHES
BEADIER
BEADLES
BEAGLES
BEAMIER
BEANIES
BEARDED
BEASLEY
BEATLES
BIALIES
BIASSED
BIASSES
BLABBED
BLABBER
BLACKED
BLACKEN
BLACKER
BLADDER
BLAKLEY
BLANDER
BLANKED
BLANKER
BLANKET
BLARNEY
BLASTED
BLASTER
BLATHER
BLATTED
BOARDED
BOARDER
BOASTED
BOASTER
BOATMEN
BRACKEN
BRACKET
BRADLEE
BRADLEY
BRAEDEN
BRAGGED
BRAGGER
BRAIDED
BRAIDER
BRAINED
BRAINER
BRAISED
BRAISES
BRAMLEY
BRANDED
BRANDER
BRASHER
BRASHES
BRASIER
BRASSES
BRAVOED
BRAVOES
BRAWLED
BRAWLER
BRAWLEY
BRAZIER
CHAFFED
CHAFFEE
CHAFFER
CHAINED
CHAINES
CHAIRED
CHAISES
CHALKED
CHAMBER
CHAMFER
CHAMPED
CHAMPER
CHANCED
CHANCEL
CHANCER
CHANCES
CHANGED
CHANGER
CHANGES
CHANNEL
CHANTED
CHANTER
CHANTEY
CHAPLET
CHAPMEN
CHAPPED
CHAPTER
CHARGED
CHARGER
CHARGES
CHARIER
CHARLES
CHARLEY
CHARMED
CHARMEN
CHARMER
CHARRED
CHARRER
CHARTED
CHARTER
CHARVET
CHASSED
CHASSES
CHASTEN
CHASTER
CHATTED
CHATTEL
CHATTER
CHAUCER
CLABBER
CLACKED
CLACKER
CLADDED
CLAIMED
CLAIMER
CLAMBER
CLAMMED
CLAMMER
CLAMPED
CLAMPER
CLANGED
CLANGER
CLANKED
CLAPPED
CLAPPER
CLAQUES
CLASHED
CLASHER
CLASHES
CLASPED
CLASPER
CLASSED
CLASSER
CLASSES
CLATTER
CLAUDEL
CLAUSES
CLAVIER
CLAYIER
COACHED
COACHES
COACTED
COAPTED
COARSEN
COARSER
COASTED
COASTER
COATEES
CRABBED
CRABBER
CRACKED
CRACKER
CRADLED
CRADLER
CRADLES
CRAFTED
CRAFTER
CRAGGED
CRAMMED
CRAMMER
CRAMPED
CRANKED
CRANMER
CRASHED
CRASHER
CRASHES
CRASSER
CRAWLED
CRAWLER
CRAWLEY
CRAZIER
CRAZIES
DEADSEA
DEADSET
DEAIRED
DEARDEN
DEARIES
DIABLES
DIALLED
DIARIES
DNAASES
DRABBER
DRAFTED
DRAFTEE
DRAFTER
DRAGEES
DRAGGED
DRAGGER
DRAGNET
DRAINED
DRAINER
DRATTED
DRAWEES
DRAWLED
DRAWLER
DRAWMEN
DRAYMEN
DWARFED
DWARVES
EBANKED
ECARTES
EDASNER
ELAINES
ELANCES
ELAPSED
ELAPSES
EMAILED
EMAILER
EMANUEL
ENABLED
ENABLER
ENABLES
ENACTED
ENARMED
EPAULET
ETAILED
ETAILER
EVACUEE
EVANDER
EVANGEL
EXACTED
EXACTER
EXALTED
EXALTER
FEASTED
FEASTER
FEATHER
FIACRES
FIANCEE
FIANCES
FLACKED
FLAGGED
FLAGGER
FLAGMEN
FLAILED
FLAKIER
FLAMBED
FLAMBES
FLAMIER
FLAMMED
FLANGES
FLANKED
FLANKEN
FLANKER
FLANNEL
FLAPPED
FLAPPER
FLASHED
FLASHER
FLASHES
FLATBED
FLATLET
FLATTED
FLATTEN
FLATTER
FLAWIER
FLAXIER
FOAMIER
FRAGGED
FRAILER
FRAISES
FRANCES
FRANKED
FRANKEN
FRANKER
FRAPPES
FRASIER
FRAWLEY
FRAZIER
GLACEED
GLACIER
GLADDEN
GLADDER
GLANCED
GLANCES
GLASSED
GLASSES
GLAZIER
GNARLED
GNARRED
GNASHED
GNASHER
GNASHES
GOAFTER
GOALIES
GOATEED
GOATEES
GRABBED
GRABBER
GRAFTED
GRAFTER
GRAINED
GRAINER
GRAMMER
GRAMMES
GRANDEE
GRANDER
GRANGER
GRANGES
GRANTED
GRANTEE
GRANTER
GRAPHED
GRAPIER
GRAPNEL
GRASPED
GRASPER
GRASSED
GRASSES
GRAVIES
GRAZIER
GUARDED
GUARDEE
GUARDER
HAARLEM
HEADIER
HEADMEN
HEADSET
HEARKEN
HEARSES
HEARTED
HEARTEN
HEATHEN
HEATHER
HEATTER
HEAVIER
HEAVIES
HOAGIES
HOARDED
HOARDER
HOARIER
HOARSEN
HOARSER
IMAGOES
INAPOEM
INAPTER
INASTEW
KEARNEY
KLAMMER
KNARRED
KRACKEL
KRAMDEN
KRASNER
KVASSES
LEACHED
LEACHER
LEACHES
LEADIER
LEADMEN
LEAFIER
LEAFLET
LEAGUED
LEAGUER
LEAGUES
LEAKIER
LEANDER
LEARJET
LEARNED
LEARNER
LEASHED
LEASHES
LEATHER
LIAISED
LIAISES
LOAMIER
LOATHED
LOATHER
LOATHES
MAARTEN
MCALLEN
MEAGLES
MEALIER
MEALIES
MEANDER
MEANIES
MEASLES
MEATIER
MEATMEN
MIAOUED
MIAOWED
NOANGEL
NUANCED
NUANCES
OMALLEY
ONADIET
OPAQUES
ORACIES
ORACLES
ORANGES
ORANGEY
ORANTES
OTARIES
OVARIES
PEACHED
PEACHES
PEAKIER
PEARLED
PEARLER
PEATIER
PHATTER
PIAFFED
PIAFFES
PIASTER
PLACKET
PLAGUED
PLAGUES
PLAICES
PLAINER
PLAINES
PLAITED
PLAITER
PLANKED
PLANNED
PLANNER
PLANTED
PLANTER
PLAQUES
PLASHED
PLASHES
PLASTER
PLATIER
PLATIES
PLATTED
PLATTER
PLAYLET
PLAYPEN
PLAYTEX
POACHED
POACHER
POACHES
PRAISED
PRAISER
PRAISES
PRANCED
PRANCER
PRANCES
PRAWNED
PSALTER
QUACKED
QUACKER
QUAFFED
QUAFFER
QUAILED
QUAKIER
QUAKIES
QUARLES
QUARREL
QUARTER
QUARTES
QUARTET
QUASHED
QUASHES
QUATRES
REACHED
REACHER
REACHES
REACTED
READDED
READIED
READIER
READIES
REAIMED
REAIRED
REALMEN
REALTER
REANNEX
REARMED
REASKED
ROACHES
ROADBED
ROADIES
ROASTED
ROASTER
RVALUES
SCALDED
SCALDER
SCALIER
SCALPED
SCALPEL
SCALPER
SCAMMED
SCAMMER
SCAMPED
SCAMPER
SCANNED
SCANNER
SCANTED
SCANTER
SCARCER
SCARFED
SCARFER
SCARIER
SCARLET
SCARPED
SCARRED
SCARVES
SCATHED
SCATHES
SCATTED
SCATTER
SEABEES
SEAGREN
SEAMIER
SEANCES
SEAWEED
SHACKED
SHADIER
SHAFFER
SHAFTED
SHAGGED
SHAKIER
SHAKOES
SHALIER
SHAMMED
SHANKED
SHANNEN
SHANTER
SHARKEY
SHARPED
SHARPEI
SHARPEN
SHARPER
SHATNER
SHATTER
SHAWLED
SHAWNEE
SLABBED
SLACKED
SLACKEN
SLACKER
SLAMMED
SLAMMER
SLANDER
SLANTED
SLAPPED
SLAPPER
SLASHED
SLASHER
SLASHES
SLATHER
SLATIER
SLATTED
SMACKED
SMACKER
SMALLER
SMARTED
SMARTEN
SMARTER
SMASHED
SMASHER
SMASHES
SMATTER
SNACKED
SNACKER
SNAFUED
SNAGGED
SNAGGER
SNAKIER
SNAPPEA
SNAPPED
SNAPPER
SNARFED
SNARLED
SNARLER
SOAPIER
SOAPNET
SPACIER
SPAMMED
SPAMMER
SPANDEX
SPANIEL
SPANKED
SPANKER
SPANNED
SPANNER
SPARKED
SPARRED
SPARRER
SPARSER
SPATHES
SPATTED
SPATTER
SPAWNED
SPAWNER
STABBED
STABBER
STABLED
STABLER
STABLES
STACKED
STACKER
STADLER
STAFFED
STAFFER
STAGGED
STAGGER
STAGIER
STAGNES
STAIDER
STAINED
STAINER
STAIRED
STALKED
STALKER
STALLED
STALLER
STAMMER
STAMPED
STAMPER
STANCES
STANDEE
STANDER
STANLEE
STANLEY
STAPLED
STAPLER
STAPLES
STARKER
STARKEY
STARLET
STARRED
STARTED
STARTER
STARVED
STARVES
STASHED
STASHES
STASSEN
STATLER
STATUES
SWABBED
SWABBER
SWAGGER
SWAGMEN
SWAMPED
SWANKED
SWANKER
SWANSEA
SWAPPED
SWAPPER
SWARMED
SWARMER
SWASHED
SWASHES
SWATHED
SWATHES
SWATTED
SWATTER
TEACHER
TEACHES
TEARIER
TEATREE
THANKED
THANKER
TIARAED
TOADIED
TOADIES
TOASTED
TOASTEE
TOASTER
TRACHEA
TRACKED
TRACKER
TRAILED
TRAILER
TRAINED
TRAINEE
TRAINER
TRAMMED
TRAMMEL
TRAMPED
TRAMPER
TRANCED
TRANCES
TRAPPED
TRAPPER
TRASHED
TRASHER
TRASHES
TRAUBEL
TRAWLED
TRAWLER
TWANGED
TWANGER
UNACTED
UNADDED
UNAIDED
UNAIMED
UNAIRED
UNARMED
UNASKED
UNAXLED
UPATREE
USABLES
USANCES
UVALUES
VEALIER
VIALLED
WEARIED
WEARIER
WEARIES
WEATHER
WHACKED
WHACKER
WHALLEY
WHAMMED
WHANGED
WHAPPED
WHARFED
WHARVES
WHAUDEN
WRACKED
WRANGEL
WRAPPED
WRAPPER
WRASSES
YEARNED
YEARNER
YEASTED

••A•••E

ABALONE
ACADEME
ADAMITE
ADAWARE
AGATINE
AHASSLE
ALADINE
ALAMODE
ALANINE
AMARONE
AMATIVE
ANALYSE
ANALYTE
ANALYZE
ANATASE
ANATOLE
APATITE
ARACHNE
ASAJOKE
ASARULE
ATATIME
AVARICE
AWARDEE
BAALITE
BEASTIE
BEATSME
BEATTIE
BLACKIE
BLANCHE
BRADLEE
BRAILLE
BRAMBLE
BRASIZE
BRASSIE
BRATTLE
BYAMILE
BYANOSE
CHAFFEE
CHALICE
CHAMBRE
CHAPPIE
CHARADE
CHARLIE
CHAYOTE
CLARICE
CLAVATE
CRACKLE
CRAIGIE
CRAPPIE
CYANIDE
DEADEYE
DEARONE
DNACODE
DRABBLE
DRAFTEE
DRAGGLE
DRAYAGE
DUALIZE
EGALITE
ELAMITE
EMANATE
ERASURE
ETAGERE
ETAMINE
EVACUEE
EVASIVE
EXABYTE
EXAMINE
EXAMPLE
FEATURE
FIANCEE
FRAGGLE
FRAGILE
FRAICHE
FRANKIE
FRAZZLE
GIAUQUE
GLADEYE
GLAVINE
GRACILE
GRACKLE
GRADATE
GRAHAME
GRANDEE
GRANITE
GRANNIE
GRANTEE
GRANULE
GRAPPLE
GRASSLE
GRAVURE
GUANINE
GUARDEE
HUANGHE
HYALITE
IMAGINE
IMAMATE
INADAZE
INAHOLE
INALINE
INAPILE
INAPOKE
INARAGE
INASHOE
INAVALE
ISADORE
IVANHOE
JEANNIE
KHANATE
LEADORE
LEAFAGE
LEAKAGE
LEAVEBE
MBABANE
MCARDLE
MEANAGE
MEANJOE
MEASURE
MEATAXE
MEATPIE
MOABITE
NBAGAME
NBALIVE
OFANAGE
OMAHANE
ONADARE
ONADATE
ONALINE
OPALINE
OXALATE
PEALIKE
PIASTRE
PLACATE
PLANATE
PRAIRIE
PRALINE
PRATTLE
QUAYAGE
RCADOME
REALINE
REALISE

REALIZE
REARGUE
REARISE
REAROSE
REAWAKE
REAWOKE
ROANOKE
SCALAGE
SCALENE
SEABLUE
SEAFARE
SEAGATE
SEALANE
SEALIFE
SEALIKE
SEAMILE
SEARACE
SEASIDE
SEATTLE
SHACKLE
SHADROE
SHALLWE
SHAMBLE
SHARPIE
SHAWNEE
SIAMESE
SNAPPLE
SOAREWE
SPACKLE
SPANGLE
SPAREME
SPARKLE
STABILE
STANDEE
STANINE
STANLEE
STARTLE
STATICE
STATURE
STATUTE
SUASIVE
SWADDLE
TEACAKE
TEAROSE
TEATIME
TEATREE
THANDIE
THATONE
TOASTEE
TRADUCE
TRAINEE
TRAIPSE
TRAMPLE
TRAPEZE
TWADDLE
ULALUME
ULANUDE
UNAGILE
UNALIKE
UNALONE
UNAWAKE
UNAWARE
UPABOVE
UPATREE
URANITE
WHATTHE
WRANGLE
YEARONE

•••AE••

ACTAEON
CELAENO
ISRAELI
MEGAERA
MEGAERG
MICAELA
PIRAEUS

•••A•E•

AARATED
ABLATED
ABLATES
ABRADED
ABRADER
ABRADES
ADDAXES
ADRATES
AERATED
AERATES
AFEARED
AFRAMES
AGNATES
AIRACES
ALIASES
ALLAGES
ALLAYED
ALLAYER
ALMADEN
ALVAREZ
ANNABEL
ANNALEE
ANNALES
ANTARES
APPAREL
ARBACES
ARCADED
ARCADES
ARIANES
ARRASES
ARRAYED
ARRAYER
ASCARED
ASHAMED
ASSAYED
ASSAYER
ATLASES
ATWATER
AUBADES
AURALEE
AVGASES
AVIATED
AVIATES
AYEAYES
BADAREA
BAHAMEN
BALASES
BANACEK
BANALER
BANANES
BAYAREA
BEDAZED
BEDAZES
BEHAVED
BEHAVES
BELATED
BELAYED
BELAYER
BENARES
BERATED
BERATER
BERATES
BETAKEN
BETAKES
BEWARED
BEWARES
BIGAPES
BLEAKER
BLEARED
BLEATED
BLEATER
BLOATED
BOBATEA
BORATES
BREADED
BREADER
BREAKER
BROADEN
BROADER
BUTANES
BYNAMES
CABARET
CADAVER
CANALED
CANAPES
CAPADES
CARAFES
CARAMEL
CARAVEL
CDCASES
CDRATES
CEDARED
CERATED
CERATES
CETANES
CHEAPEN
CHEAPER
CHEATED
CHEATER
CHIAPET
CITADEL
CLEANED
CLEANER
CLEARED
CLEARER
CLEATED
CLEAVED
CLEAVER
CLEAVES
CLOAKED
COMAKER
CREAKED
CREAMED
CREAMER
CREASED
CREASER
CREASES
CREATED
CREATES
CROAKED
CROAKER
CUBAGES
CURARES
CURATED
CURATES
DAMAGED
DAMAGES
DATASET
DEBAKEY
DEBASED
DEBASER
DEBASES
DEBATED
DEBATER
DEBATES
DECADES
DECAYED
DECAYER
DEFACED
DEFACER
DEFACES
DEFAMED
DEFAMER
DEFAMES
DEHAVEN
DELANEY
DELAYED
DELAYER
DEMARET
DERATED
DERATES
DEWATER
DEWAXED
DEWAXES
DIDASET
DILATED
DILATES
DIMAGES
DNAASES
DOGAPES
DONATED
DONATEE
DONATES
DOSAGES
DOTAGES
DOUANES
DOWAGER
DREADED
DREAMED
DREAMER
DRYADES
DUHAMEL
EFFACED
EFFACER
EFFACES
ELUATES
EMBAYED
EMPALED
EMPALES
EMPANEL
ENCAGED
ENCAGES
ENCASED
ENCASES
ENFACED
ENFACES
ENGAGED
ENGAGER
ENGAGES
ENLACED
ENLACES
ENRAGED
ENRAGES
EQUALED
EQUATED
EQUATES
ESCAPED
ESCAPEE
ESCAPER
ESCAPES
ESSAYED
ESSAYER
ESTATED
ESTATES
ETHANES
EXHALED
EXHALES
EXMATES
FABARES
FACADES
FADAYEV
FALAFEL
FATALES
FEMALES
FINALES
FIXATED
FIXATES
FLOATED
FLOATER
FOLATES
FORAGED
FORAGER
FORAGES
FORASEC
FORAYED
FREAKED
GALATEA
GALAXES
GARAGED
GARAGES
GELATED
GELATES
GEMAYEL
GLEAMED
GLEANED
GLEANER
GLOATED
GLOATER
GREASED
GREASER
GREASES
GREATEN
GREATER
GREAVES
GROANED
GROANER
GYRATED
GYRATES
HADASET
HANAPER
HASASET
HEXANES
HOMAGER
HOMAGES
HONALEE
HYRACES
HYRAXES
ICEAGES
ICEAXES
IDEAMEN
IDEATED
IDEATES
IMPALED
IMPALER
IMPALES
IMPANEL
INCASED
INCASES
INGATES
INHALED
INHALER
INHALES
INLAYER
INMATES
INNAGES
INSALES
INSANER
INTAKES
INVADED
INVADER
INVADES
IODATED
IODATES
ISRAFEL
JACALES
JANACEK
JIRASEK
JUDASES
KARASEA
KARATES
KATAYEV
KAYAKED
KAYAKER
KILAUEA
KNEADED
KNEADER
LALAKER
LAVAGES
LEGATEE
LEGATES
LEVADES
LIEABED
LIGATED
LIGATES
LILALEE
LINAGES
LIPASES
LOBATED
LOCALES
LOCATED
LOCATER
LOCATES
LOVAGES
LOYALER
LOYALES
LSHAPED
LUNATED
LUNATES
LUXATED
LUXATES
MADAMES
MADAMEX
MANAGED
MANAGER
MANAGES
MANATEE
MCCAREY
MCHALES
MCPAPER
MCRANEY
MEDALED
MEGANES
MELAMED
MENACED
MENACER
MENACES
MENAGES
METALED
METATES
MIDASES
MINARET
MIRABEL
MIRAGES
MISAVER
MOHAVES
MOJAVES
MORALES
MRHANEY
MURALED
MUTAGEN
MUTATED
MUTATES
NAIADES
NEGATED
NEGATER
NEGATES
NEWAGER
NEWAGEY
NOGALES
NONAGES
NONAMES
NOPALES
NOTATED
NOTATES
NUTATED
NUTATES
OBLATES
OCTANES
OCTAVES
OHMAGES
OLEATES
ONPAPER
ONSAGER
ONWATER
OPIATES
OSHAPED
OUTAGES
OUTAWED
OUTAWES
PALACES
PALATES
PALAVER
PANACEA
PARADED
PARADER
PARADES
PARAPET
PAVANES
PDJAMES
PEDALED
PEDALER
PELAGES
PENATES
PESADES
PETALED
PETALES
PGRATED
PHRASED
PHRASES
PILATES
PIPAGES
PIRATED
PIRATES
PLEADED
PLEADER
PLEASED
PLEASER
PLEASES
PLEATED
POLANER
POMADED
POMADES
POTAGES
PREAGED
PREAGES
PREAVER
PSHAWED
PUPATED
PUPATES
RADAMES
RAVAGED
RAVAGER
RAVAGES
REBAKED
REBAKES
REBALED
REBALES
REBATED
REBATER
REBATES
RECAGED
RECAGES
RECANED
RECANES
RECASED
RECASES
REDARED
REDARES
REDATED
REDATES
REFACED
REFACES
REFAXED
REFAXES
REGALED
REGALER
REGALES
RELABEL
RELACED
RELACES
RELANES
RELATED
RELATER
RELATES
RELAXED
RELAXER
RELAXES
RELAYED
RELAYER
REMAKES
REMATED
REMATES
RENAMED
RENAMES
REPAGED
REPAGES
REPANEL
REPAPER
REPAVED
REPAVES
RERAKED
RERAKES
RERATED
RERATES
RESALES
RESAVED
RESAVES
RESAWED
RETAKEN
RETAKER
RETAKES
RETAMED
RETAMES
RETAPED
RETAPES
RETAXED
RETAXES
REWAGER
REWAKED
REWAKEN
REWAKES
REWATER
REWAXED
REWAXES
RIVALED
ROTATED
ROTATES
ROYALES
RUTALEE
SALADES
SARACEN
SARALEE
SARAZEN
SAVAGED
SAVAGER
SAVAGES
SAYAMEN
SCHAYES
SCRAPED
SCRAPER
SCRAPES
SEDATED
SEDATER
SEDATES
SENATES
SEPALED
SERAPES
SESAMES
SHEAFED
SHEARED
SHEARER
SHEAVED
SHEAVES
SHOALED
SKIAREA
SLEAZES
SMEARED
SMEARER
SNEAKED
SNEAKER
SOFABED
SOHAVEI
SOLACED
SOLACER
SOLACES
SPEAKER
SPEARED
SPEARER
SPLAYED
SPRAYED
SPRAYER
SQUARED
SQUARER
SQUARES
SSHAPED
STEADED
STEALER
STEAMED
STEAMER
STJAMES
STRAFED
STRAFER
STRAFES
STRAYED
STRAYER
SUBAREA
SUDAFED
SUGARED
SWEARER
SWEATED
SWEATER
TABARET
TAGAMET
TAMALES
TANAGER
TENACES
THEAGES
THEATER
TINAFEY
TIRADES
TISANES
TOPAZES
TOTALED
TOTALER
TOUAREG
TOWAGES
TREADED
TREADER
TREATED
TREATER
TRIAGES
TSHAPED
TSHAPES
TULANEU
TVGAMES
TVTAPES
TWEAKED
ULLAGES
UNBAKED
UNBALED
UNBALES
UNBARED
UNBARES
UNBASED
UNBATED
UNCAGED
UNCAGES
UNCAKED
UNCAKES
UNCANED
UNCAPED
UNCASED
UNCASES
UNDARED
UNDATED
UNDAZED
UNEAGER
UNEASES
UNEATEN
UNEAVED
UNFACED
UNFADED
UNFAKED
UNFAMED
UNFATED
UNFAZED
UNGATED
UNHATED
UNHAYED
UNHAZED
UNIATES
UNJADED
UNLACED
UNLACES
UNLADED
UNLADEN
UNLADES
UNLAVED
UNLAXED
UNLAXES
UNMAKER
UNMAKES
UNMANED
UNMATED
UNMATES
UNNAMED
UNPACED
UNPAGED
UNPALED
UNPARED
UNPAVED
UNPAWED
UNRAKED
UNRATED
UNRAVEL
UNRAYED
UNRAZED
UNSAFER
UNSATED
UNSAVED
UNSAWED
UNTAKEN
UNTAMED
UNTAMES
UNTAPED
UNTAPES
UNTAXED
UNTAXES
UNWADED
UNWAGED
UNWAKED
UNWANED
UNWAVED
UNWAXED
UPDATED
UPDATER
UPDATES
UPGAZED
UPGAZES
UPRATED
UPRATES
UPTAKES
URBANER
USHAPED
USHAPES
VACATED
VACATES
VISAGED
VISAGES
VOYAGED
VOYAGER
VOYAGES
VSHAPED
VSHAPES
WAKAMES
WHEATEN
WREAKED
WREAKER
YSHAPED
YSHAPES
YUCATEC
ZAPATEO

•••A••E

AALARGE
ACTABLE
ADDABLE
ADVANCE
AFFABLE
AFFAIRE
ALCAIDE
ALCALDE
ALGARVE
ALLANTE
AMIABLE
ANDANTE
ANNALEE
ARGANTE
ARIADNE
ARRANGE
ASKANCE
ASSANTE
ASTAIRE
ASTARTE
ATLARGE
ATTACHE
AURALEE
AUSABLE
BALANCE
BECAUSE
BIVALVE
BIZARRE
BOGARDE
BOLATIE
BONAIRE
BREATHE
BUYABLE
CABALLE
CAPABLE
CAPAPIE
CENACLE
CESAIRE
CEZANNE
CHEADLE
CHEAPIE
CICADAE
CIMABUE
CITABLE
CLEANSE
CLEANTE
COCAINE
CORACLE
CURABLE
DATABLE
DEBACLE
DEBARGE
DEFARGE
DELARUE
DERALTE
DERANGE
DEVALUE
DISABLE
DOMAINE
DONAHUE
DONATEE
DRYABLE
DURABLE
DURANCE
DURANTE
EARACHE
EATABLE
ECHAPPE
EFFABLE
ELLAMAE
ENCARRE
ENDABLE
ENGARDE
ENHANCE
ENLARGE
ENMASSE
EQUABLE
ERRABLE
ESCAPEE
EXPANSE
EXPARTE
FINABLE
FINAGLE
FINANCE
FIXABLE
FLEANCE
FLYABLE
FRIABLE
FRYABLE
FTWAYNE
GALAXIE
GETABLE
GIRAFFE
GOUACHE
HATABLE
HIDABLE
HILAIRE
HIRABLE
HONALEE
IDBADGE
IGRAINE
IMPASSE
INFANTE
INHASTE
INLARGE
INRANGE
INTASTE
ITMAYBE
ITSALIE
ITSATIE
KARAOKE
LAFARGE

LAGASSE
LALANNE
LARAINE
LARAMIE
LASAGNE
LASALLE
LAVACHE
LAVAINE
LAVALSE
LECARRE
LEGATEE
LEHAVRE
LESABRE
LIKABLE
LILALEE
LINABLE
LIVABLE
LORANGE
LOSABLE
LOVABLE
LUCARNE
MACABRE
MACAQUE
MAKABLE
MALAISE
MANACLE
MANATEE
MELANGE
MELANIE
MINABLE
MIRACLE
MIXABLE
MORAINE
MORANTE
MOVABLE
MRPADRE
MUSANTE
MUTABLE
NAMABLE
NATALIE
NAVARRE
NOTABLE
NOTALIE
NOTAONE
NOTASTE
OFVALUE
ONEACRE
PALANCE
PANACHE
PARABLE
PASALLE
PAYABLE
PENANCE
PESANTE
PICANTE
PLIABLE
POSABLE
POTABLE
RAKABLE
RATABLE
REBASTE
REBATHE
RECABLE
RECARVE
REGAUGE
RELANCE
RELAPSE
REPASTE
RERAISE
RETABLE
RETASTE
REVALUE
RIDABLE
RITAMAE
ROGAINE
ROMAINE
ROMANCE
ROSALIE
ROSANNE
ROXANNE
ROYALWE
RUTALEE
SALABLE
SARALEE
SAVABLE
SAYABLE
SEEABLE
SHEATHE
SIZABLE
SKIABLE
SONANCE
STEANNE
STRANGE
STRASSE
SUSANNE
SUZANNE
SYNAPSE
TAKABLE
TAMABLE
TAXABLE
TENABLE
TENACRE
THEATRE
TITANAE
TOTABLE
TOTASTE
TOWABLE
TREACLE
TREADLE
TRIABLE
TUNABLE
TVTABLE
TWOACRE
UKRAINE
UNLARGE
UNNAIVE
UNPASTE
UNVAGUE
UPRAISE
UPVALUE
VALANCE
VENABLE
VOCABLE
VOLANTE
VOTABLE
WAXABLE
WIRABLE
WREATHE

••••AE•

CONGAED
DESTAEL
HENNAED
ISHMAEL
MAXBAER
MICHAEL
NARVAEZ
PANGAEA
POLKAED
RACHAEL
RAPHAEL
RUMBAED
SAMBAED
SAUNAED
SCUBAED
SUNDAES
TIARAED
VISTAED
VONBAER

••••A•E

ACERATE
ACETATE
ACREAGE
ACTUATE
ADAWARE
ADSPACE
ADULATE
AGEMATE
AGITATE
AIRBASE
AIRDATE
AIRFARE
AIRLANE
AIRRACE
AIRRAGE
AIRWAVE
ALIDADE
ALLMALE
ALOHAOE
AMILATE
AMYLASE
ANATASE
ANDRADE
ANIMATE
APPEASE
ARCUATE
ARTSALE
ARTWARE
ASHCAKE
ASSUAGE
ATELATE
ATGRADE
ATPEACE
ATSTAKE
AUREATE
AVERAGE
BABBAGE
BADCASE
BADNAME
BAGGAGE
BALLADE
BANDAGE
BARBATE
BARRAGE
BARWARE
BASSALE
BEBRAVE
BEDMATE
BEDRAPE
BELDAME
BELTANE
BEREAVE
BIGGAME
BIGJAKE
BIGNAME
BIGSALE
BIPLANE
BISTATE
BOBKANE
BONDAGE
BORZAGE
BOSCAGE
BREWAGE
BRIGADE
BROCADE
BROMATE
BUDVASE
BURBAGE
BUSFARE
BUSLANE
CABBAGE
CABFARE
CANDACE
CARCARE
CARFARE
CARNAGE
CARSALE
CARTAGE
CASCADE
CASEATE
CAUDATE
CAVIARE
CENTARE
CHARADE
CHELATE
CHICANE
CHORALE
CILIATE
CIRRATE
CITRATE
CLAVATE
CLIMATE
COCKADE
CODCAKE
COGNATE
COINAGE
COLGATE
COLLAGE
COLLATE
COMPARE
COMRADE
CONCAVE
CONGAME
CONNATE
CORDAGE
CORDATE
CORKAGE
CORRADE
CORSAGE
COSTATE
COTTAGE
COURAGE
COWBANE
CREMATE
CRENATE
CRUSADE
CUNEATE
CUPCAKE
CURTATE
CUSPATE
CUTRATE
DARKAGE
DAYCARE
DAYGAME
DAYMARE
DECEASE
DECIARE
DECLARE
DEFLATE
DEFRAME
DEGLAZE
DEGRADE
DENTATE
DEPLANE
DEPRAVE
DEVIATE
DICTATE
DISEASE
DISRATE
DOCKAGE
DOGBANE
DOGFACE
DOGGATE
DOGRACE
DOGSAGE
DOIDARE
DRAYAGE
DUEDATE
DUNNAGE
EATCAKE
EATLATE
ECOTAGE
EDUCATE
EGGCASE
ELEVATE
ELIYALE
EMANATE
EMBLAZE
EMBRACE
EMIRATE
EMPLACE
EMPLANE
EMULATE
ENCHASE
ENCLAVE
ENDGAME
ENDLATE
ENFLAME
ENFRAME
ENGRAVE
ENPLANE
ENSLAVE
ENSNARE
EPILATE
EUSTACE
EXCLAVE
EXPIATE
EXUDATE
EYECARE
FALCATE
FANBASE
FANFARE
FBICASE
FEEBATE
FERMATE
FERRARE
FERRATE
FLOTAGE
FLOWAGE
FOLIAGE
FOLIATE
FONTANE
FOOTAGE
FORBADE
FORGAVE
FORSAKE
FORSALE
FRIGATE
FROMAGE
FTMEADE
FURCATE
FURNACE
GALEATE
GARBAGE
GEMMATE
GERMANE
GESTATE
GINGAME
GLOBATE
GOESAPE
GONEAPE
GOSSAGE
GOSTALE
GRADATE
GRAHAME
GRENADE
GRIMACE
GUNCASE
GUNWALE
GUSTAVE
HALDANE
HANDAXE
HAULAGE
HAYBALE
HECTARE
HENBANE
HERBAGE
HESSAFE
HOECAKE
HOSCALE
HOSTAGE
HOTCAKE
HOTDATE
HOVLANE
HOWLAME
HYDRATE
ICECAVE
ILLMADE
IMAMATE
IMITATE
INADAZE
INARAGE
INAVALE
INFLAME
INFLATE
INGRATE
INPEACE
INPHASE
INPLACE
INSCALE
INSHAPE
INSPACE
INSTATE
INTRADE
INULASE
INWEAVE
IRONAGE
ISOLATE
ITERATE
ITSLATE
JANEANE
JAZZAGE
JIMDALE
KEYCASE
KHANATE
KILDARE
LABIATE
LACTASE
LACTATE
LAPLACE
LAPWARE
LAWCASE
LAYBARE
LEAFAGE
LEAKAGE
LETHAVE
LIMEADE
LINEAGE
LINEATE
LINKAGE
LIQUATE
LOCKAGE
LUGGAGE
MACRAME
MAGNATE
MALTASE
MALWARE
MANDATE
MANMADE
MARGATE
MASSAGE
MBABANE
MCSHANE
MEANAGE
MEATAXE
MEDIATE
MELTAGE
MESSAGE
METHANE
MIGRATE
MILEAGE
MILLAGE
MINTAGE
MISDATE
MISGAVE
MISMATE
MISNAME
MISPAGE
MISRATE
MISTAKE
MONDALE
MONTAGE
MONTALE
MOORAGE
MOULAGE
MRSLATE
MULHARE
MUNDANE
MYSPACE
NARRATE
NASTASE
NBAGAME
NEONATE
NESCAFE
NETCAFE
NETGAME
NETWARE
NEWFACE
NEWGATE
NEWMADE
NEWNAME
NEWWAVE
NFLGAME
NHLGAME
NICCAGE
NICTATE
NITRATE
NONBASE
NONSALE
NONSANE
NONWAGE
NOPLACE
NOTRADE
NOTRARE
NOTSAFE
OATCAKE
OBVIATE
ODDSARE
OFANAGE
OFFBASE
OILBASE
OILCAKE
OMAHANE
ONADARE
ONADATE
ONEBASE
ONELANE
ONENAME
ONEPAGE
ONLEASE
ONLEAVE
ONSTAGE
OPERATE
OUTBAKE
OUTDARE
OUTDATE
OUTFACE
OUTGAME
OUTGAVE
OUTGAZE
OUTMATE
OUTPACE
OUTRACE
OUTRAGE
OUTRATE
OUTRAVE
OUTTAKE
OUTWAVE
OVERAGE
OVERATE
OVERAWE
OXALATE
OXIDASE
OXIDATE
PACKAGE
PALEALE
PALMATE
PALPATE
PANCAKE
PARBAKE
PARKADE
PARKAVE
PARTAKE
PASSADE
PASSAGE
PAYRATE
PEERAGE
PELTATE
PENCASE
PENNAME
PENNATE
PENTANE
PEONAGE
PERCALE
PERVADE
PETCAGE
PETGATE
PETHARE
PETNAME
PICKAXE
PIESAFE
PIESALE
PILEATE
PILLAGE
PINNACE
PINNATE
PINWALE
PLACATE
PLANATE
PLICATE
PLUMAGE
POLEAXE
PORTAGE
POSTAGE
POTTAGE
PREBADE
PREBAKE
PREDATE
PREFACE
PREFADE
PREGAME
PRELATE
PREMADE
PREMAKE
PREMATE
PRENAME
PREPARE
PREPAVE
PRERACE
PRESAGE
PRESALE
PRETAPE
PRIMATE
PRIVATE
PROBATE
PROFANE
PROLATE
PRONATE
PROPANE
PRORATE
PUBGAME
PULSATE
QUAYAGE
QUINATE
RADIATE
RAILAGE
RAMPAGE
RANLATE
RATRACE
REAWAKE
REBRACE
RECLAME
RECRATE
REDFACE
REDTAPE
REFLATE
REFRAME
REGLAZE
REGRADE
REIMAGE
RELEASE
REPHASE
REPLACE
REPLANE
REPLATE
RESCALE
RESHAPE
RESHARE
RESHAVE
RESLATE
RESPACE
RESPADE
RESTAGE
RESTATE
RETRACE
RETRADE
REWEAVE
RIBCAGE
ROOFAGE
ROOTAGE
ROSEATE
ROULADE
RUINATE
RUMCAKE
RUMMAGE
RUNLATE
SACCADE
SADCAFE
SADFATE
SAIDAYE
SALVAGE
SANTAFE
SATIATE
SAUSAGE
SAYSAYE
SCALAGE
SEAFARE
SEAGATE
SEALANE
SEARACE
SEEPAGE
SELVAGE
SENSATE
SERFAGE
SERIATE
SERRATE
SETRATE
SIGNAGE
SINKAGE
SINUATE
SITUATE
SIXLANE
SKIRACE
SOILAGE
SORBATE
SOURALE
SPOKANE
SPYWARE
STORAGE
STOWAGE
STRIATE
SUBBASE
SUBCASE
SUBDATE
SUBRACE
SUCRASE
SULFATE
SUMMATE
SURFACE
SURNAME
TAGSALE
TANKAGE
TARTARE
TAXBASE
TAXRATE
TAXSALE
TEACAKE
TEENAGE
TERNATE
TERRACE
TESTATE
THEBABE
THECAPE
THEGAME
THESAME
THEWAVE
TIEGAME
TILLAGE
TIMBALE
TINWARE
TITRATE
TOBLAME
TOLEASE
TOLLAGE
TONNAGE
TOOLATE
TOPNAME
TOPRATE
TOSCALE
TOSPARE
TSQUARE
TWOBASE
TWOFACE
TWOLANE
ULULATE
UMBRAGE
UNAWAKE
UNAWARE
UNBLADE
UNBRACE
UNBRAKE
UNBRAVE
UNCRATE
UNDRAPE
UNSHADE
UNSTATE
UNWEAVE
UPGRADE
UPHEAVE
UPPHASE
UPSCALE
UPSTAGE
UPSTARE
UPSTATE
UPTRADE
USSTATE
VALUATE
VALVATE
VANTAGE
VARIATE
VCRTAPE
VENTAGE
VERSACE
VIBRATE
VILLAGE
VINTAGE
VIOLATE
VIRGATE
VITIATE
VOLTAGE
VONLAUE
VORLAGE
VOTEAYE
VULGATE
WALLACE
WANNABE
WARFARE
WARGAME
WARPAGE
WASLATE
WASTAGE
WATTAGE
WEBPAGE
WELFARE
WENTAPE
WETWARE
WINDAGE
WORDAGE
YARDAGE

•••••AE

ABOLLAE
ALUMNAE
AMOEBAE
AREOLAE
ARISTAE
AURORAE
AXILLAE
BACCHAE
CAMERAE
CANIDAE
CANULAE
CARINAE
CATENAE
CICADAE
CONCHAE
COPULAE
CORONAE
ELLAMAE
EXEDRAE
FACULAE
FASCIAE
FIBULAE
GLOSSAE
HERNIAE
LACUNAE
LAMINAE
LINGUAE
LUCIDAE
LUNULAE
MACULAE
MEDUSAE
MYCENAE
NEBULAE
PLEURAE
RETINAE
RITAMAE
SCLERAE
SHEILAE
TITANAE
UNGULAE

AF•••••

AFARCRY
AFATLOT
AFCTEAM
AFEARED
AFFABLE
AFFABLY
AFFAIRE
AFFAIRS
AFFECTS
AFFIANT
AFFINED
AFFINES
AFFIRMS
AFFIXED
AFFIXER
AFFIXES
AFFLECK
AFFLICT
AFFORDS
AFFRAYS
AFFRONT
AFGHANI
AFGHANS
AFOULOF
AFRAMES
AFRICAN
AFROPOP
AFTMOST

A•F••••

AFFABLE
AFFABLY
AFFAIRE
AFFAIRS
AFFECTS
AFFIANT
AFFINED
AFFINES
AFFIRMS
AFFIXED
AFFIXER
AFFIXES
AFFLECK
AFFLICT
AFFORDS
AFFRAYS
AFFRONT
ALFALFA
ALFEROV
ALFIERI
ALFONSE
ALFONSO
ALFORJA
ALFREDA
ALFREDE
ALFREDO
ALFREDU
ASFARAS
ATFAULT
ATFIRST

AWFULLY

A••F•••
ACTFIVE
ACTFOUR
AELFRIC
AGEFIVE
AGEFOUR
AIRFARE
AIRFLOW
AIRFOIL
AIRFONE
ALIFORM
ANTFARM
ARAFTOF
ARAFURA
ARMFULS
ARTFAIR
ARTFERN
ARTFILM
ARTFORM
ASHFORD
ASOFNOW
ATMFEES

A•••F••
ACHEFOR
ACTIFED
ACTSFOR
AIMSFOR
ALLOFIT
ALLOFME
ALLOFUS
ALOOFLY
ANTIFOG
AQUIFER
ARCHFOE
ASKSFOR
AVIDFAN

A••••F•
ABCDEFG
ACETIFY
ACIDIFY
AIRLIFT
ALEWIFE
ALFALFA
AMPLIFY
ASAGIFT
ASSTIFF

A•••••F
AFOULOF
AHEADOF
AHOSTOF
AIRWOLF
AKERLOF
ALACKOF
ALOADOF
ALTDORF
APAIROF
APECKOF
APILEOF
ARAFTOF
ASKEDOF
ASLEWOF
ASSTIFF
AWAREOF

•AF••••
BAFFERS
BAFFIES
BAFFING
BAFFLED
BAFFLER
BAFFLES
CAFTANS
DAFFIER
DAFFILY
DAFTEST
GAFFERS
GAFFING
HAFNIUM
HAFTING
LAFARGE
LAFEMME
LAFITTE
LAFLEUR
MAFIOSI
MAFIOSO
RAFFIAS
RAFFISH
RAFFLED
RAFFLER
RAFFLES
RAFTERS
RAFTING
SAFARIS
SAFEBET
SAFEWAY
SAFFRON
TAFFETA
TAFFIES
WAFERED
WAFFLED
WAFFLER
WAFFLES
WAFTERS
WAFTING

•A•F•••
BADFITS
BADFORM
BAFFERS
BAFFIES
BAFFING
BAFFLED
BAFFLER
BAFFLES
BAGFULS
BALFOUR
BARFBAG
CABFARE
CANFULS
CAPFULS
CARFARE
CARFREE
CARFULS
CATFEET
CATFISH
CATFITS
CATFLAP
CATFLEA
CATFOOD
CATFOOT
DAFFIER
DAFFILY
EARFLAP
EARFULS
EATFROM
FABFOUR
FANFARE
FANFEST
FANFICS
FANFOLD
FARFELS
FATFARM
FATFREE
GABFEST
GAFFERS
GAFFING
HADFITS
HALFBAD
HALFCUT
HALFDAY
HALFDUG
HALFFED
HALFIES
HALFMAD
HALFRAW
HALFROD
HALFSHY
HALFWAY
HALFWIT
HALFWON
HASFITS
HATFULS
HAYFORK
JARFULS
KAMFONG
KAUFMAN
LABFEES
LANFORD
LAPFULS
LAWFORD
MAHFOUZ
MANFRED
MAYFAIR
OAKFERN
PALFREY
PANFISH
PANFULS
PARFAIT
PARFIVE
PARFOUR
PARFUMS
RADFORD
RAFFIAS
RAFFISH
RAFFLED
RAFFLER
RAFFLES
RAMFANS
RANFREE
RATFINK
RAWFISH
RAWFOOD
SADFATE
SAFFRON
SANFORD
SAWFISH
TAFFETA
TAFFIES
TAXFREE
VATFULS
WAFFLED
WAFFLER
WAFFLES
WAIFISH
WARFARE
WASFAIR
WATFORD

•A••F••
BALEFUL
BANEFUL
BANKFEE
BASHFUL
BATSFOR
CALLFOR
CARAFES
CAREFOR
CAREFUL
DAREFUL
EASEFUL
FACTFUL
FAIRFAX
FAKEFUR
FALAFEL
FALLFOR
FATEFUL
FAUXFUR
GAINFUL
HADAFIT
HALFFED
HALIFAX
HANDFED
HANDFUL
HARMFUL
HASAFIT
HATEFUL
HAVEFUN
LAIDFOR
LATEFEE
LATIFAH
LAYOFFS
LAYSFOR
MADEFIT
MADEFOR
MADEFUN
MAKEFIT
MAKEFOR
MAKEFUN
MALEFIC
PACIFIC
PAIDFOR
PAILFUL
PAINFUL
PALMFUL
PASSFOR
PAYOFFS
PAYSFOR
RAGEFUL
RAMSFAN
RANGFOR
RATAFIA
SACKFUL
SANDFLY
SAVEFOR
TACTFUL
TAILFIN
TAKEFOR
TANKFUL
TARIFFS
WAILFUL
WAITFOR
WAKEFUL
YAWNFUL

•A•••F•
BACKOFF
BAILIFF
BAKEOFF
CALCIFY
CALLOFF
CAMEOFF
CARDIFF
CARTOFF
CASTOFF
DAMPOFF
DANDIFY
DARTOFF
DASHOFF
DAYSOFF
EARMUFF
EASEOFF
EASYOFF
FACEOFF
FAIROFF
FALLOFF
FALSIFY
FANCIFY
FARLEFT
GAVEOFF
HACKOFF
HANDOFF
HANGOFF
HAPPIFY
HATSOFF
HAULOFF
HAYLOFT
KARLOFF
LAIDOFF
LAYOFFS
LAYSOFF
MACDUFF
MADEOFF
MAGNIFY
MAKEOFF
MARKOFF
MASSIFS
MASTIFF
PACEOFF
PACKOFF
PAIDOFF
PAIROFF
PALMOFF
PASSOFF
PAWNOFF
PAYOFFS
PAYSOFF
QADDAFI
RAKEOFF
RANGOFF
SADCAFE
SAMHUFF
SANTAFE
SARNOFF
SATISFY
SAWNOFF
SAWSOFF
TAILOFF
TAKEOFF
TAMPAFL
TAPSOFF
TARIFFS
WALKOFF
WALLOFF
WARDOFF
WARNOFF
WASHOFF
WAVEOFF
YANKOFF

•A••••F
BACKOFF
BAILIFF
BAKEOFF
BARANOF
BAYLEAF
CALLOFF
CAMEOFF
CARDIFF
CARTOFF
CASTOFF
DAMPOFF
DARRYLF
DARTOFF
DASHOFF
DAYSOFF
EARMUFF
EASEOFF
EASYOFF
FACEOFF
FAIROFF
FALLOFF
GANDALF
GAVEOFF
HACKOFF
HANDOFF
HANGOFF
HATSOFF
HAULOFF
KARLOFF
LAIDOFF
LAYSOFF
MACDUFF
MADEOFF
MAKEOFF
MARKOFF
MASTIFF
OAKLEAF
PACEOFF
PACKOFF
PAIDOFF
PAIROFF
PALMOFF
PASSOFF
PAWNOFF
PAYSOFF
RAKEOFF
RANGOFF
SAMHUFF
SARNOFF
SAWNOFF
SAWSOFF
TAILOFF
TAKEOFF
TALKSOF
TAPSOFF
WALDORF
WALKOFF
WALLOFF
WARDOFF
WARNOFF
WARNSOF
WASHOFF
WAVEOFF
YANKOFF

••AF•••
ARAFTOF
ARAFURA
BIAFRAN
CHAFERS
CHAFFED
CHAFFEE
CHAFFER
CHAFING
CRAFTED
CRAFTER
CRAFTSY
DEAFENS
DEAFEST
DRAFTED
DRAFTEE
DRAFTER
GOAFTER
GRAFTED
GRAFTER
GRAFTON
INAFUNK
INAFURY
LEAFAGE
LEAFIER
LEAFING
LEAFLET
LEAFOUT
LOAFERS
LOAFING
LOAFPAN
OLAFIII
PEAFOWL
PIAFFED
PIAFFES
QUAFFED
QUAFFER
REAFFIX
SEAFARE
SEAFERN
SEAFOAM
SEAFOOD
SEAFOWL
SHAFFER
SHAFTED
SNAFUED
STAFFED
STAFFER
TRAFFIC

••A•F••
BOATFUL
CHAFFED
CHAFFEE
CHAFFER
CHAMFER
CLAPFOR
DWARFED
FEARFOR
FEARFUL
HEADFOR
HEADFUL
HEATFAN
HEATFUL
LEAPFOR
MOANFUL
PIAFFED
PIAFFES
PLANFOR
PLAYFUL
PRAYFOR
QUAFFED
QUAFFER
READFOR
REAFFIX
SCARFED
SCARFER
SCARFUP
SHAFFER
SNARFED
STAFFED
STAFFER
STAYFOR
TEARFUL
TRAFFIC
TRAYFUL
UNAWFUL
VIALFUL
WHARFED
WHATFOR

••A••F•
ASAGIFT
BEAROFF
BEATIFY
BEATOFF
BRANIFF
CLARIFY
DRAGOFF
DRAWOFF
GRATIFY
HEADOFF
INAHUFF
INAJIFF
LEADOFF
MIAMIFL
OCALAFL
PLAYOFF
QUALIFY
READOFF
SCARIFY
SEALIFE
SEALIFT
SEALOFF
STAYOFF
TEAROFF
WEAROFF
WHATIFS

••A•••F
ALACKOF
APAIROF
ARAFTOF
AWAREOF
BEAROFF
BEATOFF
BOASTOF
BRANIFF
DRAGOFF
DRAWOFF
HEADOFF
HEAPSOF
HEARDOF
HEARSOF
INAHUFF
INAIDOF
INAJIFF
INAWEOF
LEADOFF
LEARNOF
LOADSOF
PLAYOFF
READOFF
SCADSOF
SEALOFF
SEAWOLF
SMACKOF
STAYOFF
TEALEAF
TEAROFF
WEAROFF

•••AF••
CARAFES
FALAFEL
GIRAFFE
HADAFIT
HASAFIT
ISRAFEL
RATAFIA
SCLAFFS
SHEAFED
STRAFED
STRAFER
STRAFES
SUDAFED
TINAFEY
UNSAFER
UPWAFTS

•••A•F•
ALFALFA
GIRAFFE
SCLAFFS

•••A••F
AHEADOF
ALOADOF
BARANOF
BYWAYOF
CLEAROF
DREAMOF
SPEAKOF

••••AF•
DISTAFF
ENGRAFT
GOESAFT
GONEAFT
HESSAFE
INDRAFT
INGRAFT
MUSTAFA
NESCAFE
NETCAFE
NOTSAFE
OCALAFL
ONSTAFF
PIESAFE
POPEAFB
QADDAFI
REDRAFT
REGRAFT
RESTAFF
SADCAFE
SANTAFE
TAMPAFL
UNLEAFS
UPDRAFT
WENTAFT

••••A•F
BIGHALF
DISTAFF
GANDALF
GETSANF
METCALF
ONEHALF
ONSTAFF
PETCALF
RESTAFF

•••••AF
BAYLEAF
ENDLEAF
FIGLEAF
FLYLEAF
NEWLEAF
NONDEAF
OAKLEAF
RYELOAF
TEALEAF

AG•••••
AGAINST
AGAKHAN
AGALLOP
AGARICS
AGASSIZ
AGATINE
AGEDOUT
AGEFIVE
AGEFOUR
AGEISTS
AGELESS
AGELONG
AGEMATE
AGENCES
AGENDAS
AGENDUM
AGENINE
AGENTED
AGENTRY
AGESAGO
AGESOUT
AGGRESS
AGILELY
AGILEST
AGILITY
AGITATE
AGITATO
AGNAILS
AGNATES
AGNATIC
AGNOMEN
AGONIES
AGONISE
AGONISM
AGONIST
AGONIZE
AGOUTIS
AGREEON
AGREERS
AGREETO
AGRIBIZ
AGRIPPA
AGROUND
AGULHAS
AGUTTER

A•G••••
AEGISES
AFGHANI
AFGHANS
AGGRESS
AIGLETS
AIGRETS
ALGARVE
ALGEBRA
ALGERIA
ALGIEBA
ALGIERS
ALGREEN
ANGELAS
ANGELES
ANGELIC
ANGELOU
ANGELUS
ANGERED
ANGLAIS
ANGLERS
ANGLING
ANGOLAN
ANGORAS
ANGRIER
ANGRILY
ANGRYAT
ANGUISH
ANGULAR
ARGALIS
ARGANTE
ARGENTI
ARGENTO
ARGENTS
ARGONNE
ARGUERS
ARGUING
ARGUSES
ARGYLES
ATGRADE
AUGENDS
AUGITES
AUGMENT
AUGURAL
AUGURED
AUGURER
AUGUSTA
AUGUSTE
AUGUSTO
AUGUSTS
AVGASES

A••G•••
ABIGAIL
ADAGIOS
AIRGLOW
AIRGUNS
ALEGARS
ALEGRIA
ALIGHTS
ALIGNED
ALIGNER
ALIGOTE
ALLGONE
ALLGOOD
ANAGRAM
APOGEAL
APOGEAN
APOGEES
ARAGORN
ARIGATO
ARUGULA
ASAGIFT
ASAGRAY
AVIGNON

A•••G••
ACINGIT
ALLAGES
ALLEGED
ALLEGER
ALLEGES
ALLEGRA
ALLEGRO
ALRIGHT
AMALGAM
AMONGST
ANTIGEN
ANTIGUA
ANTIGUN
APHAGIA
APHAGIC
ASIAGOS
ASSIGNS
ATEIGHT
ATINGLE
ATNIGHT
ATSIGHT
ATSIGNS
ATTYGEN
AVENGED
AVENGER
AVENGES
AZINGER

A••••G•
AALARGE
ABRIDGE
ACEHIGH
ACREAGE
ADAYAGO
ADJUDGE
AGESAGO
AIMHIGH
AIRBAGS
AIRINGS
AIRLOGS
AIRRAGE
AIRSIGN
ALEKEGS
ALLERGY
ALLONGE
AMERIGO
ANALOGS
ANALOGY
APOLOGY
ARCINGS
ARLEDGE
ARRAIGN
ARRANGE
ASSUAGE
ATLARGE
AUBERGE
AVERAGE
AWNINGS

A•••••G
ABASING
ABATING
ABCDEFG
ABIDING
ABUSING
ACHTUNG
ADDLING
ADORING
AGELONG
ALAKING
ALAYING
ALINING
ALLYING
ALTHING
AMAZING
AMBLING
AMUSING
ANELING
ANGLING
ANTEING
ANTIFOG
ANTILOG
APPLING
ARCHING
AREARUG
ARGUING
ARISING
ARLBERG
ARTSONG
ATONING
AUTOING
AVOWING
AWAKING

•AG••••
BAGBOYS
BAGEHOT
BAGFULS
BAGGAGE
BAGGERS
BAGGIER
BAGGIES
BAGGILY
BAGGING
BAGGINS
BAGGIRL
BAGHDAD
BAGJOBS

BAGLADY
BAGLIKE
BAGNIOS
BAGNOLD
BAGPIPE
BAGWELL
BAGWIGS
CAGEDIN
CAGEDUP
CAGEPET
CAGESUP
CAGIEST
DAGGERS
DAGWOOD
EAGERER
EAGERLY
EAGLETS
EAGLING
FAGENDS
FAGOTED
GAGARIN
GAGGERS
GAGGING
GAGGLES
GAGLAWS
GAGLINE
GAGREEL
GAGRULE
GAGSTER
HAGERTY
HAGGARD
HAGGISH
HAGGLED
HAGGLER
HAGGLES
HAGLIKE
JAGGIER
JAGGIES
JAGGING
JAGLESS
JAGUARS
LAGASSE
LAGGARD
LAGGERS
LAGGING
LAGOONS
LAGUNAS
MAGALOG
MAGENTA
MAGGOTS
MAGICAL
MAGILLA
MAGINOT
MAGLEVS
MAGNANI
MAGNATE
MAGNETO
MAGNETS
MAGNIFY
MAGNUMS
MAGPIES
MAGUIRE
MAGYARS
NAGGERS
NAGGIER
NAGGING
NAGGISH
PAGEANT
PAGEBOY
PAGEONE
PAGESIX
PAGETWO
PAGINGS
PAGODAS
RAGBAGS
RAGDOLL
RAGEFUL
RAGGEDY
RAGGIER
RAGGIES
RAGGING
RAGINGS
RAGLANS
RAGMANS
RAGMOPS
RAGOUTS
RAGRUGS
RAGSHOP
RAGTIME
RAGTOPS
RAGWEED
SAGCARD
SAGEHEN
SAGETEA
SAGGIER
SAGGING
SAGIEST
SAGINAW
SAGUARO
TAGALOG
TAGAMET
TAGDAYS
TAGENDS
TAGGANT
TAGGERS
TAGGING
TAGLIKE
TAGLINE
TAGOUTS
TAGSALE
TAGSOUT
TAGTEAM
VAGRANT
VAGUELY
VAGUEST
WAGERED
WAGERER
WAGEWAR
WAGGERS
WAGGERY
WAGGING
WAGGISH
WAGGLED
WAGGLER
WAGGLES
WAGONED
WAGONER
ZAGAZIG
ZAGGING
ZAGNUTS

•A•G•••

BADGERS
BADGIRL
BADGUYS
BAGGAGE
BAGGERS
BAGGIER
BAGGIES
BAGGILY
BAGGING
BAGGINS
BAGGIRL
BANGERS
BANGING
BANGKOK
BANGLED
BANGLES
BANGOUT
BANGSON
BANGSUP
BARGAIN
BARGEIN
BARGERS
BARGING
BATGIRL
CADGERS
CADGING
CALGARY
CAMGIRL
CAPGUNS
CARGOES
CATGUTS
DAGGERS
DANGELO
DANGERS
DANGLED
DANGLER
DANGLES
DAYGAME
EADGILS
FANGING
FARGOND
FARGONE
GADGETS
GADGETY
GAGGERS
GAGGING
GAGGLES
GANGERS
GANGING
GANGLIA
GANGSAW
GANGSTA
GANGSUP
GANGTOK
GANGWAY
GARGLED
GARGLER
GARGLES
GAUGERS
GAUGING
GAUGUIN
HAGGARD
HAGGISH
HAGGLED
HAGGLER
HAGGLES
HANGARS
HANGBYS
HANGDOG
HANGERS
HANGING
HANGMAN
HANGMEN
HANGOFF
HANGOUT
HANGSBY
HANGSIN
HANGSON
HANGSUP
HANGTEN
HANGUPS
HAUGHTY
JAEGERS
JAGGIER
JAGGIES
JAGGING
JANGLED
JANGLER
JANGLES
JARGONS
JARGONY
LAGGARD
LAGGERS
LAGGING
LANGDON
LANGHAM
LANGLEY
LANGTON
LANGTRY
LANGUID
LANGUOR
LANGWAY
LARGELY
LARGENT
LARGEOJ
LARGESS
LARGEST
LARGISH
LAUGHAT
LAUGHED
LAUGHER
LAUGHIN
MACGRAW
MAGGOTS
MAIGRET
MAJGENS
MANGANO
MANGERS
MANGIER
MANGLED
MANGLER
MANGLES
MANGOES
MARGATE
MARGAUX
MARGERY
MARGINS
MARGRET
MAUGHAM
NAGGERS
NAGGIER
NAGGING
NAGGISH
NAUGHTS
NAUGHTY
PADGETT
PANGAEA
PANGRAM
PARGERS
PARGING
RAGGEDY
RAGGIER
RAGGIES
RAGGING
RANGERS
RANGFOR
RANGIER
RANGING
RANGOFF
RANGOON
RANGOUT
RAYGUNS
SAGGIER
SAGGING
SANGOUT
SANGRIA
SARGENT
TAGGANT
TAGGERS
TAGGING
TAMGLEN
TANGELO
TANGENT
TANGIER
TANGING
TANGLED
TANGLER
TANGLES
TANGOED
TANGOER
TANGRAM
TARGETS
VANGOGH
VAUGHAN
WAGGERS
WAGGERY
WAGGING
WAGGISH
WAGGLED
WAGGLER
WAGGLES
WANGLED
WANGLER
WANGLES
WARGAME
WARGODS
YANGTZE
ZAGGING

•A••G••

BABYGAP
BADEGGS
BAREGES
CAYUGAS
DAMAGED
DAMAGES
DARTGUN
FALLGUY
FARMGAL
FATIGUE
GAHAGAN
GARAGED
GARAGES
HADAGAS
HAIRGEL
HALOGEN
HANDGUN
HASAGAS
LASAGNA
LASAGNE
LASTGAS
LATIGOS
LAVAGES
MADIGAN
MALAGAN
MALAGAS
MALIGNS
MANAGED
MANAGER
MANAGES
MANAGUA
MANEGES
NAILGUN
PAANGAS
PAPAGOS
PARAGON
RAINGOD
RAREGAS
RAVAGED
RAVAGER
RAVAGES
RAWEGGS
SAVAGED
SAVAGER
SAVAGES
TANAGER

•A•••G•

AALARGE
BABBAGE
BADDOGS
BADEGGS
BADSIGN
BAGGAGE
BAGWIGS
BANDAGE
BARRAGE
CABBAGE
CABBAGY
CANINGS
CARNAGE
CARTAGE
CASINGS
CATRIGS
DARKAGE
DATINGS
EARTAGS
EARWIGS
EASTEGG
FABERGE
FACINGS
FARRAGO
GARBAGE
GARBAGY
GASBAGS
GASHOGS
GASLOGS
GATINGS
HAULAGE
HAVEAGO
HAYINGS
HAZINGS
JAZZAGE
LACINGS
LADINGS
LAFARGE
LAPDOGS
LAZONGA
MACONGA
MADDOGS
MAKESGO
MAKINGS
MARENGO
MASSAGE
MAYINGS
MAYTAGS
OAKTAGS
PACKAGE
PAGINGS
PALINGS
PANURGE
PARINGS
PASSAGE
PAVINGS
RAGBAGS
RAGINGS
RAGRUGS
RAILAGE
RALEIGH
RAMPAGE
RATINGS
RAVINGS
RAWEGGS
SALONGA
SALVAGE
SAPSAGO
SARONGS
SAUSAGE
SAVINGS
SAWLOGS
SAYINGS
TAKINGS
TANKAGE
TAPINGS
VANGOGH
VANTAGE
VANVOGT
WAKINGS
WANTAGH
WARPAGE
WASTAGE
WATTAGE
WAXINGS
WAYTOGO
YARDAGE

•A••••G

BABYING
BACHING
BACKING
BACKLOG
BAFFING
BAGGING
BAILING
BAITING
BALDING
BALKING
BAMMING
BANDING
BANGING
BANKING
BANNING
BANTING
BARBING
BARFBAG
BARGING
BARKING
BARNING
BARRING
BASHING
BASKING
BASTING
BATHING
BATTING
BATWING
BAWLING
CABBING
CABLING
CACHING
CADGING
CALKING
CALLING
CALMING
CALVING
CAMPING
CANNING
CANTING
CAPPING
CARDING
CARKING
CARLING
CARPING
CARTING
CARVING
CASHING
CASKING
CASTING
CATALOG
CAUSING
DABBING
DADOING
DAMMING
DAMNING
DAMPING
DANCING
DANNING
DAPPING
DARLING
DARNING
DARTING
DASHING
DAUBING
DAWNING
DAYLONG
EAGLING
EARNING
EARPLUG
EARRING
EASTEGG
EASTING
FABLING
FAILING
FAIRING
FALLING
FANGING
FANNING
FARCING
FARMING
FASTING
FATLING
FATTING
FAWNING
GABBING
GADDING
GAFFING
GAGGING
GAINING
GAITING
GALLING
GAMEBAG
GAMELEG
GAMMING
GANGING
GAOLING
GAPPING
GARBING
GASHING
GASPING
GASSING
GATELEG
GATLING
GAUGING
GAWKING
GAWPING
HACKING
HAFTING
HAILING
HALFDUG
HALOING
HALTING
HALVING
HAMBURG
HAMMING
HANDBAG
HANDING
HANGDOG
HANGING
HARBURG
HARDING
HARKING
HARMING
HARPING
HASHING
HASPING
HASTING
HATTING
HAULING
HAWKING
JABBING
JACKING
JAGGING
JAILING
JAMMING
JARRING
JAZZING
KACHING
KAMFONG
KAYOING
LACKING
LADADOG
LADLING
LADYBUG
LAGGING
LAIRING
LALLING
LAMBING
LAMMING
LANCING
LANDING
LANDTAG
LANSING
LAPPING
LAPSANG
LAPSING
LAPWING
LARDING
LARKING
LASHING
LASTING
LASTLEG
LATETAG
LATHING
LAUDING
MADDING
MAGALOG
MAILBAG
MAILING
MAIMING
MALEDOG
MALEHOG
MALEPIG
MALTING
MANNING
MAPPING
MARKING
MARRING
MASHING
MASKING
MASSING
MASTING
MATTING
MAULING
NABBING
NAGGING
NAILING
NAILKEG
NAMETAG
NANJING
NANKING
NAPPING
PACKING
PADDING
PAINING
PAIRING
PALLING
PALMING
PANNING
PANTING
PANTLEG
PARGING
PARKING
PARRING
PARSING
PARTING
PASSING
PASTING
PATTING
PAULING
PAUSING
PAWNING
RACKING
RAFTING
RAGGING
RAIDING
RAILING
RAINING
RAISING
RAMMING
RAMPING
RANGING
RANKING
RANTING
RAPPING
RAPSONG
RASPING
RATEDPG
RATTING
RAZZING
SACKING
SADSONG
SAGGING
SAILING
SALTING
SALVING
SAMSUNG
SANDBAG
SANDHOG
SANDING
SAPLING
SAPPING
SASHING
SASSING
SAUCING
TABBING
TABLING
TABUING
TACKING
TAGALOG
TAGGING
TAILING
TAILWAG
TALKBIG
TALKING
TAMPING
TANGING
TANKING
TANNING
TAPPING
TARRING
TARTING
TASKING
TASTING
TATTING
TAXIING
VALUING
VAMPING
VANNING
VARYING
VATTING
WADDING
WAFTING
WAGGING
WAILING
WAITING
WAIVING
WALKING
WALLING
WANNING
WANTING
WARBURG
WARDING
WARMING
WARNING
WARPING
WARRENG
WARRING
WARTHOG
WASHING
WASHRAG
WASTING
WAXWING
YAKKING
YANKING
YAOMING
YAPPING
YARDING
YARNING
YAWNING
YAWPING
ZAGAZIG
ZAGGING
ZAPPING

••AG•••

ADAGIOS
ANAGRAM
ARAGORN
ASAGIFT
ASAGRAY
BEAGLES
BRAGGED
BRAGGER
CHAGALL
CHAGRIN
COAGENT
CRAGGED
DIAGRAM
DOAGAIN
DRAGEES
DRAGGED
DRAGGER
DRAGGLE
DRAGNET
DRAGOFF
DRAGONS
DRAGOON
DRAGOTI
DRAGOUT
DRAGSIN
DRAGSON
DRAGSUP
ETAGERE
FLAGDAY
FLAGGED
FLAGGER
FLAGMAN
FLAGMEN
FLAGONS
FRAGGED
FRAGGLE
FRAGILE
HOAGIES
IMAGERS
IMAGERY
IMAGINE
IMAGING
IMAGISM
IMAGIST
IMAGOES
LEAGUED
LEAGUER
LEAGUES
MEAGLES
NBAGAME
NIAGARA
ONAGERS
PLAGUED
PLAGUES
QUAGGAS
REAGANS
REAGENT
SEAGATE
SEAGIRT
SEAGODS
SEAGRAM
SEAGREN
SEAGULL
SHAGGED
SHAGRUG
SKAGWAY
SNAGGED
SNAGGER
SNAGSUP
STAGERS
STAGGED
STAGGER
STAGIER
STAGILY
STAGING
STAGNES
SWAGGER
SWAGMAN
SWAGMEN
TEAGOWN
TRAGEDY
UNAGILE
UNAGING

••A•G••

AMALGAM
BRAGGED
BRAGGER
CHANGED
CHANGER
CHANGES
CHARGED
CHARGER
CHARGES
CLANGED
CLANGER
CLANGOR
COALGAS
CRAGGED
CRAIGIE
DEARGOD
DRAGGED
DRAGGER
DRAGGLE
DRAUGHT
EVANGEL
FLAGGED
FLAGGER
FLANGES
FRAGGED
FRAGGLE
FRAUGHT
GLASGOW
GRANGER
GRANGES
GUARGUM
HUANGHE
HUANGTI

MYALGIA
MYALGIC
NOANGEL
OKAYGUY
ORANGES
ORANGEY
OTALGIA
OTALGIC
PAANGAS
QUAGGAS
REARGUE
SHAGGED
SHANGRI
SNAGGED
SNAGGER
SPANGLE
SPANGLY
STAGGED
STAGGER
SWAGGER
TEARGAS
TRAPGUN
TWANGED
TWANGER
UNANGRY
WHANGED
WRANGEL
WRANGLE

••A••G•

ADAYAGO
ANALOGS
ANALOGY
BRANAGH
DIALOGS
DRAYAGE
IMAHOGG
INARAGE
LEAFAGE
LEAKAGE
MEANAGE
OFANAGE
QUAHOGS
QUAYAGE
REALIGN
SCALAGE
SEABAGS
SEADOGS
SEALEGS
STALAGS
TEABAGS

••A•••G

ABASING
ABATING
ALAKING
ALAYING
AMAZING
AWAKING
BEADING
BEAMING
BEANBAG
BEANING
BEARHUG
BEARING
BEATING
BIASING
BLADING
BLAMING
BLARING
BLAZING
BOATING
BRACING
BRAKING
BRAVING
BRAYING
BRAZING
CEASING
CHAFING
CHARING
CHASING
CHAWING
CLAWING
CLAYING
COALING
COATING
COAXING
CRANING
CRAPING
CRATING
CRAVING
CRAZING
DEALING
DIALING
DRAPING
DRAWING
DRAYING
ELATING
ERASING
EVADING
FEARING
FLAKING
FLAMING
FLARING
FLAWING
FLAYING
FOALING
FOAMING
FRAMING
FRAYING
GEARING
GLARING
GLAZING
GNAWING
GOADING
GOALONG
GRABBAG
GRACING
GRADING
GRATING
GRAVING
GRAYING
GRAYLAG
GRAZING
HEADING
HEALING
HEAPING
HEARING
HEATING
HEAVING
HOAXING
IMAGING
IMAHOGG
LEADDOG
LEADING
LEAFING
LEAKING
LEANING
LEAPING
LEASING
LEAVING
LOADING
LOAFING
LOAMING
LOANING
MEANING
MOANING
NEARING
NIALONG
OKAYING
ORATING
PEAKING
PEALING
PEATBOG
PHASING
PLACING
PLANING
PLATING
PLAYING
PRATING
PRAYING
QUAKING
READING
REAMING
REAPING
REARING
REAVING
ROADHOG
ROAMING
ROARING
RRATING
SCALING
SCARING
SEABORG
SEALING
SEAMING
SEARING
SEASLUG
SEATING
SHADING
SHAGRUG
SHAKING
SHAMING
SHAPING
SHARING
SHAVING
SKATING
SLAKING
SLATING
SLAVING
SLAYING
SNAKING
SNARING
SOAKING
SOAPING
SOARING
SPACING
SPADING
SPARING
SPAYING
STAGING
STAKING
STARING
STARLOG
STATING
STAVING
STAYING
SWAYING
TEAMING
TEARING
TEASING
THAWING
TRACING
TRADING
UNAGING
VIALING
WEANING
WEARING
WEAVING
WHALING
XRATING
XRAYING
YEANING
ZWANZIG

•••AG••

ALLAGES
APHAGIA
APHAGIC
ASIAGOS
CONAGRA
CUBAGES
DAMAGED
DAMAGES
DECAGON
DEMAGOG
DIMAGES
DOSAGES
DOTAGES
DOWAGER
ENCAGED
ENCAGES
ENGAGED
ENGAGER
ENGAGES
ENRAGED
ENRAGES
FINAGLE
FORAGED
FORAGER
FORAGES
GAHAGAN
GARAGED
GARAGES
HADAGAS
HASAGAS
HEXAGON
HOMAGER
HOMAGES
ICEAGES
INNAGES
LASAGNA
LASAGNE
LAVAGES
LINAGES
LISAGAY
LOVAGES
MALAGAN
MALAGAS
MANAGED
MANAGER
MANAGES
MANAGUA
MENAGES
MILAGRO
MIRAGES
MRMAGOO
MUTAGEN
NEWAGER
NEWAGEY
NONAGES
NONAGON
OCTAGON
OHMAGES
ONSAGER
OUTAGES
PAPAGOS
PARAGON
PELAGES
PELAGIC
PIPAGES
POTAGES
PREAGED
PREAGES
RAVAGED
RAVAGER
RAVAGES
RECAGED
RECAGES
REPAGED
REPAGES
REWAGER
RITAGAM
SAVAGED
SAVAGER
SAVAGES
SCRAGGY
SMEAGOL
TANAGER
THEAGES
TOWAGES
TRIAGES
ULLAGES
UNCAGED
UNCAGES
UNEAGER
UNPAGAN
UNPAGED
UNVAGUE
UNWAGED
VIRAGOS
VISAGED
VISAGES
VOYAGED
VOYAGER
VOYAGES

•••A•G•

AALARGE
ARRAIGN
ARRANGE
ATLARGE
DEBARGE
DEFANGS
DEFARGE
DERANGE
DURANGO
EMBARGO
ENLARGE
ERLANGS
HIDALGO
IDBADGE
INLARGE
INRANGE
LAFARGE
LORANGE
MELANGE
REDALGA
REGAUGE
REHANGS
SCRAGGY
STRANGE
UNLARGE

•••A••G

AREARUG
CATALOG
CUTARUG
DECALOG
DEMAGOG
EDWARDG
FLEABAG
LADADOG
MAGALOG
MEGAERG
RDLAING
TAGALOG
TOUAREG
VISAING
ZAGAZIG

••••AG•

ACREAGE
ADAYAGO
AGESAGO
AIRBAGS
AIRRAGE
ASSUAGE
AVERAGE
BABBAGE
BAGGAGE
BANDAGE
BARRAGE
BONDAGE
BORZAGE
BOSCAGE
BRANAGH
BREWAGE
BURBAGE
CABBAGE
CABBAGY
CARNAGE
CARTAGE
CHICAGO
COINAGE
COLLAGE
CORDAGE
CORKAGE
CORSAGE
COTTAGE
COURAGE
DARKAGE
DEFRAGS
DOCKAGE
DOGSAGE
DOGTAGS
DRAYAGE
DUNNAGE
EARTAGS
ECOTAGE
FARRAGO
FLOTAGE
FLOWAGE
FOLIAGE
FOOTAGE
FROMAGE
FTBRAGG
GARBAGE
GARBAGY
GASBAGS
GIGBAGS
GONZAGA
GOSSAGE
GOTTAGO
GYMBAGS
HAULAGE
HAVEAGO
HERBAGE
HOSTAGE
ICEBAGS
INARAGE
IRONAGE
ISITAGO
JAZZAGE
JETLAGS
KITBAGS
LEAFAGE
LEAKAGE
LINEAGE
LINKAGE
LOCKAGE
LONGAGO
LUGGAGE
LUMBAGO
MASSAGE
MAYTAGS
MEANAGE
MELTAGE
MESSAGE
MILEAGE
MILLAGE
MINTAGE
MISPAGE
MONTAGE
MONTAGU
MOORAGE
MOULAGE
NICCAGE
NONWAGE
OAKTAGS
OFANAGE
OLDGAGS
ONEPAGE
ONSTAGE
OUTRAGE
OVERAGE
PACKAGE
PASSAGE
PEERAGE
PEONAGE
PETCAGE
PILLAGE
PLUMAGE
PORTAGE
POSTAGE
POTTAGE
PRESAGE
QUAYAGE
RAGBAGS
RAILAGE
RAMPAGE
REDRAGS
REDTAGS
REFLAGS
REIMAGE
RESTAGE
RIBCAGE
ROOFAGE
ROOTAGE
RUMMAGE
SALVAGE
SAPSAGO
SAUSAGE
SCALAGE
SEABAGS
SEEPAGE
SELVAGE
SERFAGE
SIGNAGE
SINKAGE
SOILAGE
STALAGS
STORAGE
STOWAGE
TANKAGE
TEABAGS
TEENAGE
THEMAGI
TILLAGE
TOLLAGE
TONNAGE
UMBRAGE
UNSNAGS
UNSTAGY
UPSTAGE
USFLAGS
VANTAGE
VENTAGE
VILLAGE
VINTAGE
VOLTAGE
VORLAGE
WANTAGH
WARPAGE
WASTAGE
WATTAGE
WEBPAGE
WETRAGS
WIGWAGS
WINDAGE
WORDAGE
YARDAGE
ZHIVAGO
ZIGZAGS

••••A•G

BIGBANG
BORLAUG
DENHAAG
FTBRAGG
LAPSANG
MUSTANG
OURGANG
OUTRANG
OUTSANG
ROLVAAG
SHEBANG
THEGANG
YOURANG

•••••AG

BARFBAG
BEANBAG
BELTBAG
BOOKBAG
CHINWAG
DENHAAG
DIRTBAG
DISHRAG
DUSTRAG
FEEDBAG
FLEABAG
FOOTBAG
FREITAG
FREYTAG
GAMEBAG
GOLFBAG
GRABBAG
GRAYLAG
GREYLAG
HANDBAG
LANDTAG
LATETAG
MAILBAG
NAMETAG
NOSEBAG
OUTBRAG
OUTDRAG
POSTBAG
REDFLAG
RIKSDAG
ROLVAAG
SANDBAG
TAILWAG
TIMELAG
TOTEBAG
WASHRAG
WINDBAG

AH•••••

AHASSLE
AHCHOOS
AHEADOF
AHOSTOF

A•H••••

ACHEFOR
ACHENES
ACHERON
ACHESON
ACHIEST
ACHIEVA
ACHIEVE
ACHILLE
ACHTUNG
ADHERED
ADHERER
ADHERES
ADHIBIT
AMHARIC
AMHERST
APHAGIA
APHAGIC
APHASIA
APHASIC
APHELIA
APHIDES
APHILIP
APHONIA
APHONIC
ASHAMED
ASHANTI
ASHBERY
ASHBINS
ASHBURN
ASHBURY
ASHCAKE
ASHCANS
ASHFORD
ASHHEAP
ASHIEST
ASHIVER
ASHLAND
ASHLARS
ASHLESS
ASHPANS
ASHPITS
ASHRAMS
ASHTRAY
ASHTREE
ATHEART
ATHEISM
ATHEIST
ATHIRST
ATHLETE
ATHOMES
ATHRILL
ATHWART
AXHEADS

A••H•••

ACEHIGH
AFGHANI
AFGHANS
AHCHOOS
AIMHIGH
AIRHEAD
AIRHOLE
AIRHORN
AIRHOSE
AKIHITO
ALCHEMY
ALLHAIL
ALLHEAL
ALLHERE
ALOHAOE
ALPHARD
ALSHAIN
ALTHING
ALTHORN
AMPHION
AMPHORA
ANAHEIM
ANCHORS
ANCHOVY
ANTHEIL
ANTHEMS
ANTHERS
ANTHILL
ANTHONY
ANTHRAX
ANYHOPE
ARCHAIC
ARCHERS
ARCHERY
ARCHEST
ARCHFOE
ARCHIES
ARCHING
ARCHIVE
ARCHONS
ARCHSEE
ARCHWAY
ARMHOLE
ARSHILE
ARTHURC
ARTHURM
ARTHURS
ASHHEAP
ASPHALT
ASSHARP
ASTHMAS
ATTHIRD
ATTHREE
AUTHORS
AXEHEAD

A•••H••

ABASHED
ABASHES
ABRAHAM
AGAKHAN
AGULHAS
AINTHAY
AIRSHIP
AIRSHOW
AITCHES
ALCOHOL
ALIGHTS
ALLTHAT
ALLTHIS
ALYKHAN
AMICHAI
ANDTHEN
ANOTHER
APACHES
APISHLY
APOTHEM
ARACHNE
ARACHNO
ARTSHOP
ARTSHOW
AWASHIN

A••••H•

ACANTHI
ADELPHI
ADOLPHE
ALIYAHS
ALRIGHT
ALYOSHA
ANARCHS
ANARCHY
ARAPAHO
ARDECHE
ASEETHE
ATEIGHT
ATNIGHT
ATROPHY
ATSIGHT
ATTACHE

A•••••H

AALIYAH
ABOLISH
ABROACH
ABSINTH
ACEHIGH
AIMHIGH
AKRONOH
ALANNAH
ALDRICH
ALLCASH
ALSMITH
ALWORTH
ANDSUCH
ANGUISH
ANOUILH
ANSPACH
ANTIOCH
ASQUITH
ATLUNCH
AUTARCH
AZIMUTH

•AH••••

BAHAISM
BAHAIST
BAHAMAS
BAHAMEN
BAHIANS
BAHRAIN
BAHREIN
CAHIERS
CAHOKIA
CAHOOTS
DAHLIAS
DAHOMEY
GAHAGAN
HAHNIUM
KAHUNAS
LAHAINA
MAHALIA
MAHARIS
MAHATMA
MAHDISM
MAHDIST
MAHFOUZ
MAHONEY
MAHOUTS
MAHZORS
NAHUATL
OAHUANS
PAHLAVI
SAHARAN
TAHINIS
WAHINES
WAHWAHS
YAHTZEE

•A•H•••

BACHATA
BACHING
BACHMAN
BADHAIR
BADHAND
BADHATS
BAGHDAD
BARHOPS
BASHERS
BASHFUL
BASHING
BATHERS
BATHING
BATHMAT
BATHOIL
BATHTUB
BAUHAUS
CACHACA
CACHETS
CACHING
CALHOUN
CARHOPS
CARHORN
CASHBAR
CASHBOX
CASHCOW
CASHEWS
CASHIER
CASHING
CASHINS
CASHOUT
CATHAIR
CATHEAD
CATHODE
DABHAND
DAPHNES
DAPHNIA
DAPHNIS
DASHDOT
DASHERS
DASHIER
DASHIKI
DASHING
DASHOFF
DASHPOT
DAYHOPS
EARHART
EARHOLE
EATHERE
FASHION
FATHEAD
FATHERS
FATHOMS
GASHEAT
GASHING
GASHOGS
GATHERS
HAMHOCK
HARHARS
HASHING
HASHISH
HASHOUT
HAWHAWS
IANHOLM
JAPHETH
KACHINA
KACHING
KASHMIR
KATHRYN
LADHOOD
LASHERS
LASHING
LASHOUT

LASHUPS
LATHERS
LATHERY
LATHING
MACHAON
MACHETE
MACHINA
MACHINE
MACHONE
MACHREE
MACHSIX
MACHTWO
MANHEIM
MANHOLE
MANHOOD
MANHOUR
MANHUNT
MARHAUS
MASHERS
MASHIES
MASHING
MATHERS
MATHEWS
MATHIAS
MATHIEU
MAYHEMS
NAPHTHA
NATHANS
PACHISI
PATHAND
PATHANS
PATHWAY
PAYHEED
RACHAEL
RAMHOME
RANHOME
RAPHAEL
RASHERS
RASHEST
RASHIDA
RATHOLE
RAWHIDE
SACHEMS
SACHETS
SAMHILL
SAMHUFF
SAPHEAD
SASHAYS
SASHIMI
SASHING
SATHOME
SAXHORN
SAYHITO
TACHYON
TARHEEL
TASHLIN
TAXHIKE
WARHAWK
WARHEAD
WARHERO
WASHDAY
WASHERS
WASHIER
WASHING
WASHOFF
WASHOUT
WASHRAG
WASHTUB
WASHUPS
YACHTED
YACHTER
YACHTIE
YASHICA
YASHMAK
ZACHARY

•A••H••
BACCHAE
BACCHIC
BACCHUS
BACKHOE
BADSHOT
BAGEHOT
BALIHAI
BANSHEE
BASEHIT
BASRHIN
BATCHED
BATCHES
CAMPHOR
CANCHAS
CAPSHAW
CARSHOW
CATCHER
CATCHES
CATCHON
CATCHOW
CATCHUP
CATSHOW
CAUTHEN
DASCHLE
DAUPHIN
EARSHOT
EARTHED
EARTHEN
EARTHLY
EASTHAM
FARTHER
GALAHAD
GASOHOL
GAUCHER
GAUCHOS
HARDHAT
HARDHIT
HARSHEN
HARSHER
HARSHLY
HATCHED
HATCHER
HATCHES
HATCHET
HAUGHTY
KAISHEK
LAKSHMI
LANGHAM
LARCHEN
LARCHES
LATCHED
LATCHES
LATCHON
LAUGHAT
LAUGHED
LAUGHER
LAUGHIN
MADCHEN
MADEHAY
MAKEHAY
MALEHOG
MALTHUS
MARCHED
MARCHER
MARCHES
MARCHON
MARKHAM
MARSHAL
MARSHES
MATCHED
MATCHER
MATCHES
MATCHUP
MATTHAU
MATTHEW
MAUGHAM
NARTHEX
NARWHAL
NATCHEZ
NAUGHTS
NAUGHTY
NAVAHOS
PANCHAX
PANTHER
PARCHED
PARCHES
PASCHAL
PATCHED
PATCHEN
PATCHER
PATCHES
PATCHUP
RAGSHOP
RAINHAT
RALPHIE
RANCHED
RANCHER
RANCHES
RANCHOS
RATCHET
SAGEHEN
SALCHOW
SANDHOG
SATCHEL
SATCHMO
SAWCHUK
SAYWHAT
SAYWHEN
TAPSHOE
VAUGHAN
WALTHAM
WALTHER
WAPSHOT
WARSHIP
WARTHOG
WATCHED
WATCHER
WATCHES
WATCHIT
WATCHTV
XANTHAN
XANTHIC
YAMAHAS

•A•••H•
CALIPHS
CAMACHO
CAPUCHE
DALETHS
EARACHE
HALFSHY
HALVAHS
HAMACHI
HARRAHS
KANEOHE
KARACHI
KATISHA
LAROCHE
LAVACHE
MALACHI
MATZOHS
NAPHTHA
NATASHA
PANACHE
PARAPHS
PARIAHS
PAUNCHY
RAUNCHY
SAATCHI
SAMEKHS
SAYSWHO
TABITHA
TALLYHO
WABASHA
WAHWAHS

•A••••H
AALIYAH
BAALISH
BABYISH
BADDISH
BADITCH
BALDISH
CADDISH
CALTECH
CAPEESH
CARWASH
CATFISH
CATTISH
DAMPISH
DARKISH
FADDISH
FAIRISH
FATOUSH
FATTISH
GALUMPH
GARNISH
GAULISH
GAWKISH
HAGGISH
HAIMISH
HALAVAH
HANUKAH
HARBACH
HARDISH
HASHISH
HAWKISH
HAWORTH
JACINTH
JAPHETH
JAZZISH
KADDISH
LABTECH
LADDISH
LADYISH
LALOOSH
LAMBETH
LAPPISH
LARGISH
LARKISH
LATIFAH
LAZYISH
MACBETH
MADDASH
MADDISH
MADRUSH
MAIDISH
MAMMOTH
MANNISH
MATZOTH
MAWKISH
NAGGISH
PADUCAH
PANFISH
PARRISH
PATCASH
PAYCASH
QABALAH
RAFFISH
RALEIGH
RAMMISH
RANKISH
RANWITH
RASPISH
RATTISH
RAWFISH
SABBATH
SAIDAAH
SALTISH
SATWITH
SAWATCH
SAWFISH
SAYSAAH
TALLISH
TALLITH
TANNISH
TARNISH
TARTISH
VAMPISH
VANGOGH
VARNISH
WAGGISH
WAIFISH
WALLACH
WANNISH
WANTAGH
WARMISH
WARPATH
WASATCH
WASPISH
ZANYISH

••AH•••
ANAHEIM
BEAHERO
BRAHMAN
BRAHMAS
BRAHMIN
BYAHAIR
DIAHANN
GOAHEAD
GRAHAME
GRAHAMS
IDAHOAN
IMAHOGG
INAHEAP
INAHOLE
INAHUFF
ISAHEAD
MIAHAMM
OMAHANE
OMAHANS
PEAHENS
QUAHOGS
SEAHAWK
SEAHERO
SEAHUNT
SHAHDOM
SWAHILI
TOAHAIR
UPAHEAD
UTAHANS
YEAHBUT
YEAHMAN
YEAHYOU

••A•H••
ABASHED
ABASHES
AGAKHAN
APACHES
ARACHNE
ARACHNO
AWASHIN
BEACHAM
BEACHED
BEACHES
BEARHUG
BLATHER
BRASHER
BRASHES
BRASHLY
CHACHAS
CHACHKA
CHATHAM
CLASHED
CLASHER
CLASHES
COACHED
COACHES
CRASHAW
CRASHED
CRASHER
CRASHES
DIAPHAN
DRACHMA
FEATHER
FLASHED
FLASHER
FLASHES
FLASHON
FLATHAT
GLASHOW
GNASHED
GNASHER
GNASHES
GRAPHED
GRAPHIC
HEATHEN
HEATHER
INASHOE
IVANHOE
JOACHIM
KWACHAS
LEACHED
LEACHER
LEACHES
LEASHED
LEASHES
LEATHER
LOATHED
LOATHER
LOATHES
LOATHLY
LOATHTO
MTATHOS
ONAWHIM
PEACHED
PEACHES
PLASHED
PLASHES
POACHED
POACHER
POACHES
QUASHED
QUASHES
REACHED
REACHER
REACHES
REACHIN
REACHUP
ROACHES
ROADHOG
SCATHED
SCATHES
SLASHED
SLASHER
SLASHES
SLATHER
SMASHED
SMASHER
SMASHES
SMASHUP
SPATHES
STASHED
STASHES
SWASHED
SWASHES
SWATHED
SWATHES
TEACHER
TEACHES
TEACHIN
TEASHOP
TRACHEA
TRASHED
TRASHER
TRASHES
TRASHTV
WEATHER

••A••H•
ACANTHI
ANARCHS
ANARCHY
ARAPAHO
BIANCHI
BLANCHE
BRANCHY
DEARTHS
DRAUGHT
EPARCHS
EPARCHY
EXARCHS
FRAICHE
FRANCHI
FRAUGHT
HEALTHY
HEARTHS
HEAVEHO
HUANGHE
SAATCHI
SCACCHI
STARCHY
SWARTHY
THATCHY
WEALTHS
WEALTHY
WHATTHE
WRAITHS

••A•••H
ALANNAH
BAALISH
BEAMISH
BEARISH
BEAUISH
BOARISH
BRANAGH
CHALLAH
CLAYISH
EVANISH
GOATISH
GRAYISH
HIALEAH
INARUSH
KLAMATH
KLATSCH
KNAVISH
LEADETH
OBADIAH
OPALISH
PEAKISH
PHARAOH
PLANISH
PLAYDOH
PRADESH
SLAVISH
SPANISH
STAUNCH
TOADISH
WEAKISH

•••AH••
ABRAHAM
DONAHUE
GALAHAD
GETAHIT
GOTAHIT
ISFAHAN
ITSAHIT
MCMAHON
MEGAHIT
NAVAHOS
PERAHIA
YAMAHAS

•••A•H•
ATTACHE
BREATHE
BREATHS
BREATHY
BYPATHS
CAMACHO
EARACHE
EMPATHS
EMPATHY
GOUACHE
HAMACHI
HIBACHI
HITACHI
KARACHI
LAVACHE
MALACHI
MRMACHO
NATASHA
PANACHE
PARAPHS
PIRANHA
PREACHY
REBATHE
SERAPHS
SHEATHE
SHEATHS
SPLASHY
SQUASHY
TERAOHM
UNMACHO
WABASHA
WREATHE
WREATHS
WREATHY

•••A••H
AUTARCH
BREADTH
BYCATCH
DEBAUCH
HALAVAH
HOGARTH
INFAITH
INMARCH
JOMARCH
MONARCH
MRMARCH
NOCATCH
ONEARTH
QABALAH
RELATCH
REMATCH
REPATCH
ROMANSH
SAWATCH
SCRATCH
STEALTH
UNEARTH
UNFAITH
UNHARSH
UNLATCH
WASATCH

••••AH•
ALIYAHS
ARAPAHO
FELLAHS
GULLAHS
HALVAHS
HARRAHS
HOOHAHS
HOOKAHS
HOORAHS
HOWDAHS
HUPPAHS
HURRAHS
HUZZAHS
KENWAHL
LOOFAHS
MIZRAHI
MULCAHY
MULLAHS
OOMPAHS
PARIAHS
RUPIAHS
WAHWAHS

••••A•H
ABROACH
ALLCASH
ANSPACH
BEDBATH
BENEATH
BONEASH
BRANAGH
CARWASH
CHUMASH
COTEACH
CPEBACH
DIGRAPH
DOTDASH
DRYWASH
DYEBATH
EPITAPH
EYELASH
EYEWASH
FOREACH
GETCASH
GOLIATH
GOTCASH
GOULASH
HARBACH
HIPBATH
HOGWASH
HOTBATH
ICEBATH
IMPEACH
INREACH
JETWASH
KLAMATH
MADDASH
MESHACH
MUDBATH
NEWMATH
NONCASH
ONLEASH
OUTLASH
OUTPATH
OUTWASH
PATCASH
PAYCASH
PDQBACH
PHARAOH
PREWASH
REGRAPH
RETEACH
SABBATH
SAIDAAH
SAYSAAH
SPINACH
STOMACH
SUBCASH
SUNBATH
THEOATH
TOWPATH
UNLEASH
UNLOATH
UNTEACH
UPREACH
WALLACH
WANTAGH
WARPATH
WETWASH
XENIAOH

•••••AH
AALIYAH
ALANNAH
BOOHBAH
BUSHWAH
CHALLAH
CHEETAH
CHUPPAH
DEBORAH
DELILAH
GOOMBAH
HALAVAH
HANUKAH
HIALEAH
LATIFAH
MENORAH
MESSIAH
MEZUZAH
MISHNAH
MITZVAH
NKRUMAH
OBADIAH
PADUCAH
POOHBAH
QABALAH
REBEKAH
SAIDAAH
SAYSAAH

AI•••••
AIDLESS
AIGLETS
AIGRETS
AIKIDOS
AILERON
AILMENT
AIMEDAT
AIMHIGH
AIMLESS
AIMSFOR
AINTHAY
AIRACES
AIRBAGS
AIRBALL
AIRBASE
AIRBILL
AIRBOAT
AIRCOOL
AIRCREW
AIRDAMS
AIRDATE
AIRDRIE
AIRDROP
AIRDUCT
AIREDUP
AIRFARE
AIRFLOW
AIRFOIL
AIRFONE
AIRGLOW
AIRGUNS
AIRHEAD
AIRHOLE
AIRHORN
AIRHOSE
AIRIEST
AIRINGS
AIRKISS
AIRLANE
AIRLESS
AIRLIFT
AIRLIKE
AIRLINE
AIRLOCK
AIRLOGS
AIRMADA
AIRMAIL
AIRMASS
AIRMILE
AIRNESS
AIRPACK
AIRPARK
AIRPLAY
AIRPOPS
AIRPORT
AIRPOTS
AIRPUMP
AIRRACE
AIRRAGE
AIRRAID
AIRSACS
AIRSHIP
AIRSHOW
AIRSICK
AIRSIGN
AIRSOCK
AIRSOUT
AIRTANK
AIRTAXI
AIRTIME
AIRTRAP
AIRTUBE
AIRVENT
AIRWARS
AIRWAVE
AIRWAYS
AIRWICK
AIRWOLF
AITCHES

A•I••••
ABIDEBY
ABIDERS
ABIDING
ABIDJAN
ABIGAIL
ABILENE
ABILITY
ABINTRA
ABIOTIC
ABITIBI
ACIDIFY
ACIDITY
ACINGIT
ADIPOSE
AGILELY
AGILEST
AGILITY
AGITATE
AGITATO
AKIHITO
ALIASES
ALIBABA
ALIBIED
ALIDADE
ALIENEE
ALIENOR
ALIENTO
ALIFORM
ALIGHTS
ALIGNED
ALIGNER
ALIGOTE
ALIMENT
ALIMONY
ALINERS
ALINING
ALITTLE
ALIVETO
ALIYAHS
AMIABLE
AMIABLY
AMIBLUE
AMICHAI
AMIDALA
AMIDOLS
AMILATE
AMINUTE
AMISTAD
AMITIES
ANILINE
ANILITY
ANIMACY
ANIMALS
ANIMATE
ANIMATO
ANIMISM
ANIMIST
ANIONIC
ANISEED
ANISTON
ANITRAS
APILEOF
APISHLY
ARIADNE
ARIANES
ARIDEST
ARIDITY
ARIETTA
ARIETTE
ARIGATO
ARIKARA
ARIOSOS
ARIOSTO

ARISING
ARISTAE
ARISTAS
ARISTOS
ARIZONA
ASIAGOS
ASIATIC
ASIMMER
ASININE
ASISAID
ATINGLE
ATIPTOE
ATISSUE
AVIANCA
AVIATED
AVIATES
AVIATIC
AVIATOR
AVIDEST
AVIDFAN
AVIDITY
AVIGNON
AVIONIC
AVIVIAN
AXIALLY
AXILLAE
AXILLAR
AXILLAS
AZIMUTH
AZINGER

A••I•••

AALIYAH
AAMILNE
ABRIDGE
ABRILES
ABSINTH
ACHIEST
ACHIEVA
ACHIEVE
ACHILLE
ACRIDLY
ACTIFED
ACTINON
ACTIONS
ACTIVAS
ACTIVES
ADDIBLE
ADDICTS
ADDISON
ADHIBIT
ADMIRAL
ADMIRED
ADMIRER
ADMIRES
ADMITTO
ADMIXED
ADMIXES
ADRIANA
ADVICES
ADVISED
ADVISEE
ADVISER
ADVISES
ADVISOR
AEDILES
AEGISES
AERIALS
AERIEST
AFFIANT
AFFINED
AFFINES
AFFIRMS
AFFIXED
AFFIXER
AFFIXES
AFRICAN
AGAINST
AGEISTS
AGRIBIZ
AGRIPPA
AIKIDOS
AIRIEST
AIRINGS
AJSIMON
ALBINOS
ALBIREO
ALFIERI
ALGIEBA
ALGIERS
ALLISON
ALLIUMS
ALNICOS
ALNILAM
ALNITAK
ALNIYAT
ALPINER
ALPINES
ALRIGHT
ALTIMAS
AMBIENS
AMBIENT
AMNIONS
AMRITAS
ANCIENT
ANDIAMO
ANDIRON
ANOINTS
ANTIART
ANTIBES
ANTIFOG
ANTIGEN
ANTIGUA
ANTIGUN
ANTILOG
ANTIOCH
ANTIQUE
ANTITAX
ANTIWAR
ANXIETY
ANXIOUS
APAIROF
APHIDES
APHILIP
APLITES
APRICOT
APRIORI
APSIDES
AQUIFER
AQUINAS
AQUIVER
ARBITER
ARCINGS
ARNICAS
ARRIERE
ARRISES
ARRIVAL
ARRIVED
ARRIVER
ARRIVES
ARTICLE
ARTIEST
ARTISAN
ARTISTE
ARTISTS
ASHIEST
ASHIVER
ASPIRED
ASPIRER
ASPIRES
ASPIRIN
ASSIGNS
ASSISTS
ASSIZES
ATEIGHT
ATEINTO
ATEITUP
ATFIRST
ATHIRST
ATNIGHT
ATRIUMS
ATSIGHT
ATSIGNS
ATTICUS
ATTIMES
ATTIRED
ATTIRER
ATTIRES
AUDIBLE
AUDIBLY
AUDILES
AUDITED
AUDITEE
AUDITOR
AUGITES
AURICLE
AURISTS
AUTISTS
AVAILED
AVOIDED
AVOIDER
AWAITED
AWAITER
AWNINGS

A•••I••

ABASING
ABATING
ABIDING
ABILITY
ABITIBI
ABOLISH
ABSCISE
ABUSING
ABUSIVE
ACACIAS
ACADIAN
ACARIDS
ACEHIGH
ACETIFY
ACIDIFY
ACIDITY
ACONITE
ACQUIRE
ACQUITS
ACTFIVE
ACTLIKE
ADAGIOS
ADAMITE
ADDLING
ADELIES
ADELINA
ADELINE
ADENINE
ADJOINS
ADORING
AEOLIAN
AFFAIRE
AFFAIRS
AFFLICT
AGARICS
AGATINE
AGEFIVE
AGENINE
AGILITY
AGNAILS
AGONIES
AGONISE
AGONISM
AGONIST
AGONIZE
AIMHIGH
AIRBILL
AIRKISS
AIRLIFT
AIRLIKE
AIRLINE
AIRMILE
AIRSICK
AIRSIGN
AIRTIME
AIRWICK
AKIHITO
ALADINE
ALAKING
ALANINE
ALAYING
ALCAIDE
ALDRICH
ALEWIFE
ALIBIED
ALINING
ALLMINE
ALLRISE
ALLTIED
ALLTIME
ALLWISE
ALLYING
ALQUIST
ALSMITH
ALTHING
ALTOIDS
ALTOIST
ALUMINA
AMANITA
AMATIVE
AMAZING
AMBLING
AMBRIES
AMENITY
AMERICA
AMERIGO
AMERIKA
AMERIND
AMITIES
AMORIST
AMPHION
AMPLIFY
AMUSING
ANACINS
ANANIAS
ANELING
ANEMIAS
ANGLING
ANGRIER
ANGRILY
ANGUISH
ANILINE
ANILITY
ANIMISM
ANIMIST
ANNUITY
ANODISE
ANODIZE
ANOMIES
ANOUILH
ANTBIRD
ANTEING
ANTHILL
ANTLIKE
ANTLION
ANTOINE
ANTSIER
ANYKIND
ANYTIME
ANYWISE
APATITE
APEDIET
APELIKE
APERIES
APPLIED
APPLIER
APPLIES
APPLING
APPOINT
APPRISE
APULIAN
ARABIAN
ARABICA
ARABICS
ARABIST
ARAMIDS
ARCHIES
ARCHING
ARCHIVE
ARCSINE
ARECIBO
ARETINO
ARGUING
ARIDITY
ARISING
ARMLIKE
ARMOIRE
ARMPITS
ARRAIGN
ARSHILE
ARTFILM
ARTSIER
ASAGIFT
ASCRIBE
ASHBINS
ASHPITS
ASININE
ASOCIAL
ASQUIET
ASQUINT
ASQUITH
ASSAILS
ASSLIKE
ASSTIFF
ASTAIRE
ASTRIDE
ATATILT
ATATIME
ATAVISM
ATAVIST
ATEDIRT
ATELIER
ATHEISM
ATHEIST
ATHRILL
ATOMICS
ATOMIES
ATOMISE
ATOMISM
ATOMIST
ATOMIZE
ATONICS
ATONIES
ATONING
ATTAINS
ATTAINT
ATTHIRD
ATTRITE
ATTRITS
AUCTION
AUNTIES
AUPAIRS
AUSPICE
AUSSIES
AUSTINS
AUTOING
AVARICE
AVENIDA
AVERILL
AVIDITY
AVIVIAN
AVOWING
AWAKING
AXELIKE
AZANIAN
AZORIAN
AZURITE

A••••I•

ABIGAIL
ABIOTIC
ABOUTIT
ABSTAIN
ACCLAIM
ACERBIC
ACINGIT
ACRYLIC
ACTEDIN
ACYCLIC
ADDEDIN
ADENOID
ADHIBIT
ADONAIS
ADZUKIS
AELFRIC
AEROBIC
AGASSIZ
AGNATIC
AGOUTIS
AGRIBIZ
AIRDRIE
AIRFOIL
AIRMAIL
AIRRAID
AIRSHIP
AJACCIO
ALADDIN
ALAMEIN
ALBANIA
ALBENIZ
ALBUMIN
ALDAVIS
ALDUBIN
ALEGRIA
ALEMBIC
ALGERIA
ALKALIS
ALLELIC
ALLEWIS
ALLHAIL
ALLOFIT
ALLOWIN
ALLTHIS
ALLUVIA
ALMERIA
ALSATIA
ALSHAIN
AMANTIS
AMEBOID
AMHARIC
AMMONIA
AMMONIC
AMNERIS
AMNESIA
AMNESIC
AMOEBIC
AMRADIO
ANAEMIA
ANAEMIC
ANAHEIM
ANDROID
ANEROID
ANGELIC
ANGLAIS
ANIONIC
ANNAKIN
ANNELID
ANOSMIA
ANOSMIC
ANSONIA
ANTACID
ANTHEIL
ANTONIA
ANTONIN
ANTONIO
APESUIT
APHAGIA
APHAGIC
APHASIA
APHASIC
APHELIA
APHILIP
APHONIA
APHONIC
APPETIT
AQUARIA
AQUATIC
AQUAVIT
ARAMAIC
ARANEID
ARCADIA
ARCHAIC
ARGALIS
ARMENIA
ARSENIC
ARSENIO
ARTEMIS
ARTERIO
ARTFAIR
ASCETIC
ASEPSIS
ASEPTIC
ASIATIC
ASISAID
ASKEDIN
ASPIRIN
ASSYRIA
ASTERIX
ASTORIA
ATABOIL
ATACLIP
ATEABIT
AUSTRIA
AUTOBIO
AUTOPIA
AVANTIS
AVIATIC
AVIONIC
AWASHIN
AWEEBIT

A•••••I

ABITIBI
ABRUZZI
ACANTHI
ADELPHI
AFGHANI
AIRTAXI
ALBERTI
ALEARDI
ALEKSEI
ALFIERI
ALVEOLI
AMICHAI
ANASAZI
APRIORI
ARACARI
ARGENTI
ASHANTI

•AI••••

BAILEES
BAILERS
BAILIFF
BAILING
BAILORS
BAILOUT
BAILSON
BAINTER
BAITCAR
BAITERS
BAITING
CAILLOU
CAIMANS
CAIRENE
CAIRNED
CAISSON
DAILIES
DAIMLER
DAIRIES
DAIRYER
DAISIES
FAIENCE
FAILING
FAILLES
FAILSTO
FAILURE
FAINEST
FAINTED
FAINTER
FAINTLY
FAIREST
FAIRFAX
FAIRIES
FAIRING
FAIRISH
FAIROFF
FAIRSEX
FAIRSUP
FAIRUSE
FAIRWAY
FAISALI
GAINERS
GAINFUL
GAINING
GAINSAY
GAINSON
GAITERS
GAITING
HAIKAIS
HAILERS
HAILING
HAIMISH
HAIRCUT
HAIRDOS
HAIRDYE
HAIRGEL
HAIRIER
HAIRNET
HAIRPIN
HAITIAN
JAIALAI
JAILERS
JAILING
JAILORS
JAINISM
JAINIST
KAISERS
KAISHEK
LAICIZE
LAIDFOR
LAIDLOW
LAIDOFF
LAIDOUT
LAIRING
LAISSEZ
LAITIES
MAIDENS
MAIDISH
MAIGRET
MAILBAG
MAILBIN
MAILBOX
MAILCAR
MAILERS
MAILING
MAILINS
MAILLOL
MAILLOT
MAILMAN
MAILMEN
MAILOUT
MAILSIN
MAIMERS
MAIMING
MAIMITI
MAINERS
MAINMAN
MAINMEN
MAINTOP
MAISONS
MAISOUI
MAITAIS
MAITRED
MAITRES
NAIADES
NAILERS
NAILGUN
NAILING
NAILKEG
NAILSET
NAILSIN
NAILSIT
NAILSUP
NAILTIP
NAIPAUL
NAIROBI
NAIVELY
NAIVEST
NAIVETE
NAIVETY
PAIDADS
PAIDFOR
PAIDOFF
PAIDOUT
PAILFUL
PAINFUL
PAINING
PAINTED
PAINTER
PAIRERS
PAIRING
PAIROFF
PAIRSUP
PAISANO
PAISANS
PAISLEY
PAIUTES
RAIDERS
RAIDING
RAILAGE
RAILBUS
RAILCAR
RAILERS
RAILING
RAILMAN
RAILMEN
RAILSAT
RAILSON
RAILWAY
RAIMENT
RAINBOW
RAINGOD
RAINHAT
RAINIER
RAINILY
RAINING
RAINMAN
RAINOUT
RAINSIN
RAINSON
RAISERS
RAISEUP
RAISING
RAISINS
RAISINY
RAISONS
SAIDAAH
SAIDAYE
SAIDBOO
SAIDIDO
SAIDNAY
SAILERS
SAILING
SAILORS
SAILSON
SAILSTO
SAINTED
SAINTES
SAINTLO
SAINTLY
SAISONS
TAILEND
TAILERS
TAILFIN
TAILING
TAILOFF
TAILORS
TAILPIN
TAILWAG
TAINTED
VAINEST
WAIFISH
WAIKATO
WAIKIKI
WAILERS
WAILFUL
WAILING
WAISTED
WAITERS
WAITFOR
WAITING
WAITOUT
WAITRON
WAITSON
WAITSUP
WAIVERS
WAIVING
ZAIRIAN

•A•I•••

AALIYAH
AAMILNE
BABIEST
BABIYAR
BACILLI
BADIDEA
BADITCH
BAHIANS
BALIHAI
BARISTA
BARITES
BASILIC
BASILIO
BASINAL
BATIKED
BATISTA
BATISTE
CABINET
CACIQUE
CAGIEST
CAHIERS
CAKIEST
CALIBAN
CALIBER
CALIBRE
CALICES
CALICOS
CALIPER
CALIPHS
CALISTA
CAMILLA
CAMILLE
CAMINOS
CAMIONS
CAMISES
CANIDAE
CANIEST
CANINES
CANINGS
CANITBE
CAPITAL
CAPITAN
CAPITOL
CARIBES
CARIBOO
CARIBOU
CARINAE
CARINAS
CARIOCA
CARIOLE
CARIOUS
CASIMIR
CASINGS
CASINOS
CASITAS
CATIONS
CAVIARE
CAVIARS
CAVILAT
CAVILED
CAVILER
DANIELA
DANIELJ
DANIELS
DANIKEN
DANITES
DARIUSI
DASILVA
DATINGS
DATIVES
DAVINCI
DAVISON
EASIEST
EATINTO
EATITUP
FACIALS
FACINGS
FADIMAN
FAJITAS
FAMICOM
FAMILIA
FAMILLE
FAMINES
FANIONS
FARINAS
FATIDIC
FATIGUE
GALICIA
GALILEE
GALILEI
GALILEO
GAMIEST
GAMINES
GATINGS
GAVIALS
GAVILAN
HABILIS
HABITAT
HABITED
HABITUE
HALIBUT
HALIDES
HALIFAX
HALITES
HAMITES
HAMITIC
HAMITUP
HARICOT
HASIDIC
HASIDIM
HAYINGS
HAZIEST
HAZINGS
JACINTH
JACINTO
JALISCO
JAMISON
JANITOR
KALININ
KAPITAL
KAPITSA
KATISHA
LABIALS
LABIATE
LACIEST
LACINGS
LADIDAS
LADINGS
LADINOS
LAFITTE
LAKIEST
LAKISTS
LALIQUE
LAMINAE
LAMINAL
LAMINAR
LAMINAS

LAMINTO
LARIATS
LATICES
LATIFAH
LATIGOS
LATIMES
LATINAS
LATINII
LATINOS
LATINUS
LAVINIA
LAYINTO
LAYITON
LAZIEST
MADIGAN
MADISON
MAFIOSI
MAFIOSO
MAGICAL
MAGILLA
MAGINOT
MAKINGS
MALIANS
MALICES
MALIGNS
MANIACS
MANIKIN
MANILAS
MANILOW
MANIPLE
MANIPUR
MAOISTS
MARIANA
MARIANO
MARIDAS
MARIDOS
MARILLA
MARILYN
MARIMBA
MARINAS
MARINER
MARINES
MARITAL
MATILDA
MATINAL
MATINEE
MATISSE
MAVISES
MAXILLA
MAXIMAL
MAXIMAS
MAXIMUM
MAXIMUS
MAXIXES
MAYINGS
MAZIEST
NABISCO
NAMIBIA
NAPIERS
NATIONS
NATIVES
NAVIDAD
OAKIEST
PACIEST
PACIFIC
PAGINGS
PALINGS
PANICKY
PANICLE
PANIERS
PANINIS
PAPIERS
PAPILLA
PAPISTS
PARIAHS
PARIBUS
PARINGS
PATIENT
PATINAS
PAVIDLY
PAVINGS
PAVIORS
PAVIOUR
PAXINOU
PAYINTO
RABIDLY
RACIEST
RACINOS
RACISTS
RADIALS
RADIANS
RADIANT
RADIATE
RADICAL
RADICES
RADICLE
RADIOAD
RADIODJ
RADIOED
RADIOER
RADIOIN
RADIXES
RAGINGS
RAMINTO
RAMIREZ
RANINTO
RANITUP
RAPIDAN
RAPIDER
RAPIDLY
RAPIERS
RAPINES
RAPINIS
RARITAN
RATINES
RATINGS
RATIONS
RATITES
RAVINED
RAVINES
RAVINGS
RAVIOLI
RAWISTS
SABINES
SADISTS
SAGIEST
SAGINAW
SALIENT
SALIERI
SALINAS
SALINES
SALIVAS
SAMISEN
SANIBEL
SAPIENS
SAPIENT
SATIATE
SATIETY
SATINET
SATINON
SATIRES
SATIRIC
SATISFY
SAVINGS
SAVIORS
SAVIOUR
SAWINTO
SAYINGS
TABITHA
TACITLY
TACITUS
TAHINIS
TAKINGS
TALIBAN
TAMIAMI
TAOISTS
TAPINGS
TAPINTO
TAPIOCA
TARIFFS
TATIANA
TAXICAB
TAXIING
TAXIMAN
TAXIMEN
TAXIWAY
VALIANT
VALIDID
VALIDLY
VALINES
VALISES
VANILLA
VANILLI
VAPIDLY
VARIANT
VARIATE
VARIERS
VARIETY
VARIOUS
VARITEK
VATICAL
VATICAN
WAHINES
WAKINGS
WANIEST
WAPITIS
WARIEST
WAVICLE
WAVIEST
WAXIEST
WAXINGS
XAVIERU
YAKIMAS
ZANIEST

•A••I••

BAALISH
BAALISM
BAALIST
BAALITE
BABBITT
BABYING
BABYISH
BACHING
BACKING
BADDIES
BADDISH
BADFITS
BADGIRL
BADLIES
BADSIGN
BADTIME
BAFFIES
BAFFING
BAGGIER
BAGGIES
BAGGILY
BAGGING
BAGGINS
BAGGIRL
BAGLIKE
BAGNIOS
BAGPIPE
BAGWIGS
BAHAISM
BAHAIST
BAILIFF
BAILING
BAITING
BALDIES
BALDING
BALDISH
BALKIER
BALKILY
BALKING
BALLIOL
BALMIER
BALMILY
BAMBIII
BAMBINA
BAMBINI
BAMBINO
BAMMIES
BAMMING
BANDIDO
BANDIED
BANDIER
BANDIES
BANDING
BANDITO
BANDITS
BANGING
BANKING
BANKITS
BANNING
BANTING
BAPTISE
BAPTISM
BAPTIST
BAPTIZE
BARBIES
BARBILL
BARBING
BARGING
BARKIER
BARKING
BARLICK
BARMIER
BARNING
BARRIER
BARRING
BARRIOS
BASHING
BASKING
BASSIER
BASSIST
BASTING
BASTION
BATGIRL
BATHING
BATLIKE
BATTIER
BATTING
BATWING
BAUXITE
BAWDIER
BAWDILY
BAWLING
BAYCITY
CABBIES
CABBING
CABLING
CABRIDE
CABRINI
CABRIOS
CACHING
CADDIED
CADDIES
CADDISH
CADGING
CADMIUM
CALCIFY
CALCITE
CALCIUM
CALKING
CALKINS
CALLING
CALLINS
CALMING
CALVING
CALVINO
CAMGIRL
CAMMIES
CAMPIER
CAMPILY
CAMPING
CAMPION
CANDICE
CANDIDA
CANDIDE
CANDIDS
CANDIED
CANDIES
CANNIER
CANNILY
CANNING
CANTILY
CANTINA
CANTING
CANTINO
CAPPING
CAPRICE
CAPRINE
CAPSIZE
CAPTION
CAPTIVA
CAPTIVE
CARBIDE
CARBINE
CARDIAC
CARDIAL
CARDIFF
CARDING
CARDIUM
CARKING
CARLING
CARMINA
CARMINE
CARNIES
CARPING
CARRIED
CARRIER
CARRIES
CARTIER
CARTING
CARTIRE
CARVING
CASEINS
CASHIER
CASHING
CASHINS
CASKING
CASPIAN
CASSIAS
CASSIDY
CASSINI
CASSINO
CASSIUS
CASTILE
CASTING
CASUIST
CATBIRD
CATFISH
CATFITS
CATKINS
CATLIKE
CATMINT
CATNIPS
CATRIGS
CATSITS
CATTIER
CATTILY
CATTISH
CAUSING
CAUTION
CAVEINS
DABBING
DADAISM
DADAIST
DADDIES
DADOING
DAFFIER
DAFFILY
DAHLIAS
DAILIES
DAIRIES
DAISIES
DALLIED
DALLIER
DALLIES
DAMMING
DAMNING
DAMPING
DAMPISH
DANCING
DANDIER
DANDIES
DANDIFY
DANDILY
DANNING
DAPPING
DARKISH
DARLING
DARNING
DARTING
DASHIER
DASHIKI
DASHING
DATRILS
DAUBING
DAUMIER
DAWKINS
DAWNING
DAYLILY
DAYSIDE
DAYSINN
DAYTIME
EADGILS
EAGLING
EARLIER
EARLIES
EARLIKE
EARNING
EARRING
EARWIGS
EASTING
EATDIRT
FABLING
FABRICS
FABRIZI
FACTION
FADDIER
FADDIET
FADDISH
FADDISM
FADDIST
FADEINS
FADLIKE
FAERIES
FAILING
FAIRIES
FAIRING
FAIRISH
FAKEIDS
FALKIRK
FALLING
FALSIFY
FALSITY
FANCIED
FANCIER
FANCIES
FANCIFY
FANCILY
FANFICS
FANGING
FANLIKE
FANNING
FANTINE
FANWISE
FANZINE
FARCING
FARMING
FARRIER
FARSIDE
FASCIAE
FASCIAL
FASCIAS
FASCISM
FASCIST
FASHION
FASTING
FATCITY
FATLIKE
FATLING
FATLIPS
FATTIER
FATTILY
FATTING
FATTISH
FATUITY
FAUVISM
FAUVIST
FAWNING
GABBIER
GABBING
GABRIEL
GADDING
GAFFING
GAGGING
GAGLINE
GAINING
GAITING
GALLICO
GALLING
GALLIUM
GAMBIAN
GAMBIER
GAMBITS
GAMMING
GANGING
GAOLING
GAPKIDS
GAPPING
GARBING
GARLICS
GARLITS
GARNISH
GARPIKE
GARRICK
GASEITY
GASHING
GASLINE
GASPING
GASPIPE
GASSIER
GASSING
GATLING
GATLINS
GATWICK
GAUDIER
GAUDIES
GAUDILY
GAUGING
GAULISH
GAUTIER
GAUZIER
GAUZILY
GAWKIER
GAWKILY
GAWKING
GAWKISH
GAWPING
HACKIES
HACKING
HADFITS
HADRIAN
HADTIME
HAFNIUM
HAFTING
HAGGISH
HAGLIKE
HAHNIUM
HAILING
HAIMISH
HAIRIER
HAITIAN
HALFIES
HALOIDS
HALOING
HALTING
HALVING
HAMLINE
HAMMIER
HAMMILY
HAMMING
HANDIER
HANDILY
HANDING
HANGING
HANKIBA
HANKIES
HAPKIDO
HAPPIER
HAPPIFY
HAPPILY
HAPTICS
HARDIER
HARDILY
HARDING
HARDISH
HARKING
HARLINE
HARMING
HARNICK
HARPIES
HARPING
HARPIST
HARRIED
HARRIER
HARRIES
HARRIET
HASFITS
HASHING
HASHISH
HASPING
HASSIUM
HASTIER
HASTILY
HASTIME
HASTING
HATLIKE
HATPINS
HATSIZE
HATTING
HAULING
HAWKING
HAWKINS
HAWKISH
HAYRICK
HAYRIDE
HAYWIRE
HAZLITT
IAMBICS
IAMBIST
IATRICS
JABBING
JACKIEO
JACKING
JADEITE
JAGGIER
JAGGIES
JAGGING
JAILING
JAINISM
JAINIST
JAMAICA
JAMLIKE
JAMMIER
JAMMIES
JAMMING
JANEIRO
JANVIER
JARDINE
JARDINS
JARRING
JASMINE
JAWLIKE
JAWLINE
JAYBIRD
JAZZIER
JAZZILY
JAZZING
JAZZISH
KACHINA
KACHING
KADDISH
KANTIAN
KATRINA
KATRINE
KAYOING
LABMICE
LACKING
LACRIMO
LADDIES
LADDISH
LADLING
LADYISH
LAGGING
LAHAINA
LAICIZE
LAIRING
LAITIES
LALLING
LAMAISM
LAMAIST
LAMBING
LAMMING
LANCIAS
LANCING
LANDING
LANDINI
LANKIER
LANKILY
LANSING
LANVINS
LAOTIAN
LAPPING
LAPPISH
LAPSING
LAPWING
LARAINE
LARDIER
LARDING
LARGISH
LARKIER
LARKING
LARKINS
LARKISH
LASHING
LASSIES
LASTING
LATHING
LATRINE
LATTICE
LATVIAN
LAUDING
LAURITZ
LAVAINE
LAWLIKE
LAZYISH
MACHINA
MACHINE
MADDING
MADDISH
MADEILL
MADEIRA
MADLIBS
MAGNIFY
MAGPIES
MAGUIRE
MAHDISM
MAHDIST
MAIDISH
MAILING
MAILINS
MAIMING
MAIMITI
MAKEILL
MALAISE
MALDIVE
MALLIKA
MALTIER
MALTING
MALVINA
MANCINI
MANGIER
MANKIND
MANLIER
MANLIKE
MANNIES
MANNING
MANNISH
MANRICO
MANSION
MANSIZE
MAPPING
MARDIAN
MARGINS
MARKIII
MARKING
MARLIER
MARLINS
MARMION
MARNIER
MARRIED
MARRIES
MARRING
MARTIAL
MARTIAN
MARTINA
MARTINI
MARTINO
MARTINS
MARTINU
MARTINV
MARTIUS
MARVIER
MARXIAN
MARXISM
MARXIST
MASHIES
MASHING
MASKING
MASSIER
MASSIFS
MASSINE
MASSING
MASSIVE
MASTICS
MASTIFF
MASTING
MATHIAS
MATHIEU
MATTING
MAULING
MAURIAC
MAURIAT
MAURICE
MAWKISH
MAYTIME
MAYWINE
MAZZINI
NABBING
NAGGIER
NAGGING
NAGGISH
NAILING
NANAIMO
NANJING
NANKING
NANNIED
NANNIES
NAPKINS
NAPPIER
NAPPIES
NAPPING
NAPTIME
NASTIER
NASTIES
NASTILY
NATRIUM
NATTIER
NATTILY
NATWICK
NAUTICA
NAUTILI
NAVAIDS
OAKLIKE
OARLIKE
OATLIKE
PACHISI
PACKICE
PACKING
PADDIES
PADDING
PADSITE
PAINING
PAIRING
PALLIER
PALLING
PALMIER
PALMING
PALMIST
PAMLICO
PANDITS
PANFISH
PANNIER
PANNING
PANPIPE
PANSIES
PANTIES
PANTILE
PANTING
PAPPIES
PAPRIKA
PARAIBA
PARFIVE
PARGING
PARKING
PARKINS
PARRIED
PARRIER
PARRIES
PARRING
PARRISH
PARSING
PARTIAL
PARTIED
PARTIER
PARTIES
PARTIII
PARTING
PARTITA
PARTITE
PASSING
PASSION
PASSIVE
PASTIER
PASTIES
PASTIME
PASTINA
PASTING
PATRICE
PATRICK
PATRIES
PATRIOT
PATSIES
PATTIES
PATTING
PAUCITY
PAULIII
PAULINA
PAULINE
PAULING
PAULIST
PAUSING
PAWNING
PAYDIRT
RABBITS
RABBITT
RABBITY
RACKING
RAFFIAS
RAFFISH

RAFTING
RAGGIER
RAGGIES
RAGGING
RAGTIME
RAIDING
RAILING
RAINIER
RAINILY
RAINING
RAISING
RAISINS
RAISINY
RALEIGH
RALLIED
RALLIER
RALLIES
RAMLIKE
RAMMING
RAMMISH
RAMPING
RANDIER
RANGIER
RANGING
RANKINE
RANKING
RANKISH
RANRIOT
RANTING
RANWILD
RANWITH
RAPPING
RASHIDA
RASPIER
RASPING
RASPISH
RATFINK
RATLIKE
RATLINE
RATLINS
RATTIER
RATTING
RATTISH
RAWFISH
RAWHIDE
RAWLINS
RAWSILK
RAYLIKE
RAZZIES
RAZZING
SABRINA
SACKING
SACLIKE
SAGGIER
SAGGING
SAIDIDO
SAILING
SALLIED
SALLIER
SALLIES
SALTIER
SALTILY
SALTINE
SALTING
SALTISH
SALVING
SAMHILL
SAMWISE
SANDIER
SANDING
SANTINI
SAPLING
SAPPIER
SAPPILY
SAPPING
SARDINE
SASHIMI
SASHING
SASSIER
SASSILY
SASSING
SATWITH
SAUCIER
SAUCILY
SAUCING
SAURIAN
SAVVIED
SAVVIER
SAVVIES
SAVVILY
SAWFISH
SAWLIKE
SAWMILL
SAWPITS
SAYHITO
SAYSIDO
TABBIES
TABBING
TABLING
TABUING
TACKIER
TACKILY
TACKING
TACTICS
TACTILE
TAFFIES
TAGGING
TAGLIKE
TAGLINE
TAILING
TAKEILL
TAKEINS
TALKIER
TALKIES
TALKING
TALLIED
TALLIER
TALLIES
TALLINN
TALLISH
TALLITH
TAMPICO
TAMPING
TANGIER
TANGING
TANKING
TANKINI
TANLINE
TANNING
TANNINS
TANNISH
TANSIES
TANTIVY
TAPPING
TARDIER
TARDILY
TARNISH
TAROILS
TARPITS
TARRIED
TARRIER
TARRIES
TARRING
TARTIER
TARTILY
TARTING
TARTISH
TASKING
TASTIER
TASTILY
TASTING
TATTIER
TATTILY
TATTING
TAURINE
TAWNIER
TAWNILY
TAXHIKE
TAXIING
VACCINE
VACUITY
VALMIKI
VALUING
VAMPIER
VAMPING
VAMPIRA
VAMPIRE
VAMPISH
VANDIEN
VANDINE
VANLINE
VANNING
VANRIJN
VARMINT
VARNISH
VARRICK
VARSITY
VARYING
VASTIER
VASTITY
VATTING
WABBITS
WACKIER
WACKILY
WADDING
WADKINS
WAFTING
WAGGING
WAGGISH
WAIFISH
WAIKIKI
WAILING
WAITING
WAIVING
WALKING
WALKINS
WALLING
WANNING
WANNISH
WANTING
WARDING
WARLIKE
WARMING
WARMISH
WARNING
WARPING
WARRING
WARRIOR
WARTIER
WARTIME
WARWICK
WASHIER
WASHING
WASPIER
WASPILY
WASPISH
WASSILY
WASTING
WATKINS
WAXLIKE
WAXWING
WAYBILL
WAYSIDE
YAKKING
YANKING
YANNICK
YAOMING
YAPPING
YARDING
YARNING
YASHICA
YASMINE
YAWNIER
YAWNING
YAWPING
ZADKINE
ZAGGING
ZAIRIAN
ZAMBIAN
ZANYISH
ZANYISM
ZAPPIER
ZAPPING

•A•••I•

BABYOIL
BABYSIT
BACCHIC
BACKBIT
BACKLIT
BACKSIN
BACTRIA
BADHAIR
BADTRIP
BAHRAIN
BAHREIN
BALDRIC
BALDWIN
BALMAIN
BAMBIII
BANDAID
BANZAIS
BARGAIN
BARGEIN
BARMAID
BASEHIT
BASESIX
BASILIC
BASILIO
BASRHIN
BATAVIA
BATHOIL
BATSUIT
BAVARIA
CAGEDIN
CAHOKIA
CAKEMIX
CAKETIN
CALLSIN
CALLSIT
CALORIC
CALORIE
CAMBRIA
CAMBRIC
CAMELID
CANONIC
CANTRIP
CAPAPIE
CAPTAIN
CARAMIA
CAROLII
CAROTID
CAROTIN
CARRYIN
CARTRIP
CARTSIN
CASIMIR
CATANIA
CATHAIR
CATSUIT
CATTAIL
CAUSTIC
CAVEDIN
CAVESIN
DALASIS
DANTEII
DAPHNIA
DAPHNIS
DAUPHIN
DAYQUIL
DAYSAIL
DAYTRIP
EARCLIP
EARNSIT
EASEDIN
EASESIN
EATABIT
FACEDIT
FACESIT
FACTOID
FADEDIN
FADESIN
FAKEDIT
FAKESIT
FALLSIN
FAMILIA
FANATIC
FANEUIL
FANMAIL
FANTAIL
FARMAID
FATIDIC
GAGARIN
GALATIA
GALAXIE
GALICIA
GANGLIA
GASMAIN
GASTRIC
GAUGUIN
HABILIS
HACKSIT
HADAFIT
HADANIP
HADATIT
HAIKAIS
HAIRPIN
HALFWIT
HAMELIN
HAMITIC
HANDLIN
HANDSIN
HANGSIN
HAPLOID
HARDHIT
HARDSIX
HASAFIT
HASANIP
HASATIT
HASIDIC
HASIDIM
HATBRIM
HATEDIT
HATESIT
HAULSIN
HAZANIM
JACOBIN
JAMESII
JAMESIV
JAROMIR
JAVELIN
KABUKIS
KALININ
KASHMIR
KATYDID
LACKWIT
LACONIA
LACONIC
LACTAID
LADYKIN
LAMBKIN
LAMPLIT
LAMPOIL
LANGUID
LANOLIN
LARAMIE
LATINII
LAUGHIN
LAVINIA
LAVORIS
LAWSUIT
MACHSIX
MACNEIL
MADEFIT
MAHALIA
MAHARIS
MAILBIN
MAILSIN
MAITAIS
MAJORIN
MAKEFIT
MAKESIT
MALARIA
MALEFIC
MALEPIG
MALTBIE
MAMAMIA
MANHEIM
MANIKIN
MANOLIN
MANTRIC
MANUMIT
MAOSUIT
MARKIII
MARKVII
MARQUIS
MARRYIN
MASONIC
MASTOID
MATALIN
MAUDLIN
MAULDIN
MAUROIS
MAUVAIS
MAYALIN
MAYFAIR
MAZARIN
NAILSIN
NAILSIT
NAILTIP
NAMIBIA
NATALIA
NATALIE
NAYARIT
NAYSAID
PACIFIC
PACKSIN
PACQUIN
PADRAIC
PAGESIX
PALADIN
PALMOIL
PANINIS
PARBOIL
PARFAIT
PARKSIT
PARODIC
PAROTID
PARSNIP
PARTIII
PASSAIC
PASTEIN
PAULIII
PAYSLIP
QATARIS
RACEDIN
RADIOIN
RAINSIN
RAKEDIN
RAKESIN
RALPHIE
RAMBLIN
RAMEKIN
RANONIN
RAPINIS
RAREBIT
RATAFIA
RATTAIL
SAFARIS
SALADIN
SALAMIS
SALTPIT
SALUKIS
SAMARIA
SAMEDIS
SANDPIT
SANGRIA
SANSEIS
SATANIC
SATIRIC
SATORIS
SATYRIC
SAVARIN
SAWTOIT
SAYWAIT
TABLOID
TACONIC
TAHINIS
TAILFIN
TAILPIN
TAKEAIM
TAKENIN
TAKESIN
TAKESIT
TALARIA
TALKBIG
TASHLIN
TASTEIT
TATAMIS
TAXPAID
VALERIE
VALIDID
VANADIC
VAUDOIS
WADEDIN
WADESIN
WALLSIN
WANTSIN
WAPITIS
WAREPIC
WARSHIP
WASABIS
WASFAIR
WASSAIL
WATCHIT
WATUSIS
WAVEDIN
WAVESIN
WAYLAID
XANTHIC
YACHTIE
YANQUIS
ZAGAZIG

•A••••I

BACARDI
BACILLI
BALIHAI
BAMBIII
BAMBINI
BASENJI
BASMATI
BASSANI
CABRINI
CADUCEI
CALCULI
CAMPARI
CANETTI
CANNOLI
CANZONI
CAROLII
CASSINI
DAKTARI
DANTEII
DARIUSI
DASHIKI
DAVINCI
FABRIZI
FAISALI
FAROUKI
GALILEI
GALVANI
HAMACHI
HAROLDI
HAVARTI
JACUZZI
JAIALAI
JAMESII
JAMESVI
KARACHI
KAROLYI
LAKSHMI
LANDINI
LATINII
LAVELLI
LAZZERI
MAFIOSI
MAGNANI
MAIMITI
MAISOUI
MALACHI
MANCINI
MANDOKI
MARCONI
MARKIII
MARKVII
MARTINI
MAZZINI
NAIROBI
NAUTILI
PACHISI
PAHLAVI
PALAZZI
PARASKI
PARTIII
PASCOLI
PAULIII
QADDAFI
RAMSESI
RAPANUI
RAVIOLI
SAATCHI
SALIERI
SAMURAI
SANTINI
SASHIMI
TABOULI
TAMIAMI
TANKINI
VALENTI
VALMIKI
VANILLI
WAIKIKI
ZAMBEZI
ZAMBONI

••AI•••

AGAINST
APAIROF
AVAILED
AWAITED
AWAITER
BRAIDED
BRAIDER
BRAILLE
BRAINED
BRAINER
BRAISED
BRAISES
CHAINED
CHAINES
CHAINUP
CHAIRED
CHAISES
CLAIMED
CLAIMER
CLAIROL
CRAIGIE
CRAISIN
DEAIRED
DRAINED
DRAINER
ELAINES
EMAILED
EMAILER
ETAILED
ETAILER
FLAILAT
FLAILED
FRAICHE
FRAILER
FRAILLY
FRAILTY
FRAISES
GRAINED
GRAINER
INAIDOF
ISAIDNO
LIAISED
LIAISES
LIAISON
PLAICES
PLAINER
PLAINES
PLAINLY
PLAINTS
PLAISIR
PLAITED
PLAITER
PRAIRIE
PRAISED
PRAISER
PRAISES
QUAILED
REAIMED
REAIRED
STAIDER
STAIDLY
STAINED
STAINER
STAIRED
TRAILED
TRAILER
TRAINED
TRAINEE
TRAINER
TRAININ
TRAIPSE
TRAITOR
UNAIDED
UNAIMED
UNAIRED
WRAITHS

••A•I••

ABASING
ABATING
ACACIAS
ACADIAN
ACARIDS
ADAGIOS
ADAMITE
AGARICS
AGATINE
ALADINE
ALAKING
ALANINE
ALAYING
AMANITA
AMATIVE
AMAZING
ANACINS
ANANIAS
APATITE
ARABIAN
ARABICA
ARABICS
ARABIST
ARAMIDS
ASAGIFT
ATATILT
ATATIME
ATAVISM
ATAVIST
AVARICE
AWAKING
AZANIAN
BAALISH
BAALISM
BAALIST
BAALITE
BEADIER
BEADILY
BEADING
BEALION
BEAMIER
BEAMING
BEAMISH
BEANIES
BEANING
BEARING
BEARISH
BEATIFY
BEATING
BEAUISH
BIALIES
BIASING
BIAXIAL
BLADING
BLAMING
BLARING
BLAZING
BOARISH
BOATING
BRACING
BRAKING
BRANIFF
BRASIER
BRASIZE
BRAVING
BRAYING
BRAZIER
BRAZING
BYAMILE
CEASING
CHAFING
CHALICE
CHARIER
CHARILY
CHARING
CHARIOT
CHARITY
CHASING
CHAWING
CLARICE
CLARIFY
CLARION
CLARITY
CLAVIER
CLAWING
CLAYIER
CLAYING
CLAYISH
COALING
COATING
COAXIAL
COAXING
CRANIAL
CRANING
CRANIUM
CRAPING
CRATING
CRATION
CRAVING
CRAZIER
CRAZIES
CRAZILY
CRAZING
CYANIDE
CYANIDS
CZARINA
CZARISM
CZARIST
DEALING
DEARIES
DIALING
DIARIES
DIARIOS
DIARIST
DOASIDO
DRAPING
DRAWING
DRAYING
DUALISM
DUALIST
DUALITY
DUALIZE
EDACITY
EGALITE
ELAAIUN
ELAMITE
ELAPIDS
ELATING
ELATION
ERASING
ETALIBI
ETAMINE
EVADING
EVANISH
EVASION
EVASIVE
EXAMINE
EXANIMO
FEARING
FLAKIER
FLAKILY
FLAKING
FLAMIER
FLAMING
FLARING
FLAVIUS
FLAWIER
FLAWING
FLAXIER
FLAYING
FOALING
FOAMIER
FOAMILY
FOAMING
FRAGILE
FRAMING
FRASIER
FRAYING
FRAZIER
GEARING
GHANIAN
GLACIAL
GLACIER
GLARING
GLAVINE
GLAZIER
GLAZILY
GLAZING
GNAWING
GOADING
GOALIES
GOAMISS
GOATISH
GRACIAS
GRACILE
GRACING
GRADING
GRANITA
GRANITE
GRAPIER
GRATIAS
GRATIFY
GRATING
GRAVIES
GRAVING
GRAVITY
GRAYING
GRAYISH
GRAZIER
GRAZING
GUANINE
HEADIER
HEADILY
HEADING
HEALING
HEAPING
HEARING
HEATING
HEAVIER

HEAVIES
HEAVILY
HEAVING
HOAGIES
HOARIER
HOARILY
HOAXING
HYALITE
IMAGINE
IMAGING
IMAGISM
IMAGIST
INABIND
INAJIFF
INALINE
INANITY
INAPILE
INAWINK
IRANIAN
ITALIAN
ITALICS
IVANIII
IZATION
KIARIOS
KNAVISH
KRATION
LEADIER
LEADING
LEADINS
LEAFIER
LEAFING
LEAKIER
LEAKING
LEANING
LEAPING
LEASING
LEAVING
LOADING
LOAFING
LOAMIER
LOAMING
LOANING
MEALIER
MEALIES
MEANIES
MEANING
MEATIER
MEATILY
MIAMIAN
MIAMIFL
MOABITE
MOANING
NBALIVE
NEARING
OBADIAH
OCARINA
OFAKIND
OFAMIND
OKAYING
OLAFIII
OLAVIII
ONABIAS
ONADIET
ONAKICK
ONALINE
OPACITY
OPALINE
OPALISH

ORACIES
ORALIST
ORARION
ORARIUM
ORATING
ORATION
OTARIES
OVARIES
OVATION
PEAKIER
PEAKING
PEAKISH
PEALIKE
PEALING
PEATIER
PHASING
PIANISM
PIANIST
PLACIDO
PLACING
PLANING
PLANISH
PLATIER
PLATIES
PLATING
PLAYING
PRALINE
PRATING
PRAYING
QRATIOS
QUAKIER
QUAKIES
QUAKILY
QUAKING
QUALIFY
QUALITY
READIED
READIER
READIES
READILY
READING
REALIGN
REALINE
REALISE
REALISM
REALIST
REALITY
REALIZE
REAMING
REAPING
REARING
REARISE
REAVING
ROADIES
ROAMING
ROARING
RRATING
SCALIER
SCALING
SCARIER
SCARIFY
SCARILY
SCARING
SEABIRD
SEAGIRT
SEALIFE
SEALIFT
SEALIKE

SEALILY
SEALING
SEALION
SEAMIER
SEAMILE
SEAMING
SEAMIST
SEARING
SEASICK
SEASIDE
SEATING
SHADIER
SHADILY
SHADING
SHAKIER
SHAKILY
SHAKING
SHAKIRA
SHALIER
SHAMING
SHAPING
SHAPIRO
SHARING
SHAVIAN
SHAVING
SKATING
SLAKING
SLATIER
SLATING
SLAVING
SLAVISH
SLAYING
SNAKIER
SNAKILY
SNAKING
SNARING
SOAKING
SOAPIER
SOAPILY
SOAPING
SOARING
SPACIAL
SPACIER
SPACING
SPADING
SPANIEL
SPANISH
SPARING
SPATIAL
SPAYING
STABILE
STADIUM
STAGIER
STAGILY
STAGING
STAKING
STAMINA
STANINE
STARING
STARION
STATICE
STATICS
STATING
STATINS
STATION
STATISM
STATIST
STAVING

STAYING
SUASION
SUASIVE
SUAVITY
SWAHILI
SWAYING
TEAMING
TEARIER
TEARILY
TEARING
TEASING
TEATIME
THAWING
TOADIED
TOADIES
TOADISH
TRACING
TRADING
TSARINA
TSARISM
TSARIST
TZARINA
UNAGILE
UNAGING
UNALIKE
URACILS
URANITE
URANIUM
VEALIER
VIALING
VIATICA
WEAKISH
WEANING
WEARIED
WEARIER
WEARIES
WEARILY
WEARING
WEAVING
WHALING
WHATIFS
XRATING
XRAYING
YEANING

••A••I•

AGASSIZ
AJACCIO
ALADDIN
ALAMEIN
AMANTIS
ANAEMIA
ANAEMIC
ANAHEIM
ARAMAIC
ARANEID
ATABOIL
ATACLIP
AVANTIS
AWASHIN
BEANDIP
BEANOIL
BEARPIT
BEASTIE
BEATNIK
BEATRIX
BEATSIT
BEATTIE

BLACKIE
BRAHMIN
BRASSIE
BYAHAIR
CHABLIS
CHAGRIN
CHALCIS
CHAMOIS
CHAOTIC
CHAPLIN
CHAPPIE
CHARLIE
CHARMIN
CHARNIN
CHASMIC
CHASSIS
CHATWIN
CLAMDIP
CLASSIC
CLAUDIA
CLAUDIO
CLAYPIT
COALBIN
COALOIL
COALPIT
CRAIGIE
CRAISIN
CRAMSIN
CRAPPIE
DEADAIR
DEALSIN
DEALTIN
DEARSIR
DHARMIC
DIALSIN
DOAGAIN
DRAGSIN
DRANKIN
DRASTIC
DRAWNIN
DRAWSIN
ELASTIC
ELASTIN
FLACCID
FRANCIS
FRANKIE
FRANTIC
GRANNIE
GRAPHIC
HEADPIN
HEADSIN
HYALOID
HYANNIS
IHATEIT
IHAVEIT
IMADEIT
INAPRIL
INASNIT
INASPIN
INASTIR
INASUIT
IVANIII
IWANTIT
JEANNIE
JOACHIM
JOAQUIN
KRAMNIK
LEADSIN

LEAKSIN
LEANSIN
LEAPSIN
LEAPTIN
LEAVEIN
LEAVEIT
LOADSIN
MEANSIT
MEANTIT
MEATPIE
MIASMIC
MYALGIA
MYALGIC
NEATNIK
NIANTIC
OLAFIII
OLAVIII
ONASSIS
ONATRIP
ONAWHIM
ORATRIX
OTALGIA
OTALGIC
PHASEIN
PLAISIR
PLASMIC
PLASTIC
PLAUDIT
PRACTIC
PRAIRIE
PSALMIC
QUADRIC
QUARTIC
REACHIN
READMIT
READSIN
REAFFIX
REARLIT
REAUDIT
REAVAIL
SCARWID
SEALSIN
SEATRIP
SHAREIN
SHARPIE
SLATKIN
SOAKSIN
SPANAIR
STANDIN
STANNIC
STARLIT
STARSIN
STARTIN
STAYSIN
TEACHIN
TEARSIT
THANDIE
THATSIT
TOAHAIR
TRADEIN
TRAFFIC
TRAININ
TRANSIT
TRAVAIL
UPANDIN
WHATSIS
WHATSIT
ZWANZIG

••A•••I

ACANTHI
ANASAZI
ARACARI
BIANCHI
CHAPATI
DRAGOTI
ETALIBI
FRANCHI
GUARANI
HUANGTI
IVANIII
KHATAMI
OLAFIII
OLAVIII
PLATYPI
SAATCHI
SCACCHI
SHANGRI
SHARPEI
SHASTRI
SWAHILI
WHATAMI

•••AI••

AFFAIRE
AFFAIRS
AGNAILS
ALCAIDE
ARRAIGN
ASSAILS
ASTAIRE
ATTAINS
ATTAINT
AUPAIRS
BAHAISM
BAHAIST
BELAIRS
BEWAILS
BONAIRE
CESAIRE
COCAINE
DADAISM
DADAIST
DEHAIRS
DERAILS
DETAILS
DETAINS
DIZAINS
DOMAINE
DOMAINS
ECLAIRS
ELAAIUN
ENTAILS
GERAINT
HILAIRE
IGRAINE
IMPAIRS
INFAITH
INTAILS
JAMAICA
JUDAICA
JUDAISM
KUWAITI
LAHAINA
LAMAISM
LAMAIST
LARAINE

LAVAINE
MALAISE
MISAIMS
MOHAIRS
MORAINE
MOSAICS
NANAIMO
NAVAIDS
OBTAINS
ORDAINS
OXTAILS
PARAIBA
RDLAING
REBAITS
REGAINS
REJAILS
REMAILS
REMAINS
RENAILS
REPAINT
REPAIRS
RERAISE
RETAILS
RETAINS
ROGAINE
ROLAIDS
ROMAINE
ROMAINS
RORAIMA
SPRAINS
STRAINS
STRAITS
TUBAIST
UKRAINE
UNBAITS
UNFAITH
UNHAIRS
UNHAIRY
UNNAILS
UNNAIVE
UNRAINY
UPRAISE
VISAING
YUCAIPA

•••A•I•

AGNATIC
ALBANIA
ALDAVIS
ALKALIS
ALSATIA
AMHARIC
AMRADIO
ANNAKIN
ANTACID
APHAGIA
APHAGIC
APHASIA
APHASIC
AQUARIA
AQUATIC
AQUAVIT
ARCADIA
ARGALIS
ASIATIC
ATEABIT
AVIATIC
BATAVIA

BAVARIA
BENAZIR
BOLATIE
BONACIS
BONARIO
BOTANIC
BREAKIN
CAPAPIE
CARAMIA
CATANIA
CBRADIO
CERAMIC
CHEAPIE
CHEATIN
COHABIT
CROATIA
DALASIS
DENARII
DINARIC
DREAMIN
DRMARIO
DRYADIC
DUKAKIS
DYNAMIC
EATABIT
ERRATIC
ESTAMIN
EURASIA
FANATIC
FLEADIP
FLEAPIT
FMRADIO
FORABIT
GAGARIN
GALATIA
GALAXIE
GELATIN
GELATIS
GETAHIT
GETATIP
GIGABIT
GLOAMIN
GOTAHIT
GOTATIP
HADAFIT
HADANIP
HADATIT
HASAFIT
HASANIP
HASATIT
HAZANIM
HEMATIC
HEMATIN
HEPARIN
HEPATIC
HEXADIC
HIMALIA
HORATIO
HYPATIA
IDIAMIN
IGUANID
ILIADIC
IMEANIT
IMPAVID
INHABIT
INVALID
ISLAMIC
ITSAHIT

ITSALIE
ITSASIN
ITSATIE
KERATIN
KIWANIS
KORANIC
LARAMIE
LCHAYIM
LIPARIS
LUCANIA
LUNATIC
MAHALIA
MAHARIS
MALARIA
MAMAMIA
MATALIN
MAYALIN
MAZARIN
MCGAVIN
MEGABIT
MEGAHIT
MELANIA
MELANIC
MELANIE
MELANIN
MESAMIS
MONADIC
MORANIS
MORAVIA
NATALIA
NATALIE
NAYARIT
NEPALIS
NOMADIC
NONACID
NOTABIT
NOTALIE
NOVALIS
OCEANIA
OCEANIC
OCEANID
OCTADIC
OCTAVIA
OCTAVIO
OGHAMIC
ONTARIO
ORGANIC
OSMATIC
OTTAVIO
PALADIN
PELAGIC
PERAHIA
PERATIO
PIRATIC
PISANIO
POLARIS
PREACID
PYRAMID
QATARIS
RATAFIA
REGALIA
RITALIN
ROMAJIS
ROMANIA
ROMANIC
ROMANIS
ROSALIA
ROSALIE

ROSARIO
RUMAKIS
RUMANIA
SAFARIS
SALADIN
SALAMIS
SAMARIA
SATANIC
SAVARIN
SCIATIC
SEDALIA
SERAPIS
SNEAKIN
SOLARIA
SOMALIA
SOMALIS
SOMATIC
SQUALID
STBASIL
STEALIN
STEARIC
STEARIN
STRAPIN
SUBARID
SWEARIN
SWEATIT
TALARIA
TATAMIS
TELAVIV
THEAXIS
THIAMIN
TITANIA
TITANIC
TRIADIC
TUNAOIL
URBANII
URBANIV
VANADIC
VENATIC
VIDALIA
VISALIA
VISAVIS
VITALIS
VITAMIN
VIVARIA
VOCALIC
WASABIS
XMRADIO
ZAGAZIG

•••A••I

ALEARDI
ASHANTI
BACARDI
BUGATTI
CHIANTI
DENARII
EDWARDI
HAMACHI
HAVARTI
HIBACHI
HITACHI
ISRAELI
JAIALAI
JUMANJI
KARACHI
KUWAITI
MALACHI

PALAZZI
PARASKI
POLANYI
PULASKI
RAPANUI
SOHAVEI
STUARTI
TEBALDI
URBANII
URBANVI
VIVALDI
YOUANDI

••••AI•

ABIGAIL
ABSTAIN
ACCLAIM
ADONAIS
AIRMAIL
AIRRAID
ALLHAIL
ALSHAIN
ANGLAIS
ARAMAIC
ARCHAIC
ARTFAIR
ASISAID
BADHAIR
BAHRAIN
BALMAIN
BANDAID
BANZAIS
BARGAIN
BARMAID
BEDRAIL
BIDFAIR
BIGHAIR
BOBTAIL
BRITAIN
BYAHAIR
BYTRAIN
CAPTAIN
CATHAIR
CATTAIL
CERTAIN
COCHAIR
CONTAIN
COOLAIR
CORSAIR
CORVAIR
COSTAIN
CURTAIL
CURTAIN
DAYSAIL
DEADAIR
DECLAIM
DELTAIC
DESPAIR
DESTAIN
DETRAIN
DISDAIN
DOAGAIN
DOGHAIR
DOGTAIL
ELTRAIN
ENCHAIN
ENGRAIN
ENTRAIN

EPHRAIM
EXCLAIM
EXPLAIN
FANMAIL
FANTAIL
FARMAID
FINNAIR
FOXTAIL
FREEAIR
FUNFAIR
GASMAIN
GENNAIO
GERMAIN
GERVAIS
GOBYAIR
GOODAIM
HAIKAIS
HEBRAIC
HOBNAIL
HOTMAIL
INGRAIN
JOBFAIR
KINCAID
KINKAID
KOOLAID
LACTAID
LIVEAID
LOTHAIR
LOWPAID
LOWPAIR
LUGSAIL
MAITAIS
MAUVAIS
MAYFAIR
MERMAID
MIKHAIL
MILLAIS
MISLAID
MISSAID
NAYSAID
NETGAIN
NEWLAID
NONPAID
NOSTAIN
NOTFAIR
OLDMAID
ONEPAIR
OPENAIR
OUTGAIN
OUTLAID
OUTLAIN
OUTPAID
OUTRAIL
OUTSAID
OUTSAIL
OUTWAIT
PADRAIC
PARFAIT
PASSAIC
PERTAIN
PETHAIR
PIGTAIL
PINTAIL
PREGAIN
PREPAID
PREVAIL
PROSAIC
RATTAIL

7 AI

REAVAIL
RECLAIM
REDHAIR
REDTAIL
REFRAIN
RESNAIS
RESTAIN
RETRAIN
RITEAID
ROUBAIX
SAYWAIT
SETBAIL
SETSAIL
SPANAIR
SUNMAID
SUSTAIN
TAKEAIM
TAXPAID
TERRAIN
THINAIR
TOAHAIR
TOENAIL
TOOKAIM
TOPSAIL
TOYFAIR
TOYPAIL
TRAVAIL
TRYSAIL
TWOPAIR
UNBRAID
UNCHAIN
UNCHAIR
UNFRAIL
UNPLAIT
UNSLAIN
UNSTAID
UPBRAID
UPSTAIR
VILLAIN
VOLTAIC
WASFAIR
WASSAIL
WAYLAID
WEBMAIL
WHOSAID
WHYWAIT
YOPLAIT
ZEBRAIC

••••A•I

AFGHANI
AIRTAXI
ANASAZI
ARACARI
BASMATI
BASSANI
BENGALI
BENZALI
BHUTANI
BIRIANI
BIRYANI
BULGARI
CAMPARI
CHAPATI
DAKTARI
FAISALI
FERRARI
FORLANI
GALVANI
GOURAMI
GUARANI
HERNANI
KHATAMI
MAGNANI
MIZRAHI
MONDAVI
ONORATI
ORIGAMI
PAHLAVI
PECCAVI
PUNJABI
QADDAFI
SCOLARI
SOLLATI
SOPRANI
STEFANI
SYLLABI
TAMIAMI
THEMAGI
TIMPANI
TOPKAPI
TSUNAMI
TYMPANI
VILLARI
WHATAMI

•••••AI

AMICHAI
BALIHAI
HYUNDAI
JAIALAI
LORELAI
MOLOKAI
MTSINAI
NIKOLAI
OLDUVAI
SAMURAI

AJ•••••

AJACCIO
AJOWANS
AJSIMON

A•J••••

AAJUMBO
ABJURED
ABJURER
ABJURES
ADJOINS
ADJOURN
ADJUDGE
ADJUNCT
ADJURED
ADJURER
ADJURES
ADJUROR
ADJUSTS

A••J•••

ASAJOKE

A•••J••

ABIDJAN
ALANJAY

A••••J•

ALFORJA
AZULEJO

•AJ••••

AAJUMBO
CAJOLED
CAJOLER
CAJOLES
FAJITAS
LAJOLLA
MAJESTE
MAJESTY
MAJEURE
MAJGENS
MAJORCA
MAJORED
MAJORIN
PAJAMAS
RAJARAO

•A•J•••

BADJOKE
BAGJOBS
BANJOES
CARJACK
DAYJOBS
FANJETS
GASJETS
NANJING
PALJOEY
RAMJETS
SANJOSE
SANJUAN
VALJEAN

•A••J••

BANKJOB
EASYJOB
HADAJOB
KARAJAN
NAVAJOS

•A•••J•

BASENJI
MARUSJA
SAMMYJO
VALLEJO
VANRIJN

•A••••J

DANIELJ
LARGEOJ
RADIODJ

••AJ•••

ASAJOKE
INAJIFF
ONAJURY

••A•J••

ALANJAY
GRAYJAY
LEARJET
MEANJOE

••A••J•

PBANDJS

••A•••J

SMALLOJ

•••AJ••

ELCAJON
GETAJOB
GOTAJOB
HADAJOB
KARAJAN
NAVAJOS
ROMAJIS

•••A•J•

JUMANJI

AK•••••

AKEBONO
AKERLOF
AKIHITO
AKRONOH
AKSAKOV

A•K••••

ACKACKS
AIKIDOS
ALKALIS
ALKENES
ANKARAN
ANKLERS
ANKLETS
ASKANCE
ASKAWAY
ASKEDIN
ASKEDOF
ASKEDUP
ASKOVER
ASKSFOR
ASKSOUT
AUKLETS
AWKWARD
AYKROYD
AZKABAN

A••K•••

AGAKHAN
AIRKISS
ALAKING
ALEKEGS
ALEKSEI
ALTKEYS
ALYKHAN
ANYKIND
ARIKARA
AWAKENS
AWAKERS
AWAKING

A•••K••

ADZUKIS
AKSAKOV
ALACKOF
ALASKAN
ALASKAS
ALROKER
ANNAKIN
APECKOF

A••••K•

ACKACKS
ACTLIKE
AIRLIKE
AMERIKA
ANORAKS
ANTLIKE
APELIKE
ARENSKY
ARMLIKE
ARRACKS
ASAJOKE
ASHCAKE
ASSLIKE
ATSTAKE
ATTACKS
ATTUCKS
AUTARKY
AXELIKE

A•••••K

AFFLECK
AIRLOCK
AIRPACK
AIRPARK
AIRSICK
AIRSOCK
AIRTANK
AIRWICK
ALBORAK
ALNITAK
AMTRACK
ANYLUCK
ARAMARK
ARMLOCK
ARTBOOK
ARTROCK
ARTWORK
ASALARK
ATATURK

•AK••••

BAKEOFF
BAKEPAN
BAKERST
BAKLAVA
CAKEDUP
CAKEMIX
CAKEPAN
CAKESUP
CAKETIN
CAKIEST
DAKOTAN
DAKOTAS
DAKTARI
FAKEDIT
FAKEFUR
FAKEIDS
FAKEOUT
FAKESIT
JAKARTA
KAKAPOS
KAKUROS
LAKEBED
LAKIEST
LAKISTS
LAKOTAS
LAKSHMI
MAKABLE
MAKEDOS
MAKEFIT
MAKEFOR
MAKEFUN
MAKEHAY
MAKEILL
MAKEMAD
MAKEOFF
MAKEONE
MAKEOUT
MAKEPAR
MAKERUN
MAKESDO
MAKESGO
MAKESIT
MAKESUP
MAKEUPS
MAKEWAR
MAKEWAY
MAKINGS
NAKEDLY
OAKCASK
OAKDESK
OAKFERN
OAKIEST
OAKLAND
OAKLAWN
OAKLEAF
OAKLIKE
OAKMOSS
OAKPARK
OAKTAGS
OAKTREE
OAKWOOD
RAKABLE
RAKEDIN
RAKEDUP
RAKEOFF
RAKESIN
RAKESUP
TAKABLE
TAKEAIM
TAKEFOR
TAKEILL
TAKEINS
TAKENBY
TAKENIN
TAKENON
TAKENTO
TAKENUP
TAKEOFF
TAKEONE
TAKEOUT
TAKESIN
TAKESIT
TAKESON
TAKESTO
TAKESUP
TAKETEA
TAKETEN
TAKINGS
WAKAMES
WAKEDUP
WAKEFUL
WAKENED
WAKENER
WAKESUP
WAKEUPS
WAKINGS
WAKSMAN
YAKIMAS
YAKKERS
YAKKING
YAKUTSK
ZAKUSKA

•A•K•••

BACKBAR
BACKBAY
BACKBIT
BACKEND
BACKERS
BACKHOE
BACKING
BACKLIT
BACKLOG
BACKLOT
BACKOFF
BACKOUT
BACKPAY
BACKROW
BACKRUB
BACKSAW
BACKSIN
BACKSUP
BACKUPS
BACKWAY
BALKANS
BALKERS
BALKIER
BALKILY
BALKING
BALKSAT
BANKERS
BANKFEE
BANKING
BANKITS
BANKJOB
BANKONE
BANKSON
BANKSUP
BARKEEP
BARKERS
BARKIER
BARKING
BARKLEY
BARKSAT
BASKETS
BASKETT
BASKING
CACKLED
CACKLER
CACKLES
CALKERS
CALKING
CALKINS
CANKERS
CARKEYS
CARKING
CASKETS
CASKING
CATKINS
DANKEST
DARKAGE
DARKENS
DARKEST
DARKISH
DARKLED
DARKLES
DARKMAN
DARKRED
DARKTAN
DAWKINS
FALKIRK
GAPKIDS
GASKELL
GASKETS
GAWKERS
GAWKIER
GAWKILY
GAWKING
GAWKISH
GAWKSAT
HACKERS
HACKETT
HACKIES
HACKING
HACKLED
HACKLER
HACKLES
HACKMAN
HACKNEY
HACKOFF
HACKSAW
HACKSIT
HACKSUP
HAIKAIS
HANKERS
HANKIBA
HANKIES
HAPKIDO
HARKENS
HARKING
HASKELL
HAWKERS
HAWKEYE
HAWKING
HAWKINS
HAWKISH
HAWKMAN
JACKALS
JACKASS
JACKDAW
JACKETS
JACKIEO
JACKING
JACKPOT
JACKSON
JACKSOO
JACKSUP
JACKTAR
JANKLOW
LACKEYS
LACKING
LACKWIT
LANKEST
LANKIER
LANKILY
LARKERS
LARKIER
LARKING
LARKINS
LARKISH
MANKATO
MANKIND
MARKERS
MARKETS
MARKHAM
MARKIII
MARKING
MARKKAA
MARKOFF
MARKOUT
MARKOVA
MARKSUP
MARKUPS
MARKVII
MASKERS
MASKING
MAWKISH
NANKING
NAPKINS
PACKAGE
PACKARD
PACKERS
PACKETS
PACKICE
PACKING
PACKOFF
PACKRAT
PACKSIN
PACKSON
PACKSUP
PARKADE
PARKAVE
PARKERS
PARKING
PARKINS
PARKMAN
PARKSIT
PARKWAY
RACKERS
RACKETS
RACKETY
RACKING
RACKOUT
RACKSUP
RANKERS
RANKEST
RANKINE
RANKING
RANKISH
RANKLED
RANKLES
RANKOUT
RAYKROC
SACKERS
SACKFUL
SACKING
SACKOUT
SACKSUP
TABKEYS
TACKERS
TACKIER
TACKILY
TACKING
TACKLED
TACKLER
TACKLES
TACKSON
TACKSUP
TALKBIG
TALKERS
TALKIER
TALKIES
TALKING
TALKOUT
TALKSAT
TALKSOF
TALKSON
TALKSTO
TALKSUP
TANKAGE
TANKARD
TANKCAR
TANKERS
TANKFUL
TANKING
TANKINI
TANKSUP
TANKTOP
TASKBAR
TASKING
WACKEST
WACKIER
WACKILY
WADKINS
WAIKATO
WAIKIKI
WALKERS
WALKING
WALKINS
WALKMAN
WALKOFF
WALKONS
WALKOUT
WALKSBY
WALKSON
WALKSTO
WALKUPS
WALKURE
WALKWAY
WANKELS
WATKINS
YAKKERS
YAKKING
YANKEES
YANKERS
YANKING
YANKOFF
YANKOUT
YANKSAT
YANKSON
YANKTON
ZADKINE

•A••K••

BANGKOK
BATIKED
BAULKED
BAULKER
CAHOKIA
CARDKEY
CAULKED
CAULKER
DANIKEN
DAVEKOZ
HAECKEL
HANUKAH
JAECKEL
KABUKIS
KANAKAS
KARAKUM
KAYAKED
KAYAKER
LADYKIN
LALAKER
LAMBKIN
MANIKIN
MARKKAA
MARYKAY
NABOKOV
NAILKEG
PASSKEY
RAMEKIN
SALUKIS
SAMEKHS
TALCKED

•A•••K•

BADJOKE
BAGLIKE
BATLIKE
BAZOOKA
CANUCKS
CATLIKE
DAMASKS
DANEYKO
DASHIKI
EARLIKE
EATCAKE
FADLIKE
FANLIKE
FAROUKI
FATLIKE
GARPIKE
HAGLIKE
HATLIKE
JAMLIKE
JAWLIKE
KARAOKE
LAWLIKE
MALARKY
MALLIKA
MANDOKI
MANLIKE
MAZURKA
OAKLIKE
OARLIKE
OATCAKE
OATLIKE
PALOOKA
PANCAKE
PANICKY
PAPRIKA
PARASKI
PARBAKE
PARTAKE
RAMLIKE
RATLIKE
RAYLIKE
SACLIKE
SAWLIKE
TAGLIKE
TANOAKS
TAXHIKE
VALMIKI
VANDYKE
WAIKIKI
WARLIKE
WAXLIKE
ZAKUSKA

•A••••K

BABCOCK
BADBACK
BADLUCK
BANACEK
BANGKOK
BARLICK
BARRACK
CANNOCK
CARJACK
CARPARK
CARTALK
CASSOCK
CATWALK
DAYBOOK
DAYPACK
EARLOCK
EARMARK
FALKIRK
FARTLEK
FATBACK
GANGTOK
GARRICK
GASLEAK
GASMASK
GASTANK
GATWICK
HADDOCK
HAMHOCK
HAMMOCK
HANCOCK
HARNICK
HARTACK
HASSOCK
HATRACK
HAYFORK
HAYRACK
HAYRICK
JAMPACK
JANACEK
JAYWALK
KAISHEK
LAMARCK
LAWBOOK
LAYBACK
MADLOCK
MASARYK
MATLOCK
MATTOCK
NATWICK
OAKCASK
OAKDESK
OAKPARK
OARLOCK
PADDOCK
PADLOCK
PARTOOK
PATRICK
PAYBACK
RANAMOK
RANBACK
RANSACK
RATFINK
RATPACK
RAWSILK
SADSACK
SARAWAK
SATBACK
SAWBUCK
SAWCHUK
TANBARK
TAYBACK
VANDYCK
VANEYCK
VANWYCK
VARITEK
VARRICK
WARHAWK
WARLOCK
WARWICK
WAXWORK
WAYBACK
YAKUTSK
YANNICK
YASBECK
YASHMAK
ZATOPEK

••AK•••

AGAKHAN
ALAKING
AWAKENS
AWAKERS
AWAKING
BEAKERS
BLAKELY
BLAKLEY
BRAKING
CHAKRAS
FLAKERS
FLAKIER
FLAKILY
FLAKING
INAKNOT
KRAKENS
LEAKAGE
LEAKERS
LEAKEYS
LEAKIER
LEAKING
LEAKSIN
NDAKOTA
OFAKIND
ONAKICK
OSAKANS
PEAKIER
PEAKING
PEAKISH
PLAKATS
QUAKERS
QUAKIER
QUAKIES
QUAKILY
QUAKING
SDAKOTA
SHAKERS
SHAKEUP
SHAKIER
SHAKILY
SHAKING

SHAKIRA
SHAKOES
SLAKERS
SLAKING
SNAKERS
SNAKIER
SNAKILY
SNAKING
SOAKERS
SOAKING
SOAKSIN
SOAKSUP
STAKING
WEAKENS
WEAKEST
WEAKISH
WEAKONS

••A•K••

ALACKOF
ALASKAN
ALASKAS
BLACKED
BLACKEN
BLACKER
BLACKIE
BLACKLY
BLANKED
BLANKER
BLANKET
BLANKLY
BRACKEN
BRACKET
CHALKED
CHALKUP
CLACKED
CLACKER
CLANKED
CRACKED
CRACKER
CRACKLE
CRACKLY
CRACKUP
CRANKED
CRANKUP
DRANKIN
DRANKTO
DRANKUP
EBANKED
FLACKED
FLANKED
FLANKEN
FLANKER
FRANKED
FRANKEN
FRANKER
FRANKIE
FRANKLY
FRANKOZ
GRACKLE
HEARKEN
KHARKOV
KRACKEL
PLACKET
PLANKED
QUACKED
QUACKER
REASKED
SHACKED
SHACKLE
SHANKAR
SHANKED
SHARKEY
SLACKED
SLACKEN
SLACKER
SLACKLY
SLACKUP
SLATKIN
SMACKED
SMACKER
SMACKOF
SMACKUP
SNACKED
SNACKER
SNACKON
SPACKLE
SPANKED
SPANKER
SPARKED
SPARKLE
SPARKLY
STACKED
STACKER
STACKUP
STALKED
STALKER
STANKUP
STARKER
STARKEY
STARKLY
SWANKED
SWANKER
SWANKUP
THANKED
THANKER
TRACKED
TRACKER
UNASKED
WHACKED
WHACKER
WRACKED
WRACKUP

••A••K•

ASAJOKE
CHACHKA
INAPOKE
PEALIKE
REAWAKE
REAWOKE
ROANOKE
SEALIKE
SPASSKY
STARSKY
TEACAKE
UNALIKE
UNAWAKE

••A•••K

ARAMARK
ASALARK
ATATURK
BEATNIK
BLALOCK
BLAUBOK
BYANECK
CHARPAK
INAFUNK
INAWINK
KRAMNIK
LEACOCK
NEATNIK
ONAKICK
ONALARK
PEACOCK
SEADUCK
SEAHAWK
SEASICK
TEANECK
THATSOK

•••AK••

AKSAKOV
ANNAKIN
BETAKEN
BETAKES
BLEAKER
BLEAKLY
BREAKER
BREAKIN
BREAKUP
CLOAKED
COMAKER
CONAKRY
CREAKED
CROAKED
CROAKER
DEBAKEY
DUKAKIS
FREAKED
INTAKES
KANAKAS
KARAKUM
KAYAKED
KAYAKER
LALAKER
MEDAKAS
REBAKED
REBAKES
REMAKES
RERAKED
RERAKES
RETAKEN
RETAKER
RETAKES
REWAKED
REWAKEN
REWAKES
RUMAKIS
SNEAKBY
SNEAKED
SNEAKER
SNEAKIN
SNEAKUP
SPEAKER
SPEAKOF
SPEAKTO
SPEAKUP
TWEAKED
UNBAKED
UNCAKED
UNCAKES
UNFAKED
UNMAKER
UNMAKES
UNRAKED
UNTAKEN
UNWAKED
UPTAKES
WREAKED
WREAKER

•••A•K•

ACKACKS
ARRACKS
ATTACKS
AUTARKY
BYTALKS
CDRACKS
DAMASKS
DEBARKS
DEMARKS
EMBANKS
EMBARKS
ENRANKS
EUBANKS
EXYANKS
HIJACKS
KARAOKE
MALARKY
MOHAWKS
NYYANKS
OUTASKS
PARASKI
PULASKI
REBANKS
REMARKS
REPACKS
REPARKS
RERACKS
RERANKS
RETACKS
RVPARKS
SQUAWKS
SQUAWKY
STMARKS
THWACKS
UNCASKS
UNMASKS
UNPACKS
UNRACKS
UNTACKS
UPTALKS
UQUARKS

•••A••K

BANACEK
HOWARDK
JANACEK
JIRASEK
LAMARCK
MASARYK
MUBARAK
RANAMOK
RUNAMOK
SARAWAK

••••AK•

ANORAKS
ASHCAKE
ATSTAKE
BIGJAKE
BUNRAKU
BUROAKS
CODCAKE
CUPCAKE
EATCAKE
FORSAKE
HOECAKE
HOTCAKE
KODIAKS
MISTAKE
OATCAKE
OILCAKE
OUTBAKE
OUTTAKE
PANCAKE
PARBAKE
PARTAKE
PINOAKS
PREBAKE
PREMAKE
REAWAKE
REDOAKS
RESOAKS
RUMCAKE
SCREAKS
SLOVAKS
SQUEAKS
SQUEAKY
STREAKS
STREAKY
TANOAKS
TEACAKE
UNAWAKE
UNBRAKE
UNFLAKY
UNLEAKY
UNSNAKY

••••A•K

AIRPACK
AIRPARK
AIRTANK
AMTRACK
ARAMARK
ASALARK
BADBACK
BARRACK
BIGTALK
BULWARK
BURBANK
BUYBACK
CARJACK
CARPARK
CARTALK
CATWALK
CONRACK
CORMACK
COSSACK
CUTBACK
DAYPACK
DENMARK
DONTASK
DUNDALK
EARMARK
EYEBANK
EYEMASK
FATBACK
FINBACK
FIRBANK
FOGBANK
FUTHARK
GASMASK
GASTANK
GETBACK
GOBLANK
GOSHAWK
GOTBACK
HARTACK
HATRACK
HAYRACK
HITBACK
HOGBACK
HOLYARK
HOTPACK
ICEPACK
INBLACK
INKMARK
JAMPACK
JAYWALK
JETPACK
JOBBANK
KEYBANK
LAYBACK
LEXMARK
LIEBACK
MISMARK
MONTAUK
MUDLARK
MUDPACK
NONBANK
NONDARK
NORWALK
OAKCASK
OAKPARK
OILTANK
ONALARK
ONTRACK
OSTMARK
OUTBACK
OUTBARK
OUTRANK
OUTTALK
OUTWALK
PAYBACK
PEPTALK
POLLACK
PREDARK
PREPACK
PUTBACK
RANBACK
RANSACK
RATPACK
RECHALK
RECRANK
REDHAWK
REDJACK
RESPARK
RESTACK
RETHANK
RETRACK
RUNBACK
SADSACK
SATBACK
SEAHAWK
SETBACK
SITBACK
SIXPACK
SKIMASK
SKIRACK
SKYJACK
SKYLARK
SKYWALK
SUBBANK
SUBTASK
TANBARK
TAYBACK
TEDMACK
THELARK
THEMASK
THESACK
TIEBACK
TIERACK
TIETACK
TITLARK
TOPRANK
TULSAOK
UNFRANK
UNSLACK
UNSTACK
UNTRACK
UPQUARK
WARHAWK
WAYBACK
WIDMARK
WINBACK

•••••AK

ALBORAK
ALNITAK
BESPEAK
CHARPAK
CORKOAK
ELENIAK
GASLEAK
HOLMOAK
LEFREAK
LIVEOAK
LTKOJAK
MRNOVAK
MUBARAK
NONPEAK
OFFPEAK
ONBREAK
PRESOAK
QBSNEAK
REBREAK
RESPEAK
SARAWAK
SERIPAK
SZYSLAK
UNCLOAK
UNSPEAK
URSULAK
WOZNIAK
YASHMAK
YITZHAK

AL•••••

ALABAMA
ALABAMY
ALACKOF
ALADDIN
ALADINE
ALAKING
ALAMEDA
ALAMEIN
ALAMODE
ALAMOSA
ALANINE
ALANJAY
ALANNAH
ALARBUS
ALARCON
ALARMED
ALARMER
ALARUMS
ALASKAN
ALASKAS
ALASSAD
ALATEEN
ALAYING
ALBANIA
ALBEDOS
ALBENIZ
ALBERTA
ALBERTI
ALBERTO
ALBINOS
ALBIREO
ALBORAK
ALBSURE
ALBUMEN
ALBUMIN
ALBUNDY
ALCAIDE
ALCALDE
ALCAZAR
ALCESTE
ALCHEMY
ALCOHOL
ALCOPOP
ALCOVES
ALCYONE
ALDAVIS
ALDENTE
ALDORAY
ALDRICH
ALDUBIN
ALEARDI
ALEGARS
ALEGRIA
ALEKEGS
ALEKSEI
ALEMBIC
ALENCON
ALERTED
ALERTER
ALERTLY
ALERTTO
ALETAPS
ALETTES
ALEVELS
ALEWIFE
ALEYARD
ALFALFA
ALFEROV
ALFIERI
ALFONSE
ALFONSO
ALFORJA
ALFREDA
ALFREDE
ALFREDO
ALFREDU
ALGARVE
ALGEBRA
ALGERIA
ALGIEBA
ALGIERS
ALGREEN
ALIASES
ALIBABA
ALIBIED
ALIDADE
ALIENEE
ALIENOR
ALIENTO
ALIFORM
ALIGHTS
ALIGNED
ALIGNER
ALIGOTE
ALIMENT
ALIMONY
ALINERS
ALINING
ALITTLE
ALIVETO
ALIYAHS
ALKALIS
ALKENES
ALLAGES
ALLANTE
ALLAYED
ALLAYER
ALLBRAN
ALLCAPS
ALLCASH
ALLCLAD
ALLDONE
ALLEARS
ALLEGED
ALLEGER
ALLEGES
ALLEGRA
ALLEGRO
ALLELES
ALLELIC
ALLELSE
ALLENBY
ALLENDE
ALLERGY
ALLEWIS
ALLEYES
ALLGONE
ALLGOOD
ALLHAIL
ALLHEAL
ALLHERE
ALLISON
ALLIUMS
ALLMALE
ALLMINE
ALLNESS
ALLNEWS
ALLOFIT
ALLOFME
ALLOFUS
ALLONGE
ALLONYM
ALLOPEZ
ALLOVER
ALLOWAY
ALLOWED
ALLOWIN
ALLOWME
ALLOYED
ALLRISE
ALLSTAR
ALLSTON
ALLTHAT
ALLTHIS
ALLTIED
ALLTIME
ALLTOLD
ALLUDED
ALLUDES
ALLURED
ALLURER
ALLURES
ALLUVIA
ALLWISE
ALLYING
ALLYSON
ALMAATA
ALMADEN
ALMANAC
ALMERIA
ALMONDS
ALMONDY
ALMONER
ALMONRY
ALMSMAN
ALMSMEN
ALNICOS
ALNILAM
ALNITAK
ALNIYAT
ALOADOF
ALOHAOE
ALOOFLY
ALPACAS
ALPHARD
ALPINER
ALPINES
ALQUIST
ALREADY
ALRIGHT
ALROKER
ALROSEN
ALSATIA
ALSHAIN
ALSMITH
ALSORAN
ALTDORF
ALTERED
ALTERER
ALTHING
ALTHORN
ALTIMAS
ALTKEYS
ALTOIDS
ALTOIST
ALTOONA
ALTOSAX
ALTTABS
ALUDELS
ALUMINA
ALUMNAE
ALUMNAL
ALUMNUS
ALUNSER
ALVAREZ
ALVEOLI
ALWORTH
ALYKHAN
ALYOSHA
ALYSSUM

A•L••••

AALARGE
AALIYAH
ABLATED
ABLATES
AELFRIC
AILERON
AILMENT
ALLAGES
ALLANTE
ALLAYED
ALLAYER
ALLBRAN
ALLCAPS
ALLCASH
ALLCLAD
ALLDONE
ALLEARS
ALLEGED
ALLEGER
ALLEGES
ALLEGRA
ALLEGRO
ALLELES
ALLELIC
ALLELSE
ALLENBY
ALLENDE
ALLERGY
ALLEWIS
ALLEYES
ALLGONE
ALLGOOD
ALLHAIL
ALLHEAL
ALLHERE
ALLISON
ALLIUMS
ALLMALE
ALLMINE
ALLNESS
ALLNEWS
ALLOFIT
ALLOFME
ALLOFUS
ALLONGE
ALLONYM
ALLOPEZ
ALLOVER
ALLOWAY
ALLOWED
ALLOWIN
ALLOWME
ALLOYED
ALLRISE
ALLSTAR
ALLSTON
ALLTHAT
ALLTHIS
ALLTIED
ALLTIME
ALLTOLD
ALLUDED
ALLUDES
ALLURED
ALLURER
ALLURES
ALLUVIA
ALLWISE
ALLYING
ALLYSON
APLENTY
APLITES
APLUSES
ARLBERG
ARLEDGE
ASLEWOF
ATLANTA
ATLARGE
ATLASES
ATLEAST
ATLUNCH
AULDSOD
AULETTA
AXLROSE

A••L•••

ABALONE
ABELARD
ABILENE
ABILITY
ABOLISH
ABOLLAE
ACCLAIM
ACOLYTE
ACTLIKE
ADDLING
ADELIES
ADELINA
ADELINE
ADELPHI
ADOLLAR
ADOLPHE
ADULATE
ADULTLY
AEOLIAN
AFFLECK
AFFLICT
AGALLOP
AGELESS
AGELONG
AGILELY
AGILEST
AGILITY
AGULHAS
AIDLESS
AIGLETS
AIMLESS
AIRLANE
AIRLESS
AIRLIFT
AIRLIKE
AIRLINE
AIRLOCK
AIRLOGS
AMALGAM
AMBLERS
AMBLING
AMILATE
AMPLEST
AMPLIFY
AMULETS
AMYLASE
ANALOGS
ANALOGY
ANALYSE
ANALYST
ANALYTE
ANALYZE
ANELING
ANGLAIS
ANGLERS
ANGLING
ANILINE
ANILITY
ANKLERS
ANKLETS
ANTLERS
ANTLIKE
ANTLION
ANYLUCK
APELETS
APELIKE
APILEOF
APOLLOS
APOLOGY
APPLAUD
APPLETS
APPLIED
APPLIER
APPLIES
APPLING
APPLYTO
APULIAN
ARALSEA
ARCLAMP
ARMLESS
ARMLETS
ARMLIKE
ARMLOAD
ARMLOCK
ARTLESS
ASALARK
ASHLAND
ASHLARS
ASHLESS
ASSLIKE
ASYLUMS
ATALOSS
ATELATE
ATELESS
ATELIER
ATHLETE
AUKLETS
AUSLESE
AVALONS
AVULSED
AVULSES
AWELESS
AWNLESS
AXELIKE
AXELROD

AXILLAE
AXILLAR
AXILLAS
AXOLOTL
AZALEAS
AZULEJO

A•••L••

AACELLS
AAMILNE
ABOLLAE
ABRILES
ABSALOM
ABSOLUT
ABSOLVE
ACDELCO
ACHILLE
ACRYLIC
ACYCLIC
ADOLLAR
AEDILES
AFATLOT
AFOULOF
AGALLOP
AIRFLOW
AIRGLOW
AIRPLAY
AKERLOF
ALCALDE
ALFALFA
ALKALIS
ALLCLAD
ALLELES
ALLELIC
ALLELSE
ALNILAM
AMESLAN
AMIBLUE
AMPULES
ANGELAS
ANGELES
ANGELIC
ANGELOU
ANGELUS
ANGOLAN
ANGULAR
ANNALEE
ANNALES
ANNELID
ANNULAR
ANNULET
ANNULUS
ANSELMO
ANTILOG
APHELIA
APHILIP
APOLLOS
APPALLS
ARABLES
ARBOLES
AREOLAE
AREOLAR
AREOLAS
AREOLES
ARGALIS
ARGYLES
ARNOLDS
ASTOLAT
ATACLIP
ATEALOT
AUDILES
AURALEE
AURALLY
AVAILED
AVONLEA
AWFULLY
AXIALLY
AXILLAE
AXILLAR
AXILLAS

A••••L•

AAACELL
AACELLS
ACEROLA
ACETALS
ACHILLE
ACOUPLE
ACRIDLY
ACTABLE
ACTORLY
ACUTELY
ADDABLE
ADDEDLY
ADDIBLE
ADDSALT
ADEPTLY
ADULTLY
AERIALS
AFFABLE
AFFABLY
AGILELY
AGNAILS
AHASSLE
AIRBALL
AIRBILL
AIRHOLE
AIRMILE
AIRWOLF
ALERTLY
ALEVELS
ALITTLE
ALLMALE
ALLTOLD
ALOOFLY
ALUDELS
ALVEOLI
AMAPOLA
AMATOLS
AMIABLE
AMIABLY
AMIDALA
AMIDOLS
AMPOULE
AMSTELS
ANATOLE
ANATOLY
ANGRILY
ANIMALS
ANNEALS
ANNUALS
ANOMALY
ANOUILH
ANTHILL
APISHLY
APOSTLE
APPALLS
APPEALS
ARCWELD
ARMFULS
ARMHOLE
ARSHILE
ARTFILM
ARTICLE
ARTSALE
ARTWALL
ARUGULA
ASARULE
ASPHALT
ASSAILS
ASSAULT
ATATILT
ATFAULT
ATHRILL
ATINGLE
AUDIBLE
AUDIBLY
AURALLY
AUREOLA
AUREOLE
AURICLE
AUSABLE
AVERELL
AVERILL
AVOWALS
AWFULLY
AXIALLY

A•••••L

AAACELL
ABETTAL
ABIGAIL
ABUTTAL
ABYSMAL
ABYSSAL
ACAUDAL
ACCRUAL
ACCUSAL
ADMIRAL
ADRENAL
AEROSOL
AIRBALL
AIRBILL
AIRCOOL
AIRFOIL
AIRMAIL
ALCOHOL
ALLHAIL
ALLHEAL
ALUMNAL
ANBESOL
ANNABEL
ANTHEIL
ANTHILL
APOGEAL
APPAREL
APTERAL
AROUSAL
ARRABAL
ARRAYAL
ARRIVAL
ARSENAL
ARTWALL
ARUNDEL
ASEXUAL
ASOCIAL
ASPRAWL
ASUSUAL
ATABOIL
ATHRILL
AUGURAL
AURORAL
AUSTRAL
AVERELL
AVERILL
AVERNAL
AXOLOTL

•AL••••

AALARGE
AALIYAH
BALABAN
BALANCE
BALASES
BALATAS
BALATON
BALBOAS
BALCONY
BALDEST
BALDIES
BALDING
BALDISH
BALDRIC
BALDWIN
BALEENS
BALEFUL
BALFOUR
BALIHAI
BALKANS
BALKERS
BALKIER
BALKILY
BALKING
BALKSAT
BALLADE
BALLADS
BALLARD
BALLAST
BALLBOY
BALLETS
BALLIOL
BALLMER
BALLONE
BALLOON
BALLOTS
BALLSUP
BALLTWO
BALLUET
BALMAIN
BALMIER
BALMILY
BALONEY
BALSAMS
BALSAMY
CALABRO
CALAMAR
CALANDO
CALCIFY
CALCITE
CALCIUM
CALCULI
CALDERA
CALDERS
CALDRON
CALENDS
CALGARY
CALHOUN
CALIBAN
CALIBER
CALIBRE
CALICES
CALICOS
CALIPER
CALIPHS
CALISTA
CALKERS
CALKING
CALKINS
CALLBOX
CALLBOY
CALLEES
CALLERS
CALLFOR
CALLING
CALLINS
CALLNOW
CALLOFF
CALLOUS
CALLOUT
CALLSIN
CALLSIT
CALLSON
CALLSTO
CALLSUP
CALLUPS
CALMEST
CALMING
CALMSEA
CALORIC
CALORIE
CALOTTE
CALPOLY
CALTECH
CALUMET
CALUMNY
CALVARY
CALVERT
CALVING
CALVINO
CALYCES
CALYPSO
CALYXES
CALZONE
DALASIS
DALETHS
DALLIED
DALLIER
DALLIES
DALTONS
DALTREY
FALAFEL
FALCATE
FALCONS
FALKIRK
FALLACY
FALLALS
FALLDUE
FALLERS
FALLFOR
FALLGUY
FALLING
FALLOFF
FALLOUT
FALLOWS
FALLSIN
FALLSON
FALLSTO
FALSELY
FALSEST
FALSIFY
FALSITY
FALTERS
FALWELL
GALAHAD
GALANOS
GALANTS
GALATEA
GALATIA
GALAXES
GALAXIE
GALEATE
GALENAS
GALENTO
GALETTE
GALICIA
GALILEE
GALILEI
GALILEO
GALLANT
GALLEON
GALLERY
GALLEYS
GALLICO
GALLING
GALLIUM
GALLONS
GALLOPS
GALLOWS
GALOOTS
GALOPED
GALPALS
GALUMPH
GALVANI
GALVANO
HALALAS
HALAVAH
HALCYON
HALDANE
HALFBAD
HALFCUT
HALFDAY
HALFDUG
HALFFED
HALFIES
HALFMAD
HALFRAW
HALFROD
HALFSHY
HALFWAY
HALFWIT
HALFWON
HALIBUT
HALIDES
HALIFAX
HALITES
HALLEYS
HALLOOS
HALLOWS
HALLWAY
HALOGEN
HALOIDS
HALOING
HALSTON
HALTERS
HALTING
HALVAHS
HALVERS
HALVING
HALYARD
JALISCO
KALININ
LALAKER
LALANNE
LALIQUE
LALLING
LALOOSH
MALABAR
MALACCA
MALACHI
MALAGAN
MALAGAS
MALAISE
MALAMUD
MALARIA
MALARKY
MALAYAN
MALCOLM
MALDIVE
MALEANT
MALEBEE
MALECAT
MALEDOG
MALEFIC
MALEHOG
MALEPIG
MALIANS
MALICES
MALIGNS
MALLARD
MALLETS
MALLEUS
MALLIKA
MALLOWS
MALLRAT
MALMSEY
MALODOR
MALPASO
MALRAUX
MALTASE
MALTBIE
MALTEDS
MALTESE
MALTHUS
MALTIER
MALTING
MALTOSE
MALVINA
MALWARE
PALABRA
PALACES
PALADIN
PALAMAS
PALANCE
PALATAL
PALATES
PALAVER
PALAZZI
PALAZZO
PALEALE
PALEDRY
PALEMON
PALERMO
PALETTE
PALFREY
PALINGS
PALJOEY
PALLETS
PALLIER
PALLING
PALLORS
PALMARY
PALMATE
PALMERS
PALMFUL
PALMIER
PALMING
PALMIST
PALMOFF
PALMOIL
PALMTOP
PALMYRA
PALOMAR
PALOMAS
PALOOKA
PALPATE
PALTERS
PALTROW
PALUDAL
RALEIGH
RALLIED
RALLIER
RALLIES
RALLYES
RALLYTO
RALPHIE
RALSTON
SALAAMS
SALABLE
SALADES
SALADIN
SALAMIS
SALAZAR
SALCHOW
SALEMOR
SALERNO
SALIENT
SALIERI
SALINAS
SALINES
SALIVAS
SALLIED
SALLIER
SALLIES
SALMONP
SALMONS
SALOMON
SALONGA
SALOONS
SALSODA
SALTANT
SALTBOX
SALTERS
SALTIER
SALTILY
SALTINE
SALTING
SALTISH
SALTPIT
SALTSEA
SALUKIS
SALUTED
SALUTER
SALUTES
SALVAGE
SALVERS
SALVING
SALVOES
SALVORS
TALARIA
TALCKED
TALCUMS
TALENTS
TALIBAN
TALKBIG
TALKERS
TALKIER
TALKIES
TALKING
TALKOUT
TALKSAT
TALKSOF
TALKSON
TALKSTO
TALKSUP
TALLEST
TALLIED
TALLIER
TALLIES
TALLINN
TALLISH
TALLITH
TALLONE
TALLOWS
TALLOWY
TALLYHO
TALLYUP
TALONED
TALUSES
VALADON
VALANCE
VALENCE
VALENTE
VALENTI
VALERIE
VALETED
VALIANT
VALIDID
VALIDLY
VALINES
VALISES
VALJEAN
VALLEJO
VALLEYS
VALLONE
VALMIKI
VALOREM
VALOTTE
VALOURS
VALUATE
VALUERS
VALUING
VALVATE
VALVULA
VALVULE
WALCOTT
WALDORF
WALKERS
WALKING
WALKINS
WALKMAN
WALKOFF
WALKONS
WALKOUT
WALKSBY
WALKSON
WALKSTO
WALKUPS
WALKURE
WALKWAY
WALLABY
WALLACE
WALLACH
WALLETS
WALLEYE
WALLING
WALLMAP
WALLOFF
WALLOON
WALLOPS
WALLOWS
WALLSIN
WALLSUP
WALMART
WALNUTS
WALPOLE
WALSTON
WALTERS
WALTHAM
WALTHER
WALTONS
WALTZED
WALTZER
WALTZES
YALELAW
YALEMAN
YALEMEN

•A•L•••

BAALISH
BAALISM
BAALIST
BAALITE
BADLAND
BADLIES
BADLOTS
BADLOVE
BADLUCK
BAGLADY
BAGLIKE
BAILEES
BAILERS
BAILIFF
BAILING
BAILORS
BAILOUT
BAILSON
BAKLAVA
BALLADE
BALLADS
BALLARD
BALLAST
BALLBOY
BALLETS
BALLIOL
BALLMER
BALLONE
BALLOON
BALLOTS
BALLSUP
BALLTWO
BALLUET
BARLESS
BARLEYS
BARLICK
BATLIKE
BAULKED
BAULKER
BAWLERS
BAWLING
BAWLOUT
BAYLEAF
BAYLORU
BAYLYNX
CABLERS
CABLETS
CABLETV
CABLING
CAILLOU
CALLBOX
CALLBOY
CALLEES
CALLERS
CALLFOR
CALLING
CALLINS
CALLNOW
CALLOFF
CALLOUS
CALLOUT
CALLSIN
CALLSIT
CALLSON
CALLSTO
CALLSUP
CALLUPS
CAPLESS
CAPLETS
CARLENE
CARLESS
CARLING
CARLOAD
CARLOAN
CARLOTA
CARLOTS
CARLSON
CARLTON
CARLYLE
CATLIKE
CAULKED
CAULKER
DAHLIAS
DAILIES
DALLIED
DALLIER
DALLIES
DARLEEN
DARLENE
DARLING
DAYLILY
DAYLONG
EAGLETS
EAGLING
EARLAPS
EARLDOM
EARLESS
EARLETS
EARLIER
EARLIES
EARLIKE
EARLOBE
EARLOCK
EARLYON
EATLATE
EATLESS
FABLERS
FABLING
FADLIKE
FAILING
FAILLES
FAILSTO
FAILURE
FALLACY
FALLALS
FALLDUE
FALLERS
FALLFOR
FALLGUY
FALLING
FALLOFF
FALLOUT
FALLOWS
FALLSIN
FALLSON
FALLSTO
FANLIKE
FARLEFT
FATLESS
FATLIKE
FATLING
FATLIPS
FAULTED
FAXLORE
GAGLAWS
GAGLINE
GALLANT
GALLEON
GALLERY
GALLEYS
GALLICO
GALLING
GALLIUM
GALLONS
GALLOPS
GALLOWS
GAOLERS
GAOLING
GAPLESS
GARLAND
GARLICS
GARLITS
GASLAMP
GASLEAK
GASLESS
GASLINE
GASLOGS
GATLING
GATLINS
GAULISH
GAYLORD
HAGLIKE
HAILERS
HAILING
HALLEYS
HALLOOS
HALLOWS
HALLWAY
HAMLETS
HAMLINE
HAPLESS
HAPLOID
HARLAND
HARLEYS
HARLINE
HARLOTS
HATLESS
HATLIKE
HAULAGE
HAULERS
HAULING
HAULOFF
HAULSIN
HAULSUP
HAYLOFT
HAZLITT
IAMLOVE
JAGLESS
JAILERS
JAILING
JAILORS
JAMLIKE
JARLESS
JAWLESS
JAWLIKE
JAWLINE
JAYLENO
KARLOFF
KARLOVY
KARLSON
KAYLENZ
LADLERS
LADLING
LAFLEUR
LALLING
LAPLACA
LAPLACE
LAPLAND
LAPLATA
LAULAUS
LAWLESS
LAWLIKE
MACLEAN
MACLEOD
MADLIBS
MADLOCK
MAGLEVS
MAILBAG
MAILBIN
MAILBOX
MAILCAR
MAILERS
MAILING
MAILINS
MAILLOL
MAILLOT

MAILMAN MAILMEN MAILOUT MAILSIN MALLARD MALLETS MALLEUS MALLIKA MALLOWS MALLRAT MANLESS MANLIER MANLIKE MARLENE MARLIER MARLINS MARLOWE MATLESS MATLOCK MAULDIN MAULERS MAULING NAILERS NAILGUN NAILING NAILKEG NAILSET NAILSIN NAILSIT NAILSUP NAILTIP NAPLESS OAKLAND OAKLAWN OAKLEAF OAKLIKE OARLESS OARLIKE OARLOCK OATLIKE PABLUMS PADLOCK PAELLAS PAHLAVI PAILFUL PALLETS PALLIER PALLING PALLORS PAMLICO PARLAYS PARLEYS PARLORS PARLOUR PARLOUS PAULIII PAULINA PAULINE PAULING PAULIST PAULPRY PAULSEN PAVLOVA PAYLESS PAYLOAD RAGLANS RAILAGE RAILBUS

RAILCAR RAILERS RAILING RAILMAN RAILMEN RAILSAT RAILSON RAILWAY RALLIED RALLIER RALLIES RALLYES RALLYTO RAMLIKE RANLAPS RANLATE RATLIKE RATLINE RATLINS RAWLINS RAYLESS RAYLIKE SACLIKE SAILERS SAILING SAILORS SAILSON SAILSTO SALLIED SALLIER SALLIES SAMLETS SAMLOYD SAPLESS SAPLING SAWLIKE SAWLOGS TABLEAU TABLETS TABLING TABLOID TAGLIKE TAGLINE TAILEND TAILERS TAILFIN TAILING TAILOFF TAILORS TAILPIN TAILWAG TALLEST TALLIED TALLIER TALLIES TALLINN TALLISH TALLITH TALLONE TALLOWS TALLOWY TALLYHO TALLYUP TANLINE TAXLAWS TAXLESS TAXLEVY TAYLORS

VALLEJO VALLEYS VALLONE VANLINE VANLOAD VARLAAM VARLETS VAULTED VAULTER WAILERS WAILFUL WAILING WALLABY WALLACE WALLACH WALLETS WALLEYE WALLING WALLMAP WALLOFF WALLOON WALLOPS WALLOWS WALLSIN WALLSUP WARLESS WARLIKE WARLOCK WARLORD WASLATE WAXLIKE WAYLAID WAYLAND WAYLAYS WAYLESS

•A••L••

AACELLS AAMILNE BABBLED BABBLER BABBLES BABYLON BACILLI BACKLIT BACKLOG BACKLOT BAFFLED BAFFLER BAFFLES BANALER BANALLY BANDLET BANGLED BANGLES BARCLAY BARKLEY BAROLOS BARTLES BARTLET BASALLY BASALTS BASILIC BASILIO BATTLED BATTLER BATTLES BAUBLES

CABALAS CABALLE CACKLED CACKLER CACKLES CAILLOU CAJOLED CAJOLER CAJOLES CAMELID CAMELOT CAMILLA CAMILLE CANALED CANDLED CANDLER CANDLES CANOLAS CANTLES CANULAE CANULAS CAPELET CAPELLA CAPULET CARCLUB CAROLED CAROLER CAROLII CAROLYN CASELAW CASELLA CASELOT CASTLED CASTLES CATALAN CATALOG CATALOS CATALPA CATFLAP CATFLEA CAVALRY CAVILAT CAVILED CAVILER DABBLED DABBLER DABBLES DAIMLER DANDLED DANDLER DANDLES DANELAW DANGLED DANGLER DANGLES DAPPLED DAPPLES DARKLED DARKLES DARTLED DARTLES DASILVA DAWDLED DAWDLER DAWDLES DAZZLED DAZZLER DAZZLES

EARCLIP EARFLAP EARPLUG EASELED EATALOT FACULAE FACULTY FAILLES FAMILIA FAMILLE FAMULUS FANCLUB FANSLER FARTLEK FATALES FATALLY GABBLED GABBLES GAGGLES GALILEE GALILEI GALILEO GAMBLED GAMBLER GAMBLES GAMELAN GAMELAW GAMELEG GANGLIA GANTLET GARBLED GARBLER GARBLES GARGLED GARGLER GARGLES GATELEG GAVELED GAVILAN GAZELLE HAARLEM HABILIS HACKLED HACKLER HACKLES HAGGLED HAGGLER HAGGLES HALALAS HAMELIN HAMULUS HANDLED HANDLER HANDLES HANDLIN HAROLDI HARTLEY HASSLED HASSLES JACALES JAIALAI JANGLED JANGLER JANGLES JANKLOW JAVELIN KAROLYI KASTLER

LABELED LABELER LABELLE LAIDLOW LAJOLLA LAMPLIT LANDLER LANGLEY LANOLIN LAPALMA LAPELED LASALLE LASTLAP LASTLEG LAVALSE LAVELLI LAYSLOW MACULAE MACULAR MADALYN MADELON MAGALOG MAGILLA MAHALIA MAILLOL MAILLOT MANGLED MANGLER MANGLES MANILAS MANILOW MANOLIN MANTLED MANTLES MANTLET MARBLED MARBLER MARBLES MARILLA MARILYN MARULLO MARYLOU MATALIN MATILDA MAUDLIN MAXILLA MAYALIN NACELLE NAPALMS NASALLY NATALIA NATALIE PABULUM PACELAP PADDLED PADDLER PADDLES PAELLAS PAISLEY PANELED PANTLEG PAPELES PAPILLA PAROLED PAROLEE PAROLES PARSLEY PASALLE

PATELLA PAYOLAS PAYSLIP QABALAH QABALAS RABBLED RABBLES RAFFLED RAFFLER RAFFLES RAMBLED RAMBLER RAMBLES RAMBLIN RANKLED RANKLES RAPALLO RASSLED RASSLER RASSLES RATTLED RATTLER RATTLES RAVELED RAVELLY RAVELOE SADDLED SADDLER SADDLES SAMPLED SAMPLER SAMPLES SANBLAS SANDLER SANDLOT SARALEE SAVALAS TABULAR TACKLED TACKLER TACKLES TAGALOG TAMALES TAMBLYN TAMGLEN TANGLED TANGLER TANGLES TARTLET TASHLIN TATTLED TATTLER TATTLES VANILLA VANILLI WADDLED WADDLER WADDLES WAFFLED WAFFLER WAFFLES WAGGLED WAGGLER WAGGLES WAMBLED WAMBLES WANGLED WANGLER

WANGLES WARBLED WARBLER WARBLES WARCLUB WATTLED WATTLES WAVELET YALELAW

•A•••L•

AAACELL AACELLS BACILLI BADCALL BADCOLD BAGFULS BAGGILY BAGNOLD BAGWELL BALKILY BALMILY BANALLY BARBELL BARBILL BARBULE BARRELS BARTOLO BASALLY BASSALE BAWDILY CABALLE CABBALA CALCULI CALPOLY CAMILLA CAMILLE CAMPILY CAMRYLE CANCELS CANDELA CANFULS CANNELL CANNELS CANNILY CANNOLI CANNULA CANTALS CANTILY CAPABLE CAPABLY CAPELLA CAPFULS CAPSULE CARFULS CARIOLE CARLYLE CARMELA CARPALS CARPELS CARRELS CARROLL CARSALE CARTALK CARTELS CARVELS CASELLA CASSOLA

CASTILE CASUALS CATCALL CATTALO CATTILY CATWALK DACTYLS DAFFILY DAMSELS DANDILY DANGELO DANIELA DANIELJ DANIELS DARNELL DARRYLF DARWELL DASCHLE DATABLE DATEDLY DATRILS DAYLILY DAZEDLY EADGILS EAGERLY EARFULS EARHOLE EARTHLY EATABLE FACIALS FADEDLY FAINTLY FAISALI FALLALS FALSELY FALWELL FAMILLE FANBELT FANCILY FANFOLD FANPALM FARFELS FARRELL FATALLY FATCELL FATTILY GAGRULE GALPALS GAMBOLS GANDALF GASKELL GAUDILY GAUNTLY GAUZILY GAVIALS GAWKILY GAZELLE HADPULL HAMMILY HANDILY HANSOLO HAPPILY HARDILY HARROLD HARSHLY HARWELL HASKELL HASPULL

HASTILY HATABLE HATFULS HAYBALE IANHOLM JACKALS JADEDLY JARFULS JARRELL JAYWALK JAZZILY KABBALA KAMPALA LABELLE LABIALS LAEMMLE LAJOLLA LANKILY LAPBELT LAPFULS LARGELY LASALLE LASCALA LATRELL LAURELS LAVELLI MADEILL MAGILLA MAKABLE MAKEILL MALCOLM MAMMALS MANACLE MANDALA MANDELA MANHOLE MANIPLE MANTELS MANUALS MARCELS MARILLA MARSALA MARULLO MARVELL MARVELS MAXILLA MAXWELL MAYPOLE NACELLE NAIVELY NAKEDLY NAMABLE NAMABLY NASALLY NASTILY NATTILY NAUTILI PACBELL PALEALE PANFULS PANICLE PANOPLY PANTILE PAPILLA PARABLE PARCELS PASALLE PASCOLI

PASSELS PASTELS PATELLA PATROLS PAVIDLY PAYABLE PAYROLL PAYWELL RABIDLY RADIALS RADICLE RAGDOLL RAINILY RAKABLE RANDALL RANWILD RAPALLO RAPIDLY RAPPELS RASCALS RATABLE RATHOLE RAVELLY RAVIOLI RAWSILK RAYNELL SAINTLO SAINTLY SALABLE SALTILY SAMEOLD SAMHILL SAMUELL SANDALS SANDFLY SAPPILY SASSILY SATWELL SAUCILY SAVABLE SAVVILY SAWMILL SAYABLE TABOULI TACITLY TACKILY TACTILE TADPOLE TAGSALE TAKABLE TAKEILL TAMABLE TAMBALA TANGELO TARBELL TARDILY TAROILS TARSALS TARTILY TASSELS TASTILY TATTILY TAWNILY TAXABLE TAXSALE VACUOLE VAGUELY VALIDLY

VALVULA VALVULE VANDALS VANILLA VANILLI VANPELT VAPIDLY VASSALS VATFULS WACKILY WADDELL WALPOLE WANKELS WASPILY WASSILY WAVICLE WAXABLE WAYBILL YARNELL

•A••••L

AAACELL BABYOIL BADCALL BADGIRL BAGGIRL BAGWELL BALEFUL BALLIOL BANEFUL BARBELL BARBILL BARNOWL BASHFUL BASINAL BATGIRL BATHOIL CAMERAL CAMGIRL CANNELL CAPITAL CAPITOL CARAMEL CARAVEL CARDIAL CAREFUL CARPOOL CARROLL CASTROL CATBOWL CATCALL CATTAIL DAMOSEL DAREFUL DARNELL DARWELL DAYQUIL DAYSAIL EASEFUL FACTFUL FACTUAL FALAFEL FALWELL FANEUIL FANMAIL FANTAIL FARMGAL FARRELL

FASCIAL FATCELL FATEFUL GABRIEL GAGREEL GAINFUL GAMETAL GASKELL GASOHOL HADPULL HAECKEL HAIRGEL HANDFUL HANDSEL HARMFUL HARWELL HASKELL HASPULL HATEFUL JAECKEL JARRELL KAPITAL LACTEAL LACUNAL LAMINAL LAMPOIL LATERAL LATRELL MACNEIL MADEILL MAGICAL MAILLOL MAKEILL MANDREL MARITAL MARSHAL MARTIAL MARVELL MATINAL MAXIMAL MAXWELL MAYORAL NAHUATL NAIPAUL NARWHAL NATURAL NATUREL OATMEAL PACBELL PAILFUL PAINFUL PALATAL PALMFUL PALMOIL PALUDAL PARASOL PARBOIL PARTIAL PASCHAL PASSEUL PAYROLL PAYWELL RACHAEL RADICAL RAGDOLL RAGEFUL RANDALL RAPHAEL

7 AL

RATTAIL
RAVENAL
RAWDEAL
RAYNELL
SACKFUL
SAMHILL
SAMUELL
SANIBEL
SATCHEL
SATWELL
SAWMILL
TACTFUL
TACTUAL
TAKEILL
TAMPAFL
TANKFUL
TARBELL
TARHEEL
VANEXEL
VANPOOL
VATICAL
WADDELL
WAILFUL
WAKEFUL
WASSAIL
WASTREL
WAYBILL
WAYCOOL
YARNELL
YAWNFUL

••AL•••

ABALONE
AGALLOP
AMALGAM
ANALOGS
ANALOGY
ANALYSE
ANALYST
ANALYTE
ANALYZE
ARALSEA
ASALARK
ATALOSS
AVALONS
AZALEAS
BAALISH
BAALISM
BAALIST
BAALITE
BDALTON
BEALION
BIALIES
BLALOCK
BRALESS
CDALBUM
CHALCIS
CHALETS
CHALICE
CHALKED
CHALKUP
CHALLAH
CHALONS
CHALUPA
COALBIN
COALCAR
COALERS
COALGAS
COALING
COALOIL
COALPIT
COALTAR
DEALERS
DEALING
DEALOUT
DEALSIN
DEALSTO
DEALSUP
DEALTIN
DEALTTO
DEALTUP
DIALECT
DIALEDO
DIALERS
DIALING
DIALLED
DIALOGS
DIALOUT
DIALSIN
DIALSUP
DIALUPS
DNALABS
DUALISM
DUALIST
DUALITY
DUALIZE
EGALITE
ETALIBI
EVALUNA
EXALTED
EXALTER
FHALOAN
FOALING
GOALIES
GOALONG
HEALALL
HEALERS
HEALING
HEALSUP
HEALTHY
HIALEAH
HJALMAR
HYALITE
HYALOID
INALINE
ITALIAN
ITALICS
JEALOUS
MCALLEN
MEALIER
MEALIES
MYALGIA
MYALGIC
NBALIVE
NIALONG
OCALAFL
OMALLEY
ONALARK
ONALEAD
ONALERT
ONALINE
OPALINE
OPALISH
ORALIST
OTALGIA
OTALGIC
OXALATE
PEALIKE
PEALING
PHALANX
PRALINE
PSALMIC
PSALTER
QUALIFY
QUALITY
REALEST
REALIGN
REALINE
REALISE
REALISM
REALIST
REALITY
REALIZE
REALLOT
REALMAN
REALMEN
REALTER
REALTOR
RIALTOS
RVALUES
SCALAGE
SCALARS
SCALDED
SCALDER
SCALENE
SCALERS
SCALEUP
SCALIER
SCALING
SCALLOP
SCALPED
SCALPEL
SCALPER
SEALABS
SEALANE
SEALANT
SEALEGS
SEALERS
SEALERY
SEALIFE
SEALIFT
SEALIKE
SEALILY
SEALING
SEALION
SEALOFF
SEALSIN
SEALSUP
SHALALA
SHALIER
SHALLOT
SHALLOW
SHALLWE
SHALOMS
SLALOMS
SMALLAD
SMALLER
SMALLOJ
STALAGS
STALELY
STALEST
STALKED
STALKER
STALLED
STALLER
SWALLOW
TEALEAF
TEALESS
THALERS
TRALALA
ULALUME
UNALERT
UNALIKE
UNALONE
UVALUES
VEALIER
VIALFUL
VIALING
VIALLED
WEALTHS
WEALTHY
WHALERS
WHALING
WHALLEY
ZEALAND
ZEALOTS
ZEALOUS

••A•L••

AFATLOT
AGALLOP
ARABLES
ATACLIP
AVAILED
BEADLES
BEAGLES
BEASLEY
BEATLES
BLAKLEY
BRADLEE
BRADLEY
BRAILLE
BRAMLEY
BRAWLED
BRAWLER
BRAWLEY
CHABLIS
CHALLAH
CHAPLET
CHAPLIN
CHARLES
CHARLEY
CHARLIE
CRADLED
CRADLER
CRADLES
CRAWLED
CRAWLER
CRAWLEY
DIABLES
DIABLOS
DIALLED
DRAWLED
DRAWLER
EMAILED
EMAILER
ENABLED
ENABLER
ENABLES
EPAULET
ETAILED
ETAILER
FIATLUX
FLAILAT
FLAILED
FLATLET
FRAILER
FRAILLY
FRAILTY
FRAWLEY
GNARLED
GRAVLAX
GRAYLAG
HAARLEM
JEANLUC
LEAFLET
MCALLEN
MEAGLES
MEASLES
OHANLON
OMALLEY
ORACLES
PEARLED
PEARLER
PHARLAP
PLAYLET
QUAILED
QUARLES
REALLOT
REARLIT
SCALLOP
SCARLET
SEABLUE
SEASLUG
SHALLOT
SHALLOW
SHALLWE
SHAWLED
SMALLAD
SMALLER
SMALLOJ
SNARLAT
SNARLED
SNARLER
SNARLUP
STABLED
STABLER
STABLES
STADLER
STALLED
STALLER
STANLEE
STANLEY
STAPLED
STAPLER
STAPLES
STARLET
STARLIT
STARLOG
STATLER
SWALLOW
TRAILED
TRAILER
TRAWLED
TRAWLER
UNAXLED
USABLES
VIALLED
WHALLEY
XRAYLAB

••A••L•

AAACELL
AHASSLE
AMAPOLA
AMATOLS
ANATOLE
ANATOLY
ASARULE
ATATILT
BEADILY
BEASTLY
BEATALL
BIASPLY
BLACKLY
BLACULA
BLAKELY
BLANDLY
BLANKLY
BOATELS
BRAILLE
BRAMBLE
BRAMBLY
BRASHLY
BRATTLE
BRAVELY
BYAMILE
CHAGALL
CHANELS
CHAPALA
CHAPELS
CHARILY
CLAVELL
CRACKLE
CRACKLY
CRAPOLA
CRASSLY
CRAYOLA
CRAZILY
DIABOLO
DIAVOLO
DRABBLE
DRACULA
DRAGGLE
ENAMELS
EXACTLY
EXAMPLE
FLAKILY
FOAMILY
FRAGGLE
FRAGILE
FRAILLY
FRANKLY
FRAZZLE
GHASTLY
GLAZILY
GRACILE
GRACKLE
GRANDLY
GRANOLA
GRANULE
GRAPPLE
GRASSLE
GRAVELS
GRAVELY
HEADILY
HEALALL
HEAVILY
HOARILY
INABALL
INAHOLE
INANELY
INAPILE
INAPTLY
INAVALE
IRATELY
LOATHLY
MCARDLE
MEATILY
ONAROLL
PIANOLA
PLAINLY
PRATTLE
QUAKILY
READILY
REAPPLY
RIANTLY
SCANTLY
SCAPULA
SCARILY
SEACALM
SEAEELS
SEAGULL
SEALILY
SEAMILE
SEASALT
SEATTLE
SEAWALL
SEAWOLF
SHACKLE
SHADILY
SHAKILY
SHALALA
SHAMBLE
SHAPELY
SHARPLY
SLACKLY
SLANTLY
SMARTLY
SNAKILY
SNAPPLE
SOAPILY
SPACELY
SPACKLE
SPANGLE
SPANGLY
SPARELY
SPARKLE
SPARKLY
SPATULA
STABILE
STAGILY
STAIDLY
STALELY
STARKLY
STARTLE
STATELY
SUAVELY
SWADDLE
SWAHILI
TEABALL
TEARILY
TEASELS
TRALALA
TRAMPLE
TRAVELS
TWADDLE
UNADULT
UNAGILE
UNAPTLY
URACILS
WEARILY
WEASELS
WRANGLE

••A•••L

AAACELL
ACAUDAL
ATABOIL
BEANOIL
BEATALL
BIAXIAL
BOATFUL
CHAGALL
CHANCEL
CHANNEL
CHASMAL
CHATTEL
CLAIROL
CLAUDEL
CLAUSAL
CLAVELL
COALOIL
COASTAL
COAXIAL
CRANIAL
DOADEAL
EMANUEL
EVANGEL
FEARFUL
FLANNEL
FRACTAL
GLACIAL
GRADUAL
GRAPNEL
HEADFUL
HEALALL
HEATFUL
INABALL
INAPRIL
JCARROL
KRACKEL
MIAMIFL
MIASMAL
MOANFUL
NOANGEL
OCALAFL
ONAROLL
PEAFOWL
PLAYFUL
QUARREL
REAVAIL
SCALPEL
SCANDAL
SEAFOWL
SEAGULL
SEAWALL
SPACIAL
SPANIEL
SPATIAL
TEABALL
TEARFUL
TRAMMEL
TRAUBEL
TRAVAIL
TRAYFUL
UNAWFUL
VIALFUL
WRANGEL

•••AL••

ABSALOM
ALCALDE
ALFALFA
ALKALIS
ANNALEE
ANNALES
APPALLS
ARGALIS
ATEALOT
AURALEE
AURALLY
AXIALLY
BANALER
BANALLY
BASALLY
BASALTS
BECALMS
BEFALLS
BIVALVE
BUGALOO
BYTALKS
CABALAS
CABALLE
CANALED
CATALAN
CATALOG
CATALOS
CATALPA
CAVALRY
COBALTS
DECALOG
DEDALUS
DEFALLA
DEPALMA
DERALTE
DESALTS
DEVALUE
DUCALLY
EATALOT
ELGALLO
EMBALMS
EMPALED
EMPALES
ENDALLS
EQUALED
EQUALLY
EQUALTO
ESCALOP
ESCALUS
EXHALED
EXHALES
FATALES
FATALLY
FEMALES
FINALES
FINALLY
FUGALLY
GERALDO
GYRALLY
HALALAS
HERALDS
HIDALGO
HIMALIA
HONALEE
IDEALLY
IMPALAS
IMPALED
IMPALER
IMPALES
INGALLS
INHALED
INHALER
INHALES
INSALES
INVALID
ITSALIE
ITSALOT
JACALES
JAIALAI
LAPALMA
LASALLE
LAVALSE
LEGALLY
LILALEE
LOCALES
LOCALLY
LOYALER
LOYALES
LOYALLY
LOYALTO
LOYALTY
MADALYN
MAGALOG
MAHALIA
MATALIN
MAYALIN
MCCALLS
MCHALES
MCNALLY
MEDALED
MEGALON
METALED
MISALLY
MORALES
MORALLY
MTBALDY
MURALED
NAPALMS
NASALLY
NATALIA
NATALIE
NEPALIS
NOGALES
NOPALES
NOTALIE
NOTALOT
NOVALIS
OFVALUE
OGLALAS
PASALLE
PEDALED
PEDALER
PENALTY
PETALED
PETALES
PREALLY
QABALAH
QABALAS
RAPALLO
REBALED
REBALES
RECALLS
REDALGA
REFALLS
REGALED
REGALER
REGALES
REGALIA
REGALLY
RENALDO
RENALLY
RESALES
RESALTS
RETALLY
REVALUE
RIBALDS
RINALDO
RITALIN
RIVALED
RIVALRY
ROSALIA
ROSALIE
ROSALYN
ROYALES
ROYALLY
ROYALTY
ROYALWE
RURALLY
RUTALEE
SARALEE
SAVALAS
SEDALIA
SEEALSO
SEPALED
SHOALED
SOMALIA
SOMALIS
SQUALID
SQUALLS
SQUALLY
SQUALOR
STEALER
STEALIN
STEALTH
TAGALOG
TAMALES
TEBALDI
THEALPS
THRALLS
TIDALLY
TONALLY
TOTALED
TOTALER
TOTALLY
TOTALUP
UNBALED
UNBALES
UNPALED
UNSALTY
UNWALLS
UPTALKS
UPVALUE
USUALLY
VENALLY
VIDALIA
VISALIA
VITALIS
VITALLY
VIVALDI
VOCALIC
VOCALLY
ZOCALOS
ZONALLY

•••A•L•

ACTABLE
ADDABLE
AFFABLE
AFFABLY
AGNAILS
AMIABLE
AMIABLY
APPALLS
ASSAILS
ASSAULT
ATFAULT
AURALLY
AUSABLE
AXIALLY
BANALLY
BASALLY
BEFALLS
BEWAILS
BLEAKLY
BROADLY
BUYABLE
CABALLE
CAPABLE
CAPABLY
CENACLE
CHEADLE
CHEAPLY
CITABLE
CLEANLY
CLEARLY
CORACLE
CURABLE
CURABLY
DATABLE
DEBACLE
DECARLO
DEFALLA
DEFAULT
DEPAULU
DERAILS
DETAILS
DISABLE
DRYABLE
DUCALLY
DURABLE
DURABLY
EATABLE
EFFABLE
EFFABLY
ELGALLO
ENDABLE
ENDALLS
ENTAILS
EQUABLE
EQUABLY
EQUALLY
ERRABLE
FATALLY
FINABLE
FINAGLE
FINALLY
FIXABLE
FLYABLE
FRIABLE
FRIARLY
FRYABLE
FUGALLY
GETABLE
GREATLY
GYRALLY
HATABLE
HIDABLE
HIRABLE
HUMANLY
IDEALLY
INGALLS
INTAILS
ISRAELI
KOWADLO
LASALLE
LEGALLY
LIKABLE
LINABLE
LIVABLE
LOCALLY
LOSABLE
LOVABLE
LOVABLY
LOYALLY
MAKABLE
MANACLE
MCCALLS
MCNALLY
MICAELA
MINABLE
MIRACLE
MISALLY
MIXABLE
MORALLY
MOVABLE
MOVABLY
MUTABLE
MUTABLY
MYFAULT
NAMABLE
NAMABLY
NASALLY
NOFAULT
NOTABLE
NOTABLY
OXTAILS
PARABLE
PASALLE
PAYABLE
PLIABLE
PLIABLY
POSABLE
POTABLE
PREALLY
RAKABLE
RAPALLO
RATABLE
RECABLE
RECALLS
REFALLS
REGALLY
REHAULS
REJAILS
REMAILS

RENAILS
RENALLY
RENAULT
RETABLE
RETAILS
RETALLY
RIDABLE
ROUAULT
ROYALLY
RURALLY
SALABLE
SAVABLE
SAYABLE
SCRAWLS
SCRAWLY
SEEABLE
SIZABLE
SIZABLY
SKIABLE
SPRAWLS
SPRAWLY
SQUALLS
SQUALLY
SQUATLY
STPAULS
TAKABLE
TAMABLE
TAXABLE
TENABLE
TENABLY
THRALLS
TIDALLY
TONALLY
TOTABLE
TOTALLY
TOWABLE
TREACLE
TREACLY
TREADLE
TRIABLE
TUNABLE
TVTABLE
UNMADLY
UNMANLY
UNNAILS
UNSADLY
UNWALLS
UPEARLY
USUALLY
VENABLE
VENALLY
VITALLY
VOCABLE
VOCABLY
VOCALLY
VOTABLE
WAXABLE
WIRABLE
WOMANLY
ZONALLY

•••A••L

ANNABEL
APPAREL
ARRABAL
ARRAYAL
CARAMEL
CARAVEL
CITADEL
DUHAMEL
EMPANEL
ESPANOL
ETHANOL
FALAFEL
GEMAYEL
GIRASOL
IMPANEL
ISRAFEL
MIRABEL
MONADAL
OCTAVAL
OHCAROL
PALATAL
PARASOL
PHRASAL
RELABEL
REPANEL
SMEAGOL
STBASIL
TUNAOIL
UNNASAL
UNRAVEL

••••AL•

ACETALS
ADDSALT
AERIALS
AIRBALL
ALLMALE
AMIDALA
ANIMALS
ANNEALS
ANNUALS
ANOMALY
APPEALS
ARTSALE
ARTWALL
ASPHALT
AVOWALS
BADCALL
BASSALE
BEATALL
BEEFALO
BENGALI
BENGALS
BENZALI
BIGHALF
BIGSALE
BIGTALK
BOXBALL
BRIDALS
BUFFALO
BURIALS
CABBALA
CANTALS
CARPALS
CARSALE
CARTALK
CASUALS
CATCALL
CATTALO
CATWALK
CEMBALO
CENTALS
CEPHALO
CEPHALY
CEREALS
CHAGALL
CHAPALA
CHORALE
CHORALS
COEVALS
CORRALS
CUEBALL
CUREALL
CYMBALS
DENIALS
DENTALS
DEWFALL
DISMALS
DONNALL
DORSALS
DOSSALS
DRYWALL
DUNDALK
ELIYALE
EMERALD
ENSEALS
ESPIALS
EYEBALL
EYEWALL
FACIALS
FAISALI
FALLALS
FANPALM
FINGALS
FINIALS
FLYBALL
FORMALS
FORSALE
FURBALL
GALPALS
GANDALF
GAVIALS
GESTALT
GIMBALS
GOODALL
GOSTALE
GUMBALL
GUNWALE
GYMBALL
HAYBALE
HEALALL
HERBALS
HOGCALL
HOLDALL
HOSCALE
HYMNALS
ICEFALL
ILLCALL
INABALL
INAVALE
INGOALS
INSCALE
INSTALL
INSTALS
JACKALS
JAYWALK
JIMDALE
JONHALL
KABBALA
KAMPALA
KENDALL
KEYPALS
KIMBALL
KNOWALL
LABIALS
LASCALA
LETFALL
LIPBALM
LOWBALL
MAMMALS
MANDALA
MANUALS
MARSALA
MENIALS
MESCALS
MESSALA
METCALF
MISCALL
MISSALS
MONDALE
MONTALE
MORTALS
MUTUALS
NETBALL
NONSALE
NORMALS
NORWALK
ODDBALL
OILPALM
OLDPALS
OLDSALT
OMPHALO
ONEBALL
ONECALL
ONEHALF
OOHLALA
ORDEALS
OSTWALD
OUTCALL
OUTTALK
OUTWALK
OVERALL
PALEALE
PENPALS
PEPTALK
PERCALE
PETCALF
PIEBALD
PIESALE
PINBALL
PINWALE
PITFALL
PLURALS
PORTALS
PRESALE
PRESALT
PROBALL
RADIALS
RANDALL
RASCALS
RECHALK
RECHALL
RECOALS
REDEALS
REDEALT
REDIALS
REHEALS
RENTALS
REPEALS
RESCALE
RESEALS
REVEALS
RITUALS
RUFFALO
SANDALS
SEACALM
SEASALT
SEAWALL
SEENALL
SEESALL
SERIALS
SHALALA
SIGNALS
SIXBALL
SKYWALK
SNOBALL
SOCIALS
SOURALE
SPIRALS
SQUEALS
SUBHALL
TAGSALE
TAMBALA
TARSALS
TAXSALE
TEABALL
TELLALL
TENBALL
THEFALL
THEMALL
THEWALL
TIMBALE
TIMBALS
TOLDALL
TOOTALL
TORVALD
TOSCALE
TOYBALL
TRALALA
TWOBALL
TYNDALL
UNCIALS
UNDEALT
UNIBALL
UNSCALY
UNSEALS
UPPSALA
UPSCALE
VANDALS
VASSALS
VERBALS
VESTALS
VFWHALL
VISUALS
ZUMWALT

••••A•L

ABIGAIL
AIRBALL
AIRMAIL
ALLHAIL
ARTWALL
ASPRAWL
BADCALL
BEATALL
BEDRAIL
BOBTAIL
BOXBALL
CATCALL
CATTAIL
CHAGALL
CUEBALL
CUREALL
CURTAIL
DAYSAIL
DESTAEL
DEWFALL
DOGTAIL
DONNALL
DRYWALL
ENSNARL
EYEBALL
EYEWALL
FANMAIL
FANTAIL
FLYBALL
FOXTAIL
FURBALL
GOODALL
GUMBALL
GYMBALL
HEALALL
HOBNAIL
HOGCALL
HOLDALL
HOTMAIL
ICEFALL
ILLCALL
INABALL
INSTALL
ISHMAEL
JONHALL
KENDALL
KENWAHL
KIMBALL
KNOWALL
LESPAUL
LETFALL
LOWBALL
LUGSAIL
MICHAEL
MIKHAIL
MISCALL
MRSPAUL
NAHUATL
NAIPAUL
NETBALL
OCALAFL
ODDBALL
ONEBALL
ONECALL
OUTBAWL
OUTCALL
OUTHAUL
OUTRAIL
OUTSAIL
OVERALL
PIGTAIL
PINBALL
PINTAIL
PITFALL
PREVAIL
PROBALL
RACHAEL
RANDALL
RAPHAEL
RATTAIL
REAVAIL
RECHALL
REDTAIL
SEAWALL
SEENALL
SEESALL
SELMAAL
SETBAIL
SETSAIL
SIXBALL
SNOBALL
SUBHALL
TAMPAFL
TEABALL
TELLALL
TENBALL
THEFALL
THEMALL
THEWALL
TOENAIL
TOLDALL
TOOTALL
TOPSAIL
TOYBALL
TOYPAIL
TRAVAIL
TRYSAIL
TWOBALL
TYNDALL
UNFRAIL
UNIBALL
UNSNARL
VFWHALL
WASSAIL
WEBMAIL

•••••AL

ABETTAL
ABUTTAL
ABYSMAL
ABYSSAL
ACAUDAL
ACCRUAL
ACCUSAL
ADMIRAL
ADRENAL
ALLHEAL
ALUMNAL
APOGEAL
APTERAL
AROUSAL
ARRABAL
ARRAYAL
ARRIVAL
ARSENAL
ASEXUAL
ASOCIAL
ASUSUAL
AUGURAL
AURORAL
AUSTRAL
AVERNAL
BASINAL
BESTIAL
BIAXIAL
BIFOCAL
BIGDEAL
BIGMEAL
BIMETAL
BIMODAL
BIPEDAL
BITONAL
BORSTAL
BUMDEAL
CAMERAL
CAPITAL
CARDIAL
CENTRAL
CHASMAL
CHORDAL
CITYGAL
CLAUSAL
COASTAL
COAXIAL
COBCOAL
COEQUAL
COMICAL
CONCEAL
CONGEAL
CONICAL
CORDIAL
CORNEAL
CORONAL
CRANIAL
CREEDAL
CRUCIAL
CRUSTAL
CRYSTAL
CUBICAL
CUBITAL
CYNICAL
DECIMAL
DEPOSAL
DEXTRAL
DIGITAL
DIURNAL
DOADEAL
DOMICAL
DONEGAL
ECTYPAL
EDICTAL
ELUVIAL
ENTHRAL
EPOCHAL
ESTIVAL
ETERNAL
ETHICAL
EXCUSAL
FACTUAL
FARMGAL
FASCIAL
FEDERAL
FEMORAL
FIGURAL
FINICAL
FLOREAL
FLUIDAL
FLUVIAL
FORREAL
FRACTAL
FRONTAL
FURSEAL
GAMETAL
GENERAL
GETREAL
GLACIAL
GLOSSAL
GLOTTAL
GLUTEAL
GOTOGAL
GOTREAL
GRADUAL
HELICAL
HOTCOAL
HOTMEAL
HUMERAL
HUMORAL
ILLEGAL
IMMORAL
INITIAL
INTOTAL
ISCHIAL
JIMDIAL
JOURNAL
JUVENAL
KAPITAL
LACTEAL
LACUNAL
LAMINAL
LATERAL
LEXICAL
LIBERAL
LIMINAL
LINGUAL
LITERAL
LOGICAL
LUSTRAL
LYRICAL
MAGICAL
MARITAL
MARSHAL
MARTIAL
MATINAL
MAXIMAL
MAYORAL
MEDICAL
MIASMAL
MINERAL
MINIMAL
MISDEAL
MISDIAL
MISTRAL
MONADAL
MONDIAL
MUSICAL
NARWHAL
NATURAL
NEUTRAL
NEWDEAL
NODICAL
NOMINAL
NONORAL
NOTREAL
NUMERAL
NUPTIAL
NYMPHAL
OATMEAL
OCTAVAL
OEDIPAL
ONTRIAL
OPTICAL
OPTIMAL
ORBITAL
ORDINAL
ORTEGAL
OVOIDAL
OWNGOAL
PALATAL
PALUDAL
PARTIAL
PASCHAL
PERORAL
PERUSAL
PHRASAL
PINSEAL
PIVOTAL
PLEURAL
PLUVIAL
PREHEAL
PREORAL
PRESEAL
QUETZAL
QUINTAL
RADICAL
RAVENAL
RAWDEAL
RECITAL
RECUSAL
REFUSAL
REFUTAL
REGINAL
REMOVAL
RENEWAL
RETINAL
RETOTAL
RETRIAL
REVISAL
REVIVAL
RORQUAL
ROSTRAL
SCANDAL
SCLERAL
SEISMAL
SELMAAL
SEMINAL
SENEGAL
SENSUAL
SEVERAL
SORORAL
SOYMEAL
SPACIAL
SPATIAL
SPECIAL
SPHERAL
SPOUSAL
STERNAL
STOICAL
SUBDUAL
SUBGOAL
SUNDIAL
SURREAL
SYNODAL
TACTUAL
TEXTUAL
THERMAL
TOPICAL
TRIVIAL
TYPICAL
UNEQUAL
UNIDEAL
UNLEGAL
UNLOCAL
UNLOYAL
UNNASAL
UNREGAL
UNRURAL
UNUSUAL
UNVENAL
UNVITAL
UNVOCAL
UXORIAL
VATICAL
VEGETAL
VENTRAL
VESTRAL
VICINAL
VICTUAL
VIMINAL
VIRTUAL
WEIRDAL
WOLFGAL
XENICAL
ZOOIDAL

AM•••••

AMADEUS
AMALGAM
AMANITA
AMANTIS
AMAPOLA
AMARONE
AMASSED
AMASSER
AMASSES
AMATEUR
AMATIVE
AMATOLS
AMATORY
AMAZING
AMAZONS
AMBIENS
AMBIENT
AMBLERS
AMBLING
AMBRIES
AMBROSE
AMEBOID
AMENDED
AMENDER
AMENITY
AMERADA
AMERCED
AMERCER
AMERCES
AMERICA
AMERIGO
AMERIKA
AMERIND
AMESLAN
AMHARIC
AMHERST
AMIABLE
AMIABLY
AMIBLUE
AMICHAI
AMIDALA
AMIDOLS
AMILATE
AMINUTE
AMISTAD
AMITIES
AMMETER
AMMONIA
AMMONIC
AMNERIS
AMNESIA
AMNESIC
AMNESTY
AMNIONS
AMOEBAE
AMOEBAS
AMOEBIC
AMONGST
AMORIST
AMOROSO
AMOROUS
AMOUNTS
AMPEDUP
AMPERES
AMPHION
AMPHORA
AMPLEST
AMPLIFY
AMPOULE
AMPULES
AMRADIO
AMREETA
AMRITAS
AMSCRAY
AMSTELS
AMTRACK
AMTRACS
AMULETS
AMUSEME
AMUSERS
AMUSING
AMYLASE

A•M••••

AAMILNE
ADMIRAL
ADMIRED
ADMIRER
ADMIRES
ADMITTO
ADMIXED
ADMIXES
AIMEDAT
AIMHIGH
AIMLESS
AIMSFOR
ALMAATA
ALMADEN
ALMANAC
ALMERIA
ALMONDS
ALMONDY
ALMONER
ALMONRY
ALMSMAN
ALMSMEN
AMMETER
AMMONIA
AMMONIC
ARMADAS
ARMBAND
ARMBONE
ARMENIA
ARMFULS
ARMHOLE
ARMLESS
ARMLETS
ARMLIKE
ARMLOAD
ARMLOCK
ARMOIRE
ARMORED
ARMORER
ARMOURS
ARMOURY
ARMPITS
ARMREST
ARMYANT
ASMARAN
ATMCARD
ATMFEES

A••M•••

AAAMAPS
ACUMENS
ADAMANT
ADAMITE
ADAMSES
ADAMSON
AFTMOST
AGEMATE
AILMENT
AIRMADA
AIRMAIL
AIRMASS
AIRMILE
ALAMEDA
ALAMEIN
ALAMODE
ALAMOSA
ALEMBIC
ALIMENT
ALIMONY
ALLMALE
ALLMINE
ALSMITH
ALUMINA
ALUMNAE
ALUMNAL
ALUMNUS
ANDMORE
ANEMIAS
ANEMONE
ANIMACY
ANIMALS
ANIMATE
ANIMATO
ANIMISM
ANIMIST
ANOMALY
ANOMIES
ANYMORE
ARAMAIC
ARAMARK
ARAMEAN
ARAMIDS
ARDMORE
ASIMMER
ATAMANS
ATEMORE

ATOMICS
ATOMIES
ATOMISE
ATOMISM
ATOMIST
ATOMIZE
AUGMENT
AZIMUTH

A•••M••

AAJUMBO
ABDOMEN
ABYSMAL
ADWOMAN
ADWOMEN
AFRAMES
AGNOMEN
AJSIMON
ALARMED
ALARMER
ALBUMEN
ALBUMIN
ALMSMAN
ALMSMEN
ALTIMAS
ANAEMIA
ANAEMIC
ANDAMAN
ANNAMAY
ANOSMIA
ANOSMIC
AQUAMAN
AREAMAP
ARTEMIS
ARTEMUS
ASHAMED
ASIMMER
ASSUMED
ASSUMER
ASSUMES
ASTHMAS
ATHOMES
ATTEMPT
ATTIMES
AUTOMAT
AUTOMNE
AUTUMNS

A••••M•

ACADEME
ACADEMY
AFFIRMS
AIRDAMS
AIRPUMP
AIRTIME
ALABAMA
ALABAMY
ALARUMS
ALCHEMY
ALLIUMS
ALLOFME
ALLOWME
ALLTIME
AMUSEME
ANADEMS
ANATOMY
ANDIAMO
ANONYMS
ANSELMO
ANTHEMS
ANYTIME
ARCLAMP
ASHRAMS
ASYLUMS
ATACAMA
ATATIME
ATRIUMS
AWESOME

A•••••M

ABRAHAM
ABSALOM
ACCLAIM
ACRONYM
AFCTEAM
AGENDUM
AGONISM
ALIFORM
ALLONYM
ALNILAM
ALYSSUM
AMALGAM
ANAGRAM
ANAHEIM
ANIMISM
ANTFARM
ANTONYM
APOTHEM
ARCANUM
ARTFILM
ARTFORM
ARTHURM
ASATEAM
ASTREAM
ATAVISM
ATHEISM
ATOMISM
AUTONYM

•AM••••

AAMILNE
BAMBIII
BAMBINA
BAMBINI
BAMBINO
BAMBOOS
BAMMIES
BAMMING
CAMACHO
CAMAROS
CAMBERS
CAMBOYS
CAMBRIA
CAMBRIC
CAMEDUE
CAMELID
CAMELOT
CAMEOED
CAMEOFF
CAMEOUT
CAMERAE
CAMERAL
CAMERAS
CAMERON
CAMGIRL
CAMILLA
CAMILLE
CAMINOS
CAMIONS
CAMISES
CAMMIES
CAMPARI
CAMPBED
CAMPERS
CAMPHOR
CAMPIER
CAMPILY
CAMPING
CAMPION
CAMPOUT
CAMPSUP
CAMRYLE
DAMAGED
DAMAGES
DAMASKS
DAMASUS
DAMMERS
DAMMING
DAMNERS
DAMNING
DAMOSEL
DAMPDRY
DAMPENS
DAMPERS
DAMPEST
DAMPING
DAMPISH
DAMPMOP
DAMPOFF
DAMSELS
DAMSONS
FAMICOM
FAMILIA
FAMILLE
FAMINES
FAMULUS
GAMBADO
GAMBIAN
GAMBIER
GAMBITS
GAMBLED
GAMBLER
GAMBLES
GAMBOLS
GAMEBAG
GAMEBOY
GAMELAN
GAMELAW
GAMELEG
GAMETAL
GAMETES
GAMIEST
GAMINES
GAMMERS
GAMMING
GAMMONS
HAMACHI
HAMBONE
HAMBURG
HAMELIN
HAMHOCK
HAMITES
HAMITIC
HAMITUP
HAMLETS
HAMLINE
HAMMERS
HAMMETT
HAMMIER
HAMMILY
HAMMING
HAMMOCK
HAMMOND
HAMPERS
HAMPTON
HAMSTER
HAMULUS
IAMBICS
IAMBIST
IAMLOVE
JAMAICA
JAMBAND
JAMBEAU
JAMCAMS
JAMESII
JAMESIV
JAMESON
JAMESVI
JAMISON
JAMLIKE
JAMMERS
JAMMIER
JAMMIES
JAMMING
JAMPACK
KAMERAD
KAMFONG
KAMPALA
LAMAISM
LAMAIST
LAMARCK
LAMBADA
LAMBDAS
LAMBEAU
LAMBENT
LAMBERT
LAMBETH
LAMBING
LAMBKIN
LAMENTS
LAMINAE
LAMINAL
LAMINAR
LAMINAS
LAMINTO
LAMMING
LAMOTTA
LAMOTTE
LAMPERT
LAMPLIT
LAMPOIL
LAMPOON
LAMPREY
MAMAMIA
MAMBOED
MAMMALS
MAMMOTH
NAMABLE
NAMABLY
NAMEDAY
NAMEONE
NAMETAG
NAMIBIA
PAMLICO
PAMPERS
RAMADAN
RAMADAS
RAMBLED
RAMBLER
RAMBLES
RAMBLIN
RAMDOWN
RAMEKIN
RAMESES
RAMFANS
RAMHOME
RAMINTO
RAMIREZ
RAMJETS
RAMLIKE
RAMMERS
RAMMING
RAMMISH
RAMONES
RAMPAGE
RAMPANT
RAMPART
RAMPING
RAMPSUP
RAMRODS
RAMSESI
RAMSFAN
RAMSONS
SAMARAS
SAMARIA
SAMBAED
SAMBASS
SAMBORA
SAMBUCA
SAMEDAY
SAMEDIS
SAMEKHS
SAMEOLD
SAMHILL
SAMHUFF
SAMISEN
SAMLETS
SAMLOYD
SAMMYJO
SAMNUNN
SAMOANS
SAMOSAS
SAMOSET
SAMOVAR
SAMOYED
SAMPANS
SAMPLED
SAMPLER
SAMPLES
SAMPRAS
SAMPSON
SAMSONS
SAMSUNG
SAMUELL
SAMURAI
SAMWISE
TAMABLE
TAMALES
TAMARAC
TAMBALA
TAMBLYN
TAMGLEN
TAMIAMI
TAMMANY
TAMPAFL
TAMPERS
TAMPICO
TAMPING
TAMTAMS
VAMOOSE
VAMPERS
VAMPIER
VAMPING
VAMPIRA
VAMPIRE
VAMPISH
WAMBLED
WAMBLES
WAMPUMS
XAMOUNT
YAMAHAS
YAMMERS
ZAMBEZI
ZAMBIAN
ZAMBONI

•A•M•••

AAAMAPS
BADMOOD
BADMOVE
BALMAIN
BALMIER
BALMILY
BAMMIES
BAMMING
BARMAID
BARMIER
BASMATI
CADMIUM
CAIMANS
CALMEST
CALMING
CALMSEA
CAMMIES
CARMELA
CARMINA
CARMINE
CATMINT
CAYMANS
DAEMONS
DAIMLER
DAMMERS
DAMMING
DAUMIER
DAYMARE
EANMUND
EARMARK
EARMUFF
EATMORE
FANMAIL
FARMAID
FARMBOY
FARMERS
FARMERY
FARMGAL
FARMING
FARMORE
FARMOUT
GAMMERS
GAMMING
GAMMONS
GARMENT
GASMAIN
GASMASK
HAIMISH
HAMMERS
HAMMETT
HAMMIER
HAMMILY
HAMMING
HAMMOCK
HAMMOND
HARMERS
HARMFUL
HARMING
HARMONY
HAYMOWS
HAZMATS
JAMMERS
JAMMIER
JAMMIES
JAMMING
JASMINE
LABMICE
LAEMMLE
LAMMING
MAIMERS
MAIMING
MAIMITI
MALMSEY
MAMMALS
MAMMOTH
MANMADE
MARMARA
MARMION
MARMOTS
MAUMAUS
OAKMOSS
OATMEAL
PALMARY
PALMATE
PALMERS
PALMFUL
PALMIER
PALMING
PALMIST
PALMOFF
PALMOIL
PALMTOP
PALMYRA
PAYMENT
PAYMORE
RAGMANS
RAGMOPS
RAIMENT
RAMMERS
RAMMING
RAMMISH
RAWMEAT
RAYMOND
SALMONP
SALMONS
SAMMYJO
SAWMILL
SAYMASS
SAYMORE
TAMMANY
TARMACS
VALMIKI
VARMINT
WALMART
WARMERS
WARMEST
WARMING
WARMISH
WARMSTO
WARMSUP
WARMUPS
YAMMERS
YAOMING
YASMINE

•A••M••

AAJUMBO
BACHMAN
BADOMEN
BAHAMAS
BAHAMEN
BALLMER
BASEMAN
BASEMEN
BATEMAN
BATHMAT
BATSMAN
BATSMEN
CAKEMIX
CALAMAR
CALUMET
CALUMNY
CAPEMAY
CARAMBA
CARAMEL
CARAMIA
CAROMED
CASIMIR
CAVEMAN
CAVEMEN
DAHOMEY
DAMPMOP
DARKMAN
EASTMAN
FADIMAN
GALUMPH
GASSMAN
GATEMAN
GATEMEN
HACKMAN
HALFMAD
HANGMAN
HANGMEN
HARTMAN
HARTMUT
HAWKMAN
JACAMAR
JAROMIR
JAVAMAN
JAZZMAN
JAZZMEN
KASHMIR
KAUFMAN
LABAMBA
LAEMMLE
LAFEMME
LANDMAN
LANDMEN
LARAMIE
LASTMAY
LATIMES
MADAMES
MADAMEX
MADEMAD
MAILMAN
MAILMEN
MAINMAN
MAINMEN
MAKEMAD
MALAMUD
MAMAMIA
MANSMAN
MANUMIT
MANXMAN
MANXMEN
MARIMBA
MAXIMAL
MAXIMAS
MAXIMUM
MAXIMUS
NAVYMAN
NAVYMEN
OARSMAN
OARSMEN
PAJAMAS
PALAMAS
PALEMON
PALOMAR
PALOMAS
PANAMAS
PARAMUS
PARKMAN
RACEMES
RADAMES
RADOMES
RAILMAN
RAILMEN
RAINMAN
RANAMOK
SALAMIS
SALEMOR
SALOMON
SANDMAN
SANDMEN
SARUMAN
SAYAMEN
TACOMAS
TAGAMET
TAPEMAN
TAPEMEN
TATAMIS
TAXIMAN
TAXIMEN
WAKAMES
WAKSMAN
WALKMAN
WALLMAP
YAKIMAS
YALEMAN
YALEMEN
YARDMAN
YARDMEN
YASHMAK

•A•••M•

BADNAME
BADTIME
BALSAMS
BALSAMY
BANTAMS
BARNUMS
BAYRUMS
CATCOMB
DAYCAMP
DAYGAME
DAYTIME
FANDOMS
FATHOMS
GASLAMP
GASPUMP
GAUTAMA
HADSOME
HADTIME
HANSOMS
HASTIME
JAMCAMS
LACRIMO
LAFEMME
LAKSHMI
LANCOME
LAPALMA
LAPERMS
MACRAME
MAGNUMS
MAHATMA
MARRYME
MAYHEMS
MAYTIME
NANAIMO
NAPALMS
NAPTIME
NATSUME
PABLUMS
PALERMO
PARFUMS
PASTIME
RAGTIME
RAMHOME
RANHOME
RANSOMS
SACHEMS
SALAAMS
SANREMO
SAOTOME
SASHIMI
SATCHMO
SATCOMS
SATHOME
SATSUMA
TALCUMS
TAMIAMI
TAMTAMS
TANDEMS
VACUUMS
VANCAMP
WAMPUMS
WARGAME
WARTIME

•A••••M

BAALISM
BADFORM
BAHAISM
BAPTISM
BAREXAM
BARROOM
CACONYM
CADMIUM
CALCIUM
CARDIUM
DADAISM
DAYROOM
EARDRUM
EARLDOM
EASTHAM
EATFROM
FADDISM
FAMICOM
FANPALM
FANTASM
FASCISM
FATFARM
FAUVISM
GALLIUM
HAARLEM
HADROOM
HAFNIUM
HAHNIUM
HASIDIM
HASROOM
HASSIUM
HATBRIM
HAZANIM
IANHOLM
JAINISM
KARAKUM
LAMAISM
LANGHAM
MACADAM
MAHDISM
MALCOLM
MANHEIM
MARKHAM
MARXISM
MAUGHAM
MAXIMUM
NATRIUM
NAUSEAM
PABULUM
PANGRAM
PARONYM
SANCTUM
SARCASM
TAGTEAM
TAKEAIM
TANGRAM
TANTRUM
TAPROOM
VALOREM
VARLAAM
WALTHAM
WARROOM
YARDARM
YAYTEAM
ZANYISM

••AM•••

AAAMAPS
ADAMANT
ADAMITE
ADAMSES
ADAMSON
ALAMEDA
ALAMEIN
ALAMODE
ALAMOSA
ARAMAIC
ARAMARK
ARAMEAN
ARAMIDS
ATAMANS
BEAMERS
BEAMIER
BEAMING
BEAMISH
BEAMSUP
BLAMEON
BLAMERS
BLAMING
BRAMBLE
BRAMBLY
BRAMLEY
BYAMILE
CHAMBER
CHAMBRE
CHAMFER
CHAMOIS
CHAMPED
CHAMPER
CLAMANT
CLAMATO
CLAMBAR
CLAMBER
CLAMDIP
CLAMMED
CLAMMER
CLAMORS
CLAMOUR
CLAMPED
CLAMPER
CLAMPON
CLAMSUP
CRAMMED
CRAMMER
CRAMPED
CRAMPON
CRAMSIN
DIAMOND
DRAMADY
DRAMEDY
ELAMITE
ENAMELS
ENAMORS
ENAMOUR
ETAMINE
EXAMINE
EXAMPLE
FLAMBED
FLAMBES
FLAMERS
FLAMEUP
FLAMIER
FLAMING
FLAMMED
FOAMERS
FOAMIER
FOAMILY
FOAMING
FRAMERS
FRAMEUP
FRAMING
GLAMORS
GLAMOUR
GLAMSUP
GOAMISS
GRAMMAR
GRAMMER
GRAMMES
GRAMMYS
GRAMPAS
GRAMPUS
IMAMATE
IMAMESS
INAMESS
INAMOOD
KLAMATH
KLAMMER
KRAMDEN
KRAMNIK
LOAMIER
LOAMING
MIAMIAN
MIAMIFL
MUAMMAR
OFAMIND
REAMASS
REAMEND
REAMERS
REAMING
REAMOUT
ROAMERS
ROAMING
SCAMMED
SCAMMER
SCAMPED
SCAMPER
SEAMAPS
SEAMERS
SEAMIER
SEAMILE
SEAMING
SEAMIST
SEAMOSS
SHAMANS
SHAMBLE
SHAMING
SHAMMED
SHAMPOO
SIAMESE
SLAMMED
SLAMMER
SLAMSON
SPAMBOT
SPAMMED
SPAMMER
STAMENS
STAMINA
STAMMER
STAMPED
STAMPER
SWAMPED
TEAMING
TEAMSUP
TEAMUSA
TRAMCAR
TRAMMED

TRAMMEL
TRAMPAS
TRAMPED
TRAMPER
TRAMPLE
TRAMWAY
UNAMUNO
WHAMMED

••A•M••

ALARMED
ALARMER
ANAEMIA
ANAEMIC
BOATMAN
BOATMEN
BRAHMAN
BRAHMAS
BRAHMIN
CHAPMAN
CHAPMEN
CHARMAN
CHARMED
CHARMEN
CHARMER
CHARMIN
CHASMAL
CHASMIC
CLAIMED
CLAIMER
CLAMMED
CLAMMER
CRAMMED
CRAMMER
CRANMER
DHARMAS
DHARMIC
DRAWMAN
DRAWMEN
DRAYMAN
DRAYMEN
ENARMED
ERASMUS
FLAGMAN
FLAGMEN
FLAMMED
GRAMMAR
GRAMMER
GRAMMES
GRAMMYS
GRAUMAN
HEADMAN
HEADMEN
HJALMAR
KLAMMER
LEADMAN
LEADMEN
MEATMAN
MEATMEN
MIASMAL
MIASMAS
MIASMIC
MUAMMAR
MYANMAR
PLASMAS
PLASMIC
PSALMIC
READMIT
REAIMED
REALMAN
REALMEN
REARMED
REAUMUR
ROADMAP
SCAMMED
SCAMMER
SCATMAN
SHAMMED
SLAMMED
SLAMMER
SPAMMED
SPAMMER
STAMMER
STARMAN
STARMAP
SWAGMAN
SWAGMEN
SWARMED
SWARMER
TRAMMED
TRAMMEL
TRAUMAS
UNAIMED
UNARMED
WHAMMED
YEAHMAN

••A••M•

ACADEME
ACADEMY
ALABAMA
ALABAMY
ALARUMS
ANADEMS
ANATOMY
ATACAMA
ATATIME
BEATSME
DIADEMS
DIATOMS
DRACHMA
EXANIMO
GIACOMO
GRAHAME
GRAHAMS
GRANDMA
IPANEMA
KHATAMI
MCADAMS
MIAHAMM
MTADAMS
NBAGAME
RCADOME
SEAARMS
SHALOMS
SLALOMS
SPAREME
TEATIME
ULALUME
WHATAMI

••A•••M

AMALGAM
ANAGRAM
ANAHEIM
ASATEAM
ATAVISM
BAALISM
BEACHAM
CDALBUM
CHATHAM
CPAEXAM
CRANIUM
CZARDOM
CZARISM
DIAGRAM
DUALISM
GRANDAM
GUARGUM
HAARLEM
IMAGISM
INAPOEM
JOACHIM
KHAYYAM
MIAHAMM
NBATEAM
ONAWHIM
ORARIUM
PHANTOM
PIANISM
QUANTUM
REALISM
SEACALM
SEAFOAM
SEAGRAM
SHAHDOM
STADIUM
STANNUM
STARDOM
STATISM
TEAROOM
TRANSAM
TRANSOM
TSARDOM
TSARISM
URANIUM
YEATEAM

•••AM••

AFRAMES
ANDAMAN
ANNAMAY
AQUAMAN
AREAMAP
ASHAMED
BAHAMAS
BAHAMEN
BETAMAX
BYNAMES
CALAMAR
CARAMBA
CARAMEL
CARAMIA
CCLAMPS
CERAMIC
CREAMED
CREAMER
DECAMPS
DEFAMED
DEFAMER
DEFAMES
DREAMED
DREAMER
DREAMIN
DREAMOF
DREAMON
DREAMUP
DUHAMEL
DYNAMIC
DYNAMOS
EDNAMAY
ELCAMPO
ELLAMAE
ENCAMPS
ESTAMIN
GLEAMED
GLOAMIN
IDEAMAN
IDEAMEN
IDIAMIN
ILIAMNA
ISLAMIC
JACAMAR
JAVAMAN
JICAMAS
LABAMBA
LARAMIE
MADAMES
MADAMEX
MALAMUD
MAMAMIA
MELAMED
MESAMIS
MIRAMAR
MIRAMAX
MOGAMBO
MYMAMMY
NONAMES
OGHAMIC
ONRAMPS
PAJAMAS
PALAMAS
PANAMAS
PARAMUS
PDJAMES
POTAMUS
PREAMPS
PYRAMID
PYRAMUS
RADAMES
RANAMOK
RENAMED
RENAMES
RETAMED
RETAMES
REVAMPS
RITAMAE
RUNAMOK
SALAMIS
SAYAMEN
SESAMES
STEAMED
STEAMER
STEAMUP
STJAMES
TAGAMET
TATAMIS
THIAMIN
TINAMOU
TVGAMES
UNFAMED
UNNAMED
UNTAMED
UNTAMES
VITAMIN
WAKAMES
YOGAMAT

•••A•M•

BECALMS
DEPALMA
DISARMS
EMBALMS
LAPALMA
MAHATMA
MISAIMS
MYMAMMY
NANAIMO
NAPALMS
PREARMS
REDARMY
REWARMS
RORAIMA
SALAAMS
SEAARMS
THEARMY

•••A••M

ABRAHAM
ABSALOM
ARCANUM
BAHAISM
DADAISM
DINADAM
ERRATUM
HAZANIM
HUMANUM
JUDAISM
KARAKUM
LAMAISM
LCHAYIM
MACADAM
RITAGAM
STRATUM
TERAOHM

••••AM•

AIRDAMS
ALABAMA
ALABAMY
ANDIAMO
ARCLAMP
ASHRAMS
ATACAMA
BADNAME
BALSAMS
BALSAMY
BANTAMS
BEDLAMP
BEDLAMS
BELDAME
BELDAMS
BELLAMY
BERGAMO
BIGGAME
BIGMAMA
BIGNAME
CONGAME
CORFAMS
DAYCAMP
DAYGAME
DEFOAMS
DEFRAME
DIGRAMS
DIORAMA
DIRHAMS
DUCHAMP
EDINAMN
ENDGAME
ENFLAME
ENFRAME
ENGRAMS
EWELAMB
EXOGAMY
FOGLAMP
GASLAMP
GAUTAMA
GINGAME
GODMAMA
GOURAMI
GRAHAME
GRAHAMS
HOWLAME
ICEDAMS
INFLAME
INSEAMS
JAMCAMS
JIMJAMS
JOECAMP
KHATAMI
LOGJAMS
MACRAME
MCADAMS
MIAHAMM
MISNAME
MTADAMS
NBAGAME
NETGAME
NEWNAME
NFLGAME
NHLGAME
OFFRAMP
OILLAMP
ONENAME
ORIGAMI
OUTGAME
PENNAME
PETLAMB
PETNAME
PREGAME
PRENAME
PUBGAME
RECLAME
REFRAME
RESEAMS
RESTAMP
SALAAMS
SCREAMS
SKYCAMS
SPYCAMS
STREAMS
SUNLAMP
SURNAME
TAMIAMI
TAMTAMS
THEGAME
THELAMB
THERAMS
THESAME
TIEGAME
TOBLAME
TOPNAME
TSUNAMI
UNCLAMP
UNCRAMP
UNSEAMS
VANCAMP
WARGAME
WEBCAMS
WHATAMI
WIGWAMS
YOTEAMO

••••A•M

ACCLAIM
ANTFARM
BECHARM
DECLAIM
EPHRAIM
EXCLAIM
FANPALM
FANTASM
FATFARM
FIREARM
FOREARM
FURFARM
GETWARM
GOODAIM
GOTWARM
LEFTARM
LIPBALM
LONGARM
MIAHAMM
NONFARM
OILPALM
OVERARM
PREWARM
PROFARM
RECLAIM
SARCASM
SEACALM
SIDEARM
TAKEAIM
TONEARM
TOOKAIM
VARLAAM
YARDARM
YESMAAM

•••••AM

ABRAHAM
AFCTEAM
ALNILAM
AMALGAM
ANAGRAM
ASATEAM
ASTREAM
BAREXAM
BEACHAM
BECKHAM
BEECHAM
BENTHAM
BERTRAM
BINGHAM
BRIGHAM
BUCKRAM
BUTTRAM
CHATHAM
CPAEXAM
CULTJAM
DELIHAM
DIAGRAM
DIGICAM
DINADAM
EASTHAM
EIGHTAM
EPIGRAM
EYEEXAM
FLOTSAM
FORDHAM
GILLIAM
GINGHAM
GRANDAM
GRESHAM
GRISHAM
HEREIAM
IONBEAM
ISOGRAM
ISUREAM
JIMBEAM
KETCHAM
KHAYYAM
LANGHAM
LOWBEAM
MACADAM
MARKHAM
MAUGHAM
MERRIAM
MILLDAM
MINICAM
NAUSEAM
NBATEAM
NEEDHAM
NFCTEAM
NFLTEAM
NHLTEAM
ONECLAM
ONEGRAM
OUTBEAM
OUTSWAM
PANGRAM
PINKHAM
POTSDAM
PROGRAM
PROTEAM
QUONDAM
REDREAM
RITAGAM
SEAFOAM
SEAGRAM
SEVENAM
SUNBEAM
SUREIAM
SURINAM
TAGTEAM
TANGRAM
THREEAM
TIEBEAM
TRANSAM
TRIGRAM
VARLAAM
VIETNAM
WALTHAM
WILLIAM
WOLFRAM
WOOSNAM
WYNDHAM
YAYTEAM
YEATEAM
YESMAAM

AN•••••

ANACINS
ANADEMS
ANAEMIA
ANAEMIC
ANAGRAM
ANAHEIM
ANALOGS
ANALOGY
ANALYSE
ANALYST
ANALYTE
ANALYZE
ANANIAS
ANAPEST
ANARCHS
ANARCHY
ANASAZI
ANATASE
ANATOLE
ANATOLY
ANATOMY
ANBESOL
ANCHORS
ANCHOVY
ANCIENT
ANDAMAN
ANDANTE
ANDEANS
ANDIAMO
ANDIRON
ANDMORE
ANDORRA
ANDOVER
ANDRADE
ANDREAS
ANDRESS
ANDREWS
ANDROID
ANDROUS
ANDSOON
ANDSUCH
ANDTHEN
ANELING
ANEMIAS
ANEMONE
ANEROID
ANGELAS
ANGELES
ANGELIC
ANGELOU
ANGELUS
ANGERED
ANGLAIS
ANGLERS
ANGLING
ANGOLAN
ANGORAS
ANGRIER
ANGRILY
ANGRYAT
ANGUISH
ANGULAR
ANILINE
ANILITY
ANIMACY
ANIMALS
ANIMATE
ANIMATO
ANIMISM
ANIMIST
ANIONIC
ANISEED
ANISTON
ANITRAS
ANKARAN
ANKLERS
ANKLETS
ANNABEL
ANNAKIN
ANNALEE
ANNALES
ANNAMAY
ANNATTO
ANNEALS
ANNELID
ANNETTE
ANNEXED
ANNEXES
ANNOYED
ANNOYER
ANNUALS
ANNUITY
ANNULAR
ANNULET
ANNULUS
ANODISE
ANODIZE
ANODYNE
ANOINTS
ANOMALY
ANOMIES
ANONYMS
ANORAKS
ANOSMIA
ANOSMIC
ANOTHER
ANOUILH
ANSELMO
ANSONIA
ANSPACH
ANSWERS
ANTACID
ANTARES
ANTBEAR
ANTBIRD
ANTCOWS
ANTEDUP
ANTEING
ANTENNA
ANTERUS
ANTESUP
ANTFARM
ANTHEIL
ANTHEMS
ANTHERS
ANTHILL
ANTHONY
ANTHRAX
ANTIART
ANTIBES
ANTIFOG
ANTIGEN
ANTIGUA
ANTIGUN
ANTILOG
ANTIOCH
ANTIQUE
ANTITAX
ANTIWAR
ANTLERS
ANTLIKE
ANTLION
ANTOINE
ANTONIA
ANTONIN
ANTONIO
ANTONYM
ANTSIER
ANTWERP
ANXIETY
ANXIOUS
ANYBODY
ANYHOPE
ANYKIND
ANYLUCK
ANYMORE
ANYNEWS
ANYONES
ANYROAD
ANYTIME
ANYTOWN
ANYWAYS
ANYWISE

A•N••••

ADNOUNS
AGNAILS
AGNATES
AGNATIC
AGNOMEN
AINTHAY
ALNICOS
ALNILAM
ALNITAK
ALNIYAT
AMNERIS
AMNESIA
AMNESIC
AMNESTY
AMNIONS
ANNABEL
ANNAKIN
ANNALEE
ANNALES
ANNAMAY
ANNATTO
ANNEALS
ANNELID
ANNETTE
ANNEXED
ANNEXES
ANNOYED
ANNOYER
ANNUALS
ANNUITY
ANNULAR
ANNULET
ANNULUS
ARNICAS
ARNOLDS
ATNIGHT
AUNTBEE
AUNTIES
AWNINGS
AWNLESS
AYNRAND

A••N•••

ABANDON
ABCNEWS
ABINTRA
ACANTHI
ACINGIT
ACONITE
ADENINE
ADENOID
ADONAIS
AGENCES
AGENDAS
AGENDUM
AGENINE
AGENTED
AGENTRY
AGONIES
AGONISE
AGONISM
AGONIST
AGONIZE
AIRNESS
ALANINE
ALANJAY
ALANNAH
ALENCON
ALINERS
ALINING
ALLNESS
ALLNEWS
ALUNSER
AMANITA
AMANTIS
AMENDED
AMENDER
AMENITY
AMINUTE
AMONGST
ANANIAS
ANONYMS
ANYNEWS
APTNESS
ARANEID
ARANTXA
ARENOSE
ARENSKY
ARONNAX
ARUNDEL
ASANTES
ASININE
ASONANT
ASUNDER
ATANEND
ATINGLE
ATONERS
ATONICS
ATONIES
ATONING
AVANTIS
AVENGED
AVENGER
AVENGES
AVENIDA
AVENUEQ
AVENUES
AVONLEA
AZANIAN
AZINGER

A•••N••

ABOUNDS
ABSENCE
ABSENTS
ABSINTH
ACCENTS
ACCTNOS
ACHENES
ACORNED
ACRONYM
ACTINON
ADDENDA
ADDENDS
ADDONTO
ADJUNCT
ADORNED
ADORNER
ADRENAL
ADVANCE
ADVENTS
AFFINED
AFFINES
AGAINST
AIRINGS
AKRONOH
ALANNAH
ALBANIA
ALBENIZ
ALBINOS
ALBUNDY
ALDENTE
ALFONSE
ALFONSO
ALIENEE
ALIENOR
ALIENTO
ALIGNED
ALIGNER
ALKENES
ALLANTE
ALLENBY
ALLENDE
ALLONGE
ALLONYM
ALMANAC
ALMONDS
ALMONDY
ALMONER
ALMONRY
ALPINER
ALPINES
ALUMNAE
ALUMNAL
ALUMNUS
AMMONIA
AMMONIC

AMOUNTS
ANDANTE
ANIONIC
ANOINTS
ANSONIA
ANTENNA
ANTONIA
ANTONIN
ANTONIO
ANTONYM
ANYONES
APHONIA
APHONIC
APLENTY
APPENDS
APRONED
AQUINAS
ARCANUM
ARCINGS
ARDENCY
ARGANTE
ARGENTI
ARGENTO
ARGENTS
ARGONNE
ARIANES
ARMENIA
ARONNAX
ARRANGE
ARSENAL
ARSENIC
ARSENIO
ASCENDS
ASCENTS
ASHANTI
ASKANCE
ASOFNOW
ASPENCO
ASSANTE
ASSENTS
ASSUNTA
ATEINTO
ATLANTA
ATLUNCH
ATTENDS
ATTUNED
ATTUNES
AUGENDS
AUTONYM
AVERNAL
AVERNUS
AVIANCA
AVIGNON
AVIONIC
AWNINGS
AWOONOR

A••••N•

AAMILNE
ABALONE
ABASING
ABATING
ABEYANT
ABIDING
ABILENE
ABSCOND
ABUSING
ACCOUNT
ACETONE
ACHTUNG
ACTIONS
ACUMENS
ADAMANT
ADDLING
ADELINA
ADELINE
ADENINE
ADJOINS
ADNOUNS
ADORING
ADRIANA
AFFIANT
AFFRONT
AFGHANI
AFGHANS
AGATINE
AGELONG
AGENINE
AGROUND
AILMENT
AIRFONE
AIRGUNS
AIRLANE
AIRLINE
AIRTANK
AIRVENT
AJOWANS
AKEBONO
ALADINE
ALAKING
ALANINE
ALAYING
ALCYONE
ALIMENT
ALIMONY
ALINING
ALLDONE
ALLGONE
ALLMINE
ALLYING
ALTHING
ALTOONA
ALUMINA
AMARONE
AMAZING
AMAZONS
AMBIENS
AMBIENT
AMBLING
AMERIND
AMNIONS
AMUSING
ANACINS
ANCIENT
ANDEANS
ANELING
ANEMONE
ANGLING
ANILINE
ANODYNE
ANTEING
ANTENNA
ANTHONY
ANTOINE
ANYKIND
APPLING
APPOINT
ARACHNE
ARACHNO
ARCHING
ARCHONS
ARCSINE
ARETINO
ARGONNE
ARGUING
ARIADNE
ARISING
ARIZONA
ARMBAND
ARMBONE
ARMYANT
ARTSONG
ARUBANS
ASHBINS
ASHCANS
ASHLAND
ASHPANS
ASININE
ASONANT
ASQUINT
ASSIGNS
ASTOUND
ATAMANS
ATANEND
ATONING
ATSIGNS
ATTAINS
ATTAINT
AUBURNS
AUBURNU
AUGMENT
AUSTINS
AUTOING
AUTOMNE
AUTUMNS
AVALONS
AVOWING
AWAKENS
AWAKING
AYNRAND

A•••••N

ABANDON
ABDOMEN
ABIDJAN
ABSTAIN
ABUTSON
ACADIAN
ACHERON
ACHESON
ACTAEON
ACTEDIN
ACTEDON
ACTINON
ACTUPON
ADAMSON
ADDEDIN
ADDEDON
ADDISON
ADJOURN
ADWOMAN
ADWOMEN
AEOLIAN
AFRICAN
AGAKHAN
AGNOMEN
AGREEON
AILERON
AIRHORN
AIRSIGN
AJSIMON
ALADDIN
ALAMEIN
ALARCON
ALASKAN
ALATEEN
ALBUMEN
ALBUMIN
ALDUBIN
ALENCON
ALGREEN
ALLBRAN
ALLISON
ALLOWIN
ALLSTON
ALLYSON
ALMADEN
ALMSMAN
ALMSMEN
ALROSEN
ALSHAIN
ALSORAN
ALTHORN
ALYKHAN
AMESLAN
AMPHION
ANDAMAN
ANDIRON
ANDSOON
ANDTHEN
ANGOLAN
ANISTON
ANKARAN
ANNAKIN
ANTIGEN
ANTIGUN
ANTLION
ANTONIN
ANYTOWN
APERSON
APOGEAN
APULIAN
AQUAMAN
ARABIAN
ARAGORN
ARAMEAN
ARRAIGN
ARTFERN
ARTISAN
ASHBURN
ASKEDIN
ASMARAN
ASPIRIN
ATSEVEN
ATTYGEN
AUCTION
AUDUBON
AUTOPEN
AVESTAN
AVEYRON
AVIDFAN
AVIGNON
AVIVIAN
AWASHIN
AZANIAN
AZKABAN
AZOREAN
AZORIAN
AZTECAN

•AN••••

BANACEK
BANALER
BANALLY
BANANAS
BANANES
BANBURY
BANDAGE
BANDAID
BANDANA
BANDBOX
BANDEAU
BANDERA
BANDERS
BANDIDO
BANDIED
BANDIER
BANDIES
BANDING
BANDITO
BANDITS
BANDLET
BANDSAW
BANEFUL
BANGERS
BANGING
BANGKOK
BANGLED
BANGLES
BANGOUT
BANGSON
BANGSUP
BANJOES
BANKERS
BANKFEE
BANKING
BANKITS
BANKJOB
BANKONE
BANKSON
BANKSUP
BANNERS
BANNING
BANQUES
BANQUET
BANSHEE
BANTAMS
BANTERS
BANTING
BANYANS
BANZAIS
CANALED
CANAPES
CANARDS
CANASTA
CANCANS
CANCELS
CANCERS
CANCHAS
CANDACE
CANDELA
CANDENT
CANDICE
CANDIDA
CANDIDE
CANDIDS
CANDIED
CANDIES
CANDLED
CANDLER
CANDLES
CANDOUR
CANETTI
CANFULS
CANIDAE
CANIEST
CANINES
CANINGS
CANITBE
CANKERS
CANNELL
CANNELS
CANNERS
CANNERY
CANNIER
CANNILY
CANNING
CANNOCK
CANNOLI
CANNONS
CANNULA
CANOERS
CANOLAS
CANONIC
CANONRY
CANOPUS
CANSECO
CANTABS
CANTALS
CANTATA
CANTEEN
CANTERS
CANTILY
CANTINA
CANTING
CANTINO
CANTLES
CANTONS
CANTORS
CANTRIP
CANTSAY
CANUCKS
CANULAE
CANULAS
CANVASS
CANYONS
CANZONA
CANZONE
CANZONI
DANANAS
DANBURY
DANCERS
DANCING
DANDERS
DANDIER
DANDIES
DANDIFY
DANDILY
DANDLED
DANDLER
DANDLES
DANELAW
DANEYKO
DANGELO
DANGERS
DANGLED
DANGLER
DANGLES
DANIELA
DANIELJ
DANIELS
DANIKEN
DANITES
DANKEST
DANNING
DANSEUR
DANTEAN
DANTEII
DANVERS
EANMUND
FANATIC
FANBASE
FANBELT
FANCIED
FANCIER
FANCIES
FANCIFY
FANCILY
FANCLUB
FANCYUP
FANDOMS
FANEUIL
FANFARE
FANFEST
FANFICS
FANFOLD
FANGING
FANIONS
FANJETS
FANLIKE
FANMAIL
FANNERS
FANNING
FANOUTS
FANPALM
FANSLER
FANSOUT
FANTAIL
FANTANS
FANTASM
FANTAST
FANTASY
FANTINE
FANTODS
FANWISE
FANZINE
GANDALF
GANDERS
GANGERS
GANGING
GANGLIA
GANGSAW
GANGSTA
GANGSUP
GANGTOK
GANGWAY
GANNETS
GANNETT
GANTLET
HANAPER
HANCOCK
HANDAXE
HANDBAG
HANDCAR
HANDERS
HANDEYE
HANDFED
HANDFUL
HANDGUN
HANDIER
HANDILY
HANDING
HANDLED
HANDLER
HANDLES
HANDLIN
HANDOFF
HANDOUT
HANDSAW
HANDSEL
HANDSET
HANDSIN
HANDSON
HANDSUP
HANDYTO
HANGARS
HANGBYS
HANGDOG
HANGERS
HANGING
HANGMAN
HANGMEN
HANGOFF
HANGOUT
HANGSBY
HANGSIN
HANGSON
HANGSUP
HANGTEN
HANGUPS
HANKERS
HANKIBA
HANKIES
HANOVER
HANSARP
HANSOLO
HANSOMS
HANUKAH
IANHOLM
JANACEK
JANEANE
JANEDOE
JANEIRO
JANEWAY
JANGLED
JANGLER
JANGLES
JANITOR
JANKLOW
JANSSEN
JANSSON
JANUARY
JANVIER
KANAKAS
KANEOHE
KANSANS
KANTIAN
LANCERS
LANCETS
LANCIAS
LANCING
LANCOME
LANDAUS
LANDERS
LANDING
LANDINI
LANDLER
LANDMAN
LANDMEN
LANDSAT
LANDSUP
LANDTAG
LANDTAX
LANEONE
LANETWO
LANFORD
LANGDON
LANGHAM
LANGLEY
LANGTON
LANGTRY
LANGUID
LANGUOR
LANGWAY
LANKEST
LANKIER
LANKILY
LANOLIN
LANOTTE
LANSING
LANTANA
LANTERN
LANVINS
LANYARD
MANACLE
MANAGED
MANAGER
MANAGES
MANAGUA
MANANAS
MANATEE
MANCINI
MANCUSO
MANDALA
MANDANS
MANDATE
MANDAYS
MANDELA
MANDOKI
MANDREL
MANEGES
MANETTE
MANFRED
MANGANO
MANGERS
MANGIER
MANGLED
MANGLER
MANGLES
MANGOES
MANHEIM
MANHOLE
MANHOOD
MANHOUR
MANHUNT
MANIACS
MANIKIN
MANILAS
MANILOW
MANIPLE
MANIPUR
MANKATO
MANKIND
MANLESS
MANLIER
MANLIKE
MANMADE
MANNERS
MANNIES
MANNING
MANNISH
MANOLIN
MANOWAR
MANRICO
MANROPE
MANSARD
MANSION
MANSIZE
MANSMAN
MANTECA
MANTELS
MANTLED
MANTLES
MANTLET
MANTRAP
MANTRAS
MANTRIC
MANTUAN
MANUALS
MANUMIT
MANURED
MANURES
MANXCAT
MANXMAN
MANXMEN
MANYEAR
NANAIMO
NANETTE
NANJING
NANKING
NANNIED
NANNIES
PANACEA
PANACHE
PANADAS
PANAMAS
PANARAB
PANCAKE
PANCHAX
PANDERS
PANDITS
PANDORA
PANELED
PANETTA
PANFISH
PANFULS
PANGAEA
PANGRAM
PANICKY
PANICLE
PANIERS
PANINIS
PANNERS
PANNIER
PANNING
PANOPLY
PANPIPE
PANSIES
PANSOUT
PANTENE
PANTERA
PANTERS
PANTHER
PANTIES
PANTILE
PANTING
PANTLEG
PANTONE
PANURGE
PANZERS
RANAMOK
RANATAB
RANAWAY
RANBACK
RANCHED
RANCHER
RANCHES
RANCHOS
RANCORS
RANCOUR
RANDALL
RANDEEP
RANDIER
RANDOWN
RANFREE
RANGERS
RANGFOR
RANGIER
RANGING
RANGOFF
RANGOON
RANGOUT
RANHOME
RANINTO
RANITUP
RANKERS
RANKEST
RANKINE
RANKING
RANKISH
RANKLED
RANKLES
RANKOUT
RANLAPS
RANLATE
RANONIN
RANOVER
RANPAST
RANRIOT
RANSACK
RANSOMS
RANTERS
RANTING
RANTSAT
RANUPTO
RANWILD
RANWITH
SANBLAS
SANBORN
SANCTUM
SANCTUS
SANDALS
SANDBAG
SANDBAR
SANDBOX
SANDBUR
SANDDAB
SANDERS
SANDFLY
SANDHOG
SANDIER
SANDING
SANDLER
SANDLOT
SANDMAN
SANDMEN
SANDPIT
SANFORD
SANGOUT
SANGRIA
SANIBEL
SANJOSE
SANJUAN
SANREMO
SANSEIS
SANTAFE
SANTANA
SANTINI
TANAGER
TANBARK
TANDEMS
TANDOOR
TANGELO
TANGENT
TANGIER
TANGING
TANGLED
TANGLER
TANGLES
TANGOED
TANGOER
TANGRAM
TANKAGE
TANKARD
TANKCAR
TANKERS
TANKFUL
TANKING
TANKINI
TANKSUP
TANKTOP
TANLINE
TANNERS
TANNERY
TANNEST
TANNING
TANNINS
TANNISH
TANOAKS
TANSIES
TANTARA
TANTIVY
TANTRUM
VANADIC
VANCAMP
VANDALS
VANDIEN
VANDINE
VANDURA
VANDUYN
VANDYCK
VANDYKE
VANESSA
VANEXEL
VANEYCK
VANGOGH
VANILLA
VANILLI
VANLINE
VANLOAD
VANNING
VANOCUR
VANOWEN
VANPELT
VANPOOL
VANRIJN
VANSANT
VANTAGE
VANUATU
VANVOGT
VANWARD
VANWYCK
VANZANT
WANDERS
WANGLED
WANGLER
WANGLES
WANIEST
WANKELS
WANNABE
WANNESS
WANNEST
WANNING
WANNISH
WANTADS
WANTAGH
WANTERS
WANTING
WANTONS
WANTOUT
WANTSIN
WANTSTO
XANADUS
XANTHAN
XANTHIC
YANGTZE
YANKEES
YANKERS
YANKING
YANKOFF
YANKOUT
YANKSAT
YANKSON
YANKTON
YANNICK
YANQUIS
ZANETTO
ZANIEST
ZANYISH
ZANYISM

•A•N•••

BADNAME
BADNESS

BADNEWS
BAGNIOS
BAGNOLD
BAINTER
BANNERS
BANNING
BARNABY
BARNARD
BARNEYS
BARNING
BARNONE
BARNOWL
BARNRED
BARNUMS
BATNEXT
CANNELL
CANNELS
CANNERS
CANNERY
CANNIER
CANNILY
CANNING
CANNOCK
CANNOLI
CANNONS
CANNULA
CAPNUTS
CARNABY
CARNAGE
CARNERA
CARNETS
CARNIES
CATNAPS
CATNIPS
DAMNERS
DAMNING
DANNING
DARNELL
DARNERS
DARNING
DAUNTED
DAUNTER
DAWNING
DAWNSON
EARNERS
EARNEST
EARNING
EARNSIT
FAINEST
FAINTED
FAINTER
FAINTLY
FANNERS
FANNING
FARNESS
FATNESS
FAWNERS
FAWNING
FAWNSON
GAINERS
GAINFUL
GAINING
GAINSAY
GAINSON
GANNETS
GANNETT
GARNEAU
GARNERS
GARNETS
GARNETT
GARNISH
GAUNTER
GAUNTLY
GAYNESS
HAFNIUM
HAHNIUM
HARNESS
HARNICK
HAUNTED
HAUNTER
JAINISM
JAINIST
JAUNTED
LAENNEC
LAUNDER
LAUNDRY
LAXNESS
MAANDPA
MACNEIL
MADNESS
MAENADS
MAGNANI
MAGNATE
MAGNETO
MAGNETS
MAGNIFY
MAGNUMS
MAINERS
MAINMAN
MAINMEN
MAINTOP
MANNERS
MANNIES
MANNING
MANNISH
MARNIER
MAUNDER
MAYNARD
NANNIED
NANNIES
PAANGAS
PAINFUL
PAINING
PAINTED
PAINTER
PANNERS
PANNIER
PANNING
PATNESS
PAUNCHY
PAWNEES
PAWNERS
PAWNING
PAWNOFF
RAINBOW
RAINGOD
RAINHAT
RAINIER
RAINILY
RAINING
RAINMAN
RAINOUT
RAINSIN
RAINSON
RAUNCHY
RAWNESS
RAYNELL
SADNESS
SAINTED
SAINTES
SAINTLO
SAINTLY
SAMNUNN
SARNOFF
SAUNAED
SAUNTER
SAWNOFF
SAYNOTO
TAINTED
TANNERS
TANNERY
TANNEST
TANNING
TANNINS
TANNISH
TARNISH
TAUNTED
TAUNTER
TAUNTON
TAWNIER
TAWNILY
VAINEST
VANNING
VARNISH
VAUNTED
VAUNTER
WALNUTS
WANNABE
WANNESS
WANNEST
WANNING
WANNISH
WARNING
WARNOFF
WARNSOF
YANNICK
YARNELL
YARNING
YAWNERS
YAWNFUL
YAWNIER
YAWNING
ZAGNUTS

•A••N••

BABENCO
BADENDS
BADENOV
BALANCE
BALONEY
BANANAS
BANANES
BARANOF
BARENTS
BARONET
BASENJI
BASINAL
BAYONET
BAYONNE
CABANAS
CABINET
CACONYM
CADENCE
CADENCY
CADENZA
CAIRNED
CALANDO
CALENDS
CALLNOW
CAMINOS
CANINES
CANINGS
CANONIC
CANONRY
CARINAE
CARINAS
CASINGS
CASINOS
CATANIA
CATENAE
CATENAS
CAYENNE
DANANAS
DAPHNES
DAPHNIA
DAPHNIS
DARENOT
DATINGS
DAVINCI
EATENAT
EATENUP
EATINTO
FACINGS
FACONNE
FAGENDS
FAIENCE
FAMINES
FARINAS
FASTNET
FATONES
GALANOS
GALANTS
GALENAS
GALENTO
GAMINES
GARDNER
GARONNE
GATINGS
HACKNEY
HADANIP
HAIRNET
HAPENNY
HASANIP
HAVANAN
HAVANAS
HAVENER
HAVENOT
HAYINGS
HAZANIM
HAZINGS
JACINTH
JACINTO
JACONET
KAHUNAS
KALININ
LACINGS
LACONIA
LACONIC
LACUNAE
LACUNAL
LACUNAR
LACUNAS
LADINGS
LADINOS
LADYNAS
LAENNEC
LAGUNAS
LALANNE
LAMENTS
LAMINAE
LAMINAL
LAMINAR
LAMINAS
LAMINTO
LARDNER
LATENCY
LATENED
LATENTS
LATINAS
LATINII
LATINOS
LATINUS
LAVINIA
LAWANDA
LAYINTO
LAZENBY
LAZONGA
MACONGA
MADONNA
MAGENTA
MAGINOT
MAHONEY
MAKINGS
MANANAS
MARANTZ
MARENGO
MARINAS
MARINER
MARINES
MASONED
MASONIC
MASONRY
MATINAL
MATINEE
MAYINGS
PAGINGS
PALANCE
PALINGS
PANINIS
PARDNER
PARENTS
PARINGS
PARONYM
PARSNIP
PARTNER
PATENCY
PATENTS
PATINAS
PAVANES
PAVINGS
PAXINOU
PAYINTO
PAYSNOW
RACINOS
RAGINGS
RAMINTO
RAMONES
RANINTO
RANONIN
RAPANUI
RAPINES
RAPINIS
RATINES
RATINGS
RAVENAL
RAVENED
RAVENNA
RAVINED
RAVINES
RAVINGS
SABINES
SAGINAW
SAIDNAY
SALINAS
SALINES
SALONGA
SARANAC
SARONGS
SATANIC
SATINET
SATINON
SAVANAS
SAVANNA
SAVANTS
SAVINGS
SAWINTO
SAYINGS
SAYSNAY
TACONIC
TAGENDS
TAHINIS
TAKENBY
TAKENIN
TAKENON
TAKENTO
TAKENUP
TAKINGS
TALENTS
TALONED
TAPINGS
TAPINTO
TARANTO
VACANCY
VALANCE
VALENCE
VALENTE
VALENTI
VALINES
WAGONED
WAGONER
WAHINES
WAKENED
WAKENER
WAKINGS
WASONTO
WAXINGS
YAOUNDE

•A•••N•

AAMILNE
BABOONS
BABYING
BACHING
BACKEND
BACKING
BADHAND
BADLAND
BAFFING
BAGGING
BAGGINS
BAHIANS
BAILING
BAITING
BALCONY
BALDING
BALEENS
BALKANS
BALKING
BALLONE
BAMBINA
BAMBINI
BAMBINO
BAMMING
BANDANA
BANDING
BANGING
BANKING
BANKONE
BANNING
BANTING
BANYANS
BARBING
BARGING
BARKING
BARNING
BARNONE
BARRENS
BARRING
BARRONS
BARTEND
BARYONS
BASHING
BASKING
BASSANI
BASSANO
BASTING
BATHING
BATTENS
BATTING
BATWING
BAWLING
BAYLYNX
BAYONNE
CABBING
CABLING
CABRINI
CACHING
CADGING
CAFTANS
CAIMANS
CAIRENE
CALKING
CALKINS
CALLING
CALLINS
CALMING
CALUMNY
CALVING
CALVINO
CALZONE
CAMIONS
CAMPING
CANCANS
CANDENT
CANNING
CANNONS
CANTINA
CANTING
CANTINO
CANTONS
CANYONS
CANZONA
CANZONE
CANZONI
CAPEANN
CAPGUNS
CAPPING
CAPRINE
CAPUANA
CARBINE
CARBONS
CARDING
CAREENS
CARKING
CARLENE
CARLING
CARMINA
CARMINE
CARPING
CARTING
CARTONS
CARVING
CASEINS
CASERNE
CASERNS
CASHING
CASHINS
CASKING
CASSINI
CASSINO
CASTING
CATIONS
CATKINS
CATMINT
CAUSING
CAVEINS
CAVERNS
CAYENNE
CAYMANS
DABBING
DABHAND
DACRONS
DADOING
DAEMONS
DALTONS
DAMMING
DAMNING
DAMPENS
DAMPING
DAMSONS
DANCING
DANNING
DAPPING
DARKENS
DARLENE
DARLING
DARNING
DARTING
DASHING
DATSUNS
DAUBING
DAWKINS
DAWNING
DAYLONG
DAYSEND
DAYSINN
DAYTONA
EAGLING
EANMUND
EARBONE
EARNING
EARRING
EASTEND
EASTING
EASYONE
FABLING
FACONNE
FADEINS
FAILING
FAIRING
FALCONS
FALLING
FANGING
FANIONS
FANNING
FANTANS
FANTINE
FANZINE
FARCING
FARGOND
FARGONE
FARMING
FASTENS
FASTING
FASTONE
FATLING
FATTENS
FATTING
FAWNING
GABBANA
GABBING
GADDING
GAETANO
GAFFING
GAGGING
GAGLINE
GAINING
GAITING
GALLANT
GALLING
GALLONS
GALVANI
GALVANO
GAMMING
GAMMONS
GANGING
GAOLING
GAPPING
GARBING
GARCONS
GARDENA
GARDENS
GARLAND
GARMENT
GARONNE
GASCANS
GASCONS
GASCONY
GASHING
GASLINE
GASPING
GASSING
GASTANK
GASTONE
GATLING
GATLINS
GAUDENS
GAUGING
GAWKING
GAWPING
HACKING
HADDONE
HADRONS
HAFTING
HAILING
HALDANE
HALOING
HALTING
HALVING
HAMBONE
HAMLINE
HAMMING
HAMMOND
HANDING
HANGING
HAPENNY
HAPPENS
HARDENS
HARDING
HARKENS
HARKING
HARLAND
HARLINE
HARMING
HARMONY
HARPING
HASDONE
HASHING
HASPING
HASTENS
HASTING
HATBAND
HATPINS
HATTING
HAULING
HAVEONE
HAWKING
HAWKINS
JABBING
JACKING
JAGGING
JAILING
JAMBAND
JAMMING
JANEANE
JARDINE
JARDINS
JARGONS
JARGONY
JARRING
JASMINE
JAWBONE
JAWLINE
JAYLENO
JAZZING
KACHINA
KACHING
KAMFONG
KANSANS
KATRINA
KATRINE
KAYLENZ
KAYOING
LACKING
LADLING
LADRONE
LAGGING
LAGOONS
LAHAINA
LAIRING
LALANNE
LALLING
LAMBENT
LAMBING
LAMMING
LANCING
LANDING
LANDINI
LANEONE
LANSING
LANTANA
LANVINS
LAPLAND
LAPPING
LAPSANG
LAPSING
LAPWING
LARAINE
LARCENY
LARDING
LARDONS
LARGENT
LARKING
LARKINS
LASAGNA
LASAGNE
LASHING
LASTING
LASTONE
LATEENS
LATHING
LATRINE
LAUDING
LAURENT
LAVAINE
LAVERNE
MACHINA
MACHINE
MACHONE
MACOUNS
MACRONS
MADDENS
MADDING
MADEONE
MADONNA
MAGNANI
MAIDENS
MAILING
MAILINS
MAIMING
MAISONS
MAJGENS
MAKEONE
MALEANT
MALIANS
MALIGNS
MALTING
MALVINA
MANCINI
MANDANS
MANGANO
MANHUNT
MANKIND
MANNING
MAPPING
MARCONI
MARGINS
MARIANA
MARIANO
MARKING
MARLENE
MARLINS
MAROONS
MARRING
MARRONS
MARTENS
MARTINA
MARTINI
MARTINO
MARTINS
MARTINU
MARTINV
MARYANN
MASHING
MASKING
MASSINE
MASSING
MASTING
MATRONS
MATTING
MAULING
MAYWINE
MAZZINI
NABBING
NAGGING
NAILING
NAMEONE
NANJING
NANKING
NAPKINS
NAPPING
NASCENT
NATHANS
NATIONS
OAHUANS
OAKLAND
PACKING
PADDING
PADRONE
PADUANS
PAGEANT
PAGEONE
PAINING
PAIRING
PAISANO
PAISANS
PALLING
PALMING
PANNING
PANTENE
PANTING
PANTONE
PAPUANS
PARDONS
PARGING
PARKING
PARKINS
PARRING
PARSING
PARSONS
PARTING
PARTONE
PARVENU
PASSANT
PASSING
PASTINA
PASTING
PATERNO
PATHAND
PATHANS
PATIENT
PATRONS
PATTING
PAULINA
PAULINE
PAULING
PAUSING
PAWNING
PAYMENT
RACKING
RADIANS
RADIANT
RAFTING
RAGGING
RAGLANS
RAGMANS
RAIDING
RAILING
RAIMENT
RAINING
RAISING
RAISINS
RAISINY
RAISONS
RAMFANS
RAMMING
RAMPANT
RAMPING
RAMSONS
RANGING
RANKINE
RANKING
RANTING
RAPPING
RAPSONG
RAPTUNE
RASPING
RATFINK
RATIONS
RATLINE
RATLINS
RATTANS
RATTING
RAVENNA
RAWLINS
RAYBANS
RAYGUNS
RAYMOND
RAZZING
SABRINA
SACKING
SADDENS
SADSONG
SAGGING

SAILING
SAISONS
SALERNO
SALIENT
SALMONP
SALMONS
SALOONS
SALTANT
SALTINE
SALTING
SALVING
SAMNUNN
SAMOANS
SAMPANS
SAMSONS
SAMSUNG
SANDING
SANTANA
SANTINI
SAPIENS
SAPIENT
SAPLING
SAPPING
SARDINE
SARGENT
SASHING
SASSING
SATEENS
SATURNS
SAUCING
SAUCONY
SAVANNA
TABBING
TABLING
TABUING
TACKING
TAGGANT
TAGGING
TAGLINE
TAILEND
TAILING
TAKEINS
TAKEONE
TALKING
TALLINN
TALLONE
TAMMANY
TAMPING
TANGENT
TANGING
TANKING
TANKINI
TANLINE
TANNING
TANNINS
TAPPANS
TAPPING
TARPONS
TARRING
TARTANS
TARTING
TARZANA
TARZANS
TASKING
TASTING
TATIANA
TATTING
TAURINE
TAUTENS
TAVERNA
TAVERNS
TAXIING
VACCINE
VAGRANT
VALIANT
VALLONE
VALUING
VAMPING
VANDINE
VANLINE
VANNING
VANSANT
VANZANT
VARIANT
VARMINT
VARYING
VATTING
WADDING
WADKINS
WAFTING
WAGGING
WAILING
WAITING
WAIVING
WALKING
WALKINS
WALKONS
WALLING
WALTONS
WANNING
WANTING
WANTONS
WARBOND
WARDENS
WARDING
WARMING
WARNING
WARPING
WARRANT
WARRENG
WARRENS
WARRING
WARZONE
WASHING
WASTING
WATKINS
WAXWING
WAYLAND
XAMOUNT
YAKKING
YANKING
YAOMING
YAPPING
YARDING
YARNING
YASMINE
YAWNING
YAWPING
ZADKINE
ZAGGING
ZAMBONI
ZAPPING

•A••••N

BABYLON
BACHMAN
BACKSIN
BADOMEN
BADSIGN
BAHAMEN
BAHRAIN
BAHREIN
BAILSON
BAKEPAN
BALABAN
BALATON
BALDWIN
BALLOON
BALMAIN
BANGSON
BANKSON
BARDEEN
BARGAIN
BARGEIN
BASEDON
BASEMAN
BASEMEN
BASETEN
BASRHIN
BASSOON
BASTION
BATEMAN
BATSMAN
BATSMEN
CAGEDIN
CAISSON
CAKEPAN
CAKETIN
CALDRON
CALHOUN
CALIBAN
CALLSIN
CALLSON
CAMERON
CAMPION
CANTEEN
CAPEANN
CAPITAN
CAPSTAN
CAPTAIN
CAPTION
CARAVAN
CARBARN
CARHORN
CARLOAN
CARLSON
CARLTON
CAROLYN
CAROTIN
CARRYIN
CARRYON
CARTOON
CARTSIN
CASPIAN
CASTSON
CATALAN
CATCHON
CATSCAN
CAUTHEN
CAUTION
CAVEDIN
CAVEMAN
CAVEMEN
CAVESIN
DAKOTAN
DANIKEN
DANTEAN
DARKMAN
DARKTAN
DARLEEN
DARTGUN
DAUPHIN
DAVISON
DAWNSON
DAYSINN
EARLYON
EARTHEN
EASEDIN
EASEDON
EASESIN
EASESON
EASTERN
EASTMAN
FACEDON
FACESON
FACTION
FADEDIN
FADESIN
FADIMAN
FALLSIN
FALLSON
FASHION
FAWNSON
GADSDEN
GAGARIN
GAHAGAN
GAINSON
GALLEON
GAMBIAN
GAMELAN
GASMAIN
GASOVEN
GASSMAN
GATEMAN
GATEMEN
GAUGUIN
GAVILAN
GAZEDON
GAZESON
HACKMAN
HADBEEN
HADRIAN
HAIRPIN
HAITIAN
HALCYON
HALFWON
HALOGEN
HALSTON
HAMELIN
HAMPTON
HANDGUN
HANDLIN
HANDSIN
HANDSON
HANGMAN
HANGMEN
HANGSIN
HANGSON
HANGTEN
HARDPAN
HARDTEN
HARDWON
HARPOON
HARPSON
HARSHEN
HARTMAN
HASBEEN
HAULSIN
HAVANAN
HAVEFUN
HAWKMAN
JACKSON
JACOBIN
JAMESON
JAMISON
JANSSEN
JANSSON
JAVAMAN
JAVELIN
JAZZMAN
JAZZMEN
KALININ
KANTIAN
KARAJAN
KARLSON
KATHRYN
KAUFMAN
LACESON
LADYKIN
LAMBKIN
LAMPOON
LANDMAN
LANDMEN
LANGDON
LANGTON
LANOLIN
LANTERN
LAOCOON
LAOTIAN
LAPUTAN
LARCHEN
LASTDON
LATCHON
LATERAN
LATERON
LATVIAN
LAUGHIN
LAVERAN
LAYDOWN
LAYITON
LAYOPEN
LAYUPON
MAARTEN
MACEDON
MACHAON
MACLEAN
MADALYN
MADCHEN
MADEFUN
MADELON
MADERUN
MADIGAN
MADISON
MAILBIN
MAILMAN
MAILMEN
MAILSIN
MAINMAN
MAINMEN
MAJORIN
MAKEFUN
MAKERUN
MALAGAN
MALAYAN
MANIKIN
MANOLIN
MANSION
MANSMAN
MANTUAN
MANXMAN
MANXMEN
MARCHON
MARDIAN
MARILYN
MARMION
MARRYIN
MARSDEN
MARSTON
MARTIAN
MARXIAN
MARYANN
MATALIN
MATEWAN
MAUDLIN
MAULDIN
MAUREEN
MAXBORN
MAYALIN
MAZARIN
NAILGUN
NAILSIN
NARAYAN
NAVYMAN
NAVYMEN
OAKFERN
OAKLAWN
OARSMAN
OARSMEN
OATBRAN
OAXACAN
PACKSIN
PACKSON
PACQUIN
PALADIN
PALEMON
PARAGON
PARKMAN
PARTYON
PASSION
PASTEIN
PASTERN
PATCHEN
PATDOWN
PATROON
PATTERN
PAULSEN
RACCOON
RACEDIN
RADIOIN
RAEBURN
RAEDAWN
RAILMAN
RAILMEN
RAILSON
RAINMAN
RAINSIN
RAINSON
RAKEDIN
RAKESIN
RALSTON
RAMADAN
RAMBLIN
RAMDOWN
RAMEKIN
RAMSFAN
RANDOWN
RANGOON
RANONIN
RAPIDAN
RARITAN
RAYBURN
SAFFRON
SAGEHEN
SAHARAN
SAILSON
SALADIN
SALOMON
SAMISEN
SAMNUNN
SAMPSON
SANBORN
SANDMAN
SANDMEN
SANJUAN
SARACEN
SARAZEN
SAROYAN
SARUMAN
SASSOON
SATDOWN
SATINON
SATUPON
SAURIAN
SAVARIN
SAVEDON
SAVESON
SAXHORN
SAYAMEN
SAYWHEN
TACHYON
TACKSON
TAILFIN
TAILPIN
TAKENIN
TAKENON
TAKESIN
TAKESON
TAKETEN
TALIBAN
TALKSON
TALLINN
TAMBLYN
TAMGLEN
TAPEDON
TAPEMAN
TAPEMEN
TAPESON
TASHLIN
TAUNTON
TAUREAN
TAXIMAN
TAXIMEN
VALADON
VALJEAN
VANDIEN
VANDUYN
VANOWEN
VANRIJN
VATICAN
VAUGHAN
WADEDIN
WADESIN
WAITRON
WAITSON
WAKSMAN
WALKMAN
WALKSON
WALLOON
WALLSIN
WALSTON
WANTSIN
WARTORN
WARWORN
WAVEDIN
WAVESIN
WAXBEAN
WAYWORN
XANTHAN
YALEMAN
YALEMEN
YANKSON
YANKTON
YARDMAN
YARDMEN
ZABUTON
ZAIRIAN
ZAMBIAN

••AN•••

ABANDON
ACANTHI
ALANINE
ALANJAY
ALANNAH
AMANITA
AMANTIS
ANANIAS
ARANEID
ARANTXA
ASANTES
ATANEND
AVANTIS
AZANIAN
BEANBAG
BEANDIP
BEANERY
BEANIES
BEANING
BEANOIL
BIANCHI
BLANCHE
BLANDER
BLANDLY
BLANKED
BLANKER
BLANKET
BLANKLY
BLANTON
BRANAGH
BRANCHY
BRANDED
BRANDER
BRANDON
BRANIFF
BRANSON
BYANDBY
BYANECK
BYANOSE
CHANCED
CHANCEL
CHANCER
CHANCES
CHANELS
CHANGED
CHANGER
CHANGES
CHANNEL
CHANOYU
CHANSON
CHANTED
CHANTER
CHANTEY
CHANTRY
CLANGED
CLANGER
CLANGOR
CLANKED
CLANTON
CRANIAL
CRANING
CRANIUM
CRANKED
CRANKUP
CRANMER
CYANIDE
CYANIDS
DEANERY
DRANKIN
DRANKTO
DRANKUP
EBANKED
ELANCES
ELANETS
ELANTRA
EMANANT
EMANATE
EMANUEL
EVANDER
EVANGEL
EVANISH
EXANIMO
FIANCEE
FIANCES
FLANEUR
FLANGES
FLANKED
FLANKEN
FLANKER
FLANNEL
FRANCES
FRANCHI
FRANCIS
FRANKED
FRANKEN
FRANKER
FRANKIE
FRANKLY
FRANKOZ
FRANTIC
GHANIAN
GLANCED
GLANCES
GRANADA
GRANARY
GRANDAM
GRANDEE
GRANDER
GRANDLY
GRANDMA
GRANDPA
GRANGER
GRANGES
GRANITA
GRANITE
GRANNIE
GRANOLA
GRANPAS
GRANTED
GRANTEE
GRANTER
GRANTOR
GRANULE
GUANACO
GUANINE
HUANGHE
HUANGTI
HYANNIS
ICANNOT
INANELY
INANEST
INANITY
IPANEMA
IRANIAN
IVANHOE
IVANIII
IVANOVO
IWANTIT
IWANTTO
JEANARP
JEANLUC
JEANNIE
JEANNOT
KHANATE
KWANZAA
KWANZAS
LEANCUT
LEANDER
LEANERS
LEANEST
LEANING
LEANSIN
LEANSON
LEANSTO
LEANTOS
LLANERO
LOANERS
LOANING
LOANOUT
MAANDPA
MEANAGE
MEANDER
MEANEST
MEANIES
MEANING
MEANJOE
MEANSIT
MEANSTO
MEANTIT
MEANTTO
MOANERS
MOANFUL
MOANING
MYANMAR
NIANTIC
NOANGEL
NUANCED
NUANCES
OCANADA
OFANAGE
OHANLON
ONANDON
ORANGES
ORANGEY
ORANTES
PAANGAS
PBANDJS
PEANUTS
PHANTOM
PIANISM
PIANIST
PIANOLA
PLANATE
PLANERS
PLANETS
PLANFOR
PLANING
PLANISH
PLANKED
PLANNED
PLANNER
PLANOUT
PLANSON
PLANSTO
PLANTAR
PLANTED
PLANTER
PRANCED
PRANCER
PRANCES
PSANDQS
QUANTUM
REANNEX
RIANTLY
ROANOKE
RUANDAS
RWANDAN
SCANDAL
SCANNED
SCANNER
SCANTED
SCANTER
SCANTLY
SEANCES
SHANANA
SHANGRI
SHANKAR
SHANKED
SHANNEN
SHANNON
SHANTER
SLANDER
SLANTED
SLANTLY
SLANTUP
SOANDSO
SPANAIR
SPANDEX
SPANGLE
SPANGLY
SPANIEL
SPANISH
SPANKED
SPANKER
SPANNED
SPANNER
STANCES
STANDBY
STANDEE
STANDER
STANDIN
STANDON
STANDTO
STANDUP
STANINE
STANKUP
STANLEE
STANLEY
STANNIC
STANNUM
STANTON
STANZAS
SWANKED
SWANKER
SWANKUP
SWANSEA
SWANSON
TEANECK
THANDIE
THANKED
THANKER
TRANCED
TRANCES
TRANSAM
TRANSIT
TRANSOM
TWANGED
TWANGER
UGANDAN
ULANOVA
ULANUDE
UNANGRY
UPANDIN
URANITE
URANIUM
USANCES
WEANERS
WEANING
WHANGED
WRANGEL
WRANGLE
XSANDOS
YEANING
ZWANZIG

••A•N••

AGAINST
ALANNAH
BEATNIK
BLARNEY
BRAINED
BRAINER
CHAINED
CHAINES
CHAINUP
CHANNEL
CHARNIN
DRAGNET
DRAINED
DRAINER
DRAWNIN
DRAWNON
DRAWNTO
DRAWNUP
EDASNER
ELAINES
FEARNOT
FLANNEL
FLAUNTS
FLAUNTY
GRAINED
GRAINER
GRANNIE
GRAPNEL
HYANNIS
ICANNOT
INAKNOT
INASNAP
INASNIT
JEANNIE
JEANNOT
KEARNEY
KRAMNIK
KRASNER
LEARNED
LEARNER
LEARNOF
LEARNTO
NEATNIK
PLAINER
PLAINES
PLAINLY
PLAINTS
PLANNED
PLANNER
PRAWNED
REANNEX
SCANNED
SCANNER
SHANNEN
SHANNON
SHATNER
SHAWNEE
SOAPNET
SPANNED
SPANNER
SPAWNED
SPAWNER
STAGNES
STAINED
STAINER
STANNIC
STANNUM
STAUNCH
TRAINED
TRAINEE
TRAINER
TRAININ
TRAYNOR
WHATNOT
WHATNOW
YEARNED
YEARNER
YEARNTO

••A••N•

ABALONE
ABASING
ABATING
ADAMANT
AGATINE
ALADINE
ALAKING
ALANINE
ALAYING
AMARONE
AMAZING
AMAZONS
ANACINS
ARACHNE
ARACHNO
ATAMANS
ATANEND
AVALONS
AWAKENS
AWAKING
BEACONS
BEADING
BEAMING
BEANING
BEARING
BEATING
BIASING
BLADING
BLAMING
BLARING
BLATANT
BLAZING
BLAZONS
BOATING
BRACING
BRAKING
BRAVING
BRAYING
BRAZENS
BRAZING
CEASING
CHAFING
CHALONS
CHARING
CHASING
CHAWING
CHAZANS
CLAMANT
CLAWING
CLAYING
COAGENT
COALING
COATING
COAXING
CRANING
CRAPING
CRATING
CRAVENS
CRAVING
CRAYONS
CRAZING
CZARINA
DEACONS
DEADEND
DEADENS
DEAFENS
DEALING

DEARONE
DIAHANN
DIALING
DIAMOND
DRAGONS
DRAPING
DRAWING
DRAYING
ELATING
EMANANT
ERASING
ETAMINE
EVADING
EVALUNA
EXAMINE
FEARING
FLACONS
FLAGONS
FLAKING
FLAMING
FLARING
FLAWING
FLAYING
FOALING
FOAMING
FRAMING
FRAYING
GEARING
GLARING
GLAVINE
GLAZING
GNAWING
GOADING
GOALONG
GRACING
GRADING
GRATING
GRAVING
GRAYING
GRAZING
GUANINE
GUARANI
HEADEND
HEADING
HEALING
HEAPING
HEARING
HEATING
HEAVENS
HEAVING
HOAXING
IMAGINE
IMAGING
INABIND
INAFUNK
INALINE
INAWINK
ISAIDNO
KLAXONS
KRAKENS
LEADENS
LEADING
LEADINS
LEAFING
LEAKING
LEANING
LEAPING
LEASING

LEAVENS
LEAVING
LHASANS
LOADING
LOAFING
LOAMING
LOANING
MBABANE
MEANING
MOANING
NEARING
NEATENS
NIALONG
OCARINA
OFAKIND
OFAMIND
OKAYING
OMAHANE
OMAHANS
ONALINE
OPALINE
ORATING
OSAKANS
PEAHENS
PEAKING
PEALING
PEASANT
PHALANX
PHARYNX
PHASING
PLACING
PLANING
PLATENS
PLATING
PLAYING
PRALINE
PRATING
PRAYING
QUAKING
READING
REAGANS
REAGENT
REALINE
REAMEND
REAMING
REAPING
REAREND
REARING
REASONS
REAVING
ROAMING
ROARING
RRATING
SCALENE
SCALING
SCARING
SEAHUNT
SEALANE
SEALANT
SEALING
SEAMING
SEARING
SEASONS
SEATING
SHADING
SHAKING
SHAMANS
SHAMING

SHANANA
SHAPING
SHARING
SHARONA
SHAVING
SKATING
SLAKING
SLATING
SLAVING
SLAYING
SNAKING
SNAPONS
SNARING
SOAKING
SOAPING
SOARING
SPACING
SPADING
SPARING
SPAYING
STAGING
STAKING
STAMENS
STAMINA
STANINE
STARING
STATING
STATINS
STAVING
STAYING
SWAYING
TEAMING
TEARING
TEASING
TEAURNS
THATONE
THAWING
TRACING
TRADING
TSARINA
TZARINA
UNAGING
UNALONE
UNAMUNO
UTAHANS
VIADENT
VIALING
WEAKENS
WEAKONS
WEANING
WEAPONS
WEARING
WEAVING
WHALING
XRATING
XRAYING
YEANING
YEAREND
YEARONE
ZEALAND

••A•••N

ABANDON
ACADIAN
ADAMSON
AGAKHAN
ALADDIN
ALAMEIN
ALARCON
ALASKAN
ALATEEN
ARABIAN
ARAGORN
ARAMEAN
AWASHIN
AZANIAN
BDALTON
BEALION
BEARSON
BEATSON
BIAFRAN
BLACKEN
BLAMEON
BLANTON
BOATMAN
BOATMEN
BRACKEN
BRAEDEN
BRAHMAN
BRAHMIN
BRANDON
BRANSON
BRAXTON
CHAGRIN
CHANSON
CHAPLIN
CHAPMAN
CHAPMEN
CHARMAN
CHARMEN
CHARMIN
CHARNIN
CHASTEN
CHATWIN
CHAZZAN
CLACTON
CLAMPON
CLANTON
CLAPTON
CLARION
CLASSON
CLAYTON
COALBIN
COARSEN
CRAISIN
CRAMPON
CRAMSIN
CRATION
DEADPAN
DEALSIN
DEALTIN
DEARDEN
DIAHANN
DIALSIN
DIAPHAN
DOAGAIN
DRAGOON
DRAGSIN
DRAGSON
DRANKIN
DRAWMAN
DRAWMEN
DRAWNIN
DRAWNON
DRAWSIN
DRAWSON

DRAYMAN
DRAYMEN
DRAYTON
ELAAIUN
ELASTIN
ELATION
EVASION
FEASTON
FHALOAN
FLAGMAN
FLAGMEN
FLANKEN
FLASHON
FLATTEN
FRANKEN
GHANIAN
GLADDEN
GNAWSON
GRAFTON
GRATEON
GRAUMAN
GRAYSON
HEADMAN
HEADMEN
HEADPIN
HEADSIN
HEAPSON
HEARKEN
HEARTEN
HEATFAN
HEATHEN
HOARSEN
IDAHOAN
INASPIN
IRANIAN
ITALIAN
IZATION
JOAQUIN
KRAMDEN
KRATION
LEADMAN
LEADMEN
LEADSIN
LEADSON
LEAKSIN
LEANSIN
LEANSON
LEAPSIN
LEAPSON
LEAPTIN
LEAPTON
LEAVEIN
LEAVEON
LIAISON
LOADSIN
LOAFPAN
MAARTEN
MCALLEN
MEATMAN
MEATMEN
MIAMIAN
OHANLON
ONANDON
ORARION
ORATION
OVATION
PEABEAN
PEARSON

PHAETON
PHASEIN
PLANSON
PLATOON
PLAYPEN
PLAYSON
QUARTAN
REACHIN
READORN
READSIN
READSON
REALIGN
REALMAN
REALMEN
REARDON
RWANDAN
SCATMAN
SEAFERN
SEAGREN
SEALION
SEALSIN
SHANNEN
SHANNON
SHAREIN
SHARPEN
SHAVIAN
SLACKEN
SLAMSON
SLAPSON
SLATKIN
SLAYTON
SMARTEN
SNACKON
SNAPSON
SOAKSIN
SPARTAN
STANDIN
STANDON
STANTON
STARION
STARMAN
STARSIN
STARTIN
STARTON
STASSEN
STATION
STAYSIN
STAYSON
SUASION
SWAGMAN
SWAGMEN
SWANSON
TEACHIN
TEAGOWN
TOATURN
TRADEIN
TRADEON
TRAININ
TRAPGUN
UGANDAN
UPANDIN
WEARSON
WHARTON
WHAUDEN
YEAHMAN

•••AN••

ADVANCE
ALBANIA
ALLANTE
ALMANAC
ANDANTE
ARCANUM
ARGANTE
ARIANES
ARRANGE
ASHANTI
ASKANCE
ASSANTE
ATLANTA
AVIANCA
BALANCE
BANANAS
BANANES
BARANOF
BEGANTO
BONANZA
BOTANIC
BUTANES
CABANAS
CALANDO
CATANIA
CETANES
CEZANNE
CHIANTI
CLEANED
CLEANER
CLEANLY
CLEANSE
CLEANTE
CLEANUP
DANANAS
DECANTS
DEFANGS
DELANEY
DEMANDS
DERANGE
DOUANES
DURANCE
DURANGO
DURANTE
ELEANOR
ELUANTS
EMBANKS
EMPANEL
ENFANTS
ENHANCE
ENRANKS
ERLANGS
ERRANCY
ERRANDS
ESPANOL
ETHANES
ETHANOL
EUBANKS
EXPANDS
EXPANSE
EXYANKS
FINANCE
FLEANCE
FMBANDS
GALANOS
GALANTS
GITANOS
GLEANED
GLEANER

GROANED
GROANER
HADANIP
HASANIP
HAVANAN
HAVANAS
HAZANIM
HEXANES
HOSANNA
HUMANLY
HUMANUM
IGUANAS
IGUANID
IMEANIT
IMPANEL
INCANTS
INFANCY
INFANTA
INFANTE
INFANTS
INLANDS
INRANGE
INSANER
ISLANDS
JOHANNA
JUMANJI
KIWANIS
KOLANUT
KORANIC
LALANNE
LAWANDA
LEBANON
LEGANZA
LEPANTO
LIGANDS
LOGANUT
LORANGE
LUCANIA
MANANAS
MARANTZ
MCRANEY
MEGANES
MELANGE
MELANIA
MELANIC
MELANIE
MELANIN
MIRANDA
MORANIS
MORANTE
MRHANEY
MRNANNY
MURANOS
MUSANTE
MUTANTS
MYLANTA
NOCANDO
NOHANDS
NYYANKS
OCEANIA
OCEANIC
OCEANID
OCEANUS
OCTANES
OCTANTS
OLEANNA
OLEANNY
ORGANDY

ORGANIC
ORGANZA
ORLANDO
ORMANDY
OTRANTO
PALANCE
PAVANES
PEDANTS
PENANCE
PESANTE
PICANTE
PIRANHA
PISANIO
PLIANCY
POLANER
POLANYI
RAPANUI
REBANKS
RECANED
RECANES
RECANTS
REDANTS
REHANGS
RELANCE
RELANDS
RELANES
REMANDS
REPANEL
RERANKS
RESANDS
RIBANDS
ROMANCE
ROMANIA
ROMANIC
ROMANIS
ROMANOS
ROMANOV
ROMANSH
ROMANUS
ROSANNA
ROSANNE
ROXANNE
ROZANOV
RUMANIA
SARANAC
SATANIC
SAVANAS
SAVANNA
SAVANTS
SECANTS
SEMANAS
SONANCE
SQUANTO
STEANNE
STRANDS
STRANGE
SUSANNA
SUSANNE
SUZANNE
TARANTO
TEJANAS
TEJANOS
TENANCY
TENANTS
TETANUS
TISANES
TITANAE
TITANIA

TITANIC
TRUANCY
TRUANTS
TULANEU
TYRANNY
TYRANTS
ULYANOV
ULZANAS
UNCANED
UNCANNY
UNFANCY
UNHANDS
UNHANDY
UNMANED
UNMANLY
UNWANED
UPLANDS
URBANER
URBANII
URBANIV
URBANVI
VACANCY
VALANCE
VERANDA
VIVANTS
VOLANTE
WCHANDY
WOMANLY
YOLANDA
YOUANDI
ZENANAS

•••A•N•

ARIADNE
ATTAINS
ATTAINT
CELAENO
CEZANNE
COCAINE
DETAINS
DIZAINS
DOMAINE
DOMAINS
FTWAYNE
GERAINT
HOSANNA
IGRAINE
ILIAMNA
JOHANNA
LAHAINA
LALANNE
LARAINE
LASAGNA
LASAGNE
LAVAINE
LOCARNO
LUCARNE
MORAINE
MRNANNY
NOTAONE
OBTAINS
OLEANNA
OLEANNY
ORDAINS
RDLAING
REDARNS
REEARNS
REGAINS
REMAINS
REPAINT
RETAINS
REWARNS
ROGAINE
ROMAINE
ROMAINS
ROSANNA
ROSANNE
ROXANNE
SAVANNA
SCRAWNY
SPRAINS
STEANNE
STEARNS
STRAINS
SUKARNO
SUSANNA
SUSANNE
SUZANNE
TYRANNY
UKRAINE
UNCANNY
UNPAWNS
UNRAINY
VISAING
ZELAZNY

•••A••N

ACTAEON
ALMADEN
ANDAMAN
ANKARAN
ANNAKIN
AQUAMAN
ARRAIGN
ASMARAN
AZKABAN
BAHAMEN
BALABAN
BALATON
BETAKEN
BREAKIN
BROADEN
CARAVAN
CATALAN
CELADON
CHEAPEN
CHEATIN
CHEATON
CLEAVON
CORAZON
DECAGON
DEHAVEN
DREAMIN
DREAMON
ELAAIUN
ELCAJON
ESIASON
ESTAMIN
GAGARIN
GAHAGAN
GELATIN
GIGATON
GLEASON
GLOAMIN
GREATEN
HAVANAN
HEMATIN
HEPARIN
HEXAGON
IDEAMAN
IDEAMEN
IDIAMIN
ISFAHAN
ITHACAN
ITSASIN
JAVAMAN
KARAJAN
KERATIN
LEBANON
LEBARON
LIMACON
MADALYN
MALAGAN
MALAYAN
MATALIN
MAYALIN
MAZARIN
MCGAVIN
MCMAHON
MEGALON
MEGATON
MELANIN
MONACAN
MUTAGEN
NARAYAN
NEVADAN
NONAGON
OAXACAN
OCTAGON
OTTAWAN
PALADIN
PARAGON
RAMADAN
RETAKEN
REWAKEN
RITALIN
ROSALYN
SAHARAN
SALADIN
SARACEN
SARAZEN
SAVARIN
SAYAMEN
SMEARON
SNEAKIN
SODACAN
SPRAYON
STEALIN
STEARIN
STRAPIN
STRAPON
SWEARIN
THIAMIN
TREADON
TREASON
UNEATEN
UNLADEN
UNPAGAN
UNTAKEN
VALADON
VISAYAN
VITAMIN
WHEATEN
WHEATON

YUCATAN

••••AN•

ABEYANT
ADAMANT
ADRIANA
AFFIANT
AFGHANI
AFGHANS
AIRLANE
AIRTANK
AJOWANS
ANDEANS
ARMBAND
ARMYANT
ARUBANS
ASHCANS
ASHLAND
ASHPANS
ASONANT
ATAMANS
AYNRAND
BADHAND
BADLAND
BAHIANS
BALKANS
BANDANA
BANYANS
BASSANI
BASSANO
BELTANE
BEMOANS
BETHANY
BETTANY
BHUTANI
BIGBAND
BIGBANG
BIGFANS
BIGHAND
BIPLANE
BIRIANI
BIRMANS
BIRYANI
BLATANT
BOBKANE
BOITANO
BOYBAND
BRIGAND
BROGANS
BUOYANT
BURBANK
BURMANS
BUSLANE
BUSMANS
CAFTANS
CAIMANS
CANCANS
CAPEANN
CAPUANA
CAYMANS
CHAZANS
CHICANA
CHICANE
CHICANO
CINZANO
CLAMANT
COBRAND
COMMAND
COMPANY
COOLANT
COPLAND
COURANT
COWBANE
COWHAND
CRETANS
CRUZANS
CTSCANS
CUBFANS
CURRANT
DABHAND
DEFIANT
DEMEANS
DEPLANE
DESCANT
DEVIANT
DIAHANN
DISBAND
DISTANT
DOGBANE
DOLMANS
DORMANT
ELEGANT
ELLMANN
EMANANT
EMPLANE
ENCHANT
ENGLAND
ENPLANE
ENTRANT
EQUIANO
ETCHANT
EYEBANK
EYEHAND
FANTANS
FERNAND
FIJIANS
FINIANS
FINLAND
FIRBANK
FIREANT
FOGBANK
FONDANT
FONTANA
FONTANE
FORLANI
FRYPANS
GABBANA
GAETANO
GALLANT
GALVANI
GALVANO
GARLAND
GASCANS
GASTANK
GERMANE
GERMANS
GERMANY
GETSANA
GETSANF
GOBLANK
GUARANI
HALDANE
HARLAND
HATBAND
HENBANE
HERMANA
HERMANN
HERMANO
HERMANS
HERNANI
HEYMANS
HISPANO
HOFMANN
HOLLAND
HOTHAND
HOVLANE
HOWMANY
HUSBAND
HYDRANT
IBIZANS
ICELAND
IKEBANA
ILLEANA
ILOCANO
IMPLANT
INDIANA
INDIANS
INSPANS
INSTANT
IONIANS
IRELAND
ISSUANT
ITERANT
JAMBAND
JANEANE
JETFANS
JOBBANK
JORDANA
JUDEANS
JUGBAND
JULIANA
JUTLAND
KANSANS
KENYANS
KEYBANK
KIRMANS
KOREANS
LANTANA
LAPLAND
LAPSANG
LEBLANC
LEGRAND
LEHMANN
LENFANT
LHASANS
LIBRANS
LIBYANS
LIPMANN
LOWHAND
LOWLAND
LUCIANA
LUCIANO
MAGNANI
MALEANT
MALIANS
MANDANS
MANGANO
MARIANA
MARIANO
MARYANN
MBABANE
MCSHANE
MECCANS
MEDIANS
MEDIANT
MENSANS
METFANS
METHANE
MIDLAND
MIGRANT
MILLAND
MINOANS
MINYANS
MONTANA
MONTAND
MONTANO
MORDANT
MORGANA
MORGANS
MTBLANC
MTEVANS
MUNDANE
MUSTANG
MYGIANT
NATHANS
NEDLAND
NEUMANN
NEWHAND
NEWMANS
NIRVANA
NISSANS
NISSANZ
NITTANY
NONBANK
NONFANS
NONSANE
NORMAND
NORMANS
NOTMANY
NUBIANS
NYGIANT
OAHUANS
OAKLAND
ODORANT
OFFHAND
OHIOANS
OILCANS
OILPANS
OILSAND
OILTANK
OLDHAND
OMAHANE
OMAHANS
ONEHAND
ONELANE
OPERAND
OPERANT
OREGANO
ORLEANS
ORPHANS
ORPHANT
OSAKANS
OURGANG
OUTBANS
OUTCANT
OUTLAND
OUTMANS
OUTRANG
OUTRANK
OUTRANT
OUTSANG
OXIDANT
PADUANS
PAGEANT
PAISANO
PAISANS
PAPUANS
PASSANT
PATHAND
PATHANS
PEASANT
PECCANT
PENDANT
PENNANT
PENTANE
PEPBAND
PHALANX
PIEPANS
PIQUANT
POBLANO
POMPANO
PONTANO
PROFANE
PROPANE
RADIANS
RADIANT
RAGLANS
RAGMANS
RAMFANS
RAMPANT
RATTANS
RAYBANS
REAGANS
REBOANT
REBRAND
RECRANK
REGNANT
REGRANT
RELIANT
RELOANS
REMNANT
REPLANE
REPLANS
REPLANT
RESCANS
RESPANS
RETHANK
RIEMANN
ROLLAND
ROSSANO
ROSTAND
ROWLAND
RUTHANN
RUTLAND
RYOKANS
SALTANT
SAMOANS
SAMPANS
SANTANA
SCHWANN
SEALANE
SEALANT
SERVANT
SEXTANS
SEXTANT
SHAMANS
SHANANA
SHEBANG
SIMIANS
SIOUANS
SIXLANE
SLOGANS
SMETANA
SOPRANI
SOPRANO
SORIANO
SOXFANS
SPOKANE
STEFANI
SUBBAND
SUBBANK
SULTANA
SULTANS
SUMMAND
SUNFANS
SUNTANS
SYRIANA
SYRIANS
TAGGANT
TAMMANY
TAPPANS
TARTANS
TARZANA
TARZANS
TATIANA
TENNANT
TERRANS
THEBAND
THEBANS
THEGANG
TIFFANY
TIJUANA
TIMPANI
TINCANS
TITIANS
TONGANS
TOOMANY
TOPRANK
TOUCANS
TOYLAND
TREPANS
TROJANS
TRUMANS
TULSANS
TURBANS
TUSCANS
TUSCANY
TWOLANE
TYMPANA
TYMPANI
ULLMANN
ULULANT
UNFRANK
UNGRAND
UNMEANT
UNPLANS
UNSPANS
UPSTAND
USGRANT
UTAHANS
UTICANS
UTICANY
VAGRANT
VALIANT
VANSANT
VANZANT
VARIANT
VERDANT
VERSANT
VIBRANT
VICDANA
VINLAND
VOLCANO
VULCANS
WARRANT
WAYLAND
WELLAND
WETLAND
WICCANS
WIELAND
WYOTANA
YEOMANS
YOUMANS
YOURANG
ZEALAND
ZEELAND
ZONIANS
ZUNIANS

••••A•N

ABSTAIN
ALSHAIN
BAHRAIN
BALMAIN
BARGAIN
BRITAIN
BYTRAIN
CAPEANN
CAPTAIN
CARBARN
CERTAIN
CONTAIN
COSTAIN
CURTAIN
DESTAIN
DETRAIN
DIAHANN
DISDAIN
DOAGAIN
EDINAMN
ELLMANN
ELTRAIN
ENCHAIN
ENGRAIN
ENTRAIN
EXPLAIN
GASMAIN
GERMAIN
GOLDARN
HERMANN
HOFMANN
INDRAWN
INGRAIN
LEHMANN
LIPMANN
MACHAON
MARYANN
NETGAIN
NEUMANN
NOSTAIN
OAKLAWN
OUTEARN
OUTFAWN
OUTGAIN
OUTLAIN
PERTAIN
PREDAWN
PREGAIN
PREWARN
RAEDAWN
REDDAWN
REDRAWN
REFRAIN
RELEARN
RESTAIN
RETRAIN
RIEMANN
RIPSAWN
RUTHANN
SCHWANN
SUSTAIN
TERRAIN
ULLMANN
UNCHAIN
UNDRAWN
UNLEARN
UNSLAIN
VILLAIN

•••••AN

ABIDJAN
ACADIAN
ADWOMAN
AEOLIAN
AFRICAN
AGAKHAN
ALASKAN
ALLBRAN
ALMSMAN
ALSORAN
ALYKHAN
AMESLAN
ANDAMAN
ANGOLAN
ANKARAN
APOGEAN
APULIAN
AQUAMAN
ARABIAN
ARAMEAN
ARTISAN
ASMARAN
AVESTAN
AVIDFAN
AVIVIAN
AZANIAN
AZKABAN
AZOREAN
AZORIAN
AZTECAN
BACHMAN
BAKEPAN
BALABAN
BASEMAN
BATEMAN
BATSMAN
BEERCAN
BEHRMAN
BELGIAN
BELLMAN
BELTRAN
BERGMAN
BERIGAN
BESTMAN
BIAFRAN
BIRDMAN
BKLIBAN
BOATMAN
BOGYMAN
BONDMAN
BOOKMAN
BOOLEAN
BOORMAN
BORNEAN
BOSNIAN
BOSSMAN
BOZEMAN
BRAHMAN
BRENDAN
BRENNAN
BROSNAN
BUCHMAN
BUSHMAN
CAKEPAN
CALIBAN
CAPITAN
CAPSTAN
CARAVAN
CARLOAN
CASPIAN
CATALAN
CATSCAN
CAVEMAN
CHAPMAN
CHARMAN
CHAZZAN
CHILEAN
COCHRAN
COGHLAN
COLEMAN
COMORAN
COONCAN
COPYMAN
CREWMAN
CRIMEAN
CUBSFAN
CYPRIAN
DAKOTAN
DANTEAN
DARKMAN
DARKTAN
DEADPAN
DEEPTAN
DELIMAN
DIAPHAN
DILLMAN
DISCMAN
DISHPAN
DONEGAN
DONJUAN
DONOVAN
DOORMAN
DORFMAN
DRAWMAN
DRAYMAN
DRIPPAN
DRISTAN
DRSLOAN
DRUZEAN
DRUZIAN
DUNSTAN
DUSTMAN
DUSTPAN
EASTMAN
EIJKMAN
ELYSIAN
ESTEBAN
ESTEFAN
ETESIAN
ETONIAN
EUROVAN
EXURBAN
FADIMAN
FELDMAN
FEYNMAN
FHALOAN
FIREMAN
FIVEMAN
FLAGMAN
FLORIAN
FOOTMAN
FOREMAN
FORERAN
FORTRAN
FOURMAN
FREEMAN
FRIEDAN
FRISIAN
FROGMAN
FUJISAN
FUSTIAN
GAHAGAN
GAMBIAN
GAMELAN
GASSMAN
GATEMAN
GAVILAN
GENEVAN
GENTIAN
GHANIAN
GILLIAN
GILLMAN
GLEEMAN
GOLDMAN
GOODMAN
GORDIAN
GRAUMAN
GRECIAN
GRUMMAN
GUINEAN
HACKMAN
HADRIAN
HAITIAN
HANGMAN
HARDPAN
HARTMAN
HAVANAN
HAWKMAN
HEADMAN
HEATFAN
HECKMAN
HEISMAN
HELLMAN
HESHVAN
HESSIAN
HICKMAN
HILLMAN
HOFFMAN
HOLYMAN
HOLZMAN
HOOPMAN
HOUSMAN
HUFFMAN
IBERIAN
IDAHOAN
IDEAMAN
INHUMAN
IRANIAN
IRONMAN
ISFAHAN
ISTRIAN
ITALIAN
ITHACAN
IVORIAN
JAVAMAN
JAZZMAN
JETSFAN
JILLIAN
JOURDAN
JOYCEAN
JUNGIAN
JUNKMAN
JURYMAN
KANTIAN
KARAJAN
KAUFMAN
KEESHAN
KELLJAN
KEOGHAN
KEYSPAN
KINGMAN
KINSMAN
KLUGMAN
LANDMAN
LAOTIAN
LAPUTAN
LATERAN
LATVIAN
LAVERAN
LEADMAN
LENSMAN
LETHEAN
LILLIAN
LINEMAN
LOAFPAN
LOCKEAN
LONIGAN
LOTHIAN
LUCKMAN
MACLEAN
MADIGAN
MAILMAN
MAINMAN
MALAGAN
MALAYAN
MANSMAN
MANTUAN
MANXMAN
MARDIAN
MARTIAN
MARXIAN
MATEWAN
MCLUHAN
MEATMAN
MEDUSAN
MEGRYAN
MERCIAN
METSFAN
MEXICAN
MIAMIAN
MILKCAN
MILKMAN
MINIVAN
MISPLAN
MOHEGAN
MOHICAN
MOISSAN
MONACAN
MRCLEAN
MRISCAN
MTLOGAN
NARAYAN
NAVYMAN
NESSMAN
NEVADAN
NEWSMAN
NICEMAN
OARSMAN
OATBRAN
OAXACAN
ODESSAN
OLDBEAN
ONTKEAN
ORPHEAN
ORTOLAN
OSIRIAN
OTTAWAN
OTTOMAN
OUTPLAN
OVERMAN
OVERRAN
OVIDIAN
OXONIAN
PARKMAN
PEABEAN
PELICAN
PEORIAN
PERLMAN
PERMIAN
PERSIAN
PETEMAN
PETSCAN
PIERIAN
PISCEAN
PITTMAN
PLEBIAN
PLOWMAN
POLEMAN
PONTIAN
POOLMAN
POORMAN
PORTMAN
POSTMAN
PRELOAN
PREPLAN
PROPMAN
PROSCAN
PROTEAN
PULLMAN
PURITAN
PYTHIAN
QUARTAN
QUINLAN
RAILMAN
RAINMAN
RAMADAN
RAMSFAN
RAPIDAN
RARITAN
REALMAN
REBEGAN
RECLEAN
REDSFAN
REEDMAN
REITMAN
REPOMAN
RHODIAN
RICHMAN
RICKMAN
RIESMAN
RIORDAN
ROMULAN
ROYBEAN
RUFFIAN
RUSSIAN
RUSSLAN
RWANDAN
SAHARAN
SANDMAN
SANJUAN
SAROYAN
SARUMAN
SAURIAN
SCATMAN
SCOTIAN
SENECAN
SERBIAN
SHAVIAN
SHEEHAN
SHERMAN
SHIPMAN
SHOWMAN
SHULMAN
SIDEMAN
SIOBHAN
SNOWMAN
SODACAN
SONORAN
SOULMAN
SOUPCAN
SOYBEAN
SPARTAN
SPORRAN
STARMAN
STEWPAN
STYGIAN
SUBCLAN
SUNSFAN
SURECAN
SURFMAN
SWAGMAN
SYNGMAN
TALIBAN
TAPEMAN
TAUREAN
TAXIMAN
TEHERAN
TELERAN
TESTBAN
THESWAN
THINMAN
THURMAN
TIBETAN
TIREMAN

TOLEDAN
TOLLMAN
TOPEKAN
TRISTAN
TUBEPAN
TUCHMAN
TURFMAN
UGANDAN
UMBRIAN
UNCLEAN
UNHUMAN
UNPAGAN
UNURBAN
UTOPIAN
VALJEAN
VATICAN
VAUGHAN
VELTMAN
VENEMAN
VETERAN
VIRGOAN
VISAYAN
VOSGIAN
WAKSMAN
WALKMAN
WAXBEAN
WEIDMAN
WELLMAN
WHITMAN
WILDMAN
WINGMAN
WIREMAN
WISEMAN
WOLFMAN
WORKMAN
XANTHAN
YALEMAN
YARDMAN
YEAHMAN
YEREVAN
YESICAN
YUCATAN
YZERMAN
ZAIRIAN
ZAMBIAN

AO•••••

AOUDADS

A•O••••

ABOLISH
ABOLLAE
ABORTED
ABOUNDS
ABOUTIT
ABOUTTO
ACOLYTE
ACONITE
ACORNED
ACOUPLE
ADOLLAR
ADOLPHE
ADONAIS
ADOPTED
ADOPTEE
ADOPTER
ADORERS
ADORING
ADORNED
ADORNER
AEOLIAN
AFOULOF
AGONIES
AGONISE
AGONISM
AGONIST
AGONIZE
AGOUTIS
AHOSTOF
AJOWANS
ALOADOF
ALOHAOE
ALOOFLY
AMOEBAE
AMOEBAS
AMOEBIC
AMONGST
AMORIST
AMOROSO
AMOROUS
AMOUNTS
ANODISE
ANODIZE
ANODYNE
ANOINTS
ANOMALY
ANOMIES
ANONYMS
ANORAKS
ANOSMIA
ANOSMIC
ANOTHER
ANOUILH
APODOUS
APOGEAL
APOGEAN
APOGEES
APOLLOS
APOLOGY
APOSTLE
APOTHEM
ARONNAX
AROUSAL
AROUSED
AROUSER
AROUSES
ASOCIAL
ASOFNOW
ASONANT
ATOMICS
ATOMIES
ATOMISE
ATOMISM
ATOMIST
ATOMIZE
ATONERS
ATONICS
ATONIES
ATONING
AVOCADO
AVOCETS
AVOIDED
AVOIDER
AVONLEA
AVOWALS
AVOWERS
AVOWING
AWOONOR
AXOLOTL
AZODYES
AZOREAN
AZORIAN

A••O•••

ABBOTCY
ABDOMEN
ABIOTIC
ABROACH
ABSOLUT
ABSOLVE
ABSORBS
ACCORDS
ACCOSTS
ACCOUNT
ACROBAT
ACRONYM
ACTORLY
ADDONTO
ADJOINS
ADJOURN
ADNOUNS
ADSORBS
ADWOMAN
ADWOMEN
AEROBAT
AEROBES
AEROBIC
AEROSOL
AFFORDS
AFROPOP
AGNOMEN
AGROUND
AKRONOH
ALBORAK
ALCOHOL
ALCOPOP
ALCOVES
ALDORAY
ALFONSE
ALFONSO
ALFORJA
ALLOFIT
ALLOFME
ALLOFUS
ALLONGE
ALLONYM
ALLOPEZ
ALLOVER
ALLOWAY
ALLOWED
ALLOWIN
ALLOWME
ALLOYED
ALMONDS
ALMONDY
ALMONER
ALMONRY
ALOOFLY
ALROKER
ALROSEN
ALSORAN
ALTOIDS
ALTOIST
ALTOONA
ALTOSAX
ALWORTH
ALYOSHA
AMMONIA
AMMONIC
AMPOULE
ANDORRA
ANDOVER
ANGOLAN
ANGORAS
ANIONIC
ANNOYED
ANNOYER
ANSONIA
ANTOINE
ANTONIA
ANTONIN
ANTONIO
ANTONYM
ANYONES
APHONIA
APHONIC
APPOINT
APPOSED
APPOSES
APRONED
APROPOS
ARBOLES
ARBORED
ARBOURS
ARDOURS
AREOLAE
AREOLAR
AREOLAS
AREOLES
ARGONNE
ARIOSOS
ARIOSTO
ARMOIRE
ARMORED
ARMORER
ARMOURS
ARMOURY
ARNOLDS
ARROYOS
ASKOVER
ASSORTS
ASTOLAT
ASTORIA
ASTOUND
ATEOVER
ATHOMES
ATROPHY
ATROPOS
ATWORST
AURORAE
AURORAL
AURORAS
AUTOBIO
AUTOBUS
AUTOING
AUTOMAT
AUTOMNE
AUTONYM
AUTOPEN
AUTOPIA
AUTOPSY
AVIONIC
AWOONOR

A•••O••

ABALONE
ABATORS
ABSCOND
ACEDOUT
ACEROLA
ACEROSE
ACESOUT
ACETONE
ACTFOUR
ACTIONS
ACTSOUT
ADENOID
ADIPOSE
AFFRONT
AFTMOST
AGEDOUT
AGEFOUR
AGELONG
AGESOUT
AHCHOOS
AIRBOAT
AIRCOOL
AIRFOIL
AIRFONE
AIRHOLE
AIRHORN
AIRHOSE
AIRLOCK
AIRLOGS
AIRPOPS
AIRPORT
AIRPOTS
AIRSOCK
AIRSOUT
AIRWOLF
AKEBONO
ALAMODE
ALAMOSA
ALCYONE
ALIFORM
ALIGOTE
ALIMONY
ALLDONE
ALLGONE
ALLGOOD
ALLTOLD
ALTDORF
ALTHORN
ALTOONA
ALVEOLI
AMAPOLA
AMARONE
AMATOLS
AMATORY
AMAZONS
AMBROSE
AMEBOID
AMIDOLS
AMNIONS
AMOROSO
AMOROUS
AMPHORA
ANALOGS
ANALOGY
ANATOLE
ANATOLY
ANATOMY
ANCHORS
ANCHOVY
ANDMORE
ANDROID
ANDROUS
ANDSOON
ANEMONE
ANEROID
ANTCOWS
ANTHONY
ANTIOCH
ANXIOUS
ANYBODY
ANYHOPE
ANYMORE
ANYROAD
ANYTOWN
APODOUS
APOLOGY
APPROVE
APRIORI
AQUEOUS
ARAGORN
ARCHONS
ARDMORE
ARDUOUS
ARENOSE
ARIZONA
ARMBONE
ARMHOLE
ARMLOAD
ARMLOCK
ARTBOOK
ARTFORM
ARTROCK
ARTSONG
ARTWORK
ASABODY
ASAJOKE
ASHFORD
ASKSOUT
ATABOIL
ATACOST
ATALOSS
ATCROSS
ATEMORE
AUREOLA
AUREOLE
AUTHORS
AVALONS
AWESOME
AXLROSE
AXOLOTL
AYKROYD

A••••O•

ABANDON
ABETTOR
ABSALOM
ABUTSON
ACCTNOS
ACHEFOR
ACHERON
ACHESON
ACTAEON
ACTEDON
ACTINON
ACTSFOR
ACTUPON
ADAGIOS
ADAMSON
ADAPTOR
ADDEDON
ADDISON
ADJUROR
ADVISOR
AERATOR
AEROSOL
AFATLOT
AFOULOF
AFROPOP
AGALLOP
AGREEON
AHCHOOS
AHEADOF
AHOSTOF
AIKIDOS
AILERON
AIMSFOR
AIRCOOL
AIRDROP
AIRFLOW
AIRGLOW
AIRSHOW
AJSIMON
AKERLOF
AKRONOH
AKSAKOV
ALACKOF
ALARCON
ALBEDOS
ALBINOS
ALCOHOL
ALCOPOP
ALENCON
ALFEROV
ALIENOR
ALLGOOD
ALLISON
ALLSTON
ALLYSON
ALNICOS
ALOADOF
ALOHAOE
AMPHION
ANBESOL
ANDIRON
ANDSOON
ANGELOU
ANISTON
ANTIFOG
ANTILOG
ANTLION
APAIROF
APECKOF
APERSON
APILEOF
APOLLOS
APRICOT
APROPOS
ARAFTOF
ARCHFOE
ARIOSOS
ARISTOS
ARROYOS
ARTBOOK
ARTSHOP
ARTSHOW
ASIAGOS
ASKEDOF
ASKSFOR
ASLEWOF
ASOFNOW
ASSUROR
ATEALOT
ATECROW
ATIPTOE
ATROPOS
ATTABOY
AUCTION
AUDITOR
AUDUBON
AULDSOD
AVEYRON
AVIATOR
AVIGNON
AWAREOF
AWOONOR
AXELROD

A•••••O

AAJUMBO
ABOUTTO
ACDELCO
ADAPTTO
ADAYAGO
ADDEDTO
ADDONTO
ADDUPTO
ADMITTO
AGESAGO
AGITATO
AGREETO
AJACCIO
AKEBONO
AKIHITO
ALBERTO
ALBIREO
ALERTTO
ALFONSO
ALFREDO
ALIENTO
ALIVETO
ALLEGRO
AMERIGO
AMOROSO
AMRADIO
ANDIAMO
ANIMATO
ANNATTO
ANSELMO
ANTONIO
APPLYTO
ARACHNO
ARAPAHO
ARECIBO
ARETINO
ARGENTO
ARIGATO
ARIOSTO
ARSENIO
ARTDECO
ARTERIO
ASPENCO
ATEINTO
AUGUSTO
AUTOBIO
AVOCADO
AZULEJO

•AO••••

BAOBABS
GAOLERS
GAOLING
LAOCOON
LAOTIAN
MAOISTS
MAOSUIT
SAOTOME
TAOISTS
YAOMING
YAOUNDE

•A•O•••

BABOONS
BADOMEN
BALONEY
BAROLOS
BARONET
BAROQUE
BAYONET
BAYONNE
BAZOOKA
CABOOSE
CACONYM
CAHOKIA
CAHOOTS
CAJOLED
CAJOLER
CAJOLES
CALORIC
CALORIE
CALOTTE
CANOERS
CANOLAS
CANONIC
CANONRY
CANOPUS
CAPOTES
CAROLED
CAROLER
CAROLII
CAROLYN
CAROMED
CAROTID
CAROTIN
CAROUSE
CATORCE
CAVORTS
DACOSTA
DADOING
DAHOMEY
DAKOTAN
DAKOTAS
DAMOSEL
EATOVER
FACONNE
FAGOTED
FANOUTS
FAROESE
FAROUKI
FATONES
FATOUSH
FAVORED
FAVORER
FAVOURS
GALOOTS
GALOPED
GARONNE
GAROTTE
GASOHOL
GASOVEN
GAVOTTE
HADOVER
HALOGEN
HALOIDS
HALOING
HANOVER
HAROLDI
HASOVER
HAWORTH
IACOCCA
JACOBIN
JACONET
JAROMIR
KAROLYI
KAYOING
LABORAT
LABORED
LABORER
LABOURS
LACONIA
LACONIC
LACOSTE
LADOUCE
LAGOONS
LAJOLLA
LAKOTAS
LALOOSH
LAMOTTA
LAMOTTE
LANOLIN
LANOTTE
LAPORTE
LAROCHE
LASORDA
LATOSCA
LAVORIS
LAYODDS
LAYOFFS
LAYOPEN
LAYOUTS
LAYOVER
LAZONGA
MACONGA
MACOUNS
MADONNA
MAHONEY
MAHOUTS
MAJORCA
MAJORED
MAJORIN
MALODOR
MANOLIN
MANOWAR
MAROONS
MASONED
MASONIC
MASONRY
MAYORAL
NABOKOV
PAGODAS
PALOMAR
PALOMAS
PALOOKA
PANOPLY
PAPOOSE
PARODIC
PAROLED
PAROLEE
PAROLES
PARONYM
PAROTID
PAYOFFS
PAYOLAS
PAYOUTS
RADOMES
RAGOUTS
RAMONES
RANONIN
RANOVER
RAYOVAC
RAZORED
SALOMON
SALONGA
SALOONS
SAMOANS
SAMOSAS
SAMOSET
SAMOVAR
SAMOYED
SARONGS
SAROYAN
SATORIS
SAVORED
SAVORER
SAVOURS
SAVOURY
SAYOVER
TABOOED
TABORET
TABOULI
TACOMAS
TACONIC
TAGOUTS
TALONED
TANOAKS
TAROILS
VALOREM
VALOTTE
VALOURS
VAMOOSE
VANOCUR
VANOWEN
VAPORED
VAPORER
VAPORUB
VAPOURS
VAPOURY
WAGONED
WAGONER
WASONTO
XAMOUNT
ZAPOTEC
ZATOPEK

•A••O••

BABCOCK
BABOONS
BABYOIL
BACKOFF
BACKOUT
BADBOYS
BADCOLD
BADDOGS
BADFORM
BADJOKE
BADLOTS
BADLOVE
BADMOOD
BADMOVE
BADWORD
BAGBOYS
BAGJOBS
BAGNOLD
BAILORS
BAILOUT
BAKEOFF
BALBOAS
BALCONY
BALFOUR
BALLONE
BALLOON
BALLOTS
BAMBOOS
BANGOUT
BANJOES
BANKONE
BARCODE
BARHOPS
BARNONE
BARNOWL
BARRONS
BARROOM
BARROWS
BARSOAP
BARTOLO
BARYONS
BASSOON
BATBOYS
BATHOIL
BAWLOUT
BAYLORU
BAZOOKA
CABOOSE
CAHOOTS
CALHOUN
CALLOFF
CALLOUS
CALLOUT
CALPOLY
CALZONE
CAMBOYS
CAMEOED
CAMEOFF
CAMEOUT
CAMIONS
CAMPOUT
CANDOUR
CANNOCK
CANNOLI
CANNONS
CANTONS
CANTORS
CANYONS
CANZONA
CANZONE
CANZONI
CAPTORS
CARBONS
CARBOYS
CARCOAT
CARDOOR
CARDOZO
CARGOES
CARHOPS
CARHORN
CARIOCA
CARIOLE
CARIOUS
CARLOAD
CARLOAN
CARLOTA
CARLOTS
CARPOOL
CARPORT
CARPOUS
CARROLL
CARROTS
CARROTY
CARTOFF
CARTONS
CARTOON
CARTOPS
CASEOUS
CASEOUT
CASHOUT
CASSOCK
CASSOLA
CASTOFF
CASTOUT
CATBOAT
CATBOWL
CATCOMB
CATDOOR
CATFOOD
CATFOOT
CATHODE
CATIONS
CATTOYS
DACRONS
DAEMONS
DAEWOOS
DAGWOOD
DALTONS
DAMPOFF
DAMSONS
DARTOFF
DASBOOT
DASHOFF
DAYBOOK
DAYHOPS
DAYJOBS
DAYLONG
DAYROOM
DAYSOFF
DAYTONA
EARBONE
EARHOLE
EARLOBE
EARLOCK
EASEOFF

EASEOUT EASYOFF EASYONE EATMORE EATSOUT FABFOUR FACEOFF FACTOID FACTORS FACTORY FADEOUT FAEROES FAIROFF FAKEOUT FALCONS FALLOFF FALLOUT FALLOWS FANDOMS FANFOLD FANIONS FANSOUT FANTODS FARGOND FARGONE FARMORE FARMOUT FARROWS FASTONE FATHOMS FATUOUS FAXLORE GALLONS GALLOPS GALLOWS GALOOTS GAMBOLS GAMMONS GARCONS GARROTE GASCONS GASCONY GASEOUS GASHOGS GASLOGS GASTONE GAVEOFF GAVEOUT GAYLORD HACKOFF HADDOCK HADDONE HADRONS HADROOM HADSOME HADTOBE HALLOOS HALLOWS HAMBONE HAMHOCK HAMMOCK HAMMOND HANCOCK HANDOFF HANDOUT HANGOFF HANGOUT HANSOLO

HANSOMS HAPLOID HARBORS HARBOUR HARLOTS HARMONY HARPOON HARRODS HARROLD HARROWS HASDONE HASHOUT HASROOM HASSOCK HASTOBE HATSOFF HAULOFF HAVEONE HAVEOUT HAYFORK HAYLOFT HAYMOWS IAMLOVE IANHOLM JAILORS JARGONS JARGONY JARROTT JAWBONE KAMFONG KANEOHE KARAOKE KARLOFF KARLOVY LABCOAT LACTOSE LADHOOD LADRONE LAGOONS LAIDOFF LAIDOUT LALOOSH LAMPOIL LAMPOON LANCOME LANEONE LANFORD LAOCOON LAPDOGS LAPROBE LAPTOPS LARDONS LASHOUT LASSOED LASSOER LASSOES LASTONE LASTORY LATROBE LAWBOOK LAWFORD LAYDOWN LAYSOFF LAYSOUT LAZBOYS MACHONE MACRONS MADDOGS

MADEOFF MADEONE MADEOUT MADLOCK MAFIOSI MAFIOSO MAGGOTS MAHFOUZ MAHZORS MAILOUT MAISONS MAISOUI MAKEOFF MAKEONE MAKEOUT MALCOLM MALLOWS MALTOSE MAMBOED MAMMOTH MANDOKI MANGOES MANHOLE MANHOOD MANHOUR MANROPE MAPSOUT MARCONI MARKOFF MARKOUT MARKOVA MARLOWE MARMOTS MAROONS MARRONS MARROWS MASCOTS MASTOID MATLOCK MATRONS MATTOCK MATZOHS MATZOTH MAUROIS MAXBORN MAYPOLE NAIROBI NAMEONE NARROWS NATIONS OAKMOSS OAKWOOD OARLOCK PACEOFF PACKOFF PADDOCK PADLOCK PADRONE PAGEONE PAIDOFF PAIDOUT PAIROFF PALJOEY PALLORS PALMOFF PALMOIL PALOOKA PANDORA

PANSOUT PANTONE PAPOOSE PARBOIL PARDONS PARFOUR PARLORS PARLOUR PARLOUS PARROTS PARSONS PARTONE PARTOOK PASCOLI PASSOFF PASSOUT PASTORS PATDOWN PATROLS PATRONS PATROON PAVIORS PAVIOUR PAVLOVA PAWNOFF PAYLOAD PAYMORE PAYROLL PAYSOFF PAYSOUT RACCOON RACKOUT RADFORD RADIOAD RADIODJ RADIOED RADIOER RADIOIN RAGDOLL RAGMOPS RAGTOPS RAINOUT RAISONS RAKEOFF RAMDOWN RAMHOME RAMRODS RAMSONS RANCORS RANCOUR RANDOWN RANGOFF RANGOON RANGOUT RANHOME RANKOUT RANSOMS RAPPORT RAPSONG RAPTORS RASBORA RATHOLE RATIONS RATSOUT RAUCOUS RAVIOLI RAWFOOD RAYMOND

SACKOUT SADSONG SAILORS SAISONS SALMONP SALMONS SALOONS SALSODA SALVOES SALVORS SAMBORA SAMEOLD SAMLOYD SAMSONS SANBORN SANFORD SANGOUT SANJOSE SAOTOME SAPPORO SARNOFF SARTORS SASSOON SATCOMS SATDOWN SATHOME SAUCONY SAVIORS SAVIOUR SAWLOGS SAWNOFF SAWSOFF SAWTOIT SAWWOOD SAXHORN SAYMORE SAYNOTO TABLOID TABOOED TADPOLE TAGSOUT TAILOFF TAILORS TAKEOFF TAKEONE TAKEOUT TALKOUT TALLONE TALLOWS TALLOWY TANDOOR TANGOED TANGOER TAPIOCA TAPROOM TAPROOT TAPSOFF TAPSOUT TARPONS TATTOOS TAXCODE TAYLORS VACUOLE VACUOUS VALLONE VAMOOSE VANGOGH VANLOAD

VANPOOL VANVOGT VARIOUS VAUDOIS WAITOUT WALCOTT WALDORF WALKOFF WALKONS WALKOUT WALLOFF WALLOON WALLOPS WALLOWS WALPOLE WALTONS WANTONS WANTOUT WARBOND WARDOFF WARGODS WARLOCK WARLORD WARNOFF WARROOM WARTORN WARWORN WARZONE WASHOFF WASHOUT WATFORD WAVEOFF WAXWORK WAYCOOL WAYTOGO WAYWORN YANKOFF YANKOUT YARROWS ZAMBONI

•A•••O•

BABYBOP BABYLON BACKHOE BACKLOG BACKLOT BACKROW BADENOV BADMOOD BADSHOT BAGEHOT BAGNIOS BAILSON BALATON BALLBOY BALLIOL BALLOON BAMBOOS BANDBOX BANGKOK BANGSON BANKJOB BANKSON BARANOF BAROLOS BARRIOS BARROOM BARSTOW BASEDON BASSOON BASTION BATSFOR CABRIOS CAILLOU CAISSON CALDRON CALICOS CALLBOX CALLBOY CALLFOR CALLNOW CALLSON CAMAROS CAMELOT CAMERON CAMINOS CAMPHOR CAMPION CAPECOD CAPITOL CAPTION CARABOO CARDOOR CAREFOR CARIBOO CARIBOU CARLSON CARLTON CARPOOL CARRYON CARSHOW CARTOON CASELOT CASHBOX CASHCOW CASINOS CASTROL CASTSON CATALOG CATALOS CATCHON CATCHOW CATDOOR CATFOOD CATFOOT CATSHOW CAUTION DACAPOS DAEWOOS DAGWOOD DAMPMOP DARENOT DASBOOT DASHDOT DASHPOT DAVEKOZ DAVISON DAWNSON DAYBOOK DAYROOM EARDROP EARLDOM EARLYON EARSHOT EASEDON

EASESON EASYJOB EATALOT EATCROW EATFROM FACEDON FACESON FACTION FALLFOR FALLSON FAMICOM FAREBOX FARMBOY FASHION FAWNSON GABBROS GAINSON GALANOS GALLEON GAMEBOY GANGTOK GASOHOL GAUCHOS GAZEBOS GAZEDON GAZESON HADACOW HADAJOB HADAROW HADROOM HAIRDOS HALCYON HALFROD HALFWON HALLOOS HALSTON HAMPTON HANDSON HANGDOG HANGSON HARDTOP HARDWON HARICOT HARPOON HARPSON HASACOW HASAROW HASROOM HAUTBOY HAVENOT JACKPOT JACKSON JACKSOO JAMESON JAMISON JANEDOE JANITOR JANKLOW JANSSON JAZZBOS KAKAPOS KAKUROS KARLSON LACESON LADADOG LADHOOD LADINOS LAIDFOR

LAIDLOW LAMPOON LANGDON LANGTON LANGUOR LAOCOON LAREDOS LARGEOJ LASTDON LASTROW LATCHON LATERON LATIGOS LATINOS LAVABOS LAWBOOK LAYITON LAYSFOR LAYSLOW LAYUPON MACACOS MACEDON MACHAON MACLEOD MADEFOR MADELON MADISON MADUROS MAGALOG MAGINOT MAILBOX MAILLOL MAILLOT MAINTOP MAKEDOS MAKEFOR MALEDOG MALEHOG MALODOR MANHOOD MANILOW MANSION MARCHON MARIDOS MARMION MARSTON MARYLOU MATADOR NABOKOV NATATOR NAVAHOS NAVAJOS OAKWOOD PACKSON PAGEBOY PAIDFOR PALEMON PALMTOP PALTROW PAPADOC PAPAGOS PARADOR PARADOX PARAGON PARASOL PARTOOK PARTYON PASSFOR

PASSION PATRIOT PATROON PAXINOU PAYSFOR PAYSNOW RACCOON RACINOS RAGSHOP RAILSON RAINBOW RAINGOD RAINSON RALSTON RANAMOK RANCHOS RANGFOR RANGOON RANRIOT RAVELOE RAWFOOD RAYKROC SABADOS SAFFRON SAIDBOO SAILSON SALCHOW SALEMOR SALOMON SALTBOX SAMPSON SANDBOX SANDHOG SANDLOT SASSOON SATATOP SATINON SATUPON SAVEDON SAVEFOR SAVESON SAWWOOD SAYSBOO SAYSYOU TACHYON TACKSON TAGALOG TAKEFOR TAKENON TAKESON TALKSOF TALKSON TANDOOR TANKTOP TAPEDON TAPESON TAPROOM TAPROOT TAPSHOE TATTOOS TAUNTON VALADON VANPOOL WAITFOR WAITRON WAITSON WALKSON WALLOON

WALSTON WAPSHOT WARNSOF WARRIOR WARROOM WARTHOG WAYCOOL YANKSON YANKTON ZABUTON

•A••••O

AAJUMBO BABENCO BALLTWO BAMBINO BANDIDO BANDITO BARTOLO BASETWO BASILIO BASSANO CALABRO CALANDO CALLSTO CALVINO CALYPSO CAMACHO CANSECO CANTINO CARABOO CARDOZO CAREDTO CARESTO CARIBOO CASSINO CATERTO CATTALO DANEYKO DANGELO DARESTO DAREZZO EATINTO FAILSTO FALLSTO FARRAGO GAETANO GALENTO GALILEO GALLICO GALVANO GAMBADO GASTERO HANDYTO HANSOLO HAPKIDO HAPPYTO HAVEAGO JACINTO JACKIEO JACKSOO JALISCO JANEIRO JAYLENO LACRIMO LAMINTO LANETWO LAYINTO

MACHTWO MAESTRO MAFIOSO MAGNETO MAKESDO MAKESGO MALPASO MANCUSO MANGANO MANKATO MANRICO MARCATO MARENGO MARIANO MARTINO MARULLO MAYBESO NABISCO NABUCCO NANAIMO PAGETWO PAISANO PALAZZO PALERMO PAMLICO PARTTWO PASSADO PATERNO PAYINTO RACEDTO RACESTO RAJARAO RALLYTO RAMINTO RANINTO RANUPTO RAPALLO SAGUARO SAIDBOO SAIDIDO SAILSTO SAINTLO SALERNO SAMMYJO SANREMO SAPPORO SAPSAGO SATCHMO SAWINTO SAYHITO SAYNOTO SAYSBOO SAYSIDO SAYSWHO TABASCO TAKENTO TAKESTO TALKSTO TALLYHO TAMPICO TANGELO TAPINTO TARANTO VACCARO VALLEJO VAQUERO WAIKATO WALKSTO

WANTSTO WARHERO WARMSTO WASONTO WAVEDTO WAVESTO WAYTOGO ZANETTO ZAPATEO

••AO•••

CHAOTIC MIAOUED MIAOWED

••A•O••

ABALONE ABATORS ALAMODE ALAMOSA AMAPOLA AMARONE AMATOLS AMATORY AMAZONS ANALOGS ANALOGY ANATOLE ANATOLY ANATOMY ARAGORN ASABODY ASAJOKE ATABOIL ATACOST ATALOSS AVALONS BEACONS BEANOIL BEAROFF BEAROUT BEATOFF BEATOUT BLALOCK BLAZONS BRAVOED BRAVOES BYANOSE CHALONS CHAMOIS CHANOYU CHAYOTE CLAMORS CLAMOUR COALOIL CRAPOLA CRAPOUT CRAYOLA CRAYONS DEACONS DEALOUT DEARONE DIABOLO DIALOGS DIALOUT DIAMOND DIATOMS DIAVOLO

DNACODE
DRAGOFF
DRAGONS
DRAGOON
DRAGOTI
DRAGOUT
DRAWOFF
DRAWOUT
ENAMORS
ENAMOUR
FHALOAN
FLACONS
FLAGONS
FLATOUT
FLAVORS
FLAVORY
FLAVOUR
GIACOMO
GLAMORS
GLAMOUR
GOABOUT
GOALONG
GRANOLA
HEADOFF
HEADOUT
HEAROUT
HYALOID
IDAHOAN
IMAGOES
IMAHOGG
INAHOLE
INAMOOD
INAPOEM
INAPOKE
INAWORD
ISADORA
ISADORE
IVANOVO
JEALOUS
KLAXONS
LEACOCK
LEADOFF
LEADORE
LEADOUT
LEAFOUT
LEAWOOD
LOANOUT
MEADOWS
MEADOWY
NDAKOTA
NIALONG
OFASORT
ONAROLL
ONATOOT
ORATORS
ORATORY
PEABODY
PEACOAT
PEACOCK
PEAFOWL
PEAPODS
PEASOUP
PGATOUR
PIANOLA
PLANOUT
PLATOON
PLAYOFF
PLAYOUT
QUAHOGS
RCADOME
READOFF
READOPT
READORN
READOUT
REAMOUT
REAROSE
REASONS
REAVOWS
REAWOKE
ROANOKE
SDAKOTA
SEABOAT
SEABORG
SEACOWS
SEADOGS
SEAFOAM
SEAFOOD
SEAFOWL
SEAGODS
SEALOFF
SEAMOSS
SEAPORT
SEASONS
SEAWOLF
SHADOWS
SHADOWY
SHAKOES
SHALOMS
SHARONA
SLALOMS
SNAPONS
SPATOUT
STATORS
STAYOFF
STAYOUT
TEACOZY
TEAGOWN
TEAPOTS
TEAPOYS
TEAROFF
TEAROOM
TEAROSE
TEAROUT
THATONE
THAWOUT
ULANOVA
UNALONE
UPABOVE
WEAKONS
WEAPONS
WEAROFF
WEAROUT
YEARONE
ZEALOTS
ZEALOUS

••A••O•

ABANDON
ADAGIOS
ADAMSON
ADAPTOR
AFATLOT
AGALLOP
ALACKOF
ALARCON
APAIROF
ARAFTOF
AWAREOF
BDALTON
BEALION
BEARSON
BEATBOX
BEATCOP
BEATSON
BLAMEON
BLANTON
BLAUBOK
BOASTOF
BRANDON
BRANSON
BRAXTON
CHANSON
CHARCOT
CHARIOT
CHARROS
CLACTON
CLAIROL
CLAMPON
CLANGOR
CLANTON
CLAPFOR
CLAPTON
CLARION
CLASSON
CLAYTON
CRABPOT
CRAMPON
CRATION
CUATROS
CZARDOM
DEARGOD
DIABLOS
DIARIOS
DRAGOON
DRAGSON
DRAWNON
DRAWSON
DRAYTON
ELATION
ENACTOR
ENARBOR
EVASION
EXACTOR
FEARFOR
FEARNOT
FEASTON
FIASCOS
FLASHON
FLATTOP
FRANKOZ
GEARBOX
GLASGOW
GLASHOW
GNAWSON
GRAFTON
GRANTOR
GRATEON
GRAYSON
HEADFOR
HEAPSOF
HEAPSON
HEARDOF
HEARSOF
ICANNOT
INAIDOF
INAKNOT
INAMOOD
INASHOE
INASPOT
INAWEOF
IVANHOE
IZATION
JCARROL
JEANNOT
KHARKOV
KIARIOS
KRATION
LEADDOG
LEADSON
LEANSON
LEANTOS
LEAPFOR
LEAPSON
LEAPTON
LEARNOF
LEAVEON
LEAWOOD
LIAISON
LLADROS
LOADSOF
MEANJOE
MTATHOS
NEARYOU
OHANLON
ONANDON
ONATOOT
ORARION
ORATION
OVATION
PEARSON
PEATBOG
PEATPOT
PGAPROS
PHAETON
PHANTOM
PHARAOH
PLANFOR
PLANSON
PLATOON
PLAYBOY
PLAYDOH
PLAYSON
PRAETOR
PRAYFOR
QRATIOS
QUARTOS
REACTOR
READFOR
READSON
REALLOT
REALTOR
REARDON
RIALTOS
ROADEOS
ROADHOG
SCADSOF
SCALLOP
SEAFOOD
SEALION
SHADROE
SHAHDOM
SHALLOT
SHALLOW
SHAMPOO
SHANNON
SHAVUOT
SLAMSON
SLAPSON
SLAYTON
SMACKOF
SMALLOJ
SNACKON
SNAPSON
SOAPBOX
SPAMBOT
SPARROW
STANDON
STANTON
STARDOM
STARION
STARLOG
STARTON
STATION
STAYFOR
STAYSON
SUASION
SWALLOW
SWANSON
TEAROOM
TEASHOP
TEATROS
THATSOK
TRACTOR
TRADEON
TRAITOR
TRANSOM
TRAYNOR
TSARDOM
WEARSON
WHARTON
WHATFOR
WHATNOT
WHATNOW
XFACTOR
XSANDOS
YEAHYOU

••A•••O

ADAPTTO
ADAYAGO
AJACCIO
ARACHNO
ARAPAHO
BEAHERO
BRACERO
BRAVADO
CLAMATO
CLAUDIO
DEALSTO
DEALTTO
DIABOLO
DIALEDO
DIAVOLO
DOASIDO
DRANKTO
DRAWNTO
DRAWSTO
EXANIMO
GEARSTO
GIACOMO
GUANACO
HEADSTO
HEAVEHO
HEAVETO
ISAIDNO
IVANOVO
IWANTTO
LEADSTO
LEANSTO
LEARNTO
LEASETO
LLANERO
LOATHTO
MEANSTO
MEANTTO
PLACEBO
PLACIDO
PLANSTO
PLAYSTO
PRAYSTO
QUATTRO
REACTTO
READSTO
SEAHERO
SHAMPOO
SHAPIRO
SNAPSTO
SOANDSO
STANDTO
STARTTO
UNAMUNO
YEARNTO

•••AO••

KARAOKE
NOTAONE
TERAOHM
TUNAOIL

•••A•O•

ABSALOM
ACTAEON
AERATOR
AHEADOF
AKSAKOV
ALOADOF
ASIAGOS
ATEALOT
ATTABOY
AVIATOR
BALATON
BARANOF
BELABOR
BUGABOO
BUGALOO
BYWAYOF
CAMAROS
CARABOO
CATALOG
CATALOS
CELADON
CHEATON
CLEAROF
CLEAVON
CORAZON
CREATOR
CURATOR
DACAPOS
DECAGON
DECALOG
DECAPOD
DEMAGOG
DILATOR
DISAVOW
DONATOR
DOSADOS
DREAMOF
DREAMON
DYNAMOS
EATALOT
ECUADOR
ELCAJON
ELEANOR
EQUATOR
ESCALOP
ESIASON
ESPANOL
ESTADOS
ETHANOL
EXMAYOR
FUGATOS
GALANOS
GELATOS
GETAJOB
GIGATON
GIRASOL
GITANOS
GLEASON
GOTAJOB
GYRATOR
HADACOW
HADAJOB
HADAROW
HASACOW
HASAROW
HEXAGON
HEXAPOD
ICHABOD
IGNATOW
INFAVOR
INLABOR
ITSABOY
ITSALOT
KAKAPOS
LADADOG
LAVABOS
LEBANON
LEBARON
LEGATOR
LEGATOS
LEVATOR
LIEATOP
LIMACON
LOCATOR
MACACOS
MAGALOG
MATADOR
MCMAHON
MEGALON
MEGATON
MIKADOS
MIRADOR
MOGADOR
MOVADOS
MRMAGOO
MURANOS
NATATOR
NAVAHOS
NAVAJOS
NEGATOR
NONAGON
NOTALOT
OCTAGON
OCTAVOS
OHCAROL
PAPADOC
PAPAGOS
PARADOR
PARADOX
PARAGON
PARASOL
PICADOR
PICAROS
RANAMOK
RELATOR
ROMANOS
ROMANOV
ROTATOR
ROZANOV
RUBATOS
RUNAMOK
SABADOS
SATATOP
SENATOR
SITATOP
SMEAGOL
SMEARON
SODAPOP
SPEAKOF
SPRAYON
SQUALOR
STRAPON
TAGALOG
TEJANOS
TINAMOU
TREADON
TREASON
ULYANOV
VALADON
VIRAGOS
WHEATON
ZOCALOS

•••A••O

AMRADIO
ANNATTO
BEGANTO
BELASCO
BIZARRO
BOIARDO
BONARIO
BUGABOO
BUGALOO
CALABRO
CALANDO
CAMACHO
CARABOO
CBRADIO
CELAENO
CURACAO
DECARLO
DEFACTO
DEMARCO
DRMARIO
DURANGO
EDGARDO
EDUARDO
ELCAMPO
ELGALLO
EMBARGO
EQUALTO
ESPARTO
EXFACTO
FMRADIO
GERALDO
HIDALGO
HORATIO
IDSAYSO
IGNARRO
IMPASTO
INVACUO
IZZATSO
KOWADLO
LEPANTO
LOCARNO
LOYALTO
MILAGRO
MOGAMBO
MRMACHO
MRMAGOO
MULATTO
NANAIMO
NOCANDO
NOVARRO
OCTAVIO
ONTARIO
ORLANDO
OTRANTO
OTTAVIO
PALAZZO
PERATIO
PICARDO
PICASSO
PISANIO
PISARRO
PIZARRO
PLEADTO
RAJARAO
RAPALLO
RENALDO
RICARDO
RINALDO
ROSARIO
SEEALSO
SPEAKTO
SQUANTO
SUHARTO
SUKARNO
SWEARTO
TABASCO
TARANTO
TOBACCO
UNMACHO
XMRADIO
ZAPATEO

••••AO•

ALOHAOE
DRCHAOS
MACHAON
PHARAOH
TULSAOK
XENIAOH

••••A•O

ADAYAGO
AGESAGO
AGITATO
ANDIAMO
ANIMATO
ARAPAHO
ARIGATO
AVOCADO
BASSANO
BEEFALO
BERGAMO
BOITANO
BONIATO
BRAVADO
BUFFALO
CATTALO
CEMBALO
CENTAVO
CEPHALO
CHICAGO
CHICANO
CINZANO
CLAMATO
CRUZADO
DEODATO
DERMATO
ELPRADO
EQUIANO
FARRAGO
FERRARO
FURTADO
GAETANO
GALVANO
GAMBADO
GENNAIO
GENNARO
GESTAPO
GOTTAGO
GUANACO
HAVEAGO
HERMANO
HISPANO
ILOCANO
ISITAGO
ISOLATO
LEONATO
LONGAGO
LUCIANO
LUMBAGO
MALPASO
MANGANO
MANKATO
MARCATO
MARIANO
MERCADO
MONTANO
MOSCATO
OMPHALO
OREGANO
PAISANO
PASSADO
POBLANO
POMPANO
PONTANO
ROSSANO
RUFFALO
SAGUARO
SAPSAGO
SOPRANO
SORIANO
THEMAYO
TORNADO
VACCARO
VIBRATO
VOLCANO
WAIKATO
YOTEAMO
ZHIVAGO

•••••AO

CURACAO
LINBIAO
LINPIAO
RAJARAO

AP•••••

APACHES
APAIROF
APATITE
APECKOF
APEDIET
APELETS
APELIKE
APERCUS
APERIES
APERSON
APESUIT
APHAGIA
APHAGIC
APHASIA
APHASIC
APHELIA
APHIDES
APHILIP
APHONIA
APHONIC
APILEOF
APISHLY
APLENTY
APLITES
APLUSES
APODOUS
APOGEAL
APOGEAN
APOGEES
APOLLOS
APOLOGY
APOSTLE
APOTHEM
APPALLS
APPARAT
APPAREL
APPEALS
APPEARS
APPEASE
APPENDS
APPETIT
APPLAUD
APPLETS
APPLIED
APPLIER
APPLIES
APPLING
APPLYTO
APPOINT
APPOSED
APPOSES
APPRISE
APPROVE
APRICOT
APRIORI
APRONED
APROPOS
APSIDES
APTERAL
APTERYX
APTNESS
APULIAN

A•P••••

ALPACAS
ALPHARD
ALPINER
ALPINES
AMPEDUP
AMPERES
AMPHION
AMPHORA
AMPLEST
AMPLIFY
AMPOULE
AMPULES
APPALLS
APPARAT
APPAREL
APPEALS
APPEARS
APPEASE
APPENDS
APPETIT
APPLAUD
APPLETS
APPLIED
APPLIER
APPLIES
APPLING
APPLYTO
APPOINT
APPOSED
APPOSES
APPRISE
APPROVE
ASPECTS
ASPENCO
ASPERSE
ASPHALT
ASPIRED
ASPIRER
ASPIRES
ASPIRIN
ASPRAWL
ATPEACE
AUPAIRS

A••P•••

ADAPTED
ADAPTER
ADAPTOR
ADAPTTO
ADEPTAT
ADEPTER
ADEPTLY
ADIPOSE
ADOPTED
ADOPTEE
ADOPTER
ADSPACE
AIRPACK
AIRPARK
AIRPLAY
AIRPOPS
AIRPORT
AIRPOTS
AIRPUMP
AMAPOLA
ANAPEST
ANSPACH
ARAPAHO
ARMPITS
ASEPSIS
ASEPTIC
ASHPANS
ASHPITS
ATIPTOE
AUSPICE

A•••P••

ACCEPTS
ACOUPLE
ACTUPON
ADDUPTO
ADELPHI
ADOLPHE
AFROPOP
AGRIPPA
ALCOPOP
ALLOPEZ
APROPOS
ARUSPEX
ATROPHY
ATROPOS
AUTOPEN
AUTOPIA
AUTOPSY

A••••P•

AAAMAPS
AGRIPPA
AIRPOPS
ALETAPS
ALLCAPS
ANYHOPE
ATTEMPT

A•••••P

ACTEDUP
ADDEDUP
AFROPOP
AGALLOP
AIRDROP
AIREDUP
AIRPUMP
AIRSHIP
AIRTRAP
ALCOPOP
AMPEDUP
ANTEDUP
ANTESUP
ANTWERP

APHILIP
ARCLAMP
AREAMAP
ARTSHOP
ASHHEAP
ASKEDUP
ASSHARP
ATACLIP
ATEITUP

•AP•••••

BAPTISE
BAPTISM
BAPTIST
BAPTIZE
CAPABLE
CAPABLY
CAPADES
CAPAPIE
CAPEANN
CAPECOD
CAPEESH
CAPELET
CAPELLA
CAPEMAY
CAPERED
CAPFULS
CAPGUNS
CAPITAL
CAPITAN
CAPITOL
CAPLESS
CAPLETS
CAPNUTS
CAPOTES
CAPPERS
CAPPING
CAPRICE
CAPRINE
CAPSHAW
CAPSIZE
CAPSTAN
CAPSULE
CAPTAIN
CAPTION
CAPTIVA
CAPTIVE
CAPTORS
CAPTURE
CAPUANA
CAPUCHE
CAPULET
DAPHNES
DAPHNIA
DAPHNIS
DAPPING
DAPPLED
DAPPLES
GAPEDAT
GAPESAT
GAPKIDS
GAPLESS
GAPPING
HAPENNY
HAPKIDO
HAPLESS
HAPLOID
HAPPENS
HAPPIER
HAPPIFY
HAPPILY
HAPPYTO
HAPTICS
IAPETUS
JAPHETH
KAPITAL
KAPITSA
KAPTURE
LAPALMA
LAPBELT
LAPCATS
LAPDOGS
LAPELED
LAPERMS
LAPFULS
LAPLACA
LAPLACE
LAPLAND
LAPLATA
LAPORTE
LAPPERS
LAPPETS
LAPPING
LAPPISH
LAPROBE
LAPSANG
LAPSERS
LAPSING
LAPTOPS
LAPUTAN
LAPWARE
LAPWING
MAPPERS
MAPPING
MAPSOUT
NAPALMS
NAPHTHA
NAPIERS
NAPKINS
NAPLESS
NAPPERS
NAPPIER
NAPPIES
NAPPING
NAPSTER
NAPTIME
PAPADOC
PAPAGOS
PAPAYAS
PAPEETE
PAPELES
PAPERED
PAPERER
PAPIERS
PAPILLA
PAPISTS
PAPOOSE
PAPPIES
PAPRIKA
PAPUANS
PAPYRUS
RAPALLO
RAPANUI
RAPHAEL
RAPIDAN
RAPIDER
RAPIDLY
RAPIERS
RAPINES
RAPINIS
RAPPELS
RAPPERS
RAPPING
RAPPORT
RAPSONG
RAPSTAR
RAPTORS
RAPTUNE
RAPTURE
SAPHEAD
SAPIENS
SAPIENT
SAPLESS
SAPLING
SAPPERS
SAPPIER
SAPPILY
SAPPING
SAPPORO
SAPSAGO
TAPEDON
TAPEDUP
TAPEMAN
TAPEMEN
TAPERED
TAPESON
TAPESUP
TAPINGS
TAPINTO
TAPIOCA
TAPPANS
TAPPERS
TAPPETS
TAPPING
TAPROOM
TAPROOT
TAPSHOE
TAPSOFF
TAPSOUT
TAPSTER
VAPIDLY
VAPORED
VAPORER
VAPORUB
VAPOURS
VAPOURY
WAPITIS
WAPSHOT
YAPPERS
YAPPING
ZAPATAS
ZAPATEO
ZAPOTEC
ZAPPERS
ZAPPIER
ZAPPING

•A•P•••

BADPAST
BAGPIPE
CALPOLY
CAMPARI
CAMPBED
CAMPERS
CAMPHOR
CAMPIER
CAMPILY
CAMPING
CAMPION
CAMPOUT
CAMPSUP
CAPPERS
CAPPING
CARPALS
CARPARK
CARPELS
CARPERS
CARPETS
CARPING
CARPOOL
CARPORT
CARPOUS
CARPSAT
CASPARY
CASPIAN
DAMPDRY
DAMPENS
DAMPERS
DAMPEST
DAMPING
DAMPISH
DAMPMOP
DAMPOFF
DAPPING
DAPPLED
DAPPLES
DAUPHIN
DAYPACK
EARPLUG
FANPALM
GALPALS
GAPPING
GARPIKE
GASPARD
GASPERS
GASPING
GASPIPE
GASPUMP
GAWPERS
GAWPING
HADPULL
HAMPERS
HAMPTON
HAPPENS
HAPPIER
HAPPIFY
HAPPILY
HAPPYTO
HARPERS
HARPIES
HARPING
HARPIST
HARPOON
HARPSON
HASPING
HASPULL
HATPINS
JAMPACK
JASPERS
JASPERY
KAMPALA
LAMPERT
LAMPLIT
LAMPOIL
LAMPOON
LAMPREY
LAPPERS
LAPPETS
LAPPING
LAPPISH
MAGPIES
MALPASO
MAPPERS
MAPPING
MAUPRAT
MAYPOLE
NAIPAUL
NAPPERS
NAPPIER
NAPPIES
NAPPING
OAKPARK
PALPATE
PAMPERS
PANPIPE
PAPPIES
PAUPERS
PAWPAWS
RALPHIE
RAMPAGE
RAMPANT
RAMPART
RAMPING
RAMPSUP
RANPAST
RAPPELS
RAPPERS
RAPPING
RAPPORT
RASPERS
RASPIER
RASPING
RASPISH
RATPACK
SAMPANS
SAMPLED
SAMPLER
SAMPLES
SAMPRAS
SAMPSON
SAPPERS
SAPPIER
SAPPILY
SAPPING
SAPPORO
SAWPAST
SAWPITS
TADPOLE
TAMPAFL
TAMPERS
TAMPICO
TAMPING
TAPPANS
TAPPERS
TAPPETS
TAPPING
TARPITS
TARPONS
TAXPAID
VAMPERS
VAMPIER
VAMPING
VAMPIRA
VAMPIRE
VAMPISH
VANPELT
VANPOOL
WALPOLE
WAMPUMS
WARPAGE
WARPATH
WARPERS
WARPING
WASPIER
WASPILY
WASPISH
YAPPERS
YAPPING
YAWPERS
YAWPING
ZAPPERS
ZAPPIER
ZAPPING

•A••P••

BACKPAY
BAKEPAN
BASEPAY
CAGEPET
CAKEPAN
CALIPER
CALIPHS
CALYPSO
CANAPES
CANOPUS
CAPAPIE
CATSPAW
DACAPOS
DASHPOT
DAYSPAS
FAUXPAS
GALOPED
HAIRPIN
HANAPER
HARDPAN
HARDPUT
JACKPOT
KAKAPOS
LAYOPEN
LAYUPON
MADEPAR
MAKEPAR
MALEPIG
MANIPLE
MANIPUR
MAZEPPA
PANOPLY
PARAPET
PARAPHS
PAULPRY
RANUPTO
SALTPIT
SANDPIT
SATUPON
TAILPIN
WAREPIC
ZATOPEK

•A•••P•

AAAMAPS
BACKUPS
BADRAPS
BAGPIPE
BARHOPS
CALLUPS
CARHOPS
CARTOPS
CATALPA
CATNAPS
CATNIPS
CATSUPS
DAYHOPS
EARLAPS
FATLIPS
GALLOPS
GALUMPH
GASCAPS
GASPIPE
HANGUPS
LACEUPS
LAPTOPS
LARRUPS
LASHUPS
MAANDPA
MADCAPS
MAKEUPS
MANROPE
MARKUPS
MAZEPPA
PANPIPE
RAGMOPS
RAGTOPS
RANLAPS
RATEDPG
RAVEUPS
SATRAPS
SATRAPY
WAKEUPS
WALKUPS
WALLOPS
WARMUPS
WASHUPS

•A••••P

BABYBOP
BABYGAP
BACKSUP
BADTRIP
BALLSUP
BANGSUP
BANKSUP
BARKEEP
BARSOAP
CAGEDUP
CAGESUP
CAKEDUP
CAKESUP
CALLSUP
CAMPSUP
CANTRIP
CARTRIP
CASTSUP
CATCHUP
CATFLAP
DAMPMOP
DAYCAMP
DAYTRIP
EARCLIP
EARDROP
EARFLAP
EASEDUP
EASESUP
EATENUP
EATITUP
FAIRSUP
FANCYUP
GANGSUP
GASEDUP
GASESUP
GASLAMP
GASPUMP
HACKSUP
HADANIP
HAMITUP
HANDSUP
HANGSUP
HANSARP
HARDTOP
HASANIP
HAULSUP
JACKSUP
LACEDUP
LACESUP
LANDSUP
LASTLAP
MAINTOP
MAKESUP
MANTRAP
MARKSUP
MASTERP
MATCHUP
NAILSUP
NAILTIP
PACELAP
PACKSUP
PAIRSUP
PALMTOP
PARSNIP
PASTEUP
PATCHUP
PAYSLIP
RACEDUP
RACESUP
RACKSUP
RAGSHOP
RAISEUP
RAKEDUP
RAKESUP
RAMPSUP
RANDEEP
RANITUP
RATECAP
RATTRAP
SACKSUP
SALMONP
SATATOP
SAVEDUP
SAVESUP
TACKSUP
TAKENUP
TAKESUP
TALKSUP
TALLYUP
TANKSUP
TANKTOP
TAPEDUP
TAPESUP
TARTSUP
VANCAMP
WAITSUP
WAKEDUP
WAKESUP
WALLMAP
WALLSUP
WARMSUP
WARSHIP
WAXEDUP
WAXESUP

••AP•••

ADAPTED
ADAPTER
ADAPTOR
ADAPTTO
AMAPOLA
ANAPEST
ARAPAHO
CHAPALA
CHAPATI
CHAPEAU
CHAPELS
CHAPLET
CHAPLIN
CHAPMAN
CHAPMEN
CHAPPED
CHAPPIE
CHAPTER
CLAPFOR
CLAPPED
CLAPPER
CLAPTON
COAPTED
CRAPING
CRAPOLA
CRAPOUT
CRAPPIE
DIAPERS
DIAPHAN
DRAPERS
DRAPERY
DRAPING
ELAPIDS
ELAPSED
ELAPSES
FLAPPED
FLAPPER
FRAPPES
GRAPERY
GRAPHED
GRAPHIC
GRAPIER
GRAPNEL
GRAPPAS
GRAPPLE
HEAPERS
HEAPING
HEAPSOF
HEAPSON
HEAPSUP
INAPILE
INAPOEM
INAPOKE
INAPRIL
INAPTER
INAPTLY
LEAPDAY
LEAPERS
LEAPFOR
LEAPING
LEAPSAT
LEAPSIN
LEAPSON
LEAPSUP
LEAPTAT
LEAPTIN
LEAPTON
LEAPTUP
PEAPODS
PGAPROS
QUAPAWS
REAPERS
REAPING
REAPPLY
SCAPULA
SEAPORT
SHAPELY
SHAPERS
SHAPEUP
SHAPING
SHAPIRO
SLAPPED
SLAPPER
SLAPSON
SNAPONS
SNAPPEA
SNAPPED
SNAPPER
SNAPPLE
SNAPSAT
SNAPSON
SNAPSTO
SNAPSUP
SOAPBOX
SOAPERS
SOAPIER
SOAPILY
SOAPING
SOAPNET
SOAPPAD
SOAPSUP
STAPLED
STAPLER
STAPLES
SWAPPED
SWAPPER
TEAPOTS
TEAPOYS
TRAPEZE
TRAPGUN
TRAPPED
TRAPPER
UNAPTLY
WEAPONS
WHAPPED
WRAPPED
WRAPPER
WRAPSUP
WRAPUPS

••A•P••

BEARPAW
BEARPIT
BIASPLY
CHAMPED
CHAMPER
CHAPPED
CHAPPIE
CHARPAK
CLAMPED
CLAMPER
CLAMPON
CLAPPED
CLAPPER
CLASPED
CLASPER
CLAYPIT
COALPIT
CRABPOT
CRAMPED
CRAMPON
CRAPPIE
DEADPAN
EXAMPLE
FLAPPED
FLAPPER
FRAPPES
GRAMPAS
GRAMPUS
GRANPAS
GRAPPAS
GRAPPLE
GRASPAT
GRASPED
GRASPER
HEADPIN
INASPIN
INASPOT
LOAFPAN
MEATPIE
NEARPAR
PEATPOT
PLAYPEN
REAPPLY
SCALPED
SCALPEL
SCALPER
SCAMPED
SCAMPER
SCARPED
SHAMPOO
SHARPED
SHARPEI
SHARPEN
SHARPER
SHARPIE
SHARPLY
SLAPPED
SLAPPER
SNAPPEA
SNAPPED
SNAPPER
SNAPPLE
SOAPPAD
STAMPED
STAMPER
STAYPUT
SWAMPED
SWAPPED
SWAPPER
TRAIPSE
TRAMPAS
TRAMPED
TRAMPER
TRAMPLE
TRAPPED
TRAPPER
WHAPPED
WRAPPED
WRAPPER

••A••P•

AAAMAPS
CHALUPA
DIALUPS
GRANDPA
LEADUPS
MAANDPA
PLATYPI
READAPT
READOPT
SEAMAPS
TEACUPS
UNADEPT
WRAPUPS

••A•••P

AGALLOP
ATACLIP
BEADSUP
BEAMSUP
BEANDIP
BEARSUP
BEATCOP
BEATSUP
BLAZEUP
BOARDUP
BRACEUP
CHAINUP
CHALKUP
CHATSUP
CLAMDIP
CLAMSUP
CRACKUP
CRANKUP
CRATEUP
DEALSUP
DEALTUP
DIALSUP
DRAGSUP
DRANKUP
DRAWNUP
DRAWSUP
FLAMEUP
FLAREUP
FLATTOP
FRAMEUP
GEARSUP
GLAMSUP
GRATEUP
HEADSUP
HEALSUP
HEAPSUP
HEATSUP
INAHEAP
INASNAP
INATRAP
JEANARP
LEADSUP
LEAPSUP
LEAPTUP
LOADSUP
ONATRIP
PEASOUP
PHARLAP
PLAYSUP
REACHUP
READSUP
REARSUP
ROADMAP
SCALEUP
SCALLOP
SCAREUP
SCARFUP
SEALSUP
SEATRIP
SHAKEUP
SHAPEUP
SLACKUP
SLANTUP
SMACKUP
SMASHUP
SNAGSUP
SNAPSUP
SNARLUP
SNAZZUP
SOAKSUP
SOAPSUP
STACKUP
STANDUP
STANKUP
STARMAP
STARTUP
STAYSUP
SWANKUP
TEAMSUP
TEARSUP
TEASEUP
TEASHOP
TRADEUP
WHATSUP
WRACKUP
WRAPSUP

•••AP••

BEHAPPY
BIGAPES
CANAPES
CAPAPIE
CHEAPEN
CHEAPER
CHEAPIE
CHEAPLY
CHIAPAS
CHIAPET
DACAPOS
DECAPOD
DOGAPES
ECHAPPE
ESCAPED
ESCAPEE
ESCAPER
ESCAPES
FLEAPIT

GOKAPUT
HANAPER
HEXAPOD
IMHAPPY
KAKAPOS
LSHAPED
MCPAPER
ONPAPER
OSHAPED
PARAPET
PARAPHS
PITAPAT
RELAPSE
REPAPER
RETAPED
RETAPES
SCRAPED
SCRAPER
SCRAPES
SCRAPPY
SERAPES
SERAPHS
SERAPIS
SODAPOP
SSHAPED
STRAPIN
STRAPON
SYNAPSE
TSHAPED
TSHAPES
TVTAPES
UNCAPED
UNHAPPY
UNTAPED
UNTAPES
USHAPED
USHAPES
VSHAPED
VSHAPES
YSHAPED
YSHAPES

•••A•P•

BEHAPPY
CATALPA
CCLAMPS
DECAMPS
ECHAPPE
ELCAMPO
ENCAMPS
ESCARPS
IMHAPPY
ONRAMPS
PREAMPS
REVAMPS
SCRAPPY
THEALPS
UNHAPPY
UNHASPS
UNRASPY
YUCAIPA

•••A••P

AREAMAP
BREAKUP
CLEANUP
CLEARUP
DREAMUP
ESCALOP
FLEADIP
FLOATUP
GETATIP
GOTATIP
HADANIP
HASANIP
LIEATOP
SATATOP
SITATOP
SNEAKUP
SODAPOP
SPEAKUP
STEAMUP
TOTALUP

••••AP•

AAAMAPS
ALETAPS
ALLCAPS
BADRAPS
BEDRAPE
BITMAPS
BUMRAPS
BURLAPS
CATNAPS
DEWLAPS
DIDLAPS
DIGRAPH
DOGNAPS
EARLAPS
ENTRAPS
ENWRAPS
EPITAPH
GASCAPS
GELCAPS
GESTAPO
GODPAPA
GOESAPE
GONEAPE
GUNLAPS
HOTCAPS
HUBCAPS
ICECAPS
INSHAPE
KIDNAPS
MADCAPS
MIDCAPS
MISHAPS
OUTRAPS
PERHAPS
PERIAPT
PETNAPS
PRETAPE
RANLAPS
READAPT
REDCAPS
REDTAPE
REGRAPH
RELEAPS
RESHAPE
RESNAPS
RESOAPS
RETRAPS
REWRAPS
RIPRAPS
RUNLAPS
SATRAPS
SATRAPY
SCHNAPS
SEAMAPS
SKICAPS
SKYCAPS
SKYMAPS
SNOCAPS
THECAPE
THERAPY
TOECAPS
TOETAPS
TOPKAPI
TSTRAPS
UNDRAPE
UNSNAPS
UNTRAPS
UNWRAPS
UPHEAPS
UPLEAPS
UPLEAPT
VCRTAPE
WENTAPE
WETNAPS

••••A•P

ARCLAMP
ASSHARP
BEDLAMP
DAYCAMP
DUCHAMP
ENCLASP
EPICARP
EXOCARP
FOGLAMP
GASLAMP
HANSARP
JEANARP
JOECAMP
MUDWASP
OFFRAMP
OILLAMP
RECLASP
REGRASP
RESTAMP
SUNLAMP
UNCLAMP
UNCLASP
UNCRAMP
UNSHARP
VANCAMP

•••••AP

AIRTRAP
AREAMAP
ASHHEAP
BABYGAP
BARSOAP
BEERTAP
BELLLAP
CATFLAP
DROPCAP
EARFLAP
FLYTRAP
FURWRAP
GIDDYAP
GRIDMAP
HEELTAP
INAHEAP
INASNAP
INATRAP
INKYCAP
KNEECAP
LASTLAP
LEGTRAP
LENSCAP
LOVETAP
LYESOAP
MANTRAP
MEDIGAP
MUDFLAP
OLDCHAP
OPENTAP
OUTLEAP
OVERLAP
PACELAP
PHARLAP
PINESAP
PREWRAP
RATECAP
RATTRAP
RESTRAP
ROADMAP
ROOTCAP
SITEMAP
SNOWCAP
STARMAP
STOPGAP
TREESAP
UNSTRAP
WALLMAP
WINESAP
WIRETAP

AQ•••••

AQUAMAN
AQUARIA
AQUATIC
AQUAVIT
AQUEOUS
AQUIFER
AQUINAS
AQUIVER

A•Q••••

ACQUIRE
ACQUITS
ALQUIST
ASQUIET
ASQUINT
ASQUITH

A•••Q••

ANTIQUE

A•••••Q

AVENUEQ

•AQ••••

VAQUERO

•A•Q•••

BANQUES
BANQUET
BARQUES
BASQUES
CASQUED
CASQUES
DAYQUIL
JACQUES
LACQUER
MARQUEE
MARQUES
MARQUEZ
MARQUIS
MASQUER
MASQUES
PACQUIN
PARQUET
RACQUET
SACQUES
VASQUEZ
YANQUIS

•A••Q••

BAROQUE
CACIQUE
LALIQUE
MACAQUE

••AQ•••

CLAQUES
JOAQUIN
OPAQUES
PLAQUES

••A•Q••

GIAUQUE

••A••Q•

PSANDQS

•••AQ••

MACAQUE

••••AQ•

COMPAQS

AR•••••

ARABIAN
ARABICA
ARABICS
ARABIST
ARABLES
ARACARI
ARACHNE
ARACHNO
ARAFTOF
ARAFURA
ARAGORN
ARALSEA
ARAMAIC
ARAMARK
ARAMEAN
ARAMIDS
ARANEID
ARANTXA
ARAPAHO
ARBACES
ARBITER
ARBOLES
ARBORED
ARBOURS
ARBUTUS
ARCADED
ARCADES
ARCADIA
ARCANUM
ARCHAIC
ARCHERS
ARCHERY
ARCHEST
ARCHFOE
ARCHIES
ARCHING
ARCHIVE
ARCHONS
ARCHSEE
ARCHWAY
ARCINGS
ARCLAMP
ARCSINE
ARCUATE
ARCWELD
ARDECHE
ARDENCY
ARDMORE
ARDOURS
ARDUOUS
AREAMAP
AREARUG
AREAWAY
ARECIBO
ARENOSE
ARENSKY
AREOLAE
AREOLAR
AREOLAS
AREOLES
ARETINO
ARGALIS
ARGANTE
ARGENTI
ARGENTO
ARGENTS
ARGONNE
ARGUERS
ARGUING
ARGUSES
ARGYLES
ARIADNE
ARIANES
ARIDEST
ARIDITY
ARIETTA
ARIETTE
ARIGATO
ARIKARA
ARIOSOS
ARIOSTO
ARISING
ARISTAE
ARISTAS
ARISTOS
ARIZONA
ARLBERG
ARLEDGE
ARMADAS
ARMBAND
ARMBONE
ARMENIA
ARMFULS
ARMHOLE
ARMLESS
ARMLETS
ARMLIKE
ARMLOAD
ARMLOCK
ARMOIRE
ARMORED
ARMORER
ARMOURS
ARMOURY
ARMPITS
ARMREST
ARMYANT
ARNICAS
ARNOLDS
ARONNAX
AROUSAL
AROUSED
AROUSER
AROUSES
ARRABAL
ARRACKS
ARRAIGN
ARRANGE
ARRASES
ARRAYAL
ARRAYED
ARRAYER
ARREARS
ARRESTS
ARRIERE
ARRISES
ARRIVAL
ARRIVED
ARRIVER
ARRIVES
ARROYOS
ARSENAL
ARSENIC
ARSENIQ
ARSHILE
ARTBOOK
ARTCARS
ARTDECO
ARTEMIS
ARTEMUS
ARTERIO
ARTFAIR
ARTFERN
ARTFILM
ARTFORM
ARTHURC
ARTHURM
ARTHURS
ARTICLE
ARTIEST
ARTISAN
ARTISTE
ARTISTS
ARTLESS
ARTROCK
ARTSALE
ARTSHOP
ARTSHOW
ARTSIER
ARTSONG
ARTWALL
ARTWARE
ARTWORK
ARUBANS
ARUGULA
ARUNDEL
ARUSPEX

A•R••••

AARATED
ABRADED
ABRADER
ABRADES
ABRAHAM
ABRAXAS
ABREAST
ABRIDGE
ABRILES
ABROACH
ABRUZZI
ACREAGE
ACRIDLY
ACROBAT
ACRONYM
ACRYLIC
ADRATES
ADRENAL
ADRIANA
AERATED
AERATES
AERATOR
AERIALS
AERIEST
AEROBAT
AEROBES
AEROBIC
AEROSOL
AFRAMES
AFRICAN
AFROPOP
AGREEON
AGREERS
AGREETO
AGRIBIZ
AGRIPPA
AGROUND
AIRACES
AIRBAGS
AIRBALL
AIRBASE
AIRBILL
AIRBOAT
AIRCOOL
AIRCREW
AIRDAMS
AIRDATE
AIRDRIE
AIRDROP
AIRDUCT
AIREDUP
AIRFARE
AIRFLOW
AIRFOIL
AIRFONE
AIRGLOW
AIRGUNS
AIRHEAD
AIRHOLE
AIRHORN
AIRHOSE
AIRIEST
AIRINGS
AIRKISS
AIRLANE
AIRLESS
AIRLIFT
AIRLIKE
AIRLINE
AIRLOCK
AIRLOGS
AIRMADA
AIRMAIL
AIRMASS
AIRMILE
AIRNESS
AIRPACK
AIRPARK
AIRPLAY
AIRPOPS
AIRPORT
AIRPOTS
AIRPUMP
AIRRACE
AIRRAGE
AIRRAID
AIRSACS
AIRSHIP
AIRSHOW
AIRSICK
AIRSIGN
AIRSOCK
AIRSOUT
AIRTANK
AIRTAXI
AIRTIME
AIRTRAP
AIRTUBE
AIRVENT
AIRWARS
AIRWAVE
AIRWAYS
AIRWICK
AIRWOLF
AKRONOH
ALREADY
ALRIGHT
ALROKER
ALROSEN
AMRADIO
AMREETA
AMRITAS
APRICOT
APRIORI
APRONED
APROPOS
ARRABAL
ARRACKS
ARRAIGN
ARRANGE
ARRASES
ARRAYAL
ARRAYED
ARRAYER
ARREARS
ARRESTS
ARRIERE
ARRISES
ARRIVAL
ARRIVED
ARRIVER
ARRIVES
ARROYOS
ATRIUMS
ATROPHY
ATROPOS
AURALEE
AURALLY
AUREATE
AUREOLA
AUREOLE
AURICLE
AURISTS
AURORAE
AURORAL
AURORAS

A••R•••

ABORTED
ACARIDS
ACCRETE
ACCRUAL
ACCRUED
ACCRUES
ACERATE
ACERBIC
ACEROLA
ACEROSE
ACORNED
ACTRESS
ADDRESS
ADORERS
ADORING
ADORNED
ADORNER
AFARCRY
AFFRAYS
AFFRONT
AGARICS
AGGRESS
AIGRETS
AIRRACE
AIRRAGE
AIRRAID
AKERLOF
ALARBUS
ALARCON
ALARMED
ALARMER
ALARUMS
ALDRICH
ALERTED
ALERTER
ALERTLY
ALERTTO
ALFREDA
ALFREDE
ALFREDO
ALFREDU
ALGREEN
ALLRISE
AMARONE
AMBRIES
AMBROSE
AMERADA
AMERCED
AMERCER
AMERCES
AMERICA
AMERIGO
AMERIKA
AMERIND
AMORIST
AMOROSO
AMOROUS
AMTRACK
AMTRACS
ANARCHS
ANARCHY
ANDRADE
ANDREAS
ANDRESS
ANDREWS
ANDROID
ANDROUS
ANEROID
ANGRIER
ANGRILY
ANGRYAT
ANORAKS
ANYROAD
APERCUS
APERIES
APERSON
APPRISE
APPROVE
ARMREST
ARTROCK
ASARULE
ASCRIBE
ASHRAMS
ASPRAWL
ASTREAM
ASTRIDE
ATARAXY
ATCROSS
ATGRADE
ATHRILL
ATTRACT
ATTRITE
ATTRITS
AVARICE
AVERAGE
AVERELL
AVERILL
AVERNAL
AVERNUS
AVERRED
AVERTED
AVERTER
AWARDED
AWARDEE
AWARDER
AWAREOF
AWAREST
AXLROSE
AYKROYD
AYNRAND
AZOREAN
AZORIAN
AZURITE

A•••R••

AALARGE
ABJURED
ABJURER
ABJURES
ABSORBS
ACCORDS
ACCURST
ACHERON
ACTORLY
ADHERED
ADHERER
ADHERES
ADJURED
ADJURER
ADJURES
ADJUROR
ADMIRAL
ADMIRED
ADMIRER
ADMIRES
ADSORBS
ADVERBS
ADVERSE
ADVERTS
AELFRIC
AFEARED
AFFIRMS
AFFORDS
AILERON
AIRCREW
AIRDRIE
AIRDROP
AIRTRAP
ALBERTA
ALBERTI
ALBERTO
ALBIREO
ALBORAK
ALDORAY
ALEARDI
ALEGRIA
ALFEROV
ALFORJA
ALGARVE
ALGERIA
ALLBRAN
ALLERGY
ALLURED
ALLURER
ALLURES
ALMERIA
ALSORAN
ALTERED
ALTERER
ALVAREZ
ALWORTH
AMHARIC
AMHERST
AMNERIS
AMPERES
AMSCRAY
ANAGRAM
ANDIRON
ANDORRA
ANGERED
ANGORAS
ANITRAS
ANKARAN
ANTARES
ANTERUS
ANTHRAX
APAIROF
APPARAT
APPAREL
APTERAL
APTERYX
AQUARIA
ARBORED
AREARUG
ARMORED
ARMORER
ARTERIO
ASAGRAY
ASCARED
ASFARAS
ASHTRAY
ASHTREE
ASMARAN
ASPERSE
ASPIRED
ASPIRER
ASPIRES
ASPIRIN
ASSERTS
ASSORTS
ASSURED
ASSURER
ASSURES
ASSUROR
ASSYRIA
ASTARTE
ASTERIX
ASTORIA
ATECROW
ATFIRST
ATHIRST
ATLARGE
ATTHREE
ATTIRED
ATTIRER
ATTIRES
ATWORST
AUBERGE
AUBURNS
AUBURNU
AUGURAL
AUGURED
AUGURER
AURORAE
AURORAL
AURORAS
AUSTRAL
AUSTRIA
AUTARCH
AUTARKY
AVERRED
AVEYRON
AXELROD

A••••R•

ABASERS
ABATERS
ABATORS
ABELARD
ABIDERS
ABINTRA
ABUSERS
ACQUIRE

ACTUARY
ADAWARE
ADJOURN
ADORERS
AFARCRY
AFFAIRE
AFFAIRS
AGENTRY
AGREERS
AIRFARE
AIRHORN
AIRPARK
AIRPORT
AIRWARS
ALBSURE
ALEGARS
ALEYARD
ALFIERI
ALGEBRA
ALGIERS
ALIFORM
ALINERS
ALLEARS
ALLEGRA
ALLEGRO
ALLHERE
ALMONRY
ALPHARD
ALTDORF
ALTHORN
AMATORY
AMBLERS
AMPHORA
AMUSERS
ANCHORS
ANDMORE
ANDORRA
ANGLERS
ANKLERS
ANSWERS
ANTBIRD
ANTFARM
ANTHERS
ANTIART
ANTLERS
ANTWERP
ANYMORE
APPEARS
APRIORI
ARACARI
ARAFURA
ARAGORN
ARAMARK
ARBOURS
ARCHERS
ARCHERY
ARDMORE
ARDOURS
ARGUERS
ARIKARA
ARLBERG
ARMOIRE
ARMOURS
ARMOURY
ARREARS
ARRIERE
ARTCARS
ARTFERN
ARTFORM
ARTHURC
ARTHURM
ARTHURS
ARTWARE
ARTWORK
ASALARK
ASHBERY
ASHBURN
ASHBURY
ASHFORD
ASHLARS
ASSHARP
ASTAIRE
ATATURK
ATEDIRT
ATEMORE
ATHEART
ATHWART
ATMCARD
ATONERS
ATTHIRD
AUPAIRS
AUSTERE
AUSTERS
AUTEURS
AUTHORS
AVATARS
AVOWERS
AWAKERS
AWKWARD

A•••••R

ABETTER
ABETTOR
ABJURER
ABRADER
ABUTTER
ACCEDER
ACCUSER
ACHEFOR
ACTFOUR
ACTSFOR
ADAPTER
ADAPTOR
ADDUCER
ADEPTER
ADHERER
ADJURER
ADJUROR
ADMIRER
ADOLLAR
ADOPTER
ADORNER
ADVISER
ADVISOR
AERATOR
AFFIXER
AGEFOUR
AGUTTER
AIMSFOR
ALARMER
ALCAZAR
ALERTER
ALIENOR
ALIGNER
ALLAYER
ALLEGER
ALLOVER
ALLSTAR
ALLURER
ALMONER
ALPINER
ALROKER
ALTERER
ALUNSER
AMASSER
AMATEUR
AMENDER
AMERCER
AMMETER
ANDOVER
ANGRIER
ANGULAR
ANNOYER
ANNULAR
ANOTHER
ANTBEAR
ANTIWAR
ANTSIER
APPLIER
AQUIFER
AQUIVER
ARBITER
AREOLAR
ARMORER
AROUSER
ARRAYER
ARRIVER
ARTFAIR
ARTSIER
ASHIVER
ASIMMER
ASKOVER
ASKSFOR
ASPIRER
ASSAYER
ASSUMER
ASSURER
ASSUROR
ASTUTER
ASUNDER
ATELIER
ATEOVER
ATTIRER
ATWATER
AUDITOR
AUGURER
AVENGER
AVERTER
AVIATOR
AVOIDER
AWAITER
AWARDER
AWOONOR
AXILLAR
AZINGER

•AR••••

AARATED
BARACUS
BARANOF
BARBARA
BARBARY
BARBATE
BARBEAU
BARBELL
BARBERA
BARBERS
BARBETS
BARBIES
BARBILL
BARBING
BARBUDA
BARBULE
BARCARS
BARCLAY
BARCODE
BARDEEN
BAREGES
BARENTS
BARETTA
BAREXAM
BARFBAG
BARGAIN
BARGEIN
BARGERS
BARGING
BARHOPS
BARISTA
BARITES
BARKEEP
BARKERS
BARKIER
BARKING
BARKLEY
BARKSAT
BARLESS
BARLEYS
BARLICK
BARMAID
BARMIER
BARNABY
BARNARD
BARNEYS
BARNING
BARNONE
BARNOWL
BARNRED
BARNUMS
BAROLOS
BARONET
BAROQUE
BARQUES
BARRACK
BARRAGE
BARRELS
BARRENS
BARRETS
BARRETT
BARRIER
BARRING
BARRIOS
BARRONS
BARROOM
BARROWS
BARSOAP
BARSTOW
BARTABS
BARTEND
BARTERS
BARTLES
BARTLET
BARTOLO
BARTRAY
BARWARE
BARYONS
CARABOO
CARACAS
CARAFES
CARAMBA
CARAMEL
CARAMIA
CARAVAN
CARAVEL
CARAWAY
CARBARN
CARBIDE
CARBINE
CARBONS
CARBOYS
CARBRAS
CARCARE
CARCASS
CARCLUB
CARCOAT
CARDERS
CARDIAC
CARDIAL
CARDIFF
CARDING
CARDIUM
CARDKEY
CARDOOR
CARDOZO
CAREDTO
CAREENS
CAREERS
CAREFOR
CAREFUL
CARESTO
CARFARE
CARFREE
CARFULS
CARGOES
CARHOPS
CARHORN
CARIBES
CARIBOO
CARIBOU
CARINAE
CARINAS
CARIOCA
CARIOLE
CARIOUS
CARJACK
CARKEYS
CARKING
CARLENE
CARLESS
CARLING
CARLOAD
CARLOAN
CARLOTA
CARLOTS
CARLSON
CARLTON
CARLYLE
CARMELA
CARMINA
CARMINE
CARNABY
CARNAGE
CARNERA
CARNETS
CARNIES
CAROLED
CAROLER
CAROLII
CAROLYN
CAROMED
CAROTID
CAROTIN
CAROUSE
CARPALS
CARPARK
CARPELS
CARPERS
CARPETS
CARPING
CARPOOL
CARPORT
CARPOUS
CARPSAT
CARRARA
CARRELS
CARRERA
CARRERE
CARRIED
CARRIER
CARRIES
CARROLL
CARROTS
CARROTY
CARRYIN
CARRYON
CARSALE
CARSEAT
CARSHOW
CARTAGE
CARTALK
CARTELS
CARTERS
CARTIER
CARTING
CARTIRE
CARTOFF
CARTONS
CARTOON
CARTOPS
CARTRIP
CARTSIN
CARVELS
CARVERS
CARVING
CARWASH
DAREFUL
DARENOT
DARESAY
DARESTO
DAREZZO
DARIUSI
DARKAGE
DARKENS
DARKEST
DARKISH
DARKLED
DARKLES
DARKMAN
DARKRED
DARKTAN
DARLEEN
DARLENE
DARLING
DARNELL
DARNERS
DARNING
DARRYLF
DARTERS
DARTGUN
DARTING
DARTLED
DARTLES
DARTOFF
DARWELL
EARACHE
EARBONE
EARBUDS
EARCLIP
EARDROP
EARDRUM
EARFLAP
EARFULS
EARHART
EARHOLE
EARLAPS
EARLDOM
EARLESS
EARLETS
EARLIER
EARLIES
EARLIKE
EARLOBE
EARLOCK
EARLYON
EARMARK
EARMUFF
EARNERS
EARNEST
EARNING
EARNSIT
EARPLUG
EARRING
EARSHOT
EARTABS
EARTAGS
EARTHED
EARTHEN
EARTHLY
EARWIGS
FARADAY
FARAWAY
FARCEUR
FARCING
FAREAST
FAREBOX
FAREWAR
FARFELS
FARGOND
FARGONE
FARINAS
FARLEFT
FARMAID
FARMBOY
FARMERS
FARMERY
FARMGAL
FARMING
FARMORE
FARMOUT
FARNESS
FAROESE
FAROUKI
FARRAGO
FARRELL
FARRIER
FARROWS
FARSEER
FARSIDE
FARTHER
FARTLEK
FARWEST
GARAGED
GARAGES
GARBAGE
GARBAGY
GARBING
GARBLED
GARBLER
GARBLES
GARCONS
GARDENA
GARDENS
GARDNER
GARGLED
GARGLER
GARGLES
GARLAND
GARLICS
GARLITS
GARMENT
GARNEAU
GARNERS
GARNETS
GARNETT
GARNISH
GARONNE
GAROTTE
GARPIKE
GARRETS
GARRETT
GARRICK
GARROTE
GARTERS
HARBACH
HARBORS
HARBOUR
HARBURG
HARDDAY
HARDEES
HARDENS
HARDEST
HARDHAT
HARDHIT
HARDIER
HARDILY
HARDING
HARDISH
HARDPAN
HARDPUT
HARDSET
HARDSIX
HARDTEN
HARDTOP
HARDWAY
HARDWON
HARHARS
HARICOT
HARKENS
HARKING
HARLAND
HARLEYS
HARLINE
HARLOTS
HARMERS
HARMFUL
HARMING
HARMONY
HARNESS
HARNICK
HAROLDI
HARPERS
HARPIES
HARPING
HARPIST
HARPOON
HARPSON
HARRAHS
HARRIED
HARRIER
HARRIES
HARRIET
HARRODS
HARROLD
HARROWS
HARSHEN
HARSHER
HARSHLY
HARTACK
HARTLEY
HARTMAN
HARTMUT
HARVARD
HARVEST
HARWELL
JARDINE
JARDINS
JARFULS
JARGONS
JARGONY
JARLESS
JAROMIR
JARRELL
JARRETT
JARRING
JARROTT
KARACHI
KARAJAN
KARAKUM
KARAOKE
KARASEA
KARATES
KARLOFF
KARLOVY
KARLSON
KAROLYI
LARAINE
LARAMIE
LARCENY
LARCHEN
LARCHES
LARDERS
LARDIER
LARDING
LARDNER
LARDONS
LAREDOS
LARGELY
LARGENT
LARGEOJ
LARGESS
LARGEST
LARGISH
LARIATS
LARKERS
LARKIER
LARKING
LARKINS
LARKISH
LAROCHE
LARRUPS
LARUSSA
MARACAS
MARANTZ
MARAUDS
MARBLED
MARBLER
MARBLES
MARCATO
MARCEAU
MARCELS
MARCHED
MARCHER
MARCHES
MARCHON
MARCONI
MARCUSE
MARDIAN
MARENGO
MARGATE
MARGAUX
MARGERY
MARGINS
MARGRET
MARHAUS
MARIANA
MARIANO
MARIDAS
MARIDOS
MARILLA
MARILYN
MARIMBA
MARINAS
MARINER
MARINES
MARITAL
MARKERS
MARKETS
MARKHAM
MARKIII
MARKING
MARKKAA
MARKOFF
MARKOUT
MARKOVA
MARKSUP
MARKUPS
MARKVII
MARLENE
MARLIER
MARLINS
MARLOWE
MARMARA
MARMION
MARMOTS
MARNIER
MAROONS
MARQUEE
MARQUES
MARQUEZ
MARQUIS
MARRERS
MARRIED
MARRIES
MARRING
MARRONS
MARROWS
MARRYAT
MARRYIN
MARRYME
MARSALA
MARSBAR
MARSDEN
MARSHAL
MARSHES
MARSRED
MARSTON
MARTENS
MARTIAL
MARTIAN
MARTINA
MARTINI
MARTINO
MARTINS
MARTINU
MARTINV
MARTIUS
MARTYRS
MARULLO
MARUSJA
MARVELL
MARVELS
MARVIER
MARXIAN
MARXISM
MARXIST
MARYANN
MARYKAY
MARYLOU
MARYURE
NARAYAN
NARRATE
NARROWS
NARTHEX
NARVAEZ
NARWHAL
OARLESS
OARLIKE
OARLOCK
OARSMAN
OARSMEN
PARABLE
PARADED
PARADER
PARADES
PARADOR
PARADOX
PARAGON
PARAIBA
PARAMUS
PARAPET
PARAPHS
PARASKI
PARASOL
PARATUS
PARBAKE
PARBOIL
PARCELS
PARCHED
PARCHES
PARDNER
PARDONS
PARENTS
PARFAIT
PARFIVE
PARFOUR
PARFUMS
PARGERS
PARGING
PARIAHS
PARIBUS
PARINGS
PARKADE
PARKAVE
PARKERS
PARKING
PARKINS
PARKMAN
PARKSIT
PARKWAY
PARLAYS
PARLEYS
PARLORS
PARLOUR
PARLOUS
PARODIC
PAROLED
PAROLEE
PAROLES
PARONYM
PAROTID
PARQUET
PARRIED
PARRIER
PARRIES
PARRING
PARRISH
PARROTS
PARSECS
PARSEES
PARSERS
PARSING
PARSLEY
PARSNIP
PARSONS
PARTAKE
PARTIAL
PARTIED
PARTIER
PARTIES
PARTIII
PARTING
PARTITA
PARTITE
PARTNER
PARTONE
PARTOOK
PARTTWO
PARTWAY
PARTYER
PARTYON
PARURES
PARVENU
RAREBIT
RAREGAS
RARITAN
SARACEN
SARALEE
SARANAC
SARAWAK
SARAZEN
SARCASM
SARDINE
SARGENT
SARNOFF
SARONGS
SAROYAN
SARTORS
SARUMAN
TARANTO
TARBABY
TARBELL
TARDIER
TARDILY
TARGETS
TARHEEL
TARIFFS
TARMACS
TARNISH
TAROILS
TARPITS
TARPONS
TARRIED
TARRIER
TARRIES
TARRING
TARSALS
TARTANS
TARTARE
TARTARS
TARTEST
TARTIER
TARTILY
TARTING
TARTISH
TARTLET
TARTSUP
TARZANA
TARZANS
VARIANT
VARIATE
VARIERS
VARIETY
VARIOUS
VARITEK
VARLAAM
VARLETS
VARMINT
VARNISH
VARRICK
VARSITY
VARYING
WARBABY
WARBLED
WARBLER
WARBLES

WARBOND
WARBURG
WARCLUB
WARDENS
WARDERS
WARDING
WARDOFF
WAREPIC
WARFARE
WARGAME
WARGODS
WARHAWK
WARHEAD
WARHERO
WARIEST
WARLESS
WARLIKE
WARLOCK
WARLORD
WARMERS
WARMEST
WARMING
WARMISH
WARMSTO
WARMSUP
WARMUPS
WARNING
WARNOFF
WARNSOF
WARPAGE
WARPATH
WARPERS
WARPING
WARRANT
WARRENG
WARRENS
WARRING
WARRIOR
WARROOM
WARSHIP
WARTHOG
WARTIER
WARTIME
WARTORN
WARVETS
WARWICK
WARWORN
WARZONE
YARDAGE
YARDARM
YARDERS
YARDING
YARDMAN
YARDMEN
YARNELL
YARNING
YARROWS

•A•R•••

BADRAPS
BAHRAIN
BAHREIN
BARRACK
BARRAGE
BARRELS
BARRENS
BARRETS
BARRETT
BARRIER
BARRING
BARRIOS
BARRONS
BARROOM
BARROWS
BASRHIN
BAYRUMS
CABRIDE
CABRINI
CABRIOS
CAIRENE
CAIRNED
CAMRYLE
CAPRICE
CAPRINE
CARRARA
CARRELS
CARRERA
CARRERE
CARRIED
CARRIER
CARRIES
CARROLL
CARROTS
CARROTY
CARRYIN
CARRYON
CATRIGS
DACRONS
DAIRIES
DAIRYER
DARRYLF
DATRILS
DAYROOM
EARRING
FABRICS
FABRIZI
FAERIES
FAEROES
FAIREST
FAIRFAX
FAIRIES
FAIRING
FAIRISH
FAIROFF
FAIRSEX
FAIRSUP
FAIRUSE
FAIRWAY
FARRAGO
FARRELL
FARRIER
FARROWS
GABRIEL
GAGREEL
GAGRULE
GARRETS
GARRETT
GARRICK
GARROTE
HAARLEM
HADRIAN
HADRONS
HADROOM
HAIRCUT
HAIRDOS
HAIRDYE
HAIRGEL
HAIRIER
HAIRNET
HAIRPIN
HARRAHS
HARRIED
HARRIER
HARRIES
HARRIET
HARRODS
HARROLD
HARROWS
HASROOM
HATRACK
HATREDS
HAYRACK
HAYRICK
HAYRIDE
IATRICS
JARRELL
JARRETT
JARRING
JARROTT
KATRINA
KATRINE
LABRATS
LACRIMO
LADRONE
LAERTES
LAIRING
LAPROBE
LARRUPS
LATRELL
LATRINE
LATROBE
LAURELS
LAURENT
LAURITZ
MAARTEN
MACRAME
MACRONS
MADRUSH
MALRAUX
MANRICO
MANROPE
MARRERS
MARRIED
MARRIES
MARRING
MARRONS
MARROWS
MARRYAT
MARRYIN
MARRYME
MATRONS
MAUREEN
MAURIAC
MAURIAT
MAURICE
MAUROIS
NAIROBI
NARRATE
NARROWS
NATRIUM
PADRAIC
PADRONE
PAIRERS
PAIRING
PAIROFF
PAIRSUP
PAPRIKA
PARRIED
PARRIER
PARRIES
PARRING
PARRISH
PARROTS
PATRICE
PATRICK
PATRIES
PATRIOT
PATROLS
PATRONS
PATROON
PAYRATE
PAYROLL
RAGRUGS
RAMRODS
RANRIOT
RATRACE
SABRINA
SANREMO
SATRAPS
SATRAPY
SAURIAN
TAPROOM
TAPROOT
TARRIED
TARRIER
TARRIES
TARRING
TAUREAN
TAURINE
TAXRATE
VAGRANT
VANRIJN
VARRICK
WARRANT
WARRENG
WARRENS
WARRING
WARRIOR
WARROOM
YARROWS
ZAIRIAN

•A••R••

AALARGE
BACARDI
BACKROW
BACKRUB
BACTRIA
BADAREA
BADTRIP
BAKERST
BALDRIC
BARNRED
BARTRAY
BAVARIA
BAYAREA
BAYTREE
CABARET
CALDRON
CALORIC
CALORIE
CAMAROS
CAMBRIA
CAMBRIC
CAMERAE
CAMERAL
CAMERAS
CAMERON
CANARDS
CANTRIP
CAPERED
CARBRAS
CARFREE
CARTRIP
CASERNE
CASERNS
CASERTA
CASTROL
CATERAS
CATERED
CATERER
CATERTO
CATORCE
CAVERNS
CAVORTS
DALTREY
DARKRED
DAYTRIP
EAGERER
EAGERLY
EARDROP
EARDRUM
EATCROW
EATFROM
FABARES
FABERGE
FATFREE
FAVORED
FAVORER
FAYWRAY
GABBROS
GAGARIN
GASTRIC
HADAROW
HAGERTY
HALFRAW
HALFROD
HASAROW
HATBRIM
HAVARTI
HAWORTH
HAZARDS
JAKARTA
KAKUROS
KAMERAD
KATHRYN
LABORAT
LABORED
LABORER
LACERTA
LACUREE
LAFARGE
LAMARCK
LAMPREY
LAPERMS
LAPORTE
LASORDA
LASTROW
LATERAL
LATERAN
LATERON
LAUTREC
LAVERAN
LAVERNE
LAVORIS
LAYERED
LAZARUS
MACGRAW
MACHREE
MADERUN
MADUROS
MAHARIS
MAIGRET
MAITRED
MAITRES
MAJORCA
MAJORED
MAJORIN
MAKERUN
MALARIA
MALARKY
MALLRAT
MANDREL
MANFRED
MANTRAP
MANTRAS
MANTRIC
MANURED
MANURES
MARGRET
MARSRED
MASARYK
MATURED
MATURER
MATURES
MAUPRAT
MAYORAL
MAZARIN
MAZURKA
NATURAL
NATURED
NATUREL
NATURES
NAVARRE
NAYARIT
OAKTREE
OATBRAN
PACKRAT
PALERMO
PALFREY
PALTROW
PANARAB
PANGRAM
PANURGE
PAPERED
PAPERER
PAPYRUS
PARURES
PATERNO
QATARIS
RAJARAO
RAMIREZ
RANFREE
RASURES
RATTRAP
RAYKROC
RAZORED
SABERED
SAFARIS
SAFFRON
SAHARAN
SALERNO
SAMARAS
SAMARIA
SAMPRAS
SAMURAI
SANGRIA
SATIRES
SATIRIC
SATORIS
SATURNS
SATYRIC
SAVARIN
SAVORED
SAVORER
TABARDS
TABARET
TABORET
TALARIA
TAMARAC
TANGRAM
TANTRUM
TAPERED
TASERED
TAVERNA
TAVERNS
TAXFREE
VALERIE
VALOREM
VAPORED
VAPORER
VAPORUB
WAFERED
WAGERED
WAGERER
WAITRON
WASHRAG
WASTREL
WATERED
WATERER
WAVERED
WAVERER

•A•••R•

BACKERS
BADFORM
BADGERS
BADGIRL
BADWORD
BAFFERS
BAGGERS
BAGGIRL
BAILERS
BAILORS
BAITERS
BALKERS
BALLARD
BANBURY
BANDERA
BANDERS
BANGERS
BANKERS
BANNERS
BANTERS
BARBARA
BARBARY
BARBERA
BARBERS
BARCARS
BARGERS
BARKERS
BARNARD
BARTERS
BARWARE
BASHERS
BASTERS
BATGIRL
BATHERS
BATTERS
BATTERY
BAWLERS
BAYLORU
BAZAARS
CABFARE
CABLERS
CADBURY
CADGERS
CAESARS
CAESURA
CAHIERS
CALABRO
CALDERA
CALDERS
CALGARY
CALIBRE
CALKERS
CALLERS
CALVARY
CALVERT
CAMBERS
CAMGIRL
CAMPARI
CAMPERS
CANCERS
CANKERS
CANNERS
CANNERY
CANOERS
CANONRY
CANTERS
CANTORS
CAPPERS
CAPTORS
CAPTURE
CARBARN
CARCARE
CARDERS
CAREERS
CARFARE
CARHORN
CARNERA
CARPARK
CARPERS
CARPORT
CARRARA
CARRERA
CARRERE
CARTERS
CARTIRE
CARVERS
CASPARY
CASTERS
CATBERT
CATBIRD
CAUSERS
CAVALRY
CAVEART
CAVIARE
CAVIARS
DABBERS
DADAART
DAGGERS
DAKTARI
DAMMERS
DAMNERS
DAMPDRY
DAMPERS
DANBURY
DANCERS
DANDERS
DANGERS
DANVERS
DARNERS
DARTERS
DASHERS
DASTARD
DAUBERS
DAYCARE
DAYMARE
EARHART
EARMARK
EARNERS
EASTERN
EASTERS
EATDIRT
EATHERE
EATMORE
FABLERS
FACTORS
FACTORY
FAILURE
FALKIRK
FALLERS
FALTERS
FANFARE
FANNERS
FARMERS
FARMERY
FARMORE
FATFARM
FATHERS
FAVOURS
FAWNERS
FAXLORE
GABBERS
GADDERS
GAFFERS
GAGGERS
GAINERS
GAITERS
GALLERY
GAMMERS
GANDERS
GANGERS
GAOLERS
GARNERS
GARTERS
GASPARD
GASPERS
GASSERS
GASTERO
GASWARS
GATHERS
GAUDERY
GAUGERS
GAWKERS
GAWPERS
GAYLORD
GAZZARA
HACKERS
HAGGARD
HAILERS
HALTERS
HALVERS
HALYARD
HAMBURG
HAMMERS
HAMPERS
HANDERS
HANGARS
HANGERS
HANKERS
HANSARP
HARBORS
HARBURG
HARHARS
HARMERS
HARPERS
HARVARD
HASTERT
HATTERS
HAULERS
HAWKERS
HAWSERS
HAYFORK
HAYWARD
HAYWIRE
JABBERS
JAEGERS
JAGUARS
JAILERS
JAILORS
JAMMERS
JANEIRO
JANUARY
JASPERS
JASPERY
JAYBIRD
JAYWARD
JAZZERS
KAISERS
KAPTURE
LABOURS
LADDERS
LADLERS
LAGGARD
LAGGERS
LAMBERT
LAMPERT
LANCERS
LANDERS
LANFORD
LANGTRY
LANTERN
LANYARD
LAPPERS
LAPSERS
LAPWARE
LARDERS
LARKERS
LASCARS
LASHERS
LASTORY
LATHERS
LATHERY
LAUDERS
LAUNDRY
LAWFORD
LAWYERS
LAYBARE
LAZZERI
MACABRE
MADDERS
MADEIRA
MAESTRO
MAGUIRE
MAGYARS
MAHZORS
MAILERS
MAIMERS
MAINERS
MAJEURE
MALLARD
MALWARE
MANGERS
MANNERS
MANSARD
MAPPERS
MARGERY
MARKERS
MARMARA
MARRERS
MARTYRS
MARYURE
MASCARA
MASHERS
MASKERS
MASONRY
MASTERP
MASTERS
MASTERY
MATHERS
MATTERS
MAULERS
MAUSERS
MAXBORN
MAYNARD
NABBERS
NAGGERS
NAILERS
NAPIERS
NAPPERS
NATTERS
NAVARRE
OAKFERN
OAKPARK
PACKARD
PACKERS
PADDERS
PAIRERS
PALABRA
PALEDRY
PALLORS
PALMARY
PALMERS
PALMYRA
PALTERS
PAMPERS
PANDERS
PANDORA
PANIERS
PANNERS
PANTERA
PANTERS
PANZERS
PAPIERS
PARGERS
PARKERS
PARLORS
PARSERS
PASSERS
PASTERN
PASTERS
PASTORS
PASTURE
PATSDRY
PATTERN
PATTERS
PATZERS
PAULPRY
PAUPERS
PAUSERS
PAVIORS
PAWNERS
PAYDIRT
PAYMORE
RACKERS
RADFORD
RAEBURN
RAFTERS
RAIDERS
RAILERS
RAISERS
RAMMERS
RAMPART
RANCORS
RANGERS
RANKERS
RANTERS
RAPIERS
RAPPERS
RAPPORT
RAPTORS
RAPTURE
RASBORA
RASHERS
RASPERS
RASTERS
RATBERT
RATTERS
RAWBARS
RAYBURN
SACKERS
SAGCARD
SAGUARO
SAILERS
SAILORS
SALIERI
SALTERS
SALVERS
SALVORS
SAMBORA
SANBORN
SANDERS
SANFORD
SAPPERS
SAPPORO
SARTORS
SASSERS
SAUCERS
SAVIORS
SAVOURS
SAVOURY
SAWYERS
SAXHORN
SAYMORE
TACKERS
TAGGERS
TAILERS
TAILORS
TALKERS
TAMPERS
TANBARK
TANKARD
TANKERS
TANNERS
TANNERY
TANTARA
TAPPERS
TARTARE
TARTARS
TASTERS
TATTERS
TATTERY
TAYLORS
VACCARO
VALOURS
VALUERS
VAMPERS
VAMPIRA
VAMPIRE
VANDURA
VANWARD
VAPOURS
VAPOURY
VAQUERO
VARIERS
WADDERS
WAFTERS
WAGGERS
WAGGERY
WAILERS
WAITERS
WAIVERS
WALDORF
WALKERS
WALKURE
WALMART
WALTERS
WANDERS
WANTERS
WARBURG
WARDERS
WARFARE
WARHERO
WARLORD
WARMERS
WARPERS
WARTORN
WARWORN
WASHERS
WASSURE
WASTERS
WATFORD

WAXWORK
WAYWARD
WAYWORN
XAVIERU
YAKKERS
YAMMERS
YANKERS
YAPPERS
YARDARM
YARDERS
YATTERS
YAWNERS
YAWPERS
ZACHARY
ZAPPERS

•A••••R

BABBLER
BABIYAR
BACKBAR
BADHAIR
BAFFLER
BAGGIER
BAINTER
BAITCAR
BALFOUR
BALKIER
BALLMER
BALMIER
BANALER
BANDIER
BARKIER
BARMIER
BARRIER
BASSIER
BATSFOR
BATTIER
BATTLER
BAULKER
BAWDIER
CACKLER
CADAVER
CAJOLER
CALAMAR
CALIBER
CALIPER
CALLFOR
CAMPHOR
CAMPIER
CANDLER
CANDOUR
CANNIER
CARDOOR
CAREFOR
CAROLER
CARRIER
CARTIER
CASHBAR
CASHIER
CASIMIR
CATCHER
CATDOOR
CATERER
CATHAIR
CATTIER
CAULKER
CAVILER
DABBLER
DAFFIER
DAIMLER
DAIRYER
DALLIER
DANDIER
DANDLER
DANGLER
DANSEUR
DASHIER
DAUMIER
DAUNTER
DAWDLER
DAYSTAR
DAYWEAR
DAZZLER
EAGERER
EARLIER
EATOVER
FABFOUR
FADDIER
FAINTER
FAKEFUR
FALLFOR
FANCIER
FANSLER
FARCEUR
FAREWAR
FARRIER
FARSEER
FARTHER
FASTCAR
FATTIER
FAUXFUR
FAVORER
GABBIER
GAGSTER
GAMBIER
GAMBLER
GARBLER
GARDNER
GARGLER
GASSIER
GAUCHER
GAUDIER
GAUNTER
GAUTIER
GAUZIER
GAVEEAR
GAWKIER
HACKLER
HADOVER
HAGGLER
HAIRIER
HAMMIER
HAMSTER
HANAPER
HANDCAR
HANDIER
HANDLER
HANOVER
HAPPIER
HARBOUR
HARDIER
HARRIER
HARSHER
HASOVER
HASTIER
HATCHER
HAUNTER
HAUTEUR
HAVENER
JACAMAR
JACKTAR
JAGGIER
JAMMIER
JANGLER
JANITOR
JANVIER
JAROMIR
JAZZIER
KASHMIR
KASTLER
KAYAKER
LABELER
LABORER
LACQUER
LACUNAR
LAFLEUR
LAIDFOR
LALAKER
LAMINAR
LANDLER
LANGUOR
LANKIER
LARDIER
LARDNER
LARKIER
LASSOER
LAUGHER
LAUNDER
LAYOVER
LAYSFOR
MACULAR
MACUSER
MADEFOR
MADEPAR
MADEWAR
MAILCAR
MAKEFOR
MAKEPAR
MAKEWAR
MALABAR
MALODOR
MALTIER
MANAGER
MANGIER
MANGLER
MANHOUR
MANIPUR
MANLIER
MANOWAR
MANYEAR
MARBLER
MARCHER
MARINER
MARLIER
MARNIER
MARSBAR
MARVIER
MASQUER
MASSEUR
MASSIER
MATADOR
MATCHER
MATURER
MAUNDER
MAXBAER
MAYFAIR
NAGGIER
NAPPIER
NAPSTER
NASTIER
NATATOR
NATTIER
PACECAR
PADDLER
PAIDFOR
PAINTER
PALAVER
PALLIER
PALMIER
PALOMAR
PANNIER
PANTHER
PAPERER
PARADER
PARADOR
PARDNER
PARFOUR
PARLOUR
PARRIER
PARTIER
PARTNER
PARTYER
PASSFOR
PASTEUR
PASTIER
PATCHER
PAVIOUR
PAYSFOR
RACECAR
RADIOER
RAFFLER
RAGGIER
RAILCAR
RAINIER
RALLIER
RAMBLER
RANCHER
RANCOUR
RANDIER
RANGFOR
RANGIER
RANOVER
RAPIDER
RAPSTAR
RASPIER
RASSLER
RATTIER
RATTLER
RAVAGER
SADDLER
SAGGIER
SALAZAR
SALEMOR
SALLIER
SALTIER
SALUTER
SAMOVAR
SAMPLER
SANDBAR
SANDBUR
SANDIER
SANDLER
SAPPIER
SASSIER
SAUCIER
SAUNTER
SAVAGER
SAVEFOR
SAVIOUR
SAVORER
SAVVIER
SAYOVER
TABULAR
TACKIER
TACKLER
TAKEFOR
TALKIER
TALLIER
TANAGER
TANDOOR
TANGIER
TANGLER
TANGOER
TANKCAR
TAPSTER
TARDIER
TARRIER
TARTIER
TASKBAR
TASTIER
TATTIER
TATTLER
TAUNTER
TAWNIER
TAXYEAR
VAMPIER
VANOCUR
VAPORER
VASTIER
VAULTER
VAUNTER
WACKIER
WADDLER
WAFFLER
WAGERER
WAGEWAR
WAGGLER
WAGONER
WAITFOR
WAKENER
WALTHER
WALTZER
WANGLER
WARBLER
WARRIOR
WARTIER
WASFAIR
WASHIER
WASPIER
WATCHER
WATERER
WAVERER
YACHTER
YAWNIER
ZAPPIER

••AR•••

ACARIDS
AFARCRY
AGARICS
ALARBUS
ALARCON
ALARMED
ALARMER
ALARUMS
AMARONE
ANARCHS
ANARCHY
ASARULE
ATARAXY
AVARICE
AWARDED
AWARDEE
AWARDER
AWAREOF
AWAREST
BEARCAT
BEARCUB
BEARDED
BEARERS
BEARHUG
BEARING
BEARISH
BEAROFF
BEAROUT
BEARPAW
BEARPIT
BEARSON
BEARSUP
BLARING
BLARNEY
BOARDED
BOARDER
BOARDUP
BOARISH
CHARADE
CHARCOT
CHARGED
CHARGER
CHARGES
CHARIER
CHARILY
CHARING
CHARIOT
CHARITY
CHARLES
CHARLEY
CHARLIE
CHARMAN
CHARMED
CHARMEN
CHARMER
CHARMIN
CHARNIN
CHARPAK
CHARRED
CHARRER
CHARROS
CHARTED
CHARTER
CHARVET
CLARETS
CLARICE
CLARIFY
CLARION
CLARITY
COARSEN
COARSER
CSARDAS
CZARDAS
CZARDOM
CZARINA
CZARISM
CZARIST
DEARDEN
DEAREST
DEARGOD
DEARIES
DEARONE
DEARSIR
DEARTHS
DHARMAS
DHARMIC
DIARIES
DIARIOS
DIARIST
DWARFED
DWARVES
ECARTES
ENARBOR
ENARMED
EPARCHS
EPARCHY
EXARCHS
FEARERS
FEARFOR
FEARFUL
FEARING
FEARNOT
FLAREUP
FLARING
GEARBOX
GEARING
GEARSTO
GEARSUP
GLAREAT
GLARING
GNARLED
GNARRED
GUARANI
GUARDED
GUARDEE
GUARDER
GUARGUM
HAARLEM
HEARDOF
HEARERS
HEARING
HEARKEN
HEAROUT
HEARSAY
HEARSES
HEARSOF
HEARTED
HEARTEN
HEARTHS
HOARDED
HOARDER
HOARIER
HOARILY
HOARSEN
HOARSER
IDAREDS
IMARETS
INARAGE
INARUSH
JCARROL
KEARNEY
KHARKOV
KIARIOS
KNARRED
LEARJET
LEARNED
LEARNER
LEARNOF
LEARNTO
MAARTEN
MCARDLE
NEAREST
NEARING
NEARPAR
NEARYOU
OCARINA
ONAROLL
ORARION
ORARIUM
OTARIES
OVARIES
PEARLED
PEARLER
PEARSON
PHARAOH
PHARLAP
PHARYNX
QUARLES
QUARREL
QUARTAN
QUARTER
QUARTES
QUARTET
QUARTIC
QUARTOS
QUARTZY
REARDON
REAREND
REARERS
REARGUE
REARING
REARISE
REARLIT
REARMED
REAROSE
REARSUP
ROARERS
ROARING
ROARSAT
SCARABS
SCARCER
SCAREDY
SCARERS
SCAREUP
SCARFED
SCARFER
SCARFUP
SCARIER
SCARIFY
SCARILY
SCARING
SCARLET
SCARPED
SCARRED
SCARVES
SCARWID
SEARACE
SEARERS
SEARING
SHAREIN
SHARERS
SHARING
SHARKEY
SHARONA
SHARPED
SHARPEI
SHARPEN
SHARPER
SHARPIE
SHARPLY
SMARTED
SMARTEN
SMARTER
SMARTLY
SNARERS
SNARFED
SNARING
SNARLAT
SNARLED
SNARLER
SNARLUP
SOARERS
SOAREWE
SOARING
SPARELY
SPAREME
SPARERS
SPAREST
SPARING
SPARKED
SPARKLE
SPARKLY
SPARRED
SPARRER
SPARROW
SPARSER
SPARTAN
STARCHY
STARDOM
STAREAT
STARERS
STARING
STARION
STARKER
STARKEY
STARKLY
STARLET
STARLIT
STARLOG
STARMAN
STARMAP
STARRED
STARSIN
STARSKY
STARTED
STARTER
STARTIN
STARTLE
STARTON
STARTTO
STARTUP
STARVED
STARVES
SWARMED
SWARMER
SWARTHY
TEARERS
TEARFUL
TEARGAS
TEARIER
TEARILY
TEARING
TEAROFF
TEAROOM
TEAROSE
TEAROUT
TEARSAT
TEARSIT
TEARSUP
TIARAED
TSARDOM
TSARINA
TSARISM
TSARIST
TZARINA
UNARMED
WEARERS
WEARIED
WEARIER
WEARIES
WEARILY
WEARING
WEAROFF
WEAROUT
WEARSON
WHARFED
WHARTON
WHARVES
YEAREND
YEARNED
YEARNER
YEARNTO
YEARONE

••A•R••

ANAGRAM
APAIROF
ASAGRAY
BEATRIX
BIAFRAN
CHAGRIN
CHAIRED
CHAKRAS
CHARRED
CHARRER
CHARROS
CLAIROL
CUATROS
DEAIRED
DIAGRAM
FIACRES
GNARRED
HEATRAY
INAPRIL
INATRAP
JCARROL
KNARRED
LLADROS
ONATRIP
ORATRIX
PGAPROS
PRAIRIE
QUADRIC
QUARREL
QUATRES
REAIRED
SCARRED
SEAARMS
SEAGRAM
SEAGREN
SEATRIP
SHADROE
SHAGRUG
SPARRED
SPARRER
SPARROW
STAIRED
STARRED
TEATRAY
TEATREE
TEATROS
TEAURNS
UNAIRED
UPATREE

••A••R•

ABASERS
ABATERS
ABATORS
ADAWARE
AFARCRY
AMATORY
ARACARI
ARAFURA
ARAGORN
ARAMARK
ASALARK
ATATURK
AVATARS
AWAKERS
BEADERS
BEAHERO
BEAKERS
BEAMERS
BEANERY
BEARERS
BEATERS
BEAVERS
BLADERS
BLAMERS
BLAZERS
BOATERS
BRACERO
BRACERS
BRAVERY
BRAVURA
BRAYERS
CHAFERS
CHAMBRE
CHANTRY
CHASERS
CLAMORS
CLAWERS
COALERS
COATERS
COAXERS
CRATERS
CRAVERS
DEALERS
DEANERY
DIALERS
DIAPERS
DRAPERS
DRAPERY
DRAWERS
EBAYERS
ELANTRA
ELATERS
ENAMORS
ERASERS
ERASURE
ETAGERE
EVADERS
FEARERS
FEATURE
FLAKERS
FLAMERS
FLAVORS
FLAVORY
FLAYERS
FOAMERS
FRAMERS
FRATERS
GLAMORS
GLAZERS
GNAWERS
GRADERS
GRANARY
GRAPERY
GRATERS
GRAVERS
GRAVURE
GRAZERS
HEADERS
HEALERS
HEAPERS
HEARERS
HEATERS
HEAVERS
HOAXERS
IMAGERS
IMAGERY
INAFURY
INAWORD
ISADORA
ISADORE
JEANARP
KNAVERY
LEADERS
LEADORE
LEAKERS
LEANERS
LEAPERS
LEASERS
LLANERO
LOADERS
LOAFERS
LOANERS
MEASURE
MIASARA
MOANERS
NIAGARA
OFASORT
ONADARE
ONAGERS
ONAJURY
ONALARK
ONALERT
ORATORS
ORATORY
PHAEDRA
PHASERS
PIASTRE
PLACARD
PLACERS
PLANERS
PLATERS
PLAYERS
PRATERS
PRAYERS
QUAKERS
QUASARS
QUATTRO
QUAVERS
QUAVERY
READERS
READORN
REAMERS
REAPERS
REARERS
REAVERS
ROADERS
ROAMERS
ROARERS
SCALARS
SCALERS
SCARERS
SEABIRD
SEABORG
SEAFARE
SEAFERN
SEAGIRT
SEAHERO
SEALERS
SEALERY
SEAMERS
SEAPORT
SEARERS
SEATERS
SEAWARD
SHADERS
SHAKERS
SHAKIRA
SHANGRI
SHAPERS
SHAPIRO
SHARERS
SHASTRI
SHAVERS
SKATERS
SLAKERS
SLATERS
SLAVERS
SLAVERY
SLAYERS
SNAKERS
SNARERS
SOAKERS
SOAPERS
SOARERS
SPACERS
SPADERS
SPARERS
SPAYERS
STAGERS
STARERS
STATERS

STATORS
STATURE
STAYDRY
STAYERS
SWAYERS
TEACART
TEARERS
TEASERS
THALERS
THAWERS
TOATURN
TRABERT
TRACERS
TRACERY
TRADERS
TRAVERS
UNALERT
UNANGRY
UNAWARE
VEADARS
WEANERS
WEARERS
WEAVERS
WHALERS

••A•••R

ADAPTER
ADAPTOR
ALARMER
AMASSER
AMATEUR
AWAITER
AWARDER
BEADIER
BEAMIER
BLABBER
BLACKER
BLADDER
BLANDER
BLANKER
BLASTER
BLATHER
BOARDER
BOASTER
BRAGGER
BRAIDER
BRAINER
BRANDER
BRASHER
BRASIER
BRAWLER
BRAZIER
BYAHAIR
CHAFFER
CHAMBER
CHAMFER
CHAMPER
CHANCER
CHANGER
CHANTER
CHAPTER
CHARGER
CHARIER
CHARMER
CHARRER
CHARTER
CHASTER
CHATTER
CHAUCER
CLABBER
CLACKER
CLAIMER
CLAMBAR
CLAMBER
CLAMMER
CLAMOUR
CLAMPER
CLANGER
CLANGOR
CLAPFOR
CLAPPER
CLASHER
CLASPER
CLASSER
CLATTER
CLAVIER
CLAYIER
COALCAR
COALTAR
COARSER
COASTER
CRABBER
CRACKER
CRADLER
CRAFTER
CRAMMER
CRANMER
CRASHER
CRASSER
CRAWLER
CRAZIER
DEADAIR
DEARSIR
DRABBER
DRAFTER
DRAGGER
DRAINER
DRAWBAR
DRAWLER
EDASNER
EMAILER
ENABLER
ENACTOR
ENAMOUR
ENARBOR
ETAILER
EVANDER
EXACTER
EXACTOR
EXALTER
FEARFOR
FEASTER
FEATHER
FLAGGER
FLAKIER
FLAMIER
FLANEUR
FLANKER
FLAPPER
FLASHER
FLATCAR
FLATTER
FLAVOUR
FLAWIER
FLAXIER
FOAMIER
FRAILER
FRANKER
FRASIER
FRAZIER
GLACIER
GLADDER
GLAMOUR
GLAZIER
GNASHER
GOAFTER
GRABBAR
GRABBER
GRAFTER
GRAINER
GRAMMAR
GRAMMER
GRANDER
GRANGER
GRANTER
GRANTOR
GRAPIER
GRASPER
GRAZIER
GUARDER
HEADFOR
HEADIER
HEATHER
HEATTER
HEAVIER
HJALMAR
HOARDER
HOARIER
HOARSER
INAPTER
INASTIR
KLAMMER
KRASNER
LEACHER
LEADIER
LEAFIER
LEAGUER
LEAKIER
LEANDER
LEAPFOR
LEARNER
LEATHER
LOAMIER
LOATHER
MEALIER
MEANDER
MEATIER
MUAMMAR
MYANMAR
NEARPAR
ONATEAR
PEAKIER
PEARLER
PEATIER
PGATOUR
PHATTER
PIASTER
PLAINER
PLAISIR
PLAITER
PLANFOR
PLANNER
PLANTAR
PLANTER
PLASTER
PLATIER
PLATTER
POACHER
PRAETOR
PRAISER
PRANCER
PRAYFOR
PSALTER
QUACKER
QUAFFER
QUAKIER
QUARTER
REACHER
REACTOR
READFOR
READIER
REALTER
REALTOR
REAUMUR
ROADTAR
ROASTER
SCALDER
SCALIER
SCALPER
SCAMMER
SCAMPER
SCANNER
SCANTER
SCARCER
SCARFER
SCARIER
SCATTER
SEAMIER
SEASTAR
SHADIER
SHAFFER
SHAKIER
SHALIER
SHANKAR
SHANTER
SHARPER
SHATNER
SHATTER
SLACKER
SLAMMER
SLANDER
SLAPPER
SLASHER
SLATHER
SLATIER
SMACKER
SMALLER
SMARTER
SMASHER
SMATTER
SNACKER
SNAGGER
SNAKIER
SNAPPER
SNARLER
SOAPIER
SPACIER
SPAMMER
SPANAIR
SPANKER
SPANNER
SPARRER
SPARSER
SPATTER
SPAWNER
STABBER
STABLER
STACKER
STADLER
STAFFER
STAGGER
STAGIER
STAIDER
STAINER
STALKER
STALLER
STAMMER
STAMPER
STANDER
STAPLER
STARKER
STARTER
STATLER
STAYFOR
SWABBER
SWAGGER
SWANKER
SWAPPER
SWARMER
SWATTER
SWAYBAR
TEACHER
TEARIER
THANKER
TOAHAIR
TOASTER
TRACKER
TRACTOR
TRAILER
TRAINER
TRAITOR
TRAMCAR
TRAMPER
TRAPPER
TRASHER
TRAWLER
TRAYNOR
TWANGER
VEALIER
WEARIER
WEATHER
WHACKER
WHATFOR
WRAPPER
XFACTOR
YEARNER

•••AR••

AALARGE
AFEARED
ALEARDI
ALGARVE
ALVAREZ
AMHARIC
ANKARAN
ANTARES
APPARAT
APPAREL
AQUARIA
AREARUG
ASCARED
ASFARAS
ASMARAN
ASTARTE
ATLARGE
AUTARCH
AUTARKY
BACARDI
BADAREA
BAVARIA
BAYAREA
BELARUS
BENARES
BETARAY
BEWARED
BEWARES
BICARBS
BIZARRE
BIZARRO
BLEARED
BOGARDE
BOGARTS
BOIARDO
BONARIO
BRIARDS
CABARET
CAMAROS
CANARDS
CEDARED
CLEARED
CLEARER
CLEARLY
CLEAROF
CLEARUP
COWARDS
CURARES
CUTARUG
DEBARGE
DEBARKS
DECARLO
DEFARGE
DELARUE
DEMARCO
DEMARET
DEMARKS
DENARII
DEPARTS
DINARIC
DISARMS
DOTARDS
DRMARIO
DUBARRY
EDGARDO
EDUARDO
EDWARDG
EDWARDI
EDWARDR
EDWARDS
EDWARDV
EMBARGO
EMBARKS
ENCARRE
ENCARTA
ENGARDE
ENLARGE
ESCARPS
ESPARTO
EXPARTE
FABARES
FRIARLY
GAGARIN
GOCARTS
GOKARTS
GUJARAT
HADAROW
HASAROW
HAVARTI
HAZARDS
HEPARIN
HOGARTH
HOWARDK
HOWARDS
HOWARDU
IDCARDS
IGNARRO
IHEARYA
IMPARTS
INLARGE
INMARCH
INNARDS
INWARDS
JAKARTA
JOMARCH
LAFARGE
LAMARCK
LAZARUS
LEBARON
LECARRE
LIPARIS
LIZARDS
LOCARNO
LUCARNE
MAHARIS
MALARIA
MALARKY
MASARYK
MAZARIN
MCCAREY
MINARET
MONARCH
MRDARCY
MRMARCH
MTMARCY
MUBARAK
NAVARRE
NAYARIT
NOCARBS
NONARAB
NONARTS
NOVARRO
OHCAROL
ONEARTH
ONTARIO
ONWARDS
OXCARTS
PANARAB
PETARDS
PICARAS
PICARDO
PICARDY
PICAROS
PISARRO
PIZARRO
POLARAS
POLARIS
PREARMS
PROARAB
QATARIS
RAJARAO
RECARRY
RECARVE
REDARED
REDARES
REDARMY
REDARNS
REEARNS
REGARDS
REMARKS
REMARRY
REPARKS
RETARDS
REWARDS
REWARMS
REWARNS
RICARDO
RITARDS
ROBARDS
ROSARIO
RVPARKS
SAFARIS
SAHARAN
SAMARAS
SAMARIA
SAVARIN
SEAARMS
SEWARDS
SHEARED
SHEARER
SKIAREA
SMEARED
SMEARER
SMEARON
SOFARAS
SOLARAS
SOLARIA
SPEARED
SPEARER
SQUARED
SQUARER
SQUARES
STBARTS
STEARIC
STEARIN
STEARNS
STMARKS
STMARYS
STUARTI
SUBAREA
SUBARID
SUBARUS
SUGARED
SUHARTO
SUKARNO
SWEARAT
SWEARBY
SWEARER
SWEARIN
SWEARTO
TABARDS
TABARET
TALARIA
TAMARAC
THEARMY
THEARTS
THWARTS
TOUAREG
TOWARDS
UNBARED
UNBARES
UNDARED
UNEARTH
UNHARDY
UNHARSH
UNLARGE
UNPARED
UPCARDS
UPDARTS
UPEARLY
UPWARDS
UQUARKS
VIHARAS
VITARAS
VIVARIA
WIZARDS
ZIMARRA

•••A•R•

AFFAIRE
AFFAIRS
ASTAIRE
AUPAIRS
BAZAARS
BELAIRS
BIZARRE
BIZARRO
BONAIRE
CALABRO
CAVALRY
CESAIRE
CONAGRA
CONAKRY
DADAART
DEHAIRS
DEWAART
DRLAURA
DUBARRY
ECLAIRS
ENCARRE
HILAIRE
IGNARRO
IMPAIRS
LECARRE
LEHAVRE
LESABRE
MACABRE
MEGAERA
MEGAERG
MILAGRO
MOHAIRS
MRPADRE
NAVARRE
NOVARRO
ONEACRE
PALABRA
PISARRO
PIZARRO
RECARRY
REMARRY
REPAIRS
RIVALRY
SINATRA
SUMATRA
TENACRE
THEATRE
TWOACRE
UNHAIRS
UNHAIRY
ZIMARRA

•••A••R

ABRADER
AERATOR
ALCAZAR
ALLAYER
ARRAYER
ASSAYER
ATWATER
AVIATOR
BANALER
BELABOR
BELAYER
BENATAR
BENAZIR
BERATER
BLEAKER
BLEATER
BREADER
BREAKER
BROADER
CADAVER
CALAMAR
CHEAPER
CHEATER
CLEANER
CLEARER
CLEAVER
COMAKER
CREAMER
CREASER
CREATOR
CROAKER
CURATOR
DEBASER
DEBATER
DECATUR
DECAYER
DEFACER
DEFAMER
DELAYER
DEWATER
DILATOR
DONATOR
DOWAGER
DREAMER
ECUADOR
EDWARDR
EFFACER
ELEANOR
ELEAZAR
ENGAGER
EQUATOR
ESCAPER
ESSAYER
EXMAYOR
FLOATER
FORAGER
GLEANER
GLOATER
GREASER
GREATER
GROANER
GYRATOR
HANAPER
HOMAGER
IMPALER
INFAVOR
INHALER
INLABOR
INLAYER
INSANER
INVADER
JACAMAR
KAYAKER
KNEADER
LALAKER
LEGATOR
LEVATOR
LOCATER
LOCATOR
LOYALER
MALABAR
MANAGER
MATADOR
MCPAPER
MEDAWAR
MENACER
MIRADOR
MIRAMAR
MISAVER
MOGADOR
NATATOR
NEGATER
NEGATOR
NEWAGER
ONPAPER
ONSAGER
ONWATER
PALAVER
PARADER
PARADOR
PEDALER
PICADOR
PLEADER
PLEASER
POLANER
PREAVER
RAVAGER
REBATER
REGALER
RELATER
RELATOR
RELAXER
RELAYER
REPAPER
RETAKER
REWAGER
REWATER
ROTATOR
SALAZAR
SAVAGER
SCRAPER
SEDATER
SENATOR
SHEARER
SMEARER
SNEAKER
SOLACER
SPEAKER
SPEARER
SPRAYER
SQUALOR
SQUARER
STEALER
STEAMER
STRAFER
STRAYER
SWEARER
SWEATER
TANAGER
THEATER
TOTALER
TREADER
TREATER
UNEAGER
UNMAKER
UNSAFER
UPDATER
URBANER
VOYAGER
WREAKER

••••AR•

ABELARD
ACTUARY
ADAWARE
AIRFARE
AIRPARK
AIRWARS
ALEGARS
ALEYARD
ALLEARS
ALPHARD
ANTFARM
ANTIART
APPEARS
ARACARI
ARAMARK
ARIKARA
ARREARS
ARTCARS
ARTWARE
ASALARK
ASHLARS
ASSHARP
ATHEART
ATHWART
ATMCARD
AVATARS
AWKWARD
BALLARD
BARBARA
BARBARY
BARCARS
BARNARD
BARWARE
BAZAARS
BECHARM
BEEYARD
BEGGARS
BEGGARY
BEHEARD
BERNARD
BIGCARS
BIGEARS
BITPART
BODYART
BOKHARA
BOMBARD
BONNARD
BOWOARS
BOXCARS
BROWARD
BUKHARA
BULGARI
BULGARS
BULWARK
BURSARS
BUSFARE
BUSTARD
BUZZARD
BYHEART
CABFARE
CAESARS
CALGARY
CALVARY
CAMPARI
CARBARN
CARCARE
CARFARE
CARPARK
CARRARA
CASPARY
CAVEART
CAVIARE
CAVIARS
CELLARS
CENTARE
CILIARY
CLIPART
COLLARD
COLLARS
COMPARE
COMPART
COPCARS
COSTARD
COSTARS
COUGARS
CUECARD
CUSTARD
DADAART
DAKTARI
DASTARD
DAYCARE
DAYMARE
DEBEARD
DECIARE
DECLARE
DENMARK
DEODARS
DEWAART
DIEHARD
DIETARY
DILLARD
DISBARS
DISCARD
DISPART
DOGCART
DOGEARS
DOIDARE
DOLLARS
DULLARD
DURWARD
EARHART
EARMARK

ECKHART
EDOUARD
ELKHART
ENDEARS
ENSNARE
ENSNARL
EPICARP
ESTUARY
EXOCARP
EYECARE
FANFARE
FATFARM
FERRARA
FERRARE
FERRARI
FERRARO
FIGBARS
FINEART
FIREARM
FOLKART
FOREARM
FORWARD
FOULARD
FROWARD
FULMARS
FURFARM
FUTHARK
GASPARD
GASWARS
GAZZARA
GENNARO
GETWARM
GISCARD
GIZZARD
GODDARD
GOLDARN
GOTWARM
GRANARY
GUEVARA
GUITARS
HAGGARD
HALYARD
HANGARS
HANSARP
HARHARS
HARVARD
HAYWARD
HECKART
HECTARE
HERBART
HEYWARD
HIGHART
HILLARY
HOLYARK
HONIARA
HOTCARS
HOTWARS
HUBBARD
HUMBARD
HUNGARY
HUSSARS
HYMNARY
INBOARD
INKMARK
INTEARS
INYEARS
ISOBARS
JAGUARS
JANUARY
JAYWARD
JEANARP
JOBJARS
JUNKART
KEYCARD
KILDARE
KITHARA
LAGGARD
LANYARD
LAPWARE
LASCARS
LAYBARE
LEEWARD
LEFTARM
LEONARD
LEOPARD
LEOTARD
LEPPARD
LEXMARK
LIBRARY
LINEARA
LINEARB
LOLLARD
LOMBARD
LONGARM
LOSTART
LOWCARB
LOWCARD
LUMBARS
MAGYARS
MALLARD
MALWARE
MANSARD
MARMARA
MASCARA
MAYNARD
MCCRARY
MIASARA
MILLARD
MISMARK
MORTARS
MUDLARK
MULHARE
MUSTARD
MYSTARS
NECTARS
NECTARY
NETWARE
NEWCARS
NEWHART
NIAGARA
NONDARK
NONFARM
NONPARS
NONWARS
NOSTARS
NOTRARE
OAKPARK
OCULARS
ODDSARE
OHIOART
OLDCARS
ONADARE
ONALARK
ONBOARD
ONEPART
ONEYARD
ONGUARD
ORCHARD
OSSUARY
OSTIARY
OSTMARK
OUTBARK
OUTDARE
OUTEARN
OUTWARD
OUTWARS
OVERARM
OVIPARA
OXHEART
PACKARD
PALMARY
PECCARY
PEPPARD
PETHARE
PICCARD
PILLARS
PIPCARD
PLACARD
PLENARY
POLLARD
POMMARD
PONIARD
POPLARS
POPTART
PREDARK
PREPARE
PREWARM
PREWARN
PRIMARY
PROFARM
PSYWARS
PULSARS
QINTARS
QUASARS
QUINARY
RAMPART
RAWBARS
REBOARD
RECHART
REDCARD
REGEARS
REGNARD
REHEARD
REHEARS
RELEARN
RESHARE
RESPARK
RESTART
RETEARS
RETIARY
REWEARS
REYNARD
RHUBARB
RICHARD
ROBSART
RONSARD
RUDYARD
SAGCARD
SAGUARO
SCALARS
SCOLARI
SEAFARE
SEAWARD
SHEPARD
SHOFARS
SIDEARM
SKYLARK
SKYWARD
SPYWARE
STEWARD
STEWART
SUBWARS
SUMMARY
SUNWARD
SZILARD
TANBARK
TANKARD
TANTARA
TARTARE
TARTARS
TEACART
TERNARY
THEBARD
THECARS
THELARK
TIEBARS
TINEARS
TINWARE
TIPCART
TIPJARS
TITLARK
TOHEART
TONEARM
TOOHARD
TOPIARY
TOSPARE
TOSTART
TOWBARS
TOWCARS
TOYCARS
TOYCART
TRENARY
TRINARY
TRYHARD
TSQUARE
TVSTARS
TWOPART
UNAWARE
UNBEARD
UNCHARY
UNGUARD
UNHEARD
UNITARD
UNITARY
UNLEARN
UNSHARP
UNSMART
UNSNARL
UNWEARY
UPBEARS
UPHOARD
UPQUARK
UPREARS
UPROARS
UPSOARS
UPSTARE
UPSTART
UPTEARS
VACCARO
VANWARD
VEADARS
VILLARD
VILLARI
WALMART
WARFARE
WAYWARD
WELFARE
WETBARS
WETWARE
WIDMARK
WILLARD
WOODARD
YARDARM
ZACHARY

••••A•R

ARTFAIR
BADHAIR
BIDFAIR
BIGHAIR
BYAHAIR
CATHAIR
CENTAUR
COCHAIR
COOLAIR
CORSAIR
CORVAIR
DEADAIR
DESPAIR
DOGHAIR
FINNAIR
FREEAIR
FUNFAIR
GOBYAIR
JOBFAIR
LOTHAIR
LOWPAIR
MAXBAER
MAYFAIR
MULDAUR
NOTFAIR
ONEPAIR
OPENAIR
PETHAIR
REDHAIR
SPANAIR
THINAIR
TOAHAIR
TOYFAIR
TWOPAIR
UNCHAIR
UPSTAIR
VONBAER
WASFAIR

•••••AR

ADOLLAR
ALCAZAR
ALLSTAR
ANGULAR
ANNULAR
ANTBEAR
ANTIWAR
AREOLAR
AXILLAR
BABIYAR
BACKBAR
BAITCAR
BELLJAR
BENATAR
BESMEAR
BIGBEAR
BIGSTAR
BIPOLAR
BODYBAR
BOERWAR
BOLIVAR
BOOMCAR
BUGBEAR
BURGLAR
CALAMAR
CASHBAR
CHEDDAR
CLAMBAR
CLUBCAR
COALCAR
COALTAR
COLDWAR
COPULAR
CROWBAR
CUPULAR
DAYSTAR
DAYWEAR
DIPOLAR
DOGSEAR
DOGSTAR
DOMECAR
DOVEBAR
DRAWBAR
ELEAZAR
EVENPAR
EYEWEAR
FAREWAR
FASTCAR
FERNBAR
FIBULAR
FLATCAR
FORBEAR
GAVEEAR
GETSFAR
GIVEEAR
GOBYCAR
GOESFAR
GOLFCAR
GONEFAR
GOODBAR
GOTOWAR
GRABBAR
GRAMMAR
GULFWAR
GYROCAR
HANDCAR
HIGHBAR
HJALMAR
HOLYWAR
INDYCAR
INGEMAR
INSOFAR
INSULAR
IRONBAR
JACAMAR
JACKTAR
JETSTAR
JOCULAR
JUGULAR
JUNKCAR
KEESLAR
KILOBAR
KINNEAR
KOSOVAR
LACUNAR
LAMINAR
LEFTEAR
LEGWEAR
LESSTAR
LOWGEAR
LUNULAR
MACULAR
MADEPAR
MADEWAR
MAILCAR
MAKEPAR
MAKEWAR
MALABAR
MANOWAR
MANYEAR
MARSBAR
MEDAWAR
MENUBAR
MIDYEAR
MILKBAR
MINIBAR
MINICAR
MIRAMAR
MISHEAR
MODULAR
MUAMMAR
MYANMAR
NEARPAR
NEBULAR
NEWYEAR
NICOBAR
NODULAR
NOSUGAR
NOTNEAR
NUCLEAR
OCELLAR
OFFYEAR
ONATEAR
ONESTAR
ONEYEAR
OPENBAR
OSCULAR
OUTHEAR
OUTROAR
OUTSOAR
OUTTEAR
OUTWEAR
OVERFAR
OVERPAR
PACECAR
PALOMAR
PERYEAR
PETBEAR
PINETAR
PLANTAR
POLECAR
POPSTAR
POPULAR
POSTWAR
RACECAR
RAILCAR
RAPSTAR
REDSTAR
REGULAR
RESWEAR
ROADTAR
ROLLBAR
SALAZAR
SAMOVAR
SANDBAR
SCHMEAR
SCHOLAR
SEASTAR
SECULAR
SEMINAR
SHANKAR
SHEBEAR
SHOTPAR
SIDEBAR
SIDECAR
SIMILAR
SIXYEAR
SKIWEAR
SLOTCAR
SOWSEAR
STELLAR
SWAYBAR
TABULAR
TANKCAR
TASKBAR
TAXYEAR
TELSTAR
TEMPLAR
TENYEAR
THEBEAR
THESTAR
THUSFAR
TINSTAR
TITULAR
TOLLBAR
TOOLBAR
TOWNCAR
TRAMCAR
TRISTAR
TUBULAR
TURFWAR
TUTELAR
TWOSTAR
TWOYEAR
UNCLEAR
UNDULAR
UNGULAR
UNSWEAR
UPTOPAR
USEDCAR
VINEGAR
VIVITAR
WAGEWAR
WENTFAR
WINEBAR
WOODTAR
YESDEAR
ZONULAR

AS•••••

ASABODY
ASAGIFT
ASAGRAY
ASAJOKE
ASALARK
ASANTES
ASARULE
ASATEAM
ASBYATT
ASCARED
ASCENDS
ASCENTS
ASCETIC
ASCRIBE
ASEETHE
ASEPSIS
ASEPTIC
ASEXUAL
ASFARAS
ASHAMED
ASHANTI
ASHBERY
ASHBINS
ASHBURN
ASHBURY
ASHCAKE
ASHCANS
ASHFORD
ASHHEAP
ASHIEST
ASHIVER
ASHLAND
ASHLARS
ASHLESS
ASHPANS
ASHPITS
ASHRAMS
ASHTRAY
ASHTREE
ASIAGOS
ASIATIC
ASIMMER
ASININE
ASISAID
ASKANCE
ASKAWAY
ASKEDIN
ASKEDOF
ASKEDUP
ASKOVER
ASKSFOR
ASKSOUT
ASLEWOF
ASMARAN
ASOCIAL
ASOFNOW
ASONANT
ASPECTS
ASPENCO
ASPERSE
ASPHALT
ASPIRED
ASPIRER
ASPIRES
ASPIRIN
ASPRAWL
ASQUIET
ASQUINT
ASQUITH
ASSAILS
ASSANTE
ASSAULT
ASSAYED
ASSAYER
ASSENTS
ASSERTS
ASSHARP
ASSIGNS
ASSISTS
ASSIZES
ASSLIKE
ASSORTS
ASSTDAS
ASSTIFF
ASSUAGE
ASSUMED
ASSUMER
ASSUMES
ASSUNTA
ASSURED
ASSURER
ASSURES
ASSUROR
ASSWEET
ASSYRIA
ASTAIRE
ASTARTE
ASTERIX
ASTHMAS
ASTOLAT
ASTORIA
ASTOUND
ASTREAM
ASTRIDE
ASTUTER
ASUNDER
ASUSUAL
ASYLUMS

A•S••••

ABSALOM
ABSCISE
ABSCOND
ABSENCE
ABSENTS
ABSINTH
ABSOLUT
ABSOLVE
ABSORBS
ABSTAIN
ADSORBS
ADSPACE
AJSIMON
AKSAKOV
ALSATIA
ALSHAIN
ALSMITH
ALSORAN
AMSCRAY
AMSTELS
ANSELMO
ANSONIA
ANSPACH
ANSWERS
APSIDES
ARSENAL
ARSENIC
ARSENIO
ARSHILE
ASSAILS
ASSANTE
ASSAULT
ASSAYED
ASSAYER
ASSENTS
ASSERTS
ASSHARP
ASSIGNS
ASSISTS
ASSIZES
ASSLIKE
ASSORTS
ASSTDAS
ASSTIFF
ASSUAGE
ASSUMED
ASSUMER
ASSUMES
ASSUNTA
ASSURED
ASSURER
ASSURES
ASSUROR
ASSWEET
ASSYRIA
ATSEVEN
ATSIGHT
ATSIGNS
ATSTAKE
AUSABLE
AUSLESE
AUSPICE
AUSSIES
AUSTERE
AUSTERS
AUSTINS
AUSTRAL
AUSTRIA
AXSEEDS

A••S•••

ABASERS
ABASHED
ABASHES
ABASING
ABUSERS
ABUSING
ABUSIVE
ABYSMAL
ABYSSAL
ABYSSES
ACESOUT
ACTSFOR
ACTSOUT
ADDSALT
AGASSIZ
AGESAGO
AGESOUT
AHASSLE
AHOSTOF
AIMSFOR
AIRSACS
AIRSHIP
AIRSHOW
AIRSICK
AIRSIGN
AIRSOCK
AIRSOUT
ALASKAN
ALASKAS
ALASSAD
ALBSURE
ALLSTAR
ALLSTON
ALMSMAN
ALMSMEN
ALYSSUM
AMASSED
AMASSER
AMASSES
AMESLAN
AMISTAD
AMUSEME
AMUSERS
AMUSING
ANASAZI
ANDSOON
ANDSUCH
ANISEED
ANISTON
ANOSMIA
ANOSMIC
ANTSIER
APESUIT
APISHLY
APOSTLE
ARCSINE
ARISING
ARISTAE
ARISTAS
ARISTOS
ARTSALE
ARTSHOP
ARTSHOW
ARTSIER
ARTSONG
ARUSPEX
ASISAID
ASKSFOR
ASKSOUT
ASUSUAL
ATISSUE
AUSSIES
AVESTAN
AVESTAS
AWASHIN
AWESOME
AZUSACA

A•••S••

ABUTSON
ABYSSAL
ABYSSES
ACCOSTS
ACCUSAL
ACCUSED
ACCUSER
ACCUSES
ACHESON
ADAMSES
ADAMSON
ADDISON
ADJUSTS
ADVISED
ADVISEE
ADVISER
ADVISES
ADVISOR
AEGISES
AEROSOL
AGASSIZ
AGEISTS
AHASSLE
ALASSAD
ALCESTE
ALEKSEI
ALIASES
ALLISON
ALLYSON
ALROSEN
ALTOSAX
ALUNSER
ALYOSHA
ALYSSUM
AMASSED
AMASSER
AMASSES
AMNESIA
AMNESIC
AMNESTY
ANBESOL
ANTESUP
APERSON
APHASIA
APHASIC
APLUSES
APPOSED
APPOSES
ARALSEA
ARCHSEE
ARENSKY
ARGUSES
ARIOSOS
ARIOSTO
AROUSAL
AROUSED
AROUSER
AROUSES
ARRASES
ARRESTS
ARRISES
ARTISAN
ARTISTE
ARTISTS
ASEPSIS
ASSISTS
ATISSUE
ATLASES
ATTESTS
AUGUSTA
AUGUSTE
AUGUSTO
AUGUSTS
AULDSOD
AURISTS
AUTISTS
AVGASES
AVULSED
AVULSES

A••••S•

ABOLISH
ABREAST
ABSCISE
ACCURST
ACEROSE
ACHIEST
ACTRESS

ACUTEST
ADDRESS
ADIPOSE
ADVERSE
AERIEST
AFTMOST
AGAINST
AGELESS
AGGRESS
AGILEST
AGONISE
AGONISM
AGONIST
AIDLESS
AIMLESS
AIRBASE
AIRHOSE
AIRIEST
AIRKISS
AIRLESS
AIRMASS
AIRNESS
ALAMOSA
ALFONSE
ALFONSO
ALLCASH
ALLELSE
ALLNESS
ALLRISE
ALLWISE
ALQUIST
ALTOIST
AMBROSE
AMHERST
AMONGST
AMORIST
AMOROSO
AMPLEST
AMYLASE
ANALYSE
ANALYST
ANAPEST
ANATASE
ANDRESS
ANGUISH
ANIMISM
ANIMIST
ANODISE
ANYWISE
APPEASE
APPRISE
APTNESS
ARABIST
ARCHEST
ARENOSE
ARIDEST
ARMLESS
ARMREST
ARTIEST
ARTLESS
ASHIEST
ASHLESS
ASPERSE
ATACOST
ATALOSS
ATAVISM
ATAVIST
ATCROSS
ATELESS
ATFIRST
ATHEISM
ATHEIST
ATHIRST
ATLEAST
ATOMISE
ATOMISM
ATOMIST
ATWORST
AUSLESE
AUTOPSY
AVIDEST
AWAREST
AWELESS
AWNLESS
AXLROSE

A•••••S

AAAMAPS
AACELLS
ABASERS
ABASHES
ABATERS
ABATORS
ABCNEWS
ABDUCES
ABDUCTS
ABIDERS
ABJURES
ABLATES
ABOUNDS
ABRADES
ABRAXAS
ABRILES
ABSENTS
ABSORBS
ABUSERS
ABYSSES
ACACIAS
ACARIDS
ACCEDES
ACCENTS
ACCEPTS
ACCORDS
ACCOSTS
ACCRUES
ACCTNOS
ACCUSES
ACETALS
ACHENES
ACKACKS
ACQUITS
ACTEDAS
ACTIONS
ACTIVAS
ACTIVES
ACTRESS
ACUMENS
ADAGIOS
ADAMSES
ADDAXES
ADDENDS
ADDICTS
ADDRESS
ADDUCES
ADDUCTS
ADELIES
ADHERES
ADJOINS
ADJURES
ADJUSTS
ADMIRES
ADMIXES
ADNOUNS
ADONAIS
ADORERS
ADRATES
ADSORBS
ADVENTS
ADVERBS
ADVERTS
ADVICES
ADVISES
ADZUKIS
AEDILES
AEGISES
AERATES
AERIALS
AEROBES
AFFAIRS
AFFECTS
AFFINES
AFFIRMS
AFFIXES
AFFORDS
AFFRAYS
AFGHANS
AFRAMES
AGARICS
AGEISTS
AGELESS
AGENCES
AGENDAS
AGGRESS
AGNAILS
AGNATES
AGONIES
AGOUTIS
AGREERS
AGULHAS
AHCHOOS
AIDLESS
AIGLETS
AIGRETS
AIKIDOS
AIMLESS
AIRACES
AIRBAGS
AIRDAMS
AIRGUNS
AIRINGS
AIRKISS
AIRLESS
AIRLOGS
AIRMASS
AIRNESS
AIRPOPS
AIRPOTS
AIRSACS
AIRWARS
AIRWAYS
AITCHES
AJOWANS
ALARBUS
ALARUMS
ALASKAS
ALBEDOS
ALBINOS
ALCOVES
ALDAVIS
ALEGARS
ALEKEGS
ALETAPS
ALETTES
ALEVELS
ALGIERS
ALIASES
ALIGHTS
ALINERS
ALIYAHS
ALKALIS
ALKENES
ALLAGES
ALLCAPS
ALLEARS
ALLEGES
ALLELES
ALLEWIS
ALLEYES
ALLIUMS
ALLNESS
ALLNEWS
ALLOFUS
ALLTHIS
ALLUDES
ALLURES
ALMONDS
ALNICOS
ALPACAS
ALPINES
ALTIMAS
ALTKEYS
ALTOIDS
ALTTABS
ALUDELS
ALUMNUS
AMADEUS
AMANTIS
AMASSES
AMATOLS
AMAZONS
AMBIENS
AMBLERS
AMBRIES
AMERCES
AMIDOLS
AMITIES
AMNERIS
AMNIONS
AMOEBAS
AMOROUS
AMOUNTS
AMPERES
AMPULES
AMRITAS
AMSTELS
AMTRACS
AMULETS
AMUSERS
ANACINS
ANADEMS
ANALOGS
ANANIAS
ANARCHS
ANCHORS
ANDEANS
ANDREAS
ANDRESS
ANDREWS
ANDROUS
ANEMIAS
ANGELAS
ANGELES
ANGELUS
ANGLAIS
ANGLERS
ANGORAS
ANIMALS
ANITRAS
ANKLERS
ANKLETS
ANNALES
ANNEALS
ANNEXES
ANNUALS
ANNULUS
ANOINTS
ANOMIES
ANONYMS
ANORAKS
ANSWERS
ANTARES
ANTCOWS
ANTERUS
ANTHEMS
ANTHERS
ANTIBES
ANTLERS
ANXIOUS
ANYNEWS
ANYONES
ANYWAYS
AOUDADS
APACHES
APELETS
APERCUS
APERIES
APHIDES
APLITES
APLUSES
APODOUS
APOGEES
APOLLOS
APPALLS
APPEALS
APPEARS
APPENDS
APPLETS
APPLIES
APPOSES
APROPOS
APSIDES
APTNESS
AQUEOUS
AQUINAS
ARABICS
ARABLES
ARAMIDS
ARBACES
ARBOLES
ARBOURS
ARBUTUS
ARCADES
ARCHERS
ARCHIES
ARCHONS
ARCINGS
ARDOURS
ARDUOUS
AREOLAS
AREOLES
ARGALIS
ARGENTS
ARGUERS
ARGUSES
ARGYLES
ARIANES
ARIOSOS
ARISTAS
ARISTOS
ARMADAS
ARMFULS
ARMLESS
ARMLETS
ARMOURS
ARMPITS
ARNICAS
ARNOLDS
AROUSES
ARRACKS
ARRASES
ARREARS
ARRESTS
ARRISES
ARRIVES
ARROYOS
ARTCARS
ARTEMIS
ARTEMUS
ARTHURS
ARTISTS
ARTLESS
ARUBANS
ASANTES
ASCENDS
ASCENTS
ASEPSIS
ASFARAS
ASHBINS
ASHCANS
ASHLARS
ASHLESS
ASHPANS
ASHPITS
ASHRAMS
ASIAGOS
ASPECTS
ASPIRES
ASSAILS
ASSENTS
ASSERTS
ASSIGNS
ASSISTS
ASSIZES
ASSORTS
ASSTDAS
ASSUMES
ASSURES
ASTHMAS
ASYLUMS
ATALOSS
ATAMANS
ATCROSS
ATELESS
ATHOMES
ATLASES
ATMFEES
ATOMICS
ATOMIES
ATONERS
ATONICS
ATONIES
ATRIUMS
ATROPOS
ATSIGNS
ATTACKS
ATTAINS
ATTENDS
ATTESTS
ATTICUS
ATTIMES
ATTIRES
ATTRITS
ATTUCKS
ATTUNES
AUBADES
AUBURNS
AUDILES
AUGENDS
AUGITES
AUGUSTS
AUKLETS
AUNTIES
AUPAIRS
AURISTS
AURORAS
AUSSIES
AUSTERS
AUSTINS
AUTEURS
AUTHORS
AUTISTS
AUTOBUS
AUTUMNS
AVALONS
AVANTIS
AVATARS
AVENGES
AVENUES
AVERNUS
AVESTAS
AVGASES
AVIATES
AVOCETS
AVOWALS
AVOWERS
AVULSES
AWAKENS
AWAKERS
AWELESS
AWNINGS
AWNLESS
AXHEADS
AXILLAS
AXSEEDS
AYEAYES
AZALEAS
AZODYES

•AS••••

BASALLY
BASALTS
BASEDON
BASEHIT
BASEMAN
BASEMEN
BASENJI
BASEPAY
BASESIX
BASETEN
BASETWO
BASHERS
BASHFUL
BASHING
BASILIC
BASILIO
BASINAL
BASKETS
BASKETT
BASKING
BASMATI
BASQUES
BASRHIN
BASSALE
BASSANI
BASSANO
BASSETS
BASSETT
BASSIER
BASSIST
BASSOON
BASSSAX
BASTERS
BASTING
BASTION
CASABAS
CASAVAS
CASCADE
CASEATE
CASEINS
CASELAW
CASELLA
CASELOT
CASEOUS
CASEOUT
CASERNE
CASERNS
CASERTA
CASHBAR
CASHBOX
CASHCOW
CASHEWS
CASHIER
CASHING
CASHINS
CASHOUT
CASIMIR
CASINGS
CASINOS
CASITAS
CASKETS
CASKING
CASPARY
CASPIAN
CASQUED
CASQUES
CASSABA
CASSATT
CASSAVA
CASSIAS
CASSIDY
CASSINI
CASSINO
CASSIUS
CASSOCK
CASSOLA
CASTERS
CASTILE
CASTING
CASTLED
CASTLES
CASTOFF
CASTOUT
CASTROL
CASTSON
CASTSUP
CASUALS
CASUIST
DASBOOT
DASCHLE
DASHDOT
DASHERS
DASHIER
DASHIKI
DASHING
DASHOFF
DASHPOT
DASILVA
DASTARD
EASEDBY
EASEDIN
EASEDON
EASEDUP
EASEFUL
EASELED
EASEOFF
EASEOUT
EASESBY
EASESIN
EASESON
EASESUP
EASIEST
EASTEGG
EASTEND
EASTERN
EASTERS
EASTHAM
EASTING
EASTMAN
EASYJOB
EASYOFF
EASYONE
FASCIAE
FASCIAL
FASCIAS
FASCISM
FASCIST
FASHION
FASTCAR
FASTENS
FASTEST
FASTING
FASTNET
FASTONE
GASBAGS
GASCANS
GASCAPS
GASCONS
GASCONY
GASEDUP
GASEITY
GASEOUS
GASESUP
GASHEAT
GASHING
GASHOGS
GASJETS
GASKELL
GASKETS
GASLAMP
GASLEAK
GASLESS
GASLINE
GASLOGS
GASMAIN
GASMASK
GASOHOL
GASOVEN
GASPARD
GASPERS
GASPING
GASPIPE
GASPUMP
GASSERS
GASSIER
GASSING
GASSMAN
GASTANK
GASTERO
GASTONE
GASTRIC
GASWARS
HASACOW
HASAFIT
HASAGAS
HASANIP
HASAROW
HASASAY
HASASET
HASATIT
HASBEEN
HASDONE
HASFITS
HASHING
HASHISH
HASHOUT
HASIDIC
HASIDIM
HASKELL
HASOVER
HASPING
HASPULL
HASROOM
HASSIUM
HASSLED
HASSLES
HASSOCK
HASTENS
HASTERT
HASTIER
HASTILY
HASTIME
HASTING
HASTOBE
JASMINE
JASPERS
JASPERY
KASHMIR
KASTLER
LASAGNA
LASAGNE
LASALLE
LASCALA
LASCARS
LASCAUX
LASHERS
LASHING
LASHOUT
LASHUPS
LASORDA
LASSIES
LASSOED
LASSOER
LASSOES
LASTACT
LASTDON
LASTGAS
LASTING
LASTLAP
LASTLEG
LASTMAY
LASTONE
LASTORY
LASTROW
MASARYK
MASCARA
MASCOTS
MASHERS
MASHIES
MASHING
MASKERS
MASKING
MASONED
MASONIC
MASONRY
MASQUER
MASQUES
MASSAGE
MASSEUR
MASSIER
MASSIFS
MASSINE
MASSING
MASSIVE
MASTERP
MASTERS
MASTERY
MASTICS
MASTIFF
MASTING
MASTOID
NASALLY
NASCENT
NASTASE
NASTIER
NASTIES
NASTILY
PASALLE
PASCHAL
PASCOLI
PASSADE
PASSADO
PASSAGE
PASSAIC
PASSANT
PASSATS
PASSELS
PASSERS
PASSEUL
PASSFOR
PASSING
PASSION
PASSIVE
PASSKEY
PASSOFF
PASSOUT
PASTDUE
PASTEIN
PASTELS
PASTERN
PASTERS
PASTEUP
PASTEUR
PASTIER
PASTIES
PASTIME
PASTINA
PASTING
PASTORS
PASTURE
RASBORA
RASCALS
RASHERS
RASHEST
RASHIDA
RASPERS
RASPIER
RASPING
RASPISH
RASSLED
RASSLER
RASSLES
RASTERS
RASURES
SASHAYS
SASHIMI
SASHING
SASSERS
SASSIER
SASSILY
SASSING
SASSOON
TASERED
TASHLIN
TASKBAR
TASKING
TASSELS
TASTEIT
TASTERS
TASTIER
TASTILY
TASTING
VASQUEZ
VASSALS
VASTEST
VASTIER
VASTITY
WASABIS
WASATCH
WASFAIR
WASHDAY
WASHERS
WASHIER
WASHING
WASHOFF
WASHOUT
WASHRAG
WASHTUB
WASHUPS
WASLATE
WASONTO
WASPIER
WASPILY
WASPISH
WASSAIL
WASSILY
WASSURE
WASTAGE
WASTERS
WASTING
WASTREL
YASBECK
YASHICA
YASHMAK
YASMINE

•A•S•••

BADSHOT
BADSIGN
BALSAMS
BALSAMY
BANSHEE
BARSOAP
BARSTOW
BASSALE
BASSANI
BASSANO
BASSETS
BASSETT
BASSIER
BASSIST
BASSOON
BASSSAX
BATSFOR
BATSMAN
BATSMEN
BATSUIT
CAESARS
CAESURA
CAISSON
CANSECO
CAPSHAW
CAPSIZE
CAPSTAN
CAPSULE
CARSALE
CARSEAT
CARSHOW
CASSABA
CASSATT
CASSAVA
CASSIAS
CASSIDY
CASSINI
CASSINO

CASSIUS
CASSOCK
CASSOLA
CATSCAN
CATSEYE
CATSHOW
CATSITS
CATSPAW
CATSUIT
CATSUPS
CAUSERS
CAUSING
CAUSTIC
DAISIES
DAMSELS
DAMSONS
DANSEUR
DATSUNS
DAUSSET
DAYSAIL
DAYSEND
DAYSIDE
DAYSINN
DAYSOFF
DAYSPAS
DAYSTAR
EARSHOT
EATSOUT
FAISALI
FALSELY
FALSEST
FALSIFY
FALSITY
FANSLER
FANSOUT
FARSEER
FARSIDE
FAUSTUS
GADSDEN
GAGSTER
GASSERS
GASSIER
GASSING
GASSMAN
GAUSSES
HADSOME
HALSTON
HAMSTER
HANSARP
HANSOLO
HANSOMS
HARSHEN
HARSHER
HARSHLY
HASSIUM
HASSLED
HASSLES
HASSOCK
HATSIZE
HATSOFF
HAWSERS
HAYSEED
JANSSEN
JANSSON
KAISERS
KAISHEK
KANSANS
LAISSEZ

LAKSHMI
LANSING
LAPSANG
LAPSERS
LAPSING
LASSIES
LASSOED
LASSOER
LASSOES
LAWSUIT
LAYSFOR
LAYSLOW
LAYSOFF
LAYSOUT
MAESTRO
MAISONS
MAISOUI
MANSARD
MANSION
MANSIZE
MANSMAN
MAOSUIT
MAPSOUT
MARSALA
MARSBAR
MARSDEN
MARSHAL
MARSHES
MARSRED
MARSTON
MASSAGE
MASSEUR
MASSIER
MASSIFS
MASSINE
MASSING
MASSIVE
MAUSERS
NAPSTER
NATSUME
NAUSEAM
NAYSAID
NAYSAYS
OARSMAN
OARSMEN
PADSITE
PAISANO
PAISANS
PAISLEY
PANSIES
PANSOUT
PARSECS
PARSEES
PARSERS
PARSING
PARSLEY
PARSNIP
PARSONS
PASSADE
PASSADO
PASSAGE
PASSAIC
PASSANT
PASSATS
PASSELS
PASSERS
PASSEUL
PASSFOR

PASSING
PASSION
PASSIVE
PASSKEY
PASSOFF
PASSOUT
PATSDRY
PATSIES
PAUSERS
PAUSING
PAYSFOR
PAYSLIP
PAYSNOW
PAYSOFF
PAYSOUT
PAYSTUB
RAGSHOP
RAISERS
RAISEUP
RAISING
RAISINS
RAISINY
RAISONS
RALSTON
RAMSESI
RAMSFAN
RAMSONS
RANSACK
RANSOMS
RAPSONG
RAPSTAR
RASSLED
RASSLER
RASSLES
RATSOUT
RAWSILK
SADSACK
SADSONG
SAISONS
SALSODA
SAMSONS
SAMSUNG
SANSEIS
SAPSAGO
SASSERS
SASSIER
SASSILY
SASSING
SASSOON
SATSUMA
SAUSAGE
SAWSOFF
SAYSAAH
SAYSAYE
SAYSBOO
SAYSIDO
SAYSNAY
SAYSWHO
SAYSYES
SAYSYOU
TABSETS
TAGSALE
TAGSOUT
TANSIES
TAPSHOE
TAPSOFF
TAPSOUT
TAPSTER

TARSALS
TASSELS
TAXSALE
VANSANT
VARSITY
VASSALS
WAISTED
WAKSMAN
WALSTON
WAPSHOT
WARSHIP
WASSAIL
WASSILY
WASSURE
WAYSIDE

•A••S••

BABYSAT
BABYSIT
BACKSAW
BACKSIN
BACKSUP
BAILSON
BALASES
BALKSAT
BALLSUP
BANDSAW
BANGSON
BANGSUP
BANKSON
BANKSUP
BARISTA
BARKSAT
BASESIX
BASSSAX
BATISTA
BATISTE
CAGESUP
CAISSON
CAKESUP
CALISTA
CALLSIN
CALLSIT
CALLSON
CALLSTO
CALLSUP
CALMSEA
CAMISES
CAMPSUP
CANASTA
CANTSAY
CARESTO
CARLSON
CARPSAT
CARTSIN
CASTSON
CASTSUP
CAVESIN
CAYUSES
DACOSTA
DALASIS
DAMASKS
DAMASUS
DAMOSEL
DARESAY
DARESTO
DATASET
DAUSSET

DAVISON
DAWNSON
EARNSIT
EASESBY
EASESIN
EASESON
EASESUP
FACESIT
FACESON
FADESIN
FAILSTO
FAIRSEX
FAIRSUP
FAKESIT
FALLSIN
FALLSON
FALLSTO
FAWNSON
GAINSAY
GAINSON
GANGSAW
GANGSTA
GANGSUP
GAPESAT
GASESUP
GAUSSES
GAWKSAT
GAZESAT
GAZESON
HACKSAW
HACKSIT
HACKSUP
HADASAY
HADASET
HALFSHY
HANDSAW
HANDSEL
HANDSET
HANDSIN
HANDSON
HANDSUP
HANGSBY
HANGSIN
HANGSON
HANGSUP
HARDSET
HARDSIX
HARPSON
HASASAY
HASASET
HATESIT
HAULSIN
HAULSUP
HAYESES
JACKSON
JACKSOO
JACKSUP
JALISCO
JAMESII
JAMESIV
JAMESON
JAMESVI
JAMISON
JANSSEN
JANSSON
KARASEA
KARLSON
KATISHA

LACESON
LACESUP
LACOSTE
LAGASSE
LAISSEZ
LAKISTS
LANDSAT
LANDSUP
LARUSSA
LATOSCA
MACHSIX
MACUSER
MADISON
MAILSIN
MAJESTE
MAJESTY
MAKESDO
MAKESGO
MAKESIT
MAKESUP
MALMSEY
MAOISTS
MARKSUP
MARUSJA
MATISSE
MAVISES
NABISCO
NAILSET
NAILSIN
NAILSIT
NAILSUP
NATASHA
PACKSIN
PACKSON
PACKSUP
PAGESIX
PAIRSUP
PAPISTS
PARASKI
PARASOL
PARKSIT
PAULSEN
RACESBY
RACESTO
RACESUP
RACISTS
RACKSUP
RAILSAT
RAILSON
RAINSIN
RAINSON
RAKESIN
RAKESUP
RAMESES
RAMPSUP
RANTSAT
RAWISTS
SACKSUP
SADISTS
SAILSON
SAILSTO
SALTSEA
SAMISEN
SAMOSAS
SAMOSET
SAMPSON
SATISFY
SAVESON

SAVESUP
TABASCO
TACKSON
TACKSUP
TAKESIN
TAKESIT
TAKESON
TAKESTO
TAKESUP
TALKSAT
TALKSOF
TALKSON
TALKSTO
TALKSUP
TALUSES
TANKSUP
TAOISTS
TAPESON
TAPESUP
TARTSUP
VALISES
VANESSA
WABASHA
WADESIN
WAITSON
WAITSUP
WAKESUP
WALKSBY
WALKSON
WALKSTO
WALLSIN
WALLSUP
WANTSIN
WANTSTO
WARMSTO
WARMSUP
WARNSOF
WATUSIS
WAVESAT
WAVESIN
WAVESTO
WAXESUP
YANKSAT
YANKSON
ZAKUSKA

•A•••S•

BAALISH
BAALISM
BAALIST
BABIEST
BABYISH
BADCASE
BADDEST
BADDISH
BADNESS
BADPAST
BAHAISM
BAHAIST
BAKERST
BALDEST
BALDISH
BALLAST
BAPTISE
BAPTISM
BAPTIST
BARLESS
BASSIST

CABOOSE
CADDISH
CAGIEST
CAKIEST
CALMEST
CALYPSO
CANIEST
CANVASS
CAPEESH
CAPLESS
CARCASS
CARLESS
CAROUSE
CARWASH
CASUIST
CATFISH
CATTISH
DADAISM
DADAIST
DAFTEST
DAMPEST
DAMPISH
DANKEST
DARIUSI
DARKEST
DARKISH
EARLESS
EARNEST
EASIEST
EATLESS
FABBEST
FADDISH
FADDISM
FADDIST
FAINEST
FAIREST
FAIRISH
FAIRUSE
FALSEST
FANBASE
FANFEST
FANTASM
FANTAST
FANTASY
FANWISE
FAREAST
FARNESS
FAROESE
FARWEST
FASCISM
FASCIST
FASTEST
FATLESS
FATNESS
FATOUSH
FATTEST
FATTISH
FAUVISM
FAUVIST
GABFEST
GAMIEST
GAPLESS
GARNISH
GASLESS
GASMASK
GAULISH
GAWKISH
GAYNESS

HADBEST
HAGGISH
HAIMISH
HAPLESS
HARDEST
HARDISH
HARNESS
HARPIST
HARVEST
HASHISH
HATLESS
HAWKISH
HAZIEST
IAMBIST
JACCUSE
JACKASS
JAGLESS
JAINISM
JAINIST
JARLESS
JAWLESS
JAZZISH
KADDISH
KAPITSA
LABTEST
LACIEST
LACTASE
LACTOSE
LADDISH
LADYISH
LAGASSE
LAKIEST
LALOOSH
LAMAISM
LAMAIST
LANKEST
LAPPISH
LARGESS
LARGEST
LARGISH
LARKISH
LARUSSA
LAVALSE
LAWCASE
LAWLESS
LAXNESS
LAZIEST
LAZYISH
MADDASH
MADDEST
MADDISH
MADNESS
MADRUSH
MAEWEST
MAFIOSI
MAFIOSO
MAHDISM
MAHDIST
MAIDISH
MALAISE
MALPASO
MALTASE
MALTESE
MALTOSE
MANCUSO
MANLESS
MANNISH
MARCUSE

MARXISM
MARXIST
MATISSE
MATLESS
MAWKISH
MAYBESO
MAZIEST
NAGGISH
NAIVEST
NAPLESS
NASTASE
OAKCASK
OAKDESK
OAKIEST
OAKMOSS
OARLESS
PACHISI
PACIEST
PALMIST
PANFISH
PAPOOSE
PARRISH
PATCASH
PATNESS
PAULIST
PAYCASH
PAYLESS
RACIEST
RAFFISH
RAMMISH
RAMSESI
RANKEST
RANKISH
RANPAST
RASHEST
RASPISH
RATTISH
RAWFISH
RAWNESS
RAYLESS
SADDEST
SADNESS
SAGIEST
SALTISH
SAMBASS
SAMWISE
SANJOSE
SAPLESS
SARCASM
SAWDUST
SAWFISH
SAWPAST
SAYMASS
TALLEST
TALLISH
TANNEST
TANNISH
TARNISH
TARTEST
TARTISH
TAUTEST
TAXBASE
TAXLESS
VAGUEST
VAINEST
VAMOOSE
VAMPISH
VANESSA

VARNISH
VASTEST
WACKEST
WAGGISH
WAIFISH
WANIEST
WANNESS
WANNEST
WANNISH
WARIEST
WARLESS
WARMEST
WARMISH
WASPISH
WAVIEST
WAXIEST
WAYLESS
YAKUTSK
ZANIEST
ZANYISH
ZANYISM

•A••••S

AAAMAPS
AACELLS
BABBLES
BABOONS
BACCHUS
BACKERS
BACKUPS
BADBOYS
BADDAYS
BADDIES
BADDOGS
BADEGGS
BADENDS
BADFITS
BADGERS
BADGUYS
BADHATS
BADLIES
BADLOTS
BADNESS
BADNEWS
BADRAPS
BAFFERS
BAFFIES
BAFFLES
BAGBOYS
BAGFULS
BAGGERS
BAGGIES
BAGGINS
BAGJOBS
BAGNIOS
BAGWIGS
BAHAMAS
BAHIANS
BAILEES
BAILERS
BAILORS
BAITERS
BALASES
BALATAS
BALBOAS
BALDIES
BALEENS
BALKANS

BALKERS
BALLADS
BALLETS
BALLOTS
BALSAMS
BAMBOOS
BAMMIES
BANANAS
BANANES
BANDERS
BANDIES
BANDITS
BANGERS
BANGLES
BANJOES
BANKERS
BANKITS
BANNERS
BANQUES
BANTAMS
BANTERS
BANYANS
BANZAIS
BAOBABS
BARACUS
BARBERS
BARBETS
BARBIES
BARCARS
BAREGES
BARENTS
BARGERS
BARHOPS
BARITES
BARKERS
BARLESS
BARLEYS
BARNEYS
BARNUMS
BAROLOS
BARQUES
BARRELS
BARRENS
BARRETS
BARRIOS
BARRONS
BARROWS
BARTABS
BARTERS
BARTLES
BARYONS
BASALTS
BASHERS
BASKETS
BASQUES
BASSETS
BASTERS
BATBOYS
BATCHES
BATDAYS
BATHERS
BATTENS
BATTERS
BATTLES
BAUBLES
BAUHAUS
BAWLERS
BAYRUMS

BAZAARS
CABALAS
CABANAS
CABBIES
CABEZAS
CABLERS
CABLETS
CABRIOS
CACHETS
CACKLES
CADDIES
CADGERS
CAESARS
CAFTANS
CAHIERS
CAHOOTS
CAIMANS
CAJOLES
CALDERS
CALENDS
CALICES
CALICOS
CALIPHS
CALKERS
CALKINS
CALLEES
CALLERS
CALLINS
CALLOUS
CALLUPS
CALYCES
CALYXES
CAMAROS
CAMBERS
CAMBOYS
CAMERAS
CAMINOS
CAMIONS
CAMISES
CAMMIES
CAMPERS
CANAPES
CANARDS
CANCANS
CANCELS
CANCERS
CANCHAS
CANDIDS
CANDIES
CANDLES
CANFULS
CANINES
CANINGS
CANKERS
CANNELS
CANNERS
CANNONS
CANOERS
CANOLAS
CANOPUS
CANTABS
CANTALS
CANTERS
CANTLES
CANTONS
CANTORS
CANUCKS
CANULAS

CANVASS	CATGUTS	DATSUNS	FATONES	GATLINS	HASTENS	LADIDAS	LAZBOYS	MARCHES	NATHANS	PARFUMS	RADIXES	RAWISTS
CANYONS	CATIONS	DAUBERS	FATTENS	GAUCHOS	HATCHES	LADINGS	MACACOS	MARGINS	NATIONS	PARGERS	RADOMES	RAWLINS
CAPADES	CATKINS	DAWDLES	FATUOUS	GAUDENS	HATFULS	LADINOS	MACOUNS	MARHAUS	NATIVES	PARIAHS	RAFFIAS	RAWNESS
CAPFULS	CATNAPS	DAWKINS	FAUCETS	GAUDIES	HATLESS	LADLERS	MACRONS	MARIDAS	NATTERS	PARIBUS	RAFFLES	RAYBANS
CAPGUNS	CATNIPS	DAYBEDS	FAUSTUS	GAUGERS	HATPINS	LADYNAS	MADAMES	MARIDOS	NATURES	PARINGS	RAFTERS	RAYGUNS
CAPLESS	CATRIGS	DAYHOPS	FAUXPAS	GAUSSES	HATREDS	LAERTES	MADCAPS	MARINAS	NAUGHTS	PARKERS	RAGBAGS	RAYLESS
CAPLETS	CATSITS	DAYJOBS	FAVOURS	GAVIALS	HATTERS	LAGGERS	MADDENS	MARINES	NAVAHOS	PARKINS	RAGGIES	RAZZIES
CAPNUTS	CATSUPS	DAYSPAS	FAWNERS	GAWKERS	HAULERS	LAGOONS	MADDERS	MARKERS	NAVAIDS	PARLAYS	RAGINGS	SABADOS
CAPOTES	CATTOYS	DAZZLES	GABBERS	GAWPERS	HAVANAS	LAGUNAS	MADDOGS	MARKETS	NAVAJOS	PARLEYS	RAGLANS	SABINES
CAPPERS	CAUSERS	EADGILS	GABBLES	GAYNESS	HAWHAWS	LAITIES	MADLIBS	MARKUPS	NAYSAYS	PARLORS	RAGMANS	SACHEMS
CAPTORS	CAVEATS	EAGLETS	GABBROS	GAZEBOS	HAWKERS	LAKISTS	MADNESS	MARLINS	OAHUANS	PARLOUS	RAGMOPS	SACHETS
CARACAS	CAVEINS	EARBUDS	GADDERS	HABILIS	HAWKINS	LAKOTAS	MADUROS	MARMOTS	OAKMOSS	PAROLES	RAGOUTS	SACKERS
CARAFES	CAVERNS	EARFULS	GADGETS	HACKERS	HAWSERS	LAMBDAS	MAENADS	MAROONS	OAKTAGS	PARRIES	RAGRUGS	SACQUES
CARBONS	CAVIARS	EARLAPS	GAFFERS	HACKIES	HAYESES	LAMENTS	MAGGOTS	MARQUES	OARLESS	PARROTS	RAGTOPS	SADDENS
CARBOYS	CAVORTS	EARLESS	GAGGERS	HACKLES	HAYINGS	LAMINAS	MAGLEVS	MARQUIS	PAANGAS	PARSECS	RAIDERS	SADDLES
CARBRAS	CAYMANS	EARLETS	GAGGLES	HADAGAS	HAYMOWS	LANCERS	MAGNETS	MARRERS	PABLUMS	PARSEES	RAILBUS	SADEYES
CARCASS	CAYUGAS	EARLIES	GAGLAWS	HADFITS	HAZARDS	LANCETS	MAGNUMS	MARRIES	PACKERS	PARSERS	RAILERS	SADISTS
CARDERS	CAYUSES	EARNERS	GAINERS	HADRONS	HAZINGS	LANCIAS	MAGPIES	MARRONS	PACKETS	PARSONS	RAISERS	SADNESS
CAREENS	DABBERS	EARTABS	GAITERS	HAGGLES	HAZMATS	LANDAUS	MAGYARS	MARROWS	PADDERS	PARTIES	RAISINS	SAFARIS
CAREERS	DABBLES	EARTAGS	GALANOS	HAIKAIS	IAMBICS	LANDERS	MAHARIS	MARSHES	PADDIES	PARURES	RAISONS	SAILERS
CARFULS	DACAPOS	EARWIGS	GALANTS	HAILERS	IAPETUS	LANVINS	MAHOUTS	MARTENS	PADDLES	PASSATS	RALLIES	SAILORS
CARGOES	DACRONS	EASTERS	GALAXES	HAIRDOS	IATRICS	LAPCATS	MAHZORS	MARTINS	PADUANS	PASSELS	RALLYES	SAINTES
CARHOPS	DACTYLS	EATLESS	GALENAS	HALALAS	JABBERS	LAPDOGS	MAIDENS	MARTIUS	PAELLAS	PASSERS	RAMADAS	SAISONS
CARIBES	DADDIES	FABARES	GALLEYS	HALFIES	JACALES	LAPERMS	MAILERS	MARTYRS	PAGINGS	PASTELS	RAMBLES	SALAAMS
CARINAS	DAEMONS	FABLERS	GALLONS	HALIDES	JACKALS	LAPFULS	MAILINS	MARVELS	PAGODAS	PASTERS	RAMESES	SALADES
CARIOUS	DAEWOOS	FABRICS	GALLOPS	HALITES	JACKASS	LAPPERS	MAIMERS	MASCOTS	PAIDADS	PASTIES	RAMFANS	SALAMIS
CARKEYS	DAGGERS	FACADES	GALLOWS	HALLEYS	JACKETS	LAPPETS	MAINERS	MASHERS	PAIRERS	PASTORS	RAMJETS	SALINAS
CARLESS	DAHLIAS	FACIALS	GALOOTS	HALLOOS	JACQUES	LAPSERS	MAISONS	MASHIES	PAISANS	PATACAS	RAMMERS	SALINES
CARLOTS	DAILIES	FACINGS	GALPALS	HALLOWS	JAEGERS	LAPTOPS	MAITAIS	MASKERS	PAIUTES	PATCHES	RAMONES	SALIVAS
CARNETS	DAIRIES	FACTORS	GAMBITS	HALOIDS	JAGGIES	LARCHES	MAITRES	MASQUES	PAJAMAS	PATENTS	RAMRODS	SALLIES
CARNIES	DAISIES	FADEINS	GAMBLES	HALTERS	JAGLESS	LARDERS	MAJGENS	MASSIFS	PALACES	PATHANS	RAMSONS	SALMONS
CARPALS	DAKOTAS	FAERIES	GAMBOLS	HALVAHS	JAGUARS	LARDONS	MAKEDOS	MASTERS	PALAMAS	PATINAS	RANCHES	SALOONS
CARPELS	DALASIS	FAEROES	GAMETES	HALVERS	JAILERS	LAREDOS	MAKEUPS	MASTICS	PALATES	PATNESS	RANCHOS	SALTERS
CARPERS	DALETHS	FAGENDS	GAMINES	HAMITES	JAILORS	LARGESS	MAKINGS	MATCHES	PALINGS	PATRIES	RANCORS	SALUKIS
CARPETS	DALLIES	FAILLES	GAMMERS	HAMLETS	JAMCAMS	LARIATS	MALAGAS	MATHERS	PALLETS	PATROLS	RANGERS	SALUTES
CARPOUS	DALTONS	FAIRIES	GAMMONS	HAMMERS	JAMMERS	LARKERS	MALIANS	MATHEWS	PALLORS	PATRONS	RANKERS	SALVERS
CARRELS	DAMAGES	FAJITAS	GANDERS	HAMPERS	JAMMIES	LARKINS	MALICES	MATHIAS	PALMERS	PATSIES	RANKLES	SALVOES
CARRIES	DAMASKS	FAKEIDS	GANGERS	HAMULUS	JANGLES	LARRUPS	MALIGNS	MATLESS	PALOMAS	PATTERS	RANLAPS	SALVORS
CARROTS	DAMASUS	FALCONS	GANNETS	HANDERS	JARDINS	LASCARS	MALLETS	MATRONS	PALTERS	PATTIES	RANSOMS	SAMARAS
CARTELS	DAMMERS	FALLALS	GAOLERS	HANDLES	JARFULS	LASHERS	MALLEUS	MATTERS	PAMPERS	PATZERS	RANTERS	SAMBASS
CARTERS	DAMNERS	FALLERS	GAPKIDS	HANGARS	JARGONS	LASHUPS	MALLOWS	MATURES	PANADAS	PAUPERS	RAPIERS	SAMEDIS
CARTONS	DAMPENS	FALLOWS	GAPLESS	HANGBYS	JARLESS	LASSIES	MALTEDS	MATZOHS	PANAMAS	PAUSERS	RAPINES	SAMEKHS
CARTOPS	DAMPERS	FALTERS	GARAGES	HANGERS	JASPERS	LASSOES	MALTHUS	MAULERS	PANDERS	PAVANES	RAPINIS	SAMLETS
CARVELS	DAMSELS	FAMINES	GARBLES	HANGUPS	JAWLESS	LASTGAS	MAMMALS	MAUMAUS	PANDITS	PAVINGS	RAPPELS	SAMOANS
CARVERS	DAMSONS	FAMULUS	GARCONS	HANKERS	JAYCEES	LATCHES	MANAGES	MAUROIS	PANFULS	PAVIORS	RAPPERS	SAMOSAS
CASABAS	DANANAS	FANCIES	GARDENS	HANKIES	JAYVEES	LATEENS	MANANAS	MAUSERS	PANIERS	PAWNEES	RAPTORS	SAMPANS
CASAVAS	DANCERS	FANDOMS	GARGLES	HANSOMS	JAZZBOS	LATENTS	MANDANS	MAUVAIS	PANINIS	PAWNERS	RAREGAS	SAMPLES
CASEINS	DANDERS	FANFICS	GARLICS	HAPLESS	JAZZERS	LATEXES	MANDAYS	MAVISES	PANNERS	PAWPAWS	RASCALS	SAMPRAS
CASEOUS	DANDIES	FANIONS	GARLITS	HAPPENS	KABUKIS	LATHERS	MANEGES	MAXIMAS	PANSIES	PAYCUTS	RASHERS	SAMSONS
CASERNS	DANDLES	FANJETS	GARNERS	HAPTICS	KADETTS	LATICES	MANGERS	MAXIMUS	PANTERS	PAYDAYS	RASPERS	SANBLAS
CASHEWS	DANGERS	FANNERS	GARNETS	HARBORS	KAHUNAS	LATIGOS	MANGLES	MAXIXES	PANTIES	PAYLESS	RASSLES	SANCTUS
CASHINS	DANGLES	FANOUTS	GARRETS	HARDEES	KAISERS	LATIMES	MANGOES	MAYDAYS	PANZERS	PAYOFFS	RASTERS	SANDALS
CASINGS	DANIELS	FANTANS	GARTERS	HARDENS	KAKAPOS	LATINAS	MANIACS	MAYHEMS	PAPAGOS	PAYOLAS	RASURES	SANDERS
CASINOS	DANITES	FANTODS	GASBAGS	HARHARS	KAKUROS	LATINOS	MANILAS	MAYINGS	PAPAYAS	PAYOUTS	RATINES	SANSEIS
CASITAS	DANVERS	FARFELS	GASCANS	HARKENS	KANAKAS	LATINUS	MANLESS	MAYTAGS	PAPELES	QABALAS	RATINGS	SAPIENS
CASKETS	DAPHNES	FARINAS	GASCAPS	HARLEYS	KANSANS	LAUDERS	MANNERS	NABBERS	PAPIERS	QATARIS	RATIONS	SAPLESS
CASQUES	DAPHNIS	FARMERS	GASCONS	HARLOTS	KARATES	LAULAUS	MANNIES	NAGGERS	PAPISTS	RABBETS	RATITES	SAPPERS
CASSIAS	DAPPLES	FARNESS	GASEOUS	HARMERS	LABATTS	LAURELS	MANTELS	NAIADES	PAPPIES	RABBITS	RATLINS	SARONGS
CASSIUS	DARKENS	FARROWS	GASHOGS	HARNESS	LABFEES	LAVABOS	MANTLES	NAILERS	PAPUANS	RABBLES	RATTANS	SARTORS
CASTERS	DARKLES	FASCIAS	GASJETS	HARPERS	LABIALS	LAVAGES	MANTRAS	NANNIES	PAPYRUS	RACEMES	RATTERS	SASHAYS
CASTLES	DARNERS	FASTENS	GASKETS	HARPIES	LABOURS	LAVORIS	MANUALS	NAPALMS	PARADES	RACINOS	RATTLES	SASSERS
CASUALS	DARTERS	FATALES	GASLESS	HARRAHS	LABRATS	LAWLESS	MANURES	NAPIERS	PARAMUS	RACISTS	RAUCOUS	SATCOMS
CATALOS	DARTLES	FATCATS	GASLOGS	HARRIES	LACEUPS	LAWYERS	MAOISTS	NAPKINS	PARAPHS	RACKERS	RAVAGES	SATEENS
CATBEDS	DASHERS	FATHERS	GASPERS	HARRODS	LACINGS	LAXNESS	MAPPERS	NAPLESS	PARATUS	RACKETS	RAVEUPS	SATIRES
CATCHES	DATABUS	FATHOMS	GASSERS	HARROWS	LACKEYS	LAYODDS	MARACAS	NAPPERS	PARCELS	RADAMES	RAVINES	SATORIS
CATENAS	DATINGS	FATLESS	GASWARS	HASAGAS	LACUNAS	LAYOFFS	MARAUDS	NAPPIES	PARCHES	RADIALS	RAVINGS	SATRAPS
CATERAS	DATIVES	FATLIPS	GATHERS	HASFITS	LADDERS	LAYOUTS	MARBLES	NARROWS	PARDONS	RADIANS	RAWBARS	SATURNS
CATFITS	DATRILS	FATNESS	GATINGS	HASSLES	LADDIES	LAZARUS	MARCELS	NASTIES	PARENTS	RADICES	RAWEGGS	SAUCERS

SAVAGES
SAVALAS
SAVANAS
SAVANTS
SAVINGS
SAVIORS
SAVOURS
SAVVIES
SAWLOGS
SAWPITS
SAWYERS
SAYINGS
SAYMASS
SAYSYES
TABARDS
TABBIES
TABKEYS
TABLETS
TABSETS
TACITUS
TACKERS
TACKLES
TACOMAS
TACTICS
TAFFIES
TAGDAYS
TAGENDS
TAGGERS
TAGOUTS
TAHINIS
TAILERS
TAILORS
TAKEINS
TAKINGS
TALCUMS
TALENTS
TALKERS
TALKIES
TALLIES
TALLOWS
TALUSES
TAMALES
TAMPERS
TAMTAMS
TANDEMS
TANGLES
TANKERS
TANNERS
TANNINS
TANOAKS
TANSIES
TAOISTS
TAPINGS
TAPPANS
TAPPERS
TAPPETS
TARGETS
TARIFFS
TARMACS
TAROILS
TARPITS
TARPONS
TARRIES
TARSALS
TARTANS
TARTARS
TARZANS
TASSELS
TASTERS
TATAMIS
TATTERS
TATTLES
TATTOOS
TAUTENS
TAVERNS
TAXCUTS
TAXLAWS
TAXLESS
TAYLORS
VACATES
VACUOUS
VACUUMS
VALINES
VALISES
VALLEYS
VALOURS
VALUERS
VAMPERS
VANDALS
VAPOURS
VARIERS
VARIOUS
VARLETS
VASSALS
VATDYES
VATFULS
VAUDOIS
WABBITS
WADDERS
WADDLES
WADKINS
WAFFLES
WAFTERS
WAGGERS
WAGGLES
WAHINES
WAHWAHS
WAILERS
WAITERS
WAIVERS
WAKAMES
WAKEUPS
WAKINGS
WALKERS
WALKINS
WALKONS
WALKUPS
WALLETS
WALLOPS
WALLOWS
WALNUTS
WALTERS
WALTONS
WALTZES
WAMBLES
WAMPUMS
WANDERS
WANGLES
WANKELS
WANNESS
WANTADS
WANTERS
WANTONS
WAPITIS
WARBLES
WARDENS
WARDERS
WARGODS
WARLESS
WARMERS
WARMUPS
WARPERS
WARRENS
WARVETS
WASABIS
WASHERS
WASHUPS
WASTERS
WATCHES
WATKINS
WATTLES
WATUSIS
WAXINGS
WAYLAYS
WAYLESS
XANADUS
YAKIMAS
YAKKERS
YAMAHAS
YAMMERS
YANKEES
YANKERS
YANQUIS
YAPPERS
YARDERS
YARROWS
YATTERS
YAWNERS
YAWPERS
ZAGNUTS
ZAPATAS
ZAPPERS

••AS•••

ABASERS
ABASHED
ABASHES
ABASING
AGASSIZ
AHASSLE
ALASKAN
ALASKAS
ALASSAD
AMASSED
AMASSER
AMASSES
ANASAZI
AWASHIN
BEASLEY
BEASTIE
BEASTLY
BIASING
BIASPLY
BIASSED
BIASSES
BLASTED
BLASTER
BOASTED
BOASTER
BOASTOF
BRASHER
BRASHES
BRASHLY
BRASIER
BRASIZE
BRASSES
BRASSIE
CEASING
CHASERS
CHASING
CHASMAL
CHASMIC
CHASSED
CHASSES
CHASSIS
CHASTEN
CHASTER
CLASHED
CLASHER
CLASHES
CLASPED
CLASPER
CLASSED
CLASSER
CLASSES
CLASSIC
CLASSON
COASTAL
COASTED
COASTER
CRASHAW
CRASHED
CRASHER
CRASHES
CRASSER
CRASSLY
CRASSUS
DOASIDO
DRASTIC
EDASNER
ELASTIC
ELASTIN
ERASERS
ERASING
ERASMUS
ERASTUS
ERASURE
EVASION
EVASIVE
FEASTED
FEASTER
FEASTON
FIASCOS
FLASHED
FLASHER
FLASHES
FLASHON
FRASIER
GHASTLY
GLASGOW
GLASHOW
GLASSED
GLASSES
GNASHED
GNASHER
GNASHES
GRASPAT
GRASPED
GRASPER
GRASSED
GRASSES
GRASSLE
INASHOE
INASNAP
INASNIT
INASPIN
INASPOT
INASTEW
INASTIR
INASUIT
KRASNER
KVASSES
LEASERS
LEASETO
LEASHED
LEASHES
LEASING
LHASANS
MEASLES
MEASURE
MIASARA
MIASMAL
MIASMAS
MIASMIC
OFASORT
ONASSIS
PEASANT
PEASOUP
PHASEIN
PHASERS
PHASING
PIASTER
PIASTRE
PLASHED
PLASHES
PLASMAS
PLASMIC
PLASTER
PLASTIC
QUASARS
QUASHED
QUASHES
REASKED
REASONS
REASSAY
ROASTED
ROASTER
SEASALT
SEASICK
SEASIDE
SEASLUG
SEASONS
SEASTAR
SHASTRI
SLASHED
SLASHER
SLASHES
SMASHED
SMASHER
SMASHES
SMASHUP
SPASSKY
STASHED
STASHES
STASSEN
SUASION
SUASIVE
SWASHED
SWASHES
TEASELS
TEASERS
TEASETS
TEASEUP
TEASHOP
TEASING
TOASTED
TOASTEE
TOASTER
TRASHED
TRASHER
TRASHES
TRASHTV
UNASKED
WEASELS
WRASSES
YEASTED

••A•S••

ADAMSES
ADAMSON
AGASSIZ
AHASSLE
ALASSAD
AMASSED
AMASSER
AMASSES
ARALSEA
BEADSUP
BEAMSUP
BEARSON
BEARSUP
BEATSAT
BEATSIT
BEATSME
BEATSON
BEATSUP
BIASSED
BIASSES
BRAISED
BRAISES
BRANSON
BRASSES
BRASSIE
CHAISES
CHANSON
CHASSED
CHASSES
CHASSIS
CHATSUP
CLAMSUP
CLASSED
CLASSER
CLASSES
CLASSIC
CLASSON
CLAUSAL
CLAUSES
CLAWSAT
COARSEN
COARSER
CRAISIN
CRAMSIN
CRASSER
CRASSLY
CRASSUS
DEADSEA
DEADSET
DEALSIN
DEALSTO
DEALSUP
DEARSIR
DIALSIN
DIALSUP
DNAASES
DRAGSIN
DRAGSON
DRAGSUP
DRAWSIN
DRAWSON
DRAWSTO
DRAWSUP
ELAPSED
ELAPSES
FRAISES
GEARSTO
GEARSUP
GLAMSUP
GLASSED
GLASSES
GNAWSAT
GNAWSON
GRABSAT
GRASSED
GRASSES
GRASSLE
GRAYSON
HEADSAW
HEADSET
HEADSIN
HEADSTO
HEADSUP
HEALSUP
HEAPSOF
HEAPSON
HEAPSUP
HEARSAY
HEARSES
HEARSOF
HEATSUP
HOARSEN
HOARSER
KLATSCH
KVASSES
LEADSIN
LEADSON
LEADSTO
LEADSUP
LEAKSIN
LEANSIN
LEANSON
LEANSTO
LEAPSAT
LEAPSIN
LEAPSON
LEAPSUP
LIAISED
LIAISES
LIAISON
LOADSIN
LOADSOF
LOADSUP
MEANSIT
MEANSTO
ONASSIS
PEARSON
PLAISIR
PLANSON
PLANSTO
PLAYSAT
PLAYSBY
PLAYSON
PLAYSTO
PLAYSUP
PRAISED
PRAISER
PRAISES
PRAYSTO
READSIN
READSON
READSTO
READSUP
REARSUP
REASSAY
ROARSAT
SCADSOF
SEALSIN
SEALSUP
SLAMSON
SLAPSON
SNAGSUP
SNAPSAT
SNAPSON
SNAPSTO
SNAPSUP
SOAKSIN
SOAKSUP
SOAPSUP
SPARSER
SPASSKY
STARSIN
STARSKY
STASSEN
STAYSAT
STAYSIN
STAYSON
STAYSUP
SWANSEA
SWANSON
SWATSAT
TEAMSUP
TEARSAT
TEARSIT
TEARSUP
THATSIT
THATSOK
TRANSAM
TRANSIT
TRANSOM
WEARSON
WHATSAY
WHATSIS
WHATSIT
WHATSUP
WRAPSUP
WRASSES

••A••S•

AGAINST
ALAMOSA
ANALYSE
ANALYST
ANAPEST
ANATASE
ARABIST
ATACOST
ATALOSS
ATAVISM
ATAVIST
AWAREST
BAALISH
BAALISM
BAALIST
BEAMISH
BEARISH
BEAUISH
BOARISH
BRALESS
BRAVEST
BYANOSE
CLAYISH
CRAFTSY
CZARISM
CZARIST
DEADEST
DEAFEST
DEAREST
DIARIST
DNATEST
DUALISM
DUALIST
EVANISH
GOAMISS
GOATISH
GRAVEST
GRAYEST
GRAYISH
IMAGISM
IMAGIST
IMAMESS
INACAST
INAMESS
INANEST
INARUSH
IRATEST
KNAVISH
LEANEST
MEANEST
NEAREST
NEATEST
OPALISH
ORALIST
PEAKISH
PIANISM
PIANIST
PLANISH
PRADESH
REALEST
REALISE
REALISM
REALIST
REAMASS
REARISE
REAROSE
SEABASS
SEAMIST
SEAMOSS
SIAMESE
SLAVISH
SOANDSO
SPANISH
SPAREST
STALEST
STATISM
STATIST
SUAVEST
TEALESS
TEAMUSA
TEAROSE
TOADISH
TRAIPSE
TSARISM
TSARIST
WEAKEST
WEAKISH

••A•••S

AAAMAPS
ABASERS
ABASHES
ABATERS
ABATORS
ACACIAS
ACARIDS
ADAGIOS
ADAMSES
AGARICS
ALARBUS
ALARUMS
ALASKAS
AMADEUS
AMANTIS
AMASSES
AMATOLS
AMAZONS
ANACINS
ANADEMS
ANALOGS
ANANIAS
ANARCHS
APACHES
ARABICS
ARABLES
ARAMIDS
ASANTES
ATALOSS
ATAMANS
AVALONS
AVANTIS
AVATARS
AWAKENS
AWAKERS
AZALEAS
BEACHES
BEACONS
BEADERS
BEADLES
BEAGLES
BEAKERS
BEAMERS
BEANIES
BEARERS
BEATERS
BEATLES
BEAVERS
BIALIES
BIASSES
BLADERS
BLAMERS
BLAZERS
BLAZONS
BOATELS
BOATERS
BRACERS
BRAHMAS
BRAISES
BRALESS
BRASHES
BRASSES
BRAVOES
BRAYERS
BRAZENS
CHABLIS
CHACHAS
CHAFERS
CHAINES
CHAISES
CHAKRAS
CHALCIS
CHALETS
CHALONS
CHAMOIS
CHANCES
CHANELS
CHANGES
CHAPELS
CHARGES
CHARLES
CHARROS
CHASERS
CHASSES
CHASSIS
CHAZANS
CLAMORS
CLAQUES
CLARETS
CLASHES
CLASSES
CLAUSES
CLAWERS
COACHES
COALERS
COALGAS
COATEES
COATERS
COAXERS
CRADLES
CRASHES
CRASSUS
CRATERS
CRAVATS
CRAVENS
CRAVERS
CRAYONS
CRAZIES
CSARDAS
CUATROS
CYANIDS
CZARDAS
DEACONS
DEADENS
DEAFENS
DEALERS
DEARIES
DEARTHS
DHARMAS
DIABLES
DIABLOS
DIADEMS
DIALERS
DIALOGS
DIALUPS
DIAPERS
DIARIES
DIARIOS
DIATOMS
DNAASES
DNALABS
DRAGEES
DRAGONS
DRAPERS
DRAWEES
DRAWERS
DWARVES
EBAYERS
ECARTES
ELAINES
ELANCES
ELANETS
ELAPIDS
ELAPSES
ELATERS
ENABLES
ENAMELS
ENAMORS
EPARCHS
ERASERS
ERASMUS
ERASTUS
EVADERS
EXACTAS
EXARCHS
FEARERS
FIACRES
FIANCES
FIASCOS
FLACONS
FLAGONS
FLAKERS
FLAMBES
FLAMERS
FLANGES
FLASHES
FLATTVS
FLAUNTS
FLAUTAS
FLAVIUS
FLAVORS
FLAYERS
FOAMERS
FRAISES
FRAMERS
FRANCES
FRANCIS
FRAPPES
FRATERS
GLAMORS
GLANCES
GLASSES
GLAZERS
GNASHES
GNAWERS
GOALIES
GOAMISS
GOATEES
GRACIAS
GRADERS
GRAHAMS
GRAMMES
GRAMMYS
GRAMPAS
GRAMPUS
GRANGES
GRANPAS
GRAPPAS
GRASSES
GRATERS
GRATIAS
GRAVELS
GRAVERS
GRAVIES
GRAZERS
HEADERS
HEALERS
HEAPERS
HEARERS
HEARSES
HEARTHS
HEATERS
HEAVENS
HEAVERS
HEAVIES
HOAGIES
HOAXERS
HYANNIS
IDAREDS
IMAGERS
IMAGOES
IMAMESS
IMARETS
INAMESS
ITALICS
JEALOUS
KIARIOS
KLAXONS
KRAKENS
KVASSES
KWACHAS
KWANZAS
LEACHES
LEADENS
LEADERS
LEADINS
LEADUPS
LEAGUES
LEAKERS
LEAKEYS
LEANERS
LEANTOS
LEAPERS
LEASERS
LEASHES
LEAVENS
LHASANS
LIAISES
LLADROS
LOADERS
LOAFERS
LOANERS
LOATHES
MCADAMS
MEADOWS
MEAGLES
MEALIES
MEANIES

MEASLES
MIASMAS
MOANERS
MTADAMS
MTATHOS
NEATENS
NUANCES
OMAHANS
ONABIAS
ONAGERS
ONASSIS
OPAQUES
ORACIES
ORACLES
ORANGES
ORANTES
ORATORS
OSAKANS
OTARIES
OVARIES
PAANGAS
PBANDJS
PEACHES
PEAHENS
PEANUTS
PEAPODS
PGAPROS
PHASERS
PIAFFES
PIAZZAS
PLACERS
PLAGUES
PLAICES
PLAINES
PLAINTS
PLAKATS
PLANERS
PLANETS
PLAQUES
PLASHES
PLASMAS
PLATENS
PLATERS
PLATIES
PLAUTUS
PLAYERS
POACHES
PRAISES
PRANCES
PRATERS
PRAYERS
PSANDQS
QRATIOS
QUAGGAS
QUAHOGS
QUAKERS
QUAKIES
QUAPAWS
QUARLES
QUARTES
QUARTOS
QUASARS
QUASHES
QUATRES
QUAVERS
REACHES
READERS
READIES
REAGANS
REAMASS
REAMERS
REAPERS
REARERS
REASONS
REATTAS
REAVERS
REAVOWS
RIALTOS
ROACHES
ROADEOS
ROADERS
ROADIES
ROAMERS
ROARERS
RUANDAS
RVALUES
SCALARS
SCALERS
SCARABS
SCARERS
SCARVES
SCATHES
SEAARMS
SEABAGS
SEABASS
SEABEDS
SEABEES
SEACATS
SEACOWS
SEADOGS
SEAEELS
SEAGODS
SEALABS
SEALEGS
SEALERS
SEAMAPS
SEAMERS
SEAMOSS
SEANCES
SEARERS
SEASONS
SEATERS
SEAWAYS
SHADERS
SHADOWS
SHAKERS
SHAKOES
SHALOMS
SHAMANS
SHAPERS
SHARERS
SHAVERS
SKATERS
SLAKERS
SLALOMS
SLASHES
SLATERS
SLAVERS
SLAYERS
SMASHES
SNAKERS
SNAPONS
SNARERS
SOAKERS
SOAPERS
SOARERS
SPACERS
SPADERS
SPARERS
SPATHES
SPAYERS
STABLES
STAGERS
STAGNES
STALAGS
STAMENS
STANCES
STANZAS
STAPLES
STARERS
STARVES
STASHES
STATERS
STATICS
STATINS
STATORS
STATUES
STAYERS
SWASHES
SWATHES
SWAYERS
TEABAGS
TEACHES
TEACUPS
TEALESS
TEAPOTS
TEAPOYS
TEARERS
TEARGAS
TEASELS
TEASERS
TEASETS
TEATROS
TEAURNS
THALERS
THAWERS
TOADIES
TRACERS
TRADERS
TRAMPAS
TRANCES
TRASHES
TRAUMAS
TRAVELS
TRAVERS
URACILS
USABLES
USANCES
UTAHANS
UVALUES
VEADARS
WEAKENS
WEAKONS
WEALTHS
WEANERS
WEAPONS
WEARERS
WEARIES
WEASELS
WEAVERS
WHALERS
WHARVES
WHATIFS
WHATSIS
WRAITHS
WRAPUPS
WRASSES
XSANDOS
ZEALOTS
ZEALOUS

•••AS••

ALIASES
APHASIA
APHASIC
ARRASES
ATLASES
AVGASES
BALASES
BELASCO
BREASTS
BROASTS
CANASTA
CDCASES
CREASED
CREASER
CREASES
DALASIS
DAMASKS
DAMASUS
DATASET
DEBASED
DEBASER
DEBASES
DEMASTS
DIDASET
DNAASES
DYNASTS
DYNASTY
EMBASSY
ENCASED
ENCASES
ENMASSE
ESIASON
EURASIA
FORASEC
GIRASOL
GLEASON
GREASED
GREASER
GREASES
HADASAY
HADASET
HASASAY
HASASET
IGUASSU
IMPASSE
IMPASTO
INCASED
INCASES
INHASTE
INTASTE
ITSASIN
JIRASEK
JOCASTA
JUDASES
KARASEA
LAGASSE
LIPASES
MIDASES
MIKASAS
NATASHA
NOTASTE
OBLASTS
OUTASKS
PARASKI
PARASOL
PEGASUS
PHRASAL
PHRASED
PHRASES
PICASSO
PLEASED
PLEASER
PLEASES
PULASKI
REBASTE
RECASED
RECASES
RECASTS
REPASTE
REPASTS
RETASTE
SPLASHY
SQUASHY
STBASIL
STRASSE
TABASCO
TOTASTE
TREASON
TUNASUB
UNBASED
UNCASED
UNCASES
UNCASKS
UNEASES
UNHASPS
UNHASTY
UNMASKS
UNMASTS
UNNASAL
UNPASTE
UNRASPY
UNTASTY
UPCASTS
WABASHA

•••A•S•

BAHAISM
BAHAIST
BECAUSE
CLEANSE
DADAISM
DADAIST
DEGAUSS
EMBASSY
ENMASSE
EXHAUST
EXPANSE
IDSAYSO
IGUASSU
IMPASSE
IZZATSO
JUDAISM
KOMATSU
LAGASSE
LAMAISM
LAMAIST
LAVALSE
MALAISE
PICASSO
RELAPSE
RERAISE
ROMANSH
SEEALSO
SHIATSU
STRASSE
STRAUSS
SYNAPSE
TUBAIST
UNHARSH
UPRAISE

•••A••S

ABLATES
ABRADES
ABRAXAS
ACKACKS
ADDAXES
ADRATES
AERATES
AFFAIRS
AFRAMES
AGNAILS
AGNATES
AIRACES
ALDAVIS
ALIASES
ALKALIS
ALLAGES
ALPACAS
ANNALES
ANTARES
APPALLS
ARBACES
ARCADES
ARGALIS
ARIANES
ARMADAS
ARRACKS
ARRASES
ASFARAS
ASIAGOS
ASSAILS
ATLASES
ATTACKS
ATTAINS
AUBADES
AUPAIRS
AVGASES
AVIATES
AYEAYES
BAHAMAS
BALASES
BALATAS
BANANAS
BANANES
BARACUS
BASALTS
BAZAARS
BECALMS
BEDAUBS
BEDAZES
BEFALLS
BEHAVES
BELAIRS
BELARUS
BENARES
BERATES
BETAKES
BEWAILS
BEWARES
BICARBS
BIGAPES
BOGARTS
BONACIS
BORATES
BREASTS
BREATHS
BRIARDS
BROADAS
BROASTS
BUTANES
BYNAMES
BYPATHS
BYTALKS
CABALAS
CABANAS
CAMAROS
CANAPES
CANARDS
CAPADES
CARACAS
CARAFES
CASABAS
CASAVAS
CATALOS
CCLAMPS
CDCASES
CDRACKS
CDRATES
CERATES
CETANES
CHIAPAS
CICADAS
CLEAVES
COBALTS
COLADAS
COWARDS
CREASES
CREATES
CUBAGES
CURARES
CURATES
DACAPOS
DALASIS
DAMAGES
DAMASKS
DAMASUS
DANANAS
DATABUS
DEBARKS
DEBASES
DEBATES
DECADES
DECAMPS
DECANTS
DEDALUS
DEFACES
DEFAMES
DEFANGS
DEGAUSS
DEHAIRS
DEMANDS
DEMARKS
DEMASTS
DEPARTS
DERAILS
DERATES
DESALTS
DETAILS
DETAINS
DEWAXES
DIDACTS
DILATES
DIMAGES
DISARMS
DIZAINS
DNAASES
DOGAPES
DOMAINS
DONATES
DONATUS
DOSADOS
DOSAGES
DOTAGES
DOTARDS
DOUANES
DRYADES
DUKAKIS
DYNAMOS
DYNASTS
ECLAIRS
EDWARDS
EFFACES
ELUANTS
ELUATES
EMBALMS
EMBANKS
EMBARKS
EMPALES
EMPATHS
ENCAGES
ENCAMPS
ENCASES
ENDALLS
ENFACES
ENFANTS
ENGAGES
ENLACES
ENRAGES
ENRANKS
ENTAILS
EQUATES
ERLANGS
ERRANDS
ESCALUS
ESCAPES
ESCARPS
ESTADOS
ESTATES
ETHANES
EUBANKS
EULABUS
EXHALES
EXMATES
EXPANDS
EXYANKS
FABARES
FACADES
FATALES
FEMALES
FINALES
FIXATES
FMBANDS
FOLATES
FORAGES
FUGATOS
GALANOS
GALANTS
GALAXES
GARAGES
GELATES
GELATIS
GELATOS
GITANOS
GOCARTS
GOKARTS
GREASES
GREAVES
GYRATES
HADAGAS
HALALAS
HASAGAS
HAVANAS
HAZARDS
HERALDS
HEXANES
HIJACKS
HOMAGES
HOWARDS
HYRACES
HYRAXES
ICEAGES
ICEAXES
IDCARDS
IDEATES
IGUANAS
IMPACTS
IMPAIRS
IMPALAS
IMPALES
IMPARTS
INCANTS
INCASES
INFANTS
INGALLS
INGATES
INHALES
INLANDS
INMATES
INNAGES
INNARDS
INSALES
INTAILS
INTAKES
INVADES
INWARDS
IODATES
ISLANDS
JACALES
JICAMAS
JUDASES
JUMADAS
KAKAPOS
KANAKAS
KARATES
KIWANIS
LABATTS
LAVABOS
LAVAGES
LAZARUS
LEGATES
LEGATOS
LEVADES
LIGANDS
LIGATES
LINAGES
LIPARIS
LIPASES
LIZARDS
LOCALES
LOCATES
LOVAGES
LOYALES
LUNATES
LUXATES
MACACOS
MADAMES
MAHARIS
MALAGAS
MANAGES
MANANAS
MARACAS
MARAUDS
MCCALLS
MCHALES
MEDAKAS
MEGANES
MENACES
MENAGES
MESAMIS
METATES
MIDASES
MIKADOS
MIKASAS
MIRADAS
MIRAGES
MISACTS
MISADDS
MISAIMS
MOHAIRS
MOHAVES
MOHAWKS
MOJAVES
MORALES
MORANIS
MOSAICS
MOVADOS
MURANOS
MUTANTS
MUTATES
NAIADES
NAPALMS
NAVAHOS
NAVAIDS
NAVAJOS
NEGATES
NEPALIS
NOCARBS
NOGALES
NOHANDS
NONAGES
NONAMES
NONARTS
NOPALES
NOTATES
NOVALIS
NUTATES
NYYANKS
OBLASTS
OBLATES
OBTAINS
OCEANUS
OCTANES
OCTANTS
OCTAVES
OCTAVOS
OGLALAS
OHMAGES
OLEATES
ONEACTS
ONRAMPS
ONWARDS
OPIATES
ORDAINS
OTTAWAS
OUTACTS
OUTADDS
OUTAGES
OUTASKS
OUTAWES
OXCARTS
OXTAILS
PAJAMAS
PALACES
PALAMAS
PALATES
PANADAS
PANAMAS
PAPAGOS
PAPAYAS
PARADES
PARAMUS
PARAPHS
PARATUS
PATACAS
PAVANES
PDJAMES
PEDANTS
PEGASUS
PELAGES
PENATES
PESADES
PETALES
PETARDS
PHRASES
PICARAS
PICAROS
PILATES
PILATUS
PINATAS
PIPAGES
PIRAEUS
PIRATES
PITAYAS
PLEASES
POLARAS
POLARIS
POMADES
POSADAS
POTAGES
POTAMUS
PREACTS
PREAGES
PREAMPS
PREARMS
PUPATES
PYRAMUS
QABALAS
QATARIS
RADAMES
RAMADAS
RAVAGES
REBAITS
REBAKES
REBALES
REBANKS
REBATES
RECAGES
RECALLS
RECANES
RECANTS
RECASES
RECASTS
REDACTS
REDANTS
REDARES
REDARNS
REDATES
REEARNS
REFACES
REFALLS
REFAXES
REGAINS
REGALES
REGARDS
REHANGS
REHAULS
REJAILS
RELACES
RELANDS
RELANES
RELATES
RELAXES
REMAILS
REMAINS
REMAKES
REMANDS
REMARKS
REMATES
RENAILS
RENAMES
REPACKS
REPAGES
REPAIRS
REPARKS
REPASTS
REPAVES
RERACKS
RERAKES
RERANKS
RERATES
RESALES
RESALTS
RESANDS
RESAVES
RETACKS
RETAILS
RETAINS
RETAKES
RETAMES
RETAPES
RETARDS
RETAXES
REVAMPS
REWAKES
REWARDS
REWARMS
REWARNS
REWAXES
RIBALDS
RIBANDS
RITARDS
ROBARDS
ROLAIDS
ROMAINS
ROMAJIS
ROMANIS
ROMANOS
ROMANUS
ROTATES
ROYALES
RUBATOS
RUMAKIS
RVPARKS
SABADOS
SAFARIS
SALAAMS
SALADES
SALAMIS
SAMARAS
SAVAGES
SAVALAS
SAVANAS
SAVANTS
SCHAYES
SCLAFFS
SCRAPES
SCRAWLS
SEAARMS
SECANTS
SEDATES
SEMANAS
SENATES
SERAPES
SERAPHS
SERAPIS
SESAMES
SEWARDS
SHEATHS
SHEAVES
SLEAZES
SOFARAS
SOLACES
SOLARAS
SOMALIS
SONATAS
SPRAINS
SPRAWLS
SQUALLS
SQUARES
SQUAWKS
STBARTS
STEARNS
STJAMES
STMARKS
STMARYS
STPAULS
STRAFES
STRAINS
STRAITS
STRANDS
STRATAS

STRATUS
STRAUSS
SUBARUS
TABARDS
TAMALES
TATAMIS
TEJANAS
TEJANOS
TENACES
TENANTS
TETANUS
THEABCS
THEAGES
THEALPS
THEARTS
THEAXIS
THRALLS
THWACKS
THWARTS
TIRADES
TISANES
TOPAZES
TOWAGES
TOWARDS
TRIAGES
TRUANTS
TSHAPES
TVGAMES
TVTAPES
TWOACTS
TYRANTS
ULLAGES
ULZANAS
UMLAUTS
UNBAITS
UNBALES
UNBARES
UNCAGES
UNCAKES
UNCASES
UNCASKS
UNEASES
UNFACTS
UNHAIRS
UNHANDS
UNHASPS
UNIATES
UNLACES
UNLADES
UNLAXES
UNMAKES
UNMASKS
UNMASTS
UNMATES
UNNAILS
UNPACKS
UNPAWNS
UNRACKS
UNTACKS
UNTAMES
UNTAPES
UNTAXES
UNWALLS
UPCARDS
UPCASTS
UPDARTS
UPDATES
UPGAZES
UPLANDS
UPRATES
UPTAKES
UPTALKS
UPWAFTS
UPWARDS
UQUARKS
USHAPES
VACATES
VIHARAS
VIRAGOS
VISAGES
VISAVIS
VITALIS
VITARAS
VIVANTS
VOYAGES
VSHAPES
WAKAMES
WASABIS
WIZARDS
WREATHS
XANADUS
YAMAHAS
YSHAPES
YUKATAS
ZAPATAS
ZENANAS
ZOCALOS

••••AS•

ABREAST
AIRBASE
AIRMASS
ALLCASH
AMYLASE
ANATASE
APPEASE
ATLEAST
BADCASE
BADPAST
BALLAST
BELFAST
BIGEAST
BIGEASY
BIOMASS
BOMBAST
BONEASH
BUDVASE
BUSPASS
CANVASS
CARCASS
CARWASH
CHUMASH
COMCAST
COMPASS
CUIRASS
CUTLASS
DECEASE
DECLASS
DIECAST
DISEASE
DISMAST
DONTASK
DOTDASH
DRYWASH
DUEEAST
ECSTASY
EGGCASE
ENCHASE
ENCLASP
EYELASH
EYEMASK
EYEWASH
FANBASE
FANTASM
FANTAST
FANTASY
FAREAST
FBICASE
FLYCAST
FLYPAST
GASMASK
GETCASH
GETPAST
GOTCASH
GOTPAST
GOULASH
GUNCASE
GYMNAST
HOGWASH
ILLPASS
INACAST
INCLASS
INPHASE
INULASE
ITSEASY
JACKASS
JETWASH
KEYCASE
LACTASE
LAWCASE
LETPASS
LOWMASS
MADDASH
MALPASO
MALTASE
MIDEAST
MISCAST
MOMBASA
MRSBASS
MUDWASP
NASTASE
NOCLASS
NONBASE
NONCASH
NONPAST
NOTEASY
OAKCASK
OFFBASE
OFFCAST
OILBASE
ONEBASE
ONLEASE
ONLEASH
ONTOAST
ORGIAST
OUTCAST
OUTFAST
OUTKAST
OUTLASH
OUTLAST
OUTPASS
OUTWASH
OXIDASE
PATCASH
PAYCASH
PENCASE
PODCAST
PRECAST
PREWASH
PROEAST
QUEPASA
RANPAST
REAMASS
RECLASP
RECLASS
REGRASP
RELEASE
REPHASE
RETOAST
RUNPAST
SAMBASS
SARCASM
SAWPAST
SAYMASS
SEABASS
SEEPAST
SKIMASK
SUBBASE
SUBBASS
SUBCASE
SUBCASH
SUBCAST
SUBTASK
SUCRASE
SUNFAST
SURPASS
TAXBASE
TENPAST
THEEAST
THEMASK
TOLEASE
TOOEASY
TOPMAST
TWOBASE
UNCLASP
UNLEASH
UPCOAST
UPPHASE
WEBCAST
WETWASH
ZEBRASS

••••A•S

AAAMAPS
ACETALS
ADONAIS
AERIALS
AFFRAYS
AFGHANS
AIRBAGS
AIRDAMS
AIRMASS
AIRSACS
AIRWARS
AIRWAYS
AJOWANS
ALEGARS
ALETAPS
ALIYAHS
ALLCAPS
ALLEARS
ALLTABS
AMTRACS
ANDEANS
ANGLAIS
ANIMALS
ANNEALS
ANNUALS
ANORAKS
ANYWAYS
AOUDADS
APPEALS
APPEARS
ARREARS
ARTCARS
ARUBANS
ASHCANS
ASHLARS
ASHPANS
ASHRAMS
ATAMANS
AVATARS
AVOWALS
AXHEADS
BADDAYS
BADHATS
BADRAPS
BAHIANS
BALKANS
BALLADS
BALSAMS
BANTAMS
BANYANS
BANZAIS
BAOBABS
BARCARS
BARTABS
BATDAYS
BAUHAUS
BAZAARS
BEDLAMS
BEGGARS
BEHEADS
BELDAMS
BEMOANS
BENDAYS
BENGALS
BERNAYS
BETRAYS
BIGCARS
BIGCATS
BIGDAYS
BIGEARS
BIGFANS
BIGMACS
BIOLABS
BIOMASS
BIRMANS
BITMAPS
BOBCATS
BOWOARS
BOWSAWS
BOXCARS
BRIDALS
BROGANS
BULGARS
BUMRAPS
BUREAUS
BURIALS
BURLAPS
BURMANS
BUROAKS
BURSARS
BUSMANS
BUSPASS
BYPLAYS
BYROADS
CAESARS
CAFTANS
CAIMANS
CANCANS
CANTABS
CANTALS
CANVASS
CARCASS
CARPALS
CASUALS
CATNAPS
CAVEATS
CAVIARS
CAYMANS
CELLARS
CENTALS
CEREALS
CHAZANS
CHORALS
CLIMATS
COEVALS
COGNACS
COLLARS
COMBATS
COMPAQS
COMPASS
COMSATS
CONFABS
CONTACS
COPCARS
CORFAMS
CORRALS
COSTARS
COUGARS
CRAVATS
CRETANS
CRUZANS
CTSCANS
CUBFANS
CUIRASS
CUSHAWS
CUTLASS
CYMBALS
DECLASS
DECLAWS
DEEJAYS
DEFEATS
DEFOAMS
DEFRAGS
DEFRAYS
DELEADS
DELRAYS
DEMEANS
DENIALS
DENTALS
DEODARS
DEWLAPS
DIDLAPS
DIGRAMS
DIKTATS
DIRHAMS
DISBARS
DISMALS
DISMAYS
DNALABS
DOGDAYS
DOGEARS
DOGNAPS
DOGTAGS
DOLLARS
DOLMANS
DOODADS
DORSALS
DOSSALS
DRCHAOS
DYEVATS
EARLAPS
EARTABS
EARTAGS
EGGSACS
EMQUADS
ENDEARS
ENDWAYS
ENGRAMS
ENNEADS
ENQUADS
ENSEALS
ENSEATS
ENTRAPS
ENWRAPS
ESPIALS
ESTRAYS
FACIALS
FALLALS
FANTANS
FATCATS
FELLAHS
FERMATS
FIGBARS
FIJIANS
FINGALS
FINIALS
FINIANS
FLYWAYS
FORMALS
FORMATS
FRIDAYS
FRYPANS
FULMARS
GAGLAWS
GALPALS
GASBAGS
GASCANS
GASCAPS
GASWARS
GAVIALS
GEEGAWS
GELCAPS
GERMANS
GERVAIS
GEWGAWS
GIGBAGS
GIMBALS
GRAHAMS
GUFFAWS
GUITARS
GULLAHS
GUNLAPS
GUNLAWS
GYMBAGS
GYMRATS
HAIKAIS
HALVAHS
HANGARS
HARHARS
HARRAHS
HAWHAWS
HAZMATS
HEEHAWS
HEPCATS
HEPTADS
HERBALS
HERMANS
HEYDAYS
HEYMANS
HOOHAHS
HOOKAHS
HOORAHS
HOORAYS
HOTCAPS
HOTCARS
HOTDAYS
HOTWARS
HOWDAHS
HUBCAPS
HUPPAHS
HURRAHS
HURRAYS
HUSSARS
HUZZAHS
HYMNALS
IBIZANS
ICEBAGS
ICECAPS
ICEDAMS
ILLPASS
INCLASS
INDIANS
INGOALS
INKPADS
INKSACS
INROADS
INSEAMS
INSPANS
INSTALS
INTEARS
INTRAYS
INYEARS
IONIANS
ISOBARS
JACKALS
JACKASS
JAGUARS
JAMCAMS
JETFANS
JETLAGS
JETWAYS
JIGSAWS
JIMJAMS
JOBJARS
JOYPADS
JUDEANS
KANSANS
KENYANS
KEYPADS
KEYPALS
KEYWAYS
KIDNAPS
KIRMANS
KITBAGS
KITKATS
KODIAKS
KOREANS
LABIALS
LABRATS
LANDAUS
LAPCATS
LARIATS
LASCARS
LAULAUS
LEEWAYS
LETPASS
LHASANS
LIBRANS
LIBYANS
LOGJAMS
LOOFAHS
LOQUATS
LOWMASS
LUMBARS
MADCAPS
MAENADS
MAGYARS
MAITAIS
MALIANS
MAMMALS
MANDANS
MANDAYS
MANIACS
MANUALS
MARHAUS
MAUMAUS
MAUVAIS
MAYDAYS
MAYTAGS
MCADAMS
MECCANS
MEDIANS
MENIALS
MENSANS
MESCALS
METFANS
MICMACS
MIDCAPS
MIDDAYS
MIDWAYS
MILLAIS
MINOANS
MINYANS
MISHAPS
MISLAYS
MISSALS
MISSAYS
MONDAYS
MORGANS
MORTALS
MORTARS
MRSBASS
MTADAMS
MTEVANS
MUDCATS
MULLAHS
MUSCATS
MUTUALS
MYRIADS
MYSTARS
NATHANS
NAYSAYS
NECTARS
NEWCARS
NEWHATS
NEWMANS
NEXRADS
NIKEADS
NISSANS
NOCLASS
NOLOADS
NONFANS
NONPARS
NONWARS
NORMALS
NORMANS
NOSEATS
NOSTARS
NOUGATS
NUBIANS
NUMBATS
OAHUANS
OAKTAGS
OCICATS
OCULARS
OFFDAYS
OGDOADS
OHIOANS
OILCANS
OILPANS
OLDBATS
OLDCARS
OLDDAYS
OLDGAGS
OLDPALS
OLDSAWS
OLDWAYS
OMAHANS
ONLOADS
OOMPAHS
ORDEALS
ORGEATS
ORLEANS
ORPHANS
OSAKANS
OUTBANS
OUTBATS
OUTEATS
OUTLAWS
OUTLAYS
OUTMANS
OUTPASS
OUTPAYS
OUTRAPS
OUTSAYS
OUTWARS
OVISACS
PADUANS
PAIDADS
PAISANS
PAPUANS
PARIAHS
PARLAYS
PASSATS
PATHANS
PAWPAWS
PAYDAYS
PEDWAYS
PENPALS
PENTADS
PERHAPS
PETCATS
PETNAPS
PETRATS
PIEPANS
PILLARS
PINOAKS
PITSAWS
PLAKATS
PLURALS
POPLARS
PORTALS
PREFABS
PREPAYS
PSYWARS
PTBOATS
PULSARS
QINTARS
QUAPAWS
QUASARS
RADIALS
RADIANS
RAGBAGS
RAGLANS
RAGMANS
RAMFANS
RANLAPS
RASCALS
RATTANS
RAWBARS
RAYBANS
REAGANS
REAMASS
RECLADS
RECLASS
RECOALS
RECOATS
REDBATS
REDBAYS
REDCAPS
REDEALS
REDHATS
REDIALS
REDOAKS
REDRAGS
REDRAWS
REDTABS
REDTAGS
REFLAGS
REGEARS
REGRABS
REHEALS
REHEARS
REHEATS
RELEADS
RELEAPS
RELOADS
RELOANS
RENTALS
REPEALS
REPEATS
REPLANS
REPLAYS
REREADS
RESCANS
RESEALS
RESEAMS
RESEATS
RESEAUS
RESNAIS
RESNAPS
RESOAKS
RESOAPS
RESPANS
RESTABS
RETEARS
RETHAWS
RETRAPS
REVEALS
REWEARS
REWRAPS
REXCATS
RIBPADS
RICRACS
RIPRAPS
RIPSAWS
RITUALS
RUGRATS
RUNLAPS
RUNWAYS
RUPIAHS
RYOKANS
SALAAMS
SAMBASS
SAMOANS
SAMPANS
SANDALS
SASHAYS
SATRAPS
SAYMASS
SCALARS
SCARABS
SCHNAPS
SCREAKS
SCREAMS
SEABAGS
SEABASS
SEACATS
SEALABS
SEAMAPS
SEAWAYS
SEESAWS
SEGWAYS
SERIALS
SEXTANS
SHAMANS
SHEVATS
SHOFARS
SIGNALS
SIMIANS
SIOUANS
SKICAPS
SKIHATS
SKYCAMS
SKYCAPS
SKYMAPS
SKYWAYS
SLOGANS
SLOVAKS
SNOCAPS
SNOCATS
SOCIALS
SOSPADS
SOXFANS
SPIRALS
SPREADS
SPYCAMS
SQUEAKS
SQUEALS
STALAGS
STREAKS
STREAMS
SUBBASS
SUBWARS
SUBWAYS
SULTANS
SUNDAES
SUNDAYS
SUNFANS
SUNHATS
SUNRAYS
SUNTANS
SURPASS
SYRIANS
TAGDAYS
TAMTAMS
TANOAKS
TAPPANS
TARMACS
TARSALS
TARTANS
TARTARS
TARZANS
TAXLAWS
TEABAGS
TENDAYS
TERRANS
TETRADS
THEBANS
THECARS
THECAVS
THEMAVS
THERAMS
THREADS
THREATS
THROATS
TICTACS
TIEBARS
TIETACS
TIMBALS
TINCANS
TINEARS
TINHATS
TIPJARS
TITIANS
TOECAPS
TOETAPS
TOMCATS
TONGANS
TOPHATS
TOUCANS
TOWBARS
TOWCARS
TOYCARS
TOYHATS
TREPANS
TROJANS
TRUMANS
TSTRAPS
TULSANS
TURBANS

TUSCANS
TVSTARS
TWODAYS
TYPEABS
UNCIALS
UNDRAWS
UNIVACS
UNLEADS
UNLEAFS
UNLOADS
UNPLANS
UNSEALS
UNSEAMS
UNSEATS
UNSNAGS
UNSNAPS
UNSPANS
UNTHAWS
UNTRAPS
UNWRAPS
UPBEARS
UPBEATS
UPHEAPS
UPLEAPS
UPLOADS
UPREARS
UPROARS
UPSOARS
UPTEARS
USFLAGS
UTAHANS
UTICANS
VANDALS
VASSALS
VEADARS
VEEJAYS
VERBALS
VESTALS
VISUALS
VULCANS
WAHWAHS
WANTADS
WAYLAYS
WBYEATS
WEBCAMS
WETBARS
WETNAPS
WETRAGS
WICCANS
WIGWAGS
WIGWAMS
WINDAUS
WOMBATS
YEOMANS
YOUMANS
ZEBRASS
ZIGZAGS
ZODIACS
ZONIANS
ZUNIANS

•••••AS

ABRAXAS
ACACIAS
ACTEDAS
ACTIVAS
AGENDAS
AGULHAS

ALASKAS
ALPACAS
ALTIMAS
AMOEBAS
AMRITAS
ANANIAS
ANDREAS
ANEMIAS
ANGELAS
ANGORAS
ANITRAS
AQUINAS
AREOLAS
ARISTAS
ARMADAS
ARNICAS
ASFARAS
ASSTDAS
ASTHMAS
AURORAS
AVESTAS
AXILLAS
AZALEAS
BAHAMAS
BALATAS
BALBOAS
BANANAS
BELUGAS
BERTHAS
BODEGAS
BORGIAS
BRAHMAS
BROADAS
BUDDHAS
BULOVAS
BUQSHAS
CABALAS
CABANAS
CABEZAS
CAMERAS
CANCHAS
CANOLAS
CANULAS
CARACAS
CARBRAS
CARINAS
CASABAS
CASAVAS
CASITAS
CASSIAS
CATENAS
CATERAS
CAYUGAS
CELICAS
CESSNAS
CHACHAS
CHAKRAS
CHEETAS
CHIAPAS
CHICHAS
CHOLLAS
CHUPPAS
CICADAS
CINEMAS
COALGAS
COLADAS
COMESAS
CONTRAS

COPULAS
CORDIAS
CORNEAS
CORONAS
CORYZAS
COWPEAS
CRITIAS
CSARDAS
CUESTAS
CUMBIAS
CUPOLAS
CZARDAS
DAHLIAS
DAKOTAS
DANANAS
DAYSPAS
DEFLEAS
DHARMAS
DOUGLAS
DRESSAS
DRVEGAS
DUENNAS
ECZEMAS
EGERIAS
ENCINAS
ENIGMAS
ESPOSAS
EUREKAS
EXACTAS
EXCUSAS
FAJITAS
FARINAS
FASCIAS
FAUXPAS
FEDORAS
FIBULAS
FIESTAS
FLAUTAS
FRESCAS
FUSUMAS
FUTURAS
GALENAS
GEISHAS
GILBLAS
GLORIAS
GLOSSAS
GOTCHAS
GRACIAS
GRAMPAS
GRANPAS
GRAPPAS
GRATIAS
GUINEAS
GURKHAS
HADAGAS
HALALAS
HASAGAS
HAVANAS
HEGIRAS
HERNIAS
HOOPLAS
HOTTEAS
ICETEAS
IGUANAS
IMPALAS
JERBOAS
JICAMAS
JOGBRAS

JOJOBAS
JUDOKAS
JUMADAS
KAHUNAS
KANAKAS
KORUNAS
KWACHAS
KWANZAS
LACUNAS
LADIDAS
LADYNAS
LAGUNAS
LAKOTAS
LAMBDAS
LAMINAS
LANCIAS
LASTGAS
LATINAS
LEGOLAS
LENGUAS
LOGGIAS
LOOMPAS
LUMINAS
MALAGAS
MANANAS
MANILAS
MANTRAS
MARACAS
MARIDAS
MARINAS
MATHIAS
MAXIMAS
MEDAKAS
MEDUSAS
MEZUZAS
MIASMAS
MIKASAS
MIMOSAS
MIRADAS
MITHRAS
MIZUNAS
MODELAS
MULETAS
MYOPIAS
NEBULAS
NEONGAS
NICOLAS
NOOTKAS
NOVELAS
NOVENAS
NUBIRAS
NUTRIAS
OGLALAS
OJIBWAS
ONABIAS
ONEIDAS
OPTIMAS
OSETRAS
OTTAWAS
PAANGAS
PAELLAS
PAGODAS
PAJAMAS
PALAMAS
PALOMAS
PANADAS
PANAMAS
PAPAYAS

PATACAS
PATINAS
PAYOLAS
PELLEAS
PELOTAS
PENZIAS
PEPITAS
PESETAS
PESEWAS
PETBOAS
PHIDIAS
PHILEAS
PHINEAS
PHOBIAS
PIAZZAS
PICARAS
PINATAS
PINCHAS
PITAYAS
PLASMAS
PNEUMAS
POLARAS
POSADAS
POSEDAS
POSESAS
PREVIAS
PYTHIAS
QABALAS
QUAGGAS
QUINTAS
RAFFIAS
RAMADAS
RAREGAS
RCCOLAS
REATTAS
REGINAS
REMORAS
RETINAS
RHUMBAS
ROOMBAS
RUANDAS
RUYBLAS
SALINAS
SALIVAS
SAMARAS
SAMOSAS
SAMPRAS
SANBLAS
SAVALAS
SAVANAS
SCHEMAS
SCLERAS
SCOOBAS
SCORIAS
SEDONAS
SEMANAS
SENECAS
SENORAS
SENTRAS
SEPHIAS
SEPIRAS
SERVEAS
SHEILAS
SHERPAS
SIENNAS
SIERRAS
SIESTAS
SILICAS

SMILLAS
SOFARAS
SOLARAS
SONATAS
SPIREAS
STANZAS
STELIAS
STIGMAS
STRATAS
SUBBIAS
TACOMAS
TEARGAS
TEJANAS
TIENDAS
TIMEWAS
TOYOTAS
TRAMPAS
TRAUMAS
TREDIAS
TROIKAS
TSONGAS
TUNDRAS
ULTIMAS
ULZANAS
UTOPIAS
VECTRAS
VERITAS
VICUNAS
VIHARAS
VITARAS
VIZSLAS
WHEREAS
WHISKAS
XTERRAS
YAKIMAS
YAMAHAS
YTTRIAS
YUKATAS
ZAPATAS
ZENANAS
ZINNIAS
ZOYSIAS

AT•••••

ATABOIL
ATACAMA
ATACLIP
ATACOST
ATALOSS
ATAMANS
ATANEND
ATARAXY
ATATILT
ATATIME
ATATURK
ATAVISM
ATAVIST
ATCROSS
ATDEUCE
ATEABIT
ATEALOT
ATEAWAY
ATECROW
ATEDIRT
ATEIGHT
ATEINTO
ATEITUP
ATELATE
ATELESS
ATELIER
ATEMORE
ATEOVER
ATFAULT
ATFIRST
ATGRADE
ATHEART
ATHEISM
ATHEIST
ATHIRST
ATHLETE
ATHOMES
ATHRILL
ATHWART
ATINGLE
ATIPTOE
ATISSUE
ATLANTA
ATLARGE
ATLASES
ATLEAST
ATLUNCH
ATMCARD
ATMFEES
ATNIGHT
ATOMICS
ATOMIES
ATOMISE
ATOMISM
ATOMIST
ATOMIZE
ATONERS
ATONICS
ATONIES
ATONING
ATPEACE
ATRIUMS
ATROPHY
ATROPOS
ATSEVEN
ATSIGHT
ATSIGNS
ATSTAKE
ATTABOY
ATTACHE
ATTACKS
ATTAINS
ATTAINT
ATTEMPT
ATTENDS
ATTESTS
ATTHIRD
ATTHREE
ATTICUS
ATTIMES
ATTIRED
ATTIRER
ATTIRES
ATTRACT
ATTRITE
ATTRITS
ATTUCKS
ATTUNED
ATTUNES
ATTYGEN
ATWATER
ATWORST

A•T••••

ACTABLE
ACTAEON
ACTEDAS
ACTEDIN
ACTEDON
ACTEDUP
ACTFIVE
ACTFOUR
ACTIFED
ACTINON
ACTIONS
ACTIVAS
ACTIVES
ACTLIKE
ACTORLY
ACTRESS
ACTSFOR
ACTSOUT
ACTUARY
ACTUATE
ACTUPON
AFTMOST
AITCHES
ALTDORF
ALTERED
ALTERER
ALTHING
ALTHORN
ALTIMAS
ALTKEYS
ALTOIDS
ALTOIST
ALTOONA
ALTOSAX
ALTTABS
AMTRACK
AMTRACS
ANTACID
ANTARES
ANTBEAR
ANTBIRD
ANTCOWS
ANTEDUP
ANTEING
ANTENNA
ANTERUS
ANTESUP
ANTFARM
ANTHEIL
ANTHEMS
ANTHERS
ANTHILL
ANTHONY
ANTHRAX
ANTIART
ANTIBES
ANTIFOG
ANTIGEN
ANTIGUA
ANTIGUN
ANTILOG
ANTIOCH
ANTIQUE
ANTITAX
ANTIWAR
ANTLERS
ANTLIKE
ANTLION
ANTOINE
ANTONIA
ANTONIN
ANTONIO
ANTONYM
ANTSIER
ANTWERP
APTERAL
APTERYX
APTNESS
ARTBOOK
ARTCARS
ARTDECO
ARTEMIS
ARTEMUS
ARTERIO
ARTFAIR
ARTFERN
ARTFILM
ARTFORM
ARTHURC
ARTHURM
ARTHURS
ARTICLE
ARTIEST
ARTISAN
ARTISTE
ARTISTS
ARTLESS
ARTROCK
ARTSALE
ARTSHOP
ARTSHOW
ARTSIER
ARTSONG
ARTWALL
ARTWARE
ARTWORK
ASTAIRE
ASTARTE
ASTERIX
ASTHMAS
ASTOLAT
ASTORIA
ASTOUND
ASTREAM
ASTRIDE
ASTUTER
ATTABOY
ATTACHE
ATTACKS
ATTAINS
ATTAINT
ATTEMPT
ATTENDS
ATTESTS
ATTHIRD
ATTHREE
ATTICUS
ATTIMES
ATTIRED
ATTIRER
ATTIRES
ATTRACT
ATTRITE
ATTRITS
ATTUCKS
ATTUNED
ATTUNES
ATTYGEN
AUTARCH
AUTARKY
AUTEURS
AUTHORS
AUTISTS
AUTOBIO
AUTOBUS
AUTOING
AUTOMAT
AUTOMNE
AUTONYM
AUTOPEN
AUTOPIA
AUTOPSY
AUTUMNS
AZTECAN

A••T•••

ABATERS
ABATING
ABATORS
ABETTAL
ABETTED
ABETTER
ABETTOR
ABITIBI
ABSTAIN
ABUTSON
ABUTTAL
ABUTTED
ABUTTER
ACCTNOS
ACETALS
ACETATE
ACETIFY
ACETONE
ACHTUNG
ACUTELY
ACUTEST
AFATLOT
AFCTEAM
AGATINE
AGITATE
AGITATO
AGUTTER
AINTHAY
AIRTANK
AIRTAXI
AIRTIME
AIRTRAP
AIRTUBE
ALATEEN
ALETAPS
ALETTES
ALITTLE
ALLTHAT
ALLTHIS
ALLTIED
ALLTIME
ALLTOLD
ALTTABS
AMATEUR
AMATIVE
AMATOLS
AMATORY
AMITIES
AMSTELS
ANATASE
ANATOLE
ANATOLY
ANATOMY
ANDTHEN
ANITRAS
ANOTHER
ANYTIME
ANYTOWN
APATITE
APOTHEM
ARETINO
ASATEAM
ASHTRAY
ASHTREE
ASSTDAS
ASSTIFF
ATATILT
ATATIME
ATATURK
ATSTAKE
AUCTION
AUNTBEE
AUNTIES
AUSTERE
AUSTERS
AUSTINS
AUSTRAL
AUSTRIA
AVATARS

A•••T••

AARATED
ABBOTCY
ABETTAL
ABETTED
ABETTER
ABETTOR
ABINTRA
ABIOTIC
ABLATED
ABLATES
ABORTED
ABOUTIT
ABOUTTO
ABUTTAL
ABUTTED
ABUTTER
ACANTHI
ADAPTED
ADAPTER
ADAPTOR
ADAPTTO
ADEPTAT
ADEPTER
ADEPTLY
ADMITTO
ADOPTED
ADOPTEE
ADOPTER
ADRATES
ADULTLY
AERATED
AERATES
AERATOR
AGENTED
AGENTRY
AGNATES
AGNATIC
AGOUTIS
AGUTTER
AHOSTOF
ALERTED
ALERTER
ALERTLY
ALERTTO
ALETTES
ALITTLE
ALLSTAR
ALLSTON
ALNITAK
ALSATIA
AMANTIS
AMISTAD
AMMETER
AMRITAS
ANISTON
ANNATTO
ANNETTE
ANTITAX
APLITES
APOSTLE
APPETIT
AQUATIC
ARAFTOF
ARANTXA
ARBITER
ARBUTUS
ARIETTA
ARIETTE
ARISTAE
ARISTAS
ARISTOS
ASANTES
ASCETIC
ASEETHE
ASEPTIC
ASIATIC
ASTUTER
ATEITUP
ATIPTOE
ATWATER
AUDITED
AUDITEE
AUDITOR
AUGITES
AULETTA
AVANTIS
AVERTED
AVERTER
AVESTAN
AVESTAS
AVIATED
AVIATES
AVIATIC
AVIATOR
AWAITED
AWAITER

A••••T•

ABDUCTS
ABILITY
ABOUTTO
ABSENTS
ABSINTH
ACCENTS
ACCEPTS
ACCOSTS
ACCRETE
ACERATE
ACETATE
ACIDITY
ACOLYTE
ACONITE
ACQUITS
ACTUATE
ADAMITE
ADAPTTO
ADDEDTO
ADDICTS
ADDONTO
ADDUCTS
ADDUPTO
ADJUSTS
ADMITTO
ADULATE
ADVENTS
ADVERTS
AFFECTS
AGEISTS
AGEMATE
AGILITY
AGITATE
AGITATO
AGREETO
AIGLETS
AIGRETS
AIRDATE
AIRPOTS
AKIHITO
ALBERTA
ALBERTI
ALBERTO
ALCESTE
ALDENTE
ALERTTO
ALIENTO
ALIGHTS
ALIGOTE
ALIVETO
ALLANTE
ALMAATA
ALSMITH
ALWORTH
AMANITA
AMENITY
AMILATE
AMINUTE
AMNESTY
AMOUNTS
AMREETA
AMULETS
ANALYTE
ANDANTE
ANILITY
ANIMATE
ANIMATO
ANKLETS
ANNATTO
ANNETTE
ANNUITY
ANOINTS

ANXIETY
APATITE
APELETS
APLENTY
APPLETS
APPLYTO
ARCUATE
ARGANTE
ARGENTI
ARGENTO
ARGENTS
ARIDITY
ARIETTA
ARIETTE
ARIGATO
ARIOSTO
ARMLETS
ARMPITS
ARRESTS
ARTISTE
ARTISTS
ASBYATT
ASCENTS
ASHANTI
ASHPITS
ASPECTS
ASQUITH
ASSANTE
ASSENTS
ASSERTS
ASSISTS
ASSORTS
ASSUNTA
ASTARTE
ATEINTO
ATELATE
ATHLETE
ATLANTA
ATTESTS
ATTRITE
ATTRITS
AUGUSTA
AUGUSTE
AUGUSTO
AUGUSTS
AUKLETS
AULETTA
AUREATE
AURISTS
AUTISTS
AVIDITY
AVOCETS
AXOLOTL
AZIMUTH
AZURITE

A•••••T

ABEYANT
ABOUTIT
ABREAST
ABSOLUT
ACCOUNT
ACCURST
ACEDOUT
ACESOUT
ACHIEST
ACINGIT
ACROBAT
ACTSOUT
ACUTEST
ADAMANT
ADDSALT
ADEPTAT
ADHIBIT
ADJUNCT
AERIEST
AEROBAT
AFATLOT
AFFIANT
AFFLICT
AFFRONT
AFTMOST
AGAINST
AGEDOUT
AGESOUT
AGILEST
AGONIST
AILMENT
AIMEDAT
AIRBOAT
AIRDUCT
AIRIEST
AIRLIFT
AIRPORT
AIRSOUT
AIRVENT
ALIMENT
ALLOFIT
ALLTHAT
ALNIYAT
ALQUIST
ALRIGHT
ALTOIST
AMBIENT
AMHERST
AMONGST
AMORIST
AMPLEST
ANALYST
ANAPEST
ANCIENT
ANGRYAT
ANIMIST
ANNULET
ANTIART
APEDIET
APESUIT
APPARAT
APPETIT
APPOINT
APRICOT
AQUAVIT
ARABIST
ARCHEST
ARIDEST
ARMREST
ARMYANT
ARTIEST
ASAGIFT
ASBYATT
ASHIEST
ASKSOUT
ASONANT
ASPHALT
ASQUIET
ASQUINT
ASSAULT
ASSWEET
ASTOLAT
ATACOST
ATATILT
ATAVIST
ATEABIT
ATEALOT
ATEDIRT
ATEIGHT
ATFAULT
ATFIRST
ATHEART
ATHEIST
ATHIRST
ATHWART
ATLEAST
ATNIGHT
ATOMIST
ATSIGHT
ATTAINT
ATTEMPT
ATTRACT
ATWORST
AUGMENT
AUTOMAT
AVIDEST
AWAREST
AWEEBIT

•AT••••

BATAVIA
BATBOYS
BATCHED
BATCHES
BATDAYS
BATEAUX
BATEMAN
BATGIRL
BATHERS
BATHING
BATHMAT
BATHOIL
BATHTUB
BATIKED
BATISTA
BATISTE
BATLIKE
BATNEXT
BATSFOR
BATSMAN
BATSMEN
BATSUIT
BATTENS
BATTERS
BATTERY
BATTIER
BATTING
BATTLED
BATTLER
BATTLES
BATWING
CATALAN
CATALOG
CATALOS
CATALPA
CATANIA
CATAWBA
CATBEDS
CATBERT
CATBIRD
CATBOAT
CATBOWL
CATCALL
CATCHER
CATCHES
CATCHON
CATCHOW
CATCHUP
CATCOMB
CATDOOR
CATENAE
CATENAS
CATERAS
CATERED
CATERER
CATERTO
CATEYED
CATFEET
CATFISH
CATFITS
CATFLAP
CATFLEA
CATFOOD
CATFOOT
CATGUTS
CATHAIR
CATHEAD
CATHODE
CATIONS
CATKINS
CATLIKE
CATMINT
CATNAPS
CATNIPS
CATORCE
CATRIGS
CATSCAN
CATSEYE
CATSHOW
CATSITS
CATSPAW
CATSUIT
CATSUPS
CATTAIL
CATTALO
CATTIER
CATTILY
CATTISH
CATTOYS
CATWALK
DATABLE
DATABUS
DATASET
DATEDLY
DATINGS
DATIVES
DATRILS
DATSUNS
EATABIT
EATABLE
EATALOT
EATAWAY
EATCAKE
EATCROW
EATDIRT
EATENAT
EATENUP
EATFROM
EATHERE
EATINTO
EATITUP
EATLATE
EATLESS
EATMORE
EATOVER
EATSOUT
FATALES
FATALLY
FATBACK
FATCATS
FATCELL
FATCITY
FATEFUL
FATFARM
FATFREE
FATHEAD
FATHERS
FATHOMS
FATIDIC
FATIGUE
FATLESS
FATLIKE
FATLING
FATLIPS
FATNESS
FATONES
FATOUSH
FATTENS
FATTEST
FATTIER
FATTILY
FATTING
FATTISH
FATUITY
FATUOUS
GATEAUX
GATELEG
GATEMAN
GATEMEN
GATEWAY
GATHERS
GATINGS
GATLING
GATLINS
GATTACA
GATWICK
HATABLE
HATBAND
HATBRIM
HATCHED
HATCHER
HATCHES
HATCHET
HATEDIT
HATEFUL
HATESIT
HATFULS
HATLESS
HATLIKE
HATPINS
HATRACK
HATREDS
HATSIZE
HATSOFF
HATTERS
HATTING
IATRICS
KATAYEV
KATHRYN
KATISHA
KATRINA
KATRINE
KATYDID
LATCHED
LATCHES
LATCHON
LATEENS
LATEFEE
LATENCY
LATENED
LATENTS
LATERAL
LATERAN
LATERON
LATETAG
LATEXES
LATHERS
LATHERY
LATHING
LATICES
LATIFAH
LATIGOS
LATIMES
LATINAS
LATINII
LATINOS
LATINUS
LATOSCA
LATRELL
LATRINE
LATROBE
LATTICE
LATVIAN
MATADOR
MATALIN
MATCHED
MATCHER
MATCHES
MATCHUP
MATEWAN
MATHERS
MATHEWS
MATHIAS
MATHIEU
MATILDA
MATINAL
MATINEE
MATISSE
MATLESS
MATLOCK
MATRONS
MATTERS
MATTHAU
MATTHEW
MATTING
MATTOCK
MATURED
MATURER
MATURES
MATZOHS
MATZOTH
NATALIA
NATALIE
NATASHA
NATATOR
NATCHEZ
NATHANS
NATIONS
NATIVES
NATRIUM
NATSUME
NATTERS
NATTIER
NATTILY
NATURAL
NATURED
NATUREL
NATURES
NATWICK
OATBRAN
OATCAKE
OATLIKE
OATMEAL
PATACAS
PATCASH
PATCHED
PATCHEN
PATCHER
PATCHES
PATCHUP
PATDOWN
PATELLA
PATENCY
PATENTS
PATERNO
PATHAND
PATHANS
PATHWAY
PATIENT
PATINAS
PATNESS
PATRICE
PATRICK
PATRIES
PATRIOT
PATROLS
PATRONS
PATROON
PATSDRY
PATSIES
PATTERN
PATTERS
PATTIES
PATTING
PATZERS
QATARIS
RATABLE
RATAFIA
RATATAT
RATBERT
RATCHET
RATECAP
RATEDPG
RATFINK
RATHOLE
RATINES
RATINGS
RATIONS
RATITES
RATLIKE
RATLINE
RATLINS
RATPACK
RATRACE
RATSOUT
RATTAIL
RATTANS
RATTERS
RATTIER
RATTING
RATTISH
RATTLED
RATTLER
RATTLES
RATTRAP
SATANIC
SATATOP
SATBACK
SATCHEL
SATCHMO
SATCOMS
SATDOWN
SATEENS
SATHOME
SATIATE
SATIETY
SATINET
SATINON
SATIRES
SATIRIC
SATISFY
SATORIS
SATRAPS
SATRAPY
SATSUMA
SATUPON
SATURNS
SATWELL
SATWITH
SATYRIC
TATAMIS
TATIANA
TATTERS
TATTERY
TATTIER
TATTILY
TATTING
TATTLED
TATTLER
TATTLES
TATTOOS
VATDYED
VATDYES
VATFULS
VATICAL
VATICAN
VATTING
WATCHED
WATCHER
WATCHES
WATCHIT
WATCHTV
WATERED
WATERER
WATFORD
WATKINS
WATTAGE
WATTEAU
WATTLED
WATTLES
WATUSIS
YATTERS
ZATOPEK

•A•T•••

BACTRIA
BADTIME
BADTRIP
BAITCAR
BAITERS
BAITING
BANTAMS
BANTERS
BANTING
BAPTISE
BAPTISM
BAPTIST
BAPTIZE
BARTABS
BARTEND
BARTERS
BARTLES
BARTLET
BARTOLO
BARTRAY
BASTERS
BASTING
BASTION
BATTENS
BATTERS
BATTERY
BATTIER
BATTING
BATTLED
BATTLER
BATTLES
BAYTREE
CAFTANS
CALTECH
CANTABS
CANTALS
CANTATA
CANTEEN
CANTERS
CANTILY
CANTINA
CANTING
CANTINO
CANTLES
CANTONS
CANTORS
CANTRIP
CANTSAY
CAPTAIN
CAPTION
CAPTIVA
CAPTIVE
CAPTORS
CAPTURE
CARTAGE
CARTALK
CARTELS
CARTERS
CARTIER
CARTING
CARTIRE
CARTOFF
CARTONS
CARTOON
CARTOPS
CARTRIP
CARTSIN
CASTERS
CASTILE
CASTING
CASTLED
CASTLES
CASTOFF
CASTOUT
CASTROL
CASTSON
CASTSUP
CATTAIL
CATTALO
CATTIER
CATTILY
CATTISH
CATTOYS
CAUTHEN
CAUTION
DACTYLS
DAFTEST
DAKTARI
DALTONS
DALTREY
DANTEAN
DANTEII
DARTERS
DARTGUN
DARTING
DARTLED
DARTLES
DARTOFF
DASTARD
DAYTIME
DAYTONA
DAYTRIP
EARTABS
EARTAGS
EARTHED
EARTHEN
EARTHLY
EASTEGG
EASTEND
EASTERN
EASTERS
EASTHAM
EASTING
EASTMAN
FACTFUL
FACTION
FACTOID
FACTORS
FACTORY
FACTUAL
FALTERS
FANTAIL
FANTANS
FANTASM
FANTAST
FANTASY
FANTINE
FANTODS
FARTHER
FARTLEK
FASTCAR
FASTENS
FASTEST
FASTING
FASTNET
FASTONE
FATTENS
FATTEST
FATTIER
FATTILY
FATTING
FATTISH
GAETANO
GAITERS
GAITING
GANTLET
GARTERS
GASTANK
GASTERO
GASTONE
GASTRIC
GATTACA
GAUTAMA
GAUTIER
HADTIME
HADTOBE
HAFTING
HAITIAN
HALTERS
HALTING
HAPTICS
HARTACK
HARTLEY
HARTMAN
HARTMUT
HASTENS
HASTERT
HASTIER
HASTILY
HASTIME
HASTING
HASTOBE
HATTERS
HATTING
HAUTBOY
HAUTEUR
KANTIAN
KAPTURE
KASTLER
LABTECH
LABTEST
LABTUBE
LACTAID
LACTASE
LACTATE
LACTEAL
LACTOSE
LAITIES
LANTANA
LANTERN
LAOTIAN
LAPTOPS
LASTACT
LASTDON
LASTGAS
LASTING
LASTLAP
LASTLEG
LASTMAY
LASTONE
LASTORY
LASTROW
LATTICE
LAUTREC
MAITAIS
MAITRED
MAITRES
MALTASE
MALTBIE
MALTEDS
MALTESE
MALTHUS
MALTIER
MALTING
MALTOSE
MANTECA
MANTELS
MANTLED
MANTLES
MANTLET
MANTRAP
MANTRAS
MANTRIC
MANTUAN
MARTENS
MARTIAL
MARTIAN
MARTINA
MARTINI
MARTINO
MARTINS
MARTINU
MARTINV
MARTIUS
MARTYRS
MASTERP
MASTERS
MASTERY
MASTICS
MASTIFF
MASTING
MASTOID
MATTERS
MATTHAU
MATTHEW
MATTING
MATTOCK
MAYTAGS
MAYTIME
NAPTIME
NARTHEX
NASTASE
NASTIER
NASTIES
NASTILY
NATTERS
NATTIER
NATTILY
NAUTICA
NAUTILI
OAKTAGS
OAKTREE
PALTERS
PALTROW
PANTENE
PANTERA
PANTERS
PANTHER
PANTIES
PANTILE
PANTING
PANTLEG
PANTONE
PARTAKE
PARTIAL
PARTIED
PARTIER
PARTIES
PARTIII
PARTING
PARTITA
PARTITE
PARTNER
PARTONE
PARTOOK
PARTTWO
PARTWAY
PARTYER
PARTYON
PASTDUE
PASTEIN
PASTELS
PASTERN
PASTERS
PASTEUP
PASTEUR
PASTIER
PASTIES
PASTIME
PASTINA
PASTING
PASTORS
PASTURE
PATTERN
PATTERS
PATTIES
PATTING
RAFTERS
RAFTING
RAGTIME
RAGTOPS
RANTERS
RANTING
RANTSAT
RAPTORS
RAPTUNE
RAPTURE
RASTERS
RATTAIL
RATTANS
RATTERS
RATTIER
RATTING
RATTISH
RATTLED
RATTLER
RATTLES
RATTRAP
SAATCHI
SALTANT
SALTBOX
SALTERS

SALTIER
SALTILY
SALTINE
SALTING
SALTISH
SALTPIT
SALTSEA
SANTAFE
SANTANA
SANTINI
SAOTOME
SARTORS
SAUTEED
SAWTOIT
SAXTUBA
TACTFUL
TACTICS
TACTILE
TACTUAL
TAGTEAM
TAMTAMS
TANTARA
TANTIVY
TANTRUM
TARTANS
TARTARE
TARTARS
TARTEST
TARTIER
TARTILY
TARTING
TARTISH
TARTLET
TARTSUP
TASTEIT
TASTERS
TASTIER
TASTILY
TASTING
TATTERS
TATTERY
TATTIER
TATTILY
TATTING
TATTLED
TATTLER
TATTLES
TATTOOS
TAUTENS
TAUTEST
VANTAGE
VASTEST
VASTIER
VASTITY
VATTING
WAFTERS
WAFTING
WAITERS
WAITFOR
WAITING
WAITOUT
WAITRON
WAITSON
WAITSUP
WALTERS
WALTHAM
WALTHER
WALTONS
WALTZED
WALTZER
WALTZES
WANTADS
WANTAGH
WANTERS
WANTING
WANTONS
WANTOUT
WANTSIN
WANTSTO
WARTHOG
WARTIER
WARTIME
WARTORN
WASTAGE
WASTERS
WASTING
WASTREL
WATTAGE
WATTEAU
WATTLED
WATTLES
WAYTOGO
XANTHAN
XANTHIC
YAHTZEE
YATTERS
YAYTEAM

•A••T••

AARATED
BABETTE
BADITCH
BAINTER
BALATAS
BALATON
BALLTWO
BARETTA
BARITES
BARSTOW
BASETEN
BASETWO
BATHTUB
CADETTE
CAKETIN
CALOTTE
CANETTI
CANITBE
CAPITAL
CAPITAN
CAPITOL
CAPOTES
CAPSTAN
CARLTON
CAROTID
CAROTIN
CASITAS
CAUSTIC
DAKOTAN
DAKOTAS
DALETHS
DANITES
DARKTAN
DAUNTED
DAUNTER
DAYSTAR
EATITUP
FACETED
FAGOTED
FAINTED
FAINTER
FAINTLY
FAJITAS
FANATIC
FAULTED
FAUSTUS
FAYETTE
GAGSTER
GALATEA
GALATIA
GALETTE
GAMETAL
GAMETES
GANGTOK
GAROTTE
GAUNTER
GAUNTLY
GAVOTTE
GAZETTE
HABITAT
HABITED
HABITUE
HADATIT
HALITES
HALSTON
HAMITES
HAMITIC
HAMITUP
HAMPTON
HAMSTER
HANGTEN
HARDTEN
HARDTOP
HASATIT
HAUNTED
HAUNTER
IAPETUS
JACKTAR
JANITOR
JAUNTED
KADETTS
KAPITAL
KAPITSA
KARATES
LABATTS
LAERTES
LAFITTE
LAKOTAS
LAMOTTA
LAMOTTE
LANDTAG
LANDTAX
LANETWO
LANGTON
LANGTRY
LANOTTE
LAPUTAN
LATETAG
LAYETTE
LAYITON
MAARTEN
MACHTWO
MAESTRO
MAHATMA
MAINTOP
MANATEE
MANETTE
MARITAL
MARSTON
NAILTIP
NAMETAG
NANETTE
NAPHTHA
NAPSTER
NATATOR
PAGETWO
PAINTED
PAINTER
PAIUTES
PALATAL
PALATES
PALETTE
PALMTOP
PANETTA
PARATUS
PAROTID
PARTTWO
PAYSTUB
RALSTON
RANATAB
RANITUP
RAPSTAR
RARITAN
RATATAT
RATITES
SAGETEA
SAINTED
SAINTES
SAINTLO
SAINTLY
SALUTED
SALUTER
SALUTES
SANCTUM
SANCTUS
SATATOP
SAUNTER
SAWATCH
TABITHA
TACITLY
TACITUS
TAINTED
TAKETEA
TAKETEN
TANKTOP
TAPSTER
TAUNTED
TAUNTER
TAUNTON
VACATED
VACATES
VALETED
VALOTTE
VARITEK
VAULTED
VAULTER
VAUNTED
VAUNTER
WAISTED
WALSTON
WAPITIS
WASATCH
WASHTUB
YACHTED
YACHTER
YACHTIE
YAKUTSK
YANGTZE
YANKTON
ZABUTON
ZANETTO
ZAPATAS
ZAPATEO
ZAPOTEC

•A•••T•

BAALITE
BABBITT
BABETTE
BACHATA
BADFITS
BADHATS
BADLOTS
BALLETS
BALLOTS
BANDITO
BANDITS
BANKITS
BARBATE
BARBETS
BARENTS
BARETTA
BARISTA
BARRETS
BARRETT
BASALTS
BASKETS
BASKETT
BASMATI
BASSETS
BASSETT
BATISTA
BATISTE
BAUXITE
BAYCITY
CABLETS
CABLETV
CACHETS
CADETTE
CAHOOTS
CALCITE
CALISTA
CALLSTO
CALOTTE
CANASTA
CANETTI
CANTATA
CAPLETS
CAPNUTS
CAREDTO
CARESTO
CARLOTA
CARLOTS
CARNETS
CARPETS
CARROTS
CARROTY
CASEATE
CASERTA
CASKETS
CASSATT
CATERTO
CATFITS
CATGUTS
CATSITS
CAUDATE
CAVEATS
CAVORTS
DACOSTA
DARESTO
EAGLETS
EARLETS
EATINTO
EATLATE
FACULTY
FAILSTO
FALCATE
FALLSTO
FALSITY
FANJETS
FANOUTS
FATCATS
FATCITY
FATUITY
FAUCETS
FAWCETT
FAYETTE
GADGETS
GADGETY
GALANTS
GALEATE
GALENTO
GALETTE
GALOOTS
GAMBITS
GANGSTA
GANNETS
GANNETT
GARLITS
GARNETS
GARNETT
GAROTTE
GARRETS
GARRETT
GARROTE
GASEITY
GASJETS
GASKETS
GAVOTTE
GAZETTE
HACKETT
HADFITS
HAGERTY
HAMLETS
HAMMETT
HANDYTO
HAPPYTO
HARLOTS
HASFITS
HAUGHTY
HAVARTI
HAWORTH
HAZLITT
HAZMATS
JACINTH
JACINTO
JACKETS
JADEITE
JAKARTA
JAPHETH
JARRETT
JARROTT
KADETTS
LABATTS
LABIATE
LABRATS
LACERTA
LACOSTE
LACTATE
LAFITTE
LAKISTS
LAMBETH
LAMENTS
LAMINTO
LAMOTTA
LAMOTTE
LANCETS
LANOTTE
LAPCATS
LAPLATA
LAPORTE
LAPPETS
LARIATS
LATENTS
LAURITZ
LAYETTE
LAYINTO
LAYOUTS
MACBETH
MACHETE
MAGENTA
MAGGOTS
MAGNATE
MAGNETO
MAGNETS
MAHOUTS
MAIMITI
MAJESTE
MAJESTY
MALLETS
MAMMOTH
MANDATE
MANETTE
MANKATO
MAOISTS
MARANTZ
MARCATO
MARGATE
MARKETS
MARMOTS
MASCOTS
MATZOTH
NAHUATL
NAIVETE
NAIVETY
NANETTE
NARRATE
NAUGHTS
NAUGHTY
PACKETS
PADGETT
PADSITE
PALETTE
PALLETS
PALMATE
PALPATE
PANDITS
PANETTA
PAPEETE
PAPISTS
PARENTS
PARROTS
PARTITA
PARTITE
PASSATS
PATENTS
PAUCITY
PAYCUTS
PAYINTO
PAYOUTS
PAYRATE
RABBETS
RABBITS
RABBITT
RABBITY
RACEDTO
RACESTO
RACISTS
RACKETS
RACKETY
RADIATE
RAGOUTS
RALLYTO
RAMINTO
RAMJETS
RANINTO
RANLATE
RANUPTO
RANWITH
RAWDATA
RAWISTS
SABBATH
SACHETS
SADFATE
SADISTS
SAILSTO
SAMLETS
SATIATE
SATIETY
SATWITH
SAVANTS
SAWINTO
SAWPITS
SAYHITO
SAYNOTO
TABLETS
TABSETS
TAFFETA
TAGOUTS
TAKENTO
TAKESTO
TALENTS
TALKSTO
TALLITH
TAOISTS
TAPINTO
TAPPETS
TARANTO
TARGETS
TARPITS
TAXCUTS
TAXRATE
VACUITY
VALENTE
VALENTI
VALOTTE
VALUATE
VALVATE
VANUATU
VARIATE
VARIETY
VARLETS
VARSITY
VASTITY
WABBITS
WAIKATO
WALCOTT
WALKSTO
WALLETS
WALNUTS
WANTSTO
WARMSTO
WARPATH
WARVETS
WASLATE
WASONTO
WATCHTV
WAVEDTO
WAVESTO
ZAGNUTS
ZANETTO

•A••••T

BAALIST
BABBITT
BABIEST
BABYSAT
BABYSIT
BACKBIT
BACKLIT
BACKLOT
BACKOUT
BADDEBT
BADDEST
BADPAST
BADSHOT
BAGEHOT
BAHAIST
BAILOUT
BAKERST
BALDEST
BALKSAT
BALLAST
BALLUET
BANDLET
BANGOUT
BANQUET
BAPTIST
BARKSAT
BARONET
BARRETT
BARTLET
BASEHIT
BASKETT
BASSETT
BASSIST
BATHMAT
BATNEXT
BATSUIT
BAWLOUT
BAYEDAT
BAYONET
CABARET
CABINET
CAGEPET
CAGIEST
CAKIEST
CALLOUT
CALLSIT
CALMEST
CALUMET
CALVERT
CAMELOT
CAMEOUT
CAMPOUT
CANDENT
CANIEST
CAPELET
CAPULET
CARCOAT
CARPORT
CARPSAT
CARSEAT
CASELOT
CASEOUT
CASHOUT
CASSATT
CASTOUT
CASUIST
CATBERT
CATBOAT
CATFEET
CATFOOT
CATMINT
CATSUIT
CAVEART
CAVILAT
DADAART
DADAIST
DAFTEST
DAMPEST
DANKEST
DARENOT
DARKEST
DASBOOT
DASHDOT
DASHPOT
DATASET
DAUSSET
EARHART
EARNEST
EARNSIT
EARSHOT
EASEOUT
EASIEST
EATABIT
EATALOT
EATDIRT
EATENAT
EATSOUT
FABBEST
FACEDIT
FACESIT
FADDIET
FADDIST
FADEOUT
FAINEST
FAIREST
FAKEDIT
FAKEOUT
FAKESIT
FALLOUT
FALSEST
FANBELT
FANFEST
FANSOUT
FANTAST
FAREAST
FARLEFT
FARMOUT
FARWEST
FASCIST
FASTEST
FASTNET
FATTEST
FAUVIST
FAWCETT
GABFEST
GALLANT
GAMIEST
GANNETT
GANTLET
GAPEDAT
GAPESAT
GARMENT
GARNETT
GARRETT
GASHEAT
GAVEOUT
GAWKSAT
GAZEDAT
GAZESAT
HABITAT
HACKETT
HACKSIT
HADAFIT
HADASET
HADATIT
HADBEST
HAIRCUT
HAIRNET
HALFCUT
HALFWIT
HALIBUT
HAMMETT
HANDOUT
HANDSET
HANGOUT
HARDEST
HARDHAT
HARDHIT
HARDPUT
HARDSET
HARICOT
HARPIST
HARRIET
HARTMUT
HARVEST
HASAFIT
HASASET
HASATIT
HASHOUT
HASTERT
HATCHET
HATEDIT
HATESIT
HAVENOT
HAVEOUT
HAYLOFT
HAZIEST
HAZLITT
IAMBIST
JACKPOT
JACONET
JAINIST
JARRETT
JARROTT
JAWEDAT
LABCOAT
LABORAT
LABTEST
LACIEST
LACKWIT
LAIDOUT
LAKIEST
LAMAIST
LAMBENT
LAMBERT
LAMPERT
LAMPLIT
LANDSAT
LANKEST
LAPBELT
LARGENT
LARGEST
LASHOUT
LASTACT
LAUGHAT
LAURENT
LAWSUIT
LAYSOUT
LAZIEST
MADDEST
MADEFIT
MADEOUT
MAEWEST
MAGINOT
MAHDIST
MAIGRET
MAILLOT
MAILOUT
MAKEFIT
MAKEOUT
MAKESIT
MALEANT
MALECAT
MALLRAT
MANHUNT
MANTLET
MANUMIT
MANXCAT
MAOSUIT
MAPSOUT
MARGRET
MARKOUT
MARRYAT
MARXIST
MAUPRAT
MAURIAT
MAZIEST
NAILSET
NAILSIT
NAIVEST
NASCENT
NAYARIT
OAKIEST
PACIEST
PACKRAT
PADGETT
PAGEANT
PAIDOUT
PALMIST
PANSOUT
PARAPET
PARFAIT
PARKSIT
PARQUET
PASSANT
PASSOUT
PATIENT
PATRIOT
PAULIST
PAWEDAT
PAYDIRT
PAYMENT
PAYSOUT
RABBITT
RACIEST
RACKOUT
RACQUET
RADIANT
RAILSAT
RAIMENT
RAINHAT
RAINOUT
RAMPANT
RAMPART
RANGOUT
RANKEST
RANKOUT
RANPAST
RANRIOT
RANTSAT
RAPPORT
RAREBIT
RASHEST
RATATAT
RATBERT
RATCHET
RATSOUT
RAWMEAT
SACKOUT
SADDEST
SAFEBET
SAGIEST
SALIENT
SALTANT
SALTPIT
SAMOSET
SANDLOT
SANDPIT
SANGOUT
SAPIENT
SARGENT
SATINET
SAWDUST
SAWPAST
SAWTOIT
SAYWAIT
SAYWHAT
TABARET
TABORET
TAGAMET
TAGGANT
TAGSOUT

7 AT

TAKEOUT
TAKESIT
TALKOUT
TALKSAT
TALLEST
TANGENT
TANNEST
TAPROOT
TAPSOUT
TARTEST
TARTLET
TASTEIT
TAUTEST
VAGRANT
VAGUEST
VAINEST
VALIANT
VANPELT
VANSANT
VANVOGT
VANZANT
VARIANT
VARMINT
VASTEST
WACKEST
WAITOUT
WALCOTT
WALKOUT
WALMART
WANIEST
WANNEST
WANTOUT
WAPSHOT
WARIEST
WARMEST
WARRANT
WASHOUT
WATCHIT
WAVEDAT
WAVELET
WAVESAT
WAVIEST
WAXIEST
XAMOUNT
YANKOUT
YANKSAT
ZANIEST

••AT•••

ABATERS
ABATING
ABATORS
AFATLOT
AGATINE
ALATEEN
AMATEUR
AMATIVE
AMATOLS
AMATORY
ANATASE
ANATOLE
ANATOLY
ANATOMY
APATITE
ASATEAM
ATATILT
ATATIME
ATATURK
AVATARS
BEATALL
BEATBOX
BEATCOP
BEATERS
BEATIFY
BEATING
BEATLES
BEATNIK
BEATOFF
BEATOUT
BEATRIX
BEATSAT
BEATSIT
BEATSME
BEATSON
BEATSUP
BEATTIE
BLATANT
BLATHER
BLATTED
BOATELS
BOATERS
BOATFUL
BOATING
BOATMAN
BOATMEN
BRATTLE
CHATEAU
CHATHAM
CHATSUP
CHATTED
CHATTEL
CHATTER
CHATWIN
CLATTER
COATEES
COATERS
COATING
CRATERS
CRATEUP
CRATING
CRATION
CUATROS
DIATOMS
DNATEST
DRATTED
ELATERS
ELATING
ELATION
FEATHER
FEATURE
FIATLUX
FLATBED
FLATCAR
FLATHAT
FLATLET
FLATOUT
FLATTAX
FLATTED
FLATTEN
FLATTER
FLATTOP
FLATTVS
FRATERS
GOATEED
GOATEES
GOATISH
GRATEON
GRATERS
GRATEUP
GRATIAS
GRATIFY
GRATING
HEATERS
HEATFAN
HEATFUL
HEATHEN
HEATHER
HEATING
HEATRAY
HEATSUP
HEATTER
IHATEIT
INATRAP
IRATELY
IRATEST
IZATION
KHATAMI
KLATSCH
KRATION
LEATHER
LOATHED
LOATHER
LOATHES
LOATHLY
LOATHTO
MEATAXE
MEATIER
MEATILY
MEATMAN
MEATMEN
MEATPIE
MTATHOS
NBATEAM
NEATENS
NEATEST
NEATNIK
ONATEAR
ONATOOT
ONATRIP
ORATING
ORATION
ORATORS
ORATORY
ORATRIX
OVATION
PEATBOG
PEATIER
PEATPOT
PGATOUR
PHATTER
PLATEAU
PLATENS
PLATERS
PLATIER
PLATIES
PLATING
PLATOON
PLATTED
PLATTER
PLATYPI
PRATERS
PRATING
PRATTLE
QRATIOS
QUATRES
QUATTRO
REATTAS
RRATING
SAATCHI
SCATHED
SCATHES
SCATMAN
SCATTED
SCATTER
SEATERS
SEATING
SEATRIP
SEATTLE
SHATNER
SHATTER
SKATERS
SKATING
SLATERS
SLATHER
SLATIER
SLATING
SLATKIN
SLATTED
SMATTER
SPATHES
SPATIAL
SPATOUT
SPATTED
SPATTER
SPATULA
STATELY
STATERS
STATICE
STATICS
STATING
STATINS
STATION
STATISM
STATIST
STATLER
STATORS
STATUES
STATURE
STATUTE
SWATHED
SWATHES
SWATSAT
SWATTED
SWATTER
TEATIME
TEATRAY
TEATREE
TEATROS
THATCHY
THATONE
THATSIT
THATSOK
THATWAY
TOATURN
UPATREE
VIATICA
WEATHER
WHATAMI
WHATFOR
WHATIFS
WHATNOT
WHATNOW
WHATSAY
WHATSIS
WHATSIT
WHATSUP
WHATTHE
XRATING
YEATEAM

••A•T••

ACANTHI
ADAPTED
ADAPTER
ADAPTOR
ADAPTTO
AMANTIS
ARAFTOF
ARANTXA
ASANTES
AVANTIS
AWAITED
AWAITER
BDALTON
BEASTIE
BEASTLY
BEATTIE
BLANTON
BLASTED
BLASTER
BLATTED
BOASTED
BOASTER
BOASTOF
BRATTLE
BRAXTON
CHANTED
CHANTER
CHANTEY
CHANTRY
CHAOTIC
CHAPTER
CHARTED
CHARTER
CHASTEN
CHASTER
CHATTED
CHATTEL
CHATTER
CLACTON
CLANTON
CLAPTON
CLATTER
CLAYTON
COACTED
COALTAR
COAPTED
COASTAL
COASTED
COASTER
CRAFTED
CRAFTER
CRAFTSY
DEALTIN
DEALTTO
DEALTUP
DEARTHS
DRAFTED
DRAFTEE
DRAFTER
DRASTIC
DRATTED
DRAYTON
ECARTES
ELANTRA
ELASTIC
ELASTIN
ENACTED
ENACTOR
ERASTUS
EXACTAS
EXACTED
EXACTER
EXACTLY
EXACTOR
EXALTED
EXALTER
FEASTED
FEASTER
FEASTON
FLATTAX
FLATTED
FLATTEN
FLATTER
FLATTOP
FLATTVS
FLAUTAS
FRACTAL
FRANTIC
GHASTLY
GOAFTER
GRAFTED
GRAFTER
GRAFTON
GRANTED
GRANTEE
GRANTER
GRANTOR
HEALTHY
HEARTED
HEARTEN
HEARTHS
HEATTER
INAPTER
INAPTLY
INASTEW
INASTIR
IWANTIT
IWANTTO
LEANTOS
LEAPTAT
LEAPTIN
LEAPTON
LEAPTUP
MAARTEN
MEANTIT
MEANTTO
NIANTIC
ORANTES
PHAETON
PHANTOM
PHATTER
PIASTER
PIASTRE
PLAITED
PLAITER
PLANTAR
PLANTED
PLANTER
PLASTER
PLASTIC
PLATTED
PLATTER
PLAUTUS
PLAYTEX
PRACTIC
PRAETOR
PRATTLE
PSALTER
QUANTUM
QUARTAN
QUARTER
QUARTES
QUARTET
QUARTIC
QUARTOS
QUARTZY
QUATTRO
REACTED
REACTOR
REACTTO
REALTER
REALTOR
REATTAS
RIALTOS
RIANTLY
ROADTAR
ROADTAX
ROASTED
ROASTER
SCANTED
SCANTER
SCANTLY
SCATTED
SCATTER
SEASTAR
SEATTLE
SHAFTED
SHANTER
SHASTRI
SHATTER
SLANTED
SLANTLY
SLANTUP
SLATTED
SLAYTON
SMARTED
SMARTEN
SMARTER
SMARTLY
SMATTER
SPARTAN
SPATTED
SPATTER
STANTON
STARTED
STARTER
STARTIN
STARTLE
STARTON
STARTTO
STARTUP
SWARTHY
SWATTED
SWATTER
TOASTED
TOASTEE
TOASTER
TRACTOR
TRAITOR
UNACTED
UNAPTLY
WEALTHS
WEALTHY
WHARTON
WHATTHE
WRAITHS
XFACTOR
YEASTED

••A••T•

ADAMITE
ADAPTTO
AMANITA
ANALYTE
APATITE
BAALITE
CHALETS
CHAPATI
CHARITY
CHAYOTE
CLAMATO
CLARETS
CLARITY
CLAVATE
CRAVATS
DEALSTO
DEALTTO
DRAGOTI
DRANKTO
DRAWNTO
DRAWSTO
DUALITY
EDACITY
EGALITE
ELAMITE
ELANETS
EMANATE
EXABYTE
FLAUNTS
FLAUNTY
FRAILTY
GEARSTO
GRADATE
GRANITA
GRANITE
GRAVITY
HEADSTO
HEAVETO
HUANGTI
HYALITE
IMAMATE
IMARETS
INANITY
IWANTTO
KHANATE
KLAMATH
LEADETH
LEADSTO
LEANSTO
LEARNTO
LEASETO
LOATHTO
MEANSTO
MEANTTO
MOABITE
NDAKOTA
ONADATE
OPACITY
OXALATE
PEANUTS
PLACATE
PLAINTS
PLAKATS
PLANATE
PLANETS
PLANSTO
PLAYSTO
PRAYSTO
QUALITY
REACTTO
READSTO
REALITY
SDAKOTA
SEACATS
SEADUTY
SEAGATE
SNAPSTO
STANDTO
STARTTO
STATUTE
SUAVITY
TEAPOTS
TEASETS
TRASHTV
URANITE
YEARNTO
ZEALOTS

••A•••T

ADAMANT
AFATLOT
AGAINST
ANALYST
ANAPEST
ARABIST
ASAGIFT
ATACOST
ATATILT
ATAVIST
AWAREST
BAALIST
BEARCAT
BEAROUT
BEARPIT
BEATOUT
BEATSAT
BEATSIT
BLANKET
BLATANT
BRACKET
BRAVEST
CHAPLET
CHARCOT
CHARIOT
CHARVET
CLAMANT
CLAWSAT
CLAYPIT
COAGENT
COALPIT
CRABPOT
CRAPOUT
CZARIST
DEADEST
DEADSET
DEAFEST
DEALOUT
DEAREST
DIALECT
DIALOUT
DIARIST
DNATEST
DRAGNET
DRAGOUT
DRAUGHT
DRAWOUT
DUALIST
EMANANT
EPAULET
FEARNOT
FLAILAT
FLATHAT
FLATLET
FLATOUT
FRAUGHT
GLAREAT
GNAWSAT
GOABOUT
GRABSAT
GRASPAT
GRAVEST
GRAYEST
HEADOUT
HEADSET
HEAROUT
ICANNOT
IHATEIT
IHAVEIT
IMADEIT
IMAGIST
INACAST
INAKNOT
INANEST
INASNIT
INASPOT
INASUIT
IRATEST
IWANTIT
JEANNOT
LEADOUT
LEAFLET
LEAFOUT
LEANCUT
LEANEST
LEAPSAT
LEAPTAT
LEARJET
LEAVEIT
LOANOUT
MEANEST
MEANSIT
MEANTIT
NEAREST
NEATEST
OFASORT
ONADIET
ONALERT
ONATOOT
ORALIST
PEACOAT
PEASANT
PEATPOT
PIANIST
PLACKET
PLANOUT
PLAUDIT
PLAYACT
PLAYLET
PLAYOUT
PLAYSAT
QUARTET
READAPT
READMIT
READOPT
READOUT
REAGENT
REALEST
REALIST
REALLOT
REAMOUT
REARLIT
REAUDIT
ROARSAT
SCARLET
SEABOAT
SEAGIRT
SEAHUNT
SEALANT
SEALIFT
SEAMIST
SEAPORT
SEASALT
SHABBAT
SHALLOT
SHAVUOT
SNAPSAT
SNARLAT
SOAPNET
SPAMBOT
SPAREST
SPATOUT
STALEST
STAREAT
STARLET
STARLIT
STATIST
STAYOUT
STAYPUT
STAYSAT
SUAVEST
SWATSAT
TEACART
TEAROUT
TEARSAT
TEARSIT
THATSIT
THAWOUT
TRABERT
TRANSIT
TSARIST
UNADEPT
UNADULT
UNALERT
VIADENT
VIADUCT
WEAKEST
WEAROUT
WHATNOT
WHATSIT
YEAHBUT

•••AT••

AARATED
ABLATED
ABLATES
ADRATES
AERATED
AERATES
AERATOR
AGNATES
AGNATIC
ALSATIA
ANNATTO
AQUATIC
ASIATIC
ATWATER
AVIATED
AVIATES
AVIATIC
AVIATOR
BALATAS
BALATON
BELATED
BENATAR
BERATED
BERATER
BERATES
BLEATED
BLEATER
BLOATED
BOBATEA
BOLATIE
BORATES
BREATHE
BREATHS
BREATHY
BUGATTI
BYCATCH
BYPATHS
CDRATES
CERATED
CERATES
CHEATED
CHEATER
CHEATIN
CHEATON
CLEATED
CREATED
CREATES
CREATOR
CROATIA
CURATED
CURATES
CURATOR
DEBATED
DEBATER
DEBATES
DECATUR
DERATED
DERATES
DEWATER
DILATED
DILATES
DILATOR
DONATED
DONATEE
DONATES
DONATOR
DONATUS
ELUATES
EMPATHS
EMPATHY
EQUATED
EQUATES
EQUATOR
ERRATIC
ERRATUM
ESTATED
ESTATES
EXMATES
FANATIC
FIXATED
FIXATES
FLOATBY
FLOATED
FLOATER
FLOATUP
FOLATES
FUGATOS
GALATEA
GALATIA
GELATED
GELATES
GELATIN
GELATIS
GELATOS
GETATIP
GIGATON
GLOATED
GLOATER
GOTATIP
GREATEN
GREATER
GREATLY
GYRATED
GYRATES
GYRATOR
HADATIT
HASATIT
HEMATIC
HEMATIN
HEPATIC
HORATIO
HYPATIA
IDEATED
IDEATES
IGNATOW
INGATES
INMATES
IODATED
IODATES
ITSATIE
IZZATSO
KARATES
KERATIN
KOMATSU
LABATTS
LEGATEE
LEGATES
LEGATOR
LEGATOS
LEVATOR
LIEATOP

LIGATED
LIGATES
LOBATED
LOCATED
LOCATER
LOCATES
LOCATOR
LUNATED
LUNATES
LUNATIC
LUXATED
LUXATES
MAHATMA
MANATEE
MEGATON
METATES
MULATTO
MUTATED
MUTATES
NATATOR
NEGATED
NEGATER
NEGATES
NEGATOR
NOCATCH
NOTATED
NOTATES
NUTATED
NUTATES
OBLATES
OLEATES
ONWATER
OPIATES
OSMATIC
PALATAL
PALATES
PARATUS
PENATES
PERATIO
PGRATED
PILATES
PILATUS
PINATAS
PIRATED
PIRATES
PIRATIC
PLEATED
PUPATED
PUPATES
RANATAB
RATATAT
REBATED
REBATER
REBATES
REBATHE
REDATED
REDATES
REGATTA
RELATCH
RELATED
RELATER
RELATES
RELATOR
REMATCH
REMATED
REMATES
REPATCH
RERATED
RERATES
REWATER
ROTATED
ROTATES
ROTATOR
RUBATOS
RUNATAB
SATATOP
SAWATCH
SCIATIC
SCRATCH
SEDATED
SEDATER
SEDATES
SENATES
SENATOR
SHEATHE
SHEATHS
SHIATSU
SINATRA
SITATOP
SOMATIC
SONATAS
SQUATLY
SQUATTY
STRATAS
STRATUM
STRATUS
SUMATRA
SWEATED
SWEATER
SWEATIT
THEATER
THEATRE
TREATED
TREATER
UNBATED
UNDATED
UNEATEN
UNFATED
UNFATTY
UNGATED
UNHATED
UNIATES
UNLATCH
UNMATED
UNMATES
UNRATED
UNSATED
UPDATED
UPDATER
UPDATES
UPRATED
UPRATES
VACATED
VACATES
VENATIC
WASATCH
WHEATEN
WHEATON
WREATHE
WREATHS
WREATHY
YUCATAN
YUCATEC
YUKATAS
ZAPATAS
ZAPATEO

•••A•T•

ALLANTE
ALMAATA
ANDANTE
ANNATTO
ARGANTE
ASHANTI
ASSANTE
ASTARTE
ATLANTA
BASALTS
BEGANTO
BOGARTS
BREADTH
BREASTS
BROASTS
BUGATTI
CANASTA
CHIANTI
CLEANTE
COBALTS
DECANTS
DEFACTO
DEMASTS
DEPARTS
DERALTE
DESALTS
DIDACTS
DURANTE
DYNASTS
DYNASTY
ELUANTS
ENCARTA
ENFANTS
EQUALTO
ESPARTO
EXFACTO
EXPARTE
GALANTS
GOCARTS
GOKARTS
HAVARTI
HOGARTH
IMPACTS
IMPARTS
IMPASTO
INCANTS
INFAITH
INFANTA
INFANTE
INFANTS
INHASTE
INTASTE
JAKARTA
JOCASTA
KUWAITI
LABATTS
LEPANTO
LOYALTO
LOYALTY
MARANTZ
MISACTS
MORANTE
MULATTO
MUSANTE
MUTANTS
MYLANTA
NONARTS
NOTASTE
OBLASTS
OCTANTS
ONEACTS
ONEARTH
OTRANTO
OUTACTS
OXCARTS
PEDANTS
PENALTY
PESANTE
PICANTE
PLEADTO
PREACTS
REBAITS
REBASTE
RECANTS
RECASTS
REDACTS
REDANTS
REGATTA
REPASTE
REPASTS
RESALTS
RETASTE
ROYALTY
SAVANTS
SECANTS
SPEAKTO
SQUANTO
SQUATTY
STBARTS
STEALTH
STRAITS
STUARTI
SUHARTO
SWEARTO
TARANTO
TENANTS
THEARTS
THWARTS
TOTASTE
TRUANTS
TWOACTS
TYRANTS
UMLAUTS
UNBAITS
UNEARTH
UNFACTS
UNFAITH
UNFATTY
UNHASTY
UNMASTS
UNPASTE
UNSALTY
UNTASTY
UPCASTS
UPDARTS
UPWAFTS
VIVANTS
VOLANTE

•••A••T

APPARAT
AQUAVIT
ASSAULT
ATEABIT
ATEALOT
ATFAULT
ATTAINT
BAHAIST
CABARET
CHIAPET
COHABIT
DADAART
DADAIST
DATASET
DEFAULT
DEMARET
DEWAART
DIDASET
EATABIT
EATALOT
EXHAUST
FLEAPIT
FORABIT
GERAINT
GETAHIT
GIGABIT
GOKAPUT
GOTAHIT
GUJARAT
HADAFIT
HADASET
HADATIT
HASAFIT
HASASET
HASATIT
IMEANIT
INHABIT
ITSAHIT
ITSALOT
KOLANUT
LAMAIST
LOGANUT
MEGABIT
MEGAHIT
MINARET
MYFAULT
NAYARIT
NOFAULT
NOTABIT
NOTALOT
NUNAVUT
ONEACAT
PARAPET
PITAPAT
RATATAT
RENAULT
REPAINT
ROUAULT
SWEARAT
SWEATIT
TABARET
TAGAMET
TUBAIST
YOGAMAT

••••AT•

ACERATE
ACETATE
ACTUATE
ADULATE
AGEMATE
AGITATE
AGITATO
AIRDATE
ALMAATA
AMILATE
ANIMATE
ANIMATO
ARCUATE
ARIGATO
ASBYATT
ATELATE
AUREATE
BACHATA
BADHATS
BARBATE
BASMATI
BEDBATH
BEDMATE
BENEATH
BIGCATS
BIODATA
BISTATE
BOBCATS
BONIATO
BROMATE
CANTATA
CASEATE
CASSATT
CAUDATE
CAVEATS
CHAPATI
CHELATE
CILIATE
CIRRATE
CITRATE
CLAMATO
CLAVATE
CLIMATE
CLIMATS
COGNATE
COLGATE
COLLATE
COMBATS
COMSATS
CONNATE
CORDATE
COSTATE
CRAVATS
CREMATE
CRENATE
CUNEATE
CURTATE
CUSPATE
CUTRATE
DEFEATS
DEFLATE
DENTATE
DEODATO
DERMATO
DEVIATE
DICTATE
DIKTATS
DISRATE
DOGGATE
DOGMATA
DUEDATE
DYEBATH
DYEVATS
EATLATE
EDEMATA
EDUCATE
ELEVATE
EMANATE
EMIRATE
EMULATE
ENDLATE
ENSEATS
EPILATE
EXPIATE
EXUDATE
FALCATE
FATCATS
FEEBATE
FERMATA
FERMATE
FERMATS
FERRATE
FOLIATE
FORMATS
FRIGATE
FURCATE
GALEATE
GEMMATE
GESTATE
GLOBATE
GOLIATH
GRADATE
GYMRATS
HAZMATS
HEPCATS
HIPBATH
HOTBATH
HOTDATE
HYDRATE
ICEBATH
IMAMATE
IMITATE
INFLATE
INGRATE
INSTATE
ISOLATE
ISOLATO
ITERATE
ITSLATE
KHANATE
KITKATS
KKKKATY
KLAMATH
KOLKATA
LABIATE
LABRATS
LACTATE
LAPCATS
LAPLATA
LARIATS
LEMMATA
LEONATO
LINEATE
LIQUATE
LOQUATS
MAGNATE
MANDATE
MANKATO
MARCATO
MARGATE
MEDIATE
MIGRATE
MISDATE
MISMATE
MISRATE
MOSCATO
MRSLATE
MUDBATH
MUDCATS
MUSCATS
NAHUATL
NARRATE
NEONATE
NEWGATE
NEWHATS
NEWMATH
NICTATE
NITRATE
NOSEATS
NOUGATS
NUMBATS
OBVIATE
OCICATS
OLDBATS
ONADATE
ONORATI
OPERATE
ORGEATS
OUTBATS
OUTDATE
OUTEATS
OUTMATE
OUTPATH
OUTRATE
OVERATE
OXALATE
OXIDATE
PALMATE
PALPATE
PASSATS
PAYRATE
PELTATE
PENNATE
PETCATS
PETGATE
PETRATS
PICCATA
PILEATE
PINNATE
PLACATE
PLAKATS
PLANATE
PLICATE
PREDATA
PREDATE
PRELATE
PREMATE
PRIMATE
PRIVATE
PROBATE
PROLATE
PRONATE
PRORATA
PRORATE
PTBOATS
PULSATE
QUINATE
RADIATE
RANLATE
RAWDATA
RECOATS
RECRATE
REDBATS
REDHATS
REFLATE
REHEATS
REPEATS
REPLATE
RESEATS
RESLATE
RESTATE
REXCATS
ROSEATE
RUGRATS
RUINATE
RUNLATE
SABBATH
SADFATE
SATIATE
SEACATS
SEAGATE
SENSATE
SERIATE
SERRATE
SETRATE
SHEVATS
SINUATE
SITUATE
SKIHATS
SNOCATS
SOLLATI
SORBATE
STOMATA
STRIATE
SUBDATE
SULFATE
SUMMATE
SUNBATH
SUNHATS
TAXRATE
TERNATE
TESTATE
THEOATH
THREATS
THROATS
THROATY
TINHATS
TITRATE
TOCCATA
TOMCATS
TOOLATE
TOPHATS
TOPRATE
TOWPATH
TOYHATS
ULULATE
UNCRATE
UNLOATH
UNSEATS
UNSTATE
UPBEATS
UPSTATE
USSTATE
VALUATE
VALVATE
VANUATU
VARIATE
VIBRATE
VIBRATO
VIOLATE
VIRGATE
VITIATE
VULGATE
WAIKATO
WARPATH
WASLATE
WBYEATS
WOMBATS
ZERMATT

••••A•T

ABEYANT
ABREAST
ADAMANT
ADDSALT
AFFIANT
ANTIART
ARMYANT
ASBYATT
ASONANT
ASPHALT
ATHEART
ATHWART
ATLEAST
ATTRACT
BADPAST
BALLAST
BELFAST
BIGEAST
BITPART
BLATANT
BODYART
BOMBAST
BUOYANT
BYHEART
CASSATT
CAVEART
CLAMANT
CLIPART
COMCAST
COMPACT
COMPART
CONTACT
COOLANT
COURANT
CURRANT
DADAART
DEFIANT
DESCANT
DETRACT
DEVIANT
DEWAART
DIECAST
DISMAST
DISPART
DISTANT
DOGCART
DORMANT
DUEEAST
EARHART
ECKHART
ELEGANT
ELKHART
EMANANT
ENCHANT
ENGRAFT
ENTRANT
ETCHANT
EXTRACT
FANTAST
FAREAST
FINEART
FIREANT
FLYCAST
FLYPAST
FOLKART
FONDANT
GALLANT
GESTALT
GETPAST
GOESAFT
GONEAFT
GOTPAST
GYMNAST
HECKART
HERBART
HERBAUT
HIGHART
HYDRANT
IMPLANT
INACAST
INDRAFT
INEXACT
INFRACT
INGRAFT
INSTANT
ISSUANT
ITERANT
JIMKAAT
JUNKART
LASTACT
LENFANT
LESCAUT
LOSTART
MALEANT
MEDIANT
MIDEAST
MIGRANT
MISCAST
MORDANT
MYGIANT
NEWHART
NONFACT
NONPAST
NYGIANT
ODORANT
OFFCAST
OHIOART
OLDSALT
ONEPART
ONTOAST
OPERANT
ORGIAST
ORPHANT
OUTCANT
OUTCAST
OUTFAST
OUTKAST
OUTLAST
OUTRANT
OUTWAIT
OVERACT
OXHEART
OXIDANT
PAGEANT
PARFAIT
PASSANT
PEASANT
PECCANT
PENDANT
PENNANT
PERIAPT
PIQUANT
PLAYACT
PODCAST
POPTART
PRECAST
PRESALT
PROEAST
RADIANT
RAMPANT
RAMPART
RANPAST
READAPT
REBOANT
RECHART
REDEALT
REDRAFT
REENACT
REFRACT
REGNANT
REGRAFT
REGRANT
RELIANT
REMNANT
REPLANT
RESTART
RETOAST
RETRACT
RIOTACT
ROBSART
RUNPAST
SALTANT
SAWPAST
SAYWAIT
SEALANT
SEASALT
SEEPAST
SERVANT
SEXTANT
SOLOACT
STEWART
SUBCAST
SUNFAST
TAGGANT
TEACART
TENNANT
TENPAST
THEEAST
TIPCART
TOHEART
TOPMAST
TOSTART
TOYCART
TWOPART
ULULANT
UNDEALT
UNMEANT
UNPLAIT
UNSMART
UPCOAST
UPDRAFT
UPLEAPT
UPSTART
USGRANT
VAGRANT
VALIANT
VANSANT
VANZANT
VARIANT
VERDANT
VERSANT
VIBRANT
WALMART
WARRANT
WEBCAST
WENTAFT
WHYWAIT
YOPLAIT
ZERMATT
ZUMWALT

•••••AT

ACROBAT
ADEPTAT
AEROBAT
AIMEDAT
AIRBOAT
ALLTHAT
ALNIYAT
ANGRYAT
APPARAT
ASTOLAT
AUTOMAT
BABYSAT
BALKSAT
BARKSAT
BATHMAT
BAYEDAT
BEARCAT
BEATSAT
BEEPSAT
BIGBEAT
BLINKAT
BODYFAT
BOOEDAT
BOXCOAT
BOXSEAT
CARCOAT
CARPSAT
CARSEAT
CATBOAT
CAVILAT
CHILCAT
CHILKAT
CHROMAT
CLAWSAT
COMESAT
COOLCAT
COONCAT
COPYCAT
COWERAT
CROSSAT
CURSEAT
DEEPFAT
DIDTOAT
DINEDAT
DINESAT
DINGBAT
DOGCOAT
DOGREAT

7
AU

DOORMAT
DOWNPAT
DRIVEAT
DROVEAT
DRYHEAT
DWELLAT
EATENAT
ENDEDAT
ENDUPAT
ENTREAT
ESCHEAT
EXCELAT
FELTHAT
FIREDAT
FIREHAT
FIRESAT
FLAILAT
FLATHAT
FLIESAT
FLINGAT
FLOWNAT
FLUNGAT
FOTOMAT
FRETSAT
FROWNAT
FUMEDAT
FUMESAT
FURCOAT
GAPEDAT
GAPESAT
GASHEAT
GAWKSAT
GAZEDAT
GAZESAT
GETBEAT
GIBESAT
GLAREAT
GNAWSAT
GOINGAT
GOTBEAT
GRABSAT
GRASPAT
GREWFAT
GRINSAT
GROWFAT
GUESSAT
GUJARAT
GUNBOAT
HABITAT
HARDHAT
HELLCAT
HIGHHAT
HINTSAT
HONKSAT
HOOTSAT
HOTSEAT
HOWLSAT
ICEBOAT
IMGREAT
IREPEAT
JAWEDAT
JEERSAT
JETBOAT
JIBEDAT
JIBESAT
JIMKAAT
JUMPSAT
KEEPSAT

KIDSEAT
KINGRAT
KUMQUAT
LABCOAT
LABORAT
LANDSAT
LAUGHAT
LEAPSAT
LEAPTAT
LEERSAT
LESSFAT
LETSEAT
LIVESAT
LOOKSAT
LOSTCAT
LUNGEAT
MALECAT
MALLRAT
MANXCAT
MARRYAT
MAUPRAT
MAURIAT
MEERKAT
MISSEAT
MOLERAT
MUDFLAT
MUSKRAT
MYTREAT
NONMEAT
NOSWEAT
NOWWHAT
NUTMEAT
OFFBEAT
OILHEAT
ONEACAT
ONEOCAT
OVEREAT
OVERFAT
PACKRAT
PAWEDAT
PEACOAT
PECKSAT
PEEKSAT
PEEPSAT
PEERSAT
PETGOAT
PICKSAT
PIGMEAT
PITAPAT
PLAYSAT
PNEUMAT
POINTAT
POKEDAT
POKESAT
POLECAT
POLESAT
PREHEAT
PRESEAT
RAILSAT
RAINHAT
RANTSAT
RATATAT
RAWMEAT
REDCOAT
REDHEAT
REDMEAT
REFLOAT
RETREAT

RIBMEAT
RINKRAT
ROARSAT
ROOFRAT
ROTBLAT
ROWBOAT
SAYWHAT
SCOFFAT
SEABOAT
SHABBAT
SHEGOAT
SHOOTAT
SHOPSAT
SHOUTAT
SHOWCAT
SIGHSAT
SILKHAT
SITSPAT
SMILEAT
SNAPSAT
SNARLAT
SNEERAT
SNIFFAT
SNIPEAT
SNORTAT
SNOWCAT
SNOWHAT
STAREAT
STAYSAT
STOPSAT
SWATSAT
SWEARAT
SWINGAT
SWOREAT
SWUNGAT
TALKSAT
TEARSAT
THEBRAT
THEHEAT
THEREAT
THREWAT
THROWAT
TILTSAT
TOILSAT
TOOTSAT
TOPCOAT
TOWBOAT
TOYBOAT
TREERAT
TUGBOAT
WAVEDAT
WAVESAT
WHEREAT
WILDCAT
WINEVAT
WINKSAT
WOOLFAT
WOOLHAT
WORKSAT
YANKSAT
YELLSAT
YOGAMAT

AU•••••

AUBADES
AUBERGE
AUBURNS
AUBURNU
AUCTION
AUDIBLE
AUDIBLY
AUDILES
AUDITED
AUDITEE
AUDITOR
AUDUBON
AUGENDS
AUGITES
AUGMENT
AUGURAL
AUGURED
AUGURER
AUGUSTA
AUGUSTE
AUGUSTO
AUGUSTS
AUKLETS
AULDSOD
AULETTA
AUNTBEE
AUNTIES
AUPAIRS
AURALEE
AURALLY
AUREATE
AUREOLA
AUREOLE
AURICLE
AURISTS
AURORAE
AURORAL
AURORAS
AUSABLE
AUSLESE
AUSPICE
AUSSIES
AUSTERE
AUSTERS
AUSTINS
AUSTRAL
AUSTRIA
AUTARCH
AUTARKY
AUTEURS
AUTHORS
AUTISTS
AUTOBIO
AUTOBUS
AUTOING
AUTOMAT
AUTOMNE
AUTONYM
AUTOPEN
AUTOPIA
AUTOPSY
AUTUMNS

A•U••••

ABUSERS
ABUSING
ABUSIVE
ABUTSON
ABUTTAL
ABUTTED
ABUTTER
ACUMENS

ACUTELY
ACUTEST
ADULATE
ADULTLY
AGULHAS
AGUTTER
ALUDELS
ALUMINA
ALUMNAE
ALUMNAL
ALUMNUS
ALUNSER
AMULETS
AMUSEME
AMUSERS
AMUSING
AOUDADS
APULIAN
AQUAMAN
AQUARIA
AQUATIC
AQUAVIT
AQUEOUS
AQUIFER
AQUINAS
AQUIVER
ARUBANS
ARUGULA
ARUNDEL
ARUSPEX
ASUNDER
ASUSUAL
AVULSED
AVULSES
AZULEJO
AZURITE
AZUSACA

A••U•••

AAJUMBO
ABDUCED
ABDUCES
ABDUCTS
ABJURED
ABJURER
ABJURES
ABOUNDS
ABOUTIT
ABOUTTO
ABRUZZI
ACAUDAL
ACCURST
ACCUSAL
ACCUSED
ACCUSER
ACCUSES
ACOUPLE
ACQUIRE
ACQUITS
ACTUARY
ACTUATE
ACTUPON
ADDUCED
ADDUCER
ADDUCES
ADDUCTS
ADDUPTO
ADJUDGE

ADJUNCT
ADJURED
ADJURER
ADJURES
ADJUROR
ADJUSTS
ADZUKIS
AFOULOF
AGOUTIS
ALBUMEN
ALBUMIN
ALBUNDY
ALDUBIN
ALLUDED
ALLUDES
ALLURED
ALLURER
ALLURES
ALLUVIA
ALQUIST
AMOUNTS
AMPULES
ANGUISH
ANGULAR
ANNUALS
ANNUITY
ANNULAR
ANNULET
ANNULUS
ANOUILH
APLUSES
ARBUTUS
ARCUATE
ARDUOUS
ARGUERS
ARGUING
ARGUSES
AROUSAL
AROUSED
AROUSER
AROUSES
ASQUIET
ASQUINT
ASQUITH
ASSUAGE
ASSUMED
ASSUMER
ASSUMES
ASSUNTA
ASSURED
ASSURER
ASSURES
ASSUROR
ASTUTER
ATLUNCH
ATTUCKS
ATTUNED
ATTUNES
AUBURNS
AUBURNU
AUDUBON
AUGURAL
AUGURED
AUGURER
AUGUSTA
AUGUSTE
AUGUSTO
AUGUSTS

AUTUMNS
AWFULLY

A•••U••

ACCOUNT
ACCRUAL
ACCRUED
ACCRUES
ACHTUNG
ADJOURN
ADNOUNS
AGROUND
AIRDUCT
AIRGUNS
AIRPUMP
AIRTUBE
ALARUMS
ALBSURE
ALLIUMS
AMINUTE
AMPOULE
ANDSUCH
ANYLUCK
APESUIT
ARAFURA
ARBOURS
ARDOURS
ARMFULS
ARMOURS
ARMOURY
ARTHURC
ARTHURM
ARTHURS
ARUGULA
ASARULE
ASEXUAL
ASHBURN
ASHBURY
ASSAULT
ASTOUND
ASUSUAL
ASYLUMS
ATATURK
ATDEUCE
ATFAULT
ATRIUMS
AUTEURS
AVENUEQ
AVENUES
AZIMUTH

A••••U•

ABSOLUT
ACEDOUT
ACESOUT
ACTEDUP
ACTFOUR
ACTSOUT
ADDEDUP
AGEDOUT
AGEFOUR
AGENDUM
AGESOUT
AIREDUP
AIRSOUT
ALARBUS
ALLOFUS
ALUMNUS

ALYSSUM
AMADEUS
AMATEUR
AMIBLUE
AMOROUS
AMPEDUP
ANDROUS
ANGELUS
ANNULUS
ANTEDUP
ANTERUS
ANTESUP
ANTIGUA
ANTIGUN
ANTIQUE
ANXIOUS
APERCUS
APODOUS
APPLAUD
AQUEOUS
ARBUTUS
ARCANUM
ARDUOUS
AREARUG
ARTEMUS
ASKEDUP
ASKSOUT
ATEITUP
ATISSUE
ATTICUS
AUTOBUS
AVERNUS

A•••••U

ALFREDU
ANGELOU
AUBURNU

•AU••••

BAUBLES
BAUHAUS
BAULKED
BAULKER
BAUXITE
CAUDATE
CAULKED
CAULKER
CAUSERS
CAUSING
CAUSTIC
CAUTHEN
CAUTION
DAUBERS
DAUBING
DAUMIER
DAUNTED
DAUNTER
DAUPHIN
DAUSSET
FAUCETS
FAULTED
FAUSTUS
FAUVISM
FAUVIST
FAUXFUR
FAUXPAS
GAUCHER
GAUCHOS

GAUDENS
GAUDERY
GAUDIER
GAUDIES
GAUDILY
GAUGERS
GAUGING
GAUGUIN
GAULISH
GAUNTER
GAUNTLY
GAUSSES
GAUTAMA
GAUTIER
GAUZIER
GAUZILY
HAUGHTY
HAULAGE
HAULERS
HAULING
HAULOFF
HAULSIN
HAULSUP
HAUNTED
HAUNTER
HAUTBOY
HAUTEUR
JAUNTED
KAUFMAN
LAUDERS
LAUDING
LAUGHAT
LAUGHED
LAUGHER
LAUGHIN
LAULAUS
LAUNDER
LAUNDRY
LAURELS
LAURENT
LAURITZ
LAUTREC
MAUDLIN
MAUGHAM
MAULDIN
MAULERS
MAULING
MAUMAUS
MAUNDER
MAUPRAT
MAUREEN
MAURIAC
MAURIAT
MAURICE
MAUROIS
MAUSERS
MAUVAIS
NAUGHTS
NAUGHTY
NAUSEAM
NAUTICA
NAUTILI
PAUCITY
PAULIII
PAULINA
PAULINE
PAULING
PAULIST

PAULPRY
PAULSEN
PAUNCHY
PAUPERS
PAUSERS
PAUSING
RAUCOUS
RAUNCHY
SAUCERS
SAUCIER
SAUCILY
SAUCING
SAUCONY
SAUNAED
SAUNTER
SAURIAN
SAUSAGE
SAUTEED
TAUNTED
TAUNTER
TAUNTON
TAUREAN
TAURINE
TAUTENS
TAUTEST
VAUDOIS
VAUGHAN
VAULTED
VAULTER
VAUNTED
VAUNTER

•A•U•••

AAJUMBO
CADUCEI
CALUMET
CALUMNY
CANUCKS
CANULAE
CANULAS
CAPUANA
CAPUCHE
CAPULET
CASUALS
CASUIST
CAYUGAS
CAYUSES
FACULAE
FACULTY
FAMULUS
FATUITY
FATUOUS
GALUMPH
HAMULUS
HANUKAH
JACUZZI
JAGUARS
JANUARY
KABUKIS
KAHUNAS
KAKUROS
LACUNAE
LACUNAL
LACUNAR
LACUNAS
LACUREE
LAGUNAS
LAPUTAN

LARUSSA
LAYUPON
MACULAE
MACULAR
MACUSER
MADUROS
MAGUIRE
MANUALS
MANUMIT
MANURED
MANURES
MARULLO
MARUSJA
MATURED
MATURER
MATURES
MAZURKA
NABUCCO
NAHUATL
NATURAL
NATURED
NATUREL
NATURES
OAHUANS
PABULUM
PADUANS
PADUCAH
PAIUTES
PALUDAL
PANURGE
PAPUANS
PARURES
RANUPTO
RASURES
SAGUARO
SALUKIS
SALUTED
SALUTER
SALUTES
SAMUELL
SAMURAI
SARUMAN
SATUPON
SATURNS
TABUING
TABULAR
TALUSES
VACUITY
VACUOLE
VACUOUS
VACUUMS
VAGUELY
VAGUEST
VALUATE
VALUERS
VALUING
VANUATU
VAQUERO
WATUSIS
YAKUTSK
YAOUNDE
ZABUTON
ZAKUSKA

•A••U••

BACKUPS
BADGUYS
BADLUCK

BAGFULS
BALLUET
BANBURY
BANQUES
BANQUET
BARBUDA
BARBULE
BARNUMS
BARQUES
BASQUES
BATSUIT
BAYRUMS
CADBURY
CAESURA
CALCULI
CALLUPS
CANFULS
CANNULA
CAPFULS
CAPGUNS
CAPNUTS
CAPSULE
CAPTURE
CARFULS
CAROUSE
CASQUED
CASQUES
CATGUTS
CATSUIT
CATSUPS
DANBURY
DARIUSI
DATSUNS
DAYQUIL
EANMUND
EARBUDS
EARFULS
EARMUFF
FACTUAL
FAILURE
FAIRUSE
FANEUIL
FANOUTS
FAROUKI
FATOUSH
FAVOURS
GAGRULE
GASPUMP
GAUGUIN
HADPULL
HAMBURG
HANGUPS
HARBURG
HASPULL
HATFULS
JACCUSE
JACQUES
JARFULS
KAPTURE
LABOURS
LABTUBE
LACEUPS
LACQUER
LADOUCE
LANGUID
LANGUOR
LAPFULS
LARRUPS

LASHUPS
LAWSUIT
LAYOUTS
MACDUFF
MACOUNS
MADRUSH
MAGNUMS
MAHOUTS
MAJEURE
MAKEUPS
MANCUSO
MANHUNT
MANTUAN
MAOSUIT
MARAUDS
MARCUSE
MARKUPS
MARQUEE
MARQUES
MARQUEZ
MARQUIS
MARYURE
MASQUER
MASQUES
NATSUME
PABLUMS
PACQUIN
PANFULS
PARFUMS
PARQUET
PASTURE
PAYCUTS
PAYOUTS
RACQUET
RAEBURN
RAGOUTS
RAGRUGS
RAPTUNE
RAPTURE
RAVEUPS
RAYBURN
RAYGUNS
SACQUES
SAMBUCA
SAMHUFF
SAMNUNN
SAMSUNG
SANJUAN
SATSUMA
SAVOURS
SAVOURY
SAWBUCK
SAWDUST
SAXTUBA
TABOULI
TACTUAL
TAGOUTS
TALCUMS
TAXCUTS
VACUUMS
VALOURS
VALVULA
VALVULE
VANDURA
VANDUYN
VAPOURS
VAPOURY
VASQUEZ

VATFULS
WAKEUPS
WALKUPS
WALKURE
WALNUTS
WAMPUMS
WARBURG
WARMUPS
WASHUPS
WASSURE
XAMOUNT
YANQUIS
ZAGNUTS

•A•••U•

BACCHUS
BACKOUT
BACKRUB
BACKSUP
BAILOUT
BALEFUL
BALFOUR
BALLSUP
BANEFUL
BANGOUT
BANGSUP
BANKSUP
BARACUS
BAROQUE
BASHFUL
BATEAUX
BATHTUB
BAUHAUS
BAWLOUT
CACIQUE
CADEAUX
CADMIUM
CAGEDUP
CAGESUP
CAKEDUP
CAKESUP
CALCIUM
CALHOUN
CALLOUS
CALLOUT
CALLSUP
CAMEDUE
CAMEOUT
CAMPOUT
CAMPSUP
CANDOUR
CANOPUS
CARCLUB
CARDIUM
CAREFUL
CARIOUS
CARPOUS
CASEOUS
CASEOUT
CASHOUT
CASSIUS
CASTOUT
CASTSUP
CATCHUP
DAMASUS
DANSEUR
DAREFUL
DARTGUN
DATABUS
EARDRUM
EARPLUG
EASEDUP
EASEFUL
EASEOUT
EASESUP
EATENUP
EATITUP
EATSOUT
FABFOUR
FACTFUL
FADEOUT
FAIRSUP
FAKEFUR
FAKEOUT
FALLDUE
FALLGUY
FALLOUT
FAMULUS
FANCLUB
FANCYUP
FANSOUT
FARCEUR
FARMOUT
FATEFUL
FATIGUE
FATUOUS
FAUSTUS
FAUXFUR
GAINFUL
GALLIUM
GANGSUP
GASEDUP
GASEOUS
GASESUP
GATEAUX
GAVEOUT
HABITUE
HACKSUP
HAFNIUM
HAHNIUM
HAIRCUT
HALFCUT
HALFDUG
HALIBUT
HAMITUP
HAMULUS
HANDFUL
HANDGUN
HANDOUT
HANDSUP
HANGOUT
HANGSUP
HARBOUR
HARDPUT
HARMFUL
HARTMUT
HASHOUT
HASSIUM
HATEFUL
HAULSUP
HAUTEUR
HAVEFUN
HAVEOUT
IAPETUS
JACKSUP
KARAKUM
LACEDUP
LACESUP
LADYBUG
LAFLEUR
LAIDOUT
LALIQUE
LANDAUS
LANDSUP
LASCAUX
LASHOUT
LATINUS
LAULAUS
LAYSOUT
LAZARUS
MACAQUE
MADEFUN
MADEOUT
MADERUN
MAHFOUZ
MAILOUT
MAISOUI
MAKEFUN
MAKEOUT
MAKERUN
MAKESUP
MALAMUD
MALLEUS
MALRAUX
MALTHUS
MANAGUA
MANHOUR
MANIPUR
MAPSOUT
MARGAUX
MARHAUS
MARKOUT
MARKSUP
MARTIUS
MASSEUR
MATCHUP
MAUMAUS
MAXIMUM
MAXIMUS
NAILGUN
NAILSUP
NAIPAUL
NATRIUM
PABULUM
PACKSUP
PAIDOUT
PAILFUL
PAINFUL
PAIRSUP
PALMFUL
PANSOUT
PAPYRUS
PARAMUS
PARATUS
PARFOUR
PARIBUS
PARLOUR
PARLOUS
PASSEUL
PASSOUT
PASTDUE
PASTEUP
PASTEUR
PATCHUP
PAVIOUR
PAYSOUT
PAYSTUB
RACEDUP
RACESUP
RACKOUT
RACKSUP
RAGEFUL
RAILBUS
RAINOUT
RAISEUP
RAKEDUP
RAKESUP
RAMPSUP
RANCOUR
RANGOUT
RANITUP
RANKOUT
RAPANUI
RATSOUT
RAUCOUS
SACKFUL
SACKOUT
SACKSUP
SANCTUM
SANCTUS
SANDBUR
SANGOUT
SAVEDUP
SAVESUP
SAVIOUR
SAWCHUK
TACITUS
TACKSUP
TACTFUL
TAGSOUT
TAKENUP
TAKEOUT
TAKESUP
TALKOUT
TALKSUP
TALLYUP
TANKFUL
TANKSUP
TANTRUM
TAPEDUP
TAPESUP
TAPSOUT
TARTSUP
VACUOUS
VANOCUR
VAPORUB
VARIOUS
WAILFUL
WAITOUT
WAITSUP
WAKEDUP
WAKEFUL
WAKESUP
WALKOUT
WALLSUP
WANTOUT
WARCLUB
WARMSUP
WASHOUT
WASHTUB
WAXEDUP
WAXESUP
XANADUS
YANKOUT
YAWNFUL

•A••••U

BANDEAU
BARBEAU
BAYLORU
CAILLOU
CARIBOU
GARNEAU
JAMBEAU
LAMBEAU
MARCEAU
MARTINU
MARYLOU
MATHIEU
MATTHAU
PARVENU
PAXINOU
SAYSYOU
TABLEAU
VANUATU
WATTEAU
XAVIERU

••AU•••

ACAUDAL
BEAUISH
BLAUBOK
CHAUCER
CLAUDEL
CLAUDIA
CLAUDIO
CLAUSAL
CLAUSES
DRAUGHT
EPAULET
FLAUNTS
FLAUNTY
FLAUTAS
FRAUGHT
GIAUQUE
GRAUMAN
PLAUDIT
PLAUTUS
REAUDIT
REAUMUR
STAUNCH
TEAURNS
TRAUBEL
TRAUMAS
WHAUDEN

••A•U••

ALARUMS
ARAFURA
ASARULE
ATATURK
BLACULA
BRAVURA
CHALUPA
CLAQUES
DIALUPS
DRACULA
EMANUEL
ERASURE
EVACUEE
EVALUNA
FEATURE
GRADUAL
GRANULE
GRAVURE
INAFUNK
INAFURY
INAHUFF
INARUSH
INASUIT
JOAQUIN
LEADUPS
LEAGUED
LEAGUER
LEAGUES
MEASURE
MIAOUED
ONAJURY
OPAQUES
PEANUTS
PLAGUED
PLAGUES
PLAQUES
RVALUES
SCAPULA
SEADUCK
SEADUTY
SEAGULL
SEAHUNT
SHAVUOT
SNAFUED
SPATULA
STATUES
STATURE
STATUTE
TEACUPS
TEAMUSA
TOATURN
TRADUCE
ULALUME
ULANUDE
UNADULT
UNAMUNO
UVALUES
VIADUCT
WRAPUPS

••A••U•

ALARBUS
AMADEUS
AMATEUR
BEADSUP
BEAMSUP
BEARCUB
BEARHUG
BEAROUT
BEARSUP
BEATOUT
BEATSUP
BLAZEUP
BOARDUP
BOATFUL
BRACEUP
CDALBUM
CHAINUP
CHALKUP
CHATSUP
CLAMOUR
CLAMSUP
CRACKUP
CRANIUM
CRANKUP
CRAPOUT
CRASSUS
CRATEUP
DEALOUT
DEALSUP
DEALTUP
DIALOUT
DIALSUP
DRAGOUT
DRAGSUP
DRANKUP
DRAWNUP
DRAWOUT
DRAWSUP
ELAAIUN
ENAMOUR
ERASMUS
ERASTUS
FEARFUL
FIATLUX
FLAMEUP
FLANEUR
FLAREUP
FLATOUT
FLAVIUS
FLAVOUR
FRAMEUP
GEARSUP
GIAUQUE
GLAMOUR
GLAMSUP
GOABOUT
GRAMPUS
GRATEUP
GUARGUM
HEADFUL
HEADOUT
HEADSUP
HEALSUP
HEAPSUP
HEAROUT
HEATFUL
HEATSUP
JEALOUS
JEANLUC
LEADOUT
LEADSUP
LEAFOUT
LEANCUT
LEAPSUP
LEAPTUP
LOADSUP
LOANOUT
MOANFUL
OKAYGUY
ORARIUM
PEASOUP
PGATOUR
PLANOUT
PLAUTUS
PLAYFUL
PLAYOUT
PLAYSUP
QUANTUM
REACHUP
READOUT
READSUP
REAMOUT
REARGUE
REARSUP
REAUMUR
SCALEUP
SCAREUP
SCARFUP
SEABLUE
SEALSUP
SEASLUG
SHAGRUG
SHAKEUP
SHAPEUP
SLACKUP
SLANTUP
SMACKUP
SMASHUP
SNAGSUP
SNAPSUP
SNARLUP
SNAZZUP
SOAKSUP
SOAPSUP
SPATOUT
STACKUP
STADIUM
STANDUP
STANKUP
STANNUM
STARTUP
STAYOUT
STAYPUT
STAYSUP
SWANKUP
TEAMSUP
TEARFUL
TEAROUT
TEARSUP
TEASEUP
THAWOUT
TRADEUP
TRAPGUN
TRAYFUL
UNAWFUL
URANIUM
VIALFUL
WEAROUT
WHATSUP
WRACKUP
WRAPSUP
YEAHBUT
ZEALOUS

••A•••U

CHANOYU
CHAPEAU
CHATEAU
ISABEAU
NEARYOU
PLATEAU
YEAHYOU

•••AU••

ASSAULT
ATFAULT
BECAUSE
BEDAUBS
DEBAUCH
DEFAULT
DEGAUSS
DEPAULU
DRLAURA
EXHAUST
KILAUEA
MARAUDS
MYFAULT
NOFAULT
REGAUGE
REHAULS
RENAULT
ROUAULT
STPAULS
STRAUSS
UMLAUTS
UNGAUDY

•••A•U•

ARCANUM
AREARUG
BARACUS
BELARUS
BREAKUP
CIMABUE
CLEANUP
CLEARUP
CUTARUG
DAMASUS
DATABUS
DECATUR
DEDALUS
DELARUE
DEVALUE
DONAHUE
DONATUS
DREAMUP
ELAAIUN
ERRATUM
ESCALUS
EULABUS
FLOATUP
GOKAPUT
HUMANUM
INVACUO
KARAKUM
KOLANUT
LAZARUS
LOGANUT
MACAQUE
MALAMUD
MANAGUA
NUNAVUT
OCEANUS
OFVALUE
PARAMUS
PARATUS
PEGASUS
PILATUS
PIRAEUS
POTAMUS
PYRAMUS
RAPANUI
REVALUE
ROMANUS
ROSABUD
RUBADUB
SNEAKUP
SPEAKUP
STEAMUP
STRATUM
STRATUS
SUBARUS
TETANUS
TOTALUP
TUNASUB
UNVAGUE
UPVALUE
XANADUS

•••A••U

DEPAULU
HOWARDU
IGUASSU
KOMATSU
SHIATSU
TINAMOU
TULANEU

••••AU•

APPLAUD
BATEAUX
BAUHAUS
BORLAUG
BUREAUS
BUREAUX
CADEAUX
CENTAUR
CHEVAUX
CISEAUX
DEFRAUD
GATEAUX
HERBAUT
IBNSAUD
JOUHAUX
LANDAUS
LASCAUX
LAULAUS
LESCAUT
LESPAUL
MALRAUX
MARGAUX
MARHAUS
MAUMAUS
MICHAUX
MILHAUD
MONTAUK
MRSPAUL
MULDAUR
NAIPAUL
OISEAUX
OUTHAUL
RESEAUS
RESEAUX
REYNAUD
RIMBAUD
TUSSAUD
VONLAUE
WINDAUS

••••A•U

BUNRAKU
MONTAGU
VANUATU

•••••AU

BANDEAU
BARBEAU
BELLEAU
CHAPEAU
CHATEAU
COCTEAU
FEYDEAU
FRENEAU
GARNEAU
HOFBRAU
ISABEAU
JAMBEAU
LAMBEAU
LILINAU
LOYOLAU
MARCEAU
MATTHAU
NOUVEAU
PERREAU
PLATEAU
QUENEAU
RONDEAU
ROULEAU
TABLEAU
THOREAU
THURGAU
TONNEAU
TRUDEAU
WATTEAU
ZWICKAU

AV•••••

AVAILED
AVALONS
AVANTIS
AVARICE
AVATARS
AVENGED
AVENGER
AVENGES
AVENIDA
AVENUEQ
AVENUES
AVERAGE
AVERELL
AVERILL
AVERNAL
AVERNUS
AVERRED
AVERTED
AVERTER
AVESTAN
AVESTAS
AVEYRON
AVGASES
AVIANCA
AVIATED
AVIATES
AVIATIC
AVIATOR
AVIDEST
AVIDFAN
AVIDITY
AVIGNON
AVIONIC
AVIVIAN
AVOCADO
AVOCETS
AVOIDED
AVOIDER
AVONLEA
AVOWALS
AVOWERS
AVOWING
AVULSED
AVULSES

A•V••••

ADVANCE
ADVENTS
ADVERBS
ADVERSE
ADVERTS
ADVICES
ADVISED
ADVISEE
ADVISER
ADVISES
ADVISOR
ALVAREZ
ALVEOLI

A••V•••

AIRVENT
ALEVELS
ALIVETO
ATAVISM
ATAVIST
AVIVIAN

A•••V••

ACTIVAS
ACTIVES
ALCOVES
ALDAVIS
ALLOVER
ALLUVIA
ANDOVER
AQUAVIT
AQUIVER
ARRIVAL
ARRIVED
ARRIVER
ARRIVES
ASHIVER
ASKOVER
ATEOVER
ATSEVEN

A••••V•

ABSOLVE
ABUSIVE
ACHIEVA
ACHIEVE
ACTFIVE
AGEFIVE
AIRWAVE
ALGARVE
AMATIVE
ANCHOVY
APPROVE
ARCHIVE

A•••••V

AKSAKOV
ALFEROV

•AV••••

BAVARIA
CAVALRY
CAVEART
CAVEATS
CAVEDIN
CAVEINS
CAVEMAN
CAVEMEN
CAVERNS
CAVESIN
CAVIARE
CAVIARS
CAVILAT
CAVILED
CAVILER
CAVORTS
DAVEKOZ
DAVINCI
DAVISON
FAVORED
FAVORER
FAVOURS
GAVEEAR
GAVELED
GAVEOFF
GAVEOUT
GAVEWAY
GAVIALS
GAVILAN
GAVOTTE
HAVANAN
HAVANAS
HAVARTI
HAVEAGO
HAVEFUN
HAVENER
HAVENOT
HAVEONE
HAVEOUT
JAVAMAN
JAVELIN
LAVABOS
LAVACHE
LAVAGES
LAVAINE
LAVALSE
LAVELLI
LAVERAN
LAVERNE
LAVINIA
LAVORIS
MAVISES
NAVAHOS
NAVAIDS
NAVAJOS
NAVARRE
NAVIDAD
NAVYMAN
NAVYMEN
PAVANES
PAVIDLY
PAVINGS
PAVIORS

PAVIOUR
PAVLOVA
RAVAGED
RAVAGER
RAVAGES
RAVELED
RAVELLY
RAVELOE
RAVENAL
RAVENED
RAVENNA
RAVEUPS
RAVINED
RAVINES
RAVINGS
RAVIOLI
SAVABLE
SAVAGED
SAVAGER
SAVAGES
SAVALAS
SAVANAS
SAVANNA
SAVANTS
SAVARIN
SAVEDON
SAVEDUP
SAVEFOR
SAVESON
SAVESUP
SAVINGS
SAVIORS
SAVIOUR
SAVORED
SAVORER
SAVOURS
SAVOURY
SAVVIED
SAVVIER
SAVVIES
SAVVILY
TAVERNA
TAVERNS
WAVEDAT
WAVEDIN
WAVEDTO
WAVELET
WAVEOFF
WAVERED
WAVERER
WAVESAT
WAVESIN
WAVESTO
WAVICLE
WAVIEST
XAVIERU

•A•V•••
CALVARY
CALVERT
CALVING
CALVINO
CANVASS
CARVELS
CARVERS
CARVING
DANVERS
FAUVISM
FAUVIST
GALVANI
GALVANO
HALVAHS
HALVERS
HALVING
HARVARD
HARVEST
JANVIER
JAYVEES
LANVINS
LATVIAN
MALVINA
MARVELL
MARVELS
MARVIER
MAUVAIS
NAIVELY
NAIVEST
NAIVETE
NAIVETY
NARVAEZ
PARVENU
SALVAGE
SALVERS
SALVING
SALVOES
SALVORS
SAVVIED
SAVVIER
SAVVIES
SAVVILY
VALVATE
VALVULA
VALVULE
VANVOGT
WAIVERS
WAIVING
WARVETS

•A••V••
BATAVIA
CADAVER
CARAVAN
CARAVEL
CASAVAS
DATIVES
EATOVER
GASOVEN
HADOVER
HALAVAH
HANOVER
HASOVER
LAYOVER
MARKVII
NATIVES
PALAVER
RANOVER
RAYOVAC
SALIVAS
SAMOVAR
SAYOVER

•A•••V•
BADLOVE
BADMOVE
BAKLAVA
CAPTIVA
CAPTIVE
CASSAVA
DASILVA
IAMLOVE
JAMESVI
KARLOVY
MAGLEVS
MALDIVE
MARKOVA
MASSIVE
PAHLAVI
PARFIVE
PARKAVE
PASSIVE
PAVLOVA
TANTIVY
TAXLEVY

•A••••V
BADENOV
CABLETV
FADAYEV
JAMESIV
KATAYEV
MARTINV
NABOKOV
WATCHTV

••AV•••
ATAVISM
ATAVIST
BEAVERS
BRAVADA
BRAVADO
BRAVELY
BRAVERY
BRAVEST
BRAVING
BRAVOED
BRAVOES
BRAVURA
CLAVATE
CLAVELL
CLAVIER
CRAVATS
CRAVENS
CRAVERS
CRAVING
DIAVOLO
FLAVIUS
FLAVORS
FLAVORY
FLAVOUR
GLAVINE
GRAVELS
GRAVELY
GRAVERS
GRAVEST
GRAVIES
GRAVING
GRAVITY
GRAVLAX
GRAVURE
HEAVEHO
HEAVENS
HEAVERS
HEAVETO
HEAVIER
HEAVIES
HEAVILY
HEAVING
IHAVEIT
INAVALE
KNAVERY
KNAVISH
LEAVEBE
LEAVEIN
LEAVEIT
LEAVENS
LEAVEON
LEAVING
OLAVIII
QUAVERS
QUAVERY
REAVAIL
REAVERS
REAVING
REAVOWS
SHAVERS
SHAVIAN
SHAVING
SHAVUOT
SLAVERS
SLAVERY
SLAVING
SLAVISH
STAVING
SUAVELY
SUAVEST
SUAVITY
TRAVAIL
TRAVELS
TRAVERS
WEAVERS
WEAVING

••A•V••
CHARVET
DWARVES
SCARVES
STARVED
STARVES
WHARVES

••A••V•
AMATIVE
EVASIVE
FLATTVS
IVANOVO
NBALIVE
SUASIVE
ULANOVA
UPABOVE

••A•••V
KHARKOV
TRASHTV

•••AV••
ALDAVIS
AQUAVIT
BATAVIA
BEHAVED
BEHAVES
CADAVER
CARAVAN
CARAVEL
CASAVAS
CLEAVED
CLEAVER
CLEAVES
CLEAVON
DEHAVEN
DISAVOW
GREAVES
HALAVAH
IMPAVID
INFAVOR
LEHAVRE
MCGAVIN
MISAVER
MOHAVES
MOJAVES
MORAVIA
NUNAVUT
OCTAVAL
OCTAVES
OCTAVIA
OCTAVIO
OCTAVOS
OTTAVIO
PALAVER
PREAVER
REPAVED
REPAVES
RESAVED
RESAVES
SHEAVED
SHEAVES
SOHAVEI
TELAVIV
UNEAVED
UNLAVED
UNPAVED
UNRAVEL
UNSAVED
UNSAVVY
UNWAVED
VISAVIS

•••A•V•
ALGARVE
BIVALVE
RECARVE
UNNAIVE
UNSAVVY
URBANVI

•••A••V
AKSAKOV
EDWARDV
FADAYEV
KATAYEV
ROMANOV
ROZANOV
TELAVIV
ULYANOV
URBANIV

••••AV•
AIRWAVE
BAKLAVA
BEBRAVE
BEREAVE
CASSAVA
CENTAVO
CONCAVE
DEPRAVE
ENCLAVE
ENGRAVE
ENSLAVE
EXCLAVE
FORGAVE
GUSTAVE
ICECAVE
INWEAVE
LETHAVE
MISGAVE
MONDAVI
NEWWAVE
OLDNAVY
ONLEAVE
OSTRAVA
OUTGAVE
OUTRAVE
OUTWAVE
PAHLAVI
PARKAVE
PECCAVI
POLTAVA
PREPAVE
PRONAVY
RESHAVE
REWEAVE
THECAVS
THEMAVS
THEWAVE
UNBRAVE
UNHEAVY
UNWEAVE
UPHEAVE

AW•••••
AWAITED
AWAITER
AWAKENS
AWAKERS
AWAKING
AWARDED
AWARDEE
AWARDER
AWAREOF
AWAREST
AWASHIN
AWEEBIT
AWELESS
AWESOME
AWFULLY
AWKWARD
AWNINGS
AWNLESS
AWOONOR

A•W••••
ADWOMAN
ADWOMEN
ALWORTH
ATWATER
ATWORST

A••W•••
ADAWARE
AIRWARS
AIRWAVE
AIRWAYS
AIRWICK
AIRWOLF
AJOWANS
ALEWIFE
ALLWISE
ANSWERS
ANTWERP
ANYWAYS
ANYWISE
ARCWELD
ARTWALL
ARTWARE
ARTWORK
ASSWEET
ATHWART
AVOWALS
AVOWERS
AVOWING
AWKWARD

A•••W••
ALLEWIS
ALLOWAY
ALLOWED
ALLOWIN
ALLOWME
ANTIWAR
ARCHWAY
AREAWAY
ASKAWAY
ASLEWOF
ATEAWAY

A••••W•
ABCNEWS
ALLNEWS
ANDREWS
ANTCOWS
ANYNEWS
ANYTOWN
ASPRAWL

A•••••W
AIRCREW
AIRFLOW
AIRGLOW
AIRSHOW
ARTSHOW
ASOFNOW
ATECROW

•AW••••
BAWDIER
BAWDILY
BAWLERS
BAWLING
BAWLOUT
DAWDLED
DAWDLER
DAWDLES
DAWKINS
DAWNING
DAWNSON
FAWCETT
FAWNERS
FAWNING
FAWNSON
GAWKERS
GAWKIER
GAWKILY
GAWKING
GAWKISH
GAWKSAT
GAWPERS
GAWPING
HAWHAWS
HAWKERS
HAWKEYE
HAWKING
HAWKINS
HAWKISH
HAWKMAN
HAWORTH
HAWSERS
JAWBONE
JAWEDAT
JAWLESS
JAWLIKE
JAWLINE
LAWANDA
LAWBOOK
LAWCASE
LAWFORD
LAWLESS
LAWLIKE
LAWSUIT
LAWYERS
MAWKISH
PAWEDAT
PAWNEES
PAWNERS
PAWNING
PAWNOFF
PAWPAWS
RAWBARS
RAWDATA
RAWDEAL
RAWEGGS
RAWFISH
RAWFOOD
RAWHIDE
RAWISTS
RAWLINS
RAWMEAT
RAWNESS
RAWSILK
SAWATCH
SAWBUCK
SAWCHUK
SAWDUST
SAWFISH
SAWINTO
SAWLIKE
SAWLOGS
SAWMILL
SAWNOFF
SAWPAST
SAWPITS
SAWSOFF
SAWTOIT
SAWWOOD
SAWYERS
TAWNIER
TAWNILY
YAWNERS
YAWNFUL
YAWNIER
YAWNING
YAWPERS
YAWPING

•A•W•••
BADWORD
BAGWELL
BAGWIGS
BARWARE
BATWING
CARWASH
CATWALK
DAEWOOS
DAGWOOD
DARWELL
DAYWEAR
EARWIGS
FALWELL
FANWISE
FARWEST
FAYWRAY
GASWARS
GATWICK
HARWELL
HAYWARD
HAYWIRE
JAYWALK
JAYWARD
LAPWARE
LAPWING
MAEWEST
MALWARE
MAXWELL
MAYWINE
NARWHAL
NATWICK
OAKWOOD
PAYWELL
RAGWEED
RANWILD
RANWITH
SAMWISE
SATWELL
SATWITH
SAWWOOD
SAYWAIT
SAYWHAT
SAYWHEN
VANWARD
VANWYCK
WAHWAHS
WARWICK
WARWORN
WAXWING
WAXWORK
WAYWARD
WAYWORN

•A••W••
BACKWAY
BALDWIN
CARAWAY
CATAWBA
EATAWAY
FAIRWAY
FARAWAY
FAREWAR
GANGWAY
GATEWAY
GAVEWAY
HALFWAY
HALFWIT
HALFWON
HALLWAY
HARDWAY
HARDWON
JANEWAY
LACKWIT
LANGWAY
LAYAWAY
MADEWAR
MADEWAY
MAKEWAR
MAKEWAY
MANOWAR
MATEWAN
PARKWAY
PARTWAY
PATHWAY
RACEWAY
RAILWAY
RANAWAY
SAFEWAY
SARAWAK
SAYSWHO
TAILWAG
TAXIWAY
VANOWEN
WAGEWAR
WALKWAY

•A•••W•
BADNEWS
BALLTWO
BARNOWL
BARROWS
BASETWO
CASHEWS
CATBOWL
FALLOWS
FARROWS
GAGLAWS
GALLOWS
HALLOWS
HARROWS
HAWHAWS
HAYMOWS
LANETWO
LAYDOWN
MACHTWO
MALLOWS
MARLOWE
MARROWS
MATHEWS
NARROWS
OAKLAWN
PAGETWO
PARTTWO
PATDOWN
PAWPAWS
RAEDAWN
RAMDOWN
RANDOWN
SATDOWN
TALLOWS
TALLOWY
TAXLAWS
WALLOWS
WARHAWK
YARROWS

•A••••W
BACKROW
BACKSAW
BANDSAW
BARSTOW
CALLNOW
CAPSHAW
CARSHOW
CASELAW
CASHCOW
CATCHOW
CATSHOW
CATSPAW
DANELAW
EATCROW
GAMELAW
GANGSAW
HACKSAW
HADACOW
HADAROW
HALFRAW
HANDSAW
HASACOW
HASAROW
JACKDAW
JANKLOW
LAIDLOW
LASTROW
LAYSLOW
MACGRAW
MANILOW
MATTHEW
PALTROW
PAYSNOW
RAINBOW
SAGINAW
SALCHOW
YALELAW

••AW•••
ADAWARE
BRAWLED
BRAWLER
BRAWLEY
CHAWING
CLAWERS
CLAWING
CLAWSAT
CRAWDAD
CRAWLED
CRAWLER
CRAWLEY
DRAWBAR
DRAWEES
DRAWERS
DRAWING
DRAWLED
DRAWLER
DRAWMAN
DRAWMEN
DRAWNIN
DRAWNON
DRAWNTO
DRAWNUP
DRAWOFF
DRAWOUT
DRAWSIN
DRAWSON
DRAWSTO
DRAWSUP
FLAWIER
FLAWING
FRAWLEY
GNAWERS
GNAWING
GNAWSAT
GNAWSON
INAWEOF
INAWINK
INAWORD
LEAWOOD
ONAWHIM
PRAWNED
REAWAKE
REAWOKE
SEAWALL
SEAWARD
SEAWAYS
SEAWEED
SEAWOLF
SHAWLED
SHAWNEE
SPAWNED
SPAWNER
THAWERS
THAWING
THAWOUT
TRAWLED
TRAWLER
UNAWAKE
UNAWARE
UNAWFUL

••A•W••
CHATWIN
HEADWAY
MIAOWED
ROADWAY
SCARWID
SKAGWAY
THATWAY
TRAMWAY

••A••W•
MEADOWS
MEADOWY
PEAFOWL
QUAPAWS
REAVOWS
SEACOWS
SEAFOWL
SEAHAWK
SHADOWS
SHADOWY
SHALLWE
SOAREWE
TEAGOWN

••A•••W
BEARPAW
CRASHAW
GLASGOW
GLASHOW
HEADSAW
INASTEW
SHALLOW
SPARROW
SWALLOW
WHATNOW

•••AW••
AREAWAY
ASKAWAY
ATEAWAY
CARAWAY
CATAWBA
CUTAWAY
DIEAWAY
DUNAWAY
EATAWAY
FARAWAY
FLYAWAY
GETAWAY
GOTAWAY
HIDAWAY
LAYAWAY
LEDAWAY
MEDAWAR
MOHAWKS
OTTAWAN
OTTAWAS
OUTAWED
OUTAWES
PEGAWAY
PSHAWED
PUTAWAY
RANAWAY
RESAWED
ROTAWAY
RUNAWAY
SARAWAK
SCRAWLS
SCRAWLY
SCRAWNY
SHYAWAY
SPRAWLS
SPRAWLY
SQUAWKS
SQUAWKY
TOWAWAY
UNPAWED
UNPAWNS
UNSAWED

•••A•W•
ROYALWE

•••A••W
DISAVOW
HADACOW
HADAROW
HASACOW
HASAROW
IGNATOW

••••AW•
ASPRAWL
BOWSAWS
CUSHAWS
DECLAWS
GAGLAWS
GEEGAWS
GEWGAWS
GOSHAWK
GUFFAWS
GUNLAWS
HAWHAWS
HEEHAWS
INDRAWN
JIGSAWS
OAKLAWN
OKINAWA
OLDSAWS
OUTBAWL
OUTFAWN
OUTLAWS
OVERAWE
PAWPAWS
PITSAWS
PREDAWN
QUAPAWS
RAEDAWN
REDDAWN
REDHAWK
REDRAWN
REDRAWS
RETHAWS
RIPSAWN
RIPSAWS
SEAHAWK
SEESAWS
TAXLAWS
UNDRAWN
UNDRAWS
UNTHAWS
WARHAWK

•••••AW
BACKSAW
BANDSAW
BEARPAW
BELTSAW
BLUELAW
BUCKSAW
BUZZSAW
CAPSHAW
CASELAW
CATSPAW
CHOCTAW
CRASHAW
CUMSHAW
DANELAW
DEWCLAW
FOREPAW
FORESAW
FRETSAW
GAMELAW
GANGSAW
HACKSAW
HALFRAW
HANDSAW
HEADSAW
HINDPAW
JACKDAW
JOHNLAW
JUDELAW
KERSHAW
LOCKJAW
MACGRAW
MISDRAW
OHMSLAW
OUTDRAW
OUTGNAW
OVERSAW
POORLAW
RUBSRAW
SAGINAW
SEMIRAW
TOPDRAW
TORTLAW
WHIPSAW
WOODSAW
WROCLAW
YALELAW

AX•••••
AXEHEAD
AXELIKE
AXELROD
AXHEADS
AXIALLY
AXILLAE
AXILLAR
AXILLAS
AXLROSE
AXOLOTL
AXSEEDS

A•X••••
ANXIETY
ANXIOUS

A••X•••
ASEXUAL

A•••X••
ABRAXAS
ADDAXES
ADMIXED
ADMIXES
AFFIXED
AFFIXER
AFFIXES
ANNEXED
ANNEXES

A••••X•
AIRTAXI
ARANTXA
ATARAXY

A•••••X
ALTOSAX
ANTHRAX
ANTITAX
APTERYX
ARONNAX
ARUSPEX
ASTERIX

•AX••••
FAXLORE
LAXNESS
MAXBAER
MAXBORN
MAXILLA
MAXIMAL
MAXIMAS
MAXIMUM
MAXIMUS
MAXIXES
MAXWELL
OAXACAN
PAXINOU
SAXHORN
SAXTUBA
TAXABLE
TAXBASE
TAXCODE
TAXCUTS
TAXFREE
TAXHIKE
TAXICAB
TAXIING
TAXIMAN
TAXIMEN
TAXIWAY
TAXLAWS
TAXLESS
TAXLEVY
TAXPAID
TAXRATE
TAXSALE
TAXYEAR
WAXABLE
WAXBEAN
WAXEDUP
WAXESUP
WAXIEST
WAXINGS
WAXLIKE
WAXWING
WAXWORK

•A•X•••
BAUXITE
FAUXFUR
FAUXPAS
MANXCAT
MANXMAN
MANXMEN
MARXIAN
MARXISM
MARXIST

•A••X••
BAREXAM
CALYXES
GALAXES
GALAXIE
LATEXES
MAXIXES
RADIXES
VANEXEL

•A•••X•
BATNEXT
HANDAXE

•A••••X
BANDBOX
BASESIX
BASSSAX
BATEAUX
BAYLYNX
CADEAUX
CAKEMIX
CALLBOX
CASHBOX
FAIRFAX
FAIRSEX
FAREBOX
GATEAUX
HALIFAX
HARDSIX
LANDTAX
LASCAUX
MACHSIX
MADAMEX
MAILBOX
MALRAUX
MARGAUX
NARTHEX
PAGESIX
PANCHAX
PARADOX
SALTBOX
SANDBOX

••AX•••
BIAXIAL
BRAXTON
COAXERS
COAXIAL
COAXING
FLAXIER
HOAXERS
HOAXING
KLAXONS
UNAXLED

••A•X••
CPAEXAM

••A••X•
ARANTXA
ATARAXY
MEATAXE

••A•••X
BEATBOX
BEATRIX
FIATLUX
FLATTAX
GEARBOX
GRAVLAX
ORATRIX
PHALANX
PHARYNX
PLAYTEX
REAFFIX
REANNEX
ROADTAX
SOAPBOX
SPANDEX

•••AX••
ABRAXAS
ADDAXES
DEWAXED
DEWAXES
GALAXES
GALAXIE
HYRAXES
ICEAXES
REFAXED
REFAXES
RELAXED
RELAXER
RELAXES
RETAXED
RETAXES
REWAXED
REWAXES
THEAXIS
UNLAXED
UNLAXES
UNTAXED
UNTAXES
UNWAXED

•••A••X
BETAMAX
BROADAX
MADAMEX
MIRAMAX
PARADOX

••••AX•
AIRTAXI
ATARAXY
HANDAXE
MEATAXE
PICKAXE
POLEAXE

••••A•X
BATEAUX
BUREAUX
CADEAUX
CHEVAUX
CISEAUX
GATEAUX
JOUHAUX
LASCAUX
MALRAUX
MARGAUX
MICHAUX
OISEAUX
PHALANX
RESEAUX
ROUBAIX

•••••AX
ALTOSAX
ANTHRAX
ANTITAX
ARONNAX
BASSSAX
BEESWAX
BETAMAX
BROADAX
BROWWAX
CINEMAX
COOLMAX
EQUIFAX
FAIRFAX
FILOFAX
FLATTAX
GIFTTAX
GRAVLAX
HALIFAX
JUNKFAX
LANDTAX
MINIMAX
MIRAMAX
OMNIMAX
OVERLAX
OVERTAX
PANCHAX
PLUSTAX
POLLTAX
POORTAX
ROADTAX
STONEAX
TELEFAX

AY•••••
AYEAYES
AYKROYD
AYNRAND

A•Y••••
ABYSMAL
ABYSSAL
ABYSSES
ACYCLIC
ALYKHAN
ALYOSHA
ALYSSUM
AMYLASE
ANYBODY
ANYHOPE
ANYKIND
ANYLUCK
ANYMORE
ANYNEWS
ANYONES
ANYROAD
ANYTIME
ANYTOWN
ANYWAYS
ANYWISE
ASYLUMS

A••Y•••
ABEYANT
ACRYLIC
ADAYAGO
ALAYING
ALCYONE
ALEYARD
ALIYAHS
ALLYING
ALLYSON
ARGYLES
ARMYANT
ASBYATT
ASSYRIA
ATTYGEN
AVEYRON

A•••Y••
AALIYAH
ACOLYTE
ALLAYED
ALLAYER
ALLEYES
ALLOYED
ALNIYAT
ANALYSE
ANALYST
ANALYTE
ANALYZE
ANGRYAT
ANNOYED
ANNOYER
ANODYNE
ANONYMS
APPLYTO
ARRAYAL
ARRAYED
ARRAYER
ARROYOS
ASSAYED
ASSAYER
AYEAYES
AZODYES

A••••Y•
ACRONYM
AFFRAYS
AIRWAYS
ALLONYM
ALTKEYS
ANTONYM
ANYWAYS
APTERYX
AUTONYM
AYKROYD

A•••••Y
ABBOTCY
ABIDEBY
ABILITY
ACADEMY
ACETIFY
ACIDIFY
ACIDITY
ACRIDLY
ACTORLY
ACTUARY
ACUTELY
ADDEDLY
ADEPTLY
ADULTLY
AFARCRY
AFFABLY
AGENTRY
AGILELY
AGILITY
AINTHAY
AIRPLAY
ALABAMY
ALANJAY
ALBUNDY
ALCHEMY
ALDORAY
ALERTLY
ALIMONY
ALLENBY
ALLERGY
ALLOWAY
ALMONDY
ALMONRY
ALOOFLY
ALREADY
AMATORY
AMENITY
AMIABLY
AMNESTY
AMPLIFY
AMSCRAY
ANALOGY
ANARCHY
ANATOLY
ANATOMY
ANCHOVY
ANGRILY
ANILITY
ANIMACY
ANNAMAY
ANNUITY
ANOMALY
ANTHONY
ANXIETY
ANYBODY
APISHLY
APLENTY
APOLOGY
ARCHERY
ARCHWAY
ARDENCY
AREAWAY
ARENSKY
ARIDITY
ARMOURY
ASABODY
ASAGRAY
ASHBERY
ASHBURY
ASHTRAY
ASKAWAY
ATARAXY
ATEAWAY
ATROPHY
ATTABOY
AUDIBLY
AURALLY
AUTARKY
AUTOPSY
AVIDITY
AWFULLY
AXIALLY

•AY••••
BAYAREA
BAYCITY
BAYEDAT
BAYLEAF
BAYLORU
BAYLYNX
BAYONET
BAYONNE
BAYRUMS
BAYTREE
CAYENNE
CAYMANS
CAYUGAS
CAYUSES
DAYBEDS
DAYBOOK
DAYCAMP
DAYCARE
DAYGAME
DAYHOPS
DAYJOBS
DAYLILY
DAYLONG
DAYMARE
DAYPACK
DAYQUIL
DAYROOM
DAYSAIL
DAYSEND
DAYSIDE
DAYSINN
DAYSOFF
DAYSPAS
DAYSTAR
DAYTIME
DAYTONA
DAYTRIP
DAYWEAR
FAYETTE
FAYWRAY
GAYLORD
GAYNESS
HAYBALE
HAYESES
HAYFORK
HAYINGS
HAYLOFT
HAYMOWS
HAYRACK
HAYRICK
HAYRIDE
HAYSEED
HAYWARD
HAYWIRE
JAYBIRD
JAYCEES
JAYLENO
JAYVEES
JAYWALK
JAYWARD
KAYAKED
KAYAKER
KAYLENZ
KAYOING
LAYAWAY
LAYBACK
LAYBARE
LAYDOWN
LAYERED
LAYETTE
LAYINTO
LAYITON
LAYODDS
LAYOFFS
LAYOPEN
LAYOUTS
LAYOVER
LAYSFOR
LAYSLOW
LAYSOFF
LAYSOUT
LAYUPON
MAYALIN
MAYBESO
MAYDAYS
MAYFAIR
MAYHEMS
MAYINGS
MAYNARD
MAYORAL
MAYPOLE
MAYTAGS
MAYTIME
MAYWINE
NAYARIT
NAYSAID
NAYSAYS
PAYABLE
PAYBACK
PAYCASH
PAYCUTS
PAYDAYS
PAYDIRT
PAYHEED
PAYINTO
PAYLESS
PAYLOAD
PAYMENT
PAYMORE
PAYOFFS
PAYOLAS
PAYOUTS
PAYRATE
PAYROLL
PAYSFOR
PAYSLIP
PAYSNOW
PAYSOFF
PAYSOUT
PAYSTUB
PAYWELL
RAYBANS
RAYBURN
RAYGUNS
RAYKROC
RAYLESS
RAYLIKE
RAYMOND
RAYNELL
RAYOVAC
SAYABLE
SAYAMEN
SAYHITO
SAYINGS
SAYMASS
SAYMORE
SAYNOTO
SAYOVER
SAYSAAH
SAYSAYE
SAYSBOO
SAYSIDO
SAYSNAY
SAYSWHO
SAYSYES
SAYSYOU
SAYWAIT
SAYWHAT
SAYWHEN
TAYBACK
TAYLORS
WAYBACK
WAYBILL
WAYCOOL
WAYLAID
WAYLAND
WAYLAYS
WAYLESS
WAYSIDE
WAYTOGO
WAYWARD
WAYWORN
YAYTEAM

•A•Y•••
BABYBOP
BABYGAP
BABYING
BABYISH
BABYLON
BABYOIL
BABYSAT
BABYSIT
BANYANS
BARYONS
CALYCES
CALYPSO
CALYXES
CANYONS
EASYJOB
EASYOFF
EASYONE
HALYARD
KATYDID
LADYBUG
LADYDAY
LADYISH
LADYKIN
LADYNAS
LANYARD
LAWYERS
LAZYISH
MAGYARS
MANYEAR
MARYANN
MARYKAY
MARYLOU
MARYURE
NAVYMAN
NAVYMEN
PAPYRUS
SATYRIC
SAWYERS
TAXYEAR
VARYING
ZANYISH
ZANYISM

•A••Y••
AALIYAH
BABIYAR
BAYLYNX
CAMRYLE
CARLYLE
CARRYIN
CARRYON
CATEYED
DACTYLS
DAIRYER
DANEYKO
DARRYLF
EARLYON
FADAYEV
FANCYUP
HALCYON
HANDYTO
HAPPYTO
KATAYEV
MALAYAN
MARRYAT
MARRYIN
MARRYME
MARTYRS
NARAYAN
PALMYRA
PAPAYAS
PARTYER
PARTYON
RALLYES
RALLYTO
SADEYED
SADEYES
SAMMYJO
SAMOYED
SAROYAN
SAYSYES
SAYSYOU
TACHYON
TALLYHO
TALLYUP
VANDYCK
VANDYKE
VANEYCK
VANWYCK
VATDYED
VATDYES

•A•••Y•
BADBOYS
BADDAYS
BADGUYS
BAGBOYS
BARLEYS
BARNEYS
BATBOYS
BATDAYS
CACONYM
CAMBOYS
CARBOYS
CARKEYS
CAROLYN
CATSEYE
CATTOYS
GALLEYS
HAIRDYE
HALLEYS
HANDEYE
HANGBYS
HARLEYS
HAWKEYE
KAROLYI
KATHRYN
LACKEYS
LAZBOYS
MADALYN
MANDAYS
MARILYN
MASARYK
MAYDAYS
NAYSAYS
PARLAYS
PARLEYS
PARONYM
PAYDAYS
SAIDAYE
SAMLOYD
SASHAYS
SAYSAYE
TABKEYS
TAGDAYS
TAMBLYN
VALLEYS
VANDUYN
WALLEYE
WAYLAYS

•A••••Y
BACKBAY
BACKPAY
BACKWAY
BAGGILY
BAGLADY
BALCONY
BALKILY
BALLBOY
BALMILY
BALONEY
BALSAMY
BANALLY
BANBURY
BARBARY
BARCLAY
BARKLEY
BARNABY
BARTRAY
BASALLY
BASEPAY
BATTERY
BAWDILY
BAYCITY
CABBAGY
CADBURY
CADENCY
CALCIFY
CALGARY
CALLBOY
CALPOLY
CALUMNY
CALVARY
CAMPILY
CANNERY
CANNILY
CANONRY
CANTILY
CANTSAY
CAPABLY
CAPEMAY
CARAWAY
CARDKEY
CARNABY
CARROTY
CASPARY

CASSIDY
CATTILY
CAVALRY
DAFFILY
DAHOMEY
DALTREY
DAMPDRY
DANBURY
DANDIFY
DANDILY
DARESAY
DATEDLY
DAYLILY
DAZEDLY
EAGERLY
EARTHLY
EASEDBY
EASESBY
EATAWAY
FACTORY
FACULTY
FADEDLY
FAINTLY
FAIRWAY
FALLACY
FALLGUY
FALSELY
FALSIFY
FALSITY
FANCIFY
FANCILY
FANTASY
FARADAY
FARAWAY
FARMBOY
FARMERY
FATALLY
FATCITY
FATTILY
FATUITY
FAYWRAY
GADGETY
GAINSAY
GALLERY
GAMEBOY
GANGWAY
GARBAGY
GASCONY
GASEITY
GATEWAY
GAUDERY
GAUDILY
GAUNTLY
GAUZILY
GAVEWAY
GAWKILY
HACKNEY
HADASAY
HAGERTY
HALFDAY
HALFSHY
HALFWAY
HALLWAY
HAMMILY
HANDILY
HANGSBY
HAPENNY
HAPPIFY
HAPPILY
HARDDAY
HARDILY
HARDWAY
HARMONY
HARSHLY
HARTLEY
HASASAY
HASTILY
HAUGHTY
HAUTBOY
JADEDLY
JANEWAY
JANUARY
JARGONY
JASPERY
JAZZILY
KARLOVY
LADYDAY
LAMPREY
LANGLEY
LANGTRY
LANGWAY
LANKILY
LARCENY
LARGELY
LASTMAY
LASTORY
LATENCY
LATHERY
LAUNDRY
LAYAWAY
LAZENBY
MADEHAY
MADEWAY
MAGNIFY
MAHONEY
MAJESTY
MAKEHAY
MAKEWAY
MALARKY
MALMSEY
MARGERY
MARYKAY
MASONRY
MASTERY
NAIVELY
NAIVETY
NAKEDLY
NAMABLY
NAMEDAY
NASALLY
NASTILY
NATTILY
NAUGHTY
PAGEBOY
PAISLEY
PALEDRY
PALFREY
PALJOEY
PALMARY
PANICKY
PANOPLY
PARKWAY
PARSLEY
PARTWAY
PASSKEY
PATENCY
PATHWAY
PATSDRY
PAUCITY
PAULPRY
PAUNCHY
PAVIDLY
RABBITY
RABIDLY
RACEDBY
RACESBY
RACEWAY
RACKETY
RAGGEDY
RAILWAY
RAINILY
RAISINY
RANAWAY
RAPIDLY
RAUNCHY
RAVELLY
SAFEWAY
SAIDNAY
SAINTLY
SALTILY
SAMEDAY
SANDFLY
SAPPILY
SASSILY
SATIETY
SATISFY
SATRAPY
SAUCILY
SAUCONY
SAVOURY
SAVVILY
SAYSNAY
TACITLY
TACKILY
TAKENBY
TALLOWY
TAMMANY
TANNERY
TANTIVY
TARBABY
TARDILY
TARTILY
TASTILY
TATTERY
TATTILY
TAWNILY
TAXIWAY
TAXLEVY
VACANCY
VACUITY
VAGUELY
VALIDLY
VAPIDLY
VAPOURY
VARIETY
VARSITY
VASTITY
WACKILY
WAGGERY
WALKSBY
WALKWAY
WALLABY
WARBABY
WASHDAY
WASPILY
WASSILY
ZACHARY

••AY•••

ADAYAGO
ALAYING
BRAYERS
BRAYING
CHAYOTE
CLAYIER
CLAYING
CLAYISH
CLAYPIT
CLAYTON
CRAYOLA
CRAYONS
DRAYAGE
DRAYING
DRAYMAN
DRAYMEN
DRAYTON
EBAYERS
FLAYERS
FLAYING
FRAYING
GRAYEST
GRAYING
GRAYISH
GRAYJAY
GRAYLAG
GRAYSON
KHAYYAM
OKAYGUY
OKAYING
PLAYACT
PLAYBOY
PLAYDOH
PLAYERS
PLAYFUL
PLAYING
PLAYLET
PLAYOFF
PLAYOUT
PLAYPEN
PLAYSAT
PLAYSBY
PLAYSON
PLAYSTO
PLAYSUP
PLAYTEX
PRAYERS
PRAYFOR
PRAYING
PRAYSTO
QUAYAGE
SLAYERS
SLAYING
SLAYTON
SPAYERS
SPAYING
STAYDRY
STAYERS
STAYFOR
STAYING
STAYOFF
STAYOUT
STAYPUT
STAYSAT
STAYSIN
STAYSON
STAYSUP
SWAYBAR
SWAYERS
SWAYING
TRAYFUL
TRAYNOR
XRAYING
XRAYLAB

••A•Y••

ANALYSE
ANALYST
ANALYTE
ANALYZE
EXABYTE
KHAYYAM
NEARYOU
PHARYNX
PLATYPI
YEAHYOU

••A••Y•

CHANOYU
DEADEYE
GLADEYE
GRAMMYS
LEAKEYS
SEAWAYS
TEAPOYS

••A•••Y

ACADEMY
AFARCRY
ALABAMY
ALANJAY
AMATORY
ANALOGY
ANARCHY
ANATOLY
ANATOMY
ASABODY
ASAGRAY
ATARAXY
BEADILY
BEANERY
BEASLEY
BEASTLY
BEATIFY
BIASPLY
BLACKLY
BLAKELY
BLAKLEY
BLANDLY
BLANKLY
BLARNEY
BRADLEY
BRAMBLY
BRAMLEY
BRANCHY
BRASHLY
BRAVELY
BRAVERY
BRAWLEY
BYANDBY
CHANTEY
CHANTRY
CHARILY
CHARITY
CHARLEY
CLARIFY
CLARITY
CRACKLY
CRAFTSY
CRASSLY
CRAWLEY
CRAZILY
DEANERY
DRAMADY
DRAMEDY
DRAPERY
DUALITY
EDACITY
EPARCHY
EXACTLY
FLAGDAY
FLAKILY
FLAUNTY
FLAVORY
FOAMILY
FRAILLY
FRAILTY
FRANKLY
FRAWLEY
GHASTLY
GLAZILY
GRANARY
GRANDLY
GRAPERY
GRATIFY
GRAVELY
GRAVITY
GRAYJAY
HEADILY
HEADWAY
HEALTHY
HEARSAY
HEATRAY
HEAVILY
HOARILY
IMAGERY
INAFURY
INANELY
INANITY
INAPTLY
IRATELY
KEARNEY
KNAVERY
LEAPDAY
LOATHLY
MEADOWY
MEATILY
OKAYGUY
OMALLEY
ONAJURY
OPACITY
ORANGEY
ORATORY
PEABODY
PLAINLY
PLAYBOY
PLAYSBY
QUAKILY
QUALIFY
QUALITY
QUARTZY
QUAVERY
READILY
REALITY
REAPPLY
REASSAY
RIANTLY
ROADWAY
SCANTLY
SCAREDY
SCARIFY
SCARILY
SEADUTY
SEALERY
SEALILY
SHADILY
SHADOWY
SHAKILY
SHAPELY
SHARKEY
SHARPLY
SKAGWAY
SLACKLY
SLANTLY
SLAVERY
SMARTLY
SNAKILY
SOAPILY
SPACELY
SPANGLY
SPARELY
SPARKLY
SPASSKY
STAGILY
STAIDLY
STALELY
STANDBY
STANLEY
STARCHY
STARKEY
STARKLY
STARSKY
STATELY
STAYDRY
SUAVELY
SUAVITY
SWARTHY
TEACOZY
TEARILY
TEATRAY
THATCHY
THATWAY
TRACERY
TRAGEDY
TRAMWAY
UNANGRY
UNAPTLY
WEALTHY
WEARILY
WHALLEY
WHATSAY

•••AY••

ALLAYED
ALLAYER
ARRAYAL
ARRAYED
ARRAYER
ASSAYED
ASSAYER
AYEAYES
BELAYED
BELAYER
BYWAYOF
DECAYED
DECAYER
DELAYED
DELAYER
EMBAYED
ESSAYED
ESSAYER
EXMAYOR
FADAYEV
FORAYED
FTWAYNE
GEMAYEL
IDSAYSO
INLAYER
ITMAYBE
KATAYEV
LCHAYIM
MALAYAN
NARAYAN
PAPAYAS
PITAYAS
RELAYED
RELAYER
SCHAYES
SPLAYED
SPRAYED
SPRAYER
SPRAYON
STRAYED
STRAYER
UNHAYED
UNRAYED
VISAYAN

•••A•Y•

IHEARYA
MADALYN
MASARYK
POLANYI
ROSALYN
STMARYS

•••A••Y

AFFABLY
AMIABLY
ANNAMAY
AREAWAY
ASKAWAY
ATEAWAY
ATTABOY
AURALLY
AUTARKY
AXIALLY
BANALLY
BASALLY
BEHAPPY
BETARAY
BLEAKLY
BREATHY
BROADLY
CAPABLY
CARAWAY
CAVALRY
CHEAPLY
CLEANLY
CLEARLY
CONAKRY
CURABLY
CUTAWAY
DEBAKEY
DELANEY
DIEAWAY
DUBARRY
DUCALLY
DUNAWAY
DURABLY
DYNASTY
EATAWAY
EDNAMAY
EFFABLY
EMBASSY
EMPATHY
EQUABLY
EQUALLY
ERRANCY
FARADAY
FARAWAY
FATALLY
FINALLY
FLOATBY
FLYAWAY
FORADAY
FRIARLY
FUGALLY
GETAWAY
GOTAWAY
GREATLY
GYRALLY
HADASAY
HASASAY
HIDAWAY
HODADDY
HUMANLY
IDEALLY
IMHAPPY
INFANCY
ITSABOY
LAYAWAY
LEDAWAY
LEGALLY
LISAGAY
LOCALLY
LOVABLY
LOYALLY
LOYALTY
MALARKY
MCCAREY
MCNALLY
MCRANEY
MISALLY
MORALLY
MOVABLY
MRDARCY
MRHANEY
MRNANNY
MTBALDY
MTMARCY
MUTABLY
MYMAMMY
NAMABLY
NASALLY
NEWAGEY
NOTABLY
OLEANNY
ONEADAY
ORGANDY
ORMANDY
PEGAWAY
PENALTY
PICARDY
PLIABLY
PLIANCY
PREACHY
PREALLY
PUTAWAY
RANAWAY
RECARRY
REDARMY
REGALLY
REMARRY
RENALLY
RETALLY
RIVALRY
ROTAWAY
ROYALLY
ROYALTY
RUNAWAY
RURALLY
SCRAGGY
SCRAPPY
SCRAWLY
SCRAWNY
SHYAWAY
SIZABLY
SNEAKBY
SPLASHY
SPRAWLY
SQUALLY
SQUASHY
SQUATLY
SQUATTY
SQUAWKY
SWEARBY
TENABLY
TENANCY
THEARMY
TIDALLY
TINAFEY
TONALLY
TOTALLY
TOWAWAY
TREACLY
TRUANCY
TYRANNY
UNCANNY
UNFANCY
UNFATTY
UNGAUDY
UNHAIRY
UNHANDY
UNHAPPY
UNHARDY
UNHASTY
UNMADLY
UNMANLY
UNRAINY
UNRASPY
UNSADLY
UNSALTY
UNSAVVY
UNTASTY
UPEARLY
USUALLY
VACANCY
VENALLY
VITALLY
VOCABLY
VOCALLY
WCHANDY
WOMANLY
WREATHY
ZELAZNY
ZONALLY

••••AY•

AFFRAYS
AIRWAYS
ANYWAYS
BADDAYS
BATDAYS
BENDAYS
BERNAYS
BETRAYS
BIGDAYS
BYPLAYS
DEEJAYS
DEFRAYS
DELRAYS
DISMAYS
DOGDAYS
ENDWAYS
ESTRAYS
FLYWAYS
FRIDAYS
HEYDAYS
HOORAYS
HOTDAYS
HURRAYS
INTRAYS
JETWAYS
KEYWAYS
LEEWAYS
MANDAYS
MAYDAYS
MIDDAYS
MIDWAYS
MISLAYS
MISSAYS
MONDAYS
NAYSAYS
OFFDAYS
OLDDAYS
OLDWAYS
OUTLAYS
OUTPAYS
OUTSAYS
PARLAYS
PAYDAYS
PEDWAYS
PREPAYS
REDBAYS
REPLAYS
RUNWAYS
SAIDAYE
SASHAYS
SAYSAYE
SEAWAYS
SEGWAYS
SKYWAYS
SUBWAYS
SUNDAYS
SUNRAYS
TAGDAYS
TENDAYS
THEMAYO
TWODAYS
VEEJAYS
VOTEAYE
WAYLAYS

••••A•Y

ACTUARY
ALABAMY
ALREADY
ANIMACY
ANOMALY
ATARAXY
BAGLADY
BALSAMY
BARBARY
BARNABY
BEGGARY
BELLAMY
BETHANY
BETTANY
BIGBABY
BIGEASY
BURNABY
CABBAGY
CALGARY
CALVARY
CARNABY
CASPARY
CEPHALY
CILIARY
COMPANY
CRYBABY
DIETARY
DRAMADY
ECSTASY
EPILADY
ESTUARY
EXOGAMY
FALLACY
FANTASY
GARBAGY
GERMANY
GOCRAZY
GRANARY
HILLARY
HOWMANY
HUNGARY
HUSHABY
HYMNARY
IMREADY
ITSEASY
JANUARY
KKKKATY
LIBRARY
LULLABY
MCCRARY
MULCAHY
NECTARY
NITTANY
NOTEASY
NOTMANY
OLDLADY
OLDNAVY
OSSUARY
OSTIARY
PALMARY
PECCARY
PLENARY
PRELACY
PRIMACY
PRIMARY
PRIVACY
PRONAVY
QUINARY
RETIARY
ROCKABY
SATRAPY
SQUEAKY
STREAKY
SUMMARY
TAMMANY
TARBABY
TERNARY
TESTACY
THEBABY
THERAPY
THREADY
THROATY
TIFFANY
TOOEASY
TOOMANY
TOPIARY
TRENARY
TRINARY
TUSCANY
UNCHARY
UNCRAZY
UNFLAKY
UNHEADY
UNHEAVY
UNITARY
UNLEAKY
UNREADY
UNSCALY
UNSHADY
UNSNAKY
UNSTAGY
UNWEARY
UTICANY
WALLABY
WARBABY
ZACHARY

•••••AY

AINTHAY
AIRPLAY
ALANJAY
ALDORAY
ALLOWAY
AMSCRAY
ANNAMAY
ARCHWAY
AREAWAY
ASAGRAY
ASHTRAY
ASKAWAY

ATEAWAY
BACKBAY
BACKPAY
BACKWAY
BARCLAY
BARTRAY
BASEPAY
BELTWAY
BETARAY
BIKEWAY
BLUEJAY
BOBTWAY
CANTSAY
CAPEMAY
CARAWAY
COLDDAY
CUTAWAY
DARESAY
DEMOLAY
DIEAWAY
DISPLAY
DOORWAY
DUNAWAY
EATAWAY
EDNAMAY
ELLYMAY
ENDPLAY
EPERNAY
FAIRWAY
FARADAY
FARAWAY
FAYWRAY
FINDLAY
FIVEDAY
FIVEWAY
FLAGDAY
FLYAWAY
FMURRAY
FOLKWAY
FOOTWAY
FORADAY
FOREBAY
FOURDAY
FOURWAY
FREEWAY
FULLDAY
GAINSAY
GANGWAY
GATEWAY
GAVEWAY
GETAWAY
GIVEWAY
GOODDAY
GOODPAY
GOOMBAY
GOTAWAY
GRAYJAY
GUNPLAY
HADASAY
HALFDAY
HALFWAY
HALLWAY
HARDDAY
HARDWAY
HASASAY
HEADWAY
HEARSAY
HEATRAY

HIDAWAY
HIGHDAY
HIGHPAY
HIGHWAY
HITPLAY
HOLIDAY
HOLYDAY
HOUSSAY
ICETRAY
IFWEMAY
INNOWAY
ITSOKAY
JANEWAY
JOHNGAY
JOHNJAY
JULYDAY
JUNEDAY
LADYDAY
LANGWAY
LASTMAY
LAYAWAY
LEAPDAY
LEDAWAY
LEONDAY
LINDSAY
LISAGAY
LONGDAY
LONGWAY
MADEHAY
MADEWAY
MAKEHAY
MAKEWAY
MARYKAY
MISPLAY
MOREPAY
MOWBRAY
NAMEDAY
NEWSDAY
NEXTDAY
NICEDAY
NIKOLAY
NONPLAY
NOONDAY
NOSEGAY
OJIBWAY
ONEADAY
OUTBRAY
OUTPLAY
OUTPRAY
OUTSTAY
OUTTRAY
OVERLAY
OVERPAY
PARKWAY
PARTWAY
PATHWAY
PEGAWAY
PORTRAY
PUTAWAY
QUESNAY
RACEWAY
RAILWAY
RANAWAY
REASSAY
REDCLAY
REDECAY
RESPRAY
RIDGWAY

ROADWAY
ROLLWAY
ROSEBAY
ROTAWAY
RUNAWAY
SAFEWAY
SAIDNAY
SAMEDAY
SAYSNAY
SETPLAY
SHIPWAY
SHYAWAY
SICKBAY
SICKDAY
SICKPAY
SIDEWAY
SKAGWAY
SLOWDAY
SNOWDAY
SOMEDAY
SOMESAY
SOMEWAY
TAXIWAY
TEATRAY
THATWAY
THEYSAY
THISDAY
THISWAY
THRUWAY
TOLLWAY
TOWAWAY
TRAMWAY
TUESDAY
URUGUAY
VOTENAY
VOUVRAY
WALKWAY
WASHDAY
WEEKDAY
WHATSAY
WORKDAY

AZ•••••
AZALEAS
AZANIAN
AZIMUTH
AZINGER
AZKABAN
AZODYES
AZOREAN
AZORIAN
AZTECAN
AZULEJO
AZURITE
AZUSACA

A•Z••••
ADZUKIS

A••Z•••
AMAZING
AMAZONS
ARIZONA

A•••Z••
ABRUZZI
ALCAZAR
ASSIZES

A••••Z•
ABRUZZI
AGONIZE
ANALYZE
ANASAZI
ANODIZE
ATOMIZE

A•••••Z
AGASSIZ
AGRIBIZ
ALBENIZ
ALLOPEZ
ALVAREZ

•AZ••••
BAZAARS
BAZOOKA
DAZEDLY
DAZZLED
DAZZLER
DAZZLES
GAZEBOS
GAZEDAT
GAZEDON
GAZELLE
GAZESAT
GAZESON
GAZETTE
GAZZARA
HAZANIM
HAZARDS
HAZIEST
HAZINGS
HAZLITT
HAZMATS
JAZZAGE
JAZZBOS
JAZZERS
JAZZIER
JAZZILY
JAZZING
JAZZISH
JAZZMAN
JAZZMEN
LAZARUS
LAZBOYS
LAZENBY
LAZIEST
LAZONGA
LAZYISH
LAZZERI
MAZARIN
MAZEPPA
MAZIEST
MAZURKA
MAZZINI
RAZORED
RAZZIES
RAZZING

•A•Z•••
BANZAIS
CALZONE
CANZONA
CANZONE
CANZONI
DAZZLED
DAZZLER
DAZZLES
FANZINE
GAUZIER
GAUZILY
GAZZARA
JAZZAGE
JAZZBOS
JAZZERS
JAZZIER
JAZZILY
JAZZING
JAZZISH
JAZZMAN
JAZZMEN
LAZZERI
MAHZORS
MATZOHS
MATZOTH
MAZZINI
PANZERS
PATZERS
RAZZIES
RAZZING
TARZANA
TARZANS
VANZANT
WARZONE

•A••Z••
CABEZAS
DAREZZO
JACUZZI
PALAZZI
PALAZZO
SALAZAR
SARAZEN
WALTZED
WALTZER
WALTZES
YAHTZEE
ZAGAZIG

•A•••Z•
BAPTIZE
CADENZA
CAPSIZE
CARDOZO
DAREZZO
FABRIZI
HATSIZE
JACUZZI
LAICIZE
MANSIZE
PALAZZI
PALAZZO
YANGTZE
ZAMBEZI

•A••••Z
DAVEKOZ
KAYLENZ
LAISSEZ
LAURITZ
MAHFOUZ
MARANTZ
MARQUEZ
NARVAEZ
NATCHEZ
RAMIREZ
VASQUEZ

••AZ•••
AMAZING
AMAZONS
BLAZERS
BLAZEUP
BLAZING
BLAZONS
BRAZENS
BRAZIER
BRAZING
CHAZANS
CHAZZAN
CRAZIER
CRAZIES
CRAZILY
CRAZING
FRAZIER
FRAZZLE
GLAZERS
GLAZIER
GLAZILY
GLAZING
GRAZERS
GRAZIER
GRAZING
PIAZZAS
SNAZZUP

••A•Z••
CHAZZAN
FRAZZLE
KWANZAA
KWANZAS
PIAZZAS
SNAZZUP
STANZAS
ZWANZIG

••A••Z•
ANALYZE
ANASAZI
BRASIZE
DUALIZE
INADAZE
QUARTZY
REALIZE
TEACOZY
TRAPEZE

••A•••Z
AGASSIZ
FRANKOZ

•••AZ••
ALCAZAR
BEDAZED
BEDAZES
BENAZIR
CORAZON
ELEAZAR
PALAZZI
PALAZZO
SALAZAR
SARAZEN
SLEAZES
TOPAZES
UNDAZED
UNFAZED
UNHAZED
UNRAZED
UPGAZED
UPGAZES
ZAGAZIG
ZELAZNY

•••A•Z•
BONANZA
LEGANZA
ORGANZA
PALAZZI
PALAZZO

•••A••Z
ALVAREZ
MARANTZ

••••AZ•
ANASAZI
DEGLAZE
EMBLAZE
GOCRAZY
INADAZE
OUTGAZE
PIZZAZZ
REGLAZE
UNCRAZY

••••A•Z
NARVAEZ
NISSANZ
PIZZAZZ

•••••AZ
TEMPEAZ

BA•••••
BAALISH
BAALISM
BAALIST
BAALITE
BABBAGE
BABBITT
BABBLED
BABBLER
BABBLES
BABCOCK
BABENCO
BABETTE
BABIEST
BABIYAR
BABOONS
BABYBOP
BABYGAP
BABYING
BABYISH
BABYLON
BABYOIL
BABYSAT
BABYSIT
BACARDI
BACCHAE
BACCHIC
BACCHUS
BACHATA
BACHING
BACHMAN
BACILLI
BACKBAR
BACKBAY
BACKBIT
BACKEND
BACKERS
BACKHOE
BACKING
BACKLIT
BACKLOG
BACKLOT
BACKOFF
BACKOUT
BACKPAY
BACKROW
BACKRUB
BACKSAW
BACKSIN
BACKSUP
BACKUPS
BACKWAY
BACTRIA
BADAREA
BADBACK
BADBOYS
BADCALL
BADCASE
BADCOLD
BADDAYS
BADDEBT
BADDEED
BADDEST
BADDIES
BADDISH
BADDOGS
BADEGGS
BADENDS
BADENOV
BADFITS
BADFORM
BADGERS
BADGIRL
BADGUYS
BADHAIR
BADHAND
BADHATS
BADIDEA
BADITCH
BADJOKE
BADLAND
BADLIES
BADLOTS
BADLOVE
BADLUCK
BADMOOD
BADMOVE
BADNAME
BADNESS
BADNEWS
BADOMEN
BADPAST
BADRAPS
BADSHOT
BADSIGN
BADTIME
BADTRIP
BADWORD
BAFFERS
BAFFIES
BAFFING
BAFFLED
BAFFLER
BAFFLES
BAGBOYS
BAGEHOT
BAGFULS
BAGGAGE
BAGGERS
BAGGIER
BAGGIES
BAGGILY
BAGGING
BAGGINS
BAGGIRL
BAGHDAD
BAGJOBS
BAGLADY
BAGLIKE
BAGNIOS
BAGNOLD
BAGPIPE
BAGWELL
BAGWIGS
BAHAISM
BAHAIST
BAHAMAS
BAHAMEN
BAHIANS
BAHRAIN
BAHREIN
BAILEES
BAILERS
BAILIFF
BAILING
BAILORS
BAILOUT
BAILSON
BAINTER
BAITCAR
BAITERS
BAITING
BAKEOFF
BAKEPAN
BAKERST
BAKLAVA
BALABAN
BALANCE
BALASES
BALATAS
BALATON
BALBOAS
BALCONY
BALDEST
BALDIES
BALDING
BALDISH
BALDRIC
BALDWIN
BALEENS
BALEFUL
BALFOUR
BALIHAI
BALKANS
BALKERS
BALKIER
BALKILY
BALKING
BALKSAT
BALLADE
BALLADS
BALLARD
BALLAST
BALLBOY
BALLETS
BALLIOL
BALLMER
BALLONE
BALLOON
BALLOTS
BALLSUP
BALLTWO
BALLUET
BALMAIN
BALMIER
BALMILY
BALONEY
BALSAMS
BALSAMY
BAMBIII
BAMBINA
BAMBINI
BAMBINO
BAMBOOS
BAMMIES
BAMMING
BANACEK
BANALER
BANALLY
BANANAS
BANANES
BANBURY
BANDAGE
BANDAID
BANDANA
BANDBOX
BANDEAU
BANDERA
BANDERS
BANDIDO
BANDIED
BANDIER
BANDIES
BANDING
BANDITO
BANDITS
BANDLET
BANDSAW
BANEFUL
BANGERS
BANGING
BANGKOK
BANGLED
BANGLES
BANGOUT
BANGSON
BANGSUP
BANJOES
BANKERS
BANKFEE
BANKING
BANKITS
BANKJOB
BANKONE
BANKSON
BANKSUP
BANNERS
BANNING
BANQUES
BANQUET
BANSHEE
BANTAMS
BANTERS
BANTING
BANYANS
BANZAIS
BAOBABS
BAPTISE
BAPTISM
BAPTIST
BAPTIZE
BARACUS
BARANOF
BARBARA
BARBARY
BARBATE
BARBEAU
BARBELL
BARBERA
BARBERS
BARBETS
BARBIES
BARBILL
BARBING
BARBUDA
BARBULE
BARCARS
BARCLAY
BARCODE
BARDEEN
BAREGES
BARENTS
BARETTA
BAREXAM
BARFBAG
BARGAIN
BARGEIN
BARGERS
BARGING
BARHOPS
BARISTA
BARITES
BARKEEP
BARKERS
BARKIER
BARKING
BARKLEY
BARKSAT
BARLESS
BARLEYS
BARLICK
BARMAID
BARMIER
BARNABY
BARNARD
BARNEYS
BARNING
BARNONE
BARNOWL
BARNRED
BARNUMS
BAROLOS
BARONET
BAROQUE
BARQUES
BARRACK
BARRAGE
BARRELS
BARRENS
BARRETS
BARRETT
BARRIER
BARRING
BARRIOS
BARRONS
BARROOM
BARROWS
BARSOAP
BARSTOW
BARTABS
BARTEND
BARTERS
BARTLES
BARTLET
BARTOLO
BARTRAY
BARWARE
BARYONS
BASALLY
BASALTS
BASEDON
BASEHIT
BASEMAN
BASEMEN
BASENJI
BASEPAY
BASESIX
BASETEN
BASETWO
BASHERS
BASHFUL
BASHING
BASILIC
BASILIO
BASINAL
BASKETS
BASKETT
BASKING
BASMATI
BASQUES
BASRHIN
BASSALE
BASSANI
BASSANO
BASSETS
BASSETT
BASSIER
BASSIST
BASSOON
BASSSAX
BASTERS
BASTING
BASTION
BATAVIA
BATBOYS
BATCHED
BATCHES
BATDAYS
BATEAUX
BATEMAN
BATGIRL
BATHERS
BATHING
BATHMAT
BATHOIL
BATHTUB
BATIKED
BATISTA
BATISTE
BATLIKE
BATNEXT
BATSFOR
BATSMAN
BATSMEN
BATSUIT
BATTENS
BATTERS
BATTERY
BATTIER
BATTING
BATTLED
BATTLER
BATTLES
BATWING
BAUBLES
BAUHAUS
BAULKED
BAULKER
BAUXITE
BAVARIA
BAWDIER
BAWDILY
BAWLERS
BAWLING
BAWLOUT
BAYAREA
BAYCITY
BAYEDAT
BAYLEAF
BAYLORU
BAYLYNX
BAYONET
BAYONNE
BAYRUMS
BAYTREE
BAZAARS
BAZOOKA

B•A••••
BAALISH
BAALISM
BAALIST
BAALITE
BDALTON
BEACHAM
BEACHED
BEACHES
BEACONS
BEADERS
BEADIER
BEADILY
BEADING
BEADLES
BEADSUP
BEAGLES

BEAHERO
BEAKERS
BEALION
BEAMERS
BEAMIER
BEAMING
BEAMISH
BEAMSUP
BEANBAG
BEANDIP
BEANERY
BEANIES
BEANING
BEANOIL
BEARCAT
BEARCUB
BEARDED
BEARERS
BEARHUG
BEARING
BEARISH
BEAROFF
BEAROUT
BEARPAW
BEARPIT
BEARSON
BEARSUP
BEASLEY
BEASTIE
BEASTLY
BEATALL
BEATBOX
BEATCOP
BEATERS
BEATIFY
BEATING
BEATLES
BEATNIK
BEATOFF
BEATOUT
BEATRIX
BEATSAT
BEATSIT
BEATSME
BEATSON
BEATSUP
BEATTIE
BEAUISH
BEAVERS
BIAFRAN
BIALIES
BIANCHI
BIASING
BIASPLY
BIASSED
BIASSES
BIAXIAL
BLABBED
BLABBER
BLACKED
BLACKEN
BLACKER
BLACKIE
BLACKLY
BLACULA
BLADDER
BLADERS
BLADING
BLAKELY
BLAKLEY
BLALOCK
BLAMEON
BLAMERS
BLAMING
BLANCHE
BLANDER
BLANDLY
BLANKED
BLANKER
BLANKET
BLANKLY
BLANTON
BLARING
BLARNEY
BLASTED
BLASTER
BLATANT
BLATHER
BLATTED
BLAUBOK
BLAZERS
BLAZEUP
BLAZING
BLAZONS
BOARDED
BOARDER
BOARDUP
BOARISH
BOASTED
BOASTER
BOASTOF
BOATELS
BOATERS
BOATFUL
BOATING
BOATMAN
BOATMEN
BRACERO
BRACERS
BRACEUP
BRACING
BRACKEN
BRACKET
BRADLEE
BRADLEY
BRAEDEN
BRAGGED
BRAGGER
BRAHMAN
BRAHMAS
BRAHMIN
BRAIDED
BRAIDER
BRAILLE
BRAINED
BRAINER
BRAISED
BRAISES
BRAKING
BRALESS
BRAMBLE
BRAMBLY
BRAMLEY
BRANAGH
BRANCHY
BRANDED
BRANDER
BRANDON
BRANIFF
BRANSON
BRASHER
BRASHES
BRASHLY
BRASIER
BRASIZE
BRASSES
BRASSIE
BRATTLE
BRAVADA
BRAVADO
BRAVELY
BRAVERY
BRAVEST
BRAVING
BRAVOED
BRAVOES
BRAVURA
BRAWLED
BRAWLER
BRAWLEY
BRAXTON
BRAYERS
BRAYING
BRAZENS
BRAZIER
BRAZING
BYAHAIR
BYAMILE
BYANDBY
BYANECK
BYANOSE

B••A•••

BACARDI
BADAREA
BAHAISM
BAHAIST
BAHAMAS
BAHAMEN
BALABAN
BALANCE
BALASES
BALATAS
BALATON
BANACEK
BANALER
BANALLY
BANANAS
BANANES
BARACUS
BARANOF
BASALLY
BASALTS
BATAVIA
BAVARIA
BAYAREA
BAZAARS
BECALMS
BECAUSE
BEDAUBS
BEDAZED
BEDAZES
BEFALLS
BEGANTO
BEHAPPY
BEHAVED
BEHAVES
BELABOR
BELAIRS
BELARUS
BELASCO
BELATED
BELAYED
BELAYER
BENARES
BENATAR
BENAZIR
BERATED
BERATER
BERATES
BETAKEN
BETAKES
BETAMAX
BETARAY
BEWAILS
BEWARED
BEWARES
BICARBS
BIGAPES
BIVALVE
BIZARRE
BIZARRO
BLEAKER
BLEAKLY
BLEARED
BLEATED
BLEATER
BLOATED
BOBATEA
BOGARDE
BOGARTS
BOIARDO
BOLATIE
BONACIS
BONAIRE
BONANZA
BONARIO
BORATES
BOTANIC
BREADED
BREADER
BREADTH
BREAKER
BREAKIN
BREAKUP
BREASTS
BREATHE
BREATHS
BREATHY
BRIARDS
BROADAS
BROADAX
BROADEN
BROADER
BROADLY
BROASTS
BUGABOO
BUGALOO
BUGATTI
BUTANES
BUYABLE
BYCATCH
BYNAMES
BYPATHS
BYTALKS
BYWAYOF

B•••A••

BABBAGE
BACHATA
BADBACK
BADCALL
BADCASE
BADDAYS
BADHAIR
BADHAND
BADHATS
BADLAND
BADNAME
BADPAST
BADRAPS
BAGGAGE
BAGLADY
BAHIANS
BAHRAIN
BAKLAVA
BALKANS
BALLADE
BALLADS
BALLARD
BALLAST
BALMAIN
BALSAMS
BALSAMY
BANDAGE
BANDAID
BANDANA
BANTAMS
BANYANS
BANZAIS
BAOBABS
BARBARA
BARBARY
BARBATE
BARCARS
BARGAIN
BARMAID
BARNABY
BARNARD
BARRACK
BARRAGE
BARTABS
BARWARE
BASMATI
BASSALE
BASSANI
BASSANO
BATDAYS
BATEAUX
BAUHAUS
BAZAARS
BEATALL
BEBRAVE
BECHARM
BEDBATH
BEDLAMP
BEDLAMS
BEDMATE
BEDRAIL
BEDRAPE
BEEFALO
BEEYARD
BEGGARS
BEGGARY
BEHEADS
BEHEARD
BELDAME
BELDAMS
BELFAST
BELLAMY
BELTANE
BEMOANS
BENDAYS
BENEATH
BENGALI
BENGALS
BENZALI
BEREAVE
BERGAMO
BERNARD
BERNAYS
BETHANY
BETRAYS
BETTANY
BHUTANI
BIDFAIR
BIGBABY
BIGBAND
BIGBANG
BIGCARS
BIGCATS
BIGDAYS
BIGEARS
BIGEAST
BIGEASY
BIGFANS
BIGGAME
BIGHAIR
BIGHALF
BIGHAND
BIGJAKE
BIGMACS
BIGMAMA
BIGNAME
BIGSALE
BIGTALK
BIODATA
BIOLABS
BIOMASS
BIPLANE
BIRIANI
BIRMANS
BIRYANI
BISTATE
BITMAPS
BITPART
BLATANT
BOBCATS
BOBKANE
BOBTAIL
BODYART
BOITANO
BOKHARA
BOMBARD
BOMBAST
BONDAGE
BONEASH
BONIATO
BONNARD
BORLAUG
BORZAGE
BOSCAGE
BOWOARS
BOWSAWS
BOXBALL
BOXCARS
BOYBAND
BRANAGH
BRAVADA
BRAVADO
BREWAGE
BRIDALS
BRIGADE
BRIGAND
BRITAIN
BROCADE
BROGANS
BROMATE
BROWARD
BUDVASE
BUFFALO
BUKHARA
BULGARI
BULGARS
BULWARK
BUMRAPS
BUNRAKU
BUOYANT
BURBAGE
BURBANK
BUREAUS
BUREAUX
BURIALS
BURLAPS
BURMANS
BURNABY
BUROAKS
BURSARS
BUSFARE
BUSLANE
BUSMANS
BUSPASS
BUSTARD
BUYBACK
BUZZARD
BYAHAIR
BYHEART
BYPLAYS
BYROADS
BYTRAIN

B••••A•

BABIYAR
BABYGAP
BABYSAT
BACCHAE
BACHMAN
BACKBAR
BACKBAY
BACKPAY
BACKSAW
BACKWAY
BAGHDAD
BAHAMAS
BAITCAR
BAKEPAN
BALABAN
BALATAS
BALBOAS
BALIHAI
BALKSAT
BANANAS
BANDEAU
BANDSAW
BARBEAU
BARCLAY
BAREXAM
BARFBAG
BARKSAT
BARSOAP
BARTRAY
BASEMAN
BASEPAY
BASINAL
BASSSAX
BATEMAN
BATHMAT
BATSMAN
BAYEDAT
BAYLEAF
BEACHAM
BEANBAG
BEARCAT
BEARPAW
BEATSAT
BECKHAM
BEECHAM
BEEPSAT
BEERCAN
BEERTAP
BEESWAX
BEHRMAN
BELGIAN
BELLEAU
BELLJAR
BELLLAP
BELLMAN
BELTBAG
BELTRAN
BELTSAW
BELTWAY
BELUGAS
BENATAR
BENTHAM
BEOGRAD
BERGMAN
BERIGAN
BERTHAS
BERTRAM
BESMEAR
BESPEAK
BESTIAL
BESTMAN
BETAMAX
BETARAY
BIAFRAN
BIAXIAL
BIFOCAL
BIGBEAR
BIGBEAT
BIGDEAL
BIGHEAD
BIGLEAD
BIGMEAL
BIGSTAR
BIKEWAY
BIMETAL
BIMODAL
BINGHAM
BIPEDAL
BIPOLAR
BIRDMAN
BITONAL
BIVOUAC
BKLIBAN
BLINKAT
BLUEJAY
BLUELAW
BOATMAN
BOBTWAY
BODEGAS
BODYBAR
BODYFAT
BOERWAR
BOGYMAN
BOLIVAR
BONDMAN
BOOEDAT
BOOHBAH
BOOKBAG
BOOKMAN
BOOLEAN
BOOMCAR
BOORMAN
BORGIAS
BORNEAN
BORSTAL
BOSNIAN
BOSSMAN
BOWHEAD
BOXCOAT
BOXSEAT
BOZEMAN
BRAHMAN
BRAHMAS
BRENDAN
BRENNAN
BRIGHAM
BROADAS
BROADAX
BROSNAN
BROWWAX
BUCHMAN
BUCKRAM
BUCKSAW
BUDDHAS
BUGBEAR
BULOVAS
BUMDEAL
BUQSHAS
BURGLAR
BUSHMAN
BUSHWAH
BUSLOAD
BUTTRAM
BUZZSAW

B•••••A

BACHATA
BACTRIA
BADAREA
BADIDEA
BAKLAVA
BAMBINA
BANDANA
BANDERA
BARBARA
BARBERA
BARBUDA
BARETTA
BARISTA
BATAVIA
BATISTA
BAVARIA
BAYAREA
BAZOOKA
BEDELIA
BEEFTEA
BEGONIA
BEGORRA
BELINDA
BENBOVA
BENICIA
BERETTA
BERMUDA
BERNINA
BIENNIA
BIGIDEA
BIGMAMA
BIODATA
BIRETTA
BLACULA
BOBATEA
BOBVILA
BOFFOLA
BOHEMIA
BOKHARA
BOLIVIA
BOLOGNA
BONANZA
BONILLA
BOOTHIA
BOTHNIA
BOTTEGA
BRAVADA
BRAVURA
BRESCIA
BUKHARA
BURKINA

•BA••••

ABALONE
ABANDON
ABASERS
ABASHED
ABASHES
ABASING
ABATERS
ABATING
ABATORS
EBANKED
EBAYERS
MBABANE
NBAGAME
NBALIVE
NBATEAM
OBADIAH
PBANDJS

•B•A•••

ABLATED
ABLATES
ABRADED
ABRADER
ABRADES
ABRAHAM
ABRAXAS
ABSALOM
CBRADIO
OBLASTS
OBLATES
OBTAINS

•B••A••

ABELARD
ABEYANT
ABIGAIL
ABREAST
ABROACH
ABSTAIN
FBICASE
IBIZANS
IBNSAUD
MBABANE
NBAGAME
OBVIATE
WBYEATS

•B•••A•

ABETTAL
ABIDJAN
ABOLLAE
ABRAHAM
ABRAXAS
ABUTTAL
ABYSMAL
ABYSSAL
IBERIAN
NBATEAM
OBADIAH
QBSNEAK

•B••••A

ABINTRA
OBSCURA

••BA•••

ALBANIA
ARBACES
AUBADES
BOBATEA
CABALAS
CABALLE
CABANAS
CABARET
COBALTS
CUBAGES
DEBACLE
DEBAKEY
DEBARGE
DEBARKS
DEBASED
DEBASER
DEBASES
DEBATED
DEBATER
DEBATES
DEBAUCH
DUBARRY
EMBALMS
EMBANKS
EMBARGO
EMBARKS
EMBASSY
EMBAYED
EUBANKS
FABARES
FMBANDS
HIBACHI
IDBADGE
LABAMBA
LABATTS
LEBANON
LEBARON
LOBATED
MTBALDY
MUBARAK
QABALAH
QABALAS
REBAITS
REBAKED
REBAKES
REBALED
REBALES
REBANKS
REBASTE
REBATED
REBATER
REBATES
REBATHE
RIBALDS
RIBANDS
ROBARDS
RUBADUB
RUBATOS
SABADOS
STBARTS
STBASIL
SUBAREA
SUBARID
SUBARUS
TABARDS
TABARET
TABASCO
TEBALDI
TOBACCO
TUBAIST
UNBAITS
UNBAKED
UNBALED
UNBALES
UNBARED
UNBARES
UNBASED
UNBATED
URBANER
URBANII
URBANIV
URBANVI
WABASHA

••B•A••

ASBYATT
BABBAGE
BEBRAVE
BOBCATS
BOBKANE
BOBTAIL
CABBAGE
CABBAGY
CABBALA
CABFARE
COBRAND
CUBFANS
DABHAND
DEBEARD
EMBLAZE
EMBRACE
FTBRAGG
GABBANA
GOBLANK
GOBYAIR
HEBRAIC
HOBNAIL
HUBBARD
HUBCAPS
INBLACK
INBOARD
JOBBANK
JOBFAIR
JOBJARS
KABBALA
LABIALS
LABIATE
LABRATS
LEBLANC
LIBRANS
LIBRARY
LIBYANS
MTBLANC
NUBIANS
ONBOARD
POBLANO
PTBOATS
PUBGAME
REBOANT
REBOARD
REBRACE
REBRAND
RIBCAGE
RIBPADS
ROBSART
SABBATH
SUBBAND
SUBBANK
SUBBASE
SUBBASS
SUBCASE
SUBCASH
SUBCAST
SUBDATE
SUBHALL
SUBRACE
SUBTASK
SUBWARS
SUBWAYS
TOBLAME
UMBRAGE
UNBEARD
UNBLADE
UNBRACE
UNBRAID
UNBRAKE

UNBRAVE
UPBEARS
UPBEATS
UPBRAID
VIBRANT
VIBRATE
VIBRATO
WEBCAMS
WEBCAST
WEBMAIL
WEBPAGE
ZEBRAIC
ZEBRASS

••B••A•

ALBORAK
BABIYAR
BABYGAP
BABYSAT
BOBTWAY
CABALAS
CABANAS
CABEZAS
COBCOAL
CUBICAL
CUBITAL
CUBSFAN
DEBORAH
FIBULAE
FIBULAR
FIBULAS
GIBESAT
GOBYCAB
GOBYCAR
HABITAT
JIBEDAT
JIBESAT
LABCOAT
LABORAT
LIBERAL
MUBARAK
NEBULAE
NEBULAR
NEBULAS
NUBIRAS
ONBREAK
ORBITAL
QABALAH
QABALAS
REBEGAN
REBEKAH
REBREAK
RIBMEAT
RUBSRAW
SUBBIAS
SUBCLAN
SUBDUAL
SUBGOAL
SUBHEAD
TABLEAU
TABULAR
TIBETAN
TOBEHAD
TUBEPAN
TUBULAR
UMBRIAN

••B•••A

ALBANIA
ALBERTA
BOBATEA
BOBVILA
CABBALA
ELBERTA
GABBANA
GOBYSEA
KABBALA
LABAMBA
LIBERIA
PWBOTHA
REBECCA
ROBERTA
ROBUSTA
RUBELLA
RUBEOLA
SABRINA
SIBERIA
SUBAREA
SUBIDEA
SUBROSA
TABITHA
WABASHA

•••BA••

AIRBAGS
AIRBALL
AIRBASE
ALABAMA
ALABAMY
ALIBABA
ARMBAND
ARUBANS
BABBAGE
BADBACK
BAOBABS
BARBARA
BARBARY
BARBATE
BEDBATH
BIGBABY
BIGBAND
BIGBANG
BOMBARD
BOMBAST
BOXBALL
BOYBAND
BURBAGE
BURBANK
BUYBACK
CABBAGE
CABBAGY
CABBALA
CARBARN
CEMBALO
COMBATS
COWBANE
CPEBACH
CRYBABY
CUEBALL
CUTBACK
CYMBALS
DISBAND
DISBARS
DOGBANE
DYEBATH
EYEBALL
EYEBANK
FANBASE
FATBACK
FEEBATE
FIGBARS
FINBACK
FIRBANK
FLYBALL
FOGBANK
FORBADE
FURBALL
GABBANA
GAMBADO
GARBAGE
GARBAGY
GASBAGS
GETBACK
GIGBAGS
GIMBALS
GLOBATE
GOTBACK
GUMBALL
GYMBAGS
GYMBALL
HARBACH
HATBAND
HAYBALE
HENBANE
HERBAGE
HERBALS
HERBART
HERBAUT
HIPBATH
HITBACK
HOGBACK
HOTBATH
HUBBARD
HUMBARD
HUSBAND
ICEBAGS
ICEBATH
IKEBANA
INABALL
ISOBARS
JAMBAND
JOBBANK
JUGBAND
KABBALA
KEYBANK
KIMBALL
KITBAGS
LAMBADA
LAYBACK
LAYBARE
LIEBACK
LIPBALM
LOMBARD
LOWBALL
LUMBAGO
LUMBARS
MAXBAER
MBABANE
MOMBASA
MRSBASS
MUDBATH
NETBALL
NONBANK
NONBASE
NUMBATS
ODDBALL
OFFBASE
OILBASE
OLDBATS
ONEBALL
ONEBASE
OUTBACK
OUTBAKE
OUTBANS
OUTBARK
OUTBATS
OUTBAWL
PARBAKE
PAYBACK
PDQBACH
PEPBAND
PIEBALD
PINBALL
PREBADE
PREBAKE
PROBALL
PROBATE
PUTBACK
RAGBAGS
RANBACK
RAWBARS
RAYBANS
REDBATS
REDBAYS
RHUBARB
RIMBAUD
ROUBAIX
RUMBAED
RUNBACK
SABBATH
SAMBAED
SAMBASS
SATBACK
SCUBAED
SEABAGS
SEABASS
SETBACK
SETBAIL
SHEBANG
SITBACK
SIXBALL
SNOBALL
SORBATE
SUBBAND
SUBBANK
SUBBASE
SUBBASS
SUNBATH
TAMBALA
TANBARK
TARBABY
TAXBASE
TAYBACK
TEABAGS
TEABALL
TENBALL
THEBABE
THEBABY
THEBAND
THEBANS
THEBARD
TIEBACK
TIEBARS
TIMBALE
TIMBALS
TOWBARS
TOYBALL
TURBANS
TWOBALL
TWOBASE
UNIBALL
VERBALS
VONBAER
WARBABY
WAYBACK
WETBARS
WINBACK
WOMBATS

•••B•A•

AIRBOAT
ALLBRAN
ANTBEAR
ARABIAN
BALBOAS
BARBEAU
BIGBEAR
BIGBEAT
BUGBEAR
CARBRAS
CATBOAT
CLUBCAR
CUMBIAS
FORBEAR
GAMBIAN
GETBEAT
GILBLAS
GOTBEAT
GRABBAG
GRABBAR
GRABSAT
GUNBOAT
HOFBRAU
ICEBOAT
IONBEAM
ISABEAU
JAMBEAU
JERBOAS
JETBOAT
JIMBEAM
JOGBRAS
LAMBDAS
LAMBEAU
LINBIAO
LOWBEAM
MOWBRAY
OATBRAN
OFFBEAT
OJIBWAS
OJIBWAY
OLDBEAN
ONABIAS
OUTBEAM
OUTBRAG
OUTBRAY
PEABEAN
PETBEAR
PETBOAS
PHOBIAS
PLEBIAN
ROTBLAT
ROWBOAT
ROYBEAN
RUYBLAS
SANBLAS
SEABOAT
SERBIAN
SHABBAT
SHEBEAR
SIOBHAN
SOYBEAN
SUBBIAS
SUNBEAM
THEBEAR
THEBRAT
TIEBEAM
TOWBOAT
TOYBOAT
TUGBOAT
WAXBEAN
ZAMBIAN

•••B••A

ALABAMA
ALIBABA
ARABICA
BAMBINA
BARBARA
BARBERA
BARBUDA
BENBOVA
CABBALA
CAMBRIA
CUMBRIA
DOUBLEA
GABBANA
HERBTEA
IKEBANA
KABBALA
LAMBADA
MOMBASA
RASBORA
SAMBORA
SAMBUCA
TAMBALA
THEBIGA
TRIBECA
VERBENA

••••BA•

ACROBAT
AEROBAT
AMOEBAE
AMOEBAS
ARRABAL
AZKABAN
BACKBAR
BACKBAY
BALABAN
BARFBAG
BEANBAG
BELTBAG
BKLIBAN
BODYBAR
BOOHBAH
BOOKBAG
CALIBAN
CASABAS
CASHBAR
CLAMBAR
CROWBAR
DINGBAT
DIRTBAG
DOESBAD
DONEBAD
DOVEBAR
DRAWBAR
ESTEBAN
EXURBAN
FEEDBAG
FEELBAD
FELTBAD
FERNBAR
FLEABAG
FOOTBAG
FOREBAY
GAMEBAG
GOESBAD
GOLFBAG
GONEBAD
GOODBAR
GOOMBAH
GOOMBAY
GRABBAG
GRABBAR
HALFBAD
HANDBAG
HIGHBAR
IRONBAR
JOJOBAS
KILOBAR
MAILBAG
MALABAR
MARSBAR
MENUBAR
MILKBAR
MINIBAR
NICOBAR
NOSEBAG
OPENBAR
POOHBAH
POSTBAG
RHUMBAS
ROLLBAR
ROOMBAS
ROSEBAY
SANDBAG
SANDBAR
SCOOBAS
SHABBAT
SICKBAY
SIDEBAR
SINDBAD
SWAYBAR
TALIBAN
TASKBAR
TESTBAN
TOLLBAR
TOOLBAR
TOTEBAG
TURNBAD
UNURBAN
VERYBAD
WENTBAD
WINDBAG
WINEBAR

••••B•A

ALGEBRA
CEREBRA
EXURBIA
NAMIBIA
NOSEBRA
PALABRA
ZENOBIA

•••••BA

ALGIEBA
ALIBABA
CARAMBA
CASSABA
CATAWBA
COLUMBA
CORDOBA
HANKIBA
KOSHIBA
LABAMBA
MARIMBA
PARAIBA
SAXTUBA
TOSHIBA

BB•••••

BBQBEEF
BBQPITS
BBQPORK
BBQRIBS
BBSHOTS

B•B••••

BABBAGE
BABBITT
BABBLED
BABBLER
BABBLES
BABCOCK
BABENCO
BABETTE
BABIEST
BABIYAR
BABOONS
BABYBOP
BABYGAP
BABYING
BABYISH
BABYLON
BABYOIL
BABYSAT
BABYSIT
BEBRAVE
BIBBERS
BIBBIDI
BIBBING
BIBCOCK
BIBELOT
BIBLESS
BIBLIKE
BIBLIOG
BOBATEA
BOBBERS
BOBBIDI
BOBBIES
BOBBING
BOBBINS
BOBBLED
BOBBLER
BOBBLES
BOBBSEY
BOBCATS
BOBDOLE
BOBGOEN
BOBHOPE
BOBKANE
BOBSLED
BOBTAIL
BOBTWAY
BOBVILA
BOBWEIR
BUBBLED
BUBBLES
BYBIRTH

B••B•••

BABBAGE
BABBITT
BABBLED
BABBLER
BABBLES
BADBACK
BADBOYS
BAGBOYS
BALBOAS
BAMBIII
BAMBINA
BAMBINI
BAMBINO
BAMBOOS
BANBURY
BAOBABS
BARBARA
BARBARY
BARBATE
BARBEAU
BARBELL
BARBERA
BARBERS
BARBETS
BARBIES
BARBILL
BARBING
BARBUDA
BARBULE
BATBOYS
BAUBLES
BBQBEEF
BEDBATH
BEDBUGS
BEEBEES
BENBLUE
BENBOVA
BERBERS
BERBICK
BIBBERS
BIBBIDI
BIBBING
BIGBABY
BIGBAND
BIGBANG
BIGBEAR
BIGBEAT
BIGBEND
BIGBETS
BIGBIRD
BIGBLUE
BIGBOSS
BIGBOYS
BIMBOES
BLABBED
BLABBER
BLOBBED
BLUBBER
BOBBERS
BOBBIDI
BOBBIES
BOBBING
BOBBINS
BOBBLED
BOBBLER
BOBBLES
BOBBSEY
BOMBARD
BOMBAST
BOMBECK
BOMBERS
BOMBING
BOMBLET
BONBONS
BOOBIES
BOOBIRD
BOOBOOS
BOXBALL
BOXBEDS
BOXBOYS
BOYBAND
BRIBEES
BRIBERS
BRIBERY
BRIBING
BRUBECK
BUBBLED
BUBBLES
BUGBEAR
BUGBOYS
BULBLET
BULBOUS
BUMBLED
BUMBLER
BUMBLES
BURBAGE
BURBANK
BURBLED
BURBLER
BURBLES
BURBOTS
BUSBIES
BUSBOYS
BUYBACK
BYEBYES

B•••B••

BABYBOP
BACKBAR
BACKBAY
BACKBIT
BALABAN
BALLBOY
BANDBOX
BARFBAG
BEANBAG
BEATBOX
BELABOR
BELLBOY
BELTBAG
BESTBET
BESTBOY
BESTBUD
BESTBUY
BILOBED
BKLIBAN
BLABBED
BLABBER
BLAUBOK
BLOBBED
BLUBBER
BLUEBOY
BLURBER
BODYBAR
BOOHBAH
BOOKBAG
BOOMBOX
BOURBON
BRAMBLE
BRAMBLY
BUGABOO
BUNKBED
BUSYBEE
BUYABLE

B••••B•

BADDEBT
BAGJOBS
BAOBABS
BARNABY
BARTABS
BBQRIBS
BEDAUBS
BENUMBS
BICARBS
BIGBABY
BIOLABS
BURNABY
BYANDBY
BYTHEBY

B•••••B

BACKRUB
BANKJOB
BATHTUB
BEARCUB
BODYRUB
BREWPUB

•BB••••

ABBOTCY
EBBTIDE

•B•B•••

BBQBEEF
MBABANE
NBCBLUE

•B•••B•

ABIDEBY
ABITIBI
ABSORBS
BBQRIBS

••BB•••

BABBAGE
BABBITT
BABBLED
BABBLER
BABBLES
BIBBERS
BIBBIDI
BIBBING
BOBBERS
BOBBIDI
BOBBIES
BOBBING
BOBBINS
BOBBLED
BOBBLER
BOBBLES
BOBBSEY
BUBBLED
BUBBLES
CABBAGE
CABBAGY
CABBALA
CABBIES
CABBING
COBBLED
COBBLER
COBBLES
CUBBIES
CUBBING
CUBBINS
CUBBISH
DABBERS
DABBING
DABBLED
DABBLER
DABBLES
DIBBLED
DIBBLER
DIBBLES
DOBBINS
DUBBERS
DUBBING
DYBBUKS
FABBEST
FIBBERS
FIBBING
FOBBING
GABBANA
GABBERS
GABBIER
GABBING
GABBLED
GABBLES
GABBROS
GIBBERS
GIBBONS
GIBBOUS
GOBBLED
GOBBLER
GOBBLES
HIBBING
HIBBLER
HOBBIES
HOBBITS
HOBBLED
HOBBLER
HOBBLES
HUBBARD
HUBBELL
HUBBIES
HUBBUBS
JABBERS
JABBING
JEBBUSH
JIBBOOM
JOBBANK
JOBBERS
JOBBERY
JOBBING
KABBALA
KIBBLED
KIBBLES
KIBBUTZ
LIBBERS
LIBBING
LOBBERS
LOBBIED
LOBBIES
LOBBING
LOBBYER
LUBBERS
LUBBOCK
MOBBERS
MOBBING
MOBBISH
MOBBISM
MOBBIST
NABBERS
NABBING
NEBBISH
NIBBLED
NIBBLER
NIBBLES
NOBBIER
NUBBERS
NUBBIER
NUBBINS
NUBBLES
PEBBLED
PEBBLES
RABBETS
RABBITS
RABBITT
RABBITY
RABBLED
RABBLES
RIBBERS
RIBBIER
RIBBIES
RIBBING
RIBBONS
RIBBONY
ROBBERS
ROBBERY
ROBBING
ROBBINS
ROBBNEN
RUBBERS
RUBBERY
RUBBING
RUBBISH
RUBBLES
SABBATH
SOBBERS
SOBBING

SUBBAND
SUBBANK
SUBBASE
SUBBASS
SUBBIAS
SUBBING
TABBIES
TABBING
TIBBETT
TUBBIER
TUBBING
WABBITS
WEBBIER
WEBBING
WOBBLED
WOBBLER
WOBBLES
YOBBISH

••B•B••
BABYBOP
GOBYBUS
IMBIBED
IMBIBER
IMBIBES

••B••B•
COBWEBS
HOBNOBS
HUBBUBS
LABAMBA
LABTUBE
SUBDEBS
SUBURBS

••B•••B
GOBYCAB
LUBEJOB
RUBADUB

•••BB••
BLABBED
BLABBER
BLOBBED
BLUBBER
CLABBER
CLOBBER
CLUBBED
CLUBBER
CRABBED
CRABBER
CRIBBED
CRIBBER
DRABBER
DRABBLE
DRIBBLE
DRUBBED
DRUBBER
FLUBBED
FLUBBER
FRIBBLE
GLIBBER
GRABBAG
GRABBAR
GRABBED
GRABBER
GRUBBED
GRUBBER
KNOBBED
QUIBBLE
SHABBAT
SLABBED
SLOBBER
SNUBBED
SNUBBER
STABBED
STABBER
STUBBED
STUBBLE
STUBBLY
SWABBED
SWABBER
TRIBBLE
UNEBBED

•••B•B•
ALIBABA
BAOBABS
BIGBABY
CRYBABY
HUBBUBS
SKIBIBS
SKIBOBS
TARBABY
THEBABE
THEBABY
THEBOBO
WARBABY

•••B••B
DIMBULB
DOTBOMB
DOUBLEB
DRYBULB
FLUBDUB
RHUBARB
THEBLOB
THEBOMB
WETBULB

••••BB•
ENTEBBE
MRHOBBS
MRTIBBS
SCRUBBY
SHRUBBY

•••••BB
FREDEBB

BC•••••
BCDEFGH
BCLIONS

B•C••••
BACARDI
BACCHAE
BACCHIC
BACCHUS
BACHATA
BACHING
BACHMAN
BACILLI
BACKBAR
BACKBAY
BACKBIT
BACKEND
BACKERS
BACKHOE
BACKING
BACKLIT
BACKLOG
BACKLOT
BACKOFF
BACKOUT
BACKPAY
BACKROW
BACKRUB
BACKSAW
BACKSIN
BACKSUP
BACKUPS
BACKWAY
BACTRIA
BECALMS
BECAUSE
BECHARM
BECKETT
BECKHAM
BECKONS
BECLOUD
BECOMES
BICARBS
BICHONS
BICKERS
BICOLOR
BICORNE
BICORNS
BICYCLE
BOCCIES
BOCELLI
BOCHNER
BSCHOOL
BUCHMAN
BUCHNER
BUCKERS
BUCKETS
BUCKEYE
BUCKFOR
BUCKING
BUCKLED
BUCKLES
BUCKLEY
BUCKNER
BUCKOES
BUCKRAM
BUCKSAW
BUCKSUP
BUCOLIC
BYCATCH

B••C•••
BABCOCK
BACCHAE
BACCHIC
BACCHUS
BADCALL
BADCASE
BADCOLD
BALCONY
BARCARS
BARCLAY
BARCODE
BATCHED
BATCHES
BAYCITY
BEACHAM
BEACHED
BEACHES
BEACONS
BEECHAM
BEECHEN
BEECHER
BEECHES
BELCHED
BELCHER
BELCHES
BENCHED
BENCHER
BENCHES
BIBCOCK
BIGCARS
BIGCATS
BIGCITY
BIOCHIP
BIOCIDE
BIRCHED
BIRCHEN
BIRCHES
BISCUIT
BLACKED
BLACKEN
BLACKER
BLACKIE
BLACKLY
BLACULA
BLOCKED
BLOCKER
BLOCKUP
BOBCATS
BOCCIES
BOKCHOY
BOOCOOS
BOSCAGE
BOTCHED
BOTCHER
BOTCHES
BOTCHUP
BOUCHER
BOUCHES
BOXCARS
BOXCOAT
BOYCOTT
BRACERO
BRACERS
BRACEUP
BRACING
BRACKEN
BRACKET
BRICKED
BRICKLE
BRICKUP
BROCADE
BUNCHED
BUNCHES
BUNCHUP
BUNCOED
BUSCEMI
BUTCHER
BUTCHES

B•••C••
BAITCAR
BANACEK
BARACUS
BEARCAT
BEARCUB
BEATCOP
BEDECKS
BEERCAN
BENICIA
BENICIO
BESTCUT
BIANCHI
BICYCLE
BIFOCAL
BINOCHE
BISECTS
BLANCHE
BLOTCHY
BODICES
BONACIS
BOOMCAR
BOOTCUT
BORSCHT
BOUNCED
BOUNCER
BOUNCES
BOWECHO
BRANCHY
BRESCIA
BRIOCHE
BRITCOM
BRONCHI
BRONCHO
BRONCOS
BUZZCUT

B••••C•
BABCOCK
BABENCO
BADBACK
BADITCH
BADLUCK
BALANCE
BARLICK
BARRACK
BEDROCK
BELASCO
BEQUICK
BERBICK
BERWICK
BESEECH
BEWITCH
BEYONCE
BIBCOCK
BIGMACS
BIONICS
BIOPICS
BIOTECH
BLALOCK
BLUEICE
BOMBECK
BRUBECK
BULLOCK
BURDICK
BUYBACK
BYANECK
BYCATCH
BYFORCE

B•••••C
BACCHIC
BALDRIC
BASILIC
BENEFIC
BIVOUAC
BORONIC
BOSONIC
BOTANIC
BUCOLIC
BYRONIC

•BC••••
ABCDEFG
ABCNEWS
NBCBLUE
NBCNEWS

•B•C•••
ABSCISE
ABSCOND
FBICASE
OBSCENE
OBSCURA
OBSCURE

•B••C••
ABDUCED
ABDUCES
ABDUCTS
OBJECTS

•B•••C•
ABBOTCY
ABROACH
ABSENCE
EBONICS

•B••••C
ABIOTIC

••BC•••
BABCOCK
BIBCOCK
BOBCATS
COBCOAL
HUBCAPS
JOBCUTS
LABCOAT
RIBCAGE
RIBCUTS
SUBCASE
SUBCASH
SUBCAST
SUBCELL
SUBCLAN
SUBCODE
SUBCOOL
WEBCAMS
WEBCAST

••B•C••
ARBACES
CUBICAL
CUBICLE
CUBICLY
DEBACLE
GOBYCAB
GOBYCAR
HIBACHI
NABUCCO
REBECCA
ROBOCOP
RUBICON
SUBECHO
TOBACCO

••B••C•
ABBOTCY
BABCOCK
BABENCO
BIBCOCK
DEBAUCH
EMBRACE
FABRICS
INBLACK
IOBJECT
JOBLOCK
KUBRICK
LABMICE
LABTECH
LEBROCK
LUBBOCK
NABISCO
NABUCCO
NIBLICK
OOBLECK
PUBLICS
REBECCA
REBLOCK
REBRACE
RUBRICS
SUBDUCT
SUBJECT
SUBRACE
SUBSECT
TABASCO
TOBACCO
UNBENCH
UNBLOCK
UNBRACE

••B•••C
HEBRAIC
LEBLANC
MTBLANC
ROBOTIC
SIBYLIC
ZEBRAIC

•••BC••
CLUBCAR
CURBCUT

•••B•C•
ARABICA
ARABICS
BADBACK
BERBICK
BOMBECK
BRUBECK
BUYBACK
CPEBACH
CUTBACK
FATBACK
FINBACK
GETBACK
GOTBACK
HARBACH
HITBACK
HOGBACK
IAMBICS
JOEBUCK
JUMBUCK
LAYBACK
LIEBACK
LUBBOCK
OUTBACK
PAYBACK
PDQBACH
PHOBICS
PUTBACK
RANBACK
ROEBUCK
RUNBACK
SAMBUCA
SATBACK
SAWBUCK
SETBACK
SITBACK
TAYBACK
TIEBACK
TRIBECA
WAYBACK
WINBACK
YASBECK

•••B••C
CAMBRIC
DOUBLEC

••••BC•
THEABCS

••••B•C
ACERBIC
AEROBIC
ALEMBIC
AMOEBIC
PLUMBIC
RHOMBIC
UNCUBIC

•••••BC
EIGHTBC
FIFTYBC
FORTYBC
SEVENBC
SHOPNBC
SIXTYBC
THREEBC

BD•••••
BDALTON

B•D••••
BADAREA
BADBACK
BADBOYS
BADCALL
BADCASE
BADCOLD
BADDAYS
BADDEBT
BADDEED
BADDEST
BADDIES
BADDISH
BADDOGS
BADEGGS
BADENDS
BADENOV
BADFITS
BADFORM
BADGERS
BADGIRL
BADGUYS
BADHAIR
BADHAND
BADHATS
BADIDEA
BADITCH
BADJOKE
BADLAND
BADLIES
BADLOTS
BADLOVE
BADLUCK
BADMOOD
BADMOVE
BADNAME
BADNESS
BADNEWS
BADOMEN
BADPAST
BADRAPS
BADSHOT
BADSIGN
BADTIME
BADTRIP
BADWORD
BCDEFGH
BEDAUBS
BEDAZED
BEDAZES
BEDBATH
BEDBUGS
BEDDING
BEDDOWN
BEDECKS
BEDELIA
BEDEVIL
BEDEWED
BEDFORD
BEDIZEN
BEDLAMP
BEDLAMS
BEDLESS
BEDLIKE
BEDLOES
BEDMATE
BEDNORZ
BEDOUIN
BEDPOST
BEDRAIL
BEDRAPE
BEDREST
BEDROCK
BEDROLL
BEDROOM
BEDSIDE
BEDSITS
BEDTIME
BIDDERS
BIDDIES
BIDDING
BIDFAIR
BIDSFOR
BODEFUL
BODEGAS
BODEREK
BODICES
BODINGS
BODKINS
BODYART
BODYBAR
BODYFAT
BODYKIT
BODYRUB
BUDDERS
BUDDHAS
BUDDIED
BUDDIES
BUDDING
BUDDYUP
BUDGERS
BUDGETS
BUDGIES
BUDGING
BUDLESS
BUDLIKE
BUDTIME
BUDVASE
BUDWORM

B••D•••
BADDAYS
BADDEBT
BADDEED
BADDEST
BADDIES
BADDISH
BADDOGS
BALDEST
BALDIES
BALDING
BALDISH
BALDRIC
BALDWIN
BANDAGE
BANDAID
BANDANA
BANDBOX
BANDEAU
BANDERA
BANDERS
BANDIDO
BANDIED
BANDIER
BANDIES
BANDING
BANDITO
BANDITS
BANDLET
BANDSAW
BARDEEN
BATDAYS
BAWDIER
BAWDILY
BEADERS
BEADIER
BEADILY
BEADING
BEADLES
BEADSUP
BEDDING
BEDDOWN
BELDAME
BELDAMS
BENDAYS
BENDERS
BENDIER
BENDING
BIDDERS
BIDDIES
BIDDING
BIGDAYS
BIGDEAL
BIGDIGS
BIGDOGS
BINDERS
BINDERY
BINDING
BINDLES
BINDOFF
BINDSTO
BINDSUP
BIODATA
BIRDDOG
BIRDERS
BIRDFLU
BIRDIED
BIRDIES
BIRDING
BIRDMAN
BIRDMEN
BLADDER
BLADERS
BLADING
BLEDSOE
BLUDGED
BLUDGER
BLUDGES
BOBDOLE
BOGDOWN
BOLDEST
BONDAGE
BONDERS
BONDING
BONDMAN
BONDMEN
BOODLES
BORDERS
BORDONI
BOUDINS
BOUDOIR
BOWDLER
BOWDOIN
BOWDOWN
BRADLEE
BRADLEY
BRIDALS
BRIDGED
BRIDGER
BRIDGES
BRIDGET
BRIDLED
BRIDLER
BRIDLES
BRODIES
BRODKEY
BRODSKY
BUDDERS
BUDDHAS
BUDDIED
BUDDIES
BUDDING
BUDDYUP
BUMDEAL
BUNDLED
BUNDLER
BUNDLES
BURDENS
BURDICK
BUYDOWN

B•••D••
BADIDEA
BAGHDAD
BASEDON
BAYEDAT
BEANDIP
BEARDED
BESIDES
BETIDED
BETIDES
BIGIDEA
BIMODAL
BIPEDAL
BIRDDOG
BLADDER
BLANDER
BLANDLY
BLEEDER
BLENDED
BLENDER
BLENDES
BLENDIN
BLINDED
BLINDER
BLINDLY
BLINDTO
BLONDER
BLONDES
BLONDIE
BLOODED
BLOWDRY
BLUNDEN
BLUNDER
BOARDED
BOARDER
BOARDUP
BOLIDES
BONEDRY
BONEDUP
BOOEDAT
BOREDOM
BORIDES
BORODIN
BOULDER
BOUNDED
BOUNDER
BOUNDTO
BOUNDUP
BOWEDTO
BOXEDIN
BOXEDUP
BRAEDEN
BRAIDED
BRAIDER
BRANDED
BRANDER
BRANDON
BREADED
BREADER
BREADTH
BREEDER
BRENDAN
BRENDEL
BRENDON
BRINDLE
BROADAS
BROADAX
BROADEN
BROADER
BROADLY
BROIDER
BROODED
BROODER
BUILDER
BUILDIN
BUILDON
BUILDUP
BULLDOG
BYANDBY

B••••D•
BACARDI
BADENDS
BAGLADY
BALLADE
BALLADS
BANDIDO
BARBUDA
BARCODE
BEDSIDE
BEGIRDS
BEHEADS
BEHINDS
BEHOLDS
BELINDA
BERENDT
BERMUDA
BIBBIDI
BIGENDS
BIGKIDS
BIOCIDE
BOBBIDI
BOGARDE
BOIARDO
BOXBEDS
BRAVADA
BRAVADO
BRIARDS
BRIGADE
BROCADE
BROMIDE
BURUNDI
BUSHIDO
BUSRIDE
BYROADS
BYWORDS

B•••••D
BABBLED
BACKEND
BADCOLD
BADDEED
BADHAND
BADLAND
BADMOOD
BADWORD
BAFFLED
BAGHDAD
BAGNOLD
BALLARD
BANDAID
BANDIED
BANGLED
BARMAID
BARNARD
BARNRED
BARTEND
BATCHED
BATIKED
BATTLED
BAULKED
BEACHED
BEARDED
BECLOUD
BEDAZED
BEDEWED
BEDFORD
BEETRED
BEEYARD
BEHAVED
BEHEARD
BELATED
BELAYED
BELCHED
BELLIED
BELOVED
BEMIRED
BEMUSED
BENCHED
BENOTED
BEOGRAD
BERATED
BERNARD
BERRIED
BERTHED
BESTBUD
BETIDED
BEVELED
BEWARED
BIASSED
BIGBAND
BIGBEND
BIGBIRD
BIGEYED
BIGHAND
BIGHEAD
BIGLEAD
BIGOTED
BILOBED
BIRCHED
BIRDIED
BIRTHED
BLABBED
BLACKED
BLANKED
BLASTED
BLATTED
BLEARED
BLEATED
BLEEPED
BLENDED
BLESSED
BLINDED
BLINKED
BLIPPED
BLISSED
BLITZED
BLOATED
BLOBBED
BLOCKED
BLOGGED
BLOODED
BLOOMED
BLOOPED
BLOTTED
BLOUSED
BLOWZED
BLUDGED
BLUERED
BLUFFED
BLUNTED
BLURRED
BLURTED
BLUSHED
BOARDED
BOASTED
BOBBLED
BOBSLED
BOGEYED
BOGGLED
BOISEID
BOMBARD
BONNARD
BOOBIRD
BOOGIED
BOOKEND
BOOSTED
BOSOMED
BOTCHED
BOTTLED
BOUGHED
BOUNCED
BOUNDED
BOWERED
BOWHEAD
BOYBAND
BOYHOOD
BRAGGED
BRAIDED
BRAINED
BRAISED
BRANDED
BRAVOED
BRAWLED
BREADED
BREEZED
BRICKED
BRIDGED
BRIDLED
BRIEFED
BRIGAND
BRIMMED
BRISKED
BROILED
BRONZED
BROODED
BROOKED
BROOMED
BROWARD
BROWNED
BROWSED
BRUISED
BRUITED
BRUSHED
BUBBLED
BUCKLED
BUDDIED
BUGEYED
BULLIED
BUMBLED
BUNCHED
BUNCOED
BUNDLED
BUNGLED
BUNKBED
BUNKOED
BURBLED
BURGLED
BUSLOAD
BUSTARD
BUSTLED
BUTGOOD
BUZZARD
BYLINED

•BD••••
ABDOMEN
ABDUCED
ABDUCES
ABDUCTS

•B•D•••
ABCDEFG
ABIDEBY
ABIDERS
ABIDING
ABIDJAN
OBADIAH

•B••D••
ABANDON
ABRADED
ABRADER
ABRADES
ABRIDGE
CBRADIO
PBANDJS

•B•••D•
ABOUNDS
EBBTIDE
OBTRUDE
OBTUNDS

•B••••D
ABASHED
ABDUCED
ABELARD
ABETTED
ABJURED
ABLATED
ABORTED
ABRADED
ABSCOND
ABUTTED
EBANKED
IBNSAUD
OBLIGED

••BD•••
BOBDOLE
RUBDOWN
SUBDATE
SUBDEBS
SUBDUAL
SUBDUCT
SUBDUED
SUBDUER
SUBDUES

••B•D••
ALBEDOS
AUBADES
IDBADGE
JIBEDAT
LIBIDOS
MRBODDY
MYBUDDY
NOBODYS
RABIDLY
RUBADUB
RUBYDEE
SABADOS
SUBIDEA

••B••D•
ALBUNDY
BIBBIDI
BOBBIDI
CABRIDE
CUBOIDS
EBBTIDE
FMBANDS
HYBRIDS
KOBOLDS
MCBRIDE
MRBODDY
MTBALDY
MYBUDDY
REBENDS
REBINDS
RIBALDS
RIBANDS
RIBPADS
ROBARDS
SUBCODE
SUBGODS
SUBLIDS
SUBSIDE
SUBSIDY
TABARDS
TEBALDI
UNBELDI
UNBENDS
UNBINDS
UNBLADE

••B•••D
ARBORED
BABBLED
BOBBLED
BOBSLED
BUBBLED
COBBLED
COBRAND
DABBLED
DABHAND
DEBASED
DEBATED
DEBEARD
DEBITED
DEBONED
DEBUTED
DIBBLED
ELBOWED
EMBAYED
EMBRUED
FIBERED
FIBROID
GABBLED
GOBBLED
HABITED
HOBBLED
HUBBARD
IMBIBED
IMBORED
IMBRUED
INBOARD
INBOUND
INBREED
KIBBLED
LABELED
LABORED
LIBELED
LOBATED
LOBBIED
NIBBLED
ONBOARD
ORBITED
OXBLOOD
PEBBLED
RABBLED
REBAKED
REBALED
REBATED
REBOARD
REBORED
REBOUND
REBOXED
REBRAND
REBREED
REBUILD
REBUKED
RUBYRED
SABERED
SOBERED
SUBARID
SUBBAND
SUBDUED
SUBHEAD
SUBTEND
TABLOID
TABOOED
TOBEHAD
UMBERED
UNBAKED
UNBALED
UNBARED
UNBASED
UNBATED
UNBEARD
UNBLUED
UNBONED
UNBORED
UNBOUND
UNBOWED
UNBOXED
UNBRAID
UNBUILD
UPBOUND
UPBRAID
UPBUILD
WEBTOED
WOBBLED
ZEBROID

•••BD••
FLUBDUB
LAMBDAS

•••B•D•
ANYBODY
ASABODY
BARBUDA
BIBBIDI
BOBBIDI
BOXBEDS
CARBIDE
CATBEDS
CUEBIDS
DAYBEDS
DISBUDS
DOGBEDS
EARBUDS
FORBADE
FORBIDS
GAMBADO
HOTBEDS
LAMBADA
LOWBIDS
NONBODY
OREBODY
OUTBIDS
OUTBUDS
PEABODY
PREBADE
PREBIDS
REDBUDS
SEABEDS
THEBODY
TOPBIDS
UNIBODY
VERBIDS

•••B••D
ALIBIED
AMEBOID
ANTBIRD
ARMBAND
BABBLED
BIGBAND
BIGBEND
BIGBIRD
BLABBED
BLOBBED
BOBBLED
BOMBARD
BOOBIRD
BOYBAND
BUBBLED
BUMBLED
BURBLED
CATBIRD
CLUBBED
CLUBMED
COBBLED
COWBIRD
CRABBED
CRIBBED
DABBLED
DIBBLED
DIEBOLD
DISBAND
DOUBLED
DOUBTED
DRUBBED
ENABLED
FLUBBED
FUMBLED
GABBLED
GAMBLED
GARBLED
GLOBOID
GOBBLED
GRABBED
GRUBBED
HATBAND
HOBBLED
HUBBARD
HUMBARD
HUMBLED
HUSBAND
ILLBRED
INABIND
JAMBAND
JAYBIRD
JUGBAND
JUMBLED
KIBBLED
KNOBBED
LOBBIED
LOMBARD
LOWBRED
MAMBOED
MARBLED
MISBIND
MUMBLED
NIBBLED
OILBIRD
OUTBEND
OUTBRED
PEBBLED
PEPBAND
PETBIRD
PIEBALD
PREBIND
RABBLED
RAMBLED
REDBIRD
RIMBAUD
RUMBAED
RUMBLED
SAMBAED
SCUBAED
SEABIRD
SLABBED
SNUBBED
STABBED
STABLED
STUBBED
SUBBAND
SUNBIRD
SWABBED
THEBAND
THEBARD
TREBLED
TUMBLED
UNEBBED
WAMBLED
WARBLED
WARBOND
WOBBLED

••••B•D
BESTBUD
BILOBED
BLABBED
BLOBBED
BUNKBED
CAMPBED
CLIMBED
CLUBBED
CRABBED
CRIBBED
CRUMBED
DOESBAD
DONEBAD
DRUBBED
ENROBED
FEELBAD
FELTBAD
FLAMBED
FLATBED
FLUBBED
GOESBAD
GONEBAD
GOTOBED
GRABBED
GRUBBED
HALFBAD
ICHABOD
IMBIBED
JUMPBID
KNOBBED
LAKEBED
LIEABED
LOFTBED
LONGBED
OVERBED
OVERBID
PLUMBED
PROMBID
ROADBED
ROSABUD
ROSEBUD
SCRIBED
SEEDBED
SICKBED
SINDBAD
SLABBED
SNUBBED
SOFABED
STABBED
STUBBED
SWABBED
TENTBED
TESTBED
THUMBED
TURNBAD
TWINBED
UNEBBED
UNLOBED
UNORBED
UNROBED
VERYBAD
WENTBAD

BE•••••
BEACHAM
BEACHED
BEACHES
BEACONS
BEADERS
BEADIER
BEADILY
BEADING
BEADLES
BEADSUP
BEAGLES
BEAHERO
BEAKERS
BEALION
BEAMERS
BEAMIER
BEAMING
BEAMISH
BEAMSUP
BEANBAG
BEANDIP
BEANERY
BEANIES
BEANING
BEANOIL
BEARCAT
BEARCUB
BEARDED
BEARERS
BEARHUG
BEARING
BEARISH
BEAROFF
BEAROUT
BEARPAW
BEARPIT
BEARSON
BEARSUP
BEASLEY
BEASTIE
BEASTLY
BEATALL
BEATBOX
BEATCOP
BEATERS
BEATIFY
BEATING
BEATLES
BEATNIK
BEATOFF
BEATOUT
BEATRIX
BEATSAT
BEATSIT
BEATSME
BEATSON
BEATSUP
BEATTIE
BEAUISH
BEAVERS
BEBRAVE
BECALMS
BECAUSE
BECHARM
BECKETT
BECKHAM
BECKONS
BECLOUD
BECOMES
BEDAUBS
BEDAZED
BEDAZES
BEDBATH
BEDBUGS
BEDDING
BEDDOWN
BEDECKS
BEDELIA
BEDEVIL
BEDEWED
BEDFORD
BEDIZEN
BEDLAMP
BEDLAMS
BEDLESS
BEDLIKE
BEDLOES
BEDMATE
BEDNORZ
BEDOUIN
BEDPOST
BEDRAIL
BEDRAPE
BEDREST
BEDROCK
BEDROLL
BEDROOM
BEDSIDE
BEDSITS
BEDTIME
BEEBEES
BEECHAM
BEECHEN
BEECHER
BEECHES
BEEFALO
BEEFIER
BEEFILY
BEEFING
BEEFSUP
BEEFTEA
BEEGEES
BEEHIVE
BEELIKE
BEELINE
BEEMERS
BEEPERS
BEEPING
BEEPSAT
BEERCAN
BEERIER
BEERKEG
BEERMUG
BEERTAP
BEESWAX
BEETIER
BEETLES
BEETRED
BEETREE
BEEYARD
BEEZERS
BEFALLS
BEFOOLS
BEFOULS
BEGANTO
BEGGARS
BEGGARY
BEGGING
BEGIRDS
BEGONIA
BEGORRA
BEGRIME
BEGSFOR
BEGSOFF
BEGUILE
BEGUINE
BEHAPPY
BEHAVED
BEHAVES
BEHEADS
BEHEARD
BEHESTS
BEHINDS
BEHOLDS
BEHOOVE
BEHRENS
BEHRING
BEHRMAN
BEIGNES
BEIGNET
BEIJING
BEJEWEL
BELABOR
BELAIRS
BELARUS
BELASCO
BELATED
BELAYED
BELAYER
BELCHED
BELCHER
BELCHES
BELDAME
BELDAMS
BELEVEN
BELFAST
BELFORT
BELGIAN
BELGIUM
BELIEFS
BELIERS
BELIEVE
BELINDA
BELLAMY
BELLBOY
BELLEAU
BELLEEK
BELLHOP
BELLIED
BELLIES
BELLING
BELLINI
BELLJAR
BELLLAP
BELLMAN
BELLMEN
BELLOWS
BELLSON
BELLYUP
BELMONT
BELONGS
BELOVED
BELTANE
BELTBAG
BELTERS
BELTING
BELTOUT
BELTRAN
BELTSAW
BELTSUP
BELTWAY
BELUGAS
BELUSHI
BELVOIR
BELVOUR
BELYING
BELZONI
BEMIRED
BEMIRES
BEMOANS
BEMUSED
BEMUSES
BENARES
BENATAR
BENAZIR
BENBLUE
BENBOVA
BENCHED
BENCHER
BENCHES
BENDAYS
BENDERS
BENDIER
BENDING
BENEATH
BENEFIC
BENEFIT
BENELUX
BENGALI
BENGALS
BENGUNN
BENICIA
BENICIO
BENIGNI
BENIGNO
BENISON
BENNETT
BENNING
BENOTED
BENOTES
BENTHAM
BENTHOS
BENTLEY
BENTSEN
BENUMBS
BENZALI
BENZELL
BENZENE
BEOGRAD
BEOWULF
BEQUEST
BEQUICK
BEQUIET
BERATED
BERATER
BERATES
BERBERS
BERBICK
BEREAVE
BERENDT
BERETTA
BERGAMO
BERGERE
BERGIUS
BERGMAN
BERGSON
BERIGAN
BERKLEY
BERKNER
BERLIOZ
BERLITZ
BERMING
BERMUDA
BERNARD
BERNAYS
BERNESE
BERNINA
BERNINI
BERNSEN
BEROWNE
BERRIED
BERRIES
BERSERK
BERSUNT
BERTHAS
BERTHED
BERTOLT
BERTRAM
BERVOIX
BERWICK
BESEECH
BESIDES
BESIEGE
BESMEAR
BESPEAK
BESPOKE
BESSELL
BESTBET
BESTBOY
BESTBUD
BESTBUY
BESTCUT
BESTIAL
BESTILL
BESTING
BESTIRS
BESTMAN
BESTMEN
BESTOFF
BESTONE
BESTOWS
BESTREW
BETAKEN

BETAKES
BETAMAX
BETARAY
BETHANY
BETHELS
BETHERE
BETHINK
BETHUNE
BETIDED
BETIDES
BETIMES
BETOKEN
BETRAYS
BETROTH
BETTANY
BETTERS
BETTGER
BETTING
BETTORS
BETWEEN
BETWIXT
BEURRES
BEVELED
BEVELER
BEVERLY
BEWAILS
BEWARED
BEWARES
BEWITCH
BEYONCE
BEZIERS
BEZIQUE

B•E••••

BEEBEES
BEECHAM
BEECHEN
BEECHER
BEECHES
BEEFALO
BEEFIER
BEEFILY
BEEFING
BEEFSUP
BEEFTEA
BEEGEES
BEEHIVE
BEELIKE
BEELINE
BEEMERS
BEEPERS
BEEPING
BEEPSAT
BEERCAN
BEERIER
BEERKEG
BEERMUG
BEERTAP
BEESWAX
BEETIER
BEETLES
BEETRED
BEETREE
BEEYARD
BEEZERS
BIENNIA
BIENTOT
BLEAKER
BLEAKLY
BLEARED
BLEATED
BLEATER
BLEDSOE
BLEEDER
BLEEPED
BLEEPER
BLEMISH
BLENDED
BLENDER
BLENDES
BLENDIN
BLENTIN
BLERIOT
BLESSED
BLESSER
BLESSES
BLEWOFF
BLEWOUT
BOEINGS
BOERWAR
BREADED
BREADER
BREADTH
BREAKER
BREAKIN
BREAKUP
BREASTS
BREATHE
BREATHS
BREATHY
BREEDER
BREEZED
BREEZES
BRENDAN
BRENDEL
BRENDON
BRENGUN
BRENNAN
BRENNER
BRERFOX
BRESCIA
BRESLIN
BRETONS
BRETTON
BREVETS
BREVITY
BREWAGE
BREWERS
BREWERY
BREWING
BREWPUB
BREWSKI
BREWSUP
BREYERS
BUELLER
BYEBYES

B••E•••

BABENCO
BABETTE
BADEGGS
BADENDS
BADENOV
BAGEHOT
BAKEOFF
BAKEPAN
BAKERST
BALEENS
BALEFUL
BANEFUL
BAREGES
BARENTS
BARETTA
BAREXAM
BASEDON
BASEHIT
BASEMAN
BASEMEN
BASENJI
BASEPAY
BASESIX
BASETEN
BASETWO
BATEAUX
BATEMAN
BAYEDAT
BCDEFGH
BEDECKS
BEDELIA
BEDEVIL
BEDEWED
BEHEADS
BEHEARD
BEHESTS
BEJEWEL
BELEVEN
BENEATH
BENEFIC
BENEFIT
BENELUX
BEREAVE
BERENDT
BERETTA
BESEECH
BEVELED
BEVELER
BEVERLY
BIBELOT
BIGEARS
BIGEAST
BIGEASY
BIGELOW
BIGENDS
BIGEYED
BIGEYES
BIKEWAY
BILEVEL
BIMETAL
BIPEDAL
BIREMES
BIRETTA
BISECTS
BITEOFF
BITESIN
BITESON
BITESUP
BLEEDER
BLEEPED
BLEEPER
BLUEBOY
BLUEFIN
BLUEFLU
BLUEFOX
BLUEHEN
BLUEICE
BLUEING
BLUEISH
BLUEJAY
BLUELAW
BLUERED
BLUESKY
BLUESUN
BLUETIT
BOCELLI
BODEFUL
BODEGAS
BODEREK
BOGEYED
BOHEMIA
BOLEROS
BONEASH
BONEDRY
BONEDUP
BONELET
BONESET
BONESUP
BONEYER
BOOEDAT
BOREDOM
BOREOUT
BOWECHO
BOWEDTO
BOWERED
BOXEDIN
BOXEDUP
BOXESIN
BOXESUP
BOZEMAN
BRAEDEN
BREEDER
BREEZED
BREEZES
BRIEFED
BRIEFER
BRIEFLY
BRUEGEL
BTWELVE
BUGEYED
BUREAUS
BUREAUX
BURETTE
BUTENES
BYHEART

B•••E••

BABIEST
BACKEND
BACKERS
BADDEBT
BADDEED
BADDEST
BADGERS
BADNESS
BADNEWS
BAFFERS
BAGGERS
BAGWELL
BAHREIN
BAILEES
BAILERS
BAITERS
BALDEST
BALEENS
BALKERS
BALLETS
BANDEAU
BANDERA
BANDERS
BANGERS
BANKERS
BANNERS
BANTERS
BARBEAU
BARBELL
BARBERA
BARBERS
BARBETS
BARDEEN
BARGEIN
BARGERS
BARKEEP
BARKERS
BARLESS
BARLEYS
BARNEYS
BARRELS
BARRENS
BARRETS
BARRETT
BARTEND
BARTERS
BASHERS
BASKETS
BASKETT
BASSETS
BASSETT
BASTERS
BATHERS
BATNEXT
BATTENS
BATTERS
BATTERY
BAWLERS
BAYLEAF
BBQBEEF
BEADERS
BEAHERO
BEAKERS
BEAMERS
BEANERY
BEARERS
BEATERS
BEAVERS
BECKETT
BEDLESS
BEDREST
BEEBEES
BEEGEES
BEEMERS
BEEPERS
BEEZERS
BEHRENS
BELIEFS
BELIERS
BELIEVE
BELLEAU
BELLEEK
BELTERS
BENDERS
BENNETT
BENZELL
BENZENE
BEQUEST
BERBERS
BERGERE
BERNESE
BERSERK
BESEECH
BESIEGE
BESMEAR
BESPEAK
BESSELL
BETHELS
BETHERE
BETTERS
BETWEEN
BEZIERS
BIBBERS
BIBLESS
BICKERS
BIDDERS
BIGBEAR
BIGBEAT
BIGBEND
BIGBETS
BIGDEAL
BIGFEET
BIGGERS
BIGGEST
BIGHEAD
BIGJERK
BIGLEAD
BIGMEAL
BIGMESS
BIGNESS
BIGNEWS
BIGTENT
BILKERS
BILLERS
BILLETS
BINDERS
BINDERY
BINGERS
BIOTECH
BIRDERS
BIRLERS
BISSELL
BITLESS
BITTERN
BITTERS
BLADERS
BLAKELY
BLAMEON
BLAMERS
BLAZERS
BLAZEUP
BLOWERS
BOATELS
BOATERS
BOBBERS
BOBWEIR
BOILERS
BOISEID
BOKKENS
BOLDEST
BOLTERS
BOMBECK
BOMBERS
BONDERS
BONHEUR
BONIEST
BONKERS
BONNETS
BOOKEND
BOOKERS
BOOKERT
BOOLEAN
BOOMERS
BOOTEES
BOOTERS
BOOTERY
BOOZERS
BOPPERS
BORDERS
BORNEAN
BORNEUP
BOSWELL
BOTHERS
BOTREES
BOTTEGA
BOWHEAD
BOWLERS
BOWLESS
BOWYERS
BOXBEDS
BOXIEST
BOXSEAT
BOXSETS
BRACERO
BRACERS
BRACEUP
BRALESS
BRAVELY
BRAVERY
BRAVEST
BRAYERS
BRAZENS
BREVETS
BREWERS
BREWERY
BREYERS
BRIBEES
BRIBERS
BRIBERY
BRINERS
BROKEIN
BROKERS
BROKEUP
BRUBECK
BRUNETS
BRUTELY
BUCKERS
BUCKETS
BUCKEYE
BUDDERS
BUDGERS
BUDGETS
BUDLESS
BUFFERS
BUFFEST
BUFFETS
BUFFETT
BUGBEAR
BUGLERS
BULLETS
BUMDEAL
BUMLEGS
BUMMERS
BUMPERS
BUNGEES
BUNKERS
BUNTERS
BUNUELO
BURDENS
BURGEES
BURGEON
BURGERS
BURGESS
BURIERS
BURLERS
BURMESE
BURNERS
BURNETT
BUSCEMI
BUSHELS
BUSHERS
BUSIEST
BUSKERS
BUSSERS
BUSTERS
BUTLERS
BUTTEMT
BUTTERS
BUTTERY
BUZZELL
BUZZERS
BYANECK
BYTHEBY

B••••E•

BABBLED
BABBLER
BABBLES
BADAREA
BADDEED
BADDIES
BADIDEA
BADLIES
BADOMEN
BAFFIES
BAFFLED
BAFFLER
BAFFLES
BAGGIER
BAGGIES
BAHAMEN
BAILEES
BAINTER
BALASES
BALDIES
BALKIER
BALLMER
BALLUET
BALMIER
BALONEY
BAMMIES
BANACEK
BANALER
BANANES
BANDIED
BANDIER
BANDIES
BANDLET
BANGLED
BANGLES
BANJOES
BANKFEE
BANQUES
BANQUET
BANSHEE
BARBIES
BARDEEN
BAREGES
BARITES
BARKEEP
BARKIER
BARKLEY
BARMIER
BARNRED
BARONET
BARQUES
BARRIER
BARTLES
BARTLET
BASEMEN
BASETEN
BASQUES
BASSIER
BATCHED
BATCHES
BATIKED
BATSMEN
BATTIER
BATTLED
BATTLER
BATTLES
BAUBLES
BAULKED
BAULKER
BAWDIER
BAYAREA
BAYONET
BAYTREE
BBQBEEF
BEACHED
BEACHES
BEADIER
BEADLES
BEAGLES
BEAMIER
BEANIES
BEARDED
BEASLEY
BEATLES
BECOMES
BEDAZED
BEDAZES
BEDEWED
BEDIZEN
BEDLOES
BEEBEES
BEECHEN
BEECHER
BEECHES
BEEFIER
BEEFTEA
BEEGEES
BEERIER
BEERKEG
BEETIER
BEETLES
BEETRED
BEETREE
BEHAVED
BEHAVES
BEIGNES
BEIGNET
BEJEWEL
BELATED
BELAYED
BELAYER
BELCHED
BELCHER
BELCHES
BELEVEN
BELLEEK
BELLIED
BELLIES
BELLMEN
BELOVED
BEMIRED
BEMIRES
BEMUSED
BEMUSES
BENARES
BENCHED
BENCHER
BENCHES
BENDIER
BENOTED
BENOTES
BENTLEY
BENTSEN
BEQUIET
BERATED
BERATER
BERATES
BERKLEY
BERKNER
BERNSEN
BERRIED
BERRIES
BERTHED
BESIDES
BESTBET
BESTMEN
BESTREW
BETAKEN
BETAKES
BETIDED
BETIDES
BETIMES
BETOKEN
BETTGER
BETWEEN
BEURRES
BEVELED
BEVELER
BEWARED
BEWARES
BIALIES
BIASSED
BIASSES
BIDDIES
BIGAPES
BIGEYED
BIGEYES
BIGFEET
BIGGIES
BIGIDEA
BIGLIES
BIGONES
BIGOTED
BIGTOES
BILEVEL
BILGIER
BILLIES
BILOBED
BIMBOES
BINDLES
BINGLES
BINGOES
BIOFUEL
BIRCHED
BIRCHEN
BIRCHES
BIRDIED
BIRDIES
BIRDMEN
BIREMES
BIRTHED
BISHKEK
BISQUES
BITSIER
BITTIER
BLABBED
BLABBER
BLACKED
BLACKEN
BLACKER
BLADDER
BLAKLEY
BLANDER
BLANKED
BLANKER
BLANKET
BLARNEY
BLASTED
BLASTER
BLATHER
BLATTED
BLEAKER
BLEARED
BLEATED
BLEATER
BLEEDER
BLEEPED
BLEEPER
BLENDED
BLENDER
BLENDES
BLESSED
BLESSER
BLESSES
BLINDED
BLINDER
BLINKED
BLINKER
BLIPPED
BLISSED
BLISSES
BLISTER
BLITHER
BLITZED
BLITZEN
BLITZER
BLITZES
BLOATED
BLOBBED
BLOCKED
BLOCKER
BLOGGED
BLOGGER
BLONDER
BLONDES
BLOODED
BLOOMED
BLOOMER
BLOOPED
BLOOPER
BLOTTED
BLOTTER
BLOUSED
BLOUSES
BLOWIER
BLOWZED
BLUBBER
BLUDGED
BLUDGER
BLUDGES
BLUEHEN
BLUERED
BLUFFED
BLUFFER
BLUNDEN
BLUNDER
BLUNTED
BLUNTER
BLURBER
BLURRED
BLURTED
BLURTER
BLUSHED
BLUSHER
BLUSHES
BLUSTER
BLYNKEN
BMOVIES
BOARDED
BOARDER
BOASTED
BOASTER
BOATMEN
BOBATEA
BOBBIES
BOBBLED
BOBBLER
BOBBLES
BOBBSEY
BOBGOEN
BOBSLED
BOCCIES
BOCHNER
BODEREK
BODICES
BOGEYED
BOGGIER
BOGGLED
BOGGLER
BOGGLES
BOGYMEN
BOLIDES
BOLSTER
BOLUSES
BOMBLET
BONDMEN
BONELET
BONESET
BONEYER
BONGOES
BONNIER
BONUSES
BOOBIES
BOODLES
BOOGIED
BOOGIES
BOOKIES
BOOKLET
BOOKMEN
BOOMIER
BOOMLET
BOONIES
BOOSLER
BOOSTED
BOOSTER
BOOTEES
BOOTIES
BOOTLEG
BOOZIER
BORATES
BORIDES
BOSOMED
BOSSIER
BOSSMEN
BOTCHED
BOTCHER
BOTCHES
BOTREES
BOTTLED
BOTTLER
BOTTLES
BOUCHER
BOUCHES
BOUFFES
BOUGHED
BOULDER
BOUNCED
BOUNCER
BOUNCES
BOUNDED
BOUNDER
BOUQUET
BOURGET
BOURSES
BOUVIER
BOVINES
BOWDLER
BOWERED
BOWTIES
BOXSTEP
BOXSTER
BPLUSES
BRACKEN
BRACKET
BRADLEE
BRADLEY
BRAEDEN
BRAGGED
BRAGGER
BRAIDED
BRAIDER
BRAINED
BRAINER
BRAISED

BRAISES
BRAMLEY
BRANDED
BRANDER
BRASHER
BRASHES
BRASIER
BRASSES
BRAVOED
BRAVOES
BRAWLED
BRAWLER
BRAWLEY
BRAZIER
BREADED
BREADER
BREAKER
BREEDER
BREEZED
BREEZES
BRENDEL
BRENNER
BRIBEES
BRICKED
BRIDGED
BRIDGER
BRIDGES
BRIDGET
BRIDLED
BRIDLER
BRIDLES
BRIEFED
BRIEFER
BRIMLEY
BRIMMED
BRIMMER
BRINGER
BRINIER
BRINKER
BRIQUET
BRISKED
BRISKER
BRISKET
BRITNEY
BRITTEN
BROADEN
BROADER
BRODIES
BRODKEY
BROGUES
BROIDER
BROILED
BROILER
BRONTES
BRONWEN
BRONZED
BRONZER
BRONZES
BROODED
BROODER
BROOKED
BROOMED
BROSSES
BROTHER
BROWNED
BROWNER
BROWSED
BROWSER
BROWSES
BRUEGEL
BRUISED
BRUISER
BRUISES
BRUITED
BRUMMEL
BRUSHED
BRUSHER
BRUSHES
BRYNNER
BUBBLED
BUBBLES
BUCHNER
BUCKLED
BUCKLES
BUCKLEY
BUCKNER
BUCKOES
BUDDIED
BUDDIES
BUDGIES
BUELLER
BUGEYED
BUGFREE
BUGGIER
BUGGIES
BUGGLES
BUILDER
BUJONES
BULBLET
BULGIER
BULKIER
BULLIED
BULLIES
BULLPEN
BUMBLED
BUMBLER
BUMBLES
BUMPIER
BUNCHED
BUNCHES
BUNCOED
BUNDLED
BUNDLER
BUNDLES
BUNGEES
BUNGLED
BUNGLER
BUNGLES
BUNKBED
BUNKOED
BUNNIES
BURBLED
BURBLER
BURBLES
BURGEES
BURGHER
BURGLED
BURGLES
BURLIER
BURNLEY
BURRIER
BURSTER
BUSBIES
BUSHIER
BUSHMEN
BUSTIER
BUSTLED
BUSTLER
BUSTLES
BUSYBEE
BUTANES
BUTCHER
BUTCHES
BUTENES
BUZZIER
BYEBYES
BYFIVES
BYGONES
BYLINED
BYLINER
BYLINES
BYNAMES

B•••••E

BAALITE
BABBAGE
BABETTE
BACCHAE
BACKHOE
BADCASE
BADJOKE
BADLOVE
BADMOVE
BADNAME
BADTIME
BAGGAGE
BAGLIKE
BAGPIPE
BALANCE
BALLADE
BALLONE
BANDAGE
BANKFEE
BANKONE
BANSHEE
BAPTISE
BAPTIZE
BARBATE
BARBULE
BARCODE
BARNONE
BAROQUE
BARRAGE
BARWARE
BASSALE
BATISTE
BATLIKE
BAUXITE
BAYONNE
BAYTREE
BEASTIE
BEATSME
BEATTIE
BEBRAVE
BECAUSE
BEDLIKE
BEDMATE
BEDRAPE
BEDSIDE
BEDTIME
BEEHIVE
BEELIKE
BEELINE
BEETREE
BEGRIME
BEGUILE
BEGUINE
BEHOOVE
BELDAME
BELIEVE
BELTANE
BENBLUE
BENZENE
BEREAVE
BERGERE
BERNESE
BEROWNE
BESIEGE
BESPOKE
BESTONE
BETHERE
BETHUNE
BEYONCE
BEZIQUE
BIBLIKE
BICORNE
BICYCLE
BIGBLUE
BIGFIVE
BIGGAME
BIGJAKE
BIGLOVE
BIGNAME
BIGNOSE
BIGSALE
BIGTIME
BILLNYE
BINOCHE
BIOCIDE
BIOLITE
BIOTITE
BIOTYPE
BIPLANE
BISTATE
BITROLE
BIVALVE
BIZARRE
BLACKIE
BLANCHE
BLEDSOE
BLIMPIE
BLINTZE
BLONDIE
BLUEICE
BOBDOLE
BOBHOPE
BOBKANE
BOGARDE
BOGHOLE
BOLATIE
BOLOTIE
BONAIRE
BONDAGE
BONFIRE
BOOPSIE
BORZAGE
BOSCAGE
BOWLIKE
BOWLINE
BOXKITE
BOXLIKE
BOYLIKE
BRADLEE
BRAILLE
BRAMBLE
BRASIZE
BRASSIE
BRATTLE
BREATHE
BREWAGE
BRICKLE
BRIGADE
BRINDLE
BRIOCHE
BRISTLE
BRITTLE
BROCADE
BROMATE
BROMIDE
BROMINE
BROWNIE
BRUSQUE
BTWELVE
BUCKEYE
BUDLIKE
BUDTIME
BUDVASE
BUGFREE
BURBAGE
BURETTE
BURMESE
BUSFARE
BUSLANE
BUSLINE
BUSRIDE
BUSYBEE
BUYABLE
BUYTIME
BYAMILE
BYANOSE
BYFORCE
BYPHONE

•BE••••

ABELARD
ABETTAL
ABETTED
ABETTER
ABETTOR
ABEYANT
IBEGYOU
IBERIAN
OBELISE
OBELISK
OBELIZE
OBENTOS
OBERLIN
OBESELY
OBESITY
OBEYERS
OBEYING

•B•E•••

ABREAST
ABSENCE
ABSENTS
OBJECTS
OBSERVE
OBTESTS
OBVERSE
OBVERTS
WBYEATS

•B••E••

ABASERS
ABATERS
ABCDEFG
ABCNEWS
ABIDEBY
ABIDERS
ABILENE
ABUSERS
BBQBEEF
CBSNEWS
EBAYERS
NBATEAM
NBCNEWS
OBESELY
OBEYERS
OBSCENE
OBSNEAK

•B•••E•

ABASHED
ABASHES
ABDOMEN
ABDUCED
ABDUCES
ABETTED
ABETTER
ABJURED
ABJURER
ABJURES
ABLATED
ABLATES
ABORTED
ABRADED
ABRADER
ABRADES
ABRILES
ABUTTED
ABUTTER
ABYSSES
BBQBEEF
EBANKED
EBONIES
OBLATES
OBLIGED
OBLIGEE
OBLIGER
OBLIGES
OBTUSER

•B••••E

ABALONE
ABILENE
ABOLLAE
ABRIDGE
ABSCISE
ABSENCE
ABSOLVE
ABUSIVE
EBBTIDE
EBONITE
EBONIZE
EBWHITE
FBICASE
FBIFILE
MBABANE
NBAGAME
NBALIVE
NBCBLUE
OBELISE
OBELIZE
OBLIGEE
OBLIQUE
OBSCENE
OBSCURE
OBSERVE
OBTRUDE
OBVERSE
OBVIATE
VBLOUSE

••BE•••

ALBEDOS
ALBENIZ
ALBERTA
ALBERTI
ALBERTO
ANBESOL
AUBERGE
BABENCO
BABETTE
BIBELOT
CABEZAS
DEBEARD
DEBEERS
ELBERTA
FABERGE
FIBERED
GIBESAT
GOBELIN
GOBELOW
HIBERNO
JIBEDAT
JIBESAT
KUBELIK
LABELED
LABELER
LABELLE
LIBELED
LIBELEE
LIBELER
LIBERAL
LIBERIA
LIBERTE
LIBERTY
LUBEJOB
PUBERTY
REBECCA
REBEGAN
REBEGIN
REBEGUN
REBEKAH
REBENDS
RIBEYES
ROBERTA
ROBERTE
ROBERTF
ROBERTH
ROBERTI
ROBERTO
ROBERTS
ROBESON
RUBELLA
RUBEOLA
SABERED
SIBERIA
SOBERED
SOBERER
SOBERLY
SUBECHO
TIBETAN
TOBEHAD
TUBEPAN
TUBETOP
UMBERED
UMBERTO
UNBEARD
UNBELDI
UNBELTS
UNBENCH
UNBENDS
UNBERTH
UNBESET
UPBEARS
UPBEATS
WOBEGON

••B•E••

AMBIENS
AMBIENT
AMBLERS
BABIEST
BIBBERS
BIBLESS
BOBBERS
BOBWEIR
CABLERS
CABLETS
CABLETV
COBLENZ
COBWEBS
DABBERS
DEBEERS
DEBRETT
DEBTEES
DUBBERS
DUBIETY
EMBLEMS
FABBEST
FABLERS
FEBRERO
FIBBERS
GABBERS
GABFEST
GIBBERS
GIBLETS
GOBLETS
HEBREWS
HUBBELL
INBREED
IOBJECT
JABBERS
JOBBERS
JOBBERY
JOBLESS
KOBLENZ
LABFEES
LABTECH
LABTEST
LIBBERS
LOBBERS
LUBBERS
MOBBERS
NABBERS
NIBLETS
NOBLEST
NUBBERS
ONBREAK
OOBLECK
ORBLESS
RABBETS
REBREAK
REBREED
REBREWS
RIBBERS
RIBLESS
RIBLETS
RIBMEAT
ROBBERS
ROBBERY
RUBBERS
RUBBERY
SOBBERS
SUBCELL
SUBDEBS
SUBHEAD
SUBJECT
SUBLETS
SUBNETS
SUBSECT
SUBSETS
SUBTEEN
SUBTEND
SUBTEXT
SUBVENE
SUBVERT
SUBZERO
TABKEYS
TABLEAU
TABLETS
TABSETS
TIBBETT
UNBLENT
UNBLEST
WEBFEET
WEBLESS

••B••E•

ALBIREO
ALBUMEN
AMBRIES
ARBACES
ARBITER
ARBOLES
ARBORED
AUBADES
BABBLED
BABBLER
BABBLES
BOBATEA
BOBBIES
BOBBLED
BOBBLER
BOBBLES
BOBBSEY
BOBGOEN
BOBSLED
BUBBLED
BUBBLES
CABARET
CABBIES
CABINET
COBBLED
COBBLER
COBBLES
COBUYER
CUBAGES
CUBBIES
DABBLED
DABBLER
DABBLES
DEBAKEY
DEBASED
DEBASER
DEBASES
DEBATED
DEBATER
DEBATES
DEBITED
DEBONED
DEBONES
DEBRIEF
DEBTEES
DEBUSES
DEBUTED
DIBBLED
DIBBLER
DIBBLES
ELBOWED
ELBOWER
EMBAYED
EMBOWER
EMBRUED
EMBRUES
FABARES
FIBERED
FIBIGER
FIBSTER
FUBSIER
GABBIER
GABBLED
GABBLES
GABRIEL
GIBLUES
GIBUSES
GOBBLED
GOBBLER
GOBBLES
GOBYSEA
HABITED
HIBBLER
HOBBIES
HOBBLED
HOBBLER
HOBBLES
HOBOKEN
HUBBIES
IMBIBED
IMBIBER
IMBIBES
IMBORED
IMBRUED
IMBRUES
INBOXES
INBREED
INBRIEF
JUBILEE
KIBBLED
KIBBLES
LABELED
LABELER
LABFEES
LABORED
LABORER
LIBELED
LIBELEE
LIBELER
LOBATED
LOBBIED
LOBBIES
LOBBYER
LOBSTER
LOBULES
MOBILES
MOBSTER
MRBONES
NIBBLED
NIBBLER
NIBBLES
NOBBIER
NUBBIER
NUBBLES
ORBITED
ORBITER
PEBBLED
PEBBLES
POBOXES
RABBLED
RABBLES
REBAKED
REBAKES
REBALED
REBALES
REBATED
REBATER
REBATES
REBORED
REBORES
REBOTES
REBOXED
REBOXES
REBREED
REBUKED
REBUKER
REBUKES
REBUSES
RIBBIER
RIBBIES
RIBEYES
ROBBNEN
RUBBLES
RUBYDEE
RUBYRED
SABERED
SABINES
SOBERED
SOBERER
SUBAREA
SUBDUED
SUBDUER
SUBDUES
SUBIDEA
SUBITEM
SUBTEEN
SUBTLER
TABARET
TABBIES
TABOOED
TABORET
TUBBIER
TUBULES
UMBERED
UMBRIEL
UNBAKED
UNBALED
UNBALES
UNBARED
UNBARES
UNBASED
UNBATED
UNBESET
UNBLUED
UNBONED
UNBORED
UNBOWED
UNBOXED
UNBOXES
UNBRIEF
URBANER
WEBBIER
WEBFEET
WEBSTER
WEBTOED
WOBBLED
WOBBLER
WOBBLES

••B•••E

ALBSURE
AMBROSE
AUBERGE
BABBAGE
BABETTE
BEBRAVE
BIBLIKE
BOBDOLE
BOBHOPE
BOBKANE
CABALLE
CABBAGE
CABFARE
CABOOSE
CABRIDE
CUBICLE
DEBACLE
DEBARGE
DEBOITE
DEBOULE
DUBUQUE
EBBTIDE
EMBLAZE
EMBOITE
EMBRACE
FABERGE
FEBRILE
FIBULAE
GOBROKE
HABITUE
IDBADGE
IMBROKE
JUBILEE
LABELLE
LABIATE
LABMICE
LABTUBE
LIBELEE
LIBERTE
MCBRIDE
MOBRULE
NEBULAE
NIBLIKE
ORBLIKE
OSBORNE
PUBGAME
REBASTE
REBATHE
REBRACE
REBROKE
RIBCAGE
RIBLIKE
ROBERTE
ROBLOWE
RUBYDEE
SUBBASE
SUBCASE
SUBCODE
SUBDATE
SUBFILE
SUBLIME
SUBRACE
SUBSIDE
SUBSUME
SUBTONE
SUBTYPE
SUBVENE
SUBZONE
TOBLAME
TUBLIKE
UMBRAGE
UNBLADE
UNBORNE
UNBRACE
UNBRAKE
UNBRAVE
UNBROKE
UPBORNE
VIBRATE
WEBLIKE
WEBPAGE
WEBSITE
WEBZINE
ZEBRINE

•••BE••

ANTBEAR
ARLBERG
ASHBERY
BARBEAU
BARBELL
BARBERA
BARBERS
BARBETS
BBQBEEF
BEEBEES
BERBERS
BIBBERS
BIGBEAR
BIGBEAT
BIGBEND
BIGBETS
BOBBERS

BOMBECK
BOMBERS
BOXBEDS
BRIBEES
BRIBERS
BRIBERY
BRUBECK
BUGBEAR
CAMBERS
CATBEDS
CATBERT
COLBERT
COMBERS
CORBELS
CORBETT
COWBELL
CUMBERS
DABBERS
DAUBERS
DAYBEDS
DELBERT
DILBERT
DOGBEDS
DOGBERT
DUBBERS
DUMBEST
ESOBESO
FABBEST
FANBELT
FIBBERS
FILBERT
FORBEAR
FREBERG
GABBERS
GETBEAT
GETBENT
GIBBERS
GILBERT
GIMBELS
GOOBERS
GOTBEAT
GUNBELT
HADBEEN
HADBEST
HASBEEN
HERBERT
HILBERT
HOLBEIN
HOLBERG
HOTBEDS
HOWBEIT
HUBBELL
HUMBERT
ICEBEER
ICEBERG
IONBEAM
ISABEAU
ITSBEST
JABBERS
JAMBEAU
JIMBEAM
JOBBERS
JOBBERY
JROBERT
LAMBEAU
LAMBENT
LAMBERT
LAMBETH
LAPBELT
LIBBERS
LIMBERS
LISBETH
LOBBERS
LOWBEAM
LUBBERS
LUMBERS
MACBETH
MAYBESO
MEMBERS
MOBBERS
MOEBERG
NABBERS
NEWBERN
NEWBERY
NORBERT
NOTBEEN
NUBBERS
NUMBERS
NUMBEST
OFFBEAT
OLDBEAN
ONEBELL
OUTBEAM
OUTBEGS
OUTBEND
PACBELL
PEABEAN
PETBEAR
PROBERS
RABBETS
RATBERT
REUBENS
RIBBERS
ROBBERS
ROBBERY
ROMBERG
ROYBEAN
RUBBERS
RUBBERY
RYEBEER
SEABEDS
SEABEES
SHEBEAR
SHUBERT
SOBBERS
SORBETS
SOYBEAN
SUNBEAM
SUNBELT
TARBELL
THEBEAR
THEBELL
THEBEST
TIBBETT
TIEBEAM
TIMBERS
TIMBERY
TRABERT
TRIBECA
UNOBESE
VERBENA
WAXBEAN
WILBERT
YASBECK
ZAMBEZI

•••B•E•

ALIBIED
ARABLES
BABBLED
BABBLER
BABBLES
BARBIES
BAUBLES
BBQBEEF
BEEBEES
BIMBOES
BLABBED
BLABBER
BLOBBED
BLUBBER
BOBBIES
BOBBLED
BOBBLER
BOBBLES
BOBBSEY
BOMBLET
BOOBIES
BRIBEES
BUBBLED
BUBBLES
BULBLET
BUMBLED
BUMBLER
BUMBLES
BURBLED
BURBLER
BURBLES
BUSBIES
BYEBYES
CABBIES
CLABBER
CLOBBER
CLUBBED
CLUBBER
CLUBMED
COBBLED
COBBLER
COBBLES
COMBIEN
CRABBED
CRABBER
CRIBBED
CRIBBER
CUBBIES
DABBLED
DABBLER
DABBLES
DERBIES
DIABLES
DIBBLED
DIBBLER
DIBBLES
DOUBLEA
DOUBLEB
DOUBLEC
DOUBLED
DOUBLEE
DOUBLEF
DOUBLEG
DOUBLEH
DOUBLEI
DOUBLEJ
DOUBLEK
DOUBLEL
DOUBLEM
DOUBLEN
DOUBLEO
DOUBLEP
DOUBLEQ
DOUBLER
DOUBLES
DOUBLET
DOUBLEU
DOUBLEV
DOUBLEW
DOUBLEX
DOUBLEY
DOUBLEZ
DOUBTED
DOUBTER
DRABBER
DRIBLET
DRUBBED
DRUBBER
EDIBLES
ENABLED
ENABLER
ENABLES
FEEBLER
FLUBBED
FLUBBER
FOIBLES
FUMBLED
FUMBLER
FUMBLES
GABBIER
GABBLED
GABBLES
GAMBIER
GAMBLED
GAMBLER
GAMBLES
GARBLED
GARBLER
GARBLES
GLIBBER
GOBBLED
GOBBLER
GOBBLES
GRABBED
GRABBER
GRUBBED
GRUBBER
HADBEEN
HASBEEN
HERBIER
HERBTEA
HIBBLER
HOBBIES
HOBBLED
HOBBLER
HOBBLES
HOMBRES
HUBBIES
HUMBLED
HUMBLER
HUMBLES
ICEBEER
ILLBRED
JEEBIES
JUMBLED
JUMBLER
JUMBLES
KEEBLER
KIBBLED
KIBBLES
KNOBBED
LOBBIED
LOBBIES
LOBBYER
LOOBIES
LOWBRED
MAMBOED
MARBLED
MARBLER
MARBLES
MAXBAER
MISBREW
MUMBLED
MUMBLER
MUMBLES
MUYBIEN
NEWBIES
NIBBLED
NIBBLER
NIBBLES
NIMBLER
NOBBIER
NOMBRES
NOTBEEN
NUBBIER
NUBBLES
OUTBRED
PEBBLED
PEBBLES
PEEBLES
PROBIES
PROBLEM
RABBLED
RABBLES
RAMBLED
RAMBLER
RAMBLES
RIBBIER
RIBBIES
ROBBNEN
RUBBLES
RUMBAED
RUMBLED
RUMBLER
RUMBLES
RYEBEER
SAMBAED
SCUBAED
SEABEES
SLABBED
SLOBBER
SNUBBED
SNUBBER
STABBED
STABBER
STABLED
STABLER
STABLES
STUBBED
SWABBED
SWABBER
TABBIES
TIMBRES
TREBLED
TREBLES
TUBBIER
TUMBLED
TUMBLER
TUMBLES
TUMBREL
UNEBBED
USABLES
VONBAER
WAMBLED
WAMBLES
WARBLED
WARBLER
WARBLES
WEBBIER
WEMBLEY
WOBBLED
WOBBLER
WOBBLES
ZOMBIES

•••B••E

AIRBASE
AMIBLUE
ARMBONE
BABBAGE
BARBATE
BARBULE
BENBLUE
BIGBLUE
BURBAGE
CABBAGE
CARBIDE
CARBINE
COMBINE
COWBANE
DOGBANE
DOGBITE
DOGBONE
DOUBLEE
DRABBLE
DRIBBLE
EARBONE
EXABYTE
FANBASE
FEEBATE
FORBADE
FORBORE
FRIBBLE
GARBAGE
GLOBATE
GLOBOSE
GLOBULE
HAMBONE
HAYBALE
HENBANE
HERBAGE
HIPBONE
ICEBLUE
ILLBITE
JAWBONE
LAYBARE
LEGBONE
MBABANE
MOABITE
NBCBLUE
NIOBITE
NONBASE
OFFBASE
OILBASE
OLDBLUE
ONEBASE
ONEBYTE
OUTBAKE
PARBAKE
PREBADE
PREBAKE
PROBATE
QUIBBLE
REDBONE
SEABLUE
SKYBLUE
SORBATE
SOUBISE
STABILE
STUBBLE
SUBBASE
TAXBASE
THEBABE
TIMBALE
TMOBILE
TOYBIKE
TRIBBLE
TRIBUNE
TRIBUTE
TURBINE
TWOBASE
UNOBESE
UPABOVE
VERBOSE

••••BE•

AEROBES
ANNABEL
ANTIBES
AUNTBEE
BESTBET
BILOBED
BLABBED
BLABBER
BLOBBED
BLUBBER
BLURBER
BUNKBED
BUSYBEE
CALIBER
CAMPBED
CARIBES
CELEBES
CHAMBER
CLABBER
CLAMBER
CLIMBED
CLIMBER
CLOBBER
CLUBBED
CLUBBER
COURBET
CRABBED
CRABBER
CRIBBED
CRIBBER
CRUMBED
DECIBEL
DELIBES
DISOBEY
DONTBEE
DRABBER
DRUBBED
DRUBBER
ENROBED
ENROBES
EVENBET
FILIBEG
FLAMBED
FLAMBES
FLATBED
FLUBBED
FLUBBER
FNUMBER
FREEBEE
FRISBEE
FROEBEL
GLIBBER
GOTOBED
GRABBED
GRABBER
GRUBBED
GRUBBER
IMBIBED
IMBIBER
IMBIBES
IVTUBES
JEZEBEL
JUJUBES
KLEIBER
KNOBBED
LAKEBED
LIEABED
LOFTBED
LONGBED
MALEBEE
MIRABEL
OCTOBER
OKTOBER
OVERBED
OVERBET
PHOEBES
PLUMBED
PLUMBER
RELABEL
ROADBED
SAFEBET
SANIBEL
SCRIBED
SCRIBER
SCRIBES
SEEDBED
SHERBET
SICKBED
SIDEBET
SLABBED
SLOBBER
SLUMBER
SNUBBED
SNUBBER
SOFABED
STABBED
STABBER
STEUBEN
STROBES
STUBBED
SUREBET
SWABBED
SWABBER
TENTBED
TESTBED
THUMBED
THURBER
TOYNBEE
TRAUBEL
TWINBED
UNEBBED
UNLOBED
UNORBED
UNROBED
UNROBES
UNSOBER

••••B•E

ACTABLE
ADDABLE
ADDIBLE
AFFABLE
AMIABLE
AMOEBAE
AUDIBLE
AUNTBEE
AUSABLE
BRAMBLE
BUSYBEE
BUYABLE
CALIBRE
CAPABLE
CELEBRE
CHAMBRE
CIMABUE
CITABLE
CRUMBLE
CURABLE
DATABLE
DISABLE
DONTBEE
DRABBLE
DRIBBLE
DRYABLE
DURABLE
EATABLE
EFFABLE
ENDABLE
ENNOBLE
ENTEBBE
EQUABLE
ERRABLE
FINABLE
FIXABLE
FLYABLE
FREEBEE
FREEBIE
FRIABLE
FRIBBLE
FRISBEE
FRYABLE
FUSIBLE
GETABLE
GOODBYE
GRUMBLE
HATABLE
HIDABLE
HIRABLE
IGNOBLE
LEGIBLE
LESABRE
LIKABLE
LINABLE
LIVABLE
LOSABLE
LOVABLE
MACABRE
MAKABLE
MALEBEE
MALTBIE
MINABLE
MIXABLE
MOVABLE
MUTABLE
NAMABLE
NOTABLE
OCTOBRE
OCTUBRE
PARABLE
PAYABLE
PLIABLE
POSABLE
POTABLE
QUIBBLE
RAKABLE
RATABLE
RECABLE
RETABLE
RIDABLE
RISIBLE
SALABLE
SAVABLE
SAYABLE
SEEABLE
SHAMBLE
SIZABLE
SKIABLE
SOLUBLE
STUBBLE
STUMBLE
TAKABLE
TAMABLE
TAXABLE
TENABLE
THIMBLE
TOTABLE
TOWABLE
TOYNBEE
TREMBLE
TRIABLE
TRIBBLE
TROUBLE
TUNABLE
TVTABLE
VENABLE
VISIBLE
VOCABLE
VOLUBLE
VOTABLE
WAXABLE
WIRABLE

•••••BE

AIRTUBE
ASCRIBE
CANITBE
COULDBE
DISROBE
EARLOBE
ENTEBBE
GLORYBE
HADTOBE
HASTOBE
HEYRUBE
ICECUBE
ITMAYBE
LABTUBE
LAPROBE
LATROBE
LEAVEBE
LETITBE
LETMEBE
MICROBE
NOTTOBE
REDROBE
REPROBE
THEBABE
THEROBE
THETUBE
WANNABE
WOULDBE

B•F••••

BAFFERS
BAFFIES
BAFFING
BAFFLED
BAFFLER
BAFFLES
BEFALLS
BEFOOLS
BEFOULS
BIFFING
BIFOCAL
BOFFING
BOFFINS
BOFFOLA
BTFSPLK
BUFFALO
BUFFERS
BUFFEST
BUFFETS
BUFFETT
BUFFING
BUFFOON
BUFFSUP
BYFIVES
BYFORCE
BYFORMS

B••F•••

BADFITS
BADFORM
BAFFERS
BAFFIES
BAFFING
BAFFLED
BAFFLER
BAFFLES
BAGFULS
BALFOUR
BARFBAG
BEDFORD
BEEFALO
BEEFIER
BEEFILY
BEEFING
BEEFSUP
BEEFTEA
BELFAST
BELFORT
BIAFRAN
BIDFAIR
BIFFING
BIGFANS
BIGFEET
BIGFISH
BIGFIVE
BIGFOOT
BIGFOUR
BIOFUEL
BLUFFED
BLUFFER
BLUFFLY
BOFFING
BOFFINS
BOFFOLA
BONFIRE
BOUFFES
BOWFINS
BOXFULS
BUFFALO
BUFFERS
BUFFEST
BUFFETS
BUFFETT
BUFFING
BUFFOON
BUFFSUP
BUGFREE
BUSFARE

B•••F••

BALEFUL
BANEFUL
BANKFEE
BASHFUL
BATSFOR
BCDEFGH
BEGSFOR
BENEFIC
BENEFIT
BIDSFOR
BIRDFLU
BLOWFLY
BLUEFIN
BLUEFLU
BLUEFOX
BLUFFED
BLUFFER
BLUFFLY
BOATFUL
BODEFUL
BODYFAT
BOUFFES
BOWLFUL
BRERFOX
BRIEFED
BRIEFER
BRIEFLY
BRIMFUL
BUCKFOR
BURNFOR
BUYOFFS

B••••F•

BACKOFF
BAILIFF
BAKEOFF
BEAROFF
BEATIFY
BEATOFF
BEGSOFF
BELIEFS
BESTOFF
BINDOFF
BITEOFF
BLEWOFF
BLOWOFF
BOILOFF
BRANIFF
BUGSOFF
BURNOFF
BUYOFFS
BUYSOFF
BUZZOFF

B•••••F

BACKOFF
BAILIFF
BAKEOFF
BARANOF
BAYLEAF
BBQBEEF
BEAROFF
BEATOFF
BEGSOFF
BEOWULF
BESTOFF
BIGHALF
BINDOFF
BITEOFF
BLEWOFF
BLOWOFF
BOASTOF
BOILOFF
BRANIFF
BUGSOFF
BURNOFF
BUYSOFF
BUZZOFF
BYWAYOF

•B•F•••

FBIFILE

•B•••F•

ABCDEFG

•B••••F

BBQBEEF

••BF•••

CABFARE
CUBFANS
FABFOUR
GABFEST
JOBFAIR
LABFEES
SUBFILE
SUBFORM

TUBFULS
WEBFEET
WEBFOOT

••B•F••
CUBSFAN
REBUFFS

••B••F•
FOBSOFF
REBUFFS
RUBSOFF

••B•••F
DEBRIEF
FOBSOFF
INBRIEF
ROBERTF
RUBSOFF
UNBRIEF

•••B•F•
VERBIFY
ZOMBIFY

•••B••F
BBQBEEF
DOUBLEF

B•G••••
BAGBOYS
BAGEHOT
BAGFULS
BAGGAGE
BAGGERS
BAGGIER
BAGGIES
BAGGILY
BAGGING
BAGGINS
BAGGIRL
BAGHDAD
BAGJOBS
BAGLADY
BAGLIKE
BAGNIOS
BAGNOLD
BAGPIPE
BAGWELL
BAGWIGS
BEGANTO
BEGGARS
BEGGARY
BEGGING
BEGIRDS
BEGONIA
BEGORRA
BEGRIME
BEGSFOR
BEGSOFF
BEGUILE
BEGUINE
BIGAPES
BIGBABY
BIGBAND
BIGBANG
BIGBEAR
BIGBEAT
BIGBEND
BIGBETS
BIGBIRD
BIGBLUE
BIGBOSS
BIGBOYS
BIGCARS
BIGCATS
BIGCITY
BIGDAYS
BIGDEAL
BIGDIGS
BIGDOGS
BIGEARS
BIGEAST
BIGEASY
BIGELOW
BIGENDS
BIGEYED
BIGEYES
BIGFANS
BIGFEET
BIGFISH
BIGFIVE
BIGFOOT
BIGFOUR
BIGGAME
BIGGERS
BIGGEST
BIGGIES
BIGGIRL
BIGGISH
BIGGITY
BIGGULP
BIGGUNS
BIGHAIR
BIGHALF
BIGHAND
BIGHEAD
BIGHITS
BIGHORN
BIGHUGS
BIGIDEA
BIGJAKE
BIGJERK
BIGJOHN
BIGKIDS
BIGLEAD
BIGLIES
BIGLOTS
BIGLOVE
BIGMACS
BIGMAMA
BIGMEAL
BIGMESS
BIGNAME
BIGNESS
BIGNEWS
BIGNOSE
BIGONES
BIGOTED
BIGOTRY
BIGRIGS
BIGSALE
BIGSHOT
BIGSHOW
BIGSTAR
BIGTALK
BIGTENT
BIGTIME
BIGTOES
BIGTOPS
BIGTOWN
BIGUNIT
BIGWIGS
BIGWINS
BOGARDE
BOGARTS
BOGDOWN
BOGEYED
BOGGIER
BOGGING
BOGGISH
BOGGLED
BOGGLER
BOGGLES
BOGGUSS
BOGHOLE
BOGUSLY
BOGYMAN
BOGYMEN
BUGABOO
BUGALOO
BUGATTI
BUGBEAR
BUGBOYS
BUGEYED
BUGFREE
BUGGIER
BUGGIES
BUGGING
BUGGLES
BUGLERS
BUGLING
BUGOUTS
BUGSOFF
BUGSOUT
BYGOLLY
BYGONES

B••G•••
BADGERS
BADGIRL
BADGUYS
BAGGAGE
BAGGERS
BAGGIER
BAGGIES
BAGGILY
BAGGING
BAGGINS
BAGGIRL
BANGERS
BANGING
BANGKOK
BANGLED
BANGLES
BANGOUT
BANGSON
BANGSUP
BARGAIN
BARGEIN
BARGERS
BARGING
BATGIRL
BEAGLES
BEEGEES
BEGGARS
BEGGARY
BEGGING
BEIGNES
BEIGNET
BELGIAN
BELGIUM
BENGALI
BENGALS
BENGUNN
BEOGRAD
BERGAMO
BERGERE
BERGIUS
BERGMAN
BERGSON
BIGGAME
BIGGERS
BIGGEST
BIGGIES
BIGGIRL
BIGGISH
BIGGITY
BIGGULP
BIGGUNS
BILGIER
BINGERS
BINGHAM
BINGING
BINGLES
BINGOES
BLIGHTS
BLIGHTY
BLOGGED
BLOGGER
BOBGOEN
BOGGIER
BOGGING
BOGGISH
BOGGLED
BOGGLER
BOGGLES
BOGGUSS
BONGING
BONGOES
BOOGIED
BOOGIES
BORGIAS
BORGLUM
BOUGHED
BRAGGED
BRAGGER
BRIGADE
BRIGAND
BRIGHAM
BRIGHTS
BROGANS
BROGUES
BUDGERS
BUDGETS
BUDGIES
BUDGING
BUGGIER
BUGGIES
BUGGING
BUGGLES
BULGARI
BULGARS
BULGHUR
BULGIER
BULGING
BULGURS
BUNGEES
BUNGING
BUNGLED
BUNGLER
BUNGLES
BURGEES
BURGEON
BURGERS
BURGESS
BURGHER
BURGLAR
BURGLED
BURGLES
BURGOOS
BUSGIRL
BUTGOOD

B•••G••
BABYGAP
BADEGGS
BAREGES
BELUGAS
BENIGNI
BENIGNO
BERIGAN
BETTGER
BLOGGED
BLOGGER
BLOWGUN
BLUDGED
BLUDGER
BLUDGES
BODEGAS
BOLOGNA
BOURGET
BRAGGED
BRAGGER
BRENGUN
BRIDGED
BRIDGER
BRIDGES
BRIDGET
BRINGER
BRINGIN
BRINGIT
BRINGON
BRINGTO
BRINGUP
BROUGHT
BRUEGEL
BURPGUN
BYRIGHT

B••••G•
BABBAGE
BADDOGS
BADEGGS
BADSIGN
BAGGAGE
BAGWIGS
BANDAGE
BARRAGE
BCDEFGH
BEDBUGS
BELONGS
BESIEGE
BIGDIGS
BIGDOGS
BIGHUGS
BIGRIGS
BIGWIGS
BIOLOGY
BLTTOGO
BLUINGS
BODINGS
BOEINGS
BONDAGE
BORINGS
BOROUGH
BORZAGE
BOSCAGE
BOTTEGA
BRANAGH
BREWAGE
BUMLEGS
BURBAGE
BYJINGO

B•••••G
BABYING
BACHING
BACKING
BACKLOG
BAFFING
BAGGING
BAILING
BAITING
BALDING
BALKING
BAMMING
BANDING
BANGING
BANKING
BANNING
BANTING
BARBING
BARFBAG
BARGING
BARKING
BARNING
BARRING
BASHING
BASKING
BASTING
BATHING
BATTING
BATWING
BAWLING
BEADING
BEAMING
BEANBAG
BEANING
BEARHUG
BEARING
BEATING
BEDDING
BEEFING
BEEPING
BEERKEG
BEERMUG
BEGGING
BEHRING
BEIJING
BELLING
BELTBAG
BELTING
BELYING
BENDING
BENNING
BERMING
BESTING
BETTING
BIASING
BIBBING
BIBLIOG
BIDDING
BIFFING
BIGBANG
BILKING
BILLING
BINDING
BINGING
BINNING
BIRDDOG
BIRDING
BIRLING
BIRRING
BITTING
BLADING
BLAMING
BLARING
BLAZING
BLOWING
BLUEING
BOATING
BOBBING
BOFFING
BOGGING
BOILING
BOLLING
BOLTING
BOMBING
BONDING
BONGING
BONKING
BOOKBAG
BOOKING
BOOMING
BOOTING
BOOTLEG
BOOZING
BOPPING
BORKING
BORLAUG
BOSSING
BOWLING
BRACING
BRAKING
BRAVING
BRAYING
BRAZING
BREWING
BRIBING
BRILLIG
BRINING
BRUXING
BUCKING
BUDDING
BUDGING
BUFFING
BUGGING
BUGLING
BULGING
BULKING
BULLDOG
BULLING
BUMMING
BUMPING
BUNGING
BUNKING
BUNNING
BUNTING
BUOYING
BURLING
BURNING
BURPING
BURRING
BURYING
BUSHHOG
BUSHING
BUSHPIG
BUSKING
BUSSING
BUSTING
BUSYING
BUTTING
BUZZING

•B•G•••
ABIGAIL
IBEGYOU
NBAGAME

•B••G••
OBLIGED
OBLIGEE
OBLIGER
OBLIGES
OBLIGOR

•B•••G•
ABRIDGE
OBLONGS

•B••••G
ABASING
ABATING
ABCDEFG
ABIDING
ABUSING
OBEYING

••BG•••
BOBGOEN
PUBGAME
SUBGOAL
SUBGODS

••B•G••
BABYGAP
CUBAGES
FIBIGER
REBEGAN
REBEGIN
REBEGUN
UNBOGGY
WOBEGON

••B••G•
AUBERGE
BABBAGE
CABBAGE
CABBAGY
CYBORGS
DEBARGE
DEBURGH
EMBARGO
FABERGE
FTBRAGG
IDBADGE
RIBCAGE
UMBRAGE
UNBOGGY
WEBLOGS
WEBPAGE

••B•••G
AMBLING
BABYING
BIBBING
BIBLIOG
BOBBING
CABBING
CABLING
CUBBING
DABBING
DUBBING
FABLING
FIBBING
FOBBING
FTBRAGG
GABBING
HIBBING
HOBOING
IMBUING
JABBING
JOBBING
LIBBING
LOBBING
MOBBING
NABBING
RIBBING
ROBBING
RUBBING
SEBRING
SIBLING
SOBBING
SUBBING
SUBKING
SUBLONG
TABBING
TABLING
TABUING
TUBBING
WEBBING

•••B•G•
AIRBAGS
BABBAGE
BEDBUGS
BURBAGE
CABBAGE
CABBAGY
FLUBUGS
GARBAGE
GARBAGY
GASBAGS
GIGBAGS
GYMBAGS
HERBAGE
HUMBUGS
ICEBAGS
KITBAGS
LUMBAGO
OUTBEGS
RAGBAGS
SEABAGS
TEABAGS
THEBIGA

•••B••G
ARLBERG
BARBING
BIBBING
BIGBANG
BOBBING
BOMBING
BRIBING
CABBING
COMBING
CUBBING
CURBING
DABBING
DAUBING
DOUBLEG
DUBBING
DUMBING
FIBBING
FOBBING
FREBERG
GABBING
GARBING
GLOBING
GRABBAG
HAMBURG
HARBURG
HIBBING
HOLBERG
HOMBURG
ICEBERG
JABBING
JOBBING
LAMBING
LIBBING
LIMBING
LIMBURG
LOBBING
LONBORG
MOBBING
MOEBERG
NABBING
NEWBURG
NUMBING
OUTBRAG
PROBING
RIBBING
ROBBING
ROMBERG
RUBBING
SEABORG
SHEBANG
SIEBZIG
SOBBING
STUBING
SUBBING
TABBING
TUBBING
WARBURG
WEBBING

••••B•G
BARFBAG
BEANBAG
BELTBAG
BOOKBAG
DIRTBAG
FEEDBAG
FILIBEG
FIREBUG
FLEABAG
FOOTBAG
GAMEBAG
GOLDBUG
GOLFBAG
GRABBAG
GREWBIG
GROWBIG
HANDBAG
JUNEBUG
LADYBUG
LOSEBIG
LOSTBIG
LOVEBUG
MAILBAG
NOSEBAG
OVERBIG
PEATBOG
PILLBUG
POSTBAG
SANDBAG
TALKBIG
TOTEBAG
VERYBIG
WINDBAG
WINSBIG

BH•••••
BHUTANI

B•H••••
BAHAISM
BAHAIST
BAHAMAS
BAHAMEN
BAHIANS
BAHRAIN
BAHREIN
BEHAPPY
BEHAVED
BEHAVES
BEHEADS
BEHEARD
BEHESTS
BEHINDS
BEHOLDS
BEHOOVE
BEHRENS
BEHRING
BEHRMAN
BOHEMIA
BOHRIUM
BYHEART

B••H•••
BACHATA
BACHING
BACHMAN
BADHAIR
BADHAND
BADHATS
BAGHDAD
BARHOPS
BASHERS
BASHFUL
BASHING
BATHERS
BATHING
BATHMAT
BATHOIL
BATHTUB
BAUHAUS
BBSHOTS
BEAHERO
BECHARM
BEEHIVE
BETHANY
BETHELS
BETHERE
BETHINK
BETHUNE
BICHONS
BIGHAIR
BIGHALF
BIGHAND
BIGHEAD
BIGHITS
BIGHORN
BIGHUGS
BISHKEK
BISHOPS
BOBHOPE
BOCHNER
BOGHOLE
BOKHARA
BONHEUR
BOOHBAH
BOOHISS
BOOHOOS
BOTHERS
BOTHNIA
BOWHEAD
BOYHOOD
BRAHMAN
BRAHMAS
BRAHMIN
BSCHOOL
BUCHMAN
BUCHNER
BUKHARA
BUSHELS
BUSHERS
BUSHHOG
BUSHIDO
BUSHIER
BUSHILY
BUSHING
BUSHMAN
BUSHMEN
BUSHPIG
BUSHWAH
BYAHAIR
BYPHONE
BYTHEBY

B•••H••
BACCHAE
BACCHIC
BACCHUS
BACKHOE
BADSHOT
BAGEHOT
BALIHAI
BANSHEE
BASEHIT
BASRHIN
BATCHED
BATCHES
BEACHAM
BEACHED
BEACHES
BEARHUG
BECKHAM
BEECHAM
BEECHEN
BEECHER
BEECHES
BELCHED
BELCHER
BELCHES
BELLHOP
BENCHED
BENCHER
BENCHES
BENTHAM
BENTHOS
BERTHAS
BERTHED
BIGSHOT
BIGSHOW
BINGHAM
BIOCHIP
BIRCHED
BIRCHEN
BIRCHES
BIRTHED
BLATHER
BLIGHTS
BLIGHTY
BLITHER
BLUEHEN
BLUSHED
BLUSHER
BLUSHES
BLUSHON
BOKCHOY
BOLSHOI
BOOTHIA
BOTCHED
BOTCHER
BOTCHES
BOTCHUP
BOUCHER
BOUCHES
BOUGHED
BOWSHOT
BRASHER
BRASHES
BRASHLY
BRIGHAM

BRIGHTS
BROTHER
BRUSHED
BRUSHER
BRUSHES
BRUSHUP
BUDDHAS
BULGHUR
BUNCHED
BUNCHES
BUNCHUP
BUQSHAS
BURGHER
BUSHHOG
BUTCHER
BUTCHES

B••••H•
BELUSHI
BIANCHI
BIGJOHN
BINOCHE
BLANCHE
BLOTCHY
BORSCHT
BOWECHO
BRANCHY
BREATHE
BREATHS
BREATHY
BRIOCHE
BRONCHI
BRONCHO
BROUGHT
BYPATHS
BYRIGHT

B•••••H
BAALISH
BABYISH
BADDISH
BADITCH
BALDISH
BCDEFGH
BEAMISH
BEARISH
BEAUISH
BEDBATH
BENEATH
BESEECH
BETROTH
BEWITCH
BIGFISH
BIGGISH
BIOTECH
BISMUTH
BLEMISH
BLUEISH
BOARISH
BOGGISH
BONEASH
BOOHBAH
BOOKISH
BOORISH
BOROUGH
BRANAGH
BREADTH
BRINISH
BRITISH
BRUTISH
BULLISH
BULRUSH
BUMRUSH
BURNISH
BUSHWAH
BYBIRTH
BYCATCH
BYMOUTH

•B•H•••
BBSHOTS
EBWHITE

•B••H••
ABASHED
ABASHES
ABRAHAM

•B••••H
ABOLISH
ABROACH
ABSINTH
OBADIAH

••BH•••
BOBHOPE
DABHAND
JOBHOPS
JOBHUNT
NOBHILL
SUBHALL
SUBHEAD

••B•H••
JOBSHOP
TOBEHAD

••B••H•
HIBACHI
PWBOTHA
REBATHE
SUBECHO
TABITHA
WABASHA

••B•••H
BABYISH
BYBIRTH
CUBBISH
DEBAUCH
DEBORAH
DEBURGH
JEBBUSH
LABTECH
MOBBISH
NEBBISH
PUBLISH
QABALAH
REBEKAH
REBIRTH
REBRUSH
ROBERTH
RUBBISH
SABBATH
SUBCASH
UNBENCH
UNBERTH
YOBBISH

•••BH••
SIOBHAN

•••B•H•
NIEBUHR

•••B••H
BEDBATH
CPEBACH
CUBBISH
DOUBLEH
DYEBATH
FORBUSH
FURBISH
HARBACH
HIPBATH
HOTBATH
ICEBATH
JEBBUSH
LAMBETH
LISBETH
MACBETH
MOBBISH
MUDBATH
NEBBISH
PDQBACH
RUBBISH
SABBATH
SUNBATH
THEBUSH
YOBBISH

••••B•H
BOOHBAH
GOOMBAH
POOHBAH

BI•••••
BIAFRAN
BIALIES
BIANCHI
BIASING
BIASPLY
BIASSED
BIASSES
BIAXIAL
BIBBERS
BIBBIDI
BIBBING
BIBCOCK
BIBELOT
BIBLESS
BIBLIKE
BIBLIOG
BICARBS
BICHONS
BICKERS
BICOLOR
BICORNE
BICORNS
BICYCLE
BIDDERS
BIDDIES
BIDDING
BIDFAIR
BIDSFOR
BIENNIA
BIENTOT
BIFFING
BIFOCAL
BIGAPES
BIGBABY
BIGBAND
BIGBANG
BIGBEAR
BIGBEAT
BIGBEND
BIGBETS
BIGBIRD
BIGBLUE
BIGBOSS
BIGBOYS
BIGCARS
BIGCATS
BIGCITY
BIGDAYS
BIGDEAL
BIGDIGS
BIGDOGS
BIGEARS
BIGEAST
BIGEASY
BIGELOW
BIGENDS
BIGEYED
BIGEYES
BIGFANS
BIGFEET
BIGFISH
BIGFIVE
BIGFOOT
BIGFOUR
BIGGAME
BIGGERS
BIGGEST
BIGGIES
BIGGIRL
BIGGISH
BIGGITY
BIGGULP
BIGGUNS
BIGHAIR
BIGHALF
BIGHAND
BIGHEAD
BIGHITS
BIGHORN
BIGHUGS
BIGIDEA
BIGJAKE
BIGJERK
BIGJOHN
BIGKIDS
BIGLEAD
BIGLIES
BIGLOTS
BIGLOVE
BIGMACS
BIGMAMA
BIGMEAL
BIGMESS
BIGNAME
BIGNESS
BIGNEWS
BIGNOSE
BIGONES
BIGOTED
BIGOTRY
BIGRIGS
BIGSALE
BIGSHOT
BIGSHOW
BIGSTAR
BIGTALK
BIGTENT
BIGTIME
BIGTOES
BIGTOPS
BIGTOWN
BIGUNIT
BIGWIGS
BIGWINS
BIKEWAY
BIKINIS
BILEVEL
BILGIER
BILIOUS
BILKERS
BILKING
BILLERS
BILLETS
BILLIES
BILLING
BILLION
BILLNYE
BILLOWS
BILLOWY
BILOBED
BIMBOES
BIMETAL
BIMINIS
BIMODAL
BINDERS
BINDERY
BINDING
BINDLES
BINDOFF
BINDSTO
BINDSUP
BINGERS
BINGHAM
BINGING
BINGLES
BINGOES
BINNING
BINOCHE
BIOCHIP
BIOCIDE
BIODATA
BIOFUEL
BIOLABS
BIOLITE
BIOLOGY
BIOMASS
BIONICS
BIOPICS
BIOTECH
BIOTITE
BIOTYPE
BIPEDAL
BIPLANE
BIPOLAR
BIRCHED
BIRCHEN
BIRCHES
BIRDDOG
BIRDERS
BIRDFLU
BIRDIED
BIRDIES
BIRDING
BIRDMAN
BIRDMEN
BIREMES
BIRETTA
BIRIANI
BIRLERS
BIRLING
BIRMANS
BIRRING
BIRTHED
BIRYANI
BISCUIT
BISECTS
BISHKEK
BISHOPS
BISMUTH
BISQUES
BISSELL
BISTATE
BISTROS
BITEOFF
BITESIN
BITESON
BITESUP
BITLESS
BITMAPS
BITONAL
BITPART
BITROLE
BITSIER
BITTERN
BITTERS
BITTIER
BITTING
BIVALVE
BIVOUAC
BIZARRE
BIZARRO

B•I••••
BAILEES
BAILERS
BAILIFF
BAILING
BAILORS
BAILOUT
BAILSON
BAINTER
BAITCAR
BAITERS
BAITING
BEIGNES
BEIGNET
BEIJING
BLIGHTS
BLIGHTY
BLIMPIE
BLINDED
BLINDER
BLINDLY
BLINDTO
BLINKAT
BLINKED
BLINKER
BLINTZE
BLIPPED
BLISSED
BLISSES
BLISTER
BLITHER
BLITZED
BLITZEN
BLITZER
BLITZES
BOIARDO
BOILERS
BOILING
BOILOFF
BOILOUT
BOILSUP
BOISEID
BOITANO
BRIARDS
BRIBEES
BRIBERS
BRIBERY
BRIBING
BRICKED
BRICKLE
BRICKUP
BRIDALS
BRIDGED
BRIDGER
BRIDGES
BRIDGET
BRIDLED
BRIDLER
BRIDLES
BRIEFED
BRIEFER
BRIEFLY
BRIGADE
BRIGAND
BRIGHAM
BRIGHTS
BRILLIG
BRILLOS
BRIMFUL
BRIMLEY
BRIMMED
BRIMMER
BRINDLE
BRINERS
BRINGER
BRINGIN
BRINGIT
BRINGON
BRINGTO
BRINGUP
BRINIER
BRINING
BRINISH
BRINKER
BRIOCHE
BRIQUET
BRISKED
BRISKER
BRISKET
BRISKLY
BRISTLE
BRISTLY
BRISTOL
BRITAIN
BRITCOM
BRITISH
BRITNEY
BRITONS
BRITPOP
BRITTEN
BRITTLE
BRITTON
BUILDER
BUILDIN
BUILDON
BUILDUP
BUILTIN
BUILTON
BUILTUP
BUISSON
BUITONI

B••I•••
BABIEST
BABIYAR
BACILLI
BADIDEA
BADITCH
BAHIANS
BALIHAI
BARISTA
BARITES
BASILIC
BASILIO
BASINAL
BATIKED
BATISTA
BATISTE
BCLIONS
BEDIZEN
BEGIRDS
BEHINDS
BELIEFS
BELIERS
BELIEVE
BELINDA
BEMIRED
BEMIRES
BENICIA
BENICIO
BENIGNI
BENIGNO
BENISON
BERIGAN
BESIDES
BESIEGE
BETIDED
BETIDES
BETIMES
BEWITCH
BEZIERS
BEZIQUE
BIGIDEA
BIKINIS
BILIOUS
BIMINIS
BIRIANI
BKLIBAN
BLUINGS
BODICES
BODINGS
BOEINGS
BOLIDES
BOLIVAR
BOLIVIA
BONIATO
BONIEST
BONILLA
BONITOS
BORIDES
BORINGS
BOVINES
BOXIEST
BRAIDED
BRAIDER
BRAILLE
BRAINED
BRAINER
BRAISED
BRAISES
BROIDER
BROILED
BROILER
BRUISED
BRUISER
BRUISES
BRUITED
BUNIONS
BURIALS
BURIERS
BUSIEST
BUYINTO
BYBIRTH
BYFIVES
BYJINGO
BYLINED
BYLINER
BYLINES
BYRIGHT

B•••I••
BAALISH
BAALISM
BAALIST
BAALITE
BABBITT
BABYING
BABYISH
BACHING
BACKING
BADDIES
BADDISH
BADFITS
BADGIRL
BADLIES
BADSIGN
BADTIME
BAFFIES
BAFFING
BAGGIER
BAGGIES
BAGGILY
BAGGING
BAGGINS
BAGGIRL
BAGLIKE
BAGNIOS
BAGPIPE
BAGWIGS
BAHAISM
BAHAIST
BAILIFF
BAILING
BAITING
BALDIES
BALDING
BALDISH
BALKIER
BALKILY
BALKING
BALLIOL
BALMIER
BALMILY
BAMBIII
BAMBINA
BAMBINI
BAMBINO
BAMMIES
BAMMING
BANDIDO
BANDIED
BANDIER
BANDIES
BANDING
BANDITO
BANDITS
BANGING
BANKING
BANKITS
BANNING
BANTING
BAPTISE
BAPTISM
BAPTIST
BAPTIZE
BARBIES
BARBILL
BARBING
BARGING
BARKIER
BARKING
BARLICK
BARMIER
BARNING
BARRIER
BARRING
BARRIOS
BASHING
BASKING
BASSIER
BASSIST
BASTING
BASTION
BATGIRL
BATHING
BATLIKE
BATTIER
BATTING
BATWING
BAUXITE
BAWDIER
BAWDILY
BAWLING
BAYCITY
BBQPITS
BBQRIBS
BEADIER
BEADILY
BEADING
BEALION
BEAMIER
BEAMING
BEAMISH
BEANIES
BEANING
BEARING
BEARISH
BEATIFY
BEATING
BEAUISH
BEDDING
BEDLIKE
BEDSIDE
BEDSITS
BEDTIME
BEEFIER
BEEFILY
BEEFING
BEEHIVE
BEELIKE
BEELINE
BEEPING
BEERIER
BEETIER
BEGGING
BEGRIME
BEGUILE
BEGUINE
BEHRING
BEIJING
BELAIRS
BELGIAN
BELGIUM
BELLIED
BELLIES
BELLING
BELLINI
BELTING
BELYING
BENDIER
BENDING
BENNING
BEQUICK
BEQUIET
BERBICK
BERGIUS
BERLIOZ
BERLITZ
BERMING
BERNINA
BERNINI
BERRIED
BERRIES
BERWICK
BESTIAL
BESTILL
BESTING
BESTIRS
BETHINK
BETTING
BETWIXT
BEWAILS
BIALIES
BIASING
BIAXIAL
BIBBIDI
BIBBING
BIBLIKE
BIBLIOG
BIDDIES
BIDDING
BIFFING
BIGBIRD
BIGCITY
BIGDIGS
BIGFISH
BIGFIVE
BIGGIES
BIGGIRL
BIGGISH
BIGGITY
BIGHITS
BIGKIDS
BIGLIES
BIGRIGS
BIGTIME
BIGWIGS
BIGWINS
BILGIER
BILKING
BILLIES
BILLING
BILLION
BINDING
BINGING
BINNING
BIOCIDE
BIOLITE
BIONICS
BIOPICS
BIOTITE
BIRDIED
BIRDIES
BIRDING
BIRLING
BIRRING
BITSIER
BITTIER
BITTING
BLADING
BLAMING
BLARING
BLAZING
BLEMISH
BLERIOT
BLOWIER
BLOWING
BLUEICE
BLUEING
BLUEISH
BMOVIES
BOARISH
BOATING
BOBBIDI
BOBBIES
BOBBING
BOBBINS
BOBVILA
BOCCIES
BODKINS
BOFFING
BOFFINS
BOGGIER
BOGGING
BOGGISH
BOHRIUM
BOILING
BOLLING
BOLTING
BOMBING
BONAIRE
BONDING
BONFIRE
BONGING
BONKING
BONNIER
BONNILY
BOOBIES
BOOBIRD
BOOGIED
BOOGIES
BOOHISS
BOOKIES
BOOKIII
BOOKING
BOOKISH
BOOMIER
BOOMING
BOONIES
BOORISH
BOOTIES
BOOTING
BOOZIER
BOOZILY
BOOZING
BOPPING
BORGIAS
BORKING
BOSNIAN
BOSSIER
BOSSILY
BOSSING
BOSSISM
BOUDINS
BOUVIER
BOWFINS
BOWLIKE
BOWLINE
BOWLING
BOWTIES
BOXKITE
BOXLIKE
BOYLIKE
BRACING
BRAKING
BRANIFF
BRASIER
BRASIZE
BRAVING
BRAYING
BRAZIER
BRAZING
BREVITY
BREWING
BRIBING

BRINIER
BRINING
BRINISH
BRITISH
BRODIES
BROMIDE
BROMINE
BRUTISH
BRUXING
BRUXISM
BUCKING
BUDDIED
BUDDIES
BUDDING
BUDGIES
BUDGING
BUDLIKE
BUDTIME
BUFFING
BUGGIER
BUGGIES
BUGGING
BUGLING
BULGIER
BULGING
BULKIER
BULKING
BULLIED
BULLIES
BULLING
BULLINS
BULLION
BULLISH
BULLITT
BUMMING
BUMPIER
BUMPILY
BUMPING
BUNGING
BUNKING
BUNNIES
BUNNING
BUNTING
BUOYING
BURDICK
BURKINA
BURLIER
BURLING
BURNING
BURNISH
BURPING
BURRIER
BURRING
BURRITO
BURYING
BUSBIES
BUSGIRL
BUSHIDO
BUSHIER
BUSHILY
BUSHING
BUSKING
BUSLINE
BUSRIDE
BUSSING
BUSTIER
BUSTING
BUSYING
BUTTING
BUYTIME
BUZZIER
BUZZING
BYAMILE

B••••I•
BABYOIL
BABYSIT
BACCHIC
BACKBIT
BACKLIT
BACKSIN
BACTRIA
BADHAIR
BADTRIP
BAHRAIN
BAHREIN
BALDRIC
BALDWIN
BALMAIN
BAMBIII
BANDAID
BANZAIS
BARGAIN
BARGEIN
BARMAID
BASEHIT
BASESIX
BASILIC
BASILIO
BASRHIN
BATAVIA
BATHOIL
BATSUIT
BAVARIA
BEANDIP
BEANOIL
BEARPIT
BEASTIE
BEATNIK
BEATRIX
BEATSIT
BEATTIE
BEDELIA
BEDEVIL
BEDOUIN
BEDRAIL
BEGONIA
BELVOIR
BENAZIR
BENEFIC
BENEFIT
BENICIA
BENICIO
BERVOIX
BIDFAIR
BIENNIA
BIGHAIR
BIGUNIT
BIKINIS
BIMINIS
BIOCHIP
BISCUIT
BITESIN
BLACKIE
BLENDIN
BLENTIN
BLIMPIE
BLONDIE
BLOWNIN
BLOWSIN
BLOWSIT
BLUEFIN
BLUETIT
BOBTAIL
BOBWEIR
BODYKIT
BOHEMIA
BOISEID
BOLATIE
BOLIVIA
BOLOTIE
BONACIS
BONARIO
BONSOIR
BOOKIII
BOOKVII
BOOPSIE
BOOTHIA
BOOTSIT
BORODIN
BOROMIR
BORONIC
BORZOIS
BOSONIC
BOTANIC
BOTHNIA
BOUDOIR
BOWDOIN
BOXEDIN
BOXESIN
BRAHMIN
BRASSIE
BREAKIN
BRESCIA
BRESLIN
BRILLIG
BRINGIN
BRINGIT
BRITAIN
BROKEIN
BROWNIE
BUCOLIC
BUILDIN
BUILTIN
BUMPKIN
BURNSIN
BURNTIN
BURSTIN
BUSHPIG
BUSTRIP
BUSTSIN
BUTTSIN
BYAHAIR
BYRONIC
BYTRAIN

B•••••I
BACARDI
BACILLI
BALIHAI
BAMBIII
BAMBINI
BASENJI
BASMATI
BASSANI
BELLINI
BELUSHI
BELZONI
BENGALI
BENIGNI
BENZALI
BERNINI
BHUTANI
BIANCHI
BIBBIDI
BIRIANI
BIRYANI
BOBBIDI
BOCELLI
BOLSHOI
BONJOVI
BOOKIII
BOOKVII
BORDONI
BREWSKI
BRONCHI
BUGATTI
BUITONI
BULGARI
BURUNDI
BUSCEMI

•BI••••
ABIDEBY
ABIDERS
ABIDING
ABIDJAN
ABIGAIL
ABILENE
ABILITY
ABINTRA
ABIOTIC
ABITIBI
FBICASE
FBIFILE
IBILITY
IBIZANS
TBILISI

•B•I•••
ABRIDGE
ABRILES
ABSINTH
OBLIGED
OBLIGEE
OBLIGER
OBLIGES
OBLIGOR
OBLIQUE
OBOISTS
OBVIATE
OBVIOUS

•B••I••
ABASING
ABATING
ABIDING
ABILITY
ABITIBI
ABOLISH
ABSCISE
ABUSING
ABUSIVE
BBQPITS
BBQRIBS
EBBTIDE
EBONICS
EBONIES
EBONITE
EBONIZE
EBWHITE
FBIFILE
IBERIAN
IBILITY
NBALIVE
OBADIAH
OBELISE
OBELISK
OBELIZE
OBESITY
OBEYING
OBTAINS
TBILISI

•B•••I•
ABIGAIL
ABIOTIC
ABOUTIT
ABSTAIN
CBRADIO
OBERLIN

•B••••I
ABITIBI
ABRUZZI
TBILISI

••BI•••
ALBINOS
ALBIREO
AMBIENS
AMBIENT
ARBITER
BABIEST
BABIYAR
BYBIRTH
CABINET
CUBICAL
CUBICLE
CUBICLY
CUBISTS
CUBITAL
CUBITUS
DEBITED
DUBIETY
DUBIOUS
FIBIGER
HABILIS
HABITAT
HABITED
HABITUE
IMBIBED
IMBIBER
IMBIBES
JUBILEE
LABIALS
LABIATE
LIBIDOS
MOBILES
NABISCO
NUBIANS
NUBIRAS
ORBISON
ORBITAL
ORBITED
ORBITER
RABIDLY
REBILLS
REBINDS
REBIRTH
RUBICON
RUBIOUS
RUBITIN
SABINES
SUBIDEA
SUBITEM
TABITHA
TUBISTS
UNBINDS
VIBISTS

••B•I••
AMBLING
AMBRIES
BABBITT
BABYING
BABYISH
BIBBIDI
BIBBING
BIBLIKE
BIBLIOG
BOBBIDI
BOBBIES
BOBBING
BOBBINS
BOBVILA
CABBIES
CABBING
CABLING
CABRIDE
CABRINI
CABRIOS
CUBBIES
CUBBING
CUBBINS
CUBBISH
CUBOIDS
DABBING
DEBOITE
DEBRIEF
DOBBINS
DUBBING
DUBNIUM
EBBTIDE
EMBOITE
FABLING
FABRICS
FABRIZI
FEBRILE
FIBBING
FIBRINS
FOBBING
FTBLISS
FUBSIER
GABBIER
GABBING
GABRIEL
GOBLINS
HIBBING
HOBBIES
HOBBITS
HOBOING
HOBOISM
HUBBIES
HYBRIDS
IMBUING
INBRIEF
INBUILT
JABBING
JOBBING
KUBRICK
LABMICE
LIBBING
LOBBIED
LOBBIES
LOBBING
MCBRIDE
MOBBING
MOBBISH
MOBBISM
MOBBIST
MRBLISS
NABBING
NEBBISH
NIBLICK
NIBLIKE
NOBBIER
NOBHILL
NUBBIER
NUBBINS
ORBLIKE
PUBLICS
PUBLISH
PUBLIUS
RABBITS
RABBITT
RABBITY
REBAITS
REBOILS
REBUILD
REBUILT
RIBBIER
RIBBIES
RIBBING
RIBLIKE
ROBBING
ROBBINS
RUBBING
RUBBISH
RUBRICS
SABRINA
SEBRING
SIBLING
SOBBING
SUBBIAS
SUBBING
SUBFILE
SUBKING
SUBLIDS
SUBLIME
SUBMITS
SUBSIDE
SUBSIDY
SUBSIST
TABBIES
TABBING
TABLING
TABUING
TUBAIST
TUBBIER
TUBBING
TUBLIKE
UMBRIAN
UMBRIEL
UNBAITS
UNBRIEF
UNBUILD
UNBUILT
UPBUILD
WABBITS
WEBBIER
WEBBING
WEBLIKE
WEBSITE
WEBZINE
YOBBISH
ZEBRINE

••B••I•
ALBANIA
ALBENIZ
ALBUMIN
BABYOIL
BABYSIT
BOBTAIL
BOBWEIR
EMBROIL
FIBROID
GOBELIN
GOBYAIR
HABILIS
HEBRAIC
HOBNAIL
JOBFAIR
KABUKIS
KUBELIK
LIBERIA
REBEGIN
ROBOTIC
RUBITIN
SIBERIA
SIBYLIC
STBASIL
SUBARID
SUBJOIN
SUBSOIL
SUBUNIT
TABLOID
UNBRAID
UPBRAID
URBANII
URBANIV
WEBMAIL
ZEBRAIC
ZEBROID

••B•••I
ALBERTI
BIBBIDI
BOBBIDI
CABRINI
FABRIZI
HIBACHI
ROBERTI
TABOULI
TEBALDI
UNBELDI
URBANII
URBANVI

•••BI••
AIRBILL
ALIBIED
ANTBIRD
ARABIAN
ARABICA
ARABICS
ARABIST
ASHBINS
BABBITT
BAMBIII
BAMBINA
BAMBINI
BAMBINO
BARBIES
BARBILL
BARBING
BERBICK
BIBBIDI
BIBBING
BIGBIRD
BOBBIDI
BOBBIES
BOBBING
BOBBINS
BOMBING
BOOBIES
BOOBIRD
BRIBING
BUSBIES
CABBIES
CABBING
CARBIDE
CARBINE
CATBIRD
COMBIEN
COMBINE
COMBING
COWBIRD
CUBBIES
CUBBING
CUBBINS
CUBBISH
CUEBIDS
CUMBIAS
CURBING
DABBING
DAUBING
DERBIES
DOBBINS
DOGBITE
DUBBING
DUMBING
FIBBING
FOBBING
FORBIDS
FURBISH
GABBIER
GABBING
GAMBIAN
GAMBIER
GAMBITS
GARBING
GERBILS
GLOBING
GLOBINS
HENBITS
HERBIER
HIBBING
HOBBIES
HOBBITS
HUBBIES
IAMBICS
IAMBIST
ILLBITE
INABIND
JABBING
JAYBIRD
JEEBIES
JOBBING
LAMBING
LIBBING
LIMBING
LINBIAO
LOBBIED
LOBBIES
LOBBING
LOOBIES
LOWBIDS
MISBILL
MISBIND
MOABITE
MOBBING
MOBBISH
MOBBISM
MOBBIST
MUYBIEN
NABBING
NEBBISH
NESBITT
NEWBIES
NIOBITE
NIOBIUM
NOBBIER
NUBBIER
NUBBINS
NUMBING
OILBIRD
ONABIAS
OUTBIDS
PETBIRD
PHOBIAS
PHOBICS
PLEBIAN
PREBIDS
PREBILL
PREBIND
PROBIES
PROBING
PROBITY
RABBITS
RABBITT
RABBITY
REDBIRD
RIBBIER
RIBBIES
RIBBING
ROBBING
ROBBINS
RUBBING
RUBBISH
SEABIRD
SERBIAN
SKIBIBS
SOBBING
SOUBISE
STABILE
STUBING
SUBBIAS
SUBBING
SUNBIRD
TABBIES
TABBING
TERBIUM
THEBIGA
TIDBITS
TMOBILE
TOPBIDS
TOYBIKE
TUBBIER
TUBBING
TURBINE
TWOBITS
VERBIDS
VERBIFY
WABBITS
WAYBILL
WEBBIER
WEBBING
WEEBITS
YOBBISH
ZAMBIAN
ZOMBIES
ZOMBIFY

•••B•I•
AMEBOID
ATABOIL
BAMBIII
CAMBRIA
CAMBRIC
CHABLIS
CONBRIO
CUMBRIA
DOUBTIT
GLOBOID
HATBRIM
HOLBEIN
HOWBEIT
LAMBKIN
LEIBNIZ
PARBOIL
POTBOIL
PREBOIL
RAMBLIN
ROUBAIX
SETBAIL
SIEBZIG

•••B••I
BAMBIII
BAMBINI
BIBBIDI
BOBBIDI
DOUBLEI
ZAMBEZI
ZAMBONI

••••BI•
ACERBIC
ADHIBIT
AEROBIC
AGRIBIZ
ALDUBIN
ALEMBIC
AMOEBIC
ATEABIT
AUTOBIO
AWEEBIT
BACKBIT
CLIMBIN
COALBIN
COHABIT
CORNBIN
DEORBIT
DUSTBIN
EATABIT
EXHIBIT
EXURBIA
FEEDBIN
FORABIT
FREEBIE
GIGABIT
GREWBIG
GROWBIG
INHABIT
INHIBIT
INORBIT
JACOBIN
JUMPBID
KILOBIT
LOSEBIG
LOSTBIG
MAILBIN
MALTBIE
MEGABIT
NAMIBIA
NOTABIT
OVERBID
OVERBIG
PHILBIN
PLUMBIC
PROMBID
RAREBIT
REDEBIT
RHOMBIC
ROYGBIV
SHOWBIZ
TALKBIG
TINYBIT
UNCUBIC
VERYBIG
WASABIS
WINSBIG
WOODBIN
ZENOBIA

•••••BI
ABITIBI
ETALIBI
NAIROBI
PUNJABI
SYLLABI

B•J••••
BEJEWEL
BUJONES
BYJINGO

B••J•••
BADJOKE
BAGJOBS
BANJOES
BEIJING
BIGJAKE
BIGJERK
BIGJOHN
BONJOUR
BONJOVI

B•••J••
BANKJOB
BELLJAR
BLUEJAY

B••••J•
BASENJI

•BJ••••
ABJURED
ABJURER
ABJURES
OBJECTS

•B••J••
ABIDJAN

•B•••J•
PBANDJS

••BJ•••
IOBJECT
JOBJARS
SUBJECT
SUBJOIN

••B•J••
LUBEJOB

•••B••J
DOUBLEJ

BK•••••
BKLIBAN

B•K••••
BAKEOFF
BAKEPAN
BAKERST
BAKLAVA
BIKEWAY
BIKINIS
BOKCHOY
BOKHARA
BOKKENS
BUKHARA

B••K•••
BACKBAR
BACKBAY
BACKBIT
BACKEND
BACKERS
BACKHOE

BACKING
BACKLIT
BACKLOG
BACKLOT
BACKOFF
BACKOUT
BACKPAY
BACKROW
BACKRUB
BACKSAW
BACKSIN
BACKSUP
BACKUPS
BACKWAY
BALKANS
BALKERS
BALKIER
BALKILY
BALKING
BALKSAT
BANKERS
BANKFEE
BANKING
BANKITS
BANKJOB
BANKONE
BANKSON
BANKSUP
BARKEEP
BARKERS
BARKIER
BARKING
BARKLEY
BARKSAT
BASKETS
BASKETT
BASKING
BEAKERS
BECKETT
BECKHAM
BECKONS
BERKLEY
BERKNER
BICKERS
BIGKIDS
BILKERS
BILKING
BLAKELY
BLAKLEY
BOBKANE
BODKINS
BOKKENS
BONKERS
BONKING
BOOKBAG
BOOKEND
BOOKERS
BOOKERT
BOOKIES
BOOKIII
BOOKING
BOOKISH
BOOKLET
BOOKMAN
BOOKMEN
BOOKVII
BORKING
BOWKNOT
BOXKITE
BRAKING
BROKEIN
BROKERS
BROKEUP
BUCKERS
BUCKETS
BUCKEYE
BUCKFOR
BUCKING
BUCKLED
BUCKLES
BUCKLEY
BUCKNER
BUCKOES
BUCKRAM
BUCKSAW
BUCKSUP
BULKIER
BULKING
BULKSUP
BUNKBED
BUNKERS
BUNKING
BUNKOED
BUNKUMS
BURKINA
BUSKERS
BUSKING

B•••K••

BANGKOK
BATIKED
BAULKED
BAULKER
BEERKEG
BETAKEN
BETAKES
BETOKEN
BISHKEK
BLACKED
BLACKEN
BLACKER
BLACKIE
BLACKLY
BLANKED
BLANKER
BLANKET
BLANKLY
BLEAKER
BLEAKLY
BLINKAT
BLINKED
BLINKER
BLOCKED
BLOCKER
BLOCKUP
BLYNKEN
BODYKIT
BRACKEN
BRACKET
BREAKER
BREAKIN
BREAKUP
BRICKED
BRICKLE
BRICKUP
BRINKER
BRISKED
BRISKER
BRISKET
BRISKLY
BRODKEY
BROOKED
BUMPKIN

B••••K•

BADJOKE
BAGLIKE
BATLIKE
BAZOOKA
BEDECKS
BEDLIKE
BEELIKE
BESPOKE
BIBLIKE
BIGJAKE
BLUESKY
BOWLIKE
BOXLIKE
BOYLIKE
BREWSKI
BRODSKY
BUDLIKE
BUNRAKU
BUROAKS
BYTALKS

B•••••K

BABCOCK
BADBACK
BADLUCK
BANACEK
BANGKOK
BARLICK
BARRACK
BBQPORK
BEATNIK
BEDROCK
BELLEEK
BEQUICK
BERBICK
BERSERK
BERWICK
BESPEAK
BETHINK
BIBCOCK
BIGJERK
BIGTALK
BISHKEK
BLALOCK
BLAUBOK
BODEREK
BOMBECK
BRUBECK
BTFSPLK
BULLOCK
BULWARK
BURBANK
BURDICK
BUYBACK
BYANECK

•B••K••

EBANKED

•B••••K

BBQPORK
OBELISK
QBSNEAK

••BK•••

BOBKANE
SUBKING
TABKEYS

••B•K••

DEBAKEY
HOBOKEN
KABUKIS
NABOKOV
REBAKED
REBAKES
REBEKAH
REBUKED
REBUKER
REBUKES
UNBAKED

••B••K•

BIBLIKE
DEBARKS
DEBUNKS
DYBBUKS
EMBANKS
EMBARKS
EUBANKS
GOBROKE
IMBROKE
NIBLIKE
ORBLIKE
REBANKS
REBOOKS
REBROKE
RIBLIKE
TUBLIKE
UNBRAKE
UNBROKE
UNBULKY
WEBLIKE

••B•••K

ALBORAK
BABCOCK
BIBCOCK
GOBLANK
INBLACK
JOBBANK
JOBLOCK
KUBELIK
KUBRICK
LEBROCK
LUBBOCK
MUBARAK
NIBLICK
ONBREAK
OOBLECK
REBLOCK
REBREAK
SUBBANK
SUBTASK
UNBLOCK

•••BK••

LAMBKIN

•••B•K•

DYBBUKS
OUTBAKE
PARBAKE
PREBAKE
REEBOKS
RHEBOKS
TOYBIKE

•••B••K

ARTBOOK
BADBACK
BERBICK
BOMBECK
BRUBECK
BURBANK
BUYBACK
CUTBACK
DAYBOOK
DOUBLEK
EYEBANK
FATBACK
FINBACK
FIRBANK
FOGBANK
GETBACK
GOTBACK
HITBACK
HOGBACK
JOBBANK
JOEBUCK
JUMBUCK
KEYBANK
LAWBOOK
LAYBACK
LIEBACK
LOGBOOK
LUBBOCK
NONBANK
NONBOOK
OUTBACK
OUTBARK
OUTBULK
PAYBACK
PREBOOK
PUTBACK
RANBACK
REDBOOK
ROEBUCK
RUNBACK
SATBACK
SAWBUCK
SETBACK
SITBACK
SUBBANK
TANBARK
TAYBACK
TIEBACK
TOYBOOK
WAYBACK
WINBACK
YASBECK

••••B•K

BLAUBOK
GEMSBOK
VITEBSK

BL•••••

BLABBED
BLABBER
BLACKED
BLACKEN
BLACKER
BLACKIE
BLACKLY
BLACULA
BLADDER
BLADERS
BLADING
BLAKELY
BLAKLEY
BLALOCK
BLAMEON
BLAMERS
BLAMING
BLANCHE
BLANDER
BLANDLY
BLANKED
BLANKER
BLANKET
BLANKLY
BLANTON
BLARING
BLARNEY
BLASTED
BLASTER
BLATANT
BLATHER
BLATTED
BLAUBOK
BLAZERS
BLAZEUP
BLAZING
BLAZONS
BLEAKER
BLEAKLY
BLEARED
BLEATED
BLEATER
BLEDSOE
BLEEDER
BLEEPED
BLEEPER
BLEMISH
BLENDED
BLENDER
BLENDES
BLENDIN
BLENTIN
BLERIOT
BLESSED
BLESSER
BLESSES
BLEWOFF
BLEWOUT
BLIGHTS
BLIGHTY
BLIMPIE
BLINDED
BLINDER
BLINDLY
BLINDTO
BLINKAT
BLINKED
BLINKER
BLINTZE
BLIPPED
BLISSED
BLISSES
BLISTER
BLITHER
BLITZED
BLITZEN
BLITZER
BLITZES
BLOATED
BLOBBED
BLOCKED
BLOCKER
BLOCKUP
BLOGGED
BLOGGER
BLONDER
BLONDES
BLONDIE
BLOODED
BLOOMED
BLOOMER
BLOOPED
BLOOPER
BLOSSOM
BLOTCHY
BLOTOUT
BLOTSUP
BLOTTED
BLOTTER
BLOUSED
BLOUSES
BLOUSON
BLOWDRY
BLOWERS
BLOWFLY
BLOWGUN
BLOWIER
BLOWING
BLOWNIN
BLOWNUP
BLOWOFF
BLOWOUT
BLOWPOP
BLOWSIN
BLOWSIT
BLOWSON
BLOWSUP
BLOWUPS
BLOWZED
BLTTOGO
BLUBBER
BLUDGED
BLUDGER
BLUDGES
BLUEBOY
BLUEFIN
BLUEFLU
BLUEFOX
BLUEHEN
BLUEICE
BLUEING
BLUEISH
BLUEJAY
BLUELAW
BLUERED
BLUESKY
BLUESUN
BLUETIT
BLUFFED
BLUFFER
BLUFFLY
BLUINGS
BLUNDEN
BLUNDER
BLUNTED
BLUNTER
BLUNTLY
BLURBER
BLURRED
BLURTED
BLURTER
BLUSHED
BLUSHER
BLUSHES
BLUSHON
BLUSTER
BLYNKEN

B•L••••

BALABAN
BALANCE
BALASES
BALATAS
BALATON
BALBOAS
BALCONY
BALDEST
BALDIES
BALDING
BALDISH
BALDRIC
BALDWIN
BALEENS
BALEFUL
BALFOUR
BALIHAI
BALKANS
BALKERS
BALKIER
BALKILY
BALKING
BALKSAT
BALLADE
BALLADS
BALLARD
BALLAST
BALLBOY
BALLETS
BALLIOL
BALLMER
BALLONE
BALLOON
BALLOTS
BALLSUP
BALLTWO
BALLUET
BALMAIN
BALMIER
BALMILY
BALONEY
BALSAMS
BALSAMY
BCLIONS
BELABOR
BELAIRS
BELARUS
BELASCO
BELATED
BELAYED
BELAYER
BELCHED
BELCHER
BELCHES
BELDAME
BELDAMS
BELEVEN
BELFAST
BELFORT
BELGIAN
BELGIUM
BELIEFS
BELIERS
BELIEVE
BELINDA
BELLAMY
BELLBOY
BELLEAU
BELLEEK
BELLHOP
BELLIED
BELLIES
BELLING
BELLINI
BELLJAR
BELLLAP
BELLMAN
BELLMEN
BELLOWS
BELLSON
BELLYUP
BELMONT
BELONGS
BELOVED
BELTANE
BELTBAG
BELTERS
BELTING
BELTOUT
BELTRAN
BELTSAW
BELTSUP
BELTWAY
BELUGAS
BELUSHI
BELVOIR
BELVOUR
BELYING
BELZONI
BILEVEL
BILGIER
BILIOUS
BILKERS
BILKING
BILLERS
BILLETS
BILLIES
BILLING
BILLION
BILLNYE
BILLOWS
BILLOWY
BILOBED
BKLIBAN
BOLATIE
BOLDEST
BOLEROS
BOLIDES
BOLIVAR
BOLIVIA
BOLLING
BOLOGNA
BOLOTIE
BOLSHOI
BOLSTER
BOLTERS
BOLTING
BOLTSUP
BOLUSES
BPLUSES
BULBLET
BULBOUS
BULGARI
BULGARS
BULGHUR
BULGIER
BULGING
BULGURS
BULKIER
BULKING
BULKSUP
BULLDOG
BULLETS
BULLIED
BULLIES
BULLING
BULLINS
BULLION
BULLISH
BULLITT
BULLOCK
BULLPEN
BULLRUN
BULOVAS
BULRUSH
BULWARK
BYLINED
BYLINER
BYLINES

B••L•••

BAALISH
BAALISM
BAALIST
BAALITE
BADLAND
BADLIES
BADLOTS
BADLOVE
BADLUCK
BAGLADY
BAGLIKE
BAILEES
BAILERS
BAILIFF
BAILING
BAILORS
BAILOUT
BAILSON
BAKLAVA
BALLADE
BALLADS
BALLARD
BALLAST
BALLBOY
BALLETS
BALLIOL
BALLMER
BALLONE
BALLOON
BALLOTS
BALLSUP
BALLTWO
BALLUET
BARLESS
BARLEYS
BARLICK
BATLIKE
BAULKED
BAULKER
BAWLERS
BAWLING
BAWLOUT
BAYLEAF
BAYLORU
BAYLYNX
BDALTON
BEALION
BECLOUD
BEDLAMP
BEDLAMS
BEDLESS
BEDLIKE
BEDLOES
BEELIKE
BEELINE
BELLAMY
BELLBOY
BELLEAU
BELLEEK
BELLHOP
BELLIED
BELLIES
BELLING
BELLINI
BELLJAR
BELLLAP
BELLMAN
BELLMEN
BELLOWS
BELLSON
BELLYUP
BERLIOZ
BERLITZ
BIALIES
BIBLESS
BIBLIKE
BIBLIOG
BIGLEAD
BIGLIES
BIGLOTS
BIGLOVE
BILLERS
BILLETS
BILLIES
BILLING
BILLION
BILLNYE
BILLOWS
BILLOWY
BIOLABS
BIOLITE
BIOLOGY
BIPLANE
BIRLERS
BIRLING
BITLESS
BLALOCK
BOILERS
BOILING
BOILOFF
BOILOUT
BOILSUP
BOLLING
BOOLEAN
BORLAUG
BOULDER
BOWLERS
BOWLESS
BOWLFUL
BOWLIKE
BOWLINE
BOWLING
BOXLIKE
BOYLIKE
BRALESS
BRILLIG
BRILLOS
BUDLESS
BUDLIKE
BUELLER
BUGLERS
BUGLING
BUILDER
BUILDIN
BUILDON
BUILDUP
BUILTIN
BUILTON
BUILTUP
BULLDOG
BULLETS
BULLIED
BULLIES
BULLING
BULLINS
BULLION
BULLISH
BULLITT
BULLOCK
BULLPEN
BULLRUN
BUMLEGS
BURLAPS
BURLERS
BURLIER
BURLING
BUSLANE
BUSLINE
BUSLOAD
BUTLERS
BYPLAYS

B•••L••

BABBLED
BABBLER
BABBLES
BABYLON
BACILLI
BACKLIT
BACKLOG
BACKLOT
BAFFLED
BAFFLER
BAFFLES
BANALER
BANALLY
BANDLET
BANGLED
BANGLES
BARCLAY
BARKLEY
BAROLOS
BARTLES
BARTLET
BASALLY
BASALTS
BASILIC
BASILIO
BATTLED
BATTLER
BATTLES
BAUBLES
BEADLES
BEAGLES
BEASLEY
BEATLES
BECALMS
BEDELIA
BEETLES
BEFALLS
BEHOLDS
BELLLAP
BENBLUE
BENELUX
BENTLEY
BERKLEY
BEVELED
BEVELER
BIBELOT
BICOLOR
BIGBLUE
BIGELOW
BINDLES
BINGLES
BIPOLAR
BIVALVE
BLAKLEY
BLUELAW
BOBBLED
BOBBLER
BOBBLES
BOBSLED
BOCELLI
BOGGLED
BOGGLER
BOGGLES
BOMBLET
BONELET
BONILLA
BOODLES

BOOKLET
BOOMLET
BOOSLER
BOOTLEG
BORGLUM
BOTTLED
BOTTLER
BOTTLES
BOWDLER
BRADLEE
BRADLEY
BRAILLE
BRAMLEY
BRAWLED
BRAWLER
BRAWLEY
BRESLIN
BRIDLED
BRIDLER
BRIDLES
BRILLIG
BRILLOS
BRIMLEY
BROILED
BROILER
BTWELVE
BUBBLED
BUBBLES
BUCKLED
BUCKLES
BUCKLEY
BUCOLIC
BUELLER
BUGALOO
BUGGLES
BULBLET
BUMBLED
BUMBLER
BUMBLES
BUNDLED
BUNDLER
BUNDLES
BUNGLED
BUNGLER
BUNGLES
BURBLED
BURBLER
BURBLES
BURGLAR
BURGLED
BURGLES
BURNLEY
BUSTLED
BUSTLER
BUSTLES
BYGOLLY
BYTALKS

B••••L•

BACILLI
BADCALL
BADCOLD
BAGFULS
BAGGILY
BAGNOLD
BAGWELL
BALKILY
BALMILY
BANALLY
BARBELL
BARBILL
BARBULE
BARRELS
BARTOLO
BASALLY
BASSALE
BAWDILY
BEADILY
BEASTLY
BEATALL
BEDROLL
BEEFALO
BEEFILY
BEFALLS
BEFOOLS
BEFOULS
BEGUILE
BENGALI
BENGALS
BENZALI
BENZELL
BEOWULF
BERTOLT
BESSELL
BESTILL
BETHELS
BEVERLY
BEWAILS
BIASPLY
BICYCLE
BIGGULP
BIGHALF
BIGSALE
BIGTALK
BIRDFLU
BISSELL
BITROLE
BLACKLY
BLACULA
BLAKELY
BLANDLY
BLANKLY
BLEAKLY
BLINDLY
BLOWFLY
BLUEFLU
BLUFFLY
BLUNTLY
BOATELS
BOBDOLE
BOBVILA
BOCELLI
BOFFOLA
BOGHOLE
BOGUSLY
BONILLA
BONNILY
BOOZILY
BOSSILY
BOSWELL
BOXBALL
BOXFULS
BRAILLE
BRAMBLE
BRAMBLY
BRASHLY
BRATTLE
BRAVELY
BRICKLE
BRIDALS
BRIEFLY
BRINDLE
BRISKLY
BRISTLE
BRISTLY
BRITTLE
BROADLY
BRUTELY
BTFSPLK
BUFFALO
BUMPILY
BUNUELO
BURIALS
BUSHELS
BUSHILY
BUXOMLY
BUYABLE
BUZZELL
BYAMILE
BYGOLLY

B•••••L

BABYOIL
BADCALL
BADGIRL
BAGGIRL
BAGWELL
BALEFUL
BALLIOL
BANEFUL
BARBELL
BARBILL
BARNOWL
BASHFUL
BASINAL
BATGIRL
BATHOIL
BEANOIL
BEATALL
BEDEVIL
BEDRAIL
BEDROLL
BEJEWEL
BENZELL
BESSELL
BESTIAL
BESTILL
BIAXIAL
BIFOCAL
BIGDEAL
BIGGIRL
BIGMEAL
BILEVEL
BIMETAL
BIMODAL
BIOFUEL
BIPEDAL
BISSELL
BITONAL
BOATFUL
BOBTAIL
BODEFUL
BORSTAL
BOSWELL
BOWLFUL
BOXBALL
BRENDEL
BRIMFUL
BRISTOL
BRUEGEL
BRUMMEL
BSCHOOL
BUMDEAL
BUSGIRL
BUZZELL

•BL••••

ABLATED
ABLATES
OBLASTS
OBLATES
OBLIGED
OBLIGEE
OBLIGER
OBLIGES
OBLIGOR
OBLIQUE
OBLONGS
OBLOQUY
VBLOUSE

•B•L•••

ABALONE
ABELARD
ABILENE
ABILITY
ABOLISH
ABOLLAE
IBILITY
NBALIVE
OBELISE
OBELISK
OBELIZE
TBILISI

•B••L••

ABOLLAE
ABRILES
ABSALOM
ABSOLUT
ABSOLVE
NBCBLUE
OBERLIN

•B•••L•

FBIFILE
OBESELY

•B••••L

ABETTAL
ABIGAIL
ABUTTAL
ABYSMAL
ABYSSAL

••BL•••

AMBLERS
AMBLING
BIBLESS
BIBLIKE
BIBLIOG
CABLERS
CABLETS
CABLETV
CABLING
COBLENZ
DEBLURS
EMBLAZE
EMBLEMS
FABLERS
FABLING
FTBLISS
GIBLETS
GIBLUES
GOBLANK
GOBLETS
GOBLINS
INBLACK
INBLOOM
JOBLESS
JOBLOCK
JOBLOTS
KOBLENZ
LEBLANC
MRBLISS
MTBLANC
NIBLETS
NIBLICK
NIBLIKE
NOBLEST
OOBLECK
ORBLESS
ORBLIKE
OXBLOOD
PABLUMS
POBLANO
PUBLICS
PUBLISH
PUBLIUS
REBLOCK
REBLOOM
REBLOWN
RIBLESS
RIBLETS
RIBLIKE
ROBLOWE
SIBLING
SUBLETS
SUBLIDS
SUBLIME
SUBLONG
SUBLOTS
TABLEAU
TABLETS
TABLING
TABLOID
TOBLAME
TUBLIKE
UNBLADE
UNBLENT
UNBLEST
UNBLOCK
UNBLOWN
UNBLUED
WEBLESS
WEBLIKE
WEBLOGS

••B•L••

ARBOLES
BABBLED
BABBLER
BABBLES
BABYLON
BIBELOT
BOBBLED
BOBBLER
BOBBLES
BOBSLED
BUBBLED
BUBBLES
CABALAS
CABALLE
COBALTS
COBBLED
COBBLER
COBBLES
DABBLED
DABBLER
DABBLES
DIBBLED
DIBBLER
DIBBLES
EMBALMS
FIBULAE
FIBULAR
FIBULAS
GABBLED
GABBLES
GOBBLED
GOBBLER
GOBBLES
GOBELIN
GOBELOW
HABILIS
HIBBLER
HOBBLED
HOBBLER
HOBBLES
JUBILEE
KIBBLED
KIBBLES
KOBOLDS
KUBELIK
LABELED
LABELER
LABELLE
LIBELED
LIBELEE
LIBELER
LOBULES
MOBILES
MTBALDY
NEBULAE
NEBULAR
NEBULAS
NIBBLED
NIBBLER
NIBBLES
NUBBLES
PABULUM
PEBBLED
PEBBLES
QABALAH
QABALAS
RABBLED
RABBLES
REBALED
REBALES
REBILLS
REBOLTS
RIBALDS
RUBBLES
RUBELLA
SIBYLIC
SUBCLAN
SUBPLOT
SUBTLER
TABULAR
TEBALDI
TUBULAR
TUBULES
UNBALED
UNBALES
UNBELDI
UNBELTS
UNBOLTS
UNBULKY
WOBBLED
WOBBLER
WOBBLES
ZEBULON
ZEBULUN

••B••L•

BOBDOLE
BOBVILA
CABALLE
CABBALA
CUBICLE
CUBICLY
DEBACLE
DEBOULE
FEBRILE
HUBBELL
INBUILT
KABBALA
LABELLE
LABIALS
MOBRULE
NOBHILL
RABIDLY
REBILLS
REBOILS
REBUILD
REBUILT
RUBELLA
RUBEOLA
SOBERLY
SUBCELL
SUBFILE
SUBHALL
TABOULI
TUBFULS
UNBUILD
UNBUILT
UNBURLY
UPBUILD

••B•••L

ANBESOL
BABYOIL
BOBTAIL
COBCOAL
CUBICAL
CUBITAL
EMBROIL
GABRIEL
HOBNAIL
HUBBELL
LIBERAL
NOBHILL
ORBITAL
STBASIL
SUBCELL
SUBCOOL
SUBDUAL
SUBGOAL
SUBHALL
SUBSOIL
UMBRIEL
WEBMAIL

•••BL••

AMIBLUE
ARABLES
BABBLED
BABBLER
BABBLES
BAUBLES
BENBLUE
BIGBLUE
BOBBLED
BOBBLER
BOBBLES
BOMBLET
BUBBLED
BUBBLES
BULBLET
BUMBLED
BUMBLER
BUMBLES
BURBLED
BURBLER
BURBLES
CHABLIS
COBBLED
COBBLER
COBBLES
DABBLED
DABBLER
DABBLES
DIABLES
DIABLOS
DIBBLED
DIBBLER
DIBBLES
DOUBLEA
DOUBLEB
DOUBLEC
DOUBLED
DOUBLEE
DOUBLEF
DOUBLEG
DOUBLEH
DOUBLEI
DOUBLEJ
DOUBLEK
DOUBLEL
DOUBLEM
DOUBLEN
DOUBLEO
DOUBLEP
DOUBLEQ
DOUBLER
DOUBLES
DOUBLET
DOUBLEU
DOUBLEV
DOUBLEW
DOUBLEX
DOUBLEY
DOUBLEZ
DRIBLET
EDIBLES
ENABLED
ENABLER
ENABLES
FEEBLER
FOIBLES
FUMBLED
FUMBLER
FUMBLES
GABBLED
GABBLES
GAMBLED
GAMBLER
GAMBLES
GARBLED
GARBLER
GARBLES
GILBLAS
GOBBLED
GOBBLER
GOBBLES
HIBBLER
HOBBLED
HOBBLER
HOBBLES
HUMBLED
HUMBLER
HUMBLES
ICEBLUE
INKBLOT
JOEBLOW
JUMBLED
JUMBLER
JUMBLES
KEEBLER
KIBBLED
KIBBLES
LOWBLOW
MARBLED
MARBLER
MARBLES
MUMBLED
MUMBLER
MUMBLES
NBCBLUE
NIBBLED
NIBBLER
NIBBLES
NIMBLER
NUBBLES
OLDBLUE
OUTBLOT
OUTBLOW
PEBBLED
PEBBLES
PEEBLES
PROBLEM
PUEBLOS
RABBLED
RABBLES
RAMBLED
RAMBLER
RAMBLES
RAMBLIN
ROTBLAT
RUBBLES
RUMBLED
RUMBLER
RUMBLES
RUYBLAS
SANBLAS
SEABLUE
SKYBLUE
STABLED
STABLER
STABLES
TAMBLYN
TEMBLOR
THEBLOB
TREBLED
TREBLES
TUMBLED
TUMBLER
TUMBLES
USABLES
WAMBLED
WAMBLES
WARBLED
WARBLER
WARBLES
WEMBLEY
WOBBLED
WOBBLER
WOBBLES

•••B•L•

AIRBALL
AIRBILL
BARBELL
BARBILL
BARBULE
BOXBALL
CABBALA
CEMBALO
CORBELS
COWBELL
CUEBALL
CYMBALS
DIABOLO
DIEBOLD
DIMBULB
DRABBLE
DRIBBLE
DRYBULB
EYEBALL
EYEBOLT
FANBELT
FLYBALL
FRIBBLE
FURBALL
GAMBOLS
GERBILS
GIMBALS
GIMBELS
GLOBULE
GUMBALL
GUNBELT
GYMBALL
HAYBALE
HERBALS
HUBBELL
INABALL
KABBALA
KIMBALL
LAPBELT
LIPBALM
LOWBALL
MISBILL
NETBALL
NEWBOLT
ODDBALL
OLEBULL
ONEBALL
ONEBELL
OUTBULK
PACBELL
PIEBALD
PINBALL
PITBULL
PREBILL
PROBALL
QUIBBLE
SIXBALL
SNOBALL
STABILE
STUBBLE
STUBBLY
SUNBELT
SYMBOLS
TAMBALA
TARBELL
TEABALL
TENBALL
THEBELL
TIMBALE
TIMBALS
TMOBILE
TOYBALL
TRIBBLE
TWOBALL
UNIBALL
VERBALS
WAYBILL
WETBULB

•••B••L

AIRBALL
AIRBILL
ATABOIL
BARBELL
BARBILL
BOXBALL
CATBOWL
COWBELL
CUEBALL
DOGBOWL
DOUBLEL
EYEBALL
FLYBALL
FURBALL
GUMBALL
GYMBALL
HUBBELL
INABALL
KIMBALL
LOWBALL
MISBILL
NETBALL
ODDBALL
OLEBULL
ONEBALL
ONEBELL
OUTBAWL
OUTBOWL
PACBELL
PARBOIL
PINBALL
PITBULL
POTBOIL
PREBILL
PREBOIL
PROBALL
PROBOWL
SETBAIL
SIXBALL
SNOBALL
SUNBOWL
TARBELL
TEABALL
TENBALL
THEBELL
TOYBALL
TUMBREL
TWOBALL
UNIBALL
WAYBILL

••••BL•

ACTABLE
ADDABLE
ADDIBLE
AFFABLE
AFFABLY
AMIABLE
AMIABLY
AUDIBLE
AUDIBLY
AUSABLE
BRAMBLE
BRAMBLY
BUYABLE
CAPABLE
CAPABLY
CITABLE
CRUMBLE
CRUMBLY
CURABLE
CURABLY
DATABLE
DISABLE
DRABBLE
DRIBBLE
DRYABLE
DURABLE
DURABLY
EATABLE
EFFABLE
EFFABLY
ENDABLE
ENNOBLE
EQUABLE
EQUABLY
ERRABLE
FINABLE
FIXABLE
FLYABLE
FRIABLE
FRIBBLE
FRYABLE
FUSIBLE
GETABLE
GRUMBLE
GRUMBLY
HATABLE
HIDABLE
HIRABLE
IGNOBLE
IGNOBLY
LEGIBLE
LEGIBLY
LIKABLE
LINABLE
LIVABLE
LOSABLE
LOVABLE
LOVABLY
MAKABLE
MINABLE
MIXABLE
MOVABLE
MOVABLY
MUTABLE
MUTABLY
NAMABLE
NAMABLY
NOTABLE
NOTABLY
PARABLE
PAYABLE
PLIABLE
PLIABLY
POSABLE
POTABLE
QUIBBLE
RAKABLE
RATABLE
RECABLE
RETABLE
RIDABLE
RISIBLE
RISIBLY
SALABLE
SAVABLE
SAYABLE
SEEABLE
SHAMBLE
SIZABLE
SIZABLY
SKIABLE
SOLUBLE
STUBBLE
STUBBLY
STUMBLE
TAKABLE
TAMABLE
TAXABLE
TENABLE
TENABLY
THIMBLE
TOTABLE

TOWABLE
TREMBLE
TREMBLY
TRIABLE
TRIBBLE
TROUBLE
TUNABLE
TVTABLE
VENABLE
VISIBLE
VISIBLY
VOCABLE
VOCABLY
VOLUBLE
VOLUBLY
VOTABLE
WAXABLE
WIRABLE

••••B•L
ANNABEL
ARRABAL
DECIBEL
FROEBEL
JEZEBEL
MIRABEL
RELABEL
SANIBEL
TRAUBEL

BM•••••
BMOVIES

B•M••••
BAMBIII
BAMBINA
BAMBINI
BAMBINO
BAMBOOS
BAMMIES
BAMMING
BEMIRED
BEMIRES
BEMOANS
BEMUSED
BEMUSES
BIMBOES
BIMETAL
BIMINIS
BIMODAL
BOMBARD
BOMBAST
BOMBECK
BOMBERS
BOMBING
BOMBLET
BUMBLED
BUMBLER
BUMBLES
BUMDEAL
BUMLEGS
BUMMERS
BUMMING
BUMPERS
BUMPIER
BUMPILY
BUMPING
BUMPKIN
BUMPSUP
BUMRAPS
BUMRUSH
BUMSOUT
BYMOUTH

B••M•••
BADMOOD
BADMOVE
BALMAIN
BALMIER
BALMILY
BAMMIES
BAMMING
BARMAID
BARMIER
BASMATI
BEAMERS
BEAMIER
BEAMING
BEAMISH
BEAMSUP
BEDMATE
BEEMERS
BELMONT
BERMING
BERMUDA
BESMEAR
BIGMACS
BIGMAMA
BIGMEAL
BIGMESS
BIOMASS
BIRMANS
BISMUTH
BITMAPS
BLAMEON
BLAMERS
BLAMING
BLEMISH
BLIMPIE
BONMOTS
BOOMBOX
BOOMCAR
BOOMERS
BOOMIER
BOOMING
BOOMLET
BRAMBLE
BRAMBLY
BRAMLEY
BRIMFUL
BRIMLEY
BRIMMED
BRIMMER
BROMATE
BROMIDE
BROMINE
BRUMMEL
BRUMOUS
BUMMERS
BUMMING
BURMANS
BURMESE
BUSMANS
BYAMILE

B•••M••
BACHMAN
BADOMEN
BAHAMAS
BAHAMEN
BALLMER
BASEMAN
BASEMEN
BATEMAN
BATHMAT
BATSMAN
BATSMEN
BECOMES
BEERMUG
BEHRMAN
BELLMAN
BELLMEN
BENUMBS
BERGMAN
BESTMAN
BESTMEN
BETAMAX
BETIMES
BIRDMAN
BIRDMEN
BIREMES
BLOOMED
BLOOMER
BOATMAN
BOATMEN
BOGYMAN
BOGYMEN
BOHEMIA
BONDMAN
BONDMEN
BOOKMAN
BOOKMEN
BOORMAN
BOROMIR
BOSOMED
BOSSMAN
BOSSMEN
BOZEMAN
BRAHMAN
BRAHMAS
BRAHMIN
BRIMMED
BRIMMER
BROOMED
BRUMMEL
BUCHMAN
BUSHMAN
BUSHMEN
BUXOMLY
BYNAMES

B••••M•
BADNAME
BADTIME
BALSAMS
BALSAMY
BANTAMS
BARNUMS
BAYRUMS
BEATSME
BECALMS
BEDLAMP
BEDLAMS
BEDTIME
BEGRIME
BELDAME
BELDAMS
BELLAMY
BERGAMO
BIGGAME
BIGMAMA
BIGNAME
BIGTIME
BOTTOMS
BUDTIME
BUNKUMS
BUSCEMI
BUTTEMT
BUYTIME
BYFORMS

B•••••M
BAALISM
BADFORM
BAHAISM
BAPTISM
BAREXAM
BARROOM
BEACHAM
BECHARM
BECKHAM
BEDROOM
BEECHAM
BELGIUM
BENTHAM
BERTRAM
BINGHAM
BLOSSOM
BOHRIUM
BOREDOM
BORGLUM
BOSSISM
BRIGHAM
BRITCOM
BRUXISM
BUCKRAM
BUDWORM
BUTTRAM

•B••M••
ABDOMEN
ABYSMAL

•B•••M•
NBAGAME

•B••••M
ABRAHAM
ABSALOM
NBATEAM

••BM•••
LABMICE
RIBMEAT
SUBMITS
WEBMAIL

••B•M••
ALBUMEN
ALBUMIN
LABAMBA

••B••M•
EMBALMS
EMBLEMS
PABLUMS
PUBGAME
SUBLIME
SUBSUME
TOBLAME
WEBCAMS

••B•••M
DUBNIUM
EMBOSOM
HOBOISM
INBLOOM
JIBBOOM
MOBBISM
PABULUM
REBLOOM
SUBFORM
SUBITEM
UNBOSOM

•••BM••
CLUBMED

•••B•M•
ALABAMA
ALABAMY
DEMBUMS
DOTBOMB
SKIBUMS
THEBOMB

•••B••M
DOUBLEM
HATBRIM
IONBEAM
JIBBOOM
JIMBEAM
LIPBALM
LOWBEAM
MOBBISM
NIOBIUM
OUTBEAM
PREBOOM
PROBLEM
SUNBEAM
TERBIUM
TIEBEAM

••••B•M
CDALBUM
CRUMBUM
PLUMBUM

B•N••••
BANACEK
BANALER
BANALLY
BANANAS
BANANES
BANBURY
BANDAGE
BANDAID
BANDANA
BANDBOX
BANDEAU
BANDERA
BANDERS
BANDIDO
BANDIED
BANDIER
BANDIES
BANDING
BANDITO
BANDITS
BANDLET
BANDSAW
BANEFUL
BANGERS
BANGING
BANGKOK
BANGLED
BANGLES
BANGOUT
BANGSON
BANGSUP
BANJOES
BANKERS
BANKFEE
BANKING
BANKITS
BANKJOB
BANKONE
BANKSON
BANKSUP
BANNERS
BANNING
BANQUES
BANQUET
BANSHEE
BANTAMS
BANTERS
BANTING
BANYANS
BANZAIS
BENARES
BENATAR
BENAZIR
BENBLUE
BENBOVA
BENCHED
BENCHER
BENCHES
BENDAYS
BENDERS
BENDIER
BENDING
BENEATH
BENEFIC
BENEFIT
BENELUX
BENGALI
BENGALS
BENGUNN
BENICIA
BENICIO
BENIGNI
BENIGNO
BENISON
BENNETT
BENNING
BENOTED
BENOTES
BENTHAM
BENTHOS
BENTLEY
BENTSEN
BENUMBS
BENZALI
BENZELL
BENZENE
BINDERS
BINDERY
BINDING
BINDLES
BINDOFF
BINDSTO
BINDSUP
BINGERS
BINGHAM
BINGING
BINGLES
BINGOES
BINNING
BINOCHE
BONACIS
BONAIRE
BONANZA
BONARIO
BONBONS
BONDAGE
BONDERS
BONDING
BONDMAN
BONDMEN
BONEASH
BONEDRY
BONEDUP
BONELET
BONESET
BONESUP
BONEYER
BONFIRE
BONGING
BONGOES
BONHEUR
BONIATO
BONIEST
BONILLA
BONITOS
BONJOUR
BONJOVI
BONKERS
BONKING
BONMOTS
BONNARD
BONNETS
BONNIER
BONNILY
BONSOIR
BONUSES
BUNCHED
BUNCHES
BUNCHUP
BUNCOED
BUNDLED
BUNDLER
BUNDLES
BUNGEES
BUNGING
BUNGLED
BUNGLER
BUNGLES
BUNIONS
BUNKBED
BUNKERS
BUNKING
BUNKOED
BUNKUMS
BUNNIES
BUNNING
BUNRAKU
BUNTERS
BUNTING
BUNUELO
BYNAMES

B••N•••
BADNAME
BADNESS
BADNEWS
BAGNIOS
BAGNOLD
BAINTER
BANNERS
BANNING
BARNABY
BARNARD
BARNEYS
BARNING
BARNONE
BARNOWL
BARNRED
BARNUMS
BATNEXT
BEANBAG
BEANDIP
BEANERY
BEANIES
BEANING
BEANOIL
BEDNORZ
BENNETT
BENNING
BERNARD
BERNAYS
BERNESE
BERNINA
BERNINI
BERNSEN
BIANCHI
BIENNIA
BIENTOT
BIGNAME
BIGNESS
BIGNEWS
BIGNOSE
BINNING
BIONICS
BLANCHE
BLANDER
BLANDLY
BLANKED
BLANKER
BLANKET
BLANKLY
BLANTON
BLENDED
BLENDER
BLENDES
BLENDIN
BLENTIN
BLINDED
BLINDER
BLINDLY
BLINDTO
BLINKAT
BLINKED
BLINKER
BLINTZE
BLONDER
BLONDES
BLONDIE
BLUNDEN
BLUNDER
BLUNTED
BLUNTER
BLUNTLY
BLYNKEN
BONNARD
BONNETS
BONNIER
BONNILY
BOONIES
BORNEAN
BORNEUP
BOSNIAN
BOUNCED
BOUNCER
BOUNCES
BOUNDED
BOUNDER
BOUNDTO
BOUNDUP
BRANAGH
BRANCHY
BRANDED
BRANDER
BRANDON
BRANIFF
BRANSON
BRENDAN
BRENDEL
BRENDON
BRENGUN
BRENNAN
BRENNER
BRINDLE
BRINERS
BRINGER
BRINGIN
BRINGIT
BRINGON
BRINGTO
BRINGUP
BRINIER
BRINING
BRINISH
BRINKER
BRONCHI
BRONCHO
BRONCOS
BRONSON
BRONTES
BRONWEN
BRONZED
BRONZER
BRONZES
BRUNETS
BRYNNER
BUNNIES
BUNNING
BURNABY
BURNERS
BURNETT
BURNFOR
BURNING
BURNISH
BURNLEY
BURNOFF
BURNOUT
BURNSIN
BURNSUP
BURNTIN
BURNTUP
BYANDBY
BYANECK
BYANOSE

B•••N••
BABENCO
BADENDS
BADENOV
BALANCE
BALONEY
BANANAS
BANANES
BARANOF
BARENTS
BARONET
BASENJI
BASINAL
BAYONET
BAYONNE
BEATNIK
BEGANTO
BEGONIA
BEHINDS
BEIGNES
BEIGNET
BELINDA
BELONGS
BERENDT
BERKNER
BEYONCE
BIENNIA
BIGENDS
BIGONES
BIGUNIT
BIKINIS
BILLNYE
BIMINIS
BITONAL
BLARNEY
BLOWNIN
BLOWNUP
BLUINGS
BOCHNER
BODINGS
BOEINGS
BONANZA
BORINGS
BORONIC
BOSONIC
BOTANIC
BOTHNIA
BOVINES
BOWKNOT
BRAINED
BRAINER
BRENNAN
BRENNER
BRITNEY
BROSNAN
BROWNED
BROWNER
BROWNIE
BRYNNER
BUCHNER
BUCKNER
BUJONES
BURUNDI
BUTANES
BUTENES
BUYINTO
BYGONES
BYJINGO
BYLINED
BYLINER
BYLINES
BYRONIC

B••••N•
BABOONS
BABYING
BACHING
BACKEND
BACKING
BADHAND
BADLAND
BAFFING
BAGGING
BAGGINS
BAHIANS
BAILING
BAITING
BALCONY
BALDING
BALEENS
BALKANS
BALKING
BALLONE
BAMBINA
BAMBINI
BAMBINO
BAMMING
BANDANA
BANDING
BANGING
BANKING
BANKONE
BANNING
BANTING
BANYANS
BARBING
BARGING
BARKING
BARNING
BARNONE
BARRENS
BARRING
BARRONS
BARTEND
BARYONS
BASHING
BASKING
BASSANI
BASSANO
BASTING
BATHING
BATTENS
BATTING
BATWING
BAWLING
BAYLYNX
BAYONNE
BCLIONS
BEACONS
BEADING
BEAMING
BEANING
BEARING
BEATING
BECKONS
BEDDING
BEEFING
BEELINE
BEEPING
BEGGING
BEGUINE
BEHRENS
BEHRING
BEIJING
BELLING
BELLINI
BELMONT
BELTANE
BELTING
BELYING
BELZONI
BEMOANS
BENDING
BENGUNN
BENIGNI
BENIGNO
BENNING
BENZENE
BERMING
BERNINA
BERNINI
BEROWNE
BERSUNT
BESTING
BESTONE
BETHANY
BETHINK
BETHUNE
BETTANY
BETTING
BHUTANI
BIASING
BIBBING
BICHONS
BICORNE
BICORNS
BIDDING
BIFFING
BIGBAND
BIGBANG
BIGBEND
BIGFANS
BIGGUNS
BIGHAND
BIGTENT
BIGWINS
BILKING
BILLING
BINDING
BINGING
BINNING
BIPLANE
BIRDING
BIRIANI
BIRLING
BIRMANS
BIRRING
BIRYANI
BITTING
BLADING
BLAMING
BLARING
BLATANT
BLAZING
BLAZONS
BLOWING
BLUEING
BOATING
BOBBING
BOBBINS
BOBKANE
BODKINS
BOFFING
BOFFINS
BOGGING
BOILING
BOITANO
BOKKENS
BOLLING
BOLOGNA
BOLTING
BOMBING
BONBONS
BONDING
BONGING
BONKING
BOOKEND
BOOKING
BOOMING
BOOTING
BOOZING
BOPPING
BORDONI
BORKING
BOSSING
BOSTONS
BOSTONU
BOUDINS
BOUSONO
BOWFINS
BOWLINE
BOWLING
BOYBAND
BRACING
BRAKING
BRAVING
BRAYING
BRAZENS
BRAZING
BRETONS
BREWING

BRIBING
BRIGAND
BRINING
BRITONS
BROGANS
BROMINE
BRUXING
BUCKING
BUDDING
BUDGING
BUFFING
BUGGING
BUGLING
BUITONI
BULGING
BULKING
BULLING
BULLINS
BUMMING
BUMPING
BUNGING
BUNIONS
BUNKING
BUNNING
BUNTING
BUOYANT
BUOYING
BURBANK
BURDENS
BURKINA
BURLING
BURMANS
BURNING
BURPING
BURRING
BURYING
BUSHING
BUSKING
BUSLANE
BUSLINE
BUSMANS
BUSSING
BUSTING
BUSYING
BUTTING
BUTTONS
BUTTONY
BUZZING
BYPHONE
BYTURNS

B•••••N

BABYLON
BACHMAN
BACKSIN
BADOMEN
BADSIGN
BAHAMEN
BAHRAIN
BAHREIN
BAILSON
BAKEPAN
BALABAN
BALATON
BALDWIN
BALLOON
BALMAIN
BANGSON
BANKSON
BARDEEN
BARGAIN
BARGEIN
BASEDON
BASEMAN
BASEMEN
BASETEN
BASRHIN
BASSOON
BASTION
BATEMAN
BATSMAN
BATSMEN
BDALTON
BEALION
BEARSON
BEATSON
BEDDOWN
BEDIZEN
BEDOUIN
BEECHEN
BEERCAN
BEHRMAN
BELEVEN
BELGIAN
BELLMAN
BELLMEN
BELLSON
BELTRAN
BENGUNN
BENISON
BENTSEN
BERGMAN
BERGSON
BERIGAN
BERNSEN
BESTMAN
BESTMEN
BETAKEN
BETOKEN
BETWEEN
BIAFRAN
BIGHORN
BIGJOHN
BIGTOWN
BILLION
BIRCHEN
BIRDMAN
BIRDMEN
BITESIN
BITESON
BITTERN
BKLIBAN
BLACKEN
BLAMEON
BLANTON
BLENDIN
BLENTIN
BLITZEN
BLOUSON
BLOWGUN
BLOWNIN
BLOWSIN
BLOWSON
BLUEFIN
BLUEHEN
BLUESUN
BLUNDEN
BLUSHON
BLYNKEN
BOATMAN
BOATMEN
BOBGOEN
BOGDOWN
BOGYMAN
BOGYMEN
BONDMAN
BONDMEN
BOOKMAN
BOOKMEN
BOOLEAN
BOORMAN
BORNEAN
BORODIN
BOSNIAN
BOSSMAN
BOSSMEN
BOURBON
BOWDOIN
BOWDOWN
BOXEDIN
BOXESIN
BOZEMAN
BRACKEN
BRAEDEN
BRAHMAN
BRAHMIN
BRANDON
BRANSON
BRAXTON
BREAKIN
BRENDAN
BRENDON
BRENGUN
BRENNAN
BRESLIN
BRETTON
BRINGIN
BRINGON
BRITAIN
BRITTEN
BRITTON
BROADEN
BROKEIN
BRONSON
BRONWEN
BROSNAN
BUCHMAN
BUFFOON
BUILDIN
BUILDON
BUILTIN
BUILTON
BUISSON
BULLION
BULLPEN
BULLRUN
BUMPKIN
BURGEON
BURNSIN
BURNTIN
BURPGUN
BURSTIN
BURSTYN
BUSHMAN
BUSHMEN
BUSTSIN
BUTTSIN
BUYDOWN
BYTRAIN

•BN••••

IBNSAUD

•B•N•••

ABANDON
ABCNEWS
ABINTRA
CBSNEWS
EBANKED
EBONICS
EBONIES
EBONITE
EBONIZE
NBCNEWS
OBENTOS
PBANDJS
QBSNEAK

•B••N••

ABOUNDS
ABSENCE
ABSENTS
ABSINTH
OBLONGS
OBTUNDS

•B•••N•

ABALONE
ABASING
ABATING
ABEYANT
ABIDING
ABILENE
ABSCOND
ABUSING
IBIZANS
MBABANE
OBEYING
OBSCENE
OBTAINS

•B••••N

ABANDON
ABDOMEN
ABIDJAN
ABSTAIN
ABUTSON
IBERIAN
OBERLIN

••BN•••

COBNUTS
DUBNIUM
HOBNAIL
HOBNOBS
SUBNETS

••B•N••

ALBANIA
ALBENIZ
ALBINOS
ALBUNDY
BABENCO
CABANAS
CABINET
DEBONED
DEBONES
DEBUNKS
EMBANKS
EUBANKS
FMBANDS
LEBANON
MRBONES
REBANKS
REBENDS
REBINDS
RIBANDS
ROBBNEN
SABINES
SUBUNIT
UNBENCH
UNBENDS
UNBINDS
UNBONED
URBANER
URBANII
URBANIV
URBANVI

••B••N•

AMBIENS
AMBIENT
AMBLING
AUBURNS
AUBURNU
BABOONS
BABYING
BIBBING
BOBBING
BOBBINS
BOBKANE
CABBING
CABLING
CABRINI
COBLENZ
COBRAND
CUBBING
CUBBINS
CUBFANS
DABBING
DABHAND
DOBBINS
DUBBING
FABLING
FIBBING
FIBRINS
FOBBING
GABBANA
GABBING
GIBBONS
GIBSONS
GOBLANK
GOBLINS
HIBBING
HIBERNO
HOBOING
HOBSONS
IMBUING
INBOUND
JABBING
JOBBANK
JOBBING
JOBHUNT
KOBLENZ
LEBLANC
LIBBING
LIBRANS
LIBYANS
LOBBING
MOBBING
MRBURNS
MTBLANC
NABBING
NUBBINS
NUBIANS
OSBORNE
POBLANO
REBOANT
REBOUND
REBRAND
RIBBING
RIBBONS
RIBBONY
ROBBING
ROBBINS
RUBBING
SABRINA
SEBRING
SIBLING
SOBBING
SUBBAND
SUBBANK
SUBBING
SUBKING
SUBLONG
SUBORNS
SUBTEND
SUBTONE
SUBVENE
SUBZONE
TABBING
TABLING
TABUING
TUBBING
UNBLENT
UNBORNE
UNBOUND
UNBURNT
UPBORNE
UPBOUND
VIBRANT
WEBBING
WEBZINE
ZEBRINE

••B•••N

ALBUMEN
ALBUMIN
BABYLON
BOBGOEN
CUBSFAN
DRBROWN
EMBROWN
GOBELIN
HOBOKEN
INBROWN
LEBANON
LEBARON
MRBROWN
ORBISON
REBEGAN
REBEGIN
REBEGUN
REBLOWN
ROBBNEN
ROBESON
RUBDOWN
RUBICON
RUBITIN
RUBUPON
SUBCLAN
SUBJOIN
SUBTEEN
TIBETAN
TIBURON
TUBEPAN
UMBRIAN
UNBLOWN
WOBEGON
ZABUTON
ZEBULON
ZEBULUN

•••BN••

LEIBNIZ
ROBBNEN

•••B•N•

AKEBONO
ARMBAND
ARMBONE
ARUBANS
ASHBINS
BAMBINA
BAMBINI
BAMBINO
BARBING
BIBBING
BIGBAND
BIGBANG
BIGBEND
BOBBING
BOBBINS
BOMBING
BONBONS
BOYBAND
BRIBING
BURBANK
CABBING
CARBINE
CARBONS
COMBINE
COMBING
COWBANE
CUBBING
CUBBINS
CUIBONO
CURBING
DABBING
DAUBING
DISBAND
DOBBINS
DOGBANE
DOGBONE
DUBBING
DUMBING
EARBONE
EYEBANK
FIBBING
FIRBANK
FOBBING
FOGBANK
GABBANA
GABBING
GARBING
GETBENT
GIBBONS
GLOBING
GLOBINS
HAMBONE
HATBAND
HENBANE
HIBBING
HIPBONE
HUSBAND
IKEBANA
INABIND
JABBING
JAMBAND
JAWBONE
JOBBANK
JOBBING
JUGBAND
KEYBANK
LAMBENT
LAMBING
LEGBONE
LIBBING
LIMBING
LOBBING
MBABANE
MISBIND
MOBBING
NABBING
NONBANK
NUBBINS
NUMBING
OUTBANS
OUTBEND
PEPBAND
PREBIND
PROBING
PROBONO
RAYBANS
REDBONE
REUBENS
RIBBING
RIBBONS
RIBBONY
ROBBING
ROBBINS
RUBBING
SHEBANG
SOBBING
STUBING
SUBBAND
SUBBANK
SUBBING
TABBING
THEBAND
THEBANS
TRIBUNE
TUBBING
TURBANS
TURBINE
VERBENA
WARBOND
WEBBING
ZAMBONI

•••B••N

ALLBRAN
ARABIAN
ASHBURN
CARBARN
CLIBURN
COGBURN
COMBIEN
DOUBLEN
GAMBIAN
HADBEEN
HASBEEN
HEPBURN
HOLBEIN
LAMBKIN
LOWBORN
MAXBORN
MUYBIEN
NEWBERN
NEWBORN
NOTBEEN
OATBRAN
OLDBEAN
OUTBURN
PEABEAN
PLEBIAN
PREBORN
PREBURN
RAEBURN
RAMBLIN
RAYBURN
ROBBNEN
ROYBEAN
SANBORN
SERBIAN
SIOBHAN
SOYBEAN
SUNBURN
TAMBLYN
WAXBEAN
ZAMBIAN

••••B•N

ALDUBIN
AUDUBON
AZKABAN
BALABAN
BKLIBAN
BOURBON
CALIBAN
CLIMBIN
CLIMBON
COALBIN
CORNBIN
DUSTBIN
ESTEBAN
EXURBAN
FEEDBIN
JACOBIN
MAILBIN
PHILBIN
STEUBEN
TALIBAN
TESTBAN
UNURBAN
WOODBIN

BO•••••

BOARDED
BOARDER
BOARDUP
BOARISH
BOASTED
BOASTER
BOASTOF
BOATELS
BOATERS
BOATFUL
BOATING
BOATMAN
BOATMEN
BOBATEA
BOBBERS
BOBBIDI
BOBBIES
BOBBING
BOBBINS
BOBBLED
BOBBLER
BOBBLES
BOBBSEY
BOBCATS
BOBDOLE
BOBGOEN
BOBHOPE
BOBKANE
BOBSLED
BOBTAIL
BOBTWAY
BOBVILA
BOBWEIR
BOCCIES
BOCELLI
BOCHNER
BODEFUL
BODEGAS
BODEREK
BODICES
BODINGS
BODKINS
BODYART
BODYBAR
BODYFAT
BODYKIT
BODYRUB
BOEINGS
BOERWAR
BOFFING
BOFFINS
BOFFOLA
BOGARDE
BOGARTS
BOGDOWN
BOGEYED
BOGGIER
BOGGING
BOGGISH
BOGGLED
BOGGLER
BOGGLES
BOGGUSS
BOGHOLE
BOGUSLY
BOGYMAN
BOGYMEN
BOHEMIA
BOHRIUM
BOIARDO
BOILERS
BOILING
BOILOFF
BOILOUT
BOILSUP
BOISEID
BOITANO
BOKCHOY
BOKHARA
BOKKENS
BOLATIE
BOLDEST
BOLEROS
BOLIDES
BOLIVAR
BOLIVIA
BOLLING
BOLOGNA
BOLOTIE
BOLSHOI
BOLSTER
BOLTERS
BOLTING
BOLTSUP
BOLUSES
BOMBARD
BOMBAST
BOMBECK
BOMBERS
BOMBING
BOMBLET
BONACIS
BONAIRE
BONANZA
BONARIO
BONBONS
BONDAGE
BONDERS
BONDING
BONDMAN
BONDMEN
BONEASH
BONEDRY
BONEDUP
BONELET
BONESET
BONESUP
BONEYER
BONFIRE
BONGING
BONGOES
BONHEUR
BONIATO
BONIEST
BONILLA
BONITOS
BONJOUR
BONJOVI
BONKERS
BONKING
BONMOTS
BONNARD
BONNETS
BONNIER
BONNILY
BONSOIR
BONUSES
BOOBIES
BOOBIRD
BOOBOOS
BOOCOOS
BOODLES
BOOEDAT
BOOGIED
BOOGIES
BOOHBAH
BOOHISS
BOOHOOS
BOOKBAG
BOOKEND
BOOKERS
BOOKERT
BOOKIES
BOOKIII
BOOKING
BOOKISH
BOOKLET
BOOKMAN
BOOKMEN
BOOKVII
BOOLEAN
BOOMBOX
BOOMCAR
BOOMERS
BOOMIER
BOOMING
BOOMLET
BOONIES
BOOPSIE
BOORISH
BOORMAN
BOOSLER
BOOSTED
BOOSTER
BOOSTUP
BOOTCUT
BOOTEES
BOOTERS
BOOTERY
BOOTHIA
BOOTIES
BOOTING
BOOTLEG
BOOTOUT
BOOTSIT
BOOTSUP
BOOTTOP
BOOZERS
BOOZIER
BOOZILY
BOOZING
BOPPERS
BOPPING
BORATES
BORDERS
BORDONI
BOREDOM
BOREOUT
BORGIAS
BORGLUM
BORIDES
BORINGS
BORKING
BORLAUG
BORNEAN
BORNEUP
BORODIN
BOROMIR
BORONIC
BOROUGH
BORROWS
BORSCHT
BORSTAL
BORZAGE
BORZOIS
BOSCAGE
BOSNIAN
BOSOMED
BOSONIC
BOSSIER
BOSSILY
BOSSING
BOSSISM
BOSSMAN
BOSSMEN
BOSTONS
BOSTONU
BOSWELL
BOTANIC
BOTCHED
BOTCHER
BOTCHES
BOTCHUP
BOTHERS
BOTHNIA
BOTREES
BOTTEGA
BOTTLED
BOTTLER
BOTTLES
BOTTOMS
BOUCHER
BOUCHES
BOUDINS
BOUDOIR
BOUFFES
BOUGHED
BOULDER
BOUNCED
BOUNCER
BOUNCES
BOUNDED
BOUNDER
BOUNDTO
BOUNDUP
BOUQUET
BOURBON
BOURGET
BOURSES
BOUSONO
BOUTROS
BOUVIER
BOVINES
BOWDLER
BOWDOIN
BOWDOWN

BOWECHO
BOWEDTO
BOWERED
BOWFINS
BOWHEAD
BOWKNOT
BOWLERS
BOWLESS
BOWLFUL
BOWLIKE
BOWLINE
BOWLING
BOWOARS
BOWSAWS
BOWSHOT
BOWSOUT
BOWTIES
BOWWOWS
BOWYERS
BOXBALL
BOXBEDS
BOXBOYS
BOXCARS
BOXCOAT
BOXEDIN
BOXEDUP
BOXESIN
BOXESUP
BOXFULS
BOXIEST
BOXKITE
BOXLIKE
BOXSEAT
BOXSETS
BOXSTEP
BOXSTER
BOXTOPS
BOYBAND
BOYCOTT
BOYHOOD
BOYLIKE
BOYTOYS
BOZEMAN
BLONDER
BLONDES
BLONDIE
BLOODED
BLOOMED
BLOOMER
BLOOPED
BLOOPER
BLOSSOM
BLOTCHY
BLOTOUT
BLOTSUP
BLOTTED
BLOTTER
BLOUSED
BLOUSES
BLOUSON
BLOWDRY
BLOWERS
BLOWFLY
BLOWGUN
BLOWIER
BLOWING
BLOWNIN
BLOWNUP
BLOWOFF
BLOWOUT
BLOWPOP
BLOWSIN
BLOWSIT
BLOWSON
BLOWSUP
BLOWUPS
BLOWZED
BMOVIES
BOOBIES
BOOBIRD
BOOBOOS
BOOCOOS
BOODLES
BOOEDAT
BOOGIED
BOOGIES
BOOHBAH
BOOHISS
BOOHOOS
BOOKBAG
BOOKEND
BOOKERS
BOOKERT
BOOKIES
BOOKIII
BOOKING
BOOKISH
BOOKLET
BOOKMAN
BOOKMEN
BOOKVII
BOOLEAN
BOOMBOX
BOOMCAR
BOOMERS
BOOMIER
BOOMING
BOOMLET
BOONIES
BOOPSIE
BOORISH
BOORMAN
BOOSLER
BOOSTED
BOOSTER
BOOSTUP
BOOTCUT
BOOTEES
BOOTERS
BOOTERY
BOOTHIA
BOOTIES
BOOTING
BOOTLEG
BOOTOUT
BOOTSIT
BOOTSUP
BOOTTOP
BOOZERS
BOOZIER
BOOZILY
BOOZING
BROADAS
BROADAX
BROADEN
BROADER
BROADLY
BROASTS
BROCADE
BRODIES
BRODKEY
BRODSKY
BROGANS
BROGUES
BROIDER
BROILED
BROILER
BROKEIN
BROKERS
BROKEUP
BROMATE
BROMIDE
BROMINE
BRONCHI
BRONCHO
BRONCOS
BRONSON
BRONTES
BRONWEN
BRONZED
BRONZER
BRONZES
BROODED
BROODER
BROOKED
BROOMED
BROSNAN
BROSSES
BROTHER
BROUGHT
BROWARD
BROWNED
BROWNER
BROWNIE
BROWSED
BROWSER
BROWSES
BROWWAX
BUOYANT
BUOYING
BUOYSUP

B•O••••

BAOBABS
BEOGRAD
BEOWULF
BIOCHIP
BIOCIDE
BIODATA
BIOFUEL
BIOLABS
BIOLITE
BIOLOGY
BIOMASS
BIONICS
BIOPICS
BIOTECH
BIOTITE
BIOTYPE
BLOATED
BLOBBED
BLOCKED
BLOCKER
BLOCKUP
BLOGGED
BLOGGER

B••O•••

BABOONS
BADOMEN
BALONEY
BAROLOS
BARONET
BAROQUE
BAYONET
BAYONNE
BAZOOKA
BECOMES
BEDOUIN
BEFOOLS
BEFOULS
BEGONIA
BEGORRA
BEHOLDS
BEHOOVE
BELONGS
BELOVED
BEMOANS
BENOTED
BENOTES
BEROWNE
BETOKEN
BEYONCE
BICOLOR
BICORNE
BICORNS
BIFOCAL
BIGONES
BIGOTED
BIGOTRY
BILOBED
BIMODAL
BINOCHE
BIPOLAR
BITONAL
BIVOUAC
BLOODED
BLOOMED
BLOOMER
BLOOPED
BLOOPER
BOLOGNA
BOLOTIE
BORODIN
BOROMIR
BORONIC
BOROUGH
BOSOMED
BOSONIC
BOWOARS
BRIOCHE
BROODED
BROODER
BROOKED
BROOMED
BUCOLIC
BUGOUTS
BUJONES
BULOVAS
BUROAKS
BUXOMLY
BUYOFFS
BUYOUTS
BYFORCE
BYFORMS
BYGOLLY
BYGONES
BYMOUTH
BYROADS
BYRONIC
BYWORDS

B•••O••

BABCOCK
BABOONS
BABYOIL
BACKOFF
BACKOUT
BADBOYS
BADCOLD
BADDOGS
BADFORM
BADJOKE
BADLOTS
BADLOVE
BADMOOD
BADMOVE
BADWORD
BAGBOYS
BAGJOBS
BAGNOLD
BAILORS
BAILOUT
BAKEOFF
BALBOAS
BALCONY
BALFOUR
BALLONE
BALLOON
BALLOTS
BAMBOOS
BANGOUT
BANJOES
BANKONE
BARCODE
BARHOPS
BARNONE
BARNOWL
BARRONS
BARROOM
BARROWS
BARSOAP
BARTOLO
BARYONS
BASSOON
BATBOYS
BATHOIL
BAWLOUT
BAYLORU
BAZOOKA
BBQPORK
BBSHOTS
BCLIONS
BEACONS
BEANOIL
BEAROFF
BEAROUT
BEATOFF
BEATOUT
BECKONS
BECLOUD
BEDDOWN
BEDFORD
BEDLOES
BEDNORZ
BEDPOST
BEDROCK
BEDROLL
BEDROOM
BEFOOLS
BEGSOFF
BEHOOVE
BELFORT
BELLOWS
BELMONT
BELTOUT
BELVOIR
BELVOUR
BELZONI
BENBOVA
BERTOLT
BERVOIX
BESPOKE
BESTOFF
BESTONE
BESTOWS
BETROTH
BETTORS
BIBCOCK
BICHONS
BIGBOSS
BIGBOYS
BIGDOGS
BIGFOOT
BIGFOUR
BIGHORN
BIGJOHN
BIGLOTS
BIGLOVE
BIGNOSE
BIGTOES
BIGTOPS
BIGTOWN
BILIOUS
BILLOWS
BILLOWY
BIMBOES
BINDOFF
BINGOES
BIOLOGY
BISHOPS
BITEOFF
BITROLE
BLALOCK
BLAZONS
BLEWOFF
BLEWOUT
BLOTOUT
BLOWOFF
BLOWOUT
BLTTOGO
BOBDOLE
BOBGOEN
BOBHOPE
BOFFOLA
BOGDOWN
BOGHOLE
BOILOFF
BOILOUT
BONBONS
BONGOES
BONJOUR
BONJOVI
BONMOTS
BONSOIR
BOOBOOS
BOOCOOS
BOOHOOS
BOOTOUT
BORDONI
BOREOUT
BORROWS
BORZOIS
BOSTONS
BOSTONU
BOTTOMS
BOUDOIR
BOUSONO
BOWDOIN
BOWDOWN
BOWSOUT
BOWWOWS
BOXBOYS
BOXCOAT
BOXTOPS
BOYCOTT
BOYHOOD
BOYTOYS
BRAVOED
BRAVOES
BRETONS
BRITONS
BRUMOUS
BSCHOOL
BUCKOES
BUDWORM
BUFFOON
BUGBOYS
BUGSOFF
BUGSOUT
BUITONI
BULBOUS
BULLOCK
BUMSOUT
BUNCOED
BUNIONS
BUNKOED
BURBOTS
BURGOOS
BURNOFF
BURNOUT
BURROWS
BUSBOYS
BUSLOAD
BUSTOUR
BUSTOUT
BUTGOOD
BUTTONS
BUTTONY
BUTTOUT
BUYDOWN
BUYSOFF
BUYSOUT
BUZZOFF
BYANOSE
BYPHONE
BYPROXY

B••••O•

BABYBOP
BABYLON
BACKHOE
BACKLOG
BACKLOT
BACKROW
BADENOV
BADMOOD
BADSHOT
BAGEHOT
BAGNIOS
BAILSON
BALATON
BALLBOY
BALLIOL
BALLOON
BAMBOOS
BANDBOX
BANGKOK
BANGSON
BANKJOB
BANKSON
BARANOF
BAROLOS
BARRIOS
BARROOM
BARSTOW
BASEDON
BASSOON
BASTION
BATSFOR
BDALTON
BEALION
BEARSON
BEATBOX
BEATCOP
BEATSON
BEDROOM
BEGSFOR
BELABOR
BELLBOY
BELLHOP
BELLSON
BENISON
BENTHOS
BERGSON
BERLIOZ
BESTBOY
BIBELOT
BIBLIOG
BICOLOR
BIDSFOR
BIENTOT
BIGELOW
BIGFOOT
BIGSHOT
BIGSHOW
BILLION
BIRDDOG
BISTROS
BITESON
BLAMEON
BLANTON
BLAUBOK
BLEDSOE
BLERIOT
BLOSSOM
BLOUSON
BLOWPOP
BLOWSON
BLUEBOY
BLUEFOX
BLUSHON
BOASTOF
BOKCHOY
BOLEROS
BOLSHOI
BONITOS
BOOBOOS
BOOCOOS
BOOHOOS
BOOMBOX
BOOTTOP
BOREDOM
BOURBON
BOUTROS
BOWKNOT
BOWSHOT
BOYHOOD
BRANDON
BRANSON
BRAXTON
BRENDON
BRERFOX
BRETTON
BRILLOS
BRINGON
BRISTOL
BRITCOM
BRITPOP
BRITTON
BRONCOS
BRONSON
BRYUSOV
BSCHOOL
BUCKFOR
BUFFOON
BUGABOO
BUGALOO
BUILDON
BUILTON
BUISSON
BULLDOG
BULLION
BURGEON
BURGOOS
BURNFOR
BUSHHOG
BUSSTOP
BUTGOOD
BYWAYOF

B•••••O

BABENCO
BALLTWO
BAMBINO
BANDIDO
BANDITO
BARTOLO
BASETWO
BASILIO
BASSANO
BEAHERO
BEEFALO
BEGANTO
BELASCO
BENICIO
BENIGNO
BERGAMO
BINDSTO
BIZARRO
BLINDTO
BLTTOGO
BOIARDO
BOITANO
BONARIO
BONIATO
BOUNDTO
BOUSONO
BOWECHO
BOWEDTO
BRACERO
BRAVADO
BRINGTO
BRONCHO
BUFFALO
BUGABOO
BUGALOO
BUNUELO
BURRITO
BUSHIDO
BUYINTO
BYJINGO

•BO••••

ABOLISH
ABOLLAE
ABORTED
ABOUNDS
ABOUTIT
ABOUTTO
EBONICS
EBONIES
EBONITE
EBONIZE
OBOISTS

•B•O•••

ABBOTCY
ABDOMEN
ABIOTIC
ABROACH
ABSOLUT
ABSOLVE
ABSORBS
OBLONGS
OBLOQUY
VBLOUSE

•B••O••

ABALONE
ABATORS
ABSCOND
BBQPORK
BBSHOTS
OBVIOUS

•B•••O•

ABANDON
ABETTOR
ABSALOM
ABUTSON
IBEGYOU
OBENTOS
OBLIGOR

•B••••O

ABOUTTO
CBRADIO

••BO•••

ABBOTCY
ALBORAK
ARBOLES
ARBORED
ARBOURS
BABOONS
CABOOSE
CUBOIDS
CYBORGS
DEBOITE
DEBONED
DEBONES
DEBORAH
DEBOULE
ELBOWED
ELBOWER
EMBOITE
EMBOSOM
EMBOWER
HOBOING
HOBOISM
HOBOKEN
IMBORED
INBOARD
INBOUND
INBOXES
KOBOLDS
LABORAT
LABORED
LABORER
LABOURS
MRBODDY
MRBONES
NABOKOV
NOBODYS
ONBOARD
OSBORNE
POBOXES
PTBOATS
PWBOTHA
REBOANT
REBOARD
REBOILS
REBOLTS
REBOOKS
REBOOTS
REBORED
REBORES
REBOTES
REBOUND
REBOXED
REBOXES
REBOZOS
ROBOCOP
ROBOTIC
ROBOTRY
SUBORNS
TABOOED
TABORET
TABOULI
UNBOGGY
UNBOLTS
UNBONED
UNBORED
UNBORNE
UNBOSOM
UNBOUND
UNBOWED
UNBOXED
UNBOXES
UPBORNE
UPBOUND

••B•O••

AMBROSE
BABCOCK
BABOONS
BABYOIL
BIBCOCK
BOBDOLE
BOBGOEN
BOBHOPE
CABOOSE
COBCOAL
DEBTORS
DRBROWN
DUBIOUS
EMBROIL
EMBROWN
FABFOUR
FIBROID
FIBROUS
FOBSOFF
GIBBONS
GIBBOUS
GIBSONS
GOBROKE
HOBNOBS
HOBSONS
IMBROKE
INBLOOM
INBROWN
JIBBOOM
JOBHOPS
JOBLOCK
JOBLOTS
LABCOAT
LEBROCK
LUBBOCK
MRBROWN
OXBLOOD
REBLOCK
REBLOOM
REBLOWN
REBOOKS
REBOOTS
REBROKE
RIBBONS
RIBBONY
ROBLOWE
ROBROYS
RUBDOWN
RUBEOLA
RUBIOUS
RUBSOFF
RUBSOUT
SUBCODE
SUBCOOL
SUBFORM
SUBGOAL
SUBGODS
SUBJOIN
SUBLONG
SUBLOTS
SUBPOST
SUBROOT
SUBROSA
SUBSOIL
SUBSORT
SUBTONE
SUBZONE
TABLOID
TABOOED
UNBLOCK
UNBLOWN
UNBROKE
WEBFOOT
WEBLOGS
WEBTOED
ZEBROID

••B••O•

ALBEDOS
ALBINOS
ANBESOL
BABYBOP
BABYLON
BIBELOT
BIBLIOG
CABRIOS
EMBOSOM
EMBRYOS
GABBROS
GOBELOW
INBLOOM
JIBBOOM
JOBSHOP
LEBANON
LEBARON
LIBIDOS
LUBEJOB
NABOKOV
ORBISON
OXBLOOD
REBLOOM
REBOZOS
ROBESON
ROBOCOP
RUBATOS
RUBICON
RUBUPON
SABADOS
SUBCOOL
SUBPLOT
SUBROOT
TIBURON
TUBETOP
UNBOSOM
WEBFOOT
WOBEGON
ZABUTON
ZEBULON

••B•••O
ALBERTO
ALBIREO
BABENCO
EMBARGO
FEBRERO
HIBERNO
NABISCO
NABUCCO
POBLANO
ROBERTO
ROBUSTO
SUBECHO
SUBZERO
TABASCO
TOBACCO
UMBERTO
VIBRATO

••BO••
AIRBOAT
AKEBONO
AMEBOID
ANYBODY
ARMBONE
ARTBOOK
ASABODY
ATABOIL
BADBOYS
BAGBOYS
BALBOAS
BAMBOOS
BATBOYS
BENBOVA
BIGBOSS
BIGBOYS
BIMBOES
BONBONS
BOOBOOS
BOXBOYS
BUGBOYS
BULBOUS
BURBOTS
BUSBOYS
CAMBOYS
CARBONS
CARBOYS
CATBOAT
CATBOWL
COWBOYS
CUIBONO
DASBOOT
DAYBOOK
DIABOLO
DIEBOLD
DOGBONE
DOGBOOT
DOGBOWL
DOTBOMB
EARBONE
EYEBOLT
FEMBOTS
FLYBOYS
FOGBOWS
FORBORE
FOXBORO
GAMBOLS
GIBBONS
GIBBOUS
GLOBOID
GLOBOSE
GLOBOUS
GOABOUT
GUMBOOT
GUNBOAT
HAMBONE
HARBORS
HARBOUR
HIPBONE
HIPBOOT
ICEBOAT
JAWBONE
JERBOAS
JETBOAT
JIBBOOM
JOSBOYS
LAWBOOK
LAZBOYS
LEGBONE
LOGBOOK
LONBORG
LOWBORN
LOWBOYS
LUBBOCK
MAMBOED
MAXBORN
NEWBOLT
NEWBORN
NONBODY
NONBOOK
OLDBOYS
OREBODY
OUTBOWL
OUTBOWS
PARBOIL
PEABODY
PEPBOYS
PETBOAS
PINBOYS
PITBOSS
POTBOIL
PREBOIL
PREBOOK
PREBOOM
PREBORN
PROBONO
PROBOWL
RASBORA
REDBONE
REDBOOK
REEBOKS
RHEBOKS
RIBBONS
RIBBONY
ROWBOAT
SAMBORA
SANBORN
SEABOAT
SEABORG
SKIBOBS
SKIBOOT
SPYBOTS
SUNBOWL
SUNBOWS
SYMBOLS
THEBOBO
THEBODY
THEBOMB
THEBOSS
THEBOYS
TOMBOYS
TOPBOOT
TOWBOAT
TOYBOAT
TOYBOOK
TRIBORO
TUGBOAT
TURBOTS
UNIBODY
UPABOVE
VERBOSE
WARBOND
ZAMBONI

•••B•O•
ARTBOOK
BAMBOOS
BOOBOOS
CRABPOT
DASBOOT
DAYBOOK
DIABLOS
DOGBOOT
EYEBROW
GABBROS
GUMBOOT
HIPBOOT
INKBLOT
JIBBOOM
JOEBLOW
LAWBOOK
LOGBOOK
LOWBLOW
LOWBROW
NONBOOK
OUTBLOT
OUTBLOW
PREBOOK
PREBOOM
PUEBLOS
REDBOOK
SKIBOOT
TEMBLOR
THEBLOB
TOPBOOT
TOYBOOK

•••B••O
AKEBONO
BAMBINO
CEMBALO
CONBRIO
CUIBONO
DIABOLO
DOUBLEO
ESOBESO
FOXBORO
GAMBADO
LINBIAO
LUMBAGO
MAYBESO
PROBONO
THEBOBO
TRIBORO

••••BO•
ATTABOY
AUDUBON
BABYBOP
BALLBOY
BANDBOX
BEATBOX
BELABOR
BELLBOY
BESTBOY
BLAUBOK
BLUEBOY
BOOMBOX
BOURBON
BUGABOO
CALLBOX
CALLBOY
CARABOO
CARIBOO
CARIBOU
CASHBOX
CITYBOY
CLIMBON
COINBOX
COPYBOY
DEEDBOX
DOWNBOW
DROPBOX
ENARBOR
FAREBOX
FARMBOY
FIREBOX
FUSEBOX
GAMEBOY
GAZEBOS
GEARBOX
GEMSBOK
GIFTBOX
HAUTBOY
HELLBOY
HIGHBOY
HOMEBOY
ICHABOD
INLABOR
ITSABOY
JAZZBOS
JOHNBOY
JUKEBOX
JURYBOX
KICKBOX
LAVABOS
LOCKBOX
LONGBOW
MAILBOX
MISTBOW
MOONBOW
NEWSBOY
NICEBOY
PAGEBOY
PEATBOG
PILLBOX
PLAYBOY
PLOWBOY
POORBOX
POORBOY
POSTBOX
RAINBOW
SAIDBOO
SALTBOX
SANDBOX
SAYSBOO
SHOEBOX
SOAPBOX
SPAMBOT
TOOLBOX
WOODBOX
WORKBOX

••••B•O
AUTOBIO
BUGABOO
CALABRO
CARABOO
CARIBOO
CEREBRO
CLIMBTO
SAIDBOO
SAYSBOO

•••••BO
AAJUMBO
ARECIBO
COLOMBO
COLUMBO
INLIMBO
MOGAMBO
PLACEBO
RIOLOBO
THEBOBO

BP•••••
BPLUSES

B•P••••
BAPTISE
BAPTISM
BAPTIST
BAPTIZE
BIPEDAL
BIPLANE
BIPOLAR
BOPPERS
BOPPING
BYPATHS
BYPHONE
BYPLAYS
BYPROXY

B••P•••
BADPAST
BAGPIPE
BBQPITS
BBQPORK
BEDPOST
BEEPERS
BEEPING
BEEPSAT
BESPEAK
BESPOKE
BIOPICS
BITPART
BLIPPED
BOOPSIE
BOPPERS
BOPPING
BUMPERS
BUMPIER
BUMPILY
BUMPING
BUMPKIN
BUMPSUP
BURPGUN
BURPING
BUSPASS

B•••P••
BACKPAY
BAKEPAN
BASEPAY
BEARPAW
BEARPIT
BEHAPPY
BIASPLY
BIGAPES
BLEEPED
BLEEPER
BLIMPIE
BLIPPED
BLOOPED
BLOOPER
BLOWPOP
BREWPUB
BRITPOP
BTFSPLK
BULLPEN
BUSHPIG

B••••P•
BACKUPS
BADRAPS
BAGPIPE
BARHOPS
BEDRAPE
BEHAPPY
BIGTOPS
BIOTYPE
BISHOPS
BITMAPS
BLOWUPS
BOBHOPE
BOXTOPS
BUMRAPS
BURLAPS
BUSTUPS

B•••••P
BABYBOP
BABYGAP
BACKSUP
BADTRIP
BALLSUP
BANGSUP
BANKSUP
BARKEEP
BARSOAP
BEADSUP
BEAMSUP
BEANDIP
BEARSUP
BEATCOP
BEATSUP
BEDLAMP
BEEFSUP
BEERTAP
BELLHOP
BELLLAP
BELLYUP
BELTSUP
BIGGULP
BINDSUP
BIOCHIP
BITESUP
BLAZEUP
BLOCKUP
BLOTSUP
BLOWNUP
BLOWPOP
BLOWSUP
BOARDUP
BOILSUP
BOLTSUP
BONEDUP
BONESUP
BOOSTUP
BOOTSUP
BOOTTOP
BORNEUP
BOTCHUP
BOUNDUP
BOXEDUP
BOXESUP
BOXSTEP
BRACEUP
BREAKUP
BREWSUP
BRICKUP
BRINGUP
BRITPOP
BROKEUP
BRUSHUP
BUCKSUP
BUDDYUP
BUFFSUP
BUILDUP
BUILTUP
BULKSUP
BUMPSUP
BUNCHUP
BUOYSUP
BURNSUP
BURNTUP
BUSSTOP
BUSTRIP
BUSTSUP

•B•P•••
BBQPITS
BBQPORK

••BP•••
RIBPADS
SUBPLOT
SUBPOST
WEBPAGE

••B•P••
RUBUPON
TUBEPAN

••B••P•
BOBHOPE
HUBCAPS
JOBHOPS
SUBTYPE

••B•••P
BABYBOP
BABYGAP
JOBSHOP
ROBOCOP
TUBETOP

•••BP••
CRABPOT

•••B••P
CLUBSUP
DOUBLEP

••••B•P
BABYBOP
CLIMBUP
SCRUBUP

B•Q••••
BBQBEEF
BBQPITS
BBQPORK
BBQRIBS
BEQUEST
BEQUICK
BEQUIET
BUQSHAS

B••Q•••
BANQUES
BANQUET
BARQUES
BASQUES
BISQUES
BOUQUET
BRIQUET

B•••Q••
BAROQUE
BEZIQUE
BRUSQUE

•BQ••••
BBQBEEF
BBQPITS
BBQPORK
BBQRIBS

•B••Q••
OBLIQUE
OBLOQUY

••B•Q••
DUBUQUE

•••B••Q
DOUBLEQ

BR•••••
BRACERO
BRACERS
BRACEUP
BRACING
BRACKEN
BRACKET
BRADLEE
BRADLEY
BRAEDEN
BRAGGED
BRAGGER
BRAHMAN
BRAHMAS
BRAHMIN
BRAIDED
BRAIDER
BRAILLE
BRAINED
BRAINER
BRAISED
BRAISES
BRAKING
BRALESS
BRAMBLE
BRAMBLY
BRAMLEY
BRANAGH
BRANCHY
BRANDED
BRANDER
BRANDON
BRANIFF
BRANSON
BRASHER
BRASHES
BRASHLY
BRASIER
BRASIZE
BRASSES
BRASSIE
BRATTLE
BRAVADA
BRAVADO
BRAVELY
BRAVERY
BRAVEST
BRAVING
BRAVOED
BRAVOES
BRAVURA
BRAWLED
BRAWLER
BRAWLEY
BRAXTON
BRAYERS
BRAYING
BRAZENS
BRAZIER
BRAZING
BREADED
BREADER
BREADTH
BREAKER
BREAKIN
BREAKUP
BREASTS
BREATHE
BREATHS
BREATHY
BREEDER
BREEZED
BREEZES
BRENDAN
BRENDEL
BRENDON
BRENGUN
BRENNAN
BRENNER
BRERFOX
BRESCIA
BRESLIN
BRETONS
BRETTON
BREVETS
BREVITY
BREWAGE
BREWERS
BREWERY
BREWING
BREWPUB
BREWSKI
BREWSUP
BREYERS
BRIARDS
BRIBEES
BRIBERS
BRIBERY
BRIBING
BRICKED
BRICKLE
BRICKUP
BRIDALS
BRIDGED
BRIDGER
BRIDGES
BRIDGET
BRIDLED
BRIDLER
BRIDLES
BRIEFED
BRIEFER
BRIEFLY
BRIGADE
BRIGAND
BRIGHAM
BRIGHTS
BRILLIG
BRILLOS
BRIMFUL
BRIMLEY
BRIMMED
BRIMMER
BRINDLE
BRINERS
BRINGER
BRINGIN
BRINGIT
BRINGON
BRINGTO
BRINGUP
BRINIER
BRINING
BRINISH
BRINKER
BRIOCHE
BRIQUET
BRISKED
BRISKER
BRISKET
BRISKLY
BRISTLE
BRISTLY
BRISTOL
BRITAIN
BRITCOM
BRITISH
BRITNEY
BRITONS
BRITPOP
BRITTEN
BRITTLE
BRITTON
BROADAS
BROADAX
BROADEN
BROADER
BROADLY
BROASTS
BROCADE
BRODIES
BRODKEY
BRODSKY
BROGANS
BROGUES
BROIDER
BROILED
BROILER
BROKEIN
BROKERS
BROKEUP
BROMATE
BROMIDE
BROMINE
BRONCHI
BRONCHO
BRONCOS
BRONSON
BRONTES
BRONWEN
BRONZED
BRONZER
BRONZES
BROODED
BROODER
BROOKED
BROOMED
BROSNAN
BROSSES
BROTHER
BROUGHT
BROWARD
BROWNED
BROWNER
BROWNIE
BROWSED
BROWSER
BROWSES
BROWWAX
BRUBECK
BRUEGEL
BRUISED
BRUISER
BRUISES
BRUITED
BRUMMEL
BRUMOUS
BRUNETS
BRUSHED
BRUSHER
BRUSHES
BRUSHUP
BRUSQUE
BRUTELY
BRUTISH
BRUXING
BRUXISM
BRYNNER
BRYUSOV

B•R••••
BARACUS
BARANOF
BARBARA
BARBARY
BARBATE
BARBEAU
BARBELL
BARBERA
BARBERS
BARBETS
BARBIES
BARBILL
BARBING
BARBUDA
BARBULE
BARCARS
BARCLAY
BARCODE
BARDEEN
BAREGES
BARENTS
BARETTA
BAREXAM
BARFBAG
BARGAIN
BARGEIN
BARGERS
BARGING
BARHOPS
BARISTA
BARITES
BARKEEP
BARKERS
BARKIER
BARKING
BARKLEY
BARKSAT
BARLESS
BARLEYS
BARLICK
BARMAID
BARMIER
BARNABY
BARNARD
BARNEYS
BARNING
BARNONE
BARNOWL
BARNRED
BARNUMS
BAROLOS
BARONET
BAROQUE
BARQUES
BARRACK
BARRAGE
BARRELS
BARRENS
BARRETS
BARRETT
BARRIER
BARRING
BARRIOS
BARRONS
BARROOM
BARROWS
BARSOAP
BARSTOW
BARTABS
BARTEND
BARTERS
BARTLES
BARTLET
BARTOLO
BARTRAY
BARWARE
BARYONS
BERATED
BERATER
BERATES
BERBERS
BERBICK
BEREAVE
BERENDT
BERETTA
BERGAMO
BERGERE
BERGIUS
BERGMAN
BERGSON
BERIGAN
BERKLEY
BERKNER
BERLIOZ
BERLITZ
BERMING
BERMUDA
BERNARD
BERNAYS
BERNESE
BERNINA
BERNINI
BERNSEN
BEROWNE
BERRIED
BERRIES
BERSERK
BERSUNT
BERTHAS
BERTHED
BERTOLT
BERTRAM
BERVOIX
BERWICK
BIRCHED
BIRCHEN
BIRCHES
BIRDDOG
BIRDERS
BIRDFLU
BIRDIED
BIRDIES
BIRDING
BIRDMAN
BIRDMEN

BIREMES
BIRETTA
BIRIANI
BIRLERS
BIRLING
BIRMANS
BIRRING
BIRTHED
BIRYANI
BORATES
BORDERS
BORDONI
BOREDOM
BOREOUT
BORGIAS
BORGLUM
BORIDES
BORINGS
BORKING
BORLAUG
BORNEAN
BORNEUP
BORODIN
BOROMIR
BORONIC
BOROUGH
BORROWS
BORSCHT
BORSTAL
BORZAGE
BORZOIS
BURBAGE
BURBANK
BURBLED
BURBLER
BURBLES
BURBOTS
BURDENS
BURDICK
BUREAUS
BUREAUX
BURETTE
BURGEES
BURGEON
BURGERS
BURGESS
BURGHER
BURGLAR
BURGLED
BURGLES
BURGOOS
BURIALS
BURIERS
BURKINA
BURLAPS
BURLERS
BURLIER
BURLING
BURMANS
BURMESE
BURNABY
BURNERS
BURNETT
BURNFOR
BURNING
BURNISH
BURNLEY
BURNOFF
BURNOUT
BURNSIN
BURNSUP
BURNTIN
BURNTUP
BUROAKS
BURPGUN
BURPING
BURRIER
BURRING
BURRITO
BURROWS
BURSARS
BURSTER
BURSTIN
BURSTYN
BURUNDI
BURYING
BYRIGHT
BYROADS
BYRONIC

B••R•••

BADRAPS
BAHRAIN
BAHREIN
BARRACK
BARRAGE
BARRELS
BARRENS
BARRETS
BARRETT
BARRIER
BARRING
BARRIOS
BARRONS
BARROOM
BARROWS
BASRHIN
BAYRUMS
BBQRIBS
BEARCAT
BEARCUB
BEARDED
BEARERS
BEARHUG
BEARING
BEARISH
BEAROFF
BEAROUT
BEARPAW
BEARPIT
BEARSON
BEARSUP
BEBRAVE
BEDRAIL
BEDRAPE
BEDREST
BEDROCK
BEDROLL
BEDROOM
BEERCAN
BEERIER
BEERKEG
BEERMUG
BEERTAP
BEGRIME
BEHRENS
BEHRING
BEHRMAN
BERRIED
BERRIES
BETRAYS
BETROTH
BEURRES
BIGRIGS
BIRRING
BITROLE
BLARING
BLARNEY
BLERIOT
BLURBER
BLURRED
BLURTED
BLURTER
BOARDED
BOARDER
BOARDUP
BOARISH
BOERWAR
BOHRIUM
BOORISH
BOORMAN
BORROWS
BOTREES
BOURBON
BOURGET
BOURSES
BRERFOX
BULRUSH
BUMRAPS
BUMRUSH
BUNRAKU
BURRIER
BURRING
BURRITO
BURROWS
BUSRIDE
BYPROXY
BYTRAIN

B•••R••

BACARDI
BACKROW
BACKRUB
BACTRIA
BADAREA
BADTRIP
BAKERST
BALDRIC
BARNRED
BARTRAY
BAVARIA
BAYAREA
BAYTREE
BEATRIX
BEETRED
BEETREE
BEGIRDS
BEGORRA
BELARUS
BELTRAN
BEMIRED
BEMIRES
BENARES
BEOGRAD
BERTRAM
BESTREW
BETARAY
BEURRES
BEVERLY
BEWARED
BEWARES
BIAFRAN
BICARBS
BICORNE
BICORNS
BISTROS
BIZARRE
BIZARRO
BLEARED
BLUERED
BLURRED
BODEREK
BODYRUB
BOGARDE
BOGARTS
BOIARDO
BOLEROS
BONARIO
BOUTROS
BOWERED
BRIARDS
BUCKRAM
BUGFREE
BULLRUN
BUSTRIP
BUTTRAM
BYBIRTH
BYFORCE
BYFORMS
BYTURNS
BYWORDS

B••••R•

BACKERS
BADFORM
BADGERS
BADGIRL
BADWORD
BAFFERS
BAGGERS
BAGGIRL
BAILERS
BAILORS
BAITERS
BALKERS
BALLARD
BANBURY
BANDERA
BANDERS
BANGERS
BANKERS
BANNERS
BANTERS
BARBARA
BARBARY
BARBERA
BARBERS
BARCARS
BARGERS
BARKERS
BARNARD
BARTERS
BARWARE
BASHERS
BASTERS
BATGIRL
BATHERS
BATTERS
BATTERY
BAWLERS
BAYLORU
BAZAARS
BBQPORK
BEADERS
BEAHERO
BEAKERS
BEAMERS
BEANERY
BEARERS
BEATERS
BEAVERS
BECHARM
BEDFORD
BEDNORZ
BEEMERS
BEEPERS
BEEYARD
BEEZERS
BEGGARS
BEGGARY
BEGORRA
BEHEARD
BELAIRS
BELFORT
BELIERS
BELTERS
BENDERS
BERBERS
BERGERE
BERNARD
BERSERK
BESTIRS
BETHERE
BETTERS
BETTORS
BEZIERS
BIBBERS
BICKERS
BIDDERS
BIGBIRD
BIGCARS
BIGEARS
BIGGERS
BIGGIRL
BIGHORN
BIGJERK
BIGOTRY
BILKERS
BILLERS
BINDERS
BINDERY
BINGERS
BIRDERS
BIRLERS
BITPART
BITTERN
BITTERS
BIZARRE
BIZARRO
BLADERS
BLAMERS
BLAZERS
BLOWDRY
BLOWERS
BOATERS
BOBBERS
BODYART
BOILERS
BOKHARA
BOLTERS
BOMBARD
BOMBERS
BONAIRE
BONDERS
BONEDRY
BONFIRE
BONKERS
BONNARD
BOOBIRD
BOOKERS
BOOKERT
BOOMERS
BOOTERS
BOOTERY
BOOZERS
BOPPERS
BORDERS
BOTHERS
BOWLERS
BOWOARS
BOWYERS
BOXCARS
BRACERO
BRACERS
BRAVERY
BRAVURA
BRAYERS
BREWERS
BREWERY
BREYERS
BRIBERS
BRIBERY
BRINERS
BROKERS
BROWARD
BUCKERS
BUDDERS
BUDGERS
BUDWORM
BUFFERS
BUGLERS
BUKHARA
BULGARI
BULGARS
BULGURS
BULWARK
BUMMERS
BUMPERS
BUNKERS
BUNTERS
BURGERS
BURIERS
BURLERS
BURNERS
BURSARS
BUSFARE
BUSGIRL
BUSHERS
BUSKERS
BUSSERS
BUSTARD
BUSTERS
BUTLERS
BUTTERS
BUTTERY
BUZZARD
BUZZERS
BYHEART

B•••••R

BABBLER
BABIYAR
BACKBAR
BADHAIR
BAFFLER
BAGGIER
BAINTER
BAITCAR
BALFOUR
BALKIER
BALLMER
BALMIER
BANALER
BANDIER
BARKIER
BARMIER
BARRIER
BASSIER
BATSFOR
BATTIER
BATTLER
BAULKER
BAWDIER
BEADIER
BEAMIER
BEECHER
BEEFIER
BEERIER
BEETIER
BEGSFOR
BELABOR
BELAYER
BELCHER
BELLJAR
BELVOIR
BELVOUR
BENATAR
BENAZIR
BENCHER
BENDIER
BERATER
BERKNER
BESMEAR
BETTGER
BEVELER
BICOLOR
BIDFAIR
BIDSFOR
BIGBEAR
BIGFOUR
BIGHAIR
BIGSTAR
BILGIER
BIPOLAR
BITSIER
BITTIER
BLABBER
BLACKER
BLADDER
BLANDER
BLANKER
BLASTER
BLATHER
BLEAKER
BLEATER
BLEEDER
BLEEPER
BLENDER
BLESSER
BLINDER
BLINKER
BLISTER
BLITHER
BLITZER
BLOCKER
BLOGGER
BLONDER
BLOOMER
BLOOPER
BLOTTER
BLOWIER
BLUBBER
BLUDGER
BLUFFER
BLUNDER
BLUNTER
BLURBER
BLURTER
BLUSHER
BLUSTER
BOARDER
BOASTER
BOBBLER
BOBWEIR
BOCHNER
BODYBAR
BOERWAR
BOGGIER
BOGGLER
BOLIVAR
BOLSTER
BONEYER
BONHEUR
BONJOUR
BONNIER
BONSOIR
BOOMCAR
BOOMIER
BOOSLER
BOOSTER
BOOZIER
BOROMIR
BOSSIER
BOTCHER
BOTTLER
BOUCHER
BOUDOIR
BOULDER
BOUNCER
BOUNDER
BOUVIER
BOWDLER
BOXSTER
BRAGGER
BRAIDER
BRAINER
BRANDER
BRASHER
BRASIER
BRAWLER
BRAZIER
BREADER
BREAKER
BREEDER
BRENNER
BRIDGER
BRIDLER
BRIEFER
BRIMMER
BRINGER
BRINIER
BRINKER
BRISKER
BROADER
BROIDER
BROILER
BRONZER
BROODER
BROTHER
BROWNER
BROWSER
BRUISER
BRUSHER
BRYNNER
BUCHNER
BUCKFOR
BUCKNER
BUELLER
BUGBEAR
BUGGIER
BUILDER
BULGHUR
BULGIER
BULKIER
BUMBLER
BUMPIER
BUNDLER
BUNGLER
BURBLER
BURGHER
BURGLAR
BURLIER
BURNFOR
BURRIER
BURSTER
BUSHIER
BUSTIER
BUSTLER
BUSTOUR
BUTCHER
BUZZIER
BYAHAIR
BYLINER

•BR••••

ABRADED
ABRADER
ABRADES
ABRAHAM
ABRAXAS
ABREAST
ABRIDGE
ABRILES
ABROACH
ABRUZZI
CBRADIO

•B•R•••

ABORTED
BBQRIBS
IBERIAN
OBERLIN
OBTRUDE

•B••R••

ABJURED
ABJURER
ABJURES
ABSORBS
OBSERVE
OBVERSE
OBVERTS

•B•••R•

ABASERS
ABATERS
ABATORS
ABELARD
ABIDERS
ABINTRA
ABUSERS
BBQPORK
EBAYERS
OBEYERS
OBSCURA
OBSCURE

•B••••R

ABETTER
ABETTOR
ABJURER
ABRADER
ABUTTER
OBLIGER
OBLIGOR
OBTUSER

••BR•••

AMBRIES
AMBROSE
BEBRAVE
CABRIDE
CABRINI
CABRIOS
COBRAND
DEBRETT
DEBRIEF
DRBROWN
EMBRACE
EMBROIL
EMBROWN
EMBRUED
EMBRUES
EMBRYOS
FABRICS
FABRIZI
FEBRERO
FEBRILE
FIBRINS
FIBROID
FIBROUS
FTBRAGG
GABRIEL
GOBROKE
HEBRAIC
HEBREWS
HYBRIDS
IMBROKE
IMBRUED
IMBRUES
INBREED
INBRIEF
INBROWN
KUBRICK
LABRATS
LEBROCK
LIBRANS
LIBRARY
MCBRIDE
MOBRULE
MRBROWN
ONBREAK
REBRACE
REBRAND
REBREAK
REBREED
REBREWS
REBROKE
REBRUSH
ROBROYS
RUBRICS
SABRINA
SEBRING
SUBRACE
SUBROOT
SUBROSA
UMBRAGE
UMBRIAN
UMBRIEL
UNBRACE
UNBRAID
UNBRAKE
UNBRAVE
UNBRIEF
UNBROKE
UPBRAID
VIBRANT
VIBRATE
VIBRATO
ZEBRAIC
ZEBRASS
ZEBRINE
ZEBROID

••B•R••

ALBERTA
ALBERTI
ALBERTO
ALBIREO
ALBORAK
ARBORED
AUBERGE
AUBURNS
AUBURNU
BYBIRTH
CABARET
CYBORGS
DEBARGE
DEBARKS
DEBORAH
DEBURGH
DEBURRS
DUBARRY
ELBERTA
EMBARGO
EMBARKS
FABARES
FABERGE
FIBERED
GABBROS
HIBERNO
IMBORED
LABORAT
LABORED
LABORER
LEBARON
LIBERAL
LIBERIA
LIBERTE
LIBERTY
MRBURNS
MUBARAK
NUBIRAS
OSBORNE
PUBERTY
REBIRTH
REBORED
REBORES
ROBARDS
ROBERTA
ROBERTE
ROBERTF
ROBERTH
ROBERTI
ROBERTO
ROBERTS
RUBSRAW
RUBYRED
SABERED
SIBERIA
SOBERED
SOBERER
SOBERLY
STBARTS
SUBAREA
SUBARID
SUBARUS
SUBORNS
SUBURBS
TABARDS
TABARET
TABORET
TIBURON
UMBERED
UMBERTO
UNBARED
UNBARES
UNBERTH
UNBORED
UNBORNE
UNBURLY
UNBURNT
UNBURST
UPBORNE
UPBURST

••B••R•

ALBSURE
AMBLERS
ARBOURS
BIBBERS
BOBBERS
CABFARE
CABLERS
DABBERS
DEBEARD
DEBEERS
DEBLURS
DEBTORS
DEBURRS
DUBARRY
DUBBERS
FABLERS
FEBRERO
FIBBERS
GABBERS
GIBBERS
HUBBARD
INBOARD
JABBERS
JOBBERS
JOBBERY
JOBJARS
LABOURS
LIBBERS
LIBRARY
LOBBERS
LUBBERS
MOBBERS
NABBERS
NUBBERS
ONBOARD
REBOARD
RIBBERS
ROBBERS
ROBBERY
ROBOTRY
ROBSART
RUBBERS
RUBBERY
SOBBERS
SUBFORM
SUBSORT
SUBVERT
SUBWARS
SUBZERO
UNBEARD
UPBEARS

••B•••R

ARBITER
BABBLER
BABIYAR
BOBBLER
BOBWEIR
COBBLER
COBUYER
DABBLER
DEBASER
DEBATER
DIBBLER
ELBOWER
EMBOWER
FABFOUR

FIBIGER
FIBSTER
FIBULAR
FUBSIER
GABBIER
GOBBLER
GOBYAIR
GOBYCAR
HIBBLER
HOBBLER
IMBIBER
JOBFAIR
LABELER
LABORER
LIBELER
LOBBYER
LOBSTER
MOBSTER
NEBULAR
NIBBLER
NOBBIER
NUBBIER
ORBITER
REBATER
REBUKER
RIBBIER
SOBERER
SUBDUER
SUBTLER
TABULAR
TUBBIER
TUBULAR
URBANER
WEBBIER
WEBSTER
WOBBLER

•••BR••

ALLBRAN
CAMBRIA
CAMBRIC
CARBRAS
CONBRIO
CUMBRIA
EYEBROW
GABBROS
HATBRIM
HOFBRAU
HOMBRES
ILLBRED
JOGBRAS
LOWBRED
LOWBROW
MISBREW
MOWBRAY
NOMBRES
OATBRAN
OUTBRAG
OUTBRAY
OUTBRED
THEBRAT
TIMBRES
TUMBREL

•••B•R•

ANTBIRD
ARLBERG
ASHBERY
ASHBURN
ASHBURY
BANBURY
BARBARA
BARBARY
BARBERA
BARBERS
BERBERS
BIBBERS
BIGBIRD
BOBBERS
BOMBARD
BOMBERS
BOOBIRD
BRIBERS
BRIBERY
CADBURY
CAMBERS
CARBARN
CATBERT
CATBIRD
CLIBURN
COGBURN
COLBERT
COMBERS
COWBIRD
CUMBERS
DABBERS
DANBURY
DAUBERS
DELBERT
DILBERT
DISBARS
DOGBERT
DUBBERS
FIBBERS
FIGBARS
FILBERT
FORBORE
FOXBORO
FREBERG
GABBERS
GIBBERS
GILBERT
GOOBERS
HAMBURG
HARBORS
HARBURG
HEPBURN
HERBART
HERBERT
HILBERT
HOLBERG
HOMBURG
HUBBARD
HUMBARD
HUMBERT
ICEBERG
ISOBARS
JABBERS
JAYBIRD
JOBBERS
JOBBERY
JROBERT
LAMBERT
LAYBARE
LIBBERS
LIMBERS
LIMBURG
LOBBERS
LOMBARD
LONBORG
LOWBORN
LUBBERS
LUMBARS
LUMBERS
MAXBORN
MEMBERS
MOBBERS
MOEBERG
NABBERS
NEWBERN
NEWBERY
NEWBORN
NEWBURG
NORBERT
NUBBERS
NUMBERS
OILBIRD
OUTBARK
OUTBURN
PETBIRD
PREBORN
PREBURN
PROBERS
RAEBURN
RASBORA
RATBERT
RAWBARS
RAYBURN
REDBIRD
RHUBARB
RIBBERS
ROBBERS
ROBBERY
ROMBERG
ROXBURY
RUBBERS
RUBBERY
SAMBORA
SANBORN
SEABIRD
SEABORG
SHUBERT
SOBBERS
SUDBURY
SUNBIRD
SUNBURN
TANBARK
THEBARD
TIEBARS
TIMBERS
TIMBERY
TOWBARS
TRABERT
TRIBORO
WARBURG
WETBARS
WILBERT

•••B••R

ANTBEAR
BABBLER
BIGBEAR
BLABBER
BLUBBER
BOBBLER
BUGBEAR
BUMBLER
BURBLER
CLABBER
CLOBBER
CLUBBER
CLUBCAR
COBBLER
CRABBER
CRIBBER
DABBLER
DIBBLER
DOUBLER
DOUBTER
DRABBER
DRUBBER
ENABLER
FEEBLER
FLUBBER
FORBEAR
FUMBLER
GABBIER
GAMBIER
GAMBLER
GARBLER
GLIBBER
GOBBLER
GRABBAR
GRABBER
GRUBBER
HARBOUR
HERBIER
HIBBLER
HOBBLER
HUMBLER
ICEBEER
JUMBLER
KEEBLER
LOBBYER
MARBLER
MAXBAER
MUMBLER
NIBBLER
NIEBUHR
NIMBLER
NOBBIER
NUBBIER
PETBEAR
RAMBLER
RIBBIER
RUMBLER
RYEBEER
SHEBEAR
SLOBBER
SNUBBER
STABBER
STABLER
SWABBER
TEMBLOR
THEBEAR
TUBBIER
TUMBLER
VONBAER
WARBLER
WEBBIER
WOBBLER

••••BR•

ALGEBRA
CALABRO
CALIBRE
CELEBRE
CEREBRA
CEREBRO
CHAMBRE
LESABRE
MACABRE
NOSEBRA
OCTOBRE
OCTUBRE
PALABRA

••••B•R

BACKBAR
BELABOR
BLABBER
BLUBBER
BLURBER
BODYBAR
CALIBER
CASHBAR
CHAMBER
CLABBER
CLAMBAR
CLAMBER
CLIMBER
CLOBBER
CLUBBER
CRABBER
CRIBBER
CROWBAR
DOVEBAR
DRABBER
DRAWBAR
DRUBBER
ENARBOR
FERNBAR
FLUBBER
FNUMBER
GLIBBER
GOODBAR
GRABBAR
GRABBER
GRUBBER
HIGHBAR
IMBIBER
INLABOR
IRONBAR
KILOBAR
KLEIBER
MALABAR
MARSBAR
MENUBAR
MILKBAR
MINIBAR
NICOBAR
OCTOBER
OKTOBER
OPENBAR
PLUMBER
ROLLBAR
SANDBAR
SANDBUR
SCRIBER
SIDEBAR
SLOBBER
SLUMBER
SNUBBER
STABBER
SWABBER
SWAYBAR
TASKBAR
THURBER
TOLLBAR
TOOLBAR
UNSOBER
WINEBAR

BS•••••

BSCHOOL

B•S••••

BASALLY
BASALTS
BASEDON
BASEHIT
BASEMAN
BASEMEN
BASENJI
BASEPAY
BASESIX
BASETEN
BASETWO
BASHERS
BASHFUL
BASHING
BASILIC
BASILIO
BASINAL
BASKETS
BASKETT
BASKING
BASMATI
BASQUES
BASRHIN
BASSALE
BASSANI
BASSANO
BASSETS
BASSETT
BASSIER
BASSIST
BASSOON
BASSSAX
BASTERS
BASTING
BASTION
BBSHOTS
BESEECH
BESIDES
BESIEGE
BESMEAR
BESPEAK
BESPOKE
BESSELL
BESTBET
BESTBOY
BESTBUD
BESTBUY
BESTCUT
BESTIAL
BESTILL
BESTING
BESTIRS
BESTMAN
BESTMEN
BESTOFF
BESTONE
BESTOWS
BESTREW
BISCUIT
BISECTS
BISHKEK
BISHOPS
BISMUTH
BISQUES
BISSELL
BISTATE
BISTROS
BOSCAGE
BOSNIAN
BOSOMED
BOSONIC
BOSSIER
BOSSILY
BOSSING
BOSSISM
BOSSMAN
BOSSMEN
BOSTONS
BOSTONU
BOSWELL
BUSBIES
BUSBOYS
BUSCEMI
BUSFARE
BUSGIRL
BUSHELS
BUSHERS
BUSHHOG
BUSHIDO
BUSHIER
BUSHILY
BUSHING
BUSHMAN
BUSHMEN
BUSHPIG
BUSHWAH
BUSIEST
BUSKERS
BUSKING
BUSLANE
BUSLINE
BUSLOAD
BUSMANS
BUSPASS
BUSRIDE
BUSSERS
BUSSING
BUSSTOP
BUSTARD
BUSTERS
BUSTIER
BUSTING
BUSTLED
BUSTLER
BUSTLES
BUSTOUR
BUSTOUT
BUSTRIP
BUSTSIN
BUSTSUP
BUSTUPS
BUSYBEE
BUSYING

B••S•••

BADSHOT
BADSIGN
BALSAMS
BALSAMY
BANSHEE
BARSOAP
BARSTOW
BASSALE
BASSANI
BASSANO
BASSETS
BASSETT
BASSIER
BASSIST
BASSOON
BASSSAX
BATSFOR
BATSMAN
BATSMEN
BATSUIT
BEASLEY
BEASTIE
BEASTLY
BEDSIDE
BEDSITS
BEESWAX
BEGSFOR
BEGSOFF
BERSERK
BERSUNT
BESSELL
BIASING
BIASPLY
BIASSED
BIASSES
BIDSFOR
BIGSALE
BIGSHOT
BIGSHOW
BIGSTAR
BISSELL
BITSIER
BLASTED
BLASTER
BLESSED
BLESSER
BLESSES
BLISSED
BLISSES
BLISTER
BLOSSOM
BLUSHED
BLUSHER
BLUSHES
BLUSHON
BLUSTER
BOASTED
BOASTER
BOASTOF
BOBSLED
BOISEID
BOLSHOI
BOLSTER
BONSOIR
BOOSLER
BOOSTED
BOOSTER
BOOSTUP
BORSCHT
BORSTAL
BOSSIER
BOSSILY
BOSSING
BOSSISM
BOSSMAN
BOSSMEN
BOUSONO
BOWSAWS
BOWSHOT
BOWSOUT
BOXSEAT
BOXSETS
BOXSTEP
BOXSTER
BRASHER
BRASHES
BRASHLY
BRASIER
BRASIZE
BRASSES
BRASSIE
BRESCIA
BRESLIN
BRISKED
BRISKER
BRISKET
BRISKLY
BRISTLE
BRISTLY
BRISTOL
BROSNAN
BROSSES
BRUSHED
BRUSHER
BRUSHES
BRUSHUP
BRUSQUE
BTFSPLK
BUGSOFF
BUGSOUT
BUISSON
BUMSOUT
BUQSHAS
BURSARS
BURSTER
BURSTIN
BURSTYN
BUSSERS
BUSSING
BUSSTOP
BUYSOFF
BUYSOUT

B•••S••

BABYSAT
BABYSIT
BACKSAW
BACKSIN
BACKSUP
BAILSON
BALASES
BALKSAT
BALLSUP
BANDSAW
BANGSON
BANGSUP
BANKSON
BANKSUP
BARISTA
BARKSAT
BASESIX
BASSSAX
BATISTA
BATISTE
BEADSUP
BEAMSUP
BEARSON
BEARSUP
BEATSAT
BEATSIT
BEATSME
BEATSON
BEATSUP
BEEFSUP
BEEPSAT
BEHESTS
BELASCO
BELLSON
BELTSAW
BELTSUP
BELUSHI
BEMUSED
BEMUSES
BENISON
BENTSEN
BERGSON
BERNSEN
BIASSED
BIASSES
BINDSTO
BINDSUP
BITESIN
BITESON
BITESUP
BLEDSOE
BLESSED
BLESSER
BLESSES
BLISSED
BLISSES
BLOSSOM
BLOTSUP
BLOUSED
BLOUSES
BLOUSON
BLOWSIN
BLOWSIT
BLOWSON
BLOWSUP
BLUESKY
BLUESUN
BOBBSEY
BOGUSLY
BOILSUP
BOLTSUP
BOLUSES
BONESET
BONESUP
BONUSES
BOOPSIE
BOOTSIT
BOOTSUP
BOURSES
BOXESIN
BOXESUP
BPLUSES
BRAISED
BRAISES
BRANSON
BRASSES
BRASSIE
BREASTS
BREWSKI
BREWSUP
BROASTS
BRODSKY
BRONSON
BROSSES
BROWSED
BROWSER
BROWSES
BRUISED
BRUISER
BRUISES
BRYUSOV
BUCKSAW
BUCKSUP
BUFFSUP
BUISSON
BULKSUP
BUMPSUP
BUOYSUP
BURNSIN
BURNSUP
BUSTSIN
BUSTSUP
BUTTSIN
BUZZSAW

B••••S•

BAALISH
BAALISM
BAALIST
BABIEST
BABYISH
BADCASE
BADDEST
BADDISH
BADNESS
BADPAST
BAHAISM
BAHAIST
BAKERST
BALDEST
BALDISH
BALLAST
BAPTISE
BAPTISM
BAPTIST
BARLESS
BASSIST
BEAMISH
BEARISH
BEAUISH
BECAUSE
BEDLESS
BEDPOST
BEDREST
BELFAST
BEQUEST
BERNESE
BIBLESS
BIGBOSS
BIGEAST
BIGEASY
BIGFISH
BIGGEST
BIGGISH
BIGMESS
BIGNESS
BIGNOSE
BIOMASS
BITLESS
BLEMISH
BLUEISH
BOARISH
BOGGISH
BOGGUSS
BOLDEST
BOMBAST
BONEASH
BONIEST
BOOHISS
BOOKISH
BOORISH
BOSSISM
BOWLESS
BOXIEST
BRALESS
BRAVEST
BRINISH
BRITISH
BRUTISH
BRUXISM
BUDLESS
BUDVASE
BUFFEST
BULLISH
BULRUSH
BUMRUSH
BURGESS
BURMESE
BURNISH
BUSIEST
BUSPASS
BYANOSE

B•••••S

BABBLES
BABOONS
BACCHUS
BACKERS
BACKUPS
BADBOYS
BADDAYS
BADDIES
BADDOGS
BADEGGS
BADENDS
BADFITS
BADGERS
BADGUYS
BADHATS
BADLIES
BADLOTS
BADNESS
BADNEWS
BADRAPS
BAFFERS
BAFFIES
BAFFLES
BAGBOYS
BAGFULS
BAGGERS
BAGGIES
BAGGINS
BAGJOBS
BAGNIOS
BAGWIGS
BAHAMAS
BAHIANS
BAILEES
BAILERS
BAILORS
BAITERS
BALASES
BALATAS
BALBOAS
BALDIES
BALEENS
BALKANS
BALKERS
BALLADS
BALLETS
BALLOTS
BALSAMS
BAMBOOS
BAMMIES
BANANAS
BANANES
BANDERS
BANDIES
BANDITS
BANGERS
BANGLES
BANJOES
BANKERS
BANKITS
BANNERS
BANQUES
BANTAMS
BANTERS
BANYANS
BANZAIS
BAOBABS
BARACUS
BARBERS
BARBETS
BARBIES
BARCARS
BAREGES
BARENTS
BARGERS
BARHOPS
BARITES
BARKERS
BARLESS
BARLEYS
BARNEYS
BARNUMS
BAROLOS
BARQUES

BARRELS
BARRENS
BARRETS
BARRIOS
BARRONS
BARROWS
BARTABS
BARTERS
BARTLES
BARYONS
BASALTS
BASHERS
BASKETS
BASQUES
BASSETS
BASTERS
BATBOYS
BATCHES
BATDAYS
BATHERS
BATTENS
BATTERS
BATTLES
BAUBLES
BAUHAUS
BAWLERS
BAYRUMS
BAZAARS
BBQPITS
BBQRIBS
BBSHOTS
BCLIONS
BEACHES
BEACONS
BEADERS
BEADLES
BEAGLES
BEAKERS
BEAMERS
BEANIES
BEARERS
BEATERS
BEATLES
BEAVERS
BECALMS
BECKONS
BECOMES
BEDAUBS
BEDAZES
BEDBUGS
BEDECKS
BEDLAMS
BEDLESS
BEDLOES
BEDSITS
BEEBEES
BEECHES
BEEGEES
BEEMERS
BEEPERS
BEETLES
BEEZERS
BEFALLS
BEFOOLS
BEFOULS
BEGGARS
BEGIRDS
BEHAVES
BEHEADS
BEHESTS
BEHINDS
BEHOLDS
BEHRENS
BEIGNES
BELAIRS
BELARUS
BELCHES
BELDAMS
BELIEFS
BELIERS
BELLIES
BELLOWS
BELONGS
BELTERS
BELUGAS
BEMIRES
BEMOANS
BEMUSES
BENARES
BENCHES
BENDAYS
BENDERS
BENGALS
BENOTES
BENTHOS
BENUMBS
BERATES
BERBERS
BERGIUS
BERNAYS
BERRIES
BERTHAS
BESIDES
BESTIRS
BESTOWS
BETAKES
BETHELS
BETIDES
BETIMES
BETRAYS
BETTERS
BETTORS
BEURRES
BEWAILS
BEWARES
BEZIERS
BIALIES
BIASSES
BIBBERS
BIBLESS
BICARBS
BICHONS
BICKERS
BICORNS
BIDDERS
BIDDIES
BIGAPES
BIGBETS
BIGBOSS
BIGBOYS
BIGCARS
BIGCATS
BIGDAYS
BIGDIGS
BIGDOGS
BIGEARS
BIGENDS
BIGEYES
BIGFANS
BIGGERS
BIGGIES
BIGGUNS
BIGHITS
BIGHUGS
BIGKIDS
BIGLIES
BIGLOTS
BIGMACS
BIGMESS
BIGNESS
BIGNEWS
BIGONES
BIGRIGS
BIGTOES
BIGTOPS
BIGWIGS
BIGWINS
BIKINIS
BILIOUS
BILKERS
BILLERS
BILLETS
BILLIES
BILLOWS
BIMBOES
BIMINIS
BINDERS
BINDLES
BINGERS
BINGLES
BINGOES
BIOLABS
BIOMASS
BIONICS
BIOPICS
BIRCHES
BIRDERS
BIRDIES
BIREMES
BIRLERS
BIRMANS
BISECTS
BISHOPS
BISQUES
BISTROS
BITLESS
BITMAPS
BITTERS
BLADERS
BLAMERS
BLAZERS
BLAZONS
BLENDES
BLESSES
BLIGHTS
BLISSES
BLITZES
BLONDES
BLOUSES
BLOWERS
BLOWUPS
BLUDGES
BLUINGS
BLUSHES
BMOVIES
BOATELS
BOATERS
BOBBERS
BOBBIES
BOBBINS
BOBBLES
BOBCATS
BOCCIES
BODEGAS
BODICES
BODINGS
BODKINS
BOEINGS
BOFFINS
BOGARTS
BOGGLES
BOGGUSS
BOILERS
BOKKENS
BOLEROS
BOLIDES
BOLTERS
BOLUSES
BOMBERS
BONACIS
BONBONS
BONDERS
BONGOES
BONITOS
BONKERS
BONMOTS
BONNETS
BONUSES
BOOBIES
BOOBOOS
BOOCOOS
BOODLES
BOOGIES
BOOHISS
BOOHOOS
BOOKERS
BOOKIES
BOOMERS
BOONIES
BOOTEES
BOOTERS
BOOTIES
BOOZERS
BOPPERS
BORATES
BORDERS
BORGIAS
BORIDES
BORINGS
BORROWS
BORZOIS
BOSTONS
BOTCHES
BOTHERS
BOTREES
BOTTLES
BOTTOMS
BOUCHES
BOUDINS
BOUFFES
BOUNCES
BOURSES
BOUTROS
BOVINES
BOWFINS
BOWLERS
BOWLESS
BOWOARS
BOWSAWS
BOWTIES
BOWWOWS
BOWYERS
BOXBEDS
BOXBOYS
BOXCARS
BOXFULS
BOXSETS
BOXTOPS
BOYTOYS
BPLUSES
BRACERS
BRAHMAS
BRAISES
BRALESS
BRASHES
BRASSES
BRAVOES
BRAYERS
BRAZENS
BREASTS
BREATHS
BREEZES
BRETONS
BREVETS
BREWERS
BREYERS
BRIARDS
BRIBEES
BRIBERS
BRIDALS
BRIDGES
BRIDLES
BRIGHTS
BRILLOS
BRINERS
BRITONS
BROADAS
BROASTS
BRODIES
BROGANS
BROGUES
BROKERS
BRONCOS
BRONTES
BRONZES
BROSSES
BROWSES
BRUISES
BRUMOUS
BRUNETS
BRUSHES
BUBBLES
BUCKERS
BUCKETS
BUCKLES
BUCKOES
BUDDERS
BUDDHAS
BUDDIES
BUDGERS
BUDGETS
BUDGIES
BUDLESS
BUFFERS
BUFFETS
BUGBOYS
BUGGIES
BUGGLES
BUGLERS
BUGOUTS
BUJONES
BULBOUS
BULGARS
BULGURS
BULLETS
BULLIES
BULLINS
BULOVAS
BUMBLES
BUMLEGS
BUMMERS
BUMPERS
BUMRAPS
BUNCHES
BUNDLES
BUNGEES
BUNGLES
BUNIONS
BUNKERS
BUNKUMS
BUNNIES
BUNTERS
BUQSHAS
BURBLES
BURBOTS
BURDENS
BUREAUS
BURGEES
BURGERS
BURGESS
BURGLES
BURGOOS
BURIALS
BURIERS
BURLAPS
BURLERS
BURMANS
BURNERS
BUROAKS
BURROWS
BURSARS
BUSBIES
BUSBOYS
BUSHELS
BUSHERS
BUSKERS
BUSMANS
BUSPASS
BUSSERS
BUSTERS
BUSTLES
BUSTUPS
BUTANES
BUTCHES
BUTENES
BUTLERS
BUTTERS
BUTTONS
BUYOFFS
BUYOUTS
BUZZERS
BYEBYES
BYFIVES
BYFORMS
BYGONES
BYLINES
BYNAMES
BYPATHS
BYPLAYS
BYROADS
BYTALKS
BYTURNS
BYWORDS

•BS••••

ABSALOM
ABSCISE
ABSCOND
ABSENCE
ABSENTS
ABSINTH
ABSOLUT
ABSOLVE
ABSORBS
ABSTAIN
BBSHOTS
CBSNEWS
OBSCENE
OBSCURA
OBSCURE
OBSERVE
OBSNEAK

•B•S•••

ABASERS
ABASHED
ABASHES
ABASING
ABUSERS
ABUSING
ABUSIVE
ABYSMAL
ABYSSAL
ABYSSES
IBNSAUD
OBESELY
OBESITY

•B••S••

ABUTSON
ABYSSAL
ABYSSES
OBLASTS
OBOISTS
OBTESTS
OBTUSER

•B•••S•

ABOLISH
ABREAST
ABSCISE
FBICASE
OBELISE
OBELISK
OBVERSE
TBILISI
VBLOUSE

•B••••S

ABASERS
ABASHES
ABATERS
ABATORS
ABCNEWS
ABDUCES
ABDUCTS
ABIDERS
ABJURES
ABLATES
ABOUNDS
ABRADES
ABRAXAS
ABRILES
ABSENTS
ABSORBS
ABUSERS
ABYSSES
BBQPITS
BBQRIBS
BBSHOTS
CBSNEWS
EBAYERS
EBONICS
EBONIES
IBIZANS
NBCNEWS
OBENTOS
OBEYERS
OBJECTS
OBLASTS
OBLATES
OBLIGES
OBLONGS
OBOISTS
OBTAINS
OBTESTS
OBTUNDS
OBVERTS
OBVIOUS
PBANDJS
WBYEATS

••BS•••

ALBSURE
BOBSLED
CUBSFAN
FIBSTER
FOBSOFF
FUBSIER
GIBSONS
HOBSONS
JOBSHOP
LOBSTER
MOBSTER
ROBSART
RUBSOFF
RUBSOUT
RUBSRAW
SUBSECT
SUBSETS
SUBSIDE
SUBSIDY
SUBSIST
SUBSOIL
SUBSORT
SUBSUME
TABSETS
WEBSITE
WEBSTER

••B•S••

ANBESOL
BABYSAT
BABYSIT
BOBBSEY
CUBISTS
DEBASED
DEBASER
DEBASES
DEBUSES
DEBUSSY
EMBASSY
EMBOSOM
GIBESAT
GIBUSES
GOBYSEA
JIBESAT
NABISCO
ORBISON
REBASTE
REBUSES
ROBESON
ROBUSTA
ROBUSTO
STBASIL
TABASCO
TUBISTS
UNBASED
UNBESET
UNBOSOM
VIBISTS
WABASHA

••B••S•

AMBROSE
BABIEST
BABYISH
BIBLESS
CABOOSE
CUBBISH
DEBUSSY
EMBASSY
FABBEST
FTBLISS
GABFEST
HOBOISM
JEBBUSH
JOBLESS
LABTEST
MOBBISH
MOBBISM
MOBBIST
MRBLISS
NEBBISH
NOBLEST
ORBLESS
PUBLISH
REBRUSH
RIBLESS
RUBBISH
SUBBASE
SUBBASS
SUBCASE
SUBCASH
SUBCAST
SUBPOST
SUBROSA
SUBSIST
SUBTASK
TUBAIST
UNBLEST
UNBURST
UPBURST
WEBCAST
WEBLESS
YOBBISH
ZEBRASS

••B•••S

ALBEDOS
ALBINOS
AMBIENS
AMBLERS
AMBRIES
ARBACES
ARBOLES
ARBOURS
ARBUTUS
AUBADES
AUBURNS
BABBLES
BABOONS
BIBBERS
BIBLESS
BOBBERS
BOBBIES
BOBBINS
BOBBLES
BOBCATS
BUBBLES
CABALAS
CABANAS
CABBIES
CABEZAS
CABLERS
CABLETS
CABRIOS
COBALTS
COBBLES
COBNUTS
COBWEBS
CUBAGES
CUBBIES
CUBBINS
CUBFANS
CUBISTS
CUBITUS
CUBOIDS
CYBORGS
DABBERS
DABBLES
DEBARKS
DEBASES
DEBATES
DEBEERS
DEBLURS
DEBONES
DEBTEES
DEBTORS
DEBUNKS
DEBURRS
DEBUSES
DIBBLES
DOBBINS
DUBBERS
DUBIOUS
DYBBUKS
EMBALMS
EMBANKS
EMBARKS
EMBLEMS
EMBRUES
EMBRYOS
EUBANKS
FABARES
FABLERS
FABRICS
FIBBERS
FIBRINS
FIBROUS
FIBULAS
FMBANDS
FTBLISS
GABBERS
GABBLES
GABBROS
GIBBERS
GIBBONS
GIBBOUS
GIBLETS
GIBLUES
GIBSONS
GIBUSES
GOBBLES
GOBLETS
GOBLINS
GOBYBUS
HABILIS
HEBREWS
HOBBIES
HOBBITS
HOBBLES
HOBNOBS
HOBSONS
HUBBIES
HUBBUBS
HUBCAPS
HYBRIDS
IMBIBES
IMBRUES
INBOXES
JABBERS
JOBBERS
JOBCUTS
JOBHOPS
JOBJARS
JOBLESS
JOBLOTS
KABUKIS
KIBBLES
KOBOLDS
LABATTS
LABFEES
LABIALS
LABOURS
LABRATS
LIBBERS
LIBIDOS
LIBRANS
LIBYANS
LOBBERS
LOBBIES
LOBULES
LUBBERS
MOBBERS
MOBILES
MRBLISS
MRBONES
MRBURNS
MRBUTTS
NABBERS
NEBULAS
NIBBLES
NIBLETS
NOBODYS
NUBBERS
NUBBINS
NUBBLES
NUBIANS
NUBIRAS
ORBLESS
PABLUMS
PEBBLES
POBOXES
PTBOATS
PUBLICS
PUBLIUS
QABALAS
RABBETS
RABBITS
RABBLES
REBAITS
REBAKES
REBALES
REBANKS
REBATES
REBENDS
REBILLS
REBINDS
REBOILS
REBOLTS
REBOOKS
REBOOTS
REBORES
REBOTES
REBOXES
REBOZOS
REBREWS
REBUFFS
REBUKES
REBUSES
RIBALDS
RIBANDS
RIBBERS
RIBBIES
RIBBONS
RIBCUTS
RIBEYES
RIBLESS
RIBLETS
RIBPADS
ROBARDS
ROBBERS
ROBBINS
ROBERTS
ROBROYS
RUBATOS
RUBBERS
RUBBLES
RUBIOUS
RUBRICS
SABADOS
SABINES
SOBBERS
STBARTS
SUBARUS
SUBBASS
SUBBIAS
SUBDEBS
SUBDUES
SUBGODS
SUBLETS
SUBLIDS
SUBLOTS
SUBMITS
SUBNETS
SUBORNS
SUBSETS
SUBURBS
SUBWARS
SUBWAYS
TABARDS
TABBIES
TABKEYS
TABLETS
TABSETS
TUBFULS
TUBISTS
TUBULES
UNBAITS
UNBALES
UNBARES
UNBELTS
UNBENDS
UNBINDS
UNBOLTS
UNBOXES
UPBEARS
UPBEATS
VIBISTS
WABBITS
WEBCAMS
WEBLESS
WEBLOGS
WOBBLES
ZEBRASS

•••BS••

BOBBSEY
CLUBSUP
GRABSAT

•••B•S•

AIRBASE
ARABIST
BIGBOSS
BOMBAST
COMBUST
CUBBISH
DUMBEST
ESOBESO
FABBEST
FANBASE
FORBUSH

FURBISH
GETBUSY
GLOBOSE
GOTBUSY
HADBEST
IAMBIST
ITSBEST
JEBBUSH
MAYBESO
MOBBISH
MOBBISM
MOBBIST
MOMBASA
MRSBASS
NEBBISH
NONBASE
NONBUSY
NUMBEST
OFFBASE
OILBASE
ONEBASE
PITBOSS
RUBBISH
SAMBASS
SEABASS
SOUBISE
SUBBASE
SUBBASS
TAXBASE
THEBEST
THEBOSS
THEBUSH
TWOBASE
UNOBESE
VERBOSE
YOBBISH

•••B••S

AIRBAGS
ARABICS
ARABLES
ARUBANS
ASHBINS
BABBLES
BADBOYS
BAGBOYS
BALBOAS
BAMBOOS
BAOBABS
BARBERS
BARBETS
BARBIES
BATBOYS
BAUBLES
BEDBUGS
BEEBEES
BERBERS
BIBBERS
BIGBETS
BIGBOSS
BIGBOYS
BIMBOES
BOBBERS
BOBBIES
BOBBINS
BOBBLES
BOMBERS
BONBONS
BOOBIES
BOOBOOS
BOXBEDS
BOXBOYS
BRIBEES
BRIBERS
BUBBLES
BUGBOYS
BULBOUS
BUMBLES
BURBLES
BURBOTS
BUSBIES
BUSBOYS
BYEBYES
CABBIES
CAMBERS
CAMBOYS
CARBONS
CARBOYS
CARBRAS
CATBEDS
CHABLIS
COBBLES
COMBATS
COMBERS
CORBELS
COWBOYS
CUBBIES
CUBBINS
CUEBIDS
CUMBERS
CUMBIAS
CYMBALS
DABBERS
DABBLES
DAUBERS
DAYBEDS
DEMBUMS
DERBIES
DIABLES
DIABLOS
DIBBLES
DISBARS
DISBUDS
DOBBINS
DOGBEDS
DOUBLES
DUBBERS
DYBBUKS
EARBUDS
EDIBLES
ENABLES
FEMBOTS
FIBBERS
FIGBARS
FLUBUGS
FLYBOYS
FOGBOWS
FOIBLES
FORBIDS
FUMBLES
GABBERS
GABBLES
GABBROS
GAMBITS
GAMBLES
GAMBOLS
GARBLES
GASBAGS
GERBILS
GIBBERS
GIBBONS
GIBBOUS
GIGBAGS
GILBLAS
GIMBALS
GIMBELS
GLOBINS
GLOBOUS
GOBBLES
GOOBERS
GYMBAGS
HARBORS
HENBITS
HERBALS
HOBBIES
HOBBITS
HOBBLES
HOMBRES
HOTBEDS
HUBBIES
HUBBUBS
HUMBLES
HUMBUGS
IAMBICS
ICEBAGS
ISOBARS
JABBERS
JEEBIES
JERBOAS
JOBBERS
JOGBRAS
JOSBOYS
JUMBLES
KIBBLES
KITBAGS
LAMBDAS
LAZBOYS
LIBBERS
LIMBERS
LOBBERS
LOBBIES
LOOBIES
LOWBIDS
LOWBOYS
LUBBERS
LUMBARS
LUMBERS
MARBLES
MEMBERS
MOBBERS
MRSBASS
MUMBLES
NABBERS
NEWBIES
NIBBLES
NOMBRES
NUBBERS
NUBBINS
NUBBLES
NUMBATS
NUMBERS
OJIBWAS
OLDBATS
OLDBOYS
ONABIAS
OUTBANS
OUTBATS
OUTBEGS
OUTBIDS
OUTBOWS
OUTBUDS
OUTBUYS
PEBBLES
PEEBLES
PEPBOYS
PETBOAS
PHOBIAS
PHOBICS
PINBOYS
PITBOSS
PREBIDS
PREBUYS
PROBERS
PROBIES
PUEBLOS
RABBETS
RABBITS
RABBLES
RAGBAGS
RAMBLES
RAWBARS
RAYBANS
REDBATS
REDBAYS
REDBUDS
REEBOKS
REUBENS
RHEBOKS
RIBBERS
RIBBIES
RIBBONS
ROBBERS
ROBBINS
RUBBERS
RUBBLES
RUMBLES
RUYBLAS
SAMBASS
SANBLAS
SEABAGS
SEABASS
SEABEDS
SEABEES
SKIBIBS
SKIBOBS
SKIBUMS
SOBBERS
SORBETS
SPYBOTS
STABLES
SUBBASS
SUBBIAS
SUNBOWS
SYMBOLS
TABBIES
TEABAGS
THEBANS
THEBOSS
THEBOYS
TIDBITS
TIEBARS
TIMBALS
TIMBERS
TIMBRES
TOMBOYS
TOPBIDS
TOWBARS
TREBLES
TUMBLES
TURBANS
TURBOTS
TWOBITS
USABLES
VERBALS
VERBIDS
WABBITS
WAMBLES
WARBLES
WEEBITS
WETBARS
WOBBLES
WOMBATS
ZOMBIES

••••BS•

VITEBSK

••••B•S

AEROBES
ALARBUS
AMOEBAS
ANTIBES
AUTOBUS
CARIBES
CASABAS
CELEBES
DATABUS
DELIBES
ENROBES
EPHEBUS
EULABUS
FLAMBES
GAZEBOS
GOBYBUS
GOODBYS
HANGBYS
IMBIBES
INCUBUS
IVTUBES
JAZZBOS
JOJOBAS
JUJUBES
LAVABOS
MINIBUS
MRHOBBS
MRTIBBS
OMNIBUS
PARIBUS
PHOEBES
PHOEBUS
RAILBUS
RHOMBUS
RHUMBAS
RIDEBYS
ROOMBAS
SCOOBAS
SCRIBES
STROBES
THEABCS
TOURBUS
UNROBES
WASABIS

•••••BS

ABSORBS
ADSORBS
ADVERBS
ALTTABS
BAGJOBS
BAOBABS
BARTABS
BBQRIBS
BEDAUBS
BENUMBS
BICARBS
BIOLABS
CANTABS
CHERUBS
COBWEBS
CONFABS
CONJOBS
DAYJOBS
DNALABS
DYEJOBS
EARTABS
ENTOMBS
HERNIBS
HISNIBS
HOBNOBS
HOTTUBS
HUBBUBS
HUNNYBS
MADLIBS
MIDRIBS
MODELBS
MRHOBBS
MRTIBBS
NEWJOBS
NOCARBS
ODDJOBS
OILRUBS
OUTRIBS
PREFABS
RECOMBS
REDTABS
REGRABS
RESORBS
RESTABS
REVERBS
SCARABS
SCHLUBS
SEALABS
SKIBIBS
SKIBOBS
SUBDEBS
SUBURBS
THECUBS
TYPEABS
UNCURBS

BT•••••

BTFSPLK
BTWELVE

B•T••••

BATAVIA
BATBOYS
BATCHED
BATCHES
BATDAYS
BATEAUX
BATEMAN
BATGIRL
BATHERS
BATHING
BATHMAT
BATHOIL
BATHTUB
BATIKED
BATISTA
BATISTE
BATLIKE
BATNEXT
BATSFOR
BATSMAN
BATSMEN
BATSUIT
BATTENS
BATTERS
BATTERY
BATTIER
BATTING
BATTLED
BATTLER
BATTLES
BATWING
BETAKEN
BETAKES
BETAMAX
BETARAY
BETHANY
BETHELS
BETHERE
BETHINK
BETHUNE
BETIDED
BETIDES
BETIMES
BETOKEN
BETRAYS
BETROTH
BETTANY
BETTERS
BETTGER
BETTING
BETTORS
BETWEEN
BETWIXT
BITEOFF
BITESIN
BITESON
BITESUP
BITLESS
BITMAPS
BITONAL
BITPART
BITROLE
BITSIER
BITTERN
BITTERS
BITTIER
BITTING
BLTTOGO
BOTANIC
BOTCHED
BOTCHER
BOTCHES
BOTCHUP
BOTHERS
BOTHNIA
BOTREES
BOTTEGA
BOTTLED
BOTTLER
BOTTLES
BOTTOMS
BUTANES
BUTCHER
BUTCHES
BUTENES
BUTGOOD
BUTLERS
BUTTEMT
BUTTERS
BUTTERY
BUTTING
BUTTONS
BUTTONY
BUTTOUT
BUTTRAM
BUTTSIN
BYTALKS
BYTHEBY
BYTRAIN
BYTURNS

B••T•••

BACTRIA
BADTIME
BADTRIP
BAITCAR
BAITERS
BAITING
BANTAMS
BANTERS
BANTING
BAPTISE
BAPTISM
BAPTIST
BAPTIZE
BARTABS
BARTEND
BARTERS
BARTLES
BARTLET
BARTOLO
BARTRAY
BASTERS
BASTING
BASTION
BATTENS
BATTERS
BATTERY
BATTIER
BATTING
BATTLED
BATTLER
BATTLES
BAYTREE
BEATALL
BEATBOX
BEATCOP
BEATERS
BEATIFY
BEATING
BEATLES
BEATNIK
BEATOFF
BEATOUT
BEATRIX
BEATSAT
BEATSIT
BEATSME
BEATSON
BEATSUP
BEATTIE
BEDTIME
BEETIER
BEETLES
BEETRED
BEETREE
BELTANE
BELTBAG
BELTERS
BELTING
BELTOUT
BELTRAN
BELTSAW
BELTSUP
BELTWAY
BENTHAM
BENTHOS
BENTLEY
BENTSEN
BERTHAS
BERTHED
BERTOLT
BERTRAM
BESTBET
BESTBOY
BESTBUD
BESTBUY
BESTCUT
BESTIAL
BESTILL
BESTING
BESTIRS
BESTMAN
BESTMEN
BESTOFF
BESTONE
BESTOWS
BESTREW
BETTANY
BETTERS
BETTGER
BETTING
BETTORS
BHUTANI
BIGTALK
BIGTENT
BIGTIME
BIGTOES
BIGTOPS
BIGTOWN
BIOTECH
BIOTITE
BIOTYPE
BIRTHED
BISTATE
BISTROS
BITTERN
BITTERS
BITTIER
BITTING
BLATANT
BLATHER
BLATTED
BLITHER
BLITZED
BLITZEN
BLITZER
BLITZES
BLOTCHY
BLOTOUT
BLOTSUP
BLOTTED
BLOTTER
BLTTOGO
BOATELS
BOATERS
BOATFUL
BOATING
BOATMAN
BOATMEN
BOBTAIL
BOBTWAY
BOITANO
BOLTERS
BOLTING
BOLTSUP
BOOTCUT
BOOTEES
BOOTERS
BOOTERY
BOOTHIA
BOOTIES
BOOTING
BOOTLEG
BOOTOUT
BOOTSIT
BOOTSUP
BOOTTOP
BOSTONS
BOSTONU
BOTTEGA
BOTTLED
BOTTLER
BOTTLES
BOTTOMS
BOUTROS
BOWTIES
BOXTOPS
BOYTOYS
BRATTLE
BRETONS
BRETTON
BRITAIN
BRITCOM
BRITISH
BRITNEY
BRITONS
BRITPOP
BRITTEN
BRITTLE
BRITTON
BROTHER
BRUTELY
BRUTISH
BUDTIME
BUITONI
BUNTERS
BUNTING
BUSTARD
BUSTERS
BUSTIER
BUSTING
BUSTLED
BUSTLER
BUSTLES
BUSTOUR
BUSTOUT
BUSTRIP
BUSTSIN
BUSTSUP
BUSTUPS
BUTTEMT
BUTTERS
BUTTERY
BUTTING
BUTTONS
BUTTONY
BUTTOUT
BUTTRAM
BUTTSIN
BUYTIME

B•••T••

BABETTE
BADITCH
BAINTER
BALATAS
BALATON
BALLTWO
BARETTA
BARITES
BARSTOW
BASETEN
BASETWO
BATHTUB
BDALTON
BEASTIE
BEASTLY
BEATTIE
BEEFTEA
BEERTAP
BELATED
BENATAR
BENOTED
BENOTES
BERATED
BERATER
BERATES
BERETTA
BEWITCH
BIENTOT
BIGOTED
BIGOTRY
BIGSTAR
BIMETAL
BIRETTA
BLANTON
BLASTED
BLASTER
BLATTED
BLEATED
BLEATER
BLENTIN
BLINTZE
BLISTER
BLOATED
BLOTTED
BLOTTER
BLUETIT
BLUNTED
BLUNTER
BLUNTLY
BLURTED
BLURTER
BLUSTER
BOASTED
BOASTER
BOASTOF
BOBATEA
BOLATIE
BOLOTIE
BOLSTER
BONITOS
BOOSTED
BOOSTER
BOOSTUP
BOOTTOP
BORATES
BORSTAL
BOXSTEP
BOXSTER
BRATTLE
BRAXTON
BREATHE
BREATHS
BREATHY
BRETTON
BRISTLE
BRISTLY
BRISTOL
BRITTEN
BRITTLE
BRITTON
BRONTES
BRUITED
BUGATTI
BUILTIN
BUILTON
BUILTUP
BURETTE
BURNTIN
BURNTUP
BURSTER
BURSTIN
BURSTYN
BUSSTOP
BYCATCH
BYPATHS

B••••T•

BAALITE
BABBITT
BABETTE
BACHATA
BADFITS
BADHATS
BADLOTS
BALLETS
BALLOTS
BANDITO
BANDITS
BANKITS
BARBATE
BARBETS
BARENTS
BARETTA
BARISTA
BARRETS
BARRETT
BASALTS
BASKETS
BASKETT
BASMATI
BASSETS
BASSETT
BATISTA
BATISTE
BAUXITE
BAYCITY
BBQPITS
BBSHOTS
BECKETT
BEDBATH
BEDMATE
BEDSITS
BEGANTO
BEHESTS
BENEATH
BENNETT
BERETTA
BERLITZ
BETROTH
BIGBETS
BIGCATS
BIGCITY
BIGGITY
BIGHITS
BIGLOTS
BILLETS
BINDSTO
BIODATA
BIOLITE
BIOTITE
BIRETTA
BISECTS
BISMUTH
BISTATE
BLIGHTS
BLIGHTY
BLINDTO
BOBCATS
BOGARTS
BONIATO
BONMOTS
BONNETS
BOUNDTO
BOWEDTO
BOXKITE
BOXSETS
BOYCOTT
BREADTH
BREASTS
BREVETS
BREVITY
BRIGHTS
BRINGTO
BROASTS
BROMATE
BRUNETS

7 BT

BUCKETS
BUDGETS
BUFFETS
BUFFETT
BUGATTI
BUGOUTS
BULLETS
BULLITT
BURBOTS
BURETTE
BURNETT
BURRITO
BUYINTO
BUYOUTS
BYBIRTH
BYMOUTH

B•••••T

BAALIST
BABBITT
BABIEST
BABYSAT
BABYSIT
BACKBIT
BACKLIT
BACKLOT
BACKOUT
BADDEBT
BADDEST
BADPAST
BADSHOT
BAGEHOT
BAHAIST
BAILOUT
BAKERST
BALDEST
BALKSAT
BALLAST
BALLUET
BANDLET
BANGOUT
BANQUET
BAPTIST
BARKSAT
BARONET
BARRETT
BARTLET
BASEHIT
BASKETT
BASSETT
BASSIST
BATHMAT
BATNEXT
BATSUIT
BAWLOUT
BAYEDAT
BAYONET
BEARCAT
BEAROUT
BEARPIT
BEATOUT
BEATSAT
BEATSIT
BECKETT
BEDPOST
BEDREST
BEEPSAT
BEIGNET
BELFAST
BELFORT
BELMONT
BELTOUT
BENEFIT
BENNETT
BEQUEST
BEQUIET
BERENDT
BERSUNT
BERTOLT
BESTBET
BESTCUT
BETWIXT
BIBELOT
BIENTOT
BIGBEAT
BIGEAST
BIGFEET
BIGFOOT
BIGGEST
BIGSHOT
BIGTENT
BIGUNIT
BISCUIT
BITPART
BLANKET
BLATANT
BLERIOT
BLEWOUT
BLINKAT
BLOTOUT
BLOWOUT
BLOWSIT
BLUETIT
BODYART
BODYFAT
BODYKIT
BOILOUT
BOLDEST
BOMBAST
BOMBLET
BONELET
BONESET
BONIEST
BOOEDAT
BOOKERT
BOOKLET
BOOMLET
BOOTCUT
BOOTOUT
BOOTSIT
BOREOUT
BORSCHT
BOUQUET
BOURGET
BOWKNOT
BOWSHOT
BOWSOUT
BOXCOAT
BOXIEST
BOXSEAT
BOYCOTT
BRACKET
BRAVEST
BRIDGET
BRINGIT
BRIQUET
BRISKET
BROUGHT
BUFFEST
BUFFETT
BUGSOUT
BULBLET
BULLITT
BUMSOUT
BUOYANT
BURNETT
BURNOUT
BUSIEST
BUSTOUT
BUTTEMT
BUTTOUT
BUYSOUT
BUZZCUT
BYHEART
BYRIGHT

•BT••••

OBTAINS
OBTESTS
OBTRUDE
OBTUNDS
OBTUSER

•B•T•••

ABATERS
ABATING
ABATORS
ABETTAL
ABETTED
ABETTER
ABETTOR
ABITIBI
ABSTAIN
ABUTSON
ABUTTAL
ABUTTED
ABUTTER
EBBTIDE
NBATEAM

•B••T••

ABBOTCY
ABETTAL
ABETTED
ABETTER
ABETTOR
ABINTRA
ABIOTIC
ABLATED
ABLATES
ABORTED
ABOUTIT
ABOUTTO
ABUTTAL
ABUTTED
ABUTTER
OBENTOS
OBLATES

•B•••T•

ABDUCTS
ABILITY
ABOUTTO
ABSENTS
ABSINTH
BBQPITS
BBSHOTS
EBONITE
EBWHITE
IBILITY
OBESITY
OBJECTS
OBLASTS
OBOISTS
OBTESTS
OBVERTS
OBVIATE
WBYEATS

•B••••T

ABEYANT
ABOUTIT
ABREAST
ABSOLUT

••BT•••

BOBTAIL
BOBTWAY
DEBTEES
DEBTORS
EBBTIDE
LABTECH
LABTEST
LABTUBE
SUBTASK
SUBTEEN
SUBTEND
SUBTEXT
SUBTLER
SUBTONE
SUBTYPE
WEBTOED

••B•T••

ABBOTCY
ARBITER
ARBUTUS
BABETTE
BOBATEA
CUBITAL
CUBITUS
DEBATED
DEBATER
DEBATES
DEBITED
DEBUTED
FIBSTER
HABITAT
HABITED
HABITUE
LABATTS
LOBATED
LOBSTER
MOBSTER
MRBUTTS
ORBITAL
ORBITED
ORBITER
PWBOTHA
REBATED
REBATER
REBATES
REBATHE
REBOTES
ROBOTIC
ROBOTRY
RUBATOS
RUBITIN
SUBITEM
TABITHA
TIBETAN
TUBETOP
UNBATED
WEBSTER
ZABUTON

••B••T•

ALBERTA
ALBERTI
ALBERTO
ASBYATT
BABBITT
BABETTE
BOBCATS
BYBIRTH
CABLETS
CABLETV
COBALTS
COBNUTS
CUBISTS
DEBOITE
DEBRETT
DUBIETY
ELBERTA
EMBOITE
GIBLETS
GOBLETS
HOBBITS
JOBCUTS
JOBLOTS
KIBBUTZ
LABATTS
LABIATE
LABRATS
LIBERTE
LIBERTY
MRBUTTS
NIBLETS
PTBOATS
PUBERTY
RABBETS
RABBITS
RABBITT
RABBITY
REBAITS
REBASTE
REBIRTH
REBOLTS
REBOOTS
RIBCUTS
RIBLETS
ROBERTA
ROBERTE
ROBERTF
ROBERTH
ROBERTI
ROBERTO
ROBERTS
ROBUSTA
ROBUSTO
SABBATH
STBARTS
SUBDATE
SUBLETS
SUBLOTS
SUBMITS
SUBNETS
SUBSETS
TABLETS
TABSETS
TIBBETT
TUBISTS
UMBERTO
UNBAITS
UNBELTS
UNBERTH
UNBOLTS
UPBEATS
VIBISTS
VIBRATE
VIBRATO
WABBITS
WEBSITE

••B•••T

AMBIENT
ASBYATT
BABBITT
BABIEST
BABYSAT
BABYSIT
BIBELOT
CABARET
CABINET
DEBRETT
FABBEST
GABFEST
GIBESAT
HABITAT
INBUILT
IOBJECT
JIBEDAT
JIBESAT
JOBHUNT
LABCOAT
LABORAT
LABTEST
MOBBIST
NOBLEST
RABBITT
REBOANT
REBUILT
RIBMEAT
ROBSART
RUBSOUT
SUBCAST
SUBDUCT
SUBJECT
SUBPLOT
SUBPOST
SUBROOT
SUBSECT
SUBSIST
SUBSORT
SUBTEXT
SUBUNIT
SUBVERT
TABARET
TABORET
TIBBETT
TUBAIST
UNBESET
UNBLENT
UNBLEST
UNBUILT
UNBURNT
UNBURST
UPBURST
VIBRANT
WEBCAST
WEBFEET
WEBFOOT

•••BT••

DOUBTED
DOUBTER
DOUBTIT
HERBTEA

•••B•T•

BABBITT
BARBATE
BARBETS
BEDBATH
BIGBETS
BURBOTS
COMBATS
CORBETT
DOGBITE
DYEBATH
EXABYTE
FEEBATE
FEMBOTS
GAMBITS
GLOBATE
HENBITS
HIPBATH
HOBBITS
HOTBATH
ICEBATH
ILLBITE
KIBBUTZ
LAMBETH
LISBETH
MACBETH
MOABITE
MUDBATH
NESBITT
NIOBITE
NUMBATS
OLDBATS
ONEBYTE
OUTBATS
PROBATE
PROBITY
RABBETS
RABBITS
RABBITT
RABBITY
REDBATS
SABBATH
SORBATE
SORBETS
SPYBOTS
SUNBATH
TIBBETT
TIDBITS
TRIBUTE
TURBOTS
TWOBITS
WABBITS
WEEBITS
WOMBATS

•••B••T

AIRBOAT
ARABIST
BABBITT
BIGBEAT
BOMBAST
BOMBLET
BULBLET
CATBERT
CATBOAT
COLBERT
COMBUST
CORBETT
CRABPOT
CURBCUT
DASBOOT
DELBERT
DILBERT
DOGBERT
DOGBOOT
DOUBLET
DOUBTIT
DRIBLET
DUMBEST
EYEBOLT
FABBEST
FANBELT
FILBERT
GETBEAT
GETBENT
GILBERT
GOABOUT
GOTBEAT
GRABSAT
GUMBOOT
GUNBELT
GUNBOAT
HADBEST
HERBART
HERBAUT
HERBERT
HILBERT
HIPBOOT
HOWBEIT
HUMBERT
IAMBIST
ICEBOAT
INKBLOT
ITSBEST
JETBOAT
JROBERT
LAMBENT
LAMBERT
LAPBELT
MOBBIST
NESBITT
NEWBOLT
NORBERT
NUMBEST
OFFBEAT
OUTBLOT
RABBITT
RATBERT
ROTBLAT
ROWBOAT
SEABOAT
SHABBAT
SHUBERT
SKIBOOT
SUNBELT
THEBEST
THEBRAT
TIBBETT
TOPBOOT
TOWBOAT
TOYBOAT
TRABERT
TUGBOAT
WILBERT

••••BT•

CLIMBTO

••••B•T

ACROBAT
ADHIBIT
AEROBAT
ATEABIT
AWEEBIT
BACKBIT
BESTBET
COHABIT
COURBET
DEORBIT
DINGBAT
EATABIT
EVENBET
EXHIBIT
FORABIT
GIGABIT
HALIBUT
INHABIT
INHIBIT
INORBIT
KILOBIT
MEGABIT
NOTABIT
OVERBET
RAREBIT
REDEBIT
SAFEBET
SHABBAT
SHERBET
SIDEBET
SPAMBOT
SUREBET
TINYBIT
YEAHBUT

•••••BT

BADDEBT
INDOUBT
NODOUBT
REDOUBT

BU•••••

BUBBLED
BUBBLES
BUCHMAN
BUCHNER
BUCKERS
BUCKETS
BUCKEYE
BUCKFOR
BUCKING
BUCKLED
BUCKLES
BUCKLEY
BUCKNER
BUCKOES
BUCKRAM
BUCKSAW
BUCKSUP
BUCOLIC
BUDDERS
BUDDHAS
BUDDIED
BUDDIES
BUDDING
BUDDYUP
BUDGERS
BUDGETS
BUDGIES
BUDGING
BUDLESS
BUDLIKE
BUDTIME
BUDVASE
BUDWORM
BUELLER
BUFFALO
BUFFERS
BUFFEST
BUFFETS
BUFFETT
BUFFING
BUFFOON
BUFFSUP
BUGABOO
BUGALOO
BUGATTI
BUGBEAR
BUGBOYS
BUGEYED
BUGFREE
BUGGIER
BUGGIES
BUGGING
BUGGLES
BUGLERS
BUGLING
BUGOUTS
BUGSOFF
BUGSOUT
BUILDER
BUILDIN
BUILDON
BUILDUP
BUILTIN
BUILTON
BUILTUP
BUISSON
BUITONI
BUJONES
BUKHARA
BULBLET
BULBOUS
BULGARI
BULGARS
BULGHUR
BULGIER
BULGING
BULGURS
BULKIER
BULKING
BULKSUP
BULLDOG
BULLETS
BULLIED
BULLIES
BULLING
BULLINS
BULLION
BULLISH
BULLITT
BULLOCK
BULLPEN
BULLRUN
BULOVAS
BULRUSH
BULWARK
BUMBLED
BUMBLER
BUMBLES
BUMDEAL
BUMLEGS
BUMMERS
BUMMING
BUMPERS
BUMPIER
BUMPILY
BUMPING
BUMPKIN
BUMPSUP
BUMRAPS
BUMRUSH
BUMSOUT
BUNCHED
BUNCHES
BUNCHUP
BUNCOED
BUNDLED
BUNDLER
BUNDLES
BUNGEES
BUNGING
BUNGLED
BUNGLER
BUNGLES
BUNIONS
BUNKBED
BUNKERS
BUNKING
BUNKOED
BUNKUMS
BUNNIES
BUNNING
BUNRAKU
BUNTERS
BUNTING
BUNUELO
BUOYANT
BUOYING
BUOYSUP
BUQSHAS
BURBAGE
BURBANK
BURBLED
BURBLER
BURBLES
BURBOTS
BURDENS
BURDICK
BUREAUS
BUREAUX
BURETTE
BURGEES
BURGEON
BURGERS
BURGESS
BURGHER
BURGLAR
BURGLED
BURGLES
BURGOOS
BURIALS
BURIERS
BURKINA
BURLAPS
BURLERS
BURLIER
BURLING
BURMANS
BURMESE
BURNABY
BURNERS
BURNETT
BURNFOR
BURNING
BURNISH
BURNLEY
BURNOFF
BURNOUT
BURNSIN
BURNSUP
BURNTIN
BURNTUP
BUROAKS
BURPGUN
BURPING
BURRIER
BURRING
BURRITO
BURROWS
BURSARS
BURSTER
BURSTIN
BURSTYN
BURUNDI
BURYING
BUSBIES
BUSBOYS
BUSCEMI
BUSFARE
BUSGIRL
BUSHELS
BUSHERS
BUSHHOG
BUSHIDO
BUSHIER
BUSHILY
BUSHING
BUSHMAN
BUSHMEN
BUSHPIG
BUSHWAH
BUSIEST
BUSKERS
BUSKING
BUSLANE
BUSLINE
BUSLOAD
BUSMANS
BUSPASS
BUSRIDE
BUSSERS
BUSSING
BUSSTOP
BUSTARD
BUSTERS
BUSTIER
BUSTING
BUSTLED
BUSTLER
BUSTLES
BUSTOUR
BUSTOUT
BUSTRIP
BUSTSIN
BUSTSUP
BUSTUPS
BUSYBEE
BUSYING
BUTANES
BUTCHER
BUTCHES
BUTENES
BUTGOOD
BUTLERS
BUTTEMT
BUTTERS
BUTTERY
BUTTING
BUTTONS
BUTTONY
BUTTOUT
BUTTRAM
BUTTSIN
BUXOMLY
BUYABLE
BUYBACK
BUYDOWN
BUYINTO
BUYOFFS
BUYOUTS
BUYSOFF
BUYSOUT
BUYTIME
BUZZARD
BUZZCUT
BUZZELL
BUZZERS
BUZZIER
BUZZING
BUZZOFF
BUZZSAW

B•U••••

BAUBLES
BAUHAUS

BAULKED
BAULKER
BAUXITE
BEURRES
BHUTANI
BLUBBER
BLUDGED
BLUDGER
BLUDGES
BLUEBOY
BLUEFIN
BLUEFLU
BLUEFOX
BLUEHEN
BLUEICE
BLUEING
BLUEISH
BLUEJAY
BLUELAW
BLUERED
BLUESKY
BLUESUN
BLUETIT
BLUFFED
BLUFFER
BLUFFLY
BLUINGS
BLUNDEN
BLUNDER
BLUNTED
BLUNTER
BLUNTLY
BLURBER
BLURRED
BLURTED
BLURTER
BLUSHED
BLUSHER
BLUSHES
BLUSHON
BLUSTER
BOUCHER
BOUCHES
BOUDINS
BOUDOIR
BOUFFES
BOUGHED
BOULDER
BOUNCED
BOUNCER
BOUNCES
BOUNDED
BOUNDER
BOUNDTO
BOUNDUP
BOUQUET
BOURBON
BOURGET
BOURSES
BOUSONO
BOUTROS
BOUVIER
BRUBECK
BRUEGEL
BRUISED
BRUISER
BRUISES
BRUITED
BRUMMEL
BRUMOUS
BRUNETS
BRUSHED
BRUSHER
BRUSHES
BRUSHUP
BRUSQUE
BRUTELY
BRUTISH
BRUXING
BRUXISM

B••U•••
BEAUISH
BEGUILE
BEGUINE
BELUGAS
BELUSHI
BEMUSED
BEMUSES
BENUMBS
BEQUEST
BEQUICK
BEQUIET
BIGUNIT
BLAUBOK
BLOUSED
BLOUSES
BLOUSON
BOGUSLY
BOLUSES
BONUSES
BPLUSES
BROUGHT
BRYUSOV
BUNUELO
BURUNDI
BYTURNS

B•••U••
BACKUPS
BADGUYS
BADLUCK
BAGFULS
BALLUET
BANBURY
BANQUES
BANQUET
BARBUDA
BARBULE
BARNUMS
BARQUES
BASQUES
BATSUIT
BAYRUMS
BECAUSE
BEDAUBS
BEDBUGS
BEDOUIN
BEFOULS
BENGUNN
BEOWULF
BERMUDA
BERSUNT
BETHUNE
BIGGULP
BIGGUNS
BIGHUGS
BIOFUEL
BISCUIT
BISMUTH
BISQUES
BIVOUAC
BLACULA
BLOWUPS
BOGGUSS
BOROUGH
BOUQUET
BOXFULS
BRAVURA
BRIQUET
BROGUES
BUGOUTS
BULGURS
BULRUSH
BUMRUSH
BUNKUMS
BUSTUPS
BUYOUTS
BYMOUTH

B••••U•
BACCHUS
BACKOUT
BACKRUB
BACKSUP
BAILOUT
BALEFUL
BALFOUR
BALLSUP
BANEFUL
BANGOUT
BANGSUP
BANKSUP
BARACUS
BAROQUE
BASHFUL
BATEAUX
BATHTUB
BAUHAUS
BAWLOUT
BEADSUP
BEAMSUP
BEARCUB
BEARHUG
BEAROUT
BEARSUP
BEATOUT
BEATSUP
BECLOUD
BEEFSUP
BEERMUG
BELARUS
BELGIUM
BELLYUP
BELTOUT
BELTSUP
BELVOUR
BENBLUE
BENELUX
BERGIUS
BESTBUD
BESTBUY
BESTCUT
BEZIQUE
BIGBLUE
BIGFOUR
BILIOUS
BINDSUP
BITESUP
BLAZEUP
BLEWOUT
BLOCKUP
BLOTOUT
BLOTSUP
BLOWGUN
BLOWNUP
BLOWOUT
BLOWSUP
BLUESUN
BOARDUP
BOATFUL
BODEFUL
BODYRUB
BOHRIUM
BOILOUT
BOILSUP
BOLTSUP
BONEDUP
BONESUP
BONHEUR
BONJOUR
BOOSTUP
BOOTCUT
BOOTOUT
BOOTSUP
BOREOUT
BORGLUM
BORLAUG
BORNEUP
BOTCHUP
BOUNDUP
BOWLFUL
BOWSOUT
BOXEDUP
BOXESUP
BRACEUP
BREAKUP
BRENGUN
BREWPUB
BREWSUP
BRICKUP
BRIMFUL
BRINGUP
BROKEUP
BRUMOUS
BRUSHUP
BRUSQUE
BUCKSUP
BUDDYUP
BUFFSUP
BUGSOUT
BUILDUP
BUILTUP
BULBOUS
BULGHUR
BULKSUP
BULLRUN
BUMPSUP
BUMSOUT
BUNCHUP
BUOYSUP
BUREAUS
BUREAUX
BURNOUT
BURNSUP
BURNTUP
BURPGUN
BUSTOUR
BUSTOUT
BUSTSUP
BUTTOUT
BUYSOUT
BUZZCUT

B•••••U
BANDEAU
BARBEAU
BAYLORU
BELLEAU
BIRDFLU
BLUEFLU
BOSTONU
BUNRAKU

•BU••••
ABUSERS
ABUSING
ABUSIVE
ABUTSON
ABUTTAL
ABUTTED
ABUTTER

•B•U•••
ABDUCED
ABDUCES
ABDUCTS
ABJURED
ABJURER
ABJURES
ABOUNDS
ABOUTIT
ABOUTTO
ABRUZZI
OBTUNDS
OBTUSER

•B•U••
OBSCURA
OBSCURE
OBTRUDE
VBLOUSE

•B•••U•
ABSOLUT
IBNSAUD
NBCBLUE
OBLIQUE
OBLOQUY
OBVIOUS

•B••••U
IBEGYOU

••BU•••
ALBUMEN
ALBUMIN
ALBUNDY
ARBUTUS
AUBURNS
AUBURNU
COBUYER
DEBUNKS
DEBURGH
DEBURRS
DEBUSES
DEBUSSY
DEBUTED
DUBUQUE
FIBULAE
FIBULAR
FIBULAS
GIBUSES
IMBUING
INBUILT
KABUKIS
LOBULES
MRBURNS
MRBUTTS
MYBUDDY
NABUCCO
NEBULAE
NEBULAR
NEBULAS
PABULUM
REBUFFS
REBUILD
REBUILT
REBUKED
REBUKER
REBUKES
REBUSES
ROBUSTA
ROBUSTO
RUBUPON
SUBUNIT
SUBURBS
TABUING
TABULAR
TIBURON
TUBULAR
TUBULES
UNBUILD
UNBUILT
UNBULKY
UNBURLY
UNBURNT
UNBURST
UPBUILD
UPBURST
ZABUTON
ZEBULON
ZEBULUN

••B•U••
ALBSURE
ARBOURS
COBNUTS
DEBAUCH
DEBLURS
DEBOULE
DYBBUKS
EMBRUED
EMBRUES
GIBLUES
HUBBUBS
IMBRUED
IMBRUES
INBOUND
JEBBUSH
JOBCUTS
JOBHUNT
KIBBUTZ
LABOURS
LABTUBE
MOBRULE
PABLUMS
REBOUND
REBRUSH
RIBCUTS
SUBDUAL
SUBDUCT
SUBDUED
SUBDUER
SUBDUES
SUBSUME
TABOULI
TUBFULS
UNBLUED
UNBOUND
UPBOUND

••B••U•
ARBUTUS
CUBITUS
DUBIOUS
DUBNIUM
DUBUQUE
FABFOUR
FIBROUS
GIBBOUS
GOBYBUS
HABITUE
PABULUM
PUBLIUS
REBEGUN
RUBADUB
RUBIOUS
RUBSOUT
SUBARUS
ZEBULUN

••B•••U
AUBURNU
TABLEAU

•••BU••
ASHBURN
ASHBURY
BANBURY
BARBUDA
BARBULE
BEDBUGS
CADBURY
CLIBURN
COGBURN
COMBUST
DANBURY
DEMBUMS
DIMBULB
DISBUDS
DRYBULB
DYBBUKS
EARBUDS
FLUBUGS
FORBUSH
GETBUSY
GLOBULE
GOTBUSY
HAMBURG
HARBURG
HEPBURN
HOMBURG
HUBBUBS
HUMBUGS
JEBBUSH
JOEBUCK
JUMBUCK
KIBBUTZ
LIMBURG
NEWBURG
NIEBUHR
NONBUSY
OLEBULL
OUTBUDS
OUTBULK
OUTBURN
OUTBUYS
OUTBUZZ
PITBULL
PREBURN
PREBUYS
RAEBURN
RAYBURN
REDBUDS
ROEBUCK
ROXBURY
SAMBUCA
SAWBUCK
SKIBUMS
SUDBURY
SUNBURN
THEBUSH
TRIBUNE
TRIBUTE
WARBURG
WETBULB

•••B•U•
AMIBLUE
BENBLUE
BIGBLUE
BULBOUS
CLUBSUP
CURBCUT
FLUBDUB
GIBBOUS
GLOBOUS
GOABOUT
HARBOUR
HERBAUT
ICEBLUE
NBCBLUE
NIOBIUM
OLDBLUE
RIMBAUD
SEABLUE
SKYBLUE
TERBIUM

•••B••U
BARBEAU
DOUBLEU
HOFBRAU
ISABEAU
JAMBEAU
LAMBEAU

••••BU•
ALARBUS
AUTOBUS
BESTBUD
BESTBUY
CDALBUM
CIMABUE
CLIMBUP
CRUMBUM
DATABUS
EPHEBUS
EULABUS
FIREBUG
GOBYBUS
GOLDBUG
GOODBUY
HALIBUT
INCUBUS
JUNEBUG
LADYBUG
LOVEBUG
MINIBUS
OMNIBUS
OVERBUY
PARIBUS
PHOEBUS
PILLBUG
PLUMBUM
RAILBUS
RHOMBUS
ROSABUD
ROSEBUD
SANDBUR
SCRUBUP
TOURBUS
YEAHBUT

••••B•U
CARIBOU

B•V••••
BAVARIA
BEVELED
BEVELER
BEVERLY
BIVALVE
BIVOUAC
BOVINES

B••V•••
BEAVERS
BELVOIR
BELVOUR
BERVOIX
BMOVIES
BOBVILA
BOUVIER
BRAVADA
BRAVADO
BRAVELY
BRAVERY
BRAVEST
BRAVING
BRAVOED
BRAVOES
BRAVURA
BREVETS
BREVITY
BUDVASE

B•••V••
BATAVIA
BEDEVIL
BEHAVED
BEHAVES
BELEVEN
BELOVED
BILEVEL
BOLIVAR
BOLIVIA
BOOKVII
BULOVAS
BYFIVES

B••••V•
BADLOVE
BADMOVE
BAKLAVA
BEBRAVE
BEEHIVE
BEHOOVE
BELIEVE
BENBOVA
BEREAVE
BIGFIVE
BIGLOVE
BIVALVE
BONJOVI
BTWELVE

B•••••V
BADENOV
BRYUSOV

•BV••••
OBVERSE
OBVERTS
OBVIATE
OBVIOUS

•B•••V•
ABSOLVE
ABUSIVE
NBALIVE
OBSERVE

••BV•••
BOBVILA
SUBVENE
SUBVERT

••B••V•
BEBRAVE
UNBRAVE
URBANVI

••B•••V
CABLETV
NABOKOV
URBANIV

•••B•V•
BENBOVA
UPABOVE

•••B••V
DOUBLEV

••••B•V
ROYGBIV

B•W••••
BAWDIER
BAWDILY
BAWLERS
BAWLING
BAWLOUT
BEWAILS
BEWARED
BEWARES
BEWITCH
BOWDLER
BOWDOIN
BOWDOWN
BOWECHO
BOWEDTO
BOWERED
BOWFINS
BOWHEAD
BOWKNOT
BOWLERS
BOWLESS
BOWLFUL
BOWLIKE
BOWLINE
BOWLING
BOWOARS
BOWSAWS
BOWSHOT
BOWSOUT
BOWTIES
BOWWOWS
BOWYERS
BTWELVE
BYWAYOF
BYWORDS

B••W•••
BADWORD
BAGWELL
BAGWIGS
BARWARE
BATWING
BEOWULF
BERWICK
BETWEEN
BETWIXT
BIGWIGS
BIGWINS
BLEWOFF
BLEWOUT
BLOWDRY
BLOWERS
BLOWFLY
BLOWGUN
BLOWIER
BLOWING
BLOWNIN
BLOWNUP
BLOWOFF
BLOWOUT
BLOWPOP
BLOWSIN
BLOWSIT
BLOWSON
BLOWSUP
BLOWUPS
BLOWZED
BOBWEIR
BOSWELL
BOWWOWS
BRAWLED
BRAWLER
BRAWLEY
BREWAGE
BREWERS
BREWERY
BREWING
BREWPUB
BREWSKI
BREWSUP
BROWARD
BROWNED
BROWNER
BROWNIE
BROWSED
BROWSER
BROWSES
BROWWAX
BUDWORM
BULWARK

B•••W••
BACKWAY
BALDWIN
BEDEWED
BEESWAX
BEJEWEL
BELTWAY
BEROWNE
BIKEWAY
BOBTWAY
BOERWAR
BRONWEN
BROWWAX
BUSHWAH

B••••W•
BADNEWS
BALLTWO
BARNOWL
BARROWS
BASETWO
BEDDOWN
BELLOWS
BESTOWS
BIGNEWS
BIGTOWN
BILLOWS
BILLOWY
BOGDOWN
BORROWS
BOWDOWN
BOWSAWS
BOWWOWS
BURROWS
BUYDOWN

B•••••W
BACKROW
BACKSAW
BANDSAW
BARSTOW
BEARPAW
BELTSAW
BESTREW
BIGELOW
BIGSHOW
BLUELAW
BUCKSAW
BUZZSAW

•BW••••
EBWHITE

•B•••W•
ABCNEWS
CBSNEWS
NBCNEWS

••BW•••
BOBWEIR
COBWEBS
SUBWARS
SUBWAYS

••B•W••
BOBTWAY
ELBOWED
ELBOWER
EMBOWER
UNBOWED

••B••W•
DRBROWN
EMBROWN
HEBREWS
INBROWN
MRBROWN
REBLOWN
REBREWS
ROBLOWE
RUBDOWN
UNBLOWN

••B•••W
GOBELOW
RUBSRAW

•••BW••
OJIBWAS
OJIBWAY

•••B•W•
CATBOWL
DOGBOWL
FOGBOWS
OUTBAWL
OUTBOWL
OUTBOWS
PROBOWL
SUNBOWL
SUNBOWS

•••B••W
DOUBLEW

EYEBROW
JOEBLOW
LOWBLOW
LOWBROW
MISBREW
OUTBLOW

••••B•W
DOWNBOW
LONGBOW
MISTBOW
MOONBOW
RAINBOW

B•X••••
BOXBALL
BOXBEDS
BOXBOYS
BOXCARS
BOXCOAT
BOXEDIN
BOXEDUP
BOXESIN
BOXESUP
BOXFULS
BOXIEST
BOXKITE
BOXLIKE
BOXSEAT
BOXSETS
BOXSTEP
BOXSTER
BOXTOPS
BUXOMLY

B••X•••
BAUXITE
BIAXIAL
BRAXTON
BRUXING
BRUXISM

B•••X••
BAREXAM

B••••X•
BATNEXT
BETWIXT
BYPROXY

B•••••X
BANDBOX
BASESIX
BASSSAX
BATEAUX
BAYLYNX
BEATBOX
BEATRIX
BEESWAX
BENELUX
BERVOIX
BETAMAX
BLUEFOX
BOOMBOX
BRERFOX
BROADAX
BROWWAX
BUREAUX

•B••X••
ABRAXAS

••B•X••
INBOXES
POBOXES
REBOXED
REBOXES
UNBOXED
UNBOXES

••B••X•
SUBTEXT

•••B••X
DOUBLEX
ROUBAIX

••••B•X
BANDBOX
BEATBOX
BOOMBOX
CALLBOX
CASHBOX
COINBOX
DEEDBOX
DROPBOX
FAREBOX
FIREBOX
FUSEBOX
GEARBOX
GIFTBOX
JUKEBOX
JURYBOX
KICKBOX
LOCKBOX
MAILBOX
PILLBOX
POORBOX
POSTBOX
SALTBOX
SANDBOX
SHOEBOX
SOAPBOX
TOOLBOX
WOODBOX
WORKBOX

BY•••••
BYAHAIR
BYAMILE
BYANDBY
BYANECK
BYANOSE
BYBIRTH
BYCATCH
BYEBYES
BYFIVES
BYFORCE
BYFORMS
BYGOLLY
BYGONES
BYHEART
BYJINGO
BYLINED
BYLINER
BYLINES
BYMOUTH
BYNAMES
BYPATHS
BYPHONE
BYPLAYS
BYPROXY
BYRIGHT
BYROADS
BYRONIC
BYTALKS
BYTHEBY
BYTRAIN
BYTURNS
BYWAYOF
BYWORDS

B•Y••••
BAYAREA
BAYCITY
BAYEDAT
BAYLEAF
BAYLORU
BAYLYNX
BAYONET
BAYONNE
BAYRUMS
BAYTREE
BEYONCE
BLYNKEN
BOYBAND
BOYCOTT
BOYHOOD
BOYLIKE
BOYTOYS
BRYNNER
BRYUSOV
BUYABLE
BUYBACK
BUYDOWN
BUYINTO
BUYOFFS
BUYOUTS
BUYSOFF
BUYSOUT
BUYTIME

B••Y•••
BABYBOP
BABYGAP
BABYING
BABYISH
BABYLON
BABYOIL
BABYSAT
BABYSIT
BANYANS
BARYONS
BEEYARD
BELYING
BICYCLE
BIRYANI
BODYART
BODYBAR
BODYFAT
BODYKIT
BODYRUB
BOGYMAN
BOGYMEN
BOWYERS
BRAYERS
BRAYING
BREYERS
BUOYANT
BUOYING
BUOYSUP
BURYING
BUSYBEE
BUSYING

B•••Y••
BABIYAR
BAYLYNX
BELAYED
BELAYER
BELLYUP
BIGEYED
BIGEYES
BIOTYPE
BOGEYED
BONEYER
BUDDYUP
BUGEYED
BYEBYES
BYWAYOF

B••••Y•
BADBOYS
BADDAYS
BADGUYS
BAGBOYS
BARLEYS
BARNEYS
BATBOYS
BATDAYS
BENDAYS
BERNAYS
BETRAYS
BIGBOYS
BIGDAYS
BILLNYE
BOXBOYS
BOYTOYS
BUCKEYE
BUGBOYS
BURSTYN
BUSBOYS
BYPLAYS

B•••••Y
BACKBAY
BACKPAY
BACKWAY
BAGGILY
BAGLADY
BALCONY
BALKILY
BALLBOY
BALMILY
BALONEY
BALSAMY
BANALLY
BANBURY
BARBARY
BARCLAY
BARKLEY
BARNABY
BARTRAY
BASALLY
BASEPAY
BATTERY
BAWDILY
BAYCITY
BEADILY
BEANERY
BEASLEY
BEASTLY
BEATIFY
BEEFILY
BEGGARY
BEHAPPY
BELLAMY
BELLBOY
BELTWAY
BENTLEY
BERKLEY
BESTBOY
BESTBUY
BETARAY
BETHANY
BETTANY
BEVERLY
BIASPLY
BIGBABY
BIGCITY
BIGEASY
BIGGITY
BIGOTRY
BIKEWAY
BILLOWY
BINDERY
BIOLOGY
BLACKLY
BLAKELY
BLAKLEY
BLANDLY
BLANKLY
BLARNEY
BLEAKLY
BLIGHTY
BLINDLY
BLOTCHY
BLOWDRY
BLOWFLY
BLUEBOY
BLUEJAY
BLUESKY
BLUFFLY
BLUNTLY
BOBBSEY
BOBTWAY
BOGUSLY
BOKCHOY
BONEDRY
BONNILY
BOOTERY
BOOZILY
BOSSILY
BRADLEY
BRAMBLY
BRAMLEY
BRANCHY
BRASHLY
BRAVELY
BRAVERY
BRAWLEY
BREATHY
BREVITY
BREWERY
BRIBERY
BRIEFLY
BRIMLEY
BRISKLY
BRISTLY
BRITNEY
BROADLY
BRODKEY
BRODSKY
BRUTELY
BUCKLEY
BUMPILY
BURNABY
BURNLEY
BUSHILY
BUTTERY
BUTTONY
BUXOMLY
BYANDBY
BYGOLLY
BYPROXY
BYTHEBY

•BY••••
ABYSMAL
ABYSSAL
ABYSSES
WBYEATS

•B•Y•••
ABEYANT
EBAYERS
OBEYERS
OBEYING

•B••Y••
IBEGYOU

•B••••Y
ABBOTCY
ABIDEBY
ABILITY
IBILITY
OBESELY
OBESITY
OBLOQUY

••BY•••
ASBYATT
BABYBOP
BABYGAP
BABYING
BABYISH
BABYLON
BABYOIL
BABYSAT
BABYSIT
GOBYAIR
GOBYBUS
GOBYCAB
GOBYCAR
GOBYSEA
LIBYANS
RUBYDEE
RUBYRED
SIBYLIC

••B•Y••
BABIYAR
COBUYER
EMBAYED
EMBRYOS
LOBBYER
RIBEYES
SUBTYPE

••B••Y•
NOBODYS
ROBROYS
SUBWAYS
TABKEYS

••B•••Y
ABBOTCY
ALBUNDY
BOBBSEY
BOBTWAY
CABBAGY
CUBICLY
DEBAKEY
DEBUSSY
DUBARRY
DUBIETY
EMBASSY
JOBBERY
LIBERTY
LIBRARY
MRBODDY
MTBALDY
MYBUDDY
PUBERTY
RABBITY
RABIDLY
RIBBONY
ROBBERY
ROBOTRY
RUBBERY
SOBERLY
SUBSIDY
UNBOGGY
UNBULKY
UNBURLY

•••BY••
BYEBYES
EXABYTE
LOBBYER
ONEBYTE

•••B•Y•
BADBOYS
BAGBOYS
BATBOYS
BIGBOYS
BOXBOYS
BUGBOYS
BUSBOYS
CAMBOYS
CARBOYS
COWBOYS
FLYBOYS
JOSBOYS
LAZBOYS
LOWBOYS
OLDBOYS
OUTBUYS
PEPBOYS
PINBOYS
PREBUYS
REDBAYS
TAMBLYN
THEBOYS
TOMBOYS

•••B••Y
ALABAMY
ANYBODY
ASABODY
ASHBERY
ASHBURY
BANBURY
BARBARY
BIGBABY
BOBBSEY
BRIBERY
CABBAGY
CADBURY
CRYBABY
DANBURY
DOUBLEY
GARBAGY
GETBUSY
GOTBUSY
JOBBERY
MOWBRAY
NEWBERY
NONBODY
NONBUSY
OJIBWAY
OREBODY
OUTBRAY
PEABODY
PROBITY
RABBITY
RIBBONY
ROBBERY
ROXBURY
RUBBERY
STUBBLY
SUDBURY
TARBABY
THEBABY
THEBODY
TIMBERY
UNIBODY
VERBIFY
WARBABY
WEMBLEY
ZOMBIFY

••••BY•
GOODBYE
GOODBYS
HANGBYS
RIDEBYS

••••B•Y
AFFABLY
AMIABLY
ATTABOY
AUDIBLY
BACKBAY
BALLBOY
BELLBOY
BESTBOY
BESTBUY
BLUEBOY
BRAMBLY
CALLBOY
CAPABLY
CITYBOY
COPYBOY
CRUMBLY
CURABLY
DISOBEY
DURABLY
EFFABLY
EQUABLY
FARMBOY
FOREBAY
GAMEBOY
GOODBUY
GOOMBAY
GRUMBLY
HAUTBOY
HELLBOY
HIGHBOY
HOMEBOY
IGNOBLY
ITSABOY
JOHNBOY
LEGIBLY
LOVABLY
MOVABLY
MUTABLY
NAMABLY
NEWSBOY
NICEBOY
NOTABLY
OVERBUY
PAGEBOY
PLAYBOY
PLIABLY
PLOWBOY
POORBOY
RISIBLY
ROSEBAY
SCRUBBY
SHRUBBY
SICKBAY
SIZABLY
STUBBLY
TENABLY
TREMBLY
VISIBLY
VOCABLY
VOLUBLY

•••••BY
ABIDEBY
ALLENBY
BARNABY
BIGBABY
BURNABY
BYANDBY
BYTHEBY
CARNABY
CLOSEBY
COMESBY
CREEPBY
CRYBABY
DRIVEBY
DROPSBY
DROVEBY
DRWELBY
EASEDBY
EASESBY
EKINGBY
ENDERBY
FILEDBY
FILESBY
FLIESBY
FLITSBY
FLOATBY
FLOWNBY
GIVENBY
GLIDEBY
GOINGBY
GRIMSBY
HANGSBY
HORNSBY
HUSHABY
LAZENBY
LETGOBY
LULLABY
LYINGBY
MORESBY
PLAYSBY
RACEDBY
RACESBY
RIDESBY
ROCKABY
ROLLSBY
RULEDBY
SCRUBBY
SENDSBY
SHOOTBY
SHRUBBY
SKIPSBY
SLIDEBY
SLIPSBY
SNEAKBY
SOTHEBY
STANDBY
STICKBY
STOODBY
STOPSBY
STUCKBY
SWEARBY
SWINGBY
SWOREBY
SWUNGBY
TAKENBY
TARBABY
THEBABY
THEREBY
TICKSBY
WALKSBY
WALLABY
WARBABY
WHEREBY

B•Z••••
BAZAARS
BAZOOKA
BEZIERS
BEZIQUE
BIZARRE
BIZARRO
BOZEMAN
BUZZARD
BUZZCUT
BUZZELL
BUZZERS
BUZZIER
BUZZING
BUZZOFF
BUZZSAW

B••Z•••
BANZAIS
BEEZERS
BELZONI
BENZALI
BENZELL
BENZENE
BLAZERS
BLAZEUP
BLAZING
BLAZONS
BOOZERS
BOOZIER
BOOZILY
BOOZING
BORZAGE
BORZOIS
BRAZENS
BRAZIER
BRAZING
BUZZARD
BUZZCUT
BUZZELL
BUZZERS
BUZZIER
BUZZING
BUZZOFF
BUZZSAW

B•••Z••
BEDAZED
BEDAZES
BEDIZEN
BENAZIR
BLITZED
BLITZEN
BLITZER
BLITZES
BLOWZED
BREEZED
BREEZES
BRONZED
BRONZER
BRONZES

B••••Z•
BAPTIZE
BLINTZE
BONANZA
BRASIZE

B•••••Z
BEDNORZ
BERLIOZ
BERLITZ

•B•Z•••
IBIZANS

•B••Z••
ABRUZZI

•B•••Z•
ABRUZZI
EBONIZE
OBELIZE

••BZ•••
SUBZERO
SUBZONE
WEBZINE

••B•Z••
CABEZAS
REBOZOS

••B••Z•
EMBLAZE
FABRIZI

••B•••Z
ALBENIZ
COBLENZ
KIBBUTZ
KOBLENZ

•••BZ••
SIEBZIG

•••B•Z•
OUTBUZZ
ZAMBEZI

•••B••Z
DOUBLEZ
KIBBUTZ
LEIBNIZ
OUTBUZZ

••••B•Z
AGRIBIZ
SHOWBIZ

CA•••••
CABALAS
CABALLE
CABANAS
CABARET
CABBAGE
CABBAGY
CABBALA
CABBIES
CABBING
CABEZAS
CABFARE
CABINET
CABLERS
CABLETS
CABLETV
CABLING
CABOOSE
CABRIDE
CABRINI
CABRIOS
CACHACA
CACHETS
CACHING
CACIQUE
CACKLED
CACKLER
CACKLES
CACONYM
CADAVER
CADBURY
CADDIED
CADDIES
CADDISH
CADEAUX
CADENCE
CADENCY
CADENZA
CADETTE
CADGERS
CADGING
CADMIUM
CADUCEI
CAESARS
CAESURA
CAFTANS
CAGEDIN
CAGEDUP
CAGEPET
CAGESUP
CAGIEST
CAHIERS
CAHOKIA
CAHOOTS
CAILLOU
CAIMANS
CAIRENE
CAIRNED
CAISSON
CAJOLED
CAJOLER
CAJOLES
CAKEDUP
CAKEMIX
CAKEPAN
CAKESUP
CAKETIN
CAKIEST
CALABRO
CALAMAR
CALANDO
CALCIFY
CALCITE
CALCIUM
CALCULI
CALDERA
CALDERS
CALDRON
CALENDS
CALGARY
CALHOUN
CALIBAN
CALIBER
CALIBRE
CALICES
CALICOS
CALIPER
CALIPHS
CALISTA

CALKERS
CALKING
CALKINS
CALLBOX
CALLBOY
CALLEES
CALLERS
CALLFOR
CALLING
CALLINS
CALLNOW
CALLOFF
CALLOUS
CALLOUT
CALLSIN
CALLSIT
CALLSON
CALLSTO
CALLSUP
CALLUPS
CALMEST
CALMING
CALMSEA
CALORIC
CALORIE
CALOTTE
CALPOLY
CALTECH
CALUMET
CALUMNY
CALVARY
CALVERT
CALVING
CALVINO
CALYCES
CALYPSO
CALYXES
CALZONE
CAMACHO
CAMAROS
CAMBERS
CAMBOYS
CAMBRIA
CAMBRIC
CAMEDUE
CAMELID
CAMELOT
CAMEOED
CAMEOFF
CAMEOUT
CAMERAE
CAMERAL
CAMERAS
CAMERON
CAMGIRL
CAMILLA
CAMILLE
CAMINOS
CAMIONS
CAMISES
CAMMIES
CAMPARI
CAMPBED
CAMPERS
CAMPHOR
CAMPIER
CAMPILY
CAMPING
CAMPION
CAMPOUT
CAMPSUP
CAMRYLE
CANALED
CANAPES
CANARDS
CANASTA
CANCANS
CANCELS
CANCERS
CANCHAS
CANDACE
CANDELA
CANDENT
CANDICE
CANDIDA
CANDIDE
CANDIDS
CANDIED
CANDIES
CANDLED
CANDLER
CANDLES
CANDOUR
CANETTI
CANFULS
CANIDAE
CANIEST
CANINES
CANINGS
CANITBE
CANKERS
CANNELL
CANNELS
CANNERS
CANNERY
CANNIER
CANNILY
CANNING
CANNOCK
CANNOLI
CANNONS
CANNULA
CANOERS
CANOLAS
CANONIC
CANONRY
CANOPUS
CANSECO
CANTABS
CANTALS
CANTATA
CANTEEN
CANTERS
CANTILY
CANTINA
CANTING
CANTINO
CANTLES
CANTONS
CANTORS
CANTRIP
CANTSAY
CANUCKS
CANULAE
CANULAS
CANVASS
CANYONS
CANZONA
CANZONE
CANZONI
CAPABLE
CAPABLY
CAPADES
CAPAPIE
CAPEANN
CAPECOD
CAPEESH
CAPELET
CAPELLA
CAPEMAY
CAPERED
CAPFULS
CAPGUNS
CAPITAL
CAPITAN
CAPITOL
CAPLESS
CAPLETS
CAPNUTS
CAPOTES
CAPPERS
CAPPING
CAPRICE
CAPRINE
CAPSHAW
CAPSIZE
CAPSTAN
CAPSULE
CAPTAIN
CAPTION
CAPTIVA
CAPTIVE
CAPTORS
CAPTURE
CAPUANA
CAPUCHE
CAPULET
CARABOO
CARACAS
CARAFES
CARAMBA
CARAMEL
CARAMIA
CARAVAN
CARAVEL
CARAWAY
CARBARN
CARBIDE
CARBINE
CARBONS
CARBOYS
CARBRAS
CARCARE
CARCASS
CARCLUB
CARCOAT
CARDERS
CARDIAC
CARDIAL
CARDIFF
CARDING
CARDIUM
CARDKEY
CARDOOR
CARDOZO
CAREDTO
CAREENS
CAREERS
CAREFOR
CAREFUL
CARESTO
CARFARE
CARFREE
CARFULS
CARGOES
CARHOPS
CARHORN
CARIBES
CARIBOO
CARIBOU
CARINAE
CARINAS
CARIOCA
CARIOLE
CARIOUS
CARJACK
CARKEYS
CARKING
CARLENE
CARLESS
CARLING
CARLOAD
CARLOAN
CARLOTA
CARLOTS
CARLSON
CARLTON
CARLYLE
CARMELA
CARMINA
CARMINE
CARNABY
CARNAGE
CARNERA
CARNETS
CARNIES
CAROLED
CAROLER
CAROLII
CAROLYN
CAROMED
CAROTID
CAROTIN
CAROUSE
CARPALS
CARPARK
CARPELS
CARPERS
CARPETS
CARPING
CARPOOL
CARPORT
CARPOUS
CARPSAT
CARRARA
CARRELS
CARRERA
CARRERE
CARRIED
CARRIER
CARRIES
CARROLL
CARROTS
CARROTY
CARRYIN
CARRYON
CARSALE
CARSEAT
CARSHOW
CARTAGE
CARTALK
CARTELS
CARTERS
CARTIER
CARTING
CARTIRE
CARTOFF
CARTONS
CARTOON
CARTOPS
CARTRIP
CARTSIN
CARVELS
CARVERS
CARVING
CARWASH
CASABAS
CASAVAS
CASCADE
CASEATE
CASEINS
CASELAW
CASELLA
CASELOT
CASEOUS
CASEOUT
CASERNE
CASERNS
CASERTA
CASHBAR
CASHBOX
CASHCOW
CASHEWS
CASHIER
CASHING
CASHINS
CASHOUT
CASIMIR
CASINGS
CASINOS
CASITAS
CASKETS
CASKING
CASPARY
CASPIAN
CASQUED
CASQUES
CASSABA
CASSATT
CASSAVA
CASSIAS
CASSIDY
CASSINI
CASSINO
CASSIUS
CASSOCK
CASSOLA
CASTERS
CASTILE
CASTING
CASTLED
CASTLES
CASTOFF
CASTOUT
CASTROL
CASTSON
CASTSUP
CASUALS
CASUIST
CATALAN
CATALOG
CATALOS
CATALPA
CATANIA
CATAWBA
CATBEDS
CATBERT
CATBIRD
CATBOAT
CATBOWL
CATCALL
CATCHER
CATCHES
CATCHON
CATCHOW
CATCHUP
CATCOMB
CATDOOR
CATENAE
CATENAS
CATERAS
CATERED
CATERER
CATERTO
CATEYED
CATFEET
CATFISH
CATFITS
CATFLAP
CATFLEA
CATFOOD
CATFOOT
CATGUTS
CATHAIR
CATHEAD
CATHODE
CATIONS
CATKINS
CATLIKE
CATMINT
CATNAPS
CATNIPS
CATORCE
CATRIGS
CATSCAN
CATSEYE
CATSHOW
CATSITS
CATSPAW
CATSUIT
CATSUPS
CATTAIL
CATTALO
CATTIER
CATTILY
CATTISH
CATTOYS
CATWALK
CAUDATE
CAULKED
CAULKER
CAUSERS
CAUSING
CAUSTIC
CAUTHEN
CAUTION
CAVALRY
CAVEART
CAVEATS
CAVEDIN
CAVEINS
CAVEMAN
CAVEMEN
CAVERNS
CAVESIN
CAVIARE
CAVIARS
CAVILAT
CAVILED
CAVILER
CAVORTS
CAYENNE
CAYMANS
CAYUGAS
CAYUSES

C•A••••

CDALBUM
CEASING
CHABLIS
CHACHAS
CHACHKA
CHAFERS
CHAFFED
CHAFFEE
CHAFFER
CHAFING
CHAGALL
CHAGRIN
CHAINED
CHAINES
CHAINUP
CHAIRED
CHAISES
CHAKRAS
CHALCIS
CHALETS
CHALICE
CHALKED
CHALKUP
CHALLAH
CHALONS
CHALUPA
CHAMBER
CHAMBRE
CHAMFER
CHAMOIS
CHAMPED
CHAMPER
CHANCED
CHANCEL
CHANCER
CHANCES
CHANELS
CHANGED
CHANGER
CHANGES
CHANNEL
CHANOYU
CHANSON
CHANTED
CHANTER
CHANTEY
CHANTRY
CHAOTIC
CHAPALA
CHAPATI
CHAPEAU
CHAPELS
CHAPLET
CHAPLIN
CHAPMAN
CHAPMEN
CHAPPED
CHAPPIE
CHAPTER
CHARADE
CHARCOT
CHARGED
CHARGER
CHARGES
CHARIER
CHARILY
CHARING
CHARIOT
CHARITY
CHARLES
CHARLEY
CHARLIE
CHARMAN
CHARMED
CHARMEN
CHARMER
CHARMIN
CHARNIN
CHARPAK
CHARRED
CHARRER
CHARROS
CHARTED
CHARTER
CHARVET
CHASERS
CHASING
CHASMAL
CHASMIC
CHASSED
CHASSES
CHASSIS
CHASTEN
CHASTER
CHATEAU
CHATHAM
CHATSUP
CHATTED
CHATTEL
CHATTER
CHATWIN
CHAUCER
CHAWING
CHAYOTE
CHAZANS
CHAZZAN
CLABBER
CLACKED
CLACKER
CLACTON
CLADDED
CLAIMED
CLAIMER
CLAIROL
CLAMANT
CLAMATO
CLAMBAR
CLAMBER
CLAMDIP
CLAMMED
CLAMMER
CLAMORS
CLAMOUR
CLAMPED
CLAMPER
CLAMPON
CLAMSUP
CLANGED
CLANGER
CLANGOR
CLANKED
CLANTON
CLAPFOR
CLAPPED
CLAPPER
CLAPTON
CLAQUES
CLARETS
CLARICE
CLARIFY
CLARION
CLARITY
CLASHED
CLASHER
CLASHES
CLASPED
CLASPER
CLASSED
CLASSER
CLASSES
CLASSIC
CLASSON
CLATTER
CLAUDEL
CLAUDIA
CLAUDIO
CLAUSAL
CLAUSES
CLAVATE
CLAVELL
CLAVIER
CLAWERS
CLAWING
CLAWSAT
CLAYIER
CLAYING
CLAYISH
CLAYPIT
CLAYTON
COACHED
COACHES
COACTED
COAGENT
COALBIN
COALCAR
COALERS
COALGAS
COALING
COALOIL
COALPIT
COALTAR
COAPTED
COARSEN
COARSER
COASTAL
COASTED
COASTER
COATEES
COATERS
COATING
COAXERS
COAXIAL
COAXING
CPAEXAM
CRABBED
CRABBER
CRABPOT
CRACKED
CRACKER
CRACKLE
CRACKLY
CRACKUP
CRADLED
CRADLER
CRADLES
CRAFTED
CRAFTER
CRAFTSY
CRAGGED
CRAIGIE
CRAISIN
CRAMMED
CRAMMER
CRAMPED
CRAMPON
CRAMSIN
CRANIAL
CRANING
CRANIUM
CRANKED
CRANKUP
CRANMER
CRAPING
CRAPOLA
CRAPOUT
CRAPPIE
CRASHAW
CRASHED
CRASHER
CRASHES
CRASSER
CRASSLY
CRASSUS
CRATERS
CRATEUP
CRATING
CRATION
CRAVATS
CRAVENS
CRAVERS
CRAVING
CRAWDAD
CRAWLED
CRAWLER
CRAWLEY
CRAYOLA
CRAYONS
CRAZIER
CRAZIES
CRAZILY
CRAZING
CSARDAS
CUATROS
CYANIDE
CYANIDS
CZARDAS
CZARDOM
CZARINA
CZARISM
CZARIST

C••A•••

CABALAS
CABALLE
CABANAS
CABARET
CADAVER
CALABRO
CALAMAR
CALANDO
CAMACHO
CAMAROS
CANALED
CANAPES
CANARDS
CANASTA
CAPABLE
CAPABLY
CAPADES
CAPAPIE
CARABOO
CARACAS
CARAFES
CARAMBA
CARAMEL
CARAMIA
CARAVAN
CARAVEL
CARAWAY
CASABAS
CASAVAS
CATALAN
CATALOG
CATALOS
CATALPA
CATANIA
CATAWBA
CAVALRY
CBRADIO
CCLAMPS
CDCASES
CDRACKS
CDRATES
CEDARED
CELADON
CELAENO
CENACLE
CERAMIC
CERATED
CERATES
CESAIRE
CETANES
CEZANNE
CHEADLE
CHEAPEN
CHEAPER
CHEAPIE
CHEAPLY
CHEATED
CHEATER
CHEATIN
CHEATON
CHIANTI
CHIAPAS
CHIAPET
CICADAE
CICADAS
CIMABUE
CITABLE
CITADEL
CLEANED
CLEANER
CLEANLY
CLEANSE
CLEANTE
CLEANUP
CLEARED
CLEARER
CLEARLY
CLEAROF
CLEARUP
CLEATED
CLEAVED
CLEAVER
CLEAVES
CLEAVON
CLOAKED
COBALTS
COCAINE
COHABIT
COLADAS
COMAKER
CONAGRA
CONAKRY
CORACLE
CORAZON
COWARDS
CREAKED
CREAMED
CREAMER
CREASED
CREASER
CREASES
CREATED
CREATES
CREATOR
CROAKED
CROAKER
CROATIA
CUBAGES
CURABLE
CURABLY
CURACAO
CURARES
CURATED
CURATES
CURATOR
CUTARUG
CUTAWAY

C•••A••

CABBAGE
CABBAGY
CABBALA
CABFARE
CACHACA
CADEAUX
CAESARS
CAFTANS
CAIMANS
CALGARY
CALVARY
CAMPARI
CANCANS
CANDACE
CANTABS
CANTALS
CANTATA
CANVASS
CAPEANN
CAPTAIN
CAPUANA
CARBARN
CARCARE
CARCASS
CARFARE
CARJACK
CARNABY
CARNAGE
CARPALS
CARPARK
CARRARA
CARSALE
CARTAGE
CARTALK
CARWASH
CASCADE
CASEATE
CASPARY
CASSABA
CASSATT
CASSAVA
CASUALS
CATCALL
CATHAIR
CATNAPS
CATTAIL
CATTALO
CATWALK
CAUDATE
CAVEART
CAVEATS
CAVIARE
CAVIARS
CAYMANS
CELLARS
CEMBALO
CENTALS
CENTARE
CENTAUR
CENTAVO
CEPHALO
CEPHALY
CEREALS
CERTAIN
CHAGALL
CHAPALA
CHAPATI

CHARADE
CHAZANS
CHELATE
CHEVAUX
CHICAGO
CHICANA
CHICANE
CHICANO
CHORALE
CHORALS
CHUMASH
CILIARY
CILIATE
CINZANO
CIRRATE
CISEAUX
CITRATE
CLAMANT
CLAMATO
CLAVATE
CLIMATE
CLIMATS
CLIPART
COBRAND
COCHAIR
COCKADE
CODCAKE
COEVALS
COGNACS
COGNATE
COINAGE
COLGATE
COLLAGE
COLLARD
COLLARS
COLLATE
COMBATS
COMCAST
COMMAND
COMPACT
COMPANY
COMPAQS
COMPARE
COMPART
COMPASS
COMRADE
COMSATS
CONCAVE
CONFABS
CONGAED
CONGAME
CONNATE
CONRACK
CONTACS
CONTACT
CONTAIN
COOLAIR
COOLANT
COPCARS
COPLAND
CORDAGE
CORDATE
CORFAMS
CORKAGE
CORMACK
CORRADE
CORRALS
CORSAGE
CORSAIR
CORVAIR
COSSACK
COSTAIN
COSTARD
COSTARS
COSTATE
COTEACH
COTTAGE
COUGARS
COURAGE
COURANT
COWBANE
COWHAND
CPEBACH
CRAVATS
CREMATE
CRENATE
CRETANS
CRUSADE
CRUZADO
CRUZANS
CRYBABY
CTSCANS
CUBFANS
CUEBALL
CUECARD
CUIRASS
CUNEATE
CUPCAKE
CUREALL
CURRANT
CURTAIL
CURTAIN
CURTATE
CUSHAWS
CUSPATE
CUSTARD
CUTBACK
CUTLASS
CUTRATE
CYMBALS

C••••A•

CABALAS
CABANAS
CABEZAS
CAKEPAN
CALAMAR
CALIBAN
CAMERAE
CAMERAL
CAMERAS
CANCHAS
CANIDAE
CANOLAS
CANTSAY
CANULAE
CANULAS
CAPEMAY
CAPITAL
CAPITAN
CAPSHAW
CAPSTAN
CARACAS
CARAVAN
CARAWAY
CARBRAS
CARCOAT
CARDIAC
CARDIAL
CARINAE
CARINAS
CARLOAD
CARLOAN
CARPSAT
CARSEAT
CASABAS
CASAVAS
CASELAW
CASHBAR
CASITAS
CASPIAN
CASSIAS
CATALAN
CATBOAT
CATENAE
CATENAS
CATERAS
CATFLAP
CATHEAD
CATSCAN
CATSPAW
CAVEMAN
CAVILAT
CAYUGAS
CELICAS
CENTRAL
CESSNAS
CHACHAS
CHAKRAS
CHALLAH
CHAPEAU
CHAPMAN
CHARMAN
CHARPAK
CHASMAL
CHATEAU
CHATHAM
CHAZZAN
CHEDDAR
CHEETAH
CHEETAS
CHEMLAB
CHIAPAS
CHICHAS
CHILCAT
CHILEAN
CHILIAD
CHILKAT
CHINWAG
CHOCTAW
CHOLLAS
CHORDAL
CHROMAT
CHUPPAH
CHUPPAS
CICADAE
CICADAS
CINEMAS
CINEMAX
CITYGAL
CLAMBAR
CLAUSAL
CLAWSAT
CLUBCAR
COALCAR
COALGAS
COALTAR
COASTAL
COAXIAL
COBCOAL
COCHRAN
COCTEAU
COEQUAL
COGHLAN
COLADAS
COLDDAY
COLDWAR
COLEMAN
COMESAS
COMESAT
COMICAL
COMORAN
CONCEAL
CONCHAE
CONGEAL
CONICAL
CONTRAS
COOLCAT
COOLMAX
COONCAN
COONCAT
COPULAE
COPULAR
COPULAS
COPYCAT
COPYMAN
CORDIAL
CORDIAS
CORKOAK
CORNEAL
CORNEAS
CORONAE
CORONAL
CORONAS
CORYZAS
COWERAT
COWPEAS
CPAEXAM
CRANIAL
CRASHAW
CRAWDAD
CREEDAL
CREWMAN
CRIMEAN
CRITIAS
CROSSAT
CROWBAR
CRUCIAL
CRUSTAL
CRYSTAL
CSARDAS
CUBICAL
CUBITAL
CUBSFAN
CUESTAS
CULTJAM
CUMBIAS
CUMSHAW
CUPOLAS
CUPULAR
CURACAO
CURSEAT
CUTAWAY
CYNICAL
CYPRIAN
CZARDAS

C•••••A

CABBALA
CACHACA
CADENZA
CAESURA
CAHOKIA
CALDERA
CALISTA
CALMSEA
CAMBRIA
CAMILLA
CANASTA
CANDELA
CANDIDA
CANNULA
CANTATA
CANTINA
CANZONA
CAPELLA
CAPTIVA
CAPUANA
CARAMBA
CARAMIA
CARIOCA
CARLOTA
CARMELA
CARMINA
CARNERA
CARRARA
CARRERA
CASELLA
CASERTA
CASSABA
CASSAVA
CASSOLA
CATALPA
CATANIA
CATAWBA
CATFLEA
CECILIA
CEDILLA
CELESTA
CEREBRA
CERVEZA
CHACHKA
CHALUPA
CHAPALA
CHELSEA
CHICANA
CHIMERA
CHOLERA
CHRISTA
CHUTZPA
CINESIA
CLAUDIA
COCHLEA
COLONNA
COLUMBA
COMEDIA
CONAGRA
COPPOLA
COQUINA
CORDOBA
CORETTA
COROLLA
CORPORA
CORRIDA
CORSICA
CORTINA
CORVINA
CRAPOLA
CRAYOLA
CREMONA
CREMORA
CROATIA
CRUELLA
CUMBRIA
CURIOSA
CYNTHIA
CZARINA

•CA••••

ACACIAS
ACADEME
ACADEMY
ACADIAN
ACANTHI
ACARIDS
ACAUDAL
ECARTES
ICANNOT
JCARROL
MCADAMS
MCALLEN
MCARDLE
OCALAFL
OCANADA
OCARINA
RCADOME
SCACCHI
SCADSOF
SCALAGE
SCALARS
SCALDED
SCALDER
SCALENE
SCALERS
SCALEUP
SCALIER
SCALING
SCALLOP
SCALPED
SCALPEL
SCALPER
SCAMMED
SCAMMER
SCAMPED
SCAMPER
SCANDAL
SCANNED
SCANNER
SCANTED
SCANTER
SCANTLY
SCAPULA
SCARABS
SCARCER
SCAREDY
SCARERS
SCAREUP
SCARFED
SCARFER
SCARFUP
SCARIER
SCARIFY
SCARILY
SCARING
SCARLET
SCARPED
SCARRED
SCARVES
SCARWID
SCATHED
SCATHES
SCATMAN
SCATTED
SCATTER

•C•A•••

ACKACKS
ACTABLE
ACTAEON
CCLAMPS
ECHAPPE
ECLAIRS
ECUADOR
ICEAGES
ICEAXES
ICHABOD
LCHAYIM
MCCALLS
MCCAREY
MCGAVIN
MCHALES
MCMAHON
MCNALLY
MCPAPER
MCRANEY
OCEANIA
OCEANIC
OCEANID
OCEANUS
OCTADIC
OCTAGON
OCTANES
OCTANTS
OCTAVAL
OCTAVES
OCTAVIA
OCTAVIO
OCTAVOS
SCHAYES
SCIATIC
SCLAFFS
SCRAGGY
SCRAPED
SCRAPER
SCRAPES
SCRAPPY
SCRATCH
SCRAWLS
SCRAWLY
SCRAWNY
WCHANDY

•C••A••

ACCLAIM
ACERATE
ACETALS
ACETATE
ACREAGE
ACTUARY
ACTUATE
ECKHART
ECOTAGE
ECSTASY
ICEBAGS
ICEBATH
ICECAPS
ICECAVE
ICEDAMS
ICEFALL
ICELAND
ICEPACK
MCADAMS
MCCRARY
MCSHANE
OCALAFL
OCANADA
OCICATS
OCULARS
SCALAGE
SCALARS
SCARABS
SCHNAPS
SCHWANN
SCOLARI
SCREAKS
SCREAMS
SCUBAED
VCRTAPE

•C•••A•

ACACIAS
ACADIAN
ACAUDAL
ACCRUAL
ACCUSAL
ACROBAT
ACTEDAS
ACTIVAS
ECTYPAL
ECZEMAS
ICEBOAT
ICETEAS
ICETRAY
MCLUHAN
OCELLAR
OCTAVAL
RCCOLAS
SCANDAL
SCATMAN
SCHEMAS
SCHMEAR
SCHOLAR
SCLERAE
SCLERAL
SCLERAS
SCOFFAT
SCOOBAS
SCORIAS
SCOTIAN

•C••••A

ACEROLA
ACHIEVA
ECHIDNA
ICEDTEA
MCKENNA
OCANADA
OCARINA
OCEANIA
OCHENTA
OCTAVIA
SCAPULA
SCHIRRA
SCIORRA

••CA•••

ALCAIDE
ALCALDE
ALCAZAR
ARCADED
ARCADES
ARCADIA
ARCANUM
ASCARED
BACARDI
BECALMS
BECAUSE
BICARBS
BYCATCH
CDCASES
CICADAE
CICADAS
COCAINE
DACAPOS
DECADES
DECAGON
DECALOG
DECAMPS
DECANTS
DECAPOD
DECARLO
DECATUR
DECAYED
DECAYER
DUCALLY
ELCAJON
ELCAMPO
ENCAGED
ENCAGES
ENCAMPS
ENCARRE
ENCARTA
ENCASED
ENCASES
ESCALOP
ESCALUS
ESCAPED
ESCAPEE
ESCAPER
ESCAPES
ESCARPS
FACADES
GOCARTS
IDCARDS
INCANTS
INCASED
INCASES
JACALES
JACAMAR
JICAMAS
JOCASTA
LECARRE
LOCALES
LOCALLY
LOCARNO
LOCATED
LOCATER
LOCATES
LOCATOR
LUCANIA
LUCARNE
MACABRE
MACACOS
MACADAM
MACAQUE
MCCALLS
MCCAREY
MICAELA
NOCANDO
NOCARBS
NOCATCH
OHCAROL
OXCARTS
PICADOR
PICANTE
PICARAS
PICARDO
PICARDY
PICAROS
PICASSO
RECABLE
RECAGED
RECAGES
RECALLS
RECANED
RECANES
RECANTS
RECARRY
RECARVE
RECASED
RECASES
RECASTS
RICARDO
SECANTS
UNCAGED
UNCAGES
UNCAKED
UNCAKES
UNCANED
UNCANNY
UNCAPED
UNCASED
UNCASES
UNCASKS
UPCARDS
UPCASTS
VACANCY
VACATED
VACATES
VOCABLE
VOCABLY
VOCALIC
VOCALLY
YUCAIPA
YUCATAN
YUCATEC
ZOCALOS

••C•A••

ACCLAIM
ARCHAIC
ARCLAMP
ARCUATE
BACHATA
BECHARM
CACHACA
COCHAIR
COCKADE
DECEASE
DECIARE
DECLAIM
DECLARE
DECLASS
DECLAWS
DICTATE
DOCKAGE
DRCHAOS
DUCHAMP
ENCHAIN
ENCHANT
ENCHASE
ENCLASP
ENCLAVE
ETCHANT
EXCLAIM
EXCLAVE
FACIALS
GOCRAZY
HECKART
HECTARE
INCLASS
JACKALS
JACKASS
LACTAID
LACTASE
LACTATE
LOCKAGE
LUCIANA
LUCIANO
MACHAON
MACRAME
MCCRARY
MECCANS
MICHAEL
MICHAUX
MICMACS
NECTARS
NECTARY
NICCAGE
NICTATE
NOCLASS
ORCHARD
PACKAGE
PACKARD
PECCANT
PECCARY
PECCAVI
PICCARD
PICCATA
PICKAXE
RACHAEL
RECHALK
RECHALL
RECHART
RECLADS
RECLAIM
RECLAME
RECLASP
RECLASS
RECOALS
RECOATS
RECRANK
RECRATE
RICHARD
RICRACS
ROCKABY
SACCADE
SOCIALS
SUCRASE
TICTACS
TOCCATA
UNCHAIN
UNCHAIR
UNCHARY
UNCIALS
UNCLAMP
UNCLASP
UNCRAMP
UNCRATE
UNCRAZY
UPCOAST
VACCARO
VICDANA
WICCANS
ZACHARY

••C••A•

ACCRUAL
ACCUSAL
AFCTEAM
ALCAZAR
ARCHWAY
BACCHAE
BACHMAN
BACKBAR
BACKBAY
BACKPAY
BACKSAW
BACKWAY
BECKHAM
BUCHMAN
BUCKRAM
BUCKSAW
CICADAE
CICADAS
COCHRAN
COCTEAU
DECIMAL
ENCINAS
ESCHEAT
EXCELAT
EXCUSAL
EXCUSAS
FACTUAL
FACULAE
HACKMAN
HACKSAW
HECKMAN
HICKMAN
ISCHIAL
JACAMAR
JACKDAW
JACKTAR
JICAMAS
JOCULAR
LACTEAL
LACUNAE
LACUNAL
LACUNAR
LACUNAS
LOCKEAN
LOCKJAW
LUCIDAE
LUCKMAN
MACADAM
MACGRAW
MACLEAN
MACULAE
MACULAR
MRCLEAN
MYCENAE
NFCTEAM
NICEDAY
NICEMAN
NICOBAR
NICOLAS
NUCLEAR
OSCULAR
PACECAR
PACELAP
PACKRAT
PECKSAT
PICARAS
PICKSAT
RACECAR
RACEWAY
RCCOLAS
RECITAL
RECLEAN
RECUSAL
RICHMAN
RICKMAN
SECULAR
SICKBAY
SICKDAY
SICKPAY
TACOMAS
TACTUAL
TUCHMAN
UNCLEAN
UNCLEAR
UNCLOAK
VECTRAS
VICINAL
VICTUAL
VICUNAS
YUCATAN

••C•••A

ARCADIA
BACHATA
BACTRIA
CACHACA
CECILIA
COCHLEA
DACOSTA
ENCARTA
ENCOMIA
ESCUELA
FUCHSIA
HECKUVA
IACOCCA
JOCASTA
KACHINA

LACERTA
LACONIA
LECUONA
LUCANIA
LUCETTA
LUCIANA
LUCINDA
MACHINA
MACONGA
MICAELA
NICOSIA
OSCEOLA
PICCATA
RICKSHA
RICOTTA
SICILIA
TOCCATA
TOCELIA
VICDANA
VICENZA
WICHITA
YUCAIPA

•••CA••

ALLCAPS
ALLCASH
ARACARI
ARTCARS
ASHCAKE
ASHCANS
ATACAMA
ATMCARD
AVOCADO
BADCALL
BADCASE
BARCARS
BIGCARS
BIGCATS
BOBCATS
BOSCAGE
BOXCARS
BROCADE
CANCANS
CARCARE
CARCASS
CASCADE
CATCALL
CHICAGO
CHICANA
CHICANE
CHICANO
CODCAKE
COMCAST
CONCAVE
COPCARS
CTSCANS
CUECARD
CUPCAKE
DAYCAMP
DAYCARE
DESCANT
DIECAST
DISCARD
DOGCART
EATCAKE
EDUCATE
EGGCASE
EPICARP
EXOCARP
EYECARE
FALCATE
FATCATS
FBICASE
FLYCAST
FURCATE
GASCANS
GASCAPS
GELCAPS
GETCASH
GISCARD
GOTCASH
GUNCASE
HEPCATS
HOECAKE
HOGCALL
HOSCALE
HOTCAKE
HOTCAPS
HOTCARS
HUBCAPS
ICECAPS
ICECAVE
ILLCALL
ILOCANO
INACAST
INSCALE
JAMCAMS
JOECAMP
KEYCARD
KEYCASE
KINCAID
LAPCATS
LASCALA
LASCARS
LASCAUX
LAWCASE
LESCAUT
LOWCARB
LOWCARD
MADCAPS
MARCATO
MASCARA
MECCANS
MERCADO
MESCALS
METCALF
MIDCAPS
MISCALL
MISCAST
MOSCATO
MUDCATS
MULCAHY
MUSCATS
NESCAFE
NETCAFE
NEWCARS
NICCAGE
NONCASH
OAKCASK
OATCAKE
OCICATS
OFFCAST
OILCAKE
OILCANS
OLDCARS
ONECALL
OUTCALL
OUTCANT
OUTCAST
PANCAKE
PATCASH
PAYCASH
PECCANT
PECCARY
PECCAVI
PENCASE
PERCALE
PETCAGE
PETCALF
PETCATS
PICCARD
PICCATA
PIPCARD
PLACARD
PLACATE
PLICATE
PODCAST
PRECAST
RASCALS
REDCAPS
REDCARD
RESCALE
RESCANS
REXCATS
RIBCAGE
RUMCAKE
SACCADE
SADCAFE
SAGCARD
SARCASM
SEACALM
SEACATS
SKICAPS
SKYCAMS
SKYCAPS
SNOCAPS
SNOCATS
SPYCAMS
SUBCASE
SUBCASH
SUBCAST
TEACAKE
TEACART
THECAPE
THECARS
THECAVS
TINCANS
TIPCART
TOCCATA
TOECAPS
TOMCATS
TOSCALE
TOUCANS
TOWCARS
TOYCARS
TOYCART
TUSCANS
TUSCANY
UNSCALY
UPSCALE
UTICANS
UTICANY
VACCARO
VANCAMP
VOLCANO
VULCANS
WEBCAMS
WEBCAST
WICCANS

•••C•A•

ACACIAS
ALLCLAD
AMICHAI
AMSCRAY
ASOCIAL
BACCHAE
BARCLAY
BEACHAM
BEECHAM
BOXCOAT
CANCHAS
CARCOAT
CHACHAS
CHICHAS
CHOCTAW
COBCOAL
CONCEAL
CONCHAE
CRUCIAL
DEWCLAW
DISCMAN
DOGCOAT
EDICTAL
EPOCHAL
EXACTAS
FASCIAE
FASCIAL
FASCIAS
FRACTAL
FURCOAT
GLACIAL
GOTCHAS
GRACIAS
GRECIAN
HOTCOAL
ILLCLAD
JOYCEAN
KETCHAM
KWACHAS
LABCOAT
LANCIAS
MARCEAU
MERCIAN
OLDCHAP
ONECLAM
PANCHAX
PASCHAL
PEACOAT
PINCHAS
PISCEAN
REDCLAY
REDCOAT
SHECRAB
SPACIAL
SPECIAL
SUBCLAN
THECRAB
TOPCOAT
WROCLAW
ZWICKAU

•••C••A

ATACAMA
BLACULA
CHACHKA
CHICANA
DRACHMA
DRACULA
ELECTRA
INOCULA
KOSCINA
LASCALA
MASCARA
MUSCIDA
NONCOLA
OBSCURA
PICCATA
PLECTRA
QUECHUA
SPECTRA
TOCCATA
TRACHEA
VINCULA
VISCERA

••••CA•

AFRICAN
ALPACAS
ARNICAS
AZTECAN
BAITCAR
BEARCAT
BEERCAN
BIFOCAL
BOOMCAR
CARACAS
CATSCAN
CELICAS
CHILCAT
CLUBCAR
COALCAR
COMICAL
CONICAL
COOLCAT
COONCAN
COONCAT
COPYCAT
CUBICAL
CURACAO
CYNICAL
DIGICAM
DOMECAR
DOMICAL
DROPCAP
ETHICAL
FASTCAR
FINICAL
FLATCAR
FRESCAS
GOBYCAB
GOBYCAR
GOLFCAR
GYROCAR
HANDCAR
HELICAL
HELLCAT
HOPACAB
INDYCAR
INKYCAP
ITHACAN
JUNKCAR
KNEECAP
LENSCAP
LEXICAL
LOGICAL
LOSTCAT
LYRICAL
MAGICAL
MAILCAR
MALECAT
MANXCAT
MARACAS
MEDICAL
MEXICAN
MILKCAN
MINICAB
MINICAM
MINICAR
MOHICAN
MONACAN
MRISCAN
MUSICAL
NODICAL
OAXACAN
ONEACAT
ONEOCAT
OPTICAL
PACECAR
PADUCAH
PATACAS
PEDICAB
PELICAN
PETSCAN
POLECAR
POLECAT
PROSCAN
RACECAR
RADICAL
RAILCAR
RATECAP
REDECAY
ROOTCAP
SENECAN
SENECAS
SHOWCAT
SIDECAR
SILICAS
SLOTCAR
SNOWCAP
SNOWCAT
SODACAN
SOUPCAN
STOICAL
SURECAN
TANKCAR
TAXICAB
TOPICAL
TOWNCAR
TRAMCAR
TYPICAL
UNLOCAL
UNVOCAL
USEDCAR
VATICAL
VATICAN
VIVICAA
WILDCAT
XENICAL
YESICAN

••••C•A

BENICIA
BRESCIA
FELICIA
GALICIA
IACOCCA
IGOTCHA
INDICIA
INSECTA
INVICTA
MALACCA
MOLUCCA
PANACEA
REBECCA
RUZICKA
STLUCIA
VIVICAA

•••••CA

AMERICA
ARABICA
AVIANCA
AZUSACA
CACHACA
CARIOCA
CORSICA
EROTICA
EXOTICA
FORMICA
GATTACA
HENDECA
IACOCCA
JAMAICA
JESSICA
JUDAICA
LAPLACA
LATOSCA
MAJORCA
MALACCA
MANTECA
MENORCA
MINORCA
MOLUCCA
NAUTICA
NORDICA
POETICA
REBECCA
REPLICA
SAMBUCA
TAPIOCA
TRIBECA
VERRUCA
VIATICA
YASHICA

CB•••••

CBRADIO
CBSNEWS

C•B••••

CABALAS
CABALLE
CABANAS
CABARET
CABBAGE
CABBAGY
CABBALA
CABBIES
CABBING
CABEZAS
CABFARE
CABINET
CABLERS
CABLETS
CABLETV
CABLING
CABOOSE
CABRIDE
CABRINI
CABRIOS
COBALTS
COBBLED
COBBLER
COBBLES
COBCOAL
COBLENZ
COBNUTS
COBRAND
COBUYER
COBWEBS
CUBAGES
CUBBIES
CUBBING
CUBBINS
CUBBISH
CUBFANS
CUBICAL
CUBICLE
CUBICLY
CUBISTS
CUBITAL
CUBITUS
CUBOIDS
CUBSFAN
CYBORGS

C••B•••

CABBAGE
CABBAGY
CABBALA
CABBIES
CABBING
CADBURY
CAMBERS
CAMBOYS
CAMBRIA
CAMBRIC
CARBARN
CARBIDE
CARBINE
CARBONS
CARBOYS
CARBRAS
CATBEDS
CATBERT
CATBIRD
CATBOAT
CATBOWL
CEMBALO
CHABLIS
CLABBER
CLIBURN
CLOBBER
CLUBBED
CLUBBER
CLUBCAR
CLUBMED
CLUBSUP
COBBLED
COBBLER
COBBLES
COGBURN
COLBERT
COMBATS
COMBERS
COMBIEN
COMBINE
COMBING
COMBUST
CONBRIO
CORBELS
CORBETT
COWBANE
COWBELL
COWBIRD
COWBOYS
CPEBACH
CRABBED
CRABBER
CRABPOT
CRIBBED
CRIBBER
CRYBABY
CUBBIES
CUBBING
CUBBINS
CUBBISH
CUEBALL
CUEBIDS
CUIBONO
CUMBERS
CUMBIAS
CUMBRIA
CURBCUT
CURBING
CUTBACK
CYMBALS

C•••B••

CALABRO
CALIBAN
CALIBER
CALIBRE
CALLBOX
CALLBOY
CAMPBED
CAPABLE
CAPABLY
CARABOO
CARIBES
CARIBOO
CARIBOU
CASABAS
CASHBAR
CASHBOX
CDALBUM
CELEBES
CELEBRE
CEREBRA
CEREBRO
CHAMBER
CHAMBRE
CIMABUE
CITABLE
CITYBOY
CLABBER
CLAMBAR
CLAMBER
CLIMBED
CLIMBER
CLIMBIN
CLIMBON
CLIMBTO
CLIMBUP
CLOBBER
CLUBBED
CLUBBER
COALBIN
COHABIT
COINBOX
COPYBOY
CORNBIN
COURBET
CRABBED
CRABBER
CRIBBED
CRIBBER
CROWBAR
CRUMBED
CRUMBLE
CRUMBLY
CRUMBUM
CURABLE
CURABLY

C••••B•

CANITBE
CANTABS
CARAMBA
CARNABY
CASSABA
CATAWBA
CHERUBS
CLOSEBY
COBWEBS
COLOMBO
COLUMBA
COLUMBO
COMESBY
CONFABS
CONJOBS
CORDOBA
COULDBE
CREEPBY
CRYBABY

C•••••B

CARCLUB
CATCOMB
CHEMLAB
CORNCOB
COULOMB
COXCOMB

•CB••••

MCBRIDE

•C•B•••

ICEBAGS
ICEBATH
ICEBEER
ICEBERG
ICEBLUE
ICEBOAT
SCUBAED

•C••B••

ACERBIC
ACROBAT
ACTABLE
ICHABOD
OCTOBER
OCTOBRE
OCTUBRE
SCOOBAS
SCRIBED
SCRIBER
SCRIBES
SCRUBBY
SCRUBUP

•C•••B•

ICECUBE
SCARABS
SCHLUBS
SCRUBBY

•C••••B

MCCRUMB

••CB•••

MACBETH
NBCBLUE
PACBELL

••C•B••

BACKBAR
BACKBAY
BACKBIT
DECIBEL
INCUBUS
JACOBIN
KICKBOX
LOCKBOX
MACABRE
NICEBOY
NICOBAR
RECABLE
SICKBAY
SICKBED
UNCUBIC
VOCABLE
VOCABLY

••C••B•

ASCRIBE
BICARBS
MICROBE
NOCARBS
RACEDBY
RACESBY
RECOMBS
ROCKABY
TICKSBY
UNCURBS

••C•••B

BACKRUB
DECRUMB
MCCRUMB
NICEJOB
RECLIMB
SUCCUMB
UPCLIMB

•••C•B•

ARECIBO
ICECUBE
PLACEBO
STICKBY
STUCKBY
THECUBS

•••C••B

CARCLUB
CATCOMB
COXCOMB
DOGCOMB
FANCLUB
GYMCLUB
HOTCOMB
KEYCLUB
LOWCARB
ONECLUB
PETCOMB
RESCRUB
SHECRAB
SUCCUMB
THECRAB
WARCLUB

••••C•B

BEARCUB
CORNCOB
GOBYCAB
HOPACAB
LIONCUB
MINICAB
PEDICAB
TAXICAB
WOLFCUB

CC•••••

CCLAMPS
CCRIDER

C•C••••

CACHACA
CACHETS
CACHING
CACIQUE
CACKLED
CACKLER
CACKLES
CACONYM
CDCASES
CECILIA
CICADAE
CICADAS
CICCONE
CICHLID
COCAINE
COCCOID
COCHAIR
COCHISE
COCHLEA
COCHRAN
COCKADE
COCKERS
COCKIER
COCKILY
COCKING
COCKISH
COCKLED
COCKLES
COCKNEY
COCKPIT
COCONUT
COCOONS
COCTEAU
CUCKOOS
CYCLERS
CYCLING
CYCLIST
CYCLOID
CYCLONE
CYCLOPS

C••C•••

CALCIFY
CALCITE
CALCIUM
CALCULI
CANCANS
CANCELS
CANCERS
CANCHAS
CARCARE
CARCASS
CARCLUB
CARCOAT
CASCADE
CATCALL
CATCHER
CATCHES
CATCHON
CATCHOW
CATCHUP
CATCOMB
CHACHAS
CHACHKA
CHECHEN
CHECKED
CHECKER
CHECKIN
CHECKON
CHECKUP
CHICAGO
CHICANA
CHICANE
CHICANO
CHICEST
CHICHAS
CHICHEN
CHICHIS
CHICKEN
CHICLES
CHICLET
CHICORY
CHOCKED
CHOCTAW
CHUCKED

CHUCKIT
CHUCKLE
CICCONE
CINCHED
CINCHES
CIRCLED
CIRCLER
CIRCLES
CIRCLET
CIRCUIT
CIRCUSY
CISCOES
CLACKED
CLACKER
CLACTON
CLICHED
CLICHES
CLICKED
CLICKER
CLICKON
CLOCHES
CLOCKED
CLOCKER
CLOCKIN
CLUCKED
CLUCKER
COACHED
COACHES
COACTED
COBCOAL
COCCOID
CODCAKE
COLCHIS
COMCAST
CONCAVE
CONCEAL
CONCEDE
CONCEIT
CONCEPT
CONCERN
CONCERT
CONCHAE
CONCHES
CONCHOS
CONCISE
CONCOCT
CONCORD
CONCURS
CONCUSS
COPCARS
COUCHED
COUCHES
COXCOMB
CRACKED
CRACKER
CRACKLE
CRACKLY
CRACKUP
CRECHES
CRICKED
CRICKET
CROCHET
CROCKED
CROCKER
CROCKET
CRUCIAL
CTSCANS
CUECARD
CULCHES
CUPCAKE

C•••C••

CADUCEI
CALICES
CALICOS
CALYCES
CAMACHO
CANUCKS
CAPECOD
CAPUCHE
CARACAS
CASHCOW
CATSCAN
CDRACKS
CELICAS
CENACLE
CEVICHE
CHALCIS
CHANCED
CHANCEL
CHANCER
CHANCES
CHARCOT
CHAUCER
CHILCAT
CHOICER
CHOICES
CHURCHY
CLUBCAR
CLUTCHY
COALCAR
CODICES
CODICIL
COERCED
COERCER
COERCES
COLDCUP
COLDCUT
COLICKY
COMICAL
COMICES
CONICAL
COOLCAT
COONCAN
COONCAT
COPYCAT
CORACLE
CORNCOB
COUNCIL
CREWCUT
CRUNCHY
CUBICAL
CUBICLE
CUBICLY
CURACAO
CURBCUT
CUTICLE
CYNICAL

C••••C•

CACHACA
CADENCE
CADENCY
CALTECH
CANDACE
CANDICE
CANNOCK
CANSECO
CAPRICE
CARIOCA
CARJACK
CASSOCK
CATORCE
CELTICS
CHALICE
CHIRICO
CLARICE
CLERICS
CLINICS
COGENCY
COGNACS
COLLECT
COMPACT
CONCOCT
CONDUCE
CONDUCT
CONFECT
CONNECT
CONNICK
CONRACK
CONTACS
CONTACT
CONVECT
CONVICT
COPPICE
CORMACK
CORNICE
CORRECT
CORSICA
CORTICO
COSSACK
COTEACH
COWLICK
CPEBACH
CREVICE
CRITICS
CUTBACK
CYMRICS

C•••••C

CALORIC
CAMBRIC
CANONIC
CARDIAC
CAUSTIC
CENTRIC
CERAMIC
CHAOTIC
CHASMIC
CHLORIC
CHROMIC
CHRONIC
CLASSIC
COMEDIC
CROSTIC
CRYPTIC

•CC••••

ACCEDED
ACCEDER
ACCEDES
ACCENTS
ACCEPTS
ACCLAIM
ACCORDS
ACCOSTS
ACCOUNT
ACCRETE
ACCRUAL
ACCRUED
ACCRUES
ACCTNOS
ACCURST
ACCUSAL
ACCUSED
ACCUSER
ACCUSES
ECCLESI
MCCALLS
MCCAREY
MCCLOUD
MCCLURE
MCCLURG
MCCOURT
MCCOVEY
MCCOWEN
MCCRARY
MCCRUMB
OCCIPUT
OCCLUDE
OCCULTS
OCCURTO
PCCLONE
RCCOLAS
UCCELLO

•C•C•••

ACACIAS
ACYCLIC
ECOCIDE
ICECAPS
ICECAVE
ICECOLD
ICECUBE
ICICLES
OCICATS
SCACCHI

•C••C••

ACKACKS
SCACCHI
SCARCER
SCHICKS
SCONCES

•C•••C•

ACDELCO
ICEPACK
ICEPICK
SCENICS
SCHLOCK
SCHTICK
SCIENCE
SCITECH
SCOOTCH
SCRATCH
SCREECH
SCRUNCH

•C••••C

ACERBIC
ACRYLIC
ACYCLIC
OCEANIC
OCTADIC
SCEPTIC
SCIATIC

••CC•••

BACCHAE
BACCHIC
BACCHUS
BOCCIES
CICCONE
COCCOID
HICCUPS
JACCUSE
MECCANS
NICCAGE
NICCOLO
PECCANT
PECCARY
PECCAVI
PICCARD
PICCATA
PICCOLO
PUCCINI
RACCOON
SACCADE
SICCING
SUCCEED
SUCCESS
SUCCORS
SUCCOTH
SUCCOUR
SUCCUMB
TICCING
TOCCATA
UPCCODE
VACCARO
VACCINE
WICCANS

••C•C••

BICYCLE
DECOCTS
DICECUP
IACOCCA
MACACOS
PACECAR
RACECAR
RECOCKS
RECYCLE
ROCKCOD
ROCOCOS

••C••C•

BYCATCH
CACHACA
DECENCY
ESCENCE
IACOCCA
INCHECK
LICENCE
LUCENCY
MICMACS
NOCATCH
PACKICE
PICNICS
RECENCY
RECHECK
RICRACS
SECRECY
TACTICS
TICTACS
UNCHECK
UNCINCH
VACANCY

••C•••C

ARCHAIC
ASCETIC
BACCHIC
BUCOLIC
LACONIC
LECTRIC
NUCLEIC
PACIFIC
TACONIC
UNCIVIC
UNCOMIC
UNCUBIC
VOCALIC
YUCATEC

•••CC••

AJACCIO
DRMCCOY
FLACCID
GNOCCHI
REOCCUR
SCACCHI
STUCCOS

•••C•C•

BABCOCK
BIBCOCK
CONCOCT
HANCOCK
LEACOCK
PEACOCK
PETCOCK

•••C••C

ACYCLIC
BACCHIC
ORECTIC
PRACTIC
PSYCHIC

••••CC•

IACOCCA
MALACCA
MOLUCCA
MOROCCO
NABUCCO
REBECCA
SIROCCO
TOBACCO

CD•••••

CDALBUM
CDCASES
CDEFGHI
CDRACKS
CDRATES
CDSTORE
CDTOWER

C•D••••

CADAVER
CADBURY
CADDIED
CADDIES
CADDISH
CADEAUX
CADENCE
CADENCY
CADENZA
CADETTE
CADGERS
CADGING
CADMIUM
CADUCEI
CEDARED
CEDILLA
CODCAKE
CODDLED
CODDLER
CODDLES
CODEINE
CODERED
CODFISH
CODGERS
CODICES
CODICIL
CUDDIES
CUDDLED
CUDDLES
CUDGELS

C••D•••

CADDIED
CADDIES
CADDISH
CALDERA
CALDERS
CALDRON
CANDACE
CANDELA
CANDENT
CANDICE
CANDIDA
CANDIDE
CANDIDS
CANDIED
CANDIES
CANDLED
CANDLER
CANDLES
CANDOUR
CARDERS
CARDIAC
CARDIAL
CARDIFF
CARDING
CARDIUM
CARDKEY
CARDOOR
CARDOZO
CATDOOR
CAUDATE
CHEDDAR
CHEDERS
CHIDDEN
CHIDERS
CHIDING
CINDERS
CINDERY
CLADDED
CODDLED
CODDLER
CODDLES
COEDITS
COLDCUP
COLDCUT
COLDDAY
COLDEST
COLDISH
COLDONE
COLDWAR
CONDEMN
CONDIGN
CONDOLE
CONDONE
CONDORS
CONDUCE
CONDUCT
CONDUIT
CORDAGE
CORDATE
CORDELL
CORDERO
CORDERS
CORDIAL
CORDIAS
CORDING
CORDITE
CORDOBA
CORDONS
COYDOGS
CRADLED
CRADLER
CRADLES
CREDITS
CRUDELY
CRUDEST
CRUDITY
CRUDSUP
CRYDOWN
CUDDIES
CUDDLED
CUDDLES
CURDIER
CURDING
CURDLED
CURDLER
CURDLES
CUTDOWN

C•••D••

CAGEDIN
CAGEDUP
CAKEDUP
CAMEDUE
CANIDAE
CAPADES
CAREDTO
CAVEDIN
CBRADIO
CCRIDER
CELADON
CHEADLE
CHEDDAR
CHIDDEN
CHORDAL
CHORDED
CHOWDER
CICADAE
CICADAS
CITADEL
CLADDED
CLAMDIP
CLAUDEL
CLAUDIA
CLAUDIO
CLOUDED
CLOUDUP
CLOWDER
CLUEDIN
COLADAS
COLDDAY
COMEDIA
COMEDIC
COMEDIE
COMEDUE
COONDOG
CORNDOG
COTEDOR
COULDBE
COULDNT
CRAWDAD
CREEDAL
CRIEDUP
CROWDED
CROWDER
CROWDIN
CSARDAS
CZARDAS
CZARDOM

C••••D•

CABRIDE
CALANDO
CALENDS
CANARDS
CANDIDA
CANDIDE
CANDIDS
CARBIDE
CASCADE
CASSIDY
CATBEDS
CATHODE
CERVIDS
CHARADE
COCKADE
COLLIDE
COLLODI
COLLUDE
COMMODE
COMRADE
CONCEDE
CONFIDE
CONOIDS
CORRADE
CORRIDA
CORRODE
CORVIDS
COWARDS
COWHIDE
CRUSADE
CRUZADO
CUBOIDS
CUEBIDS
CUSPIDS
CUSTODY
CYANIDE
CYANIDS

C•••••D

CACKLED
CADDIED
CAIRNED
CAJOLED
CAMELID
CAMEOED
CAMPBED
CANALED
CANDIED
CANDLED
CAPECOD
CAPERED
CARLOAD
CAROLED
CAROMED
CAROTID
CARRIED
CASQUED
CASTLED
CATBIRD
CATERED
CATEYED
CATFOOD
CATHEAD
CAULKED
CAVILED
CEDARED
CENTRED
CERATED
CHAFFED
CHAINED
CHAIRED
CHALKED
CHAMPED
CHANCED
CHANGED
CHANTED
CHAPPED
CHARGED
CHARMED
CHARRED
CHARTED
CHASSED
CHATTED
CHEATED
CHECKED
CHEEKED
CHEEPED
CHEERED
CHEESED
CHESTED
CHILIAD
CHILLED
CHINKED
CHINNED
CHIPPED
CHIRPED
CHIRRED
CHIVIED
CHOCKED
CHOIRED
CHOMPED
CHOPPED
CHORDED
CHROMED
CHUCKED
CHUFFED
CHUGGED
CHUMMED
CHUMPED
CHUNKED
CHURNED
CICHLID
CINCHED
CIRCLED
CLACKED
CLADDED
CLAIMED
CLAMMED
CLAMPED
CLANGED
CLANKED
CLAPPED
CLASHED
CLASPED
CLASSED
CLEANED
CLEARED
CLEATED
CLEAVED
CLERKED
CLICHED
CLICKED
CLIMBED
CLINKED
CLIPPED
CLIQUED
CLOAKED
CLOCKED
CLOGGED
CLOMPED
CLONKED
CLOPPED
CLOTHED
CLOTTED
CLOUDED
CLOUTED
CLOWNED
CLUBBED
CLUBMED
CLUCKED
CLUMPED
CLUNKED
COACHED
COACTED
COAPTED
COASTED
COBBLED
COBRAND
COCCOID
COCKLED
CODDLED
CODERED
COERCED
COFOUND
COHERED
COIFFED
COIGNED
COLLARD
COLLOID
COLORED
COMMAND
COMMEND
COMPEND
CONCORD
CONGAED
CONRIED
CONTEND
COOPTED
COOWNED
COPLAND
CORNFED
COSTARD
COUCHED
COUGHED
COUNTED
COUPLED
COURSED
COURTED
COVERED
COVETED
COWBIRD
COWERED
COWHAND
COWHERD
COWSHED
COZENED
CRABBED
CRACKED
CRADLED
CRAFTED
CRAGGED
CRAMMED
CRAMPED
CRANKED
CRASHED
CRAWDAD
CRAWLED
CREAKED
CREAMED
CREASED
CREATED
CREEPED
CRESTED
CRIBBED
CRICKED
CRIMPED
CRINGED
CRISPED
CROAKED
CROCKED
CROOKED
CROONED
CROPPED
CROSSED
CROWDED
CROWNED
CRUISED
CRUMBED
CRUMPED
CRUSHED
CRUSTED
CTENOID
CUDDLED
CUECARD
CULLIED
CUPELED
CURATED
CURDLED
CURRIED
CUSTARD
CYCLOID

•CD••••

ACDELCO
BCDEFGH
ECDYSES
ECDYSIS

•C•D•••

ACADEME
ACADEMY
ACADIAN
ACEDOUT
ACIDIFY
ACIDITY
ICEDAMS
ICEDOUT
ICEDOWN
ICEDTEA
ICHDIEN
MCADAMS
RCADOME
SCADSOF
SCUDDED
SCUDDER

•C••D••

ACAUDAL
ACCEDED
ACCEDER
ACCEDES
ACRIDLY
ACTEDAS
ACTEDIN
ACTEDON
ACTEDUP
CCRIDER
ECHIDNA
ECUADOR
MCARDLE
OCTADIC
SCALDED
SCALDER
SCANDAL
SCOLDED
SCOLDER
SCUDDED
SCUDDER

•C•••D•

ACARIDS
ACCORDS
ECOCIDE
MCBRIDE
MCMURDO
OCANADA
OCCLUDE
SCAREDY
SCHELDT
SCHMIDT
SCREEDS
WCHANDY

•C••••D
ACCEDED
ACCRUED
ACCUSED
ACORNED
ACTIFED
ICECOLD
ICELAND
ICHABOD
ICYWIND
MCCLOUD
OCEANID
OCHROID
OCTOPOD
PCWORLD
SCALDED
SCALPED
SCAMMED
SCAMPED
SCANNED
SCANTED
SCARFED
SCARPED
SCARRED
SCARWID
SCATHED
SCATTED
SCENTED
SCHEMED
SCOFFED
SCOLDED
SCOOPED
SCOOTED
SCORNED
SCOURED
SCOUTED
SCOWLED
SCRAPED
SCREWED
SCRIBED
SCUBAED
SCUDDED
SCUFFED
SCULLED
SCULPED
SCYTHED

••CD•••
ABCDEFG
MACDUFF
VICDANA

••C•D••
ACCEDED
ACCEDER
ACCEDES
ARCADED
ARCADES
ARCADIA
CICADAE
CICADAS
DECADES
DECIDED
DECIDER
DECIDES
DECODED
DECODER
DECODES
ENCODED
ENCODER
ENCODES
ESCUDOS
EXCIDED
EXCIDES
FACADES
FACEDIT
FACEDON
INCUDES
JACKDAW
LACEDUP
LUCIDAE
LUCIDLY
MACADAM
MACEDON
NICEDAY
NICEDOG
PICADOR
RACEDBY
RACEDIN
RACEDTO
RACEDUP
RECEDED
RECEDES
RECODED
RECODES
SECEDED
SECEDER
SECEDES
SICKDAY
SUCKDRY
UNCEDED
UNCODED
VOCODER

••C••D•
ACCORDS
ALCAIDE
ALCALDE
ASCENDS
BACARDI
COCKADE
EXCEEDS
EXCLUDE
IDCARDS
INCLUDE
LUCINDA
NOCANDO
NUCLIDE
OCCLUDE
ORCHIDS
PICARDO
PICARDY
RECLADS
RECORDS
RICARDO
SACCADE
SECLUDE
SECONDI
SECONDO
SECONDR
SECONDS
UNCRUDE
UPCARDS
UPCCODE

••C•••D
ACCEDED
ACCRUED
ACCUSED
ARCADED
ARCWELD
ASCARED
BACKEND
BECLOUD
BUCKLED
CACKLED
CICHLID
COCCOID
COCKLED
CYCLOID
DECAPOD
DECAYED
DECIDED
DECKLED
DECODED
DECOYED
DECREED
DECRIED
ENCAGED
ENCASED
ENCODED
ENCORED
ESCAPED
EUCHRED
EXCIDED
EXCISED
EXCITED
EXCUSED
FACETED
FACTOID
FOCUSED
HACKLED
HECKLED
HOCUSED
INCASED
INCISED
INCITED
INCROWD
INCUSED
LACTAID
LOCATED
MACLEOD
MCCLOUD
NICEKID
ORCHARD
PACKARD
PICCARD
PICKLED
PICOTED
RECAGED
RECANED
RECASED
RECEDED
RECITED
RECODED
RECURED
RECUSED
RICHARD
ROCKCOD
SECEDED
SECURED
SICKBED
STCLOUD
SUCCEED
TACKLED
TICKLED
UNCAGED
UNCAKED
UNCANED
UNCAPED
UNCASED
UNCEDED
UNCITED
UNCLOUD
UNCODED
UNCORED
UNCOWED
UNCRIED
UNCURED
VACATED
YACHTED

•••C•D•
AVOCADO
BARCODE
BIOCIDE
BROCADE
CASCADE
CONCEDE
DNACODE
ECOCIDE
GEOCODE
MERCADO
MISCODE
MUSCIDA
PEPCIDS
PLACIDO
PRECEDE
PRECODE
REDCODS
SACCADE
SUBCODE
TAXCODE
TENCODE
UNICODE
UPCCODE
ZIPCODE

•••C••D
ABSCOND
ALLCLAD
ATMCARD
BADCOLD
BATCHED
BEACHED
BELCHED
BENCHED
BIRCHED
BLACKED
BLOCKED
BOTCHED
BRICKED
BUNCHED
BUNCOED
CHECKED
CHOCKED
CHUCKED
CINCHED
CIRCLED
CLACKED
CLICHED
CLICKED
CLOCKED
CLUCKED
COACHED
COACTED
COCCOID
CONCORD
COUCHED
CRACKED
CRICKED
CROCKED
CUECARD
DESCEND
DISCARD
DISCOED
DISCOID
DISCORD
DITCHED
EDUCTED
EJECTED
ELECTED
ENACTED
ERECTED
ERUCTED
EVICTED
EXACTED
EXSCIND
FANCIED
FETCHED
FILCHED
FLACCID
FLACKED
FLECKED
FLICKED
FLOCKED
FROCKED
GETCOLD
GISCARD
GLACEED
GOTCOLD
HATCHED
HITCHED
HUNCHED
ICECOLD
ILLCLAD
ISECOND
ITSCOLD
KEYCARD
KINCAID
KNOCKED
LATCHED
LEACHED
LEECHED
LOWCARD
LUNCHED
LURCHED
MARCHED
MATCHED
MISCUED
MOOCHED
MULCHED
MULCTED
MUNCHED
MUSCLED
NOTCHED
OUTCOLD
PARCHED
PATCHED
PEACHED
PERCHED
PICCARD
PINCHED
PIPCARD
PITCHED
PLACARD
PLUCKED
POACHED
POUCHED
PRICKED
PROCEED
PSYCHED
PUNCHED
QUACKED
RANCHED
REACHED
REACTED
REDCARD
RESCIND
RESCUED
RIPCORD
SAGCARD
SHACKED
SHOCKED
SHUCKED
SLACKED
SLICKED
SMACKED
SNACKED
SPECKED
STACKED
STOCKED
SUCCEED
SYNCHED
TALCKED
TINCTED
TORCHED
TOUCHED
TRACKED
TRICKED
TRUCKED
UNACTED
VNECKED
VOUCHED
WATCHED
WHACKED
WINCHED
WITCHED
WRACKED
WRECKED
ZINCKED

••••CD•
USEDCDS

••••C•D
ABDUCED
ADDUCED
AMERCED
ANTACID
BOUNCED
CAPECOD
CHANCED
COERCED
DEDUCED
DEFACED
EFFACED
ENFACED
ENLACED
ENTICED
EVINCED
FLACCID
FLEECED
GLANCED
INDUCED
JOUNCED
LINGCOD
MENACED
NONACID
NOTICED
NUANCED
PIERCED
POLICED
POUNCED
PRANCED
PREACID
PUMICED
REDUCED
REFACED
RELACED
ROCKCOD
SEDUCED
SLUICED
SOLACED
SOURCED
SPLICED
SPRUCED
TRANCED
UNFACED
UNLACED
UNLUCID
UNPACED

CE•••••
CEASING
CECILIA
CEDARED
CEDILLA
CEILING
CELADON
CELAENO
CELEBES
CELEBRE
CELESTA
CELESTE
CELICAS
CELLARS
CELLINI
CELLIST
CELLULE
CELOTEX
CELSIUS
CELTICS
CEMBALO
CEMENTS
CENACLE
CENSERS
CENSING
CENSORS
CENSURE
CENTALS
CENTARE
CENTAUR
CENTAVO
CENTERS
CENTIME
CENTIMO
CENTRAL
CENTRED
CENTRES
CENTRIC
CENTRUM
CENTURY
CEPHALO
CEPHALY
CEPHEUS
CERAMIC
CERATED
CERATES
CEREALS
CEREBRA
CEREBRO
CERISES
CERTAIN
CERTIFY
CERUMEN
CERVEZA
CERVIDS
CERVINE
CESAIRE
CESSING
CESSION
CESSNAS
CESSPIT
CESTMOI
CETANES
CETERIS
CEVICHE
CEZANNE

C•E••••
CAESARS
CAESURA
CDEFGHI
CHEADLE
CHEAPEN
CHEAPER
CHEAPIE
CHEAPLY
CHEATED
CHEATER
CHEATIN
CHEATON
CHECHEN
CHECKED
CHECKER
CHECKIN
CHECKON
CHECKUP
CHEDDAR
CHEDERS
CHEEKED
CHEEPED
CHEEPER
CHEERED
CHEERER
CHEERIO
CHEERON
CHEERUP
CHEESED
CHEESES
CHEETAH
CHEETAS
CHEETOS
CHEEVER
CHEEZIT
CHEFING
CHEKHOV
CHELATE
CHELSEA
CHEMISE
CHEMIST
CHEMLAB
CHENIER
CHEQUER
CHEQUES
CHERISH
CHEROOT
CHERUBS
CHERVIL
CHESTED
CHESTER
CHETRUM
CHEVAUX
CHEVETS
CHEVIOT
CHEVONS
CHEVRES
CHEVRET
CHEVRON
CHEWERS
CHEWGUM
CHEWIER
CHEWING
CHEWOUT
CHEWSON
CHEWSUP
CHEWTOY
CHEXMIX
CHEZMOI
CLEANED
CLEANER
CLEANLY
CLEANSE
CLEANTE
CLEANUP
CLEARED
CLEARER
CLEARLY
CLEAROF
CLEARUP
CLEATED
CLEAVED
CLEAVER
CLEAVES
CLEAVON
CLEMENS
CLEMENT
CLEMSON
CLERICS
CLERISY
CLERKED
CLERKLY
CLEWING
COEDITS
COEPTIS
COEQUAL
COERCED
COERCER
COERCES
COETZEE
COEVALS
COEXIST
CPEBACH
CREAKED
CREAMED
CREAMER
CREASED
CREASER
CREASES
CREATED
CREATES
CREATOR
CRECHES
CREDITS
CREEDAL
CREELEY
CREEPBY
CREEPED
CREEPER
CREEPIN
CREEPOS
CREEPUP
CREMATE
CREMINI
CREMONA
CREMORA
CRENATE
CRENELS
CREOLES
CREOSOL
CREPING
CREPTIN
CREPTUP
CRESPIN
CRESSES
CRESSET
CRESTED
CRESTON
CRETANS
CRETINS
CREVICE
CREWCUT
CREWELS
CREWING
CREWMAN
CREWMEN
CTENOID
CUEBALL
CUEBIDS
CUECARD
CUESTAS
CUETIPS

C••E•••
CABEZAS
CADEAUX
CADENCE
CADENCY
CADENZA
CADETTE
CAGEDIN
CAGEDUP
CAGEPET
CAGESUP
CAKEDUP
CAKEMIX
CAKEPAN
CAKESUP
CAKETIN
CALENDS
CAMEDUE
CAMELID
CAMELOT
CAMEOED
CAMEOFF
CAMEOUT
CAMERAE
CAMERAL
CAMERAS
CAMERON
CANETTI
CAPEANN
CAPECOD
CAPEESH
CAPELET
CAPELLA
CAPEMAY
CAPERED
CAREDTO
CAREENS
CAREERS
CAREFOR
CAREFUL
CARESTO
CASEATE
CASEINS
CASELAW
CASELLA
CASELOT
CASEOUS
CASEOUT
CASERNE
CASERNS
CASERTA
CATENAE
CATENAS
CATERAS
CATERED
CATERER
CATERTO
CATEYED
CAVEART
CAVEATS
CAVEDIN
CAVEINS
CAVEMAN
CAVEMEN
CAVERNS
CAVESIN
CAYENNE
CELEBES
CELEBRE
CELESTA
CELESTE
CEMENTS
CEREALS
CEREBRA
CEREBRO
CETERIS
CHEEKED
CHEEPED
CHEEPER
CHEERED
CHEERER
CHEERIO
CHEERON
CHEERUP
CHEESED
CHEESES
CHEETAH
CHEETAS
CHEETOS
CHEEVER
CHEEZIT
CHIEFLY
CILENTO
CINEMAS
CINEMAX
CINEOLE
CINERGY
CINESIA
CISEAUX
CLIENTS
CLUEDIN
CLUEFUL
CLUEING
CLUESIN
CODEINE
CODERED
COGENCY
COHEIRS
COHERED
COHERER
COHERES
COLEMAN
COLETTE
COMEDIA
COMEDIC
COMEDIE
COMEDUE
COMENOW
COMEOFF
COMEONS
COMEOUT
COMESAS
COMESAT
COMESBY
COMESIN
COMESON
COMESTO
COMESUP
CONELET
CORELLI
CORETTA
COSETTE
COTEACH
COTEDOR
COTERIE
COVERED
COVERER
COVERME
COVERTS
COVERUP
COVETED
COVETER
COWERAT
COWERED
COZENED
COZENER
CPAEXAM
CREEDAL
CREELEY
CREEPBY
CREEPED
CREEPER
CREEPIN
CREEPOS
CREEPUP
CRIEDUP
CRIESUP
CROESUS
CRUELER
CRUELLA
CRUELLY
CRUELTY
CSLEWIS
CULEXES
CUNEATE
CUPELED
CUPELER
CUREALL
CURETTE
CUVETTE

C•••E••
CABLERS
CABLETS
CABLETV
CACHETS
CADGERS
CAGIEST
CAHIERS
CAIRENE
CAKIEST
CALDERA
CALDERS
CALKERS
CALLEES
CALLERS
CALMEST
CALTECH
CALVERT
CAMBERS
CAMPERS
CANCELS
CANCERS
CANDELA
CANDENT
CANIEST
CANKERS
CANNELL
CANNELS
CANNERS
CANNERY
CANOERS
CANSECO
CANTEEN
CANTERS
CAPEESH
CAPLESS
CAPLETS
CAPPERS
CARDERS
CAREENS
CAREERS
CARKEYS
CARLENE
CARLESS
CARMELA
CARNERA
CARNETS
CARPELS

CARPERS
CARPETS
CARRELS
CARRERA
CARRERE
CARSEAT
CARTELS
CARTERS
CARVELS
CARVERS
CASHEWS
CASKETS
CASTERS
CATBEDS
CATBERT
CATFEET
CATHEAD
CATSEYE
CAUSERS
CBSNEWS
CELAENO
CENSERS
CENTERS
CEPHEUS
CERVEZA
CHAFERS
CHALETS
CHANELS
CHAPEAU
CHAPELS
CHASERS
CHATEAU
CHEDERS
CHEVETS
CHEWERS
CHICEST
CHIDERS
CHILEAN
CHIMEIN
CHIMERA
CHIMERS
CHINESE
CHISELS
CHOKEON
CHOKERS
CHOKEUP
CHOLERA
CHOLERS
CHOSEUP
CINDERS
CINDERY
CIPHERS
CISTERN
CLARETS
CLAVELL
CLAWERS
CLEMENS
CLEMENT
CLONERS
CLORETS
CLOSEBY
CLOSEIN
CLOSELY
CLOSERS
CLOSEST
CLOSETO
CLOSETS
CLOSEUP
CLOVERS
CLOVERY
COAGENT
COALERS
COATEES
COATERS
COAXERS
COBLENZ
COBWEBS
COCKERS
COCTEAU
CODGERS
COFFEES
COFFERS
COILERS
COINERS
COKIEST
COLBERT
COLDEST
COLLECT
COLLEEN
COLLEGE
COLLETS
COMBERS
COMMEND
COMMENT
COMPEER
COMPELS
COMPEND
COMPERE
COMPETE
CONCEAL
CONCEDE
CONCEIT
CONCEPT
CONCERN
CONCERT
CONDEMN
CONFECT
CONFERS
CONFESS
CONGEAL
CONGERS
CONGEST
CONKERS
CONNECT
CONNERY
CONSENT
CONTEMN
CONTEND
CONTENT
CONTEST
CONTEXT
CONVECT
CONVENE
CONVENT
CONVERT
CONVEYS
COOKERS
COOKERY
COOLERS
COOLEST
COOPERS
COOPERY
COOTERS
COPIERS
COPPERS
COPPERY
COPTERS
CORBELS
CORBETT
CORDELL
CORDERO
CORDERS
CORKERS
CORNEAL
CORNEAS
CORNELL
CORNERS
CORNETS
CORRECT
CORSETS
CORTEGE
CORVEES
CORYELL
COSHERS
COSIEST
COSSETS
COTTERS
COULEES
COUTERS
COWBELL
COWHERD
COWIEST
COWPEAS
COXLESS
COYNESS
COZIEST
COZZENS
CRATERS
CRATEUP
CRAVENS
CRAVERS
CRENELS
CREWELS
CRIMEAN
CROWELL
CROWERS
CRUDELY
CRUDEST
CUDGELS
CULLERS
CULLETS
CULVERT
CUMBERS
CURFEWS
CURLERS
CURLEWS
CURRENT
CURSEAT
CURSERS
CURTEST
CURVETS
CUSSERS
CUSTERS
CUTLERS
CUTLERY
CUTLETS
CUTTERS
CYCLERS
CYGNETS
CYPHERS
CYPRESS

C••••E•

CABARET
CABBIES
CABINET
CACKLED
CACKLER
CACKLES
CADAVER
CADDIED
CADDIES
CADUCEI
CAGEPET
CAIRNED
CAJOLED
CAJOLER
CAJOLES
CALIBER
CALICES
CALIPER
CALLEES
CALMSEA
CALUMET
CALYCES
CALYXES
CAMEOED
CAMISES
CAMMIES
CAMPBED
CAMPIER
CANALED
CANAPES
CANDIED
CANDIES
CANDLED
CANDLER
CANDLES
CANINES
CANNIER
CANTEEN
CANTLES
CAPADES
CAPELET
CAPERED
CAPOTES
CAPULET
CARAFES
CARAMEL
CARAVEL
CARDKEY
CARFREE
CARGOES
CARIBES
CARNIES
CAROLED
CAROLER
CAROMED
CARRIED
CARRIER
CARRIES
CARTIER
CASHIER
CASQUED
CASQUES
CASTLED
CASTLES
CATCHER
CATCHES
CATERED
CATERER
CATEYED
CATFEET
CATFLEA
CATTIER
CAULKED
CAULKER
CAUTHEN
CAVEMEN
CAVILED
CAVILER
CAYUSES
CCRIDER
CDCASES
CDRATES
CDTOWER
CEDARED
CELEBES
CELOTEX
CENTRED
CENTRES
CERATED
CERATES
CERISES
CERUMEN
CETANES
CHAFFED
CHAFFEE
CHAFFER
CHAINED
CHAINES
CHAIRED
CHAISES
CHALKED
CHAMBER
CHAMFER
CHAMPED
CHAMPER
CHANCED
CHANCEL
CHANCER
CHANCES
CHANGED
CHANGER
CHANGES
CHANNEL
CHANTED
CHANTER
CHANTEY
CHAPLET
CHAPMEN
CHAPPED
CHAPTER
CHARGED
CHARGER
CHARGES
CHARIER
CHARLES
CHARLEY
CHARMED
CHARMEN
CHARMER
CHARRED
CHARRER
CHARTED
CHARTER
CHARVET
CHASSED
CHASSES
CHASTEN
CHASTER
CHATTED
CHATTEL
CHATTER
CHAUCER
CHEAPEN
CHEAPER
CHEATED
CHEATER
CHECHEN
CHECKED
CHECKER
CHEEKED
CHEEPED
CHEEPER
CHEERED
CHEERER
CHEESED
CHEESES
CHEEVER
CHELSEA
CHENIER
CHEQUER
CHEQUES
CHESTED
CHESTER
CHEVRES
CHEVRET
CHEWIER
CHIAPET
CHICHEN
CHICKEN
CHICLES
CHICLET
CHIDDEN
CHIGGER
CHIGOES
CHILIES
CHILLED
CHILLER
CHIMNEY
CHINKED
CHINNED
CHIPPED
CHIPPER
CHIRPED
CHIRPER
CHIRRED
CHITTER
CHIVIED
CHIVIES
CHOCKED
CHOICER
CHOICES
CHOIRED
CHOKIER
CHOMPED
CHOOSER
CHOOSES
CHOOSEY
CHOPPED
CHOPPER
CHORDED
CHOWDER
CHROMED
CHROMES
CHUCKED
CHUFFED
CHUGGED
CHUGGER
CHUKKER
CHUMMED
CHUMPED
CHUNKED
CHUNNEL
CHURNED
CHURNER
CHUTNEY
CINCHED
CINCHES
CINQUES
CIRCLED
CIRCLER
CIRCLES
CIRCLET
CIRQUES
CISCOES
CITADEL
CITIZEN
CITROEN
CIVVIES
CLABBER
CLACKED
CLACKER
CLADDED
CLAIMED
CLAIMER
CLAMBER
CLAMMED
CLAMMER
CLAMPED
CLAMPER
CLANGED
CLANGER
CLANKED
CLAPPED
CLAPPER
CLAQUES
CLASHED
CLASHER
CLASHES
CLASPED
CLASPER
CLASSED
CLASSER
CLASSES
CLATTER
CLAUDEL
CLAUSES
CLAVIER
CLAYIER
CLEANED
CLEANER
CLEARED
CLEARER
CLEATED
CLEAVED
CLEAVER
CLEAVES
CLERKED
CLICHED
CLICHES
CLICKED
CLICKER
CLIMBED
CLIMBER
CLINGER
CLINKED
CLINKER
CLIPPED
CLIPPER
CLIQUED
CLIQUES
CLIQUEY
CLOAKED
CLOBBER
CLOCHES
CLOCKED
CLOCKER
CLOGGED
CLOMPED
CLONKED
CLOONEY
CLOPPED
CLOTHED
CLOTHES
CLOTTED
CLOUDED
CLOUTED
CLOUTER
CLOWDER
CLOWNED
CLUBBED
CLUBBER
CLUBMED
CLUCKED
CLUCKER
CLUMPED
CLUNKED
CLUNKER
CLUSTER
CLUTTER
CNTOWER
COACHED
COACHES
COACTED
COAPTED
COARSEN
COARSER
COASTED
COASTER
COATEES
COBBLED
COBBLER
COBBLES
COBUYER
COCHLEA
COCKIER
COCKLED
COCKLES
COCKNEY
CODDLED
CODDLER
CODDLES
CODERED
CODICES
COERCED
COERCER
COERCES
COETZEE
COFFEES
COGGLES
COHERED
COHERER
COHERES
COIFFED
COIGNED
COIGNES
COLLEEN
COLLIER
COLLIES
COLLYER
COLONEL
COLONES
COLORED
COLORER
COMAKER
COMBIEN
COMFIER
COMICES
COMPEER
COMPLEX
COMTREX
CONCHES
CONELET
CONFREY
CONGAED
CONIFER
CONQUER
CONRIED
CONURES
COOKIES
COOLIES
COOPTED
COOTIES
COOWNED
COPYMEN
CORKIER
CORNFED
CORNIER
CORONER
CORONET
CORPSES
CORVEES
COSINES
COSTNER
COUCHED
COUCHES
COUGHED
COULEES
COULTER
COUNSEL
COUNTED
COUNTEE
COUNTEM
COUNTER
COUPLED
COUPLER
COUPLES
COUPLET
COURBET
COURIER
COURSED
COURSER
COURSES
COURTED
COVERED
COVERER
COVETED
COVETER
COWERED
COWRIES
COWSHED
COYOTES
COZENED
COZENER
COZUMEL
CPLUSES
CRABBED
CRABBER
CRACKED
CRACKER
CRADLED
CRADLER
CRADLES
CRAFTED
CRAFTER
CRAGGED
CRAMMED
CRAMMER
CRAMPED
CRANKED
CRANMER
CRASHED
CRASHER
CRASHES
CRASSER
CRAWLED
CRAWLER
CRAWLEY
CRAZIER
CRAZIES
CREAKED
CREAMED
CREAMER
CREASED
CREASER
CREASES
CREATED
CREATES
CRECHES
CREELEY
CREEPED
CREEPER
CREOLES
CRESSES
CRESSET
CRESTED
CREWMEN
CRIBBED
CRIBBER
CRICKED
CRICKET
CRIMPED
CRIMPER
CRINGED
CRINGES
CRISPED
CRISPEN
CRISPER
CRITTER
CROAKED
CROAKER
CROCHET
CROCKED
CROCKER
CROCKET
CROFTER
CRONIES
CROOKED
CROOKES
CROONED
CROONER
CROPPED
CROPPER
CROQUET
CROSIER
CROSSED
CROSSER
CROSSES
CROUTES
CROWDED
CROWDER
CROWLEY
CROWNED
CROWNER
CROZIER
CRUELER
CRUGUET
CRUISED
CRUISER
CRUISES
CRULLER
CRUMBED
CRUMPED
CRUMPET
CRUPPER
CRUSHED
CRUSHER
CRUSHES
CRUSTED
CRUTZEN
CRYOGEN
CRYOVER
CUBAGES
CUBBIES
CUDDIES
CUDDLED
CUDDLES
CULCHES
CULEXES
CULLIED
CULLIES
CUPELED
CUPELER
CUPPIER
CUPULES
CURARES
CURATED
CURATES
CURDIER
CURDLED
CURDLER
CURDLES
CURLIER
CURRIED
CURRIER
CURRIES
CURTSEY
CURVIER
CUSHIER
CUSSLER
CUTISES
CUTOPEN
CUTOVER

C•••••E

CABALLE
CABBAGE
CABFARE
CABOOSE
CABRIDE
CACIQUE
CADENCE
CADETTE
CAIRENE
CALCITE
CALIBRE
CALORIE
CALOTTE
CALZONE
CAMEDUE
CAMERAE
CAMILLE
CAMRYLE
CANDACE
CANDICE
CANDIDE
CANIDAE
CANITBE
CANULAE
CANZONE
CAPABLE
CAPAPIE
CAPRICE
CAPRINE
CAPSIZE
CAPSULE
CAPTIVE
CAPTURE
CAPUCHE
CARBIDE
CARBINE
CARCARE
CARFARE
CARFREE
CARINAE
CARIOLE
CARLENE
CARLYLE
CARMINE
CARNAGE
CAROUSE
CARRERE
CARSALE
CARTAGE
CARTIRE
CASCADE
CASEATE
CASERNE
CASTILE
CATENAE
CATHODE
CATLIKE
CATORCE
CATSEYE
CAUDATE
CAVIARE
CAYENNE
CDSTORE
CELEBRE
CELESTE
CELLULE
CENACLE
CENSURE
CENTARE
CENTIME
CERVINE
CESAIRE
CEVICHE
CEZANNE
CHAFFEE
CHALICE
CHAMBRE
CHAPPIE
CHARADE
CHARLIE
CHAYOTE
CHEADLE
CHEAPIE
CHELATE
CHEMISE
CHICANE
CHINESE
CHOLINE
CHOPINE
CHORALE
CHORINE
CHORTLE
CHUCKLE
CICADAE
CICCONE
CILIATE
CIMABUE
CINEOLE
CIRRATE
CITABLE
CITRATE
CITRINE
CLARICE
CLAVATE
CLEANSE
CLEANTE
CLIMATE
CLOSURE
CLOTURE
COCAINE
COCHISE
COCKADE
CODCAKE
CODEINE
COETZEE
COGNATE
COGNIZE
COINAGE
COLDONE
COLETTE
COLGATE
COLLAGE
COLLATE
COLLEGE
COLLIDE
COLLINE
COLLUDE
COLOGNE
COMBINE
COMEDIE
COMEDUE
COMIQUE
COMMODE
COMMOVE
COMMUNE
COMMUTE
COMPARE

COMPERE
COMPETE
COMPILE
COMPOSE
COMPOTE
COMPUTE
COMRADE
CONCAVE
CONCEDE
CONCHAE
CONCISE
CONDOLE
CONDONE
CONDUCE
CONFIDE
CONFINE
CONFUSE
CONFUTE
CONGAME
CONJURE
CONNATE
CONNIVE
CONNOTE
CONSOLE
CONSUME
CONTUSE
CONVENE
CONVOKE
COPPICE
COPULAE
CORACLE
CORDAGE
CORDATE
CORDITE
CORINNE
CORKAGE
CORNICE
CORNUTE
CORONAE
CORRADE
CORRODE
CORSAGE
CORTEGE
CORVINE
CORZINE
COSETTE
COSTATE
COSTIVE
COSTUME
COTERIE
COTTAGE
COULDBE
COUNTEE
COURAGE
COUSINE
COUTURE
COVERME
COWBANE
COWHIDE
COWLIKE
COWPOKE
COWRITE
COWROTE
CRACKLE
CRAIGIE
CRAPPIE
CREMATE
CRENATE
CREVICE
CRINKLE
CRIPPLE
CRUMBLE
CRUMPLE
CRUSADE
CUBICLE
CUISINE
CULOTTE
CULTURE
CUNEATE
CUPCAKE
CUPLIKE
CUPRITE
CURABLE
CURETTE
CURLIKE
CURSIVE
CURTATE
CUSPATE
CUTICLE
CUTRATE
CUTTIME
CUVETTE
CYANIDE
CYCLONE

•CE••••

ACEDOUT
ACEHIGH
ACERATE
ACERBIC
ACEROLA
ACEROSE
ACESOUT
ACETALS
ACETATE
ACETIFY
ACETONE
ICEAGES
ICEAXES
ICEBAGS
ICEBATH
ICEBEER
ICEBERG
ICEBLUE
ICEBOAT
ICECAPS
ICECAVE
ICECOLD
ICECUBE
ICEDAMS
ICEDOUT
ICEDOWN
ICEDTEA
ICEFALL
ICEFLOE
ICEFOGS
ICEFREE
ICEHOLE
ICELAND
ICELESS
ICELIKE
ICELINE
ICEMILK
ICEOUTS
ICEOVER
ICEPACK
ICEPICK
ICEPOPS
ICERINK
ICERUNS
ICESHOW
ICESOUT
ICETEAS
ICETRAY
ICEWINE
MCENROE
OCEANIA
OCEANIC
OCEANID
OCEANUS
OCELLAR
OCELLUS
OCELOTS
SCENEII
SCENEIV
SCENERY
SCENEVI
SCENICS
SCENTED
SCENTER
SCEPTER
SCEPTIC
SCEPTRE

•C•E•••

ACCEDED
ACCEDER
ACCEDES
ACCENTS
ACCEPTS
ACDELCO
ACHEFOR
ACHENES
ACHERON
ACHESON
ACREAGE
ACTEDAS
ACTEDIN
ACTEDON
ACTEDUP
BCDEFGH
ECHELON
ECUELLE
ECZEMAS
ICTERUS
MCHENRY
MCKENNA
MCNEILL
OCHENTA
OCTETTE
SCHELDT
SCHEMAS
SCHEMED
SCHEMER
SCHEMES
SCHERZI
SCHERZO
SCIENCE
SCLERAE
SCLERAL
SCLERAS
SCREAKS
SCREAMS
SCREECH
SCREEDS
SCREENS
SCREWED
SCREWUP
UCCELLO

•C••E••

ACADEME
ACADEMY
ACCRETE
ACHIEST
ACHIEVA
ACHIEVE
ACTAEON
ACTRESS
ACUMENS
ACUTELY
ACUTEST
ECCLESI
ECHOERS
ECOTEUR
ICEBEER
ICEBERG
ICELESS
ICETEAS
ICINESS
ICKIEST
MCQUEEN
NCWYETH
PCUSERS
SCALENE
SCALERS
SCALEUP
SCAREDY
SCARERS
SCAREUP
SCENEII
SCENEIV
SCENERY
SCENEVI
SCHLEPP
SCHLEPS
SCHMEAR
SCHMEER
SCITECH
SCORERS
SCOTERS
SCREECH
SCREEDS
SCREENS
SCUSEME

•C•••E•

ACCEDED
ACCEDER
ACCEDES
ACCRUED
ACCRUES
ACCUSED
ACCUSER
ACCUSES
ACHENES
ACORNED
ACTIFED
ACTIVES
CCRIDER
ECARTES
ECDYSES
ECTYPES
ICEAGES
ICEAXES
ICEBEER
ICEDTEA
ICEFREE
ICEOVER
ICHDIEN
ICICLES
ICTUSES
KCJONES
MCALLEN
MCCAREY
MCCOVEY
MCCOWEN
MCHALES
MCPAPER
MCQUEEN
MCRANEY
OCTANES
OCTAVES
OCTOBER
SCALDED
SCALDER
SCALIER
SCALPED
SCALPEL
SCALPER
SCAMMED
SCAMMER
SCAMPED
SCAMPER
SCANNED
SCANNER
SCANTED
SCANTER
SCARCER
SCARFED
SCARFER
SCARIER
SCARLET
SCARPED
SCARRED
SCARVES
SCATHED
SCATHES
SCATTED
SCATTER
SCENTED
SCENTER
SCEPTER
SCHAYES
SCHEMED
SCHEMER
SCHEMES
SCHMEER
SCHMOES
SCHOLES
SCHUMER
SCOFFED
SCOFFER
SCOLDED
SCOLDER
SCONCES
SCOOPED
SCOOPER
SCOOTED
SCOOTER
SCORNED
SCORNER
SCOUPES
SCOURED
SCOURER
SCOUTED
SCOUTER
SCOWLED
SCOWLER
SCRAPED
SCRAPER
SCRAPES
SCREWED
SCRIBED
SCRIBER
SCRIBES
SCUBAED
SCUDDED
SCUDDER
SCUFFED
SCUFFER
SCULLED
SCULLER
SCULPED
SCUPPER
SCURVES
SCUZZES
SCYTHED
SCYTHES

•C••••E

ACADEME
ACCRETE
ACERATE
ACEROSE
ACETATE
ACETONE
ACHIEVE
ACHILLE
ACOLYTE
ACONITE
ACOUPLE
ACQUIRE
ACREAGE
ACTABLE
ACTFIVE
ACTLIKE
ACTUATE
ECHAPPE
ECLIPSE
ECLOGUE
ECOCIDE
ECOTAGE
ECOTYPE
ECUELLE
ICEBLUE
ICECAVE
ICECUBE
ICEFLOE
ICEFREE
ICEHOLE
ICELIKE
ICELINE
ICEWINE
MCARDLE
MCBRIDE
MCCLURE
MCENROE
MCGUIRE
MCGWIRE
MCSHANE
MCSWINE
OCCLUDE
OCTETTE
OCTOBRE
OCTUBRE
OCTUPLE
PCCLONE
RCADOME
SCALAGE
SCALENE
SCEPTRE
SCIENCE
SCLERAE
SCOTTIE
SCOURGE
SCROOGE
SCRUPLE
SCUFFLE
SCUSEME
SCUTTLE
VCRTAPE

••CE•••

AACELLS
ACCEDED
ACCEDER
ACCEDES
ACCENTS
ACCEPTS
ALCESTE
ASCENDS
ASCENTS
ASCETIC
BOCELLI
DECEASE
DECEITS
DECEIVE
DECENCY
DICECUP
DOCENTS
ESCENCE
EUCERIN
EXCEEDS
EXCELAT
EXCELIN
EXCEPTS
EXCERPT
FACEDIT
FACEDON
FACEOFF
FACESIT
FACESON
FACETED
INCENSE
INCENTS
INCEPTS
JOCELYN
LACEDUP
LACERTA
LACESON
LACESUP
LACEUPS
LICENCE
LICENSE
LUCENCY
LUCERNE
LUCETTA
LYCEUMS
MACEDON
MYCENAE
NACELLE
NICEBOY
NICEDAY
NICEDOG
NICEGUY
NICEJOB
NICEKID
NICEMAN
NICEMEN
NICEONE
NICETRY
OSCEOLA
PACECAR
PACELAP
PACEOFF
PICEOUS
RACECAR
RACEDBY
RACEDIN
RACEDTO
RACEDUP
RACEMES
RACESBY
RACESTO
RACESUP
RACEWAY
RECEDED
RECEDES
RECEIPT
RECEIVE
RECENCY
SECEDED
SECEDER
SECEDES
TOCELIA
UCCELLO
UNCEDED
VICENTE
VICENZA
VICEROY

••C•E••

ABCDEFG
ABCNEWS
ACCRETE
AFCTEAM
ALCHEMY
ANCIENT
ARCHERS
ARCHERY
ARCHEST
ARCWELD
BACKEND
BACKERS
BECKETT
BICKERS
BUCKERS
BUCKETS
BUCKEYE
CACHETS
COCKERS
COCTEAU
CYCLERS
DECKERS
DECREED
DECREER
DECREES
DICIEST
DICKENS
DICKERS
DICKEYS
DOCKERS
DOCKETS
DUCHESS
DUCKERS
ECCLESI
ESCHEAT
ESCHERS
ESCHEWS
ESCUELA
ETCHERS
EXCEEDS
EXCRETE
HACKERS
HACKETT
HICKEYS
HOCKERS
INCHECK
INCHERS
IPCRESS
JACKETS
JOCKEYS
KICKERS
KUCHENS
LACIEST
LACKEYS
LACTEAL
LECHERS
LECTERN
LICHEES
LICHENS
LICKERS
LICKETY
LOCKEAN
LOCKERS
LOCKETS
MACBETH
MACHETE
MACLEAN
MACLEOD
MACNEIL
MICAELA
MICKEYS
MOCKERS
MOCKERY
MRCLEAN
MUCKERS
NBCNEWS
NECKERS
NFCTEAM
NICKELS
NICKERS
NUCLEAR
NUCLEIC
NUCLEON
NUCLEUS
PACBELL
PACIEST
PACKERS
PACKETS
PICKENS
PICKERS
PICKETS
PICKETT
POCKETS
PUCKERS
PUCKERY
PUCKETT
RACIEST
RACKERS
RACKETS
RACKETY
RECHECK
RECHEWS
RECLEAN
RICHENS
RICHEST
RICKETY
RICKEYS
ROCHETS
ROCKERS
ROCKERY
ROCKETS
RUCKERT
SACHEMS
SACHETS
SACKERS
SECKELS
SECRECY
SECRETE
SECRETS
SICKENS
SICKEST
SOCIETY
SOCKETS
SOCKEYE
SUCCEED
SUCCESS
SUCKERS
TACKERS
TICKERS
TICKETS
TUCKERS
TVCREWS
UNCHECK
UNCLEAN
UNCLEAR
UNCLEFT
VICKERS
WACKEST
WICKERS
WICKETS

••C••E•

ACCEDED
ACCEDER
ACCEDES
ACCRUED
ACCRUES
ACCUSED
ACCUSER
ACCUSES
ALCOVES
ARCADED
ARCADES
ARCHIES
ARCHSEE
ASCARED
BECOMES
BOCCIES
BOCHNER
BUCHNER
BUCKLED
BUCKLES
BUCKLEY
BUCKNER
BUCKOES
CACKLED
CACKLER
CACKLES
CDCASES
COCHLEA
COCKIER
COCKLED
COCKLES
COCKNEY
DECADES
DECAYED
DECAYER
DECIBEL
DECIDED
DECIDER
DECIDES
DECILES
DECKLED
DECKLES
DECODED
DECODER
DECODES
DECOYED
DECOYER
DECREED
DECREER
DECREES
DECRIED
DECRIER
DECRIES
DICHTER
DICKIES
DUCHIES
DUCKIER
DUCKIES
ENCAGED
ENCAGES
ENCASED
ENCASES
ENCODED
ENCODER
ENCODES
ENCORED
ENCORES
ESCAPED
ESCAPEE
ESCAPER
ESCAPES
EUCHRED
EUCHRES
EXCIDED
EXCIDES
EXCISED
EXCISES
EXCITED
EXCITER
EXCITES
EXCUSED
EXCUSER
EXCUSES
EXCUSEZ
FACADES
FACETED
FECHNER
FICKLER
FICUSES
FOCSLES
FOCUSED
FOCUSER
FOCUSES
GECKOES
GUCKIER
HACKIES
HACKLED
HACKLER
HACKLES
HACKNEY
HECKLED
HECKLER
HECKLES
HECKYES
HOCUSED
INCASED
INCASES
INCISED
INCISES
INCITED
INCITER
INCITES
INCOMER
INCOMES
INCUDES
INCUSED
INCUSES
ITCHIER
JACALES
JACKIEO
JACONET
JACQUES
KICKIER
LACQUER
LACUREE
LICHEES
LOCALES
LOCATED
LOCATER
LOCATES
LOCKLET
LOCKSET
LUCIFER
LUCITES
LUCKIER
MACHREE
MACUSER
MCCAREY
MCCOVEY
MCCOWEN
MICHAEL
MUCKIER
NECKLET
NICEMEN
NICKLES
NICOLET
OOCYTES
OSCINES
OSCULES
PICKIER
PICKLED
PICKLES
PICOTED
RACEMES
RACHAEL
RACQUET
RECAGED
RECAGES
RECANED
RECANES
RECASED
RECASES
RECEDED
RECEDES
RECIPES
RECITED
RECITER
RECITES
RECODED
RECODES
RECOVER
RECURED
RECURES
RECUSED
RECUSES
RICHLER
RICHMEN
RICHTER
RICKLES
ROCKIER
ROCKIES
SACQUES
SECEDED
SECEDER
SECEDES
SECURED
SECURER
SECURES
SICKBED
SICKLES
SUCCEED
SUCKIER
TACKIER
TACKLED
TACKLER
TACKLES
TECHIES
TICKLED
TICKLER
TICKLES
UNCAGED
UNCAGES
UNCAKED
UNCAKES
UNCANED
UNCAPED
UNCASED
UNCASES
UNCEDED
UNCITED
UNCODED
UNCORED
UNCORES
UNCOVER
UNCOWED
UNCOYER
UNCRIED
UNCRUEL
UNCURED

VACATED
VACATES
VECHTEN
VICKREY
VOCODER
WACKIER
YACHTED
YACHTER
YUCATEC
YUCKIER

••C•••E

ACCRETE
ALCAIDE
ALCALDE
ALCESTE
ALCYONE
ARCHFOE
ARCHIVE
ARCHSEE
ARCSINE
ARCUATE
ASCRIBE
BACCHAE
BACKHOE
BECAUSE
BICORNE
BICYCLE
BUCKEYE
CACIQUE
CICADAE
CICCONE
COCAINE
COCHISE
COCKADE
CYCLONE
DECEASE
DECEIVE
DECIARE
DECLARE
DECLINE
DECUPLE
DICTATE
DOCKAGE
DUCTILE
ENCARRE
ENCHASE
ENCLAVE
ENCLOSE
ESCAPEE
ESCENCE
EXCLAVE
EXCLUDE
EXCRETE
EXCURSE
FACONNE
FACULAE
FICTILE
FICTIVE
HECTARE
INCENSE
INCLINE
INCLOSE
INCLUDE
INCURVE
JACCUSE
LACOSTE
LACTASE
LACTATE
LACTOSE
LACUNAE
LACUREE
LECARRE
LECONTE
LECTURE
LICENCE
LICENSE
LOCKAGE
LUCARNE
LUCERNE
LUCIDAE
LUCILLE
MACABRE
MACAQUE
MACHETE
MACHINE
MACHONE
MACHREE
MACRAME
MACULAE
MCCLURE
MICROBE
MOCHRIE
MYCENAE
NACELLE
NBCBLUE
NECKTIE
NICCAGE
NICEONE
NICOISE
NICOLLE
NICTATE
NUCLIDE
OCCLUDE
PACKAGE
PACKICE
PCCLONE
PICANTE
PICKAXE
PICTURE
PVCPIPE
RECABLE
RECARVE
RECEIVE
RECHOSE
RECLAME
RECLINE
RECLUSE
RECRATE
RECURVE
RECYCLE
SACCADE
SACLIKE
SECLUDE
SECRETE
SOCKEYE
SUCRASE
SUCROSE
TACTILE
UNCHOKE
UNCLOSE
UNCRATE
UNCRUDE
UPCCODE
UPCLOSE
UPCURVE
VACCINE
VACUOLE
VICENTE
VICOMTE
VOCABLE
YACHTIE

•••CE••

AAACELL
AVOCETS
BRACERO
BRACERS
BRACEUP
BUSCEMI
CANCELS
CANCERS
CHICEST
CONCEAL
CONCEDE
CONCEIT
CONCEPT
CONCERN
CONCERT
DANCERS
DEICERS
DESCEND
DESCENT
DIOCESE
DISCERN
DOUCEUR
DRYCELL
EPICENE
EXOCETS
FARCEUR
FATCELL
FAUCETS
FAWCETT
FENCEIN
FENCERS
FENCEUP
FORCEIN
FORCEON
FORCEPS
FORCERS
FORCEUP
GLACEED
GROCERS
GROCERY
JAYCEES
JOYCEAN
JUICERS
JUICEUP
LANCERS
LANCETS
LARCENY
LYOCELL
MARCEAU
MARCELS
MERCERS
MERCERY
MINCERS
MIOCENE
MORCERF
NASCENT
NEOCENE
OBSCENE
ONECELL
ONECENT
PARCELS
PERCENT
PERCEPT
PIECERS
PINCERS
PISCEAN
PLACEBO
PLACERS
PRECEDE
PRECEPT
PRICERS
PROCEED
PROCESS
PURCELL
REDCELL
REDCENT
SAUCERS
SINCERE
SLICERS
SLICEUP
SORCERY
SPACELY
SPACERS
SPICERS
SPICERY
SPICEUP
SUBCELL
SUCCEED
SUCCESS
TENCENT
TERCELS
TRACERS
TRACERY
TRICEPS
VINCENT
VISCERA
VOICERS
WETCELL
WINCERS

•••C•E•

AIRCREW
AITCHES
APACHES
BATCHED
BATCHES
BEACHED
BEACHES
BEECHEN
BEECHER
BEECHES
BELCHED
BELCHER
BELCHES
BENCHED
BENCHER
BENCHES
BIRCHED
BIRCHEN
BIRCHES
BLACKED
BLACKEN
BLACKER
BLOCKED
BLOCKER
BOCCIES
BOTCHED
BOTCHER
BOTCHES
BOUCHER
BOUCHES
BRACKEN
BRACKET
BRICKED
BUNCHED
BUNCHES
BUNCOED
BUTCHER
BUTCHES
CATCHER
CATCHES
CHECHEN
CHECKED
CHECKER
CHICHEN
CHICKEN
CHICLES
CHICLET
CHOCKED
CHUCKED
CINCHED
CINCHES
CIRCLED
CIRCLER
CIRCLES
CIRCLET
CISCOES
CLACKED
CLACKER
CLICHED
CLICHES
CLICKED
CLICKER
CLOCHES
CLOCKED
CLOCKER
CLUCKED
CLUCKER
COACHED
COACHES
COACTED
CONCHES
COUCHED
COUCHES
CRACKED
CRACKER
CRECHES
CRICKED
CRICKET
CROCHET
CROCKED
CROCKER
CROCKET
CULCHES
DISCOED
DITCHED
DITCHER
DITCHES
DOGCHEW
DRUCKER
EDUCTED
EJECTED
ELECTED
ELECTEE
ENACTED
ERECTED
ERECTER
ERUCTED
ETICKET
EVACUEE
EVICTED
EVICTEE
EXACTED
EXACTER
FANCIED
FANCIER
FANCIES
FESCUES
FETCHED
FETCHER
FETCHES
FIACRES
FILCHED
FILCHER
FILCHES
FINCHES
FISCHER
FLACKED
FLECHES
FLECKED
FLICKED
FLICKER
FLOCKED
FRICKER
FROCKED
GAUCHER
GLACEED
GLACIER
GULCHES
HAECKEL
HATCHED
HATCHER
HATCHES
HATCHET
HITCHED
HITCHER
HITCHES
HOOCHES
HUNCHED
HUNCHES
HUTCHES
ICICLES
JAECKEL
JAYCEES
JIMCHEE
JUICIER
JUNCOES
KETCHES
KIMCHEE
KITCHEN
KNOCKED
KNOCKER
KRACKEL
KUTCHER
LARCHEN
LARCHES
LATCHED
LATCHES
LEACHED
LEACHER
LEACHES
LEECHED
LEECHEE
LEECHES
LOWCHEN
LUNCHED
LUNCHER
LUNCHES
LURCHED
LURCHER
LURCHES
MADCHEN
MARCHED
MARCHER
MARCHES
MATCHED
MATCHER
MATCHES
MENCKEN
MERCHES
MERCIES
MISCUED
MISCUES
MOOCHED
MOOCHER
MOOCHES
MULCHED
MULCHES
MULCTED
MUNCHED
MUNCHEN
MUNCHER
MUNCHES
MUSCLED
MUSCLES
NATCHEZ
NOTCHED
NOTCHER
NOTCHES
ORACIES
ORACLES
PARCHED
PARCHES
PATCHED
PATCHEN
PATCHER
PATCHES
PEACHED
PEACHES
PERCHED
PERCHER
PERCHES
PETCHEW
PINCHED
PINCHER
PINCHES
PITCHED
PITCHER
PITCHES
PITCREW
PLACKET
PLUCKED
POACHED
POACHER
POACHES
POOCHES
PORCHES
POUCHED
POUCHES
PRICIER
PRICKED
PROCEED
PROCTER
PSYCHED
PSYCHES
PUNCHED
PUNCHER
PUNCHES
QUACKED
QUACKER
QUICHES
QUICKEN
QUICKER
RANCHED
RANCHER
RANCHES
RATCHET
REACHED
REACHER
REACHES
REACTED
RESCUED
RESCUER
RESCUES
ROACHES
ROSCOES
SATCHEL
SAUCIER
SHACKED
SHOCKED
SHOCKER
SHUCKED
SHUCKER
SLACKED
SLACKEN
SLACKER
SLICKED
SLICKER
SMACKED
SMACKER
SMUCKER
SNACKED
SNACKER
SNICKER
SNICKET
SPACIER
SPECIES
SPECKED
SPECTER
SPICIER
STACKED
STACKER
STICKER
STOCKED
STOCKER
SUCCEED
SYNCHED
TALCKED
TEACHER
TEACHES
TEICHER
TENCHES
THICKEN
THICKER
THICKET
TINCTED
TORCHED
TORCHER
TORCHES
TOUCHED
TOUCHER
TOUCHES
TRACHEA
TRACKED
TRACKER
TRICKED
TRICKER
TROCHEE
TROCHES
TRUCKED
TRUCKEE
TRUCKER
UNACTED
UNSCREW
VETCHES
VNECKED
VOLCKER
VOUCHED
VOUCHER
VOUCHES
WATCHED
WATCHER
WATCHES
WENCHES
WHACKED
WHACKER
WINCHED
WINCHER
WINCHES
WITCHED
WITCHES
WRACKED
WRECKED
WRECKER
ZILCHES
ZINCKED

•••C••E

ABSCISE
ARACHNE
ASHCAKE
BACCHAE
BADCASE
BARCODE
BIOCIDE
BLACKIE
BOSCAGE
BRICKLE
BROCADE
CALCITE
CARCARE
CASCADE
CHICANE
CHUCKLE
CICCONE
CODCAKE
CONCAVE
CONCEDE
CONCHAE
CONCISE
CRACKLE
CUPCAKE
DASCHLE
DAYCARE
DIOCESE
DNACODE
EATCAKE
ECOCIDE
EDUCATE
EGGCASE
ELECTEE
ELECTME
ELOCUTE
EPICENE
EPICURE
EVACUEE
EVICTEE
EXECUTE
EYECARE
FALCATE
FASCIAE
FBICASE
FRECKLE
FURCATE
GEOCODE
GETCUTE
GLUCOSE
GLYCINE
GOTCUTE
GRACILE
GRACKLE
GRECIZE
GUNCASE
HERCULE
HIRCINE
HOECAKE
HOSCALE
HOTCAKE
HOWCOME
ICECAVE
ICECUBE
INSCALE
JACCUSE
JIMCHEE
KEYCASE
KIMCHEE
KNUCKLE
LAICIZE
LANCOME
LAWCASE
LEECHEE
LEUCINE
MARCUSE
MERCURE
MIOCENE
MISCITE
MISCODE
MUNCHIE
NEOCENE
NESCAFE
NETCAFE
NICCAGE
NONCORE
NOSCORE
OATCAKE
OBSCENE
OBSCURE
OILCAKE
OUTCOME
OUTCURE
PANCAKE
PENCASE
PERCALE
PETCAGE
PINCHME
PISCINE
PLACATE
PLICATE
POOCHIE
PORCINE
PRECEDE
PRECISE
PRECITE
PRECODE
PRECURE
PRICKLE
PROCURE
QUICKIE
RESCALE
RESCORE
RIBCAGE
RITCHIE
RUMCAKE
SACCADE
SADCAFE
SHACKLE
SINCERE
SNOCONE
SPACKLE
SPECKLE
SPECTRE
SUBCASE
SUBCODE
SYNCOPE
TAXCODE
TEACAKE
TENCODE
THECAPE
TOSCALE
TRICKLE
TROCHEE
TRUCKEE
TRUCKLE
UNICODE
UPCCODE
UPSCALE
VACCINE
WELCOME
ZINCITE
ZIPCODE

••••CE•

ABDUCED
ABDUCES
ADDUCED
ADDUCER
ADDUCES
ADVICES
AGENCES
AIRACES
AMERCED
AMERCER
AMERCES
ARBACES
BANACEK
BODICES
BOUNCED
BOUNCER
BOUNCES
CADUCEI
CALICES
CALYCES
CHANCED
CHANCEL
CHANCER
CHANCES
CHAUCER
CHOICER
CHOICES
CODICES
COERCED
COERCER
COERCES
COMICES
DEDUCED
DEDUCER
DEDUCES
DEFACED
DEFACER
DEFACES
DEVICES
EFFACED
EFFACER
EFFACES
ELANCES
ENFACED
ENFACES
ENLACED
ENLACES
ENTICED
ENTICER
ENTICES
EVINCED
EVINCES
FIANCEE
FIANCES
FIERCER
FLEECED
FLEECER
FLEECES
FRANCES
GFORCES
GLANCED
GLANCES
HELICES
HYRACES
INDICES
INDUCED
INDUCER
INDUCES
JANACEK
JOUNCED
JOUNCES
LATICES
MALICES
MENACED
MENACER
MENACES
NOTICED
NOTICER
NOTICES
NOVICES
NUANCED
NUANCES
OFFICER
OFFICES
PALACES
PANACEA
PIERCED
PIERCER
PIERCES
PLAICES
POLICED
POLICER
POLICES
POUNCED
POUNCER
POUNCES
PRANCED
PRANCER
PRANCES
PRINCES
PUMICED
PUMICES
QUINCES
QUINCEY
RADICES
REDUCED
REDUCER
REDUCES
REFACED
REFACES
RELACED
RELACES
SARACEN
SCARCER
SCONCES
SEANCES
SEDUCED
SEDUCER
SEDUCES
SLUICED
SLUICES
SOLACED
SOLACER
SOLACES
SOURCED
SOURCES
SPENCER
SPLICED
SPLICER
SPLICES
SPRUCED
SPRUCER
SPRUCES
STANCES
TENACES
TIERCES
TRANCED
TRANCES
UNFACED
UNLACED
UNLACES
UNPACED
USANCES

••••C•E

ARDECHE
ARTICLE
ATTACHE
AURICLE
BICYCLE
BINOCHE
BLANCHE
BRIOCHE
CAPUCHE
CENACLE
CEVICHE
CORACLE
CUBICLE

CUTICLE
DEBACLE
DEPECHE
EARACHE
FIANCEE
FRAICHE
GLENCOE
GOUACHE
LAROCHE
LAVACHE
MANACLE
MIRACLE
MONOCLE
ONEACRE
OSSICLE
PANACHE
PANICLE
PENUCHE
POOLCUE
PORSCHE
RADICLE
RECYCLE
RETICLE
TENACRE
TREACLE
TUNICLE
TWOACRE
VEHICLE
VESICLE
WAVICLE

•••••CE

ABSENCE
ADSPACE
ADVANCE
AIRRACE
ASKANCE
ATDEUCE
ATPEACE
AUSPICE
AVARICE
BALANCE
BEYONCE
BLUEICE
BYFORCE
CADENCE
CANDACE
CANDICE
CAPRICE
CATORCE
CHALICE
CLARICE
CONDUCE
COPPICE
CORNICE
CREVICE
DEFENCE
DEHISCE
DENIECE
DIVORCE
DOGFACE
DOGRACE
DORMICE
DOTRICE
DURANCE
EDIFICE
EMBRACE
EMPLACE
ENFORCE
ENHANCE
ENOUNCE
ESCENCE
ESSENCE
EUSTACE
FAIENCE
FINANCE
FIREICE
FLEANCE
FLOUNCE
FORONCE
FURNACE
GRIMACE
HOMEICE
HOSPICE
HOWNICE
INFORCE
INPEACE
INPLACE
INSPACE
INVOICE
JIMRICE
JUSTICE
LABMICE
LADOUCE
LAPLACE
LATTICE
LETTUCE
LICENCE
LIKEICE
MAURICE
MORTICE
MYSPACE
NEWFACE
NOPLACE
NOTNICE
NOTONCE
OFFENCE
ORIFICE
OUTFACE
OUTPACE
OUTRACE
OVERICE
PACKICE
PALANCE
PATRICE
PENANCE
PETMICE
PINNACE
POTENCE
PREFACE
PRERACE
PRODUCE
RATRACE
REBRACE
REDFACE
REFENCE
REJOICE
RELANCE
REPLACE
REPRICE
RESPACE
RESPICE
RETRACE
REVOICE
ROMANCE
SCIENCE
SEARACE
SENESCE
SERVICE
SILENCE
SKIRACE
SONANCE
STATICE
SUBRACE
SUFFICE
SURFACE
TERENCE
TERRACE
THINICE
TIMRICE
TITMICE
TRADUCE
TROUNCE
TUMESCE
TWOFACE
UNBRACE
UNFENCE
UNVOICE
VALANCE
VALENCE
VERSACE
WALLACE

C•F••••

CAFTANS
COFFEES
COFFERS
COFFINS
COFOUND
CUFFING

C••F•••

CABFARE
CANFULS
CAPFULS
CARFARE
CARFREE
CARFULS
CATFEET
CATFISH
CATFITS
CATFLAP
CATFLEA
CATFOOD
CATFOOT
CDEFGHI
CHAFERS
CHAFFED
CHAFFEE
CHAFFER
CHAFING
CHEFING
CHIFFON
CHUFFED
CLIFTON
CODFISH
COFFEES
COFFERS
COFFINS
COIFFED
COIFING
COMFIER
COMFITS
COMFORT
CONFABS
CONFECT
CONFERS
CONFESS
CONFIDE
CONFINE
CONFIRM
CONFITS
CONFORM
CONFREY
CONFUSE
CONFUTE
CORFAMS
COWFISH
CRAFTED
CRAFTER
CRAFTSY
CROFTER
CUBFANS
CUFFING
CUPFULS
CURFEWS

C•••F••

CALLFOR
CARAFES
CAREFOR
CAREFUL
CHAFFED
CHAFFEE
CHAFFER
CHAMFER
CHIEFLY
CHIFFON
CHUFFED
CLAPFOR
CLUEFUL
COIFFED
CONIFER
CORNFED
CUBSFAN
CUTOFFS

C••••F•

CALCIFY
CALLOFF
CAMEOFF
CARDIFF
CARTOFF
CASTOFF
CERTIFY
CHOPOFF
CLARIFY
CLIPOFF
COMEOFF
CONKOFF
CONNIFF
COOKOFF
CUTOFFS
CUTSOFF

C•••••F

CALLOFF
CAMEOFF
CARDIFF
CARTOFF
CASTOFF
CHOPOFF
CLEAROF
CLIPOFF
COMEOFF
CONKOFF
CONNIFF
COOKOFF
CRYWOLF
CUTSOFF

•C•F•••

ACTFIVE
ACTFOUR
ICEFALL
ICEFLOE
ICEFOGS
ICEFREE
SCOFFAT
SCOFFED
SCOFFER
SCUFFED
SCUFFER
SCUFFLE

•C••F••

ACHEFOR
ACTIFED
ACTSFOR
BCDEFGH
SCARFED
SCARFER
SCARFUP
SCLAFFS
SCOFFAT
SCOFFED
SCOFFER
SCRUFFS
SCRUFFY
SCUFFED
SCUFFER
SCUFFLE

•C•••F•

ACETIFY
ACIDIFY
ICONIFY
MCGRIFF
MCGRUFF
OCALAFL
SCARIFY
SCLAFFS
SCRUFFS
SCRUFFY

•C••••F

MCGRIFF
MCGRUFF
SCADSOF

••C•F••

ARCHFOE
BUCKFOR
FACTFUL
ITCHFOR
LUCIFER
PACIFIC
SACKFUL
TACTFUL
UNCUFFS

••C••F•

ABCDEFG
BACKOFF
FACEOFF
HACKOFF
KICKOFF
MACDUFF
MYCROFT
PACEOFF
PACKOFF
PICKOFF
RECTIFY
TICKOFF
UNCLEFT
UNCUFFS

••C•••F

BACKOFF
FACEOFF
HACKOFF
KICKOFF
MACDUFF
PACEOFF
PACKOFF
PICKOFF
TICKOFF

•••C•F•

CALCIFY
DULCIFY
FANCIFY
NESCAFE
NETCAFE
SADCAFE
SPECIFY
ZINCIFY
ZIPCUFF

•••C••F

ALACKOF
APECKOF
METCALF
MORCERF
PETCALF
SMACKOF
ZIPCUFF

C•G••••

CAGEDIN
CAGEDUP
CAGEPET
CAGESUP
CAGIEST
COGBURN
COGENCY
COGGING
COGGLES
COGHLAN
COGNACS
COGNATE
COGNIZE
CYGNETS

C••G•••

CADGERS
CADGING
CALGARY
CAMGIRL
CAPGUNS
CARGOES
CATGUTS
CHAGALL
CHAGRIN
CHIGGER
CHIGNON
CHIGOES
CHUGGED
CHUGGER
CLOGGED
CLOGSUP
COAGENT
CODGERS
COGGING
COGGLES
COIGNED
COIGNES
COLGATE
CONGAED
CONGAME
CONGEAL
CONGERS
CONGEST
CONGOUS
COUGARS
COUGHED
COUGHUP
COWGIRL
CRAGGED
CRUGUET
CUDGELS

C•••G••

CAYUGAS
CDEFGHI
CHANGED
CHANGER
CHANGES
CHARGED
CHARGER
CHARGES
CHEWGUM
CHIGGER
CHOUGHS
CHUGGED
CHUGGER
CITYGAL
CLANGED
CLANGER
CLANGOR
CLINGER
CLINGTO
CLOGGED
CLUNGTO
COALGAS
COLOGNE
CONAGRA
COSIGNS
CRAGGED
CRAIGIE
CRINGED
CRINGES
CRYOGEN
CUBAGES
CUINGIN

C••••G•

CABBAGE
CABBAGY
CANINGS
CARNAGE
CARTAGE
CASINGS
CATRIGS
CHICAGO
CINERGY
COINAGE
COLLAGE
COLLEGE
COMINGS
CONDIGN
CONSIGN
CORDAGE
CORKAGE
CORSAGE
CORTEGE
COTTAGE
COURAGE
COYDOGS
CYBORGS

C•••••G

CABBING
CABLING
CACHING
CADGING
CALKING
CALLING
CALMING
CALVING
CAMPING
CANNING
CANTING
CAPPING
CARDING
CARKING
CARLING
CARPING
CARTING
CARVING
CASHING
CASKING
CASTING
CATALOG
CAUSING
CEASING
CEILING
CENSING
CESSING
CHAFING
CHARING
CHASING
CHAWING
CHEFING
CHEWING
CHIDING
CHIMING
CHINWAG
CHOKING
CHOWING
CHUTING
CLAWING
CLAYING
CLEWING
CLONING
CLOSING
CLOYING
CLUEING
COALING
COATING
COAXING
COCKING
COGGING
COIFING
COILING
COINING
COMBING
COMPING
CONKING
CONNING
COOKING
COOLING
COONDOG
COOPING
COPPING
COPYING
CORDING
CORKING
CORNDOG
CORNING
COSHING
COSTING
COSYING
COUPING
COWLING
COZYING
CRANING
CRAPING
CRATING
CRAVING
CRAZING
CREPING
CREWING
CROWING
CUBBING
CUFFING
CULLING
CUNNING
CUPPING
CURBING
CURDING
CURLING
CURRING
CURSING
CURVING
CUSHING
CUSSING
CUTARUG
CUTTING
CYCLING
CYYOUNG

•CG••••

MCGAVIN
MCGRIFF
MCGRORY
MCGRUFF
MCGUIRE
MCGWIRE

•C••G••

ACINGIT
ECLOGUE
ICEAGES
ICINGIN
ICINGIT
ICINGUP
OCTAGON
SCRAGGY
SCRUGGS

•C•••G•

ACEHIGH
ACREAGE
BCDEFGH
ECOLOGY
ECOTAGE
ICEBAGS
ICEFOGS
SCALAGE
SCOURGE
SCRAGGY
SCROOGE
SCRUGGS

•C••••G

ACHTUNG
ECHOING
ICEBERG
MCCLURG
SCALING
SCARING
SCOPING
SCORING

••CG•••

MACGRAW

••C•G••

DECAGON
ENCAGED
ENCAGES
NICEGUY
RECAGED
RECAGES
UNCAGED
UNCAGES

••C••G•

ARCINGS
DOCKAGE
FACINGS
LACINGS
LOCKAGE
MACONGA
NICCAGE
PACKAGE
UNCLOGS

••C•••G

ABCDEFG
ARCHING
BACHING
BACKING
BACKLOG
BUCKING
CACHING
COCKING
CYCLING
DECALOG
DECKING
DOCKING
DUCKING
DUCTING
ETCHING
HACKING
HOCKING
INCHING
ITCHING
JACKING
KACHING
KICKING
LACKING
LICKING
LOCKING
LUCKING
MCCLURG
MOCKING
MUCKING
NECKING
NICEDOG
NICHING
NICKING
NOCKING
PACKING
PECKING
PICKING
RACKING
ROCKING
RUCHING
RUCKING
SACKING
SECHZIG
SICCING
SOCKING
SUCKING
TACKING
TICCING
TICKING
TUCKING
WICKING

•••C•G•

BOSCAGE
CHICAGO
NICCAGE
PETCAGE
RIBCAGE

•••C••G

BRACING
DANCING
DEICING
DEUCING
DISCING
EDUCING
FARCING
FENCING
FORCING
GRACING
JUICING
LANCING
MINCING
PIECING
PLACING
PRICING
REICING
SAUCING
SICCING
SLICING
SPACING
SPECING
SPICING
SYNCING
TICCING
TRACING
VOICING
WINCING
ZINCING

CH•••••

CHABLIS
CHACHAS
CHACHKA
CHAFERS
CHAFFED
CHAFFEE
CHAFFER
CHAFING
CHAGALL
CHAGRIN
CHAINED
CHAINES
CHAINUP
CHAIRED
CHAISES
CHAKRAS
CHALCIS
CHALETS
CHALICE
CHALKED
CHALKUP
CHALLAH
CHALONS
CHALUPA
CHAMBER
CHAMBRE
CHAMFER
CHAMOIS
CHAMPED
CHAMPER
CHANCED
CHANCEL
CHANCER
CHANCES
CHANELS
CHANGED
CHANGER
CHANGES
CHANNEL
CHANOYU
CHANSON
CHANTED
CHANTER
CHANTEY
CHANTRY
CHAOTIC
CHAPALA
CHAPATI
CHAPEAU
CHAPELS
CHAPLET
CHAPLIN
CHAPMAN
CHAPMEN
CHAPPED
CHAPPIE
CHAPTER
CHARADE
CHARCOT
CHARGED
CHARGER
CHARGES
CHARIER
CHARILY
CHARING
CHARIOT
CHARITY
CHARLES
CHARLEY
CHARLIE
CHARMAN
CHARMED
CHARMEN
CHARMER
CHARMIN
CHARNIN
CHARPAK
CHARRED
CHARRER
CHARROS
CHARTED
CHARTER
CHARVET
CHASERS
CHASING
CHASMAL
CHASMIC
CHASSED
CHASSES
CHASSIS
CHASTEN
CHASTER
CHATEAU
CHATHAM
CHATSUP
CHATTED
CHATTEL
CHATTER
CHATWIN
CHAUCER
CHAWING
CHAYOTE
CHAZANS
CHAZZAN
CHEADLE
CHEAPEN
CHEAPER
CHEAPIE
CHEAPLY
CHEATED
CHEATER
CHEATIN
CHEATON
CHECHEN
CHECKED
CHECKER
CHECKIN
CHECKON
CHECKUP
CHEDDAR
CHEDERS
CHEEKED
CHEEPED

7 CH

CHEEPER
CHEERED
CHEERER
CHEERIO
CHEERON
CHEERUP
CHEESED
CHEESES
CHEETAH
CHEETAS
CHEETOS
CHEEVER
CHEEZIT
CHEFING
CHEKHOV
CHELATE
CHELSEA
CHEMISE
CHEMIST
CHEMLAB
CHENIER
CHEQUER
CHEQUES
CHERISH
CHEROOT
CHERUBS
CHERVIL
CHESTED
CHESTER
CHETRUM
CHEVAUX
CHEVETS
CHEVIOT
CHEVONS
CHEVRES
CHEVRET
CHEVRON
CHEWERS
CHEWGUM
CHEWIER
CHEWING
CHEWOUT
CHEWSON
CHEWSUP
CHEWTOY
CHEXMIX
CHEZMOI
CHIANTI
CHIAPAS
CHIAPET
CHICAGO
CHICANA
CHICANE
CHICANO
CHICEST
CHICHAS
CHICHEN
CHICHIS
CHICKEN
CHICLES
CHICLET
CHICORY
CHIDDEN
CHIDERS
CHIDING
CHIEFLY
CHIFFON
CHIGGER
CHIGNON
CHIGOES
CHILCAT
CHILEAN
CHILIAD
CHILIES
CHILKAT
CHILLED
CHILLER
CHILLIS
CHILLUM
CHIMEIN
CHIMERA
CHIMERS
CHIMING
CHIMINH
CHIMNEY
CHINESE
CHINKED
CHINNED
CHINOIS
CHINOOK
CHINTZY
CHINUPS
CHINWAG
CHIPPED
CHIPPER
CHIPSIN
CHIPSUP
CHIRICO
CHIRPED
CHIRPER
CHIRRED
CHIRRUP
CHISELS
CHITLIN
CHITONS
CHITOWN
CHITTER
CHIVIED
CHIVIES
CHLORIC
CHOCKED
CHOCTAW
CHOICER
CHOICES
CHOIRED
CHOKEON
CHOKERS
CHOKEUP
CHOKIER
CHOKING
CHOLERA
CHOLERS
CHOLINE
CHOLLAS
CHOMPED
CHOMPON
CHOMSKY
CHOOSER
CHOOSES
CHOOSEY
CHOPINE
CHOPOFF
CHOPPED
CHOPPER
CHOPSUP
CHORALE
CHORALS
CHORDAL
CHORDED
CHORINE
CHORIST
CHORIZO
CHORTLE
CHOSEUP
CHOUGHS
CHOWDER
CHOWING
CHRISMS
CHRISOM
CHRISTA
CHRISTI
CHRISTO
CHRISTY
CHROMAT
CHROMED
CHROMES
CHROMIC
CHRONIC
CHUCKED
CHUCKIT
CHUCKLE
CHUFFED
CHUGGED
CHUGGER
CHUKKER
CHUMASH
CHUMMED
CHUMPED
CHUNKED
CHUNNEL
CHUPPAH
CHUPPAS
CHURCHY
CHURNED
CHURNER
CHURNUP
CHURROS
CHUTING
CHUTIST
CHUTNEY
CHUTZPA
CHYRONS

C•H••••

CAHIERS
CAHOKIA
CAHOOTS
COHABIT
COHEIRS
COHERED
COHERER
COHERES
COHORTS
COHOSTS

C••H•••

CACHACA
CACHETS
CACHING
CALHOUN
CARHOPS
CARHORN
CASHBAR
CASHBOX
CASHCOW
CASHEWS
CASHIER
CASHING
CASHINS
CASHOUT
CATHAIR
CATHEAD
CATHODE
CEPHALO
CEPHALY
CEPHEUS
CICHLID
CIPHERS
COCHAIR
COCHISE
COCHLEA
COCHRAN
COGHLAN
COSHERS
COSHING
COWHAND
COWHERD
COWHIDE
CUSHAWS
CUSHIER
CUSHILY
CUSHING
CUSHION
CYPHERS

C•••H••

CAMPHOR
CANCHAS
CAPSHAW
CARSHOW
CATCHER
CATCHES
CATCHON
CATCHOW
CATCHUP
CATSHOW
CAUTHEN
CHACHAS
CHACHKA
CHATHAM
CHECHEN
CHEKHOV
CHICHAS
CHICHEN
CHICHIS
CINCHED
CINCHES
CLASHED
CLASHER
CLASHES
CLICHED
CLICHES
CLOCHES
CLOTHED
CLOTHES
COACHED
COACHES
COLCHIS
CONCHAE
CONCHES
CONCHOS
COPSHOP
COUCHED
COUCHES
COUGHED
COUGHUP
COWSHED
CRASHAW
CRASHED
CRASHER
CRASHES
CRECHES
CROCHET
CRUSHED
CRUSHER
CRUSHES
CULCHES
CUMSHAW
CYNTHIA

C••••H•

CALIPHS
CAMACHO
CAPUCHE
CDEFGHI
CEVICHE
CHOUGHS
CHURCHY
CLUTCHY
CRUNCHY

C•••••H

CADDISH
CALTECH
CAPEESH
CARWASH
CATFISH
CATTISH
CHALLAH
CHEETAH
CHERISH
CHIMINH
CHUMASH
CHUPPAH
CLAYISH
COCKISH
CODFISH
COLDISH
COLTISH
COMMISH
COOLISH
CORINTH
CORNISH
COTEACH
COWFISH
CPEBACH
CUBBISH
CULTISH
CURRISH

•CH••••

ACHEFOR
ACHENES
ACHERON
ACHESON
ACHIEST
ACHIEVA
ACHIEVE
ACHILLE
ACHTUNG
ECHAPPE
ECHELON
ECHIDNA
ECHOERS
ECHOING
ECHOISM
ICHABOD
ICHDIEN
LCHAYIM
MCHALES
MCHENRY
OCHENTA
OCHROID
OCHROUS
SCHAYES
SCHELDT
SCHEMAS
SCHEMED
SCHEMER
SCHEMES
SCHERZI
SCHERZO
SCHICKS
SCHIRRA
SCHISMS
SCHISTS
SCHLEPP
SCHLEPS
SCHLITZ
SCHLOCK
SCHLUBS
SCHLUMP
SCHMEAR
SCHMEER
SCHMIDT
SCHMITT
SCHMOES
SCHNAPS
SCHNOOK
SCHNOZZ
SCHOLAR
SCHOLES
SCHOOLS
SCHTICK
SCHULTZ
SCHUMER
SCHWANN
SCHWINN
WCHANDY

•C•H•••

ACEHIGH
ECKHART
ICEHOLE
MCSHANE

•C••H••

ICESHOW
MCLUHAN
MCMAHON
SCATHED
SCATHES
SCYTHED
SCYTHES

•C•••H•

ACANTHI
SCACCHI

•C••••H

ACEHIGH
BCDEFGH
ICEBATH
NCWYETH
SCITECH
SCOOTCH
SCRATCH
SCREECH
SCRUNCH

••CH•••

AHCHOOS
ALCHEMY
ANCHORS
ANCHOVY
ARCHAIC
ARCHERS
ARCHERY
ARCHEST
ARCHFOE
ARCHIES
ARCHING
ARCHIVE
ARCHONS
ARCHSEE
ARCHWAY
BACHATA
BACHING
BACHMAN
BECHARM
BICHONS
BOCHNER
BSCHOOL
BUCHMAN
BUCHNER
CACHACA
CACHETS
CACHING
CICHLID
COCHAIR
COCHISE
COCHLEA
COCHRAN
DICHTER
DRCHAOS
DUCHAMP
DUCHESS
DUCHIES
ENCHAIN
ENCHANT
ENCHASE
ESCHEAT
ESCHERS
ESCHEWS
ETCHANT
ETCHERS
ETCHING
EUCHRED
EUCHRES
FECHNER
FUCHSIA
INCHECK
INCHERS
INCHING
ISCHIAL
ISCHIUM
ITCHFOR
ITCHIER
ITCHING
KACHINA
KACHING
KUCHENS
LECHERS
LICHEES
LICHENS
LUCHINO
MACHAON
MACHETE
MACHINA
MACHINE
MACHONE
MACHREE
MACHSIX
MACHTWO
MECHLIN
MICHAEL
MICHAUX
MOCHRIE
MRCHIPS
NICHING
NICHOLS
ORCHARD
ORCHIDS
PACHISI
QSCHOOL
RACHAEL
RECHALK
RECHALL
RECHART
RECHECK
RECHEWS
RECHOSE
RICHARD
RICHENS
RICHEST
RICHLER
RICHMAN
RICHMEN
RICHTER
ROCHETS
RUCHING
SACHEMS
SACHETS
SECHZIG
TACHYON
TECHIES
TECHNOS
TUCHMAN
UNCHAIN
UNCHAIR
UNCHARY
UNCHECK
UNCHOKE
UNCHURN
URCHINS
VECHTEN
WICHITA
YACHTED
YACHTER
YACHTIE
ZACHARY

••C•H••

ALCOHOL
BACCHAE
BACCHIC
BACCHUS
BACKHOE
BECKHAM
SOCKHOP

••C••H•

RICKSHA

••C•••H

BYCATCH
COCKISH
JACINTH
MACBETH
NOCATCH
PECKISH
PICTISH
PUCKISH
SICKISH
SUCCOTH
UNCINCH
UNCOUTH

•••CH••

AITCHES
AMICHAI
APACHES
ARACHNE
ARACHNO
BACCHAE
BACCHIC
BACCHUS
BATCHED
BATCHES
BEACHAM
BEACHED
BEACHES
BEECHAM
BEECHEN
BEECHER
BEECHES
BELCHED
BELCHER
BELCHES
BENCHED
BENCHER
BENCHES
BIOCHIP
BIRCHED
BIRCHEN
BIRCHES
BOKCHOY
BOTCHED
BOTCHER
BOTCHES
BOTCHUP
BOUCHER
BOUCHES
BUNCHED
BUNCHES
BUNCHUP
BUTCHER
BUTCHES
CANCHAS
CATCHER
CATCHES
CATCHON
CATCHOW
CATCHUP
CHACHAS
CHACHKA
CHECHEN
CHICHAS
CHICHEN
CHICHIS
CINCHED
CINCHES
CLICHED
CLICHES
CLOCHES
COACHED
COACHES
COLCHIS
CONCHAE
CONCHES
CONCHOS
COUCHED
COUCHES
CRECHES
CROCHET
CULCHES
DASCHLE
DITCHED
DITCHER
DITCHES
DOGCHEW
DOGCHOW
DRACHMA
EPOCHAL
FETCHED
FETCHER
FETCHES
FILCHED
FILCHER
FILCHES
FINCHES
FISCHER
FLECHES
GAUCHER
GAUCHOS
GOTCHAS
GULCHES
HATCHED
HATCHER
HATCHES
HATCHET
HITCHED
HITCHER
HITCHES
HITCHON
HITCHUP
HONCHOS
HOOCHES
HUNCHED
HUNCHES
HUTCHES
JIMCHEE
JOACHIM
KETCHAM
KETCHES
KETCHUM
KETCHUP
KIMCHEE
KITCHEN
KUTCHER
KWACHAS
LARCHEN
LARCHES
LATCHED
LATCHES
LATCHON
LEACHED
LEACHER
LEACHES
LEECHED
LEECHEE
LEECHES
LITCHIS
LOWCHEN
LUNCHED
LUNCHER
LUNCHES
LURCHED
LURCHER
LURCHES
MADCHEN
MARCHED
MARCHER
MARCHES
MARCHON
MATCHED
MATCHER
MATCHES
MATCHUP
MERCHES
MITCHUM
MOOCHED
MOOCHER
MOOCHES
MULCHED
MULCHES
MUNCHED
MUNCHEN
MUNCHER
MUNCHES
MUNCHIE
MUNCHON
NATCHEZ
NOTCHED
NOTCHER
NOTCHES
OLDCHAP
ONECHIP
PANCHAX
PARCHED
PARCHES
PASCHAL
PATCHED
PATCHEN
PATCHER
PATCHES
PATCHUP
PEACHED
PEACHES
PERCHED
PERCHER
PERCHES
PERCHIK
PETCHEW
PINCHAS
PINCHED
PINCHER
PINCHES
PINCHME
PINCHOT
PITCHED
PITCHER
PITCHES
PITCHIN
PITCHTO
POACHED
POACHER
POACHES
PONCHOS
POOCHES
POOCHIE
PORCHES
POUCHED
POUCHES
PSYCHED
PSYCHES
PSYCHIC
PSYCHOS
PSYCHUP
PUNCHED
PUNCHER
PUNCHES
PUNCHIN
PUNCHUP
PYNCHON
QUECHUA
QUICHES
RANCHED
RANCHER
RANCHES
RANCHOS
RATCHET
REACHED
REACHER
REACHES
REACHIN
REACHUP
REDCHIP
RITCHIE
ROACHES
SALCHOW
SATCHEL
SATCHMO
SAWCHUK
SYNCHED
TEACHER
TEACHES
TEACHIN
TEICHER
TENCHES
TORCHED
TORCHER
TORCHES
TOUCHED
TOUCHER
TOUCHES
TOUCHON
TOUCHUP
TRACHEA
TROCHEE
TROCHES
VETCHES
VOUCHED
VOUCHER
VOUCHES
WATCHED
WATCHER
WATCHES
WATCHIT
WATCHTV
WENCHES
WINCHED
WINCHER
WINCHES
WITCHED
WITCHES
ZILCHES

•••C•H•

GNOCCHI
MULCAHY
ROYCOHN
SCACCHI

•••C••H

ALLCASH
DUNCISH
GETCASH
GOTCASH
NONCASH
PATCASH
PAYCASH
SUBCASH
SUCCOTH

••••CH•

ANARCHS
ANARCHY
ARDECHE
ATTACHE
BIANCHI
BINOCHE
BLANCHE
BLOTCHY
BORSCHT
BOWECHO
BRANCHY
BRIOCHE
BRONCHI
BRONCHO
CAMACHO
CAPUCHE
CEVICHE
CHURCHY
CLUTCHY
CRUNCHY
DEPECHE
DERECHO
EARACHE
EPARCHS
EPARCHY
EXARCHS
FRAICHE
FRANCHI
FRENCHI
FRENCHS
GLITCHY
GNOCCHI
GOUACHE
GROUCHO
GROUCHY
HAMACHI
HIBACHI
HITACHI
IGOTCHA

JERICHO
KARACHI
KENICHI
KITSCHY
KVETCHY
LAROCHE
LAVACHE
MALACHI
MENSCHY
MRMACHO
NOGUCHI
OUTECHO
PANACHE
PAUNCHY
PENUCHE
PORSCHE
PREACHY
RAUNCHY
SAATCHI
SCACCHI
SKETCHY
SLOUCHY
STARCHY
SUBECHO
THATCHY
TWITCHY
UNMACHO
UTRECHT
VOTECHS

••••C•H

PADUCAH

•••••CH

ABROACH
ALDRICH
ANDSUCH
ANSPACH
ANTIOCH
ATLUNCH
AUTARCH
BADITCH
BESEECH
BEWITCH
BIOTECH
BYCATCH
CALTECH
COTEACH
CPEBACH
DEBAUCH
DEUTSCH
DIPTYCH
DISTICH
DOLUNCH
DRIESCH
EHRLICH
ELDRICH
ERDRICH
FOREACH
GODUTCH
HARBACH
HENRICH
HOWMUCH
IMPEACH
INDUTCH
INMARCH
INREACH
INSYNCH
INTOUCH
IPSWICH
JOMARCH
KLATSCH
KLENSCH
LABTECH
LELOUCH
LOWTECH
MESHACH
MIRISCH
MONARCH
MRMARCH
MURDOCH
NEWRICH
NIDETCH
NOCATCH
NONSUCH
NORWICH
NOTMUCH
OILRICH
ONEINCH
OSTRICH
PDQBACH
REHITCH
RELATCH
REMATCH
REPATCH
RETEACH
RETOUCH
SAWATCH
SCITECH
SCOOTCH
SCRATCH
SCREECH
SCRUNCH
SNEETCH
SPINACH
SPLOTCH
SQUELCH
SQUINCH
STAUNCH
STOMACH
STRETCH
STRITCH
TOOMUCH
UNBENCH
UNCINCH
UNHITCH
UNLATCH
UNTEACH
UPREACH
WALLACH
WASATCH

CI•••••

CICADAE
CICADAS
CICCONE
CICHLID
CILENTO
CILIARY
CILIATE
CIMABUE
CINCHED
CINCHES
CINDERS
CINDERY
CINEMAS
CINEMAX
CINEOLE
CINERGY
CINESIA
CINQUES
CINZANO
CIPHERS
CIRCLED
CIRCLER
CIRCLES
CIRCLET
CIRCUIT
CIRCUSY
CIRQUES
CIRRATE
CISCOES
CISEAUX
CISTERN
CITABLE
CITADEL
CITIZEN
CITRATE
CITRINE
CITROEN
CITRONS
CITROUS
CITYBOY
CITYGAL
CIVILLY
CIVVIES

C•I••••

CAILLOU
CAIMANS
CAIRENE
CAIRNED
CAISSON
CEILING
CHIANTI
CHIAPAS
CHIAPET
CHICAGO
CHICANA
CHICANE
CHICANO
CHICEST
CHICHAS
CHICHEN
CHICHIS
CHICKEN
CHICLES
CHICLET
CHICORY
CHIDDEN
CHIDERS
CHIDING
CHIEFLY
CHIFFON
CHIGGER
CHIGNON
CHIGOES
CHILCAT
CHILEAN
CHILIAD
CHILIES
CHILKAT
CHILLED
CHILLER
CHILLIS
CHILLUM
CHIMEIN
CHIMERA
CHIMERS
CHIMING
CHIMINH
CHIMNEY
CHINESE
CHINKED
CHINNED
CHINOIS
CHINOOK
CHINTZY
CHINUPS
CHINWAG
CHIPPED
CHIPPER
CHIPSIN
CHIPSUP
CHIRICO
CHIRPED
CHIRPER
CHIRRED
CHIRRUP
CHISELS
CHITLIN
CHITONS
CHITOWN
CHITTER
CHIVIED
CHIVIES
CLIBURN
CLICHED
CLICHES
CLICKED
CLICKER
CLICKON
CLIENTS
CLIFTON
CLIMATE
CLIMATS
CLIMBED
CLIMBER
CLIMBIN
CLIMBON
CLIMBTO
CLIMBUP
CLINGER
CLINGTO
CLINICS
CLINKED
CLINKER
CLINTON
CLIPART
CLIPOFF
CLIPONS
CLIPOUT
CLIPPED
CLIPPER
CLIPSON
CLIQUED
CLIQUES
CLIQUEY
COIFFED
COIFING
COIGNED
COIGNES
COILERS
COILING
COILSUP
COINAGE
COINBOX
COINERS
COINING
COINOPS
CRIBBED
CRIBBER
CRICKED
CRICKET
CRIEDUP
CRIESUP
CRIMEAN
CRIMINY
CRIMPED
CRIMPER
CRIMSON
CRINGED
CRINGES
CRINKLE
CRINKLY
CRIPPLE
CRISPED
CRISPEN
CRISPER
CRISPIN
CRISPIX
CRISPLY
CRISPUS
CRITIAS
CRITICS
CRITTER
CRITTUR
CUIBONO
CUINGIN
CUIRASS
CUISINE

C••I•••

CABINET
CACIQUE
CAGIEST
CAHIERS
CAKIEST
CALIBAN
CALIBER
CALIBRE
CALICES
CALICOS
CALIPER
CALIPHS
CALISTA
CAMILLA
CAMILLE
CAMINOS
CAMIONS
CAMISES
CANIDAE
CANIEST
CANINES
CANINGS
CANITBE
CAPITAL
CAPITAN
CAPITOL
CARIBES
CARIBOO
CARIBOU
CARINAE
CARINAS
CARIOCA
CARIOLE
CARIOUS
CASIMIR
CASINGS
CASINOS
CASITAS
CATIONS
CAVIARE
CAVIARS
CAVILAT
CAVILED
CAVILER
CCRIDER
CECILIA
CEDILLA
CELICAS
CERISES
CEVICHE
CHAINED
CHAINES
CHAINUP
CHAIRED
CHAISES
CHOICER
CHOICES
CHOIRED
CHRISMS
CHRISOM
CHRISTA
CHRISTI
CHRISTO
CHRISTY
CILIARY
CILIATE
CITIZEN
CIVILLY
CLAIMED
CLAIMER
CLAIROL
CODICES
CODICIL
COKIEST
COLICKY
COMICAL
COMICES
COMINGS
COMIQUE
CONICAL
CONIFER
COPIERS
COPILOT
COPIOUS
CORINNE
CORINTH
COSIEST
COSIGNS
COSINES
COWIEST
COZIEST
CRAIGIE
CRAISIN
CRUISED
CRUISER
CRUISES
CUBICAL
CUBICLE
CUBICLY
CUBISTS
CUBITAL
CUBITUS
CURIOSA
CURIOUS
CUTICLE
CUTINON
CUTINTO
CUTISES
CYNICAL

C•••I••

CABBIES
CABBING
CABLING
CABRIDE
CABRINI
CABRIOS
CACHING
CADDIED
CADDIES
CADDISH
CADGING
CADMIUM
CALCIFY
CALCITE
CALCIUM
CALKING
CALKINS
CALLING
CALLINS
CALMING
CALVING
CALVINO
CAMGIRL
CAMMIES
CAMPIER
CAMPILY
CAMPING
CAMPION
CANDICE
CANDIDA
CANDIDE
CANDIDS
CANDIED
CANDIES
CANNIER
CANNILY
CANNING
CANTILY
CANTINA
CANTING
CANTINO
CAPPING
CAPRICE
CAPRINE
CAPSIZE
CAPTION
CAPTIVA
CAPTIVE
CARBIDE
CARBINE
CARDIAC
CARDIAL
CARDIFF
CARDING
CARDIUM
CARKING
CARLING
CARMINA
CARMINE
CARNIES
CARPING
CARRIED
CARRIER
CARRIES
CARTIER
CARTING
CARTIRE
CARVING
CASEINS
CASHIER
CASHING
CASHINS
CASKING
CASPIAN
CASSIAS
CASSIDY
CASSINI
CASSINO
CASSIUS
CASTILE
CASTING
CASUIST
CATBIRD
CATFISH
CATFITS
CATKINS
CATLIKE
CATMINT
CATNIPS
CATRIGS
CATSITS
CATTIER
CATTILY
CATTISH
CAUSING
CAUTION
CAVEINS
CEASING
CEILING
CELLINI
CELLIST
CELSIUS
CELTICS
CENSING
CENTIME
CENTIMO
CERTIFY
CERVIDS
CERVINE
CESAIRE
CESSING
CESSION
CHAFING
CHALICE
CHARIER
CHARILY
CHARING
CHARIOT
CHARITY
CHASING
CHAWING
CHEFING
CHEMISE
CHEMIST
CHENIER
CHERISH
CHEVIOT
CHEWIER
CHEWING
CHIDING
CHILIAD
CHILIES
CHIMING
CHIMINH
CHIRICO
CHIVIED
CHIVIES
CHOKIER
CHOKING
CHOLINE
CHOPINE
CHORINE
CHORIST
CHORIZO
CHOWING
CHUTING
CHUTIST
CITRINE
CIVVIES
CLARICE
CLARIFY
CLARION
CLARITY
CLAVIER
CLAWING
CLAYIER
CLAYING
CLAYISH
CLERICS
CLERISY
CLEWING
CLINICS
CLONING
CLOSING
CLOYING
CLUEING
COALING
COATING
COAXIAL
COAXING
COCAINE
COCHISE
COCKIER
COCKILY
COCKING
COCKISH
CODEINE
CODFISH
COEDITS
COEXIST
COFFINS
COGGING
COGNIZE
COHEIRS
COIFING
COILING
COINING
COLDISH
COLLIDE
COLLIER
COLLIES
COLLINE
COLLINS
COLTISH
COMBIEN
COMBINE
COMBING
COMFIER
COMFITS
COMMISH
COMMITS
COMPILE
COMPING
COMTISM
COMTIST
CONCISE
CONDIGN
CONFIDE
CONFINE
CONFIRM
CONFITS
CONKING
CONNICK
CONNIFF
CONNING
CONNIVE
CONOIDS
CONRIED
CONSIGN
CONSIST
CONVICT
COOKIES
COOKING
COOLIES
COOLING
COOLISH
COOPING
COOTIES
COPPICE
COPPING
COPYING
COPYIST
COQUINA
CORDIAL
CORDIAS
CORDING
CORDITE
CORKIER
CORKING
CORNICE
CORNIER
CORNILY
CORNING
CORNISH
CORRIDA
CORSICA
CORTICO
CORTINA
CORVIDS
CORVINA
CORVINE
CORZINE
COSHING
COSTING
COSTIVE
COSYING
COUPING
COURIER
COUSINE
COUSINS
COWBIRD
COWFISH
COWGIRL
COWHIDE
COWLICK
COWLIKE
COWLING
COWRIES
COWRITE
COZYING
CRANIAL
CRANING
CRANIUM
CRAPING
CRATING
CRATION
CRAVING
CRAZIER
CRAZIES
CRAZILY
CRAZING
CREDITS
CREMINI
CREPING
CRETINS
CREVICE
CREWING
CRIMINY
CRITIAS
CRITICS
CRONIES
CROSIER
CROWING
CROZIER
CRUCIAL
CRUDITY
CUBBIES
CUBBING
CUBBINS
CUBBISH
CUBOIDS
CUDDIES
CUEBIDS
CUETIPS
CUFFING
CUISINE
CULLIED
CULLIES
CULLING
CULTISH
CULTISM
CULTIST
CUMBIAS
CUNNING
CUPLIKE
CUPPIER
CUPPING
CUPRITE
CURBING
CURDIER
CURDING
CURLIER
CURLIKE
CURLING
CURRIED
CURRIER
CURRIES
CURRING
CURRISH
CURSING
CURSIVE
CURTISS
CURVIER
CURVING
CUSHIER
CUSHILY
CUSHING
CUSHION
CUSPIDS
CUSSING
CUTTIME
CUTTING
CYANIDE
CYANIDS
CYCLING
CYCLIST
CYMRICS
CYPRIAN
CYPRIOT
CZARINA
CZARISM
CZARIST

C••••I•

CAGEDIN
CAHOKIA
CAKEMIX
CAKETIN
CALLSIN
CALLSIT
CALORIC
CALORIE
CAMBRIA
CAMBRIC
CAMELID
CANONIC
CANTRIP
CAPAPIE
CAPTAIN
CARAMIA
CAROLII
CAROTID
CAROTIN
CARRYIN
CARTRIP
CARTSIN
CASIMIR
CATANIA
CATHAIR
CATSUIT
CATTAIL
CAUSTIC
CAVEDIN
CAVESIN
CBRADIO
CECILIA
CENTRIC
CERAMIC
CERTAIN
CESSPIT
CETERIS
CHABLIS
CHAGRIN
CHALCIS
CHAMOIS
CHAOTIC
CHAPLIN
CHAPPIE
CHARLIE
CHARMIN
CHARNIN
CHASMIC
CHASSIS
CHATWIN
CHEAPIE
CHEATIN
CHECKIN
CHEERIO
CHEEZIT
CHERVIL
CHEXMIX
CHICHIS
CHILLIS
CHIMEIN
CHINOIS
CHIPSIN
CHITLIN
CHLORIC
CHROMIC
CHRONIC
CHUCKIT
CICHLID
CINESIA
CIRCUIT
CLAMDIP
CLASSIC
CLAUDIA
CLAUDIO
CLAYPIT
CLIMBIN
CLOCKIN
CLOSEIN
CLUEDIN
CLUESIN
COALBIN
COALOIL
COALPIT
COCCOID
COCHAIR
COCKPIT
CODICIL
COEPTIS
COHABIT
COLCHIS
COLLOID
COMEDIA
COMEDIC
COMEDIE
COMESIN
COMPLIN
CONBRIO
CONCEIT
CONDUIT
CONJOIN
CONKLIN
CONTAIN
COOLAIR
COOLPIX
COOLSIT
CORNBIN

7 CI

CORNOIL
CORSAIR
CORVAIR
COSTAIN
COTERIE
COUNCIL
COUNTIN
COWSKIN
COWSLIP
CRAIGIE
CRAISIN
CRAMSIN
CRAPPIE
CREEPIN
CREPTIN
CRESPIN
CRISPIN
CRISPIX
CROATIA
CROQUIS
CROSTIC
CROWDIN
CRYPTIC
CSLEWIS
CTENOID
CUINGIN
CULPRIT
CUMBRIA
CURLSIN
CURTAIL
CURTAIN
CYCLOID
CYNTHIA
CYRUSII

C•••••I

CABRINI
CADUCEI
CALCULI
CAMPARI
CANETTI
CANNOLI
CANZONI
CAROLII
CASSINI
CDEFGHI
CELLINI
CESTMOI
CHAPATI
CHEZMOI
CHIANTI
CHRISTI
COLLODI
COLOSSI
CORELLI
CREMINI
CYRUSII

•CI••••

ACIDIFY
ACIDITY
ACINGIT
ICICLES
ICINESS
ICINGIN
ICINGIT
ICINGUP
OCICATS
SCIATIC
SCIENCE
SCIORRA
SCISSOR
SCITECH

•C•I•••

ACHIEST
ACHIEVA
ACHIEVE
ACHILLE
ACRIDLY
ACTIFED
ACTINON
ACTIONS
ACTIVAS
ACTIVES
BCLIONS
CCRIDER
ECHIDNA
ECLIPSE
ICKIEST
ICTINUS
OCCIPUT
SCHICKS
SCHIRRA
SCHISMS
SCHISTS
SCRIBED
SCRIBER
SCRIBES
SCRIMPS
SCRIMPY
SCRIPPS
SCRIPTS

•C••I••

ACACIAS
ACADIAN
ACARIDS
ACEHIGH
ACETIFY
ACIDIFY
ACIDITY
ACONITE
ACQUIRE
ACQUITS
ACTFIVE
ACTLIKE
ECHOING
ECHOISM
ECLAIRS
ECOCIDE
ICELIKE
ICELINE
ICEMILK
ICEPICK
ICERINK
ICEWINE
ICHDIEN
ICONIFY
ICYWIND
MCBRIDE
MCGRIFF
MCGUIRE
MCGWIRE
MCNEILL
MCSWINE
OCARINA
OCULIST
SCALIER
SCALING
SCARIER
SCARIFY
SCARILY
SCARING
SCENICS
SCHLITZ
SCHMIDT
SCHMITT
SCHTICK
SCHWINN
SCOPING
SCORIAS
SCORING
SCOTIAN

•C•••I•

ACCLAIM
ACERBIC
ACINGIT
ACRYLIC
ACTEDIN
ACYCLIC
ECDYSIS
ECOTRIN
ICINGIN
ICINGIT
LCHAYIM
MCGAVIN
OCEANIA
OCEANIC
OCEANID
OCHROID
OCTADIC
OCTAVIA
OCTAVIO
OCTROIS
SCARWID
SCENEII
SCENEIV
SCEPTIC
SCIATIC
SCORPIO
SCOTTIE

•C••••I

ACANTHI
ECCLESI
SCACCHI
SCENEII
SCENEVI
SCHERZI
SCOLARI

••CI•••

ANCIENT
ARCINGS
BACILLI
CACIQUE
CECILIA
DECIARE
DECIBEL
DECIDED
DECIDER
DECIDES
DECILES
DECIMAL
DICIEST
DICILLO
ENCINAS
EXCIDED
EXCIDES
EXCISED
EXCISES
EXCITED
EXCITER
EXCITES
EXCITOR
FACIALS
FACINGS
INCISED
INCISES
INCISOR
INCITED
INCITER
INCITES
INCIVIL
JACINTH
JACINTO
LACIEST
LACINGS
LICITLY
LUCIANA
LUCIANO
LUCIDAE
LUCIDLY
LUCIFER
LUCILLE
LUCINDA
LUCITES
LUCIUSI
OCCIPUT
OSCINES
PACIEST
PACIFIC
RACIEST
RACINOS
RACISTS
RECIPES
RECITAL
RECITED
RECITER
RECITES
SICILIA
SOCIALS
SOCIETY
TACITLY
TACITUS
UNCIALS
UNCINCH
UNCITED
UNCIVIC
UNCIVIL
VICINAL
VICIOUS

••C•I••

ALCAIDE
ARCHIES
ARCHING
ARCHIVE
ARCSINE
ASCRIBE
AUCTION
BACHING
BACKING
BOCCIES
BUCKING
CACHING
COCAINE
COCHISE
COCKIER
COCKILY
COCKING
COCKISH
CYCLING
CYCLIST
DECEITS
DECEIVE
DECKING
DECLINE
DECRIED
DECRIER
DECRIES
DICKIES
DICTION
DOCKING
DUCHIES
DUCKIER
DUCKIES
DUCKING
DUCTILE
DUCTING
ETCHING
FACTION
FICTILE
FICTION
FICTIVE
GUCKIER
HACKIES
HACKING
HOCKING
INCHING
INCLINE
ISCHIAL
ISCHIUM
ITCHIER
ITCHING
JACKIEO
JACKING
KACHINA
KACHING
KICKIER
KICKING
LACKING
LACRIMO
LICKING
LOCKING
LOCKINS
LUCHINO
LUCKIER
LUCKILY
LUCKING
MACHINA
MACHINE
MOCKING
MRCHIPS
MUCKIER
MUCKING
NECKING
NICHING
NICKING
NICOISE
NOCKING
NUCLIDE
ORCHIDS
PACHISI
PACKICE
PACKING
PECKING
PECKISH
PECTINS
PICKIER
PICKING
PICNICS
PICTISH
PUCCINI
PUCKISH
PVCPIPE
RACKING
RECEIPT
RECEIVE
RECLIMB
RECLINE
RECOILS
RECOINS
RECTIFY
ROCKIER
ROCKIES
ROCKILY
ROCKING
RUCHING
RUCKING
RUCTION
SACKING
SACLIKE
SECTION
SICCING
SICKISH
SOCKING
SUCKIER
SUCKING
SUCTION
TACKIER
TACKILY
TACKING
TACTICS
TACTILE
TECHIES
TICCING
TICKING
TOCSINS
TUCKING
UNCLIPS
UNCLIPT
UNCOILS
UNCRIED
UNCTION
UPCLIMB
UPCOILS
URCHINS
VACCINE
VACUITY
VICTIMS
WACKIER
WACKILY
WICHITA
WICKING
WICKIUP
YUCAIPA
YUCKIER

••C••I•

ACCLAIM
ARCADIA
ARCHAIC
ASCETIC
BACCHIC
BACKBIT
BACKLIT
BACKSIN
BACTRIA
BUCOLIC
CECILIA
CICHLID
COCCOID
COCHAIR
COCKPIT
CYCLOID
DECLAIM
DUCKPIN
ENCHAIN
ENCOMIA
EUCERIN
EXCELIN
EXCLAIM
FACEDIT
FACESIT
FACTOID
FUCHSIA
HACKSIT
INCIVIL
JACOBIN
KICKSIN
LACKWIT
LACONIA
LACONIC
LACTAID
LECTRIC
LOCKLIN
LOCKSIN
LUCANIA
LUCYLIU
MACHSIX
MACNEIL
MECHLIN
MOCHRIE
NECKTIE
NICEKID
NICOSIA
NUCLEIC
PACIFIC
PACKSIN
PACQUIN
RACEDIN
RECLAIM
RECRUIT
ROCKOIL
ROCKYII
ROCKYIV
SECHZIG
SICILIA
SOCKSIN
STCROIX
SUCKSIN
TACONIC
TICOTIN
TOCELIA
TUCKSIN
UNCHAIN
UNCHAIR
UNCIVIC
UNCIVIL
UNCOMIC
UNCUBIC
VICTRIX
VOCALIC
YACHTIE

••C•••I

BACARDI
BACILLI
BOCELLI
ECCLESI
JACUZZI
LUCIUSI
PACHISI
PECCAVI
PUCCINI
ROCKYII
SECONDI

•••CI••

ABSCISE
ACACIAS
ANACINS
ARECIBO
ASOCIAL
BAYCITY
BIGCITY
BIOCIDE
BOCCIES
BRACING
CALCIFY
CALCITE
CALCIUM
CONCISE
CRUCIAL
DANCING
DEICING
DELCITY
DEUCING
DISCING
DULCIFY
DUNCISH
ECOCIDE
EDACITY
EDUCING
ELICITS
ELMCITY
EXSCIND
FANCIED
FANCIER
FANCIES
FANCIFY
FANCILY
FARCING
FASCIAE
FASCIAL
FASCIAS
FASCISM
FASCIST
FATCITY
FENCING
FOGCITY
FORCING
GLACIAL
GLACIER
GLYCINE
GRACIAS
GRACILE
GRACING
GRECIAN
GRECISM
GRECIZE
HIRCINE
JUICIER
JUICILY
JUICING
KOSCINA
LAICIZE
LANCIAS
LANCING
LEUCINE
MANCINI
MENCIUS
MERCIAN
MERCIES
MINCING
MISCITE
MUSCIDA
NUNCIOS
OLDCITY
OPACITY
ORACIES
OUTCITY
PAUCITY
PENCILS
PEPCIDS
PIECING
PISCINE
PLACIDO
PLACING
PORCINE
PRECISE
PRECITE
PRICIER
PRICILY
PRICING
PROCITY
PUCCINI
REICING
RESCIND
SAUCIER
SAUCILY
SAUCING
SICCING
SIMCITY
SINCITY
SLICING
SPACIAL
SPACIER
SPACING
SPECIAL
SPECIES
SPECIFY
SPECING
SPICIER
SPICILY
SPICING
SUNCITY
SYNCING
THECITY
TICCING
TRACING
URACILS
VACCINE
VOICING
WINCING
ZINCIFY
ZINCING
ZINCITE

•••C•I•

ACYCLIC
AJACCIO
ATACLIP
BACCHIC
BIOCHIP
BISCUIT
BLACKIE
CHECKIN
CHICHIS
CHUCKIT
CIRCUIT
CLOCKIN
COCCOID
COLCHIS
CONCEIT
DISCOID
EARCLIP
FENCEIN
FLACCID
FORCEIN
JOACHIM
KINCAID
LITCHIS
LITCRIT
MISCOIN
MUNCHIE
ONECHIP
ORECTIC
PERCHIK
PITCHIN
POOCHIE
PRACTIC
PRECOIL
PSYCHIC
PUNCHIN
QUICKIE
REACHIN
REDCHIP
RITCHIE
STICKIN
STUCKIN
TEACHIN
TIECLIP
WATCHIT

•••C••I

AMICHAI
ARACARI
BUSCEMI
CALCULI
GNOCCHI
MANCINI
MARCONI
MOSCONI
PASCOLI
PECCAVI
PUCCINI
SCACCHI

••••CI•

AJACCIO
ANTACID
BENICIA
BENICIO
BONACIS
BRESCIA
CHALCIS
CODICIL
COUNCIL
DEFICIT
DOMICIL
FELICIA
FLACCID
FRANCIS
GALICIA
ILLICIT
INDICIA
NONACID
OFFICIO
PREACID
SOLICIT
STENCIL
STLUCIA
UNLUCID

••••C•I

BIANCHI
BRONCHI
CADUCEI
DELICTI
FRANCHI
FRENCHI
GNOCCHI
HAMACHI
HIBACHI
HITACHI
KARACHI
KENICHI
MALACHI
NOGUCHI
SAATCHI
SCACCHI

•••••CI

DAVINCI
MENISCI
POLISCI
POLYSCI

C•J••••

CAJOLED
CAJOLER
CAJOLES
COJUROR

C••J•••

CARJACK
CONJOBS
CONJOIN
CONJURE
CONJURY

C•••J••

CULTJAM

•CJ••••

KCJONES

••C•J••

ELCAJON
LOCKJAW
NICEJOB

••C•••J

LLCOOLJ

C•K••••

CAKEDUP
CAKEMIX
CAKEPAN
CAKESUP
CAKETIN
CAKIEST
COKIEST

C••K•••

CACKLED
CACKLER
CACKLES
CALKERS
CALKING
CALKINS
CANKERS
CARKEYS
CARKING
CASKETS
CASKING
CATKINS
CHAKRAS
CHEKHOV
CHOKEON
CHOKERS
CHOKEUP
CHOKIER
CHOKING
CHUKKER
COCKADE
COCKERS
COCKIER
COCKILY
COCKING
COCKISH
COCKLED
COCKLES
COCKNEY
COCKPIT
CONKERS
CONKING
CONKLIN
CONKOFF
CONKOUT
COOKERS
COOKERY
COOKIES
COOKING
COOKOFF
COOKOUT
COOKPOT
COOKSUP
COOKTOP
CORKAGE
CORKERS
CORKIER
CORKING
CORKOAK
CORKSUP
CUCKOOS

C•••K••

CAHOKIA
CARDKEY
CAULKED
CAULKER
CHALKED
CHALKUP
CHECKED
CHECKER
CHECKIN
CHECKON
CHECKUP
CHEEKED
CHICKEN
CHILKAT
CHINKED
CHOCKED
CHUCKED
CHUCKIT
CHUCKLE
CHUKKER
CHUNKED
CLACKED
CLACKER
CLANKED
CLERKED
CLERKLY
CLICKED
CLICKER
CLICKON
CLINKED
CLINKER
CLOAKED
CLOCKED
CLOCKER
CLOCKIN
CLONKED
CLUCKED
CLUCKER
CLUNKED
CLUNKER
COMAKER
CONAKRY
COWSKIN
CRACKED
CRACKER
CRACKLE
CRACKLY
CRACKUP
CRANKED
CRANKUP
CREAKED
CRICKED
CRICKET
CRINKLE
CRINKLY
CROAKED
CROAKER
CROCKED
CROCKER
CROCKET
CROOKED
CROOKES

C••••K•
CANUCKS CATLIKE CDRACKS CHACHKA CHOMSKY CODCAKE COLICKY CONVOKE COWLIKE COWPOKE CUPCAKE CUPLIKE CURLIKE

C•••••K
CANNOCK CARJACK CARPARK CARTALK CASSOCK CATWALK CHARPAK CHINOOK CONNICK CONRACK CORKOAK CORMACK COSSACK COWLICK CUTBACK CUTWORK

•CK••••
ACKACKS ECKHART ICKIEST ICKYPOO MCKENNA

•C•••K•
ACKACKS ACTLIKE ICELIKE SCHICKS SCREAKS

•C••••K
ICEMILK ICEPACK ICEPICK ICERINK SCHLOCK SCHNOOK SCHTICK

••CK•••
BACKBAR BACKBAY BACKBIT BACKEND BACKERS BACKHOE BACKING BACKLIT BACKLOG BACKLOT BACKOFF BACKOUT BACKPAY BACKROW BACKRUB BACKSAW BACKSIN BACKSUP BACKUPS BACKWAY BECKETT BECKHAM BECKONS BICKERS BUCKERS BUCKETS BUCKEYE BUCKFOR BUCKING BUCKLED BUCKLES BUCKLEY BUCKNER BUCKOES BUCKRAM BUCKSAW BUCKSUP CACKLED CACKLER CACKLES COCKADE COCKERS COCKIER COCKILY COCKING COCKISH COCKLED COCKLES COCKNEY COCKPIT CUCKOOS DECKERS DECKING DECKLED DECKLES DECKOUT DICKENS DICKERS DICKEYS DICKIES DICKORY DICKSON DOCKAGE DOCKERS DOCKETS DOCKING DUCKERS DUCKIER DUCKIES DUCKING DUCKOUT DUCKPIN FICKLER GECKOES GUCKIER HACKERS HACKETT HACKIES HACKING HACKLED HACKLER HACKLES HACKMAN HACKNEY HACKOFF HACKSAW HACKSIT HACKSUP HECKART HECKLED HECKLER HECKLES HECKMAN HECKUVA HECKYES HICKEYS HICKMAN HICKORY HOCKERS HOCKING JACKALS JACKASS JACKDAW JACKETS JACKIEO JACKING JACKPOT JACKSON JACKSOO JACKSUP JACKTAR JOCKEYS KICKBOX KICKERS KICKIER KICKING KICKOFF KICKOUT KICKSIN KICKSUP KICKUPS LACKEYS LACKING LACKWIT LICKERS LICKETY LICKING LICKSUP LOCKAGE LOCKBOX LOCKEAN LOCKERS LOCKETS LOCKING LOCKINS LOCKJAW LOCKLET LOCKLIN LOCKNUT LOCKOUT LOCKSET LOCKSIN LOCKSON LOCKSUP LOCKUPS LUCKIER LUCKILY LUCKING LUCKMAN LUCKNOW LUCKOUT MICKEYS MOCKERS MOCKERY MOCKING MOCKSUP MOCKUPS MUCKERS MUCKIER MUCKING MUCKSUP NECKERS NECKING NECKLET NECKTIE NICKELS NICKERS NICKING NICKLES NOCKING PACKAGE PACKARD PACKERS PACKETS PACKICE PACKING PACKOFF PACKRAT PACKSIN PACKSON PACKSUP PECKING PECKISH PECKSAT PICKAXE PICKENS PICKERS PICKETS PICKETT PICKIER PICKING PICKLED PICKLES PICKOFF PICKOUT PICKSAT PICKSON PICKSUP PICKUPS POCKETS PUCKERS PUCKERY PUCKETT PUCKISH RACKERS RACKETS RACKETY RACKING RACKOUT RACKSUP RECKONS RICKETY RICKEYS RICKLES RICKMAN RICKSHA ROCKABY ROCKCOD ROCKERS ROCKERY ROCKETS ROCKIER ROCKIES ROCKILY ROCKING ROCKOIL ROCKOON ROCKYII ROCKYIV RUCKERT RUCKING RUCKSUP SACKERS SACKFUL SACKING SACKOUT SACKSUP SECKELS SICKBAY SICKBED SICKDAY SICKENS SICKEST SICKISH SICKLES SICKOUT SICKPAY SOCKETS SOCKEYE SOCKHOP SOCKING SOCKSIN SUCKDRY SUCKERS SUCKIER SUCKING SUCKSIN SUCKSUP TACKERS TACKIER TACKILY TACKING TACKLED TACKLER TACKLES TACKSON TACKSUP TICKERS TICKETS TICKING TICKLED TICKLER TICKLES TICKOFF TICKSBY TUCKERS TUCKING TUCKSIN VICKERS VICKREY WACKEST WACKIER WACKILY WICKERS WICKETS WICKING WICKIUP WICKLOW YUCKIER

••C•K••
NICEKID UNCAKED UNCAKES

••C••K•
RECOCKS RECOOKS RECORKS SACLIKE UNCASKS UNCHOKE UNCORKS

••C•••K
INCHECK RECHALK RECHECK RECRANK UNCHECK UNCLOAK

•••CK••
ALACKOF APECKOF BLACKED BLACKEN BLACKER BLACKIE BLACKLY BLOCKED BLOCKER BLOCKUP BRACKEN BRACKET BRICKED BRICKLE BRICKUP CHECKED CHECKER CHECKIN CHECKON CHECKUP CHICKEN CHOCKED CHUCKED CHUCKIT CHUCKLE CLACKED CLACKER CLICKED CLICKER CLICKON CLOCKED CLOCKER CLOCKIN CLUCKED CLUCKER CRACKED CRACKER CRACKLE CRACKLY CRACKUP CRICKED CRICKET CROCKED CROCKER CROCKET DRUCKER ETICKET FLACKED FLECKED FLICKED FLICKER FLOCKED FLOCKTO FRECKLE FRECKLY FRICKER FROCKED GRACKLE HAECKEL IRECKON JAECKEL KNOCKED KNOCKER KNOCKON KNUCKLE KNUCKLY KRACKEL MENCKEN PLACKET PLUCKED PRICKED PRICKLE PRICKLY PRICKUP QUACKED QUACKER QUICKEN QUICKER QUICKIE QUICKLY SHACKED SHACKLE SHOCKED SHOCKER SHUCKED SHUCKER SLACKED SLACKEN SLACKER SLACKLY SLACKUP SLICKED SLICKER SLICKLY SMACKED SMACKER SMACKOF SMACKUP SMUCKER SNACKED SNACKER SNACKON SNICKER SNICKET SNUCKUP SPACKLE SPECKED SPECKLE STACKED STACKER STACKUP STICKBY STICKER STICKIN STICKON STICKTO STICKUM STICKUP STOCKED STOCKER STOCKUP STUCKBY STUCKIN STUCKON STUCKTO STUCKUP TALCKED THICKEN THICKER THICKET THICKLY TRACKED TRACKER TRICKED TRICKER TRICKLE TRUCKED TRUCKEE TRUCKER TRUCKLE VNECKED VOLCKER WHACKED WHACKER WRACKED WRACKUP WRECKED WRECKER ZINCKED ZWICKAU

•••C•K•
ASHCAKE CHACHKA CODCAKE CUPCAKE EATCAKE HOECAKE HOTCAKE OATCAKE OILCAKE PANCAKE RUMCAKE TEACAKE

•••C••K
BABCOCK BIBCOCK FRYCOOK HANCOCK LEACOCK OAKCASK OLICOOK OUTCOOK PEACOCK PERCHIK PETCOCK PRECOOK SAWCHUK

••••CK•
ACKACKS ARRACKS ATTACKS ATTUCKS BEDECKS CANUCKS CDRACKS COLICKY FINICKY HIJACKS KOPECKS MRLUCKY MUSICKS OPTICKS PANICKY RECOCKS REDOCKS REKICKS RELOCKS REPACKS REPICKS RERACKS RETACKS RUZICKA SCHICKS SHLOCKY SHTICKS SHTICKY THWACKS UNDOCKS UNLOCKS UNLUCKY UNPACKS UNPICKS UNRACKS UNROCKY UNTACKS UNTUCKS UPTICKS

••••C•K
BANACEK JANACEK

•••••CK
AFFLECK AIRLOCK AIRPACK AIRSICK AIRSOCK AIRWICK AMTRACK ANYLUCK ARMLOCK ARTROCK BABCOCK BADBACK BADLUCK BARLICK BARRACK BEDROCK BEQUICK BERBICK BERWICK BIBCOCK BLALOCK BOMBECK BRUBECK BULLOCK BURDICK BUYBACK BYANECK CANNOCK CARJACK CASSOCK CONNICK CONRACK CORMACK COSSACK COWLICK CUTBACK DAYPACK DEFROCK DERRICK DESTOCK DOGTICK DRSPOCK DRYDOCK EARLOCK ELDRICK ELFLOCK EWENECK EYETUCK FATBACK FETLOCK FINBACK FOSDICK GARRICK GATWICK GEDRICK GENLOCK GEODUCK GETBACK GIMMICK GOTBACK GUNLOCK GYMSOCK HADDOCK HAMHOCK HAMMOCK HANCOCK HARNICK HARTACK HASSOCK HATRACK HAYRACK HAYRICK HEMLOCK HENPECK HERRICK HILLOCK HITBACK HOGBACK HOTLICK HOTPACK ICEPACK ICEPICK ILLLUCK INBLACK INCHECK INSHOCK INSTOCK JAMPACK JETPACK JOBLOCK JOEBUCK JUMBUCK KEYLOCK KIDROCK KUBRICK LAMARCK LAYBACK LEACOCK LEBROCK LIEBACK LOWNECK LUBBOCK MADLOCK MATLOCK MATTOCK MEDWICK MERRICK MESSICK MORLOCK MRSPOCK MUDPACK NATWICK NIBLICK NIPMUCK NITPICK NOKNOCK NUMLOCK OARLOCK ODDDUCK ODDSOCK OLDNICK ONAKICK ONESOCK ONTRACK OOBLECK OUTBACK OUTKICK OUTPICK OUTROCK PADDOCK PADLOCK PATRICK PAYBACK PEACOCK PENNOCK PETCOCK PETDUCK PETROCK POLLACK POLLOCK POPROCK POTLUCK PREPACK PREROCK PUTBACK RANBACK RANSACK RATPACK REBLOCK RECHECK REDJACK REDNECK REKNOCK RENWICK RESTACK RESTICK RESTOCK RETRACK RIDDICK RIMROCK RODDICK ROEBUCK ROLLICK ROSTOCK RUNBACK SADSACK SATBACK SAWBUCK SCHLOCK SCHTICK SEADUCK SEASICK SELLECK SETBACK SHYLOCK SITBACK SIXPACK SKIRACK SKYJACK SUNDECK TAYBACK TEANECK TEDMACK THEMICK THEROCK THESACK TIEBACK TIERACK TIETACK TOEPICK TOPKICK TUSSOCK UNBLOCK UNCHECK UNFROCK UNQUICK UNSLACK UNSLICK UNSTACK UNSTICK UNSTUCK UNTHICK UNTRACK VANDYCK VANEYCK VANWYCK VARRICK VEENECK WARLOCK WARWICK WAYBACK WEDLOCK WINBACK WOZZECK YANNICK YASBECK ZIPLOCK

CL•••••
CLABBER CLACKED CLACKER CLACTON CLADDED CLAIMED CLAIMER CLAIROL CLAMANT CLAMATO CLAMBAR CLAMBER CLAMDIP CLAMMED CLAMMER CLAMORS CLAMOUR CLAMPED CLAMPER CLAMPON CLAMSUP CLANGED CLANGER CLANGOR CLANKED CLANTON CLAPFOR CLAPPED CLAPPER CLAPTON CLAQUES CLARETS CLARICE CLARIFY CLARION CLARITY CLASHED CLASHER CLASHES CLASPED CLASPER CLASSED CLASSER CLASSES CLASSIC CLASSON CLATTER CLAUDEL CLAUDIA CLAUDIO CLAUSAL CLAUSES CLAVATE CLAVELL CLAVIER CLAWERS CLAWING CLAWSAT CLAYIER CLAYING CLAYISH CLAYPIT CLAYTON CLEANED CLEANER CLEANLY CLEANSE CLEANTE CLEANUP

CLEARED
CLEARER
CLEARLY
CLEAROF
CLEARUP
CLEATED
CLEAVED
CLEAVER
CLEAVES
CLEAVON
CLEMENS
CLEMENT
CLEMSON
CLERICS
CLERISY
CLERKED
CLERKLY
CLEWING
CLIBURN
CLICHED
CLICHES
CLICKED
CLICKER
CLICKON
CLIENTS
CLIFTON
CLIMATE
CLIMATS
CLIMBED
CLIMBER
CLIMBIN
CLIMBON
CLIMBTO
CLIMBUP
CLINGER
CLINGTO
CLINICS
CLINKED
CLINKER
CLINTON
CLIPART
CLIPOFF
CLIPONS
CLIPOUT
CLIPPED
CLIPPER
CLIPSON
CLIQUED
CLIQUES
CLIQUEY
CLOAKED
CLOBBER
CLOCHES
CLOCKED
CLOCKER
CLOCKIN
CLOGGED
CLOGSUP
CLOMPED
CLONERS
CLONING
CLONKED
CLOONEY
CLOPPED
CLORETS
CLOSEBY
CLOSEIN
CLOSELY
CLOSERS
CLOSEST
CLOSETO
CLOSETS
CLOSEUP
CLOSING
CLOSURE
CLOTHED
CLOTHES
CLOTSUP
CLOTTED
CLOTURE
CLOUDED
CLOUDUP
CLOUTED
CLOUTER
CLOVERS
CLOVERY
CLOWDER
CLOWNED
CLOYING
CLUBBED
CLUBBER
CLUBCAR
CLUBMED
CLUBSUP
CLUCKED
CLUCKER
CLUEDIN
CLUEFUL
CLUEING
CLUESIN
CLUMPED
CLUNGTO
CLUNKED
CLUNKER
CLUSTER
CLUTCHY
CLUTTER

C•L••••

CALABRO
CALAMAR
CALANDO
CALCIFY
CALCITE
CALCIUM
CALCULI
CALDERA
CALDERS
CALDRON
CALENDS
CALGARY
CALHOUN
CALIBAN
CALIBER
CALIBRE
CALICES
CALICOS
CALIPER
CALIPHS
CALISTA
CALKERS
CALKING
CALKINS
CALLBOX
CALLBOY
CALLEES
CALLERS
CALLFOR
CALLING
CALLINS
CALLNOW
CALLOFF
CALLOUS
CALLOUT
CALLSIN
CALLSIT
CALLSON
CALLSTO
CALLSUP
CALLUPS
CALMEST
CALMING
CALMSEA
CALORIC
CALORIE
CALOTTE
CALPOLY
CALTECH
CALUMET
CALUMNY
CALVARY
CALVERT
CALVING
CALVINO
CALYCES
CALYPSO
CALYXES
CALZONE
CCLAMPS
CELADON
CELAENO
CELEBES
CELEBRE
CELESTA
CELESTE
CELICAS
CELLARS
CELLINI
CELLIST
CELLULE
CELOTEX
CELSIUS
CELTICS
CHLORIC
CILENTO
CILIARY
CILIATE
COLADAS
COLBERT
COLCHIS
COLDCUP
COLDCUT
COLDDAY
COLDEST
COLDISH
COLDONE
COLDWAR
COLEMAN
COLETTE
COLGATE
COLICKY
COLLAGE
COLLARD
COLLARS
COLLATE
COLLECT
COLLEEN
COLLEGE
COLLETS
COLLIDE
COLLIER
COLLIES
COLLINE
COLLINS
COLLODI
COLLOID
COLLOPS
COLLUDE
COLLYER
COLOGNE
COLOMBO
COLONEL
COLONES
COLONNA
COLONUS
COLORED
COLORER
COLORTV
COLOSSI
COLOURS
COLTISH
COLUMBA
COLUMBO
COLUMNS
CPLUSES
CSLEWIS
CULCHES
CULEXES
CULLERS
CULLETS
CULLIED
CULLIES
CULLING
CULOTTE
CULPRIT
CULTISH
CULTISM
CULTIST
CULTJAM
CULTURE
CULVERT

C••L•••

CABLERS
CABLETS
CABLETV
CABLING
CAILLOU
CALLBOX
CALLBOY
CALLEES
CALLERS
CALLFOR
CALLING
CALLINS
CALLNOW
CALLOFF
CALLOUS
CALLOUT
CALLSIN
CALLSIT
CALLSON
CALLSTO
CALLSUP
CALLUPS
CAPLESS
CAPLETS
CARLENE
CARLESS
CARLING
CARLOAD
CARLOAN
CARLOTA
CARLOTS
CARLSON
CARLTON
CARLYLE
CATLIKE
CAULKED
CAULKER
CDALBUM
CEILING
CELLARS
CELLINI
CELLIST
CELLULE
CHALCIS
CHALETS
CHALICE
CHALKED
CHALKUP
CHALLAH
CHALONS
CHALUPA
CHELATE
CHELSEA
CHILCAT
CHILEAN
CHILIAD
CHILIES
CHILKAT
CHILLED
CHILLER
CHILLIS
CHILLUM
CHOLERA
CHOLERS
CHOLINE
CHOLLAS
COALBIN
COALCAR
COALERS
COALGAS
COALING
COALOIL
COALPIT
COALTAR
COBLENZ
COILERS
COILING
COILSUP
COLLAGE
COLLARD
COLLARS
COLLATE
COLLECT
COLLEEN
COLLEGE
COLLETS
COLLIDE
COLLIER
COLLIES
COLLINE
COLLINS
COLLODI
COLLOID
COLLOPS
COLLUDE
COLLYER
COOLAIR
COOLANT
COOLCAT
COOLERS
COOLEST
COOLIES
COOLING
COOLISH
COOLMAX
COOLOUT
COOLPIX
COOLSIT
COPLAND
COULDBE
COULDNT
COULEES
COULOMB
COULTER
COWLICK
COWLIKE
COWLING
COXLESS
CRULLER
CULLERS
CULLETS
CULLIED
CULLIES
CULLING
CUPLIKE
CURLERS
CURLEWS
CURLIER
CURLIKE
CURLING
CURLSIN
CURLSUP
CUTLASS
CUTLERS
CUTLERY
CUTLETS
CYCLERS
CYCLING
CYCLIST
CYCLOID
CYCLONE
CYCLOPS

C•••L••

CABALAS
CABALLE
CACKLED
CACKLER
CACKLES
CAILLOU
CAJOLED
CAJOLER
CAJOLES
CAMELID
CAMELOT
CAMILLA
CAMILLE
CANALED
CANDLED
CANDLER
CANDLES
CANOLAS
CANTLES
CANULAE
CANULAS
CAPELET
CAPELLA
CAPULET
CARCLUB
CAROLED
CAROLER
CAROLII
CAROLYN
CASELAW
CASELLA
CASELOT
CASTLED
CASTLES
CATALAN
CATALOG
CATALOS
CATALPA
CATFLAP
CATFLEA
CAVALRY
CAVILAT
CAVILED
CAVILER
CECILIA
CEDILLA
CHABLIS
CHALLAH
CHAPLET
CHAPLIN
CHARLES
CHARLEY
CHARLIE
CHEMLAB
CHICLES
CHICLET
CHILLED
CHILLER
CHILLIS
CHILLUM
CHITLIN
CHOLLAS
CICHLID
CIRCLED
CIRCLER
CIRCLES
CIRCLET
CIVILLY
COBALTS
COBBLED
COBBLER
COBBLES
COCHLEA
COCKLED
COCKLES
CODDLED
CODDLER
CODDLES
COGGLES
COGHLAN
COMPLEX
COMPLIN
CONELET
CONKLIN
COPILOT
COPULAE
COPULAR
COPULAS
CORELLI
COROLLA
COUPLED
COUPLER
COUPLES
COUPLET
COWSLIP
CRADLED
CRADLER
CRADLES
CRAWLED
CRAWLER
CRAWLEY
CREELEY
CREOLES
CROWLEY
CRUELER
CRUELLA
CRUELLY
CRUELTY
CRULLER
CUDDLED
CUDDLES
CUMULUS
CUPELED
CUPELER
CUPOLAS
CUPULAR
CUPULES
CURDLED
CURDLER
CURDLES
CUSSLER

C••••L•

CABALLE
CABBALA
CALCULI
CALPOLY
CAMILLA
CAMILLE
CAMPILY
CAMRYLE
CANCELS
CANDELA
CANFULS
CANNELL
CANNELS
CANNILY
CANNOLI
CANNULA
CANTALS
CANTILY
CAPABLE
CAPABLY
CAPELLA
CAPFULS
CAPSULE
CARFULS
CARIOLE
CARLYLE
CARMELA
CARPALS
CARPELS
CARRELS
CARROLL
CARSALE
CARTALK
CARTELS
CARVELS
CASELLA
CASSOLA
CASTILE
CASUALS
CATCALL
CATTALO
CATTILY
CATWALK
CEDILLA
CELLULE
CEMBALO
CENACLE
CENTALS
CEPHALO
CEPHALY
CEREALS
CHAGALL
CHANELS
CHAPALA
CHAPELS
CHARILY
CHEADLE
CHEAPLY
CHIEFLY
CHISELS
CHORALE
CHORALS
CHORTLE
CHUCKLE
CINEOLE
CITABLE
CIVILLY
CLAVELL
CLEANLY
CLEARLY
CLERKLY
CLOSELY
COCKILY
COEVALS
COMPELS
COMPILE
CONDOLE
CONSOLE
CONSULS
CONSULT
COPPOLA
CORACLE
CORBELS
CORDELL
CORELLI
CORNELL
CORNILY
COROLLA
CORRALS
CORYELL
COURTLY
COWBELL
CRACKLE
CRACKLY
CRAPOLA
CRASSLY
CRAYOLA
CRAZILY
CRENELS
CREWELS
CRINKLE
CRINKLY
CRIPPLE
CRISPLY
CROSSLY
CROWELL
CRUDELY
CRUELLA
CRUELLY
CRUMBLE
CRUMBLY
CRUMPLE
CRUMPLY
CRYWOLF
CUBICLE
CUBICLY
CUDGELS
CUEBALL
CUPFULS
CURABLE
CURABLY
CUREALL
CUSHILY
CUTICLE
CYMBALS

C•••••L

CAMERAL
CAMGIRL
CANNELL
CAPITAL
CAPITOL
CARAMEL
CARAVEL
CARDIAL
CAREFUL
CARPOOL
CARROLL
CASTROL
CATBOWL
CATCALL
CATTAIL
CENTRAL
CHAGALL
CHANCEL
CHANNEL
CHASMAL
CHATTEL
CHERVIL
CHORDAL
CHUNNEL
CITADEL
CITYGAL
CLAIROL
CLAUDEL
CLAUSAL
CLAVELL
CLUEFUL
COALOIL
COASTAL
COAXIAL
COBCOAL
CODICIL
COEQUAL
COLONEL
COMICAL
CONCEAL
CONGEAL
CONICAL
CONTROL
CORDELL
CORDIAL
CORNEAL
CORNELL
CORNOIL
CORONAL
CORYELL
COUNCIL
COUNSEL
COWBELL
COWGIRL
COZUMEL
CRANIAL
CREEDAL
CREOSOL
CROWELL
CRUCIAL
CRUSTAL
CRYSTAL
CUBICAL
CUBITAL
CUEBALL
CUREALL
CURTAIL
CYNICAL

•CL••••

BCLIONS
CCLAMPS
ECLAIRS
ECLIPSE
ECLOGUE
MCLUHAN
SCLAFFS
SCLERAE
SCLERAL
SCLERAS

•C•L•••

ACCLAIM
ACOLYTE
ACTLIKE
ECCLESI
ECOLOGY
ICELAND
ICELESS
ICELIKE
ICELINE
MCALLEN
MCCLOUD
MCCLURE
MCCLURG
OCALAFL
OCCLUDE
OCELLAR
OCELLUS
OCELOTS
OCULARS
OCULIST
PCCLONE
SCALAGE
SCALARS
SCALDED
SCALDER
SCALENE
SCALERS
SCALEUP
SCALIER
SCALING
SCALLOP
SCALPED
SCALPEL
SCALPER
SCHLEPP
SCHLEPS
SCHLITZ
SCHLOCK
SCHLUBS
SCHLUMP
SCOLARI
SCOLDED
SCOLDER
SCULLED
SCULLER
SCULPED
SCULPTS

•C••L••

ACDELCO
ACHILLE
ACRYLIC
ACYCLIC
ECHELON
ECUELLE
ICEBLUE
ICEFLOE
ICICLES
MCALLEN
MCCALLS
MCHALES
MCNALLY
OCCULTS
OCELLAR
OCELLUS
RCCOLAS
SCALLOP
SCARLET
SCHELDT
SCHOLAR
SCHOLES
SCHULTZ
SCOWLED
SCOWLER
SCROLLS
SCULLED
SCULLER
UCCELLO

•C•••L•

ACEROLA
ACETALS
ACHILLE
ACOUPLE
ACRIDLY
ACTABLE
ACTORLY
ACUTELY
ECUELLE
ICECOLD
ICEFALL
ICEHOLE
ICEMILK
MCARDLE
MCCALLS
MCNALLY
MCNEILL
OCTUPLE
OCTUPLY
PCWORLD
SCANTLY
SCAPULA
SCARILY
SCHOOLS
SCRAWLS
SCRAWLY
SCROLLS
SCRUPLE
SCUFFLE
SCUTTLE
UCCELLO

•C••••L

ACAUDAL
ACCRUAL
ACCUSAL
ECTYPAL
ICEFALL
JCARROL
MCNEILL
OCALAFL
OCTAVAL
SCALPEL
SCANDAL
SCLERAL

••CL•••

ACCLAIM
ARCLAMP
BECLOUD
CYCLERS
CYCLING
CYCLIST
CYCLOID
CYCLONE
CYCLOPS
DECLAIM
DECLARE
DECLASS
DECLAWS
DECLINE
DECLOTS
ECCLESI
ENCLASP
ENCLAVE
ENCLOSE
EXCLAIM
EXCLAVE
EXCLUDE
INCLASS
INCLINE
INCLOSE
INCLUDE
MACLEAN
MACLEOD

MCCLOUD
MCCLURE
MCCLURG
MRCLEAN
NOCLASS
NUCLEAR
NUCLEIC
NUCLEON
NUCLEUS
NUCLIDE
OCCLUDE
PCCLONE
RECLADS
RECLAIM
RECLAME
RECLASP
RECLASS
RECLEAN
RECLIMB
RECLINE
RECLUSE
SACLIKE
SECLUDE
STCLOUD
UNCLAMP
UNCLASP
UNCLEAN
UNCLEAR
UNCLEFT
UNCLIPS
UNCLIPT
UNCLOAK
UNCLOGS
UNCLOSE
UNCLOUD
UPCLIMB
UPCLOSE

••C•L••

AACELLS
ALCALDE
BACILLI
BACKLIT
BACKLOG
BACKLOT
BECALMS
BICOLOR
BOCELLI
BUCKLED
BUCKLES
BUCKLEY
BUCOLIC
CACKLED
CACKLER
CACKLES
CECILIA
CICHLID
COCHLEA
COCKLED
COCKLES
DECALOG
DECILES
DECKLED
DECKLES
DECOLOR
DICILLO
DUCALLY
ESCALOP
ESCALUS
EXCELAT
EXCELIN
FACULAE
FACULTY
FICKLER
FOCSLES
HACKLED
HACKLER
HACKLES
HECKLED
HECKLER
HECKLES
INCOLOR
JACALES
JOCELYN
JOCULAR
LOCALES
LOCALLY
LOCKLET
LOCKLIN
LOCULUS
LUCILLE
LUCYLIU
MACULAE
MACULAR
MCCALLS
MECHLIN
NACELLE
NBCBLUE
NECKLET
NICKLES
NICOLAS
NICOLET
NICOLLE
OCCULTS
OSCULAR
OSCULES
PACELAP
PICKLED
PICKLES
RCCOLAS
RECALLS
RECOLOR
RICHLER
RICKLES
SECULAR
SICILIA
SICKLES
TACKLED
TACKLER
TACKLES
TICKLED
TICKLER
TICKLES
TOCELIA
UCCELLO
VOCALIC
VOCALLY
WICKLOW
ZOCALOS

••C••L•

AACELLS
ARCWELD
BACILLI
BICYCLE
BOCELLI
COCKILY
DACTYLS
DECARLO
DECUPLE
DICILLO
DUCALLY
DUCTILE
ESCUELA
FACIALS
FICTILE
JACKALS
LICITLY
LLCOOLJ
LOCALLY
LUCIDLY
LUCILLE
LUCKILY
MCCALLS
MICAELA
NACELLE
NICCOLO
NICHOLS
NICKELS
NICOLLE
OSCEOLA
PACBELL
PICCOLO
RECABLE
RECALLS
RECHALK
RECHALL
RECOALS
RECOILS
RECOOLS
RECURLS
RECYCLE
ROCKILY
SECKELS
SOCIALS
TACITLY
TACKILY
TACTILE
UCCELLO
UNCIALS
UNCOILS
UNCOYLY
UNCURLS
UPCOILS
UPCURLS
VACUOLE
VOCABLE
VOCABLY
VOCALLY
WACKILY

••C•••L

ACCRUAL
ACCUSAL
ALCOHOL
BSCHOOL
DECIBEL
DECIMAL
EXCUSAL
FACTFUL
FACTUAL
INCIVIL
ISCHIAL
LACTEAL
LACUNAL
MACNEIL
MICHAEL
OHCAROL
PACBELL
QSCHOOL
RACHAEL
RECHALL
RECITAL
RECUSAL
ROCKOIL
SACKFUL
TACTFUL
TACTUAL
UNCIVIL
UNCRUEL
VICINAL
VICTUAL

•••CL••

ACYCLIC
ALLCLAD
ATACLIP
BARCLAY
CARCLUB
CHICLES
CHICLET
CIRCLED
CIRCLER
CIRCLES
CIRCLET
DEWCLAW
EARCLIP
FANCLUB
GYMCLUB
ICICLES
ILLCLAD
KEYCLUB
MUSCLED
MUSCLES
ONECLAM
ONECLUB
ORACLES
PROCLUS
REDCLAY
SUBCLAN
TIECLIP
WARCLUB
WROCLAW

•••C•L•

AAACELL
BADCALL
BADCOLD
BLACKLY
BLACULA
BRICKLE
CALCULI
CANCELS
CATCALL
CHUCKLE
CRACKLE
CRACKLY
DASCHLE
DRACULA
DRYCELL
ERECTLY
EXACTLY
FANCILY
FATCELL
FOSCOLO
FRECKLE
FRECKLY
GETCOLD
GLYCOLS
GOTCOLD
GRACILE
GRACKLE
HERCULE
HOGCALL
HOSCALE
ICECOLD
ILLCALL
INOCULA
INSCALE
ITSCOLD
JUICILY
KNUCKLE
KNUCKLY
LASCALA
LINCOLN
LYOCELL
MALCOLM
MARCELS
MESCALS
METCALF
MISCALL
NICCOLO
NONCOLA
ONECALL
ONECELL
OUTCALL
OUTCOLD
OUTCULL
PARCELS
PASCOLI
PENCILS
PERCALE
PETCALF
PICCOLO
PRICILY
PRICKLE
PRICKLY
PURCELL
QUICKLY
RASCALS
REDCELL
RESCALE
SAUCILY
SEACALM
SHACKLE
SLACKLY
SLICKLY
SPACELY
SPACKLE
SPECKLE
SPICILY
SUBCELL
TERCELS
THICKLY
TOSCALE
TRICKLE
TRUCKLE
UNSCALY
UPSCALE
URACILS
VINCULA
WETCELL

•••C••L

AAACELL
AIRCOOL
ASOCIAL
BADCALL
CATCALL
COBCOAL
CONCEAL
CRUCIAL
DRYCELL
EDICTAL
EPOCHAL
FASCIAL
FATCELL
FRACTAL
GLACIAL
HAECKEL
HOGCALL
HOTCOAL
ILLCALL
JAECKEL
JOECOOL
KRACKEL
LYOCELL
MISCALL
ONECALL
ONECELL
OUTCALL
OUTCULL
PASCHAL
PINCURL
PRECOIL
PRECOOL
PURCELL
REDCELL
SATCHEL
SPACIAL
SPECIAL
SUBCELL
SUBCOOL
WAYCOOL
WETCELL

••••CL•

ARTICLE
AURICLE
BICYCLE
CENACLE
CORACLE
CUBICLE
CUBICLY
CUTICLE
DEBACLE
MANACLE
MIRACLE
MONOCLE
OSSICLE
PANICLE
RADICLE
RECYCLE
RETICLE
TREACLE
TREACLY
TUNICLE
VEHICLE
VESICLE
WAVICLE

••••C•L

BIFOCAL
CHANCEL
CODICIL
COMICAL
CONICAL
COUNCIL
CUBICAL
CYNICAL
DOMICAL
DOMICIL
ETHICAL
FINICAL
HELICAL
LEXICAL
LOGICAL
LYRICAL
MAGICAL
MEDICAL
MUSICAL
NODICAL
OPTICAL
RADICAL
STENCIL
STOICAL
TOPICAL
TYPICAL
UNLOCAL
UNVOCAL
VATICAL
XENICAL

C•M••••

CAMACHO
CAMAROS
CAMBERS
CAMBOYS
CAMBRIA
CAMBRIC
CAMEDUE
CAMELID
CAMELOT
CAMEOED
CAMEOFF
CAMEOUT
CAMERAE
CAMERAL
CAMERAS
CAMERON
CAMGIRL
CAMILLA
CAMILLE
CAMINOS
CAMIONS
CAMISES
CAMMIES
CAMPARI
CAMPBED
CAMPERS
CAMPHOR
CAMPIER
CAMPILY
CAMPING
CAMPION
CAMPOUT
CAMPSUP
CAMRYLE
CEMBALO
CEMENTS
CIMABUE
COMAKER
COMBATS
COMBERS
COMBIEN
COMBINE
COMBING
COMBUST
COMCAST
COMEDIA
COMEDIC
COMEDIE
COMEDUE
COMENOW
COMEOFF
COMEONS
COMEOUT
COMESAS
COMESAT
COMESBY
COMESIN
COMESON
COMESTO
COMESUP
COMFIER
COMFITS
COMFORT
COMICAL
COMICES
COMINGS
COMIQUE
COMMAND
COMMEND
COMMENT
COMMISH
COMMITS
COMMODE
COMMONS
COMMOVE
COMMUNE
COMMUTE
COMORAN
COMOROS
COMPACT
COMPANY
COMPAQS
COMPARE
COMPART
COMPASS
COMPEER
COMPELS
COMPEND
COMPERE
COMPETE
COMPILE
COMPING
COMPLEX
COMPLIN
COMPORT
COMPOSE
COMPOST
COMPOTE
COMPTON
COMPUTE
COMRADE
COMSATS
COMTISM
COMTIST
COMTREX
CUMBERS
CUMBIAS
CUMBRIA
CUMSHAW
CUMULUS
CYMBALS
CYMRICS

C••M•••

CADMIUM
CAIMANS
CALMEST
CALMING
CALMSEA
CAMMIES
CARMELA
CARMINA
CARMINE
CATMINT
CAYMANS
CHAMBER
CHAMBRE
CHAMFER
CHAMOIS
CHAMPED
CHAMPER
CHEMISE
CHEMIST
CHEMLAB
CHIMEIN
CHIMERA
CHIMERS
CHIMING
CHIMINH
CHIMNEY
CHOMPED
CHOMPON
CHOMSKY
CHUMASH
CHUMMED
CHUMPED
CLAMANT
CLAMATO
CLAMBAR
CLAMBER
CLAMDIP
CLAMMED
CLAMMER
CLAMORS
CLAMOUR
CLAMPED
CLAMPER
CLAMPON
CLAMSUP
CLEMENS
CLEMENT
CLEMSON
CLIMATE
CLIMATS
CLIMBED
CLIMBER
CLIMBIN
CLIMBON
CLIMBTO
CLIMBUP
CLOMPED
CLUMPED
COMMAND
COMMEND
COMMENT
COMMISH
COMMITS
COMMODE
COMMONS
COMMOVE
COMMUNE
COMMUTE
CONMOTO
CORMACK
CRAMMED
CRAMMER
CRAMPED
CRAMPON
CRAMSIN
CREMATE
CREMINI
CREMONA
CREMORA
CRIMEAN
CRIMINY
CRIMPED
CRIMPER
CRIMSON
CRUMBED
CRUMBLE
CRUMBLY
CRUMBUM
CRUMPED
CRUMPET
CRUMPLE
CRUMPLY

C•••M••

CAKEMIX
CALAMAR
CALUMET
CALUMNY
CAPEMAY
CARAMBA
CARAMEL
CARAMIA
CAROMED
CASIMIR
CAVEMAN
CAVEMEN
CCLAMPS
CERAMIC
CERUMEN
CESTMOI
CHAPMAN
CHAPMEN
CHARMAN
CHARMED
CHARMEN
CHARMER
CHARMIN
CHASMAL
CHASMIC
CHEXMIX
CHEZMOI
CHROMAT
CHROMED
CHROMES
CHROMIC
CHUMMED
CINEMAS
CINEMAX
CLAIMED
CLAIMER
CLAMMED
CLAMMER
CLUBMED
COLEMAN
COLOMBO
COLUMBA
COLUMBO
COLUMNS
COOLMAX
COPYMAN
COPYMEN
COZUMEL
CRAMMED
CRAMMER
CRANMER
CREAMED
CREAMER
CREWMAN
CREWMEN

C••••M•

CATCOMB
CENTIME
CENTIMO
CHRISMS
CONDEMN
CONGAME
CONSUME
CONTEMN
CORFAMS
COSTUME
COULOMB
COVERME
COXCOMB
CUSTOMS
CUTTIME

C•••••M

CACONYM
CADMIUM
CALCIUM
CARDIUM
CDALBUM
CENTRUM
CHATHAM
CHETRUM
CHEWGUM
CHILLUM
CHRISOM
COMTISM
CONFIRM
CONFORM
COUNTEM
CPAEXAM
CRANIUM
CRUMBUM
CULTISM
CULTJAM
CUTWORM
CZARDOM
CZARISM

•CM••••

MCMAHON
MCMURDO

•C•M•••

ACUMENS
ICEMILK
SCAMMED
SCAMMER
SCAMPED
SCAMPER
SCHMEAR
SCHMEER
SCHMIDT
SCHMITT
SCHMOES

•C••M••

CCLAMPS
ECZEMAS
SCAMMED
SCAMMER
SCATMAN
SCHEMAS
SCHEMED
SCHEMER
SCHEMES
SCHUMER
SCRIMPS
SCRIMPY

•C•••M•

ACADEME
ACADEMY
ECONOMY
ICEDAMS
MCADAMS
MCCRUMB
RCADOME
SCHISMS
SCHLUMP
SCREAMS
SCUSEME

•C••••M

ACCLAIM
ACRONYM
ECHOISM
LCHAYIM

••CM•••

MICMACS

••C•M••

BACHMAN
BECOMES
BUCHMAN
DECAMPS
DECIMAL
ELCAMPO
ENCAMPS
ENCOMIA
HACKMAN
HECKMAN
HICKMAN
INCOMER
INCOMES
JACAMAR
JICAMAS
LUCKMAN
NICEMAN
NICEMEN
RACEMES
RECOMBS
RICHMAN
RICHMEN
RICKMAN
TACOMAS
TUCHMAN
UNCOMIC
VICOMTE

••C••M•

ALCHEMY
ARCLAMP
BECALMS
DECRUMB
DICTUMS
DUCHAMP
LACRIMO
LYCEUMS
MACRAME
MCCRUMB
RECLAME
RECLIMB
SACHEMS
SUCCUMB
UNCLAMP
UNCRAMP
UPCLIMB
VACUUMS
VICTIMS

••C•••M

ACCLAIM
AFCTEAM
ARCANUM
BECHARM
BECKHAM
BUCKRAM
CACONYM
DECLAIM
DECORUM
EXCLAIM
ISCHIUM
MACADAM
NFCTEAM
RECLAIM
RECROOM

•••CM••

DISCMAN

•••C•M•

ATACAMA
BUSCEMI
CATCOMB
COXCOMB
DAYCAMP
DOGCOMB
DOTCOMS
DRACHMA
ELECTME
GIACOMO

HOTCOMB
HOWCOME
JAMCAMS
JOECAMP
KIDCOMS
LANCOME
NONCOMS
OUTCOME
PETCOMB
PINCHME
ROMCOMS
SATCHMO
SATCOMS
SITCOMS
SKYCAMS
SPYCAMS
SUCCUMB
TALCUMS
VANCAMP
WEBCAMS
WELCOME
ZITCOMS

•••C••M

BEACHAM
BEECHAM
CALCIUM
FASCISM
FULCRUM
GRECISM
JOACHIM
KETCHAM
KETCHUM
MALCOLM
MITCHUM
ONECLAM
SANCTUM
SARCASM
SEACALM
STICKUM

••••C•M

BRITCOM
DIGICAM
FAMICOM
MINICAM
MODICUM
TELECOM

CN•••••

CNOSSUS
CNTOWER

C•N••••

CANALED
CANAPES
CANARDS
CANASTA
CANCANS
CANCELS
CANCERS
CANCHAS
CANDACE
CANDELA
CANDENT
CANDICE
CANDIDA
CANDIDE
CANDIDS
CANDIED
CANDIES
CANDLED
CANDLER
CANDLES
CANDOUR
CANETTI
CANFULS
CANIDAE
CANIEST
CANINES
CANINGS
CANITBE
CANKERS
CANNELL
CANNELS
CANNERS
CANNERY
CANNIER
CANNILY
CANNING
CANNOCK
CANNOLI
CANNONS
CANNULA
CANOERS
CANOLAS
CANONIC
CANONRY
CANOPUS
CANSECO
CANTABS
CANTALS
CANTATA
CANTEEN
CANTERS
CANTILY
CANTINA
CANTING
CANTINO
CANTLES
CANTONS
CANTORS
CANTRIP
CANTSAY
CANUCKS
CANULAE
CANULAS
CANVASS
CANYONS
CANZONA
CANZONE
CANZONI
CENACLE
CENSERS
CENSING
CENSORS
CENSURE
CENTALS
CENTARE
CENTAUR
CENTAVO
CENTERS
CENTIME
CENTIMO
CENTRAL
CENTRED
CENTRES
CENTRIC
CENTRUM
CENTURY
CINCHED
CINCHES
CINDERS
CINDERY
CINEMAS
CINEMAX
CINEOLE
CINERGY
CINESIA
CINQUES
CINZANO
CONAGRA
CONAKRY
CONBRIO
CONCAVE
CONCEAL
CONCEDE
CONCEIT
CONCEPT
CONCERN
CONCERT
CONCHAE
CONCHES
CONCHOS
CONCISE
CONCOCT
CONCORD
CONCURS
CONCUSS
CONDEMN
CONDIGN
CONDOLE
CONDONE
CONDORS
CONDUCE
CONDUCT
CONDUIT
CONELET
CONFABS
CONFECT
CONFERS
CONFESS
CONFIDE
CONFINE
CONFIRM
CONFITS
CONFORM
CONFREY
CONFUSE
CONFUTE
CONGAED
CONGAME
CONGEAL
CONGERS
CONGEST
CONGOUS
CONICAL
CONIFER
CONJOBS
CONJOIN
CONJURE
CONJURY
CONKERS
CONKING
CONKLIN
CONKOFF
CONKOUT
CONMOTO
CONNATE
CONNECT
CONNERY
CONNICK
CONNIFF
CONNING
CONNIVE
CONNORS
CONNOTE
CONOIDS
CONQUER
CONRACK
CONRIED
CONSENT
CONSIGN
CONSIST
CONSOLE
CONSORT
CONSULS
CONSULT
CONSUME
CONTACS
CONTACT
CONTAIN
CONTEMN
CONTEND
CONTENT
CONTEST
CONTEXT
CONTORT
CONTOUR
CONTRAS
CONTROL
CONTUSE
CONURES
CONVECT
CONVENE
CONVENT
CONVERT
CONVEYS
CONVICT
CONVOKE
CONVOYS
CUNEATE
CUNNING
CYNICAL
CYNTHIA

C••N•••

CANNELL
CANNELS
CANNERS
CANNERY
CANNIER
CANNILY
CANNING
CANNOCK
CANNOLI
CANNONS
CANNULA
CAPNUTS
CARNABY
CARNAGE
CARNERA
CARNETS
CARNIES
CATNAPS
CATNIPS
CBSNEWS
CHANCED
CHANCEL
CHANCER
CHANCES
CHANELS
CHANGED
CHANGER
CHANGES
CHANNEL
CHANOYU
CHANSON
CHANTED
CHANTER
CHANTEY
CHANTRY
CHENIER
CHINESE
CHINKED
CHINNED
CHINOIS
CHINOOK
CHINTZY
CHINUPS
CHINWAG
CHUNKED
CHUNNEL
CLANGED
CLANGER
CLANGOR
CLANKED
CLANTON
CLINGER
CLINGTO
CLINICS
CLINKED
CLINKER
CLINTON
CLONERS
CLONING
CLONKED
CLUNGTO
CLUNKED
CLUNKER
COBNUTS
COGNACS
COGNATE
COGNIZE
COINAGE
COINBOX
COINERS
COINING
COINOPS
CONNATE
CONNECT
CONNERY
CONNICK
CONNIFF
CONNING
CONNIVE
CONNORS
CONNOTE
COONCAN
COONCAT
COONDOG
CORNBIN
CORNCOB
CORNDOG
CORNEAL
CORNEAS
CORNELL
CORNERS
CORNETS
CORNFED
CORNICE
CORNIER
CORNILY
CORNING
CORNISH
CORNOIL
CORNROW
CORNUTE
COUNCIL
COUNSEL
COUNTED
COUNTEE
COUNTEM
COUNTER
COUNTIN
COUNTON
COUNTRY
COUNTUP
COYNESS
CRANIAL
CRANING
CRANIUM
CRANKED
CRANKUP
CRANMER
CRENATE
CRENELS
CRINGED
CRINGES
CRINKLE
CRINKLY
CRONIES
CRUNCHY
CTENOID
CUINGIN
CUNNING
CYANIDE
CYANIDS
CYGNETS

C•••N••

CABANAS
CABINET
CACONYM
CADENCE
CADENCY
CADENZA
CAIRNED
CALANDO
CALENDS
CALLNOW
CAMINOS
CANINES
CANINGS
CANONIC
CANONRY
CARINAE
CARINAS
CASINGS
CASINOS
CATANIA
CATENAE
CATENAS
CAYENNE
CEMENTS
CESSNAS
CETANES
CEZANNE
CHAINED
CHAINES
CHAINUP
CHANNEL
CHARNIN
CHIANTI
CHIGNON
CHIMNEY
CHINNED
CHRONIC
CHUNNEL
CHURNED
CHURNER
CHURNUP
CHUTNEY
CILENTO
CLEANED
CLEANER
CLEANLY
CLEANSE
CLEANTE
CLEANUP
CLIENTS
CLOONEY
CLOWNED
COCKNEY
COCONUT
COGENCY
COIGNED
COIGNES
COLONEL
COLONES
COLONNA
COLONUS
COMENOW
COMINGS
COOWNED
CORINNE
CORINTH
CORONAE
CORONAL
CORONAS
CORONER
CORONET
COSINES
COSTNER
COZENED
COZENER
CROONED
CROONER
CROWNED
CROWNER
CUTINON
CUTINTO

C••••N•

CABBING
CABLING
CABRINI
CACHING
CADGING
CAFTANS
CAIMANS
CAIRENE
CALKING
CALKINS
CALLING
CALLINS
CALMING
CALUMNY
CALVING
CALVINO
CALZONE
CAMIONS
CAMPING
CANCANS
CANDENT
CANNING
CANNONS
CANTINA
CANTING
CANTINO
CANTONS
CANYONS
CANZONA
CANZONE
CANZONI
CAPEANN
CAPGUNS
CAPPING
CAPRINE
CAPUANA
CARBINE
CARBONS
CARDING
CAREENS
CARKING
CARLENE
CARLING
CARMINA
CARMINE
CARPING
CARTING
CARTONS
CARVING
CASEINS
CASERNE
CASERNS
CASHING
CASHINS
CASKING
CASSINI
CASSINO
CASTING
CATIONS
CATKINS
CATMINT
CAUSING
CAVEINS
CAVERNS
CAYENNE
CAYMANS
CEASING
CEILING
CELAENO
CELLINI
CENSING
CERVINE
CESSING
CEZANNE
CHAFING
CHALONS
CHARING
CHASING
CHAWING
CHAZANS
CHEFING
CHEVONS
CHEWING
CHICANA
CHICANE
CHICANO
CHIDING
CHIMING
CHIMINH
CHITONS
CHOKING
CHOLINE
CHOPINE
CHORINE
CHOWING
CHUTING
CHYRONS
CICCONE
CINZANO
CITRINE
CITRONS
CLAMANT
CLAWING
CLAYING
CLEMENS
CLEMENT
CLEWING
CLIPONS
CLONING
CLOSING
CLOYING
CLUEING
COAGENT
COALING
COATING
COAXING
COBLENZ
COBRAND
COCAINE
COCKING
COCOONS
CODEINE
COFFINS
COFOUND
COGGING
COIFING
COILING
COINING
COLDONE
COLLINE
COLLINS
COLOGNE
COLONNA
COLUMNS
COMBINE
COMBING
COMEONS
COMMAND
COMMEND
COMMENT
COMMONS
COMMUNE
COMPANY
COMPEND
COMPING
CONDONE
CONFINE
CONKING
CONNING
CONSENT
CONTEND
CONTENT
CONVENE
CONVENT
COOKING
COOLANT
COOLING
COOPING
COPLAND
COPPING
COPYING
COQUINA
CORDING
CORDONS
CORINNE
CORKING
CORNING
CORTINA
CORVINA
CORVINE
CORZINE
COSHING
COSIGNS
COSTING
COSYING
COTTONS
COTTONY
COULDNT
COUPING
COUPONS
COURANT
COUSINE
COUSINS
COWBANE
COWHAND
COWLING
COWPONY
COZYING
COZZENS
CRANING
CRAPING
CRATING
CRAVENS
CRAVING
CRAYONS
CRAZING
CREMINI
CREMONA
CREPING
CRETANS
CRETINS
CREWING
CRIMINY
CROTONS
CROWING
CRUZANS
CTSCANS
CUBBING
CUBBINS
CUBFANS
CUFFING
CUIBONO
CUISINE
CULLING
CUNNING
CUPPING
CURBING
CURDING
CURLING
CURRANT
CURRENT
CURRING
CURSING
CURVING
CUSHING
CUSSING
CUTTING
CYCLING
CYCLONE
CYYOUNG
CZARINA

C•••••N

CAGEDIN
CAISSON
CAKEPAN
CAKETIN
CALDRON
CALHOUN
CALIBAN
CALLSIN
CALLSON
CAMERON
CAMPION
CANTEEN
CAPEANN
CAPITAN
CAPSTAN
CAPTAIN
CAPTION
CARAVAN
CARBARN
CARHORN
CARLOAN
CARLSON
CARLTON
CAROLYN
CAROTIN
CARRYIN
CARRYON
CARTOON
CARTSIN
CASPIAN
CASTSON
CATALAN
CATCHON
CATSCAN
CAUTHEN
CAUTION
CAVEDIN
CAVEMAN
CAVEMEN
CAVESIN
CELADON
CERTAIN
CERUMEN
CESSION
CHAGRIN
CHANSON
CHAPLIN
CHAPMAN
CHAPMEN
CHARMAN
CHARMEN
CHARMIN
CHARNIN
CHASTEN
CHATWIN
CHAZZAN
CHEAPEN
CHEATIN
CHEATON
CHECHEN
CHECKIN
CHECKON
CHEERON
CHEVRON
CHEWSON
CHICHEN
CHICKEN
CHIDDEN
CHIFFON
CHIGNON
CHILEAN
CHIMEIN
CHIPSIN
CHITLIN
CHITOWN
CHOKEON
CHOMPON
CISTERN
CITIZEN
CITROEN
CLACTON
CLAMPON
CLANTON
CLAPTON
CLARION
CLASSON
CLAYTON
CLEAVON
CLEMSON
CLIBURN
CLICKON
CLIFTON
CLIMBIN
CLIMBON
CLINTON
CLIPSON
CLOCKIN
CLOSEIN
CLUEDIN
CLUESIN
COALBIN
COARSEN
COCHRAN
COGBURN
COGHLAN
COLEMAN
COLLEEN
COMBIEN
COMESIN
COMESON
COMORAN
COMPLIN
COMPTON
CONCERN
CONDEMN
CONDIGN
CONJOIN
CONKLIN
CONSIGN
CONTAIN
CONTEMN
COONCAN
COPYMAN
COPYMEN
CORAZON
CORNBIN
COSTAIN
COUNTIN
COUNTON
COWSKIN
COWTOWN
CRAISIN
CRAMPON
CRAMSIN
CRATION
CREEPIN
CREPTIN
CRESPIN
CRESTON
CREWMAN
CREWMEN
CRIMEAN
CRIMSON
CRISPEN
CRISPIN
CROUTON
CROWDIN
CRUTZEN
CRYDOWN
CRYOGEN
CUBSFAN
CUINGIN
CURLSIN
CURTAIN
CUSHION
CUTDOWN
CUTINON
CUTOPEN
CYPRIAN

•CN••••

MCNALLY
MCNEILL

•C•N•••

ACANTHI
ACINGIT
ACONITE
ECONOMY
ICANNOT
ICINESS
ICINGIN
ICINGIT
ICINGUP
ICONIFY
MCENROE
OCANADA

OCONNOR
SCANDAL
SCANNED
SCANNER
SCANTED
SCANTER
SCANTLY
SCENEII
SCENEIV
SCENERY
SCENEVI
SCENICS
SCENTED
SCENTER
SCHNAPS
SCHNOOK
SCHNOZZ
SCONCES

•C••N••

ACCENTS
ACCTNOS
ACHENES
ACORNED
ACRONYM
ACTINON
ICANNOT
ICTINUS
KCJONES
MCHENRY
MCKENNA
MCRANEY
OCEANIA
OCEANIC
OCEANID
OCEANUS
OCHENTA
OCONNOR
OCTANES
OCTANTS
SCANNED
SCANNER
SCIENCE
SCORNED
SCORNER
SCRUNCH
WCHANDY

•C•••N•

ACCOUNT
ACETONE
ACHTUNG
ACTIONS
ACUMENS
BCLIONS
ECHIDNA
ECHOING
ICELAND
ICELINE
ICERINK
ICERUNS
ICEWINE
ICYWIND
MCKENNA
MCSHANE
MCSWINE
OCARINA
PCCLONE
SCALENE
SCALING
SCARING
SCHWANN
SCHWINN
SCOPING
SCORING
SCRAWNY
SCREENS

•C••••N

ACADIAN
ACHERON
ACHESON
ACTAEON
ACTEDIN
ACTEDON
ACTINON
ACTUPON
ECHELON
ECOTRIN
ICEDOWN
ICHDIEN
ICINGIN
MCALLEN
MCCOWEN
MCGAVIN
MCLUHAN
MCMAHON
MCQUEEN
OCTAGON
SCATMAN
SCHWANN
SCHWINN
SCOTIAN

••CN•••

ABCNEWS
MACNEIL
NBCNEWS
PICNICS

••C•N••

ACCENTS
ACCTNOS
ARCANUM
ARCINGS
ASCENDS
ASCENTS
BOCHNER
BUCHNER
BUCKNER
CACONYM
COCKNEY
COCONUT
DECANTS
DECENCY
DOCENTS
ENCINAS
ESCENCE
FACINGS
FACONNE
FECHNER
HACKNEY
INCANTS
INCENSE
INCENTS
JACINTH
JACINTO
JACONET
LACINGS
LACONIA
LACONIC
LACUNAE
LACUNAL
LACUNAR
LACUNAS
LECONTE
LICENCE
LICENSE
LOCKNUT
LUCANIA
LUCENCY
LUCINDA
LUCKNOW
MACONGA
MYCENAE
NOCANDO
OSCINES
PICANTE
POCONOS
RACINOS
RECANED
RECANES
RECANTS
RECENCY
SECANTS
SECONDI
SECONDO
SECONDR
SECONDS
TACONIC
TECHNOS
UNCANED
UNCANNY
UNCINCH
VACANCY
VICENTE
VICENZA
VICINAL
VICUNAS

••C••N•

ACCOUNT
ALCYONE
ANCIENT
ARCHING
ARCHONS
ARCSINE
BACHING
BACKEND
BACKING
BECKONS
BICHONS
BICORNE
BICORNS
BUCKING
CACHING
CICCONE
COCAINE
COCKING
COCOONS
CYCLING
CYCLONE
DACRONS
DECKING
DECLINE
DICKENS
DOCKING
DUCKING
DUCTING
ENCHANT
ETCHANT
ETCHING
FACONNE
HACKING
HOCKING
INCHING
INCLINE
ITCHING
JACKING
KACHINA
KACHING
KICKING
KUCHENS
LACKING
LECUONA
LICHENS
LICKING
LOCARNO
LOCKING
LOCKINS
LUCARNE
LUCERNE
LUCHINO
LUCIANA
LUCIANO
LUCKING
MACHINA
MACHINE
MACHONE
MACOUNS
MACRONS
MECCANS
MICRONS
MOCKING
MUCKING
NECKING
NICEONE
NICHING
NICKING
NOCKING
NOCOUNT
PACKING
PCCLONE
PECCANT
PECKING
PECTINS
PICKENS
PICKING
PUCCINI
RACKING
RECKONS
RECLINE
RECOINS
RECOUNT
RECRANK
RICHENS
ROCKING
RUCHING
RUCKING
SACKING
SICCING
SICKENS
SOCKING
SUCKING
TACKING
TICCING
TICKING
TOCSINS
TUCKING
TUCSONS
TYCOONS
UNCANNY
URCHINS
VACCINE
VICDANA
WICCANS
WICKING

••C•••N

AUCTION
BACHMAN
BACKSIN
BUCHMAN
COCHRAN
DECAGON
DICKSON
DICTION
DUCKPIN
ELCAJON
ENCHAIN
EUCERIN
EXCELIN
FACEDON
FACESON
FACTION
FICTION
FOCUSON
HACKMAN
HECKMAN
HICKMAN
JACKSON
JACOBIN
JOCELYN
KICKSIN
LACESON
LECTERN
LOCKEAN
LOCKLIN
LOCKSIN
LOCKSON
LUCKMAN
MACEDON
MACHAON
MACLEAN
MCCOWEN
MECHLIN
MRCLEAN
NICEMAN
NICEMEN
NUCLEON
PACKSIN
PACKSON
PACQUIN
PICKSON
RACCOON
RACEDIN
RECLEAN
RECROWN
RICHMAN
RICHMEN
RICKMAN
ROCKOON
RUCTION
SECTION
SOCKSIN
SUCKSIN
SUCTION
TACHYON
TACKSON
TICOTIN
TUCHMAN
TUCKSIN
UNCHAIN
UNCHURN
UNCLEAN
UNCROWN
UNCTION
VECHTEN
YUCATAN

•••C•N•

ABSCOND
ANACINS
ARACHNE
ARACHNO
ASHCANS
BALCONY
BEACONS
BRACING
CANCANS
CHICANA
CHICANE
CHICANO
CICCONE
CTSCANS
DANCING
DEACONS
DEFCONS
DEICING
DESCANT
DESCEND
DESCENT
DEUCING
DISCING
EDUCING
EPICENE
EXSCIND
FALCONS
FARCING
FENCING
FLACONS
FORCING
GARCONS
GASCANS
GASCONS
GASCONY
GLYCINE
GRACING
HIRCINE
ILOCANO
ISECOND
JUICING
KOSCINA
LANCING
LARCENY
LEUCINE
MANCINI
MARCONI
MECCANS
MINCING
MIOCENE
MOSCONI
NASCENT
NEOCENE
NEOCONS
OBSCENE
OILCANS
ONECENT
OUTCANT
PECCANT
PERCENT
PIECING
PISCINE
PLACING
PORCINE
PRICING
PUCCINI
REDCENT
REICING
RESCANS
RESCIND
SAUCING
SAUCONY
SICCING
SLICING
SNOCONE
SPACING
SPECING
SPICING
SYNCING
TENCENT
TICCING
TINCANS
TOUCANS
TRACING
TUSCANS
TUSCANY
UTICANS
UTICANY
VACCINE
VINCENT
VOICING
VOLCANO
VULCANS
WICCANS
WINCING
ZINCING
ZIRCONS

•••C••N

BEECHEN
BIRCHEN
BLACKEN
BRACKEN
CATCHON
CHECHEN
CHECKIN
CHECKON
CHICHEN
CHICKEN
CLACTON
CLICKON
CLOCKIN
CONCERN
DISCERN
DISCMAN
ERICSON
FENCEIN
FORCEIN
FORCEON
GRECIAN
HALCYON
HITCHON
IRECKON
JOYCEAN
KITCHEN
KNOCKON
LAOCOON
LARCHEN
LATCHON
LINCOLN
LOWCHEN
MADCHEN
MARCHON
MENCKEN
MERCIAN
MISCOIN
MONCTON
MUNCHEN
MUNCHON
OMICRON
PATCHEN
PISCEAN
PITCHIN
POPCORN
PROCYON
PUNCHIN
PYNCHON
QUICKEN
RACCOON
REACHIN
ROYCOHN
SLACKEN
SNACKON
STICKIN
STICKON
STUCKIN
STUCKON
SUBCLAN
TEACHIN
THICKEN
TOUCHON
TRICORN
UNICORN

••••C•N

AFRICAN
ALARCON
ALENCON
AZTECAN
BEERCAN
CATSCAN
COONCAN
HELICON
ITHACAN
LEXICON
LIMACON
LYRICON
MEXICAN
MILKCAN
MOHICAN
MONACAN
MRISCAN
OAXACAN
PELICAN
PETSCAN
PROSCAN
RUBICON
SARACEN
SENECAN
SILICON
SODACAN
SOUPCAN
SOUPCON
SURECAN
VATICAN
VIDICON
YESICAN

CO•••••

COACHED
COACHES
COACTED
COAGENT
COALBIN
COALCAR
COALERS
COALGAS
COALING
COALOIL
COALPIT
COALTAR
COAPTED
COARSEN
COARSER
COASTAL
COASTED
COASTER
COATEES
COATERS
COATING
COAXERS
COAXIAL
COAXING
COBALTS
COBBLED
COBBLER
COBBLES
COBCOAL
COBLENZ
COBNUTS
COBRAND
COBUYER
COBWEBS
COCAINE
COCCOID
COCHAIR
COCHISE
COCHLEA
COCHRAN
COCKADE
COCKERS
COCKIER
COCKILY
COCKING
COCKISH
COCKLED
COCKLES
COCKNEY
COCKPIT
COCONUT
COCOONS
COCTEAU
CODCAKE
CODDLED
CODDLER
CODDLES
CODEINE
CODERED
CODFISH
CODGERS
CODICES
CODICIL
COEDITS
COEPTIS
COEQUAL
COERCED
COERCER
COERCES
COETZEE
COEVALS
COEXIST
COFFEES
COFFERS
COFFINS
COFOUND
COGBURN
COGENCY
COGGING
COGGLES
COGHLAN
COGNACS
COGNATE
COGNIZE
COHABIT
COHEIRS
COHERED
COHERER
COHERES
COHORTS
COHOSTS
COIFFED
COIFING
COIGNED
COIGNES
COILERS
COILING
COILSUP
COINAGE
COINBOX
COINERS
COINING
COINOPS
COJUROR
COKIEST
COLADAS
COLBERT
COLCHIS
COLDCUP
COLDCUT
COLDDAY
COLDEST
COLDISH
COLDONE
COLDWAR
COLEMAN
COLETTE
COLGATE
COLICKY
COLLAGE
COLLARD
COLLARS
COLLATE
COLLECT
COLLEEN
COLLEGE
COLLETS
COLLIDE
COLLIER
COLLIES
COLLINE
COLLINS
COLLODI
COLLOID
COLLOPS
COLLUDE
COLLYER
COLOGNE
COLOMBO
COLONEL
COLONES
COLONNA
COLONUS
COLORED
COLORER
COLORTV
COLOSSI
COLOURS
COLTISH
COLUMBA
COLUMBO
COLUMNS
COMAKER
COMBATS
COMBERS
COMBIEN
COMBINE
COMBING
COMBUST
COMCAST
COMEDIA
COMEDIC
COMEDIE
COMEDUE
COMENOW
COMEOFF
COMEONS
COMEOUT
COMESAS
COMESAT
COMESBY
COMESIN
COMESON
COMESTO
COMESUP
COMFIER
COMFITS
COMFORT
COMICAL
COMICES
COMINGS
COMIQUE
COMMAND
COMMEND
COMMENT
COMMISH
COMMITS
COMMODE
COMMONS
COMMOVE
COMMUNE
COMMUTE
COMORAN
COMOROS
COMPACT
COMPANY
COMPAQS
COMPARE
COMPART
COMPASS
COMPEER
COMPELS
COMPEND
COMPERE
COMPETE
COMPILE
COMPING
COMPLEX
COMPLIN
COMPORT
COMPOSE
COMPOST
COMPOTE
COMPTON
COMPUTE
COMRADE
COMSATS
COMTISM
COMTIST
COMTREX
CONAGRA
CONAKRY
CONBRIO
CONCAVE
CONCEAL
CONCEDE
CONCEIT
CONCEPT
CONCERN
CONCERT
CONCHAE
CONCHES
CONCHOS
CONCISE
CONCOCT
CONCORD
CONCURS
CONCUSS
CONDEMN
CONDIGN
CONDOLE
CONDONE
CONDORS
CONDUCE
CONDUCT
CONDUIT
CONELET
CONFABS
CONFECT
CONFERS
CONFESS
CONFIDE
CONFINE
CONFIRM
CONFITS
CONFORM
CONFREY
CONFUSE
CONFUTE
CONGAED
CONGAME
CONGEAL
CONGERS
CONGEST
CONGOUS
CONICAL
CONIFER
CONJOBS
CONJOIN
CONJURE
CONJURY
CONKERS
CONKING
CONKLIN
CONKOFF
CONKOUT
CONMOTO
CONNATE
CONNECT
CONNERY
CONNICK
CONNIFF
CONNING
CONNIVE
CONNORS
CONNOTE
CONOIDS
CONQUER
CONRACK
CONRIED
CONSENT
CONSIGN
CONSIST
CONSOLE
CONSORT
CONSULS
CONSULT
CONSUME
CONTACS
CONTACT
CONTAIN
CONTEMN
CONTEND
CONTENT
CONTEST
CONTEXT
CONTORT
CONTOUR
CONTRAS
CONTROL
CONTUSE
CONURES
CONVECT
CONVENE
CONVENT
CONVERT
CONVEYS
CONVICT
CONVOKE
CONVOYS
COOKERS
COOKERY
COOKIES
COOKING

COOKOFF
COOKOUT
COOKPOT
COOKSUP
COOKTOP
COOLAIR
COOLANT
COOLCAT
COOLERS
COOLEST
COOLIES
COOLING
COOLISH
COOLMAX
COOLOUT
COOLPIX
COOLSIT
COONCAN
COONCAT
COONDOG
COOPERS
COOPERY
COOPING
COOPSUP
COOPTED
COOTERS
COOTIES
COOWNED
COPCARS
COPIERS
COPILOT
COPIOUS
COPLAND
COPOUTS
COPPERS
COPPERY
COPPICE
COPPING
COPPOLA
COPSHOP
COPSOUT
COPTERS
COPULAE
COPULAR
COPULAS
COPYBOY
COPYCAT
COPYING
COPYIST
COPYMAN
COPYMEN
COQUINA
CORACLE
CORAZON
CORBELS
CORBETT
CORDAGE
CORDATE
CORDELL
CORDERO
CORDERS
CORDIAL
CORDIAS
CORDING
CORDITE
CORDOBA
CORDONS
CORELLI
CORETTA
CORFAMS
CORINNE
CORINTH
CORKAGE
CORKERS
CORKIER
CORKING
CORKOAK
CORKSUP
CORMACK
CORNBIN
CORNCOB
CORNDOG
CORNEAL
CORNEAS
CORNELL
CORNERS
CORNETS
CORNFED
CORNICE
CORNIER
CORNILY
CORNING
CORNISH
CORNOIL
CORNROW
CORNUTE
COROLLA
CORONAE
CORONAL
CORONAS
CORONER
CORONET
CORPORA
CORPSES
CORRADE
CORRALS
CORRECT
CORRIDA
CORRODE
CORRUPT
CORSAGE
CORSAIR
CORSETS
CORSICA
CORTEGE
CORTICO
CORTINA
CORVAIR
CORVEES
CORVIDS
CORVINA
CORVINE
CORYELL
CORYZAS
CORZINE
COSETTE
COSHERS
COSHING
COSIEST
COSIGNS
COSINES
COSSACK
COSSETS
COSTAIN
COSTARD
COSTARS
COSTATE
COSTING
COSTIVE
COSTNER
COSTUME
COSYING
COTEACH
COTEDOR
COTERIE
COTTAGE
COTTERS
COTTONS
COTTONY
COUCHED
COUCHES
COUGARS
COUGHED
COUGHUP
COULDBE
COULDNT
COULEES
COULOMB
COULTER
COUNCIL
COUNSEL
COUNTED
COUNTEE
COUNTEM
COUNTER
COUNTIN
COUNTON
COUNTRY
COUNTUP
COUPING
COUPLED
COUPLER
COUPLES
COUPLET
COUPONS
COURAGE
COURANT
COURBET
COURIER
COURSED
COURSER
COURSES
COURTED
COURTLY
COURTTV
COUSINE
COUSINS
COUTERS
COUTURE
COVERED
COVERER
COVERME
COVERTS
COVERUP
COVETED
COVETER
COWARDS
COWBANE
COWBELL
COWBIRD
COWBOYS
COWERAT
COWERED
COWFISH
COWGIRL
COWHAND
COWHERD
COWHIDE
COWIEST
COWLICK
COWLIKE
COWLING
COWPEAS
COWPOKE
COWPONY
COWRIES
COWRITE
COWROTE
COWSHED
COWSKIN
COWSLIP
COWTOWN
COXCOMB
COXLESS
COYDOGS
COYNESS
COYOTES
COZENED
COZENER
COZIEST
COZUMEL
COZYING
COZZENS

C•O••••

CHOCKED
CHOCTAW
CHOICER
CHOICES
CHOIRED
CHOKEON
CHOKERS
CHOKEUP
CHOKIER
CHOKING
CHOLERA
CHOLERS
CHOLINE
CHOLLAS
CHOMPED
CHOMPON
CHOMSKY
CHOOSER
CHOOSES
CHOOSEY
CHOPINE
CHOPOFF
CHOPPED
CHOPPER
CHOPSUP
CHORALE
CHORALS
CHORDAL
CHORDED
CHORINE
CHORIST
CHORIZO
CHORTLE
CHOSEUP
CHOUGHS
CHOWDER
CHOWING
CLOAKED
CLOBBER
CLOCHES
CLOCKED
CLOCKER
CLOCKIN
CLOGGED
CLOGSUP
CLOMPED
CLONERS
CLONING
CLONKED
CLOONEY
CLOPPED
CLORETS
CLOSEBY
CLOSEIN
CLOSELY
CLOSERS
CLOSEST
CLOSETO
CLOSETS
CLOSEUP
CLOSING
CLOSURE
CLOTHED
CLOTHES
CLOTSUP
CLOTTED
CLOTURE
CLOUDED
CLOUDUP
CLOUTED
CLOUTER
CLOVERS
CLOVERY
CLOWDER
CLOWNED
CLOYING
CNOSSUS
COOKERS
COOKERY
COOKIES
COOKING
COOKOFF
COOKOUT
COOKPOT
COOKSUP
COOKTOP
COOLAIR
COOLANT
COOLCAT
COOLERS
COOLEST
COOLIES
COOLING
COOLISH
COOLMAX
COOLOUT
COOLPIX
COOLSIT
COONCAN
COONCAT
COONDOG
COOPERS
COOPERY
COOPING
COOPSUP
COOPTED
COOTERS
COOTIES
COOWNED
CROAKED
CROAKER
CROATIA
CROCHET
CROCKED
CROCKER
CROCKET
CROESUS
CROFTER
CRONIES
CROOKED
CROOKES
CROONED
CROONER
CROPPED
CROPPER
CROPSUP
CROPTOP
CROQUET
CROQUIS
CROSIER
CROSSAT
CROSSED
CROSSER
CROSSES
CROSSLY
CROSSUP
CROSTIC
CROTONS
CROUTES
CROUTON
CROWBAR
CROWDED
CROWDER
CROWDIN
CROWELL
CROWERS
CROWING
CROWLEY
CROWNED
CROWNER
CROZIER

C••O•••

CABOOSE
CACONYM
CAHOKIA
CAHOOTS
CAJOLED
CAJOLER
CAJOLES
CALORIC
CALORIE
CALOTTE
CANOERS
CANOLAS
CANONIC
CANONRY
CANOPUS
CAPOTES
CAROLED
CAROLER
CAROLII
CAROLYN
CAROMED
CAROTID
CAROTIN
CAROUSE
CATORCE
CAVORTS
CDTOWER
CELOTEX
CHAOTIC
CHLORIC
CHOOSER
CHOOSES
CHOOSEY
CHROMAT
CHROMED
CHROMES
CHROMIC
CHRONIC
CLOONEY
CNTOWER
COCONUT
COCOONS
COFOUND
COHORTS
COHOSTS
COLOGNE
COLOMBO
COLONEL
COLONES
COLONNA
COLONUS
COLORED
COLORER
COLORTV
COLOSSI
COLOURS
COMORAN
COMOROS
CONOIDS
COPOUTS
COROLLA
CORONAE
CORONAL
CORONAS
CORONER
CORONET
COYOTES
CREOLES
CREOSOL
CROOKED
CROOKES
CROONED
CROONER
CRYOGEN
CRYOVER
CUBOIDS
CULOTTE
CUPOLAS
CUTOFFS
CUTOPEN
CUTOUTS
CUTOVER
CYBORGS
CYYOUNG

C•••O••

CABOOSE
CAHOOTS
CALHOUN
CALLOFF
CALLOUS
CALLOUT
CALPOLY
CALZONE
CAMBOYS
CAMEOED
CAMEOFF
CAMEOUT
CAMIONS
CAMPOUT
CANDOUR
CANNOCK
CANNOLI
CANNONS
CANTONS
CANTORS
CANYONS
CANZONA
CANZONE
CANZONI
CAPTORS
CARBONS
CARBOYS
CARCOAT
CARDOOR
CARDOZO
CARGOES
CARHOPS
CARHORN
CARIOCA
CARIOLE
CARIOUS
CARLOAD
CARLOAN
CARLOTA
CARLOTS
CARPOOL
CARPORT
CARPOUS
CARROLL
CARROTS
CARROTY
CARTOFF
CARTONS
CARTOON
CARTOPS
CASEOUS
CASEOUT
CASHOUT
CASSOCK
CASSOLA
CASTOFF
CASTOUT
CATBOAT
CATBOWL
CATCOMB
CATDOOR
CATFOOD
CATFOOT
CATHODE
CATIONS
CATTOYS
CDSTORE
CENSORS
CHALONS
CHAMOIS
CHANOYU
CHAYOTE
CHEROOT
CHEVONS
CHEWOUT
CHICORY
CHIGOES
CHINOIS
CHINOOK
CHITONS
CHITOWN
CHOPOFF
CHYRONS
CICCONE
CINEOLE
CISCOES
CITROEN
CITRONS
CITROUS
CLAMORS
CLAMOUR
CLIPOFF
CLIPONS
CLIPOUT
COALOIL
COBCOAL
COCCOID
COCOONS
COINOPS
COLDONE
COLLODI
COLLOID
COLLOPS
COMEOFF
COMEONS
COMEOUT
COMFORT
COMMODE
COMMONS
COMMOVE
COMPORT
COMPOSE
COMPOST
COMPOTE
CONCOCT
CONCORD
CONDOLE
CONDONE
CONDORS
CONFORM
CONGOUS
CONJOBS
CONJOIN
CONKOFF
CONKOUT
CONMOTO
CONNORS
CONNOTE
CONSOLE
CONSORT
CONTORT
CONTOUR
CONVOKE
CONVOYS
COOKOFF
COOKOUT
COOLOUT
COPIOUS
COPPOLA
COPSOUT
CORDOBA
CORDONS
CORKOAK
CORNOIL
CORPORA
CORRODE
COTTONS
COTTONY
COULOMB
COUPONS
COWBOYS
COWPOKE
COWPONY
COWROTE
COWTOWN
COXCOMB
COYDOGS
CRAPOLA
CRAPOUT
CRAYOLA
CRAYONS
CREMONA
CREMORA
CROTONS
CRYDOWN
CRYWOLF
CTENOID
CUCKOOS
CUIBONO
CUPROUS
CURIOSA
CURIOUS
CURSORS
CURSORY
CUSTODY
CUSTOMS
CUTDOWN
CUTSOFF
CUTSOUT
CUTWORK
CUTWORM
CYCLOID
CYCLONE
CYCLOPS

C••••O•

CABRIOS
CAILLOU
CAISSON
CALDRON
CALICOS
CALLBOX
CALLBOY
CALLFOR
CALLNOW
CALLSON
CAMAROS
CAMELOT
CAMERON
CAMINOS
CAMPHOR
CAMPION
CAPECOD
CAPITOL
CAPTION
CARABOO
CARDOOR
CAREFOR
CARIBOO
CARIBOU
CARLSON
CARLTON
CARPOOL
CARRYON
CARSHOW
CARTOON
CASELOT
CASHBOX
CASHCOW
CASINOS
CASTROL
CASTSON
CATALOG
CATALOS
CATCHON
CATCHOW
CATDOOR
CATFOOD
CATFOOT
CATSHOW
CAUTION
CELADON
CESSION
CESTMOI
CHANSON
CHARCOT
CHARIOT
CHARROS
CHEATON
CHECKON
CHEERON
CHEETOS
CHEKHOV
CHEROOT
CHEVIOT
CHEVRON
CHEWSON
CHEWTOY
CHEZMOI
CHIFFON
CHIGNON
CHINOOK
CHOKEON
CHOMPON
CHRISOM
CHURROS
CITYBOY
CLACTON
CLAIROL
CLAMPON
CLANGOR
CLANTON
CLAPFOR
CLAPTON
CLARION
CLASSON
CLAYTON
CLEAROF
CLEAVON
CLEMSON
CLICKON
CLIFTON
CLIMBON
CLINTON
CLIPSON
COINBOX
COJUROR
COMENOW
COMESON
COMOROS
COMPTON
CONCHOS
CONTROL
COOKPOT
COOKTOP
COONDOG
COPILOT
COPSHOP
COPYBOY
CORAZON
CORNCOB
CORNDOG
CORNROW
COTEDOR
COUNTON
CRABPOT
CRAMPON
CRATION
CREATOR
CREEPOS
CREOSOL
CRESTON
CRIMSON
CROPTOP
CROUTON
CRYPTOS
CUATROS
CUCKOOS
CURATOR
CUSHION
CUTINON
CYPRIOT
CZARDOM

C•••••O

CALABRO
CALANDO
CALLSTO
CALVINO
CALYPSO
CAMACHO
CANSECO
CANTINO
CARABOO
CARDOZO
CAREDTO
CARESTO
CARIBOO
CASSINO
CATERTO
CATTALO
CBRADIO
CELAENO
CEMBALO
CENTAVO
CENTIMO
CEPHALO
CEREBRO
CHEERIO
CHICAGO
CHICANO
CHIRICO
CHORIZO
CHRISTO
CILENTO
CINZANO
CLAMATO
CLAUDIO
CLIMBTO
CLINGTO
CLOSETO
CLUNGTO
COLOMBO
COLUMBO
COMESTO
CONBRIO
CONMOTO
CORDERO
CORTICO
CRUZADO
CUIBONO
CURACAO
CUTINTO

•CO••••

ACOLYTE
ACONITE
ACORNED
ACOUPLE
ECOCIDE
ECOLOGY
ECONOMY
ECOTAGE
ECOTEUR
ECOTRIN
ECOTYPE
ICONIFY
OCONNOR
SCOFFAT
SCOFFED
SCOFFER
SCOLARI
SCOLDED
SCOLDER
SCONCES
SCOOBAS
SCOOPED
SCOOPER
SCOOTCH
SCOOTED
SCOOTER
SCOPING
SCORERS
SCORIAS
SCORING
SCORNED
SCORNER
SCORPIO
SCOTERS
SCOTIAN
SCOTTIE
SCOUPES
SCOURED
SCOURER
SCOURGE
SCOUTED
SCOUTER
SCOUTUP
SCOWLED
SCOWLER

•C•O•••
ACCORDS ACCOSTS ACCOUNT ACROBAT ACRONYM ACTORLY ECHOERS ECHOING ECHOISM ECLOGUE ICEOUTS ICEOVER JCPOWYS KCJONES MCCOURT MCCOVEY MCCOWEN OCTOBER OCTOBRE OCTOPOD OCTOPUS PCWORLD RCCOLAS SCHOLAR SCHOLES SCHOOLS SCIORRA SCOOBAS SCOOPED SCOOPER SCOOTCH SCOOTED SCOOTER SCROLLS SCROOGE

•C••O••
ACEDOUT ACEROLA ACEROSE ACESOUT ACETONE ACTFOUR ACTIONS ACTSOUT BCLIONS ECOLOGY ECONOMY ICEBOAT ICECOLD ICEDOUT ICEDOWN ICEFOGS ICEHOLE ICEPOPS ICESOUT MCCLOUD MCGRORY OCELOTS OCHROID OCHROUS OCTROIS PCCLONE RCADOME SCHLOCK SCHMOES SCHNOOK SCHNOZZ SCHOOLS SCROOGE

•C•••O•
ACCTNOS ACHEFOR ACHERON ACHESON ACTAEON ACTEDON ACTINON ACTSFOR ACTUPON ECHELON ECUADOR ICANNOT ICEFLOE ICESHOW ICHABOD ICKYPOO JCARROL MCENROE MCMAHON OCONNOR OCTAGON OCTAVOS OCTOPOD SCADSOF SCALLOP SCHNOOK SCISSOR

•C••••O
ACDELCO ICKYPOO MCMURDO OCCURTO OCTAVIO SCHERZO SCORPIO UCCELLO

••CO•••
ACCORDS ACCOSTS ACCOUNT ALCOHOL ALCOPOP ALCOVES BECOMES BICOLOR BICORNE BICORNS BUCOLIC CACONYM COCONUT COCOONS DACOSTA DECOCTS DECODED DECODER DECODES DECOLOR DECORUM DECOYED DECOYER ENCODED ENCODER ENCODES ENCOMIA ENCORED ENCORES ESCORTS FACONNE IACOCCA INCOLOR INCOMER INCOMES INCOURT JACOBIN JACONET LACONIA LACONIC LACOSTE LECONTE LLCOOLJ MACONGA MACOUNS MCCOURT MCCOVEY MCCOWEN NICOBAR NICOISE NICOLAS NICOLET NICOLLE NICOSIA NOCOUNT PICOTED POCONOS RCCOLAS RECOALS RECOATS RECOCKS RECODED RECODES RECOILS RECOINS RECOLOR RECOMBS RECOOKS RECOOLS RECORDS RECORKS RECOSTS RECOUNT RECOUPS RECOVER RICOTTA ROCOCOS SECONDI SECONDO SECONDR SECONDS TACOMAS TACONIC TICOTIN TYCOONS UNCODED UNCOILS UNCOMIC UNCOOPS UNCORED UNCORES UNCORKS UNCOUTH UNCOVER UNCOWED UNCOYER UNCOYLY UPCOAST UPCOILS UPCOURT VICOMTE VOCODER

••C•O••
AHCHOOS ALCYONE ANCHORS ANCHOVY ARCHONS ATCROSS BACKOFF BACKOUT BECKONS BECLOUD BICHONS BSCHOOL BUCKOES CICCONE COCCOID COCOONS CUCKOOS CYCLOID CYCLONE CYCLOPS DACRONS DECKOUT DECLOTS DICKORY DOCTORS DUCKOUT ENCLOSE ESCROWS FACEOFF FACTOID FACTORS FACTORY GECKOES HACKOFF HECTORS HICKORY INCLOSE INCROWD KICKOFF KICKOUT LACTOSE LECTORS LECUONA LLCOOLJ LOCKOUT LUCKOUT MACHONE MACRONS MCCLOUD MICROBE MICRONS MYCROFT NICCOLO NICEONE NICHOLS NOCUOUS OSCEOLA PACEOFF PACKOFF PCCLONE PICCOLO PICEOUS PICKOFF PICKOUT QSCHOOL RACCOON RACKOUT RECHOSE RECKONS RECOOKS RECOOLS RECROOM RECROSS RECROWN RECTORS RECTORY ROCKOIL ROCKOON SACKOUT SECTORS SICKOUT STCLOUD STCROIX SUCCORS SUCCOTH SUCCOUR SUCROSE TICKOFF TUCSONS TYCOONS UNCHOKE UNCLOAK UNCLOGS UNCLOSE UNCLOUD UNCOOPS UNCROSS UNCROWN UPCCODE UPCLOSE VACUOLE VACUOUS VECTORS VICIOUS VICTORS VICTORY

••C••O•
ACCTNOS AHCHOOS ALCOHOL ALCOPOP ARCHFOE AUCTION BACKHOE BACKLOG BACKLOT BACKROW BICOLOR BSCHOOL BUCKFOR CUCKOOS DACAPOS DECAGON DECALOG DECAPOD DECOLOR DICKSON DICTION DRCHAOS ELCAJON ESCALOP ESCUDOS EXCITOR FACEDON FACESON FACTION FICTION FOCUSON INCISOR INCOLOR ITCHFOR JACKPOT JACKSON JACKSOO KICKBOX LACESON LOCATOR LOCKBOX LOCKSON LUCKNOW MACACOS MACEDON MACHAON MACLEOD NICEBOY NICEDOG NICEJOB NUCLEON OHCAROL PACKSON PICADOR PICAROS PICKSON POCONOS QSCHOOL RACCOON RACINOS RECOLOR RECROOM ROCKCOD ROCKOON ROCOCOS RUCTION SECTION SOCKHOP SUCTION TACHYON TACKSON TECHNOS UNCTION VICEROY WICKLOW ZOCALOS

••C•••O
DECARLO DICILLO ELCAMPO JACINTO JACKIEO JACKSOO LACRIMO LOCARNO LUCHINO LUCIANO MACHTWO NICCOLO NOCANDO OCCURTO PICARDO PICASSO PICCOLO RACEDTO RACESTO RICARDO SECONDO UCCELLO VACCARO

•••CO••
ABSCOND AIRCOOL ANTCOWS ATACOST BABCOCK BADCOLD BALCONY BARCODE BEACONS BIBCOCK BOOCOOS BOXCOAT BOYCOTT BUNCOED CARCOAT CATCOMB CHICORY CICCONE CISCOES COBCOAL COCCOID CONCOCT CONCORD COXCOMB DEACONS DEFCONS DISCOED DISCOID DISCORD DNACODE DOGCOAT DOGCOMB DOTCOMS FALCONS FLACONS FOSCOLO FRYCOOK FURCOAT GARCONS GASCONS GASCONY GEOCODE GETCOLD GIACOMO GIOCOSO GLUCOSE GLYCOLS GOTCOLD HANCOCK HENCOOP HOTCOAL HOTCOMB HOWCOME ICECOLD ISECOND ITSCOLD JOECOOL JUNCOES KIDCOMS LABCOAT LANCOME LAOCOON LEACOCK LINCOLN LOWCOST MALCOLM MARCONI MASCOTS MISCODE MISCOIN MISCOPY MOOCOWS MOSCONI MRSCOTT NEOCONS NETCOST NICCOLO NONCOLA NONCOMS NONCORE NOSCORE OLICOOK OUTCOLD OUTCOME OUTCOOK PASCOLI PEACOAT PEACOCK PETCOCK PETCOMB PETCOWS PICCOLO PISCOPO POPCORN PRECODE PRECOIL PRECOOK PRECOOL PRECOUP RACCOON RANCORS RANCOUR RAUCOUS REDCOAT REDCODS RESCORE RIPCORD ROMCOMS ROSCOES ROYCOHN SATCOMS SAUCONY SEACOWS SITCOMS SNOCONE SPECOUT SUBCODE SUBCOOL SUCCORS SUCCOTH SUCCOUR SYNCOPE TAXCODE TEACOZY TENCODE TOPCOAT TRICORN TRICOTS UNICODE UNICORN UPCCODE VISCOUS WALCOTT WAYCOOL WELCOME WESCOTT ZINCOUS ZIPCODE ZIRCONS ZITCOMS

•••C•O•
AIRCOOL ALACKOF APECKOF ATECROW BOKCHOY BOOCOOS CATCHON CATCHOW CHECKON CLACTON CLICKON CONCHOS DOGCHOW DRMCCOY EATCROW EDUCTOR EJECTOR ELECTOR ENACTOR ERECTOR ERICSON EVICTOR EXACTOR FORCEON FRYCOOK GAUCHOS HALCYON HENCOOP HITCHON HONCHOS IRECKON JOECOOL KNOCKON LAOCOON LATCHON MARCHON MONCTON MUNCHON NONCROP NUNCIOS OLICOOK OMICRON OUTCOOK OUTCROP OUTCROW PETCROW PILCROW PINCHOT PONCHOS PRECOOK PRECOOL PROCTOR PROCYON PSYCHOS PYNCHON RACCOON RANCHOS REACTOR SALCHOW SMACKOF SNACKON SPECTOR STICKON STUCCOS STUCKON SUBCOOL THECROW TOUCHON TRACTOR VELCROS WAYCOOL XFACTOR

•••C••O
AJACCIO ARACHNO ARECIBO AVOCADO BRACERO CHICAGO CHICANO ELECTRO FLOCKTO FOSCOLO GIACOMO GIOCOSO ILOCANO MANCUSO MARCATO MERCADO MOSCATO NICCOLO PICCOLO PISCOPO PITCHTO PLACEBO PLACIDO REACTTO SATCHMO STICKTO STUCKTO VACCARO VISCUSO VOLCANO

••••CO•
ALARCON ALENCON ALNICOS APRICOT BEATCOP BRITCOM BRONCOS CALICOS CAPECOD CASHCOW CHARCOT CORNCOB DOVECOT DRMCCOY FAMICOM FIASCOS FRESCOS GLENCOE HADACOW HARICOT HASACOW HELICON HOLYCOW LEXICON LIMACON LINGCOD LYRICON MACACOS MEDICOS MILKCOW OVERCOY PHILCOS PLUMCOT ROBOCOP ROCKCOD ROCOCOS RUBICON SILICON SOUPCON STUCCOS TELECOM TIMECOP VIDICON ZYDECOS

••••C•O
AJACCIO BENICIO BOWECHO BRONCHO CAMACHO CURACAO DEFACTO DELICTO DERECHO DETECTO EXFACTO GROUCHO INVACUO JERICHO MOROCCO MRMACHO NABUCCO OFFICIO OUTECHO SIROCCO SUBECHO TOBACCO UNMACHO

•••••CO
ACDELCO ARTDECO ASPENCO BABENCO BELASCO CANSECO CHIRICO CORTICO DEMARCO DERRICO ELGRECO GALLICO GUANACO IONESCO JALISCO MANRICO MOROCCO NABISCO NABUCCO NORELCO ORINOCO PAMLICO PEPSICO PIMLICO PORTICO SERPICO SIROCCO TABASCO TAMPICO TENNECO TOBACCO

CP•••••
CPAEXAM CPEBACH CPLUSES

C•P••••
CAPABLE CAPABLY CAPADES CAPAPIE CAPEANN CAPECOD CAPEESH CAPELET CAPELLA CAPEMAY CAPERED CAPFULS CAPGUNS CAPITAL CAPITAN CAPITOL CAPLESS CAPLETS CAPNUTS CAPOTES CAPPERS CAPPING CAPRICE CAPRINE CAPSHAW CAPSIZE CAPSTAN CAPSULE CAPTAIN CAPTION CAPTIVA CAPTIVE CAPTORS CAPTURE CAPUANA CAPUCHE CAPULET CEPHALO CEPHALY CEPHEUS CIPHERS COPCARS COPIERS COPILOT COPIOUS COPLAND COPOUTS COPPERS COPPERY COPPICE COPPING COPPOLA COPSHOP COPSOUT COPTERS COPULAE COPULAR COPULAS COPYBOY COPYCAT COPYING COPYIST COPYMAN COPYMEN CUPCAKE CUPELED CUPELER CUPFULS CUPLIKE CUPOLAS CUPPIER CUPPING CUPRITE CUPROUS CUPULAR CUPULES CYPHERS CYPRESS CYPRIAN CYPRIOT

C••P•••
CALPOLY CAMPARI CAMPBED CAMPERS CAMPHOR CAMPIER CAMPILY CAMPING CAMPION CAMPOUT CAMPSUP CAPPERS CAPPING CARPALS CARPARK CARPELS CARPERS CARPETS

CARPING
CARPOOL
CARPORT
CARPOUS
CARPSAT
CASPARY
CASPIAN
CHAPALA
CHAPATI
CHAPEAU
CHAPELS
CHAPLET
CHAPLIN
CHAPMAN
CHAPMEN
CHAPPED
CHAPPIE
CHAPTER
CHIPPED
CHIPPER
CHIPSIN
CHIPSUP
CHOPINE
CHOPOFF
CHOPPED
CHOPPER
CHOPSUP
CHUPPAH
CHUPPAS
CLAPFOR
CLAPPED
CLAPPER
CLAPTON
CLIPART
CLIPOFF
CLIPONS
CLIPOUT
CLIPPED
CLIPPER
CLIPSON
CLOPPED
COAPTED
COEPTIS
COMPACT
COMPANY
COMPAQS
COMPARE
COMPART
COMPASS
COMPEER
COMPELS
COMPEND
COMPERE
COMPETE
COMPILE
COMPING
COMPLEX
COMPLIN
COMPORT
COMPOSE
COMPOST
COMPOTE
COMPTON
COMPUTE
COOPERS
COOPERY
COOPING
COOPSUP
COOPTED
COPPERS
COPPERY
COPPICE
COPPING
COPPOLA
CORPORA
CORPSES
COUPING
COUPLED
COUPLER
COUPLES
COUPLET
COUPONS
COWPEAS
COWPOKE
COWPONY
CRAPING
CRAPOLA
CRAPOUT
CRAPPIE
CREPING
CREPTIN
CREPTUP
CRIPPLE
CROPPED
CROPPER
CROPSUP
CROPTOP
CRUPPER
CRYPTIC
CRYPTOS
CULPRIT
CUPPIER
CUPPING
CUSPATE
CUSPIDS

C•••P••

CAGEPET
CAKEPAN
CALIPER
CALIPHS
CALYPSO
CANAPES
CANOPUS
CAPAPIE
CATSPAW
CESSPIT
CHAMPED
CHAMPER
CHAPPED
CHAPPIE
CHARPAK
CHEAPEN
CHEAPER
CHEAPIE
CHEAPLY
CHEEPED
CHEEPER
CHIAPAS
CHIAPET
CHIPPED
CHIPPER
CHIRPED
CHIRPER
CHOMPED
CHOMPON
CHOPPED
CHOPPER
CHUMPED
CHUPPAH
CHUPPAS
CLAMPED
CLAMPER
CLAMPON
CLAPPED
CLAPPER
CLASPED
CLASPER
CLAYPIT
CLIPPED
CLIPPER
CLOMPED
CLOPPED
CLUMPED
COALPIT
COCKPIT
COOKPOT
COOLPIX
CRABPOT
CRAMPED
CRAMPON
CRAPPIE
CREEPBY
CREEPED
CREEPER
CREEPIN
CREEPOS
CREEPUP
CRESPIN
CRIMPED
CRIMPER
CRIPPLE
CRISPED
CRISPEN
CRISPER
CRISPIN
CRISPIX
CRISPLY
CRISPUS
CROPPED
CROPPER
CRUMPED
CRUMPET
CRUMPLE
CRUMPLY
CRUPPER
CUTOPEN

C••••P•

CALLUPS
CARHOPS
CARTOPS
CATALPA
CATNAPS
CATNIPS
CATSUPS
CCLAMPS
CHALUPA
CHINUPS
CHUTZPA
COINOPS
COLLOPS
CONCEPT
CORRUPT
CUETIPS
CYCLOPS

C•••••P

CAGEDUP
CAGESUP
CAKEDUP
CAKESUP
CALLSUP
CAMPSUP
CANTRIP
CARTRIP
CASTSUP
CATCHUP
CATFLAP
CHAINUP
CHALKUP
CHATSUP
CHECKUP
CHEERUP
CHEWSUP
CHIPSUP
CHIRRUP
CHOKEUP
CHOPSUP
CHOSEUP
CHURNUP
CLAMDIP
CLAMSUP
CLEANUP
CLEARUP
CLIMBUP
CLOGSUP
CLOSEUP
CLOTSUP
CLOUDUP
CLUBSUP
COILSUP
COLDCUP
COMESUP
COOKSUP
COOKTOP
COOPSUP
COPSHOP
CORKSUP
COUGHUP
COUNTUP
COVERUP
COWSLIP
CRACKUP
CRANKUP
CRATEUP
CREEPUP
CREPTUP
CRIEDUP
CRIESUP
CROPSUP
CROPTOP
CROSSUP
CRUDSUP
CURLSUP

•CP••••

JCPOWYS
MCPAPER

•C•P•••

ICEPACK
ICEPICK
ICEPOPS
SCAPULA
SCEPTER
SCEPTIC
SCEPTRE
SCOPING
SCUPPER

•C••P••

ACCEPTS
ACOUPLE
ACTUPON
ECHAPPE
ECLIPSE
ECTYPAL
ECTYPES
ICKYPOO
MCPAPER
OCCIPUT
OCTOPOD
OCTOPUS
OCTUPLE
OCTUPLY
SCALPED
SCALPEL
SCALPER
SCAMPED
SCAMPER
SCARPED
SCOOPED
SCOOPER
SCORPIO
SCOUPES
SCRAPED
SCRAPER
SCRAPES
SCRAPPY
SCRIPPS
SCRIPTS
SCRUPLE
SCULPED
SCULPTS
SCUPPER

•C•••P•

CCLAMPS
ECHAPPE
ECOTYPE
ICECAPS
ICEPOPS
SCHLEPP
SCHLEPS
SCHNAPS
SCRAPPY
SCRIMPS
SCRIMPY
SCRIPPS
VCRTAPE

•C••••P

ACTEDUP
ICINGUP
SCALEUP
SCALLOP
SCAREUP
SCARFUP
SCHLEPP
SCHLUMP
SCOUTUP
SCREWUP
SCRUBUP

••CP•••

PVCPIPE

••C•P••

ACCEPTS
ALCOPOP
BACKPAY
COCKPIT
DACAPOS
DECAPOD
DECUPLE
DUCKPIN
ESCAPED
ESCAPEE
ESCAPER
ESCAPES
EXCEPTS
INCEPTS
JACKPOT
OCCIPUT
RECIPES
SICKPAY
UNCAPED

••C••P•

BACKUPS
CYCLOPS
DECAMPS
DECRYPT
ELCAMPO
ENCAMPS
ENCRYPT
ESCARPS
EXCERPT
HICCUPS
KICKUPS
LACEUPS
LOCKUPS
MOCKUPS
MRCHIPS
PICKUPS
PVCPIPE
RECEIPT
RECOUPS
UNCLIPS
UNCLIPT
UNCOOPS
YUCAIPA

••C•••P

ALCOPOP
ARCLAMP
BACKSUP
BUCKSUP
DICECUP
DUCHAMP
ENCLASP
ESCALOP
HACKSUP
JACKSUP
KICKSUP
LACEDUP
LACESUP
LICKSUP
LOCKSUP
MOCKSUP
MUCKSUP
PACELAP
PACKSUP
PICKSUP
RACEDUP
RACESUP
RACKSUP
RECLASP
RUCKSUP
SACKSUP
SOCKHOP
SUCKSUP
TACKSUP
UNCLAMP
UNCLASP
UNCRAMP
WICKIUP

•••C•P•

ALLCAPS
CONCEPT
EGGCUPS
EYECUPS
FORCEPS
GASCAPS
GELCAPS
HICCUPS
HOTCAPS
HOTCUPS
HUBCAPS
ICECAPS
MADCAPS
MIDCAPS
MISCOPY
OILCUPS
PERCEPT
PISCOPO
PRECEPT
REDCAPS
SKICAPS
SKYCAPS
SNOCAPS
SYNCOPE
TEACUPS
THECAPE
TOECAPS
TRICEPS

•••C••P

ATACLIP
BIOCHIP
BLOCKUP
BOTCHUP
BRACEUP
BRICKUP
BUNCHUP
CATCHUP
CHECKUP
CRACKUP
DAYCAMP
EARCLIP
EPICARP
EXOCARP
FANCYUP
FENCEUP
FORCEUP
HENCOOP
HITCHUP
JOECAMP
JUICEUP
KETCHUP
MATCHUP
NONCROP
OLDCHAP
ONECHIP
OUTCROP
PATCHUP
PRECOUP
PRICKUP
PSYCHUP
PUNCHUP
REACHUP
REDCHIP
SLACKUP
SLICEUP
SMACKUP
SNUCKUP
SPICEUP
STACKUP
STICKUP
STOCKUP
STUCKUP
TIECLIP
TOUCHUP
VANCAMP
WRACKUP

••••C•P

BEATCOP
COLDCUP
DICECUP
DROPCAP
GREYCUP
INKYCAP
KNEECAP
LENSCAP
RATECAP
ROBOCOP
ROOTCAP
SNOWCAP
TIMECOP

C•Q••••

COQUINA

C••Q•••

CASQUED
CASQUES
CHEQUER
CHEQUES
CINQUES
CIRQUES
CLAQUES
CLIQUED
CLIQUES
CLIQUEY
COEQUAL
CONQUER
CROQUET
CROQUIS

C•••Q••

CACIQUE
COMIQUE

C••••Q•

COMPAQS

•CQ••••

ACQUIRE
ACQUITS
MCQUEEN

••CQ•••

JACQUES
LACQUER
PACQUIN
RACQUET
SACQUES

••C•Q••

CACIQUE
MACAQUE

CR•••••

CRABBED
CRABBER
CRABPOT
CRACKED
CRACKER
CRACKLE
CRACKLY
CRACKUP
CRADLED
CRADLER
CRADLES
CRAFTED
CRAFTER
CRAFTSY
CRAGGED
CRAIGIE
CRAISIN
CRAMMED
CRAMMER
CRAMPED
CRAMPON
CRAMSIN
CRANIAL
CRANING
CRANIUM
CRANKED
CRANKUP
CRANMER
CRAPING
CRAPOLA
CRAPOUT
CRAPPIE
CRASHAW
CRASHED
CRASHER
CRASHES
CRASSER
CRASSLY
CRASSUS
CRATERS
CRATEUP
CRATING
CRATION
CRAVATS
CRAVENS
CRAVERS
CRAVING
CRAWDAD
CRAWLED
CRAWLER
CRAWLEY
CRAYOLA
CRAYONS
CRAZIER
CRAZIES
CRAZILY
CRAZING
CREAKED
CREAMED
CREAMER
CREASED
CREASER
CREASES
CREATED
CREATES
CREATOR
CRECHES
CREDITS
CREEDAL
CREELEY
CREEPBY
CREEPED
CREEPER
CREEPIN
CREEPOS
CREEPUP
CREMATE
CREMINI
CREMONA
CREMORA
CRENATE
CRENELS
CREOLES
CREOSOL
CREPING
CREPTIN
CREPTUP
CRESPIN
CRESSES
CRESSET
CRESTED
CRESTON
CRETANS
CRETINS
CREVICE
CREWCUT
CREWELS
CREWING
CREWMAN
CREWMEN
CRIBBED
CRIBBER
CRICKED
CRICKET
CRIEDUP
CRIESUP
CRIMEAN
CRIMINY
CRIMPED
CRIMPER
CRIMSON
CRINGED
CRINGES
CRINKLE
CRINKLY
CRIPPLE
CRISPED
CRISPEN
CRISPER
CRISPIN
CRISPIX
CRISPLY
CRISPUS
CRITIAS
CRITICS
CRITTER
CRITTUR
CROAKED
CROAKER
CROATIA
CROCHET
CROCKED
CROCKER
CROCKET
CROESUS
CROFTER
CRONIES
CROOKED
CROOKES
CROONED
CROONER
CROPPED
CROPPER
CROPSUP
CROPTOP
CROQUET
CROQUIS
CROSIER
CROSSAT
CROSSED
CROSSER
CROSSES
CROSSLY
CROSSUP
CROSTIC
CROTONS
CROUTES
CROUTON
CROWBAR
CROWDED
CROWDER
CROWDIN
CROWELL
CROWERS
CROWING
CROWLEY
CROWNED
CROWNER
CROZIER
CRUCIAL
CRUDELY
CRUDEST
CRUDITY
CRUDSUP
CRUELER
CRUELLA
CRUELLY
CRUELTY
CRUGUET
CRUISED
CRUISER
CRUISES
CRULLER
CRUMBED
CRUMBLE
CRUMBLY
CRUMBUM
CRUMPED
CRUMPET
CRUMPLE
CRUMPLY
CRUNCHY
CRUPPER
CRUSADE
CRUSHED
CRUSHER
CRUSHES
CRUSTAL
CRUSTED
CRUTZEN
CRUZADO
CRUZANS
CRYBABY
CRYDOWN
CRYOGEN
CRYOVER
CRYPTIC
CRYPTOS
CRYSTAL
CRYWOLF

C•R••••

CARABOO
CARACAS
CARAFES
CARAMBA
CARAMEL
CARAMIA
CARAVAN
CARAVEL
CARAWAY
CARBARN
CARBIDE
CARBINE
CARBONS
CARBOYS
CARBRAS
CARCARE
CARCASS
CARCLUB
CARCOAT
CARDERS
CARDIAC
CARDIAL
CARDIFF
CARDING
CARDIUM
CARDKEY
CARDOOR
CARDOZO
CAREDTO
CAREENS
CAREERS
CAREFOR
CAREFUL
CARESTO
CARFARE
CARFREE
CARFULS
CARGOES
CARHOPS
CARHORN
CARIBES
CARIBOO
CARIBOU
CARINAE
CARINAS
CARIOCA
CARIOLE
CARIOUS
CARJACK
CARKEYS
CARKING
CARLENE
CARLESS
CARLING
CARLOAD
CARLOAN
CARLOTA
CARLOTS
CARLSON
CARLTON
CARLYLE
CARMELA
CARMINA
CARMINE
CARNABY
CARNAGE
CARNERA
CARNETS
CARNIES
CAROLED
CAROLER
CAROLII
CAROLYN
CAROMED
CAROTID
CAROTIN
CAROUSE
CARPALS
CARPARK
CARPELS
CARPERS
CARPETS
CARPING
CARPOOL
CARPORT
CARPOUS
CARPSAT
CARRARA
CARRELS
CARRERA
CARRERE
CARRIED
CARRIER
CARRIES
CARROLL
CARROTS
CARROTY
CARRYIN
CARRYON
CARSALE
CARSEAT
CARSHOW
CARTAGE
CARTALK
CARTELS
CARTERS

CARTIER
CARTING
CARTIRE
CARTOFF
CARTONS
CARTOON
CARTOPS
CARTRIP
CARTSIN
CARVELS
CARVERS
CARVING
CARWASH
CBRADIO
CCRIDER
CDRACKS
CDRATES
CERAMIC
CERATED
CERATES
CEREALS
CEREBRA
CEREBRO
CERISES
CERTAIN
CERTIFY
CERUMEN
CERVEZA
CERVIDS
CERVINE
CHRISMS
CHRISOM
CHRISTA
CHRISTI
CHRISTO
CHRISTY
CHROMAT
CHROMED
CHROMES
CHROMIC
CHRONIC
CIRCLED
CIRCLER
CIRCLES
CIRCLET
CIRCUIT
CIRCUSY
CIRQUES
CIRRATE
CORACLE
CORAZON
CORBELS
CORBETT
CORDAGE
CORDATE
CORDELL
CORDERO
CORDERS
CORDIAL
CORDIAS
CORDING
CORDITE
CORDOBA
CORDONS
CORELLI
CORETTA
CORFAMS
CORINNE
CORINTH
CORKAGE
CORKERS
CORKIER
CORKING
CORKOAK
CORKSUP
CORMACK
CORNBIN
CORNCOB
CORNDOG
CORNEAL
CORNEAS
CORNELL
CORNERS
CORNETS
CORNFED
CORNICE
CORNIER
CORNILY
CORNING
CORNISH
CORNOIL
CORNROW
CORNUTE
COROLLA
CORONAE
CORONAL
CORONAS
CORONER
CORONET
CORPORA
CORPSES
CORRADE
CORRALS
CORRECT
CORRIDA
CORRODE
CORRUPT
CORSAGE
CORSAIR
CORSETS
CORSICA
CORTEGE
CORTICO
CORTINA
CORVAIR
CORVEES
CORVIDS
CORVINA
CORVINE
CORYELL
CORYZAS
CORZINE
CURABLE
CURABLY
CURACAO
CURARES
CURATED
CURATES
CURATOR
CURBCUT
CURBING
CURDIER
CURDING
CURDLED
CURDLER
CURDLES
CUREALL
CURETTE
CURFEWS
CURIOSA
CURIOUS
CURLERS
CURLEWS
CURLIER
CURLIKE
CURLING
CURLSIN
CURLSUP
CURRANT
CURRENT
CURRIED
CURRIER
CURRIES
CURRING
CURRISH
CURSEAT
CURSERS
CURSING
CURSIVE
CURSORS
CURSORY
CURTAIL
CURTAIN
CURTATE
CURTEST
CURTISS
CURTSEY
CURVETS
CURVIER
CURVING
CYRUSII

C••R•••

CABRIDE
CABRINI
CABRIOS
CAIRENE
CAIRNED
CAMRYLE
CAPRICE
CAPRINE
CARRARA
CARRELS
CARRERA
CARRERE
CARRIED
CARRIER
CARRIES
CARROLL
CARROTS
CARROTY
CARRYIN
CARRYON
CATRIGS
CHARADE
CHARCOT
CHARGED
CHARGER
CHARGES
CHARIER
CHARILY
CHARING
CHARIOT
CHARITY
CHARLES
CHARLEY
CHARLIE
CHARMAN
CHARMED
CHARMEN
CHARMER
CHARMIN
CHARNIN
CHARPAK
CHARRED
CHARRER
CHARROS
CHARTED
CHARTER
CHARVET
CHERISH
CHEROOT
CHERUBS
CHERVIL
CHIRICO
CHIRPED
CHIRPER
CHIRRED
CHIRRUP
CHORALE
CHORALS
CHORDAL
CHORDED
CHORINE
CHORIST
CHORIZO
CHORTLE
CHURCHY
CHURNED
CHURNER
CHURNUP
CHURROS
CHYRONS
CIRRATE
CITRATE
CITRINE
CITROEN
CITRONS
CITROUS
CLARETS
CLARICE
CLARIFY
CLARION
CLARITY
CLERICS
CLERISY
CLERKED
CLERKLY
CLORETS
COARSEN
COARSER
COBRAND
COERCED
COERCER
COERCES
COMRADE
CONRACK
CONRIED
CORRADE
CORRALS
CORRECT
CORRIDA
CORRODE
CORRUPT
COURAGE
COURANT
COURBET
COURIER
COURSED
COURSER
COURSES
COURTED
COURTLY
COURTTV
COWRIES
COWRITE
COWROTE
CSARDAS
CUIRASS
CUPRITE
CUPROUS
CURRANT
CURRENT
CURRIED
CURRIER
CURRIES
CURRING
CURRISH
CUTRATE
CYMRICS
CYPRESS
CYPRIAN
CYPRIOT
CZARDAS
CZARDOM
CZARINA
CZARISM
CZARIST

C•••R••

CABARET
CALDRON
CALORIC
CALORIE
CAMAROS
CAMBRIA
CAMBRIC
CAMERAE
CAMERAL
CAMERAS
CAMERON
CANARDS
CANTRIP
CAPERED
CARBRAS
CARFREE
CARTRIP
CASERNE
CASERNS
CASERTA
CASTROL
CATERAS
CATERED
CATERER
CATERTO
CATORCE
CAVERNS
CAVORTS
CEDARED
CENTRAL
CENTRED
CENTRES
CENTRIC
CENTRUM
CETERIS
CHAGRIN
CHAIRED
CHAKRAS
CHARRED
CHARRER
CHARROS
CHEERED
CHEERER
CHEERIO
CHEERON
CHEERUP
CHETRUM
CHEVRES
CHEVRET
CHEVRON
CHIRRED
CHIRRUP
CHLORIC
CHOIRED
CHURROS
CINERGY
CLAIROL
CLEARED
CLEARER
CLEARLY
CLEAROF
CLEARUP
COCHRAN
CODERED
COHERED
COHERER
COHERES
COHORTS
COJUROR
COLORED
COLORER
COLORTV
COMORAN
COMOROS
COMTREX
CONBRIO
CONFREY
CONTRAS
CONTROL
CONURES
CORNROW
COTERIE
COVERED
COVERER
COVERME
COVERTS
COVERUP
COWARDS
COWERAT
COWERED
CUATROS
CULPRIT
CUMBRIA
CURARES
CUTARUG
CYBORGS

C••••R•

CABFARE
CABLERS
CADBURY
CADGERS
CAESARS
CAESURA
CAHIERS
CALABRO
CALDERA
CALDERS
CALGARY
CALIBRE
CALKERS
CALLERS
CALVARY
CALVERT
CAMBERS
CAMGIRL
CAMPARI
CAMPERS
CANCERS
CANKERS
CANNERS
CANNERY
CANOERS
CANONRY
CANTERS
CANTORS
CAPPERS
CAPTORS
CAPTURE
CARBARN
CARCARE
CARDERS
CAREERS
CARFARE
CARHORN
CARNERA
CARPARK
CARPERS
CARPORT
CARRARA
CARRERA
CARRERE
CARTERS
CARTIRE
CARVERS
CASPARY
CASTERS
CATBERT
CATBIRD
CAUSERS
CAVALRY
CAVEART
CAVIARE
CAVIARS
CDSTORE
CELEBRE
CELLARS
CENSERS
CENSORS
CENSURE
CENTARE
CENTERS
CENTURY
CEREBRA
CEREBRO
CESAIRE
CHAFERS
CHAMBRE
CHANTRY
CHASERS
CHEDERS
CHEWERS
CHICORY
CHIDERS
CHIMERA
CHIMERS
CHOKERS
CHOLERA
CHOLERS
CILIARY
CINDERS
CINDERY
CIPHERS
CISTERN
CLAMORS
CLAWERS
CLIBURN
CLIPART
CLONERS
CLOSERS
CLOSURE
CLOTURE
CLOVERS
CLOVERY
COALERS
COATERS
COAXERS
COCKERS
CODGERS
COFFERS
COGBURN
COHEIRS
COILERS
COINERS
COLBERT
COLLARD
COLLARS
COLOURS
COMBERS
COMFORT
COMPARE
COMPART
COMPERE
COMPORT
CONAGRA
CONAKRY
CONCERN
CONCERT
CONCORD
CONCURS
CONDORS
CONFERS
CONFIRM
CONFORM
CONGERS
CONJURE
CONJURY
CONKERS
CONNERY
CONNORS
CONSORT
CONTORT
CONVERT
COOKERS
COOKERY
COOLERS
COOPERS
COOPERY
COOTERS
COPCARS
COPIERS
COPPERS
COPPERY
COPTERS
CORDERO
CORDERS
CORKERS
CORNERS
CORPORA
COSHERS
COSTARD
COSTARS
COTTERS
COUGARS
COUNTRY
COUTERS
COUTURE
COWBIRD
COWGIRL
COWHERD
CRATERS
CRAVERS
CREMORA
CROWERS
CUECARD
CULLERS
CULTURE
CULVERT
CUMBERS
CURLERS
CURSERS
CURSORS
CURSORY
CUSSERS
CUSTARD
CUSTERS
CUTLERS
CUTLERY
CUTTERS
CUTWORK
CUTWORM
CYCLERS
CYPHERS

C•••••R

CACKLER
CADAVER
CAJOLER
CALAMAR
CALIBER
CALIPER
CALLFOR
CAMPHOR
CAMPIER
CANDLER
CANDOUR
CANNIER
CARDOOR
CAREFOR
CAROLER
CARRIER
CARTIER
CASHBAR
CASHIER
CASIMIR
CATCHER
CATDOOR
CATERER
CATHAIR
CATTIER
CAULKER
CAVILER
CCRIDER
CDTOWER
CENTAUR
CHAFFER
CHAMBER
CHAMFER
CHAMPER
CHANCER
CHANGER
CHANTER
CHAPTER
CHARGER
CHARIER
CHARMER
CHARRER
CHARTER
CHASTER
CHATTER
CHAUCER
CHEAPER
CHEATER
CHECKER
CHEDDAR
CHEEPER
CHEERER
CHEEVER
CHENIER
CHEQUER
CHESTER
CHEWIER
CHIGGER
CHILLER
CHIPPER
CHIRPER
CHITTER
CHOICER
CHOKIER
CHOOSER
CHOPPER
CHOWDER
CHUGGER
CHUKKER
CHURNER
CIRCLER
CLABBER
CLACKER
CLAIMER
CLAMBAR
CLAMBER
CLAMMER
CLAMOUR
CLAMPER
CLANGER
CLANGOR
CLAPFOR
CLAPPER
CLASHER
CLASPER
CLASSER
CLATTER
CLAVIER
CLAYIER
CLEANER
CLEARER
CLEAVER
CLICKER
CLIMBER
CLINGER
CLINKER
CLIPPER
CLOBBER
CLOCKER
CLOUTER
CLOWDER
CLUBBER
CLUBCAR
CLUCKER
CLUNKER
CLUSTER
CLUTTER
CNTOWER
COALCAR
COALTAR
COARSER
COASTER
COBBLER
COBUYER
COCHAIR
COCKIER
CODDLER
COERCER
COHERER
COJUROR
COLDWAR
COLLIER
COLLYER
COLORER
COMAKER
COMFIER
COMPEER
CONIFER
CONQUER
CONTOUR
COOLAIR
COPULAR
CORKIER
CORNIER
CORONER
CORSAIR
CORVAIR
COSTNER
COTEDOR
COULTER
COUNTER
COUPLER
COURIER
COURSER
COVERER
COVETER
COZENER
CRABBER
CRACKER
CRADLER
CRAFTER
CRAMMER
CRANMER
CRASHER
CRASSER
CRAWLER
CRAZIER
CREAMER
CREASER
CREATOR
CREEPER
CRIBBER
CRIMPER
CRISPER
CRITTER
CRITTUR
CROAKER
CROCKER
CROFTER
CROONER
CROPPER
CROSIER
CROSSER
CROWBAR
CROWDER
CROWNER
CROZIER
CRUELER
CRUISER
CRULLER
CRUPPER
CRUSHER
CRYOVER
CUPELER
CUPPIER
CUPULAR
CURATOR
CURDIER
CURDLER
CURLIER
CURRIER
CURVIER
CUSHIER
CUSSLER
CUTOVER

•CR••••

ACREAGE
ACRIDLY
ACROBAT
ACRONYM
ACRYLIC
CCRIDER
MCRANEY
SCRAGGY
SCRAPED
SCRAPER
SCRAPES
SCRAPPY
SCRATCH
SCRAWLS
SCRAWLY
SCRAWNY
SCREAKS
SCREAMS
SCREECH
SCREEDS
SCREENS
SCREWED
SCREWUP
SCRIBED
SCRIBER
SCRIBES
SCRIMPS
SCRIMPY
SCRIPPS
SCRIPTS
SCROLLS
SCROOGE
SCRUBBY
SCRUBUP
SCRUFFS
SCRUFFY
SCRUGGS
SCRUNCH
SCRUPLE
VCRTAPE

•C•R•••

ACARIDS
ACCRETE
ACCRUAL
ACCRUED
ACCRUES
ACERATE
ACERBIC
ACEROLA
ACEROSE
ACORNED
ACTRESS
ECARTES
ICERINK
ICERUNS
JCARROL
MCARDLE
MCBRIDE
MCCRARY
MCCRUMB
MCGRIFF
MCGRORY
MCGRUFF
OCARINA
OCHROID
OCHROUS
OCTROIS
SCARABS
SCARCER
SCAREDY
SCARERS
SCAREUP
SCARFED
SCARFER
SCARFUP
SCARIER
SCARIFY
SCARILY
SCARING
SCARLET
SCARPED
SCARRED
SCARVES
SCARWID
SCORERS
SCORIAS
SCORING
SCORNED
SCORNER
SCORPIO

SCURVES

•C••R••
ACCORDS
ACCURST
ACHERON
ACTORLY
ECOTRIN
ICEFREE
ICETRAY
ICTERUS
JCARROL
MCCAREY
MCENROE
MCMURDO
OCCURTO
PCWORLD
SCARRED
SCHERZI
SCHERZO
SCHIRRA
SCIORRA
SCLERAE
SCLERAL
SCLERAS
SCOURED
SCOURER
SCOURGE

•C•••R•
ACQUIRE
ACTUARY
ECHOERS
ECKHART
ECLAIRS
ICEBERG
MCCLURE
MCCLURG
MCCOURT
MCCRARY
MCGRORY
MCGUIRE
MCGWIRE
MCHENRY
OCTOBRE
OCTUBRE
OCULARS
PCUSERS
SCALARS
SCALERS
SCARERS
SCENERY
SCEPTRE
SCHIRRA
SCIORRA
SCOLARI
SCORERS
SCOTERS

•C••••R
ACCEDER
ACCUSER
ACHEFOR
ACTFOUR
ACTSFOR
CCRIDER
ECOTEUR
ECUADOR
ICEBEER
ICEOVER
MCPAPER
OCELLAR
OCONNOR
OCTOBER
SCALDER
SCALIER
SCALPER
SCAMMER
SCAMPER
SCANNER
SCANTER
SCARCER
SCARFER
SCARIER
SCATTER
SCENTER
SCEPTER
SCHEMER
SCHMEAR
SCHMEER
SCHOLAR
SCHUMER
SCISSOR
SCOFFER
SCOLDER
SCOOPER
SCOOTER
SCORNER
SCOURER
SCOUTER
SCOWLER
SCRAPER
SCRIBER
SCUDDER
SCUFFER
SCULLER
SCUPPER

••CR•••
ACCRETE
ACCRUAL
ACCRUED
ACCRUES
ASCRIBE
ATCROSS
DACRONS
DECREED
DECREER
DECREES
DECRIED
DECRIER
DECRIES
DECRUMB
DECRYPT
ENCRUST
ENCRYPT
ESCROWS
EXCRETE
GOCRAZY
INCROWD
INCRUST
IPCRESS
LACRIMO
MACRAME
MACRONS
MCCRARY
MCCRUMB
MICROBE
MICRONS
MYCROFT
RECRANK
RECRATE
RECROOM
RECROSS
RECROWN
RECRUIT
RICRACS
SECRECY
SECRETE
SECRETS
STCROIX
SUCRASE
SUCROSE
TVCREWS
UNCRAMP
UNCRATE
UNCRAZY
UNCRIED
UNCROSS
UNCROWN
UNCRUDE
UNCRUEL

••C•R••
ACCORDS
ACCURST
ASCARED
BACARDI
BACKROW
BACKRUB
BACTRIA
BICARBS
BICORNE
BICORNS
BUCKRAM
COCHRAN
DECARLO
DECORUM
ENCARRE
ENCARTA
ENCORED
ENCORES
ESCARPS
ESCORTS
EUCERIN
EUCHRED
EUCHRES
EXCERPT
EXCURSE
GOCARTS
IDCARDS
INCURVE
LACERTA
LACUREE
LECARRE
LECTRIC
LOCARNO
LUCARNE
LUCERNE
MACGRAW
MACHREE
MCCAREY
MOCHRIE
NOCARBS
OCCURTO
OHCAROL
OXCARTS
PACKRAT
PICARAS
PICARDO
PICARDY
PICAROS
RECARRY
RECARVE
RECORDS
RECORKS
RECURED
RECURES
RECURLS
RECURVE
RICARDO
SECURED
SECURER
SECURES
UNCORED
UNCORES
UNCORKS
UNCURBS
UNCURED
UNCURLS
UPCARDS
UPCURLS
UPCURVE
VECTRAS
VICEROY
VICKREY
VICTRIX

••C••R•
ANCHORS
ARCHERS
ARCHERY
BACKERS
BECHARM
BICKERS
BUCKERS
COCKERS
CYCLERS
DECIARE
DECKERS
DECLARE
DICKERS
DICKORY
DOCKERS
DOCTORS
DUCKERS
ENCARRE
ESCHERS
ETCHERS
FACTORS
FACTORY
HACKERS
HECKART
HECTARE
HECTORS
HICKORY
HOCKERS
INCHERS
INCOURT
KICKERS
LECARRE
LECHERS
LECTERN
LECTORS
LECTURE
LICKERS
LOCKERS
MACABRE
MCCLURE
MCCLURG
MCCOURT
MCCRARY
MOCKERS
MOCKERY
MUCKERS
NECKERS
NECTARS
NECTARY
NICETRY
NICKERS
ORCHARD
PACKARD
PACKERS
PECCARY
PICCARD
PICKERS
PICTURE
PUCKERS
PUCKERY
RACKERS
RECARRY
RECHART
RECTORS
RECTORY
RICHARD
ROCKERS
ROCKERY
RUCKERT
SACKERS
SECTORS
SUCCORS
SUCKDRY
SUCKERS
TACKERS
TICKERS
TUCKERS
UNCHARY
UNCHURN
UPCOURT
VACCARO
VECTORS
VICKERS
VICTORS
VICTORY
WICKERS
ZACHARY

••C•••R
ACCEDER
ACCUSER
ALCAZAR
BACKBAR
BICOLOR
BOCHNER
BUCHNER
BUCKFOR
BUCKNER
CACKLER
COCHAIR
COCKIER
DECATUR
DECAYER
DECIDER
DECODER
DECOLOR
DECOYER
DECREER
DECRIER
DICHTER
DUCKIER
ENCODER
ESCAPER
EXCITER
EXCITOR
EXCUSER
FECHNER
FICKLER
FOCUSER
GUCKIER
HACKLER
HECKLER
INCISOR
INCITER
INCOLOR
INCOMER
ITCHFOR
ITCHIER
JACAMAR
JACKTAR
JOCULAR
KICKIER
LACQUER
LACUNAR
LOCATER
LOCATOR
LUCIFER
LUCKIER
MACULAR
MACUSER
MUCKIER
NICOBAR
NUCLEAR
OSCULAR
PACECAR
PICADOR
PICKIER
RACECAR
RECITER
RECOLOR
RECOVER
RICHLER
RICHTER
ROCKIER
SECEDER
SECONDR
SECULAR
SECURER
SUCCOUR
SUCKIER
TACKIER
TACKLER
TICKLER
UNCHAIR
UNCLEAR
UNCOVER
UNCOYER
VOCODER
WACKIER
YACHTER
YUCKIER

•••CR••
AIRCREW
AMSCRAY
ATECROW
EATCROW
FIACRES
FULCRUM
LITCRIT
NONCROP
OMICRON
OUTCROP
OUTCROW
PETCROW
PILCROW
PITCREW
RESCRUB
SHECRAB
THECRAB
THECROW
UNSCREW
VELCROS

•••C•R•
ARACARI
ARTCARS
ATMCARD
BARCARS
BIGCARS
BOXCARS
BRACERO
BRACERS
CANCERS
CARCARE
CHICORY
CONCERN
CONCERT
CONCORD
CONCURS
COPCARS
CUECARD
DANCERS
DAYCARE
DEICERS
DISCARD
DISCERN
DISCORD
DOGCART
ELECTRA
ELECTRO
EPICARP
EPICURE
EXOCARP
EYECARE
FENCERS
FORCERS
GISCARD
GROCERS
GROCERY
HOTCARS
JUICERS
KEYCARD
LANCERS
LASCARS
LOWCARB
LOWCARD
MASCARA
MERCERS
MERCERY
MERCURE
MERCURY
MINCERS
MORCERF
NEWCARS
NONCORE
NOSCORE
OBSCURA
OBSCURE
OLDCARS
OUTCURE
PECCARY
PICCARD
PIECERS
PINCERS
PINCURL
PIPCARD
PLACARD
PLACERS
PLECTRA
POPCORN
PRECURE
PRICERS
PROCURE
RANCORS
REDCARD
RESCORE
RIPCORD
SAGCARD
SAUCERS
SINCERE
SLICERS
SORCERY
SPACERS
SPECTRA
SPECTRE
SPICERS
SPICERY
SUCCORS
TEACART
THECARS
TIPCART
TOWCARS
TOYCARS
TOYCART
TRACERS
TRACERY
TRICORN
UNICORN
VACCARO
VISCERA
VOICERS
WINCERS

•••C••R
BEECHER
BELCHER
BENCHER
BLACKER
BLOCKER
BOTCHER
BOUCHER
BUTCHER
CATCHER
CHECKER
CIRCLER
CLACKER
CLICKER
CLOCKER
CLUCKER
CRACKER
CROCKER
DITCHER
DOUCEUR
DRUCKER
EDUCTOR
EJECTOR
ELECTOR
ENACTOR
ERECTER
ERECTOR
EVICTOR
EXACTER
EXACTOR
FANCIER
FARCEUR
FETCHER
FILCHER
FISCHER
FLICKER
FRICKER
GAUCHER
GLACIER
HATCHER
HITCHER
JUICIER
KNOCKER
KUTCHER
LEACHER
LUNCHER
LURCHER
MARCHER
MATCHER
MOOCHER
MUNCHER
NOTCHER
PATCHER
PERCHER
PINCHER
PITCHER
POACHER
PRICIER
PROCTER
PROCTOR
PUNCHER
QUACKER
QUICKER
RANCHER
RANCOUR
REACHER
REACTOR
REOCCUR
RESCUER
SAUCIER
SHOCKER
SHUCKER
SLACKER
SLICKER
SMACKER
SMUCKER
SNACKER
SNICKER
SPACIER
SPECTER
SPECTOR
SPICIER
STACKER
STICKER
STOCKER
SUCCOUR
TEACHER
TEICHER
THICKER
TORCHER
TOUCHER
TRACKER
TRACTOR
TRICKER
TRUCKER
VOLCKER
VOUCHER
WATCHER
WHACKER
WINCHER
WRECKER
XFACTOR

••••CR•
AFARCRY
DONTCRY
MIMICRY
ONEACRE
TENACRE
TWOACRE

••••C•R
ADDUCER
AMERCER
BAITCAR
BOOMCAR
BOUNCER
CHANCER
CHAUCER
CHOICER
CLUBCAR
COALCAR
COERCER
DEDUCER
DEFACER
DOMECAR
EFFACER
ENTICER
FASTCAR
FIERCER
FLATCAR
FLEECER
GOBYCAR
GOLFCAR
GYROCAR
HANDCAR
INDUCER
INDYCAR
JUNKCAR
MAILCAR
MENACER
MINICAR
NOTICER
OFFICER
PACECAR
PIERCER
POLECAR
POLICER
POUNCER
PRANCER
RACECAR
RAILCAR
REDUCER
REOCCUR
SCARCER
SEDUCER
SIDECAR
SLOTCAR
SOLACER
SPENCER
SPLICER
SPRUCER
TANKCAR
TOWNCAR
TRAMCAR
USEDCAR
VANOCUR

CS•••••
CSARDAS
CSLEWIS

C•S••••
CASABAS
CASAVAS
CASCADE
CASEATE
CASEINS
CASELAW
CASELLA
CASELOT
CASEOUS
CASEOUT
CASERNE
CASERNS
CASERTA
CASHBAR
CASHBOX
CASHCOW
CASHEWS
CASHIER
CASHING
CASHINS
CASHOUT
CASIMIR
CASINGS
CASINOS
CASITAS
CASKETS
CASKING
CASPARY
CASPIAN
CASQUED
CASQUES
CASSABA
CASSATT
CASSAVA
CASSIAS
CASSIDY
CASSINI
CASSINO
CASSIUS
CASSOCK
CASSOLA
CASTERS
CASTILE
CASTING
CASTLED
CASTLES
CASTOFF
CASTOUT
CASTROL
CASTSON
CASTSUP
CASUALS
CASUIST
CBSNEWS
CDSTORE
CESAIRE
CESSING
CESSION
CESSNAS
CESSPIT
CESTMOI
CISCOES
CISEAUX
CISTERN
COSETTE
COSHERS
COSHING
COSIEST
COSIGNS
COSINES
COSSACK
COSSETS
COSTAIN
COSTARD
COSTARS
COSTATE
COSTING
COSTIVE
COSTNER
COSTUME
COSYING
CTSCANS
CUSHAWS
CUSHIER
CUSHILY
CUSHING
CUSHION
CUSPATE
CUSPIDS
CUSSERS
CUSSING
CUSSLER
CUSTARD
CUSTERS
CUSTODY
CUSTOMS

C••S•••
CAESARS
CAESURA
CAISSON
CANSECO
CAPSHAW
CAPSIZE
CAPSTAN
CAPSULE
CARSALE
CARSEAT
CARSHOW
CASSABA
CASSATT
CASSAVA
CASSIAS
CASSIDY
CASSINI
CASSINO
CASSIUS
CASSOCK
CASSOLA
CATSCAN
CATSEYE
CATSHOW
CATSITS
CATSPAW
CATSUIT
CATSUPS
CAUSERS
CAUSING
CAUSTIC
CEASING
CELSIUS
CENSERS
CENSING
CENSORS
CENSURE
CESSING
CESSION
CESSNAS
CESSPIT
CHASERS
CHASING
CHASMAL
CHASMIC
CHASSED
CHASSES
CHASSIS
CHASTEN
CHASTER
CHESTED
CHESTER
CHISELS
CHOSEUP
CLASHED
CLASHER
CLASHES
CLASPED
CLASPER
CLASSED
CLASSER
CLASSES
CLASSIC
CLASSON
CLOSEBY
CLOSEIN
CLOSELY
CLOSERS
CLOSEST
CLOSETO
CLOSETS
CLOSEUP
CLOSING
CLOSURE
CLUSTER
CNOSSUS
COASTAL
COASTED
COASTER
COMSATS

CONSENT
CONSIGN
CONSIST
CONSOLE
CONSORT
CONSULS
CONSULT
CONSUME
COPSHOP
COPSOUT
CORSAGE
CORSAIR
CORSETS
CORSICA
COSSACK
COSSETS
COUSINE
COUSINS
COWSHED
COWSKIN
COWSLIP
CRASHAW
CRASHED
CRASHER
CRASHES
CRASSER
CRASSLY
CRASSUS
CRESPIN
CRESSES
CRESSET
CRESTED
CRESTON
CRISPED
CRISPEN
CRISPER
CRISPIN
CRISPIX
CRISPLY
CRISPUS
CROSIER
CROSSAT
CROSSED
CROSSER
CROSSES
CROSSLY
CROSSUP
CROSTIC
CRUSADE
CRUSHED
CRUSHER
CRUSHES
CRUSTAL
CRUSTED
CRYSTAL
CUBSFAN
CUESTAS
CUISINE
CUMSHAW
CURSEAT
CURSERS
CURSING
CURSIVE
CURSORS
CURSORY
CUSSERS
CUSSING
CUSSLER
CUTSOFF
CUTSOUT

C•••S••

CAGESUP
CAISSON
CAKESUP
CALISTA
CALLSIN
CALLSIT
CALLSON
CALLSTO
CALLSUP
CALMSEA
CAMISES
CAMPSUP
CANASTA
CANTSAY
CARESTO
CARLSON
CARPSAT
CARTSIN
CASTSON
CASTSUP
CAVESIN
CAYUSES
CDCASES
CELESTA
CELESTE
CERISES
CHAISES
CHANSON
CHASSED
CHASSES
CHASSIS
CHATSUP
CHEESED
CHEESES
CHELSEA
CHEWSON
CHEWSUP
CHIPSIN
CHIPSUP
CHOMSKY
CHOOSER
CHOOSES
CHOOSEY
CHOPSUP
CHRISMS
CHRISOM
CHRISTA
CHRISTI
CHRISTO
CHRISTY
CINESIA
CLAMSUP
CLASSED
CLASSER
CLASSES
CLASSIC
CLASSON
CLAUSAL
CLAUSES
CLAWSAT
CLEMSON
CLIPSON
CLOGSUP
CLOTSUP
CLUBSUP
CLUESIN
CNOSSUS
COARSEN
COARSER
COHOSTS
COILSUP
COLOSSI
COMESAS
COMESAT
COMESBY
COMESIN
COMESON
COMESTO
COMESUP
COOKSUP
COOLSIT
COOPSUP
CORKSUP
CORPSES
COUNSEL
COURSED
COURSER
COURSES
CPLUSES
CRAISIN
CRAMSIN
CRASSER
CRASSLY
CRASSUS
CREASED
CREASER
CREASES
CREOSOL
CRESSES
CRESSET
CRIESUP
CRIMSON
CROESUS
CROPSUP
CROSSAT
CROSSED
CROSSER
CROSSES
CROSSLY
CROSSUP
CRUDSUP
CRUISED
CRUISER
CRUISES
CUBISTS
CURLSIN
CURLSUP
CURTSEY
CUTISES
CYRUSII

C••••S•

CABOOSE
CADDISH
CAGIEST
CAKIEST
CALMEST
CALYPSO
CANIEST
CANVASS
CAPEESH
CAPLESS
CARCASS
CARLESS
CAROUSE
CARWASH
CASUIST
CATFISH
CATTISH
CELLIST
CHEMISE
CHEMIST
CHERISH
CHICEST
CHINESE
CHORIST
CHUMASH
CHUTIST
CIRCUSY
CLAYISH
CLEANSE
CLERISY
CLOSEST
COCHISE
COCKISH
CODFISH
COEXIST
COKIEST
COLDEST
COLDISH
COLOSSI
COLTISH
COMBUST
COMCAST
COMMISH
COMPASS
COMPOSE
COMPOST
COMTISM
COMTIST
CONCISE
CONCUSS
CONFESS
CONFUSE
CONGEST
CONSIST
CONTEST
CONTUSE
COOLEST
COOLISH
COPYIST
CORNISH
COSIEST
COWFISH
COWIEST
COXLESS
COYNESS
COZIEST
CRAFTSY
CRUDEST
CUBBISH
CUIRASS
CULTISH
CULTISM
CULTIST
CURIOSA
CURRISH
CURTEST
CURTISS
CUTLASS
CYCLIST
CYPRESS
CZARISM
CZARIST

C•••••S

CABALAS
CABANAS
CABBIES
CABEZAS
CABLERS
CABLETS
CABRIOS
CACHETS
CACKLES
CADDIES
CADGERS
CAESARS
CAFTANS
CAHIERS
CAHOOTS
CAIMANS
CAJOLES
CALDERS
CALENDS
CALICES
CALICOS
CALIPHS
CALKERS
CALKINS
CALLEES
CALLERS
CALLINS
CALLOUS
CALLUPS
CALYCES
CALYXES
CAMAROS
CAMBERS
CAMBOYS
CAMERAS
CAMINOS
CAMIONS
CAMISES
CAMMIES
CAMPERS
CANAPES
CANARDS
CANCANS
CANCELS
CANCERS
CANCHAS
CANDIDS
CANDIES
CANDLES
CANFULS
CANINES
CANINGS
CANKERS
CANNELS
CANNERS
CANNONS
CANOERS
CANOLAS
CANOPUS
CANTABS
CANTALS
CANTERS
CANTLES
CANTONS
CANTORS
CANUCKS
CANULAS
CANVASS
CANYONS
CAPADES
CAPFULS
CAPGUNS
CAPLESS
CAPLETS
CAPNUTS
CAPOTES
CAPPERS
CAPTORS
CARACAS
CARAFES
CARBONS
CARBOYS
CARBRAS
CARCASS
CARDERS
CAREENS
CAREERS
CARFULS
CARGOES
CARHOPS
CARIBES
CARINAS
CARIOUS
CARKEYS
CARLESS
CARLOTS
CARNETS
CARNIES
CARPALS
CARPELS
CARPERS
CARPETS
CARPOUS
CARRELS
CARRIES
CARROTS
CARTELS
CARTERS
CARTONS
CARTOPS
CARVELS
CARVERS
CASABAS
CASAVAS
CASEINS
CASEOUS
CASERNS
CASHEWS
CASHINS
CASINGS
CASINOS
CASITAS
CASKETS
CASQUES
CASSIAS
CASSIUS
CASTERS
CASTLES
CASUALS
CATALOS
CATBEDS
CATCHES
CATENAS
CATERAS
CATFITS
CATGUTS
CATIONS
CATKINS
CATNAPS
CATNIPS
CATRIGS
CATSITS
CATSUPS
CATTOYS
CAUSERS
CAVEATS
CAVEINS
CAVERNS
CAVIARS
CAVORTS
CAYMANS
CAYUGAS
CAYUSES
CBSNEWS
CCLAMPS
CDCASES
CDRACKS
CDRATES
CELEBES
CELICAS
CELLARS
CELSIUS
CELTICS
CEMENTS
CENSERS
CENSORS
CENTALS
CENTERS
CENTRES
CEPHEUS
CERATES
CEREALS
CERISES
CERVIDS
CESSNAS
CETANES
CETERIS
CHABLIS
CHACHAS
CHAFERS
CHAINES
CHAISES
CHAKRAS
CHALCIS
CHALETS
CHALONS
CHAMOIS
CHANCES
CHANELS
CHANGES
CHAPELS
CHARGES
CHARLES
CHARROS
CHASERS
CHASSES
CHASSIS
CHAZANS
CHEDERS
CHEESES
CHEETAS
CHEETOS
CHEQUES
CHERUBS
CHEVETS
CHEVONS
CHEVRES
CHEWERS
CHIAPAS
CHICHAS
CHICHIS
CHICLES
CHIDERS
CHIGOES
CHILIES
CHILLIS
CHIMERS
CHINOIS
CHINUPS
CHISELS
CHITONS
CHIVIES
CHOICES
CHOKERS
CHOLERS
CHOLLAS
CHOOSES
CHORALS
CHOUGHS
CHRISMS
CHROMES
CHUPPAS
CHURROS
CHYRONS
CICADAS
CINCHES
CINDERS
CINEMAS
CINQUES
CIPHERS
CIRCLES
CIRQUES
CISCOES
CITRONS
CITROUS
CIVVIES
CLAMORS
CLAQUES
CLARETS
CLASHES
CLASSES
CLAUSES
CLAWERS
CLEAVES
CLEMENS
CLERICS
CLICHES
CLIENTS
CLIMATS
CLINICS
CLIPONS
CLIQUES
CLOCHES
CLONERS
CLORETS
CLOSERS
CLOSETS
CLOTHES
CLOVERS
CNOSSUS
COACHES
COALERS
COALGAS
COATEES
COATERS
COAXERS
COBALTS
COBBLES
COBNUTS
COBWEBS
COCKERS
COCKLES
COCOONS
CODDLES
CODGERS
CODICES
COEDITS
COEPTIS
COERCES
COEVALS
COFFEES
COFFERS
COFFINS
COGGLES
COGNACS
COHEIRS
COHERES
COHORTS
COHOSTS
COIGNES
COILERS
COINERS
COINOPS
COLADAS
COLCHIS
COLLARS
COLLETS
COLLIES
COLLINS
COLLOPS
COLONES
COLONUS
COLOURS
COLUMNS
COMBATS
COMBERS
COMEONS
COMESAS
COMFITS
COMICES
COMINGS
COMMITS
COMMONS
COMOROS
COMPAQS
COMPASS
COMPELS
COMSATS
CONCHES
CONCHOS
CONCURS
CONCUSS
CONDORS
CONFABS
CONFERS
CONFESS
CONFITS
CONGERS
CONGOUS
CONJOBS
CONKERS
CONNORS
CONOIDS
CONSULS
CONTACS
CONTRAS
CONURES
CONVEYS
CONVOYS
COOKERS
COOKIES
COOLERS
COOLIES
COOPERS
COOTERS
COOTIES
COPCARS
COPIERS
COPIOUS
COPOUTS
COPPERS
COPTERS
COPULAS
CORBELS
CORDERS
CORDIAS
CORDONS
CORFAMS
CORKERS
CORNEAS
CORNERS
CORNETS
CORONAS
CORPSES
CORRALS
CORSETS
CORVEES
CORVIDS
CORYZAS
COSHERS
COSIGNS
COSINES
COSSETS
COSTARS
COTTERS
COTTONS
COUCHES
COUGARS
COULEES
COUPLES
COUPONS
COURSES
COUSINS
COUTERS
COVERTS
COWARDS
COWBOYS
COWPEAS
COWRIES
COXLESS
COYDOGS
COYNESS
COYOTES
COZZENS
CPLUSES
CRADLES
CRASHES
CRASSUS
CRATERS
CRAVATS
CRAVENS
CRAVERS
CRAYONS
CRAZIES
CREASES
CREATES
CRECHES
CREDITS
CREEPOS
CRENELS
CREOLES
CRESSES
CRETANS
CRETINS
CREWELS
CRINGES
CRISPUS
CRITIAS
CRITICS
CROESUS
CRONIES
CROOKES
CROQUIS
CROSSES
CROTONS
CROUTES
CROWERS
CRUISES
CRUSHES
CRUZANS
CRYPTOS
CSARDAS
CSLEWIS
CTSCANS
CUATROS
CUBAGES
CUBBIES
CUBBINS
CUBFANS
CUBISTS
CUBITUS
CUBOIDS
CUCKOOS
CUDDIES
CUDDLES
CUDGELS
CUEBIDS
CUESTAS
CUETIPS
CUIRASS
CULCHES
CULEXES
CULLERS
CULLETS
CULLIES
CUMBERS
CUMBIAS
CUMULUS
CUPFULS
CUPOLAS
CUPROUS
CUPULES
CURARES
CURATES
CURDLES
CURFEWS
CURIOUS
CURLERS
CURLEWS
CURRIES
CURSERS
CURSORS
CURTISS
CURVETS
CUSHAWS
CUSPIDS
CUSSERS
CUSTERS
CUSTOMS
CUTISES
CUTLASS
CUTLERS
CUTLETS
CUTOFFS
CUTOUTS
CUTTERS
CYANIDS
CYBORGS
CYCLERS
CYCLOPS
CYGNETS
CYMBALS
CYMRICS
CYPHERS
CYPRESS
CZARDAS

•CS••••

ECSTASY
MCSHANE
MCSWINE

•C•S•••

ACESOUT
ACTSFOR
ACTSOUT
ICESHOW
ICESOUT
PCUSERS
SCISSOR
SCUSEME

•C••S••

ACCOSTS
ACCUSAL
ACCUSED
ACCUSER
ACCUSES
ACHESON
ECDYSES
ECDYSIS
ICTUSES
SCADSOF
SCHISMS
SCHISTS
SCISSOR

•C•••S•

ACCURST
ACEROSE
ACHIEST
ACTRESS
ACUTEST
ECCLESI
ECHOISM
ECLIPSE
ECSTASY
ICELESS
ICINESS
ICKIEST
OCULIST

•C••••S

ACACIAS
ACARIDS
ACCEDES
ACCENTS
ACCEPTS
ACCORDS
ACCOSTS
ACCRUES
ACCTNOS
ACCUSES
ACETALS
ACHENES
ACKACKS
ACQUITS
ACTEDAS
ACTIONS
ACTIVAS
ACTIVES
ACTRESS
ACUMENS
BCLIONS
CCLAMPS
ECARTES
ECDYSES
ECDYSIS
ECHOERS
ECLAIRS
ECTYPES
ECZEMAS
ICEAGES
ICEAXES
ICEBAGS
ICECAPS
ICEDAMS
ICEFOGS
ICELESS
ICEOUTS
ICEPOPS
ICERUNS
ICETEAS
ICICLES
ICINESS
ICTERUS
ICTINUS
ICTUSES
JCPOWYS
KCJONES
MCADAMS
MCCALLS
MCHALES
OCCULTS
OCEANUS

OCELLUS
OCELOTS
OCHROUS
OCICATS
OCTANES
OCTANTS
OCTAVES
OCTAVOS
OCTOPUS
OCTROIS
OCULARS
PCUSERS
RCCOLAS
SCALARS
SCALERS
SCARABS
SCARERS
SCARVES
SCATHES
SCENICS
SCHAYES
SCHEMAS
SCHEMES
SCHICKS
SCHISMS
SCHISTS
SCHLEPS
SCHLUBS
SCHMOES
SCHNAPS
SCHOLES
SCHOOLS
SCLAFFS
SCLERAS
SCONCES
SCOOBAS
SCORERS
SCORIAS
SCOTERS
SCOUPES
SCRAPES
SCRAWLS
SCREAKS
SCREAMS
SCREEDS
SCREENS
SCRIBES
SCRIMPS
SCRIPPS
SCRIPTS
SCROLLS
SCRUFFS
SCRUGGS
SCULPTS
SCURVES
SCUZZES
SCYTHES

••CS•••

ARCSINE
FOCSLES
TOCSINS
TUCSONS

••C•S••

ACCOSTS
ACCUSAL
ACCUSED
ACCUSER
ACCUSES
ALCESTE
ARCHSEE
BACKSAW
BACKSIN
BACKSUP
BUCKSAW
BUCKSUP
CDCASES
DACOSTA
DICKSON
ENCASED
ENCASES
EXCISED
EXCISES
EXCUSAL
EXCUSAS
EXCUSED
EXCUSER
EXCUSES
EXCUSEZ
FACESIT
FACESON
FICUSES
FOCUSED
FOCUSER
FOCUSES
FOCUSON
FUCHSIA
HACKSAW
HACKSIT
HACKSUP
HOCUSED
INCASED
INCASES
INCISED
INCISES
INCISOR
INCUSED
INCUSES
JACKSON
JACKSOO
JACKSUP
JOCASTA
KICKSIN
KICKSUP
LACESON
LACESUP
LACOSTE
LICKSUP
LOCKSET
LOCKSIN
LOCKSON
LOCKSUP
LOCUSTS
MACHSIX
MACUSER
MOCKSUP
MUCKSUP
NICOSIA
PACKSIN
PACKSON
PACKSUP
PECKSAT
PICASSO
PICKSAT
PICKSON
PICKSUP
RACESBY
RACESTO
RACESUP
RACISTS
RACKSUP
RECASED
RECASES
RECASTS
RECOSTS
RECUSAL
RECUSED
RECUSES
RICKSHA
RUCKSUP
SACKSUP
SOCKSIN
SUCKSIN
SUCKSUP
TACKSON
TACKSUP
TICKSBY
TUCKSIN
UNCASED
UNCASES
UNCASKS
UPCASTS

••C••S•

ACCURST
ARCHEST
ATCROSS
BECAUSE
COCHISE
COCKISH
CYCLIST
DECEASE
DECLASS
DICIEST
DUCHESS
ECCLESI
ENCHASE
ENCLASP
ENCLOSE
ENCRUST
EXCURSE
INCENSE
INCLASS
INCLOSE
INCRUST
IPCRESS
JACCUSE
JACKASS
LACIEST
LACTASE
LACTOSE
LICENSE
LUCIUSI
NICOISE
NOCLASS
PACHISI
PACIEST
PECKISH
PICASSO
PICTISH
PUCKISH
RACIEST
RECHOSE
RECLASP
RECLASS
RECLUSE
RECROSS
RICHEST
SICKEST
SICKISH
SUCCESS
SUCRASE
SUCROSE
UNCLASP
UNCLOSE
UNCROSS
UPCLOSE
UPCOAST
WACKEST

••C•••S

AACELLS
ABCNEWS
ACCEDES
ACCENTS
ACCEPTS
ACCORDS
ACCOSTS
ACCRUES
ACCTNOS
ACCUSES
AHCHOOS
ALCOVES
ANCHORS
ARCADES
ARCHERS
ARCHIES
ARCHONS
ARCINGS
ASCENDS
ASCENTS
ATCROSS
BACCHUS
BACKERS
BACKUPS
BECALMS
BECKONS
BECOMES
BICARBS
BICHONS
BICKERS
BICORNS
BOCCIES
BUCKERS
BUCKETS
BUCKLES
BUCKOES
CACHETS
CACKLES
CDCASES
CICADAS
COCKERS
COCKLES
COCOONS
CUCKOOS
CYCLERS
CYCLOPS
DACAPOS
DACRONS
DACTYLS
DECADES
DECAMPS
DECANTS
DECEITS
DECIDES
DECILES
DECKERS
DECKLES
DECLASS
DECLAWS
DECLOTS
DECOCTS
DECODES
DECREES
DECRIES
DICKENS
DICKERS
DICKEYS
DICKIES
DICTUMS
DOCENTS
DOCKERS
DOCKETS
DOCTORS
DRCHAOS
DUCHESS
DUCHIES
DUCKERS
DUCKIES
ENCAGES
ENCAMPS
ENCASES
ENCINAS
ENCODES
ENCORES
ESCALUS
ESCAPES
ESCARPS
ESCHERS
ESCHEWS
ESCORTS
ESCROWS
ESCUDOS
ETCHERS
EUCHRES
EXCEEDS
EXCEPTS
EXCIDES
EXCISES
EXCITES
EXCUSAS
EXCUSES
FACADES
FACIALS
FACINGS
FACTORS
FICUSES
FOCSLES
FOCUSES
GECKOES
GOCARTS
HACKERS
HACKIES
HACKLES
HECKLES
HECKYES
HECTORS
HICCUPS
HICKEYS
HOCKERS
IDCARDS
INCANTS
INCASES
INCENTS
INCEPTS
INCHERS
INCISES
INCITES
INCLASS
INCOMES
INCUBUS
INCUDES
INCUSES
IPCRESS
JACALES
JACKALS
JACKASS
JACKETS
JACQUES
JICAMAS
JOCKEYS
KICKERS
KICKUPS
KUCHENS
LACEUPS
LACINGS
LACKEYS
LACUNAS
LECHERS
LECTORS
LICHEES
LICHENS
LICKERS
LOCALES
LOCATES
LOCKERS
LOCKETS
LOCKINS
LOCKUPS
LOCULUS
LOCUSTS
LUCITES
LYCEUMS
MACACOS
MACOUNS
MACRONS
MCCALLS
MECCANS
MICKEYS
MICMACS
MICRONS
MOCKERS
MOCKUPS
MRCHIPS
MUCKERS
NBCNEWS
NECKERS
NECTARS
NICHOLS
NICKELS
NICKERS
NICKLES
NICOLAS
NOCARBS
NOCLASS
NOCUOUS
NUCLEUS
OCCULTS
OOCYTES
ORCHIDS
OSCINES
OSCULES
OXCARTS
PACKERS
PACKETS
PECTINS
PICARAS
PICAROS
PICEOUS
PICKENS
PICKERS
PICKETS
PICKLES
PICKUPS
PICNICS
POCKETS
POCONOS
PUCKERS
RACEMES
RACINOS
RACISTS
RACKERS
RACKETS
RCCOLAS
RECAGES
RECALLS
RECANES
RECANTS
RECASES
RECASTS
RECEDES
RECHEWS
RECIPES
RECITES
RECKONS
RECLADS
RECLASS
RECOALS
RECOATS
RECOCKS
RECODES
RECOILS
RECOINS
RECOMBS
RECOOKS
RECOOLS
RECORDS
RECORKS
RECOSTS
RECOUPS
RECROSS
RECTORS
RECURES
RECURLS
RECUSES
RICHENS
RICKEYS
RICKLES
RICRACS
ROCHETS
ROCKERS
ROCKETS
ROCKIES
ROCOCOS
SACHEMS
SACHETS
SACKERS
SACQUES
SECANTS
SECEDES
SECKELS
SECONDS
SECRETS
SECTORS
SECURES
SICKENS
SICKLES
SOCIALS
SOCKETS
SUCCESS
SUCCORS
SUCKERS
TACITUS
TACKERS
TACKLES
TACOMAS
TACTICS
TECHIES
TECHNOS
TICKERS
TICKETS
TICKLES
TICTACS
TOCSINS
TUCKERS
TUCSONS
TVCREWS
TYCOONS
UNCAGES
UNCAKES
UNCASES
UNCASKS
UNCIALS
UNCLIPS
UNCLOGS
UNCOILS
UNCOOPS
UNCORES
UNCORKS
UNCROSS
UNCUFFS
UNCURBS
UNCURLS
UPCARDS
UPCASTS
UPCOILS
UPCURLS
URCHINS
VACATES
VACUOUS
VACUUMS
VECTORS
VECTRAS
VICIOUS
VICKERS
VICTIMS
VICTORS
VICUNAS
WICCANS
WICKERS
WICKETS
ZOCALOS

•••CS••

ERICSON

•••C•S•

ABSCISE
ALLCASH
ATACOST
BADCASE
CARCASS
CHICEST
CIRCUSY
COMCAST
CONCISE
CONCUSS
DIECAST
DIOCESE
DISCUSS
DUNCISH
EGGCASE
FASCISM
FASCIST
FBICASE
FLYCAST
GETCASH
GIOCOSO
GLUCOSE
GOTCASH
GRECISM
GUNCASE
INACAST
JACCUSE
KEYCASE
LAWCASE
LOWCOST
MANCUSO
MARCUSE
MISCAST
NETCOST
NONCASH
OAKCASK
OFFCAST
OUTCAST
PATCASH
PAYCASH
PENCASE
PERCUSS
PODCAST
PRECAST
PRECISE
PROCESS
SARCASM
SUBCASE
SUBCASH
SUBCAST
SUCCESS
VISCUSO
WEBCAST

•••C••S

ACACIAS
AITCHES
ALLCAPS
ANACINS
ANTCOWS
APACHES
ARTCARS
ASHCANS
AVOCETS
BACCHUS
BARCARS
BATCHES
BEACHES
BEACONS
BEECHES
BELCHES
BENCHES
BIGCARS
BIGCATS
BIRCHES
BOBCATS
BOCCIES
BOOCOOS
BOTCHES
BOUCHES
BOXCARS
BRACERS
BUNCHES
BUTCHES
CANCANS
CANCELS
CANCERS
CANCHAS
CARCASS
CATCHES
CHACHAS
CHICHAS
CHICHIS
CHICLES
CINCHES
CIRCLES
CISCOES
CLICHES
CLOCHES
COACHES
COLCHIS
CONCHES
CONCHOS
CONCURS
CONCUSS
COPCARS
COUCHES
CRECHES
CTSCANS
CULCHES
DANCERS
DEACONS
DEFCONS
DEICERS
DIECUTS
DISCUSS
DITCHES
DOTCOMS
EGGCUPS
ELICITS
ENDCUTS
ERECTUS
EXACTAS
EXOCETS
EYECUPS
FALCONS
FANCIES
FASCIAS
FATCATS
FAUCETS
FENCERS
FESCUES
FETCHES
FIACRES
FILCHES
FINCHES
FLACONS
FLECHES
FORCEPS
FORCERS
GARCONS
GASCANS
GASCAPS
GASCONS
GAUCHOS
GELCAPS
GLYCOLS
GOTCHAS
GRACIAS
GROCERS
GULCHES
HATCHES
HEPCATS
HICCUPS
HITCHES
HONCHOS
HOOCHES
HOTCAPS
HOTCARS
HOTCUPS
HUBCAPS
HUNCHES
HUTCHES
ICECAPS
ICICLES
JAMCAMS
JAYCEES
JOBCUTS
JUICERS
JUNCOES
KETCHES
KIDCOMS
KWACHAS
LANCERS
LANCETS
LANCIAS
LAPCATS
LARCHES
LASCARS
LATCHES
LEACHES
LEECHES
LITCHIS
LUNCHES
LURCHES
MADCAPS
MARCELS
MARCHES
MASCOTS
MATCHES
MECCANS
MENCIUS
MERCERS
MERCHES
MERCIES
MESCALS
MIDCAPS
MINCERS
MISCUES
MISCUTS
MOOCHES
MOOCOWS
MUDCATS
MULCHES
MUNCHES
MUSCATS
MUSCLES
NEOCONS
NEWCARS
NONCOMS
NOTCHES
NUNCIOS
OCICATS
OILCANS
OILCUPS
OLDCARS
ORACIES
ORACLES
OUTCUTS
PARCELS
PARCHES
PATCHES
PAYCUTS
PEACHES
PENCILS
PEPCIDS
PERCHES
PERCUSS
PETCATS
PETCOWS
PIECERS
PINCERS
PINCHAS
PINCHES
PITCHES
PLACERS
POACHES
PONCHOS
POOCHES
PORCHES
POUCHES
PRECUTS
PRICERS
PROCESS
PROCLUS
PSYCHES
PSYCHOS
PUNCHES
QUICHES
RANCHES
RANCHOS
RANCORS
RASCALS
RAUCOUS
REACHES
REDCAPS
REDCODS
RESCANS
RESCUES
REXCATS
RIBCUTS
ROACHES
ROMCOMS
ROSCOES
SANCTUS
SATCOMS
SAUCERS
SEACATS
SEACOWS
SITCOMS
SKICAPS
SKYCAMS
SKYCAPS
SLICERS
SNOCAPS
SNOCATS
SPACERS
SPECIES
SPICERS
SPYCAMS
STUCCOS
SUCCESS
SUCCORS
TALCUMS
TAXCUTS
TEACHES
TEACUPS
TENCHES
TERCELS
THECARS
THECAVS
THECUBS
TINCANS
TOECAPS
TOMCATS
TORCHES
TOUCANS
TOUCHES
TOWCARS
TOYCARS
TRACERS
TRICEPS
TRICOTS
TROCHES
TUSCANS
URACILS
UTICANS
VELCROS
VETCHES
VISCOUS
VOICERS
VOUCHES
VULCANS
WATCHES
WEBCAMS
WENCHES
WICCANS
WINCERS
WINCHES
WITCHES
ZILCHES
ZINCOUS
ZIRCONS
ZITCOMS

••••C•S

ABDUCES
ABDUCTS
ACKACKS
ADDICTS
ADDUCES
ADDUCTS
ADVICES
AFFECTS
AGENCES
AIRACES

ALNICOS
ALPACAS
AMERCES
ANARCHS
APERCUS
ARBACES
ARNICAS
ARRACKS
ASPECTS
ATTACKS
ATTICUS
ATTUCKS
BARACUS
BEDECKS
BISECTS
BODICES
BONACIS
BOUNCES
BRONCOS
CALICES
CALICOS
CALYCES
CANUCKS
CARACAS
CDRACKS
CELICAS
CHALCIS
CHANCES
CHOICES
CODICES
COERCES
COMICES
DECOCTS
DEDUCES
DEDUCTS
DEFACES
DEFECTS
DEFOCUS
DEJECTS
DELICTS
DEPICTS
DETECTS
DEVICES
DIDACTS
DIRECTS
EFFACES
EFFECTS
ELANCES
ENFACES
ENLACES
ENTICES
EPARCHS
EVINCES
EXARCHS
EXPECTS
EXSECTS
FIANCES
FIASCOS
FLEECES
FRANCES
FRANCIS
FRENCHS
FRESCAS
FRESCOS
GFORCES
GLANCES
HELICES
HIJACKS
HYRACES
IMPACTS
INDICES
INDICTS
INDUCES
INDUCTS
INFECTS
INFOCUS
INJECTS
INSECTS
JOUNCES
KOPECKS
LATICES
MACACOS
MALICES
MARACAS
MEDICOS
MENACES
MISACTS
MUSICKS
NOTICES
NOVICES
NUANCES
OBJECTS
OFFICES
ONEACTS
OPTICKS
OUTACTS
PALACES
PATACAS
PHILCOS
PIERCES
PLAICES
POLICES
POUNCES
PRANCES
PREACTS
PRINCES
PUMICES
QUINCES
RADICES
RECOCKS
REDACTS
REDOCKS
REDUCES
REFACES
REFOCUS
REJECTS
REKICKS
RELACES
RELICTS
RELOCKS
RELUCTS
REPACKS
REPICKS
RERACKS
RESECTS
RETACKS
RHOECUS
ROCOCOS
SCHICKS
SCONCES
SEANCES
SEDUCES
SELECTS
SENECAS
SHTICKS
SILICAS
SLUICES
SOLACES
SOURCES
SPLICES
SPRUCES
STANCES
STUCCOS
TENACES
THWACKS
TIERCES
TRANCES
TWOACTS
UNDOCKS
UNFACTS
UNLACES
UNLOCKS
UNPACKS
UNPICKS
UNRACKS
UNTACKS
UNTUCKS
UPTICKS
USANCES
USEDCDS
VOTECHS
ZYDECOS

•••••CS

AGARICS
AIRSACS
AMTRACS
ARABICS
ATOMICS
ATONICS
BIGMACS
BIONICS
BIOPICS
CELTICS
CLERICS
CLINICS
COGNACS
CONTACS
CRITICS
CYMRICS
EBONICS
EGGSACS
EMETICS
EROTICS
ETHNICS
ETONICS
EXOTICS
FABRICS
FANFICS
FROLICS
GARLICS
GOTHICS
HAPTICS
HEROICS
IAMBICS
IATRICS
INKSACS
IRENICS
ITALICS
MANIACS
MASTICS
METRICS
MICMACS
MIXTECS
MOSAICS
MYSTICS
NOETICS
NORDICS
OVISACS
PARSECS
PEPTICS
PHOBICS
PHONICS
PHOTICS
PHYSICS
PICNICS
POETICS
PUBLICS
RICRACS
RUBRICS
RUSTICS
SCENICS
STATICS
SYNDICS
TACTICS
TARMACS
THEABCS
TICTACS
TIETACS
TOLTECS
TROPICS
UNIVACS
VITRICS
ZIPLOCS
ZODIACS

CT•••••

CTENOID
CTSCANS

C•T••••

CATALAN
CATALOG
CATALOS
CATALPA
CATANIA
CATAWBA
CATBEDS
CATBERT
CATBIRD
CATBOAT
CATBOWL
CATCALL
CATCHER
CATCHES
CATCHON
CATCHOW
CATCHUP
CATCOMB
CATDOOR
CATENAE
CATENAS
CATERAS
CATERED
CATERER
CATERTO
CATEYED
CATFEET
CATFISH
CATFITS
CATFLAP
CATFLEA
CATFOOD
CATFOOT
CATGUTS
CATHAIR
CATHEAD
CATHODE
CATIONS
CATKINS
CATLIKE
CATMINT
CATNAPS
CATNIPS
CATORCE
CATRIGS
CATSCAN
CATSEYE
CATSHOW
CATSITS
CATSPAW
CATSUIT
CATSUPS
CATTAIL
CATTALO
CATTIER
CATTILY
CATTISH
CATTOYS
CATWALK
CDTOWER
CETANES
CETERIS
CITABLE
CITADEL
CITIZEN
CITRATE
CITRINE
CITROEN
CITRONS
CITROUS
CITYBOY
CITYGAL
CNTOWER
COTEACH
COTEDOR
COTERIE
COTTAGE
COTTERS
COTTONS
COTTONY
CUTARUG
CUTAWAY
CUTBACK
CUTDOWN
CUTICLE
CUTINON
CUTINTO
CUTISES
CUTLASS
CUTLERS
CUTLERY
CUTLETS
CUTOFFS
CUTOPEN
CUTOUTS
CUTOVER
CUTRATE
CUTSOFF
CUTSOUT
CUTTERS
CUTTIME
CUTTING
CUTWORK
CUTWORM

C••T•••

CAFTANS
CALTECH
CANTABS
CANTALS
CANTATA
CANTEEN
CANTERS
CANTILY
CANTINA
CANTING
CANTINO
CANTLES
CANTONS
CANTORS
CANTRIP
CANTSAY
CAPTAIN
CAPTION
CAPTIVA
CAPTIVE
CAPTORS
CAPTURE
CARTAGE
CARTALK
CARTELS
CARTERS
CARTIER
CARTING
CARTIRE
CARTOFF
CARTONS
CARTOON
CARTOPS
CARTRIP
CARTSIN
CASTERS
CASTILE
CASTING
CASTLED
CASTLES
CASTOFF
CASTOUT
CASTROL
CASTSON
CASTSUP
CATTAIL
CATTALO
CATTIER
CATTILY
CATTISH
CATTOYS
CAUTHEN
CAUTION
CDSTORE
CELTICS
CENTALS
CENTARE
CENTAUR
CENTAVO
CENTERS
CENTIME
CENTIMO
CENTRAL
CENTRED
CENTRES
CENTRIC
CENTRUM
CENTURY
CERTAIN
CERTIFY
CESTMOI
CHATEAU
CHATHAM
CHATSUP
CHATTED
CHATTEL
CHATTER
CHATWIN
CHETRUM
CHITLIN
CHITONS
CHITOWN
CHITTER
CHUTING
CHUTIST
CHUTNEY
CHUTZPA
CISTERN
CLATTER
CLOTHED
CLOTHES
CLOTSUP
CLOTTED
CLOTURE
CLUTCHY
CLUTTER
COATEES
COATERS
COATING
COCTEAU
COETZEE
COLTISH
COMTISM
COMTIST
COMTREX
CONTACS
CONTACT
CONTAIN
CONTEMN
CONTEND
CONTENT
CONTEST
CONTEXT
CONTORT
CONTOUR
CONTRAS
CONTROL
CONTUSE
COOTERS
COOTIES
COPTERS
CORTEGE
CORTICO
CORTINA
COSTAIN
COSTARD
COSTARS
COSTATE
COSTING
COSTIVE
COSTNER
COSTUME
COTTAGE
COTTERS
COTTONS
COTTONY
COUTERS
COUTURE
COWTOWN
CRATERS
CRATEUP
CRATING
CRATION
CRETANS
CRETINS
CRITIAS
CRITICS
CRITTER
CRITTUR
CROTONS
CRUTZEN
CUATROS
CUETIPS
CULTISH
CULTISM
CULTIST
CULTJAM
CULTURE
CURTAIL
CURTAIN
CURTATE
CURTEST
CURTISS
CURTSEY
CUSTARD
CUSTERS
CUSTODY
CUSTOMS
CUTTERS
CUTTIME
CUTTING
CYNTHIA

C•••T••

CADETTE
CAKETIN
CALOTTE
CANETTI
CANITBE
CAPITAL
CAPITAN
CAPITOL
CAPOTES
CAPSTAN
CARLTON
CAROTID
CAROTIN
CASITAS
CAUSTIC
CDRATES
CELOTEX
CERATED
CERATES
CHANTED
CHANTER
CHANTEY
CHANTRY
CHAOTIC
CHAPTER
CHARTED
CHARTER
CHASTEN
CHASTER
CHATTED
CHATTEL
CHATTER
CHEATED
CHEATER
CHEATIN
CHEATON
CHEETAH
CHEETAS
CHEETOS
CHESTED
CHESTER
CHEWTOY
CHINTZY
CHITTER
CHOCTAW
CHORTLE
CLACTON
CLANTON
CLAPTON
CLATTER
CLAYTON
CLEATED
CLIFTON
CLINTON
CLOTTED
CLOUTED
CLOUTER
CLUSTER
CLUTTER
COACTED
COALTAR
COAPTED
COASTAL
COASTED
COASTER
COEPTIS
COLETTE
COMPTON
COOKTOP
COOPTED
CORETTA
COSETTE
COULTER
COUNTED
COUNTEE
COUNTEM
COUNTER
COUNTIN
COUNTON
COUNTRY
COUNTUP
COURTED
COURTLY
COURTTV
COVETED
COVETER
COYOTES
CRAFTED
CRAFTER
CRAFTSY
CREATED
CREATES
CREATOR
CREPTIN
CREPTUP
CRESTED
CRESTON
CRITTER
CRITTUR
CROATIA
CROFTER
CROPTOP
CROSTIC
CROUTES
CROUTON
CRUSTAL
CRUSTED
CRYPTIC
CRYPTOS
CRYSTAL
CUBITAL
CUBITUS
CUESTAS
CULOTTE
CURATED
CURATES
CURATOR
CURETTE
CUVETTE

C••••T•

CABLETS
CABLETV
CACHETS
CADETTE
CAHOOTS
CALCITE
CALISTA
CALLSTO
CALOTTE
CANASTA
CANETTI
CANTATA
CAPLETS
CAPNUTS
CAREDTO
CARESTO
CARLOTA
CARLOTS
CARNETS
CARPETS
CARROTS
CARROTY
CASEATE
CASERTA
CASKETS
CASSATT
CATERTO
CATFITS
CATGUTS
CATSITS
CAUDATE
CAVEATS
CAVORTS
CELESTA
CELESTE
CEMENTS
CHALETS
CHAPATI
CHARITY
CHAYOTE
CHELATE
CHEVETS
CHIANTI
CHRISTA
CHRISTI
CHRISTO
CHRISTY
CILENTO
CILIATE
CIRRATE
CITRATE
CLAMATO
CLARETS
CLARITY
CLAVATE
CLEANTE
CLIENTS
CLIMATE
CLIMATS
CLIMBTO
CLINGTO
CLORETS
CLOSETO
CLOSETS
CLUNGTO
COBALTS
COBNUTS
COEDITS
COGNATE
COHORTS
COHOSTS
COLETTE
COLGATE
COLLATE
COLLETS
COLORTV
COMBATS
COMESTO
COMFITS
COMMITS
COMMUTE
COMPETE
COMPOTE
COMPUTE
COMSATS
CONFITS
CONFUTE
CONMOTO
CONNATE
CONNOTE
COPOUTS
CORBETT
CORDATE
CORDITE
CORETTA
CORINTH
CORNETS
CORNUTE
CORSETS
COSETTE
COSSETS
COSTATE
COURTTV
COVERTS
COWRITE
COWROTE
CRAVATS
CREDITS
CREMATE
CRENATE
CRUDITY
CRUELTY
CUBISTS
CULLETS
CULOTTE
CUNEATE
CUPRITE
CURETTE
CURTATE
CURVETS
CUSPATE
CUTINTO
CUTLETS
CUTOUTS
CUTRATE
CUVETTE
CYGNETS

C•••••T

CABARET
CABINET
CAGEPET
CAGIEST
CAKIEST
CALLOUT
CALLSIT
CALMEST
CALUMET
CALVERT
CAMELOT
CAMEOUT
CAMPOUT
CANDENT
CANIEST
CAPELET
CAPULET
CARCOAT
CARPORT
CARPSAT
CARSEAT
CASELOT
CASEOUT
CASHOUT
CASSATT
CASTOUT
CASUIST
CATBERT
CATBOAT
CATFEET
CATFOOT
CATMINT
CATSUIT
CAVEART
CAVILAT
CELLIST
CESSPIT
CHAPLET
CHARCOT
CHARIOT
CHARVET
CHEEZIT
CHEMIST
CHEROOT
CHEVIOT
CHEVRET
CHEWOUT
CHIAPET
CHICEST
CHICLET
CHILCAT
CHILKAT
CHORIST
CHROMAT
CHUCKIT
CHUTIST
CIRCLET
CIRCUIT
CLAMANT
CLAWSAT
CLAYPIT
CLEMENT
CLIPART
CLIPOUT
CLOSEST
COAGENT
COALPIT
COCKPIT
COCONUT
COEXIST
COHABIT
COKIEST
COLBERT
COLDCUT
COLDEST
COLLECT
COMBUST
COMCAST
COMEOUT
COMESAT
COMFORT
COMMENT
COMPACT
COMPART
COMPORT
COMPOST
COMTIST
CONCEIT
CONCEPT
CONCERT
CONCOCT
CONDUCT
CONDUIT
CONELET
CONFECT
CONGEST
CONKOUT
CONNECT
CONSENT
CONSIST
CONSORT
CONSULT
CONTACT
CONTENT
CONTEST
CONTEXT
CONTORT
CONVECT
CONVENT
CONVERT
CONVICT
COOKOUT
COOKPOT

COOLANT
COOLCAT
COOLEST
COOLOUT
COOLSIT
COONCAT
COPILOT
COPSOUT
COPYCAT
COPYIST
CORBETT
CORONET
CORRECT
CORRUPT
COSIEST
COULDNT
COUPLET
COURANT
COURBET
COWERAT
COWIEST
COZIEST
CRABPOT
CRAPOUT
CRESSET
CREWCUT
CRICKET
CROCHET
CROCKET
CROQUET
CROSSAT
CRUDEST
CRUGUET
CRUMPET
CULPRIT
CULTIST
CULVERT
CURBCUT
CURRANT
CURRENT
CURSEAT
CURTEST
CUTSOUT
CYCLIST
CYPRIOT
CZARIST

•CT••••

ACTABLE
ACTAEON
ACTEDAS
ACTEDIN
ACTEDON
ACTEDUP
ACTFIVE
ACTFOUR
ACTIFED
ACTINON
ACTIONS
ACTIVAS
ACTIVES
ACTLIKE
ACTORLY
ACTRESS
ACTSFOR
ACTSOUT
ACTUARY
ACTUATE
ACTUPON
ECTYPAL
ECTYPES
ICTERUS
ICTINUS
ICTUSES
OCTADIC
OCTAGON
OCTANES
OCTANTS
OCTAVAL
OCTAVES
OCTAVIA
OCTAVIO
OCTAVOS
OCTETTE
OCTOBER
OCTOBRE
OCTOPOD
OCTOPUS
OCTROIS
OCTUBRE
OCTUPLE
OCTUPLY

•C•T•••

ACCTNOS
ACETALS
ACETATE
ACETIFY
ACETONE
ACHTUNG
ACUTELY
ACUTEST
ECOTAGE
ECOTEUR
ECOTRIN
ECOTYPE
ECSTASY
ICETEAS
ICETRAY
SCATHED
SCATHES
SCATMAN
SCATTED
SCATTER
SCHTICK
SCITECH
SCOTERS
SCOTIAN
SCOTTIE
SCUTTLE
SCYTHED
SCYTHES
VCRTAPE

•C••T••

ACANTHI
ECARTES
ICEDTEA
OCTETTE
SCANTED
SCANTER
SCANTLY
SCATTED
SCATTER
SCENTED
SCENTER
SCEPTER
SCEPTIC
SCEPTRE
SCIATIC
SCOOTCH
SCOOTED
SCOOTER
SCOTTIE
SCOUTED
SCOUTER
SCOUTUP
SCRATCH
SCUTTLE

•C•••T•

ACCENTS
ACCEPTS
ACCOSTS
ACCRETE
ACERATE
ACETATE
ACIDITY
ACOLYTE
ACONITE
ACQUITS
ACTUATE
ICEBATH
ICEOUTS
NCWYETH
OCCULTS
OCCURTO
OCELOTS
OCHENTA
OCICATS
OCTANTS
OCTETTE
SCHISTS
SCHLITZ
SCHMITT
SCHULTZ
SCRIPTS
SCULPTS

•C••••T

ACCOUNT
ACCURST
ACEDOUT
ACESOUT
ACHIEST
ACINGIT
ACROBAT
ACTSOUT
ACUTEST
ECKHART
ICANNOT
ICEBOAT
ICEDOUT
ICESOUT
ICINGIT
ICKIEST
MCCOURT
OCCIPUT
OCULIST
SCARLET
SCHELDT
SCHMIDT
SCHMITT
SCOFFAT

••CT•••

ACCTNOS
AFCTEAM
AUCTION
BACTRIA
COCTEAU
DACTYLS
DICTATE
DICTION
DICTUMS
DOCTORS
DUCTILE
DUCTING
FACTFUL
FACTION
FACTOID
FACTORS
FACTORY
FACTUAL
FICTILE
FICTION
FICTIVE
HECTARE
HECTORS
LACTAID
LACTASE
LACTATE
LACTEAL
LACTOSE
LECTERN
LECTORS
LECTRIC
LECTURE
NECTARS
NECTARY
NFCTEAM
NICTATE
PECTINS
PICTISH
PICTURE
RECTIFY
RECTORS
RECTORY
RUCTION
SECTION
SECTORS
SUCTION
TACTFUL
TACTICS
TACTILE
TACTUAL
TICTACS
UNCTION
VECTORS
VECTRAS
VICTIMS
VICTORS
VICTORY
VICTRIX
VICTUAL

••C•T••

ASCETIC
BYCATCH
DECATUR
DICHTER
EXCITED
EXCITER
EXCITES
EXCITOR
FACETED
INCITED
INCITER
INCITES
JACKTAR
LICITLY
LOCATED
LOCATER
LOCATES
LOCATOR
LUCETTA
LUCITES
MACHTWO
NECKTIE
NICETRY
NOCATCH
OOCYTES
PICOTED
RECITAL
RECITED
RECITER
RECITES
RICHTER
RICOTTA
TACITLY
TACITUS
TICOTIN
UNCITED
VACATED
VACATES
VECHTEN
YACHTED
YACHTER
YACHTIE
YUCATAN
YUCATEC

••C••T•

ACCENTS
ACCEPTS
ACCOSTS
ACCRETE
ALCESTE
ARCUATE
ASCENTS
BACHATA
BECKETT
BUCKETS
CACHETS
DACOSTA
DECANTS
DECEITS
DECLOTS
DECOCTS
DICTATE
DOCENTS
DOCKETS
ENCARTA
ESCORTS
EXCEPTS
EXCRETE
FACULTY
GOCARTS
HACKETT
INCANTS
INCENTS
INCEPTS
JACINTH
JACINTO
JACKETS
JOCASTA
LACERTA
LACOSTE
LACTATE
LECONTE
LICKETY
LOCKETS
LOCUSTS
LUCETTA
MACBETH
MACHETE
NICTATE
OCCULTS
OCCURTO
OXCARTS
PACKETS
PICANTE
PICCATA
PICKETS
PICKETT
POCKETS
PUCKETT
RACEDTO
RACESTO
RACISTS
RACKETS
RACKETY
RECANTS
RECASTS
RECOATS
RECOSTS
RECRATE
RICKETY
RICOTTA
ROCHETS
ROCKETS
SACHETS
SECANTS
SECRETE
SECRETS
SOCIETY
SOCKETS
SUCCOTH
TICKETS
TOCCATA
UNCOUTH
UNCRATE
UPCASTS
VACUITY
VICENTE
VICOMTE
WICHITA
WICKETS

••C•••T

ACCOUNT
ACCURST
ANCIENT
ARCHEST
BACKBIT
BACKLIT
BACKLOT
BACKOUT
BECKETT
COCKPIT
COCONUT
CYCLIST
DECKOUT
DECRYPT
DICIEST
DUCKOUT
ENCHANT
ENCRUST
ENCRYPT
ESCHEAT
ETCHANT
EXCELAT
EXCERPT
FACEDIT
FACESIT
HACKETT
HACKSIT
HECKART
INCOURT
INCRUST
JACKPOT
JACONET
KICKOUT
LACIEST
LACKWIT
LOCKLET
LOCKNUT
LOCKOUT
LOCKSET
LUCKOUT
MCCOURT
MYCROFT
NECKLET
NICOLET
NOCOUNT
OCCIPUT
PACIEST
PACKRAT
PECCANT
PECKSAT
PICKETT
PICKOUT
PICKSAT
PUCKETT
RACIEST
RACKOUT
RACQUET
RECEIPT
RECHART
RECOUNT
RECRUIT
RICHEST
RUCKERT
SACKOUT
SICKEST
SICKOUT
UNCLEFT
UNCLIPT
UPCOAST
UPCOURT
WACKEST

•••CT••

CHOCTAW
CLACTON
COACTED
EDICTAL
EDUCTED
EDUCTOR
EJECTED
EJECTOR
ELECTED
ELECTEE
ELECTME
ELECTOR
ELECTRA
ELECTRO
ENACTED
ENACTOR
ERECTED
ERECTER
ERECTLY
ERECTOR
ERECTUS
ERUCTED
EVICTED
EVICTEE
EVICTOR
EXACTAS
EXACTED
EXACTER
EXACTLY
EXACTOR
FRACTAL
MONCTON
MULCTED
ORECTIC
PLECTRA
PRACTIC
PROCTER
PROCTOR
REACTED
REACTOR
REACTTO
SANCTUM
SANCTUS
SPECTER
SPECTOR
SPECTRA
SPECTRE
TINCTED
TRACTOR
UNACTED
XFACTOR

•••C•T•

AVOCETS
BAYCITY
BIGCATS
BIGCITY
BOBCATS
BOYCOTT
CALCITE
DELCITY
DIECUTS
EDACITY
EDUCATE
ELICITS
ELMCITY
ELOCUTE
ENDCUTS
EXECUTE
EXOCETS
FALCATE
FATCATS
FATCITY
FAUCETS
FAWCETT
FLOCKTO
FOGCITY
FURCATE
GETCUTE
GOTCUTE
HEPCATS
JOBCUTS
LANCETS
LAPCATS
MARCATO
MASCOTS
MISCITE
MISCUTS
MOSCATO
MRSCOTT
MUDCATS
MUSCATS
OCICATS
OLDCITY
OPACITY
OUTCITY
OUTCUTS
PAUCITY
PAYCUTS
PETCATS
PICCATA
PITCHTO
PLACATE
PLICATE
PRECITE
PRECUTS
PROCITY
REACTTO
REXCATS
RIBCUTS
SEACATS
SIMCITY
SINCITY
SNOCATS
STICKTO
STUCKTO
SUCCOTH
SUNCITY
TAXCUTS
THECITY
TOCCATA
TOMCATS
TRICOTS
WALCOTT
WATCHTV
WESCOTT
ZINCITE

•••C••T

ATACOST
BISCUIT
BOXCOAT
BOYCOTT
BRACKET
CARCOAT
CHICEST
CHICLET
CHUCKIT
CIRCLET
CIRCUIT
COMCAST
CONCEIT
CONCEPT
CONCERT
CONCOCT
CRICKET
CROCHET
CROCKET
DESCANT
DESCENT
DIECAST
DOGCART
DOGCOAT
ETICKET
FASCIST
FAWCETT
FLYCAST
FURCOAT
HATCHET
INACAST
LABCOAT
LESCAUT
LITCRIT
LOWCOST
MISCAST
MRSCOTT
NASCENT
NETCOST
OFFCAST
ONECENT
OUTCANT
OUTCAST
PEACOAT
PECCANT
PERCENT
PERCEPT
PINCHOT
PLACKET
PODCAST
PRECAST
PRECEPT
RATCHET
REDCENT
REDCOAT
SNICKET
SPECOUT
SUBCAST
TEACART
TENCENT
THICKET
TIPCART
TOPCOAT
TOYCART
VINCENT
WALCOTT
WATCHIT
WEBCAST
WESCOTT

••••CT•

ABDUCTS
ADDICTS
ADDUCTS
AFFECTS
ASPECTS
BISECTS
DECOCTS
DEDUCTS
DEFACTO
DEFECTS
DEJECTS
DELICTI
DELICTO
DELICTS
DEPICTS
DETECTO
DETECTS
DIDACTS
DIRECTS
DIRECTV
EFFECTS
EXFACTO
EXPECTS
EXSECTS
IMPACTS
INDICTS
INDUCTS
INFECTS
INJECTS
INSECTA
INSECTS
INVICTA
MISACTS
OBJECTS
ONEACTS
OUTACTS
PREACTS
REDACTS
REJECTS
RELICTS
RELUCTS
RESECTS
SELECTS
TWOACTS
UNFACTS

••••C•T

APRICOT
BEARCAT
BESTCUT
BOOTCUT
BORSCHT
BUZZCUT
CHARCOT
CHILCAT
COLDCUT
COOLCAT
COONCAT
COPYCAT
CREWCUT
CURBCUT
DEFICIT
DOVECOT
HAIRCUT
HALFCUT
HARICOT
HELLCAT
ILLICIT
JUMPCUT
LEANCUT
LINECUT
LOSTCAT
MALECAT
MANXCAT
ONEACAT
ONEOCAT
OVERCUT
PLUMCOT
POLECAT
SHOWCAT
SNOWCAT
SOLICIT
UTRECHT
WELLCUT
WILDCAT
WOODCUT

•••••CT

ADJUNCT
AFFLICT
AIRDUCT
ATTRACT
COLLECT
COMPACT
CONCOCT
CONDUCT
CONFECT
CONNECT
CONTACT
CONVECT
CONVICT
CORRECT
DEFLECT
DEFUNCT
DETRACT
DIALECT
DISSECT
EXTINCT
EXTRACT
INEXACT
INFLECT
INFLICT
INFRACT
INSPECT
IOBJECT
LASTACT
NEGLECT
NONFACT
OVERACT
OVIDUCT
PERFECT
PLAYACT
PREDICT
PREFECT
PRODUCT
PROJECT
PROTECT
REEJECT
REELECT
REENACT
REERECT
REEVICT
REFLECT
REFRACT
RESPECT
RETRACT
RIOTACT
SOLOACT
SUBDUCT
SUBJECT
SUBSECT
SUSPECT
TRISECT
UNERECT
VERDICT
VIADUCT

CU•••••

CUATROS
CUBAGES
CUBBIES
CUBBING
CUBBINS
CUBBISH
CUBFANS
CUBICAL
CUBICLE
CUBICLY
CUBISTS
CUBITAL
CUBITUS
CUBOIDS
CUBSFAN
CUCKOOS
CUDDIES
CUDDLED
CUDDLES
CUDGELS
CUEBALL
CUEBIDS
CUECARD
CUESTAS
CUETIPS
CUFFING
CUIBONO
CUINGIN
CUIRASS
CUISINE
CULCHES
CULEXES
CULLERS
CULLETS
CULLIED
CULLIES
CULLING
CULOTTE
CULPRIT
CULTISH
CULTISM
CULTIST
CULTJAM
CULTURE
CULVERT
CUMBERS
CUMBIAS
CUMBRIA
CUMSHAW
CUMULUS
CUNEATE
CUNNING
CUPCAKE
CUPELED
CUPELER
CUPFULS
CUPLIKE
CUPOLAS
CUPPIER
CUPPING
CUPRITE
CUPROUS
CUPULAR
CUPULES

CURABLE
CURABLY
CURACAO
CURARES
CURATED
CURATES
CURATOR
CURBCUT
CURBING
CURDIER
CURDING
CURDLED
CURDLER
CURDLES
CUREALL
CURETTE
CURFEWS
CURIOSA
CURIOUS
CURLERS
CURLEWS
CURLIER
CURLIKE
CURLING
CURLSIN
CURLSUP
CURRANT
CURRENT
CURRIED
CURRIER
CURRIES
CURRING
CURRISH
CURSEAT
CURSERS
CURSING
CURSIVE
CURSORS
CURSORY
CURTAIL
CURTAIN
CURTATE
CURTEST
CURTISS
CURTSEY
CURVETS
CURVIER
CURVING
CUSHAWS
CUSHIER
CUSHILY
CUSHING
CUSHION
CUSPATE
CUSPIDS
CUSSERS
CUSSING
CUSSLER
CUSTARD
CUSTERS
CUSTODY
CUSTOMS
CUTARUG
CUTAWAY
CUTBACK
CUTDOWN
CUTICLE
CUTINON
CUTINTO
CUTISES
CUTLASS
CUTLERS
CUTLERY
CUTLETS
CUTOFFS
CUTOPEN
CUTOUTS
CUTOVER
CUTRATE
CUTSOFF
CUTSOUT
CUTTERS
CUTTIME
CUTTING
CUTWORK
CUTWORM
CUVETTE

C•U••••

CAUDATE
CAULKED
CAULKER
CAUSERS
CAUSING
CAUSTIC
CAUTHEN
CAUTION
CHUCKED
CHUCKIT
CHUCKLE
CHUFFED
CHUGGED
CHUGGER
CHUKKER
CHUMASH
CHUMMED
CHUMPED
CHUNKED
CHUNNEL
CHUPPAH
CHUPPAS
CHURCHY
CHURNED
CHURNER
CHURNUP
CHURROS
CHUTING
CHUTIST
CHUTNEY
CHUTZPA
CLUBBED
CLUBBER
CLUBCAR
CLUBMED
CLUBSUP
CLUCKED
CLUCKER
CLUEDIN
CLUEFUL
CLUEING
CLUESIN
CLUMPED
CLUNGTO
CLUNKED
CLUNKER
CLUSTER
CLUTCHY
CLUTTER
COUCHED
COUCHES
COUGARS
COUGHED
COUGHUP
COULDBE
COULDNT
COULEES
COULOMB
COULTER
COUNCIL
COUNSEL
COUNTED
COUNTEE
COUNTEM
COUNTER
COUNTIN
COUNTON
COUNTRY
COUNTUP
COUPING
COUPLED
COUPLER
COUPLES
COUPLET
COUPONS
COURAGE
COURANT
COURBET
COURIER
COURSED
COURSER
COURSES
COURTED
COURTLY
COURTTV
COUSINE
COUSINS
COUTERS
COUTURE
CRUCIAL
CRUDELY
CRUDEST
CRUDITY
CRUDSUP
CRUELER
CRUELLA
CRUELLY
CRUELTY
CRUGUET
CRUISED
CRUISER
CRUISES
CRULLER
CRUMBED
CRUMBLE
CRUMBLY
CRUMBUM
CRUMPED
CRUMPET
CRUMPLE
CRUMPLY
CRUNCHY
CRUPPER
CRUSADE
CRUSHED
CRUSHER
CRUSHES
CRUSTAL
CRUSTED
CRUTZEN
CRUZADO
CRUZANS

C••U•••

CADUCEI
CALUMET
CALUMNY
CANUCKS
CANULAE
CANULAS
CAPUANA
CAPUCHE
CAPULET
CASUALS
CASUIST
CAYUGAS
CAYUSES
CERUMEN
CHAUCER
CHOUGHS
CLAUDEL
CLAUDIA
CLAUDIO
CLAUSAL
CLAUSES
CLOUDED
CLOUDUP
CLOUTED
CLOUTER
COBUYER
COJUROR
COLUMBA
COLUMBO
COLUMNS
CONURES
COPULAE
COPULAR
COPULAS
COQUINA
COZUMEL
CPLUSES
CROUTES
CROUTON
CUMULUS
CUPULAR
CUPULES
CYRUSII

C•••U••

CADBURY
CAESURA
CALCULI
CALLUPS
CANFULS
CANNULA
CAPFULS
CAPGUNS
CAPNUTS
CAPSULE
CAPTURE
CARFULS
CAROUSE
CASQUED
CASQUES
CATGUTS
CATSUIT
CATSUPS
CELLULE
CENSURE
CENTURY
CHALUPA
CHEQUER
CHEQUES
CHERUBS
CHINUPS
CINQUES
CIRCUIT
CIRCUSY
CIRQUES
CLAQUES
CLIBURN
CLIQUED
CLIQUES
CLIQUEY
CLOSURE
CLOTURE
COBNUTS
COEQUAL
COFOUND
COGBURN
COLLUDE
COLOURS
COMBUST
COMMUNE
COMMUTE
COMPUTE
CONCURS
CONCUSS
CONDUCE
CONDUCT
CONDUIT
CONFUSE
CONFUTE
CONJURE
CONJURY
CONQUER
CONSULS
CONSULT
CONSUME
CONTUSE
COPOUTS
CORNUTE
CORRUPT
COSTUME
COUTURE
CROQUET
CROQUIS
CRUGUET
CULTURE
CUPFULS
CUTOUTS
CYYOUNG

C••••U•

CACIQUE
CADEAUX
CADMIUM
CAGEDUP
CAGESUP
CAKEDUP
CAKESUP
CALCIUM
CALHOUN
CALLOUS
CALLOUT
CALLSUP
CAMEDUE
CAMEOUT
CAMPOUT
CAMPSUP
CANDOUR
CANOPUS
CARCLUB
CARDIUM
CAREFUL
CARIOUS
CARPOUS
CASEOUS
CASEOUT
CASHOUT
CASSIUS
CASTOUT
CASTSUP
CATCHUP
CDALBUM
CELSIUS
CENTAUR
CENTRUM
CEPHEUS
CHAINUP
CHALKUP
CHATSUP
CHECKUP
CHEERUP
CHETRUM
CHEVAUX
CHEWGUM
CHEWOUT
CHEWSUP
CHILLUM
CHIPSUP
CHIRRUP
CHOKEUP
CHOPSUP
CHOSEUP
CHURNUP
CIMABUE
CISEAUX
CITROUS
CLAMOUR
CLAMSUP
CLEANUP
CLEARUP
CLIMBUP
CLIPOUT
CLOGSUP
CLOSEUP
CLOTSUP
CLOUDUP
CLUBSUP
CLUEFUL
CNOSSUS
COCONUT
COILSUP
COLDCUP
COLDCUT
COLONUS
COMEDUE
COMEOUT
COMESUP
COMIQUE
CONGOUS
CONKOUT
CONTOUR
COOKOUT
COOKSUP
COOLOUT
COOPSUP
COPIOUS
COPSOUT
CORKSUP
COUGHUP
COUNTUP
COVERUP
CRACKUP
CRANIUM
CRANKUP
CRAPOUT
CRASSUS
CRATEUP
CREEPUP
CREPTUP
CREWCUT
CRIEDUP
CRIESUP
CRISPUS
CRITTUR
CROESUS
CROPSUP
CROSSUP
CRUDSUP
CRUMBUM
CUBITUS
CUMULUS
CUPROUS
CURBCUT
CURIOUS
CURLSUP
CUTARUG
CUTSOUT

C•••••U

CAILLOU
CARIBOU
CHANOYU
CHAPEAU
CHATEAU
COCTEAU

•CU••••

ACUMENS
ACUTELY
ACUTEST
ECUADOR
ECUELLE
OCULARS
OCULIST
PCUSERS
SCUBAED
SCUDDED
SCUDDER
SCUFFED
SCUFFER
SCUFFLE
SCULLED
SCULLER
SCULPED
SCULPTS
SCUPPER
SCURVES
SCUSEME
SCUTTLE
SCUZZES

•C•U•••

ACAUDAL
ACCURST
ACCUSAL
ACCUSED
ACCUSER
ACCUSES
ACOUPLE
ACQUIRE
ACQUITS
ACTUARY
ACTUATE
ACTUPON
ICTUSES
MCGUIRE
MCLUHAN
MCMURDO
MCQUEEN
OCCULTS
OCCURTO
OCTUBRE
OCTUPLE
OCTUPLY
SCHULTZ
SCHUMER
SCOUPES
SCOURED
SCOURER
SCOURGE
SCOUTED
SCOUTER
SCOUTUP
SCRUBBY
SCRUBUP
SCRUFFS
SCRUFFY
SCRUGGS
SCRUNCH
SCRUPLE

•C••U••

ACCOUNT
ACCRUAL
ACCRUED
ACCRUES
ACHTUNG
ICECUBE
ICEOUTS
ICERUNS
MCCLURE
MCCLURG
MCCOURT
MCCRUMB
MCGRUFF
OCCLUDE
SCAPULA
SCHLUBS
SCHLUMP

•C•••U•

ACEDOUT
ACESOUT
ACTEDUP
ACTFOUR
ACTSOUT
ECLOGUE
ECOTEUR
ICEBLUE
ICEDOUT
ICESOUT
ICINGUP
ICTERUS
ICTINUS
MCCLOUD
OCCIPUT
OCEANUS
OCELLUS
OCHROUS
OCTOPUS
SCALEUP
SCAREUP
SCARFUP
SCOUTUP
SCREWUP
SCRUBUP

••CU•••

ACCURST
ACCUSAL
ACCUSED
ACCUSER
ACCUSES
ARCUATE
DECUPLE
ESCUDOS
ESCUELA
EXCURSE
EXCUSAL
EXCUSAS
EXCUSED
EXCUSER
EXCUSES
EXCUSEZ
FACULAE
FACULTY
FICUSES
FOCUSED
FOCUSER
FOCUSES
FOCUSON
HOCUSED
INCUBUS
INCUDES
INCURVE
INCUSED
INCUSES
JACUZZI
JOCULAR
LACUNAE
LACUNAL
LACUNAR
LACUNAS
LACUREE
LECUONA
LOCULUS
LOCUSTS
MACULAE
MACULAR
MACUSER
NOCUOUS
OCCULTS
OCCURTO
OSCULAR
OSCULES
RECURED
RECURES
RECURLS
RECURVE
RECUSAL
RECUSED
RECUSES
SECULAR
SECURED
SECURER
SECURES
UNCUBIC
UNCUFFS
UNCURBS
UNCURED
UNCURLS
UPCURLS
UPCURVE
VACUITY
VACUOLE
VACUOUS
VACUUMS
VICUNAS

••C•U••

ACCOUNT
ACCRUAL
ACCRUED
ACCRUES
BACKUPS
BECAUSE
DECRUMB
DICTUMS
ENCRUST
EXCLUDE
FACTUAL
HECKUVA
HICCUPS
INCLUDE
INCOURT
INCRUST
JACCUSE
JACQUES
KICKUPS
LACEUPS
LACQUER
LECTURE
LOCKUPS
LUCIUSI
LYCEUMS
MACDUFF
MACOUNS
MCCLURE
MCCLURG
MCCOURT
MCCRUMB
MOCKUPS
NOCOUNT
OCCLUDE
PACQUIN
PICKUPS
PICTURE
RACQUET
RECLUSE
RECOUNT
RECOUPS
RECRUIT
SACQUES
SECLUDE
SUCCUMB
TACTUAL
UNCHURN
UNCOUTH
UNCRUDE
UNCRUEL
UPCOURT
VACUUMS
VICTUAL

••C••U•

ARCANUM
BACCHUS
BACKOUT
BACKRUB
BACKSUP
BECLOUD
BUCKSUP
CACIQUE
COCONUT
DECATUR
DECKOUT
DECORUM
DICECUP
DUCKOUT
ESCALUS
FACTFUL
HACKSUP
INCUBUS
ISCHIUM
JACKSUP
KICKOUT
KICKSUP
LACEDUP
LACESUP
LICKSUP
LOCKNUT
LOCKOUT
LOCKSUP
LOCULUS
LUCKOUT
MACAQUE
MCCLOUD
MICHAUX
MOCKSUP
MUCKSUP
NBCBLUE
NICEGUY
NOCUOUS
NUCLEUS
OCCIPUT
PACKSUP
PICEOUS
PICKOUT
PICKSUP
RACEDUP
RACESUP
RACKOUT
RACKSUP
RUCKSUP
SACKFUL
SACKOUT
SACKSUP
SICKOUT
STCLOUD
SUCCOUR
SUCKSUP
TACITUS
TACKSUP
TACTFUL
UNCLOUD
VACUOUS
VICIOUS
WICKIUP

••C•••U

COCTEAU
LUCYLIU

•••CU••

BISCUIT
BLACULA
CALCULI
CIRCUIT
CIRCUSY
CONCURS
CONCUSS
DIECUTS
DISCUSS
DRACULA
EGGCUPS
ELOCUTE
ENDCUTS
EPICURE
EVACUEE
EXECUTE
EYECUPS
FESCUES
GETCUTE
GOTCUTE
HERCULE
HICCUPS
HOTCUPS
ICECUBE
INOCULA
JACCUSE
JOBCUTS
MANCUSO
MARCUSE
MERCURE
MERCURY
MISCUED
MISCUES
MISCUTS
OBSCURA
OBSCURE
OILCUPS
OUTCULL
OUTCURE
OUTCUTS
PAYCUTS
PERCUSS
PINCURL
PRECURE
PRECUTS
PROCURE
RESCUED
RESCUER
RESCUES
RIBCUTS
SUCCUMB
TALCUMS
TAXCUTS
TEACUPS
THECUBS
VINCULA
VISCUSO
ZIPCUFF

•••C•U•

BACCHUS
BLOCKUP
BOTCHUP
BRACEUP
BRICKUP
BUNCHUP
CALCIUM
CARCLUB
CATCHUP
CHECKUP
CRACKUP
DOUCEUR
ERECTUS
FANCLUB
FANCYUP
FARCEUR
FENCEUP
FORCEUP
FULCRUM
GYMCLUB
HITCHUP
JUICEUP
KETCHUM
KETCHUP
KEYCLUB
LASCAUX
LESCAUT
MATCHUP
MENCIUS
MITCHUM
ONECLUB
PATCHUP
PRECOUP
PRICKUP
PROCLUS
PSYCHUP
PUNCHUP
QUECHUA
RANCOUR
RAUCOUS
REACHUP
REOCCUR
RESCRUB
SANCTUM
SANCTUS
SAWCHUK
SLACKUP
SLICEUP
SMACKUP
SNUCKUP
SPECOUT
SPICEUP
STACKUP
STICKUM
STICKUP
STOCKUP
STUCKUP
SUCCOUR

TOUCHUP
VISCOUS
WARCLUB
WRACKUP
ZINCOUS

•••C••U

MARCEAU
ZWICKAU

••••CU•

APERCUS
ATTICUS
BARACUS
BEARCUB
BESTCUT
BOOTCUT
BUZZCUT
COLDCUP
COLDCUT
CREWCUT
CURBCUT
DEFOCUS
DICECUP
GREYCUP
HAIRCUT
HALFCUT
INFOCUS
INVACUO
JUMPCUT
LEANCUT
LINECUT
LIONCUB
MODICUM
OVERCUT
POOLCUE
REFOCUS
REOCCUR
RHOECUS
VANOCUR
WELLCUT
WOLFCUB
WOODCUT

•••••CU

ILIESCU

C•V••••

CAVALRY
CAVEART
CAVEATS
CAVEDIN
CAVEINS
CAVEMAN
CAVEMEN
CAVERNS
CAVESIN
CAVIARE
CAVIARS
CAVILAT
CAVILED
CAVILER
CAVORTS
CEVICHE
CIVILLY
CIVVIES
COVERED
COVERER
COVERME
COVERTS
COVERUP
COVETED
COVETER
CUVETTE

C••V•••

CALVARY
CALVERT
CALVING
CALVINO
CANVASS
CARVELS
CARVERS
CARVING
CERVEZA
CERVIDS
CERVINE
CHEVAUX
CHEVETS
CHEVIOT
CHEVONS
CHEVRES
CHEVRET
CHEVRON
CHIVIED
CHIVIES
CIVVIES
CLAVATE
CLAVELL
CLAVIER
CLOVERS
CLOVERY
COEVALS
CONVECT
CONVENE
CONVENT
CONVERT
CONVEYS
CONVICT
CONVOKE
CONVOYS
CORVAIR
CORVEES
CORVIDS
CORVINA
CORVINE
CRAVATS
CRAVENS
CRAVERS
CRAVING
CREVICE
CULVERT
CURVETS
CURVIER
CURVING

C•••V••

CADAVER
CARAVAN
CARAVEL
CASAVAS
CHARVET
CHEEVER
CHERVIL
CLEAVED
CLEAVER
CLEAVES
CLEAVON
CRYOVER
CUTOVER

C••••V•

CAPTIVA
CAPTIVE
CASSAVA
CENTAVO
COMMOVE
CONCAVE
CONNIVE
COSTIVE
CURSIVE

C•••••V

CABLETV
CHEKHOV
COLORTV
COURTTV

•C••V••

ACTIVAS
ACTIVES
ICEOVER
MCCOVEY
MCGAVIN
OCTAVAL
OCTAVES
OCTAVIA
OCTAVIO
OCTAVOS
SCARVES
SCURVES

•C•••V•

ACHIEVA
ACHIEVE
ACTFIVE
ICECAVE
SCENEVI

•C••••V

SCENEIV

••C•V••

ALCOVES
INCIVIL
MCCOVEY
RECOVER
UNCIVIC
UNCIVIL
UNCOVER

••C••V•

ANCHOVY
ARCHIVE
DECEIVE
ENCLAVE
EXCLAVE
FICTIVE
HECKUVA
INCURVE
PECCAVI
RECARVE
RECEIVE
RECURVE
UPCURVE

••C•••V

ROCKYIV

•••C•V•

CONCAVE
ICECAVE
PECCAVI
THECAVS

•••C••V

WATCHTV

••••C•V

DIRECTV

C•W••••

COWARDS
COWBANE
COWBELL
COWBIRD
COWBOYS
COWERAT
COWERED
COWFISH
COWGIRL
COWHAND
COWHERD
COWHIDE
COWIEST
COWLICK
COWLIKE
COWLING
COWPEAS
COWPOKE
COWPONY
COWRIES
COWRITE
COWROTE
COWSHED
COWSKIN
COWSLIP
COWTOWN

C••W•••

CARWASH
CATWALK
CHAWING
CHEWERS
CHEWGUM
CHEWIER
CHEWING
CHEWOUT
CHEWSON
CHEWSUP
CHEWTOY
CHOWDER
CHOWING
CLAWERS
CLAWING
CLAWSAT
CLEWING
CLOWDER
CLOWNED
COBWEBS
COOWNED
CRAWDAD
CRAWLED
CRAWLER
CRAWLEY
CREWCUT
CREWELS
CREWING
CREWMAN
CREWMEN
CROWBAR
CROWDED
CROWDER
CROWDIN
CROWELL
CROWERS
CROWING
CROWLEY
CROWNED
CROWNER
CRYWOLF
CUTWORK
CUTWORM

C•••W••

CARAWAY
CATAWBA
CDTOWER
CHATWIN
CHINWAG
CNTOWER
COLDWAR
CSLEWIS
CUTAWAY

C••••W•

CASHEWS
CATBOWL
CBSNEWS
CHITOWN
COWTOWN
CRYDOWN
CURFEWS
CURLEWS
CUSHAWS
CUTDOWN

C•••••W

CALLNOW
CAPSHAW
CARSHOW
CASELAW
CASHCOW
CATCHOW
CATSHOW
CATSPAW
CHOCTAW
COMENOW
CORNROW
CRASHAW
CUMSHAW

•CW••••

NCWYETH
PCWORLD

•C•W•••

ICEWINE
ICYWIND
MCGWIRE
MCSWINE
SCHWANN
SCHWINN
SCOWLED
SCOWLER

•C••W••

JCPOWYS
MCCOWEN
SCARWID
SCRAWLS
SCRAWLY
SCRAWNY
SCREWED
SCREWUP

•C•••W•

ICEDOWN

•C••••W

ICESHOW

••CW•••

ARCWELD

••C•W••

ARCHWAY
BACKWAY
LACKWIT
MCCOWEN
RACEWAY
UNCOWED

••C••W•

ABCNEWS
DECLAWS
ESCHEWS
ESCROWS
INCROWD
MACHTWO
NBCNEWS
RECHEWS
RECROWN
TVCREWS
UNCROWN

••C•••W

BACKROW
BACKSAW
BUCKSAW
HACKSAW
JACKDAW
LOCKJAW
LUCKNOW
MACGRAW
WICKLOW

•••C•W•

ANTCOWS
MOOCOWS
PETCOWS
SEACOWS

•••C••W

AIRCREW
ATECROW
CATCHOW
CHOCTAW
DEWCLAW
DOGCHEW
DOGCHOW
EATCROW
OUTCROW
PETCHEW
PETCROW
PILCROW
PITCREW
SALCHOW
THECROW
UNSCREW
WROCLAW

••••C•W

CASHCOW
HADACOW
HASACOW
HOLYCOW
MILKCOW

C•X••••

COXCOMB
COXLESS

C••X•••

CHEXMIX
COAXERS
COAXIAL
COAXING
COEXIST

C•••X••

CALYXES
CPAEXAM
CULEXES

C••••X•

CONTEXT

C•••••X

CADEAUX
CAKEMIX
CALLBOX
CASHBOX
CELOTEX
CHEVAUX
CHEXMIX
CINEMAX
CISEAUX
COINBOX
COMPLEX
COMTREX
COOLMAX
COOLPIX
CRISPIX

•C••X••

ICEAXES

••C••X•

PICKAXE

••C•••X

KICKBOX
LOCKBOX
MACHSIX
MICHAUX
STCROIX
VICTRIX

•••C••X

LASCAUX
PANCHAX

CY•••••

CYANIDE
CYANIDS
CYBORGS
CYCLERS
CYCLING
CYCLIST
CYCLOID
CYCLONE
CYCLOPS
CYGNETS
CYMBALS
CYMRICS
CYNICAL
CYNTHIA
CYPHERS
CYPRESS
CYPRIAN
CYPRIOT
CYRUSII
CYYOUNG

C•Y••••

CAYENNE
CAYMANS
CAYUGAS
CAYUSES
CHYRONS
COYDOGS
COYNESS
COYOTES
CRYBABY
CRYDOWN
CRYOGEN
CRYOVER
CRYPTIC
CRYPTOS
CRYSTAL
CRYWOLF
CYYOUNG

C••Y•••

CALYCES
CALYPSO
CALYXES
CANYONS
CHAYOTE
CITYBOY
CITYGAL
CLAYIER
CLAYING
CLAYISH
CLAYPIT
CLAYTON
CLOYING
COPYBOY
COPYCAT
COPYING
COPYIST
COPYMAN
COPYMEN
CORYELL
CORYZAS
COSYING
COZYING
CRAYOLA
CRAYONS

C•••Y••

CAMRYLE
CARLYLE
CARRYIN
CARRYON
CATEYED
COBUYER
COLLYER

C••••Y•

CACONYM
CAMBOYS
CARBOYS
CARKEYS
CAROLYN
CATSEYE
CATTOYS
CHANOYU
CONVEYS
CONVOYS
COWBOYS

C•••••Y

CABBAGY
CADBURY
CADENCY
CALCIFY
CALGARY
CALLBOY
CALPOLY
CALUMNY
CALVARY
CAMPILY
CANNERY
CANNILY
CANONRY
CANTILY
CANTSAY
CAPABLY
CAPEMAY
CARAWAY
CARDKEY
CARNABY
CARROTY
CASPARY
CASSIDY
CATTILY
CAVALRY
CENTURY
CEPHALY
CERTIFY
CHANTEY
CHANTRY
CHARILY
CHARITY
CHARLEY
CHEAPLY
CHEWTOY
CHICORY
CHIEFLY
CHIMNEY
CHINTZY
CHOMSKY
CHOOSEY
CHRISTY
CHURCHY
CHUTNEY
CILIARY
CINDERY
CINERGY
CIRCUSY
CITYBOY
CIVILLY
CLARIFY
CLARITY
CLEANLY
CLEARLY
CLERISY
CLERKLY
CLIQUEY
CLOONEY
CLOSEBY
CLOSELY
CLOVERY
CLUTCHY
COCKILY
COCKNEY
COGENCY
COLDDAY
COLICKY
COMESBY
COMPANY
CONAKRY
CONFREY
CONJURY
CONNERY
COOKERY
COOPERY
COPPERY
COPYBOY
CORNILY
COTTONY
COUNTRY
COURTLY
COWPONY
CRACKLY
CRAFTSY
CRASSLY
CRAWLEY
CRAZILY
CREELEY
CREEPBY
CRIMINY
CRINKLY
CRISPLY
CROSSLY
CROWLEY
CRUDELY
CRUDITY
CRUELLY
CRUELTY
CRUMBLY
CRUMPLY
CRUNCHY
CRYBABY
CUBICLY
CURABLY
CURSORY
CURTSEY
CUSHILY
CUSTODY
CUTAWAY
CUTLERY

•CY••••

ACYCLIC
ICYWIND
SCYTHED
SCYTHES

•C•Y•••

ACRYLIC
ECDYSES
ECDYSIS
ECTYPAL
ECTYPES
ICKYPOO
NCWYETH

•C••Y••

ACOLYTE
ECOTYPE
LCHAYIM
SCHAYES

•C•••Y•

ACRONYM
JCPOWYS

•C••••Y

ACADEMY
ACETIFY
ACIDIFY
ACIDITY
ACRIDLY
ACTORLY
ACTUARY
ACUTELY
ECOLOGY
ECONOMY
ECSTASY
ICETRAY
ICONIFY
MCCAREY
MCCOVEY
MCCRARY
MCGRORY
MCHENRY
MCNALLY
MCRANEY
OCTUPLY
SCANTLY
SCAREDY
SCARIFY
SCARILY
SCENERY
SCRAGGY
SCRAPPY
SCRAWLY
SCRAWNY
SCRIMPY
SCRUBBY
SCRUFFY
WCHANDY

••CY•••

ALCYONE
BICYCLE
LUCYLIU
OOCYTES
RECYCLE

••C•Y••

DACTYLS
DECAYED
DECAYER
DECOYED
DECOYER
DECRYPT
ENCRYPT
HECKYES
ROCKYII
ROCKYIV
TACHYON
UNCOYER
UNCOYLY

••C••Y•

BUCKEYE
CACONYM
DICKEYS
HICKEYS
JOCELYN
JOCKEYS
LACKEYS
MICKEYS
RICKEYS
SOCKEYE

••C•••Y

ALCHEMY
ANCHOVY
ARCHERY
ARCHWAY
BACKBAY
BACKPAY
BACKWAY
BUCKLEY
COCKILY
COCKNEY
DECENCY
DICKORY
DUCALLY
FACTORY
FACULTY
GOCRAZY
HACKNEY
HICKORY
LICITLY
LICKETY
LOCALLY
LUCENCY
LUCIDLY
LUCKILY
MCCAREY
MCCOVEY
MCCRARY
MOCKERY
NECTARY
NICEBOY
NICEDAY
NICEGUY
NICETRY
PECCARY
PICARDY
PUCKERY
RACEDBY
RACESBY
RACEWAY
RACKETY
RECARRY
RECENCY
RECTIFY
RECTORY
RICKETY
ROCKABY
ROCKERY
ROCKILY
SECRECY
SICKBAY
SICKDAY
SICKPAY
SOCIETY
SUCKDRY
TACITLY
TACKILY
TICKSBY
UNCANNY
UNCHARY
UNCOYLY
UNCRAZY
VACANCY
VACUITY
VICEROY
VICKREY
VICTORY
VOCABLY
VOCALLY
WACKILY
ZACHARY

•••CY••

FANCYUP
HALCYON
PROCYON

•••C••Y

AMSCRAY
BALCONY
BARCLAY
BAYCITY
BIGCITY
BLACKLY
BOKCHOY
CALCIFY
CHICORY
CIRCUSY
CRACKLY
DELCITY
DRMCCOY
DULCIFY
EDACITY
ELMCITY
ERECTLY
EXACTLY
FANCIFY
FANCILY
FATCITY
FOGCITY
FRECKLY
GASCONY
GROCERY
JUICILY

KNUCKLY
LARCENY
MERCERY
MERCURY
MISCOPY
MULCAHY
OLDCITY
OPACITY
OUTCITY
PAUCITY
PECCARY
PRICILY
PRICKLY
PROCITY
QUICKLY
REDCLAY
SAUCILY
SAUCONY
SIMCITY
SINCITY
SLACKLY
SLICKLY
SORCERY
SPACELY
SPECIFY
SPICERY
SPICILY
STICKBY
STUCKBY
SUNCITY
TEACOZY
THECITY
THICKLY
TRACERY
TUSCANY
UNSCALY
UTICANY
ZINCIFY

••••C•Y
AFARCRY
ANARCHY
BLOTCHY
BRANCHY
CHURCHY
CLUTCHY
COLICKY
CRUNCHY
CUBICLY
DONTCRY
DRMCCOY
EPARCHY
FINICKY
GLITCHY
GROUCHY
KITSCHY
KVETCHY
MENSCHY
MIMICRY
MRLUCKY
OVERCOY
PANICKY
PAUNCHY
PREACHY
QUINCEY
RAUNCHY
REDECAY
SHLOCKY

SHTICKY
SKETCHY
SLOUCHY
STARCHY
THATCHY
TREACLY
TWITCHY
UNLUCKY
UNROCKY

•••••CY
ABBOTCY
ANIMACY
ARDENCY
CADENCY
COGENCY
DECENCY
ERRANCY
FALLACY
FLOUNCY
FLUENCY
INFANCY
LATENCY
LUCENCY
MRDARCY
MTMARCY
NOMERCY
PATENCY
PLIANCY
POTENCY
PRELACY
PRIMACY
PRIVACY
PUDENCY
RECENCY
REGENCY
SECRECY
TENANCY
TESTACY
TRUANCY
UNFANCY
UNJUICY
UNSPICY
URGENCY
VACANCY

CZ•••••
CZARDAS
CZARDOM
CZARINA
CZARISM
CZARIST

C•Z••••
CEZANNE
COZENED
COZENER
COZIEST
COZUMEL
COZYING
COZZENS

C••Z•••
CALZONE
CANZONA
CANZONE
CANZONI
CHAZANS

CHAZZAN
CHEZMOI
CINZANO
CORZINE
COZZENS
CRAZIER
CRAZIES
CRAZILY
CRAZING
CROZIER
CRUZADO
CRUZANS

C•••Z••
CABEZAS
CHAZZAN
CHEEZIT
CHUTZPA
CITIZEN
COETZEE
CORAZON
CORYZAS
CRUTZEN

C••••Z•
CADENZA
CAPSIZE
CARDOZO
CERVEZA
CHINTZY
CHORIZO
COGNIZE

C•••••Z
COBLENZ

•CZ••••
ECZEMAS

•C•Z•••
SCUZZES

•C••Z••
SCUZZES

•C•••Z•
SCHERZI
SCHERZO
SCHNOZZ

•C••••Z
SCHLITZ
SCHNOZZ
SCHULTZ

••C•Z••
ALCAZAR
JACUZZI
SECHZIG

••C••Z•
GOCRAZY
JACUZZI
UNCRAZY
VICENZA

••C•••Z
EXCUSEZ

•••C•Z•
GRECIZE
LAICIZE
TEACOZY

•••C••Z
NATCHEZ

DA•••••
DABBERS
DABBING
DABBLED
DABBLER
DABBLES
DABHAND
DACAPOS
DACOSTA
DACRONS
DACTYLS
DADAART
DADAISM
DADAIST
DADDIES
DADOING
DAEMONS
DAEWOOS
DAFFIER
DAFFILY
DAFTEST
DAGGERS
DAGWOOD
DAHLIAS
DAHOMEY
DAILIES
DAIMLER
DAIRIES
DAIRYER
DAISIES
DAKOTAN
DAKOTAS
DAKTARI
DALASIS
DALETHS
DALLIED
DALLIER
DALLIES
DALTONS
DALTREY
DAMAGED
DAMAGES
DAMASKS
DAMASUS
DAMMERS
DAMMING
DAMNERS
DAMNING
DAMOSEL
DAMPDRY
DAMPENS
DAMPERS
DAMPEST
DAMPING
DAMPISH
DAMPMOP
DAMPOFF
DAMSELS
DAMSONS
DANANAS

DANBURY
DANCERS
DANCING
DANDERS
DANDIER
DANDIES
DANDIFY
DANDILY
DANDLED
DANDLER
DANDLES
DANELAW
DANEYKO
DANGELO
DANGERS
DANGLED
DANGLER
DANGLES
DANIELA
DANIELJ
DANIELS
DANIKEN
DANITES
DANKEST
DANNING
DANSEUR
DANTEAN
DANTEII
DANVERS
DAPHNES
DAPHNIA
DAPHNIS
DAPPING
DAPPLED
DAPPLES
DAREFUL
DARENOT
DARESAY
DARESTO
DAREZZO
DARIUSI
DARKAGE
DARKENS
DARKEST
DARKISH
DARKLED
DARKLES
DARKMAN
DARKRED
DARKTAN
DARLEEN
DARLENE
DARLING
DARNELL
DARNERS
DARNING
DARRYLF
DARTERS
DARTGUN
DARTING
DARTLED
DARTLES
DARTOFF
DARWELL
DASBOOT
DASCHLE
DASHDOT
DASHERS

DASHIER
DASHIKI
DASHING
DASHOFF
DASHPOT
DASILVA
DASTARD
DATABLE
DATABUS
DATASET
DATEDLY
DATINGS
DATIVES
DATRILS
DATSUNS
DAUBERS
DAUBING
DAUMIER
DAUNTED
DAUNTER
DAUPHIN
DAUSSET
DAVEKOZ
DAVINCI
DAVISON
DAWDLED
DAWDLER
DAWDLES
DAWKINS
DAWNING
DAWNSON
DAYBEDS
DAYBOOK
DAYCAMP
DAYCARE
DAYGAME
DAYHOPS
DAYJOBS
DAYLILY
DAYLONG
DAYMARE
DAYPACK
DAYQUIL
DAYROOM
DAYSAIL
DAYSEND
DAYSIDE
DAYSINN
DAYSOFF
DAYSPAS
DAYSTAR
DAYTIME
DAYTONA
DAYTRIP
DAYWEAR
DAZEDLY
DAZZLED
DAZZLER
DAZZLES

D•A••••
DEACONS
DEADAIR
DEADEND
DEADENS
DEADEST
DEADEYE
DEADPAN

DEADSEA
DEADSET
DEAFENS
DEAFEST
DEAIRED
DEALERS
DEALING
DEALOUT
DEALSIN
DEALSTO
DEALSUP
DEALTIN
DEALTTO
DEALTUP
DEANERY
DEARDEN
DEAREST
DEARGOD
DEARIES
DEARONE
DEARSIR
DEARTHS
DHARMAS
DHARMIC
DIABLES
DIABLOS
DIABOLO
DIADEMS
DIAGRAM
DIAHANN
DIALECT
DIALEDO
DIALERS
DIALING
DIALLED
DIALOGS
DIALOUT
DIALSIN
DIALSUP
DIALUPS
DIAMOND
DIAPERS
DIAPHAN
DIARIES
DIARIOS
DIARIST
DIATOMS
DIAVOLO
DNAASES
DNACODE
DNALABS
DNATEST
DOADEAL
DOAGAIN
DOASIDO
DRABBER
DRABBLE
DRACHMA
DRACULA
DRAFTED
DRAFTEE
DRAFTER
DRAGEES
DRAGGED
DRAGGER
DRAGGLE
DRAGNET
DRAGOFF

DRAGONS
DRAGOON
DRAGOTI
DRAGOUT
DRAGSIN
DRAGSON
DRAGSUP
DRAINED
DRAINER
DRAMADY
DRAMEDY
DRANKIN
DRANKTO
DRANKUP
DRAPERS
DRAPERY
DRAPING
DRASTIC
DRATTED
DRAUGHT
DRAWBAR
DRAWEES
DRAWERS
DRAWING
DRAWLED
DRAWLER
DRAWMAN
DRAWMEN
DRAWNIN
DRAWNON
DRAWNTO
DRAWNUP
DRAWOFF
DRAWOUT
DRAWSIN
DRAWSON
DRAWSTO
DRAWSUP
DRAYAGE
DRAYING
DRAYMAN
DRAYMEN
DRAYTON
DUALISM
DUALIST
DUALITY
DUALIZE
DWARFED
DWARVES

D••A•••
DACAPOS
DADAART
DADAISM
DADAIST
DALASIS
DAMAGED
DAMAGES
DAMASKS
DAMASUS
DANANAS
DATABLE
DATABUS
DATASET
DEBACLE
DEBAKEY
DEBARGE
DEBARKS

DEBASED
DEBASER
DEBASES
DEBATED
DEBATER
DEBATES
DEBAUCH
DECADES
DECAGON
DECALOG
DECAMPS
DECANTS
DECAPOD
DECARLO
DECATUR
DECAYED
DECAYER
DEDALUS
DEFACED
DEFACER
DEFACES
DEFACTO
DEFALLA
DEFAMED
DEFAMER
DEFAMES
DEFANGS
DEFARGE
DEFAULT
DEGAUSS
DEHAIRS
DEHAVEN
DELANEY
DELARUE
DELAYED
DELAYER
DEMAGOG
DEMANDS
DEMARCO
DEMARET
DEMARKS
DEMASTS
DENARII
DEPALMA
DEPARTS
DEPAULU
DERAILS
DERALTE
DERANGE
DERATED
DERATES
DESALTS
DETAILS
DETAINS
DEVALUE
DEWAART
DEWATER
DEWAXED
DEWAXES
DIDACTS
DIDASET
DIEAWAY
DILATED
DILATES
DILATOR
DIMAGES
DINADAM
DINARIC

DISABLE
DISARMS
DISAVOW
DIZAINS
DNAASES
DOGAPES
DOMAINE
DOMAINS
DONAHUE
DONATED
DONATEE
DONATES
DONATOR
DONATUS
DOSADOS
DOSAGES
DOTAGES
DOTARDS
DOUANES
DOWAGER
DREADED
DREAMED
DREAMER
DREAMIN
DREAMOF
DREAMON
DREAMUP
DRLAURA
DRMARIO
DRYABLE
DRYADES
DRYADIC
DUBARRY
DUCALLY
DUHAMEL
DUKAKIS
DUNAWAY
DURABLE
DURABLY
DURANCE
DURANGO
DURANTE
DYNAMIC
DYNAMOS
DYNASTS
DYNASTY

D•••A••
DABHAND
DADAART
DAKTARI
DARKAGE
DASTARD
DAYCAMP
DAYCARE
DAYGAME
DAYMARE
DAYPACK
DAYSAIL
DEADAIR
DEBEARD
DECEASE
DECIARE
DECLAIM
DECLARE
DECLASS
DECLAWS
DEEJAYS

DEFEATS
DEFIANT
DEFLATE
DEFOAMS
DEFRAGS
DEFRAME
DEFRAUD
DEFRAYS
DEGLAZE
DEGRADE
DELEADS
DELRAYS
DELTAIC
DEMEANS
DENHAAG
DENIALS
DENMARK
DENTALS
DENTATE
DEODARS
DEODATO
DEPLANE
DEPRAVE
DERMATO
DESCANT
DESPAIR
DESTAEL
DESTAIN
DETRACT
DETRAIN
DEVIANT
DEVIATE
DEWAART
DEWFALL
DEWLAPS
DIAHANN
DICTATE
DIDLAPS
DIECAST
DIEHARD
DIETARY
DIGRAMS
DIGRAPH
DIKTATS
DILLARD
DIORAMA
DIRHAMS
DISBAND
DISBARS
DISCARD
DISDAIN
DISEASE
DISMALS
DISMAST
DISMAYS
DISPART
DISRATE
DISTAFF
DISTANT
DNALABS
DOAGAIN
DOCKAGE
DOGBANE
DOGCART
DOGDAYS
DOGEARS
DOGFACE
DOGGATE

DOGHAIR
DOGMATA
DOGNAPS
DOGRACE
DOGSAGE
DOGTAGS
DOGTAIL
DOIDARE
DOLLARS
DOLMANS
DONNALL
DONTASK
DOODADS
DORMANT
DORSALS
DOSSALS
DOTDASH
DRAMADY
DRAYAGE
DRCHAOS
DRYWALL
DRYWASH
DUCHAMP
DUEDATE
DUEEAST
DULLARD
DUNDALK
DUNNAGE
DURWARD
DYEBATH
DYEVATS

D••••A•
DAHLIAS
DAKOTAN
DAKOTAS
DANANAS
DANELAW
DANTEAN
DARESAY
DARKMAN
DARKTAN
DAYSPAS
DAYSTAR
DAYWEAR
DEADPAN
DEBORAH
DECIMAL
DEEPFAT
DEEPTAN
DEFLEAS
DELIHAM
DELILAH
DELIMAN
DEMOLAY
DENHAAG
DEPOSAL
DEWCLAW
DEXTRAL
DHARMAS
DIAGRAM
DIAPHAN
DIDTOAT
DIEAWAY
DIGICAM
DIGITAL
DILLMAN
DINADAM

DINEDAT
DINESAT
DINGBAT
DIPOLAR
DIRTBAG
DISCMAN
DISHPAN
DISHRAG
DISPLAY
DIURNAL
DOADEAL
DOESBAD
DOGCOAT
DOGREAT
DOGSEAR
DOGSTAR
DOMECAR
DOMICAL
DONEBAD
DONEGAL
DONEGAN
DONJUAN
DONOVAN
DOORMAN
DOORMAT
DOORWAY
DORFMAN
DOUGLAS
DOVEBAR
DOWNPAT
DRAWBAR
DRAWMAN
DRAYMAN
DRESSAS
DRIPPAN
DRISTAN
DRIVEAT
DROPCAP
DROVEAT
DRSLOAN
DRUZEAN
DRUZIAN
DRVEGAS
DRYHEAT
DUENNAS
DUNAWAY
DUNSTAN
DUSTMAN
DUSTPAN
DUSTRAG
DWELLAT

D•••••A
DACOSTA
DANIELA
DAPHNIA
DASILVA
DAYTONA
DEADSEA
DEEPSEA
DEFALLA
DELEDDA
DELIRIA
DELTONA
DEPALMA
DERONDA
DERRIDA
DESPINA

DESYLVA
DILEMMA
DIORAMA
DIOTIMA
DIPLOMA
DOGFLEA
DOGMATA
DOUBLEA
DRACHMA
DRACULA
DRLAURA
DRYIDEA
DUODENA
DYKSTRA

•DA••••

ADAGIOS
ADAMANT
ADAMITE
ADAMSES
ADAMSON
ADAPTED
ADAPTER
ADAPTOR
ADAPTTO
ADAWARE
ADAYAGO
BDALTON
CDALBUM
EDACITY
EDASNER
IDAHOAN
IDAREDS
NDAKOTA
SDAKOTA

•D•A•••

ADDABLE
ADDAXES
ADRATES
ADVANCE
CDCASES
CDRACKS
CDRATES
EDGARDO
EDNAMAY
EDUARDO
EDWARDG
EDWARDI
EDWARDR
EDWARDS
EDWARDV
IDBADGE
IDCARDS
IDEALLY
IDEAMAN
IDEAMEN
IDEATED
IDEATES
IDIAMIN
IDSAYSO
PDJAMES
RDLAING

•D••A••

ADAMANT
ADAWARE
ADAYAGO
ADDSALT
ADONAIS
ADRIANA
ADSPACE
ADULATE
EDEMATA
EDINAMN
EDOUARD
EDUCATE
ODDBALL
ODDSARE
ODORANT
PDQBACH

•D•••A•

ADEPTAT
ADMIRAL
ADOLLAR
ADRENAL
ADWOMAN
EDICTAL
EDNAMAY
IDAHOAN
IDEAMAN
ODESSAN

•D••••A

ADDENDA
ADELINA
ADRIANA
EDEMATA
NDAKOTA
ODONTIA
SDAKOTA

••DA•••

ADDABLE
ADDAXES
ALDAVIS
ANDAMAN
ANDANTE
BADAREA
BEDAUBS
BEDAZED
BEDAZES
CADAVER
CEDARED
DADAART
DADAISM
DADAIST
DEDALUS
DIDACTS
DIDASET
ENDABLE
ENDALLS
FADAYEV
HADACOW
HADAFIT
HADAGAS
HADAJOB
HADANIP
HADAROW
HADASAY
HADASET
HADATIT
HIDABLE
HIDALGO
HIDAWAY
HODADDY
IODATED
IODATES
JUDAICA
JUDAISM
JUDASES
LADADOG
LEDAWAY
MADALYN
MADAMES
MADAMEX
MEDAKAS
MEDALED
MEDAWAR
MIDASES
MRDARCY
ORDAINS
PEDALED
PEDALER
PEDANTS
RADAMES
REDACTS
REDALGA
REDANTS
REDARED
REDARES
REDARMY
REDARNS
REDATED
REDATES
RIDABLE
SEDALIA
SEDATED
SEDATER
SEDATES
SODACAN
SODAPOP
SUDAFED
TIDALLY
UNDARED
UNDATED
UNDAZED
UPDARTS
UPDATED
UPDATER
UPDATES
VIDALIA

••D•A••

ADDSALT
ANDEANS
ANDIAMO
ANDRADE
BADBACK
BADCALL
BADCASE
BADDAYS
BADHAIR
BADHAND
BADHATS
BADLAND
BADNAME
BADPAST
BADRAPS
BEDBATH
BEDLAMP
BEDLAMS
BEDMATE
BEDRAIL
BEDRAPE
BIDFAIR
BODYART
BUDVASE
CADEAUX
CODCAKE
DADAART
DIDLAPS
ENDEARS
ENDGAME
ENDLATE
ENDWAYS
GODDARD
GODMAMA
GODPAPA
HYDRANT
HYDRATE
INDIANA
INDIANS
INDRAFT
INDRAWN
JUDEANS
KIDNAPS
KODIAKS
MADCAPS
MADDASH
MEDIANS
MEDIANT
MEDIATE
MIDCAPS
MIDDAYS
MIDEAST
MIDLAND
MIDWAYS
MUDBATH
MUDCATS
MUDLARK
MUDPACK
MUDWASP
NEDLAND
ODDBALL
ODDSARE
OGDOADS
OLDBATS
OLDCARS
OLDDAYS
OLDGAGS
OLDHAND
OLDLADY
OLDMAID
OLDNAVY
OLDPALS
OLDSALT
OLDSAWS
OLDWAYS
ORDEALS
PADRAIC
PADUANS
PEDWAYS
PODCAST
QADDAFI
RADIALS
RADIANS
RADIANT
RADIATE
REDBATS
REDBAYS
REDCAPS
REDCARD
REDDAWN
REDEALS
REDEALT
REDFACE
REDHAIR
REDHATS
REDHAWK
REDIALS
REDJACK
REDOAKS
REDRAFT
REDRAGS
REDRAWN
REDRAWS
REDTABS
REDTAGS
REDTAIL
REDTAPE
RUDYARD
SADCAFE
SADFATE
SADSACK
SIDEARM
TEDMACK
UNDEALT
UNDRAPE
UNDRAWN
UNDRAWS
UPDRAFT
WIDMARK
ZODIACS

••D••A•

ALDORAY
ANDAMAN
ANDREAS
BODEGAS
BODYBAR
BODYFAT
BUDDHAS
DIDTOAT
ENDEDAT
ENDLEAF
ENDPLAY
ENDUPAT
FADIMAN
FEDERAL
FEDORAS
GIDDYAP
GODHEAD
GODTHAB
HADAGAS
HADASAY
HADRIAN
HIDAWAY
INDYCAR
JUDELAW
JUDOKAS
KIDSEAT
LADIDAS
LADYDAY
LADYNAS
LEDAWAY
MADEHAY
MADEMAD
MADEPAR
MADEWAR
MADEWAY
MADIGAN
MEDAKAS
MEDAWAR
MEDEVAC
MEDICAL
MEDIGAP
MEDIVAC
MEDUSAE
MEDUSAN
MEDUSAS
MIDYEAR
MODELAS
MODULAR
MUDFLAP
MUDFLAT
NODICAL
NODULAR
OEDIPAL
OLDBEAN
OLDCHAP
OLDUVAI
ORDINAL
PADUCAH
PEDICAB
RADICAL
RADIOAD
REDCLAY
REDCOAT
REDECAY
REDFLAG
REDHEAD
REDHEAT
REDMEAT
REDREAM
REDSFAN
REDSTAR
RIDGWAY
SEDONAS
SIDEBAR
SIDECAR
SIDEMAN
SIDEWAY
SODACAN
UNDULAR

••D•••A

ADDENDA
ANDORRA
BADAREA
BADIDEA
BEDELIA
CADENZA
CEDILLA
FIDELIA
GODMAMA
GODPAPA
INDIANA
INDICIA
JUDAICA
KEDROVA
LIDWINA
MADEIRA
MADONNA
MEDULLA
PODRIDA
REDALGA
SEDALIA
VIDALIA

•••DA••

AIRDAMS
AIRDATE
ALIDADE
AMIDALA
AOUDADS
BADDAYS
BANDAGE
BANDAID
BANDANA
BATDAYS
BELDAME
BELDAMS
BENDAYS
BIGDAYS
BIODATA
BONDAGE
BRIDALS
CANDACE
CAUDATE
CORDAGE
CORDATE
DEADAIR
DEODARS
DEODATO
DISDAIN
DOGDAYS
DOIDARE
DOODADS
DOTDASH
DUEDATE
DUNDALK
EXUDATE
FONDANT
FRIDAYS
GANDALF
GODDARD
GOLDARN
GOODAIM
GOODALL
GRADATE
HALDANE
HANDAXE
HEYDAYS
HOLDALL
HOTDATE
HOTDAYS
HOWDAHS
ICEDAMS
INADAZE
JIMDALE
JORDANA
KENDALL
KILDARE
LANDAUS
MADDASH
MANDALA
MANDANS
MANDATE
MANDAYS
MAYDAYS
MCADAMS
MIDDAYS
MISDATE
MONDALE
MONDAVI
MONDAYS
MORDANT
MTADAMS
MULDAUR
MUNDANE
NONDARK
OFFDAYS
OLDDAYS
ONADARE
ONADATE
OUTDARE
OUTDATE
OXIDANT
OXIDASE
OXIDATE
PAIDADS
PAYDAYS
PENDANT
PREDARK
PREDATA
PREDATE
PREDAWN
QADDAFI
RAEDAWN
RANDALL
RAWDATA
READAPT
REDDAWN
SAIDAAH
SAIDAYE
SANDALS
SUBDATE
SUNDAES
SUNDAYS
TAGDAYS
TENDAYS
TOLDALL
TWODAYS
TYNDALL
VANDALS
VEADARS
VERDANT
VICDANA
WINDAGE
WINDAUS
WOODARD
WORDAGE
YARDAGE
YARDARM

•••D•A•

ABIDJAN
ACADIAN
AVIDFAN
BANDEAU
BANDSAW
BIGDEAL
BIRDMAN
BONDMAN
BUDDHAS
BUMDEAL
CARDIAC
CARDIAL
CHEDDAR
COLDDAY
COLDWAR
CORDIAL
CORDIAS
DEADPAN
DOADEAL
EXEDRAE
FEEDBAG
FELDMAN
FEYDEAU
FINDLAY
FORDHAM
GIDDYAP
GOLDMAN
GOODBAR
GOODDAY
GOODMAN
GOODPAY
GORDIAN
GRADEAA
GRADUAL
GRIDMAP
HANDBAG
HANDCAR
HANDSAW
HARDDAY
HARDHAT
HARDPAN
HARDWAY
HEADMAN
HEADSAW
HEADWAY
HINDPAW
JIMDIAL
LANDMAN
LANDSAT
LANDTAG
LANDTAX
LEADMAN
LINDSAY
MARDIAN
MISDEAL
MISDIAL
MISDRAW
MONDIAL
NEEDHAM
NEWDEAL
NONDEAF
OBADIAH
OUTDRAG
OUTDRAW
OVIDIAN
PHIDIAS
RAWDEAL
REEDMAN
RHODIAN
ROADMAP
ROADTAR
ROADTAX
ROADWAY
RONDEAU
SAIDAAH
SAIDNAY
SANDBAG
SANDBAR
SANDDAB
SANDMAN
SINDBAD
SUBDUAL
SUNDIAL
TOPDRAW
TREDIAS
TRUDEAU
TUNDRAS
UNIDEAL
USEDCAR
WEIDMAN
WILDCAT
WILDMAN
WINDBAG
WOODSAW
WOODTAR
WYNDHAM
YARDMAN
YESDEAR

•••D••A

AMIDALA
BANDANA
BANDERA
BIODATA
CALDERA
CANDELA
CANDIDA
CORDOBA
DEADSEA
DUODENA
GARDENA
GONDOLA
GORDITA
GRADEAA
HENDECA
ICEDTEA
INEDITA
ISADORA
JORDANA
KUNDERA
MANDALA
MANDELA
MOLDOVA
NORDICA
PANDORA
PERDITA
POPDIVA
PREDATA
RAWDATA
VANDURA
VICDANA

••••DA•

ACAUDAL
ACTEDAS
AGENDAS
AIMEDAT
ARMADAS
ASSTDAS
BAGHDAD
BAYEDAT
BIMODAL
BIPEDAL
BOOEDAT
BRENDAN
BROADAS
BROADAX
CANIDAE
CHEDDAR
CHORDAL
CICADAE
CICADAS
COLADAS
COLDDAY
CRAWDAD
CREEDAL
CSARDAS
CZARDAS
DINADAM
DINEDAT
ENDEDAT
FARADAY
FIREDAT
FIVEDAY
FLAGDAY
FLUIDAL
FORADAY
FOURDAY
FRIEDAN
FULLDAY
FUMEDAT
GAPEDAT
GAZEDAT
GOODDAY
GRANDAM
HALFDAY
HARDDAY
HIGHDAY
HOLIDAY
HOLYDAY
HYUNDAI
JACKDAW
JAWEDAT
JIBEDAT
JOURDAN
JULYDAY
JUMADAS
JUNEDAY
LADIDAS
LADYDAY
LAMBDAS
LEAPDAY
LEONDAY
LONGDAY
LUCIDAE
MACADAM
MARIDAS
MILLDAM
MIRADAS
MONADAL
NAMEDAY
NAVIDAD
NEVADAN
NEWSDAY
NEXTDAY
NICEDAY
NOONDAY
ONEADAY
ONEIDAS
OVOIDAL
PAGODAS
PALUDAL
PANADAS
PAWEDAT
POKEDAT
POSADAS
POSEDAS
POTSDAM
QUONDAM
RAMADAN
RAMADAS
RAPIDAN
RIKSDAG
RIORDAN
RUANDAS
RWANDAN
SAMEDAY
SANDDAB
SCANDAL
SICKDAY
SLOWDAY
SNOWDAY
SOLEDAD
SOMEDAY
STEPDAD
SYNODAL
THISDAY
TIENDAS
TOLEDAN
TUESDAY
UGANDAN
WASHDAY
WAVEDAT
WEEKDAY
WEIRDAL
WORKDAY
ZOOIDAL

••••D•A

ARCADIA
BADIDEA
BIGIDEA
CLAUDIA
COMEDIA
DELEDDA
DRYIDEA
ECHIDNA
EPHEDRA
EXHEDRA
EXORDIA
GRANDMA
GRANDPA
HEREDIA
JUNKDNA
MAANDPA
MELODIA
NEWIDEA
PHAEDRA
PREIDEA
RESIDUA
SUBIDEA
THEIDEA

•••••DA

ADDENDA
AIRMADA
ALAMEDA
ALFREDA
AMERADA
AVENIDA
BARBUDA
BELINDA
BERMUDA
BRAVADA
CANDIDA
CORRIDA
DELEDDA
DERONDA
DERRIDA
ENTRADA
ESTRADA
FLORIDA
GRANADA
GRENADA
LAMBADA
LASORDA
LAWANDA
LUCINDA
MATILDA
MELINDA
MIRANDA
MUSCIDA
OCANADA
PODRIDA
QUERIDA
RASHIDA
RIGVEDA
ROLONDA
ROTUNDA
SALSODA
SHOULDA
SPLENDA
TOSTADA
VERANDA
YOLANDA

D•B••••

DABBERS
DABBING
DABBLED
DABBLER
DABBLES
DABHAND
DEBACLE
DEBAKEY
DEBARGE
DEBARKS
DEBASED
DEBASER
DEBASES
DEBATED
DEBATER
DEBATES
DEBAUCH
DEBEARD
DEBEERS
DEBITED
DEBLURS
DEBOITE
DEBONED
DEBONES
DEBORAH
DEBOULE
DEBRETT
DEBRIEF
DEBTEES
DEBTORS
DEBUNKS
DEBURGH
DEBURRS
DEBUSES
DEBUSSY
DEBUTED
DIBBLED
DIBBLER
DIBBLES

DOBBINS
DRBROWN
DUBARRY
DUBBERS
DUBBING
DUBIETY
DUBIOUS
DUBNIUM
DUBUQUE
DYBBUKS

D••B•••
DABBERS
DABBING
DABBLED
DABBLER
DABBLES
DANBURY
DASBOOT
DAUBERS
DAUBING
DAYBEDS
DAYBOOK
DELBERT
DEMBUMS
DERBIES
DIABLES
DIABLOS
DIABOLO
DIBBLED
DIBBLER
DIBBLES
DIEBOLD
DILBERT
DIMBULB
DISBAND
DISBARS
DISBUDS
DOBBINS
DOGBANE
DOGBEDS
DOGBERT
DOGBITE
DOGBONE
DOGBOOT
DOGBOWL
DOTBOMB
DOUBLEA
DOUBLEB
DOUBLEC
DOUBLED
DOUBLEE
DOUBLEF
DOUBLEG
DOUBLEH
DOUBLEI
DOUBLEJ
DOUBLEK
DOUBLEL
DOUBLEM
DOUBLEN
DOUBLEO
DOUBLEP
DOUBLEQ
DOUBLER
DOUBLES
DOUBLET
DOUBLEU
DOUBLEV
DOUBLEW
DOUBLEX
DOUBLEY
DOUBLEZ
DOUBTED
DOUBTER
DOUBTIT
DRABBER
DRABBLE
DRIBBLE
DRIBLET
DRUBBED
DRUBBER
DRYBULB
DUBBERS
DUBBING
DUMBEST
DUMBING
DYBBUKS
DYEBATH

D•••B••
DATABLE
DATABUS
DECIBEL
DEEDBOX
DELIBES
DEORBIT
DINGBAT
DIRTBAG
DISABLE
DISOBEY
DOESBAD
DONEBAD
DONTBEE
DOVEBAR
DOWNBOW
DRABBER
DRABBLE
DRAWBAR
DRIBBLE
DROPBOX
DRUBBED
DRUBBER
DRYABLE
DURABLE
DURABLY
DUSTBIN

D••••B•
DAYJOBS
DISROBE
DNALABS
DRIVEBY
DROPSBY
DROVEBY
DRWELBY
DYEJOBS

D•••••B
DECRUMB
DIMBULB
DISTURB
DOGCOMB
DOTBOMB
DOUBLEB
DRYBULB

•DB••••
IDBADGE

•D•B•••
EDIBLES
ODDBALL
PDQBACH

•D••B••
ADDABLE
ADDIBLE
ADHIBIT
CDALBUM

•D•••B•
ADSORBS
ADVERBS
ODDJOBS

••DB•••
BADBACK
BADBOYS
BEDBATH
BEDBUGS
CADBURY
HADBEEN
HADBEST
MUDBATH
ODDBALL
OLDBATS
OLDBEAN
OLDBLUE
OLDBOYS
REDBATS
REDBAYS
REDBIRD
REDBONE
REDBOOK
REDBUDS
SUDBURY
TIDBITS

••D•B••
ADDABLE
ADDIBLE
ALDUBIN
AUDIBLE
AUDIBLY
AUDUBON
BODYBAR
ENDABLE
HIDABLE
LADYBUG
REDEBIT
RIDABLE
RIDEBYS
SIDEBAR
SIDEBET

••D••B•
BADDEBT
BEDAUBS
ENDERBY
HADTOBE
INDOUBT
MADLIBS
MIDRIBS
MODELBS
NODOUBT
ODDJOBS
REDOUBT
REDROBE
REDTABS
RIDESBY

••D•••B
BODYRUB
GODTHAB
HADAJOB
PEDICAB

•••DB••
BANDBOX
DEEDBOX
FEEDBAG
FEEDBIN
GOLDBUG
GOODBAR
GOODBUY
GOODBYE
GOODBYS
HANDBAG
ROADBED
SAIDBOO
SANDBAG
SANDBAR
SANDBOX
SANDBUR
SEEDBED
SINDBAD
WINDBAG
WOODBIN
WOODBOX

•••D•B•
ABIDEBY
BADDEBT
CORDOBA
FREDEBB
GLIDEBY
SENDSBY
SLIDEBY
SUBDEBS

•••D••B
FOODWEB
FREDEBB
GOODJOB
LYNDONB
SANDDAB

••••DB•
BYANDBY
COULDBE
EASEDBY
FILEDBY
RACEDBY
RULEDBY
STANDBY
STOODBY
WOULDBE

••••D•B
FLUBDUB
OVERDUB
RUBADUB
SANDDAB

D•C••••
DACAPOS
DACOSTA
DACRONS
DACTYLS
DECADES
DECAGON
DECALOG
DECAMPS
DECANTS
DECAPOD
DECARLO
DECATUR
DECAYED
DECAYER
DECEASE
DECEITS
DECEIVE
DECENCY
DECIARE
DECIBEL
DECIDED
DECIDER
DECIDES
DECILES
DECIMAL
DECKERS
DECKING
DECKLED
DECKLES
DECKOUT
DECLAIM
DECLARE
DECLASS
DECLAWS
DECLINE
DECLOTS
DECOCTS
DECODED
DECODER
DECODES
DECOLOR
DECORUM
DECOYED
DECOYER
DECREED
DECREER
DECREES
DECRIED
DECRIER
DECRIES
DECRUMB
DECRYPT
DECUPLE
DICECUP
DICHTER
DICIEST
DICILLO
DICKENS
DICKERS
DICKEYS
DICKIES
DICKORY
DICKSON
DICTATE
DICTION
DICTUMS
DOCENTS
DOCKAGE
DOCKERS
DOCKETS
DOCKING
DOCTORS
DRCHAOS
DUCALLY
DUCHAMP
DUCHESS
DUCHIES
DUCKERS
DUCKIER
DUCKIES
DUCKING
DUCKOUT
DUCKPIN
DUCTILE
DUCTING

D••C•••
DANCERS
DANCING
DASCHLE
DAYCAMP
DAYCARE
DEACONS
DEFCONS
DEICERS
DEICING
DELCITY
DESCANT
DESCEND
DESCENT
DEUCING
DEWCLAW
DIECAST
DIECUTS
DIOCESE
DISCARD
DISCERN
DISCING
DISCMAN
DISCOED
DISCOID
DISCORD
DISCUSS
DITCHED
DITCHER
DITCHES
DNACODE
DOGCART
DOGCHEW
DOGCHOW
DOGCOAT
DOGCOMB
DOTCOMS
DOUCEUR
DRACHMA
DRACULA
DRMCCOY
DRUCKER
DRYCELL
DULCIFY
DUNCISH

D•••C••
DEBACLE
DECOCTS
DEDUCED
DEDUCER
DEDUCES
DEDUCTS
DEFACED
DEFACER
DEFACES
DEFACTO
DEFECTS
DEFICIT
DEFOCUS
DEJECTS
DELICTI
DELICTO
DELICTS
DEPECHE
DEPICTS
DERECHO
DETECTO
DETECTS
DEVICES
DICECUP
DIDACTS
DIGICAM
DIRECTS
DIRECTV
DOMECAR
DOMICAL
DOMICIL
DONTCRY
DOVECOT
DRMCCOY
DROPCAP

D••••C•
DAVINCI
DAYPACK
DEBAUCH
DECENCY
DEFENCE
DEFLECT
DEFROCK
DEFUNCT
DEHISCE
DEMARCO
DENIECE
DERRICK
DERRICO
DESTOCK
DETRACT
DEUTSCH
DIALECT
DIPTYCH
DISSECT
DISTICH
DIVORCE
DOGFACE
DOGRACE
DOGTICK
DOLUNCH
DORMICE
DOTRICE
DRIESCH
DRSPOCK
DRYDOCK
DURANCE

D•••••C
DEISTIC
DELPHIC
DELTAIC
DEMONIC
DEMOTIC
DHARMIC
DINARIC
DOMINIC
DOUBLEC
DRASTIC
DRUIDIC
DRYADIC
DYNAMIC

•DC••••
CDCASES
IDCARDS

•D•C•••
EDACITY
EDICTAL
EDUCATE
EDUCING
EDUCTED
EDUCTOR

•D••C••
ADDICTS
ADDUCED
ADDUCER
ADDUCES
ADDUCTS
ADVICES
CDRACKS

•D•••C•
ADJUNCT
ADSPACE
ADVANCE
EDIFICE
ODDDUCK
ODDSOCK
PDQBACH

•D••••C
IDENTIC
IDIOTIC
IDYLLIC

••DC•••
BADCALL
BADCASE
BADCOLD
CODCAKE
ENDCUTS
KIDCOMS
MADCAPS
MADCHEN
MIDCAPS
MUDCATS
OLDCARS
OLDCHAP
OLDCITY
PODCAST
REDCAPS
REDCARD
REDCELL
REDCENT
REDCHIP
REDCLAY
REDCOAT
REDCODS
SADCAFE

••D•C••
ABDUCED
ABDUCES
ABDUCTS
ADDICTS
ADDUCED
ADDUCER
ADDUCES
ADDUCTS
ARDECHE
BEDECKS
BODICES
CADUCEI
CODICES
CODICIL
DEDUCED
DEDUCER
DEDUCES
DEDUCTS
DIDACTS
HADACOW
INDICES
INDICIA
INDICTS
INDUCED
INDUCER
INDUCES
INDUCTS
INDYCAR
MEDICAL
MEDICOS
MODICUM
NODICAL
PADUCAH
PEDICAB
RADICAL
RADICES
RADICLE
REDACTS
REDECAY
REDOCKS
REDUCED
REDUCER
REDUCES
SEDUCED
SEDUCER
SEDUCES
SIDECAR
SODACAN
UNDOCKS
VIDICON
ZYDECOS

••D••C•
ACDELCO
ALDRICH
ANDSUCH
ARDENCY
ATDEUCE
BADBACK
BADITCH
BADLUCK
BEDROCK
CADENCE
CADENCY
ELDRICH
ELDRICK
ERDRICH
GEDRICK
GODUTCH
HADDOCK
INDUTCH
JUDAICA
KIDROCK
LADOUCE
MADLOCK
MEDWICK
MRDARCY
MUDPACK
NIDETCH
ODDDUCK
ODDSOCK
OLDNICK
PADDOCK
PADLOCK
PUDENCY
REDFACE
REDJACK
REDNECK
RIDDICK
RODDICK
SADSACK
TEDMACK
WEDLOCK
ZODIACS

••D•••C
EIDETIC
EIDOLIC
ENDEMIC
HEDONIC
MEDEVAC
MEDIVAC
MIDDLEC
PADRAIC

•••DC••
COLDCUP
COLDCUT
HANDCAR
USEDCAR
USEDCDS
WILDCAT
WOODCUT

•••D•C•
AIRDUCT
ARTDECO
BURDICK
CANDACE
CANDICE
CONDUCE
CONDUCT
DRYDOCK
FOSDICK
GEODUCK
HADDOCK
HENDECA
MURDOCH
NORDICA
NORDICS
ODDDUCK
OVIDUCT
PADDOCK
PETDUCK
PREDICT
PRODUCE
PRODUCT
RIDDICK
RODDICK
SEADUCK
SUBDUCT
SUNDECK
SYNDICS
TRADUCE
VANDYCK
VERDICT
VIADUCT

•••D••C
BALDRIC
CARDIAC
FREDRIC
MIDDLEC
QUADRIC

••••D•C
COMEDIC
DRUIDIC
DRYADIC
FATIDIC
FJORDIC
FLUIDIC
HASIDIC
HEXADIC
ILIADIC
JURIDIC
LIPIDIC
MELODIC
MONADIC
MONODIC
NOMADIC
OCTADIC
PAPADOC
PARODIC
POSTDOC
SYNODIC
TRIADIC
VANADIC
VERIDIC

D•D••••
DADAART
DADAISM
DADAIST
DADDIES
DADOING
DEDALUS
DEDUCED
DEDUCER
DEDUCES
DEDUCTS
DIDACTS
DIDASET
DIDDLED
DIDDLER
DIDDLES
DIDDLEY
DIDEROT
DIDFINE
DIDGOOD
DIDLAPS
DIDLIKE
DIDOVER
DIDSUMS
DIDTIME
DIDTOAT
DIDWELL
DODDERS
DODDERY
DODGEMS
DODGERS
DODGIER
DODGING
DODGSON
DUDEDUP
DUDESUP
DUDGEON

D••D•••
DADDIES
DANDERS
DANDIER
DANDIES
DANDIFY
DANDILY
DANDLED
DANDLER
DANDLES
DAWDLED
DAWDLER
DAWDLES
DEADAIR
DEADEND
DEADENS
DEADEST
DEADEYE
DEADPAN
DEADSEA
DEADSET
DEEDBOX
DEEDING
DENDRON
DEODARS
DEODATO
DEWDROP
DIADEMS
DIDDLED
DIDDLER
DIDDLES
DIDDLEY
DIEDFOR
DIEDOFF
DIEDOUT
DIEDOWN
DIKDIKS
DINDINS
DISDAIN
DOADEAL
DODDERS
DODDERY
DOGDAYS
DOGDOOR
DOIDARE
DOODADS
DOODLED
DOODLER
DOODLES
DOTDASH
DOWDIER
DOWDIES
DOWDILY
DREDGED
DREDGER
DREDGES
DRUDGED
DRUDGER
DRUDGES
DRYDOCK
DUEDATE
DUMDUMS
DUNDALK
DUODENA

D•••D••
DAMPDRY
DASHDOT
DATEDLY
DAZEDLY
DEARDEN
DECADES
DECIDED
DECIDER
DECIDES
DECODED
DECODER
DECODES
DEIRDRE
DELEDDA
DELUDED
DELUDER
DELUDES
DENUDED
DENUDER
DENUDES
DERIDED
DERIDER
DERIDES
DINADAM
DINEDAT
DINEDIN
DINEDON
DIRNDLS
DIVEDIN
DIVIDED
DIVIDER
DIVIDES
DOORDIE
DOSADOS
DOSIDOS
DOTEDON
DREADED
DREIDEL
DRESDEN
DRIEDUP
DRIPDRY
DRUIDIC
DRYADES
DRYADIC
DRYIDEA
DUDEDUP

DUKEDOM
DUNEDIN
DWINDLE
DYNODES

D••••D•

DAYBEDS
DAYSIDE
DEFENDS
DEFUNDS
DEGRADE
DELEADS
DELEDDA
DEMANDS
DEPENDS
DERONDA
DERRIDA
DESEEDS
DETRUDE
DEWILDE
DIALEDO
DIOMEDE
DIOXIDE
DISBUDS
DNACODE
DOASIDO
DOGBEDS
DOODADS
DOTARDS
DOVERDE
DRAMADY
DRAMEDY

D•••••D

DABBLED
DABHAND
DAGWOOD
DALLIED
DAMAGED
DANDLED
DANGLED
DAPPLED
DARKLED
DARKRED
DARTLED
DASTARD
DAUNTED
DAWDLED
DAYSEND
DAZZLED
DEADEND
DEAIRED
DEARGOD
DEBASED
DEBATED
DEBEARD
DEBITED
DEBONED
DEBUTED
DECAPOD
DECAYED
DECIDED
DECKLED
DECODED
DECOYED
DECREED
DECRIED
DEDUCED
DEEPEND
DEEPRED
DEFACED
DEFAMED
DEFILED
DEFINED
DEFRAUD
DEFUSED
DEGREED
DEHEXED
DEHIRED
DEIFIED
DEIGNED
DELAYED
DELETED
DELTOID
DELUDED
DELUGED
DEMIGOD
DEMISED
DEMOTED
DENIMED
DENOTED
DENTOID
DENUDED
DEPONED
DEPOSED
DEPUTED
DERATED
DERIDED
DERIVED
DESCEND
DESEXED
DESIRED
DESMOND
DESPOND
DETOXED
DETUNED
DEVILED
DEVISED
DEVOTED
DEWAXED
DEWIRED
DIALLED
DIAMOND
DIBBLED
DIDDLED
DIDGOOD
DIEBOLD
DIEHARD
DILATED
DILLARD
DILUTED
DIMPLED
DIPLOID
DIRTIED
DISBAND
DISCARD
DISCOED
DISCOID
DISCORD
DISTEND
DISUSED
DITCHED
DITTOED
DIVIDED
DIVINED
DIVVIED
DIZZIED
DOEEYED
DOESBAD
DOGFOOD
DOGSLED
DOGWOOD
DOLLIED
DONATED
DONEBAD
DOODLED
DOUBLED
DOUBTED
DOWERED
DRAFTED
DRAGGED
DRAINED
DRATTED
DRAWLED
DREADED
DREAMED
DREDGED
DRESSED
DRFREUD
DRIFTED
DRILLED
DRIPPED
DROOLED
DROOPED
DROPPED
DROWNED
DROWSED
DRUBBED
DRUDGED
DRUGGED
DRUMMED
DRYEYED
DUELLED
DUETTED
DULLARD
DUMMIED
DURWARD
DWARFED
DWELLED
DWIGHTD
DYEWOOD

•DD••••

ADDABLE
ADDAXES
ADDEDIN
ADDEDLY
ADDEDON
ADDEDTO
ADDEDUP
ADDENDA
ADDENDS
ADDIBLE
ADDICTS
ADDISON
ADDLING
ADDONTO
ADDRESS
ADDSALT
ADDUCED
ADDUCER
ADDUCES
ADDUCTS
ADDUPTO
EDDYING
ODDBALL
ODDDUCK
ODDJOBS
ODDLOTS
ODDMENT
ODDNESS
ODDSARE
ODDSHOE
ODDSOCK

•D•D•••

IDIDTOO
ODDDUCK

•D••D••

ADDEDIN
ADDEDLY
ADDEDON
ADDEDTO
ADDEDUP
ADJUDGE
EDGEDIN
IDBADGE
IDOODIT

•D•••D•

ADDENDA
ADDENDS
EDGARDO
EDMONDS
EDMUNDI
EDMUNDS
EDUARDO
EDWARDG
EDWARDI
EDWARDR
EDWARDS
EDWARDV
IDAREDS
IDCARDS

•D••••D

ADAPTED
ADDUCED
ADENOID
ADHERED
ADJURED
ADMIRED
ADMIXED
ADOPTED
ADORNED
ADVISED
EDIFIED
EDOUARD
EDUCTED
IDEATED

••DD•••

BADDAYS
BADDEBT
BADDEED
BADDEST
BADDIES
BADDISH
BADDOGS
BEDDING
BEDDOWN
BIDDERS
BIDDIES
BIDDING
BUDDERS
BUDDHAS
BUDDIED
BUDDIES
BUDDING
BUDDYUP
CADDIED
CADDIES
CADDISH
CODDLED
CODDLER
CODDLES
CUDDIES
CUDDLED
CUDDLES
DADDIES
DIDDLED
DIDDLER
DIDDLES
DIDDLEY
DODDERS
DODDERY
FADDIER
FADDIET
FADDISH
FADDISM
FADDIST
FEDDERS
FIDDLED
FIDDLER
FIDDLES
FODDERS
FUDDIES
FUDDLED
FUDDLES
GADDERS
GADDING
GIDDIED
GIDDIER
GIDDIES
GIDDILY
GIDDYAP
GIDDYUP
GODDARD
GODDESS
HADDOCK
HADDONE
HODDING
HUDDLED
HUDDLER
HUDDLES
KADDISH
KIDDERS
KIDDIES
KIDDING
KIDDISH
LADDERS
LADDIES
LADDISH
LUDDISM
LUDDITE
LYDDITE
MADDASH
MADDENS
MADDERS
MADDEST
MADDING
MADDISH
MADDOGS
MEDDLED
MEDDLER
MEDDLES
MIDDAYS
MIDDIES
MIDDLEC
MIDDLED
MIDDLER
MIDDLES
MUDDERS
MUDDIED
MUDDIER
MUDDIES
MUDDILY
MUDDING
MUDDLED
MUDDLER
MUDDLES
NODDERS
NODDIES
NODDING
ODDDUCK
OLDDAYS
OLDDOGS
PADDERS
PADDIES
PADDING
PADDLED
PADDLER
PADDLES
PADDOCK
PEDDLED
PEDDLER
PEDDLES
PIDDLED
PIDDLES
PUDDING
PUDDLED
PUDDLES
QADDAFI
REDDAWN
REDDEER
REDDENS
REDDEST
REDDING
REDDISH
REDDOGS
REDDOTS
REDDUST
REDDYES
RIDDERS
RIDDICK
RIDDING
RIDDLED
RIDDLER
RIDDLES
RODDICK
RODDING
RUDDERS
RUDDIED
RUDDIER
RUDDILY
SADDENS
SADDEST
SADDLED
SADDLER
SADDLES
SIDDONS
SIDDURS
SODDIER
SODDING
TEDDIES
TODDIES
TODDLED
TODDLER
TODDLES
WADDELL
WADDERS
WADDING
WADDLED
WADDLER
WADDLES
WEDDELL
WEDDERS
WEDDING
YIDDISH

••D•D••

ADDEDIN
ADDEDLY
ADDEDON
ADDEDTO
ADDEDUP
BADIDEA
DUDEDUP
ENDEDAT
ENDEDIN
ENDEDIT
ENDEDON
ENDEDUP
FADEDIN
FADEDLY
FTDODGE
GADSDEN
HODADDY
IODIDES
JADEDLY
LADADOG
LADIDAS
LADYDAY
SODIDWE
WADEDIN
WEDIDIT

••D••D•

ADDENDA
ADDENDS
ANDRADE
BADENDS
BEDSIDE
HODADDY
HYDRIDE
INDEEDY
KIDVIDS
MRDEEDS
OGDOADS
OLDLADY
PODRIDA
RADIODJ
REDBUDS
REDCODS
REDEEDS
REDONDO
REDTIDE
UNDERDO

••D•••D

ABDUCED
ADDUCED
ANDROID
AUDITED
BADCOLD
BADDEED
BADHAND
BADLAND
BADMOOD
BADWORD
BEDAZED
BEDEWED
BEDFORD
BUDDIED
CADDIED
CEDARED
CODDLED
CODERED
CUDDLED
DEDUCED
DIDDLED
DIDGOOD
ENDOWED
ENDURED
FEDEXED
FIDDLED
FUDDLED
GIDDIED
GODDARD
GODHEAD
GODHOOD
GODSEND
HUDDLED
INDEXED
INDITED
INDUCED
IODATED
IODISED
IODIZED
LADHOOD
MADEMAD
MEDALED
MEDDLED
MEDFORD
MIDDLED
MIDLAND
MODELED
MODEMED
MUDDIED
MUDDLED
NEDLAND
NODULED
NUDZHED
OLDGOLD
OLDHAND
OLDMAID
ORDERED
PADDLED
PEDALED
PEDDLED
PIDDLED
PUDDLED
RADFORD
RADIOAD
RADIOED
REDARED
REDATED
REDBIRD
REDCARD
REDEYED
REDFORD
REDHEAD
REDMOND
REDOSED
REDOUND
REDRIED
REDUCED
REDWOOD
RIDDLED
RUDDIED
RUDYARD
SADDLED
SADEYED
SEDATED
SEDUCED
SUDAFED
TODDLED
UNDARED
UNDATED
UNDAZED
UNDEWED
UNDIKED
UNDOMED
UNDRIED
UNDUPED
UPDATED
UPDIVED
UPDRIED
VIDEOED
WADDLED
WEDELED
WIDENED
WIDOWED
YODELED

•••DD••

ALADDIN
BIRDDOG
BLADDER
CHEDDAR
CHIDDEN
CLADDED
COLDDAY
FREDDIE
GLADDEN
GLADDER
GOODDAY
GOODDOG
GRIDDED
GRIDDER
GRIDDLE
HARDDAY
LEADDOG
PLODDED
PLODDER
PRODDED
PRODDER
READDED
SANDDAB
SCUDDED
SCUDDER
SHEDDER
SHODDEN
SHUDDER
SKIDDED
SKIDDER
SKIDDOO
SLEDDED
SLEDDER
SLEDDOG
STUDDED
SWADDLE
THUDDED
TRODDEN
TWADDLE
TWIDDLE
UNADDED
WILDDOG

•••D•D•

ALIDADE
AOUDADS
BANDIDO
CANDIDA
CANDIDE
CANDIDS
DOODADS
HOWDEDO
HOWDYDO
PAIDADS
PERDIDO
SAIDIDO
USEDCDS

•••D••D

AULDSOD
BADDEED
BANDAID
BANDIED
BIRDIED
BLUDGED
BRIDGED
BRIDLED
BUDDIED
BUNDLED
CADDIED
CANDIED
CANDLED
CLADDED
CODDLED
CRADLED
CUDDLED
CURDLED
DANDLED
DAWDLED
DEADEND
DIDDLED
DOODLED
DREDGED
DRUDGED
FIDDLED
FLEDGED
FONDLED
FONDUED
FORDLTD
FUDDLED
GIDDIED
GIRDLED
GODDARD
GOODKID
GRIDDED
GRUDGED
HANDFED
HANDLED
HEADEND
HUDDLED
HUNDRED
HURDLED
KINDLED
KINDRED
KLUDGED
LINDIED
MEDDLED
MIDDLED
MILDRED
MISDEED
MORDRED
MUDDIED
MUDDLED
NEEDLED
NOODGED
NOODLED
PADDLED
PEDDLED
PIDDLED
PLEDGED
PLODDED
PRODDED
PUDDLED
READDED
READIED
RIDDLED
ROADBED
RUDDIED
SADDLED
SCUDDED
SEEDBED
SEEDPOD
SINDBAD
SKIDDED
SKIDLID
SLEDDED
SLEDGED
SMUDGED
STODGED
STUDDED
STUDIED
SUBDUED
THUDDED
TIEDYED
TOADIED
TODDLED
TRUDGED
UNADDED
UNEDGED
VATDYED
WADDLED
WINDGOD
WOODARD

••••DD•

DELEDDA
HODADDY
LAYODDS
MISADDS
MRBODDY
MYBUDDY
OUTADDS
UNGIDDY
UNMUDDY

••••D•D

ABRADED
ACCEDED
ALLUDED
AMENDED
ARCADED
AVOIDED
AWARDED
BAGHDAD
BEARDED
BETIDED
BLENDED
BLINDED
BLOODED
BOARDED
BOUNDED
BRAIDED
BRANDED
BREADED
BROODED
CHORDED
CLADDED
CLOUDED
CRAWDAD
CROWDED
DECIDED
DECODED
DELUDED
DENUDED
DERIDED
DIVIDED
DREADED
EMENDED
ENCODED
EXCIDED
FIELDED
FLOODED
FOUNDED
GRIDDED
GUARDED
HOARDED
HOUNDED
ILLUDED
IMPEDED
INVADED
KATYDID
KNEADED
MILKDUD
MOULDED
MOUNDED
NAVIDAD
OVERDID
PARADED
PLEADED
PLODDED
POMADED
POUNDED
PRODDED
READDED
RECEDED
RECODED
RESIDED
ROUNDED
SCALDED
SCOLDED
SCUDDED
SECEDED
SKIDDED
SLEDDED
SOLEDAD
SOUNDED
SPEEDED
STEADED
STEPDAD
STUDDED
THUDDED
TREADED
TRENDED
UNADDED
UNAIDED
UNCEDED
UNCODED
UNENDED
UNFADED
UNJADED
UNLADED
UNSIDED
UNWADED
UPENDED
VALIDID
WEIRDED
WIELDED
WOUNDED
YESIDID
YIELDED

•••••DD

JOEKIDD
VERYODD

DE•••••

DEACONS
DEADAIR
DEADEND
DEADENS
DEADEST
DEADEYE
DEADPAN
DEADSEA
DEADSET
DEAFENS
DEAFEST
DEAIRED
DEALERS
DEALING
DEALOUT
DEALSIN
DEALSTO
DEALSUP
DEALTIN
DEALTTO
DEALTUP
DEANERY
DEARDEN
DEAREST
DEARGOD
DEARIES
DEARONE
DEARSIR
DEARTHS
DEBACLE
DEBAKEY

DEBARGE
DEBARKS
DEBASED
DEBASER
DEBASES
DEBATED
DEBATER
DEBATES
DEBAUCH
DEBEARD
DEBEERS
DEBITED
DEBLURS
DEBOITE
DEBONED
DEBONES
DEBORAH
DEBOULE
DEBRETT
DEBRIEF
DEBTEES
DEBTORS
DEBUNKS
DEBURGH
DEBURRS
DEBUSES
DEBUSSY
DEBUTED
DECADES
DECAGON
DECALOG
DECAMPS
DECANTS
DECAPOD
DECARLO
DECATUR
DECAYED
DECAYER
DECEASE
DECEITS
DECEIVE
DECENCY
DECIARE
DECIBEL
DECIDED
DECIDER
DECIDES
DECILES
DECIMAL
DECKERS
DECKING
DECKLED
DECKLES
DECKOUT
DECLAIM
DECLARE
DECLASS
DECLAWS
DECLINE
DECLOTS
DECOCTS
DECODED
DECODER
DECODES
DECOLOR
DECORUM
DECOYED
DECOYER
DECREED
DECREER
DECREES
DECRIED
DECRIER
DECRIES
DECRUMB
DECRYPT
DECUPLE
DEDALUS
DEDUCED
DEDUCER
DEDUCES
DEDUCTS
DEEDBOX
DEEDING
DEEJAYS
DEEMING
DEEPEND
DEEPENS
DEEPEST
DEEPFAT
DEEPFRY
DEEPISH
DEEPRED
DEEPSEA
DEEPSET
DEEPSIX
DEEPSKY
DEEPTAN
DEERFLY
DEFACED
DEFACER
DEFACES
DEFACTO
DEFALLA
DEFAMED
DEFAMER
DEFAMES
DEFANGS
DEFARGE
DEFAULT
DEFCONS
DEFEATS
DEFECTS
DEFENCE
DEFENDS
DEFENSE
DEFERTO
DEFFEST
DEFGHIJ
DEFIANT
DEFICIT
DEFIERS
DEFILED
DEFILER
DEFILES
DEFINED
DEFINER
DEFINES
DEFLATE
DEFLEAS
DEFLECT
DEFOAMS
DEFOCUS
DEFORMS
DEFRAGS
DEFRAME
DEFRAUD
DEFRAYS
DEFROCK
DEFROST
DEFTEST
DEFUELS
DEFUNCT
DEFUNDS
DEFUSED
DEFUSER
DEFUSES
DEFYING
DEGAUSS
DEGERMS
DEGHOST
DEGLAZE
DEGRADE
DEGREED
DEGREES
DEGUSTS
DEHAIRS
DEHAVEN
DEHEXED
DEHEXES
DEHIRED
DEHIRES
DEHISCE
DEHMELT
DEHORNS
DEICERS
DEICING
DEIFIED
DEIFIER
DEIFIES
DEIGNED
DEIGNTO
DEIRDRE
DEISTIC
DEITIES
DEJECTS
DEJUNKS
DEKEING
DEKLERK
DELANEY
DELARUE
DELAYED
DELAYER
DELBERT
DELCITY
DELEADS
DELEDDA
DELEING
DELETED
DELETES
DELIBES
DELICTI
DELICTO
DELICTS
DELIGHT
DELIHAM
DELILAH
DELILLO
DELIMAN
DELIMEN
DELIMIT
DELINTS
DELIRIA
DELISTS
DELIVER
DELKEYS
DELMONT
DELMORE
DELORIS
DELORME
DELOUSE
DELPHIC
DELRAYS
DELRUTH
DELSOLS
DELTAIC
DELTOID
DELTONA
DELTORO
DELUDED
DELUDER
DELUDES
DELUGED
DELUGES
DELUISE
DELVERS
DELVING
DEMAGOG
DEMANDS
DEMARCO
DEMARET
DEMARKS
DEMASTS
DEMBUMS
DEMEANS
DEMENTO
DEMERGE
DEMERIT
DEMEROL
DEMESNE
DEMETER
DEMIGOD
DEMILLE
DEMISED
DEMISES
DEMISTS
DEMOING
DEMOLAY
DEMONIC
DEMONYM
DEMOTED
DEMOTES
DEMOTHS
DEMOTIC
DEMOUNT
DEMPSEY
DEMURER
DENARII
DENDRON
DENEUVE
DENHAAG
DENIALS
DENIECE
DENIERS
DENIMED
DENISON
DENIZEN
DENMARK
DENMOMS
DENNEHY
DENNING
DENOTED
DENOTES
DENSELY
DENSEST
DENSIFY
DENSITY
DENTALS
DENTATE
DENTINE
DENTING
DENTINS
DENTIST
DENTOID
DENTONS
DENTURE
DENTYNE
DENUDED
DENUDER
DENUDES
DENYING
DEODARS
DEODATO
DEORBIT
DEPALMA
DEPARTS
DEPAULU
DEPECHE
DEPENDS
DEPESTS
DEPICTS
DEPLANE
DEPLETE
DEPLORE
DEPLOYS
DEPONED
DEPONER
DEPONES
DEPORTS
DEPOSAL
DEPOSED
DEPOSER
DEPOSES
DEPOSIT
DEPOWER
DEPRAVE
DEPRESS
DEPRIVE
DEPULPS
DEPUTED
DEPUTES
DEQUEUE
DERAILS
DERALTE
DERANGE
DERATED
DERATES
DERBIES
DERECHO
DERIDED
DERIDER
DERIDES
DERIVED
DERIVER
DERIVES
DERMATO
DERNIER
DERONDA
DERRICK
DERRICO
DERRIDA
DERRING
DERUSTS
DERVISH
DERWENT
DESALTS
DESCANT
DESCEND
DESCENT
DESEEDS
DESERET
DESERTS
DESERVE
DESEXED
DESEXES
DESHELL
DESIGNS
DESILTS
DESIRED
DESIREE
DESIRER
DESIRES
DESISTS
DESKFUL
DESKSET
DESKTOP
DESLUMS
DESMOGS
DESMOND
DESOTOS
DESPAIR
DESPINA
DESPISE
DESPITE
DESPOIL
DESPOND
DESPOTS
DESSERT
DESTAEL
DESTAIN
DESTEMS
DESTINE
DESTINO
DESTINY
DESTOCK
DESTROY
DESYLVA
DETAILS
DETAINS
DETECTO
DETECTS
DETENTE
DETENTS
DETERGE
DETESTS
DETOURS
DETOXED
DETOXES
DETRACT
DETRAIN
DETROIT
DETRUDE
DETUNED
DETUNES
DEUCING
DEUTERO
DEUTSCH
DEVALUE
DEVEINS
DEVELOP
DEVESTS
DEVIANT
DEVIATE
DEVICES
DEVILED
DEVILLE
DEVILRY
DEVIOUS
DEVISED
DEVISEE
DEVISER
DEVISES
DEVISOR
DEVOIRS
DEVOLVE
DEVORES
DEVOTED
DEVOTEE
DEVOTES
DEVOURS
DEVRIES
DEWAART
DEWATER
DEWAXED
DEWAXES
DEWCLAW
DEWDROP
DEWFALL
DEWIEST
DEWILDE
DEWIRED
DEWIRES
DEWLAPS
DEWLESS
DEWLINE
DEWORMS
DEXTRAL
DEXTRIN
DEYOUNG

D•E••••

DAEMONS
DAEWOOS
DEEDBOX
DEEDING
DEEJAYS
DEEMING
DEEPEND
DEEPENS
DEEPEST
DEEPFAT
DEEPFRY
DEEPISH
DEEPRED
DEEPSEA
DEEPSET
DEEPSIX
DEEPSKY
DEEPTAN
DEERFLY
DIEAWAY
DIEBOLD
DIECAST
DIECUTS
DIEDFOR
DIEDOFF
DIEDOUT
DIEDOWN
DIEHARD
DIEMENS
DIEOFFS
DIESELS
DIESFOR
DIESOFF
DIESOUT
DIETARY
DIETERS
DIETING
DOEEYED
DOESBAD
DOESFOR
DOESKIN
DOESNOT
DOESTOO
DOEUVRE
DREADED
DREAMED
DREAMER
DREAMIN
DREAMOF
DREAMON
DREAMUP
DREDGED
DREDGER
DREDGES
DREGION
DREIDEL
DREISER
DRESDEN
DRESSAS
DRESSED
DRESSER
DRESSES
DRESSIN
DRESSUP
DREWOFF
DREWOUT
DREXELU
DREXLER
DREYFUS
DUEDATE
DUEEAST
DUELERS
DUELING
DUELIST
DUELLED
DUENNAS
DUETING
DUETTED
DUETTOS
DUEWEST
DWEEZIL
DWELLAT
DWELLED
DWELLER
DWELLIN
DWELLON
DWELTON
DYEBATH
DYEJOBS
DYELOTS
DYEVATS
DYEWOOD

D••E•••

DALETHS
DANELAW
DANEYKO
DAREFUL
DARENOT
DARESAY
DARESTO
DAREZZO
DATEDLY
DAVEKOZ
DAZEDLY
DEBEARD
DEBEERS
DECEASE
DECEITS
DECEIVE
DECENCY
DEFEATS
DEFECTS
DEFENCE
DEFENDS
DEFENSE
DEFERTO
DEGERMS
DEHEXED
DEHEXES
DEJECTS
DEKEING
DELEADS
DELEDDA
DELEING
DELETED
DELETES
DEMEANS
DEMENTO
DEMERGE
DEMERIT
DEMEROL
DEMESNE
DEMETER
DENEUVE
DEPECHE
DEPENDS
DEPESTS
DERECHO
DESEEDS
DESERET
DESERTS
DESERVE
DESEXED
DESEXES
DETECTO
DETECTS
DETENTE
DETENTS
DETERGE
DETESTS
DEVEINS
DEVELOP
DEVESTS
DICECUP
DIDEROT
DIGESTS
DILEMMA
DIMETER
DINEDAT
DINEDIN
DINEDON
DINEOUT
DINESAT
DINESEN
DINESIN
DINESON
DINETTE
DIRECTS
DIRECTV
DIREFUL
DISEASE
DISEURS
DISEUSE
DIVEDIN
DIVERGE
DIVERSE
DIVERTS
DIVESIN
DIVESTS
DNIEPER
DOCENTS
DOEEYED
DOGEARS
DOHERTY
DOLEFUL
DOLEOUT
DOMECAR
DONEBAD
DONEFOR
DONEGAL
DONEGAN
DONETSK
DOPEOUT
DOTEDON
DOTESON
DOVEBAR
DOVECOT
DOVELET
DOVERDE
DOWERED
DOYENNE
DOZENTH
DOZEOFF
DRIEDUP
DRIESCH
DRIESUP
DRMELFI
DRSEUSS
DRTEETH
DRVEGAS
DRWELBY
DRYEYED
DRYEYES
DUDEDUP
DUDESUP
DUEEAST
DUKEDOM
DUNEDIN
DUTEOUS
DWEEZIL

D•••E••

DABBERS
DAFTEST
DAGGERS
DAMMERS
DAMNERS
DAMPENS
DAMPERS
DAMPEST
DAMSELS
DANCERS
DANDERS
DANGELO
DANGERS
DANIELA
DANIELJ
DANIELS
DANKEST
DANSEUR
DANTEAN
DANTEII
DANVERS
DARKENS
DARKEST
DARLEEN
DARLENE
DARNELL
DARNERS
DARTERS
DARWELL
DASHERS
DAUBERS
DAYBEDS
DAYSEND
DAYWEAR
DEADEND
DEADENS
DEADEST
DEADEYE
DEAFENS
DEAFEST
DEALERS
DEANERY
DEAREST
DEBEERS
DEBRETT
DEBTEES
DECKERS
DECREED
DECREER
DECREES
DEEPEND
DEEPENS
DEEPEST
DEFFEST
DEFIERS
DEFLEAS
DEFLECT
DEFTEST
DEFUELS
DEGREED
DEGREES
DEHMELT
DEICERS
DEKLERK
DELBERT
DELKEYS
DELVERS
DENIECE
DENIERS
DENNEHY
DENSELY
DENSEST
DEPLETE
DEPRESS
DEQUEUE
DERWENT
DESCEND
DESCENT
DESEEDS
DESHELL
DESSERT
DESTEMS
DEUTERO
DEWIEST
DEWLESS
DIADEMS
DIALECT
DIALEDO
DIALERS
DIAPERS
DICIEST
DICKENS
DICKERS
DICKEYS
DIDWELL
DIEMENS
DIESELS
DIETERS
DIFFERS
DIGGERS
DIGRESS
DILBERT
DILUENT
DIMMERS
DIMMEST
DIMNESS
DINGERS
DINNERS
DIOCESE
DIOMEDE
DIPNETS
DIPPERS
DISCERN
DISPELS
DISSECT
DISSENT
DISSERT
DISTEND
DITHERS
DITHERY
DNATEST
DOADEAL
DOCKERS
DOCKETS
DODDERS
DODDERY
DODGEMS
DODGERS
DOFFERS
DOGBEDS
DOGBERT
DOGGETT
DOGLEGS
DOGLESS
DOGREAT
DOGSEAR
DOGVEST
DONKEYS
DONLEVY
DOONEIN
DOOVERS
DOOZERS
DOPIEST
DORMERS
DORSETT
DORSEYS
DOTTERS
DOUCEUR
DOUREST
DOUSERS
DOWNERS
DOWSERS
DOZIEST
DRAGEES
DRAMEDY
DRAPERS
DRAPERY
DRAWEES
DRAWERS
DREXELU
DRFREUD
DRIVEAT
DRIVEBY
DRIVEIN
DRIVELS
DRIVERS
DRIVETO
DRIVEUP
DRONEON
DRONERS
DROVEAT
DROVEBY
DROVEIN
DROVERS
DROVETO
DROVEUP
DRTEETH
DRUZEAN
DRYCELL
DRYHEAT
DRYNESS
DRYPERS
DRYWELL
DUBBERS
DUBIETY
DUCHESS
DUCKERS
DUDGEON
DUELERS
DUEWEST
DUFFELS
DUFFERS
DULLEST
DUMBEST
DUMPERS
DUNGEON
DUNKERS
DUNNERS
DUODENA
DURRELL
DURWENT
DUSTERS

D••••E•

DABBLED
DABBLER
DABBLES
DADDIES
DAFFIER
DAHOMEY

DAILIES
DAIMLER
DAIRIES
DAIRYER
DAISIES
DALLIED
DALLIER
DALLIES
DALTREY
DAMAGED
DAMAGES
DAMOSEL
DANDIER
DANDIES
DANDLED
DANDLER
DANDLES
DANGLED
DANGLER
DANGLES
DANIKEN
DANITES
DAPHNES
DAPPLED
DAPPLES
DARKLED
DARKLES
DARKRED
DARLEEN
DARTLED
DARTLES
DASHIER
DATASET
DATIVES
DAUMIER
DAUNTED
DAUNTER
DAUSSET
DAWDLED
DAWDLER
DAWDLES
DAZZLED
DAZZLER
DAZZLES
DEADSEA
DEADSET
DEAIRED
DEARDEN
DEARIES
DEBAKEY
DEBASED
DEBASER
DEBASES
DEBATED
DEBATER
DEBATES
DEBITED
DEBONED
DEBONES
DEBRIEF
DEBTEES
DEBUSES
DEBUTED
DECADES
DECAYED
DECAYER
DECIBEL
DECIDED
DECIDER
DECIDES
DECILES
DECKLED
DECKLES
DECODED
DECODER
DECODES
DECOYED
DECOYER
DECREED
DECREER
DECREES
DECRIED
DECRIER
DECRIES
DEDUCED
DEDUCER
DEDUCES
DEEPRED
DEEPSEA
DEEPSET
DEFACED
DEFACER
DEFACES
DEFAMED
DEFAMER
DEFAMES
DEFILED
DEFILER
DEFILES
DEFINED
DEFINER
DEFINES
DEFUSED
DEFUSER
DEFUSES
DEGREED
DEGREES
DEHAVEN
DEHEXED
DEHEXES
DEHIRED
DEHIRES
DEIFIED
DEIFIER
DEIFIES
DEIGNED
DEITIES
DELANEY
DELAYED
DELAYER
DELETED
DELETES
DELIBES
DELIMEN
DELIVER
DELUDED
DELUDER
DELUDES
DELUGED
DELUGES
DEMARET
DEMETER
DEMISED
DEMISES
DEMOTED
DEMOTES
DEMPSEY
DEMURER
DENIMED
DENIZEN
DENOTED
DENOTES
DENUDED
DENUDER
DENUDES
DEPONED
DEPONER
DEPONES
DEPOSED
DEPOSER
DEPOSES
DEPOWER
DEPUTED
DEPUTES
DERATED
DERATES
DERBIES
DERIDED
DERIDER
DERIDES
DERIVED
DERIVER
DERIVES
DERNIER
DESERET
DESEXED
DESEXES
DESIRED
DESIREE
DESIRER
DESIRES
DESKSET
DESTAEL
DETOXED
DETOXES
DETUNED
DETUNES
DEVICES
DEVILED
DEVISED
DEVISEE
DEVISER
DEVISES
DEVORES
DEVOTED
DEVOTEE
DEVOTES
DEVRIES
DEWATER
DEWAXED
DEWAXES
DEWIRED
DEWIRES
DIABLES
DIALLED
DIARIES
DIBBLED
DIBBLER
DIBBLES
DICHTER
DICKIES
DIDASET
DIDDLED
DIDDLER
DIDDLES
DIDDLEY
DIDOVER
DIGIPET
DILATED
DILATES
DILLIES
DILUTED
DILUTER
DILUTES
DIMAGES
DIMETER
DIMPLED
DIMPLES
DIMVIEW
DINESEN
DINGIER
DINGLES
DINGOES
DINKIER
DIOPTER
DIPOLES
DIPPIER
DIRKSEN
DIRTIED
DIRTIER
DIRTIES
DISCOED
DISHIER
DISOBEY
DISUSED
DISUSES
DITCHED
DITCHER
DITCHES
DITSIER
DITTIES
DITTOED
DITZIER
DIVIDED
DIVIDER
DIVIDES
DIVINED
DIVINER
DIVINES
DIVVIED
DIVVIES
DIZZIED
DIZZIER
DIZZIES
DNAASES
DNIEPER
DODGIER
DOEEYED
DOGAPES
DOGCHEW
DOGFLEA
DOGGIER
DOGGIES
DOGSLED
DOILIES
DOLLIED
DOLLIES
DOLORES
DONATED
DONATEE
DONATES
DONGLES
DONTBEE
DOODLED
DOODLER
DOODLES
DOOLIES
DOOMIER
DOORMEN
DOOZIES
DOPPLER
DORKIER
DOSAGES
DOSSIER
DOTAGES
DOTTIER
DOTTLES
DOUANES
DOUBLEA
DOUBLEB
DOUBLEC
DOUBLED
DOUBLEE
DOUBLEF
DOUBLEG
DOUBLEH
DOUBLEI
DOUBLEJ
DOUBLEK
DOUBLEL
DOUBLEM
DOUBLEN
DOUBLEO
DOUBLEP
DOUBLEQ
DOUBLER
DOUBLES
DOUBLET
DOUBLEU
DOUBLEV
DOUBLEW
DOUBLEX
DOUBLEY
DOUBLEZ
DOUBTED
DOUBTER
DOVELET
DOWAGER
DOWDIER
DOWDIES
DOWERED
DOWNIER
DOWRIES
DPLUSES
DRABBER
DRAFTED
DRAFTEE
DRAFTER
DRAGEES
DRAGGED
DRAGGER
DRAGNET
DRAINED
DRAINER
DRATTED
DRAWEES
DRAWLED
DRAWLER
DRAWMEN
DRAYMEN
DREADED
DREAMED
DREAMER
DREDGED
DREDGER
DREDGES
DREIDEL
DREISER
DRESDEN
DRESSED
DRESSER
DRESSES
DREXLER
DRIBLET
DRIFTED
DRIFTER
DRILLED
DRILLER
DRINKER
DRIPPED
DRIPPER
DROGUES
DROLLER
DROOLED
DROOLER
DROOPED
DROPLET
DROPNET
DROPPED
DROPPER
DROSSES
DROWNED
DROWSED
DROWSES
DROXIES
DRUBBED
DRUBBER
DRUCKER
DRUDGED
DRUDGER
DRUDGES
DRUGGED
DRUMMED
DRUMMER
DRUMSET
DRUNKEN
DRUNKER
DRYADES
DRYEYED
DRYEYES
DRYIDEA
DUCHIES
DUCKIER
DUCKIES
DUELLED
DUETTED
DUFFLES
DUFUSES
DUHAMEL
DUMMIED
DUMMIES
DUMPIER
DUSKIER
DUSTIER
DUSTMEN
DWARFED
DWARVES
DWELLED
DWELLER
DYNODES

D•••••E

DARKAGE
DARLENE
DASCHLE
DATABLE
DAYCARE
DAYGAME
DAYMARE
DAYSIDE
DAYTIME
DEADEYE
DEARONE
DEBACLE
DEBARGE
DEBOITE
DEBOULE
DECEASE
DECEIVE
DECIARE
DECLARE
DECLINE
DECUPLE
DEFARGE
DEFENCE
DEFENSE
DEFLATE
DEFRAME
DEGLAZE
DEGRADE
DEHISCE
DEIRDRE
DELARUE
DELMORE
DELORME
DELOUSE
DELUISE
DEMERGE
DEMESNE
DEMILLE
DENEUVE
DENIECE
DENTATE
DENTINE
DENTURE
DENTYNE
DEPECHE
DEPLANE
DEPLETE
DEPLORE
DEPRAVE
DEPRIVE
DEQUEUE
DERALTE
DERANGE
DESERVE
DESIREE
DESPISE
DESPITE
DESTINE
DETENTE
DETERGE
DETRUDE
DEVALUE
DEVIATE
DEVILLE
DEVISEE
DEVOLVE
DEVOTEE
DEWILDE
DEWLINE
DHURRIE
DICTATE
DIDFINE
DIDLIKE
DIDTIME
DIFFUSE
DINETTE
DIOCESE
DIOMEDE
DIORITE
DIOXIDE
DISABLE
DISEASE
DISEUSE
DISLIKE
DISPOSE
DISPUTE
DISRATE
DISROBE
DIVERGE
DIVERSE
DIVORCE
DIVULGE
DIVULSE
DNACODE
DOCKAGE
DOEUVRE
DOGBANE
DOGBITE
DOGBONE
DOGFACE
DOGGATE
DOGGONE
DOGLIKE
DOGPILE
DOGRACE
DOGROSE
DOGSAGE
DOIDARE
DOMAINE
DONAHUE
DONATEE
DONJOSE
DONOHOE
DONTBEE
DONTLIE
DOORDIE
DORMICE
DOTLIKE
DOTRICE
DOUBLEE
DOVERDE
DOYENNE
DRABBLE
DRAFTEE
DRAGGLE
DRAYAGE
DRIBBLE
DRINKME
DRIZZLE
DRYABLE
DRYHOLE
DUALIZE
DUBUQUE
DUCTILE
DUEDATE
DUNNAGE
DUOTONE
DURABLE
DURANCE
DURANTE
DWINDLE

•DE••••

ADELIES
ADELINA
ADELINE
ADELPHI
ADENINE
ADENOID
ADEPTAT
ADEPTER
ADEPTLY
CDEFGHI
EDEMATA
IDEALLY
IDEAMAN
IDEAMEN
IDEATED
IDEATES
IDENTIC
ODELETS
ODESSAN

•D•E•••

ADDEDIN
ADDEDLY
ADDEDON
ADDEDTO
ADDEDUP
ADDENDA
ADDENDS
ADHERED
ADHERER
ADHERES
ADRENAL
ADVENTS
ADVERBS
ADVERSE
ADVERTS
EDGEDIN
EDGEOUT
EDGESIN
EDMEESE
IDLESSE

•D••E••

ADDRESS
ADORERS
EDGIEST
EDMEESE
IDAREDS
IDTHEFT
ODDMENT
ODDNESS
ODELETS

•D•••E•

ADAMSES
ADAPTED
ADAPTER
ADDAXES
ADDUCED
ADDUCER
ADDUCES
ADELIES
ADEPTER
ADHERED
ADHERER
ADHERES
ADJURED
ADJURER
ADJURES
ADMIRED
ADMIRER
ADMIRES
ADMIXED
ADMIXES
ADOPTED
ADOPTEE
ADOPTER
ADORNED
ADORNER
ADRATES
ADVICES
ADVISED
ADVISEE
ADVISER
ADVISES
ADWOMEN
CDCASES
CDRATES
CDTOWER
EDASNER
EDIBLES
EDIFIED
EDIFIER
EDIFIES
EDUCTED
HDTVSET
IDEAMEN
IDEATED
IDEATES
IDOTTER
JDPOWER
ODYSSEY
PDJAMES

•D••••E

ADAMITE
ADAWARE
ADDABLE
ADDIBLE
ADELINE
ADENINE
ADIPOSE
ADJUDGE
ADOLPHE
ADOPTEE
ADSPACE
ADULATE
ADVANCE
ADVERSE
ADVISEE
CDSTORE
EDIFICE
EDMEESE
EDOMITE
EDUCATE
IDBADGE
IDLESSE
IDOLISE
IDOLIZE
ODDSARE
ODDSHOE
ODORIZE

••DE•••

ACDELCO
ADDEDIN
ADDEDLY
ADDEDON
ADDEDTO
ADDEDUP
ADDENDA
ADDENDS
ALDENTE
ANDEANS
ARDECHE
ARDENCY
ATDEUCE
BADEGGS
BADENDS
BADENOV
BCDEFGH
BEDECKS
BEDELIA
BEDEVIL
BEDEWED
BODEFUL
BODEGAS
BODEREK
CADEAUX
CADENCE
CADENCY
CADENZA
CADETTE
CODEINE
CODERED
DIDEROT
DUDEDUP
DUDESUP
EIDETIC
ELDERLY
ENDEARS
ENDEDAT
ENDEDIN
ENDEDIT
ENDEDON
ENDEDUP
ENDEMIC
ENDERBY
EUDEMON
FADEDIN
FADEDLY
FADEINS
FADEOUT
FADESIN
FEDERAL
FEDERKO
FEDEXED
FEDEXES
FIDELES
FIDELIA
FIDELIO
FIDELIS
GIDEONS
GODEVIL
HIDEOUS
HIDEOUT
INDEEDY
INDENTS
INDEPTH
INDEXED
INDEXER
INDEXES
JADEDLY
JADEITE
JUDEANS
JUDELAW
KADETTS
LEDERER
MADEFIT
MADEFOR
MADEFUN
MADEHAY
MADEILL
MADEIRA
MADELON
MADEMAD
MADEOFF
MADEONE
MADEOUT
MADEPAR
MADERUN
MADEWAR
MADEWAY
MEDELES
MEDEVAC
MIDEAST
MODELAS
MODELBS
MODELED
MODELER
MODELTS
MODEMED
MODERNE
MODERNS
MODESTO
MODESTY
MRDEEDS
MUDEELS
NIDETCH
OGDENUT
ORDEALS
ORDERED
ORDERER
ORDERIN
ORDERLY
ORDERUP
PUDENCY
REDEALS
REDEALT
REDEBIT
REDECAY
REDEEDS
REDEEMS
REDEYED
REDEYES
RIDEBYS
RIDEOFF
RIDEOUT
RIDESBY
RIDESIN
RIDESTO
RIDESUP
RODENTS
RODEOFF
RODEOUT
SADEYED
SADEYES
SIDEARM
SIDEBAR
SIDEBET
SIDECAR
SIDEMAN
SIDEMEN
SIDEONE
SIDETWO
SIDEWAY
STDENIS
TEDEUMS
TIDERIP
UNDEALT
UNDERDO
UNDERGO
UNDEWED
VEDETTE
VIDEOED
VIDETTE
WADEDIN
WADESIN
WEDELED
WEDELNS
WIDENED
WIDENER
YODELED
YODELER
ZYDECOS

••D•E••

ADDRESS
AIDLESS
ANDREAS
ANDRESS
ANDREWS
BADDEBT
BADDEED
BADDEST
BADGERS
BADNESS
BADNEWS
BEDLESS
BEDREST
BIDDERS
BUDDERS
BUDGERS
BUDGETS
BUDLESS
CADGERS
CODGERS
CUDGELS
DIDWELL
DODDERS
DODDERY
DODGEMS
DODGERS
DUDGEON
ENDLEAF
ENDLESS
FEDDERS
FIDGETS
FIDGETY

FODDERS	REDMEAT	CUDDLES	LEDERER	REDOSES	ADDIBLE	MODISTE	BIRDERS	GRADEAA	POWDERS	WARDENS	CODDLER	GIRDLER
FUDGERS	REDNECK	DADDIES	LEDGIER	REDOXES	ALDENTE	MUDHOLE	BLADERS	GRADERS	POWDERY	WARDERS	CODDLES	GIRDLES
GADDERS	REDNESS	DEDUCED	MADAMES	REDRIED	ANDANTE	ODDSARE	BOLDEST	GUIDERS	PRADESH	WEDDELL	CRADLED	GLADDEN
GADGETS	REDREAM	DEDUCER	MADAMEX	REDRIES	ANDMORE	ODDSHOE	BONDERS	GULDENS	PREDEFY	WEDDERS	CRADLER	GLADDER
GADGETY	REDRESS	DEDUCES	MADCHEN	REDTIES	ANDRADE	OLDBLUE	BORDERS	HANDERS	PREDENY	WEEDERS	CRADLES	GOODIES
GODDESS	RIDDERS	DIDASET	MEDALED	REDUCED	ARDECHE	OLDJOKE	BUDDERS	HANDEYE	PRUDENT	WELDERS	CUDDIES	GOODMEN
GODHEAD	RODGERS	DIDDLED	MEDDLED	REDUCER	ARDMORE	OLDLINE	BUMDEAL	HARDEES	PRUDERY	WENDELL	CUDDLED	GRIDDED
GODLESS	RODLESS	DIDDLER	MEDDLER	REDUCES	ATDEUCE	OLDLYME	BURDENS	HARDENS	RAIDERS	WENDERS	CUDDLES	GRIDDER
GODSEND	RUDDERS	DIDDLES	MEDDLES	RIDDLED	AUDIBLE	OLDROSE	CALDERA	HARDEST	RANDEEP	WILDEST	CURDIER	GRODIER
GODSENT	SADDENS	DIDDLEY	MEDELES	RIDDLER	AUDITEE	OLDSHOE	CALDERS	HEADEND	RAWDEAL	WINDERS	CURDLED	GRUDGED
GUDGEON	SADDEST	DIDOVER	MIDASES	RIDDLES	BADCASE	OLDTIME	CANDELA	HEADERS	READERS	WONDERS	CURDLER	GRUDGER
HADBEEN	SADNESS	DODGIER	MIDDIES	RIDGIER	BADJOKE	PADRONE	CANDENT	HEEDERS	REDDEER	YARDERS	CURDLES	GRUDGES
HADBEST	SODLESS	ECDYSES	MIDDLEC	RUDDIED	BADLOVE	PADSITE	CARDERS	HENDECA	REDDENS	YESDEAR	DADDIES	HANDFED
HEDGERS	SUDSERS	ENDIVES	MIDDLED	RUDDIER	BADMOVE	PODLIKE	CHEDERS	HERDERS	REDDEST		DANDIER	HANDIER
INDEEDY	TIDIEST	ENDOWED	MIDDLER	SADDLED	BADNAME	RADIATE	CHIDERS	HINDERS	RENDELL	•••D•E•	DANDIES	HANDLED
INDWELL	UNDOERS	ENDOWER	MIDDLES	SADDLER	BADTIME	RADICLE	CINDERS	HOLDERS	RENDERS	APEDIET	DANDLED	HANDLER
INDWELT	UNDRESS	ENDURED	MIDTEEN	SADDLES	BEDLIKE	REDBONE	CINDERY	HOWDEDO	RIDDERS	AZODYES	DANDLER	HANDLES
JODRELL	WADDELL	ENDURER	MIDWEEK	SADEYED	BEDMATE	REDFACE	COLDEST	HOYDENS	ROADEOS	BADDEED	DANDLES	HANDSEL
JUDGERS	WADDERS	ENDURES	MODELED	SADEYES	BEDRAPE	REDFIVE	CONDEMN	IMADEIT	ROADERS	BADDIES	DAWDLED	HANDSET
KEDGERS	WEDDELL	ENDUSER	MODELER	SEDATED	BEDSIDE	REDLINE	CORDELL	KEYDETS	ROEDEER	BALDIES	DAWDLER	HARDEES
KIDDERS	WEDDERS	ENDUSES	MODEMED	SEDATER	BEDTIME	REDNINE	CORDERO	KIDDERS	RONDEAU	BANDIED	DAWDLES	HARDIER
KIDNEYS	WEDGEIN	FADAYEV	MODULES	SEDATES	BUDLIKE	REDNOSE	CORDERS	KINDEST	RONDELS	BANDIER	DEADSEA	HARDSET
KIDSEAT	WIDGEON	FADDIER	MUDDIED	SEDGIER	BUDTIME	REDPINE	CRUDELY	KORDELL	RUDDERS	BANDIES	DEADSET	HARDTEN
LADDERS	WIDGETS	FADDIET	MUDDIER	SEDUCED	BUDVASE	REDRIVE	CRUDEST	KUNDERA	RUNDEEP	BANDLET	DIDDLED	HEADIER
LADLERS		FEDEXED	MUDDIES	SEDUCER	CADENCE	REDROBE	DANDERS	LADDERS	SADDENS	BARDEEN	DIDDLER	HEADMEN
LEDGERS	••D••E•	FEDEXES	MUDDLED	SEDUCES	CADETTE	REDROSE	DEADEND	LANDERS	SADDEST	BAWDIER	DIDDLES	HEADSET
LIDLESS	ABDOMEN	FIDDLED	MUDDLER	SIDEBET	CODCAKE	REDTAPE	DEADENS	LARDERS	SANDERS	BEADIER	DIDDLEY	HINDLEG
LODGEIN	ABDUCED	FIDDLER	MUDDLES	SIDEMEN	CODEINE	REDTIDE	DEADEST	LAUDERS	SEEDERS	BEADLES	DOODLED	HOODIES
LODGERS	ABDUCES	FIDDLES	MUDPIES	SODDIER	DIDFINE	REDWINE	DEADEYE	LEADENS	SENDEES	BENDIER	DOODLER	HUDDLED
MADDENS	ADDAXES	FIDELES	NODDIES	SUDAFED	DIDLIKE	REDZONE	DIADEMS	LEADERS	SENDERS	BIDDIES	DOODLES	HUDDLER
MADDERS	ADDUCED	FUDDIES	NODULED	SUDSIER	DIDTIME	RIDABLE	DOADEAL	LEADETH	SHADERS	BINDLES	DOWDIER	HUDDLES
MADDEST	ADDUCER	FUDDLED	NODULES	TEDDIES	ENDABLE	RODLIKE	DODDERS	LENDERS	SLIDEBY	BIRDIED	DOWDIES	HUNDRED
MADNESS	ADDUCES	FUDDLES	NUDZHED	TODDIES	ENDGAME	SADCAFE	DODDERY	LEWDEST	SLIDEIN	BIRDIES	DREDGED	HURDLED
MEDLEYS	AEDILES	GADSDEN	NUDZHES	TODDLED	ENDLATE	SADFATE	DUODENA	LINDENS	SLIDERS	BIRDMEN	DREDGER	HURDLER
MIDGETS	ANDOVER	GIDDIED	OLDSTER	TODDLER	ENDLINE	SIDEONE	ELIDERS	LOADERS	SNIDELY	BLADDER	DREDGES	HURDLES
MIDLEGS	ANDTHEN	GIDDIER	ORDERED	TODDLES	ENDNOTE	SODIDWE	ELUDERS	LOUDENS	SNIDEST	BLUDGED	DRUDGED	ICEDTEA
MIDTEEN	AUDILES	GIDDIES	ORDERER	UNDARED	ENDORSE	TADPOLE	EPIDERM	LOUDEST	SOLDERS	BLUDGER	DRUDGER	ICHDIEN
MIDTERM	AUDITED	GODFREY	ORDINES	UNDATED	ENDWISE	UNDRAPE	ERODENT	MADDENS	SPADERS	BLUDGES	DRUDGES	KENDREW
MIDWEEK	AUDITEE	GODLIER	ORDONEZ	UNDAZED	ENDZONE	VEDETTE	ERODERS	MADDERS	SPIDERS	BONDMEN	FADDIER	KIDDIES
MIDWEST	BADAREA	HADASET	PADDIES	UNDEWED	FADLIKE	VIDETTE	EVADERS	MADDEST	SPIDERY	BOODLES	FADDIET	KINDLED
MIDYEAR	BADDEED	HADBEEN	PADDLED	UNDIKED	FTDODGE	ZADKINE	EVIDENT	MAIDENS	SPYDERS	BOWDLER	FIDDLED	KINDLER
MRDEEDS	BADDIES	HADOVER	PADDLER	UNDINES	GODLIKE		FEDDERS	MANDELA	STUDENT	BRADLEE	FIDDLER	KINDLES
MUDDERS	BADIDEA	HEDGIER	PADDLES	UNDOMED	HADDONE	•••DE••	FEEDERS	MELDERS	SUBDEBS	BRADLEY	FIDDLES	KINDRED
MUDEELS	BADLIES	HUDDLED	PEDALED	UNDRIED	HADSOME	ABCDEFG	FENDERS	MENDELS	SUNDECK	BRIDGED	FIEDLER	KLUDGED
MUDHENS	BADOMEN	HUDDLER	PEDALER	UNDUPED	HADTIME	ABIDEBY	FEYDEAU	MENDERS	SUNDERS	BRIDGER	FINDLEY	KLUDGES
NODDERS	BEDAZED	HUDDLES	PEDDLED	UPDATED	HADTOBE	ABIDERS	FINDERS	MILDEST	TANDEMS	BRIDGES	FLEDGED	LADDIES
NUDGERS	BEDAZES	INDEXED	PEDDLER	UPDATER	HIDABLE	ACADEME	FODDERS	MILDEWS	TENDERS	BRIDGET	FLEDGES	LANDLER
ODDMENT	BEDEWED	INDEXER	PEDDLES	UPDATES	HYDRATE	ACADEMY	FOLDERS	MILDEWY	THEDEEP	BRIDLED	FONDLED	LANDMEN
ODDNESS	BEDIZEN	INDEXES	PIDDLED	UPDIVED	HYDRIDE	ALUDELS	FONDEST	MINDERS	THEDELL	BRIDLER	FONDLER	LARDIER
OLDBEAN	BEDLOES	INDICES	PIDDLES	UPDIVES	INDORSE	AMADEUS	FREDEBB	MISDEAL	TINDERS	BRIDLES	FONDLES	LARDNER
OLDNESS	BIDDIES	INDIGEN	PUDDLED	UPDRIED	INDULGE	ANADEMS	FUNDERS	MISDEED	TINDERY	BRODIES	FONDUED	LEADIER
OLDNEWS	BODEREK	INDITED	PUDDLES	UPDRIES	JADEITE	ARIDEST	GADDERS	MISDEEM	TRADEIN	BRODKEY	FONDUES	LEADMEN
OLDWEST	BODICES	INDITER	PUDGIER	VIDEOED	KIDLIKE	ARTDECO	GANDERS	MOLDERS	TRADEON	BUDDIED	FOODIES	LINDIED
PADDERS	BUDDIED	INDITES	RADAMES	WADDLED	LADOUCE	AVIDEST	GARDENA	MONDESI	TRADERS	BUDDIES	FOODWEB	LINDIES
PADGETT	BUDDIES	INDUCED	RADICES	WADDLER	LADRONE	BADDEBT	GARDENS	MORDENT	TRADEUP	BUNDLED	FORDOES	LINDNER
PIDGEON	BUDGIES	INDUCER	RADIOED	WADDLES	LUDDITE	BADDEED	GAUDENS	MUDDERS	TRIDENT	BUNDLER	FOUDRES	LINDSEY
REDCELL	CADAVER	INDUCES	RADIOER	WEDELED	LYDDITE	BADDEST	GAUDERY	MURDERS	TRUDEAU	BUNDLES	FRIDGES	LONDRES
REDCENT	CADDIED	IODATED	RADIXES	WEDGIER	MADEONE	BALDEST	GENDERS	NEEDERS	TWODEEP	CADDIED	FRIDLEY	MANDREL
REDDEER	CADDIES	IODATES	RADOMES	WEDGIES	MEDIATE	BANDEAU	GEODESY	NEWDEAL	UNADEPT	CADDIES	FUDDIES	MEDDLED
REDDENS	CADUCEI	IODIDES	REDARED	WIDENED	MEDUSAE	BANDERA	GILDERS	NODDERS	UNIDEAL	CANDIED	FUDDLED	MEDDLER
REDDEST	CEDARED	IODISED	REDARES	WIDENER	MIDJUNE	BANDERS	GIRDERS	NONDEAF	VENDEES	CANDIES	FUDDLES	MEDDLES
REDEEDS	CODDLED	IODISES	REDATED	WIDOWED	MIDLIFE	BARDEEN	GLADEYE	NONDEEP	VENDERS	CANDLED	GARDNER	MIDDIES
REDEEMS	CODDLER	IODIZED	REDATES	WIDOWER	MIDLINE	BEADERS	GLIDEBY	OAKDESK	VERDELL	CANDLER	GAUDIER	MIDDLEC
REDFERN	CODDLES	IODIZER	REDDEER	YODELED	MIDRISE	BENDERS	GLIDEIN	PADDERS	VIADENT	CANDLES	GAUDIES	MIDDLED
REDHEAD	CODERED	IODIZES	REDDYES	YODELER	MIDSIZE	BIDDERS	GLIDERS	PANDERS	VOIDERS	CARDKEY	GIDDIED	MIDDLER
REDHEAT	CODICES	JUDASES	REDEYED		MIDSOLE	BIGDEAL	GODDESS	PENDENT	WADDELL	CHIDDEN	GIDDIER	MIDDLES
REDHENS	CUDDIES	KIDDIES	REDEYES	••D•••E	MIDWIFE	BINDERS	GOODEGG	PETDEER	WADDERS	CLADDED	GIDDIES	MILDRED
REDLEGS	CUDDLED	LADDIES	REDOSED	ADDABLE	MODERNE	BINDERY	GOODERS	PONDERS	WANDERS	CODDLED	GIRDLED	MINDSET

MISDEED
MISDEEM
MISDOER
MISDOES
MISDREW
MOLDIER
MONDIEU
MOODIER
MORDRED
MUDDIED
MUDDIER
MUDDIES
MUDDLED
MUDDLER
MUDDLES
NEEDIER
NEEDLED
NEEDLER
NEEDLES
NERDIER
NODDIES
NONDEEP
NONDIET
NOODGED
NOODGES
NOODLED
NOODLES
ONADIET
OUTDOER
OUTDOES
OUTDREW
OUTDUEL
PADDIES
PADDLED
PADDLER
PADDLES
PARDNER
PEDDLED
PEDDLER
PEDDLES
PERDIEM
PETDEER
PIDDLED
PIDDLES
PLEDGED
PLEDGEE
PLEDGER
PLEDGES
PLODDED
PLODDER
POODLES
POUDRES
PREDIET
PRODDED
PRODDER
PUDDLED
PUDDLES
PURDUEU
RANDEEP
RANDIER
READDED
READIED
READIER
READIES
REDDEER
REDDYES
REEDIER
REEDMEN
RIDDLED
RIDDLER
RIDDLES
RINDIER
RITDYES
ROADBED
ROADIES
ROEDEER
ROWDIER
ROWDIES
RUDDIED
RUDDIER
RUNDEEP
RUNDLES
SADDLED
SADDLER
SADDLES
SANDIER
SANDLER
SANDMEN
SCUDDED
SCUDDER
SEEDBED
SEEDIER
SEEDLET
SENDEES
SHADIER
SHEDDER
SHODDEN
SHUDDER
SKIDDED
SKIDDER
SLEDDED
SLEDDER
SLEDGED
SLEDGES
SLUDGES
SMIDGEN
SMIDGES
SMUDGED
SMUDGES
SODDIER
SOLDIER
STADLER
STODGED
STODGES
STUDDED
STUDIED
STUDIER
STUDIES
SUBDUED
SUBDUER
SUBDUES
SUNDAES
TARDIER
TEDDIES
THEDEEP
THEDIET
THUDDED
TIEDYED
TIEDYES
TOADIED
TOADIES
TODDIES
TODDLED
TODDLER
TODDLES
TOODLES
TRODDEN
TRUDGED
TRUDGEN
TRUDGER
TRUDGES
TWODEEP
UNADDED
UNEDGED
UNEDGES
VANDIEN
VATDYED
VATDYES
VENDEES
VENDUES
WADDLED
WADDLER
WADDLES
WEEDIER
WILDMEN
WINDIER
WINDTEE
WOODIER
WOODIES
WOODLEY
WORDIER
YARDMEN

•••D••E

ACADEME
AIRDATE
AIRDRIE
ALADINE
ALIDADE
ALLDONE
ANODISE
ANODIZE
ANODYNE
BANDAGE
BELDAME
BLEDSOE
BOBDOLE
BONDAGE
BRADLEE
CANDACE
CANDICE
CANDIDE
CAUDATE
COLDONE
CONDOLE
CONDONE
CONDUCE
CORDAGE
CORDATE
CORDITE
DEADEYE
DOIDARE
DUEDATE
EPIDOTE
ERUDITE
EXEDRAE
EXUDATE
FORDONE
FREDDIE
GETDONE
GLADEYE
GOODBYE
GOODJOE
GOODONE
GOODUSE
GOTDONE
GRADATE
GRIDDLE
HADDONE
HALDANE
HANDAXE
HANDEYE
HASDONE
HOTDATE
ILLDONE
INADAZE
ISADORE
ISIDORE
ITSDONE
JARDINE
JIMDALE
KHEDIVE
KILDARE
LEADORE
LOWDIVE
LUDDITE
LYDDITE
MALDIVE
MANDATE
MISDATE
MISDONE
MONDALE
MUNDANE
NORDOWE
NOTDONE
ONADARE
ONADATE
ONEDIME
OUTDARE
OUTDATE
OUTDONE
OXIDASE
OXIDATE
OXIDISE
OXIDIZE
PERDURE
PETDOVE
PLEDGEE
PREDATE
PREDIVE
PRODUCE
PRUDHOE
RCADOME
RONDURE
SAIDAYE
SARDINE
SHADROE
SIRDUKE
SKYDIVE
SKYDOME
SUBDATE
SWADDLE
THEDOLE
THEDUKE
TRADUCE
TWADDLE
TWIDDLE
VANDINE
VANDYKE
VENDOME
VERDURE
WILDONE
WINDAGE
WINDTEE
WORDAGE
WORDONE
YARDAGE

••••DE•

ABRADED
ABRADER
ABRADES
ACCEDED
ACCEDER
ACCEDES
ALLUDED
ALLUDES
ALMADEN
AMENDED
AMENDER
APHIDES
APSIDES
ARCADED
ARCADES
ARUNDEL
ASUNDER
AUBADES
AVOIDED
AVOIDER
AWARDED
AWARDEE
AWARDER
BADIDEA
BEARDED
BESIDES
BETIDED
BETIDES
BIGIDEA
BLADDER
BLANDER
BLEEDER
BLENDED
BLENDER
BLENDES
BLINDED
BLINDER
BLONDER
BLONDES
BLOODED
BLUNDEN
BLUNDER
BOARDED
BOARDER
BOLIDES
BORIDES
BOULDER
BOUNDED
BOUNDER
BRAEDEN
BRAIDED
BRAIDER
BRANDED
BRANDER
BREADED
BREADER
BREEDER
BRENDEL
BROADEN
BROADER
BROIDER
BROODED
BROODER
BUILDER
CAPADES
CCRIDER
CHIDDEN
CHORDED
CHOWDER
CITADEL
CLADDED
CLAUDEL
CLOUDED
CLOWDER
CROWDED
CROWDER
DEARDEN
DECADES
DECIDED
DECIDER
DECIDES
DECODED
DECODER
DECODES
DELUDED
DELUDER
DELUDES
DENUDED
DENUDER
DENUDES
DERIDED
DERIDER
DERIDES
DIVIDED
DIVIDER
DIVIDES
DREADED
DREIDEL
DRESDEN
DRYADES
DRYIDEA
DYNODES
EMENDED
EMENDER
ENCODED
ENCODER
ENCODES
EVANDER
EXCIDED
EXCIDES
FACADES
FIELDED
FIELDER
FLOODED
FOUNDED
FOUNDER
GADSDEN
GLADDEN
GLADDER
GOUNDER
GOURDES
GQMODEL
GRANDEE
GRANDER
GRENDEL
GRIDDED
GRIDDER
GRINDER
GUARDED
GUARDEE
GUARDER
GUILDER
HALIDES
HOARDED
HOARDER
HOUNDED
HOUNDER
HUMIDEX
ILLUDED
ILLUDES
IMPEDED
IMPEDER
IMPEDES
INCUDES
INFIDEL
INORDER
INSIDER
INSIDES
INVADED
INVADER
INVADES
IODIDES
IWONDER
JOEYDEE
JOINDER
KIKIDEE
KNEADED
KNEADER
KRAMDEN
LAUNDER
LEANDER
LEVADES
LONGDEN
LOURDES
MARSDEN
MAUNDER
MEANDER
MERIDEN
MOULDED
MOULDER
MOUNDED
NAIADES
NEWIDEA
ONORDER
ONSIDES
ONVIDEO
OXHIDES
PARADED
PARADER
PARADES
PESADES
PLEADED
PLEADER
PLODDED
PLODDER
PLUNDER
POMADED
POMADES
POUNDED
POUNDER
PREIDEA
PRODDED
PRODDER
PROUDER
RAPIDER
READDED
RECEDED
RECEDES
RECODED
RECODES
REHIDES
REINDEX
REMODEL
REORDER
RERIDES
RESIDED
RESIDER
RESIDES
REWIDEN
ROLODEX
ROUNDED
ROUNDEL
ROUNDER
RUBYDEE
SALADES
SCALDED
SCALDER
SCOLDED
SCOLDER
SCUDDED
SCUDDER
SECEDED
SECEDER
SECEDES
SHEDDER
SHODDEN
SHUDDER
SKIDDED
SKIDDER
SLANDER
SLEDDED
SLEDDER
SLENDER
SMOLDER
SOLIDER
SOUNDED
SOUNDER
SPANDEX
SPEEDED
SPEEDER
SPENDER
SPONDEE
STAIDER
STANDEE
STANDER
STEADED
STRIDER
STRIDES
STRUDEL
STUDDED
SUBIDEA
THEIDEA
THUDDED
THUNDER
TIMIDER
TIRADES
TIREDER
TOORDER
TREADED
TREADER
TRENDED
TRIODES
TRODDEN
UNADDED
UNAIDED
UNCEDED
UNCODED
UNENDED
UNFADED
UNJADED
UNLADED
UNLADEN
UNLADES
UNSIDED
UNWADED
UPENDED
UPSIDES
USTEDES
UVINDEX
VIVIDER
VOCODER
WEIRDED
WEIRDER
WHAUDEN
WIELDED
WIELDER
WOUNDED
WOWEDEM
YIELDED
YIELDER

••••D•E

ABRIDGE
ADJUDGE
ARIADNE
ARLEDGE
AWARDEE
BLONDIE
BRINDLE
CAMEDUE
CANIDAE
CHEADLE
CICADAE
COMEDIE
COMEDUE
COULDBE
DEIRDRE
DOORDIE
DWINDLE
ELFUDGE
FALLDUE
FELLDUE
FREDDIE
FTDODGE
GRANDEE
GRIDDLE
GUARDEE
HAIRDYE
IDBADGE
IFITDIE
IPLEDGE
JANEDOE
JOEYDEE
JOHNDOE
KIKIDEE
KYOODLE
LUCIDAE
MCARDLE
MRPADRE
OHFUDGE
OUTEDGE
OVERDUE
OVERDYE
PASTDUE
REJUDGE
RESIDUE
RUBYDEE
RUSHDIE
SINEDIE
SODIDWE
SPINDLE
SPONDEE
STANDEE
SWADDLE
SWINDLE
THANDIE
THEEDGE
TREADLE
TRUNDLE
TWADDLE
TWEEDLE
TWIDDLE
UNWEDGE
WHEEDLE
WOULDBE

•••••DE

ALAMODE
ALCAIDE
ALCALDE
ALFREDE
ALIDADE
ALLENDE
ANDRADE
ASTRIDE
ATGRADE
BALLADE
BARCODE
BEDSIDE
BIOCIDE
BOGARDE
BRIGADE
BROCADE
BROMIDE
BUSRIDE
CABRIDE
CANDIDE
CARBIDE
CASCADE
CATHODE
CHARADE
COCKADE
COLLIDE
COLLUDE
COMMODE
COMRADE
CONCEDE
CONFIDE
CORRADE
CORRODE
COWHIDE
CRUSADE
CYANIDE
DAYSIDE
DEGRADE
DETRUDE
DEWILDE
DIOMEDE
DIOXIDE
DNACODE
DOVERDE
EBBTIDE
ECOCIDE
ENGARDE
EPISODE
EXCLUDE
EXPLODE
EXTRUDE
FARSIDE
FORBADE
FTMEADE
GEOCODE
GIRONDE
GRENADE
HAYRIDE
HEYJUDE
HYDRIDE
ILLMADE
IMPLODE
INCLUDE
INTRADE
INTRUDE
JOYRIDE
LEETIDE
LEMONDE
LETRIDE
LIMEADE
LOWSIDE
LOWTIDE
MANMADE
MCBRIDE
MISCODE
NEWMADE
NITRIDE
NOTRADE
NUCLIDE
OBTRUDE
OCCLUDE
OFFSIDE
OUTMODE
OUTRIDE
OUTRODE
OUTSIDE
PARKADE
PASSADE
PEPTIDE
PERVADE
PREBADE
PRECEDE
PRECODE
PREFADE
PRELUDE
PREMADE
PRESIDE
PROVIDE
RAWHIDE
REDTIDE
REGRADE
REGUIDE
RESPADE
RETRADE
RIPTIDE
ROULADE
SACCADE
SEASIDE
SECLUDE
SUBCODE
SUBSIDE
SULFIDE
TAXCODE
TENCODE
TETRODE
TOPSIDE
TVGUIDE
ULANUDE
UNBLADE
UNCRUDE
UNICODE
UNSHADE
UPCCODE
UPGRADE
UPTRADE
WAYSIDE
YAOUNDE
ZIPCODE

D•F••••

DAFFIER
DAFFILY
DAFTEST
DEFACED
DEFACER
DEFACES
DEFACTO
DEFALLA
DEFAMED
DEFAMER
DEFAMES
DEFANGS
DEFARGE
DEFAULT
DEFCONS
DEFEATS
DEFECTS
DEFENCE
DEFENDS
DEFENSE
DEFERTO
DEFFEST
DEFGHIJ
DEFIANT
DEFICIT
DEFIERS
DEFILED
DEFILER
DEFILES
DEFINED
DEFINER
DEFINES
DEFLATE
DEFLEAS
DEFLECT
DEFOAMS
DEFOCUS
DEFORMS
DEFRAGS
DEFRAME
DEFRAUD
DEFRAYS
DEFROCK
DEFROST
DEFTEST
DEFUELS
DEFUNCT
DEFUNDS
DEFUSED
DEFUSER
DEFUSES
DEFYING
DIFFERS
DIFFUSE
DOFFERS
DOFFING
DRFREUD
DRFRIST
DUFFELS
DUFFERS
DUFFLES
DUFUSES

D••F•••

DAFFIER
DAFFILY
DEAFENS
DEAFEST
DEFFEST
DEIFIED
DEIFIER
DEIFIES
DEWFALL
DIDFINE
DIFFERS
DIFFUSE
DOFFERS
DOFFING
DOGFACE
DOGFISH
DOGFLEA
DOGFOOD
DORFMAN
DRAFTED
DRAFTEE
DRAFTER
DRIFTED
DRIFTER
DRIFTIN
DRIFTUP
DRYFOGS
DUFFELS
DUFFERS
DUFFLES

D•••F••

DAREFUL
DEEPFAT
DEEPFRY
DEERFLY
DESKFUL
DIEDFOR
DIEOFFS
DIESFOR
DIGSFOR
DIREFUL
DISHFUL
DOESFOR
DOLEFUL
DONEFOR
DOOMFUL
DREYFUS
DUTIFUL
DWARFED

D••••F•

DAMPOFF
DANDIFY

DARTOFF
DASHOFF
DAYSOFF
DENSIFY
DIEDOFF
DIEOFFS
DIESOFF
DIGNIFY
DISTAFF
DOZEOFF
DRAGOFF
DRAWOFF
DREWOFF
DRMELFI
DROPOFF
DULCIFY
DUSTOFF

D•••••F

DAMPOFF
DARRYLF
DARTOFF
DASHOFF
DAYSOFF
DEBRIEF
DIEDOFF
DIESOFF
DISTAFF
DOOUTOF
DOUBLEF
DOZEOFF
DRAGOFF
DRAWOFF
DREAMOF
DREWOFF
DROPOFF
DUSTOFF

•D•F•••

CDEFGHI
EDIFICE
EDIFIED
EDIFIER
EDIFIES

•D••F••

ODORFUL

•D•••F•

IDTHEFT

••DF•••

BADFITS
BADFORM
BEDFORD
BIDFAIR
CODFISH
DIDFINE
GODFREY
HADFITS
MEDFORD
MUDFISH
MUDFLAP
MUDFLAT
MUDFLOW
OLDFILM
OLDFOGY
RADFORD
REDFACE
REDFERN
REDFINS
REDFIRS
REDFISH
REDFIVE
REDFLAG
REDFORD
REDFOUR
SADFATE

••D•F••

BCDEFGH
BIDSFOR
BODEFUL
BODYFAT
HADAFIT
MADEFIT
MADEFOR
MADEFUN
MIDOFFS
REDSFAN
SUDAFED

••D••F•

INDRAFT
MADEOFF
MIDLIFE
MIDOFFS
MIDRIFF
MIDWIFE
NODSOFF
QADDAFI
REDRAFT
RIDEOFF
RODEOFF
RODOLFO
RUDOLFI
SADCAFE
SYDHOFF
UPDRAFT
UPDRIFT

••D•••F

ENDLEAF
MADEOFF
MIDRIFF
NODSOFF
REDWOLF
RIDEOFF
RODEOFF
SYDHOFF

•••DF••

AVIDFAN
BIRDFLU
DIEDFOR
GOODFOR
HANDFED
HANDFUL
HEADFOR
HEADFUL
HEEDFUL
LAIDFOR
LIEDFOR
MINDFUL
NEEDFUL
PAIDFOR
READFOR
SANDFLY
SENDFOR
SLEDFUL
SOLDFOR
SUEDFOR
USEDFOR
VIEDFOR

•••D•F•

ABCDEFG
ACIDIFY
BINDOFF
CARDIFF
DANDIFY
DIEDOFF
FENDOFF
HANDOFF
HEADOFF
HELDOFF
HOLDOFF
LAIDOFF
LEADOFF
MACDUFF
NORDOFF
PAIDOFF
PREDEFY
QADDAFI
READOFF
SENDOFF
SLIDOFF
SOLDOFF
SPEDOFF
TEEDOFF
TIEDOFF
TOLDOFF
WARDOFF

•••D••F

ALTDORF
BINDOFF
CARDIFF
DIEDOFF
FENDOFF
GANDALF
HANDOFF
HEADOFF
HELDOFF
HOLDOFF
LAIDOFF
LEADOFF
LINDORF
LOADSOF
MACDUFF
NONDEAF
NORDOFF
PAIDOFF
READOFF
SCADSOF
SENDOFF
SLIDOFF
SOLDOFF
SPEDOFF
TEEDOFF
TIEDOFF
TOLDOFF
WALDORF
WARDOFF

••••D•F

AHEADOF
ALOADOF
ASKEDOF
FREEDOF
HEARDOF
INAIDOF
NOENDOF
PROUDOF
TIREDOF

D•G••••

DAGGERS
DAGWOOD
DEGAUSS
DEGERMS
DEGHOST
DEGLAZE
DEGRADE
DEGREED
DEGREES
DEGUSTS
DIGESTS
DIGGERS
DIGGING
DIGGITY
DIGGORY
DIGICAM
DIGINTO
DIGIPET
DIGITAL
DIGLOTS
DIGNIFY
DIGNITY
DIGRAMS
DIGRAPH
DIGRESS
DIGSFOR
DIGSOUT
DOGAPES
DOGBANE
DOGBEDS
DOGBERT
DOGBITE
DOGBONE
DOGBOOT
DOGBOWL
DOGCART
DOGCHEW
DOGCHOW
DOGCOAT
DOGCOMB
DOGDAYS
DOGDOOR
DOGEARS
DOGFACE
DOGFISH
DOGFLEA
DOGFOOD
DOGGATE
DOGGETT
DOGGIER
DOGGIES
DOGGING
DOGGISH
DOGGONE
DOGHAIR
DOGLEGS
DOGLESS
DOGLIKE
DOGMATA
DOGNAPS
DOGPILE
DOGRACE
DOGREAT
DOGROSE
DOGRUNS
DOGSAGE
DOGSEAR
DOGSHOW
DOGSITS
DOGSLED
DOGSTAR
DOGTAGS
DOGTAIL
DOGTICK
DOGTOYS
DOGTROT
DOGVEST
DOGWOOD
DUGINTO
DUGONGS
DUGOUTS

D••G•••

DAGGERS
DANGELO
DANGERS
DANGLED
DANGLER
DANGLES
DAYGAME
DEFGHIJ
DEIGNED
DEIGNTO
DIAGRAM
DIDGOOD
DIGGERS
DIGGING
DIGGITY
DIGGORY
DINGBAT
DINGERS
DINGIER
DINGILY
DINGING
DINGLES
DINGOES
DISGUST
DOAGAIN
DODGEMS
DODGERS
DODGIER
DODGING
DODGSON
DOGGATE
DOGGETT
DOGGIER
DOGGIES
DOGGING
DOGGISH
DOGGONE
DONGLES
DOUGHTY
DOUGLAS
DRAGEES
DRAGGED
DRAGGER
DRAGGLE
DRAGNET
DRAGOFF
DRAGONS
DRAGOON
DRAGOTI
DRAGOUT
DRAGSIN
DRAGSON
DRAGSUP
DREGION
DROGUES
DRUGGED
DUDGEON
DUNGEON
DWIGHTD

D•••G••

DAMAGED
DAMAGES
DARTGUN
DEARGOD
DECAGON
DELIGHT
DELUGED
DELUGES
DEMAGOG
DEMIGOD
DESIGNS
DIMAGES
DOINGIN
DOINGOK
DOINGSO
DOINGTO
DOINGUP
DONEGAL
DONEGAN
DORIGHT
DOSAGES
DOTAGES
DOWAGER
DRAGGED
DRAGGER
DRAGGLE
DRAUGHT
DREDGED
DREDGER
DREDGES
DROUGHT
DRUDGED
DRUDGER
DRUDGES
DRUGGED
DRVEGAS
DUSTGUN

D••••G•

DARKAGE
DATINGS
DEBARGE
DEBURGH
DEFANGS
DEFARGE
DEFRAGS
DEMERGE
DERANGE
DESMOGS
DETERGE
DIALOGS
DIVERGE
DIVULGE
DOCKAGE
DOGLEGS
DOGSAGE
DOGTAGS
DOMINGO
DONOTGO
DRAYAGE
DRYFOGS
DUGONGS
DUNNAGE
DURANGO

D•••••G

DABBING
DADOING
DAMMING
DAMNING
DAMPING
DANCING
DANNING
DAPPING
DARLING
DARNING
DARTING
DASHING
DAUBING
DAWNING
DAYLONG
DEALING
DECALOG
DECKING
DEEDING
DEEMING
DEFYING
DEICING
DEKEING
DELEING
DELVING
DEMAGOG
DEMOING
DENHAAG
DENNING
DENTING
DENYING
DERRING
DEUCING
DEYOUNG
DIALING
DIETING
DIGGING
DIMMING
DINGING
DINNING
DINTING
DIPPING
DIRKING
DIRTBAG
DISCING
DISHING
DISHRAG
DISKING
DISSING
DOCKING
DODGING
DOFFING
DOGGING
DOLLING
DONKING
DONNING
DOOMING
DOSSING
DOTTING
DOUBLEG
DOUSING
DOWLING
DOWNING
DOWRONG
DOWSING
DRAPING
DRAWING
DRAYING
DRIVING
DRONING
DUBBING
DUCKING
DUCTING
DUELING
DUETING
DULLING
DUMBING
DUMPING
DUNKING
DUNNING
DURNING
DUSKING
DUSTING
DUSTRAG

•DG••••

EDGARDO
EDGEDIN
EDGEOUT
EDGESIN
EDGIEST
EDGINGS

•D•G•••

ADAGIOS

•D••G••

CDEFGHI
ODINGON

•D•••G•

ADAYAGO
ADJUDGE
EDGINGS
IDBADGE

•D••••G

ADDLING
ADORING
EDDYING
EDITING
EDUCING
EDWARDG
RDLAING

••DG•••

BADGERS
BADGIRL
BADGUYS
BUDGERS
BUDGETS
BUDGIES
BUDGING
CADGERS
CADGING
CODGERS
CUDGELS
DIDGOOD
DODGEMS
DODGERS
DODGIER
DODGING
DODGSON
DUDGEON
EADGILS
ENDGAME
FIDGETS
FIDGETY
FUDGERS
FUDGING
GADGETS
GADGETY
GUDGEON
HEDGERS
HEDGIER
HEDGING
JUDGERS
JUDGING
KEDGERS
KEDGING
LEDGERS
LEDGIER
LODGEIN
LODGERS
LODGING
MIDGETS
NUDGERS
NUDGING
OLDGAGS
OLDGIRL
OLDGOLD
PADGETT
PIDGEON
PIDGINS
PUDGIER
PUDGILY
RIDGIER
RIDGING
RIDGWAY
RODGERS
SEDGIER
WEDGEIN
WEDGIER
WEDGIES
WEDGING
WIDGEON
WIDGETS

••D•G••

BADEGGS
BODEGAS
HADAGAS
INDIGEN
INDIGOS
MADIGAN
MEDIGAP

••D••G•

BADDOGS
BADEGGS
BADSIGN
BCDEFGH
BEDBUGS
BODINGS
ENDINGS
FTDODGE
HIDALGO
HIDINGS
INDULGE
LADINGS
MADDOGS
MIDLEGS
OLDDOGS
OLDFOGY
OLDGAGS
REDALGA
REDDOGS
REDLEGS
REDRAGS
REDTAGS
RIDINGS
RODRIGO
SIDINGS
TIDINGS
UNDERGO

••D•••G

ADDLING
BEDDING
BIDDING
BUDDING
BUDGING
CADGING
DADOING
DODGING
EDDYING
ENDLONG
ENDUING
FUDGING
GADDING
GODLING
HEDGING
HODDING
JUDGING
KEDGING
KIDDING
LADADOG
LADLING
LADYBUG
LODGING
MADDING
MUDDING
NODDING
NUDGING
OLDSONG
PADDING
PUDDING
REDDING
REDFLAG
REDKING
REDOING
REDWING
REDYING
RIDDING
RIDGING
RODDING
SADSONG
SIDLING
SODDING
SUDSING
TIDYING
UNDOING
UNDYING
WADDING
WEDDING
WEDGING

•••DG••

BLUDGED
BLUDGER
BLUDGES
BRIDGED
BRIDGER
BRIDGES
BRIDGET
DREDGED
DREDGER
DREDGES
DRUDGED
DRUDGER
DRUDGES
FLEDGED
FLEDGES
FORDGTS
FRIDGES
GOODGUY
GRUDGED
GRUDGER
GRUDGES
HANDGUN
KLUDGED
KLUDGES
NOODGED
NOODGES
PLEDGED
PLEDGEE
PLEDGER
PLEDGES
SLEDGED
SLEDGES
SLUDGES
SMIDGEN
SMIDGES
SMUDGED
SMUDGES
STODGED
STODGES
TRUDGED
TRUDGEN
TRUDGER
TRUDGES
UNEDGED
UNEDGES
WINDGOD

•••D•G•

BADDOGS
BANDAGE
BIGDIGS
BIGDOGS
BONDAGE
CONDIGN
CORDAGE
COYDOGS
FOGDOGS
GOODEGG
GUNDOGS
HOTDOGS
LAPDOGS
MADDOGS
OLDDOGS
PETDOGS
PRODIGY
PYEDOGS
REDDOGS
SEADOGS
SUNDOGS
TOPDOGS
TOYDOGS
VERDUGO
WINDAGE
WINDIGO
WORDAGE
YARDAGE

•••D••G

ABCDEFG
ABIDING
BALDING
BANDING
BEADING
BEDDING
BENDING
BIDDING
BINDING
BIRDDOG
BIRDING
BLADING
BONDING
BUDDING
CARDING
CHIDING
CORDING
CURDING
DEEDING
ELIDING
ELUDING
ERODING
EVADING
EXUDING
FEEDBAG
FEEDING
FENDING
FEUDING
FINDING
FOLDING
FORDING
FRODING
FUNDING
GADDING
GELDING
GILDING
GIRDING
GLIDING
GOADING
GOLDBUG
GOLDING
GOODDOG
GOODEGG
GOODING
GRADING
GUIDING
HANDBAG
HANDING
HARDING
HEADING
HEEDING
HERDING
HINDLEG
HODDING
HOLDING
HOODING
HORDING
KIDDING
LANDING
LANDTAG
LARDING
LAUDING
LEADDOG
LEADING
LENDING
LOADING
LOIDING
LORDING
MADDING
MELDING
MENDING
MINDING
MOLDING
MUDDING
NEEDING
NODDING
NONDRUG
OUTDRAG
PADDING
PENDING
PONDING
PRIDING
PUDDING
RAIDING
READING
REDDING
REEDING
RENDING
RIDDING
ROADHOG
RODDING
SANDBAG
SANDHOG
SANDING
SEEDING
SENDING
SHADING
SLEDDOG
SLIDING
SODDING
SPADING
TENDING
TRADING
VENDING
VOIDING
WADDING
WARDING
WEDDING
WEEDING
WELDING
WENDING
WILDDOG
WILDING

WILDPIG
WINDBAG
WINDING
WOODING
WORDING
YARDING

••••DG•
ABRIDGE
ADJUDGE
ARLEDGE
ELFUDGE
FTDODGE
IDBADGE
IPLEDGE
OHFUDGE
OUTEDGE
REJUDGE
THEEDGE
UNWEDGE

••••D•G
BIRDDOG
BULLDOG
COONDOG
CORNDOG
FIREDOG
GOODDOG
HALFDUG
HANGDOG
LADADOG
LEADDOG
LOSTDOG
MALEDOG
MOONDOG
NICEDOG
OVERDOG
RATEDPG
RIKSDAG
SHINDIG
SHOWDOG
SLEDDOG
WILDDOG
WOLFDOG

•••••DG
EDWARDG

DH•••••
DHARMAS
DHARMIC
DHURRIE

D•H••••
DAHLIAS
DAHOMEY
DEHAIRS
DEHAVEN
DEHEXED
DEHEXES
DEHIRED
DEHIRES
DEHISCE
DEHMELT
DEHORNS
DOHERTY
DUHAMEL

D••H•••
DABHAND
DAPHNES
DAPHNIA
DAPHNIS
DASHDOT
DASHERS
DASHIER
DASHIKI
DASHING
DASHOFF
DASHPOT
DAYHOPS
DEGHOST
DENHAAG
DESHELL
DIAHANN
DICHTER
DIEHARD
DIRHAMS
DISHFUL
DISHIER
DISHING
DISHOUT
DISHPAN
DISHRAG
DITHERS
DITHERY
DOGHAIR
DOSHOTS
DRCHAOS
DRYHEAT
DRYHOLE
DUCHAMP
DUCHESS
DUCHIES

D•••H••
DASCHLE
DAUPHIN
DEFGHIJ
DELIHAM
DELPHIC
DIAPHAN
DITCHED
DITCHER
DITCHES
DOGCHEW
DOGCHOW
DOGSHOW
DOLPHIN
DONAHUE
DONOHOE
DOUGHTY
DRACHMA
DWIGHTD

D••••H•
DALETHS
DEARTHS
DELIGHT
DEMOTHS
DENNEHY
DEPECHE
DERECHO
DORIGHT
DOROTHY
DRAUGHT
DROUGHT

D•••••H
DAMPISH
DARKISH
DEBAUCH
DEBORAH
DEBURGH
DEEPISH
DELILAH
DELRUTH
DERVISH
DEUTSCH
DIGRAPH
DIPTYCH
DISTICH
DOGFISH
DOGGISH
DOLLISH
DOLTISH
DOLUNCH
DONNISH
DOTDASH
DOUBLEH
DOZENTH
DRIESCH
DRONISH
DRTEETH
DRYWASH
DULLISH
DUMPISH
DUNCISH
DUSKISH
DYEBATH

•DH••••
ADHERED
ADHERER
ADHERES
ADHIBIT

•D•H•••
IDAHOAN
IDTHEFT

•D••H••
ODDSHOE

•D•••H•
ADELPHI
ADOLPHE
CDEFGHI

•D••••H
PDQBACH

••DH•••
BADHAIR
BADHAND
BADHATS
GODHEAD
GODHOOD
JODHPUR
LADHOOD
MUDHENS
MUDHOLE
OLDHAND
REDHAIR
REDHATS
REDHAWK
REDHEAD
REDHEAT
REDHENS
REDHOTS
SYDHOFF

••D•H••
ANDTHEN
BADSHOT
BUDDHAS
GODTHAB
MADCHEN
MADEHAY
MIDSHIP
NUDZHED
NUDZHES
ODDSHOE
OLDCHAP
OLDSHOE
REDCHIP

••D••H•
ARDECHE

••D•••H
ALDRICH
ANDSUCH
BADDISH
BADITCH
BCDEFGH
BEDBATH
CADDISH
CODFISH
ELDRICH
ERDRICH
FADDISH
GODUTCH
INDEPTH
INDUTCH
KADDISH
KIDDISH
LADDISH
LADYISH
MADDASH
MADDISH
MADRUSH
MUDBATH
MUDFISH
NIDETCH
PADUCAH
REDDISH
REDFISH
RUDOLPH
YIDDISH

•••DH••
BUDDHAS
FORDHAM
HARDHAT
HARDHIT
NEEDHAM
PRUDHOE
ROADHOG
SANDHOG
WYNDHAM

•••D•H•
HOWDAHS

•••D••H
BADDISH
BALDISH
CADDISH
COLDISH
DOTDASH
FADDISH
GOODISH
HARDISH
KADDISH
KIDDISH
KURDISH
LADDISH
LEADETH
LOUDISH
MADDASH
MADDISH
MAIDISH
MURDOCH
NERDISH
OBADIAH
PRADESH
PRUDISH
REDDISH
SAIDAAH
SWEDISH
TOADISH
WILDISH
YIDDISH

••••D•H
BREADTH
PLAYDOH

DI•••••
DIABLES
DIABLOS
DIABOLO
DIADEMS
DIAGRAM
DIAHANN
DIALECT
DIALEDO
DIALERS
DIALING
DIALLED
DIALOGS
DIALOUT
DIALSIN
DIALSUP
DIALUPS
DIAMOND
DIAPERS
DIAPHAN
DIARIES
DIARIOS
DIARIST
DIATOMS
DIAVOLO
DIBBLED
DIBBLER
DIBBLES
DICECUP
DICHTER
DICIEST
DICILLO
DICKENS
DICKERS
DICKEYS
DICKIES
DICKORY
DICKSON
DICTATE
DICTION
DICTUMS
DIDACTS
DIDASET
DIDDLED
DIDDLER
DIDDLES
DIDDLEY
DIDEROT
DIDFINE
DIDGOOD
DIDLAPS
DIDLIKE
DIDOVER
DIDSUMS
DIDTIME
DIDTOAT
DIDWELL
DIEAWAY
DIEBOLD
DIECAST
DIECUTS
DIEDFOR
DIEDOFF
DIEDOUT
DIEDOWN
DIEHARD
DIEMENS
DIEOFFS
DIESELS
DIESFOR
DIESOFF
DIESOUT
DIETARY
DIETERS
DIETING
DIFFERS
DIFFUSE
DIGESTS
DIGGERS
DIGGING
DIGGITY
DIGGORY
DIGICAM
DIGINTO
DIGIPET
DIGITAL
DIGLOTS
DIGNIFY
DIGNITY
DIGRAMS
DIGRAPH
DIGRESS
DIGSFOR
DIGSOUT
DIKDIKS
DIKTATS
DILATED
DILATES
DILATOR
DILBERT
DILEMMA
DILLARD
DILLIES
DILLMAN
DILUENT
DILUTED
DILUTER
DILUTES
DILUTOR
DIMAGES
DIMBULB
DIMETER
DIMITRI
DIMMERS
DIMMEST
DIMMING
DIMNESS
DIMOUTS
DIMPLED
DIMPLES
DIMSOUT
DIMVIEW
DIMWITS
DINADAM
DINARIC
DINDINS
DINEDAT
DINEDIN
DINEDON
DINEOUT
DINESAT
DINESEN
DINESIN
DINESON
DINETTE
DINGBAT
DINGERS
DINGIER
DINGILY
DINGING
DINGLES
DINGOES
DINKIER
DINMONT
DINNERS
DINNING
DINTING
DIOCESE
DIOMEDE
DIOPTER
DIORAMA
DIORITE
DIOTIMA
DIOXIDE
DIOXINS
DIPINTO
DIPLOID
DIPLOMA
DIPNETS
DIPOLAR
DIPOLES
DIPPERS
DIPPIER
DIPPING
DIPTYCH
DIRECTS
DIRECTV
DIREFUL
DIRHAMS
DIRKING
DIRKSEN
DIRNDLS
DIRTBAG
DIRTIED
DIRTIER
DIRTIES
DIRTILY
DISABLE
DISARMS
DISAVOW
DISBAND
DISBARS
DISBUDS
DISCARD
DISCERN
DISCING
DISCMAN
DISCOED
DISCOID
DISCORD
DISCUSS
DISDAIN
DISEASE
DISEURS
DISEUSE
DISGUST
DISHFUL
DISHIER
DISHING
DISHOUT
DISHPAN
DISHRAG
DISJOIN
DISKING
DISLIKE
DISMALS
DISMAST
DISMAYS
DISMISS
DISOBEY
DISOWNS
DISPART
DISPELS
DISPLAY
DISPORT
DISPOSE
DISPUTE
DISRATE
DISROBE
DISRUPT
DISSECT
DISSENT
DISSERT
DISSING
DISTAFF
DISTANT
DISTEND
DISTICH
DISTILL
DISTILS
DISTORT
DISTROS
DISTURB
DISUSED
DISUSES
DITCHED
DITCHER
DITCHES
DITHERS
DITHERY
DITSIER
DITTIES
DITTOED
DITZIER
DIURNAL
DIVEDIN
DIVERGE
DIVERSE
DIVERTS
DIVESIN
DIVESTS
DIVIDED
DIVIDER
DIVIDES
DIVINED
DIVINER
DIVINES
DIVISOR
DIVORCE
DIVULGE
DIVULSE
DIVVIED
DIVVIES
DIVVYUP
DIZAINS
DIZZIED
DIZZIER
DIZZIES
DIZZILY

D•I••••
DAILIES
DAIMLER
DAIRIES
DAIRYER
DAISIES
DEICERS
DEICING
DEIFIED
DEIFIER
DEIFIES
DEIGNED
DEIGNTO
DEIRDRE
DEISTIC
DEITIES
DJINNIS
DNIEPER
DOIDARE
DOILIES
DOINGIN
DOINGOK
DOINGSO
DOINGTO
DOINGUP
DOITNOW
DRIBBLE
DRIBLET
DRIEDUP
DRIESCH
DRIESUP
DRIFTED
DRIFTER
DRIFTIN
DRIFTUP
DRILLED
DRILLER
DRINKER
DRINKIN
DRINKME
DRINKTO
DRINKUP
DRIPDRY
DRIPPAN
DRIPPED
DRIPPER
DRIPSON
DRISTAN
DRIVEAT
DRIVEBY
DRIVEIN
DRIVELS
DRIVERS
DRIVETO
DRIVEUP
DRIVING
DRIZZLE
DRIZZLY
DWIGHTD
DWINDLE

D••I•••
DANIELA
DANIELJ
DANIELS
DANIKEN
DANITES
DARIUSI
DASILVA
DATINGS
DATIVES
DAVINCI
DAVISON
DEAIRED
DEBITED
DECIARE
DECIBEL
DECIDED
DECIDER
DECIDES
DECILES
DECIMAL
DEFIANT
DEFICIT
DEFIERS
DEFILED
DEFILER
DEFILES
DEFINED
DEFINER
DEFINES
DEHIRED
DEHIRES
DEHISCE
DELIBES
DELICTI
DELICTO
DELICTS
DELIGHT
DELIHAM
DELILAH
DELILLO
DELIMAN
DELIMEN
DELIMIT
DELINTS
DELIRIA
DELISTS
DELIVER
DEMIGOD
DEMILLE
DEMISED
DEMISES
DEMISTS
DENIALS
DENIECE
DENIERS
DENIMED
DENISON
DENIZEN
DEPICTS
DERIDED
DERIDER
DERIDES
DERIVED
DERIVER
DERIVES
DESIGNS
DESILTS
DESIRED
DESIREE
DESIRER
DESIRES
DESISTS
DEVIANT
DEVIATE
DEVICES
DEVILED
DEVILLE
DEVILRY
DEVIOUS
DEVISED
DEVISEE
DEVISER
DEVISES
DEVISOR
DEWIEST
DEWILDE
DEWIRED
DEWIRES
DICIEST
DICILLO
DIGICAM
DIGINTO
DIGIPET
DIGITAL
DIMITRI
DIPINTO
DIVIDED
DIVIDER
DIVIDES
DIVINED
DIVINER
DIVINES
DIVISOR
DOMICAL
DOMICIL
DOMINGO
DOMINIC
DOMINOS
DOMINUS
DONIMUS
DOPIEST
DORIGHT
DORITOS
DOSIDOS
DOZIEST
DRAINED
DRAINER
DREIDEL
DREISER
DRUIDIC
DRYIDEA
DUBIETY
DUBIOUS
DUGINTO
DUTIFUL

D•••I••
DABBING
DADAISM
DADAIST
DADDIES
DADOING
DAFFIER
DAFFILY
DAHLIAS
DAILIES
DAIRIES
DAISIES
DALLIED
DALLIER
DALLIES
DAMMING
DAMNING
DAMPING
DAMPISH
DANCING
DANDIER
DANDIES
DANDIFY
DANDILY
DANNING
DAPPING
DARKISH
DARLING
DARNING
DARTING
DASHIER
DASHIKI
DASHING
DATRILS
DAUBING
DAUMIER
DAWKINS
DAWNING
DAYLILY
DAYSIDE
DAYSINN
DAYTIME
DEALING
DEARIES
DEBOITE
DEBRIEF
DECEITS
DECEIVE
DECKING
DECLINE
DECRIED
DECRIER
DECRIES
DEEDING
DEEMING
DEEPISH
DEFYING
DEHAIRS
DEICING
DEIFIED
DEIFIER
DEIFIES
DEITIES
DEKEING
DELCITY
DELEING
DELUISE
DELVING
DEMOING
DENNING
DENSIFY
DENSITY
DENTINE
DENTING
DENTINS
DENTIST
DENYING
DEPRIVE
DERAILS
DERBIES
DERNIER
DERRICK
DERRICO
DERRIDA
DERRING
DERVISH
DESPINA
DESPISE
DESPITE
DESTINE
DESTINO
DESTINY
DETAILS
DETAINS
DEUCING
DEVEINS
DEVOIRS
DEVRIES
DEWLINE
DIALING
DIARIES
DIARIOS
DIARIST
DICKIES
DICTION
DIDFINE
DIDLIKE
DIDTIME
DIETING
DIGGING
DIGGITY
DIGNIFY
DIGNITY
DIKDIKS
DILLIES
DIMMING
DIMVIEW

DIMWITS
DINDINS
DINGIER
DINGILY
DINGING
DINKIER
DINNING
DINTING
DIORITE
DIOTIMA
DIOXIDE
DIOXINS
DIPPIER
DIPPING
DIRKING
DIRTIED
DIRTIER
DIRTIES
DIRTILY
DISCING
DISHIER
DISHING
DISKING
DISLIKE
DISMISS
DISSING
DISTICH
DISTILL
DISTILS
DITSIER
DITTIES
DITZIER
DIVVIED
DIVVIES
DIZAINS
DIZZIED
DIZZIER
DIZZIES
DIZZILY
DOASIDO
DOBBINS
DOCKING
DODGIER
DODGING
DOFFING
DOGBITE
DOGFISH
DOGGIER
DOGGIES
DOGGING
DOGGISH
DOGLIKE
DOGPILE
DOGSITS
DOGTICK
DOILIES
DOLLIED
DOLLIES
DOLLING
DOLLISH
DOLTISH
DOMAINE
DOMAINS
DONKING
DONNING
DONNISH
DOOLIES
DOOMIER
DOOMING
DOOZIES
DORKIER
DORMICE
DOSSIER
DOSSING
DOTLIKE
DOTRICE
DOTTIER
DOTTILY
DOTTING
DOUSING
DOWDIER
DOWDIES
DOWDILY
DOWLING
DOWNIER
DOWNING
DOWRIES
DOWSING
DRAPING
DRAWING
DRAYING
DREGION
DRFRIST
DRIVING
DRONING
DRONISH
DROPINS
DROXIES
DRQUINN
DRUZIAN
DUALISM
DUALIST
DUALITY
DUALIZE
DUBBING
DUBNIUM
DUCHIES
DUCKIER
DUCKIES
DUCKING
DUCTILE
DUCTING
DUELING
DUELIST
DUETING
DULCIFY
DULLING
DULLISH
DUMBING
DUMMIED
DUMMIES
DUMPIER
DUMPILY
DUMPING
DUMPISH
DUNCISH
DUNKING
DUNKIRK
DUNLINS
DUNNING
DURNING
DUSKIER
DUSKILY
DUSKING
DUSKISH
DUSTIER
DUSTILY
DUSTING

D••••I•

DALASIS
DANTEII
DAPHNIA
DAPHNIS
DAUPHIN
DAYQUIL
DAYSAIL
DAYTRIP
DEADAIR
DEALSIN
DEALTIN
DEARSIR
DECLAIM
DEEPSIX
DEFGHIJ
DEFICIT
DEISTIC
DELIMIT
DELIRIA
DELORIS
DELPHIC
DELTAIC
DELTOID
DEMERIT
DEMONIC
DEMOTIC
DENARII
DENTOID
DEORBIT
DEPOSIT
DESPAIR
DESPOIL
DESTAIN
DETRAIN
DETROIT
DEXTRIN
DHARMIC
DHURRIE
DIALSIN
DINARIC
DINEDIN
DINESIN
DIPLOID
DISCOID
DISDAIN
DISJOIN
DIVEDIN
DIVESIN
DJINNIS
DOAGAIN
DOESKIN
DOGHAIR
DOGTAIL
DOINGIN
DOLPHIN
DOMICIL
DOMINIC
DONTLIE
DOONEIN
DOORDIE
DOUBTIT
DRAGSIN
DRANKIN
DRASTIC
DRAWNIN
DRAWSIN
DREAMIN
DRESSIN
DRIFTIN
DRINKIN
DRIVEIN
DRMARIO
DROPSIN
DROPSIT
DROVEIN
DRUIDIC
DRUMLIN
DRYADIC
DRYSUIT
DUCKPIN
DUKAKIS
DUNEDIN
DUSTBIN
DUUMVIR
DWEEZIL
DWELLIN
DYNAMIC

D•••••I

DAKTARI
DANTEII
DARIUSI
DASHIKI
DAVINCI
DELICTI
DENARII
DIMITRI
DOUBLEI
DRAGOTI
DRMELFI

•DI••••

ADIPOSE
EDIBLES
EDICTAL
EDIFICE
EDIFIED
EDIFIER
EDIFIES
EDINAMN
EDITING
EDITION
EDITORS
EDITOUT
EDITRIX
IDIAMIN
IDIDTOO
IDIOTIC
ODINGON

•D•I•••

ADDIBLE
ADDICTS
ADDISON
ADHIBIT
ADMIRAL
ADMIRED
ADMIRER
ADMIRES
ADMITTO
ADMIXED
ADMIXES
ADRIANA
ADVICES
ADVISED
ADVISEE
ADVISER
ADVISES
ADVISOR
EDGIEST
EDGINGS

•D••I••

ADAGIOS
ADAMITE
ADDLING
ADELIES
ADELINA
ADELINE
ADENINE
ADJOINS
ADORING
EDACITY
EDDYING
EDIFICE
EDIFIED
EDIFIER
EDIFIES
EDITING
EDITION
EDOMITE
EDUCING
IDOLISE
IDOLIST
IDOLIZE
IDYLIST
ODORIZE
RDLAING

•D•••I•

ADDEDIN
ADENOID
ADHIBIT
ADONAIS
ADZUKIS
EDGEDIN
EDGESIN
EDITRIX
IDENTIC
IDIAMIN
IDIOTIC
IDOODIT
IDYLLIC
ODONTIA

•D••••I

ADELPHI
CDEFGHI
EDMUNDI
EDWARDI

••DI•••

ADDIBLE
ADDICTS
ADDISON
AEDILES
ANDIAMO
ANDIRON
AUDIBLE
AUDIBLY
AUDILES
AUDITED
AUDITEE
AUDITOR
BADIDEA
BADITCH
BEDIZEN
BODICES
BODINGS
CEDILLA
CODICES
CODICIL
ENDINGS
ENDIVES
FADIMAN
FEDINTO
FTDIXNJ
HEDISON
HIDINGS
INDIANA
INDIANS
INDICES
INDICIA
INDICTS
INDIGEN
INDIGOS
INDITED
INDITER
INDITES
IODIDES
IODISED
IODISES
IODIZED
IODIZER
IODIZES
KODIAKS
LADIDAS
LADINGS
LADINOS
LEDINTO
MADIGAN
MADISON
MEDIANS
MEDIANT
MEDIATE
MEDICAL
MEDICOS
MEDIGAP
MEDIUMS
MEDIVAC
MIDIRON
MODICUM
MODISTE
NODICAL
NUDISTS
OEDIPAL
OEDIPUS
ORDINAL
ORDINES
PEDICAB
PODIUMS
RADIALS
RADIANS
RADIANT
RADIATE
RADICAL
RADICES
RADICLE
RADIOAD
RADIODJ
RADIOED
RADIOER
RADIOIN
RADIXES
REDIALS
RIDINGS
SADISTS
SIDINGS
SIDIOUS
SODIDWE
TEDIOUS
TEDIUMS
TIDIEST
TIDINGS
UNDIKED
UNDINES
UPDIVED
UPDIVES
VEDISTS
VIDICON
VIDIOTS
WEDIDIT
ZEDILLO
ZODIACS

••D•I••

ADDLING
ALDRICH
BADDIES
BADDISH
BADFITS
BADGIRL
BADLIES
BADSIGN
BADTIME
BEDDING
BEDLIKE
BEDSIDE
BEDSITS
BEDTIME
BIDDIES
BIDDING
BODKINS
BUDDIED
BUDDIES
BUDDING
BUDGIES
BUDGING
BUDLIKE
BUDTIME
CADDIED
CADDIES
CADDISH
CADGING
CADMIUM
CODEINE
CODFISH
CUDDIES
DADAISM
DADAIST
DADDIES
DADOING
DIDFINE
DIDLIKE
DIDTIME
DODGIER
DODGING
EADGILS
EDDYING
ELDRICH
ELDRICK
ENDLINE
ENDPINS
ENDUING
ENDWISE
ERDRICH
FADDIER
FADDIET
FADDISH
FADDISM
FADDIST
FADEINS
FADLIKE
FUDDIES
FUDGING
GADDING
GEDRICK
GIDDIED
GIDDIER
GIDDIES
GIDDILY
GODLIER
GODLIKE
GODLING
GODWITS
HADFITS
HADRIAN
HADTIME
HEDGIER
HEDGING
HODDING
HYDRIDE
JADEITE
JUDAICA
JUDAISM
JUDGING
JUDOIST
KADDISH
KEDGING
KIDDIES
KIDDING
KIDDISH
KIDLIKE
KIDVIDS
LADDIES
LADDISH
LADLING
LADYISH
LEDGIER
LIDWINA
LODGING
LUDDISM
LUDDITE
LYDDITE
MADDING
MADDISH
MADEILL
MADEIRA
MADLIBS
MEDWICK
MIDDIES
MIDLIFE
MIDLINE
MIDLIST
MIDRIBS
MIDRIFF
MIDRISE
MIDSIZE
MIDWIFE
MUDDIED
MUDDIER
MUDDIES
MUDDILY
MUDDING
MUDFISH
MUDPIES
NODDIES
NODDING
NUDGING
NUDNIKS
OLDCITY
OLDFILM
OLDGIRL
OLDLINE
OLDNICK
OLDTIME
ORDAINS
PADDIES
PADDING
PADSITE
PIDGINS
PODLIKE
PODRIDA
PUDDING
PUDGIER
PUDGILY
REDBIRD
REDDING
REDDISH
REDFINS
REDFIRS
REDFISH
REDFIVE
REDKING
REDLINE
REDNINE
REDOING
REDPINE
REDRIED
REDRIES
REDRILL
REDRIVE
REDTIDE
REDTIES
REDWINE
REDWING
REDYING
RIDDICK
RIDDING
RIDGIER
RIDGING
RODDICK
RODDING
RODLIKE
RODRIGO
RUDDIED
RUDDIER
RUDDILY
SEDGIER
SIDLING
SODDIER
SODDING
SUDSIER
SUDSING
TEDDIES
TIDBITS
TIDYING
TODDIES
UNDOING
UNDRIED
UNDYING
UPDRIED
UPDRIES
UPDRIFT
WADDING
WADKINS
WEDDING
WEDGIER
WEDGIES
WEDGING
YIDDISH
ZADKINE

••D••I•

ADDEDIN
ALDAVIS
ALDUBIN
ANDROID
BADHAIR
BADTRIP
BEDELIA
BEDEVIL
BEDOUIN
BEDRAIL
BIDFAIR
BODYKIT
CODICIL
ECDYSIS
EIDETIC
EIDOLIC
ENDEDIN
ENDEDIT
ENDEMIC
FADEDIN
FADESIN
FIDELIA
FIDELIO
FIDELIS
GODEVIL
HADAFIT
HADANIP
HADATIT
HEDONIC
INDICIA
KIDSKIN
LADYKIN
LODGEIN
MADEFIT
MIDSHIP
OLDMAID
ORDERIN
PADRAIC
RADIOIN
REDCHIP
REDEBIT
REDHAIR
REDSKIN
REDSUIT
REDTAIL
RIDESIN
SEDALIA
STDENIS
TIDERIP
VIDALIA
WADEDIN
WADESIN
WEDGEIN
WEDIDIT

••D•••I

CADUCEI
OLDUVAI
QADDAFI
RUDOLFI

•••DI••

ABIDING
ACADIAN
ACIDIFY
ACIDITY
ALADINE
ANODISE
ANODIZE
APEDIET
ARIDITY
ATEDIRT
AVIDITY
BADDIES
BADDISH
BALDIES
BALDING
BALDISH
BANDIDO
BANDIED
BANDIER
BANDIES
BANDING
BANDITO
BANDITS
BAWDIER
BAWDILY
BEADIER
BEADILY
BEADING
BEDDING
BENDIER
BENDING
BIDDIES
BIDDING
BIGDIGS
BINDING
BIRDIED
BIRDIES
BIRDING
BLADING
BONDING
BOUDINS
BRODIES
BUDDIED
BUDDIES
BUDDING
BURDICK
CADDIED
CADDIES
CADDISH
CANDICE
CANDIDA
CANDIDE
CANDIDS
CANDIED
CANDIES
CARDIAC
CARDIAL
CARDIFF
CARDING
CARDIUM
CHIDING
COEDITS
COLDISH
CONDIGN
CORDIAL
CORDIAS
CORDING
CORDITE
CREDITS
CRUDITY
CUDDIES
CURDIER
CURDING
DADDIES
DANDIER
DANDIES
DANDIFY
DANDILY
DEEDING
DIKDIKS
DINDINS
DOWDIER
DOWDIES
DOWDILY
EATDIRT
ELIDING
ELUDING
ERODING
ERUDITE
EVADING
EXUDING
FADDIER
FADDIET
FADDISH
FADDISM
FADDIST
FEEDING
FENDING
FEUDING
FEUDIST
FINDING
FOLDING
FOODIES
FORDING
FOSDICK
FRODING
FUDDIES
FUNDING
GADDING
GAUDIER
GAUDIES
GAUDILY
GELDING
GIDDIED
GIDDIER
GIDDIES
GIDDILY
GILDING
GIRDING
GLIDING
GOADING
GOLDING
GOODIES
GOODING
GOODISH
GORDIAN
GORDITA
GORDIUS
GRADING
GRODIER
GUIDING
HANDIER
HANDILY
HANDING
HARDIER
HARDILY
HARDING
HARDISH
HEADIER
HEADILY
HEADING
HEEDING
HERDING
HODDING
HOLDING
HOODIES
HOODING
HORDING
HOUDINI
ICHDIEN
INEDITA
IRIDIUM
JARDINE
JARDINS
JIMDIAL
KADDISH
KHEDIVE
KIDDIES
KIDDING
KIDDISH
KURDISH
LADDIES
LADDISH
LANDING
LANDINI
LARDIER
LARDING
LAUDING
LEADIER
LEADING
LEADINS
LENDING
LINDIED
LINDIES
LOADING
LOIDING
LORDING
LOUDISH
LOWDIVE
LUDDISM
LUDDITE
LYDDITE
MADDING
MADDISH
MAHDISM
MAHDIST
MAIDISH
MALDIVE

MARDIAN
MELDING
MENDING
MIDDIES
MINDING
MISDIAL
MOLDIER
MOLDING
MONDIAL
MONDIEU
MOODIER
MOODILY
MUDDIED
MUDDIER
MUDDIES
MUDDILY
MUDDING
NEEDIER
NEEDILY
NEEDING
NERDIER
NERDISH
NODDIES
NODDING
NONDIET
NORDICA
NORDICS
OBADIAH
ONADIET
ONEDIME
OVIDIAN
OXIDISE
OXIDIZE
PADDIES
PADDING
PANDITS
PAYDIRT
PENDING
PERDIDO
PERDIEM
PERDITA
PHIDIAS
PONDING
POPDIVA
PREDICT
PREDIET
PREDIVE
PRIDING
PRODIGY
PRUDISH
PUDDING
PUNDITS
RAIDING
RANDIER
READIED
READIER
READIES
READILY
READING
REDDING
REDDISH
REEDIER
REEDING
REEDITS
RENDING
RHODIAN
RHODIUM
RIDDICK
RIDDING
RINDIER
ROADIES
RODDICK
RODDING
ROWDIER
ROWDIES
ROWDILY
RUDDIED
RUDDIER
RUDDILY
SAIDIDO
SANDIER
SANDING
SARDINE
SEEDIER
SEEDILY
SEEDING
SENDING
SHADIER
SHADILY
SHADING
SKYDIVE
SLIDING
SODDIER
SODDING
SOLDIER
SORDINI
SORDINO
SPADING
STADIUM
STUDIED
STUDIER
STUDIES
STUDIOS
SUNDIAL
SWEDISH
SYNDICS
TARDIER
TARDILY
TEDDIES
TENDING
THEDIET
TOADIED
TOADIES
TOADISH
TODDIES
TRADING
TREDIAS
VANDIEN
VANDINE
VENDING
VERDICT
VERDINS
VOIDING
WADDING
WARDING
WEDDING
WEEDIER
WEEDILY
WEEDING
WELDING
WENDING
WILDING
WILDISH
WINDIER
WINDIGO
WINDILY
WINDING
WOODIER
WOODIES
WOODING
WORDIER
WORDILY
WORDING
YARDING
YIDDISH
ZIPDISK

•••D•I•

AIRDRIE
ALADDIN
BALDRIC
BALDWIN
BANDAID
BOUDOIR
BOWDOIN
CONDUIT
DEADAIR
DISDAIN
FEEDBIN
FEEDSIN
FOLDSIN
FREDDIE
FREDRIC
GLIDEIN
GOLDTIP
GOODAIM
GOODKID
GOODNIK
GOODWIN
HANDLIN
HANDSIN
HARDHIT
HARDSIX
HEADPIN
HEADSIN
HENDRIX
HOLDSIN
HOLDSIT
ILLDOIT
IMADEIT
LEADSIN
LOADSIN
LORDJIM
LORDSIT
MAUDLIN
NONDRIP
QUADRIC
READM1T
READSIN
SANDPIT
SENDSIN
SKIDLID
SLIDEIN
TENDRIL
TRADEIN
VAUDOIS
WILDPIG
WOODBIN

•••D••I

BORDONI
FEODORI
GOLDONI
HOUDINI
LANDINI
MANDOKI
MONDAVI
MONDESI
QADDAFI
SORDINI

••••DI•

ACTEDIN
ADDEDIN
ALADDIN
AMRADIO
ARCADIA
ASKEDIN
BEANDIP
BLENDIN
BLONDIE
BORODIN
BOXEDIN
BUILDIN
CAGEDIN
CAVEDIN
CBRADIO
CLAMDIP
CLAUDIA
CLAUDIO
CLUEDIN
COMEDIA
COMEDIC
COMEDIE
CROWDIN
DINEDIN
DIVEDIN
DOORDIE
DRUIDIC
DRYADIC
DUNEDIN
EASEDIN
EDGEDIN
ENDEDIN
ENDEDIT
EXORDIA
FACEDIT
FADEDIN
FAKEDIT
FATIDIC
FILEDIN
FJORDIC
FLEADIP
FLUIDIC
FMRADIO
FORTDIX
FREDDIE
GREWDIM
GROWDIM
HASIDIC
HASIDIM
HATEDIT
HEREDIA
HEXADIC
HOMEDIN
HONEDIN
IDOODIT
IFITDIE
ILIADIC
INKEDIN
JURIDIC
KATYDID
KEYEDIN
LIPIDIC
LIVEDIN
LOVEDIT
LUREDIN
MAULDIN
MELODIA
MELODIC
MISEDIT
MIXEDIN
MONADIC
MONODIC
MOVEDIN
MOVEDIT
NOMADIC
NOSEDIN
OCTADIC
OPTEDIN
OVERDID
PALADIN
PARODIC
PILEDIN
PIPEDIN
PLAUDIT
PLOVDIV
PREEDIT
RACEDIN
RAKEDIN
REAUDIT
ROPEDIN
RUSHDIE
SALADIN
SAMEDIS
SHINDIG
SINEDIE
STANDIN
STOODIN
SYNODIC
THANDIE
TOWEDIN
TRIADIC
TRIEDIT
TUNEDIN
TYPEDIN
UPANDIN
VALIDID
VANADIC
VERIDIC
VOTEDIN
WADEDIN
WAVEDIN
WEDIDIT
WIREDIN
XMRADIO
YESIDID

••••D•I

HYUNDAI

•••••DI

ALEARDI
BACARDI
BIBBIDI
BOBBIDI
BURUNDI
COLLODI
EDMUNDI
EDWARDI
EFFENDI
HAROLDI
SECONDI
SHOULDI
TEBALDI
UNBELDI
VIVALDI
VIVENDI
YOUANDI

DJ•••••

DJINNIS

D•J••••

DEJECTS
DEJUNKS

D••J•••

DAYJOBS
DEEJAYS
DISJOIN
DONJONS
DONJOSE
DONJUAN
DYEJOBS

D•••••J

DANIELJ
DEFGHIJ
DOUBLEJ

•DJ••••

ADJOINS
ADJOURN
ADJUDGE
ADJUNCT
ADJURED
ADJURER
ADJURES
ADJUROR
ADJUSTS
PDJAMES

•D•J•••

ODDJOBS

••DJ•••

BADJOKE
MIDJULY
MIDJUNE
ODDJOBS
OLDJOKE
REDJACK

••D•J••

HADAJOB

••D•••J

FTDIXNJ
RADIODJ

•••DJ••

ABIDJAN
GOODJOB
GOODJOE
LORDJIM

••••DJ•

PBANDJS

•••••DJ

HEYMRDJ
RADIODJ

D•K••••

DAKOTAN
DAKOTAS
DAKTARI
DEKEING
DEKLERK
DIKDIKS
DIKTATS
DUKAKIS
DUKEDOM
DYKSTRA

D••K•••

DANKEST
DARKAGE
DARKENS
DARKEST
DARKISH
DARKLED
DARKLES
DARKMAN
DARKRED
DARKTAN
DAWKINS
DECKERS
DECKING
DECKLED
DECKLES
DECKOUT
DELKEYS
DESKFUL
DESKSET
DESKTOP
DICKENS
DICKERS
DICKEYS
DICKIES
DICKORY
DICKSON
DINKIER
DIRKING
DIRKSEN
DISKING
DOCKAGE
DOCKERS
DOCKETS
DOCKING
DONKEYS
DONKING
DORKIER
DUCKERS
DUCKIER
DUCKIES
DUCKING
DUCKOUT
DUCKPIN
DUNKERS
DUNKING
DUNKIRK
DUSKIER
DUSKILY
DUSKING
DUSKISH

D•••K••

DANIKEN
DAVEKOZ
DEBAKEY
DOESKIN
DRANKIN
DRANKTO
DRANKUP
DRINKER
DRINKIN
DRINKME
DRINKTO
DRINKUP
DRUCKER
DRUNKEN
DRUNKER
DUKAKIS

D••••K•

DAMASKS
DANEYKO
DASHIKI
DEBARKS
DEBUNKS
DEEPSKY
DEJUNKS
DEMARKS
DIDLIKE
DIKDIKS
DISLIKE
DOGLIKE
DOTLIKE
DYBBUKS

D•••••K

DAYBOOK
DAYPACK
DEFROCK
DEKLERK
DENMARK
DERRICK
DESTOCK
DMYTRYK
DOGTICK
DOINGOK
DONETSK
DONTASK
DOUBLEK
DRSPOCK
DRYDOCK
DUNDALK
DUNKIRK

•D•K•••

NDAKOTA
SDAKOTA

•D••K••

ADZUKIS

•D•••K•

CDRACKS

•D••••K

ODDDUCK
ODDSOCK

••DK•••

BODKINS
REDKING
WADKINS
ZADKINE

••D•K••

BODYKIT
JUDOKAS
KIDSKIN
LADYKIN
MEDAKAS
REDSKIN
SUDOKUS
UNDIKED

••D••K•

BADJOKE
BEDECKS
BEDLIKE
BUDLIKE
CODCAKE
DIDLIKE
FADLIKE
FEDERKO
GODLIKE
KIDLIKE
KODIAKS
NUDNIKS
OLDJOKE
PODLIKE
REDOAKS
REDOCKS
RODLIKE
UNDOCKS
ZEDONKS

••D•••K

BADBACK
BADLUCK
BEDROCK
BODEREK
ELDRICK
GEDRICK
HADDOCK
KIDROCK
MADLOCK
MEDWICK
MIDWEEK
MUDLARK
MUDPACK
ODDDUCK
ODDSOCK
OLDNICK
PADDOCK
PADLOCK
REDBOOK
REDHAWK
REDJACK
REDNECK
RIDDICK
RODDICK
SADSACK
TEDMACK
UNDRUNK
WEDLOCK
WIDMARK

•••DK••

BRODKEY
CARDKEY
GOODKID
WENDKOS

•••D•K•

BRODSKY
DIKDIKS
MANDOKI
SIRDUKE
THEDUKE
VANDYKE

•••D••K

BURDICK
DRYDOCK
DUNDALK
FOSDICK
GEODUCK
GOODNIK
HADDOCK
NONDARK
OAKDESK
ODDDUCK
PADDOCK
PETDUCK
PREDARK
PREDUSK
RIDDICK
RODDICK
SEADUCK
SUNDECK
VANDYCK
ZIPDISK

•••••DK

HOWARDK

D•L••••

DALASIS
DALETHS
DALLIED
DALLIER
DALLIES
DALTONS
DALTREY
DELANEY
DELARUE
DELAYED
DELAYER
DELBERT
DELCITY
DELEADS
DELEDDA
DELEING
DELETED
DELETES
DELIBES
DELICTI
DELICTO
DELICTS
DELIGHT
DELIHAM
DELILAH
DELILLO
DELIMAN
DELIMEN
DELIMIT
DELINTS
DELIRIA
DELISTS
DELIVER
DELKEYS
DELMONT
DELMORE
DELORIS
DELORME
DELOUSE
DELPHIC
DELRAYS
DELRUTH
DELSOLS
DELTAIC
DELTOID
DELTONA
DELTORO
DELUDED
DELUDER
DELUDES
DELUGED
DELUGES
DELUISE
DELVERS
DELVING
DILATED
DILATES
DILATOR
DILBERT
DILEMMA
DILLARD
DILLIES
DILLMAN
DILUENT
DILUTED
DILUTER
DILUTES
DILUTOR
DOLEFUL
DOLEOUT
DOLLARS
DOLLIED
DOLLIES
DOLLING
DOLLISH
DOLLOPS
DOLLSUP
DOLMANS
DOLORES
DOLOURS
DOLPHIN
DOLTISH
DOLUNCH
DPLUSES
DRLAURA
DULCIFY
DULLARD
DULLEST
DULLING
DULLISH

D••L•••

DAHLIAS
DAILIES
DALLIED
DALLIER
DALLIES
DARLEEN
DARLENE
DARLING
DAYLILY
DAYLONG
DEALERS
DEALING
DEALOUT
DEALSIN
DEALSTO
DEALSUP
DEALTIN
DEALTTO
DEALTUP
DEBLURS
DECLAIM
DECLARE
DECLASS
DECLAWS
DECLINE
DECLOTS
DEFLATE
DEFLEAS
DEFLECT
DEGLAZE
DEKLERK
DEPLANE
DEPLETE
DEPLORE
DEPLOYS
DESLUMS
DEWLAPS
DEWLESS
DEWLINE
DIALECT
DIALEDO
DIALERS
DIALING
DIALLED
DIALOGS
DIALOUT
DIALSIN
DIALSUP
DIALUPS
DIDLAPS
DIDLIKE
DIGLOTS
DILLARD
DILLIES
DILLMAN
DIPLOID
DIPLOMA
DISLIKE
DNALABS
DOGLEGS
DOGLESS
DOGLIKE
DOILIES
DOLLARS
DOLLIED
DOLLIES
DOLLING
DOLLISH
DOLLOPS
DOLLSUP
DONLEVY
DOOLIES
DOTLIKE
DOWLING
DRILLED
DRILLER
DROLLER
DRSLOAN
DUALISM
DUALIST
DUALITY
DUALIZE
DUELERS
DUELING
DUELIST
DUELLED
DULLARD
DULLEST
DULLING
DULLISH
DUNLINS
DUNLOPS
DWELLAT
DWELLED
DWELLER
DWELLIN
DWELLON
DWELTON
DYELOTS

D•••L••

DABBLED
DABBLER
DABBLES
DAIMLER
DANDLED
DANDLER
DANDLES
DANELAW
DANGLED
DANGLER
DANGLES
DAPPLED
DAPPLES
DARKLED
DARKLES
DARTLED
DARTLES
DASILVA
DAWDLED
DAWDLER
DAWDLES
DAZZLED
DAZZLER
DAZZLES
DECALOG
DECILES
DECKLED
DECKLES
DECOLOR
DEDALUS
DEFALLA
DEFILED
DEFILER
DEFILES
DELILAH
DELILLO
DEMILLE

DEMOLAY
DEPALMA
DEPULPS
DERALTE
DESALTS
DESILTS
DESYLVA
DEVALUE
DEVELOP
DEVILED
DEVILLE
DEVILRY
DEVOLVE
DEWCLAW
DEWILDE
DIABLES
DIABLOS
DIALLED
DIBBLED
DIBBLER
DIBBLES
DICILLO
DIDDLED
DIDDLER
DIDDLES
DIDDLEY
DIMPLED
DIMPLES
DINGLES
DIPOLAR
DIPOLES
DISPLAY
DIVULGE
DIVULSE
DOGFLEA
DOGSLED
DONGLES
DONTLIE
DOODLED
DOODLER
DOODLES
DOPPLER
DOTTLES
DOUBLEA
DOUBLEB
DOUBLEC
DOUBLED
DOUBLEE
DOUBLEF
DOUBLEG
DOUBLEH
DOUBLEI
DOUBLEJ
DOUBLEK
DOUBLEL
DOUBLEM
DOUBLEN
DOUBLEO
DOUBLEP
DOUBLEQ
DOUBLER
DOUBLES
DOUBLET
DOUBLEU
DOUBLEV
DOUBLEW
DOUBLEX
DOUBLEY
DOUBLEZ
DOUGLAS
DOVELET
DRAWLED
DRAWLER
DREXLER
DRIBLET
DRILLED
DRILLER
DRMELFI
DROLLER
DROOLED
DROOLER
DROPLET
DRUMLIN
DRWELBY
DUCALLY
DUELLED
DUFFLES
DWELLAT
DWELLED
DWELLER
DWELLIN
DWELLON

D••••L•
DACTYLS
DAFFILY
DAMSELS
DANDILY
DANGELO
DANIELA
DANIELJ
DANIELS
DARNELL
DARRYLF
DARWELL
DASCHLE
DATABLE
DATEDLY
DATRILS
DAYLILY
DAZEDLY
DEBACLE
DEBOULE
DECARLO
DECUPLE
DEERFLY
DEFALLA
DEFAULT
DEFUELS
DEHMELT
DELILLO
DELSOLS
DEMILLE
DENIALS
DENSELY
DENTALS
DEPAULU
DERAILS
DESHELL
DETAILS
DEVILLE
DEWFALL
DIABOLO
DIAVOLO
DICILLO
DIDWELL
DIEBOLD
DIESELS
DIMBULB
DINGILY
DIRNDLS
DIRTILY
DISABLE
DISMALS
DISPELS
DISTILL
DISTILS
DIZZILY
DOGPILE
DONNALL
DORSALS
DOSSALS
DOTTILY
DOWDILY
DRABBLE
DRACULA
DRAGGLE
DREXELU
DRIBBLE
DRIVELS
DRIZZLE
DRIZZLY
DRYABLE
DRYBULB
DRYCELL
DRYHOLE
DRYWALL
DRYWELL
DUCALLY
DUCTILE
DUFFELS
DUMPILY
DUNDALK
DUOPOLY
DURABLE
DURABLY
DURRELL
DUSKILY
DUSTILY
DWINDLE

D•••••L
DAMOSEL
DAREFUL
DARNELL
DARWELL
DAYQUIL
DAYSAIL
DECIBEL
DECIMAL
DEMEROL
DEPOSAL
DESHELL
DESKFUL
DESPOIL
DESTAEL
DEWFALL
DEXTRAL
DIDWELL
DIGITAL
DIREFUL
DISHFUL
DISTILL
DIURNAL
DOADEAL
DOGBOWL
DOGTAIL
DOLEFUL
DOMICAL
DOMICIL
DONEGAL
DONNALL
DOOMFUL
DOUBLEL
DREIDEL
DRYCELL
DRYWALL
DRYWELL
DUHAMEL
DURRELL
DUTIFUL
DWEEZIL

•DL••••
IDLESSE
RDLAING

•D•L•••
ADDLING
ADELIES
ADELINA
ADELINE
ADELPHI
ADOLLAR
ADOLPHE
ADULATE
ADULTLY
BDALTON
CDALBUM
IDOLISE
IDOLIST
IDOLIZE
IDYLIST
IDYLLIC
ODDLOTS
ODELETS

•D••L••
ADOLLAR
EDIBLES
IDEALLY
IDYLLIC

•D•••L•
ADDABLE
ADDEDLY
ADDIBLE
ADDSALT
ADEPTLY
ADULTLY
IDEALLY
ODDBALL

•D••••L
ADMIRAL
ADRENAL
EDICTAL
ODDBALL
ODORFUL

••DL•••
ADDLING
AIDLESS
BADLAND
BADLIES
BADLOTS
BADLOVE
BADLUCK
BEDLAMP
BEDLAMS
BEDLESS
BEDLIKE
BEDLOES
BUDLESS
BUDLIKE
DIDLAPS
DIDLIKE
ENDLATE
ENDLEAF
ENDLESS
ENDLINE
ENDLONG
FADLIKE
GODLESS
GODLIER
GODLIKE
GODLING
KIDLIKE
LADLERS
LADLING
LIDLESS
MADLIBS
MADLOCK
MEDLEYS
MIDLAND
MIDLEGS
MIDLIFE
MIDLINE
MIDLIST
MUDLARK
NEDLAND
ODDLOTS
OLDLADY
OLDLINE
OLDLYME
PADLOCK
PODLIKE
REDLEGS
REDLINE
RODLESS
RODLIKE
SIDLING
SODLESS
WEDLOCK

••D•L••
ACDELCO
AEDILES
AUDILES
BEDELIA
CEDILLA
CODDLED
CODDLER
CODDLES
CUDDLED
CUDDLES
DEDALUS
DIDDLED
DIDDLER
DIDDLES
DIDDLEY
EIDOLIC
EIDOLON
ENDALLS
ENDPLAY
FIDDLED
FIDDLER
FIDDLES
FIDELES
FIDELIA
FIDELIO
FIDELIS
FUDDLED
FUDDLES
HIDALGO
HUDDLED
HUDDLER
HUDDLES
INDULGE
JUDELAW
KIDULTS
MADALYN
MADELON
MEDALED
MEDDLED
MEDDLER
MEDDLES
MEDELES
MEDULLA
MIDDLEC
MIDDLED
MIDDLER
MIDDLES
MODELAS
MODELBS
MODELED
MODELER
MODELTS
MODULAR
MODULES
MODULUS
MUDDLED
MUDDLER
MUDDLES
MUDFLAP
MUDFLAT
MUDFLOW
NODULAR
NODULED
NODULES
OLDBLUE
PADDLED
PADDLER
PADDLES
PEDALED
PEDALER
PEDDLED
PEDDLER
PEDDLES
PIDDLED
PIDDLES
PUDDLED
PUDDLES
REDALGA
REDCLAY
REDFLAG
RIDDLED
RIDDLER
RIDDLES
RODOLFO
RUDOLFI
RUDOLPH
SADDLED
SADDLER
SADDLES
SEDALIA
TIDALLY
TODDLED
TODDLER
TODDLES
UNDULAR
VIDALIA
WADDLED
WADDLER
WADDLES
WEDELED
WEDELNS
YODELED
YODELER
ZEDILLO

••D••L•
ADDABLE
ADDEDLY
ADDIBLE
ADDSALT
AUDIBLE
AUDIBLY
BADCALL
BADCOLD
BEDROLL
CEDILLA
CUDGELS
DIDWELL
EADGILS
ELDERLY
ENDABLE
ENDALLS
FADEDLY
GIDDILY
HADPULL
HIDABLE
INDWELL
INDWELT
JADEDLY
JODRELL
MADEILL
MEDULLA
MIDJULY
MIDSOLE
MUDDILY
MUDEELS
MUDHOLE
ODDBALL
OLDFILM
OLDGOLD
OLDPALS
OLDSALT
ORDEALS
ORDERLY
PUDGILY
RADIALS
RADICLE
REDCELL
REDEALS
REDEALT
REDIALS
REDPOLL
REDRILL
REDWOLF
RIDABLE
RUDDILY
TADPOLE
TIDALLY
UNDEALT
WADDELL
WEDDELL
ZEDILLO

••D•••L
BADCALL
BADGIRL
BEDEVIL
BEDRAIL
BEDROLL
BODEFUL
CODICIL
DIDWELL
FEDERAL
GODEVIL
HADPULL
INDWELL
JODRELL
MADEILL
MEDICAL
NODICAL
ODDBALL
OEDIPAL
OLDGIRL
ORDINAL
RADICAL
REDCELL
REDPOLL
REDRILL
REDTAIL
WADDELL
WEDDELL

•••DL••
BANDLET
BEADLES
BINDLES
BOODLES
BOWDLER
BRADLEE
BRADLEY
BRIDLED
BRIDLER
BRIDLES
BUNDLED
BUNDLER
BUNDLES
CANDLED
CANDLER
CANDLES
CODDLED
CODDLER
CODDLES
CRADLED
CRADLER
CRADLES
CUDDLED
CUDDLES
CURDLED
CURDLER
CURDLES
DANDLED
DANDLER
DANDLES
DAWDLED
DAWDLER
DAWDLES
DIDDLED
DIDDLER
DIDDLES
DIDDLEY
DOODLED
DOODLER
DOODLES
FEEDLOT
FIDDLED
FIDDLER
FIDDLES
FIEDLER
FINDLAY
FINDLEY
FONDLED
FONDLER
FONDLES
FORDLTD
FRIDLEY
FUDDLED
FUDDLES
GIRDLED
GIRDLER
GIRDLES
HANDLED
HANDLER
HANDLES
HANDLIN
HINDLEG
HOODLUM
HUDDLED
HUDDLER
HUDDLES
HURDLED
HURDLER
HURDLES
KINDLED
KINDLER
KINDLES
LAIDLOW
LANDLER
MAUDLIN
MEDDLED
MEDDLER
MEDDLES
MIDDLEC
MIDDLED
MIDDLER
MIDDLES
MUDDLED
MUDDLER
MUDDLES
NEEDLED
NEEDLER
NEEDLES
NOODLED
NOODLES
PADDLED
PADDLER
PADDLES
PEDDLED
PEDDLER
PEDDLES
PIDDLED
PIDDLES
POODLES
PUDDLED
PUDDLES
RIDDLED
RIDDLER
RIDDLES
RUNDLES
SADDLED
SADDLER
SADDLES
SANDLER
SANDLOT
SEEDLET
SKIDLID
STADLER
TODDLED
TODDLER
TODDLES
TOODLES
WADDLED
WADDLER
WADDLES
WOODLEY
WOODLOT

•••D•L•
ALUDELS
AMIDALA
AMIDOLS
BAWDILY
BEADILY
BIRDFLU
BOBDOLE
BRIDALS
CANDELA
CONDOLE
CORDELL
CRUDELY
DANDILY
DOWDILY
DUNDALK
GANDALF
GAUDILY
GIDDILY
GONDOLA
GOODALL
GRIDDLE
HANDILY
HARDILY
HEADILY
HOLDALL
HOWDULL
JIMDALE
KENDALL
KENDOLL
KORDELL
MANDALA
MANDELA
MENDELS
MONDALE
MOODILY
MUDDILY
NEEDILY
RAGDOLL
RANDALL
READILY
RENDELL
RONDELS
ROWDILY
RUDDILY
SANDALS
SANDFLY
SEEDILY
SHADILY
SNIDELY
SWADDLE
TARDILY
THEDELL
THEDOLE
TOLDALL
TOYDOLL
TVIDOLS
TWADDLE
TWIDDLE
TYNDALL
UNADULT
VANDALS
VERDELL
WADDELL
WEDDELL
WEEDILY
WENDELL
WINDILY
WORDILY

•••D••L
BIGDEAL
BUMDEAL
CARDIAL
CORDELL
CORDIAL
DOADEAL
GOODALL
GRADUAL
HANDFUL
HANDSEL
HEADFUL
HEEDFUL
HOLDALL
HOWDULL
JIMDIAL
KENDALL
KENDOLL
KORDELL
MANDREL
MINDFUL
MISDEAL
MISDIAL
MONDIAL
NEEDFUL
NEWDEAL
OUTDUEL
RAGDOLL
RANDALL
RAWDEAL
RENDELL
SLEDFUL
SUBDUAL
SUNDIAL
TENDRIL
THEDELL
TOLDALL
TOYDOLL
TYNDALL
UNIDEAL
VERDELL
WADDELL
WEDDELL
WENDELL

••••DL•
ACRIDLY
ADDEDLY
BLANDLY
BLINDLY
BRINDLE
BROADLY
CHEADLE
DATEDLY
DAZEDLY
DIRNDLS
DWINDLE
FADEDLY
FETIDLY
FIXEDLY
FLUIDLY
GELIDLY
GRANDLY
GRIDDLE
HUMIDLY
JADEDLY
KOWADLO
KYOODLE
LIVIDLY
LUCIDLY
LURIDLY
MCARDLE
MIXEDLY
MUTEDLY
NAKEDLY
NOTEDLY
PAVIDLY
PROUDLY
RABIDLY
RAPIDLY
RIGIDLY
ROUNDLY
SOLIDLY
SOUNDLY
SPINDLE
SPINDLY
STAIDLY
SWADDLE
SWINDLE
TEPIDLY
THIRDLY
TIMIDLY
TIREDLY
TREADLE
TRUNDLE
TWADDLE
TWEEDLE
TWIDDLE
UNGODLY
UNMADLY
UNSADLY
VALIDLY
VAPIDLY
VEXEDLY
VIVIDLY
WEIRDLY
WHEEDLE
WORLDLY

••••D•L
ACAUDAL
ARUNDEL
BIMODAL
BIPEDAL
BRENDEL
CHORDAL
CITADEL
CLAUDEL
CREEDAL
DREIDEL
FLUIDAL
GOMODEL
GRENDEL
INFIDEL
MONADAL
OVOIDAL
PALUDAL
REMODEL
ROUNDEL
SCANDAL
STRUDEL
SYNODAL
WEIRDAL
ZOOIDAL

•••••DL
ONTHEDL

DM•••••
DMYTRYK

D•M••••
DAMAGED
DAMAGES
DAMASKS
DAMASUS
DAMMERS
DAMMING
DAMNERS
DAMNING
DAMOSEL
DAMPDRY
DAMPENS
DAMPERS
DAMPEST
DAMPING
DAMPISH
DAMPMOP
DAMPOFF
DAMSELS
DAMSONS
DEMAGOG
DEMANDS
DEMARCO
DEMARET
DEMARKS
DEMASTS
DEMBUMS
DEMEANS
DEMENTO
DEMERGE
DEMERIT

DEMEROL
DEMESNE
DEMETER
DEMIGOD
DEMILLE
DEMISED
DEMISES
DEMISTS
DEMOING
DEMOLAY
DEMONIC
DEMONYM
DEMOTED
DEMOTES
DEMOTHS
DEMOTIC
DEMOUNT
DEMPSEY
DEMURER
DIMAGES
DIMBULB
DIMETER
DIMITRI
DIMMERS
DIMMEST
DIMMING
DIMNESS
DIMOUTS
DIMPLED
DIMPLES
DIMSOUT
DIMVIEW
DIMWITS
DOMAINE
DOMAINS
DOMECAR
DOMICAL
DOMICIL
DOMINGO
DOMINIC
DOMINOS
DOMINUS
DRMARIO
DRMCCOY
DRMELFI
DUMBEST
DUMBING
DUMDUMS
DUMMIED
DUMMIES
DUMMYUP
DUMPERS
DUMPIER
DUMPILY
DUMPING
DUMPISH
DUMPOUT
DUMPSON

D••M•••

DAEMONS
DAIMLER
DAMMERS
DAMMING
DAUMIER
DAYMARE
DEEMING
DEHMELT
DELMONT
DELMORE
DENMARK
DENMOMS
DERMATO
DESMOGS
DESMOND
DIAMOND
DIEMENS
DIMMERS
DIMMEST
DIMMING
DINMONT
DIOMEDE
DISMALS
DISMAST
DISMAYS
DISMISS
DOGMATA
DOLMANS
DOOMFUL
DOOMIER
DOOMING
DOOMSTO
DORMANT
DORMERS
DORMICE
DRAMADY
DRAMEDY
DRUMLIN
DRUMMED
DRUMMER
DRUMOUT
DRUMSET
DRUMSUP
DRYMOPS
DUMMIED
DUMMIES
DUMMYUP
DUUMVIR

D•••M••

DAHOMEY
DAMPMOP
DARKMAN
DECAMPS
DECIMAL
DEFAMED
DEFAMER
DEFAMES
DELIMAN
DELIMEN
DELIMIT
DENIMED
DHARMAS
DHARMIC
DILEMMA
DILLMAN
DISCMAN
DONIMUS
DOORMAN
DOORMAT
DOORMEN
DORFMAN
DRAWMAN
DRAWMEN
DRAYMAN
DRAYMEN
DREAMED
DREAMER
DREAMIN
DREAMOF
DREAMON
DREAMUP
DRUMMED
DRUMMER
DUHAMEL
DUSTMAN
DUSTMEN
DUSTMOP
DYNAMIC
DYNAMOS

D••••M•

DAYCAMP
DAYGAME
DAYTIME
DECRUMB
DEFOAMS
DEFORMS
DEFRAME
DEGERMS
DELORME
DEMBUMS
DENMOMS
DEPALMA
DESLUMS
DESTEMS
DEWORMS
DIADEMS
DIATOMS
DICTUMS
DIDSUMS
DIDTIME
DIGRAMS
DILEMMA
DIORAMA
DIOTIMA
DIPLOMA
DIRHAMS
DISARMS
DODGEMS
DOGCOMB
DOTBOMB
DOTCOMS
DRACHMA
DRINKME
DUCHAMP
DUMDUMS

D•••••M

DADAISM
DAYROOM
DECLAIM
DECORUM
DELIHAM
DEMONYM
DIAGRAM
DIGICAM
DINADAM
DOUBLEM
DUALISM
DUBNIUM
DUKEDOM

•DM••••

ADMIRAL
ADMIRED
ADMIRER
ADMIRES
ADMITTO
ADMIXED
ADMIXES
EDMEESE
EDMONDS
EDMUNDI
EDMUNDS

•D•M•••

ADAMANT
ADAMITE
ADAMSES
ADAMSON
EDEMATA
EDOMITE
ODDMENT

•D••M••

ADWOMAN
ADWOMEN
EDNAMAY
IDEAMAN
IDEAMEN
IDIAMIN
PDJAMES

•D•••M•

EDINAMN

•D••••M

CDALBUM

••DM•••

ANDMORE
ARDMORE
BADMOOD
BADMOVE
BEDMATE
CADMIUM
ENDMOST
GODMAMA
MIDMORN
MIDMOST
ODDMENT
OLDMAID
OLDMOON
REDMEAT
REDMOND
TEDMACK
WIDMARK

••D•M••

ABDOMEN
ANDAMAN
BADOMEN
ENDEMIC
EUDEMON
FADIMAN
MADAMES
MADAMEX
MADEMAD
MODEMED
RADAMES
RADOMES
SIDEMAN
SIDEMEN
UNDOMED

••D••M•

ANDIAMO
BADNAME
BADTIME
BEDLAMP
BEDLAMS
BEDTIME
BUDTIME
DIDSUMS
DIDTIME
DODGEMS
ENDGAME
GODMAMA
HADSOME
HADTIME
KIDCOMS
MEDIUMS
OLDLYME
OLDTIME
PODIUMS
REDARMY
REDEEMS
TEDEUMS
TEDIUMS

••D•••M

BADFORM
BEDROOM
BUDWORM
CADMIUM
DADAISM
FADDISM
HADROOM
JUDAISM
LUDDISM
MIDTERM
MODICUM
MUDROOM
OLDFILM
REDREAM
REDWORM
SIDEARM
TIDYSUM

•••DM••

BIRDMAN
BIRDMEN
BONDMAN
BONDMEN
FELDMAN
GOLDMAN
GOODMAN
GOODMEN
GRIDMAP
HEADMAN
HEADMEN
LANDMAN
LANDMEN
LEADMAN
LEADMEN
READMIT
REEDMAN
REEDMEN
ROADMAP
SANDMAN
SANDMEN
WEIDMAN
WILDMAN
WILDMEN
YARDMAN
YARDMEN

•••D•M•

ACADEME
ACADEMY
AIRDAMS
ANADEMS
BELDAME
BELDAMS
CONDEMN
DIADEMS
DUMDUMS
FANDOMS
ICEDAMS
MCADAMS
MTADAMS
ONEDIME
RCADOME
SKYDOME
TANDEMS
VENDOME
WINDOMS
WISDOMS

•••D••M

CARDIUM
EARDRUM
EPIDERM
FADDISM
FORDHAM
GOODAIM
HOODLUM
HUMDRUM
IRIDIUM
LORDJIM
LUDDISM
MAHDISM
MISDEEM
NEEDHAM
OILDRUM
PERDIEM
PREDOOM
RHODIUM
STADIUM
WYNDHAM
YARDARM

••••DM•

GRANDMA

••••D•M

AGENDUM
BOREDOM
CZARDOM
DINADAM
DUKEDOM
EARLDOM
FIEFDOM
FILMDOM
FREEDOM
GEEKDOM
GRANDAM
GREWDIM
GROWDIM
HASIDIM
HEIRDOM
KINGDOM
MACADAM
MILLDAM
POPEDOM
POTSDAM
QUONDAM
SERFDOM
SHAHDOM
STARDOM
TSARDOM
WOWEDEM

DN•••••

DNAASES
DNACODE
DNALABS
DNATEST
DNIEPER

D•N••••

DANANAS
DANBURY
DANCERS
DANCING
DANDERS
DANDIER
DANDIES
DANDIFY
DANDILY
DANDLED
DANDLER
DANDLES
DANELAW
DANEYKO
DANGELO
DANGERS
DANGLED
DANGLER
DANGLES
DANIELA
DANIELJ
DANIELS
DANIKEN
DANITES
DANKEST
DANNING
DANSEUR
DANTEAN
DANTEII
DANVERS
DENARII
DENDRON
DENEUVE
DENHAAG
DENIALS
DENIECE
DENIERS
DENIMED
DENISON
DENIZEN
DENMARK
DENMOMS
DENNEHY
DENNING
DENOTED
DENOTES
DENSELY
DENSEST
DENSIFY
DENSITY
DENTALS
DENTATE
DENTINE
DENTING
DENTINS
DENTIST
DENTOID
DENTONS
DENTURE
DENTYNE
DENUDED
DENUDER
DENUDES
DENYING
DINADAM
DINARIC
DINDINS
DINEDAT
DINEDIN
DINEDON
DINEOUT
DINESAT
DINESEN
DINESIN
DINESON
DINETTE
DINGBAT
DINGERS
DINGIER
DINGILY
DINGING
DINGLES
DINGOES
DINKIER
DINMONT
DINNERS
DINNING
DINTING
DONAHUE
DONATED
DONATEE
DONATES
DONATOR
DONATUS
DONEBAD
DONEFOR
DONEGAL
DONEGAN
DONETSK
DONGLES
DONIMUS
DONJONS
DONJOSE
DONJUAN
DONKEYS
DONKING
DONLEVY
DONNALL
DONNING
DONNISH
DONOHOE
DONOTGO
DONOVAN
DONRUSS
DONTASK
DONTBEE
DONTCRY
DONTLIE
DUNAWAY
DUNCISH
DUNDALK
DUNEDIN
DUNGEON
DUNKERS
DUNKING
DUNKIRK
DUNLINS
DUNLOPS
DUNNAGE
DUNNERS
DUNNING
DUNSTAN
DYNAMIC
DYNAMOS
DYNASTS
DYNASTY
DYNODES

D••N•••

DAMNERS
DAMNING
DANNING
DARNELL
DARNERS
DARNING
DAUNTED
DAUNTER
DAWNING
DAWNSON
DEANERY
DENNEHY
DENNING
DERNIER
DIGNIFY
DIGNITY
DIMNESS
DINNERS
DINNING
DIPNETS
DIRNDLS
DJINNIS
DOGNAPS
DOINGIN
DOINGOK
DOINGSO
DOINGTO
DOINGUP
DONNALL
DONNING
DONNISH
DOONEIN
DOWNBOW
DOWNERS
DOWNIER
DOWNING
DOWNPAT
DRANKIN
DRANKTO
DRANKUP
DRINKER
DRINKIN
DRINKME
DRINKTO
DRINKUP
DRONEON
DRONERS
DRONING
DRONISH
DRUNKEN
DRUNKER
DRYNESS
DUBNIUM
DUENNAS
DUNNAGE
DUNNERS
DUNNING
DURNING
DWINDLE

D•••N••

DANANAS
DAPHNES
DAPHNIA
DAPHNIS
DARENOT
DATINGS
DAVINCI
DEBONED
DEBONES
DEBUNKS
DECANTS
DECENCY
DEFANGS
DEFENCE
DEFENDS
DEFENSE
DEFINED
DEFINER
DEFINES
DEFUNCT
DEFUNDS
DEIGNED
DEIGNTO
DEJUNKS
DELANEY
DELINTS
DEMANDS
DEMENTO
DEMONIC
DEMONYM
DEPENDS
DEPONED
DEPONER
DEPONES
DERANGE
DERONDA
DETENTE
DETENTS
DETUNED
DETUNES
DIGINTO
DIPINTO
DIURNAL
DIVINED
DIVINER
DIVINES
DJINNIS
DOCENTS
DOESNOT
DOITNOW
DOLUNCH
DOMINGO
DOMINIC
DOMINOS
DOMINUS
DOUANES
DOYENNE
DOZENTH
DRAGNET
DRAINED
DRAINER
DRAWNIN
DRAWNON
DRAWNTO
DRAWNUP
DROPNET
DROWNED
DUENNAS
DUGINTO
DUGONGS
DURANCE
DURANGO
DURANTE

D••••N•

DABBING
DABHAND
DACRONS
DADOING
DAEMONS
DALTONS
DAMMING
DAMNING
DAMPENS
DAMPING
DAMSONS
DANCING
DANNING
DAPPING
DARKENS
DARLENE
DARLING
DARNING
DARTING
DASHING
DATSUNS
DAUBING
DAWKINS
DAWNING
DAYLONG
DAYSEND
DAYSINN
DAYTONA
DEACONS
DEADEND
DEADENS
DEAFENS
DEALING
DEARONE
DECKING
DECLINE
DEEDING
DEEMING
DEEPEND
DEEPENS
DEFCONS
DEFIANT
DEFYING
DEHORNS
DEICING
DEKEING
DELEING
DELMONT
DELTONA
DELVING
DEMEANS
DEMESNE
DEMOING
DEMOUNT
DENNING
DENTINE
DENTING
DENTINS
DENTONS
DENTYNE
DENYING
DEPLANE
DERRING
DERWENT
DESCANT
DESCEND
DESCENT
DESIGNS
DESMOND
DESPINA
DESPOND
DESTINE
DESTINO
DESTINY
DETAINS
DEUCING
DEVEINS
DEVIANT
DEWLINE
DEYOUNG
DIAHANN
DIALING
DIAMOND
DICKENS
DIDFINE
DIEMENS
DIETING
DIGGING
DILUENT
DIMMING
DINDINS
DINGING
DINMONT
DINNING
DINTING
DIOXINS
DIPPING
DIRKING
DISBAND
DISCING
DISHING
DISKING
DISOWNS
DISSENT
DISSING
DISTANT
DISTEND
DIZAINS
DOBBINS
DOCKING
DODGING
DOFFING
DOGBANE
DOGBONE
DOGGING
DOGGONE
DOGRUNS
DOLLING
DOLMANS
DOMAINE
DOMAINS
DONJONS
DONKING
DONNING
DOOMING
DORMANT
DOSSING
DOTTING
DOUSING
DOWLING
DOWNING
DOWRONG
DOWSING
DOYENNE
DRAGONS
DRAPING
DRAWING
DRAYING
DRIVING
DRONING
DROPINS
DRQUINN
DRYRUNS
DUBBING
DUCKING
DUCTING
DUELING
DUETING
DULLING
DUMBING
DUMPING
DUNKING
DUNLINS
DUNNING
DUODENA
DUOTONE
DURNING
DURWENT
DUSKING
DUSTING

D•••••N

DAKOTAN
DANIKEN
DANTEAN
DARKMAN
DARKTAN
DARLEEN
DARTGUN
DAUPHIN
DAVISON
DAWNSON
DAYSINN
DEADPAN
DEALSIN
DEALTIN

DEARDEN
DECAGON
DEEPTAN
DEHAVEN
DELIMAN
DELIMEN
DENDRON
DENISON
DENIZEN
DESTAIN
DETRAIN
DEXTRIN
DIAHANN
DIALSIN
DIAPHAN
DICKSON
DICTION
DIEDOWN
DILLMAN
DINEDIN
DINEDON
DINESEN
DINESIN
DINESON
DIRKSEN
DISCERN
DISCMAN
DISDAIN
DISHPAN
DISJOIN
DIVEDIN
DIVESIN
DOAGAIN
DODGSON
DOESKIN
DOINGIN
DOLPHIN
DONEGAN
DONJUAN
DONOVAN
DOONEIN
DOORMAN
DOORMEN
DORFMAN
DOTEDON
DOTESON
DOUBLEN
DRAGOON
DRAGSIN
DRAGSON
DRANKIN
DRAWMAN
DRAWMEN
DRAWNIN
DRAWNON
DRAWSIN
DRAWSON
DRAYMAN
DRAYMEN
DRAYTON
DRBROWN
DREAMIN
DREAMON
DREGION
DRESDEN
DRESSIN
DRIFTIN
DRINKIN
DRIPPAN
DRIPSON
DRISTAN
DRIVEIN
DRONEON
DROPSIN
DROVEIN
DRQUINN
DRSLOAN
DRUMLIN
DRUNKEN
DRUZEAN
DRUZIAN
DUCKPIN
DUDGEON
DUMPSON
DUNEDIN
DUNGEON
DUNSTAN
DUSTBIN
DUSTGUN
DUSTMAN
DUSTMEN
DUSTPAN
DWELLIN
DWELLON
DWELTON

•DN••••

ADNOUNS
EDNAMAY

•D•N•••

ADENINE
ADENOID
ADONAIS
EDINAMN
IDENTIC
ODDNESS
ODINGON
ODONTIA

•D••N••

ADDENDA
ADDENDS
ADDONTO
ADJUNCT
ADORNED
ADORNER
ADRENAL
ADVANCE
ADVENTS
EDASNER
EDGINGS
EDMONDS
EDMUNDI
EDMUNDS

•D•••N•

ADAMANT
ADDLING
ADELINA
ADELINE
ADENINE
ADJOINS
ADNOUNS
ADORING
ADRIANA
EDDYING
EDITING
EDUCING
ODDMENT
ODORANT
RDLAING

•D••••N

ADAMSON
ADDEDIN
ADDEDON
ADDISON
ADJOURN
ADWOMAN
ADWOMEN
BDALTON
EDGEDIN
EDGESIN
EDINAMN
EDITION
IDAHOAN
IDEAMAN
IDEAMEN
IDIAMIN
ODESSAN
ODINGON

••DN•••

BADNAME
BADNESS
BADNEWS
BEDNORZ
ENDNOTE
KIDNAPS
KIDNEYS
MADNESS
MIDNOON
NUDNIKS
ODDNESS
OLDNAVY
OLDNESS
OLDNEWS
OLDNICK
REDNECK
REDNESS
REDNINE
REDNOSE
SADNESS

••D•N••

ADDENDA
ADDENDS
ADDONTO
ALDENTE
ANDANTE
ARDENCY
BADENDS
BADENOV
BODINGS
CADENCE
CADENCY
CADENZA
ENDINGS
FEDINTO
GODUNOV
HADANIP
HEDONIC
HIDINGS
INDENTS
LADINGS
LADINOS
LADYNAS
LEDINTO
MADONNA
OGDENUT
ORDINAL
ORDINES
ORDONEZ
PEDANTS
PUDENCY
REDANTS
REDONDO
RIDINGS
RODENTS
SEDONAS
SIDINGS
STDENIS
TIDINGS
UNDINES
WIDENED
WIDENER
ZEDONKS

••D••N•

ADDLING
ANDEANS
BADHAND
BADLAND
BEDDING
BIDDING
BODKINS
BUDDING
BUDGING
CADGING
CODEINE
DADOING
DIDFINE
DODGING
EDDYING
ENDLINE
ENDLONG
ENDPINS
ENDRUNS
ENDUING
ENDZONE
FADEINS
FTDIXNJ
FUDGING
GADDING
GIDEONS
GODLING
GODSEND
GODSENT
GODSONS
HADDONE
HADRONS
HEDGING
HODDING
HYDRANT
INDIANA
INDIANS
JUDEANS
JUDGING
KEDGING
KIDDING
LADLING
LADRONE
LIDWINA
LODGING
MADDENS
MADDING
MADEONE
MADONNA
MEDIANS
MEDIANT
MIDJUNE
MIDLAND
MIDLINE
MODERNE
MODERNS
MUDDING
MUDHENS
NEDLAND
NODDING
NUDGING
ODDMENT
OLDHAND
OLDLINE
OLDSONG
ORDAINS
PADDING
PADRONE
PADUANS
PIDGINS
PUDDING
RADIANS
RADIANT
REDARNS
REDBONE
REDCENT
REDDENS
REDDING
REDFINS
REDHENS
REDKING
REDLINE
REDMOND
REDNINE
REDOING
REDOUND
REDPINE
REDPONY
REDSUNS
REDWINE
REDWING
REDYING
REDZONE
RIDDING
RIDGING
RODDING
SADDENS
SADSONG
SIDDONS
SIDEONE
SIDLING
SODDING
SUDSING
TIDYING
UNDOING
UNDRUNK
UNDYING
WADDING
WADKINS
WEDDING
WEDELNS
WEDGING
ZADKINE

••D•••N

ABDOMEN
ADDEDIN
ADDEDON
ADDISON
ALDUBIN
ANDAMAN
ANDIRON
ANDSOON
ANDTHEN
AUDUBON
BADOMEN
BADSIGN
BEDDOWN
BEDIZEN
BEDOUIN
DODGSON
DUDGEON
EIDOLON
ENDEDIN
ENDEDON
EUDEMON
FADEDIN
FADESIN
FADIMAN
GADSDEN
GUDGEON
HADBEEN
HADRIAN
HEDISON
INDIGEN
INDRAWN
KIDSKIN
LADYKIN
LODGEIN
MADALYN
MADCHEN
MADEFUN
MADELON
MADERUN
MADIGAN
MADISON
MEDUSAN
MIDIRON
MIDMORN
MIDNOON
MIDTEEN
MIDTOWN
OLDBEAN
OLDMOON
OLDTOWN
ORDERIN
PIDGEON
RADIOIN
REDDAWN
REDFERN
REDRAWN
REDSFAN
REDSKIN
RIDESIN
SIDEMAN
SIDEMEN
SODACAN
UNDRAWN
VIDICON
WADEDIN
WADESIN
WEDGEIN
WIDGEON

•••DN••

GARDNER
GOODNIK
LARDNER
LINDNER
NEEDNOT
PARDNER
SAIDNAY

•••D•N•

ABIDING
ALADINE
ALLDONE
ANODYNE
BALDING
BANDANA
BANDING
BEADING
BEDDING
BENDING
BIDDING
BINDING
BIRDING
BLADING
BONDING
BORDONI
BOUDINS
BUDDING
BURDENS
CANDENT
CARDING
CHIDING
COLDONE
CONDONE
CORDING
CORDONS
CURDING
DEADEND
DEADENS
DEEDING
DINDINS
DUODENA
ELIDING
ELUDING
ERODENT
ERODING
EVADING
EVIDENT
EXUDING
FEEDING
FENDING
FEUDING
FINDING
FOLDING
FONDANT
FORDING
FORDONE
FRODING
FUNDING
GADDING
GARDENA
GARDENS
GAUDENS
GELDING
GETDONE
GILDING
GIRDING
GLIDING
GOADING
GOLDING
GOLDONI
GOODING
GOODONE
GOTDONE
GRADING
GUIDING
GULDENS
HADDONE
HALDANE
HANDING
HARDENS
HARDING
HASDONE
HEADEND
HEADING
HEEDING
HERDING
HODDING
HOLDING
HOODING
HORDING
HOUDINI
HOYDENS
ILLDONE
ITSDONE
JARDINE
JARDINS
JORDANA
KIDDING
LANDING
LANDINI
LARDING
LARDONS
LAUDING
LEADENS
LEADING
LEADINS
LENDING
LINDENS
LOADING
LOIDING
LORDING
LOUDENS
LYNDONB
MADDENS
MADDING
MAIDENS
MANDANS
MELDING
MENDING
MINDING
MISDONE
MOLDING
MORDANT
MORDENT
MUDDING
MUNDANE
NEEDING
NODDING
NOTDONE
OUTDONE
OXIDANT
PADDING
PARDONS
PENDANT
PENDENT
PENDING
PONDING
PREDENY
PRIDING
PRUDENT
PUDDING
RAIDING
READING
REDDENS
REDDING
REEDING
RENDING
RIDDING
RODDING
SADDENS
SANDING
SARDINE
SEEDING
SENDING
SHADING
SIDDONS
SLIDING
SODDING
SORDINI
SORDINO
SPADING
STUDENT
TENDING
TENDONS
TRADING
TRIDENT
VANDINE
VENDING
VERDANT
VERDINS
VIADENT
VICDANA
VOIDING
WADDING
WARDENS
WARDING
WEDDING
WEEDING
WELDING
WENDING
WILDING
WILDONE
WINDING
WOODING
WORDING
WORDONE
YARDING

•••D••N

ABIDJAN
ACADIAN
ALADDIN
AVIDFAN
BALDWIN
BARDEEN
BEDDOWN
BIRDMAN
BIRDMEN
BOGDOWN
BONDMAN
BONDMEN
BOWDOIN
BOWDOWN
BUYDOWN
CALDRON
CHIDDEN
CONDEMN
CONDIGN
CRYDOWN
CUTDOWN
DEADPAN
DENDRON
DIEDOWN
DISDAIN
FEEDBIN
FEEDSIN
FEEDSON
FELDMAN
FOLDSIN
GETDOWN
GLADDEN
GLIDEIN
GOLDARN
GOLDMAN
GOLDWYN
GOODMAN
GOODMEN
GOODSON
GOODWIN
GORDIAN
GOTDOWN
HANDGUN
HANDLIN
HANDSIN
HANDSON
HARDPAN
HARDTEN
HARDWON
HEADMAN
HEADMEN
HEADPIN
HEADSIN
HOEDOWN
HOLDSIN
HOLDSON
ICEDOWN
ICHDIEN
JOTDOWN
LANDMAN
LANDMEN
LAYDOWN
LEADMAN
LEADMEN
LEADSIN
LEADSON
LETDOWN
LIEDOWN
LOADSIN
LOWDOWN
MARDIAN
MAUDLIN
MOWDOWN
MULDOON
ONEDOWN
OVIDIAN
PATDOWN
PINDOWN
PREDAWN
PRODSON
PUTDOWN
RAEDAWN
RAMDOWN
RANDOWN
READORN
READSIN
READSON
REDDAWN
REEDMAN
REEDMEN
RHODIAN
RUBDOWN
RUNDOWN
SANDMAN
SANDMEN
SATDOWN
SENDSIN
SENDSON
SETDOWN
SHEDSON
SHODDEN
SITDOWN
SLIDEIN
SMIDGEN
SUNDOWN
TIEDOWN
TIPDOWN
TOPDOWN
TRADEIN
TRADEON
TRODDEN
TRUDGEN
VANDIEN
VANDUYN
WEIDMAN
WETDOWN
WILDMAN
WILDMEN
WOODBIN
WOODSON
YARDMAN
YARDMEN

••••DN•

ARIADNE
COULDNT
ECHIDNA
ISAIDNO
JUNKDNA
VOTEDNO
WOULDNT

••••D•N

ABANDON
ACTEDIN
ACTEDON
ADDEDIN
ADDEDON
ALADDIN
ALMADEN
ASKEDIN
BASEDON
BLENDIN
BLUNDEN
BORODIN
BOXEDIN
BRAEDEN
BRANDON
BRENDAN
BRENDON
BROADEN
BUILDIN
BUILDON
CAGEDIN
CAVEDIN
CELADON
CHIDDEN
CLUEDIN
CROWDIN
DEARDEN
DINEDIN
DINEDON
DIVEDIN
DOTEDON
DRESDEN
DUNEDIN
EASEDIN
EASEDON
EDGEDIN
EGGEDON
ENDEDIN
ENDEDON
FACEDON
FADEDIN
FILEDIN
FIREDON
FIXEDON
FRIEDAN
GADSDEN
GAZEDON
GGORDON
GLADDEN
GLUEDON
GUERDON
HERNDON
HIREDON
HOMEDIN
HONEDIN
INKEDIN
JOURDAN
KEYEDIN
KEYEDON
KRAMDEN
LANGDON
LASTDON
LIVEDIN
LIVEDON
LONGDEN
LUREDIN
MACEDON
MARSDEN
MAULDIN
MERIDEN
MIXEDIN
MOVEDIN
MOVEDON
MUSEDON
NEVADAN
NOSEDIN
ONANDON
OPTEDIN
PALADIN
PILEDIN
PILEDON
PIPEDIN
RACEDIN
RAKEDIN
RAMADAN
RAPIDAN
REARDON
REWIDEN
RIORDAN
ROPEDIN
ROUNDON
RULEDON
RWANDAN
SALADIN
SAVEDON
SEWEDON
SHELDON
SHODDEN
SNOWDON
SPENDON
SPIEDON
STANDIN
STANDON
STOODIN
STOODON
TAPEDON
TOLEDAN
TOWEDIN
TREADON
TRIEDON
TRODDEN
TUNEDIN
TYPEDIN
UGANDAN
UNLADEN
UPANDIN
URGEDON
VALADON
VOTEDIN
VOTEDON
WADEDIN
WAVEDIN
WHAUDEN
WIREDIN

DO•••••

DOADEAL
DOAGAIN
DOASIDO
DOBBINS
DOCENTS
DOCKAGE
DOCKERS
DOCKETS
DOCKING
DOCTORS
DODDERS
DODDERY
DODGEMS
DODGERS
DODGIER
DODGING
DODGSON
DOEEYED
DOESBAD
DOESFOR
DOESKIN

DOESNOT
DOESTOO
DOEUVRE
DOFFERS
DOFFING
DOGAPES
DOGBANE
DOGBEDS
DOGBERT
DOGBITE
DOGBONE
DOGBOOT
DOGBOWL
DOGCART
DOGCHEW
DOGCHOW
DOGCOAT
DOGCOMB
DOGDAYS
DOGDOOR
DOGEARS
DOGFACE
DOGFISH
DOGFLEA
DOGFOOD
DOGGATE
DOGGETT
DOGGIER
DOGGIES
DOGGING
DOGGISH
DOGGONE
DOGHAIR
DOGLEGS
DOGLESS
DOGLIKE
DOGMATA
DOGNAPS
DOGPILE
DOGRACE
DOGREAT
DOGROSE
DOGRUNS
DOGSAGE
DOGSEAR
DOGSHOW
DOGSITS
DOGSLED
DOGSTAR
DOGTAGS
DOGTAIL
DOGTICK
DOGTOYS
DOGTROT
DOGVEST
DOGWOOD
DOHERTY
DOIDARE
DOILIES
DOINGIN
DOINGOK
DOINGSO
DOINGTO
DOINGUP
DOITNOW
DOLEFUL
DOLEOUT
DOLLARS
DOLLIED
DOLLIES
DOLLING
DOLLISH
DOLLOPS
DOLLSUP
DOLMANS
DOLORES
DOLOURS
DOLPHIN
DOLTISH
DOLUNCH
DOMAINE
DOMAINS
DOMECAR
DOMICAL
DOMICIL
DOMINGO
DOMINIC
DOMINOS
DOMINUS
DONAHUE
DONATED
DONATEE
DONATES
DONATOR
DONATUS
DONEBAD
DONEFOR
DONEGAL
DONEGAN
DONETSK
DONGLES
DONIMUS
DONJONS
DONJOSE
DONJUAN
DONKEYS
DONKING
DONLEVY
DONNALL
DONNING
DONNISH
DONOHOE
DONOTGO
DONOVAN
DONRUSS
DONTASK
DONTBEE
DONTCRY
DONTLIE
DOODADS
DOODLED
DOODLER
DOODLES
DOOLIES
DOOMFUL
DOOMIER
DOOMING
DOOMSTO
DOONEIN
DOORDIE
DOORMAN
DOORMAT
DOORMEN
DOORWAY
DOOUTOF
DOOVERS
DOOWOPS
DOOZERS
DOOZIES
DOPEOUT
DOPIEST
DOPPLER
DORFMAN
DORIGHT
DORITOS
DORKIER
DORMANT
DORMERS
DORMICE
DOROTHY
DORSALS
DORSETT
DORSEYS
DOSADOS
DOSAGES
DOSHOTS
DOSIDOS
DOSSALS
DOSSIER
DOSSING
DOTAGES
DOTARDS
DOTBOMB
DOTCOMS
DOTDASH
DOTEDON
DOTESON
DOTLIKE
DOTRICE
DOTTERS
DOTTIER
DOTTILY
DOTTING
DOTTLES
DOUANES
DOUBLEA
DOUBLEB
DOUBLEC
DOUBLED
DOUBLEE
DOUBLEF
DOUBLEG
DOUBLEH
DOUBLEI
DOUBLEJ
DOUBLEK
DOUBLEL
DOUBLEM
DOUBLEN
DOUBLEO
DOUBLEP
DOUBLEQ
DOUBLER
DOUBLES
DOUBLET
DOUBLEU
DOUBLEV
DOUBLEW
DOUBLEX
DOUBLEY
DOUBLEZ
DOUBTED
DOUBTER
DOUBTIT
DOUCEUR
DOUGHTY
DOUGLAS
DOUREST
DOUSERS
DOUSING
DOVEBAR
DOVECOT
DOVELET
DOVERDE
DOWAGER
DOWDIER
DOWDIES
DOWDILY
DOWERED
DOWLING
DOWNBOW
DOWNERS
DOWNIER
DOWNING
DOWNPAT
DOWRIES
DOWRONG
DOWSERS
DOWSING
DOYENNE
DOZENTH
DOZEOFF
DOZIEST

D•O••••

DEODARS
DEODATO
DEORBIT
DIOCESE
DIOMEDE
DIOPTER
DIORAMA
DIORITE
DIOTIMA
DIOXIDE
DIOXINS
DOODADS
DOODLED
DOODLER
DOODLES
DOOLIES
DOOMFUL
DOOMIER
DOOMING
DOOMSTO
DOONEIN
DOORDIE
DOORMAN
DOORMAT
DOORMEN
DOORWAY
DOOUTOF
DOOVERS
DOOWOPS
DOOZERS
DOOZIES
DROGUES
DROLLER
DRONEON
DRONERS
DRONING
DRONISH
DROOLED
DROOLER
DROOPED
DROPBOX
DROPCAP
DROPINS
DROPLET
DROPNET
DROPOFF
DROPOUT
DROPPED
DROPPER
DROPSBY
DROPSIN
DROPSIT
DROPTOP
DROSSES
DROUGHT
DROVEAT
DROVEBY
DROVEIN
DROVERS
DROVETO
DROVEUP
DROWNED
DROWSED
DROWSES
DROXIES
DUODENA
DUOPOLY
DUOTONE

D••O•••

DACOSTA
DADOING
DAHOMEY
DAKOTAN
DAKOTAS
DAMOSEL
DEBOITE
DEBONED
DEBONES
DEBORAH
DEBOULE
DECOCTS
DECODED
DECODER
DECODES
DECOLOR
DECORUM
DECOYED
DECOYER
DEFOAMS
DEFOCUS
DEFORMS
DEHORNS
DELORIS
DELORME
DELOUSE
DEMOING
DEMOLAY
DEMONIC
DEMONYM
DEMOTED
DEMOTES
DEMOTHS
DEMOTIC
DEMOUNT
DENOTED
DENOTES
DEPONED
DEPONER
DEPONES
DEPORTS
DEPOSAL
DEPOSED
DEPOSER
DEPOSES
DEPOSIT
DEPOWER
DERONDA
DESOTOS
DETOURS
DETOXED
DETOXES
DEVOIRS
DEVOLVE
DEVORES
DEVOTED
DEVOTEE
DEVOTES
DEVOURS
DEWORMS
DEYOUNG
DIDOVER
DIEOFFS
DIMOUTS
DIPOLAR
DIPOLES
DISOBEY
DISOWNS
DIVORCE
DOLORES
DOLOURS
DONOHOE
DONOTGO
DONOVAN
DOROTHY
DROOLED
DROOLER
DROOPED
DUGONGS
DUGOUTS
DYNODES

D•••O••

DACRONS
DAEMONS
DAEWOOS
DAGWOOD
DALTONS
DAMPOFF
DAMSONS
DARTOFF
DASBOOT
DASHOFF
DAYBOOK
DAYHOPS
DAYJOBS
DAYLONG
DAYROOM
DAYSOFF
DAYTONA
DEACONS
DEALOUT
DEARONE
DEBTORS
DECKOUT
DECLOTS
DEFCONS
DEFROCK
DEFROST
DEGHOST
DELMONT
DELMORE
DELSOLS
DELTOID
DELTONA
DELTORO
DENMOMS
DENTOID
DENTONS
DEPLORE
DEPLOYS
DESMOGS
DESMOND
DESPOIL
DESPOND
DESPOTS
DESTOCK
DETROIT
DEVIOUS
DIABOLO
DIALOGS
DIALOUT
DIAMOND
DIATOMS
DIAVOLO
DICKORY
DIDGOOD
DIDTOAT
DIEBOLD
DIEDOFF
DIEDOUT
DIEDOWN
DIESOFF
DIESOUT
DIGGORY
DIGLOTS
DIGSOUT
DIMSOUT
DINEOUT
DINGOES
DINMONT
DIPLOID
DIPLOMA
DISCOED
DISCOID
DISCORD
DISHOUT
DISJOIN
DISPORT
DISPOSE
DISROBE
DISTORT
DITTOED
DNACODE
DOCTORS
DOGBONE
DOGBOOT
DOGBOWL
DOGCOAT
DOGCOMB
DOGDOOR
DOGFOOD
DOGGONE
DOGROSE
DOGTOYS
DOGWOOD
DOLEOUT
DOLLOPS
DONJONS
DONJOSE
DOOWOPS
DOPEOUT
DOSHOTS
DOTBOMB
DOTCOMS
DOWRONG
DOZEOFF
DRAGOFF
DRAGONS
DRAGOON
DRAGOTI
DRAGOUT
DRAWOFF
DRAWOUT
DRBROWN
DREWOFF
DREWOUT
DROPOFF
DROPOUT
DRSLOAN
DRSPOCK
DRUMOUT
DRYDOCK
DRYFOGS
DRYHOLE
DRYMOPS
DRYROTS
DUBIOUS
DUCKOUT
DUMPOUT
DUNLOPS
DUOPOLY
DUOTONE
DUSTOFF
DUTEOUS
DYEJOBS
DYELOTS
DYEWOOD

D••••O•

DACAPOS
DAEWOOS
DAGWOOD
DAMPMOP
DARENOT
DASBOOT
DASHDOT
DASHPOT
DAVEKOZ
DAVISON
DAWNSON
DAYBOOK
DAYROOM
DEARGOD
DECAGON
DECALOG
DECAPOD
DECOLOR
DEEDBOX
DEMAGOG
DEMEROL
DEMIGOD
DENDRON
DENISON
DESKTOP
DESOTOS
DESTROY
DEVELOP
DEVISOR
DEWDROP
DIABLOS
DIARIOS
DICKSON
DICTION
DIDEROT
DIDGOOD
DIEDFOR
DIESFOR
DIGSFOR
DILATOR
DILUTOR
DINEDON
DINESON
DISAVOW
DISTROS
DIVISOR
DODGSON
DOESFOR
DOESNOT
DOESTOO
DOGBOOT
DOGCHOW
DOGDOOR
DOGFOOD
DOGSHOW
DOGTROT
DOGWOOD
DOINGOK
DOITNOW
DOMINOS
DONATOR
DONEFOR
DONOHOE
DOOUTOF
DORITOS
DOSADOS
DOSIDOS
DOTEDON
DOTESON
DOVECOT
DOWNBOW
DRAGOON
DRAGSON
DRAWNON
DRAWSON
DRAYTON
DRCHAOS
DREAMOF
DREAMON
DREGION
DRIPSON
DRMCCOY
DRONEON
DROPBOX
DROPTOP
DUDGEON
DUETTOS
DUKEDOM
DUMPSON
DUNGEON
DUSTMOP
DWELLON
DWELTON
DYEWOOD
DYNAMOS

D•••••O

DANEYKO
DANGELO
DARESTO
DAREZZO
DEALSTO
DEALTTO
DECARLO
DEFACTO
DEFERTO
DEIGNTO
DELICTO
DELILLO
DELTORO
DEMARCO
DEMENTO
DEODATO
DERECHO
DERMATO
DERRICO
DESTINO
DETECTO
DEUTERO
DIABOLO
DIALEDO
DIAVOLO
DICILLO
DIGINTO
DIPINTO
DOASIDO
DOESTOO
DOINGSO
DOINGTO
DOMINGO
DONOTGO
DOOMSTO
DOUBLEO
DRANKTO
DRAWNTO
DRAWSTO
DRINKTO
DRIVETO
DRMARIO
DROVETO
DUGINTO
DURANGO

•DO••••

ADOLLAR
ADOLPHE
ADONAIS
ADOPTED
ADOPTEE
ADOPTER
ADORERS
ADORING
ADORNED
ADORNER
EDOMITE
EDOUARD
IDOLISE
IDOLIST
IDOLIZE
IDOODIT
IDOTTER
ODONTIA
ODORANT
ODORFUL
ODORIZE
ODOROUS

•D•O•••

ADDONTO
ADJOINS
ADJOURN
ADNOUNS
ADSORBS
ADWOMAN
ADWOMEN
CDTOWER
EDMONDS
IDIOTIC
IDOODIT
JDPOWER

•D••O••

ADENOID
ADIPOSE
CDSTORE
EDGEOUT
EDITORS
EDITOUT
IDAHOAN
NDAKOTA
ODDJOBS
ODDLOTS
ODDSOCK
ODOROUS
SDAKOTA

•D•••O•

ADAGIOS
ADAMSON
ADAPTOR
ADDEDON
ADDISON
ADJUROR
ADVISOR
BDALTON
EDITION
EDUCTOR
IDIDTOO
ODDSHOE
ODINGON

•D••••O

ADAPTTO
ADAYAGO
ADDEDTO
ADDONTO
ADDUPTO
ADMITTO
EDGARDO
EDUARDO
IDIDTOO
IDSAYSO

••DO•••

ABDOMEN
ADDONTO
ALDORAY
ANDORRA
ANDOVER
ARDOURS
BADOMEN
BEDOUIN
DADOING
DIDOVER
EIDOLIC
EIDOLON
ENDORSE
ENDOWED
ENDOWER
FEDORAS
FEDOROV
FTDODGE
HADOVER
HEDONIC
INDOORS
INDORSE
INDOUBT
JUDOIST
JUDOKAS
LADOUCE
MADONNA
MIDOFFS
NODOUBT
OGDOADS
ORDONEZ
RADOMES
REDOAKS
REDOCKS
REDOING
REDONDO
REDOSED
REDOSES
REDOUBT
REDOUND
REDOUTS
REDOXES
RIDOTTO
RODOLFO
RUDOLFI
RUDOLPH
SEDONAS
SUDOKUS
UNDOCKS
UNDOERS
UNDOING
UNDOMED
WIDOWED
WIDOWER
ZEDONKS

••D•O••

ANDMORE
ANDROID
ANDROUS
ANDSOON
ARDMORE
ARDUOUS
BADBOYS
BADCOLD
BADDOGS
BADFORM
BADJOKE
BADLOTS
BADLOVE
BADMOOD
BADMOVE
BADWORD
BEDDOWN
BEDFORD
BEDLOES
BEDNORZ
BEDPOST
BEDROCK
BEDROLL
BEDROOM
BUDWORM
DIDGOOD
DIDTOAT
ENDLONG
ENDMOST
ENDNOTE
ENDZONE
FADEOUT
GIDEONS
GODHOOD
GODSONS
HADDOCK
HADDONE
HADRONS
HADROOM
HADSOME
HADTOBE
HIDEOUS
HIDEOUT
HYDROUS
INDOORS
KEDROVA
KIDCOMS
KIDROCK
LADHOOD
LADRONE
MADDOGS
MADEOFF
MADEONE
MADEOUT
MADLOCK
MEDFORD
MIDMORN
MIDMOST
MIDNOON
MIDSOLE
MIDTOWN
MUDHOLE
MUDROOM
NODSOFF
ODDJOBS
ODDLOTS
ODDSOCK
OLDBOYS
OLDDOGS
OLDFOGY
OLDGOLD
OLDJOKE
OLDMOON
OLDROSE
OLDSONG
OLDTOWN
PADDOCK
PADLOCK

PADRONE
RADFORD
RADIOAD
RADIODJ
RADIOED
RADIOER
RADIOIN
REDBONE
REDBOOK
REDCOAT
REDCODS
REDDOGS
REDDOTS
REDFORD
REDFOUR
REDHOTS
REDMOND
REDNOSE
REDPOLL
REDPONY
REDROBE
REDROOP
REDROOT
REDROSE
REDTOPS
REDWOLF
REDWOOD
REDWORM
REDZONE
RIDEOFF
RIDEOUT
RODEOFF
RODEOUT
SADSONG
SIDDONS
SIDEONE
SIDIOUS
SYDHOFF
TADPOLE
TEDIOUS
VIDEOED
VIDIOTS
WEDLOCK

••D••O•
ADDEDON
ADDISON
ANDIRON
ANDSOON
AUDITOR
AUDUBON
BADENOV
BADMOOD
BADSHOT
BEDROOM
BIDSFOR
DIDEROT
DIDGOOD
DODGSON
DUDGEON
EIDOLON
ENDEDON
ENDUROS
EUDEMON
FEDOROV
GODHOOD
GODUNOV
GUDGEON
HADACOW
HADAJOB
HADAROW
HADROOM
HEDISON
INDIGOS
LADADOG
LADHOOD
LADINOS
MADEFOR
MADELON
MADISON
MADUROS
MEDICOS
MIDIRON
MIDNOON
MUDFLOW
MUDROOM
ODDSHOE
OLDMOON
OLDPROS
OLDSHOE
PIDGEON
REDBOOK
REDROOP
REDROOT
REDSPOT
REDWOOD
SODAPOP
VIDICON
WIDGEON
ZYDECOS

••D•••O
ACDELCO
ADDEDTO
ADDONTO
ADDUPTO
ANDIAMO
FEDERKO
FEDINTO
FIDELIO
HIDALGO
LEDINTO
LEDUPTO
MODESTO
REDONDO
RIDESTO
RIDOTTO
RODOLFO
RODRIGO
SIDETWO
UNDERDO
UNDERGO
ZEDILLO

•••DO••
ACEDOUT
AGEDOUT
ALLDONE
ALTDORF
AMIDOLS
APODOUS
BADDOGS
BEDDOWN
BIGDOGS
BINDOFF
BOBDOLE
BOGDOWN
BORDONI
BOUDOIR
BOWDOIN
BOWDOWN
BUYDOWN
CANDOUR
CARDOOR
CARDOZO
CATDOOR
COLDONE
CONDOLE
CONDONE
CONDORS
CORDOBA
CORDONS
COYDOGS
CRYDOWN
CUTDOWN
DIEDOFF
DIEDOUT
DIEDOWN
DOGDOOR
DRYDOCK
EKEDOUT
EPIDOTE
FANDOMS
FENDOFF
FEODORI
FINDOUT
FOGDOGS
FOLDOUT
FORDOES
FORDONE
GETDONE
GETDOWN
GOLDONI
GONDOLA
GOODONE
GOTDONE
GOTDOWN
GUNDOGS
HADDOCK
HADDONE
HANDOFF
HANDOUT
HASDONE
HEADOFF
HEADOUT
HELDOFF
HELDOUT
HOEDOWN
HOLDOFF
HOLDOUT
HOODOOS
HOTDOGS
ICEDOUT
ICEDOWN
ILLDOIT
ILLDONE
ISADORA
ISADORE
ISIDORE
ITSDONE
JOTDOWN
KENDOLL
LAIDOFF
LAIDOUT
LAPDOGS
LARDONS
LAYDOWN
LEADOFF
LEADORE
LEADOUT
LENDOUT
LETDOWN
LIEDOWN
LINDORF
LOWDOWN
LYNDONB
MADDOGS
MANDOKI
MEADOWS
MEADOWY
MINDORO
MISDOER
MISDOES
MISDONE
MOLDOVA
MOWDOWN
MULDOON
MURDOCH
NORDOFF
NORDOWE
NOTDONE
OLDDOGS
ONEDOWN
OUTDOER
OUTDOES
OUTDONE
OUTDOOR
PADDOCK
PAIDOFF
PAIDOUT
PANDORA
PARDONS
PATDOWN
PETDOGS
PETDOOR
PETDOVE
PINDOWN
PREDOOM
PUTDOWN
PYEDOGS
RAGDOLL
RAMDOWN
RANDOWN
RCADOME
READOFF
READOPT
READORN
READOUT
REDDOGS
REDDOTS
RUBDOWN
RUNDOWN
SATDOWN
SEADOGS
SENDOFF
SENDOUT
SETDOWN
SHADOWS
SHADOWY
SIDDONS
SITDOWN
SKIDOOS
SKYDOME
SLIDOFF
SLIDOUT
SOLDOFF
SOLDOUT
SPEDOFF
SUNDOGS
SUNDOWN
TANDOOR
TEEDOFF
TENDONS
THEDOLE
TIEDOFF
TIEDOWN
TIPDOWN
TOLDOFF
TOPDOGS
TOPDOWN
TOYDOGS
TOYDOLL
TVIDOLS
TWODOOR
VAUDOIS
VENDOME
VENDORS
VERDOUX
VOIDOUT
VOODOOS
WALDORF
WARDOFF
WEEDOUT
WETDOWN
WILDONE
WINDOMS
WINDOWS
WINDOWY
WISDOMS
WORDONE

•••D•O•
AIRDROP
AULDSOD
BANDBOX
BIRDDOG
BLEDSOE
CALDRON
CARDOOR
CATDOOR
DEEDBOX
DENDRON
DEWDROP
DIEDFOR
DOGDOOR
EARDROP
EGGDROP
EYEDROP
FEEDLOT
FEEDSON
GOODDOG
GOODFOR
GOODJOB
GOODJOE
GOODSON
GUMDROP
HANDSON
HARDTOP
HARDWON
HEADFOR
HOLDSON
HOODOOS
IDIDTOO
LAIDFOR
LAIDLOW
LEADDOG
LEADSON
LETDROP
LIEDFOR
LINDROS
LLADROS
LOADSOF
MULDOON
NEEDNOT
OUTDOOR
OUTDROP
PAIDFOR
PETDOOR
PREDOOM
PRODSON
PRUDHOE
READFOR
READSON
ROADEOS
ROADHOG
SAIDBOO
SANDBOX
SANDHOG
SANDLOT
SCADSOF
SEEDPOD
SENDFOR
SENDSON
SHADROE
SHEDSON
SKIDDOO
SKIDOOS
SKIDROW
SLEDDOG
SOLDFOR
STUDIOS
SUEDFOR
TANDOOR
TRADEON
TWODOOR
USEDFOR
VIEDFOR
VOODOOS
WENDKOS
WILDDOG
WINDGOD
WINDSOR
WOODBOX
WOODLOT
WOODROW
WOODSON

•••D••O
ARTDECO
BANDIDO
BANDITO
BINDSTO
CARDOZO
CORDERO
DEODATO
FEEDSTO
HANDYTO
HEADSTO
HOLDSTO
HOWDEDO
HOWDYDO
IDIDTOO
LEADSTO
MINDORO
NEEDSTO
PERDIDO
READSTO
SAIDBOO
SAIDIDO
SENDSTO
SKIDDOO
SORDINO
TENDSTO
VERDUGO
WINDIGO

••••DO•
ABANDON
ACTEDON
ADDEDON
AHEADOF
AIKIDOS
ALBEDOS
ALOADOF
ASKEDOF
BASEDON
BIRDDOG
BOREDOM
BRANDON
BRENDON
BUILDON
BULLDOG
CELADON
COONDOG
CORNDOG
COTEDOR
CZARDOM
DASHDOT
DINEDON
DOSADOS
DOSIDOS
DOTEDON
DUKEDOM
EARLDOM
EASEDON
ECUADOR
EGGEDON
ENDEDON
ESCUDOS
ESTADOS
FACEDON
FIEFDOM
FILMDOM
FIREDOG
FIREDON
FIXEDON
FREEDOF
FREEDOM
GAZEDON
GEEKDOM
GGORDON
GLUEDON
GOODDOG
GUERDON
HAIRDOS
HANGDOG
HEARDOF
HEIRDOM
HERNDON
HIREDON
HUMIDOR
INAIDOF
JANEDOE
JOHNDOE
KEMIDOV
KEYEDON
KINGDOM
LADADOG
LANGDON
LAREDOS
LASTDON
LEADDOG
LIBIDOS
LIVEDON
LOSTDOG
MACEDON
MAKEDOS
MALEDOG
MALODOR
MARIDOS
MATADOR
MENUDOS
MIKADOS
MIRADOR
MOGADOR
MOONDOG
MOVADOS
MOVEDON
MUSEDON
MUSTDOS
NICEDOG
NOENDOF
ONANDON
OVERDOG
PAPADOC
PARADOR
PARADOX
PERIDOT
PICADOR
PILEDON
PLAYDOH
POPEDOM
POSTDOC
PROUDOF
REARDON
REENDOW
REREDOS
ROUNDON
RULEDON
SABADOS
SAVEDON
SERFDOM
SEWEDON
SHAHDOM
SHELDON
SHOWDOG
SKIDDOO
SLEDDOG
SNOWDON
SPEEDOS
SPENDON
SPIEDON
STANDON
STARDOM
STOODON
TAPEDON
THEODOR
TIREDOF
TOLEDOS
TONYDOW
TREADON
TRIEDON
TSARDOM
TUXEDOS
URGEDON
VALADON
VOTEDON
WEIRDOS
WILDDOG
WOLFDOG
XSANDOS

••••D•O
ADDEDTO
AMRADIO
BLINDTO
BOUNDTO
BOWEDTO
CAREDTO
CBRADIO
CLAUDIO
FLIEDTO
FMRADIO
GLUEDTO
HEWEDTO
HOPEDSO
HOPEDTO
ISAIDNO
KOWADLO
LOVEDTO
MOVEDTO
NOENDTO
ONVIDEO
OPTEDTO
PLEADTO
RACEDTO
SKIDDOO
SOANDSO
STANDTO
STOODTO
TRIEDTO
TUNEDTO
VOTEDNO
WAVEDTO
XMRADIO
YIELDTO

•••••DO
ALFREDO
AVOCADO
BANDIDO
BOIARDO
BRAVADO
BUSHIDO
CALANDO
CRUZADO
DIALEDO
DOASIDO
EDGARDO
EDUARDO
ELMUNDO
ELPRADO
FURTADO
GAMBADO
GERALDO
HAPKIDO
HOWDEDO
HOWDYDO
ISUREDO
MAKESDO
MCMURDO
MERCADO
NOCANDO
ORLANDO
PASSADO
PERDIDO
PICARDO
PLACIDO
QUERIDO
REDONDO
RENALDO
RICARDO
RINALDO
SAIDIDO
SAYSIDO
SECONDO
SUREIDO
TORNADO
TORPEDO
UNDERDO

DP•••••
DPLUSES

D•P••••
DAPHNES
DAPHNIA
DAPHNIS
DAPPING
DAPPLED
DAPPLES
DEPALMA
DEPARTS
DEPAULU
DEPECHE
DEPENDS
DEPESTS
DEPICTS
DEPLANE
DEPLETE
DEPLORE
DEPLOYS
DEPONED
DEPONER
DEPONES
DEPORTS
DEPOSAL
DEPOSED
DEPOSER
DEPOSES
DEPOSIT
DEPOWER
DEPRAVE
DEPRESS
DEPRIVE
DEPULPS
DEPUTED
DEPUTES
DIPINTO
DIPLOID
DIPLOMA
DIPNETS
DIPOLAR
DIPOLES
DIPPERS
DIPPIER
DIPPING
DIPTYCH
DOPEOUT
DOPIEST
DOPPLER

D••P•••
DAMPDRY
DAMPENS
DAMPERS
DAMPEST
DAMPING
DAMPISH
DAMPMOP
DAMPOFF
DAPPING
DAPPLED
DAPPLES
DAUPHIN
DAYPACK
DEEPEND
DEEPENS
DEEPEST
DEEPFAT
DEEPFRY
DEEPISH
DEEPRED
DEEPSEA
DEEPSET
DEEPSIX
DEEPSKY
DEEPTAN
DELPHIC
DEMPSEY
DESPAIR
DESPINA
DESPISE
DESPITE
DESPOIL
DESPOND
DESPOTS
DIAPERS
DIAPHAN
DIMPLED
DIMPLES
DIOPTER
DIPPERS
DIPPIER
DIPPING
DISPART
DISPELS
DISPLAY
DISPORT
DISPOSE
DISPUTE
DOGPILE
DOLPHIN
DOPPLER
DRAPERS
DRAPERY
DRAPING
DRIPDRY
DRIPPAN
DRIPPED
DRIPPER
DRIPSON
DROPBOX
DROPCAP
DROPINS
DROPLET
DROPNET
DROPOFF
DROPOUT
DROPPED
DROPPER
DROPSBY
DROPSIN
DROPSIT
DROPTOP
DRSPOCK
DRYPERS
DUMPERS
DUMPIER
DUMPILY
DUMPING
DUMPISH
DUMPOUT
DUMPSON
DUOPOLY

D•••P••
DACAPOS
DASHPOT
DAYSPAS
DEADPAN
DECAPOD
DECUPLE
DIGIPET
DISHPAN
DNIEPER
DOGAPES
DOWNPAT
DRIPPAN
DRIPPED
DRIPPER
DROOPED
DROPPED
DROPPER
DUCKPIN
DUSTPAN

D••••P•
DAYHOPS
DECAMPS
DECRYPT
DEPULPS
DEWLAPS
DIALUPS
DIDLAPS
DIGRAPH
DISRUPT
DOGNAPS
DOLLOPS
DOOWOPS
DRYMOPS
DUNLOPS
DUSTUPS

D•••••P
DAMPMOP
DAYCAMP
DAYTRIP
DEALSUP
DEALTUP
DESKTOP
DEVELOP
DEWDROP
DIALSUP
DICECUP
DIVVYUP
DOINGUP
DOLLSUP
DOUBLEP
DRAGSUP
DRANKUP
DRAWNUP
DRAWSUP
DREAMUP
DRESSUP
DRIEDUP
DRIESUP
DRIFTUP
DRINKUP
DRIVEUP
DROPCAP
DROPTOP
DROVEUP
DRUMSUP
DUCHAMP
DUDEDUP
DUDESUP
DUMMYUP
DUSTMOP

•DP••••
JDPOWER

•D•P•••
ADAPTED
ADAPTER
ADAPTOR
ADAPTTO
ADEPTAT
ADEPTER
ADEPTLY
ADIPOSE
ADOPTED
ADOPTEE
ADOPTER
ADSPACE

•D••P••
ADDUPTO
ADELPHI
ADOLPHE

•D••••P
ADDEDUP

••DP•••
BADPAST
BEDPOST
ENDPINS
ENDPLAY
GODPAPA
HADPULL
MUDPACK
MUDPIES

OLDPALS
OLDPROS
REDPINE
REDPOLL
REDPONY
TADPOLE

••D•P••

ADDUPTO
ENDUPAT
INDEPTH
JODHPUR
LEDUPTO
MADEPAR
OEDIPAL
OEDIPUS
REDSPOT
SODAPOP
UNDUPED

••D••P•

BADRAPS
BEDRAPE
DIDLAPS
GODPAPA
KIDNAPS
MADCAPS
MIDCAPS
REDCAPS
REDTAPE
REDTOPS
RUDOLPH
UNDRAPE

••D•••P

ADDEDUP
BADTRIP
BEDLAMP
BUDDYUP
DUDEDUP
DUDESUP
ENDEDUP
GIDDYAP
GIDDYUP
HADANIP
MEDIGAP
MIDSHIP
MUDFLAP
MUDWASP
OLDCHAP
ORDERUP
REDCHIP
REDROOP
RIDESUP
SODAPOP
TIDERIP

•••DP••

DEADPAN
GOODPAY
HARDPAN
HARDPUT
HEADPIN
HINDPAW
SANDPIT
SEEDPOD
WILDPIG

•••D•P•

FOLDUPS
HOLDUPS
LEADUPS
READAPT
READOPT
SENDUPS
UNADEPT
WINDUPS

•••D••P

AIRDROP
BEADSUP
BINDSUP
BUDDYUP
COLDCUP
CRUDSUP
DEWDROP
EARDROP
EGGDROP
EYEDROP
FOLDSUP
GIDDYAP
GIDDYUP
GOLDTIP
GRIDMAP
GUMDROP
HANDSUP
HARDTOP
HEADSUP
HOLDSUP
LANDSUP
LEADSUP
LETDROP
LOADSUP
NONDEEP
NONDRIP
OUTDROP
RANDEEP
READSUP
ROADMAP
RUNDEEP
SENDSUP
THEDEEP
TRADEUP
TWODEEP
WINDSUP

••••DP•

GRANDPA
MAANDPA
RATEDPG

••••D•P

ACTEDUP
ADDEDUP
AIREDUP
AMPEDUP
ANTEDUP
ASKEDUP
BEANDIP
BOARDUP
BONEDUP
BOUNDUP
BOXEDUP
BUILDUP
CAGEDUP
CAKEDUP
CLAMDIP
CLOUDUP
CRIEDUP
DRIEDUP
DUDEDUP
EASEDUP
ENDEDUP
FIREDUP
FIXEDUP
FLEADIP
FREEDUP
FRIEDUP
GASEDUP
HIKEDUP
HOLEDUP
HYPEDUP
KEYEDUP
LACEDUP
LINEDUP
MIXEDUP
MOVEDUP
NOSEDUP
OWNEDUP
PILEDUP
PIPEDUP
RACEDUP
RAKEDUP
RILEDUP
ROPEDUP
ROUNDUP
SAVEDUP
SEWEDUP
SIZEDUP
SPEEDUP
STANDUP
STOODUP
TAPEDUP
TONEDUP
TRUEDUP
TUNEDUP
TYPEDUP
WAKEDUP
WAXEDUP
WIPEDUP
WIREDUP
WISEDUP
WOUNDUP

D•Q••••

DEQUEUE
DRQUINN

D••Q•••

DAYQUIL

D•••Q••

DUBUQUE

D•••••Q

DOUBLEQ

•DQ••••

PDQBACH

••••DQ•

PSANDQS

DR•••••

DRABBER
DRABBLE
DRACHMA
DRACULA
DRAFTED
DRAFTEE
DRAFTER
DRAGEES
DRAGGED
DRAGGER
DRAGGLE
DRAGNET
DRAGOFF
DRAGONS
DRAGOON
DRAGOTI
DRAGOUT
DRAGSIN
DRAGSON
DRAGSUP
DRAINED
DRAINER
DRAMADY
DRAMEDY
DRANKIN
DRANKTO
DRANKUP
DRAPERS
DRAPERY
DRAPING
DRASTIC
DRATTED
DRAUGHT
DRAWBAR
DRAWEES
DRAWERS
DRAWING
DRAWLED
DRAWLER
DRAWMAN
DRAWMEN
DRAWNIN
DRAWNON
DRAWNTO
DRAWNUP
DRAWOFF
DRAWOUT
DRAWSIN
DRAWSON
DRAWSTO
DRAWSUP
DRAYAGE
DRAYING
DRAYMAN
DRAYMEN
DRAYTON
DRBROWN
DRCHAOS
DREADED
DREAMED
DREAMER
DREAMIN
DREAMOF
DREAMON
DREAMUP
DREDGED
DREDGER
DREDGES
DREGION
DREIDEL
DREISER
DRESDEN
DRESSAS
DRESSED
DRESSER
DRESSES
DRESSIN
DRESSUP
DREWOFF
DREWOUT
DREXELU
DREXLER
DREYFUS
DRFREUD
DRFRIST
DRIBBLE
DRIBLET
DRIEDUP
DRIESCH
DRIESUP
DRIFTED
DRIFTER
DRIFTIN
DRIFTUP
DRILLED
DRILLER
DRINKER
DRINKIN
DRINKME
DRINKTO
DRINKUP
DRIPDRY
DRIPPAN
DRIPPED
DRIPPER
DRIPSON
DRISTAN
DRIVEAT
DRIVEBY
DRIVEIN
DRIVELS
DRIVERS
DRIVETO
DRIVEUP
DRIVING
DRIZZLE
DRIZZLY
DRLAURA
DRMARIO
DRMCCOY
DRMELFI
DROGUES
DROLLER
DRONEON
DRONERS
DRONING
DRONISH
DROOLED
DROOLER
DROOPED
DROPBOX
DROPCAP
DROPINS
DROPLET
DROPNET
DROPOFF
DROPOUT
DROPPED
DROPPER
DROPSBY
DROPSIN
DROPSIT
DROPTOP
DROSSES
DROUGHT
DROVEAT
DROVEBY
DROVEIN
DROVERS
DROVETO
DROVEUP
DROWNED
DROWSED
DROWSES
DROXIES
DRQUINN
DRSEUSS
DRSLOAN
DRSPOCK
DRTEETH
DRUBBED
DRUBBER
DRUCKER
DRUDGED
DRUDGER
DRUDGES
DRUGGED
DRUIDIC
DRUMLIN
DRUMMED
DRUMMER
DRUMOUT
DRUMSET
DRUMSUP
DRUNKEN
DRUNKER
DRUZEAN
DRUZIAN
DRVEGAS
DRWELBY
DRYABLE
DRYADES
DRYADIC
DRYBULB
DRYCELL
DRYDOCK
DRYEYED
DRYEYES
DRYFOGS
DRYHEAT
DRYHOLE
DRYIDEA
DRYMOPS
DRYNESS
DRYPERS
DRYROTS
DRYRUNS
DRYSUIT
DRYWALL
DRYWASH
DRYWELL

D•R••••

DAREFUL
DARENOT
DARESAY
DARESTO
DAREZZO
DARIUSI
DARKAGE
DARKENS
DARKEST
DARKISH
DARKLED
DARKLES
DARKMAN
DARKRED
DARKTAN
DARLEEN
DARLENE
DARLING
DARNELL
DARNERS
DARNING
DARRYLF
DARTERS
DARTGUN
DARTING
DARTLED
DARTLES
DARTOFF
DARWELL
DERAILS
DERALTE
DERANGE
DERATED
DERATES
DERBIES
DERECHO
DERIDED
DERIDER
DERIDES
DERIVED
DERIVER
DERIVES
DERMATO
DERNIER
DERONDA
DERRICK
DERRICO
DERRIDA
DERRING
DERUSTS
DERVISH
DERWENT
DIRECTS
DIRECTV
DIREFUL
DIRHAMS
DIRKING
DIRKSEN
DIRNDLS
DIRTBAG
DIRTIED
DIRTIER
DIRTIES
DIRTILY
DORFMAN
DORIGHT
DORITOS
DORKIER
DORMANT
DORMERS
DORMICE
DOROTHY
DORSALS
DORSETT
DORSEYS
DURABLE
DURABLY
DURANCE
DURANGO
DURANTE
DURNING
DURRELL
DURWARD
DURWENT

D••R•••

DACRONS
DAIRIES
DAIRYER
DARRYLF
DATRILS
DAYROOM
DEARDEN
DEAREST
DEARGOD
DEARIES
DEARONE
DEARSIR
DEARTHS
DEBRETT
DEBRIEF
DECREED
DECREER
DECREES
DECRIED
DECRIER
DECRIES
DECRUMB
DECRYPT
DEERFLY
DEFRAGS
DEFRAME
DEFRAUD
DEFRAYS
DEFROCK
DEFROST
DEGRADE
DEGREED
DEGREES
DEIRDRE
DELRAYS
DELRUTH
DEORBIT
DEPRAVE
DEPRESS
DEPRIVE
DERRICK
DERRICO
DERRIDA
DERRING
DETRACT
DETRAIN
DETROIT
DETRUDE
DEVRIES
DHARMAS
DHARMIC
DHURRIE
DIARIES
DIARIOS
DIARIST
DIGRAMS
DIGRAPH
DIGRESS
DIORAMA
DIORITE
DISRATE
DISROBE
DISRUPT
DIURNAL
DOGRACE
DOGREAT
DOGROSE
DOGRUNS
DONRUSS
DOORDIE
DOORMAN
DOORMAT
DOORMEN
DOORWAY
DOTRICE
DOUREST
DOWRIES
DOWRONG
DRBROWN
DRFREUD
DRFRIST
DRYROTS
DRYRUNS
DURRELL
DWARFED
DWARVES

D•••R••

DALTREY
DARKRED
DAYTRIP
DEAIRED
DEBARGE
DEBARKS
DEBORAH
DEBURGH
DEBURRS
DECARLO
DECORUM
DEEPRED
DEFARGE
DEFERTO
DEFORMS
DEGERMS
DEHIRED
DEHIRES
DEHORNS
DELARUE
DELIRIA
DELORIS
DELORME
DEMARCO
DEMARET
DEMARKS
DEMERGE
DEMERIT
DEMEROL
DEMURER
DENARII
DENDRON
DEPARTS
DEPORTS
DESERET
DESERTS
DESERVE
DESIRED
DESIREE
DESIRER
DESIRES
DESTROY
DETERGE
DEVORES
DEWDROP
DEWIRED
DEWIRES
DEWORMS
DEXTRAL
DEXTRIN
DHURRIE
DIAGRAM
DIDEROT
DINARIC
DISARMS
DISHRAG
DISTROS
DIVERGE
DIVERSE
DIVERTS
DIVORCE
DMYTRYK
DOGTROT
DOHERTY
DOLORES
DOTARDS
DOVERDE
DOWERED
DRMARIO
DUBARRY
DUSTRAG

D••••R•

DABBERS
DADAART
DAGGERS
DAKTARI
DAMMERS
DAMNERS
DAMPDRY
DAMPERS
DANBURY
DANCERS
DANDERS
DANGERS
DANVERS
DARNERS
DARTERS
DASHERS
DASTARD
DAUBERS
DAYCARE
DAYMARE
DEALERS
DEANERY
DEBEARD
DEBEERS
DEBLURS
DEBTORS
DEBURRS
DECIARE
DECKERS
DECLARE
DEEPFRY
DEFIERS
DEHAIRS
DEICERS
DEIRDRE
DEKLERK
DELBERT
DELMORE
DELTORO
DELVERS
DENIERS
DENMARK
DENTURE
DEODARS
DEPLORE
DESSERT
DETOURS
DEUTERO
DEVILRY
DEVOIRS
DEVOURS
DEWAART
DIALERS
DIAPERS
DICKERS
DICKORY
DIEHARD
DIETARY
DIETERS
DIFFERS
DIGGERS
DIGGORY
DILBERT
DILLARD
DIMITRI
DIMMERS
DINGERS
DINNERS
DIPPERS
DISBARS
DISCARD
DISCERN
DISCORD
DISEURS
DISPART
DISPORT
DISSERT
DISTORT
DISTURB
DITHERS
DITHERY
DOCKERS
DOCTORS
DODDERS
DODDERY
DODGERS
DOEUVRE
DOFFERS
DOGBERT
DOGCART
DOGEARS
DOIDARE
DOLLARS
DOLOURS
DONTCRY
DOOVERS
DOOZERS
DORMERS
DOTTERS
DOUSERS
DOWNERS
DOWSERS
DRAPERS
DRAPERY
DRAWERS
DRIPDRY
DRIVERS
DRLAURA
DRONERS
DROVERS
DRYPERS
DUBARRY
DUBBERS
DUCKERS
DUELERS
DUFFERS
DULLARD
DUMPERS
DUNKERS
DUNKIRK
DUNNERS
DURWARD
DUSTERS
DYKSTRA

D•••••R

DABBLER
DAFFIER
DAIMLER
DAIRYER
DALLIER
DANDIER
DANDLER
DANGLER
DANSEUR
DASHIER
DAUMIER
DAUNTER
DAWDLER
DAYSTAR
DAYWEAR
DAZZLER
DEADAIR
DEARSIR
DEBASER
DEBATER
DECATUR
DECAYER
DECIDER
DECODER
DECOLOR
DECOYER
DECREER
DECRIER
DEDUCER
DEFACER
DEFAMER
DEFILER
DEFINER
DEFUSER
DEIFIER
DELAYER
DELIVER
DELUDER
DEMETER
DEMURER
DENUDER
DEPONER
DEPOSER
DEPOWER
DERIDER
DERIVER
DERNIER
DESIRER
DESPAIR
DEVISER
DEVISOR
DEWATER
DIBBLER
DICHTER
DIDDLER
DIDOVER
DIEDFOR
DIESFOR
DIGSFOR
DILATOR
DILUTER
DILUTOR
DIMETER
DINGIER
DINKIER
DIOPTER
DIPOLAR
DIPPIER
DIRTIER
DISHIER
DITCHER
DITSIER
DITZIER
DIVIDER
DIVINER
DIVISOR
DIZZIER
DNIEPER
DODGIER
DOESFOR
DOGDOOR
DOGGIER
DOGHAIR
DOGSEAR
DOGSTAR
DOMECAR
DONATOR
DONEFOR
DOODLER
DOOMIER
DOPPLER
DORKIER
DOSSIER
DOTTIER
DOUBLER
DOUBTER
DOUCEUR
DOVEBAR
DOWAGER
DOWDIER
DOWNIER
DRABBER

DRAFTER
DRAGGER
DRAINER
DRAWBAR
DRAWLER
DREAMER
DREDGER
DREISER
DRESSER
DREXLER
DRIFTER
DRILLER
DRINKER
DRIPPER
DROLLER
DROOLER
DROPPER
DRUBBER
DRUCKER
DRUDGER
DRUMMER
DRUNKER
DUCKIER
DUMPIER
DUSKIER
DUSTIER
DUUMVIR
DWELLER

•DR••••

ADRATES
ADRENAL
ADRIANA
CDRACKS
CDRATES

•D•R•••

ADDRESS
ADORERS
ADORING
ADORNED
ADORNER
IDAREDS
ODORANT
ODORFUL
ODORIZE
ODOROUS

•D••R••

ADHERED
ADHERER
ADHERES
ADJURED
ADJURER
ADJURES
ADJUROR
ADMIRAL
ADMIRED
ADMIRER
ADMIRES
ADSORBS
ADVERBS
ADVERSE
ADVERTS
EDGARDO
EDITRIX
EDUARDO
EDWARDG
EDWARDI
EDWARDR
EDWARDS
EDWARDV
IDCARDS

•D•••R•

ADAWARE
ADJOURN
ADORERS
CDSTORE
EDITORS
EDOUARD
ODDSARE

•D••••R

ADAPTER
ADAPTOR
ADDUCER
ADEPTER
ADHERER
ADJURER
ADJUROR
ADMIRER
ADOLLAR
ADOPTER
ADORNER
ADVISER
ADVISOR
CDTOWER
EDASNER
EDIFIER
EDUCTOR
EDWARDR
IDOTTER
JDPOWER

••DR•••

ADDRESS
ALDRICH
ANDRADE
ANDREAS
ANDRESS
ANDREWS
ANDROID
ANDROUS
BADRAPS
BEDRAIL
BEDRAPE
BEDREST
BEDROCK
BEDROLL
BEDROOM
ELDRICH
ELDRICK
ENDRUNS
ERDRICH
GEDRICK
HADRIAN
HADRONS
HADROOM
HYDRANT
HYDRATE
HYDRIDE
HYDROUS
INDRAFT
INDRAWN
JODRELL
KEDROVA
KIDROCK
LADRONE
MADRUSH
MIDRIBS
MIDRIFF
MIDRISE
MUDROOM
OLDROSE
PADRAIC
PADRONE
PODRIDA
REDRAFT
REDRAGS
REDRAWN
REDRAWS
REDREAM
REDRESS
REDRIED
REDRIES
REDRILL
REDRIVE
REDROBE
REDROOP
REDROOT
REDROSE
RODRIGO
UNDRAPE
UNDRAWN
UNDRAWS
UNDRESS
UNDRIED
UNDRUNK
UPDRAFT
UPDRIED
UPDRIES
UPDRIFT

••D•R••

ALDORAY
ANDIRON
ANDORRA
BADAREA
BADTRIP
BODEREK
BODYRUB
CEDARED
CODERED
DIDEROT
ELDERLY
ENDERBY
ENDORSE
ENDURED
ENDURER
ENDURES
ENDUROS
FEDERAL
FEDERKO
FEDORAS
FEDOROV
GODFREY
HADAROW
INDORSE
KIDSRUS
LEDERER
MADERUN
MADUROS
MIDIRON
MODERNE
MODERNS
MRDARCY
OLDPROS
ORDERED
ORDERER
ORDERIN
ORDERLY
ORDERUP
REDARED
REDARES
REDARMY
REDARNS
TIDERIP
UNDARED
UNDERDO
UNDERGO
UPDARTS

••D••R•

ANDMORE
ANDORRA
ARDMORE
ARDOURS
BADFORM
BADGERS
BADGIRL
BADWORD
BEDFORD
BEDNORZ
BIDDERS
BODYART
BUDDERS
BUDGERS
BUDWORM
CADBURY
CADGERS
CODGERS
DADAART
DODDERS
DODDERY
DODGERS
ENDEARS
FEDDERS
FODDERS
FUDGERS
GADDERS
GODDARD
HEDGERS
INDOORS
JUDGERS
KEDGERS
KIDDERS
LADDERS
LADLERS
LEDGERS
LODGERS
MADDERS
MADEIRA
MEDFORD
MIDMORN
MIDTERM
MUDDERS
MUDLARK
NODDERS
NUDGERS
ODDSARE
OLDCARS
OLDGIRL
PADDERS
RADFORD
REDBIRD
REDCARD
REDFERN
REDFIRS
REDFORD
REDWORM
RIDDERS
RODGERS
RUDDERS
RUDYARD
SIDDURS
SIDEARM
SUDBURY
SUDSERS
UNDOERS
WADDERS
WEDDERS
WIDMARK

••D•••R

ADDUCER
ANDOVER
AUDITOR
BADHAIR
BIDFAIR
BIDSFOR
BODYBAR
CADAVER
CODDLER
DEDUCER
DIDDLER
DIDOVER
DODGIER
ENDOWER
ENDURER
ENDUSER
FADDIER
FIDDLER
GIDDIER
GODLIER
HADOVER
HEDGIER
HUDDLER
INDEXER
INDITER
INDUCER
INDYCAR
IODIZER
JODHPUR
LEDERER
LEDGIER
MADEFOR
MADEPAR
MADEWAR
MEDAWAR
MEDDLER
MIDDLER
MIDYEAR
MODELER
MODULAR
MUDDIER
MUDDLER
NODULAR
OLDSTER
ORDERER
PADDLER
PEDALER
PEDDLER
PUDGIER
RADIOER
REDDEER
REDFOUR
REDHAIR
REDSTAR
REDUCER
RIDDLER
RIDGIER
RUDDIER
SADDLER
SEDATER
SEDGIER
SEDUCER
SIDEBAR
SIDECAR
SODDIER
SUDSIER
TODDLER
UNDULAR
UPDATER
WADDLER
WEDGIER
WIDENER
WIDOWER
YODELER

•••DR••

AIRDRIE
AIRDROP
BALDRIC
CALDRON
DENDRON
DEWDROP
EARDROP
EARDRUM
EGGDROP
EXEDRAE
EYEDROP
FOUDRES
FREDRIC
GUMDROP
HENDRIX
HENDRYX
HUMDRUM
HUNDRED
KENDREW
KINDRED
LETDROP
LINDROS
LLADROS
LONDRES
MANDREL
MILDRED
MISDRAW
MISDREW
MORDRED
NONDRIP
NONDRUG
OILDRUM
OUTDRAG
OUTDRAW
OUTDREW
OUTDROP
POUDRES
QUADRIC
SHADROE
SKIDROW
TENDRIL
TOPDRAW
TUNDRAS
WOODROW

•••D•R•

ABIDERS
ALTDORF
ATEDIRT
BANDERA
BANDERS
BEADERS
BENDERS
BIDDERS
BINDERS
BINDERY
BIRDERS
BLADERS
BONDERS
BORDERS
BUDDERS
CALDERA
CALDERS
CARDERS
CHEDERS
CHIDERS
CINDERS
CINDERY
CONDORS
CORDERO
CORDERS
DANDERS
DEODARS
DODDERS
DODDERY
DOIDARE
EATDIRT
ELIDERS
ELUDERS
EPIDERM
ERODERS
EVADERS
FEDDERS
FEEDERS
FENDERS
FEODORI
FINDERS
FODDERS
FOLDERS
FUNDERS
GADDERS
GANDERS
GAUDERY
GENDERS
GILDERS
GIRDERS
GLIDERS
GODDARD
GOLDARN
GOODERS
GOODTRY
GRADERS
GUIDERS
HANDERS
HEADERS
HEEDERS
HERDERS
HINDERS
HOLDERS
ISADORA
ISADORE
ISIDORE
KIDDERS
KILDARE
KUNDERA
LADDERS
LANDERS
LARDERS
LAUDERS
LEADERS
LEADORE
LENDERS
LINDORF
LOADERS
MADDERS
MELDERS
MENDERS
MINDERS
MINDORO
MOLDERS
MUDDERS
MURDERS
NEEDERS
NODDERS
NONDARK
ONADARE
OUTDARE
PADDERS
PANDERS
PANDORA
PAYDIRT
PERDURE
PONDERS
POWDERS
POWDERY
PREDARK
PRUDERY
RAIDERS
READERS
READORN
RENDERS
RIDDERS
ROADERS
RONDURE
RUDDERS
SANDERS
SEEDERS
SENDERS
SHADERS
SIDDURS
SLIDERS
SOLDERS
SPADERS
SPIDERS
SPIDERY
SPYDERS
SUNDERS
TENDERS
TINDERS
TINDERY
TRADERS
VANDURA
VEADARS
VENDERS
VENDORS
VERDURE
VOIDERS
WADDERS
WALDORF
WANDERS
WARDERS
WEDDERS
WEEDERS
WELDERS
WENDERS
WINDERS
WONDERS
WOODARD
YARDARM
YARDERS

•••D••R

BANDIER
BAWDIER
BEADIER
BENDIER
BLADDER
BLUDGER
BOUDOIR
BOWDLER
BRIDGER
BRIDLER
BUNDLER
CANDLER
CANDOUR
CARDOOR
CATDOOR
CHEDDAR
CODDLER
COLDWAR
CRADLER
CURDIER
CURDLER
DANDIER
DANDLER
DAWDLER
DEADAIR
DIDDLER
DIEDFOR
DOGDOOR
DOODLER
DOWDIER
DREDGER
DRUDGER
FADDIER
FIDDLER
FIEDLER
FONDLER
GARDNER
GAUDIER
GIDDIER
GIRDLER
GLADDER
GOODBAR
GOODFOR
GRIDDER
GRODIER
GRUDGER
HANDCAR
HANDIER
HANDLER
HARDIER
HEADFOR
HEADIER
HUDDLER
HURDLER
KINDLER
LAIDFOR
LANDLER
LARDIER
LARDNER
LEADIER
LIEDFOR
LINDNER
MEDDLER
MIDDLER
MISDOER
MOLDIER
MOODIER
MUDDIER
MUDDLER
MULDAUR
NEEDIER
NEEDLER
NERDIER
OUTDOER
OUTDOOR
PADDLER
PAIDFOR
PARDNER
PEDDLER
PETDEER
PETDOOR
PLEDGER
PLODDER
PRODDER
RANDIER
READFOR
READIER
REDDEER
REEDIER
RIDDLER
RINDIER
ROADTAR
ROEDEER
ROWDIER
RUDDIER
SADDLER
SANDBAR
SANDBUR
SANDIER
SANDLER
SCUDDER
SEEDIER
SENDFOR
SHADIER
SHEDDER
SHUDDER
SKIDDER
SLEDDER
SODDIER
SOLDFOR
SOLDIER
STADLER
STUDIER
SUBDUER
SUEDFOR
TANDOOR
TARDIER
TODDLER
TRUDGER
TWODOOR
USEDCAR
USEDFOR
VIEDFOR
WADDLER
WEEDIER
WINDIER
WINDSOR
WOODIER
WOODTAR
WORDIER
YESDEAR

••••DR•

BLOWDRY
BONEDRY
DAMPDRY
DEIRDRE
DRIPDRY
EPHEDRA
EXHEDRA
FOUNDRY
KILNDRY
LAUNDRY
LINEDRY
MRPADRE
OVERDRY
PALEDRY
PATSDRY
PHAEDRA
RUNSDRY
SEMIDRY
SPINDRY
STAYDRY
SUCKDRY
VERYDRY

••••D•R

ABRADER
ACCEDER
AMENDER
ASUNDER
AVOIDER
AWARDER
BLADDER
BLANDER
BLEEDER
BLENDER
BLINDER
BLONDER
BLUNDER
BOARDER
BOULDER
BOUNDER
BRAIDER
BRANDER
BREADER
BREEDER
BROADER
BROIDER
BROODER
BUILDER
CCRIDER
CHEDDAR
CHOWDER
CLOWDER
COTEDOR
CROWDER
DECIDER
DECODER
DELUDER
DENUDER
DERIDER
DIVIDER
ECUADOR
EMENDER
ENCODER
EVANDER
EVERDUR
FIELDER
FOUNDER
GLADDER
GOUNDER
GRANDER
GRIDDER
GRINDER
GUARDER
GUILDER
HOARDER
HOUNDER
HUMIDOR
IMPEDER
INORDER
INSIDER
INVADER
IWONDER
JOINDER
KNEADER
LAUNDER
LEANDER
MALODOR
MATADOR
MAUNDER
MEANDER
MIRADOR
MOGADOR
MOULDER
ONORDER
PARADER
PARADOR
PICADOR
PLEADER
PLODDER
PLUNDER
POUNDER
PRODDER
PROUDER
RAPIDER
REORDER
RESIDER
ROUNDER
SCALDER
SCOLDER
SCUDDER
SECEDER
SHEDDER
SHUDDER
SKIDDER
SLANDER
SLEDDER
SLENDER
SMOLDER
SOLIDER
SOUNDER
SPEEDER
SPENDER
STAIDER
STANDER
STRIDER
THEODOR
THUNDER
TIMIDER
TIREDER
TOORDER
TREADER
VIVIDER
VOCODER
WEIRDER
WIELDER
YIELDER

•••••DR

EDWARDR
SECONDR

D•S••••

DASBOOT
DASCHLE
DASHDOT
DASHERS
DASHIER
DASHIKI
DASHING
DASHOFF
DASHPOT
DASILVA
DASTARD
DESALTS
DESCANT
DESCEND
DESCENT
DESEEDS
DESERET
DESERTS
DESERVE
DESEXED
DESEXES
DESHELL
DESIGNS
DESILTS
DESIRED
DESIREE
DESIRER
DESIRES
DESISTS
DESKFUL
DESKSET
DESKTOP
DESLUMS
DESMOGS
DESMOND
DESOTOS
DESPAIR
DESPINA
DESPISE
DESPITE
DESPOIL
DESPOND
DESPOTS
DESSERT
DESTAEL
DESTAIN

DESTEMS
DESTINE
DESTINO
DESTINY
DESTOCK
DESTROY
DESYLVA
DISABLE
DISARMS
DISAVOW
DISBAND
DISBARS
DISBUDS
DISCARD
DISCERN
DISCING
DISCMAN
DISCOED
DISCOID
DISCORD
DISCUSS
DISDAIN
DISEASE
DISEURS
DISEUSE
DISGUST
DISHFUL
DISHIER
DISHING
DISHOUT
DISHPAN
DISHRAG
DISJOIN
DISKING
DISLIKE
DISMALS
DISMAST
DISMAYS
DISMISS
DISOBEY
DISOWNS
DISPART
DISPELS
DISPLAY
DISPORT
DISPOSE
DISPUTE
DISRATE
DISROBE
DISRUPT
DISSECT
DISSENT
DISSERT
DISSING
DISTAFF
DISTANT
DISTEND
DISTICH
DISTILL
DISTILS
DISTORT
DISTROS
DISTURB
DISUSED
DISUSES
DOSADOS
DOSAGES
DOSHOTS
DOSIDOS
DOSSALS
DOSSIER
DOSSING
DRSEUSS
DRSLOAN
DRSPOCK
DUSKIER
DUSKILY
DUSKING
DUSKISH
DUSTBIN
DUSTERS
DUSTGUN
DUSTIER
DUSTILY
DUSTING
DUSTMAN
DUSTMEN
DUSTMOP
DUSTOFF
DUSTPAN
DUSTRAG
DUSTUPS

D••S•••

DAISIES
DAMSELS
DAMSONS
DANSEUR
DATSUNS
DAUSSET
DAYSAIL
DAYSEND
DAYSIDE
DAYSINN
DAYSOFF
DAYSPAS
DAYSTAR
DEISTIC
DELSOLS
DENSELY
DENSEST
DENSIFY
DENSITY
DESSERT
DIDSUMS
DIESELS
DIESFOR
DIESOFF
DIESOUT
DIGSFOR
DIGSOUT
DIMSOUT
DISSECT
DISSENT
DISSERT
DISSING
DITSIER
DOASIDO
DOESBAD
DOESFOR
DOESKIN
DOESNOT
DOESTOO
DOGSAGE
DOGSEAR
DOGSHOW
DOGSITS
DOGSLED
DOGSTAR
DORSALS
DORSETT
DORSEYS
DOSSALS
DOSSIER
DOSSING
DOUSERS
DOUSING
DOWSERS
DOWSING
DRASTIC
DRESDEN
DRESSAS
DRESSED
DRESSER
DRESSES
DRESSIN
DRESSUP
DRISTAN
DROSSES
DRYSUIT
DUNSTAN
DYKSTRA

D•••S••

DACOSTA
DALASIS
DAMASKS
DAMASUS
DAMOSEL
DARESAY
DARESTO
DATASET
DAUSSET
DAVISON
DAWNSON
DEADSEA
DEADSET
DEALSIN
DEALSTO
DEALSUP
DEARSIR
DEBASED
DEBASER
DEBASES
DEBUSES
DEBUSSY
DEEPSEA
DEEPSET
DEEPSIX
DEEPSKY
DEFUSED
DEFUSER
DEFUSES
DEGUSTS
DEHISCE
DELISTS
DEMASTS
DEMESNE
DEMISED
DEMISES
DEMISTS
DEMPSEY
DENISON
DEPESTS
DEPOSAL
DEPOSED
DEPOSER
DEPOSES
DEPOSIT
DERUSTS
DESISTS
DESKSET
DETESTS
DEUTSCH
DEVESTS
DEVISED
DEVISEE
DEVISER
DEVISES
DEVISOR
DIALSIN
DIALSUP
DICKSON
DIDASET
DIGESTS
DINESAT
DINESEN
DINESIN
DINESON
DIRKSEN
DISUSED
DISUSES
DIVESIN
DIVESTS
DIVISOR
DNAASES
DODGSON
DOLLSUP
DOOMSTO
DOTESON
DPLUSES
DRAGSIN
DRAGSON
DRAGSUP
DRAWSIN
DRAWSON
DRAWSTO
DRAWSUP
DREISER
DRESSAS
DRESSED
DRESSER
DRESSES
DRESSIN
DRESSUP
DRIESCH
DRIESUP
DRIPSON
DROPSBY
DROPSIN
DROPSIT
DROSSES
DROWSED
DROWSES
DRUMSET
DRUMSUP
DUDESUP
DUFUSES
DUMPSON
DYNASTS
DYNASTY

D••••S•

DADAISM
DADAIST
DAFTEST
DAMPEST
DAMPISH
DANKEST
DARIUSI
DARKEST
DARKISH
DEADEST
DEAFEST
DEAREST
DEBUSSY
DECEASE
DECLASS
DEEPEST
DEEPISH
DEFENSE
DEFFEST
DEFROST
DEFTEST
DEGAUSS
DEGHOST
DELOUSE
DELUISE
DENSEST
DENTIST
DEPRESS
DERVISH
DESPISE
DEWIEST
DEWLESS
DIARIST
DICIEST
DIECAST
DIFFUSE
DIGRESS
DIMMEST
DIMNESS
DIOCESE
DISCUSS
DISEASE
DISEUSE
DISGUST
DISMAST
DISMISS
DISPOSE
DIVERSE
DIVULSE
DNATEST
DOGFISH
DOGGISH
DOGLESS
DOGROSE
DOGVEST
DOINGSO
DOLLISH
DOLTISH
DONETSK
DONJOSE
DONNISH
DONRUSS
DONTASK
DOPIEST
DOTDASH
DOUREST
DOZIEST
DRFRIST
DRONISH
DRSEUSS
DRYNESS
DRYWASH
DUALISM
DUALIST
DUCHESS
DUEEAST
DUELIST
DUEWEST
DULLEST
DULLISH
DUMBEST
DUMPISH
DUNCISH
DUSKISH

D•••••S

DABBERS
DABBLES
DACAPOS
DACRONS
DACTYLS
DADDIES
DAEMONS
DAEWOOS
DAGGERS
DAHLIAS
DAILIES
DAIRIES
DAISIES
DAKOTAS
DALASIS
DALETHS
DALLIES
DALTONS
DAMAGES
DAMASKS
DAMASUS
DAMMERS
DAMNERS
DAMPENS
DAMPERS
DAMSELS
DAMSONS
DANANAS
DANCERS
DANDERS
DANDIES
DANDLES
DANGERS
DANGLES
DANIELS
DANITES
DANVERS
DAPHNES
DAPHNIS
DAPPLES
DARKENS
DARKLES
DARNERS
DARTERS
DARTLES
DASHERS
DATABUS
DATINGS
DATIVES
DATRILS
DATSUNS
DAUBERS
DAWDLES
DAWKINS
DAYBEDS
DAYHOPS
DAYJOBS
DAYSPAS
DAZZLES
DEACONS
DEADENS
DEAFENS
DEALERS
DEARIES
DEARTHS
DEBARKS
DEBASES
DEBATES
DEBEERS
DEBLURS
DEBONES
DEBTEES
DEBTORS
DEBUNKS
DEBURRS
DEBUSES
DECADES
DECAMPS
DECANTS
DECEITS
DECIDES
DECILES
DECKERS
DECKLES
DECLASS
DECLAWS
DECLOTS
DECOCTS
DECODES
DECREES
DECRIES
DEDALUS
DEDUCES
DEDUCTS
DEEJAYS
DEEPENS
DEFACES
DEFAMES
DEFANGS
DEFCONS
DEFEATS
DEFECTS
DEFENDS
DEFIERS
DEFILES
DEFINES
DEFLEAS
DEFOAMS
DEFOCUS
DEFORMS
DEFRAGS
DEFRAYS
DEFUELS
DEFUNDS
DEFUSES
DEGAUSS
DEGERMS
DEGREES
DEGUSTS
DEHAIRS
DEHEXES
DEHIRES
DEHORNS
DEICERS
DEIFIES
DEITIES
DEJECTS
DEJUNKS
DELEADS
DELETES
DELIBES
DELICTS
DELINTS
DELISTS
DELKEYS
DELORIS
DELRAYS
DELSOLS
DELUDES
DELUGES
DELVERS
DEMANDS
DEMARKS
DEMASTS
DEMBUMS
DEMEANS
DEMISES
DEMISTS
DEMOTES
DEMOTHS
DENIALS
DENIERS
DENMOMS
DENOTES
DENTALS
DENTINS
DENTONS
DENUDES
DEODARS
DEPARTS
DEPENDS
DEPESTS
DEPICTS
DEPLOYS
DEPONES
DEPORTS
DEPOSES
DEPRESS
DEPULPS
DEPUTES
DERAILS
DERATES
DERBIES
DERIDES
DERIVES
DERUSTS
DESALTS
DESEEDS
DESERTS
DESEXES
DESIGNS
DESILTS
DESIRES
DESISTS
DESLUMS
DESMOGS
DESOTOS
DESPOTS
DESTEMS
DETAILS
DETAINS
DETECTS
DETENTS
DETESTS
DETOURS
DETOXES
DETUNES
DEVEINS
DEVESTS
DEVICES
DEVIOUS
DEVISES
DEVOIRS
DEVORES
DEVOTES
DEVOURS
DEVRIES
DEWAXES
DEWIRES
DEWLAPS
DEWLESS
DEWORMS
DHARMAS
DIABLES
DIABLOS
DIADEMS
DIALERS
DIALOGS
DIALUPS
DIAPERS
DIARIES
DIARIOS
DIATOMS
DIBBLES
DICKENS
DICKERS
DICKEYS
DICKIES
DICTUMS
DIDACTS
DIDDLES
DIDLAPS
DIDSUMS
DIECUTS
DIEMENS
DIEOFFS
DIESELS
DIETERS
DIFFERS
DIGESTS
DIGGERS
DIGLOTS
DIGRAMS
DIGRESS
DIKDIKS
DIKTATS
DILATES
DILLIES
DILUTES
DIMAGES
DIMMERS
DIMNESS
DIMOUTS
DIMPLES
DIMWITS
DINDINS
DINGERS
DINGLES
DINGOES
DINNERS
DIOXINS
DIPNETS
DIPOLES
DIPPERS
DIRECTS
DIRHAMS
DIRNDLS
DIRTIES
DISARMS
DISBARS
DISBUDS
DISCUSS
DISEURS
DISMALS
DISMAYS
DISMISS
DISOWNS
DISPELS
DISTILS
DISTROS
DISUSES
DITCHES
DITHERS
DITTIES
DIVERTS
DIVESTS
DIVIDES
DIVINES
DIVVIES
DIZAINS
DIZZIES
DJINNIS
DNAASES
DNALABS
DOBBINS
DOCENTS
DOCKERS
DOCKETS
DOCTORS
DODDERS
DODGEMS
DODGERS
DOFFERS
DOGAPES
DOGBEDS
DOGDAYS
DOGEARS
DOGGIES
DOGLEGS
DOGLESS
DOGNAPS
DOGRUNS
DOGSITS
DOGTAGS
DOGTOYS
DOILIES
DOLLARS
DOLLIES
DOLLOPS
DOLMANS
DOLORES
DOLOURS
DOMAINS
DOMINOS
DOMINUS
DONATES
DONATUS
DONGLES
DONIMUS
DONJONS
DONKEYS
DONRUSS
DOODADS
DOODLES
DOOLIES
DOOVERS
DOOWOPS
DOOZERS
DOOZIES
DORITOS
DORMERS
DORSALS
DORSEYS
DOSADOS
DOSAGES
DOSHOTS
DOSIDOS
DOSSALS
DOTAGES
DOTARDS
DOTCOMS
DOTTERS
DOTTLES
DOUANES
DOUBLES
DOUGLAS
DOUSERS
DOWDIES
DOWNERS
DOWRIES
DOWSERS
DPLUSES
DRAGEES
DRAGONS
DRAPERS
DRAWEES
DRAWERS
DRCHAOS
DREDGES
DRESSAS
DRESSES
DREYFUS
DRIVELS
DRIVERS
DROGUES
DRONERS
DROPINS
DROSSES
DROVERS
DROWSES
DROXIES
DRSEUSS
DRUDGES
DRVEGAS
DRYADES
DRYEYES
DRYFOGS
DRYMOPS
DRYNESS
DRYPERS
DRYROTS
DRYRUNS
DUBBERS
DUBIOUS
DUCHESS
DUCHIES
DUCKERS
DUCKIES
DUELERS
DUENNAS
DUETTOS
DUFFELS
DUFFERS
DUFFLES
DUFUSES
DUGONGS
DUGOUTS
DUKAKIS
DUMDUMS
DUMMIES
DUMPERS
DUNKERS
DUNLINS
DUNLOPS
DUNNERS
DUSTERS
DUSTUPS
DUTEOUS
DWARVES
DYBBUKS
DYEJOBS
DYELOTS
DYEVATS
DYNAMOS
DYNASTS
DYNODES

•DS••••

ADSORBS
ADSPACE
CDSTORE
IDSAYSO

•D•S•••

ADDSALT
EDASNER
ODDSARE
ODDSHOE
ODDSOCK
ODESSAN
ODYSSEY

•D••S••

ADAMSES
ADAMSON
ADDISON
ADJUSTS
ADVISED
ADVISEE
ADVISER
ADVISES
ADVISOR
CDCASES
EDGESIN
HDTVSET
IDLESSE
ODESSAN
ODYSSEY

•D•••S•

ADDRESS
ADIPOSE
ADVERSE
EDGIEST
EDMEESE
IDLESSE
IDOLISE
IDOLIST
IDSAYSO
IDYLIST
ODDNESS

•D••••S

ADAGIOS
ADAMSES
ADDAXES
ADDENDS
ADDICTS
ADDRESS
ADDUCES
ADDUCTS
ADELIES
ADHERES
ADJOINS
ADJURES
ADJUSTS
ADMIRES
ADMIXES
ADNOUNS
ADONAIS
ADORERS
ADRATES
ADSORBS
ADVENTS
ADVERBS
ADVERTS
ADVICES
ADVISES
ADZUKIS
CDCASES
CDRACKS
CDRATES
EDGINGS
EDIBLES
EDIFIES
EDITORS
EDMONDS
EDMUNDS
EDWARDS
IDAREDS
IDCARDS
IDEATES
ODDJOBS
ODDLOTS
ODDNESS
ODELETS
ODOROUS
PDJAMES

••DS•••

ADDSALT
ANDSOON
ANDSUCH
BADSHOT
BADSIGN

BEDSIDE
BEDSITS
BIDSFOR
DIDSUMS
GADSDEN
GODSEND
GODSENT
GODSONS
HADSOME
KIDSEAT
KIDSKIN
KIDSRUS
MIDSHIP
MIDSIZE
MIDSOLE
NODSOFF
ODDSARE
ODDSHOE
ODDSOCK
OLDSALT
OLDSAWS
OLDSHOE
OLDSONG
OLDSTER
PADSITE
REDSFAN
REDSKIN
REDSPOT
REDSTAR
REDSUIT
REDSUNS
SADSACK
SADSONG
SUDSERS
SUDSIER
SUDSING

••D•S••

ADDISON
DIDASET
DODGSON
DUDESUP
ECDYSES
ECDYSIS
ENDUSER
ENDUSES
FADESIN
HADASAY
HADASET
HEDISON
IODISED
IODISES
JUDASES
MADISON
MEDUSAE
MEDUSAN
MEDUSAS
MIDASES
MODESTO
MODESTY
MODISTE
NUDISTS
REDOSED
REDOSES
REDUSTS
RIDESBY
RIDESIN
RIDESTO
RIDESUP
SADISTS
TIDYSUM
UNDUSTY
VEDISTS
WADESIN

••D••S•

ADDRESS
AIDLESS
ANDRESS
BADCASE
BADDEST
BADDISH
BADNESS
BADPAST
BEDLESS
BEDPOST
BEDREST
BUDLESS
BUDVASE
CADDISH
CODFISH
DADAISM
DADAIST
ENDLESS
ENDMOST
ENDORSE
ENDWISE
FADDISH
FADDISM
FADDIST
GODDESS
GODLESS
HADBEST
INDORSE
JUDAISM
JUDOIST
KADDISH
KIDDISH
LADDISH
LADYISH
LIDLESS
LUDDISM
MADDASH
MADDEST
MADDISH
MADNESS
MADRUSH
MIDEAST
MIDLIST
MIDMOST
MIDRISE
MIDWEST
MUDFISH
MUDWASP
ODDNESS
OLDNESS
OLDROSE
OLDWEST
PODCAST
REDDEST
REDDISH
REDDUST
REDFISH
REDNESS
REDNOSE
REDRESS
REDROSE
RODLESS
SADDEST
SADNESS
SODLESS
TIDIEST
UNDRESS
YIDDISH

••D•••S

ABDUCES
ABDUCTS
ADDAXES
ADDENDS
ADDICTS
ADDRESS
ADDUCES
ADDUCTS
AEDILES
AIDLESS
ALDAVIS
ANDEANS
ANDREAS
ANDRESS
ANDREWS
ANDROUS
ARDOURS
ARDUOUS
AUDILES
BADBOYS
BADDAYS
BADDIES
BADDOGS
BADEGGS
BADENDS
BADFITS
BADGERS
BADGUYS
BADHATS
BADLIES
BADLOTS
BADNESS
BADNEWS
BADRAPS
BEDAUBS
BEDAZES
BEDBUGS
BEDECKS
BEDLAMS
BEDLESS
BEDLOES
BEDSITS
BIDDERS
BIDDIES
BODEGAS
BODICES
BODINGS
BODKINS
BUDDERS
BUDDHAS
BUDDIES
BUDGERS
BUDGETS
BUDGIES
BUDLESS
CADDIES
CADGERS
CODDLES
CODGERS
CODICES
CUDDIES
CUDDLES
CUDGELS
DADDIES
DEDALUS
DEDUCES
DEDUCTS
DIDACTS
DIDDLES
DIDLAPS
DIDSUMS
DODDERS
DODGEMS
DODGERS
EADGILS
ECDYSES
ECDYSIS
ENDALLS
ENDCUTS
ENDEARS
ENDINGS
ENDIVES
ENDLESS
ENDPINS
ENDRUNS
ENDURES
ENDUROS
ENDUSES
ENDWAYS
FADEINS
FEDDERS
FEDEXES
FEDORAS
FIDDLES
FIDELES
FIDELIS
FIDGETS
FODDERS
FUDDIES
FUDDLES
FUDGERS
GADDERS
GADGETS
GIDDIES
GIDEONS
GODDESS
GODLESS
GODSONS
GODWITS
HADAGAS
HADFITS
HADRONS
HEDGERS
HIDEOUS
HIDINGS
HUDDLES
HYDROUS
INDENTS
INDEXES
INDIANS
INDICES
INDICTS
INDIGOS
INDITES
INDOORS
INDUCES
INDUCTS
IODATES
IODIDES
IODISES
IODIZES
JUDASES
JUDEANS
JUDGERS
JUDOKAS
KADETTS
KEDGERS
KIDCOMS
KIDDERS
KIDDIES
KIDNAPS
KIDNEYS
KIDSRUS
KIDULTS
KIDVIDS
KODIAKS
LADDERS
LADDIES
LADIDAS
LADINGS
LADINOS
LADLERS
LADYNAS
LEDGERS
LIDLESS
LODGERS
MADAMES
MADCAPS
MADDENS
MADDERS
MADDOGS
MADLIBS
MADNESS
MADUROS
MEDAKAS
MEDDLES
MEDELES
MEDIANS
MEDICOS
MEDIUMS
MEDLEYS
MEDUSAS
MIDASES
MIDCAPS
MIDDAYS
MIDDIES
MIDDLES
MIDGETS
MIDLEGS
MIDOFFS
MIDRIBS
MIDWAYS
MODELAS
MODELBS
MODELTS
MODERNS
MODULES
MODULUS
MRDEEDS
MUDCATS
MUDDERS
MUDDIES
MUDDLES
MUDEELS
MUDHENS
MUDPIES
NODDERS
NODDIES
NODULES
NUDGERS
NUDISTS
NUDNIKS
NUDZHES
ODDJOBS
ODDLOTS
ODDNESS
OEDIPUS
OGDOADS
OLDBATS
OLDBOYS
OLDCARS
OLDDAYS
OLDDOGS
OLDGAGS
OLDNESS
OLDNEWS
OLDPALS
OLDPROS
OLDSAWS
OLDWAYS
ORDAINS
ORDEALS
ORDINES
PADDERS
PADDIES
PADDLES
PADUANS
PEDANTS
PEDDLES
PEDWAYS
PIDDLES
PIDGINS
PODIUMS
PUDDLES
RADAMES
RADIALS
RADIANS
RADICES
RADIXES
RADOMES
REDACTS
REDANTS
REDARES
REDARNS
REDATES
REDBATS
REDBAYS
REDBUDS
REDCAPS
REDCODS
REDDENS
REDDOGS
REDDOTS
REDDYES
REDEALS
REDEEDS
REDEEMS
REDEYES
REDFINS
REDFIRS
REDHATS
REDHENS
REDHOTS
REDIALS
REDLEGS
REDNESS
REDOAKS
REDOCKS
REDOSES
REDOUTS
REDOXES
REDRAGS
REDRAWS
REDRESS
REDRIES
REDSUNS
REDTABS
REDTAGS
REDTIES
REDTOPS
REDUCES
REDUSTS
RIDDERS
RIDDLES
RIDEBYS
RIDINGS
RODENTS
RODGERS
RODLESS
RUDDERS
SADDENS
SADDLES
SADEYES
SADISTS
SADNESS
SEDATES
SEDONAS
SEDUCES
SIDDONS
SIDDURS
SIDINGS
SIDIOUS
SODLESS
STDENIS
SUDOKUS
SUDSERS
TEDDIES
TEDEUMS
TEDIOUS
TEDIUMS
TIDBITS
TIDINGS
TODDIES
TODDLES
UNDINES
UNDOCKS
UNDOERS
UNDRAWS
UNDRESS
UPDARTS
UPDATES
UPDIVES
UPDRIES
VEDISTS
VIDIOTS
WADDERS
WADDLES
WADKINS
WEDDERS
WEDELNS
WEDGIES
WIDGETS
ZEDONKS
ZODIACS
ZYDECOS

•••DS••

AULDSOD
BANDSAW
BEADSUP
BINDSTO
BINDSUP
BLEDSOE
BRODSKY
CRUDSUP
DEADSEA
DEADSET
FEEDSIN
FEEDSON
FEEDSTO
FOLDSIN
FOLDSUP
GOODSON
HANDSAW
HANDSEL
HANDSET
HANDSIN
HANDSON
HANDSUP
HARDSET
HARDSIX
HEADSAW
HEADSET
HEADSIN
HEADSTO
HEADSUP
HOLDSIN
HOLDSIT
HOLDSON
HOLDSTO
HOLDSUP
LANDSAT
LANDSUP
LEADSIN
LEADSON
LEADSTO
LEADSUP
LINDSAY
LINDSEY
LOADSIN
LOADSOF
LOADSUP
LORDSIT
MINDSET
NEEDSTO
PRODSON
READSIN
READSON
READSTO
READSUP
SCADSOF
SENDSBY
SENDSIN
SENDSON
SENDSTO
SENDSUP
SHEDSON
TENDSTO
WINDSOR
WINDSUP
WOODSAW
WOODSON

•••D•S•

ANODISE
ARIDEST
AVIDEST
BADDEST
BADDISH
BALDEST
BALDISH
BOLDEST
CADDISH
COLDEST
COLDISH
CRUDEST
DEADEST
DOTDASH
FADDISH
FADDISM
FADDIST
FEUDIST
FONDEST
GEODESY
GODDESS
GOODISH
GOODUSE
HARDEST
HARDISH
KADDISH
KIDDISH
KINDEST
KURDISH
LADDISH
LEWDEST
LOUDEST
LOUDISH
LUDDISM
MADDASH
MADDEST
MADDISH
MAHDISM
MAHDIST
MAIDISH
MILDEST
MONDESI
NERDISH
OAKDESK
OXIDASE
OXIDISE
PRADESH
PREDUSK
PRUDISH
REDDEST
REDDISH
REDDUST
SADDEST
SAWDUST
SNIDEST
SWEDISH
TOADISH
WILDEST
WILDISH
YIDDISH
ZIPDISK

•••D••S

ABIDERS
AIRDAMS
ALUDELS
AMADEUS
AMIDOLS
ANADEMS
AOUDADS
APODOUS
AZODYES
BADDAYS
BADDIES
BADDOGS
BALDIES
BANDERS
BANDIES
BANDITS
BATDAYS
BEADERS
BEADLES
BELDAMS
BENDAYS
BENDERS
BIDDERS
BIDDIES
BIGDAYS
BIGDIGS
BIGDOGS
BINDERS
BINDLES
BIRDERS
BIRDIES
BLADERS
BLUDGES
BONDERS
BOODLES
BORDERS
BOUDINS
BRIDALS
BRIDGES
BRIDLES
BRODIES
BUDDERS
BUDDHAS
BUDDIES
BUNDLES
BURDENS
CADDIES
CALDERS
CANDIDS
CANDIES
CANDLES
CARDERS
CHEDERS
CHIDERS
CINDERS
CODDLES
COEDITS
CONDORS
CORDERS
CORDIAS
CORDONS
COYDOGS
CRADLES
CREDITS
CUDDIES
CUDDLES
CURDLES
DADDIES
DANDERS
DANDIES
DANDLES
DAWDLES
DEADENS
DEODARS
DIADEMS
DIDDLES
DIKDIKS
DINDINS
DODDERS
DOGDAYS
DOODADS
DOODLES
DOWDIES
DREDGES
DRUDGES
DUMDUMS
ELIDERS
ELUDERS
ERODERS
EVADERS
FANDOMS
FEDDERS
FEEDERS
FENDERS
FIDDLES
FINDERS
FLEDGES
FODDERS
FOGDOGS
FOLDERS
FOLDUPS
FONDLES
FONDUES
FOODIES
FORDGTS
FORDOES
FOUDRES
FRIDAYS
FRIDGES
FUDDIES
FUDDLES
FUNDERS
GADDERS
GANDERS
GARDENS
GAUDENS
GAUDIES
GENDERS
GIDDIES
GILDERS
GIRDERS
GIRDLES
GLIDERS
GODDESS
GOODBYS
GOODERS
GOODIES
GORDIUS
GRADERS
GRUDGES
GUIDERS
GULDENS
GUNDOGS
HANDERS
HANDLES
HARDEES
HARDENS
HEADERS
HEEDERS
HERDERS
HEYDAYS
HINDERS
HOLDERS
HOLDUPS
HOODIES
HOODOOS
HOTDAYS
HOTDOGS
HOWDAHS
HOYDENS
HUDDLES
HURDLES
ICEDAMS
JARDINS
KEYDETS
KIDDERS
KIDDIES
KINDLES
KLUDGES
LADDERS
LADDIES
LANDAUS
LANDERS
LAPDOGS
LARDERS
LARDONS
LAUDERS
LEADENS
LEADERS
LEADINS
LEADUPS
LENDERS
LINDENS
LINDIES
LINDROS
LLADROS
LOADERS
LONDRES
LOUDENS
MADDENS
MADDERS
MADDOGS
MAIDENS
MANDANS
MANDAYS
MAYDAYS
MCADAMS
MEADOWS
MEDDLES
MELDERS
MENDELS
MENDERS
MIDDAYS
MIDDIES
MIDDLES
MILDEWS
MINDERS
MISDOES
MOLDERS
MONDAYS
MTADAMS
MUDDERS
MUDDIES
MUDDLES
MURDERS
NEEDERS
NEEDLES
NODDERS
NODDIES
NOODGES
NOODLES
NORDICS
OFFDAYS
OLDDAYS
OLDDOGS
OUTDOES
PADDERS
PADDIES
PADDLES
PAIDADS
PANDERS
PANDITS
PARDONS
PAYDAYS
PEDDLES
PETDOGS
PHIDIAS
PIDDLES
PLEDGES
PONDERS
POODLES
POUDRES
POWDERS
PUDDLES
PUNDITS
PYEDOGS
RAIDERS
READERS
READIES
REDDENS
REDDOGS
REDDOTS
REDDYES
REEDITS
RENDERS
RIDDERS
RIDDLES
RITDYES
ROADEOS
ROADERS
ROADIES
RONDELS
ROWDIES
RUDDERS
RUNDLES
SADDENS
SADDLES
SANDALS
SANDERS
SEADOGS
SEEDERS
SENDEES
SENDERS
SENDUPS
SHADERS
SHADOWS
SIDDONS
SIDDURS
SKIDOOS
SLEDGES
SLIDERS

SLUDGES
SMIDGES
SMUDGES
SOLDERS
SPADERS
SPIDERS
SPYDERS
STODGES
STUDIES
STUDIOS
SUBDEBS
SUBDUES
SUNDAES
SUNDAYS
SUNDERS
SUNDOGS
SYNDICS
TAGDAYS
TANDEMS
TEDDIES
TENDAYS
TENDERS
TENDONS
TIEDYES
TINDERS
TOADIES
TODDIES
TODDLES
TOODLES
TOPDOGS
TOYDOGS
TRADERS
TREDIAS
TRUDGES
TUNDRAS
TVIDOLS
TWODAYS
UNEDGES
USEDCDS
VANDALS
VATDYES
VAUDOIS
VEADARS
VENDEES
VENDERS
VENDORS
VENDUES
VERDINS
VOIDERS
VOODOOS
WADDERS
WADDLES
WANDERS
WARDENS
WARDERS
WEDDERS
WEEDERS
WELDERS
WENDERS
WENDKOS
WINDAUS
WINDERS
WINDOMS
WINDOWS
WINDUPS
WISDOMS
WONDERS
WOODIES
YARDERS

••••DS•

HOPEDSO
SOANDSO
WOULDST

••••D•S

ABRADES
ACCEDES
ACTEDAS
AGENDAS
AIKIDOS
ALBEDOS
ALLUDES
APHIDES
APSIDES
ARCADES
ARMADAS
ASSTDAS
AUBADES
BESIDES
BETIDES
BLENDES
BLONDES
BOLIDES
BORIDES
BROADAS
CAPADES
CICADAS
COLADAS
CSARDAS
CZARDAS
DECADES
DECIDES
DECODES
DELUDES
DENUDES
DERIDES
DIRNDLS
DIVIDES
DOSADOS
DOSIDOS
DRYADES
DYNODES
ENCODES
ESCUDOS
ESTADOS
EXCIDES
FACADES
GOURDES
HAIRDOS
HALIDES
ILLUDES
IMPEDES
INCUDES
INSIDES
INVADES
IODIDES
JUMADAS
LADIDAS
LAMBDAS
LAREDOS
LAYODDS
LEPIDUS
LEVADES
LIBIDOS
LOURDES
MAKEDOS
MARIDAS
MARIDOS
MENUDOS
MIKADOS
MIRADAS
MISADDS
MOVADOS
MUSTDOS
NAIADES
NOBODYS
ONEIDAS
ONSIDES
OUTADDS
OXHIDES
PAGODAS
PANADAS
PARADES
PBANDJS
PESADES
POMADES
POSADAS
POSEDAS
PSANDQS
RAMADAS
RECEDES
RECODES
REHIDES
REREDOS
RERIDES
RESIDES
RUANDAS
SABADOS
SALADES
SAMEDIS
SECEDES
SPEEDOS
STRIDES
TIENDAS
TIRADES
TOLEDOS
TRIODES
TUXEDOS
UNLADES
UPSIDES
USTEDES
WEIRDOS
XANADUS
XSANDOS

•••••DS

ABOUNDS
ACARIDS
ACCORDS
ADDENDS
AFFORDS
ALMONDS
ALTOIDS
AOUDADS
APPENDS
ARAMIDS
ARNOLDS
ASCENDS
ATTENDS
AUGENDS
AXHEADS
AXSEEDS
BADENDS
BALLADS
BEGIRDS
BEHEADS
BEHINDS
BEHOLDS
BIGENDS
BIGKIDS
BOXBEDS
BRIARDS
BYROADS
BYWORDS
CALENDS
CANARDS
CANDIDS
CATBEDS
CERVIDS
CONOIDS
CORVIDS
COWARDS
CUBOIDS
CUEBIDS
CUSPIDS
CYANIDS
DAYBEDS
DEFENDS
DEFUNDS
DELEADS
DEMANDS
DEPENDS
DESEEDS
DISBUDS
DOGBEDS
DOODADS
DOTARDS
EARBUDS
EDMONDS
EDMUNDS
EDWARDS
ELAPIDS
EMQUADS
ENFOLDS
ENGILDS
ENGIRDS
ENNEADS
ENQUADS
ENWINDS
ERRANDS
EXCEEDS
EXPANDS
EXPENDS
EXTENDS
EYELIDS
FAGENDS
FAKEIDS
FANTODS
FLYRODS
FMBANDS
FORBIDS
FRIENDS
GAPKIDS
GERUNDS
GROUNDS
HALOIDS
HARRODS
HATREDS
HAZARDS
HEPTADS
HERALDS
HOTBEDS
HOTRODS
HOWARDS
HYBRIDS
IDAREDS
IDCARDS
IMPENDS
INFOLDS
INKPADS
INLANDS
INNARDS
INROADS
INTENDS
INWARDS
ISLANDS
ISOPODS
JOYPADS
KEYPADS
KIDVIDS
KOBOLDS
LAYODDS
LEGENDS
LEONIDS
LIGANDS
LIQUIDS
LIZARDS
LOWBIDS
MAENADS
MALTEDS
MARAUDS
METHODS
MILORDS
MISADDS
MRDEEDS
MRWORDS
MYRIADS
NAVAIDS
NEREIDS
NEWKIDS
NEXRADS
NIKEADS
NIMRODS
NOGOODS
NOHANDS
NOLOADS
OBTUNDS
OFFENDS
OGDOADS
ONLOADS
ONWARDS
ORCHIDS
OSMONDS
OSMUNDS
OUTADDS
OUTBIDS
OUTBUDS
OXFORDS
PAIDADS
PEAPODS
PENTADS
PEPCIDS
PERIODS
PETARDS
PONGIDS
POTLIDS
PREBIDS
PREMEDS
PROKEDS
RAMRODS
REBENDS
REBINDS
RECLADS
RECORDS
REDBUDS
REDCODS
REDEEDS
REFEEDS
REFINDS
REFOLDS
REFUNDS
REGARDS
REGILDS
REGIRDS
RELANDS
RELEADS
RELENDS
RELOADS
REMANDS
REMENDS
REMINDS
REMOLDS
REREADS
RESANDS
RESEEDS
RESENDS
RETARDS
REVENDS
REWARDS
REWELDS
REWINDS
REWORDS
RIBALDS
RIBANDS
RIBPADS
RITARDS
ROBARDS
ROLAIDS
SCREEDS
SEABEDS
SEAGODS
SECONDS
SEWARDS
SHIELDS
SHROUDS
SOSPADS
SPREADS
SPYKIDS
STRANDS
STUPIDS
SUBGODS
SUBLIDS
SUNGODS
TABARDS
TAGENDS
TETRADS
THEFEDS
THEREDS
THREADS
TIERODS
TINGODS
TOPBIDS
TOROIDS
TOWARDS
TRIPODS
UNBENDS
UNBINDS
UNFOLDS
UNGIRDS
UNHANDS
UNHEEDS
UNHOODS
UNIPODS
UNLEADS
UNLOADS
UNMOLDS
UNWINDS
UPCARDS
UPFOLDS
UPGIRDS
UPHOLDS
UPLANDS
UPLOADS
UPSENDS
UPWARDS
UPWINDS
USEDCDS
USERIDS
VERBIDS
VESPIDS
WANTADS
WARGODS
WHWORDS
WIZARDS

D•T••••

DATABLE
DATABUS
DATASET
DATEDLY
DATINGS
DATIVES
DATRILS
DATSUNS
DETAILS
DETAINS
DETECTO
DETECTS
DETENTE
DETENTS
DETERGE
DETESTS
DETOURS
DETOXED
DETOXES
DETRACT
DETRAIN
DETROIT
DETRUDE
DETUNED
DETUNES
DITCHED
DITCHER
DITCHES
DITHERS
DITHERY
DITSIER
DITTIES
DITTOED
DITZIER
DOTAGES
DOTARDS
DOTBOMB
DOTCOMS
DOTDASH
DOTEDON
DOTESON
DOTLIKE
DOTRICE
DOTTERS
DOTTIER
DOTTILY
DOTTING
DOTTLES
DRTEETH
DUTEOUS
DUTIFUL

D••T•••

DACTYLS
DAFTEST
DAKTARI
DALTONS
DALTREY
DANTEAN
DANTEII
DARTERS
DARTGUN
DARTING
DARTLED
DARTLES
DARTOFF
DASTARD
DAYTIME
DAYTONA
DAYTRIP
DEBTEES
DEBTORS
DEFTEST
DEITIES
DELTAIC
DELTOID
DELTONA
DELTORO
DENTALS
DENTATE
DENTINE
DENTING
DENTINS
DENTIST
DENTOID
DENTONS
DENTURE
DENTYNE
DESTAEL
DESTAIN
DESTEMS
DESTINE
DESTINO
DESTINY
DESTOCK
DESTROY
DEUTERO
DEUTSCH
DEXTRAL
DEXTRIN
DIATOMS
DICTATE
DICTION
DICTUMS
DIDTIME
DIDTOAT
DIETARY
DIETERS
DIETING
DIKTATS
DINTING
DIOTIMA
DIPTYCH
DIRTBAG
DIRTIED
DIRTIER
DIRTIES
DIRTILY
DISTAFF
DISTANT
DISTEND
DISTICH
DISTILL
DISTILS
DISTORT
DISTROS
DISTURB
DITTIES
DITTOED
DMYTRYK
DNATEST
DOCTORS
DOGTAGS
DOGTAIL
DOGTICK
DOGTOYS
DOGTROT
DOITNOW
DOLTISH
DONTASK
DONTBEE
DONTCRY
DONTLIE
DOTTERS
DOTTIER
DOTTILY
DOTTING
DOTTLES
DRATTED
DUCTILE
DUCTING
DUETING
DUETTED
DUETTOS
DUOTONE
DUSTBIN
DUSTERS
DUSTGUN
DUSTIER
DUSTILY
DUSTING
DUSTMAN
DUSTMEN
DUSTMOP
DUSTOFF
DUSTPAN
DUSTRAG
DUSTUPS

D•••T••

DAKOTAN
DAKOTAS
DALETHS
DANITES
DARKTAN
DAUNTED
DAUNTER
DAYSTAR
DEALTIN
DEALTTO
DEALTUP
DEARTHS
DEBATED
DEBATER
DEBATES
DEBITED
DEBUTED
DECATUR
DEEPTAN
DEISTIC
DELETED
DELETES
DEMETER
DEMOTED
DEMOTES
DEMOTHS
DEMOTIC
DENOTED
DENOTES
DEPUTED
DEPUTES
DERATED
DERATES
DESKTOP
DESOTOS
DEVOTED
DEVOTEE
DEVOTES
DEWATER
DICHTER
DIGITAL
DILATED
DILATES
DILATOR
DILUTED
DILUTER
DILUTES
DILUTOR
DIMETER
DIMITRI
DINETTE
DIOPTER
DOESTOO
DOGSTAR
DONATED
DONATEE
DONATES
DONATOR
DONATUS
DONETSK
DONOTGO
DOOUTOF
DORITOS
DOROTHY
DOUBTED
DOUBTER
DOUBTIT
DRAFTED
DRAFTEE
DRAFTER
DRASTIC
DRATTED
DRAYTON
DRIFTED
DRIFTER
DRIFTIN
DRIFTUP
DRISTAN
DROPTOP
DUETTED
DUETTOS
DUNSTAN
DWELTON
DYKSTRA

D••••T•

DACOSTA
DARESTO
DEALSTO
DEALTTO
DEBOITE
DEBRETT
DECANTS
DECEITS
DECLOTS
DECOCTS
DEDUCTS
DEFACTO
DEFEATS
DEFECTS
DEFERTO
DEFLATE
DEGUSTS
DEIGNTO
DEJECTS
DELCITY
DELICTI
DELICTO
DELICTS
DELINTS
DELISTS
DELRUTH
DEMASTS
DEMENTO
DEMISTS
DENSITY
DENTATE
DEODATO
DEPARTS
DEPESTS
DEPICTS
DEPLETE
DEPORTS
DERALTE
DERMATO
DERUSTS
DESALTS
DESERTS
DESILTS
DESISTS
DESPITE
DESPOTS
DETECTO
DETECTS
DETENTE
DETENTS
DETESTS
DEVESTS
DEVIATE
DICTATE
DIDACTS
DIECUTS
DIGESTS
DIGGITY
DIGINTO
DIGLOTS
DIGNITY
DIKTATS
DIMOUTS
DIMWITS
DINETTE
DIORITE
DIPINTO
DIPNETS
DIRECTS
DIRECTV
DISPUTE
DISRATE
DIVERTS
DIVESTS
DOCENTS
DOCKETS
DOGBITE
DOGGATE
DOGGETT
DOGMATA
DOGSITS
DOHERTY
DOINGTO
DOOMSTO
DORSETT
DOSHOTS
DOUGHTY
DOZENTH
DRAGOTI
DRANKTO
DRAWNTO
DRAWSTO
DRINKTO
DRIVETO
DROVETO
DRTEETH
DRYROTS
DUALITY
DUBIETY
DUEDATE
DUGINTO
DUGOUTS
DURANTE
DWIGHTD
DYEBATH
DYELOTS
DYEVATS
DYNASTS
DYNASTY

D•••••T

DADAART
DADAIST
DAFTEST
DAMPEST
DANKEST
DARENOT
DARKEST
DASBOOT
DASHDOT
DASHPOT
DATASET
DAUSSET
DEADEST
DEADSET
DEAFEST
DEALOUT
DEAREST
DEBRETT
DECKOUT
DECRYPT
DEEPEST
DEEPFAT
DEEPSET
DEFAULT
DEFFEST
DEFIANT
DEFICIT
DEFLECT
DEFROST
DEFTEST
DEFUNCT
DEGHOST
DEHMELT
DELBERT
DELIGHT
DELIMIT
DELMONT
DEMARET
DEMERIT
DEMOUNT
DENSEST
DENTIST
DEORBIT
DEPOSIT
DERWENT
DESCANT
DESCENT
DESERET
DESKSET
DESSERT
DETRACT
DETROIT
DEVIANT
DEWAART
DEWIEST
DIALECT
DIALOUT
DIARIST
DICIEST
DIDASET
DIDEROT
DIDTOAT
DIECAST
DIEDOUT
DIESOUT
DIGIPET
DIGSOUT
DILBERT
DILUENT
DIMMEST
DIMSOUT
DINEDAT
DINEOUT
DINESAT
DINGBAT
DINMONT
DISGUST
DISHOUT
DISMAST
DISPART

DISPORT
DISRUPT
DISSECT
DISSENT
DISSERT
DISTANT
DISTORT
DNATEST
DOESNOT
DOGBERT
DOGBOOT
DOGCART
DOGCOAT
DOGGETT
DOGREAT
DOGTROT
DOGVEST
DOLEOUT
DOORMAT
DOPEOUT
DOPIEST
DORIGHT
DORMANT
DORSETT
DOUBLET
DOUBTIT
DOUREST
DOVECOT
DOVELET
DOWNPAT
DOZIEST
DRAGNET
DRAGOUT
DRAUGHT
DRAWOUT
DREWOUT
DRFRIST
DRIBLET
DRIVEAT
DROPLET
DROPNET
DROPOUT
DROPSIT
DROUGHT
DROVEAT
DRUMOUT
DRUMSET
DRYHEAT
DRYSUIT
DUALIST
DUCKOUT
DUEEAST
DUELIST
DUEWEST
DULLEST
DUMBEST
DUMPOUT
DURWENT
DWELLAT

•DT••••

CDTOWER
HDTVSET
IDTHEFT

•D•T•••

CDSTORE
EDITING
EDITION
EDITORS
EDITOUT
EDITRIX
IDOTTER

•D••T••

ADAPTED
ADAPTER
ADAPTOR
ADAPTTO
ADEPTAT
ADEPTER
ADEPTLY
ADMITTO
ADOPTED
ADOPTEE
ADOPTER
ADRATES
ADULTLY
BDALTON
CDRATES
EDICTAL
EDUCTED
EDUCTOR
IDEATED
IDEATES
IDENTIC
IDIDTOO
IDIOTIC
IDOTTER
ODONTIA

•D•••T•

ADAMITE
ADAPTTO
ADDEDTO
ADDICTS
ADDONTO
ADDUCTS
ADDUPTO
ADJUSTS
ADMITTO
ADULATE
ADVENTS
ADVERTS
EDACITY
EDEMATA
EDOMITE
EDUCATE
NDAKOTA
ODDLOTS
ODELETS
SDAKOTA

•D••••T

ADAMANT
ADDSALT
ADEPTAT
ADHIBIT
ADJUNCT
EDGEOUT
EDGIEST
EDITOUT
HDTVSET
IDOLIST
IDOODIT
IDTHEFT
IDYLIST
ODDMENT
ODORANT

••DT•••

ANDTHEN
BADTIME
BADTRIP
BEDTIME
BUDTIME
DIDTIME
DIDTOAT
GODTHAB
HADTIME
HADTOBE
MIDTEEN
MIDTERM
MIDTOWN
OLDTIME
OLDTOWN
REDTABS
REDTAGS
REDTAIL
REDTAPE
REDTIDE
REDTIES
REDTOPS

••D•T••

AUDITED
AUDITEE
AUDITOR
BADITCH
CADETTE
EIDETIC
GODUTCH
HADATIT
INDITED
INDITER
INDITES
INDUTCH
IODATED
IODATES
KADETTS
NIDETCH
OLDSTER
REDATED
REDATES
REDSTAR
RIDOTTO
SEDATED
SEDATER
SEDATES
SIDETWO
UNDATED
UPDATED
UPDATER
UPDATES
VEDETTE
VIDETTE

••D••T•

ABDUCTS
ADDEDTO
ADDICTS
ADDONTO
ADDUCTS
ADDUPTO
ALDENTE
ANDANTE
BADFITS
BADHATS
BADLOTS
BEDBATH
BEDMATE
BEDSITS
BUDGETS
CADETTE
DEDUCTS
DIDACTS
ENDCUTS
ENDLATE
ENDNOTE
FEDINTO
FIDGETS
FIDGETY
GADGETS
GADGETY
GODWITS
HADFITS
HYDRATE
INDENTS
INDEPTH
INDICTS
INDUCTS
JADEITE
KADETTS
KIDULTS
LEDINTO
LEDUPTO
LUDDITE
LYDDITE
MEDIATE
MIDGETS
MODELTS
MODESTO
MODESTY
MODISTE
MUDBATH
MUDCATS
NUDISTS
ODDLOTS
OLDBATS
OLDCITY
PADGETT
PADSITE
PEDANTS
RADIATE
REDACTS
REDANTS
REDBATS
REDDOTS
REDHATS
REDHOTS
REDOUTS
REDUSTS
RIDESTO
RIDOTTO
RODENTS
SADFATE
SADISTS
TIDBITS
UNDUSTY
UPDARTS
VEDETTE
VEDISTS
VIDETTE
VIDIOTS
WIDGETS

••D•••T

ADDSALT
BADDEBT
BADDEST
BADPAST
BADSHOT
BEDPOST
BEDREST
BODYART
BODYFAT
BODYKIT
DADAART
DADAIST
DIDASET
DIDEROT
DIDTOAT
ENDEDAT
ENDEDIT
ENDMOST
ENDUPAT
FADDIET
FADDIST
FADEOUT
GODSENT
HADAFIT
HADASET
HADATIT
HADBEST
HIDEOUT
HYDRANT
INDOUBT
INDRAFT
INDWELT
JUDOIST
KIDSEAT
MADDEST
MADEFIT
MADEOUT
MEDIANT
MIDEAST
MIDLIST
MIDMOST
MIDWEST
MUDFLAT
NODOUBT
ODDMENT
OGDENUT
OLDSALT
OLDWEST
PADGETT
PODCAST
RADIANT
REDCENT
REDCOAT
REDDEST
REDDUST
REDEALT
REDEBIT
REDHEAT
REDMEAT
REDOUBT
REDRAFT
REDROOT
REDSPOT
REDSUIT
RIDEOUT
RODEOUT
SADDEST
SIDEBET
TIDIEST
UNDEALT
UPDRAFT
UPDRIFT
WEDIDIT

•••DT••

GOLDTIP
GOODTRY
HARDTEN
HARDTOP
ICEDTEA
IDIDTOO
LANDTAG
LANDTAX
ROADTAR
ROADTAX
WINDTEE
WOODTAR

•••D•T•

ACIDITY
AIRDATE
ARIDITY
AVIDITY
BANDITO
BANDITS
BINDSTO
BIODATA
CAUDATE
COEDITS
CORDATE
CORDITE
CREDITS
CRUDITY
DEODATO
DUEDATE
EPIDOTE
ERUDITE
EXUDATE
FEEDSTO
FORDGTS
FORDLTD
GORDITA
GRADATE
HANDYTO
HEADSTO
HOLDSTO
HOTDATE
INEDITA
KEYDETS
LEADETH
LEADSTO
LUDDITE
LYDDITE
MANDATE
MISDATE
NEEDSTO
OFFDUTY
ONADATE
OUTDATE
OXIDATE
PANDITS
PERDITA
PREDATA
PREDATE
PUNDITS
RAWDATA
READSTO
REDDOTS
REEDITS
SEADUTY
SENDSTO
SUBDATE
TENDSTO

•••D••T

ACEDOUT
AGEDOUT
AIRDUCT
APEDIET
ARIDEST
ATEDIRT
AVIDEST
BADDEBT
BADDEST
BALDEST
BANDLET
BOLDEST
BRIDGET
CANDENT
COLDCUT
COLDEST
CONDUCT
CONDUIT
CRUDEST
DEADEST
DEADSET
DIEDOUT
EATDIRT
EKEDOUT
ERODENT
EVIDENT
FADDIET
FADDIST
FEEDLOT
FEUDIST
FINDOUT
FOLDOUT
FONDANT
FONDEST
HANDOUT
HANDSET
HARDEST
HARDHAT
HARDHIT
HARDPUT
HARDSET
HEADOUT
HEADSET
HELDOUT
HOLDOUT
HOLDSIT
ICEDOUT
ILLDOIT
IMADEIT
KINDEST
LAIDOUT
LANDSAT
LEADOUT
LENDOUT
LEWDEST
LORDSIT
LOUDEST
MADDEST
MAHDIST
MILDEST
MINDSET
MORDANT
MORDENT
NEEDNOT
NONDIET
ONADIET
OVIDUCT
OXIDANT
PAIDOUT
PAYDIRT
PENDANT
PENDENT
PREDICT
PREDIET
PRODUCT
PRUDENT
READAPT
READMIT
READOPT
READOUT
REDDEST
REDDUST
SADDEST
SANDLOT
SANDPIT
SAWDUST
SEEDLET
SENDOUT
SLIDOUT
SNIDEST
SOLDOUT
STUDENT
SUBDUCT
THEDIET
TRIDENT
UNADEPT
UNADULT
VERDANT
VERDICT
VIADENT
VIADUCT
VOIDOUT
WEEDOUT
WILDCAT
WILDEST
WOODCUT
WOODLOT

••••DT•

ADDEDTO
BLINDTO
BOUNDTO
BOWEDTO
BREADTH
CAREDTO
FLIEDTO
GLUEDTO
HEWEDTO
HOPEDTO
LOVEDTO
MOVEDTO
NOENDTO
OPTEDTO
PLEADTO
RACEDTO
STANDTO
STOODTO
TRIEDTO
TUNEDTO
WAVEDTO
YIELDTO

••••D•T

AIMEDAT
BAYEDAT
BOOEDAT
COULDNT
DASHDOT
DINEDAT
ENDEDAT
ENDEDIT
FACEDIT
FAKEDIT
FIREDAT
FUMEDAT
GAPEDAT
GAZEDAT
HATEDIT
IDOODIT
JAWEDAT
JIBEDAT
LOVEDIT
MISEDIT
MOVEDIT
PAWEDAT
PERIDOT
PLAUDIT
POKEDAT
PREEDIT
REAUDIT
TRIEDIT
WAVEDAT
WEDIDIT
WOULDNT
WOULDST

•••••DT

BERENDT
SCHELDT
SCHMIDT

DU•••••

DUALISM
DUALIST
DUALITY
DUALIZE
DUBARRY
DUBBERS
DUBBING
DUBIETY
DUBIOUS
DUBNIUM
DUBUQUE
DUCALLY
DUCHAMP
DUCHESS
DUCHIES
DUCKERS
DUCKIER
DUCKIES
DUCKING
DUCKOUT
DUCKPIN
DUCTILE
DUCTING
DUDEDUP
DUDESUP
DUDGEON
DUEDATE
DUEEAST
DUELERS
DUELING
DUELIST
DUELLED
DUENNAS
DUETING
DUETTED
DUETTOS
DUEWEST
DUFFELS
DUFFERS
DUFFLES
DUFUSES
DUGINTO
DUGONGS
DUGOUTS
DUHAMEL
DUKAKIS
DUKEDOM
DULCIFY
DULLARD
DULLEST
DULLING
DULLISH
DUMBEST
DUMBING
DUMDUMS
DUMMIED
DUMMIES
DUMMYUP
DUMPERS
DUMPIER
DUMPILY
DUMPING
DUMPISH
DUMPOUT
DUMPSON
DUNAWAY
DUNCISH
DUNDALK
DUNEDIN
DUNGEON
DUNKERS
DUNKING
DUNKIRK
DUNLINS
DUNLOPS
DUNNAGE
DUNNERS
DUNNING
DUNSTAN
DUODENA
DUOPOLY
DUOTONE
DURABLE
DURABLY
DURANCE
DURANGO
DURANTE
DURNING
DURRELL
DURWARD
DURWENT
DUSKIER
DUSKILY
DUSKING
DUSKISH
DUSTBIN
DUSTERS
DUSTGUN
DUSTIER
DUSTILY
DUSTING
DUSTMAN
DUSTMEN
DUSTMOP
DUSTOFF
DUSTPAN
DUSTRAG
DUSTUPS
DUTEOUS
DUTIFUL
DUUMVIR

D•U••••

DAUBERS
DAUBING
DAUMIER
DAUNTED
DAUNTER
DAUPHIN
DAUSSET
DEUCING
DEUTERO
DEUTSCH
DHURRIE
DIURNAL
DOUANES
DOUBLEA
DOUBLEB
DOUBLEC
DOUBLED
DOUBLEE
DOUBLEF
DOUBLEG
DOUBLEH
DOUBLEI
DOUBLEJ
DOUBLEK
DOUBLEL
DOUBLEM
DOUBLEN
DOUBLEO
DOUBLEP
DOUBLEQ
DOUBLER
DOUBLES
DOUBLET
DOUBLEU
DOUBLEV
DOUBLEW
DOUBLEX
DOUBLEY
DOUBLEZ
DOUBTED
DOUBTER
DOUBTIT
DOUCEUR
DOUGHTY
DOUGLAS
DOUREST
DOUSERS
DOUSING
DRUBBED
DRUBBER
DRUCKER
DRUDGED
DRUDGER
DRUDGES
DRUGGED
DRUIDIC
DRUMLIN
DRUMMED
DRUMMER
DRUMOUT
DRUMSET
DRUMSUP
DRUNKEN
DRUNKER
DRUZEAN
DRUZIAN
DUUMVIR

D••U•••

DEBUNKS
DEBURGH
DEBURRS
DEBUSES
DEBUSSY
DEBUTED
DECUPLE
DEDUCED
DEDUCER
DEDUCES
DEDUCTS
DEFUELS
DEFUNCT
DEFUNDS
DEFUSED
DEFUSER
DEFUSES
DEGUSTS
DEJUNKS
DELUDED
DELUDER
DELUDES
DELUGED
DELUGES
DELUISE
DEMURER
DENUDED
DENUDER
DENUDES
DEPULPS
DEPUTED
DEPUTES
DEQUEUE
DERUSTS
DETUNED
DETUNES
DILUENT
DILUTED
DILUTER
DILUTES
DILUTOR
DISUSED
DISUSES
DIVULGE
DIVULSE
DOEUVRE
DOLUNCH
DOOUTOF
DPLUSES
DRAUGHT
DROUGHT
DROUINN
DUBUQUE
DUFUSES

D•••U••

DANBURY
DARIUSI
DATSUNS
DAYQUIL
DEBAUCH
DEBLURS
DEBOULE
DECRUMB
DEFAULT
DEGAUSS
DELOUSE
DELRUTH
DEMBUMS
DEMOUNT
DENEUVE
DENTURE
DEPAULU
DESLUMS
DETOURS
DETRUDE
DEVOURS
DEYOUNG
DIALUPS
DICTUMS
DIDSUMS
DIECUTS
DIFFUSE
DIMBULB
DIMOUTS
DISBUDS
DISCUSS
DISEURS
DISEUSE
DISGUST
DISPUTE
DISRUPT
DISTURB
DOGRUNS
DOLOURS
DONJUAN
DONRUSS
DRACULA
DRLAURA
DROGUES
DRSEUSS
DRYBULB
DRYRUNS
DRYSUIT
DUGOUTS
DUMDUMS
DUSTUPS
DYBBUKS

D••••U•
DAMASUS
DANSEUR
DAREFUL
DARTGUN
DATABUS
DEALOUT
DEALSUP
DEALTUP
DECATUR
DECKOUT
DECORUM
DEDALUS
DEFOCUS
DEFRAUD
DELARUE
DEQUEUE
DESKFUL
DEVALUE
DEVIOUS
DIALOUT
DIALSUP
DICECUP
DIEDOUT
DIESOUT
DIGSOUT
DIMSOUT
DINEOUT
DIREFUL
DISHFUL
DISHOUT
DIVVYUP
DOINGUP
DOLEFUL
DOLEOUT
DOLLSUP
DOMINUS
DONAHUE
DONATUS
DONIMUS
DOOMFUL
DOPEOUT
DOUCEUR
DRAGOUT
DRAGSUP
DRANKUP
DRAWNUP
DRAWOUT
DRAWSUP
DREAMUP
DRESSUP
DREWOUT
DREYFUS
DRFREUD
DRIEDUP
DRIESUP
DRIFTUP
DRINKUP
DRIVEUP
DROPOUT
DROVEUP
DRUMOUT
DRUMSUP
DUBIOUS
DUBNIUM
DUBUQUE
DUCKOUT
DUDEDUP
DUDESUP
DUMMYUP
DUMPOUT
DUSTGUN
DUTEOUS
DUTIFUL

D•••••U
DEPAULU
DOUBLEU
DREXELU

•DU••••
ADULATE
ADULTLY
EDUARDO
EDUCATE
EDUCING
EDUCTED
EDUCTOR

•D•U•••
ADDUCED
ADDUCER
ADDUCES
ADDUCTS
ADDUPTO
ADJUDGE
ADJUNCT
ADJURED
ADJURER
ADJURES
ADJUROR
ADJUSTS
ADZUKIS
EDMUNDI
EDMUNDS
EDOUARD

•D••U••
ADJOURN
ADNOUNS
ODDDUCK

•D•••U•
ADDEDUP
CDALBUM
EDGEOUT
EDITOUT
ODORFUL
ODOROUS

••DU•••
ABDUCED
ABDUCES
ABDUCTS
ADDUCED
ADDUCER
ADDUCES
ADDUCTS
ADDUPTO
ALDUBIN
ARDUOUS
AUDUBON
CADUCEI
DEDUCED
DEDUCER
DEDUCES
DEDUCTS
ENDUING
ENDUPAT
ENDURED
ENDURER
ENDURES
ENDUROS
ENDUSER
ENDUSES
GODUNOV
GODUTCH
INDUCED
INDUCER
INDUCES
INDUCTS
INDULGE
INDUTCH
KIDULTS
LEDUPTO
MADUROS
MEDULLA
MEDUSAE
MEDUSAN
MEDUSAS
MODULAR
MODULES
MODULUS
NODULAR
NODULED
NODULES
OLDUVAI
PADUANS
PADUCAH
REDUCED
REDUCER
REDUCES
REDUSTS
SEDUCED
SEDUCER
SEDUCES
UNDULAR
UNDUPED
UNDUSTY

••D•U••
ANDSUCH
ARDOURS
ATDEUCE
BADGUYS
BADLUCK
BEDAUBS
BEDBUGS
BEDOUIN
CADBURY
DIDSUMS
ENDCUTS
ENDRUNS
HADPULL
INDOUBT
LADOUCE
MADRUSH
MEDIUMS
MIDJULY
MIDJUNE
NODOUBT
ODDDUCK
PODIUMS
REDBUDS
REDDUST
REDOUBT
REDOUND
REDOUTS
REDSUIT
REDSUNS
SIDDURS
SUDBURY
TEDEUMS
TEDIUMS
UNDRUNK

••D••U•
ADDEDUP
ANDROUS
ARDUOUS
BODEFUL
BODYRUB
BUDDYUP
CADEAUX
CADMIUM
DEDALUS
DUDEDUP
DUDESUP
ENDEDUP
FADEOUT
GIDDYUP
HIDEOUS
HIDEOUT
HYDROUS
JODHPUR
KIDSRUS
LADYBUG
MADEFUN
MADEOUT
MADERUN
MODICUM
MODULUS
OEDIPUS
OGDENUT
OLDBLUE
ORDERUP
REDFOUR
RIDEOUT
RIDESUP
RODEOUT
SIDIOUS
SUDOKUS
TEDIOUS
TIDYSUM

•••DU••
AIRDUCT
CONDUCE
CONDUCT
CONDUIT
DUMDUMS
FOLDUPS
FONDUED
FONDUES
GEODUCK
GOODUSE
GRADUAL
HOLDUPS
HOWDULL
LEADUPS
MACDUFF
ODDDUCK
OFFDUTY
OUTDUEL
OVIDUCT
PERDURE
PETDUCK
PREDUSK
PRODUCE
PRODUCT
PURDUEU
REDDUST
RONDURE
SAWDUST
SEADUCK
SEADUTY
SENDUPS
SIDDURS
SIRDUKE
SUBDUAL
SUBDUCT
SUBDUED
SUBDUER
SUBDUES
THEDUKE
TRADUCE
UNADULT
VANDURA
VANDUYN
VENDUES
VERDUGO
VERDURE
VIADUCT
WINDUPS

•••D•U•
ACEDOUT
AGEDOUT
AMADEUS
APODOUS
BEADSUP
BINDSUP
BUDDYUP
CANDOUR
CARDIUM
COLDCUP
COLDCUT
CRUDSUP
DIEDOUT
EARDRUM
EKEDOUT
FINDOUT
FOLDOUT
FOLDSUP
GIDDYUP
GOLDBUG
GOODBUY
GOODGUY
GORDIUS
HANDFUL
HANDGUN
HANDOUT
HANDSUP
HARDPUT
HEADFUL
HEADOUT
HEADSUP
HEEDFUL
HELDOUT
HOLDOUT
HOLDSUP
HOODLUM
HUMDRUM
ICEDOUT
IRIDIUM
LAIDOUT
LANDAUS
LANDSUP
LEADOUT
LEADSUP
LENDOUT
LOADSUP
MINDFUL
MULDAUR
NEEDFUL
NONDRUG
OILDRUM
PAIDOUT
READOUT
READSUP
RHODIUM
SANDBUR
SENDOUT
SENDSUP
SLEDFUL
SLIDOUT
SOLDOUT
STADIUM
TRADEUP
VERDOUX
VOIDOUT
WEEDOUT
WINDAUS
WINDSUP
WOODCUT

•••D••U
BANDEAU
BIRDFLU
FEYDEAU
MONDIEU
PURDUEU
RONDEAU
TRUDEAU

••••DU•
ACTEDUP
ADDEDUP
AGENDUM
AIREDUP
AMPEDUP
ANTEDUP
ASKEDUP
BOARDUP
BONEDUP
BOUNDUP
BOXEDUP
BUILDUP
CAGEDUP
CAKEDUP
CAMEDUE
CLOUDUP
COMEDUE
CRIEDUP
DRIEDUP
DUDEDUP
EASEDUP
ENDEDUP
EVERDUR
FALLDUE
FELLDUE
FIREDUP
FIXEDUP
FLUBDUB
FREEDUP
FRIEDUP
GASEDUP
HALFDUG
HIKEDUP
HOLEDUP
HYPEDUP
KEYEDUP
LACEDUP
LEPIDUS
LINEDUP
MILKDUD
MIXEDUP
MOVEDUP
NOSEDUP
OVERDUB
OVERDUE
OWNEDUP
PASTDUE
PILEDUP
PIPEDUP
RACEDUP
RAKEDUP
RESIDUA
RESIDUE
RILEDUP
ROPEDUP
ROUNDUP
RUBADUB
SAVEDUP
SEWEDUP
SIZEDUP
SPEEDUP
STANDUP
STOODUP
TAPEDUP
TONEDUP
TRUEDUP
TUNEDUP
TYPEDUP
WAKEDUP
WAXEDUP
WIPEDUP
WIREDUP
WISEDUP
WOUNDUP
XANADUS

•••••DU
ALFREDU
HOWARDU

D•V••••
DAVEKOZ
DAVINCI
DAVISON
DEVALUE
DEVEINS
DEVELOP
DEVESTS
DEVIANT
DEVIATE
DEVICES
DEVILED
DEVILLE
DEVILRY
DEVIOUS
DEVISED
DEVISEE
DEVISER
DEVISES
DEVISOR
DEVOIRS
DEVOLVE
DEVORES
DEVOTED
DEVOTEE
DEVOTES
DEVOURS
DEVRIES
DIVEDIN
DIVERGE
DIVERSE
DIVERTS
DIVESIN
DIVESTS
DIVIDED
DIVIDER
DIVIDES
DIVINED
DIVINER
DIVINES
DIVISOR
DIVORCE
DIVULGE
DIVULSE
DIVVIED
DIVVIES
DIVVYUP
DOVEBAR
DOVECOT
DOVELET
DOVERDE
DRVEGAS

D••V•••
DANVERS
DELVERS
DELVING
DERVISH
DIAVOLO
DIMVIEW
DIVVIED
DIVVIES
DIVVYUP
DOGVEST
DOOVERS
DRIVEAT
DRIVEBY
DRIVEIN
DRIVELS
DRIVERS
DRIVETO
DRIVEUP
DRIVING
DROVEAT
DROVEBY
DROVEIN
DROVERS
DROVETO
DROVEUP
DYEVATS

D•••V••
DATIVES
DEHAVEN
DELIVER
DERIVED
DERIVER
DERIVES
DIDOVER
DISAVOW
DOEUVRE
DONOVAN
DUUMVIR
DWARVES

D••••V•
DASILVA
DECEIVE
DENEUVE
DEPRAVE
DEPRIVE
DESERVE
DESYLVA
DEVOLVE
DONLEVY

D•••••V
DIRECTV
DOUBLEV

•DV••••
ADVANCE
ADVENTS
ADVERBS
ADVERSE
ADVERTS
ADVICES
ADVISED
ADVISEE
ADVISER
ADVISES
ADVISOR

•D•V•••
HDTVSET

•D••••V
EDWARDV

••DV•••
BUDVASE
KIDVIDS

••D•V••
ALDAVIS
ANDOVER
BEDEVIL
CADAVER
DIDOVER
ENDIVES
GODEVIL
HADOVER
MEDEVAC
MEDIVAC
OLDUVAI
UPDIVED
UPDIVES

••D••V•
BADLOVE
BADMOVE
KEDROVA
OLDNAVY
REDFIVE
REDRIVE

••D•••V
BADENOV
FADAYEV
FEDOROV
GODUNOV

•••D•V•
KHEDIVE
LOWDIVE
MALDIVE
MOLDOVA
MONDAVI
PETDOVE
POPDIVA
PREDIVE
SKYDIVE

••••D•V
KEMIDOV
PLOVDIV

•••••DV
EDWARDV

DW•••••
DWARFED
DWARVES
DWEEZIL
DWELLAT
DWELLED
DWELLER
DWELLIN
DWELLON
DWELTON
DWIGHTD
DWINDLE

D•W••••
DAWDLED
DAWDLER
DAWDLES
DAWKINS
DAWNING
DAWNSON
DEWAART
DEWATER
DEWAXED
DEWAXES
DEWCLAW
DEWDROP
DEWFALL
DEWIEST
DEWILDE
DEWIRED
DEWIRES
DEWLAPS
DEWLESS
DEWLINE
DEWORMS
DOWAGER
DOWDIER
DOWDIES
DOWDILY
DOWERED
DOWLING
DOWNBOW
DOWNERS
DOWNIER
DOWNING
DOWNPAT
DOWRIES
DOWRONG
DOWSERS
DOWSING
DRWELBY

D••W•••
DAEWOOS
DAGWOOD
DARWELL
DAYWEAR
DERWENT
DIDWELL
DIMWITS
DOGWOOD
DOOWOPS
DRAWBAR
DRAWEES
DRAWERS
DRAWING
DRAWLED
DRAWLER
DRAWMAN
DRAWMEN
DRAWNIN
DRAWNON
DRAWNTO
DRAWNUP
DRAWOFF
DRAWOUT
DRAWSIN
DRAWSON
DRAWSTO
DRAWSUP
DREWOFF
DREWOUT
DROWNED
DROWSED
DROWSES
DRYWALL
DRYWASH
DRYWELL
DUEWEST
DURWARD
DURWENT
DYEWOOD

D•••W••
DEPOWER
DIEAWAY
DISOWNS
DOORWAY
DUNAWAY

D••••W•
DECLAWS
DIEDOWN
DOGBOWL
DRBROWN

D•••••W
DANELAW
DEWCLAW
DIMVJEW
DISAVOW
DOGCHEW
DOGCHOW
DOGSHOW
DOITNOW
DOUBLEW
DOWNBOW

•DW••••
ADWOMAN
ADWOMEN
EDWARDG
EDWARDI
EDWARDR
EDWARDS
EDWARDV

•D•W•••
ADAWARE

•D••W••
CDTOWER
JDPOWER

••DW•••
BADWORD
BUDWORM
DIDWELL
ENDWAYS
ENDWISE
GODWITS
INDWELL
INDWELT
LIDWINA
MEDWICK
MIDWAYS
MIDWEEK
MIDWEST
MIDWIFE
MUDWASP
OLDWAYS
OLDWEST
PEDWAYS
REDWINE
REDWING
REDWOLF
REDWOOD
REDWORM

••D•W••
BEDEWED
ENDOWED
ENDOWER
HIDAWAY
LEDAWAY
MADEWAR
MADEWAY
MEDAWAR
RIDGWAY
SIDEWAY
UNDEWED
WIDOWED
WIDOWER

••D••W•
ANDREWS
BADNEWS
BEDDOWN
INDRAWN
MIDTOWN
OLDNEWS
OLDSAWS
OLDTOWN
REDDAWN
REDHAWK
REDRAWN
REDRAWS
SIDETWO
SODIDWE
UNDRAWN
UNDRAWS

••D•••W
HADACOW
HADAROW
JUDELAW
MUDFLOW

•••DW••
BALDWIN
COLDWAR
FOODWEB
GOLDWYN
GOODWIN
HARDWAY
HARDWON
HEADWAY
ROADWAY

•••D•W•
BEDDOWN
BOGDOWN
BOWDOWN
BUYDOWN
CRYDOWN
CUTDOWN
DIEDOWN
GETDOWN
GOTDOWN
HOEDOWN
ICEDOWN
JOTDOWN
LAYDOWN
LETDOWN
LIEDOWN
LOWDOWN
MEADOWS
MEADOWY
MILDEWS
MILDEWY
MOWDOWN
NORDOWE
ONEDOWN
PATDOWN
PINDOWN
PREDAWN
PUTDOWN
RAEDAWN

RAMDOWN
RANDOWN
REDDAWN
RUBDOWN
RUNDOWN
SATDOWN
SETDOWN
SHADOWS
SHADOWY
SITDOWN
SUNDOWN
TIEDOWN
TIPDOWN
TOPDOWN
WETDOWN
WINDOWS
WINDOWY

•••D••W
BANDSAW
HANDSAW
HEADSAW
HINDPAW
KENDREW
LAIDLOW
MISDRAW
MISDREW
OUTDRAW
OUTDREW
SKIDROW
TOPDRAW
WOODROW
WOODSAW

••••DW•
SODIDWE

••••D•W
JACKDAW
REENDOW
TONYDOW

D•X••••
DEXTRAL
DEXTRIN

D••X•••
DIOXIDE
DIOXINS
DREXELU
DREXLER
DROXIES

D•••X••
DEHEXED
DEHEXES
DESEXED
DESEXES
DETOXED
DETOXES
DEWAXED
DEWAXES

D•••••X
DEEDBOX
DEEPSIX
DOUBLEX
DROPBOX

•D••X••
ADDAXES
ADMIXED
ADMIXES

•D••••X
EDITRIX

••D•X••
ADDAXES
FEDEXED
FEDEXES
FTDIXNJ
INDEXED
INDEXER
INDEXES
RADIXES
REDOXES

••D•••X
CADEAUX
MADAMEX

•••D•X•
HANDAXE

•••D••X
BANDBOX
DEEDBOX
HARDSIX
HENDRIX
HENDRYX
LANDTAX
ROADTAX
SANDBOX
VERDOUX
WOODBOX

••••D•X
BROADAX
FORTDIX
HUMIDEX
PARADOX
REINDEX
ROLODEX
SPANDEX
UVINDEX

DY•••••
DYBBUKS
DYEBATH
DYEJOBS
DYELOTS
DYEVATS
DYEWOOD
DYKSTRA
DYNAMIC
DYNAMOS
DYNASTS
DYNASTY
DYNODES

D•Y••••
DAYBEDS
DAYBOOK
DAYCAMP
DAYCARE
DAYGAME
DAYHOPS
DAYJOBS
DAYLILY
DAYLONG
DAYMARE
DAYPACK
DAYQUIL
DAYROOM
DAYSAIL
DAYSEND
DAYSIDE
DAYSINN
DAYSOFF
DAYSPAS
DAYSTAR
DAYTIME
DAYTONA
DAYTRIP
DAYWEAR
DEYOUNG
DMYTRYK
DOYENNE
DRYABLE
DRYADES
DRYADIC
DRYBULB
DRYCELL
DRYDOCK
DRYEYED
DRYEYES
DRYFOGS
DRYHEAT
DRYHOLE
DRYIDEA
DRYMOPS
DRYNESS
DRYPERS
DRYROTS
DRYRUNS
DRYSUIT
DRYWALL
DRYWASH
DRYWELL

D••Y•••
DEFYING
DENYING
DESYLVA
DRAYAGE
DRAYING
DRAYMAN
DRAYMEN
DRAYTON
DREYFUS

D•••Y••
DACTYLS
DAIRYER
DANEYKO
DARRYLF
DECAYED
DECAYER
DECOYED
DECOYER
DECRYPT
DELAYED
DELAYER
DENTYNE
DIPTYCH
DIVVYUP
DOEEYED
DRYEYED
DRYEYES
DUMMYUP

D••••Y•
DEADEYE
DEEJAYS
DEFRAYS
DELKEYS
DELRAYS
DEMONYM
DEPLOYS
DICKEYS
DISMAYS
DMYTRYK
DOGDAYS
DOGTOYS
DONKEYS
DORSEYS

D•••••Y
DAFFILY
DAHOMEY
DALTREY
DAMPDRY
DANBURY
DANDIFY
DANDILY
DARESAY
DATEDLY
DAYLILY
DAZEDLY
DEANERY
DEBAKEY
DEBUSSY
DECENCY
DEEPFRY
DEEPSKY
DEERFLY
DELANEY
DELCITY
DEMOLAY
DEMPSEY
DENNEHY
DENSELY
DENSIFY
DENSITY
DESTINY
DESTROY
DEVILRY
DICKORY
DIDDLEY
DIEAWAY
DIETARY
DIGGITY
DIGGORY
DIGNIFY
DIGNITY
DINGILY
DIRTILY
DISOBEY
DISPLAY
DITHERY
DIZZILY
DODDERY
DOHERTY
DONLEVY
DONTCRY
DOORWAY
DOROTHY
DOTTILY
DOUBLEY
DOUGHTY
DOWDILY
DRAMADY
DRAMEDY
DRAPERY
DRIPDRY
DRIVEBY
DRIZZLY
DRMCCOY
DROPSBY
DROVEBY
DRWELBY
DUALITY
DUBARRY
DUBIETY
DUCALLY
DULCIFY
DUMPILY
DUNAWAY
DUOPOLY
DURABLY
DUSKILY
DUSTILY
DYNASTY

•DY••••
IDYLIST
IDYLLIC
ODYSSEY

•D•Y•••
ADAYAGO
EDDYING

•D••Y••
IDSAYSO

•D••••Y
ADDEDLY
ADEPTLY
ADULTLY
EDACITY
EDNAMAY
IDEALLY
ODYSSEY

••DY•••
BODYART
BODYBAR
BODYFAT
BODYKIT
BODYRUB
ECDYSES
ECDYSIS
EDDYING
INDYCAR
LADYBUG
LADYDAY
LADYISH
LADYKIN
LADYNAS
MIDYEAR
REDYING
RUDYARD
TIDYING
TIDYSUM
UNDYING

••D•Y••
BUDDYUP
FADAYEV
GIDDYAP
GIDDYUP
OLDLYME
REDDYES
REDEYED
REDEYES
SADEYED
SADEYES

••D••Y•
BADBOYS
BADDAYS
BADGUYS
ENDWAYS
KIDNEYS
MADALYN
MEDLEYS
MIDDAYS
MIDWAYS
OLDBOYS
OLDDAYS
OLDWAYS
PEDWAYS
REDBAYS
RIDEBYS

••D•••Y
ADDEDLY
ALDORAY
ARDENCY
AUDIBLY
CADBURY
CADENCY
DIDDLEY
DODDERY
ELDERLY
ENDERBY
ENDPLAY
FADEDLY
FIDGETY
GADGETY
GIDDILY
GODFREY
HADASAY
HIDAWAY
HODADDY
INDEEDY
JADEDLY
LADYDAY
LEDAWAY
MADEHAY
MADEWAY
MIDJULY
MODESTY
MRDARCY
MUDDILY
OLDCITY
OLDFOGY
OLDLADY
OLDNAVY
ORDERLY
PUDENCY
PUDGILY
REDARMY
REDCLAY
REDECAY
REDPONY
RIDESBY
RIDGWAY
RUDDILY
SIDEWAY
SUDBURY
TIDALLY
UNDUSTY

•••DY••
ANODYNE
AZODYES
BUDDYUP
GIDDYAP
GIDDYUP
HANDYTO
HOWDYDO
REDDYES
RITDYES
TIEDYED
TIEDYES
VANDYCK
VANDYKE
VATDYED
VATDYES

•••D•Y•
BADDAYS
BATDAYS
BENDAYS
BIGDAYS
DEADEYE
DOGDAYS
FRIDAYS
GLADEYE
GOLDWYN
GOODBYE
GOODBYS
HANDEYE
HENDRYX
HEYDAYS
HOTDAYS
MANDAYS
MAYDAYS
MIDDAYS
MONDAYS
OFFDAYS
OLDDAYS
PAYDAYS
SAIDAYE
SUNDAYS
TAGDAYS
TENDAYS
TWODAYS
VANDUYN

•••D••Y
ABIDEBY
ACADEMY
ACIDIFY
ACIDITY
ARIDITY
AVIDITY
BAWDILY
BEADILY
BINDERY
BRADLEY
BRODKEY
BRODSKY
CARDKEY
CINDERY
COLDDAY
CRUDELY
CRUDITY
DANDIFY
DANDILY
DIDDLEY
DODDERY
DOWDILY
FINDLAY
FINDLEY
FRIDLEY
GAUDERY
GAUDILY
GEODESY
GIDDILY
GLIDEBY
GOODBUY
GOODDAY
GOODGUY
GOODPAY
GOODTRY
HANDILY
HARDDAY
HARDILY
HARDWAY
HEADILY
HEADWAY
LINDSAY
LINDSEY
MEADOWY
MILDEWY
MOODILY
MUDDILY
NEEDILY
OFFDUTY
POWDERY
PREDEFY
PREDENY
PRODIGY
PRUDERY
READILY
ROADWAY
ROWDILY
RUDDILY
SAIDNAY
SANDFLY
SEADUTY
SEEDILY
SENDSBY
SHADILY
SHADOWY
SLIDEBY
SNIDELY
SPIDERY
TARDILY
TINDERY
WEEDILY
WINDILY
WINDOWY
WOODLEY
WORDILY

••••DY•
HAIRDYE
NOBODYS
OVERDYE

••••D•Y
ACRIDLY
ADDEDLY
BLANDLY
BLINDLY
BLOWDRY
BONEDRY
BROADLY
BYANDBY
COLDDAY
DAMPDRY
DATEDLY
DAZEDLY
DRIPDRY
EASEDBY
FADEDLY
FARADAY
FETIDLY
FILEDBY
FIVEDAY
FIXEDLY
FLAGDAY
FLUIDLY
FORADAY
FOUNDRY
FOURDAY
FULLDAY
GELIDLY
GOODDAY
GRANDLY
HALFDAY
HARDDAY
HIGHDAY
HODADDY
HOLIDAY
HOLYDAY
HUMIDLY
JADEDLY
JULYDAY
JUNEDAY
KILNDRY
LADYDAY
LAUNDRY
LEAPDAY
LEONDAY
LINEDRY
LIVIDLY
LONGDAY
LUCIDLY
LURIDLY
MIXEDLY
MRBODDY
MUTEDLY
MYBUDDY
NAKEDLY
NAMEDAY
NEWSDAY
NEXTDAY
NICEDAY
NOONDAY
NOTEDLY
ONEADAY
OVERDRY
PALEDRY
PATSDRY
PAVIDLY
PROUDLY
RABIDLY
RACEDBY
RAPIDLY
RIGIDLY
ROUNDLY
RULEDBY
RUNSDRY
SAMEDAY
SEMIDRY
SICKDAY
SLOWDAY
SNOWDAY
SOLIDLY
SOMEDAY
SOUNDLY
SPINDLY
SPINDRY
STAIDLY
STANDBY
STAYDRY
STOODBY
SUCKDRY
TEPIDLY
THIRDLY
THISDAY
TIMIDLY
TIREDLY
TUESDAY
UNGIDDY
UNGODLY
UNMADLY
UNMUDDY
UNSADLY
VALIDLY
VAPIDLY
VERYDRY
VEXEDLY
VIVIDLY
WASHDAY
WEEKDAY
WEIRDLY
WORKDAY
WORLDLY

•••••DY
ALBUNDY
ALMONDY
ALREADY
ANYBODY
ASABODY
BAGLADY
CASSIDY
CUSTODY
DRAMADY
DRAMEDY
EPILADY
HODADDY
HYMNODY
IMREADY
INDEEDY
KENNEDY
MRBODDY
MTBALDY
MYBUDDY
NONBODY
OLDLADY
OREBODY
ORGANDY
ORMANDY
PEABODY
PERFIDY
PICARDY
PROSODY
RAGGEDY
RESTUDY
REVERDY
SCAREDY
SUBSIDY
THEBODY
THREADY
TRAGEDY
UNGAUDY
UNGIDDY
UNHANDY
UNHARDY
UNHEADY
UNIBODY
UNMOLDY
UNMOODY
UNMUDDY
UNNEEDY
UNREADY
UNROWDY
UNSHADY
UNWINDY
WCHANDY

D•Z••••
DAZEDLY
DAZZLED
DAZZLER
DAZZLES
DIZAINS
DIZZIED
DIZZIER
DIZZIES
DIZZILY
DOZENTH
DOZEOFF
DOZIEST

D••Z•••
DAZZLED
DAZZLER
DAZZLES
DITZIER
DIZZIED
DIZZIER
DIZZIES
DIZZILY
DOOZERS
DOOZIES
DRIZZLE
DRIZZLY
DRUZEAN
DRUZIAN

D•••Z••
DAREZZO
DENIZEN
DRIZZLE
DRIZZLY
DWEEZIL

D••••Z•
DAREZZO
DEGLAZE
DUALIZE

D•••••Z
DAVEKOZ
DOUBLEZ

•DZ••••
ADZUKIS

•D•••Z•
IDOLIZE
ODORIZE

••DZ•••
ENDZONE
NUDZHED
NUDZHES
REDZONE

••D•Z••
BEDAZED
BEDAZES
BEDIZEN
IODIZED
IODIZER
IODIZES
UNDAZED

••D••Z•
CADENZA
MIDSIZE

••D•••Z
BEDNORZ
ORDONEZ

•••D•Z•
ANODIZE
CARDOZO
INADAZE
OXIDIZE

EA•••••
EADGILS
EAGERER
EAGERLY
EAGLETS
EAGLING
EANMUND
EARACHE
EARBONE
EARBUDS
EARCLIP
EARDROP
EARDRUM
EARFLAP
EARFULS
EARHART
EARHOLE
EARLAPS
EARLDOM
EARLESS
EARLETS
EARLIER
EARLIES
EARLIKE
EARLOBE
EARLOCK
EARLYON
EARMARK
EARMUFF
EARNERS
EARNEST
EARNING
EARNSIT
EARPLUG
EARRING
EARSHOT
EARTABS
EARTAGS
EARTHED
EARTHEN
EARTHLY
EARWIGS
EASEDBY
EASEDIN
EASEDON
EASEDUP
EASEFUL
EASELED
EASEOFF
EASEOUT
EASESBY
EASESIN
EASESON
EASESUP
EASIEST
EASTEGG
EASTEND
EASTERN
EASTERS
EASTHAM
EASTING
EASTMAN
EASYJOB
EASYOFF
EASYONE
EATABIT
EATABLE
EATALOT
EATAWAY
EATCAKE
EATCROW
EATDIRT
EATENAT
EATENUP
EATFROM
EATHERE
EATINTO
EATITUP
EATLATE
EATLESS
EATMORE
EATOVER
EATSOUT

E•A••••

EBANKED
EBAYERS
ECARTES
EDACITY
EDASNER
EGALITE
ELAAIUN
ELAINES
ELAMITE
ELANCES
ELANETS
ELANTRA
ELAPIDS
ELAPSED
ELAPSES
ELASTIC
ELASTIN
ELATERS
ELATING
ELATION
EMAILED
EMAILER
EMANANT
EMANATE
EMANUEL
ENABLED
ENABLER
ENABLES
ENACTED
ENACTOR
ENAMELS
ENAMORS
ENAMOUR
ENARBOR
ENARMED
EPARCHS
EPARCHY
EPAULET
ERASERS
ERASING
ERASMUS
ERASTUS
ERASURE
ETAGERE
ETAILED
ETAILER
ETALIBI
ETAMINE
EVACUEE
EVADERS
EVADING
EVALUNA
EVANDER
EVANGEL
EVANISH
EVASION
EVASIVE
EXABYTE
EXACTAS
EXACTED
EXACTER
EXACTLY
EXACTOR
EXALTED
EXALTER
EXAMINE
EXAMPLE
EXANIMO
EXARCHS

E••A•••

EARACHE
EATABIT
EATABLE
EATALOT
EATAWAY
ECHAPPE
ECLAIRS
ECUADOR
EDGARDO
EDNAMAY
EDUARDO
EDWARDG
EDWARDI
EDWARDR
EDWARDS
EDWARDV
EFFABLE
EFFABLY
EFFACED
EFFACER
EFFACES
ELAAIUN
ELCAJON
ELCAMPO
ELEANOR
ELEAZAR
ELGALLO
ELLAMAE
ELUANTS
ELUATES
EMBALMS
EMBANKS
EMBARGO
EMBARKS
EMBASSY
EMBAYED
EMPALED
EMPALES
EMPANEL
EMPATHS
EMPATHY
ENCAGED
ENCAGES
ENCAMPS
ENCARRE
ENCARTA
ENCASED
ENCASES
ENDABLE
ENDALLS
ENFACED
ENFACES
ENFANTS
ENGAGED
ENGAGER
ENGAGES
ENGARDE
ENHANCE
ENLACED
ENLACES
ENLARGE
ENMASSE
ENRAGED
ENRAGES
ENRANKS
ENTAILS
EQUABLE
EQUABLY
EQUALED
EQUALLY
EQUALTO
EQUATED
EQUATES
EQUATOR
ERLANGS
ERRABLE
ERRANCY
ERRANDS
ERRATIC
ERRATUM
ESCALOP
ESCALUS
ESCAPED
ESCAPEE
ESCAPER
ESCAPES
ESCARPS
ESIASON
ESPANOL
ESPARTO
ESSAYED
ESSAYER
ESTADOS
ESTAMIN
ESTATED
ESTATES
ETHANES
ETHANOL
EUBANKS
EULABUS
EURASIA
EXFACTO
EXHALED
EXHALES
EXHAUST
EXMATES
EXMAYOR
EXPANDS
EXPANSE
EXPARTE
EXYANKS

E•••A••

EARHART
EARLAPS
EARMARK
EARTABS
EARTAGS
EATCAKE
EATLATE
ECKHART
ECOTAGE
ECSTASY
EDEMATA
EDINAMN
EDOUARD
EDUCATE
EGGCASE
EGGSACS
ELEGANT
ELEVATE
ELIYALE
ELKHART
ELLMANN
ELPRADO
ELTRAIN
EMANANT
EMANATE
EMBLAZE
EMBRACE
EMERALD
EMIRATE
EMPLACE
EMPLANE
EMQUADS
EMULATE
ENCHAIN
ENCHANT
ENCHASE
ENCLASP
ENCLAVE
ENDEARS
ENDGAME
ENDLATE
ENDWAYS
ENFLAME
ENFRAME
ENGLAND
ENGRAFT
ENGRAIN
ENGRAMS
ENGRAVE
ENNEADS
ENPLANE
ENQUADS
ENSEALS
ENSEATS
ENSLAVE
ENSNARE
ENSNARL
ENTRADA
ENTRAIN
ENTRANT
ENTRAPS
ENWRAPS
EPHRAIM
EPICARP
EPILADY
EPILATE
EPITAPH
EQUIANO
ESPIALS
ESTRADA
ESTRAYS
ESTUARY
ETCHANT
EUSTACE
EWELAMB
EXCLAIM
EXCLAVE
EXOCARP
EXOGAMY
EXPIATE
EXPLAIN
EXTRACT
EXUDATE
EYEBALL
EYEBANK
EYECARE
EYEHAND
EYELASH
EYEMASK
EYEWALL
EYEWASH

E••••A•

EARFLAP
EASTHAM
EASTMAN
EATAWAY
EATENAT
ECTYPAL
ECZEMAS
EDICTAL
EDNAMAY
EGERIAS
EGGHEAD
EIGHTAD
EIGHTAM
EIJKMAN
ELEAZAR
ELEGIAC
ELENIAK
ELLAMAE
ELLYMAY
ELUVIAL
ELYSIAN
ENCINAS
ENDEDAT
ENDLEAF
ENDPLAY
ENDUPAT
ENIGMAS
ENTHRAL
ENTREAT
EPERNAY
EPIGRAM
EPOCHAL
EQUIFAX
ESCHEAT
ESPOSAS
ESTEBAN
ESTEFAN
ESTIVAL
ETERNAL
ETESIAN
ETHICAL
ETONIAN
EUREKAS
EUROVAN
EVENPAR
EXACTAS
EXCELAT
EXCUSAL
EXCUSAS
EXEDRAE
EXURBAN
EYEEXAM
EYEWEAR

E•••••A

ECHIDNA
EDEMATA
ELANTRA
ELBERTA
ELECTRA
ELEKTRA
ELEVENA
EMERITA
EMMUSKA
EMPORIA
ENCARTA
ENCOMIA
ENTRADA
EPHEDRA
ERIGENA
ERITREA
ERMINIA
ERNESTA
EROTICA
ESCUELA
ESTELLA
ESTONIA
ESTRADA
ETRURIA
ETVOILA
EUGENIA
EUGLENA
EUNOMIA
EURASIA
EVALUNA
EXEMPLA
EXHEDRA
EXORDIA
EXOTICA
EXURBIA

•EA••••

BEACHAM
BEACHED
BEACHES
BEACONS
BEADERS
BEADIER
BEADILY
BEADING
BEADLES
BEADSUP
BEAGLES
BEAHERO
BEAKERS
BEALION
BEAMERS
BEAMIER
BEAMING
BEAMISH
BEAMSUP
BEANBAG
BEANDIP
BEANERY
BEANIES
BEANING
BEANOIL
BEARCAT
BEARCUB
BEARDED
BEARERS
BEARHUG
BEARING
BEARISH
BEAROFF
BEAROUT
BEARPAW
BEARPIT
BEARSON
BEARSUP
BEASLEY
BEASTIE
BEASTLY
BEATALL
BEATBOX
BEATCOP
BEATERS
BEATIFY
BEATING
BEATLES
BEATNIK
BEATOFF
BEATOUT
BEATRIX
BEATSAT
BEATSIT
BEATSME
BEATSON
BEATSUP
BEATTIE
BEAUISH
BEAVERS
CEASING
DEACONS
DEADAIR
DEADEND
DEADENS
DEADEST
DEADEYE
DEADPAN
DEADSEA
DEADSET
DEAFENS
DEAFEST
DEAIRED
DEALERS
DEALING
DEALOUT
DEALSIN
DEALSTO
DEALSUP
DEALTIN
DEALTTO
DEALTUP
DEANERY
DEARDEN
DEAREST
DEARGOD
DEARIES
DEARONE
DEARSIR
DEARTHS
FEARERS
FEARFOR
FEARFUL
FEARING
FEARNOT
FEASTED
FEASTER
FEASTON
FEATHER
FEATURE
GEARBOX
GEARING
GEARSTO
GEARSUP
HEADEND
HEADERS
HEADFOR
HEADFUL
HEADIER
HEADILY
HEADING
HEADMAN
HEADMEN
HEADOFF
HEADOUT
HEADPIN
HEADSAW
HEADSET
HEADSIN
HEADSTO
HEADSUP
HEADWAY
HEALALL
HEALERS
HEALING
HEALSUP
HEALTHY
HEAPERS
HEAPING
HEAPSOF
HEAPSON
HEAPSUP
HEARDOF
HEARERS
HEARING
HEARKEN
HEAROUT
HEARSAY
HEARSES
HEARSOF
HEARTED
HEARTEN
HEARTHS
HEATERS
HEATFAN
HEATFUL
HEATHEN
HEATHER
HEATING
HEATRAY
HEATSUP
HEATTER
HEAVEHO
HEAVENS
HEAVERS
HEAVETO
HEAVIER
HEAVIES
HEAVILY
HEAVING
JEALOUS
JEANARP
JEANLUC
JEANNIE
JEANNOT
KEARNEY
LEACHED
LEACHER
LEACHES
LEACOCK
LEADDOG
LEADENS
LEADERS
LEADETH
LEADIER
LEADING
LEADINS
LEADMAN
LEADMEN
LEADOFF
LEADORE
LEADOUT
LEADSIN
LEADSON
LEADSTO
LEADSUP
LEADUPS
LEAFAGE
LEAFIER
LEAFING
LEAFLET
LEAFOUT
LEAGUED
LEAGUER
LEAGUES
LEAKAGE
LEAKERS
LEAKEYS
LEAKIER
LEAKING
LEAKSIN
LEANCUT
LEANDER
LEANERS
LEANEST
LEANING
LEANSIN
LEANSON
LEANSTO
LEANTOS
LEAPDAY
LEAPERS
LEAPFOR
LEAPING
LEAPSAT
LEAPSIN
LEAPSON
LEAPSUP
LEAPTAT
LEAPTIN
LEAPTON
LEAPTUP
LEARJET
LEARNED
LEARNER
LEARNOF
LEARNTO
LEASERS
LEASETO
LEASHED
LEASHES
LEASING
LEATHER
LEAVEBE
LEAVEIN
LEAVEIT
LEAVENS
LEAVEON
LEAVING
LEAWOOD
MEADOWS
MEADOWY
MEAGLES
MEALIER
MEALIES
MEANAGE
MEANDER
MEANEST
MEANIES
MEANING
MEANJOE
MEANSIT
MEANSTO
MEANTIT
MEANTTO
MEASLES
MEASURE
MEATAXE
MEATIER
MEATILY
MEATMAN
MEATMEN
MEATPIE
NEAREST
NEARING
NEARPAR
NEARYOU
NEATENS
NEATEST
NEATNIK
PEABEAN
PEABODY
PEACHED
PEACHES
PEACOAT
PEACOCK
PEAFOWL
PEAHENS
PEAKIER
PEAKING
PEAKISH
PEALIKE
PEALING
PEANUTS
PEAPODS
PEARLED
PEARLER
PEARSON
PEASANT
PEASOUP
PEATBOG
PEATIER
PEATPOT
REACHED
REACHER
REACHES
REACHIN
REACHUP
REACTED
REACTOR
REACTTO
READAPT
READDED
READERS
READFOR
READIED
READIER
READIES
READILY
READING
READMIT
READOFF
READOPT
READORN
READOUT
READSIN
READSON
READSTO
READSUP
REAFFIX
REAGANS
REAGENT
REAIMED
REAIRED
REALEST
REALIGN
REALINE
REALISE
REALISM
REALIST
REALITY
REALIZE
REALLOT
REALMAN
REALMEN
REALTER
REALTOR
REAMASS
REAMEND
REAMERS
REAMING
REAMOUT
REANNEX
REAPERS
REAPING
REAPPLY
REARDON
REAREND
REARERS
REARGUE
REARING
REARISE
REARLIT
REARMED
REAROSE
REARSUP
REASKED
REASONS
REASSAY
REATTAS
REAUDIT
REAUMUR
REAVAIL
REAVERS
REAVING
REAVOWS
REAWAKE
REAWOKE
SEAARMS
SEABAGS
SEABASS
SEABEDS
SEABEES
SEABIRD
SEABLUE
SEABOAT
SEABORG
SEACALM
SEACATS
SEACOWS
SEADOGS
SEADUCK
SEADUTY
SEAEELS
SEAFARE
SEAFERN
SEAFOAM
SEAFOOD
SEAFOWL
SEAGATE
SEAGIRT
SEAGODS
SEAGRAM
SEAGREN
SEAGULL
SEAHAWK
SEAHERO
SEAHUNT
SEALABS
SEALANE
SEALANT
SEALEGS
SEALERS
SEALERY
SEALIFE
SEALIFT
SEALIKE
SEALILY
SEALING
SEALION
SEALOFF
SEALSIN
SEALSUP
SEAMAPS
SEAMERS
SEAMIER
SEAMILE
SEAMING
SEAMIST
SEAMOSS
SEANCES
SEAPORT
SEARACE
SEARERS
SEARING
SEASALT
SEASICK
SEASIDE
SEASLUG
SEASONS
SEASTAR
SEATERS
SEATING
SEATRIP
SEATTLE
SEAWALL
SEAWARD
SEAWAYS
SEAWEED
SEAWOLF
TEABAGS
TEABALL
TEACAKE
TEACART
TEACHER
TEACHES
TEACHIN
TEACOZY
TEACUPS
TEAGOWN
TEALEAF
TEALESS
TEAMING
TEAMSUP
TEAMUSA
TEANECK
TEAPOTS
TEAPOYS
TEARERS
TEARFUL
TEARGAS
TEARIER
TEARILY
TEARING
TEAROFF
TEAROOM
TEAROSE
TEAROUT
TEARSAT
TEARSIT
TEARSUP
TEASELS
TEASERS
TEASETS
TEASEUP
TEASHOP
TEASING
TEATIME
TEATRAY
TEATREE
TEATROS
TEAURNS
VEADARS
VEALIER
WEAKENS
WEAKEST
WEAKISH
WEAKONS
WEALTHS
WEALTHY
WEANERS
WEANING
WEAPONS
WEARERS
WEARIED
WEARIER
WEARIES
WEARILY
WEARING
WEAROFF
WEAROUT
WEARSON
WEASELS
WEATHER
WEAVERS
WEAVING
YEAHBUT
YEAHMAN
YEAHYOU
YEANING
YEAREND
YEARNED
YEARNER
YEARNTO

YEARONE
YEASTED
YEATEAM
ZEALAND
ZEALOTS
ZEALOUS

•E•A•••

AERATED
AERATES
AERATOR
BECALMS
BECAUSE
BEDAUBS
BEDAZED
BEDAZES
BEFALLS
BEGANTO
BEHAPPY
BEHAVED
BEHAVES
BELABOR
BELAIRS
BELARUS
BELASCO
BELATED
BELAYED
BELAYER
BENARES
BENATAR
BENAZIR
BERATED
BERATER
BERATES
BETAKEN
BETAKES
BETAMAX
BETARAY
BEWAILS
BEWARED
BEWARES
CEDARED
CELADON
CELAENO
CENACLE
CERAMIC
CERATED
CERATES
CESAIRE
CETANES
CEZANNE
DEBACLE
DEBAKEY
DEBARGE
DEBARKS
DEBASED
DEBASER
DEBASES
DEBATED
DEBATER
DEBATES
DEBAUCH
DECADES
DECAGON
DECALOG
DECAMPS
DECANTS
DECAPOD
DECARLO
DECATUR
DECAYED
DECAYER
DEDALUS
DEFACED
DEFACER
DEFACES
DEFACTO
DEFALLA
DEFAMED
DEFAMER
DEFAMES
DEFANGS
DEFARGE
DEFAULT
DEGAUSS
DEHAIRS
DEHAVEN
DELANEY
DELARUE
DELAYED
DELAYER
DEMAGOG
DEMANDS
DEMARCO
DEMARET
DEMARKS
DEMASTS
DENARII
DEPALMA
DEPARTS
DEPAULU
DERAILS
DERALTE
DERANGE
DERATED
DERATES
DESALTS
DETAILS
DETAINS
DEVALUE
DEWAART
DEWATER
DEWAXED
DEWAXES
FEMALES
GELATED
GELATES
GELATIN
GELATIS
GELATOS
GEMAYEL
GERAINT
GERALDO
GETABLE
GETAHIT
GETAJOB
GETATIP
GETAWAY
HEMATIC
HEMATIN
HEPARIN
HEPATIC
HERALDS
HEXADIC
HEXAGON
HEXANES
HEXAPOD
KERATIN
LEBANON
LEBARON
LECARRE
LEDAWAY
LEGALLY
LEGANZA
LEGATEE
LEGATES
LEGATOR
LEGATOS
LEHAVRE
LEPANTO
LESABRE
LEVADES
LEVATOR
MEDAKAS
MEDALED
MEDAWAR
MEGABIT
MEGAERA
MEGAERG
MEGAHIT
MEGALON
MEGANES
MEGATON
MELAMED
MELANGE
MELANIA
MELANIC
MELANIE
MELANIN
MENACED
MENACER
MENACES
MENAGES
MESAMIS
METALED
METATES
NEGATED
NEGATER
NEGATES
NEGATOR
NEPALIS
NEVADAN
NEWAGER
NEWAGEY
PEDALED
PEDALER
PEDANTS
PEGASUS
PEGAWAY
PELAGES
PELAGIC
PENALTY
PENANCE
PENATES
PERAHIA
PERATIO
PESADES
PESANTE
PETALED
PETALES
PETARDS
REBAITS
REBAKED
REBAKES
REBALED
REBALES
REBANKS
REBASTE
REBATED
REBATER
REBATES
REBATHE
RECABLE
RECAGED
RECAGES
RECALLS
RECANED
RECANES
RECANTS
RECARRY
RECARVE
RECASED
RECASES
RECASTS
REDACTS
REDALGA
REDANTS
REDARED
REDARES
REDARMY
REDARNS
REDATED
REDATES
REEARNS
REFACED
REFACES
REFALLS
REFAXED
REFAXES
REGAINS
REGALED
REGALER
REGALES
REGALIA
REGALLY
REGARDS
REGATTA
REGAUGE
REHANGS
REHAULS
REJAILS
RELABEL
RELACED
RELACES
RELANCE
RELANDS
RELANES
RELAPSE
RELATCH
RELATED
RELATER
RELATES
RELATOR
RELAXED
RELAXER
RELAXES
RELAYED
RELAYER
REMAILS
REMAINS
REMAKES
REMANDS
REMARKS
REMARRY
REMATCH
REMATED
REMATES
RENAILS
RENALDO
RENALLY
RENAMED
RENAMES
RENAULT
REPACKS
REPAGED
REPAGES
REPAINT
REPAIRS
REPANEL
REPAPER
REPARKS
REPASTE
REPASTS
REPATCH
REPAVED
REPAVES
RERACKS
RERAISE
RERAKED
RERAKES
RERANKS
RERATED
RERATES
RESALES
RESALTS
RESANDS
RESAVED
RESAVES
RESAWED
RETABLE
RETACKS
RETAILS
RETAINS
RETAKEN
RETAKER
RETAKES
RETALLY
RETAMED
RETAMES
RETAPED
RETAPES
RETARDS
RETASTE
RETAXED
RETAXES
REVALUE
REVAMPS
REWAGER
REWAKED
REWAKEN
REWAKES
REWARDS
REWARMS
REWARNS
REWATER
REWAXED
REWAXES
SEAARMS
SECANTS
SEDALIA
SEDATED
SEDATER
SEDATES
SEEABLE
SEEALSO
SEMANAS
SENATES
SENATOR
SEPALED
SERAPES
SERAPHS
SERAPIS
SESAMES
SEWARDS
TEBALDI
TEJANAS
TEJANOS
TELAVIV
TENABLE
TENABLY
TENACES
TENACRE
TENANCY
TENANTS
TERAOHM
TETANUS
VENABLE
VENALLY
VENATIC
VERANDA
ZELAZNY
ZENANAS

•E••A••

AERIALS
BEATALL
BEBRAVE
BECHARM
BEDBATH
BEDLAMP
BEDLAMS
BEDMATE
BEDRAIL
BEDRAPE
BEEFALO
BEEYARD
BEGGARS
BEGGARY
BEHEADS
BEHEARD
BELDAME
BELDAMS
BELFAST
BELLAMY
BELTANE
BEMOANS
BENDAYS
BENEATH
BENGALI
BENGALS
BENZALI
BEREAVE
BERGAMO
BERNARD
BERNAYS
BETHANY
BETRAYS
BETTANY
CELLARS
CEMBALO
CENTALS
CENTARE
CENTAUR
CENTAVO
CEPHALO
CEPHALY
CEREALS
CERTAIN
DEADAIR
DEBEARD
DECEASE
DECIARE
DECLAIM
DECLARE
DECLASS
DECLAWS
DEEJAYS
DEFEATS
DEFIANT
DEFLATE
DEFOAMS
DEFRAGS
DEFRAME
DEFRAUD
DEFRAYS
DEGLAZE
DEGRADE
DELEADS
DELRAYS
DELTAIC
DEMEANS
DENHAAG
DENIALS
DENMARK
DENTALS
DENTATE
DEODARS
DEODATO
DEPLANE
DEPRAVE
DERMATO
DESCANT
DESPAIR
DESTAEL
DESTAIN
DETRACT
DETRAIN
DEVIANT
DEVIATE
DEWAART
DEWFALL
DEWLAPS
FEEBATE
FELLAHS
FERMATA
FERMATE
FERMATS
FERNAND
FERRARA
FERRARE
FERRARI
FERRARO
FERRATE
GEEGAWS
GELCAPS
GEMMATE
GENNAIO
GENNARO
GERMAIN
GERMANE
GERMANS
GERMANY
GERVAIS
GESTALT
GESTAPO
GESTATE
GETBACK
GETCASH
GETPAST
GETSANA
GETSANF
GETWARM
GEWGAWS
HEALALL
HEBRAIC
HECKART
HECTARE
HEEHAWS
HENBANE
HENNAED
HEPCATS
HEPTADS
HERBAGE
HERBALS
HERBART
HERBAUT
HERMANA
HERMANN
HERMANO
HERMANS
HERNANI
HESSAFE
HEYDAYS
HEYMANS
HEYWARD
JEANARP
JETFANS
JETLAGS
JETPACK
JETWASH
JETWAYS
KENDALL
KENWAHL
KENYANS
KEYBANK
KEYCARD
KEYCASE
KEYPADS
KEYPALS
KEYWAYS
LEAFAGE
LEAKAGE
LEBLANC
LEEWARD
LEEWAYS
LEFTARM
LEGRAND
LEHMANN
LEMMATA
LENFANT
LEONARD
LEONATO
LEOPARD
LEOTARD
LEPPARD
LESCAUT
LESPAUL
LETFALL
LETHAVE
LETPASS
LEXMARK
MEANAGE
MEATAXE
MECCANS
MEDIANS
MEDIANT
MEDIATE
MELTAGE
MENIALS
MENSANS
MERCADO
MERMAID
MESCALS
MESHACH
MESSAGE
MESSALA
METCALF
METFANS
METHANE
NECTARS
NECTARY
NEDLAND
NEONATE
NESCAFE
NETBALL
NETCAFE
NETGAIN
NETGAME
NETWARE
NEUMANN
NEWCARS
NEWFACE
NEWGATE
NEWHAND
NEWHART
NEWHATS
NEWLAID
NEWMADE
NEWMANS
NEWMATH
NEWNAME
NEWWAVE
NEXRADS
PEASANT
PECCANT
PECCARY
PECCAVI
PEDWAYS
PEERAGE
PELTATE
PENCASE
PENDANT
PENNAME
PENNANT
PENNATE
PENPALS
PENTADS
PENTANE
PEONAGE
PEPBAND
PEPPARD
PEPTALK
PERCALE
PERHAPS
PERIAPT
PERTAIN
PERVADE
PETCAGE
PETCALF
PETCATS
PETGATE
PETHAIR
PETHARE
PETLAMB
PETNAME
PETNAPS
PETRATS
READAPT
REAGANS
REAMASS
REAVAIL
REAWAKE
REBOANT
REBOARD
REBRACE
REBRAND
RECHALK
RECHALL
RECHART
RECLADS
RECLAIM
RECLAME
RECLASP
RECLASS
RECOALS
RECOATS
RECRANK
RECRATE
REDBATS
REDBAYS
REDCAPS
REDCARD
REDDAWN
REDEALS
REDEALT
REDFACE
REDHAIR
REDHATS
REDHAWK
REDIALS
REDJACK
REDOAKS
REDRAFT
REDRAGS
REDRAWN
REDRAWS
REDTABS
REDTAGS
REDTAIL
REDTAPE
REENACT
REFLAGS
REFLATE
REFRACT
REFRAIN
REFRAME
REGEARS
REGLAZE
REGNANT
REGNARD
REGRABS
REGRADE
REGRAFT
REGRANT
REGRAPH
REGRASP
REHEALS
REHEARD
REHEARS
REHEATS
REIMAGE
RELEADS
RELEAPS
RELEARN
RELEASE
RELIANT
RELOADS
RELOANS
REMNANT
RENTALS
REPEALS
REPEATS
REPHASE
REPLACE
REPLANE
REPLANS
REPLANT
REPLATE
REPLAYS
REREADS
RESCALE
RESCANS
RESEALS
RESEAMS
RESEATS
RESEAUS
RESEAUX
RESHAPE
RESHARE
RESHAVE
RESLATE
RESNAIS
RESNAPS
RESOAKS
RESOAPS
RESPACE
RESPADE
RESPANS
RESPARK
RESTABS
RESTACK
RESTAFF
RESTAGE
RESTAIN
RESTAMP
RESTART
RESTATE
RETEACH
RETEARS
RETHANK
RETHAWS
RETIARY
RETOAST
RETRACE
RETRACK
RETRACT
RETRADE
RETRAIN
RETRAPS
REVEALS
REWEARS
REWEAVE
REWRAPS
REXCATS
REYNARD
REYNAUD
SEABAGS
SEABASS
SEACALM
SEACATS
SEAFARE
SEAGATE
SEAHAWK
SEALABS
SEALANE
SEALANT
SEAMAPS
SEARACE
SEASALT
SEAWALL
SEAWARD
SEAWAYS
SEENALL
SEEPAGE
SEEPAST
SEESALL
SEESAWS
SEGWAYS
SELMAAL
SELVAGE
SENSATE
SERFAGE
SERIALS
SERIATE
SERRATE
SERVANT
SETBACK
SETBAIL
SETRATE
SETSAIL
SEXTANS
SEXTANT
TEABAGS
TEABALL
TEACAKE
TEACART
TEDMACK
TEENAGE
TELLALL
TENBALL
TENDAYS
TENNANT
TENPAST
TERNARY
TERNATE
TERRACE
TERRAIN
TERRANS
TESTACY
TESTATE
TETRADS
VEADARS
VEEJAYS
VENTAGE
VERBALS
VERDANT
VERSACE
VERSANT
VESTALS
WEBCAMS
WEBCAST
WEBMAIL
WEBPAGE
WELFARE
WELLAND
WENTAFT
WENTAPE
WETBARS
WETLAND
WETNAPS
WETRAGS
WETWARE
WETWASH
XENIAOH
YEOMANS
YESMAAM
ZEALAND
ZEBRAIC
ZEBRASS
ZEELAND
ZERMATT

•E•••A•

AEOLIAN
AEROBAT
BEACHAM
BEANBAG
BEARCAT
BEARPAW
BEATSAT
BECKHAM
BEECHAM
BEEPSAT
BEERCAN
BEERTAP
BEESWAX
BEHRMAN
BELGIAN
BELLEAU
BELLJAR
BELLLAP
BELLMAN
BELTBAG
BELTRAN
BELTSAW
BELTWAY
BELUGAS
BENATAR
BENTHAM
BEOGRAD
BERGMAN
BERIGAN
BERTHAS
BERTRAM
BESMEAR
BESPEAK
BESTIAL
BESTMAN
BETAMAX
BETARAY
CELICAS
CENTRAL
CESSNAS
DEADPAN

DEBORAH
DECIMAL
DEEPFAT
DEEPTAN
DEFLEAS
DELIHAM
DELILAH
DELIMAN
DEMOLAY
DENHAAG
DEPOSAL
DEWCLAW
DEXTRAL
FEDERAL
FEDORAS
FEEDBAG
FEELBAD
FELDMAN
FELTBAD
FELTHAT
FEMORAL
FERNBAR
FEYDEAU
FEYNMAN
GEISHAS
GENERAL
GENEVAN
GENTIAN
GETAWAY
GETBEAT
GETREAL
GETSFAR
GETSMAD
HEADMAN
HEADSAW
HEADWAY
HEARSAY
HEATFAN
HEATRAY
HECKMAN
HEELPAD
HEELTAP
HEGIRAS
HEISMAN
HELICAL
HELIPAD
HELLCAT
HELLMAN
HEREIAM
HERNIAE
HERNIAS
HESHVAN
HESSIAN
JEERSAT
JERBOAS
JETBOAT
JETSFAN
JETSTAR
KEEPSAT
KEESHAN
KEESLAR
KELLJAN
KEOGHAN
KEROUAC
KERSHAW
KETCHAM
KEYSPAN
LEADMAN
LEAPDAY
LEAPSAT
LEAPTAT
LEDAWAY
LEERSAT
LEFREAK
LEFTEAR
LEFTJAB
LEGOLAS
LEGTRAP
LEGWEAR
LENGUAS
LENSCAP
LENSMAN
LEONDAY
LESSFAT
LESSTAR
LETHEAN
LETSEAT
LEWHOAD
LEXICAL
MEATMAN
MEDAKAS
MEDAWAR
MEDEVAC
MEDICAL
MEDIGAP
MEDIVAC
MEDUSAE
MEDUSAN
MEDUSAS
MEERKAT
MEGRYAN
MEMOPAD
MENORAH
MENUBAR
MERCIAN
MERRIAM
MESSIAH
METSFAN
MEXICAN
MEZUZAH
MEZUZAS
NEARPAR
NEBULAE
NEBULAR
NEBULAS
NEEDHAM
NEONGAS
NESSMAN
NEUTRAL
NEVADAN
NEWDEAL
NEWLEAF
NEWSDAY
NEWSMAN
NEWYEAR
NEXTDAY
OEDIPAL
PEABEAN
PEACOAT
PECKSAT
PEDICAB
PEEKSAT
PEEPSAT
PEERSAT
PEGAWAY
PELICAN
PELLEAS
PELOTAS
PENZIAS
PEORIAN
PEPITAS
PERLMAN
PERMIAN
PERORAL
PERREAU
PERSIAN
PERUSAL
PERYEAR
PESETAS
PESEWAS
PETBEAR
PETBOAS
PETEMAN
PETGOAT
PETSCAN
REALMAN
REASSAY
REATTAS
REBEGAN
REBEKAH
REBREAK
RECITAL
RECLEAN
RECUSAL
REDCLAY
REDCOAT
REDECAY
REDFLAG
REDHEAD
REDHEAT
REDMEAT
REDREAM
REDSFAN
REDSTAR
REEDMAN
REFLOAT
REFUSAL
REFUTAL
REGINAL
REGINAS
REGULAR
REITMAN
REKNEAD
REMORAS
REMOVAL
RENEWAL
REPLEAD
REPOMAN
RESPEAK
RESPRAY
RESTRAP
RESWEAR
RETINAE
RETINAL
RETINAS
RETOTAL
RETREAD
RETREAT
RETRIAL
REVISAL
REVIVAL
SEABOAT
SEAFOAM
SEAGRAM
SEASTAR
SECULAR
SEDONAS
SEISMAL
SELMAAL
SEMANAS
SEMINAL
SEMINAR
SEMIRAW
SENECAN
SENECAS
SENEGAL
SENORAS
SENSUAL
SENTRAS
SEPHIAS
SEPIRAS
SERBIAN
SERIPAK
SERVEAS
SETPLAY
SEVENAD
SEVENAM
SEVERAL
TEALEAF
TEARGAS
TEARSAT
TEATRAY
TEHERAN
TEJANAS
TELEFAX
TELERAN
TELSTAR
TEMPEAZ
TEMPLAR
TENYEAR
TESTBAN
TESTLAB
TEXTUAL
VECTRAS
VEGETAL
VELTMAN
VENEMAN
VENTRAD
VENTRAL
VERITAS
VERYBAD
VERYMAD
VERYSAD
VESTRAL
VETERAN
WEEKDAY
WEIDMAN
WEIRDAL
WELLMAN
WENTBAD
WENTFAR
WENTMAD
XENICAL
YEAHMAN
YEATEAM
YELLSAT
YEREVAN
YESDEAR
YESICAN
YESMAAM
ZENANAS

•E•••A

BEDELIA
BEEFTEA
BEGONIA
BEGORRA
BELINDA
BENBOVA
BENICIA
BERETTA
BERMUDA
BERNINA
CECILIA
CEDILLA
CELESTA
CEREBRA
CERVEZA
DEADSEA
DEEPSEA
DEFALLA
DELEDDA
DELIRIA
DELTONA
DEPALMA
DERONDA
DERRIDA
DESPINA
DESYLVA
FELICIA
FERMATA
FERRARA
FESTINA
FESTIVA
GEHENNA
GEORGIA
GETSANA
HECKUVA
HELLUVA
HENDECA
HERBTEA
HEREDIA
HERMANA
HERMOSA
JEPHTHA
JERITZA
JESSICA
KEDROVA
KELOWNA
KENOSHA
LECUONA
LEGANZA
LEMMATA
LEMPIRA
LEONORA
LETITIA
LETTERA
MEDULLA
MEGAERA
MEGILLA
MELANIA
MELINDA
MELISMA
MELISSA
MELITTA
MELODIA
MENORCA
MESHUGA
MESSALA
MESSINA
NERISSA
NEWIDEA
PERAHIA
PERDITA
PERGOLA
PERISSA
PERSONA
PERUGIA
PETULIA
PETUNIA
REBECCA
REDALGA
REGALIA
REGATTA
REPLICA
RESIDUA
RETSINA
REVERSA
REYNOSA
SEDALIA
SEGOVIA
SENHORA
SEQUOIA
SEQUOYA
SESTINA
SETENTA
SEVILLA
TEAMUSA
TEMPERA
TEMPURA
TEQUILA
TESSERA
VENEZIA
VENTURA
VERANDA
VERBENA
VERONIA
VERRUCA
YESHIVA
ZENOBIA

••EA•••

AFEARED
AHEADOF
ALEARDI
AREAMAP
AREARUG
AREAWAY
ATEABIT
ATEALOT
ATEAWAY
AYEAYES
BLEAKER
BLEAKLY
BLEARED
BLEATED
BLEATER
BREADED
BREADER
BREADTH
BREAKER
BREAKIN
BREAKUP
BREASTS
BREATHE
BREATHS
BREATHY
CHEADLE
CHEAPEN
CHEAPER
CHEAPIE
CHEAPLY
CHEATED
CHEATER
CHEATIN
CHEATON
CLEANED
CLEANER
CLEANLY
CLEANSE
CLEANTE
CLEANUP
CLEARED
CLEARER
CLEARLY
CLEAROF
CLEARUP
CLEATED
CLEAVED
CLEAVER
CLEAVES
CLEAVON
CREAKED
CREAMED
CREAMER
CREASED
CREASER
CREASES
CREATED
CREATES
CREATOR
DIEAWAY
DREADED
DREAMED
DREAMER
DREAMIN
DREAMOF
DREAMON
DREAMUP
ELEANOR
ELEAZAR
FLEABAG
FLEADIP
FLEANCE
FLEAPIT
FREAKED
GLEAMED
GLEANED
GLEANER
GLEASON
GREASED
GREASER
GREASES
GREATEN
GREATER
GREATLY
GREAVES
ICEAGES
ICEAXES
IDEALLY
IDEAMAN
IDEAMEN
IDEATED
IDEATES
IHEARYA
IMEANIT
KNEADED
KNEADER
LIEABED
LIEATOP
OCEANIA
OCEANIC
OCEANID
OCEANUS
OLEANNA
OLEANNY
OLEATES
ONEACAT
ONEACRE
ONEACTS
ONEADAY
ONEARTH
PLEADED
PLEADER
PLEADTO
PLEASED
PLEASER
PLEASES
PLEATED
PREACHY
PREACID
PREACTS
PREAGED
PREAGES
PREALLY
PREAMPS
PREARMS
PREAVER
REEARNS
SEEABLE
SEEALSO
SHEAFED
SHEARED
SHEARER
SHEATHE
SHEATHS
SHEAVED
SHEAVES
SLEAZES
SMEAGOL
SMEARED
SMEARER
SMEARON
SNEAKBY
SNEAKED
SNEAKER
SNEAKIN
SNEAKUP
SPEAKER
SPEAKOF
SPEAKTO
SPEAKUP
SPEARED
SPEARER
STEADED
STEALER
STEALIN
STEALTH
STEAMED
STEAMER
STEAMUP
STEANNE
STEARIC
STEARIN
STEARNS
SWEARAT
SWEARBY
SWEARER
SWEARIN
SWEARTO
SWEATED
SWEATER
SWEATIT
THEABCS
THEAGES
THEALPS
THEARMY
THEARTS
THEATER
THEATRE
THEAXIS
TREACLE
TREACLY
TREADED
TREADER
TREADLE
TREADON
TREASON
TREATED
TREATER
TWEAKED
UNEAGER
UNEARTH
UNEASES
UNEATEN
UNEAVED
UPEARLY
WHEATEN
WHEATON
WREAKED
WREAKER
WREATHE
WREATHS
WREATHY

••E•A••

ABELARD
ABEYANT
ACERATE
ACETALS
ACETATE
AGEMATE
AGESAGO
ALEGARS
ALETAPS
ALEYARD
AMERADA
ATELATE
AVERAGE
BEEFALO
BEEYARD
BREWAGE
CAESARS
CHELATE
CHEVAUX
COEVALS
CPEBACH
CREMATE
CRENATE
CRETANS
CUEBALL
CUECARD
DEEJAYS
DIECAST
DIEHARD
DIETARY
DUEDATE
DUEEAST
DYEBATH
DYEVATS
EDEMATA
ELEGANT
ELEVATE
EMERALD
EWELAMB
EYEBALL
EYEBANK
EYECARE
EYEHAND
EYELASH
EYEMASK
EYEWALL
EYEWASH
FEEBATE
FREEAIR
GAETANO
GEEGAWS
GOESAFT
GOESAPE
GRENADA
GRENADE
GUEVARA
HEEHAWS
HOECAKE
ICEBAGS
ICEBATH
ICECAPS
ICECAVE
ICEDAMS
ICEFALL
ICELAND
ICEPACK
IKEBANA
INEXACT
IRELAND
ITERANT
ITERATE
JOECAMP
LEEWARD
LEEWAYS
LIEBACK
MAENADS
MTEVANS
ONEBALL
ONEBASE
ONECALL
ONEHALF
ONEHAND
ONELANE
ONENAME
ONEPAGE
ONEPAIR
ONEPART
ONEYARD
OPENAIR
OPERAND
OPERANT
OPERATE
OREGANO
OVERACT
OVERAGE
OVERALL
OVERARM
OVERATE
OVERAWE
PEERAGE
PIEBALD
PIEPANS
PIESAFE
PIESALE
PLENARY
PREBADE
PREBAKE
PRECAST
PREDARK
PREDATA
PREDATE
PREDAWN
PREFABS
PREFACE
PREFADE
PREGAIN
PREGAME
PRELACY
PRELATE
PREMADE
PREMAKE
PREMATE
PRENAME
PREPACK
PREPAID
PREPARE
PREPAVE
PREPAYS
PRERACE
PRESAGE
PRESALE
PRESALT
PRETAPE
PREVAIL
PREWARM
PREWARN
PREWASH
QUEPASA
RAEDAWN
REENACT
RIEMANN
SEENALL
SEEPAGE
SEEPAST
SEESALL
SEESAWS
SHEBANG
SHEPARD
SHEVATS
SMETANA
STEFANI
STEWARD
STEWART
TEENAGE
THEBABE
THEBABY
THEBAND
THEBANS
THEBARD
THECAPE
THECARS
THECAVS
THEEAST
THEFALL
THEGAME
THEGANG
THELAMB
THELARK
THEMAGI
THEMALL
THEMASK
THEMAVS
THEMAYO
THEOATH
THERAMS
THERAPY
THESACK
THESAME
THEWALL
THEWAVE
TIEBACK
TIEBARS
TIEGAME
TIERACK
TIETACK
TIETACS
TOECAPS
TOENAIL
TOETAPS
TRENARY
TREPANS
VEEJAYS
WIELAND
ZEELAND

••E••A•

ABETTAL
ADEPTAT
AGENDAS
AMESLAN
ANEMIAS
AREAMAP
AREAWAY
AREOLAE
AREOLAR
AREOLAS
ASEXUAL
ATEAWAY
AVERNAL
AVESTAN
AVESTAS
AXEHEAD
BEECHAM
BEEPSAT
BEERCAN
BEERTAP
BEESWAX
BOERWAR
BRENDAN
BRENNAN
CHEDDAR
CHEETAH
CHEETAS
CHEMLAB
COEQUAL
CREEDAL
CREWMAN
CUESTAS
DEEPFAT
DEEPTAN
DIEAWAY
DOESBAD
DRESSAS
DUENNAS
DWELLAT
EGERIAS
ELEAZAR
ELEGIAC
ELENIAK
EPERNAY
ETERNAL
ETESIAN
EVENPAR
EXEDRAE
EYEEXAM
EYEWEAR
FEEDBAG
FEELBAD
FIESTAS
FLEABAG
FREEMAN
FREEWAY
FREITAG
FRENEAU
FRESCAS
FRETSAT
FRETSAW
FREYTAG
GLEEMAN
GOESBAD
GOESFAR
GOESMAD
GRECIAN
GRESHAM
GREWFAT
GREYLAG
GUESSAT
HEELPAD
HEELTAP
IBERIAN
ICEBOAT
ICETEAS
ICETRAY
IDEAMAN
IREPEAT
JEERSAT
KEEPSAT
KEESHAN
KEESLAR
KNEECAP
KNEEPAD
LEERSAT
LYESOAP
MEERKAT
NEEDHAM
OCELLAR
ODESSAN
ONEACAT
ONEADAY
ONECLAM
ONEGRAM
ONEIDAS
ONEOCAT
ONESTAR
ONEYEAR
OPENBAR
OPENTAP
OSETRAS

OVEREAT
OVERFAR
OVERFAT
OVERLAP
OVERLAX
OVERLAY
OVERMAN
OVERPAR
OVERPAY
OVERRAN
OVERSAD
OVERSAW
OVERTAX
PAELLAS
PEEKSAT
PEEPSAT
PEERSAT
PIERIAN
PLEBIAN
PLEURAE
PLEURAL
PNEUMAS
PNEUMAT
PREHEAL
PREHEAT
PRELOAD
PRELOAN
PREORAL
PREPLAN
PRESEAL
PRESEAT
PRESOAK
PREVIAS
PREWRAP
QUENEAU
QUESNAY
QUETZAL
REEDMAN
RIESMAN
RYELOAF
SHEBEAR
SHECRAB
SHEEHAN
SHEGOAT
SHEILAE
SHEILAS
SHELLAC
SHERMAN
SHERPAS
SIENNAS
SIERRAS
SIESTAS
SNEERAT
SPECIAL
STELIAS
STELLAR
STEPDAD
STERNAL
STEWPAN
SWEARAT
THEBEAR
THEBRAT
THECRAB
THEHEAT
THEREAT
THERIAC
THERMAL
THESTAR

THESWAN
THEYSAY
TIEBEAM
TIENDAS
TREDIAS
TREERAT
TREESAP
TUESDAY
UNEQUAL
USEDCAR
VIETNAM
WEEKDAY
WHEREAS
WHEREAT
XTERRAS
YZERMAN

••E•••A

ACEROLA
ADELINA
ALEGRIA
AMERADA
AMERICA
AMERIKA
AVENIDA
BEEFTEA
BIENNIA
BRESCIA
CAESURA
CHELSEA
CREMONA
CREMORA
DEEPSEA
EDEMATA
ELECTRA
ELEKTRA
ELEVENA
EMERITA
EXEMPLA
FREESIA
GRENADA
GUEVARA
ICEDTEA
IHEARYA
IKEBANA
INEDITA
INERTIA
NUESTRA
OCEANIA
OLEANNA
OLESTRA
ONEIOTA
ONELIRA
ONEONTA
OPENSEA
OVERSEA
PLECTRA
POETICA
PREDATA
PREIDEA
PREPUPA
QUECHUA
QUEPASA
QUERIDA
QUESERA
SMETANA
SPECTRA
SWEEPEA

THEBIGA
THEFLEA
THEIDEA
THERESA
TREINTA
TWELVEA

•••EA••

ABREAST
ACREAGE
ALLEARS
ALREADY
ANDEANS
ANNEALS
APPEALS
APPEARS
APPEASE
ARREARS
ATHEART
ATLEAST
ATPEACE
AUREATE
AXHEADS
BATEAUX
BEHEADS
BEHEARD
BENEATH
BEREAVE
BIGEARS
BIGEAST
BIGEASY
BONEASH
BUREAUS
BUREAUX
BYHEART
CADEAUX
CAPEANN
CASEATE
CAVEART
CAVEATS
CEREALS
CISEAUX
COTEACH
CUNEATE
CUREALL
DEBEARD
DECEASE
DEFEATS
DELEADS
DEMEANS
DISEASE
DOGEARS
DUEEAST
ENDEARS
ENNEADS
ENSEALS
ENSEATS
FAREAST
FINEART
FIREANT
FIREARM
FIVEAAA
FOREACH
FOREARM
FREEAIR
FTMEADE
GALEATE
GATEAUX

GONEAFT
GONEAPE
HAVEAGO
ILLEANA
IMPEACH
IMREADY
INPEACE
INREACH
INSEAMS
INTEARS
INWEAVE
*INYEARS
ITSEASY
JANEANE
JUDEANS
KOREANS
LIMEADE
LINEAGE
LINEARA
LINEARB
LINEATE
LIVEAID
MALEANT
MIDEAST
MILEAGE
NIKEADS
NOSEATS
NOTEASY
OISEAUX
ONLEASE
ONLEASH
ONLEAVE
ORDEALS
ORGEATS
ORLEANS
OUTEARN
OUTEATS
OXHEART
PAGEANT
PALEALE
PILEATE
POLEAXE
POPEAFB
PROEAST
REDEALS
REDEALT
REGEARS
REHEALS
REHEARD
REHEARS
REHEATS
RELEADS
RELEAPS
RELEARN
RELEASE
REPEALS
REPEATS
REREADS
RESEALS
RESEAMS
RESEATS
RESEAUS
RESEAUX
RETEACH
RETEARS
REVEALS
REWEARS
REWEAVE

RITEAID
ROSEATE
SCREAKS
SCREAMS
SIDEARM
SPREADS
SQUEAKS
SQUEAKY
SQUEALS
STREAKS
STREAKY
STREAMS
TAKEAIM
THEEAST
THREADS
THREADY
THREATS
TINEARS
TOHEART
TOLEASE
TONEARM
TOOEASY
TYPEABS
UNBEARD
UNDEALT
UNHEADY
UNHEARD
UNHEAVY
UNLEADS
UNLEAFS
UNLEAKY
UNLEARN
UNLEASH
UNMEANT
UNREADY
UNSEALS
UNSEAMS
UNSEATS
UNTEACH
UNWEARY
UNWEAVE
UPBEARS
UPBEATS
UPHEAPS
UPHEAVE
UPLEAPS
UPLEAPT
UPREACH
UPREARS
UPTEARS
VOTEAYE
WBYEATS
YOTEAMO

•••E•A•

ACTEDAS
ADRENAL
AIMEDAT
AMOEBAE
AMOEBAS
ANGELAS
APTERAL
ARSENAL
AZTECAN
BAKEPAN
BAREXAM
BASEMAN
BASEPAY

BATEMAN
BAYEDAT
BIKEWAY
BIMETAL
BIPEDAL
BLUEJAY
BLUELAW
BODEGAS
BOOEDAT
BOZEMAN
CABEZAS
CAKEPAN
CAMERAE
CAMERAL
CAMERAS
CAPEMAY
CASELAW
CATENAE
CATENAS
CATERAS
CAVEMAN
CHEETAH
CHEETAS
CINEMAS
CINEMAX
COLEMAN
COMESAS
COMESAT
COWERAT
CPAEXAM
CREEDAL
DANELAW
DARESAY
DINEDAT
DINESAT
DOMECAR
DONEBAD
DONEGAL
DONEGAN
DOVEBAR
DRVEGAS
EATENAT
ECZEMAS
ENDEDAT
ESTEBAN
ESTEFAN
EUREKAS
EXCELAT
EYEEXAM
FAREWAR
FEDERAL
FIREDAT
FIREHAT
FIREMAN
FIRESAT
FIVEAAA
FIVEDAY
FIVEMAN
FIVEWAY
FLIESAT
FOREBAY
FOREMAN
FOREPAW
FORERAN
FORESAW
FREEMAN
FREEWAY
FRIEDAN

FUMEDAT
FUMESAT
GALENAS
GAMEBAG
GAMELAN
GAMELAW
GAMETAL
GAPEDAT
GAPESAT
GATEMAN
GATEWAY
GAVEEAR
GAVEWAY
GAZEDAT
GAZESAT
GENERAL
GENEVAN
GIBESAT
GIVEEAR
GIVEWAY
GLEEMAN
GONEBAD
GONEFAR
GONEMAD
HEREIAM
HOMELAB
HUMERAL
HYGELAC
IFWEMAY
ILLEGAL
INGEMAR
JANEWAY
JAWEDAT
JIBEDAT
JIBESAT
JUDELAW
JUNEDAY
JUVENAL
KAMERAD
KNEECAP
KNEEPAD
LATERAL
LATERAN
LATETAG
LAVERAN
LIBERAL
LIKEMAD
LINEMAN
LITERAL
LIVEOAK
LIVESAT
LORELAI
LOVETAP
MADEHAY
MADEMAD
MADEPAR
MADEWAR
MADEWAY
MAKEHAY
MAKEMAD
MAKEPAR
MAKEWAR
MAKEWAY
MALECAT
MATEWAN
MEDEVAC
MINERAL
MODELAS

MOHEGAN
MOLERAT
MOREPAY
MULETAS
MYCENAE
NAMEDAY
NAMETAG
NICEDAY
NICEMAN
NOSEBAG
NOSEGAY
NOTEPAD
NOVELAS
NOVENAS
NUMERAL
ORTEGAL
PACECAR
PACELAP
PAWEDAT
PESETAS
PESEWAS
PETEMAN
PINESAP
PINETAR
POKEDAT
POKESAT
POLECAR
POLECAT
POLEMAN
POLESAT
POSEDAS
POSESAS
RACECAR
RACEWAY
RAREGAS
RATECAP
RAVENAL
REBEGAN
REBEKAH
REDECAY
RENEWAL
ROSEBAY
SAFEWAY
SAMEDAY
SCHEMAS
SCLERAE
SCLERAL
SCLERAS
SENECAN
SENECAS
SENEGAL
SEVENAD
SEVENAM
SEVERAL
SHEEHAN
SHOEPAC
SIDEBAR
SIDECAR
SIDEMAN
SIDEWAY
SITEMAP
SNEERAT
SOLEDAD
SOMEDAY
SOMESAY
SOMEWAY
SPHERAL
SURECAN

SUREIAM
TAPEMAN
TEHERAN
TELEFAX
TELERAN
THREEAD
THREEAM
THREWAT
TIBETAN
TIMELAG
TIMEWAS
TIREMAN
TOBEHAD
TOLEDAN
TOPEKAN
TOTEBAG
TREERAT
TREESAP
TUBEPAN
TUTELAR
UNLEGAL
UNREGAL
UNVENAL
VEGETAL
VENEMAN
VETERAN
VINEGAR
VOTENAY
WAGEWAR
WAVEDAT
WAVESAT
WINEBAR
WINESAP
WINEVAT
WIREMAN
WIRETAP
WISEMAN
YALELAW
YALEMAN
YEREVAN

•••E••A

ADDENDA
ALBERTA
ALGEBRA
ALGERIA
ALLEGRA
ALMERIA
AMNESIA
AMREETA
ANAEMIA
ANTENNA
APHELIA
ARIETTA
ARMENIA
AULETTA
AUREOLA
BARETTA
BEDELIA
BERETTA
BIRETTA
BOHEMIA
CADENZA
CAPELLA
CASELLA
CASERTA
CELESTA
CEREBRA

CINESIA
COMEDIA
CORETTA
CRUELLA
DELEDDA
DILEMMA
ELBERTA
EPHEDRA
ERNESTA
ESTELLA
EUGENIA
EXHEDRA
FIDELIA
FIRENZA
FIVEAAA
FORENZA
FREESIA
GEHENNA
HEREDIA
ILLEANA
INGESTA
INSECTA
INTEGRA
JOSEPHA
LACERTA
LIBERIA
LINEARA
LORETTA
LOUELLA
LUCETTA
LUNESTA
LUTETIA
MADEIRA
MAGENTA
MAZEPPA
MCKENNA
MINEOLA
MINERVA
MOMENTA
MORELLA
MOZETTA
MTKENYA
MUSETTA
NIGERIA
NOSEBRA
NOVELLA
OCHENTA
OPHELIA
OSCEOLA
OSSETRA
PANETTA
PATELLA
PHAEDRA
POLENTA
PYREXIA
RAVENNA
REBECCA
REVERSA
ROBERTA
ROSELLA
ROSEOLA
ROSETEA
ROSETTA
ROVETTA
RUBELLA
RUBEOLA
SAGETEA
SETENTA

SIBERIA
SILENTA
SILESIA
SPLENDA
SWEEPEA
TAKETEA
TAVERNA
TOCELIA
VANESSA
VENEZIA
VICENZA
VOTEYEA

••••EA•

AFCTEAM
AIRHEAD
ALLHEAL
ANDREAS
ANTBEAR
APOGEAL
APOGEAN
ARAMEAN
ASATEAM
ASHHEAP
ASTREAM
AXEHEAD
AZALEAS
AZOREAN
BANDEAU
BARBEAU
BAYLEAF
BELLEAU
BESMEAR
BESPEAK
BIGBEAR
BIGBEAT
BIGDEAL
BIGHEAD
BIGLEAD
BIGMEAL
BOOLEAN
BORNEAN
BOWHEAD
BOXSEAT
BUGBEAR
BUMDEAL
CARSEAT
CATHEAD
CHAPEAU
CHATEAU
CHILEAN
COCTEAU
CONCEAL
CONGEAL
CORNEAL
CORNEAS
COWPEAS
CRIMEAN
CURSEAT
DANTEAN
DAYWEAR
DEFLEAS
DOADEAL
DOGREAT
DOGSEAR
DRIVEAT
DROVEAT
DRUZEAN

DRYHEAT
EGGHEAD
ENDLEAF
ENTREAT
ESCHEAT
EYEWEAR
FATHEAD
FEYDEAU
FIGLEAF
FLOREAL
FLYLEAF
FORBEAR
FORREAL
FRENEAU
FURSEAL
GARNEAU
GASHEAT
GASLEAK
GAVEEAR
GETBEAT
GETREAL
GIVEEAR
GLAREAT
GLUTEAL
GOAHEAD
GODHEAD
GOTBEAT
GOTREAL
GRADEAA
GUINEAN
GUINEAS
HIALEAH
HOTHEAD
HOTLEAD
HOTMEAL
HOTSEAT
HOTTEAS
ICETEAS
IMGREAT
IMPLEAD
INAHEAP
INSTEAD
IONBEAM
IREPEAT
ISABEAU
ISAHEAD
ISSUEAD
ISUREAM
JAMBEAU
JIMBEAM
JOYCEAN
JUGHEAD
KIDSEAT
KINNEAR
LACTEAL
LAMBEAU
LEFREAK
LEFTEAR
LEGWEAR
LETHEAN
LETSEAT
LIPREAD
LOCKEAN
LOWBEAM
LOWGEAR
LUNGEAT
MACLEAN
MANYEAR

MARCEAU
MIDYEAR
MISDEAL
MISHEAR
MISLEAD
MISREAD
MISSEAT
MOPHEAD
MRCLEAN
MYTREAT
NAUSEAM
NBATEAM
NEWDEAL
NEWLEAF
NEWYEAR
NFCTEAM
NFLTEAM
NHLTEAM
NONDEAF
NONMEAT
NONPEAK
NOSWEAT
NOTNEAR
NOTREAL
NOUVEAU
NUCLEAR
NUTMEAT
OAKLEAF
OATMEAL
OFFBEAT
OFFPEAK
OFFYEAR
OILHEAT
OLDBEAN
ONALEAD
ONATEAR
ONBREAK
ONEYEAR
ONTKEAN
ORPHEAN
OUTBEAM
OUTHEAR
OUTLEAD
OUTLEAP
OUTREAD
OUTTEAR
OUTWEAR
OVEREAT
PEABEAN
PELLEAS
PERREAU
PERYEAR
PETBEAR
PHILEAS
PHINEAS
PIGMEAT
PINHEAD
PINSEAL
PISCEAN
PITHEAD
PLATEAU
PREHEAL
PREHEAT
PRESEAL
PRESEAT
PROTEAM
PROTEAN
OBSNEAK

7 EA

QUENEAU
RAWDEAL
RAWMEAT
REBREAK
RECLEAN
REDHEAD
REDHEAT
REDMEAT
REDREAM
REKNEAD
REPLEAD
RESPEAK
RESWEAR
RETREAD
RETREAT
RIBMEAT
RONDEAU
ROULEAU
ROYBEAN
SAPHEAD
SCHMEAR
SERVEAS
SHEBEAR
SIXYEAR
SKIWEAR
SMILEAT
SNIPEAT
SOWSEAR
SOYBEAN
SOYMEAL
SPIREAS
STAREAT
STONEAX
SUBHEAD
SUNBEAM
SURREAL
SWOREAT
TABLEAU
TAGTEAM
TAUREAN
TAXYEAR
TEALEAF
TEMPEAZ
TENYEAR
THEBEAR
THEHEAT
THEREAT
THOREAU
THREEAD
THREEAM
TIEBEAM
TONNEAU
TOWHEAD
TRUDEAU
TWOYEAR
UNCLEAN
UNCLEAR
UNIDEAL
UNSPEAK
UNSWEAR
UNTREAD
UPAHEAD
VALJEAN
WARHEAD
WATTEAU
WAXBEAN
WHEREAS
WHEREAT
YAYTEAM
YEATEAM
YESDEAR

••••E•A

ACHIEVA
ALAMEDA
ALFREDA
ALGIEBA
AMREETA
BANDERA
BARBERA
BOTTEGA
CALDERA
CANDELA
CARMELA
CARNERA
CARRERA
CERVEZA
CHIMERA
CHOLERA
DANIELA
DUODENA
ELEVENA
ERIGENA
ESCUELA
EUGLENA
GARDENA
GRADEAA
HENDECA
HYGIEIA
ILOVELA
IMPREZA
IPANEMA
KUNDERA
LETTERA
MANDELA
MANTECA
MEGAERA
MICAELA
NORIEGA
NOXZEMA
PANTERA
POLLERA
POMPEIA
PORSENA
PRIMERA
QUESERA
QUINELA
RIGVEDA
RIVIERA
TAFFETA
TEMPERA
TESSERA
THERESA
TRIBECA
VERBENA
VISCERA

•••••EA

ARALSEA
AVONLEA
BADAREA
BADIDEA
BAYAREA
BEEFTEA
BIGIDEA
BOBATEA
CALMSEA
CATFLEA
CHELSEA
COCHLEA
DEADSEA
DEEPSEA
DOGFLEA
DOUBLEA
DRYIDEA
ERITREA
GALATEA
GOBYSEA
GOTOSEA
HERBTEA
HIGHSEA
HIGHTEA
ICEDTEA
KARASEA
KILAUEA
MINTTEA
NEWIDEA
OPENSEA
OVERSEA
PANACEA
PANGAEA
PREIDEA
ROSETEA
ROSSSEA
SAGETEA
SALTSEA
SKIAREA
SNAPPEA
SNOWPEA
SUBAREA
SUBIDEA
SULUSEA
SWANSEA
SWEEPEA
TAKETEA
THEFLEA
THEIDEA
TRACHEA
TRIPLEA
TWELVEA
VOTEYEA

EB•••••

EBANKED
EBAYERS
EBBTIDE
EBONICS
EBONIES
EBONITE
EBONIZE
EBWHITE

E•B••••

EBBTIDE
ELBERTA
ELBOWED
ELBOWER
EMBALMS
EMBANKS
EMBARGO
EMBARKS
EMBASSY
EMBAYED
EMBLAZE
EMBLEMS
EMBOITE
EMBOSOM
EMBOWER
EMBRACE
EMBROIL
EMBROWN
EMBRUED
EMBRUES
EMBRYOS
EUBANKS

E••B•••

EARBONE
EARBUDS
EDIBLES
ENABLED
ENABLER
ENABLES
ESOBESO
EXABYTE
EYEBALL
EYEBANK
EYEBOLT
EYEBROW

E•••B••

EATABIT
EATABLE
EFFABLE
EFFABLY
ENARBOR
ENDABLE
ENNOBLE
ENROBED
ENROBES
ENTEBBE
EPHEBUS
EQUABLE
EQUABLY
ERRABLE
ESTEBAN
EULABUS
EVENBET
EXHIBIT
EXURBAN
EXURBIA

E••••B•

EARLOBE
EARTABS
EASEDBY
EASESBY
EIGHTBC
EKINGBY
ENDERBY
ENTEBBE
ENTOMBS
ETALIBI

E•••••B

EASYJOB
ELEVENB
EWELAMB

•EB••••

BEBRAVE
DEBACLE
DEBAKEY
DEBARGE
DEBARKS
DEBASED
DEBASER
DEBASES
DEBATED
DEBATER
DEBATES
DEBAUCH
DEBEARD
DEBEERS
DEBITED
DEBLURS
DEBOITE
DEBONED
DEBONES
DEBORAH
DEBOULE
DEBRETT
DEBRIEF
DEBTEES
DEBTORS
DEBUNKS
DEBURGH
DEBURRS
DEBUSES
DEBUSSY
DEBUTED
FEBRERO
FEBRILE
HEBRAIC
HEBREWS
JEBBUSH
LEBANON
LEBARON
LEBLANC
LEBROCK
NEBBISH
NEBULAE
NEBULAR
NEBULAS
PEBBLED
PEBBLES
REBAITS
REBAKED
REBAKES
REBALED
REBALES
REBANKS
REBASTE
REBATED
REBATER
REBATES
REBATHE
REBECCA
REBEGAN
REBEGIN
REBEGUN
REBEKAH
REBENDS
REBILLS
REBINDS
REBIRTH
REBLOCK
REBLOOM
REBLOWN
REBOANT
REBOARD
REBOILS
REBOLTS
REBOOKS
REBOOTS
REBORED
REBORES
REBOTES
REBOUND
REBOXED
REBOXES
REBOZOS
REBRACE
REBRAND
REBREAK
REBREED
REBREWS
REBROKE
REBRUSH
REBUFFS
REBUILD
REBUILT
REBUKED
REBUKER
REBUKES
REBUSES
SEBRING
TEBALDI
WEBBIER
WEBBING
WEBCAMS
WEBCAST
WEBFEET
WEBFOOT
WEBLESS
WEBLIKE
WEBLOGS
WEBMAIL
WEBPAGE
WEBSITE
WEBSTER
WEBTOED
WEBZINE
ZEBRAIC
ZEBRASS
ZEBRINE
ZEBROID
ZEBULON
ZEBULUN

•E•B•••

BEDBATH
BEDBUGS
BEEBEES
BENBLUE
BENBOVA
BERBERS
BERBICK
CEMBALO
DELBERT
DEMBUMS
DERBIES
FEEBATE
FEEBLER
FEMBOTS
GERBILS
GETBACK
GETBEAT
GETBENT
GETBUSY
HENBANE
HENBITS
HEPBURN
HERBAGE
HERBALS
HERBART
HERBAUT
HERBERT
HERBIER
HERBTEA
JEBBUSH
JEEBIES
JERBOAS
JETBOAT
KEEBLER
KEYBANK
LEGBONE
LEIBNIZ
MEMBERS
NEBBISH
NESBITT
NETBALL
NEWBERN
NEWBERY
NEWBIES
NEWBOLT
NEWBORN
NEWBURG
PEABEAN
PEABODY
PEBBLED
PEBBLES
PEEBLES
PEPBAND
PEPBOYS
PETBEAR
PETBIRD
PETBOAS
REDBATS
REDBAYS
REDBIRD
REDBONE
REDBOOK
REDBUDS
REEBOKS
REUBENS
SEABAGS
SEABASS
SEABEDS
SEABEES
SEABIRD
SEABLUE
SEABOAT
SEABORG
SERBIAN
SETBACK
SETBAIL
TEABAGS
TEABALL
TEMBLOR
TENBALL
TERBIUM
VERBALS
VERBENA
VERBIDS
VERBIFY
VERBOSE
WEBBIER
WEBBING
WEEBITS
WEMBLEY
WETBARS
WETBULB

•E••B••

AEROBAT
AEROBES
AEROBIC
BEANBAG
BEATBOX
BELABOR
BELLBOY
BELTBAG
BESTBET
BESTBOY
BESTBUD
BESTBUY
CELEBES
CELEBRE
CEREBRA
CEREBRO
DECIBEL
DEEDBOX
DELIBES
DEORBIT
FEEDBAG
FEEDBIN
FEELBAD
FELTBAD
FERNBAR
GEARBOX
GEMSBOK
GETABLE
HELLBOY
JEZEBEL
LEGIBLE
LEGIBLY
LESABRE
MEGABIT
MENUBAR
NEWSBOY
PEATBOG
RECABLE
REDEBIT
RELABEL
RETABLE
SEEABLE
SEEDBED
TENABLE
TENABLY
TENTBED
TESTBAN
TESTBED
VENABLE
VERYBAD
VERYBIG
WENTBAD
YEAHBUT
ZENOBIA

•E•••B•

BEDAUBS
BENUMBS
HERNIBS
HEYRUBE
LEAVEBE
LETGOBY
LETITBE
LETMEBE
NEWJOBS
RECOMBS
REDOUBT
REDROBE
REDTABS
REGRABS
REPROBE
RESORBS
RESTABS
REVERBS
SEALABS
SENDSBY
SEVENBC

•E••••B

BEARCUB
DECRUMB
GETAJOB
KEYCLUB
LEFTJAB
LETTERB
PEDICAB
PERTURB
PETCOMB
PETLAMB
RECLIMB
REPLUMB
RESCRUB
TEMPJOB
TESTLAB
WETBULB

••EB•••

AKEBONO
AMEBOID
BEEBEES
BYEBYES
CPEBACH
CUEBALL
CUEBIDS
DIEBOLD
DYEBATH
EYEBALL
EYEBANK
EYEBOLT
EYEBROW
FEEBATE
FEEBLER
FREBERG
ICEBAGS
ICEBATH
ICEBEER
ICEBERG
ICEBLUE
ICEBOAT
IKEBANA
JEEBIES
JOEBLOW
JOEBUCK
KEEBLER
LIEBACK
MOEBERG
NIEBUHR
OLEBULL
ONEBALL
ONEBASE
ONEBELL
ONEBYTE
OREBODY
PEEBLES
PIEBALD
PLEBIAN
PREBADE
PREBAKE
PREBIDS
PREBILL
PREBIND
PREBOIL
PREBOOK
PREBOOM
PREBORN
PREBURN
PREBUYS
PUEBLOS
RAEBURN
REEBOKS
RHEBOKS
ROEBUCK
RYEBEER
SHEBANG
SHEBEAR
SIEBZIG
THEBABE
THEBABY
THEBAND
THEBANS
THEBARD
THEBEAR
THEBELL
THEBEST
THEBIGA
THEBLOB
THEBOBO
THEBODY
THEBOMB
THEBOSS
THEBOYS
THEBRAT
THEBUSH
TIEBACK
TIEBARS
TIEBEAM
TREBLED
TREBLES
UNEBBED
WEEBITS

••E•B••

ACERBIC
ALEMBIC
ATEABIT
AWEEBIT
DEEDBOX
DOESBAD
EVENBET
FEEDBAG
FEEDBIN
FEELBAD
FLEABAG
FREEBEE
FREEBIE
GOESBAD
GREWBIG
KLEIBER
LIEABED
OPENBAR
OVERBED
OVERBET
OVERBID
OVERBIG
OVERBUY
SEEABLE
SEEDBED
SHERBET
STEUBEN
THEABCS
TREMBLE
TREMBLY
UNEBBED

••E••B•

ARECIBO
CHERUBS
CREEPBY
DYEJOBS
FREDEBB
ICECUBE
PREFABS
SNEAKBY
SWEARBY
THEBABE
THEBABY
THEBOBO
THECUBS
THEREBY
THEROBE
THETUBE
WHEREBY

••E•••B

BREWPUB
CHEMLAB
ELEVENB
EWELAMB
FREDEBB
ONECLUB
OVERDUB
PREVERB
SHECRAB
THEBLOB
THEBOMB
THECRAB
THELAMB
THETRIB
TWELVEB

•••EB••

ALGEBRA
AMOEBAE
AMOEBAS
AMOEBIC
AWEEBIT
BLUEBOY
CELEBES
CELEBRE
CEREBRA
CEREBRO
DONEBAD
DOVEBAR
ENTEBBE
EPHEBUS
ESTEBAN
FAREBOX
FIREBOX
FIREBUG
FOREBAY
FREEBEE
FREEBIE
FROEBEL
FUSEBOX
GAMEBAG
GAMEBOY
GAZEBOS
GONEBAD
HOMEBOY
JEZEBEL
JUKEBOX
JUNEBUG
LAKEBED
LOSEBIG
LOVEBUG
MALEBEE
NICEBOY
NOSEBAG
NOSEBRA
PAGEBOY
PHOEBES
PHOEBUS
RAREBIT
REDEBIT
RIDEBYS
ROSEBAY
ROSEBUD
SAFEBET
SHOEBOX
SIDEBAR
SIDEBET
SUREBET
TOTEBAG
VITEBSK
WINEBAR

•••E•B•

ADVERBS
ALLENBY
COMESBY
CREEPBY
DRWELBY
EASEDBY
EASESBY
ENDERBY
ENTEBBE
FILEDBY
FILESBY
FLIESBY
GIVENBY
LAZENBY
MODELBS
MORESBY
RACEDBY
RACESBY
REVERBS
RIDESBY
RULEDBY
SEVENBC
TAKENBY
THREEBC
TYPEABS

•••E••B

HOMELAB
LINEARB
LUBEJOB
NICEJOB
NOSEJOB
POPEAFB
SILENTB
TRUERIB

••••EB•

ABIDEBY
ALGIEBA
BADDEBT
BYTHEBY
CLOSEBY
COBWEBS
DRIVEBY
DROVEBY
FREDEBB
GLIDEBY
LEAVEBE
LETMEBE
PLACEBO
SLIDEBY
SOTHEBY
SUBDEBS
SWOREBY
THEREBY
THREEBC
WHEREBY

••••E•B

ELEVENB
FREDEBB
LETTERB
POTHERB
PREVERB
PROVERB

•••••EB

DOUBLEB
FOODWEB
TWELVEB

EC•••••

ECARTES
ECCLESI
ECDYSES
ECDYSIS
ECHAPPE
ECHELON
ECHIDNA
ECHOERS
ECHOING
ECHOISM
ECKHART
ECLAIRS
ECLIPSE
ECLOGUE
ECOCIDE
ECOLOGY
ECONOMY
ECOTAGE
ECOTEUR
ECOTRIN

7 EC

ECOTYPE
ECSTASY
ECTYPAL
ECTYPES
ECUADOR
ECUELLE
ECZEMAS

E•C••••

ECCLESI
ELCAJON
ELCAMPO
ENCAGED
ENCAGES
ENCAMPS
ENCARRE
ENCARTA
ENCASED
ENCASES
ENCHAIN
ENCHANT
ENCHASE
ENCINAS
ENCLASP
ENCLAVE
ENCLOSE
ENCODED
ENCODER
ENCODES
ENCOMIA
ENCORED
ENCORES
ENCRUST
ENCRYPT
ESCALOP
ESCALUS
ESCAPED
ESCAPEE
ESCAPER
ESCAPES
ESCARPS
ESCENCE
ESCHEAT
ESCHERS
ESCHEWS
ESCORTS
ESCROWS
ESCUDOS
ESCUELA
ETCHANT
ETCHERS
ETCHING
EUCERIN
EUCHRED
EUCHRES
EXCEEDS
EXCELAT
EXCELIN
EXCEPTS
EXCERPT
EXCIDED
EXCIDES
EXCISED
EXCISES
EXCITED
EXCITER
EXCITES
EXCITOR
EXCLAIM
EXCLAVE
EXCLUDE
EXCRETE
EXCURSE
EXCUSAL
EXCUSAS
EXCUSED
EXCUSER
EXCUSES
EXCUSEZ

E••C•••

EARCLIP
EATCAKE
EATCROW
ECOCIDE
EDACITY
EDICTAL
EDUCATE
EDUCING
EDUCTED
EDUCTOR
EGGCASE
EGGCUPS
EJECTED
EJECTOR
ELECTED
ELECTEE
ELECTME
ELECTOR
ELECTRA
ELECTRO
ELICITS
ELMCITY
ELOCUTE
ENACTED
ENACTOR
ENDCUTS
EPICARP
EPICENE
EPICURE
EPOCHAL
ERECTED
ERECTER
ERECTLY
ERECTOR
ERECTUS
ERICSON
ERUCTED
ETICKET
EVACUEE
EVICTED
EVICTEE
EVICTOR
EXACTAS
EXACTED
EXACTER
EXACTLY
EXACTOR
EXECUTE
EXOCARP
EXOCETS
EXSCIND
EYECARE
EYECUPS

E•••C••

EARACHE
EFFACED
EFFACER
EFFACES
EFFECTS
ELANCES
ENFACED
ENFACES
ENLACED
ENLACES
ENTICED
ENTICER
ENTICES
EPARCHS
EPARCHY
ETHICAL
EVINCED
EVINCES
EXARCHS
EXFACTO
EXPECTS
EXSECTS

E••••C•

EARLOCK
EBONICS
EDIFICE
EGGSACS
EHRLICH
ELDRICH
ELDRICK
ELFLOCK
ELGRECO
EMBRACE
EMETICS
EMPLACE
ENFORCE
ENHANCE
ENOUNCE
ERDRICH
EROTICA
EROTICS
ERRANCY
ESCENCE
ESSENCE
ETHNICS
ETONICS
EUSTACE
EWENECK
EXOTICA
EXOTICS
EXTINCT
EXTRACT
EYETUCK

E•••••C

EIDETIC
EIDOLIC
EIGHTBC
EKISTIC
ELASTIC
ELEGIAC
ELEVENC
EMPIRIC
ENDEMIC
ENTERIC
ENZYMIC
ERGOTIC
ERISTIC
ERRATIC
ETHERIC
EUGENIC

•EC••••

BECALMS
BECAUSE
BECHARM
BECKETT
BECKHAM
BECKONS
BECLOUD
BECOMES
CECILIA
DECADES
DECAGON
DECALOG
DECAMPS
DECANTS
DECAPOD
DECARLO
DECATUR
DECAYED
DECAYER
DECEASE
DECEITS
DECEIVE
DECENCY
DECIARE
DECIBEL
DECIDED
DECIDER
DECIDES
DECILES
DECIMAL
DECKERS
DECKING
DECKLED
DECKLES
DECKOUT
DECLAIM
DECLARE
DECLASS
DECLAWS
DECLINE
DECLOTS
DECOCTS
DECODED
DECODER
DECODES
DECOLOR
DECORUM
DECOYED
DECOYER
DECREED
DECREER
DECREES
DECRIED
DECRIER
DECRIES
DECRUMB
DECRYPT
DECUPLE
FECHNER
GECKOES
HECKART
HECKLED
HECKLER
HECKLES
HECKMAN
HECKUVA
HECKYES
HECTARE
HECTORS
LECARRE
LECHERS
LECONTE
LECTERN
LECTORS
LECTRIC
LECTURE
LECUONA
MECCANS
MECHLIN
NECKERS
NECKING
NECKLET
NECKTIE
NECTARS
NECTARY
PECCANT
PECCARY
PECCAVI
PECKING
PECKISH
PECKSAT
PECTINS
RECABLE
RECAGED
RECAGES
RECALLS
RECANED
RECANES
RECANTS
RECARRY
RECARVE
RECASED
RECASES
RECASTS
RECEDED
RECEDES
RECEIPT
RECEIVE
RECENCY
RECHALK
RECHALL
RECHART
RECHECK
RECHEWS
RECHOSE
RECIPES
RECITAL
RECITED
RECITER
RECITES
RECKONS
RECLADS
RECLAIM
RECLAME
RECLASP
RECLASS
RECLEAN
RECLIMB
RECLINE
RECLUSE
RECOALS
RECOATS
RECOCKS
RECODED
RECODES
RECOILS
RECOINS
RECOLOR
RECOMBS
RECOOKS
RECOOLS
RECORDS
RECORKS
RECOSTS
RECOUNT
RECOUPS
RECOVER
RECRANK
RECRATE
RECROOM
RECROSS
RECROWN
RECRUIT
RECTIFY
RECTORS
RECTORY
RECURED
RECURES
RECURLS
RECURVE
RECUSAL
RECUSED
RECUSES
RECYCLE
SECANTS
SECEDED
SECEDER
SECEDES
SECHZIG
SECKELS
SECLUDE
SECONDI
SECONDO
SECONDR
SECONDS
SECRECY
SECRETE
SECRETS
SECTION
SECTORS
SECULAR
SECURED
SECURER
SECURES
TECHIES
TECHNOS
VECHTEN
VECTORS
VECTRAS

•E•C•••

BEACHAM
BEACHED
BEACHES
BEACONS
BEECHAM
BEECHEN
BEECHER
BEECHES
BELCHED
BELCHER
BELCHES
BENCHED
BENCHER
BENCHES
DEACONS
DEFCONS
DEICERS
DEICING
DELCITY
DESCANT
DESCEND
DESCENT
DEUCING
DEWCLAW
FENCEIN
FENCERS
FENCEUP
FENCING
FESCUES
FETCHED
FETCHER
FETCHES
GELCAPS
GEOCODE
GETCASH
GETCOLD
GETCUTE
HENCOOP
HEPCATS
HERCULE
KETCHAM
KETCHES
KETCHUM
KETCHUP
KEYCARD
KEYCASE
KEYCLUB
LEACHED
LEACHER
LEACHES
LEACOCK
LEECHED
LEECHEE
LEECHES
LESCAUT
LEUCINE
MECCANS
MENCIUS
MENCKEN
MERCADO
MERCERS
MERCERY
MERCHES
MERCIAN
MERCIES
MERCURE
MERCURY
MESCALS
METCALF
NEOCENE
NEOCONS
NESCAFE
NETCAFE
NETCOST
NEWCARS
PEACHED
PEACHES
PEACOAT
PEACOCK
PECCANT
PECCARY
PECCAVI
PENCASE
PENCILS
PEPCIDS
PERCALE
PERCENT
PERCEPT
PERCHED
PERCHER
PERCHES
PERCHIK
PERCUSS
PETCAGE
PETCALF
PETCATS
PETCHEW
PETCOCK
PETCOMB
PETCOWS
PETCROW
REACHED
REACHER
REACHES
REACHIN
REACHUP
REACTED
REACTOR
REACTTO
REDCAPS
REDCARD
REDCELL
REDCENT
REDCHIP
REDCLAY
REDCOAT
REDCODS
REICING
REOCCUR
RESCALE
RESCANS
RESCIND
RESCORE
RESCRUB
RESCUED
RESCUER
RESCUES
REXCATS
SEACALM
SEACATS
SEACOWS
TEACAKE
TEACART
TEACHER
TEACHES
TEACHIN
TEACOZY
TEACUPS
TEICHER
TENCENT
TENCHES
TENCODE
TERCELS
VELCROS
VETCHES
WEBCAMS
WEBCAST
WELCOME
WENCHES
WESCOTT
WETCELL

•E••C••

BEARCAT
BEARCUB
BEATCOP
BEDECKS
BEERCAN
BENICIA
BENICIO
BESTCUT
CELICAS
CENACLE
CEVICHE
DEBACLE
DECOCTS
DEDUCED
DEDUCER
DEDUCES
DEDUCTS
DEFACED
DEFACER
DEFACES
DEFACTO
DEFECTS
DEFICIT
DEFOCUS
DEJECTS
DELICTI
DELICTO
DELICTS
DEPECHE
DEPICTS
DERECHO
DETECTO
DETECTS
DEVICES
FELICIA
HELICAL
HELICES
HELICON
HELLCAT
JERICHO
KENICHI
LEANCUT
LENSCAP
LEXICAL
LEXICON
MEDICAL
MEDICOS
MENACED
MENACER
MENACES
MENSCHY
MEXICAN
PEDICAB
PELICAN
PENUCHE
PETSCAN
REBECCA
RECOCKS
RECYCLE
REDACTS
REDECAY
REDOCKS
REDUCED
REDUCER
REDUCES
REFACED
REFACES
REFOCUS
REJECTS
REKICKS
RELACED
RELACES
RELICTS
RELOCKS
RELUCTS
REOCCUR
REPACKS
REPICKS
RERACKS
RESECTS
RETACKS
RETICLE
SEANCES
SEDUCED
SEDUCER
SEDUCES
SELECTS
SENECAN
SENECAS
TELECOM
TENACES
TENACRE
VEHICLE
VESICLE
WELLCUT
XENICAL
YESICAN

•E•••C•

BEDROCK
BELASCO
BEQUICK
BERBICK
BERWICK
BESEECH
BEWITCH
BEYONCE
CELTICS
DEBAUCH
DECENCY
DEFENCE
DEFLECT
DEFROCK
DEFUNCT
DEHISCE
DEMARCO
DENIECE
DERRICK
DERRICO
DESTOCK
DETRACT
DEUTSCH
FETLOCK
GEDRICK
GENLOCK
GEODUCK
GETBACK
HEMLOCK
HENDECA
HENPECK
HENRICH
HEROICS
HERRICK
JESSICA
JETPACK
KEYLOCK
LEACOCK
LEBROCK
LELOUCH
LETTUCE
MEDWICK
MENISCI
MENORCA
MERRICK
MESHACH
MESSICK
METRICS
NEGLECT
NEWFACE
NEWRICH
PEACOCK
PENANCE
PENNOCK
PEPSICO
PEPTICS
PERFECT
PETCOCK
PETDUCK
PETMICE
PETROCK
REBECCA
REBLOCK
REBRACE
RECENCY
RECHECK
REDFACE
REDJACK
REDNECK
REEJECT
REELECT
REENACT
REERECT
REEVICT
REFENCE
REFLECT
REFRACT
REGENCY
REHITCH
REJOICE
REKNOCK
RELANCE
RELATCH
REMATCH
RENWICK
REPATCH
REPLACE
REPLICA
REPRICE
RESPACE
RESPECT
RESPICE
RESTACK
RESTICK
RESTOCK
RETEACH
RETOUCH
RETRACE
RETRACK
RETRACT
REVOICE
SEADUCK
SEARACE
SEASICK
SECRECY
SELLECK
SENESCE
SERPICO
SERVICE
SETBACK
TEANECK
TEDMACK
TENANCY
TENNECO
TERENCE
TERRACE
TESTACY
VEENECK
VERDICT
VERRUCA
VERSACE
WEDLOCK

•E••••C

AELFRIC
AEROBIC
BENEFIC
CENTRIC
CERAMIC
DEISTIC
DELPHIC
DELTAIC
DEMONIC
DEMOTIC
GENERIC
GENETIC
GENOMIC
GEORGEC
GEORGIC
HEBRAIC
HEDONIC
HEMATIC
HEPATIC
HERETIC
HEXADIC
JEANLUC
KEROUAC
KETONIC
LEBLANC
LECTRIC
LETTERC
LEVITIC
LEXUSSC
MEDEVAC
MEDIVAC
MEIOTIC
MELANIC
MELODIC
MESONIC
NEPHRIC
NEPOTIC
PELAGIC
SEISMIC
SELENIC
SEMITIC
SEVENBC
TELEPIC
VENATIC
VERIDIC
XEROTIC
ZEBRAIC

••EC•••

APECKOF
ARECIBO
ATECROW
BEECHAM
BEECHEN
BEECHER
BEECHES
CHECHEN
CHECKED
CHECKER
CHECKIN
CHECKON
CHECKUP
CRECHES
CUECARD
DIECAST
DIECUTS
EJECTED
EJECTOR
ELECTED
ELECTEE
ELECTME
ELECTOR
ELECTRA
ELECTRO
ERECTED
ERECTER
ERECTLY
ERECTOR
ERECTUS
EXECUTE
EYECARE
EYECUPS
FLECHES
FLECKED
FRECKLE
FRECKLY
GRECIAN
GRECISM
GRECIZE
HAECKEL
HOECAKE
ICECAPS
ICECAVE
ICECOLD
ICECUBE
IRECKON
ISECOND
JAECKEL
JOECAMP
JOECOOL
LEECHED
LEECHEE
LEECHES
ONECALL
ONECELL
ONECENT

ONECHIP
ONECLAM
ONECLUB
ORECTIC
PIECERS
PIECING
PLECTRA
PRECAST
PRECEDE
PRECEPT
PRECISE
PRECITE
PRECODE
PRECOIL
PRECOOK
PRECOOL
PRECOUP
PRECURE
PRECUTS
QUECHUA
SHECRAB
SPECIAL
SPECIES
SPECIFY
SPECING
SPECKED
SPECKLE
SPECOUT
SPECTER
SPECTOR
SPECTRA
SPECTRE
THECAPE
THECARS
THECAVS
THECITY
THECRAB
THECROW
THECUBS
TIECLIP
TOECAPS
VNECKED
WRECKED
WRECKER

••E•C••

AGENCES
ALENCON
AMERCED
AMERCER
AMERCES
APERCUS
BEERCAN
BRESCIA
COERCED
COERCER
COERCES
CREWCUT
FIERCER
FLEECED
FLEECER
FLEECES
FRENCHI
FRENCHS
FRESCAS
FRESCOS
GLENCOE
GREYCUP
KNEECAP
KVETCHY
ONEACAT
ONEACRE
ONEACTS
ONEOCAT
OVERCOY
OVERCUT
PIERCED
PIERCER
PIERCES
PREACHY
PREACID
PREACTS
SKETCHY
SPENCER
STENCIL
TIERCES
TREACLE
TREACLY
USEDCAR
USEDCDS

••E••C•

AMERICA
CLERICS
CPEBACH
CREVICE
EMETICS
EWENECK
EYETUCK
FLEANCE
ICEPACK
ICEPICK
INEXACT
IRENICS
JOEBUCK
KLENSCH
LIEBACK
NOETICS
ONEINCH
ONESOCK
OVERACT
OVERICE
POETICA
POETICS
PREDICT
PREFACE
PREFECT
PRELACY
PREPACK
PRERACE
PREROCK
REEJECT
REELECT
REENACT
REERECT
REEVICT
ROEBUCK
SCENICS
SNEETCH
THEABCS
THEMICK
THEROCK
THESACK
TIEBACK
TIERACK
TIETACK
TIETACS
TOEPICK
UNERECT
VEENECK

••E•••C

ACERBIC
ALEMBIC
ASEPTIC
ELEGIAC
ELEVENC
FREDRIC
IDENTIC
LAENNEC
OCEANIC
ONEIRIC
ORECTIC
RHEUMIC
SCEPTIC
SHELLAC
SKEPTIC
STEARIC
THERIAC
THERMIC
TWELVEC

•••EC••

AFFECTS
ARDECHE
ASPECTS
AZTECAN
BEDECKS
BISECTS
BOWECHO
CAPECOD
DEFECTS
DEJECTS
DEPECHE
DERECHO
DETECTO
DETECTS
DICECUP
DIRECTS
DIRECTV
DOMECAR
DOVECOT
EFFECTS
EXPECTS
EXSECTS
FLEECED
FLEECER
FLEECES
INFECTS
INJECTS
INSECTA
INSECTS
KNEECAP
KOPECKS
LINECUT
MALECAT
OBJECTS
OUTECHO
PACECAR
POLECAR
POLECAT
RACECAR
RATECAP
REBECCA
REDECAY
REJECTS
RESECTS
RHOECUS
SELECTS
SENECAN
SENECAS
SIDECAR
SUBECHO
SURECAN
TELECOM
TIMECOP
UTRECHT
VOTECHS
ZYDECOS

•••E•C•

ABSENCE
ACDELCO
ARDENCY
ASPENCO
ATDEUCE
ATPEACE
BABENCO
BESEECH
BLUEICE
CADENCE
CADENCY
COGENCY
COTEACH
DECENCY
DEFENCE
DRIESCH
ESCENCE
ESSENCE
FAIENCE
FIREICE
FLUENCY
FOREACH
HOMEICE
ILIESCU
IMPEACH
INPEACE
INREACH
IONESCO
LATENCY
LICENCE
LIKEICE
LUCENCY
NIDETCH
NOMERCY
NORELCO
OFFENCE
PATENCY
POTENCE
POTENCY
PUDENCY
REBECCA
RECENCY
REFENCE
REGENCY
RETEACH
SCIENCE
SCREECH
SENESCE
SILENCE
SNEETCH
SQUELCH
STRETCH
TERENCE
TUMESCE
UNBENCH
UNFENCE
UNTEACH
UPREACH
URGENCY
VALENCE
VANEYCK

•••E••C

ALLELIC
AMNESIC
AMOEBIC
ANAEMIC
ANGELIC
ARSENIC
ASCETIC
BENEFIC
COMEDIC
EIDETIC
ENDEMIC
ENTERIC
ETHERIC
EUGENIC
GENERIC
GENETIC
HERETIC
HOMERIC
HYGELAC
KINESIC
KINETIC
MALEFIC
MEDEVAC
MIMETIC
NONEPIC
NUMERIC
PHRENIC
POLEMIC
PYRETIC
SELENIC
SEVENBC
SHOEPAC
SILENTC
SPHERIC
TELEPIC
THREEBC
TONELOC
TOTEMIC
WAREPIC

••••EC•

AFFLECK
ARTDECO
BESEECH
BIOTECH
BOMBECK
BRUBECK
BYANECK
CALTECH
CANSECO
COLLECT
CONFECT
CONNECT
CONVECT
CORRECT
DEFLECT
DENIECE
DIALECT
DISSECT
ELGRECO
EWENECK
HENDECA
HENPECK
INCHECK
INFLECT
INSPECT
IOBJECT
LABTECH
LOWNECK
LOWTECH
MANTECA
MIXTECS
NEGLECT
OOBLECK
PARSECS
PERFECT
PREFECT
PROJECT
PROTECT
RECHECK
REDNECK
REEJECT
REELECT
REERECT
REFLECT
RESPECT
SCITECH
SCREECH
SECRECY
SELLECK
SUBJECT
SUBSECT
SUNDECK
SUSPECT
TEANECK
TENNECO
TOLTECS
TRIBECA
TRISECT
UNCHECK
UNERECT
VEENECK
WOZZECK
YASBECK

••••E•C

ELEVENC
LETTERC
NUCLEIC
POULENC
THREEBC

•••••EC

DOUBLEC
FORASEC
GEORGEC
LAENNEC
LAUTREC
MIDDLEC
TWELVEC
YUCATEC
ZAPOTEC

ED•••••

EDACITY
EDASNER
EDDYING
EDEMATA
EDGARDO
EDGEDIN
EDGEOUT
EDGESIN
EDGIEST
EDGINGS
EDIBLES
EDICTAL
EDIFICE
EDIFIED
EDIFIER
EDIFIES
EDINAMN
EDITING
EDITION
EDITORS
EDITOUT
EDITRIX
EDMEESE
EDMONDS
EDMUNDI
EDMUNDS
EDNAMAY
EDOMITE
EDOUARD
EDUARDO
EDUCATE
EDUCING
EDUCTED
EDUCTOR
EDWARDG
EDWARDI
EDWARDR
EDWARDS
EDWARDV

E•D••••

EADGILS
ECDYSES
ECDYSIS
EDDYING
EIDETIC
EIDOLIC
EIDOLON
ELDERLY
ELDRICH
ELDRICK
ENDABLE
ENDALLS
ENDCUTS
ENDEARS
ENDEDAT
ENDEDIN
ENDEDIT
ENDEDON
ENDEDUP
ENDEMIC
ENDERBY
ENDGAME
ENDINGS
ENDIVES
ENDLATE
ENDLEAF
ENDLESS
ENDLINE
ENDLONG
ENDMOST
ENDNOTE
ENDORSE
ENDOWED
ENDOWER
ENDPINS
ENDPLAY
ENDRUNS
ENDUING
ENDUPAT
ENDURED
ENDURER
ENDURES
ENDUROS
ENDUSER
ENDUSES
ENDWAYS
ENDWISE
ENDZONE
ERDRICH
EUDEMON

E••D•••

EARDROP
EARDRUM
EATDIRT
EGGDROP
EKEDOUT
ELIDERS
ELIDING
ELUDERS
ELUDING
EPIDERM
EPIDOTE
ERODENT
ERODERS
ERODING
ERUDITE
EVADERS
EVADING
EVIDENT
EXEDRAE
EXUDATE
EXUDING
EYEDROP

E•••D••

EARLDOM
EASEDBY
EASEDIN
EASEDON
EASEDUP
ECHIDNA
ECUADOR
EDGEDIN
EGGEDON
ELFUDGE
EMENDED
EMENDER
ENCODED
ENCODER
ENCODES
ENDEDAT
ENDEDIN
ENDEDIT
ENDEDON
ENDEDUP
EPHEDRA
ESCUDOS
ESTADOS
EVANDER
EVERDUR
EXCIDED
EXCIDES
EXHEDRA
EXORDIA

E••••D•

EARBUDS
EBBTIDE
ECOCIDE
EDGARDO
EDMONDS
EDMUNDI
EDMUNDS
EDUARDO
EDWARDG
EDWARDI
EDWARDR
EDWARDS
EDWARDV
EFFENDI
ELAPIDS
ELMUNDO
ELPRADO
EMQUADS
ENFOLDS
ENGARDE
ENGILDS
ENGIRDS
ENNEADS
ENQUADS
ENTRADA
ENWINDS
EPILADY
EPISODE
ERRANDS
ESTRADA
EXCEEDS
EXCLUDE
EXPANDS
EXPENDS
EXPLODE
EXTENDS
EXTRUDE
EYELIDS

E•••••D

EANMUND
EARTHED
EASELED
EASTEND
EBANKED
EDIFIED
EDOUARD
EDUCTED
EFFACED
EFFUSED
EGESTED
EGGHEAD
EIGHTAD
EJECTED
ELAPSED
ELBOWED
ELECTED
ELEVEND
ELMWOOD
EMAILED
EMBAYED
EMBRUED
EMENDED
EMERALD
EMERGED
EMERSED
EMITTED
EMPALED
EMPTIED
ENABLED
ENACTED
ENARMED
ENCAGED
ENCASED
ENCODED
ENCORED
ENDOWED
ENDURED
ENFACED
ENFIELD
ENGAGED
ENGINED
ENGLAND
ENGLUND
ENISLED
ENJOYED
ENLACED
ENOILED
ENRAGED
ENROBED
ENSILED
ENSKIED
ENSURED
ENTERED
ENTICED
ENWOUND
EPOXIED
EQUALED
EQUATED
ERECTED
ERMINED
ERUCTED
ERUPTED
ESCAPED
ESSAYED
ESTATED
ETAILED
ETHMOID
EUCHRED
EVERTED
EVICTED
EVINCED
EVOLVED
EVULSED
EXACTED
EXALTED
EXCIDED
EXCISED
EXCITED
EXCUSED
EXERTED
EXHALED
EXHUMED
EXISTED
EXPIRED
EXPOSED
EXPOUND
EXSCIND
EXULTED
EYEFOLD
EYEHAND

•ED••••

AEDILES
BEDAUBS
BEDAZED
BEDAZES
BEDBATH
BEDBUGS
BEDDING
BEDDOWN
BEDECKS
BEDELIA
BEDEVIL
BEDEWED
BEDFORD
BEDIZEN
BEDLAMP
BEDLAMS
BEDLESS
BEDLIKE
BEDLOES
BEDMATE
BEDNORZ
BEDOUIN
BEDPOST
BEDRAIL
BEDRAPE
BEDREST
BEDROCK
BEDROLL
BEDROOM
BEDSIDE
BEDSITS
BEDTIME
CEDARED
CEDILLA
DEDALUS
DEDUCED
DEDUCER
DEDUCES
DEDUCTS
FEDDERS
FEDERAL
FEDERKO
FEDEXED
FEDEXES
FEDINTO
FEDORAS
FEDOROV
GEDRICK
HEDGERS
HEDGIER
HEDGING
HEDISON
HEDONIC
KEDGERS
KEDGING
KEDROVA
LEDAWAY
LEDERER
LEDGERS
LEDGIER
LEDINTO
LEDUPTO
MEDAKAS
MEDALED
MEDAWAR
MEDDLED
MEDDLER
MEDDLES
MEDELES
MEDEVAC
MEDFORD
MEDIANS
MEDIANT
MEDIATE
MEDICAL
MEDICOS
MEDIGAP
MEDIUMS
MEDIVAC
MEDLEYS
MEDULLA
MEDUSAE
MEDUSAN
MEDUSAS
MEDWICK
NEDLAND
OEDIPAL
OEDIPUS
PEDALED
PEDALER
PEDANTS
PEDDLED
PEDDLER
PEDDLES
PEDICAB
PEDWAYS
REDACTS
REDALGA
REDANTS
REDARED
REDARES
REDARMY
REDARNS
REDATED
REDATES
REDBATS
REDBAYS
REDBIRD
REDBONE
REDBOOK
REDBUDS
REDCAPS
REDCARD
REDCELL
REDCENT
REDCHIP
REDCLAY
REDCOAT
REDCODS
REDDAWN
REDDEER
REDDENS
REDDEST
REDDING
REDDISH
REDDOGS
REDDOTS
REDDUST
REDDYES
REDEALS
REDEALT
REDEBIT
REDECAY
REDEEDS
REDEEMS
REDEYED
REDEYES
REDFACE
REDFERN
REDFINS
REDFIRS
REDFISH
REDFIVE
REDFLAG
REDFORD
REDFOUR
REDHAIR
REDHATS
REDHAWK
REDHEAD
REDHEAT
REDHENS
REDHOTS
REDIALS
REDJACK
REDKING
REDLEGS
REDLINE
REDMEAT
REDMOND
REDNECK
REDNESS
REDNINE
REDNOSE
REDOAKS
REDOCKS
REDOING
REDONDO
REDOSED
REDOSES
REDOUBT
REDOUND
REDOUTS
REDOXES
REDPINE
REDPOLL
REDPONY
REDRAFT
REDRAGS
REDRAWN
REDRAWS
REDREAM
REDRESS
REDRIED
REDRIES
REDRILL
REDRIVE
REDROBE
REDROOP
REDROOT
REDROSE
REDSFAN
REDSKIN
REDSPOT

REDSTAR
REDSUIT
REDSUNS
REDTABS
REDTAGS
REDTAIL
REDTAPE
REDTIDE
REDTIES
REDTOPS
REDUCED
REDUCER
REDUCES
REDUSTS
REDWINE
REDWING
REDWOLF
REDWOOD
REDWORM
REDYING
REDZONE
SEDALIA
SEDATED
SEDATER
SEDATES
SEDGIER
SEDONAS
SEDUCED
SEDUCER
SEDUCES
TEDDIES
TEDEUMS
TEDIOUS
TEDIUMS
TEDMACK
VEDETTE
VEDISTS
WEDDELL
WEDDERS
WEDDING
WEDELED
WEDELNS
WEDGEIN
WEDGIER
WEDGIES
WEDGING
WEDIDIT
WEDLOCK
ZEDILLO
ZEDONKS

•E•D•••

BEADERS
BEADIER
BEADILY
BEADING
BEADLES
BEADSUP
BEDDING
BEDDOWN
BELDAME
BELDAMS
BENDAYS
BENDERS
BENDIER
BENDING
DEADAIR
DEADEND
DEADENS
DEADEST
DEADEYE
DEADPAN
DEADSEA
DEADSET
DEEDBOX
DEEDING
DENDRON
DEODARS
DEODATO
DEWDROP
FEDDERS
FEEDBAG
FEEDBIN
FEEDERS
FEEDING
FEEDLOT
FEEDSIN
FEEDSON
FEEDSTO
FELDMAN
FENDERS
FENDING
FENDOFF
FEODORI
FEUDING
FEUDIST
FEYDEAU
GELDING
GENDERS
GEODESY
GEODUCK
GETDONE
GETDOWN
HEADEND
HEADERS
HEADFOR
HEADFUL
HEADIER
HEADILY
HEADING
HEADMAN
HEADMEN
HEADOFF
HEADOUT
HEADPIN
HEADSAW
HEADSET
HEADSIN
HEADSTO
HEADSUP
HEADWAY
HEEDERS
HEEDFUL
HEEDING
HELDOFF
HELDOUT
HENDECA
HENDRIX
HENDRYX
HERDERS
HERDING
HEYDAYS
KENDALL
KENDOLL
KENDREW
KEYDETS
LEADDOG
LEADENS
LEADERS
LEADETH
LEADIER
LEADING
LEADINS
LEADMAN
LEADMEN
LEADOFF
LEADORE
LEADOUT
LEADSIN
LEADSON
LEADSTO
LEADSUP
LEADUPS
LENDERS
LENDING
LENDOUT
LETDOWN
LETDROP
LEWDEST
MEADOWS
MEADOWY
MEDDLED
MEDDLER
MEDDLES
MELDERS
MELDING
MENDELS
MENDERS
MENDING
NEEDERS
NEEDFUL
NEEDHAM
NEEDIER
NEEDILY
NEEDING
NEEDLED
NEEDLER
NEEDLES
NEEDNOT
NEEDSTO
NERDIER
NERDISH
NEWDEAL
PEDDLED
PEDDLER
PEDDLES
PENDANT
PENDENT
PENDING
PERDIDO
PERDIEM
PERDITA
PERDURE
PETDEER
PETDOGS
PETDOOR
PETDOVE
PETDUCK
READAPT
READDED
READERS
READFOR
READIED
READIER
READIES
READILY
READING
READMIT
READOFF
READOPT
READORN
READOUT
READSIN
READSON
READSTO
READSUP
REDDAWN
REDDEER
REDDENS
REDDEST
REDDING
REDDISH
REDDOGS
REDDOTS
REDDUST
REDDYES
REEDIER
REEDING
REEDITS
REEDMAN
REEDMEN
RENDELL
RENDERS
RENDING
SEADOGS
SEADUCK
SEADUTY
SEEDBED
SEEDERS
SEEDIER
SEEDILY
SEEDING
SEEDLET
SEEDPOD
SENDEES
SENDERS
SENDFOR
SENDING
SENDOFF
SENDOUT
SENDSBY
SENDSIN
SENDSON
SENDSTO
SENDSUP
SENDUPS
SETDOWN
TEDDIES
TEEDOFF
TENDAYS
TENDERS
TENDING
TENDONS
TENDRIL
TENDSTO
VEADARS
VENDEES
VENDERS
VENDING
VENDOME
VENDORS
VENDUES
VERDANT
VERDELL
VERDICT
VERDINS
VERDOUX
VERDUGO
VERDURE
WEDDELL
WEDDERS
WEDDING
WEEDERS
WEEDIER
WEEDILY
WEEDING
WEEDOUT
WEIDMAN
WELDERS
WELDING
WENDELL
WENDERS
WENDING
WENDKOS
WETDOWN
YESDEAR

•E••D••

BEANDIP
BEARDED
BESIDES
BETIDED
BETIDES
CELADON
DEARDEN
DECADES
DECIDED
DECIDER
DECIDES
DECODED
DECODER
DECODES
DEIRDRE
DELEDDA
DELUDED
DELUDER
DELUDES
DENUDED
DENUDER
DENUDES
DERIDED
DERIDER
DERIDES
FELLDUE
FETIDLY
GEEKDOM
GELIDLY
HEARDOF
HEIRDOM
HEREDIA
HERNDON
HEWEDTO
HEXADIC
KEMIDOV
KEYEDIN
KEYEDON
KEYEDUP
LEADDOG
LEANDER
LEAPDAY
LEONDAY
LEPIDUS
LEVADES
MEANDER
MELODIA
MELODIC
MENUDOS
MERIDEN
NEVADAN
NEWIDEA
NEWSDAY
NEXTDAY
PERIDOT
PESADES
READDED
REARDON
REAUDIT
RECEDED
RECEDES
RECODED
RECODES
REENDOW
REHIDES
REINDEX
REJUDGE
REMODEL
REORDER
REREDOS
RERIDES
RESIDED
RESIDER
RESIDES
RESIDUA
RESIDUE
REWIDEN
SECEDED
SECEDER
SECEDES
SEMIDRY
SERFDOM
SEWEDON
SEWEDUP
TEPIDLY
VERIDIC
VERYDRY
VEXEDLY
WEDIDIT
WEEKDAY
WEIRDAL
WEIRDED
WEIRDER
WEIRDLY
WEIRDOS
YESIDID

•E•••D•

BEDSIDE
BEGIRDS
BEHEADS
BEHINDS
BEHOLDS
BELINDA
BERENDT
BERMUDA
CERVIDS
DEFENDS
DEFUNDS
DEGRADE
DELEADS
DELEDDA
DEMANDS
DEPENDS
DERONDA
DERRIDA
DESEEDS
DETRUDE
DEWILDE
GEOCODE
GERALDO
GERUNDS
HEPTADS
HERALDS
HEYJUDE
HEYMRDJ
KENNEDY
KEYPADS
LEETIDE
LEGENDS
LEMONDE
LEONIDS
LETRIDE
MELINDA
MERCADO
METHODS
NEREIDS
NEWKIDS
NEWMADE
NEXRADS
PEABODY
PEAPODS
PENTADS
PEPCIDS
PEPTIDE
PERDIDO
PERFIDY
PERIODS
PERVADE
PETARDS
REBENDS
REBINDS
RECLADS
RECORDS
REDBUDS
REDCODS
REDEEDS
REDONDO
REDTIDE
REFEEDS
REFINDS
REFOLDS
REFUNDS
REGARDS
REGILDS
REGIRDS
REGRADE
REGUIDE
RELANDS
RELEADS
RELENDS
RELOADS
REMANDS
REMENDS
REMINDS
REMOLDS
RENALDO
REREADS
RESANDS
RESEEDS
RESENDS
RESPADE
RESTUDY
RETARDS
RETRADE
REVENDS
REVERDY
REWARDS
REWELDS
REWINDS
REWORDS
SEABEDS
SEAGODS
SEASIDE
SECLUDE
SECONDI
SECONDO
SECONDR
SECONDS
SEWARDS
TEBALDI
TENCODE
TETRADS
TETRODE
VERANDA
VERBIDS
VERYODD
VESPIDS

•E••••D

AERATED
BEACHED
BEARDED
BECLOUD
BEDAZED
BEDEWED
BEDFORD
BEETRED
BEEYARD
BEHAVED
BEHEARD
BELATED
BELAYED
BELCHED
BELLIED
BELOVED
BEMIRED
BEMUSED
BENCHED
BENOTED
BEOGRAD
BERATED
BERNARD
BERRIED
BERTHED
BESTBUD
BETIDED
BEVELED
BEWARED
CEDARED
CENTRED
CERATED
DEADEND
DEAIRED
DEARGOD
DEBASED
DEBATED
DEBEARD
DEBITED
DEBONED
DEBUTED
DECAPOD
DECAYED
DECIDED
DECKLED
DECODED
DECOYED
DECREED
DECRIED
DEDUCED
DEEPEND
DEEPRED
DEFACED
DEFAMED
DEFILED
DEFINED
DEFRAUD
DEFUSED
DEGREED
DEHEXED
DEHIRED
DEIFIED
DEIGNED
DELAYED
DELETED
DELTOID
DELUDED
DELUGED
DEMIGOD
DEMISED
DEMOTED
DENIMED
DENOTED
DENTOID
DENUDED
DEPONED
DEPOSED
DEPUTED
DERATED
DERIDED
DERIVED
DESCEND
DESEXED
DESIRED
DESMOND
DESPOND
DETOXED
DETUNED
DEVILED
DEVISED
DEVOTED
DEWAXED
DEWIRED
FEASTED
FEDEXED
FEELBAD
FEIGNED
FEINTED
FELTBAD
FEOFFED
FERNAND
FERRIED
FETCHED
FEVERED
GELATED
GENTLED
GESSOED
GETCOLD
GETGOOD
GETSMAD
GETSOLD
GETSRID
GETWORD
HEADEND
HEARTED
HECKLED
HEELPAD
HEISTED
HELIPAD
HELLOED
HELMOND
HENNAED
HENREID
HEXAPOD
HEYWARD
HEYWOOD
JELLIED
JETTIED
JEWELED
KEYCARD
KEYWORD
LEACHED
LEAGUED
LEARNED
LEASHED
LEAWOOD
LEECHED
LEEFORD
LEEWARD
LEFTEND
LEGRAND
LEONARD
LEOPARD
LEOPOLD
LEOTARD
LEPPARD
LETTERD
LEVELED
LEVERED
LEWHOAD
MEDALED
MEDDLED
MEDFORD
MELAMED
MEMOPAD
MENACED
MERITED
MERMAID
METALED
METERED
NEDLAND
NEEDLED
NEGATED
NEIGHED
NESTLED
NETTLED
NEWHAND
NEWLAID
NEWWORD
OERSTED
PEACHED
PEARLED
PEBBLED
PEDALED
PEDDLED
PEOPLED
PEPBAND
PEPPARD
PERCHED
PERILED
PERSEID
PERUSED
PESTLED
PETALED
PETBIRD
PETERED
REACHED
REACTED
READDED
READIED
REAIMED
REAIRED
REAMEND
REAREND
REARMED
REASKED
REBAKED
REBALED
REBATED
REBOARD
REBORED
REBOUND
REBOXED
REBRAND
REBREED
REBUILD
REBUKED
RECAGED
RECANED
RECASED
RECEDED
RECITED
RECODED
RECURED
RECUSED
REDARED
REDATED
REDBIRD
REDCARD
REDEYED
REDFORD
REDHEAD
REDMOND
REDOSED
REDOUND
REDRIED
REDUCED
REDWOOD
REFACED
REFAXED
REFILED
REFINED
REFIRED
REFIXED
REFLOOD
REFOUND
REFRIED
REFUGED
REFUSED
REFUTED
REGALED
REGLUED
REGNARD
REGRIND
REHEARD
REHIRED
REHONED
REIFIED
REIGNED
REINKED
REKEYED
REKNEAD
RELACED
RELATED
RELAXED
RELAYED
RELINED
RELIVED
RELUMED
REMATED
REMINED
REMISED
REMIXED
REMOVED
REMOWED
RENAMED
RENEGED
RENEWED
RENOTED
REOILED
REOWNED
REPAGED
REPAVED
REPINED
REPLEAD
REPLIED
REPOSED
REPUTED
RERAKED
RERATED
RESAVED
RESAWED
RESCIND
RESCUED
RESEWED
RESIDED
RESILED
RESINED
RESITED
RESIZED
RESOLED
RESOUND
RESOWED
RESPOND
RESUMED
RETAMED
RETAPED
RETAXED
RETILED
RETIMED
RETIRED
RETONED
RETOWED
RETREAD
RETRIED
RETUNED
RETYPED
REUPPED
REURGED
REVELED
REVERED
REVILED
REVISED
REVIVED
REVOKED
REVOTED
REWAKED
REWAXED
REWIPED
REWIRED
REWOUND
REXREED
REYNARD
REYNAUD
REYOKED
REZONED
SEABIRD
SEAFOOD
SEAWARD
SEAWEED
SECEDED
SECURED
SEDATED
SEDUCED
SEEDBED
SEEDPOD
SEESRED
SEETHED
SEPALED
SETTLED
SEVENAD
SEVERED
TEEHEED
TEETHED
TELEXED
TEMPLED
TEMPTED
TENFOLD
TENONED
TENTBED
TENURED
TESTBED
VENTRAD
VERYBAD
VERYMAD
VERYODD
VERYOLD
VERYRED
VERYSAD
WEARIED
WEBTOED
WEDELED
WEEKEND
WEIGHED
WEIRDED
WELLAND
WELLFED
WELLHID
WELLLED
WENTBAD
WENTMAD
WESTEND
WETEYED
WETLAND
WEXFORD
XEROXED

YEAREND
YEARNED
YEASTED
YESIDID
ZEALAND
ZEBROID
ZEELAND

••ED•••

ACEDOUT
AGEDOUT
APEDIET
ATEDIRT
BLEDSOE
CHEDDAR
CHEDERS
COEDITS
CREDITS
DEEDBOX
DEEDING
DIEDFOR
DIEDOFF
DIEDOUT
DIEDOWN
DREDGED
DREDGER
DREDGES
DUEDATE
EKEDOUT
EXEDRAE
EYEDROP
FEEDBAG
FEEDBIN
FEEDERS
FEEDING
FEEDLOT
FEEDSIN
FEEDSON
FEEDSTO
FIEDLER
FLEDGED
FLEDGES
FREDDIE
FREDEBB
FREDRIC
HEEDERS
HEEDFUL
HEEDING
HOEDOWN
ICEDAMS
ICEDOUT
ICEDOWN
ICEDTEA
INEDITA
KHEDIVE
LIEDFOR
LIEDOWN
NEEDERS
NEEDFUL
NEEDHAM
NEEDIER
NEEDILY
NEEDING
NEEDLED
NEEDLER
NEEDLES
NEEDNOT
NEEDSTO
ONEDIME
ONEDOWN
PLEDGED
PLEDGEE
PLEDGER
PLEDGES
PREDARK
PREDATA
PREDATE
PREDAWN
PREDEFY
PREDENY
PREDICT
PREDIET
PREDIVE
PREDOOM
PREDUSK
PYEDOGS
RAEDAWN
REEDIER
REEDING
REEDITS
REEDMAN
REEDMEN
ROEDEER
SEEDBED
SEEDERS
SEEDIER
SEEDILY
SEEDING
SEEDLET
SEEDPOD
SHEDDER
SHEDSON
SLEDDED
SLEDDER
SLEDDOG
SLEDFUL
SLEDGED
SLEDGES
SPEDOFF
SUEDFOR
SWEDISH
TEEDOFF
THEDEEP
THEDELL
THEDIET
THEDOLE
THEDUKE
TIEDOFF
TIEDOWN
TIEDYED
TIEDYES
TREDIAS
UNEDGED
UNEDGES
USEDCAR
USEDCDS
USEDFOR
VIEDFOR
WEEDERS
WEEDIER
WEEDILY
WEEDING
WEEDOUT

••E•D••

AGENDAS
AGENDUM
AHEADOF
AMENDED
AMENDER
BLEEDER
BLENDED
BLENDER
BLENDES
BLENDIN
BREADED
BREADER
BREADTH
BREEDER
BRENDAN
BRENDEL
BRENDON
CHEADLE
CHEDDAR
CREEDAL
DREADED
DREIDEL
DRESDEN
EMENDED
EMENDER
EVERDUR
FIEFDOM
FIELDED
FIELDER
FLEADIP
FREDDIE
FREEDOF
FREEDOM
FREEDUP
GEEKDOM
GRENDEL
GREWDIM
GUERDON
JOEYDEE
KNEADED
KNEADER
NOENDOF
NOENDTO
ONEADAY
ONEIDAS
OVERDID
OVERDOG
OVERDRY
OVERDUB
OVERDUE
OVERDYE
PLEADED
PLEADER
PLEADTO
PREEDIT
PREIDEA
REENDOW
SHEDDER
SHELDON
SLEDDED
SLEDDER
SLEDDOG
SLENDER
SPEEDED
SPEEDER
SPEEDOS
SPEEDUP
SPENDER
SPENDON
STEADED
STEPDAD
THEEDGE
THEIDEA
THEODOR
TIENDAS
TREADED
TREADER
TREADLE
TREADON
TRENDED
TUESDAY
TWEEDLE
UNENDED
UPENDED
WEEKDAY
WHEEDLE
WIELDED
WIELDER
YIELDED
YIELDER
YIELDTO

••E••D•

ALEARDI
AMERADA
AVENIDA
CUEBIDS
EYELIDS
GRENADA
GRENADE
JOEKIDD
LEETIDE
MAENADS
OREBODY
PREBADE
PREBIDS
PRECEDE
PRECODE
PREFADE
PRELUDE
PREMADE
PREMEDS
PRESIDE
QUERIDA
QUERIDO
THEBODY
THEFEDS
THEREDS
TIERODS
USEDCDS
USERIDS

••E•••D

ABELARD
ABETTED
ADENOID
AFEARED
AGENTED
ALERTED
ALEYARD
AMEBOID
AMENDED
AMERCED
AMERIND
ANEROID
AVENGED
AVERRED
AVERTED
AXEHEAD
AXELROD
BEETRED
BEEYARD
BLEARED
BLEATED
BLEEPED
BLENDED
BLESSED
BREADED
BREEZED
CHEATED
CHECKED
CHEEKED
CHEEPED
CHEERED
CHEESED
CHESTED
CLEANED
CLEARED
CLEATED
CLEAVED
CLERKED
COERCED
CREAKED
CREAMED
CREASED
CREATED
CREEPED
CRESTED
CTENOID
CUECARD
DEEPEND
DEEPRED
DIEBOLD
DIEHARD
DOEEYED
DOESBAD
DREADED
DREAMED
DREDGED
DRESSED
DUELLED
DUETTED
DWELLED
DYEWOOD
EGESTED
EJECTED
ELECTED
ELEVEND
EMENDED
EMERALD
EMERGED
EMERSED
ERECTED
EVERTED
EXERTED
EYEFOLD
EYEHAND
FEELBAD
FIELDED
FLECKED
FLEDGED
FLEECED
FLEERED
FLEETED
FLENSED
FLESHED
FREAKED
FRESHED
FRESSED
FRETTED
FUELLED
FUELROD
GIELGUD
GLEAMED
GLEANED
GOESBAD
GOESMAD
GREASED
GREENED
GREETED
GREWOLD
GUESSED
GUESTED
HEELPAD
ICECOLD
ICELAND
IDEATED
IRELAND
ISECOND
JOEKIDD
KNEADED
KNEELED
KNEEPAD
KNELLED
KVELLED
LEECHED
LEEFORD
LEEWARD
LIEABED
NEEDLED
OCEANID
ONEEYED
ONEFOLD
ONEHAND
ONEWOOD
ONEYARD
OPENEND
OPERAND
OVERBED
OVERBID
OVERDID
OVERFED
OVERSAD
PIEBALD
PIEEYED
PIERCED
PLEADED
PLEASED
PLEATED
PLEDGED
PREACID
PREAGED
PREBIND
PREENED
PREFUND
PRELOAD
PREPAID
PREPPED
PRESOLD
PRESSED
PRETEND
PRETOLD
PREVOID
PREVUED
QUEENED
QUEERED
QUELLED
QUERIED
QUESTED
SCENTED
SEEDBED
SEEDPOD
SEESRED
SEETHED
SHEAFED
SHEARED
SHEAVED
SHEERED
SHEETED
SHELLED
SHELVED
SHEPARD
SLEDDED
SLEDGED
SLEEKED
SLEETED
SLEEVED
SMEARED
SMELLED
SMELTED
SNEAKED
SNEERED
SNEEZED
SPEARED
SPECKED
SPEEDED
SPELLED
STEADED
STEAMED
STEELED
STEEPED
STEERED
STEEVED
STEMMED
STEPDAD
STEPPED
STEROID
STETTED
STEWARD
SWEATED
SWELLED
SWERVED
TEEHEED
TEETHED
THEBAND
THEBARD
THEGOLD
THEHOOD
THEPOND
THEWIND
TIEDYED
TOEHOLD
TREADED
TREATED
TREBLED
TREKKED
TRENDED
TRESSED
TWEAKED
TWEETED
TWEEZED
TWELVED
UNEAVED
UNEBBED
UNEDGED
UNENDED
UPENDED
VNECKED
WEEKEND
WHEELED
WHEEZED
WHELMED
WHELPED
WHETTED
WIELAND
WIELDED
WREAKED
WRECKED
WRESTED
YIELDED
ZEELAND

•••ED••

ACCEDED
ACCEDER
ACCEDES
ACTEDAS
ACTEDIN
ACTEDON
ACTEDUP
ADDEDIN
ADDEDLY
ADDEDON
ADDEDTO
ADDEDUP
AIMEDAT
AIREDUP
ALBEDOS
AMPEDUP
ANTEDUP
ARLEDGE
ASKEDIN
ASKEDOF
ASKEDUP
BASEDON
BAYEDAT
BIPEDAL
BLEEDER
BONEDRY
BONEDUP
BOOEDAT
BOREDOM
BOWEDTO
BOXEDIN
BOXEDUP
BRAEDEN
BREEDER
CAGEDIN
CAGEDUP
CAKEDUP
CAMEDUE
CAREDTO
CAVEDIN
CLUEDIN
COMEDIA
COMEDIC
COMEDIE
COMEDUE
COTEDOR
CREEDAL
CRIEDUP
DATEDLY
DAZEDLY
DELEDDA
DINEDAT
DINEDIN
DINEDON
DIVEDIN
DOTEDON
DRIEDUP
DUDEDUP
DUKEDOM
DUNEDIN
EASEDBY
EASEDIN
EASEDON
EASEDUP
EDGEDIN
EGGEDON
ENDEDAT
ENDEDIN
ENDEDIT
ENDEDON
ENDEDUP
EPHEDRA
EXHEDRA
FACEDIT
FACEDON
FADEDIN
FADEDLY
FAKEDIT
FILEDBY
FILEDIN
FIREDAT
FIREDOG
FIREDON
FIREDUP
FIVEDAY
FIXEDLY
FIXEDON
FIXEDUP
FLIEDTO
FREEDOF
FREEDOM
FREEDUP
FRIEDAN
FRIEDUP
FUMEDAT
GAPEDAT
GASEDUP
GAZEDAT
GAZEDON
GLUEDON
GLUEDTO
HATEDIT
HEREDIA
HEWEDTO
HIKEDUP
HIREDON
HOLEDUP
HOMEDIN
HONEDIN
HOPEDSO
HOPEDTO
HYPEDUP
IMPEDED
IMPEDER
IMPEDES
INKEDIN
IPLEDGE
JADEDLY
JANEDOE
JAWEDAT
JIBEDAT
JUNEDAY
KEYEDIN
KEYEDON
KEYEDUP
LACEDUP
LAREDOS
LINEDRY
LINEDUP
LIVEDIN
LIVEDON
LOVEDIT
LOVEDTO
LUREDIN
MACEDON
MAKEDOS
MALEDOG
MISEDIT
MIXEDIN
MIXEDLY
MIXEDUP
MOVEDIN
MOVEDIT
MOVEDON
MOVEDTO
MOVEDUP
MUSEDON
MUTEDLY
NAKEDLY
NAMEDAY
NICEDAY
NICEDOG
NOSEDIN
NOSEDUP
NOTEDLY
OPTEDIN
OPTEDTO
OUTEDGE
OWNEDUP
PALEDRY
PAWEDAT
PHAEDRA
PILEDIN
PILEDON
PILEDUP
PIPEDIN
PIPEDUP
POKEDAT
POPEDOM
POSEDAS
PREEDIT
RACEDBY
RACEDIN
RACEDTO
RACEDUP
RAKEDIN
RAKEDUP
RATEDPG
RECEDED
RECEDES
REREDOS
RILEDUP
ROPEDIN
ROPEDUP
RULEDBY
RULEDON
SAMEDAY
SAMEDIS
SAVEDON
SAVEDUP
SECEDED
SECEDER
SECEDES
SEWEDON
SEWEDUP
SINEDIE
SIZEDUP
SOLEDAD
SOMEDAY
SPEEDED
SPEEDER
SPEEDOS
SPEEDUP
SPIEDON
TAPEDON
TAPEDUP
THEEDGE
TIREDER
TIREDLY
TIREDOF
TOLEDAN
TOLEDOS
TONEDUP
TOWEDIN
TRIEDIT
TRIEDON
TRIEDTO
TRUEDUP
TUNEDIN
TUNEDTO
TUNEDUP
TUXEDOS
TWEEDLE
TYPEDIN
TYPEDUP
UNCEDED
UNWEDGE
URGEDON
USTEDES
VEXEDLY
VOTEDIN
VOTEDNO
VOTEDON
WADEDIN
WAKEDUP
WAVEDAT
WAVEDIN
WAVEDTO
WAXEDUP
WHEEDLE
WIPEDUP
WIREDIN
WIREDUP
WISEDUP
WOWEDEM

•••E•D•

ADDENDA
ADDENDS
ALLENDE
ALREADY
APPENDS
ASCENDS
ATTENDS
AUGENDS
AXHEADS
AXSEEDS
BADENDS
BEHEADS
BERENDT
BIGENDS
CALENDS
DEFENDS
DELEADS
DELEDDA
DEPENDS
DESEEDS
DOVERDE
EFFENDI
ENNEADS
EXCEEDS
EXPENDS
EXTENDS
FAGENDS
FAKEIDS
FRIENDS
FTMEADE
IMPENDS
IMREADY
INDEEDY
INTENDS
LEGENDS
LIMEADE
MAKESDO
MRDEEDS
NEREIDS
NIKEADS
OFFENDS
REBENDS
REDEEDS
REFEEDS
RELEADS
RELENDS
REMENDS
REREADS
RESEEDS
RESENDS
REVENDS
REVERDY
REWELDS
SCHELDT
SCREEDS
SHIELDS
SPLENDA
SPREADS
SUREIDO
TAGENDS
THREADS
THREADY
UNBELDI
UNBENDS
UNDERDO
UNHEADY
UNHEEDS
UNLEADS
UNNEEDY
UNREADY
UPSENDS
VIVENDI

•••E••D

ACCEDED
ADHERED
ALLEGED
ALTERED
ANGERED
ANNELID
ANNEXED
BEDEWED
BEHEARD
BEVELED
BIGEYED
BLEEPED
BLUERED
BOGEYED
BOWERED
BREEZED
BRIEFED
BUGEYED
CAMELID
CAMEOED
CAPECOD
CAPERED
CATERED
CATEYED
CHEEKED
CHEEPED
CHEERED
CHEESED
CODERED
COHERED
COVERED
COVETED
COWERED
COZENED
CREEPED
CUPELED
DEBEARD
DEHEXED
DELETED
DESEXED
DOEEYED
DONEBAD
DOWERED
DRYEYED
EASELED
ENTERED
FACETED
FEDEXED
FEVERED
FIBERED
FLEECED
FLEERED
FLEETED
GAVELED
GONEBAD
GONEMAD
GREENED
GREETED
GRIEVED
HOMERED
HONEYED
HOVERED
IMPEDED
INDEXED
INHERED

ISLETED
JEWELED
JONESED
KAMERAD
KNEELED
KNEEPAD
LABELED
LAKEBED
LAPELED
LATENED
LAYERED
LEVELED
LEVERED
LIBELED
LIKEMAD
LIKENED
LIVEAID
LIVENED
LIVERED
LOWERED
MADEMAD
MAKEMAD
METERED
MIMEOED
MITERED
MODELED
MODEMED
MONEYED
MOSEYED
NICEKID
NOTEPAD
OFFERED
ONEEYED
ORDERED
OSIERED
OSTEOID
OWLEYED
PANELED
PAPERED
PETERED
PIEEYED
PIGEYED
POPEYED
POWERED
PREENED
QUEENED
QUEERED
QUIETED
RAVELED
RAVENED
RECEDED
REDEYED
REHEARD
REKEYED
RENEGED
RENEWED
RESEWED
REVELED
REVERED
RIPENED
RITEAID
RIVETED
ROGERED
ROSEBUD
ROSERED
ROWELED
SABERED
SADEYED
SAMEOLD
SCHEMED
SCREWED
SECEDED
SEVENAD
SEVERED
SHEERED
SHEETED
SILENTD
SINEWED
SIRENED
SLEEKED
SLEETED
SLEEVED
SNEERED
SNEEZED
SOBERED
SOLEDAD
SPEEDED
SPHERED
SPIELED
STEELED
STEEPED
STEERED
STEEVED
STREWED
TAPERED
TASERED
TELEXED
THIEVED
THREEAD
TOBEHAD
TOKENED
TOWELED
TOWERED
TWEETED
TWEEZED
UMBERED
UNBEARD
UNCEDED
UNDEWED
UNFETED
UNHEARD
UNHEWED
UNKEYED
UNMEWED
UNSEWED
UNVEXED
USHERED
UTTERED
VALETED
VIDEOED
WAFERED
WAGERED
WAKENED
WATERED
WAVERED
WEDELED
WETEYED
WHEELED
WHEEZED
WIDENED
WINERED
WIZENED
YODELED

••••ED•

ALAMEDA
ALFREDA
ALFREDE
ALFREDO
ALFREDU
AXSEEDS
BOXBEDS
CATBEDS
CONCEDE
DAYBEDS
DESEEDS
DIALEDO
DIOMEDE
DOGBEDS
DRAMEDY
EXCEEDS
HATREDS
HOTBEDS
HOWDEDO
IDAREDS
INDEEDY
ISUREDO
KENNEDY
MALTEDS
MRDEEDS
ONTHEDL
PRECEDE
PREMEDS
PROKEDS
RAGGEDY
REDEEDS
REFEEDS
RESEEDS
RIGVEDA
SCAREDY
SCREEDS
SEABEDS
THEFEDS
THEREDS
TORPEDO
TRAGEDY
UNHEEDS
UNNEEDY

••••E•D

AIRHEAD
ANISEED
ARANEID
ARCWELD
ATANEND
AXEHEAD
BACKEND
BADDEED
BARTEND
BIGBEND
BIGHEAD
BIGLEAD
BOISEID
BOOKEND
BOWHEAD
CATHEAD
COMMEND
COMPEND
CONTEND
COWHERD
DAYSEND
DEADEND
DECREED
DEEPEND
DEGREED
DESCEND
DISTEND
DRFREUD
EASTEND
EGGHEAD
ELEVEND
ENFIELD
FATHEAD
FORFEND
GLACEED
GOAHEAD
GOATEED
GODHEAD
GODSEND
HAYSEED
HEADEND
HENREID
HIGHEND
HISPEED
HOGWEED
HOTHEAD
HOTLEAD
IMPLEAD
INBREED
INFIELD
INSTEAD
ISAHEAD
ISSUEAD
JUGHEAD
LEFTEND
LETTERD
LINSEED
LIPREAD
LOUREED
MACLEOD
MILLEND
MINUEND
MISDEED
MISFEED
MISLEAD
MISREAD
MISSEND
MOPHEAD
OILSEED
ONALEAD
OPENEND
OUTBEND
OUTFEED
OUTLEAD
OUTREAD
OUTWEED
PAYHEED
PERSEID
PIGWEED
PINHEAD
PITHEAD
PORTEND
PRETEND
PROCEED
RAGWEED
REAMEND
REAREND
REBREED
REDHEAD
REKNEAD
REPLEAD
RETREAD
REXREED
RUMPEND
SAPHEAD
SAUTEED
SEAWEED
SOTWEED
STIPEND
SUBHEAD
SUBTEND
SUCCEED
SUSPEND
TAILEND
TEEHEED
THREEAD
TIMREID
TOPSEED
TOWHEAD
UNFREED
UNTREAD
UNTREED
UPAHEAD
UPFIELD
UPTREND
WARHEAD
WEEKEND
WESTEND
WITSEND
YEAREND

•••••ED

AARATED
ABASHED
ABDUCED
ABETTED
ABJURED
ABLATED
ABORTED
ABRADED
ABUTTED
ACCEDED
ACCRUED
ACCUSED
ACORNED
ACTIFED
ADAPTED
ADDUCED
ADHERED
ADJURED
ADMIRED
ADMIXED
ADOPTED
ADORNED
ADVISED
AERATED
AFEARED
AFFINED
AFFIXED
AGENTED
ALARMED
ALERTED
ALIBIED
ALIGNED
ALLAYED
ALLEGED
ALLOWED
ALLOYED
ALLTIED
ALLUDED
ALLURED
ALTERED
AMASSED
AMENDED
AMERCED
ANGERED
ANISEED
ANNEXED
ANNOYED
APPLIED
APPOSED
APRONED
ARBORED
ARCADED
ARMORED
AROUSED
ARRAYED
ARRIVED
ASCARED
ASHAMED
ASPIRED
ASSAYED
ASSUMED
ASSURED
ATTIRED
ATTUNED
AUDITED
AUGURED
AVAILED
AVENGED
AVERRED
AVERTED
AVIATED
AVOIDED
AVULSED
AWAITED
AWARDED
BABBLED
BADDEED
BAFFLED
BANDIED
BANGLED
BARNRED
BATCHED
BATIKED
BATTLED
BAULKED
BEACHED
BEARDED
BEDAZED
BEDEWED
BEETRED
BEHAVED
BELATED
BELAYED
BELCHED
BELLIED
BELOVED
BEMIRED
BEMUSED
BENCHED
BENOTED
BERATED
BERRIED
BERTHED
BETIDED
BEVELED
BEWARED
BIASSED
BIGEYED
BIGOTED
BILOBED
BIRCHED
BIRDIED
BIRTHED
BLABBED
BLACKED
BLANKED
BLASTED
BLATTED
BLEARED
BLEATED
BLEEPED
BLENDED
BLESSED
BLINDED
BLINKED
BLIPPED
BLISSED
BLITZED
BLOATED
BLOBBED
BLOCKED
BLOGGED
BLOODED
BLOOMED
BLOOPED
BLOTTED
BLOUSED
BLOWZED
BLUDGED
BLUERED
BLUFFED
BLUNTED
BLURRED
BLURTED
BLUSHED
BOARDED
BOASTED
BOBBLED
BOBSLED
BOGEYED
BOGGLED
BOOGIED
BOOSTED
BOSOMED
BOTCHED
BOTTLED
BOUGHED
BOUNCED
BOUNDED
BOWERED
BRAGGED
BRAIDED
BRAINED
BRAISED
BRANDED
BRAVOED
BRAWLED
BREADED
BREEZED
BRICKED
BRIDGED
BRIDLED
BRIEFED
BRIMMED
BRISKED
BROILED
BRONZED
BROODED
BROOKED
BROOMED
BROWNED
BROWSED
BRUISED
BRUITED
BRUSHED
BUBBLED
BUCKLED
BUDDIED
BUGEYED
BULLIED
BUMBLED
BUNCHED
BUNCOED
BUNDLED
BUNGLED
BUNKBED
BUNKOED
BURBLED
BURGLED
BUSTLED
BYLINED
CACKLED
CADDIED
CAIRNED
CAJOLED
CAMEOED
CAMPBED
CANALED
CANDIED
CANDLED
CAPERED
CAROLED
CAROMED
CARRIED
CASQUED
CASTLED
CATERED
CATEYED
CAULKED
CAVILED
CEDARED
CENTRED
CERATED
CHAFFED
CHAINED
CHAIRED
CHALKED
CHAMPED
CHANCED
CHANGED
CHANTED
CHAPPED
CHARGED
CHARMED
CHARRED
CHARTED
CHASSED
CHATTED
CHEATED
CHECKED
CHEEKED
CHEEPED
CHEERED
CHEESED
CHESTED
CHILLED
CHINKED
CHINNED
CHIPPED
CHIRPED
CHIRRED
CHIVIED
CHOCKED
CHOIRED
CHOMPED
CHOPPED
CHORDED
CHROMED
CHUCKED
CHUFFED
CHUGGED
CHUMMED
CHUMPED
CHUNKED
CHURNED
CINCHED
CIRCLED
CLACKED
CLADDED
CLAIMED
CLAMMED
CLAMPED
CLANGED
CLANKED
CLAPPED
CLASHED
CLASPED
CLASSED
CLEANED
CLEARED
CLEATED
CLEAVED
CLERKED
CLICHED
CLICKED
CLIMBED
CLINKED
CLIPPED
CLIQUED
CLOAKED
CLOCKED
CLOGGED
CLOMPED
CLONKED
CLOPPED
CLOTHED
CLOTTED
CLOUDED
CLOUTED
CLOWNED
CLUBBED
CLUBMED
CLUCKED
CLUMPED
CLUNKED
COACHED
COACTED
COAPTED
COASTED
COBBLED
COCKLED
CODDLED
CODERED
COERCED
COHERED
COIFFED
COIGNED
COLORED
CONGAED
CONRIED
COOPTED
COOWNED
CORNFED
COUCHED
COUGHED
COUNTED
COUPLED
COURSED
COURTED
COVERED
COVETED
COWERED
COWSHED
COZENED
CRABBED
CRACKED
CRADLED
CRAFTED
CRAGGED
CRAMMED
CRAMPED
CRANKED
CRASHED
CRAWLED
CREAKED
CREAMED
CREASED
CREATED
CREEPED
CRESTED
CRIBBED
CRICKED
CRIMPED
CRINGED
CRISPED
CROAKED
CROCKED
CROOKED
CROONED
CROPPED
CROSSED
CROWDED
CROWNED
CRUISED
CRUMBED
CRUMPED
CRUSHED
CRUSTED
CUDDLED
CULLIED
CUPELED
CURATED
CURDLED
CURRIED
DABBLED
DALLIED
DAMAGED
DANDLED
DANGLED
DAPPLED
DARKLED
DARKRED
DARTLED
DAUNTED
DAWDLED
DAZZLED
DEAIRED
DEBASED
DEBATED
DEBITED
DEBONED
DEBUTED
DECAYED
DECIDED
DECKLED
DECODED
DECOYED
DECREED
DECRIED
DEDUCED
DEEPRED
DEFACED
DEFAMED
DEFILED
DEFINED
DEFUSED
DEGREED
DEHEXED
DEHIRED
DEIFIED
DEIGNED
DELAYED
DELETED
DELUDED
DELUGED
DEMISED
DEMOTED
DENIMED
DENOTED
DENUDED
DEPONED
DEPOSED
DEPUTED
DERATED
DERIDED
DERIVED
DESEXED
DESIRED
DETOXED
DETUNED
DEVILED
DEVISED
DEVOTED
DEWAXED
DEWIRED
DIALLED
DIBBLED
DIDDLED
DILATED
DILUTED
DIMPLED
DIRTIED
DISCOED
DISUSED
DITCHED
DITTOED
DIVIDED
DIVINED
DIVVIED
DIZZIED
DOEEYED
DOGSLED
DOLLIED
DONATED
DOODLED
DOUBLED
DOUBTED
DOWERED
DRAFTED
DRAGGED
DRAINED
DRATTED
DRAWLED
DREADED
DREAMED
DREDGED
DRESSED
DRIFTED
DRILLED
DRIPPED
DROOLED
DROOPED
DROPPED
DROWNED
DROWSED
DRUBBED
DRUDGED
DRUGGED
DRUMMED
DRYEYED
DUELLED
DUETTED
DUMMIED
DWARFED
DWELLED
EARTHED
EASELED
EBANKED
EDIFIED
EDUCTED
EFFACED
EFFUSED
EGESTED
EJECTED
ELAPSED
ELBOWED
ELECTED
EMAILED
EMBAYED
EMBRUED
EMENDED
EMERGED
EMERSED
EMITTED
EMPALED
EMPTIED
ENABLED
ENACTED
ENARMED
ENCAGED
ENCASED
ENCODED
ENCORED
ENDOWED
ENDURED
ENFACED
ENGAGED
ENGINED
ENISLED
ENJOYED
ENLACED
ENOILED
ENRAGED
ENROBED
ENSILED
ENSKIED
ENSURED
ENTERED
ENTICED
EPOXIED
EQUALED
EQUATED
ERECTED
ERMINED
ERUCTED
ERUPTED
ESCAPED
ESSAYED
ESTATED
ETAILED
EUCHRED
EVERTED
EVICTED
EVINCED
EVOLVED
EVULSED
EXACTED
EXALTED
EXCIDED
EXCISED
EXCITED
EXCUSED
EXERTED
EXHALED
EXHUMED
EXISTED
EXPIRED
EXPOSED
EXULTED
FACETED
FAGOTED
FAINTED
FANCIED
FAULTED
FAVORED
FEASTED
FEDEXED
FEIGNED
FEINTED
FEOFFED
FERRIED
FETCHED
FEVERED
FIBERED
FIDDLED
FIELDED
FIGURED
FILCHED
FIXATED
FIZZLED
FLACKED
FLAGGED

FLAILED
FLAMBED
FLAMMED
FLANKED
FLAPPED
FLASHED
FLATBED
FLATTED
FLECKED
FLEDGED
FLEECED
FLEERED
FLEETED
FLENSED
FLESHED
FLICKED
FLIPPED
FLIRTED
FLITTED
FLOATED
FLOCKED
FLOGGED
FLOODED
FLOORED
FLOPPED
FLOSSED
FLOURED
FLOUTED
FLUBBED
FLUFFED
FLUNKED
FLUSHED
FOCUSED
FOISTED
FOLIOED
FONDLED
FONDUED
FOOTLED
FOOZLED
FORAGED
FORAYED
FOUNDED
FRAGGED
FRANKED
FREAKED
FRESHED
FRESSED
FRETTED
FRILLED
FRINGED
FRISKED
FRITTED
FRIZZED
FROCKED
FRONTED
FROSTED
FROTHED
FROWNED
FRUITED
FUDDLED
FUELLED
FUMBLED
GABBLED
GALOPED
GAMBLED
GARAGED
GARBLED
GARGLED
GAVELED
GELATED
GENTLED
GESSOED
GHOSTED
GIDDIED
GIGGLED
GIRDLED
GIRTHED
GLACEED
GLANCED
GLASSED
GLEAMED
GLEANED
GLINTED
GLITZED
GLOATED
GLOMMED
GLOOMED
GLORIED
GLOSSED
GLUGGED
GLUMMED
GLUTTED
GNARLED
GNARRED
GNASHED
GOATEED
GOBBLED
GOGGLED
GOOGLED
GOTOBED
GRABBED
GRAFTED
GRAINED
GRANTED
GRAPHED
GRASPED
GRASSED
GREASED
GREENED
GREETED
GRIDDED
GRIEVED
GRIFTED
GRILLED
GRINNED
GRIPPED
GRITTED
GROANED
GROINED
GROKKED
GROOMED
GROOVED
GROSSED
GROUPED
GROUSED
GROUTED
GROWLED
GRUBBED
GRUDGED
GRUMPED
GRUNTED
GUARDED
GUESSED
GUESTED
GULLIED
GURGLED
GUSSIED
GUZZLED
GYRATED
HABITED
HACKLED
HAGGLED
HALFFED
HANDFED
HANDLED
HARRIED
HASSLED
HATCHED
HAUNTED
HAYSEED
HEARTED
HECKLED
HEISTED
HELLOED
HENNAED
HIGGLED
HISPEED
HITCHED
HOARDED
HOBBLED
HOCUSED
HOGTIED
HOGWEED
HOISTED
HOMERED
HONEYED
HONORED
HOUNDED
HOVERED
HUDDLED
HULLOED
HUMBLED
HUMORED
HUMPHED
HUNCHED
HUNDRED
HURDLED
HURRIED
HURTLED
HUSTLED
IDEATED
IGNITED
IGNORED
IGOOFED
ILLBRED
ILLUDED
ILLUMED
ILLUSED
IMBIBED
IMBORED
IMBRUED
IMMIXED
IMMURED
IMPALED
IMPEDED
IMPLIED
IMPOSED
IMPUTED
IMTIRED
INBREED
INCASED
INCISED
INCITED
INCUSED
INDEXED
INDITED
INDUCED
INFIXED
INFUSED
INHALED
INHERED
INHUMED
INJURED
INSURED
INTONED
INVADED
INVITED
INVOKED
IODATED
IODISED
IODIZED
IONISED
IONIZED
ISLETED
JANGLED
JAUNTED
JELLIED
JETTIED
JEWELED
JIGGLED
JIMMIED
JINGLED
JOGGLED
JOINTED
JOISTED
JOLLIED
JONESED
JOSTLED
JOUNCED
JOUSTED
JUGGLED
JUMBLED
KAYAKED
KIBBLED
KINDLED
KINDRED
KLUDGED
KNARRED
KNEADED
KNEELED
KNELLED
KNITTED
KNOBBED
KNOCKED
KNOTTED
KNOUTED
KNURLED
KVELLED
LABELED
LABORED
LAKEBED
LAPELED
LASSOED
LATCHED
LATENED
LAUGHED
LAYERED
LEACHED
LEAGUED
LEARNED
LEASHED
LEECHED
LEVELED
LEVERED
LIAISED
LIBELED
LIEABED
LIGATED
LIGHTED
LIKENED
LIMITED
LINDIED
LINSEED
LIVENED
LIVERED
LOATHED
LOBATED
LOBBIED
LOCATED
LOFTBED
LONGBED
LOUNGED
LOUREED
LOUVRED
LOWBRED
LOWERED
LSHAPED
LUNATED
LUNCHED
LURCHED
LUSTRED
LUXATED
MAITRED
MAJORED
MAMBOED
MANAGED
MANFRED
MANGLED
MANTLED
MANURED
MARBLED
MARCHED
MARRIED
MARSRED
MASONED
MATCHED
MATURED
MEDALED
MEDDLED
MELAMED
MENACED
MERITED
METALED
METERED
MIAOUED
MIAOWED
MIDDLED
MILDRED
MILKFED
MIMEOED
MINGLED
MINORED
MINUTED
MISCUED
MISDEED
MISFEED
MISUSED
MITERED
MIZZLED
MODELED
MODEMED
MONEYED
MOOCHED
MORDRED
MORPHED
MOSEYED
MOTIVED
MOTORED
MOTTLED
MOULDED
MOULTED
MOUNDED
MOUNTED
MOURNED
MOUSSED
MOUTHED
MUDDIED
MUDDLED
MUFFLED
MULCHED
MULCTED
MUMBLED
MUNCHED
MURALED
MUSCLED
MUTATED
MUZZLED
MYRRHED
NANNIED
NATURED
NEEDLED
NEGATED
NEIGHED
NESTLED
NETTLED
NIBBLED
NIGGLED
NODULED
NONSKED
NOODGED
NOODLED
NOTATED
NOTCHED
NOTICED
NOTUSED
NUANCED
NUDZHED
NUTATED
NUZZLED
OBLIGED
OERSTED
OFFERED
OILSEED
OLMSTED
OMITTED
ONEEYED
OPPOSED
ORBITED
ORDERED
OSHAPED
OSIERED
OSMOSED
OUTAWED
OUTBRED
OUTFEED
OUTSPED
OUTVIED
OUTWEED
OVERBED
OVERFED
OWLEYED
PADDLED
PAINTED
PANELED
PAPERED
PARADED
PARCHED
PAROLED
PARRIED
PARTIED
PATCHED
PAYHEED
PEACHED
PEARLED
PEBBLED
PEDALED
PEDDLED
PEOPLED
PERCHED
PERILED
PERUSED
PESTLED
PETALED
PETERED
PGRATED
PHISHED
PHRASED
PIAFFED
PICKLED
PICOTED
PIDDLED
PIEEYED
PIERCED
PIFFLED
PIGEYED
PIGWEED
PILOTED
PIMPLED
PINCHED
PIRATED
PITCHED
PIVOTED
PLAGUED
PLAITED
PLANKED
PLANNED
PLANTED
PLASHED
PLATTED
PLEADED
PLEASED
PLEATED
PLEDGED
PLINKED
PLODDED
PLONKED
PLOPPED
PLOTTED
PLOTZED
PLUCKED
PLUGGED
PLUMBED
PLUMPED
PLUNGED
PLUNKED
POACHED
POINTED
POLICED
POLKAED
POLYPED
POMADED
POPEYED
POPPLED
POSITED
POUCHED
POUNCED
POUNDED
POWERED
PRAISED
PRANCED
PRAWNED
PREAGED
PREENED
PREPPED
PRESSED
PREVUED
PRICKED
PRIMMED
PRIMPED
PRINKED
PRINTED
PROCEED
PRODDED
PROMOED
PRONGED
PROOFED
PROPPED
PROWLED
PSHAWED
PSYCHED
PUDDLED
PUMICED
PUNCHED
PUPATED
PURFLED
PURPLED
PURSUED
PUTTIED
PUZZLED
QUACKED
QUAFFED
QUAILED
QUASHED
QUEENED
QUEERED
QUELLED
QUERIED
QUESTED
QUIETED
QUILLED
QUILTED
QUIPPED
QUIRTED
QUITTED
QUIZZED
QUOINED
QUOITED
RABBLED
RADIOED
RAFFLED
RAGWEED
RALLIED
RAMBLED
RANCHED
RANKLED
RASSLED
RATTLED
RAVAGED
RAVELED
RAVENED
RAVINED
RAZORED
REACHED
REACTED
READDED
READIED
REAIMED
REAIRED
REARMED
REASKED
REBAKED
REBALED
REBATED
REBORED
REBOXED
REBREED
REBUKED
RECAGED
RECANED
RECASED
RECEDED
RECITED
RECODED
RECURED
RECUSED
REDARED
REDATED
REDEYED
REDOSED
REDRIED
REDUCED
REFACED
REFAXED
REFILED
REFINED
REFIRED
REFIXED
REFRIED
REFUGED
REFUSED
REFUTED
REGALED
REGLUED
REHIRED
REHONED
REIFIED
REIGNED
REINKED
REKEYED
RELACED
RELATED
RELAXED
RELAYED
RELINED
RELIVED
RELUMED
REMATED
REMINED
REMISED
REMIXED
REMOVED
REMOWED
RENAMED
RENEGED
RENEWED
RENOTED
REOILED
REOWNED
REPAGED
REPAVED
REPINED
REPLIED
REPOSED
REPUTED
RERAKED
RERATED
RESAVED
RESAWED
RESCUED
RESEWED
RESIDED
RESILED
RESINED
RESITED
RESIZED
RESOLED
RESOWED
RESUMED
RETAMED
RETAPED
RETAXED
RETILED
RETIMED
RETIRED
RETONED
RETOWED
RETRIED
RETUNED
RETYPED
REUPPED
REURGED
REVELED
REVERED
REVILED
REVISED
REVIVED
REVOKED
REVOTED
REWAKED
REWAXED
REWIPED
REWIRED
REXREED
REYOKED
REZONED
RIDDLED
RIFFLED
RIGHTED
RIMPLED
RIPENED
RIPPLED
RIVALED
RIVETED
ROADBED
ROASTED
ROGERED
ROOSTED
ROOTLED
ROSERED
ROSINED
ROTATED
ROUGHED
ROUNDED
ROUSTED
ROWELED
RUBYRED
RUDDIED
RUFFLED
RUMBAED
RUMBLED
RUMORED
RUMPLED
RUSTLED
SABERED
SADDLED
SADEYED
SAINTED
SALLIED
SALUTED
SAMBAED
SAMOYED
SAMPLED
SAUNAED
SAUTEED
SAVAGED
SAVORED
SAVVIED
SCALDED
SCALPED
SCAMMED
SCAMPED
SCANNED
SCANTED
SCARFED
SCARPED
SCARRED
SCATHED
SCATTED
SCENTED
SCHEMED
SCOFFED
SCOLDED
SCOOPED
SCOOTED
SCORNED
SCOURED
SCOUTED
SCOWLED
SCRAPED
SCREWED
SCRIBED
SCUBAED
SCUDDED
SCUFFED
SCULLED
SCULPED
SCYTHED
SEAWEED
SECEDED
SECURED
SEDATED
SEDUCED
SEEDBED
SEESRED
SEETHED
SEPALED
SETTLED
SEVERED
SHACKED
SHAFTED
SHAGGED
SHAMMED
SHANKED
SHARPED
SHAWLED
SHEAFED
SHEARED
SHEAVED
SHEERED
SHEETED
SHELLED
SHELVED
SHIFTED
SHILLED
SHINNED
SHIPPED
SHIRKED
SHIRRED
SHOALED
SHOCKED
SHOPPED
SHORTED
SHOUTED
SHRINED
SHUCKED
SHUNNED
SHUNTED
SHUSHED
SICKBED
SIGHTED
SINEWED
SINGLED
SIRENED
SIZZLED
SKIDDED
SKIFFED
SKILLED
SKIMMED
SKIMPED
SKINNED
SKIPPED
SKIRLED
SKIRTED
SKULKED
SKULLED
SKUNKED
SLABBED
SLACKED
SLAMMED
SLANTED
SLAPPED
SLASHED
SLATTED
SLEDDED
SLEDGED
SLEEKED
SLEETED
SLEEVED
SLICKED
SLIMMED
SLINKED
SLIPPED
SLITTED
SLOGGED
SLOPPED
SLOSHED
SLOTTED
SLUGGED
SLUICED
SLUMMED
SLUMPED
SLURPED
SLURRED
SLUSHED
SMACKED
SMARTED
SMASHED
SMEARED
SMELLED
SMELTED
SMIRKED
SMITHED
SMUDGED
SMUSHED
SNACKED
SNAFUED
SNAGGED
SNAPPED
SNARFED
SNARLED
SNEAKED
SNEERED
SNEEZED
SNIFFED
SNIPPED
SNOOPED
SNOOTED
SNOOZED
SNORTED
SNOUTED
SNUBBED
SNUFFED
SNUGGED
SOBERED
SOFABED
SOLACED
SOOTHED
SORTIED
SOTWEED
SOUNDED
SOURCED
SPAMMED
SPANKED
SPANNED
SPARKED
SPARRED
SPATTED
SPAWNED
SPEARED
SPECKED
SPEEDED
SPELLED
SPHERED
SPIELED
SPIFFED
SPILLED
SPLAYED
SPLICED
SPOILED
SPONGED
SPOOFED
SPOOKED
SPOOLED
SPOONED

SPORTED
SPOTTED
SPOUTED
SPRAYED
SPRUCED
SPURNED
SPURRED
SPURTED
SQUARED
SQUIRED
SSHAPED
STABBED
STABLED
STACKED
STAFFED
STAGGED
STAINED
STAIRED
STALKED
STALLED
STAMPED
STAPLED
STARRED
STARTED
STARVED
STASHED
STEADED
STEAMED
STEELED
STEEPED
STEERED
STEEVED
STEMMED
STEPPED
STETTED
STIFFED
STIFLED
STILLED
STILTED
STINTED
STIRRED
STOCKED
STODGED
STOMPED
STOOGED
STOOLED
STOOPED
STOPPED
STORIED
STORMED
STRAFED
STRAYED
STREWED
STRIPED
STRIVED
STROKED
STUBBED
STUDDED
STUDIED
STUFFED
STUMPED
STUNNED
STUNTED
STYMIED
SUBDUED
SUCCEED
SUDAFED
SUGARED
SULLIED
SUPPLED
SUTURED
SWABBED
SWAMPED
SWANKED
SWAPPED
SWARMED
SWASHED
SWATHED
SWATTED
SWEATED
SWELLED
SWERVED
SWIGGED
SWILLED
SWIRLED
SWISHED
SWOONED
SWOOPED
SYNCHED
TABOOED
TACKLED
TAINTED
TALCKED
TALLIED
TALONED
TANGLED
TANGOED
TAPERED
TARRIED
TASERED
TATTLED
TAUNTED
TEEHEED
TEETHED
TELEXED
TEMPLED
TEMPTED
TENONED
TENTBED
TENURED
TESTBED
THANKED
THIEVED
THINNED
THORNED
THRIVED
THUDDED
THUMBED
THUMPED
THUNKED
TIARAED
TICKLED
TIEDYED
TINCTED
TINGLED
TINKLED
TIPPLED
TIPTOED
TOADIED
TOASTED
TODDLED
TOGGLED
TOKENED
TOOTHED
TOOTLED
TOPPLED
TOPSEED
TORCHED
TORQUED
TOTALED
TOUCHED
TOUSLED
TOWELED
TOWERED
TOYSLED
TRACKED
TRAILED
TRAINED
TRAMMED
TRAMPED
TRANCED
TRAPPED
TRASHED
TRAWLED
TREADED
TREATED
TREBLED
TREKKED
TRENDED
TRESSED
TRICKED
TRIFLED
TRILLED
TRIMMED
TRIPLED
TRIPPED
TROLLED
TROMPED
TROOPED
TROTHED
TROTTED
TROUPED
TRUCKED
TRUDGED
TRUMPED
TRUSSED
TRUSTED
TRYSTED
TSHAPED
TUMBLED
TURNRED
TURTLED
TUSSLED
TUTORED
TWANGED
TWEAKED
TWEETED
TWEEZED
TWELVED
TWILLED
TWINBED
TWINGED
TWINNED
TWIRLED
TWISTED
TWITTED
TWOTOED
UMBERED
UMPIRED
UNACTED
UNADDED
UNAIDED
UNAIMED
UNAIRED
UNARMED
UNASKED
UNAXLED
UNBAKED
UNBALED
UNBARED
UNBASED
UNBATED
UNBLUED
UNBONED
UNBORED
UNBOWED
UNBOXED
UNCAGED
UNCAKED
UNCANED
UNCAPED
UNCASED
UNCEDED
UNCITED
UNCODED
UNCORED
UNCOWED
UNCRIED
UNCURED
UNDARED
UNDATED
UNDAZED
UNDEWED
UNDIKED
UNDOMED
UNDRIED
UNDUPED
UNEAVED
UNEBBED
UNEDGED
UNENDED
UNFACED
UNFADED
UNFAKED
UNFAMED
UNFATED
UNFAZED
UNFETED
UNFILED
UNFINED
UNFIRED
UNFIXED
UNFOXED
UNFREED
UNFRIED
UNFUSED
UNGATED
UNGLUED
UNGORED
UNGUYED
UNGYVED
UNHATED
UNHAYED
UNHAZED
UNHEWED
UNHIRED
UNHONED
UNHOPED
UNIFIED
UNINKED
UNJADED
UNJOYED
UNKEYED
UNLACED
UNLADED
UNLAVED
UNLAXED
UNLIKED
UNLINED
UNLIVED
UNLOBED
UNLOVED
UNLURED
UNMANED
UNMATED
UNMEWED
UNMIKED
UNMINED
UNMIRED
UNMIXED
UNMOVED
UNMOWED
UNMUTED
UNNAMED
UNNOSED
UNNOTED
UNOGLED
UNOILED
UNOPTED
UNORBED
UNOWNED
UNPACED
UNPAGED
UNPALED
UNPARED
UNPAVED
UNPAWED
UNPILED
UNPIPED
UNPLIED
UNPOLED
UNPOSED
UNRAKED
UNRATED
UNRAYED
UNRAZED
UNRILED
UNRIMED
UNRIVED
UNROBED
UNROPED
UNRULED
UNSATED
UNSAVED
UNSAWED
UNSEWED
UNSHOED
UNSIDED
UNSIZED
UNSOLED
UNSOWED
UNSPIED
UNTAMED
UNTAPED
UNTAXED
UNTILED
UNTIMED
UNTIRED
UNTONED
UNTREED
UNTRIED
UNTUNED
UNTYPED
UNURGED
UNVEXED
UNVOTED
UNVOWED
UNWADED
UNWAGED
UNWAKED
UNWANED
UNWAVED
UNWAXED
UNWIPED
UNWIRED
UNWOOED
UNYOKED
UNZONED
UPDATED
UPDIVED
UPDRIED
UPENDED
UPGAZED
UPPILED
UPRATED
UPSIZED
USHAPED
USHERED
USURPED
UTTERED
VACATED
VALETED
VAPORED
VATDYED
VAULTED
VAUNTED
VERYRED
VIALLED
VIDEOED
VISAGED
VISITED
VISORED
VISTAED
VIZORED
VNECKED
VOLUMED
VOLUTED
VOUCHED
VOYAGED
VROOMED
VSHAPED
WADDLED
WAFERED
WAFFLED
WAGERED
WAGGLED
WAGONED
WAISTED
WAKENED
WALTZED
WAMBLED
WANGLED
WARBLED
WATCHED
WATERED
WATTLED
WAVERED
WEARIED
WEBTOED
WEDELED
WEIGHED
WEIRDED
WELLFED
WELLLED
WETEYED
WHACKED
WHAMMED
WHANGED
WHAPPED
WHARFED
WHEELED
WHEEZED
WHELMED
WHELPED
WHETTED
WHIFFED
WHIPPED
WHIRLED
WHIRRED
WHISHED
WHISKED
WHIZZED
WHOMPED
WHOOPED
WHOPPED
WHORLED
WHUPPED
WIDENED
WIDOWED
WIELDED
WIGGLED
WILFRED
WIMPLED
WINCHED
WINERED
WITCHED
WIZENED
WOBBLED
WOOSHED
WORRIED
WORSTED
WOUNDED
WRACKED
WRAPPED
WREAKED
WRECKED
WRESTED
WRITHED
WRONGED
XEROXED
YACHTED
YEARNED
YEASTED
YIELDED
YODELED
YSHAPED
ZINCKED

EE•••••

EELIEST
EELLIKE
EELPOTS
EELPOUT
EELSKIN
EELWORM
EERIEST

E•E••••

EDEMATA
EGERIAS
EGESTED
EJECTED
EJECTOR
EJEMPLO
EKEDOUT
EKESOUT
ELEANOR
ELEAZAR
ELECTED
ELECTEE
ELECTME
ELECTOR
ELECTRA
ELECTRO
ELEGANT
ELEGIAC
ELEGIES
ELEGIST
ELEGITS
ELEGIZE
ELEISON
ELEKTRA
ELEMENT
ELENIAK
ELEVATE
ELEVENA
ELEVENB
ELEVENC
ELEVEND
ELEVENE
ELEVENS
ELEVONS
EMENDED
EMENDER
EMERALD
EMERGED
EMERGES
EMERIES
EMERITA
EMERITI
EMERSED
EMERSON
EMETICS
ENEMIES
EPEEIST
EPERGNE
EPERNAY
ERECTED
ERECTER
ERECTLY
ERECTOR
ERECTUS
ERELONG
EREMITE
EREWHON
ETERNAL
ETESIAN
EVELONG
EVENBET
EVENERS
EVENEST
EVENING
EVENNOW
EVENOFF
EVENOUT
EVENPAR
EVENSUP
EVERDUR
EVEREST
EVERETT
EVERLYS
EVERTED
EVERTOR
EWELAMB
EWENECK
EWERIES
EXECUTE
EXEDRAE
EXEGETE
EXEMPLA
EXEMPTS
EXENEMY
EXERTED
EXERTER
EXEUNTS
EYEBALL
EYEBANK
EYEBOLT
EYEBROW
EYECARE
EYECUPS
EYEDROP
EYEEXAM
EYEFOLD
EYEFULS
EYEHAND
EYEHOLE
EYEHOOK
EYELASH
EYELESS
EYELETS
EYELIDS
EYELIFT
EYELIKE
EYELINE
EYEMASK
EYEPITS
EYEROLL
EYESHOT
EYESORE
EYESPOT
EYETEST
EYETUCK
EYEWALL
EYEWASH
EYEWEAR
EYEWINK
EZEKIEL

E••E•••

EAGERER
EAGERLY
EASEDBY
EASEDIN
EASEDON
EASEDUP
EASEFUL
EASELED
EASEOFF
EASEOUT
EASESBY
EASESIN
EASESON
EASESUP
EATENAT
EATENUP
ECHELON
ECUELLE
ECZEMAS
EDGEDIN
EDGEOUT
EDGESIN
EDMEESE
EFFECTS
EFFENDI
EGGEDON
EIDETIC
EKUELES
EKWENSI
ELBERTA
ELDERLY
ELIEZER
EMPEROR
ENDEARS
ENDEDAT
ENDEDIN
ENDEDIT
ENDEDON
ENDEDUP
ENDEMIC
ENDERBY
ENNEADS
ENSEALS
ENSEATS
ENTEBBE
ENTENTE
ENTERED
ENTERER
ENTERIC
ENTERIN
ENTERON
ENVEILS
ENVELOP
ENVENOM
EPEEIST
EPHEBUS
EPHEDRA
EPHESUS
EPPERLY
EQUERRY
ERNESTA
ERNESTO
ERTEGUN
ESCENCE
ESSENCE
ESSENES
ESTEBAN
ESTEEMS
ESTEFAN
ESTELLA
ESTELLE
ESTEVEZ
ETHENES
ETHERIC
ETIENNE
EUCERIN
EUDEMON
EUGENIA
EUGENIC
EUGENIE
EUREKAS
EUTERPE
EXCEEDS
EXCELAT
EXCELIN
EXCEPTS
EXCERPT
EXHEDRA
EXPECTS
EXPENDS
EXPENSE
EXPERTS
EXSECTS
EXSERTS
EXTENDS
EXTENSO
EXTENTS
EXTERNE
EXTERNS
EYEEXAM

E•••E••

EAGLETS
EARLESS
EARLETS
EARNERS
EARNEST
EASIEST
EASTEGG
EASTEND
EASTERN
EASTERS
EATHERE
EATLESS
EBAYERS
ECCLESI
ECHOERS
ECOTEUR
EDGIEST
EDMEESE
EELIEST
EERIEST
EGGHEAD
EGGIEST
EGGLERS
EGGLESS
ELANETS
ELATERS
ELEMENT
ELEVENA
ELEVENB
ELEVENC
ELEVEND
ELEVENE
ELEVENS
ELGRECO
ELIDERS
ELITEST
ELMIEST
ELOPERS
ELUDERS
ELYSEES
EMBLEMS
EMINENT
EMOTERS
EMPRESS
ENAMELS
ENDLEAF
ENDLESS
ENFIELD
ENQUEUE
ENTREAT
ENTREES
ENVIERS
EPICENE
EPIDERM
EPOPEES
EPSTEIN
ERASERS
ERIGENA
ERODENT
ERODERS
EROSELY
ESCHEAT
ESCHERS
ESCHEWS
ESCUELA
ESOBESO
ESOTERY
ESPNEWS
ESTEEMS
ESTHETE
ETAGERE
ETCHERS
EUGLENA
EVADERS
EVENERS
EVENEST
EVEREST
EVERETT
EVIDENT
EVILEST
EVILEYE
EVOKERS
EWENECK
EXCEEDS
EXCRETE
EXEGETE
EXENEMY
EXIGENT
EXILERS
EXOCETS
EXPRESS
EXTREME
EXUPERY
EYELESS
EYELETS
EYETEST
EYEWEAR

E••••E•

EAGERER
EARLIER
EARLIES
EARTHED
EARTHEN
EASELED
EATOVER
EBANKED
EBONIES
ECARTES
ECDYSES
ECTYPES
EDASNER
EDIBLES
EDIFIED
EDIFIER
EDIFIES
EDUCTED
EFFACED
EFFACER
EFFACES
EFFUSED
EFFUSES
EGESTED
EGLISES
EIGHTEE
EJECTED
EKUELES
ELAINES
ELANCES
ELAPSED
ELAPSES
ELBOWED
ELBOWER
ELECTED
ELECTEE
ELEGIES
ELIEZER
ELMTREE
ELUATES
ELYSEES
EMAILED
EMAILER
EMANUEL
EMBAYED
EMBOWER
EMBRUED
EMBRUES
EMENDED
EMENDER
EMERGED
EMERGES
EMERIES
EMERSED
EMIGREE
EMIGRES
EMITTED
EMITTER
EMPALED
EMPALES
EMPANEL
EMPIRES
EMPOWER
EMPTIED
EMPTIER
EMPTIES
ENABLED
ENABLER
ENABLES
ENACTED
ENARMED
ENCAGED
ENCAGES
ENCASED
ENCASES
ENCODED
ENCODER
ENCODES
ENCORED
ENCORES
ENDIVES
ENDOWED
ENDOWER
ENDURED

ENDURER
ENDURES
ENDUSER
ENDUSES
ENEMIES
ENFACED
ENFACES
ENGAGED
ENGAGER
ENGAGES
ENGINED
ENGINES
ENISLED
ENISLES
ENJOYED
ENJOYER
ENLACED
ENLACES
ENLIVEN
ENOILED
ENRAGED
ENRAGES
ENROBED
ENROBES
ENSILED
ENSILES
ENSKIED
ENSKIES
ENSURED
ENSURER
ENSURES
ENTERED
ENTERER
ENTICED
ENTICER
ENTICES
ENTIRES
ENTREES
ENTRIES
ENZYMES
EOSINES
EPAULET
EPITHET
EPOPEES
EPOQUES
EPOXIED
EPOXIES
EQUALED
EQUATED
EQUATES
EQUINES
ERECTED
ERECTER
ERINYES
ERITREA
ERMINED
ERMINES
ERUCTED
ERUPTED
ERUPTER
ESCAPED
ESCAPEE
ESCAPER
ESCAPES
ESSAYED
ESSAYER
ESSENES
ESTATED
ESTATES
ESTEVEZ
ETAILED
ETAILER
ETHANES
ETHENES
ETICKET
ETOILES
EUCHRED
EUCHRES
EVACUEE
EVANDER
EVANGEL
EVENBET
EVERTED
EVICTED
EVICTEE
EVILLER
EVINCED
EVINCES
EVOLVED
EVOLVER
EVOLVES
EVULSED
EVULSES
EWERIES
EXACTED
EXACTER
EXALTED
EXALTER
EXCIDED
EXCIDES
EXCISED
EXCISES
EXCITED
EXCITER
EXCITES
EXCUSED
EXCUSER
EXCUSES
EXCUSEZ
EXERTED
EXERTER
EXHALED
EXHALES
EXHUMED
EXHUMER
EXHUMES
EXISTED
EXITFEE
EXMATES
EXOILER
EXPIRED
EXPIRES
EXPOSED
EXPOSER
EXPOSES
EXULTED
EXWIVES
EZEKIEL

E•••••E

EARACHE
EARBONE
EARHOLE
EARLIKE
EARLOBE
EASYONE
EATABLE
EATCAKE
EATHERE
EATLATE
EATMORE
EBBTIDE
EBONITE
EBONIZE
EBWHITE
ECHAPPE
ECLIPSE
ECLOGUE
ECOCIDE
ECOTAGE
ECOTYPE
ECUELLE
EDIFICE
EDMEESE
EDOMITE
EDUCATE
EELLIKE
EFFABLE
EGALITE
EGGCASE
EGGLIKE
EGOISTE
EIGHTEE
ELAMITE
ELECTEE
ELECTME
ELEGIZE
ELEVATE
ELEVENE
ELFLIKE
ELFUDGE
ELIYALE
ELLAMAE
ELLIPSE
ELMONTE
ELMTREE
ELNORTE
ELOCUTE
ELUSIVE
EMANATE
EMBLAZE
EMBOITE
EMBRACE
EMIGREE
EMIRATE
EMOTIVE
EMPLACE
EMPLANE
EMPRISE
EMULATE
ENCARRE
ENCHASE
ENCLAVE
ENCLOSE
ENDABLE
ENDGAME
ENDLATE
ENDLINE
ENDNOTE
ENDORSE
ENDWISE
ENDZONE
ENFLAME
ENFORCE
ENFRAME
ENGARDE
ENGORGE
ENGRAVE
ENHANCE
ENLARGE
ENMASSE
ENNOBLE
ENOUNCE
ENPLANE
ENPRISE
ENQUEUE
ENQUIRE
ENRIQUE
ENROUTE
ENSLAVE
ENSNARE
ENSUITE
ENTEBBE
ENTENTE
ENTHUSE
ENTITLE
ENTWINE
ENVOGUE
EONLINE
EPERGNE
EPICENE
EPICURE
EPIDOTE
EPIGONE
EPILATE
EPISODE
EPISTLE
EPITOME
EPONINE
EQUABLE
ERASURE
EREMITE
EROSIVE
ERRABLE
ERSKINE
ERUDITE
ESCAPEE
ESCENCE
ESPOUSE
ESQUIRE
ESSENCE
ESTELLE
ESTHETE
ETAGERE
ETAMINE
ETIENNE
EUGENIE
EUSTACE
EUTERPE
EVACUEE
EVASIVE
EVICTEE
EVILEYE
EVILONE
EVOLUTE
EXABYTE
EXAMINE
EXAMPLE
EXCLAVE
EXCLUDE
EXCRETE
EXCURSE
EXECUTE
EXEDRAE
EXEGETE
EXITFEE
EXPANSE
EXPARTE
EXPENSE
EXPIATE
EXPLODE
EXPLORE
EXPUNGE
EXTERNE
EXTREME
EXTRUDE
EXUDATE
EYECARE
EYEHOLE
EYELIKE
EYELINE
EYESORE

•EE••••

BEEBEES
BEECHAM
BEECHEN
BEECHER
BEECHES
BEEFALO
BEEFIER
BEEFILY
BEEFING
BEEFSUP
BEEFTEA
BEEGEES
BEEHIVE
BEELIKE
BEELINE
BEEMERS
BEEPERS
BEEPING
BEEPSAT
BEERCAN
BEERIER
BEERKEG
BEERMUG
BEERTAP
BEESWAX
BEETIER
BEETLES
BEETRED
BEETREE
BEEYARD
BEEZERS
DEEDBOX
DEEDING
DEEJAYS
DEEMING
DEEPEND
DEEPENS
DEEPEST
DEEPFAT
DEEPFRY
DEEPISH
DEEPRED
DEEPSEA
DEEPSET
DEEPSIX
DEEPSKY
DEEPTAN
DEERFLY
FEEBATE
FEEBLER
FEEDBAG
FEEDBIN
FEEDERS
FEEDING
FEEDLOT
FEEDSIN
FEEDSON
FEEDSTO
FEEFREE
FEELBAD
FEELERS
FEELESS
FEELFOR
FEELILL
FEELING
FEELOFF
FEELOUT
FEELSOK
GEEGAWS
GEEKDOM
GEEKIER
GEEWHIZ
GEEZERS
HEEDERS
HEEDFUL
HEEDING
HEEHAWS
HEELERS
HEELING
HEELPAD
HEELTAP
JEEBIES
JEEPERS
JEERERS
JEERING
JEERSAT
KEEBLER
KEELING
KEENENH
KEENERS
KEENEST
KEENING
KEEPERS
KEEPFIT
KEEPING
KEEPMUM
KEEPOFF
KEEPOUT
KEEPSAT
KEEPSIN
KEEPSON
KEEPSTO
KEEPSUP
KEESHAN
KEESLAR
KEESLER
LEECHED
LEECHEE
LEECHES
LEEFORD
LEERERS
LEERIER
LEERILY
LEERING
LEERSAT
LEETIDE
LEEWARD
LEEWAYS
MEEKEST
MEEMIES
MEERKAT
MEETERS
MEETING
MEETSUP
NEEDERS
NEEDFUL
NEEDHAM
NEEDIER
NEEDILY
NEEDING
NEEDLED
NEEDLER
NEEDLES
NEEDNOT
NEEDSTO
PEEBLES
PEEKERS
PEEKING
PEEKOUT
PEEKSAT
PEEKSIN
PEELERS
PEELING
PEELOFF
PEELOUT
PEENING
PEEPERS
PEEPING
PEEPLES
PEEPOUT
PEEPSAT
PEERAGE
PEERESS
PEERING
PEEROUT
PEERSAT
PEERSIN
PEEVING
PEEVISH
PEEWEES
REEARNS
REEBOKS
REEDIER
REEDING
REEDITS
REEDMAN
REEDMEN
REEFERS
REEFIER
REEFING
REEJECT
REEKERS
REEKIER
REEKING
REEKSOF
REELECT
REELERS
REELING
REELOFF
REELOUT
REELSIN
REELSUP
REEMITS
REENACT
REENDOW
REENJOY
REENTER
REENTRY
REEQUIP
REERECT
REERUPT
REEVICT
REEVING
REEVOKE
REEXPEL
SEEABLE
SEEALSO
SEEDBED
SEEDERS
SEEDIER
SEEDILY
SEEDING
SEEDLET
SEEDPOD
SEEHERE
SEEINTO
SEEKERS
SEEKING
SEEKOUT
SEEMING
SEEMSTO
SEENALL
SEENFIT
SEENOFF
SEENOUT
SEEPAGE
SEEPAST
SEEPIER
SEEPING
SEEPOUT
SEEPSIN
SEERESS
SEESALL
SEESAWS
SEESFIT
SEESOFF
SEESOUT
SEESRED
SEETHED
SEETHES
SEETHRU
SEETOIT
TEEDOFF
TEEHEED
TEEHEES
TEEITUP
TEEMING
TEENAGE
TEENERS
TEENIER
TEENSIE
TEEOFFS
TEEPEES
TEESHOT
TEESOFF
TEETERS
TEETHED
TEETHER
TEETHES
TEETIME
TEEVEES
VEEJAYS
VEENECK
VEERIES
VEERING
VEEROFF
WEEBITS
WEEDERS
WEEDIER
WEEDILY
WEEDING
WEEDOUT
WEEFOLK
WEEHOUR
WEEKDAY
WEEKEND
WEENESS
WEENIES
WEEONES
WEEPERS
WEEPFOR
WEEPIER
WEEPING
WEEVILS
ZEELAND

•E•E•••

BEDECKS
BEDELIA
BEDEVIL
BEDEWED
BEHEADS
BEHEARD
BEHESTS
BEJEWEL
BELEVEN
BENEATH
BENEFIC
BENEFIT
BENELUX
BEREAVE
BERENDT
BERETTA
BESEECH
BEVELED
BEVELER
BEVERLY
CELEBES
CELEBRE
CELESTA
CELESTE
CEMENTS
CEREALS
CEREBRA
CEREBRO
CETERIS
DEBEARD
DEBEERS
DECEASE
DECEITS
DECEIVE
DECENCY
DEFEATS
DEFECTS
DEFENCE
DEFENDS
DEFENSE
DEFERTO
DEGERMS
DEHEXED
DEHEXES
DEJECTS
DEKEING
DELEADS
DELEDDA
DELEING
DELETED
DELETES
DEMEANS
DEMENTO
DEMERGE
DEMERIT
DEMEROL
DEMESNE
DEMETER
DENEUVE
DEPECHE
DEPENDS
DEPESTS
DERECHO
DESEEDS
DESERET
DESERTS
DESERVE
DESEXED
DESEXES
DETECTO
DETECTS
DETENTE
DETENTS
DETERGE
DETESTS
DEVEINS
DEVELOP
DEVESTS
FEDERAL
FEDERKO
FEDEXED
FEDEXES
FENELON
FENETRE
FEVERED
GEHENNA
GEMELLI
GENERAL
GENERIC
GENERIS
GENESEE
GENESES
GENESET
GENESIS
GENETIC
GENEVAN
GERENTS
GETEVEN
HEREDIA
HEREIAM
HERENOW
HERESTO
HERETIC
HEWEDTO
JEWELED
JEWELER
JEWELRY
JEZEBEL
KEYEDIN
KEYEDON
KEYEDUP
LEDERER
LEGENDS
LEJEUNE
LETEMIN
LEVELED
LEVELER
LEVELLY
LEVERED
LEVERET
MEDELES
MEDEVAC
MEMENTO
MESEEMS
METEORS
METEOUT
METERED
NEMEROV
NEMESES
NEMESIS
NEREIDS
PEKEPOO
PERETTI
PESETAS
PESEWAS
PETEMAN
PETEMEN
PETERED
PETERII
REBECCA
REBEGAN
REBEGIN
REBEGUN
REBEKAH
REBENDS
RECEDED
RECEDES
RECEIPT
RECEIVE
RECENCY
REDEALS
REDEALT
REDEBIT
REDECAY
REDEEDS
REDEEMS
REDEYED
REDEYES
REFEEDS
REFENCE
REFEREE
REFERTO
REGEARS
REGENCY
REGENTS
REHEALS
REHEARD
REHEARS
REHEATS
REHEELS
REJECTS
REKEYED
RELEADS
RELEAPS
RELEARN
RELEASE
RELENDS
RELENTS
RELEVEL
RELEVER
RELEVES
REMEETS
REMELTS
REMENDS
REMERGE
RENEGED
RENEGER
RENEGES
RENESTS
RENEWAL
RENEWED
RENEWER
REPEALS
REPEATS
REPENTS
REPERKS
REREADS
REREDOS
REREELS
RERENTS
RESEALS
RESEAMS
RESEATS
RESEAUS
RESEAUX
RESECTS
RESEEDS
RESEEKS
RESEIZE
RESELLS
RESENDS
RESENTS
RESERVE
RESEWED
RETEACH
RETEARS
RETELLS
RETESTS
REVEALS
REVELED
REVELER
REVELIN
REVELRY
REVENDS
REVENGE
REVENUE
REVERBS
REVERDY
REVERED
REVERER
REVERES
REVERIE
REVERSA
REVERSE
REVERTS
REVESTS
REWEARS
REWEAVE
REWEIGH
REWELDS
REZEROS
SEAEELS
SECEDED
SECEDER
SECEDES
SEFERIS
SELECTS
SELENIC
SENECAN
SENECAS
SENEGAL
SENESCE
SERENER
SETENTA
SEVENAD
SEVENAM
SEVENBC
SEVENEE
SEVENNO
SEVENPM
SEVENTH
SEVENTY
SEVENUP
SEVERAL
SEVERED
SEVERER
SEVERUS
SEWEDON
SEWEDUP
TEDEUMS
TEHERAN
TELECOM
TELEFAX
TELEPIC
TELEPIX
TELERAN
TELESTO
TELEXED
TELEXES
TENEEEE
TERENCE
VEDETTE
VEGETAL
VENEERS
VENEMAN
VENEZIA
VEREINE
VETERAN
VEXEDLY
WEDELED
WEDELNS
WEGENER
WETEYED
YEMENIS
YEREVAN

•E••E••

AERIEST
BEADERS
BEAHERO
BEAKERS
BEAMERS
BEANERY
BEARERS
BEATERS
BEAVERS
BECKETT
BEDLESS
BEDREST
BEEBEES
BEEGEES
BEEMERS
BEEPERS

BEEZERS
BEHRENS
BELIEFS
BELIERS
BELIEVE
BELLEAU
BELLEEK
BELTERS
BENDERS
BENNETT
BENZELL
BENZENE
BEQUEST
BERBERS
BERGERE
BERNESE
BERSERK
BESEECH
BESIEGE
BESMEAR
BESPEAK
BESSELL
BETHELS
BETHERE
BETTERS
BETWEEN
BEZIERS
CELAENO
CENSERS
CENTERS
CEPHEUS
CERVEZA
DEADEND
DEADENS
DEADEST
DEADEYE
DEAFENS
DEAFEST
DEALERS
DEANERY
DEAREST
DEBEERS
DEBRETT
DEBTEES
DECKERS
DECREED
DECREER
DECREES
DEEPEND
DEEPENS
DEEPEST
DEFFEST
DEFIERS
DEFLEAS
DEFLECT
DEFTEST
DEFUELS
DEGREED
DEGREES
DEHMELT
DEICERS
DEKLERK
DELBERT
DELKEYS
DELVERS
DENIECE
DENIERS
DENNEHY
DENSELY
DENSEST
DEPLETE
DEPRESS
DEQUEUE
DERWENT
DESCEND
DESCENT
DESEEDS
DESHELL
DESSERT
DESTEMS
DEUTERO
DEWIEST
DEWLESS
EELIEST
EERIEST
FEARERS
FEBRERO
FEDDERS
FEEDERS
FEELERS
FEELESS
FELLERS
FENCEIN
FENCERS
FENCEUP
FENDERS
FENNELS
FERMENT
FERNERY
FERRETS
FERRETY
FERVENT
FESTERS
FETTERS
FEWNESS
FEYDEAU
FEYNESS
GEEZERS
GELPENS
GEMLESS
GENDERS
GENOESE
GENTEEL
GENXERS
GEODESY
GETBEAT
GETBENT
GETHELP
GETREAL
GETTERS
GETWELL
GEYSERS
HEADEND
HEADERS
HEALERS
HEAPERS
HEARERS
HEATERS
HEAVEHO
HEAVENS
HEAVERS
HEAVETO
HEBREWS
HEDGERS
HEEDERS
HEELERS
HEFTERS
HEHHEHS
HEIFERS
HEIFETZ
HEIRESS
HELLENE
HELLENO
HELMETS
HELPERS
HEMMERS
HENDECA
HENNERY
HENPECK
HENREID
HEPPEST
HERBERT
HERDERS
HERPETO
HERSELF
HEWLETT
JEEPERS
JEERERS
JEFFERS
JENNETS
JERGENS
JERKERS
JERSEYS
JESTERS
JETSETS
KEDGERS
KEENENH
KEENERS
KEENEST
KEEPERS
KEGGERS
KEGLERS
KENNEDY
KENNELS
KENNETH
KERNELS
KERTESZ
KEYDETS
KEYLESS
KEYWEST
LEADENS
LEADERS
LEADETH
LEAKERS
LEAKEYS
LEANERS
LEANEST
LEAPERS
LEASERS
LEASETO
LEAVEBE
LEAVEIN
LEAVEIT
LEAVENS
LEAVEON
LECHERS
LECTERN
LEDGERS
LEERERS
LEFREAK
LEFTEAR
LEFTEND
LEFTEST
LEFTEYE
LEGLESS
LEGREST
LEGWEAR
LEMIEUX
LENDERS
LENIENT
LEOGENN
LESSEES
LESSENS
LESSEPS
LETHEAN
LETMEBE
LETMEGO
LETMEIN
LETSEAT
LETTERA
LETTERB
LETTERC
LETTERD
LETTERE
LETTERF
LETTERG
LETTERH
LETTERI
LETTERJ
LETTERK
LETTERL
LETTERM
LETTERN
LETTERO
LETTERP
LETTERQ
LETTERR
LETTERS
LETTERT
LETTERU
LETTERV
LETTERW
LETTERX
LETTERY
LETTERZ
LEVIERS
LEWDEST
MEANEST
MEDLEYS
MEEKEST
MEETERS
MEGAERA
MEGAERG
MELDERS
MELTERS
MEMBERS
MENDELS
MENDERS
MENTEES
MEOWERS
MERCERS
MERCERY
MERGEES
MERGERS
MESEEMS
METIERS
MEWLERS
MEYNELL
NEAREST
NEATENS
NEATEST
NECKERS
NEEDERS
NEGLECT
NEOCENE
NEOGENE
NEPHEWS
NESTEGG
NESTERS
NETLESS
NETTERS
NETZERO
NEUTERS
NEWBERN
NEWBERY
NEWDEAL
NEWLEAF
NEWLEFT
NEWNESS
NEWWEEK
NEWYEAR
PEABEAN
PEAHENS
PEEKERS
PEELERS
PEEPERS
PEERESS
PEEWEES
PEGLEGS
PEGLESS
PELLEAS
PELLETS
PELTERS
PENDENT
PENNERS
PENNEYS
PENSEES
PENTELS
PEPPERS
PEPPERY
PERCENT
PERCEPT
PERFECT
PERREAU
PERSEID
PERSEUS
PERTEST
PERWEEK
PERYEAR
PESTERS
PETBEAR
PETDEER
PETRELS
PETTERS
PEUGEOT
PEWTERS
READERS
REAGENT
REALEST
REAMEND
REAMERS
REAPERS
REAREND
REARERS
REAVERS
REBREAK
REBREED
REBREWS
RECHECK
RECHEWS
RECLEAN
REDCELL
REDCENT
REDDEER
REDDENS
REDDEST
REDEEDS
REDEEMS
REDFERN
REDHEAD
REDHEAT
REDHENS
REDLEGS
REDMEAT
REDNECK
REDNESS
REDREAM
REDRESS
REEFERS
REEJECT
REEKERS
REELECT
REELERS
REERECT
REFEEDS
REFLECT
REFRESH
REFUELS
REGREET
REGRESS
REGRETS
REHEELS
REKNEAD
RELIEFS
RELIERS
RELIEVE
RELLENO
REMEETS
RENDELL
RENDERS
RENNETS
RENTEES
RENTERS
REOPENS
REPLEAD
REPLETE
REPRESS
REQUEST
REREELS
RESEEDS
RESEEKS
RESMELT
RESPEAK
RESPECT
RESPELL
RESPELT
RESTERS
RESWEAR
RESWEEP
RETREAD
RETREAT
REUBENS
REUNERS
REUSERS
REUTERS
REVIEWS
REXREED
SEABEDS
SEABEES
SEAEELS
SEAFERN
SEAHERO
SEALEGS
SEALERS
SEALERY
SEAMERS
SEARERS
SEATERS
SEAWEED
SECKELS
SECRECY
SECRETE
SECRETS
SEEDERS
SEEHERE
SEEKERS
SEERESS
SEGMENT
SEINERS
SEIZEON
SEIZERS
SELLECK
SELLERS
SENDEES
SENDERS
SENNETT
SENSEIS
SENSENS
SEPTETS
SEQUELS
SERIESE
SERIESF
SERIESG
SERIESH
SERIESI
SERIESJ
SERIESK
SERPENS
SERPENT
SERVEAS
SERVERS
SERVEUP
SESTETS
SETFEES
SETTEES
SETTERS
SEXIEST
SEXLESS
SEXTETS
TEALEAF
TEALESS
TEANECK
TEARERS
TEASELS
TEASERS
TEASETS
TEASEUP
TEEHEED
TEEHEES
TEENERS
TEEPEES
TEETERS
TEEVEES
TELLERS
TEMPEAZ
TEMPEHS
TEMPERA
TEMPERS
TEMPEST
TENCENT
TENDERS
TENEEEE
TENFEET
TENNECO
TENNERS
TENSELY
TENSEST
TENSEUP
TENTERS
TENWEEK
TENYEAR
TERCELS
TERRELL
TERRENE
TERRETS
TERSELY
TERSEST
TESSERA
TESTEES
TESTERS
TETHERS
VEENECK
VEILERS
VELVETS
VELVETY
VENDEES
VENDERS
VENEERS
VENTERS
VERBENA
VERDELL
VERGEON
VERGERS
VERIEST
VERMEER
VERMEIL
VERSETS
VESPERS
VESSELS
VESTEES
VETOERS
VETTERS
WEAKENS
WEAKEST
WEANERS
WEARERS
WEASELS
WEAVERS
WEBFEET
WEBLESS
WEDDELL
WEDDERS
WEDGEIN
WEEDERS
WEEKEND
WEENESS
WEEPERS
WELDERS
WELTERS
WENDELL
WENDERS
WESTEGG
WESTEND
WESTERN
WESTERS
WETCELL
WETNESS
WETTEST
XERXESI
YEAREND
YEATEAM
YELLERS
YELPERS
YESDEAR
YESLETS
YEVGENY
ZESTERS

•E•••E•

AEDILES
AEGISES
AERATED
AERATES
AEROBES
BEACHED
BEACHES
BEADIER
BEADLES
BEAGLES
BEAMIER
BEANIES
BEARDED
BEASLEY
BEATLES
BECOMES
BEDAZED
BEDAZES
BEDEWED
BEDIZEN
BEDLOES
BEEBEES
BEECHEN
BEECHER
BEECHES
BEEFIER
BEEFTEA
BEEGEES
BEERIER
BEERKEG
BEETIER
BEETLES
BEETRED
BEETREE
BEHAVED
BEHAVES
BEIGNES
BEIGNET
BEJEWEL
BELATED
BELAYED
BELAYER
BELCHED
BELCHER
BELCHES
BELEVEN
BELLEEK
BELLIED
BELLIES
BELLMEN
BELOVED
BEMIRED
BEMIRES
BEMUSED
BEMUSES
BENARES
BENCHED
BENCHER
BENCHES
BENDIER
BENOTED
BENOTES
BENTLEY
BENTSEN
BEQUIET
BERATED
BERATER
BERATES
BERKLEY
BERKNER
BERNSEN
BERRIED
BERRIES
BERTHED
BESIDES
BESTBET
BESTMEN
BESTREW
BETAKEN
BETAKES
BETIDED
BETIDES
BETIMES
BETOKEN
BETTGER
BETWEEN
BEURRES
BEVELED
BEVELER
BEWARED
BEWARES
CEDARED
CELEBES
CELOTEX
CENTRED
CENTRES
CERATED
CERATES
CERISES
CERUMEN
CETANES
DEADSEA
DEADSET
DEAIRED
DEARDEN
DEARIES
DEBAKEY
DEBASED
DEBASER
DEBASES
DEBATED
DEBATER
DEBATES
DEBITED
DEBONED
DEBONES
DEBRIEF
DEBTEES
DEBUSES
DEBUTED
DECADES
DECAYED
DECAYER
DECIBEL
DECIDED
DECIDER
DECIDES
DECILES
DECKLED
DECKLES
DECODED
DECODER
DECODES
DECOYED
DECOYER
DECREED
DECREER
DECREES
DECRIED
DECRIER
DECRIES
DEDUCED
DEDUCER
DEDUCES
DEEPRED
DEEPSEA
DEEPSET
DEFACED
DEFACER
DEFACES
DEFAMED
DEFAMER
DEFAMES
DEFILED
DEFILER
DEFILES
DEFINED
DEFINER
DEFINES
DEFUSED
DEFUSER
DEFUSES
DEGREED
DEGREES
DEHAVEN
DEHEXED
DEHEXES
DEHIRED
DEHIRES
DEIFIED
DEIFIER
DEIFIES
DEIGNED
DEITIES
DELANEY
DELAYED
DELAYER
DELETED
DELETES
DELIBES
DELIMEN
DELIVER
DELUDED
DELUDER
DELUDES
DELUGED
DELUGES
DEMARET
DEMETER
DEMISED
DEMISES
DEMOTED
DEMOTES
DEMPSEY
DEMURER
DENIMED
DENIZEN
DENOTED
DENOTES
DENUDED
DENUDER
DENUDES
DEPONED
DEPONER
DEPONES
DEPOSED
DEPOSER
DEPOSES
DEPOWER
DEPUTED
DEPUTES
DERATED
DERATES
DERBIES
DERIDED
DERIDER
DERIDES
DERIVED
DERIVER
DERIVES
DERNIER
DESERET
DESEXED
DESEXES
DESIRED
DESIREE
DESIRER
DESIRES
DESKSET
DESTAEL
DETOXED
DETOXES
DETUNED
DETUNES
DEVICES
DEVILED
DEVISED
DEVISEE
DEVISER
DEVISES
DEVORES
DEVOTED
DEVOTEE
DEVOTES
DEVRIES
DEWATER
DEWAXED
DEWAXES
DEWIRED
DEWIRES
FEASTED
FEASTER
FEATHER
FECHNER
FEDEXED
FEDEXES
FEEBLER
FEEFREE
FEIFFER
FEIGNED
FEIGNER
FEINTED
FELINES
FELTPEN
FEMALES
FENNIER
FEOFFED
FERNIER
FERRIED
FERRIES
FERULES
FESCUES
FETCHED
FETCHER
FETCHES
FETTLES
FETUSES
FEVERED
FEVRIER
GECKOES
GEEKIER
GELATED
GELATES
GEMAYEL
GEMMIER
GENESEE
GENESES
GENESET
GENOMES
GENTEEL
GENTLED
GENTLER
GENTLES
GENUSES
GEORGEC
GEORGEI
GEORGEM
GEORGES
GEORGEV
GEORGEW
GERMIER
GESSOED
GESSOES
GETEVEN
GETFREE
GETOVER
GETSHEP
GETSSET
GETSWET
HEADIER
HEADMEN
HEADSET
HEARKEN
HEARSES
HEARTED
HEARTEN
HEATHEN
HEATHER
HEATTER
HEAVIER
HEAVIES
HECKLED
HECKLER
HECKLES
HECKYES

HEDGIER
HEFTIER
HEISTED
HELICES
HELIXES
HELLOED
HELLOES
HELLYES
HEMPIER
HEMSLEY
HENNAED
HENRIES
HENSLEY
HERBIER
HERBTEA
HERSHEY
HEXANES
HEXOSES
JEEBIES
JEFFREY
JELLIED
JELLIES
JERKIER
JERKIES
JETTIED
JETTIES
JEWELED
JEWELER
JEZEBEL
KEARNEY
KEEBLER
KEESLER
KEISTER
KELPIES
KENDREW
KESTREL
KETCHES
KETONES
KETTLES
KEWPIES
LEACHED
LEACHER
LEACHES
LEADIER
LEADMEN
LEAFIER
LEAFLET
LEAGUED
LEAGUER
LEAGUES
LEAKIER
LEANDER
LEARJET
LEARNED
LEARNER
LEASHED
LEASHES
LEATHER
LEDERER
LEDGIER
LEECHED
LEECHEE
LEECHES
LEERIER
LEFTIES
LEFTLEG
LEGATEE
LEGATES

LEGGIER
LEGOSET
LEGUMES
LEISTER
LENSMEN
LESSEES
LETSSEE
LETTRES
LEVADES
LEVELED
LEVELER
LEVERED
LEVERET
LEVITES
LEXISES
LEXUSES
MEAGLES
MEALIER
MEALIES
MEANDER
MEANIES
MEASLES
MEATIER
MEATMEN
MEDALED
MEDDLED
MEDDLER
MEDDLES
MEDELES
MEEMIES
MEGANES
MEIOSES
MEISSEN
MEISTER
MEITNER
MELAMED
MEMOREX
MENACED
MENACER
MENACES
MENAGES
MENCKEN
MENTEES
MENZIES
MERCHES
MERCIES
MERGEES
MERIDEN
MERIMEE
MERITED
MERRIER
MESHIER
MESSIER
METALED
METATES
METERED
METOOER
METTLER
METTLES
NECKLET
NEEDIER
NEEDLED
NEEDLER
NEEDLES
NEGATED
NEGATER
NEGATES
NEGUSES

NEIGHED
NEITHER
NEMESES
NERDIER
NERVIER
NESTLED
NESTLER
NESTLES
NETIZEN
NETSTER
NETTLED
NETTLES
NEWAGER
NEWAGEY
NEWBIES
NEWIDEA
NEWSIER
NEWSIES
NEWSMEN
NEWSPEG
NEWWEEK
NEXUSES
OERSTED
OEUVRES
PEACHED
PEACHES
PEAKIER
PEARLED
PEARLER
PEATIER
PEBBLED
PEBBLES
PEDALED
PEDALER
PEDDLED
PEDDLER
PEDDLES
PEEBLES
PEEPLES
PEEWEES
PELAGES
PENATES
PENNIES
PENSEES
PEONIES
PEOPLED
PEOPLES
PEPPIER
PERCHED
PERCHER
PERCHES
PERDIEM
PERIGEE
PERILED
PERKIER
PERPLEX
PERRIER
PERUKES
PERUSED
PERUSER
PERUSES
PERWEEK
PESADES
PESKIER
PESTLED
PESTLES
PETALED
PETALES

PETCHEW
PETDEER
PETEMEN
PETERED
PETITES
PETTIER
PEYOTES
REACHED
REACHER
REACHES
REACTED
READDED
READIED
READIER
READIES
REAIMED
REAIRED
REALMEN
REALTER
REANNEX
REARMED
REASKED
REBAKED
REBAKES
REBALED
REBALES
REBATED
REBATER
REBATES
REBORED
REBORES
REBOTES
REBOXED
REBOXES
REBREED
REBUKED
REBUKER
REBUKES
REBUSES
RECAGED
RECAGES
RECANED
RECANES
RECASED
RECASES
RECEDED
RECEDES
RECIPES
RECITED
RECITER
RECITES
RECODED
RECODES
RECOVER
RECURED
RECURES
RECUSED
RECUSES
REDARED
REDARES
REDATED
REDATES
REDDEER
REDDYES
REDEYED
REDEYES
REDOSED
REDOSES

REDOXES
REDRIED
REDRIES
REDTIES
REDUCED
REDUCER
REDUCES
REEDIER
REEDMEN
REEFIER
REEKIER
REENTER
REEXPEL
REFACED
REFACES
REFAXED
REFAXES
REFEREE
REFILED
REFILES
REFINED
REFINER
REFINES
REFIRED
REFIRES
REFIXED
REFIXES
REFLIES
REFRIED
REFRIES
REFUGED
REFUGEE
REFUGES
REFUSED
REFUSER
REFUSES
REFUTED
REFUTER
REFUTES
REGALED
REGALER
REGALES
REGIMEN
REGIMES
REGIVEN
REGIVES
REGLUED
REGLUES
REGNIER
REGREET
REHIDES
REHIRED
REHIRES
REHONED
REHONES
REIFIED
REIFIES
REIGNED
REINDEX
REINKED
REKEYED
RELABEL
RELACED
RELACES
RELANES
RELATED
RELATER
RELATES

RELAXED
RELAXER
RELAXES
RELAYED
RELAYER
RELEVEL
RELEVER
RELEVES
RELINED
RELINES
RELIVED
RELIVES
RELOSES
RELUMED
RELUMES
REMAKES
REMATED
REMATES
REMINED
REMINES
REMISED
REMISES
REMIXED
REMIXES
REMODEL
REMOTER
REMOTES
REMOVED
REMOVER
REMOVES
REMOWED
RENAMED
RENAMES
RENEGED
RENEGER
RENEGES
RENEWED
RENEWER
RENFREW
RENOTED
RENOTES
RENTEES
RENTIER
REOFFER
REOILED
REORDER
REOWNED
REPAGED
REPAGES
REPANEL
REPAPER
REPAVED
REPAVES
REPINED
REPINER
REPINES
REPLIED
REPLIER
REPLIES
REPOSED
REPOSER
REPOSES
REPOWER
REPUTED
REPUTES
REQUIEM
RERAKED
RERAKES

RERATED
RERATES
RERIDES
RERISEN
RERISES
RESALES
RESAVED
RESAVES
RESAWED
RESCUED
RESCUER
RESCUES
RESEWED
RESHOES
RESIDED
RESIDER
RESIDES
RESILED
RESILES
RESINED
RESITED
RESIZED
RESIZER
RESIZES
RESOJET
RESOLED
RESOLER
RESOLES
RESOWED
RESTREW
RESUMED
RESUMES
RESWEEP
RETAKEN
RETAKER
RETAKES
RETAMED
RETAMES
RETAPED
RETAPES
RETAXED
RETAXES
RETILED
RETILES
RETIMED
RETIMES
RETIRED
RETIREE
RETIRES
RETONED
RETONES
RETOWED
RETRIED
RETRIES
RETUNED
RETUNES
RETYPED
RETYPES
REUPPED
REURGED
REURGES
REUTHER
REUTTER
REVELED
REVELER
REVERED
REVERER
REVERES

REVILED
REVILER
REVILES
REVISED
REVISER
REVISES
REVIVED
REVIVER
REVIVES
REVOKED
REVOKER
REVOKES
REVOTED
REVOTES
REWAGER
REWAKED
REWAKEN
REWAKES
REWATER
REWAXED
REWAXES
REWIDEN
REWIPED
REWIPES
REWIRED
REWIRES
REWOKEN
REWOVEN
REXREED
REYOKED
REYOKES
REZONED
REZONES
SEABEES
SEAGREN
SEAMIER
SEANCES
SEAWEED
SECEDED
SECEDER
SECEDES
SECURED
SECURER
SECURES
SEDATED
SEDATER
SEDATES
SEDGIER
SEDUCED
SEDUCER
SEDUCES
SEEDBED
SEEDIER
SEEDLET
SEEPIER
SEESRED
SEETHED
SEETHES
SELTZER
SEMITES
SENATES
SENDEES
SENORES
SEPALED
SERAPES
SERENER
SESAMES
SETFEES

SETFREE
SETTEES
SETTLED
SETTLER
SETTLES
SEVENEE
SEVERED
SEVERER
TEACHER
TEACHES
TEARIER
TEATREE
TECHIES
TEDDIES
TEEHEED
TEEHEES
TEENIER
TEEPEES
TEETHED
TEETHER
TEETHES
TEEVEES
TEICHER
TEKKIES
TELEXED
TELEXES
TELLIES
TEMPLED
TEMPLES
TEMPTED
TEMPTER
TENACES
TENCHES
TENEEEE
TENFEET
TENNIEL
TENNIES
TENONED
TENONER
TENTBED
TENTPEG
TENURED
TENURES
TENWEEK
TERRIER
TERRIES
TESTBED
TESTEES
TESTIER
VEALIER
VECHTEN
VEERIES
VEGGIES
VEINIER
VEINLET
VEINTES
VELOXES
VELURES
VENDEES
VENDUES
VENULES
VENUSES
VERMEER
VERNIER
VERYFEW
VERYNEW
VERYRED
VERYWET

VESTEES
VETCHES
WEARIED
WEARIER
WEARIES
WEATHER
WEBBIER
WEBFEET
WEBSTER
WEBTOED
WEDELED
WEDGIER
WEDGIES
WEEDIER
WEENIES
WEEONES
WEEPIER
WEGENER
WEIGHED
WEIGHER
WEIRDED
WEIRDER
WELLFED
WELLLED
WELLSEE
WELLSET
WELLYES
WEMBLEY
WENCHES
WERNHER
WERTHER
WESTIES
WETEYED
WETONES
XEROSES
XEROXED
XEROXES
YEARNED
YEARNER
YEASTED
YESISEE
YETTIES
YEWTREE
ZESTIER

•E••••E

BEASTIE
BEATSME
BEATTIE
BEBRAVE
BECAUSE
BEDLIKE
BEDMATE
BEDRAPE
BEDSIDE
BEDTIME
BEEHIVE
BEELIKE
BEELINE
BEETREE
BEGRIME
BEGUILE
BEGUINE
BEHOOVE
BELDAME
BELIEVE
BELTANE
BENBLUE

BENZENE
BEREAVE
BERGERE
BERNESE
BEROWNE
BESIEGE
BESPOKE
BESTONE
BETHERE
BETHUNE
BEYONCE
BEZIQUE
CELEBRE
CELESTE
CELLULE
CENACLE
CENSURE
CENTARE
CENTIME
CERVINE
CESAIRE
CEVICHE
CEZANNE
DEADEYE
DEARONE
DEBACLE
DEBARGE
DEBOITE
DEBOULE
DECEASE
DECEIVE
DECIARE
DECLARE
DECLINE
DECUPLE
DEFARGE
DEFENCE
DEFENSE
DEFLATE
DEFRAME
DEGLAZE
DEGRADE
DEHISCE
DEIRDRE
DELARUE
DELMORE
DELORME
DELOUSE
DELUISE
DEMERGE
DEMESNE
DEMILLE
DENEUVE
DENIECE
DENTATE
DENTINE
DENTURE
DENTYNE
DEPECHE
DEPLANE
DEPLETE
DEPLORE
DEPRAVE
DEPRIVE
DEQUEUE
DERALTE
DERANGE
DESERVE

DESIREE
DESPISE
DESPITE
DESTINE
DETENTE
DETERGE
DETRUDE
DEVALUE
DEVIATE
DEVILLE
DEVISEE
DEVOLVE
DEVOTEE
DEWILDE
DEWLINE
EELLIKE
FEATURE
FEBRILE
FEEBATE
FEEFREE
FELLDUE
FENETRE
FERMATE
FERRARE
FERRATE
FERRITE
FERRULE
FERTILE
FESTIVE
GEFILTE
GEMLIKE
GEMMATE
GENESEE
GENOESE
GENOISE
GENTILE
GENUINE
GENZYME
GEOCODE
GEORGIE
GERMANE
GESTATE
GESTURE
GETABLE
GETCUTE
GETDONE
GETFREE
GETSORE
GETWISE
HECTARE
HELLENE
HELOISE
HEMLINE
HENBANE
HENLIKE
HERBAGE
HERCULE
HERNIAE
HEROINE
HESSAFE
HEURIGE
HEYJUDE
HEYRUBE
JEANNIE
JETFIRE
KENMORE
KEYCASE
KEYHOLE

KEYLIME
KEYNOTE
LEADORE
LEAFAGE
LEAKAGE
LEAVEBE
LECARRE
LECONTE
LECTURE
LEECHEE
LEETIDE
LEFTEYE
LEGATEE
LEGBONE
LEGIBLE
LEGLIKE
LEGROPE
LEHAVRE
LEISURE
LEJEUNE
LEMONDE
LEMOYNE
LEONINE
LEONORE
LESABRE
LETHAVE
LETITBE
LETLIVE
LETMEBE
LETRIDE
LETSSEE
LETSUSE
LETTERE
LETTUCE
LEUCINE
MEANAGE
MEANJOE
MEASURE
MEATAXE
MEATPIE
MEDIATE
MEDUSAE
MELANGE
MELANIE
MELROSE
MELTAGE
MEMOIRE
MERCURE
MERIMEE
MESSAGE
METHANE
METLIFE
NEBULAE
NECKTIE
NEOCENE
NEOGENE
NEOLYTE
NEONATE
NEPTUNE
NERVINE
NERVULE
NESCAFE
NETCAFE
NETGAME
NETLIKE
NETSUKE
NETWARE
NEURONE

NEVILLE
NEWFACE
NEWGATE
NEWHIRE
NEWHOPE
NEWLIFE
NEWLINE
NEWLOVE
NEWMADE
NEWNAME
NEWSOME
NEWWAVE
PEALIKE
PEERAGE
PEGLIKE
PELISSE
PELTATE
PENANCE
PENCASE
PENLIKE
PENLITE
PENNAME
PENNATE
PENNINE
PENROSE
PENSIVE
PENTANE
PENUCHE
PEONAGE
PEPTIDE
PEPTONE
PERCALE
PERDURE
PERFUME
PERFUSE
PERIGEE
PERJURE
PERLITE
PERMUTE
PERRINE
PERVADE
PESANTE
PETCAGE
PETDOVE
PETGATE
PETHARE
PETIOLE
PETMICE
PETMULE
PETNAME
REALINE
REALISE
REALIZE
REARGUE
REARISE
REAROSE
REAWAKE
REAWOKE
REBASTE
REBATHE
REBRACE
REBROKE
RECABLE
RECARVE
RECEIVE
RECHOSE
RECLAME
RECLINE

RECLUSE
RECRATE
RECURVE
RECYCLE
REDBONE
REDFACE
REDFIVE
REDLINE
REDNINE
REDNOSE
REDPINE
REDRIVE
REDROBE
REDROSE
REDTAPE
REDTIDE
REDWINE
REDZONE
REEVOKE
REFENCE
REFEREE
REFLATE
REFORGE
REFRAME
REFUGEE
REGAUGE
REGLAZE
REGRADE
REGUIDE
REHINGE
REHOUSE
REIMAGE
REISSUE
REJOICE
REJUDGE
RELANCE
RELAPSE
RELEASE
RELIEVE
REMERGE
REMORSE
REPASTE
REPHASE
REPHONE
REPLACE
REPLANE
REPLATE
REPLETE
REPLUME
REPRICE
REPRIME
REPRISE
REPROBE
REPROVE
REPRUNE
REPTILE
REPULSE
REQUIRE
REQUITE
REQUOTE
RERAISE
RERINSE
REROUTE
RESCALE
RESCORE
RESEIZE
RESERVE
RESHAPE

RESHARE
RESHAVE
RESHINE
RESIDUE
RESLATE
RESOLVE
RESPACE
RESPADE
RESPICE
RESPIRE
RESPITE
RESPOKE
RESTAGE
RESTATE
RESTIVE
RESTOKE
RESTORE
RESTYLE
RESURGE
RESWORE
RETABLE
RETASTE
RETICLE
RETINAE
RETINGE
RETINUE
RETIREE
RETITLE
RETRACE
RETRADE
RETWINE
REUNITE
REVALUE
REVENGE
REVENUE
REVERIE
REVERSE
REVOICE
REVOLVE
REWEAVE
REWRITE
REWROTE
SEABLUE
SEAFARE
SEAGATE
SEALANE
SEALIFE
SEALIKE
SEAMILE
SEARACE
SEASIDE
SEATTLE
SECLUDE
SECRETE
SEEABLE
SEEHERE
SEEPAGE
SEIZURE
SELVAGE
SENESCE
SENSATE
SERFAGE
SERIATE
SERIESE
SERRATE
SERVICE
SERVILE
SESSILE

SETFREE
SETRATE
SETTYPE
SEVENEE
SEVILLE
TEACAKE
TEAROSE
TEATIME
TEATREE
TEENAGE
TEENSIE
TEETIME
TEMPORE
TENABLE
TENACRE
TENCODE
TENEEEE
TENMILE
TENSILE
TENSIVE
TERENCE
TERHUNE
TERMITE
TERNATE
TERRACE
TERRENE
TERRINE
TESTATE
TETRODE
TEXTILE
TEXTURE
VEDETTE
VEHICLE
VEINULE
VELOUTE
VENABLE
VENDOME
VENTAGE
VENTURE
VERBOSE
VERDURE
VEREINE
VERSACE
VESICLE
VESTIGE
VESTURE
WEBLIKE
WEBPAGE
WEBSITE
WEBZINE
WELCOME
WELFARE
WELLSEE
WENTAPE
WETWARE
YEARONE
YESISEE
YESSIRE
YESVOTE
YEWTREE
ZEBRINE
ZEPPOLE
ZERNIKE

••EE•••

ASEETHE
AWEEBIT
BLEEDER

BLEEPED
BLEEPER
BREEDER
BREEZED
BREEZES
CHEEKED
CHEEPED
CHEEPER
CHEERED
CHEERER
CHEERIO
CHEERON
CHEERUP
CHEESED
CHEESES
CHEETAH
CHEETAS
CHEETOS
CHEEVER
CHEEZIT
CREEDAL
CREELEY
CREEPBY
CREEPED
CREEPER
CREEPIN
CREEPOS
CREEPUP
DOEEYED
DUEEAST
DWEEZIL
EPEEIST
EYEEXAM
FLEECED
FLEECER
FLEECES
FLEEGLE
FLEEING
FLEERED
FLEETED
FLEETER
FLEETLY
FREEAIR
FREEBEE
FREEBIE
FREEDOF
FREEDOM
FREEDUP
FREEING
FREEMAN
FREEMEN
FREESIA
FREESOF
FREESUP
FREETOY
FREEWAY
FREEZER
FREEZES
GLEEFUL
GLEEMAN
GLEEMEN
GREELEY
GREENED
GREENER
GREENLY
GREETED
GREETER
ISEENOW

ISEEYOU
KLEENEX
KNEECAP
KNEEING
KNEELED
KNEELER
KNEEPAD
KNEESUP
OKEEFFE
ONEEEEE
ONEEYED
PIEEYED
PREEDIT
PREEMIE
PREEMPT
PREENED
PREENER
QUEENED
QUEENIE
QUEENIT
QUEENLY
QUEERED
QUEERER
QUEERLY
SHEEHAN
SHEERED
SHEERER
SHEERLY
SHEETED
SKEETER
SKEEZIX
SLEEKED
SLEEKEN
SLEEKER
SLEEKLY
SLEEPER
SLEEPIN
SLEEPON
SLEETED
SLEEVED
SLEEVES
SNEERAT
SNEERED
SNEERER
SNEETCH
SNEEZED
SNEEZER
SNEEZES
SPEEDED
SPEEDER
SPEEDOS
SPEEDUP
STEELED
STEELER
STEELIE
STEEPED
STEEPEN
STEEPER
STEEPIN
STEEPLE
STEEPLY
STEERED
STEERER
STEEVED
STEEVES
SWEENEY
SWEEPEA
SWEEPER

SWEEPUP
SWEETEN
SWEETER
SWEETIE
SWEETLY
SWEETON
THEEAST
THEEDGE
TREEING
TREELET
TREERAT
TREESAP
TREETOP
TWEEDLE
TWEENER
TWEETED
TWEETER
TWEEZED
TWEEZER
TWEEZES
WHEEDLE
WHEELED
WHEELER
WHEELIE
WHEELIN
WHEEZED
WHEEZER
WHEEZES

••E•E••

AGELESS
ALEKEGS
ALEVELS
APELETS
ATELESS
AVERELL
AWELESS
AXEHEAD
BEEBEES
BEEGEES
BEEMERS
BEEPERS
BEEZERS
BREVETS
BREWERS
BREWERY
BREYERS
CHEDERS
CHEVETS
CHEWERS
CLEMENS
CLEMENT
CRENELS
CREWELS
DEEPEND
DEEPENS
DEEPEST
DIEMENS
DIESELS
DIETERS
DREXELU
DUELERS
DUEWEST
ELEMENT
ELEVENA
ELEVENB
ELEVENC
ELEVEND

ELEVENE
ELEVENS
EVENERS
EVENEST
EVEREST
EVERETT
EWENECK
EXEGETE
EXENEMY
EYELESS
EYELETS
EYETEST
EYEWEAR
FEEDERS
FEELERS
FEELESS
FOELESS
FREBERG
FREDEBB
FRELENG
FRENEAU
FRENEMY
FRENESI
FUELERS
GEEZERS
GREYEST
HEEDERS
HEELERS
HUELESS
ICEBEER
ICEBERG
ICELESS
ICETEAS
IRELESS
IREPEAT
JAEGERS
JEEPERS
JEERERS
KEENENH
KEENERS
KEENEST
KEEPERS
LEERERS
LIEFEST
LIENEES
LIETEST
MAEWEST
MEEKEST
MEETERS
MOEBERG
NEEDERS
OBESELY
OBEYERS
ODELETS
OLEVELS
OMELETS
ONEBELL
ONECELL
ONECENT
ONEEEEE
ONENESS
ONEREEL
ONESELF
ONETERM
ONEWEEK
ONEYEAR
OPENEND
OPENERS

ORELESS
OVEREAT
PEEKERS
PEELERS
PEEPERS
PEERESS
PEEWEES
PIECERS
POETESS
PRECEDE
PRECEPT
PREDEFY
PREDENY
PREFECT
PREFERS
PREHEAL
PREHEAT
PREMEDS
PREMEET
PRERENT
PRESEAL
PRESEAT
PRESELL
PRESENT
PRESETS
PRETEEN
PRETELL
PRETEND
PRETERM
PRETEST
PRETEXT
PREVENT
PREVERB
PREVERT
PREVETO
PREYERS
QUENEAU
QUESERA
QUEUERS
QUEUEUP
REEFERS
REEJECT
REEKERS
REELECT
REELERS
REERECT
RIEGERT
RIESENS
ROEDEER
RYEBEER
SCENEII
SCENEIV
SCENERY
SCENEVI
SEEDERS
SEEHERE
SEEKERS
SEERESS
SHEBEAR
SHEKELS
SIEMENS
SIENESE
SKEWERS
SPEWERS
STEREOS
STEVENS
STEWERS
TEEHEED

TEEHEES
TEENERS
TEEPEES
TEETERS
TEEVEES
THEBEAR
THEBELL
THEBEST
THEDEEP
THEDELL
THEFEDS
THEHEAT
THEHELP
THEHERO
THEJERK
THEJETS
THELEFT
THEMETS
THENETS
THENEWS
THEREAT
THEREBY
THEREDS
THEREIN
THERENT
THEREOF
THEREON
THERESA
THERETO
THESELF
THESEUS
TIEBEAM
TIELESS
TOELESS
TWERENT
UKELELE
UNERECT
USELESS
VEENECK
VIEWERS
WEEDERS
WEEKEND
WEENESS
WEEPERS
WHEREAS
WHEREAT
WHEREBY
WHEREIN
WHERELL
WHEREOF
WHEREON
WHERERE
WHERETO
WHEREVE
WIENERS

••E••E•

ABETTED
ABETTER
ADELIES
ADEPTER
AFEARED
AGENCES
AGENTED
ALEKSEI
ALERTED
ALERTER
ALETTES

AMENDED
AMENDER
AMERCED
AMERCER
AMERCES
APEDIET
APERIES
AREOLES
ATELIER
ATEOVER
AVENGED
AVENGER
AVENGES
AVENUEQ
AVENUES
AVERRED
AVERTED
AVERTER
AYEAYES
BEEBEES
BEECHEN
BEECHER
BEECHES
BEEFIER
BEEFTEA
BEEGEES
BEERIER
BEERKEG
BEETIER
BEETLES
BEETRED
BEETREE
BLEAKER
BLEARED
BLEATED
BLEATER
BLEEDER
BLEEPED
BLEEPER
BLENDED
BLENDER
BLENDES
BLESSED
BLESSER
BLESSES
BREADED
BREADER
BREAKER
BREEDER
BREEZED
BREEZES
BRENDEL
BRENNER
BUELLER
BYEBYES
CHEAPEN
CHEAPER
CHEATED
CHEATER
CHECHEN
CHECKED
CHECKER
CHEEKED
CHEEPED
CHEEPER
CHEERED
CHEERER
CHEESED

CHEESES
CHEEVER
CHELSEA
CHENIER
CHEQUER
CHEQUES
CHESTED
CHESTER
CHEVRES
CHEVRET
CHEWIER
CLEANED
CLEANER
CLEARED
CLEARER
CLEATED
CLEAVED
CLEAVER
CLEAVES
CLERKED
COERCED
COERCER
COERCES
COETZEE
CREAKED
CREAMED
CREAMER
CREASED
CREASER
CREASES
CREATED
CREATES
CRECHES
CREELEY
CREEPED
CREEPER
CREOLES
CRESSES
CRESSET
CRESTED
CREWMEN
DEEPRED
DEEPSEA
DEEPSET
DOEEYED
DREADED
DREAMED
DREAMER
DREDGED
DREDGER
DREDGES
DREIDEL
DREISER
DRESDEN
DRESSED
DRESSER
DRESSES
DREXLER
DUELLED
DUETTED
DWELLED
DWELLER
EGESTED
EJECTED
ELECTED
ELECTEE
ELEGIES
EMENDED

EMENDER
EMERGED
EMERGES
EMERIES
EMERSED
ENEMIES
ERECTED
ERECTER
EVENBET
EVERTED
EWERIES
EXERTED
EXERTER
EZEKIEL
FAERIES
FAEROES
FEEBLER
FEEFREE
FIEDLER
FIELDED
FIELDER
FIENNES
FIERCER
FIERIER
FLECHES
FLECKED
FLEDGED
FLEDGES
FLEECED
FLEECER
FLEECES
FLEERED
FLEETED
FLEETER
FLENSED
FLENSER
FLENSES
FLESHED
FLESHES
FLEXNER
FREAKED
FREEBEE
FREEMEN
FREEZER
FREEZES
FRESHED
FRESHEN
FRESHER
FRESHES
FRESHET
FRESNEL
FRESSED
FRESSES
FRETTED
FRETTER
FUELLED
FUENTES
GEEKIER
GLEAMED
GLEANED
GLEANER
GLEEMEN
GREASED
GREASER
GREASES
GREATEN
GREATER
GREAVES

GREELEY
GREENED
GREENER
GREETED
GREETER
GRENDEL
GREYHEN
GUESSED
GUESSER
GUESSES
GUESTED
HAECKEL
HRETHEL
ICEAGES
ICEAXES
ICEBEER
ICEDTEA
ICEFREE
ICEOVER
IDEAMEN
IDEATED
IDEATES
JAECKEL
JEEBIES
JOEYDEE
KEEBLER
KEESLER
KIEFFER
KLEENEX
KLEIBER
KLEISER
KLEZMER
KNEADED
KNEADER
KNEELED
KNEELER
KNELLED
KNESSET
KOEHLER
KVELLED
LAENNEC
LAERTES
LEECHED
LEECHEE
LEECHES
LEERIER
LIEABED
LIENEES
LIEOVER
LOESSER
LOESSES
MEEMIES
MUELLER
NEEDIER
NEEDLED
NEEDLER
NEEDLES
NIELSEN
OKELLEY
OLEATES
ONEEEEE
ONEEYED
ONEOVER
ONEREEL
ONESTEP
ONEWEEK
OPENNET
OPENSEA
ORESTES
OVERBED
OVERBET
OVERFED
OVERFEE
OVERFEW
OVERLET
OVERNEW
OVERSEA
OVERSEE
OVERSET
OVERSEW
OVERWET
PEEBLES
PEEPLES
PEEWEES
PIEEYED
PIERCED
PIERCER
PIERCES
PIETIES
PLEADED
PLEADER
PLEASED
PLEASER
PLEASES
PLEATED
PLEDGED
PLEDGEE
PLEDGER
PLEDGES
POESIES
PREAGED
PREAGES
PREAVER
PREDIET
PREENED
PREENER
PREIDEA
PREMEET
PREMIER
PREMIES
PREOPEN
PREPPED
PREQUEL
PRESLEY
PRESSED
PRESSEL
PRESSER
PRESSES
PRETEEN
PRETZEL
PREVIEW
PREVUED
PREVUES
PREXIES
QUEENED
QUEERED
QUEERER
QUELLED
QUELLER
QUERIED
QUERIER
QUERIES
QUESTED
QUESTER
REEDIER
REEDMEN
REEFIER
REEKIER
REENTER
REEXPEL
RIESSEN
ROEDEER
RYEBEER
SCENTED
SCENTER
SCEPTER
SEEDBED
SEEDIER
SEEDLET
SEEPIER
SEESRED
SEETHED
SEETHES
SHEAFED
SHEARED
SHEARER
SHEAVED
SHEAVES
SHEDDER
SHEERED
SHEERER
SHEETED
SHEFFER
SHELLED
SHELLER
SHELLEY
SHELTER
SHELVED
SHELVER
SHELVES
SHERBET
SKEETER
SKELTER
SLEAZES
SLEDDED
SLEDDER
SLEDGED
SLEDGES
SLEEKED
SLEEKEN
SLEEKER
SLEEPER
SLEETED
SLEEVED
SLEEVES
SLENDER
SMEARED
SMEARER
SMELLED
SMELLER
SMELTED
SMELTER
SNEAKED
SNEAKER
SNEERED
SNEERER
SNEEZED
SNEEZER
SNEEZES
SNELLEN
SPEAKER
SPEARED
SPEARER
SPECIES
SPECKED
SPECTER
SPEEDED
SPEEDER
SPELLED
SPELLER
SPENCER
SPENDER
SPENSER
STEADED
STEALER
STEAMED
STEAMER
STEELED
STEELER
STEEPED
STEEPEN
STEEPER
STEERED
STEERER
STEEVED
STEEVES
STEIGER
STEINEM
STEINER
STEMMED
STEMPEL
STENGEL
STEPHEN
STEPPED
STEPPER
STEPPES
STERNER
STETTED
STEUBEN
STEWIER
SUELLEN
SVELTER
SWEARER
SWEATED
SWEATER
SWEENEY
SWEEPEA
SWEEPER
SWEETEN
SWEETER
SWELLED
SWELLER
SWELTER
SWERVED
SWERVES
TEEHEED
TEEHEES
TEENIER
TEEPEES
TEETHED
TEETHER
TEETHES
TEEVEES
THEAGES
THEATER
THEDEEP
THEDIET
THEFLEA
THEIDEA
THEOMEN
THEOREM
THETREE
THEVIEW
TIEDYED
TIEDYES
TIERCES
TIERNEY
TREADED
TREADER
TREATED
TREATER
TREBLED
TREBLES
TREELET
TREIZES
TREKKED
TREKKER
TRENDED
TRESSED
TRESSES
TSETSES
TWEAKED
TWEENER
TWEETED
TWEETER
TWEEZED
TWEEZER
TWEEZES
TWELVEA
TWELVEB
TWELVEC
TWELVED
TWELVEE
TWELVES
UNEAGER
UNEASES
UNEATEN
UNEAVED
UNEBBED
UNEDGED
UNEDGES
UNENDED
UPENDED
USERFEE
VEERIES
VIELLES
VIERNES
VIEWIER
VNECKED
WEEDIER
WEENIES
WEEONES
WEEPIER
WHEATEN
WHEELED
WHEELER
WHEEZED
WHEEZER
WHEEZES
WHELMED
WHELPED
WHETHER
WHETTED
WHETTER
WIELDED
WIELDER
WIENIES
WREAKED
WREAKER
WRECKED
WRECKER
WRESTED
WRESTER
YIELDED
YIELDER
ZIEGLER
ZOELLER

••E•••E

ACERATE
ACEROSE
ACETATE
ACETONE
ADELINE
ADENINE
AGEFIVE
AGEMATE
AGENINE
ALEWIFE
ANEMONE
APELIKE
ARENOSE
AREOLAE
ASEETHE
ATELATE
ATEMORE
AVERAGE
AWESOME
AXELIKE
BEEHIVE
BEELIKE
BEELINE
BEETREE
BLEDSOE
BREATHE
BREWAGE
CHEADLE
CHEAPIE
CHELATE
CHEMISE
CLEANSE
CLEANTE
COETZEE
CREMATE
CRENATE
CREVICE
DOEUVRE
DUEDATE
ELECTEE
ELECTME
ELEGIZE
ELEVATE
ELEVENE
EPERGNE
EREMITE
EXECUTE
EXEDRAE
EXEGETE
EYECARE
EYEHOLE
EYELIKE
EYELINE
EYESORE
FEEBATE
FEEFREE
FLEANCE
FLEEGLE
FLEXILE
FLEXURE
FRECKLE
FREDDIE
FREEBEE
FREEBIE
GLENCOE
GOESAPE
GRECIZE
GRENADE
HOECAKE
ICEBLUE
ICECAVE
ICECUBE
ICEFLOE
ICEFREE
ICEHOLE
ICELIKE
ICELINE
ICEWINE
IMEMINE
INEXILE
IREFUSE
ITEMISE
ITEMIZE
ITEMONE
ITERATE
JOEYDEE
KHEDIVE
LAEMMLE
LEECHEE
LEETIDE
MCENROE
OBELISE
OBELIZE
OKEEFFE
ONEACRE
ONEBASE
ONEBYTE
ONEDIME
ONEEEEE
ONELANE
ONELOVE
ONEMILE
ONEMORE
ONENAME
ONENOTE
ONEPAGE
ONESHOE
ONESIZE
ONETIME
ONEVOTE
OPENTOE
OPERATE
OPEROSE
OVERAGE
OVERATE
OVERAWE
OVERDUE
OVERDYE
OVERFEE
OVERICE
OVERLIE
OVERSEE
OVERUSE
PEERAGE
PIEHOLE
PIELIKE
PIESAFE
PIESALE
PLEDGEE
PLEURAE
POETISE
POETIZE
PREBADE
PREBAKE
PRECEDE
PRECISE
PRECITE
PRECODE
PRECURE
PREDATE
PREDIVE
PREEMIE
PREFACE
PREFADE
PREFILE
PREGAME
PRELATE
PRELIFE
PRELUDE
PREMADE
PREMAKE
PREMATE
PREMISE
PRENAME
PREPARE
PREPAVE
PREPPIE
PRERACE
PRESAGE
PRESALE
PRESIDE
PRESQUE
PRESUME
PRETAPE
PRETIRE
PRETYPE
PREWIRE
PUERILE
QUEENIE
QUELQUE
REEVOKE
ROETHKE
SCEPTRE
SEEABLE
SEEHERE
SEEPAGE
SHEATHE
SHEILAE
SHELTIE
SIENESE
SPECKLE
SPECTRE
STEANNE
STEELIE
STEEPLE
STEPONE
STERILE
SVERIGE
SWEETIE
TEENAGE
TEENSIE
TEETIME
THEATRE
THEBABE
THECAPE
THEDOLE
THEDUKE
THEEDGE
THEFIVE
THEGAME
THEHOPE
THELIKE
THENILE
THEPOPE
THEROBE
THEROPE
THEROSE
THERULE
THESAME
THETREE
THETUBE
THEWAVE
TIEGAME
TIELINE
TIEROPE
TOELIKE
TOESHOE
TREACLE
TREADLE
TREKKIE
TREMBLE
TRESTLE
TWEEDLE
TWELVEE
UKELELE
USERFEE
WHEEDLE
WHEELIE
WHERERE
WHEREVE
WOEISME
WREATHE
WRESTLE

•••EE••

AGREEON
AGREERS
AGREETO
AMREETA
AXSEEDS
BALEENS
BESEECH
CAPEESH
CAREENS
CAREERS
DEBEERS
DESEEDS
DRTEETH
EDMEESE
ESTEEMS
EXCEEDS
FIVEEEE
GAVEEAR
GIVEEAR
INDEEDY
LATEENS
LOWEEZY
MESEEMS
MOREENS
MRDEEDS
MUDEELS
NINEEEE
NOSEEUM
ONEEEEE
PAPEETE
POTEENS
REDEEDS
REDEEMS
REFEEDS
REHEELS
REMEETS
REREELS
RESEEDS
RESEEKS
SATEENS
SCREECH
SCREEDS
SCREENS
SEAEELS
SIXEEEE
SPLEENS
SPLEENY
SQUEERS
SQUEEZE
STREETS
TENEEEE
THREEAD
THREEAM
THREEBC
THREEEE
THREENO
THREEPM
THREERS
THREEUP
TUREENS
TWOEEEE
UNHEEDS
UNNEEDY
UNPEELS
UNREELS
UPKEEPS
VENEERS

•••E•E•

ACCEDED
ACCEDER
ACCEDES
ACHENES
ADHERED
ADHERER
ADHERES
ALIENEE
ALKENES
ALLEGED
ALLEGER
ALLEGES
ALLELES
ALLEYES
ALTERED
ALTERER
AMMETER
AMPERES
ANGELES
ANGERED
ANNEXED
ANNEXES
ATSEVEN
BAREGES
BASEMEN
BASETEN
BEDEWED
BEJEWEL
BELEVEN
BEVELED
BEVELER
BIGEYED
BIGEYES
BILEVEL
BIREMES
BLEEDER
BLEEPED
BLEEPER
BLUEHEN
BLUERED
BODEREK
BOGEYED
BONELET
BONESET
BONEYER
BOWERED
BRAEDEN
BREEDER
BREEZED
BREEZES
BRIEFED
BRIEFER
BRUEGEL
BUGEYED
BUTENES
CAGEPET
CAMEOED
CAPELET
CAPERED
CATERED
CATERER
CATEYED
CAVEMEN
CELEBES
CHEEKED
CHEEPED
CHEEPER
CHEERED
CHEERER
CHEESED
CHEESES
CHEEVER
CODERED
COHERED
COHERER
COHERES
CONELET
COVERED
COVERER
COVETED
COVETER
COWERED
COZENED
COZENER
CREELEY
CREEPED
CREEPER
CRUELER
CULEXES
CUPELED
CUPELER
DEHEXED
DEHEXES
DELETED
DELETES
DEMETER
DESERET
DESEXED
DESEXES
DIMETER
DINESEN
DNIEPER
DOEEYED
DOVELET
DOWERED
DRYEYED
DRYEYES
EAGERER
EASELED
EKUELES
ELIEZER
ENTERED
ENTERER
ESSENES
ESTEVEZ
ETHENES
FACETED
FEDEXED
FEDEXES
FEVERED
FIBERED
FIDELES
FILENES
FIREMEN
FIVEEEE
FIVETEN
FLEECED
FLEECER
FLEECES
FLEERED
FLEETED
FLEETER
FORELEG
FOREMEN
FORESEE
FOREVER
FREEBEE
FREEMEN
FREEZER
FREEZES
FRIEZES
FROEBEL
GAMELEG
GAMETES
GATELEG
GATEMEN
GAVELED
GENESEE
GENESES
GENESET
GETEVEN
GLEEMEN
GOGETEM
GORETEX
GOTEVEN
GREELEY
GREENED
GREENER
GREETED
GREETER
GRIEVED
GRIEVER
GRIEVES
GYRENES
HAVENER
HAYESES
HOMEIER
HOMERED
HONEYED
HOVERED
HOVERER
HOWEVER
IIPETER
IMPEDED
IMPEDER
IMPEDES
INDEXED
INDEXER
INDEXES
INHERED
INHERES
INTEGER
ISLETED
JEWELED
JEWELER
JEZEBEL
JIMENEZ
JONESED
JONESES
KINESES
KLEENEX
KNEELED
KNEELER
KNIEVEL
KROEMER
KRUEGER
LABELED
LABELER
LAKEBED
LAPELED
LATEFEE
LATENED
LATEXES
LAYERED
LEDERER
LEVELED
LEVELER
LEVERED
LEVERET
LIBELED
LIBELEE
LIBELER
LIFENET
LIKENED
LIKENEW
LILETEE
LINEMEN
LIVENED
LIVENER
LIVERED
LIVESET
LIVESEY
LORELEI
LOVESET
LOWERED
LUREXES
MALEBEE
MANEGES
MEDELES
METERED
MIGENES

MIMEOED
MIMESES
MITERED
MODELED
MODELER
MODEMED
MONEYED
MOSEYED
MTPELEE
MUJERES
NEMESES
NICEMEN
NINEEEE
NINEVEH
NONEVER
NOTEVEN
NOTEVER
NUREYEV
OFFERED
OFFEREE
OFFERER
OFTENER
ONEEEEE
ONEEYED
ORDERED
ORDERER
OSIERED
OWLEYED
PANELED
PAPELES
PAPERED
PAPERER
PETEMEN
PETERED
PHOEBES
PIEEYED
PIGEYED
POLEMEN
POPELEO
POPEYED
POPEYES
POWERED
PREENED
PREENER
QUEENED
QUEERED
QUEERER
QUIETED
QUIETEN
QUIETER
RACEMES
RAMESES
RAVELED
RAVENED
RECEDED
RECEDES
REDEYED
REDEYES
REFEREE
REKEYED
RELEVEL
RELEVER
RELEVES
RENEGED
RENEGER
RENEGES
RENEWED
RENEWER
RESEWED
REVELED
REVELER
REVERED
REVERER
REVERES
RIBEYES
RIPENED
RIPENER
RIVETED
RIVETER
ROGERED
ROLEXES
ROSERED
ROSETEA
ROWELED
SABERED
SADEYED
SADEYES
SAFEBET
SAGEHEN
SAGETEA
SCHEMED
SCHEMER
SCHEMES
SCREWED
SECEDED
SECEDER
SECEDES
SERENER
SEVENEE
SEVERED
SEVERER
SHEERED
SHEERER
SHEETED
SIDEBET
SIDEMEN
SINEWED
SIRENED
SIXEEEE
SIZETEN
SKEETER
SLEEKED
SLEEKEN
SLEEKER
SLEEPER
SLEETED
SLEEVED
SLEEVES
SNEERED
SNEERER
SNEEZED
SNEEZER
SNEEZES
SOBERED
SOBERER
SPEEDED
SPEEDER
SPHERED
SPHERES
SPIEGEL
SPIELED
SPIELER
STEELED
STEELER
STEEPED
STEEPEN
STEEPER
STEERED
STEERER
STEEVED
STEEVES
STPETER
STREWED
STREWER
SUREBET
SWEENEY
SWEEPEA
SWEEPER
SWEETEN
SWEETER
TAKETEA
TAKETEN
TAPEMEN
TAPERED
TASERED
TELEXED
TELEXES
TENEEEE
THIEVED
THIEVES
THREEEE
TIMEXES
TIREDER
TIREMEN
TOHELEN
TOKENED
TONEMES
TOWELED
TOWERED
TREELET
TWEENER
TWEETED
TWEETER
TWEEZED
TWEEZER
TWEEZES
TWOEEEE
TYPESET
UMBERED
UNBESET
UNCEDED
UNDEWED
UNFETED
UNHEWED
UNKEYED
UNLEVEL
UNMEWED
UNSEWED
UNVEXED
USHERED
USTEDES
UTTERED
UTTERER
VALETED
VANEXEL
VIDEOED
VOTEYEA
VOTEYES
VUMETER
WAFERED
WAGERED
WAGERER
WAKENED
WAKENER
WATERED
WATERER
WAVELET
WAVERED
WAVERER
WEDELED
WEGENER
WETEYED
WHEELED
WHEELER
WHEEZED
WHEEZER
WHEEZES
WHOEVER
WHYEVER
WIDENED
WIDENER
WINERED
WIREMEN
WISEMEN
WIZENED
WOWEDEM
XIMENES
YALEMEN
YODELED
YODELER

•••E••E

ABSENCE
ACREAGE
ADVERSE
ALCESTE
ALDENTE
ALIENEE
ALLELSE
ALLENDE
AMOEBAE
ANNETTE
APPEASE
ARDECHE
ARIETTE
ARLEDGE
ASEETHE
ASPERSE
ATDEUCE
ATPEACE
AUBERGE
AUREATE
AUREOLE
BABETTE
BEREAVE
BLUEICE
BTWELVE
BURETTE
CADENCE
CADETTE
CAMEDUE
CAMERAE
CASEATE
CASERNE
CATENAE
CAYENNE
CELEBRE
CELESTE
CINEOLE
CODEINE
COLETTE
COMEDIE
COMEDUE
COSETTE
COTERIE
COVERME
CUNEATE
CURETTE
CUVETTE
DECEASE
DECEIVE
DEFENCE
DEFENSE
DEMERGE
DEMESNE
DENEUVE
DEPECHE
DESERVE
DETENTE
DETERGE
DINETTE
DISEASE
DISEUSE
DIVERGE
DIVERSE
DOVERDE
DOYENNE
ECUELLE
EDMEESE
ENTEBBE
ENTENTE
ESCENCE
ESSENCE
ESTELLE
ETIENNE
EUGENIE
EUTERPE
EXPENSE
EXTERNE
FABERGE
FAIENCE
FAYETTE
FENETRE
FINESSE
FIREICE
FIRENZE
FIVEEEE
FIVEONE
FLEEGLE
FORESEE
FOUETTE
FREEBEE
FREEBIE
FTMEADE
GALEATE
GALETTE
GAZELLE
GAZETTE
GENESEE
GISELLE
GONEAPE
HAVEONE
HOMEICE
HOWELSE
IDLESSE
IMMENSE
IMMERGE
IMMERSE
INCENSE
INGENUE
INNERVE
INPEACE
INTENSE
INTERNE
INTERSE
INVERSE
INWEAVE
IPLEDGE
ITWELVE
JADEITE
JANEANE
JANEDOE
KANEOHE
LABELLE
LAFEMME
LANEONE
LATEFEE
LAVERNE
LAYETTE
LEJEUNE
LIBELEE
LIBERTE
LICENCE
LICENSE
LIKEICE
LILETEE
LIMEADE
LIMEPIE
LINEAGE
LINEATE
LINEONE
LISENTE
LIVEONE
LIZETTE
LONETTE
LOZENGE
LUCERNE
LUNETTE
LYNETTE
MADEONE
MAJESTE
MAJEURE
MAKEONE
MALEBEE
MANETTE
MILEAGE
MODERNE
MOSELLE
MTPELEE
MUSETTE
MYCENAE
NACELLE
NAMEONE
NANETTE
NICEONE
NINEEEE
NOMERGE
NONETTE
NOVELLE
OBSERVE
OBVERSE
OCTETTE
OFFENCE
OFFENSE
OFFEREE
OKEEFFE
ONEEEEE
ONLEASE
ONLEAVE
ONSERVE
ORIENTE
ORNETTE
OUTEDGE
PAGEONE
PALEALE
PALETTE
PAPEETE
PILEATE
PIPETTE
POLEAXE
POSEUSE
POTENCE
PREEMIE
QUEENIE
RAVELOE
RECEIVE
REFENCE
REFEREE
RELEASE
REMERGE
RESEIZE
RESERVE
REVENGE
REVENUE
REVERIE
REVERSE
REWEAVE
ROBERTE
RONETTE
ROSEATE
ROSELLE
ROSETTE
ROTELLE
ROZELLE
RULEONE
SCIENCE
SCLERAE
SENESCE
SEVENEE
SIDEONE
SILENCE
SILENTE
SINEDIE
SIXEEEE
SIZEONE
SOMEONE
SQUEEZE
STEELIE
STEEPLE
SUZETTE
SWEETIE
TAKEONE
TENEEEE
TERENCE
THEEDGE
THREEEE
TOLEASE
TONETTE
TRIESTE
TUMESCE
TWEEDLE
TWOEEEE
UNFENCE
UNMERGE
UNNERVE
UNTENSE
UNTERSE
UNWEAVE
UNWEDGE
UPHEAVE
VALENCE
VALENTE
VALERIE
VEDETTE
VEREINE
VICENTE
VIDETTE
VOLENTE
VOTEAYE
WHEEDLE
WHEELIE
WISEONE
WYNETTE

••••EE•

ALATEEN
ALGREEN
ANISEED
APOGEES
ASSWEET
ATMFEES
BADDEED
BAILEES
BARDEEN
BARKEEP
BBQBEEF
BEEBEES
BEEGEES
BELLEEK
BETWEEN
BIGFEET
BOOTEES
BOTREES
BRIBEES
BUNGEES
BURGEES
CALLEES
CANTEEN
CATFEET
COATEES
COFFEES
COLLEEN
COMPEER
CORVEES
COULEES
DARLEEN
DEBTEES
DECREED
DECREER
DECREES
DEGREED
DEGREES
DRAGEES
DRAWEES
ELYSEES
ENTREES
EPOPEES
FARSEER
FIFTEEN
FIVEEEE
FOUREEE
GAGREEL
GENTEEL
GIFTEES
GLACEED
GOATEED
GOATEES
HADBEEN
HARDEES
HASBEEN
HAYSEED
HISPEED
HOGWEED
HUMVEES
ICEBEER
INBREED
INGREEN
JAYCEES
JAYVEES
KILLEEN
LABFEES
LESSEES
LICHEES
LIENEES
LINSEED
LISTEES
LOUREED
LOWHEEL
LURLEEN
MAUREEN
MCQUEEN
MENTEES
MERGEES
MIDTEEN
MIDWEEK
MISDEED
MISDEEM
MISFEED
MONKEES
MRGREEN
MRSPEEL
MYNHEER
NEWWEEK
NINEEEE
NONDEEP
NOTBEEN
OILSEED
ONEEEEE
ONEREEL
ONEWEEK
OUTFEED
OUTFEEL
OUTKEEP
OUTPEEP
OUTSEEK
OUTSEEN
OUTSEES
OUTWEED
OUTWEEP
PARSEES
PAWNEES
PAYHEED
PEEWEES
PENSEES
PERWEEK
PETDEER
PIGWEED
PIONEER
POLLEES
PONGEES
PREMEET
PRETEEN
PROCEED
PUTTEES
QUOTEES
RAGWEED
RANDEEP
REBREED
REDDEER
REGREET
RENTEES
RESWEEP
REXREED
ROEDEER
RUNDEEP
RUSHEES
RYEBEER
SAUTEED
SCHMEER
SEABEES
SEAWEED
SENDEES
SETFEES
SETTEES
SIGNEES
SIXEEEE
SIXFEET
SIXTEEN
SIXWEEK
SOIREES
SOTWEED
SUBTEEN
SUCCEED
TARHEEL
TEEHEED
TEEHEES
TEEPEES
TEEVEES
TENEEEE
TENFEET
TENWEEK
TESTEES
THEDEEP
THREEEE
TIPPEES
TOFFEES
TOPSEED
TOUPEES
TOWHEES
TWODEEP
TWOEEEE
TWOFEET
TWOWEEK
UMPTEEN
UNFREED
UNFREES
UNGREEN
UNSHEER
UNSLEEK
UNSTEEL
UNSWEET
UNTREED
UNWHEEL
UPSWEEP
USSTEEL
VENDEES
VERMEER
VESTEES
WEBFEET
YANKEES

••••E•E

ABILENE
ACADEME
ACCRETE
ACHIEVE
ALFREDE
ALLHERE
AMUSEME
ARRIERE
ATHLETE
AUSLESE
AUSTERE
BELIEVE
BENZENE
BERGERE
BERNESE
BESIEGE
BETHERE
BUCKEYE
BURMESE
CAIRENE
CARLENE
CARRERE
CATSEYE
CHINESE
COLLEGE
COMPERE
COMPETE
CONCEDE
CONVENE
CORTEGE
DARLENE
DEADEYE
DENIECE
DEPLETE
DEQUEUE
DIOCESE
DIOMEDE
EATHERE
EDMEESE
ELEVENE
ENQUEUE
EPICENE
ESTHETE
ETAGERE
EVILEYE
EXCRETE
EXEGETE
EXTREME
FAROESE
FISHEYE
FIVEEEE
FOUREEE
GENOESE
GLADEYE
GRUYERE
HANDEYE
HAWKEYE
HELLENE
HITHERE
HYGIENE
IMOGENE
IMTHERE
INGLESE
INTHERE
ITSHERE
LEAVEBE
LEFTEYE
LETMEBE
LETTERE
LUMIERE
MACHETE
MALTESE
MARLENE
MIOCENE
MOLIERE
MOONEYE
NAIVETE
NEOCENE
NEOGENE
NINEEEE
NOTHERE
NOWHERE
OBSCENE
ONEEEEE
OUTHERE
PANTENE
PAPEETE
PHONEME
PRECEDE
PROTEGE
RELIEVE
REPLETE
RIVIERE
SCALENE
SCUSEME
SECRETE
SEEHERE
SERIESE
SHUTEYE
SIAMESE
SIENESE
SINCERE
SIXEEEE
SLOVENE
SOAREWE
SOCKEYE
SOLFEGE
SOSUEME
SOTHERE
SPAREME
SQUEEZE
STYRENE
SUBVENE
SUPREME
TENEEEE
TERRENE
THREEEE
TOLUENE
TRAPEZE
TRIREME
TWOEEEE
UKELELE
UKULELE
UNOBESE
UPTHERE
WALLEYE
WHERERE
WHEREVE
WRITEME

•••••EE

ADOPTEE
ADVISEE
ALIENEE
ANNALEE
ARCHSEE
ASHTREE
ATTHREE
AUDITEE
AUNTBEE
AURALEE
AWARDEE
BANKFEE
BANSHEE
BAYTREE
BEETREE
BRADLEE
BUGFREE
BUSYBEE
CARFREE
CHAFFEE
COETZEE
COUNTEE
DESIREE
DEVISEE
DEVOTEE
DONATEE
DONTBEE
DOUBLEE
DRAFTEE
EIGHTEE
ELECTEE
ELMTREE
EMIGREE
ESCAPEE
EVACUEE
EVICTEE
EXITFEE
FATFREE
FEEFREE
FIANCEE
FIGTREE
FIRTREE
FIVEEEE
FORESEE
FORFREE
FORTLEE
FOUREEE
FREEBEE
FRISBEE
GALILEE
GENESEE
GETFREE
GOLFTEE
GOTFREE
GOTOSEE
GRANDEE
GRANTEE
GUARDEE
GUMTREE
HOLYSEE
HONALEE
HONOREE
ICEFREE
INTHREE
INVITEE
JIMCHEE
JOEYDEE
JOHNLEE
JOURNEE
JUBILEE
KIKIDEE
KILLFEE

KIMCHEE
LACUREE
LATEFEE
LEECHEE
LEGATEE
LETSSEE
LIBELEE
LILALEE
LILETEE
LOOKSEE
MACHREE
MALEBEE
MANATEE
MARQUEE
MATINEE
MERIMEE
MPTHREE
MTPELEE
MUSTSEE
NINEEEE
NOMINEE
NOSIREE
NOWISEE
NUTTREE
OAKTREE
OBLIGEE
OFFEREE
ONEEEEE
ONTHREE
OSSIPEE
OUTFLEE
OVERFEE
OVERSEE
PAROLEE
PERIGEE
PLEDGEE
PRITHEE
RANFREE
REFEREE
REFUGEE
RETIREE
RUBYDEE
RUNFREE
RUTALEE
SARALEE
SETFREE
SEVENEE
SHAWNEE
SIXEEEE
SLURPEE
SOIGNEE
SPONDEE
STANDEE
STANLEE
TAXFREE
TEATREE
TENEEEE
THETREE
THREEEE
TOASTEE
TOYNBEE
TRAINEE
TROCHEE
TRUCKEE
TRUSTEE
TWELVEE
TWOEEEE
UPATREE
USERFEE
WELLSEE
WHOOPEE
WINDTEE
WOOKIEE
YAHTZEE
YESISEE
YEWTREE

EF•••••

EFFABLE
EFFABLY
EFFACED
EFFACER
EFFACES
EFFECTS
EFFENDI
EFFORTS
EFFUSED
EFFUSES
EFGHIJK

E•F••••

EFFABLE
EFFABLY
EFFACED
EFFACER
EFFACES
EFFECTS
EFFENDI
EFFORTS
EFFUSED
EFFUSES
ELFLIKE
ELFLOCK
ELFOWLS
ELFUDGE
ENFACED
ENFACES
ENFANTS
ENFIELD
ENFLAME
ENFOLDS
ENFORCE
ENFRAME
EXFACTO

E••F•••

EARFLAP
EARFULS
EATFROM
EDIFICE
EDIFIED
EDIFIER
EDIFIES
EYEFOLD
EYEFULS

E•••F••

EASEFUL
EQUIFAX
ESTEFAN
EXITFEE

E••••F•

EARMUFF
EASEOFF
EASYOFF
ENGRAFT
ENGULFS
EVENOFF
EYELIFT

E•••••F

EARMUFF
EASEOFF
EASYOFF
EGOSURF
ENDLEAF
EVENOFF

•EF••••

BEFALLS
BEFOOLS
BEFOULS
DEFACED
DEFACER
DEFACES
DEFACTO
DEFALLA
DEFAMED
DEFAMER
DEFAMES
DEFANGS
DEFARGE
DEFAULT
DEFCONS
DEFEATS
DEFECTS
DEFENCE
DEFENDS
DEFENSE
DEFERTO
DEFFEST
DEFGHIJ
DEFIANT
DEFICIT
DEFIERS
DEFILED
DEFILER
DEFILES
DEFINED
DEFINER
DEFINES
DEFLATE
DEFLEAS
DEFLECT
DEFOAMS
DEFOCUS
DEFORMS
DEFRAGS
DEFRAME
DEFRAUD
DEFRAYS
DEFROCK
DEFROST
DEFTEST
DEFUELS
DEFUNCT
DEFUNDS
DEFUSED
DEFUSER
DEFUSES
DEFYING
GEFILTE
HEFTERS
HEFTIER
HEFTILY
HEFTING
JEFFERS
JEFFREY
LEFREAK
LEFTARM
LEFTEAR
LEFTEND
LEFTEST
LEFTEYE
LEFTFOR
LEFTHIP
LEFTIES
LEFTISH
LEFTISM
LEFTIST
LEFTJAB
LEFTLEG
LEFTOFF
LEFTOUT
MEFIRST
REFACED
REFACES
REFALLS
REFAXED
REFAXES
REFEEDS
REFENCE
REFEREE
REFERTO
REFFING
REFIGHT
REFILED
REFILES
REFILLS
REFILMS
REFINDS
REFINED
REFINER
REFINES
REFIRED
REFIRES
REFIXED
REFIXES
REFLAGS
REFLATE
REFLECT
REFLIES
REFLIPS
REFLOAT
REFLOOD
REFLOWN
REFLOWS
REFOCUS
REFOLDS
REFORGE
REFORMS
REFOUND
REFRACT
REFRAIN
REFRAME
REFRESH
REFRIED
REFRIES
REFRONT
REFUELS
REFUGED
REFUGEE
REFUGES
REFUNDS
REFUSAL
REFUSED
REFUSER
REFUSES
REFUTAL
REFUTED
REFUTER
REFUTES
REFYING
SEFERIS
TEFLONS

•E•F•••

AELFRIC
BEDFORD
BEEFALO
BEEFIER
BEEFILY
BEEFING
BEEFSUP
BEEFTEA
BELFAST
BELFORT
DEAFENS
DEAFEST
DEFFEST
DEIFIED
DEIFIER
DEIFIES
DEWFALL
FEEFREE
FEIFFER
FEOFFED
GETFREE
GETFROM
HEIFERS
HEIFETZ
JEFFERS
JEFFREY
JETFANS
JETFIRE
JETFOIL
KERFLOP
LEAFAGE
LEAFIER
LEAFING
LEAFLET
LEAFOUT
LEEFORD
LENFANT
LETFALL
MEDFORD
MENFOLK
METFANS
NETFLIX
NETFULS
NEWFACE
PEAFOWL
PERFECT
PERFIDY
PERFORM
PERFUME
PERFUMY
PERFUSE
PETFISH
PETFROG
REAFFIX
REDFACE
REDFERN
REDFINS
REDFIRS
REDFISH
REDFIVE
REDFLAG
REDFORD
REDFOUR
REEFERS
REEFIER
REEFING
REFFING
REIFIED
REIFIES
RENFREW
REOFFER
SEAFARE
SEAFERN
SEAFOAM
SEAFOOD
SEAFOWL
SELFISH
SERFAGE
SERFDOM
SETFEES
SETFREE
TENFEET
TENFOLD
TENFOOT
TENFOUR
WEBFEET
WEBFOOT
WEEFOLK
WELFARE
WEXFORD

•E••F••

BEGSFOR
BENEFIC
BENEFIT
DEEPFAT
DEEPFRY
DEERFLY
DESKFUL
FEARFOR
FEARFUL
FEELFOR
FEIFFER
FELLFOR
FELTFOR
FEOFFED
GETSFAR
GETSFIT
HEADFOR
HEADFUL
HEATFAN
HEATFUL
HEEDFUL
HELPFUL
JETSFAN
KEEPFIT
KEPTFIT
LEAPFOR
LEFTFOR
LESSFAT
LETSFLY
METSFAN
NEEDFUL
NESTFUL
READFOR
REAFFIX
REBUFFS
REDSFAN
REGIFTS
REOFFER
REPSFOR
RESIFTS
RESTFUL
SEENFIT
SEESFIT
SELLFOR
SENDFOR
SENTFOR
SETOFFS
TEARFUL
TEEOFFS
TELEFAX
TENTFUL
TESTFLY
TESTFOR
VERYFEW
VERYFIT
WEEPFOR
WELLFED
WENTFAR
WENTFOR
YELLFOR
YENSFOR
ZESTFUL

•E•••F•

BEAROFF
BEATIFY
BEATOFF
BEGSOFF
BELIEFS
BESTOFF
CERTIFY
DENSIFY
FEELOFF
FELLOFF
FELTOFF
FENDOFF
GETSOFF
GETSOFT
HEADOFF
HELDOFF
HENTOFF
HESSAFE
JELLIFY
KEEPOFF
KEPTOFF
LEADOFF
LEFTOFF
LETSOFF
METLIFE
NESCAFE
NETCAFE
NEWLEFT
NEWLIFE
PEELOFF
PERSOFF
PETRIFY
READOFF
REBUFFS
RECTIFY
REDRAFT
REELOFF
REGRAFT
RELIEFS
REROOFS
RESHIFT
RESTAFF
RESTUFF
RETURFS
REUNIFY
SEALIFE
SEALIFT
SEALOFF
SEENOFF
SEESOFF
SELLOFF
SENDOFF
SENTOFF
SETOFFS
SETSOFF
TEAROFF
TEEDOFF
TEEOFFS
TEESOFF
TELLOFF
TERRIFY
TESTIFY
VEEROFF
VERBIFY
VERSIFY
WEAROFF
WELLOFF
WENTAFT
WENTOFF

•E••••F

BEAROFF
BEATOFF
BEGSOFF
BEOWULF
BESTOFF
DEBRIEF
FEELOFF
FELLOFF
FELTOFF
FENDOFF
GETSANF
GETSOFF
HEADOFF
HEAPSOF
HEARDOF
HEARSOF
HELDOFF
HENTOFF
HERSELF
KEEPOFF
KEPTOFF
LEADOFF
LEARNOF
LEFTOFF
LETGOOF
LETSOFF
LETTERF
METCALF
NETSURF
NEWLEAF
PEELOFF
PERSOFF
PETCALF
READOFF
REDWOLF
REEKSOF
REELOFF
REPROOF
RESTAFF
RESTUFF
SEALOFF
SEAWOLF
SEENOFF
SEESOFF
SELLOFF
SENDOFF
SENTOFF
SERIESF
SETSOFF
TEALEAF
TEAROFF
TEEDOFF
TEESOFF
TELLOFF
VEEROFF
WEAROFF
WELLOFF
WENTOFF

••EF•••

AGEFIVE
AGEFOUR
BEEFALO
BEEFIER
BEEFILY
BEEFING
BEEFSUP
BEEFTEA
CDEFGHI
CHEFING
EYEFOLD
EYEFULS
FEEFREE
FIEFDOM
ICEFALL
ICEFLOE
ICEFOGS
ICEFREE
IREFUSE
KIEFFER
LEEFORD
LIEFEST
OLEFINS
ONEFOLD
ONEFOOT
PREFABS
PREFACE
PREFADE
PREFECT
PREFERS
PREFILE
PREFORM
PREFUND
REEFERS
REEFIER
REEFING
SHEFFER
STEFANI
THEFALL
THEFEDS
THEFIRM
THEFIVE
THEFLEA
THEFLOP
THEFONZ
THEFOOL
THEFRUG
TREFOIL
WEEFOLK

••E•F••

BRERFOX
DEEPFAT
DEEPFRY
DEERFLY
DIEDFOR
DIEOFFS
DIESFOR
DOESFOR
DREYFUS
FEELFOR
FRETFUL
GLEEFUL
GOESFAR
GOESFOR
GREWFAT
HEEDFUL
KEEPFIT
KIEFFER
LIEDFOR
LIESFOR
NEEDFUL
OKEEFFE
ONEOFFS
ONEOFUS
OVERFAR
OVERFAT
OVERFED
OVERFEE
OVERFEW
OVERFIT
OVERFIX
OVERFLY
SEENFIT
SEESFIT
SHEAFED
SHEFFER
SLEDFUL
SUEDFOR
SUESFOR
TEEOFFS
TWELFTH
USEDFOR
USERFEE
USESFOR
VIEDFOR
VIESFOR
WEEPFOR

••E••F•

ACETIFY
ALEWIFE
BLEWOFF
DIEDOFF
DIEOFFS
DIESOFF
DREWOFF
EVENOFF
EYELIFT
FEELOFF
GOESAFT
GOESOFF
KEEPOFF
OKEEFFE
ONEOFFS
PEELOFF
PIESAFE
PREDEFY
PRELIFE
PRESIFT
REELOFF
SEENOFF
SEESOFF
SHERIFF
SHERIFS
SPECIFY
SPEDOFF
STEPOFF
TEEDOFF
TEEOFFS
TEESOFF
THEGIFT
THELEFT
TIEDOFF
TIESOFF
VEEROFF

••E•••F

AHEADOF
AKERLOF
APECKOF
BLEWOFF
CLEAROF
DIEDOFF
DIESOFF
DREAMOF
DREWOFF
EVENOFF
FEELOFF
FREEDOF
FREESOF
GOESOFF
KEEPOFF
NOENDOF
ONEHALF
ONESELF
PEELOFF
REEKSOF
REELOFF
RYELOAF
SEENOFF
SEESOFF
SHERIFF
SHEWOLF
SPEAKOF
SPEDOFF
STEPOFF
TEEDOFF
TEESOFF
THEREOF
THESELF
TIEDOFF
TIESOFF
VEEROFF
WHEREOF

•••EF••

ACHEFOR
BALEFUL
BANEFUL
BCDEFGH
BENEFIC
BENEFIT
BLUEFIN
BLUEFLU
BLUEFOX
BODEFUL
BRIEFED
BRIEFER
BRIEFLY
CAREFOR
CAREFUL
CHIEFLY
CLUEFUL
DAREFUL
DIREFUL
DOLEFUL
DONEFOR
EASEFUL
ESTEFAN
FAKEFUR
FATEFUL
FIREFLY
FIREFOX
GLEEFUL
GONEFAR
GONEFOR
HATEFUL
HAVEFUN
HOPEFOR
HOPEFUL
LATEFEE
LIFEFUL
LIVEFOR
MADEFIT
MADEFOR
MADEFUN
MAKEFIT
MAKEFOR
MAKEFUN
MALEFIC
MUSEFUL
OKEEFFE
PINEFOR
PIPEFUL
POKEFUN
RAGEFUL
SAVEFOR
TAKEFOR
TELEFAX
TUNEFUL
VOTEFOR
WAKEFUL

•••E•F•

BAKEOFF
BITEOFF
CAMEOFF
COMEOFF
DOZEOFF
DRMELFI
EASEOFF
FACEOFF
FIREOFF
GAVEOFF
GIVEOFF
GONEAFT
GONEOFF
HIVEOFF
MADEOFF
MAKEOFF
MOVEOFF
OKEEFFE
PACEOFF
POPEAFB
RAKEOFF
RIDEOFF
RODEOFF
ROPEOFF
TAKEOFF
TIMEOFF
TOREOFF
UNLEAFS
WAVEOFF
WIPEOFF
WOREOFF

•••E••F

ASKEDOF
ASLEWOF
BAKEOFF
BITEOFF
CAMEOFF
COMEOFF
DOZEOFF
EASEOFF
FACEOFF
FIREOFF
FREEDOF
FREESOF
GAVEOFF
GIVENOF
GIVEOFF
GIVESOF
GONEOFF
HIVEOFF
MADEOFF
MAKEOFF
MOVEOFF
PACEOFF
PILESOF
RAKEOFF
RIDEOFF
ROBERTF
RODEOFF
ROPEOFF
SILENTF
SUREROF
TAKEOFF
TIMEOFF
TIREDOF
TIRESOF
TOREOFF
WAVEOFF
WIPEOFF
WOREOFF

••••EF•
ABCDEFG
BELIEFS
FARLEFT
IDTHEFT
LIQUEFY
NEWLEFT
PREDEFY
PUTREFY
RELIEFS
STUPEFY
THELEFT
TORREFY
UNCLEFT

••••E•F
APILEOF
AWAREOF
BAYLEAF
BBQBEEF
ENDLEAF
FIGLEAF
FLYLEAF
HERSELF
HIMSELF
INAWEOF
LETTERF
MORCERF
NEWLEAF
NONDEAF
NONSELF
OAKLEAF
ONESELF
OURSELF
SERIESF
SPOKEOF
TEALEAF
THEREOF
THESELF
THYSELF
WHEREOF

•••••EF
BBQBEEF
DEBRIEF
DOUBLEF
INBRIEF
UNBRIEF

EG•••••
EGALITE
EGERIAS
EGESTED
EGGCASE
EGGCUPS
EGGDROP
EGGEDON
EGGHEAD
EGGHUNT
EGGIEST
EGGLERS
EGGLESS
EGGLIKE
EGGNOGS
EGGROLL
EGGSACS
EGGTOSS
EGLISES
EGOISTE
EGOISTS
EGOSURF
EGOTISM
EGOTIST
EGOTRIP

E•G••••
EAGERER
EAGERLY
EAGLETS
EAGLING
EDGARDO
EDGEDIN
EDGEOUT
EDGESIN
EDGIEST
EDGINGS
EFGHIJK
EGGCASE
EGGCUPS
EGGDROP
EGGEDON
EGGHEAD
EGGHUNT
EGGIEST
EGGLERS
EGGLESS
EGGLIKE
EGGNOGS
EGGROLL
EGGSACS
EGGTOSS
EIGHTAD
EIGHTAM
EIGHTBC
EIGHTEE
EIGHTHS
EIGHTPM
EIGHTUP
ELGALLO
ELGRECO
ENGAGED
ENGAGER
ENGAGES
ENGARDE
ENGILDS
ENGINED
ENGINES
ENGIRDS
ENGLAND
ENGLISH
ENGLUND
ENGLUTS
ENGORGE
ENGRAFT
ENGRAIN
ENGRAMS
ENGRAVE
ENGROSS
ENGULFS
ERGOTIC
EUGENIA
EUGENIC
EUGENIE
EUGLENA

E••G•••
EADGILS
ELEGANT
ELEGIAC
ELEGIES
ELEGIST
ELEGITS
ELEGIZE
ELIGIUS
EMIGREE
EMIGRES
ENDGAME
ENIGMAS
EPIGONE
EPIGRAM
ERIGENA
ETAGERE
EXEGETE
EXIGENT
EXOGAMY

E•••G••
ECLOGUE
EKINGBY
EMERGED
EMERGES
ENCAGED
ENCAGES
ENGAGED
ENGAGER
ENGAGES
ENRAGED
ENRAGES
ENRIGHT
ENSIGNS
ENVOGUE
EPERGNE
ERTEGUN
ERYNGOS
EVANGEL

E••••G•
EARTAGS
EARWIGS
EASTEGG
ECOLOGY
ECOTAGE
EDGINGS
EGGNOGS
ELFUDGE
EMBARGO
ENDINGS
ENGORGE
ENLARGE
ENOLOGY
EPILOGS
ERLANGS
EXPUNGE

E•••••G
EAGLING
EARNING
EARPLUG
EARRING
EASTEGG
EASTING
ECHOING
EDDYING
EDITING
EDUCING
EDWARDG
ELATING
ELIDING
ELOPING
ELUDING
ELUTING
EMOTING
ENDLONG
ENDUING
ENSUING
ENURING
ENVYING
ERASING
ERELONG
ERODING
ESPYING
ESTRING
ETCHING
EVADING
EVELONG
EVENING
EVOKING
EXILING
EXITING
EXUDING

•EG••••
AEGISES
BEGANTO
BEGGARS
BEGGARY
BEGGING
BEGIRDS
BEGONIA
BEGORRA
BEGRIME
BEGSFOR
BEGSOFF
BEGUILE
BEGUINE
DEGAUSS
DEGERMS
DEGHOST
DEGLAZE
DEGRADE
DEGREED
DEGREES
DEGUSTS
HEGIRAS
KEGGERS
KEGGING
KEGLERS
LEGALLY
LEGANZA
LEGATEE
LEGATES
LEGATOR
LEGATOS
LEGBONE
LEGENDS
LEGGIER
LEGGING
LEGHORN
LEGIBLE
LEGIBLY
LEGIONS
LEGIRON
LEGISTS
LEGLESS
LEGLIKE
LEGOLAS
LEGOSET
LEGPULL
LEGRAND
LEGREST
LEGROOM
LEGROPE
LEGTRAP
LEGUMES
LEGWEAR
LEGWORK
MEGABIT
MEGAERA
MEGAERG
MEGAHIT
MEGALON
MEGANES
MEGATON
MEGILLA
MEGOHMS
MEGRIMS
MEGRYAN
NEGATED
NEGATER
NEGATES
NEGATOR
NEGLECT
NEGRONI
NEGUSES
PEGASUS
PEGAWAY
PEGGING
PEGLEGS
PEGLESS
PEGLIKE
PEGTOPS
REGAINS
REGALED
REGALER
REGALES
REGALIA
REGALLY
REGARDS
REGATTA
REGAUGE
REGEARS
REGENCY
REGENTS
REGIFTS
REGILDS
REGIMEN
REGIMES
REGINAL
REGINAS
REGIONS
REGIRDS
REGIVEN
REGIVES
REGLAZE
REGLOSS
REGLOWS
REGLUED
REGLUES
REGNANT
REGNARD
REGNIER
REGRABS
REGRADE
REGRAFT
REGRANT
REGRAPH
REGRASP
REGREET
REGRESS
REGRETS
REGRIND
REGRIPS
REGROOM
REGROUP
REGROWN
REGROWS
REGUIDE
REGULAR
REGULUS
SEGMENT
SEGOVIA
SEGWAYS
VEGETAL
VEGGIES
VEGGING
WEGENER

•E•G•••
BEAGLES
BEEGEES
BEGGARS
BEGGARY
BEGGING
BEIGNES
BEIGNET
BELGIAN
BELGIUM
BENGALI
BENGALS
BENGUNN
BEOGRAD
BERGAMO
BERGERE
BERGIUS
BERGMAN
BERGSON
DEFGHIJ
DEIGNED
DEIGNTO
FEIGNED
FEIGNER
GEEGAWS
GENGHIS
GETGOOD
GEWGAWS
HEDGERS
HEDGIER
HEDGING
HEIGHHO
HEIGHTS
IEIGHTY
JERGENS
JETGUNS
KEDGERS
KEDGING
KEGGERS
KEGGING
KEOGHAN
KEYGRIP
LEAGUED
LEAGUER
LEAGUES
LEDGERS
LEDGIER
LEGGIER
LEGGING
LENGTHS
LENGTHY
LENGUAS
LEOGENN
LETGOBY
LETGOOF
MEAGLES
MERGEES
MERGERS
MERGING
NEIGHED
NEOGENE
NETGAIN
NETGAME
NEWGATE
PEGGING
PENGUIN
PERGOLA
PETGATE
PETGOAT
PEUGEOT
REAGANS
REAGENT
REIGNED
SEAGATE
SEAGIRT
SEAGODS
SEAGRAM
SEAGREN
SEAGULL
SEDGIER
TEAGOWN
VEGGIES
VEGGING
VEIGHTS
VERGEON
VERGERS
VERGING
WEDGEIN
WEDGIER
WEDGIES
WEDGING
WEIGHED
WEIGHER
WEIGHIN
WEIGHON
WEIGHTS
WEIGHTY
WEIGHUP
YEVGENY

•E••G••
BELUGAS
BENIGNI
BENIGNO
BERIGAN
BETTGER
DEARGOD
DECAGON
DELIGHT
DELUGED
DELUGES
DEMAGOG
DEMIGOD
DESIGNS
GEORGEC
GEORGEI
GEORGEM
GEORGES
GEORGEV
GEORGEW
GEORGIA
GEORGIC
GEORGIE
HEXAGON
LEHIGHU
MEDIGAP
MENAGES
NEONGAS
NEWAGER
NEWAGEY
PELAGES
PELAGIC
PERIGEE
PERUGIA
REARGUE
REBEGAN
REBEGIN
REBEGUN
RECAGED
RECAGES
REFIGHT
REFUGED
REFUGEE
REFUGES
RELIGHT
RENEGED
RENEGER
RENEGES
REPAGED
REPAGES
REPUGNS
RESIGHT
RESIGNS
REURGED
REURGES
REWAGER
SENEGAL
SEVIGNY
TEARGAS

•E•••G•
BEDBUGS
BELONGS
BESIEGE
DEBARGE
DEBURGH
DEFANGS
DEFARGE
DEFRAGS
DEMERGE
DERANGE
DESMOGS
DETERGE
GEOLOGY
HERBAGE
HEURIGE
HEXSIGN
JETLAGS
KELLOGG
LEAFAGE
LEAKAGE
LENTIGO
LETITGO
LETMEGO
LEXUSGS
LEXUSGX
MEANAGE
MELANGE
MELTAGE
MESHUGA
MESSAGE
NEOLOGY
NESTEGG
PEERAGE
PEGLEGS
PEONAGE
PETCAGE
PETDOGS
PETPIGS
REALIGN
REDALGA
REDDOGS
REDLEGS
REDRAGS
REDTAGS
REFLAGS
REFORGE
REGAUGE
REHANGS
REHINGE
REIMAGE
REJUDGE
REMERGE
RESINGS
RESTAGE
RESURGE
RETINGE
REVENGE
REWEIGH
SEABAGS
SEADOGS
SEALEGS
SEEPAGE
SELVAGE
SERFAGE
TEABAGS
TEENAGE
VENTAGE
VERDUGO
VERTIGO
VESTIGE
WEBLOGS
WEBPAGE
WESTEGG
WETRAGS

•E••••G
BEADING
BEAMING
BEANBAG
BEANING
BEARHUG
BEARING
BEATING
BEDDING
BEEFING
BEEPING
BEERKEG
BEERMUG
BEGGING
BEHRING
BEIJING
BELLING
BELTBAG
BELTING
BELYING
BENDING
BENNING
BERMING
BESTING
BETTING
CEASING
CEILING
CENSING
CESSING
DEALING
DECALOG
DECKING
DEEDING
DEEMING
DEFYING
DEICING
DEKEING
DELEING
DELVING
DEMAGOG
DEMOING
DENHAAG
DENNING
DENTING
DENYING
DERRING
DEUCING
DEYOUNG
FEARING
FEEDBAG
FEEDING
FEELING
FELLING
FELTING
FENCING
FENDING
FESSING
FEUDING
GEARING
GELDING
GELLING
GETTING
HEADING
HEALING
HEAPING
HEARING
HEATING
HEAVING
HEDGING
HEEDING
HEELING
HEFTING
HELMING
HELPING
HELSING
HEMMING
HERDING
HERRING
JEERING
JELLING
JERKING
JESTING
JETTING
KEDGING
KEELING
KEENING
KEEPING
KEGGING
KELLOGG
KENNING
KEYRING
LEADDOG
LEADING
LEAFING
LEAKING
LEANING
LEAPING
LEASING
LEAVING
LEERING
LEFTLEG
LEGGING
LEIPZIG
LEMMING
LENDING
LESSING
LETTERG
LETTING
LEVYING
MEANING
MEETING
MEGAERG
MELDING
MELTING
MEMLING
MENDING
MEOWING
MERGING
MESHING
MESSING
MEWLING
NEARING
NECKING
NEEDING
NERVING
NESTEGG
NESTING
NETTING
NEWBURG
NEWSPEG
PEAKING
PEALING
PEATBOG
PECKING
PEEKING
PEELING
PEENING
PEEPING
PEERING
PEEVING
PEGGING
PEIPING
PELTING
PENDING
PENNING
PEPPING
PERIWIG
PERKING
PERMING
PETFROG
PETTING
READING
REAMING
REAPING
REARING
REAVING
REDDING
REDFLAG
REDKING
REDOING
REDWING
REDYING
REEDING
REEFING
REEKING
REELING
REEVING
REFFING
REFYING
REICING
REINING
RELYING
RENDING
RENTING
REPPING
RESTING
RETTING
REUSING
REVVING
SEABORG
SEALING
SEAMING
SEARING
SEASLUG
SEATING
SEBRING
SECHZIG
SEEDING
SEEKING
SEEMING
SEEPING
SEINING
SEIZING
SELLING
SEMILOG
SENDING
SENSING
SERIESG
SERLING
SERVING
SETTING
TEAMING
TEARING
TEASING
TEEMING
TELLING
TEMPING
TENDING
TENSING
TENTING
TENTPEG
TENZING
TERMING
TESTING
TEXTING
VEERING
VEGGING
VEILING
VEINING
VENDING
VENTING
VERGING
VERSING
VERYBIG
VESTING
VETOING
VETTING
WEANING
WEARING
WEAVING
WEBBING
WEDDING
WEDGING
WEEDING
WEEPING
WELDING
WELLING
WELTING
WENDING
WESTEGG
WETTING
YEANING
YELLING
YELPING
YENNING
YESSING
ZEITUNG
ZEROING
ZESTING

••EG•••
ALEGARS
ALEGRIA
BEEGEES
DREGION
ELEGANT
ELEGIAC
ELEGIES
ELEGIST
ELEGITS
ELEGIZE
EXEGETE
GEEGAWS
GREGORY
IBEGYOU
JAEGERS
ONEGRAM
OREGANO
PREGAIN
PREGAME
RIEGERT
SHEGOAT
SIEGING
THEGAME
THEGANG
THEGIFT
THEGOLD
TIEGAME
ZIEGLER

••E•G••
ATEIGHT
AVENGED
AVENGER
AVENGES
BRENGUN
CDEFGHI
CHEWGUM
DREDGED
DREDGER
DREDGES
EMERGED
EMERGES
EPERGNE
FLEDGED
FLEDGES
FLEEGLE
FREIGHT
GIELGUD
ICEAGES
PLEDGED
PLEDGEE
PLEDGER
PLEDGES
PREAGED
PREAGES
SLEDGED
SLEDGES
SLEIGHS
SLEIGHT
SMEAGOL
STEIGER
STENGEL
STENGUN
THEAGES
UNEAGER
UNEDGED
UNEDGES

••E••G•
ACEHIGH
AGESAGO
ALEKEGS
AMERIGO
AVERAGE
BOEINGS
BREWAGE
ICEBAGS
ICEFOGS
IRESIGN
ONEPAGE
ONETOGO
OVERAGE
PEERAGE
PRESAGE
PYEDOGS
SEEPAGE
SVERIGE
TEENAGE
THEBIGA
THEEDGE
THEHOGS
THEMAGI

••E•••G
AGELONG
ANELING
AREARUG
BEEFING
BEEPING
BEERKEG
BEERMUG
BREWING
CHEFING
CHEWING
CLEWING
CREPING
CREWING
DEEDING
DEEMING
DIETING
DUELING
DUETING
ERELONG
EVELONG
EVENING
FEEDBAG
FEEDING
FEELING
FLEABAG
FLEEING
FLEMING
FLEXING
FREBERG
FREEING
FREITAG
FRELENG
FREYTAG
FUELING
GREWBIG
GREYING
GREYLAG
HEEDING
HEELING
ICEBERG
ITEMING
JEERING
JREWING
KEELING
KEENING
KEEPING
KNEEING
LEERING
MEETING
MOEBERG
NEEDING
OBEYING
OMENING
OPENING
OVERBIG
OVERDOG
PEEKING
PEELING
PEENING
PEEPING
PEERING
PEEVING
PFENNIG
PIECING
PRESONG
PREYING
QUEUING
REEDING
REEFING
REEKING
REELING
REEVING
SEEDING
SEEKING
SEEMING
SEEPING
SHEBANG
SIEBZIG
SIEGING
SIEVING
SKEWING
SLEDDOG
SLEWING
SPECING
SPEWING
STEWING
TEEMING
THEFRUG
THEGANG
THEKING
THERING
TIERING
TREEING
TSETUNG
VEERING
VIERZIG
VIEWING
WEEDING
WEEPING
ZIERING

•••EG••
ALLEGED
ALLEGER
ALLEGES
ALLEGRA
ALLEGRO
BADEGGS
BAREGES
BODEGAS
BRUEGEL
DONEGAL
DONEGAN
DRVEGAS
ERTEGUN
FLEEGLE
GLUEGUN
ILLEGAL
ILLEGIT
INTEGER
INTEGRA
KRUEGER
MANEGES
MOHEGAN
NICEGUY
NOSEGAY
ORTEGAL
OWLEGGS
PHLEGMY
PILEGGI
RAREGAS
RAWEGGS
REBEGAN
REBEGIN
REBEGUN
RENEGED
RENEGER
RENEGES
SENEGAL
SLOEGIN
SPIEGEL
STREGIS
TWOEGGS
UNLEGAL
UNREGAL
VINEGAR
WISEGUY
WOBEGON

•••E•G•
ACREAGE
ALLERGY
ARLEDGE
AUBERGE
BADEGGS
BCDEFGH
CINERGY
DEMERGE
DETERGE
DIVERGE
FABERGE
FOLENGO
FOREIGN
HAVEAGO
IMMERGE
INVEIGH
IPLEDGE
LINEAGE
LOZENGE
MAKESGO
MARENGO
MILEAGE
NOMERGE
OUTEDGE
OWLEGGS
PILEGGI
RALEIGH
RAWEGGS
REMERGE
REVENGE
REWEIGH
SUPERGS
SYNERGY
THEEDGE
TWOEGGS
UNDERGO
UNMERGE
UNWEDGE

•••E••G
ANTEING
BLUEING
CLUEING
DEKEING
DELEING
FIREBUG
FIREDOG
FLEEING
FORELEG
FREEING
GAMEBAG
GAMELEG
GATELEG
JUNEBUG
KNEEING
LATETAG
LOSEBIG
LOVEBUG
MALEDOG
MALEHOG
MALEPIG
NAMETAG
NICEDOG
NOSEBAG
RATEDPG
SHOEING
SILENTG
TIMELAG
TOTEBAG
TREEING
TRUEING
YULELOG

••••EG•
ALEKEGS
BESIEGE
BOTTEGA
BUMLEGS
COLLEGE
CORTEGE
DOGLEGS
EASTEGG
GOODEGG
LETMEGO
MIDLEGS
MONTEGO
MUSKEGO
NESTEGG
NORIEGA
NUTMEGS
OFFWEGO
ONTHEGO
OUTBEGS
PEGLEGS
PROTEGE
REDLEGS
SEALEGS
SOLFEGE
WESTEGG

••••E•G
ABCDEFG
ARLBERG
EASTEGG
FREBERG
FRELENG
GINSENG
GOODEGG
HOLBERG
ICEBERG
LETTERG
MEGAERG
MOEBERG
NESTEGG
ROMBERG
SERIESG
WARRENG
WESTEGG

•••••EG
BEERKEG
BOOTLEG
DOUBLEG
FILIBEG
FORELEG
FROGLEG
GAMELEG
GATELEG
HINDLEG
LASTLEG
LEFTLEG
NAILKEG
NEWSPEG
PANTLEG
PONYKEG
TENTPEG
TOUAREG

EH•••••
EHRLICH

E•H••••
ECHAPPE
ECHELON
ECHIDNA
ECHOERS
ECHOING
ECHOISM
ENHANCE
EPHEBUS
EPHEDRA
EPHESUS
EPHRAIM
ETHANES
ETHANOL
ETHENES
ETHERIC
ETHICAL
ETHMOID
ETHNICS
EXHALED
EXHALES
EXHAUST
EXHEDRA
EXHIBIT
EXHORTS
EXHUMED
EXHUMER
EXHUMES

E••H•••
EARHART
EARHOLE
EATHERE
EBWHITE
ECKHART
EFGHIJK
EGGHEAD
EGGHUNT
EIGHTAD
EIGHTAM
EIGHTBC
EIGHTEE
EIGHTHS
EIGHTPM
EIGHTUP
ELKHART
ENCHAIN
ENCHANT
ENCHASE
ENTHRAL
ENTHUSE
ESCHEAT
ESCHERS
ESCHEWS
ESTHETE
ETCHANT
ETCHERS
ETCHING
EUCHRED
EUCHRES
EUPHONY
EYEHAND
EYEHOLE
EYEHOOK

E•••H••
EARSHOT
EARTHED
EARTHEN
EARTHLY
EASTHAM
EPITHET
EPOCHAL
EREWHON
ERYTHRO
EYESHOT

E••••H•
EARACHE
EIGHTHS
EMPATHS
EMPATHY
ENRIGHT
EOLITHS
EPARCHS
EPARCHY
EXARCHS

E•••••H
EHRLICH
ELDRICH
ENGLISH
EPITAPH
ERDRICH
EVANISH
EYELASH
EYEWASH

•EH••••
BEHAPPY
BEHAVED
BEHAVES
BEHEADS
BEHEARD
BEHESTS
BEHINDS
BEHOLDS
BEHOOVE
BEHRENS
BEHRING
BEHRMAN
DEHAIRS
DEHAVEN
DEHEXED
DEHEXES
DEHIRED
DEHIRES
DEHISCE
DEHMELT
DEHORNS
GEHENNA
HEHHEHS
LEHAVRE
LEHIGHU
LEHMANN
REHANGS
REHAULS
REHEALS
REHEARD
REHEARS
REHEATS
REHEELS
REHIDES
REHINGE
REHIRED
REHIRES
REHITCH
REHONED
REHONES
REHONOR
REHOOKS
REHOUSE
TEHERAN
VEHICLE

•E•H•••
BEAHERO
BECHARM
BEEHIVE
BETHANY
BETHELS
BETHERE
BETHINK
BETHUNE
CEPHALO
CEPHALY
CEPHEUS
DEGHOST
DENHAAG
DESHELL
FECHNER
GETHELP
GETHURT
HEEHAWS
HEHHEHS
HESHVAN
JEPHTHA
KEYHOLE
LECHERS
LEGHORN
LETHAVE
LETHEAN
LEWHOAD
MECHLIN
MESHACH
MESHIER
MESHING
MESHUGA
METHANE
METHODS
NEPHEWS
NEPHRIC
NEWHAND
NEWHART
NEWHATS
NEWHIRE
NEWHOPE
PEAHENS
PERHAPS
PETHAIR
PETHARE
RECHALK
RECHALL
RECHART
RECHECK
RECHEWS
RECHOSE
REDHAIR
REDHATS
REDHAWK
REDHEAD
REDHEAT
REDHENS
REDHOTS
REPHASE
REPHONE
RESHAPE
RESHARE
RESHAVE
RESHIFT
RESHINE
RESHIPS
RESHOES
RESHOOT
RESHOWN
RESHOWS
RESHUTS
RETHANK
RETHAWS
RETHINK
SEAHAWK
SEAHERO
SEAHUNT
SECHZIG
SEEHERE
SENHORA
SEPHIAS
TECHIES
TECHNOS
TEEHEED
TEEHEES
TERHUNE
TETHERS
VECHTEN
WEEHOUR
YEAHBUT
YEAHMAN
YEAHYOU
YESHIVA
ZEPHYRS

•E••H••
BEACHAM
BEACHED
BEACHES
BEARHUG
BECKHAM
BEECHAM
BEECHEN
BEECHER
BEECHES
BELCHED
BELCHER
BELCHES
BELLHOP
BENCHED
BENCHER
BENCHES
BENTHAM
BENTHOS
BERTHAS
BERTHED
DEFGHIJ
DELIHAM
DELPHIC
FEATHER
FELTHAT
FETCHED
FETCHER
FETCHES
GEEWHIZ
GEISHAS
GENGHIS
GERSHON
GETAHIT
GETSHEP
GETSHIP
GETSHOT
GETTHIS
HEATHEN
HEATHER
HEIGHHO
HEIGHTS
HERSHEY
IEIGHTY
KEESHAN
KEOGHAN
KERSHAW
KETCHAM
KETCHES
KETCHUM
KETCHUP
LEACHED
LEACHER
LEACHES
LEASHED
LEASHES
LEATHER
LEECHED
LEECHEE
LEECHES
LEFTHIP
MEGAHIT
MEGOHMS
MEMPHIS
MENTHOL
MENUHIN
MERCHES
NEEDHAM
NEIGHED
NEITHER
PEACHED
PEACHES
PERAHIA
PERCHED
PERCHER
PERCHES
PERCHIK
PETCHEW
PETSHOP
REACHED
REACHER
REACHES
REACHIN
REACHUP
REDCHIP
REUTHER
SEETHED
SEETHES
SEETHRU
SETSHOT
TEACHER
TEACHES
TEACHIN
TEASHOP
TEESHOT
TEETHED
TEETHER
TEETHES
TEICHER
TENCHES
TENTHLY
VEIGHTS
VERYHIP
VERYHOT
VETCHES
WEATHER
WEIGHED
WEIGHER
WEIGHIN
WEIGHON
WEIGHTS
WEIGHTY
WEIGHUP
WELLHID
WELLHIT
WENCHES
WERNHER
WERTHER

•E•••H•
BELUSHI
CEVICHE
DEARTHS
DELIGHT
DEMOTHS
DENNEHY
DEPECHE
DERECHO
FELLAHS
HEALTHY
HEARTHS
HEAVEHO
HEHHEHS
HEIGHHO
JEPHTHA
JERICHO
KENICHI
KENOSHA
KENWAHL
LEHIGHU
LENGTHS
LENGTHY
LESOTHO
MENSCHY
PENUCHE
REBATHE
REFIGHT
RELIGHT
RESIGHT
SERAPHS
TEMPEHS
TERAOHM
VERYSHY
WEALTHS
WEALTHY
ZENITHS

•E••••H
BEAMISH
BEARISH
BEAUISH
BEDBATH
BENEATH
BESEECH
BETROTH
BEWITCH
DEBAUCH
DEBORAH
DEBURGH
DEEPISH
DELILAH
DELRUTH
DERVISH
DEUTSCH
GETCASH
HELLISH
HENNISH
HENRICH
JEBBUSH
JETWASH
KEENENH
KENNETH
KENTISH
LEADETH
LEFTISH
LELOUCH
LETTERH
LETTISH
MENORAH
MESHACH
MESSIAH
METWITH
MEZUZAH
NEBBISH
NEOLITH
NERDISH
NESMITH
NEWMATH
NEWRICH
PEAKISH
PECKISH
PEEVISH
PELTISH
PERKISH
PETFISH
PETTISH
REBEKAH
REBIRTH
REBRUSH
REDDISH
REDFISH
REFRESH
REGRAPH
REHITCH
RELATCH
REMATCH
REPATCH
RETEACH
RETOUCH
REWEIGH
REXROTH
SELFISH
SERIESH
SEVENTH
WEAKISH
WETTISH
WETWASH
XENIAOH
YERKISH

••EH•••
ACEHIGH
AXEHEAD
BEEHIVE
DIEHARD
EYEHAND
EYEHOLE
EYEHOOK
HEEHAWS
ICEHOLE
JOEHILL
KOEHLER
ONEHALF
ONEHAND
ONEHOUR
PIEHOLE
PREHEAL
PREHEAT
SEEHERE
TEEHEED
TEEHEES
THEHEAT
THEHELP
THEHERO
THEHILL
THEHOGS
THEHOOD
THEHOPE
THEHULK
TOEHOLD
WEEHOUR

••E•H••
BEECHAM
BEECHEN
BEECHER
BEECHES
CHECHEN
CHEKHOV
CRECHES
EREWHON
EYESHOT
FLECHES
FLESHED
FLESHES
FLESHLY
FRESHED
FRESHEN
FRESHER
FRESHES
FRESHET
FRESHLY
GEEWHIZ
GRESHAM
GREYHEN
HRETHEL
ICESHOW

KEESHAN
KNEWHOW
LEECHED
LEECHEE
LEECHES
NEEDHAM
ONECHIP
ONESHOE
ONESHOT
ONEWHIT
OVERHOT
PRESHIP
PRESHOW
PREWHIP
QUECHUA
ROETHKE
SEETHED
SEETHES
SEETHRU
SHEEHAN
STEPHEN
TEESHOT
TEETHED
TEETHER
TEETHES
THESHOW
TOESHOE
WHETHER

••E••H•

ADELPHI
ASEETHE
ATEIGHT
BREATHE
BREATHS
BREATHY
CDEFGHI
FREIGHT
FRENCHI
FRENCHS
KVETCHY
NIEBUHR
PREACHY
SHEATHE
SHEATHS
SHEIKHS
SKETCHY
SLEIGHS
SLEIGHT
SLEUTHS
WREATHE
WREATHS
WREATHY

••E•••H

ACEHIGH
BLEMISH
BREADTH
CHEETAH
CHERISH
CPEBACH
DEEPISH
DYEBATH
EYELASH
EYEWASH
FLEMISH
GREYISH
ICEBATH
JOEROTH
KEENENH
KLENSCH
ONEARTH
ONEINCH
PEEVISH
PLENISH
PREWASH
RHENISH
SNEETCH
STEALTH
SWEDISH
THEBUSH
THEOATH
THEPOOH
TWELFTH
UNEARTH
VIEWITH
WHEYISH

•••EH••

BAGEHOT
BASEHIT
BLUEHEN
FIREHAT
MADEHAY
MAKEHAY
MALEHOG
ROSEHIP
SAGEHEN
SHEEHAN
SOMEHOW
TOBEHAD

•••E•H•

ARDECHE
ASEETHE
BOWECHO
DALETHS
DEPECHE
DERECHO
JOSEPHA
JOSEPHI
KANEOHE
OUTECHO
SAMEKHS
SUBECHO
UTRECHT
VOTECHS

•••E••H

BCDEFGH
BENEATH
BESEECH
BLUEISH
BONEASH
CAPEESH
CHEETAH
COTEACH
DOZENTH
DRIESCH
DRTEETH
FOREACH
IMPEACH
INDEPTH
INREACH
INVEIGH
NIDETCH
NILESOH
NINEVEH
OGREISH
ONLEASH
RALEIGH
REBEKAH
RETEACH
REWEIGH
ROBERTH
SCREECH
SEVENTH
SILENTH
SNEETCH
SQUELCH
STRETCH
UNBENCH
UNBERTH
UNFERTH
UNLEASH
UNTEACH
UPREACH

••••EH•

DENNEHY
HEAVEHO
HEHHEHS
TEMPEHS

••••E•H

BESEECH
BIOTECH
CALTECH
CAPEESH
DRTEETH
GWYNETH
HIALEAH
JAPHETH
KEENENH
KENNETH
KNOWETH
LABTECH
LAMBETH
LEADETH
LETTERH
LISBETH
LOWTECH
MACBETH
MISMESH
NCWYETH
PRADESH
REFRESH
RUNNETH
SCITECH
SCREECH
SERIESH

•••••EH

DOUBLEH
NINEVEH
WIMOWEH

EI•••••

EIDETIC
EIDOLIC
EIDOLON
EIGHTAD
EIGHTAM
EIGHTBC
EIGHTEE
EIGHTHS
EIGHTPM
EIGHTUP
EIJKMAN

E•I••••

EDIBLES
EDICTAL
EDIFICE
EDIFIED
EDIFIER
EDIFIES
EDINAMN
EDITING
EDITION
EDITORS
EDITOUT
EDITRIX
EKINGBY
EKISTIC
ELICITS
ELIDERS
ELIDING
ELIEZER
ELIGIUS
ELISION
ELITEST
ELITISM
ELITIST
ELIXIRS
ELIYALE
EMIGREE
EMIGRES
EMINENT
EMIRATE
EMITTED
EMITTER
ENIGMAS
ENISLED
ENISLES
EPICARP
EPICENE
EPICURE
EPIDERM
EPIDOTE
EPIGONE
EPIGRAM
EPILADY
EPILATE
EPILOGS
EPISODE
EPISTLE
EPITAPH
EPITHET
EPITOME
ERICSON
ERIGENA
ERIKSON
ERINYES
ERISTIC
ERITREA
ESIASON
ETICKET
ETIENNE
EVICTED
EVICTEE
EVICTOR
EVIDENT
EVILEST
EVILEYE
EVILLER
EVILONE
EVINCED
EVINCES
EXIGENT
EXILERS
EXILING
EXISTED
EXITFEE
EXITING
EXITNOW

E••I•••

EASIEST
EATINTO
EATITUP
ECHIDNA
ECLIPSE
EDGIEST
EDGINGS
EELIEST
EERIEST
EGGIEST
EGLISES
EGOISTE
EGOISTS
ELAINES
ELEISON
ELLIOTT
ELLIPSE
ELLISON
ELMIEST
ELMISTI
ELNINOS
EMAILED
EMAILER
EMPIRES
EMPIRIC
EMPIRIN
ENCINAS
ENDINGS
ENDIVES
ENFIELD
ENGILDS
ENGINED
ENGINES
ENGIRDS
ENLINKS
ENLISTS
ENLIVEN
ENOILED
ENRIGHT
ENRIQUE
ENSIGNS
ENSILED
ENSILES
ENTICED
ENTICER
ENTICES
ENTIRES
ENTITLE
ENVIERS
ENVIOUS
ENVIRON
ENVIROS
ENWINDS
EOLITHS
EOSINES
EPSILON
EQUIANO
EQUIFAX
EQUINES
EQUINOX
ERMINED
ERMINES
ERMINIA
ESKIMOS
ESPIALS
ESTIVAL
ETAILED
ETAILER
ETHICAL
ETOILES
EXCIDED
EXCIDES
EXCISED
EXCISES
EXCITED
EXCITER
EXCITES
EXCITOR
EXHIBIT
EXOILER
EXPIATE
EXPIRED
EXPIRES
EXTINCT
EXWIVES

E•••I••

EADGILS
EAGLING
EARLIER
EARLIES
EARLIKE
EARNING
EARRING
EARWIGS
EASTING
EATDIRT
EBBTIDE
EBONICS
EBONIES
EBONITE
EBONIZE
EBWHITE
ECHOING
ECHOISM
ECLAIRS
ECOCIDE
EDACITY
EDDYING
EDIFICE
EDIFIED
EDIFIER
EDIFIES
EDITING
EDITION
EDOMITE
EDUCING
EELLIKE
EFGHIJK
EGALITE
EGERIAS
EGGLIKE
EGOTISM
EGOTIST
EHRLICH
ELAAIUN
ELAMITE
ELAPIDS
ELATING
ELATION
ELDRICH
ELDRICK
ELEGIAC
ELEGIES
ELEGIST
ELEGITS
ELEGIZE
ELENIAK
ELFLIKE
ELICITS
ELIDING
ELIGIUS
ELISION
ELITISM
ELITIST
ELIXIRS
ELMCITY
ELOPING
ELUDING
ELUSIVE
ELUTING
ELUTION
ELUVIAL
ELUVIUM
ELYSIAN
ELYSIUM
EMBOITE
EMERIES
EMERITA
EMERITI
EMETICS
EMOTING
EMOTION
EMOTIVE
EMPRISE
EMPTIED
EMPTIER
EMPTIES
EMPTILY
ENDLINE
ENDPINS
ENDUING
ENDWISE
ENEMIES
ENGLISH
ENJOINS
ENPRISE
ENQUIRE
ENQUIRY
ENSKIED
ENSKIES
ENSUING
ENSUITE
ENTAILS
ENTRIES
ENTWINE
ENTWIST
ENURING
ENVEILS
ENVYING
EONLINE
EPEEIST
EPONINE
EPOXIED
EPOXIES
ERASING
ERDRICH
EREMITE
ERODING
EROSION
EROSIVE
EROTICA
EROTICS
ERSKINE
ERUDITE
ESPRITS
ESPYING
ESQUIRE
ESTRING
ETALIBI
ETAMINE
ETCHING
ETESIAN
ETHNICS
ETONIAN
ETONICS
ETVOILA
EVADING
EVANISH
EVASION
EVASIVE
EVENING
EVOKING
EWERIES
EXAMINE
EXANIMO
EXILING
EXITING
EXOTICA
EXOTICS
EXOTISM
EXSCIND
EXUDING
EYELIDS
EYELIFT
EYELIKE
EYELINE
EYEPITS
EYEWINK
EZEKIEL

E••••I•

EARCLIP
EARNSIT
EASEDIN
EASESIN
EATABIT
ECDYSIS
ECOTRIN
EDGEDIN
EDGESIN
EDITRIX
EELSKIN
EGOTRIP
EIDETIC
EIDOLIC
EKISTIC
ELASTIC
ELASTIN
ELTRAIN
EMBROIL
EMPIRIC
EMPIRIN
EMPORIA
ENCHAIN
ENCOMIA
ENDEDIN
ENDEDIT
ENDEMIC
ENGRAIN
ENTERIC
ENTERIN
ENTRAIN
ENZYMIC
EPHRAIM
EPSTEIN
ERGOTIC
ERISTIC
ERMINIA
ERRATIC
ESTAMIN
ESTONIA
ESTORIL
ETHERIC
ETHMOID
ETRURIA
EUCERIN
EUGENIA
EUGENIC
EUGENIE
EUNOMIA
EURASIA
EXCELIN
EXCLAIM
EXHIBIT
EXORDIA
EXPLAIN
EXPLOIT
EXPOSIT
EXURBIA

E•••••I

ECCLESI
EDMUNDI
EDWARDI
EFFENDI
EKWENSI
ELMISTI
EMERITI
ETALIBI

•EI••••

BEIGNES
BEIGNET
BEIJING
CEILING
DEICERS
DEICING
DEIFIED
DEIFIER
DEIFIES
DEIGNED
DEIGNTO
DEIRDRE
DEISTIC
DEITIES
FEIFFER
FEIGNED
FEIGNER
FEINTED
GEISHAS
HEIFERS
HEIFETZ
HEIGHHO
HEIGHTS
HEINOUS
HEIRDOM
HEIRESS
HEISMAN
HEISTED
IEIGHTY
KEILLOR
KEISTER
LEIBNIZ
LEIPZIG
LEISTER
LEISURE
LEITRIM
MEIOSES
MEIOSIS
MEIOTIC
MEISSEN
MEISTER
MEITNER
NEIGHED
NEITHER
PEIPING
REICING
REIFIED
REIFIES
REIGNED
REIMAGE
REIMPLY
REINDEX
REINING
REINKED
REINSIN
REISSUE
REITMAN
SEINERS
SEINING
SEISMAL
SEISMIC
SEIZEON
SEIZERS
SEIZING
SEIZORS
SEIZURE
TEICHER
VEIGHTS
VEILERS
VEILING
VEINIER
VEINING
VEINLET
VEINTES
VEINULE
WEIDMAN
WEIGHED
WEIGHER
WEIGHIN
WEIGHON
WEIGHTS
WEIGHTY
WEIGHUP
WEIRDAL
WEIRDED
WEIRDER
WEIRDLY
WEIRDOS
WEIRTON
ZEITUNG

•E•I•••

AEDILES
AEGISES
AERIALS
AERIEST
BEDIZEN
BEGIRDS
BEHINDS
BELIEFS
BELIERS
BELIEVE
BELINDA
BEMIRED
BEMIRES
BENICIA
BENICIO
BENIGNI
BENIGNO
BENISON
BERIGAN
BESIDES
BESIEGE
BETIDED
BETIDES
BETIMES
BEWITCH
BEZIERS
BEZIQUE
CECILIA
CEDILLA
CELICAS
CERISES
CEVICHE
DEAIRED
DEBITED
DECIARE
DECIBEL
DECIDED
DECIDER
DECIDES
DECILES
DECIMAL
DEFIANT
DEFICIT
DEFIERS
DEFILED
DEFILER
DEFILES
DEFINED
DEFINER
DEFINES
DEHIRED
DEHIRES
DEHISCE
DELIBES
DELICTI
DELICTO
DELICTS
DELIGHT
DELIHAM
DELILAH
DELILLO
DELIMAN
DELIMEN
DELIMIT
DELINTS
DELIRIA
DELISTS
DELIVER
DEMIGOD
DEMILLE
DEMISED
DEMISES
DEMISTS
DENIALS
DENIECE
DENIERS
DENIMED
DENISON
DENIZEN
DEPICTS
DERIDED
DERIDER
DERIDES
DERIVED
DERIVER
DERIVES
DESIGNS
DESILTS
DESIRED
DESIREE
DESIRER
DESIRES
DESISTS
DEVIANT
DEVIATE
DEVICES
DEVILED
DEVILLE
DEVILRY
DEVIOUS
DEVISED
DEVISEE
DEVISER
DEVISES
DEVISOR
DEWIEST
DEWILDE
DEWIRED
DEWIRES
EELIEST
EERIEST
FEDINTO
FELICIA
FELINES
FEMINUM
FETIDLY
GEFILTE
GELIDLY
GEMINIS
GENITOR
GERITOL
GETINON
GETINTO
GETITON
HEDISON
HEGIRAS
HELICAL
HELICES
HELICON
HELIPAD
HELIXES
HERITOR
JEMISON
JERICHO
JERILYN
JERITZA
JEWISON
KEMIDOV
KENICHI
KEYINON
LEDINTO
LEGIBLE
LEGIBLY
LEGIONS
LEGIRON
LEGISTS
LEHIGHU
LEMIEUX
LENIENT
LEPIDUS
LESIONS
LETINON
LETITBE
LETITGO
LETITIA
LEVIERS
LEVILLI
LEVITES
LEVITIC
LEXICAL
LEXICON
LEXISES
MEDIANS
MEDIANT
MEDIATE
MEDICAL
MEDICOS
MEDIGAP
MEDIUMS
MEDIVAC
MEFIRST
MEGILLA
MELINDA
MELISMA
MELISSA
MELITTA
MENIALS
MENISCI
MERIDEN
MERIMEE
MERINOS
MERITED
METIERS
MEXICAN
NERISSA
NETIZEN
NEUILLY
NEVILLE
NEWIDEA
OEDIPAL
OEDIPUS
PEDICAB

PELICAN PELISSE PEPITAS PERIAPT PERIDOT PERIGEE PERILED PERIODS PERISSA PERITUS PERIWIG PETIOLE PETITES REAIMED REAIRED REBILLS REBINDS REBIRTH RECIPES RECITAL RECITED RECITER RECITES REDIALS REFIGHT REFILED REFILES REFILLS REFILMS REFINDS REFINED REFINER REFINES REFIRED REFIRES REFIXED REFIXES REGIFTS REGILDS REGIMEN REGIMES REGINAL REGINAS REGIONS REGIRDS REGIVEN REGIVES REHIDES REHINGE REHIRED REHIRES REHITCH REKICKS RELIANT RELICTS RELIEFS RELIERS RELIEVE RELIGHT RELIMIT RELINED RELINES RELINKS RELISTS RELIVED RELIVES REMILLS REMINDS

REMINED REMINES REMINTS REMISED REMISES REMIXED REMIXES REOILED REPICKS REPINED REPINER REPINES RERIDES RERINSE RERISEN RERISES RESIDED RESIDER RESIDES RESIDUA RESIDUE RESIFTS RESIGHT RESIGNS RESILED RESILES RESINED RESINGS RESINKS RESISTS RESITED RESIZED RESIZER RESIZES RETIARY RETICLE RETILED RETILES RETILLS RETIMED RETIMES RETINAE RETINAL RETINAS RETINGE RETINOL RETINTS RETINUE RETIRED RETIREE RETIRES RETITLE REVIEWS REVILED REVILER REVILES REVISAL REVISED REVISER REVISES REVISIT REVISOR REVITUP REVIVAL REVIVED REVIVER REVIVES REWIDEN

REWINDS REWIPED REWIPES REWIRED REWIRES SEEINTO SEMIDRY SEMILOG SEMINAL SEMINAR SEMIPRO SEMIRAW SEMITES SEMITIC SENIORS SEPIRAS SERIALS SERIATE SERIESE SERIESF SERIESG SERIESH SERIESI SERIESJ SERIESK SERIOUS SERIPAK SETINTO SEVIGNY SEVILLA SEVILLE SEWISTS SEXIEST SEXISTS TEDIOUS TEDIUMS TEEITUP TEPIDLY VEDISTS VEHICLE VENISON VERIDIC VERIEST VERISMO VERISTS VERITAS VERIZON VESICLE WEDIDIT XENIAOH XENICAL YESICAN YESIDID YESISEE YESITIS ZEDILLO ZENISTS ZENITHS

•E••I••

AEOLIAN BEADIER BEADILY BEADING BEALION BEAMIER BEAMING BEAMISH

BEANIES BEANING BEARING BEARISH BEATIFY BEATING BEAUISH BEDDING BEDLIKE BEDSIDE BEDSITS BEDTIME BEEFIER BEEFILY BEEFING BEEHIVE BEELIKE BEELINE BEEPING BEERIER BEETIER BEGGING BEGRIME BEGUILE BEGUINE BEHRING BEIJING BELAIRS BELGIAN BELGIUM BELLIED BELLIES BELLING BELLINI BELTING BELYING BENDIER BENDING BENNING BEQUICK BEQUIET BERBICK BERGIUS BERLIOZ BERLITZ BERMING BERNINA BERNINI BERRIED BERRIES BERWICK BESTIAL BESTILL BESTING BESTIRS BETHINK BETTING BETWIXT BEWAILS CEASING CEILING CELLINI CELLIST CELSIUS CELTICS CENSING CENTIME CENTIMO

CERTIFY CERVIDS CERVINE CESAIRE CESSING CESSION DEALING DEARIES DEBOITE DEBRIEF DECEITS DECEIVE DECKING DECLINE DECRIED DECRIER DECRIES DEEDING DEEMING DEEPISH DEFYING DEHAIRS DEICING DEIFIED DEIFIER DEIFIES DEITIES DEKEING DELCITY DELEING DELUISE DELVING DEMOING DENNING DENSIFY DENSITY DENTINE DENTING DENTINS DENTIST DENYING DEPRIVE DERAILS DERBIES DERNIER DERRICK DERRICO DERRIDA DERRING DERVISH DESPINA DESPISE DESPITE DESTINE DESTINO DESTINY DETAILS DETAINS DEUCING DEVEINS DEVOIRS DEVRIES DEWLINE EELLIKE FEARING FEBRILE FEEDING FEELILL

FEELING FELLING FELLINI FELTILL FELTING FENCING FENDING FENNIER FERMION FERMIUM FERNIER FERRIED FERRIES FERRITE FERTILE FESSING FESTINA FESTIVA FESTIVE FEUDING FEUDIST FEVRIER GEARING GEDRICK GEEKIER GELDING GELLING GEMLIKE GEMMIER GENOISE GENTIAN GENTILE GENUINE GERAINT GERBILS GERMIER GETTING GETWISE HEADIER HEADILY HEADING HEALING HEAPING HEARING HEATING HEAVIER HEAVIES HEAVILY HEAVING HEDGIER HEDGING HEEDING HEELING HEFTIER HEFTILY HEFTING HELLION HELLISH HELMING HELOISE HELPING HELSING HEMLINE HEMMING HEMPIER HENBITS HENLIKE HENNISH

HENRICH HENRIES HERBIER HERDING HEREIAM HERMITS HERNIAE HERNIAS HERNIBS HEROICS HEROINE HEROISM HERRICK HERRING HERRIOT HESSIAN HEURIGE HEXSIGN JEEBIES JEERING JELLIED JELLIES JELLIFY JELLING JENKINS JERKIER JERKIES JERKILY JERKING JERKINS JESSICA JESTING JESUITS JETFIRE JETTIED JETTIES JETTING KEDGING KEELING KEENING KEEPING KEGGING KELPIES KELVINS KENNING KENTISH KEWPIES KEYLIME KEYRING LEADIER LEADING LEADINS LEAFIER LEAFING LEAKIER LEAKING LEANING LEAPING LEASING LEAVING LEDGIER LEERIER LEERILY LEERING LEETIDE LEFTIES LEFTISH LEFTISM

LEFTIST LEGGIER LEGGING LEGLIKE LEMMING LEMPIRA LENDING LENTIGO LENTILS LEONIDS LEONINE LEOVIII LEOXIII LESSING LETLIVE LETRIDE LETTING LETTISH LEUCINE LEVYING MEALIER MEALIES MEANIES MEANING MEATIER MEATILY MEDWICK MEEMIES MEETING MEGRIMS MELDING MELTING MEMLING MEMOIRE MEMOIRS MENCIUS MENDING MENTION MENZIES MEOWING MERCIAN MERCIES MERGING MERLINS MERRIAM MERRICK MERRIER MERRILL MERRILY MESHIER MESHING MESSIAH MESSICK MESSIER MESSILY MESSINA MESSING METLIFE METRICS METRIST METWITH MEWLING NEARING NEBBISH NECKING NEEDIER NEEDILY NEEDING

NENNIUS NEOLITH NERDIER NERDISH NEREIDS NERVIER NERVILY NERVINE NERVING NESBITT NESMITH NESTING NETLIKE NETTING NEWBIES NEWHIRE NEWKIDS NEWLIFE NEWLINE NEWMINT NEWRICH NEWSIER NEWSIES PEAKIER PEAKING PEAKISH PEALIKE PEALING PEATIER PECKING PECKISH PECTINS PEEKING PEELING PEENING PEEPING PEERING PEEVING PEEVISH PEGGING PEGLIKE PEIPING PELTING PELTISH PENCILS PENDING PENLIKE PENLITE PENNIES PENNINE PENNING PENSION PENSIVE PENTIUM PENZIAS PEONIES PEORIAN PEPCIDS PEPPIER PEPPILL PEPPILY PEPPING PEPPINO PEPSICO PEPSINS PEPTICS PEPTIDE PERDIDO

PERDIEM PERDITA PERFIDY PERKIER PERKILY PERKING PERKINS PERKISH PERLITE PERMIAN PERMING PERMITS PERRIER PERRINE PERRINS PERSIAN PERSIST PERSIUS PESKIER PESKILY PETBIRD PETFISH PETLION PETMICE PETPIGS PETRIFY PETSITS PETTIER PETTILY PETTING PETTISH READIED READIER READIES READILY READING REALIGN REALINE REALISE REALISM REALIST REALITY REALIZE REAMING REAPING REARING REARISE REAVING REBAITS REBOILS REBUILD REBUILT RECEIPT RECEIVE RECLIMB RECLINE RECOILS RECOINS RECTIFY REDBIRD REDDING REDDISH REDFINS REDFIRS REDFISH REDFIVE REDKING REDLINE

REDNINE REDOING REDPINE REDRIED REDRIES REDRILL REDRIVE REDTIDE REDTIES REDWINE REDWING REDYING REEDIER REEDING REEDITS REEFIER REEFING REEKIER REEKING REELING REEMITS REEVICT REEVING REFFING REFLIES REFLIPS REFRIED REFRIES REFYING REGAINS REGNIER REGRIND REGRIPS REGUIDE REICING REIFIED REIFIES REINING REJAILS REJOICE REJOINS REKNITS RELYING REMAILS REMAINS RENAILS RENDING RENNINS RENOIRS RENTIER RENTING RENWICK REPAINT REPAIRS REPLICA REPLIED REPLIER REPLIES REPOINT REPPING REPRICE REPRIME REPRINT REPRISE REPTILE REQUIEM REQUIRE REQUITE

RERAISE RESCIND RESEIZE RESHIFT RESHINE RESHIPS RESOILS RESPICE RESPINS RESPIRE RESPITE RESTICK RESTING RESTIRS RESTIVE RESUITS RESWIMS RETAILS RETAINS RETHINK RETRIAL RETRIED RETRIES RETRIMS RETSINA RETTING RETWINE RETWIST REUNIFY REUNION REUNITE REUSING REVOICE REVVING REWEIGH REWRITE SEABIRD SEAGIRT SEALIFE SEALIFT SEALIKE SEALILY SEALING SEALION SEAMIER SEAMILE SEAMING SEAMIST SEARING SEASICK SEASIDE SEATING SEBRING SECTION SEDGIER SEEDIER SEEDILY SEEDING SEEKING SEEMING SEEPIER SEEPING SEINING SEIZING SELFISH SELKIRK SELLING SENDING

SENSING SEPHIAS SEQUINS SERBIAN SERLING SERPICO SERVICE SERVILE SERVING SESSILE SESSION SESTINA SETTING TEAMING TEARIER TEARILY TEARING TEASING TEATIME TECHIES TEDDIES TEEMING TEENIER TEETIME TEKKIES TELLIES TELLING TEMPING TENDING TENMILE TENNIEL TENNIES TENPINS TENSILE TENSING TENSION TENSITY TENSIVE TENTING TENUITY TENZING TEQUILA TERBIUM TERMING TERMINI TERMITE TERRIER TERRIES TERRIFY TERRINE TESTIER TESTIFY TESTILY TESTING TEXTILE TEXTING VEALIER VEERIES VEERING VEGGIES VEGGING VEILING VEINIER VEINING VENDING VENTING VERBIDS VERBIFY

VERDICT
VERDINS
VEREINE
VERGING
VERMINY
VERNIER
VERSIFY
VERSING
VERSION
VERTIGO
VERYILL
VESPIDS
VESTIGE
VESTING
VETOING
VETTING
WEAKISH
WEANING
WEARIED
WEARIER
WEARIES
WEARILY
WEARING
WEAVING
WEBBIER
WEBBING
WEBLIKE
WEBSITE
WEBZINE
WEDDING
WEDGIER
WEDGIES
WEDGING
WEEBITS
WEEDIER
WEEDILY
WEEDING
WEENIES
WEEPIER
WEEPING
WEEVILS
WELDING
WELLING
WELTING
WENDING
WESKITS
WESTIES
WESTINS
WETKISS
WETTING
WETTISH
YEANING
YELLING
YELPING
YENNING
YERKISH
YESHIVA
YESSING
YESSIRE
YETTIES
ZEBRINE
ZERNIKE
ZEROING
ZESTIER
ZESTILY
ZESTING

•E•••I•

AELFRIC
AEROBIC
BEANDIP
BEANOIL
BEARPIT
BEASTIE
BEATNIK
BEATRIX
BEATSIT
BEATTIE
BEDELIA
BEDEVIL
BEDOUIN
BEDRAIL
BEGONIA
BELVOIR
BENAZIR
BENEFIC
BENEFIT
BENICIA
BENICIO
BERVOIX
CECILIA
CENTRIC
CERAMIC
CERTAIN
CESSPIT
CETERIS
DEADAIR
DEALSIN
DEALTIN
DEARSIR
DECLAIM
DEEPSIX
DEFGHIJ
DEFICIT
DEISTIC
DELIMIT
DELIRIA
DELORIS
DELPHIC
DELTAIC
DELTOID
DEMERIT
DEMONIC
DEMOTIC
DENARII
DENTOID
DEORBIT
DEPOSIT
DESPAIR
DESPOIL
DESTAIN
DETRAIN
DETROIT
DEXTRIN
EELSKIN
FEEDBIN
FEEDSIN
FELICIA
FELTTIP
FEMORIS
FENCEIN
GEEWHIZ
GELATIN
GELATIS
GELUSIL
GEMINIS
GENERIC
GENERIS
GENESIS
GENETIC
GENGHIS
GENNAIO
GENOMIC
GEORGIA
GEORGIC
GEORGIE
GERMAIN
GERVAIS
GETAHIT
GETATIP
GETONIT
GETSFIT
GETSHIP
GETSRID
GETTHIS
GETTOIT
HEADPIN
HEADSIN
HEBRAIC
HEDONIC
HELPSIN
HEMATIC
HEMATIN
HENDRIX
HENREID
HENRYII
HENRYIV
HEPARIN
HEPATIC
HEREDIA
HERETIC
HEXADIC
JEANNIE
JETFOIL
JETSKIS
KEEPFIT
KEEPSIN
KENOLIN
KEPTFIT
KERATIN
KETONIC
KEYEDIN
KEYGRIP
LEADSIN
LEAKSIN
LEANSIN
LEAPSIN
LEAPTIN
LEAVEIN
LEAVEIT
LECTRIC
LEFTHIP
LEIBNIZ
LEIPZIG
LEITRIM
LEOVIII
LEOXIII
LESTOIL
LETEMIN
LETITIA
LETMEIN
LETSLIP
LETSRIP
LEVITIC
LEXUSIS
MEANSIT
MEANTIT
MEATPIE
MECHLIN
MEGABIT
MEGAHIT
MEIOSIS
MEIOTIC
MELANIA
MELANIC
MELANIE
MELANIN
MELODIA
MELODIC
MEMPHIS
MENUHIN
MEOWMIX
MERMAID
MESAMIS
MESONIC
MESSKIT
NEATNIK
NECKTIE
NEMESIS
NEPALIS
NEPHRIC
NEPOTIC
NESQUIK
NESTSIN
NETFLIX
NETGAIN
NEWLAID
PEEKSIN
PEERSIN
PELAGIC
PENGUIN
PERAHIA
PERATIO
PERCHIK
PERIWIG
PERSEID
PERTAIN
PERUGIA
PETERII
PETHAIR
PETULIA
PETUNIA
REACHIN
READMIT
READSIN
REAFFIX
REARLIT
REAUDIT
REAVAIL
REBEGIN
RECLAIM
RECRUIT
REDCHIP
REDEBIT
REDHAIR
REDSKIN
REDSUIT
REDTAIL
REELSIN
REEQUIP
REFRAIN
REGALIA
REINSIN
RELIMIT
RENUZIT
RENVOIS
REPOSIT
RESNAIS
RESPLIT
RESTAIN
RESTRIP
RESTSIN
RETRAIN
REVELIN
REVERIE
REVISIT
SEALSIN
SEATRIP
SECHZIG
SEDALIA
SEENFIT
SEEPSIN
SEESFIT
SEETOIT
SEFERIS
SEGOVIA
SEISMIC
SELENIC
SELLSIT
SEMITIC
SENDSIN
SENSEIS
SEQUOIA
SERAPIS
SETBAIL
SETSAIL
TEACHIN
TEARSIT
TEENSIE
TELAVIV
TELEPIC
TELEPIX
TELLSIT
TENDRIL
TERRAIN
TERROIR
TESTKIT
VENATIC
VENEZIA
VENTRIS
VERIDIC
VERMEIL
VERONIA
VERYBIG
VERYFIT
VERYHIP
WEBMAIL
WEDGEIN
WEDIDIT
WEIGHIN
WELLHID
WELLHIT
WELLLIT
WETSUIT
XEROSIS
XEROTIC
YELTSIN
YEMENIS
YESIDID
YESITIS
ZEBRAIC
ZEBROID
ZENOBIA
ZEROSIN

•E••••I

BELLINI
BELUSHI
BELZONI
BENGALI
BENIGNI
BENZALI
BERNINI
CELLINI
CESTMOI
DELICTI
DENARII
FELLINI
FEODORI
FERRARI
GEMELLI
GEORGEI
HENRYII
HENRYVI
HERNANI
KENICHI
LEOVIII
LEOXIII
LETTERI
LEVILLI
MENISCI
MENOTTI
NEGRONI
PECCAVI
PERETTI
PETERII
SECONDI
SERIESI
TEBALDI
TERMINI
VENTURI
XERXESI
ZEPPOLI

••EI•••

AGEISTS
ATEIGHT
ATEINTO
ATEITUP
BOEINGS
DREIDEL
DREISER
ELEISON
FREIGHT
FREITAG
KLEIBER
KLEISER
ONEIDAS
ONEINCH
ONEIOTA
ONEIRIC
ONEIRON
OREILLY
PREIDEA
QUEIROS
SEEINTO
SHEIKHS
SHEILAE
SHEILAS
SLEIGHS
SLEIGHT
STEIGER
STEINEM
STEINER
TEEITUP
THEIDEA
THEISMS
THEISTS
TIEINTO
TREINTA
TREIZES
WOEISME

••E•I••

ACEHIGH
ACETIFY
ADELIES
ADELINA
ADELINE
ADENINE
AGEFIVE
AGENINE
ALEWIFE
AMENITY
AMERICA
AMERIGO
AMERIKA
AMERIND
ANELING
ANEMIAS
APEDIET
APELIKE
APERIES
ARECIBO
ARETINO
ATEDIRT
ATELIER
AVENIDA
AVERILL
AXELIKE
BEEFIER
BEEFILY
BEEFING
BEEHIVE
BEELIKE
BEELINE
BEEPING
BEERIER
BEETIER
BLEMISH
BLERIOT
BREVITY
BREWING
CHEFING
CHEMISE
CHEMIST
CHENIER
CHERISH
CHEVIOT
CHEWIER
CHEWING
CLERICS
CLERISY
CLEWING
COEDITS
COEXIST
CREDITS
CREMINI
CREPING
CRETINS
CREVICE
CREWING
CUEBIDS
CUETIPS
DEEDING
DEEMING
DEEPISH
DIETING
DREGION
DUELING
DUELIST
DUETING
EGERIAS
ELEGIAC
ELEGIES
ELEGIST
ELEGITS
ELEGIZE
ELENIAK
EMERIES
EMERITA
EMERITI
EMETICS
ENEMIES
EPEEIST
EREMITE
ETESIAN
EVENING
EWERIES
EYELIDS
EYELIFT
EYELIKE
EYELINE
EYEPITS
EYEWINK
EZEKIEL
FAERIES
FEEDING
FEELILL
FEELING
FIERIER
FIERILY
FLEEING
FLEMING
FLEMISH
FLEXILE
FLEXING
FLEXION
FREEING
FUELING
GEEKIER
GRECIAN
GRECISM
GRECIZE
GREYING
GREYISH
HEEDING
HEELING
IBERIAN
ICELIKE
ICELINE
ICEMILK
ICEPICK
ICERINK
ICEWINE
IMEMINE
INEDITA
INEXILE
IRENICS
IRESIGN
ITEMING
ITEMISE
ITEMIZE
JEEBIES
JEERING
JOEHILL
JOEKIDD
JREWING
KEELING
KEENING
KEEPING
KHEDIVE
KNEEING
LEERIER
LEERILY
LEERING
LEETIDE
MEEMIES
MEETING
NEEDIER
NEEDILY
NEEDING
NOETICS
OBELISE
OBELISK
OBELIZE
OBESITY
OBEYING
OLEFINS
OLEMISS
OMENING
ONEDIME
ONEKILO
ONELIRA
ONEMILE
ONEPINT
ONESIZE
ONETIME
OPENING
OVERICE
PEEKING
PEELING
PEENING
PEEPING
PEERING
PEEVING
PEEVISH
PHEMIUS
PIECING
PIELIKE
PIERIAN
PIETIES
PIETINS
PLEBIAN
PLENISH
POESIES
POETICA
POETICS
POETISE
POETIZE
PREBIDS
PREBILL
PREBIND
PRECISE
PRECITE
PREDICT
PREDIET
PREDIVE
PREFILE
PRELIFE
PRELIMS
PREMIER
PREMIES
PREMISE
PREMISS
PREMIUM
PRERIOT
PRESIDE
PRESIFT
PRETIRE
PREVIAS
PREVIEW
PREWIRE
PREWITT
PREXIES
PREYING
PUERILE
QUERIDA
QUERIDO
QUERIED
QUERIER
QUERIES
QUERIST
QUEUING
REEDIER
REEDING
REEDITS
REEFIER
REEFING
REEKIER
REEKING
REELING
REEMITS
REEVICT
REEVING
RHENISH
RHENIUM
SCENICS
SEEDIER
SEEDILY
SEEDING
SEEKING
SEEMING
SEEPIER
SEEPING
SHERIFF
SHERIFS
SIEGING
SIEVING
SKEWING
SLEWING
SPECIAL
SPECIES
SPECIFY
SPECING
SPEWING
STELIAS
STEPINS
STERILE
STEWIER
STEWING
SVERIGE
SWEDISH
TEEMING
TEENIER
TEETIME
THEBIGA
THECITY
THEDIET
THEFIRM
THEFIVE
THEGIFT
THEHILL
THEKING
THEKISS
THELIKE
THEMICK
THENILE
THEPIPS
THEPITS
THERIAC
THERING
THERINK
THERITZ
THESIMS
THEVIEW
THEVIPS
THEWIND
THEYIPS
TIELINE
TIEPINS
TIERING
TOELIKE
TOEPICK
TREDIAS
TREEING
TREVINO
TSELIOT
USERIDS
VEERIES
VEERING
VIEWIER
VIEWING
VIEWITH
WEEBITS
WEEDIER
WEEDILY
WEEDING
WEENIES
WEEPIER
WEEPING
WEEVILS
WHEYISH
WIENIES
ZIERING

••E••I•

ACERBIC
ADENOID
ALEGRIA
ALEMBIC
AMEBOID
ANEROID
APESUIT
ASEPSIS
ASEPTIC
ATEABIT
AWEEBIT
BIENNIA
BLENDIN
BLENTIN
BREAKIN
BRESCIA
BRESLIN
CHEAPIE
CHEATIN
CHECKIN
CHEERIO
CHEEZIT
CHERVIL
CHEXMIX
COEPTIS
CREEPIN
CREPTIN
CRESPIN
CTENOID
DEEPSIX
DOESKIN
DREAMIN
DRESSIN
DWEEZIL
DWELLIN
FEEDBIN
FEEDSIN
FLEADIP
FLEAPIT
FREDDIE
FREDRIC
FREEAIR
FREEBIE
FREESIA
FUELOIL
GEEWHIZ
GHERKIN
GREMLIN
GREWBIG
GREWDIM
IDENTIC
IMEANIT
INERTIA
KEEPFIT
KEEPSIN
KJELLIN
KREMLIN
KRESKIN
MUESLIS
MUESLIX
MUEZZIN
OBERLIN
OCEANIA
OCEANIC
OCEANID
OLEOOIL
ONECHIP
ONEIRIC
ONEPAIR
ONEUNIT
ONEWHIT
OPENAIR
OPENPIT
ORECTIC
OVERBID
OVERBIG
OVERDID
OVERFIT
OVERFIX
OVERLIE
OVERLIT
OVERMIX
OVERTIP
PEEKSIN
PEERSIN
PFENNIG
PREACID
PREBOIL
PRECOIL
PREEDIT
PREEMIE
PREGAIN
PREOMIT
PREPAID
PREPPIE
PRESHIP
PRETRIM
PREVAIL
PREVOID
PREWHIP
QUEENIE
QUEENIT
QUENTIN
REELSIN
REEQUIP
RHEUMIC
SCENEII
SCENEIV
SCEPTIC
SEENFIT
SEEPSIN
SEESFIT
SEETOIT
SHELTIE
SHERWIN
SIEBZIG
SKEEZIX
SKEPTIC
SLEEPIN
SLEPTIN
SNEAKIN
STEALIN
STEARIC
STEARIN
STEELIE
STEEPIN
STENCIL
STENNIS
STEPSIN
STEROID
SWEARIN
SWEATIT
SWEETIE
TEENSIE
THEAXIS
THEREIN
THERMIC
THESPIS
THETRIB
TIECLIP
TOENAIL
TREFOIL
TREKKIE
TRELLIS
UTENSIL
VIERZIG

WHEELIE
WHEELIN
WHEREIN

••E•••I
ADELPHI
ALEARDI
ALEKSEI
BREWSKI
CDEFGHI
CHEZMOI
CREMINI
EMERITI
FRENCHI
FRENESI
SCENEII
SCENEVI
STEFANI
THEMAGI
THEOMNI

•••EI••
ANTEING
ATHEISM
ATHEIST
BLUEICE
BLUEING
BLUEISH
CASEINS
CAVEINS
CLUEING
CODEINE
COHEIRS
DECEITS
DECEIVE
DEKEING
DELEING
DEVEINS
ENVEILS
EPEEIST
FADEINS
FAKEIDS
FIREICE
FLEEING
FOREIGN
FREEING
GASEITY
HEREIAM
HJHEINZ
HOMEICE
HOMEIER
INVEIGH
JADEITE
JANEIRO
KNEEING
LIKEICE
LOVEINS
MADEILL
MADEIRA
MAKEILL
MCNEILL
NEREIDS
OGREISH
RALEIGH
RECEIPT
RECEIVE
RESEIZE
REWEIGH
SHOEING
SUREIAM
SUREIDO
TAKEILL
TAKEINS
TREEING
TRUEING
UNVEILS
VEREINE

•••E•I•
ACTEDIN
ADDEDIN
ALBENIZ
ALGERIA
ALLELIC
ALLEWIS
ALMERIA
AMNERIS
AMNESIA
AMNESIC
AMOEBIC
ANAEMIA
ANAEMIC
ANGELIC
ANNELID
APHELIA
APPETIT
ARMENIA
ARSENIC
ARSENIO
ARTEMIS
ARTERIO
ASCETIC
ASKEDIN
ASTERIX
AWEEBIT
BASEHIT
BASESIX
BEDELIA
BEDEVIL
BENEFIC
BENEFIT
BITESIN
BLUEFIN
BLUETIT
BOHEMIA
BOXEDIN
BOXESIN
CAGEDIN
CAKEMIX
CAKETIN
CAMELID
CAVEDIN
CAVESIN
CETERIS
CHEERIO
CHEEZIT
CINESIA
CLUEDIN
CLUESIN
COMEDIA
COMEDIC
COMEDIE
COMESIN
COTERIE
CREEPIN
CSLEWIS
DEMERIT
DINEDIN
DINESIN
DIVEDIN
DIVESIN
DUNEDIN
DWEEZIL
EASEDIN
EASESIN
EDGEDIN
EDGESIN
EIDETIC
ENDEDIN
ENDEDIT
ENDEMIC
ENTERIC
ENTERIN
ETHERIC
EUCERIN
EUGENIA
EUGENIC
EUGENIE
EXCELIN
FACEDIT
FACESIT
FADEDIN
FADESIN
FAKEDIT
FAKESIT
FANEUIL
FIDELIA
FIDELIO
FIDELIS
FILEDIN
FILESIN
FIRELIT
FIREPIT
FIVEPIN
FIVESIX
FLIESIN
FREEAIR
FREEBIE
FREESIA
GENERIC
GENERIS
GENESIS
GENETIC
GIVENIN
GIVESIN
GOBELIN
GODEVIL
GONERIL
HAMELIN
HATEDIT
HATESIT
HEREDIA
HERETIC
HOMEDIN
HOMERIC
HOMESIN
HONEDIN
HONESIN
IKNEWIT
ILLEGIT
IMPERIL
INHERIT
INKEDIN
INPERIL
INTERIM
JAMESII
JAMESIV
JAVELIN
JONERIK
KEYEDIN
KINESIC
KINESIS
KINETIC
KUBELIK
LETEMIN
LIBERIA
LIMEPIE
LIVEAID
LIVEDIN
LIVESIN
LOSEBIG
LOSESIT
LOVEDIT
LOVESIT
LUREDIN
LURESIN
LUTETIA
MADEFIT
MAKEFIT
MAKESIT
MALEFIC
MALEPIG
MIMESIS
MIMETIC
MINEPIT
MISEDIT
MIXEDIN
MIXESIN
MOVEDIN
MOVEDIT
MOVESIN
MOVESIT
NEMESIS
NICEKID
NIGERIA
NINEPIN
NONEPIC
NONEVIL
NOSEDIN
NOSESIN
NUMERIC
OPHELIA
OPTEDIN
ORDERIN
OSTEOID
PAGESIX
PETERII
PHOENIX
PHRENIC
PILEDIN
PILESIN
PINEOIL
PIPEDIN
PIPESIN
POLEMIC
POLESIT
PREEDIT
PREEMIE
PYRETIC
PYREXIA
QUEENIE
QUEENIT
RACEDIN
RAKEDIN
RAKESIN
RAMEKIN
RAREBIT
REBEGIN
REDEBIT
REVELIN
REVERIE
RIDESIN
RITEAID
ROPEDIN
ROPESIN
ROSEHIP
ROSEOIL
SAMEDIS
SEFERIS
SELENIC
SIBERIA
SILESIA
SINEDIE
SIZESIX
SKEEZIX
SLEEPIN
SLOEGIN
SPHERIC
STDENIS
STEELIE
STEEPIN
STREGIS
SWEETIE
TAKEAIM
TAKENIN
TAKESIN
TAKESIT
TELEPIC
TELEPIX
THREWIN
TIDERIP
TOCELIA
TOTEMIC
TOWEDIN
TRIEDIT
TRIESIT
TRUERIB
TUNEDIN
TUNESIN
TYPEDIN
TYPESIN
USHERIN
VALERIE
VENEZIA
VOTEDIN
VOTESIN
WADEDIN
WADESIN
WAREPIC
WAVEDIN
WAVESIN
WHEELIE
WHEELIN
WIREDIN
WIRESIN
YEMENIS

•••E••I
ALBERTI
ALVEOLI
ARGENTI
BASENJI
BOCELLI
CANETTI
CORELLI
DRMELFI
EFFENDI
EKWENSI
GEMELLI
JAMESII
JAMESVI
JOSEPHI
LAVELLI
LORELAI
LORELEI
MORETTI
PERETTI
PETERII
PILEGGI
PIRELLI
PLOESTI
ROBERTI
SCHERZI
SILENTI
STRETTI
UNBELDI
VALENTI
VIVENDI

••••EI•
ALAMEIN
ANAHEIM
ANTHEIL
ARANEID
BAHREIN
BARGEIN
BOBWEIR
BOISEID
BROKEIN
CHIMEIN
CLOSEIN
CONCEIT
DANTEII
DOONEIN
DRIVEIN
DROVEIN
EPSTEIN
FENCEIN
FORCEIN
FORFEIT
GLIDEIN
HENREID
HOLBEIN
HOWBEIT
HUSSEIN
HYGIEIA
IHATEIT
IHAVEIT
ILIKEIT
ILOVEIT
IMADEIT
LEAVEIN
LEAVEIT
LETMEIN
LODGEIN
MACNEIL
MANHEIM
NUCLEIC
PASTEIN
PERSEID
PHASEIN
PHONEIN
POMPEIA
POMPEII
PROTEIN
PROVEIT
ROLLEIS
SANSEIS
SCENEII
SCENEIV
SENSEIS
SHAREIN
SHOVEIN
SLIDEIN
SOLVEIT
STOLEIN
SURFEIT
SURVEIL
SWOREIN
TASTEIT
THEREIN
TIMREID
TRADEIN
VERMEIL
VILLEIN
WEDGEIN
WHEREIN
WRITEIN
WROTEIN
YOUREIT

••••E•I
ALFIERI
BUSCEMI
DANTEII
ECCLESI
FRENESI
ISRAELI
LAZZERI
LETTERI
MONDESI
POMPEII
RAMSESI
RIPIENI
SALIERI
SCENEII
SCENEVI
SERIESI
XERXESI
ZAMBEZI

•••••EI
ALEKSEI
CADUCEI
DOUBLEI
GALILEI
GEORGEI
LORELEI
SHARPEI
SOHAVEI

EJ•••••
EJECTED
EJECTOR
EJEMPLO

E•J••••
EIJKMAN
ENJOINS
ENJOYED
ENJOYER

E•••J••
EASYJOB
ELCAJON

E••••J•
EFGHIJK

•EJ••••
BEJEWEL
DEJECTS
DEJUNKS
JEJUNUM
LEJEUNE
REJAILS
REJECTS
REJOICE
REJOINS
REJUDGE
TEJANAS
TEJANOS

•E•J•••
BEIJING
DEEJAYS
HEYJUDE
NEWJOBS
PERJURE
PERJURY
REDJACK
REEJECT
VEEJAYS

•E••J••
BELLJAR
GETAJOB
KELLJAN
LEARJET
LEFTJAB
MEANJOE
REENJOY
RESOJET
TEMPJOB

•E••••J
DEFGHIJ
HEYMRDJ
LETTERJ
SERIESJ

••EJ•••
DEEJAYS
DYEJOBS
REEJECT
THEJERK
THEJETS
VEEJAYS

••E•J••
OVERJOY
REENJOY

•••EJ••
BLUEJAY
LOVEJOY
LUBEJOB
NICEJOB
NOSEJOB

•••E•J•
BASENJI

•••E••J
SILENTJ

••••EJ•
AZULEJO
VALLEJO

••••E•J
DANIELJ
LARGEOJ
LETTERJ
SERIESJ

•••••EJ
DOUBLEJ

EK•••••
EKEDOUT
EKESOUT
EKINGBY
EKISTIC
EKUELES
EKWENSI

E•K••••
ECKHART
ELKHART
ESKIMOS

E••K•••
EIJKMAN
ELEKTRA
ENSKIED
ENSKIES
ERIKSON
ERSKINE
EVOKERS
EVOKING
EZEKIEL

E•••K••
EBANKED
EELSKIN
ETICKET
EUREKAS

E••••K•
EARLIKE
EATCAKE
EELLIKE
EGGLIKE
ELFLIKE
EMBANKS
EMBARKS
EMMUSKA
ENLINKS
ENRANKS
EUBANKS
EXWORKS
EXYANKS
EYELIKE

E•••••K
EARLOCK
EARMARK
EFGHIJK
ELDRICK
ELENIAK
ELFLOCK
EWENECK
EYEBANK
EYEHOOK
EYEMASK
EYETUCK
EYEWINK

•EK••••
DEKEING
DEKLERK
PEKEPOO
REKEYED
REKICKS
REKNEAD
REKNITS
REKNOCK
REKNOTS
TEKKIES

•E•K•••
BEAKERS
BECKETT
BECKHAM
BECKONS
BERKLEY
BERKNER
DECKERS
DECKING
DECKLED
DECKLES
DECKOUT
DELKEYS
DESKFUL
DESKSET
DESKTOP
GECKOES
GEEKDOM
GEEKIER
HECKART
HECKLED
HECKLER
HECKLES
HECKMAN
HECKUVA
HECKYES
JENKINS
JERKERS
JERKIER
JERKIES
JERKILY
JERKING
JERKINS
JERKOUT
JERKSUP
LEAKAGE
LEAKERS
LEAKEYS
LEAKIER
LEAKING
LEAKSIN
LETKNOW
MEEKEST
NECKERS
NECKING
NECKLET
NECKTIE
NEWKIDS
PEAKIER
PEAKING
PEAKISH
PECKING
PECKISH
PECKSAT
PEEKERS
PEEKING
PEEKOUT
PEEKSAT
PEEKSIN
PERKIER
PERKILY
PERKING
PERKINS
PERKISH
PERKSUP
PESKIER
PESKILY
RECKONS
REDKING
REEKERS
REEKIER
REEKING
REEKSOF
SECKELS
SEEKERS
SEEKING
SEEKOUT
SELKIRK
TEKKIES
TENKRUN
WEAKENS
WEAKEST
WEAKISH
WEAKONS
WEEKDAY
WEEKEND
WESKITS
WETKISS
YERKISH

•E••K••
BEERKEG
BETAKEN
BETAKES
BETOKEN
DEBAKEY
EELSKIN
HEARKEN
JETSKIS
MEDAKAS
MEERKAT
MENCKEN
MESSKIT
PERUKES
REASKED
REBAKED
REBAKES
REBEKAH
REBUKED
REBUKER
REBUKES
REDSKIN
REINKED
REMAKES
RERAKED
RERAKES
RETAKEN
RETAKER
RETAKES
REVOKED
REVOKER
REVOKES
REWAKED
REWAKEN
REWAKES
REWOKEN
REYOKED
REYOKES
TESTKIT
WENDKOS

•E•••K•
BEDECKS
BEDLIKE
BEELIKE
BESPOKE
DEBARKS
DEBUNKS
DEEPSKY
DEJUNKS
DEMARKS
EELLIKE
FEDERKO
GEMLIKE
HENLIKE
LEGLIKE
NETLIKE
NETSUKE
PEALIKE
PEGLIKE
PENLIKE
REAWAKE
REAWOKE
REBANKS
REBOOKS
REBROKE
RECOCKS
RECOOKS
RECORKS
REDOAKS
REDOCKS
REEBOKS
REEVOKE
REHOOKS
REKICKS
RELINKS
RELOCKS
RELOOKS
REMARKS
REPACKS
REPARKS
REPERKS
REPICKS
RERACKS
RERANKS
RESEEKS
RESINKS
RESOAKS
RESPOKE
RESTOKE
RETACKS
REWORKS
SEALIKE
TEACAKE
WEBLIKE
ZEDONKS
ZERNIKE

•E••••K
BEATNIK
BEDROCK
BELLEEK
BEQUICK
BERBICK
BERSERK
BERWICK
BESPEAK
BETHINK
DEFROCK
DEKLERK
DENMARK
DERRICK
DESTOCK
FEELSOK
FETLOCK
GEDRICK
GEMSBOK
GENLOCK
GEODUCK
GETBACK
HEMLOCK
HENPECK
HERRICK
HEYLOOK
JETPACK
KEYBANK
KEYLOCK
LEACOCK
LEBROCK
LEFREAK
LEGWORK
LETTERK
LEXMARK
MEDWICK
MENFOLK
MERRICK
MESSICK
NEATNIK
NESQUIK
NETWORK
NEWLOOK
NEWWEEK
NEWYORK
PEACOCK
PENNOCK
PEPTALK
PERCHIK
PERWEEK
PETCOCK
PETDUCK
PETROCK
REBLOCK

REBREAK
RECHALK
RECHECK
RECRANK
REDBOOK
REDHAWK
REDJACK
REDNECK
REKNOCK
RENWICK
RESPARK
RESPEAK
RESTACK
RESTICK
RESTOCK
RETHANK
RETHINK
RETRACK
SEADUCK
SEAHAWK
SEASICK
SELKIRK
SELLECK
SERIESK
SERIPAK
SETBACK
TEANECK
TEDMACK
TENWEEK
VEENECK
WEDLOCK
WEEFOLK
WETLOOK

••EK•••

ALEKEGS
ALEKSEI
CHEKHOV
ELEKTRA
EZEKIEL
GEEKDOM
GEEKIER
JOEKIDD
MEEKEST
ONEKILO
PEEKERS
PEEKING
PEEKOUT
PEEKSAT
PEEKSIN
REEKERS
REEKIER
REEKING
REEKSOF
SEEKERS
SEEKING
SEEKOUT
SHEKELS
THEKING
THEKISS
TREKKED
TREKKER
TREKKIE
WEEKDAY
WEEKEND

••E•K••

APECKOF
BEERKEG
BLEAKER
BLEAKLY
BREAKER
BREAKIN
BREAKUP
CHECKED
CHECKER
CHECKIN
CHECKON
CHECKUP
CHEEKED
CLERKED
CLERKLY
CREAKED
DOESKIN
FLECKED
FREAKED
FRECKLE
FRECKLY
GHERKIN
HAECKEL
IRECKON
JAECKEL
KRESKIN
MEERKAT
SHEIKHS
SLEEKED
SLEEKEN
SLEEKER
SLEEKLY
SNEAKBY
SNEAKED
SNEAKER
SNEAKIN
SNEAKUP
SPEAKER
SPEAKOF
SPEAKTO
SPEAKUP
SPECKED
SPECKLE
TREKKED
TREKKER
TREKKIE
TWEAKED
VNECKED
WREAKED
WREAKER
WRECKED
WRECKER

••E••K•

AMERIKA
APELIKE
ARENSKY
AXELIKE
BEELIKE
BREWSKI
DEEPSKY
EYELIKE
GRETZKY
HOECAKE
ICELIKE
PIELIKE
PREBAKE
PREMAKE
REEBOKS
REEVOKE
RHEBOKS
ROETHKE
THEDUKE
THELIKE
TOELIKE

••E•••K

ELENIAK
EWENECK
EYEBANK
EYEHOOK
EYEMASK
EYETUCK
EYEWINK
FEELSOK
ICEMILK
ICEPACK
ICEPICK
ICERINK
JOEBUCK
LIEBACK
OBELISK
ONELOOK
ONESOCK
ONEWEEK
PREBOOK
PRECOOK
PREDARK
PREDUSK
PREPACK
PREROCK
PRESOAK
PREWORK
ROEBUCK
SPELUNK
THEHULK
THEJERK
THELARK
THELOOK
THEMASK
THEMICK
THERINK
THEROCK
THESACK
TIEBACK
TIERACK
TIETACK
TOEPICK
VEENECK
WEEFOLK

•••EK••

CHEEKED
DAVEKOZ
EUREKAS
NICEKID
RAMEKIN
REBEKAH
SAMEKHS
SLEEKED
SLEEKEN
SLEEKER
SLEEKLY
TOPEKAN

•••E•K•

BEDECKS
BLUESKY
DANEYKO
FEDERKO
KOPECKS
LYSENKO
REPERKS
RESEEKS
SCREAKS
SQUEAKS
SQUEAKY
STREAKS
STREAKY
UNLEAKY

•••E••K

BODEREK
DONETSK
JONERIK
KUBELIK
LIVEOAK
SILENTK
VANEYCK
VITEBSK

••••EK•

RESEEKS
SHRIEKS

••••E•K

AFFLECK
BELLEEK
BERSERK
BESPEAK
BIGJERK
BOMBECK
BRUBECK
BYANECK
DEKLERK
EWENECK
GASLEAK
HENPECK
INCHECK
LEFREAK
LETTERK
LOWNECK
MIDWEEK
NEWWEEK
NONPEAK
OAKDESK
OFFPEAK
ONBREAK
ONEWEEK
OOBLECK
OUTSEEK
PERWEEK
QBSNEAK
REBREAK
RECHECK
REDNECK
RESPEAK
SELLECK
SERIESK
SIXWEEK
SUNDECK
TEANECK
TENWEEK
THEJERK
TWOWEEK
UNCHECK
UNSLEEK
UNSPEAK
VEENECK
WOZZECK
YASBECK

•••••EK

BANACEK
BELLEEK
BISHKEK
BODEREK
DOUBLEK
FARTLEK
JANACEK
JIRASEK
KAISHEK
MIDWEEK
NEWWEEK
ONEWEEK
OUTSEEK
PERWEEK
SIXWEEK
TENWEEK
TWOWEEK
UNSLEEK
VARITEK
ZATOPEK

EL•••••

ELAAIUN
ELAINES
ELAMITE
ELANCES
ELANETS
ELANTRA
ELAPIDS
ELAPSED
ELAPSES
ELASTIC
ELASTIN
ELATERS
ELATING
ELATION
ELBERTA
ELBOWED
ELBOWER
ELCAJON
ELCAMPO
ELDERLY
ELDRICH
ELDRICK
ELEANOR
ELEAZAR
ELECTED
ELECTEE
ELECTME
ELECTOR
ELECTRA
ELECTRO
ELEGANT
ELEGIAC
ELEGIES
ELEGIST
ELEGITS
ELEGIZE
ELEISON
ELEKTRA
ELEMENT
ELENIAK
ELEVATE
ELEVENA
ELEVENB
ELEVENC
ELEVEND
ELEVENE
ELEVENS
ELEVONS
ELFLIKE
ELFLOCK
ELFOWLS
ELFUDGE
ELGALLO
ELGRECO
ELICITS
ELIDERS
ELIDING
ELIEZER
ELIGIUS
ELISION
ELITEST
ELITISM
ELITIST
ELIXIRS
ELIYALE
ELKHART
ELLAMAE
ELLIOTT
ELLIPSE
ELLISON
ELLMANN
ELLYMAY
ELMCITY
ELMIEST
ELMISTI
ELMONTE
ELMTREE
ELMUNDO
ELMWOOD
ELNINOS
ELNORTE
ELOCUTE
ELOPERS
ELOPING
ELPRADO
ELTRAIN
ELUANTS
ELUATES
ELUDERS
ELUDING
ELUSIVE
ELUSORY
ELUTING
ELUTION
ELUVIAL
ELUVIUM
ELYSEES
ELYSIAN
ELYSIUM

E•L••••

ECLAIRS
ECLIPSE
ECLOGUE
EELIEST
EELLIKE
EELPOTS
EELPOUT
EELSKIN
EELWORM
EGLISES
ELLAMAE
ELLIOTT
ELLIPSE
ELLISON
ELLMANN
ELLYMAY
ENLACED
ENLACES
ENLARGE
ENLINKS
ENLISTS
ENLIVEN
EOLITHS
ERLANGS
EULABUS

E••L•••

EAGLETS
EAGLING
EARLAPS
EARLDOM
EARLESS
EARLETS
EARLIER
EARLIES
EARLIKE
EARLOBE
EARLOCK
EARLYON
EATLATE
EATLESS
ECCLESI
ECOLOGY
EELLIKE
EGALITE
EGGLERS
EGGLESS
EGGLIKE
EHRLICH
ELFLIKE
ELFLOCK
EMBLAZE
EMBLEMS
EMPLACE
EMPLANE
EMPLOYS
EMULATE
EMULOUS
ENCLASP
ENCLAVE
ENCLOSE
ENDLATE
ENDLEAF
ENDLESS
ENDLINE
ENDLONG
ENFLAME
ENGLAND
ENGLISH
ENGLUND
ENGLUTS
ENOLOGY
ENPLANE
ENSLAVE
EONLINE
EPILADY
EPILATE
EPILOGS
ERELONG
ETALIBI
EUGLENA
EVALUNA
EVELONG
EVILEST
EVILEYE
EVILLER
EVILONE
EVOLUTE
EVOLVED
EVOLVER
EVOLVES
EVULSED
EVULSES
EWELAMB
EXALTED
EXALTER
EXCLAIM
EXCLAVE
EXCLUDE
EXILERS
EXILING
EXPLAIN
EXPLODE
EXPLOIT
EXPLORE
EXULTED
EYELASH
EYELESS
EYELETS
EYELIDS
EYELIFT
EYELIKE
EYELINE

E•••L••

EARCLIP
EARFLAP
EARPLUG
EASELED
EATALOT
ECHELON
ECUELLE
EDIBLES
EIDOLIC
EIDOLON
EKUELES
ELGALLO
EMAILED
EMAILER
EMBALMS
EMMYLOU
EMPALED
EMPALES
ENABLED
ENABLER
ENABLES
ENDALLS
ENDPLAY
ENFOLDS
ENGILDS
ENGULFS
ENISLED
ENISLES
ENOILED
ENROLLS
ENSILED
ENSILES
ENVELOP
EPAULET
EPSILON
EQUALED
EQUALLY
EQUALTO
ESCALOP
ESCALUS
ESTELLA
ESTELLE
ETAILED
ETAILER
ETOILES
EVERLYS
EVILLER
EXCELAT
EXCELIN
EXHALED
EXHALES
EXOILER
EXTOLLS

E••••L•

EADGILS
EAGERLY
EARFULS
EARHOLE
EARTHLY
EATABLE
ECUELLE
EFFABLE
EFFABLY
EGGROLL
EJEMPLO
ELDERLY
ELFOWLS
ELGALLO
ELIYALE
EMERALD
EMPTILY
ENAMELS
ENDABLE
ENDALLS
ENFIELD
ENNOBLE
ENROLLS
ENSEALS
ENSOULS
ENTAILS
ENTITLE
ENVEILS
EPISTLE
EPPERLY
EQUABLE
EQUABLY
EQUALLY
ERECTLY
EROSELY
ERRABLE
ESCUELA
ESPIALS
ESTELLA
ESTELLE
ETVOILA
EXACTLY
EXAMPLE
EXEMPLA
EXTOLLS
EYEBALL
EYEBOLT
EYEFOLD
EYEFULS
EYEHOLE
EYEROLL
EYEWALL

E•••••L

EASEFUL
ECTYPAL
EDICTAL
EGGROLL
ELUVIAL
EMANUEL
EMBROIL
EMPANEL
ENSNARL
ENTHRAL
EPOCHAL
ESPANOL
ESTIVAL
ESTORIL
ETERNAL
ETHANOL
ETHICAL
EVANGEL
EXCUSAL
EYEBALL
EYEROLL
EYEWALL
EZEKIEL

•EL••••

AELFRIC
BELABOR
BELAIRS
BELARUS
BELASCO
BELATED
BELAYED
BELAYER
BELCHED
BELCHER
BELCHES
BELDAME
BELDAMS
BELEVEN
BELFAST
BELFORT
BELGIAN
BELGIUM
BELIEFS
BELIERS
BELIEVE
BELINDA
BELLAMY
BELLBOY
BELLEAU
BELLEEK
BELLHOP
BELLIED
BELLIES
BELLING
BELLINI
BELLJAR
BELLLAP
BELLMAN
BELLMEN
BELLOWS
BELLSON
BELLYUP
BELMONT
BELONGS
BELOVED
BELTANE
BELTBAG
BELTERS
BELTING
BELTOUT
BELTRAN
BELTSAW
BELTSUP
BELTWAY
BELUGAS
BELUSHI
BELVOIR
BELVOUR
BELYING
BELZONI
CELADON
CELAENO
CELEBES
CELEBRE
CELESTA
CELESTE
CELICAS
CELLARS
CELLINI
CELLIST
CELLULE
CELOTEX
CELSIUS
CELTICS
DELANEY
DELARUE
DELAYED
DELAYER
DELBERT
DELCITY
DELEADS
DELEDDA
DELEING
DELETED
DELETES
DELIBES
DELICTI
DELICTO
DELICTS
DELIGHT
DELIHAM
DELILAH
DELILLO
DELIMAN
DELIMEN
DELIMIT
DELINTS
DELIRIA
DELISTS
DELIVER
DELKEYS
DELMONT
DELMORE
DELORIS
DELORME
DELOUSE
DELPHIC
DELRAYS
DELRUTH
DELSOLS
DELTAIC
DELTOID
DELTONA
DELTORO
DELUDED
DELUDER
DELUDES
DELUGED
DELUGES
DELUISE
DELVERS
DELVING
EELIEST
EELLIKE
EELPOTS
EELPOUT
EELSKIN
EELWORM
FELDMAN
FELICIA
FELINES
FELLAHS
FELLDUE
FELLERS
FELLFOR
FELLING
FELLINI
FELLOFF
FELLOUT
FELLOWS
FELONRY
FELTBAD
FELTFOR
FELTHAT
FELTILL
FELTING
FELTOFF
FELTOUT
FELTPEN
FELTTIP
GELATED
GELATES
GELATIN
GELATIS
GELATOS
GELCAPS
GELDING
GELIDLY
GELLING
GELPENS
GELUSIL
HELDOFF
HELDOUT
HELICAL
HELICES
HELICON
HELIPAD
HELIXES
HELLBOY
HELLCAT
HELLENE
HELLENO
HELLION
HELLISH
HELLMAN
HELLOED
HELLOES
HELLUVA
HELLYES
HELMETS
HELMING
HELMOND
HELOISE
HELOTRY
HELPERS
HELPFUL
HELPING
HELPOUT
HELPSIN
HELPSON
HELPSUP
HELSING
JELLIED
JELLIES
JELLIFY
JELLING
KELLJAN
KELLOGG
KELOWNA
KELPIES
KELVINS
LELOUCH
MELAMED
MELANGE
MELANIA
MELANIC
MELANIE
MELANIN
MELDERS
MELDING
MELINDA
MELISMA
MELISSA
MELITTA
MELLOWS
MELODIA
MELODIC
MELROSE
MELTAGE
MELTERS
MELTING
NELSONS
PELAGES
PELAGIC
PELICAN
PELISSE
PELLEAS
PELLETS
PELOTAS
PELOTON
PELTATE
PELTERS
PELTING
PELTISH
RELABEL
RELACED

RELACES	TELESTO	BELLBOY	FELLOUT	NETLIKE	REFLOWN	WEALTHY	DELILLO	MEGILLA	REMILLS	•E•••L•	GETWELL	REBILLS
RELANCE	TELEXED	BELLEAU	FELLOWS	NETLOSS	REFLOWS	WEBLESS	DEMILLE	METALED	REMOLDS	AERIALS	HEADILY	REBOILS
RELANDS	TELEXES	BELLEEK	FETLOCK	NEWLAID	REGLAZE	WEBLIKE	DEMOLAY	METTLER	RENALDO	BEADILY	HEALALL	REBUILD
RELANES	TELLALL	BELLHOP	GELLING	NEWLEAF	REGLOSS	WEBLOGS	DEPALMA	METTLES	RENALLY	BEASTLY	HEAVILY	REBUILT
RELAPSE	TELLERS	BELLIED	GEMLESS	NEWLEFT	REGLOWS	WEDLOCK	DEPULPS	NEBULAE	REOILED	BEATALL	HEFTILY	RECABLE
RELATCH	TELLIES	BELLIES	GEMLIKE	NEWLIFE	REGLUED	WELLAND	DERALTE	NEBULAR	REPOLLS	BEDROLL	HERBALS	RECALLS
RELATED	TELLING	BELLING	GENLOCK	NEWLINE	REGLUES	WELLCUT	DESALTS	NEBULAS	REPULSE	BEEFALO	HERCULE	RECHALK
RELATER	TELLOFF	BELLINI	GEOLOGY	NEWLOOK	RELLENO	WELLFED	DESILTS	NECKLET	REROLLS	BEEFILY	HERSELF	RECHALL
RELATES	TELLSIT	BELLJAR	GETLOST	NEWLOVE	REPLACE	WELLHID	DESYLVA	NEEDLED	RESALES	BEFALLS	JERKILY	RECOALS
RELATOR	TELLSOF	BELLLAP	HEALALL	PEALIKE	REPLANE	WELLHIT	DEVALUE	NEEDLER	RESALTS	BEFOOLS	KENDALL	RECOILS
RELAXED	TELLSON	BELLMAN	HEALERS	PEALING	REPLANS	WELLING	DEVELOP	NEEDLES	RESELLS	BEFOULS	KENDOLL	RECOOLS
RELAXER	TELSTAR	BELLMEN	HEALING	PEELERS	REPLANT	WELLLED	DEVILED	NEPALIS	RESILED	BEGUILE	KENNELS	RECURLS
RELAXES	VELCROS	BELLOWS	HEALSUP	PEELING	REPLATE	WELLLIT	DEVILLE	NESTLED	RESILES	BENGALI	KERNELS	RECYCLE
RELAYED	VELLUMS	BELLSON	HEALTHY	PEELOFF	REPLAYS	WELLMAN	DEVILRY	NESTLER	RESOLED	BENGALS	KEYHOLE	REDCELL
RELAYER	VELOURS	BELLYUP	HEELERS	PEELOUT	REPLEAD	WELLOFF	DEVOLVE	NESTLES	RESOLER	BENZALI	KEYPALS	REDEALS
RELEADS	VELOUTE	BERLIOZ	HEELING	PEGLEGS	REPLETE	WELLPUT	DEWCLAW	NETFLIX	RESOLES	BENZELL	LEERILY	REDEALT
RELEAPS	VELOXES	BERLITZ	HEELPAD	PEGLESS	REPLICA	WELLRUN	DEWILDE	NETTLED	RESOLVE	BEOWULF	LEGALLY	REDIALS
RELEARN	VELTMAN	CEILING	HEELTAP	PEGLIKE	REPLIED	WELLSEE	FEEBLER	NETTLES	RESPLIT	BERTOLT	LEGIBLE	REDPOLL
RELEASE	VELURES	CELLARS	HELLBOY	PELLEAS	REPLIER	WELLSET	FEEDLOT	NEUILLY	RESULTS	BESSELL	LEGIBLY	REDRILL
RELENDS	VELVETS	CELLINI	HELLCAT	PELLETS	REPLIES	WELLSUP	FEMALES	NEVILLE	RETALLY	BESTILL	LEGPULL	REDWOLF
RELENTS	VELVETY	CELLIST	HELLENE	PENLIKE	REPLOTS	WELLWON	FENELON	PEARLED	RETELLS	BETHELS	LENTILS	REFALLS
RELEVEL	WELCOME	CELLULE	HELLENO	PENLITE	REPLOWS	WELLYES	FERULES	PEARLER	RETILED	BEVERLY	LEOPOLD	REFILLS
RELEVER	WELDERS	DEALERS	HELLION	PEPLUMS	REPLUMB	WETLAND	FETTLES	PEBBLED	RETILES	BEWAILS	LETFALL	REFUELS
RELEVES	WELDING	DEALING	HELLISH	PERLITE	REPLUME	WETLOOK	GEFILTE	PEBBLES	RETILLS	CEDILLA	LETROLL	REGALLY
RELIANT	WELFARE	DEALOUT	HELLMAN	PERLMAN	REPLYTO	YELLERS	GEMELLI	PEDALED	REVALUE	CELLULE	LETSFLY	REHAULS
RELICTS	WELLAND	DEALSIN	HELLOED	PETLAMB	RESLATE	YELLFOR	GENTLED	PEDALER	REVELED	CEMBALO	LEVELLY	REHEALS
RELIEFS	WELLCUT	DEALSTO	HELLOES	PETLION	SEALABS	YELLING	GENTLER	PEDDLED	REVELER	CENACLE	LEVILLI	REHEELS
RELIERS	WELLFED	DEALSUP	HELLUVA	REALEST	SEALANE	YELLOUT	GENTLES	PEDDLER	REVELIN	CENTALS	LEXUSLS	REIMPLY
RELIEVE	WELLHID	DEALTIN	HELLYES	REALIGN	SEALANT	YELLOWS	GERALDO	PEDDLES	REVELRY	CEPHALO	LEXUSLX	REJAILS
RELIGHT	WELLHIT	DEALTTO	HEMLINE	REALINE	SEALEGS	YELLOWY	HECKLED	PEEBLES	REVILED	CEPHALY	MEATILY	REMAILS
RELIMIT	WELLING	DEALTUP	HEMLOCK	REALISE	SEALERS	YELLSAT	HECKLER	PEEPLES	REVILER	CEREALS	MEDULLA	REMILLS
RELINED	WELLLED	DEBLURS	HENLIKE	REALISM	SEALERY	YESLETS	HECKLES	PENALTY	REVILES	DEBACLE	MEGILLA	RENAILS
RELINES	WELLLIT	DECLAIM	HEWLETT	REALIST	SEALIFE	ZEALAND	HEMSLEY	PENULTS	REVOLTS	DEBOULE	MENDELS	RENALLY
RELINKS	WELLMAN	DECLARE	HEYLOOK	REALITY	SEALIFT	ZEALOTS	HENSLEY	PEOPLED	REVOLVE	DECARLO	MENFOLK	RENAULT
RELISTS	WELLOFF	DECLASS	JEALOUS	REALIZE	SEALIKE	ZEALOUS	HERALDS	PEOPLES	REWELDS	DECUPLE	MENIALS	RENDELL
RELIVED	WELLPUT	DECLAWS	JELLIED	REALLOT	SEALILY	ZEELAND	JEANLUC	PERILED	SEABLUE	DEERFLY	MERRILL	RENTALS
RELIVES	WELLRUN	DECLINE	JELLIES	REALMAN	SEALING		JERILYN	PERPLEX	SEASLUG	DEFALLA	MERRILY	REPEALS
RELLENO	WELLSEE	DECLOTS	JELLIFY	REALMEN	SEALION	•E••L••	JEWELED	PESTLED	SECULAR	DEFAULT	MESCALS	REPOLLS
RELOADS	WELLSET	DEFLATE	JELLING	REALTER	SEALOFF	AEDILES	JEWELER	PESTLES	SEDALIA	DEFUELS	MESSALA	REPTILE
RELOANS	WELLSUP	DEFLEAS	JETLAGS	REALTOR	SEALSIN	BEADLES	JEWELRY	PETALED	SEEALSO	DEHMELT	MESSILY	REREELS
RELOCKS	WELLWON	DEFLECT	KEELING	REBLOCK	SEALSUP	BEAGLES	KEEBLER	PETALES	SEEDLET	DELILLO	METCALF	REROLLS
RELOOKS	WELLYES	DEGLAZE	KEGLERS	REBLOOM	SECLUDE	BEASLEY	KEESLAR	PETULIA	SEMILOG	DELSOLS	MEYNELL	RESCALE
RELOSES	WELTERS	DEKLERK	KEILLOR	REBLOWN	SELLECK	BEATLES	KEESLER	REALLOT	SEPALED	DEMILLE	NEEDILY	RESEALS
RELUCTS	WELTING	DEPLANE	KELLJAN	RECLADS	SELLERS	BECALMS	KEILLOR	REARLIT	SETPLAY	DENIALS	NERVILY	RESELLS
RELUMED	YELLERS	DEPLETE	KELLOGG	RECLAIM	SELLFOR	BEDELIA	KENOLIN	REBALED	SETTLED	DENSELY	NERVULE	RESMELT
RELUMES	YELLFOR	DEPLORE	KEYLESS	RECLAME	SELLING	BEETLES	KERFLOP	REBALES	SETTLER	DENTALS	NETBALL	RESOILS
RELYING	YELLING	DEPLOYS	KEYLIME	RECLASP	SELLOFF	BEFALLS	KERPLOP	REBILLS	SETTLES	DEPAULU	NETFULS	RESPELL
SELECTS	YELLOUT	DESLUMS	KEYLOCK	RECLASS	SELLOUT	BEHOLDS	KETTLES	REBOLTS	SETTLOR	DERAILS	NEUILLY	RESPELT
SELENIC	YELLOWS	DEWLAPS	LEBLANC	RECLEAN	SELLSIT	BELLLAP	KEYCLUB	RECALLS	SEVILLA	DESHELL	NEVILLE	RESTYLE
SELFISH	YELLOWY	DEWLESS	LEGLESS	RECLIMB	SELLSTO	BENBLUE	LEAFLET	RECOLOR	SEVILLE	DETAILS	NEWBOLT	RETABLE
SELKIRK	YELLSAT	DEWLINE	LEGLIKE	RECLINE	SERLING	BENELUX	LEFTLEG	REDALGA	TEBALDI	DEVILLE	PENCILS	RETAILS
SELLECK	YELPERS	EELLIKE	LETLIVE	RECLUSE	SEXLESS	BENTLEY	LEGALLY	REDCLAY	TEMBLOR	DEWFALL	PENPALS	RETALLY
SELLERS	YELPING	FEELBAD	MEALIER	REDLEGS	TEALEAF	BERKLEY	LEGOLAS	REDFLAG	TEMPLAR	FEBRILE	PENTELS	RETELLS
SELLFOR	YELTSIN	FEELERS	MEALIES	REDLINE	TEALESS	BEVELED	LETSLIP	REFALLS	TEMPLED	FEELILL	PEPPILL	RETICLE
SELLING	ZELAZNY	FEELESS	MEDLEYS	REELECT	TEFLONS	BEVELER	LEVELED	REFILED	TEMPLES	FELTILL	PEPPILY	RETILLS
SELLOFF		FEELFOR	MELLOWS	REELERS	TELLALL	CECILIA	LEVELER	REFILES	TESTLAB	FENNELS	PEPTALK	RETITLE
SELLOUT	•E•L•••	FEELILL	MEMLING	REELING	TELLERS	CEDILLA	LEVELLY	REFILLS	VEINLET	FERRULE	PERCALE	RETOOLS
SELLSIT	AEOLIAN	FEELING	MERLINS	REELOFF	TELLIES	DECALOG	LEVILLI	REFILMS	VENALLY	FERTILE	PERGOLA	REVEALS
SELLSTO	BEALION	FEELOFF	MERLOTS	REELOUT	TELLING	DECILES	MEAGLES	REFOLDS	VENULES	FETIDLY	PERKILY	SEACALM
SELMAAL	BECLOUD	FEELOUT	METLIFE	REELSIN	TELLOFF	DECKLED	MEASLES	REGALED	VERYLOW	GELIDLY	PESKILY	SEAEELS
SELTZER	BEDLAMP	FEELSOK	MEWLERS	REELSUP	TELLSIT	DECKLES	MECHLIN	REGALER	WEDELED	GEMELLI	PETCALF	SEAGULL
SELVAGE	BEDLAMS	FELLAHS	MEWLING	REFLAGS	TELLSOF	DECOLOR	MEDALED	REGALES	WEDELNS	GENTILE	PETIOLE	SEALILY
TELAVIV	BEDLESS	FELLDUE	NEDLAND	REFLATE	TELLSON	DEDALUS	MEDDLED	REGALIA	WELLLED	GERBILS	PETMULE	SEAMILE
TELECOM	BEDLIKE	FELLERS	NEGLECT	REFLECT	VEALIER	DEFALLA	MEDDLER	REGALLY	WELLLIT	GESTALT	PETRELS	SEASALT
TELEFAX	BEDLOES	FELLFOR	NEOLITH	REFLIES	VEILERS	DEFILED	MEDDLES	REGILDS	WEMBLEY	GETABLE	PETROLS	SEATTLE
TELEPIC	BEELIKE	FELLING	NEOLOGY	REFLIPS	VEILING	DEFILER	MEDELES	REGULAR	ZEBULON	GETCOLD	PETTILY	SEAWALL
TELEPIX	BEELINE	FELLINI	NEOLYTE	REFLOAT	VELLUMS	DEFILES	MEDULLA	REGULUS	ZEBULUN	GETHELP	READILY	SEAWOLF
TELERAN	BELLAMY	FELLOFF	NETLESS	REFLOOD	WEALTHS	DELILAH	MEGALON	REMELTS	ZEDILLO	GETSOLD	REAPPLY	SECKELS

SEEABLE
SEEDILY
SEENALL
SEESALL
SEQUELS
SERIALS
SERVILE
SESSILE
SEVILLA
SEVILLE
TEABALL
TEARILY
TEASELS
TELLALL
TENABLE
TENABLY
TENBALL
TENFOLD
TENMILE
TENSELY
TENSILE
TENTHLY
TEPIDLY
TEQUILA
TERCELS
TERRELL
TERSELY
TESTFLY
TESTILY
TEXTILE
VEHICLE
VEINULE
VENABLE
VENALLY
VERBALS
VERDELL
VERYILL
VERYOLD
VESICLE
VESSELS
VESTALS
VEXEDLY
WEARILY
WEASELS
WEDDELL
WEEDILY
WEEFOLK
WEEVILS
WEIRDLY
WENDELL
WETBULB
WETCELL
ZEDILLO
ZEPPOLE
ZEPPOLI
ZESTILY

•E••••L

AEROSOL
BEANOIL
BEATALL
BEDEVIL
BEDRAIL
BEDROLL
BEJEWEL
BENZELL
BESSELL
BESTIAL
BESTILL
CENTRAL
DECIBEL
DECIMAL
DEMEROL
DEPOSAL
DESHELL
DESKFUL
DESPOIL
DESTAEL
DEWFALL
DEXTRAL
FEARFUL
FEDERAL
FEELILL
FELTILL
FEMORAL
GELUSIL
GEMAYEL
GENERAL
GENTEEL
GERITOL
GETREAL
GETWELL
HEADFUL
HEALALL
HEATFUL
HEEDFUL
HELICAL
HELPFUL
JETFOIL
JEZEBEL
KENDALL
KENDOLL
KENWAHL
KESTREL
LEGPULL
LESPAUL
LESTOIL
LETFALL
LETROLL
LETTERL
LEXICAL
MEDICAL
MENTHOL
MERRILL
MEYNELL
NEEDFUL
NESTFUL
NETBALL
NEUTRAL
NEWDEAL
OEDIPAL
PEAFOWL
PEPPILL
PERORAL
PERUSAL
REAVAIL
RECHALL
RECITAL
RECUSAL
REDCELL
REDPOLL
REDRILL
REDTAIL
REEXPEL
REFUSAL
REFUTAL
REGINAL
RELABEL
RELEVEL
REMODEL
REMOVAL
RENDELL
RENEWAL
REPANEL
RESPELL
RESPOOL
RESTFUL
RETINAL
RETINOL
RETOTAL
RETRIAL
REVISAL
REVIVAL
SEAFOWL
SEAGULL
SEAWALL
SEENALL
SEESALL
SEISMAL
SELMAAL
SEMINAL
SENEGAL
SENSUAL
SETBAIL
SETSAIL
SEVERAL
TEABALL
TEARFUL
TELLALL
TENBALL
TENDRIL
TENNIEL
TENTFUL
TERRELL
TEXTUAL
VEGETAL
VENTRAL
VERDELL
VERMEIL
VERYILL
VESTRAL
WEBMAIL
WEDDELL
WEIRDAL
WENDELL
WETCELL
XENICAL
ZESTFUL

••EL•••

ABELARD
ADELIES
ADELINA
ADELINE
ADELPHI
AGELESS
AGELONG
ANELING
APELETS
APELIKE
ATELATE
ATELESS
ATELIER
AWELESS
AXELIKE
AXELROD
BEELIKE
BEELINE
BUELLER
CHELATE
CHELSEA
DUELERS
DUELING
DUELIST
DUELLED
DWELLAT
DWELLED
DWELLER
DWELLIN
DWELLON
DWELTON
DYELOTS
ERELONG
EVELONG
EWELAMB
EYELASH
EYELESS
EYELETS
EYELIDS
EYELIFT
EYELIKE
EYELINE
FEELBAD
FEELERS
FEELESS
FEELFOR
FEELILL
FEELING
FEELOFF
FEELOUT
FEELSOK
FIELDED
FIELDER
FOELESS
FRELENG
FUELERS
FUELING
FUELLED
FUELOIL
FUELROD
FUELSUP
GIELGUD
HEELERS
HEELING
HEELPAD
HEELTAP
HUELESS
ICELAND
ICELESS
ICELIKE
ICELINE
IRELAND
IRELESS
KEELING
KJELLIN
KNELLED
KVELLED
MUELLER
NIELSEN
OBELISE
OBELISK
OBELIZE
OCELLAR
OCELLUS
OCELOTS
ODELETS
OKELLEY
OMELETS
ONELANE
ONELIRA
ONELOOK
ONELOVE
ONELUMP
ORELESS
PAELLAS
PEELERS
PEELING
PEELOFF
PEELOUT
PIELIKE
PRELACY
PRELATE
PRELIFE
PRELIMS
PRELOAD
PRELOAN
PRELOSS
PRELUDE
QUELLED
QUELLER
QUELQUE
REELECT
REELERS
REELING
REELOFF
REELOUT
REELSIN
REELSUP
RYELOAF
SHELDON
SHELLAC
SHELLED
SHELLER
SHELLEY
SHELTER
SHELTIE
SHELVED
SHELVER
SHELVES
SKELTER
SKELTON
SMELLED
SMELLER
SMELTED
SMELTER
SNELLEN
SPELLED
SPELLER
SPELUNK
STELIAS
STELLAR
SUELLEN
SUELYON
SVELTER
SWELLED
SWELLER
SWELLUP
SWELTER
SWELTRY
THELAMB
THELARK
THELEFT
THELIKE
THELOOK
THELOOP
TIELESS
TIELINE
TOELESS
TOELIKE
TOELOOP
TRELLIS
TSELIOT
TWELFTH
TWELVEA
TWELVEB
TWELVEC
TWELVED
TWELVEE
TWELVES
UKELELE
USELESS
VIELLES
WHELMED
WHELPED
WIELAND
WIELDED
WIELDER
YIELDED
YIELDER
YIELDTO
ZEELAND
ZOELLER

••E•L••

AKERLOF
AMESLAN
AREOLAE
AREOLAR
AREOLAS
AREOLES
ATEALOT
BEETLES
BRESLIN
BUELLER
CHEMLAB
CREELEY
CREOLES
DREXLER
DUELLED
DWELLAT
DWELLED
DWELLER
DWELLIN
DWELLON
EVERLYS
FEEBLER
FEEDLOT
FIEDLER
FUELLED
GREELEY
GREMLIN
GREYLAG
ICEBLUE
ICEFLOE
IDEALLY
JOEBLOW
KEEBLER
KEESLAR
KEESLER
KJELLIN
KNEELED
KNEELER
KNELLED
KOEHLER
KREMLIN
KVELLED
LIESLOW
MUELLER
MUESLIS
MUESLIX
NEEDLED
NEEDLER
NEEDLES
OBERLIN
OCELLAR
OCELLUS
OKELLEY
ONECLAM
ONECLUB
OREILLY
OVERLAP
OVERLAX
OVERLAY
OVERLET
OVERLIE
OVERLIT
PAELLAS
PEEBLES
PEEPLES
PREALLY
PREPLAN
PREPLOT
PRESLEY
PUEBLOS
QUELLED
QUELLER
SEEALSO
SEEDLET
SHEILAE
SHEILAS
SHELLAC
SHELLED
SHELLER
SHELLEY
SMELLED
SMELLER
SNELLEN
SPELLED
SPELLER
STEALER
STEALIN
STEALTH
STEELED
STEELER
STEELIE
STELLAR
SUELLEN
SWELLED
SWELLER
SWELLUP
THEALPS
THEBLOB
THEFLEA
THEFLOP
TIECLIP
TREBLED
TREBLES
TREELET
TRELLIS
VIELLES
WHEELED
WHEELER
WHEELIE
WHEELIN
ZIEGLER
ZOELLER

••E••L•

ACEROLA
ACETALS
ADEPTLY
ALERTLY
ALEVELS
AVERELL
AVERILL
BEEFALO
BEEFILY
BLEAKLY
CHEADLE
CHEAPLY
CLEANLY
CLEARLY
CLERKLY
COEVALS
CRENELS
CREWELS
CUEBALL
DEERFLY
DIEBOLD
DIESELS
DREXELU
EJEMPLO
EMERALD
ERECTLY
EXEMPLA
EYEBALL
EYEBOLT
EYEFOLD
EYEFULS
EYEHOLE
EYEROLL
EYEWALL
FEELILL
FIERILY
FLEEGLE
FLEETLY
FLESHLY
FLEXILE
FRECKLE
FRECKLY
FRESHLY
GREATLY
GREENLY
GREWOLD
ICECOLD
ICEFALL
ICEHOLE
ICEMILK
IDEALLY
INEPTLY
INERTLY
INEXILE
JOEHILL
LAEMMLE
LEERILY
NEEDILY
OBESELY
OLEBULL
OLEVELS
ONEBALL
ONEBELL
ONECALL
ONECELL
ONEFOLD
ONEHALF
ONEKILO
ONEMILE
ONESELF
OREILLY
OVERALL
OVERFLY
OVERPLY
OVERTLY
PHENOLS
PIEBALD
PIEHOLE
PIESALE
PREALLY
PREBILL
PREFILE
PRESALE
PRESALT
PRESELL
PRESOLD
PRETELL
PRETOLD
PUERILE
QUEENLY
QUEERLY
SEEABLE
SEEDILY
SEENALL
SEESALL
SHEERLY
SHEKELS
SHEWOLF
SLEEKLY
SPECKLE
STEEPLE
STEEPLY
STERILE
STERNLY
STEROLS
SWEETLY
THEBELL
THEDELL
THEDOLE
THEFALL
THEGOLD
THEHELP
THEHILL
THEHULK
THEMALL
THENILE
THERULE
THESELF
THEWALL
TIEPOLO
TOEHOLD
TREACLE
TREACLY
TREADLE
TREMBLE
TREMBLY
TREMOLO
TRESTLE
TWEEDLE
UKELELE
UPEARLY
WEEDILY
WEEFOLK
WEEVILS
WHEEDLE
WHERELL
WRESTLE

••E•••L

ABETTAL
ASEXUAL
AVERELL
AVERILL
AVERNAL
BRENDEL
CHERVIL
COEQUAL
CREEDAL
CREOSOL
CUEBALL
DREIDEL
DWEEZIL
ETERNAL
EYEBALL
EYEROLL
EYEWALL
EZEKIEL
FEELILL
FRESNEL
FRETFUL
FUELOIL
GLEEFUL
GRENDEL
HAECKEL
HEEDFUL
HRETHEL
ICEFALL
JAECKEL
JOECOOL
JOEHILL
NEEDFUL
OLEBULL
OLEOOIL
ONEBALL
ONEBELL
ONECALL
ONECELL
ONEREEL
OVERALL
PLEURAL
PREBILL
PREBOIL
PRECOIL
PRECOOL
PREHEAL
PREORAL
PREQUEL
PRESEAL
PRESELL
PRESSEL
PRETELL
PRETZEL
PREVAIL
QUETZAL
REEXPEL
SEENALL
SEESALL
SLEDFUL
SMEAGOL
SPECIAL
STEMPEL
STENCIL
STENGEL
STERNAL
THEBELL
THEDELL
THEFALL
THEFOOL
THEHILL
THEMALL
THERMAL
THEWALL
TOENAIL
TREFOIL
UNEQUAL
UTENSIL
WHERELL

•••EL••

AACELLS
ACDELCO
ALLELES
ALLELIC
ALLELSE
ANGELAS
ANGELES
ANGELIC
ANGELOU
ANGELUS
ANNELID
ANSELMO
APHELIA
BEDELIA
BENELUX
BEVELED
BEVELER
BIBELOT
BIGELOW
BLUELAW
BOCELLI
BONELET
BTWELVE
CAMELID
CAMELOT
CAPELET
CAPELLA
CASELAW
CASELLA
CASELOT
CONELET
CORELLI
CREELEY
CRUELER
CRUELLA
CRUELLY
CRUELTY
CUPELED
CUPELER
DANELAW
DEVELOP
DOVELET
DRMELFI
DRWELBY
EASELED
ECHELON
ECUELLE
EKUELES
ENVELOP
ESTELLA
ESTELLE
EXCELAT
EXCELIN
FENELON
FIDELES
FIDELIA
FIDELIO
FIDELIS
FIRELIT
FORELEG
GAMELAN
GAMELAW
GAMELEG
GATELEG
GAVELED
GAZELLE
GEMELLI
GISELLE
GOBELIN
GOBELOW
GREELEY
HAMELIN
HGWELLS
HOMELAB
HOWELLS
HOWELSE
HYGELAC
ITWELVE
JAVELIN
JEWELED
JEWELER
JEWELRY
JOCELYN
JUDELAW
KNEELED
KNEELER
KUBELIK
LABELED
LABELER
LABELLE
LAPELED
LAVELLI
LEVELED
LEVELER
LEVELLY
LIBELED
LIBELEE
LIBELER
LORELAI
LORELEI
LOUELLA
MADELON
MEDELES
MODELAS
MODELBS
MODELED
MODELER
MODELTS
MORELLA
MORELLO
MORELOS
MOSELLE
MTPELEE
NACELLE
NORELCO
NOVELAS
NOVELLA
NOVELLE
NOVELLO
NOVELTY
OPHELIA
OTHELLO
PACELAP
PANELED
PAPELES
PATELLA
PIRELLI
POMELOS
POPELEO
RAVELED
RAVELLY
RAVELOE
REMELTS
RESELLS
RETELLS
REVELED
REVELER
REVELIN
REVELRY
REWELDS
ROSELLA
ROSELLE
ROTELLE
ROWELED
ROZELLE
RUBELLA
SCHELDT
SHIELDS
SPIELED
SPIELER
SQUELCH
STEELED
STEELER
STEELIE
TIMELAG
TOCELIA
TOHELEN
TONELOC
TOWELED
TREELET
TUPELOS
TUTELAR
UCCELLO
UNBELDI
UNBELTS
UNHELMS
UNSELLS
UPWELLS
VOWELLY
WAVELET
WEDELED
WEDELNS
WHEELED
WHEELER
WHEELIE
WHEELIN
YALELAW

YODELED
YODELER
YULELOG

•••E•L•

AACELLS
ADDEDLY
ALVEOLI
ANNEALS
APPEALS
AUREOLA
AUREOLE
BEVERLY
BLUEFLU
BOCELLI
BRIEFLY
CAPELLA
CASELLA
CEREALS
CHIEFLY
CINEOLE
CORELLI
CRUELLA
CRUELLY
CUREALL
DATEDLY
DAZEDLY
EAGERLY
ECUELLE
ELDERLY
ENSEALS
ENVEILS
EPPERLY
ESTELLA
ESTELLE
FADEDLY
FIREFLY
FIXEDLY
FLEEGLE
FLEETLY
GAZELLE
GEMELLI
GISELLE
GREENLY
HGWELLS
HOWELLS
INNERLY
JADEDLY
LABELLE
LAVELLI
LEVELLY
LOUELLA
LOVERLY
MADEILL
MAKEILL
MCNEILL
MINEOLA
MISERLY
MIXEDLY
MORELLA
MORELLO
MOSELLE
MUDEELS
MUTEDLY
NACELLE
NAKEDLY
NOTEDLY
NOVELLA
NOVELLE
NOVELLO
ORDEALS
ORDERLY
OSCEOLA
OTHELLO
PALEALE
PATELLA
PIRELLI
QUEENLY
QUEERLY
QUIETLY
RAVELLY
REDEALS
REDEALT
REHEALS
REHEELS
REPEALS
REREELS
RESEALS
RESELLS
RETELLS
REVEALS
ROSELLA
ROSELLE
ROSEOLA
ROTELLE
ROZELLE
RUBELLA
RUBEOLA
SAMEOLD
SEAEELS
SHEERLY
SHTETLS
SLEEKLY
SOBERLY
SQUEALS
STEEPLE
STEEPLY
SWEETLY
TAKEILL
TIREDLY
TWEEDLE
UCCELLO
UNDEALT
UNPEELS
UNREELS
UNSEALS
UNSELLS
UNVEILS
UPWELLS
UTTERLY
VEXEDLY
VIXENLY
VOWELLY
WHEEDLE

•••E••L

ADRENAL
ANBESOL
APTERAL
ARSENAL
BALEFUL
BANEFUL
BEDEVIL
BEJEWEL
BILEVEL
BIMETAL
BIPEDAL
BODEFUL
BRUEGEL
CAMERAL
CAREFUL
CLUEFUL
CREEDAL
CUREALL
DAREFUL
DEMEROL
DIREFUL
DOLEFUL
DONEGAL
DWEEZIL
EASEFUL
FANEUIL
FATEFUL
FEDERAL
FROEBEL
GAMETAL
GENERAL
GLEEFUL
GODEVIL
GONERIL
HATEFUL
HOPEFUL
HUMERAL
ILLEGAL
IMPERIL
INPERIL
JEZEBEL
JUVENAL
KNIEVEL
LATERAL
LIBERAL
LIFEFUL
LITERAL
MADEILL
MAKEILL
MCNEILL
MINERAL
MUSEFUL
NONEVIL
NUMERAL
ORTEGAL
PINEOIL
PINESOL
PIPEFUL
RAGEFUL
RAVENAL
RELEVEL
RENEWAL
ROSEOIL
SCLERAL
SENEGAL
SEVERAL
SILENTL
SPHERAL
SPIEGEL
TAKEILL
TUNEFUL
TYLENOL
UNLEGAL
UNLEVEL
UNREGAL
UNVENAL
VANEXEL
VEGETAL
WAKEFUL

••••EL•

AAACELL
ACUTELY
AGILELY
ALEVELS
ALUDELS
AMSTELS
ARCWELD
AVERELL
BAGWELL
BARBELL
BARRELS
BENZELL
BESSELL
BETHELS
BISSELL
BLAKELY
BOATELS
BOSWELL
BRAVELY
BRUTELY
BUNUELO
BUSHELS
BUZZELL
CANCELS
CANDELA
CANNELL
CANNELS
CARMELA
CARPELS
CARRELS
CARTELS
CARVELS
CHANELS
CHAPELS
CHISELS
CLAVELL
CLOSELY
COMPELS
CORBELS
CORDELL
CORNELL
CORYELL
COWBELL
CRENELS
CREWELS
CROWELL
CRUDELY
CUDGELS
DAMSELS
DANGELO
DANIELA
DANIELJ
DANIELS
DARNELL
DARWELL
DEFUELS
DEHMELT
DENSELY
DESHELL
DIDWELL
DIESELS
DISPELS
DREXELU
DRIVELS
DRYCELL
DRYWELL
DUFFELS
DURRELL
ENAMELS
ENFIELD
EROSELY
ESCUELA
FALSELY
FALWELL
FANBELT
FARFELS
FARRELL
FATCELL
FENNELS
FITWELL
FUNNELS
GASKELL
GETHELP
GETWELL
GIMBELS
GOSPELS
GOTHELP
GOTWELL
GRAVELS
GRAVELY
GROVELS
GUNBELT
GUNSELS
HARWELL
HASKELL
HERSELF
HIMSELF
HOSTELS
HUBBELL
HUMMELS
IFIFELL
ILLTELL
ILOVELA
IMSWELL
INANELY
INDWELL
INDWELT
INFIELD
INKWELL
IRATELY
ISOHELS
ISRAELI
JARRELL
JODRELL
KENNELS
KERNELS
KINNELL
KISSELS
KORDELL
KUMMELS
LAPBELT
LARGELY
LATRELL
LAURELS
LINTELS
LIONELL
LIONELS
LITHELY
LOOSELY
LYOCELL
LYONELL
MANDELA
MANTELS
MARCELS
MARVELL
MARVELS
MAXWELL
MENDELS
MEYNELL
MICAELA
MISRELY
MISTELL
MORSELS
MUDEELS
MURIELS
MUSSELS
NAIVELY
NICKELS
NONSELF
NOTWELL
OBESELY
OILWELL
OLEVELS
ONEBELL
ONECELL
ONESELF
OURSELF
OUTSELL
OUTTELL
OUTWELL
OUTYELL
OUTYELP
PACBELL
PARCELS
PASSELS
PASTELS
PAYWELL
PENTELS
PETRELS
POMMELS
PRESELL
PRETELL
PRIMELY
PRONELY
PROPELS
PUMMELS
PURCELL
QUINELA
RAPPELS
RAYNELL
REDCELL
REFUELS
REHEELS
RENDELL
REREELS
RESMELT
RESPELL
RESPELT
RONDELS
ROSWELL
RUNNELS
RUSSELL
SAMUELL
SATWELL
SEAEELS
SECKELS
SEQUELS
SHAPELY
SHEKELS
SHOVELS
SITWELL
SNIDELY
SNIVELS
SORRELL
SORRELS
SPACELY
SPARELY
SPINELS
STALELY
STATELY
STOKELY
SUAVELY
SUBCELL
SUNBELT
SWIVELS
TANGELO
TARBELL
TASSELS
TEASELS
TENSELY
TERCELS
TERRELL
TERSELY
THEBELL
THEDELL
THEHELP
THESELF
THYSELF
TINSELS
TRAVELS
TRITELY
TROWELS
TUNNELS
UKELELE
UKULELE
UNPEELS
UNREELS
UNSHELL
UNSPELT
UPFIELD
UPSWELL
VAGUELY
VANPELT
VERDELL
VESSELS
VONZELL
WADDELL
WANKELS
WEASELS
WEDDELL
WENDELL
WETCELL
WHERELL
WHITELY
WILHELM
WORRELL
YARNELL

••••E•L

AAACELL
ALLHEAL
ANTHEIL
APOGEAL
AVERELL
BAGWELL
BARBELL
BENZELL
BESSELL
BIGDEAL
BIGMEAL
BISSELL
BOSWELL
BUMDEAL
BUZZELL
CANNELL
CLAVELL
CONCEAL
CONGEAL
CORDELL
CORNEAL
CORNELL
CORYELL
COWBELL
CROWELL
DARNELL
DARWELL
DESHELL
DIDWELL
DOADEAL
DRYCELL
DRYWELL
DURRELL
FALWELL
FARRELL
FATCELL
FITWELL
FLOREAL
FORREAL
FURSEAL
GAGREEL
GASKELL
GENTEEL
GETREAL
GETWELL
GLUTEAL
GOTREAL
GOTWELL
HARWELL
HASKELL
HOTMEAL
HUBBELL
HUSSERL
IFIFELL
ILLTELL
IMSWELL
INDWELL
INKWELL
JARRELL
JODRELL
KINNELL
KORDELL
LACTEAL
LATRELL
LETTERL
LIONELL
LOWHEEL
LYOCELL
LYONELL
MACNEIL
MARVELL
MAXWELL
MEYNELL
MISDEAL
MISTELL
MRSPEEL
NEWDEAL
NOTREAL
NOTWELL
OATMEAL
OILWELL
ONEBELL
ONECELL
ONEREEL
ONTHEDL
OUTFEEL
OUTSELL
OUTTELL
OUTWELL
OUTYELL
PACBELL
PASSEUL
PAYWELL
PINSEAL
PREHEAL
PRESEAL
PRESELL
PRETELL
PURCELL
RAWDEAL
RAYNELL
REDCELL
RENDELL
RESPELL
ROSWELL
RUSSELL
SAMUELL
SATWELL
SITWELL
SORRELL
SOYMEAL
SUBCELL
SURREAL
SURVEIL
TARBELL
TARHEEL
TERRELL
THEBELL
THEDELL
UNIDEAL
UNSHELL
UNSTEEL
UNWHEEL
UPSWELL
USSTEEL
VERDELL
VERMEIL
VONZELL
WADDELL
WEDDELL
WENDELL
WETCELL
WHERELL
WORRELL
YARNELL

•••••EL

ANNABEL
APPAREL
ARUNDEL
BEJEWEL
BILEVEL
BIOFUEL
BRENDEL
BRUEGEL
BRUMMEL
CARAMEL
CARAVEL
CHANCEL
CHANNEL
CHATTEL
CHUNNEL
CITADEL
CLAUDEL
COLONEL
COUNSEL
COZUMEL
DAMOSEL
DECIBEL
DESTAEL
DOUBLEL
DREIDEL
DUHAMEL
EMANUEL
EMPANEL
EVANGEL
EZEKIEL
FALAFEL
FLANNEL
FRESNEL
FROEBEL
GABRIEL
GAGREEL
GEMAYEL
GENTEEL
GQMODEL
GRAPNEL
GRENDEL
HAECKEL
HAIRGEL
HANDSEL
HRETHEL
IMPANEL
INFIDEL
ISHMAEL
ISRAFEL
JAECKEL
JEZEBEL
KESTREL
KNIEVEL
KRACKEL
LOWHEEL
MANDREL
MICHAEL
MIRABEL
MONGREL
MRSPEEL
NATUREL
NOANGEL
NONFUEL
ONEREEL
OUTDUEL
OUTFEEL
PREQUEL
PRESSEL
PRETZEL
QUARREL
RACHAEL
RAPHAEL
REEXPEL
RELABEL
RELEVEL
REMODEL
REPANEL
ROUNDEL
SANIBEL
SATCHEL
SCALPEL
SHRIVEL
SNORKEL
SOFTGEL
SPANIEL
SPIEGEL
STEMPEL
STENGEL
STIFFEL
STRUDEL
SYNFUEL
TARHEEL
TENNIEL
TRAMMEL
TRAUBEL
TUMBREL
UMBRIEL
UNCRUEL
UNLEVEL
UNNOVEL
UNRAVEL
UNSTEEL
UNWHEEL
USSTEEL
VANEXEL
VONOPEL
WASTREL
WRANGEL

EM•••••

EMAILED
EMAILER
EMANANT
EMANATE
EMANUEL
EMBALMS
EMBANKS
EMBARGO
EMBARKS
EMBASSY
EMBAYED
EMBLAZE
EMBLEMS
EMBOITE
EMBOSOM
EMBOWER
EMBRACE
EMBROIL
EMBROWN
EMBRUED
EMBRUES
EMBRYOS
EMENDED
EMENDER
EMERALD
EMERGED
EMERGES
EMERIES
EMERITA
EMERITI
EMERSED
EMERSON
EMETICS
EMIGREE
EMIGRES
EMINENT
EMIRATE
EMITTED
EMITTER
EMMUSKA
EMMYLOU
EMOTERS
EMOTING
EMOTION
EMOTIVE
EMPALED
EMPALES
EMPANEL
EMPATHS
EMPATHY
EMPEROR
EMPIRES
EMPIRIC
EMPIRIN
EMPLACE
EMPLANE
EMPLOYS
EMPORIA
EMPOWER
EMPRESS
EMPRISE
EMPTIED
EMPTIER
EMPTIES
EMPTILY
EMQUADS
EMULATE
EMULOUS

E•M••••

EDMEESE
EDMONDS
EDMUNDI
EDMUNDS
ELMCITY
ELMIEST
ELMISTI
ELMONTE
ELMTREE
ELMUNDO
ELMWOOD
EMMUSKA
EMMYLOU
ENMASSE
ERMINED
ERMINES
ERMINIA
EXMATES
EXMAYOR

E••M•••

EANMUND
EARMARK
EARMUFF
EATMORE
EDEMATA
EDOMITE
EJEMPLO
ELAMITE
ELEMENT
ELLMANN
ENAMELS
ENAMORS
ENAMOUR
ENDMOST
ENEMIES
EREMITE
ETAMINE
ETHMOID
ETYMONS
EXAMINE
EXAMPLE
EXEMPLA
EXEMPTS
EYEMASK

E•••M••

EASTMAN
ECZEMAS
EDNAMAY
EIJKMAN
ELCAMPO
ELLAMAE
ELLYMAY
ENARMED
ENCAMPS
ENCOMIA
ENDEMIC
ENIGMAS
ENTOMBS
ENZYMES
ENZYMIC
ERASMUS
ESKIMOS
ESTAMIN
EUDEMON
EUNOMIA
EXHUMED
EXHUMER
EXHUMES

E••••M•

ECONOMY
EDINAMN
ELECTME
EMBALMS
EMBLEMS
ENDGAME
ENFLAME
ENFRAME
ENGRAMS
EPITOME
EPONYMS
EPONYMY
ESTEEMS
EUONYMS
EWELAMB
EXANIMO
EXENEMY
EXOGAMY
EXONYMS
EXTREME

E•••••M

EARDRUM
EARLDOM
EASTHAM
EATFROM
ECHOISM
EELWORM
EGOTISM

EIGHTAM
EIGHTPM
ELITISM
ELUVIUM
ELYSIUM
EMBOSOM
ENVENOM
EPHRAIM
EPIDERM
EPIGRAM
ERRATUM
EXCLAIM
EXOTISM
EYEEXAM

•EM••••

BEMIRED
BEMIRES
BEMOANS
BEMUSED
BEMUSES
CEMBALO
CEMENTS
DEMAGOG
DEMANDS
DEMARCO
DEMARET
DEMARKS
DEMASTS
DEMBUMS
DEMEANS
DEMENTO
DEMERGE
DEMERIT
DEMEROL
DEMESNE
DEMETER
DEMIGOD
DEMILLE
DEMISED
DEMISES
DEMISTS
DEMOING
DEMOLAY
DEMONIC
DEMONYM
DEMOTED
DEMOTES
DEMOTHS
DEMOTIC
DEMOUNT
DEMPSEY
DEMURER
FEMALES
FEMBOTS
FEMINUM
FEMORAL
FEMORIS
GEMAYEL
GEMELLI
GEMINIS
GEMLESS
GEMLIKE
GEMMATE
GEMMIER
GEMSBOK
HEMATIC
HEMATIN
HEMLINE
HEMLOCK
HEMMERS
HEMMING
HEMPIER
HEMSLEY
JEMISON
KEMIDOV
KEMPTON
LEMIEUX
LEMMATA
LEMMING
LEMONDE
LEMOYNE
LEMPIRA
MEMBERS
MEMENTO
MEMLING
MEMOIRE
MEMOIRS
MEMOPAD
MEMOREX
MEMPHIS
NEMEROV
NEMESES
NEMESIS
REMAILS
REMAINS
REMAKES
REMANDS
REMARKS
REMARRY
REMATCH
REMATED
REMATES
REMEETS
REMELTS
REMENDS
REMERGE
REMILLS
REMINDS
REMINED
REMINES
REMINTS
REMISED
REMISES
REMIXED
REMIXES
REMNANT
REMODEL
REMOLDS
REMORAS
REMORSE
REMOTER
REMOTES
REMOUNT
REMOVAL
REMOVED
REMOVER
REMOVES
REMOWED
SEMANAS
SEMIDRY
SEMILOG
SEMINAL
SEMINAR
SEMIPRO
SEMIRAW
SEMITES
SEMITIC
TEMBLOR
TEMPEAZ
TEMPEHS
TEMPERA
TEMPERS
TEMPEST
TEMPING
TEMPJOB
TEMPLAR
TEMPLED
TEMPLES
TEMPORE
TEMPTED
TEMPTER
TEMPURA
WEMBLEY
YEMENIS
ZEMSTVO

•E•M•••

BEAMERS
BEAMIER
BEAMING
BEAMISH
BEAMSUP
BEDMATE
BEEMERS
BELMONT
BERMING
BERMUDA
BESMEAR
DEEMING
DEHMELT
DELMONT
DELMORE
DENMARK
DENMOMS
DERMATO
DESMOGS
DESMOND
FERMATA
FERMATE
FERMATS
FERMENT
FERMION
FERMIUM
GEMMATE
GEMMIER
GERMAIN
GERMANE
GERMANS
GERMANY
GERMIER
HELMETS
HELMING
HELMOND
HEMMERS
HEMMING
HERMANA
HERMANN
HERMANO
HERMANS
HERMITS
HERMOSA
HERMOSO
HEYMANS
HEYMRDJ
KENMORE
LEHMANN
LEMMATA
LEMMING
LETMEBE
LETMEGO
LETMEIN
LEXMARK
MEEMIES
MERMAID
NESMITH
NEUMANN
NEWMADE
NEWMANS
NEWMATH
NEWMINT
NEWMONT
NEWMOON
NEWMOWN
PERMIAN
PERMING
PERMITS
PERMUTE
PETMICE
PETMULE
REAMASS
REAMEND
REAMERS
REAMING
REAMOUT
REDMEAT
REDMOND
REEMITS
REIMAGE
REIMPLY
RESMELT
REYMONT
SEAMAPS
SEAMERS
SEAMIER
SEAMILE
SEAMING
SEAMIST
SEAMOSS
SEEMING
SEEMSTO
SEGMENT
SELMAAL
SERMONS
SEYMOUR
TEAMING
TEAMSUP
TEAMUSA
TEDMACK
TEEMING
TENMILE
TERMING
TERMINI
TERMITE
VERMEER
VERMEIL
VERMINY
VERMONT
WEBMAIL
WETMOPS
YEOMANS
YESMAAM
ZERMATT

•E••M••

BECOMES
BEERMUG
BEHRMAN
BELLMAN
BELLMEN
BENUMBS
BERGMAN
BESTMAN
BESTMEN
BETAMAX
BETIMES
CERAMIC
CERUMEN
CESTMOI
DECAMPS
DECIMAL
DEFAMED
DEFAMER
DEFAMES
DELIMAN
DELIMEN
DELIMIT
DENIMED
FELDMAN
FEYNMAN
GENOMES
GENOMIC
GETSMAD
HEADMAN
HEADMEN
HECKMAN
HEISMAN
HELLMAN
KEEPMUM
KEPTMUM
LEADMAN
LEADMEN
LEGUMES
LENSMAN
LENSMEN
LETEMIN
MEATMAN
MEATMEN
MELAMED
MEOWMIX
MERIMEE
MESAMIS
NESSMAN
NEWSMAN
NEWSMEN
PERLMAN
PETEMAN
PETEMEN
READMIT
REAIMED
REALMAN
REALMEN
REARMED
REAUMUR
RECOMBS
REEDMAN
REEDMEN
REGIMEN
REGIMES
REITMAN
RELIMIT
RELUMED
RELUMES
RENAMED
RENAMES
REPOMAN
REPUMPS
RESUMED
RESUMES
RETAMED
RETAMES
RETIMED
RETIMES
REVAMPS
SEISMAL
SEISMIC
SESAMES
VELTMAN
VENEMAN
VERYMAD
WEIDMAN
WELLMAN
WENTMAD
YEAHMAN

•E•••M•

BEATSME
BECALMS
BEDLAMP
BEDLAMS
BEDTIME
BEGRIME
BELDAME
BELDAMS
BELLAMY
BERGAMO
CENTIME
CENTIMO
DECRUMB
DEFOAMS
DEFORMS
DEFRAME
DEGERMS
DELORME
DEMBUMS
DENMOMS
DEPALMA
DESLUMS
DESTEMS
DEWORMS
GENZYME
KEYLIME
MEDIUMS
MEGOHMS
MEGRIMS
MELISMA
MESEEMS
NETGAME
NEWNAME
NEWSOME
PENNAME
PEPLUMS
PERFUME
PERFUMY
PETCOMB
PETLAMB
PETNAME
RECLAME
RECLIMB
REDARMY
REDEEMS
REFILMS
REFORMS
REFRAME
REPLUMB
REPLUME
REPRIME
RESEAMS
RESTAMP
RESWIMS
RETRIMS
REWARMS
SEAARMS
TEATIME
TEDEUMS
TEDIUMS
TEETIME
VELLUMS
VENDOME
VERISMO
WEBCAMS
WELCOME

•E••••M

BEACHAM
BECHARM
BECKHAM
BEDROOM
BEECHAM
BELGIUM
BENTHAM
BERTRAM
CENTRUM
DECLAIM
DECORUM
DELIHAM
DEMONYM
EELWORM
FEMINUM
FERMIUM
GEEKDOM
GEORGEM
GETFROM
GETWARM
HEIRDOM
HEREIAM
HEROISM
JEJUNUM
KEEPMUM
KEPTMUM
KETCHAM
KETCHUM
LEFTARM
LEFTISM
LEGROOM
LEITRIM
LETTERM
MERRIAM
NEEDHAM
PENTIUM
PERDIEM
PERFORM
REALISM
REBLOOM
RECLAIM
RECROOM
REDREAM
REDWORM
REGROOM
REQUIEM
SEACALM
SEAFOAM
SEAGRAM
SERFDOM
SEVENAM
SEVENPM
TEAROOM
TELECOM
TERAOHM
TERBIUM
YEATEAM
YESMAAM
ZEROSUM

••EM•••

AGEMATE
ALEMBIC
ANEMIAS
ANEMONE
ATEMORE
BEEMERS
BLEMISH
CHEMISE
CHEMIST
CHEMLAB
CLEMENS
CLEMENT
CLEMSON
CREMATE
CREMINI
CREMONA
CREMORA
DAEMONS
DEEMING
DIEMENS
EDEMATA
EJEMPLO
ELEMENT
ENEMIES
EREMITE
EXEMPLA
EXEMPTS
EYEMASK
FLEMING
FLEMISH
FREMONT
GREMLIN
ICEMILK
IMEMINE
ITEMING
ITEMISE
ITEMIZE
ITEMONE
KREMLIN
LAEMMLE
MEEMIES
OLEMISS
ONEMILE
ONEMORE
ONEMPTY
PHEMIUS
PREMADE
PREMAKE
PREMATE
PREMEDS
PREMEET
PREMIER
PREMIES
PREMISE
PREMISS
PREMIUM
REEMITS
RIEMANN
SEEMING
SEEMSTO
SIEMENS
STEMMED
STEMPEL
TEEMING
THEMAGI
THEMALL
THEMASK
THEMAVS
THEMAYO
THEMETS
THEMICK
THEMOON
THEMOST
TIEMPOS
TREMBLE
TREMBLY
TREMOLO
TREMORS
UNEMPTY

••E•M••

AREAMAP
BEERMUG
CHEXMIX
CHEZMOI
CREAMED
CREAMER
CREWMAN
CREWMEN
DREAMED
DREAMER
DREAMIN
DREAMOF
DREAMON
DREAMUP
FREEMAN
FREEMEN
GLEAMED
GLEEMAN
GLEEMEN
GOESMAD
IDEAMAN
IDEAMEN
KEEPMUM
KLEZMER
LAEMMLE
OVERMAN
OVERMIX
PNEUMAS
PNEUMAT
PNEUMON
PREAMPS
PREEMIE
PREEMPT
PREOMIT
REEDMAN
REEDMEN
RHEUMIC
RIESMAN
SHERMAN
STEAMED
STEAMER
STEAMUP
STEMMED
STEPMOM
THEOMEN
THEOMNI
THERMAL
THERMIC
THERMOS
WHELMED
YZERMAN

••E••M•

AWESOME
ELECTME
EWELAMB
EXENEMY
FRENEMY
ICEDAMS
JOECAMP
ONEDIME
ONELUMP
ONENAME
ONETIME
PHENOMS
PLENUMS
PREARMS
PREGAME
PRELIMS
PRENAME
PRESUME
TEETIME
THEARMY
THEBOMB
THEGAME
THEISMS
THELAMB
THEPUMP
THERAMS
THESAME
THESIMS
TIEGAME
WOEISME

••E•••M

AGENDUM
BEECHAM
CHETRUM
CHEWGUM
EYEEXAM
FIEFDOM
FREEDOM
GEEKDOM
GRECISM
GRESHAM
GREWDIM
KEEPMUM
NEEDHAM
ONECLAM
ONEGRAM
ONEROOM
ONETERM
OVERARM
PREBOOM
PREDOOM
PREFORM
PREMIUM
PRETERM
PRETRIM
PREWARM
RHENIUM
STEINEM
STEPMOM
STERNUM
THEFIRM
THEOREM
THEROOM
TIEBEAM
VIETNAM

•••EM••

ANAEMIA
ANAEMIC
ARTEMIS
ARTEMUS
ATTEMPT
BASEMAN
BASEMEN
BATEMAN
BIREMES
BOHEMIA
BOZEMAN
CAKEMIX
CAPEMAY
CAVEMAN
CAVEMEN
CINEMAS
CINEMAX
COLEMAN
DILEMMA
ECZEMAS
ENDEMIC
EUDEMON
FIREMAN
FIREMEN
FIVEMAN
FOREMAN
FOREMEN
FREEMAN
FREEMEN
GATEMAN
GATEMEN
GLEEMAN
GLEEMEN
GONEMAD
IFWEMAY
INGEMAR
KROEMER
LAFEMME
LETEMIN
LIKEMAD
LINEMAN
LINEMEN
MADEMAD
MAKEMAD
MODEMED
NICEMAN
NICEMEN
PALEMON
PETEMAN
PETEMEN
POKEMON
POLEMAN
POLEMEN
POLEMIC
PREEMIE
PREEMPT
PUTEMUP
RACEMES
SALEMOR
SCHEMAS
SCHEMED
SCHEMER
SCHEMES
SIDEMAN
SIDEMEN
SITEMAP
TAPEMAN
TAPEMEN
TIREMAN
TIREMEN
TONEMES
TOTEMIC
UNKEMPT
UPTEMPO
VENEMAN
WIREMAN
WIREMEN
WISEMAN
WISEMEN
YALEMAN
YALEMEN

•••E•M•

ANSELMO
COVERME
DEGERMS
DILEMMA
ESTEEMS
INSEAMS
LAFEMME
LAPERMS
LYCEUMS
MESEEMS
MUSEUMS
PALERMO
PHLEGMY
REDEEMS
RESEAMS
SCREAMS
STREAMS
TEDEUMS
UNHELMS
UNSEAMS
YOTEAMO

•••E••M

ATHEISM
BAREXAM
BOREDOM
CPAEXAM
DUKEDOM
ENVENOM
EYEEXAM
FIREARM
FOREARM
FREEDOM
GOGETEM
HEREIAM
INTERIM
NOSEEUM
PINETUM
POPEDOM
SEVENAM
SEVENPM
SIDEARM
SILENTM
SUREIAM
TAKEAIM
TELECOM
THREEAM
THREEPM
TONEARM
WOWEDEM

••••EM•

ACADEME
ACADEMY
ALCHEMY
AMUSEME
ANADEMS
ANTHEMS
BUSCEMI
BUTTEMT
CONDEMN
CONTEMN
DESTEMS
DIADEMS
DODGEMS
EMBLEMS
ESTEEMS
EXENEMY
EXTREME
FRENEMY
IPANEMA
MAYHEMS
MESEEMS
MOSLEMS
NOXZEMA
PHLOEMS
PHONEME
PTOLEMY
REDEEMS
SACHEMS
SANREMO
SCUSEME
SOSUEME
SPAREME
SUPREME
SYSTEMS
TANDEMS
TRIREME
WRITEME

••••E•M

AFCTEAM
ANAHEIM
ASATEAM
ASTREAM
EPIDERM
IONBEAM
ISUREAM
JIMBEAM
LETTERM
LOWBEAM
MANHEIM
MIDTERM
MISDEEM

MISTERM
NAUSEAM
NBATEAM
NFCTEAM
NFLTEAM
NHLTEAM
NOSEEUM
ONETERM
ORPHEUM
OUTBEAM
PRETERM
PROTEAM
REDREAM
SUNBEAM
TAGTEAM
THREEAM
THREEPM
TIEBEAM
TWOTERM
WILHELM
YAYTEAM
YEATEAM

•••••EM

APOTHEM
COUNTEM
DOUBLEM
GEORGEM
GOGETEM
HAARLEM
HOTITEM
INAPOEM
MISDEEM
PERDIEM
PROBLEM
REQUIEM
STEINEM
SUBITEM
THEOREM
VALOREM
WOWEDEM

EN•••••

ENABLED
ENABLER
ENABLES
ENACTED
ENACTOR
ENAMELS
ENAMORS
ENAMOUR
ENARBOR
ENARMED
ENCAGED
ENCAGES
ENCAMPS
ENCARRE
ENCARTA
ENCASED
ENCASES
ENCHAIN
ENCHANT
ENCHASE
ENCINAS
ENCLASP
ENCLAVE
ENCLOSE
ENCODED
ENCODER
ENCODES
ENCOMIA
ENCORED
ENCORES
ENCRUST
ENCRYPT
ENDABLE
ENDALLS
ENDCUTS
ENDEARS
ENDEDAT
ENDEDIN
ENDEDIT
ENDEDON
ENDEDUP
ENDEMIC
ENDERBY
ENDGAME
ENDINGS
ENDIVES
ENDLATE
ENDLEAF
ENDLESS
ENDLINE
ENDLONG
ENDMOST
ENDNOTE
ENDORSE
ENDOWED
ENDOWER
ENDPINS
ENDPLAY
ENDRUNS
ENDUING
ENDUPAT
ENDURED
ENDURER
ENDURES
ENDUROS
ENDUSER
ENDUSES
ENDWAYS
ENDWISE
ENDZONE
ENEMIES
ENFACED
ENFACES
ENFANTS
ENFIELD
ENFLAME
ENFOLDS
ENFORCE
ENFRAME
ENGAGED
ENGAGER
ENGAGES
ENGARDE
ENGILDS
ENGINED
ENGINES
ENGIRDS
ENGLAND
ENGLISH
ENGLUND
ENGLUTS
ENGORGE
ENGRAFT
ENGRAIN
ENGRAMS
ENGRAVE
ENGROSS
ENGULFS
ENHANCE
ENIGMAS
ENISLED
ENISLES
ENJOINS
ENJOYED
ENJOYER
ENLACED
ENLACES
ENLARGE
ENLINKS
ENLISTS
ENLIVEN
ENMASSE
ENNEADS
ENNOBLE
ENOILED
ENOLOGY
ENOUNCE
ENPLANE
ENPRISE
ENQUADS
ENQUEUE
ENQUIRE
ENQUIRY
ENRAGED
ENRAGES
ENRANKS
ENRIGHT
ENRIQUE
ENROBED
ENROBES
ENROLLS
ENROOTS
ENROUTE
ENSEALS
ENSEATS
ENSIGNS
ENSILED
ENSILES
ENSKIED
ENSKIES
ENSLAVE
ENSNARE
ENSNARL
ENSOULS
ENSUING
ENSUITE
ENSURED
ENSURER
ENSURES
ENTAILS
ENTEBBE
ENTENTE
ENTERED
ENTERER
ENTERIC
ENTERIN
ENTERON
ENTHRAL
ENTHUSE
ENTICED
ENTICER
ENTICES
ENTIRES
ENTITLE
ENTOMBS
ENTRADA
ENTRAIN
ENTRANT
ENTRAPS
ENTREAT
ENTREES
ENTRIES
ENTROPY
ENTRUST
ENTWINE
ENTWIST
ENURING
ENVEILS
ENVELOP
ENVENOM
ENVIERS
ENVIOUS
ENVIRON
ENVIROS
ENVOGUE
ENVYING
ENWINDS
ENWOUND
ENWRAPS
ENZYMES
ENZYMIC

E•N••••

EANMUND
EDNAMAY
ELNINOS
ELNORTE
ENNEADS
ENNOBLE
EONLINE
ERNESTA
ERNESTO
EUNOMIA

E••N•••

EARNERS
EARNEST
EARNING
EARNSIT
EBANKED
EBONICS
EBONIES
EBONITE
EBONIZE
ECONOMY
EDINAMN
EGGNOGS
EKINGBY
ELANCES
ELANETS
ELANTRA
ELENIAK
EMANANT
EMANATE
EMANUEL
EMENDED
EMENDER
EMINENT
ENDNOTE
ENSNARE
ENSNARL
EPONINE
EPONYMS
EPONYMY
ERINYES
ERYNGOS
ESPNEWS
ETHNICS
ETONIAN
ETONICS
EUONYMS
EVANDER
EVANGEL
EVANISH
EVENBET
EVENERS
EVENEST
EVENING
EVENNOW
EVENOFF
EVENOUT
EVENPAR
EVENSUP
EVINCED
EVINCES
EWENECK
EXANIMO
EXENEMY
EXONYMS

E•••N••

EATENAT
EATENUP
EATINTO
EDASNER
EDGINGS
EDMONDS
EDMUNDI
EDMUNDS
EFFENDI
EKWENSI
ELAINES
ELEANOR
ELMONTE
ELMUNDO
ELNINOS
ELUANTS
EMBANKS
EMPANEL
ENCINAS
ENDINGS
ENFANTS
ENGINED
ENGINES
ENHANCE
ENLINKS
ENOUNCE
ENRANKS
ENTENTE
ENVENOM
ENWINDS
EOSINES
EPERNAY
EQUINES
EQUINOX
ERLANGS
ERMINED
ERMINES
ERMINIA
ERRANCY
ERRANDS
ESCENCE
ESPANOL
ESSENCE
ESSENES
ESTONIA
ETERNAL
ETHANES
ETHANOL
ETHENES
ETIENNE
EUBANKS
EUGENIA
EUGENIC
EUGENIE
EVENNOW
EXEUNTS
EXITNOW
EXPANDS
EXPANSE
EXPENDS
EXPENSE
EXPUNGE
EXTENDS
EXTENSO
EXTENTS
EXTINCT
EXYANKS

E••••N•

EAGLING
EANMUND
EARBONE
EARNING
EARRING
EASTEND
EASTING
EASYONE
ECHIDNA
ECHOING
EDDYING
EDITING
EDUCING
EGGHUNT
ELATING
ELEGANT
ELEMENT
ELEVENA
ELEVENB
ELEVENC
ELEVEND
ELEVENE
ELEVENS
ELEVONS
ELIDING
ELLMANN
ELOPING
ELUDING
ELUTING
EMANANT
EMINENT
EMOTING
EMPLANE
ENCHANT
ENDLINE
ENDLONG
ENDPINS
ENDRUNS
ENDUING
ENDZONE
ENGLAND
ENGLUND
ENJOINS
ENPLANE
ENSIGNS
ENSUING
ENTRANT
ENTWINE
ENURING
ENVYING
ENWOUND
EONLINE
EPERGNE
EPICENE
EPIGONE
EPONINE
EQUIANO
ERASING
ERELONG
ERIGENA
ERODENT
ERODING
ERSKINE
ESPYING
ESTRING
ETAMINE
ETCHANT
ETCHING
ETIENNE
ETYMONS
EUGLENA
EUPHONY
EVADING
EVALUNA
EVELONG
EVENING
EVIDENT
EVILONE
EVOKING
EXAMINE
EXIGENT
EXILING
EXITING
EXPOUND
EXSCIND
EXTERNE
EXTERNS
EXUDING
EYEBANK
EYEHAND
EYELINE
EYEWINK

E•••••N

EARLYON
EARTHEN
EASEDIN
EASEDON
EASESIN
EASESON
EASTERN
EASTMAN
ECHELON
ECOTRIN
EDGEDIN
EDGESIN
EDINAMN
EDITION
EELSKIN
EGGEDON
EIDOLON
EIJKMAN
ELAAIUN
ELASTIN
ELATION
ELCAJON
ELEISON
ELISION
ELLISON
ELLMANN
ELTRAIN
ELUTION
ELYSIAN
EMBROWN
EMERSON
EMOTION
EMPIRIN
ENCHAIN
ENDEDIN
ENDEDON
ENGRAIN
ENLIVEN
ENTERIN
ENTERON
ENTRAIN
ENVIRON
EPSILON
EPSTEIN
EREWHON
ERICSON
ERIKSON
EROSION
ERTEGUN
ESIASON
ESTAMIN
ESTEBAN
ESTEFAN
ETESIAN
ETONIAN
EUCERIN
EUDEMON
EUROVAN
EVASION
EXCELIN
EXPLAIN
EXURBAN

•EN••••

BENARES
BENATAR
BENAZIR
BENBLUE
BENBOVA
BENCHED
BENCHER
BENCHES
BENDAYS
BENDERS
BENDIER
BENDING
BENEATH
BENEFIC
BENEFIT
BENELUX
BENGALI
BENGALS
BENGUNN
BENICIA
BENICIO
BENIGNI
BENIGNO
BENISON
BENNETT
BENNING
BENOTED
BENOTES
BENTHAM
BENTHOS
BENTLEY
BENTSEN
BENUMBS
BENZALI
BENZELL
BENZENE
CENACLE
CENSERS
CENSING
CENSORS
CENSURE
CENTALS
CENTARE
CENTAUR
CENTAVO
CENTERS
CENTIME
CENTIMO
CENTRAL
CENTRED
CENTRES
CENTRIC
CENTRUM
CENTURY
DENARII
DENDRON
DENEUVE
DENHAAG
DENIALS
DENIECE
DENIERS
DENIMED
DENISON
DENIZEN
DENMARK
DENMOMS
DENNEHY
DENNING
DENOTED
DENOTES
DENSELY
DENSEST
DENSIFY
DENSITY
DENTALS
DENTATE
DENTINE
DENTING
DENTINS
DENTIST
DENTOID
DENTONS
DENTURE
DENTYNE
DENUDED
DENUDER
DENUDES
DENYING
FENCEIN
FENCERS
FENCEUP
FENCING
FENDERS
FENDING
FENDOFF
FENELON
FENETRE
FENNELS
FENNIER
GENDERS
GENERAL
GENERIC
GENERIS
GENESEE
GENESES
GENESET
GENESIS
GENETIC
GENEVAN
GENGHIS
GENITOR
GENLOCK
GENNAIO
GENNARO
GENOESE
GENOISE
GENOMES
GENOMIC
GENTEEL
GENTIAN
GENTILE
GENTLED
GENTLER
GENTLES
GENUINE
GENUSES
GENXERS
GENZYME
HENBANE
HENBITS
HENCOOP
HENDECA
HENDRIX
HENDRYX
HENLIKE
HENNAED
HENNERY
HENNISH
HENPECK
HENREID
HENRICH
HENRIES
HENRYII
HENRYIV
HENRYVI
HENSLEY
HENTOFF
JENKINS
JENNETS
KENDALL
KENDOLL
KENDREW
KENICHI
KENMORE
KENNEDY
KENNELS
KENNETH
KENNING
KENOLIN
KENOSHA
KENTISH
KENWAHL
KENYANS
LENDERS
LENDING
LENDOUT
LENFANT
LENGTHS
LENGTHY
LENGUAS
LENIENT
LENNONS
LENOVOS
LENSCAP
LENSMAN
LENSMEN
LENTIGO
LENTILS
MENACED
MENACER
MENACES
MENAGES
MENCIUS
MENCKEN
MENDELS
MENDERS
MENDING
MENFOLK
MENIALS
MENISCI
MENORAH
MENORCA
MENOTTI
MENSANS
MENSCHY
MENTEES
MENTHOL
MENTION
MENTORS
MENUBAR
MENUDOS
MENUHIN
MENZIES
NENNIUS
PENALTY
PENANCE
PENATES
PENCASE
PENCILS
PENDANT
PENDENT
PENDING
PENGUIN
PENLIKE
PENLITE
PENNAME
PENNANT
PENNATE
PENNERS
PENNEYS
PENNIES
PENNINE
PENNING
PENNOCK
PENNONS
PENPALS
PENROSE
PENSEES
PENSION
PENSIVE
PENTADS
PENTANE
PENTELS
PENTIUM
PENUCHE
PENULTS
PENZIAS
RENAILS
RENALDO
RENALLY
RENAMED
RENAMES
RENAULT
RENDELL
RENDERS
RENDING
RENEGED
RENEGER
RENEGES
RENESTS
RENEWAL
RENEWED
RENEWER
RENFREW
RENNETS
RENNINS
RENOIRS
RENOTED
RENOTES
RENOWNS
RENTALS
RENTEES
RENTERS
RENTIER
RENTING
RENTOUT
RENTSTO
RENUZIT
RENVOIS
RENWICK
SENATES
SENATOR
SENDEES
SENDERS
SENDFOR
SENDING
SENDOFF
SENDOUT
SENDSBY
SENDSIN
SENDSON
SENDSTO
SENDSUP
SENDUPS
SENECAN
SENECAS
SENEGAL
SENESCE
SENHORA
SENIORS
SENNETT
SENORAS
SENORES
SENSATE
SENSEIS
SENSENS
SENSING
SENSORS
SENSORY
SENSUAL
SENTFOR
SENTOFF
SENTOUT
SENTRAS
TENABLE
TENABLY
TENACES
TENACRE
TENANCY
TENANTS
TENBALL
TENCENT
TENCHES
TENCODE
TENDAYS
TENDERS
TENDING
TENDONS
TENDRIL
TENDSTO
TENEEEE
TENFEET
TENFOLD
TENFOOT
TENFOUR
TENKRUN
TENMILE
TENNANT
TENNECO
TENNERS
TENNIEL
TENNIES
TENONED
TENONER
TENPAST
TENPINS
TENSELY
TENSEST
TENSEUP
TENSILE
TENSING
TENSION
TENSITY
TENSIVE
TENSORS
TENSPOT
TENTBED
TENTERS
TENTFUL
TENTHLY
TENTING
TENTONS
TENTPEG

TENUITY
TENUOUS
TENURED
TENURES
TENWEEK
TENYEAR
TENZING
VENABLE
VENALLY
VENATIC
VENDEES
VENDERS
VENDING
VENDOME
VENDORS
VENDUES
VENEERS
VENEMAN
VENEZIA
VENISON
VENTAGE
VENTERS
VENTING
VENTNOR
VENTRAD
VENTRAL
VENTRIS
VENTURA
VENTURE
VENTURI
VENULES
VENUSES
WENCHES
WENDELL
WENDERS
WENDING
WENDKOS
WENTAFT
WENTAPE
WENTBAD
WENTFAR
WENTFOR
WENTMAD
WENTOFF
WENTOUT
WENTPRO
XENIAOH
XENICAL
YENNING
YENSFOR
ZENANAS
ZENISTS
ZENITHS
ZENOBIA

•E•N•••

BEANBAG
BEANDIP
BEANERY
BEANIES
BEANING
BEANOIL
BEDNORZ
BENNETT
BENNING
BERNARD
BERNAYS
BERNESE
BERNINA
BERNINI
BERNSEN
DEANERY
DENNEHY
DENNING
DERNIER
FEINTED
FENNELS
FENNIER
FERNAND
FERNBAR
FERNERY
FERNIER
FEWNESS
FEYNESS
FEYNMAN
GENNAIO
GENNARO
HEINOUS
HENNAED
HENNERY
HENNISH
HERNANI
HERNDON
HERNIAE
HERNIAS
HERNIBS
HEXNUTS
JEANARP
JEANLUC
JEANNIE
JEANNOT
JENNETS
KEENENH
KEENERS
KEENEST
KEENING
KENNEDY
KENNELS
KENNETH
KENNING
KERNELS
KEYNOTE
LEANCUT
LEANDER
LEANERS
LEANEST
LEANING
LEANSIN
LEANSON
LEANSTO
LEANTOS
LENNONS
LEONARD
LEONATO
LEONDAY
LEONIDS
LEONINE
LEONORA
LEONORE
MEANAGE
MEANDER
MEANEST
MEANIES
MEANING
MEANJOE
MEANSIT
MEANSTO
MEANTIT
MEANTTO
MEYNELL
NENNIUS
NEONATE
NEONGAS
NEWNAME
NEWNESS
PEANUTS
PEENING
PENNAME
PENNANT
PENNATE
PENNERS
PENNEYS
PENNIES
PENNINE
PENNING
PENNOCK
PENNONS
PEONAGE
PEONIES
PETNAME
PETNAPS
REANNEX
REDNECK
REDNESS
REDNINE
REDNOSE
REENACT
REENDOW
REENJOY
REENTER
REENTRY
REGNANT
REGNARD
REGNIER
REINDEX
REINING
REINKED
REINSIN
REKNEAD
REKNITS
REKNOCK
REKNOTS
REMNANT
RENNETS
RENNINS
RESNAIS
RESNAPS
REUNERS
REUNIFY
REUNION
REUNITE
REYNARD
REYNAUD
REYNOSA
SEANCES
SEENALL
SEENFIT
SEENOFF
SEENOUT
SEINERS
SEINING
SENNETT
TEANECK
TEENAGE
TEENERS
TEENIER
TEENSIE
TENNANT
TENNECO
TENNERS
TENNIEL
TENNIES
TERNARY
TERNATE
VEENECK
VEINIER
VEINING
VEINLET
VEINTES
VEINULE
VERNIER
WEANERS
WEANING
WEENESS
WEENIES
WERNHER
WETNAPS
WETNESS
YEANING
YENNING
ZERNIKE

•E••N••

BEATNIK
BEGANTO
BEGONIA
BEHINDS
BEIGNES
BEIGNET
BELINDA
BELONGS
BERENDT
BERKNER
BEYONCE
CEMENTS
CESSNAS
CETANES
CEZANNE
DEBONED
DEBONES
DEBUNKS
DECANTS
DECENCY
DEFANGS
DEFENCE
DEFENDS
DEFENSE
DEFINED
DEFINER
DEFINES
DEFUNCT
DEFUNDS
DEIGNED
DEIGNTO
DEJUNKS
DELANEY
DELINTS
DEMANDS
DEMENTO
DEMONIC
DEMONYM
DEPENDS
DEPONED
DEPONER
DEPONES
DERANGE
DERONDA
DETENTE
DETENTS
DETUNED
DETUNES
FEARNOT
FECHNER
FEDINTO
FEIGNED
FEIGNER
FELINES
FELONRY
FEMINUM
GEHENNA
GEMINIS
GERENTS
GERUNDS
GETINON
GETINTO
GETONIT
GETONTO
HEDONIC
HERENOW
HERONRY
HEXANES
JEANNIE
JEANNOT
JEJUNUM
KEARNEY
KETONES
KETONIC
KEYINON
LEARNED
LEARNER
LEARNOF
LEARNTO
LEBANON
LECONTE
LEDINTO
LEGANZA
LEGENDS
LEIBNIZ
LEMONDE
LEPANTO
LETINON
LETKNOW
LETSNOT
MEGANES
MEITNER
MELANGE
MELANIA
MELANIC
MELANIE
MELANIN
MELINDA
MEMENTO
MERINOS
MESONIC
NEATNIK
NEEDNOT
PEDANTS
PENANCE
PESANTE
PETUNIA
REANNEX
REBANKS
REBENDS
REBINDS
RECANED
RECANES
RECANTS
RECENCY
REDANTS
REDONDO
REFENCE
REFINDS
REFINED
REFINER
REFINES
REFUNDS
REGENCY
REGENTS
REGINAL
REGINAS
REHANGS
REHINGE
REHONED
REHONES
REHONOR
REIGNED
RELANCE
RELANDS
RELANES
RELENDS
RELENTS
RELINED
RELINES
RELINKS
REMANDS
REMENDS
REMINDS
REMINED
REMINES
REMINTS
REOWNED
REPANEL
REPENTS
REPINED
REPINER
REPINES
RERANKS
RERENTS
RERINSE
RESANDS
RESENDS
RESENTS
RESINED
RESINGS
RESINKS
RETINAE
RETINAL
RETINAS
RETINGE
RETINOL
RETINTS
RETINUE
RETONED
RETONES
RETUNED
RETUNES
REVENDS
REVENGE
REVENUE
REWINDS
REZONED
REZONES
SECANTS
SECONDI
SECONDO
SECONDR
SECONDS
SEDONAS
SEEINTO
SELENIC
SEMANAS
SEMINAL
SEMINAR
SERENER
SETENTA
SETINTO
SEVENAD
SEVENAM
SEVENBC
SEVENEE
SEVENNO
SEVENPM
SEVENTH
SEVENTY
SEVENUP
TECHNOS
TEJANAS
TEJANOS
TENANCY
TENANTS
TENONED
TENONER
TERENCE
TETANUS
VENTNOR
VERANDA
VERONIA
VERYNEW
WEEONES
WEGENER
WETONES
YEARNED
YEARNER
YEARNTO
YEMENIS
ZEDONKS
ZENANAS

•E•••N•

BEACONS
BEADING
BEAMING
BEANING
BEARING
BEATING
BECKONS
BEDDING
BEEFING
BEELINE
BEEPING
BEGGING
BEGUINE
BEHRENS
BEHRING
BEIJING
BELLING
BELLINI
BELMONT
BELTANE
BELTING
BELYING
BELZONI
BEMOANS
BENDING
BENGUNN
BENIGNI
BENIGNO
BENNING
BENZENE
BERMING
BERNINA
BERNINI
BEROWNE
BERSUNT
BESTING
BESTONE
BETHANY
BETHINK
BETHUNE
BETTANY
BETTING
CEASING
CEILING
CELAENO
CELLINI
CENSING
CERVINE
CESSING
CEZANNE
DEACONS
DEADEND
DEADENS
DEAFENS
DEALING
DEARONE
DECKING
DECLINE
DEEDING
DEEMING
DEEPEND
DEEPENS
DEFCONS
DEFIANT
DEFYING
DEHORNS
DEICING
DEKEING
DELEING
DELMONT
DELTONA
DELVING
DEMEANS
DEMESNE
DEMOING
DEMOUNT
DENNING
DENTINE
DENTING
DENTINS
DENTONS
DENTYNE
DENYING
DEPLANE
DERRING
DERWENT
DESCANT
DESCEND
DESCENT
DESIGNS
DESMOND
DESPINA
DESPOND
DESTINE
DESTINO
DESTINY
DETAINS
DEUCING
DEVEINS
DEVIANT
DEWLINE
DEYOUNG
FEARING
FEEDING
FEELING
FELLING
FELLINI
FELTING
FENCING
FENDING
FERMENT
FERNAND
FERVENT
FESSING
FESTINA
FEUDING
GEARING
GEHENNA
GELDING
GELLING
GELPENS
GENUINE
GERAINT
GERMANE
GERMANS
GERMANY
GETBENT
GETDONE
GETSANA
GETSANF
GETTING
HEADEND
HEADING
HEALING
HEAPING
HEARING
HEATING
HEAVENS
HEAVING
HEDGING
HEEDING
HEELING
HEFTING
HELLENE
HELLENO
HELMING
HELMOND
HELPING
HELSING
HEMLINE
HEMMING
HENBANE
HERDING
HERMANA
HERMANN
HERMANO
HERMANS
HERNANI
HEROINE
HERRING
HEYMANS
JEERING
JELLING
JENKINS
JERGENS
JERKING
JERKINS
JESTING
JETFANS
JETGUNS
JETSONS
JETTING
KEDGING
KEELING
KEENENH
KEENING
KEEPING
KEGGING
KELOWNA
KELVINS
KENNING
KENYANS
KEYBANK
KEYRING
LEADENS
LEADING
LEADINS
LEAFING
LEAKING
LEANING
LEAPING
LEASING
LEAVENS
LEAVING
LEBLANC
LECUONA
LEERING
LEFTEND
LEGBONE
LEGGING
LEGIONS
LEGRAND
LEHMANN
LEJEUNE
LEMMING
LEMOYNE
LENDING
LENFANT
LENIENT
LENNONS
LEOGENN
LEONINE
LEPTONS
LESIONS
LESSENS
LESSING
LESSONS
LETTING
LEUCINE
LEVYING
MEANING
MECCANS
MEDIANS
MEDIANT
MEETING
MELDING
MELTING
MEMLING
MENDING
MENSANS
MEOWING
MERGING
MERLINS
MESHING
MESSINA
MESSING
METFANS
METHANE
MEWLING
NEARING
NEATENS
NECKING
NEDLAND
NEEDING
NEGRONI
NELSONS
NEOCENE
NEOCONS
NEOGENE
NEPTUNE
NERVINE
NERVING
NESTING
NETTING
NETTONS
NEUMANN
NEURONE
NEURONS
NEWHAND
NEWLINE
NEWMANS
NEWMINT
NEWMONT
NEWTONS
PEAHENS
PEAKING
PEALING
PEASANT
PECCANT
PECKING
PECTINS
PEEKING
PEELING
PEENING
PEEPING
PEERING
PEEVING
PEGGING
PEIPING
PELTING
PENDANT
PENDENT
PENDING
PENNANT
PENNINE
PENNING
PENNONS
PENTANE
PEPBAND
PEPPING
PEPPINO
PEPSINS
PEPTONE
PERCENT
PERKING
PERKINS
PERMING
PERRINE
PERRINS
PERSONA
PERSONS
PETPONY
PETTING
READING
REAGANS
REAGENT
REALINE
REAMEND
REAMING
REAPING
REAREND
REARING
REASONS
REAVING
REBOANT
REBOUND
REBRAND
RECKONS
RECLINE
RECOINS
RECOUNT
RECRANK
REDARNS
REDBONE
REDCENT
REDDENS
REDDING
REDFINS
REDHENS
REDKING
REDLINE
REDMOND
REDNINE
REDOING
REDOUND
REDPINE
REDPONY
REDSUNS
REDWINE
REDWING
REDYING
REDZONE
REEARNS
REEDING
REEFING
REEKING
REELING
REEVING
REFFING
REFOUND
REFRONT
REFYING
REGAINS
REGIONS
REGNANT
REGRANT
REGRIND
REICING
REINING
REJOINS
RELIANT
RELLENO
RELOANS
RELYING
REMAINS
REMNANT
REMOUNT
RENDING
RENNINS
RENOWNS
RENTING
REOPENS
REPAINT
REPHONE
REPLANE
REPLANS
REPLANT
REPOINT
REPPING
REPRINT
REPRUNE
REPUGNS
RESCANS
RESCIND
RESHINE
RESIGNS
RESOUND
RESPANS
RESPINS
RESPOND
RESTING
RETAINS
RETHANK
RETHINK
RETSINA
RETTING
RETURNS
RETWINE
REUBENS
REUSING
REVVING
REWARNS
REWOUND
REYMONT
SEAHUNT
SEALANE
SEALANT
SEALING
SEAMING
SEARING
SEASONS
SEATING
SEBRING
SEEDING
SEEKING
SEEMING
SEEPING
SEGMENT
SEINING
SEIZING
SELLING
SENDING
SENSENS
SENSING
SEQUINS

SERLING
SERMONS
SERPENS
SERPENT
SERVANT
SERVING
SESTINA
SETTING
SEVENNO
SEVIGNY
SEXTANS
SEXTANT
SEXTONS
TEAMING
TEARING
TEASING
TEAURNS
TEEMING
TEFLONS
TELLING
TEMPING
TENCENT
TENDING
TENDONS
TENNANT
TENPINS
TENSING
TENTING
TENTONS
TENZING
TERHUNE
TERMING
TERMINI
TERRANS
TERRENE
TERRINE
TESTING
TEUTONS
TEXTING
VEERING
VEGGING
VEILING
VEINING
VENDING
VENTING
VERBENA
VERDANT
VERDINS
VEREINE
VERGING
VERMINY
VERMONT
VERSANT
VERSING
VESTING
VETOING
VETTING
WEAKENS
WEAKONS
WEANING
WEAPONS
WEARING
WEAVING
WEBBING
WEBZINE
WEDDING
WEDELNS
WEDGING
WEEDING
WEEKEND
WEEPING
WELDING
WELLAND
WELLING
WELTING
WENDING
WESTEND
WESTINS
WETLAND
WETTING
YEANING
YEAREND
YEARONE
YELLING
YELPING
YENNING
YEOMANS
YESORNO
YESSING
YEVGENY
ZEALAND
ZEBRINE
ZEELAND
ZEITUNG
ZELAZNY
ZEROING
ZESTING

•E•••N

AEOLIAN
BEALION
BEARSON
BEATSON
BEDDOWN
BEDIZEN
BEDOUIN
BEECHEN
BEERCAN
BEHRMAN
BELEVEN
BELGIAN
BELLMAN
BELLMEN
BELLSON
BELTRAN
BENGUNN
BENISON
BENTSEN
BERGMAN
BERGSON
BERIGAN
BERNSEN
BESTMAN
BESTMEN
BETAKEN
BETOKEN
BETWEEN
CELADON
CERTAIN
CERUMEN
CESSION
DEADPAN
DEALSIN
DEALTIN
DEARDEN
DECAGON
DEEPTAN
DEHAVEN
DELIMAN
DELIMEN
DENDRON
DENISON
DENIZEN
DESTAIN
DETRAIN
DEXTRIN
EELSKIN
FEASTON
FEEDBIN
FEEDSIN
FEEDSON
FELDMAN
FELTPEN
FENCEIN
FENELON
FERMION
FESTOON
FEYNMAN
GELATIN
GENEVAN
GENTIAN
GERMAIN
GERSHON
GETDOWN
GETEVEN
GETINON
GETITON
GETUPON
HEADMAN
HEADMEN
HEADPIN
HEADSIN
HEAPSON
HEARKEN
HEARTEN
HEATFAN
HEATHEN
HECKMAN
HEDISON
HEISMAN
HELICON
HELLION
HELLMAN
HELPSIN
HELPSON
HEMATIN
HEPARIN
HEPBURN
HERMANN
HERNDON
HESHVAN
HESSIAN
HEXAGON
HEXSIGN
JEMISON
JERILYN
JETSFAN
JEWISON
KEEPSIN
KEEPSON
KEESHAN
KELLJAN
KEMPTON
KENOLIN
KEOGHAN
KERATIN
KEYEDIN
KEYEDON
KEYINON
KEYSPAN
LEADMAN
LEADMEN
LEADSIN
LEADSON
LEAKSIN
LEANSIN
LEANSON
LEAPSIN
LEAPSON
LEAPTIN
LEAPTON
LEAVEIN
LEAVEON
LEBANON
LEBARON
LECTERN
LEGHORN
LEGIRON
LEHMANN
LENSMAN
LENSMEN
LEOGENN
LETDOWN
LETEMIN
LETHEAN
LETINON
LETMEIN
LETTERN
LETUPON
LEXICON
MEATMAN
MEATMEN
MECHLIN
MEDUSAN
MEGALON
MEGATON
MEGRYAN
MEISSEN
MELANIN
MENCKEN
MENTION
MENUHIN
MERCIAN
MERIDEN
METSFAN
MEXICAN
NESSMAN
NESTSIN
NETGAIN
NETIZEN
NEUMANN
NEUTRON
NEVADAN
NEWBERN
NEWBORN
NEWMOON
NEWMOWN
NEWSMAN
NEWSMEN
NEWTOWN
PEABEAN
PEARSON
PEEKSIN
PEERSIN
PELICAN
PELOTON
PENGUIN
PENSION
PEORIAN
PERLMAN
PERMIAN
PERSIAN
PERSSON
PERTAIN
PETEMAN
PETEMEN
PETLION
PETSCAN
REACHIN
READORN
READSIN
READSON
REALIGN
REALMAN
REALMEN
REARDON
REBEGAN
REBEGIN
REBEGUN
REBLOWN
RECLEAN
RECROWN
REDDAWN
REDFERN
REDRAWN
REDSFAN
REDSKIN
REEDMAN
REEDMEN
REELSIN
REFLOWN
REFRAIN
REGIMEN
REGIVEN
REGROWN
REINSIN
REITMAN
RELEARN
REPOMAN
RERISEN
RESHOWN
RESTAIN
RESTSIN
RESTSON
RESWORN
RETAKEN
RETRAIN
REUNION
REVELIN
REWAKEN
REWIDEN
REWOKEN
REWOVEN
SEAFERN
SEAGREN
SEALION
SEALSIN
SECTION
SEEPSIN
SEIZEON
SENDSIN
SENDSON
SENECAN
SERBIAN
SESSION
SETDOWN
SETUPON
SEWEDON
TEACHIN
TEAGOWN
TEHERAN
TELERAN
TELLSON
TENKRUN
TENSION
TERRAIN
TESTBAN
TESTRUN
TEXTRON
VECHTEN
VELTMAN
VENEMAN
VENISON
VERGEON
VERIZON
VERSION
VESTRON
VETERAN
WEARSON
WEDGEIN
WEIDMAN
WEIGHIN
WEIGHON
WEIRTON
WELLMAN
WELLRUN
WELLWON
WESTERN
WETDOWN
YEAHMAN
YELTSIN
YEREVAN
YESICAN
ZEBULON
ZEBULUN
ZEROSIN

••EN•••

ADENINE
ADENOID
AGENCES
AGENDAS
AGENDUM
AGENINE
AGENTED
AGENTRY
ALENCON
AMENDED
AMENDER
AMENITY
ARENOSE
ARENSKY
AVENGED
AVENGER
AVENGES
AVENIDA
AVENUEQ
AVENUES
BIENNIA
BIENTOT
BLENDED
BLENDER
BLENDES
BLENDIN
BLENTIN
BRENDAN
BRENDEL
BRENDON
BRENGUN
BRENNAN
BRENNER
CHENIER
CRENATE
CRENELS
CTENOID
DUENNAS
ELENIAK
EMENDED
EMENDER
EVENBET
EVENERS
EVENEST
EVENING
EVENNOW
EVENOFF
EVENOUT
EVENPAR
EVENSUP
EWENECK
EXENEMY
FIENNES
FLENSED
FLENSER
FLENSES
FRENCHI
FRENCHS
FRENEAU
FRENEMY
FRENESI
FUENTES
GLENCOE
GRENADA
GRENADE
GRENDEL
IDENTIC
IRENICS
KEENENH
KEENERS
KEENEST
KEENING
KLENSCH
LAENNEC
LIENEES
LIENORS
MAENADS
MCENROE
NOENDOF
NOENDTO
NOENTRY
OBENTOS
OMENING
ONENAME
ONENESS
ONENOTE
OPENAIR
OPENBAR
OPENEND
OPENERS
OPENING
OPENNET
OPENOUT
OPENPIT
OPENSEA
OPENSUP
OPENTAP
OPENTOE
OPENTOP
PEENING
PFENNIG
PHENOLS
PHENOMS
PLENARY
PLENISH
PLENUMS
PRENAME
PRENOON
PRENUPS
QUENEAU
QUENTIN
REENACT
REENDOW
REENJOY
REENTER
REENTRY
RHENISH
RHENIUM
SCENEII
SCENEIV
SCENERY
SCENEVI
SCENICS
SCENTED
SCENTER
SEENALL
SEENFIT
SEENOFF
SEENOUT
SIENESE
SIENNAS
SLENDER
SPENCER
SPENDER
SPENDON
SPENSER
SPENTON
STENCIL
STENGEL
STENGUN
STENNIS
STENTOR
SWENSON
TEENAGE
TEENERS
TEENIER
TEENSIE
THENETS
THENEWS
THENILE
TIENDAS
TOENAIL
TRENARY
TRENDED
TRENTON
UNENDED
UPENDED
UTENSIL
VEENECK
WEENESS
WEENIES
WIENERS
WIENIES

••E•N••

ATEINTO
AVERNAL
AVERNUS
BIENNIA
BOEINGS
BRENNAN
BRENNER
CLEANED
CLEANER
CLEANLY
CLEANSE
CLEANTE
CLEANUP
DOESNOT
DUENNAS
ELEANOR
EPERNAY
ETERNAL
EVENNOW
EXEUNTS
FIENNES
FLEANCE
FLEXNER
FRESNEL
GLEANED
GLEANER
GREENED
GREENER
GREENLY
IMEANIT
ISEENOW
KLEENEX
LAENNEC
NEEDNOT
OCEANIA
OCEANIC
OCEANID
OCEANUS
OLEANNA
OLEANNY
ONEINCH
ONEONTA
ONEUNIT
OPENNET
OVERNEW
PFENNIG
PREENED
PREENER
QUEENED
QUEENIE
QUEENIT
QUEENLY
QUESNAY
SEEINTO
SIENNAS
STEANNE
STEINEM
STEINER
STENNIS
STERNAL
STERNER
STERNLY
STERNOS
STERNUM
SWEENEY
TIEINTO
TIERNEY
TREINTA
TWEENER
VIERNES
VIETNAM
WEEONES

••E••N•

ABEYANT
ACETONE
ADELINA
ADELINE
ADENINE
AGELONG
AGENINE
AKEBONO
AMERIND
ANELING
ANEMONE
ARETINO
BEEFING
BEELINE
BEEPING
BRETONS
BREWING
CHEFING
CHEVONS
CHEWING
CLEMENS
CLEMENT
CLEWING
CREMINI
CREMONA
CREPING
CRETANS
CRETINS
CREWING
DAEMONS
DEEDING
DEEMING
DEEPEND
DEEPENS
DIEMENS
DIETING
DUELING
DUETING
ELEGANT
ELEMENT
ELEVENA
ELEVENB
ELEVENC
ELEVEND
ELEVENE
ELEVENS
ELEVONS
EPERGNE
ERELONG
EVELONG
EVENING
EYEBANK
EYEHAND
EYELINE
EYEWINK
FEEDING
FEELING
FLEEING
FLEMING
FLEXING
FREEING
FRELENG
FREMONT
FUELING
GAETANO
GREYING
HEEDING
HEELING
ICELAND
ICELINE
ICERINK
ICERUNS
ICEWINE
IKEBANA
IMEMINE
IRELAND
ISECOND
ITEMING
ITEMONE
ITERANT
JEERING
JREWING
KEELING
KEENENH
KEENING
KEEPING
KMESONS
KNEEING
LEERING
MEETING
MTEVANS
NEEDING
OBEYING
OLEANNA
OLEANNY
OLEFINS
OMENING
ONECENT
ONEHAND
ONELANE
ONEPINT
OPENEND
OPENING
OPERAND
OPERANT
OREGANO
PEEKING
PEELING
PEENING
PEEPING
PEERING
PEEVING
PIECING
PIEPANS
PIETINS
PREBIND
PREDENY
PREFUND
PRERENT
PRESENT
PRESONG
PRETEND
PREVENT
PREYING
QUEUING
REEARNS
REEDING
REEFING
REEKING
REELING
REEVING
RIEMANN
RIESENS
SEEDING
SEEKING
SEEMING
SEEPING
SHEBANG
SIEGING
SIEMENS
SIEVING
SKEWING
SLEWING
SMETANA
SPECING
SPELUNK
SPEWING
STEANNE
STEARNS
STEFANI
STEPINS
STEPONE
STEVENS
STEWING
TEEMING
THEBAND
THEBANS
THEFONZ
THEGANG
THEKING
THEOMNI
THEPOND
THERENT
THERING
THERINK
THESUNS
THEWIND
TIELINE
TIEPINS
TIERING
TREEING
TREPANS
TREVINO
TSETUNG
TWERENT
VEERING
VIEWING
WEEDING
WEEKEND
WEEPING
WIELAND
ZEELAND
ZIERING

••E•••N

ALENCON
AMESLAN
APERSON
AVESTAN
AVEYRON
BEECHEN
BEERCAN
BLENDIN
BLENTIN
BREAKIN
BRENDAN
BRENDON
BRENGUN
BRENNAN
BRESLIN
BRETTON
CHEAPEN
CHEATIN
CHEATON
CHECHEN
CHECKIN
CHECKON
CHEERON
CHEVRON
CHEWSON
CLEAVON
CLEMSON
CREEPIN
CREPTIN
CRESPIN
CRESTON
CREWMAN
CREWMEN
DEEPTAN
DIEDOWN
DOESKIN
DREAMIN
DREAMON
DREGION
DRESDEN
DRESSIN
DWELLIN
DWELLON
DWELTON
ELEISON
EMERSON
EREWHON
ETESIAN
FEEDBIN
FEEDSIN
FEEDSON
FLEURON
FLEXION
FREEMAN
FREEMEN
FRESHEN
GHERKIN
GLEASON
GLEEMAN
GLEEMEN
GREATEN
GRECIAN
GREMLIN
GREYHEN
GUERDON
HOEDOWN
IBERIAN
ICEDOWN
IDEAMAN
IDEAMEN
IRECKON
IRESIGN

- IVERSON
- KEEPSIN
- KEEPSON
- KEESHAN
- KJELLIN
- KREMLIN
- KRESKIN
- LIEDOWN
- LLEYTON
- MUEZZIN
- MYERSON
- NIELSEN
- OBERLIN
- ODESSAN
- ONEDOWN
- ONEIRON
- OVERMAN
- OVERRAN
- OVERRUN
- PEEKSIN
- PEERSIN
- PIERIAN
- PLEBIAN
- PNEUMON
- PREBORN
- PREBURN
- PREDAWN
- PREGAIN
- PRELOAN
- PRENOON
- PREOPEN
- PREPLAN
- PRESSON
- PRESTON
- PRETEEN
- PREWARN
- PREWORN
- PREYSON
- QUENTIN
- RAEBURN
- RAEDAWN
- REEDMAN
- REEDMEN
- REELSIN
- RIEMANN
- RIESMAN
- RIESSEN
- SEEPSIN
- SHEDSON
- SHEEHAN
- SHELDON
- SHERMAN
- SHERWIN
- SKELTON
- SLEEKEN
- SLEEPIN
- SLEEPON
- SLEPTIN
- SLEPTON
- SMEARON
- SNEAKIN
- SNELLEN
- SPENDON
- SPENTON
- STEALIN
- STEARIN
- STEEPEN
- STEEPIN
- STENGUN
- STEPHEN
- STEPSIN
- STEPSON
- STETSON
- STEUBEN
- STEWPAN
- SUELLEN
- SUELYON
- SWEARIN
- SWEETEN
- SWEETON
- SWENSON
- THEMOON
- THEOMEN
- THEREIN
- THEREON
- THESWAN
- THETURN
- TIEDOWN
- TREADON
- TREASON
- TRENTON
- UNEATEN
- WHEATEN
- WHEATON
- WHEELIN
- WHEREIN
- WHEREON
- YZERMAN

•••EN••

- ABSENCE
- ABSENTS
- ACCENTS
- ACHENES
- ADDENDA
- ADDENDS
- ADRENAL
- ADVENTS
- ALBENIZ
- ALDENTE
- ALIENEE
- ALIENOR
- ALIENTO
- ALKENES
- ALLENBY
- ALLENDE
- ANTENNA
- APLENTY
- APPENDS
- ARDENCY
- ARGENTI
- ARGENTO
- ARGENTS
- ARMENIA
- ARSENAL
- ARSENIC
- ARSENIO
- ASCENDS
- ASCENTS
- ASPENCO
- ASSENTS
- ATTENDS
- AUGENDS
- BABENCO
- BADENDS
- BADENOV
- BARENTS
- BASENJI
- BERENDT
- BIGENDS
- BUTENES
- CADENCE
- CADENCY
- CADENZA
- CALENDS
- CATENAE
- CATENAS
- CAYENNE
- CEMENTS
- CILENTO
- CLIENTS
- COGENCY
- COMENOW
- COZENED
- COZENER
- DARENOT
- DECENCY
- DEFENCE
- DEFENDS
- DEFENSE
- DEMENTO
- DEPENDS
- DETENTE
- DETENTS
- DOCENTS
- DOYENNE
- DOZENTH
- EATENAT
- EATENUP
- EFFENDI
- EKWENSI
- ENTENTE
- ENVENOM
- ESCENCE
- ESSENCE
- ESSENES
- ETHENES
- ETIENNE
- EUGENIA
- EUGENIC
- EUGENIE
- EXPENDS
- EXPENSE
- EXTENDS
- EXTENSO
- EXTENTS
- FAGENDS
- FAIENCE
- FILENES
- FIRENZA
- FIRENZE
- FLUENCY
- FOLENGO
- FOMENTS
- FORENZA
- FRIENDS
- FTHENRY
- GALENAS
- GALENTO
- GEHENNA
- GERENTS
- GIVENBY
- GIVENIN
- GIVENOF
- GIVENON
- GIVENTO
- GIVENUP
- GREENED
- GREENER
- GREENLY
- GYRENES
- HAPENNY
- HAVENER
- HAVENOT
- HERENOW
- HOPENOT
- IMMENSE
- IMPENDS
- INCENSE
- INCENTS
- INDENTS
- INGENUE
- INTENDS
- INTENSE
- INTENTS
- INVENTS
- ISEENOW
- ITWENTY
- JIMENEZ
- JUVENAL
- KLEENEX
- LAMENTS
- LATENCY
- LATENED
- LATENTS
- LAZENBY
- LEGENDS
- LICENCE
- LICENSE
- LIFENET
- LIKENED
- LIKENEW
- LIKENTO
- LISENTE
- LIVENED
- LIVENER
- LIVENUP
- LORENTZ
- LORENZO
- LOZENGE
- LUCENCY
- LYSENKO
- MAGENTA
- MARENGO
- MCHENRY
- MCKENNA
- MEMENTO
- MIGENES
- MOMENTA
- MOMENTS
- MTKENYA
- MYCENAE
- NOVENAS
- OCHENTA
- OFFENCE
- OFFENDS
- OFFENSE
- OFTENER
- OGDENUT
- ORIENTE
- ORIENTS
- PARENTS
- PATENCY
- PATENTS
- PHOENIX
- PHRENIC
- PIMENTO
- PINENUT
- POLENTA
- POTENCE
- POTENCY
- PREENED
- PREENER
- PUDENCY
- QUEENED
- QUEENIE
- QUEENIT
- QUEENLY
- RAVENAL
- RAVENED
- RAVENNA
- REBENDS
- RECENCY
- REFENCE
- REGENCY
- REGENTS
- RELENDS
- RELENTS
- REMENDS
- REPENTS
- RERENTS
- RESENDS
- RESENTS
- REVENDS
- REVENGE
- REVENUE
- RIPENED
- RIPENER
- RISENTO
- RODENTS
- SCIENCE
- SELENIC
- SERENER
- SETENTA
- SEVENAD
- SEVENAM
- SEVENBC
- SEVENEE
- SEVENNO
- SEVENPM
- SEVENTH
- SEVENTY
- SEVENUP
- SILENCE
- SILENTA
- SILENTB
- SILENTC
- SILENTD
- SILENTE
- SILENTF
- SILENTG
- SILENTH
- SILENTI
- SILENTJ
- SILENTK
- SILENTL
- SILENTM
- SILENTN
- SILENTO
- SILENTP
- SILENTQ
- SILENTR
- SILENTS
- SILENTT
- SILENTU
- SILENTV
- SILENTW
- SILENTX
- SILENTY
- SILENTZ
- SIMENON
- SIRENED
- SISENOR
- SORENTO
- SPLENDA
- STDENIS
- SWEENEY
- TAGENDS
- TAKENBY
- TAKENIN
- TAKENON
- TAKENTO
- TAKENUP
- TALENTS
- TERENCE
- TOKENED
- TWEENER
- TYLENOL
- UNBENCH
- UNBENDS
- UNFENCE
- UNTENSE
- UNVENAL
- UPSENDS
- URGENCY
- VALENCE
- VALENTE
- VALENTI
- VICENTE
- VICENZA
- VIVENDI
- VIXENLY
- VOLENTE
- VOTENAY
- WAKENED
- WAKENER
- WEGENER
- WIDENED
- WIDENER
- WIZENED
- WOKENUP
- XIMENES
- YEMENIS

•••E•N•

- ANDEANS
- ANTEING
- ANTENNA
- BALEENS
- BLUEING
- CAPEANN
- CAREENS
- CASEINS
- CASERNE
- CASERNS
- CAVEINS
- CAVERNS
- CAYENNE
- CLUEING
- CODEINE
- COMEONS
- DEKEING
- DELEING
- DEMEANS
- DEMESNE
- DEVEINS
- DOYENNE
- ETIENNE
- EXTERNE
- EXTERNS
- FADEINS
- FIREANT
- FIVEONE
- FLEEING
- FREEING
- GEHENNA
- GIDEONS
- GOVERNS
- HAPENNY
- HAVEONE
- HIBERNO
- HJHEINZ
- ILLEANA
- INFERNO
- INTERNE
- INTERNS
- JANEANE
- JUDEANS
- KNEEING
- KOREANS
- LANEONE
- LATEENS
- LAVERNE
- LEJEUNE
- LINEONE
- LIVEONE
- LOVEINS
- LUCERNE
- MADEONE
- MAKEONE
- MALEANT
- MCKENNA
- MODERNE
- MODERNS
- MOREENS
- NAMEONE
- NICEONE
- ORLEANS
- PAGEANT
- PAGEONE
- PATERNO
- PIGEONS
- POTEENS
- RAVENNA
- RULEONE
- SALERNO
- SATEENS
- SCREENS
- SEVENNO
- SHOEING
- SIDEONE
- SIZEONE
- SOMEONE
- SPLEENS
- SPLEENY
- TAKEINS
- TAKEONE
- TAVERNA
- TAVERNS
- THREENO
- TREEING
- TRUEING
- TUREENS
- UNMEANT
- VEREINE
- VOTEDNO
- VOTESNO
- WEDELNS
- WISEONE
- WYVERNS

•••E••N

- ACHERON
- ACHESON
- ACTEDIN
- ACTEDON
- ADDEDIN
- ADDEDON
- AGREEON
- AILERON
- ASKEDIN
- ATSEVEN
- AZTECAN
- BAKEPAN
- BASEDON
- BASEMAN
- BASEMEN
- BASETEN
- BATEMAN
- BELEVEN
- BITESIN
- BITESON
- BLUEFIN
- BLUEHEN
- BLUESUN
- BOXEDIN
- BOXESIN
- BOZEMAN
- BRAEDEN
- CAGEDIN
- CAKEPAN
- CAKETIN
- CAMERON
- CAPEANN
- CAVEDIN
- CAVEMAN
- CAVEMEN
- CAVESIN
- CHEERON
- CLUEDIN
- CLUESIN
- COLEMAN
- COMESIN
- COMESON
- CREEPIN
- DINEDIN
- DINEDON
- DINESEN
- DINESIN
- DINESON
- DIVEDIN
- DIVESIN
- DONEGAN
- DOTEDON
- DOTESON
- DUNEDIN
- EASEDIN
- EASEDON
- EASESIN
- EASESON
- ECHELON
- EDGEDIN
- EDGESIN
- EGGEDON
- ENDEDIN
- ENDEDON
- ENTERIN
- ENTERON
- ERTEGUN
- ESTEBAN
- ESTEFAN
- EUCERIN
- EUDEMON
- EXCELIN
- FACEDON
- FACESON
- FADEDIN
- FADESIN
- FENELON
- FILEDIN
- FILESIN
- FIREDON
- FIREMAN
- FIREMEN
- FIRESON
- FIVEMAN
- FIVEPIN
- FIVETEN
- FIXEDON
- FIXESON
- FLIESIN
- FLIESON
- FOREIGN
- FOREMAN
- FOREMEN
- FORERAN
- FORERUN
- FREEMAN
- FREEMEN
- FRIEDAN
- GAMELAN
- GATEMAN
- GATEMEN
- GAZEDON
- GAZESON
- GENEVAN
- GETEVEN
- GIVENIN
- GIVENON
- GIVESIN
- GIVESON
- GLEEMAN
- GLEEMEN
- GLUEDON
- GLUEGUN
- GLUESON
- GOBELIN
- GOTEVEN
- HAMELIN
- HAVEFUN
- HIREDON
- HIRESON
- HOMEDIN
- HOMERUN
- HOMESIN
- HONEDIN
- HONESIN
- HYPERON
- INKEDIN
- JAMESON
- JAVELIN
- JOCELYN
- KEYEDIN
- KEYEDON
- LACESON
- LATERAN
- LATERON
- LAVERAN
- LETEMIN
- LINEMAN
- LINEMEN
- LIVEDIN
- LIVEDON
- LIVESIN
- LIVESON
- LUREDIN
- LURESIN
- MACEDON
- MADEFUN
- MADELON
- MADERUN
- MAKEFUN
- MAKERUN
- MATEWAN
- MILERUN
- MIXEDIN
- MIXESIN
- MOHEGAN
- MOVEDIN
- MOVEDON
- MOVESIN
- MOVESON
- MUMESON
- MUSEDON
- MUSESON
- NICEMAN
- NICEMEN
- NINEPIN
- NOSEDIN
- NOSESIN
- NOTEVEN
- OPTEDIN
- ORDERIN
- OUTEARN
- PALEMON
- PETEMAN
- PETEMEN
- PHAETON
- PILEDIN
- PILEDON
- PILESIN
- PILESON
- PIMESON
- PIPEDIN
- PIPESIN
- POKEFUN
- POKEMON
- POLEMAN
- POLEMEN
- QUIETEN
- RACEDIN
- RAKEDIN
- RAKESIN
- RAMEKIN
- REBEGAN
- REBEGIN
- REBEGUN
- RELEARN
- REVELIN
- RIDESIN
- ROBESON
- ROPEDIN
- ROPESIN
- RULEDON
- RULESON
- SAGEHEN
- SAVEDON
- SAVESON
- SENECAN
- SEWEDON
- SHEEHAN
- SIDEMAN
- SIDEMEN
- SILENTN
- SIMENON
- SIZETEN
- SLEEKEN
- SLEEPIN
- SLEEPON
- SLOEGIN
- SPIEDON
- SPIESON
- STEEPEN
- STEEPIN
- SURECAN
- SWEETEN
- SWEETON
- TAKENIN
- TAKENON
- TAKESIN
- TAKESON
- TAKETEN
- TAPEDON
- TAPEMAN
- TAPEMEN
- TAPESON
- TEHERAN
- TELERAN
- THREWIN
- THREWON
- TIBETAN
- TIREMAN
- TIREMEN
- TOHELEN
- TOLEDAN
- TOPEKAN
- TOWEDIN
- TRIEDON
- TRIESON
- TUBEPAN
- TUNEDIN
- TUNESIN
- TYPEDIN
- TYPESIN
- UNLEARN
- URGEDON
- URGESON
- USHERIN
- VENEMAN
- VETERAN
- VOTEDIN
- VOTEDON
- VOTESIN
- VOTESON
- WADEDIN
- WADESIN
- WAVEDIN
- WAVESIN
- WHEELIN
- WIREDIN
- WIREMAN
- WIREMEN
- WIRESIN
- WISEMAN
- WISEMEN
- WOBEGON
- YALEMAN
- YALEMEN
- YEREVAN

••••EN•

- ABILENE
- ACUMENS
- AILMENT
- AIRVENT
- ALIMENT
- AMBIENS
- AMBIENT
- ANCIENT
- ATANEND
- AUGMENT
- AWAKENS
- BACKEND
- BALEENS
- BARRENS
- BARTEND
- BATTENS
- BEHRENS
- BENZENE
- BIGBEND
- BIGTENT
- BOKKENS
- BOOKEND
- BRAZENS
- BURDENS
- CAIRENE
- CANDENT
- CAREENS
- CARLENE
- CELAENO
- CLEMENS
- CLEMENT
- COAGENT
- COBLENZ
- COMMEND
- COMMENT
- COMPEND
- CONSENT
- CONTEND
- CONTENT
- CONVENE
- CONVENT
- COZZENS
- CRAVENS
- CURRENT
- DAMPENS
- DARKENS
- DARLENE
- DAYSEND
- DEADEND
- DEADENS
- DEAFENS
- DEEPEND
- DEEPENS
- DERWENT
- DESCEND
- DESCENT
- DICKENS
- DIEMENS
- DILUENT
- DISSENT
- DISTEND
- DUODENA
- DURWENT
- EASTEND
- ELEMENT
- ELEVENA
- ELEVENB
- ELEVENC
- ELEVEND
- ELEVENE
- ELEVENS
- EMINENT
- EPICENE
- ERIGENA
- ERODENT
- EUGLENA
- EVIDENT
- EXIGENT
- FASTENS
- FATTENS
- FERMENT
- FERVENT
- FIGMENT
- FLORENZ
- FORFEND
- FORRENT
- FORWENT
- FRELENG
- FULGENT
- GARDENA
- GARDENS
- GARMENT
- GAUDENS
- GELPENS
- GETBENT
- GINSENG
- GLUTENS
- GODSEND
- GODSENT
- GULDENS
- HAPPENS
- HARDENS
- HARKENS
- HASTENS
- HEADEND
- HEAVENS
- HELLENE
- HELLENO
- HIGHEND
- HOYDENS
- HUYGENS
- HYGIENE
- HYPHENS

IMOGENE
JAYLENO
JERGENS
JURGENS
KAYLENZ
KEENENH
KITTENS
KOBLENZ
KRAKENS
KUCHENS
KURRENT
LAMBENT
LARCENY
LARGENT
LATEENS
LAURENT
LEADENS
LEAVENS
LEFTEND
LENIENT
LEOGENN
LESSENS
LICHENS
LINDENS
LISTENS
LOOSENS
LORIENT
LOUDENS
LOWRENT
MADDENS
MAIDENS
MAJGENS
MARLENE
MARTENS
MILLEND
MINUEND
MIOCENE
MISSEND
MISSENT
MITTENS
MIZZENS
MORDENT
MOREENS
MUDHENS
NASCENT
NEATENS
NEOCENE
NEOGENE
OBSCENE
ODDMENT
ONECENT
OPENEND
OPULENT
OROGENY
OUTBEND
OUTWENT
PANTENE
PARVENU
PATIENT
PAYMENT
PEAHENS
PENDENT
PERCENT
PHONENO
PICKENS
PIGMENT
PIGPENS
PINKENS
PLATENS
POLLENS
PORSENA
PORTEND
PORTENT
POTEENS
POULENC
PREDENY
PRERENT
PRESENT
PRETEND
PREVENT
PROGENY
PRUDENT
PUNGENT
PUPTENT
RAIMENT
REAGENT
REAMEND
REAREND
REDCENT
REDDENS
REDHENS
RELLENO
REOPENS
REUBENS
RICHENS
RIESENS
RIPIENI
RIPIENO
RUMPEND
SADDENS
SALIENT
SAPIENS
SAPIENT
SARGENT
SATEENS
SCALENE
SCREENS
SEGMENT
SENSENS
SERPENS
SERPENT
SICKENS
SIEMENS
SLOVENE
SLOVENS
SOFTENS
SOLVENT
SOYLENT
SPLEENS
SPLEENY
STAMENS
STEVENS
STIPEND
STUDENT
STYRENE
SUBTEND
SUBVENE
SUSPEND
TAILEND
TANGENT
TAUTENS
TENCENT
TERRENE
THERENT
THREENO
TOLUENE
TOPTENS
TORMENT
TORRENT
TRIDENT
TUREENS
TWERENT
UNBLENT
UNGUENT
UNSPENT
UPTREND
USOPENS
VERBENA
VIADENT
VINCENT
VIOLENT
WARDENS
WARRENG
WARRENS
WEAKENS
WEEKEND
WESTEND
WHITENS
WILKENS
WITSEND
WOOLENS
WORSENS
YEAREND
YEVGENY

••••E•N

ACTAEON
AGREEON
ALAMEIN
ALATEEN
ALGREEN
APOGEAN
ARAMEAN
ARTFERN
AZOREAN
BAHREIN
BARDEEN
BARGEIN
BETWEEN
BITTERN
BLAMEON
BOOLEAN
BORNEAN
BROKEIN
BURGEON
CANTEEN
CHILEAN
CHIMEIN
CHOKEON
CISTERN
CLOSEIN
COLLEEN
CONCERN
CONDEMN
CONTEMN
CRIMEAN
DANTEAN
DARLEEN
DISCERN
DOONEIN
DRIVEIN
DRONEON
DROVEIN
DRUZEAN
DUDGEON
DUNGEON
EASTERN
EPSTEIN
FENCEIN
FIFTEEN
FONTEYN
FORCEIN
FORCEON
GALLEON
GLIDEIN
GRATEON
GUDGEON
GUINEAN
HADBEEN
HASBEEN
HINGEON
HOLBEIN
HUSSEIN
INGREEN
JOYCEAN
KILLEEN
LANTERN
LEAVEIN
LEAVEON
LECTERN
LEOGENN
LETHEAN
LETMEIN
LETTERN
LOCKEAN
LODGEIN
LURLEEN
MACLEAN
MAUREEN
MCQUEEN
MIDTEEN
MRCLEAN
MRGREEN
NEWBERN
NOTBEEN
NUCLEON
OAKFERN
OLDBEAN
ONTKEAN
ORPHEAN
OUTSEEN
PASTEIN
PASTERN
PATTERN
PEABEAN
PHASEIN
PHONEIN
PIDGEON
PISCEAN
POSTERN
PRETEEN
PROTEAN
PROTEIN
RECLEAN
REDFERN
ROYBEAN
SEAFERN
SEIZEON
SHAREIN
SHINEON
SHOVEIN
SIXTEEN
SLIDEIN
SMILEON
SOTHERN
SOYBEAN
STOLEIN
SUBTEEN
SURGEON
SWOREIN
TAUREAN
THEREIN
THEREON
TINTERN
TRADEIN
TRADEON
UMPTEEN
UNCLEAN
UNGREEN
UNSTERN
VALJEAN
VERGEON
VILLEIN
VISTEON
WAXBEAN
WEDGEIN
WESTERN
WHEREIN
WHEREON
WIDGEON
WRITEIN
WRITEON
WROTEIN
WROTEON
YOUREON

•••••EN

ABDOMEN
ADWOMEN
AGNOMEN
ALATEEN
ALBUMEN
ALGREEN
ALMADEN
ALMSMEN
ALROSEN
ANDTHEN
ANTIGEN
ATSEVEN
ATTYGEN
AUTOPEN
BADOMEN
BAHAMEN
BARDEEN
BASEMEN
BASETEN
BATSMEN
BEDIZEN
BEECHEN
BELEVEN
BELLMEN
BENTSEN
BERNSEN
BESTMEN
BETAKEN
BETOKEN
BETWEEN
BIRCHEN
BIRDMEN
BLACKEN
BLITZEN
BLUEHEN
BLUNDEN
BLYNKEN
BOATMEN
BOBGOEN
BOGYMEN
BONDMEN
BOOKMEN
BOSSMEN
BRACKEN
BRAEDEN
BRITTEN
BROADEN
BRONWEN
BULLPEN
BUSHMEN
CANTEEN
CAUTHEN
CAVEMEN
CERUMEN
CHAPMEN
CHARMEN
CHASTEN
CHEAPEN
CHECHEN
CHICHEN
CHICKEN
CHIDDEN
CITIZEN
CITROEN
COARSEN
COLLEEN
COMBIEN
COPYMEN
CREWMEN
CRISPEN
CRUTZEN
CRYOGEN
CUTOPEN
DANIKEN
DARLEEN
DEARDEN
DEHAVEN
DELIMEN
DENIZEN
DINESEN
DIRKSEN
DOORMEN
DOUBLEN
DRAWMEN
DRAYMEN
DRESDEN
DRUNKEN
DUSTMEN
EARTHEN
ENLIVEN
FELTPEN
FIFTEEN
FIREMEN
FIVETEN
FLAGMEN
FLANKEN
FLATTEN
FLIPPEN
FLYOPEN
FOOTMEN
FOREMEN
FRANKEN
FREEMEN
FRESHEN
FROGMEN
GADSDEN
GASOVEN
GATEMEN
GETEVEN
GLADDEN
GLEEMEN
GLISTEN
GOODMEN
GOTEVEN
GREATEN
GREYHEN
HADBEEN
HALOGEN
HANGMEN
HANGTEN
HARDTEN
HARSHEN
HASBEEN
HEADMEN
HEARKEN
HEARTEN
HEATHEN
HILLMEN
HOARSEN
HOBOKEN
HOLYMEN
HOOPMEN
HOWTHEN
HUNGTEN
ICHDIEN
IDEAMEN
INDIGEN
INGREEN
INWOVEN
IRONMEN
ITSOPEN
JANSSEN
JAZZMEN
JUNKMEN
JURYMEN
KILLEEN
KINSMEN
KIRSTEN
KITCHEN
KRAMDEN
LANDMEN
LARCHEN
LAYOPEN
LEADMEN
LENSMEN
LIGHTEN
LINEMEN
LONGDEN
LOWCHEN
LURLEEN
MAARTEN
MADCHEN
MAILMEN
MAINMEN
MANXMEN
MARSDEN
MAUREEN
MCALLEN
MCCOWEN
MCQUEEN
MEATMEN
MEISSEN
MENCKEN
MERIDEN
MIDTEEN
MILKMEN
MOISTEN
MOMMSEN
MOORHEN
MRGREEN
MUNCHEN
MUTAGEN
MUYBIEN
NAVYMEN
NETIZEN
NEWSMEN
NICEMEN
NIELSEN
NOTBEEN
NOTEVEN
NOTOPEN
NOWTHEN
NUNGWEN
OARSMEN
OUTSEEN
PATCHEN
PAULSEN
PETEMEN
PIROGEN
PLAYPEN
PLOWMEN
POLEMEN
POOLMEN
POORMEN
POSTMEN
PREOPEN
PRETEEN
PROPMEN
PRYOPEN
QUICKEN
QUIETEN
RAILMEN
REALMEN
REEDMEN
REGIMEN
REGIVEN
RERISEN
RETAKEN
REWAKEN
REWIDEN
REWOKEN
REWOVEN
RICHMEN
RIESSEN
RIPOPEN
ROBBNEN
RONTGEN
ROUGHEN
SAGEHEN
SAMISEN
SANDMEN
SARACEN
SARAZEN
SAYAMEN
SAYWHEN
SEAGREN
SHANNEN
SHARPEN
SHIPMEN
SHODDEN
SHORTEN
SHOWMEN
SIDEMEN
SIXTEEN
SIZETEN
SLACKEN
SLEEKEN
SMARTEN
SMIDGEN
SMITTEN
SNELLEN
SNOWMEN
STASSEN
STEEPEN
STEPHEN
STEUBEN
STIFFEN
STOLLEN
STOUTEN
STRIVEN
SUBTEEN
SUELLEN
SURFMEN
SWAGMEN
SWEETEN
SWOLLEN
TAKETEN
TAMGLEN
TAPEMEN
TAXIMEN
THEOMEN
THICKEN
THIGPEN
THRIVEN
TIGHTEN
TIREMEN
TOHELEN
TOLKIEN
TOLLMEN
TOOKTEN
TOUGHEN
TRODDEN
TRUDGEN
TURFMEN
UMPTEEN
UNEATEN
UNGIVEN
UNGREEN
UNLADEN
UNOFTEN
UNRISEN
UNRIVEN
UNTAKEN
UNWOVEN
UPRISEN
VANDIEN
VANOWEN
VECHTEN
WHAUDEN
WHEATEN
WILDMEN
WINGMEN
WIREMEN
WISEMEN
WOLFMEN
WOOLLEN
WORKMEN
WRITTEN
YALEMEN
YARDMEN
YOUTHEN

EO•••••

EOLITHS
EONLINE
EOSINES

E•O••••

EBONICS
EBONIES
EBONITE
EBONIZE
ECOCIDE
ECOLOGY
ECONOMY
ECOTAGE
ECOTEUR
ECOTRIN
ECOTYPE
EDOMITE
EDOUARD
EGOISTE
EGOISTS
EGOSURF
EGOTISM
EGOTIST
EGOTRIP
ELOCUTE
ELOPERS
ELOPING
EMOTERS
EMOTING
EMOTION
EMOTIVE
ENOILED
ENOLOGY
ENOUNCE
EPOCHAL
EPONINE
EPONYMS
EPONYMY
EPOPEES
EPOQUES
EPOXIED
EPOXIES
ERODENT
ERODERS
ERODING
EROSELY
EROSION
EROSIVE
EROTICA
EROTICS
ESOBESO
ESOTERY
ETOILES
ETONIAN
ETONICS
EUONYMS
EVOKERS
EVOKING
EVOLUTE
EVOLVED
EVOLVER
EVOLVES
EXOCARP
EXOCETS
EXOGAMY
EXOILER
EXONYMS
EXORDIA
EXOTICA
EXOTICS
EXOTISM

E••O•••

EATOVER
ECHOERS
ECHOING
ECHOISM
ECLOGUE
EDMONDS
EFFORTS
EIDOLIC
EIDOLON
ELBOWED
ELBOWER
ELFOWLS
ELMONTE
ELNORTE
EMBOITE
EMBOSOM
EMBOWER
EMPORIA
EMPOWER
ENCODED
ENCODER
ENCODES
ENCOMIA
ENCORED
ENCORES
ENDORSE
ENDOWED
ENDOWER
ENFOLDS
ENFORCE
ENGORGE
ENJOINS
ENJOYED
ENJOYER
ENNOBLE
ENROBED
ENROBES
ENROLLS
ENROOTS
ENROUTE
ENSOULS
ENTOMBS
ENVOGUE
ENWOUND
ERGOTIC
ESCORTS
ESPOSAS
ESPOSOS
ESPOUSE
ESTONIA
ESTORIL
ETVOILA
EUNOMIA
EUROPOP
EUROVAN
EXHORTS
EXPORTS
EXPOSED
EXPOSER
EXPOSES
EXPOSIT
EXPOUND
EXTOLLS
EXTORTS
EXWORKS

E•••O••

EARBONE
EARHOLE
EARLOBE
EARLOCK
EASEOFF
EASEOUT
EASYOFF
EASYONE
EATMORE
EATSOUT
ECOLOGY
ECONOMY
EDGEOUT
EDITORS
EDITOUT
EELPOTS
EELPOUT
EELWORM
EGGNOGS
EGGROLL
EGGTOSS
EKEDOUT
EKESOUT
ELEVONS
ELFLOCK
ELLIOTT
ELMWOOD
ELUSORY
EMBROIL
EMBROWN
EMPLOYS
EMULOUS
ENAMORS
ENAMOUR
ENCLOSE
ENDLONG
ENDMOST
ENDNOTE
ENDZONE
ENGROSS
ENOLOGY
ENROOTS
ENTROPY
ENVIOUS
EPIDOTE
EPIGONE
EPILOGS
EPISODE
EPITOME
ERELONG
ESCROWS
ETHMOID
ETYMONS
EUPHONY
EVELONG
EVENOFF
EVENOUT
EVILONE
EXPLODE
EXPLOIT
EXPLORE
EYEBOLT
EYEFOLD
EYEHOLE
EYEHOOK
EYEROLL
EYESORE

E••••O•

EARDROP
EARLDOM
EARLYON
EARSHOT
EASEDON
EASESON
EASYJOB
EATALOT
EATCROW
EATFROM
ECHELON
ECUADOR
EDITION
EDUCTOR
EGGDROP
EGGEDON
EIDOLON
EJECTOR
ELATION
ELCAJON
ELEANOR
ELECTOR
ELEISON
ELISION
ELLISON
ELMWOOD
ELNINOS
ELUTION
EMBOSOM
EMBRYOS
EMERSON
EMMYLOU
EMOTION
EMPEROR
ENACTOR
ENARBOR
ENDEDON
ENDUROS
ENTERON
ENVELOP
ENVENOM
ENVIRON
ENVIROS
EPSILON
EQUATOR
EQUINOX
ERECTOR
EREWHON
ERICSON
ERIKSON
EROSION
ERYNGOS
ESCALOP
ESCUDOS
ESIASON

ESKIMOS ESPANOL ESPOSOS ESTADOS ETHANOL EUDEMON EUROPOP EVASION EVENNOW EVERTOR EVICTOR EXACTOR EXCITOR EXITNOW EXMAYOR EYEBROW EYEDROP EYEHOOK EYESHOT EYESPOT

E•••••O

EATINTO EDGARDO EDUARDO EJEMPLO ELCAMPO ELECTRO ELGALLO ELGRECO ELMUNDO ELPRADO EMBARGO EQUALTO EQUIANO ERNESTO ERYTHRO ESOBESO ESPARTO EXANIMO EXFACTO EXTENSO

•EO••••

AEOLIAN BEOGRAD BEOWULF DEODARS DEODATO DEORBIT FEODORI FEOFFED GEOCODE GEODESY GEODUCK GEOLOGY GEORGEC GEORGEI GEORGEM GEORGES GEORGEV GEORGEW GEORGIA GEORGIC GEORGIE KEOGHAN LEOGENN LEONARD

LEONATO LEONDAY LEONIDS LEONINE LEONORA LEONORE LEOPARD LEOPOLD LEOTARD LEOVIII LEOXIII MEOWERS MEOWING MEOWMIX NEOCENE NEOCONS NEOGENE NEOLITH NEOLOGY NEOLYTE NEONATE NEONGAS PEONAGE PEONIES PEOPLED PEOPLES PEORIAN REOCCUR REOFFER REOILED REOPENS REORDER REOWNED YEOMANS

•E•O•••

AEROBAT AEROBES AEROBIC AEROSOL BECOMES BEDOUIN BEFOOLS BEFOULS BEGONIA BEGORRA BEHOLDS BEHOOVE BELONGS BELOVED BEMOANS BENOTED BENOTES BEROWNE BETOKEN BEYONCE CELOTEX DEBOITE DEBONED DEBONES DEBORAH DEBOULE DECOCTS DECODED DECODER DECODES DECOLOR DECORUM

DECOYED DECOYER DEFOAMS DEFOCUS DEFORMS DEHORNS DELORIS DELORME DELOUSE DEMOING DEMOLAY DEMONIC DEMONYM DEMOTED DEMOTES DEMOTHS DEMOTIC DEMOUNT DENOTED DENOTES DEPONED DEPONER DEPONES DEPORTS DEPOSAL DEPOSED DEPOSER DEPOSES DEPOSIT DEPOWER DERONDA DESOTOS DETOURS DETOXED DETOXES DEVOIRS DEVOLVE DEVORES DEVOTED DEVOTEE DEVOTES DEVOURS DEWORMS DEYOUNG FEDORAS FEDOROV FELONRY FEMORAL FEMORIS GENOESE GENOISE GENOMES GENOMIC GETONIT GETONTO GETOVER HEDONIC HELOISE HELOTRY HEROICS HEROINE HEROISM HERONRY HEXOSES KELOWNA KENOLIN KENOSHA KEROUAC

KETONES KETONIC LECONTE LEGOLAS LEGOSET LELOUCH LEMONDE LEMOYNE LENOVOS LESOTHO MEGOHMS MEIOSES MEIOSIS MEIOTIC MELODIA MELODIC MEMOIRE MEMOIRS MEMOPAD MEMOREX MENORAH MENORCA MENOTTI MESONIC METOOER NEPOTIC PELOTAS PELOTON PERORAL PEYOTES REBOANT REBOARD REBOILS REBOLTS REBOOKS REBOOTS REBORED REBORES REBOTES REBOUND REBOXED REBOXES REBOZOS RECOALS RECOATS RECOCKS RECODED RECODES RECOILS RECOINS RECOLOR RECOMBS RECOOKS RECOOLS RECORDS RECORKS RECOSTS RECOUNT RECOUPS RECOVER REDOAKS REDOCKS REDOING REDONDO REDOSED REDOSES REDOUBT REDOUND

REDOUTS REDOXES REFOCUS REFOLDS REFORGE REFORMS REFOUND REHONED REHONES REHONOR REHOOKS REHOUSE REJOICE REJOINS RELOADS RELOANS RELOCKS RELOOKS RELOSES REMODEL REMOLDS REMORAS REMORSE REMOTER REMOTES REMOUNT REMOVAL REMOVED REMOVER REMOVES REMOWED RENOIRS RENOTED RENOTES RENOWNS REPOINT REPOLLS REPOMAN REPORTS REPOSED REPOSER REPOSES REPOSIT REPOSTS REPOURS REPOWER REROLLS REROOFS REROOTS REROUTE RESOAKS RESOAPS RESOILS RESOJET RESOLED RESOLER RESOLES RESOLVE RESORBS RESORTS RESOUND RESOWED RETOAST RETONED RETONES RETOOLS RETORTS RETOTAL

RETOUCH RETOURS RETOWED REVOICE REVOKED REVOKER REVOKES REVOLTS REVOLVE REVOTED REVOTES REWOKEN REWORDS REWORKS REWOUND REWOVEN REYOKED REYOKES REZONED REZONES SECONDI SECONDO SECONDR SECONDS SEDONAS SEGOVIA SENORAS SENORES SETOFFS SETOUTS TEEOFFS TENONED TENONER VELOURS VELOUTE VELOXES VERONIA VETOERS VETOING WEEONES WETONES XEROSES XEROSIS XEROTIC XEROXED XEROXES YESORNO ZEDONKS ZENOBIA ZEROING ZEROOUT ZEROSIN ZEROSUM

•E••O••

BEACONS BEANOIL BEAROFF BEAROUT BEATOFF BEATOUT BECKONS BECLOUD BEDDOWN BEDFORD BEDLOES BEDNORZ BEDPOST

BEDROCK BEDROLL BEDROOM BEFOOLS BEGSOFF BEHOOVE BELFORT BELLOWS BELMONT BELTOUT BELVOIR BELVOUR BELZONI BENBOVA BERTOLT BERVOIX BESPOKE BESTOFF BESTONE BESTOWS BETROTH BETTORS CENSORS DEACONS DEALOUT DEARONE DEBTORS DECKOUT DECLOTS DEFCONS DEFROCK DEFROST DEGHOST DELMONT DELMORE DELSOLS DELTOID DELTONA DELTORO DENMOMS DENTOID DENTONS DEPLORE DEPLOYS DESMOGS DESMOND DESPOIL DESPOND DESPOTS DESTOCK DETROIT DEVIOUS EELPOTS EELPOUT EELWORM FEELOFF FEELOUT FELLOFF FELLOUT FELLOWS FELTOFF FELTOUT FEMBOTS FENDOFF FEODORI FERROUS FERVORS FERVOUR

FESTOON FESTOSO FETLOCK GECKOES GENLOCK GEOCODE GEOLOGY GESSOED GESSOES GETCOLD GETDONE GETDOWN GETGOOD GETLOST GETSOFF GETSOFT GETSOLD GETSORE GETSOUT GETTOIT GETWORD HEADOFF HEADOUT HEAROUT HECTORS HEINOUS HELDOFF HELDOUT HELLOED HELLOES HELMOND HELPOUT HEMLOCK HENCOOP HENTOFF HERMOSA HERMOSO HEYLOOK HEYWOOD JEALOUS JERBOAS JERKOUT JETBOAT JETFOIL JETPORT JETSONS KEDROVA KEEPOFF KEEPOUT KELLOGG KENDOLL KENMORE KEPTOFF KEPTOUT KEYHOLE KEYLOCK KEYNOTE KEYWORD LEACOCK LEADOFF LEADORE LEADOUT LEAFOUT LEAWOOD LEBROCK LECTORS LECUONA LEEFORD

LEFTOFF LEFTOUT LEGBONE LEGHORN LEGIONS LEGROOM LEGROPE LEGWORK LENDOUT LENNONS LEONORA LEONORE LEOPOLD LEPTONS LESIONS LESSONS LESSORS LESTOIL LETDOWN LETGOBY LETGOOF LETROLL LETSOFF LETSOUT LEWHOAD MEADOWS MEADOWY MEDFORD MELLOWS MELROSE MENFOLK MENTORS MERLOTS METEORS METEOUT METHODS METOOER NEGRONI NELSONS NEOCONS NEOLOGY NERVOUS NESTORS NETCOST NETLOSS NETTONS NETWORK NEURONE NEURONS NEWBOLT NEWBORN NEWHOPE NEWJOBS NEWLOOK NEWLOVE NEWMONT NEWMOON NEWMOWN NEWPORT NEWSOME NEWTONS NEWTOWN NEWTOYS NEWWORD NEWYORK PEABODY PEACOAT PEACOCK

PEAFOWL PEAPODS PEASOUP PEEKOUT PEELOFF PEELOUT PEEPOUT PEEROUT PEGTOPS PENNOCK PENNONS PENROSE PEPBOYS PEPTONE PEQUOTS PERFORM PERGOLA PERIODS PERSOFF PERSONA PERSONS PETBOAS PETCOCK PETCOMB PETCOWS PETDOGS PETDOOR PETDOVE PETGOAT PETIOLE PETPONY PETROCK PETROLS PETROUS PETTOYS READOFF READOPT READORN READOUT REAMOUT REAROSE REASONS REAVOWS REAWOKE REBLOCK REBLOOM REBLOWN REBOOKS REBOOTS REBROKE RECHOSE RECKONS RECOOKS RECOOLS RECROOM RECROSS RECROWN RECTORS RECTORY REDBONE REDBOOK REDCOAT REDCODS REDDOGS REDDOTS REDFORD REDFOUR REDHOTS

REDMOND REDNOSE REDPOLL REDPONY REDROBE REDROOP REDROOT REDROSE REDTOPS REDWOLF REDWOOD REDWORM REDZONE REEBOKS REELOFF REELOUT REEVOKE REFLOAT REFLOOD REFLOWN REFLOWS REFRONT REGIONS REGLOSS REGLOWS REGROOM REGROUP REGROWN REGROWS REHOOKS REKNOCK REKNOTS RELOOKS RENTOUT RENVOIS REPHONE REPLOTS REPLOWS REPROBE REPROOF REPROVE REQUOTE REROOFS REROOTS RESCORE RESHOES RESHOOT RESHOWN RESHOWS RESPOKE RESPOND RESPOOL RESPOTS RESTOCK RESTOKE RESTORE RESTOWS RESWORE RESWORN RETOOLS REWROTE REXROTH REYMONT REYNOSA SEABOAT SEABORG SEACOWS SEADOGS

SEAFOAM SEAFOOD SEAFOWL SEAGODS SEALOFF SEAMOSS SEAPORT SEASONS SEAWOLF SECTORS SEEKOUT SEENOFF SEENOUT SEEPOUT SEESOFF SEESOUT SEETOIT SEIZORS SELLOFF SELLOUT SENDOFF SENDOUT SENHORA SENIORS SENSORS SENSORY SENTOFF SENTOUT SEQUOIA SEQUOYA SERIOUS SERMONS SETDOWN SETSOFF SETSOUT SEXPOTS SEXTONS SEYMOUR TEACOZY TEAGOWN TEAPOTS TEAPOYS TEAROFF TEAROOM TEAROSE TEAROUT TEDIOUS TEEDOFF TEESOFF TEFLONS TELLOFF TEMPORE TENCODE TENDONS TENFOLD TENFOOT TENFOUR TENSORS TENTONS TENUOUS TERAOHM TERROIR TERRORS TESTOUT TETRODE TEUTONS VECTORS VEEROFF

VENDOME VENDORS VERBOSE VERDOUX VERMONT VERYODD VERYOLD WEAKONS WEAPONS WEAROFF WEAROUT WEBFOOT WEBLOGS WEBTOED WEDLOCK WEEDOUT WEEFOLK WEEHOUR WELCOME WELLOFF WENTOFF WENTOUT WESCOTT WETDOWN WETLOOK WETMOPS WEXFORD YEARONE YELLOUT YELLOWS YELLOWY YESVOTE ZEALOTS ZEALOUS ZEBROID ZEPPOLE ZEPPOLI ZEROOUT

•E•••O•

AERATOR AEROSOL BEALION BEARSON BEATBOX BEATCOP BEATSON BEDROOM BEGSFOR BELABOR BELLBOY BELLHOP BELLSON BENISON BENTHOS BERGSON BERLIOZ BESTBOY CELADON CESSION CESTMOI DEARGOD DECAGON DECALOG DECAPOD DECOLOR DEEDBOX DEMAGOG

DEMEROL
DEMIGOD
DENDRON
DENISON
DESKTOP
DESOTOS
DESTROY
DEVELOP
DEVISOR
DEWDROP
FEARFOR
FEARNOT
FEASTON
FEDOROV
FEEDLOT
FEEDSON
FEELFOR
FEELSOK
FELLFOR
FELTFOR
FENELON
FERMION
FESTOON
GEARBOX
GEEKDOM
GELATOS
GEMSBOK
GENITOR
GERITOL
GERSHON
GETAJOB
GETFROM
GETGOOD
GETINON
GETITON
GETSHOT
GETUPON
HEADFOR
HEAPSOF
HEAPSON
HEARDOF
HEARSOF
HEDISON
HEIRDOM
HELICON
HELLBOY
HELLION
HELPSON
HENCOOP
HERENOW
HERITOR
HERNDON
HERRIOT
HEXAGON
HEXAPOD
HEYLOOK
HEYWOOD
JEANNOT
JEMISON
JEWISON
KEEPSON
KEILLOR
KEMIDOV
KEMPTON
KERFLOP
KERPLOP
KEYEDON
KEYINON
LEADDOG
LEADSON
LEANSON
LEANTOS
LEAPFOR
LEAPSON
LEAPTON
LEARNOF
LEAVEON
LEAWOOD
LEBANON
LEBARON
LEFTFOR
LEGATOR
LEGATOS
LEGIRON
LEGROOM
LENOVOS
LETDROP
LETGOOF
LETINON
LETKNOW
LETSNOT
LETUPON
LEVATOR
LEXICON
MEANJOE
MEDICOS
MEGALON
MEGATON
MENTHOL
MENTION
MENUDOS
MERINOS
NEARYOU
NEEDNOT
NEGATOR
NEMEROV
NEUTRON
NEWLOOK
NEWMOON
NEWSBOY
PEARSON
PEATBOG
PEATPOT
PEKEPOO
PELOTON
PENSION
PERIDOT
PERSSON
PETCROW
PETDOOR
PETFROG
PETLION
PETSHOP
PEUGEOT
REACTOR
READFOR
READSON
REALLOT
REALTOR
REARDON
REBLOOM
REBOZOS
RECOLOR
RECROOM
REDBOOK
REDROOP
REDROOT
REDSPOT
REDWOOD
REEKSOF
REENDOW
REENJOY
REFLOOD
REGROOM
REHONOR
RELATOR
REPROOF
REPSFOR
REREDOS
RESHOOT
RESPOOL
RESTSON
RETINOL
REUNION
REVISOR
REZEROS
SEAFOOD
SEALION
SECTION
SEEDPOD
SEIZEON
SELLFOR
SEMILOG
SENATOR
SENDFOR
SENDSON
SENTFOR
SERFDOM
SESSION
SETSHOT
SETTLOR
SETUPON
SEWEDON
TEAROOM
TEASHOP
TEATROS
TECHNOS
TEESHOT
TEJANOS
TELECOM
TELLSOF
TELLSON
TEMBLOR
TEMPJOB
TENFOOT
TENSION
TENSPOT
TESTFOR
TEXTRON
VELCROS
VENISON
VENTNOR
VERGEON
VERIZON
VERSION
VERYHOT
VERYLOW
VESTRON
WEARSON
WEBFOOT
WEEPFOR
WEIGHON
WEIRDOS
WEIRTON
WELLWON
WENDKOS
WENTFOR
WETLOOK
XENIAOH
YEAHYOU
YELLFOR
YENSFOR
ZEBULON

•E••••O

BEAHERO
BEEFALO
BEGANTO
BELASCO
BENICIO
BENIGNO
BERGAMO
CELAENO
CEMBALO
CENTAVO
CENTIMO
CEPHALO
CEREBRO
DEALSTO
DEALTTO
DECARLO
DEFACTO
DEFERTO
DEIGNTO
DELICTO
DELILLO
DELTORO
DEMARCO
DEMENTO
DEODATO
DERECHO
DERMATO
DERRICO
DESTINO
DETECTO
DEUTERO
FEBRERO
FEDERKO
FEDINTO
FEEDSTO
FERRARO
FESTOSO
GEARSTO
GENNAIO
GENNARO
GERALDO
GESTAPO
GETINTO
GETONTO
HEADSTO
HEAVEHO
HEAVETO
HEIGHHO
HELLENO
HERESTO
HERMANO
HERMOSO
HERPETO
HEWEDTO
JERICHO
KEEPSTO
LEADSTO
LEANSTO
LEARNTO
LEASETO
LEDINTO
LEDUPTO
LENTIGO
LEONATO
LEPANTO
LESOTHO
LETITGO
LETMEGO
LETTERO
MEANSTO
MEANTTO
MEMENTO
MERCADO
NEEDSTO
NETZERO
PEKEPOO
PEPPINO
PEPSICO
PERATIO
PERDIDO
REACTTO
READSTO
REDONDO
REFERTO
RELLENO
RENALDO
RENTSTO
REPLYTO
SEAHERO
SECONDO
SEEALSO
SEEINTO
SEEMSTO
SELLSTO
SEMIPRO
SENDSTO
SERPICO
SETINTO
SEVENNO
TELESTO
TENDSTO
TENNECO
VERDUGO
VERISMO
VERTIGO
WENTPRO
YEARNTO
YESORNO
ZEDILLO
ZEMSTVO

••EO•••

AREOLAE
AREOLAR
AREOLAS
AREOLES
ATEOVER
CREOLES
CREOSOL
DIEOFFS
ICEOUTS
ICEOVER
LIEOVER
OLEOOIL
ONEOCAT
ONEOFFS
ONEOFUS
ONEONTA
ONEOVER
PREOMIT
PREOPEN
PREORAL
TEEOFFS
THEOATH
THEODOR
THEOMEN
THEOMNI
THEOREM
WEEONES

••E•O••

ACEDOUT
ACEROLA
ACEROSE
ACESOUT
ACETONE
ADENOID
AGEDOUT
AGEFOUR
AGELONG
AGESOUT
AKEBONO
AMEBOID
ANEMONE
ANEROID
ARENOSE
ATEMORE
AWESOME
BLEWOFF
BLEWOUT
BRETONS
CHEROOT
CHEVONS
CHEWOUT
CREMONA
CREMORA
CTENOID
DAEMONS
DAEWOOS
DIEBOLD
DIEDOFF
DIEDOUT
DIEDOWN
DIESOFF
DIESOUT
DREWOFF
DREWOUT
DYEJOBS
DYELOTS
DYEWOOD
EKEDOUT
EKESOUT
ELEVONS
ERELONG
EVELONG
EVENOFF
EVENOUT
EYEBOLT
EYEFOLD
EYEHOLE
EYEHOOK
EYEROLL
EYESORE
FAEROES
FEELOFF
FEELOUT
FLEXORS
FREMONT
FUELOIL
GJETOST
GOESOFF
GOESOUT
GREGORY
GREWOLD
HOEDOWN
ICEBOAT
ICECOLD
ICEDOUT
ICEDOWN
ICEFOGS
ICEHOLE
ICEPOPS
ICESOUT
ISECOND
ITEMONE
JOECOOL
JOEROTH
KEEPOFF
KEEPOUT
KMESONS
LEEFORD
LIEDOWN
LIENORS
LYESOAP
OCELOTS
OLEOOIL
ONEDOWN
ONEFOLD
ONEFOOT
ONEHOUR
ONEIOTA
ONELOOK
ONELOVE
ONEMORE
ONENOTE
ONEROOM
ONEROUS
ONESOCK
ONETOGO
ONEVOTE
ONEWOOD
OPENOUT
OPEROSE
OREBODY
PEEKOUT
PEELOFF
PEELOUT
PEEPOUT
PEEROUT
PHENOLS
PHENOMS
PIEHOLE
PIETOSO
PLEXORS
PREBOIL
PREBOOK
PREBOOM
PREBORN
PRECODE
PRECOIL
PRECOOK
PRECOOL
PRECOUP
PREDOOM
PREFORM
PRELOAD
PRELOAN
PRELOSS
PRENOON
PREROCK
PRESOAK
PRESOLD
PRESONG
PRESORT
PRETOLD
PRETORS
PREVOID
PREVOST
PREWORK
PREWORN
PTEROUS
PYEDOGS
REEBOKS
REELOFF
REELOUT
REEVOKE
RHEBOKS
RHETORS
RYELOAF
SEEKOUT
SEENOFF
SEENOUT
SEEPOUT
SEESOFF
SEESOUT
SEETOIT
SHEGOAT
SHEWOLF
SPECOUT
SPEDOFF
SPEWOUT
STEPOFF
STEPONE
STEPOUT
STEROID
STEROLS
TEEDOFF
TEESOFF
THEBOBO
THEBODY
THEBOMB
THEBOSS
THEBOYS
THEDOLE
THEFONZ
THEFOOL
THEGOLD
THEHOGS
THEHOOD
THEHOPE
THELOOK
THELOOP
THEMOON
THEMOST
THEPOND
THEPOOH
THEPOPE
THEPOST
THEROBE
THEROCK
THEROOM
THEROPE
THEROSE
THEROUX
THETOUR
TIEDOFF
TIEDOWN
TIEPOLO
TIERODS
TIEROPE
TIESOFF
TOEHOLD
TOELOOP
TREFOIL
TREMOLO
TREMORS
VEEROFF
WEEDOUT
WEEFOLK
WEEHOUR

••E••O•

ABETTOR
AHEADOF
AKERLOF
ALENCON
APECKOF
APERSON
ATEALOT
ATECROW
AVEYRON
AXELROD
BIENTOT
BLEDSOE
BLERIOT
BRENDON
BRERFOX
BRETTON
CHEATON
CHECKON
CHEERON
CHEETOS
CHEKHOV
CHEROOT
CHEVIOT
CHEVRON
CHEWSON
CHEWTOY
CHEZMOI
CLEAROF
CLEAVON
CLEMSON
CREATOR
CREEPOS
CREOSOL
CRESTON
DAEWOOS
DEEDBOX
DIEDFOR
DIESFOR
DOESFOR
DOESNOT
DOESTOO
DREAMOF
DREAMON
DREGION
DUETTOS
DWELLON
DWELTON
DYEWOOD
EJECTOR
ELEANOR
ELECTOR
ELEISON
EMERSON
ERECTOR
EREWHON
EVENNOW
EVERTOR
EYEBROW
EYEDROP
EYEHOOK
EYESHOT
EYESPOT
FEEDLOT
FEEDSON
FEELFOR
FEELSOK
FIEFDOM
FLEURON
FLEXION
FREEDOF
FREEDOM
FREESOF
FREETOY
FRESCOS
FUELROD
GEEKDOM
GHETTOS
GLEASON
GLENCOE
GOESFOR
GUERDON
IBEGYOU
ICEFLOE
ICESHOW
INERROR
IRECKON
ISEENOW
ISEEYOU
IVERSON
JOEBLOW
JOECOOL
KEEPSON
KLEPTOS
KNEWHOW
LIEATOP
LIEDFOR
LIESFOR
LIESLOW
LLEYTON
MCENROE
MYERSON
NEEDNOT
NOENDOF
OBENTOS
ONEFOOT
ONEIRON
ONELOOK
ONEROOM
ONESHOE
ONESHOT
ONESPOT
ONESTOP
ONETWOS
ONEWOOD
OPENTOE
OPENTOP
OVERCOY
OVERDOG
OVERHOT
OVERJOY
OVERTOP
PIERROT
PIETROS
PNEUMON
PREBOOK
PREBOOM
PRECOOK
PRECOOL
PREDOOM
PRENOON
PREPLOT
PRERIOT
PRESHOW
PRESSON
PRESTON
PRESTOS
PREYSON
PUEBLOS
QUEIROS
REEKSOF
REENDOW
REENJOY
SEEDPOD
SHEDSON
SHELDON
SKELTON
SLEDDOG
SLEEPON
SLEPTON
SMEAGOL
SMEARON
SPEAKOF
SPECTOR
SPEEDOS
SPENDON
SPENTON
STENTOR
STEPMOM
STEPSON
STEREOS
STERNOS
STERTOR
STETSON
STEWPOT
SUEDFOR
SUELYON
SUESFOR
SWEETON
SWENSON
TEESHOT
THEBLOB
THECROW
THEFLOP
THEFOOL
THEHOOD
THELOOK
THELOOP
THEMOON
THEODOR
THEPOOH
THEREOF
THEREON
THERMOS
THEROOM
THESHOW
TIEMPOS
TOELOOP
TOESHOE
TREADON
TREASON
TREETOP
TRENTON
TSELIOT
USEDFOR
USESFOR
VIEDFOR
VIESFOR
WEEPFOR
WHEATON
WHEREOF
WHEREON

••E•••O

AGESAGO
AKEBONO
ALERTTO
AMERIGO
ARECIBO
ARETINO
ATEINTO
BEEFALO
CHEERIO
DOESTOO
EJEMPLO
ELECTRO
FEEDSTO
GAETANO
GOESPRO
GUESSSO
KEEPSTO
MAESTRO
NEEDSTO
NOENDTO
NUESTRO
ONEKILO
ONETOGO
OREGANO
PIETOSO
PLEADTO
PREVETO
QUERIDO
SEEALSO
SEEINTO
SEEMSTO
SPEAKTO
STEPTWO
SWEARTO
THEBOBO
THEHERO
THEMAYO
THERETO
TIEINTO
TIEPOLO
TREMOLO
TREVINO
WHERETO
YIELDTO

•••EO••

ALVEOLI
AQUEOUS
AUREOLA
AUREOLE
BAKEOFF
BITEOFF
BOREOUT
CAMEOED
CAMEOFF
CAMEOUT
CASEOUS
CASEOUT
CINEOLE
COMEOFF
COMEONS
COMEOUT
DINEOUT
DOLEOUT
DOPEOUT
DOZEOFF
DUTEOUS
EASEOFF
EASEOUT
EDGEOUT
FACEOFF
FADEOUT
FAKEOUT
FILEOUT
FIREOFF
FIVEONE
GASEOUS
GAVEOFF
GAVEOUT
GIDEONS
GIVEOFF
GIVEOUT
GONEOFF
GONEOUT
HAVEONE
HAVEOUT
HIDEOUS
HIDEOUT
HIKEOUT
HIREOUT
HIVEOFF
HOLEOUT
IGNEOUS
KANEOHE
LANEONE
LINEONE
LINEOUT
LIVEOAK
LIVEONE
LIVEOUT
LOSEOUT
MADEOFF
MADEONE
MADEOUT
MAKEOFF
MAKEONE
MAKEOUT
METEORS
METEOUT
MIMEOED
MINEOLA
MOVEOFF
MOVEOUT

NAMEONE
NICEONE
NIVEOUS
NOSEOUT
OOZEOUT
OSCEOLA
OSSEOUS
OSTEOID
PACEOFF
PAGEONE
PICEOUS
PIGEONS
PILEOUS
PINEOIL
PITEOUS
POKEOUT
RAKEOFF
RIDEOFF
RIDEOUT
RODEOFF
RODEOUT
ROPEOFF
ROSEOIL
ROSEOLA
RUBEOLA
RULEONE
RULEOUT
SAMEOLD
SIDEONE
SIZEONE
SOMEONE
TAKEOFF
TAKEONE
TAKEOUT
TIMEOFF
TIMEOUT
TIREOUT
TOREOFF
TOREOUT
TUNEOUT
VIDEOED
VOTEOUT
WAVEOFF
WIPEOFF
WIPEOUT
WISEONE
WITEOUT
WOREOFF
WOREOUT
ZONEOUT

•••E•O•

ACHEFOR
ACHERON
ACHESON
ACTEDON
ADDEDON
AGREEON
AILERON
ALBEDOS
ALFEROV
ALIENOR
ANBESOL
ANGELOU
ASKEDOF
ASLEWOF
BADENOV
BAGEHOT
BASEDON
BIBELOT
BIGELOW
BITESON
BLUEBOY
BLUEFOX
BOLEROS
BOREDOM
CAMELOT
CAMERON
CAPECOD
CAREFOR
CASELOT
CHEERON
CHEETOS
COMENOW
COMESON
COTEDOR
CREEPOS
DARENOT
DAVEKOZ
DEMEROL
DEVELOP
DIDEROT
DINEDON
DINESON
DONEFOR
DOTEDON
DOTESON
DOVECOT
DUKEDOM
EASEDON
EASESON
ECHELON
EGGEDON
EMPEROR
ENDEDON
ENTERON
ENVELOP
ENVENOM
EUDEMON
FACEDON
FACESON
FAREBOX
FENELON
FIREBOX
FIREDOG
FIREDON
FIREFOX
FIRESON
FIXEDON
FIXESON
FLIESON
FORETOP
FREEDOF
FREEDOM
FREESOF
FREETOY
FUSEBOX
GAMEBOY
GAZEBOS
GAZEDON
GAZESON
GIVENOF
GIVENON
GIVESOF
GIVESON
GLUEDON
GLUESON
GOBELOW
GONEFOR
HAVENOT
HERENOW
HIREDON
HIRESON
HOMEBOY
HOPEFOR
HOPENOT
HYPERON
IOWEYOU
ISEENOW
ISEEYOU
JAMESON
JANEDOE
JUKEBOX
KEYEDON
LACESON
LAREDOS
LATERON
LIKEWOW
LIVEDON
LIVEFOR
LIVESON
LOVEJOY
LOVEYOU
LUBEJOB
MACEDON
MADEFOR
MADELON
MAKEDOS
MAKEFOR
MALEDOG
MALEHOG
MORELOS
MOVEDON
MOVESON
MUMESON
MUSEDON
MUSESON
NEMEROV
NICEBOY
NICEDOG
NICEJOB
NILESOH
NOSEJOB
NUMEROS
OFFEROR
PAGEBOY
PALEMON
PEKEPOO
PHAETON
PILEDON
PILESOF
PILESON
PIMESON
PINEFOR
PINESOL
PINETOP
POKEMON
POMELOS
POPEDOM
PRAETOR
RAVELOE
REREDOS
REZEROS
ROBESON
ROPETOW
RULEDON
RULESON
SALEMOR
SAVEDON
SAVEFOR
SAVESON
SEWEDON
SHOEBOX
SIMENON
SISENOR
SLEEPON
SOMEHOW
SPEEDOS
SPIEDON
SPIESON
SUREROF
SWEETON
TAKEFOR
TAKENON
TAKESON
TAPEDON
TAPESON
TELECOM
THREWON
TIMECOP
TIREDOF
TIRESOF
TOLEDOS
TONELOC
TONEROW
TOREROS
TREETOP
TRIEDON
TRIESON
TUBETOP
TUPELOS
TUXEDOS
TYLENOL
URGEDON
URGESON
VICEROY
VOTEDON
VOTEFOR
VOTESON
WOBEGON
YULELOG
ZYDECOS

•••E••O

ACDELCO
ADDEDTO
AGREETO
ALBERTO
ALIENTO
ALLEGRO
ANSELMO
ARGENTO
ARSENIO
ARTERIO
ASPENCO
BABENCO
BASETWO
BOWECHO
BOWEDTO
CAREDTO
CARESTO
CATERTO
CEREBRO
CHEERIO
CILENTO
COMESTO
DANEYKO
DARESTO
DAREZZO
DEFERTO
DEMENTO
DERECHO
DETECTO
ERNESTO
EXTENSO
FEDERKO
FIDELIO
FIVETWO
FLIEDTO
FLIESTO
FOLENGO
GALENTO
GIVENTO
GIVESTO
GLUEDTO
GLUESTO
GONEPRO
HAVEAGO
HERESTO
HEWEDTO
HIBERNO
HOPEDSO
HOPEDTO
HOPESSO
HOPESTO
INFERNO
IONESCO
JANEIRO
LANETWO
LIKENTO
LINETWO
LORENZO
LOSESTO
LOVEDTO
LOVESTO
LYSENKO
MAKESDO
MAKESGO
MARENGO
MEMENTO
MODESTO
MORELLO
MOVEDTO
MOVESTO
NORELCO
NOVELLO
OPTEDTO
OTHELLO
OUTECHO
PAGETWO
PALERMO
PATERNO
PEKEPOO
PIMENTO
POPELEO
RACEDTO
RACESTO
REFERTO
RIDESTO
RISENTO
RISESTO
RIVERPO
ROBERTO
SALERNO
SCHERZO
SEVENNO
SIDETWO
SILENTO
SIZETWO
SORENTO
STRETTO
SUBECHO
SUREIDO
TAKENTO
TAKESTO
TELESTO
THREENO
TRIEDTO
TRIESTO
TRUERTO
TUNEDTO
TUNESTO
UCCELLO
UMBERTO
UNDERDO
UNDERGO
UPTEMPO
VOTEDNO
VOTESNO
WAVEDTO
WAVESTO
YOTEAMO
ZANETTO

••••EO•

ACTAEON
AGREEON
APILEOF
AWAREOF
BLAMEON
BURGEON
CHOKEON
DRONEON
DUDGEON
DUNGEON
FORCEON
GALLEON
GRATEON
GUDGEON
HINGEON
INAWEOF
LARGEOJ
LEAVEON
MACLEOD
NUCLEON
PEUGEOT
PIDGEON
ROADEOS
SEIZEON
SHINEON
SMILEON
SPOKEOF
STEREOS
SURGEON
THEREOF
THEREON
TRADEON
VERGEON
VISTEON
WHEREOF
WHEREON
WIDGEON
WRITEON
WROTEON
YOUREON

••••E•O

AGREETO
ALFREDO
ALIVETO
ARTDECO
AZULEJO
BEAHERO
BRACERO
BUNUELO
CANSECO
CELAENO
CLOSETO
CORDERO
DANGELO
DEUTERO
DIALEDO
DRIVETO
DROVETO
ELGRECO
ESOBESO
FEBRERO
GASTERO
HEAVEHO
HEAVETO
HELLENO
HERPETO
HOWDEDO
IHOPESO
INUTERO
ISUREDO
JAYLENO
LEASETO
LETMEGO
LETTERO
LLANERO
MAGNETO
MAYBESO
MONTEGO
MONTERO
MUSKEGO
NETZERO
NONHERO
NONZERO
OFFWEGO
ONTHEGO
ORVIETO
PHONENO
PLACEBO
PREVETO
PRIMERO
PRONETO
QUITESO
RELLENO
RILIEVO
RIPIENO
SANREMO
SEAHERO
SPOKETO
SUBZERO
SWORETO
TANGELO
TENNECO
THEHERO
THERETO
THREENO
TORPEDO
VALLEJO
VAQUERO
WARHERO
WHERETO
WRITETO
WROTETO

•••••EO

ALBIREO
DOUBLEO
GALILEO
JACKIEO
ONVIDEO
POPELEO
ZAPATEO

EP•••••

EPARCHS
EPARCHY
EPAULET
EPEEIST
EPERGNE
EPERNAY
EPHEBUS
EPHEDRA
EPHESUS
EPHRAIM
EPICARP
EPICENE
EPICURE
EPIDERM
EPIDOTE
EPIGONE
EPIGRAM
EPILADY
EPILATE
EPILOGS
EPISODE
EPISTLE
EPITAPH
EPITHET
EPITOME
EPOCHAL
EPONINE
EPONYMS
EPONYMY
EPOPEES
EPOQUES
EPOXIED
EPOXIES
EPPERLY
EPSILON
EPSTEIN

E•P••••

ELPRADO
EMPALED
EMPALES
EMPANEL
EMPATHS
EMPATHY
EMPEROR
EMPIRES
EMPIRIC
EMPIRIN
EMPLACE
EMPLANE
EMPLOYS
EMPORIA
EMPOWER
EMPRESS
EMPRISE
EMPTIED
EMPTIER
EMPTIES
EMPTILY
ENPLANE
ENPRISE
EPPERLY
ESPANOL
ESPARTO
ESPIALS
ESPNEWS
ESPOSAS
ESPOSOS
ESPOUSE
ESPRITS
ESPYING
EUPHONY
EXPANDS
EXPANSE
EXPARTE
EXPECTS
EXPENDS
EXPENSE
EXPERTS
EXPIATE
EXPIRED
EXPIRES
EXPLAIN
EXPLODE
EXPLOIT
EXPLORE
EXPORTS
EXPOSED
EXPOSER
EXPOSES
EXPOSIT
EXPOUND
EXPRESS
EXPUNGE

E••P•••

EARPLUG
EELPOTS
EELPOUT
ELAPIDS
ELAPSED
ELAPSES
ELOPERS
ELOPING
ENDPINS
ENDPLAY
EPOPEES
ERUPTED
ERUPTER
EXUPERY
EYEPITS

E•••P••

ECHAPPE
ECLIPSE
ECTYPAL
ECTYPES
EJEMPLO
ELLIPSE
ENDUPAT
ESCAPED
ESCAPEE
ESCAPER
ESCAPES
EUROPOP
EVENPAR
EXAMPLE
EXCEPTS
EXEMPLA
EXEMPTS
EYESPOT

E••••P•

EARLAPS
ECHAPPE
ECOTYPE
EGGCUPS
EIGHTPM
ELCAMPO
ENCAMPS
ENCRYPT
ENTRAPS
ENTROPY
ENWRAPS
EPITAPH
ESCARPS
EUTERPE
EXCERPT
EYECUPS

E•••••P

EARCLIP
EARDROP
EARFLAP
EASEDUP
EASESUP
EATENUP
EATITUP
EGGDROP
EGOTRIP
EIGHTUP
ENCLASP
ENDEDUP
ENVELOP
EPICARP
ESCALOP
EUROPOP
EVENSUP
EXOCARP
EYEDROP

•EP••••

CEPHALO
CEPHALY
CEPHEUS
DEPALMA
DEPARTS
DEPAULU
DEPECHE
DEPENDS
DEPESTS
DEPICTS
DEPLANE
DEPLETE
DEPLORE
DEPLOYS
DEPONED
DEPONER
DEPONES
DEPORTS
DEPOSAL
DEPOSED
DEPOSER
DEPOSES
DEPOSIT
DEPOWER
DEPRAVE
DEPRESS
DEPRIVE
DEPULPS
DEPUTED
DEPUTES
HEPARIN
HEPATIC
HEPBURN
HEPCATS
HEPPEST
HEPTADS
JEPHTHA
KEPTFIT
KEPTMUM
KEPTOFF
KEPTOUT
LEPANTO
LEPIDUS
LEPPARD
LEPTONS
NEPALIS
NEPHEWS
NEPHRIC
NEPOTIC
NEPTUNE
PEPBAND
PEPBOYS
PEPCIDS
PEPITAS
PEPLUMS
PEPPARD
PEPPERS
PEPPERY
PEPPIER
PEPPILL
PEPPILY
PEPPING
PEPPINO
PEPSICO
PEPSINS
PEPTALK
PEPTICS
PEPTIDE
PEPTONE
REPACKS
REPAGED
REPAGES
REPAINT
REPAIRS
REPANEL
REPAPER
REPARKS
REPASTE
REPASTS
REPATCH
REPAVED
REPAVES
REPEALS
REPEATS
REPENTS
REPERKS
REPHASE
REPHONE
REPICKS
REPINED
REPINER
REPINES
REPLACE
REPLANE
REPLANS
REPLANT
REPLATE
REPLAYS
REPLEAD
REPLETE
REPLICA
REPLIED
REPLIER
REPLIES
REPLOTS
REPLOWS
REPLUMB
REPLUME
REPLYTO
REPOINT
REPOLLS
REPOMAN
REPORTS
REPOSED
REPOSER
REPOSES
REPOSIT
REPOSTS
REPOURS
REPOWER
REPPING
REPRESS
REPRICE
REPRIME
REPRINT
REPRISE
REPROBE
REPROOF
REPROVE
REPRUNE
REPSFOR
REPTILE
REPUGNS
REPULSE
REPUMPS
REPUTED
REPUTES
SEPALED
SEPHIAS
SEPIRAS
SEPTETS
TEPIDLY
ZEPHYRS
ZEPPOLE
ZEPPOLI

•E•P•••

BEDPOST
BEEPERS
BEEPING
BEEPSAT
BESPEAK
BESPOKE
DEEPEND
DEEPENS
DEEPEST
DEEPFAT
DEEPFRY
DEEPISH
DEEPRED
DEEPSEA
DEEPSET
DEEPSIX
DEEPSKY
DEEPTAN
DELPHIC
DEMPSEY
DESPAIR
DESPINA
DESPISE
DESPITE
DESPOIL
DESPOND
DESPOTS
EELPOTS
EELPOUT
GELPENS
GETPAST
HEAPERS
HEAPING
HEAPSOF
HEAPSON
HEAPSUP
HELPERS
HELPFUL
HELPING
HELPOUT
HELPSIN
HELPSON
HELPSUP
HEMPIER
HENPECK
HEPPEST
HERPETO
JEEPERS
JETPACK
JETPORT
KEEPERS
KEEPFIT
KEEPING
KEEPMUM
KEEPOFF
KEEPOUT
KEEPSAT
KEEPSIN
KEEPSON
KEEPSTO
KEEPSUP
KELPIES
KEMPTON
KERPLOP
KEWPIES

KEYPADS
KEYPALS
LEAPDAY
LEAPERS
LEAPFOR
LEAPING
LEAPSAT
LEAPSIN
LEAPSON
LEAPSUP
LEAPTAT
LEAPTIN
LEAPTON
LEAPTUP
LEGPULL
LEIPZIG
LEMPIRA
LEOPARD
LEOPOLD
LEPPARD
LESPAUL
LETPASS
MEMPHIS
NEWPORT
PEAPODS
PEEPERS
PEEPING
PEEPLES
PEEPOUT
PEEPSAT
PEIPING
PENPALS
PEOPLED
PEOPLES
PEPPARD
PEPPERS
PEPPERY
PEPPIER
PEPPILL
PEPPILY
PEPPING
PEPPINO
PERPLEX
PETPIGS
PETPONY
PETPUPS
REAPERS
REAPING
REAPPLY
REDPINE
REDPOLL
REDPONY
REOPENS
REPPING
RESPACE
RESPADE
RESPANS
RESPARK
RESPEAK
RESPECT
RESPELL
RESPELT
RESPICE
RESPINS
RESPIRE
RESPITE
RESPLIT
RESPOKE
RESPOND
RESPOOL
RESPOTS
RESPRAY
REUPPED
SEAPORT
SEEPAGE
SEEPAST
SEEPIER
SEEPING
SEEPOUT
SEEPSIN
SERPENS
SERPENT
SERPICO
SETPLAY
SEXPOTS
TEAPOTS
TEAPOYS
TEEPEES
TEMPEAZ
TEMPEHS
TEMPERA
TEMPERS
TEMPEST
TEMPING
TEMPJOB
TEMPLAR
TEMPLED
TEMPLES
TEMPORE
TEMPTED
TEMPTER
TEMPURA
TENPAST
TENPINS
VESPERS
VESPIDS
WEAPONS
WEBPAGE
WEEPERS
WEEPFOR
WEEPIER
WEEPING
YELPERS
YELPING
ZEPPOLE
ZEPPOLI

•E••P••

BEARPAW
BEARPIT
BEHAPPY
CESSPIT
DEADPAN
DECAPOD
DECUPLE
FELTPEN
GETUPON
HEADPIN
HEELPAD
HELIPAD
HEXAPOD
KEYSPAN
LEDUPTO
LETUPON
MEATPIE
MEMOPAD
NEARPAR
NEWSPEG
OEDIPAL
OEDIPUS
PEATPOT
PEKEPOO
REAPPLY
RECIPES
REDSPOT
REEXPEL
REIMPLY
RELAPSE
REPAPER
RETAPED
RETAPES
RETYPED
RETYPES
REUPPED
REWIPED
REWIPES
SEEDPOD
SEMIPRO
SERAPES
SERAPHS
SERAPIS
SERIPAK
SETUPON
TELEPIC
TELEPIX
TENSPOT
TENTPEG
WELLPUT
WENTPRO

•E•••P•

BEDRAPE
BEHAPPY
DECAMPS
DECRYPT
DEPULPS
DEWLAPS
GELCAPS
GESTAPO
LEADUPS
LEGROPE
LESSEPS
MESSUPS
NEWHOPE
PEGTOPS
PERCEPT
PERHAPS
PERIAPT
PETNAPS
PETPUPS
READAPT
READOPT
RECEIPT
RECOUPS
REDCAPS
REDTAPE
REDTOPS
REERUPT
REFLIPS
REGRAPH
REGRIPS
RELEAPS
REPUMPS
RESHAPE
RESHIPS
RESNAPS
RESOAPS
RETRAPS
REVAMPS
REWRAPS
SEAMAPS
SENDUPS
SETTYPE
SEVENPM
TEACUPS
WENTAPE
WETMOPS
WETNAPS

•E••••P

BEADSUP
BEAMSUP
BEANDIP
BEARSUP
BEATCOP
BEATSUP
BEDLAMP
BEEFSUP
BEERTAP
BELLHOP
BELLLAP
BELLYUP
BELTSUP
DEALSUP
DEALTUP
DESKTOP
DEVELOP
DEWDROP
FELTTIP
FENCEUP
GEARSUP
GETATIP
GETHELP
GETSHEP
GETSHIP
HEADSUP
HEALSUP
HEAPSUP
HEATSUP
HEELTAP
HELPSUP
HENCOOP
JEANARP
JERKSUP
KEEPSUP
KERFLOP
KERPLOP
KETCHUP
KEYEDUP
KEYGRIP
LEADSUP
LEAPSUP
LEAPTUP
LEFTHIP
LEGTRAP
LENSCAP
LETDROP
LETSLIP
LETSRIP
LETTERP
MEDIGAP
MEETSUP
PEASOUP
PERKSUP
PETSHOP
REACHUP
READSUP
REARSUP
RECLASP
REDCHIP
REDROOP
REELSUP
REEQUIP
REGRASP
REGROUP
RESTAMP
RESTRAP
RESTRIP
RESTSUP
RESWEEP
REVITUP
SEALSUP
SEATRIP
SENDSUP
SERVEUP
SEVENUP
SEWEDUP
TEAMSUP
TEARSUP
TEASEUP
TEASHOP
TEEITUP
TENSEUP
VERYHIP
WEIGHUP
WELLSUP

••EP•••

ADEPTAT
ADEPTER
ADEPTLY
ASEPSIS
ASEPTIC
BEEPERS
BEEPING
BEEPSAT
COEPTIS
CREPING
CREPTIN
CREPTUP
DEEPEND
DEEPENS
DEEPEST
DEEPFAT
DEEPFRY
DEEPISH
DEEPRED
DEEPSEA
DEEPSET
DEEPSIX
DEEPSKY
DEEPTAN
EYEPITS
ICEPACK
ICEPICK
ICEPOPS
INEPTLY
IREPEAT
JEEPERS
KEEPERS
KEEPFIT
KEEPING
KEEPMUM
KEEPOFF
KEEPOUT
KEEPSAT
KEEPSIN
KEEPSON
KEEPSTO
KEEPSUP
KLEPTOS
ONEPAGE
ONEPAIR
ONEPART
ONEPINT
PEEPERS
PEEPING
PEEPLES
PEEPOUT
PEEPSAT
PIEPANS
PREPACK
PREPAID
PREPARE
PREPAVE
PREPAYS
PREPLAN
PREPLOT
PREPPED
PREPPIE
PREPUPA
QUEPASA
SCEPTER
SCEPTIC
SCEPTRE
SEEPAGE
SEEPAST
SEEPIER
SEEPING
SEEPOUT
SEEPSIN
SHEPARD
SKEPTIC
SLEPTIN
SLEPTON
STEPDAD
STEPHEN
STEPINS
STEPMOM
STEPOFF
STEPONE
STEPOUT
STEPPED
STEPPER
STEPPES
STEPSIN
STEPSON
STEPSUP
STEPTWO
STEPUPS
SWEPTUP
TEEPEES
THEPIPS
THEPITS
THEPOND
THEPOOH
THEPOPE
THEPOST
THEPUMP
TIEPINS
TIEPOLO
TOEPICK
TREPANS
WEEPERS
WEEPFOR
WEEPIER
WEEPING

••E•P••

ADELPHI
BLEEPED
BLEEPER
BREWPUB
CHEAPEN
CHEAPER
CHEAPIE
CHEAPLY
CHEEPED
CHEEPER
CREEPBY
CREEPED
CREEPER
CREEPIN
CREEPOS
CREEPUP
CRESPIN
EJEMPLO
EVENPAR
EXEMPLA
EXEMPTS
EYESPOT
FLEAPIT
GOESPRO
HEELPAD
KNEEPAD
ONEMPTY
ONESPOT
OPENPIT
OVERPAR
OVERPAY
OVERPLY
PREOPEN
PREPPED
PREPPIE
PRESPUR
REEXPEL
SEEDPOD
SHERPAS
SLEEPER
SLEEPIN
SLEEPON
STEEPED
STEEPEN
STEEPER
STEEPIN
STEEPLE
STEEPLY
STEMPEL
STEPPED
STEPPER
STEPPES
STEWPAN
STEWPOT
SWEEPEA
SWEEPER
SWEEPUP
THESPIS
TIEMPOS
UNEMPTY
WHELPED

••E••P•

ALETAPS
CUETIPS
EYECUPS
GOESAPE
ICECAPS
ICEPOPS
PREAMPS
PRECEPT
PREEMPT
PRENUPS
PREPUPA
PRETAPE
PRETYPE
REERUPT
STEPUPS
THEALPS
THECAPE
THEHOPE
THEPIPS
THEPOPE
THERAPY
THEROPE
THEVIPS
THEYIPS
TIEROPE
TOECAPS
TOETAPS

••E•••P

AREAMAP
ATEITUP
BEEFSUP
BEERTAP
BREAKUP
BREWSUP
CHECKUP
CHEERUP
CHEWSUP
CLEANUP
CLEARUP
CREEPUP
CREPTUP
DREAMUP
DRESSUP
EVENSUP
EYEDROP
FLEADIP
FREEDUP
FREESUP
FUELSUP
GREYCUP
HEELTAP
JOECAMP
KEEPSUP
KNEECAP
KNEESUP
LIEATOP
LYESOAP
MEETSUP
ONECHIP
ONELUMP
ONESTEP
ONESTOP
OPENSUP
OPENTAP
OPENTOP
OVERLAP
OVERSUP
OVERTIP
OVERTOP
PRECOUP
PRESHIP
PRESSUP
PREWHIP
PREWRAP
QUEUEUP
REELSUP
REEQUIP
SNEAKUP
SPEAKUP
SPEEDUP
STEAMUP
STEPSUP
SWEEPUP
SWELLUP
SWEPTUP
TEEITUP
THEDEEP
THEFLOP
THEHELP
THELOOP
THEPUMP
TIECLIP
TOELOOP
TREESAP
TREETOP

•••EP••

ACCEPTS
BAKEPAN
BASEPAY
BLEEPED
BLEEPER
CAGEPET
CAKEPAN
CHEEPED
CHEEPER
CREEPBY
CREEPED
CREEPER
CREEPIN
CREEPOS
CREEPUP
DNIEPER
EXCEPTS
FIREPIT
FIVEPIN
FOREPAW
GONEPRO
INCEPTS
INDEPTH
JOSEPHA
JOSEPHI
KNEEPAD
LIMEPIE
MADEPAR
MAKEPAR
MALEPIG
MAZEPPA
MINEPIT
MOREPAY
NINEPIN
NONEPIC
NOTEPAD
PEKEPOO
SHOEPAC
SLEEPER
SLEEPIN
SLEEPON
STEEPED
STEEPEN
STEEPER
STEEPIN
STEEPLE
STEEPLY
SWEEPEA
SWEEPER
SWEEPUP
TELEPIC
TELEPIX
TUBEPAN
WAREPIC

•••E•P•

ATTEMPT
EUTERPE
EXCERPT
GIVEUPS
GONEAPE
LACEUPS
LINEUPS
MAKEUPS
MAZEPPA
PILEUPS
PREEMPT
RATEDPG
RAVEUPS
RECEIPT
RELEAPS
RIVERPO
SEVENPM
THREEPM
TUNEUPS
UNKEMPT
UPHEAPS
UPKEEPS
UPLEAPS
UPLEAPT
UPTEMPO
WAKEUPS

•••E••P

ACTEDUP
ADDEDUP
AIREDUP
AMPEDUP
ANTEDUP
ANTESUP
ASKEDUP
BITESUP
BONEDUP
BONESUP
BOXEDUP
BOXESUP
CAGEDUP
CAGESUP
CAKEDUP
CAKESUP
CHEERUP
COMESUP
COVERUP
CREEPUP
CRIEDUP
CRIESUP
DEVELOP
DICECUP
DRIEDUP
DRIESUP
DUDEDUP
DUDESUP
EASEDUP
EASESUP
EATENUP
ENDEDUP
ENVELOP
FIREDUP
FIRESUP
FIXEDUP
FIXESUP
FLIESUP
FORETOP
FREEDUP
FREESUP
FRIEDUP
FRIESUP
GASEDUP
GASESUP
GIVENUP
GIVESUP
HIKEDUP
HIKESUP
HOLEDUP
HOLESUP
HYPEDUP
HYPESUP
KEYEDUP
KNEECAP
KNEESUP
LACEDUP
LACESUP
LINEDUP
LINESUP
LIVENUP
LOVETAP
MAKESUP
MIXEDUP
MIXESUP
MOVEDUP
MOVESUP
NOSEDUP
NOSESUP
OFFERUP
ORDERUP
OWNEDUP
PACELAP
PILEDUP
PILESUP
PINESAP
PINETOP
PIPEDUP
PIPESUP
POWERUP
PUTEMUP
RACEDUP
RACESUP
RAKEDUP
RAKESUP
RATECAP
RIDESUP
RILEDUP
RILESUP
RISESUP
ROPEDUP
ROPESUP
ROSEHIP
SAVEDUP
SAVESUP
SCREWUP
SEVENUP
SEWEDUP
SILENTP
SITEMAP
SIZEDUP
SIZESUP
SPEEDUP
SWEEPUP
TAKENUP
TAKESUP
TAPEDUP
TAPESUP
THREEUP
THREWUP
TIDERIP
TIMECOP
TIMESUP
TONEDUP
TONESUP
TOTESUP
TREESAP
TREETOP
TRUEDUP
TRUESUP
TUBETOP
TUNEDUP
TUNESUP
TYPEDUP
TYPESUP
WAKEDUP
WAKESUP
WAXEDUP
WAXESUP
WINESAP
WIPEDUP
WIPESUP
WIREDUP
WIRESUP
WIRETAP
WISEDUP
WISESUP
WOKENUP

••••EP•

CONCEPT
FORCEPS
INSTEPS
INSWEPT
LESSEPS
OUTKEPT
OUTWEPT
PERCEPT
PRECEPT
SCHLEPP
SCHLEPS
THREEPM
TRICEPS
UNADEPT
UNSTEPS
UNSWEPT
UPKEEPS
UPSTEPS
UPSWEPT

••••E•P

ANTWERP
ASHHEAP
BARKEEP
BLAZEUP
BORNEUP
BRACEUP
BROKEUP
CHOKEUP
CHOSEUP
CLOSEUP
CRATEUP
DRIVEUP
DROVEUP
FENCEUP
FLAMEUP
FLAREUP
FORCEUP
FRAMEUP
FROZEUP
GETHELP
GOTHELP
GRATEUP
IGIVEUP
INAHEAP
JUICEUP
LETTERP
LOUSEUP
MASTERP
NONDEEP
OUTKEEP
OUTLEAP
OUTPEEP
OUTWEEP
OUTYELP
PASTEUP
QUEUEUP
RAISEUP
RANDEEP
RESWEEP
RUNDEEP
SCALEUP
SCAREUP
SCHLEPP
SERVEUP
SHAKEUP
SHAPEUP
SHINEUP
SHOREUP
SLICEUP
SMOKEUP
SPICEUP
SPIKEUP
SPOKEUP
STOKEUP
STOREUP
TEASEUP
TENSEUP
THEDEEP
THEHELP

THREEUP
TRADEUP
TWODEEP
UPSWEEP
WRITEUP
WROTEUP

•••••EP
BARKEEP
BOXSTEP
DOUBLEP
GETSHEP
IMHOTEP
MISSTEP
NONDEEP
ONESTEP
OUTKEEP
OUTPEEP
OUTSTEP
OUTWEEP
RANDEEP
RESWEEP
RUNDEEP
THEDEEP
TWODEEP
TWOSTEP
UPSWEEP

EQ•••••
EQUABLE
EQUABLY
EQUALED
EQUALLY
EQUALTO
EQUATED
EQUATES
EQUATOR
EQUERRY
EQUIANO
EQUIFAX
EQUINES
EQUINOX

E•Q••••
EMQUADS
ENQUADS
ENQUEUE
ENQUIRE
ENQUIRY
ESQUIRE

E••Q•••
EPOQUES

E•••Q••
ENRIQUE

•EQ••••
BEQUEST
BEQUICK
BEQUIET
DEQUEUE
PEQUOTS
REQUEST
REQUIEM
REQUIRE
REQUITE
REQUOTE
SEQUELS
SEQUINS
SEQUOIA
SEQUOYA
TEQUILA

•E•Q•••
NESQUIK
REEQUIP

•E••Q••
BEZIQUE

•E••••Q
LETTERQ

••EQ•••
CHEQUER
CHEQUES
COEQUAL
PREQUEL
REEQUIP
UNEQUAL

••E•Q••
PRESQUE
QUELQUE

••E•••Q
AVENUEQ

•••E••Q
SILENTQ

••••EQ•
ONTHEQT

••••E•Q
LETTERQ

•••••EQ
AVENUEQ
DOUBLEQ

ER•••••
ERASERS
ERASING
ERASMUS
ERASTUS
ERASURE
ERDRICH
ERECTED
ERECTER
ERECTLY
ERECTOR
ERECTUS
ERELONG
EREMITE
EREWHON
ERGOTIC
ERICSON
ERIGENA
ERIKSON
ERINYES
ERISTIC
ERITREA
ERLANGS
ERMINED
ERMINES
ERMINIA
ERNESTA
ERNESTO
ERODENT
ERODERS
ERODING
EROSELY
EROSION
EROSIVE
EROTICA
EROTICS
ERRABLE
ERRANCY
ERRANDS
ERRATIC
ERRATUM
ERSKINE
ERTEGUN
ERUCTED
ERUDITE
ERUPTED
ERUPTER
ERYNGOS
ERYTHRO

E•R••••
EARACHE
EARBONE
EARBUDS
EARCLIP
EARDROP
EARDRUM
EARFLAP
EARFULS
EARHART
EARHOLE
EARLAPS
EARLDOM
EARLESS
EARLETS
EARLIER
EARLIES
EARLIKE
EARLOBE
EARLOCK
EARLYON
EARMARK
EARMUFF
EARNERS
EARNEST
EARNING
EARNSIT
EARPLUG
EARRING
EARSHOT
EARTABS
EARTAGS
EARTHED
EARTHEN
EARTHLY
EARWIGS
EERIEST
EHRLICH
ENRAGED
ENRAGES
ENRANKS
ENRIGHT
ENRIQUE
ENROBED
ENROBES
ENROLLS
ENROOTS
ENROUTE
ERRABLE
ERRANCY
ERRANDS
ERRATIC
ERRATUM
ETRURIA
EURASIA
EUREKAS
EUROPOP
EUROVAN

E••R•••
EARRING
ECARTES
EGERIAS
EGGROLL
ELDRICH
ELDRICK
ELGRECO
ELPRADO
ELTRAIN
EMBRACE
EMBROIL
EMBROWN
EMBRUED
EMBRUES
EMBRYOS
EMERALD
EMERGED
EMERGES
EMERIES
EMERITA
EMERITI
EMERSED
EMERSON
EMIRATE
EMPRESS
EMPRISE
ENARBOR
ENARMED
ENCRUST
ENCRYPT
ENDRUNS
ENFRAME
ENGRAFT
ENGRAIN
ENGRAMS
ENGRAVE
ENGROSS
ENPRISE
ENTRADA
ENTRAIN
ENTRANT
ENTRAPS
ENTREAT
ENTREES
ENTRIES
ENTROPY
ENTRUST
ENURING
ENWRAPS
EPARCHS
EPARCHY
EPERGNE
EPERNAY
EPHRAIM
ERDRICH
ESCROWS
ESPRITS
ESTRADA
ESTRAYS
ESTRING
ETERNAL
EVERDUR
EVEREST
EVERETT
EVERLYS
EVERTED
EVERTOR
EWERIES
EXARCHS
EXCRETE
EXERTED
EXERTER
EXORDIA
EXPRESS
EXTRACT
EXTREME
EXTRUDE
EXURBAN
EXURBIA
EYEROLL

E•••R••
EAGERER
EAGERLY
EARDROP
EARDRUM
EATCROW
EATFROM
ECOTRIN
EDGARDO
EDITRIX
EDUARDO
EDWARDG
EDWARDI
EDWARDR
EDWARDS
EDWARDV
EFFORTS
EGGDROP
EGOTRIP
ELBERTA
ELDERLY
ELMTREE
ELNORTE
EMBARGO
EMBARKS
EMIGREE
EMIGRES
EMPEROR
EMPIRES
EMPIRIC
EMPIRIN
EMPORIA
ENCARRE
ENCARTA
ENCORED
ENCORES
ENDERBY
ENDORSE
ENDURED
ENDURER
ENDURES
ENDUROS
ENFORCE
ENGARDE
ENGIRDS
ENGORGE
ENLARGE
ENSURED
ENSURER
ENSURES
ENTERED
ENTERER
ENTERIC
ENTERIN
ENTERON
ENTHRAL
ENTIRES
ENVIRON
ENVIROS
EPIGRAM
EPPERLY
EQUERRY
ERITREA
ESCARPS
ESCORTS
ESPARTO
ESTORIL
ETHERIC
ETRURIA
EUCERIN
EUCHRED
EUCHRES
EUTERPE
EXCERPT
EXCURSE
EXEDRAE
EXHORTS
EXPARTE
EXPERTS
EXPIRED
EXPIRES
EXPORTS
EXSERTS
EXTERNE
EXTERNS
EXTORTS
EXWORKS
EYEBROW
EYEDROP

E••••R•
EARHART
EARMARK
EARNERS
EASTERN
EASTERS
EATDIRT
EATHERE
EATMORE
EBAYERS
ECHOERS
ECKHART
ECLAIRS
EDITORS
EDOUARD
EELWORM
EGGLERS
EGOSURF
ELANTRA
ELATERS
ELECTRA
ELECTRO
ELEKTRA
ELIDERS
ELIXIRS
ELKHART
ELOPERS
ELUDERS
ELUSORY
EMOTERS
ENAMORS
ENCARRE
ENDEARS
ENQUIRE
ENQUIRY
ENSNARE
ENSNARL
ENVIERS
EPHEDRA
EPICARP
EPICURE
EPIDERM
EQUERRY
ERASERS
ERASURE
ERODERS
ERYTHRO
ESCHERS
ESOTERY
ESQUIRE
ESTUARY
ETAGERE
ETCHERS
EVADERS
EVENERS
EVOKERS
EXHEDRA
EXILERS
EXOCARP
EXPLORE
EXUPERY
EYECARE
EYESORE

E•••••R
EAGERER
EARLIER
EATOVER
ECOTEUR
ECUADOR
EDASNER
EDIFIER
EDUCTOR
EDWARDR
EFFACER
EJECTOR
ELBOWER
ELEANOR
ELEAZAR
ELECTOR
ELIEZER
EMAILER
EMBOWER
EMENDER
EMITTER
EMPEROR
EMPOWER
EMPTIER
ENABLER
ENACTOR
ENAMOUR
ENARBOR
ENCODER
ENDOWER
ENDURER
ENDUSER
ENGAGER
ENJOYER
ENSURER
ENTERER
ENTICER
EQUATOR
ERECTER
ERECTOR
ERUPTER
ESCAPER
ESSAYER
ETAILER
EVANDER
EVENPAR
EVERDUR
EVERTOR
EVICTOR
EVILLER
EVOLVER
EXACTER
EXACTOR
EXALTER
EXCITER
EXCITOR
EXCUSER
EXERTER
EXHUMER
EXMAYOR
EXOILER
EXPOSER
EYEWEAR

•ER••••
AERATED
AERATES
AERATOR
AERIALS
AERIEST
AEROBAT
AEROBES
AEROBIC
AEROSOL
BERATED
BERATER
BERATES
BERBERS
BERBICK
BEREAVE
BERENDT
BERETTA
BERGAMO
BERGERE
BERGIUS
BERGMAN
BERGSON
BERIGAN
BERKLEY
BERKNER
BERLIOZ
BERLITZ
BERMING
BERMUDA
BERNARD
BERNAYS
BERNESE
BERNINA
BERNINI
BERNSEN
BEROWNE
BERRIED
BERRIES
BERSERK
BERSUNT
BERTHAS
BERTHED
BERTOLT
BERTRAM
BERVOIX
BERWICK
CERAMIC
CERATED
CERATES
CEREALS
CEREBRA
CEREBRO
CERISES
CERTAIN
CERTIFY
CERUMEN
CERVEZA
CERVIDS
CERVINE
DERAILS
DERALTE
DERANGE
DERATED
DERATES
DERBIES
DERECHO
DERIDED
DERIDER
DERIDES
DERIVED
DERIVER
DERIVES
DERMATO
DERNIER
DERONDA
DERRICK
DERRICO
DERRIDA
DERRING
DERUSTS
DERVISH
DERWENT
EERIEST
FERMATA
FERMATE
FERMATS
FERMENT
FERMION
FERMIUM
FERNAND
FERNBAR
FERNERY
FERNIER
FERRARA
FERRARE
FERRARI
FERRARO
FERRATE
FERRETS
FERRETY
FERRIED
FERRIES
FERRITE
FERROUS
FERRULE
FERTILE
FERULES
FERVENT
FERVORS
FERVOUR
GERAINT
GERALDO
GERBILS
GERENTS
GERITOL
GERMAIN
GERMANE
GERMANS
GERMANY
GERMIER
GERSHON
GERUNDS
GERVAIS
HERALDS
HERBAGE
HERBALS
HERBART
HERBAUT
HERBERT
HERBIER
HERBTEA
HERCULE
HERDERS
HERDING
HEREDIA
HEREIAM
HERENOW
HERESTO
HERETIC
HERITOR
HERMANA
HERMANN
HERMANO
HERMANS
HERMITS
HERMOSA
HERMOSO
HERNANI
HERNDON
HERNIAE
HERNIAS
HERNIBS
HEROICS
HEROINE
HEROISM
HERONRY
HERPETO
HERRICK
HERRING
HERRIOT
HERSELF
HERSHEY
JERBOAS
JERGENS
JERICHO
JERILYN
JERITZA
JERKERS
JERKIER
JERKIES
JERKILY
JERKING
JERKINS
JERKOUT
JERKSUP
JERSEYS
KERATIN
KERFLOP
KERNELS
KEROUAC
KERPLOP
KERSHAW
KERTESZ
MERCADO
MERCERS
MERCERY
MERCHES
MERCIAN
MERCIES
MERCURE
MERCURY
MERGEES
MERGERS
MERGING
MERIDEN
MERIMEE
MERINOS
MERITED
MERLINS
MERLOTS
MERMAID
MERRIAM
MERRICK
MERRIER
MERRILL
MERRILY
NERDIER
NERDISH
NEREIDS
NERISSA
NERVIER
NERVILY
NERVINE
NERVING
NERVOUS
NERVULE
OERSTED
PERAHIA
PERATIO
PERCALE
PERCENT
PERCEPT
PERCHED
PERCHER
PERCHES
PERCHIK
PERCUSS
PERDIDO
PERDIEM
PERDITA
PERDURE
PERETTI
PERFECT
PERFIDY
PERFORM
PERFUME
PERFUMY
PERFUSE
PERGOLA
PERHAPS
PERIAPT
PERIDOT
PERIGEE
PERILED
PERIODS
PERISSA
PERITUS
PERIWIG
PERJURE
PERJURY
PERKIER
PERKILY
PERKING
PERKINS
PERKISH
PERKSUP
PERLITE
PERLMAN
PERMIAN
PERMING
PERMITS
PERMUTE
PERORAL
PERPLEX
PERREAU
PERRIER
PERRINE
PERRINS
PERSEID
PERSEUS
PERSIAN
PERSIST
PERSIUS
PERSOFF
PERSONA
PERSONS
PERSSON
PERTAIN
PERTEST
PERTURB
PERUGIA
PERUKES
PERUSAL
PERUSED
PERUSER
PERUSES
PERVADE
PERWEEK
PERYEAR
RERACKS
RERAISE
RERAKED
RERAKES
RERANKS
RERATED
RERATES
REREADS
REREDOS
REREELS
RERENTS
RERIDES
RERINSE
RERISEN
RERISES
REROLLS
REROOFS
REROOTS
REROUTE
SERAPES
SERAPHS
SERAPIS
SERBIAN
SERENER
SERFAGE
SERFDOM
SERIALS
SERIATE
SERIESE
SERIESF
SERIESG
SERIESH
SERIESI
SERIESJ
SERIESK
SERIOUS
SERIPAK
SERLING
SERMONS
SERPENS
SERPENT
SERPICO
SERRATE
SERVANT
SERVEAS
SERVERS
SERVEUP
SERVICE
SERVILE
SERVING
TERAOHM
TERBIUM
TERCELS
TERENCE
TERHUNE
TERMING
TERMINI
TERMITE
TERNARY
TERNATE
TERRACE
TERRAIN
TERRANS
TERRELL
TERRENE
TERRETS
TERRIER
TERRIES
TERRIFY
TERRINE
TERROIR
TERRORS
TERSELY

TERSEST
VERANDA
VERBALS
VERBENA
VERBIDS
VERBIFY
VERBOSE
VERDANT
VERDELL
VERDICT
VERDINS
VERDOUX
VERDUGO
VERDURE
VEREINE
VERGEON
VERGERS
VERGING
VERIDIC
VERIEST
VERISMO
VERISTS
VERITAS
VERIZON
VERMEER
VERMEIL
VERMINY
VERMONT
VERNIER
VERONIA
VERRUCA
VERSACE
VERSANT
VERSETS
VERSIFY
VERSING
VERSION
VERTIGO
VERYBAD
VERYBIG
VERYDRY
VERYFEW
VERYFIT
VERYHIP
VERYHOT
VERYILL
VERYLOW
VERYMAD
VERYNEW
VERYODD
VERYOLD
VERYRED
VERYSAD
VERYSHY
VERYWET
WERNHER
WERTHER
XEROSES
XEROSIS
XEROTIC
XEROXED
XEROXES
XERXESI
YEREVAN
YERKISH
ZERMATT
ZERNIKE
ZEROING
ZEROOUT
ZEROSIN
ZEROSUM

•E•R•••

BEARCAT
BEARCUB
BEARDED
BEARERS
BEARHUG
BEARING
BEARISH
BEAROFF
BEAROUT
BEARPAW
BEARPIT
BEARSON
BEARSUP
BEBRAVE
BEDRAIL
BEDRAPE
BEDREST
BEDROCK
BEDROLL
BEDROOM
BEERCAN
BEERIER
BEERKEG
BEERMUG
BEERTAP
BEGRIME
BEHRENS
BEHRING
BEHRMAN
BERRIED
BERRIES
BETRAYS
BETROTH
BEURRES
DEARDEN
DEAREST
DEARGOD
DEARIES
DEARONE
DEARSIR
DEARTHS
DEBRETT
DEBRIEF
DECREED
DECREER
DECREES
DECRIED
DECRIER
DECRIES
DECRUMB
DECRYPT
DEERFLY
DEFRAGS
DEFRAME
DEFRAUD
DEFRAYS
DEFROCK
DEFROST
DEGRADE
DEGREED
DEGREES
DEIRDRE
DELRAYS
DELRUTH
DEORBIT
DEPRAVE
DEPRESS
DEPRIVE
DERRICK
DERRICO
DERRIDA
DERRING
DETRACT
DETRAIN
DETROIT
DETRUDE
DEVRIES
FEARERS
FEARFOR
FEARFUL
FEARING
FEARNOT
FEBRERO
FEBRILE
FERRARA
FERRARE
FERRARI
FERRARO
FERRATE
FERRETS
FERRETY
FERRIED
FERRIES
FERRITE
FERROUS
FERRULE
FEVRIER
GEARBOX
GEARING
GEARSTO
GEARSUP
GEDRICK
GEORGEC
GEORGEI
GEORGEM
GEORGES
GEORGEV
GEORGEW
GEORGIA
GEORGIC
GEORGIE
GETREAL
HEARDOF
HEARERS
HEARING
HEARKEN
HEAROUT
HEARSAY
HEARSES
HEARSOF
HEARTED
HEARTEN
HEARTHS
HEBRAIC
HEBREWS
HEIRDOM
HEIRESS
HENREID
HENRICH
HENRIES
HENRYII
HENRYIV
HENRYVI
HERRICK
HERRING
HERRIOT
HEURIGE
HEYRUBE
JEERERS
JEERING
JEERSAT
KEARNEY
KEDROVA
KEYRING
LEARJET
LEARNED
LEARNER
LEARNOF
LEARNTO
LEBROCK
LEERERS
LEERIER
LEERILY
LEERING
LEERSAT
LEFREAK
LEGRAND
LEGREST
LEGROOM
LEGROPE
LETRIDE
LETROLL
MEERKAT
MEGRIMS
MEGRYAN
MELROSE
MERRIAM
MERRICK
MERRIER
MERRILL
MERRILY
METRICS
METRIST
NEAREST
NEARING
NEARPAR
NEARYOU
NEGRONI
NEURONE
NEURONS
NEWRICH
NEXRADS
PEARLED
PEARLER
PEARSON
PEERAGE
PEERESS
PEERING
PEEROUT
PEERSAT
PEERSIN
PENROSE
PEORIAN
PERREAU
PERRIER
PERRINE
PERRINS
PETRATS
PETRELS
PETRIFY
PETROCK
PETROLS
PETROUS
REARDON
REAREND
REARERS
REARGUE
REARING
REARISE
REARLIT
REARMED
REAROSE
REARSUP
REBRACE
REBRAND
REBREAK
REBREED
REBREWS
REBROKE
REBRUSH
RECRANK
RECRATE
RECROOM
RECROSS
RECROWN
RECRUIT
REDRAFT
REDRAGS
REDRAWN
REDRAWS
REDREAM
REDRESS
REDRIED
REDRIES
REDRILL
REDRIVE
REDROBE
REDROOP
REDROOT
REDROSE
REERECT
REERUPT
REFRACT
REFRAIN
REFRAME
REFRESH
REFRIED
REFRIES
REFRONT
REGRABS
REGRADE
REGRAFT
REGRANT
REGRAPH
REGRASP
REGREET
REGRESS
REGRETS
REGRIND
REGRIPS
REGROOM
REGROUP
REGROWN
REGROWS
REORDER
REPRESS
REPRICE
REPRIME
REPRINT
REPRISE
REPROBE
REPROOF
REPROVE
REPRUNE
RETRACE
RETRACK
RETRACT
RETRADE
RETRAIN
RETRAPS
RETREAD
RETREAT
RETRIAL
RETRIED
RETRIES
RETRIMS
REURGED
REURGES
REWRAPS
REWRITE
REWROTE
REXREED
REXROTH
SEARACE
SEARERS
SEARING
SEBRING
SECRECY
SECRETE
SECRETS
SEERESS
SERRATE
SETRATE
TEARERS
TEARFUL
TEARGAS
TEARIER
TEARILY
TEARING
TEAROFF
TEAROOM
TEAROSE
TEAROUT
TEARSAT
TEARSIT
TEARSUP
TERRACE
TERRAIN
TERRANS
TERRELL
TERRENE
TERRETS
TERRIER
TERRIES
TERRIFY
TERRINE
TERROIR
TERRORS
TETRADS
TETRODE
VEERIES
VEERING
VEEROFF
VERRUCA
WEARERS
WEARIED
WEARIER
WEARIES
WEARILY
WEARING
WEAROFF
WEAROUT
WEARSON
WEIRDAL
WEIRDED
WEIRDER
WEIRDLY
WEIRDOS
WEIRTON
WETRAGS
YEAREND
YEARNED
YEARNER
YEARNTO
YEARONE
ZEBRAIC
ZEBRASS
ZEBRINE
ZEBROID

•E••R••

AELFRIC
BEATRIX
BEETRED
BEETREE
BEGIRDS
BEGORRA
BELARUS
BELTRAN
BEMIRED
BEMIRES
BENARES
BEOGRAD
BERTRAM
BESTREW
BETARAY
BEURRES
BEVERLY
BEWARED
BEWARES
CEDARED
CENTRAL
CENTRED
CENTRES
CENTRIC
CENTRUM
CETERIS
DEAIRED
DEBARGE
DEBARKS
DEBORAH
DEBURGH
DEBURRS
DECARLO
DECORUM
DEEPRED
DEFARGE
DEFERTO
DEFORMS
DEGERMS
DEHIRED
DEHIRES
DEHORNS
DELARUE
DELIRIA
DELORIS
DELORME
DEMARCO
DEMARET
DEMARKS
DEMERGE
DEMERIT
DEMEROL
DEMURER
DENARII
DENDRON
DEPARTS
DEPORTS
DESERET
DESERTS
DESERVE
DESIRED
DESIREE
DESIRER
DESIRES
DESTROY
DETERGE
DEVORES
DEWDROP
DEWIRED
DEWIRES
DEWORMS
DEXTRAL
DEXTRIN
FEDERAL
FEDERKO
FEDORAS
FEDOROV
FEEFREE
FEMORAL
FEMORIS
FEVERED
GENERAL
GENERIC
GENERIS
GETFREE
GETFROM
GETSRID
HEATRAY
HEGIRAS
HENDRIX
HENDRYX
HEPARIN
HEYMRDJ
JEFFREY
KENDREW
KESTREL
KEYGRIP
LEBARON
LECARRE
LECTRIC
LEDERER
LEGIRON
LEGTRAP
LEITRIM
LETDROP
LETSRIP
LETTRES
LEVERED
LEVERET
MEFIRST
MEMOREX
MENORAH
MENORCA
METERED
NEMEROV
NEPHRIC
NEUTRAL
NEUTRON
OEUVRES
PERORAL
PETARDS
PETCROW
PETERED
PETERII
PETFROG
REAIRED
REBIRTH
REBORED
REBORES
RECARRY
RECARVE
RECORDS
RECORKS
RECURED
RECURES
RECURLS
RECURVE
REDARED
REDARES
REDARMY
REDARNS
REEARNS
REFEREE
REFERTO
REFIRED
REFIRES
REFORGE
REFORMS
REGARDS
REGIRDS
REHIRED
REHIRES
REMARKS
REMARRY
REMERGE
REMORAS
REMORSE
RENFREW
REPARKS
REPERKS
REPORTS
RESCRUB
RESERVE
RESORBS
RESORTS
RESPRAY
RESTRAP
RESTREW
RESTRIP
RESURGE
RETARDS
RETIRED
RETIREE
RETIRES
RETORTS
RETURFS
RETURNS
REVERBS
REVERDY
REVERED
REVERER
REVERES
REVERIE
REVERSA
REVERSE
REVERTS
REWARDS
REWARMS
REWARNS
REWIRED
REWIRES
REWORDS
REWORKS
REZEROS
SEAARMS
SEAGRAM
SEAGREN
SEATRIP
SECURED
SECURER
SECURES
SEESRED
SEFERIS
SEMIRAW
SENORAS
SENORES
SENTRAS
SEPIRAS
SETFREE
SEVERAL
SEVERED
SEVERER
SEVERUS
SEWARDS
TEATRAY
TEATREE
TEATROS
TEAURNS
TEHERAN
TELERAN
TENDRIL
TENKRUN
TENURED
TENURES
TESTRUN
TEXTRON
VECTRAS
VELCROS
VELURES
VENTRAD
VENTRAL
VENTRIS
VERYRED
VESTRAL
VESTRON
VETERAN
WELLRUN
YESORNO
YEWTREE

•E•••R•

BEADERS
BEAHERO
BEAKERS
BEAMERS
BEANERY
BEARERS
BEATERS
BEAVERS
BECHARM
BEDFORD
BEDNORZ
BEEMERS
BEEPERS
BEEYARD
BEEZERS
BEGGARS
BEGGARY
BEGORRA
BEHEARD
BELAIRS
BELFORT
BELIERS
BELTERS
BENDERS
BERBERS
BERGERE
BERNARD
BERSERK
BESTIRS
BETHERE
BETTERS
BETTORS
BEZIERS
CELEBRE
CELLARS
CENSERS
CENSORS
CENSURE
CENTARE
CENTERS
CENTURY
CEREBRA
CEREBRO
CESAIRE
DEALERS
DEANERY
DEBEARD
DEBEERS
DEBLURS
DEBTORS
DEBURRS
DECIARE
DECKERS
DECLARE
DEEPFRY
DEFIERS
DEHAIRS
DEICERS
DEIRDRE
DEKLERK
DELBERT
DELMORE
DELTORO
DELVERS
DENIERS
DENMARK
DENTURE
DEODARS
DEPLORE
DESSERT
DETOURS
DEUTERO
DEVILRY
DEVOIRS
DEVOURS
DEWAART
EELWORM
FEARERS
FEATURE
FEBRERO
FEDDERS
FEEDERS
FEELERS
FELLERS
FELONRY
FENCERS
FENDERS
FENETRE
FEODORI
FERNERY
FERRARA
FERRARE
FERRARI
FERRARO
FERVORS
FESTERS
FETTERS
GEEZERS
GENDERS
GENNARO
GENXERS
GESTURE
GETHURT
GETSORE
GETTERS
GETWARM
GETWORD
GEYSERS
HEADERS
HEALERS
HEAPERS
HEARERS
HEATERS
HEAVERS
HECKART
HECTARE
HECTORS
HEDGERS
HEEDERS
HEELERS
HEFTERS
HEIFERS
HELOTRY
HELPERS
HEMMERS
HENNERY
HEPBURN
HERBART
HERBERT
HERDERS
HERONRY
HEYWARD
JEANARP
JEEPERS
JEERERS
JEFFERS
JERKERS
JESTERS
JETFIRE
JETPORT
JEWELRY
KEDGERS
KEENERS
KEEPERS
KEGGERS
KEGLERS
KENMORE
KEYCARD
KEYWORD
LEADERS
LEADORE
LEAKERS
LEANERS
LEAPERS
LEASERS
LECARRE
LECHERS
LECTERN
LECTORS
LECTURE
LEDGERS
LEEFORD
LEERERS
LEEWARD
LEFTARM
LEGHORN
LEGWORK
LEHAVRE
LEISURE
LEMPIRA
LENDERS
LEONARD
LEONORA
LEONORE
LEOPARD
LEOTARD
LEPPARD
LESABRE
LESSORS
LETTERA
LETTERB
LETTERC
LETTERD
LETTERE
LETTERF
LETTERG
LETTERH
LETTERI
LETTERJ
LETTERK
LETTERL
LETTERM
LETTERN
LETTERO
LETTERP
LETTERQ
LETTERR
LETTERS
LETTERT
LETTERU
LETTERV
LETTERW
LETTERX
LETTERY
LETTERZ
LEVIERS
LEXMARK
LEXUSRX
MEASURE

MEDFORD
MEETERS
MEGAERA
MEGAERG
MELDERS
MELTERS
MEMBERS
MEMOIRE
MEMOIRS
MENDERS
MENTORS
MEOWERS
MERCERS
MERCERY
MERCURE
MERCURY
MERGERS
METEORS
METIERS
MEWLERS
NECKERS
NECTARS
NECTARY
NEEDERS
NESTERS
NESTORS
NETSURF
NETTERS
NETWARE
NETWORK
NETZERO
NEUTERS
NEWBERN
NEWBERY
NEWBORN
NEWBURG
NEWCARS
NEWHART
NEWHIRE
NEWPORT
NEWWORD
NEWYORK
PECCARY
PEEKERS
PEELERS
PEEPERS
PELTERS
PENNERS
PEPPARD
PEPPERS
PEPPERY
PERDURE
PERFORM
PERJURE
PERJURY
PERTURB
PESTERS
PETBIRD
PETHARE
PETTERS
PEWTERS
READERS
READORN
REAMERS
REAPERS
REARERS
REAVERS
REBOARD
RECARRY
RECHART
RECTORS
RECTORY
REDBIRD
REDCARD
REDFERN
REDFIRS
REDFORD
REDWORM
REEFERS
REEKERS
REELERS
REENTRY
REGEARS
REGNARD
REHEARD
REHEARS
RELEARN
RELIERS
REMARRY
RENDERS
RENOIRS
RENTERS
REPAIRS
REPOURS
REQUIRE
RESCORE
RESHARE
RESPARK
RESPIRE
RESTART
RESTERS
RESTIRS
RESTORE
RESWORE
RESWORN
RETEARS
RETIARY
RETOURS
REUNERS
REUSERS
REUTERS
REVELRY
REWEARS
REYNARD
SEABIRD
SEABORG
SEAFARE
SEAFERN
SEAGIRT
SEAHERO
SEALERS
SEALERY
SEAMERS
SEAPORT
SEARERS
SEATERS
SEAWARD
SECTORS
SEEDERS
SEEHERE
SEEKERS
SEETHRU
SEINERS
SEIZERS
SEIZORS
SEIZURE
SELKIRK
SELLERS
SEMIDRY
SEMIPRO
SENDERS
SENHORA
SENIORS
SENSORS
SENSORY
SERVERS
SETTERS
TEACART
TEARERS
TEASERS
TEENERS
TEETERS
TELLERS
TEMPERA
TEMPERS
TEMPORE
TEMPURA
TENACRE
TENDERS
TENNERS
TENSORS
TENTERS
TERNARY
TERRORS
TESSERA
TESTERS
TETHERS
TEXTURE
VEADARS
VECTORS
VEILERS
VELOURS
VENDERS
VENDORS
VENEERS
VENTERS
VENTURA
VENTURE
VENTURI
VERDURE
VERGERS
VERYDRY
VESPERS
VESTURE
VETOERS
VETTERS
WEANERS
WEARERS
WEAVERS
WEDDERS
WEEDERS
WEEPERS
WELDERS
WELFARE
WELTERS
WENDERS
WENTPRO
WESTERN
WESTERS
WETBARS
WETWARE
WEXFORD
YELLERS
YELPERS
YESSIRE
ZEPHYRS
ZESTERS

•E•••R

AERATOR
BEADIER
BEAMIER
BEECHER
BEEFIER
BEERIER
BEETIER
BEGSFOR
BELABOR
BELAYER
BELCHER
BELLJAR
BELVOIR
BELVOUR
BENATAR
BENAZIR
BENCHER
BENDIER
BERATER
BERKNER
BESMEAR
BETTGER
BEVELER
CENTAUR
DEADAIR
DEARSIR
DEBASER
DEBATER
DECATUR
DECAYER
DECIDER
DECODER
DECOLOR
DECOYER
DECREER
DECRIER
DEDUCER
DEFACER
DEFAMER
DEFILER
DEFINER
DEFUSER
DEIFIER
DELAYER
DELIVER
DELUDER
DEMETER
DEMURER
DENUDER
DEPONER
DEPOSER
DEPOWER
DERIDER
DERIVER
DERNIER
DESIRER
DESPAIR
DEVISER
DEVISOR
DEWATER
FEARFOR
FEASTER
FEATHER
FECHNER
FEEBLER
FEELFOR
FEIFFER
FEIGNER
FELLFOR
FELTFOR
FENNIER
FERNBAR
FERNIER
FERVOUR
FETCHER
FEVRIER
GEEKIER
GEMMIER
GENITOR
GENTLER
GERMIER
GETOVER
GETSFAR
HEADFOR
HEADIER
HEATHER
HEATTER
HEAVIER
HECKLER
HEDGIER
HEFTIER
HEMPIER
HERBIER
HERITOR
JERKIER
JETSTAR
JEWELER
KEEBLER
KEESLAR
KEESLER
KEILLOR
KEISTER
LEACHER
LEADIER
LEAFIER
LEAGUER
LEAKIER
LEANDER
LEAPFOR
LEARNER
LEATHER
LEDERER
LEDGIER
LEERIER
LEFTEAR
LEFTFOR
LEGATOR
LEGGIER
LEGWEAR
LEISTER
LESSTAR
LETTERR
LEVATOR
LEVELER
MEALIER
MEANDER
MEATIER
MEDAWAR
MEDDLER
MEISTER
MEITNER
MENACER
MENUBAR
MERRIER
MESHIER
MESSIER
METOOER
METTLER
NEARPAR
NEBULAR
NEEDIER
NEEDLER
NEGATER
NEGATOR
NEITHER
NERDIER
NERVIER
NESTLER
NETSTER
NEWAGER
NEWSIER
NEWYEAR
PEAKIER
PEARLER
PEATIER
PEDALER
PEDDLER
PEPPIER
PERCHER
PERKIER
PERRIER
PERUSER
PERYEAR
PESKIER
PETBEAR
PETDEER
PETDOOR
PETHAIR
PETTIER
REACHER
REACTOR
READFOR
READIER
REALTER
REALTOR
REAUMUR
REBATER
REBUKER
RECITER
RECOLOR
RECOVER
REDDEER
REDFOUR
REDHAIR
REDSTAR
REDUCER
REEDIER
REEFIER
REEKIER
REENTER
REFINER
REFUSER
REFUTER
REGALER
REGNIER
REGULAR
REHONOR
RELATER
RELATOR
RELAXER
RELAYER
RELEVER
REMOTER
REMOVER
RENEGER
RENEWER
RENTIER
REOCCUR
REOFFER
REORDER
REPAPER
REPINER
REPLIER
REPOSER
REPOWER
REPSFOR
RESCUER
RESIDER
RESIZER
RESOLER
RESWEAR
RETAKER
REUTHER
REUTTER
REVELER
REVERER
REVILER
REVISER
REVISOR
REVIVER
REVOKER
REWAGER
REWATER
SEAMIER
SEASTAR
SECEDER
SECONDR
SECULAR
SECURER
SEDATER
SEDGIER
SEDUCER
SEEDIER
SEEPIER
SELLFOR
SELTZER
SEMINAR
SENATOR
SENDFOR
SENTFOR
SERENER
SETTLER
SETTLOR
SEVERER
SEYMOUR
TEACHER
TEARIER
TEENIER
TEETHER
TEICHER
TELSTAR
TEMBLOR
TEMPLAR
TEMPTER
TENFOUR
TENONER
TENYEAR
TERRIER
TERROIR
TESTFOR
TESTIER
VEALIER
VEINIER
VENTNOR
VERMEER
VERNIER
WEARIER
WEATHER
WEBBIER
WEBSTER
WEDGIER
WEEDIER
WEEHOUR
WEEPFOR
WEEPIER
WEGENER
WEIGHER
WEIRDER
WENTFAR
WENTFOR
WERNHER
WERTHER
YEARNER
YELLFOR
YENSFOR
YESDEAR
ZESTIER

••ER•••

ACERATE
ACERBIC
ACEROLA
ACEROSE
AKERLOF
ALERTED
ALERTER
ALERTLY
ALERTTO
AMERADA
AMERCED
AMERCER
AMERCES
AMERICA
AMERIGO
AMERIKA
AMERIND
ANEROID
APERCUS
APERIES
APERSON
AVERAGE
AVERELL
AVERILL
AVERNAL
AVERNUS
AVERRED
AVERTED
AVERTER
BEERCAN
BEERIER
BEERKEG
BEERMUG
BEERTAP
BLERIOT
BOERWAR
BRERFOX
CHERISH
CHEROOT
CHERUBS
CHERVIL
CLERICS
CLERISY
CLERKED
CLERKLY
COERCED
COERCER
COERCES
DEERFLY
EGERIAS
EMERALD
EMERGED
EMERGES
EMERIES
EMERITA
EMERITI
EMERSED
EMERSON
EPERGNE
EPERNAY
ETERNAL
EVERDUR
EVEREST
EVERETT
EVERLYS
EVERTED
EVERTOR
EWERIES
EXERTED
EXERTER
EYEROLL
FAERIES
FAEROES
FIERCER
FIERIER
FIERILY
GHERKIN
GUERDON
IBERIAN
ICERINK
ICERUNS
INERROR
INERTIA
INERTLY
ITERANT
ITERATE
IVERSON
JEERERS
JEERING
JEERSAT
JOEROTH
LAERTES
LEERERS
LEERIER
LEERILY
LEERING
LEERSAT
MEERKAT
MYERSON
OBERLIN
ONEREEL
ONEROOM
ONEROUS
OPERAND
OPERANT
OPERATE
OPEROSE
OVERACT
OVERAGE
OVERALL
OVERARM
OVERATE
OVERAWE
OVERBED
OVERBET
OVERBID
OVERBIG
OVERBUY
OVERCOY
OVERCUT
OVERDID
OVERDOG
OVERDRY
OVERDUB
OVERDUE
OVERDYE
OVEREAT
OVERFAR
OVERFAT
OVERFED
OVERFEE
OVERFEW
OVERFIT
OVERFIX
OVERFLY
OVERHOT
OVERICE
OVERJOY
OVERLAP
OVERLAX
OVERLAY
OVERLET
OVERLIE
OVERLIT
OVERMAN
OVERMIX
OVERNEW
OVERPAR
OVERPAY
OVERPLY
OVERRAN
OVERRUN
OVERSAD
OVERSAW
OVERSEA
OVERSEE
OVERSET
OVERSEW
OVERSUP
OVERTAX
OVERTIP
OVERTLY
OVERTOP
OVERUSE
OVERWET
PEERAGE
PEERESS
PEERING
PEEROUT
PEERSAT
PEERSIN
PIERCED
PIERCER
PIERCES
PIERIAN
PIERROT
PRERACE
PRERENT
PRERIOT
PREROCK
PTEROUS
PUERILE
QUERIDA
QUERIDO
QUERIED
QUERIER
QUERIES
QUERIST
REERECT
REERUPT
SEERESS
SHERBET
SHERIFF
SHERIFS
SHERMAN
SHERPAS
SHERWIN
SIERRAS
STEREOS
STERILE
STERNAL
STERNER
STERNLY
STERNOS
STERNUM
STEROID
STEROLS
STERTOR
SVERIGE
SWERVED
SWERVES
THERAMS
THERAPY
THEREAT
THEREBY
THEREDS
THEREIN
THERENT
THEREOF
THEREON
THERESA
THERETO
THERIAC
THERING
THERINK
THERITZ
THERMAL
THERMIC
THERMOS
THEROBE
THEROCK
THEROOM
THEROPE
THEROSE
THEROUX
THERULE
TIERACK
TIERCES
TIERING
TIERNEY
TIERODS
TIEROPE
TWERENT
UNERECT
USERFEE
USERIDS
VEERIES
VEERING
VEEROFF
VIERNES
VIERZIG
WHEREAS
WHEREAT
WHEREBY
WHEREIN
WHERELL
WHEREOF
WHEREON
WHERERE
WHERETO
WHEREVE
XTERRAS
YZERMAN
ZIERING

••E•R••

AFEARED
ALEARDI
ALEGRIA
AREARUG
ATECROW
AVERRED
AVEYRON
AXELROD
BEETRED
BEETREE
BLEARED
CHEERED
CHEERER
CHEERIO
CHEERON
CHEERUP
CHETRUM
CHEVRES
CHEVRET
CHEVRON
CLEARED
CLEARER
CLEARLY
CLEAROF
CLEARUP
DEEPRED
EXEDRAE
EYEBROW
EYEDROP
FEEFREE
FLEERED
FLEURON
FREDRIC
FUELROD
ICEFREE
ICETRAY
IHEARYA
INERROR
MCENROE
ONEARTH
ONEGRAM
ONEIRIC
ONEIRON
OSETRAS
OVERRAN
OVERRUN
PIERROT
PIETROS
PLEURAE
PLEURAL
PREARMS
PREORAL
PRETRIM
PREWRAP
QUEERED
QUEERER
QUEERLY
QUEIROS
REEARNS
SEESRED
SHEARED
SHEARER
SHECRAB
SHEERED
SHEERER
SHEERLY
SIERRAS
SMEARED
SMEARER
SMEARON
SNEERAT
SNEERED
SNEERER
SPEARED
SPEARER
STEARIC
STEARIN
STEARNS
STEERED
STEERER
SWEARAT
SWEARBY
SWEARER
SWEARIN
SWEARTO
THEARMY
THEARTS
THEBRAT
THECRAB
THECROW
THEFRUG
THEOREM
THETREE
THETRIB
TREERAT
UNEARTH
UPEARLY
XTERRAS

••E••R•

ABELARD
AGENTRY
ALEGARS
ALEYARD
ATEDIRT
ATEMORE
BEEMERS
BEEPERS
BEEYARD
BEEZERS

BREWERS
BREWERY
BREYERS
CAESARS
CAESURA
CHEDERS
CHEWERS
CREMORA
CUECARD
DEEPFRY
DIEHARD
DIETARY
DIETERS
DOEUVRE
DUELERS
ELECTRA
ELECTRO
ELEKTRA
EVENERS
EYECARE
EYESORE
FEEDERS
FEELERS
FLEXORS
FLEXURE
FREBERG
FUELERS
GEEZERS
GOESPRO
GREGORY
GUEVARA
HEEDERS
HEELERS
ICEBERG
JAEGERS
JEEPERS
JEERERS
KEENERS
KEEPERS
LEEFORD
LEERERS
LEEWARD
LIENORS
MAESTRO
MEETERS
MOEBERG
NEEDERS
NOENTRY
NUESTRA
NUESTRO
OBEYERS
OLESTRA
ONEACRE
ONELIRA
ONEMORE
ONEPART
ONETERM
ONEYARD
OPENERS
OVERARM
OVERDRY
PEEKERS
PEELERS
PEEPERS
PIECERS
PLECTRA
PLENARY
PLEXORS
PREBORN
PREBURN
PRECURE
PREDARK
PREFERS
PREFORM
PREPARE
PRESORT
PRETERM
PRETIRE
PRETORS
PREVERB
PREVERT
PREWARM
PREWARN
PREWIRE
PREWORK
PREWORN
PREYERS
QUESERA
QUEUERS
RAEBURN
REEFERS
REEKERS
REELERS
REENTRY
RHETORS
RIEGERT
SCENERY
SCEPTRE
SEEDERS
SEEHERE
SEEKERS
SEETHRU
SHEPARD
SKEWERS
SPECTRA
SPECTRE
SPEWERS
STEWARD
STEWART
STEWERS
SWELTRY
TEENERS
TEETERS
THEATRE
THEBARD
THECARS
THEFIRM
THEHERO
THEJERK
THELARK
THETURN
TIEBARS
TREMORS
TRENARY
VIEWERS
WEEDERS
WEEPERS
WHERERE
WIENERS

••E•••R

ABETTER
ABETTOR
ADEPTER
AGEFOUR
ALERTER
AMENDER
AMERCER
AREOLAR
ATELIER
ATEOVER
AVENGER
AVERTER
BEECHER
BEEFIER
BEERIER
BEETIER
BLEAKER
BLEATER
BLEEDER
BLEEPER
BLENDER
BLESSER
BOERWAR
BREADER
BREAKER
BREEDER
BRENNER
BUELLER
CHEAPER
CHEATER
CHECKER
CHEDDAR
CHEEPER
CHEERER
CHEEVER
CHENIER
CHEQUER
CHESTER
CHEWIER
CLEANER
CLEARER
CLEAVER
COERCER
CREAMER
CREASER
CREATOR
CREEPER
DIEDFOR
DIESFOR
DOESFOR
DREAMER
DREDGER
DREISER
DRESSER
DREXLER
DWELLER
EJECTOR
ELEANOR
ELEAZAR
ELECTOR
EMENDER
ERECTER
ERECTOR
EVENPAR
EVERDUR
EVERTOR
EXERTER
EYEWEAR
FEEBLER
FEELFOR
FIEDLER
FIELDER
FIERCER
FIERIER
FLEECER
FLEETER
FLENSER
FLEXNER
FREEAIR
FREEZER
FRESHER
FRETTER
GEEKIER
GLEANER
GOESFAR
GOESFOR
GREASER
GREATER
GREENER
GREETER
GUESSER
ICEBEER
ICEOVER
INERROR
KEEBLER
KEESLAR
KEESLER
KIEFFER
KLEIBER
KLEISER
KLEZMER
KNEADER
KNEELER
KOEHLER
LEERIER
LIEDFOR
LIEOVER
LIESFOR
LOESSER
MUELLER
NEEDIER
NEEDLER
NIEBUHR
OCELLAR
ONEHOUR
ONEOVER
ONEPAIR
ONESTAR
ONEYEAR
OPENAIR
OPENBAR
OVERFAR
OVERPAR
PIERCER
PLEADER
PLEASER
PLEDGER
PREAVER
PREENER
PREMIER
PRESPUR
PRESSER
QUEERER
QUELLER
QUERIER
QUESTER
REEDIER
REEFIER
REEKIER
REENTER
ROEDEER
RYEBEER
SCENTER
SCEPTER
SEEDIER
SEEPIER
SHEARER
SHEBEAR
SHEDDER
SHEERER
SHEFFER
SHELLER
SHELTER
SHELVER
SKEETER
SKELTER
SLEDDER
SLEEKER
SLEEPER
SLENDER
SMEARER
SMELLER
SMELTER
SNEAKER
SNEERER
SNEEZER
SPEAKER
SPEARER
SPECTER
SPECTOR
SPEEDER
SPELLER
SPENCER
SPENDER
SPENSER
STEALER
STEAMER
STEELER
STEEPER
STEERER
STEIGER
STEINER
STELLAR
STENTOR
STEPPER
STERNER
STERTOR
STEWIER
SUEDFOR
SUESFOR
SVELTER
SWEARER
SWEATER
SWEEPER
SWEETER
SWELLER
SWELTER
TEENIER
TEETHER
THEATER
THEBEAR
THEODOR
THESTAR
THETOUR
THEUSSR
TREADER
TREATER
TREKKER
TWEENER
TWEETER
TWEEZER
UNEAGER
USEDCAR
USEDFOR
USESFOR
VIEDFOR
VIESFOR
VIEWIER
WEEDIER
WEEHOUR
WEEPFOR
WEEPIER
WHEELER
WHEEZER
WHETHER
WHETTER
WIELDER
WREAKER
WRECKER
WRESTER
YIELDER
ZIEGLER
ZOELLER

•••ER••

ACHERON
ADHERED
ADHERER
ADHERES
ADVERBS
ADVERSE
ADVERTS
AILERON
ALBERTA
ALBERTI
ALBERTO
ALFEROV
ALGERIA
ALLERGY
ALMERIA
ALTERED
ALTERER
AMHERST
AMNERIS
AMPERES
ANGERED
ANTERUS
APTERAL
APTERYX
ARTERIO
ASPERSE
ASSERTS
ASTERIX
AUBERGE
BAKERST
BEVERLY
BLUERED
BODEREK
BOLEROS
BOWERED
CAMERAE
CAMERAL
CAMERAS
CAMERON
CAPERED
CASERNE
CASERNS
CASERTA
CATERAS
CATERED
CATERER
CATERTO
CAVERNS
CETERIS
CHEERED
CHEERER
CHEERIO
CHEERON
CHEERUP
CINERGY
CODERED
COHERED
COHERER
COHERES
COTERIE
COVERED
COVERER
COVERME
COVERTS
COVERUP
COWERAT
COWERED
DEFERTO
DEGERMS
DEMERGE
DEMERIT
DEMEROL
DESERET
DESERTS
DESERVE
DETERGE
DIDEROT
DIVERGE
DIVERSE
DIVERTS
DOHERTY
DOVERDE
DOWERED
EAGERER
EAGERLY
ELBERTA
ELDERLY
EMPEROR
ENDERBY
ENTERED
ENTERER
ENTERIC
ENTERIN
ENTERON
EPPERLY
EQUERRY
ETHERIC
EUCERIN
EUTERPE
EXCERPT
EXPERTS
EXSERTS
EXTERNE
EXTERNS
FABERGE
FEDERAL
FEDERKO
FEVERED
FIBERED
FLEERED
FOGERTY
FORERAN
FORERUN
GENERAL
GENERIC
GENERIS
GONERIL
GOVERNS
HAGERTY
HIBERNO
HOMERED
HOMERIC
HOMERUN
HOVERED
HOVERER
HUMERAL
HUMERUS
HYPERON
ICTERUS
IMMERGE
IMMERSE
IMPERIL
INFERNO
INHERED
INHERES
INHERIT
INNERLY
INNERVE
INPERIL
INSERTS
INTERIM
INTERNE
INTERNS
INTERSE
INVERSE
INVERTS
JONERIK
KAMERAD
LACERTA
LAPERMS
LATERAL
LATERAN
LATERON
LAVERAN
LAVERNE
LAYERED
LEDERER
LEVERED
LEVERET
LIBERAL
LIBERIA
LIBERTE
LIBERTY
LITERAL
LIVERED
LOVERLY
LOWERED
LUCERNE
MADERUN
MAKERUN
METERED
MILERUN
MINERAL
MINERVA
MISERLY
MITERED
MODERNE
MODERNS
MOLERAT
MUJERES
NEMEROV
NIGERIA
NOMERCY
NOMERGE
NUMERAL
NUMERIC
NUMEROS
OBSERVE
OBVERSE
OBVERTS
OFFERED
OFFEREE
OFFERER
OFFEROR
OFFERUP
ONSERVE
ORDERED
ORDERER
ORDERIN
ORDERLY
ORDERUP
OSIERED
PALERMO
PAPERED
PAPERER
PATERNO
PETERED
PETERII
POVERTY
POWERED
POWERUP
PUBERTY
QUEERED
QUEERER
QUEERLY
REFEREE
REFERTO
REMERGE
REPERKS
RESERVE
REVERBS
REVERDY
REVERED
REVERER
REVERES
REVERIE
REVERSA
REVERSE
REVERTS
REZEROS
RIVERPO
ROBERTA
ROBERTE
ROBERTF
ROBERTH
ROBERTI
ROBERTO
ROBERTS
ROGERED
ROSERED
SABERED
SALERNO
SCHERZI
SCHERZO
SCLERAE
SCLERAL
SCLERAS
SEFERIS
SEVERAL
SEVERED
SEVERER
SEVERUS
SHEERED
SHEERER
SHEERLY
SIBERIA
SNEERAT
SNEERED
SNEERER
SOBERED
SOBERER
SOBERLY
SPHERAL
SPHERED
SPHERES
SPHERIC
STEERED
STEERER
SUPERGS
SUREROF
SYNERGY
TAPERED
TASERED
TAVERNA
TAVERNS
TEHERAN
TELERAN
THIERRY
TIDERIP
TONEROW
TOREROS
TOWERED
TREERAT
TRUERIB
TRUERTO
UMBERED
UMBERTO
UNBERTH
UNDERDO
UNDERGO
UNFERTH
UNMERGE
UNMERRY
UNNERVE
UNTERSE
USHERED
USHERIN
UTTERED
UTTERER
UTTERLY
VALERIE
VETERAN
VICEROY
WAFERED
WAGERED
WAGERER
WATERED
WATERER
WAVERED
WAVERER
WINERED
WYVERNS

•••E•R•

AGREERS
ALGEBRA
ALLEARS
ALLEGRA
ALLEGRO
APPEARS
ARREARS
ATHEART
AUTEURS
BEHEARD
BIGEARS
BONEDRY
BYHEART
CAREERS
CAVEART
CELEBRE
CEREBRA
CEREBRO
COHEIRS
DEBEARD
DEBEERS
DISEURS
DOGEARS
ENDEARS
EPHEDRA
EQUERRY
EXHEDRA
FENETRE
FINEART
FIREARM
FOREARM
FTHENRY
GONEPRO
INTEARS
INTEGRA
INYEARS
JANEIRO
JEWELRY
LINEARA
LINEARB
LINEDRY
MADEIRA
MAJEURE
MCHENRY
METEORS
MSIEURS
NICETRY
NOSEBRA
OSSETRA
OUTEARN
OXHEART
PALEDRY
PHAEDRA
POSEURS
REGEARS
REHEARD
REHEARS
RELEARN
RETEARS
REVELRY
REWEARS
SIDEARM
SQUEERS
THIERRY
THREERS
TINEARS
TOHEART
TONEARM
UNBEARD
UNHEARD
UNLEARN
UNMERRY
UNWEARY
UPBEARS
UPREARS
UPTEARS
VENEERS

•••E••R

ACCEDER
ACHEFOR
ADHERER
ALIENOR
ALLEGER
ALTERER
AMMETER
BEVELER
BLEEDER
BLEEPER
BONEYER
BREEDER
BRIEFER
CAREFOR
CATERER
CHEEPER
CHEERER
CHEEVER
COHERER
COTEDOR
COVERER
COVETER
COZENER
CREEPER
CRUELER
CUPELER
DEMETER
DIMETER
DNIEPER
DOMECAR
DONEFOR
DOVEBAR
EAGERER
ELIEZER
EMPEROR
ENTERER
FAKEFUR
FAREWAR
FLEECER
FLEETER
FOREVER
FREEAIR
FREEZER
GAVEEAR
GIVEEAR
GONEFAR
GONEFOR
GREENER
GREETER
GRIEVER
HAVENER
HOMEIER
HOPEFOR
HOVERER
HOWEVER
IIPETER
IMPEDER
INDEXER
INGEMAR
INTEGER
JEWELER
KNEELER
KROEMER
KRUEGER
LABELER
LEDERER
LEVELER
LIBELER
LIVEFOR
LIVENER
MADEFOR
MADEPAR
MADEWAR
MAKEFOR
MAKEPAR
MAKEWAR
MODELER
NONEVER
NOTEVER
OFFERER
OFFEROR
OFTENER
ORDERER
PACECAR
PAPERER
PINEFOR
PINETAR
POLECAR
PRAETOR
PREENER
QUEERER
QUIETER
RACECAR
RELEVER
RENEGER
RENEWER
REVELER
REVERER
RIPENER
RIVETER
SALEMOR
SAVEFOR
SCHEMER
SECEDER
SERENER
SEVERER
SHEERER
SIDEBAR
SIDECAR
SILENTR
SISENOR
SKEETER
SLEEKER
SLEEPER
SNEERER
SNEEZER
SOBERER
SPEEDER
SPIELER
STEELER
STEEPER
STEERER
STPETER
STREWER

SWEEPER
SWEETER
TAKEFOR
TIREDER
TUTELAR
TWEENER
TWEETER
TWEEZER
UTTERER
VINEGAR
VOTEFOR
VUMETER
WAGERER
WAGEWAR
WAKENER
WATERER
WAVERER
WEGENER
WHEELER
WHEEZER
WHOEVER
WHYEVER
WIDENER
WINEBAR
YODELER

••••ER•

ABASERS
ABATERS
ABIDERS
ABUSERS
ADORERS
AGREERS
ALFIERI
ALGIERS
ALINERS
ALLHERE
AMBLERS
AMUSERS
ANGLERS
ANKLERS
ANSWERS
ANTHERS
ANTLERS
ANTWERP
ARCHERS
ARCHERY
ARGUERS
ARLBERG
ARRIERE
ARTFERN
ASHBERY
ATONERS
AUSTERE
AUSTERS
AVOWERS
AWAKERS
BACKERS
BADGERS
BAFFERS
BAGGERS
BAILERS
BAITERS
BALKERS
BANDERA
BANDERS
BANGERS
BANKERS
BANNERS
BANTERS
BARBERA
BARBERS
BARGERS
BARKERS
BARTERS
BASHERS
BASTERS
BATHERS
BATTERS
BATTERY
BAWLERS
BEADERS
BEAHERO
BEAKERS
BEAMERS
BEANERY
BEARERS
BEATERS
BEAVERS
BEEMERS
BEEPERS
BEEZERS
BELIERS
BELTERS
BENDERS
BERBERS
BERGERE
BERSERK
BETHERE
BETTERS
BEZIERS
BIBBERS
BICKERS
BIDDERS
BIGGERS
BIGJERK
BILKERS
BILLERS
BINDERS
BINDERY
BINGERS
BIRDERS
BIRLERS
BITTERN
BITTERS
BLADERS
BLAMERS
BLAZERS
BLOWERS
BOATERS
BOBBERS
BOILERS
BOLTERS
BOMBERS
BONDERS
BONKERS
BOOKERS
BOOKERT
BOOMERS
BOOTERS
BOOTERY
BOOZERS
BOPPERS
BORDERS
BOTHERS
BOWLERS
BOWYERS
BRACERO
BRACERS
BRAVERY
BRAYERS
BREWERS
BREWERY
BREYERS
BRIBERS
BRIBERY
BRINERS
BROKERS
BUCKERS
BUDDERS
BUDGERS
BUFFERS
BUGLERS
BUMMERS
BUMPERS
BUNKERS
BUNTERS
BURGERS
BURIERS
BURLERS
BURNERS
BUSHERS
BUSKERS
BUSSERS
BUSTERS
BUTLERS
BUTTERS
BUTTERY
BUZZERS
CABLERS
CADGERS
CAHIERS
CALDERA
CALDERS
CALKERS
CALLERS
CALVERT
CAMBERS
CAMPERS
CANCERS
CANKERS
CANNERS
CANNERY
CANOERS
CANTERS
CAPPERS
CARDERS
CAREERS
CARNERA
CARPERS
CARRERA
CARRERE
CARTERS
CARVERS
CASTERS
CATBERT
CAUSERS
CENSERS
CENTERS
CHAFERS
CHASERS
CHEDERS
CHEWERS
CHIDERS
CHIMERA
CHIMERS
CHOKERS
CHOLERA
CHOLERS
CINDERS
CINDERY
CIPHERS
CISTERN
CLAWERS
CLONERS
CLOSERS
CLOVERS
CLOVERY
COALERS
COATERS
COAXERS
COCKERS
CODGERS
COFFERS
COILERS
COINERS
COLBERT
COMBERS
COMPERE
CONCERN
CONCERT
CONFERS
CONGERS
CONKERS
CONNERY
CONVERT
COOKERS
COOKERY
COOLERS
COOPERS
COOPERY
COOTERS
COPIERS
COPPERS
COPPERY
COPTERS
CORDERO
CORDERS
CORKERS
CORNERS
COSHERS
COTTERS
COUTERS
COWHERD
CRATERS
CRAVERS
CROWERS
CULLERS
CULVERT
CUMBERS
CURLERS
CURSERS
CUSSERS
CUSTERS
CUTLERS
CUTLERY
CUTTERS
CYCLERS
CYPHERS
DABBERS
DAGGERS
DAMMERS
DAMNERS
DAMPERS
DANCERS
DANDERS
DANGERS
DANVERS
DARNERS
DARTERS
DASHERS
DAUBERS
DEALERS
DEANERY
DEBEERS
DECKERS
DEFIERS
DEICERS
DEKLERK
DELBERT
DELVERS
DENIERS
DESSERT
DEUTERO
DIALERS
DIAPERS
DICKERS
DIETERS
DIFFERS
DIGGERS
DILBERT
DIMMERS
DINGERS
DINNERS
DIPPERS
DISCERN
DISSERT
DITHERS
DITHERY
DOCKERS
DODDERS
DODDERY
DODGERS
DOFFERS
DOGBERT
DOOVERS
DOOZERS
DORMERS
DOTTERS
DOUSERS
DOWNERS
DOWSERS
DRAPERS
DRAPERY
DRAWERS
DRIVERS
DRONERS
DROVERS
DRYPERS
DUBBERS
DUCKERS
DUELERS
DUFFERS
DUMPERS
DUNKERS
DUNNERS
DUSTERS
EARNERS
EASTERN
EASTERS
EATHERE
EBAYERS
ECHOERS
EGGLERS
ELATERS
ELIDERS
ELOPERS
ELUDERS
EMOTERS
ENVIERS
EPIDERM
ERASERS
ERODERS
ESCHERS
ESOTERY
ETAGERE
ETCHERS
EVADERS
EVENERS
EVOKERS
EXILERS
EXUPERY
FABLERS
FALLERS
FALTERS
FANNERS
FARMERS
FARMERY
FATHERS
FAWNERS
FEARERS
FEBRERO
FEDDERS
FEEDERS
FEELERS
FELLERS
FENCERS
FENDERS
FERNERY
FESTERS
FETTERS
FIBBERS
FILBERT
FILLERS
FILTERS
FINDERS
FINGERS
FISHERS
FISHERY
FITTERS
FIZZERS
FLAKERS
FLAMERS
FLAYERS
FLOWERS
FLOWERY
FLUTERS
FOAMERS
FODDERS
FOGGERS
FOKKERS
FOLDERS
FOLGERS
FOOLERS
FOOLERY
FOOTERS
FOPPERY
FORCERS
FORGERS
FORGERY
FORKERS
FORMERS
FOSTERS
FOWLERS
FRAMERS
FRATERS
FREBERG
FTMYERS
FUDGERS
FUELERS
FUNDERS
FURLERS
FUSSERS
GABBERS
GADDERS
GAFFERS
GAGGERS
GAINERS
GAITERS
GALLERY
GAMMERS
GANDERS
GANGERS
GAOLERS
GARNERS
GARTERS
GASPERS
GASSERS
GASTERO
GATHERS
GAUDERY
GAUGERS
GAWKERS
GAWPERS
GEEZERS
GENDERS
GENXERS
GETTERS
GEYSERS
GIBBERS
GILBERT
GILDERS
GINGERS
GINGERY
GIRDERS
GLAZERS
GLIDERS
GLOWERS
GNAWERS
GOITERS
GOLFERS
GOMPERS
GOOBERS
GOODERS
GOPHERS
GORGERS
GOUGERS
GRADERS
GRAPERY
GRATERS
GRAVERS
GRAZERS
GRIPERS
GROCERS
GROCERY
GROPERS
GROVERS
GROWERS
GRUYERE
GUIDERS
GULPERS
GUNNERS
GUNNERY
GUSHERS
GUTTERS
GYPPERS
HACKERS
HAILERS
HALTERS
HALVERS
HAMMERS
HAMPERS
HANDERS
HANGERS
HANKERS
HARMERS
HARPERS
HASTERT
HATTERS
HAULERS
HAWKERS
HAWSERS
HEADERS
HEALERS
HEAPERS
HEARERS
HEATERS
HEAVERS
HEDGERS
HEEDERS
HEELERS
HEFTERS
HEIFERS
HELPERS
HEMMERS
HENNERY
HERBERT
HERDERS
HILBERT
HINDERS
HINTERS
HISSERS
HITHERE
HITTERS
HOAXERS
HOCKERS
HOGGERY
HOHNERS
HOLBERG
HOLDERS
HOLLERS
HONKERS
HOOFERS
HOOPERS
HOOTERS
HOOVERS
HOPPERS
HOSIERS
HOSIERY
HOWLERS
HUGGERS
HULLERS
HUMBERT
HUMMERS
HUNGERS
HUNKERS
HUNTERS
HUPPERT
HURLERS
HURTERS
HUSKERS
HUSSERL
ICEBERG
IMAGERS
IMAGERY
IMTHERE
INCHERS
INTHERE
INUTERO
IRONERS
ISOMERS
ISSUERS
ITSHERE
JABBERS
JAEGERS
JAILERS
JAMMERS
JASPERS
JASPERY
JAZZERS
JEEPERS
JEERERS
JEFFERS
JERKERS
JESTERS
JIGGERS
JIGGERY
JILTERS
JINXERS
JITTERS
JITTERY
JOBBERS
JOBBERY
JOGGERS
JOINERS
JOINERY
JOLTERS
JOSHERS
JOTTERS
JROBERT
JUDGERS
JUICERS
JUMPERS
JUNKERS
KAISERS
KEDGERS
KEENERS
KEEPERS
KEGGERS
KEGLERS
KICKERS
KIDDERS
KILLERS
KIPPERS
KISSERS
KITTERY
KNAVERY
KNIFERS
KNOWERS
KOSHERS
KUNDERA
LADDERS
LADLERS
LAGGERS
LAMBERT
LAMPERT
LANCERS
LANDERS
LANTERN
LAPPERS
LAPSERS
LARDERS
LARKERS
LASHERS
LATHERS
LATHERY
LAUDERS
LAWYERS
LAZZERI
LEADERS
LEAKERS
LEANERS
LEAPERS
LEASERS
LECHERS
LECTERN
LEDGERS
LEERERS
LENDERS
LETTERA
LETTERB
LETTERC
LETTERD
LETTERE
LETTERF
LETTERG
LETTERH
LETTERI
LETTERJ
LETTERK
LETTERL
LETTERM
LETTERN
LETTERO
LETTERP
LETTERQ
LETTERR
LETTERS
LETTERT
LETTERU
LETTERV
LETTERW
LETTERX
LETTERY
LETTERZ
LEVIERS
LIBBERS
LICKERS
LIFTERS
LIMBERS
LIMNERS
LINGERS
LINKERS
LINTERS
LIPPERS
LISPERS
LISTERS
LITTERS
LITTERY
LLANERO
LOADERS
LOAFERS
LOANERS
LOBBERS
LOCKERS
LODGERS
LOFTERS
LOGGERS
LOITERS
LOLLERS
LOOKERS
LOOPERS
LOOTERS
LOPPERS
LOTTERS
LOTTERY
LOUVERS
LUBBERS
LUGGERS
LULLERS
LUMBERS
LUMIERE
LUMPERS
LUNGERS
LUNKERS
LURKERS
LUSTERS
MADDERS
MAILERS
MAIMERS
MAINERS
MANGERS
MANNERS
MAPPERS
MARGERY
MARKERS
MARRERS
MASHERS
MASKERS
MASTERP
MASTERS
MASTERY
MATHERS
MATTERS
MAULERS
MAUSERS
MEETERS
MEGAERA
MEGAERG
MELDERS
MELTERS
MEMBERS
MENDERS
MEOWERS
MERCERS
MERCERY
MERGERS
METIERS
MEWLERS
MIDTERM
MILKERS
MILLERS
MINCERS
MINDERS
MINTERS
MISTERM
MISTERS
MISTERX
MOANERS
MOBBERS
MOCKERS
MOCKERY
MOEBERG
MOILERS
MOLDERS
MOLIERE
MOLTERS
MONGERS
MONTERO
MOONERS
MOOTERS
MOPPERS
MORCERF
MOSHERS
MOTHERS
MOTHERY
MOUSERS
MUCKERS
MUDDERS
MUGGERS
MULLERS
MUMMERS
MUMMERY
MURDERS
MUSHERS
MUSTERS
MUTTERS
MYSTERY
NABBERS
NAGGERS
NAILERS
NAPIERS
NAPPERS
NATTERS
NECKERS
NEEDERS
NESTERS
NETTERS
NETZERO
NEUTERS
NEWBERN
NEWBERY
NICKERS
NIPPERS
NODDERS
NONHERO
NONZERO
NOONERS
NOOSERS
NORBERT
NOSHERS
NOTHERE
NOWHERE
NUBBERS
NUDGERS
NUMBERS
NUNNERY
NURSERS
NURSERY
NUTTERS
OAKFERN
OBEYERS
OINKERS
ONAGERS
ONALERT
ONETERM
OPENERS
OPINERS
OSTLERS
OUSTERS
OUTHERE
OUTSERT
OYSTERS
PACKERS
PADDERS
PAIRERS
PALMERS
PALTERS
PAMPERS
PANDERS
PANIERS
PANNERS
PANTERA
PANTERS
PANZERS
PAPIERS
PARGERS
PARKERS
PARSERS
PASSERS
PASTERN
PASTERS
PATTERN
PATTERS
PATZERS
PAUPERS
PAUSERS
PAWNERS
PCUSERS
PEEKERS
PEELERS
PEEPERS
PELTERS
PENNERS
PEPPERS
PEPPERY
PESTERS
PETTERS
PEWTERS
PHASERS
PHONERS
PICKERS
PIECERS
PIGGERY
PILFERS
PINCERS
PINGERS
PINNERS
PITIERS
PLACERS
PLANERS
PLATERS
PLAYERS
PLOVERS
PLOWERS
POISERS
POLLERA
POLLERS
PONDERS
POOLERS
POPPERS
PORKERS
PORTERS
POSTERN

POSTERS
POTHERB
POTHERS
POTTERS
POTTERY
POURERS
POUTERS
POWDERS
POWDERY
PRATERS
PRAYERS
PREFERS
PRETERM
PREVERB
PREVERT
PREYERS
PRICERS
PRIMERA
PRIMERO
PRIMERS
PROBERS
PROSERS
PROVERB
PROVERS
PRUDERY
PRUNERS
PUCKERS
PUCKERY
PUFFERS
PUFFERY
PULLERS
PULPERS
PUMPERS
PUNKERS
PUNNERS
PUNTERS
PURRERS
PURSERS
PUSHERS
PUTTERS
QUAKERS
QUAVERS
QUAVERY
QUESERA
QUEUERS
QUIVERS
QUIVERY
QUOTERS
RACKERS
RAFTERS
RAIDERS
RAILERS
RAISERS
RAMMERS
RANGERS
RANKERS
RANTERS
RAPIERS
RAPPERS
RASHERS
RASPERS
RASTERS
RATBERT
RATTERS
READERS
REAMERS
REAPERS
REARERS
REAVERS
REDFERN
REEFERS
REEKERS
REELERS
RELIERS
RENDERS
RENTERS
RESTERS
REUNERS
REUSERS
REUTERS
RHYMERS
RIBBERS
RIDDERS
RIEGERT
RIFLERS
RIFLERY
RIGGERS
RINGERS
RINSERS
RIOTERS
RIPPERS
RISKERS
RIVIERA
RIVIERE
ROADERS
ROAMERS
ROARERS
ROBBERS
ROBBERY
ROCKERS
ROCKERY
RODGERS
ROGUERY
ROLFERS
ROLLERS
ROMBERG
ROMPERS
ROOFERS
ROOKERY
ROOMERS
ROOTERS
ROSTERS
ROTTERS
ROUSERS
ROUTERS
RUBBERS
RUBBERY
RUCKERT
RUDDERS
RUINERS
RUMMERS
RUNNERS
RUSHERS
RUSSERT
RUTGERS
RUTTERS
SACKERS
SAILERS
SALIERI
SALTERS
SALVERS
SANDERS
SAPPERS
SASSERS
SAUCERS
SAWYERS
SCALERS
SCARERS
SCENERY
SCORERS
SCOTERS
SEAFERN
SEAHERO
SEALERS
SEALERY
SEAMERS
SEARERS
SEATERS
SEEDERS
SEEHERE
SEEKERS
SEINERS
SEIZERS
SELLERS
SENDERS
SERVERS
SETTERS
SHADERS
SHAKERS
SHAPERS
SHARERS
SHAVERS
SHINERS
SHIVERS
SHIVERY
SHOVERS
SHOWERS
SHOWERY
SHUBERT
SIFTERS
SIGHERS
SIGNERS
SILVERS
SILVERY
SIMMERS
SIMPERS
SINCERE
SINGERS
SINKERS
SINNERS
SIPPERS
SISTERS
SITTERS
SKATERS
SKEWERS
SLAKERS
SLATERS
SLAVERS
SLAVERY
SLAYERS
SLICERS
SLIDERS
SLIVERS
SLOPERS
SMILERS
SMITERS
SMOKERS
SNAKERS
SNARERS
SNIPERS
SNORERS
SOAKERS
SOAPERS
SOARERS
SOBBERS
SOLDERS
SOLVERS
SOONERS
SORCERY
SORTERS
SOTHERE
SOTHERN
SOUPERS
SPACERS
SPADERS
SPARERS
SPAYERS
SPEWERS
SPICERS
SPICERY
SPIDERS
SPIDERY
SPIKERS
SPYDERS
SQUEERS
STAGERS
STARERS
STATERS
STAYERS
STEWERS
STOKERS
STONERS
STORERS
STOWERS
STYLERS
SUBVERT
SUBZERO
SUCKERS
SUDSERS
SUFFERS
SULKERS
SUMMERS
SUMMERY
SUNDERS
SUPPERS
SURFERS
SURGERY
SWAYERS
SWIGERT
SWINERY
SWIPERS
TACKERS
TAGGERS
TAILERS
TALKERS
TAMPERS
TANKERS
TANNERS
TANNERY
TAPPERS
TASTERS
TATTERS
TATTERY
TEARERS
TEASERS
TEENERS
TEETERS
TELLERS
TEMPERA
TEMPERS
TENDERS
TENNERS
TENTERS
TESSERA
TESTERS
TETHERS
THALERS
THAWERS
THEHERO
THEJERK
THREERS
TICKERS
TILLERS
TILTERS
TIMBERS
TIMBERY
TINDERS
TINDERY
TINKERS
TINNERS
TINTERN
TINTERS
TIPPERS
TITHERS
TITTERS
TOGGERY
TOILERS
TOLLERS
TOOLERS
TOOTERS
TOPPERS
TOSSERS
TOTTERS
TOTTERY
TOURERS
TOUTERS
TOWNERS
TRABERT
TRACERS
TRACERY
TRADERS
TRAVERS
TUCKERS
TUGGERS
TURNERS
TURNERY
TUSHERY
TUSKERS
TWINERS
TWOFERS
TWOTERM
ULSTERS
UNALERT
UNDOERS
UNFIERY
UNINERT
UNITERS
UNOVERT
UNSTERN
UNTIERS
UPTHERE
USURERS
VALUERS
VAMPERS
VAQUERO
VARIERS
VEILERS
VENDERS
VENEERS
VENTERS
VERGERS
VESPERS
VETOERS
VETTERS
VICKERS
VIEWERS
VISCERA
VIZIERS
VOGUERS
VOICERS
VOIDERS
WADDERS
WAFTERS
WAGGERS
WAGGERY
WAILERS
WAITERS
WAIVERS
WALKERS
WALTERS
WANDERS
WANTERS
WARDERS
WARHERO
WARMERS
WARPERS
WASHERS
WASTERS
WEANERS
WEARERS
WEAVERS
WEDDERS
WEEDERS
WEEPERS
WELDERS
WELTERS
WENDERS
WESTERN
WESTERS
WHALERS
WHERERE
WHINERS
WICKERS
WIENERS
WIGGERY
WILBERT
WILLERS
WINCERS
WINDERS
WINGERS
WINKERS
WINNERS
WINTERS
WINTERY
WISHERS
WITHERS
WONDERS
WOOFERS
WOOLERY
WORKERS
WORMERS
WRITERS
XAVIERU
XYSTERS
YAKKERS
YAMMERS
YANKERS
YAPPERS
YARDERS
YATTERS
YAWNERS
YAWPERS
YELLERS
YELPERS
YONKERS
YORKERS
YOTHERS
YOWLERS
ZAPPERS
ZESTERS
ZINGERS
ZIPPERS
ZITHERS

••••E•R

AMATEUR
ANTBEAR
BESMEAR
BIGBEAR
BOBWEIR
BONHEUR
BUGBEAR
COMPEER
DANSEUR
DAYWEAR
DECREER
DOGSEAR
DOUCEUR
ECOTEUR
EYEWEAR
FARCEUR
FARSEER
FLANEUR
FORBEAR
FRISEUR
GAVEEAR
GIVEEAR
HAUTEUR
ICEBEER
KINNEAR
LAFLEUR
LEFTEAR
LEGWEAR
LETTERR
LIQUEUR
LOWGEAR
MANYEAR
MASSEUR
MIDYEAR
MISHEAR
MYNHEER
NEWYEAR
NOTNEAR
NUCLEAR
OFFYEAR
ONATEAR
ONEYEAR
OUTHEAR
OUTTEAR
OUTWEAR
PASTEUR
PERYEAR
PETBEAR
PETDEER
PIONEER
REDDEER
RESWEAR
RIGUEUR
ROEDEER
RYEBEER
SCHMEAR
SCHMEER
SHEBEAR
SIXYEAR
SKIWEAR
SOWSEAR
TAXYEAR
TENYEAR
THEBEAR
TWOYEAR
UNCLEAR
UNSHEER
UNSWEAR
VERMEER
YESDEAR

•••••ER

ABETTER
ABJURER
ABRADER
ABUTTER
ACCEDER
ACCUSER
ADAPTER
ADDUCER
ADEPTER
ADHERER
ADJURER
ADMIRER
ADOPTER
ADORNER
ADVISER
AFFIXER
AGUTTER
ALARMER
ALERTER
ALIGNER
ALLAYER
ALLEGER
ALLOVER
ALLURER
ALMONER
ALPINER
ALROKER
ALTERER
ALUNSER
AMASSER
AMENDER
AMERCER
AMMETER
ANDOVER
ANGRIER
ANNOYER
ANOTHER
ANTSIER
APPLIER
AQUIFER
AQUIVER
ARBITER
ARMORER
AROUSER
ARRAYER
ARRIVER
ARTSIER
ASHIVER
ASIMMER
ASKOVER
ASPIRER
ASSAYER
ASSUMER
ASSURER
ASTUTER
ASUNDER
ATELIER
ATEOVER
ATTIRER
ATWATER
AUGURER
AVENGER
AVERTER
AVOIDER
AWAITER
AWARDER
AZINGER
BABBLER
BAFFLER
BAGGIER
BAINTER
BALKIER
BALLMER
BALMIER
BANALER
BANDIER
BARKIER
BARMIER
BARRIER
BASSIER
BATTIER
BATTLER
BAULKER
BAWDIER
BEADIER
BEAMIER
BEECHER
BEEFIER
BEERIER
BEETIER
BELAYER
BELCHER
BENCHER
BENDIER
BERATER
BERKNER
BETTGER
BEVELER
BILGIER
BITSIER
BITTIER
BLABBER
BLACKER
BLADDER
BLANDER
BLANKER
BLASTER
BLATHER
BLEAKER
BLEATER
BLEEDER
BLEEPER
BLENDER
BLESSER
BLINDER
BLINKER
BLISTER
BLITHER
BLITZER
BLOCKER
BLOGGER
BLONDER
BLOOMER
BLOOPER
BLOTTER
BLOWIER
BLUBBER
BLUDGER
BLUFFER
BLUNDER
BLUNTER
BLURBER
BLURTER
BLUSHER
BLUSTER
BOARDER
BOASTER
BOBBLER
BOCHNER
BOGGIER
BOGGLER
BOLSTER
BONEYER
BONNIER
BOOMIER
BOOSLER
BOOSTER
BOOZIER
BOSSIER
BOTCHER
BOTTLER
BOUCHER
BOULDER
BOUNCER
BOUNDER
BOUVIER
BOWDLER
BOXSTER
BRAGGER
BRAIDER
BRAINER
BRANDER
BRASHER
BRASIER
BRAWLER
BRAZIER
BREADER
BREAKER
BREEDER
BRENNER
BRIDGER
BRIDLER
BRIEFER
BRIMMER
BRINGER
BRINIER
BRINKER
BRISKER
BROADER
BROIDER
BROILER
BRONZER
BROODER
BROTHER
BROWNER
BROWSER
BRUISER
BRUSHER
BRYNNER
BUCHNER
BUCKNER
BUELLER
BUGGIER
BUILDER
BULGIER
BULKIER
BUMBLER
BUMPIER
BUNDLER
BUNGLER
BURBLER
BURGHER
BURLIER
BURRIER
BURSTER
BUSHIER
BUSTIER
BUSTLER
BUTCHER
BUZZIER
BYLINER
CACKLER
CADAVER
CAJOLER
CALIBER
CALIPER
CAMPIER
CANDLER
CANNIER
CAROLER
CARRIER
CARTIER
CASHIER
CATCHER
CATERER
CATTIER
CAULKER
CAVILER
CCRIDER
CDTOWER
CHAFFER
CHAMBER
CHAMFER
CHAMPER
CHANCER
CHANGER
CHANTER
CHAPTER
CHARGER
CHARIER
CHARMER
CHARRER
CHARTER
CHASTER
CHATTER
CHAUCER
CHEAPER
CHEATER
CHECKER
CHEEPER
CHEERER
CHEEVER
CHENIER
CHEQUER
CHESTER
CHEWIER
CHIGGER
CHILLER
CHIPPER
CHIRPER
CHITTER
CHOICER
CHOKIER
CHOOSER
CHOPPER
CHOWDER
CHUGGER
CHUKKER
CHURNER
CIRCLER
CLABBER
CLACKER
CLAIMER
CLAMBER
CLAMMER
CLAMPER
CLANGER
CLAPPER
CLASHER
CLASPER
CLASSER
CLATTER
CLAVIER
CLAYIER
CLEANER
CLEARER
CLEAVER
CLICKER
CLIMBER
CLINGER
CLINKER
CLIPPER
CLOBBER
CLOCKER
CLOUTER
CLOWDER
CLUBBER
CLUCKER
CLUNKER
CLUSTER
CLUTTER
CNTOWER
COARSER
COASTER
COBBLER
COBUYER
COCKIER
CODDLER
COERCER
COHERER
COLLIER
COLLYER
COLORER
COMAKER
COMFIER
COMPEER
CONIFER
CONQUER
CORKIER
CORNIER
CORONER
COSTNER
COULTER
COUNTER
COUPLER
COURIER
COURSER
COVERER
COVETER
COZENER
CRABBER
CRACKER
CRADLER
CRAFTER
CRAMMER
CRANMER
CRASHER
CRASSER
CRAWLER
CRAZIER
CREAMER
CREASER
CREEPER
CRIBBER
CRIMPER
CRISPER
CRITTER
CROAKER
CROCKER
CROFTER
CROONER
CROPPER
CROSIER
CROSSER
CROWDER
CROWNER
CROZIER
CRUELER
CRUISER
CRULLER
CRUPPER
CRUSHER
CRYOVER
CUPELER
CUPPIER
CURDIER
CURDLER
CURLIER
CURRIER
CURVIER
CUSHIER
CUSSLER
CUTOVER
DABBLER
DAFFIER
DAIMLER
DAIRYER
DALLIER
DANDIER
DANDLER
DANGLER
DASHIER
DAUMIER
DAUNTER
DAWDLER
DAZZLER
DEBASER

DEBATER	DREISER	FAVORER	FOLKIER	GLOATER	GUTSIER	ICEBEER	KEEBLER	LOONIER	MOONIER	OFFICER	PLEDGER	QUICKER
DECAYER	DRESSER	FEASTER	FONDLER	GLOSSER	GUTTIER	ICEOVER	KEESLER	LOOPIER	MOORIER	OFTENER	PLODDER	QUIETER
DECIDER	DREXLER	FEATHER	FOOTLER	GLUMMER	GUZZLER	IDOTTER	KEISTER	LOPPIER	MOSSIER	OKTOBER	PLOTTER	QUILLER
DECODER	DRIFTER	FECHNER	FOOZLER	GNASHER	HACKLER	IGNITER	KICKIER	LOUNGER	MOTHIER	OLDSTER	PLUGGER	QUILTER
DECOYER	DRILLER	FEEBLER	FORAGER	GOAFTER	HADOVER	IGNORER	KIEFFER	LOUSIER	MOULDER	OLIVIER	PLUMBER	QUIPPER
DECREER	DRINKER	FEIFFER	FOREVER	GOBBLER	HAGGLER	IIPETER	KINDLER	LOWLIER	MOUNTER	OMITTER	PLUMIER	QUITTER
DECRIER	DRIPPER	FEIGNER	FORGOER	GODLIER	HAIRIER	IMBIBER	KINKIER	LOYALER	MOURNER	ONEOVER	PLUMMER	QUIZZER
DEDUCER	DROLLER	FENNIER	FORKIER	GOGGLER	HAMMIER	IMPALER	KLAMMER	LUCIFER	MOUSIER	ONORDER	PLUMPER	RADIOER
DEFACER	DROOLER	FERNIER	FORSTER	GOOFIER	HAMSTER	IMPEDER	KLEIBER	LUCKIER	MOUTHER	ONPAPER	PLUNDER	RAFFLER
DEFAMER	DROPPER	FETCHER	FOUNDER	GOOGLER	HANAPER	IMPOSER	KLEISER	LUMPIER	MRTIGER	ONSAGER	PLUNGER	RAGGIER
DEFILER	DRUBBER	FEVRIER	FOURIER	GOONIER	HANDIER	IMPURER	KLEZMER	LUNCHER	MUCKIER	ONWATER	PLUNKER	RAINIER
DEFINER	DRUCKER	FIBIGER	FRAILER	GOOPIER	HANDLER	IMPUTER	KLINGER	LURCHER	MUDDIER	OPPOSER	PLUSHER	RALLIER
DEFUSER	DRUDGER	FIBSTER	FRANKER	GOOSIER	HANOVER	INAPTER	KLINKER	LUSHIER	MUDDLER	ORBITER	POACHER	RAMBLER
DEIFIER	DRUMMER	FICKLER	FRASIER	GORSIER	HAPPIER	INCITER	KLISTER	LUSTIER	MUELLER	ORDERER	POINTER	RANCHER
DELAYER	DRUNKER	FIDDLER	FRAZIER	GORTNER	HARDIER	INCOMER	KNEADER	LUTHIER	MUFFLER	OUTDOER	POITIER	RANDIER
DELIVER	DUCKIER	FIEDLER	FREEZER	GOTOVER	HARRIER	INDEXER	KNEELER	MACUSER	MUGGIER	OUTLIER	POLANER	RANGIER
DELUDER	DUMPIER	FIELDER	FRESHER	GOUNDER	HARSHER	INDITER	KNITTER	MALTIER	MUMBLER	PADDLER	POLICER	RANOVER
DEMETER	DUSKIER	FIERCER	FRETTER	GOUTIER	HASOVER	INDUCER	KNOCKER	MANAGER	MUNCHER	PAINTER	POLITER	RAPIDER
DEMURER	DUSTIER	FIERIER	FRICKER	GRABBER	HASTIER	INFUSER	KNOTTER	MANGIER	MUNSTER	PALAVER	POLYMER	RASPIER
DENUDER	DWELLER	FIGHTER	FRISKER	GRAFTER	HATCHER	INHALER	KOEHLER	MANGLER	MURKIER	PALLIER	POPOVER	RASSLER
DEPONER	EAGERER	FIGURER	FRITTER	GRAINER	HAUNTER	INHUMER	KOOKIER	MANLIER	MUSHIER	PALMIER	PORIVER	RATTIER
DEPOSER	EARLIER	FILCHER	FRIZZER	GRAMMER	HAVENER	INJURER	KRASNER	MARBLER	MUSKIER	PANNIER	PORKIER	RATTLER
DEPOWER	EATOVER	FILMIER	FROGGER	GRANDER	HEADIER	INKSTER	KROEMER	MARCHER	MUSSIER	PANTHER	POTTIER	RAVAGER
DERIDER	EDASNER	FINNIER	FROMMER	GRANGER	HEATHER	INLAYER	KRUEGER	MARINER	MUSTIER	PAPERER	POUNCER	REACHER
DERIVER	EDIFIER	FIRRIER	FROSTER	GRANTER	HEATTER	INORDER	KUTCHER	MARLIER	MUZZIER	PARADER	POUNDER	READIER
DERNIER	EFFACER	FISCHER	FROTHER	GRAPIER	HEAVIER	INPOWER	LABELER	MARNIER	MUZZLER	PARDNER	POUTIER	REALTER
DESIRER	ELBOWER	FISHIER	FROWNER	GRASPER	HECKLER	INSANER	LABORER	MARVIER	MYNHEER	PARRIER	PRAISER	REBATER
DEVISER	ELIEZER	FIZZIER	FUBSIER	GRAZIER	HEDGIER	INSIDER	LACQUER	MASQUER	NAGGIER	PARTIER	PRANCER	REBUKER
DEWATER	EMAILER	FIZZLER	FUMBLER	GREASER	HEFTIER	INSURER	LALAKER	MASSIER	NAPPIER	PARTNER	PREAVER	RECITER
DIBBLER	EMBOWER	FLAGGER	FUNKIER	GREATER	HEMPIER	INTEGER	LANDLER	MATCHER	NAPSTER	PARTYER	PREENER	RECOVER
DICHTER	EMENDER	FLAKIER	FUNNIER	GREENER	HERBIER	INTONER	LANKIER	MATURER	NASTIER	PASTIER	PREMIER	REDDEER
DIDDLER	EMITTER	FLAMIER	FUNSTER	GREETER	HIBBLER	INVADER	LARDIER	MAUNDER	NATTIER	PATCHER	PRESSER	REDUCER
DIDOVER	EMPOWER	FLANKER	FURRIER	GRIDDER	HIGGLER	INVITER	LARDNER	MAXBAER	NEEDIER	PEAKIER	PRICIER	REEDIER
DILUTER	EMPTIER	FLAPPER	FURTHER	GRIEVER	HILLIER	INVOKER	LARKIER	MCPAPER	NEEDLER	PEARLER	PRIMMER	REEFIER
DIMETER	ENABLER	FLASHER	FUSSIER	GRIFTER	HINKIER	IODIZER	LASSOER	MEALIER	NEGATER	PEATIER	PRINKER	REEKIER
DINGIER	ENCODER	FLATTER	FUSTIER	GRILLER	HIPPIER	IONISER	LAUGHER	MEANDER	NEITHER	PEDALER	PRINTER	REENTER
DINKIER	ENDOWER	FLAWIER	FUZZIER	GRIMIER	HIPSTER	IONIZER	LAUNDER	MEATIER	NERDIER	PEDDLER	PRIVIER	REFINER
DIOPTER	ENDURER	FLAXIER	GABBIER	GRIMMER	HISSIER	IRISHER	LAYOVER	MEDDLER	NERVIER	PEPPIER	PROCTER	REFUSER
DIPPIER	ENDUSER	FLEECER	GAGSTER	GRINDER	HITCHER	ITCHIER	LEACHER	MEISTER	NESTLER	PERCHER	PRODDER	REFUTER
DIRTIER	ENGAGER	FLEETER	GAMBIER	GRINNER	HOARDER	ITSOVER	LEADIER	MEITNER	NETSTER	PERKIER	PROFFER	REGALER
DISHIER	ENJOYER	FLENSER	GAMBLER	GRIPPER	HOARIER	IWONDER	LEAFIER	MENACER	NEWAGER	PERRIER	PROOFER	REGNIER
DITCHER	ENSURER	FLEXNER	GARBLER	GRISTER	HOARSER	JAGGIER	LEAGUER	MERRIER	NEWSIER	PERUSER	PROSIER	RELATER
DITSIER	ENTERER	FLICKER	GARDNER	GRITTER	HOBBLER	JAMMIER	LEAKIER	MESHIER	NIBBLER	PESKIER	PROSPER	RELAXER
DITZIER	ENTICER	FLINGER	GARGLER	GROANER	HOISTER	JANGLER	LEANDER	MESSIER	NIFTIER	PETDEER	PROUDER	RELAYER
DIVIDER	ERECTER	FLIPPER	GASSIER	GRODIER	HOLSTER	JANVIER	LEARNER	METOOER	NIGGLER	PETTIER	PROWLER	RELEVER
DIVINER	ERUPTER	FLIRTER	GAUCHER	GROLIER	HOMAGER	JAZZIER	LEATHER	METTLER	NIGHTER	PHATTER	PSALTER	REMOTER
DIZZIER	ESCAPER	FLITTER	GAUDIER	GROOMER	HOMEIER	JDPOWER	LEDERER	MIDDLER	NIMBLER	PHILTER	PUDGIER	REMOVER
DNIEPER	ESSAYER	FLIVVER	GAUNTER	GROSSER	HONORER	JERKIER	LEDGIER	MIFFIER	NIPPIER	PHISHER	PUFFIER	RENEGER
DODGIER	ETAILER	FLOATER	GAUTIER	GROUPER	HOOSIER	JEWELER	LEERIER	MILKIER	NITTIER	PHONIER	PULPIER	RENEWER
DOGGIER	EVANDER	FLOGGER	GAUZIER	GROUSER	HOPOVER	JIGGIER	LEGGIER	MINGIER	NOBBIER	PIASTER	PUNCHER	RENTIER
DOODLER	EVILLER	FLOORER	GAWKIER	GROUTER	HOPPIER	JINGLER	LEISTER	MINGLER	NOISIER	PICKIER	PUNKIER	REOFFER
DOOMIER	EVOLVER	FLOPPER	GEEKIER	GROWLER	HORNIER	JOGGLER	LEVELER	MINIVER	NONEVER	PIERCER	PUNNIER	REORDER
DOPPLER	EXACTER	FLOSSER	GEMMIER	GRUBBER	HORSIER	JOINDER	LIBELER	MINSTER	NONUSER	PIGGIER	PUNSTER	REPAPER
DORKIER	EXALTER	FLOUTER	GENTLER	GRUDGER	HOSTLER	JOINTER	LIEOVER	MINTIER	NOOTHER	PILSNER	PURFLER	REPINER
DOSSIER	EXCITER	FLUBBER	GERMIER	GRUFFER	HOTOVER	JOLLIER	LIGHTER	MINUTER	NORTHER	PINCHER	PURSIER	REPLIER
DOTTIER	EXCUSER	FLUFFER	GETOVER	GRUNGER	HOUNDER	JOLTIER	LIMITER	MISAVER	NOTCHER	PIONEER	PURSUER	REPOSER
DOUBLER	EXERTER	FLUKIER	GIDDIER	GRUNTER	HOVERER	JOSTLER	LINDNER	MISDOER	NOTEVER	PITCHER	PURTIER	REPOWER
DOUBTER	EXHUMER	FLUNKER	GIGGLER	GUARDER	HOWEVER	JOUSTER	LINTIER	MISTIER	NOTICER	PITHIER	PUSHIER	RESCUER
DOWAGER	EXOILER	FLUSHER	GIRDLER	GUCKIER	HUDDLER	JOWLIER	LIPPIER	MISUSER	NOTOVER	PIVOTER	PUTOVER	RESIDER
DOWDIER	EXPOSER	FLUSTER	GIRLIER	GUESSER	HUFFIER	JUGGLER	LITTLER	MOBSTER	NOWISER	PLAINER	PUZZLER	RESIZER
DOWNIER	FADDIER	FLUTIER	GLACIER	GUILDER	HULKIER	JUICIER	LIVENER	MODELER	NUBBIER	PLAITER	QUACKER	RESOLER
DRABBER	FAINTER	FLUTTER	GLADDER	GULPIER	HUMBLER	JUMBLER	LOAMIER	MOISTER	NUTSIER	PLANNER	QUAFFER	RETAKER
DRAFTER	FANCIER	FLYOVER	GLAZIER	GUMMIER	HUMPIER	JUMPIER	LOATHER	MOLDIER	NUTTIER	PLANTER	QUAKIER	REUTHER
DRAGGER	FANSLER	FLYTIER	GLEANER	GUNKIER	HUNKIER	JUNIPER	LOBBYER	MONIKER	NUZZLER	PLASTER	QUARTER	REUTTER
DRAINER	FARRIER	FNUMBER	GLIBBER	GUNTHER	HURDLER	JUNKIER	LOBSTER	MONOMER	OBLIGER	PLATIER	QUEERER	REVELER
DRAWLER	FARSEER	FOAMIER	GLIMMER	GUNUSER	HURRIER	JUPITER	LOCATER	MONSTER	OBTUSER	PLATTER	QUELLER	REVERER
DREAMER	FARTHER	FOCUSER	GLISTER	GUSHIER	HUSKIER	KASTLER	LOESSER	MOOCHER	OCTOBER	PLEADER	QUERIER	REVILER
DREDGER	FATTIER	FOGGIER	GLITTER	GUSTIER	HUSTLER	KAYAKER	LOFTIER	MOODIER	OFFERER	PLEASER	QUESTER	REVISER

REVIVER
REVOKER
REWAGER
REWATER
RIBBIER
RICHLER
RICHTER
RIDDLER
RIDGIER
RIFFLER
RIGHTER
RINDIER
RIPENER
RISKIER
RITZIER
RIVETER
ROASTER
ROCKIER
ROEDEER
ROILIER
ROISTER
ROOKIER
ROOMIER
ROOSTER
ROOTIER
ROSSNER
ROTIFER
ROUGHER
ROUNDER
ROUSTER
ROWDIER
RUDDIER
RUFFLER
RUMBLER
RUNNIER
RUNOVER
RUNTIER
RUSHIER
RUSTIER
RUSTLER
RUTTIER
RYEBEER
SADDLER
SAGGIER
SALLIER
SALTIER
SALUTER
SAMPLER
SANDIER
SANDLER
SAPPIER
SASSIER
SAUCIER
SAUNTER
SAVAGER
SAVORER
SAVVIER
SAYOVER
SCALDER
SCALIER
SCALPER
SCAMMER
SCAMPER
SCANNER
SCANTER
SCARCER
SCARFER
SCARIER
SCATTER
SCENTER
SCEPTER
SCHEMER
SCHMEER
SCHUMER
SCOFFER
SCOLDER
SCOOPER
SCOOTER
SCORNER
SCOURER
SCOUTER
SCOWLER
SCRAPER
SCRIBER
SCUDDER
SCUFFER
SCULLER
SCUPPER
SEAMIER
SECEDER
SECURER
SEDATER
SEDGIER
SEDUCER
SEEDIER
SEEPIER
SELTZER
SERENER
SETTLER
SEVERER
SHADIER
SHAFFER
SHAKIER
SHALIER
SHANTER
SHARPER
SHATNER
SHATTER
SHEARER
SHEDDER
SHEERER
SHEFFER
SHELLER
SHELTER
SHELVER
SHIFTER
SHIMMER
SHINIER
SHIPPER
SHIRKER
SHOCKER
SHOOTER
SHOPPER
SHORTER
SHOUTER
SHOWIER
SHRINER
SHRIVER
SHUCKER
SHUDDER
SHUNTER
SHUSTER
SHUTTER
SHYSTER
SIGHTER
SILKIER
SILLIER
SILTIER
SIMPLER
SISSIER
SIZZLER
SKEETER
SKELTER
SKIDDER
SKIMMER
SKINNER
SKIPPER
SKIRTER
SKITTER
SKULKER
SLACKER
SLAMMER
SLANDER
SLAPPER
SLASHER
SLATHER
SLATIER
SLEDDER
SLEEKER
SLEEPER
SLENDER
SLICKER
SLIMIER
SLIMMER
SLINGER
SLINKER
SLIPPER
SLITHER
SLITTER
SLOBBER
SLOGGER
SLOTTER
SLUGGER
SLUMBER
SLUMMER
SLURPER
SMACKER
SMALLER
SMARTER
SMASHER
SMATTER
SMEARER
SMELLER
SMELTER
SMIRKER
SMOKIER
SMOLDER
SMOTHER
SMUCKER
SMUGGER
SNACKER
SNAGGER
SNAKIER
SNAPPER
SNARLER
SNEAKER
SNEERER
SNEEZER
SNICKER
SNIFFER
SNIFTER
SNIPPER
SNOOKER
SNOOPER
SNOOZER
SNORTER
SNOWIER
SNUBBER
SNUFFER
SNUGGER
SOAPIER
SOBERER
SODDIER
SOGGIER
SOLACER
SOLDIER
SOLIDER
SOOTHER
SOOTIER
SOPPIER
SORRIER
SOUNDER
SOUPIER
SPACIER
SPAMMER
SPANKER
SPANNER
SPARRER
SPARSER
SPATTER
SPAWNER
SPEAKER
SPEARER
SPECTER
SPEEDER
SPELLER
SPENCER
SPENDER
SPENSER
SPICIER
SPIELER
SPIKIER
SPILLER
SPINIER
SPINNER
SPIRIER
SPITTER
SPLICER
SPOILER
SPONGER
SPOOFER
SPOOLER
SPOONER
SPOTTER
SPOUTER
SPRAYER
SPRUCER
SPUMIER
SPURNER
SPUTTER
SQUARER
STABBER
STABLER
STACKER
STADLER
STAFFER
STAGGER
STAGIER
STAIDER
STAINER
STALKER
STALLER
STAMMER
STAMPER
STANDER
STAPLER
STARKER
STARTER
STATLER
STEALER
STEAMER
STEELER
STEEPER
STEERER
STEIGER
STEINER
STEPPER
STERNER
STEWIER
STICKER
STIFFER
STILLER
STINGER
STINKER
STINTER
STIRRER
STOCKER
STONIER
STOOPER
STOPPER
STOUTER
STPETER
STRAFER
STRAYER
STREWER
STRIDER
STRIKER
STRIPER
STRIVER
STROKER
STUDIER
STUFFER
STUMPER
STUNNER
STUTTER
SUBDUER
SUBTLER
SUCKIER
SUDSIER
SULKIER
SUNNIER
SUPPLER
SURFIER
SURLIER
SVELTER
SWABBER
SWAGGER
SWANKER
SWAPPER
SWARMER
SWATTER
SWEARER
SWEATER
SWEEPER
SWEETER
SWELLER
SWELTER
SWIFTER
SWILLER
SWIMMER
SWINGER
SWITZER
SWOONER
SWOOPER
TACKIER
TACKLER
TALKIER
TALLIER
TANAGER
TANGIER
TANGLER
TANGOER
TAPSTER
TARDIER
TARRIER
TARTIER
TASTIER
TATTIER
TATTLER
TAUNTER
TAWNIER
TEACHER
TEARIER
TEENIER
TEETHER
TEICHER
TEMPTER
TENONER
TERRIER
TESTIER
THANKER
THEATER
THICKER
THINKER
THINNER
THITHER
THRIVER
THROWER
THUMPER
THUNDER
THURBER
TICKLER
TIGHTER
TIMIDER
TINGLER
TINKLER
TINNIER
TIPOVER
TIPPIER
TIPPLER
TIPSIER
TIPSTER
TIREDER
TOASTER
TODDLER
TOFFLER
TOGGLER
TOHOMER
TOORDER
TOOTLER
TORCHER
TOTALER
TOUCHER
TOUGHER
TRACKER
TRAILER
TRAINER
TRAMPER
TRAPPER
TRASHER
TRAWLER
TREADER
TREATER
TREKKER
TRICKER
TRIFLER
TRIGGER
TRILLER
TRIMMER
TRIPPER
TROLLER
TROOPER
TROTTER
TROUPER
TROUSER
TRUCKER
TRUDGER
TRUSTER
TRYSTER
TUBBIER
TUFTIER
TUMBLER
TUMMLER
TURFIER
TWANGER
TWEENER
TWEETER
TWEEZER
TWINIER
TWIRLER
TWISTER
TWITTER
UNCOVER
UNCOYER
UNEAGER
UNIFIER
UNMAKER
UNMITER
UNRIPER
UNSAFER
UNSHEER
UNSHIER
UNSHYER
UNSLIER
UNSLYER
UNSOBER
UNTRUER
UNWISER
UPDATER
UPRISER
UPRIVER
URBANER
USURPER
UTTERER
VAMPIER
VAPORER
VASTIER
VAULTER
VAUNTER
VEALIER
VEINIER
VERMEER
VERNIER
VIEWIER
VINTNER
VIVIDER
VOCODER
VOLCKER
VONBAER
VORSTER
VOUCHER
VOYAGER
VUMETER
WACKIER
WADDLER
WAFFLER
WAGERER
WAGGLER
WAGONER
WAKENER
WALTHER
WALTZER
WANGLER
WARBLER
WARTIER
WASHIER
WASPIER
WATCHER
WATERER
WAVERER
WEARIER
WEATHER
WEBBIER
WEBSTER
WEDGIER
WEEDIER
WEEPIER
WEGENER
WEIGHER
WEIRDER
WERNHER
WERTHER
WHACKER
WHEELER
WHEEZER
WHETHER
WHETTER
WHIFFER
WHIMPER
WHINIER
WHIPPER
WHIRLER
WHISKER
WHISPER
WHITHER
WHIZZER
WHOEVER
WHOOPER
WHOPPER
WHYEVER
WIDENER
WIDOWER
WIELDER
WIGGIER
WIGGLER
WIMPIER
WINCHER
WINDIER
WINKLER
WINOVER
WISPIER
WITTIER
WOBBLER
WONOVER
WOODIER
WOOLIER
WOOSTER
WOOZIER
WORDIER
WORMIER
WORRIER
WRAPPER
WREAKER
WRECKER
WRESTER
WRINGER
WRITHER
WRONGER
YACHTER
YAWNIER
YEARNER
YIELDER
YODELER
YOUNGER
YUCKIER
YUMMIER
ZAPPIER
ZESTIER
ZIEGLER
ZINGIER
ZINKIER
ZIPPIER
ZOELLER

ES•••••

ESCALOP
ESCALUS
ESCAPED
ESCAPEE
ESCAPER
ESCAPES
ESCARPS
ESCENCE
ESCHEAT
ESCHERS
ESCHEWS
ESCORTS
ESCROWS
ESCUDOS
ESCUELA
ESIASON
ESKIMOS
ESOBESO
ESOTERY
ESPANOL
ESPARTO
ESPIALS
ESPNEWS
ESPOSAS
ESPOSOS
ESPOUSE
ESPRITS
ESPYING
ESQUIRE
ESSAYED
ESSAYER
ESSENCE
ESSENES
ESTADOS
ESTAMIN
ESTATED
ESTATES
ESTEBAN
ESTEEMS
ESTEFAN
ESTELLA
ESTELLE
ESTEVEZ
ESTHETE
ESTIVAL
ESTONIA
ESTORIL
ESTRADA
ESTRAYS
ESTRING
ESTUARY

E•S••••

EASEDBY
EASEDIN
EASEDON
EASEDUP
EASEFUL
EASELED
EASEOFF
EASEOUT
EASESBY
EASESIN
EASESON
EASESUP
EASIEST
EASTEGG
EASTEND
EASTERN
EASTERS
EASTHAM
EASTING
EASTMAN
EASYJOB
EASYOFF
EASYONE
ECSTASY
ENSEALS
ENSEATS
ENSIGNS
ENSILED
ENSILES
ENSKIED
ENSKIES
ENSLAVE
ENSNARE
ENSNARL
ENSOULS
ENSUING
ENSUITE
ENSURED
ENSURER
ENSURES
EOSINES
EPSILON
EPSTEIN
ERSKINE
ESSAYED
ESSAYER
ESSENCE
ESSENES
EUSTACE
EXSCIND
EXSECTS
EXSERTS

E••S•••

EARSHOT
EATSOUT
EDASNER
EELSKIN
EGESTED
EGGSACS
EGOSURF
EKESOUT
EKISTIC
ELASTIC
ELASTIN
ELISION
ELUSIVE
ELUSORY
ELYSEES
ELYSIAN
ELYSIUM
ENISLED
ENISLES
EPISODE
EPISTLE
ERASERS
ERASING
ERASMUS
ERASTUS
ERASURE
ERISTIC
EROSELY
EROSION
EROSIVE
ETESIAN
EVASION
EVASIVE
EXISTED
EYESHOT
EYESORE
EYESPOT

E•••S••

EARNSIT
EASESBY
EASESIN
EASESON
EASESUP
ECDYSES
ECDYSIS
EDGESIN
EFFUSED
EFFUSES
EGLISES
EGOISTE
EGOISTS
ELAPSED
ELAPSES
ELEISON
ELLISON
ELMISTI
EMBASSY
EMBOSOM
EMERSED
EMERSON
EMMUSKA
ENCASED
ENCASES
ENDUSER
ENDUSES
ENLISTS
ENMASSE
EPHESUS
ERICSON
ERIKSON
ERNESTA
ERNESTO
ESIASON
ESPOSAS
ESPOSOS
EURASIA
EVENSUP
EVULSED
EVULSES
EXCISED
EXCISES
EXCUSAL
EXCUSAS
EXCUSED
EXCUSER
EXCUSES
EXCUSEZ
EXPOSED
EXPOSER
EXPOSES
EXPOSIT

E••••S•

EARLESS
EARNEST
EASIEST
EATLESS
ECCLESI
ECHOISM
ECLIPSE
ECSTASY
EDGIEST
EDMEESE
EELIEST
EERIEST
EGGCASE
EGGIEST
EGGLESS
EGGTOSS
EGOTISM
EGOTIST
EKWENSI
ELEGIST
ELITEST
ELITISM
ELITIST
ELLIPSE
ELMIEST
EMBASSY
EMPRESS
EMPRISE
ENCHASE
ENCLASP
ENCLOSE
ENCRUST
ENDLESS
ENDMOST
ENDORSE
ENDWISE
ENGLISH
ENGROSS
ENMASSE
ENPRISE
ENTHUSE
ENTRUST
ENTWIST
EPEEIST
ESOBESO
ESPOUSE
EVANISH
EVENEST
EVEREST
EVILEST
EXCURSE
EXHAUST
EXOTISM
EXPANSE
EXPENSE
EXPRESS
EXTENSO
EYELASH
EYELESS
EYEMASK
EYETEST
EYEWASH

E•••••S

EADGILS
EAGLETS
EARBUDS
EARFULS
EARLAPS
EARLESS
EARLETS
EARLIES
EARNERS
EARTABS
EARTAGS
EARWIGS
EASTERS
EATLESS
EBAYERS
EBONICS
EBONIES
ECARTES
ECDYSES
ECDYSIS
ECHOERS
ECLAIRS
ECTYPES
ECZEMAS
EDGINGS
EDIBLES
EDIFIES
EDITORS
EDMONDS
EDMUNDS
EDWARDS
EELPOTS
EFFACES
EFFECTS
EFFORTS
EFFUSES
EGERIAS
EGGCUPS
EGGLERS
EGGLESS
EGGNOGS
EGGSACS
EGGTOSS
EGLISES
EGOISTS

EIGHTHS
EKUELES
ELAINES
ELANCES
ELANETS
ELAPIDS
ELAPSES
ELATERS
ELEGIES
ELEGITS
ELEVENS
ELEVONS
ELFOWLS
ELICITS
ELIDERS
ELIGIUS
ELIXIRS
ELNINOS
ELOPERS
ELUANTS
ELUATES
ELUDERS
ELYSEES
EMBALMS
EMBANKS
EMBARKS
EMBLEMS
EMBRUES
EMBRYOS
EMERGES
EMERIES
EMETICS
EMIGRES
EMOTERS
EMPALES
EMPATHS
EMPIRES
EMPLOYS
EMPRESS
EMPTIES
EMQUADS
EMULOUS
ENABLES
ENAMELS
ENAMORS
ENCAGES
ENCAMPS
ENCASES
ENCINAS
ENCODES
ENCORES
ENDALLS
ENDCUTS
ENDEARS
ENDINGS
ENDIVES
ENDLESS
ENDPINS
ENDRUNS
ENDURES
ENDUROS
ENDUSES
ENDWAYS
ENEMIES
ENFACES
ENFANTS
ENFOLDS
ENGAGES

ENGILDS
ENGINES
ENGIRDS
ENGLUTS
ENGRAMS
ENGROSS
ENGULFS
ENIGMAS
ENISLES
ENJOINS
ENLACES
ENLINKS
ENLISTS
ENNEADS
ENQUADS
ENRAGES
ENRANKS
ENROBES
ENROLLS
ENROOTS
ENSEALS
ENSEATS
ENSIGNS
ENSILES
ENSKIES
ENSOULS
ENSURES
ENTAILS
ENTICES
ENTIRES
ENTOMBS
ENTRAPS
ENTREES
ENTRIES
ENVEILS
ENVIERS
ENVIOUS
ENVIROS
ENWINDS
ENWRAPS
ENZYMES
EOLITHS
EOSINES
EPARCHS
EPHEBUS
EPHESUS
EPILOGS
EPONYMS
EPOPEES
EPOQUES
EPOXIES
EQUATES
EQUINES
ERASERS
ERASMUS
ERASTUS
ERECTUS
ERINYES
ERLANGS
ERMINES
ERODERS
EROTICS
ERRANDS
ERYNGOS
ESCALUS
ESCAPES
ESCARPS
ESCHERS

ESCHEWS
ESCORTS
ESCROWS
ESCUDOS
ESKIMOS
ESPIALS
ESPNEWS
ESPOSAS
ESPOSOS
ESPRITS
ESSENES
ESTADOS
ESTATES
ESTEEMS
ESTRAYS
ETCHERS
ETHANES
ETHENES
ETHNICS
ETOILES
ETONICS
ETYMONS
EUBANKS
EUCHRES
EULABUS
EUONYMS
EUREKAS
EVADERS
EVENERS
EVERLYS
EVINCES
EVOKERS
EVOLVES
EVULSES
EWERIES
EXACTAS
EXARCHS
EXCEEDS
EXCEPTS
EXCIDES
EXCISES
EXCITES
EXCUSAS
EXCUSES
EXEMPTS
EXEUNTS
EXHALES
EXHORTS
EXHUMES
EXILERS
EXMATES
EXOCETS
EXONYMS
EXOTICS
EXPANDS
EXPECTS
EXPENDS
EXPERTS
EXPIRES
EXPORTS
EXPOSES
EXPRESS
EXSECTS
EXSERTS
EXTENDS
EXTENTS
EXTERNS
EXTOLLS

EXTORTS
EXWIVES
EXWORKS
EXYANKS
EYECUPS
EYEFULS
EYELESS
EYELETS
EYELIDS
EYEPITS

•ES••••

BESEECH
BESIDES
BESIEGE
BESMEAR
BESPEAK
BESPOKE
BESSELL
BESTBET
BESTBOY
BESTBUD
BESTBUY
BESTCUT
BESTIAL
BESTILL
BESTING
BESTIRS
BESTMAN
BESTMEN
BESTOFF
BESTONE
BESTOWS
BESTREW
CESAIRE
CESSING
CESSION
CESSNAS
CESSPIT
CESTMOI
DESALTS
DESCANT
DESCEND
DESCENT
DESEEDS
DESERET
DESERTS
DESERVE
DESEXED
DESEXES
DESHELL
DESIGNS
DESILTS
DESIRED
DESIREE
DESIRER
DESIRES
DESISTS
DESKFUL
DESKSET
DESKTOP
DESLUMS
DESMOGS
DESMOND
DESOTOS
DESPAIR
DESPINA
DESPISE

DESPITE
DESPOIL
DESPOND
DESPOTS
DESSERT
DESTAEL
DESTAIN
DESTEMS
DESTINE
DESTINO
DESTINY
DESTOCK
DESTROY
DESYLVA
FESCUES
FESSING
FESTERS
FESTINA
FESTIVA
FESTIVE
FESTOON
FESTOSO
GESSOED
GESSOES
GESTALT
GESTAPO
GESTATE
GESTURE
HESHVAN
HESSAFE
HESSIAN
JESSICA
JESTERS
JESTING
JESUITS
KESTREL
LESABRE
LESCAUT
LESIONS
LESOTHO
LESPAUL
LESSEES
LESSENS
LESSEPS
LESSFAT
LESSING
LESSONS
LESSORS
LESSTAR
LESTOIL
MESAMIS
MESCALS
MESEEMS
MESHACH
MESHIER
MESHING
MESHUGA
MESONIC
MESSAGE
MESSALA
MESSIAH
MESSICK
MESSIER
MESSILY
MESSINA
MESSING
MESSKIT
MESSUPS

NESBITT
NESCAFE
NESMITH
NESQUIK
NESSMAN
NESTEGG
NESTERS
NESTFUL
NESTING
NESTLED
NESTLER
NESTLES
NESTORS
NESTSIN
PESADES
PESANTE
PESETAS
PESEWAS
PESKIER
PESKILY
PESTERS
PESTLED
PESTLES
RESALES
RESALTS
RESANDS
RESAVED
RESAVES
RESAWED
RESCALE
RESCANS
RESCIND
RESCORE
RESCRUB
RESCUED
RESCUER
RESCUES
RESEALS
RESEAMS
RESEATS
RESEAUS
RESEAUX
RESECTS
RESEEDS
RESEEKS
RESEIZE
RESELLS
RESENDS
RESENTS
RESERVE
RESEWED
RESHAPE
RESHARE
RESHAVE
RESHIFT
RESHINE
RESHIPS
RESHOES
RESHOOT
RESHOWN
RESHOWS
RESHUTS
RESIDED
RESIDER
RESIDES
RESIDUA
RESIDUE
RESIFTS

RESIGHT
RESIGNS
RESILED
RESILES
RESINED
RESINGS
RESINKS
RESISTS
RESITED
RESIZED
RESIZER
RESIZES
RESLATE
RESMELT
RESNAIS
RESNAPS
RESOAKS
RESOAPS
RESOILS
RESOJET
RESOLED
RESOLER
RESOLES
RESOLVE
RESORBS
RESORTS
RESOUND
RESOWED
RESPACE
RESPADE
RESPANS
RESPARK
RESPEAK
RESPECT
RESPELL
RESPELT
RESPICE
RESPINS
RESPIRE
RESPITE
RESPLIT
RESPOKE
RESPOND
RESPOOL
RESPOTS
RESPRAY
RESTABS
RESTACK
RESTAFF
RESTAGE
RESTAIN
RESTAMP
RESTART
RESTATE
RESTERS
RESTFUL
RESTICK
RESTING
RESTIRS
RESTIVE
RESTOCK
RESTOKE
RESTORE
RESTOWS
RESTRAP
RESTREW
RESTRIP
RESTSIN

RESTSON
RESTSUP
RESTUDY
RESTUFF
RESTYLE
RESUITS
RESULTS
RESUMED
RESUMES
RESURGE
RESWEAR
RESWEEP
RESWIMS
RESWORE
RESWORN
SESAMES
SESSILE
SESSION
SESTETS
SESTINA
TESSERA
TESTACY
TESTATE
TESTBAN
TESTBED
TESTEES
TESTERS
TESTFLY
TESTFOR
TESTIER
TESTIFY
TESTILY
TESTING
TESTKIT
TESTLAB
TESTOUT
TESTRUN
VESICLE
VESPERS
VESPIDS
VESSELS
VESTALS
VESTEES
VESTIGE
VESTING
VESTRAL
VESTRON
VESTURE
WESCOTT
WESKITS
WESTEGG
WESTEND
WESTERN
WESTERS
WESTIES
WESTINS
YESDEAR
YESHIVA
YESICAN
YESIDID
YESISEE
YESITIS
YESLETS
YESMAAM
YESORNO
YESSING
YESSIRE
YESVOTE

ZESTERS
ZESTFUL
ZESTIER
ZESTILY
ZESTING

•E•S•••

BEASLEY
BEASTIE
BEASTLY
BEDSIDE
BEDSITS
BEESWAX
BEGSFOR
BEGSOFF
BERSERK
BERSUNT
BESSELL
CEASING
CELSIUS
CENSERS
CENSING
CENSORS
CENSURE
CESSING
CESSION
CESSNAS
CESSPIT
DEISTIC
DELSOLS
DENSELY
DENSEST
DENSIFY
DENSITY
DESSERT
EELSKIN
FEASTED
FEASTER
FEASTON
FESSING
GEISHAS
GEMSBOK
GERSHON
GESSOED
GESSOES
GETSANA
GETSANF
GETSFAR
GETSFIT
GETSHEP
GETSHIP
GETSHOT
GETSMAD
GETSOFF
GETSOFT
GETSOLD
GETSORE
GETSOUT
GETSRID
GETSSET
GETSWET
GEYSERS
HEISMAN
HEISTED
HELSING
HEMSLEY
HENSLEY
HERSELF

HERSHEY
HESSAFE
HESSIAN
HEXSIGN
JERSEYS
JESSICA
JETSETS
JETSFAN
JETSKIS
JETSONS
JETSTAR
KEESHAN
KEESLAR
KEESLER
KEISTER
KERSHAW
KEYSPAN
LEASERS
LEASETO
LEASHED
LEASHES
LEASING
LEISTER
LEISURE
LENSCAP
LENSMAN
LENSMEN
LESSEES
LESSENS
LESSEPS
LESSFAT
LESSING
LESSONS
LESSORS
LESSTAR
LETSEAT
LETSFLY
LETSLIP
LETSNOT
LETSOFF
LETSOUT
LETSRIP
LETSSEE
LETSUSE
MEASLES
MEASURE
MEISSEN
MEISTER
MENSANS
MENSCHY
MESSAGE
MESSALA
MESSIAH
MESSICK
MESSIER
MESSILY
MESSINA
MESSING
MESSKIT
MESSUPS
METSFAN
NELSONS
NESSMAN
NETSTER
NETSUKE
NETSURF
NEWSBOY
NEWSDAY

NEWSIER
NEWSIES
NEWSMAN
NEWSMEN
NEWSOME
NEWSPEG
OERSTED
PEASANT
PEASOUP
PENSEES
PENSION
PENSIVE
PEPSICO
PEPSINS
PERSEID
PERSEUS
PERSIAN
PERSIST
PERSIUS
PERSOFF
PERSONA
PERSONS
PERSSON
PETSCAN
PETSHOP
PETSITS
REASKED
REASONS
REASSAY
REDSFAN
REDSKIN
REDSPOT
REDSTAR
REDSUIT
REDSUNS
REISSUE
REPSFOR
RETSINA
REUSERS
REUSING
SEASALT
SEASICK
SEASIDE
SEASLUG
SEASONS
SEASTAR
SEESALL
SEESAWS
SEESFIT
SEESOFF
SEESOUT
SEESRED
SEISMAL
SEISMIC
SENSATE
SENSEIS
SENSENS
SENSING
SENSORS
SENSORY
SENSUAL
SESSILE
SESSION
SETSAIL
SETSHOT
SETSOFF
SETSOUT
TEASELS

TEASERS
TEASETS
TEASEUP
TEASHOP
TEASING
TEESHOT
TEESOFF
TELSTAR
TENSELY
TENSEST
TENSEUP
TENSILE
TENSING
TENSION
TENSITY
TENSIVE
TENSORS
TENSPOT
TERSELY
TERSEST
TESSERA
VERSACE
VERSANT
VERSETS
VERSIFY
VERSING
VERSION
VESSELS
WEASELS
WEBSITE
WEBSTER
WETSUIT
YEASTED
YENSFOR
YESSING
YESSIRE
ZEMSTVO

•E••S••

AEGISES
AEROSOL
BEADSUP
BEAMSUP
BEARSON
BEARSUP
BEATSAT
BEATSIT
BEATSME
BEATSON
BEATSUP
BEEFSUP
BEEPSAT
BEHESTS
BELASCO
BELLSON
BELTSAW
BELTSUP
BELUSHI
BEMUSED
BEMUSES
BENISON
BENTSEN
BERGSON
BERNSEN
CELESTA
CELESTE
CERISES
DEADSEA

DEADSET
DEALSIN
DEALSTO
DEALSUP
DEARSIR
DEBASED
DEBASER
DEBASES
DEBUSES
DEBUSSY
DEEPSEA
DEEPSET
DEEPSIX
DEEPSKY
DEFUSED
DEFUSER
DEFUSES
DEGUSTS
DEHISCE
DELISTS
DEMASTS
DEMESNE
DEMISED
DEMISES
DEMISTS
DEMPSEY
DENISON
DEPESTS
DEPOSAL
DEPOSED
DEPOSER
DEPOSES
DEPOSIT
DERUSTS
DESISTS
DESKSET
DETESTS
DEUTSCH
DEVESTS
DEVISED
DEVISEE
DEVISER
DEVISES
DEVISOR
FEEDSIN
FEEDSON
FEEDSTO
FEELSOK
FETUSES
GEARSTO
GEARSUP
GELUSIL
GENESEE
GENESES
GENESET
GENESIS
GENUSES
GETSSET
HEADSAW
HEADSET
HEADSIN
HEADSTO
HEADSUP
HEALSUP
HEAPSOF
HEAPSON
HEAPSUP
HEARSAY

HEARSES
HEARSOF
HEATSUP
HEDISON
HELPSIN
HELPSON
HELPSUP
HERESTO
HEXOSES
JEERSAT
JEMISON
JERKSUP
JEWISON
KEEPSAT
KEEPSIN
KEEPSON
KEEPSTO
KEEPSUP
KENOSHA
LEADSIN
LEADSON
LEADSTO
LEADSUP
LEAKSIN
LEANSIN
LEANSON
LEANSTO
LEAPSAT
LEAPSIN
LEAPSON
LEAPSUP
LEERSAT
LEGISTS
LEGOSET
LETSSEE
LEXISES
LEXUSES
LEXUSGS
LEXUSGX
LEXUSIS
LEXUSLS
LEXUSLX
LEXUSRX
LEXUSSC
MEANSIT
MEANSTO
MEDUSAE
MEDUSAN
MEDUSAS
MEETSUP
MEIOSES
MEIOSIS
MEISSEN
MELISMA
MELISSA
MENISCI
NEEDSTO
NEGUSES
NEMESES
NEMESIS
NERISSA
NESTSIN
NEXUSES
PEARSON
PECKSAT
PEEKSAT
PEEKSIN
PEEPSAT
PEERSAT
PEERSIN
PEGASUS
PELISSE
PERISSA
PERKSUP
PERSSON
PERUSAL
PERUSED
PERUSER
PERUSES
READSIN
READSON
READSTO
READSUP
REARSUP
REASSAY
REBASTE
REBUSES
RECASED
RECASES
RECASTS
RECOSTS
RECUSAL
RECUSED
RECUSES
REDOSED
REDOSES
REDUSTS
REEKSOF
REELSIN
REELSUP
REFUSAL
REFUSED
REFUSER
REFUSES
REINSIN
REISSUE
RELISTS
RELOSES
REMISED
REMISES
RENESTS
RENTSTO
REPASTE
REPASTS
REPOSED
REPOSER
REPOSES
REPOSIT
REPOSTS
RERISEN
RERISES
RESISTS
RESTSIN
RESTSON
RESTSUP
RETASTE
RETESTS
REVESTS
REVISAL
REVISED
REVISER
REVISES
REVISIT
REVISOR
SEALSIN
SEALSUP
SEEMSTO
SEEPSIN
SELLSIT
SELLSTO
SENDSBY
SENDSIN
SENDSON
SENDSTO
SENDSUP
SENESCE
SEWISTS
SEXISTS
TEAMSUP
TEARSAT
TEARSIT
TEARSUP
TEENSIE
TELESTO
TELLSIT
TELLSOF
TELLSON
TENDSTO
VEDISTS
VENISON
VENUSES
VERISMO
VERISTS
VERYSAD
VERYSHY
WEARSON
WELLSEE
WELLSET
WELLSUP
XEROSES
XEROSIS
YELLSAT
YELTSIN
YESISEE
ZENISTS
ZEROSIN
ZEROSUM

•E•••S•

AERIEST
BEAMISH
BEARISH
BEAUISH
BECAUSE
BEDLESS
BEDPOST
BEDREST
BELFAST
BEQUEST
BERNESE
CELLIST
DEADEST
DEAFEST
DEAREST
DEBUSSY
DECEASE
DECLASS
DEEPEST
DEEPISH
DEFENSE
DEFFEST
DEFROST
DEFTEST
DEGAUSS
DEGHOST
DELOUSE
DELUISE
DENSEST
DENTIST
DEPRESS
DERVISH
DESPISE
DEWIEST
DEWLESS
EELIEST
EERIEST
FEELESS
FESTOSO
FEUDIST
FEWNESS
FEYNESS
GEMLESS
GENOESE
GENOISE
GEODESY
GETBUSY
GETCASH
GETLOST
GETPAST
GETWISE
HEIRESS
HELLISH
HELOISE
HENNISH
HEPPEST
HERMOSA
HERMOSO
HEROISM
JEBBUSH
JETWASH
KEENEST
KENTISH
KERTESZ
KEYCASE
KEYLESS
KEYWEST
LEANEST
LEFTEST
LEFTISH
LEFTISM
LEFTIST
LEGLESS
LEGREST
LETPASS
LETSUSE
LETTISH
LEWDEST
LEXUSSC
MEANEST
MEEKEST
MEFIRST
MELISSA
MELROSE
METRIST
NEAREST
NEATEST
NEBBISH
NERDISH
NERISSA
NETCOST
NETLESS
NETLOSS
NEWNESS
PEAKISH
PECKISH
PEERESS
PEEVISH
PEGLESS
PELISSE
PELTISH
PENCASE
PENROSE
PERCUSS
PERFUSE
PERISSA
PERKISH
PERSIST
PERTEST
PETFISH
PETTISH
REALEST
REALISE
REALISM
REALIST
REAMASS
REARISE
REAROSE
REBRUSH
RECHOSE
RECLASP
RECLASS
RECLUSE
RECROSS
REDDEST
REDDISH
REDDUST
REDFISH
REDNESS
REDNOSE
REDRESS
REDROSE
REFRESH
REGLOSS
REGRASP
REGRESS
REHOUSE
RELAPSE
RELEASE
REMORSE
REPHASE
REPRESS
REPRISE
REPULSE
REQUEST
RERAISE
RERINSE
RETOAST
RETWIST
REVERSA
REVERSE
REYNOSA
SEABASS
SEAMIST
SEAMOSS
SEEALSO
SEEPAST
SEERESS
SELFISH
SERIESE
SERIESF
SERIESG
SERIESH
SERIESI
SERIESJ
SERIESK
SEXIEST
SEXLESS
TEALESS
TEAMUSA
TEAROSE
TEMPEST
TENPAST
TENSEST
TERSEST
VERBOSE
VERIEST
WEAKEST
WEAKISH
WEBCAST
WEBLESS
WEENESS
WETKISS
WETNESS
WETTEST
WETTISH
WETWASH
XERXESI
YERKISH
ZEBRASS

•E••••S

AEDILES
AEGISES
AERATES
AERIALS
AEROBES
BEACHES
BEACONS
BEADERS
BEADLES
BEAGLES
BEAKERS
BEAMERS
BEANIES
BEARERS
BEATERS
BEATLES
BEAVERS
BECALMS
BECKONS
BECOMES
BEDAUBS
BEDAZES
BEDBUGS
BEDECKS
BEDLAMS
BEDLESS
BEDLOES
BEDSITS
BEEBEES
BEECHES
BEEGEES
BEEMERS
BEEPERS
BEETLES
BEEZERS
BEFALLS
BEFOOLS
BEFOULS
BEGGARS
BEGIRDS
BEHAVES
BEHEADS
BEHESTS
BEHINDS
BEHOLDS
BEHRENS
BEIGNES
BELAIRS
BELARUS
BELCHES
BELDAMS
BELIEFS
BELIERS
BELLIES
BELLOWS
BELONGS
BELTERS
BELUGAS
BEMIRES
BEMOANS
BEMUSES
BENARES
BENCHES
BENDAYS
BENDERS
BENGALS
BENOTES
BENTHOS
BENUMBS
BERATES
BERBERS
BERGIUS
BERNAYS
BERRIES
BERTHAS
BESIDES
BESTIRS
BESTOWS
BETAKES
BETHELS
BETIDES
BETIMES
BETRAYS
BETTERS
BETTORS
BEURRES
BEWAILS
BEWARES
BEZIERS
CELEBES
CELICAS
CELLARS
CELSIUS
CELTICS
CEMENTS
CENSERS
CENSORS
CENTALS
CENTERS
CENTRES
CEPHEUS
CERATES
CEREALS
CERISES
CERVIDS
CESSNAS
CETANES
CETERIS
DEACONS
DEADENS
DEAFENS
DEALERS
DEARIES
DEARTHS
DEBARKS
DEBASES
DEBATES
DEBEERS
DEBLURS
DEBONES
DEBTEES
DEBTORS
DEBUNKS
DEBURRS
DEBUSES
DECADES
DECAMPS
DECANTS
DECEITS
DECIDES
DECILES
DECKERS
DECKLES
DECLASS
DECLAWS
DECLOTS
DECOCTS
DECODES
DECREES
DECRIES
DEDALUS
DEDUCES
DEDUCTS
DEEJAYS
DEEPENS
DEFACES
DEFAMES
DEFANGS
DEFCONS
DEFEATS
DEFECTS
DEFENDS
DEFIERS
DEFILES
DEFINES
DEFLEAS
DEFOAMS
DEFOCUS
DEFORMS
DEFRAGS
DEFRAYS
DEFUELS
DEFUNDS
DEFUSES
DEGAUSS
DEGERMS
DEGREES
DEGUSTS
DEHAIRS
DEHEXES
DEHIRES
DEHORNS
DEICERS
DEIFIES
DEITIES
DEJECTS
DEJUNKS
DELEADS
DELETES
DELIBES
DELICTS
DELINTS
DELISTS
DELKEYS
DELORIS
DELRAYS
DELSOLS
DELUDES
DELUGES
DELVERS
DEMANDS
DEMARKS
DEMASTS
DEMBUMS
DEMEANS
DEMISES
DEMISTS
DEMOTES
DEMOTHS
DENIALS
DENIERS
DENMOMS
DENOTES
DENTALS
DENTINS
DENTONS
DENUDES
DEODARS
DEPARTS
DEPENDS
DEPESTS
DEPICTS
DEPLOYS
DEPONES
DEPORTS
DEPOSES
DEPRESS
DEPULPS
DEPUTES
DERAILS
DERATES
DERBIES
DERIDES
DERIVES
DERUSTS
DESALTS
DESEEDS
DESERTS
DESEXES
DESIGNS
DESILTS
DESIRES
DESISTS
DESLUMS
DESMOGS
DESOTOS
DESPOTS
DESTEMS
DETAILS
DETAINS
DETECTS
DETENTS
DETESTS
DETOURS
DETOXES
DETUNES
DEVEINS
DEVESTS
DEVICES
DEVIOUS
DEVISES
DEVOIRS
DEVORES
DEVOTES
DEVOURS
DEVRIES
DEWAXES
DEWIRES
DEWLAPS
DEWLESS
DEWORMS
EELPOTS
FEARERS
FEDDERS
FEDEXES
FEDORAS
FEEDERS
FEELERS
FEELESS
FELINES
FELLAHS
FELLERS
FELLOWS
FEMALES
FEMBOTS
FEMORIS
FENCERS
FENDERS
FENNELS
FERMATS
FERRETS
FERRIES
FERROUS
FERULES
FERVORS
FESCUES
FESTERS
FETCHES
FETTERS
FETTLES
FETUSES
FEWNESS
FEYNESS
GECKOES
GEEGAWS
GEEZERS
GEISHAS
GELATES
GELATIS
GELATOS
GELCAPS
GELPENS
GEMINIS
GEMLESS
GENDERS
GENERIS
GENESES
GENESIS
GENGHIS
GENOMES
GENTLES
GENUSES
GENXERS
GEORGES
GERBILS
GERENTS
GERMANS
GERUNDS
GERVAIS
GESSOES
GETTERS
GETTHIS
GEWGAWS
GEYSERS
HEADERS
HEALERS
HEAPERS
HEARERS
HEARSES
HEARTHS
HEATERS
HEAVENS
HEAVERS
HEAVIES
HEBREWS
HECKLES
HECKYES
HECTORS
HEDGERS
HEEDERS
HEEHAWS
HEELERS
HEFTERS
HEGIRAS
HEHHEHS
HEIFERS
HEIGHTS
HEINOUS
HEIRESS
HELICES
HELIXES
HELLOES
HELLYES
HELMETS
HELPERS
HEMMERS
HENBITS
HENRIES
HEPCATS
HEPTADS
HERALDS
HERBALS
HERDERS
HERMANS
HERMITS
HERNIAS
HERNIBS
HEROICS
HEXANES
HEXNUTS
HEXOSES
HEYDAYS
HEYMANS
JEALOUS
JEEBIES
JEEPERS
JEERERS
JEFFERS
JELLIES
JENKINS
JENNETS
JERBOAS
JERGENS
JERKERS
JERKIES
JERKINS
JERSEYS
JESTERS
JESUITS
JETFANS
JETGUNS
JETLAGS
JETSETS
JETSKIS
JETSONS
JETTIES
JETWAYS
KEDGERS
KEENERS
KEEPERS
KEGGERS
KEGLERS
KELPIES
KELVINS
KENNELS
KENYANS
KERNELS
KETCHES
KETONES
KETTLES
KEWPIES
KEYDETS
KEYLESS
KEYPADS
KEYPALS
KEYWAYS
LEACHES
LEADENS
LEADERS
LEADINS
LEADUPS
LEAGUES
LEAKERS
LEAKEYS
LEANERS
LEANTOS
LEAPERS
LEASERS
LEASHES
LEAVENS
LECHERS
LECTORS
LEDGERS
LEECHES
LEERERS
LEEWAYS
LEFTIES
LEGATES
LEGATOS
LEGENDS
LEGIONS
LEGISTS
LEGLESS
LEGOLAS
LEGUMES
LENDERS
LENGTHS
LENGUAS
LENNONS
LENOVOS
LENTILS
LEONIDS
LEPIDUS
LEPTONS
LESIONS
LESSEES
LESSENS
LESSEPS
LESSONS
LESSORS
LETPASS
LETTERS
LETTRES
LEVADES
LEVIERS
LEVITES
LEXISES
LEXUSES
LEXUSGS
LEXUSIS
LEXUSLS
MEADOWS
MEAGLES
MEALIES
MEANIES
MEASLES
MECCANS
MEDAKAS
MEDDLES
MEDELES
MEDIANS
MEDICOS
MEDIUMS
MEDLEYS
MEDUSAS
MEEMIES
MEETERS
MEGANES
MEGOHMS
MEGRIMS
MEIOSES
MEIOSIS
MELDERS
MELLOWS
MELTERS
MEMBERS
MEMOIRS
MEMPHIS
MENACES
MENAGES
MENCIUS
MENDELS
MENDERS
MENIALS
MENSANS
MENTEES
MENTORS
MENUDOS
MENZIES
MEOWERS
MERCERS
MERCHES
MERCIES

MERGEES
MERGERS
MERINOS
MERLINS
MERLOTS
MESAMIS
MESCALS
MESEEMS
MESSUPS
METATES
METEORS
METFANS
METHODS
METIERS
METRICS
METTLES
MEWLERS
MEZUZAS
NEATENS
NEBULAS
NECKERS
NECTARS
NEEDERS
NEEDLES
NEGATES
NEGUSES
NELSONS
NEMESES
NEMESIS
NENNIUS
NEOCONS
NEONGAS
NEPALIS
NEPHEWS
NEREIDS
NERVOUS
NESTERS
NESTLES
NESTORS
NETFULS
NETLESS
NETLOSS
NETTERS
NETTLES
NETTONS
NEURONS
NEUTERS
NEWBIES
NEWCARS
NEWHATS
NEWJOBS
NEWKIDS
NEWMANS
NEWNESS
NEWSIES
NEWTONS
NEWTOYS
NEXRADS
NEXUSES
OEDIPUS
OEUVRES
PEACHES
PEAHENS
PEANUTS
PEAPODS
PEBBLES
PECTINS
PEDANTS
PEDDLES
PEDWAYS
PEEBLES
PEEKERS
PEELERS
PEEPERS
PEEPLES
PEERESS
PEEWEES
PEGASUS
PEGLEGS
PEGLESS
PEGTOPS
PELAGES
PELLEAS
PELLETS
PELOTAS
PELTERS
PENATES
PENCILS
PENNERS
PENNEYS
PENNIES
PENNONS
PENPALS
PENSEES
PENTADS
PENTELS
PENULTS
PENZIAS
PEONIES
PEOPLES
PEPBOYS
PEPCIDS
PEPITAS
PEPLUMS
PEPPERS
PEPSINS
PEPTICS
PEQUOTS
PERCHES
PERCUSS
PERHAPS
PERIODS
PERITUS
PERKINS
PERMITS
PERRINS
PERSEUS
PERSIUS
PERSONS
PERUKES
PERUSES
PESADES
PESETAS
PESEWAS
PESTERS
PESTLES
PETALES
PETARDS
PETBOAS
PETCATS
PETCOWS
PETDOGS
PETITES
PETNAPS
PETPIGS
PETPUPS
PETRATS
PETRELS
PETROLS
PETROUS
PETSITS
PETTERS
PETTOYS
PEWTERS
PEYOTES
REACHES
READERS
READIES
REAGANS
REAMASS
REAMERS
REAPERS
REARERS
REASONS
REATTAS
REAVERS
REAVOWS
REBAITS
REBAKES
REBALES
REBANKS
REBATES
REBENDS
REBILLS
REBINDS
REBOILS
REBOLTS
REBOOKS
REBOOTS
REBORES
REBOTES
REBOXES
REBOZOS
REBREWS
REBUFFS
REBUKES
REBUSES
RECAGES
RECALLS
RECANES
RECANTS
RECASES
RECASTS
RECEDES
RECHEWS
RECIPES
RECITES
RECKONS
RECLADS
RECLASS
RECOALS
RECOATS
RECOCKS
RECODES
RECOILS
RECOINS
RECOMBS
RECOOKS
RECOOLS
RECORDS
RECORKS
RECOSTS
RECOUPS
RECROSS
RECTORS
RECURES
RECURLS
RECUSES
REDACTS
REDANTS
REDARES
REDARNS
REDATES
REDBATS
REDBAYS
REDBUDS
REDCAPS
REDCODS
REDDENS
REDDOGS
REDDOTS
REDDYES
REDEALS
REDEEDS
REDEEMS
REDEYES
REDFINS
REDFIRS
REDHATS
REDHENS
REDHOTS
REDIALS
REDLEGS
REDNESS
REDOAKS
REDOCKS
REDOSES
REDOUTS
REDOXES
REDRAGS
REDRAWS
REDRESS
REDRIES
REDSUNS
REDTABS
REDTAGS
REDTIES
REDTOPS
REDUCES
REDUSTS
REEARNS
REEBOKS
REEDITS
REEFERS
REEKERS
REELERS
REEMITS
REFACES
REFALLS
REFAXES
REFEEDS
REFILES
REFILLS
REFILMS
REFINDS
REFINES
REFIRES
REFIXES
REFLAGS
REFLIES
REFLIPS
REFLOWS
REFOCUS
REFOLDS
REFORMS
REFRIES
REFUELS
REFUGES
REFUNDS
REFUSES
REFUTES
REGAINS
REGALES
REGARDS
REGEARS
REGENTS
REGIFTS
REGILDS
REGIMES
REGINAS
REGIONS
REGIRDS
REGIVES
REGLOSS
REGLOWS
REGLUES
REGRABS
REGRESS
REGRETS
REGRIPS
REGROWS
REGULUS
REHANGS
REHAULS
REHEALS
REHEARS
REHEATS
REHEELS
REHIDES
REHIRES
REHONES
REHOOKS
REIFIES
REJAILS
REJECTS
REJOINS
REKICKS
REKNITS
REKNOTS
RELACES
RELANDS
RELANES
RELATES
RELAXES
RELEADS
RELEAPS
RELENDS
RELENTS
RELEVES
RELICTS
RELIEFS
RELIERS
RELINES
RELINKS
RELISTS
RELIVES
RELOADS
RELOANS
RELOCKS
RELOOKS
RELOSES
RELUCTS
RELUMES
REMAILS
REMAINS
REMAKES
REMANDS
REMARKS
REMATES
REMEETS
REMELTS
REMENDS
REMILLS
REMINDS
REMINES
REMINTS
REMISES
REMIXES
REMOLDS
REMORAS
REMOTES
REMOVES
RENAILS
RENAMES
RENDERS
RENEGES
RENESTS
RENNETS
RENNINS
RENOIRS
RENOTES
RENOWNS
RENTALS
RENTEES
RENTERS
RENVOIS
REOPENS
REPACKS
REPAGES
REPAIRS
REPARKS
REPASTS
REPAVES
REPEALS
REPEATS
REPENTS
REPERKS
REPICKS
REPINES
REPLANS
REPLAYS
REPLIES
REPLOTS
REPLOWS
REPOLLS
REPORTS
REPOSES
REPOSTS
REPOURS
REPRESS
REPUGNS
REPUMPS
REPUTES
RERACKS
RERAKES
RERANKS
RERATES
REREADS
REREDOS
REREELS
RERENTS
RERIDES
RERISES
REROLLS
REROOFS
REROOTS
RESALES
RESALTS
RESANDS
RESAVES
RESCANS
RESCUES
RESEALS
RESEAMS
RESEATS
RESEAUS
RESECTS
RESEEDS
RESEEKS
RESELLS
RESENDS
RESENTS
RESHIPS
RESHOES
RESHOWS
RESHUTS
RESIDES
RESIFTS
RESIGNS
RESILES
RESINGS
RESINKS
RESISTS
RESIZES
RESNAIS
RESNAPS
RESOAKS
RESOAPS
RESOILS
RESOLES
RESORBS
RESORTS
RESPANS
RESPINS
RESPOTS
RESTABS
RESTERS
RESTIRS
RESTOWS
RESUITS
RESULTS
RESUMES
RESWIMS
RETACKS
RETAILS
RETAINS
RETAKES
RETAMES
RETAPES
RETARDS
RETAXES
RETEARS
RETELLS
RETESTS
RETHAWS
RETILES
RETILLS
RETIMES
RETINAS
RETINTS
RETIRES
RETONES
RETOOLS
RETORTS
RETOURS
RETRAPS
RETRIES
RETRIMS
RETUNES
RETURFS
RETURNS
RETYPES
REUBENS
REUNERS
REURGES
REUSERS
REUTERS
REVAMPS
REVEALS
REVENDS
REVERBS
REVERES
REVERTS
REVESTS
REVIEWS
REVILES
REVISES
REVIVES
REVOKES
REVOLTS
REVOTES
REWAKES
REWARDS
REWARMS
REWARNS
REWAXES
REWEARS
REWELDS
REWINDS
REWIPES
REWIRES
REWORDS
REWORKS
REWRAPS
REXCATS
REYOKES
REZEROS
REZONES
SEAARMS
SEABAGS
SEABASS
SEABEDS
SEABEES
SEACATS
SEACOWS
SEADOGS
SEAEELS
SEAGODS
SEALABS
SEALEGS
SEALERS
SEAMAPS
SEAMERS
SEAMOSS
SEANCES
SEARERS
SEASONS
SEATERS
SEAWAYS
SECANTS
SECEDES
SECKELS
SECONDS
SECRETS
SECTORS
SECURES
SEDATES
SEDONAS
SEDUCES
SEEDERS
SEEKERS
SEERESS
SEESAWS
SEETHES
SEFERIS
SEGWAYS
SEINERS
SEIZERS
SEIZORS
SELECTS
SELLERS
SEMANAS
SEMITES
SENATES
SENDEES
SENDERS
SENDUPS
SENECAS
SENIORS
SENORAS
SENORES
SENSEIS
SENSENS
SENSORS
SENTRAS
SEPHIAS
SEPIRAS
SEPTETS
SEQUELS
SEQUINS
SERAPES
SERAPHS
SERAPIS
SERIALS
SERIOUS
SERMONS
SERPENS
SERVEAS
SERVERS
SESAMES
SESTETS
SETFEES
SETOFFS
SETOUTS
SETTEES
SETTERS
SETTLES
SEVERUS
SEWARDS
SEWISTS
SEXISTS
SEXLESS
SEXPOTS
SEXTANS
SEXTETS
SEXTONS
TEABAGS
TEACHES
TEACUPS
TEALESS
TEAPOTS
TEAPOYS
TEARERS
TEARGAS
TEASELS
TEASERS
TEASETS
TEATROS
TEAURNS
TECHIES
TECHNOS
TEDDIES
TEDEUMS
TEDIOUS
TEDIUMS
TEEHEES
TEENERS
TEEOFFS
TEEPEES
TEETERS
TEETHES
TEEVEES
TEFLONS
TEJANAS
TEJANOS
TEKKIES
TELEXES
TELLERS
TELLIES
TEMPEHS
TEMPERS
TEMPLES
TENACES
TENANTS
TENCHES
TENDAYS
TENDERS
TENDONS
TENNERS
TENNIES
TENPINS
TENSORS
TENTERS
TENTONS
TENUOUS
TENURES
TERCELS
TERRANS
TERRETS
TERRIES
TERRORS
TESTEES
TESTERS
TETANUS
TETHERS
TETRADS
TEUTONS
VEADARS
VECTORS
VECTRAS
VEDISTS
VEEJAYS
VEERIES
VEGGIES
VEIGHTS
VEILERS
VEINTES
VELCROS
VELLUMS
VELOURS
VELOXES
VELURES
VELVETS
VENDEES
VENDERS
VENDORS
VENDUES
VENEERS
VENTERS
VENTRIS
VENULES
VENUSES
VERBALS
VERBIDS
VERDINS
VERGERS
VERISTS
VERITAS
VERSETS
VESPERS
VESPIDS
VESSELS
VESTALS
VESTEES
VETCHES
VETOERS
VETTERS
WEAKENS
WEAKONS
WEALTHS
WEANERS
WEAPONS
WEARERS
WEARIES
WEASELS
WEAVERS
WEBCAMS
WEBLESS
WEBLOGS
WEDDERS
WEDELNS
WEDGIES
WEEBITS
WEEDERS
WEENESS
WEENIES
WEEONES
WEEPERS
WEEVILS
WEIGHTS
WEIRDOS
WELDERS
WELLYES
WELTERS
WENCHES
WENDERS
WENDKOS
WESKITS
WESTERS
WESTIES
WESTINS
WETBARS
WETKISS
WETMOPS
WETNAPS
WETNESS
WETONES
WETRAGS
XEROSES
XEROSIS
XEROXES
YELLERS
YELLOWS
YELPERS
YEMENIS
YEOMANS
YESITIS
YESLETS
YETTIES
ZEALOTS
ZEALOUS
ZEBRASS
ZEDONKS
ZENANAS
ZENISTS
ZENITHS
ZEPHYRS
ZESTERS

••ES•••

ACESOUT
AGESAGO
AGESOUT
AMESLAN
APESUIT
AVESTAN
AVESTAS
AWESOME
BEESWAX
BLESSED
BLESSER
BLESSES
BRESCIA
BRESLIN
CAESARS
CAESURA
CHESTED
CHESTER
CRESPIN
CRESSES
CRESSET
CRESTED
CRESTON
CUESTAS
DIESELS
DIESFOR
DIESOFF
DIESOUT
DOESBAD
DOESFOR
DOESKIN
DOESNOT
DOESTOO
DRESDEN
DRESSAS
DRESSED
DRESSER
DRESSES
DRESSIN
DRESSUP
EGESTED
EKESOUT
ETESIAN
EYESHOT
EYESORE
EYESPOT
FIESTAS
FLESHED
FLESHES
FLESHLY
FRESCAS
FRESCOS
FRESHED
FRESHEN
FRESHER
FRESHES
FRESHET
FRESHLY
FRESNEL
FRESSED
FRESSES
GOESAFT
GOESAPE
GOESBAD
GOESFAR
GOESFOR
GOESMAD
GOESOFF
GOESOUT
GOESPRO
GRESHAM
GUESSAT
GUESSED
GUESSER
GUESSES
GUESSSO
GUESTED
ICESHOW
ICESOUT
IRESIGN
KEESHAN
KEESLAR
KEESLER
KMESONS
KNESSET
KRESKIN
LIESFOR
LIESLOW
LOESSER
LOESSES
LYESOAP
MAESTRO
MUESLIS
MUESLIX
NUESTRA
NUESTRO
OBESELY
OBESITY
ODESSAN
OLESTRA
ONESELF
ONESHOE
ONESHOT
ONESIZE

ONESOCK
ONESPOT
ONESTAR
ONESTEP
ONESTOP
ORESTES
PIESAFE
PIESALE
POESIES
PRESAGE
PRESALE
PRESALT
PRESEAL
PRESEAT
PRESELL
PRESENT
PRESETS
PRESHIP
PRESHOW
PRESIDE
PRESIFT
PRESLEY
PRESOAK
PRESOLD
PRESONG
PRESORT
PRESPUR
PRESQUE
PRESSED
PRESSEL
PRESSER
PRESSES
PRESSON
PRESSUP
PRESTON
PRESTOS
PRESUME
QUESERA
QUESNAY
QUESTED
QUESTER
RIESENS
RIESMAN
RIESSEN
SEESALL
SEESAWS
SEESFIT
SEESOFF
SEESOUT
SEESRED
SIESTAS
SUESFOR
TEESHOT
TEESOFF
THESACK
THESAME
THESELF
THESEUS
THESHOW
THESIMS
THESPIS
THESTAR
THESUNS
THESWAN
TIESOFF
TOESHOE
TRESSED
TRESSES
TRESTLE
TUESDAY
USESFOR
VIESFOR
WRESTED
WRESTER
WRESTLE

••E•S••

AGEISTS
ALEKSEI
APERSON
ARENSKY
ASEPSIS
BEEFSUP
BEEPSAT
BLEDSOE
BLESSED
BLESSER
BLESSES
BREASTS
BREWSKI
BREWSUP
CHEESED
CHEESES
CHELSEA
CHEWSON
CHEWSUP
CLEMSON
CREASED
CREASER
CREASES
CREOSOL
CRESSES
CRESSET
DEEPSEA
DEEPSET
DEEPSIX
DEEPSKY
DREISER
DRESSAS
DRESSED
DRESSER
DRESSES
DRESSIN
DRESSUP
ELEISON
EMERSED
EMERSON
EVENSUP
FEEDSIN
FEEDSON
FEEDSTO
FEELSOK
FLENSED
FLENSER
FLENSES
FREESIA
FREESOF
FREESUP
FRESSED
FRESSES
FRETSAT
FRETSAW
FUELSUP
GLEASON
GREASED
GREASER
GREASES
GUESSAT
GUESSED
GUESSER
GUESSES
GUESSSO
IVERSON
JEERSAT
KEEPSAT
KEEPSIN
KEEPSON
KEEPSTO
KEEPSUP
KLEISER
KLENSCH
KNEESUP
KNESSET
LEERSAT
LOESSER
LOESSES
MEETSUP
MYERSON
NEEDSTO
NIELSEN
ODESSAN
OPENSEA
OPENSUP
OVERSAD
OVERSAW
OVERSEA
OVERSEE
OVERSET
OVERSEW
OVERSUP
PEEKSAT
PEEKSIN
PEEPSAT
PEERSAT
PEERSIN
PLEASED
PLEASER
PLEASES
PRESSED
PRESSEL
PRESSER
PRESSES
PRESSON
PRESSUP
PREYSON
REEKSOF
REELSIN
REELSUP
RIESSEN
SEEMSTO
SEEPSIN
SHEDSON
SPENSER
STEPSIN
STEPSON
STEPSUP
STETSON
SWENSON
TEENSIE
THEISMS
THEISTS
THEUSSR
THEYSAY
TREASON
TREESAP
TRESSED
TRESSES
TSETSES
UNEASES
UTENSIL
WOEISME

••E••S•

ACEROSE
AGELESS
ARENOSE
ATELESS
AWELESS
BLEMISH
CHEMISE
CHEMIST
CHERISH
CLEANSE
CLERISY
COEXIST
DEEPEST
DEEPISH
DIECAST
DUEEAST
DUELIST
DUEWEST
ELEGIST
EPEEIST
EVENEST
EVEREST
EYELASH
EYELESS
EYEMASK
EYETEST
EYEWASH
FEELESS
FLEMISH
FOELESS
FRENESI
GJETOST
GRECISM
GREYEST
GREYISH
GUESSSO
HUELESS
ICELESS
IREFUSE
IRELESS
ITEMISE
KEENEST
LIEFEST
LIETEST
MAEWEST
MEEKEST
OBELISE
OBELISK
OLEMISS
ONEBASE
ONENESS
OPEROSE
ORELESS
OVERUSE
PEERESS
PEEVISH
PIETOSO
PLENISH
POETESS
POETISE
PRECAST
PRECISE
PREDUSK
PRELOSS
PREMISE
PREMISS
PRETEST
PREVOST
PREWASH
QUEPASA
QUERIST
RHENISH
SEEALSO
SEEPAST
SEERESS
SIENESE
SWEDISH
THEBEST
THEBOSS
THEBUSH
THEEAST
THEKISS
THEMASK
THEMOST
THEPOST
THERESA
THEROSE
THEUSSR
TIELESS
TOELESS
USELESS
WEENESS
WHEYISH

••E•••S

ACETALS
ADELIES
AGEISTS
AGELESS
AGENCES
AGENDAS
ALEGARS
ALEKEGS
ALETAPS
ALETTES
ALEVELS
AMERCES
ANEMIAS
APELETS
APERCUS
APERIES
AREOLAS
AREOLES
ASEPSIS
ATELESS
AVENGES
AVENUES
AVERNUS
AVESTAS
AWELESS
AYEAYES
BEEBEES
BEECHES
BEEGEES
BEEMERS
BEEPERS
BEETLES
BEEZERS
BLENDES
BLESSES
BOEINGS
BREASTS
BREATHS
BREEZES
BRETONS
BREVETS
BREWERS
BREYERS
BYEBYES
CAESARS
CHEDERS
CHEESES
CHEETAS
CHEETOS
CHEQUES
CHERUBS
CHEVETS
CHEVONS
CHEVRES
CHEWERS
CLEAVES
CLEMENS
CLERICS
COEDITS
COEPTIS
COERCES
COEVALS
CREASES
CREATES
CRECHES
CREDITS
CREEPOS
CRENELS
CREOLES
CRESSES
CRETANS
CRETINS
CREWELS
CUEBIDS
CUESTAS
CUETIPS
DAEMONS
DAEWOOS
DEEJAYS
DEEPENS
DIECUTS
DIEMENS
DIEOFFS
DIESELS
DIETERS
DREDGES
DRESSAS
DRESSES
DREYFUS
DUELERS
DUENNAS
DUETTOS
DYEJOBS
DYELOTS
DYEVATS
EGERIAS
ELEGIES
ELEGITS
ELEVENS
ELEVONS
EMERGES
EMERIES
EMETICS
ENEMIES
ERECTUS
EVENERS
EVERLYS
EWERIES
EXEMPTS
EXEUNTS
EYECUPS
EYEFULS
EYELESS
EYELETS
EYELIDS
EYEPITS
FAERIES
FAEROES
FEEDERS
FEELERS
FEELESS
FIENNES
FIESTAS
FLECHES
FLEDGES
FLEECES
FLENSES
FLESHES
FLEXORS
FOELESS
FREEZES
FRENCHS
FRESCAS
FRESCOS
FRESHES
FRESSES
FUELERS
FUENTES
GEEGAWS
GEEZERS
GHETTOS
GREASES
GREAVES
GUESSES
HEEDERS
HEEHAWS
HEELERS
HUELESS
ICEAGES
ICEAXES
ICEBAGS
ICECAPS
ICEDAMS
ICEFOGS
ICELESS
ICEOUTS
ICEPOPS
ICERUNS
ICETEAS
IDEATES
IRELESS
IRENICS
JAEGERS
JEEBIES
JEEPERS
JEERERS
KEENERS
KEEPERS
KLEPTOS
KMESONS
LAERTES
LEECHES
LEERERS
LEEWAYS
LIENEES
LIENORS
LOESSES
MAENADS
MEEMIES
MEETERS
MTEVANS
MUESLIS
NEEDERS
NEEDLES
NOETICS
OBENTOS
OBEYERS
OCEANUS
OCELLUS
OCELOTS
ODELETS
OLEATES
OLEFINS
OLEMISS
OLEVELS
OMELETS
ONEACTS
ONEIDAS
ONENESS
ONEOFFS
ONEOFUS
ONEROUS
ONETWOS
OPENERS
ORELESS
ORESTES
OSETRAS
PAELLAS
PEEBLES
PEEKERS
PEELERS
PEEPERS
PEEPLES
PEERESS
PEEWEES
PHEMIUS
PHENOLS
PHENOMS
PIECERS
PIEPANS
PIERCES
PIETIES
PIETINS
PIETROS
PLEASES
PLEDGES
PLENUMS
PLEXORS
PNEUMAS
POESIES
POETESS
POETICS
PREACTS
PREAGES
PREAMPS
PREARMS
PREBIDS
PREBUYS
PRECUTS
PREFABS
PREFERS
PRELIMS
PRELOSS
PREMEDS
PREMIES
PREMISS
PRENUPS
PREPAYS
PRESETS
PRESSES
PRESTOS
PRETORS
PREVIAS
PREVUES
PREXIES
PREYERS
PTEROUS
PUEBLOS
PYEDOGS
QUEIROS
QUERIES
QUEUERS
REEARNS
REEBOKS
REEDITS
REEFERS
REEKERS
REELERS
REEMITS
RHEBOKS
RHETORS
RIESENS
SCENICS
SEEDERS
SEEKERS
SEERESS
SEESAWS
SEETHES
SHEATHS
SHEAVES
SHEIKHS
SHEILAS
SHEKELS
SHELVES
SHERIFS
SHERPAS
SHEVATS
SIEMENS
SIENNAS
SIERRAS
SIESTAS
SKEWERS
SLEAZES
SLEDGES
SLEEVES
SLEIGHS
SLEUTHS
SNEEZES
SPECIES
SPEEDOS
SPEWERS
STEARNS
STEEVES
STELIAS
STENNIS
STEPINS
STEPPES
STEPUPS
STEREOS
STERNOS
STEROLS
STEVENS
STEWERS
SWERVES
TEEHEES
TEENERS
TEEOFFS
TEEPEES
TEETERS
TEETHES
TEEVEES
THEABCS
THEAGES
THEALPS
THEARTS
THEAXIS
THEBANS
THEBOSS
THEBOYS
THECARS
THECAVS
THECUBS
THEFEDS
THEHOGS
THEISMS
THEISTS
THEJETS
THEKISS
THEMAVS
THEMETS
THENETS
THENEWS
THEPIPS
THEPITS
THERAMS
THEREDS
THERMOS
THESEUS
THESIMS
THESPIS
THESUNS
THEVIPS
THEYIPS
TIEBARS
TIEDYES
TIELESS
TIEMPOS
TIENDAS
TIEPINS
TIERCES
TIERODS
TIETACS
TOECAPS
TOELESS
TOETAPS
TREBLES
TREDIAS
TREIZES
TRELLIS
TREMORS
TREPANS
TRESSES
TSETSES
TWEEZES
TWELVES
UNEASES
UNEDGES
USEDCDS
USELESS
USERIDS
VEEJAYS
VEERIES
VIELLES
VIERNES
VIEWERS
WEEBITS
WEEDERS
WEENESS
WEENIES
WEEONES
WEEPERS
WEEVILS
WHEEZES
WHEREAS
WIENERS
WIENIES
WREATHS
XTERRAS

•••ES••

ACHESON
ALCESTE
AMNESIA
AMNESIC
AMNESTY
ANBESOL
ANTESUP
ARRESTS
ATTESTS
BASESIX
BEHESTS
BITESIN
BITESON
BITESUP
BLUESKY
BLUESUN
BONESET
BONESUP
BOXESIN
BOXESUP
CAGESUP
CAKESUP
CARESTO
CAVESIN
CELESTA
CELESTE
CHEESED
CHEESES
CINESIA
CLUESIN
COMESAS
COMESAT
COMESBY
COMESIN
COMESON
COMESTO
COMESUP
CRIESUP
CROESUS
DARESAY
DARESTO
DEMESNE
DEPESTS
DETESTS
DEVESTS
DIGESTS
DINESAT
DINESEN
DINESIN
DINESON
DIVESIN
DIVESTS
DOTESON
DRIESCH
DRIESUP
DUDESUP
EASESBY
EASESIN
EASESON
EASESUP
EDGESIN
EPHESUS
ERNESTA
ERNESTO
FACESIT
FACESON
FADESIN
FAKESIT
FILESBY
FILESIN
FINESSE
FIRESAT
FIRESON
FIRESUP
FIVESIX
FIXESON
FIXESUP
FLIESAT
FLIESBY
FLIESIN
FLIESON
FLIESTO
FLIESUP
FORESAW
FORESEE
FORESTS
FREESIA
FREESOF
FREESUP
FRIESUP
FUMESAT
GAPESAT
GASESUP
GAZESAT
GAZESON
GENESEE
GENESES
GENESET
GENESIS
GIBESAT
GIVESIN
GIVESOF
GIVESON
GIVESTO
GIVESUP
GLUESON
GLUESTO
HATESIT
HAYESES
HERESTO
HIKESUP
HIRESON
HOLESUP
HOMESIN
HONESIN
HONESTY
HOPESSO
HOPESTO
HYPESUP
IDLESSE
ILIESCU
INFESTS
INGESTA
INGESTS
INVESTS
IONESCO
IQTESTS
JAMESII
JAMESIV
JAMESON
JAMESVI
JIBESAT
JONESED
JONESES
KINESES
KINESIC
KINESIS
KNEESUP
LACESON
LACESUP
LINESUP
LIVESAT
LIVESET
LIVESEY
LIVESIN
LIVESON
LOSESIT
LOSESTO
LOVESET
LOVESIT
LOVESTO
LUNESTA
LURESIN
MAJESTE
MAJESTY
MAKESDO
MAKESGO
MAKESIT
MAKESUP
MIMESES
MIMESIS
MIXESIN
MIXESUP
MODESTO
MODESTY
MOLESTS
MORESBY
MOVESIN
MOVESIT
MOVESON
MOVESTO
MOVESUP
MUMESON
MUSESON
NEMESES
NEMESIS

NILESOH
NOSESIN
NOSESUP
OBTESTS
PAGESIX
PILESIN
PILESOF
PILESON
PILESUP
PIMESON
PINESAP
PINESOL
PIPESIN
PIPESUP
PLOESTI
POKESAT
POLESAT
POLESIT
POSESAS
PRIESTS
RACESBY
RACESTO
RACESUP
RAKESIN
RAKESUP
RAMESES
RENESTS
RETESTS
REVESTS
RIDESBY
RIDESIN
RIDESTO
RIDESUP
RILESUP
RISESTO
RISESUP
ROBESON
ROPESIN
ROPESUP
RULESON
SAVESON
SAVESUP
SENESCE
SILESIA
SIZESIX
SIZESUP
SOMESAY
SPIESON
TAKESIN
TAKESIT
TAKESON
TAKESTO
TAKESUP
TAPESON
TAPESUP
TELESTO
TIMESUP
TIRESOF
TONESUP
TOTESUP
TREESAP
TRIESIT
TRIESON
TRIESTE
TRIESTO
TRUESUP
TUMESCE
TUNESIN
TUNESTO
TUNESUP
TYPESET
TYPESIN
TYPESUP
UNBESET
UNRESTS
URGESON
VANESSA
VOTESIN
VOTESNO
VOTESON
WADESIN
WAKESUP
WAVESAT
WAVESIN
WAVESTO
WAXESUP
WINESAP
WIPESUP
WIRESIN
WIRESUP
WISESUP

•••E•S•

ABREAST
ADVERSE
ALLELSE
AMHERST
APPEASE
ASPERSE
ATHEISM
ATHEIST
ATLEAST
BAKERST
BIGEAST
BIGEASY
BLUEISH
BONEASH
CAPEESH
DECEASE
DEFENSE
DISEASE
DISEUSE
DIVERSE
DONETSK
DRSEUSS
DUEEAST
EDMEESE
EKWENSI
EPEEIST
EXPENSE
EXTENSO
FAREAST
FINESSE
HOPEDSO
HOPESSO
HOWELSE
IDLESSE
IMMENSE
IMMERSE
INCENSE
INTENSE
INTERSE
INVERSE
ITSEASY
LICENSE
MIDEAST
NOTEASY
OBVERSE
OFFENSE
OGREISH
ONLEASE
ONLEASH
POSEUSE
PROEAST
RELEASE
REVERSA
REVERSE
THEEAST
TOLEASE
TOOEASY
UNLEASH
UNTENSE
UNTERSE
VANESSA
VITEBSK

•••E••S

AACELLS
ABSENTS
ACCEDES
ACCENTS
ACCEPTS
ACHENES
ACTEDAS
ADDENDS
ADHERES
ADVENTS
ADVERBS
ADVERTS
AFFECTS
AGREERS
ALBEDOS
ALKENES
ALLEARS
ALLEGES
ALLELES
ALLEWIS
ALLEYES
AMNERIS
AMOEBAS
AMPERES
ANDEANS
ANGELAS
ANGELES
ANGELUS
ANNEALS
ANNEXES
ANTERUS
APPEALS
APPEARS
APPENDS
AQUEOUS
ARGENTS
ARREARS
ARRESTS
ARTEMIS
ARTEMUS
ASCENDS
ASCENTS
ASPECTS
ASSENTS
ASSERTS
ATTENDS
ATTESTS
AUGENDS
AUTEURS
AXHEADS
AXSEEDS
BADEGGS
BADENDS
BALEENS
BAREGES
BARENTS
BEDECKS
BEHEADS
BEHESTS
BIGEARS
BIGENDS
BIGEYES
BIREMES
BISECTS
BODEGAS
BOLEROS
BREEZES
BUREAUS
BUTENES
CABEZAS
CALENDS
CAMERAS
CAREENS
CAREERS
CASEINS
CASEOUS
CASERNS
CATENAS
CATERAS
CAVEATS
CAVEINS
CAVERNS
CELEBES
CEMENTS
CEREALS
CETERIS
CHEESES
CHEETAS
CHEETOS
CINEMAS
CLIENTS
COHEIRS
COHERES
COMEONS
COMESAS
COVERTS
CREEPOS
CROESUS
CSLEWIS
CULEXES
DALETHS
DEBEERS
DECEITS
DEFEATS
DEFECTS
DEFENDS
DEGERMS
DEHEXES
DEJECTS
DELEADS
DELETES
DEMEANS
DEPENDS
DEPESTS
DESEEDS
DESERTS
DESEXES
DETECTS
DETENTS
DETESTS
DEVEINS
DEVESTS
DIGESTS
DIRECTS
DISEURS
DIVERTS
DIVESTS
DOCENTS
DOGEARS
DRSEUSS
DRVEGAS
DRYEYES
DUTEOUS
ECZEMAS
EFFECTS
EKUELES
ENDEARS
ENNEADS
ENSEALS
ENSEATS
ENVEILS
EPHEBUS
EPHESUS
ESSENES
ESTEEMS
ETHENES
EUREKAS
EXCEEDS
EXCEPTS
EXPECTS
EXPENDS
EXPERTS
EXSECTS
EXSERTS
EXTENDS
EXTENTS
EXTERNS
FADEINS
FAGENDS
FAKEIDS
FEDEXES
FIDELES
FIDELIS
FILENES
FLEECES
FOMENTS
FORESTS
FREEZES
FRIENDS
FRIEZES
GALENAS
GAMETES
GASEOUS
GAZEBOS
GENERIS
GENESES
GENESIS
GERENTS
GIDEONS
GIVEUPS
GOVERNS
GRIEVES
GYRENES
HAYESES
HGWELLS
HIDEOUS
HOWELLS
HUMERUS
IAPETUS
ICTERUS
IGNEOUS
IMPEDES
IMPENDS
IMPETUS
INCENTS
INCEPTS
INDENTS
INDEXES
INFECTS
INFESTS
INGESTS
INHERES
INJECTS
INSEAMS
INSECTS
INSERTS
INTEARS
INTENDS
INTENTS
INTERNS
INVENTS
INVERTS
INVESTS
INYEARS
IQTESTS
JONESES
JUDEANS
KADETTS
KINESES
KINESIS
KOPECKS
KOREANS
LACEUPS
LAMENTS
LAPERMS
LAREDOS
LATEENS
LATENTS
LATEXES
LEGENDS
LINEUPS
LOVEINS
LUREXES
LYCEUMS
MAKEDOS
MAKEUPS
MANEGES
MEDELES
MESEEMS
METEORS
MIGENES
MIMESES
MIMESIS
MODELAS
MODELBS
MODELTS
MODERNS
MOLESTS
MOMENTS
MOREENS
MORELOS
MRDEEDS
MSIEURS
MUDEELS
MUJERES
MULETAS
MUSEUMS
NEMESES
NEMESIS
NEREIDS
NIKEADS
NIVEOUS
NOSEATS
NOVELAS
NOVENAS
NUMEROS
OBJECTS
OBTESTS
OBVERTS
OFFENDS
ORDEALS
ORGEATS
ORIENTS
ORLEANS
OSSEOUS
OUTEATS
OWLEGGS
PAPELES
PARENTS
PATENTS
PESETAS
PESEWAS
PHOEBES
PHOEBUS
PICEOUS
PIGEONS
PILEOUS
PILEUPS
PITEOUS
POMELOS
POPEYES
POSEDAS
POSESAS
POSEURS
POTEENS
PRIESTS
QUIETUS
RACEMES
RAMESES
RAREGAS
RAVEUPS
RAWEGGS
REBENDS
RECEDES
REDEALS
REDEEDS
REDEEMS
REDEYES
REFEEDS
REGEARS
REGENTS
REHEALS
REHEARS
REHEATS
REHEELS
REJECTS
RELEADS
RELEAPS
RELENDS
RELENTS
RELEVES
REMEETS
REMELTS
REMENDS
RENEGES
RENESTS
REPEALS
REPEATS
REPENTS
REPERKS
REREADS
REREDOS
REREELS
RERENTS
RESEALS
RESEAMS
RESEATS
RESEAUS
RESECTS
RESEEDS
RESEEKS
RESELLS
RESENDS
RESENTS
RETEARS
RETELLS
RETESTS
REVEALS
REVENDS
REVERBS
REVERES
REVERTS
REVESTS
REWEARS
REWELDS
REZEROS
RHOECUS
RIBEYES
RIDEBYS
ROBERTS
RODENTS
ROLEXES
SADEYES
SAMEDIS
SAMEKHS
SATEENS
SCHEMAS
SCHEMES
SCLERAS
SCREAKS
SCREAMS
SCREEDS
SCREENS
SEAEELS
SECEDES
SEFERIS
SELECTS
SENECAS
SEVERUS
SHIELDS
SHTETLS
SILENTS
SLEEVES
SNEEZES
SPEEDOS
SPHERES
SPLEENS
SPREADS
SQUEAKS
SQUEALS
SQUEERS
STDENIS
STEEVES
STREAKS
STREAMS
STREETS
STREGIS
SUPERGS
TAGENDS
TAKEINS
TALENTS
TAVERNS
TEDEUMS
TELEXES
THIEVES
THREADS
THREATS
THREERS
TIMEWAS
TIMEXES
TINEARS
TOLEDOS
TONEMES
TOREROS
TUNEUPS
TUPELOS
TUREENS
TUXEDOS
TWEEZES
TWOEGGS
TYPEABS
UNBELTS
UNBENDS
UNHEEDS
UNHELMS
UNLEADS
UNLEAFS
UNPEELS
UNREELS
UNRESTS
UNSEALS
UNSEAMS
UNSEATS
UNSELLS
UNVEILS
UPBEARS
UPBEATS
UPHEAPS
UPKEEPS
UPLEAPS
UPREARS
UPSENDS
UPTEARS
UPWELLS
URTEXTS
USTEDES
VENEERS
VOTECHS
VOTEYES
WAKEUPS
WBYEATS
WEDELNS
WHEEZES
WYVERNS
XIMENES
YEMENIS
ZYDECOS

••••ES•

ACHIEST
ACTRESS
ACUTEST
ADDRESS
AERIEST
AGELESS
AGGRESS
AGILEST
AIDLESS
AIMLESS
AIRIEST
AIRLESS
AIRNESS
ALLNESS
AMPLEST
ANAPEST
ANDRESS
APTNESS
ARCHEST
ARIDEST
ARMLESS
ARMREST
ARTIEST
ARTLESS
ASHIEST
ASHLESS
ATELESS
AUSLESE
AVIDEST
AWAREST
AWELESS
AWNLESS
BABIEST
BADDEST
BADNESS
BALDEST
BARLESS
BEDLESS
BEDREST
BEQUEST
BERNESE
BIBLESS
BIGGEST
BIGMESS
BIGNESS
BITLESS
BOLDEST
BONIEST
BOWLESS
BOXIEST
BRALESS
BRAVEST
BUDLESS
BUFFEST
BURGESS
BURMESE
BUSIEST
CAGIEST
CAKIEST
CALMEST
CANIEST
CAPEESH
CAPLESS
CARLESS
CHICEST
CHINESE
CLOSEST
COKIEST
COLDEST
CONFESS
CONGEST
CONTEST
COOLEST
COSIEST
COWIEST
COXLESS
COYNESS
COZIEST
CRUDEST
CURTEST
CYPRESS
DAFTEST
DAMPEST
DANKEST
DARKEST
DEADEST
DEAFEST
DEAREST
DEEPEST
DEFFEST
DEFTEST
DENSEST
DEPRESS
DEWIEST
DEWLESS
DICIEST
DIGRESS
DIMMEST
DIMNESS
DIOCESE
DNATEST
DOGLESS
DOGVEST
DOPIEST
DOUREST
DOZIEST
DRYNESS
DUCHESS
DUEWEST
DULLEST
DUMBEST
EARLESS
EARNEST
EASIEST
EATLESS
ECCLESI
EDGIEST
EDMEESE
EELIEST
EERIEST
EGGIEST
EGGLESS
ELITEST
ELMIEST
EMPRESS
ENDLESS
ESOBESO
EVENEST
EVEREST
EVILEST
EXPRESS
EYELESS
EYETEST
FABBEST
FAINEST
FAIREST
FALSEST
FANFEST
FARNESS
FAROESE
FARWEST
FASTEST
FATLESS
FATNESS
FATTEST
FEELESS
FEWNESS
FEYNESS
FINLESS
FIRMEST
FITNESS
FITTEST
FLYLESS
FOELESS
FOGLESS
FONDEST
FORREST
FOULEST
FOXIEST
FRENESI
FULLEST
FULNESS
FUMIEST
FUNFEST
FURLESS
FURNESS
GABFEST
GAMIEST
GAPLESS
GASLESS
GAYNESS
GEMLESS
GENOESE
GEODESY
GLUIEST
GODDESS
GODLESS
GOOIEST
GORIEST
GRAVEST
GRAYEST
GREYEST
GUMLESS
GUNLESS
GUTLESS
HADBEST
HAPLESS
HARDEST
HARNESS
HARVEST
HATLESS
HAZIEST
HEIRESS
HEPPEST
HIGHEST
HIPLESS
HIPNESS
HIPPEST
HITLESS
HOKIEST
HOLIEST
HOMIEST
HOSTESS
HOTNESS
HOTTEST
HUELESS
ICELESS
ICINESS
ICKIEST
IFFIEST
IHOPESO
ILLNESS
IMAMESS
IMPRESS
IMPREST
INAMESS
INANEST
INGLESE
INGRESS
INKIEST
INKLESS
INNLESS
INQUEST
IPCRESS
IRATEST
IRELESS
ITSBEST
JAGLESS
JARLESS
JAWLESS
JIVIEST
JOBLESS
JOKIEST
JOYLESS
JUSTEST
KEENEST
KERTESZ
KEYLESS
KEYWEST
KINDEST
KINLESS
LABTEST
LACIEST
LAKIEST
LANKEST
LARGESS
LARGEST
LAWLESS
LAXNESS
LAZIEST
LEANEST
LEFTEST
LEGLESS
LEGREST
LEWDEST
LIDLESS
LIEFEST
LIETEST
LIMIEST
LIMPEST
LINIEST
LIONESS
LIPLESS
LITHEST
LOGIEST
LONGEST
LOOSEST
LOUDEST

LOWNESS
LUSHEST
MADDEST
MADNESS
MAEWEST
MALTESE
MANLESS
MATLESS
MAYBESO
MAZIEST
MEANEST
MEEKEST
MIDWEST
MILDEST
MIRIEST
MISMESH
MONDESI
MOPIEST
NAIVEST
NAPLESS
NEAREST
NEATEST
NETLESS
NEWNESS
NIGHEST
NOBLEST
NOSIEST
NOWNESS
NUMBEST
OAKDESK
OAKIEST
OARLESS
ODDNESS
OILIEST
OILLESS
OLDNESS
OLDWEST
ONENESS
ONLIEST
OOZIEST
OPPRESS
ORBLESS
ORELESS
OUTJEST
OUTWEST
OWLIEST
OZZFEST
PACIEST
PATNESS
PAYLESS
PEERESS
PEGLESS
PERTEST
PINIEST
PINKEST
PINLESS
PIPIEST
PIPLESS
POETESS
POKIEST
POOREST
POSHEST
POSSESS
PRADESH
PRETEST
PROCESS
PROFESS
PROTEST

PROWESS
PROWEST
PUNIEST
PUNLESS
QUITESO
RACIEST
RAMSESI
RANKEST
RASHEST
RAWNESS
RAYLESS
REALEST
REDDEST
REDNESS
REDRESS
REFRESH
REGRESS
REPRESS
REQUEST
RIBLESS
RICHEST
RIMIEST
RIMLESS
RODLESS
ROPIEST
ROSIEST
RULIEST
RUMLESS
RUNLESS
SADDEST
SADNESS
SAGIEST
SAPLESS
SEERESS
SERIESE
SERIESF
SERIESG
SERIESH
SERIESI
SERIESJ
SERIESK
SEXIEST
SEXLESS
SHYNESS
SIAMESE
SICKEST
SIENESE
SINLESS
SKIVEST
SKYLESS
SLOWEST
SLYNESS
SNIDEST
SODLESS
SOFTEST
SOLNESS
SONLESS
SOONEST
SOUREST
SPAREST
SPRIEST
SPRYEST
STALEST
SUAVEST
SUCCESS
SUGGEST
SUMLESS
SUNLESS

TALLEST
TANNEST
TARTEST
TAUTEST
TAXLESS
TEALESS
TEMPEST
TENSEST
TERSEST
THEBEST
THERESA
TIDIEST
TIELESS
TIGRESS
TINIEST
TIPLESS
TOELESS
TONIEST
TOPLESS
TOYLESS
TRITEST
TUGLESS
UGLIEST
UNBLEST
UNDRESS
UNOBESE
USELESS
VAGUEST
VAINEST
VASTEST
VERIEST
VINIEST
VOWLESS
WACKEST
WANIEST
WANNESS
WANNEST
WARIEST
WARLESS
WARMEST
WAVIEST
WAXIEST
WAYLESS
WEAKEST
WEBLESS
WEENESS
WETNESS
WETTEST
WHITEST
WIGLESS
WILDEST
WILIEST
WINIEST
WINLESS
WIRIEST
WITLESS
WITNESS
WRYNESS
XERXESI
ZANIEST
ZOOIEST

••••E•S

ABASERS
ABATERS
ABCNEWS
ABIDERS
ABUSERS

ACTRESS
ACUMENS
ADDRESS
ADORERS
AGELESS
AGGRESS
AGREERS
AIDLESS
AIGLETS
AIGRETS
AIMLESS
AIRLESS
AIRNESS
ALEKEGS
ALEVELS
ALGIERS
ALINERS
ALLNESS
ALLNEWS
ALTKEYS
ALUDELS
AMADEUS
AMBIENS
AMBLERS
AMSTELS
AMULETS
AMUSERS
ANADEMS
ANDREAS
ANDRESS
ANDREWS
ANGLERS
ANKLERS
ANKLETS
ANSWERS
ANTHEMS
ANTHERS
ANTLERS
ANYNEWS
APELETS
APOGEES
APPLETS
APTNESS
ARCHERS
ARGUERS
ARMLESS
ARMLETS
ARTLESS
ASHLESS
ATELESS
ATMFEES
ATONERS
AUKLETS
AUSTERS
AVOCETS
AVOWERS
AWAKENS
AWAKERS
AWELESS
AWNLESS
AXSEEDS
AZALEAS
BACKERS
BADGERS
BADNESS
BADNEWS
BAFFERS
BAGGERS

BAILEES
BAILERS
BAITERS
BALEENS
BALKERS
BALLETS
BANDERS
BANGERS
BANKERS
BANNERS
BANTERS
BARBERS
BARBETS
BARGERS
BARKERS
BARLESS
BARLEYS
BARNEYS
BARRELS
BARRENS
BARRETS
BARTERS
BASHERS
BASKETS
BASSETS
BASTERS
BATHERS
BATTENS
BATTERS
BAWLERS
BEADERS
BEAKERS
BEAMERS
BEARERS
BEATERS
BEAVERS
BEDLESS
BEEBEES
BEEGEES
BEEMERS
BEEPERS
BEEZERS
BEHRENS
BELIEFS
BELIERS
BELTERS
BENDERS
BERBERS
BETHELS
BETTERS
BEZIERS
BIBBERS
BIBLESS
BICKERS
BIDDERS
BIGBETS
BIGGERS
BIGMESS
BIGNESS
BIGNEWS
BILKERS
BILLERS
BILLETS
BINDERS
BINGERS
BIRDERS
BIRLERS
BITLESS

BITTERS
BLADERS
BLAMERS
BLAZERS
BLOWERS
BOATELS
BOATERS
BOBBERS
BOILERS
BOKKENS
BOLTERS
BOMBERS
BONDERS
BONKERS
BONNETS
BOOKERS
BOOMERS
BOOTEES
BOOTERS
BOOZERS
BOPPERS
BORDERS
BOTHERS
BOTREES
BOWLERS
BOWLESS
BOWYERS
BOXBEDS
BOXSETS
BRACERS
BRALESS
BRAYERS
BRAZENS
BREVETS
BREWERS
BREYERS
BRIBEES
BRIBERS
BRINERS
BROKERS
BRUNETS
BUCKERS
BUCKETS
BUDDERS
BUDGERS
BUDGETS
BUDLESS
BUFFERS
BUFFETS
BUGLERS
BULLETS
BUMLEGS
BUMMERS
BUMPERS
BUNGEES
BUNKERS
BUNTERS
BURDENS
BURGEES
BURGERS
BURGESS
BURIERS
BURLERS
BURNERS
BUSHELS
BUSHERS
BUSKERS
BUSSERS

BUSTERS
BUTLERS
BUTTERS
BUZZERS
CABLERS
CABLETS
CACHETS
CADGERS
CAHIERS
CALDERS
CALKERS
CALLEES
CALLERS
CAMBERS
CAMPERS
CANCELS
CANCERS
CANKERS
CANNELS
CANNERS
CANOERS
CANTERS
CAPLESS
CAPLETS
CAPPERS
CARDERS
CAREENS
CAREERS
CARKEYS
CARLESS
CARNETS
CARPELS
CARPERS
CARPETS
CARRELS
CARTELS
CARTERS
CARVELS
CARVERS
CASHEWS
CASKETS
CASTERS
CATBEDS
CAUSERS
CBSNEWS
CENSERS
CENTERS
CEPHEUS
CHAFERS
CHALETS
CHANELS
CHAPELS
CHASERS
CHEDERS
CHEVETS
CHEWERS
CHIDERS
CHIMERS
CHISELS
CHOKERS
CHOLERS
CINDERS
CIPHERS
CLARETS
CLAWERS
CLEMENS
CLONERS
CLORETS

CLOSERS
CLOSETS
CLOVERS
COALERS
COATEES
COATERS
COAXERS
COBWEBS
COCKERS
CODGERS
COFFEES
COFFERS
COILERS
COINERS
COLLETS
COMBERS
COMPELS
CONFERS
CONFESS
CONGERS
CONKERS
CONVEYS
COOKERS
COOLERS
COOPERS
COOTERS
COPIERS
COPPERS
COPTERS
CORBELS
CORDERS
CORKERS
CORNEAS
CORNERS
CORNETS
CORSETS
CORVEES
COSHERS
COSSETS
COTTERS
COULEES
COUTERS
COWPEAS
COXLESS
COYNESS
COZZENS
CRATERS
CRAVENS
CRAVERS
CRENELS
CREWELS
CROWERS
CUDGELS
CULLERS
CULLETS
CUMBERS
CURFEWS
CURLERS
CURLEWS
CURSERS
CURVETS
CUSSERS
CUSTERS
CUTLERS
CUTLETS
CUTTERS
CYCLERS
CYGNETS

CYPHERS
CYPRESS
DABBERS
DAGGERS
DAMMERS
DAMNERS
DAMPENS
DAMPERS
DAMSELS
DANCERS
DANDERS
DANGERS
DANIELS
DANVERS
DARKENS
DARNERS
DARTERS
DASHERS
DAUBERS
DAYBEDS
DEADENS
DEAFENS
DEALERS
DEBEERS
DEBTEES
DECKERS
DECREES
DEEPENS
DEFIERS
DEFLEAS
DEFUELS
DEGREES
DEICERS
DELKEYS
DELVERS
DENIERS
DEPRESS
DESEEDS
DESTEMS
DEWLESS
DIADEMS
DIALERS
DIAPERS
DICKENS
DICKERS
DICKEYS
DIEMENS
DIESELS
DIETERS
DIFFERS
DIGGERS
DIGRESS
DIMMERS
DIMNESS
DINGERS
DINNERS
DIPNETS
DIPPERS
DISPELS
DITHERS
DOCKERS
DOCKETS
DODDERS
DODGEMS
DODGERS
DOFFERS
DOGBEDS
DOGLEGS

DOGLESS
DONKEYS
DOOVERS
DOOZERS
DORMERS
DORSEYS
DOTTERS
DOUSERS
DOWNERS
DOWSERS
DRAGEES
DRAPERS
DRAWEES
DRAWERS
DRIVELS
DRIVERS
DRONERS
DROVERS
DRYNESS
DRYPERS
DUBBERS
DUCHESS
DUCKERS
DUELERS
DUFFELS
DUFFERS
DUMPERS
DUNKERS
DUNNERS
DUSTERS
EAGLETS
EARLESS
EARLETS
EARNERS
EASTERS
EATLESS
EBAYERS
ECHOERS
EGGLERS
EGGLESS
ELANETS
ELATERS
ELEVENS
ELIDERS
ELOPERS
ELUDERS
ELYSEES
EMBLEMS
EMOTERS
EMPRESS
ENAMELS
ENDLESS
ENTREES
ENVIERS
EPOPEES
ERASERS
ERODERS
ESCHERS
ESCHEWS
ESPNEWS
ESTEEMS
ETCHERS
EVADERS
EVENERS
EVOKERS
EXCEEDS
EXILERS
EXOCETS

EXPRESS
EYELESS
EYELETS
FABLERS
FALLERS
FALTERS
FANJETS
FANNERS
FARFELS
FARMERS
FARNESS
FASTENS
FATHERS
FATLESS
FATNESS
FATTENS
FAUCETS
FAWNERS
FEARERS
FEDDERS
FEEDERS
FEELERS
FEELESS
FELLERS
FENCERS
FENDERS
FENNELS
FERRETS
FESTERS
FETTERS
FEWNESS
FEYNESS
FIBBERS
FIDGETS
FILLERS
FILLETS
FILTERS
FINDERS
FINGERS
FINLESS
FISHERS
FITNESS
FITTERS
FIZZERS
FLAKERS
FLAMERS
FLAYERS
FLORETS
FLOWERS
FLUTERS
FLYLESS
FLYNETS
FOAMERS
FODDERS
FOELESS
FOGGERS
FOGLESS
FOKKERS
FOLDERS
FOLGERS
FOOLERS
FOOTERS
FORCEPS
FORCERS
FORGERS
FORGETS
FORKERS
FORMERS

FOSTERS
FOWLERS
FOXNEWS
FRAMERS
FRATERS
FTMYERS
FUDGERS
FUELERS
FULNESS
FUNDERS
FUNNELS
FURLERS
FURLESS
FURNESS
FUSSERS
GABBERS
GADDERS
GADGETS
GAFFERS
GAGGERS
GAINERS
GAITERS
GALLEYS
GAMMERS
GANDERS
GANGERS
GANNETS
GAOLERS
GAPLESS
GARDENS
GARNERS
GARNETS
GARRETS
GARTERS
GASJETS
GASKETS
GASLESS
GASPERS
GASSERS
GATHERS
GAUDENS
GAUGERS
GAWKERS
GAWPERS
GAYNESS
GEEZERS
GELPENS
GEMLESS
GENDERS
GENXERS
GETTERS
GEYSERS
GIBBERS
GIBLETS
GIFTEES
GILDERS
GIMBELS
GIMLETS
GINGERS
GIRDERS
GLAZERS
GLIDERS
GLOWERS
GLUTENS
GLUTEUS
GNAWERS
GOATEES
GOBLETS

GODDESS
GODLESS
GOITERS
GOLFERS
GOMPERS
GOOBERS
GOODERS
GOONEYS
GOPHERS
GORGERS
GOSPELS
GOUGERS
GRADERS
GRATERS
GRAVELS
GRAVERS
GRAZERS
GRIPERS
GROCERS
GROPERS
GROVELS
GROVERS
GROWERS
GUIDERS
GUINEAS
GULDENS
GULLETS
GULPERS
GUMLESS
GUNLESS
GUNNERS
GUNSELS
GURNEYS
GUSHERS
GUSSETS
GUTLESS
GUTTERS
GYPPERS
HACKERS
HAILERS
HALLEYS
HALTERS
HALVERS
HAMLETS
HAMMERS
HAMPERS
HANDERS
HANGERS
HANKERS
HAPLESS
HAPPENS
HARDEES
HARDENS
HARKENS
HARLEYS
HARMERS
HARNESS
HARPERS
HASTENS
HATLESS
HATREDS
HATTERS
HAULERS
HAWKERS
HAWSERS
HEADERS
HEALERS
HEAPERS

HEARERS
HEATERS
HEAVENS
HEAVERS
HEBREWS
HEDGERS
HEEDERS
HEELERS
HEFTERS
HEHHEHS
HEIFERS
HEIRESS
HELMETS
HELPERS
HEMMERS
HERDERS
HICKEYS
HINDERS
HINTERS
HIPLESS
HIPNESS
HISSERS
HITLESS
HITTERS
HOAXERS
HOCKERS
HOHNERS
HOLDERS
HOLLERS
HONKERS
HOOFERS
HOOPERS
HOOTERS
HOOVERS
HOPPERS
HORNETS
HOSIERS
HOSTELS
HOSTESS
HOTBEDS
HOTKEYS
HOTNESS
HOTTEAS
HOWLERS
HOYDENS
HUELESS
HUGGERS
HULLERS
HUMMELS
HUMMERS
HUMVEES
HUNGERS
HUNKERS
HUNTERS
HURLERS
HURTERS
HUSKERS
HUYGENS
HYPHENS
ICELESS
ICETEAS
ICINESS
IDAREDS
ILLNESS
IMAGERS
IMAMESS
IMARETS
IMPRESS

INAMESS
INCHERS
INGRESS
INKJETS
INKLESS
INNLESS
INSTEPS
IPCRESS
IRELESS
IRONERS
ISOHELS
ISOMERS
ISSUERS
JABBERS
JACKETS
JAEGERS
JAGLESS
JAILERS
JAMMERS
JARLESS
JASPERS
JAWLESS
JAYCEES
JAYVEES
JAZZERS
JEEPERS
JEERERS
JEFFERS
JENNETS
JERGENS
JERKERS
JERSEYS
JESTERS
JETSETS
JIGGERS
JILTERS
JINXERS
JITNEYS
JITTERS
JOBBERS
JOBLESS
JOCKEYS
JOGGERS
JOINERS
JOLTERS
JOSHERS
JOTTERS
JOYLESS
JUDGERS
JUICERS
JUMPERS
JUNKERS
JUNKETS
JURGENS
KAISERS
KEDGERS
KEENERS
KEEPERS
KEGGERS
KEGLERS
KENNELS
KERNELS
KEYDETS
KEYLESS
KICKERS
KIDDERS
KIDNEYS
KILLERS

KINLESS
KIPPERS
KISLEVS
KISMETS
KISSELS
KISSERS
KITTENS
KNIFERS
KNOWERS
KOSHERS
KRAKENS
KUCHENS
KUMMELS
KUZNETS
LABFEES
LACKEYS
LADDERS
LADLERS
LAGGERS
LANCERS
LANCETS
LANDERS
LAPPERS
LAPPETS
LAPSERS
LARDERS
LARGESS
LARKERS
LASHERS
LATEENS
LATHERS
LAUDERS
LAURELS
LAWLESS
LAWYERS
LAXNESS
LEADENS
LEADERS
LEAKERS
LEAKEYS
LEANERS
LEAPERS
LEASERS
LEAVENS
LECHERS
LEDGERS
LEERERS
LEGLESS
LENDERS
LESSEES
LESSENS
LESSEPS
LETTERS
LEVIERS
LIBBERS
LICHEES
LICHENS
LICKERS
LIDLESS
LIENEES
LIFTERS
LIMBERS
LIMNERS
LIMPETS
LINDENS
LINGERS
LINKERS
LINNETS

LINTELS
LINTERS
LIONELS
LIONESS
LIONETS
LIPLESS
LIPPERS
LISPERS
LISTEES
LISTENS
LISTERS
LITTERS
LOADERS
LOAFERS
LOANERS
LOBBERS
LOCKERS
LOCKETS
LODGERS
LOFTERS
LOGGERS
LOITERS
LOLLERS
LOOKERS
LOOPERS
LOOSENS
LOOTERS
LOPPERS
LOTTERS
LOUDENS
LOUVERS
LOWNESS
LUBBERS
LUGGERS
LULLERS
LUMBERS
LUMPERS
LUNGERS
LUNKERS
LURKERS
LUSTERS
MADDENS
MADDERS
MADNESS
MAGLEVS
MAGNETS
MAIDENS
MAILERS
MAIMERS
MAINERS
MAJGENS
MALLETS
MALLEUS
MALTEDS
MANGERS
MANLESS
MANNERS
MANTELS
MAPPERS
MARCELS
MARKERS
MARKETS
MARRERS
MARTENS
MARVELS
MASHERS
MASKERS
MASTERS

MATHERS
MATHEWS
MATLESS
MATTERS
MAULERS
MAUSERS
MAYHEMS
MEDLEYS
MEETERS
MELDERS
MELTERS
MEMBERS
MENDELS
MENDERS
MENTEES
MEOWERS
MERCERS
MERGEES
MERGERS
MESEEMS
METIERS
MEWLERS
MICKEYS
MIDGETS
MIDLEGS
MILDEWS
MILIEUS
MILKERS
MILLERS
MILLETS
MINCERS
MINDERS
MINTERS
MINUETS
MISKEYS
MISSETS
MISTERS
MITTENS
MIXTECS
MIZZENS
MOANERS
MOBBERS
MOCKERS
MOILERS
MOLDERS
MOLTERS
MONGERS
MONKEES
MONKEYS
MOONERS
MOOTERS
MOPPERS
MOPPETS
MOREENS
MORSELS
MOSHERS
MOSLEMS
MOTHERS
MOTLEYS
MOUSERS
MRDEEDS
MUCKERS
MUDDERS
MUDEELS
MUDHENS
MUGGERS
MULLERS
MULLETS

MUMMERS
MUPPETS
MURDERS
MURIELS
MUSHERS
MUSKETS
MUSSELS
MUSTERS
MUTTERS
NABBERS
NAGGERS
NAILERS
NAPIERS
NAPLESS
NAPPERS
NATTERS
NBCNEWS
NEATENS
NECKERS
NEEDERS
NEPHEWS
NESTERS
NETLESS
NETTERS
NEUTERS
NEWNESS
NIBLETS
NICKELS
NICKERS
NIPPERS
NODDERS
NONJEWS
NONNEWS
NOONERS
NOOSERS
NOSHERS
NOWNESS
NUBBERS
NUCLEUS
NUDGERS
NUGGETS
NUMBERS
NURSERS
NUTLETS
NUTMEGS
NUTTERS
OARLESS
OBEYERS
ODDNESS
ODELETS
OFFSETS
OILLESS
OINKERS
OLDNESS
OLDNEWS
OLEVELS
OMELETS
ONAGERS
ONENESS
OPENERS
OPINERS
OPPRESS
ORBLESS
ORELESS
ORKNEYS
ORPHEUS
OSPREYS
OSTLERS

OUSTERS
OUTBEGS
OUTJETS
OUTLETS
OUTSEES
OUTSETS
OYSTERS
PACKERS
PACKETS
PADDERS
PAIRERS
PALLETS
PALMERS
PALTERS
PAMPERS
PANDERS
PANIERS
PANNERS
PANTERS
PANZERS
PAPIERS
PARCELS
PARGERS
PARKERS
PARLEYS
PARSECS
PARSEES
PARSERS
PASSELS
PASSERS
PASTELS
PASTERS
PATNESS
PATTERS
PATZERS
PAUPERS
PAUSERS
PAWNEES
PAWNERS
PAYLESS
PCUSERS
PEAHENS
PEEKERS
PEELERS
PEEPERS
PEERESS
PEEWEES
PEGLEGS
PEGLESS
PELLEAS
PELLETS
PELTERS
PENNERS
PENNEYS
PENSEES
PENTELS
PEPPERS
PERSEUS
PESTERS
PETRELS
PETTERS
PEWTERS
PHASERS
PHILEAS
PHINEAS
PHLOEMS
PHONERS
PHONEYS

PICKENS
PICKERS
PICKETS
PIECERS
PIGLETS
PIGPENS
PILFERS
PINCERS
PINGERS
PINKENS
PINLESS
PINNERS
PIOLETS
PIPLESS
PIRAEUS
PITIERS
PLACERS
PLANERS
PLANETS
PLATENS
PLATERS
PLAYERS
PLOVERS
PLOWERS
POCKETS
POETESS
POISERS
POLLEES
POLLENS
POLLERS
POMMELS
PONDERS
PONGEES
POOLERS
POPPERS
PORKERS
PORTERS
POSSESS
POSTERS
POTEENS
POTHERS
POTTERS
POURERS
POUTERS
POWDERS
PRATERS
PRAYERS
PREFERS
PREMEDS
PRESETS
PREYERS
PRICERS
PRIMERS
PRIVETS
PROBERS
PROCESS
PROFESS
PROJETS
PROKEDS
PROPELS
PROSERS
PROTEUS
PROVERS
PROWESS
PRUNERS
PUCKERS
PUFFERS
PULLERS

PULLETS
PULLEYS
PULPERS
PUMMELS
PUMPERS
PUNKERS
PUNLESS
PUNNERS
PUNTERS
PUPPETS
PURRERS
PURSERS
PURVEYS
PUSHERS
PUTTEES
PUTTERS
QUAKERS
QUAVERS
QUEUERS
QUIVERS
QUOTEES
QUOTERS
RABBETS
RACKERS
RACKETS
RAFTERS
RAIDERS
RAILERS
RAISERS
RAMJETS
RAMMERS
RANGERS
RANKERS
RANTERS
RAPIERS
RAPPELS
RAPPERS
RASHERS
RASPERS
RASTERS
RATTERS
RAWNESS
RAYLESS
READERS
REAMERS
REAPERS
REARERS
REAVERS
REBREWS
RECHEWS
REDDENS
REDEEDS
REDEEMS
REDHENS
REDLEGS
REDNESS
REDRESS
REEFERS
REEKERS
REELERS
REFEEDS
REFUELS
REGRESS
REGRETS
REHEELS
RELIEFS
RELIERS
REMEETS

RENDERS
RENNETS
RENTEES
RENTERS
REOPENS
REPRESS
REREELS
RESEEDS
RESEEKS
RESTERS
REUBENS
REUNERS
REUSERS
REUTERS
REVIEWS
RHYMERS
RIBBERS
RIBLESS
RIBLETS
RICHENS
RICKEYS
RIDDERS
RIESENS
RIFLERS
RIGGERS
RILLETS
RIMLESS
RINGERS
RINSERS
RIOTERS
RIPPERS
RISKERS
ROADEOS
ROADERS
ROAMERS
ROARERS
ROBBERS
ROCHETS
ROCKERS
ROCKETS
RODGERS
RODLESS
ROLFERS
ROLLEIS
ROLLERS
ROMNEYS
ROMPERS
RONDELS
ROOFERS
ROOMERS
ROOTERS
ROSTERS
ROTTERS
ROUSERS
ROUTERS
RUBBERS
RUDDERS
RUINERS
RUMLESS
RUMMERS
RUNLESS
RUNLETS
RUNNELS
RUNNERS
RUSHEES
RUSHERS
RUSSETS
RUTGERS

RUTTERS
SACHEMS
SACHETS
SACKERS
SADDENS
SADNESS
SAILERS
SALTERS
SALVERS
SAMLETS
SANDERS
SANSEIS
SAPIENS
SAPLESS
SAPPERS
SASSERS
SATEENS
SAUCERS
SAWYERS
SCALERS
SCARERS
SCHLEPS
SCORERS
SCOTERS
SCREEDS
SCREENS
SEABEDS
SEABEES
SEAEELS
SEALEGS
SEALERS
SEAMERS
SEARERS
SEATERS
SECKELS
SECRETS
SEEDERS
SEEKERS
SEERESS
SEINERS
SEIZERS
SELLERS
SENDEES
SENDERS
SENSEIS
SENSENS
SEPTETS
SEQUELS
SERPENS
SERVEAS
SERVERS
SESTETS
SETFEES
SETTEES
SETTERS
SEXLESS
SEXTETS
SHADERS
SHAKERS
SHAPERS
SHARERS
SHAVERS
SHEKELS
SHINERS
SHIVERS
SHOVELS
SHOVERS
SHOWERS

SHRIEKS
SHYNESS
SICKENS
SIEMENS
SIFTERS
SIGHERS
SIGNEES
SIGNERS
SIGNETS
SILVERS
SIMMERS
SIMPERS
SINGERS
SINKERS
SINLESS
SINNERS
SIPPERS
SISTERS
SITTERS
SKATERS
SKEWERS
SKYLESS
SLAKERS
SLATERS
SLAVERS
SLAYERS
SLICERS
SLIDERS
SLIVERS
SLOPERS
SLOVENS
SLYNESS
SMILERS
SMILEYS
SMITERS
SMOKERS
SMOKEYS
SNAKERS
SNARERS
SNIPERS
SNIVELS
SNORERS
SOAKERS
SOAPERS
SOARERS
SOBBERS
SOCKETS
SODLESS
SOFTENS
SOIREES
SOLDERS
SOLNESS
SOLVERS
SONLESS
SONNETS
SOONERS
SORBETS
SORRELS
SORTERS
SOUPERS
SOVIETS
SPACERS
SPADERS
SPARERS
SPAYERS
SPEWERS
SPICERS
SPIDERS

SPIKERS
SPINELS
SPINETS
SPIREAS
SPLEENS
SPYDERS
SQUEERS
STAGERS
STAMENS
STARERS
STATERS
STAYERS
STEREOS
STEVENS
STEWERS
STOKERS
STONERS
STORERS
STOWERS
STREETS
STYLERS
STYLETS
SUBDEBS
SUBLETS
SUBNETS
SUBSETS
SUCCESS
SUCKERS
SUDSERS
SUFFERS
SULKERS
SUMLESS
SUMMERS
SUNDERS
SUNLESS
SUNSETS
SUPPERS
SURFERS
SURREYS
SURVEYS
SWAYERS
SWIPERS
SWIVELS
SWIVETS
SYSTEMS
TABKEYS
TABLETS
TABSETS
TACKERS
TAGGERS
TAILERS
TALKERS
TAMPERS
TANDEMS
TANKERS
TANNERS
TAPPERS
TAPPETS
TARGETS
TASSELS
TASTERS
TATTERS
TAUTENS
TAXLESS
TEALESS
TEARERS
TEASELS
TEASERS

TEASETS
TEEHEES
TEENERS
TEEPEES
TEETERS
TEEVEES
TELLERS
TEMPEHS
TEMPERS
TENDERS
TENNERS
TENTERS
TERCELS
TERRETS
TESTEES
TESTERS
TETHERS
THALERS
THAWERS
THEFEDS
THEJETS
THEMETS
THENETS
THENEWS
THEREDS
THESEUS
THREERS
TICKERS
TICKETS
TIELESS
TIGRESS
TILLERS
TILLETS
TILTERS
TIMBERS
TINDERS
TINKERS
TINNERS
TINSELS
TINTERS
TIPLESS
TIPPEES
TIPPERS
TIPPETS
TITHERS
TITTERS
TOELESS
TOFFEES
TOILERS
TOILETS
TOLLERS
TOLTECS
TOOLERS
TOOTERS
TOPLESS
TOPPERS
TOPTENS
TOSSERS
TOTTERS
TOUPEES
TOURERS
TOUTERS
TOWHEES
TOWNERS
TOYLESS
TRACERS
TRADERS
TRAVELS

TRAVERS
TRICEPS
TRIJETS
TRIVETS
TROWELS
TUCKERS
TUFFETS
TUGGERS
TUGLESS
TUNNELS
TUREENS
TURKEYS
TURNERS
TURRETS
TUSKERS
TVCREWS
TWINERS
TWOFERS
ULSTERS
UNDOERS
UNDRESS
UNFREES
UNHEEDS
UNITERS
UNPEELS
UNREELS
UNSKEWS
UNSTEPS
UNTIERS
UPKEEPS
UPSTEPS
USELESS
USOPENS
USURERS
VALLEYS
VALUERS
VAMPERS
VARIERS
VARLETS
VEILERS
VELVETS
VENDEES
VENDERS
VENEERS
VENTERS
VERGERS
VERSETS
VESPERS
VESSELS
VESTEES
VETOERS
VETTERS
VICKERS
VIEWERS
VIOLETS
VIZIERS
VOGUERS
VOICERS
VOIDERS
VOLLEYS
VOWLESS
WADDERS
WAFTERS
WAGGERS
WAILERS
WAITERS
WAIVERS
WALKERS

WALLETS
WALTERS
WANDERS
WANKELS
WANNESS
WANTERS
WARDENS
WARDERS
WARLESS
WARMERS
WARPERS
WARRENS
WARVETS
WASHERS
WASTERS
WAYLESS
WEAKENS
WEANERS
WEARERS
WEASELS
WEAVERS
WEBLESS
WEDDERS
WEEDERS
WEENESS
WEEPERS
WELDERS
WELTERS
WENDERS
WESTERS
WETNESS
WHALERS
WHEREAS
WHINERS
WHITENS
WICKERS
WICKETS
WIDGETS
WIENERS
WIGLESS
WIGLETS
WILKENS
WILLERS
WINCERS
WINDERS
WINGERS
WINKERS
WINLESS
WINNERS
WINTERS
WISHERS
WITHERS
WITLESS
WITNESS
WONDERS
WOOFERS
WOOLENS
WORKERS
WORMERS
WORSENS
WRITERS
WRYNESS
XYSTERS
YAKKERS
YAMMERS
YANKEES
YANKERS
YAPPERS

YARDERS
YATTERS
YAWNERS
YAWPERS
YELLERS
YELPERS
YESLETS
YONKERS
YORKERS
YOTHERS
YOWLERS
ZAPPERS
ZESTERS
ZINGERS
ZIPPERS
ZITHERS

•••••ES

ABASHES
ABDUCES
ABJURES
ABLATES
ABRADES
ABRILES
ABYSSES
ACCEDES
ACCRUES
ACCUSES
ACHENES
ACTIVES
ADAMSES
ADDAXES
ADDUCES
ADELIES
ADHERES
ADJURES
ADMIRES
ADMIXES
ADRATES
ADVICES
ADVISES
AEDILES
AEGISES
AERATES
AEROBES
AFFINES
AFFIXES
AFRAMES
AGENCES
AGNATES
AGONIES
AIRACES
AITCHES
ALCOVES
ALETTES
ALIASES
ALKENES
ALLAGES
ALLEGES
ALLELES
ALLEYES
ALLUDES
ALLURES
ALPINES
AMASSES
AMBRIES
AMERCES
AMITIES

AMPERES
AMPULES
ANGELES
ANNALES
ANNEXES
ANOMIES
ANTARES
ANTIBES
ANYONES
APACHES
APERIES
APHIDES
APLITES
APLUSES
APOGEES
APPLIES
APPOSES
APSIDES
ARABLES
ARBACES
ARBOLES
ARCADES
ARCHIES
AREOLES
ARGUSES
ARGYLES
ARIANES
AROUSES
ARRASES
ARRISES
ARRIVES
ASANTES
ASPIRES
ASSIZES
ASSUMES
ASSURES
ATHOMES
ATLASES
ATMFEES
ATOMIES
ATONIES
ATTIMES
ATTIRES
ATTUNES
AUBADES
AUDILES
AUGITES
AUNTIES
AUSSIES
AVENGES
AVENUES
AVGASES
AVIATES
AVULSES
AYEAYES
AZODYES
BABBLES
BADDIES
BADLIES
BAFFIES
BAFFLES
BAGGIES
BAILEES
BALASES
BALDIES
BAMMIES
BANANES
BANDIES

BANGLES
BANJOES
BANQUES
BARBIES
BAREGES
BARITES
BARQUES
BARTLES
BASQUES
BATCHES
BATTLES
BAUBLES
BEACHES
BEADLES
BEAGLES
BEANIES
BEATLES
BECOMES
BEDAZES
BEDLOES
BEEBEES
BEECHES
BEEGEES
BEETLES
BEHAVES
BEIGNES
BELCHES
BELLIES
BEMIRES
BEMUSES
BENARES
BENCHES
BENOTES
BERATES
BERRIES
BESIDES
BETAKES
BETIDES
BETIMES
BEURRES
BEWARES
BIALIES
BIASSES
BIDDIES
BIGAPES
BIGEYES
BIGGIES
BIGLIES
BIGONES
BIGTOES
BILLIES
BIMBOES
BINDLES
BINGLES
BINGOES
BIRCHES
BIRDIES
BIREMES
BISQUES
BLENDES
BLESSES
BLISSES
BLITZES
BLONDES
BLOUSES
BLUDGES
BLUSHES
BMOVIES

BOBBIES
BOBBLES
BOCCIES
BODICES
BOGGLES
BOLIDES
BOLUSES
BONGOES
BONUSES
BOOBIES
BOODLES
BOOGIES
BOOKIES
BOONIES
BOOTEES
BOOTIES
BORATES
BORIDES
BOTCHES
BOTREES
BOTTLES
BOUCHES
BOUFFES
BOUNCES
BOURSES
BOVINES
BOWTIES
BPLUSES
BRAISES
BRASHES
BRASSES
BRAVOES
BREEZES
BRIBEES
BRIDGES
BRIDLES
BRODIES
BROGUES
BRONTES
BRONZES
BROSSES
BROWSES
BRUISES
BRUSHES
BUBBLES
BUCKLES
BUCKOES
BUDDIES
BUDGIES
BUGGIES
BUGGLES
BUJONES
BULLIES
BUMBLES
BUNCHES
BUNDLES
BUNGEES
BUNGLES
BUNNIES
BURBLES
BURGEES
BURGLES
BUSBIES
BUSTLES
BUTANES
BUTCHES
BUTENES
BYEBYES

BYFIVES
BYGONES
BYLINES
BYNAMES
CABBIES
CACKLES
CADDIES
CAJOLES
CALICES
CALLEES
CALYCES
CALYXES
CAMISES
CAMMIES
CANAPES
CANDIES
CANDLES
CANINES
CANTLES
CAPADES
CAPOTES
CARAFES
CARGOES
CARIBES
CARNIES
CARRIES
CASQUES
CASTLES
CATCHES
CAYUSES
CDCASES
CDRATES
CELEBES
CENTRES
CERATES
CERISES
CETANES
CHAINES
CHAISES
CHANCES
CHANGES
CHARGES
CHARLES
CHASSES
CHEESES
CHEQUES
CHEVRES
CHICLES
CHIGOES
CHILIES
CHIVIES
CHOICES
CHOOSES
CHROMES
CINCHES
CINQUES
CIRCLES
CIRQUES
CISCOES
CIVVIES
CLAQUES
CLASHES
CLASSES
CLAUSES
CLEAVES
CLICHES
CLIQUES
CLOCHES

CLOTHES
COACHES
COATEES
COBBLES
COCKLES
CODDLES
CODICES
COERCES
COFFEES
COGGLES
COHERES
COIGNES
COLLIES
COLONES
COMICES
CONCHES
CONURES
COOKIES
COOLIES
COOTIES
CORPSES
CORVEES
COSINES
COUCHES
COULEES
COUPLES
COURSES
COWRIES
COYOTES
CPLUSES
CRADLES
CRASHES
CRAZIES
CREASES
CREATES
CRECHES
CREOLES
CRESSES
CRINGES
CRONIES
CROOKES
CROSSES
CROUTES
CRUISES
CRUSHES
CUBAGES
CUBBIES
CUDDIES
CUDDLES
CULCHES
CULEXES
CULLIES
CUPULES
CURARES
CURATES
CURDLES
CURRIES
CUTISES
DABBLES
DADDIES
DAILIES
DAIRIES
DAISIES
DALLIES
DAMAGES
DANDIES
DANDLES
DANGLES

DANITES
DAPHNES
DAPPLES
DARKLES
DARTLES
DATIVES
DAWDLES
DAZZLES
DEARIES
DEBASES
DEBATES
DEBONES
DEBTEES
DEBUSES
DECADES
DECIDES
DECILES
DECKLES
DECODES
DECREES
DECRIES
DEDUCES
DEFACES
DEFAMES
DEFILES
DEFINES
DEFUSES
DEGREES
DEHEXES
DEHIRES
DEIFIES
DEITIES
DELETES
DELIBES
DELUDES
DELUGES
DEMISES
DEMOTES
DENOTES
DENUDES
DEPONES
DEPOSES
DEPUTES
DERATES
DERBIES
DERIDES
DERIVES
DESEXES
DESIRES
DETOXES
DETUNES
DEVICES
DEVISES
DEVORES
DEVOTES
DEVRIES
DEWAXES
DEWIRES
DIABLES
DIARIES
DIBBLES
DICKIES
DIDDLES
DILATES
DILLIES
DILUTES
DIMAGES
DIMPLES

DINGLES
DINGOES
DIPOLES
DIRTIES
DISUSES
DITCHES
DITTIES
DIVIDES
DIVINES
DIVVIES
DIZZIES
DNAASES
DOGAPES
DOGGIES
DOILIES
DOLLIES
DOLORES
DONATES
DONGLES
DOODLES
DOOLIES
DOOZIES
DOSAGES
DOTAGES
DOTTLES
DOUANES
DOUBLES
DOWDIES
DOWRIES
DPLUSES
DRAGEES
DRAWEES
DREDGES
DRESSES
DROGUES
DROSSES
DROWSES
DROXIES
DRUDGES
DRYADES
DRYEYES
DUCHIES
DUCKIES
DUFFLES
DUFUSES
DUMMIES
DWARVES
DYNODES
EARLIES
EBONIES
ECARTES
ECDYSES
ECTYPES
EDIBLES
EDIFIES
EFFACES
EFFUSES
EGLISES
EKUELES
ELAINES
ELANCES
ELAPSES
ELEGIES
ELUATES
ELYSEES
EMBRUES
EMERGES
EMERIES

EMIGRES
EMPALES
EMPIRES
EMPTIES
ENABLES
ENCAGES
ENCASES
ENCODES
ENCORES
ENDIVES
ENDURES
ENDUSES
ENEMIES
ENFACES
ENGAGES
ENGINES
ENISLES
ENLACES
ENRAGES
ENROBES
ENSILES
ENSKIES
ENSURES
ENTICES
ENTIRES
ENTREES
ENTRIES
ENZYMES
EOSINES
EPOPEES
EPOQUES
EPOXIES
EQUATES
EQUINES
ERINYES
ERMINES
ESCAPES
ESSENES
ESTATES
ETHANES
ETHENES
ETOILES
EUCHRES
EVINCES
EVOLVES
EVULSES
EWERIES
EXCIDES
EXCISES
EXCITES
EXCUSES
EXHALES
EXHUMES
EXMATES
EXPIRES
EXPOSES
EXWIVES
FABARES
FACADES
FAERIES
FAEROES
FAILLES
FAIRIES
FAMINES
FANCIES
FATALES
FATONES
FEDEXES

FELINES
FEMALES
FERRIES
FERULES
FESCUES
FETCHES
FETTLES
FETUSES
FIACRES
FIANCES
FICUSES
FIDDLES
FIDELES
FIENNES
FIFTIES
FIGURES
FILCHES
FILENES
FILLIES
FINALES
FINCHES
FINITES
FIPPLES
FIXATES
FIZZLES
FLAMBES
FLANGES
FLASHES
FLECHES
FLEDGES
FLEECES
FLENSES
FLESHES
FLOSSES
FLUSHES
FLUTIES
FOCSLES
FOCUSES
FOIBLES
FOLATES
FOLKIES
FOLLIES
FONDLES
FONDUES
FOODIES
FOOTLES
FOOZLES
FORAGES
FORDOES
FORGOES
FORTIES
FOUDRES
FRAISES
FRANCES
FRAPPES
FREEZES
FRESHES
FRESSES
FRIDGES
FRIEZES
FRINGES
FRIZZES
FUDDIES
FUDDLES
FUENTES
FUMBLES
FUNGOES
FUNNIES

FURORES	GUZZLES	IGNITES	JETTIES	LIMOGES	MEEMIES	NEEDLES	OUTAWES	PINKOES	PUTTEES	REDUCES	RETUNES	SCRAPES
FUTURES	GYPSIES	IGNORES	JIFFIES	LINAGES	MEGANES	NEGATES	OUTDOES	PINONES	PUTTIES	REFACES	RETYPES	SCRIBES
GABBLES	GYRATES	ILLUDES	JIGGLES	LINDIES	MEIOSES	NEGUSES	OUTGOES	PIPAGES	PUZZLES	REFAXES	REURGES	SCURVES
GAGGLES	GYRENES	ILLUMES	JIMMIES	LINGOES	MENACES	NEMESES	OUTLIES	PIRATES	PYGMIES	REFILES	REVERES	SCUZZES
GALAXES	HACKIES	ILLUSES	JINGLES	LIPASES	MENAGES	NESTLES	OUTSEES	PITCHES	PYRITES	REFINES	REVILES	SCYTHES
GAMBLES	HACKLES	IMAGOES	JINGOES	LISTEES	MENTEES	NETTLES	OUTVIES	PLAGUES	QUAKIES	REFIRES	REVISES	SEABEES
GAMETES	HAGGLES	IMBIBES	JOGGLES	LITOTES	MENZIES	NEWBIES	OVARIES	PLAICES	QUARLES	REFIXES	REVIVES	SEANCES
GAMINES	HALFIES	IMBRUES	JOLLIES	LITTLES	MERCHES	NEWSIES	OXHIDES	PLAINES	QUARTES	REFLIES	REVOKES	SECEDES
GARAGES	HALIDES	IMMIXES	JONESES	LIZZIES	MERCIES	NEXUSES	PADDIES	PLAQUES	QUASHES	REFRIES	REVOTES	SECURES
GARBLES	HALITES	IMMUNES	JOSTLES	LOATHES	MERGEES	NIBBLES	PADDLES	PLASHES	QUATRES	REFUGES	REWAKES	SEDATES
GARGLES	HAMITES	IMMURES	JOUNCES	LOBBIES	METATES	NICKLES	PAIUTES	PLATIES	QUERIES	REFUSES	REWAXES	SEDUCES
GAUDIES	HANDLES	IMPALES	JUDASES	LOBULES	METTLES	NIFTIES	PALACES	PLEASES	QUICHES	REFUTES	REWIPES	SEETHES
GAUSSES	HANKIES	IMPEDES	JUGGLES	LOCALES	MIDASES	NIGGLES	PALATES	PLEDGES	QUINCES	REGALES	REWIRES	SEMITES
GECKOES	HARDEES	IMPLIES	JUJUBES	LOCATES	MIDDIES	NINNIES	PANSIES	PLISSES	QUINTES	REGIMES	REYOKES	SENATES
GELATES	HARPIES	IMPOSES	JUMBLES	LOESSES	MIDDLES	NIPPLES	PANTIES	PLOTZES	QUINZES	REGIVES	REZONES	SENDEES
GENESES	HARRIES	IMPUTES	JUNCOES	LOLLIES	MIGENES	NODDIES	PAPELES	PLUNGES	QUIZZES	REGLUES	RIBBIES	SENORES
GENOMES	HASSLES	INBOXES	JUNGLES	LONDRES	MIMESES	NODULES	PAPPIES	PLUSHES	QUOTEES	REHIDES	RIBEYES	SERAPES
GENTLES	HATCHES	INCASES	JUNKIES	LONGIES	MINGLES	NOGALES	PARADES	PLUSSES	RABBLES	REHIRES	RICKLES	SESAMES
GENUSES	HAYESES	INCISES	KARATES	LONGUES	MINUSES	NOMBRES	PARCHES	POACHES	RACEMES	REHONES	RIDDLES	SETFEES
GEORGES	HEARSES	INCITES	KCJONES	LOOBIES	MINUTES	NONAGES	PAROLES	POBOXES	RADAMES	REIFIES	RIFFLES	SETTEES
GESSOES	HEAVIES	INCOMES	KELPIES	LOONIES	MIRAGES	NONAMES	PARRIES	POESIES	RADICES	RELACES	RIMPLES	SETTLES
GFORCES	HECKLES	INCUDES	KETCHES	LORISES	MISCUES	NONUKES	PARSEES	POINTES	RADIXES	RELANES	RIPPLES	SHAKOES
GIBLUES	HECKYES	INCUSES	KETONES	LORRIES	MISDOES	NOODGES	PARTIES	POIVRES	RADOMES	RELATES	RITDYES	SHEAVES
GIBUSES	HELICES	INDEXES	KETTLES	LORUSES	MISSIES	NOODLES	PARURES	POLICES	RAFFLES	RELAXES	ROACHES	SHELVES
GIDDIES	HELIXES	INDICES	KEWPIES	LOTUSES	MISUSES	NOOGIES	PASTIES	POLLEES	RAGGIES	RELEVES	ROADIES	SHIITES
GIFTEES	HELLOES	INDITES	KIBBLES	LOUNGES	MITOSES	NOPALES	PATCHES	POMADES	RALLIES	RELINES	ROCKIES	SHOPPES
GIGGLES	HELLYES	INDUCES	KIDDIES	LOURDES	MIZZLES	NORITES	PATRIES	PONGEES	RALLYES	RELIVES	ROLEXES	SHRIKES
GIPSIES	HENRIES	INFIVES	KILTIES	LOUVRES	MOBILES	NOTATES	PATSIES	POOCHES	RAMBLES	RELOSES	ROOKIES	SHRINES
GIRDLES	HEXANES	INFIXES	KINDLES	LOVAGES	MODULES	NOTCHES	PATTIES	POODLES	RAMESES	RELUMES	ROOMIES	SHRIVES
GIRLIES	HEXOSES	INFUSES	KINESES	LOYALES	MOHAVES	NOTICES	PAVANES	POPEYES	RAMONES	REMAKES	ROOTLES	SHUSHES
GLANCES	HIGGLES	INGATES	KISHKES	LUCITES	MOJAVES	NOVICES	PAWNEES	POPPIES	RANCHES	REMATES	ROSCOES	SICKLES
GLASSES	HIGHRES	INHALES	KITTIES	LUNATES	MOLLIES	NOVOTES	PDJAMES	POPPLES	RANKLES	REMINES	ROTATES	SIGNEES
GLITZES	HINNIES	INHERES	KLUDGES	LUNCHES	MOMMIES	NOZZLES	PEACHES	PORCHES	RAPINES	REMISES	ROWDIES	SILLIES
GLORIES	HIPPIES	INHUMES	KLUTZES	LUPINES	MOMUSES	NTUPLES	PEBBLES	PORGIES	RASSLES	REMIXES	ROYALES	SIMILES
GLOSSES	HITCHES	INJOKES	KNISHES	LURCHES	MONKEES	NUANCES	PEDDLES	POSOLES	RASURES	REMOTES	RUBBLES	SIMPLES
GLURGES	HOAGIES	INJURES	KNOWLES	LUREXES	MONROES	NUBBLES	PEEBLES	POSTIES	RATINES	REMOVES	RUFFLES	SINGLES
GNASHES	HOBBIES	INLINES	KOOSHES	LUSTRES	MOOCHES	NUDZHES	PEEPLES	POTAGES	RATITES	RENAMES	RUGGLES	SINUSES
GOALIES	HOBBLES	INMATES	KURILES	LUXATES	MOONIES	NUTATES	PEEWEES	POTPIES	RATTLES	RENEGES	RUMBLES	SISSIES
GOATEES	HOGTIES	INNAGES	KVASSES	MADAMES	MORALES	NUZZLES	PELAGES	POTTIES	RAVAGES	RENOTES	RUMMIES	SIXTIES
GOBBLES	HOLLIES	INSALES	LABFEES	MAGPIES	MORGUES	NYTIMES	PENATES	POUCHES	RAVINES	RENTEES	RUMPLES	SIZZLES
GOGGLES	HOMAGES	INSIDES	LADDIES	MAITRES	MOSQUES	OBLATES	PENNIES	POUDRES	RAZZIES	REPAGES	RUNDLES	SKOSHES
GOODIES	HOMBRES	INSOLES	LAERTES	MALICES	MOTIVES	OBLIGES	PENSEES	POUNCES	REACHES	REPAVES	RUSHEES	SLASHES
GOOGLES	HOOCHES	INSURES	LAITIES	MANAGES	MOTTLES	OCTANES	PEONIES	POZOLES	READIES	REPINES	RUSTLES	SLEAZES
GOONIES	HOODIES	INTAKES	LARCHES	MANEGES	MOTTOES	OCTAVES	PEOPLES	PRAISES	REBAKES	REPLIES	RUTILES	SLEDGES
GOURDES	HOOPOES	INTONES	LASSIES	MANGLES	MOUSSES	OEUVRES	PERCHES	PRANCES	REBALES	REPOSES	RVALUES	SLEEVES
GRAMMES	HOTONES	INVADES	LASSOES	MANGOES	MRBONES	OFFICES	PERUKES	PREAGES	REBATES	REPUTES	SABINES	SLOSHES
GRANGES	HOTTIES	INVITES	LATCHES	MANNIES	MRJONES	OHMAGES	PERUSES	PREMIES	REBORES	RERAKES	SACQUES	SLUDGES
GRASSES	HUBBIES	INVOKES	LATEXES	MANTLES	MUDDIES	OLEATES	PESADES	PRESSES	REBOTES	RERATES	SADDLES	SLUICES
GRAVIES	HUDDLES	IODATES	LATICES	MANURES	MUDDLES	OLOGIES	PESTLES	PREVUES	REBOXES	RERIDES	SADEYES	SLUSHES
GREASES	HUGGIES	IODIDES	LATIMES	MARBLES	MUDPIES	ONSIDES	PETALES	PREXIES	REBUKES	RERISES	SAINTES	SMASHES
GREAVES	HUMBLES	IODISES	LAVAGES	MARCHES	MUFFLES	OOCYTES	PETITES	PRINCES	REBUSES	RESALES	SALADES	SMIDGES
GRIEVES	HUMUSES	IODIZES	LEACHES	MARINES	MUGGLES	OOLITES	PEYOTES	PRISSES	RECAGES	RESAVES	SALINES	SMOKIES
GRILLES	HUMVEES	IONISES	LEAGUES	MARQUES	MUJERES	OPAQUES	PHISHES	PRIUSES	RECANES	RESCUES	SALLIES	SMUDGES
GRIPPES	HUNCHES	IONIZES	LEASHES	MARRIES	MULCHES	OPIATES	PHLOXES	PRIVIES	RECASES	RESHOES	SALUTES	SMUSHES
GROOVES	HURDLES	IONONES	LEECHES	MARSHES	MUMBLES	OPPOSES	PHOEBES	PROBIES	RECEDES	RESIDES	SALVOES	SNEEZES
GROSSES	HURRIES	IRONIES	LEFTIES	MASHIES	MUMMIES	ORACIES	PHONIES	PROXIES	RECIPES	RESILES	SAMPLES	SNOOZES
GROUSES	HURTLES	IVORIES	LEGATES	MASQUES	MUNCHES	ORACLES	PHRASES	PSYCHES	RECITES	RESIZES	SATIRES	SOFTIES
GRUDGES	HUSKIES	IVTUBES	LEGUMES	MATCHES	MUSCLES	ORANGES	PIAFFES	PUDDLES	RECODES	RESOLES	SAVAGES	SOIREES
GRUNGES	HUSSIES	JACALES	LESSEES	MATURES	MUSKIES	ORANTES	PICKLES	PUGGLES	RECURES	RESUMES	SAVVIES	SOLACES
GUESSES	HUSTLES	JACQUES	LETTRES	MAVISES	MUTATES	ORDINES	PIDDLES	PUMICES	RECUSES	RETAKES	SAYSYES	SOLUTES
GULCHES	HUTCHES	JAGGIES	LEVADES	MAXIXES	MUZZLES	ORESTES	PIERCES	PUNCHES	REDARES	RETAMES	SCARVES	SOOTHES
GULLIES	HYRACES	JAMMIES	LEVITES	MCHALES	MYRTLES	ORIOLES	PIETIES	PUNKIES	REDATES	RETAPES	SCATHES	SOPHIES
GUNITES	HYRAXES	JANGLES	LEXISES	MEAGLES	NAIADES	ORRISES	PIFFLES	PUPATES	REDDYES	RETAXES	SCHAYES	SORTIES
GUNNIES	ICEAGES	JAYCEES	LEXUSES	MEALIES	NANNIES	OSCINES	PIGGIES	PUPPIES	REDEYES	RETILES	SCHEMES	SOURCES
GUPPIES	ICEAXES	JAYVEES	LIAISES	MEANIES	NAPPIES	OSCULES	PILATES	PURFLES	REDOSES	RETIMES	SCHMOES	SPATHES
GURGLES	ICICLES	JEEBIES	LICHEES	MEASLES	NASTIES	OSMOSES	PIMPLES	PURPLES	REDOXES	RETIRES	SCHOLES	SPECIES
GUSSIES	ICTUSES	JELLIES	LIENEES	MEDDLES	NATIVES	OTARIES	PINCHES	PURSUES	REDRIES	RETONES	SCONCES	SPHERES
GUSTOES	IDEATES	JERKIES	LIGATES	MEDELES	NATURES	OUTAGES	PINKIES	PUSSIES	REDTIES	RETRIES	SCOUPES	SPITZES

SPLICES
SPLINES
SPONGES
SPOUSES
SPRITES
SPRUCES
SQUARES
SQUIRES
STABLES
STAGNES
STANCES
STAPLES
STARVES
STASHES
STATUES
STEEVES
STEPPES
STIFLES
STJAMES
STLUKES
STODGES
STOGIES
STOOGES
STORIES
STRAFES
STRIDES
STRIFES
STRIKES
STRIPES
STRIVES
STROBES
STROKES
STUDIES
STURGES
STUTZES
STYMIES
SUBDUES
SULKIES
SULLIES
SUNDAES
SUPPLES
SUTURES
SWASHES
SWATHES
SWERVES
SWISHES
TABBIES
TACKLES
TAFFIES
TALKIES
TALLIES
TALUSES
TAMALES
TANGLES
TANSIES
TARRIES
TATTLES
TEACHES
TECHIES
TEDDIES
TEEHEES
TEEPEES
TEETHES
TEEVEES
TEKKIES
TELEXES
TELLIES
TEMPLES
TENACES
TENCHES
TENNIES
TENURES
TERRIES
TESTEES
THEAGES
THIEVES
THRIVES
THRONES
TICKLES
TIEDYES
TIERCES
TIMBRES
TIMEXES
TINGLES
TINKLES
TINORES
TIPPEES
TIPPLES
TIPTOES
TIRADES
TISANES
TISSUES
TITTLES
TIZZIES
TOADIES
TODDIES
TODDLES
TOFFEES
TOGGLES
TONEMES
TONGUES
TONUSES
TOODLES
TOONIES
TOOTLES
TOPAZES
TOPPLES
TORCHES
TORQUES
TOUCHES
TOUPEES
TOUSLES
TOWAGES
TOWHEES
TOWNIES
TRANCES
TRASHES
TREBLES
TREIZES
TRESSES
TRIAGES
TRIFLES
TRIODES
TRIPLES
TROCHES
TROUPES
TRUDGES
TRUSSES
TSETSES
TSHAPES
TUBULES
TUILLES
TUMBLES
TUMMIES
TURTLES
TUSHIES
TUSSLES
TVGAMES
TVTAPES
TWEEZES
TWELVES
TWINGES
TZIMMES
ULLAGES
ULYSSES
UMPIRES
UNBALES
UNBARES
UNBOXES
UNCAGES
UNCAKES
UNCASES
UNCORES
UNDINES
UNEASES
UNEDGES
UNFILES
UNFINES
UNFIXES
UNFREES
UNGLUES
UNHIRES
UNIATES
UNIFIES
UNIQUES
UNITIES
UNLACES
UNLADES
UNLAXES
UNLIKES
UNLIVES
UNMAKES
UNMATES
UNMIXES
UNPILES
UNROBES
UNROPES
UNSHOES
UNSOLES
UNTAMES
UNTAPES
UNTAXES
UNTUNES
UNYOKES
UNZONES
UPDATES
UPDIVES
UPDRIES
UPGAZES
UPPILES
UPRATES
UPRISES
UPSIDES
UPSIZES
UPTAKES
UPTIMES
USABLES
USANCES
USHAPES
USTEDES
USURIES
UVALUES
VACATES
VALINES
VALISES
VATDYES
VEERIES
VEGGIES
VEINTES
VELOXES
VELURES
VENDEES
VENDUES
VENULES
VENUSES
VESTEES
VETCHES
VIELLES
VIERNES
VIRTUES
VIRUSES
VISAGES
VITTLES
VOLUMES
VOLUTES
VOTEYES
VOTIVES
VOUCHES
VOYAGES
VSHAPES
WADDLES
WAFFLES
WAGGLES
WAHINES
WAKAMES
WALTZES
WAMBLES
WANGLES
WARBLES
WATCHES
WATTLES
WEARIES
WEDGIES
WEENIES
WEEONES
WELLYES
WENCHES
WESTIES
WETONES
WHARVES
WHEEZES
WHISHES
WHIZZES
WIENIES
WIGGLES
WILLIES
WIMPLES
WINCHES
WITCHES
WITHIES
WOBBLES
WOODIES
WOOLIES
WOOSHES
WORRIES
WRASSES
WRITHES
XEROSES
XEROXES
XIMENES
XYLOSES
YANKEES
YETTIES
YIPPIES
YORKIES
YSHAPES
YUPPIES
ZILCHES
ZOMBIES
ZONULES
ZYGOTES

ET•••••

ETAGERE
ETAILED
ETAILER
ETALIBI
ETAMINE
ETCHANT
ETCHERS
ETCHING
ETERNAL
ETESIAN
ETHANES
ETHANOL
ETHENES
ETHERIC
ETHICAL
ETHMOID
ETHNICS
ETICKET
ETIENNE
ETOILES
ETONIAN
ETONICS
ETRURIA
ETVOILA
ETYMONS

E•T••••

EATABIT
EATABLE
EATALOT
EATAWAY
EATCAKE
EATCROW
EATDIRT
EATENAT
EATENUP
EATFROM
EATHERE
EATINTO
EATITUP
EATLATE
EATLESS
EATMORE
EATOVER
EATSOUT
ECTYPAL
ECTYPES
ELTRAIN
ENTAILS
ENTEBBE
ENTENTE
ENTERED
ENTERER
ENTERIC
ENTERIN
ENTERON
ENTHRAL
ENTHUSE
ENTICED
ENTICER
ENTICES
ENTIRES
ENTITLE
ENTOMBS
ENTRADA
ENTRAIN
ENTRANT
ENTRAPS
ENTREAT
ENTREES
ENTRIES
ENTROPY
ENTRUST
ENTWINE
ENTWIST
ERTEGUN
ESTADOS
ESTAMIN
ESTATED
ESTATES
ESTEBAN
ESTEEMS
ESTEFAN
ESTELLA
ESTELLE
ESTEVEZ
ESTHETE
ESTIVAL
ESTONIA
ESTORIL
ESTRADA
ESTRAYS
ESTRING
ESTUARY
EUTERPE
EXTENDS
EXTENSO
EXTENTS
EXTERNE
EXTERNS
EXTINCT
EXTOLLS
EXTORTS
EXTRACT
EXTREME
EXTRUDE

E••T•••

EARTABS
EARTAGS
EARTHED
EARTHEN
EARTHLY
EASTEGG
EASTEND
EASTERN
EASTERS
EASTHAM
EASTING
EASTMAN
EBBTIDE
ECOTAGE
ECOTEUR
ECOTRIN
ECOTYPE
ECSTASY
EDITING
EDITION
EDITORS
EDITOUT
EDITRIX
EGGTOSS
EGOTISM
EGOTIST
EGOTRIP
ELATERS
ELATING
ELATION
ELITEST
ELITISM
ELITIST
ELMTREE
ELUTING
ELUTION
EMETICS
EMITTED
EMITTER
EMOTERS
EMOTING
EMOTION
EMOTIVE
EMPTIED
EMPTIER
EMPTIES
EMPTILY
EPITAPH
EPITHET
EPITOME
EPSTEIN
ERITREA
EROTICA
EROTICS
ERYTHRO
ESOTERY
EUSTACE
EXITFEE
EXITING
EXITNOW
EXOTICA
EXOTICS
EXOTISM
EYETEST
EYETUCK

E•••T••

EATITUP
ECARTES
EDICTAL
EDUCTED
EDUCTOR
EGESTED
EIDETIC
EIGHTAD
EIGHTAM
EIGHTBC
EIGHTEE
EIGHTHS
EIGHTPM
EIGHTUP
EJECTED
EJECTOR
EKISTIC
ELANTRA
ELASTIC
ELASTIN
ELECTED
ELECTEE
ELECTME
ELECTOR
ELECTRA
ELECTRO
ELEKTRA
ELUATES
EMITTED
EMITTER
EMPATHS
EMPATHY
ENACTED
ENACTOR
ENTITLE
EOLITHS
EPISTLE
EQUATED
EQUATES
EQUATOR
ERASTUS
ERECTED
ERECTER
ERECTLY
ERECTOR
ERECTUS
ERGOTIC
ERISTIC
ERRATIC
ERRATUM
ERUCTED
ERUPTED
ERUPTER
ESTATED
ESTATES
EVERTED
EVERTOR
EVICTED
EVICTEE
EVICTOR
EXACTAS
EXACTED
EXACTER
EXACTLY
EXACTOR
EXALTED
EXALTER
EXCITED
EXCITER
EXCITES
EXCITOR
EXERTED
EXERTER
EXISTED
EXMATES
EXULTED

E••••T•

EAGLETS
EARLETS
EATINTO
EATLATE
EBONITE
EBWHITE
EDACITY
EDEMATA
EDOMITE
EDUCATE
EELPOTS
EFFECTS
EFFORTS
EGALITE
EGOISTE
EGOISTS
ELAMITE
ELANETS
ELBERTA
ELEGITS
ELEVATE
ELICITS
ELLIOTT
ELMCITY
ELMISTI
ELMONTE
ELNORTE
ELOCUTE
ELUANTS
EMANATE
EMBOITE
EMERITA
EMERITI
EMIRATE
EMULATE
ENCARTA
ENDCUTS
ENDLATE
ENDNOTE
ENFANTS
ENGLUTS
ENLISTS
ENROOTS
ENROUTE
ENSEATS
ENSUITE
ENTENTE
EPIDOTE
EPILATE
EQUALTO
EREMITE
ERNESTA
ERNESTO
ERUDITE
ESCORTS
ESPARTO
ESPRITS
ESTHETE
EVERETT
EVOLUTE
EXABYTE
EXCEPTS
EXCRETE
EXECUTE
EXEGETE
EXEMPTS
EXEUNTS
EXFACTO
EXHORTS
EXOCETS
EXPARTE
EXPECTS
EXPERTS
EXPIATE
EXPORTS
EXSECTS
EXSERTS
EXTENTS
EXTORTS
EXUDATE
EYELETS
EYEPITS

E•••••T

EARHART
EARNEST
EARNSIT
EARSHOT
EASEOUT
EASIEST
EATABIT
EATALOT
EATDIRT
EATENAT
EATSOUT
ECKHART
EDGEOUT
EDGIEST
EDITOUT
EELIEST
EELPOUT
EERIEST
EGGHUNT
EGGIEST
EGOTIST
EKEDOUT
EKESOUT
ELEGANT
ELEGIST
ELEMENT
ELITEST
ELITIST
ELKHART
ELLIOTT
ELMIEST
EMANANT
EMINENT
ENCHANT
ENCRUST
ENCRYPT
ENDEDAT
ENDEDIT
ENDMOST
ENDUPAT
ENGRAFT
ENRIGHT
ENTRANT
ENTREAT
ENTRUST
ENTWIST
EPAULET
EPEEIST
EPITHET
ERODENT
ESCHEAT
ETCHANT
ETICKET
EVENBET
EVENEST
EVENOUT
EVEREST
EVERETT
EVIDENT
EVILEST
EXCELAT
EXCERPT
EXHAUST
EXHIBIT
EXIGENT
EXPLOIT
EXPOSIT
EXTINCT
EXTRACT
EYEBOLT
EYELIFT
EYESHOT
EYESPOT
EYETEST

•ET••••

BETAKEN
BETAKES
BETAMAX
BETARAY
BETHANY
BETHELS
BETHERE
BETHINK
BETHUNE
BETIDED
BETIDES
BETIMES
BETOKEN
BETRAYS
BETROTH
BETTANY
BETTERS
BETTGER
BETTING
BETTORS
BETWEEN
BETWIXT
CETANES
CETERIS
DETAILS
DETAINS
DETECTO
DETECTS
DETENTE
DETENTS
DETERGE
DETESTS
DETOURS
DETOXED
DETOXES
DETRACT
DETRAIN
DETROIT
DETRUDE
DETUNED
DETUNES
FETCHED
FETCHER
FETCHES
FETIDLY
FETLOCK
FETTERS
FETTLES
FETUSES
GETABLE
GETAHIT
GETAJOB
GETATIP
GETAWAY
GETBACK
GETBEAT
GETBENT
GETBUSY
GETCASH
GETCOLD
GETCUTE
GETDONE
GETDOWN
GETEVEN
GETFREE
GETFROM
GETGOOD
GETHELP
GETHURT
GETINON
GETINTO
GETITON
GETLOST
GETONIT
GETONTO
GETOVER
GETPAST
GETREAL
GETSANA
GETSANF
GETSFAR
GETSFIT
GETSHEP
GETSHIP
GETSHOT
GETSMAD
GETSOFF
GETSOFT
GETSOLD
GETSORE
GETSOUT
GETSRID
GETSSET
GETSWET
GETTERS
GETTHIS
GETTING
GETTOIT
GETUPON
GETWARM
GETWELL
GETWISE
GETWORD
JETBOAT
JETFANS
JETFIRE
JETFOIL
JETGUNS
JETLAGS
JETPACK
JETPORT
JETSETS
JETSFAN
JETSKIS
JETSONS
JETSTAR
JETTIED
JETTIES
JETTING
JETWASH
JETWAYS
KETCHAM
KETCHES
KETCHUM
KETCHUP
KETONES
KETONIC
KETTLES
LETDOWN
LETDROP
LETEMIN
LETFALL
LETGOBY
LETGOOF
LETHAVE
LETHEAN
LETINON
LETITBE
LETITGO
LETITIA
LETKNOW
LETLIVE
LETMEBE
LETMEGO
LETMEIN
LETPASS
LETRIDE
LETROLL
LETSEAT
LETSFLY
LETSLIP
LETSNOT
LETSOFF
LETSOUT
LETSRIP
LETSSEE
LETSUSE
LETTERA
LETTERB
LETTERC
LETTERD
LETTERE
LETTERF
LETTERG
LETTERH
LETTERI
LETTERJ
LETTERK
LETTERL
LETTERM
LETTERN
LETTERO
LETTERP
LETTERQ
LETTERR
LETTERS
LETTERT
LETTERU
LETTERV
LETTERW
LETTERX
LETTERY
LETTERZ
LETTING
LETTISH
LETTRES
LETTUCE
LETUPON

METALED
METATES
METCALF
METEORS
METEOUT
METERED
METFANS
METHANE
METHODS
METIERS
METLIFE
METOOER
METRICS
METRIST
METSFAN
METTLER
METTLES
METWITH
NETBALL
NETCAFE
NETCOST
NETFLIX
NETFULS
NETGAIN
NETGAME
NETIZEN
NETLESS
NETLIKE
NETLOSS
NETSTER
NETSUKE
NETSURF
NETTERS
NETTING
NETTLED
NETTLES
NETTONS
NETWARE
NETWORK
NETZERO
PETALED
PETALES
PETARDS
PETBEAR
PETBIRD
PETBOAS
PETCAGE
PETCALF
PETCATS
PETCHEW
PETCOCK
PETCOMB
PETCOWS
PETCROW
PETDEER
PETDOGS
PETDOOR
PETDOVE
PETDUCK
PETEMAN
PETEMEN
PETERED
PETERII
PETFISH
PETFROG
PETGATE
PETGOAT
PETHAIR
PETHARE
PETIOLE
PETITES
PETLAMB
PETLION
PETMICE
PETMULE
PETNAME
PETNAPS
PETPIGS
PETPONY
PETPUPS
PETRATS
PETRELS
PETRIFY
PETROCK
PETROLS
PETROUS
PETSCAN
PETSHOP
PETSITS
PETTERS
PETTIER
PETTILY
PETTING
PETTISH
PETTOYS
PETULIA
PETUNIA
RETABLE
RETACKS
RETAILS
RETAINS
RETAKEN
RETAKER
RETAKES
RETALLY
RETAMED
RETAMES
RETAPED
RETAPES
RETARDS
RETASTE
RETAXED
RETAXES
RETEACH
RETEARS
RETELLS
RETESTS
RETHANK
RETHAWS
RETHINK
RETIARY
RETICLE
RETILED
RETILES
RETILLS
RETIMED
RETIMES
RETINAE
RETINAL
RETINAS
RETINGE
RETINOL
RETINTS
RETINUE
RETIRED
RETIREE
RETIRES
RETITLE
RETOAST
RETONED
RETONES
RETOOLS
RETORTS
RETOTAL
RETOUCH
RETOURS
RETOWED
RETRACE
RETRACK
RETRACT
RETRADE
RETRAIN
RETRAPS
RETREAD
RETREAT
RETRIAL
RETRIED
RETRIES
RETRIMS
RETSINA
RETTING
RETUNED
RETUNES
RETURFS
RETURNS
RETWINE
RETWIST
RETYPED
RETYPES
SETBACK
SETBAIL
SETDOWN
SETENTA
SETFEES
SETFREE
SETINTO
SETOFFS
SETOUTS
SETPLAY
SETRATE
SETSAIL
SETSHOT
SETSOFF
SETSOUT
SETTEES
SETTERS
SETTING
SETTLED
SETTLER
SETTLES
SETTLOR
SETTYPE
SETUPON
TETANUS
TETHERS
TETRADS
TETRODE
VETCHES
VETERAN
VETOERS
VETOING
VETTERS
VETTING
WETBARS
WETBULB
WETCELL
WETDOWN
WETEYED
WETKISS
WETLAND
WETLOOK
WETMOPS
WETNAPS
WETNESS
WETONES
WETRAGS
WETSUIT
WETTEST
WETTING
WETTISH
WETWARE
WETWASH
YETTIES

•E•T•••

BEATALL
BEATBOX
BEATCOP
BEATERS
BEATIFY
BEATING
BEATLES
BEATNIK
BEATOFF
BEATOUT
BEATRIX
BEATSAT
BEATSIT
BEATSME
BEATSON
BEATSUP
BEATTIE
BEDTIME
BEETIER
BEETLES
BEETRED
BEETREE
BELTANE
BELTBAG
BELTERS
BELTING
BELTOUT
BELTRAN
BELTSAW
BELTSUP
BELTWAY
BENTHAM
BENTHOS
BENTLEY
BENTSEN
BERTHAS
BERTHED
BERTOLT
BERTRAM
BESTBET
BESTBOY
BESTBUD
BESTBUY
BESTCUT
BESTIAL
BESTILL
BESTING
BESTIRS
BESTMAN
BESTMEN
BESTOFF
BESTONE
BESTOWS
BESTREW
BETTANY
BETTERS
BETTGER
BETTING
BETTORS
CELTICS
CENTALS
CENTARE
CENTAUR
CENTAVO
CENTERS
CENTIME
CENTIMO
CENTRAL
CENTRED
CENTRES
CENTRIC
CENTRUM
CENTURY
CERTAIN
CERTIFY
CESTMOI
DEBTEES
DEBTORS
DEFTEST
DEITIES
DELTAIC
DELTOID
DELTONA
DELTORO
DENTALS
DENTATE
DENTINE
DENTING
DENTINS
DENTIST
DENTOID
DENTONS
DENTURE
DENTYNE
DESTAEL
DESTAIN
DESTEMS
DESTINE
DESTINO
DESTINY
DESTOCK
DESTROY
DEUTERO
DEUTSCH
DEXTRAL
DEXTRIN
FEATHER
FEATURE
FELTBAD
FELTFOR
FELTHAT
FELTILL
FELTING
FELTOFF
FELTOUT
FELTPEN
FELTTIP
FERTILE
FESTERS
FESTINA
FESTIVA
FESTIVE
FESTOON
FESTOSO
FETTERS
FETTLES
GENTEEL
GENTIAN
GENTILE
GENTLED
GENTLER
GENTLES
GESTALT
GESTAPO
GESTATE
GESTURE
GETTERS
GETTHIS
GETTING
GETTOIT
HEATERS
HEATFAN
HEATFUL
HEATHEN
HEATHER
HEATING
HEATRAY
HEATSUP
HEATTER
HECTARE
HECTORS
HEFTERS
HEFTIER
HEFTILY
HEFTING
HENTOFF
HEPTADS
JESTERS
JESTING
JETTIED
JETTIES
JETTING
KENTISH
KEPTFIT
KEPTMUM
KEPTOFF
KEPTOUT
KERTESZ
KESTREL
KETTLES
LEATHER
LECTERN
LECTORS
LECTRIC
LECTURE
LEETIDE
LEFTARM
LEFTEAR
LEFTEND
LEFTEST
LEFTEYE
LEFTFOR
LEFTHIP
LEFTIES
LEFTISH
LEFTISM
LEFTIST
LEFTJAB
LEFTLEG
LEFTOFF
LEFTOUT
LEGTRAP
LEITRIM
LENTIGO
LENTILS
LEOTARD
LEPTONS
LESTOIL
LETTERA
LETTERB
LETTERC
LETTERD
LETTERE
LETTERF
LETTERG
LETTERH
LETTERI
LETTERJ
LETTERK
LETTERL
LETTERM
LETTERN
LETTERO
LETTERP
LETTERQ
LETTERR
LETTERS
LETTERT
LETTERU
LETTERV
LETTERW
LETTERX
LETTERY
LETTERZ
LETTING
LETTISH
LETTRES
LETTUCE
MEATAXE
MEATIER
MEATILY
MEATMAN
MEATMEN
MEATPIE
MEETERS
MEETING
MEETSUP
MEITNER
MELTAGE
MELTERS
MELTING
MENTEES
MENTHOL
MENTION
MENTORS
METTLER
METTLES
NEATENS
NEATEST
NEATNIK
NECTARS
NECTARY
NEITHER
NEPTUNE
NESTEGG
NESTERS
NESTFUL
NESTING
NESTLED
NESTLER
NESTLES
NESTORS
NESTSIN
NETTERS
NETTING
NETTLED
NETTLES
NETTONS
NEUTERS
NEUTRAL
NEUTRON
NEWTONS
NEWTOWN
NEWTOYS
NEXTDAY
PEATBOG
PEATIER
PEATPOT
PECTINS
PEGTOPS
PELTATE
PELTERS
PELTING
PELTISH
PENTADS
PENTANE
PENTELS
PENTIUM
PEPTALK
PEPTICS
PEPTIDE
PEPTONE
PERTAIN
PERTEST
PERTURB
PESTERS
PESTLED
PESTLES
PETTERS
PETTIER
PETTILY
PETTING
PETTISH
PETTOYS
PEWTERS
REATTAS
RECTIFY
RECTORS
RECTORY
REDTABS
REDTAGS
REDTAIL
REDTAPE
REDTIDE
REDTIES
REDTOPS
REITMAN
RENTALS
RENTEES
RENTERS
RENTIER
RENTING
RENTOUT
RENTSTO
REPTILE
RESTABS
RESTACK
RESTAFF
RESTAGE
RESTAIN
RESTAMP
RESTART
RESTATE
RESTERS
RESTFUL
RESTICK
RESTING
RESTIRS
RESTIVE
RESTOCK
RESTOKE
RESTORE
RESTOWS
RESTRAP
RESTREW
RESTRIP
RESTSIN
RESTSON
RESTSUP
RESTUDY
RESTUFF
RESTYLE
RETTING
REUTERS
REUTHER
REUTTER
SEATERS
SEATING
SEATRIP
SEATTLE
SECTION
SECTORS
SEETHED
SEETHES
SEETHRU
SEETOIT
SELTZER
SENTFOR
SENTOFF
SENTOUT
SENTRAS
SEPTETS
SESTETS
SESTINA
SETTEES
SETTERS
SETTING
SETTLED
SETTLER
SETTLES
SETTLOR
SETTYPE
SEXTANS
SEXTANT
SEXTETS
SEXTONS
TEATIME
TEATRAY
TEATREE
TEATROS
TEETERS
TEETHED
TEETHER
TEETHES
TEETIME
TENTBED
TENTERS
TENTFUL
TENTHLY
TENTING
TENTONS
TENTPEG
TESTACY
TESTATE
TESTBAN
TESTBED
TESTEES
TESTERS
TESTFLY
TESTFOR
TESTIER
TESTIFY
TESTILY
TESTING
TESTKIT
TESTLAB
TESTOUT
TESTRUN
TEUTONS
TEXTILE
TEXTING
TEXTRON
TEXTUAL
TEXTURE
VECTORS
VECTRAS
VELTMAN
VENTAGE
VENTERS
VENTING
VENTNOR
VENTRAD
VENTRAL
VENTRIS
VENTURA
VENTURE
VENTURI
VERTIGO
VESTALS
VESTEES
VESTIGE
VESTING
VESTRAL
VESTRON
VESTURE
VETTERS
VETTING
WEATHER
WEBTOED
WELTERS
WELTING
WENTAFT
WENTAPE
WENTBAD
WENTFAR
WENTFOR
WENTMAD
WENTOFF
WENTOUT
WENTPRO
WERTHER
WESTEGG
WESTEND
WESTERN
WESTERS
WESTIES
WESTINS
WETTEST
WETTING
WETTISH
YEATEAM
YELTSIN
YETTIES
YEWTREE
ZEITUNG
ZESTERS
ZESTFUL
ZESTIER
ZESTILY
ZESTING

•E••T•

AERATED
AERATES
AERATOR
BEASTIE
BEASTLY
BEATTIE
BEEFTEA
BEERTAP
BELATED
BENATAR
BENOTED
BENOTES
BERATED
BERATER
BERATES
BERETTA
BEWITCH
CELOTEX
CERATED
CERATES
DEALTIN
DEALTTO
DEALTUP
DEARTHS
DEBATED
DEBATER
DEBATES
DEBITED
DEBUTED
DECATUR
DEEPTAN
DEISTIC
DELETED
DELETES
DEMETER
DEMOTED
DEMOTES
DEMOTHS
DEMOTIC
DENOTED
DENOTES
DEPUTED
DEPUTES
DERATED
DERATES
DESKTOP
DESOTOS
DEVOTED
DEVOTEE
DEVOTES
DEWATER
FEASTED
FEASTER
FEASTON
FEINTED
FELTTIP
FENETRE
GELATED
GELATES
GELATIN
GELATIS
GELATOS
GENETIC
GENITOR
GERITOL
GETATIP
GETITON
HEALTHY
HEARTED
HEARTEN
HEARTHS
HEATTER
HEELTAP
HEISTED
HELOTRY
HEMATIC
HEMATIN
HEPATIC
HERBTEA
HERETIC
HERITOR
JEPHTHA
JERITZA
JETSTAR
KEISTER
KEMPTON
KERATIN
LEANTOS
LEAPTAT
LEAPTIN
LEAPTON
LEAPTUP
LEGATEE
LEGATES
LEGATOR
LEGATOS
LEISTER
LENGTHS
LENGTHY
LESOTHO
LESSTAR
LETITBE
LETITGO
LETITIA
LEVATOR
LEVITES
LEVITIC
MEANTIT
MEANTTO
MEGATON
MEIOTIC
MEISTER
MELITTA
MENOTTI
MERITED
METATES
NECKTIE
NEGATED
NEGATER
NEGATES
NEGATOR
NEPOTIC
NETSTER
OERSTED
PELOTAS
PELOTON
PENATES
PEPITAS
PERATIO
PERETTI
PERITUS
PESETAS
PETITES
PEYOTES
REACTED
REACTOR
REACTTO
REALTER
REALTOR
REATTAS
REBATED
REBATER
REBATES
REBATHE
REBOTES
RECITAL
RECITED
RECITER
RECITES
REDATED
REDATES
REDSTAR
REENTER
REENTRY
REFUTAL
REFUTED
REFUTER
REFUTES
REGATTA
REHITCH
RELATCH
RELATED
RELATER
RELATES
RELATOR
REMATCH
REMATED
REMATES
REMOTER
REMOTES
RENOTED
RENOTES
REPATCH
REPUTED
REPUTES
RERATED
RERATES

7 ET

RESITED
RETITLE
RETOTAL
REUTTER
REVITUP
REVOTED
REVOTES
REWATER
SEASTAR
SEATTLE
SEDATED
SEDATER
SEDATES
SEMITES
SEMITIC
SENATES
SENATOR
TEEITUP
TELSTAR
TEMPTED
TEMPTER
VECHTEN
VEDETTE
VEGETAL
VEINTES
VENATIC
VERITAS
WEALTHS
WEALTHY
WEBSTER
WEIRTON
XEROTIC
YEASTED
YESITIS
ZEMSTVO
ZENITHS

•E••T•

BECKETT
BEDBATH
BEDMATE
BEDSITS
BEGANTO
BEHESTS
BENEATH
BENNETT
BERETTA
BERLITZ
BETROTH
CELESTA
CELESTE
CEMENTS
DEALSTO
DEALTTO
DEBOITE
DEBRETT
DECANTS
DECEITS
DECLOTS
DECOCTS
DEDUCTS
DEFACTO
DEFEATS
DEFECTS
DEFERTO
DEFLATE
DEGUSTS
DEIGNTO
DEJECTS
DELCITY
DELICTI
DELICTO
DELICTS
DELINTS
DELISTS
DELRUTH
DEMASTS
DEMENTO
DEMISTS
DENSITY
DENTATE
DEODATO
DEPARTS
DEPESTS
DEPICTS
DEPLETE
DEPORTS
DERALTE
DERMATO
DERUSTS
DESALTS
DESERTS
DESILTS
DESISTS
DESPITE
DESPOTS
DETECTO
DETECTS
DETENTE
DETENTS
DETESTS
DEVESTS
DEVIATE
EELPOTS
FEDINTO
FEEBATE
FEEDSTO
FEMBOTS
FERMATA
FERMATE
FERMATS
FERRATE
FERRETS
FERRETY
FERRITE
GEARSTO
GEFILTE
GEMMATE
GERENTS
GESTATE
GETCUTE
GETINTO
GETONTO
HEADSTO
HEAVETO
HEIFETZ
HEIGHTS
HELMETS
HENBITS
HEPCATS
HERESTO
HERMITS
HERPETO
HEWEDTO
HEWLETT
HEXNUTS
IEIGHTY
JENNETS
JESUITS
JETSETS
KEEPSTO
KENNETH
KEYDETS
KEYNOTE
LEADETH
LEADSTO
LEANSTO
LEARNTO
LEASETO
LECONTE
LEDINTO
LEDUPTO
LEGISTS
LEMMATA
LEONATO
LEPANTO
MEANSTO
MEANTTO
MEDIATE
MELITTA
MEMENTO
MENOTTI
MERLOTS
METWITH
NEEDSTO
NEOLITH
NEOLYTE
NEONATE
NESBITT
NESMITH
NEWGATE
NEWHATS
NEWMATH
PEANUTS
PEDANTS
PELLETS
PELTATE
PENALTY
PENLITE
PENNATE
PENULTS
PEQUOTS
PERDITA
PERETTI
PERLITE
PERMITS
PERMUTE
PESANTE
PETCATS
PETGATE
PETRATS
PETSITS
REACTTO
READSTO
REALITY
REBAITS
REBASTE
REBIRTH
REBOLTS
REBOOTS
RECANTS
RECASTS
RECOATS
RECOSTS
RECRATE
REDACTS
REDANTS
REDBATS
REDDOTS
REDHATS
REDHOTS
REDOUTS
REDUSTS
REEDITS
REEMITS
REFERTO
REFLATE
REGATTA
REGENTS
REGIFTS
REGRETS
REHEATS
REJECTS
REKNITS
REKNOTS
RELENTS
RELICTS
RELISTS
RELUCTS
REMEETS
REMELTS
REMINTS
RENESTS
RENNETS
RENTSTO
REPASTE
REPASTS
REPEATS
REPENTS
REPLATE
REPLETE
REPLOTS
REPLYTO
REPORTS
REPOSTS
REQUITE
REQUOTE
RERENTS
REROOTS
REROUTE
RESALTS
RESEATS
RESECTS
RESENTS
RESHUTS
RESIFTS
RESISTS
RESLATE
RESORTS
RESPITE
RESPOTS
RESTATE
RESUITS
RESULTS
RETASTE
RETESTS
RETINTS
RETORTS
REUNITE
REVERTS
REVESTS
REVOLTS
REWRITE
REWROTE
REXCATS
REXROTH
SEACATS
SEADUTY
SEAGATE
SECANTS
SECRETE
SECRETS
SEEINTO
SEEMSTO
SELECTS
SELLSTO
SENDSTO
SENNETT
SENSATE
SEPTETS
SERIATE
SERRATE
SESTETS
SETENTA
SETINTO
SETOUTS
SETRATE
SEVENTH
SEVENTY
SEWISTS
SEXISTS
SEXPOTS
SEXTETS
TEAPOTS
TEASETS
TELESTO
TENANTS
TENDSTO
TENSITY
TENUITY
TERMITE
TERNATE
TERRETS
TESTATE
VEDETTE
VEDISTS
VEIGHTS
VELOUTE
VELVETS
VELVETY
VERISTS
VERSETS
WEBSITE
WEEBITS
WEIGHTS
WEIGHTY
WESCOTT
WESKITS
YEARNTO
YESLETS
YESVOTE
ZEALOTS
ZENISTS
ZERMATT

•E••••T

AERIEST
AEROBAT
BEARCAT
BEAROUT
BEARPIT
BEATOUT
BEATSAT
BEATSIT
BECKETT
BEDPOST
BEDREST
BEEPSAT
BEIGNET
BELFAST
BELFORT
BELMONT
BELTOUT
BENEFIT
BENNETT
BEQUEST
BEQUIET
BERENDT
BERSUNT
BERTOLT
BESTBET
BESTCUT
BETWIXT
CELLIST
CESSPIT
DEADEST
DEADSET
DEAFEST
DEALOUT
DEAREST
DEBRETT
DECKOUT
DECRYPT
DEEPEST
DEEPFAT
DEEPSET
DEFAULT
DEFFEST
DEFIANT
DEFICIT
DEFLECT
DEFROST
DEFTEST
DEFUNCT
DEGHOST
DEHMELT
DELBERT
DELIGHT
DELIMIT
DELMONT
DEMARET
DEMERIT
DEMOUNT
DENSEST
DENTIST
DEORBIT
DEPOSIT
DERWENT
DESCANT
DESCENT
DESERET
DESKSET
DESSERT
DETRACT
DETROIT
DEVIANT
DEWAART
DEWIEST
EELIEST
EELPOUT
EERIEST
FEARNOT
FEEDLOT
FEELOUT
FELLOUT
FELTHAT
FELTOUT
FERMENT
FERVENT
FEUDIST
GENESET
GERAINT
GESTALT
GETAHIT
GETBEAT
GETBENT
GETHURT
GETLOST
GETONIT
GETPAST
GETSFIT
GETSHOT
GETSOFT
GETSOUT
GETSSET
GETSWET
GETTOIT
HEADOUT
HEADSET
HEAROUT
HECKART
HELDOUT
HELLCAT
HELPOUT
HEPPEST
HERBART
HERBAUT
HERBERT
HERRIOT
HEWLETT
JEANNOT
JEERSAT
JERKOUT
JETBOAT
JETPORT
KEENEST
KEEPFIT
KEEPOUT
KEEPSAT
KEPTFIT
KEPTOUT
KEYWEST
LEADOUT
LEAFLET
LEAFOUT
LEANCUT
LEANEST
LEAPSAT
LEAPTAT
LEARJET
LEAVEIT
LEERSAT
LEFTEST
LEFTIST
LEFTOUT
LEGOSET
LEGREST
LENDOUT
LENFANT
LENIENT
LESCAUT
LESSFAT
LETSEAT
LETSNOT
LETSOUT
LETTERT
LEVERET
LEWDEST
MEANEST
MEANSIT
MEANTIT
MEDIANT
MEEKEST
MEERKAT
MEFIRST
MEGABIT
MEGAHIT
MESSKIT
METEOUT
METRIST
NEAREST
NEATEST
NECKLET
NEEDNOT
NEGLECT
NESBITT
NETCOST
NEWBOLT
NEWHART
NEWLEFT
NEWMINT
NEWMONT
NEWPORT
PEACOAT
PEASANT
PEATPOT
PECCANT
PECKSAT
PEEKOUT
PEEKSAT
PEELOUT
PEEPOUT
PEEPSAT
PEEROUT
PEERSAT
PENDANT
PENDENT
PENNANT
PERCENT
PERCEPT
PERFECT
PERIAPT
PERIDOT
PERSIST
PERTEST
PETGOAT
PEUGEOT
READAPT
READMIT
READOPT
READOUT
REAGENT
REALEST
REALIST
REALLOT
REAMOUT
REARLIT
REAUDIT
REBOANT
REBUILT
RECEIPT
RECHART
RECOUNT
RECRUIT
REDCENT
REDCOAT
REDDEST
REDDUST
REDEALT
REDEBIT
REDHEAT
REDMEAT
REDOUBT
REDRAFT
REDROOT
REDSPOT
REDSUIT
REEJECT
REELECT
REELOUT
REENACT
REERECT
REERUPT
REEVICT
REFIGHT
REFLECT
REFLOAT
REFRACT
REFRONT
REGNANT
REGRAFT
REGRANT
REGREET
RELIANT
RELIGHT
RELIMIT
REMNANT
REMOUNT
RENAULT
RENTOUT
RENUZIT
REPAINT
REPLANT
REPOINT
REPOSIT
REPRINT
REQUEST
RESHIFT
RESHOOT
RESIGHT
RESMELT
RESOJET
RESPECT
RESPELT
RESPLIT
RESTART
RETOAST
RETRACT
RETREAT
RETWIST
REVISIT
REYMONT
SEABOAT
SEAGIRT
SEAHUNT
SEALANT
SEALIFT
SEAMIST
SEAPORT
SEASALT
SEEDLET
SEEKOUT
SEENFIT
SEENOUT
SEEPAST
SEEPOUT
SEESFIT
SEESOUT
SEETOIT
SEGMENT
SELLOUT
SELLSIT
SENDOUT
SENNETT
SENTOUT
SERPENT
SERVANT
SETSHOT
SETSOUT
SEXIEST
SEXTANT
TEACART
TEAROUT
TEARSAT
TEARSIT
TEESHOT
TELLSIT
TEMPEST
TENCENT
TENFEET
TENFOOT
TENNANT
TENPAST
TENSEST
TENSPOT
TERSEST
TESTKIT
TESTOUT
VEINLET
VERDANT
VERDICT
VERIEST
VERMONT
VERSANT
VERYFIT
VERYHOT
VERYWET
WEAKEST
WEAROUT
WEBCAST
WEBFEET
WEBFOOT
WEDIDIT
WEEDOUT
WELLCUT
WELLHIT
WELLLIT
WELLPUT
WELLSET
WENTAFT
WENTOUT
WESCOTT
WETSUIT
WETTEST
YEAHBUT
YELLOUT
YELLSAT
ZERMATT
ZEROOUT

••ET•••

ABETTAL
ABETTED
ABETTER
ABETTOR
ACETALS
ACETATE
ACETIFY
ACETONE
ALETAPS
ALETTES
ARETINO
BEETIER
BEETLES
BEETRED
BEETREE
BRETONS
BRETTON
CHETRUM
COETZEE
CRETANS
CRETINS
CUETIPS
DIETARY
DIETERS
DIETING
DUETING
DUETTED
DUETTOS
EMETICS
EYETEST
EYETUCK
FRETFUL
FRETSAT
FRETSAW
FRETTED
FRETTER
GAETANO
GHETTOS
GJETOST
GRETZKY
HRETHEL
ICETEAS
ICETRAY
KVETCHY
LEETIDE
LIETEST
MEETERS
MEETING
MEETSUP
NOETICS
ONETERM
ONETIME
ONETOGO
ONETWOS
OSETRAS
PIETIES
PIETINS
PIETOSO
PIETROS
POETESS
POETICA
POETICS
POETISE
POETIZE
PRETAPE
PRETEEN
PRETELL
PRETEND
PRETERM
PRETEST
PRETEXT
PRETIRE
PRETOLD
PRETORS
PRETRIM
PRETYPE
PRETZEL
QUETZAL
RHETORS
ROETHKE
SEETHED
SEETHES
SEETHRU
SEETOIT
SKETCHY
SMETANA
STETSON
STETTED
TEETERS
TEETHED
TEETHER
TEETHES
TEETIME
THETOUR
THETREE
THETRIB
THETUBE
THETURN
TIETACK
TIETACS
TOETAPS
TSETSES
TSETUNG
VIETNAM
WHETHER
WHETTED
WHETTER

••E•T••

ABETTAL
ABETTED
ABETTER
ABETTOR
ADEPTAT
ADEPTER
ADEPTLY
AGENTED
AGENTRY
ALERTED
ALERTER
ALERTLY
ALERTTO
ALETTES
ASEETHE
ASEPTIC
ATEITUP
AVERTED
AVERTER
AVESTAN
AVESTAS
BEEFTEA
BEERTAP
BIENTOT
BLEATED
BLEATER
BLENTIN
BREATHE
BREATHS
BREATHY
BRETTON
CHEATED
CHEATER
CHEATIN
CHEATON
CHEETAH
CHEETAS
CHEETOS
CHESTED
CHESTER
CHEWTOY
CLEATED
COEPTIS
CREATED
CREATES
CREATOR
CREPTIN
CREPTUP
CRESTED
CRESTON
CUESTAS
DEEPTAN
DOESTOO
DUETTED
DUETTOS
DWELTON
EGESTED
EJECTED
EJECTOR
ELECTED
ELECTEE
ELECTME
ELECTOR
ELECTRA
ELECTRO
ELEKTRA
ERECTED
ERECTER
ERECTLY
ERECTOR
ERECTUS
EVERTED
EVERTOR
EXERTED
EXERTER
FIESTAS
FLEETED
FLEETER
FLEETLY
FREETOY
FREITAG
FRETTED
FRETTER
FREYTAG

FUENTES
GHETTOS
GREATEN
GREATER
GREATLY
GREETED
GREETER
GUESTED
HEELTAP
ICEDTEA
IDEATED
IDEATES
IDENTIC
INEPTLY
INERTIA
INERTLY
KLEPTOS
LAERTES
LIEATOP
LLEYTON
MAESTRO
NOENTRY
NUESTRA
NUESTRO
OBENTOS
OLEATES
OLESTRA
ONESTAR
ONESTEP
ONESTOP
OPENTAP
OPENTOE
OPENTOP
ORECTIC
ORESTES
OVERTAX
OVERTIP
OVERTLY
OVERTOP
PLEATED
PLECTRA
PRESTON
PRESTOS
QUENTIN
QUESTED
QUESTER
REENTER
REENTRY
SCENTED
SCENTER
SCEPTER
SCEPTIC
SCEPTRE
SHEATHE
SHEATHS
SHEETED
SHELTER
SHELTIE
SIESTAS
SKEETER
SKELTER
SKELTON
SKEPTIC
SLEETED
SLEPTIN
SLEPTON
SLEUTHS
SMELTED
SMELTER
SNEETCH
SPECTER
SPECTOR
SPECTRA
SPECTRE
SPENTON
STENTOR
STEPTWO
STERTOR
STETTED
SVELTER
SWEATED
SWEATER
SWEATIT
SWEETEN
SWEETER
SWEETIE
SWEETLY
SWEETON
SWELTER
SWELTRY
SWEPTUP
TEEITUP
THEATER
THEATRE
THESTAR
TREATED
TREATER
TREETOP
TRENTON
TRESTLE
TWEETED
TWEETER
UNEATEN
WHEATEN
WHEATON
WHETTED
WHETTER
WREATHE
WREATHS
WREATHY
WRESTED
WRESTER
WRESTLE

••E••T•

ACERATE
ACETATE
AGEISTS
AGEMATE
ALERTTO
AMENITY
APELETS
ATEINTO
ATELATE
BREADTH
BREASTS
BREVETS
BREVITY
CHELATE
CHEVETS
CLEANTE
COEDITS
CREDITS
CREMATE
CRENATE
DIECUTS
DUEDATE
DYEBATH
DYELOTS
DYEVATS
EDEMATA
ELEGITS
ELEVATE
EMERITA
EMERITI
EREMITE
EVERETT
EXECUTE
EXEGETE
EXEMPTS
EXEUNTS
EYELETS
EYEPITS
FEEBATE
FEEDSTO
ICEBATH
ICEOUTS
INEDITA
ITERATE
JOEROTH
KEEPSTO
NEEDSTO
NOENDTO
OBESITY
OCELOTS
ODELETS
OMELETS
ONEACTS
ONEARTH
ONEBYTE
ONEIOTA
ONEMPTY
ONENOTE
ONEONTA
ONEVOTE
OPERATE
OVERATE
PLEADTO
PREACTS
PRECITE
PRECUTS
PREDATA
PREDATE
PRELATE
PREMATE
PRESETS
PREVETO
PREWITT
REEDITS
REEMITS
SEEINTO
SEEMSTO
SHEVATS
SPEAKTO
STEALTH
SWEARTO
THEARTS
THECITY
THEISTS
THEJETS
THEMETS
THENETS
THEOATH
THEPITS
THERETO
THERITZ
TIEINTO
TREINTA
TWELFTH
UNEARTH
UNEMPTY
VIEWITH
WEEBITS
WHERETO
YIELDTO

••E•••T

ABEYANT
ACEDOUT
ACESOUT
ADEPTAT
AGEDOUT
AGESOUT
APEDIET
APESUIT
ATEABIT
ATEALOT
ATEDIRT
ATEIGHT
AWEEBIT
BEEPSAT
BIENTOT
BLERIOT
BLEWOUT
CHEEZIT
CHEMIST
CHEROOT
CHEVIOT
CHEVRET
CHEWOUT
CLEMENT
COEXIST
CRESSET
CREWCUT
DEEPEST
DEEPFAT
DEEPSET
DIECAST
DIEDOUT
DIESOUT
DOESNOT
DREWOUT
DUEEAST
DUELIST
DUEWEST
DWELLAT
EKEDOUT
EKESOUT
ELEGANT
ELEGIST
ELEMENT
EPEEIST
EVENBET
EVENEST
EVENOUT
EVEREST
EVERETT
EYEBOLT
EYELIFT
EYESHOT
EYESPOT
EYETEST
FEEDLOT
FEELOUT
FLEAPIT
FREIGHT
FREMONT
FRESHET
FRETSAT
GJETOST
GOESAFT
GOESOUT
GREWFAT
GREYEST
GUESSAT
ICEBOAT
ICEDOUT
ICESOUT
IMEANIT
INEXACT
IREPEAT
ITERANT
JEERSAT
KEENEST
KEEPFIT
KEEPOUT
KEEPSAT
KNESSET
LEERSAT
LIEFEST
LIETEST
MAEWEST
MEEKEST
MEERKAT
NEEDNOT
ONEACAT
ONECENT
ONEFOOT
ONEOCAT
ONEPART
ONEPINT
ONESHOT
ONESPOT
ONEUNIT
ONEWHIT
OPENNET
OPENOUT
OPENPIT
OPERANT
OVERACT
OVERBET
OVERCUT
OVEREAT
OVERFAT
OVERFIT
OVERHOT
OVERLET
OVERLIT
OVERSET
OVERWET
PEEKOUT
PEEKSAT
PEELOUT
PEEPOUT
PEEPSAT
PEEROUT
PEERSAT
PIERROT
PNEUMAT
PRECAST
PRECEPT
PREDICT
PREDIET
PREEDIT
PREEMPT
PREFECT
PREHEAT
PREMEET
PREOMIT
PREPLOT
PRERENT
PRERIOT
PRESALT
PRESEAT
PRESENT
PRESIFT
PRESORT
PRETEST
PRETEXT
PREVENT
PREVERT
PREVOST
PREWITT
QUEENIT
QUERIST
REEJECT
REELECT
REELOUT
REENACT
REERECT
REERUPT
REEVICT
RIEGERT
SEEDLET
SEEKOUT
SEENFIT
SEENOUT
SEEPAST
SEEPOUT
SEESFIT
SEESOUT
SEETOIT
SHEGOAT
SHERBET
SLEIGHT
SNEERAT
SPECOUT
SPEWOUT
STEPOUT
STEWART
STEWPOT
SWEARAT
SWEATIT
TEESHOT
THEBEST
THEBRAT
THEDIET
THEEAST
THEGIFT
THEHEAT
THELEFT
THEMOST
THEPOST
THEREAT
THERENT
TREELET
TREERAT
TSELIOT
TWERENT
UNERECT
WEEDOUT
WHEREAT

•••ET••

AMMETER
ANNETTE
APPETIT
ARIETTA
ARIETTE
ASCETIC
ASEETHE
AULETTA
BABETTE
BARETTA
BASETEN
BASETWO
BERETTA
BIMETAL
BIRETTA
BLUETIT
BURETTE
CADETTE
CAKETIN
CANETTI
CHEETAH
CHEETAS
CHEETOS
COLETTE
CORETTA
COSETTE
COVETED
COVETER
CURETTE
CUVETTE
DALETHS
DELETED
DELETES
DEMETER
DIMETER
DINETTE
DONETSK
EIDETIC
FACETED
FAYETTE
FENETRE
FIVETEN
FIVETWO
FLEETED
FLEETER
FLEETLY
FORETOP
FOUETTE
FREETOY
GALETTE
GAMETAL
GAMETES
GAZETTE
GENETIC
GOGETEM
GORETEX
GREETED
GREETER
HERETIC
IAPETUS
IIPETER
IMPETUS
ISLETED
KADETTS
KINETIC
LANETWO
LATETAG
LAYETTE
LILETEE
LINETWO
LIZETTE
LONETTE
LORETTA
LOVETAP
LUCETTA
LUNETTE
LUTETIA
LYNETTE
MANETTE
MIMETIC
MORETTI
MOZETTA
MULETAS
MUSETTA
MUSETTE
NAMETAG
NANETTE
NICETRY
NIDETCH
NONETTE
OCTETTE
ORNETTE
OSSETRA
PAGETWO
PALETTE
PANETTA
PERETTI
PESETAS
PHAETON
PINETAR
PINETOP
PINETUM
PIPETTE
PRAETOR
PYRETIC
QUIETED
QUIETEN
QUIETER
QUIETLY
QUIETUS
RIVETED
RIVETER
RONETTE
ROPETOW
ROSETEA
ROSETTA
ROSETTE
ROVETTA
SAGETEA
SHEETED
SHTETLS
SIDETWO
SIZETEN
SIZETWO
SKEETER
SLEETED
SNEETCH
STPETER
STRETCH
STRETTI
STRETTO
SUZETTE
SWEETEN
SWEETER
SWEETIE
SWEETLY
SWEETON
TAKETEA
TAKETEN
TIBETAN
TONETTE
TREETOP
TUBETOP
TWEETED
TWEETER
UNFETED
VALETED
VEDETTE
VEGETAL
VIDETTE
VUMETER
WIRETAP
WYNETTE
ZANETTO

•••E•T•

ABSENTS
ACCENTS
ACCEPTS
ADDEDTO
ADVENTS
ADVERTS
AFFECTS
AGREETO
ALBERTA
ALBERTI
ALBERTO
ALCESTE
ALDENTE
ALIENTO
AMNESTY
AMREETA
ANNETTE
APLENTY
ARGENTI
ARGENTO
ARGENTS
ARIETTA
ARIETTE
ARRESTS
ASCENTS
ASPECTS
ASSENTS
ASSERTS
ATTESTS
AULETTA
AUREATE
BABETTE
BARENTS
BARETTA
BEHESTS
BENEATH
BERETTA
BIRETTA
BISECTS
BOWEDTO
BURETTE
CADETTE
CANETTI
CAREDTO
CARESTO
CASEATE
CASERTA
CATERTO
CAVEATS
CELESTA
CELESTE
CEMENTS
CILENTO
CLIENTS
COLETTE
COMESTO
CORETTA
COSETTE
COVERTS
CRUELTY
CUNEATE
CURETTE
CUVETTE
DARESTO
DECEITS
DEFEATS
DEFECTS
DEFERTO
DEJECTS
DEMENTO
DEPESTS
DESERTS
DETECTO
DETECTS
DETENTE
DETENTS
DETESTS
DEVESTS
DIGESTS
DINETTE
DIRECTS
DIRECTV
DIVERTS
DIVESTS
DOCENTS
DOHERTY
DOZENTH
DRTEETH
EFFECTS
ELBERTA
ENSEATS
ENTENTE
ERNESTA
ERNESTO
EXCEPTS
EXPECTS
EXPERTS
EXSECTS
EXSERTS
EXTENTS
FAYETTE
FLIEDTO
FLIESTO
FOGERTY
FOMENTS
FORESTS
FOUETTE
GALEATE
GALENTO
GALETTE
GASEITY
GAZETTE
GERENTS
GIVENTO
GIVESTO
GLUEDTO
GLUESTO
HAGERTY
HERESTO
HEWEDTO
HONESTY
HOPEDTO
HOPESTO
INCENTS
INCEPTS
INDENTS
INDEPTH
INFECTS
INFESTS
INGESTA
INGESTS
INJECTS
INSECTA
INSECTS
INSERTS
INTENTS
INVENTS
INVERTS
INVESTS
IQTESTS
ITWENTY
JADEITE
KADETTS
LACERTA
LAMENTS
LATENTS
LAYETTE
LIBERTE
LIBERTY
LIKENTO
LINEATE
LISENTE
LIZETTE
LONETTE
LORENTZ
LORETTA
LOSESTO
LOVEDTO
LOVESTO
LUCETTA
LUNESTA
LUNETTE
LYNETTE
MAGENTA
MAJESTE
MAJESTY
MANETTE
MEMENTO
MODELTS
MODESTO
MODESTY
MOLESTS
MOMENTA
MOMENTS
MORETTI
MOVEDTO
MOVESTO
MOZETTA
MUSETTA
MUSETTE
NANETTE
NONETTE
NOSEATS
NOVELTY
OBJECTS
OBTESTS
OBVERTS
OCHENTA
OCTETTE
OPTEDTO
ORGEATS
ORIENTE
ORIENTS
ORNETTE
OUTEATS
PALETTE
PANETTA
PAPEETE
PARENTS
PATENTS
PERETTI
PILEATE
PIMENTO
PIPETTE
PLOESTI
POLENTA
POVERTY
PRIESTS
PUBERTY
RACEDTO
RACESTO
REFERTO
REGENTS
REHEATS
REJECTS
RELENTS
REMEETS
REMELTS
RENESTS
REPEATS
REPENTS
RERENTS
RESEATS
RESECTS
RESENTS
RETESTS
REVERTS
REVESTS
RIDESTO
RISENTO
RISESTO
ROBERTA
ROBERTE
ROBERTF
ROBERTH
ROBERTI
ROBERTO
ROBERTS
RODENTS
RONETTE
ROSEATE
ROSETTA
ROSETTE
ROVETTA
SELECTS
SETENTA
SEVENTH
SEVENTY
SILENTA
SILENTB
SILENTC
SILENTD
SILENTE
SILENTF
SILENTG
SILENTH
SILENTI
SILENTJ
SILENTK
SILENTL
SILENTM
SILENTN
SILENTO
SILENTP
SILENTQ
SILENTR
SILENTS
SILENTT
SILENTU
SILENTV
SILENTW
SILENTX
SILENTY
SILENTZ
SORENTO
STREETS
STRETTI
STRETTO
SUZETTE
TAKENTO
TAKESTO
TALENTS
TELESTO
THREATS
TONETTE
TRIEDTO
TRIESTE
TRIESTO
TRUERTO
TUNEDTO
TUNESTO
UMBERTO
UNBELTS
UNBERTH
UNFERTH
UNRESTS
UNSEATS
UPBEATS
URTEXTS
VALENTE
VALENTI
VEDETTE
VICENTE
VIDETTE
VOLENTE
WAVEDTO
WAVESTO
WBYEATS
WYNETTE
ZANETTO

•••E••T

ABREAST
AIMEDAT

AMHERST
APPETIT
ATHEART
ATHEIST
ATLEAST
ATTEMPT
AWEEBIT
BAGEHOT
BAKERST
BASEHIT
BAYEDAT
BENEFIT
BERENDT
BIBELOT
BIGEAST
BLUETIT
BONELET
BONESET
BOOEDAT
BOREOUT
BYHEART
CAGEPET
CAMELOT
CAMEOUT
CAPELET
CASELOT
CASEOUT
CAVEART
CHEEZIT
COMEOUT
COMESAT
CONELET
COWERAT
DARENOT
DEMERIT
DESERET
DIDEROT
DINEDAT
DINEOUT
DINESAT
DOLEOUT
DOPEOUT
DOVECOT
DOVELET
DUEEAST
EASEOUT
EATENAT
EDGEOUT
ENDEDAT
ENDEDIT
EPEEIST
EXCELAT
EXCERPT
FACEDIT
FACESIT
FADEOUT
FAKEDIT
FAKEOUT
FAKESIT
FAREAST
FILEOUT
FINEART
FIREANT
FIREDAT
FIREHAT
FIRELIT
FIREPIT
FIRESAT

FLIESAT
FUMEDAT
FUMESAT
GAPEDAT
GAPESAT
GAVEOUT
GAZEDAT
GAZESAT
GENESET
GIBESAT
GIVEOUT
GONEAFT
GONEOUT
HATEDIT
HATESIT
HAVENOT
HAVEOUT
HIDEOUT
HIKEOUT
HIREOUT
HOLEOUT
HOPENOT
IKNEWIT
ILLEGIT
INHERIT
JAWEDAT
JIBEDAT
JIBESAT
LEVERET
LIFENET
LINECUT
LINEOUT
LIVEOUT
LIVESAT
LIVESET
LOSEOUT
LOSESIT
LOVEDIT
LOVESET
LOVESIT
MADEFIT
MADEOUT
MAKEFIT
MAKEOUT
MAKESIT
MALEANT
MALECAT
METEOUT
MIDEAST
MINEPIT
MISEDIT
MOLERAT
MOVEDIT
MOVEOUT
MOVESIT
NOSEOUT
OGDENUT
OOZEOUT
OXHEART
PAGEANT
PAWEDAT
PINENUT
POKEDAT
POKEOUT
POKESAT
POLECAT
POLESAT
POLESIT

PREEDIT
PREEMPT
PROEAST
QUEENIT
RAREBIT
RECEIPT
REDEALT
REDEBIT
RIDEOUT
RODEOUT
RULEOUT
SAFEBET
SCHELDT
SIDEBET
SILENTT
SNEERAT
SUREBET
TAKEOUT
TAKESIT
THEEAST
THREWAT
TIMEOUT
TIREOUT
TOHEART
TOREOUT
TREELET
TREERAT
TRIEDIT
TRIESIT
TUNEOUT
TYPESET
UNBESET
UNDEALT
UNKEMPT
UNMEANT
UPLEAPT
UTRECHT
VOTEOUT
WAVEDAT
WAVELET
WAVESAT
WINEVAT
WIPEOUT
WITEOUT
WOREOUT
ZONEOUT

••••ET•

ACCRETE
AGREETO
AIGLETS
AIGRETS
ALIVETO
AMREETA
AMULETS
ANKLETS
ANXIETY
APELETS
APPLETS
ARMLETS
ATHLETE
AUKLETS
AVOCETS
BALLETS
BARBETS
BARRETS
BARRETT
BASKETS

BASKETT
BASSETS
BASSETT
BECKETT
BENNETT
BIGBETS
BILLETS
BONNETS
BOXSETS
BREVETS
BRUNETS
BUCKETS
BUDGETS
BUFFETS
BUFFETT
BULLETS
BURNETT
CABLETS
CABLETV
CACHETS
CAPLETS
CARNETS
CARPETS
CASKETS
CHALETS
CHEVETS
CLARETS
CLORETS
CLOSETO
CLOSETS
COLLETS
COMPETE
CORBETT
CORNETS
CORSETS
COSSETS
CULLETS
CURVETS
CUTLETS
CYGNETS
DEBRETT
DEPLETE
DIPNETS
DOCKETS
DOGGETT
DORSETT
DRIVETO
DROVETO
DRTEETH
DUBIETY
EAGLETS
EARLETS
ELANETS
ESTHETE
EVERETT
EXCRETE
EXEGETE
EXOCETS
EYELETS
FANJETS
FAUCETS
FAWCETT
FERRETS
FERRETY
FIDGETS
FIDGETY
FILLETS
FLORETS

FLYNETS
FOLLETT
FORGETS
GADGETS
GADGETY
GANNETS
GANNETT
GARNETS
GARNETT
GARRETS
GARRETT
GASJETS
GASKETS
GIBLETS
GIMLETS
GOBLETS
GOSSETT
GULLETS
GUSSETS
GWYNETH
HACKETT
HAMLETS
HAMMETT
HEAVETO
HEIFETZ
HELMETS
HERPETO
HEWLETT
HORNETS
IMARETS
IMPIETY
ININETY
INKJETS
JACKETS
JAPHETH
JARRETT
JENNETS
JETSETS
JUNKETS
KENNETH
KEYDETS
KISMETS
KNOWETH
KUZNETS
LAMBETH
LANCETS
LAPPETS
LEADETH
LEASETO
LICKETY
LIGGETT
LIMPETS
LINNETS
LIONETS
LISBETH
LOCKETS
MACBETH
MACHETE
MAGNETO
MAGNETS
MALLETS
MARKETS
MIDGETS
MILLETS
MILLETT
MINUETS
MISSETS
MOPPETS

MULLETS
MUPPETS
MUSKETS
NAIVETE
NAIVETY
NCWYETH
NIBLETS
NIMIETY
NUGGETS
NUGGETY
NUTLETS
ODELETS
OFFSETS
OMELETS
ORVIETO
OUTJETS
OUTLETS
OUTSETS
PACKETS
PADGETT
PALLETS
PAPEETE
PELLETS
PICKETS
PICKETT
PIGLETS
PINKETT
PIOLETS
PLANETS
POCKETS
PRESETS
PREVETO
PRIVETS
PROJETS
PRONETO
PUCKETT
PULLETS
PUPPETS
RABBETS
RACKETS
RACKETY
RAMJETS
REGRETS
REMEETS
RENNETS
REPLETE
RIBLETS
RICKETY
RILLETS
ROCHETS
ROCKETS
RUNLETS
RUNNETH
RUSSETS
RUSSETY
SACHETS
SAMLETS
SATIETY
SECRETE
SECRETS
SENNETT
SEPTETS
SESTETS
SEXTETS
SIGNETS
SOCIETY
SOCKETS
SONNETS

SORBETS
SOVIETS
SPIKETV
SPINETS
SPOKETO
STREETS
STYLETS
SUBLETS
SUBNETS
SUBSETS
SUNSETS
SWIVETS
SWORETO
TABLETS
TABSETS
TAFFETA
TAPPETS
TARGETS
TEASETS
TERRETS
THEJETS
THEMETS
THENETS
THERETO
TIBBETT
TICKETS
TILLETS
TIPPETS
TOILETS
TRIJETS
TRIVETS
TUFFETS
TURRETS
UNPIETY
VARIETY
VARLETS
VELVETS
VELVETY
VERSETS
VIOLETS
WALLETS
WARVETS
WHERETO
WICKETS
WIDGETS
WIGLETS
WRITETO
WROTETO
YESLETS

••••E•T

ACHIEST
ACUTEST
AERIEST
AGILEST
AILMENT
AIRIEST
AIRVENT
ALIMENT
AMBIENT
AMPLEST
ANAPEST
ANCIENT
ARCHEST
ARIDEST
ARMREST
ARTIEST
ASHIEST

ASSWEET
AUGMENT
AVIDEST
AWAREST
BABIEST
BADDEBT
BADDEST
BALDEST
BARRETT
BASKETT
BASSETT
BATNEXT
BECKETT
BEDREST
BENNETT
BEQUEST
BIGBEAT
BIGFEET
BIGGEST
BIGTENT
BOLDEST
BONIEST
BOOKERT
BOXIEST
BOXSEAT
BRAVEST
BUFFEST
BUFFETT
BURNETT
BUSIEST
BUTTEMT
CAGIEST
CAKIEST
CALMEST
CALVERT
CANDENT
CANIEST
CARSEAT
CATBERT
CATFEET
CHICEST
CLEMENT
CLOSEST
COAGENT
COKIEST
COLBERT
COLDEST
COLLECT
COMMENT
CONCEIT
CONCEPT
CONCERT
CONFECT
CONGEST
CONNECT
CONSENT
CONTENT
CONTEST
CONTEXT
CONVECT
CONVENT
CONVERT
COOLEST
CORBETT
CORRECT
COSIEST
COWIEST
COZIEST

CRUDEST
CULVERT
CURRENT
CURSEAT
CURTEST
DAFTEST
DAMPEST
DANKEST
DARKEST
DEADEST
DEAFEST
DEAREST
DEBRETT
DEEPEST
DEFFEST
DEFLECT
DEFTEST
DEHMELT
DELBERT
DENSEST
DERWENT
DESCENT
DESSERT
DEWIEST
DIALECT
DICIEST
DILBERT
DILUENT
DIMMEST
DISSECT
DISSENT
DISSERT
DNATEST
DOGBERT
DOGGETT
DOGREAT
DOGVEST
DOPIEST
DORSETT
DOUREST
DOZIEST
DRIVEAT
DROVEAT
DRYHEAT
DUEWEST
DULLEST
DUMBEST
DURWENT
EARNEST
EASIEST
EDGIEST
EELIEST
EERIEST
EGGIEST
ELEMENT
ELITEST
ELMIEST
EMINENT
ENTREAT
ERODENT
ESCHEAT
EVENEST
EVEREST
EVERETT
EVIDENT
EVILEST
EXIGENT
EYETEST

FABBEST
FAINEST
FAIREST
FALSEST
FANBELT
FANFEST
FARLEFT
FARWEST
FASTEST
FATTEST
FAWCETT
FERMENT
FERVENT
FIGMENT
FILBERT
FIRMEST
FITTEST
FOLLETT
FONDEST
FORFEIT
FORRENT
FORREST
FORWENT
FOULEST
FOXIEST
FULGENT
FULLEST
FUMIEST
FUNFEST
GABFEST
GAMIEST
GANNETT
GARMENT
GARNETT
GARRETT
GASHEAT
GETBEAT
GETBENT
GILBERT
GLAREAT
GLUIEST
GODSENT
GOOIEST
GORIEST
GOSSETT
GOTBEAT
GRAVEST
GRAYEST
GREYEST
GUNBELT
HACKETT
HADBEST
HAMMETT
HARDEST
HARVEST
HASTERT
HAZIEST
HEPPEST
HERBERT
HEWLETT
HIGHEST
HILBERT
HIPPEST
HOKIEST
HOLIEST
HOMIEST
HOTSEAT
HOTTEST

HOWBEIT
HUMBERT
HUPPERT
ICKIEST
IDTHEFT
IFFIEST
IHATEIT
IHAVEIT
ILIKEIT
ILOVEIT
IMADEIT
IMGREAT
IMPREST
INANEST
INDWELT
INFLECT
INKIEST
INQUEST
INSPECT
INSWEPT
IOBJECT
IRATEST
IREPEAT
ITSBEST
JARRETT
JIVIEST
JOKIEST
JROBERT
JUSTEST
KEENEST
KEYWEST
KIDSEAT
KINDEST
KURRENT
LABTEST
LACIEST
LAKIEST
LAMBENT
LAMBERT
LAMPERT
LANKEST
LAPBELT
LARGENT
LARGEST
LAURENT
LAZIEST
LEANEST
LEAVEIT
LEFTEST
LEGREST
LENIENT
LETSEAT
LETTERT
LEWDEST
LIEFEST
LIETEST
LIGGETT
LIMIEST
LIMPEST
LINIEST
LITHEST
LOGIEST
LONGEST
LOOSEST
LORIENT
LOUDEST
LOWRENT
LUNGEAT

LUSHEST
MADDEST
MAEWEST
MAZIEST
MEANEST
MEEKEST
MIDWEST
MILDEST
MILLETT
MIRIEST
MISSEAT
MISSENT
MOPIEST
MORDENT
MYTREAT
NAIVEST
NASCENT
NEAREST
NEATEST
NEGLECT
NEWLEFT
NIGHEST
NOBLEST
NONMEAT
NORBERT
NOSIEST
NOSWEAT
NUMBEST
NUTMEAT
OAKIEST
ODDMENT
OFFBEAT
OILHEAT
OILIEST
OLDWEST
ONALERT
ONECENT
ONLIEST
ONTHEQT
OOZIEST
OPULENT
OUTJEST
OUTKEPT
OUTSERT
OUTWENT
OUTWEPT
OUTWEST
OVEREAT
OWLIEST
OZZFEST
PACIEST
PADGETT
PATIENT
PAYMENT
PENDENT
PERCENT
PERCEPT
PERFECT
PERTEST
PEUGEOT
PICKETT
PIGMEAT
PIGMENT
PINIEST
PINKEST
PINKETT
PIPIEST
POKIEST

POOREST
PORTENT
POSHEST
PRECEPT
PREFECT
PREHEAT
PREMEET
PRERENT
PRESEAT
PRESENT
PRETEST
PRETEXT
PREVENT
PREVERT
PROJECT
PROTECT
PROTEST
PROVEIT
PROWEST
PRUDENT
PUCKETT
PUNGENT
PUNIEST
PUPTENT
RACIEST
RAIMENT
RANKEST
RASHEST
RATBERT
RAWMEAT
REAGENT
REALEST
REDCENT
REDDEST
REDHEAT
REDMEAT
REEJECT
REELECT
REERECT
REFLECT
REGREET
REQUEST
RESMELT
RESPECT
RESPELT
RETREAT
RIBMEAT
RICHEST
RIEGERT
RIMIEST
ROPIEST
ROSIEST
RUCKERT
RULIEST
RUSSERT
SADDEST
SAGIEST
SALIENT
SAPIENT
SARGENT
SEGMENT
SENNETT
SERPENT
SEXIEST
SHUBERT
SICKEST
SIXFEET
SKIVEST

SLOWEST
SMILEAT
SNIDEST
SNIPEAT
SOFTEST
SOLVEIT
SOLVENT
SOONEST
SOUREST
SOYLENT
SPAREST
SPRIEST
SPRYEST
STALEST
STAREAT
STUDENT
SUAVEST
SUBJECT
SUBSECT
SUBTEXT
SUBVERT
SUGGEST
SUNBELT
SURFEIT
SUSPECT
SWIGERT
SWOREAT
TALLEST
TANGENT
TANNEST
TARTEST
TASTEIT
TAUTEST
TEMPEST
TENCENT
TENFEET
TENSEST
TERSEST
THEBEST
THEHEAT
THELEFT
THEREAT
THERENT
TIBBETT
TIDIEST
TINIEST
TONIEST
TORMENT
TORRENT
TRABERT
TRIDENT
TRISECT
TRITEST
TWERENT
TWOFEET
UGLIEST
UNADEPT
UNALERT
UNBLENT
UNBLEST
UNCLEFT
UNERECT
UNGUENT
UNINERT
UNOVERT
UNSPELT
UNSPENT
UNSWEET
UNSWEPT
UPSWEPT
VAGUEST
VAINEST
VANPELT
VASTEST
VERIEST
VIADENT
VINCENT
VINIEST
VIOLENT
WACKEST
WANIEST
WANNEST
WARIEST
WARMEST
WAVIEST
WAXIEST
WEAKEST
WEBFEET
WETTEST
WHEREAT
WHITEST
WILBERT
WILDEST
WILIEST
WINIEST
WIRIEST
YOUREIT
ZANIEST
ZOOIEST

•••••ET

ANNULET
APEDIET
ASQUIET
ASSWEET
BALLUET
BANDLET
BANQUET
BARONET
BARTLET
BAYONET
BEIGNET
BEQUIET
BESTBET
BIGFEET
BLANKET
BOMBLET
BONELET
BONESET
BOOKLET
BOOMLET
BOUQUET
BOURGET
BRACKET
BRIDGET
BRIQUET
BRISKET
BULBLET
CABARET
CABINET
CAGEPET
CALUMET
CAPELET
CAPULET
CATFEET
CHAPLET
CHARVET
CHEVRET
CHIAPET
CHICLET
CIRCLET
CONELET
CORONET
COUPLET
COURBET
CRESSET
CRICKET
CROCHET
CROCKET
CROQUET
CRUGUET
CRUMPET
DATASET
DAUSSET
DEADSET
DEEPSET
DEMARET
DESERET
DESKSET
DIDASET
DIGIPET
DOUBLET
DOVELET
DRAGNET
DRIBLET
DROPLET
DROPNET
DRUMSET
EPAULET
EPITHET
ETICKET
EVENBET
FADDIET
FASTNET
FILMSET
FISHNET
FLATLET
FOOTLET
FRESHET
FROGLET
GANTLET
GENESET
GETSSET
GETSWET
GIFTSET
GILLNET
GOURMET
GRISLET
GROMMET
HADASET
HAIRNET
HANDSET
HARDSET
HARRIET
HASASET
HATCHET
HDTVSET
HEADSET
IFORGET
JACONET
JOLLIET
JUILLET
KINGLET
KNESSET
LEAFLET
LEARJET
LEGOSET
LEVERET
LIFENET
LIVESET
LOCKLET
LOCKSET
LOSTPET
LOVESET
MAIGRET
MANTLET
MARGRET
MINARET
MINDSET
MOONLET
MOONSET
NAILSET
NECKLET
NICOLET
NONDIET
NONPOET
NULLSET
ONADIET
OPENNET
OVERBET
OVERLET
OVERSET
OVERWET
PARAPET
PARQUET
PLACKET
PLAYLET
PLUMMET
PREDIET
PREMEET
PROPHET
PROPJET
QUARTET
QUINTET
QUONSET
RACQUET
RATCHET
REGREET
RESOJET
RINGLET
RIPPLET
RIVULET
ROOTLET
SAFEBET
SAMOSET
SATINET
SCARLET
SEEDLET
SHERBET
SIDEBET
SINGLET
SIXFEET
SKILLET
SNICKET
SNIGLET
SNIPPET
SOAPNET
STARLET
SUREBET
TABARET
TABORET
TAGAMET
TARTLET
TENFEET
THEDIET
THICKET
TOOLSET
TOWNLET
TREELET
TRINKET
TRIOLET
TRIPLET
TRIPPET
TRUMPET
TWINJET
TWINSET
TWOFEET
TYPESET
UNBESET
UNQUIET
UNSWEET
VEINLET
VERYWET
WAVELET
WEBFEET
WELLSET
WHIPPET
WINGLET
WINSLET

EU•••••

EUBANKS
EUCERIN
EUCHRED
EUCHRES
EUDEMON
EUGENIA
EUGENIC
EUGENIE
EUGLENA
EULABUS
EUNOMIA
EUONYMS
EUPHONY
EURASIA
EUREKAS
EUROPOP
EUROVAN
EUSTACE
EUTERPE

E•U••••

ECUADOR
ECUELLE
EDUARDO
EDUCATE
EDUCING
EDUCTED
EDUCTOR
EKUELES
ELUANTS
ELUATES
ELUDERS
ELUDING
ELUSIVE
ELUSORY
ELUTING
ELUTION
ELUVIAL
ELUVIUM
EMULATE
EMULOUS
ENURING
EQUABLE
EQUABLY
EQUALED
EQUALLY
EQUALTO
EQUATED
EQUATES
EQUATOR
EQUERRY
EQUIANO
EQUIFAX
EQUINES
EQUINOX
ERUCTED
ERUDITE
ERUPTED
ERUPTER
EVULSED
EVULSES
EXUDATE
EXUDING
EXULTED
EXUPERY
EXURBAN
EXURBIA

E••U•••

EDMUNDI
EDMUNDS
EDOUARD
EFFUSED
EFFUSES
ELFUDGE
ELMUNDO
EMMUSKA
EMQUADS
ENDUING
ENDUPAT
ENDURED
ENDURER
ENDURES
ENDUROS
ENDUSER
ENDUSES
ENGULFS
ENOUNCE
ENQUADS
ENQUEUE
ENQUIRE
ENQUIRY
ENSUING
ENSUITE
ENSURED
ENSURER
ENSURES
EPAULET
ESCUDOS
ESCUELA
ESQUIRE
ESTUARY
ETRURIA
EXCURSE
EXCUSAL
EXCUSAS
EXCUSED
EXCUSER
EXCUSES
EXCUSEZ
EXEUNTS
EXHUMED
EXHUMER
EXHUMES
EXPUNGE

E•••U••

EANMUND
EARBUDS
EARFULS
EARMUFF
EGGCUPS
EGGHUNT
EGOSURF
ELOCUTE
EMANUEL
EMBRUED
EMBRUES
ENCRUST
ENDCUTS
ENDRUNS
ENGLUND
ENGLUTS
ENROUTE
ENSOULS
ENTHUSE
ENTRUST
ENWOUND
EPICURE
EPOQUES
ERASURE
ESPOUSE
EVACUEE
EVALUNA
EVOLUTE
EXCLUDE
EXECUTE
EXHAUST
EXPOUND
EXTRUDE
EYECUPS
EYEFULS
EYETUCK

E••••U•

EARDRUM
EARPLUG
EASEDUP
EASEFUL
EASEOUT
EASESUP
EATENUP
EATITUP
EATSOUT
ECLOGUE
ECOTEUR
EDGEOUT
EDITOUT
EELPOUT
EIGHTUP
EKEDOUT
EKESOUT
ELAAIUN
ELIGIUS
ELUVIUM
ELYSIUM
EMULOUS
ENAMOUR
ENDEDUP
ENQUEUE
ENRIQUE
ENVIOUS
ENVOGUE
EPHEBUS
EPHESUS
ERASMUS
ERASTUS
ERECTUS
ERRATUM
ERTEGUN
ESCALUS
EULABUS
EVENOUT
EVENSUP
EVERDUR

E•••••U

EMMYLOU

•EU••••

BEURRES
DEUCING
DEUTERO
DEUTSCH
FEUDING
FEUDIST
HEURIGE
LEUCINE
NEUILLY
NEUMANN
NEURONE
NEURONS
NEUTERS
NEUTRAL
NEUTRON
OEUVRES
PEUGEOT
REUBENS
REUNERS
REUNIFY
REUNION
REUNITE
REUPPED
REURGED
REURGES
REUSERS
REUSING
REUTERS
REUTHER
REUTTER
TEUTONS

•E•U•••

BEAUISH
BEGUILE
BEGUINE
BELUGAS
BELUSHI
BEMUSED
BEMUSES
BENUMBS
BEQUEST
BEQUICK
BEQUIET
CERUMEN
DEBUNKS
DEBURGH
DEBURRS
DEBUSES
DEBUSSY
DEBUTED
DECUPLE
DEDUCED
DEDUCER
DEDUCES
DEDUCTS
DEFUELS
DEFUNCT
DEFUNDS
DEFUSED
DEFUSER
DEFUSES
DEGUSTS
DEJUNKS
DELUDED
DELUDER
DELUDES
DELUGED
DELUGES
DELUISE
DEMURER
DENUDED
DENUDER
DENUDES
DEPULPS
DEPUTED
DEPUTES
DEQUEUE
DERUSTS
DETUNED
DETUNES
FERULES
FETUSES
GELUSIL
GENUINE
GENUSES
GERUNDS
GETUPON
JEJUNUM
JESUITS
LECUONA
LEDUPTO
LEGUMES
LETUPON
LEXUSES
LEXUSGS
LEXUSGX
LEXUSIS
LEXUSLS
LEXUSLX
LEXUSRX
LEXUSSC
MEDULLA
MEDUSAE
MEDUSAN
MEDUSAS
MENUBAR
MENUDOS
MENUHIN
MEZUZAH
MEZUZAS
NEBULAE
NEBULAR
NEBULAS
NEGUSES
NEXUSES
PENUCHE
PENULTS
PEQUOTS
PERUGIA
PERUKES
PERUSAL
PERUSED
PERUSER
PERUSES
PETULIA
PETUNIA
REAUDIT
REAUMUR
REBUFFS
REBUILD
REBUILT
REBUKED
REBUKER
REBUKES
REBUSES
RECURED
RECURES
RECURLS
RECURVE
RECUSAL
RECUSED
RECUSES
REDUCED
REDUCER
REDUCES
REDUSTS
REFUELS
REFUGED
REFUGEE
REFUGES
REFUNDS
REFUSAL
REFUSED
REFUSER
REFUSES
REFUTAL
REFUTED
REFUTER
REFUTES
REGUIDE
REGULAR
REGULUS
REJUDGE
RELUCTS
RELUMED
RELUMES
RENUZIT
REPUGNS
REPULSE
REPUMPS
REPUTED
REPUTES
REQUEST
REQUIEM
REQUIRE
REQUITE
REQUOTE
RESUITS
RESULTS
RESUMED
RESUMES
RESURGE
RETUNED
RETUNES
RETURFS
RETURNS
SECULAR
SECURED
SECURER
SECURES
SEDUCED
SEDUCER
SEDUCES
SEQUELS
SEQUINS
SEQUOIA
SEQUOYA
SETUPON
TEAURNS
TENUITY
TENUOUS
TENURED
TENURES
TEQUILA
VELURES
VENULES
VENUSES
ZEBULON
ZEBULUN

•E••U••

BECAUSE
BEDAUBS
BEDBUGS
BEDOUIN
BEFOULS
BENGUNN
BEOWULF
BERMUDA
BERSUNT
BETHUNE
CELLULE
CENSURE
CENTURY
DEBAUCH
DEBLURS
DEBOULE
DECRUMB
DEFAULT
DEGAUSS
DELOUSE
DELRUTH
DEMBUMS
DEMOUNT
DENEUVE
DENTURE
DEPAULU
DESLUMS
DETOURS
DETRUDE
DEVOURS
DEYOUNG
FEATURE
FERRULE
FESCUES
GEODUCK
GESTURE
GETBUSY
GETCUTE
GETHURT
HECKUVA
HELLUVA
HEPBURN
HERCULE
HEXNUTS
HEYJUDE
HEYRUBE
JEBBUSH
JETGUNS
KEROUAC
LEADUPS
LEAGUED
LEAGUER
LEAGUES
LECTURE
LEGPULL
LEISURE
LEJEUNE
LELOUCH
LENGUAS
LETSUSE
LETTUCE
MEASURE
MEDIUMS
MERCURE
MERCURY
MESHUGA
MESSUPS
NEPTUNE
NERVULE
NESQUIK
NETFULS
NETSUKE
NETSURF
NEWBURG
PEANUTS
PENGUIN
PEPLUMS
PERCUSS
PERDURE
PERFUME
PERFUMY
PERFUSE
PERJURE
PERJURY
PERMUTE
PERTURB
PETDUCK
PETMULE
PETPUPS
REBOUND
REBRUSH
RECLUSE
RECOUNT
RECOUPS
RECRUIT
REDBUDS
REDDUST
REDOUBT
REDOUND
REDOUTS
REDSUIT
REDSUNS
REEQUIP
REERUPT
REFOUND
REGAUGE
REGLUED
REGLUES
REHAULS
REHOUSE
REMOUNT
RENAULT
REPLUMB
REPLUME
REPOURS
REPRUNE
REROUTE
RESCUED
RESCUER
RESCUES
RESHUTS
RESOUND
RESTUDY
RESTUFF
RETOUCH
RETOURS
REWOUND
SEADUCK
SEADUTY
SEAGULL
SEAHUNT
SECLUDE
SEIZURE
SENDUPS
SENSUAL
SETOUTS
TEACUPS
TEAMUSA
TEDEUMS
TEDIUMS
TEMPURA
TERHUNE
TEXTUAL
TEXTURE
VEINULE
VELLUMS
VELOURS
VELOUTE
VENDUES
VENTURA
VENTURE
VENTURI
VERDUGO
VERDURE
VERRUCA
VESTURE
WETBULB
WETSUIT
ZEITUNG

•E•••U•

BEADSUP
BEAMSUP
BEARCUB
BEARHUG
BEAROUT
BEARSUP
BEATOUT
BEATSUP
BECLOUD
BEEFSUP

BEERMUG
BELARUS
BELGIUM
BELLYUP
BELTOUT
BELTSUP
BELVOUR
BENBLUE
BENELUX
BERGIUS
BESTBUD
BESTBUY
BESTCUT
BEZIQUE
CELSIUS
CENTAUR
CENTRUM
CEPHEUS
DEALOUT
DEALSUP
DEALTUP
DECATUR
DECKOUT
DECORUM
DEDALUS
DEFOCUS
DEFRAUD
DELARUE
DEQUEUE
DESKFUL
DEVALUE
DEVIOUS
EELPOUT
FEARFUL
FEELOUT
FELLDUE
FELLOUT
FELTOUT
FEMINUM
FENCEUP
FERMIUM
FERROUS
FERVOUR
GEARSUP
GETSOUT
HEADFUL
HEADOUT
HEADSUP
HEALSUP
HEAPSUP
HEAROUT
HEATFUL
HEATSUP
HEEDFUL
HEINOUS
HELDOUT
HELPFUL
HELPOUT
HELPSUP
HERBAUT
JEALOUS
JEANLUC
JEJUNUM
JERKOUT
JERKSUP
KEEPMUM
KEEPOUT
KEEPSUP
KEPTMUM
KEPTOUT
KETCHUM
KETCHUP
KEYCLUB
KEYEDUP
LEADOUT
LEADSUP
LEAFOUT
LEANCUT
LEAPSUP
LEAPTUP
LEFTOUT
LEMIEUX
LENDOUT
LEPIDUS
LESCAUT
LESPAUL
LETSOUT
MEETSUP
MENCIUS
METEOUT
NEEDFUL
NENNIUS
NERVOUS
NESTFUL
OEDIPUS
PEASOUP
PEEKOUT
PEELOUT
PEEPOUT
PEEROUT
PEGASUS
PENTIUM
PERITUS
PERKSUP
PERSEUS
PERSIUS
PETROUS
REACHUP
READOUT
READSUP
REAMOUT
REARGUE
REARSUP
REAUMUR
REBEGUN
REDFOUR
REELOUT
REELSUP
REFOCUS
REGROUP
REGULUS
REISSUE
RENTOUT
REOCCUR
RESCRUB
RESEAUS
RESEAUX
RESIDUA
RESIDUE
RESTFUL
RESTSUP
RETINUE
REVALUE
REVENUE
REVITUP
REYNAUD
SEABLUE
SEALSUP
SEASLUG
SEEKOUT
SEENOUT
SEEPOUT
SEESOUT
SELLOUT
SENDOUT
SENDSUP
SENTOUT
SERIOUS
SERVEUP
SETSOUT
SEVENUP
SEVERUS
SEWEDUP
SEYMOUR
TEAMSUP
TEARFUL
TEAROUT
TEARSUP
TEASEUP
TEDIOUS
TEEITUP
TENFOUR
TENKRUN
TENSEUP
TENTFUL
TENUOUS
TERBIUM
TESTOUT
TESTRUN
TETANUS
VERDOUX
WEAROUT
WEEDOUT
WEEHOUR
WEIGHUP
WELLCUT
WELLPUT
WELLRUN
WELLSUP
WENTOUT
YEAHBUT
YELLOUT
ZEALOUS
ZEBULUN
ZEROOUT
ZEROSUM
ZESTFUL

•E••••U

BELLEAU
DEPAULU
FEYDEAU
LEHIGHU
LETTERU
NEARYOU
PERREAU
SEETHRU
YEAHYOU

••EU•••

DOEUVRE
EXEUNTS
FLEURON
ONEUNIT
PLEURAE
PLEURAL
PNEUMAS
PNEUMAT
PNEUMON
QUEUERS
QUEUEUP
QUEUING
RHEUMIC
SLEUTHS
STEUBEN
THEUSSR

••E•U••

APESUIT
ASEXUAL
AVENUEQ
AVENUES
CAESURA
CHEQUER
CHEQUES
CHERUBS
COEQUAL
DIECUTS
EXECUTE
EYECUPS
EYEFULS
EYETUCK
FLEXURE
ICECUBE
ICEOUTS
ICERUNS
IREFUSE
JOEBUCK
NIEBUHR
OLEBULL
ONELUMP
OVERUSE
PLENUMS
PREBURN
PREBUYS
PRECURE
PRECUTS
PREDUSK
PREFUND
PRELUDE
PRENUPS
PREPUPA
PREQUEL
PRESUME
PREVUED
PREVUES
RAEBURN
REEQUIP
REERUPT
ROEBUCK
SPELUNK
STEPUPS
THEBUSH
THECUBS
THEDUKE
THEHULK
THEPUMP
THERULE
THESUNS
THETUBE
THETURN
TSETUNG
UNEQUAL

••E••U•

ACEDOUT
ACESOUT
AGEDOUT
AGEFOUR
AGENDUM
AGESOUT
APERCUS
AREARUG
ATEITUP
AVERNUS
BEEFSUP
BEERMUG
BLEWOUT
BREAKUP
BRENGUN
BREWPUB
BREWSUP
CHECKUP
CHEERUP
CHETRUM
CHEVAUX
CHEWGUM
CHEWOUT
CHEWSUP
CLEANUP
CLEARUP
CREEPUP
CREPTUP
CREWCUT
DIEDOUT
DIESOUT
DREAMUP
DRESSUP
DREWOUT
DREYFUS
EKEDOUT
EKESOUT
ERECTUS
EVENOUT
EVENSUP
EVERDUR
FEELOUT
FREEDUP
FREESUP
FRETFUL
FUELSUP
GIELGUD
GLEEFUL
GOESOUT
GREYCUP
HEEDFUL
ICEBLUE
ICEDOUT
ICESOUT
KEEPMUM
KEEPOUT
KEEPSUP
KNEESUP
MEETSUP
NEEDFUL
OCEANUS
OCELLUS
ONECLUB
ONEHOUR
ONEOFUS
ONEROUS
OPENOUT
OPENSUP
OVERBUY
OVERCUT
OVERDUB
OVERDUE
OVERRUN
OVERSUP
PEEKOUT
PEELOUT
PEEPOUT
PEEROUT
PHEMIUS
PRECOUP
PREMIUM
PRESPUR
PRESQUE
PRESSUP
PTEROUS
QUECHUA
QUELQUE
QUEUEUP
REELOUT
REELSUP
RHENIUM
SEEKOUT
SEENOUT
SEEPOUT
SEESOUT
SLEDFUL
SNEAKUP
SPEAKUP
SPECOUT
SPEEDUP
SPEWOUT
STEAMUP
STENGUN
STEPOUT
STEPSUP
STERNUM
SWEEPUP
SWELLUP
SWEPTUP
TEEITUP
THEFRUG
THEROUX
THESEUS
THETOUR
WEEDOUT
WEEHOUR

••E•••U

DREXELU
FRENEAU
IBEGYOU
ISEEYOU
QUENEAU
SEETHRU

•••EU••

ATDEUCE
AUTEURS
DENEUVE
DISEURS
DISEUSE
DRSEUSS
FANEUIL
GIVEUPS
LACEUPS
LEJEUNE
LINEUPS
LYCEUMS
MAJEURE
MAKEUPS
MSIEURS
MUSEUMS
PILEUPS
POSEURS
POSEUSE
RAVEUPS
TEDEUMS
TUNEUPS
WAKEUPS

•••E•U•

ACTEDUP
ADDEDUP
AIREDUP
AMPEDUP
ANGELUS
ANTEDUP
ANTERUS
ANTESUP
AQUEOUS
ARTEMUS
ASKEDUP
BALEFUL
BANEFUL
BATEAUX
BENELUX
BITESUP
BLUESUN
BODEFUL
BONEDUP
BONESUP
BOREOUT
BOXEDUP
BOXESUP
BUREAUS
BUREAUX
CADEAUX
CAGEDUP
CAGESUP
CAKEDUP
CAKESUP
CAMEDUE
CAMEOUT
CAREFUL
CASEOUS
CASEOUT
CHEERUP
CISEAUX
CLUEFUL
COMEDUE
COMEOUT
COMESUP
COVERUP
CREEPUP
CRIEDUP
CRIESUP
CROESUS
DAREFUL
DICECUP
DINEOUT
DIREFUL
DOLEFUL
DOLEOUT
DOPEOUT
DRIEDUP
DRIESUP
DUDEDUP
DUDESUP
DUTEOUS
EASEDUP
EASEFUL
EASEOUT
EASESUP
EATENUP
EDGEOUT
ENDEDUP
EPHEBUS
EPHESUS
ERTEGUN
FADEOUT
FAKEFUR
FAKEOUT
FATEFUL
FILEOUT
FIREBUG
FIREDUP
FIRESUP
FIXEDUP
FIXESUP
FLIESUP
FORERUN
FREEDUP
FREESUP
FRIEDUP
FRIESUP
GASEDUP
GASEOUS
GASESUP
GATEAUX
GAVEOUT
GIVENUP
GIVEOUT
GIVESUP
GLEEFUL
GLUEGUN
GONEOUT
HATEFUL
HAVEFUN
HAVEOUT
HIDEOUS
HIDEOUT
HIKEDUP
HIKEOUT
HIKESUP
HIREOUT
HOLEDUP
HOLEOUT
HOLESUP
HOMERUN
HOPEFUL
HUMERUS
HYPEDUP
HYPESUP
IAPETUS
ICTERUS
IGNEOUS
IMPETUS
INGENUE
JUNEBUG
KEYEDUP
KNEESUP
LACEDUP
LACESUP
LIFEFUL
LINECUT
LINEDUP
LINEOUT
LINESUP
LIVENUP
LIVEOUT
LOSEOUT
LOVEBUG
MADEFUN
MADEOUT
MADERUN
MAKEFUN
MAKEOUT
MAKERUN
MAKESUP
METEOUT
MILERUN
MIXEDUP
MIXESUP
MOVEDUP
MOVEOUT
MOVESUP
MUSEFUL
NICEGUY
NIVEOUS
NOSEDUP
NOSEEUM
NOSEOUT
NOSESUP
OFFERUP
OGDENUT
OISEAUX
OOZEOUT
ORDERUP
OSSEOUS
OWNEDUP
PHOEBUS
PICEOUS
PILEDUP
PILEOUS
PILESUP
PINENUT
PINETUM
PIPEDUP
PIPEFUL
PIPESUP
PITEOUS
POKEFUN
POKEOUT
POWERUP
PUTEMUP
QUIETUS
RACEDUP
RACESUP
RAGEFUL
RAKEDUP
RAKESUP
REBEGUN
RESEAUS
RESEAUX
REVENUE
RHOECUS
RIDEOUT
RIDESUP
RILEDUP
RILESUP
RISESUP
RODEOUT
ROPEDUP
ROPESUP
ROSEBUD
RULEOUT
SAVEDUP
SAVESUP
SCREWUP
SEVENUP
SEVERUS
SEWEDUP
SIZEDUP
SIZESUP
SPEEDUP
SWEEPUP
TAKENUP
TAKEOUT
TAKESUP
TAPEDUP
TAPESUP
THREEUP
THREWUP
TIMEOUT
TIMESUP
TIREOUT
TONEDUP
TONESUP
TOREOUT
TOTESUP
TRUEDUP
TRUESUP
TUNEDUP
TUNEFUL
TUNEOUT
TUNESUP
TYPEDUP
TYPESUP
VOTEOUT
WAKEDUP
WAKEFUL
WAKESUP
WAXEDUP
WAXESUP
WIPEDUP
WIPEOUT
WIPESUP
WIREDUP
WIRESUP
WISEDUP
WISEGUY
WISESUP
WITEOUT
WOKENUP
WOREOUT
ZONEOUT

•••E••U

ANGELOU
BLUEFLU
ILIESCU
IOWEYOU
ISEEYOU
LOVEYOU
SILENTU

••••EU•

AMADEUS
AMATEUR
BLAZEUP
BONHEUR
BORNEUP
BRACEUP
BROKEUP
CEPHEUS
CHOKEUP
CHOSEUP
CLOSEUP
CRATEUP
DANSEUR
DEQUEUE
DOUCEUR
DRFREUD
DRIVEUP
DROVEUP
ECOTEUR
ENQUEUE
FARCEUR
FENCEUP
FLAMEUP
FLANEUR
FLAREUP
FORCEUP
FRAMEUP
FRISEUR
FROZEUP
GLUTEUS
GRATEUP
HAUTEUR
IGIVEUP
JUICEUP
LAFLEUR
LEMIEUX
LIQUEUR
LOUSEUP
MALLEUS
MASSEUR
MILIEUS
MILIEUX
MIMIEUX
MONTEUX
NOSEEUM
NUCLEUS
ORPHEUM
ORPHEUS
PASSEUL
PASTEUP
PASTEUR
PERSEUS
PIRAEUS
PROTEUS
QUEUEUP
RAISEUP
RIGUEUR
SCALEUP
SCAREUP
SERVEUP
SHAKEUP
SHAPEUP
SHINEUP
SHOREUP
SLICEUP
SMOKEUP
SPICEUP
SPIKEUP
SPOKEUP
STOKEUP
STOREUP
TEASEUP
TENSEUP
THESEUS
THREEUP
TRADEUP
WRITEUP
WROTEUP

••••E•U

ALFREDU
BANDEAU
BARBEAU
BELLEAU
CHAPEAU
CHATEAU
COCTEAU
DREXELU
FEYDEAU
FRENEAU
GARNEAU
ISABEAU
JAMBEAU
LAMBEAU
LETTERU
MARCEAU
NOUVEAU
PARVENU
PERREAU
PLATEAU
QUENEAU
RONDEAU
ROULEAU
TABLEAU
THOREAU
TONNEAU
TRUDEAU
WATTEAU
XAVIERU

•••••EU

DOUBLEU
MATHIEU
MONDIEU
PURDUEU
PURLIEU
TULANEU

EV•••••

EVACUEE
EVADERS
EVADING
EVALUNA
EVANDER
EVANGEL
EVANISH
EVASION
EVASIVE
EVELONG
EVENBET
EVENERS
EVENEST
EVENING
EVENNOW
EVENOFF
EVENOUT
EVENPAR
EVENSUP
EVERDUR
EVEREST
EVERETT
EVERLYS
EVERTED
EVERTOR
EVICTED
EVICTEE
EVICTOR
EVIDENT
EVILEST
EVILEYE
EVILLER
EVILONE
EVINCED
EVINCES
EVOKERS
EVOKING
EVOLUTE
EVOLVED
EVOLVER
EVOLVES
EVULSED
EVULSES

E•V••••

ENVEILS
ENVELOP
ENVENOM
ENVIERS
ENVIOUS
ENVIRON
ENVIROS
ENVOGUE
ENVYING
ETVOILA

E••V•••

ELEVATE
ELEVENA
ELEVENB
ELEVENC
ELEVEND
ELEVENE
ELEVENS
ELEVONS
ELUVIAL
ELUVIUM

E•••V••

EATOVER
ENDIVES
ENLIVEN
ESTEVEZ
ESTIVAL
EUROVAN
EVOLVED
EVOLVER
EVOLVES
EXWIVES

E••••V•

ELUSIVE
EMOTIVE
ENCLAVE

ENGRAVE
ENSLAVE
EROSIVE
EVASIVE
EXCLAVE

E•••••V
EDWARDV

•EV••••
BEVELED
BEVELER
BEVERLY
CEVICHE
DEVALUE
DEVEINS
DEVELOP
DEVESTS
DEVIANT
DEVIATE
DEVICES
DEVILED
DEVILLE
DEVILRY
DEVIOUS
DEVISED
DEVISEE
DEVISER
DEVISES
DEVISOR
DEVOIRS
DEVOLVE
DEVORES
DEVOTED
DEVOTEE
DEVOTES
DEVOURS
DEVRIES
FEVERED
FEVRIER
LEVADES
LEVATOR
LEVELED
LEVELER
LEVELLY
LEVERED
LEVERET
LEVIERS
LEVILLI
LEVITES
LEVITIC
LEVYING
NEVADAN
NEVILLE
REVALUE
REVAMPS
REVEALS
REVELED
REVELER
REVELIN
REVELRY
REVENDS
REVENGE
REVENUE
REVERBS
REVERDY
REVERED
REVERER
REVERES
REVERIE
REVERSA
REVERSE
REVERTS
REVESTS
REVIEWS
REVILED
REVILER
REVILES
REVISAL
REVISED
REVISER
REVISES
REVISIT
REVISOR
REVITUP
REVIVAL
REVIVED
REVIVER
REVIVES
REVOICE
REVOKED
REVOKER
REVOKES
REVOLTS
REVOLVE
REVOTED
REVOTES
REVVING
SEVENAD
SEVENAM
SEVENBC
SEVENEE
SEVENNO
SEVENPM
SEVENTH
SEVENTY
SEVENUP
SEVERAL
SEVERED
SEVERER
SEVERUS
SEVIGNY
SEVILLA
SEVILLE
YEVGENY

•E•V•••
BEAVERS
BELVOIR
BELVOUR
BERVOIX
CERVEZA
CERVIDS
CERVINE
DELVERS
DELVING
DERVISH
FERVENT
FERVORS
FERVOUR
GERVAIS
HEAVEHO
HEAVENS
HEAVERS
HEAVETO
HEAVIER
HEAVIES
HEAVILY
HEAVING
KELVINS
LEAVEBE
LEAVEIN
LEAVEIT
LEAVENS
LEAVEON
LEAVING
LEOVIII
NERVIER
NERVILY
NERVINE
NERVING
NERVOUS
NERVULE
OEUVRES
PEEVING
PEEVISH
PERVADE
REAVAIL
REAVERS
REAVING
REAVOWS
REEVICT
REEVING
REEVOKE
RENVOIS
REVVING
SELVAGE
SERVANT
SERVEAS
SERVERS
SERVEUP
SERVICE
SERVILE
SERVING
TEEVEES
VELVETS
VELVETY
WEAVERS
WEAVING
WEEVILS
YESVOTE

•E••V••
BEDEVIL
BEHAVED
BEHAVES
BELEVEN
BELOVED
DEHAVEN
DELIVER
DERIVED
DERIVER
DERIVES
GENEVAN
GETEVEN
GETOVER
HESHVAN
LEHAVRE
LENOVOS
MEDEVAC
MEDIVAC
RECOVER
REGIVEN
REGIVES
RELEVEL
RELEVER
RELEVES
RELIVED
RELIVES
REMOVAL
REMOVED
REMOVER
REMOVES
REPAVED
REPAVES
RESAVED
RESAVES
REVIVAL
REVIVED
REVIVER
REVIVES
REWOVEN
SEGOVIA
TELAVIV
YEREVAN

•E•••V•
BEBRAVE
BEEHIVE
BEHOOVE
BELIEVE
BENBOVA
BEREAVE
CENTAVO
DECEIVE
DENEUVE
DEPRAVE
DEPRIVE
DESERVE
DESYLVA
DEVOLVE
FESTIVA
FESTIVE
HECKUVA
HELLUVA
HENRYVI
KEDROVA
LETHAVE
LETLIVE
NEWLOVE
NEWWAVE
PECCAVI
PENSIVE
PETDOVE
RECARVE
RECEIVE
RECURVE
REDFIVE
REDRIVE
RELIEVE
REPROVE
RESERVE
RESHAVE
RESOLVE
RESTIVE
REVOLVE
REWEAVE
TENSIVE
YESHIVA
ZEMSTVO

•E••••V
FEDOROV
GEORGEV
HENRYIV
KEMIDOV
LETTERV
NEMEROV
TELAVIV

••EV•••
ALEVELS
BREVETS
BREVITY
CHEVAUX
CHEVETS
CHEVIOT
CHEVONS
CHEVRES
CHEVRET
CHEVRON
COEVALS
CREVICE
DYEVATS
ELEVATE
ELEVENA
ELEVENB
ELEVENC
ELEVEND
ELEVENE
ELEVENS
ELEVONS
GUEVARA
MTEVANS
OLEVELS
ONEVOTE
PEEVING
PEEVISH
PREVAIL
PREVENT
PREVERB
PREVERT
PREVETO
PREVIAS
PREVIEW
PREVOID
PREVOST
PREVUED
PREVUES
REEVICT
REEVING
REEVOKE
SHEVATS
SIEVING
STEVENS
TEEVEES
THEVIEW
THEVIPS
TREVINO
WEEVILS

••E•V••
ATEOVER
CHEEVER
CHERVIL
CLEAVED
CLEAVER
CLEAVES
CLEAVON
DOEUVRE
GREAVES
ICEOVER
LIEOVER
ONEOVER
PREAVER
SHEAVED
SHEAVES
SHELVED
SHELVER
SHELVES
SLEEVED
SLEEVES
STEEVED
STEEVES
SWERVED
SWERVES
TWELVEA
TWELVEB
TWELVEC
TWELVED
TWELVEE
TWELVES
UNEAVED

••E••V•
AGEFIVE
BEEHIVE
ICECAVE
KHEDIVE
ONELOVE
PREDIVE
PREPAVE
SCENEVI
THECAVS
THEFIVE
THEMAVS
THEWAVE
WHEREVE

••E•••V
CHEKHOV
SCENEIV

•••EV••
ATSEVEN
BEDEVIL
BELEVEN
BILEVEL
CHEEVER
ESTEVEZ
FOREVER
GENEVAN
GETEVEN
GODEVIL
GOTEVEN
GRIEVED
GRIEVER
GRIEVES
HOWEVER
KNIEVEL
MEDEVAC
NINEVEH
NONEVER
NONEVIL
NOTEVEN
NOTEVER
RELEVEL
RELEVER
RELEVES
SLEEVED
SLEEVES
STEEVED
STEEVES
THIEVED
THIEVES
UNLEVEL
WHOEVER
WHYEVER
WINEVAT
YEREVAN

•••E•V•
BEREAVE
BTWELVE
DECEIVE
DENEUVE
DESERVE
INNERVE
INWEAVE
ITWELVE
JAMESVI
MINERVA
OBSERVE
ONLEAVE
ONSERVE
RECEIVE
RESERVE
REWEAVE
UNHEAVY
UNNERVE
UNWEAVE
UPHEAVE

•••E••V
ALFEROV
BADENOV
DIRECTV
JAMESIV
NEMEROV
NUREYEV
SILENTV

••••EV•
ACHIEVA
ACHIEVE
BELIEVE
DONLEVY
KISLEVS
MAGLEVS
RELIEVE
RILIEVO
SCENEVI
TAXLEVY
WHEREVE

••••E•V
CABLETV
LETTERV
SCENEIV
SPIKETV

•••••EV
DOUBLEV
FADAYEV
GEORGEV
KATAYEV
NUREYEV
TUPOLEV

EW•••••
EWELAMB
EWENECK
EWERIES

E•W••••
EBWHITE
EDWARDG
EDWARDI
EDWARDR
EDWARDS
EDWARDV
EKWENSI
ENWINDS
ENWOUND
ENWRAPS
EXWIVES
EXWORKS

E••W•••
EARWIGS
EELWORM
ELMWOOD
ENDWAYS
ENDWISE
ENTWINE
ENTWIST
EREWHON
EYEWALL
EYEWASH
EYEWEAR
EYEWINK

E•••W••
EATAWAY
ELBOWED
ELBOWER
ELFOWLS
EMBOWER
EMPOWER
ENDOWED
ENDOWER

E••••W•
EMBROWN
ESCHEWS
ESCROWS
ESPNEWS

E•••••W
EATCROW
EVENNOW
EXITNOW
EYEBROW

•EW••••
BEWAILS
BEWARED
BEWARES
BEWITCH
DEWAART
DEWATER
DEWAXED
DEWAXES
DEWCLAW
DEWDROP
DEWFALL
DEWIEST
DEWILDE
DEWIRED
DEWIRES
DEWLAPS
DEWLESS
DEWLINE
DEWORMS
FEWNESS
GEWGAWS
HEWEDTO
HEWLETT
JEWELED
JEWELER
JEWELRY
JEWISON
KEWPIES
LEWDEST
LEWHOAD
MEWLERS
MEWLING
NEWAGER
NEWAGEY
NEWBERN
NEWBERY
NEWBIES
NEWBOLT
NEWBORN
NEWBURG
NEWCARS
NEWDEAL
NEWFACE
NEWGATE
NEWHAND
NEWHART
NEWHATS
NEWHIRE
NEWHOPE
NEWIDEA
NEWJOBS
NEWKIDS
NEWLAID
NEWLEAF
NEWLEFT
NEWLIFE
NEWLINE
NEWLOOK
NEWLOVE
NEWMADE
NEWMANS
NEWMATH
NEWMINT
NEWMONT
NEWMOON
NEWMOWN
NEWNAME
NEWNESS
NEWPORT
NEWRICH
NEWSBOY
NEWSDAY
NEWSIER
NEWSIES
NEWSMAN
NEWSMEN
NEWSOME
NEWSPEG
NEWTONS
NEWTOWN
NEWTOYS
NEWWAVE
NEWWEEK
NEWWORD
NEWYEAR
NEWYORK
PEWTERS
REWAGER
REWAKED
REWAKEN
REWAKES
REWARDS
REWARMS
REWARNS
REWATER
REWAXED
REWAXES
REWEARS
REWEAVE
REWEIGH
REWELDS
REWIDEN
REWINDS
REWIPED
REWIPES
REWIRED
REWIRES
REWOKEN
REWORDS
REWORKS
REWOUND
REWOVEN
REWRAPS
REWRITE
REWROTE
SEWARDS
SEWEDON
SEWEDUP
SEWISTS
YEWTREE

•E•W•••
BEOWULF
BERWICK
BETWEEN
BETWIXT
DERWENT
EELWORM
GEEWHIZ
GETWARM
GETWELL
GETWISE
GETWORD
HEYWARD
HEYWOOD
JETWASH
JETWAYS
KENWAHL
KEYWAYS
KEYWEST
KEYWORD
LEAWOOD
LEEWARD
LEEWAYS
LEGWEAR
LEGWORK
MEDWICK
MEOWERS
MEOWING
MEOWMIX
METWITH
NETWARE
NETWORK
NEWWAVE
NEWWEEK
NEWWORD
PEDWAYS
PEEWEES
PERWEEK
REAWAKE
REAWOKE
REDWINE
REDWING
REDWOLF
REDWOOD
REDWORM
RENWICK
REOWNED
RESWEAR
RESWEEP
RESWIMS
RESWORE
RESWORN
RETWINE
RETWIST
SEAWALL
SEAWARD
SEAWAYS
SEAWEED
SEAWOLF
SEGWAYS
TENWEEK
WETWARE
WETWASH

•E••W••
BEDEWED
BEESWAX
BEJEWEL
BELTWAY
BEROWNE
DEPOWER
GETAWAY
GETSWET
HEADWAY
KELOWNA
LEDAWAY
MEDAWAR
PEGAWAY
PERIWIG
PESEWAS
REMOWED
RENEWAL
RENEWED
RENEWER
RENOWNS
REPOWER
RESAWED
RESEWED
RESOWED
RETOWED
VERYWET
WELLWON

•E•••W•
BEDDOWN
BELLOWS
BESTOWS
DECLAWS
FELLOWS
GEEGAWS
GETDOWN
GEWGAWS
HEBREWS
HEEHAWS
LETDOWN
MEADOWS
MEADOWY
MELLOWS
NEPHEWS
NEWMOWN
NEWTOWN
PEAFOWL
PETCOWS
REAVOWS
REBLOWN
REBREWS
RECHEWS
RECROWN
REDDAWN
REDHAWK
REDRAWN
REDRAWS
REFLOWN
REFLOWS
REGLOWS
REGROWN
REGROWS
REPLOWS
RESHOWN
RESHOWS
RESTOWS
RETHAWS
REVIEWS
SEACOWS
SEAFOWL
SEAHAWK
SEESAWS
SETDOWN
TEAGOWN
WETDOWN
YELLOWS
YELLOWY

•E••••W
BEARPAW
BELTSAW
BESTREW
DEWCLAW
GEORGEW
HEADSAW
HERENOW
KENDREW
KERSHAW
LETKNOW
LETTERW
PETCHEW
PETCROW
REENDOW
RENFREW
RESTREW
SEMIRAW
VERYFEW
VERYLOW
VERYNEW

••EW•••
ALEWIFE
BLEWOFF
BLEWOUT
BREWAGE
BREWERS
BREWERY
BREWING
BREWPUB
BREWSKI
BREWSUP
CHEWERS
CHEWGUM
CHEWIER
CHEWING
CHEWOUT
CHEWSON
CHEWSUP
CHEWTOY
CLEWING
CREWCUT
CREWELS
CREWING
CREWMAN
CREWMEN
DAEWOOS
DREWOFF
DREWOUT
DUEWEST
DYEWOOD
EREWHON
EYEWALL
EYEWASH
EYEWEAR
EYEWINK
GEEWHIZ
GREWBIG
GREWDIM
GREWFAT
GREWOLD
ICEWINE
JREWING
KNEWHOW
LEEWARD
LEEWAYS
MAEWEST
ONEWEEK
ONEWHIT
ONEWOOD
PEEWEES
PREWARM
PREWARN
PREWASH
PREWHIP
PREWIRE
PREWITT
PREWORK
PREWORN
PREWRAP
SHEWOLF
SKEWERS
SKEWING

SLEWING
SPEWERS
SPEWING
SPEWOUT
STEWARD
STEWART
STEWERS
STEWIER
STEWING
STEWPAN
STEWPOT
THEWALL
THEWAVE
THEWIND
VIEWERS
VIEWIER
VIEWING
VIEWITH

••E•W••
AREAWAY
ATEAWAY
BEESWAX
BOERWAR
DIEAWAY
FREEWAY
ONETWOS
OVERWET
SHERWIN
THESWAN

••E••W•
DIEDOWN
GEEGAWS
HEEHAWS
HOEDOWN
ICEDOWN
LIEDOWN
ONEDOWN
OVERAWE
PREDAWN
RAEDAWN
SEESAWS
STEPTWO
THENEWS
TIEDOWN

••E•••W
ATECROW
EVENNOW
EYEBROW
FRETSAW
ICESHOW
ISEENOW
JOEBLOW
KNEWHOW
LIESLOW
OVERFEW
OVERNEW
OVERSAW
OVERSEW
PRESHOW
PREVIEW
REENDOW
THECROW
THESHOW
THEVIEW

•••EW••
ALLEWIS
ASLEWOF
BEDEWED
BEJEWEL
BIKEWAY
CSLEWIS
FAREWAR
FIVEWAY
FREEWAY
GATEWAY
GAVEWAY
GIVEWAY
IKNEWIT
JANEWAY
LIKEWOW
MADEWAR
MADEWAY
MAKEWAR
MAKEWAY
MATEWAN
PESEWAS
RACEWAY
RENEWAL
RENEWED
RENEWER
RESEWED
SAFEWAY
SCREWED
SCREWUP
SIDEWAY
SINEWED
SOMEWAY
STREWED
STREWER
THREWAT
THREWIN
THREWON
THREWUP
TIMEWAS
UNDEWED
UNHEWED
UNMEWED
UNSEWED
WAGEWAR

•••E•W•
BASETWO
FIVETWO
LANETWO
LINETWO
PAGETWO
SIDETWO
SIZETWO

•••E••W
BIGELOW
BLUELAW
CASELAW
COMENOW
DANELAW
FOREPAW
FORESAW
GAMELAW
GOBELOW
HERENOW
ISEENOW
JUDELAW
LIKENEW
LIKEWOW
ROPETOW
SILENTW
SOMEHOW
TONEROW
YALELAW

••••EW•
ABCNEWS
ALLNEWS
ANDREWS
ANYNEWS
BADNEWS
BIGNEWS
CASHEWS
CBSNEWS
CURFEWS
CURLEWS
ESCHEWS
ESPNEWS
FOXNEWS
HEBREWS
MATHEWS
MILDEWS
MILDEWY
NBCNEWS
NEPHEWS
NONJEWS
NONNEWS
OLDNEWS
REBREWS
RECHEWS
REVIEWS
SOAREWE
THENEWS
TVCREWS
UNSKEWS

••••E•W
LETTERW

•••••EW
AIRCREW
BESTREW
DIMVIEW
DOGCHEW
DOUBLEW
GEORGEW
INASTEW
KENDREW
LIKENEW
MATTHEW
MISBREW
MISDREW
MISKNEW
MULGREW
OUTDREW
OUTGREW
OVERFEW
OVERNEW
OVERSEW
PETCHEW
PITCREW
PREVIEW
PURVIEW
RENFREW
RESTREW
THEVIEW
UNSCREW
VERYFEW
VERYNEW
WHOKNEW

EX•••••
EXABYTE
EXACTAS
EXACTED
EXACTER
EXACTLY
EXACTOR
EXALTED
EXALTER
EXAMINE
EXAMPLE
EXANIMO
EXARCHS
EXCEEDS
EXCELAT
EXCELIN
EXCEPTS
EXCERPT
EXCIDED
EXCIDES
EXCISED
EXCISES
EXCITED
EXCITER
EXCITES
EXCITOR
EXCLAIM
EXCLAVE
EXCLUDE
EXCRETE
EXCURSE
EXCUSAL
EXCUSAS
EXCUSED
EXCUSER
EXCUSES
EXCUSEZ
EXECUTE
EXEDRAE
EXEGETE
EXEMPLA
EXEMPTS
EXENEMY
EXERTED
EXERTER
EXEUNTS
EXFACTO
EXHALED
EXHALES
EXHAUST
EXHEDRA
EXHIBIT
EXHORTS
EXHUMED
EXHUMER
EXHUMES
EXIGENT
EXILERS
EXILING
EXISTED
EXITFEE
EXITING
EXITNOW
EXMATES
EXMAYOR
EXOCARP
EXOCETS
EXOGAMY
EXOILER
EXONYMS
EXORDIA
EXOTICA
EXOTICS
EXOTISM
EXPANDS
EXPANSE
EXPARTE
EXPECTS
EXPENDS
EXPENSE
EXPERTS
EXPIATE
EXPIRED
EXPIRES
EXPLAIN
EXPLODE
EXPLOIT
EXPLORE
EXPORTS
EXPOSED
EXPOSER
EXPOSES
EXPOSIT
EXPOUND
EXPRESS
EXPUNGE
EXSCIND
EXSECTS
EXSERTS
EXTENDS
EXTENSO
EXTENTS
EXTERNE
EXTERNS
EXTINCT
EXTOLLS
EXTORTS
EXTRACT
EXTREME
EXTRUDE
EXUDATE
EXUDING
EXULTED
EXUPERY
EXURBAN
EXURBIA
EXWIVES
EXWORKS
EXYANKS

E••X•••
ELIXIRS
EPOXIED
EPOXIES

E•••X••
EYEEXAM

E•••••X
EDITRIX
EQUIFAX
EQUINOX

•EX••••
DEXTRAL
DEXTRIN
HEXADIC
HEXAGON
HEXANES
HEXAPOD
HEXNUTS
HEXOSES
HEXSIGN
LEXICAL
LEXICON
LEXISES
LEXMARK
LEXUSES
LEXUSGS
LEXUSGX
LEXUSIS
LEXUSLS
LEXUSLX
LEXUSRX
LEXUSSC
MEXICAN
NEXRADS
NEXTDAY
NEXUSES
REXCATS
REXREED
REXROTH
SEXIEST
SEXISTS
SEXLESS
SEXPOTS
SEXTANS
SEXTANT
SEXTETS
SEXTONS
TEXTILE
TEXTING
TEXTRON
TEXTUAL
TEXTURE
VEXEDLY
WEXFORD

•E•X•••
GENXERS
LEOXIII
REEXPEL
XERXESI

•E••X••
DEHEXED
DEHEXES
DESEXED
DESEXES
DETOXED
DETOXES
DEWAXED
DEWAXES
FEDEXED
FEDEXES
HELIXES
REBOXED
REBOXES
REDOXES
REFAXED
REFAXES
REFIXED
REFIXES
RELAXED
RELAXER
RELAXES
REMIXED
REMIXES
RETAXED
RETAXES
REWAXED
REWAXES
TELEXED
TELEXES
VELOXES
XEROXED
XEROXES

•E•••X•
BETWIXT
MEATAXE

•E••••X
BEATBOX
BEATRIX
BEESWAX
BENELUX
BERVOIX
BETAMAX
CELOTEX
DEEDBOX
DEEPSIX
GEARBOX
HENDRIX
HENDRYX
LEMIEUX
LETTERX
LEXUSGX
LEXUSLX
LEXUSRX
MEMOREX
MEOWMIX
NETFLIX
PERPLEX
REAFFIX
REANNEX
REINDEX
RESEAUX
TELEFAX
TELEPIX
VERDOUX

••EX•••
ASEXUAL
CHEXMIX
COEXIST
DREXELU
DREXLER
FLEXILE
FLEXING
FLEXION
FLEXNER
FLEXORS
FLEXURE
INEXACT
INEXILE
PLEXORS
PREXIES
REEXPEL

••E•X••
EYEEXAM
ICEAXES
THEAXIS

••E••X•
PRETEXT

••E•••X
BEESWAX
BRERFOX
CHEVAUX
CHEXMIX
DEEDBOX
DEEPSIX
KLEENEX
MUESLIX
OVERFIX
OVERLAX
OVERMIX
OVERTAX
SKEEZIX
THEROUX

•••EX••
ANNEXED
ANNEXES
BAREXAM
CPAEXAM
CULEXES
DEHEXED
DEHEXES
DESEXED
DESEXES
EYEEXAM
FEDEXED
FEDEXES
INDEXED
INDEXER
INDEXES
LATEXES
LUREXES
PYREXIA
ROLEXES
TELEXED
TELEXES
TIMEXES
UNVEXED
URTEXTS
VANEXEL

•••E•X•
POLEAXE

•••E••X
APTERYX
ASTERIX
BASESIX
BATEAUX
BENELUX
BLUEFOX
BUREAUX
CADEAUX
CAKEMIX
CINEMAX
CISEAUX
FAREBOX
FIREBOX
FIREFOX
FIVESIX
FUSEBOX
GATEAUX
GORETEX
JUKEBOX
KLEENEX
OISEAUX
PAGESIX
PHOENIX
RESEAUX
SHOEBOX
SILENTX
SIZESIX
SKEEZIX
TELEFAX
TELEPIX

••••EX•
BATNEXT
CONTEXT
PRETEXT
SUBTEXT

••••E•X
LEMIEUX
LETTERX
MILIEUX
MIMIEUX
MISTERX
MONTEUX
STONEAX

•••••EX
ARUSPEX
CELOTEX
COMPLEX
COMTREX
DOUBLEX
FAIRSEX
FUNPLEX
GORETEX
HUMIDEX
KLEENEX
MADAMEX
MEMOREX
NARTHEX
PERPLEX
PLAYTEX
REANNEX
REINDEX
ROLODEX
SIMPLEX
SOMINEX
SPANDEX
TRIPLEX
UNIPLEX
UVINDEX

EY•••••
EYEBALL
EYEBANK
EYEBOLT
EYEBROW
EYECARE
EYECUPS
EYEDROP
EYEEXAM
EYEFOLD
EYEFULS
EYEHAND
EYEHOLE
EYEHOOK
EYELASH
EYELESS
EYELETS
EYELIDS
EYELIFT
EYELIKE
EYELINE
EYEMASK
EYEPITS
EYEROLL
EYESHOT
EYESORE
EYESPOT
EYETEST
EYETUCK
EYEWALL
EYEWASH
EYEWEAR
EYEWINK

E•Y••••
ELYSEES
ELYSIAN
ELYSIUM
ERYNGOS
ERYTHRO
ETYMONS
EXYANKS

E••Y•••
EASYJOB
EASYOFF
EASYONE
EBAYERS
ECDYSES
ECDYSIS
ECTYPAL
ECTYPES
EDDYING
ELIYALE
ELLYMAY
EMMYLOU
ENVYING
ENZYMES
ENZYMIC
ESPYING

E•••Y••
EARLYON
ECOTYPE
EMBAYED
EMBRYOS
ENCRYPT
ENJOYED
ENJOYER
EPONYMS
EPONYMY
ERINYES
ESSAYED
ESSAYER
EUONYMS
EXABYTE
EXMAYOR
EXONYMS

E••••Y•
EMPLOYS
ENDWAYS
ESTRAYS
EVERLYS
EVILEYE

E•••••Y
EAGERLY
EARTHLY
EASEDBY
EASESBY
EATAWAY
ECOLOGY
ECONOMY
ECSTASY
EDACITY
EDNAMAY
EFFABLY
EKINGBY
ELDERLY
ELLYMAY
ELMCITY
ELUSORY
EMBASSY
EMPATHY
EMPTILY
ENDERBY
ENDPLAY
ENOLOGY
ENQUIRY
ENTROPY
EPARCHY
EPERNAY
EPILADY
EPONYMY
EPPERLY
EQUABLY
EQUALLY
EQUERRY
ERECTLY
EROSELY
ERRANCY
ESOTERY
ESTUARY
EUPHONY
EXACTLY
EXENEMY
EXOGAMY
EXUPERY

•EY••••
BEYONCE
DEYOUNG
FEYDEAU
FEYNESS
FEYNMAN
GEYSERS
HEYDAYS
HEYJUDE
HEYLOOK
HEYMANS
HEYMRDJ
HEYRUBE
HEYWARD
HEYWOOD
KEYBANK
KEYCARD
KEYCASE
KEYCLUB
KEYDETS
KEYEDIN
KEYEDON
KEYEDUP
KEYGRIP
KEYHOLE
KEYINON
KEYLESS
KEYLIME
KEYLOCK
KEYNOTE
KEYPADS
KEYPALS
KEYRING
KEYSPAN
KEYWAYS
KEYWEST
KEYWORD
MEYNELL
PEYOTES
REYMONT
REYNARD
REYNAUD
REYNOSA
REYOKED
REYOKES
SEYMOUR

•E•Y•••
BEEYARD
BELYING
DEFYING
DENYING
DESYLVA
KENYANS
LEVYING
NEWYEAR
NEWYORK
PERYEAR
RECYCLE
REDYING
REFYING
RELYING
RETYPED
RETYPES
TENYEAR
VERYBAD
VERYBIG
VERYDRY
VERYFEW
VERYFIT
VERYHIP
VERYHOT
VERYILL
VERYLOW
VERYMAD
VERYNEW
VERYODD
VERYOLD
VERYRED
VERYSAD
VERYSHY
VERYWET

•E••Y••
BELAYED
BELAYER
BELLYUP
DECAYED
DECAYER
DECOYED
DECOYER
DECRYPT
DELAYED
DELAYER
DENTYNE
GEMAYEL
GENZYME
HECKYES
HELLYES
HENRYII
HENRYIV
HENRYVI
LEMOYNE
MEGRYAN
NEARYOU
NEOLYTE
REDDYES
REDEYED
REDEYES
REKEYED
RELAYED
RELAYER
REPLYTO
RESTYLE
SETTYPE
WELLYES
WETEYED
YEAHYOU
ZEPHYRS

•E•••Y•
BENDAYS
BERNAYS
BETRAYS
DEADEYE
DEEJAYS
DEFRAYS
DELKEYS
DELRAYS
DEMONYM
DEPLOYS
HENDRYX
HEYDAYS
JERILYN
JERSEYS
JETWAYS
KEYWAYS
LEAKEYS
LEEWAYS
LEFTEYE
MEDLEYS
NEWTOYS
PEDWAYS
PENNEYS
PEPBOYS
PETTOYS
REDBAYS

REPLAYS
SEAWAYS
SEGWAYS
SEQUOYA
TEAPOYS
TENDAYS
VEEJAYS

•E•••Y

BEADILY
BEANERY
BEASLEY
BEASTLY
BEATIFY
BEEFILY
BEGGARY
BEHAPPY
BELLAMY
BELLBOY
BELTWAY
BENTLEY
BERKLEY
BESTBOY
BESTBUY
BETARAY
BETHANY
BETTANY
BEVERLY
CENTURY
CEPHALY
CERTIFY
DEANERY
DEBAKEY
DEBUSSY
DECENCY
DEEPFRY
DEEPSKY
DEERFLY
DELANEY
DELCITY
DEMOLAY
DEMPSEY
DENNEHY
DENSELY
DENSIFY
DENSITY
DESTINY
DESTROY
DEVILRY
FELONRY
FERNERY
FERRETY
FETIDLY
GELIDLY
GEODESY
GEOLOGY
GERMANY
GETAWAY
GETBUSY
HEADILY
HEADWAY
HEALTHY
HEARSAY
HEATRAY
HEAVILY
HEFTILY
HELLBOY
HELOTRY

HEMSLEY
HENNERY
HENSLEY
HERONRY
HERSHEY
IEIGHTY
JEFFREY
JELLIFY
JERKILY
JEWELRY
KEARNEY
KENNEDY
LEAPDAY
LEDAWAY
LEERILY
LEGALLY
LEGIBLY
LENGTHY
LEONDAY
LETGOBY
LETSFLY
LETTERY
LEVELLY
MEADOWY
MEATILY
MENSCHY
MERCERY
MERCURY
MERRILY
MESSILY
NECTARY
NEEDILY
NEOLOGY
NERVILY
NEUILLY
NEWAGEY
NEWBERY
NEWSBOY
NEWSDAY
NEXTDAY
PEABODY
PECCARY
PEGAWAY
PENALTY
PEPPERY
PEPPILY
PERFIDY
PERFUMY
PERJURY
PERKILY
PESKILY
PETPONY
PETRIFY
PETTILY
READILY
REALITY
REAPPLY
REASSAY
RECARRY
RECENCY
RECTIFY
RECTORY
REDARMY
REDCLAY
REDECAY
REDPONY
REENJOY
REENTRY

REGALLY
REGENCY
REIMPLY
REMARRY
RENALLY
RESPRAY
RESTUDY
RETALLY
RETIARY
REUNIFY
REVELRY
REVERDY
SEADUTY
SEALERY
SEALILY
SECRECY
SEEDILY
SEMIDRY
SENDSBY
SENSORY
SETPLAY
SEVENTY
SEVIGNY
TEACOZY
TEARILY
TEATRAY
TENABLY
TENANCY
TENSELY
TENSITY
TENTHLY
TENUITY
TEPIDLY
TERNARY
TERRIFY
TERSELY
TESTACY
TESTFLY
TESTIFY
TESTILY
VELVETY
VENALLY
VERBIFY
VERMINY
VERSIFY
VERYDRY
VERYSHY
VEXEDLY
WEALTHY
WEARILY
WEEDILY
WEEKDAY
WEIGHTY
WEIRDLY
WEMBLEY
YELLOWY
YEVGENY
ZELAZNY
ZESTILY

••EY•••

ABEYANT
ALEYARD
AVEYRON
BEEYARD
BREYERS
DREYFUS
FREYTAG

GREYCUP
GREYEST
GREYHEN
GREYING
GREYISH
GREYLAG
JOEYDEE
LLEYTON
OBEYERS
OBEYING
ONEYARD
ONEYEAR
PREYERS
PREYING
PREYSON
THEYIPS
THEYSAY
WHEYISH

••E•Y••

AYEAYES
BYEBYES
DOEEYED
IBEGYOU
ISEEYOU
ONEBYTE
ONEEYED
PIEEYED
PRETYPE
SUELYON
TIEDYED
TIEDYES

••E••Y•

DEEJAYS
EVERLYS
IHEARYA
LEEWAYS
OVERDYE
PREBUYS
PREPAYS
THEBOYS
THEMAYO
VEEJAYS

••E•••Y

ACETIFY
ADEPTLY
AGENTRY
ALERTLY
AMENITY
AREAWAY
ARENSKY
ATEAWAY
BEEFILY
BLEAKLY
BREATHY
BREVITY
BREWERY
CHEAPLY
CHEWTOY
CLEANLY
CLEARLY
CLERISY
CLERKLY
CREELEY
CREEPBY
DEEPFRY

DEEPSKY
DEERFLY
DIEAWAY
DIETARY
EPERNAY
ERECTLY
EXENEMY
FIERILY
FLEETLY
FLESHLY
FRECKLY
FREETOY
FREEWAY
FRENEMY
FRESHLY
GREATLY
GREELEY
GREENLY
GREGORY
GRETZKY
ICETRAY
IDEALLY
INEPTLY
INERTLY
KVETCHY
LEERILY
NEEDILY
NOENTRY
OBESELY
OBESITY
OKELLEY
OLEANNY
ONEADAY
ONEMPTY
OREBODY
OREILLY
OVERBUY
OVERCOY
OVERDRY
OVERFLY
OVERJOY
OVERLAY
OVERPAY
OVERPLY
OVERTLY
PLENARY
PREACHY
PREALLY
PREDEFY
PREDENY
PRELACY
PRESLEY
QUEENLY
QUEERLY
QUESNAY
REENJOY
REENTRY
SCENERY
SEEDILY
SHEERLY
SHELLEY
SKETCHY
SLEEKLY
SNEAKBY
SPECIFY
STEEPLY
STERNLY
SWEARBY

SWEENEY
SWEETLY
SWELTRY
THEARMY
THEBABY
THEBODY
THECITY
THERAPY
THEREBY
THEYSAY
TIERNEY
TREACLY
TREMBLY
TRENARY
TUESDAY
UNEMPTY
UPEARLY
WEEDILY
WEEKDAY
WHEREBY
WREATHY

•••EY••

ALLEYES
BIGEYED
BIGEYES
BOGEYED
BONEYER
BUGEYED
CATEYED
DANEYKO
DOEEYED
DRYEYED
DRYEYES
HONEYED
IOWEYOU
ISEEYOU
LOVEYOU
MONEYED
MOSEYED
NUREYEV
ONEEYED
OWLEYED
PIEEYED
PIGEYED
POPEYED
POPEYES
REDEYED
REDEYES
REKEYED
RIBEYES
SADEYED
SADEYES
UNKEYED
VANEYCK
VOTEYEA
VOTEYES
WETEYED

•••E•Y•

APTERYX
JOCELYN
MTKENYA
RIDEBYS
VOTEAYE

•••E••Y

ADDEDLY

ALLENBY
ALLERGY
ALREADY
AMNESTY
APLENTY
ARDENCY
BASEPAY
BEVERLY
BIGEASY
BIKEWAY
BLUEBOY
BLUEJAY
BLUESKY
BONEDRY
BRIEFLY
CADENCY
CAPEMAY
CHIEFLY
CINERGY
COGENCY
COMESBY
CREELEY
CREEPBY
CRUELLY
CRUELTY
DARESAY
DATEDLY
DAZEDLY
DECENCY
DOHERTY
DRWELBY
EAGERLY
EASEDBY
EASESBY
ELDERLY
ENDERBY
EPPERLY
EQUERRY
FADEDLY
FILEDBY
FILESBY
FIREFLY
FIVEDAY
FIVEWAY
FIXEDLY
FLEETLY
FLIESBY
FLUENCY
FOGERTY
FOREBAY
FREETOY
FREEWAY
FTHENRY
GAMEBOY
GASEITY
GATEWAY
GAVEWAY
GIVENBY
GIVEWAY
GREELEY
GREENLY
HAGERTY
HAPENNY
HOMEBOY
HONESTY
IFWEMAY
IMREADY
INDEEDY

INNERLY
ITSEASY
ITWENTY
JADEDLY
JANEWAY
JEWELRY
JUNEDAY
LATENCY
LAZENBY
LEVELLY
LIBERTY
LINEDRY
LIVESEY
LOVEJOY
LOVERLY
LOWEEZY
LUCENCY
MADEHAY
MADEWAY
MAJESTY
MAKEHAY
MAKEWAY
MCHENRY
MISERLY
MIXEDLY
MODESTY
MOREPAY
MORESBY
MUTEDLY
NAKEDLY
NAMEDAY
NICEBOY
NICEDAY
NICEGUY
NICETRY
NOMERCY
NOSEGAY
NOTEASY
NOTEDLY
NOVELTY
ORDERLY
PAGEBOY
PALEDRY
PATENCY
PHLEGMY
POTENCY
POVERTY
PUBERTY
PUDENCY
QUEENLY
QUEERLY
QUIETLY
RACEDBY
RACESBY
RACEWAY
RAVELLY
RECENCY
REDECAY
REGENCY
REVELRY
REVERDY
RIDESBY
ROSEBAY
RULEDBY
SAFEWAY
SAMEDAY
SEVENTY
SHEERLY

SIDEWAY
SILENTY
SLEEKLY
SOBERLY
SOMEDAY
SOMESAY
SOMEWAY
SPLEENY
SQUEAKY
STEEPLY
STREAKY
SWEENEY
SWEETLY
SYNERGY
TAKENBY
THIERRY
THREADY
TIREDLY
TOOEASY
UNHEADY
UNHEAVY
UNLEAKY
UNMERRY
UNNEEDY
UNREADY
UNWEARY
URGENCY
UTTERLY
VEXEDLY
VICEROY
VIXENLY
VOTENAY
VOWELLY
WISEGUY

••••EY•

ALTKEYS
BARLEYS
BARNEYS
BUCKEYE
CARKEYS
CATSEYE
CONVEYS
DEADEYE
DELKEYS
DICKEYS
DONKEYS
DORSEYS
EVILEYE
FISHEYE
FONTEYN
GALLEYS
GLADEYE
GOONEYS
GURNEYS
HALLEYS
HANDEYE
HARLEYS
HAWKEYE
HICKEYS
HOTKEYS
JERSEYS
JITNEYS
JOCKEYS
KIDNEYS
LACKEYS
LEAKEYS
LEFTEYE

MEDLEYS
MICKEYS
MISKEYS
MONKEYS
MOONEYE
MOTLEYS
ORKNEYS
OSPREYS
PARLEYS
PENNEYS
PHONEYS
PULLEYS
PURVEYS
RICKEYS
ROMNEYS
SHUTEYE
SMILEYS
SMOKEYS
SOCKEYE
SURREYS
SURVEYS
TABKEYS
TURKEYS
VALLEYS
VOLLEYS
WALLEYE

••••E•Y

ABIDEBY
ACADEMY
ACUTELY
AGILELY
ALCHEMY
ANXIETY
ARCHERY
ASHBERY
BATTERY
BEANERY
BINDERY
BLAKELY
BOOTERY
BRAVELY
BRAVERY
BREWERY
BRIBERY
BRUTELY
BUTTERY
BYTHEBY
CANNERY
CINDERY
CLOSEBY
CLOSELY
CLOVERY
CONNERY
COOKERY
COOPERY
COPPERY
CRUDELY
CUTLERY
DEANERY
DENNEHY
DENSELY
DITHERY
DODDERY
DONLEVY
DRAMEDY
DRAPERY
DRIVEBY

DROVEBY
DUBIETY
EROSELY
ESOTERY
EXENEMY
EXUPERY
FALSELY
FARMERY
FERNERY
FERRETY
FIDGETY
FISHERY
FLOWERY
FOOLERY
FOPPERY
FORGERY
FRENEMY
GADGETY
GALLERY
GAUDERY
GEODESY
GINGERY
GLIDEBY
GRAPERY
GRAVELY
GROCERY
GUNNERY
HENNERY
HOGGERY
HOSIERY
IMAGERY
IMPIETY
INANELY
INDEEDY
ININETY
IRATELY
JASPERY
JIGGERY
JITTERY
JOBBERY
JOINERY
KENNEDY
KITTERY
KNAVERY
LARCENY
LARGELY
LATHERY
LETTERY
LICKETY
LIQUEFY
LITHELY
LITTERY
LOOSELY
LOTTERY
LOWEEZY
MARGERY
MASTERY
MERCERY
MILDEWY
MISRELY
MOCKERY
MOTHERY
MUMMERY
MYSTERY
NAIVELY
NAIVETY
NEWBERY
NIMIETY

NUGGETY
NUNNERY
NURSERY
OBESELY
OROGENY
PEPPERY
PIGGERY
POTTERY
POWDERY
PREDEFY
PREDENY
PRIMELY
PROGENY
PRONELY
PRUDERY
PTOLEMY
PUCKERY
PUFFERY
PUTREFY
QUAVERY
QUIVERY
RACKETY
RAGGEDY
RICKETY
RIFLERY
ROBBERY
ROCKERY
ROGUERY
ROOKERY
RUBBERY
RUSSETY
SATIETY
SCAREDY
SCENERY
SEALERY
SECRECY
SHAPELY
SHIVERY
SHOWERY
SILVERY
SLAVERY
SLIDEBY
SNIDELY
SOCIETY
SORCERY
SOTHEBY
SPACELY
SPARELY
SPICERY
SPIDERY
SPLEENY
STALELY
STATELY
STOKELY
STUPEFY
SUAVELY
SUMMERY
SURGERY
SWINERY
SWOREBY
TANNERY
TATTERY
TAXLEVY
TENSELY
TERSELY
THEREBY
TIMBERY
TINDERY

TOGGERY
TORREFY
TOTTERY
TRACERY
TRAGEDY
TRITELY
TURNERY
TUSHERY
UNFIERY
UNNEEDY
UNPIETY
VAGUELY
VARIETY
VELVETY
WAGGERY
WHEREBY
WHITELY
WIGGERY
WINTERY
WOOLERY
YEVGENY

•••••EY

BALONEY
BARKLEY
BEASLEY
BENTLEY
BERKLEY
BLAKLEY
BLARNEY
BOBBSEY
BRADLEY
BRAMLEY
BRAWLEY
BRIMLEY
BRITNEY
BRODKEY
BUCKLEY
BURNLEY
CARDKEY
CHANTEY
CHARLEY
CHIMNEY
CHOOSEY
CHUTNEY
CLIQUEY
CLOONEY
COCKNEY
CONFREY
CRAWLEY
CREELEY
CROWLEY
CURTSEY
DAHOMEY
DALTREY
DEBAKEY
DELANEY
DEMPSEY
DIDDLEY
DISOBEY
DOUBLEY
FINDLEY
FRAWLEY
FRIDLEY
FTRILEY
GODFREY
GREELEY
GRIFFEY

HACKNEY
HARTLEY
HEMSLEY
HENSLEY
HERSHEY
HORSLEY
HUNTLEY
JEFFREY
JOFFREY
JOURNEY
JTMONEY
KEARNEY
LAMPREY
LANGLEY
LINDSEY
LIVESEY
MAHONEY
MALMSEY
MCCAREY
MCCOVEY
MCRANEY
MOMONEY
MRHANEY
NEWAGEY
ODYSSEY
OKELLEY
OMALLEY
ORANGEY
PAISLEY
PALFREY
PALJOEY
PARSLEY
PASSKEY
PRESLEY
PUGSLEY
QUIGLEY
QUINCEY
SHARKEY
SHELLEY
SHIRLEY
SOUTHEY
SPINNEY
STANLEY
STARKEY
STOOKEY
SWEENEY
TIERNEY
TINAFEY
TISSUEY
TOURNEY
TROLLEY
TURNKEY
VICKREY
WEMBLEY
WHALLEY
WHISKEY
WHITNEY
WINFREY
WOODLEY
WOOLLEY
WOOLSEY
WORSLEY
WRIGLEY

EZ•••••
EZEKIEL

E•Z••••
ECZEMAS
ENZYMES
ENZYMIC

E••Z•••
ENDZONE

E•••Z••
ELEAZAR
ELIEZER

E••••Z•
EBONIZE
ELEGIZE
EMBLAZE

E•••••Z
ESTEVEZ
EXCUSEZ

•EZ••••
BEZIERS
BEZIQUE
CEZANNE
JEZEBEL
MEZUZAH
MEZUZAS
REZEROS
REZONED
REZONES

•E•Z•••
BEEZERS
BELZONI
BENZALI
BENZELL
BENZENE
GEEZERS
GENZYME
MENZIES
NETZERO
PENZIAS
REDZONE
SEIZEON
SEIZERS
SEIZING
SEIZORS
SEIZURE
TENZING
WEBZINE

•E••Z••
BEDAZED
BEDAZES
BEDIZEN
BENAZIR
DENIZEN
LEIPZIG
MEZUZAH
MEZUZAS
NETIZEN
REBOZOS
RENUZIT
RESIZED
RESIZER
RESIZES
SECHZIG
SELTZER
VENEZIA
VERIZON
ZELAZNY

•E•••Z•
CERVEZA
DEGLAZE
JERITZA
LEGANZA
REALIZE
REGLAZE
RESEIZE
TEACOZY

•E••••Z
BEDNORZ
BERLIOZ
BERLITZ
GEEWHIZ
HEIFETZ
KERTESZ
LEIBNIZ
LETTERZ
TEMPEAZ

••EZ•••
BEEZERS
CHEZMOI
GEEZERS
KLEZMER
MUEZZIN

••E•Z••
BREEZED
BREEZES
CHEEZIT
COETZEE
DWEEZIL
ELEAZAR
FREEZER
FREEZES
GRETZKY
MUEZZIN
PRETZEL
QUETZAL
SIEBZIG
SKEEZIX
SLEAZES
SNEEZED
SNEEZER
SNEEZES
TREIZES
TWEEZED
TWEEZER
TWEEZES
VIERZIG
WHEEZED
WHEEZER
WHEEZES

••E••Z•
ELEGIZE
GRECIZE
ITEMIZE
OBELIZE
ONESIZE
POETIZE

••E•••Z
GEEWHIZ
THEFONZ
THERITZ

•••EZ••
BREEZED
BREEZES
CABEZAS
CHEEZIT
DAREZZO
DWEEZIL
ELIEZER
FREEZER
FREEZES
FRIEZES
SKEEZIX
SNEEZED
SNEEZER
SNEEZES
TWEEZED
TWEEZER
TWEEZES
VENEZIA
WHEEZED
WHEEZER
WHEEZES

•••E•Z•
CADENZA
DAREZZO
FIRENZA
FIRENZE
FORENZA
LORENZO
LOWEEZY
RESEIZE
SCHERZI
SCHERZO
SQUEEZE
VICENZA

•••E••Z
ALBENIZ
DAVEKOZ
ESTEVEZ
HJHEINZ
JIMENEZ
LORENTZ
SILENTZ

••••EZ•
CERVEZA
IMPREZA
LOWEEZY
SQUEEZE
TRAPEZE
ZAMBEZI

••••E•Z
COBLENZ
FLORENZ
HEIFETZ
KAYLENZ
KERTESZ
KOBLENZ
LETTERZ
TEMPEAZ

•••••EZ
ALLOPEZ
ALVAREZ
DOUBLEZ
ESTEVEZ
EXCUSEZ
GRISNEZ
JIMENEZ
JIMINEZ
LAISSEZ
MARQUEZ
NARVAEZ
NATCHEZ
ORDONEZ
RAMIREZ
VASQUEZ

FA•••••
FABARES
FABBEST
FABERGE
FABFOUR
FABLERS
FABLING
FABRICS
FABRIZI
FACADES
FACEDIT
FACEDON
FACEOFF
FACESIT
FACESON
FACETED
FACIALS
FACINGS
FACONNE
FACTFUL
FACTION
FACTOID
FACTORS
FACTORY
FACTUAL
FACULAE
FACULTY
FADAYEV
FADDIER
FADDIET
FADDISH
FADDISM
FADDIST
FADEDIN
FADEDLY
FADEINS
FADEOUT
FADESIN
FADIMAN
FADLIKE
FAERIES
FAEROES
FAGENDS
FAGOTED
FAIENCE
FAILING
FAILLES
FAILSTO
FAILURE
FAINEST
FAINTED
FAINTER
FAINTLY
FAIREST
FAIRFAX
FAIRIES
FAIRING
FAIRISH
FAIROFF
FAIRSEX
FAIRSUP
FAIRUSE
FAIRWAY
FAISALI
FAJITAS
FAKEDIT
FAKEFUR
FAKEIDS
FAKEOUT
FAKESIT
FALAFEL
FALCATE
FALCONS
FALKIRK
FALLACY
FALLALS
FALLDUE
FALLERS
FALLFOR
FALLGUY
FALLING
FALLOFF
FALLOUT
FALLOWS
FALLSIN
FALLSON
FALLSTO
FALSELY
FALSEST
FALSIFY
FALSITY
FALTERS
FALWELL
FAMICOM
FAMILIA
FAMILLE
FAMINES
FAMULUS
FANATIC
FANBASE
FANBELT
FANCIED
FANCIER
FANCIES
FANCIFY
FANCILY
FANCLUB
FANCYUP
FANDOMS
FANEUIL
FANFARE
FANFEST
FANFICS
FANFOLD
FANGING
FANIONS
FANJETS
FANLIKE
FANMAIL
FANNERS
FANNING
FANOUTS
FANPALM
FANSLER
FANSOUT
FANTAIL
FANTANS
FANTASM
FANTAST
FANTASY
FANTINE
FANTODS
FANWISE
FANZINE
FARADAY
FARAWAY
FARCEUR
FARCING
FAREAST
FAREBOX
FAREWAR
FARFELS
FARGOND
FARGONE
FARINAS
FARLEFT
FARMAID
FARMBOY
FARMERS
FARMERY
FARMGAL
FARMING
FARMORE
FARMOUT
FARNESS
FAROESE
FAROUKI
FARRAGO
FARRELL
FARRIER
FARROWS
FARSEER
FARSIDE
FARTHER
FARTLEK
FARWEST
FASCIAE
FASCIAL
FASCIAS
FASCISM
FASCIST
FASHION
FASTCAR
FASTENS
FASTEST
FASTING
FASTNET
FASTONE
FATALES
FATALLY
FATBACK
FATCATS
FATCELL
FATCITY
FATEFUL
FATFARM
FATFREE
FATHEAD
FATHERS
FATHOMS
FATIDIC
FATIGUE
FATLESS
FATLIKE
FATLING
FATLIPS
FATNESS
FATONES
FATOUSH
FATTENS
FATTEST
FATTIER
FATTILY
FATTING
FATTISH
FATUITY
FATUOUS
FAUCETS
FAULTED
FAUSTUS
FAUVISM
FAUVIST
FAUXFUR
FAUXPAS
FAVORED
FAVORER
FAVOURS
FAWCETT
FAWNERS
FAWNING
FAWNSON
FAXLORE
FAYETTE
FAYWRAY

F•A••••
FEARERS
FEARFOR
FEARFUL
FEARING
FEARNOT
FEASTED
FEASTER
FEASTON
FEATHER
FEATURE
FHALOAN
FIACRES
FIANCEE
FIANCES
FIASCOS
FIATLUX
FLACCID
FLACKED
FLACONS
FLAGDAY
FLAGGED
FLAGGER
FLAGMAN
FLAGMEN
FLAGONS
FLAILAT
FLAILED
FLAKERS
FLAKIER
FLAKILY
FLAKING
FLAMBED
FLAMBES
FLAMERS
FLAMEUP
FLAMIER
FLAMING
FLAMMED
FLANEUR
FLANGES
FLANKED
FLANKEN
FLANKER
FLANNEL
FLAPPED
FLAPPER
FLAREUP
FLARING
FLASHED
FLASHER
FLASHES
FLASHON
FLATBED
FLATCAR
FLATHAT
FLATLET
FLATOUT
FLATTAX
FLATTED
FLATTEN
FLATTER
FLATTOP
FLATTVS
FLAUNTS
FLAUNTY
FLAUTAS
FLAVIUS
FLAVORS
FLAVORY
FLAVOUR
FLAWIER
FLAWING
FLAXIER
FLAYERS
FLAYING
FOALING
FOAMERS
FOAMIER
FOAMILY
FOAMING
FRACTAL
FRAGGED
FRAGGLE
FRAGILE
FRAICHE
FRAILER
FRAILLY
FRAILTY
FRAISES
FRAMERS
FRAMEUP
FRAMING
FRANCES
FRANCHI
FRANCIS
FRANKED
FRANKEN
FRANKER
FRANKIE
FRANKLY
FRANKOZ
FRANTIC
FRAPPES
FRASIER
FRATERS
FRAUGHT
FRAWLEY
FRAYING
FRAZIER
FRAZZLE

F••A•••
FABARES
FACADES
FADAYEV
FALAFEL
FANATIC
FARADAY
FARAWAY
FATALES
FATALLY
FEMALES
FINABLE
FINAGLE
FINALES
FINALLY
FINANCE
FIXABLE
FIXATED
FIXATES
FLEABAG
FLEADIP
FLEANCE
FLEAPIT
FLOATBY
FLOATED
FLOATER
FLOATUP
FLYABLE
FLYAWAY
FMBANDS
FMRADIO
FOLATES
FORABIT
FORADAY
FORAGED
FORAGER
FORAGES
FORASEC
FORAYED
FREAKED
FRIABLE
FRIARLY
FRYABLE
FTWAYNE
FUGALLY
FUGATOS

F•••A••
FACIALS
FAISALI
FALCATE
FALLACY
FALLALS
FANBASE
FANFARE
FANMAIL
FANPALM
FANTAIL
FANTANS
FANTASM
FANTAST
FANTASY
FAREAST
FARMAID
FARRAGO
FATBACK
FATCATS
FATFARM
FBICASE
FEEBATE
FELLAHS
FERMATA
FERMATE
FERMATS
FERNAND
FERRARA
FERRARE
FERRARI
FERRARO
FERRATE
FIGBARS
FIJIANS
FINBACK
FINEART
FINGALS
FINIALS
FINIANS
FINLAND
FINNAIR
FIRBANK
FIREANT
FIREARM
FIVEAAA
FLOTAGE
FLOWAGE
FLYBALL
FLYCAST
FLYPAST
FLYWAYS
FOGBANK
FOGLAMP
FOLIAGE
FOLIATE
FOLKART
FONDANT
FONTANA
FONTANE
FOOTAGE
FORBADE
FOREACH
FOREARM
FORGAVE
FORLANI
FORMALS
FORMATS
FORSAKE
FORSALE
FORWARD
FOULARD
FOURAAA
FOXTAIL
FREEAIR
FRIDAYS
FRIGATE
FROMAGE
FROWARD
FRYPANS
FTBRAGG
FTMEADE
FULMARS
FUNFAIR
FURBALL
FURCATE
FURFARM
FURNACE
FURTADO
FUTHARK

F••••A•
FACTUAL
FACULAE
FADIMAN
FAIRFAX
FAIRWAY
FAJITAS
FARADAY
FARAWAY
FAREWAR
FARINAS
FARMGAL
FASCIAE
FASCIAL
FASCIAS
FASTCAR
FATHEAD
FAUXPAS
FAYWRAY
FEDERAL
FEDORAS
FEEDBAG
FEELBAD
FELDMAN
FELTBAD
FELTHAT
FEMORAL
FERNBAR
FEYDEAU
FEYNMAN
FHALOAN
FIBULAE
FIBULAR
FIBULAS
FIESTAS
FIFTYAD
FIGLEAF
FIGURAL
FILOFAX
FINDLAY
FINICAL
FIREDAT
FIREHAT
FIREMAN
FIRESAT
FIVEAAA
FIVEDAY
FIVEMAN
FIVEWAY
FLAGDAY
FLAGMAN
FLAILAT
FLATCAR
FLATHAT
FLATTAX
FLAUTAS
FLEABAG
FLIESAT
FLINGAT
FLOREAL
FLORIAN
FLOTSAM
FLOWNAT
FLUIDAL
FLUNGAT
FLUVIAL
FLYAWAY
FLYLEAF
FLYTRAP
FMURRAY
FOLKWAY
FOOTBAG
FOOTMAN
FOOTPAD
FOOTWAY
FORADAY
FORBEAR
FORDHAM
FOREBAY
FOREMAN
FOREPAW
FORERAN
FORESAW
FORREAL
FORTRAN
FORTYAD
FOTOMAT
FOURAAA
FOURDAY
FOURMAN
FOURWAY
FRACTAL
FREEMAN
FREEWAY
FREITAG
FRENEAU
FRESCAS
FRETSAT
FRETSAW
FREYTAG
FRIEDAN
FRISIAN
FROGMAN
FRONTAL
FROWNAT
FUJISAN
FULLDAY
FUMEDAT
FUMESAT
FURCOAT
FURSEAL
FURWRAP
FUSTIAN
FUSUMAS
FUTURAS

F•••••A
FAMILIA
FELICIA
FERMATA

FERRARA FESTINA FESTIVA FIDELIA FIORINA FIRENZA FIVEAAA FLORIDA FONTANA FONTINA FORENZA FORMICA FORMOSA FORMULA FORTUNA FOURAAA FREESIA FUCHSIA

•FA••••

AFARCRY AFATLOT OFAKIND OFAMIND OFANAGE OFASORT XFACTOR

•F•A•••

AFEARED AFFABLE AFFABLY AFFAIRE AFFAIRS AFRAMES EFFABLE EFFABLY EFFACED EFFACER EFFACES OFVALUE

•F••A••

AFFIANT AFFRAYS AFGHANI AFGHANS NFLGAME OFANAGE OFFBASE OFFCAST OFFDAYS OFFHAND OFFRAMP VFWHALL

•F•••A•

AFCTEAM AFRICAN IFWEMAY NFCTEAM NFLTEAM OFFBEAT OFFLOAD OFFPEAK OFFROAD OFFYEAR

••FA•••

AFFABLE AFFABLY AFFAIRE AFFAIRS ALFALFA ASFARAS ATFAULT BEFALLS DEFACED DEFACER DEFACES DEFACTO DEFALLA DEFAMED DEFAMER DEFAMES DEFANGS DEFARGE DEFAULT EFFABLE EFFABLY EFFACED EFFACER EFFACES ENFACED ENFACES ENFANTS EXFACTO INFAITH INFANCY INFANTA INFANTE INFANTS INFAVOR ISFAHAN LAFARGE MYFAULT NOFAULT REFACED REFACES REFALLS REFAXED REFAXES SAFARIS SOFABED SOFARAS UNFACED UNFACTS UNFADED UNFAITH UNFAKED UNFAMED UNFANCY UNFATED UNFATTY UNFAZED

••F•A••

AFFIANT AFFRAYS BUFFALO CAFTANS DEFEATS DEFIANT DEFLATE DEFOAMS DEFRAGS DEFRAME DEFRAUD DEFRAYS ENFLAME ENFRAME GUFFAWS HOFMANN INFLAME INFLATE INFRACT LEFTARM OFFBASE OFFCAST OFFDAYS OFFHAND OFFRAMP REFLAGS REFLATE REFRACT REFRAIN REFRAME RUFFALO TIFFANY UNFLAKY UNFRAIL UNFRANK USFLAGS

••F••A•

ASFARAS BIFOCAL DEFLEAS FIFTYAD GIFTTAX HOFBRAU HOFFMAN HUFFMAN ISFAHAN LEFREAK LEFTEAR LEFTJAB OFFBEAT OFFLOAD OFFPEAK OFFROAD OFFYEAR RAFFIAS REFLOAT REFUSAL REFUTAL RUFFIAN RUFIYAA SAFEWAY SOFARAS

••F•••A

ALFALFA ALFORJA ALFREDA BOFFOLA DEFALLA HOFSTRA INFANTA RUFIYAA TAFFETA

•••FA••

AIRFARE ANTFARM ARTFAIR BEEFALO BELFAST BIDFAIR BIGFANS BUFFALO BUSFARE CABFARE CARFARE CONFABS CORFAMS CUBFANS DEWFALL DOGFACE FANFARE FATFARM FUNFAIR FURFARM GUFFAWS ICEFALL JETFANS JOBFAIR LEAFAGE LENFANT LETFALL LOOFAHS MAYFAIR METFANS NEWFACE NONFACT NONFANS NONFARM NOTFAIR OUTFACE OUTFAST OUTFAWN PARFAIT PITFALL PREFABS PREFACE PREFADE PROFANE PROFARM RAMFANS REDFACE ROOFAGE RUFFALO SADFATE SEAFARE SERFAGE SHOFARS SOXFANS STEFANI SULFATE SUNFANS SUNFAST SURFACE THEFALL TIFFANY TOYFAIR TWOFACE WARFARE WASFAIR WELFARE

•••F•A•

BARFBAG BIAFRAN CATFLAP DORFMAN EARFLAP GOLFBAG GOLFCAR GULFWAR HALFBAD HALFDAY HALFMAD HALFRAW HALFWAY HOFFMAN HUFFMAN KAUFMAN LOAFPAN MUDFLAP MUDFLAT RAFFIAS REDFLAG ROOFRAT RUFFIAN SCOFFAT SEAFOAM SNIFFAT SURFMAN TURFMAN TURFWAR WOLFGAL WOLFMAN WOLFRAM

•••F••A

ARAFURA BEEFTEA BOFFOLA CATFLEA DOGFLEA TAFFETA THEFLEA

••••FA•

AVIDFAN BODYFAT CUBSFAN DEEPFAT EQUIFAX ESTEFAN FAIRFAX FILOFAX GETSFAR GOESFAR GONEFAR GREWFAT GROWFAT HALIFAX HEATFAN INSOFAR JETSFAN JUNKFAX LATIFAH LESSFAT METSFAN OVERFAR OVERFAT RAMSFAN REDSFAN SCOFFAT SNIFFAT SUNSFAN TELEFAX THUSFAR WENTFAR WOOLFAT

••••F•A

RATAFIA

•••••FA

ALFALFA MUSTAFA

FB•••••

FBICASE FBIFILE

F•B••••

FABARES FABBEST FABERGE FABFOUR FABLERS FABLING FABRICS FABRIZI FEBRERO FEBRILE FIBBERS FIBBING FIBERED FIBIGER FIBRINS FIBROID FIBROUS FIBSTER FIBULAE FIBULAR FIBULAS FMBANDS FOBBING FOBSOFF FTBLISS FTBRAGG FUBSIER

F••B•••

FABBEST FANBASE FANBELT FATBACK FEEBATE FEEBLER FEMBOTS FIBBERS FIBBING FIGBARS FILBERT FINBACK FIRBANK FLUBBED FLUBBER FLUBDUB FLUBUGS FLYBALL FLYBOYS FOBBING FOGBANK FOGBOWS FOIBLES FORBADE FORBEAR FORBIDS FORBORE FORBUSH FOXBORO FREBERG FRIBBLE FUMBLED FUMBLER FUMBLES FURBALL FURBISH

F•••B••

FAREBOX FARMBOY FEEDBAG FEEDBIN FEELBAD FELTBAD FERNBAR FILIBEG FINABLE FIREBOX FIREBUG FIXABLE FLAMBED FLAMBES FLATBED FLEABAG FLUBBED FLUBBER FLYABLE FNUMBER FOOTBAG FORABIT FOREBAY FREEBEE FREEBIE FRIABLE FRIBBLE FRISBEE FROEBEL FRYABLE FUSEBOX FUSIBLE

F••••B•

FIFTYBC FILEDBY FILESBY FLIESBY FLITSBY FLOATBY FLOWNBY FORTYBC FREDEBB

F•••••B

FANCLUB FLUBDUB FOODWEB FOOTRUB FREDEBB

•F•B•••

OFFBASE OFFBEAT

•F••B••

AFFABLE AFFABLY EFFABLE EFFABLY

••FB•••

HOFBRAU OFFBASE OFFBEAT

••F•B••

AFFABLE AFFABLY EFFABLE EFFABLY GIFTBOX LOFTBED SAFEBET SOFABED

••F••B•

FIFTYBC

••F•••B

LEFTJAB

•••FB••

BARFBAG GOLFBAG HALFBAD

•••F•B•

CONFABS PREFABS

•••F••B

WOLFCUB

•••••FB

POPEAFB

F•C••••

FACADES FACEDIT FACEDON FACEOFF FACESIT FACESON FACETED FACIALS FACINGS FACONNE FACTFUL FACTION FACTOID FACTORS FACTORY FACTUAL FACULAE FACULTY FECHNER FICKLER FICTILE FICTION FICTIVE FICUSES FOCSLES FOCUSED FOCUSER FOCUSES FOCUSON FUCHSIA

F••C•••

FALCATE FALCONS FANCIED FANCIER FANCIES FANCIFY FANCILY FANCLUB FANCYUP FARCEUR FARCING FASCIAE FASCIAL FASCIAS FASCISM FASCIST FATCATS FATCELL FATCITY FAUCETS FAWCETT FBICASE FENCEIN FENCERS FENCEUP FENCING FESCUES FETCHED FETCHER FETCHES FIACRES FILCHED FILCHER FILCHES FINCHES FISCHER FLACCID FLACKED FLACONS FLECHES FLECKED FLICKED FLICKER FLOCKED FLOCKTO FLYCAST FOGCITY FORCEIN FORCEON FORCEPS FORCERS FORCEUP FORCING FOSCOLO FRACTAL FRECKLE FRECKLY FRICKER FROCKED FRYCOOK FULCRUM FURCATE FURCOAT

F•••C••

FAMICOM FASTCAR FELICIA FIANCEE FIANCES FIASCOS FIERCER FINICAL FINICKY FLACCID FLATCAR FLEECED FLEECER FLEECES FRAICHE FRANCES FRANCHI FRANCIS FRENCHI FRENCHS FRESCAS FRESCOS

F••••C•

FABRICS FAIENCE FALLACY FANFICS FATBACK FETLOCK FINANCE FINBACK FIREICE FLEANCE FLOUNCE FLOUNCY FLUENCY FOREACH FORMICA FORONCE FOSDICK FROLICS FURNACE

F•••••C

FANATIC FATIDIC FIFTYBC FJORDIC FLUIDIC FORASEC FORTYBC FRANTIC FREDRIC

•FC••••

AFCTEAM NFCTEAM

•F•C•••

OFFCAST XFACTOR

•F••C••

AFARCRY AFFECTS AFRICAN EFFACED EFFACER EFFACES EFFECTS GFORCES OFFICER OFFICES OFFICIO

•F•••C•

AFFLECK AFFLICT OFFENCE

••FC•••

DEFCONS OFFCAST

••F•C••

AFFECTS BIFOCAL DEFACED DEFACER DEFACES DEFACTO DEFECTS DEFICIT DEFOCUS EFFACED EFFACER EFFACES EFFECTS ENFACED ENFACES EXFACTO INFECTS INFOCUS OFFICER OFFICES OFFICIO REFACED REFACES REFOCUS UNFACED UNFACTS

••F••C•

AFFLECK AFFLICT BYFORCE DEFENCE DEFLECT DEFROCK DEFUNCT ELFLOCK ENFORCE INFANCY INFLECT INFLICT INFORCE INFRACT OFFENCE REFENCE REFLECT REFRACT SUFFICE UNFANCY UNFENCE UNFROCK

••F•••C

FIFTYBC

•••FC••

GOLFCAR HALFCUT WOLFCUB

•••F•C•

CONFECT DOGFACE EDIFICE FANFICS NEWFACE NONFACT ORIFICE OUTFACE PERFECT PREFACE PREFECT REDFACE SUFFICE SURFACE TWOFACE

•••F••C

AELFRIC TRAFFIC

••••F•C

BENEFIC MALEFIC OSSIFIC PACIFIC TRAFFIC

F•D••••

FADAYEV FADDIER FADDIET FADDISH FADDISM FADDIST FADEDIN FADEDLY FADEINS FADEOUT FADESIN FADIMAN FADLIKE FEDDERS FEDERAL FEDERKO FEDEXED FEDEXES FEDINTO FEDORAS FEDOROV FIDDLED FIDDLER FIDDLES FIDELES FIDELIA FIDELIO FIDELIS FIDGETS FIDGETY FODDERS FTDIXNJ FTDODGE FUDDIES FUDDLED FUDDLES FUDGERS FUDGING

F••D•••

FADDIER FADDIET FADDISH FADDISM FADDIST FANDOMS FEDDERS FEEDBAG FEEDBIN FEEDERS FEEDING FEEDLOT FEEDSIN FEEDSON FEEDSTO FELDMAN FENDERS FENDING FENDOFF FEODORI FEUDING FEUDIST FEYDEAU FIDDLED FIDDLER FIDDLES FIEDLER FINDERS FINDING FINDLAY FINDLEY FINDOUT FLEDGED FLEDGES FODDERS FOGDOGS FOLDERS FOLDING FOLDOUT FOLDSIN FOLDSUP FOLDUPS FONDANT FONDEST FONDLED FONDLER FONDLES FONDUED FONDUES

FOODIES
FOODWEB
FORDGTS
FORDHAM
FORDING
FORDLTD
FORDOES
FORDONE
FOSDICK
FOUDRES
FREDDIE
FREDEBB
FREDRIC
FRIDAYS
FRIDGES
FRIDLEY
FRODING
FUDDIES
FUDDLED
FUDDLES
FUNDERS
FUNDING

F•••D••

FACADES
FACEDIT
FACEDON
FADEDIN
FADEDLY
FAKEDIT
FALLDUE
FARADAY
FATIDIC
FELLDUE
FETIDLY
FIEFDOM
FIELDED
FIELDER
FILEDBY
FILEDIN
FILMDOM
FIREDAT
FIREDOG
FIREDON
FIREDUP
FIVEDAY
FIXEDLY
FIXEDON
FIXEDUP
FJORDIC
FLAGDAY
FLEADIP
FLIEDTO
FLOODED
FLUBDUB
FLUIDAL
FLUIDIC
FLUIDLY
FMRADIO
FORADAY
FORTDIX
FOUNDED
FOUNDER
FOUNDRY
FOURDAY
FREDDIE
FREEDOF
FREEDOM
FREEDUP
FRIEDAN
FRIEDUP
FTDODGE
FULLDAY
FUMEDAT

F••••D•

FAGENDS
FAKEIDS
FANTODS
FARSIDE
FLORIDA
FLYRODS
FMBANDS
FORBADE
FORBIDS
FRIENDS
FTMEADE
FURTADO

F•••••D

FACETED
FACTOID
FAGOTED
FAINTED
FANCIED
FANFOLD
FARGOND
FARMAID
FATHEAD
FAULTED
FAVORED
FEASTED
FEDEXED
FEELBAD
FEIGNED
FEINTED
FELTBAD
FEOFFED
FERNAND
FERRIED
FETCHED
FEVERED
FIBERED
FIBROID
FIDDLED
FIELDED
FIFTYAD
FIGURED
FILCHED
FINISHD
FINLAND
FIXATED
FIZZLED
FLACCID
FLACKED
FLAGGED
FLAILED
FLAMBED
FLAMMED
FLANKED
FLAPPED
FLASHED
FLATBED
FLATTED
FLECKED
FLEDGED
FLEECED
FLEERED
FLEETED
FLENSED
FLESHED
FLICKED
FLIPPED
FLIRTED
FLITTED
FLOATED
FLOCKED
FLOGGED
FLOODED
FLOORED
FLOPPED
FLOSSED
FLOURED
FLOUTED
FLUBBED
FLUFFED
FLUNKED
FLUSHED
FOCUSED
FOISTED
FOLIOED
FONDLED
FONDUED
FOOTLED
FOOTPAD
FOOZLED
FORAGED
FORAYED
FORDLTD
FORFEND
FORGOOD
FORTORD
FORTYAD
FORWARD
FOULARD
FOUNDED
FRAGGED
FRANKED
FREAKED
FRESHED
FRESSED
FRETTED
FRILLED
FRINGED
FRISKED
FRITTED
FRIZZED
FROCKED
FRONTED
FROSTED
FROTHED
FROWARD
FROWNED
FRUITED
FUDDLED
FUELLED
FUELROD
FUMBLED

•F•D•••

OFFDAYS
OFFDUTY

•F••D••

IFITDIE

•F•••D•

AFFORDS
EFFENDI
OFFENDS
OFFSIDE

•F••••D

AFEARED
AFFINED
AFFIXED
EFFACED
EFFUSED
OFAKIND
OFAMIND
OFFERED
OFFHAND
OFFLOAD
OFFROAD

••FD•••

OFFDAYS
OFFDUTY

••F•D••

ELFUDGE
INFIDEL
OHFUDGE
UNFADED

••F••D•

AFFORDS
ALFREDA
ALFREDE
ALFREDO
ALFREDU
DEFENDS
DEFUNDS
EFFENDI
ENFOLDS
INFOLDS
OFFENDS
OFFSIDE
OXFORDS
REFEEDS
REFINDS
REFOLDS
REFUNDS
UNFOLDS
UPFOLDS

••F•••D

AFFINED
AFFIXED
BAFFLED
COFOUND
DEFACED
DEFAMED
DEFILED
DEFINED
DEFRAUD
DEFUSED
DRFREUD
EFFACED
EFFUSED
ENFACED
ENFIELD
FIFTYAD
GIFFORD
INFIELD
INFIXED
INFUSED
LEFTEND
LOFTBED
MUFFLED
OFFERED
OFFHAND
OFFLOAD
OFFROAD
PIFFLED
RAFFLED
REFACED
REFAXED
REFILED
REFINED
REFIRED
REFIXED
REFLOOD
REFOUND
REFRIED
REFUGED
REFUSED
REFUTED
RIFFLED
RUFFLED
SOFABED
UNFACED
UNFADED
UNFAKED
UNFAMED
UNFATED
UNFAZED
UNFETED
UNFILED
UNFINED
UNFIRED
UNFIXED
UNFLUID
UNFOUND
UNFOXED
UNFREED
UNFRIED
UNFUSED
UPFIELD
WAFERED
WAFFLED

•••FD••

FIEFDOM
HALFDAY
HALFDUG
SERFDOM
WOLFDOG

•••F•D•

CONFIDE
PERFIDY
PREFADE
SULFIDE
THEFEDS

•••F••D

ASHFORD
BAFFLED
BEDFORD
BLUFFED
CATFOOD
CHAFFED
CHUFFED
COIFFED
CRAFTED
DEIFIED
DOGFOOD
DRAFTED
DRIFTED
EDIFIED
EYEFOLD
FANFOLD
FEOFFED
FLUFFED
FORFEND
GIFFORD
GILFORD
GOSFORD
GRAFTED
GRIFTED
HALFBAD
HALFFED
HALFMAD
HALFROD
ILLFOLD
LANFORD
LAWFORD
LEEFORD
MANFRED
MEDFORD
MISFEED
MITFORD
MUFFLED
MUMFORD
NONFOOD
ONEFOLD
OUTFEED
OUTFIND
PIAFFED
PIFFLED
PINFOLD
PREFUND
PURFLED
QUAFFED
RADFORD
RAFFLED
RAWFOOD
REDFORD
REIFIED
RIFFLED
RUFFLED
RUMFORD
SANFORD
SCOFFED
SCUFFED
SEAFOOD
SHAFTED
SHIFTED
SIXFOLD
SKIFFED
SNAFUED
SNIFFED
SNUFFED
SPIFFED
STAFFED
STIFFED
STIFLED
STUFFED
TENFOLD
TRIFFID
TRIFLED
TRIFOLD
TWOFOLD
UNIFIED
WAFFLED
WATFORD
WEXFORD
WHIFFED
WILFORD
WILFRED

••••F•D

ACTIFED
BLUFFED
BRIEFED
CHAFFED
CHUFFED
COIFFED
CORNFED
DWARFED
FEOFFED
FLUFFED
HALFFED
HANDFED
IGOOFED
MILKFED
OVERFED
PIAFFED
PROOFED
QUAFFED
SCARFED
SCOFFED
SCUFFED
SHEAFED
SKIFFED
SNARFED
SNIFFED
SNUFFED
SPIFFED
SPOOFED
STAFFED
STIFFED
STRAFED
STUFFED
SUDAFED
TRIFFID
WELLFED
WHARFED
WHIFFED

FE•••••

FEARERS
FEARFOR
FEARFUL
FEARING
FEARNOT
FEASTED
FEASTER
FEASTON
FEATHER
FEATURE
FEBRERO
FEBRILE
FECHNER
FEDDERS
FEDERAL
FEDERKO
FEDEXED
FEDEXES
FEDINTO
FEDORAS
FEDOROV
FEEBATE
FEEBLER
FEEDBAG
FEEDBIN
FEEDERS
FEEDING
FEEDLOT
FEEDSIN
FEEDSON
FEEDSTO
FEEFREE
FEELBAD
FEELERS
FEELESS
FEELFOR
FEELILL
FEELING
FEELOFF
FEELOUT
FEELSOK
FEIFFER
FEIGNED
FEIGNER
FEINTED
FELDMAN
FELICIA
FELINES
FELLAHS
FELLDUE
FELLERS
FELLFOR
FELLING
FELLINI
FELLOFF
FELLOUT
FELLOWS
FELONRY
FELTBAD
FELTFOR
FELTHAT
FELTILL
FELTING
FELTOFF
FELTOUT
FELTPEN
FELTTIP
FEMALES
FEMBOTS
FEMINUM
FEMORAL
FEMORIS
FENCEIN
FENCERS
FENCEUP
FENCING
FENDERS
FENDING
FENDOFF
FENELON
FENETRE
FENNELS
FENNIER
FEODORI
FEOFFED
FERMATA
FERMATE
FERMATS
FERMENT
FERMION
FERMIUM
FERNAND
FERNBAR
FERNERY
FERNIER
FERRARA
FERRARE
FERRARI
FERRARO
FERRATE
FERRETS
FERRETY
FERRIED
FERRIES
FERRITE
FERROUS
FERRULE
FERTILE
FERULES
FERVENT
FERVORS
FERVOUR
FESCUES
FESSING
FESTERS
FESTINA
FESTIVA
FESTIVE
FESTOON
FESTOSO
FETCHED
FETCHER
FETCHES
FETIDLY
FETLOCK
FETTERS
FETTLES
FETUSES
FEUDING
FEUDIST
FEVERED
FEVRIER
FEWNESS
FEYDEAU
FEYNESS
FEYNMAN

F•E••••

FAERIES
FAEROES
FEEBATE
FEEBLER
FEEDBAG
FEEDBIN
FEEDERS
FEEDING
FEEDLOT
FEEDSIN
FEEDSON
FEEDSTO
FEEFREE
FEELBAD
FEELERS
FEELESS
FEELFOR
FEELILL
FEELING
FEELOFF
FEELOUT
FEELSOK
FIEDLER
FIEFDOM
FIELDED
FIELDER
FIENNES
FIERCER
FIERIER
FIERILY
FIESTAS
FLEABAG
FLEADIP
FLEANCE
FLEAPIT
FLECHES
FLECKED
FLEDGED
FLEDGES
FLEECED
FLEECER
FLEECES
FLEEGLE
FLEEING
FLEERED
FLEETED
FLEETER
FLEETLY
FLEMING
FLEMISH
FLENSED
FLENSER
FLENSES
FLESHED
FLESHES
FLESHLY
FLEURON
FLEXILE
FLEXING
FLEXION
FLEXNER
FLEXORS
FLEXURE
FOELESS
FREAKED
FREBERG
FRECKLE
FRECKLY
FREDDIE
FREDEBB
FREDRIC
FREEAIR
FREEBEE
FREEBIE
FREEDOF
FREEDOM
FREEDUP
FREEING
FREEMAN
FREEMEN
FREESIA
FREESOF
FREESUP
FREETOY
FREEWAY
FREEZER
FREEZES
FREIGHT
FREITAG
FRELENG
FREMONT
FRENCHI
FRENCHS
FRENEAU
FRENEMY
FRENESI
FRESCAS
FRESCOS
FRESHED
FRESHEN
FRESHER
FRESHES
FRESHET
FRESHLY
FRESNEL
FRESSED
FRESSES
FRETFUL
FRETSAT
FRETSAW
FRETTED
FRETTER
FREYTAG
FUELERS
FUELING
FUELLED
FUELOIL
FUELROD
FUELSUP
FUENTES

F••E•••

FABERGE
FACEDIT
FACEDON
FACEOFF
FACESIT
FACESON
FACETED
FADEDIN
FADEDLY
FADEINS
FADEOUT
FADESIN
FAGENDS
FAIENCE
FAKEDIT
FAKEFUR
FAKEIDS
FAKEOUT
FAKESIT
FANEUIL
FAREAST
FAREBOX
FAREWAR
FATEFUL
FAYETTE
FEDERAL
FEDERKO
FEDEXED
FEDEXES
FENELON
FENETRE
FEVERED
FIBERED
FIDELES
FIDELIA
FIDELIO
FIDELIS
FILEDBY
FILEDIN
FILENES
FILEOUT
FILESBY
FILESIN
FINEART
FINESSE
FIREANT
FIREARM
FIREBOX
FIREBUG
FIREDAT
FIREDOG
FIREDON
FIREDUP
FIREFLY
FIREFOX
FIREHAT
FIREICE
FIRELIT
FIREMAN
FIREMEN
FIRENZA
FIRENZE
FIREOFF
FIREPIT
FIRESAT
FIRESON
FIRESUP
FIVEAAA
FIVEDAY
FIVEEEE
FIVEMAN
FIVEONE
FIVEPIN
FIVESIX
FIVETEN
FIVETWO
FIVEWAY
FIXEDLY
FIXEDON
FIXEDUP
FIXESON
FIXESUP
FLEECED
FLEECER
FLEECES
FLEEGLE
FLEEING
FLEERED
FLEETED
FLEETER
FLEETLY
FLIEDTO
FLIESAT
FLIESBY
FLIESIN
FLIESON
FLIESTO
FLIESUP
FLUENCY
FOGERTY
FOLENGO
FOMENTS
FOREACH
FOREARM
FOREBAY
FOREIGN
FORELEG
FOREMAN
FOREMEN
FORENZA
FOREPAW
FORERAN
FORERUN
FORESAW
FORESEE
FORESTS
FORETOP
FOREVER
FOUETTE
FREEAIR
FREEBEE
FREEBIE
FREEDOF
FREEDOM
FREEDUP
FREEING
FREEMAN
FREEMEN
FREESIA
FREESOF
FREESUP
FREETOY
FREEWAY
FREEZER
FREEZES
FRIEDAN
FRIEDUP
FRIENDS
FRIESUP
FRIEZES
FROEBEL
FTHENRY
FTMEADE
FUMEDAT
FUMESAT
FUSEBOX

F•••E••

FABBEST
FABLERS
FAINEST
FAIREST
FALLERS
FALSELY
FALSEST
FALTERS
FALWELL
FANBELT
FANFEST
FANJETS
FANNERS

FARCEUR
FARFELS
FARLEFT
FARMERS
FARMERY
FARNESS
FAROESE
FARRELL
FARSEER
FARWEST
FASTENS
FASTEST
FATCELL
FATHEAD
FATHERS
FATLESS
FATNESS
FATTENS
FATTEST
FAUCETS
FAWCETT
FAWNERS
FEARERS
FEBRERO
FEDDERS
FEEDERS
FEELERS
FEELESS
FELLERS
FENCEIN
FENCERS
FENCEUP
FENDERS
FENNELS
FERMENT
FERNERY
FERRETS
FERRETY
FERVENT
FESTERS
FETTERS
FEWNESS
FEYDEAU
FEYNESS
FIBBERS
FIDGETS
FIDGETY
FIFTEEN
FIGLEAF
FIGMENT
FILBERT
FILLERS
FILLETS
FILTERS
FINDERS
FINGERS
FINLESS
FIRMEST
FISHERS
FISHERY
FISHEYE
FITNESS
FITTERS
FITTEST
FITWELL
FIVEEEE
FIZZERS
FLAKERS
FLAMERS
FLAMEUP
FLANEUR
FLAREUP
FLAYERS
FLOREAL
FLORENZ
FLORETS
FLOWERS
FLOWERY
FLUTERS
FLYLEAF
FLYLESS
FLYNETS
FOAMERS
FODDERS
FOELESS
FOGGERS
FOGLESS
FOKKERS
FOLDERS
FOLGERS
FOLLETT
FONDEST
FONTEYN
FOOLERS
FOOLERY
FOOTERS
FOPPERY
FORBEAR
FORCEIN
FORCEON
FORCEPS
FORCERS
FORCEUP
FORFEIT
FORFEND
FORGERS
FORGERY
FORGETS
FORKERS
FORMERS
FORREAL
FORRENT
FORREST
FORWENT
FOSTERS
FOULEST
FOUREEE
FOWLERS
FOXIEST
FOXNEWS
FRAMERS
FRAMEUP
FRATERS
FREBERG
FREDEBB
FRELENG
FRENEAU
FRENEMY
FRENESI
FRISEUR
FROZEUP
FTMYERS
FUDGERS
FUELERS
FULGENT
FULLEST
FULNESS
FUMIEST
FUNDERS
FUNFEST
FUNNELS
FURLERS
FURLESS
FURNESS
FURSEAL
FUSSERS

F••••E•

FABARES
FACADES
FACETED
FADAYEV
FADDIER
FADDIET
FAERIES
FAEROES
FAGOTED
FAILLES
FAINTED
FAINTER
FAIRIES
FAIRSEX
FALAFEL
FAMINES
FANCIED
FANCIER
FANCIES
FANSLER
FARRIER
FARSEER
FARTHER
FARTLEK
FASTNET
FATALES
FATFREE
FATONES
FATTIER
FAULTED
FAVORED
FAVORER
FEASTED
FEASTER
FEATHER
FECHNER
FEDEXED
FEDEXES
FEEBLER
FEEFREE
FEIFFER
FEIGNED
FEIGNER
FEINTED
FELINES
FELTPEN
FEMALES
FENNIER
FEOFFED
FERNIER
FERRIED
FERRIES
FERULES
FESCUES
FETCHED
FETCHER
FETCHES
FETTLES
FETUSES
FEVERED
FEVRIER
FIACRES
FIANCEE
FIANCES
FIBERED
FIBIGER
FIBSTER
FICKLER
FICUSES
FIDDLED
FIDDLER
FIDDLES
FIDELES
FIEDLER
FIELDED
FIELDER
FIENNES
FIERCER
FIERIER
FIFTEEN
FIFTIES
FIGHTER
FIGTREE
FIGURED
FIGURER
FIGURES
FILCHED
FILCHER
FILCHES
FILENES
FILIBEG
FILLIES
FILMIER
FILMSET
FINALES
FINCHES
FINDLEY
FINITES
FINNIER
FIPPLES
FIREMEN
FIRRIER
FIRTREE
FISCHER
FISHIER
FISHNET
FIVEEEE
FIVETEN
FIXATED
FIXATES
FIZZIER
FIZZLED
FIZZLER
FIZZLES
FLACKED
FLAGGED
FLAGGER
FLAGMEN
FLAILED
FLAKIER
FLAMBED
FLAMBES
FLAMIER
FLAMMED
FLANGES
FLANKED
FLANKEN
FLANKER
FLANNEL
FLAPPED
FLAPPER
FLASHED
FLASHER
FLASHES
FLATBED
FLATLET
FLATTED
FLATTEN
FLATTER
FLAWIER
FLAXIER
FLECHES
FLECKED
FLEDGED
FLEDGES
FLEECED
FLEECER
FLEECES
FLEERED
FLEETED
FLEETER
FLENSED
FLENSER
FLENSES
FLESHED
FLESHES
FLEXNER
FLICKED
FLICKER
FLINGER
FLIPPED
FLIPPEN
FLIPPER
FLIRTED
FLIRTER
FLITTED
FLITTER
FLIVVER
FLOATED
FLOATER
FLOCKED
FLOGGED
FLOGGER
FLOODED
FLOORED
FLOORER
FLOPPED
FLOPPER
FLOSSED
FLOSSER
FLOSSES
FLOURED
FLOUTED
FLOUTER
FLUBBED
FLUBBER
FLUFFED
FLUFFER
FLUKIER
FLUNKED
FLUNKER
FLUSHED
FLUSHER
FLUSHES
FLUSTER
FLUTIER
FLUTIES
FLUTTER
FLYOPEN
FLYOVER
FLYTIER
FNUMBER
FOAMIER
FOCSLES
FOCUSED
FOCUSER
FOCUSES
FOGGIER
FOIBLES
FOISTED
FOLATES
FOLIOED
FOLKIER
FOLKIES
FOLLIES
FONDLED
FONDLER
FONDLES
FONDUED
FONDUES
FOODIES
FOODWEB
FOOTLED
FOOTLER
FOOTLES
FOOTLET
FOOTMEN
FOOZLED
FOOZLER
FOOZLES
FORAGED
FORAGER
FORAGES
FORASEC
FORAYED
FORDOES
FORELEG
FOREMEN
FORESEE
FOREVER
FORFREE
FORGOER
FORGOES
FORKIER
FORSTER
FORTIES
FORTLEE
FOUDRES
FOUNDED
FOUNDER
FOUREEE
FOURIER
FRAGGED
FRAILER
FRAISES
FRANCES
FRANKED
FRANKEN
FRANKER
FRAPPES
FRASIER
FRAWLEY
FRAZIER
FREAKED
FREEBEE
FREEMEN
FREEZER
FREEZES
FRESHED
FRESHEN
FRESHER
FRESHES
FRESHET
FRESNEL
FRESSED
FRESSES
FRETTED
FRETTER
FRICKER
FRIDGES
FRIDLEY
FRIEZES
FRILLED
FRINGED
FRINGES
FRISBEE
FRISKED
FRISKER
FRITTED
FRITTER
FRIZZED
FRIZZER
FRIZZES
FROCKED
FROEBEL
FROGGER
FROGLEG
FROGLET
FROGMEN
FROMMER
FRONTED
FROSTED
FROSTER
FROTHED
FROTHER
FROWNED
FROWNER
FRUITED
FTRILEY
FUBSIER
FUDDIES
FUDDLED
FUDDLES
FUELLED
FUENTES
FUMBLED
FUMBLER
FUMBLES
FUNGOES
FUNKIER
FUNNIER
FUNNIES
FUNPLEX
FUNSTER
FURORES
FURRIER
FURTHER
FUSSIER
FUSTIER
FUTURES
FUZZIER

F•••••E

FABERGE
FACONNE
FACULAE
FADLIKE
FAIENCE
FAILURE
FAIRUSE
FALCATE
FALLDUE
FAMILLE
FANBASE
FANFARE
FANLIKE
FANTINE
FANWISE
FANZINE
FARGONE
FARMORE
FAROESE
FARSIDE
FASCIAE
FASTONE
FATFREE
FATIGUE
FATLIKE
FAXLORE
FAYETTE
FBICASE
FBIFILE
FEATURE
FEBRILE
FEEBATE
FEEFREE
FELLDUE
FENETRE
FERMATE
FERRARE
FERRATE
FERRITE
FERRULE
FERTILE
FESTIVE
FIANCEE
FIBULAE
FICTILE
FICTIVE
FIGTREE
FINABLE
FINAGLE
FINANCE
FINESSE
FINLIKE
FIREICE
FIRENZE
FIRTREE
FISHEYE
FISSILE
FISSURE
FIVEEEE
FIVEONE
FIXABLE
FIXTURE
FLEANCE
FLEEGLE
FLEXILE
FLEXURE
FLOSSIE
FLOTAGE
FLOUNCE
FLOWAGE
FLYABLE
FOLIAGE
FOLIATE
FOLIOSE
FONTANE
FOOTAGE
FOOTSIE
FORBADE
FORBORE
FORDONE
FORESEE
FORFREE
FORGAVE
FORGIVE
FORGONE
FORHIRE
FORLIFE
FORLOVE
FORONCE
FORSAKE
FORSALE
FORSIZE
FORSURE
FORSYTE
FORTLEE
FORTUNE
FOUETTE
FOUREEE
FOXFIRE
FOXHOLE
FOXLIKE
FRAGGLE
FRAGILE
FRAICHE
FRANKIE
FRAZZLE
FRECKLE
FREDDIE
FREEBEE
FREEBIE
FRIABLE
FRIBBLE
FRIGATE
FRIJOLE
FRISBEE
FRIZZLE
FROMAGE
FROOGLE
FROZONE
FRYABLE
FTDODGE
FTMEADE
FTWAYNE
FULSOME
FUNTIME
FURCATE
FURNACE
FURTIVE
FUSIBLE

•FE••••

AFEARED
PFENNIG

•F•E•••

AFFECTS
EFFECTS
EFFENDI
IFWEMAY
OFFENCE
OFFENDS
OFFENSE
OFFERED
OFFEREE
OFFERER
OFFEROR
OFFERUP
OFTENER

•F••E••

AFCTEAM
AFFLECK
IFFIEST
IFIFELL
NFCTEAM
NFLTEAM
OFFBEAT
OFFPEAK
OFFSETS
OFFWEGO
OFFYEAR

•F•••E•

AFEARED
AFFINED
AFFINES
AFFIXED
AFFIXER
AFFIXES
AFRAMES
EFFACED
EFFACER
EFFACES
EFFUSED
EFFUSES
GFORCES
IFORGET
OFFERED
OFFEREE
OFFERER
OFFICER
OFFICES
OFTENER

•F••••E

AFFABLE
AFFAIRE
EFFABLE
IFITDIE
IFORONE
IFSTONE
NFLGAME
OFANAGE
OFFBASE
OFFENCE
OFFENSE
OFFEREE
OFFLINE
OFFSIDE
OFFSITE
OFNOUSE
OFVALUE

••FE•••

AFFECTS
ALFEROV
DEFEATS
DEFECTS
DEFENCE
DEFENDS
DEFENSE
DEFERTO
EFFECTS
EFFENDI
INFECTS
INFERNO
INFESTS
LAFEMME
LIFEFUL
LIFENET
OFFENCE
OFFENDS
OFFENSE
OFFERED
OFFEREE
OFFERER
OFFEROR
OFFERUP
REFEEDS
REFENCE
REFEREE
REFERTO
SAFEBET
SAFEWAY
SEFERIS
UNFENCE
UNFERTH
UNFETED
WAFERED

••F•E••

AFFLECK
ALFIERI
ALFREDA
ALFREDE
ALFREDO
ALFREDU
BAFFERS
BUFFERS
BUFFEST
BUFFETS
BUFFETT
COFFEES
COFFERS
DAFTEST
DEFFEST
DEFIERS
DEFLEAS
DEFLECT
DEFTEST
DEFUELS
DIFFERS
DOFFERS
DRFREUD
DUFFELS
DUFFERS
ENFIELD
FIFTEEN
GAFFERS
GIFTEES
HEFTERS
IFFIEST
INFIELD
INFLECT
JEFFERS
LAFLEUR
LEFREAK
LEFTEAR
LEFTEND
LEFTEST
LEFTEYE
LIFTERS
LOFTERS
OFFBEAT
OFFPEAK
OFFSETS
OFFWEGO
OFFYEAR
PUFFERS
PUFFERY
RAFTERS
REFEEDS
REFLECT
REFRESH
REFUELS
RIFLERS
RIFLERY
SIFTERS
SOFTENS
SOFTEST
SUFFERS
TAFFETA
TOFFEES
TUFFETS
UNFIERY
UNFREED
UNFREES
UPFIELD
WAFTERS

••F••E•

AFFINED
AFFINES
AFFIXED
AFFIXER
AFFIXES
BAFFIES
BAFFLED
BAFFLER
BAFFLES
BYFIVES
COFFEES
DAFFIER
DEFACED
DEFACER
DEFACES
DEFAMED
DEFAMER
DEFAMES
DEFILED
DEFILER
DEFILES
DEFINED
DEFINER
DEFINES
DEFUSED
DEFUSER
DEFUSES
DUFFLES
DUFUSES
EFFACED
EFFACER
EFFACES
EFFUSED
EFFUSES
ENFACED
ENFACES
FIFTEEN
FIFTIES
GIFTEES
GIFTSET
HEFTIER
HUFFIER
INFIDEL
INFIVES
INFIXED
INFIXES
INFUSED
INFUSER
INFUSES
JEFFREY
JIFFIES
JOFFREY
LEFTIES
LEFTLEG
LIFENET
LOFTBED
LOFTIER
MIFFIER
MUFFLED
MUFFLER
MUFFLES
NIFTIER
NIFTIES
OFFERED
OFFEREE
OFFERER
OFFICER
OFFICES
PIFFLED
PIFFLES
PUFFIER
RAFFLED
RAFFLER
RAFFLES
REFACED
REFACES
REFAXED
REFAXES
REFEREE
REFILED
REFILES
REFINED
REFINER
REFINES
REFIRED
REFIRES
REFIXED
REFIXES
REFLIES
REFRIED
REFRIES

REFUGED
REFUGEE
REFUGES
REFUSED
REFUSER
REFUSES
REFUTED
REFUTER
REFUTES
RIFFLED
RIFFLER
RIFFLES
RUFFLED
RUFFLER
RUFFLES
SAFEBET
SOFABED
SOFTGEL
SOFTIES
TAFFIES
TOFFEES
TOFFLER
TUFTIER
UNFACED
UNFADED
UNFAKED
UNFAMED
UNFATED
UNFAZED
UNFETED
UNFILED
UNFILES
UNFINED
UNFINES
UNFIRED
UNFIXED
UNFIXES
UNFOXED
UNFREED
UNFREES
UNFRIED
UNFUSED
WAFERED
WAFFLED
WAFFLER
WAFFLES

••F•••E

AFFABLE
AFFAIRE
ALFONSE
ALFREDE
BYFORCE
DEFARGE
DEFENCE
DEFENSE
DEFLATE
DEFRAME
DIFFUSE
EFFABLE
ELFLIKE
ELFUDGE
ENFLAME
ENFORCE
ENFRAME
GEFILTE
INFANTE
INFLAME
INFLATE
INFORCE
LAFARGE
LAFEMME
LAFITTE
LEFTEYE
OFFBASE
OFFENCE
OFFENSE
OFFEREE
OFFLINE
OFFSIDE
OFFSITE
OHFUDGE
REFENCE
REFEREE
REFLATE
REFORGE
REFRAME
REFUGEE
SUFFICE
SUFFUSE
UNFENCE
UNFROZE

•••FE••

ARTFERN
ATMFEES
BAFFERS
BIGFEET
BUFFERS
BUFFEST
BUFFETS
BUFFETT
CATFEET
CHAFERS
COFFEES
COFFERS
CONFECT
CONFERS
CONFESS
CURFEWS
DEAFENS
DEAFEST
DEFFEST
DIFFERS
DOFFERS
DUFFELS
DUFFERS
FANFEST
FARFELS
FORFEIT
FORFEND
FUNFEST
GABFEST
GAFFERS
GOLFERS
HEIFERS
HEIFETZ
HOOFERS
IFIFELL
JEFFERS
KNIFERS
LABFEES
LIEFEST
LOAFERS
MISFEED
OAKFERN
OUTFEED
OUTFEEL
OZZFEST
PERFECT
PILFERS
PREFECT
PREFERS
PROFESS
PUFFERS
PUFFERY
REDFERN
REEFERS
ROLFERS
ROOFERS
SEAFERN
SETFEES
SIXFEET
SOLFEGE
SUFFERS
SURFEIT
SURFERS
TAFFETA
TENFEET
THEFEDS
TOFFEES
TUFFETS
TWOFEET
TWOFERS
WEBFEET
WOOFERS

•••F•E•

ATMFEES
BAFFIES
BAFFLED
BAFFLER
BAFFLES
BEEFIER
BEEFTEA
BIGFEET
BIOFUEL
BLUFFED
BLUFFER
BOUFFES
BUGFREE
CARFREE
CATFEET
CATFLEA
CHAFFED
CHAFFEE
CHAFFER
CHUFFED
COFFEES
COIFFED
COMFIER
CONFREY
CRAFTED
CRAFTER
CROFTER
DAFFIER
DEIFIED
DEIFIER
DEIFIES
DOGFLEA
DRAFTED
DRAFTEE
DRAFTER
DRIFTED
DRIFTER
DUFFLES
EDIFIED
EDIFIER
EDIFIES
FATFREE
FEEFREE
FEIFFER
FEOFFED
FLUFFED
FLUFFER
FORFREE
GETFREE
GOAFTER
GODFREY
GOLFTEE
GOOFIER
GOTFREE
GRAFTED
GRAFTER
GRIFFEY
GRIFTED
GRIFTER
GRUFFER
HALFFED
HALFIES
HUFFIER
ICEFREE
JEFFREY
JIFFIES
JOFFREY
KIEFFER
LABFEES
LEAFIER
LEAFLET
MANFRED
MIFFIER
MISFEED
MUFFLED
MUFFLER
MUFFLES
NONFUEL
OUTFEED
OUTFEEL
OUTFLEE
PALFREY
PIAFFED
PIAFFES
PIFFLED
PIFFLES
PROFFER
PUFFIER
PURFLED
PURFLER
PURFLES
QUAFFED
QUAFFER
RAFFLED
RAFFLER
RAFFLES
RANFREE
REEFIER
REIFIED
REIFIES
RENFREW
REOFFER
RIFFLED
RIFFLER
RIFFLES
RUFFLED
RUFFLER
RUFFLES
RUNFREE
SCOFFED
SCOFFER
SCUFFED
SCUFFER
SETFEES
SETFREE
SHAFFER
SHAFTED
SHEFFER
SHIFTED
SHIFTER
SIXFEET
SKIFFED
SNAFUED
SNIFFED
SNIFFER
SNIFTER
SNUFFED
SNUFFER
SPIFFED
STAFFED
STAFFER
STIFFED
STIFFEL
STIFFEN
STIFFER
STIFLED
STIFLES
STUFFED
STUFFER
SURFIER
SURFMEN
SWIFTER
SYNFUEL
TAFFIES
TAXFREE
TENFEET
THEFLEA
TOFFEES
TOFFLER
TRIFLED
TRIFLER
TRIFLES
TURFIER
TURFMEN
TWOFEET
UNIFIED
UNIFIER
UNIFIES
UNOFTEN
WAFFLED
WAFFLER
WAFFLES
WEBFEET
WHIFFED
WHIFFER
WILFRED
WINFREY
WOLFMEN

•••F••E

ACTFIVE
AGEFIVE
AIRFARE
AIRFONE
BIGFIVE
BONFIRE
BUGFREE
BUSFARE
CABFARE
CARFARE
CARFREE
CHAFFEE
CONFIDE
CONFINE
CONFUSE
CONFUTE
DIDFINE
DIFFUSE
DOGFACE
DRAFTEE
EDIFICE
FANFARE
FATFREE
FBIFILE
FEEFREE
FORFREE
FOXFIRE
GETFREE
GOLFTEE
GOTFREE
GUNFIRE
ICEFLOE
ICEFREE
IREFUSE
ITSFINE
JETFIRE
LEAFAGE
MISFILE
MISFIRE
NEWFACE
ORIFICE
OUTFACE
OUTFIRE
OUTFLEE
PARFIVE
PERFUME
PERFUSE
PREFACE
PREFADE
PREFILE
PROFANE
PROFILE
PROFUSE
RANFREE
REDFACE
REDFIVE
ROOFAGE
RUNFREE
SADFATE
SCUFFLE
SEAFARE
SERFAGE
SETFREE
SHUFFLE
SIXFIVE
SKIFFLE
SNIFFLE
SNUFFLE
SOLFEGE
SOUFFLE
SUBFILE
SUFFICE
SUFFUSE
SULFATE
SULFIDE
SULFITE
SUNFIRE
SURFACE
TAXFREE
THEFIVE
TOPFIVE
TRUFFLE
TURFTOE
TWOFACE
WARFARE
WELFARE
WHIFFLE

••••FE•

ACTIFED
AQUIFER
BANKFEE
BLUFFED
BLUFFER
BOUFFES
BRIEFED
BRIEFER
CARAFES
CHAFFED
CHAFFEE
CHAFFER
CHAMFER
CHUFFED
COIFFED
CONIFER
CORNFED
DWARFED
EXITFEE
FALAFEL
FEIFFER
FEOFFED
FLUFFED
FLUFFER
GRIFFEY
GRUFFER
HALFFED
HANDFED
IGOOFED
ISRAFEL
KIEFFER
KILLFEE
LATEFEE
LUCIFER
MILKFED
OVERFED
OVERFEE
OVERFEW
PIAFFED
PIAFFES
PROFFER
PROOFED
PROOFER
QUAFFED
QUAFFER
REOFFER
ROTIFER
SCARFED
SCARFER
SCOFFED
SCOFFER
SCUFFED
SCUFFER
SHAFFER
SHEAFED
SHEFFER
SKIFFED
SNARFED
SNIFFED
SNIFFER
SNUFFED
SNUFFER
SPIFFED
SPOOFED
SPOOFER
STAFFED
STAFFER
STIFFED
STIFFEL
STIFFEN
STIFFER
STRAFED
STRAFER
STRAFES
STRIFES
STUFFED
STUFFER
SUDAFED
TINAFEY
UNSAFER
USERFEE
VERYFEW
WELLFED
WHARFED
WHIFFED
WHIFFER

••••F•E

ALLOFME
ARCHFOE
BANKFEE
CHAFFEE
EXITFEE
GIRAFFE
KILLFEE
LATEFEE
OKEEFFE
OVERFEE
SCUFFLE
SHUFFLE
SKIFFLE
SNIFFLE
SNUFFLE
SOUFFLE
TRUFFLE
USERFEE
WHIFFLE

•••••FE

ALEWIFE
FORLIFE
GIRAFFE
HESSAFE
LOWLIFE
METLIFE
MIDLIFE
MIDWIFE
NESCAFE
NETCAFE
NEWLIFE
NONLIFE
NOTSAFE
OKEEFFE
PIESAFE
PRELIFE
PROLIFE
SADCAFE
SANTAFE
SEALIFE

F•F••••

FIFTEEN
FIFTHLY
FIFTIES
FIFTYAD
FIFTYBC

F••F•••

FABFOUR
FANFARE
FANFEST
FANFICS
FANFOLD
FARFELS
FATFARM
FATFREE
FBIFILE
FEEFREE
FEIFFER
FEOFFED
FIEFDOM
FLUFFED
FLUFFER
FLUFFUP
FLYFISH
FORFEIT
FORFEND
FORFREE
FOXFIRE
FULFILL
FULFILS
FUNFAIR
FUNFEST
FUNFURS
FUNFZIG
FURFARM

F•••F••

FACTFUL
FAIRFAX
FAKEFUR
FALAFEL
FALLFOR
FATEFUL
FAUXFUR
FEARFOR
FEARFUL
FEELFOR
FEIFFER
FELLFOR
FELTFOR
FEOFFED
FILOFAX
FIREFLY
FIREFOX
FISHFOR
FISHFRY
FISTFUL
FLUFFED
FLUFFER
FLUFFUP
FORKFUL
FORMFUL
FRETFUL

F••••F•

FACEOFF
FAIROFF
FALLOFF
FALSIFY
FANCIFY
FARLEFT
FEELOFF
FELLOFF
FELTOFF
FENDOFF
FIREOFF
FOBSOFF
FORLIFE
FORTIFY

F•••••F

FACEOFF
FAIROFF
FALLOFF
FEELOFF
FELLOFF
FELTOFF
FENDOFF
FIGLEAF
FIREOFF
FLYLEAF
FOBSOFF
FREEDOF
FREESOF

•FF••••

AFFABLE
AFFABLY
AFFAIRE
AFFAIRS
AFFECTS
AFFIANT
AFFINED
AFFINES
AFFIRMS
AFFIXED
AFFIXER
AFFIXES
AFFLECK
AFFLICT
AFFORDS
AFFRAYS
AFFRONT
EFFABLE
EFFABLY
EFFACED
EFFACER
EFFACES
EFFECTS
EFFENDI
EFFORTS
EFFUSED
EFFUSES
IFFIEST
OFFBASE
OFFBEAT
OFFCAST
OFFDAYS
OFFDUTY
OFFENCE
OFFENDS
OFFENSE
OFFERED
OFFEREE
OFFERER
OFFEROR
OFFERUP
OFFHAND
OFFHOUR
OFFICER
OFFICES
OFFICIO
OFFINGS
OFFLINE
OFFLOAD
OFFPEAK
OFFRAMP
OFFROAD
OFFSETS
OFFSIDE
OFFSITE
OFFWEGO
OFFYEAR

•F•F•••

IFIFELL

•F••••F

AFOULOF

••FF•••

BAFFERS
BAFFIES
BAFFING
BAFFLED
BAFFLER
BAFFLES
BIFFING
BOFFING
BOFFINS
BOFFOLA
BUFFALO
BUFFERS
BUFFEST
BUFFETS
BUFFETT
BUFFING
BUFFOON
BUFFSUP
COFFEES
COFFERS
COFFINS
CUFFING
DAFFIER
DAFFILY
DEFFEST
DIFFERS
DIFFUSE
DOFFERS
DOFFING
DUFFELS
DUFFERS
DUFFLES
GAFFERS
GAFFING
GIFFORD
GUFFAWS
HOFFMAN
HUFFIER
HUFFILY
HUFFING
HUFFISH
HUFFMAN
JEFFERS
JEFFREY
JIFFIES
JOFFREY
LUFFING
MIFFIER
MIFFING
MIFFLIN
MUFFING
MUFFINS
MUFFLED
MUFFLER
MUFFLES
PIFFLED
PIFFLES
PUFFERS
PUFFERY
PUFFIER
PUFFILY
PUFFING
PUFFINS
PUFFOUT
PUFFSUP
RAFFIAS
RAFFISH
RAFFLED
RAFFLER
RAFFLES
REFFING
RIFFING
RIFFLED
RIFFLER
RIFFLES
RUFFALO
RUFFIAN
RUFFING
RUFFLED
RUFFLER
RUFFLES
SAFFRON
SOFFITS
SUFFERS
SUFFICE
SUFFOLK
SUFFUSE
TAFFETA
TAFFIES
TIFFANY
TIFFING
TIFFINS
TOFFEES
TOFFLER
TUFFETS
WAFFLED
WAFFLER
WAFFLES

••F•F••

LEFTFOR
LIFEFUL

••F••F•

ALFALFA
LEFTOFF
LIFTOFF

••F•••F

LEFTOFF
LIFTOFF

•••FF••

BLUFFED
BLUFFER
BLUFFLY
BOUFFES
CHAFFED
CHAFFEE
CHAFFER
CHIFFON
CHUFFED
COIFFED
FEIFFER
FEOFFED
FLUFFED
FLUFFER
FLUFFUP
GRIFFEY
GRIFFIN
GRIFFON
GRUFFER
GRUFFLY
HALFFED
KIEFFER
PIAFFED
PIAFFES
PROFFER
QUAFFED
QUAFFER
REAFFIX
REOFFER
SCOFFAT
SCOFFED
SCOFFER
SCUFFED
SCUFFER
SCUFFLE
SHAFFER
SHEFFER
SHUFFLE
SKIFFED
SKIFFLE
SNIFFAT
SNIFFED
SNIFFER
SNIFFLE
SNIFFLY
SNIFFUP
SNUFFED
SNUFFER
SNUFFLE
SOUFFLE
SPIFFED
SPIFFUP

STAFFED
STAFFER
STIFFED
STIFFEL
STIFFEN
STIFFER
STIFFLY
STUFFED
STUFFER
STUFFIN
TRAFFIC
TRIFFID
TRUFFLE
WHIFFED
WHIFFER
WHIFFLE

•••F•F•

GOOFOFF

•••F••F

ARAFTOF
GOOFOFF

••••FF•

BUYOFFS
CUTOFFS
DIEOFFS
GIRAFFE
LAYOFFS
LOGOFFS
MIDOFFS
OKEEFFE
ONEOFFS
PAYOFFS
POPOFFS
PUTOFFS
REBUFFS
RIPOFFS
RUNOFFS
SCLAFFS
SCRUFFS
SCRUFFY
SETOFFS
TARIFFS
TEEOFFS
TIPOFFS
UNCUFFS

•••••FF

ASSTIFF
BACKOFF
BAILIFF
BAKEOFF
BEAROFF
BEATOFF
BEGSOFF
BESTOFF
BINDOFF
BITEOFF
BLEWOFF
BLOWOFF
BOILOFF
BRANIFF
BUGSOFF
BURNOFF
BUYSOFF
BUZZOFF
CALLOFF
CAMEOFF
CARDIFF
CARTOFF
CASTOFF
CHOPOFF
CLIPOFF
COMEOFF
CONKOFF
CONNIFF
COOKOFF
CUTSOFF
DAMPOFF
DARTOFF
DASHOFF
DAYSOFF
DIEDOFF
DIESOFF
DISTAFF
DOZEOFF
DRAGOFF
DRAWOFF
DREWOFF
DROPOFF
DUSTOFF
EARMUFF
EASEOFF
EASYOFF
EVENOFF
FACEOFF
FAIROFF
FALLOFF
FEELOFF
FELLOFF
FELTOFF
FENDOFF
FIREOFF
FOBSOFF
GAVEOFF
GETSOFF
GIVEOFF
GOESOFF
GONEOFF
GOOFOFF
HACKOFF
HANDOFF
HANGOFF
HATSOFF
HAULOFF
HEADOFF
HELDOFF
HENTOFF
HITSOFF
HIVEOFF
HOLDOFF
HOPSOFF
HUNGOFF
INAHUFF
INAJIFF
JUMPOFF
KARLOFF
KEEPOFF
KEPTOFF
KICKOFF
KISSOFF
LAIDOFF
LAYSOFF
LEADOFF
LEFTOFF
LETSOFF
LIFTOFF
LIPSOFF
LOGSOFF
LOPSOFF
MACDUFF
MADEOFF
MAKEOFF
MARKOFF
MASTIFF
MCGRIFF
MCGRUFF
MIDRIFF
MOVEOFF
NODSOFF
NORDOFF
ONSTAFF
PACEOFF
PACKOFF
PAIDOFF
PAIROFF
PALMOFF
PASSOFF
PAWNOFF
PAYSOFF
PEELOFF
PERSOFF
PICKOFF
PLAYOFF
PONTIFF
POPSOFF
PULLOFF
PUSHOFF
PUTSOFF
RAKEOFF
RANGOFF
READOFF
REELOFF
RESTAFF
RESTUFF
RIDEOFF
RINGOFF
RIPSOFF
RODEOFF
ROLLOFF
ROPEOFF
RUBSOFF
RUNGOFF
RUNSOFF
RUSHOFF
SAMHUFF
SARNOFF
SAWNOFF
SAWSOFF
SEALOFF
SEENOFF
SEESOFF
SELLOFF
SENDOFF
SENTOFF
SETSOFF
SHERIFF
SHONUFF
SHOOOFF
SHOWOFF
SHUTOFF
SIGNOFF
SLIDOFF
SLIPOFF
SNIPOFF
SOLDOFF
SPEDOFF
SPINOFF
SPUNOFF
STAYOFF
STEPOFF
STOPOFF
SYDHOFF
TAILOFF
TAKEOFF
TAPSOFF
TEAROFF
TEEDOFF
TEESOFF
TELLOFF
TICKOFF
TIEDOFF
TIESOFF
TIMEOFF
TIPSOFF
TOLDOFF
TOOKOFF
TOPSOFF
TOREOFF
TORNOFF
TOSSOFF
TRIMOFF
TROTOFF
TURNOFF
UNGRUFF
UNSTIFF
VEEROFF
WALKOFF
WALLOFF
WARDOFF
WARNOFF
WASHOFF
WAVEOFF
WEAROFF
WELLOFF
WENTOFF
WIPEOFF
WOREOFF
WORKOFF
WORNOFF
YANKOFF
ZIPCUFF
ZIPSOFF

FG•••••

FGHIJKL

F•G••••

FAGENDS
FAGOTED
FIGBARS
FIGHTER
FIGLEAF
FIGMENT
FIGTREE
FIGURAL
FIGURED
FIGURER
FIGURES
FOGBANK
FOGBOWS
FOGCITY
FOGDOGS
FOGERTY
FOGGERS
FOGGIER
FOGGILY
FOGGING
FOGHORN
FOGLAMP
FOGLESS
FOGYISH
FOGYISM
FUGALLY
FUGATOS

F••G•••

FANGING
FARGOND
FARGONE
FEIGNED
FEIGNER
FIDGETS
FIDGETY
FINGALS
FINGERS
FIZGIGS
FLAGDAY
FLAGGED
FLAGGER
FLAGMAN
FLAGMEN
FLAGONS
FLIGHTS
FLIGHTY
FLOGGED
FLOGGER
FLYGIRL
FOGGERS
FOGGIER
FOGGILY
FOGGING
FOLGERS
FORGAVE
FORGERS
FORGERY
FORGETS
FORGING
FORGIVE
FORGOER
FORGOES
FORGONE
FORGOOD
FRAGGED
FRAGGLE
FRAGILE
FRIGATE
FRIGHTS
FROGGER
FROGLEG
FROGLET
FROGMAN
FROGMEN
FUDGERS
FUDGING
FULGENT
FULGHUM
FUNGOES

F•••G••

FALLGUY
FARMGAL
FATIGUE
FIBIGER
FINAGLE
FLAGGED
FLAGGER
FLANGES
FLEDGED
FLEDGES
FLEEGLE
FLINGAT
FLINGER
FLOGGED
FLOGGER
FLUNGAT
FORAGED
FORAGER
FORAGES
FORDGTS
FRAGGED
FRAGGLE
FRAUGHT
FREIGHT
FRIDGES
FRINGED
FRINGES
FROGGER
FROOGLE

F••••G•

FABERGE
FACINGS
FARRAGO
FILINGS
FIRINGS
FIXINGS
FIZGIGS
FLOTAGE
FLOWAGE
FLUBUGS
FLYHIGH
FOGDOGS
FOLENGO
FOLIAGE
FOOTAGE
FOREIGN
FROMAGE
FTBRAGG
FTDODGE

F•••••G

FABLING
FAILING
FAIRING
FALLING
FANGING
FANNING
FARCING
FARMING
FASTING
FATLING
FATTING
FAWNING
FEARING
FEEDBAG
FEEDING
FEELING
FELLING
FELTING
FENCING
FENDING
FESSING
FEUDING
FIBBING
FILIBEG
FILLING
FILMING
FINDING
FINKING
FIREBUG
FIREDOG
FIRMING
FISHING
FITTING
FIZZING
FLAKING
FLAMING
FLARING
FLAWING
FLAYING
FLEABAG
FLEEING
FLEMING
FLEXING
FLOWING
FLUTING
FLUXING
FOALING
FOAMING
FOBBING
FOGGING
FOILING
FOLDING
FOOLING
FOOTBAG
FOOTING
FORCING
FORDING
FORELEG
FORGING
FORKING
FORMING
FOULING
FOWLING
FRAMING
FRAYING
FREBERG
FREEING
FREITAG
FRELENG
FREYTAG
FRODING
FROGLEG
FTBRAGG
FUDGING
FUELING
FUNDING
FUNFZIG
FUNKING
FUNNING
FURLING
FURLONG
FURRING
FUSSING
FUTZING
FUZZING

•FG••••

AFGHANI
AFGHANS
EFGHIJK

•F•G•••

NFLGAME

•F••G••

IFORGET
IFORGOT

•F•••G•

IFYOUGO
OFANAGE
OFFINGS
OFFWEGO
UFOLOGY

•F••••G

PFENNIG

••FG•••

DEFGHIJ

••F•G••

REFIGHT
REFUGED
REFUGEE
REFUGES
SOFTGEL
UNFOGGY

••F••G•

DEFANGS
DEFARGE
DEFRAGS
ELFUDGE
LAFARGE
OFFINGS
OFFWEGO
OHFUDGE
REFLAGS
REFORGE
UNFOGGY
USFLAGS

••F•••G

BAFFING
BIFFING
BOFFING
BUFFING
CUFFING
DEFYING
DOFFING
GAFFING
GIFTING
HAFTING
HEFTING
HUFFING
LEFTLEG
LIFTING
LOFTING
LUFFING
MIFFING
MUFFING
PUFFING
RAFTING
REFFING
REFYING
RIFFING
RIFLING
RIFTING
RUFFING
SIFTING
TIFFING
TUFTING
UPFLING
WAFTING
WIFYING

•••FG••

CDEFGHI
WOLFGAL

•••F•G•

DRYFOGS
ICEFOGS
LEAFAGE
OLDFOGY
ROOFAGE
SERFAGE
SOLFEGE

•••F••G

BAFFING
BARFBAG
BEEFING
BIFFING
BOFFING
BUFFING
CHAFING
CHEFING
COIFING
CUFFING
DOFFING
FUNFZIG
GAFFING
GOLFBAG
GOLFING
GOOFING
GULFING
HALFDUG
HOOFING
HUFFING
KAMFONG
KNIFING
LEAFING
LOAFING
LUFFING
MIFFING
MUFFING
PETFROG
PUFFING
REDFLAG
REEFING
REFFING
RIFFING
ROLFING
ROOFING
RUFFING
SURFING
THEFRUG
TIFFING
TURFING
WOLFDOG
WOLFING
WOOFING

••••FG•

BCDEFGH

••••F•G

ANTIFOG

•••••FG

ABCDEFG

FH•••••

FHALOAN

F•H••••

FGHIJKL
FTHENRY

F••H•••

FASHION
FATHEAD
FATHERS
FATHOMS
FECHNER
FIGHTER
FISHERS
FISHERY
FISHEYE
FISHFOR
FISHFRY
FISHIER
FISHILY
FISHING
FISHNET
FISHOIL
FISHOUT
FLYHIGH
FOGHORN
FORHIRE
FOXHOLE
FOXHUNT
FUCHSIA
FUTHARK

F•••H••

FARTHER
FEATHER
FELTHAT
FETCHED
FETCHER
FETCHES
FIFTHLY
FILCHED
FILCHER
FILCHES
FINCHES
FIREHAT
FISCHER
FLASHED
FLASHER
FLASHES
FLASHON
FLATHAT
FLECHES
FLESHED
FLESHES
FLESHLY
FLIGHTS
FLIGHTY
FLUSHED
FLUSHER
FLUSHES
FLUSHOT
FORDHAM
FORSHOW
FRESHED
FRESHEN
FRESHER
FRESHES
FRESHET
FRESHLY
FRIGHTS
FROTHED
FROTHER
FROTHUP
FULGHUM
FURTHER

F••••H•

FELLAHS
FINISHD
FOURTHS
FRAICHE
FRANCHI
FRAUGHT
FREIGHT
FRENCHI
FRENCHS

F•••••H

FADDISH
FAIRISH
FATOUSH
FATTISH
FINNISH
FLEMISH
FLYFISH
FLYHIGH
FOGYISH
FOLKISH
FOOLISH
FOPPISH
FORBUSH
FOREACH
FORSYTH
FTWORTH
FURBISH
FURNISH

•F•H•••

AFGHANI
AFGHANS
EFGHIJK
OFFHAND
OFFHOUR
VFWHALL

••FH•••

OFFHAND
OFFHOUR

••F•H••

DEFGHIJ
FIFTHLY
ISFAHAN
LEFTHIP

••F••H•

REFIGHT

••F•••H

GOFORTH
HUFFISH
INFAITH
LEFTISH
RAFFISH
REFRESH
SOFTISH
UNFAITH
UNFERTH

•••F•H•

CDEFGHI
HALFSHY
LOOFAHS

•••F••H

BIGFISH
CATFISH
CODFISH
COWFISH
DOGFISH
FLYFISH
HUFFISH
MUDFISH
OUTFISH
PANFISH
PETFISH
PIGFISH
RAFFISH
RAWFISH
REDFISH
SAWFISH
SELFISH
SUNFISH
TINFISH
WAIFISH
WOLFISH

••••F•H

BCDEFGH
LATIFAH
TWELFTH

FI•••••

FIACRES
FIANCEE
FIANCES
FIASCOS
FIATLUX
FIBBERS
FIBBING
FIBERED
FIBIGER
FIBRINS
FIBROID
FIBROUS
FIBSTER
FIBULAE
FIBULAR
FIBULAS
FICKLER
FICTILE
FICTION
FICTIVE
FICUSES
FIDDLED
FIDDLER
FIDDLES
FIDELES
FIDELIA
FIDELIO
FIDELIS
FIDGETS
FIDGETY
FIEDLER
FIEFDOM
FIELDED
FIELDER
FIENNES
FIERCER
FIERIER
FIERILY
FIESTAS
FIFTEEN
FIFTHLY
FIFTIES
FIFTYAD
FIFTYBC
FIGBARS
FIGHTER
FIGLEAF
FIGMENT
FIGTREE
FIGURAL
FIGURED
FIGURER
FIGURES
FIJIANS
FILBERT
FILCHED
FILCHER
FILCHES
FILEDBY
FILEDIN
FILENES
FILEOUT
FILESBY
FILESIN
FILIBEG
FILINGS
FILIPPO
FILLERS
FILLETS
FILLIES
FILLING
FILLINS
FILLIPS
FILLOUT
FILLSIN
FILLSUP
FILLUPS
FILMDOM
FILMIER
FILMILY
FILMING
FILMSET

FILOFAX
FILTERS
FINABLE
FINAGLE
FINALES
FINALLY
FINANCE
FINBACK
FINCHES
FINDERS
FINDING
FINDLAY
FINDLEY
FINDOUT
FINEART
FINESSE
FINGALS
FINGERS
FINIALS
FINIANS
FINICAL
FINICKY
FINISHD
FINITES
FINKING
FINKSON
FINLAND
FINLESS
FINLIKE
FINNAIR
FINNIER
FINNISH
FIORINA
FIPPLES
FIRBANK
FIREANT
FIREARM
FIREBOX
FIREBUG
FIREDAT
FIREDOG
FIREDON
FIREDUP
FIREFLY
FIREFOX
FIREHAT
FIREICE
FIRELIT
FIREMAN
FIREMEN
FIRENZA
FIRENZE
FIREOFF
FIREPIT
FIRESAT
FIRESON
FIRESUP
FIRINGS
FIRKINS
FIRMEST
FIRMING
FIRMSUP
FIRRIER
FIRSTLY
FIRSTUP
FIRTREE
FISCHER
FISHERS
FISHERY
FISHEYE
FISHFOR
FISHFRY
FISHIER
FISHILY
FISHING
FISHNET
FISHOIL
FISHOUT
FISSILE
FISSION
FISSURE
FISTFUL
FITINTO
FITNESS
FITTERS
FITTEST
FITTING
FITWELL
FITZROY
FIVEAAA
FIVEDAY
FIVEEEE
FIVEMAN
FIVEONE
FIVEPIN
FIVESIX
FIVETEN
FIVETWO
FIVEWAY
FIXABLE
FIXATED
FIXATES
FIXEDLY
FIXEDON
FIXEDUP
FIXESON
FIXESUP
FIXINGS
FIXTURE
FIXUPON
FIZGIGS
FIZZERS
FIZZIER
FIZZING
FIZZLED
FIZZLER
FIZZLES

F•I••••

FAIENCE
FAILING
FAILLES
FAILSTO
FAILURE
FAINEST
FAINTED
FAINTER
FAINTLY
FAIREST
FAIRFAX
FAIRIES
FAIRING
FAIRISH
FAIROFF
FAIRSEX
FAIRSUP
FAIRUSE
FAIRWAY
FAISALI
FBICASE
FBIFILE
FEIFFER
FEIGNED
FEIGNER
FEINTED
FLICKED
FLICKER
FLIEDTO
FLIESAT
FLIESBY
FLIESIN
FLIESON
FLIESTO
FLIESUP
FLIGHTS
FLIGHTY
FLINGAT
FLINGER
FLINTMI
FLIPOUT
FLIPPED
FLIPPEN
FLIPPER
FLIPTOP
FLIPUPS
FLIRTED
FLIRTER
FLITSBY
FLITSIN
FLITTED
FLITTER
FLIVVER
FOIBLES
FOILING
FOISTED
FOISTON
FRIABLE
FRIARLY
FRIBBLE
FRICKER
FRIDAYS
FRIDGES
FRIDLEY
FRIEDAN
FRIEDUP
FRIENDS
FRIESUP
FRIEZES
FRIGATE
FRIGHTS
FRIJOLE
FRILLED
FRINGED
FRINGES
FRISBEE
FRISEUR
FRISIAN
FRISKED
FRISKER
FRISSON
FRITTED
FRITTER
FRIVOLS
FRIZZED
FRIZZER
FRIZZES
FRIZZLE
FRIZZLY

F••I•••

FACIALS
FACINGS
FADIMAN
FAJITAS
FAMICOM
FAMILIA
FAMILLE
FAMINES
FANIONS
FARINAS
FATIDIC
FATIGUE
FEDINTO
FELICIA
FELINES
FEMINUM
FETIDLY
FGHIJKL
FIBIGER
FIJIANS
FILIBEG
FILINGS
FILIPPO
FINIALS
FINIANS
FINICAL
FINICKY
FINISHD
FINITES
FIRINGS
FITINTO
FIXINGS
FLAILAT
FLAILED
FLUIDAL
FLUIDIC
FLUIDLY
FLYINTO
FOLIAGE
FOLIATE
FOLIOED
FOLIOSE
FORINTS
FOXIEST
FRAICHE
FRAILER
FRAILLY
FRAILTY
FRAISES
FREIGHT
FREITAG
FRUITED
FTDIXNJ
FTRILEY
FUJISAN
FUJITSU
FUMIEST
FURILLO
FURIOSO
FURIOUS
FUSIBLE
FUSILLI
FUSIONS

F•••I••

FABLING
FABRICS
FABRIZI
FACTION
FADDIER
FADDIET
FADDISH
FADDISM
FADDIST
FADEINS
FADLIKE
FAERIES
FAILING
FAIRIES
FAIRING
FAIRISH
FAKEIDS
FALKIRK
FALLING
FALSIFY
FALSITY
FANCIED
FANCIER
FANCIES
FANCIFY
FANCILY
FANFICS
FANGING
FANLIKE
FANNING
FANTINE
FANWISE
FANZINE
FARCING
FARMING
FARRIER
FARSIDE
FASCIAE
FASCIAL
FASCIAS
FASCISM
FASCIST
FASHION
FASTING
FATCITY
FATLIKE
FATLING
FATLIPS
FATTIER
FATTILY
FATTING
FATTISH
FATUITY
FAUVISM
FAUVIST
FAWNING
FBIFILE
FEARING
FEBRILE
FEEDING
FEELILL
FEELING
FELLING
FELLINI
FELTILL
FELTING
FENCING
FENDING
FENNIER
FERMION
FERMIUM
FERNIER
FERRIED
FERRIES
FERRITE
FERTILE
FESSING
FESTINA
FESTIVA
FESTIVE
FEUDING
FEUDIST
FEVRIER
FIBBING
FIBRINS
FICTILE
FICTION
FICTIVE
FIERIER
FIERILY
FIFTIES
FILLIES
FILLING
FILLINS
FILLIPS
FILMIER
FILMILY
FILMING
FINDING
FINKING
FINLIKE
FINNIER
FINNISH
FIORINA
FIREICE
FIRKINS
FIRMING
FIRRIER
FISHIER
FISHILY
FISHING
FISSILE
FISSION
FITTING
FIZGIGS
FIZZIER
FIZZING
FLAKIER
FLAKILY
FLAKING
FLAMIER
FLAMING
FLARING
FLAVIUS
FLAWIER
FLAWING
FLAXIER
FLAYING
FLEEING
FLEMING
FLEMISH
FLEXILE
FLEXING
FLEXION
FLORIAN
FLORIDA
FLORINS
FLORIST
FLOWING
FLUKIER
FLUKILY
FLUTIER
FLUTIES
FLUTING
FLUTIST
FLUVIAL
FLUXING
FLUXION
FLYFISH
FLYGIRL
FLYHIGH
FLYTIER
FOALING
FOAMIER
FOAMILY
FOAMING
FOBBING
FOGCITY
FOGGIER
FOGGILY
FOGGING
FOGYISH
FOGYISM
FOILING
FOLDING
FOLKIER
FOLKIES
FOLKISH
FOLLIES
FONTINA
FOODIES
FOOLING
FOOLISH
FOOTING
FOPPISH
FORBIDS
FORCING
FORDING
FOREIGN
FORGING
FORGIVE
FORHIRE
FORKIER
FORKING
FORLIFE
FORMICA
FORMING
FORSIZE
FORTIES
FORTIFY
FORTIUS
FOSDICK
FOSSILS
FOULING
FOURIER
FOWLING
FOXFIRE
FOXLIKE
FRAGILE
FRAMING
FRASIER
FRAYING
FRAZIER
FREEING
FRISIAN
FRODING
FROLICS
FTBLISS
FUBSIER
FUDDIES
FUDGING
FUELING
FULFILL
FULFILS
FUNDING
FUNKIER
FUNKILY
FUNKING
FUNNIER
FUNNIES
FUNNILY
FUNNING
FUNTIME
FURBISH
FURLING
FURNISH
FURRIER
FURRING
FURTIVE
FUSSIER
FUSSILY
FUSSING
FUSTIAN
FUSTIER
FUSTILY
FUTZING
FUZZIER
FUZZILY
FUZZING

F••••I•

FACEDIT
FACESIT
FACTOID
FADEDIN
FADESIN
FAKEDIT
FAKESIT
FALLSIN
FAMILIA
FANATIC
FANEUIL
FANMAIL
FANTAIL
FARMAID
FATIDIC
FEEDBIN
FEEDSIN
FELICIA
FELTTIP
FEMORIS
FENCEIN
FIBROID
FIDELIA
FIDELIO
FIDELIS
FILEDIN
FILESIN
FILLSIN
FINNAIR
FIRELIT
FIREPIT
FISHOIL
FIVEPIN
FIVESIX
FJORDIC
FLACCID
FLEADIP
FLEAPIT
FLIESIN
FLITSIN
FLOORIT
FLOSSIE
FLOWNIN
FLOWSIN
FLUIDIC
FMRADIO
FOLDSIN
FOOTSIE
FOOTSIT
FORABIT
FORCEIN
FORFEIT
FORTDIX
FOULTIP
FOURPIN
FOXTAIL
FRANCIS
FRANKIE
FRANTIC
FREDDIE
FREDRIC
FREEAIR
FREEBIE
FREESIA
FUCHSIA
FUELOIL
FUNFAIR
FUNFZIG

F•••••I

FABRIZI
FAISALI
FAROUKI
FELLINI
FEODORI
FERRARI
FLINTMI
FORLANI
FRANCHI
FRENCHI
FRENESI
FUSILLI

•FI••••

IFIFELL
IFITDIE

•F•I•••

AFFIANT
AFFINED
AFFINES
AFFIRMS
AFFIXED
AFFIXER
AFFIXES
AFRICAN
IFFIEST
OFFICER
OFFICES
OFFICIO
OFFINGS

•F••I••

AFFAIRE
AFFAIRS
AFFLICT
EFGHIJK
OFAKIND
OFAMIND
OFFLINE
OFFSIDE
OFFSITE

•F•••I•

IFITDIE
OFFICIO
PFENNIG

•F••••I

AFGHANI
EFFENDI

••FI•••

AFFIANT
AFFINED
AFFINES
AFFIRMS
AFFIXED
AFFIXER
AFFIXES
ALFIERI
ATFIRST
BYFIVES
DEFIANT
DEFICIT
DEFIERS
DEFILED
DEFILER
DEFILES
DEFINED
DEFINER
DEFINES
ENFIELD
GEFILTE
GOFIRST
IFFIEST
INFIDEL
INFIELD
INFIRST
INFIVES
INFIXED
INFIXES
LAFITTE
MAFIOSI
MAFIOSO
MEFIRST
MRFIXIT
OFFICER
OFFICES
OFFICIO
OFFINGS
ONFIRST
PRFIRMS
REFIGHT
REFILED
REFILES
REFILLS
REFILMS
REFINDS
REFINED
REFINER
REFINES
REFIRED
REFIRES
REFIXED
REFIXES
RUFIYAA
UNFIERY
UNFILED
UNFILES
UNFINED
UNFINES
UNFIRED
UNFITLY
UNFIXED
UNFIXES
UPFIELD
UPFIRST

••F•I••

AFFAIRE
AFFAIRS
AFFLICT
BAFFIES
BAFFING
BIFFING
BOFFING
BOFFINS
BUFFING
COFFINS
CUFFING
DAFFIER
DAFFILY
DEFYING
DOFFING
DRFRIST
ELFLIKE
FIFTIES
GAFFING
GIFTING
HAFNIUM
HAFTING
HEFTIER
HEFTILY
HEFTING
HUFFIER
HUFFILY
HUFFING
HUFFISH
INFAITH
INFLICT
JIFFIES
LEFTIES
LEFTISH
LEFTISM
LEFTIST
LIFTING
LOFTIER
LOFTILY
LOFTING
LUFFING
MIFFIER
MIFFING
MUFFING
MUFFINS
NIFTIER
NIFTIES
NIFTILY
OFFLINE
OFFSIDE
OFFSITE
PUFFIER
PUFFILY
PUFFING
PUFFINS
RAFFIAS
RAFFISH
RAFTING
REFFING
REFLIES
REFLIPS
REFRIED
REFRIES
REFYING
RIFFING
RIFLING
RIFTING
RUFFIAN
RUFFING
SIFTING
SOFFITS
SOFTIES
SOFTISH
SUFFICE
TAFFIES
TIFFING
TIFFINS
TUFTIER
TUFTING
UNFAITH
UNFRIED
UNFRILL
UPFLING
WAFTING
WIFYING

••F••I•

DEFGHIJ
DEFICIT
GOFORIT
IMFORIT
INFORIT
LEFTHIP
MIFFLIN
MRFIXIT
OFFICIO
REFRAIN
SAFARIS
SEFERIS
UNFLUID
UNFRAIL
UPFORIT

••F•••I

ALFIERI
EFFENDI
MAFIOSI
TOFUTTI

•••FI••

ACTFIVE
AGEFIVE
ARTFILM
BADFITS
BAFFIES
BAFFING
BEEFIER
BEEFILY
BEEFING
BIFFING
BIGFISH
BIGFIVE
BOFFING
BOFFINS
BONFIRE
BOWFINS
BUFFING
CATFISH
CATFITS
CHAFING
CHEFING
CODFISH
COFFINS
COIFING
COMFIER
COMFITS
CONFIDE
CONFINE
CONFIRM
CONFITS
COWFISH
CUFFING
DAFFIER
DAFFILY
DEIFIED
DEIFIER
DEIFIES
DIDFINE
DOFFING
DOGFISH
EDIFICE
EDIFIED
EDIFIER
EDIFIES
FANFICS
FBIFILE
FLYFISH
FOXFIRE
FULFILL
FULFILS
GAFFING
GINFIZZ
GOLFING
GOOFIER
GOOFILY
GOOFING
GULFING
GUNFIRE
HADFITS
HALFIES
HASFITS
HITFILM
HOOFING
HUFFIER
HUFFILY
HUFFING
HUFFISH

ITSFINE
JETFIRE
JIFFIES
JIMFIXX
KNIFING
LEAFIER
LEAFING
LOAFING
LUFFING
MIFFIER
MIFFING
MISFILE
MISFIRE
MISFITS
MUDFISH
MUFFING
MUFFINS
OLAFIII
OLDFILM
OLEFINS
ORIFICE
OUTFIND
OUTFIRE
OUTFISH
OUTFITS
PANFISH
PARFIVE
PERFIDY
PETFISH
PIGFISH
PREFILE
PROFILE
PROFITS
PUFFIER
PUFFILY
PUFFING
PUFFINS
RAFFIAS
RAFFISH
RATFINK
RAWFISH
REDFINS
REDFIRS
REDFISH
REDFIVE
REEFIER
REEFING
REFFING
REIFIED
REIFIES
RIFFING
ROLFING
ROOFING
RUFFIAN
RUFFING
SAWFISH
SELFISH
SIXFIVE
SOFFITS
SUBFILE
SUFFICE
SULFIDE
SULFITE
SUNFIRE
SUNFISH
SURFIER
SURFING
TAFFIES
THEFIRM
THEFIVE
TIFFING
TIFFINS
TINFISH
TOPFIVE
TURFIER
TURFING
UNIFIED
UNIFIER
UNIFIES
WAIFISH
WOLFING
WOLFISH
WOOFING

•••F•I•

AELFRIC
AIRFOIL
ARTFAIR
BIDFAIR
DRIFTIN
FORFEIT
FUNFAIR
FUNFZIG
GRIFFIN
GULFOIL
HALFWIT
HOOFSIT
JETFOIL
JOBFAIR
MAYFAIR
MIFFLIN
NETFLIX
NOTFAIR
OLAFIII
PARFAIT
REAFFIX
STUFFIN
SURFEIT
TINFOIL
TOYFAIR
TRAFFIC
TREFOIL
TRIFFID
WASFAIR

•••F••I

CDEFGHI
OLAFIII
STEFANI
TURFSKI

••••FI•

ALLOFIT
BENEFIC
BENEFIT
BLUEFIN
GETSFIT
GRIFFIN
HADAFIT
HASAFIT
KEEPFIT
KEPTFIT
MADEFIT
MAKEFIT
MALEFIC
OSSIFIC
OUTOFIT
OVERFIT
OVERFIX
PACIFIC
POSTFIX
RATAFIA
REAFFIX
SEENFIT
SEESFIT
SNUGFIT
STUFFIN
TAILFIN
TRAFFIC
TRIFFID
VERYFIT

•••••FI

DRMELFI
QADDAFI
RUDOLFI

FJ•••••

FJORDIC

F•J••••

FAJITAS
FIJIANS
FUJISAN
FUJITSU

F••J•••

FANJETS
FRIJOLE

F•••J••

FGHIJKL

F•••••J

FTDIXNJ

•F•••J•

EFGHIJK

••F•J••

LEFTJAB

••F••J•

ALFORJA

••F•••J

DEFGHIJ

F•K••••

FAKEDIT
FAKEFUR
FAKEIDS
FAKEOUT
FAKESIT
FOKKERS

F••K•••

FALKIRK
FICKLER
FINKING
FINKSON
FIRKINS
FLAKERS
FLAKIER
FLAKILY
FLAKING
FLUKIER
FLUKILY
FOKKERS
FOLKART
FOLKIER
FOLKIES
FOLKISH
FOLKWAY
FORKERS
FORKFUL
FORKIER
FORKING
FORKOUT
FORKSUP
FUNKIER
FUNKILY
FUNKING

F•••K••

FLACKED
FLANKED
FLANKEN
FLANKER
FLECKED
FLICKED
FLICKER
FLOCKED
FLOCKTO
FLUNKED
FLUNKER
FRANKED
FRANKEN
FRANKER
FRANKIE
FRANKLY
FRANKOZ
FREAKED
FRECKLE
FRECKLY
FRICKER
FRISKED
FRISKER
FROCKED

F••••K•

FADLIKE
FANLIKE
FAROUKI
FATLIKE
FEDERKO
FGHIJKL
FINICKY
FINLIKE
FORSAKE
FOXLIKE

F•••••K

FALKIRK
FARTLEK
FATBACK
FEELSOK
FETLOCK
FINBACK
FIRBANK
FOGBANK
FORSOOK
FOSDICK
FRYCOOK
FUTHARK

•F•K•••

OFAKIND

•F••••K

AFFLECK
EFGHIJK
OFFPEAK

••F•K••

UNFAKED

••F••K•

ELFLIKE
UNFLAKY
UNFORKS

••F•••K

AFFLECK
BTFSPLK
DEFROCK
ELFLOCK
LEFREAK
OFFPEAK
SUFFOLK
UNFRANK
UNFROCK

•••F•K•

TURFSKI

•••F••K

HAYFORK
INAFUNK
KINFOLK
MENFOLK
NORFOLK
RATFINK
SUFFOLK
WEEFOLK

FL•••••

FLACCID
FLACKED
FLACONS
FLAGDAY
FLAGGED
FLAGGER
FLAGMAN
FLAGMEN
FLAGONS
FLAILAT
FLAILED
FLAKERS
FLAKIER
FLAKILY
FLAKING
FLAMBED
FLAMBES
FLAMERS
FLAMEUP
FLAMIER
FLAMING
FLAMMED
FLANEUR
FLANGES
FLANKED
FLANKEN
FLANKER
FLANNEL
FLAPPED
FLAPPER
FLAREUP
FLARING
FLASHED
FLASHER
FLASHES
FLASHON
FLATBED
FLATCAR
FLATHAT
FLATLET
FLATOUT
FLATTAX
FLATTED
FLATTEN
FLATTER
FLATTOP
FLATTVS
FLAUNTS
FLAUNTY
FLAUTAS
FLAVIUS
FLAVORS
FLAVORY
FLAVOUR
FLAWIER
FLAWING
FLAXIER
FLAYERS
FLAYING
FLEABAG
FLEADIP
FLEANCE
FLEAPIT
FLECHES
FLECKED
FLEDGED
FLEDGES
FLEECED
FLEECER
FLEECES
FLEEGLE
FLEEING
FLEERED
FLEETED
FLEETER
FLEETLY
FLEMING
FLEMISH
FLENSED
FLENSER
FLENSES
FLESHED
FLESHES
FLESHLY
FLEURON
FLEXILE
FLEXING
FLEXION
FLEXNER
FLEXORS
FLEXURE
FLICKED
FLICKER
FLIEDTO
FLIESAT
FLIESBY
FLIESIN
FLIESON
FLIESTO
FLIESUP
FLIGHTS
FLIGHTY
FLINGAT
FLINGER
FLINTMI
FLIPOUT
FLIPPED
FLIPPEN
FLIPPER
FLIPTOP
FLIPUPS
FLIRTED
FLIRTER
FLITSBY
FLITSIN
FLITTED
FLITTER
FLIVVER
FLOATBY
FLOATED
FLOATER
FLOATUP
FLOCKED
FLOCKTO
FLOGGED
FLOGGER
FLOODED
FLOORED
FLOORER
FLOORIT
FLOPPED
FLOPPER
FLOREAL
FLORENZ
FLORETS
FLORIAN
FLORIDA
FLORINS
FLORIST
FLOSSED
FLOSSER
FLOSSES
FLOSSIE
FLOTAGE
FLOTSAM
FLOUNCE
FLOUNCY
FLOURED
FLOUTED
FLOUTER
FLOWAGE
FLOWERS
FLOWERY
FLOWING
FLOWNAT
FLOWNBY
FLOWNIN
FLOWNON
FLOWNTO
FLOWNUP
FLOWOUT
FLOWSIN
FLUBBED
FLUBBER
FLUBDUB
FLUBUGS
FLUENCY
FLUFFED
FLUFFER
FLUFFUP
FLUIDAL
FLUIDIC
FLUIDLY
FLUKIER
FLUKILY
FLUMMOX
FLUNGAT
FLUNKED
FLUNKER
FLUSHED
FLUSHER
FLUSHES
FLUSHOT
FLUSTER
FLUTERS
FLUTIER
FLUTIES
FLUTING
FLUTIST
FLUTTER
FLUVIAL
FLUXING
FLUXION
FLYABLE
FLYAWAY
FLYBALL
FLYBOYS
FLYCAST
FLYFISH
FLYGIRL
FLYHIGH
FLYINTO
FLYLEAF
FLYLESS
FLYNETS
FLYOPEN
FLYOVER
FLYPAST
FLYRODS
FLYSOLO
FLYTIER
FLYTRAP
FLYWAYS

F•L••••

FALAFEL
FALCATE
FALCONS
FALKIRK
FALLACY
FALLALS
FALLDUE
FALLERS
FALLFOR
FALLGUY
FALLING
FALLOFF
FALLOUT
FALLOWS
FALLSIN
FALLSON
FALLSTO
FALSELY
FALSEST
FALSIFY
FALSITY
FALTERS
FALWELL
FELDMAN
FELICIA
FELINES
FELLAHS
FELLDUE
FELLERS
FELLFOR
FELLING
FELLINI
FELLOFF
FELLOUT
FELLOWS
FELONRY
FELTBAD
FELTFOR
FELTHAT
FELTILL
FELTING
FELTOFF
FELTOUT
FELTPEN
FELTTIP
FILBERT
FILCHED
FILCHER
FILCHES
FILEDBY
FILEDIN
FILENES
FILEOUT
FILESBY
FILESIN
FILIBEG
FILINGS
FILIPPO
FILLERS
FILLETS
FILLIES
FILLING
FILLINS
FILLIPS
FILLOUT
FILLSIN
FILLSUP
FILLUPS
FILMDOM
FILMIER
FILMILY
FILMING
FILMSET
FILOFAX
FILTERS
FOLATES
FOLDERS
FOLDING
FOLDOUT
FOLDSIN
FOLDSUP
FOLDUPS
FOLENGO
FOLGERS
FOLIAGE
FOLIATE
FOLIOED
FOLIOSE
FOLKART
FOLKIER
FOLKIES
FOLKISH
FOLKWAY
FOLLETT
FOLLIES
FOLLOWS
FULCRUM
FULFILL
FULFILS
FULGENT
FULGHUM
FULLDAY
FULLEST
FULLLOT
FULLOUT
FULMARS
FULNESS
FULSOME

F••L•••

FABLERS
FABLING
FADLIKE
FAILING
FAILLES
FAILSTO
FAILURE
FALLACY
FALLALS
FALLDUE
FALLERS
FALLFOR
FALLGUY
FALLING
FALLOFF
FALLOUT
FALLOWS
FALLSIN
FALLSON
FALLSTO
FANLIKE
FARLEFT
FATLESS
FATLIKE
FATLING
FATLIPS
FAULTED
FAXLORE
FEELBAD
FEELERS
FEELESS
FEELFOR
FEELILL
FEELING
FEELOFF
FEELOUT
FEELSOK
FELLAHS
FELLDUE
FELLERS
FELLFOR
FELLING
FELLINI
FELLOFF
FELLOUT
FELLOWS
FETLOCK
FHALOAN
FIELDED
FIELDER
FIGLEAF
FILLERS
FILLETS
FILLIES
FILLING
FILLINS
FILLIPS
FILLOUT
FILLSIN
FILLSUP
FILLUPS
FINLAND
FINLESS
FINLIKE
FLYLEAF
FLYLESS
FOALING
FOELESS
FOGLAMP
FOGLESS
FOILING
FOLLETT
FOLLIES
FOLLOWS
FOOLERS
FOOLERY
FOOLING
FOOLISH
FORLANI
FORLIFE
FORLORN
FORLOVE
FOULARD
FOULEST
FOULING
FOULOUT
FOULSUP
FOULTIP
FOULUPS
FOWLERS
FOWLING
FOXLIKE
FRELENG
FRILLED
FROLICS
FTBLISS
FUELERS
FUELING
FUELLED
FUELOIL
FUELROD
FUELSUP
FULLDAY
FULLEST
FULLLOT
FULLOUT
FURLERS
FURLESS
FURLING
FURLONG

F•••L••

FACULAE
FACULTY
FAILLES
FAMILIA
FAMILLE
FAMULUS
FANCLUB
FANSLER
FARTLEK
FATALES
FATALLY
FEEBLER
FEEDLOT
FEMALES
FENELON
FERULES
FETTLES
FIATLUX
FIBULAE
FIBULAR
FIBULAS
FICKLER
FIDDLED
FIDDLER
FIDDLES
FIDELES
FIDELIA
FIDELIO
FIDELIS
FIEDLER
FINALES
FINALLY
FINDLAY
FINDLEY
FIPPLES
FIRELIT
FIZZLED
FIZZLER
FIZZLES
FLAILAT
FLAILED
FLATLET
FOCSLES
FOIBLES
FONDLED
FONDLER
FONDLES
FOOTLED
FOOTLER
FOOTLES
FOOTLET
FOOZLED
FOOZLER
FOOZLES
FORDLTD
FORELEG
FORTLEE
FRAILER
FRAILLY
FRAILTY
FRAWLEY
FRIDLEY
FRILLED
FROGLEG
FROGLET
FTRILEY
FUDDLED
FUDDLES
FUELLED
FUGALLY
FULLLOT
FUMBLED
FUMBLER
FUMBLES
FUNPLEX
FURILLO
FUSILLI

F••••L•

FACIALS
FADEDLY
FAINTLY
FAISALI
FALLALS
FALSELY
FALWELL
FAMILLE
FANBELT
FANCILY
FANFOLD
FANPALM
FARFELS
FARRELL
FATALLY
FATCELL
FATTILY
FBIFILE
FEBRILE
FEELILL
FELTILL
FENNELS
FERRULE
FERTILE
FETIDLY
FICTILE
FIERILY
FIFTHLY
FILMILY
FINABLE
FINAGLE
FINALLY
FINGALS
FINIALS
FIREFLY
FIRSTLY
FISHILY
FISSILE
FITWELL
FIXABLE
FIXEDLY
FLAKILY
FLEEGLE
FLEETLY
FLESHLY
FLEXILE
FLUIDLY
FLUKILY
FLYABLE
FLYBALL
FLYSOLO

FOAMILY FOGGILY FORMALS FORMULA FORSALE FOSCOLO FOSSILS FOXHOLE FRAGGLE FRAGILE FRAILLY FRANKLY FRAZZLE FRECKLE FRECKLY FRESHLY FRIABLE FRIARLY FRIBBLE FRIJOLE FRIVOLS FRIZZLE FRIZZLY FROOGLE FRYABLE FUGALLY FULFILL FULFILS FUNKILY FUNNELS FUNNILY FURBALL FURILLO FUSIBLE FUSILLI FUSSILY FUSTILY FUZZILY

F•••••L

FACTFUL FACTUAL FALAFEL FALWELL FANEUIL FANMAIL FANTAIL FARMGAL FARRELL FASCIAL FATCELL FATEFUL FEARFUL FEDERAL FEELILL FELTILL FEMORAL FGHIJKL FIGURAL FINICAL FISHOIL FISTFUL FITWELL FLANNEL FLOREAL FLUIDAL FLUVIAL FLYBALL FLYGIRL FORKFUL FORMFUL FORREAL FOXTAIL FRACTAL FRESNEL FRETFUL FROEBEL FRONTAL FUELOIL FULFILL FURBALL FURSEAL

•FL••••

NFLGAME NFLTEAM

•F•L•••

AFFLECK AFFLICT OFFLINE OFFLOAD UFOLOGY

•F••L••

AFATLOT AFOULOF OFVALUE

•F•••L•

AFFABLE AFFABLY EFFABLE EFFABLY IFIFELL VFWHALL

•F••••L

IFIFELL VFWHALL

••FL•••

AFFLECK AFFLICT DEFLATE DEFLEAS DEFLECT ELFLIKE ELFLOCK ENFLAME INFLAME INFLATE INFLECT INFLICT INFLOWS LAFLEUR OFFLINE OFFLOAD REFLAGS REFLATE REFLECT REFLIES REFLIPS REFLOAT REFLOOD REFLOWN REFLOWS RIFLERS RIFLERY RIFLING TEFLONS UNFLAKY UNFLOOR UNFLOWN UNFLUID UPFLING UPFLOWS USFLAGS

••F•L••

ALFALFA AWFULLY BAFFLED BAFFLER BAFFLES BEFALLS DEFALLA DEFILED DEFILER DEFILES DUFFLES ENFOLDS GEFILTE INFOLDS LEFTLEG MIFFLIN MUFFLED MUFFLER MUFFLES PIFFLED PIFFLES RAFFLED RAFFLER RAFFLES REFALLS REFILED REFILES REFILLS REFILMS REFOLDS RIFFLED RIFFLER RIFFLES RUFFLED RUFFLER RUFFLES TOFFLER UNFILED UNFILES UNFOLDS UNFULLY UPFOLDS WAFFLED WAFFLER WAFFLES

••F••L•

AFFABLE AFFABLY ATFAULT AWFULLY BEFALLS BEFOOLS BEFOULS BOFFOLA BTFSPLK BUFFALO DAFFILY DEFALLA DEFAULT DEFUELS DUFFELS EFFABLE EFFABLY ELFOWLS ENFIELD FIFTHLY HEFTILY HUFFILY INFIELD LOFTILY MYFAULT NIFTILY NOFAULT PUFFILY REFALLS REFILLS REFUELS RUFFALO SUFFOLK UNFITLY UNFRILL UNFULLY UNFURLS UPFIELD

••F•••L

BIFOCAL INFIDEL LIFEFUL REFUSAL REFUTAL SOFTGEL UNFRAIL UNFRILL

•••FL••

AIRFLOW BAFFLED BAFFLER BAFFLES CATFLAP CATFLEA DOGFLEA DUFFLES EARFLAP ICEFLOE KERFLOP LEAFLET MIFFLIN MUDFLAP MUDFLAT MUDFLOW MUFFLED MUFFLER MUFFLES NETFLIX NONFLUX OUTFLEE OUTFLOW OUTFLUX PIFFLED PIFFLES PURFLED PURFLER PURFLES RAFFLED RAFFLER RAFFLES REDFLAG RIFFLED RIFFLER RIFFLES RUFFLED RUFFLER RUFFLES STIFLED STIFLES THEFLEA THEFLOP TOFFLER TRIFLED TRIFLER TRIFLES WAFFLED WAFFLER WAFFLES

•••F•L•

ARMFULS ARTFILM BAGFULS BEEFALO BEEFILY BLUFFLY BOFFOLA BOXFULS BUFFALO CANFULS CAPFULS CARFULS CUPFULS DAFFILY DEWFALL DUFFELS EARFULS EYEFOLD EYEFULS FANFOLD FARFELS FBIFILE FULFILL FULFILS GOOFILY GRUFFLY HATFULS HITFILM HUFFILY ICEFALL IFIFELL ILLFOLD JARFULS JUGFULS KINFOLK LAPFULS LETFALL MENFOLK MISFILE MUGFULS NETFULS NORFOLK OLDFILM ONEFOLD PANFULS PINFOLD PITFALL POTFULS PREFILE PROFILE PUFFILY RUFFALO SCUFFLE SHUFFLE SIXFOLD SKIFFLE SNIFFLE SNIFFLY SNUFFLE SOUFFLE STIFFLY SUBFILE SUFFOLK SWIFTLY TENFOLD THEFALL TRIFOLD TRUFFLE TUBFULS TWOFOLD URNFULS VATFULS WEEFOLK WHIFFLE

•••F••L

AIRFOIL BIOFUEL DEWFALL FULFILL GULFOIL ICEFALL IFIFELL JETFOIL LETFALL NONFUEL OUTFEEL OUTFOOL PEAFOWL PITFALL SEAFOWL STIFFEL SYNFUEL THEFALL THEFOOL TINFOIL TOMFOOL TREFOIL WOLFGAL

••••FL•

ALOOFLY BIRDFLU BLOWFLY BLUEFLU BLUFFLY BRIEFLY CHIEFLY DEERFLY FIREFLY GRUFFLY LETSFLY OVERFLY SANDFLY SCUFFLE SHOOFLY SHUFFLE SKIFFLE SNIFFLE SNIFFLY SNUFFLE SOUFFLE STIFFLY TESTFLY TRUFFLE WHIFFLE

••••F•L

BALEFUL BANEFUL BASHFUL BOATFUL BODEFUL BOWLFUL BRIMFUL CAREFUL CLUEFUL DAREFUL DESKFUL DIREFUL DISHFUL DOLEFUL DOOMFUL DUTIFUL EASEFUL FACTFUL FALAFEL FATEFUL FEARFUL FISTFUL FORKFUL FORMFUL FRETFUL GAINFUL GLEEFUL HANDFUL HARMFUL HATEFUL HEADFUL HEATFUL HEEDFUL HELPFUL HOPEFUL HURTFUL HUSHFUL ISRAFEL LIFEFUL LUSTFUL MINDFUL MOANFUL MUSEFUL NEEDFUL NESTFUL ODORFUL PAILFUL PAINFUL PALMFUL PIPEFUL PITIFUL PLAYFUL PLOTFUL POUTFUL PUSHFUL RAGEFUL RESTFUL ROOMFUL RUTHFUL SACKFUL SHIPFUL SHOPFUL SIGHFUL SKILFUL SLEDFUL SONGFUL SOULFUL STIFFEL TACTFUL TANKFUL TEARFUL TENTFUL TOILFUL TRAYFUL TUNEFUL UNAWFUL VIALFUL WAILFUL WAKEFUL WILLFUL WISHFUL WISTFUL YAWNFUL ZESTFUL

•••••FL

MIAMIFL OCALAFL TAMPAFL

FM•••••

FMBANDS FMRADIO FMURRAY

F•M••••

FAMICOM FAMILIA FAMILLE FAMINES FAMULUS FEMALES FEMBOTS FEMINUM FEMORAL FEMORIS FOMENTS FTMEADE FTMYERS FUMBLED FUMBLER FUMBLES FUMEDAT FUMESAT FUMIEST

F••M•••

FANMAIL FARMAID FARMBOY FARMERS FARMERY FARMGAL FARMING FARMORE FARMOUT FERMATA FERMATE FERMATS FERMENT FERMION FERMIUM FIGMENT FILMDOM FILMIER FILMILY FILMING FILMSET FIRMEST FIRMING FIRMSUP FLAMBED FLAMBES FLAMERS FLAMEUP FLAMIER FLAMING FLAMMED FLEMING FLEMISH FLUMMOX FNUMBER FOAMERS FOAMIER FOAMILY FOAMING FORMALS FORMATS FORMERS FORMFUL FORMICA FORMING FORMOSA FORMULA FRAMERS FRAMEUP FRAMING FREMONT FROMAGE FROMMER FULMARS

F•••M••

FADIMAN FELDMAN FEYNMAN FIREMAN FIREMEN FIVEMAN FLAGMAN FLAGMEN FLAMMED FLUMMOX FOOTMAN FOOTMEN FOREMAN FOREMEN FOTOMAT FOURMAN FREEMAN FREEMEN FROGMAN FROGMEN FROMMER FUSUMAS

F••••M•

FANDOMS FATHOMS FLINTMI FOGLAMP FRENEMY FULSOME FUNTIME

F•••••M

FADDISM FAMICOM FANPALM FANTASM FASCISM FATFARM FAUVISM FEMINUM FERMIUM FIEFDOM FILMDOM FIREARM FLOTSAM FOGYISM FORDHAM FOREARM FREEDOM FRUSTUM FULCRUM FULGHUM FURFARM

•F•M•••

AFTMOST OFAMIND

•F••M••

AFRAMES IFWEMAY

•F•••M•

AFFIRMS NFLGAME OFFRAMP

•F••••M

AFCTEAM NFCTEAM NFLTEAM

••FM•••

HOFMANN

••F•M••

DEFAMED DEFAMER DEFAMES HOFFMAN HUFFMAN LAFEMME UNFAMED

••F••M•

AFFIRMS BYFORMS DEFOAMS DEFORMS DEFRAME ENFLAME ENFRAME INFLAME INFORMS LAFEMME OFFRAMP PRFIRMS REFILMS REFORMS REFRAME

••F•••M

HAFNIUM LEFTARM LEFTISM

•••FM••

DORFMAN HALFMAD HOFFMAN HUFFMAN KAUFMAN SURFMAN SURFMEN TURFMAN TURFMEN WOLFMAN WOLFMEN

•••F•M•

CORFAMS PARFUMS PERFUME PERFUMY

•••F••M

ALIFORM ANTFARM ARTFILM ARTFORM BADFORM CONFIRM CONFORM EATFROM FATFARM FIEFDOM FURFARM GETFROM HITFILM IRSFORM MISFORM NONFARM NONFORM OLDFILM OVIFORM PERFORM PREFORM PROFARM SEAFOAM SERFDOM SHYFROM SUBFORM THEFIRM TOPFORM TRIFORM UNIFORM WOLFRAM

••••FM•

ALLOFME

FN•••••

FNUMBER

F•N••••

FANATIC FANBASE FANBELT FANCIED FANCIER FANCIES FANCIFY FANCILY FANCLUB FANCYUP FANDOMS FANEUIL FANFARE FANFEST FANFICS FANFOLD FANGING FANIONS FANJETS FANLIKE FANMAIL FANNERS FANNING FANOUTS FANPALM FANSLER FANSOUT FANTAIL FANTANS FANTASM FANTAST FANTASY FANTINE FANTODS FANWISE FANZINE FENCEIN FENCERS FENCEUP FENCING FENDERS FENDING FENDOFF FENELON FENETRE FENNELS FENNIER FINABLE FINAGLE FINALES FINALLY FINANCE FINBACK FINCHES FINDERS FINDING FINDLAY FINDLEY FINDOUT FINEART FINESSE FINGALS FINGERS FINIALS FINIANS FINICAL FINICKY FINISHD FINITES FINKING FINKSON FINLAND FINLESS FINLIKE FINNAIR FINNIER FINNISH FONDANT FONDEST FONDLED FONDLER FONDLES FONDUED FONDUES FONTANA FONTANE FONTEYN FONTINA FUNDERS FUNDING FUNFAIR FUNFEST FUNFURS FUNFZIG FUNGOES FUNKIER FUNKILY FUNKING FUNNELS FUNNIER FUNNIES FUNNILY FUNNING FUNPLEX FUNRUNS FUNSTER FUNTIME

F••N•••

FAINEST FAINTED FAINTER FAINTLY FANNERS FANNING FARNESS FATNESS

FAWNERS
FAWNING
FAWNSON
FEINTED
FENNELS
FENNIER
FERNAND
FERNBAR
FERNERY
FERNIER
FEWNESS
FEYNESS
FEYNMAN
FIANCEE
FIANCES
FIENNES
FINNAIR
FINNIER
FINNISH
FITNESS
FLANEUR
FLANGES
FLANKED
FLANKEN
FLANKER
FLANNEL
FLENSED
FLENSER
FLENSES
FLINGAT
FLINGER
FLINTMI
FLUNGAT
FLUNKED
FLUNKER
FLYNETS
FOUNDED
FOUNDER
FOUNDRY
FOXNEWS
FRANCES
FRANCHI
FRANCIS
FRANKED
FRANKEN
FRANKER
FRANKIE
FRANKLY
FRANKOZ
FRANTIC
FRENCHI
FRENCHS
FRENEAU
FRENEMY
FRENESI
FRINGED
FRINGES
FRONTAL
FRONTED
FRONTON
FUENTES
FULNESS
FUNNELS
FUNNIER
FUNNIES
FUNNILY
FUNNING
FURNACE
FURNESS
FURNISH

F•••N••

FACINGS
FACONNE
FAGENDS
FAIENCE
FAMINES
FARINAS
FASTNET
FATONES
FEARNOT
FECHNER
FEDINTO
FEIGNED
FEIGNER
FELINES
FELONRY
FEMINUM
FIENNES
FILENES
FILINGS
FINANCE
FIRENZA
FIRENZE
FIRINGS
FISHNET
FITINTO
FIXINGS
FLANNEL
FLAUNTS
FLAUNTY
FLEANCE
FLEXNER
FLOUNCE
FLOUNCY
FLOWNAT
FLOWNBY
FLOWNIN
FLOWNON
FLOWNTO
FLOWNUP
FLUENCY
FLYINTO
FMBANDS
FOLENGO
FOMENTS
FORENZA
FORINTS
FORONCE
FRESNEL
FRIENDS
FROWNAT
FROWNED
FROWNER
FROWNON
FTHENRY

F••••N•

FABLING
FACONNE
FADEINS
FAILING
FAIRING
FALCONS
FALLING
FANGING
FANIONS
FANNING
FANTANS
FANTINE
FANZINE
FARCING
FARGOND
FARGONE
FARMING
FASTENS
FASTING
FASTONE
FATLING
FATTENS
FATTING
FAWNING
FEARING
FEEDING
FEELING
FELLING
FELLINI
FELTING
FENCING
FENDING
FERMENT
FERNAND
FERVENT
FESSING
FESTINA
FEUDING
FIBBING
FIBRINS
FIGMENT
FIJIANS
FILLING
FILLINS
FILMING
FINDING
FINIANS
FINKING
FINLAND
FIORINA
FIRBANK
FIREANT
FIRKINS
FIRMING
FISHING
FITTING
FIVEONE
FIZZING
FLACONS
FLAGONS
FLAKING
FLAMING
FLARING
FLAWING
FLAYING
FLEEING
FLEMING
FLEXING
FLORENZ
FLORINS
FLOWING
FLUTING
FLUXING
FOALING
FOAMING
FOBBING
FOGBANK
FOGGING
FOILING
FOLDING
FONDANT
FONTANA
FONTANE
FONTINA
FOOLING
FOOTING
FORCING
FORDING
FORDONE
FORFEND
FORGING
FORGONE
FORKING
FORLANI
FORMING
FORRENT
FORTUNA
FORTUNE
FORWENT
FOULING
FOWLING
FOXHUNT
FRAMING
FRAYING
FREEING
FRELENG
FREMONT
FRODING
FROZONE
FRYPANS
FTDIXNJ
FTWAYNE
FUDGING
FUELING
FULGENT
FUNDING
FUNKING
FUNNING
FUNRUNS
FURLING
FURLONG
FURRING
FUSIONS
FUSSING
FUTZING
FUZZING

F•••••N

FACEDON
FACESON
FACTION
FADEDIN
FADESIN
FADIMAN
FALLSIN
FALLSON
FASHION
FAWNSON
FEASTON
FEEDBIN
FEEDSIN
FEEDSON
FELDMAN
FELTPEN
FENCEIN
FENELON
FERMION
FESTOON
FEYNMAN
FHALOAN
FICTION
FIFTEEN
FILEDIN
FILESIN
FILLSIN
FINKSON
FIREDON
FIREMAN
FIREMEN
FIRESON
FISSION
FIVEMAN
FIVEPIN
FIVETEN
FIXEDON
FIXESON
FIXUPON
FLAGMAN
FLAGMEN
FLANKEN
FLASHON
FLATTEN
FLEURON
FLEXION
FLIESIN
FLIESON
FLIPPEN
FLITSIN
FLORIAN
FLOWNIN
FLOWNON
FLOWSIN
FLUXION
FLYOPEN
FOCUSON
FOGHORN
FOISTON
FOLDSIN
FONTEYN
FOOTMAN
FOOTMEN
FORCEIN
FORCEON
FOREIGN
FOREMAN
FOREMEN
FORERAN
FORERUN
FORLORN
FORTRAN
FOURMAN
FOURPIN
FRANKEN
FREEMAN
FREEMEN
FRESHEN
FRIEDAN
FRISIAN
FRISSON
FROGMAN
FROGMEN
FRONTON
FROWNON
FUJISAN
FUSTIAN

•FN••••

OFNOUSE

•F•N•••

OFANAGE
PFENNIG

•F••N••

AFFINED
AFFINES
EFFENDI
OFFENCE
OFFENDS
OFFENSE
OFFINGS
OFTENER
PFENNIG

•F•••N•

AFFIANT
AFFRONT
AFGHANI
AFGHANS
IFORONE
IFSTONE
OFAKIND
OFAMIND
OFFHAND
OFFLINE

•F••••N

AFRICAN

••FN•••

HAFNIUM

••F•N••

AFFINED
AFFINES
ALFONSE
ALFONSO
DEFANGS
DEFENCE
DEFENDS
DEFENSE
DEFINED
DEFINER
DEFINES
DEFUNCT
DEFUNDS
EFFENDI
ENFANTS
INFANCY
INFANTA
INFANTE
INFANTS
LIFENET
OFFENCE
OFFENDS
OFFENSE
OFFINGS
REFENCE
REFINDS
REFINED
REFINER
REFINES
REFUNDS
UNFANCY
UNFENCE
UNFINED
UNFINES
UNFUNNY

••F••N•

AFFIANT
AFFRONT
BAFFING
BIFFING
BOFFING
BOFFINS
BUFFING
CAFTANS
COFFINS
COFOUND
CUFFING
DEFCONS
DEFIANT
DEFYING
DOFFING
GAFFING
GIFTING
HAFTING
HEFTING
HOFMANN
HUFFING
INFERNO
INFRONT
LEFTEND
LIFTING
LOFTING
LUFFING
MIFFING
MUFFING
MUFFINS
OFFHAND
OFFLINE
PUFFING
PUFFINS
RAFTING
REFFING
REFOUND
REFRONT
REFYING
RIFFING
RIFLING
RIFTING
RUFFING
SIFTING
SOFTENS
TEFLONS
TIFFANY
TIFFING
TIFFINS
TUFTING
UNFOUND
UNFRANK
UNFUNNY
UPFLING
UPFRONT
WAFTING
WIFYING

••F•••N

BUFFOON
FIFTEEN
HOFFMAN
HOFMANN
HUFFMAN
ISFAHAN
MIFFLIN
REFLOWN
REFRAIN
RUFFIAN
SAFFRON
UNFLOWN

•••FN••

ASOFNOW

•••F•N•

AIRFONE
BAFFING
BEEFING
BIFFING
BIGFANS
BOFFING
BOFFINS
BOWFINS
BUFFING
CHAFING
CHEFING
COFFINS
COIFING
CONFINE
CUBFANS
CUFFING
DEAFENS
DIDFINE
DOFFING
FORFEND
GAFFING
GOLFING
GOOFING
GULFING
HOOFING
HUFFING
INAFUNK
ITSFINE
JETFANS
KAMFONG
KNIFING
LEAFING
LENFANT
LOAFING
LUFFING
METFANS
MIFFING
MUFFING
MUFFINS
NONFANS
OLEFINS
OUTFIND
PREFUND
PROFANE
PUFFING
PUFFINS
RAMFANS
RATFINK
REDFINS
REEFING
REFFING
RIFFING
ROLFING
ROOFING
RUFFING
SOXFANS
STEFANI
SUNFANS
SURFING
THEFONZ
TIFFANY
TIFFING
TIFFINS
TURFING
WOLFING
WOOFING

•••F••N

ARTFERN
BIAFRAN
BUFFOON
CHIFFON
CLIFTON
DORFMAN
DRIFTIN
GRAFTON
GRIFFIN
GRIFFON
HALFWON
HOFFMAN
HUFFMAN
KAUFMAN
LOAFPAN
MIFFLIN
OAKFERN
OUTFAWN
REDFERN
RUFFIAN
SAFFRON
SEAFERN
STIFFEN
STUFFIN
SURFMAN
SURFMEN
TURFMAN
TURFMEN
UNOFTEN
WOLFMAN
WOLFMEN

••••F•N

AVIDFAN
BLUEFIN
CHIFFON
CUBSFAN
ESTEFAN
GRIFFIN
GRIFFON
HAVEFUN
HEATFAN
JETSFAN
MADEFUN
MAKEFUN
METSFAN
POKEFUN
RAMSFAN
REDSFAN
STIFFEN
STUFFIN
SUNSFAN
TAILFIN

FO•••••

FOALING
FOAMERS
FOAMIER
FOAMILY
FOAMING
FOBBING
FOBSOFF
FOCSLES
FOCUSED
FOCUSER
FOCUSES
FOCUSON
FODDERS
FOELESS
FOGBANK
FOGBOWS
FOGCITY
FOGDOGS
FOGERTY
FOGGERS
FOGGIER
FOGGILY
FOGGING
FOGHORN
FOGLAMP
FOGLESS
FOGYISH
FOGYISM
FOIBLES
FOILING
FOISTED
FOISTON
FOKKERS
FOLATES
FOLDERS
FOLDING
FOLDOUT
FOLDSIN
FOLDSUP
FOLDUPS
FOLENGO
FOLGERS
FOLIAGE
FOLIATE
FOLIOED
FOLIOSE
FOLKART
FOLKIER
FOLKIES
FOLKISH
FOLKWAY
FOLLETT
FOLLIES
FOLLOWS
FOMENTS
FONDANT
FONDEST
FONDLED
FONDLER
FONDLES
FONDUED
FONDUES
FONTANA
FONTANE
FONTEYN
FONTINA
FOODIES
FOODWEB
FOOLERS
FOOLERY
FOOLING
FOOLISH
FOOTAGE
FOOTBAG
FOOTERS
FOOTING
FOOTLED
FOOTLER
FOOTLES
FOOTLET
FOOTMAN
FOOTMEN
FOOTPAD
FOOTRUB
FOOTSIE
FOOTSIT
FOOTSUP
FOOTWAY
FOOZLED
FOOZLER
FOOZLES
FOPPERY
FOPPISH
FORABIT
FORADAY
FORAGED
FORAGER
FORAGES
FORASEC
FORAYED
FORBADE
FORBEAR
FORBIDS
FORBORE
FORBUSH
FORCEIN
FORCEON
FORCEPS
FORCERS
FORCEUP
FORCING
FORDGTS
FORDHAM
FORDING
FORDLTD
FORDOES
FORDONE
FOREACH
FOREARM
FOREBAY
FOREIGN
FORELEG
FOREMAN
FOREMEN
FORENZA
FOREPAW
FORERAN
FORERUN
FORESAW
FORESEE
FORESTS
FORETOP
FOREVER
FORFEIT
FORFEND
FORFREE
FORGAVE
FORGERS
FORGERY
FORGETS
FORGING
FORGIVE
FORGOER
FORGOES
FORGONE
FORGOOD
FORHIRE
FORINTS
FORKERS
FORKFUL
FORKIER
FORKING
FORKOUT
FORKSUP
FORLANI
FORLIFE
FORLORN
FORLOVE
FORMALS
FORMATS
FORMERS
FORMFUL
FORMICA
FORMING
FORMOSA
FORMULA
FORONCE
FORREAL
FORRENT
FORREST
FORSAKE
FORSALE
FORSHOW
FORSIZE
FORSOOK
FORSTER
FORSURE
FORSYTE
FORSYTH
FORTDIX
FORTIES
FORTIFY
FORTIUS
FORTLEE
FORTORD
FORTRAN
FORTUNA
FORTUNE
FORTYAD
FORTYBC
FORWARD
FORWENT
FOSCOLO
FOSDICK
FOSSILS
FOSTERS
FOTOMAT
FOUDRES
FOUETTE
FOULARD
FOULEST
FOULING
FOULOUT
FOULSUP
FOULTIP
FOULUPS
FOUNDED
FOUNDER
FOUNDRY
FOURAAA
FOURDAY
FOUREEE
FOURIER
FOURMAN
FOURPIN
FOURTHS
FOURWAY
FOWLERS
FOWLING
FOXBORO
FOXFIRE
FOXHOLE
FOXHUNT
FOXIEST
FOXLIKE
FOXNEWS
FOXTAIL
FOXTROT

F•O••••

FEODORI
FEOFFED
FIORINA
FJORDIC
FLOATBY
FLOATED
FLOATER
FLOATUP
FLOCKED
FLOCKTO
FLOGGED
FLOGGER
FLOODED
FLOORED
FLOORER
FLOORIT
FLOPPED
FLOPPER
FLOREAL
FLORENZ
FLORETS
FLORIAN
FLORIDA
FLORINS
FLORIST
FLOSSED
FLOSSER
FLOSSES
FLOSSIE
FLOTAGE
FLOTSAM
FLOUNCE
FLOUNCY
FLOURED
FLOUTED
FLOUTER
FLOWAGE

FLOWERS
FLOWERY
FLOWING
FLOWNAT
FLOWNBY
FLOWNIN
FLOWNON
FLOWNTO
FLOWNUP
FLOWOUT
FLOWSIN
FOODIES
FOODWEB
FOOLERS
FOOLERY
FOOLING
FOOLISH
FOOTAGE
FOOTBAG
FOOTERS
FOOTING
FOOTLED
FOOTLER
FOOTLES
FOOTLET
FOOTMAN
FOOTMEN
FOOTPAD
FOOTRUB
FOOTSIE
FOOTSIT
FOOTSUP
FOOTWAY
FOOZLED
FOOZLER
FOOZLES
FROCKED
FRODING
FROEBEL
FROGGER
FROGLEG
FROGLET
FROGMAN
FROGMEN
FROLICS
FROMAGE
FROMMER
FRONTAL
FRONTED
FRONTON
FROOGLE
FROSTED
FROSTER
FROTHED
FROTHER
FROTHUP
FROWARD
FROWNAT
FROWNED
FROWNER
FROWNON
FROZEUP
FROZONE

F••O•••

FACONNE
FAGOTED
FANOUTS
FAROESE
FAROUKI
FATONES
FATOUSH
FAVORED
FAVORER
FAVOURS
FEDORAS
FEDOROV
FELONRY
FEMORAL
FEMORIS
FILOFAX
FLOODED
FLOORED
FLOORER
FLOORIT
FLYOPEN
FLYOVER
FORONCE
FOTOMAT
FROOGLE
FTDODGE
FTWORTH
FURORES

F•••O••

FABFOUR
FACEOFF
FACTOID
FACTORS
FACTORY
FADEOUT
FAEROES
FAIROFF
FAKEOUT
FALCONS
FALLOFF
FALLOUT
FALLOWS
FANDOMS
FANFOLD
FANIONS
FANSOUT
FANTODS
FARGOND
FARGONE
FARMORE
FARMOUT
FARROWS
FASTONE
FATHOMS
FATUOUS
FAXLORE
FEELOFF
FEELOUT
FELLOFF
FELLOUT
FELLOWS
FELTOFF
FELTOUT
FEMBOTS
FENDOFF
FEODORI
FERROUS
FERVORS
FERVOUR
FESTOON
FESTOSO
FETLOCK
FHALOAN
FIBROID
FIBROUS
FILEOUT
FILLOUT
FINDOUT
FIREOFF
FISHOIL
FISHOUT
FIVEONE
FLACONS
FLAGONS
FLATOUT
FLAVORS
FLAVORY
FLAVOUR
FLEXORS
FLIPOUT
FLOWOUT
FLYBOYS
FLYRODS
FLYSOLO
FOBSOFF
FOGBOWS
FOGDOGS
FOGHORN
FOLDOUT
FOLIOED
FOLIOSE
FOLLOWS
FORBORE
FORDOES
FORDONE
FORGOER
FORGOES
FORGONE
FORGOOD
FORKOUT
FORLORN
FORLOVE
FORMOSA
FORSOOK
FORTORD
FOSCOLO
FOULOUT
FOXBORO
FOXHOLE
FREMONT
FRIJOLE
FRIVOLS
FROZONE
FRYCOOK
FUELOIL
FULLOUT
FULSOME
FUNGOES
FURCOAT
FURIOSO
FURIOUS
FURLONG
FURROWS
FUSIONS

F••••O•

FACEDON
FACESON
FACTION
FALLFOR
FALLSON
FAMICOM
FAREBOX
FARMBOY
FASHION
FAWNSON
FEARFOR
FEARNOT
FEASTON
FEDOROV
FEEDLOT
FEEDSON
FEELFOR
FEELSOK
FELLFOR
FELTFOR
FENELON
FERMION
FESTOON
FIASCOS
FICTION
FIEFDOM
FILMDOM
FINKSON
FIREBOX
FIREDOG
FIREDON
FIREFOX
FIRESON
FISHFOR
FISSION
FITZROY
FIXEDON
FIXESON
FIXUPON
FLASHON
FLATTOP
FLEURON
FLEXION
FLIESON
FLIPTOP
FLOWNON
FLUMMOX
FLUSHOT
FLUXION
FOCUSON
FOISTON
FORCEON
FORETOP
FORGOOD
FORSHOW
FORSOOK
FOXTROT
FRANKOZ
FREEDOF
FREEDOM
FREESOF
FREETOY
FRESCOS
FRISSON
FRONTON
FROWNON
FRYCOOK
FUELROD
FUGATOS
FULLLOT
FUSEBOX
FUSSPOT

F•••••O

FAILSTO
FALLSTO
FARRAGO
FEBRERO
FEDERKO
FEDINTO
FEEDSTO
FERRARO
FESTOSO
FIDELIO
FILIPPO
FITINTO
FIVETWO
FLIEDTO
FLIESTO
FLOCKTO
FLOWNTO
FLYINTO
FLYSOLO
FMRADIO
FOLENGO
FOSCOLO
FOXBORO
FRUSTRO
FURILLO
FURIOSO
FURTADO

•FO••••

AFOULOF
GFORCES
IFORGET
IFORGOT
IFORONE
UFOLOGY

•F•O•••

AFFORDS
AFROPOP
EFFORTS
IFYOUGO
OFNOUSE
OFSORTS
TFPOWYS

•F••O••

AFFRONT
AFTMOST
IFORONE
IFSTONE
OFASORT
OFFHOUR
OFFLOAD
OFFROAD
UFOLOGY
VFWPOST

•F•••O•

AFATLOT
AFOULOF
AFROPOP
IFORGOT
OFFEROR
XFACTOR

•F••••O

IFYOUGO
OFFICIO
OFFWEGO

••FO•••

AFFORDS
ALFONSE
ALFONSO
ALFORJA
BEFOOLS
BEFOULS
BIFOCAL
BYFORCE
BYFORMS
COFOUND
DEFOAMS
DEFOCUS
DEFORMS
EFFORTS
ELFOWLS
ENFOLDS
ENFORCE
GOFORIT
GOFORTH
IMFORIT
INFOCUS
INFOLDS
INFORCE
INFORIT
INFORMS
OXFORDS
REFOCUS
REFOLDS
REFORGE
REFORMS
REFOUND
UNFOGGY
UNFOLDS
UNFORKS
UNFOUND
UNFOXED
UPFOLDS
UPFORIT

••F•O••

AFFRONT
BEFOOLS
BOFFOLA
BUFFOON
DEFCONS
DEFROCK
DEFROST
ELFLOCK
GIFFORD
INFLOWS
INFRONT
LEFTOFF
LEFTOUT
LIFTOFF
MAFIOSI
MAFIOSO
OFFHOUR
OFFLOAD
OFFROAD
PUFFOUT
REFLOAT
REFLOOD
REFLOWN
REFLOWS
REFRONT
SUFFOLK
TEFLONS
UNFLOOR
UNFLOWN
UNFROCK
UNFROST
UNFROZE
UPFLOWS
UPFRONT

••F••O•

ALFEROV
BUFFOON
GIFTBOX
INFAVOR
LEFTFOR
OFFEROR
REFLOOD
SAFFRON
SOFTTOP
UNFLOOR

••F•••O

ALFONSO
ALFREDO
BUFFALO
DEFACTO
DEFERTO
EXFACTO
INFERNO
MAFIOSO
OFFICIO
OFFWEGO
REFERTO
RUFFALO

•••FO••

ACTFOUR
AGEFOUR
AIRFOIL
AIRFONE
ALIFORM
ARTFORM
ASHFORD
BADFORM
BALFOUR
BEDFORD
BELFORT
BIGFOOT
BIGFOUR
BOFFOLA
BUFFOON
CATFOOD
CATFOOT
COMFORT
CONFORM
DOGFOOD
DRYFOGS
EYEFOLD
FABFOUR
FANFOLD
GIFFORD
GILFORD
GOOFOFF
GOSFORD
GULFOIL
HAYFORK
HOTFOOT
ICEFOGS
ILLFOLD
IRSFORM
JETFOIL
KAMFONG
KINFOLK
LANFORD
LAWFORD
LEAFOUT
LEEFORD
MAHFOUZ
MEDFORD
MENFOLK
MISFORM
MITFORD
MUMFORD
NONFOOD
NONFORM
NORFOLK
OLDFOGY
ONEFOLD
ONEFOOT
OUTFOOL
OUTFOOT
OVIFORM
PARFOUR
PEAFOWL
PERFORM
PINFOLD
PREFORM
PUFFOUT
RADFORD
RAWFOOD
REDFORD
REDFOUR
RUMFORD
SANFORD
SEAFOAM
SEAFOOD
SEAFOWL
SIXFOLD
SIXFOOT
SIXFOUR
SUBFORM
SUFFOLK
TENFOLD
TENFOOT
TENFOUR
THEFONZ
THEFOOL
TINFOIL
TOMFOOL
TOPFORM
TREFOIL
TRIFOLD
TRIFORM
TWOFOLD
TWOFOOT
UNIFORM
WATFORD
WEBFOOT
WEEFOLK
WEXFORD
WILFORD

•••F•O•

AIRFLOW
ARAFTOF
ASOFNOW
BIGFOOT
BUFFOON
CATFOOD
CATFOOT
CHIFFON
CLIFTON
DOGFOOD
EATFROM
FIEFDOM
GETFROM
GRAFTON
GRIFFON
HALFROD
HALFWON
HOTFOOT
ICEFLOE
KERFLOP
MUDFLOW
NONFOOD
ONEFOOT
OUTFLOW
OUTFOOL
OUTFOOT
PETFROG
RAWFOOD
ROOFTOP
SAFFRON
SEAFOOD
SERFDOM
SHYFROM
SIXFOOT
TENFOOT
THEFLOP
THEFOOL
TOMFOOL
TURFTOE
TWOFOOT
WEBFOOT
WOLFDOG

•••F••O

BEEFALO
BUFFALO
GOLFPRO
RUFFALO

••••FO•

ACHEFOR
ACTSFOR
AIMSFOR
ANTIFOG
ARCHFOE
ASKSFOR
BATSFOR
BEGSFOR
BIDSFOR
BLUEFOX
BRERFOX
BUCKFOR
BURNFOR
CALLFOR
CAREFOR
CHIFFON
CLAPFOR
DIEDFOR
DIESFOR
DIGSFOR
DOESFOR
DONEFOR
FALLFOR
FEARFOR
FEELFOR
FELLFOR
FELTFOR
FIREFOX
FISHFOR
GOESFOR
GOINFOR
GONEFOR
GOODFOR
GRIFFON
GUNSFOR
HEADFOR
HITSFOR
HOPEFOR
HUNTFOR
HURTFOR
ITCHFOR
LAIDFOR
LAYSFOR
LEAPFOR
LEFTFOR
LIEDFOR
LIESFOR
LIVEFOR
LONGFOR
LOOKFOR
MADEFOR
MAKEFOR
OPTSFOR
PAIDFOR
PASSFOR
PAYSFOR
PINEFOR
PLANFOR
PRAYFOR
PULLFOR
PUSHFOR
RANGFOR
READFOR
REPSFOR
RINGFOR
ROOTFOR
RUNGFOR
RUNSFOR
SAVEFOR
SELLFOR
SENDFOR
SENTFOR
SHOPFOR
SHOTFOR
SIGHFOR
SIGNFOR
SITSFOR
SOLDFOR
STAYFOR
STOPFOR
SUEDFOR
SUESFOR
TAKEFOR
TESTFOR
TOOKFOR
USEDFOR
USESFOR
VIEDFOR
VIESFOR
VOTEFOR
WAITFOR
WEEPFOR
WENTFOR
WHATFOR
WISHFOR
WORKFOR
YELLFOR
YENSFOR

•••••FO

RODOLFO

F•P••••

FIPPLES
FOPPERY
FOPPISH

F••P•••

FANPALM
FIPPLES
FLAPPED
FLAPPER
FLIPOUT
FLIPPED
FLIPPEN
FLIPPER
FLIPTOP
FLIPUPS
FLOPPED
FLOPPER
FLYPAST
FOPPERY
FOPPISH
FRAPPES
FRYPANS
FUNPLEX

F•••P••

FAUXPAS
FELTPEN
FILIPPO
FIREPIT
FIVEPIN
FIXUPON
FLAPPED
FLAPPER
FLEAPIT
FLIPPED
FLIPPEN
FLIPPER
FLOPPED
FLOPPER
FLYOPEN
FOOTPAD
FOREPAW
FOURPIN
FRAPPES
FUSSPOT

F••••P•

FATLIPS
FILIPPO
FILLIPS
FILLUPS
FLIPUPS
FOLDUPS
FORCEPS
FOULUPS

F•••••P

FAIRSUP
FANCYUP
FELTTIP
FENCEUP
FILLSUP
FIREDUP
FIRESUP
FIRMSUP
FIRSTUP
FIXEDUP
FIXESUP
FLAMEUP
FLAREUP
FLATTOP
FLEADIP
FLIESUP
FLIPTOP
FLOATUP
FLOWNUP
FLUFFUP
FLYTRAP
FOGLAMP
FOLDSUP
FOOTSUP
FORCEUP
FORETOP
FORKSUP
FOULSUP
FOULTIP
FRAMEUP
FREEDUP
FREESUP
FRIEDUP
FRIESUP
FROTHUP
FROZEUP
FUELSUP
FURWRAP

•FP••••

TFPOWYS

•F•P•••

OFFPEAK
VFWPOST

•F••P••

AFROPOP

•F••••P

AFROPOP
OFFERUP
OFFRAMP

••FP•••

OFFPEAK

••F•P••

BTFSPLK

••F••P•

REFLIPS

••F•••P

BUFFSUP
LEFTHIP
LIFTSUP
OFFERUP
OFFRAMP
PUFFSUP
SOFTTOP

•••FP••

GOLFPRO
LOAFPAN

•••F•P•

GOOFUPS

•••F••P

BEEFSUP
BUFFSUP
CATFLAP
DRIFTUP
EARFLAP
FLUFFUP
GOOFSUP
KERFLOP
MUDFLAP
PUFFSUP
ROOFTOP
SNIFFUP
SPIFFUP
SURFSUP
THEFLOP

••••F•P

FLUFFUP
SCARFUP
SNIFFUP
SPIFFUP

FR•••••

FRACTAL
FRAGGED
FRAGGLE
FRAGILE
FRAICHE
FRAILER
FRAILLY
FRAILTY
FRAISES
FRAMERS
FRAMEUP
FRAMING
FRANCES
FRANCHI
FRANCIS
FRANKED
FRANKEN
FRANKER
FRANKIE
FRANKLY
FRANKOZ
FRANTIC
FRAPPES
FRASIER
FRATERS

FRAUGHT
FRAWLEY
FRAYING
FRAZIER
FRAZZLE
FREAKED
FREBERG
FRECKLE
FRECKLY
FREDDIE
FREDEBB
FREDRIC
FREEAIR
FREEBEE
FREEBIE
FREEDOF
FREEDOM
FREEDUP
FREEING
FREEMAN
FREEMEN
FREESIA
FREESOF
FREESUP
FREETOY
FREEWAY
FREEZER
FREEZES
FREIGHT
FREITAG
FRELENG
FREMONT
FRENCHI
FRENCHS
FRENEAU
FRENEMY
FRENESI
FRESCAS
FRESCOS
FRESHED
FRESHEN
FRESHER
FRESHES
FRESHET
FRESHLY
FRESNEL
FRESSED
FRESSES
FRETFUL
FRETSAT
FRETSAW
FRETTED
FRETTER
FREYTAG
FRIABLE
FRIARLY
FRIBBLE
FRICKER
FRIDAYS
FRIDGES
FRIDLEY
FRIEDAN
FRIEDUP
FRIENDS
FRIESUP
FRIEZES
FRIGATE
FRIGHTS
FRIJOLE
FRILLED
FRINGED
FRINGES
FRISBEE
FRISEUR
FRISIAN
FRISKED
FRISKER
FRISSON
FRITTED
FRITTER
FRIVOLS
FRIZZED
FRIZZER
FRIZZES
FRIZZLE
FRIZZLY
FROCKED
FRODING
FROEBEL
FROGGER
FROGLEG
FROGLET
FROGMAN
FROGMEN
FROLICS
FROMAGE
FROMMER
FRONTAL
FRONTED
FRONTON
FROOGLE
FROSTED
FROSTER
FROTHED
FROTHER
FROTHUP
FROWARD
FROWNAT
FROWNED
FROWNER
FROWNON
FROZEUP
FROZONE
FRUITED
FRUSTRO
FRUSTUM
FRYABLE
FRYCOOK
FRYPANS

F•R••••

FARADAY
FARAWAY
FARCEUR
FARCING
FAREAST
FAREBOX
FAREWAR
FARFELS
FARGOND
FARGONE
FARINAS
FARLEFT
FARMAID
FARMBOY
FARMERS
FARMERY
FARMGAL
FARMING
FARMORE
FARMOUT
FARNESS
FAROESE
FAROUKI
FARRAGO
FARRELL
FARRIER
FARROWS
FARSEER
FARSIDE
FARTHER
FARTLEK
FARWEST
FERMATA
FERMATE
FERMATS
FERMENT
FERMION
FERMIUM
FERNAND
FERNBAR
FERNERY
FERNIER
FERRARA
FERRARE
FERRARI
FERRARO
FERRATE
FERRETS
FERRETY
FERRIED
FERRIES
FERRITE
FERROUS
FERRULE
FERTILE
FERULES
FERVENT
FERVORS
FERVOUR
FIRBANK
FIREANT
FIREARM
FIREBOX
FIREBUG
FIREDAT
FIREDOG
FIREDON
FIREDUP
FIREFLY
FIREFOX
FIREHAT
FIREICE
FIRELIT
FIREMAN
FIREMEN
FIRENZA
FIRENZE
FIREOFF
FIREPIT
FIRESAT
FIRESON
FIRESUP
FIRINGS
FIRKINS
FIRMEST
FIRMING
FIRMSUP
FIRRIER
FIRSTLY
FIRSTUP
FIRTREE
FMRADIO
FORABIT
FORADAY
FORAGED
FORAGER
FORAGES
FORASEC
FORAYED
FORBADE
FORBEAR
FORBIDS
FORBORE
FORBUSH
FORCEIN
FORCEON
FORCEPS
FORCERS
FORCEUP
FORCING
FORDGTS
FORDHAM
FORDING
FORDLTD
FORDOES
FORDONE
FOREACH
FOREARM
FOREBAY
FOREIGN
FORELEG
FOREMAN
FOREMEN
FORENZA
FOREPAW
FORERAN
FORERUN
FORESAW
FORESEE
FORESTS
FORETOP
FOREVER
FORFEIT
FORFEND
FORFREE
FORGAVE
FORGERS
FORGERY
FORGETS
FORGING
FORGIVE
FORGOER
FORGOES
FORGONE
FORGOOD
FORHIRE
FORINTS
FORKERS
FORKFUL
FORKIER
FORKING
FORKOUT
FORKSUP
FORLANI
FORLIFE
FORLORN
FORLOVE
FORMALS
FORMATS
FORMERS
FORMFUL
FORMICA
FORMING
FORMOSA
FORMULA
FORONCE
FORREAL
FORRENT
FORREST
FORSAKE
FORSALE
FORSHOW
FORSIZE
FORSOOK
FORSTER
FORSURE
FORSYTE
FORSYTH
FORTDIX
FORTIES
FORTIFY
FORTIUS
FORTLEE
FORTORD
FORTRAN
FORTUNA
FORTUNE
FORTYAD
FORTYBC
FORWARD
FORWENT
FTRILEY
FURBALL
FURBISH
FURCATE
FURCOAT
FURFARM
FURILLO
FURIOSO
FURIOUS
FURLERS
FURLESS
FURLING
FURLONG
FURNACE
FURNESS
FURNISH
FURORES
FURRIER
FURRING
FURROWS
FURSEAL
FURTADO
FURTHER
FURTIVE
FURWRAP

F••R•••

FABRICS
FABRIZI
FAERIES
FAEROES
FAIREST
FAIRFAX
FAIRIES
FAIRING
FAIRISH
FAIROFF
FAIRSEX
FAIRSUP
FAIRUSE
FAIRWAY
FARRAGO
FARRELL
FARRIER
FARROWS
FEARERS
FEARFOR
FEARFUL
FEARING
FEARNOT
FEBRERO
FEBRILE
FERRARA
FERRARE
FERRARI
FERRARO
FERRATE
FERRETS
FERRETY
FERRIED
FERRIES
FERRITE
FERROUS
FERRULE
FEVRIER
FIBRINS
FIBROID
FIBROUS
FIERCER
FIERIER
FIERILY
FIORINA
FIRRIER
FJORDIC
FLAREUP
FLARING
FLIRTED
FLIRTER
FLOREAL
FLORENZ
FLORETS
FLORIAN
FLORIDA
FLORINS
FLORIST
FLYRODS
FMURRAY
FORREAL
FORRENT
FORREST
FOURAAA
FOURDAY
FOUREEE
FOURIER
FOURMAN
FOURPIN
FOURTHS
FOURWAY
FTBRAGG
FUNRUNS
FURRIER
FURRING
FURROWS

F•••R••

FABARES
FABERGE
FATFREE
FAVORED
FAVORER
FAYWRAY
FEDERAL
FEDERKO
FEDORAS
FEDOROV
FEEFREE
FEMORAL
FEMORIS
FEVERED
FIACRES
FIBERED
FIGTREE
FIGURAL
FIGURED
FIGURER
FIGURES
FIRTREE
FITZROY
FLEERED
FLEURON
FLOORED
FLOORER
FLOORIT
FLOURED
FLYTRAP
FMURRAY
FOGERTY
FOOTRUB
FORERAN
FORERUN
FORFREE
FORTRAN
FOUDRES
FOXTROT
FREDRIC
FRIARLY
FTWORTH
FUELROD
FULCRUM
FURORES
FURWRAP
FUTURAS
FUTURES

F••••R•

FABLERS
FACTORS
FACTORY
FAILURE
FALKIRK
FALLERS
FALTERS
FANFARE
FANNERS
FARMERS
FARMERY
FARMORE
FATFARM
FATHERS
FAVOURS
FAWNERS
FAXLORE
FEARERS
FEATURE
FEBRERO
FEDDERS
FEEDERS
FEELERS
FELLERS
FELONRY
FENCERS
FENDERS
FENETRE
FEODORI
FERNERY
FERRARA
FERRARE
FERRARI
FERRARO
FERVORS
FESTERS
FETTERS
FIBBERS
FIGBARS
FILBERT
FILLERS
FILTERS
FINDERS
FINEART
FINGERS
FIREARM
FISHERS
FISHERY
FISHFRY
FISSURE
FITTERS
FIXTURE
FIZZERS
FLAKERS
FLAMERS
FLAVORS
FLAVORY
FLAYERS
FLEXORS
FLEXURE
FLOWERS
FLOWERY
FLUTERS
FLYGIRL
FOAMERS
FODDERS
FOGGERS
FOGHORN
FOKKERS
FOLDERS
FOLGERS
FOLKART
FOOLERS
FOOLERY
FOOTERS
FOPPERY
FORBORE
FORCERS
FOREARM
FORGERS
FORGERY
FORHIRE
FORKERS
FORLORN
FORMERS
FORSURE
FORTORD
FORWARD
FOSTERS
FOULARD
FOUNDRY
FOWLERS
FOXBORO
FOXFIRE
FRAMERS
FRATERS
FREBERG
FROWARD
FRUSTRO
FTHENRY
FTMYERS
FUDGERS
FUELERS
FULMARS
FUNDERS
FUNFURS
FURFARM
FURLERS
FUSSERS
FUTHARK

F•••••R

FABFOUR
FADDIER
FAINTER
FAKEFUR
FALLFOR
FANCIER
FANSLER
FARCEUR
FAREWAR
FARRIER
FARSEER
FARTHER
FASTCAR
FATTIER
FAUXFUR
FAVORER
FEARFOR
FEASTER
FEATHER
FECHNER
FEEBLER
FEELFOR
FEIFFER
FEIGNER
FELLFOR
FELTFOR
FENNIER
FERNBAR
FERNIER
FERVOUR
FETCHER
FEVRIER
FIBIGER
FIBSTER
FIBULAR
FICKLER
FIDDLER
FIEDLER
FIELDER
FIERCER
FIERIER
FIGHTER
FIGURER
FILCHER
FILMIER
FINNAIR
FINNIER
FIRRIER
FISCHER
FISHFOR
FISHIER
FIZZIER
FIZZLER
FLAGGER
FLAKIER
FLAMIER
FLANEUR
FLANKER
FLAPPER
FLASHER
FLATCAR
FLATTER
FLAVOUR
FLAWIER
FLAXIER
FLEECER
FLEETER
FLENSER
FLEXNER
FLICKER
FLINGER
FLIPPER
FLIRTER
FLITTER
FLIVVER
FLOATER
FLOGGER
FLOORER
FLOPPER
FLOSSER
FLOUTER
FLUBBER
FLUFFER
FLUKIER
FLUNKER
FLUSHER
FLUSTER
FLUTIER
FLUTTER
FLYOVER
FLYTIER
FNUMBER
FOAMIER
FOCUSER
FOGGIER
FOLKIER
FONDLER
FOOTLER
FOOZLER
FORAGER
FORBEAR
FOREVER
FORGOER
FORKIER
FORSTER
FOUNDER
FOURIER
FRAILER
FRANKER
FRASIER
FRAZIER
FREEAIR
FREEZER
FRESHER
FRETTER
FRICKER
FRISEUR
FRISKER
FRITTER
FRIZZER
FROGGER
FROMMER
FROSTER
FROTHER
FROWNER
FUBSIER
FUMBLER
FUNFAIR
FUNKIER
FUNNIER
FUNSTER
FURRIER
FURTHER
FUSSIER
FUSTIER
FUZZIER

•FR••••

AFRAMES
AFRICAN
AFROPOP

•F•R•••

AFARCRY
AFFRAYS
AFFRONT
GFORCES
IFORGET
IFORGOT
IFORONE
OFFRAMP
OFFROAD

•F••R••

AFEARED
AFFIRMS
AFFORDS
EFFORTS
OFFERED
OFFEREE
OFFERER
OFFEROR
OFFERUP
OFSORTS

•F•••R•

AFARCRY
AFFAIRE
AFFAIRS
OFASORT

•F••••R

AFFIXER
EFFACER
OFFERER
OFFEROR
OFFHOUR
OFFICER
OFFYEAR
OFTENER
XFACTOR

••FR•••

AFFRAYS
AFFRONT
ALFREDA
ALFREDE
ALFREDO
ALFREDU
DEFRAGS
DEFRAME
DEFRAUD
DEFRAYS
DEFROCK
DEFROST
DRFREUD
DRFRIST
ENFRAME
INFRACT
INFRONT
LEFREAK
OFFRAMP
OFFROAD
REFRACT
REFRAIN
REFRAME
REFRESH
REFRIED
REFRIES
REFRONT
UNFRAIL
UNFRANK
UNFREED
UNFREES
UNFRIED
UNFRILL
UNFROCK
UNFROST
UNFROZE
UPFRONT

••F•R••

AFFIRMS
AFFORDS
ALFEROV
ALFORJA
ASFARAS
ATFIRST
BYFORCE
BYFORMS
DEFARGE
DEFERTO
DEFORMS
EFFORTS
ENFORCE
GOFIRST
GOFORIT
GOFORTH
HOFBRAU
IMFORIT
INFERNO
INFIRST
INFORCE
INFORIT
INFORMS
JEFFREY
JOFFREY
LAFARGE
MEFIRST
OFFERED
OFFEREE
OFFERER
OFFEROR
OFFERUP
ONFIRST
OXFORDS
PRFIRMS
REFEREE
REFERTO
REFIRED
REFIRES
REFORGE
REFORMS
SAFARIS
SAFFRON
SEFERIS
SOFARAS
UNFERTH
UNFIRED
UNFORKS
UNFURLS
UPFIRST
UPFORIT
WAFERED

••F••R•

AFFAIRE
AFFAIRS
ALFIERI
BAFFERS
BUFFERS
COFFERS
DEFIERS
DIFFERS
DOFFERS
DUFFERS
GAFFERS
GIFFORD
HEFTERS
HOFSTRA
JEFFERS
LEFTARM
LIFTERS
LOFTERS
PUFFERS
PUFFERY
RAFTERS
RIFLERS
RIFLERY
SIFTERS
SUFFERS
UNFIERY
WAFTERS

••F•••R
AFFIXER
BAFFLER
DAFFIER
DEFACER
DEFAMER
DEFILER
DEFINER
DEFUSER
EFFACER
HEFTIER
HUFFIER
INFAVOR
INFUSER
LAFLEUR
LEFTEAR
LEFTFOR
LOFTIER
MIFFIER
MUFFLER
NIFTIER
OFFERER
OFFEROR
OFFHOUR
OFFICER
OFFYEAR
PUFFIER
RAFFLER
REFINER
REFUSER
REFUTER
RIFFLER
RUFFLER
TOFFLER
TUFTIER
UNFLOOR
WAFFLER

•••FR••
AELFRIC
BIAFRAN
BUGFREE
CARFREE
CONFREY
EATFROM
FATFREE
FEEFREE
FORFREE
GETFREE
GETFROM
GODFREY
GOTFREE
HALFRAW
HALFROD
ICEFREE
JEFFREY
JOFFREY
MANFRED
PALFREY
PETFROG
RANFREE
RENFREW
ROOFRAT
RUNFREE
SAFFRON
SETFREE
SHYFROM
TAXFREE
THEFRUG
WILFRED
WINFREY
WOLFRAM

•••F•R•
AIRFARE
ALLFORM
ANTFARM
ARAFURA
ARTFERN
ARTFORM
ASHFORD
BADFORM
BAFFERS
BEDFORD
BELFORT
BONFIRE
BUFFERS
BUSFARE
CABFARE
CARFARE
CHAFERS
COFFERS
COMFORT
CONFERS
CONFIRM
CONFORM
DIFFERS
DOFFERS
DUFFERS
FANFARE
FATFARM
FOXFIRE
FUNFURS
FURFARM
GAFFERS
GIFFORD
GILFORD
GOLFERS
GOLFPRO
GOSFORD
GUNFIRE
HAYFORK
HEIFERS
HOOFERS
INAFURY
IRSFORM
JEFFERS
JETFIRE
KNIFERS
LANFORD
LAWFORD
LEEFORD
LOAFERS
MEDFORD
MISFIRE
MISFORM
MITFORD
MUMFORD
NONFARM
NONFORM
OAKFERN
OUTFIRE
OVIFORM
PERFORM
PILFERS
PREFERS
PREFORM
PROFARM
PUFFERS
PUFFERY
RADFORD
REDFERN
REDFIRS
REDFORD
REEFERS
ROLFERS
ROOFERS
RUMFORD
SANFORD
SEAFARE
SEAFERN
SHOFARS
SUBFORM
SUFFERS
SUNFIRE
SURFERS
THEFIRM
TOPFORM
TRIFORM
TWOFERS
UNIFORM
WARFARE
WATFORD
WELFARE
WEXFORD
WILFORD
WOOFERS

•••F•R
ACTFOUR
AGEFOUR
ARTFAIR
BAFFLER
BALFOUR
BEEFIER
BIDFAIR
BIGFOUR
BLUFFER
CHAFFER
COMFIER
CRAFTER
CROFTER
DAFFIER
DEIFIER
DRAFTER
DRIFTER
EDIFIER
FABFOUR
FEIFFER
FLUFFER
FUNFAIR
GOAFTER
GOLFCAR
GOOFIER
GRAFTER
GRIFTER
GRUFFER
GULFWAR
HUFFIER
JOBFAIR
KIEFFER
LEAFIER
MAYFAIR
MIFFIER
MUFFLER
NOTFAIR
PARFOUR
PROFFER
PUFFIER
PURFLER
QUAFFER
RAFFLER
REDFOUR
REEFIER
REOFFER
RIFFLER
RUFFLER
SCOFFER
SCUFFER
SHAFFER
SHEFFER
SHIFTER
SIXFOUR
SNIFFER
SNIFTER
SNUFFER
STAFFER
STIFFER
STUFFER
SURFIER
SWIFTER
TENFOUR
TOFFLER
TOYFAIR
TRIFLER
TURFIER
TURFWAR
UNIFIER
WAFFLER
WASFAIR
WHIFFER

••••FR•
DEEPFRY
FISHFRY
STIRFRY

••••F•R
ACHEFOR
ACTSFOR
AIMSFOR
AQUIFER
ASKSFOR
BATSFOR
BEGSFOR
BIDSFOR
BLUFFER
BRIEFER
BUCKFOR
BURNFOR
CALLFOR
CAREFOR
CHAFFER
CHAMFER
CLAPFOR
CONIFER
DIEDFOR
DIESFOR
DIGSFOR
DOESFOR
DONEFOR
FAKEFUR
FALLFOR
FAUXFUR
FEARFOR
FEELFOR
FEIFFER
FELLFOR
FELTFOR
FISHFOR
FLUFFER
GETSFAR
GOESFAR
GOESFOR
GOINFOR
GONEFAR
GONEFOR
GOODFOR
GRUFFER
GUNSFOR
HEADFOR
HITSFOR
HOPEFOR
HUNTFOR
HURTFOR
INSOFAR
ITCHFOR
KIEFFER
LAIDFOR
LAYSFOR
LEAPFOR
LEFTFOR
LIEDFOR
LIESFOR
LIVEFOR
LONGFOR
LOOKFOR
LUCIFER
MADEFOR
MAKEFOR
OPTSFOR
OVERFAR
PAIDFOR
PASSFOR
PAYSFOR
PINEFOR
PLANFOR
PRAYFOR
PROFFER
PROOFER
PULLFOR
PUSHFOR
QUAFFER
RANGFOR
READFOR
REOFFER
REPSFOR
RINGFOR
ROOTFOR
ROTIFER
RUNGFOR
RUNSFOR
SAVEFOR
SCARFER
SCOFFER
SCUFFER
SELLFOR
SENDFOR
SENTFOR
SHAFFER
SHEFFER
SHOPFOR
SHOTFOR
SIGHFOR
SIGNFOR
SITSFOR
SNIFFER
SNUFFER
SOLDFOR
SPOOFER
STAFFER
STAYFOR
STIFFER
STOPFOR
STRAFER
STUFFER
SUEDFOR
SUESFOR
TAKEFOR
TESTFOR
THUSFAR
TOOKFOR
UNSAFER
USEDFOR
USESFOR
VIEDFOR
VIESFOR
VOTEFOR
WAITFOR
WEEPFOR
WENTFAR
WENTFOR
WHATFOR
WHIFFER
WISHFOR
WORKFOR
YELLFOR
YENSFOR

F•S••••
FASCIAE
FASCIAL
FASCIAS
FASCISM
FASCIST
FASHION
FASTCAR
FASTENS
FASTEST
FASTING
FASTNET
FASTONE
FESCUES
FESSING
FESTERS
FESTINA
FESTIVA
FESTIVE
FESTOON
FESTOSO
FISCHER
FISHERS
FISHERY
FISHEYE
FISHFOR
FISHFRY
FISHIER
FISHILY
FISHING
FISHNET
FISHOIL
FISHOUT
FISSILE
FISSION
FISSURE
FISTFUL
FOSCOLO
FOSDICK
FOSSILS
FOSTERS
FUSEBOX
FUSIBLE
FUSILLI
FUSIONS
FUSSERS
FUSSIER
FUSSILY
FUSSING
FUSSPOT
FUSTIAN
FUSTIER
FUSTILY
FUSUMAS

F••S•••
FAISALI
FALSELY
FALSEST
FALSIFY
FALSITY
FANSLER
FANSOUT
FARSEER
FARSIDE
FAUSTUS
FEASTED
FEASTER
FEASTON
FESSING
FIASCOS
FIBSTER
FIESTAS
FIRSTLY
FIRSTUP
FISSILE
FISSION
FISSURE
FLASHED
FLASHER
FLASHES
FLASHON
FLESHED
FLESHES
FLESHLY
FLOSSED
FLOSSER
FLOSSES
FLOSSIE
FLUSHED
FLUSHER
FLUSHES
FLUSHOT
FLUSTER
FLYSOLO
FOBSOFF
FOCSLES
FOISTED
FOISTON
FORSAKE
FORSALE
FORSHOW
FORSIZE
FORSOOK
FORSTER
FORSURE
FORSYTE
FORSYTH
FOSSILS
FRASIER
FRESCAS
FRESCOS
FRESHED
FRESHEN
FRESHER
FRESHES
FRESHET
FRESHLY
FRESNEL
FRESSED
FRESSES
FRISBEE
FRISEUR
FRISIAN
FRISKED
FRISKER
FRISSON
FROSTED
FROSTER
FRUSTRO
FRUSTUM
FUBSIER
FULSOME
FUNSTER
FURSEAL
FUSSERS
FUSSIER
FUSSILY
FUSSING
FUSSPOT

F•••S••
FACESIT
FACESON
FADESIN
FAILSTO
FAIRSEX
FAIRSUP
FAKESIT
FALLSIN
FALLSON
FALLSTO
FAWNSON
FEEDSIN
FEEDSON
FEEDSTO
FEELSOK
FETUSES
FICUSES
FILESBY
FILESIN
FILLSIN
FILLSUP
FILMSET
FINESSE
FINISHD
FINKSON
FIRESAT
FIRESON
FIRESUP
FIRMSUP
FIVESIX
FIXESON
FIXESUP
FLENSED
FLENSER
FLENSES
FLIESAT
FLIESBY
FLIESIN
FLIESON
FLIESTO
FLIESUP
FLITSBY
FLITSIN
FLOSSED
FLOSSER
FLOSSES
FLOSSIE
FLOTSAM
FLOWSIN
FOCUSED
FOCUSER
FOCUSES
FOCUSON
FOLDSIN
FOLDSUP
FOOTSIE
FOOTSIT
FOOTSUP
FORASEC
FORESAW
FORESEE
FORESTS
FORKSUP
FOULSUP
FRAISES
FREESIA
FREESOF
FREESUP
FRESSED
FRESSES
FRETSAT
FRETSAW
FRIESUP
FRISSON
FUCHSIA
FUELSUP
FUJISAN
FUMESAT

F••••S•
FABBEST
FADDISH
FADDISM
FADDIST
FAINEST
FAIREST
FAIRISH
FAIRUSE
FALSEST
FANBASE
FANFEST
FANTASM
FANTAST
FANTASY
FANWISE
FAREAST
FARNESS
FAROESE
FARWEST
FASCISM
FASCIST
FASTEST
FATLESS
FATNESS
FATOUSH
FATTEST
FATTISH
FAUVISM
FAUVIST
FBICASE
FEELESS
FESTOSO
FEUDIST
FEWNESS
FEYNESS
FINESSE
FINLESS
FINNISH
FIRMEST
FITNESS
FITTEST
FLEMISH
FLORIST
FLUTIST
FLYCAST
FLYFISH
FLYLESS
FLYPAST
FOELESS
FOGLESS
FOGYISH
FOGYISM
FOLIOSE
FOLKISH
FONDEST
FOOLISH
FOPPISH
FORBUSH
FORMOSA
FORREST
FOULEST
FOXIEST
FRENESI
FTBLISS
FUJITSU
FULLEST
FULNESS
FUMIEST
FUNFEST
FURBISH
FURIOSO
FURLESS
FURNESS
FURNISH

F•••••S
FABARES
FABLERS
FABRICS
FACADES
FACIALS
FACINGS
FACTORS
FADEINS
FAERIES
FAEROES
FAGENDS
FAILLES
FAIRIES
FAJITAS
FAKEIDS
FALCONS
FALLALS
FALLERS
FALLOWS
FALTERS
FAMINES
FAMULUS
FANCIES
FANDOMS
FANFICS
FANIONS
FANJETS
FANNERS
FANOUTS
FANTANS
FANTODS
FARFELS
FARINAS
FARMERS
FARNESS
FARROWS
FASCIAS
FASTENS
FATALES
FATCATS
FATHERS
FATHOMS
FATLESS
FATLIPS
FATNESS
FATONES
FATTENS
FATUOUS
FAUCETS
FAUSTUS
FAUXPAS
FAVOURS
FAWNERS
FEARERS
FEDDERS
FEDEXES
FEDORAS
FEEDERS
FEELERS
FEELESS
FELINES
FELLAHS
FELLERS
FELLOWS
FEMALES
FEMBOTS
FEMORIS
FENCERS
FENDERS
FENNELS
FERMATS
FERRETS
FERRIES
FERROUS
FERULES
FERVORS
FESCUES
FESTERS
FETCHES
FETTERS
FETTLES
FETUSES
FEWNESS
FEYNESS
FIACRES
FIANCES
FIASCOS
FIBBERS
FIBRINS
FIBROUS
FIBULAS
FICUSES
FIDDLES
FIDELES
FIDELIS
FIDGETS
FIENNES
FIESTAS
FIFTIES
FIGBARS
FIGURES
FIJIANS
FILCHES
FILENES
FILINGS
FILLERS
FILLETS
FILLIES
FILLINS
FILLIPS
FILLUPS
FILTERS
FINALES
FINCHES
FINDERS
FINGALS
FINGERS
FINIALS
FINIANS
FINITES
FINLESS
FIPPLES
FIRINGS
FIRKINS
FISHERS
FITNESS
FITTERS
FIXATES
FIXINGS
FIZGIGS
FIZZERS
FIZZLES
FLACONS
FLAGONS
FLAKERS
FLAMBES
FLAMERS
FLANGES
FLASHES
FLATTVS
FLAUNTS
FLAUTAS
FLAVIUS
FLAVORS
FLAYERS
FLECHES
FLEDGES
FLEECES
FLENSES
FLESHES
FLEXORS
FLIGHTS
FLIPUPS
FLORETS
FLORINS
FLOSSES
FLOWERS
FLUBUGS
FLUSHES
FLUTERS
FLUTIES
FLYBOYS
FLYLESS
FLYNETS
FLYRODS
FLYWAYS
FMBANDS
FOAMERS
FOCSLES
FOCUSES
FODDERS
FOELESS
FOGBOWS
FOGDOGS
FOGGERS
FOGLESS
FOIBLES
FOKKERS
FOLATES
FOLDERS
FOLDUPS
FOLGERS
FOLKIES
FOLLIES
FOLLOWS
FOMENTS
FONDLES
FONDUES
FOODIES
FOOLERS
FOOTERS
FOOTLES
FOOZLES
FORAGES
FORBIDS
FORCEPS
FORCERS
FORDGTS
FORDOES
FORESTS
FORGERS
FORGETS
FORGOES
FORINTS
FORKERS
FORMALS
FORMATS

FORMERS
FORTIES
FORTIUS
FOSSILS
FOSTERS
FOUDRES
FOULUPS
FOURTHS
FOWLERS
FOXNEWS
FRAISES
FRAMERS
FRANCES
FRANCIS
FRAPPES
FRATERS
FREEZES
FRENCHS
FRESCAS
FRESCOS
FRESHES
FRESSES
FRIDAYS
FRIDGES
FRIENDS
FRIEZES
FRIGHTS
FRINGES
FRIVOLS
FRIZZES
FROLICS
FRYPANS
FTBLISS
FTMYERS
FUDDIES
FUDDLES
FUDGERS
FUELERS
FUENTES
FUGATOS
FULFILS
FULMARS
FULNESS
FUMBLES
FUNDERS
FUNFURS
FUNGOES
FUNNELS
FUNNIES
FUNRUNS
FURIOUS
FURLERS
FURLESS
FURNESS
FURORES
FURROWS
FUSIONS
FUSSERS
FUSUMAS
FUTURAS
FUTURES

•FS••••
IFSTONE
OFSORTS

•F•S•••
OFASORT
OFFSETS
OFFSIDE
OFFSITE

•F••S••
EFFUSED
EFFUSES

•F•••S•
AFTMOST
IFFIEST
OFFBASE
OFFCAST
OFFENSE
OFNOUSE
VFWPOST

•F••••S
AFFAIRS
AFFECTS
AFFINES
AFFIRMS
AFFIXES
AFFORDS
AFFRAYS
AFGHANS
AFRAMES
EFFACES
EFFECTS
EFFORTS
EFFUSES
GFORCES
OFFDAYS
OFFENDS
OFFICES
OFFINGS
OFFSETS
OFSORTS
TFPOWYS

••FS•••
BTFSPLK
HOFSTRA
OFFSETS
OFFSIDE
OFFSITE

••F•S••
BUFFSUP
DEFUSED
DEFUSER
DEFUSES
DUFUSES
EFFUSED
EFFUSES
GIFTSET
INFESTS
INFUSED
INFUSER
INFUSES
LIFTSUP
PUFFSUP
REFUSAL
REFUSED
REFUSER
REFUSES
UNFUSED
UNFUSSY

••F••S•
ALFONSE
ALFONSO
ATFIRST
BUFFEST
DAFTEST
DEFENSE
DEFFEST
DEFROST
DEFTEST
DIFFUSE
DRFRIST
GOFIRST
HUFFISH
IFFIEST
INFIRST
LEFTEST
LEFTISH
LEFTISM
LEFTIST
MAFIOSI
MAFIOSO
MEFIRST
OFFBASE
OFFCAST
OFFENSE
ONFIRST
RAFFISH
REFRESH
SOFTEST
SOFTISH
SUFFUSE
UNFROST
UNFUSSY
UPFIRST

••F•••S
AFFAIRS
AFFECTS
AFFINES
AFFIRMS
AFFIXES
AFFORDS
AFFRAYS
ASFARAS
BAFFERS
BAFFIES
BAFFLES
BEFALLS
BEFOOLS
BEFOULS
BOFFINS
BUFFERS
BUFFETS
BYFIVES
BYFORMS
CAFTANS
COFFEES
COFFERS
COFFINS
DEFACES
DEFAMES
DEFANGS
DEFCONS
DEFEATS
DEFECTS
DEFENDS
DEFIERS
DEFILES
DEFINES
DEFLEAS
DEFOAMS
DEFOCUS
DEFORMS
DEFRAGS
DEFRAYS
DEFUELS
DEFUNDS
DEFUSES
DIFFERS
DOFFERS
DUFFELS
DUFFERS
DUFFLES
DUFUSES
EFFACES
EFFECTS
EFFORTS
EFFUSES
ELFOWLS
ENFACES
ENFANTS
ENFOLDS
FIFTIES
GAFFERS
GIFTEES
GUFFAWS
HEFTERS
INFANTS
INFECTS
INFESTS
INFIVES
INFIXES
INFLOWS
INFOCUS
INFOLDS
INFORMS
INFUSES
JEFFERS
JIFFIES
LEFTIES
LIFTERS
LOFTERS
MUFFINS
MUFFLES
NIFTIES
OFFDAYS
OFFENDS
OFFICES
OFFINGS
OFFSETS
OXFORDS
PIFFLES
PRFIRMS
PUFFERS
PUFFINS
RAFFIAS
RAFFLES
RAFTERS
REFACES
REFALLS
REFAXES
REFEEDS
REFILES
REFILLS
REFILMS
REFINDS
REFINES
REFIRES
REFIXES
REFLAGS
REFLIES
REFLIPS
REFLOWS
REFOCUS
REFOLDS
REFORMS
REFRIES
REFUELS
REFUGES
REFUNDS
REFUSES
REFUTES
RIFFLES
RIFLERS
RUFFLES
SAFARIS
SEFERIS
SIFTERS
SOFARAS
SOFFITS
SOFTENS
SOFTIES
SUFFERS
TAFFIES
TEFLONS
TIFFINS
TOFFEES
TUFFETS
UNFACTS
UNFILES
UNFINES
UNFIXES
UNFOLDS
UNFORKS
UNFREES
UNFURLS
UPFLOWS
UPFOLDS
USFLAGS
WAFFLES
WAFTERS

•••FS••
BEEFSUP
BUFFSUP
GOOFSUP
HALFSHY
HOOFSIT
PUFFSUP
SURFSUP
TURFSKI

•••F•S•
BELFAST
BIGFISH
BUFFEST
CATFISH
CODFISH
CONFESS
CONFUSE
COWFISH
CRAFTSY
DEAFEST
DEFFEST
DIFFUSE
DOGFISH
FANFEST
FLYFISH
FUNFEST
GABFEST
HUFFISH
IREFUSE
LIEFEST
MUDFISH
OUTFAST
OUTFISH
OZZFEST
PANFISH
PERFUSE
PETFISH
PIGFISH
PROFESS
PROFUSE
RAFFISH
RAWFISH
REDFISH
SAWFISH
SELFISH
SUFFUSE
SUNFAST
SUNFISH
TINFISH
WAIFISH
WOLFISH

•••F••S
ARMFULS
ATMFEES
BADFITS
BAFFERS
BAFFIES
BAFFLES
BAGFULS
BIGFANS
BOFFINS
BOUFFES
BOWFINS
BOXFULS
BUFFERS
BUFFETS
CANFULS
CAPFULS
CARFULS
CATFITS
CHAFERS
COFFEES
COFFERS
COFFINS
COMFITS
CONFABS
CONFERS
CONFESS
CONFITS
CORFAMS
CUBFANS
CUPFULS
CURFEWS
DEAFENS
DEIFIES
DIFFERS
DOFFERS
DRYFOGS
DUFFELS
DUFFERS
DUFFLES
EARFULS
EDIFIES
EYEFULS
FANFICS
FARFELS
FULFILS
FUNFURS
GAFFERS
GOLFERS
GOOFUPS
GUFFAWS
HADFITS
HALFIES
HASFITS
HATFULS
HEIFERS
HOOFERS
ICEFOGS
JARFULS
JEFFERS
JETFANS
JIFFIES
JUGFULS
KNIFERS
LABFEES
LAPFULS
LOAFERS
LOOFAHS
METFANS
MISFITS
MUFFINS
MUFFLES
MUGFULS
NETFULS
NONFANS
OLEFINS
OUTFITS
PANFULS
PARFUMS
PIAFFES
PIFFLES
PILFERS
POTFULS
PREFABS
PREFERS
PROFESS
PROFITS
PUFFERS
PUFFINS
PURFLES
RAFFIAS
RAFFLES
RAMFANS
REDFINS
REDFIRS
REEFERS
REIFIES
RIFFLES
ROLFERS
ROOFERS
RUFFLES
SETFEES
SHOFARS
SOFFITS
SOXFANS
STIFLES
SUFFERS
SUNFANS
SURFERS
TAFFIES
THEFEDS
TIFFINS
TOFFEES
TRIFLES
TUBFULS
TUFFETS
TWOFERS
UNIFIES
URNFULS
VATFULS
WAFFLES
WOOFERS

••••F•S
ALLOFUS
BOUFFES
BUYOFFS
CARAFES
CUTOFFS
DIEOFFS
DREYFUS
LAYOFFS
LOGOFFS
MIDOFFS
NOGIFTS
ONEOFFS
ONEOFUS
PAYOFFS
PIAFFES
POPOFFS
PUTOFFS
REBUFFS
REGIFTS
RESIFTS
RIPOFFS
RUNOFFS
SCLAFFS
SCRUFFS
SETOFFS
STRAFES
STRIFES
TARIFFS
TEEOFFS
THRIFTS
TIPOFFS
UNCUFFS
UPLIFTS
UPWAFTS

•••••FS
BELIEFS
BUYOFFS
CUTOFFS
DIEOFFS
ENGULFS
INGULFS
LAYOFFS
LOGOFFS
MASSIFS
MIDOFFS
ONEOFFS
PAYOFFS
POPOFFS
PUTOFFS
REBUFFS
RELIEFS
REROOFS
RETURFS
RIPOFFS
RUNOFFS
SCLAFFS
SCRUFFS
SETOFFS
SHERIFS
TARIFFS
TEEOFFS
TIPOFFS
UNCUFFS
UNLEAFS
UNROOFS
WHATIFS

FT•••••
FTBLISS
FTBRAGG
FTDIXNJ
FTDODGE
FTHENRY
FTMEADE
FTMYERS
FTRILEY
FTWAYNE
FTWORTH

F•T••••
FATALES
FATALLY
FATBACK
FATCATS
FATCELL
FATCITY
FATEFUL
FATFARM
FATFREE
FATHEAD
FATHERS
FATHOMS
FATIDIC
FATIGUE
FATLESS
FATLIKE
FATLING
FATLIPS
FATNESS
FATONES
FATOUSH
FATTENS
FATTEST
FATTIER
FATTILY
FATTING
FATTISH
FATUITY
FATUOUS
FETCHED
FETCHER
FETCHES
FETIDLY
FETLOCK
FETTERS
FETTLES
FETUSES
FITINTO
FITNESS
FITTERS
FITTEST
FITTING
FITWELL
FITZROY
FOTOMAT
FUTHARK
FUTURAS
FUTURES
FUTZING

F••T•••
FACTFUL
FACTION
FACTOID
FACTORS
FACTORY
FACTUAL
FALTERS
FANTAIL
FANTANS
FANTASM
FANTAST
FANTASY
FANTINE
FANTODS
FARTHER
FARTLEK
FASTCAR
FASTENS
FASTEST
FASTING
FASTNET
FASTONE
FATTENS
FATTEST
FATTIER
FATTILY
FATTING
FATTISH
FEATHER
FEATURE
FELTBAD
FELTFOR
FELTHAT
FELTILL
FELTING
FELTOFF
FELTOUT
FELTPEN
FELTTIP
FERTILE
FESTERS
FESTINA
FESTIVA
FESTIVE
FESTOON
FESTOSO
FETTERS
FETTLES
FIATLUX
FICTILE
FICTION
FICTIVE
FIFTEEN
FIFTHLY
FIFTIES
FIFTYAD
FIFTYBC
FIGTREE
FILTERS
FIRTREE
FISTFUL
FITTERS
FITTEST
FITTING
FIXTURE
FLATBED
FLATCAR
FLATHAT
FLATLET
FLATOUT
FLATTAX
FLATTED
FLATTEN
FLATTER
FLATTOP
FLATTVS
FLITSBY
FLITSIN
FLITTED
FLITTER
FLOTAGE
FLOTSAM
FLUTERS
FLUTIER
FLUTIES
FLUTING
FLUTIST
FLUTTER
FLYTIER
FLYTRAP
FONTANA
FONTANE
FONTEYN
FONTINA
FOOTAGE
FOOTBAG
FOOTERS
FOOTING
FOOTLED
FOOTLER
FOOTLES
FOOTLET
FOOTMAN
FOOTMEN
FOOTPAD
FOOTRUB
FOOTSIE
FOOTSIT
FOOTSUP
FOOTWAY
FORTDIX
FORTIES
FORTIFY
FORTIUS
FORTLEE
FORTORD
FORTRAN
FORTUNA
FORTUNE
FORTYAD
FORTYBC
FOSTERS
FOXTAIL
FOXTROT
FRATERS
FRETFUL
FRETSAT
FRETSAW
FRETTED
FRETTER
FRITTED
FRITTER
FROTHED
FROTHER
FROTHUP
FUNTIME
FURTADO
FURTHER
FURTIVE
FUSTIAN
FUSTIER
FUSTILY

F•••T••
FACETED
FAGOTED
FAINTED
FAINTER
FAINTLY
FAJITAS
FANATIC
FAULTED
FAUSTUS
FAYETTE
FEASTED
FEASTER
FEASTON
FEINTED
FELTTIP
FENETRE
FIBSTER
FIESTAS
FIGHTER
FINITES
FIRSTLY
FIRSTUP
FIVETEN
FIVETWO
FIXATED
FIXATES
FLATTAX
FLATTED
FLATTEN
FLATTER
FLATTOP
FLATTVS
FLAUTAS
FLEETED
FLEETER
FLEETLY
FLINTMI
FLIPTOP
FLIRTED
FLIRTER
FLITTED
FLITTER
FLOATBY
FLOATED
FLOATER
FLOATUP
FLOUTED
FLOUTER
FLUSTER
FLUTTER
FOISTED
FOISTON
FOLATES
FORETOP
FORSTER
FOUETTE
FOULTIP
FOURTHS
FRACTAL
FRANTIC
FREETOY
FREITAG
FRETTED
FRETTER
FREYTAG
FRITTED
FRITTER
FRONTAL
FRONTED
FRONTON
FROSTED
FROSTER
FRUITED
FRUSTRO
FRUSTUM
FUENTES
FUGATOS
FUJITSU
FUNSTER

F••••T•
FACULTY
FAILSTO
FALCATE
FALLSTO
FALSITY
FANJETS
FANOUTS
FATCATS
FATCITY
FATUITY
FAUCETS
FAWCETT
FAYETTE
FEDINTO
FEEBATE
FEEDSTO
FEMBOTS
FERMATA
FERMATE
FERMATS
FERRATE
FERRETS
FERRETY
FERRITE
FIDGETS
FIDGETY
FILLETS
FITINTO
FLAUNTS
FLAUNTY
FLIEDTO

FLIESTO
FLIGHTS
FLIGHTY
FLOCKTO
FLORETS
FLOWNTO
FLYINTO
FLYNETS
FOGCITY
FOGERTY
FOLIATE
FOLLETT
FOMENTS
FORDGTS
FORDLTD
FORESTS
FORGETS
FORINTS
FORMATS
FORSYTE
FORSYTH
FOUETTE
FRAILTY
FRIGATE
FRIGHTS
FTWORTH
FURCATE

F•••••T

FABBEST
FACEDIT
FACESIT
FADDIET
FADDIST
FADEOUT
FAINEST
FAIREST
FAKEDIT
FAKEOUT
FAKESIT
FALLOUT
FALSEST
FANBELT
FANFEST
FANSOUT
FANTAST
FAREAST
FARLEFT
FARMOUT
FARWEST
FASCIST
FASTEST
FASTNET
FATTEST
FAUVIST
FAWCETT
FEARNOT
FEEDLOT
FEELOUT
FELLOUT
FELTHAT
FELTOUT
FERMENT
FERVENT
FEUDIST
FIGMENT
FILBERT
FILEOUT
FILLOUT
FILMSET
FINDOUT
FINEART
FIREANT
FIREDAT
FIREHAT
FIRELIT
FIREPIT
FIRESAT
FIRMEST
FISHNET
FISHOUT
FITTEST
FLAILAT
FLATHAT
FLATLET
FLATOUT
FLEAPIT
FLIESAT
FLINGAT
FLIPOUT
FLOORIT
FLORIST
FLOWNAT
FLOWOUT
FLUNGAT
FLUSHOT
FLUTIST
FLYCAST
FLYPAST
FOLDOUT
FOLKART
FOLLETT
FONDANT
FONDEST
FOOTLET
FOOTSIT
FORABIT
FORFEIT
FORKOUT
FORRENT
FORREST
FORWENT
FOTOMAT
FOULEST
FOULOUT
FOXHUNT
FOXIEST
FOXTROT
FRAUGHT
FREIGHT
FREMONT
FRESHET
FRETSAT
FROGLET
FROWNAT
FULGENT
FULLEST
FULLLOT
FULLOUT
FUMEDAT
FUMESAT
FUMIEST
FUNFEST
FURCOAT
FUSSPOT

•FT••••

AFTMOST
OFTENER

•F•T•••

AFATLOT
AFCTEAM
IFITDIE
IFSTONE
NFCTEAM
NFLTEAM

•F••T••

XFACTOR

•F•••T•

AFFECTS
EFFECTS
EFFORTS
OFFDUTY
OFFSETS
OFFSITE
OFSORTS

•F••••T

AFATLOT
AFFIANT
AFFLICT
AFFRONT
AFTMOST
IFFIEST
IFORGET
IFORGOT
OFASORT
OFFBEAT
OFFCAST
VFWPOST

••FT•••

CAFTANS
DAFTEST
DEFTEST
FIFTEEN
FIFTHLY
FIFTIES
FIFTYAD
FIFTYBC
GIFTBOX
GIFTEES
GIFTING
GIFTSET
GIFTTAX
HAFTING
HEFTERS
HEFTIER
HEFTILY
HEFTING
LEFTARM
LEFTEAR
LEFTEND
LEFTEST
LEFTEYE
LEFTFOR
LEFTHIP
LEFTIES
LEFTISH
LEFTISM
LEFTIST
LEFTJAB
LEFTLEG
LEFTOFF
LEFTOUT
LIFTERS
LIFTING
LIFTOFF
LIFTSUP
LOFTBED
LOFTERS
LOFTIER
LOFTILY
LOFTING
NIFTIER
NIFTIES
NIFTILY
RAFTERS
RAFTING
RIFTING
SIFTERS
SIFTING
SOFTENS
SOFTEST
SOFTGEL
SOFTIES
SOFTISH
SOFTTOP
TUFTIER
TUFTING
WAFTERS
WAFTING

••F•T••

GIFTTAX
HOFSTRA
LAFITTE
REFUTAL
REFUTED
REFUTER
REFUTES
SOFTTOP
TOFUTTI
UNFATED
UNFATTY
UNFETED
UNFITLY

••F••T•

AFFECTS
BUFFETS
BUFFETT
DEFACTO
DEFEATS
DEFECTS
DEFERTO
DEFLATE
EFFECTS
EFFORTS
ENFANTS
EXFACTO
GEFILTE
GOFORTH
INFAITH
INFANTA
INFANTE
INFANTS
INFECTS
INFESTS
INFLATE
LAFITTE
OFFDUTY
OFFSETS
OFFSITE
REFERTO
REFLATE
SOFFITS
TAFFETA
TOFUTTI
TUFFETS
UNFACTS
UNFAITH
UNFATTY
UNFERTH

••F•••T

AFFIANT
AFFLICT
AFFRONT
ATFAULT
ATFIRST
BUFFEST
BUFFETT
DAFTEST
DEFAULT
DEFFEST
DEFIANT
DEFICIT
DEFLECT
DEFROST
DEFTEST
DEFUNCT
DRFRIST
GIFTSET
GOFIRST
GOFORIT
IFFIEST
IMFORIT
INFIRST
INFLECT
INFLICT
INFORIT
INFRACT
INFRONT
LEFTEST
LEFTIST
LEFTOUT
LIFENET
MEFIRST
MRFIXIT
MYFAULT
NOFAULT
OFFBEAT
OFFCAST
ONFIRST
PUFFOUT
REFIGHT
REFLECT
REFLOAT
REFRACT
REFRONT
SAFEBET
SOFTEST
UNFROST
UPFIRST
UPFORIT
UPFRONT

•••FT••

ARAFTOF
BEEFTEA
CLIFTON
CRAFTED
CRAFTER
CRAFTSY
CROFTER
DRAFTED
DRAFTEE
DRAFTER
DRIFTED
DRIFTER
DRIFTIN
DRIFTUP
GOAFTER
GOLFTEE
GRAFTED
GRAFTER
GRAFTON
GRIFTED
GRIFTER
ROOFTOP
SHAFTED
SHIFTED
SHIFTER
SNIFTER
SWIFTER
SWIFTLY
TURFTOE
UNOFTEN

•••F•T•

BADFITS
BUFFETS
BUFFETT
CATFITS
COMFITS
CONFITS
CONFUTE
HADFITS
HASFITS
HEIFETZ
MISFITS
OUTFITS
PROFITS
SADFATE
SOFFITS
SULFATE
SULFITE
TAFFETA
TUFFETS

•••F••T

BELFAST
BELFORT
BIGFEET
BIGFOOT
BUFFEST
BUFFETT
CATFEET
CATFOOT
COMFORT
CONFECT
DEAFEST
DEFFEST
FANFEST
FORFEIT
FUNFEST
GABFEST
HALFCUT
HALFWIT
HOOFSIT
HOTFOOT
LEAFLET
LEAFOUT
LENFANT
LIEFEST
MUDFLAT
NONFACT
ONEFOOT
OUTFAST
OUTFOOT
OZZFEST
PARFAIT
PERFECT
PREFECT
PUFFOUT
ROOFRAT
SCOFFAT
SIXFEET
SIXFOOT
SNIFFAT
SUNFAST
SURFEIT
TENFEET
TENFOOT
TWOFEET
TWOFOOT
WEBFEET
WEBFOOT

••••FT•

NOGIFTS
REGIFTS
RESIFTS
THRIFTS
THRIFTY
TWELFTH
UNLOFTY
UPLIFTS
UPWAFTS

••••F•T

ALLOFIT
BENEFIT
BODYFAT
DEEPFAT
GETSFIT
GREWFAT
GROWFAT
HADAFIT
HASAFIT
KEEPFIT
KEPTFIT
LESSFAT
MADEFIT
MAKEFIT
OUTOFIT
OVERFAT
OVERFIT
SCOFFAT
SEENFIT
SEESFIT
SNIFFAT
SNUGFIT
VERYFIT
WOOLFAT

•••••FT

AIRLIFT
ASAGIFT
ENGRAFT
EYELIFT
FARLEFT
GETSOFT
GOESAFT
GONEAFT
GOTSOFT
HAYLOFT
IDTHEFT
INDRAFT
INGRAFT
MYCROFT
NEWLEFT
OUTSIFT
PRESIFT
REDRAFT
REGRAFT
RESHIFT
SEALIFT
SKILIFT
THEGIFT
THELEFT
UNCLEFT
UNSHIFT
UPDRAFT
UPDRIFT
UPSHIFT
WENTAFT

FU•••••

FUBSIER
FUCHSIA
FUDDIES
FUDDLED
FUDDLES
FUDGERS
FUDGING
FUELERS
FUELING
FUELLED
FUELOIL
FUELROD
FUELSUP
FUENTES
FUGALLY
FUGATOS
FUJISAN
FUJITSU
FULCRUM
FULFILL
FULFILS
FULGENT
FULGHUM
FULLDAY
FULLEST
FULLLOT
FULLOUT
FULMARS
FULNESS
FULSOME
FUMBLED
FUMBLER
FUMBLES
FUMEDAT
FUMESAT
FUMIEST
FUNDERS
FUNDING
FUNFAIR
FUNFEST
FUNFURS
FUNFZIG
FUNGOES
FUNKIER
FUNKILY
FUNKING
FUNNELS
FUNNIER
FUNNIES
FUNNILY
FUNNING
FUNPLEX
FUNRUNS
FUNSTER
FUNTIME
FURBALL
FURBISH
FURCATE
FURCOAT
FURFARM
FURILLO
FURIOSO
FURIOUS
FURLERS
FURLESS
FURLING
FURLONG
FURNACE
FURNESS
FURNISH
FURORES
FURRIER
FURRING
FURROWS
FURSEAL
FURTADO
FURTHER
FURTIVE
FURWRAP
FUSEBOX
FUSIBLE
FUSILLI
FUSIONS
FUSSERS
FUSSIER
FUSSILY
FUSSING
FUSSPOT
FUSTIAN
FUSTIER
FUSTILY
FUSUMAS
FUTHARK
FUTURAS
FUTURES
FUTZING
FUZZIER
FUZZILY
FUZZING

F•U••••

FAUCETS
FAULTED
FAUSTUS
FAUVISM
FAUVIST
FAUXFUR
FAUXPAS
FEUDING
FEUDIST
FLUBBED
FLUBBER
FLUBDUB
FLUBUGS
FLUENCY
FLUFFED
FLUFFER
FLUFFUP
FLUIDAL
FLUIDIC
FLUIDLY
FLUKIER
FLUKILY
FLUMMOX
FLUNGAT
FLUNKED
FLUNKER
FLUSHED
FLUSHER
FLUSHES
FLUSHOT
FLUSTER
FLUTERS
FLUTIER
FLUTIES
FLUTING
FLUTIST
FLUTTER
FLUVIAL
FLUXING
FLUXION
FMURRAY
FNUMBER
FOUDRES
FOUETTE
FOULARD
FOULEST
FOULING
FOULOUT
FOULSUP
FOULTIP
FOULUPS
FOUNDED
FOUNDER
FOUNDRY
FOURAAA
FOURDAY
FOUREEE
FOURIER
FOURMAN
FOURPIN
FOURTHS
FOURWAY
FRUITED
FRUSTRO
FRUSTUM

F••U•••

FACULAE
FACULTY
FAMULUS
FATUITY
FATUOUS
FERULES
FETUSES
FIBULAE
FIBULAR
FIBULAS
FICUSES
FIGURAL
FIGURED
FIGURER
FIGURES
FIXUPON
FLAUNTS
FLAUNTY
FLAUTAS
FLEURON
FLOUNCE
FLOUNCY
FLOURED
FLOUTED
FLOUTER
FOCUSED
FOCUSER
FOCUSES
FOCUSON
FRAUGHT
FUSUMAS
FUTURAS
FUTURES

F•••U••

FACTUAL
FAILURE
FAIRUSE
FANEUIL
FANOUTS
FAROUKI
FATOUSH
FAVOURS
FEATURE
FERRULE
FESCUES
FILLUPS
FISSURE
FIXTURE
FLEXURE
FLIPUPS
FLUBUGS
FOLDUPS
FONDUED
FONDUES
FORBUSH
FORMULA
FORSURE
FORTUNA
FORTUNE
FOULUPS
FOXHUNT
FUNFURS
FUNRUNS

F••••U•

FABFOUR
FACTFUL
FADEOUT
FAIRSUP
FAKEFUR
FAKEOUT
FALLDUE
FALLGUY
FALLOUT
FAMULUS
FANCLUB
FANCYUP
FANSOUT
FARCEUR
FARMOUT
FATEFUL
FATIGUE
FATUOUS
FAUSTUS
FAUXFUR
FEARFUL
FEELOUT
FELLDUE
FELLOUT
FELTOUT
FEMINUM
FENCEUP
FERMIUM
FERROUS
FERVOUR
FIATLUX
FIBROUS
FILEOUT
FILLOUT
FILLSUP
FINDOUT
FIREBUG
FIREDUP
FIRESUP
FIRMSUP
FIRSTUP
FISHOUT
FISTFUL
FIXEDUP
FIXESUP
FLAMEUP
FLANEUR
FLAREUP
FLATOUT
FLAVIUS
FLAVOUR
FLIESUP
FLIPOUT
FLOATUP
FLOWNUP
FLOWOUT
FLUBDUB
FLUFFUP
FOLDOUT
FOLDSUP
FOOTRUB
FOOTSUP
FORCEUP
FORERUN
FORKFUL
FORKOUT
FORKSUP
FORMFUL
FORTIUS
FOULOUT
FOULSUP
FRAMEUP
FREEDUP
FREESUP
FRETFUL
FRIEDUP
FRIESUP
FRISEUR
FROTHUP
FROZEUP
FRUSTUM
FUELSUP
FULCRUM
FULGHUM
FULLOUT
FURIOUS

F•••••U

FEYDEAU
FRENEAU
FUJITSU

•F•U•••

AFOULOF
EFFUSED
EFFUSES

•F••U••

IFYOUGO
OFFDUTY
OFNOUSE

•F•••U•

OFFERUP
OFFHOUR
OFVALUE

••FU•••

AWFULLY
DEFUELS
DEFUNCT
DEFUNDS
DEFUSED
DEFUSER
DEFUSES
DUFUSES
EFFUSED
EFFUSES
ELFUDGE
INFUSED
INFUSER
INFUSES
OHFUDGE
REFUELS
REFUGED
REFUGEE
REFUGES
REFUNDS
REFUSAL
REFUSED
REFUSER
REFUSES
REFUTAL
REFUTED
REFUTER
REFUTES
TOFUTTI

UNFULLY
UNFUNNY
UNFURLS
UNFUSED
UNFUSSY

••F•U••
ATFAULT
BEFOULS
COFOUND
DEFAULT
DIFFUSE
MYFAULT
NOFAULT
OFFDUTY
REFOUND
SUFFUSE
UNFLUID
UNFOUND

••F••U•
BUFFSUP
DEFOCUS
DEFRAUD
DRFREUD
HAFNIUM
INFOCUS
LAFLEUR
LEFTOUT
LIFEFUL
LIFTSUP
OFFERUP
OFFHOUR
PUFFOUT
PUFFSUP
REFOCUS

••F•••U
ALFREDU
HOFBRAU

•••FU••
ARAFURA
ARMFULS
BAGFULS
BIOFUEL
BOXFULS
CANFULS
CAPFULS
CARFULS
CONFUSE
CONFUTE
CUPFULS
DIFFUSE
EARFULS
EYEFULS
FUNFURS
GOOFUPS
HATFULS
INAFUNK
INAFURY
IREFUSE
JARFULS
JUGFULS
LAPFULS
MUGFULS
NETFULS
NONFUEL
PANFULS
PARFUMS
PERFUME
PERFUMY
PERFUSE
POTFULS
PREFUND
PROFUSE
SNAFUED
SUFFUSE
SYNFUEL
TUBFULS
URNFULS
VATFULS

•••F•U•
ACTFOUR
AGEFOUR
BALFOUR
BEEFSUP
BIGFOUR
BUFFSUP
DRIFTUP
FABFOUR
FLUFFUP
GOOFSUP
HALFCUT
HALFDUG
LEAFOUT
MAHFOUZ
NONFLUX
OUTFLUX
PARFOUR
PUFFOUT
PUFFSUP
REDFOUR
SIXFOUR
SNIFFUP
SPIFFUP
SURFSUP
TENFOUR
THEFRUG
WOLFCUB

••••FU•
ALLOFUS
BALEFUL
BANEFUL
BASHFUL
BOATFUL
BODEFUL
BOWLFUL
BRIMFUL
CAREFUL
CLUEFUL
DAREFUL
DESKFUL
DIREFUL
DISHFUL
DOLEFUL
DOOMFUL
DREYFUS
DUTIFUL
EASEFUL
FACTFUL
FAKEFUR
FATEFUL
FAUXFUR
FEARFUL
FISTFUL
FLUFFUP
FORKFUL
FORMFUL
FRETFUL
GAINFUL
GLEEFUL
HANDFUL
HARMFUL
HATEFUL
HAVEFUN
HEADFUL
HEATFUL
HEEDFUL
HELPFUL
HOPEFUL
HURTFUL
HUSHFUL
LIFEFUL
LUSTFUL
MADEFUN
MAKEFUN
MINDFUL
MOANFUL
MUSEFUL
NEEDFUL
NESTFUL
ODORFUL
ONEOFUS
PAILFUL
PAINFUL
PALMFUL
PIPEFUL
PITIFUL
PLAYFUL
PLOTFUL
POKEFUN
POUTFUL
PUSHFUL
RAGEFUL
RESTFUL
ROOMFUL
RUTHFUL
SACKFUL
SCARFUP
SHIPFUL
SHOPFUL
SIGHFUL
SKILFUL
SLEDFUL
SNIFFUP
SONGFUL
SOULFUL
SPIFFUP
TACTFUL
TANKFUL
TEARFUL
TENTFUL
TOILFUL
TRAYFUL
TUNEFUL
UNAWFUL
VIALFUL
WAILFUL
WAKEFUL
WILLFUL
WISHFUL
WISTFUL
YAWNFUL
ZESTFUL

•••••FU
BIRDFLU
BLUEFLU

F•V••••
FAVORED
FAVORER
FAVOURS
FEVERED
FEVRIER
FIVEAAA
FIVEDAY
FIVEEEE
FIVEMAN
FIVEONE
FIVEPIN
FIVESIX
FIVETEN
FIVETWO
FIVEWAY

F••V•••
FAUVISM
FAUVIST
FERVENT
FERVORS
FERVOUR
FLAVIUS
FLAVORS
FLAVORY
FLAVOUR
FLIVVER
FLUVIAL
FRIVOLS

F•••V••
FLIVVER
FLYOVER
FOREVER

F••••V•
FESTIVA
FESTIVE
FICTIVE
FLATTVS
FORGAVE
FORGIVE
FORLOVE
FURTIVE

F•••••V
FADAYEV
FEDOROV

•FV••••
OFVALUE

••F•V••
BYFIVES
INFAVOR
INFIVES

••F•••V
ALFEROV

•••F•V•
ACTFIVE
AGEFIVE
BIGFIVE
PARFIVE
REDFIVE
SIXFIVE
THEFIVE
TOPFIVE

F•W••••
FAWCETT
FAWNERS
FAWNING
FAWNSON
FEWNESS
FOWLERS
FOWLING
FTWAYNE
FTWORTH

F••W•••
FALWELL
FANWISE
FARWEST
FAYWRAY
FITWELL
FLAWIER
FLAWING
FLOWAGE
FLOWERS
FLOWERY
FLOWING
FLOWNAT
FLOWNBY
FLOWNIN
FLOWNON
FLOWNTO
FLOWNUP
FLOWOUT
FLOWSIN
FLYWAYS
FORWARD
FORWENT
FRAWLEY
FROWARD
FROWNAT
FROWNED
FROWNER
FROWNON
FURWRAP

F•••W••
FAIRWAY
FARAWAY
FAREWAR
FIVEWAY
FLYAWAY
FOLKWAY
FOODWEB
FOOTWAY
FOURWAY
FREEWAY

F••••W•
FALLOWS
FARROWS
FELLOWS
FIVETWO
FOGBOWS
FOLLOWS
FOXNEWS
FURROWS

F•••••W
FOREPAW
FORESAW
FORSHOW
FRETSAW

•FW••••
IFWEMAY
VFWHALL
VFWPOST

•F•W•••
OFFWEGO

•F••W••
TFPOWYS

••FW•••
OFFWEGO

••F•W••
ELFOWLS
SAFEWAY

••F••W•
GUFFAWS
INFLOWS
REFLOWN
REFLOWS
UNFLOWN
UPFLOWS

•••FW••
GULFWAR
HALFWAY
HALFWIT
HALFWON
TURFWAR

•••F•W•
CURFEWS
GUFFAWS
OUTFAWN
PEAFOWL
SEAFOWL

•••F••W
AIRFLOW
ASOFNOW
HALFRAW
MUDFLOW
OUTFLOW
RENFREW

••••F•W
OVERFEW
VERYFEW

F•X••••
FAXLORE
FIXABLE
FIXATED
FIXATES
FIXEDLY
FIXEDON
FIXEDUP
FIXESON
FIXESUP
FIXINGS
FIXTURE
FIXUPON
FOXBORO
FOXFIRE
FOXHOLE
FOXHUNT
FOXIEST
FOXLIKE
FOXNEWS
FOXTAIL
FOXTROT

F••X•••
FAUXFUR
FAUXPAS
FLAXIER
FLEXILE
FLEXING
FLEXION
FLEXNER
FLEXORS
FLEXURE
FLUXING
FLUXION

F•••X••
FEDEXED
FEDEXES
FTDIXNJ

F•••••X
FAIRFAX
FAIRSEX
FAREBOX
FIATLUX
FILOFAX
FIREBOX
FIREFOX
FIVESIX
FLATTAX
FLUMMOX
FORTDIX
FUNPLEX
FUSEBOX

•F••X••
AFFIXED
AFFIXER
AFFIXES

••F•X••
AFFIXED
AFFIXER
AFFIXES
INFIXED
INFIXES
MRFIXIT
REFAXED
REFAXES
REFIXED
REFIXES
UNFIXED
UNFIXES
UNFOXED

••F•••X
GIFTBOX
GIFTTAX

•••F•X•
JIMFIXX

•••F••X
JIMFIXX
NETFLIX
NONFLUX
OUTFLUX
REAFFIX

••••F•X
BLUEFOX
BRERFOX
EQUIFAX
FAIRFAX
FILOFAX
FIREFOX
HALIFAX
JUNKFAX
OVERFIX
POSTFIX
REAFFIX
TELEFAX

F•Y••••
FAYETTE
FAYWRAY
FEYDEAU
FEYNESS
FEYNMAN
FLYABLE
FLYAWAY
FLYBALL
FLYBOYS
FLYCAST
FLYFISH
FLYGIRL
FLYHIGH
FLYINTO
FLYLEAF
FLYLESS
FLYNETS
FLYOPEN
FLYOVER
FLYPAST
FLYRODS
FLYSOLO
FLYTIER
FLYTRAP
FLYWAYS
FRYABLE
FRYCOOK
FRYPANS

F••Y•••
FLAYERS
FLAYING
FOGYISH
FOGYISM
FRAYING
FREYTAG
FTMYERS

F•••Y••
FADAYEV
FANCYUP
FIFTYAD
FIFTYBC
FORAYED
FORSYTE
FORSYTH
FORTYAD
FORTYBC
FTWAYNE

F••••Y•
FISHEYE
FLYBOYS
FLYWAYS
FONTEYN
FRIDAYS

F•••••Y
FACTORY
FACULTY
FADEDLY
FAINTLY
FAIRWAY
FALLACY
FALLGUY
FALSELY
FALSIFY
FALSITY
FANCIFY
FANCILY
FANTASY
FARADAY
FARAWAY
FARMBOY
FARMERY
FATALLY
FATCITY
FATTILY
FATUITY
FAYWRAY
FELONRY
FERNERY
FERRETY
FETIDLY
FIDGETY
FIERILY
FIFTHLY
FILEDBY
FILESBY
FILMILY
FINALLY
FINDLAY
FINDLEY
FINICKY
FIREFLY
FIRSTLY
FISHERY
FISHFRY
FISHILY
FITZROY
FIVEDAY
FIVEWAY
FIXEDLY
FLAGDAY
FLAKILY
FLAUNTY
FLAVORY
FLEETLY
FLESHLY
FLIESBY
FLIGHTY
FLITSBY
FLOATBY
FLOUNCY
FLOWERY
FLOWNBY
FLUENCY
FLUIDLY
FLUKILY
FLYAWAY
FMURRAY
FOAMILY
FOGCITY
FOGERTY
FOGGILY
FOLKWAY
FOOLERY
FOOTWAY
FOPPERY
FORADAY
FOREBAY
FORGERY
FORTIFY
FOUNDRY
FOURDAY
FOURWAY
FRAILLY
FRAILTY
FRANKLY
FRAWLEY
FRECKLY
FREETOY
FREEWAY
FRENEMY
FRESHLY
FRIARLY
FRIDLEY
FRIZZLY
FTHENRY
FTRILEY
FUGALLY
FULLDAY
FUNKILY
FUNNILY
FUSSILY
FUSTILY
FUZZILY

•FY••••
IFYOUGO

•F•Y•••
OFFYEAR

•F•••Y•
AFFRAYS
OFFDAYS
TFPOWYS

•F••••Y
AFARCRY
AFFABLY
EFFABLY
IFWEMAY
OFFDUTY
UFOLOGY

••FY•••
DEFYING
OFFYEAR
REFYING
WIFYING

••F•Y••
FIFTYAD
FIFTYBC
RUFIYAA

••F••Y•
AFFRAYS
DEFRAYS
LEFTEYE
OFFDAYS

••F•••Y
AFFABLY
AWFULLY
DAFFILY
EFFABLY
FIFTHLY
HEFTILY
HUFFILY
INFANCY
JEFFREY
JOFFREY
LOFTILY
NIFTILY
OFFDUTY
PUFFERY
PUFFILY
RIFLERY
SAFEWAY
TIFFANY
UNFANCY
UNFATTY
UNFIERY
UNFITLY
UNFLAKY
UNFOGGY
UNFULLY
UNFUNNY
UNFUSSY

•••F••Y
BEEFILY
BLUFFLY
CONFREY
CRAFTSY
DAFFILY
GODFREY
GOOFILY
GRIFFEY
GRUFFLY
HALFDAY
HALFSHY
HALFWAY
HUFFILY
INAFURY
JEFFREY
JOFFREY
OLDFOGY
PALFREY
PERFIDY
PERFUMY
PUFFERY
PUFFILY
SNIFFLY
STIFFLY
SWIFTLY
TIFFANY
WINFREY

••••F•Y
ALOOFLY
BLOWFLY
BLUFFLY
BRIEFLY
CHIEFLY
DEEPFRY
DEERFLY
FIREFLY
FISHFRY
GRIFFEY
GRUFFLY
LETSFLY
OVERFLY
SANDFLY
SCRUFFY
SHOOFLY
SNIFFLY
STIFFLY
STIRFRY
TESTFLY
THRIFTY
TINAFEY
UNLOFTY

•••••FY
ACETIFY
ACIDIFY
AMPLIFY
BEATIFY
CALCIFY
CERTIFY
CLARIFY
DANDIFY
DENSIFY
DIGNIFY
DULCIFY
FALSIFY
FANCIFY
FORTIFY
GLORIFY
GRATIFY
HAPPIFY
HORRIFY
ICONIFY
JELLIFY
JOLLIFY
JUSTIFY
LIGNIFY
LIQUEFY
MAGNIFY
MOLLIFY
MORTIFY
MUMMIFY
MYSTIFY
MYTHIFY
NITRIFY
NULLIFY
PETRIFY
PREDEFY
PULPIFY
PUTREFY
QUALIFY
RECTIFY
REUNIFY
SATISFY
SCARIFY
SCRUFFY
SIGNIFY
SPECIFY
STUPEFY
TERRIFY
TESTIFY
TORREFY
VERBIFY
VERSIFY
VITRIFY
YUPPIFY
ZINCIFY
ZOMBIFY

F•Z••••
FIZGIGS
FIZZERS
FIZZIER
FIZZING
FIZZLED
FIZZLER
FIZZLES
FUZZIER
FUZZILY
FUZZING

F••Z•••
FANZINE
FITZROY
FIZZERS
FIZZIER
FIZZING
FIZZLED
FIZZLER
FIZZLES
FOOZLED
FOOZLER
FOOZLES
FRAZIER
FRAZZLE
FRIZZED
FRIZZER
FRIZZES
FRIZZLE
FRIZZLY
FROZEUP
FROZONE
FUTZING
FUZZIER
FUZZILY
FUZZING

F•••Z••
FRAZZLE
FREEZER
FREEZES

FRIEZES
FRIZZED
FRIZZER
FRIZZES
FRIZZLE
FRIZZLY
FUNFZIG

F••••Z•
FABRIZI
FIRENZA
FIRENZE
FORENZA
FORSIZE

F•••••Z
FLORENZ
FRANKOZ

••F•Z••
UNFAZED

••F••Z•
UNFROZE

•••FZ••
FUNFZIG

•••F•Z•
GINFIZZ

•••F••Z
GINFIZZ
HEIFETZ
MAHFOUZ
THEFONZ

GA•••••
GABBANA
GABBERS
GABBIER
GABBING
GABBLED
GABBLES
GABBROS
GABFEST
GABRIEL
GADDERS
GADDING
GADGETS
GADGETY
GADSDEN
GAETANO
GAFFERS
GAFFING
GAGARIN
GAGGERS
GAGGING
GAGGLES
GAGLAWS
GAGLINE
GAGREEL
GAGRULE
GAGSTER
GAHAGAN
GAINERS
GAINFUL
GAINING
GAINSAY
GAINSON
GAITERS
GAITING
GALAHAD
GALANOS
GALANTS
GALATEA
GALATIA
GALAXES
GALAXIE
GALEATE
GALENAS
GALENTO
GALETTE
GALICIA
GALILEE
GALILEI
GALILEO
GALLANT
GALLEON
GALLERY
GALLEYS
GALLICO
GALLING
GALLIUM
GALLONS
GALLOPS
GALLOWS
GALOOTS
GALOPED
GALPALS
GALUMPH
GALVANI
GALVANO
GAMBADO
GAMBIAN
GAMBIER
GAMBITS
GAMBLED
GAMBLER
GAMBLES
GAMBOLS
GAMEBAG
GAMEBOY
GAMELAN
GAMELAW
GAMELEG
GAMETAL
GAMETES
GAMIEST
GAMINES
GAMMERS
GAMMING
GAMMONS
GANDALF
GANDERS
GANGERS
GANGING
GANGLIA
GANGSAW
GANGSTA
GANGSUP
GANGTOK
GANGWAY
GANNETS
GANNETT
GANTLET
GAOLERS
GAOLING
GAPEDAT
GAPESAT
GAPKIDS
GAPLESS
GAPPING
GARAGED
GARAGES
GARBAGE
GARBAGY
GARBING
GARBLED
GARBLER
GARBLES
GARCONS
GARDENA
GARDENS
GARDNER
GARGLED
GARGLER
GARGLES
GARLAND
GARLICS
GARLITS
GARMENT
GARNEAU
GARNERS
GARNETS
GARNETT
GARNISH
GARONNE
GAROTTE
GARPIKE
GARRETS
GARRETT
GARRICK
GARROTE
GARTERS
GASBAGS
GASCANS
GASCAPS
GASCONS
GASCONY
GASEDUP
GASEITY
GASEOUS
GASESUP
GASHEAT
GASHING
GASHOGS
GASJETS
GASKELL
GASKETS
GASLAMP
GASLEAK
GASLESS
GASLINE
GASLOGS
GASMAIN
GASMASK
GASOHOL
GASOVEN
GASPARD
GASPERS
GASPING
GASPIPE
GASPUMP
GASSERS
GASSIER
GASSING
GASSMAN
GASTANK
GASTERO
GASTONE
GASTRIC
GASWARS
GATEAUX
GATELEG
GATEMAN
GATEMEN
GATEWAY
GATHERS
GATINGS
GATLING
GATLINS
GATTACA
GATWICK
GAUCHER
GAUCHOS
GAUDENS
GAUDERY
GAUDIER
GAUDIES
GAUDILY
GAUGERS
GAUGING
GAUGUIN
GAULISH
GAUNTER
GAUNTLY
GAUSSES
GAUTAMA
GAUTIER
GAUZIER
GAUZILY
GAVEEAR
GAVELED
GAVEOFF
GAVEOUT
GAVEWAY
GAVIALS
GAVILAN
GAVOTTE
GAWKERS
GAWKIER
GAWKILY
GAWKING
GAWKISH
GAWKSAT
GAWPERS
GAWPING
GAYLORD
GAYNESS
GAZEBOS
GAZEDAT
GAZEDON
GAZELLE
GAZESAT
GAZESON
GAZETTE
GAZZARA

G•A••••
GEARBOX
GEARING
GEARSTO
GEARSUP
GHANIAN
GHASTLY
GIACOMO
GIAUQUE
GLACEED
GLACIAL
GLACIER
GLADDEN
GLADDER
GLADEYE
GLAMORS
GLAMOUR
GLAMSUP
GLANCED
GLANCES
GLAREAT
GLARING
GLASGOW
GLASHOW
GLASSED
GLASSES
GLAVINE
GLAZERS
GLAZIER
GLAZILY
GLAZING
GNARLED
GNARRED
GNASHED
GNASHER
GNASHES
GNAWERS
GNAWING
GNAWSAT
GNAWSON
GOABOUT
GOADING
GOAFTER
GOAHEAD
GOALIES
GOALONG
GOAMISS
GOATEED
GOATEES
GOATISH
GRABBAG
GRABBAR
GRABBED
GRABBER
GRABSAT
GRACIAS
GRACILE
GRACING
GRACKLE
GRADATE
GRADEAA
GRADERS
GRADING
GRADUAL
GRAFTED
GRAFTER
GRAFTON
GRAHAME
GRAHAMS
GRAINED
GRAINER
GRAMMAR
GRAMMER
GRAMMES
GRAMMYS
GRAMPAS
GRAMPUS
GRANADA
GRANARY
GRANDAM
GRANDEE
GRANDER
GRANDLY
GRANDMA
GRANDPA
GRANGER
GRANGES
GRANITA
GRANITE
GRANNIE
GRANOLA
GRANPAS
GRANTED
GRANTEE
GRANTER
GRANTOR
GRANULE
GRAPERY
GRAPHED
GRAPHIC
GRAPIER
GRAPNEL
GRAPPAS
GRAPPLE
GRASPAT
GRASPED
GRASPER
GRASSED
GRASSES
GRASSLE
GRATEON
GRATERS
GRATEUP
GRATIAS
GRATIFY
GRATING
GRAUMAN
GRAVELS
GRAVELY
GRAVERS
GRAVEST
GRAVIES
GRAVING
GRAVITY
GRAVLAX
GRAVURE
GRAYEST
GRAYING
GRAYISH
GRAYJAY
GRAYLAG
GRAYSON
GRAZERS
GRAZIER
GRAZING
GUANACO
GUANINE
GUARANI
GUARDED
GUARDEE
GUARDER
GUARGUM

G••A•••
GAGARIN
GAHAGAN
GALAHAD
GALANOS
GALANTS
GALATEA
GALATIA
GALAXES
GALAXIE
GARAGED
GARAGES
GELATED
GELATES
GELATIN
GELATIS
GELATOS
GEMAYEL
GERAINT
GERALDO
GETABLE
GETAHIT
GETAJOB
GETATIP
GETAWAY
GIGABIT
GIGATON
GIRAFFE
GIRASOL
GITANOS
GLEAMED
GLEANED
GLEANER
GLEASON
GLOAMIN
GLOATED
GLOATER
GOCARTS
GOKAPUT
GOKARTS
GOTAHIT
GOTAJOB
GOTATIP
GOTAWAY
GOUACHE
GREASED
GREASER
GREASES
GREATEN
GREATER
GREATLY
GREAVES
GROANED
GROANER
GUJARAT
GYRALLY
GYRATED
GYRATES
GYRATOR

G•••A••
GABBANA
GAETANO
GAGLAWS
GALEATE
GALLANT
GALPALS
GALVANI
GALVANO
GAMBADO
GANDALF
GARBAGE
GARBAGY
GARLAND
GASBAGS
GASCANS
GASCAPS
GASLAMP
GASMAIN
GASMASK
GASPARD
GASTANK
GASWARS
GATEAUX
GATTACA
GAUTAMA
GAVIALS
GAZZARA
GEEGAWS
GELCAPS
GEMMATE
GENNAIO
GENNARO
GERMAIN
GERMANE
GERMANS
GERMANY
GERVAIS
GESTALT
GESTAPO
GESTATE
GETBACK
GETCASH
GETPAST
GETSANA
GETSANF
GETWARM
GEWGAWS
GIGBAGS
GIMBALS
GINGAME
GISCARD
GIZZARD
GLOBATE
GOBLANK
GOBYAIR
GOCRAZY
GODDARD
GODMAMA
GODPAPA
GOESAFT
GOESAPE
GOLDARN
GOLIATH
GONEAFT
GONEAPE
GONZAGA
GOODAIM
GOODALL
GOSHAWK
GOSSAGE
GOSTALE
GOTBACK
GOTCASH
GOTPAST
GOTTAGO
GOTWARM
GOULASH
GOURAMI
GRADATE
GRAHAME
GRAHAMS
GRANADA
GRANARY
GRENADA
GRENADE
GRIMACE
GUANACO
GUARANI
GUEVARA
GUFFAWS
GUITARS
GULLAHS
GUMBALL
GUNCASE
GUNLAPS
GUNLAWS
GUNWALE
GUSTAVE
GYMBAGS
GYMBALL
GYMNAST
GYMRATS

G••••A•
GAHAGAN
GAINSAY
GALAHAD
GALENAS
GAMBIAN
GAMEBAG
GAMELAN
GAMELAW
GAMETAL
GANGSAW
GANGWAY
GAPEDAT
GAPESAT
GARNEAU
GASHEAT
GASLEAK
GASSMAN
GATEMAN
GATEWAY
GAVEEAR
GAVEWAY
GAVILAN
GAWKSAT
GAZEDAT
GAZESAT
GEISHAS
GENERAL
GENEVAN
GENTIAN
GETAWAY
GETBEAT
GETREAL
GETSFAR
GETSMAD
GHANIAN
GIBESAT
GIDDYAP
GIFTTAX
GILBLAS
GILLIAM
GILLIAN
GILLMAN
GINGHAM
GIVEEAR
GIVEWAY
GLACIAL
GLAREAT
GLEEMAN
GLORIAS
GLOSSAE
GLOSSAL
GLOSSAS
GLOTTAL
GLUTEAL
GNAWSAT
GOAHEAD
GOBYCAB
GOBYCAR
GODHEAD
GODTHAB
GOESBAD
GOESFAR
GOESMAD
GOINGAT
GOLDMAN
GOLFBAG
GOLFCAR
GONEBAD
GONEFAR
GONEMAD
GOODBAR
GOODDAY
GOODMAN
GOODPAY
GOOMBAH
GOOMBAY
GORDIAN
GOTAWAY
GOTBEAT
GOTCHAS
GOTOGAL
GOTOWAR
GOTREAL
GRABBAG
GRABBAR
GRABSAT
GRACIAS
GRADEAA
GRADUAL
GRAMMAR
GRAMPAS
GRANDAM
GRANPAS
GRAPPAS
GRASPAT
GRATIAS
GRAUMAN
GRAVLAX
GRAYJAY
GRAYLAG
GRECIAN
GRESHAM
GREWFAT
GREYLAG
GRIDMAP
GRINSAT
GRISHAM
GROWFAT
GRUMMAN
GUESSAT
GUINEAN
GUINEAS
GUJARAT
GULFWAR
GUNBOAT
GUNPLAY
GURKHAS
GYROCAR

G•••••A
GABBANA
GALATEA
GALATIA
GALICIA
GANGLIA
GANGSTA
GARDENA
GATTACA
GAUTAMA
GAZZARA
GEHENNA
GEORGIA
GETSANA
GINGIVA
GOBYSEA
GODMAMA
GODPAPA
GONDOLA
GONGORA
GONZAGA
GORDITA
GORILLA
GOTHIKA
GOTOSEA
GRADEAA
GRANADA
GRANDMA
GRANDPA
GRANITA
GRANOLA
GRENADA
GUEVARA

•GA••••
AGAINST
AGAKHAN
AGALLOP
AGARICS
AGASSIZ
AGATINE
EGALITE
PGAPROS
PGATOUR
UGANDAN

•G•A•••
AGNAILS
AGNATES
AGNATIC
IGNARRO
IGNATOW
IGRAINE
IGUANAS
IGUANID
IGUASSU
OGHAMIC
OGLALAS
PGRATED

•G••A••
AGEMATE
AGESAGO
AGITATE
AGITATO
EGGCASE
EGGSACS
OGDOADS

•G•••A•
AGAKHAN
AGENDAS
AGULHAS
EGERIAS
EGGHEAD
IGUANAS
OGLALAS
UGANDAN

•G••••A
AGRIPPA
IGOTCHA

••GA•••
ALGARVE
ARGALIS
ARGANTE
AVGASES
BEGANTO
BIGAPES
BOGARDE
BOGARTS
BUGABOO
BUGALOO
BUGATTI
DEGAUSS
DOGAPES
EDGARDO
ELGALLO
ENGAGED
ENGAGER
ENGAGES
ENGARDE
FUGALLY
FUGATOS
GAGARIN
GIGABIT
GIGATON
HOGARTH
INGALLS
INGATES
LAGASSE
LEGALLY
LEGANZA
LEGATEE
LEGATES
LEGATOR
LEGATOS
LIGANDS
LIGATED
LIGATES
LOGANUT
MAGALOG
MCGAVIN
MEGABIT
MEGAERA
MEGAERG
MEGAHIT
MEGALON
MEGANES
MEGATON
MOGADOR
MOGAMBO
NEGATED
NEGATER
NEGATES
NEGATOR
NOGALES
ORGANDY
ORGANIC
ORGANZA
PEGASUS
PEGAWAY
REGAINS
REGALED
REGALER
REGALES
REGALIA
REGALLY
REGARDS
REGATTA
REGAUGE
ROGAINE
SUGARED
TAGALOG
TAGAMET
TVGAMES
UNGATED
UNGAUDY
UPGAZED
UPGAZES
YOGAMAT
ZAGAZIG

••G•A••
AFGHANI
AFGHANS
ANGLAIS
ATGRADE
BAGGAGE
BAGLADY
BEGGARS
BEGGARY
BIGBABY
BIGBAND
BIGBANG
BIGCARS
BIGCATS
BIGDAYS
BIGEARS
BIGEAST
BIGEASY
BIGFANS
BIGGAME
BIGHAIR
BIGHALF
BIGHAND
BIGJAKE

BIGMACS
BIGMAMA
BIGNAME
BIGSALE
BIGTALK
COGNACS
COGNATE
DEGLAZE
DEGRADE
DIGRAMS
DIGRAPH
DOGBANE
DOGCART
DOGDAYS
DOGEARS
DOGFACE
DOGGATE
DOGHAIR
DOGMATA
DOGNAPS
DOGRACE
DOGSAGE
DOGTAGS
DOGTAIL
EGGCASE
EGGSACS
ENGLAND
ENGRAFT
ENGRAIN
ENGRAMS
ENGRAVE
FIGBARS
FOGBANK
FOGLAMP
GAGLAWS
GIGBAGS
HAGGARD
HIGHART
HOGBACK
HOGCALL
HOGWASH
INGOALS
INGRAFT
INGRAIN
INGRATE
JAGUARS
JIGSAWS
JUGBAND
LAGGARD
LEGRAND
LOGJAMS
LUGGAGE
LUGSAIL
MAGNANI
MAGNATE
MAGYARS
MIGRANT
MIGRATE
MYGIANT
NYGIANT
ONGUARD
ORGEATS
ORGIAST
PAGEANT
PIGTAIL
RAGBAGS
RAGLANS
RAGMANS
REGEARS
REGLAZE
REGNANT
REGNARD
REGRABS
REGRADE
REGRAFT
REGRANT
REGRAPH
REGRASP
RUGRATS
SAGCARD
SAGUARO
SEGWAYS
SIGNAGE
SIGNALS
TAGDAYS
TAGGANT
TAGSALE
UNGRAND
UNGUARD
UPGRADE
USGRANT
VAGRANT
WIGWAGS
WIGWAMS
ZIGZAGS

••G••A•

ANGELAS
ANGOLAN
ANGORAS
ANGRYAT
ANGULAR
AUGURAL
BAGHDAD
BIGBEAR
BIGBEAT
BIGDEAL
BIGHEAD
BIGLEAD
BIGMEAL
BIGSTAR
BOGYMAN
BUGBEAR
COGHLAN
DIGICAM
DIGITAL
DOGCOAT
DOGREAT
DOGSEAR
DOGSTAR
EGGHEAD
EIGHTAD
EIGHTAM
FIGLEAF
FIGURAL
HEGIRAS
HIGHBAR
HIGHDAY
HIGHHAT
HIGHPAY
HIGHWAY
HYGELAC
IMGREAT
INGEMAR
JOGBRAS
JUGHEAD
JUGULAR
LAGUNAS
LEGOLAS
LEGTRAP
LEGWEAR
LOGGIAS
LOGICAL
MAGICAL
MEGRYAN
PAGODAS
PEGAWAY
PIGMEAT
REGINAL
REGINAS
REGULAR
SAGINAW
SIGHSAT
TAGTEAM
TUGBOAT
UNGULAE
UNGULAR
VEGETAL
WAGEWAR
YOGAMAT

••G•••A

ALGEBRA
ALGERIA
ALGIEBA
AUGUSTA
BEGONIA
BEGORRA
BIGIDEA
BIGMAMA
DOGFLEA
DOGMATA
EUGENIA
EUGLENA
HIGHSEA
HIGHTEA
HYGIEIA
INGESTA
LEGANZA
LIGURIA
MAGENTA
MAGILLA
MEGAERA
MEGILLA
NIGERIA
ORGANZA
OUGUIYA
REGALIA
REGATTA
RIGVEDA
SAGETEA
SEGOVIA
SIGNORA
VIGNOLA

•••GA••

ABIGAIL
ALEGARS
ARIGATO
BAGGAGE
BARGAIN
BEGGARS
BEGGARY
BENGALI
BENGALS
BERGAMO
BIGGAME
BRIGADE
BRIGAND
BROGANS
BULGARI
BULGARS
CALGARY
CHAGALL
COLGATE
CONGAED
CONGAME
COUGARS
DAYGAME
DOAGAIN
DOGGATE
ELEGANT
ENDGAME
EXOGAMY
FINGALS
FORGAVE
FRIGATE
GEEGAWS
GEWGAWS
GINGAME
HAGGARD
HANGARS
HUNGARY
LAGGARD
LONGAGO
LONGARM
LUGGAGE
MANGANO
MARGATE
MARGAUX
MISGAVE
MORGANA
MORGANS
NBAGAME
NETGAIN
NETGAME
NEWGATE
NFLGAME
NHLGAME
NIAGARA
NOUGATS
OLDGAGS
OREGANO
ORIGAMI
OURGANG
OUTGAIN
OUTGAME
OUTGAVE
OUTGAZE
PANGAEA
PETGATE
PREGAIN
PREGAME
PUBGAME
REAGANS
SEAGATE
SLOGANS
TAGGANT
THEGAME
THEGANG
TIEGAME
TONGANS
VIRGATE
VULGATE
WARGAME

•••G•A•

ANAGRAM
APOGEAL
APOGEAN
ASAGRAY
BELGIAN
BEOGRAD
BERGMAN
BINGHAM
BORGIAS
BRIGHAM
BURGLAR
CONGEAL
DIAGRAM
DINGBAT
DOUGLAS
ELEGIAC
ENIGMAS
EPIGRAM
FLAGDAY
FLAGMAN
FROGMAN
GANGSAW
GANGWAY
GINGHAM
HANGMAN
ISOGRAM
JUNGIAN
KEOGHAN
KINGMAN
KINGRAT
KLUGMAN
LANGHAM
LANGWAY
LAUGHAT
LENGUAS
LINGUAE
LINGUAL
LOGGIAS
LONGDAY
LONGWAY
LOWGEAR
LUNGEAT
MACGRAW
MAUGHAM
ONEGRAM
OUTGNAW
OWNGOAL
PANGRAM
PETGOAT
PROGRAM
QUAGGAS
RIDGWAY
SEAGRAM
SHEGOAT
SKAGWAY
STIGMAS
STYGIAN
SUBGOAL
SWAGMAN
SYNGMAN
TANGRAM
TRIGRAM
URUGUAY
VAUGHAN
VIRGOAN
VOSGIAN
WINGMAN

•••G••A

ALEGRIA
ARUGULA
ERIGENA
GANGLIA
GANGSTA
GINGIVA
GONGORA
LINGULA
MORGANA
NIAGARA
PANGAEA
PERGOLA
PLUGOLA
SANGRIA
TOMGOLA

••••GA•

AMALGAM
BABYGAP
BELUGAS
BERIGAN
BODEGAS
CAYUGAS
CITYGAL
COALGAS
DONEGAL
DONEGAN
DRVEGAS
FARMGAL
FLINGAT
FLUNGAT
GAHAGAN
GOINGAT
GOTOGAL
HADAGAS
HASAGAS
ILLEGAL
JOHNGAY
LASTGAS
LISAGAY
LONIGAN
MADIGAN
MALAGAN
MALAGAS
MEDIGAP
MOHEGAN
MTLOGAN
NEONGAS
NOSEGAY
NOSUGAR
ORTEGAL
PAANGAS
QUAGGAS
RAREGAS
REBEGAN
RITAGAM
SENEGAL
STOPGAP
SWINGAT
SWUNGAT
TEARGAS
THURGAU
TSONGAS
UNLEGAL
UNPAGAN
UNREGAL
VINEGAR
WOLFGAL

••••G•A

ALLEGRA
ANTIGUA
APHAGIA
BOLOGNA
CONAGRA
GEORGIA
INTEGRA
LASAGNA
MANAGUA
MYALGIA
OTALGIA
PERUGIA
PHRYGIA

•••••GA

BOTTEGA
GONZAGA
LAZONGA
MACONGA
MESHUGA
NORIEGA
REDALGA
SALONGA
THEBIGA
TORTUGA

G•B••••

GABBANA
GABBERS
GABBIER
GABBING
GABBLED
GABBLES
GABBROS
GABFEST
GABRIEL
GIBBERS
GIBBONS
GIBBOUS
GIBESAT
GIBLETS
GIBLUES
GIBSONS
GIBUSES
GOBBLED
GOBBLER
GOBBLES
GOBELIN
GOBELOW
GOBLANK
GOBLETS
GOBLINS
GOBROKE
GOBYAIR
GOBYBUS
GOBYCAB
GOBYCAR
GOBYSEA

G••B•••

GABBANA
GABBERS
GABBIER
GABBING
GABBLED
GABBLES
GABBROS
GAMBADO
GAMBIAN
GAMBIER
GAMBITS
GAMBLED
GAMBLER
GAMBLES
GAMBOLS
GARBAGE
GARBAGY
GARBING
GARBLED
GARBLER
GARBLES
GASBAGS
GERBILS
GETBACK
GETBEAT
GETBENT
GETBUSY
GIBBERS
GIBBONS
GIBBOUS
GIGBAGS
GILBERT
GILBLAS
GIMBALS
GIMBELS
GLIBBER
GLOBATE
GLOBING
GLOBINS
GLOBOID
GLOBOSE
GLOBOUS
GLOBULE
GOABOUT
GOBBLED
GOBBLER
GOBBLES
GOOBERS
GOTBACK
GOTBEAT
GOTBUSY
GRABBAG
GRABBAR
GRABBED
GRABBER
GRABSAT
GRUBBED
GRUBBER
GUMBALL
GUMBOOT
GUNBELT
GUNBOAT
GYMBAGS
GYMBALL

G•••B••

GAMEBAG
GAMEBOY
GAZEBOS
GEARBOX
GEMSBOK
GETABLE
GIFTBOX
GIGABIT
GLIBBER
GOBYBUS
GOESBAD
GOLDBUG
GOLFBAG
GONEBAD
GOODBAR
GOODBUY
GOODBYE
GOODBYS
GOOMBAH
GOOMBAY
GOTOBED
GRABBAG
GRABBAR
GRABBED
GRABBER
GREWBIG
GROWBIG
GRUBBED
GRUBBER
GRUMBLE
GRUMBLY

G••••B•

GIVENBY
GLIDEBY
GLORYBE
GOINGBY
GRIMSBY

G•••••B

GETAJOB
GOBYCAB
GODTHAB
GOODJOB
GOTAJOB
GYMCLUB

•G••B••

AGRIBIZ
IGNOBLE
IGNOBLY

••GB•••

BAGBOYS
BIGBABY
BIGBAND
BIGBANG
BIGBEAR
BIGBEAT
BIGBEND
BIGBETS
BIGBIRD
BIGBLUE
BIGBOSS
BIGBOYS
BUGBEAR
BUGBOYS
COGBURN
DOGBANE
DOGBEDS
DOGBERT
DOGBITE
DOGBONE
DOGBOOT
DOGBOWL
FIGBARS
FOGBANK
FOGBOWS
GIGBAGS
HOGBACK
JOGBRAS
JUGBAND
LEGBONE
LOGBOOK
RAGBAGS
TUGBOAT

••G•B••

ALGEBRA
BUGABOO
GIGABIT
HIGHBAR
HIGHBOY
LEGIBLE
LEGIBLY
MEGABIT
PAGEBOY

••G••B•

ALGIEBA
BAGJOBS
BIGBABY
EIGHTBC
MOGAMBO
REGRABS

••G•••B

DOGCOMB

•••GB••

DINGBAT
HANGBYS
LONGBED
LONGBOW
ROYGBIV

•••G•B•

HANGSBY
LETGOBY

••••GB•

EKINGBY
GOINGBY
LYINGBY
SWINGBY
SWUNGBY

G•C••••

GECKOES
GOCARTS
GOCRAZY
GUCKIER

G••C•••

GARCONS
GASCANS
GASCAPS
GASCONS
GASCONY
GAUCHER
GAUCHOS
GELCAPS
GEOCODE
GETCASH
GETCOLD
GETCUTE
GIACOMO
GIOCOSO
GISCARD
GLACEED
GLACIAL
GLACIER
GLUCOSE
GLYCINE
GLYCOLS
GNOCCHI
GOTCASH
GOTCHAS
GOTCOLD
GOTCUTE
GRACIAS
GRACILE
GRACING
GRACKLE
GRECIAN
GRECISM
GRECIZE
GROCERS
GROCERY
GULCHES
GUNCASE
GYMCLUB

G•••C••

GALICIA
GFORCES
GLANCED
GLANCES
GLENCOE
GLITCHY
GNOCCHI
GOBYCAB
GOBYCAR
GOLFCAR
GOUACHE
GREYCUP
GROUCHO
GROUCHY
GYROCAR

G••••C•

GALLICO
GARLICS
GARRICK
GATTACA
GATWICK
GEDRICK
GENLOCK
GEODUCK
GETBACK
GIMMICK
GODUTCH
GOTBACK
GOTHICS
GRIMACE
GUANACO
GUNLOCK
GYMSOCK

G•••••C

GASTRIC
GENERIC
GENETIC
GENOMIC
GEORGEC
GEORGIC
GLYPHIC
GLYPTIC
GNOSTIC
GRAPHIC

•G•C•••

EGGCASE
EGGCUPS

•G••C••

AGENCES
IGOTCHA

•G•••C•

AGARICS
EGGSACS

•G••••C

AGNATIC
OGHAMIC

••GC•••

BIGCARS
BIGCATS
BIGCITY
DOGCART
DOGCHEW
DOGCHOW
DOGCOAT
DOGCOMB
EGGCASE
EGGCUPS
FOGCITY
HOGCALL
SAGCARD

••G•C••

DIGICAM
LOGICAL
MAGICAL
NOGUCHI

••G••C•

BIGMACS
COGENCY
COGNACS
DOGFACE
DOGRACE
DOGTICK
EGGSACS
ELGRECO
HOGBACK
NEGLECT
REGENCY
URGENCY

••G•••C

ANGELIC
EIGHTBC
ERGOTIC
EUGENIC
HYGELAC
ORGANIC

•••GC••

LINGCOD

•••G••C

ELEGIAC

••••G•C

APHAGIC
GEORGEC
GEORGIC
ILLOGIC
MYALGIC
OTALGIC
PELAGIC
YOUNGMC

G•D••••

GADDERS
GADDING
GADGETS
GADGETY
GADSDEN
GEDRICK
GIDDIED
GIDDIER
GIDDIES
GIDDILY
GIDDYAP
GIDDYUP
GIDEONS
GODDARD
GODDESS
GODEVIL
GODFREY
GODHEAD
GODHOOD
GODLESS
GODLIER
GODLIKE
GODLING
GODMAMA
GODPAPA
GODSEND
GODSENT
GODSONS
GODTHAB
GODUNOV
GODUTCH
GODWITS
GUDGEON

G••D•••

GADDERS
GADDING
GANDALF
GANDERS
GARDENA
GARDENS
GARDNER
GAUDENS

GAUDERY
GAUDIER
GAUDIES
GAUDILY
GELDING
GENDERS
GEODESY
GEODUCK
GETDONE
GETDOWN
GIDDIED
GIDDIER
GIDDIES
GIDDILY
GIDDYAP
GIDDYUP
GILDERS
GILDING
GIRDERS
GIRDING
GIRDLED
GIRDLER
GIRDLES
GLADDEN
GLADDER
GLADEYE
GLIDEBY
GLIDEIN
GLIDERS
GLIDING
GOADING
GODDARD
GODDESS
GOLDARN
GOLDBUG
GOLDING
GOLDMAN
GOLDONI
GOLDTIP
GOLDWYN
GONDOLA
GOODAIM
GOODALL
GOODBAR
GOODBUY
GOODBYE
GOODBYS
GOODDAY
GOODDOG
GOODEGG
GOODERS
GOODFOR
GOODGUY
GOODIES
GOODING
GOODISH
GOODJOB
GOODJOE
GOODKID
GOODMAN
GOODMEN
GOODNIK
GOODONE
GOODPAY
GOODSON
GOODTRY
GOODUSE
GOODWIN
GORDIAN
GORDITA
GORDIUS
GOTDONE
GOTDOWN
GRADATE
GRADEAA
GRADERS
GRADING
GRADUAL
GRIDDED
GRIDDER
GRIDDLE
GRIDMAP
GRODIER
GRUDGED
GRUDGER
GRUDGES
GUIDERS
GUIDING
GULDENS
GUMDROP
GUNDOGS

G•••D••

GADSDEN
GAPEDAT
GASEDUP
GAZEDAT
GAZEDON
GEEKDOM
GELIDLY
GGORDON
GLADDEN
GLADDER
GLUEDON
GLUEDTO
GOODDAY
GOODDOG
GOUNDER
GOURDES
GQMODEL
GRANDAM
GRANDEE
GRANDER
GRANDLY
GRANDMA
GRANDPA
GRENDEL
GREWDIM
GRIDDED
GRIDDER
GRIDDLE
GRINDER
GROWDIM
GUARDED
GUARDEE
GUARDER
GUERDON
GUILDER

G••••D•

GAMBADO
GAPKIDS
GEOCODE
GERALDO
GERUNDS
GIRONDE
GRANADA
GRENADA
GRENADE
GROUNDS

G•••••D

GABBLED
GALAHAD
GALOPED
GAMBLED
GARAGED
GARBLED
GARGLED
GARLAND
GASPARD
GAVELED
GAYLORD
GELATED
GENTLED
GESSOED
GETCOLD
GETGOOD
GETSMAD
GETSOLD
GETSRID
GETWORD
GHOSTED
GIDDIED
GIELGUD
GIFFORD
GIGGLED
GILFORD
GINGOLD
GIRDLED
GIRTHED
GISCARD
GIZZARD
GLACEED
GLANCED
GLASSED
GLEAMED
GLEANED
GLINTED
GLITZED
GLOATED
GLOBOID
GLOMMED
GLOOMED
GLORIED
GLOSSED
GLUGGED
GLUMMED
GLUTTED
GNARLED
GNARRED
GNASHED
GOAHEAD
GOATEED
GOBBLED
GODDARD
GODHEAD
GODHOOD
GODSEND
GOESBAD
GOESMAD
GOGGLED
GONEBAD
GONEMAD
GOODKID
GOOGLED
GOROUND
GOSFORD
GOTCOLD
GOTGOOD
GOTOBED
GOTWORD
GRABBED
GRAFTED
GRAINED
GRANTED
GRAPHED
GRASPED
GRASSED
GREASED
GREENED
GREETED
GREWOLD
GRIDDED
GRIEVED
GRIFTED
GRILLED
GRINNED
GRIPPED
GRITTED
GROANED
GROINED
GROKKED
GROOMED
GROOVED
GROSSED
GROUPED
GROUSED
GROUTED
GROWLED
GROWOLD
GRUBBED
GRUDGED
GRUMPED
GRUNTED
GUARDED
GUESSED
GUESTED
GULLIED
GUMWOOD
GURGLED
GUSSIED
GUZZLED
GYRATED

•GD••••

OGDENUT
OGDOADS

•G•D•••

AGEDOUT
EGGDROP

•G••D••

AGENDAS
AGENDUM
EGGEDON
GGORDON
UGANDAN

•G•••D•

OGDOADS

•G••••D

AGENTED
AGROUND
EGESTED
EGGHEAD
IGNITED
IGNORED
IGOOFED
IGUANID
PGRATED

••GD•••

BIGDAYS
BIGDEAL
BIGDIGS
BIGDOGS
BOGDOWN
DOGDAYS
DOGDOOR
EGGDROP
FOGDOGS
RAGDOLL
TAGDAYS

••G•D••

BAGHDAD
BIGIDEA
CAGEDIN
CAGEDUP
EDGEDIN
EGGEDON
HIGHDAY
MOGADOR
PAGODAS
RIGIDLY
UNGIDDY
UNGODLY
URGEDON

••G••D•

ATGRADE
AUGENDS
BAGLADY
BEGIRDS
BIGENDS
BIGKIDS
BOGARDE
DEGRADE
DOGBEDS
EDGARDO
ENGARDE
ENGILDS
ENGIRDS
FAGENDS
LEGENDS
LIGANDS
NOGOODS
ORGANDY
RAGGEDY
REGARDS
REGILDS
REGIRDS
REGRADE
REGUIDE
RIGVEDA
TAGENDS
TVGUIDE
UNGAUDY
UNGIDDY
UNGIRDS
UPGIRDS
UPGRADE

••G•••D

ANGERED
AUGURED
BAGHDAD
BAGNOLD
BIGBAND
BIGBEND
BIGBIRD
BIGEYED
BIGHAND
BIGHEAD
BIGLEAD
BIGOTED
BOGEYED
BOGGLED
BUGEYED
DAGWOOD
DEGREED
DOGFOOD
DOGSLED
DOGWOOD
EGGHEAD
EIGHTAD
ENGAGED
ENGINED
ENGLAND
ENGLUND
FAGOTED
FIGURED
GIGGLED
GOGGLED
HAGGARD
HAGGLED
HIGGLED
HIGHEND
HOGTIED
HOGWEED
HOGWILD
JIGGLED
JOGGLED
JUGBAND
JUGGLED
JUGHEAD
LAGGARD
LEGRAND
LIGATED
LIGHTED
NEGATED
NIGGLED
ONGUARD
PIGEYED
PIGWEED
RAGWEED
REGALED
REGLUED
REGNARD
REGRIND
RIGHTED
ROGERED
SAGCARD
SIGHTED
SIGMOID
SIGMUND
SUGARED
TOGGLED
UNGATED
UNGLUED
UNGORED
UNGRAND
UNGUARD
UNGUYED
UNGYVED
UPGAZED
WAGERED
WAGGLED
WAGONED
WIGGLED

•••GD••

FLAGDAY
HANGDOG
KINGDOM
LANGDON
LONGDAY
LONGDEN

•••G•D•

BRIGADE
PONGIDS
RAGGEDY
SEAGODS
SUBGODS
SUNGODS
TINGODS
TRAGEDY
WARGODS

•••G••D

ALIGNED
ALLGOOD
BANGLED
BEOGRAD
BLOGGED
BOGGLED
BOOGIED
BOUGHED
BRAGGED
BRIGAND
BUNGLED
BURGLED
BUTGOOD
CHUGGED
CLOGGED
COIGNED
CONGAED
COUGHED
CRAGGED
DANGLED
DEIGNED
DIDGOOD
DRAGGED
DRUGGED
DWIGHTD
FARGOND
FEIGNED
FLAGGED
FLOGGED
FORGOOD
FRAGGED
GARGLED
GETGOOD
GIGGLED
GINGOLD
GLUGGED
GOGGLED
GOOGLED
GOTGOOD
GURGLED
HAGGARD
HAGGLED
HIGGLED
JANGLED
JIGGLED
JINGLED
JOGGLED
JUGGLED
LAGGARD
LANGUID
LAUGHED
LEAGUED
LINGCOD
LONGBED
MANGLED
MINGLED
NEIGHED
NIGGLED
NONGOLD
NOTGOOD
OLDGOLD
PINGUID
PLAGUED
PLUGGED
REIGNED
ROUGHED
SHAGGED
SINGLED
SLOGGED
SLUGGED
SNAGGED
SNUGGED
STAGGED
SWIGGED
TANGLED
TANGOED
THEGOLD
TINGLED
TOGGLED
UNOGLED
WAGGLED
WANGLED
WEIGHED
WIGGLED

••••G•D

ALLEGED
AVENGED
BLOGGED
BLUDGED
BRAGGED
BRIDGED
CHANGED
CHARGED
CHUGGED
CLANGED
CLOGGED
CRAGGED
CRINGED
DAMAGED
DEARGOD
DELUGED
DEMIGOD
DRAGGED
DREDGED
DRUDGED
DRUGGED
EMERGED
ENCAGED
ENGAGED
ENRAGED
FLAGGED
FLEDGED
FLOGGED
FORAGED
FRAGGED
FRINGED
GARAGED
GIELGUD
GLUGGED
GRUDGED
KLUDGED
LOUNGED
MANAGED
MOONGOD
NOODGED
OBLIGED
PLEDGED
PLUGGED
PLUNGED
PREAGED
PRONGED
RAINGOD
RAVAGED
RECAGED
REFUGED
RENEGED
REPAGED
REURGED
SAVAGED
SHAGGED
SLEDGED
SLOGGED
SLUGGED
SMUDGED
SNAGGED
SNUGGED
SPONGED
STAGGED
STODGED
STOOGED
SWIGGED
TRUDGED
TWANGED
TWINGED
UNCAGED
UNEDGED
UNPAGED
UNRIGID
UNURGED
UNWAGED
VISAGED
VOYAGED
WHANGED
WINDGOD
WRONGED

GE•••••

GEARBOX
GEARING
GEARSTO
GEARSUP
GECKOES
GEDRICK
GEEGAWS
GEEKDOM
GEEKIER
GEEWHIZ
GEEZERS
GEFILTE
GEHENNA
GEISHAS
GELATED
GELATES
GELATIN
GELATIS
GELATOS
GELCAPS
GELDING
GELIDLY
GELLING
GELPENS
GELUSIL
GEMAYEL
GEMELLI
GEMINIS
GEMLESS
GEMLIKE
GEMMATE
GEMMIER
GEMSBOK
GENDERS
GENERAL
GENERIC
GENERIS
GENESEE
GENESES
GENESET
GENESIS
GENETIC
GENEVAN
GENGHIS
GENITOR
GENLOCK
GENNAIO
GENNARO
GENOESE
GENOISE
GENOMES
GENOMIC
GENTEEL
GENTIAN
GENTILE
GENTLED
GENTLER
GENTLES
GENUINE
GENUSES
GENXERS
GENZYME
GEOCODE
GEODESY
GEODUCK
GEOLOGY
GEORGEC
GEORGEI
GEORGEM
GEORGES
GEORGEV
GEORGEW
GEORGIA
GEORGIC
GEORGIE
GERAINT
GERALDO
GERBILS
GERENTS
GERITOL
GERMAIN
GERMANE
GERMANS
GERMANY
GERMIER
GERSHON
GERUNDS
GERVAIS
GESSOED
GESSOES
GESTALT
GESTAPO
GESTATE
GESTURE
GETABLE
GETAHIT
GETAJOB
GETATIP
GETAWAY
GETBACK
GETBEAT
GETBENT
GETBUSY
GETCASH
GETCOLD
GETCUTE
GETDONE
GETDOWN
GETEVEN
GETFREE
GETFROM
GETGOOD
GETHELP
GETHURT
GETINON
GETINTO
GETITON
GETLOST
GETONIT
GETONTO
GETOVER
GETPAST
GETREAL
GETSANA
GETSANF
GETSFAR
GETSFIT
GETSHEP
GETSHIP
GETSHOT
GETSMAD
GETSOFF
GETSOFT
GETSOLD
GETSORE
GETSOUT
GETSRID
GETSSET
GETSWET
GETTERS
GETTHIS
GETTING
GETTOIT
GETUPON
GETWARM
GETWELL
GETWISE
GETWORD
GEWGAWS
GEYSERS

G•E••••

GAETANO
GEEGAWS
GEEKDOM
GEEKIER
GEEWHIZ
GEEZERS
GHERKIN
GHETTOS
GIELGUD
GJETOST
GLEAMED
GLEANED
GLEANER
GLEASON
GLEEFUL
GLEEMAN
GLEEMEN
GLENCOE
GOESAFT
GOESAPE
GOESBAD
GOESFAR
GOESFOR
GOESMAD
GOESOFF
GOESOUT
GOESPRO
GREASED
GREASER
GREASES
GREATEN
GREATER
GREATLY
GREAVES
GRECIAN
GRECISM
GRECIZE
GREELEY
GREENED
GREENER
GREENLY
GREETED
GREETER
GREGORY
GREMLIN
GRENADA
GRENADE
GRENDEL
GRESHAM
GRETZKY
GREWBIG
GREWDIM
GREWFAT
GREWOLD
GREYCUP
GREYEST
GREYHEN
GREYING
GREYISH
GREYLAG
GUERDON
GUESSAT
GUESSED
GUESSER
GUESSES
GUESSSO
GUESTED
GUEVARA

G••E•••

GALEATE
GALENAS
GALENTO
GALETTE
GAMEBAG
GAMEBOY
GAMELAN
GAMELAW
GAMELEG
GAMETAL
GAMETES
GAPEDAT
GAPESAT
GASEDUP
GASEITY
GASEOUS
GASESUP
GATEAUX
GATELEG
GATEMAN
GATEMEN
GATEWAY
GAVEEAR
GAVELED
GAVEOFF
GAVEOUT
GAVEWAY
GAZEBOS
GAZEDAT
GAZEDON
GAZELLE
GAZESAT
GAZESON
GAZETTE
GEHENNA
GEMELLI
GENERAL
GENERIC
GENERIS
GENESEE
GENESES
GENESET
GENESIS
GENETIC
GENEVAN
GERENTS
GETEVEN
GIBESAT
GIDEONS
GISELLE
GIVEEAR

GIVENBY
GIVENIN
GIVENOF
GIVENON
GIVENTO
GIVENUP
GIVEOFF
GIVEOUT
GIVESIN
GIVESOF
GIVESON
GIVESTO
GIVESUP
GIVEUPS
GIVEWAY
GLEEFUL
GLEEMAN
GLEEMEN
GLUEDON
GLUEDTO
GLUEGUN
GLUESON
GLUESTO
GOBELIN
GOBELOW
GODEVIL
GOGETEM
GONEAFT
GONEAPE
GONEBAD
GONEFAR
GONEFOR
GONEMAD
GONEOFF
GONEOUT
GONEPRO
GONERIL
GORETEX
GOTEVEN
GOVERNS
GREELEY
GREENED
GREENER
GREENLY
GREETED
GREETER
GRIEVED
GRIEVER
GRIEVES
GYRENES

G•••E••

GABBERS
GABFEST
GADDERS
GADGETS
GADGETY
GAFFERS
GAGGERS
GAGREEL
GAINERS
GAITERS
GALLEON
GALLERY
GALLEYS
GAMIEST
GAMMERS
GANDERS
GANGERS
GANNETS
GANNETT
GAOLERS
GAPLESS
GARDENA
GARDENS
GARMENT
GARNEAU
GARNERS
GARNETS
GARNETT
GARRETS
GARRETT
GARTERS
GASHEAT
GASJETS
GASKELL
GASKETS
GASLEAK
GASLESS
GASPERS
GASSERS
GASTERO
GATHERS
GAUDENS
GAUDERY
GAUGERS
GAVEEAR
GAWKERS
GAWPERS
GAYNESS
GEEZERS
GELPENS
GEMLESS
GENDERS
GENOESE
GENTEEL
GENXERS
GEODESY
GETBEAT
GETBENT
GETHELP
GETREAL
GETTERS
GETWELL
GEYSERS
GIBBERS
GIBLETS
GIFTEES
GILBERT
GILDERS
GIMBELS
GIMLETS
GINGERS
GINGERY
GINSENG
GIRDERS
GIVEEAR
GLACEED
GLADEYE
GLAREAT
GLAZERS
GLIDEBY
GLIDEIN
GLIDERS
GLOWERS
GLUIEST
GLUTEAL
GLUTENS
GLUTEUS
GNAWERS
GOAHEAD
GOATEED
GOATEES
GOBLETS
GODDESS
GODHEAD
GODLESS
GODSEND
GODSENT
GOITERS
GOLFERS
GOMPERS
GOOBERS
GOODEGG
GOODERS
GOOIEST
GOONEYS
GOPHERS
GORGERS
GORIEST
GOSPELS
GOSSETT
GOTBEAT
GOTHELP
GOTREAL
GOTWELL
GOUGERS
GRADEAA
GRADERS
GRAPERY
GRATEON
GRATERS
GRATEUP
GRAVELS
GRAVELY
GRAVERS
GRAVEST
GRAYEST
GRAZERS
GREYEST
GRIPERS
GROCERS
GROCERY
GROPERS
GROVELS
GROVERS
GROWERS
GRUYERE
GUDGEON
GUIDERS
GUINEAN
GUINEAS
GULDENS
GULLETS
GULPERS
GUMLESS
GUNBELT
GUNLESS
GUNNERS
GUNNERY
GUNSELS
GURNEYS
GUSHERS
GUSSETS
GUTLESS
GUTTERS
GWYNETH
GYPPERS

G••••E•

GABBIER
GABBLED
GABBLES
GABRIEL
GADSDEN
GAGGLES
GAGREEL
GAGSTER
GALATEA
GALAXES
GALILEE
GALILEI
GALILEO
GALOPED
GAMBIER
GAMBLED
GAMBLER
GAMBLES
GAMELEG
GAMETES
GAMINES
GANTLET
GARAGED
GARAGES
GARBLED
GARBLER
GARBLES
GARDNER
GARGLED
GARGLER
GARGLES
GASOVEN
GASSIER
GATELEG
GATEMEN
GAUCHER
GAUDIER
GAUDIES
GAUNTER
GAUSSES
GAUTIER
GAUZIER
GAVELED
GAWKIER
GECKOES
GEEKIER
GELATED
GELATES
GEMAYEL
GEMMIER
GENESEE
GENESES
GENESET
GENOMES
GENTEEL
GENTLED
GENTLER
GENTLES
GENUSES
GEORGEC
GEORGEI
GEORGEM
GEORGES
GEORGEV
GEORGEW
GERMIER
GESSOED
GESSOES
GETEVEN
GETFREE
GETOVER
GETSHEP
GETSSET
GETSWET
GFORCES
GHOSTED
GIBLUES
GIBUSES
GIDDIED
GIDDIER
GIDDIES
GIFTEES
GIFTSET
GIGGLED
GIGGLER
GIGGLES
GILLNET
GIPSIES
GIRDLED
GIRDLER
GIRDLES
GIRLIER
GIRLIES
GIRTHED
GLACEED
GLACIER
GLADDEN
GLADDER
GLANCED
GLANCES
GLASSED
GLASSES
GLAZIER
GLEAMED
GLEANED
GLEANER
GLEEMEN
GLIBBER
GLIMMER
GLINTED
GLISTEN
GLISTER
GLITTER
GLITZED
GLITZES
GLOATED
GLOATER
GLOMMED
GLOOMED
GLORIED
GLORIES
GLOSSED
GLOSSER
GLOSSES
GLUGGED
GLUMMED
GLUMMER
GLURGES
GLUTTED
GNARLED
GNARRED
GNASHED
GNASHER
GNASHES
GOAFTER
GOALIES
GOATEED
GOATEES
GOBBLED
GOBBLER
GOBBLES
GOBYSEA
GODFREY
GODLIER
GOGETEM
GOGGLED
GOGGLER
GOGGLES
GOLFTEE
GOODIES
GOODMEN
GOOFIER
GOOGLED
GOOGLER
GOOGLES
GOONIER
GOONIES
GOOPIER
GOOSIER
GORETEX
GORSIER
GORTNER
GOTEVEN
GOTFREE
GOTOBED
GOTOSEA
GOTOSEE
GOTOVER
GOUNDER
GOURDES
GOURMET
GOUTIER
GQMODEL
GRABBED
GRABBER
GRAFTED
GRAFTER
GRAINED
GRAINER
GRAMMER
GRAMMES
GRANDEE
GRANDER
GRANGER
GRANGES
GRANTED
GRANTEE
GRANTER
GRAPHED
GRAPIER
GRAPNEL
GRASPED
GRASPER
GRASSED
GRASSES
GRAVIES
GRAZIER
GREASED
GREASER
GREASES
GREATEN
GREATER
GREAVES
GREELEY
GREENED
GREENER
GREETED
GREETER
GRENDEL
GREYHEN
GRIDDED
GRIDDER
GRIEVED
GRIEVER
GRIEVES
GRIFFEY
GRIFTED
GRIFTER
GRILLED
GRILLER
GRILLES
GRIMIER
GRIMMER
GRINDER
GRINNED
GRINNER
GRIPPED
GRIPPER
GRIPPES
GRISLET
GRISNEZ
GRISTER
GRITTED
GRITTER
GROANED
GROANER
GRODIER
GROINED
GROKKED
GROLIER
GROMMET
GROOMED
GROOMER
GROOVED
GROOVES
GROSSED
GROSSER
GROSSES
GROUPED
GROUPER
GROUSED
GROUSER
GROUSES
GROUTED
GROUTER
GROWLED
GROWLER
GRUBBED
GRUBBER
GRUDGED
GRUDGER
GRUDGES
GRUFFER
GRUMPED
GRUNGER
GRUNGES
GRUNTED
GRUNTER
GUARDED
GUARDEE
GUARDER
GUCKIER
GUESSED
GUESSER
GUESSES
GUESTED
GUILDER
GULCHES
GULLIED
GULLIES
GULPIER
GUMMIER
GUMTREE
GUNITES
GUNKIER
GUNNIES
GUNTHER
GUNUSER
GUPPIES
GURGLED
GURGLES
GUSHIER
GUSSIED
GUSSIES
GUSTIER
GUSTOES
GUTSIER
GUTTIER
GUZZLED
GUZZLER
GUZZLES
GYPSIES
GYRATED
GYRATES
GYRENES

G•••••E

GAGLINE
GAGRULE
GALAXIE
GALEATE
GALETTE
GALILEE
GARBAGE
GARONNE
GAROTTE
GARPIKE
GARROTE
GASLINE
GASPIPE
GASTONE
GAVOTTE
GAZELLE
GAZETTE
GEFILTE
GEMLIKE
GEMMATE
GENESEE
GENOESE
GENOISE
GENTILE
GENUINE
GENZYME
GEOCODE
GEORGIE
GERMANE
GESTATE
GESTURE
GETABLE
GETCUTE
GETDONE
GETFREE
GETSORE
GETWISE
GIAUQUE
GILMORE
GINGAME
GIRAFFE
GIROLLE
GIRONDE
GISELLE
GLADEYE
GLAVINE
GLENCOE
GLIMPSE
GLOBATE
GLOBOSE
GLOBULE
GLORYBE
GLOSSAE
GLUCOSE
GLYCINE
GOBROKE
GODLIKE
GOESAPE
GOLFTEE
GONEAPE
GOODBYE
GOODJOE
GOODONE
GOODUSE
GOSSAGE
GOSTALE
GOTCUTE
GOTDONE
GOTFREE
GOTOSEE
GOTSORE
GOTWISE
GOUACHE
GRACILE
GRACKLE
GRADATE
GRAHAME
GRANDEE
GRANITE
GRANNIE
GRANTEE
GRANULE
GRAPPLE
GRASSLE
GRAVURE
GRECIZE
GRENADE
GRIDDLE
GRIMACE
GRISTLE
GRIZZLE
GROUPIE
GRUMBLE
GRUYERE
GUANINE
GUARDEE
GUMLIKE
GUMSHOE
GUMTREE
GUNCASE
GUNFIRE
GUNWALE
GUSTAVE
GUTHRIE
GUYROPE
GYMSHOE

•GE••••

AGEDOUT
AGEFIVE
AGEFOUR
AGEISTS
AGELESS
AGELONG
AGEMATE
AGENCES
AGENDAS
AGENDUM
AGENINE
AGENTED
AGENTRY
AGESAGO
AGESOUT
EGERIAS
EGESTED

•G•E•••

AGREEON
AGREERS
AGREETO
EGGEDON
HGWELLS
IGNEOUS
OGDENUT
OGREISH

•G••E••

AGELESS
AGGRESS
AGILELY
AGILEST
AGREEON
AGREERS
AGREETO
EGGHEAD
EGGIEST
EGGLERS
EGGLESS
IGIVEUP
UGLIEST

•G•••E•

AGENCES
AGENTED
AGNATES
AGNOMEN
AGONIES
AGUTTER
EGESTED
EGLISES
IGNITED
IGNITER
IGNITES
IGNORED
IGNORER
IGNORES
IGOOFED
PGRATED

•G••••E

AGATINE
AGEFIVE
AGEMATE
AGENINE
AGITATE
AGONISE
AGONIZE
EGALITE
EGGCASE
EGGLIKE
EGOISTE
IGNOBLE
IGRAINE

••GE•••

ALGEBRA
ALGERIA
ANGELAS
ANGELES
ANGELIC
ANGELOU
ANGELUS
ANGERED
ARGENTI
ARGENTO
ARGENTS
AUGENDS
BAGEHOT
BIGEARS
BIGEAST
BIGEASY
BIGELOW
BIGENDS
BIGEYED
BIGEYES
BOGEYED
BUGEYED
CAGEDIN
CAGEDUP
CAGEPET
CAGESUP
COGENCY
DEGERMS
DIGESTS
DOGEARS
EAGERER
EAGERLY
EDGEDIN
EDGEOUT
EDGESIN
EGGEDON
EUGENIA
EUGENIC
EUGENIE
FAGENDS
FOGERTY
GOGETEM
HAGERTY
HYGELAC
INGEMAR
INGENUE
INGESTA
INGESTS
LEGENDS
MAGENTA
MIGENES
NIGERIA
ORGEATS
PAGEANT
PAGEBOY
PAGEONE
PAGESIX
PAGETWO
PIGEONS
PIGEYED
RAGEFUL
REGEARS
REGENCY
REGENTS
ROGERED
SAGEHEN
SAGETEA
TAGENDS
URGEDON
URGENCY
URGESON
VEGETAL
WAGERED
WAGERER
WAGEWAR
WEGENER

••G•E••

AGGRESS
AIGLETS
AIGRETS
ALGIEBA
ALGIERS
ALGREEN
ANGLERS
ARGUERS
AUGMENT
BAGGERS
BAGWELL
BIGBEAR
BIGBEAT
BIGBEND
BIGBETS
BIGDEAL
BIGFEET
BIGGERS
BIGGEST
BIGHEAD
BIGJERK
BIGLEAD
BIGMEAL
BIGMESS
BIGNESS
BIGNEWS
BIGTENT
BUGBEAR
BUGLERS
CAGIEST
CYGNETS
DAGGERS
DEGREED
DEGREES
DIGGERS
DIGRESS
DOGBEDS
DOGBERT
DOGGETT
DOGLEGS
DOGLESS
DOGREAT
DOGSEAR
DOGVEST
EAGLETS
EDGIEST
EGGHEAD
EGGIEST
EGGLERS
EGGLESS
ELGRECO
EUGLENA
FIGLEAF
FIGMENT
FOGGERS
FOGLESS
GAGGERS
GAGREEL
HIGHEND
HIGHEST
HOGGERY
HOGWEED
HUGGERS
HYGIEIA
HYGIENE
IMGREAT
INGLESE
INGREEN
INGRESS
JAGLESS
JIGGERS
JIGGERY
JOGGERS
JUGHEAD
KEGGERS
KEGLERS
LAGGERS
LEGLESS
LEGREST
LEGWEAR
LIGGETT
LOGGERS
LOGIEST
LUGGERS
MAGLEVS
MAGNETO
MAGNETS
MEGAERA
MEGAERG
MRGREEN
MUGGERS
NAGGERS
NEGLECT
NIGHEST
NUGGETS
NUGGETY
PEGLEGS
PEGLESS
PIGGERY
PIGLETS
PIGMEAT
PIGMENT
PIGPENS
PIGWEED

RAGGEDY
RAGWEED
REGREET
REGRESS
REGRETS
RIGGERS
RIGUEUR
RIGVEDA
ROGUERY
SAGIEST
SEGMENT
SIGHERS
SIGNEES
SIGNERS
SIGNETS
SUGGEST
TAGGERS
TAGTEAM
TIGRESS
TOGGERY
TUGGERS
TUGLESS
UNGREEN
UNGUENT
VAGUELY
VAGUEST
VOGUERS
WAGGERS
WAGGERY
WIGGERY
WIGLESS
WIGLETS

••G••E•

AEGISES
ALGREEN
ANGELES
ANGERED
ANGRIER
ARGUSES
ARGYLES
AUGITES
AUGURED
AUGURER
AVGASES
BAGGIER
BAGGIES
BIGAPES
BIGEYED
BIGEYES
BIGFEET
BIGGIES
BIGIDEA
BIGLIES
BIGONES
BIGOTED
BIGTOES
BOGEYED
BOGGIER
BOGGLED
BOGGLER
BOGGLES
BOGYMEN
BUGEYED
BUGFREE
BUGGIER
BUGGIES
BUGGLES
BYGONES
CAGEPET
COGGLES
DEGREED
DEGREES
DIGIPET
DOGAPES
DOGCHEW
DOGFLEA
DOGGIER
DOGGIES
DOGSLED
EAGERER
EIGHTEE
ENGAGED
ENGAGER
ENGAGES
ENGINED
ENGINES
FAGOTED
FIGHTER
FIGTREE
FIGURED
FIGURER
FIGURES
FOGGIER
GAGGLES
GAGREEL
GAGSTER
GIGGLED
GIGGLER
GIGGLES
GOGETEM
GOGGLED
GOGGLER
GOGGLES
HAGGLED
HAGGLER
HAGGLES
HIGGLED
HIGGLER
HIGGLES
HIGHRES
HIGHSEA
HIGHTEA
HOGTIED
HOGTIES
HOGWEED
HUGGIES
INGATES
INGREEN
JAGGIER
JAGGIES
JIGGIER
JIGGLED
JIGGLES
JOGGLED
JOGGLER
JOGGLES
JUGGLED
JUGGLER
JUGGLES
LEGATEE
LEGATES
LEGGIER
LEGOSET
LEGUMES
LIGATED
LIGATES
LIGHTED
LIGHTEN
LIGHTER
MAGPIES
MEGANES
MIGENES
MRGREEN
MUGGIER
MUGGLES
NAGGIER
NEGATED
NEGATER
NEGATES
NEGUSES
NIGGLED
NIGGLER
NIGGLES
NIGHTER
NOGALES
PIGEYED
PIGGIER
PIGGIES
PIGWEED
PUGGLES
PUGSLEY
PYGMIES
RAGGIER
RAGGIES
RAGWEED
REGALED
REGALER
REGALES
REGIMEN
REGIMES
REGIVEN
REGIVES
REGLUED
REGLUES
REGNIER
REGREET
RIGHTED
RIGHTER
ROGERED
RUGGLES
SAGEHEN
SAGETEA
SAGGIER
SIGHTED
SIGHTER
SIGNEES
SOGGIER
SUGARED
TAGAMET
TIGHTEN
TIGHTER
TOGGLED
TOGGLER
TOGGLES
TVGAMES
UNGATED
UNGIVEN
UNGLUED
UNGLUES
UNGORED
UNGREEN
UNGUYED
UNGYVED
UPGAZED
UPGAZES
VEGGIES
WAGERED
WAGERER
WAGGLED
WAGGLER
WAGGLES
WAGONED
WAGONER
WEGENER
WIGGIER
WIGGLED
WIGGLER
WIGGLES
ZYGOTES

••G•••E

ALGARVE
ARGANTE
ARGONNE
ATGRADE
AUGUSTE
BAGGAGE
BAGLIKE
BAGPIPE
BEGRIME
BEGUILE
BEGUINE
BIGBLUE
BIGFIVE
BIGGAME
BIGJAKE
BIGLOVE
BIGNAME
BIGNOSE
BIGSALE
BIGTIME
BOGARDE
BOGHOLE
BUGFREE
COGNATE
COGNIZE
DEGLAZE
DEGRADE
DOGBANE
DOGBITE
DOGBONE
DOGFACE
DOGGATE
DOGGONE
DOGLIKE
DOGPILE
DOGRACE
DOGROSE
DOGSAGE
EGGCASE
EGGLIKE
EIGHTEE
ENGARDE
ENGORGE
ENGRAVE
EUGENIE
FIGTREE
GAGLINE
GAGRULE
HAGLIKE
HOGLIKE
HOGNOSE
HYGIENE
INGENUE
INGLESE
INGRATE
JIGLIKE
JIGTIME
JUGWINE
LAGASSE
LEGATEE
LEGBONE
LEGIBLE
LEGLIKE
LEGROPE
LIGNITE
LUGGAGE
MAGNATE
MAGUIRE
MCGUIRE
MCGWIRE
MIGRATE
NIGHTIE
PAGEONE
PEGLIKE
PIGLIKE
PUGNOSE
RAGTIME
REGAUGE
REGLAZE
REGRADE
REGUIDE
ROGAINE
RUGLIKE
SIGNAGE
SIGNORE
TAGLIKE
TAGLINE
TAGSALE
TVGUIDE
UNGLOVE
UNGULAE
UPGRADE
WIGLIKE

•••GE••

APOGEAL
APOGEAN
APOGEES
BADGERS
BAGGERS
BANGERS
BARGEIN
BARGERS
BEEGEES
BERGERE
BIGGERS
BIGGEST
BINGERS
BUDGERS
BUDGETS
BUNGEES
BURGEES
BURGEON
BURGERS
BURGESS
CADGERS
COAGENT
CODGERS
CONGEAL
CONGERS
CONGEST
CUDGELS
DAGGERS
DANGELO
DANGERS
DIGGERS
DINGERS
DODGEMS
DODGERS
DOGGETT
DRAGEES
DUDGEON
DUNGEON
ERIGENA
ETAGERE
EXEGETE
EXIGENT
FIDGETS
FIDGETY
FINGERS
FOGGERS
FOLGERS
FORGERS
FORGERY
FORGETS
FUDGERS
FULGENT
GADGETS
GADGETY
GAGGERS
GANGERS
GAUGERS
GINGERS
GINGERY
GORGERS
GOUGERS
GUDGEON
HANGERS
HEDGERS
HINGEON
HOGGERY
HUGGERS
HUNGERS
HUYGENS
IMAGERS
IMAGERY
IMOGENE
JAEGERS
JERGENS
JIGGERS
JIGGERY
JOGGERS
JUDGERS
JURGENS
KEDGERS
KEGGERS
LAGGERS
LARGELY
LARGENT
LARGEOJ
LARGESS
LARGEST
LEDGERS
LEOGENN
LIGGETT
LINGERS
LODGEIN
LODGERS
LOGGERS
LONGEST
LOWGEAR
LUGGERS
LUNGEAT
LUNGERS
MAJGENS
MANGERS
MARGERY
MERGEES
MERGERS
MIDGETS
MONGERS
MUGGERS
NAGGERS
NEOGENE
NUDGERS
NUGGETS
NUGGETY
ONAGERS
OROGENY
PADGETT
PARGERS
PEUGEOT
PIDGEON
PIGGERY
PINGERS
PONGEES
PROGENY
PUNGENT
RAGGEDY
RANGERS
REAGENT
RIEGERT
RIGGERS
RINGERS
RODGERS
RUTGERS
SARGENT
SINGERS
STAGERS
SUGGEST
SURGEON
SURGERY
SWIGERT
TAGGERS
TANGELO
TANGENT
TARGETS
TOGGERY
TRAGEDY
TUGGERS
VERGEON
VERGERS
WAGGERS
WAGGERY
WEDGEIN
WIDGEON
WIDGETS
WIGGERY
WINGERS
YEVGENY
ZINGERS

•••G•E•

ALIGNED
ALIGNER
APOGEES
BAGGIER
BAGGIES
BANGLED
BANGLES
BEAGLES
BEEGEES
BEIGNES
BEIGNET
BIGGIES
BILGIER
BINGLES
BINGOES
BLOGGED
BLOGGER
BOBGOEN
BOGGIER
BOGGLED
BOGGLER
BOGGLES
BONGOES
BOOGIED
BOOGIES
BOUGHED
BRAGGED
BRAGGER
BROGUES
BUDGIES
BUGGIER
BUGGIES
BUGGLES
BULGIER
BUNGEES
BUNGLED
BUNGLER
BUNGLES
BURGEES
BURGHER
BURGLED
BURGLES
CARGOES
CHIGGER
CHIGOES
CHUGGED
CHUGGER
CLOGGED
COGGLES
COIGNED
COIGNES
CONGAED
COUGHED
CRAGGED
CRUGUET
DANGLED
DANGLER
DANGLES
DEIGNED
DINGIER
DINGLES
DINGOES
DODGIER
DOGGIER
DOGGIES
DONGLES
DRAGEES
DRAGGED
DRAGGER
DRAGNET
DROGUES
DRUGGED
ELEGIES
EMIGREE
EMIGRES
FEIGNED
FEIGNER
FLAGGED
FLAGGER
FLAGMEN
FLOGGED
FLOGGER
FOGGIER
FORGOER
FORGOES
FRAGGED
FROGGER
FROGLEG
FROGLET
FROGMEN
FUNGOES
GAGGLES
GARGLED
GARGLER
GARGLES
GIGGLED
GIGGLER
GIGGLES
GLUGGED
GOGGLED
GOGGLER
GOGGLES
GOOGLED
GOOGLER
GOOGLES
GURGLED
GURGLES
HAGGLED
HAGGLER
HAGGLES
HANGMEN
HANGTEN
HEDGIER
HIGGLED
HIGGLER
HIGGLES
HOAGIES
HUGGIES
HUNGTEN
IMAGOES
JAGGIER
JAGGIES
JANGLED
JANGLER
JANGLES
JIGGIER
JIGGLED
JIGGLES
JINGLED
JINGLER
JINGLES
JINGOES
JOGGLED
JOGGLER
JOGGLES
JUGGLED
JUGGLER
JUGGLES
JUNGLES
KINGLET
LANGLEY
LAUGHED
LAUGHER
LEAGUED
LEAGUER
LEAGUES
LEDGIER
LEGGIER
LINGOES
LONGBED
LONGDEN
LONGIES
LONGUES
MAIGRET
MANGIER
MANGLED
MANGLER
MANGLES
MANGOES
MARGRET
MEAGLES
MERGEES
MINGIER
MINGLED
MINGLER
MINGLES
MONGREL
MORGUES
MUGGIER
MUGGLES
MULGREW
NAGGIER
NEIGHED
NIGGLED
NIGGLER
NIGGLES
NOOGIES
NUNGWEN
OLOGIES
OUTGOES
OUTGREW
PANGAEA
PIGGIER
PIGGIES
PLAGUED
PLAGUES
PLUGGED
PLUGGER
PONGEES
PORGIES
PUDGIER
PUGGLES
QUIGLEY
RAGGIER
RAGGIES
RANGIER
REIGNED
RIDGIER
RINGLET
ROUGHED
ROUGHEN
ROUGHER
RUGGLES
SAGGIER
SEAGREN
SEDGIER
SHAGGED
SINGLED
SINGLES
SINGLET
SLOGGED
SLOGGER
SLUGGED
SLUGGER
SMUGGER
SNAGGED
SNAGGER
SNIGLET
SNUGGED
SNUGGER
SOGGIER
SOIGNEE
STAGGED
STAGGER
STAGIER
STAGNES
STOGIES
SWAGGER
SWAGMEN
SWIGGED
TAMGLEN
TANGIER
TANGLED
TANGLER
TANGLES
TANGOED
TANGOER
THIGPEN
TINGLED
TINGLER
TINGLES
TOGGLED
TOGGLER
TOGGLES
TONGUES
TOUGHEN
TOUGHER
TRIGGER
UNOGLED
VEGGIES
WAGGLED
WAGGLER
WAGGLES
WANGLED
WANGLER
WANGLES
WEDGIER
WEDGIES
WEIGHED
WEIGHER
WIGGIER
WIGGLED
WIGGLER
WIGGLES
WINGLET
WINGMEN
WRIGLEY
ZIEGLER
ZINGIER

•••G••E

ALIGOTE
ALLGONE
BAGGAGE
BERGERE
BIGGAME
BRIGADE
COLGATE
CONGAME
DAYGAME
DOGGATE
DOGGONE
DRAGGLE
ELEGIZE
EMIGREE
ENDGAME
EPIGONE
ETAGERE
EXEGETE
FARGONE
FORGAVE
FORGIVE
FORGONE
FRAGGLE
FRAGILE
FRIGATE
GINGAME
HOTGLUE
IMAGINE
IMOGENE
ITSGONE
LINGUAE
LUGGAGE
MARGATE
MISGAVE
MISGIVE
NBAGAME
NEOGENE
NETGAME
NEWGATE
NFLGAME
NHLGAME
ORIGINE
OUTGAME
OUTGAVE
OUTGAZE
OUTGIVE
PETGATE
PREGAME
PUBGAME
SEAGATE
SMUGGLE
SNUGGLE
SOIGNEE
THEGAME
TIEGAME
TOUGHIE
UNAGILE
VIRGATE
VIRGULE
VULGATE
WARGAME
WRIGGLE
YANGTZE

••••GE•

ALLAGES
ALLEGED
ALLEGER
ALLEGES
ANTIGEN
ATTYGEN
AVENGED
AVENGER
AVENGES
AZINGER
BAREGES
BETTGER
BLOGGED
BLOGGER
BLUDGED
BLUDGER
BLUDGES
BOURGET
BRAGGED
BRAGGER
BRIDGED
BRIDGER
BRIDGES
BRIDGET
BRINGER
BRUEGEL
CHANGED
CHANGER
CHANGES
CHARGED
CHARGER
CHARGES
CHIGGER
CHUGGED
CHUGGER
CLANGED
CLANGER
CLINGER
CLOGGED
CRAGGED
CRINGED
CRINGES
CRYOGEN
CUBAGES
DAMAGED
DAMAGES
DELUGED
DELUGES
DIMAGES
DOSAGES
DOTAGES
DOWAGER
DRAGGED
DRAGGER
DREDGED
DREDGER
DREDGES
DRUDGED
DRUDGER
DRUDGES
DRUGGED
EMERGED
EMERGES
ENCAGED
ENCAGES
ENGAGED
ENGAGER
ENGAGES
ENRAGED
ENRAGES
EVANGEL
FIBIGER
FLAGGED

FLAGGER
FLANGES
FLEDGED
FLEDGES
FLINGER
FLOGGED
FLOGGER
FORAGED
FORAGER
FORAGES
FRAGGED
FRIDGES
FRINGED
FRINGES
FROGGER
GARAGED
GARAGES
GEORGEC
GEORGEI
GEORGEM
GEORGES
GEORGEV
GEORGEW
GLUGGED
GLURGES
GRANGER
GRANGES
GRUDGED
GRUDGER
GRUDGES
GRUNGER
GRUNGES
HAIRGEL
HALOGEN
HOMAGER
HOMAGES
ICEAGES
IFORGET
INDIGEN
INNAGES
INTEGER
KLINGER
KLUDGED
KLUDGES
KRUEGER
LAVAGES
LIMOGES
LINAGES
LOUNGED
LOUNGER
LOUNGES
LOVAGES
MANAGED
MANAGER
MANAGES
MANEGES
MENAGES
MIRAGES
MRTIGER
MUTAGEN
NEWAGER
NEWAGEY
NOANGEL
NONAGES
NOODGED
NOODGES
OBLIGED
OBLIGEE
OBLIGER
OBLIGES
OHMAGES
ONSAGER
ORANGES
ORANGEY
OUTAGES
PELAGES
PERIGEE
PIPAGES
PIROGEN
PLEDGED
PLEDGEE
PLEDGER
PLEDGES
PLUGGED
PLUGGER
PLUNGED
PLUNGER
PLUNGES
POTAGES
PREAGED
PREAGES
PRONGED
RAVAGED
RAVAGER
RAVAGES
RECAGED
RECAGES
REFUGED
REFUGEE
REFUGES
RENEGED
RENEGER
RENEGES
REPAGED
REPAGES
REURGED
REURGES
REWAGER
RONTGEN
SAVAGED
SAVAGER
SAVAGES
SHAGGED
SLEDGED
SLEDGES
SLINGER
SLOGGED
SLOGGER
SLUDGES
SLUGGED
SLUGGER
SMIDGEN
SMIDGES
SMUDGED
SMUDGES
SMUGGER
SNAGGED
SNAGGER
SNUGGED
SNUGGER
SOFTGEL
SPIEGEL
SPONGED
SPONGER
SPONGES
STAGGED
STAGGER
STEIGER
STENGEL
STINGER
STODGED
STODGES
STOOGED
STOOGES
STURGES
SWAGGER
SWIGGED
SWINGER
TANAGER
THEAGES
TOWAGES
TRIAGES
TRIGGER
TRUDGED
TRUDGEN
TRUDGER
TRUDGES
TWANGED
TWANGER
TWINGED
TWINGES
ULLAGES
UNCAGED
UNCAGES
UNEAGER
UNEDGED
UNEDGES
UNPAGED
UNURGED
UNWAGED
VISAGED
VISAGES
VOYAGED
VOYAGER
VOYAGES
WHANGED
WRANGEL
WRINGER
WRONGED
WRONGER
YOUNGER

••••G•E

ATINGLE
COLOGNE
CRAIGIE
DRAGGLE
ECLOGUE
ENVOGUE
EPERGNE
FATIGUE
FINAGLE
FLEEGLE
FRAGGLE
FROOGLE
GEORGIE
HUANGHE
INSIGNE
INVOGUE
KRINGLE
LASAGNE
MINOGUE
OBLIGEE
PERIGEE
PIROGUE
PLEDGEE
PRINGLE
REARGUE
REFUGEE
SHINGLE
SMUGGLE
SNUGGLE
SPANGLE
UNVAGUE
WRANGLE
WRIGGLE

•••••GE

AALARGE
ABRIDGE
ACREAGE
ADJUDGE
AIRRAGE
ALLONGE
ARLEDGE
ARRANGE
ASSUAGE
ATLARGE
AUBERGE
AVERAGE
BABBAGE
BAGGAGE
BANDAGE
BARRAGE
BESIEGE
BONDAGE
BORZAGE
BOSCAGE
BREWAGE
BURBAGE
CABBAGE
CARNAGE
CARTAGE
COINAGE
COLLAGE
COLLEGE
CORDAGE
CORKAGE
CORSAGE
CORTEGE
COTTAGE
COURAGE
DARKAGE
DEBARGE
DEFARGE
DEMERGE
DERANGE
DETERGE
DIVERGE
DIVULGE
DOCKAGE
DOGSAGE
DRAYAGE
DUNNAGE
ECOTAGE
ELFUDGE
ENGORGE
ENLARGE
EXPUNGE
FABERGE
FLOTAGE
FLOWAGE
FOLIAGE
FOOTAGE
FROMAGE
FTDODGE
GARBAGE
GOSSAGE
HAULAGE
HERBAGE
HEURIGE
HOSTAGE
IDBADGE
IMMERGE
IMPINGE
INARAGE
INDULGE
INLARGE
INRANGE
IPLEDGE
IRONAGE
JAZZAGE
LAFARGE
LEAFAGE
LEAKAGE
LINEAGE
LINKAGE
LOCKAGE
LORANGE
LOZENGE
LUGGAGE
MASSAGE
MEANAGE
MELANGE
MELTAGE
MESSAGE
MILEAGE
MILLAGE
MINTAGE
MISPAGE
MONTAGE
MOORAGE
MOULAGE
NICCAGE
NOMERGE
NONWAGE
OFANAGE
OHFUDGE
ONEPAGE
ONSTAGE
OUTEDGE
OUTRAGE
OVERAGE
PACKAGE
PANURGE
PASSAGE
PEERAGE
PEONAGE
PETCAGE
PILLAGE
PLUMAGE
PORTAGE
POSTAGE
POTTAGE
PRESAGE
PROTEGE
QUAYAGE
RAILAGE
RAMPAGE
REFORGE
REGAUGE
REHINGE
REIMAGE
REJUDGE
REMERGE
RESTAGE
RESURGE
RETINGE
REVENGE
RIBCAGE
ROOFAGE
ROOTAGE
RUMMAGE
SALVAGE
SAUSAGE
SCALAGE
SCOURGE
SCROOGE
SEEPAGE
SELVAGE
SERFAGE
SIGNAGE
SINKAGE
SOILAGE
SOLFEGE
SPLURGE
STORAGE
STOWAGE
STRANGE
SVERIGE
SYRINGE
TANKAGE
TEENAGE
THEEDGE
TILLAGE
TOLLAGE
TONNAGE
UMBRAGE
UNHINGE
UNLARGE
UNMERGE
UNWEDGE
UPSTAGE
UPSURGE
VANTAGE
VENTAGE
VESTIGE
VILLAGE
VINTAGE
VOLTAGE
VORLAGE
WARPAGE
WASTAGE
WATTAGE
WEBPAGE
WINDAGE
WORDAGE
YARDAGE

GF•••••

GFORCES

G•F••••

GAFFERS
GAFFING
GEFILTE
GIFFORD
GIFTBOX
GIFTEES
GIFTING
GIFTSET
GIFTTAX
GOFIRST
GOFORIT
GOFORTH
GUFFAWS

G••F•••

GABFEST
GAFFERS
GAFFING
GETFREE
GETFROM
GIFFORD
GILFORD
GINFIZZ
GOAFTER
GODFREY
GOLFBAG
GOLFCAR
GOLFERS
GOLFING
GOLFPRO
GOLFTEE
GOOFIER
GOOFILY
GOOFING
GOOFOFF
GOOFSUP
GOOFUPS
GOSFORD
GOTFREE
GRAFTED
GRAFTER
GRAFTON
GRIFFEY
GRIFFIN
GRIFFON
GRIFTED
GRIFTER
GRUFFER
GRUFFLY
GUFFAWS
GULFING
GULFOIL
GULFWAR
GUNFIRE

G•••F••

GAINFUL
GETSFAR
GETSFIT
GIRAFFE
GLEEFUL
GOESFAR
GOESFOR
GOINFOR
GONEFAR
GONEFOR
GOODFOR
GREWFAT
GRIFFEY
GRIFFIN
GRIFFON
GROWFAT
GRUFFER
GRUFFLY
GUNSFOR

G••••F•

GAVEOFF
GETSOFF
GETSOFT
GIRAFFE
GIVEOFF
GLORIFY
GOESAFT
GOESOFF
GONEAFT
GONEOFF
GOOFOFF
GOTSOFT
GRATIFY

G•••••F

GANDALF
GAVEOFF
GETSANF
GETSOFF
GIVENOF
GIVEOFF
GIVESOF
GOESOFF
GONEOFF
GOOFOFF

•G•F•••

AGEFIVE
AGEFOUR

•G••F••

IGOOFED

•G••••F

EGOSURF

••GF•••

BAGFULS
BIGFANS
BIGFEET
BIGFISH
BIGFIVE
BIGFOOT
BIGFOUR
BUGFREE
DOGFACE
DOGFISH
DOGFLEA
DOGFOOD
JUGFULS
MUGFULS
PIGFISH

••G•F••

BEGSFOR
DIGSFOR
LOGOFFS
NOGIFTS
RAGEFUL
REGIFTS
SIGHFOR
SIGHFUL
SIGNFOR

••G••F•

BEGSOFF
BUGSOFF
DIGNIFY
ENGRAFT
ENGULFS
INGRAFT
INGULFS
LIGNIFY
LOGOFFS
LOGSOFF
MAGNIFY
MCGRIFF
MCGRUFF
REGRAFT
SIGNIFY
SIGNOFF
UNGRUFF

••G•••F

BEGSOFF
BIGHALF
BUGSOFF
FIGLEAF
LOGSOFF
MCGRIFF
MCGRUFF
SIGNOFF
UNGRUFF

•••GF••

LONGFOR
RANGFOR
RINGFOR
RUNGFOR
SNUGFIT
SONGFUL

•••G•F•

ASAGIFT
DRAGOFF
HANGOFF
HUNGOFF
RANGOFF
RINGOFF
RUNGOFF
THEGIFT

•••G••F

DRAGOFF
HANGOFF
HUNGOFF
LETGOOF
RANGOFF
RINGOFF
RUNGOFF

GG•••••

GGORDON

G•G••••

GAGARIN
GAGGERS
GAGGING
GAGGLES
GAGLAWS
GAGLINE
GAGREEL
GAGRULE
GAGSTER
GIGABIT
GIGATON
GIGBAGS
GIGGING
GIGGLED
GIGGLER
GIGGLES
GIGOLOS
GOGETEM
GOGGLED
GOGGLER
GOGGLES
GOGIRLS

G••G•••

GADGETS
GADGETY
GAGGERS
GAGGING
GAGGLES
GANGERS
GANGING
GANGLIA
GANGSAW
GANGSTA
GANGSUP
GANGTOK
GANGWAY
GARGLED
GARGLER
GARGLES
GAUGERS
GAUGING
GAUGUIN
GEEGAWS
GENGHIS
GETGOOD
GEWGAWS
GIGGING
GIGGLED
GIGGLER
GIGGLES
GINGAME
GINGERS
GINGERY
GINGHAM
GINGIVA
GINGKOS
GINGOLD
GLUGGED
GOGGLED
GOGGLER
GOGGLES
GONGING
GONGORA
GOOGLED
GOOGLER
GOOGLES
GOOGOLS
GORGERS
GORGING
GORGONS
GOTGOOD
GOUGERS
GOUGING
GREGORY
GRIGRIS
GUDGEON
GUIGNOL
GURGLED
GURGLES

G•••G••

GAHAGAN
GARAGED
GARAGES
GEORGEC
GEORGEI
GEORGEM
GEORGES
GEORGEV
GEORGEW
GEORGIA
GEORGIC
GEORGIE
GIELGUD
GINKGOS
GIORGIO
GIORGOS
GLASGOW
GLUEGUN
GLUGGED
GLURGES
GOINGAT
GOINGBY
GOINGIN
GOINGON
GOINGTO
GOINGUP
GOODGUY
GOTOGAL
GOTOGUY
GRANGER
GRANGES
GRINGOS
GRUDGED
GRUDGER
GRUDGES
GRUNGER
GRUNGES
GUARGUM

G••••G•

GARBAGE
GARBAGY
GASBAGS
GASHOGS
GASLOGS
GATINGS
GEOLOGY
GIGBAGS
GONZAGA
GOODEGG
GOSSAGE
GOTTAGO
GUNDOGS
GYMBAGS

G•••••G

GABBING
GADDING
GAFFING
GAGGING
GAINING
GAITING
GALLING
GAMEBAG
GAMELEG
GAMMING
GANGING
GAOLING
GAPPING
GARBING
GASHING
GASPING
GASSING
GATELEG
GATLING
GAUGING
GAWKING
GAWPING
GEARING
GELDING
GELLING
GETTING
GIFTING
GIGGING
GILDING
GILLING
GIMPING
GINNING
GINSENG
GIRDING
GIRTING
GISSING
GITTING
GLARING
GLAZING
GLIDING
GLOBING
GLOVING
GLOWING
GNAWING
GOADING
GOALONG
GODLING
GOLDBUG
GOLDING
GOLFBAG
GOLFING
GONGING
GOODDOG
GOODEGG
GOODING
GOOFING
GOOSING
GORGING
GORMING
GOSLING
GOUGING
GOWNING
GOWRONG
GRABBAG
GRACING
GRADING
GRATING
GRAVING
GRAYING
GRAYLAG
GRAZING
GREWBIG
GREYING
GREYLAG
GRIMING
GRIPING
GROPING
GROWBIG
GROWING
GSTRING
GUIDING
GUILING
GULFING
GULLING
GULPING
GUMMING
GUNNING
GUSHING
GUSTING
GUTTING
GYPPING

•GG••••

AGGRESS
EGGCASE
EGGCUPS
EGGDROP
EGGEDON
EGGHEAD
EGGHUNT
EGGIEST
EGGLERS
EGGLESS
EGGLIKE
EGGNOGS
EGGROLL
EGGSACS
EGGTOSS
IGGYPOP

•G•••G•

AGESAGO
EGGNOGS

•G••••G

AGELONG

••GG•••

BAGGAGE
BAGGERS
BAGGIER
BAGGIES
BAGGILY
BAGGING
BAGGINS
BAGGIRL
BEGGARS
BEGGARY
BEGGING
BIGGAME
BIGGERS
BIGGEST
BIGGIES
BIGGIRL
BIGGISH
BIGGITY
BIGGULP
BIGGUNS
BOGGIER
BOGGING
BOGGISH

BOGGLED
BOGGLER
BOGGLES
BOGGUSS
BUGGIER
BUGGIES
BUGGING
BUGGLES
COGGING
COGGLES
DAGGERS
DIGGERS
DIGGING
DIGGITY
DIGGORY
DOGGATE
DOGGETT
DOGGIER
DOGGIES
DOGGING
DOGGISH
DOGGONE
FOGGERS
FOGGIER
FOGGILY
FOGGING
GAGGERS
GAGGING
GAGGLES
GIGGING
GIGGLED
GIGGLER
GIGGLES
GOGGLED
GOGGLER
GOGGLES
HAGGARD
HAGGISH
HAGGLED
HAGGLER
HAGGLES
HIGGINS
HIGGLED
HIGGLER
HIGGLES
HOGGERY
HOGGING
HOGGISH
HUGGERS
HUGGIES
HUGGING
HUGGINS
JAGGIER
JAGGIES
JAGGING
JIGGERS
JIGGERY
JIGGIER
JIGGING
JIGGISH
JIGGLED
JIGGLES
JOGGERS
JOGGING
JOGGLED
JOGGLER
JOGGLES
JUGGING
JUGGLED
JUGGLER
JUGGLES
KEGGERS
KEGGING
LAGGARD
LAGGERS
LAGGING
LEGGIER
LEGGING
LIGGETT
LOGGERS
LOGGIAS
LOGGING
LOGGINS
LOGGISH
LUGGAGE
LUGGERS
LUGGING
MAGGOTS
MUGGERS
MUGGIER
MUGGING
MUGGISH
MUGGLES
NAGGERS
NAGGIER
NAGGING
NAGGISH
NIGGLED
NIGGLER
NIGGLES
NOGGINS
NUGGETS
NUGGETY
PEGGING
PIGGERY
PIGGIER
PIGGIES
PIGGING
PIGGISH
PUGGISH
PUGGLES
RAGGEDY
RAGGIER
RAGGIES
RAGGING
RIGGERS
RIGGING
RUGGLES
SAGGIER
SAGGING
SOGGIER
SOGGILY
SUGGEST
TAGGANT
TAGGERS
TAGGING
TOGGERY
TOGGING
TOGGLED
TOGGLER
TOGGLES
TUGGERS
TUGGING
VEGGIES
VEGGING
WAGGERS
WAGGERY
WAGGING
WAGGISH
WAGGLED
WAGGLER
WAGGLES
WIGGERY
WIGGIER
WIGGING
WIGGLED
WIGGLER
WIGGLES
ZAGGING
ZIGGING

••G•G••

ENGAGED
ENGAGER
ENGAGES

••G••G•

BAGGAGE
BAGWIGS
BIGDIGS
BIGDOGS
BIGHUGS
BIGRIGS
BIGWIGS
DOGLEGS
DOGSAGE
DOGTAGS
DUGONGS
EDGINGS
EGGNOGS
ENGORGE
FOGDOGS
GIGBAGS
LUGGAGE
PAGINGS
PEGLEGS
RAGBAGS
RAGINGS
RAGRUGS
REGAUGE
SIGNAGE
URGINGS
WIGWAGS
ZIGZAGS

••G•••G

ANGLING
ARGUING
BAGGING
BEGGING
BIGBANG
BOGGING
BUGGING
BUGLING
COGGING
DIGGING
DOGGING
EAGLING
FOGGING
GAGGING
GIGGING
HOGGING
HUGGING
IMGOING
INGOING
JAGGING
JIGGING
JOGGING
JUGGING
KEGGING
LAGGING
LEGGING
LOGGING
LUGGING
MAGALOG
MEGAERG
MUGGING
NAGGING
ONGOING
PEGGING
PIGGING
RAGGING
RIGGING
ROGUING
SAGGING
SIGHING
SIGNING
TAGALOG
TAGGING
TOGGING
TUGGING
UPGOING
VEGGING
VOGUING
WAGGING
WIGGING
ZAGAZIG
ZAGGING
ZIGGING

•••GG••

BLOGGED
BLOGGER
BRAGGED
BRAGGER
CHIGGER
CHUGGED
CHUGGER
CLOGGED
CRAGGED
DRAGGED
DRAGGER
DRAGGLE
DRUGGED
FLAGGED
FLAGGER
FLOGGED
FLOGGER
FRAGGED
FRAGGLE
FROGGER
GLUGGED
PLUGGED
PLUGGER
QUAGGAS
SHAGGED
SLOGGED
SLOGGER
SLUGGED
SLUGGER
SMUGGER
SMUGGLE
SNAGGED
SNAGGER
SNUGGED
SNUGGER
SNUGGLE
SNUGGLY
STAGGED
STAGGER
SWAGGER
SWIGGED
TRIGGER
WRIGGLE
WRIGGLY

•••G•G•

BAGGAGE
FIZGIGS
LONGAGO
LUGGAGE
NONGOGO
OLDGAGS
ROUGHGO
VANGOGH

•••G••G

BAGGING
BANGING
BARGING
BEGGING
BINGING
BOGGING
BONGING
BUDGING
BUGGING
BULGING
BUNGING
CADGING
COGGING
DIGGING
DINGING
DODGING
DOGGING
FANGING
FOGGING
FORGING
FROGLEG
FUDGING
GAGGING
GANGING
GAUGING
GIGGING
GONGING
GORGING
GOUGING
HANGDOG
HANGING
HEDGING
HINGING
HOGGING
HUGGING
IMAGING
JAGGING
JIGGING
JOGGING
JUDGING
JUGGING
KEDGING
KEGGING
KINGING
LAGGING
LEGGING
LODGING
LOGGING
LONGING
LUGGING
LUNGING
MERGING
MUGGING
NAGGING
NUDGING
OURGANG
PARGING
PEGGING
PIGGING
PINGING
PURGING
RAGGING
RANGING
RIDGING
RIGGING
RINGING
ROUGING
SAGGING
SHAGRUG
SIEGING
SINGING
STAGING
SURGING
TAGGING
TANGING
THEGANG
TINGING
TOGGING
TONGING
TUGGING
UNAGING
VEGGING
VERGING
WAGGING
WEDGING
WIGGING
WINGING
ZAGGING
ZIGGING
ZINGING

••••GG•

BADEGGS
OWLEGGS
PILEGGI
RAWEGGS
SCRAGGY
SCRUGGS
TWOEGGS
UNBOGGY
UNFOGGY
UNSOGGY

••••G•G

DEMAGOG

•••••GG

EASTEGG
FTBRAGG
GOODEGG
IMAHOGG
JIMHOGG
KELLOGG
NESTEGG
WESTEGG

GH•••••

GHANIAN
GHASTLY
GHERKIN
GHETTOS
GHIJKLM
GHOSTED
GHOSTLY

G•H••••

GAHAGAN
GEHENNA

G••H•••

GASHEAT
GASHING
GASHOGS
GATHERS
GETHELP
GETHURT
GOAHEAD
GODHEAD
GODHOOD
GOPHERS
GOSHAWK
GOTHELP
GOTHICS
GOTHIKA
GOTHURT
GRAHAME
GRAHAMS
GUSHERS
GUSHIER
GUSHILY
GUSHING
GUSHOUT
GUTHRIE

G•••H••

GALAHAD
GASOHOL
GAUCHER
GAUCHOS
GEEWHIZ
GEISHAS
GENGHIS
GERSHON
GETAHIT
GETSHEP
GETSHIP
GETSHOT
GETTHIS
GINGHAM
GIRTHED
GLASHOW
GLYPHIC
GNASHED
GNASHER
GNASHES
GODTHAB
GOTAHIT
GOTCHAS
GRAPHED
GRAPHIC
GRESHAM
GREYHEN
GRISHAM
GRYPHON
GULCHES
GUMSHOE
GUNSHIP
GUNSHOT
GUNTHER
GURKHAS
GYMSHOE

G••••H•

GIRLSHY
GLITCHY
GNOCCHI
GOUACHE
GROUCHO
GROUCHY
GROWTHS
GULLAHS

G•••••H

GALUMPH
GARNISH
GAULISH
GAWKISH
GETCASH
GIRLISH
GNOMISH
GOATISH
GODUTCH
GOFORTH
GOIRISH
GOLIATH
GOODISH
GOOMBAH
GOSOUTH
GOTCASH
GOULASH
GOUTISH
GRAYISH
GREYISH
GWYNETH

•GH••••

FGHIJKL
OGHAMIC

•G•H•••

EGGHEAD
EGGHUNT

•G••H••

AGAKHAN
AGULHAS

•G•••H•

IGOTCHA

•G••••H

OGREISH

••GH•••

AFGHANI
AFGHANS
BAGHDAD
BIGHAIR
BIGHALF
BIGHAND
BIGHEAD
BIGHITS
BIGHORN
BIGHUGS
BOGHOLE
COGHLAN
DEGHOST
DOGHAIR
EFGHIJK
EGGHEAD
EGGHUNT
EIGHTAD
EIGHTAM
EIGHTBC
EIGHTEE
EIGHTHS
EIGHTPM
EIGHTUP
FIGHTER
FOGHORN
HIGHART
HIGHBAR
HIGHBOY
HIGHDAY
HIGHEND
HIGHEST
HIGHHAT
HIGHIQS
HIGHISH
HIGHLOW
HIGHPAY
HIGHRES
HIGHSEA
HIGHTEA
HIGHTOP
HIGHWAY
JUGHEAD
LEGHORN
LIGHTED
LIGHTEN
LIGHTER
LIGHTLY
LIGHTON
LIGHTUP
MIGHTNT
NIGHEST
NIGHTER
NIGHTIE
NIGHTLY
OUGHTNT
OUGHTTO
RIGHTED
RIGHTER
RIGHTLY
RIGHTON
SIGHERS
SIGHFOR
SIGHFUL
SIGHING
SIGHSAT
SIGHTED
SIGHTER
SIGHTLY
TIGHTEN
TIGHTER
TIGHTLY
YOGHURT

••G•H••

BAGEHOT
BIGSHOT
BIGSHOW
DOGCHEW
DOGCHOW
DOGSHOW
HIGHHAT
MEGAHIT
MEGOHMS
MUGSHOT
RAGSHOP
SAGEHEN

••G••H•

BIGJOHN
EIGHTHS
NOGUCHI

••G•••H

ANGUISH
BIGFISH
BIGGISH
BOGGISH
DIGRAPH
DOGFISH
DOGGISH
ENGLISH
FOGYISH
HAGGISH
HIGHISH
HOGARTH
HOGGISH
HOGWASH
JIGGISH
LOGGISH
MUGGISH
NAGGISH
PIGFISH
PIGGISH
PUGGISH
REGRAPH
ROGUISH
VOGUISH
WAGGISH

•••GH••

ALIGHTS
BINGHAM
BLIGHTS
BLIGHTY
BOUGHED
BRIGHAM
BRIGHTS
BULGHUR
BURGHER
COUGHED
COUGHUP
DEFGHIJ
DOUGHTY
DWIGHTD
FLIGHTS
FLIGHTY
FRIGHTS
FULGHUM
GENGHIS
GINGHAM
HAUGHTY
HEIGHHO
HEIGHTS
IEIGHTY
KEOGHAN
KNIGHTS
LANGHAM
LAUGHAT
LAUGHED
LAUGHER
LAUGHIN
MAUGHAM
NAUGHTS
NAUGHTY
NEIGHED
NOUGHTS
PLIGHTS
ROUGHED
ROUGHEN
ROUGHER
ROUGHGO
ROUGHIT
ROUGHLY
ROUGHUP
SLIGHTS
SORGHUM
TOUGHEN
TOUGHER
TOUGHIE
TOUGHLY
VAUGHAN
VEIGHTS
WEIGHED
WEIGHER
WEIGHIN
WEIGHON
WEIGHTS
WEIGHTY
WEIGHUP
WRIGHTS

•••G•H•

HEIGHHO
LENGTHS
LENGTHY

•••G••H

BIGGISH
BOGGISH
DOGGISH
HAGGISH
HOGGISH
JIGGISH
LARGISH
LOGGISH
LONGISH
MUGGISH
NAGGISH
OMIGOSH
OUTGUSH
PIGGISH
PUGGISH
VANGOGH
WAGGISH

••••GH•

ALRIGHT
ATEIGHT
ATNIGHT
ATSIGHT
BROUGHT
BYRIGHT
CDEFGHI
CHOUGHS
DELIGHT
DORIGHT
DRAUGHT
DROUGHT
ENRIGHT
FRAUGHT
FREIGHT
HUANGHE
INSIGHT
LEHIGHU
MRRIGHT
ONSIGHT
PLOUGHS
REFIGHT
RELIGHT
RESIGHT
SLEIGHS
SLEIGHT
SLOUGHS
THOUGHT
TONIGHT
TROUGHS
UNLIGHT
UNSIGHT
UPLIGHT
UPRIGHT
UPTIGHT
WROUGHT

•••••GH

ACEHIGH
AIMHIGH
BCDEFGH
BOROUGH
BRANAGH
DEBURGH
FLYHIGH
HOWHIGH
INVEIGH
OUTSIGH
RALEIGH
REWEIGH
SKYHIGH
THROUGH
TOOHIGH
UNTOUGH
VANGOGH
WANTAGH

GI•••••

GIACOMO
GIAUQUE
GIBBERS
GIBBONS
GIBBOUS
GIBESAT
GIBLETS
GIBLUES
GIBSONS
GIBUSES
GIDDIED
GIDDIER
GIDDIES
GIDDILY
GIDDYAP
GIDDYUP
GIDEONS
GIELGUD
GIFFORD
GIFTBOX
GIFTEES
GIFTING
GIFTSET
GIFTTAX
GIGABIT
GIGATON
GIGBAGS
GIGGING
GIGGLED
GIGGLER
GIGGLES
GIGOLOS
GILBERT
GILBLAS
GILDERS
GILDING
GILFORD
GILLIAM
GILLIAN
GILLING
GILLMAN
GILLNET
GILMORE
GIMBALS
GIMBELS
GIMLETS
GIMMICK
GIMPING
GINFIZZ
GINGAME
GINGERS
GINGERY
GINGHAM
GINGIVA
GINGKOS
GINGOLD
GINKGOS
GINMILL
GINNING
GINSENG
GIOCOSO
GIORGIO
GIORGOS
GIPSIES
GIRAFFE
GIRASOL
GIRDERS
GIRDING
GIRDLED
GIRDLER
GIRDLES
GIRLIER
GIRLIES
GIRLISH
GIRLSHY
GIROLLE
GIRONDE

GIRTHED
GIRTING
GISCARD
GISELLE
GISSING
GITANOS
GITTING
GIVEEAR
GIVENBY
GIVENIN
GIVENOF
GIVENON
GIVENTO
GIVENUP
GIVEOFF
GIVEOUT
GIVESIN
GIVESOF
GIVESON
GIVESTO
GIVESUP
GIVEUPS
GIVEWAY
GIZZARD

G•I••••

GAINERS
GAINFUL
GAINING
GAINSAY
GAINSON
GAITERS
GAITING
GEISHAS
GHIJKLM
GLIBBER
GLIDEBY
GLIDEIN
GLIDERS
GLIDING
GLIMMER
GLIMPSE
GLINTED
GLISTEN
GLISTER
GLITCHY
GLITTER
GLITZED
GLITZES
GOINFOR
GOINGAT
GOINGBY
GOINGIN
GOINGON
GOINGTO
GOINGUP
GOIRISH
GOITERS
GRIDDED
GRIDDER
GRIDDLE
GRIDMAP
GRIEVED
GRIEVER
GRIEVES
GRIFFEY
GRIFFIN
GRIFFON
GRIFTED
GRIFTER
GRIGRIS
GRILLED
GRILLER
GRILLES
GRIMACE
GRIMIER
GRIMILY
GRIMING
GRIMMER
GRIMSBY
GRINDER
GRINGOS
GRINKOV
GRINNED
GRINNER
GRINSAT
GRIPERS
GRIPING
GRIPPED
GRIPPER
GRIPPES
GRISHAM
GRISLET
GRISNEZ
GRISSOM
GRISTER
GRISTLE
GRISTLY
GRITTED
GRITTER
GRIZZLE
GRIZZLY
GUIDERS
GUIDING
GUIGNOL
GUILDER
GUILING
GUINEAN
GUINEAS
GUITARS

G••I•••

GALICIA
GALILEE
GALILEI
GALILEO
GAMIEST
GAMINES
GATINGS
GAVIALS
GAVILAN
GEFILTE
GELIDLY
GEMINIS
GENITOR
GERITOL
GETINON
GETINTO
GETITON
GLUIEST
GOFIRST
GOGIRLS
GOLIATH
GOOIEST
GORIEST
GORILLA
GOTINON
GOTINTO
GOTITON
GRAINED
GRAINER
GROINED
GUNITES

G•••I••

GABBIER
GABBING
GABRIEL
GADDING
GAFFING
GAGGING
GAGLINE
GAINING
GAITING
GALLICO
GALLING
GALLIUM
GAMBIAN
GAMBIER
GAMBITS
GAMMING
GANGING
GAOLING
GAPKIDS
GAPPING
GARBING
GARLICS
GARLITS
GARNISH
GARPIKE
GARRICK
GASEITY
GASHING
GASLINE
GASPING
GASPIPE
GASSIER
GASSING
GATLING
GATLINS
GATWICK
GAUDIER
GAUDIES
GAUDILY
GAUGING
GAULISH
GAUTIER
GAUZIER
GAUZILY
GAWKIER
GAWKILY
GAWKING
GAWKISH
GAWPING
GEARING
GEDRICK
GEEKIER
GELDING
GELLING
GEMLIKE
GEMMIER
GENOISE
GENTIAN
GENTILE
GENUINE
GERAINT
GERBILS
GERMIER
GETTING
GETWISE
GHANIAN
GIDDIED
GIDDIER
GIDDIES
GIDDILY
GIFTING
GIGGING
GILDING
GILLIAM
GILLIAN
GILLING
GIMMICK
GIMPING
GINFIZZ
GINGIVA
GINMILL
GINNING
GIPSIES
GIRDING
GIRLIER
GIRLIES
GIRLISH
GIRTING
GISSING
GITTING
GLACIAL
GLACIER
GLARING
GLAVINE
GLAZIER
GLAZILY
GLAZING
GLIDING
GLOBING
GLOBINS
GLORIAS
GLORIED
GLORIES
GLORIFY
GLOVING
GLOWING
GLYCINE
GNAWING
GNOMISH
GNOMIST
GOADING
GOALIES
GOAMISS
GOATISH
GOBLINS
GODLIER
GODLIKE
GODLING
GODWITS
GOIRISH
GOLDING
GOLFING
GONGING
GOODIES
GOODING
GOODISH
GOOFIER
GOOFILY
GOOFING
GOONIER
GOONIES
GOONILY
GOOPIER
GOOSIER
GOOSING
GORDIAN
GORDITA
GORDIUS
GORGING
GORMING
GORSIER
GOSLING
GOSSIPS
GOSSIPY
GOTHICS
GOTHIKA
GOTMILK
GOTWISE
GOUGING
GOUTIER
GOUTILY
GOUTISH
GOWNING
GRACIAS
GRACILE
GRACING
GRADING
GRANITA
GRANITE
GRAPIER
GRATIAS
GRATIFY
GRATING
GRAVIES
GRAVING
GRAVITY
GRAYING
GRAYISH
GRAZIER
GRAZING
GRECIAN
GRECISM
GRECIZE
GREYING
GREYISH
GRIMIER
GRIMILY
GRIMING
GRIPING
GRODIER
GROLIER
GROPING
GROPIUS
GROTIUS
GROWING
GRUNION
GSTRING
GUANINE
GUCKIER
GUIDING
GUILING
GULFING
GULLIED
GULLIES
GULLING
GULPIER
GULPING
GUMLIKE
GUMMIER
GUMMING
GUNFIRE
GUNKIER
GUNNIES
GUNNING
GUPPIES
GUSHIER
GUSHILY
GUSHING
GUSSIED
GUSSIES
GUSTIER
GUSTILY
GUSTING
GUTSIER
GUTSILY
GUTTIER
GUTTING
GYPPING
GYPSIES

G••••I•

GAGARIN
GALATIA
GALAXIE
GALICIA
GANGLIA
GASMAIN
GASTRIC
GAUGUIN
GEEWHIZ
GELATIN
GELATIS
GELUSIL
GEMINIS
GENERIC
GENERIS
GENESIS
GENETIC
GENGHIS
GENNAIO
GENOMIC
GEORGIA
GEORGIC
GEORGIE
GERMAIN
GERVAIS
GETAHIT
GETATIP
GETONIT
GETSFIT
GETSHIP
GETSRID
GETTHIS
GETTOIT
GHERKIN
GIGABIT
GIORGIO
GIVENIN
GIVESIN
GLIDEIN
GLOAMIN
GLOBOID
GLOTTIS
GLYNNIS
GLYPHIC
GLYPTIC
GNOSTIC
GOBELIN
GOBYAIR
GODEVIL
GOFORIT
GOINGIN
GOLDTIP
GONERIL
GOODAIM
GOODKID
GOODNIK
GOODWIN
GOTAHIT
GOTATIP
GOTONIT
GOTTOIT
GRANNIE
GRAPHIC
GREMLIN
GREWBIG
GREWDIM
GRIFFIN
GRIGRIS
GROOVIN
GROUPIE
GROWBIG
GROWDIM
GULFOIL
GUNSHIP
GUTHRIE
GYMSUIT

G•••••I

GALILEI
GALVANI
GEMELLI
GEORGEI
GNOCCHI
GOLDONI
GOURAMI
GUARANI

•GI••••

AGILELY
AGILEST
AGILITY
AGITATE
AGITATO
IGIVEUP

•G•I•••

AGAINST
AGEISTS
AGRIBIZ
AGRIPPA
EGGIEST
EGLISES
EGOISTE
EGOISTS
FGHIJKL
IGNITED
IGNITER
IGNITES
IGNITOR
UGLIEST

•G••I••

AGARICS
AGATINE
AGEFIVE
AGENINE
AGILITY
AGNAILS
AGONIES
AGONISE
AGONISM
AGONIST
AGONIZE
EGALITE
EGERIAS
EGGLIKE
EGOTISM
EGOTIST
IGRAINE
MGMLION
OGREISH
UGOLINO

•G•••I•

AGASSIZ
AGNATIC
AGOUTIS
AGRIBIZ
EGOTRIP
IGUANID
OGHAMIC

••GI•••

AEGISES
ALGIEBA
ALGIERS
AUGITES
BEGIRDS
BIGIDEA
CAGIEST
DIGICAM
DIGINTO
DIGIPET
DIGITAL
DUGINTO
EDGIEST
EDGINGS
EGGIEST
ENGILDS
ENGINED
ENGINES
ENGIRDS
GOGIRLS
HEGIRAS
HYGIEIA
HYGIENE
HYGINUS
ITGIRLS
LEGIBLE
LEGIBLY
LEGIONS
LEGIRON
LEGISTS
LOGICAL
LOGIEST
MAGICAL
MAGILLA
MAGINOT
MEGILLA
MYGIANT
NOGIFTS
NYGIANT
ORGIAST
PAGINGS
PIGIRON
RAGINGS
REGIFTS
REGILDS
REGIMEN
REGIMES
REGINAL
REGINAS
REGIONS
REGIRDS
REGIVEN
REGIVES
RIGIDLY
SAGIEST
SAGINAW
UNGIDDY
UNGIRDS
UNGIVEN
UPGIRDS
URGINGS
YOGIISM
YOGINIS

••G•I••

ANGLING
ANGRIER
ANGRILY
ANGUISH
ARGUING
BAGGIER
BAGGIES
BAGGILY
BAGGING
BAGGINS
BAGGIRL
BAGLIKE
BAGNIOS
BAGPIPE
BAGWIGS
BEGGING
BEGRIME
BEGUILE
BEGUINE
BIGBIRD
BIGCITY
BIGDIGS
BIGFISH
BIGFIVE
BIGGIES
BIGGIRL
BIGGISH
BIGGITY
BIGHITS
BIGKIDS
BIGLIES
BIGRIGS
BIGTIME
BIGWIGS
BIGWINS
BOGGIER
BOGGING
BOGGISH
BUGGIER
BUGGIES
BUGGING
BUGLING
COGGING
COGNIZE
DIGGING
DIGGITY
DIGNIFY
DIGNITY
DOGBITE
DOGFISH
DOGGIER
DOGGIES
DOGGING
DOGGISH
DOGLIKE
DOGPILE
DOGSITS
DOGTICK
EAGLING
EFGHIJK
EGGLIKE
ENGLISH
FOGCITY
FOGGIER
FOGGILY
FOGGING
FOGYISH
FOGYISM
GAGGING
GAGLINE
GIGGING
HAGGISH
HAGLIKE
HIGGINS
HIGHIQS
HIGHISH
HOGGING
HOGGISH
HOGLIKE
HOGTIED
HOGTIES
HOGWILD
HUGGIES
HUGGING
HUGGINS
IMGOING
INGOING
JAGGIER
JAGGIES
JAGGING
JIGGIER
JIGGING
JIGGISH
JIGLIKE
JIGTIME
JOGGING
JUGGING
JUGWINE
KEGGING
LAGGING
LEGGIER
LEGGING
LEGLIKE
LIGNIFY
LIGNINS
LIGNITE
LOGGIAS
LOGGING
LOGGINS
LOGGISH
LUGGING
MAGNIFY
MAGPIES
MAGUIRE
MCGRIFF
MCGUIRE
MCGWIRE
MEGRIMS
MUGGIER
MUGGING
MUGGISH
NAGGIER
NAGGING
NAGGISH
NOGGINS
ONGOING
OUGUIYA
PEGGING
PEGLIKE
PIGFISH
PIGGIER
PIGGIES
PIGGING
PIGGISH
PIGLIKE
PUGGISH
PYGMIES
RAGGIER
RAGGIES
RAGGING
RAGTIME
REGAINS
REGNIER
REGRIND
REGRIPS
REGUIDE
RIGGING
ROGAINE
ROGUING
ROGUISH
RUGLIKE
SAGGIER
SAGGING
SIGHING
SIGNIFY
SIGNING
SOGGIER
SOGGILY
TAGGING
TAGLIKE
TAGLINE
TOGGING
TUGGING
TUGRIKS
TVGUIDE
UNGRIPS
UPGOING
VEGGIES
VEGGING
VOGUING
VOGUISH
WAGGING
WAGGISH
WIGGIER
WIGGING
WIGLIKE
YOGIISM
ZAGGING
ZIGGING

••G••I•

ALGERIA
ANGELIC
ANGLAIS
ARGALIS
BEGONIA
BIGHAIR
BIGUNIT
CAGEDIN
DOGHAIR
DOGTAIL
EDGEDIN
EDGESIN
ENGRAIN
ERGOTIC
EUGENIA
EUGENIC
EUGENIE
GAGARIN
GIGABIT
HYGIEIA
INGRAIN
LIGURIA
LUGSAIL
MCGAVIN
MEGABIT
MEGAHIT
NIGERIA
NIGHTIE
ORGANIC
PAGESIX
PIGSKIN
PIGTAIL
REGALIA
SEGOVIA
SIGMOID
SIGNSIN
YOGINIS
ZAGAZIG

••G•••I

AFGHANI
ARGENTI
BUGATTI
MAGNANI
NEGRONI
NOGUCHI

•••GI••

ADAGIOS
ASAGIFT
BADGIRL
BAGGIER
BAGGIES
BAGGILY
BAGGING
BAGGINS
BAGGIRL
BANGING
BARGING
BATGIRL
BEGGING
BELGIAN
BELGIUM
BERGIUS
BIGGIES
BIGGIRL
BIGGISH
BIGGITY
BILGIER
BINGING
BOGGIER
BOGGING
BOGGISH
BONGING
BOOGIED
BOOGIES
BORGIAS
BUDGIES
BUDGING
BUGGIER
BUGGIES
BUGGING
BULGIER
BULGING
BUNGING
BUSGIRL
CADGING
CAMGIRL
COGGING
COWGIRL
DIGGING
DIGGITY
DINGIER
DINGILY
DINGING
DODGIER
DODGING
DOGGIER
DOGGIES
DOGGING
DOGGISH
DREGION
EADGILS
ELEGIAC
ELEGIES
ELEGIST
ELEGITS
ELEGIZE
ELIGIUS
FANGING
FIZGIGS
FLYGIRL
FOGGIER
FOGGILY
FOGGING
FORGING
FORGIVE
FRAGILE
FUDGING
GAGGING
GANGING
GAUGING
GIGGING
GINGIVA
GONGING
GORGING
GOUGING
HAGGISH
HANGING
HEDGIER

HEDGING
HIGGINS
HINGING
HOAGIES
HOGGING
HOGGISH
HUGGIES
HUGGING
HUGGINS
IMAGINE
IMAGING
IMAGISM
IMAGIST
JAGGIER
JAGGIES
JAGGING
JIGGIER
JIGGING
JIGGISH
JOGGING
JUDGING
JUGGING
JUNGIAN
KEDGING
KEGGING
KINGING
LAGGING
LARGISH
LEDGIER
LEGGIER
LEGGING
LODGING
LOGGIAS
LOGGING
LOGGINS
LOGGISH
LONGIES
LONGING
LONGISH
LUGGING
LUNGING
MANGIER
MARGINS
MERGING
MINGIER
MISGIVE
MUGGIER
MUGGING
MUGGISH
NAGGIER
NAGGING
NAGGISH
NOGGINS
NOOGIES
NUDGING
OLDGIRL
OLOGIES
ORIGINE
ORIGINS
OUTGIVE
PARGING
PEGGING
PIDGINS
PIGGIER
PIGGIES
PIGGING
PIGGISH
PINGING
PLUGINS
PONGIDS
PORGIES
PUDGIER
PUDGILY
PUGGISH
PURGING
RAGGIER
RAGGIES
RAGGING
RANGIER
RANGING
RIDGIER
RIDGING
RIGGING
RINGING
ROUGING
SAGGIER
SAGGING
SEAGIRT
SEDGIER
SIEGING
SINGING
SOGGIER
SOGGILY
STAGIER
STAGILY
STAGING
STOGIES
STYGIAN
SURGING
TAGGING
TANGIER
TANGING
THEGIFT
TINGING
TOGGING
TONGING
TUGGING
UNAGILE
UNAGING
VEGGIES
VEGGING
VERGING
VIRGINS
VOSGIAN
WAGGING
WAGGISH
WEDGIER
WEDGIES
WEDGING
WIGGIER
WIGGING
WINGING
ZAGGING
ZIGGING
ZINGIER
ZINGING

•••G•I•
ABIGAIL
ALEGRIA
BARGAIN
BARGEIN
CHAGRIN
DEFGHIJ
DOAGAIN
DRAGSIN
GANGLIA
GAUGUIN
GENGHIS
GRIGRIS
HANGSIN
KEYGRIP
KINGPIN
LANGUID
LAUGHIN
LODGEIN
NETGAIN
OUTGAIN
OUTGRIN
PENGUIN
PILGRIM
PINGUID
PLUGSIN
PREGAIN
RINGSIN
ROUGHIT
ROYGBIV
SANGRIA
SNUGFIT
SNUGLIS
TOUGHIE
TUNGOIL
WEDGEIN
WEIGHIN
WINGSIT
WINGTIP

•••G••I
BENGALI
BULGARI
DRAGOTI
ORIGAMI

••••GI•
ACINGIT
APHAGIA
APHAGIC
BRINGIN
BRINGIT
CRAIGIE
CUINGIN
DOINGIN
GEORGIA
GEORGIC
GEORGIE
GIORGIO
GOINGIN
ICINGIN
ICINGIT
ILLEGIT
ILLOGIC
KOSYGIN
MYALGIA
MYALGIC
OTALGIA
OTALGIC
PELAGIC
PERUGIA
PHRYGIA
REBEGIN
SLOEGIN
STREGIS
SWINGIT
SWUNGIT
TLINGIT
TYINGIN
UNRIGID
USINGIN

••••G•I
BENIGNI
CDEFGHI
GEORGEI
HUANGTI
PILEGGI
SHANGRI
ZWINGLI

•••••GI
PILEGGI
THEMAGI

GJ•••••
GJETOST

G•J••••
GUJARAT

G••J•••
GASJETS
GHIJKLM

G•••J••
GETAJOB
GOODJOB
GOODJOE
GOTAJOB
GRAYJAY

•G••J••
FGHIJKL

••GJ•••
BAGJOBS
BIGJAKE
BIGJERK
BIGJOHN
LOGJAMS

••G••J•
EFGHIJK

•••G••J
DEFGHIJ
LARGEOJ

G•K••••
GOKAPUT
GOKARTS

G••K•••
GAPKIDS
GASKELL
GASKETS
GAWKERS
GAWKIER
GAWKILY
GAWKING
GAWKISH
GAWKSAT
GECKOES
GEEKDOM
GEEKIER
GINKGOS
GROKKED
GUCKIER
GUNKIER
GURKHAS

G•••K••
GHERKIN
GHIJKLM
GINGKOS
GOODKID
GRACKLE
GRINKOV
GROKKED

G••••K•
GARPIKE
GEMLIKE
GOBROKE
GODLIKE
GOTHIKA
GRETZKY
GROMYKO
GUMLIKE

G•••••K
GANGTOK
GARRICK
GASLEAK
GASMASK
GASTANK
GATWICK
GEDRICK
GEMSBOK
GENLOCK
GEODUCK
GETBACK
GIMMICK
GOBLANK
GOODNIK
GOSHAWK
GOTBACK
GOTMILK
GUNLOCK
GYMSOCK

•G•K•••
AGAKHAN

•G•••K•
EGGLIKE
FGHIJKL

••GK•••
BIGKIDS

••G•K••
PIGSKIN

••G••K•
BAGLIKE
BIGJAKE
DOGLIKE
EGGLIKE
HAGLIKE
HOGLIKE
JIGLIKE
LEGLIKE
PEGLIKE
PIGLIKE
RUGLIKE
TAGLIKE
TUGRIKS
WIGLIKE

••G•••K
BIGJERK
BIGTALK
DOGTICK
EFGHIJK
FOGBANK
HOGBACK
LEGWORK
LOGBOOK

•••GK••
BANGKOK
GINGKOS
MONGKUT

•••G••K
BANGKOK
GANGTOK

••••G•K
DOINGOK

GL•••••
GLACEED
GLACIAL
GLACIER
GLADDEN
GLADDER
GLADEYE
GLAMORS
GLAMOUR
GLAMSUP
GLANCED
GLANCES
GLAREAT
GLARING
GLASGOW
GLASHOW
GLASSED
GLASSES
GLAVINE
GLAZERS
GLAZIER
GLAZILY
GLAZING
GLEAMED
GLEANED
GLEANER
GLEASON
GLEEFUL
GLEEMAN
GLEEMEN
GLENCOE
GLIBBER
GLIDEBY
GLIDEIN
GLIDERS
GLIDING
GLIMMER
GLIMPSE
GLINTED
GLISTEN
GLISTER
GLITCHY
GLITTER
GLITZED
GLITZES
GLOAMIN
GLOATED
GLOATER
GLOBATE
GLOBING
GLOBINS
GLOBOID
GLOBOSE
GLOBOUS
GLOBULE
GLOMMED
GLOOMED
GLORIAS
GLORIED
GLORIES
GLORIFY
GLORYBE
GLOSSAE
GLOSSAL
GLOSSAS
GLOSSED
GLOSSER
GLOSSES
GLOTTAL
GLOTTIS
GLOVING
GLOWERS
GLOWING
GLUCOSE
GLUEDON
GLUEDTO
GLUEGUN
GLUESON
GLUESTO
GLUGGED
GLUIEST
GLUMMED
GLUMMER
GLURGES
GLUTEAL
GLUTENS
GLUTEUS
GLUTTED
GLUTTON
GLYCINE
GLYCOLS
GLYNNIS
GLYPHIC
GLYPTIC

G•L••••
GALAHAD
GALANOS
GALANTS
GALATEA
GALATIA
GALAXES
GALAXIE
GALEATE
GALENAS
GALENTO
GALETTE
GALICIA
GALILEE
GALILEI
GALILEO
GALLANT
GALLEON
GALLERY
GALLEYS
GALLICO
GALLING
GALLIUM
GALLONS
GALLOPS
GALLOWS
GALOOTS
GALOPED
GALPALS
GALUMPH
GALVANI
GALVANO
GELATED
GELATES
GELATIN
GELATIS
GELATOS
GELCAPS
GELDING
GELIDLY
GELLING
GELPENS
GELUSIL
GILBERT
GILBLAS
GILDERS
GILDING
GILFORD
GILLIAM
GILLIAN
GILLING
GILLMAN
GILLNET
GILMORE
GOLDARN
GOLDBUG
GOLDING
GOLDMAN
GOLDONI
GOLDTIP
GOLDWYN
GOLFBAG
GOLFCAR
GOLFERS
GOLFING
GOLFPRO
GOLFTEE
GOLIATH
GULCHES
GULDENS
GULFING
GULFOIL
GULFWAR
GULLAHS
GULLETS
GULLIED
GULLIES
GULLING
GULPERS
GULPIER
GULPING

G••L•••
GAGLAWS
GAGLINE
GALLANT
GALLEON
GALLERY
GALLEYS
GALLICO
GALLING
GALLIUM
GALLONS
GALLOPS
GALLOWS
GAOLERS
GAOLING
GAPLESS
GARLAND
GARLICS
GARLITS
GASLAMP
GASLEAK
GASLESS
GASLINE
GASLOGS
GATLING
GATLINS
GAULISH
GAYLORD
GELLING
GEMLESS
GEMLIKE
GENLOCK
GEOLOGY
GETLOST
GIBLETS
GIBLUES
GIELGUD
GILLIAM
GILLIAN
GILLING
GILLMAN
GILLNET
GIMLETS
GIRLIER
GIRLIES
GIRLISH
GIRLSHY
GOALIES
GOALONG
GOBLANK
GOBLETS
GOBLINS
GODLESS
GODLIER
GODLIKE
GODLING
GOSLING
GOTLOST
GOULASH
GRILLED
GRILLER
GRILLES
GROLIER
GUILDER
GUILING
GULLAHS
GULLETS
GULLIED
GULLIES
GULLING
GUMLESS
GUMLIKE
GUNLAPS
GUNLAWS
GUNLESS
GUNLOCK
GUTLESS

G•••L••
GABBLED
GABBLES
GAGGLES
GALILEE
GALILEI
GALILEO
GAMBLED
GAMBLER
GAMBLES
GAMELAN
GAMELAW
GAMELEG
GANGLIA
GANTLET
GARBLED
GARBLER
GARBLES
GARGLED
GARGLER
GARGLES
GATELEG
GAVELED
GAVILAN
GAZELLE
GEFILTE
GEMELLI
GENTLED
GENTLER
GENTLES
GERALDO
GIGGLED
GIGGLER
GIGGLES
GIGOLOS
GILBLAS
GIRDLED
GIRDLER
GIRDLES
GIROLLE
GISELLE
GNARLED
GOBBLED
GOBBLER
GOBBLES
GOBELIN
GOBELOW
GOGGLED
GOGGLER
GOGGLES
GOOGLED
GOOGLER
GOOGLES
GORILLA
GRAVLAX
GRAYLAG
GREELEY
GREMLIN
GREYLAG
GRILLED
GRILLER
GRILLES
GRISLET
GROWLED
GROWLER
GUNPLAY
GURGLED
GURGLES
GUZZLED
GUZZLER
GUZZLES
GYMCLUB
GYRALLY

G••••L•
GAGRULE
GALPALS
GAMBOLS
GANDALF
GASKELL
GAUDILY
GAUNTLY
GAUZILY
GAVIALS
GAWKILY
GAZELLE
GELIDLY
GEMELLI
GENTILE
GERBILS
GESTALT
GETABLE
GETCOLD
GETHELP
GETSOLD
GETWELL
GHASTLY
GHIJKLM
GHOSTLY
GIDDILY
GIMBALS
GIMBELS
GINGOLD
GINMILL
GIROLLE
GISELLE
GLAZILY
GLOBULE
GLYCOLS
GOGIRLS
GONDOLA
GOODALL
GOOFILY
GOOGOLS
GOONILY
GORILLA
GOSPELS
GOSTALE
GOTCOLD
GOTHELP
GOTMILK
GOTWELL
GOUTILY
GRACILE
GRACKLE
GRANDLY
GRANOLA
GRANULE
GRAPPLE
GRASSLE
GRAVELS
GRAVELY
GREATLY
GREENLY
GREWOLD
GRIDDLE
GRIMILY
GRISTLE
GRISTLY
GRIZZLE
GRIZZLY
GROSSLY
GROVELS
GROWOLD
GRUFFLY
GRUMBLE
GRUMBLY
GUMBALL
GUNBELT
GUNMOLL
GUNSELS
GUNWALE
GUSHILY
GUSTILY
GUTSILY
GYMBALL
GYRALLY

G•••••L
GABRIEL
GAGREEL
GAINFUL
GAMETAL
GASKELL
GASOHOL
GELUSIL
GEMAYEL
GENERAL
GENTEEL
GERITOL
GETREAL
GETWELL
GINMILL
GIRASOL
GLACIAL
GLEEFUL
GLOSSAL
GLOTTAL
GLUTEAL
GODEVIL
GONERIL
GOODALL
GOTOGAL
GOTREAL
GOTWELL
GQMODEL
GRADUAL
GRAPNEL
GRENDEL
GUIGNOL
GULFOIL
GUMBALL
GUNMOLL
GYMBALL

•GL••••
EGLISES
OGLALAS
UGLIEST

•G•L•••
AGALLOP
AGELESS
AGELONG
AGILELY
AGILEST
AGILITY
AGULHAS
EGALITE
EGGLERS
EGGLESS
EGGLIKE
MGMLION
UGOLINO

•G••L••
AGALLOP
HGWELLS
OGLALAS

•G•••L•
AGILELY
AGNAILS
EGGROLL
HGWELLS
IGNOBLE
IGNOBLY

•G••••L
EGGROLL
FGHIJKL

••GL•••
AIGLETS
ANGLAIS
ANGLERS
ANGLING
BAGLADY
BAGLIKE
BIGLEAD
BIGLIES
BIGLOTS
BIGLOVE
BUGLERS
BUGLING
DEGLAZE
DIGLOTS
DOGLEGS
DOGLESS
DOGLIKE
EAGLETS
EAGLING
EGGLERS
EGGLESS
EGGLIKE
ENGLAND
ENGLISH
ENGLUND
ENGLUTS

EUGLENA
FIGLEAF
FOGLAMP
FOGLESS
GAGLAWS
GAGLINE
HAGLIKE
HOGLIKE
INGLESE
JAGLESS
JIGLIKE
KEGLERS
LEGLESS
LEGLIKE
MAGLEVS
NEGLECT
PEGLEGS
PEGLESS
PEGLIKE
PIGLETS
PIGLIKE
RAGLANS
REGLAZE
REGLOSS
REGLOWS
REGLUED
REGLUES
RUGLIKE
TAGLIKE
TAGLINE
TIGLONS
TUGLESS
UNGLOVE
UNGLUED
UNGLUES
WIGLESS
WIGLETS
WIGLIKE

••G•L••

ANGELAS
ANGELES
ANGELIC
ANGELOU
ANGELUS
ANGOLAN
ANGULAR
ARGALIS
ARGYLES
BIGBLUE
BIGELOW
BOGGLED
BOGGLER
BOGGLES
BUGALOO
BUGGLES
BYGOLLY
COGGLES
COGHLAN
DOGFLEA
DOGSLED
ELGALLO
ENGILDS
ENGULFS
FUGALLY
GAGGLES
GIGGLED
GIGGLER
GIGGLES
GIGOLOS
GOGGLED
GOGGLER
GOGGLES
HAGGLED
HAGGLER
HAGGLES
HIGGLED
HIGGLER
HIGGLES
HIGHLOW
HYGELAC
INGALLS
INGULFS
JIGGLED
JIGGLES
JOGGLED
JOGGLER
JOGGLES
JUGGLED
JUGGLER
JUGGLES
JUGULAR
LEGALLY
LEGOLAS
MAGALOG
MAGILLA
MEGALON
MEGILLA
MUGGLES
NIGGLED
NIGGLER
NIGGLES
NOGALES
PUGGLES
PUGSLEY
REGALED
REGALER
REGALES
REGALIA
REGALLY
REGILDS
REGULAR
REGULUS
RUGGLES
TAGALOG
TOGGLED
TOGGLER
TOGGLES
UNGULAE
UNGULAR
WAGGLED
WAGGLER
WAGGLES
WIGGLED
WIGGLER
WIGGLES

••G••L•

ANGRILY
BAGFULS
BAGGILY
BAGNOLD
BAGWELL
BEGUILE
BIGGULP
BIGHALF
BIGSALE
BIGTALK
BOGHOLE
BOGUSLY
BYGOLLY
DOGPILE
EAGERLY
EGGROLL
ELGALLO
FOGGILY
FUGALLY
GAGRULE
GOGIRLS
HOGCALL
HOGWILD
INGALLS
INGOALS
ITGIRLS
JUGFULS
LEGALLY
LEGIBLE
LEGIBLY
LEGPULL
LIGHTLY
LOGROLL
MAGILLA
MEGILLA
MUGFULS
NIGHTLY
RAGDOLL
REGALLY
RIGHTLY
RIGIDLY
SIGHTLY
SIGNALS
SOGGILY
TAGSALE
TIGHTLY
UNGODLY
VAGUELY
VIGNOLA

••G•••L

AUGURAL
BAGGIRL
BAGWELL
BIGDEAL
BIGGIRL
BIGMEAL
DIGITAL
DOGBOWL
DOGTAIL
EGGROLL
FIGURAL
GAGREEL
HOGCALL
LEGPULL
LOGICAL
LOGROLL
LUGSAIL
MAGICAL
PIGTAIL
RAGDOLL
RAGEFUL
REGINAL
SIGHFUL
VEGETAL

•••GL••

AIRGLOW
BANGLED
BANGLES
BEAGLES
BINGLES
BOGGLED
BOGGLER
BOGGLES
BORGLUM
BUGGLES
BUNGLED
BUNGLER
BUNGLES
BURGLAR
BURGLED
BURGLES
COGGLES
DANGLED
DANGLER
DANGLES
DINGLES
DONGLES
DOUGLAS
FROGLEG
FROGLET
GAGGLES
GANGLIA
GARGLED
GARGLER
GARGLES
GIGGLED
GIGGLER
GIGGLES
GOGGLED
GOGGLER
GOGGLES
GOOGLED
GOOGLER
GOOGLES
GURGLED
GURGLES
HAGGLED
HAGGLER
HAGGLES
HIGGLED
HIGGLER
HIGGLES
HOTGLUE
JANGLED
JANGLER
JANGLES
JIGGLED
JIGGLES
JINGLED
JINGLER
JINGLES
JOGGLED
JOGGLER
JOGGLES
JUGGLED
JUGGLER
JUGGLES
JUNGLES
KINGLET
LANGLEY
MANGLED
MANGLER
MANGLES
MEAGLES
MINGLED
MINGLER
MINGLES
MUGGLES
NIGGLED
NIGGLER
NIGGLES
OUTGLOW
PUGGLES
QUIGLEY
RINGLET
RUGGLES
SINGLED
SINGLES
SINGLET
SNIGLET
SNUGLIS
SUNGLOW
TAMGLEN
TANGLED
TANGLER
TANGLES
TINGLED
TINGLER
TINGLES
TOGGLED
TOGGLER
TOGGLES
UNOGLED
WAGGLED
WAGGLER
WAGGLES
WANGLED
WANGLER
WANGLES
WIGGLED
WIGGLER
WIGGLES
WINGLET
WRIGLEY
ZIEGLER

•••G•L•

ARUGULA
BAGGILY
BENGALI
BENGALS
BIGGULP
CHAGALL
CUDGELS
DANGELO
DINGILY
DRAGGLE
EADGILS
FINGALS
FOGGILY
FRAGGLE
FRAGILE
GINGOLD
GOOGOLS
LARGELY
LINGULA
MONGOLS
NONGOLD
OLDGOLD
PERGOLA
PLUGOLA
PUDGILY
ROUGHLY
SEAGULL
SMUGGLE
SNUGGLE
SNUGGLY
SOGGILY
STAGILY
TANGELO
THEGOLD
TOMGOLA
TOUGHLY
UNAGILE
VIRGULE
WRIGGLE
WRIGGLY

•••G••L

ABIGAIL
APOGEAL
BADGIRL
BAGGIRL
BATGIRL
BIGGIRL
BUSGIRL
CAMGIRL
CHAGALL
CONGEAL
COWGIRL
FLYGIRL
GUIGNOL
LINGUAL
MONGREL
OLDGIRL
OWNGOAL
SEAGULL
SONGFUL
SUBGOAL
TUNGOIL

••••GL•

ATINGLE
DRAGGLE
FINAGLE
FLEEGLE
FRAGGLE
FROOGLE
KRINGLE
PRINGLE
SHINGLE
SHINGLY
SMUGGLE
SNUGGLE
SNUGGLY
SPANGLE
SPANGLY
WRANGLE
WRIGGLE
WRIGGLY
WRONGLY
ZWINGLI

••••G•L

BRUEGEL
CITYGAL
DONEGAL
EVANGEL
FARMGAL
GOTOGAL
HAIRGEL
ILLEGAL
NOANGEL
ORTEGAL
SENEGAL
SMEAGOL
SOFTGEL
SPIEGEL
STENGEL
UNLEGAL
UNREGAL
WOLFGAL
WRANGEL

G•M••••

GAMBADO
GAMBIAN
GAMBIER
GAMBITS
GAMBLED
GAMBLER
GAMBLES
GAMBOLS
GAMEBAG
GAMEBOY
GAMELAN
GAMELAW
GAMELEG
GAMETAL
GAMETES
GAMIEST
GAMINES
GAMMERS
GAMMING
GAMMONS
GEMAYEL
GEMELLI
GEMINIS
GEMLESS
GEMLIKE
GEMMATE
GEMMIER
GEMSBOK
GIMBALS
GIMBELS
GIMLETS
GIMMICK
GIMPING
GOMPERS
GOMODEL
GUMBALL
GUMBOOT
GUMDROP
GUMLESS
GUMLIKE
GUMMIER
GUMMING
GUMSHOE
GUMTREE
GUMWOOD
GYMBAGS
GYMBALL
GYMCLUB
GYMNAST
GYMRATS
GYMSHOE
GYMSOCK
GYMSUIT

G••M•••

GAMMERS
GAMMING
GAMMONS
GARMENT
GASMAIN
GASMASK
GEMMATE
GEMMIER
GERMAIN
GERMANE
GERMANS
GERMANY
GERMIER
GILMORE
GIMMICK
GINMILL
GLAMORS
GLAMOUR
GLAMSUP
GLIMMER
GLIMPSE
GLOMMED
GLUMMED
GLUMMER
GNOMISH
GNOMIST
GNOMONS
GOAMISS
GODMAMA
GOOMBAH
GOOMBAY
GORMING
GOTMILK
GRAMMAR
GRAMMER
GRAMMES
GRAMMYS
GRAMPAS
GRAMPUS
GREMLIN
GRIMACE
GRIMIER
GRIMILY
GRIMING
GRIMMER
GRIMSBY
GROMMET
GROMYKO
GRUMBLE
GRUMBLY
GRUMMAN
GRUMPED
GUMMIER
GUMMING
GUNMOLL

G•••M••

GALUMPH
GASSMAN
GATEMAN
GATEMEN
GENOMES
GENOMIC
GETSMAD
GILLMAN
GLEAMED
GLEEMAN
GLEEMEN
GLIMMER
GLOAMIN
GLOMMED
GLOOMED
GLUMMED
GLUMMER
GOESMAD
GOLDMAN
GONEMAD
GOODMAN
GOODMEN
GOURMET
GRAMMAR
GRAMMER
GRAMMES
GRAMMYS
GRAUMAN
GRIDMAP
GRIMMER
GROMMET
GROOMED
GROOMER
GRUMMAN

G••••M•

GASLAMP
GASPUMP
GAUTAMA
GENZYME
GIACOMO
GINGAME
GODMAMA
GOURAMI
GRAHAME
GRAHAMS
GRANDMA
GYPSUMS

G•••••M

GALLIUM
GEEKDOM
GEORGEM
GETFROM
GETWARM
GHIJKLM
GILLIAM
GINGHAM
GOGETEM
GOODAIM
GOTWARM
GRANDAM
GRECISM
GRESHAM
GREWDIM
GRISHAM
GRISSOM
GROWDIM
GUARGUM
GUNROOM

•GM••••

MGMLION

•G•M•••

AGEMATE

•G••M••

AGNOMEN
OGHAMIC

•G••••M

AGENDUM
AGONISM
EGOTISM

••GM•••

AUGMENT
BIGMACS
BIGMAMA
BIGMEAL
BIGMESS
DOGMATA
FIGMENT
PIGMEAT
PIGMENT
PYGMIES
RAGMANS
RAGMOPS
SEGMENT
SIGMOID
SIGMUND

••G•M••

BOGYMAN
BOGYMEN
INGEMAR
LEGUMES
MOGAMBO
REGIMEN
REGIMES
TAGAMET
TVGAMES
YOGAMAT

••G••M•

BEGRIME
BIGGAME
BIGMAMA
BIGNAME
BIGTIME
DEGERMS
DIGRAMS
DOGCOMB
ENGRAMS
FOGLAMP
JIGTIME
LOGJAMS
MAGNUMS
MEGOHMS
MEGRIMS
MUGWUMP
RAGTIME
WIGWAMS

••G•••M

DIGICAM
EIGHTAM
EIGHTPM
FOGYISM
GOGETEM
LEGROOM
LUGWORM
REGROOM
TAGTEAM
YOGIISM

•••GM••

BERGMAN
ENIGMAS
FLAGMAN
FLAGMEN
FROGMAN
FROGMEN
HANGMAN
HANGMEN
KINGMAN
KLUGMAN
STIGMAS
SWAGMAN
SWAGMEN
SYNGMAN
WINGMAN
WINGMEN

•••G•M•

BERGAMO
BIGGAME
CONGAME
DAYGAME
DODGEMS
ENDGAME
EXOGAMY
GINGAME
NBAGAME
NETGAME
NFLGAME
NHLGAME
ORIGAMI
OUTGAME
PREGAME
PUBGAME
THEGAME
TIEGAME
WARGAME

•••G••M

ANAGRAM
BELGIUM
BINGHAM
BORGLUM
BRIGHAM
DIAGRAM
EPIGRAM
FULGHUM
GINGHAM
IMAGISM
ISOGRAM
KINGDOM
LANGHAM
LONGARM
LONGTOM
MAUGHAM
ONEGRAM
PANGRAM
PILGRIM
PROGRAM
SEAGRAM
SORGHUM
TANGRAM
TRIGRAM

••••GM•

PHLEGMY
YOUNGMC

••••G•M

AMALGAM
CHEWGUM
GEORGEM
GUARGUM
RITAGAM

GN•••••

GNARLED
GNARRED
GNASHED
GNASHER
GNASHES
GNAWERS
GNAWING
GNAWSAT
GNAWSON
GNOCCHI
GNOMISH
GNOMIST
GNOMONS
GNOSSUS
GNOSTIC

G•N••••

GANDALF
GANDERS
GANGERS
GANGING
GANGLIA
GANGSAW
GANGSTA
GANGSUP
GANGTOK
GANGWAY
GANNETS
GANNETT
GANTLET
GENDERS
GENERAL
GENERIC
GENERIS
GENESEE
GENESES
GENESET
GENESIS
GENETIC
GENEVAN
GENGHIS
GENITOR
GENLOCK
GENNAIO
GENNARO
GENOESE
GENOISE
GENOMES
GENOMIC
GENTEEL
GENTIAN
GENTILE
GENTLED
GENTLER
GENTLES
GENUINE
GENUSES
GENXERS
GENZYME
GINFIZZ
GINGAME
GINGERS
GINGERY
GINGHAM
GINGIVA
GINGKOS
GINGOLD
GINKGOS
GINMILL
GINNING
GINSENG
GONDOLA
GONEAFT
GONEAPE
GONEBAD
GONEFAR
GONEFOR
GONEMAD
GONEOFF
GONEOUT
GONEPRO
GONERIL
GONGING
GONGORA
GONZAGA
GUNBELT
GUNBOAT
GUNCASE
GUNDOGS
GUNFIRE
GUNITES
GUNKIER
GUNLAPS
GUNLAWS
GUNLESS
GUNLOCK
GUNMOLL
GUNNERS
GUNNERY
GUNNIES
GUNNING
GUNPLAY
GUNROOM
GUNSELS
GUNSFOR
GUNSHIP
GUNSHOT
GUNTHER
GUNUSER
GUNWALE

G••N•••

GAINERS
GAINFUL
GAINING
GAINSAY
GAINSON
GANNETS
GANNETT
GARNEAU
GARNERS
GARNETS

GARNETT
GARNISH
GAUNTER
GAUNTLY
GAYNESS
GENNAIO
GENNARO
GHANIAN
GINNING
GLANCED
GLANCES
GLENCOE
GLINTED
GLYNNIS
GOINFOR
GOINGAT
GOINGBY
GOINGIN
GOINGON
GOINGTO
GOINGUP
GOONEYS
GOONIER
GOONIES
GOONILY
GOUNDER
GOWNING
GRANADA
GRANARY
GRANDAM
GRANDEE
GRANDER
GRANDLY
GRANDMA
GRANDPA
GRANGER
GRANGES
GRANITA
GRANITE
GRANNIE
GRANOLA
GRANPAS
GRANTED
GRANTEE
GRANTER
GRANTOR
GRANULE
GRENADA
GRENADE
GRENDEL
GRINDER
GRINGOS
GRINKOV
GRINNED
GRINNER
GRINSAT
GRUNGER
GRUNGES
GRUNION
GRUNTED
GRUNTER
GUANACO
GUANINE
GUINEAN
GUINEAS
GUNNERS
GUNNERY
GUNNIES
GUNNING
GURNEYS
GUVNORS
GWYNETH
GYMNAST

G•••N••

GALANOS
GALANTS
GALENAS
GALENTO
GAMINES
GARDNER
GARONNE
GATINGS
GEHENNA
GEMINIS
GERENTS
GERUNDS
GETINON
GETINTO
GETONIT
GETONTO
GILLNET
GIRONDE
GITANOS
GIVENBY
GIVENIN
GIVENOF
GIVENON
GIVENTO
GIVENUP
GLEANED
GLEANER
GLYNNIS
GODUNOV
GOODNIK
GORTNER
GOTINON
GOTINTO
GOTONIT
GOTONTO
GRAINED
GRAINER
GRANNIE
GRAPNEL
GREENED
GREENER
GREENLY
GRINNED
GRINNER
GRISNEZ
GROANED
GROANER
GROINED
GROUNDS
GROWNON
GROWNUP
GUIGNOL
GYRENES

G••••N•

GABBANA
GABBING
GADDING
GAETANO
GAFFING
GAGGING
GAGLINE
GAINING
GAITING
GALLANT
GALLING
GALLONS
GALVANI
GALVANO
GAMMING
GAMMONS
GANGING
GAOLING
GAPPING
GARBING
GARCONS
GARDENA
GARDENS
GARLAND
GARMENT
GARONNE
GASCANS
GASCONS
GASCONY
GASHING
GASLINE
GASPING
GASSING
GASTANK
GASTONE
GATLING
GATLINS
GAUDENS
GAUGING
GAWKING
GAWPING
GEARING
GEHENNA
GELDING
GELLING
GELPENS
GENUINE
GERAINT
GERMANE
GERMANS
GERMANY
GETBENT
GETDONE
GETSANA
GETSANF
GETTING
GIBBONS
GIBSONS
GIDEONS
GIFTING
GIGGING
GILDING
GILLING
GIMPING
GINNING
GINSENG
GIRDING
GIRTING
GISSING
GITTING
GLARING
GLAVINE
GLAZING
GLIDING
GLOBING
GLOBINS
GLOVING
GLOWING
GLUTENS
GLYCINE
GNAWING
GNOMONS
GOADING
GOALONG
GOBLANK
GOBLINS
GODLING
GODSEND
GODSENT
GODSONS
GOLDING
GOLDONI
GOLFING
GONGING
GOODING
GOODONE
GOOFING
GOOSING
GORGING
GORGONS
GORMING
GOROUND
GOSLING
GOTDONE
GOUGING
GOVERNS
GOWNING
GOWRONG
GRACING
GRADING
GRATING
GRAVING
GRAYING
GRAZING
GREYING
GRIMING
GRIPING
GROPING
GROWING
GSTRING
GUANINE
GUARANI
GUIDING
GUILING
GULDENS
GULFING
GULLING
GULPING
GUMMING
GUNNING
GUSHING
GUSTING
GUTTING
GYPPING

G•••••N

GADSDEN
GAGARIN
GAHAGAN
GAINSON
GALLEON
GAMBIAN
GAMELAN
GASMAIN
GASOVEN
GASSMAN
GATEMAN
GATEMEN
GAUGUIN
GAVILAN
GAZEDON
GAZESON
GELATIN
GENEVAN
GENTIAN
GERMAIN
GERSHON
GETDOWN
GETEVEN
GETINON
GETITON
GETUPON
GGORDON
GHANIAN
GHERKIN
GIGATON
GILLIAN
GILLMAN
GIVENIN
GIVENON
GIVESIN
GIVESON
GLADDEN
GLEASON
GLEEMAN
GLEEMEN
GLIDEIN
GLISTEN
GLOAMIN
GLUEDON
GLUEGUN
GLUESON
GLUTTON
GNAWSON
GOBELIN
GOINGIN
GOINGON
GOLDARN
GOLDMAN
GOLDWYN
GOODMAN
GOODMEN
GOODSON
GOODWIN
GORDIAN
GOTDOWN
GOTEVEN
GOTINON
GOTITON
GOTUPON
GRAFTON
GRATEON
GRAUMAN
GRAYSON
GREATEN
GRECIAN
GREMLIN
GREYHEN
GRIFFIN
GRIFFON
GROOVIN
GROWNON
GROWSON
GRUMMAN
GRUNION
GRYPHON
GUDGEON
GUERDON
GUINEAN

•GN••••

AGNAILS
AGNATES
AGNATIC
AGNOMEN
IGNARRO
IGNATOW
IGNEOUS
IGNITED
IGNITER
IGNITES
IGNITOR
IGNOBLE
IGNOBLY
IGNORED
IGNORER
IGNORES

•G•N•••

AGENCES
AGENDAS
AGENDUM
AGENINE
AGENTED
AGENTRY
AGONIES
AGONISE
AGONISM
AGONIST
AGONIZE
EGGNOGS
UGANDAN

•G••N••

AGAINST
IGUANAS
IGUANID
OGDENUT

•G•••N•

AGATINE
AGELONG
AGENINE
AGROUND
EGGHUNT
IGRAINE
UGOLINO

•G••••N

AGAKHAN
AGNOMEN
AGREEON
EGGEDON
GGORDON
MGMLION
UGANDAN

••GN•••

BAGNIOS
BAGNOLD
BIGNAME
BIGNESS
BIGNEWS
BIGNOSE
COGNACS
COGNATE
COGNIZE
CYGNETS
DIGNIFY
DIGNITY
DOGNAPS
EGGNOGS
HOGNOSE
HOGNUTS
LIGNIFY
LIGNINS
LIGNITE
LUGNUTS
MAGNANI
MAGNATE
MAGNETO
MAGNETS
MAGNIFY
MAGNUMS
MIGNONS
PIGNUTS
PUGNOSE
REGNANT
REGNARD
REGNIER
SIGNAGE
SIGNALS
SIGNEES
SIGNERS
SIGNETS
SIGNFOR
SIGNIFY
SIGNING
SIGNOFF
SIGNORA
SIGNORE
SIGNORS
SIGNOUT
SIGNSIN
SIGNSON
SIGNSUP
SIGNUPS
VIGNOLA
ZAGNUTS

••G•N••

ARGANTE
ARGENTI
ARGENTO
ARGENTS
ARGONNE
AUGENDS
BEGANTO
BEGONIA
BIGENDS
BIGONES
BIGUNIT
BYGONES
COGENCY
DIGINTO
DUGINTO
DUGONGS
EDGINGS
ENGINED
ENGINES
EUGENIA
EUGENIC
EUGENIE
FAGENDS
HYGINUS
INGENUE
LAGUNAS
LEGANZA
LEGENDS
LIGANDS
LOGANUT
LOGONTO
MAGENTA
MAGINOT
MEGANES
MIGENES
ORGANDY
ORGANIC
ORGANZA
PAGINGS
RAGINGS
REGENCY
REGENTS
REGINAL
REGINAS
SAGINAW
TAGENDS
URGENCY
URGINGS
WAGONED
WAGONER
WEGENER
YOGINIS

••G••N•

AFGHANI
AFGHANS
ANGLING
ARGONNE
ARGUING
AUGMENT
BAGGING
BAGGINS
BEGGING
BEGUINE
BIGBAND
BIGBANG
BIGBEND
BIGFANS
BIGGUNS
BIGHAND
BIGTENT
BIGWINS
BOGGING
BUGGING
BUGLING
COGGING
DIGGING
DOGBANE
DOGBONE
DOGGING
DOGGONE
DOGRUNS
EAGLING
EGGHUNT
ENGLAND
ENGLUND
EUGLENA
FIGMENT
FOGBANK
FOGGING
GAGGING
GAGLINE
GIGGING
HIGGINS
HIGHEND
HOGGING
HUGGING
HUGGINS
HYGIENE
IMGOING
INGOING
JAGGING
JIGGING
JOGGING
JUGBAND
JUGGING
JUGWINE
KEGGING
LAGGING
LAGOONS
LEGBONE
LEGGING
LEGIONS
LEGRAND
LIGNINS
LOGGING
LOGGINS
LUGGING
MAGNANI
MIGHTNT
MIGNONS
MIGRANT
MUGGING
MYGIANT
NAGGING
NEGRONI
NOGGINS
NYGIANT
ONGOING
OUGHTNT
PAGEANT
PAGEONE
PEGGING
PIGEONS
PIGGING
PIGMENT
PIGPENS
RAGGING
RAGLANS
RAGMANS
REGAINS
REGIONS
REGNANT
REGRANT
REGRIND
RIGGING
ROGAINE
ROGUING
SAGGING
SEGMENT
SIGHING
SIGMUND
SIGNING
TAGGANT
TAGGING
TAGLINE
TIGLONS
TOGGING
TUGGING
UNGRAND
UNGUENT
UPGOING
USGRANT
VAGRANT
VEGGING
VOGUING
WAGGING
WIGGING
ZAGGING
ZIGGING

••G•••N

ALGREEN
ANGOLAN
BIGHORN
BIGJOHN
BIGTOWN
BOGDOWN
BOGYMAN
BOGYMEN
CAGEDIN
COGBURN
COGHLAN
EDGEDIN
EDGESIN
EGGEDON
ENGRAIN
FOGHORN
GAGARIN
GIGATON
INGRAIN
INGREEN
INGROWN
LEGHORN
LEGIRON
LIGHTEN
LIGHTON
MCGAVIN
MEGALON
MEGATON
MEGRYAN
MRGREEN
PIGIRON
PIGSKIN
REGIMEN
REGIVEN
REGROWN
RIGHTON
SAGEHEN
SIGNSIN
SIGNSON
TIGHTEN
UNGIVEN
UNGREEN
UNGROWN
UPGROWN
URGEDON
URGESON

•••GN••

ALIGNED
ALIGNER
AVIGNON
BEIGNES
BEIGNET
CHIGNON
COIGNED
COIGNES
DEIGNED
DEIGNTO
DRAGNET
FEIGNED
FEIGNER
GUIGNOL
LORGNON
OUTGNAW
REIGNED
SOIGNEE
STAGNES
WINGNUT

•••G•N•

AIRGUNS
ALLGONE
BAGGING
BAGGINS
BANGING
BARGING
BEGGING
BENGUNN
BIGGUNS
BINGING
BOGGING
BONGING
BRIGAND
BROGANS
BUDGING
BUGGING
BULGING
BUNGING
CADGING
CAPGUNS
COAGENT
COGGING
DIGGING
DINGING
DODGING
DOGGING
DOGGONE
DRAGONS
ELEGANT
EPIGONE
ERIGENA
EXIGENT
FANGING
FARGOND
FARGONE
FLAGONS
FOGGING
FORGING
FORGONE
FUDGING
FULGENT
GAGGING
GANGING
GAUGING
GIGGING
GONGING
GORGING
GORGONS
GOUGING
HANGING
HEDGING
HIGGINS
HINGING
HOGGING
HUGGING
HUGGINS
HUYGENS
IMAGINE
IMAGING
IMOGENE
ISOGONS
ITSGONE
JAGGING
JARGONS
JARGONY
JERGENS
JETGUNS
JIGGING
JOGGING
JUDGING
JUGGING
JURGENS
KEDGING
KEGGING
KINGING
LAGGING
LARGENT
LEGGING
LEOGENN
LODGING
LOGGING
LOGGINS
LONGING
LUGGING
LUNGING
MAJGENS
MANGANO
MARGINS
MERGING
MORGANA
MORGANS
MUGGING
NAGGING
NEOGENE
NOGGINS
NUDGING
OREGANO
ORIGINE
ORIGINS
OROGENY
OURGANG
OUTGUNS
PARGING
PEGGING
PIDGINS
PIGGING
PINGING
PLUGINS
POPGUNS
PROGENY
PUNGENT
PURGING
RAGGING
RANGING
RAYGUNS
REAGANS
REAGENT
RIDGING
RIGGING
RINGING
ROUGING
SAGGING
SARGENT
SHOGUNS
SIEGING
SINGING
SIXGUNS
SLOGANS
STAGING
SURGING
TAGGANT
TAGGING
TANGENT
TANGING
THEGANG
TINGING
TOGGING
TONGANS
TONGING
TOPGUNS
TOYGUNS
TRIGONS
TUGGING
UNAGING
VEGGING
VERGING
VIRGINS
WAGGING
WEDGING
WIGGING
WINGING
YEVGENY
ZAGGING
ZIGGING
ZINGING
ZIPGUNS

•••G••N

APOGEAN
ARAGORN
AVIGNON
BANGSON
BARGAIN
BARGEIN
BELGIAN
BENGUNN
BERGMAN
BERGSON
BOBGOEN
BURGEON
CHAGRIN
CHIGNON
DOAGAIN
DODGSON
DRAGOON
DRAGSIN
DRAGSON
DREGION
DUDGEON
DUNGEON
FLAGMAN

FLAGMEN
FROGMAN
FROGMEN
GAUGUIN
GUDGEON
HANGMAN
HANGMEN
HANGSIN
HANGSON
HANGTEN
HINGEON
HUNGTEN
JUNGIAN
KEOGHAN
KINGMAN
KINGPIN
KLUGMAN
LANGDON
LANGTON
LAUGHIN
LEOGENN
LODGEIN
LONGDEN
LONGRUN
LONGTON
LORGNON
NETGAIN
NUNGWEN
OUTGAIN
OUTGRIN
PENGUIN
PIDGEON
PLUGSIN
PREGAIN
RANGOON
RINGSIN
ROUGHEN
SEAGREN
STYGIAN
SURGEON
SWAGMAN
SWAGMEN
SYNGMAN
TAMGLEN
TEAGOWN
THIGPEN
TOUGHEN
VAUGHAN
VERGEON
VIRGOAN
VOSGIAN
WEDGEIN
WEIGHIN
WEIGHON
WIDGEON
WINGMAN
WINGMEN

••••GN•

ASSIGNS
ATSIGNS
BENIGNI
BENIGNO
BOLOGNA
COLOGNE
COSIGNS
DESIGNS
ENSIGNS
EPERGNE
IMPUGNS
INSIGNE
LASAGNA
LASAGNE
MALIGNS
MUSIGNY
OPPUGNS
REPUGNS
RESIGNS
SEVIGNY

••••G•N

ANTIGEN
ANTIGUN
ATTYGEN
BERIGAN
BLOWGUN
BRENGUN
BRINGIN
BRINGON
BURPGUN
CRYOGEN
CUINGIN
DARTGUN
DECAGON
DOINGIN
DONEGAN
DUSTGUN
ERTEGUN
GAHAGAN
GLUEGUN
GOINGIN
GOINGON
HALOGEN
HANDGUN
HEXAGON
ICINGIN
INDIGEN
KLINGON
KOSYGIN
LONIGAN
LYINGON
MADIGAN
MALAGAN
MOHEGAN
MTLOGAN
MUTAGEN
NAILGUN
NIPIGON
NONAGON
OCTAGON
ODINGON
OWINGON
PARAGON
PIROGEN
POLYGON
REBEGAN
REBEGIN
REBEGUN
RIOTGUN
RONTGEN
SHOTGUN
SLOEGIN
SMIDGEN
STENGUN
STUNGUN
TRAPGUN
TRUDGEN
TYINGIN
TYINGON
UNPAGAN
USINGIN
WOBEGON
YOUNGUN

•••••GN

AIRSIGN
ARRAIGN
BADSIGN
CONDIGN
CONSIGN
FOREIGN
HEXSIGN
IRESIGN
REALIGN

GO•••••

GOABOUT
GOADING
GOAFTER
GOAHEAD
GOALIES
GOALONG
GOAMISS
GOATEED
GOATEES
GOATISH
GOBBLED
GOBBLER
GOBBLES
GOBELIN
GOBELOW
GOBLANK
GOBLETS
GOBLINS
GOBROKE
GOBYAIR
GOBYBUS
GOBYCAB
GOBYCAR
GOBYSEA
GOCARTS
GOCRAZY
GODDARD
GODDESS
GODEVIL
GODFREY
GODHEAD
GODHOOD
GODLESS
GODLIER
GODLIKE
GODLING
GODMAMA
GODPAPA
GODSEND
GODSENT
GODSONS
GODTHAB
GODUNOV
GODUTCH
GODWITS
GOESAFT
GOESAPE
GOESBAD
GOESFAR
GOESFOR
GOESMAD
GOESOFF
GOESOUT
GOESPRO
GOFIRST
GOFORIT
GOFORTH
GOGETEM
GOGGLED
GOGGLER
GOGGLES
GOGIRLS
GOINFOR
GOINGAT
GOINGBY
GOINGIN
GOINGON
GOINGTO
GOINGUP
GOIRISH
GOITERS
GOKAPUT
GOKARTS
GOLDARN
GOLDBUG
GOLDING
GOLDMAN
GOLDONI
GOLDTIP
GOLDWYN
GOLFBAG
GOLFCAR
GOLFERS
GOLFING
GOLFPRO
GOLFTEE
GOLIATH
GOMPERS
GONDOLA
GONEAFT
GONEAPE
GONEBAD
GONEFAR
GONEFOR
GONEMAD
GONEOFF
GONEOUT
GONEPRO
GONERIL
GONGING
GONGORA
GONZAGA
GOOBERS
GOODAIM
GOODALL
GOODBAR
GOODBUY
GOODBYE
GOODBYS
GOODDAY
GOODDOG
GOODEGG
GOODERS
GOODFOR
GOODGUY
GOODIES
GOODING
GOODISH
GOODJOB
GOODJOE
GOODKID
GOODMAN
GOODMEN
GOODNIK
GOODONE
GOODPAY
GOODSON
GOODTRY
GOODUSE
GOODWIN
GOOFIER
GOOFILY
GOOFING
GOOFOFF
GOOFSUP
GOOFUPS
GOOGLED
GOOGLER
GOOGLES
GOOGOLS
GOOIEST
GOOMBAH
GOOMBAY
GOONEYS
GOONIER
GOONIES
GOONILY
GOOPIER
GOOSIER
GOOSING
GOPHERS
GORDIAN
GORDITA
GORDIUS
GORETEX
GORGERS
GORGING
GORGONS
GORIEST
GORILLA
GORMING
GOROUND
GORSIER
GORTNER
GOSFORD
GOSHAWK
GOSLING
GOSOUTH
GOSPELS
GOSSAGE
GOSSETT
GOSSIPS
GOSSIPY
GOSTALE
GOTAHIT
GOTAJOB
GOTATIP
GOTAWAY
GOTBACK
GOTBEAT
GOTBUSY
GOTCASH
GOTCHAS
GOTCOLD
GOTCUTE
GOTDONE
GOTDOWN
GOTEVEN
GOTFREE
GOTGOOD
GOTHELP
GOTHICS
GOTHIKA
GOTHURT
GOTINON
GOTINTO
GOTITON
GOTLOST
GOTMILK
GOTOBED
GOTOGAL
GOTOGUY
GOTONIT
GOTONTO
GOTOPOT
GOTOSEA
GOTOSEE
GOTOVER
GOTOWAR
GOTPAST
GOTREAL
GOTSOFT
GOTSORE
GOTTAGO
GOTTOIT
GOTUPON
GOTUPTO
GOTWARM
GOTWELL
GOTWISE
GOTWORD
GOUACHE
GOUGERS
GOUGING
GOULASH
GOUNDER
GOURAMI
GOURDES
GOURMET
GOUTIER
GOUTILY
GOUTISH
GOVERNS
GOWNING
GOWRONG

G•O••••

GAOLERS
GAOLING
GEOCODE
GEODESY
GEODUCK
GEOLOGY
GEORGEC
GEORGEI
GEORGEM
GEORGES
GEORGEV
GEORGEW
GEORGIA
GEORGIC
GEORGIE
GFORCES
GGORDON
GHOSTED
GHOSTLY
GIOCOSO
GIORGIO
GIORGOS
GLOAMIN
GLOATED
GLOATER
GLOBATE
GLOBING
GLOBINS
GLOBOID
GLOBOSE
GLOBOUS
GLOBULE
GLOMMED
GLOOMED
GLORIAS
GLORIED
GLORIES
GLORIFY
GLORYBE
GLOSSAE
GLOSSAL
GLOSSAS
GLOSSED
GLOSSER
GLOSSES
GLOTTAL
GLOTTIS
GLOVING
GLOWERS
GLOWING
GNOCCHI
GNOMISH
GNOMIST
GNOMONS
GNOSSUS
GNOSTIC
GOOBERS
GOODAIM
GOODALL
GOODBAR
GOODBUY
GOODBYE
GOODBYS
GOODDAY
GOODDOG
GOODEGG
GOODERS
GOODFOR
GOODGUY
GOODIES
GOODING
GOODISH
GOODJOB
GOODJOE
GOODKID
GOODMAN
GOODMEN
GOODNIK
GOODONE
GOODPAY
GOODSON
GOODTRY
GOODUSE
GOODWIN
GOOFIER
GOOFILY
GOOFING
GOOFOFF
GOOFSUP
GOOFUPS
GOOGLED
GOOGLER
GOOGLES
GOOGOLS
GOOIEST
GOOMBAH
GOOMBAY
GOONEYS
GOONIER
GOONIES
GOONILY
GOOPIER
GOOSIER
GOOSING
GROANED
GROANER
GROCERS
GROCERY
GRODIER
GROINED
GROKKED
GROLIER
GROMMET
GROMYKO
GROOMED
GROOMER
GROOVED
GROOVES
GROOVIN
GROPERS
GROPING
GROPIUS
GROSSED
GROSSER
GROSSES
GROSSLY
GROTIUS
GROTTOS
GROUCHO
GROUCHY
GROUNDS
GROUPED
GROUPER
GROUPIE
GROUSED
GROUSER
GROUSES
GROUTED
GROUTER
GROVELS
GROVERS
GROWBIG
GROWDIM
GROWERS
GROWFAT
GROWING
GROWLED
GROWLER
GROWNON
GROWNUP
GROWOLD
GROWSON
GROWSUP
GROWTHS

G••O•••

GALOOTS
GALOPED
GARONNE
GAROTTE
GASOHOL
GASOVEN
GAVOTTE
GENOESE
GENOISE
GENOMES
GENOMIC
GETONIT
GETONTO
GETOVER
GIGOLOS
GIROLLE
GIRONDE
GLOOMED
GOFORIT
GOFORTH
GOROUND
GOSOUTH
GOTOBED
GOTOGAL
GOTOGUY
GOTONIT
GOTONTO
GOTOPOT
GOTOSEA
GOTOSEE
GOTOVER
GOTOWAR
GQMODEL
GROOMED
GROOMER
GROOVED
GROOVES
GROOVIN
GYROCAR

G•••O••

GALLONS
GALLOPS
GALLOWS
GALOOTS
GAMBOLS
GAMMONS
GARCONS
GARROTE
GASCONS
GASCONY
GASEOUS
GASHOGS
GASLOGS
GASTONE
GAVEOFF
GAVEOUT
GAYLORD
GECKOES
GENLOCK
GEOCODE
GEOLOGY
GESSOED
GESSOES
GETCOLD
GETDONE
GETDOWN
GETGOOD
GETLOST
GETSOFF
GETSOFT
GETSOLD
GETSORE
GETSOUT
GETTOIT
GETWORD
GIACOMO
GIBBONS
GIBBOUS
GIBSONS
GIDEONS
GIFFORD
GILFORD
GILMORE
GINGOLD
GIOCOSO
GIVEOFF
GIVEOUT
GJETOST
GLAMORS
GLAMOUR
GLOBOID
GLOBOSE
GLOBOUS
GLUCOSE
GLYCOLS
GNOMONS
GOABOUT
GOALONG
GOBROKE
GODHOOD
GODSONS
GOESOFF
GOESOUT
GOLDONI
GONDOLA
GONEOFF
GONEOUT
GONGORA
GOODONE
GOOFOFF
GOOGOLS
GORGONS
GOSFORD
GOTCOLD
GOTDONE
GOTDOWN
GOTGOOD
GOTLOST
GOTSOFT
GOTSORE
GOTTOIT
GOTWORD
GOWRONG
GRANOLA
GREGORY
GREWOLD
GROWOLD
GULFOIL
GUMBOOT
GUMWOOD
GUNBOAT
GUNDOGS
GUNLOCK
GUNMOLL
GUNROOM
GUSHOUT
GUSTOES
GUVNORS
GUYROPE
GYMSOCK

G••••O•

GABBROS
GAINSON
GALANOS
GALLEON
GAMEBOY
GANGTOK
GASOHOL
GAUCHOS
GAZEBOS
GAZEDON
GAZESON
GEARBOX
GEEKDOM
GELATOS
GEMSBOK
GENITOR
GERITOL
GERSHON
GETAJOB
GETFROM
GETGOOD
GETINON
GETITON
GETSHOT
GETUPON
GGORDON
GHETTOS
GIFTBOX
GIGATON
GIGOLOS
GINGKOS
GINKGOS
GIORGOS
GIRASOL
GITANOS
GIVENOF
GIVENON
GIVESOF
GIVESON
GLASGOW
GLASHOW
GLEASON
GLENCOE
GLUEDON
GLUESON
GLUTTON
GNAWSON
GOBELOW
GODHOOD
GODUNOV
GOESFOR
GOINFOR
GOINGON
GONEFOR
GOODDOG
GOODFOR
GOODJOB
GOODJOE
GOODSON
GOTAJOB
GOTGOOD
GOTINON
GOTITON
GOTOPOT
GOTUPON
GRAFTON
GRANTOR
GRATEON
GRAYSON
GRIFFON
GRINGOS
GRINKOV
GRISSOM
GROTTOS
GROWNON
GROWSON
GRUNION
GRYPHON
GUDGEON
GUERDON
GUIGNOL
GUMBOOT
GUMDROP
GUMSHOE
GUMWOOD
GUNROOM
GUNSFOR
GUNSHOT
GYMSHOE
GYRATOR

G•••••O

GAETANO
GALENTO
GALILEO
GALLICO
GALVANO
GAMBADO
GASTERO
GEARSTO
GENNAIO
GENNARO
GERALDO
GESTAPO
GETINTO
GETONTO
GIACOMO
GIOCOSO
GIORGIO
GIVENTO
GIVESTO
GLUEDTO
GLUESTO
GOESPRO
GOINGTO
GOLFPRO
GONEPRO
GOTINTO
GOTONTO
GOTTAGO
GOTUPTO
GROMYKO
GROUCHO
GUANACO
GUESSSO

•GO••••

AGONIES
AGONISE
AGONISM
AGONIST
AGONIZE
AGOUTIS
EGOISTE
EGOISTS
EGOSURF
EGOTISM
EGOTIST
EGOTRIP
GGORDON
IGOOFED
IGOROTS
IGOTCHA
IGOTYOU
UGOLINO

•G•O•••

AGNOMEN
AGROUND
IGNOBLE
IGNOBLY
IGNORED
IGNORER
IGNORES
IGOOFED
OGDOADS

•G••O••

AGEDOUT
AGEFOUR
AGELONG
AGESOUT
EGGNOGS
EGGROLL
EGGTOSS
IGNEOUS
IGOROTS
PGATOUR

•G•••O•

AGALLOP
AGREEON
EGGDROP
EGGEDON
GGORDON
IGGYPOP
IGNATOW
IGNITOR
IGOTYOU
MGMLION
PGAPROS

•G••••O

AGESAGO
AGITATO
AGREETO
IGNARRO
UGOLINO

••GO•••

ANGOLAN
ANGORAS

ARGONNE
BEGONIA
BEGORRA
BIGONES
BIGOTED
BIGOTRY
BUGOUTS
BYGOLLY
BYGONES
DUGONGS
DUGOUTS
ENGORGE
ERGOTIC
FAGOTED
GIGOLOS
IMGOING
INGOALS
INGOING
LAGOONS
LEGOLAS
LEGOSET
LOGOFFS
LOGONTO
LOGOUTS
MEGOHMS
NOGOODS
ONGOING
PAGODAS
PIGOUTS
RAGOUTS
RIGOURS
SEGOVIA
TAGOUTS
UNGODLY
UNGORED
UPGOING
VIGOURS
WAGONED
WAGONER
ZYGOTES

••G•O••

BAGBOYS
BAGJOBS
BAGNOLD
BEGSOFF
BIGBOSS
BIGBOYS
BIGDOGS
BIGFOOT
BIGFOUR
BIGHORN
BIGJOHN
BIGLOTS
BIGLOVE
BIGNOSE
BIGTOES
BIGTOPS
BIGTOWN
BOGDOWN
BOGHOLE
BUGBOYS
BUGSOFF
BUGSOUT
DAGWOOD
DEGHOST
DIGGORY
DIGLOTS
DIGSOUT
DOGBONE
DOGBOOT
DOGBOWL
DOGCOAT
DOGCOMB
DOGDOOR
DOGFOOD
DOGGONE
DOGROSE
DOGTOYS
DOGWOOD
EDGEOUT
EGGNOGS
EGGROLL
EGGTOSS
ENGROSS
FOGBOWS
FOGDOGS
FOGHORN
HOGNOSE
INGROUP
INGROWN
LAGOONS
LEGBONE
LEGHORN
LEGIONS
LEGROOM
LEGROPE
LEGWORK
LOGBOOK
LOGROLL
LOGSOFF
LOGSOUT
LUGSOUT
LUGWORM
MAGGOTS
MCGRORY
MIGNONS
NEGRONI
NOGOODS
PAGEONE
PEGTOPS
PIGEONS
PIGSOUT
PUGNOSE
RAGDOLL
RAGMOPS
RAGTOPS
REGIONS
REGLOSS
REGLOWS
REGROOM
REGROUP
REGROWN
REGROWS
RIGSOUT
SIGMOID
SIGNOFF
SIGNORA
SIGNORE
SIGNORS
SIGNOUT
TAGSOUT
TIGLONS
TOGSOUT
TUGBOAT
UNGLOVE
UNGROSS
UNGROWN
UPGROWN
UPGROWS
VIGNOLA
WIGSOUT

••G••O•

ANGELOU
BAGEHOT
BAGNIOS
BEGSFOR
BIGELOW
BIGFOOT
BIGSHOT
BIGSHOW
BUGABOO
BUGALOO
DAGWOOD
DIGSFOR
DOGBOOT
DOGCHOW
DOGDOOR
DOGFOOD
DOGSHOW
DOGTROT
DOGWOOD
EGGDROP
EGGEDON
FUGATOS
GIGATON
GIGOLOS
HIGHBOY
HIGHLOW
HIGHTOP
IGGYPOP
JOGTROT
LEGATOR
LEGATOS
LEGIRON
LEGROOM
LIGHTON
LOGBOOK
MAGALOG
MAGINOT
MEGALON
MEGATON
MOGADOR
MUGSHOT
NEGATOR
PAGEBOY
PIGIRON
RAGSHOP
REGROOM
RIGHTON
SIGHFOR
SIGNFOR
SIGNSON
TAGALOG
URGEDON
URGESON

••G•••O

ARGENTO
AUGUSTO
BEGANTO
BUGABOO
BUGALOO
DIGINTO
DUGINTO
EDGARDO
ELGALLO
ELGRECO
LOGONTO
MAGNETO
MOGAMBO
OUGHTTO
PAGETWO
SAGUARO

•••GO••

ALIGOTE
ALLGONE
ALLGOOD
ARAGORN
BANGOUT
BINGOES
BOBGOEN
BONGOES
BURGOOS
BUTGOOD
CARGOES
CHIGOES
CONGOUS
DIDGOOD
DIGGORY
DINGOES
DOGGONE
DRAGOFF
DRAGONS
DRAGOON
DRAGOTI
DRAGOUT
EPIGONE
FARGOND
FARGONE
FLAGONS
FORGOER
FORGOES
FORGONE
FORGOOD
FUNGOES
GETGOOD
GINGOLD
GONGORA
GOOGOLS
GORGONS
GOTGOOD
GREGORY
HANGOFF
HANGOUT
HUNGOFF
HUNGOUT
IMAGOES
ISOGONS
ITSGONE
JARGONS
JARGONY
JINGOES
LETGOBY
LETGOOF
LINGOES
MAGGOTS
MANGOES
MONGOLS
NONGOGO
NONGOLD
NOTGOOD
OLDGOLD
OMIGOSH
OUTGOES
OWNGOAL
PERGOLA
PETGOAT
PLUGOLA
RANGOFF
RANGOON
RANGOUT
RINGOFF
RINGOUT
RUNGOFF
RUNGOUT
SANGOUT
SEAGODS
SHEGOAT
SINGOUT
SPIGOTS
SUBGOAL
SUBGODS
SUNGODS
TANGOED
TANGOER
TEAGOWN
THEGOLD
TINGODS
TOMGOLA
TRIGONS
TUNGOIL
VANGOGH
VIRGOAN
WARGODS
XINGOUT

•••G•O•

ADAGIOS
AIRGLOW
ALLGOOD
AVIGNON
BANGKOK
BANGSON
BERGSON
BURGEON
BURGOOS
BUTGOOD
CHIGNON
DIDGOOD
DODGSON
DRAGOON
DRAGSON
DREGION
DUDGEON
DUNGEON
FORGOOD
GANGTOK
GETGOOD
GINGKOS
GOTGOOD
GUDGEON
GUIGNOL
HANGDOG
HANGSON
HINGEON
IBEGYOU
KINGDOM
LANGDON
LANGTON
LANGUOR
LARGEOJ
LETGOOF
LINGCOD
LONGBOW
LONGFOR
LONGTOM
LONGTON
LORGNON
NOTGOOD
OUTGLOW
OUTGROW
PEUGEOT
PIDGEON
RANGFOR
RANGOON
RINGFOR
RUNGFOR
SUNGLOW
SURGEON
VERGEON
WEIGHON
WIDGEON

•••G••O

ARIGATO
BERGAMO
DANGELO
DEIGNTO
HEIGHHO
LONGAGO
MANGANO
NONGOGO
OREGANO
ROUGHGO
SINGSTO
TANGELO

••••GO•

ASIAGOS
BRINGON
CLANGOR
DEARGOD
DECAGON
DEMAGOG
DEMIGOD
DOINGOK
ERYNGOS
GINKGOS
GIORGOS
GLASGOW
GOINGON
GRINGOS
HEXAGON
IFORGOT
INDIGOS
KLINGON
LATIGOS
LITHGOW
LYINGON
MOONGOD
MRMAGOO
NIPIGON
NONAGON
OBLIGOR
OCTAGON
ODINGON
OWINGON
PAPAGOS
PARAGON
POLYGON
RAINGOD
SMEAGOL
TYINGON
VIRAGOS
WINDGOD
WOBEGON

••••G•O

ALLEGRO
BENIGNO
BRINGTO
CLINGTO
CLUNGTO
DOINGSO
DOINGTO
GIORGIO
GOINGTO
LYINGTO
MILAGRO
MRMAGOO
OWINGTO
TYINGTO

•••••GO

ADAYAGO
AGESAGO
AMERIGO
BLTTOGO
BYJINGO
CHICAGO
DOMINGO
DONOTGO
DURANGO
EMBARGO
FARRAGO
FOLENGO
GOTTAGO
HAVEAGO
HIDALGO
IFYOUGO
IMUSTGO
ISITAGO
LENTIGO
LETITGO
LETMEGO
LONGAGO
LUMBAGO
MAKESGO
MARENGO
MONTEGO
MUSKEGO
NONGOGO
OFFWEGO
ONETOGO
ONTHEGO
RODRIGO
ROUGHGO
SAPSAGO
UNDERGO
VERDUGO
VERTIGO
WAYTOGO
WINDIGO
ZHIVAGO

G•P••••

GAPEDAT
GAPESAT
GAPKIDS
GAPLESS
GAPPING
GIPSIES
GOPHERS
GUPPIES
GYPPERS
GYPPING
GYPSIES
GYPSUMS

G••P•••

GALPALS
GAPPING
GARPIKE
GASPARD
GASPERS
GASPING
GASPIPE
GASPUMP
GAWPERS
GAWPING
GELPENS
GETPAST
GIMPING
GLYPHIC
GLYPTIC
GODPAPA
GOMPERS
GOOPIER
GOSPELS
GOTPAST
GRAPERY
GRAPHED
GRAPHIC
GRAPIER
GRAPNEL
GRAPPAS
GRAPPLE
GRIPERS
GRIPING
GRIPPED
GRIPPER
GRIPPES
GROPERS
GROPING
GROPIUS
GRYPHON
GULPERS
GULPIER
GULPING
GUNPLAY
GUPPIES
GYPPERS
GYPPING

G•••P••

GALOPED
GETUPON
GLIMPSE
GOESPRO
GOKAPUT
GOLFPRO
GONEPRO
GOODPAY
GOTOPOT
GOTUPON
GOTUPTO
GRAMPAS
GRAMPUS
GRANPAS
GRAPPAS
GRAPPLE
GRASPAT
GRASPED
GRASPER
GRIPPED
GRIPPER
GRIPPES
GROUPED
GROUPER
GROUPIE
GRUMPED

G••••P•

GALLOPS
GALUMPH
GASCAPS
GASPIPE
GELCAPS
GESTAPO
GIVEUPS
GODPAPA
GOESAPE
GONEAPE
GOOFUPS
GOSSIPS
GOSSIPY
GRANDPA
GUNLAPS
GUYROPE

G•••••P

GANGSUP
GASEDUP
GASESUP
GASLAMP
GASPUMP
GEARSUP
GETATIP
GETHELP
GETSHEP
GETSHIP
GIDDYAP
GIDDYUP
GIVENUP
GIVESUP
GLAMSUP
GOINGUP
GOLDTIP
GOOFSUP
GOTATIP
GOTHELP
GRATEUP
GREYCUP
GRIDMAP
GROWNUP
GROWSUP
GUMDROP
GUNSHIP
GUSSYUP

•G•P•••

PGAPROS

•G••P••

AGRIPPA
IGGYPOP

•G•••P•

AGRIPPA
EGGCUPS

•G••••P

AGALLOP
EGGDROP
EGOTRIP
IGGYPOP
IGIVEUP

••GP•••

BAGPIPE
DOGPILE
LEGPULL
MAGPIES
PIGPENS

••G•P••

BIGAPES
CAGEPET
DIGIPET
DOGAPES
HIGHPAY
IGGYPOP

••G••P•

BAGPIPE
BIGTOPS
DIGRAPH
DOGNAPS
EGGCUPS
EIGHTPM
LEGROPE
PEGTOPS
RAGMOPS
RAGTOPS
REGRAPH
REGRIPS
SIGNUPS
UNGRIPS

••G•••P

BIGGULP
CAGEDUP
CAGESUP
EGGDROP
EIGHTUP
FOGLAMP
HIGHTOP
IGGYPOP
INGROUP
LEGTRAP
LIGHTUP
MUGWUMP
RAGSHOP
REGRASP
REGROUP
SIGNSUP

•••GP••

KINGPIN
THIGPEN

•••G•P•

HANGUPS

•••G••P

BANGSUP
BIGGULP
CLOGSUP
COUGHUP
DRAGSUP
GANGSUP
HANGSUP
KEYGRIP
PLUGSUP
RINGSUP
ROUGHUP
SNAGSUP
WEIGHUP
WINGTIP

••••G•P

BABYGAP
BRINGUP
DOINGUP
GOINGUP
ICINGUP
LYINGUP
MEDIGAP
STOPGAP
TYINGUP
USINGUP

GQ•••••

GQMODEL

G•••Q••

GIAUQUE

••G••Q•

HIGHIQS

GR•••••

GRABBAG
GRABBAR
GRABBED
GRABBER
GRABSAT
GRACIAS
GRACILE
GRACING
GRACKLE
GRADATE
GRADEAA
GRADERS
GRADING
GRADUAL
GRAFTED
GRAFTER
GRAFTON
GRAHAME
GRAHAMS
GRAINED
GRAINER
GRAMMAR
GRAMMER
GRAMMES
GRAMMYS
GRAMPAS
GRAMPUS
GRANADA
GRANARY
GRANDAM
GRANDEE
GRANDER
GRANDLY
GRANDMA
GRANDPA
GRANGER
GRANGES
GRANITA
GRANITE
GRANNIE
GRANOLA
GRANPAS
GRANTED
GRANTEE
GRANTER
GRANTOR
GRANULE
GRAPERY
GRAPHED
GRAPHIC
GRAPIER
GRAPNEL
GRAPPAS
GRAPPLE
GRASPAT
GRASPED
GRASPER
GRASSED
GRASSES
GRASSLE
GRATEON
GRATERS
GRATEUP
GRATIAS
GRATIFY
GRATING
GRAUMAN
GRAVELS
GRAVELY
GRAVERS
GRAVEST
GRAVIES
GRAVING
GRAVITY
GRAVLAX
GRAVURE
GRAYEST
GRAYING
GRAYISH
GRAYJAY
GRAYLAG
GRAYSON
GRAZERS
GRAZIER
GRAZING
GREASED
GREASER
GREASES
GREATEN
GREATER
GREATLY
GREAVES
GRECIAN
GRECISM
GRECIZE
GREELEY
GREENED
GREENER
GREENLY
GREETED
GREETER
GREGORY
GREMLIN
GRENADA
GRENADE
GRENDEL
GRESHAM
GRETZKY
GREWBIG
GREWDIM
GREWFAT
GREWOLD
GREYCUP
GREYEST
GREYHEN
GREYING
GREYISH
GREYLAG
GRIDDED
GRIDDER
GRIDDLE
GRIDMAP
GRIEVED
GRIEVER
GRIEVES
GRIFFEY
GRIFFIN
GRIFFON
GRIFTED
GRIFTER
GRIGRIS
GRILLED
GRILLER
GRILLES
GRIMACE
GRIMIER
GRIMILY
GRIMING
GRIMMER
GRIMSBY
GRINDER
GRINGOS
GRINKOV
GRINNED
GRINNER
GRINSAT
GRIPERS
GRIPING
GRIPPED
GRIPPER
GRIPPES
GRISHAM
GRISLET
GRISNEZ
GRISSOM
GRISTER
GRISTLE
GRISTLY
GRITTED

GRITTER GRIZZLE GRIZZLY GROANED GROANER GROCERS GROCERY GRODIER GROINED GROKKED GROLIER GROMMET GROMYKO GROOMED GROOMER GROOVED GROOVES GROOVIN GROPERS GROPING GROPIUS GROSSED GROSSER GROSSES GROSSLY GROTIUS GROTTOS GROUCHO GROUCHY GROUNDS GROUPED GROUPER GROUPIE GROUSED GROUSER GROUSES GROUTED GROUTER GROVELS GROVERS GROWBIG GROWDIM GROWERS GROWFAT GROWING GROWLED GROWLER GROWNON GROWNUP GROWOLD GROWSON GROWSUP GROWTHS GRUBBED GRUBBER GRUDGED GRUDGER GRUDGES GRUFFER GRUFFLY GRUMBLE GRUMBLY GRUMMAN GRUMPED GRUNGER GRUNGES GRUNION GRUNTED GRUNTER GRUYERE GRYPHON

G•R••••

GARAGED GARAGES GARBAGE GARBAGY GARBING GARBLED GARBLER GARBLES GARCONS GARDENA GARDENS GARDNER GARGLED GARGLER GARGLES GARLAND GARLICS GARLITS GARMENT GARNEAU GARNERS GARNETS GARNETT GARNISH GARONNE GAROTTE GARPIKE GARRETS GARRETT GARRICK GARROTE GARTERS GERAINT GERALDO GERBILS GERENTS GERITOL GERMAIN GERMANE GERMANS GERMANY GERMIER GERSHON GERUNDS GERVAIS GIRAFFE GIRASOL GIRDERS GIRDING GIRDLED GIRDLER GIRDLES GIRLIER GIRLIES GIRLISH GIRLSHY GIROLLE GIRONDE GIRTHED GIRTING GORDIAN GORDITA GORDIUS GORETEX GORGERS GORGING GORGONS GORIEST GORILLA GORMING GOROUND GORSIER GORTNER GURGLED GURGLES GURKHAS GURNEYS GYRALLY GYRATED GYRATES GYRATOR GYRENES GYROCAR

G••R•••

GABRIEL GAGREEL GAGRULE GARRETS GARRETT GARRICK GARROTE GEARBOX GEARING GEARSTO GEARSUP GEDRICK GEORGEC GEORGEI GEORGEM GEORGES GEORGEV GEORGEW GEORGIA GEORGIC GEORGIE GETREAL GFORCES GGORDON GHERKIN GIORGIO GIORGOS GLAREAT GLARING GLORIAS GLORIED GLORIES GLORIFY GLORYBE GLURGES GNARLED GNARRED GOBROKE GOCRAZY GOIRISH GOTREAL GOURAMI GOURDES GOURMET GOWRONG GSTRING GUARANI GUARDED GUARDEE GUARDER GUARGUM GUERDON GUNROOM GUYROPE GYMRATS

G•••R••

GABBROS GAGARIN GASTRIC GENERAL GENERIC GENERIS GETFREE GETFROM GETSRID GNARRED GOCARTS GODFREY GOFIRST GOFORIT GOFORTH GOGIRLS GOKARTS GONERIL GOTFREE GOVERNS GRIGRIS GUJARAT GUMDROP GUMTREE GUTHRIE

G••••R•

GABBERS GADDERS GAFFERS GAGGERS GAINERS GAITERS GALLERY GAMMERS GANDERS GANGERS GAOLERS GARNERS GARTERS GASPARD GASPERS GASSERS GASTERO GASWARS GATHERS GAUDERY GAUGERS GAWKERS GAWPERS GAYLORD GAZZARA GEEZERS GENDERS GENNARO GENXERS GESTURE GETHURT GETSORE GETTERS GETWARM GETWORD GEYSERS GIBBERS GIFFORD GILBERT GILDERS GILFORD GILMORE GINGERS GINGERY GIRDERS GISCARD GIZZARD GLAMORS GLAZERS GLIDERS GLOWERS GNAWERS GODDARD GOESPRO GOITERS GOLDARN GOLFERS GOLFPRO GOMPERS GONEPRO GONGORA GOOBERS GOODERS GOODTRY GOPHERS GORGERS GOSFORD GOTHURT GOTSORE GOTWARM GOTWORD GOUGERS GRADERS GRANARY GRAPERY GRATERS GRAVERS GRAVURE GRAZERS GREGORY GRIPERS GROCERS GROCERY GROPERS GROVERS GROWERS GRUYERE GUEVARA GUIDERS GUITARS GULPERS GUNFIRE GUNNERS GUNNERY GUSHERS GUTTERS GUVNORS GYPPERS

G•••••R

GABBIER GAGSTER GAMBIER GAMBLER GARBLER GARDNER GARGLER GASSIER GAUCHER GAUDIER GAUNTER GAUTIER GAUZIER GAVEEAR GAWKIER GEEKIER GEMMIER GENITOR GENTLER GERMIER GETOVER GETSFAR GIDDIER GIGGLER GIRDLER GIRLIER GIVEEAR GLACIER GLADDER GLAMOUR GLAZIER GLEANER GLIBBER GLIMMER GLISTER GLITTER GLOATER GLOSSER GLUMMER GNASHER GOAFTER GOBBLER GOBYAIR GOBYCAR GODLIER GOESFAR GOESFOR GOGGLER GOINFOR GOLFCAR GONEFAR GONEFOR GOODBAR GOODFOR GOOFIER GOOGLER GOONIER GOOPIER GOOSIER GORSIER GORTNER GOTOVER GOTOWAR GOUNDER GOUTIER GRABBAR GRABBER GRAFTER GRAINER GRAMMAR GRAMMER GRANDER GRANGER GRANTER GRANTOR GRAPIER GRASPER GRAZIER GREASER GREATER GREENER GREETER GRIDDER GRIEVER GRIFTER GRILLER GRIMIER GRIMMER GRINDER GRINNER GRIPPER GRISTER GRITTER GROANER GRODIER GROLIER GROOMER GROSSER GROUPER GROUSER GROUTER GROWLER GRUBBER GRUDGER GRUFFER GRUNGER GRUNTER GUARDER GUCKIER GUESSER GUILDER GULFWAR GULPIER GUMMIER GUNKIER GUNSFOR GUNTHER GUNUSER GUSHIER GUSTIER GUTSIER GUTTIER GUZZLER GYRATOR GYROCAR

•GR••••

AGREEON AGREERS AGREETO AGRIBIZ AGRIPPA AGROUND IGRAINE OGREISH PGRATED

•G•R•••

AGARICS AGGRESS EGERIAS EGGROLL GGORDON IGOROTS

•G••R••

EGGDROP EGOTRIP IGNARRO IGNORED IGNORER IGNORES PGAPROS

•G•••R•

AGENTRY AGREERS EGGLERS EGOSURF IGNARRO

•G••••R

AGEFOUR AGUTTER IGNITER IGNITOR IGNORER PGATOUR

••GR•••

AGGRESS AIGRETS ALGREEN ANGRIER ANGRILY ANGRYAT ATGRADE BEGRIME BIGRIGS DEGRADE DEGREED DEGREES DIGRAMS DIGRAPH DIGRESS DOGRACE DOGREAT DOGROSE DOGRUNS EGGROLL ELGRECO ENGRAFT ENGRAIN ENGRAMS ENGRAVE ENGROSS GAGREEL GAGRULE IMGREAT INGRAFT INGRAIN INGRATE INGREEN INGRESS INGROUP INGROWN LEGRAND LEGREST LEGROOM LEGROPE LOGROLL MCGRIFF MCGRORY MCGRUFF MEGRIMS MEGRYAN MIGRANT MIGRATE MRGREEN NEGRONI RAGRUGS REGRABS REGRADE REGRAFT REGRANT REGRAPH REGRASP REGREET REGRESS REGRETS REGRIND REGRIPS REGROOM REGROUP REGROWN REGROWS RUGRATS TIGRESS TUGRIKS UNGRAND UNGREEN UNGRIPS UNGROSS UNGROWN UNGRUFF UPGRADE UPGROWN UPGROWS USGRANT VAGRANT

••G•R••

ALGARVE ALGERIA ANGERED ANGORAS AUGURAL AUGURED AUGURER BEGIRDS BEGORRA BOGARDE BOGARTS BUGFREE DEGERMS DOGTROT EAGERER EAGERLY EDGARDO EGGDROP ENGARDE ENGIRDS ENGORGE FIGTREE FIGURAL FIGURED FIGURER FIGURES FOGERTY GAGARIN GOGIRLS HAGERTY HEGIRAS HIGHRES HOGARTH ITGIRLS JOGBRAS JOGTROT LEGIRON LEGTRAP LIGURIA NIGERIA PIGIRON REGARDS REGIRDS ROGERED SUGARED UNGIRDS UNGORED UPGIRDS WAGERED WAGERER YOGURTS

••G••R•

ALGEBRA ALGIERS ANGLERS ARGUERS BAGGERS BAGGIRL BEGGARS BEGGARY BEGORRA BIGBIRD BIGCARS BIGEARS BIGGERS BIGGIRL BIGHORN BIGJERK BIGOTRY BUGLERS COGBURN DAGGERS DIGGERS DIGGORY DOGBERT DOGCART DOGEARS EGGLERS FIGBARS FOGGERS FOGHORN GAGGERS HAGGARD HIGHART HOGGERY HUGGERS JAGUARS JIGGERS JIGGERY JOGGERS KEGGERS KEGLERS LAGGARD LAGGERS LEGHORN LEGWORK LOGGERS LUGGERS LUGWORM MAGUIRE MAGYARS MCGRORY MCGUIRE MCGWIRE MEGAERA MEGAERG MUGGERS NAGGERS ONGUARD PIGGERY REGEARS REGNARD RIGGERS RIGOURS ROGUERY SAGCARD SAGUARO SIGHERS SIGNERS SIGNORA SIGNORE SIGNORS TAGGERS TOGGERY TUGGERS UNGUARD VIGOURS VOGUERS WAGGERS WAGGERY WIGGERY YOGHURT

••G•••R

ANGRIER ANGULAR AUGURER BAGGIER BEGSFOR BIGBEAR BIGFOUR BIGHAIR BIGSTAR BOGGIER BOGGLER BUGBEAR BUGGIER DIGSFOR DOGDOOR DOGGIER DOGHAIR DOGSEAR DOGSTAR EAGERER ENGAGER FIGHTER FIGURER FOGGIER GAGSTER GIGGLER GOGGLER HAGGLER HIGGLER HIGHBAR INGEMAR JAGGIER JIGGIER JOGGLER JUGGLER JUGULAR LEGATOR LEGGIER LEGWEAR LIGHTER MOGADOR MUGGIER NAGGIER NEGATER NEGATOR NIGGLER NIGHTER PIGGIER RAGGIER REGALER REGNIER REGULAR RIGHTER RIGUEUR SAGGIER SIGHFOR SIGHTER SIGNFOR SOGGIER TIGHTER TOGGLER UNGULAR WAGERER WAGEWAR WAGGLER WAGONER WEGENER WIGGIER WIGGLER

•••GR••

ALEGRIA ANAGRAM ASAGRAY BEOGRAD CHAGRIN DIAGRAM EMIGREE EMIGRES EPIGRAM GRIGRIS ISOGRAM KEYGRIP KINGRAT LONGRUN MACGRAW MAIGRET MARGRET MONGREL MULGREW ONEGRAM OUTGREW OUTGRIN OUTGROW PANGRAM PILGRIM PROGRAM SANGRIA SEAGRAM SEAGREN SHAGRUG TANGRAM TRIGRAM

•••G•R•

ALEGARS ARAGORN BADGERS BADGIRL BAGGERS BAGGIRL BANGERS BARGERS BATGIRL BEGGARS BEGGARY BERGERE BIGGERS BIGGIRL BINGERS BUDGERS BULGARI BULGARS BULGURS BURGERS BUSGIRL CADGERS CALGARY CAMGIRL CODGERS CONGERS COUGARS COWGIRL DAGGERS DANGERS DIGGERS DIGGORY DINGERS DODGERS ETAGERE FINGERS FLYGIRL FOGGERS FOLGERS FORGERS FORGERY FUDGERS GAGGERS GANGERS GAUGERS GINGERS GINGERY GONGORA GORGERS GOUGERS GREGORY

HAGGARD
HANGARS
HANGERS
HEDGERS
HOGGERY
HUGGERS
HUNGARY
HUNGERS
IMAGERS
IMAGERY
JAEGERS
JIGGERS
JIGGERY
JOGGERS
JUDGERS
KEDGERS
KEGGERS
LAGGARD
LAGGERS
LANGTRY
LEDGERS
LINGERS
LODGERS
LOGGERS
LONGARM
LUGGERS
LUNGERS
MANGERS
MARGERY
MERGERS
MONGERS
MUGGERS
NAGGERS
NIAGARA
NUDGERS
OLDGIRL
ONAGERS
PARGERS
PIGGERY
PINGERS
RANGERS
RIEGERT
RIGGERS
RINGERS
RODGERS
RUTGERS
SEAGIRT
SINGERS
STAGERS
SURGERY
SWIGERT
TAGGERS
TOGGERY
TUGGERS
VERGERS
WAGGERS
WAGGERY
WIGGERY
WINGERS
ZINGERS

•••G••R

ALIGNER
BAGGIER
BILGIER
BLOGGER
BOGGIER
BOGGLER
BRAGGER
BUGGIER
BULGHUR
BULGIER
BUNGLER
BURGHER
BURGLAR
CHIGGER
CHUGGER
DANGLER
DINGIER
DODGIER
DOGGIER
DRAGGER
FEIGNER
FLAGGER
FLOGGER
FOGGIER
FORGOER
FROGGER
GARGLER
GIGGLER
GOGGLER
GOOGLER
HAGGLER
HEDGIER
HIGGLER
JAGGIER
JANGLER
JIGGIER
JINGLER
JOGGLER
JUGGLER
LANGUOR
LAUGHER
LEAGUER
LEDGIER
LEGGIER
LONGFOR
LOWGEAR
MANGIER
MANGLER
MINGIER
MINGLER
MUGGIER
NAGGIER
NIGGLER
PIGGIER
PLUGGER
PUDGIER
RAGGIER
RANGFOR
RANGIER
RIDGIER
RINGFOR
ROUGHER
RUNGFOR
SAGGIER
SEDGIER
SLOGGER
SLUGGER
SMUGGER
SNAGGER
SNUGGER
SOGGIER
STAGGER
STAGIER
SWAGGER
TANGIER
TANGLER
TANGOER
TINGLER
TOGGLER
TOUGHER
TRIGGER
WAGGLER
WANGLER
WEDGIER
WEIGHER
WIGGIER
WIGGLER
ZIEGLER
ZINGIER

••••GR•

ALLEGRA
ALLEGRO
CONAGRA
INTEGRA
MILAGRO
SHANGRI
UNANGRY

••••G•R

ALLEGER
AVENGER
AZINGER
BETTGER
BLOGGER
BLUDGER
BRAGGER
BRIDGER
BRINGER
CHANGER
CHARGER
CHIGGER
CHUGGER
CLANGER
CLANGOR
CLINGER
DOWAGER
DRAGGER
DREDGER
DRUDGER
ENGAGER
FIBIGER
FLAGGER
FLINGER
FLOGGER
FORAGER
FROGGER
GRANGER
GRUDGER
GRUNGER
HOMAGER
INTEGER
KLINGER
KRUEGER
LOUNGER
MANAGER
MRTIGER
NEWAGER
NOSUGAR
OBLIGER
OBLIGOR
ONSAGER
PLEDGER
PLUGGER
PLUNGER
RAVAGER
RENEGER
REWAGER
SAVAGER
SLINGER
SLOGGER
SLUGGER
SMUGGER
SNAGGER
SNUGGER
SPONGER
STAGGER
STEIGER
STINGER
SWAGGER
SWINGER
TANAGER
TRIGGER
TRUDGER
TWANGER
UNEAGER
VINEGAR
VOYAGER
WRINGER
WRONGER
YOUNGER

GS•••••

GSTRING

G•S••••

GASBAGS
GASCANS
GASCAPS
GASCONS
GASCONY
GASEDUP
GASEJTY
GASEOUS
GASESUP
GASHEAT
GASHING
GASHOGS
GASJETS
GASKELL
GASKETS
GASLAMP
GASLEAK
GASLESS
GASLINE
GASLOGS
GASMAIN
GASMASK
GASOHOL
GASOVEN
GASPARD
GASPERS
GASPING
GASPIPE
GASPUMP
GASSERS
GASSIER
GASSING
GASSMAN
GASTANK
GASTERO
GASTONE
GASTRIC
GASWARS
GESSOED
GESSOES
GESTALT
GESTAPO
GESTATE
GESTURE
GISCARD
GISELLE
GISSING
GOSFORD
GOSHAWK
GOSLING
GOSOUTH
GOSPELS
GOSSAGE
GOSSETT
GOSSIPS
GOSSIPY
GOSTALE
GUSHERS
GUSHIER
GUSHILY
GUSHING
GUSHOUT
GUSSETS
GUSSIED
GUSSIES
GUSSYUP
GUSTAVE
GUSTIER
GUSTILY
GUSTING
GUSTOES

G••S•••

GADSDEN
GAGSTER
GASSERS
GASSIER
GASSING
GASSMAN
GAUSSES
GEISHAS
GEMSBOK
GERSHON
GESSOED
GESSOES
GETSANA
GETSANF
GETSFAR
GETSFIT
GETSHEP
GETSHIP
GETSHOT
GETSMAD
GETSOFF
GETSOFT
GETSOLD
GETSORE
GETSOUT
GETSRID
GETSSET
GETSWET
GEYSERS
GHASTLY
GHOSTED
GHOSTLY
GIBSONS
GINSENG
GIPSIES
GISSING
GLASGOW
GLASHOW
GLASSED
GLASSES
GLISTEN
GLISTER
GLOSSAE
GLOSSAL
GLOSSAS
GLOSSED
GLOSSER
GLOSSES
GNASHED
GNASHER
GNASHES
GNOSSUS
GNOSTIC
GODSEND
GODSENT
GODSONS
GOESAFT
GOESAPE
GOESBAD
GOESFAR
GOESFOR
GOESMAD
GOESOFF
GOESOUT
GOESPRO
GOOSIER
GOOSING
GORSIER
GOSSAGE
GOSSETT
GOSSIPS
GOSSIPY
GOTSOFT
GOTSORE
GRASPAT
GRASPED
GRASPER
GRASSED
GRASSES
GRASSLE
GRESHAM
GRISHAM
GRISLET
GRISNEZ
GRISSOM
GRISTER
GRISTLE
GRISTLY
GROSSED
GROSSER
GROSSES
GROSSLY
GUESSAT
GUESSED
GUESSER
GUESSES
GUESSSO
GUESTED
GUMSHOE
GUNSELS
GUNSFOR
GUNSHIP
GUNSHOT
GUSSETS
GUSSIED
GUSSIES
GUSSYUP
GUTSIER
GUTSILY
GYMSHOE
GYMSOCK
GYMSUIT
GYPSIES
GYPSUMS

G•••S••

GAINSAY
GAINSON
GANGSAW
GANGSTA
GANGSUP
GAPESAT
GASESUP
GAUSSES
GAWKSAT
GAZESAT
GAZESON
GEARSTO
GEARSUP
GELUSIL
GENESEE
GENESES
GENESET
GENESIS
GENUSES
GETSSET
GIBESAT
GIBUSES
GIFTSET
GIRASOL
GIRLSHY
GIVESIN
GIVESOF
GIVESON
GIVESTO
GIVESUP
GLAMSUP
GLASSED
GLASSES
GLEASON
GLOSSAE
GLOSSAL
GLOSSAS
GLOSSED
GLOSSER
GLOSSES
GLUESON
GLUESTO
GNAWSAT
GNAWSON
GNOSSUS
GOBYSEA
GOODSON
GOOFSUP
GOTOSEA
GOTOSEE
GRABSAT
GRASSED
GRASSES
GRASSLE
GRAYSON
GREASED
GREASER
GREASES
GRIMSBY
GRINSAT
GRISSOM
GROSSED
GROSSER
GROSSES
GROSSLY
GROUSED
GROUSER
GROUSES
GROWSON
GROWSUP
GUESSAT
GUESSED
GUESSER
GUESSES
GUESSSO
GUNUSER

G••••S•

GABFEST
GAMIEST
GAPLESS
GARNISH
GASLESS
GASMASK
GAULISH
GAWKISH
GAYNESS
GEMLESS
GENOESE
GENOISE
GEODESY
GETBUSY
GETCASH
GETLOST
GETPAST
GETWISE
GIOCOSO
GIRLISH
GJETOST
GLIMPSE
GLOBOSE
GLUCOSE
GLUIEST
GNOMISH
GNOMIST
GOAMISS
GOATISH
GODDESS
GODLESS
GOFIRST
GOIRISH
GOODISH
GOODUSE
GOOIEST
GORIEST
GOTBUSY
GOTCASH
GOTLOST
GOTPAST
GOTWISE
GOULASH
GOUTISH
GRAVEST
GRAYEST
GRAYISH
GRECISM
GREYEST
GREYISH
GUESSSO
GUMLESS
GUNCASE
GUNLESS
GUTLESS
GYMNAST

G•••••S

GABBERS
GABBLES
GABBROS
GADDERS
GADGETS
GAFFERS
GAGGERS
GAGGLES
GAGLAWS
GAINERS
GAITERS
GALANOS
GALANTS
GALAXES
GALENAS
GALLEYS
GALLONS
GALLOPS
GALLOWS
GALOOTS
GALPALS
GAMBITS
GAMBLES
GAMBOLS
GAMETES
GAMINES
GAMMERS
GAMMONS
GANDERS
GANGERS
GANNETS
GAOLERS
GAPKIDS
GAPLESS
GARAGES
GARBLES
GARCONS
GARDENS
GARGLES
GARLICS
GARLITS
GARNERS
GARNETS
GARRETS
GARTERS
GASBAGS
GASCANS
GASCAPS
GASCONS
GASEOUS
GASHOGS
GASJETS
GASKETS
GASLESS
GASLOGS
GASPERS
GASSERS
GASWARS
GATHERS
GATINGS
GATLINS
GAUCHOS
GAUDENS
GAUDIES
GAUGERS
GAUSSES
GAVIALS
GAWKERS
GAWPERS
GAYNESS
GAZEBOS
GECKOES
GEEGAWS
GEEZERS
GEISHAS
GELATES
GELATIS
GELATOS
GELCAPS
GELPENS
GEMINIS
GEMLESS
GENDERS
GENERIS
GENESES
GENESIS
GENGHIS
GENOMES
GENTLES
GENUSES
GENXERS
GEORGES
GERBILS
GERENTS
GERMANS
GERUNDS
GERVAIS
GESSOES
GETTERS
GETTHIS
GEWGAWS
GEYSERS
GFORCES
GHETTOS
GIBBERS
GIBBONS
GIBBOUS
GIBLETS
GIBLUES
GIBSONS
GIBUSES
GIDDIES
GIDEONS
GIFTEES
GIGBAGS
GIGGLES
GIGOLOS
GILBLAS
GILDERS
GIMBALS
GIMBELS
GIMLETS
GINGERS
GINGKOS
GINKGOS
GIORGOS
GIPSIES
GIRDERS
GIRDLES
GIRLIES
GITANOS
GIVEUPS
GLAMORS
GLANCES
GLASSES
GLAZERS
GLIDERS
GLITZES
GLOBINS
GLOBOUS
GLORIAS
GLORIES
GLOSSAS
GLOSSES
GLOTTIS
GLOWERS
GLURGES
GLUTENS
GLUTEUS
GLYCOLS
GLYNNIS
GNASHES
GNAWERS
GNOMONS
GNOSSUS
GOALIES
GOAMISS
GOATEES
GOBBLES
GOBLETS
GOBLINS
GOBYBUS
GOCARTS
GODDESS
GODLESS
GODSONS
GODWITS
GOGGLES
GOGIRLS
GOITERS
GOKARTS
GOLFERS
GOMPERS
GOOBERS
GOODBYS
GOODERS
GOODIES
GOOFUPS
GOOGLES
GOOGOLS
GOONEYS
GOONIES
GOPHERS
GORDIUS
GORGERS
GORGONS
GOSPELS
GOSSIPS
GOTCHAS
GOTHICS
GOUGERS
GOURDES
GOVERNS
GRACIAS
GRADERS
GRAHAMS
GRAMMES
GRAMMYS
GRAMPAS
GRAMPUS
GRANGES
GRANPAS
GRAPPAS
GRASSES
GRATERS
GRATIAS
GRAVELS
GRAVERS
GRAVIES
GRAZERS
GREASES
GREAVES
GRIEVES
GRIGRIS
GRILLES
GRINGOS
GRIPERS
GRIPPES
GROCERS
GROOVES
GROPERS
GROPIUS
GROSSES
GROTIUS
GROTTOS
GROUNDS
GROUSES
GROVELS
GROVERS
GROWERS
GROWTHS
GRUDGES
GRUNGES
GUESSES
GUFFAWS
GUIDERS
GUINEAS
GUITARS
GULCHES
GULDENS
GULLAHS
GULLETS
GULLIES
GULPERS
GUMLESS
GUNDOGS
GUNITES
GUNLAPS
GUNLAWS
GUNLESS
GUNNERS
GUNNIES
GUNSELS
GUPPIES
GURGLES
GURKHAS
GURNEYS
GUSHERS
GUSSETS
GUSSIES
GUSTOES
GUTLESS
GUTTERS
GUVNORS
GUZZLES
GYMBAGS
GYMRATS
GYPPERS
GYPSIES
GYPSUMS
GYRATES
GYRENES

•G•S•••

AGASSIZ
AGESAGO
AGESOUT
EGESTED
EGGSACS
EGOSURF

•G••S••

AGASSIZ
AGEISTS
EGLISES
EGOISTE
EGOISTS
IGUASSU

•G•••S•

AGAINST
AGELESS
AGGRESS
AGILEST
AGONISE
AGONISM
AGONIST
EGGCASE
EGGIEST
EGGLESS
EGGTOSS
EGOTISM
EGOTIST
IGUASSU
OGREISH
UGLIEST

•G••••S

AGARICS
AGEISTS
AGELESS
AGENCES
AGENDAS
AGGRESS
AGNAILS
AGNATES
AGONIES
AGOUTIS
AGREERS
AGULHAS
EGERIAS

EGGCUPS
EGGLERS
EGGLESS
EGGNOGS
EGGSACS
EGGTOSS
EGLISES
EGOISTS
HGWELLS
IGNEOUS
IGNITES
IGNORES
IGOROTS
IGUANAS
OGDOADS
OGLALAS
PGAPROS

••GS•••

BEGSFOR
BEGSOFF
BIGSALE
BIGSHOT
BIGSHOW
BIGSTAR
BUGSOFF
BUGSOUT
DIGSFOR
DIGSOUT
DOGSAGE
DOGSEAR
DOGSHOW
DOGSITS
DOGSLED
DOGSTAR
EGGSACS
GAGSTER
JIGSAWS
LOGSOFF
LOGSOUT
LUGSAIL
LUGSOUT
MUGSHOT
PIGSKIN
PIGSOUT
PUGSLEY
RAGSHOP
RIGSOUT
TAGSALE
TAGSOUT
TOGSOUT
WIGSOUT

••G•S••

AEGISES
ARGUSES
AUGUSTA
AUGUSTE
AUGUSTO
AUGUSTS
AVGASES
BOGUSLY
CAGESUP
DEGUSTS
DIGESTS
EDGESIN
HIGHSEA
INGESTA
INGESTS
LAGASSE
LEGISTS
LEGOSET
NEGUSES
PAGESIX
PEGASUS
SIGHSAT
SIGNSIN
SIGNSON
SIGNSUP
URGESON

••G••S•

AGGRESS
ANGUISH
BIGBOSS
BIGEAST
BIGEASY
BIGFISH
BIGGEST
BIGGISH
BIGMESS
BIGNESS
BIGNOSE
BOGGISH
BOGGUSS
CAGIEST
DEGAUSS
DEGHOST
DIGRESS
DOGFISH
DOGGISH
DOGLESS
DOGROSE
DOGVEST
EDGIEST
EGGCASE
EGGIEST
EGGLESS
EGGTOSS
ENGLISH
ENGROSS
FOGLESS
FOGYISH
FOGYISM
HAGGISH
HIGHEST
HIGHISH
HOGGISH
HOGNOSE
HOGWASH
INGLESE
INGRESS
JAGLESS
JIGGISH
LAGASSE
LEGLESS
LEGREST
LOGGISH
LOGIEST
MUGGISH
NAGGISH
NIGHEST
ORGIAST
PEGLESS
PIGFISH
PIGGISH
PUGGISH
PUGNOSE
REGLOSS
REGRASP
REGRESS
ROGUISH
SAGIEST
SUGGEST
TIGRESS
TUGLESS
UNGROSS
VAGUEST
VOGUISH
WAGGISH
WIGLESS
YOGIISM

••G•••S

AEGISES
AFGHANS
AGGRESS
AIGLETS
AIGRETS
ALGIERS
ANGELAS
ANGELES
ANGELUS
ANGLAIS
ANGLERS
ANGORAS
ARGALIS
ARGENTS
ARGUERS
ARGUSES
ARGYLES
AUGENDS
AUGITES
AUGUSTS
AVGASES
BAGBOYS
BAGFULS
BAGGERS
BAGGIES
BAGGINS
BAGJOBS
BAGNIOS
BAGWIGS
BEGGARS
BEGIRDS
BIGAPES
BIGBETS
BIGBOSS
BIGBOYS
BIGCARS
BIGCATS
BIGDAYS
BIGDIGS
BIGDOGS
BIGEARS
BIGENDS
BIGEYES
BIGFANS
BIGGERS
BIGGIES
BIGGUNS
BIGHITS
BIGHUGS
BIGKIDS
BIGLIES
BIGLOTS
BIGMACS
BIGMESS
BIGNESS
BIGNEWS
BIGONES
BIGRIGS
BIGTOES
BIGTOPS
BIGWIGS
BIGWINS
BOGARTS
BOGGLES
BOGGUSS
BUGBOYS
BUGGIES
BUGGLES
BUGLERS
BUGOUTS
BYGONES
COGGLES
COGNACS
CYGNETS
DAGGERS
DEGAUSS
DEGERMS
DEGREES
DEGUSTS
DIGESTS
DIGGERS
DIGLOTS
DIGRAMS
DIGRESS
DOGAPES
DOGBEDS
DOGDAYS
DOGEARS
DOGGIES
DOGLEGS
DOGLESS
DOGNAPS
DOGRUNS
DOGSITS
DOGTAGS
DOGTOYS
DUGONGS
DUGOUTS
EAGLETS
EDGINGS
EGGCUPS
EGGLERS
EGGLESS
EGGNOGS
EGGSACS
EGGTOSS
EIGHTHS
ENGAGES
ENGILDS
ENGINES
ENGIRDS
ENGLUTS
ENGRAMS
ENGROSS
ENGULFS
FAGENDS
FIGBARS
FIGURES
FOGBOWS
FOGDOGS
FOGGERS
FOGLESS
FUGATOS
GAGGERS
GAGGLES
GAGLAWS
GIGBAGS
GIGGLES
GIGOLOS
GOGGLES
GOGIRLS
HAGGLES
HEGIRAS
HIGGINS
HIGGLES
HIGHIQS
HIGHRES
HOGNUTS
HOGTIES
HUGGERS
HUGGIES
HUGGINS
HYGINUS
INGALLS
INGATES
INGESTS
INGOALS
INGRESS
INGULFS
ITGIRLS
JAGGIES
JAGLESS
JAGUARS
JIGGERS
JIGGLES
JIGSAWS
JOGBRAS
JOGGERS
JOGGLES
JUGFULS
JUGGLES
KEGGERS
KEGLERS
LAGGERS
LAGOONS
LAGUNAS
LEGATES
LEGATOS
LEGENDS
LEGIONS
LEGISTS
LEGLESS
LEGOLAS
LEGUMES
LIGANDS
LIGATES
LIGNINS
LOGGERS
LOGGIAS
LOGGINS
LOGJAMS
LOGOFFS
LOGOUTS
LUGGERS
LUGNUTS
MAGGOTS
MAGLEVS
MAGNETS
MAGNUMS
MAGPIES
MAGYARS
MEGANES
MEGOHMS
MEGRIMS
MIGENES
MIGNONS
MUGFULS
MUGGERS
MUGGLES
NAGGERS
NEGATES
NEGUSES
NIGGLES
NOGALES
NOGGINS
NOGIFTS
NOGOODS
NUGGETS
ORGEATS
PAGINGS
PAGODAS
PEGASUS
PEGLEGS
PEGLESS
PEGTOPS
PIGEONS
PIGGIES
PIGLETS
PIGNUTS
PIGOUTS
PIGPENS
PUGGLES
PYGMIES
RAGBAGS
RAGGIES
RAGINGS
RAGLANS
RAGMANS
RAGMOPS
RAGOUTS
RAGRUGS
RAGTOPS
REGAINS
REGALES
REGARDS
REGEARS
REGENTS
REGIFTS
REGILDS
REGIMES
REGINAS
REGIONS
REGIRDS
REGIVES
REGLOSS
REGLOWS
REGLUES
REGRABS
REGRESS
REGRETS
REGRIPS
REGROWS
REGULUS
RIGGERS
RIGOURS
RUGGLES
RUGRATS
SEGWAYS
SIGHERS
SIGNALS
SIGNEES
SIGNERS
SIGNETS
SIGNORS
SIGNUPS
TAGDAYS
TAGENDS
TAGGERS
TAGOUTS
TIGLONS
TIGRESS
TOGGLES
TUGGERS
TUGLESS
TUGRIKS
TVGAMES
UNGIRDS
UNGLUES
UNGRIPS
UNGROSS
UPGAZES
UPGIRDS
UPGROWS
URGINGS
VEGGIES
VIGOURS
VOGUERS
WAGGERS
WAGGLES
WIGGLES
WIGLESS
WIGLETS
WIGWAGS
WIGWAMS
YOGINIS
YOGURTS
ZAGNUTS
ZIGZAGS
ZYGOTES

•••GS••

BANGSON
BANGSUP
BERGSON
CLOGSUP
DODGSON
DRAGSIN
DRAGSON
DRAGSUP
GANGSAW
GANGSTA
GANGSUP
HANGSBY
HANGSIN
HANGSON
HANGSUP
PLUGSIN
PLUGSUP
RINGSIN
RINGSUP
SINGSTO
SNAGSUP
WINGSIT

•••G•S•

BIGGEST
BIGGISH
BOGGISH
BOGGUSS
BURGESS
CONGEST
DISGUST
DOGGISH
ELEGIST
HAGGISH
HOGGISH
IMAGISM
IMAGIST
JIGGISH
LARGESS
LARGEST
LARGISH
LOGGISH
LONGEST
LONGISH
MUGGISH
NAGGISH
OMIGOSH
OUTGUSH
PIGGISH
PUGGISH
SUGGEST
WAGGISH

•••G••S

ADAGIOS
AIRGUNS
ALEGARS
ALIGHTS
APOGEES
BADGERS
BADGUYS
BAGGERS
BAGGIES
BAGGINS
BANGERS
BANGLES
BARGERS
BEAGLES
BEEGEES
BEGGARS
BEIGNES
BENGALS
BERGIUS
BIGGERS
BIGGIES
BIGGUNS
BINGERS
BINGLES
BINGOES
BLIGHTS
BOGGLES
BOGGUSS
BONGOES
BOOGIES
BORGIAS
BRIGHTS
BROGANS
BROGUES
BUDGERS
BUDGETS
BUDGIES
BUGGIES
BUGGLES
BULGARS
BULGURS
BUNGEES
BUNGLES
BURGESS
BURGEES
BURGERS
BURGESS
BURGLES
BURGOOS
CADGERS
CAPGUNS
CARGOES
CATGUTS
CHIGOES
CODGERS
COGGLES
COIGNES
CONGERS
CONGOUS
COUGARS
CUDGELS
DAGGERS
DANGERS
DANGLES
DIGGERS
DINGERS
DINGLES
DINGOES
DODGEMS
DODGERS
DOGGIES
DONGLES
DOUGLAS
DRAGEES
DRAGONS
DROGUES
EADGILS
ELEGIES
ELEGITS
ELIGIUS
EMIGRES
ENIGMAS
FIDGETS
FINGALS
FINGERS
FIZGIGS
FLAGONS
FLIGHTS
FOGGERS
FOLGERS
FORGERS
FORGETS
FORGOES
FRIGHTS
FUDGERS
FUNGOES
GADGETS
GAGGERS
GAGGLES
GANGERS
GARGLES
GAUGERS
GEEGAWS
GENGHIS
GEWGAWS
GIGGLES
GINGERS
GINGKOS
GOGGLES
GOOGLES
GOOGOLS
GORGERS
GORGONS
GOUGERS
GRIGRIS
GURGLES
HAGGLES
HANGARS
HANGBYS
HANGERS
HANGUPS
HEDGERS
HEIGHTS
HIGGINS
HIGGLES
HOAGIES
HUGGERS
HUGGIES
HUGGINS
HUNGERS
HUYGENS
IMAGERS
IMAGOES
ISOGONS
JAEGERS
JAGGIES
JANGLES
JARGONS
JERGENS
JETGUNS
JIGGERS
JIGGLES
JINGLES
JINGOES
JOGGERS
JOGGLES
JUDGERS
JUGGLES
JUNGLES
JURGENS
KEDGERS
KEGGERS
KNIGHTS
LAGGERS
LARGESS
LEAGUES
LEDGERS
LENGTHS
LENGUAS
LINGERS
LINGOES
LODGERS
LOGGERS
LOGGIAS
LOGGINS
LONGIES
LONGUES
LUGGERS
LUNGERS
MAGGOTS
MAJGENS
MANGERS
MANGLES
MANGOES
MARGINS
MEAGLES
MERGEES
MERGERS
MIDGETS
MINGLES
MONGERS
MONGOLS
MORGANS
MORGUES
MUGGERS
MUGGLES
NAGGERS
NAUGHTS
NIGGLES
NOGGINS
NOOGIES
NOUGATS
NOUGHTS
NUDGERS
NUGGETS
OLDGAGS
OLOGIES
ONAGERS
ORIGINS
OUTGOES
OUTGUNS
PARGERS
PIDGINS
PIGGIES
PINGERS
PLAGUES
PLIGHTS
PLUGINS
PONGEES
PONGIDS
POPGUNS
PORGIES
PUGGLES
QUAGGAS
RAGGIES
RANGERS
RAYGUNS
REAGANS
RIGGERS
RINGERS
RODGERS
ROTGUTS
RUGGLES
RUTGERS
SEAGODS
SHOGUNS
SINGERS
SINGLES
SIXGUNS
SLIGHTS
SLOGANS
SNUGLIS
SPIGOTS
STAGERS
STAGNES
STIGMAS
STOGIES
SUBGODS
SUNGODS
TAGGERS
TANGLES
TARGETS
TINGLES
TINGODS
TOGGLES
TONGANS
TONGUES
TOPGUNS
TOYGUNS
TRIGONS
TUGGERS
VEGGIES
VEIGHTS
VERGERS
VIRGINS
WAGGERS
WAGGLES
WANGLES
WARGODS
WEDGIES
WEIGHTS
WIDGETS
WIGGLES
WINGERS
WRIGHTS
ZINGERS
ZIPGUNS

••••GS•

AMONGST
DOINGSO

••••G•S

ALLAGES
ALLEGES
ASIAGOS
ASSIGNS
ATSIGNS
AVENGES
BADEGGS
BAREGES
BELUGAS
BLUDGES
BODEGAS
BRIDGES
CAYUGAS
CHANGES
CHARGES
CHOUGHS
COALGAS
COSIGNS
CRINGES
CUBAGES
DAMAGES
DELUGES
DESIGNS
DIMAGES
DOSAGES
DOTAGES
DREDGES
DRUDGES
DRVEGAS
EMERGES
ENCAGES
ENGAGES
ENRAGES
ENSIGNS
ERYNGOS
FLANGES
FLEDGES
FORAGES
FORDGTS
FRIDGES
FRINGES
GARAGES
GEORGES
GINKGOS
GIORGOS
GLURGES
GRANGES
GRINGOS
GRUDGES
GRUNGES
HADAGAS
HASAGAS
HOMAGES
ICEAGES
IMPUGNS
INDIGOS
INNAGES
KLUDGES
LASTGAS
LATIGOS
LAVAGES
LIMOGES
LINAGES
LOUNGES
LOVAGES
MALAGAS
MALIGNS
MANAGES
MANEGES
MENAGES
MIRAGES
NEONGAS
NONAGES
NOODGES
OBLIGES
OHMAGES
OPPUGNS
ORANGES
OUTAGES
OWLEGGS
PAANGAS
PAPAGOS
PELAGES
PIPAGES
PLEDGES
PLOUGHS
PLUNGES
POTAGES
PREAGES
QUAGGAS
RAREGAS
RAVAGES
RAWEGGS
RECAGES
REFUGES
RENEGES
REPAGES
REPUGNS
RESIGNS
REURGES
SAVAGES
SCRUGGS
SLEDGES

SLEIGHS
SLOUGHS
SLUDGES
SMIDGES
SMUDGES
SPONGES
STODGES
STOOGES
STREGIS
STURGES
TEARGAS
THEAGES
TOWAGES
TRIAGES
TROUGHS
TRUDGES
TSONGAS
TWINGES
TWOEGGS
ULLAGES
UNCAGES
UNEDGES
VIRAGOS
VISAGES
VOYAGES

•••••GS

AIRBAGS
AIRINGS
AIRLOGS
ALEKEGS
ANALOGS
ARCINGS
AWNINGS
BADDOGS
BADEGGS
BAGWIGS
BEDBUGS
BELONGS
BIGDIGS
BIGDOGS
BIGHUGS
BIGRIGS
BIGWIGS
BLUINGS
BODINGS
BOEINGS
BORINGS
BUMLEGS
CANINGS
CASINGS
CATRIGS
COMINGS
COYDOGS
CYBORGS
DATINGS
DEFANGS
DEFRAGS
DESMOGS
DIALOGS
DOGLEGS
DOGTAGS
DRYFOGS
DUGONGS
EARTAGS
EARWIGS
EDGINGS
EGGNOGS
ENDINGS
EPILOGS
ERLANGS
FACINGS
FILINGS
FIRINGS
FIXINGS
FIZGIGS
FLUBUGS
FOGDOGS
GASBAGS
GASHOGS
GASLOGS
GATINGS
GIGBAGS
GUNDOGS
GYMBAGS
HAYINGS
HAZINGS
HIDINGS
HOTDOGS
HUMBUGS
ICEBAGS
ICEFOGS
IIKINGS
INKINGS
INNINGS
JETLAGS
KITBAGS
LACINGS
LADINGS
LAPDOGS
LEXUSGS
LIKINGS
LININGS
LIVINGS
LOSINGS
MADDOGS
MAKINGS
MAYINGS
MAYTAGS
MIDLEGS
MININGS
MOWINGS
MUSINGS
NUTMEGS
OAKTAGS
OBLONGS
OFFINGS
OILRIGS
OLDDOGS
OLDGAGS
OOLONGS
OUTBEGS
OUTINGS
OUTRIGS
OWLEGGS
PAGINGS
PALINGS
PARINGS
PAVINGS
PEGLEGS
PETDOGS
PETPIGS
PHOTOGS
PILINGS
PIPINGS
PROLOGS
PYEDOGS
QUAHOGS
RAGBAGS
RAGINGS
RAGRUGS
RATINGS
RAVINGS
RAWEGGS
REDDOGS
REDLEGS
REDRAGS
REDTAGS
REFLAGS
REHANGS
RESINGS
RIDINGS
RISINGS
ROVINGS
RULINGS
SARONGS
SAVINGS
SAWLOGS
SAYINGS
SCRUGGS
SEABAGS
SEADOGS
SEALEGS
SIDINGS
SPRINGS
SPYINGS
STALAGS
STRINGS
SUNDOGS
SUPERGS
TAKINGS
TAPINGS
TEABAGS
THEHOGS
THRONGS
TIDINGS
TILINGS
TIMINGS
TOPDOGS
TOWINGS
TOYDOGS
TWOEGGS
UNCLOGS
UNPLUGS
UNSNAGS
URGINGS
USFLAGS
VIKINGS
WAKINGS
WAXINGS
WEBLOGS
WETRAGS
WIGWAGS
WIRINGS
ZIGZAGS

G•T••••

GATEAUX
GATELEG
GATEMAN
GATEMEN
GATEWAY
GATHERS
GATINGS
GATLING
GATLINS
GATTACA
GATWICK
GETABLE
GETAHIT
GETAJOB
GETATIP
GETAWAY
GETBACK
GETBEAT
GETBENT
GETBUSY
GETCASH
GETCOLD
GETCUTE
GETDONE
GETDOWN
GETEVEN
GETFREE
GETFROM
GETGOOD
GETHELP
GETHURT
GETINON
GETINTO
GETITON
GETLOST
GETONIT
GETONTO
GETOVER
GETPAST
GETREAL
GETSANA
GETSANF
GETSFAR
GETSFIT
GETSHEP
GETSHIP
GETSHOT
GETSMAD
GETSOFF
GETSOFT
GETSOLD
GETSORE
GETSOUT
GETSRID
GETSSET
GETSWET
GETTERS
GETTHIS
GETTING
GETTOIT
GETUPON
GETWARM
GETWELL
GETWISE
GETWORD
GITANOS
GITTING
GOTAHIT
GOTAJOB
GOTATIP
GOTAWAY
GOTBACK
GOTBEAT
GOTBUSY
GOTCASH
GOTCHAS
GOTCOLD
GOTCUTE
GOTDONE
GOTDOWN
GOTEVEN
GOTFREE
GOTGOOD
GOTHELP
GOTHICS
GOTHIKA
GOTHURT
GOTINON
GOTINTO
GOTITON
GOTLOST
GOTMILK
GOTOBED
GOTOGAL
GOTOGUY
GOTONIT
GOTONTO
GOTOPOT
GOTOSEA
GOTOSEE
GOTOVER
GOTOWAR
GOTPAST
GOTREAL
GOTSOFT
GOTSORE
GOTTAGO
GOTTOIT
GOTUPON
GOTUPTO
GOTWARM
GOTWELL
GOTWISE
GOTWORD
GSTRING
GUTHRIE
GUTLESS
GUTSIER
GUTSILY
GUTTERS
GUTTIER
GUTTING

G••T•••

GAETANO
GAITERS
GAITING
GANTLET
GARTERS
GASTANK
GASTERO
GASTONE
GASTRIC
GATTACA
GAUTAMA
GAUTIER
GENTEEL
GENTIAN
GENTILE
GENTLED
GENTLER
GENTLES
GESTALT
GESTAPO
GESTATE
GESTURE
GETTERS
GETTHIS
GETTING
GETTOIT
GHETTOS
GIFTBOX
GIFTEES
GIFTING
GIFTSET
GIFTTAX
GIRTHED
GIRTING
GITTING
GJETOST
GLITCHY
GLITTER
GLITZED
GLITZES
GLOTTAL
GLOTTIS
GLUTEAL
GLUTENS
GLUTEUS
GLUTTED
GLUTTON
GOATEED
GOATEES
GOATISH
GODTHAB
GOITERS
GORTNER
GOSTALE
GOTTAGO
GOTTOIT
GOUTIER
GOUTILY
GOUTISH
GRATEON
GRATERS
GRATEUP
GRATIAS
GRATIFY
GRATING
GRETZKY
GRITTED
GRITTER
GROTIUS
GROTTOS
GUITARS
GUMTREE
GUNTHER
GUSTAVE
GUSTIER
GUSTILY
GUSTING
GUSTOES
GUTTERS
GUTTIER
GUTTING

G•••T••

GAGSTER
GALATEA
GALATIA
GALETTE
GAMETAL
GAMETES
GANGTOK
GAROTTE
GAUNTER
GAUNTLY
GAVOTTE
GAZETTE
GELATED
GELATES
GELATIN
GELATIS
GELATOS
GENETIC
GENITOR
GERITOL
GETATIP
GETITON
GHASTLY
GHETTOS
GHOSTED
GHOSTLY
GIFTTAX
GIGATON
GLINTED
GLISTEN
GLISTER
GLITTER
GLOATED
GLOATER
GLOTTAL
GLOTTIS
GLUTTED
GLUTTON
GLYPTIC
GNOSTIC
GOAFTER
GODUTCH
GOGETEM
GOLDTIP
GOLFTEE
GOODTRY
GORETEX
GOTATIP
GOTITON
GRAFTED
GRAFTER
GRAFTON
GRANTED
GRANTEE
GRANTER
GRANTOR
GREATEN
GREATER
GREATLY
GREETED
GREETER
GRIFTED
GRIFTER
GRISTER
GRISTLE
GRISTLY
GRITTED
GRITTER
GROTTOS
GROUTED
GROUTER
GROWTHS
GRUNTED
GRUNTER
GUESTED
GUNITES
GYRATED
GYRATES
GYRATOR

G••••T•

GADGETS
GADGETY
GALANTS
GALEATE
GALENTO
GALETTE
GALOOTS
GAMBITS
GANGSTA
GANNETS
GANNETT
GARLITS
GARNETS
GARNETT
GAROTTE
GARRETS
GARRETT
GARROTE
GASEITY
GASJETS
GASKETS
GAVOTTE
GAZETTE
GEARSTO
GEFILTE
GEMMATE
GERENTS
GESTATE
GETCUTE
GETINTO
GETONTO
GIBLETS
GIMLETS
GIVENTO
GIVESTO
GLOBATE
GLUEDTO
GLUESTO
GOBLETS
GOCARTS
GODWITS
GOFORTH
GOINGTO
GOKARTS
GOLIATH
GORDITA
GOSOUTH
GOSSETT
GOTCUTE
GOTINTO
GOTONTO
GOTUPTO
GRADATE
GRANITA
GRANITE
GRAVITY
GULLETS
GUSSETS
GWYNETH
GYMRATS

G•••••T

GABFEST
GALLANT
GAMIEST
GANNETT
GANTLET
GAPEDAT
GAPESAT
GARMENT
GARNETT
GARRETT
GASHEAT
GAVEOUT
GAWKSAT
GAZEDAT
GAZESAT
GENESET
GERAINT
GESTALT
GETAHIT
GETBEAT
GETBENT
GETHURT
GETLOST
GETONIT
GETPAST
GETSFIT
GETSHOT
GETSOFT
GETSOUT
GETSSET
GETSWET
GETTOIT
GIBESAT
GIFTSET
GIGABIT
GILBERT
GILLNET
GIVEOUT
GJETOST
GLAREAT
GLUIEST
GNAWSAT
GNOMIST
GOABOUT
GODSENT
GOESAFT
GOESOUT
GOFIRST
GOFORIT
GOINGAT
GOKAPUT
GONEAFT
GONEOUT
GOOIEST
GORIEST
GOSSETT
GOTAHIT
GOTBEAT
GOTHURT
GOTLOST
GOTONIT
GOTOPOT
GOTPAST
GOTSOFT
GOTTOIT
GOURMET
GRABSAT
GRASPAT
GRAVEST
GRAYEST
GREWFAT
GREYEST
GRINSAT
GRISLET
GROMMET
GROWFAT
GUESSAT
GUJARAT
GUMBOOT
GUNBELT
GUNBOAT
GUNSHOT
GUSHOUT
GYMNAST
GYMSUIT

•G•T•••

AGATINE
AGITATE
AGITATO
AGUTTER
EGGTOSS
EGOTISM
EGOTIST
EGOTRIP
IGOTCHA
IGOTYOU
PGATOUR

•G••T••

AGENTED
AGENTRY
AGNATES
AGNATIC
AGOUTIS
AGUTTER
EGESTED
IGNATOW
IGNITED
IGNITER
IGNITES
IGNITOR
PGRATED

•G•••T•

AGEISTS
AGEMATE
AGILITY
AGITATE
AGITATO
AGREETO
EGALITE
EGOISTE
EGOISTS
IGOROTS

•G••••T

AGAINST
AGEDOUT
AGESOUT
AGILEST
AGONIST
EGGHUNT
EGGIEST
EGOTIST
OGDENUT
UGLIEST

••GT•••

BIGTALK
BIGTENT
BIGTIME
BIGTOES
BIGTOPS
BIGTOWN
DOGTAGS
DOGTAIL
DOGTICK
DOGTOYS
DOGTROT
EGGTOSS
FIGTREE
HOGTIED
HOGTIES
JIGTIME
JOGTROT
LEGTRAP
PEGTOPS
PIGTAIL
RAGTIME
RAGTOPS
TAGTEAM

••G•T••

AUGITES
BIGOTED
BIGOTRY
BIGSTAR
BUGATTI
DIGITAL
DOGSTAR
EIGHTAD
EIGHTAM
EIGHTBC
EIGHTEE
EIGHTHS
EIGHTPM
EIGHTUP
ERGOTIC
FAGOTED
FIGHTER
FUGATOS
GAGSTER
GIGATON
GOGETEM
HIGHTEA
HIGHTOP
INGATES
LEGATEE
LEGATES
LEGATOR
LEGATOS
LIGATED
LIGATES
LIGHTED
LIGHTEN
LIGHTER
LIGHTLY
LIGHTON
LIGHTUP
MEGATON
MIGHTNT
NEGATED
NEGATER
NEGATES
NEGATOR
NIGHTER
NIGHTIE
NIGHTLY
OUGHTNT
OUGHTTO
PAGETWO
REGATTA
RIGHTED
RIGHTER
RIGHTLY
RIGHTON
SAGETEA
SIGHTED
SIGHTER
SIGHTLY
TIGHTEN
TIGHTER
TIGHTLY
UNGATED
VEGETAL
ZYGOTES

••G••T•

AIGLETS
AIGRETS
ARGANTE
ARGENTI
ARGENTO
ARGENTS
AUGUSTA
AUGUSTE
AUGUSTO
AUGUSTS
BEGANTO
BIGBETS
BIGCATS
BIGCITY
BIGGITY
BIGHITS
BIGLOTS
BOGARTS
BUGATTI
BUGOUTS
COGNATE
CYGNETS
DEGUSTS
DIGESTS
DIGGITY
DIGINTO
DIGLOTS
DIGNITY
DOGBITE
DOGGATE
DOGGETT
DOGMATA
DOGSITS
DUGINTO
DUGOUTS
EAGLETS
ENGLUTS
FOGCITY
FOGERTY
HAGERTY
HOGARTH
HOGNUTS
INGESTA
INGESTS
INGRATE
LEGISTS
LIGGETT
LIGNITE
LOGONTO
LOGOUTS
LUGNUTS
MAGENTA
MAGGOTS
MAGNATE
MAGNETO
MAGNETS
MIGRATE
NOGIFTS
NUGGETS
NUGGETY
ORGEATS
OUGHTTO
PIGLETS
PIGNUTS
PIGOUTS
RAGOUTS
REGATTA
REGENTS
REGIFTS
REGRETS
RUGRATS
SIGNETS
TAGOUTS
WIGLETS
YOGURTS
ZAGNUTS

••G•••T

ANGRYAT
AUGMENT
BAGEHOT
BIGBEAT
BIGEAST
BIGFEET
BIGFOOT
BIGGEST
BIGSHOT
BIGTENT
BIGUNIT
BUGSOUT
CAGEPET
CAGIEST
DEGHOST
DIGIPET
DIGSOUT
DOGBERT
DOGBOOT
DOGCART
DOGCOAT
DOGGETT
DOGREAT
DOGTROT
DOGVEST
EDGEOUT
EDGIEST
EGGHUNT
EGGIEST
ENGRAFT

FIGMENT
GIGABIT
HIGHART
HIGHEST
HIGHHAT
IMGREAT
INGRAFT
JOGTROT
LEGOSET
LEGREST
LIGGETT
LOGANUT
LOGIEST
LOGSOUT
LUGSOUT
MAGINOT
MEGABIT
MEGAHIT
MIGHTNT
MIGRANT
MUGSHOT
MYGIANT
NEGLECT
NIGHEST
NYGIANT
ORGIAST
OUGHTNT
PAGEANT
PIGMEAT
PIGMENT
PIGSOUT
REGNANT
REGRAFT
REGRANT
REGREET
RIGSOUT
SAGIEST
SEGMENT
SIGHSAT
SIGNOUT
SUGGEST
TAGAMET
TAGGANT
TAGSOUT
TOGSOUT
TUGBOAT
UNGUENT
USGRANT
VAGRANT
VAGUEST
WIGSOUT
YOGAMAT
YOGHURT

•••GT••

GANGTOK
HANGTEN
HUNGTEN
KINGTUT
LANGTON
LANGTRY
LENGTHS
LENGTHY
LONGTOM
LONGTON
WINGTIP
YANGTZE

•••G•T•

ALIGHTS
ALIGOTE
ARIGATO
BIGGITY
BLIGHTS
BLIGHTY
BRIGHTS
BUDGETS
CATGUTS
COLGATE
DEIGNTO
DIGGITY
DOGGATE
DOGGETT
DOUGHTY
DRAGOTI
DWIGHTD
ELEGITS
EXEGETE
FIDGETS
FIDGETY
FLIGHTS
FLIGHTY
FORGETS
FRIGATE
FRIGHTS
GADGETS
GADGETY
GANGSTA
HAUGHTY
HEIGHTS
IEIGHTY
KNIGHTS
LIGGETT
MAGGOTS
MARGATE
MIDGETS
NAUGHTS
NAUGHTY
NEWGATE
NOUGATS
NOUGHTS
NUGGETS
NUGGETY
PADGETT
PETGATE
PLIGHTS
ROTGUTS
SEAGATE
SINGSTO
SLIGHTS
SPIGOTS
TARGETS
VEIGHTS
VIRGATE
VULGATE
WEIGHTS
WEIGHTY
WIDGETS
WRIGHTS

•••G••T

ASAGIFT
BANGOUT
BEIGNET
BIGGEST
COAGENT
CONGEST
CRUGUET
DINGBAT
DISGUST
DOGGETT
DRAGNET
DRAGOUT
ELEGANT
ELEGIST
EXIGENT
FROGLET
FULGENT
HANGOUT
HUNGOUT
IMAGIST
KINGLET
KINGRAT
KINGTUT
LARGENT
LARGEST
LAUGHAT
LIGGETT
LONGEST
LUNGEAT
MAIGRET
MARGRET
MONGKUT
PADGETT
PETGOAT
PEUGEOT
PUNGENT
RANGOUT
REAGENT
RIEGERT
RINGLET
RINGOUT
ROUGHIT
RUNGOUT
SANGOUT
SARGENT
SEAGIRT
SHEGOAT
SINGLET
SINGOUT
SNIGLET
SNUGFIT
SUGGEST
SWIGERT
TAGGANT
TANGENT
THEGIFT
WINGLET
WINGNUT
WINGSIT
XINGOUT

••••GT•

BRINGTO
CLINGTO
CLUNGTO
DOINGTO
FORDGTS
GOINGTO
HUANGTI
LYINGTO
OWINGTO
TYINGTO

••••G•T

ACINGIT
ALRIGHT
AMONGST
ATEIGHT
ATNIGHT
ATSIGHT
BOURGET
BRIDGET
BRINGIT
BROUGHT
BYRIGHT
DELIGHT
DORIGHT
DRAUGHT
DROUGHT
ENRIGHT
FLINGAT
FLUNGAT
FRAUGHT
FREIGHT
GOINGAT
ICINGIT
IFORGET
IFORGOT
ILLEGIT
INSIGHT
MRRIGHT
ONSIGHT
REFIGHT
RELIGHT
RESIGHT
SLEIGHT
SWINGAT
SWINGIT
SWUNGAT
SWUNGIT
THOUGHT
TLINGIT
TONIGHT
UNLIGHT
UNSIGHT
UPLIGHT
UPRIGHT
UPTIGHT
WROUGHT

•••••GT

VANVOGT

GU•••••

GUANACO
GUANINE
GUARANI
GUARDED
GUARDEE
GUARDER
GUARGUM
GUCKIER
GUDGEON
GUERDON
GUESSAT
GUESSED
GUESSER
GUESSES
GUESSSO
GUESTED
GUEVARA
GUFFAWS
GUIDERS
GUIDING
GUIGNOL
GUILDER
GUILING
GUINEAN
GUINEAS
GUITARS
GUJARAT
GULCHES
GULDENS
GULFING
GULFOIL
GULFWAR
GULLAHS
GULLETS
GULLIED
GULLIES
GULLING
GULPERS
GULPIER
GULPING
GUMBALL
GUMBOOT
GUMDROP
GUMLESS
GUMLIKE
GUMMIER
GUMMING
GUMSHOE
GUMTREE
GUMWOOD
GUNBELT
GUNBOAT
GUNCASE
GUNDOGS
GUNFIRE
GUNITES
GUNKIER
GUNLAPS
GUNLAWS
GUNLESS
GUNLOCK
GUNMOLL
GUNNERS
GUNNERY
GUNNIES
GUNNING
GUNPLAY
GUNROOM
GUNSELS
GUNSFOR
GUNSHIP
GUNSHOT
GUNTHER
GUNUSER
GUNWALE
GUPPIES
GURGLED
GURGLES
GURKHAS
GURNEYS
GUSHERS
GUSHIER
GUSHILY
GUSHING
GUSHOUT
GUSSETS
GUSSIED
GUSSIES
GUSSYUP
GUSTAVE
GUSTIER
GUSTILY
GUSTING
GUSTOES
GUTHRIE
GUTLESS
GUTSIER
GUTSILY
GUTTERS
GUTTIER
GUTTING
GUVNORS
GUYROPE
GUZZLED
GUZZLER
GUZZLES

G•U••••

GAUCHER
GAUCHOS
GAUDENS
GAUDERY
GAUDIER
GAUDIES
GAUDILY
GAUGERS
GAUGING
GAUGUIN
GAULISH
GAUNTER
GAUNTLY
GAUSSES
GAUTAMA
GAUTIER
GAUZIER
GAUZILY
GLUCOSE
GLUEDON
GLUEDTO
GLUEGUN
GLUESON
GLUESTO
GLUGGED
GLUIEST
GLUMMED
GLUMMER
GLURGES
GLUTEAL
GLUTENS
GLUTEUS
GLUTTED
GLUTTON
GOUACHE
GOUGERS
GOUGING
GOULASH
GOUNDER
GOURAMI
GOURDES
GOURMET
GOUTIER
GOUTILY
GOUTISH
GRUBBED
GRUBBER
GRUDGED
GRUDGER
GRUDGES
GRUFFER
GRUFFLY
GRUMBLE
GRUMBLY
GRUMMAN
GRUMPED
GRUNGER
GRUNGES
GRUNION
GRUNTED
GRUNTER
GRUYERE

G••U•••

GALUMPH
GELUSIL
GENUINE
GENUSES
GERUNDS
GETUPON
GIAUQUE
GIBUSES
GODUNOV
GODUTCH
GOTUPON
GOTUPTO
GRAUMAN
GROUCHO
GROUCHY
GROUNDS
GROUPED
GROUPER
GROUPIE
GROUSED
GROUSER
GROUSES
GROUTED
GROUTER
GUNUSER

G•••U••

GAGRULE
GASPUMP
GAUGUIN
GEODUCK
GESTURE
GETBUSY
GETCUTE
GETHURT
GIBLUES
GIVEUPS
GLOBULE
GOODUSE
GOOFUPS
GOROUND
GOSOUTH
GOTBUSY
GOTCUTE
GOTHURT
GRADUAL
GRANULE
GRAVURE
GYMSUIT
GYPSUMS

G••••U•

GAINFUL
GALLIUM
GANGSUP
GASEDUP
GASEOUS
GASESUP
GATEAUX
GAVEOUT
GEARSUP
GETSOUT
GIAUQUE
GIBBOUS
GIDDYUP
GIELGUD
GIVENUP
GIVEOUT
GIVESUP
GLAMOUR
GLAMSUP
GLEEFUL
GLOBOUS
GLUEGUN
GLUTEUS
GNOSSUS
GOABOUT
GOBYBUS
GOESOUT
GOINGUP
GOKAPUT
GOLDBUG
GONEOUT
GOODBUY
GOODGUY
GOOFSUP
GORDIUS
GOTOGUY
GRAMPUS
GRATEUP
GREYCUP
GROPIUS
GROTIUS
GROWNUP
GROWSUP
GUARGUM
GUSHOUT
GUSSYUP
GYMCLUB

G•••••U

GARNEAU

•GU••••

AGULHAS
AGUTTER
IGUANAS
IGUANID
IGUASSU

•G•U•••

AGOUTIS

•G••U••

AGROUND
EGGCUPS
EGGHUNT
EGOSURF

•G•••U•

AGEDOUT
AGEFOUR
AGENDUM
AGESOUT
IGIVEUP
IGNEOUS
OGDENUT
PGATOUR

•G••••U

IGOTYOU
IGUASSU

••GU•••

ANGUISH
ANGULAR
ARGUERS
ARGUING
ARGUSES
AUGURAL
AUGURED
AUGURER
AUGUSTA
AUGUSTE
AUGUSTO
AUGUSTS
BEGUILE
BEGUINE
BIGUNIT
BOGUSLY
DEGUSTS
ENGULFS
FIGURAL
FIGURED
FIGURER
FIGURES
INGULFS
JAGUARS
JUGULAR
LAGUNAS
LEGUMES
LIGURIA
MAGUIRE
MCGUIRE
NEGUSES
NOGUCHI
ONGUARD
OUGUIYA
REGUIDE
REGULAR
REGULUS
RIGUEUR
ROGUERY
ROGUING
ROGUISH
SAGUARO
TVGUIDE
UNGUARD
UNGUENT
UNGULAE
UNGULAR
UNGUYED
VAGUELY
VAGUEST
VOGUERS
VOGUING
VOGUISH
YOGURTS

••G•U••

BAGFULS
BIGGULP
BIGGUNS
BIGHUGS
BOGGUSS
BUGOUTS
COGBURN
DEGAUSS
DOGRUNS
DUGOUTS
EGGCUPS
EGGHUNT
ENGLUND
ENGLUTS
GAGRULE
HOGNUTS
JUGFULS
LEGPULL
LOGOUTS
LUGNUTS
MAGNUMS
MCGRUFF
MUGFULS
MUGWUMP
PIGNUTS
PIGOUTS
RAGOUTS
RAGRUGS
REGAUGE
REGLUED
REGLUES
RIGOURS
SIGMUND
SIGNUPS
TAGOUTS
UNGAUDY
UNGLUED
UNGLUES
UNGRUFF
VIGOURS
YOGHURT
ZAGNUTS

••G••U•

ANGELUS
BIGBLUE
BIGFOUR
BUGSOUT
CAGEDUP
CAGESUP
DIGSOUT
EDGEOUT
EIGHTUP
HYGINUS
INGENUE
INGROUP
LIGHTUP
LOGANUT
LOGSOUT
LUGSOUT
PEGASUS
PIGSOUT
RAGEFUL
REGROUP
REGULUS
RIGSOUT
RIGUEUR
SIGHFUL
SIGNOUT
SIGNSUP
TAGSOUT
TOGSOUT
WIGSOUT

••G•••U

ANGELOU

•••GU••

AIRGUNS
ARUGULA
BADGUYS
BENGUNN
BIGGULP
BIGGUNS
BOGGUSS
BROGUES
BULGURS
CAPGUNS
CATGUTS
CRUGUET
DISGUST
DROGUES
GAUGUIN
HANGUPS
JETGUNS
LANGUID
LANGUOR
LEAGUED
LEAGUER
LEAGUES
LENGUAS
LINGUAE
LINGUAL
LINGULA
LONGUES
MORGUES
OUTGUNS
OUTGUSH
PENGUIN
PINGUID
PLAGUED
PLAGUES
POPGUNS
RAYGUNS
ROTGUTS
SEAGULL
SHOGUNS
SIXGUNS
TONGUES
TOPGUNS
TOYGUNS
URUGUAY
VIRGULE
ZIPGUNS

•••G•U•

BANGOUT
BANGSUP
BELGIUM
BERGIUS
BORGLUM
BULGHUR
CLOGSUP
CONGOUS
COUGHUP
DRAGOUT
DRAGSUP
ELIGIUS
FULGHUM
GANGSUP
HANGOUT
HANGSUP
HOTGLUE
HUNGOUT
KINGTUT
LONGRUN
MARGAUX
MONGKUT
PLUGSUP
RANGOUT
RINGOUT
RINGSUP
ROUGHUP
RUNGOUT
SANGOUT
SHAGRUG
SINGOUT
SNAGSUP
SONGFUL
SORGHUM
WEIGHUP
WINGNUT
XINGOUT

•••G••U

IBEGYOU

••••GU•

ANTIGUA
ANTIGUN
BLOWGUN
BRENGUN
BRINGUP
BURPGUN
CHEWGUM
DARTGUN
DOINGUP
DUSTGUN
ECLOGUE
ENVOGUE
ERTEGUN
FALLGUY
FATIGUE
GIELGUD
GLUEGUN
GOINGUP
GOODGUY
GOTOGUY
GUARGUM
HANDGUN
ICINGUP
INVOGUE
LYINGUP
MANAGUA
MINOGUE
NAILGUN
NICEGUY
OKAYGUY
PIROGUE
REARGUE
REBEGUN
RIOTGUN
SHOTGUN
STENGUN
STUNGUN
TRAPGUN
TYINGUP
UNVAGUE
USINGUP
WISEGUY
YOUNGUN

••••G•U

LEHIGHU
THURGAU

•••••GU

MONTAGU

G•V••••

GAVEEAR
GAVELED
GAVEOFF
GAVEOUT
GAVEWAY
GAVIALS
GAVILAN
GAVOTTE
GIVEEAR
GIVENBY
GIVENIN
GIVENOF
GIVENON
GIVENTO
GIVENUP
GIVEOFF
GIVEOUT
GIVESIN
GIVESOF
GIVESON
GIVESTO
GIVESUP
GIVEUPS
GIVEWAY
GOVERNS
GUVNORS

G••V•••

GALVANI
GALVANO
GERVAIS
GLAVINE
GLOVING
GRAVELS
GRAVELY
GRAVERS
GRAVEST
GRAVIES
GRAVING
GRAVITY
GRAVLAX
GRAVURE
GROVELS
GROVERS
GUEVARA

7 GV

G•••V••
GASOVEN
GENEVAN
GETEVEN
GETOVER
GODEVIL
GOTEVEN
GOTOVER
GREAVES
GRIEVED
GRIEVER
GRIEVES
GROOVED
GROOVES
GROOVIN

G••••V•
GINGIVA
GUSTAVE

G•••••V
GEORGEV
GODUNOV
GRINKOV

•G•V•••
IGIVEUP

•G•••V•
AGEFIVE

••GV•••
DOGVEST
RIGVEDA

••G•V••
MCGAVIN
REGIVEN
REGIVES
SEGOVIA
UNGIVEN
UNGYVED

••G••V•
ALGARVE
BIGFIVE
BIGLOVE
ENGRAVE
MAGLEVS
UNGLOVE

•••G•V•
FORGAVE
FORGIVE
GINGIVA
MISGAVE
MISGIVE
OUTGAVE
OUTGIVE

•••G••V
ROYGBIV

••••G•V
GEORGEV

GW•••••
GWYNETH

G•W••••
GAWKERS
GAWKIER
GAWKILY
GAWKING
GAWKISH
GAWKSAT
GAWPERS
GAWPING
GEWGAWS
GOWNING
GOWRONG

G••W•••
GASWARS
GATWICK
GEEWHIZ
GETWARM
GETWELL
GETWISE
GETWORD
GLOWERS
GLOWING
GNAWERS
GNAWING
GNAWSAT
GNAWSON
GODWITS
GOTWARM
GOTWELL
GOTWISE
GOTWORD
GREWBIG
GREWDIM
GREWFAT
GREWOLD
GROWBIG
GROWDIM
GROWERS
GROWFAT
GROWING
GROWLED
GROWLER
GROWNON
GROWNUP
GROWOLD
GROWSON
GROWSUP
GROWTHS
GUMWOOD
GUNWALE

G•••W••
GANGWAY
GATEWAY
GAVEWAY
GETAWAY
GETSWET
GIVEWAY
GOLDWYN
GOODWIN
GOTAWAY
GOTOWAR
GULFWAR

G••••W•
GAGLAWS
GALLOWS
GEEGAWS
GETDOWN
GEWGAWS
GOSHAWK
GOTDOWN
GUFFAWS
GUNLAWS

G•••••W
GAMELAW
GANGSAW
GEORGEW
GLASGOW
GLASHOW
GOBELOW
BIGSHOW
DOGCHEW
DOGCHOW
DOGSHOW
HIGHLOW
SAGINAW

•GW••••
HGWELLS

•G••••W
IGNATOW

••GW•••
BAGWELL
BAGWIGS
BIGWIGS
BIGWINS
DAGWOOD
DOGWOOD
HOGWASH
HOGWEED
HOGWILD
JUGWINE
LEGWEAR
LEGWORK
LUGWORM
MCGWIRE
MUGWUMP
PIGWEED
RAGWEED
SEGWAYS
WIGWAGS
WIGWAMS

••G•W••
HIGHWAY
PEGAWAY
WAGEWAR

••G••W•
BIGNEWS
BIGTOWN
BOGDOWN
DOGBOWL
FOGBOWS
GAGLAWS
INGROWN
JIGSAWS
PAGETWO
REGLOWS
REGROWN
REGROWS
UNGROWN
UPGROWN
UPGROWS

••G•••W
BIGELOW

•••GW••
GANGWAY
LANGWAY
LONGWAY
NUNGWEN
RIDGWAY
SKAGWAY

•••G•W•
GEEGAWS
GEWGAWS
TEAGOWN

•••G••W
AIRGLOW
GANGSAW
LONGBOW
MACGRAW
MULGREW
OUTGLOW
OUTGNAW
OUTGREW
OUTGROW
SUNGLOW

••••G•W
GEORGEW
GLASGOW
LITHGOW

G••X•••
GENXERS

G•••X••
GALAXES
GALAXIE

G•••••X
GATEAUX
GEARBOX
GIFTBOX
GIFTTAX
GORETEX
GRAVLAX

••G•••X
PAGESIX

•••G••X
MARGAUX

•••••GX
LEXUSGX

GY•••••
GYMBAGS
GYMBALL
GYMCLUB
GYMNAST
GYMRATS
GYMSHOE
GYMSOCK
GYMSUIT
GYPPERS
GYPPING
GYPSIES
GYPSUMS
GYRALLY
GYRATED
GYRATES
GYRATOR
GYRENES
GYROCAR

G•Y••••
GAYLORD
GAYNESS
GEYSERS
GLYCINE
GLYCOLS
GLYNNIS
GLYPHIC
GLYPTIC
GRYPHON
GUYROPE
GWYNETH

G••Y•••
GOBYAIR
GOBYBUS
GOBYCAB
GOBYCAR
GOBYSEA
GRAYEST
GRAYING
GRAYISH
GRAYJAY
GRAYLAG
GRAYSON
GREYCUP
GREYEST
GREYHEN
GREYING
GREYISH
GREYLAG
GRUYERE

G•••Y••
GEMAYEL
GENZYME
GIDDYAP
GIDDYUP
GLORYBE
GROMYKO
GUSSYUP

G••••Y•
GALLEYS
GLADEYE
GOLDWYN
GOODBYE
GOODBYS
GOONEYS
GRAMMYS
GURNEYS

G•••••Y
GADGETY
GAINSAY
GALLERY
GAMEBOY
GANGWAY
GARBAGY
GASCONY
GASEITY
GATEWAY
GAUDERY
GAUDILY
GAUNTLY
GAUZILY
GAVEWAY
GAWKILY
GELIDLY
GEODESY
GEOLOGY
GERMANY
GETAWAY
GETBUSY
GHASTLY
GHOSTLY
GIDDILY
GINGERY
GIRLSHY
GIVENBY
GIVEWAY
GLAZILY
GLIDEBY
GLITCHY
GLORIFY
GOCRAZY
GODFREY
GOINGBY
GOODBUY
GOODDAY
GOODGUY
GOODPAY
GOODTRY
GOOFILY
GOOMBAY
GOONILY
GOSSIPY
GOTAWAY
GOTBUSY
GOTOGUY
GOUTILY
GRANARY
GRANDLY
GRAPERY
GRATIFY
GRAVELY
GRAVITY
GRAYJAY
GREATLY
GREELEY
GREENLY
GREGORY
GRETZKY
GRIFFEY
GRIMILY
GRIMSBY
GRISTLY
GRIZZLY
GROCERY
GROSSLY
GROUCHY
GRUFFLY
GRUMBLY
GUNNERY
GUNPLAY
GUSHILY
GUSTILY
GUTSILY
GYRALLY

•G•Y•••
IGGYPOP

•G••Y••
IGOTYOU

•G••••Y
AGENTRY
AGILELY
AGILITY
IGNOBLY

••GY•••
ARGYLES
BOGYMAN
BOGYMEN
FOGYISH
FOGYISM
IGGYPOP
MAGYARS
UNGYVED

••G•Y••
ANGRYAT
BIGEYED
BIGEYES
BOGEYED
BUGEYED
MEGRYAN
PIGEYED
UNGUYED

••G••Y•
BAGBOYS
BIGBOYS
BIGDAYS
BUGBOYS
DOGDAYS
DOGTOYS
OUGUIYA
SEGWAYS
TAGDAYS

••G•••Y
ANGRILY
BAGGILY
BAGLADY
BEGGARY
BIGBABY
BIGCITY
BIGEASY
BIGGITY
BIGOTRY
BOGUSLY
BYGOLLY
COGENCY
DIGGITY
DIGGORY
DIGNIFY
DIGNITY
EAGERLY
FOGCITY
FOGERTY
FOGGILY
FUGALLY
HAGERTY
HIGHBOY
HIGHDAY
HIGHPAY
HIGHWAY
HOGGERY
JIGGERY
LEGALLY
LEGIBLY
LIGHTLY
LIGNIFY
MAGNIFY
MCGRORY
NIGHTLY
NUGGETY
ORGANDY
PAGEBOY
PEGAWAY
PIGGERY
PUGSLEY
RAGGEDY
REGALLY
REGENCY
RIGHTLY
RIGIDLY
ROGUERY
SIGHTLY
SIGNIFY
SOGGILY
TIGHTLY
TOGGERY
UNGAUDY
UNGIDDY
UNGODLY
URGENCY
VAGUELY
WAGGERY
WIGGERY

•••GY••
IBEGYOU

•••G•Y•
BADGUYS
HANGBYS

•••G••Y
ASAGRAY
BAGGILY
BEGGARY
BIGGITY
BLIGHTY
CALGARY
DIGGITY
DIGGORY
DINGILY
DOUGHTY
EXOGAMY
FIDGETY
FLAGDAY
FLIGHTY
FOGGILY
FORGERY
GADGETY
GANGWAY
GINGERY
GREGORY
HANGSBY
HAUGHTY
HOGGERY
HUNGARY
IEIGHTY
IMAGERY
JARGONY
JIGGERY
LANGLEY
LANGTRY
LANGWAY
LARGELY
LENGTHY
LETGOBY
LONGDAY
LONGWAY
MARGERY
NAUGHTY
NUGGETY
OROGENY
PIGGERY
PROGENY
PUDGILY
QUIGLEY
RAGGEDY
RIDGWAY
ROUGHLY
SKAGWAY
SNUGGLY
SOGGILY
STAGILY
SURGERY
TOGGERY
TOUGHLY
TRAGEDY
URUGUAY
WAGGERY
WEIGHTY
WIGGERY
WRIGGLY
WRIGLEY
YEVGENY

••••G•Y
EKINGBY
FALLGUY
GOINGBY
GOODGUY
GOTOGUY
JOHNGAY
LISAGAY
LYINGBY
MUSIGNY
NEWAGEY
NICEGUY
NOSEGAY
OKAYGUY
ORANGEY
PHLEGMY
SCRAGGY
SEVIGNY
SHINGLY
SNUGGLY
SPANGLY
SWINGBY
SWUNGBY
UNANGRY
UNBOGGY
UNFOGGY
UNSOGGY
WISEGUY
WRIGGLY
WRONGLY

•••••GY
ALLERGY
ANALOGY
APOLOGY
BIOLOGY
CABBAGY
CINERGY
ECOLOGY
ENOLOGY
GARBAGY
GEOLOGY
LITURGY
MYOLOGY
NEOLOGY
OLDFOGY
OROLOGY
OTOLOGY
PRODIGY
SCRAGGY
SPRINGY
STRINGY
SYNERGY
TRILOGY
UFOLOGY
UNBOGGY
UNFOGGY
UNSOGGY
UNSTAGY
UROLOGY
ZOOLOGY
ZYMURGY

G•Z••••
GAZEBOS
GAZEDAT
GAZEDON
GAZELLE
GAZESAT
GAZESON
GAZETTE
GAZZARA
GIZZARD
GUZZLED
GUZZLER
GUZZLES

G••Z•••
GAUZIER
GAUZILY
GAZZARA
GEEZERS
GENZYME
GIZZARD
GLAZERS
GLAZIER
GLAZILY
GLAZING
GONZAGA
GRAZERS
GRAZIER
GRAZING
GRIZZLE
GRIZZLY
GUZZLED
GUZZLER
GUZZLES

G•••Z••
GLITZED
GLITZES
GRETZKY
GRIZZLE
GRIZZLY

G••••Z•
GINFIZZ
GOCRAZY
GRECIZE

G•••••Z
GEEWHIZ
GINFIZZ
GRISNEZ

•G•••Z•
AGONIZE

•G••••Z
AGASSIZ
AGRIBIZ

••GZ•••
ZIGZAGS

••G•Z••
UPGAZED
UPGAZES
ZAGAZIG

••G••Z•
COGNIZE
DEGLAZE
LEGANZA
ORGANZA
REGLAZE

•••G•Z•
ELEGIZE
OUTGAZE
YANGTZE

HA•••••
HAARLEM
HABILIS
HABITAT
HABITED
HABITUE
HACKERS
HACKETT
HACKIES
HACKING
HACKLED
HACKLER
HACKLES
HACKMAN
HACKNEY
HACKOFF
HACKSAW
HACKSIT
HACKSUP
HADACOW
HADAFIT
HADAGAS
HADAJOB
HADANIP
HADAROW
HADASAY
HADASET
HADATIT
HADBEEN
HADBEST
HADDOCK
HADDONE
HADFITS
HADOVER
HADPULL
HADRIAN
HADRONS
HADROOM
HADSOME
HADTIME
HADTOBE
HAECKEL
HAFNIUM
HAFTING
HAGERTY
HAGGARD
HAGGISH
HAGGLED
HAGGLER
HAGGLES
HAGLIKE
HAHNIUM
HAIKAIS
HAILERS
HAILING
HAIMISH
HAIRCUT
HAIRDOS
HAIRDYE
HAIRGEL
HAIRIER
HAIRNET
HAIRPIN
HAITIAN
HALALAS
HALAVAH
HALCYON
HALDANE
HALFBAD
HALFCUT
HALFDAY
HALFDUG
HALFFED
HALFIES
HALFMAD
HALFRAW
HALFROD
HALFSHY
HALFWAY
HALFWIT
HALFWON
HALIBUT
HALIDES
HALIFAX
HALITES
HALLEYS
HALLOOS
HALLOWS
HALLWAY
HALOGEN
HALOIDS
HALOING
HALSTON
HALTERS
HALTING
HALVAHS
HALVERS
HALVING
HALYARD
HAMACHI
HAMBONE
HAMBURG
HAMELIN
HAMHOCK
HAMITES
HAMITIC
HAMITUP
HAMLETS
HAMLINE
HAMMERS
HAMMETT
HAMMIER
HAMMILY
HAMMING
HAMMOCK
HAMMOND
HAMPERS
HAMPTON
HAMSTER
HAMULUS
HANAPER
HANCOCK
HANDAXE
HANDBAG
HANDCAR
HANDERS
HANDEYE
HANDFED
HANDFUL
HANDGUN
HANDIER
HANDILY
HANDING
HANDLED
HANDLER
HANDLES
HANDLIN
HANDOFF
HANDOUT
HANDSAW
HANDSEL
HANDSET
HANDSIN
HANDSON
HANDSUP
HANDYTO
HANGARS
HANGBYS
HANGDOG
HANGERS
HANGING
HANGMAN

HANGMEN
HANGOFF
HANGOUT
HANGSBY
HANGSIN
HANGSON
HANGSUP
HANGTEN
HANGUPS
HANKERS
HANKIBA
HANKIES
HANOVER
HANSARP
HANSOLO
HANSOMS
HANUKAH
HAPENNY
HAPKIDO
HAPLESS
HAPLOID
HAPPENS
HAPPIER
HAPPIFY
HAPPILY
HAPPYTO
HAPTICS
HARBACH
HARBORS
HARBOUR
HARBURG
HARDDAY
HARDEES
HARDENS
HARDEST
HARDHAT
HARDHIT
HARDIER
HARDILY
HARDING
HARDISH
HARDPAN
HARDPUT
HARDSET
HARDSIX
HARDTEN
HARDTOP
HARDWAY
HARDWON
HARHARS
HARICOT
HARKENS
HARKING
HARLAND
HARLEYS
HARLINE
HARLOTS
HARMERS
HARMFUL
HARMING
HARMONY
HARNESS
HARNICK
HAROLDI
HARPERS
HARPIES
HARPING
HARPIST
HARPOON
HARPSON
HARRAHS
HARRIED
HARRIER
HARRIES
HARRIET
HARRODS
HARROLD
HARROWS
HARSHEN
HARSHER
HARSHLY
HARTACK
HARTLEY
HARTMAN
HARTMUT
HARVARD
HARVEST
HARWELL
HASACOW
HASAFIT
HASAGAS
HASANIP
HASAROW
HASASAY
HASASET
HASATIT
HASBEEN
HASDONE
HASFITS
HASHING
HASHISH
HASHOUT
HASIDIC
HASIDIM
HASKELL
HASOVER
HASPING
HASPULL
HASROOM
HASSIUM
HASSLED
HASSLES
HASSOCK
HASTENS
HASTERT
HASTIER
HASTILY
HASTIME
HASTING
HASTOBE
HATABLE
HATBAND
HATBRIM
HATCHED
HATCHER
HATCHES
HATCHET
HATEDIT
HATEFUL
HATESIT
HATFULS
HATLESS
HATLIKE
HATPINS
HATRACK
HATREDS
HATSIZE
HATSOFF
HATTERS
HATTING
HAUGHTY
HAULAGE
HAULERS
HAULING
HAULOFF
HAULSIN
HAULSUP
HAUNTED
HAUNTER
HAUTBOY
HAUTEUR
HAVANAN
HAVANAS
HAVARTI
HAVEAGO
HAVEFUN
HAVENER
HAVENOT
HAVEONE
HAVEOUT
HAWHAWS
HAWKERS
HAWKEYE
HAWKING
HAWKINS
HAWKISH
HAWKMAN
HAWORTH
HAWSERS
HAYBALE
HAYESES
HAYFORK
HAYINGS
HAYLOFT
HAYMOWS
HAYRACK
HAYRICK
HAYRIDE
HAYSEED
HAYWARD
HAYWIRE
HAZANIM
HAZARDS
HAZIEST
HAZINGS
HAZLITT
HAZMATS

H•A••••

HAARLEM
HEADEND
HEADERS
HEADFOR
HEADFUL
HEADIER
HEADILY
HEADING
HEADMAN
HEADMEN
HEADOFF
HEADOUT
HEADPIN
HEADSAW
HEADSET
HEADSIN
HEADSTO
HEADSUP
HEADWAY
HEALALL
HEALERS
HEALING
HEALSUP
HEALTHY
HEAPERS
HEAPING
HEAPSOF
HEAPSON
HEAPSUP
HEARDOF
HEARERS
HEARING
HEARKEN
HEAROUT
HEARSAY
HEARSES
HEARSOF
HEARTED
HEARTEN
HEARTHS
HEATERS
HEATFAN
HEATFUL
HEATHEN
HEATHER
HEATING
HEATRAY
HEATSUP
HEATTER
HEAVEHO
HEAVENS
HEAVERS
HEAVETO
HEAVIER
HEAVIES
HEAVILY
HEAVING
HIALEAH
HJALMAR
HOAGIES
HOARDED
HOARDER
HOARIER
HOARILY
HOARSEN
HOARSER
HOAXERS
HOAXING
HUANGHE
HUANGTI
HYALITE
HYALOID
HYANNIS

H••A•••

HADACOW
HADAFIT
HADAGAS
HADAJOB
HADANIP
HADAROW
HADASAY
HADASET
HADATIT
HALALAS
HALAVAH
HAMACHI
HANAPER
HASACOW
HASAFIT
HASAGAS
HASANIP
HASAROW
HASASAY
HASASET
HASATIT
HATABLE
HAVANAN
HAVANAS
HAVARTI
HAZANIM
HAZARDS
HEMATIC
HEMATIN
HEPARIN
HEPATIC
HERALDS
HEXADIC
HEXAGON
HEXANES
HEXAPOD
HIBACHI
HIDABLE
HIDALGO
HIDAWAY
HIJACKS
HILAIRE
HIMALIA
HIRABLE
HITACHI
HODADDY
HOGARTH
HOMAGER
HOMAGES
HONALEE
HOPACAB
HORATIO
HOSANNA
HOWARDK
HOWARDS
HOWARDU
HUMANLY
HUMANUM
HYPATIA
HYRACES
HYRAXES

H•••A••

HAGGARD
HAIKAIS
HALDANE
HALVAHS
HALYARD
HANDAXE
HANGARS
HANSARP
HARBACH
HARHARS
HARLAND
HARRAHS
HARTACK
HARVARD
HATBAND
HATRACK
HAULAGE
HAVEAGO
HAWHAWS
HAYBALE
HAYRACK
HAYWARD
HAZMATS
HEALALL
HEBRAIC
HECKART
HECTARE
HEEHAWS
HENBANE
HENNAED
HEPCATS
HEPTADS
HERBAGE
HERBALS
HERBART
HERBAUT
HERMANA
HERMANN
HERMANO
HERMANS
HERNANI
HESSAFE
HEYDAYS
HEYMANS
HEYWARD
HIGHART
HILLARY
HIPBATH
HISPANO
HITBACK
HOBNAIL
HOECAKE
HOFMANN
HOGBACK
HOGCALL
HOGWASH
HOLDALL
HOLLAND
HOLYARK
HONIARA
HOOHAHS
HOOKAHS
HOORAHS
HOORAYS
HOSCALE
HOSTAGE
HOTBATH
HOTCAKE
HOTCAPS
HOTCARS
HOTDATE
HOTDAYS
HOTHAND
HOTMAIL
HOTPACK
HOTWARS
HOVLANE
HOWDAHS
HOWLAME
HOWMANY
HUBBARD
HUBCAPS
HUMBARD
HUNGARY
HUPPAHS
HURRAHS
HURRAYS
HUSBAND
HUSHABY
HUSSARS
HUZZAHS
HYDRANT
HYDRATE
HYMNALS
HYMNARY

H••••A•

HABITAT
HACKMAN
HACKSAW
HADAGAS
HADASAY
HADRIAN
HAITIAN
HALALAS
HALAVAH
HALFBAD
HALFDAY
HALFMAD
HALFRAW
HALFWAY
HALIFAX
HALLWAY
HANDBAG
HANDCAR
HANDSAW
HANGMAN
HANUKAH
HARDDAY
HARDHAT
HARDPAN
HARDWAY
HARTMAN
HASAGAS
HASASAY
HAVANAN
HAVANAS
HAWKMAN
HEADMAN
HEADSAW
HEADWAY
HEARSAY
HEATFAN
HEATRAY
HECKMAN
HEELPAD
HEELTAP
HEGIRAS
HEISMAN
HELICAL
HELIPAD
HELLCAT
HELLMAN
HEREIAM
HERNIAE
HERNIAS
HESHVAN
HESSIAN
HIALEAH
HICKMAN
HIDAWAY
HIGHBAR
HIGHDAY
HIGHHAT
HIGHPAY
HIGHWAY
HILLMAN
HINDPAW
HINTSAT
HITPLAY
HJALMAR
HOFBRAU
HOFFMAN
HOLIDAY
HOLMOAK
HOLYDAY
HOLYMAN
HOLYWAR
HOLZMAN
HOMELAB
HONKSAT
HOOPLAS
HOOPMAN
HOOTSAT
HOPACAB
HOTCOAL
HOTHEAD
HOTLEAD
HOTMEAL
HOTSEAT
HOTTEAS
HOUSMAN
HOUSSAY
HOWLSAT
HUFFMAN
HUMERAL
HUMORAL
HYGELAC
HYUNDAI

H•••••A

HANKIBA
HECKUVA
HELLUVA
HENDECA
HERBTEA
HEREDIA
HERMANA
HERMOSA
HIGHSEA
HIGHTEA
HIMALIA
HOFSTRA
HONIARA
HOSANNA
HOTTUNA
HRYVNIA
HYGIEIA
HYPATIA

•HA••••

AHASSLE
CHABLIS
CHACHAS
CHACHKA
CHAFERS
CHAFFED
CHAFFEE
CHAFFER
CHAFING
CHAGALL
CHAGRIN
CHAINED
CHAINES
CHAINUP
CHAIRED
CHAISES
CHAKRAS
CHALCIS
CHALETS
CHALICE
CHALKED
CHALKUP
CHALLAH
CHALONS
CHALUPA
CHAMBER
CHAMBRE
CHAMFER
CHAMOIS
CHAMPED
CHAMPER
CHANCED
CHANCEL
CHANCER
CHANCES
CHANELS
CHANGED
CHANGER
CHANGES
CHANNEL
CHANOYU
CHANSON
CHANTED
CHANTER
CHANTEY
CHANTRY
CHAOTIC
CHAPALA
CHAPATI
CHAPEAU
CHAPELS
CHAPLET
CHAPLIN
CHAPMAN
CHAPMEN
CHAPPED
CHAPPIE
CHAPTER
CHARADE
CHARCOT
CHARGED
CHARGER
CHARGES
CHARIER
CHARILY
CHARING
CHARIOT
CHARITY
CHARLES
CHARLEY
CHARLIE
CHARMAN
CHARMED
CHARMEN
CHARMER
CHARMIN
CHARNIN
CHARPAK
CHARRED
CHARRER
CHARROS
CHARTED
CHARTER
CHARVET
CHASERS
CHASING
CHASMAL
CHASMIC
CHASSED
CHASSES
CHASSIS
CHASTEN
CHASTER
CHATEAU
CHATHAM
CHATSUP
CHATTED
CHATTEL
CHATTER
CHATWIN
CHAUCER
CHAWING
CHAYOTE
CHAZANS
CHAZZAN
DHARMAS
DHARMIC
FHALOAN
GHANIAN
GHASTLY
IHATEIT
IHAVEIT
KHANATE
KHARKOV
KHATAMI
KHAYYAM
LHASANS
OHANLON
PHAEDRA
PHAETON
PHALANX
PHANTOM
PHARAOH
PHARLAP
PHARYNX
PHASEIN
PHASERS
PHASING
PHATTER
SHABBAT
SHACKED
SHACKLE
SHADERS
SHADIER
SHADILY
SHADING
SHADOWS
SHADOWY
SHADROE
SHAFFER
SHAFTED
SHAGGED
SHAGRUG
SHAHDOM
SHAKERS
SHAKEUP
SHAKIER
SHAKILY
SHAKING
SHAKIRA
SHAKOES
SHALALA
SHALIER
SHALLOT
SHALLOW
SHALLWE
SHALOMS
SHAMANS
SHAMBLE
SHAMING
SHAMMED
SHAMPOO
SHANANA
SHANGRI
SHANKAR
SHANKED
SHANNEN
SHANNON
SHANTER
SHAPELY
SHAPERS
SHAPEUP
SHAPING
SHAPIRO
SHAREIN
SHARERS
SHARING
SHARKEY
SHARONA
SHARPED
SHARPEI
SHARPEN
SHARPER
SHARPIE
SHARPLY
SHASTRI
SHATNER
SHATTER
SHAVERS
SHAVIAN
SHAVING
SHAVUOT
SHAWLED
SHAWNEE
THALERS
THANDIE
THANKED
THANKER
THATCHY
THATONE
THATSIT
THATSOK
THATWAY
THAWERS
THAWING
THAWOUT
WHACKED
WHACKER
WHALERS
WHALING
WHALLEY
WHAMMED
WHANGED
WHAPPED
WHARFED
WHARTON
WHARVES
WHATAMI
WHATFOR
WHATIFS
WHATNOT
WHATNOW
WHATSAY
WHATSIS
WHATSIT
WHATSUP
WHATTHE
WHAUDEN

•H•A•••

AHEADOF
CHEADLE
CHEAPEN
CHEAPER
CHEAPIE
CHEAPLY
CHEATED
CHEATER
CHEATIN
CHEATON
CHIANTI
CHIAPAS
CHIAPET
IHEARYA
OHCAROL
OHMAGES
PHRASAL
PHRASED
PHRASES
SHEAFED
SHEARED
SHEARER
SHEATHE
SHEATHS
SHEAVED
SHEAVES
SHIATSU
SHOALED
SHYAWAY
THEABCS
THEAGES
THEALPS
THEARMY
THEARTS
THEATER
THEATRE
THEAXIS
THIAMIN
THRALLS
THWACKS
THWARTS
WHEATEN
WHEATON

•H••A••

BHUTANI
CHAGALL
CHAPALA
CHAPATI
CHARADE
CHAZANS
CHELATE
CHEVAUX
CHICAGO
CHICANA
CHICANE
CHICANO
CHORALE
CHORALS
CHUMASH
KHANATE
KHATAMI
LHASANS
NHLGAME
OHIOANS
OHIOART
PHALANX
PHARAOH
RHUBARB
SHALALA
SHAMANS
SHANANA
SHEBANG
SHEPARD
SHEVATS
SHOFARS
THEBABE
THEBABY
THEBAND
THEBANS
THEBARD
THECAPE
THECARS
THECAVS
THEEAST
THEFALL
THEGAME
THEGANG
THELAMB
THELARK
THEMAGI
THEMALL
THEMASK
THEMAVS
THEMAYO
THEOATH
THERAMS
THERAPY
THESACK
THESAME
THEWALL
THEWAVE
THINAIR
THREADS
THREADY
THREATS
THROATS
THROATY
WHATAMI
WHOSAID
WHYWAIT
ZHIVAGO

•H•••A•

CHACHAS
CHAKRAS

CHALLAH
CHAPEAU
CHAPMAN
CHARMAN
CHARPAK
CHASMAL
CHATEAU
CHATHAM
CHAZZAN
CHEDDAR
CHEETAH
CHEETAS
CHEMLAB
CHIAPAS
CHICHAS
CHILCAT
CHILEAN
CHILIAD
CHILKAT
CHINWAG
CHOCTAW
CHOLLAS
CHORDAL
CHROMAT
CHUPPAH
CHUPPAS
DHARMAS
FHALOAN
GHANIAN
KHAYYAM
NHLTEAM
OHMSLAW
PHARLAP
PHIDIAS
PHILEAS
PHINEAS
PHOBIAS
PHRASAL
RHODIAN
RHUMBAS
SHABBAT
SHANKAR
SHAVIAN
SHEBEAR
SHECRAB
SHEEHAN
SHEGOAT
SHEILAE
SHEILAS
SHELLAC
SHERMAN
SHERPAS
SHINPAD
SHIPMAN
SHIPWAY
SHOEPAC
SHOOTAT
SHOPSAT
SHOTPAR
SHOUTAT
SHOWCAT
SHOWMAN
SHULMAN
SHYAWAY
THATWAY
THEBEAR
THEBRAT
THECRAB
THEHEAT
THEREAT
THERIAC
THERMAL
THESTAR
THESWAN
THEYSAY
THINMAN
THISDAY
THISWAY
THOREAU
THREEAD
THREEAM
THREWAT
THROWAT
THRUWAY
THURGAU
THURMAN
THUSFAR
WHATSAY
WHEREAS
WHEREAT
WHIPSAW
WHISKAS
WHITMAN

•H••••A

CHACHKA
CHALUPA
CHAPALA
CHELSEA
CHICANA
CHIMERA
CHOLERA
CHRISTA
CHUTZPA
IHEARYA
PHAEDRA
PHRYGIA
SHAKIRA
SHALALA
SHANANA
SHARONA
SHINOLA
SHOULDA
THEBIGA
THEFLEA
THEIDEA
THERESA
THRILLA

••HA•••

AMHARIC
APHAGIA
APHAGIC
APHASIA
APHASIC
ASHAMED
ASHANTI
BAHAISM
BAHAIST
BAHAMAS
BAHAMEN
BEHAPPY
BEHAVED
BEHAVES
COHABIT
DEHAIRS
DEHAVEN
DUHAMEL
ECHAPPE
ENHANCE
ETHANES
ETHANOL
EXHALED
EXHALES
EXHAUST
GAHAGAN
ICHABOD
IMHAPPY
INHABIT
INHALED
INHALER
INHALES
INHASTE
ITHACAN
JOHANNA
LAHAINA
LCHAYIM
LEHAVRE
LSHAPED
MAHALIA
MAHARIS
MAHATMA
MCHALES
MOHAIRS
MOHAVES
MOHAWKS
MRHANEY
NOHANDS
OGHAMIC
OSHAPED
PSHAWED
REHANGS
REHAULS
SAHARAN
SCHAYES
SOHAVEI
SSHAPED
SUHARTO
TSHAPED
TSHAPES
UNHAIRS
UNHAIRY
UNHANDS
UNHANDY
UNHAPPY
UNHARDY
UNHARSH
UNHASPS
UNHASTY
UNHATED
UNHAYED
UNHAZED
USHAPED
USHAPES
VIHARAS
VSHAPED
VSHAPES
WCHANDY
YSHAPED
YSHAPES

••H•A••

ASHCAKE
ASHCANS
ASHLAND
ASHLARS
ASHPANS
ASHRAMS
ATHEART
ATHWART
AXHEADS
BAHIANS
BAHRAIN
BEHEADS
BEHEARD
BYHEART
EPHRAIM
ISHMAEL
LEHMANN
NAHUATL
OAHUANS
OOHLALA
OXHEART
PAHLAVI
REHEALS
REHEARD
REHEARS
REHEATS
SCHNAPS
SCHWANN
TOHEART
UNHEADY
UNHEARD
UNHEAVY
UPHEAPS
UPHEAVE
UPHOARD
WAHWAHS

••H••A•

ASHHEAP
ASHTRAY
BAHAMAS
BEHRMAN
DAHLIAS
ETHICAL
GAHAGAN
INHUMAN
ITHACAN
JOHNGAY
JOHNJAY
JOHNLAW
KAHUNAS
MOHEGAN
MOHICAN
SAHARAN
SCHEMAS
SCHMEAR
SCHOLAR
SPHERAL
TEHERAN
UNHUMAN
VIHARAS

••H•••A

ACHIEVA
APHAGIA
APHASIA
APHELIA
APHONIA
BOHEMIA
CAHOKIA
ECHIDNA
EPHEDRA
EXHEDRA
GEHENNA
JOHANNA
LAHAINA
MAHALIA
MAHATMA
OCHENTA
OOHLALA
OPHELIA
SCHIRRA

•••HA••

AFGHANI
AFGHANS
ALLHAIL
ALOHAOE
ALPHARD
ALSHAIN
ARCHAIC
ASPHALT
ASSHARP
BACHATA
BADHAIR
BADHAND
BADHATS
BAUHAUS
BECHARM
BETHANY
BIGHAIR
BIGHALF
BIGHAND
BOKHARA
BUKHARA
BYAHAIR
CACHACA
CATHAIR
CEPHALO
CEPHALY
COCHAIR
COWHAND
CUSHAWS
DABHAND
DENHAAG
DIAHANN
DIEHARD
DIRHAMS
DOGHAIR
DRCHAOS
DUCHAMP
EARHART
ECKHART
ELKHART
ENCHAIN
ENCHANT
ENCHASE
ETCHANT
EYEHAND
FUTHARK
GOSHAWK
GRAHAME
GRAHAMS
HARHARS
HAWHAWS
HEEHAWS
HIGHART
HOOHAHS
HOTHAND
HUSHABY
INPHASE
INSHAPE
JONHALL
JOUHAUX
KITHARA
LETHAVE
LOTHAIR
LOWHAND
MACHAON
MARHAUS
MCSHANE
MESHACH
METHANE
MIAHAMM
MICHAEL
MICHAUX
MIKHAIL
MILHAUD
MISHAPS
MULHARE
NATHANS
NEWHAND
NEWHART
NEWHATS
OFFHAND
OLDHAND
OMAHANE
OMAHANS
OMPHALO
ONEHALF
ONEHAND
ORCHARD
ORPHANS
ORPHANT
OUTHAUL
PATHAND
PATHANS
PERHAPS
PETHAIR
PETHARE
RACHAEL
RAPHAEL
RECHALK
RECHALL
RECHART
REDHAIR
REDHATS
REDHAWK
REPHASE
RESHAPE
RESHARE
RESHAVE
RETHANK
RETHAWS
RICHARD
RUTHANN
SASHAYS
SEAHAWK
SKIHATS
SUBHALL
SUNHATS
TINHATS
TOAHAIR
TOOHARD
TOPHATS
TOYHATS
TRYHARD
UNCHAIN
UNCHAIR
UNCHARY
UNSHADE
UNSHADY
UNSHARP
UNTHAWS
UPPHASE
UTAHANS
VFWHALL
WARHAWK
ZACHARY

•••H•A•

AIRHEAD
ALLHEAL
ANTHRAX
ARCHWAY
ASHHEAP
ASTHMAS
AXEHEAD
BACHMAN
BAGHDAD
BATHMAT
BIGHEAD
BOOHBAH
BOWHEAD
BRAHMAN
BRAHMAS
BUCHMAN
BUSHMAN
BUSHWAH
CASHBAR
CATHEAD
COCHRAN
COGHLAN
DENHAAG
DISHPAN
DISHRAG
DRYHEAT
EGGHEAD
EIGHTAD
EIGHTAM
ENTHRAL
ESCHEAT
FATHEAD
GASHEAT
GOAHEAD
GODHEAD
HESHVAN
HIGHBAR
HIGHDAY
HIGHHAT
HIGHPAY
HIGHWAY
HOTHEAD
IDAHOAN
INAHEAP
ISAHEAD
ISCHIAL
JUGHEAD
LETHEAN
LEWHOAD
LOTHIAN
MATHIAS
MISHEAR
MISHNAH
MITHRAS
MOPHEAD
OILHEAT
ORPHEAN
OUTHEAR
PATHWAY
PINHEAD
PITHEAD
POOHBAH
PREHEAL
PREHEAT
PYTHIAN
PYTHIAS
REDHEAD
REDHEAT
RICHMAN
SAPHEAD
SEPHIAS
SIGHSAT
SUBHEAD
THEHEAT
TOWHEAD
TUCHMAN
UPAHEAD
WARHEAD
WASHDAY
WASHRAG
YASHMAK
YEAHMAN

•••H••A

AMPHORA
BACHATA
BOKHARA
BOTHNIA
BUKHARA
CACHACA
COCHLEA
DAPHNIA
FUCHSIA
GOTHIKA
HIGHSEA
HIGHTEA
JEPHTHA
KACHINA
KITHARA
KOSHIBA
MACHINA
MESHUGA
MISHIMA
NAPHTHA
RASHIDA
ROTHIRA
SENHORA
TOSHIBA
WICHITA
YASHICA
YESHIVA

••••HA•

ABRAHAM
AGAKHAN
AGULHAS
AINTHAY
ALLTHAT
ALYKHAN
AMICHAI
BACCHAE
BALIHAI
BEACHAM
BECKHAM
BEECHAM
BENTHAM
BERTHAS
BINGHAM
BRIGHAM
BUDDHAS
BUQSHAS
CANCHAS
CAPSHAW
CHACHAS
CHATHAM
CHICHAS
CONCHAE
CRASHAW
CUMSHAW
DELIHAM
DIAPHAN
EASTHAM
EPOCHAL
FELTHAT
FIREHAT
FLATHAT
FORDHAM
GALAHAD
GEISHAS
GINGHAM
GODTHAB
GOTCHAS
GRESHAM
GRISHAM
GURKHAS
HARDHAT
HIGHHAT
ISFAHAN
KEESHAN
KEOGHAN
KERSHAW
KETCHAM
KWACHAS
LANGHAM
LAUGHAT
MADEHAY
MAKEHAY
MARKHAM
MARSHAL
MATTHAU
MAUGHAM
MCLUHAN
NARWHAL
NEEDHAM
NOWWHAT
NYMPHAL
OLDCHAP
PANCHAX
PASCHAL
PINCHAS
PINKHAM
RAINHAT
SAYWHAT
SHEEHAN
SILKHAT
SIOBHAN
SNOWHAT
TOBEHAD
VAUGHAN
WALTHAM
WOOLHAT
WYNDHAM
XANTHAN
YAMAHAS
YITZHAK

••••H•A

BOOTHIA
CHACHKA
CYNTHIA
DRACHMA
KRISHNA
PERAHIA
QUECHUA
TRACHEA

•••••HA

ALYOSHA
IGOTCHA
JEPHTHA
JOSEPHA
KATISHA
KENOSHA
NAPHTHA
NATASHA
PIRANHA
PWBOTHA
RICKSHA
TABITHA
WABASHA

H•B••••

HABILIS
HABITAT
HABITED
HABITUE
HEBRAIC
HEBREWS
HIBACHI
HIBBING
HIBBLER
HIBERNO
HOBBIES
HOBBITS
HOBBLED
HOBBLER
HOBBLES
HOBNAIL
HOBNOBS
HOBOING
HOBOISM
HOBOKEN
HOBSONS
HUBBARD
HUBBELL
HUBBIES
HUBBUBS
HUBCAPS
HYBRIDS

H••B•••

HADBEEN
HADBEST
HAMBONE
HAMBURG
HARBACH
HARBORS
HARBOUR
HARBURG
HASBEEN
HATBAND
HATBRIM
HAYBALE
HENBANE
HENBITS
HEPBURN
HERBAGE
HERBALS
HERBART
HERBAUT
HERBERT
HERBIER
HERBTEA
HIBBING
HIBBLER
HILBERT
HIPBATH
HIPBONE
HIPBOOT
HITBACK
HOBBIES
HOBBITS
HOBBLED
HOBBLER
HOBBLES
HOFBRAU
HOGBACK
HOLBEIN
HOLBERG
HOMBRES
HOMBURG
HOTBATH
HOTBEDS
HOWBEIT
HUBBARD
HUBBELL
HUBBIES
HUBBUBS
HUMBARD
HUMBERT
HUMBLED
HUMBLER
HUMBLES
HUMBUGS
HUSBAND

H•••B••

HALFBAD
HALIBUT
HANDBAG
HANGBYS
HATABLE
HAUTBOY
HELLBOY
HIDABLE
HIGHBAR
HIGHBOY
HIRABLE
HOMEBOY

H••••B•

HADTOBE
HANGSBY
HANKIBA
HASTOBE
HERNIBS
HEYRUBE
HISNIBS
HOBNOBS
HORNSBY
HOTTUBS
HUBBUBS
HUNNYBS
HUSHABY

H•••••B

HADAJOB
HOMELAB
HOPACAB
HOTCOMB

•H•B•••

CHABLIS
PHOBIAS
PHOBICS
RHEBOKS
RHUBARB
SHABBAT
SHEBANG
SHEBEAR
SHUBERT
THEBABE
THEBABY
THEBAND
THEBANS
THEBARD
THEBEAR
THEBELL
THEBEST
THEBIGA
THEBLOB
THEBOBO
THEBODY
THEBOMB
THEBOSS
THEBOYS
THEBRAT
THEBUSH

•H••B••

CHAMBER
CHAMBRE
PHILBIN
PHOEBES
PHOEBUS
RHOMBIC
RHOMBUS
RHUMBAS
SHABBAT
SHAMBLE
SHERBET
SHOEBOX
SHOWBIZ
SHRUBBY
THEABCS
THIMBLE
THUMBED
THURBER

•H•••B•

CHERUBS
SHOOTBY
SHOPNBC
SHRUBBY
THEBABE
THEBABY
THEBOBO
THECUBS
THEREBY
THEROBE
THETUBE
THREEBC
WHEREBY

•H••••B

CHEMLAB
RHUBARB
SHECRAB
THEBLOB
THEBOMB
THECRAB
THELAMB
THETRIB

••HB•••

ASHBERY
ASHBINS
ASHBURN
ASHBURY

••H•B••

ADHIBIT
COHABIT
EPHEBUS
EXHIBIT
ICHABOD
INHABIT
INHIBIT
JOHNBOY
MRHOBBS

••H••B•

MRHOBBS
SCHLUBS

••H•••B

JOHNNYB

•••HB••

BOOHBAH
CASHBAR
CASHBOX
HIGHBAR
HIGHBOY
POOHBAH
YEAHBUT

•••H•B•

BYTHEBY
EIGHTBC
HUSHABY
KOSHIBA
SOTHEBY
TOSHIBA

•••H••B

BATHTUB
POTHERB
WASHTUB

••••H•B
GODTHAB

H•C••••
HACKERS
HACKETT
HACKIES
HACKING
HACKLED
HACKLER
HACKLES
HACKMAN
HACKNEY
HACKOFF
HACKSAW
HACKSIT
HACKSUP
HECKART
HECKLED
HECKLER
HECKLES
HECKMAN
HECKUVA
HECKYES
HECTARE
HECTORS
HICCUPS
HICKEYS
HICKMAN
HICKORY
HOCKERS
HOCKING
HOCUSED

H••C•••
HAECKEL
HALCYON
HANCOCK
HATCHED
HATCHER
HATCHES
HATCHET
HENCOOP
HEPCATS
HERCULE
HICCUPS
HIRCINE
HITCHED
HITCHER
HITCHES
HITCHON
HITCHUP
HOECAKE
HOGCALL
HONCHOS
HOOCHES
HOSCALE
HOTCAKE
HOTCAPS
HOTCARS
HOTCOAL
HOTCOMB
HOTCUPS
HOWCOME
HUBCAPS
HUNCHED
HUNCHES
HUTCHES

H•••C••
HADACOW
HAIRCUT
HALFCUT
HAMACHI
HANDCAR
HARICOT
HASACOW
HELICAL
HELICES
HELICON
HELLCAT
HIBACHI
HIJACKS
HITACHI
HOLYCOW
HOPACAB
HYRACES

H••••C•
HADDOCK
HAMHOCK
HAMMOCK
HANCOCK
HAPTICS
HARBACH
HARNICK
HARTACK
HASSOCK
HATRACK
HAYRACK
HAYRICK
HEMLOCK
HENDECA
HENPECK
HENRICH
HEROICS
HERRICK
HILLOCK
HITBACK
HOGBACK
HOMEICE
HOSPICE
HOTLICK
HOTPACK
HOWMUCH
HOWNICE

H•••••C
HAMITIC
HASIDIC
HEBRAIC
HEDONIC
HEMATIC
HEPATIC
HERETIC
HEXADIC
HOMERIC
HYGELAC

•HC••••
AHCHOOS
OHCAROL

•H•C•••
CHACHAS
CHACHKA
CHECHEN
CHECKED
CHECKER
CHECKIN
CHECKON
CHECKUP
CHICAGO
CHICANA
CHICANE
CHICANO
CHICEST
CHICHAS
CHICHEN
CHICHIS
CHICKEN
CHICLES
CHICLET
CHICORY
CHOCKED
CHOCTAW
CHUCKED
CHUCKIT
CHUCKLE
SHACKED
SHACKLE
SHECRAB
SHOCKED
SHOCKER
SHUCKED
SHUCKER
THECAPE
THECARS
THECAVS
THECITY
THECRAB
THECROW
THECUBS
THICKEN
THICKER
THICKET
THICKLY
WHACKED
WHACKER

•H••C••
CHALCIS
CHANCED
CHANCEL
CHANCER
CHANCES
CHARCOT
CHAUCER
CHILCAT
CHOICER
CHOICES
CHURCHY
PHILCOS
RHOECUS
SHLOCKY
SHOWCAT
SHTICKS
SHTICKY
THATCHY
THWACKS

•H•••C•
CHALICE
CHIRICO
EHRLICH
PHOBICS
PHONICS
PHOTICS
PHYSICS
SHYLOCK
THEABCS
THEMICK
THEROCK
THESACK
THINICE

•H••••C
CHAOTIC
CHASMIC
CHLORIC
CHROMIC
CHRONIC
DHARMIC
PHRENIC
RHEUMIC
RHOMBIC
SHELLAC
SHOEPAC
SHOPNBC
THERIAC
THERMIC
THREEBC

••HC•••
ASHCAKE
ASHCANS

••H•C••
ETHICAL
ITHACAN
MOHICAN
SCHICKS
VEHICLE

••H••C•
DEHISCE
ENHANCE
ETHNICS
REHITCH
SCHLOCK
SCHTICK
UNHITCH

••H•••C
AMHARIC
APHAGIC
APHASIC
APHONIC
ETHERIC
OGHAMIC
SPHERIC

•••HC••
CASHCOW

•••H•C•
CACHACA
GOTHICS
HAMHOCK
INCHECK
INSHOCK
MESHACH
RECHECK
UNCHECK
UNTHICK
YASHICA

•••H••C
ARCHAIC
ARTHURC
EIGHTBC
NEPHRIC

••••H•C
BACCHIC
DELPHIC
GLYPHIC
GRAPHIC
MORPHIC
MYRRHIC
NYMPHIC
POSTHOC
PSYCHIC
PYRRHIC
SYLPHIC
XANTHIC

HD•••••
HDTVSET

H•D••••
HADACOW
HADAFIT
HADAGAS
HADAJOB
HADANIP
HADAROW
HADASAY
HADASET
HADATIT
HADBEEN
HADBEST
HADDOCK
HADDONE
HADFITS
HADOVER
HADPULL
HADRIAN
HADRONS
HADROOM
HADSOME
HADTIME
HADTOBE
HEDGERS
HEDGIER
HEDGING
HEDISON
HEDONIC
HIDABLE
HIDALGO
HIDAWAY
HIDEOUS
HIDEOUT
HIDINGS
HODADDY
HODDING
HUDDLED
HUDDLER
HUDDLES
HYDRANT
HYDRATE
HYDRIDE
HYDROUS

H••D•••
HADDOCK
HADDONE
HALDANE
HANDAXE
HANDBAG
HANDCAR
HANDERS
HANDEYE
HANDFED
HANDFUL
HANDGUN
HANDIER
HANDILY
HANDING
HANDLED
HANDLER
HANDLES
HANDLIN
HANDOFF
HANDOUT
HANDSAW
HANDSEL
HANDSET
HANDSIN
HANDSON
HANDSUP
HANDYTO
HARDDAY
HARDEES
HARDENS
HARDEST
HARDHAT
HARDHIT
HARDIER
HARDILY
HARDING
HARDISH
HARDPAN
HARDPUT
HARDSET
HARDSIX
HARDTEN
HARDTOP
HARDWAY
HARDWON
HASDONE
HEADEND
HEADERS
HEADFOR
HEADFUL
HEADIER
HEADILY
HEADING
HEADMAN
HEADMEN
HEADOFF
HEADOUT
HEADPIN
HEADSAW
HEADSET
HEADSIN
HEADSTO
HEADSUP
HEADWAY
HEEDERS
HEEDFUL
HEEDING
HELDOFF
HELDOUT
HENDECA
HENDRIX
HENDRYX
HERDERS
HERDING
HEYDAYS
HINDERS
HINDLEG
HINDPAW
HODDING
HOEDOWN
HOLDALL
HOLDERS
HOLDING
HOLDOFF
HOLDOUT
HOLDSIN
HOLDSIT
HOLDSON
HOLDSTO
HOLDSUP
HOLDUPS
HOODIES
HOODING
HOODLUM
HOODOOS
HORDING
HOTDATE
HOTDAYS
HOTDOGS
HOUDINI
HOWDAHS
HOWDEDO
HOWDULL
HOWDYDO
HOYDENS
HUDDLED
HUDDLER
HUDDLES
HUMDRUM
HUNDRED
HURDLED
HURDLER
HURDLES

H•••D••
HAIRDOS
HAIRDYE
HALFDAY
HALFDUG
HALIDES
HANGDOG
HARDDAY
HASIDIC
HASIDIM
HATEDIT
HEARDOF
HEIRDOM
HEREDIA
HERNDON
HEWEDTO
HEXADIC
HIGHDAY
HIKEDUP
HIREDON
HOARDED
HOARDER
HODADDY
HOLEDUP
HOLIDAY
HOLYDAY
HOMEDIN
HONEDIN
HOPEDSO
HOPEDTO
HOUNDED
HOUNDER
HUMIDEX
HUMIDLY
HUMIDOR
HYPEDUP
HYUNDAI

H••••D•
HALOIDS
HAPKIDO
HAROLDI
HARRODS
HATREDS
HAYRIDE
HAZARDS
HEPTADS
HERALDS
HEYJUDE
HEYMRDJ
HODADDY
HOTBEDS
HOTRODS
HOWARDK
HOWARDS
HOWARDU
HOWDEDO
HOWDYDO
HYBRIDS
HYDRIDE
HYMNODY

H•••••D
HABITED
HACKLED
HAGGARD
HAGGLED
HALFBAD
HALFFED
HALFMAD
HALFROD
HALYARD
HAMMOND
HANDFED
HANDLED
HAPLOID
HARLAND
HARRIED
HARROLD
HARVARD
HASSLED
HATBAND
HATCHED
HAUNTED
HAYSEED
HAYWARD
HEADEND
HEARTED
HECKLED
HEELPAD
HEISTED
HELIPAD
HELLOED
HELMOND
HENNAED
HENREID
HEXAPOD
HEYWARD
HEYWOOD
HIGGLED
HIGHEND
HISPEED
HITCHED
HOARDED
HOBBLED
HOCUSED
HOGTIED
HOGWEED
HOGWILD
HOISTED
HOLLAND
HOMERED
HOMINID
HONEYED
HONORED
HOTHAND
HOTHEAD
HOTLEAD
HOUNDED
HOVERED
HUBBARD
HUDDLED
HULLOED
HUMBARD
HUMBLED
HUMORED
HUMPHED
HUNCHED
HUNDRED
HURDLED
HURRIED
HURTLED
HUSBAND
HUSTLED
HYALOID
HYPNOID

•H•D•••
CHEDDAR
CHEDERS
CHIDDEN
CHIDERS
CHIDING
KHEDIVE
PHIDIAS
RHODIAN
RHODIUM
SHADERS
SHADIER
SHADILY
SHADING
SHADOWS
SHADOWY
SHADROE
SHEDDER
SHEDSON
SHODDEN
SHUDDER
THEDEEP
THEDELL
THEDIET
THEDOLE
THEDUKE
THUDDED

•H••D••
AHEADOF
CHEADLE
CHEDDAR
CHIDDEN
CHORDAL
CHORDED
CHOWDER
OHFUDGE
PHAEDRA
SHAHDOM
SHEDDER
SHELDON
SHINDIG
SHODDEN
SHOWDOG
SHUDDER
THANDIE
THEEDGE
THEIDEA
THEODOR
THIRDLY
THISDAY
THUDDED
THUNDER
WHAUDEN
WHEEDLE

•H•••D•
CHARADE
SHIELDS
SHOULDA
SHOULDI
SHROUDS
THEBODY
THEFEDS
THEREDS
THREADS
THREADY
WHWORDS

•H••••D
CHAFFED
CHAINED
CHAIRED
CHALKED
CHAMPED
CHANCED
CHANGED
CHANTED
CHAPPED
CHARGED
CHARMED
CHARRED
CHARTED
CHASSED
CHATTED
CHEATED
CHECKED
CHEEKED
CHEEPED
CHEERED
CHEESED
CHESTED
CHILIAD
CHILLED
CHINKED
CHINNED
CHIPPED
CHIRPED
CHIRRED
CHIVIED
CHOCKED
CHOIRED
CHOMPED
CHOPPED
CHORDED
CHROMED
CHUCKED
CHUFFED
CHUGGED
CHUMMED
CHUMPED
CHUNKED
CHURNED
GHOSTED
PHISHED
PHOTOID
PHRASED
SHACKED
SHAFTED
SHAGGED
SHAMMED
SHANKED
SHARPED
SHAWLED
SHEAFED
SHEARED
SHEAVED
SHEERED
SHEETED
SHELLED
SHELVED
SHEPARD
SHIFTED
SHILLED
SHINNED
SHINPAD
SHIPPED
SHIRKED
SHIRRED
SHOALED
SHOCKED
SHOPPED
SHORTED
SHOUTED
SHRINED
SHUCKED
SHUNNED
SHUNTED
SHUSHED
THANKED
THEBAND
THEBARD
THEGOLD
THEHOOD
THEPOND
THEWIND
THIEVED
THINNED
THORNED
THREEAD
THRIVED
THUDDED
THUMBED
THUMPED
THUNKED
THYROID
WHACKED
WHAMMED
WHANGED
WHAPPED
WHARFED
WHEELED
WHEEZED
WHELMED
WHELPED
WHETTED
WHIFFED
WHIPPED
WHIRLED
WHIRRED
WHISHED
WHISKED
WHIZKID
WHIZZED
WHOMPED
WHOOPED
WHOPPED
WHORLED
WHOSAID
WHUPPED

••HD•••
ICHDIEN
MAHDISM
MAHDIST

••H•D••
APHIDES
ECHIDNA
EPHEDRA
EXHEDRA
JOHNDOE
OXHIDES
REHIDES

••H••D•
AXHEADS
BEHEADS
BEHINDS
BEHOLDS
NOHANDS
SCHELDT
SCHMIDT
UNHANDS
UNHANDY
UNHARDY
UNHEADY
UNHEEDS
UNHOODS
UPHOLDS
WCHANDY

••H•••D
ADHERED
ASHAMED
ASHFORD
ASHLAND
BEHAVED
BEHEARD
COHERED
DEHEXED
DEHIRED
ETHMOID
EXHALED
EXHUMED
ICHABOD
INHALED
INHERED
INHUMED
LSHAPED
OCHROID
OSHAPED
PSHAWED
REHEARD
REHIRED
REHONED
SCHEMED
SPHERED
SSHAPED
TSHAPED
UNHATED
UNHAYED
UNHAZED
UNHEARD
UNHEWED
UNHIRED
UNHONED
UNHOPED
UNHUMID
UPHOARD
USHAPED
USHERED
VSHAPED
YSHAPED

•••HD••
BAGHDAD
DASHDOT
HIGHDAY
RUSHDIE
SHAHDOM
WASHDAY

•••H•D•
BUSHIDO
CATHODE
COWHIDE
METHODS
ONTHEDL
ORCHIDS
RASHIDA
RAWHIDE
UNSHADE
UNSHADY

••••H•D
AIRHEAD
ALPHARD
ATTHIRD
AXEHEAD

BADHAND
BAGHDAD
BIGHAND
BIGHEAD
BOWHEAD
BOYHOOD
CATHEAD
CICHLID
COWHAND
COWHERD
DABHAND
DIEHARD
EGGHEAD
EIGHTAD
EUCHRED
EYEHAND
FATHEAD
GOAHEAD
GODHEAD
GODHOOD
HIGHEND
HOTHAND
HOTHEAD
INTHIRD
ISAHEAD
JUGHEAD
LADHOOD
LEWHOAD
LIGHTED
LITHOID
LOWHAND
MANHOOD
MILHAUD
MOPHEAD
NEWHAND
NUNHOOD
OFFHAND
OLDHAND
ONEHAND
ORCHARD
PATHAND
PAYHEED
PINHEAD
PITHEAD
PUSHROD
REDHEAD
RICHARD
RIGHTED
SAPHEAD
SIGHTED
SUBHEAD
TEEHEED
THEHOOD
TOEHOLD
TOOHARD
TOWHEAD
TRYHARD
TYPHOID
UNSHOED
UPAHEAD
WARHEAD
XIPHOID
YACHTED

••••H•D

ABASHED
BATCHED
BEACHED
BELCHED
BENCHED
BERTHED
BIRCHED
BIRTHED
BLUSHED
BOTCHED
BOUGHED
BRUSHED
BUNCHED
CINCHED
CLASHED
CLICHED
CLOTHED
COACHED
COUCHED
COUGHED
COWSHED
CRASHED
CRUSHED
DITCHED
DWIGHTD
EARTHED
FETCHED
FILCHED
FLASHED
FLESHED
FLUSHED
FRESHED
FROTHED
GALAHAD
GIRTHED
GNASHED
GRAPHED
HATCHED
HITCHED
HUMPHED
HUNCHED
LATCHED
LAUGHED
LEACHED
LEASHED
LEECHED
LOATHED
LUNCHED
LURCHED
MARCHED
MATCHED
MOOCHED
MORPHED
MOUTHED
MULCHED
MUNCHED
MYRRHED
NEIGHED
NOTCHED
NUDZHED
PARCHED
PATCHED
PEACHED
PERCHED
PHISHED
PINCHED
PITCHED
PLASHED
POACHED
POUCHED
PSYCHED
PUNCHED
QUASHED
RANCHED
REACHED
ROUGHED
SCATHED
SCYTHED
SEETHED
SHUSHED
SLASHED
SLOSHED
SLUSHED
SMASHED
SMITHED
SMUSHED
SOOTHED
STASHED
SWASHED
SWATHED
SWISHED
SYNCHED
TEETHED
TOBEHAD
TOOTHED
TORCHED
TOUCHED
TRASHED
TROTHED
VOSKHOD
VOUCHED
WATCHED
WEIGHED
WELLHID
WHISHED
WINCHED
WITCHED
WOOSHED
WRITHED

•••••HD

FINISHD

HE•••••

HEADEND
HEADERS
HEADFOR
HEADFUL
HEADIER
HEADILY
HEADING
HEADMAN
HEADMEN
HEADOFF
HEADOUT
HEADPIN
HEADSAW
HEADSET
HEADSIN
HEADSTO
HEADSUP
HEADWAY
HEALALL
HEALERS
HEALING
HEALSUP
HEALTHY
HEAPERS
HEAPING
HEAPSOF
HEAPSON
HEAPSUP
HEARDOF
HEARERS
HEARING
HEARKEN
HEAROUT
HEARSAY
HEARSES
HEARSOF
HEARTED
HEARTEN
HEARTHS
HEATERS
HEATFAN
HEATFUL
HEATHEN
HEATHER
HEATING
HEATRAY
HEATSUP
HEATTER
HEAVEHO
HEAVENS
HEAVERS
HEAVETO
HEAVIER
HEAVIES
HEAVILY
HEAVING
HEBRAIC
HEBREWS
HECKART
HECKLED
HECKLER
HECKLES
HECKMAN
HECKUVA
HECKYES
HECTARE
HECTORS
HEDGERS
HEDGIER
HEDGING
HEDISON
HEDONIC
HEEDERS
HEEDFUL
HEEDING
HEEHAWS
HEELERS
HEELING
HEELPAD
HEELTAP
HEFTERS
HEFTIER
HEFTILY
HEFTING
HEGIRAS
HEHHEHS
HEIFERS
HEIFETZ
HEIGHHO
HEIGHTS
HEINOUS
HEIRDOM
HEIRESS
HEISMAN
HEISTED
HELDOFF
HELDOUT
HELICAL
HELICES
HELICON
HELIPAD
HELIXES
HELLBOY
HELLCAT
HELLENE
HELLENO
HELLION
HELLISH
HELLMAN
HELLOED
HELLOES
HELLUVA
HELLYES
HELMETS
HELMING
HELMOND
HELOISE
HELOTRY
HELPERS
HELPFUL
HELPING
HELPOUT
HELPSIN
HELPSON
HELPSUP
HELSING
HEMATIC
HEMATIN
HEMLINE
HEMLOCK
HEMMERS
HEMMING
HEMPIER
HEMSLEY
HENBANE
HENBITS
HENCOOP
HENDECA
HENDRIX
HENDRYX
HENLIKE
HENNAED
HENNERY
HENNISH
HENPECK
HENREID
HENRICH
HENRIES
HENRYII
HENRYIV
HENRYVI
HENSLEY
HENTOFF
HEPARIN
HEPATIC
HEPBURN
HEPCATS
HEPPEST
HEPTADS
HERALDS
HERBAGE
HERBALS
HERBART
HERBAUT
HERBERT
HERBIER
HERBTEA
HERCULE
HERDERS
HERDING
HEREDIA
HEREIAM
HERENOW
HERESTO
HERETIC
HERITOR
HERMANA
HERMANN
HERMANO
HERMANS
HERMITS
HERMOSA
HERMOSO
HERNANI
HERNDON
HERNIAE
HERNIAS
HERNIBS
HEROICS
HEROINE
HEROISM
HERONRY
HERPETO
HERRICK
HERRING
HERRIOT
HERSELF
HERSHEY
HESHVAN
HESSAFE
HESSIAN
HEURIGE
HEWEDTO
HEWLETT
HEXADIC
HEXAGON
HEXANES
HEXAPOD
HEXNUTS
HEXOSES
HEXSIGN
HEYDAYS
HEYJUDE
HEYLOOK
HEYMANS
HEYMRDJ
HEYRUBE
HEYWARD
HEYWOOD

H•E••••

HAECKEL
HEEDERS
HEEDFUL
HEEDING
HEEHAWS
HEELERS
HEELING
HEELPAD
HEELTAP
HOECAKE
HOEDOWN
HRETHEL
HUELESS

H••E•••

HAGERTY
HAMELIN
HAPENNY
HATEDIT
HATEFUL
HATESIT
HAVEAGO
HAVEFUN
HAVENER
HAVENOT
HAVEONE
HAVEOUT
HAYESES
HEREDIA
HEREIAM
HERENOW
HERESTO
HERETIC
HEWEDTO
HGWELLS
HIBERNO
HIDEOUS
HIDEOUT
HIKEDUP
HIKEOUT
HIKESUP
HIREDON
HIREOUT
HIRESON
HIVEOFF
HJHEINZ
HOLEDUP
HOLEOUT
HOLESUP
HOMEBOY
HOMEDIN
HOMEICE
HOMEIER
HOMELAB
HOMERED
HOMERIC
HOMERUN
HOMESIN
HONEDIN
HONESIN
HONESTY
HONEYED
HOPEDSO
HOPEDTO
HOPEFOR
HOPEFUL
HOPENOT
HOPESSO
HOPESTO
HOVERED
HOVERER
HOWELLS
HOWELSE
HOWEVER
HUMERAL
HUMERUS
HYGELAC
HYPEDUP
HYPERON
HYPESUP

H•••E••

HACKERS
HACKETT
HADBEEN
HADBEST
HAILERS
HALLEYS
HALTERS
HALVERS
HAMLETS
HAMMERS
HAMMETT
HAMPERS
HANDERS
HANDEYE
HANGERS
HANKERS
HAPLESS
HAPPENS
HARDEES
HARDENS
HARDEST
HARKENS
HARLEYS
HARMERS
HARNESS
HARPERS
HARVEST
HARWELL
HASBEEN
HASKELL
HASTENS
HASTERT
HATLESS
HATREDS
HATTERS
HAULERS
HAUTEUR
HAWKERS
HAWKEYE
HAWSERS
HAYSEED
HAZIEST
HEADEND
HEADERS
HEALERS
HEAPERS
HEARERS
HEATERS
HEAVEHO
HEAVENS
HEAVERS
HEAVETO
HEBREWS
HEDGERS
HEEDERS
HEELERS
HEFTERS
HEHHEHS
HEIFERS
HEIFETZ
HEIRESS
HELLENE
HELLENO
HELMETS
HELPERS
HEMMERS
HENDECA
HENNERY
HENPECK
HENREID
HEPPEST
HERBERT
HERDERS
HERPETO
HERSELF
HEWLETT
HIALEAH
HICKEYS
HIGHEND
HIGHEST
HILBERT
HIMSELF
HINDERS
HINGEON
HINTERS
HIPLESS
HIPNESS
HIPPEST
HISPEED
HISSERS
HITHERE
HITLESS
HITTERS
HOAXERS
HOCKERS
HOGGERY
HOGWEED
HOHNERS
HOKIEST
HOLBEIN
HOLBERG
HOLDERS
HOLIEST
HOLLERS
HOMIEST
HONKERS
HOOFERS
HOOPERS
HOOTERS
HOOVERS
HOPPERS
HORNETS
HOSIERS
HOSIERY
HOSTELS
HOSTESS
HOTBEDS
HOTHEAD
HOTKEYS
HOTLEAD
HOTMEAL
HOTNESS
HOTSEAT
HOTTEAS
HOTTEST
HOWBEIT
HOWDEDO
HOWLERS
HOYDENS
HUBBELL
HUELESS
HUGGERS
HULLERS
HUMBERT
HUMMELS
HUMMERS
HUMVEES
HUNGERS
HUNKERS
HUNTERS
HUPPERT
HURLERS
HURTERS
HUSKERS
HUSSEIN
HUSSERL
HUYGENS
HYGIEIA
HYGIENE
HYPHENS

H••••E•

HAARLEM
HABITED
HACKIES
HACKLED
HACKLER
HACKLES
HACKNEY
HADASET
HADBEEN
HADOVER
HAECKEL
HAGGLED
HAGGLER
HAGGLES
HAIRGEL
HAIRIER
HAIRNET
HALFFED
HALFIES
HALIDES
HALITES
HALOGEN
HAMITES
HAMMIER
HAMSTER
HANAPER
HANDFED
HANDIER
HANDLED
HANDLER
HANDLES
HANDSEL
HANDSET
HANGMEN
HANGTEN
HANKIES
HANOVER
HAPPIER
HARDEES
HARDIER
HARDSET
HARDTEN
HARPIES
HARRIED
HARRIER
HARRIES
HARRIET
HARSHEN
HARSHER
HARTLEY
HASASET
HASBEEN
HASOVER
HASSLED
HASSLES
HASTIER
HATCHED
HATCHER
HATCHES
HATCHET
HAUNTED
HAUNTER
HAVENER
HAYESES
HAYSEED
HDTVSET
HEADIER
HEADMEN
HEADSET
HEARKEN
HEARSES
HEARTED
HEARTEN
HEATHEN
HEATHER
HEATTER
HEAVIER
HEAVIES
HECKLED
HECKLER
HECKLES
HECKYES
HEDGIER
HEFTIER
HEISTED
HELICES
HELIXES
HELLOED
HELLOES
HELLYES
HEMPIER
HEMSLEY
HENNAED
HENRIES
HENSLEY
HERBIER
HERBTEA
HERSHEY
HEXANES
HEXOSES
HIBBLER
HIGGLED
HIGGLER
HIGGLES
HIGHRES
HIGHSEA
HIGHTEA
HILLIER
HILLMEN
HINDLEG
HINKIER
HINNIES
HIPPIER
HIPPIES
HIPSTER
HISPEED
HISSIER
HITCHED
HITCHER
HITCHES
HOAGIES
HOARDED
HOARDER
HOARIER
HOARSEN
HOARSER
HOBBIES
HOBBLED
HOBBLER
HOBBLES
HOBOKEN
HOCUSED
HOGTIED
HOGTIES
HOGWEED
HOISTED
HOISTER
HOLLIES
HOLSTER
HOLYMEN
HOLYSEE
HOMAGER
HOMAGES
HOMBRES
HOMEIER
HOMERED
HONALEE
HONEYED
HONORED
HONOREE
HONORER
HOOCHES
HOODIES
HOOPMEN
HOOPOES
HOOSIER
HOPOVER
HOPPIER
HORNIER
HORSIER
HORSLEY
HOSTLER
HOTITEM
HOTONES
HOTOVER
HOTTIES
HOUNDED
HOUNDER
HOVERED
HOVERER
HOWEVER
HOWTHEN
HRETHEL
HUBBIES
HUDDLED
HUDDLER
HUDDLES
HUFFIER
HUGGIES
HULKIER
HULLOED
HUMBLED
HUMBLER
HUMBLES
HUMIDEX
HUMORED
HUMPHED
HUMPIER
HUMUSES
HUMVEES
HUNCHED
HUNCHES
HUNDRED
HUNGTEN
HUNKIER
HUNTLEY
HURDLED
HURDLER
HURDLES
HURRIED
HURRIER
HURRIES
HURTLED
HURTLES
HUSKIER
HUSKIES
HUSSIES
HUSTLED
HUSTLER
HUSTLES
HUTCHES
HYRACES
HYRAXES

H•••••E

HABITUE
HADDONE
HADSOME
HADTIME
HADTOBE
HAGLIKE
HAIRDYE
HALDANE
HAMBONE
HAMLINE
HANDAXE
HANDEYE
HARLINE
HASDONE
HASTIME
HASTOBE
HATABLE
HATLIKE
HATSIZE
HAULAGE
HAVEONE
HAWKEYE
HAYBALE
HAYRIDE
HAYWIRE
HECTARE
HELLENE
HELOISE
HEMLINE
HENBANE
HENLIKE
HERBAGE
HERCULE
HERNIAE
HEROINE

HESSAFE
HEURIGE
HEYJUDE
HEYRUBE
HIDABLE
HILAIRE
HIPBONE
HIPLIKE
HIRABLE
HIRCINE
HIRSUTE
HITHERE
HITHOME
HITTITE
HITTUNE
HOECAKE
HOGLIKE
HOGNOSE
HOLYJOE
HOLYOKE
HOLYONE
HOLYSEE
HOMEICE
HONALEE
HONOREE
HOPLITE
HORMONE
HOSCALE
HOSPICE
HOSTAGE
HOSTILE
HOTCAKE
HOTDATE
HOTGLUE
HOTLINE
HOTTIME
HOTWIRE
HOTZONE
HOVLANE
HOWCOME
HOWELSE
HOWLAME
HOWNICE
HUANGHE
HUMORME
HUNLIKE
HUSSITE
HUTLIKE
HYALITE
HYDRATE
HYDRIDE
HYGIENE

•HE••••

AHEADOF
CHEADLE
CHEAPEN
CHEAPER
CHEAPIE
CHEAPLY
CHEATED
CHEATER
CHEATIN
CHEATON
CHECHEN
CHECKED
CHECKER
CHECKIN
CHECKON
CHECKUP
CHEDDAR
CHEDERS
CHEEKED
CHEEPED
CHEEPER
CHEERED
CHEERER
CHEERIO
CHEERON
CHEERUP
CHEESED
CHEESES
CHEETAH
CHEETAS
CHEETOS
CHEEVER
CHEEZIT
CHEFING
CHEKHOV
CHELATE
CHELSEA
CHEMISE
CHEMIST
CHEMLAB
CHENIER
CHEQUER
CHEQUES
CHERISH
CHEROOT
CHERUBS
CHERVIL
CHESTED
CHESTER
CHETRUM
CHEVAUX
CHEVETS
CHEVIOT
CHEVONS
CHEVRES
CHEVRET
CHEVRON
CHEWERS
CHEWGUM
CHEWIER
CHEWING
CHEWOUT
CHEWSON
CHEWSUP
CHEWTOY
CHEXMIX
CHEZMOI
GHERKIN
GHETTOS
IHEARYA
KHEDIVE
PHEMIUS
PHENOLS
PHENOMS
RHEBOKS
RHENISH
RHENIUM
RHETORS
RHEUMIC
SHEAFED
SHEARED
SHEARER
SHEATHE
SHEATHS
SHEAVED
SHEAVES
SHEBANG
SHEBEAR
SHECRAB
SHEDDER
SHEDSON
SHEEHAN
SHEERED
SHEERER
SHEERLY
SHEETED
SHEFFER
SHEGOAT
SHEIKHS
SHEILAE
SHEILAS
SHEKELS
SHELDON
SHELLAC
SHELLED
SHELLER
SHELLEY
SHELTER
SHELTIE
SHELVED
SHELVER
SHELVES
SHEPARD
SHERBET
SHERIFF
SHERIFS
SHERMAN
SHERPAS
SHERWIN
SHEVATS
SHEWOLF
THEABCS
THEAGES
THEALPS
THEARMY
THEARTS
THEATER
THEATRE
THEAXIS
THEBABE
THEBABY
THEBAND
THEBANS
THEBARD
THEBEAR
THEBELL
THEBEST
THEBIGA
THEBLOB
THEBOBO
THEBODY
THEBOMB
THEBOSS
THEBOYS
THEBRAT
THEBUSH
THECAPE
THECARS
THECAVS
THECITY
THECRAB
THECROW
THECUBS
THEDEEP
THEDELL
THEDIET
THEDOLE
THEDUKE
THEEAST
THEEDGE
THEFALL
THEFEDS
THEFIRM
THEFIVE
THEFLEA
THEFLOP
THEFONZ
THEFOOL
THEFRUG
THEGAME
THEGANG
THEGIFT
THEGOLD
THEHEAT
THEHELP
THEHERO
THEHILL
THEHOGS
THEHOOD
THEHOPE
THEHULK
THEIDEA
THEISMS
THEISTS
THEJERK
THEJETS
THEKING
THEKISS
THELAMB
THELARK
THELEFT
THELIKE
THELOOK
THELOOP
THEMAGI
THEMALL
THEMASK
THEMAVS
THEMAYO
THEMETS
THEMICK
THEMOON
THEMOST
THENETS
THENEWS
THENILE
THEOATH
THEODOR
THEOMEN
THEOMNI
THEOREM
THEPIPS
THEPITS
THEPOND
THEPOOH
THEPOPE
THEPOST
THEPUMP
THERAMS
THERAPY
THEREAT
THEREBY
THEREDS
THEREIN
THERENT
THEREOF
THEREON
THERESA
THERETO
THERIAC
THERING
THERINK
THERITZ
THERMAL
THERMIC
THERMOS
THEROBE
THEROCK
THEROOM
THEROPE
THEROSE
THEROUX
THERULE
THESACK
THESAME
THESELF
THESEUS
THESHOW
THESIMS
THESPIS
THESTAR
THESUNS
THESWAN
THETOUR
THETREE
THETRIB
THETUBE
THETURN
THEUSSR
THEVIEW
THEVIPS
THEWALL
THEWAVE
THEWIND
THEYIPS
THEYSAY
WHEATEN
WHEATON
WHEEDLE
WHEELED
WHEELER
WHEELIE
WHEELIN
WHEEZED
WHEEZER
WHEEZES
WHELMED
WHELPED
WHEREAS
WHEREAT
WHEREBY
WHEREIN
WHERELL
WHEREOF
WHEREON
WHERERE
WHERETO
WHEREVE
WHETHER
WHETTED
WHETTER
WHEYISH

•H•E•••

CHEEKED
CHEEPED
CHEEPER
CHEERED
CHEERER
CHEERIO
CHEERON
CHEERUP
CHEESED
CHEESES
CHEETAH
CHEETAS
CHEETOS
CHEEVER
CHEEZIT
CHIEFLY
PHAEDRA
PHAETON
PHLEGMY
PHOEBES
PHOEBUS
PHOENIX
PHRENIC
RHOECUS
SHEEHAN
SHEERED
SHEERER
SHEERLY
SHEETED
SHIELDS
SHOEBOX
SHOEING
SHOEPAC
SHTETLS
THEEAST
THEEDGE
THIERRY
THIEVED
THIEVES
THREADS
THREADY
THREATS
THREEAD
THREEAM
THREEBC
THREEEE
THREENO
THREEPM
THREERS
THREEUP
THREWAT
THREWIN
THREWON
THREWUP
WHEEDLE
WHEELED
WHEELER
WHEELIE
WHEELIN
WHEEZED
WHEEZER
WHEEZES
WHOEVER
WHYEVER

•H••E••

CHAFERS
CHALETS
CHANELS
CHAPEAU
CHAPELS
CHASERS
CHATEAU
CHEDERS
CHEVETS
CHEWERS
CHICEST
CHIDERS
CHILEAN
CHIMEIN
CHIMERA
CHIMERS
CHINESE
CHISELS
CHOKEON
CHOKERS
CHOKEUP
CHOLERA
CHOLERS
CHOSEUP
IHATEIT
IHAVEIT
IHOPESO
NHLTEAM
PHASEIN
PHASERS
PHILEAS
PHINEAS
PHLOEMS
PHONEIN
PHONEME
PHONENO
PHONERS
PHONEYS
RHYMERS
SHADERS
SHAKERS
SHAKEUP
SHAPELY
SHAPERS
SHAPEUP
SHAREIN
SHARERS
SHAVERS
SHEBEAR
SHEKELS
SHINEON
SHINERS
SHINEUP
SHIVERS
SHIVERY
SHOREUP
SHOVEIN
SHOVELS
SHOVERS
SHOWERS
SHOWERY
SHRIEKS
SHUBERT
SHUTEYE
SHYNESS
THALERS
THAWERS
THEBEAR
THEBELL
THEBEST
THEDEEP
THEDELL
THEFEDS
THEHEAT
THEHELP
THEHERO
THEJERK
THEJETS
THELEFT
THEMETS
THENETS
THENEWS
THEREAT
THEREBY
THEREDS
THEREIN
THERENT
THEREOF
THEREON
THERESA
THERETO
THESELF
THESEUS
THOREAU
THREEAD
THREEAM
THREEBC
THREEEE
THREENO
THREEPM
THREERS
THREEUP
THYSELF
WHALERS
WHEREAS
WHEREAT
WHEREBY
WHEREIN
WHERELL
WHEREOF
WHEREON
WHERERE
WHERETO
WHEREVE
WHINERS
WHITELY
WHITENS
WHITEST

•H•••E•

CHAFFED
CHAFFEE
CHAFFER
CHAINED
CHAINES
CHAIRED
CHAISES
CHALKED
CHAMBER
CHAMFER
CHAMPED
CHAMPER
CHANCED
CHANCEL
CHANCER
CHANCES
CHANGED
CHANGER
CHANGES
CHANNEL
CHANTED
CHANTER
CHANTEY
CHAPLET
CHAPMEN
CHAPPED
CHAPTER
CHARGED
CHARGER
CHARGES
CHARIER
CHARLES
CHARLEY
CHARMED
CHARMEN
CHARMER
CHARRED
CHARRER
CHARTED
CHARTER
CHARVET
CHASSED
CHASSES
CHASTEN
CHASTER
CHATTED
CHATTEL
CHATTER
CHAUCER
CHEAPEN
CHEAPER
CHEATED
CHEATER
CHECHEN
CHECKED
CHECKER
CHEEKED
CHEEPED
CHEEPER
CHEERED
CHEERER
CHEESED
CHEESES
CHEEVER
CHELSEA
CHENIER
CHEQUER
CHEQUES
CHESTED
CHESTER
CHEVRES
CHEVRET
CHEWIER
CHIAPET
CHICHEN
CHICKEN
CHICLES
CHICLET
CHIDDEN
CHIGGER
CHIGOES
CHILIES
CHILLED
CHILLER
CHIMNEY
CHINKED
CHINNED
CHIPPED
CHIPPER
CHIRPED
CHIRPER
CHIRRED
CHITTER
CHIVIED
CHIVIES
CHOCKED
CHOICER
CHOICES
CHOIRED
CHOKIER
CHOMPED
CHOOSER
CHOOSES
CHOOSEY
CHOPPED
CHOPPER
CHORDED
CHOWDER
CHROMED
CHROMES
CHUCKED
CHUFFED
CHUGGED
CHUGGER
CHUKKER
CHUMMED
CHUMPED
CHUNKED
CHUNNEL
CHURNED
CHURNER
CHUTNEY
GHOSTED
OHMAGES
PHATTER
PHILTER
PHISHED
PHISHER
PHISHES
PHLOXES
PHOEBES
PHONIER
PHONIES
PHRASED
PHRASES
SHACKED
SHADIER
SHAFFER
SHAFTED
SHAGGED
SHAKIER
SHAKOES
SHALIER
SHAMMED
SHANKED
SHANNEN
SHANTER
SHARKEY
SHARPED
SHARPEI
SHARPEN
SHARPER
SHATNER
SHATTER
SHAWLED
SHAWNEE
SHEAFED
SHEARED
SHEARER
SHEAVED
SHEAVES
SHEDDER
SHEERED
SHEERER
SHEETED
SHEFFER
SHELLED
SHELLER
SHELLEY
SHELTER
SHELVED
SHELVER
SHELVES
SHERBET
SHIFTED
SHIFTER
SHIITES
SHILLED
SHIMMER
SHINIER
SHINNED
SHIPMEN
SHIPPED
SHIPPER
SHIRKED
SHIRKER
SHIRLEY
SHIRRED
SHOALED
SHOCKED
SHOCKER
SHODDEN
SHOOTER
SHOPPED
SHOPPER
SHOPPES
SHORTED
SHORTEN
SHORTER
SHOUTED
SHOUTER
SHOWIER
SHOWMEN
SHRIKES
SHRINED
SHRINER
SHRINES
SHRIVEL
SHRIVER
SHRIVES
SHUCKED
SHUCKER
SHUDDER
SHUNNED
SHUNTED
SHUNTER
SHUSHED
SHUSHES
SHUSTER
SHUTTER
SHYSTER
THANKED
THANKER
THEAGES
THEATER
THEDEEP
THEDIET
THEFLEA
THEIDEA
THEOMEN
THEOREM
THETREE
THEVIEW
THICKEN
THICKER
THICKET
THIEVED
THIEVES
THIGPEN
THINKER
THINNED
THINNER
THITHER
THORNED
THREEEE
THRIVED
THRIVEN
THRIVER
THRIVES
THRONES
THROWER
THUDDED
THUMBED
THUMPED
THUMPER
THUNDER
THUNKED
THURBER
WHACKED
WHACKER
WHALLEY
WHAMMED
WHANGED
WHAPPED
WHARFED
WHARVES
WHAUDEN
WHEATEN
WHEELED
WHEELER
WHEEZED
WHEEZER
WHEEZES
WHELMED
WHELPED
WHETHER
WHETTED
WHETTER
WHIFFED
WHIFFER
WHIMPER
WHINIER
WHIPPED
WHIPPER
WHIPPET
WHIRLED
WHIRLER
WHIRRED
WHISHED
WHISHES
WHISKED
WHISKER
WHISKEY
WHISPER
WHITHER
WHITNEY
WHIZZED
WHIZZER
WHIZZES
WHOEVER
WHOKNEW
WHOMPED
WHOOPED
WHOOPEE
WHOOPER
WHOPPED
WHOPPER
WHORLED
WHUPPED
WHYEVER

•H••••E

AHASSLE
CHAFFEE
CHALICE
CHAMBRE
CHAPPIE
CHARADE
CHARLIE
CHAYOTE
CHEADLE
CHEAPIE
CHELATE
CHEMISE
CHICANE
CHINESE
CHOLINE
CHOPINE
CHORALE
CHORINE
CHORTLE
CHUCKLE
DHURRIE
KHANATE
KHEDIVE
NHLGAME
OHFUDGE
PHILLIE
PHILTRE
PHONEME
RHIZOME
SHACKLE
SHADROE
SHALLWE
SHAMBLE
SHARPIE
SHAWNEE
SHEATHE
SHEILAE
SHELTIE

SHINGLE
SHORTIE
SHUFFLE
SHUTEYE
SHUTTLE
THANDIE
THATONE
THEATRE
THEBABE
THECAPE
THEDOLE
THEDUKE
THEEDGE
THEFIVE
THEGAME
THEHOPE
THELIKE
THENILE
THEPOPE
THEROBE
THEROPE
THEROSE
THERULE
THESAME
THETREE
THETUBE
THEWAVE
THIMBLE
THINICE
THISONE
THISTLE
THREEEE
THWHITE
THYMINE
WHATTHE
WHEEDLE
WHEELIE
WHERERE
WHEREVE
WHIFFLE
WHIPPLE
WHISTLE
WHITTLE
WHOOPEE
WHOOPIE

••HE•••

ACHEFOR
ACHENES
ACHERON
ACHESON
ADHERED
ADHERER
ADHERES
AMHERST
APHELIA
ATHEART
ATHEISM
ATHEIST
AXHEADS
BEHEADS
BEHEARD
BEHESTS
BOHEMIA
BYHEART
COHEIRS
COHERED
COHERER
COHERES
DEHEXED
DEHEXES
DOHERTY
ECHELON
EPHEBUS
EPHEDRA
EPHESUS
ETHENES
ETHERIC
EXHEDRA
FTHENRY
GEHENNA
HJHEINZ
INHERED
INHERES
INHERIT
MCHENRY
MOHEGAN
OCHENTA
OPHELIA
OTHELLO
OXHEART
REHEALS
REHEARD
REHEARS
REHEATS
REHEELS
SCHELDT
SCHEMAS
SCHEMED
SCHEMER
SCHEMES
SCHERZI
SCHERZO
SPHERAL
SPHERED
SPHERES
SPHERIC
TEHERAN
TOHEART
TOHELEN
UNHEADY
UNHEARD
UNHEAVY
UNHEEDS
UNHELMS
UNHEWED
UPHEAPS
UPHEAVE
USHERED
USHERIN

••H•E••

ACHIEST
ACHIEVA
ACHIEVE
ASHBERY
ASHHEAP
ASHIEST
ASHLESS
ATHLETE
BAHREIN
BEHRENS
CAHIERS
DEHMELT
ECHOERS
HEHHEHS
HOHNERS
REHEELS
SCHLEPP
SCHLEPS
SCHMEAR
SCHMEER
UNHEEDS

••H••E•

ACHENES
ADHERED
ADHERER
ADHERES
APHIDES
ASHAMED
ASHIVER
ASHTREE
ATHOMES
BAHAMEN
BEHAVED
BEHAVES
COHERED
COHERER
COHERES
DAHOMEY
DEHAVEN
DEHEXED
DEHEXES
DEHIRED
DEHIRES
DUHAMEL
ETHANES
ETHENES
EXHALED
EXHALES
EXHUMED
EXHUMER
EXHUMES
ICHDIEN
IMHOTEP
INHALED
INHALER
INHALES
INHERED
INHERES
INHUMED
INHUMER
INHUMES
ISHMAEL
JOHNLEE
LSHAPED
MAHONEY
MCHALES
MOHAVES
MRHANEY
OSHAPED
OXHIDES
PSHAWED
REHIDES
REHIRED
REHIRES
REHONED
REHONES
SCHAYES
SCHEMED
SCHEMER
SCHEMES
SCHMEER
SCHMOES
SCHOLES
SCHUMER
SOHAVEI
SPHERED
SPHERES
SSHAPED
TOHELEN
TOHOMER
TSHAPED
TSHAPES
UNHATED
UNHAYED
UNHAZED
UNHEWED
UNHIRED
UNHIRES
UNHONED
UNHOPED
USHAPED
USHAPES
USHERED
VSHAPED
VSHAPES
WAHINES
YAHTZEE
YSHAPED
YSHAPES

••H•••E

ACHIEVE
ACHILLE
ASHCAKE
ASHTREE
ATHLETE
BEHOOVE
DEHISCE
ECHAPPE
ENHANCE
INHASTE
INHOUSE
JOHNDOE
JOHNLEE
JOHNNIE
LEHAVRE
MRHORSE
REHINGE
REHOUSE
TOHORSE
UNHINGE
UNHORSE
UNHOUSE
UPHEAVE
VEHICLE
YAHTZEE

•••HE••

AIRHEAD
ALCHEMY
ALLHEAL
ALLHERE
ANAHEIM
ANTHEIL
ANTHEMS
ANTHERS
ARCHERS
ARCHERY
ARCHEST
ASHHEAP
AXEHEAD
BASHERS
BATHERS
BEAHERO
BETHELS
BETHERE
BIGHEAD
BONHEUR
BOTHERS
BOWHEAD
BUSHELS
BUSHERS
BYTHEBY
CACHETS
CASHEWS
CATHEAD
CEPHEUS
CIPHERS
COSHERS
COWHERD
CYPHERS
DASHERS
DESHELL
DITHERS
DITHERY
DRYHEAT
DUCHESS
EATHERE
EGGHEAD
ESCHEAT
ESCHERS
ESCHEWS
ESTHETE
ETCHERS
FATHEAD
FATHERS
FISHERS
FISHERY
FISHEYE
GASHEAT
GATHERS
GETHELP
GOAHEAD
GODHEAD
GOPHERS
GOTHELP
GUSHERS
HEHHEHS
HIGHEND
HIGHEST
HITHERE
HOTHEAD
HYPHENS
IDTHEFT
IMTHERE
INAHEAP
INCHECK
INCHERS
INTHERE
ISAHEAD
ISOHELS
ITSHERE
JAPHETH
JOSHERS
JUGHEAD
KOSHERS
KUCHENS
LASHERS
LATHERS
LATHERY
LECHERS
LETHEAN
LICHEES
LICHENS
LITHELY
LITHEST
LOWHEEL
LUSHEST
MACHETE
MANHEIM
MASHERS
MATHERS
MATHEWS
MAYHEMS
MISHEAR
MOPHEAD
MOSHERS
MOTHERS
MOTHERY
MUDHENS
MUSHERS
MYNHEER
NEPHEWS
NIGHEST
NONHERO
NOSHERS
NOTHERE
NOWHERE
OILHEAT
ONTHEDL
ONTHEGO
ONTHEQT
ORPHEAN
ORPHEUM
ORPHEUS
OUTHEAR
OUTHERE
PAYHEED
PEAHENS
PINHEAD
PITHEAD
POSHEST
POTHERB
POTHERS
PREHEAL
PREHEAT
PUSHERS
RASHERS
RASHEST
RECHECK
RECHEWS
REDHEAD
REDHEAT
REDHENS
RICHENS
RICHEST
ROCHETS
RUSHEES
RUSHERS
SACHEMS
SACHETS
SAPHEAD
SEAHERO
SEEHERE
SIGHERS
SOTHEBY
SOTHERE
SOTHERN
SUBHEAD
TARHEEL
TEEHEED
TEEHEES
TETHERS
THEHEAT
THEHELP
THEHERO
TITHERS
TOWHEAD
TOWHEES
TUSHERY
UNCHECK
UNSHEER
UNSHELL
UNWHEEL
UPAHEAD
UPTHERE
WARHEAD
WARHERO
WASHERS
WILHELM
WISHERS
WITHERS
YOTHERS
ZITHERS

•••H•E•

ARCHIES
ARCHSEE
ATTHREE
BISHKEK
BOCHNER
BUCHNER
BUSHIER
BUSHMEN
CASHIER
COCHLEA
CUSHIER
DAPHNES
DASHIER
DICHTER
DISHIER
DUCHIES
EIGHTEE
EUCHRED
EUCHRES
FECHNER
FIGHTER
FISHIER
FISHNET
GUSHIER
HIGHRES
HIGHSEA
HIGHTEA
INTHREE
ITCHIER
KISHKES
KOEHLER
LICHEES
LIGHTED
LIGHTEN
LIGHTER
LOWHEEL
LUSHIER
LUTHIER
MACHREE
MASHIES
MATHIEU
MESHIER
MICHAEL
MOTHIER
MPTHREE
MUSHIER
MYNHEER
NIGHTER
ONTHREE
PAYHEED
PITHIER
PUSHIER
RACHAEL
RAPHAEL
RESHOES
RICHLER
RICHMEN
RICHTER
RIGHTED
RIGHTER
RUSHEES
RUSHIER
SIGHTED
SIGHTER
SOPHIES
TARHEEL
TECHIES
TEEHEED
TEEHEES
TIGHTEN
TIGHTER
TOWHEES
TUSHIES
UNSHEER
UNSHIER
UNSHOED
UNSHOES
UNSHYER
UNWHEEL
VECHTEN
WASHIER
WITHIES
YACHTED
YACHTER

•••H••E

AIRHOLE
AIRHOSE
ALLHERE
ALOHAOE
ANYHOPE
ARCHFOE
ARCHIVE
ARCHSEE
ARMHOLE
ARSHILE
ATTHREE
BEEHIVE
BETHERE
BETHUNE
BOBHOPE
BOGHOLE
BYPHONE
CATHODE
COCHISE
COWHIDE
DRYHOLE
EARHOLE
EATHERE
EBWHITE
EIGHTEE
ENCHASE
ENTHUSE
ESTHETE
EYEHOLE
FISHEYE
FORHIRE
FOXHOLE
GRAHAME
GUTHRIE
HITHERE
HITHOME
ICEHOLE
IMTHERE
INAHOLE
INPHASE
INSHAPE
INSHORE
INTHERE
INTHREE
INWHITE
ITSHERE
KEYHOLE
LETHAVE
MACHETE
MACHINE
MACHONE
MACHREE
MANHOLE
MCSHANE
METHANE
MOCHRIE
MPTHREE
MUDHOLE
MULHARE
NEWHIRE
NEWHOPE
NIGHTIE
NONHOME
NOTHERE
NOTHOME
NOWHERE
OMAHANE
ONSHORE
ONTHREE
OUTHERE
OUTHIRE
PETHARE
PIEHOLE
PINHOLE
POTHOLE
RAMHOME
RANHOME
RATHOLE
RAWHIDE
RECHOSE
REPHASE
REPHONE
RESHAPE
RESHARE
RESHAVE
RESHINE
RUNHOME
RUSHDIE
SATHOME
SEEHERE
SITHOME
SOTHERE
SPYHOLE
TAXHIKE
TERHUNE
THEHOPE
THWHITE
TOPHOLE
UNCHOKE
UNRHYME
UNSHADE
UNWHITE
UNWHOLE
UPPHASE
UPTHERE
YACHTIE

••••HE•

ABASHED
ABASHES
AITCHES
ANDTHEN
ANOTHER
APACHES
APOTHEM
BANSHEE
BATCHED
BATCHES
BEACHED
BEACHES
BEECHEN
BEECHER
BEECHES
BELCHED
BELCHER
BELCHES
BENCHED
BENCHER
BENCHES
BERTHED
BIRCHED
BIRCHEN
BIRCHES
BIRTHED
BLATHER
BLITHER
BLUEHEN
BLUSHED
BLUSHER
BLUSHES
BOTCHED
BOTCHER
BOTCHES
BOUCHER
BOUCHES
BOUGHED
BRASHER
BRASHES
BROTHER
BRUSHED
BRUSHER
BRUSHES
BUNCHED
BUNCHES
BURGHER
BUTCHER
BUTCHES
CATCHER
CATCHES
CAUTHEN
CHECHEN
CHICHEN
CINCHED
CINCHES
CLASHED
CLASHER
CLASHES
CLICHED
CLICHES
CLOCHES
CLOTHED
CLOTHES
COACHED
COACHES
CONCHES
COUCHED
COUCHES
COUGHED
COWSHED
CRASHED
CRASHER
CRASHES
CRECHES
CROCHET
CRUSHED
CRUSHER
CRUSHES
CULCHES
DITCHED
DITCHER
DITCHES
DOGCHEW
EARTHED
EARTHEN
EPITHET
FARTHER
FEATHER
FETCHED
FETCHER
FETCHES
FILCHED
FILCHER
FILCHES
FINCHES
FISCHER
FLASHED
FLASHER
FLASHES
FLECHES
FLESHED
FLESHES
FLUSHED
FLUSHER
FLUSHES
FRESHED
FRESHEN
FRESHER
FRESHES
FRESHET
FROTHED
FROTHER
FURTHER
GAUCHER
GETSHEP
GIRTHED
GNASHED
GNASHER
GNASHES
GRAPHED
GREYHEN
GULCHES
GUNTHER
HARSHEN
HARSHER
HATCHED
HATCHER
HATCHES
HATCHET
HEATHEN
HEATHER
HERSHEY
HITCHED
HITCHER
HITCHES
HOOCHES
HOWTHEN
HRETHEL
HUMPHED
HUNCHED
HUNCHES
HUTCHES
IRISHER
JIMCHEE
KAISHEK
KETCHES
KIMCHEE
KITCHEN
KNISHES
KOOSHES
KUTCHER
LARCHEN
LARCHES
LATCHED
LATCHES
LAUGHED
LAUGHER
LEACHED
LEACHER
LEACHES
LEASHED
LEASHES
LEATHER
LEECHED
LEECHEE
LEECHES
LOATHED
LOATHER
LOATHES
LOWCHEN
LUNCHED
LUNCHER
LUNCHES
LURCHED
LURCHER
LURCHES
MADCHEN
MARCHED
MARCHER
MARCHES
MARSHES
MATCHED
MATCHER
MATCHES
MATTHEW
MERCHES
MOOCHED
MOOCHER
MOOCHES
MOORHEN
MORPHED
MOUTHED
MOUTHER
MULCHED
MULCHES
MUNCHED
MUNCHEN
MUNCHER
MUNCHES
MYRRHED
NARTHEX
NATCHEZ
NEIGHED
NEITHER
NOOTHER
NORTHER
NOTCHED
NOTCHER
NOTCHES
NOWTHEN
NUDZHED
NUDZHES
PANTHER
PARCHED
PARCHES
PATCHED
PATCHEN
PATCHER
PATCHES
PEACHED
PEACHES
PERCHED
PERCHER
PERCHES
PETCHEW
PHISHED
PHISHER
PHISHES
PINCHED
PINCHER
PINCHES
PITCHED
PITCHER
PITCHES
PLASHED
PLASHES
PLUSHER
PLUSHES
POACHED
POACHER
POACHES
POOCHES
PORCHES
POUCHED
POUCHES
PRITHEE
PROPHET
PSYCHED
PSYCHES
PUNCHED

PUNCHER
PUNCHES
QUASHED
QUASHES
QUICHES
RANCHED
RANCHER
RANCHES
RATCHET
REACHED
REACHER
REACHES
REUTHER
ROACHES
ROUGHED
ROUGHEN
ROUGHER
SAGEHEN
SATCHEL
SAYWHEN
SCATHED
SCATHES
SCYTHED
SCYTHES
SEETHED
SEETHES
SHUSHED
SHUSHES
SKOSHES
SLASHED
SLASHER
SLASHES
SLATHER
SLITHER
SLOSHED
SLOSHES
SLUSHED
SLUSHES
SMASHED
SMASHER
SMASHES
SMITHED
SMOTHER
SMUSHED
SMUSHES
SOOTHED
SOOTHER
SOOTHES
SOUTHEY
SPATHES
STASHED
STASHES
STEPHEN
SWASHED
SWASHES
SWATHED
SWATHES
SWISHED
SWISHES
SYNCHED
TEACHER
TEACHES
TEETHED
TEETHER
TEETHES
TEICHER
TENCHES
THITHER

TOOTHED
TORCHED
TORCHER
TORCHES
TOUCHED
TOUCHER
TOUCHES
TOUGHEN
TOUGHER
TRACHEA
TRASHED
TRASHER
TRASHES
TROCHEE
TROCHES
TROTHED
VETCHES
VOUCHED
VOUCHER
VOUCHES
WALTHER
WATCHED
WATCHER
WATCHES
WEATHER
WEIGHED
WEIGHER
WENCHES
WERNHER
WERTHER
WHETHER
WHISHED
WHISHES
WHITHER
WINCHED
WINCHER
WINCHES
WITCHED
WITCHES
WOOSHED
WOOSHES
WRITHED
WRITHER
WRITHES
YOUTHEN
ZILCHES

••••H•E
ARACHNE
BACCHAE
BACKHOE
BANSHEE
CONCHAE
DASCHLE
DONAHUE
DONOHOE
GUMSHOE
GYMSHOE
INASHOE
IVANHOE
JIMCHEE
KIMCHEE
LEECHEE
MUNCHIE
ODDSHOE
OLDSHOE
ONESHOE
PINCHME

POOCHIE
PRITHEE
PRUDHOE
RALPHIE
RITCHIE
ROETHKE
TAPSHOE
TOESHOE
TOUGHIE
TROCHEE

•••••HE
ADOLPHE
ARDECHE
ASEETHE
ATTACHE
BINOCHE
BLANCHE
BREATHE
BRIOCHE
CAPUCHE
CEVICHE
DEPECHE
EARACHE
FRAICHE
GOUACHE
HUANGHE
KANEOHE
LAROCHE
LAVACHE
PANACHE
PENUCHE
PORSCHE
REBATHE
SHEATHE
STROPHE
WHATTHE
WREATHE

H•F••••
HAFNIUM
HAFTING
HEFTERS
HEFTIER
HEFTILY
HEFTING
HOFBRAU
HOFFMAN
HOFMANN
HOFSTRA
HUFFIER
HUFFILY
HUFFING
HUFFISH
HUFFMAN

H••F•••
HADFITS
HALFBAD
HALFCUT
HALFDAY
HALFDUG
HALFFED
HALFIES
HALFMAD
HALFRAW
HALFROD
HALFSHY
HALFWAY
HALFWIT
HALFWON
HASFITS
HATFULS
HAYFORK
HEIFERS
HEIFETZ
HITFILM
HOFFMAN
HOOFERS
HOOFING
HOOFSIT
HOTFOOT
HUFFIER
HUFFILY
HUFFING
HUFFISH
HUFFMAN

H•••F••
HADAFIT
HALFFED
HALIFAX
HANDFED
HANDFUL
HARMFUL
HASAFIT
HATEFUL
HAVEFUN
HEADFOR
HEADFUL
HEATFAN
HEATFUL
HEEDFUL
HELPFUL
HITSFOR
HOPEFOR
HOPEFUL
HUNTFOR
HURTFOR
HURTFUL
HUSHFUL

H••••F•
HACKOFF
HANDOFF
HANGOFF
HAPPIFY
HATSOFF
HAULOFF
HAYLOFT
HEADOFF
HELDOFF
HENTOFF
HESSAFE
HITSOFF
HIVEOFF
HOLDOFF
HOPSOFF
HORRIFY
HUNGOFF

H•••••F
HACKOFF
HANDOFF
HANGOFF
HATSOFF
HAULOFF
HEADOFF
HEAPSOF
HEARDOF
HEARSOF
HELDOFF
HENTOFF
HERSELF
HIMSELF
HIPROOF
HITSOFF
HIVEOFF
HOLDOFF
HOPSOFF
HUNGOFF

•HF••••
OHFUDGE

•H•F•••
CHAFERS
CHAFFED
CHAFFEE
CHAFFER
CHAFING
CHEFING
CHIFFON
CHUFFED
SHAFFER
SHAFTED
SHEFFER
SHIFTED
SHIFTER
SHOFARS
SHUFFLE
SHYFROM
THEFALL
THEFEDS
THEFIRM
THEFIVE
THEFLEA
THEFLOP
THEFONZ
THEFOOL
THEFRUG
WHIFFED
WHIFFER
WHIFFLE

•H••F••
CHAFFED
CHAFFEE
CHAFFER
CHAMFER
CHIEFLY
CHIFFON
CHUFFED
SHAFFER
SHEAFED
SHEFFER
SHIPFUL
SHOOFLY
SHOPFOR
SHOPFUL
SHOTFOR
SHUFFLE
THRIFTS
THRIFTY
THUSFAR
WHARFED
WHATFOR
WHIFFED
WHIFFER
WHIFFLE

•H•••F•
CHOPOFF
SHERIFF
SHERIFS
SHONUFF
SHOOOFF
SHOWOFF
SHUTOFF
THEGIFT
THELEFT
WHATIFS

•H••••F
AHEADOF
AHOSTOF
CHOPOFF
SHERIFF
SHEWOLF
SHONUFF
SHOOOFF
SHORTOF
SHOWOFF
SHUTOFF
THEREOF
THESELF
THINKOF
THYSELF
WHEREOF

••HF•••
ASHFORD
MAHFOUZ

••H•F••
ACHEFOR

•••HF••
ARCHFOE
BASHFUL
DISHFUL
FISHFOR
FISHFRY
HUSHFUL
ITCHFOR
PUSHFOR
PUSHFUL
RUTHFUL
SIGHFOR
SIGHFUL
WISHFOR
WISHFUL

•••H•F•
DASHOFF
IDTHEFT
INAHUFF
MYTHIFY
PUSHOFF
RESHIFT
RUSHOFF
SAMHUFF
SYDHOFF
UNSHIFT
UPSHIFT
WASHOFF

•••H••F
BIGHALF
DASHOFF
INAHUFF
ONEHALF
PUSHOFF
RUSHOFF
SAMHUFF
SYDHOFF
WASHOFF

••••H•F
NORTHOF
SOUTHOF

HG•••••
HGWELLS

H•G••••
HAGERTY
HAGGARD
HAGGISH
HAGGLED
HAGGLER
HAGGLES
HAGLIKE
HEGIRAS
HIGGINS
HIGGLED
HIGGLER
HIGGLES
HIGHART
HIGHBAR
HIGHBOY
HIGHDAY
HIGHEND
HIGHEST
HIGHHAT
HIGHIQS
HIGHISH
HIGHLOW
HIGHPAY
HIGHRES
HIGHSEA
HIGHTEA
HIGHTOP
HIGHWAY
HOGARTH
HOGBACK
HOGCALL
HOGGERY
HOGGING
HOGGISH
HOGLIKE
HOGNOSE
HOGNUTS
HOGTIED
HOGTIES
HOGWASH
HOGWEED
HOGWILD
HUGGERS
HUGGIES
HUGGING
HUGGINS
HYGELAC
HYGIEIA
HYGIENE
HYGINUS

H••G•••
HAGGARD
HAGGISH
HAGGLED
HAGGLER
HAGGLES
HANGARS
HANGBYS
HANGDOG
HANGERS
HANGING
HANGMAN
HANGMEN
HANGOFF
HANGOUT
HANGSBY
HANGSIN
HANGSON
HANGSUP
HANGTEN
HANGUPS
HAUGHTY
HEDGERS
HEDGIER
HEDGING
HEIGHHO
HEIGHTS
HIGGINS
HIGGLED
HIGGLER
HIGGLES
HINGEON
HINGING
HOAGIES
HOGGERY
HOGGING
HOGGISH
HOTGLUE
HUGGERS
HUGGIES
HUGGING
HUGGINS
HUNGARY
HUNGERS
HUNGOFF
HUNGOUT
HUNGTEN
HUYGENS

H•••G••
HADAGAS
HAIRGEL
HALOGEN
HANDGUN
HASAGAS
HEXAGON
HOMAGER
HOMAGES
HUANGHE
HUANGTI

H••••G•
HAULAGE
HAVEAGO
HAYINGS
HAZINGS
HERBAGE
HEURIGE
HEXSIGN
HIDALGO
HIDINGS
HOSTAGE
HOTDOGS
HOWHIGH
HUMBUGS

H•••••G
HACKING
HAFTING
HAILING
HALFDUG
HALOING
HALTING
HALVING
HAMBURG
HAMMING
HANDBAG
HANDING
HANGDOG
HANGING
HARBURG
HARDING
HARKING
HARMING
HARPING
HASHING
HASPING
HASTING
HATTING
HAULING
HAWKING
HEADING
HEALING
HEAPING
HEARING
HEATING
HEAVING
HEDGING
HEEDING
HEELING
HEFTING
HELMING
HELPING
HELSING
HEMMING
HERDING
HERRING
HIBBING
HILLING
HILTING
HINDLEG
HINGING
HINTING
HISSING
HITSONG
HITTING
HOAXING
HOBOING
HOCKING
HODDING
HOGGING
HOLBERG
HOLDING
HOMBURG
HONKING
HOODING
HOOFING
HOOKING
HOOPING
HOOTING
HOPPING
HOPSING
HORDING
HORNING
HORNUNG
HORSING
HOSTING
HOUSING
HOWLING
HOWLONG
HUFFING
HUGGING
HULKING
HULLING
HUMMING
HUNTING
HURLING
HURTING
HUSHING
HUSKING
HUTTING
HYMNING
HYPOING

•H•G•••
CHAGALL
CHAGRIN
CHIGGER
CHIGNON
CHIGOES
CHUGGED
CHUGGER
NHLGAME
SHAGGED
SHAGRUG
SHEGOAT
SHOGUNS
THEGAME
THEGANG
THEGIFT
THEGOLD
THIGPEN

•H••G••
CHANGED
CHANGER
CHANGES
CHARGED
CHARGER
CHARGES
CHEWGUM
CHIGGER
CHOUGHS
CHUGGED
CHUGGER
OHMAGES
PHLEGMY
PHRYGIA
SHAGGED
SHANGRI
SHINGLE
SHINGLY
SHOTGUN
THEAGES
THOUGHT
THURGAU
WHANGED

•H•••G•
CHICAGO
OHFUDGE
PHOTOGS
THEBIGA
THEEDGE
THEHOGS
THEMAGI
THRONGS
THROUGH
ZHIVAGO

•H••••G
CHAFING
CHARING
CHASING
CHAWING
CHEFING
CHEWING
CHIDING
CHIMING
CHINWAG
CHOKING
CHOWING
CHUTING
PHASING
PHONING
RHYMING
SHADING
SHAGRUG
SHAKING
SHAMING
SHAPING
SHARING
SHAVING
SHEBANG
SHINDIG
SHINING
SHOEING
SHOOING
SHORING
SHOVING
SHOWDOG
SHOWING
THAWING
THEFRUG
THEGANG
THEKING
THERING
WHALING
WHILING
WHINING
WHITING

••H•G••
APHAGIA
APHAGIC
GAHAGAN
JOHNGAY
LEHIGHU
MOHEGAN

••H••G•
REHANGS
REHINGE
UNHINGE

••H•••G
ACHTUNG
BEHRING
ECHOING

•••HG••
LITHGOW

•••H•G•
ACEHIGH
AIMHIGH
BIGHUGS
FLYHIGH
GASHOGS
HOWHIGH
IMAHOGG
JIMHOGG
MESHUGA
ONTHEGO
QUAHOGS
SKYHIGH
THEHOGS
TOOHIGH

•••H••G
ALTHING
ARCHING
BACHING
BASHING
BATHING
BUSHHOG
BUSHING
BUSHPIG
CACHING
CASHING
COSHING
CUSHING
DASHING
DENHAAG
DISHING
DISHRAG
ETCHING
FISHING
GASHING
GUSHING
HASHING
HUSHING
IMAHOGG
INCHING
INTHING
ITCHING
JIMHOGG
JOSHING
KACHING
LASHING
LATHING
MASHING
MESHING
MOSHING
MUSHING
NICHING
NOSHING
NOTHING
PISHING
PITHING
PUSHING
RUCHING
RUSHING
SASHING
SECHZIG
SIGHING
TITHING
WASHING
WASHRAG
WISHING

••••HG•
ROUGHGO

••••H•G
BEARHUG
BUSHHOG
MALEHOG
ROADHOG
SANDHOG
WARTHOG

HH•••••
HHMUNRO

H•H••••
HAHNIUM
HEHHEHS
HJHEINZ
HOHNERS

H••H•••
HAMHOCK
HARHARS
HASHING
HASHISH
HASHOUT
HAWHAWS
HEEHAWS
HEHHEHS
HESHVAN
HIGHART
HIGHBAR
HIGHBOY
HIGHDAY
HIGHEND
HIGHEST
HIGHHAT
HIGHIQS
HIGHISH
HIGHLOW
HIGHPAY
HIGHRES
HIGHSEA
HIGHTEA
HIGHTOP
HIGHWAY
HITHERE
HITHOME
HOOHAHS
HOTHAND

HOTHEAD
HOWHIGH
HUSHABY
HUSHFUL
HUSHING
HYPHENS

H•••H••
HARDHAT
HARDHIT
HARSHEN
HARSHER
HARSHLY
HATCHED
HATCHER
HATCHES
HATCHET
HAUGHTY
HEATHEN
HEATHER
HEIGHHO
HEIGHTS
HERSHEY
HIGHHAT
HITCHED
HITCHER
HITCHES
HITCHON
HITCHUP
HITSHOW
HONCHOS
HOOCHES
HOTSHOT
HOWTHEN
HRETHEL
HUMPHED
HUMPHRY
HUNCHED
HUNCHES
HUTCHES

H••••H•
HALFSHY
HALVAHS
HAMACHI
HARRAHS
HEALTHY
HEARTHS
HEAVEHO
HEHHEHS
HEIGHHO
HIBACHI
HITACHI
HOOHAHS
HOOKAHS
HOORAHS
HOWDAHS
HUANGHE
HUPPAHS
HURRAHS
HUZZAHS

H•••••H
HAGGISH
HAIMISH
HALAVAH
HANUKAH
HARBACH
HARDISH
HASHISH
HAWKISH
HAWORTH
HELLISH
HENNISH
HENRICH
HIALEAH
HIGHISH
HIPBATH
HIPPISH
HOGARTH
HOGGISH
HOGWASH
HORNISH
HOTBATH
HOWHIGH
HOWMUCH
HUFFISH
HUNNISH

•HH••••
SHHHHHH

•H•H•••
AHCHOOS
SHAHDOM
SHHHHHH
SHIHTZU
THEHEAT
THEHELP
THEHERO
THEHILL
THEHOGS
THEHOOD
THEHOPE
THEHULK
THWHITE

•H••H••
CHACHAS
CHACHKA
CHATHAM
CHECHEN
CHEKHOV
CHICHAS
CHICHEN
CHICHIS
PHISHED
PHISHER
PHISHES
RHYTHMS
SHEEHAN
SHHHHHH
SHOWHOW
SHUSHED
SHUSHES
THESHOW
THITHER
WHETHER
WHISHED
WHISHES
WHITHER

•H•••H•
CHOUGHS
CHURCHY
SHEATHE
SHEATHS
SHEIKHS
SHHHHHH
THATCHY
THIMPHU
THOUGHT
WHATTHE
WHOSWHO

•H••••H
CHALLAH
CHEETAH
CHERISH
CHIMINH
CHUMASH
CHUPPAH
EHRLICH
PHARAOH
RHENISH
SHHHHHH
THEBUSH
THEOATH
THEPOOH
THROUGH
WHEYISH
WHITISH

••HH•••
ASHHEAP
HEHHEHS
SHHHHHH

••H•H••
SHHHHHH

••H••H•
HEHHEHS
LEHIGHU
SHHHHHH
WAHWAHS

••H•••H
OSHKOSH
REHITCH
SHHHHHH
UNHARSH
UNHITCH

•••HH••
BUSHHOG
HIGHHAT
SHHHHHH

•••H•H•
EIGHTHS
HEHHEHS
HOOHAHS
JEPHTHA
NAPHTHA
SHHHHHH

•••H••H
ACEHIGH
AIMHIGH
BOOHBAH
BUSHWAH
FLYHIGH
HASHISH
HIGHISH
HOWHIGH
JAPHETH
MESHACH
MISHNAH
POOHBAH
SHHHHHH
SKYHIGH
TOOHIGH

••••HH•
HEIGHHO
SHHHHHH

••••H•H
SHHHHHH

•••••HH
SHHHHHH

HI•••••
HIALEAH
HIBACHI
HIBBING
HIBBLER
HIBERNO
HICCUPS
HICKEYS
HICKMAN
HICKORY
HIDABLE
HIDALGO
HIDAWAY
HIDEOUS
HIDEOUT
HIDINGS
HIGGINS
HIGGLED
HIGGLER
HIGGLES
HIGHART
HIGHBAR
HIGHBOY
HIGHDAY
HIGHEND
HIGHEST
HIGHHAT
HIGHIQS
HIGHISH
HIGHLOW
HIGHPAY
HIGHRES
HIGHSEA
HIGHTEA
HIGHTOP
HIGHWAY
HIJACKS
HIJINKS
HIJKLMN
HIKEDUP
HIKEOUT
HIKESUP
HILAIRE
HILBERT
HILLARY
HILLIER
HILLING
HILLMAN
HILLMEN
HILLOCK
HILLTOP
HILTING
HILTONS
HIMALIA
HIMSELF
HINDERS
HINDLEG
HINDPAW
HINGEON
HINGING
HINKIER
HINNIES
HINTERS
HINTING
HINTSAT
HIPBATH
HIPBONE
HIPBOOT
HIPLESS
HIPLIKE
HIPNESS
HIPPEST
HIPPIER
HIPPIES
HIPPISH
HIPPITY
HIPROOF
HIPSTER
HIRABLE
HIRCINE
HIREDON
HIREOUT
HIRESON
HIRSUTE
HISNIBS
HISPANO
HISPEED
HISSERS
HISSIER
HISSING
HISTORY
HITACHI
HITBACK
HITCHED
HITCHER
HITCHES
HITCHON
HITCHUP
HITFILM
HITHERE
HITHOME
HITINTO
HITLESS
HITLIST
HITPLAY
HITSFOR
HITSHOW
HITSOFF
HITSONG
HITSOUT
HITTERS
HITTING
HITTITE
HITTOWN
HITTUNE
HITUPON
HIVEOFF

H•I••••
HAIKAIS
HAILERS
HAILING
HAIMISH
HAIRCUT
HAIRDOS
HAIRDYE
HAIRGEL
HAIRIER
HAIRNET
HAIRPIN
HAITIAN
HEIFERS
HEIFETZ
HEIGHHO
HEIGHTS
HEINOUS
HEIRDOM
HEIRESS
HEISMAN
HEISTED
HOISTED
HOISTER
HOISTUP

H••I•••
HABILIS
HABITAT
HABITED
HABITUE
HALIBUT
HALIDES
HALIFAX
HALITES
HAMITES
HAMITIC
HAMITUP
HARICOT
HASIDIC
HASIDIM
HAYINGS
HAZIEST
HAZINGS
HEDISON
HEGIRAS
HELICAL
HELICES
HELICON
HELIPAD
HELIXES
HERITOR
HIDINGS
HIJINKS
HITINTO
HOKIEST
HOLIDAY
HOLIEST
HOLISTS
HOMIEST
HOMINID
HONIARA
HOPINTO
HORIZON
HOSIERS
HOSIERY
HOTITEM
HUMIDEX
HUMIDLY
HUMIDOR
HYGIEIA
HYGIENE
HYGINUS

H•••I••
HACKIES
HACKING
HADFITS
HADRIAN
HADTIME
HAFNIUM
HAFTING
HAGGISH
HAGLIKE
HAHNIUM
HAILING
HAIMISH
HAIRIER
HAITIAN
HALFIES
HALOIDS
HALOING
HALTING
HALVING
HAMLINE
HAMMIER
HAMMILY
HAMMING
HANDIER
HANDILY
HANDING
HANGING
HANKIBA
HANKIES
HAPKIDO
HAPPIER
HAPPIFY
HAPPILY
HAPTICS
HARDIER
HARDILY
HARDING
HARDISH
HARKING
HARLINE
HARMING
HARNICK
HARPIES
HARPING
HARPIST
HARRIED
HARRIER
HARRIES
HARRIET
HASFITS
HASHING
HASHISH
HASPING
HASSIUM
HASTIER
HASTILY
HASTIME
HASTING
HATLIKE
HATPINS
HATSIZE
HATTING
HAULING
HAWKING
HAWKINS
HAWKISH
HAYRICK
HAYRIDE
HAYWIRE
HAZLITT
HEADIER
HEADILY
HEADING
HEALING
HEAPING
HEARING
HEATING
HEAVIER
HEAVIES
HEAVILY
HEAVING
HEDGIER
HEDGING
HEEDING
HEELING
HEFTIER
HEFTILY
HEFTING
HELLION
HELLISH
HELMING
HELOISE
HELPING
HELSING
HEMLINE
HEMMING
HEMPIER
HENBITS
HENLIKE
HENNISH
HENRICH
HENRIES
HERBIER
HERDING
HEREIAM
HERMITS
HERNIAE
HERNIAS
HERNIBS
HEROICS
HEROINE
HEROISM
HERRICK
HERRING
HERRIOT
HESSIAN
HEURIGE
HEXSIGN
HIBBING
HIGGINS
HIGHIQS
HIGHISH
HILAIRE
HILLIER
HILLING
HILTING
HINGING
HINKIER
HINNIES
HINTING
HIPLIKE
HIPPIER
HIPPIES
HIPPISH
HIPPITY
HIRCINE
HISNIBS
HISSIER
HISSING
HITFILM
HITLIST
HITTING
HITTITE
HJHEINZ
HOAGIES
HOARIER
HOARILY
HOAXING
HOBBIES
HOBBITS
HOBOING
HOBOISM
HOCKING
HODDING
HOGGING
HOGGISH
HOGLIKE
HOGTIED
HOGTIES
HOGWILD
HOLDING
HOLLIES
HOLMIUM
HOMEICE
HOMEIER
HONKING
HOODIES
HOODING
HOOFING
HOOKING
HOOPING
HOOSIER
HOOTING
HOPKINS
HOPLITE
HOPPIER
HOPPING
HOPSING
HORDING
HORNIER
HORNING
HORNISH
HORNIST
HORRIFY
HORSIER
HORSILY
HORSING
HORVITZ
HOSKINS
HOSPICE
HOSTILE
HOSTING
HOTLICK
HOTLINE
HOTLINK
HOTLIPS
HOTMILK
HOTPINK
HOTTIES
HOTTIME
HOTTIPS
HOTWIRE
HOUDINI
HOUSING
HOWHIGH
HOWLING
HOWNICE
HUBBIES
HUFFIER
HUFFILY
HUFFING
HUFFISH
HUGGIES
HUGGING
HUGGINS
HULKIER
HULKING
HULLING
HUMMING
HUMPIER
HUNKIER
HUNLIKE
HUNNISH
HUNTING
HURLING
HURRIED
HURRIER
HURRIES
HURTING
HUSHING
HUSKIER
HUSKIES
HUSKILY
HUSKING
HUSSIES
HUSSITE
HUTLIKE
HUTTING
HYALITE
HYBRIDS
HYDRIDE
HYMNING
HYPOING

H••••I•
HABILIS
HACKSIT
HADAFIT
HADANIP
HADATIT
HAIKAIS
HAIRPIN
HALFWIT
HAMELIN
HAMITIC
HANDLIN
HANDSIN
HANGSIN
HAPLOID
HARDHIT
HARDSIX
HASAFIT
HASANIP
HASATIT
HASIDIC
HASIDIM
HATBRIM
HATEDIT
HATESIT
HAULSIN
HAZANIM
HEADPIN
HEADSIN
HEBRAIC
HEDONIC
HELPSIN
HEMATIC
HEMATIN
HENDRIX
HENREID
HENRYII
HENRYIV
HEPARIN
HEPATIC
HEREDIA
HERETIC
HEXADIC
HIMALIA
HOBNAIL
HOLBEIN
HOLDSIN
HOLDSIT
HOLYOIL
HOMEDIN
HOMERIC
HOMESIN
HOMINID
HONEDIN
HONESIN
HOOFSIT
HOPTOIT
HORATIO
HORNSIN
HOTMAIL
HOWBEIT
HRYVNIA
HUSSEIN
HYALOID
HYANNIS
HYGIEIA
HYPATIA
HYPNOID

H•••••I
HAMACHI
HAROLDI
HAVARTI
HENRYII
HENRYVI
HERNANI
HIBACHI
HITACHI
HOUDINI
HUANGTI
HYUNDAI

•HI••••
CHIANTI
CHIAPAS
CHIAPET
CHICAGO
CHICANA
CHICANE
CHICANO
CHICEST
CHICHAS
CHICHEN
CHICHIS
CHICKEN
CHICLES
CHICLET
CHICORY
CHIDDEN
CHIDERS
CHIDING
CHIEFLY
CHIFFON
CHIGGER
CHIGNON
CHIGOES
CHILCAT
CHILEAN
CHILIAD
CHILIES
CHILKAT
CHILLED
CHILLER
CHILLIS
CHILLUM
CHIMEIN
CHIMERA
CHIMERS
CHIMING
CHIMINH
CHIMNEY
CHINESE
CHINKED
CHINNED
CHINOIS
CHINOOK
CHINTZY
CHINUPS
CHINWAG
CHIPPED
CHIPPER
CHIPSIN
CHIPSUP
CHIRICO
CHIRPED
CHIRPER
CHIRRED
CHIRRUP
CHISELS
CHITLIN
CHITONS
CHITOWN
CHITTER
CHIVIED
CHIVIES
GHIJKLM
OHIOANS
OHIOART
PHIDIAS
PHILBIN
PHILCOS
PHILEAS
PHILIPK
PHILIPS
PHILIPV
PHILLIE
PHILLIP
PHILOUS
PHILTER
PHILTRE
PHINEAS
PHISHED
PHISHER
PHISHES
RHIZOME
SHIATSU
SHIELDS
SHIFTED
SHIFTER
SHIHTZU
SHIITES
SHIKOKU
SHILLED
SHIMMER
SHINDIG
SHINEON
SHINERS
SHINEUP
SHINGLE
SHINGLY
SHINIER
SHINILY
SHINING
SHINNED
SHINOLA
SHINPAD
SHIPFUL
SHIPMAN
SHIPMEN
SHIPOUT
SHIPPED
SHIPPER
SHIPWAY
SHIRKED
SHIRKER
SHIRLEY
SHIRRED
SHIVERS
SHIVERY
THIAMIN
THICKEN
THICKER
THICKET
THICKLY
THIERRY
THIEVED
THIEVES
THIGPEN
THIMBLE
THIMPHU
THINAIR
THINICE
THINKER
THINKOF
THINKSO
THINKUP
THINMAN
THINNED
THINNER
THINOUT
THIRDLY
THIRSTS
THIRSTY

THISDAY
THISONE
THISTLE
THISTLY
THISWAY
THITHER
WHIFFED
WHIFFER
WHIFFLE
WHILING
WHIMPER
WHINERS
WHINIER
WHINING
WHIPPED
WHIPPER
WHIPPET
WHIPPLE
WHIPSAW
WHIPSIN
WHIPSUP
WHIRLED
WHIRLER
WHIRRED
WHISHED
WHISHES
WHISKAS
WHISKED
WHISKER
WHISKEY
WHISPER
WHISTLE
WHITELY
WHITENS
WHITEST
WHITHER
WHITING
WHITISH
WHITMAN
WHITNEY
WHITSUN
WHITTLE
WHIZKID
WHIZZED
WHIZZER
WHIZZES
ZHIVAGO

•H•I•••

CHAINED
CHAINES
CHAINUP
CHAIRED
CHAISES
CHOICER
CHOICES
CHOIRED
CHRISMS
CHRISOM
CHRISTA
CHRISTI
CHRISTO
CHRISTY
SHEIKHS
SHEILAE
SHEILAS
SHIITES
SHRIEKS
SHRIKES
SHRILLS
SHRILLY
SHRIMPS
SHRIMPY
SHRINED
SHRINER
SHRINES
SHRINKS
SHRIVEL
SHRIVER
SHRIVES
SHTICKS
SHTICKY
THEIDEA
THEISMS
THEISTS
THRIFTS
THRIFTY
THRILLA
THRILLS
THRIVED
THRIVEN
THRIVER
THRIVES
WHOISIT
WHYISIT

•H••I••

CHAFING
CHALICE
CHARIER
CHARILY
CHARING
CHARIOT
CHARITY
CHASING
CHAWING
CHEFING
CHEMISE
CHEMIST
CHENIER
CHERISH
CHEVIOT
CHEWIER
CHEWING
CHIDING
CHILIAD
CHILIES
CHIMING
CHIMINH
CHIRICO
CHIVIED
CHIVIES
CHOKIER
CHOKING
CHOLINE
CHOPINE
CHORINE
CHORIST
CHORIZO
CHOWING
CHUTING
CHUTIST
EHRLICH
GHANIAN
KHEDIVE
PHASING
PHEMIUS
PHIDIAS
PHILIPK
PHILIPS
PHILIPV
PHOBIAS
PHOBICS
PHONICS
PHONIER
PHONIES
PHONILY
PHONING
PHOTICS
PHYSICS
RHENISH
RHENIUM
RHODIAN
RHODIUM
RHYMING
RHYMIST
SHADIER
SHADILY
SHADING
SHAKIER
SHAKILY
SHAKING
SHAKIRA
SHALIER
SHAMING
SHAPING
SHAPIRO
SHARING
SHAVIAN
SHAVING
SHERIFF
SHERIFS
SHINIER
SHINILY
SHINING
SHOEING
SHOOING
SHOOINS
SHORING
SHOVING
SHOWIER
SHOWILY
SHOWING
SHUTINS
THAWING
THEBIGA
THECITY
THEDIET
THEFIRM
THEFIVE
THEGIFT
THEHILL
THEKING
THEKISS
THELIKE
THEMICK
THENILE
THEPIPS
THEPITS
THERIAC
THERING
THERINK
THERITZ
THESIMS
THEVIEW
THEVIPS
THEWIND
THEYIPS
THINICE
THORIUM
THULIUM
THWHITE
THYMINE
WHALING
WHATIFS
WHEYISH
WHILING
WHINIER
WHINING
WHITING
WHITISH

•H•••I•

CHABLIS
CHAGRIN
CHALCIS
CHAMOIS
CHAOTIC
CHAPLIN
CHAPPIE
CHARLIE
CHARMIN
CHARNIN
CHASMIC
CHASSIS
CHATWIN
CHEAPIE
CHEATIN
CHECKIN
CHEERIO
CHEEZIT
CHERVIL
CHEXMIX
CHICHIS
CHILLIS
CHIMEIN
CHINOIS
CHIPSIN
CHITLIN
CHLORIC
CHROMIC
CHRONIC
CHUCKIT
DHARMIC
DHURRIE
GHERKIN
IHATEIT
IHAVEIT
PHASEIN
PHILBIN
PHILLIE
PHILLIP
PHOENIX
PHONEIN
PHOTOID
PHRENIC
PHRYGIA
PHYLLIS
RHEUMIC
RHOMBIC
SHAREIN
SHARPIE
SHELTIE
SHERWIN
SHINDIG
SHOOSIN
SHORTIE
SHOVEIN
SHOWBIZ
SHOWNIN
SHOWSIN
SHUTSIN
THANDIE
THATSIT
THEAXIS
THEREIN
THERMIC
THESPIS
THETRIB
THIAMIN
THINAIR
THREWIN
THROWIN
THYROID
WHATSIS
WHATSIT
WHEELIE
WHEELIN
WHEREIN
WHIPSIN
WHIZKID
WHOISIT
WHOOPIE
WHOOSIS
WHOSAID
WHYISIT
WHYWAIT

•H••••I

BHUTANI
CHAPATI
CHEZMOI
CHIANTI
CHRISTI
KHATAMI
SHANGRI
SHARPEI
SHASTRI
SHOULDI
THEMAGI
THEOMNI
WHATAMI

••HI•••

ACHIEST
ACHIEVA
ACHIEVE
ACHILLE
ADHIBIT
APHIDES
APHILIP
ASHIEST
ASHIVER
ATHIRST
BAHIANS
BEHINDS
CAHIERS
DEHIRED
DEHIRES
DEHISCE
ECHIDNA
ETHICAL
EXHIBIT
FGHIJKL
INHIBIT
ITHIRTY
LEHIGHU
MOHICAN
OXHIDES
REHIDES
REHINGE
REHIRED
REHIRES
REHITCH
SCHICKS
SCHIRRA
SCHISMS
SCHISTS
TAHINIS
TSHIRTS
UNHILLY
UNHINGE
UNHIRED
UNHIRES
UNHITCH
UPHILLS
VEHICLE
WAHINES

••H•I••

ASHBINS
ASHPITS
ATHEISM
ATHEIST
ATHRILL
BAHAISM
BAHAIST
BEHRING
BOHRIUM
COHEIRS
DAHLIAS
DEHAIRS
ECHOING
ECHOISM
ETHNICS
HAHNIUM
HJHEINZ
ICHDIEN
JOHNIII
LAHAINA
MAHDISM
MAHDIST
MOHAIRS
SCHLITZ
SCHMIDT
SCHMITT
SCHTICK
SCHWINN
UNHAIRS
UNHAIRY

••H••I•

ADHIBIT
AMHARIC
APHAGIA
APHAGIC
APHASIA
APHASIC
APHELIA
APHILIP
APHONIA
APHONIC
BAHRAIN
BAHREIN
BOHEMIA
CAHOKIA
COHABIT
EPHRAIM
ETHERIC
ETHMOID
EXHIBIT
INHABIT
INHERIT
INHIBIT
JOHNIII
JOHNNIE
JOHNVII
JOHNXII
JOHNXIV
JOHNXIX
LCHAYIM
MAHALIA
MAHARIS
OCHROID
OGHAMIC
OPHELIA
SPHERIC
TAHINIS
UNHUMID
USHERIN

••H•••I

ASHANTI
JOHNIII
JOHNVII
JOHNXII
JOHNXVI
JOHNXXI
PAHLAVI
SCHERZI
SOHAVEI

•••HI••

ACEHIGH
AIMHIGH
AKIHITO
ALTHING
AMPHION
ANTHILL
ARCHIES
ARCHING
ARCHIVE
ARSHILE
ATTHIRD
BACHING
BASHING
BATHING
BEEHIVE
BETHINK
BIGHITS
BOOHISS
BUSHIDO
BUSHIER
BUSHILY
BUSHING
CACHING
CASHIER
CASHING
CASHINS
COCHISE
COSHING
COWHIDE
CUSHIER
CUSHILY
CUSHING
CUSHION
DASHIER
DASHIKI
DASHING
DISHIER
DISHING
DUCHIES
EBWHITE
EFGHIJK
ETCHING
FASHION
FISHIER
FISHILY
FISHING
FLYHIGH
FORHIRE
GASHING
GOTHICS
GOTHIKA
GUSHIER
GUSHILY
GUSHING
HASHING
HASHISH
HIGHIQS
HIGHISH
HOWHIGH
HUSHING
INCHING
INTHING
INTHIRD
INWHITE
ISCHIAL
ISCHIUM
ITCHIER
ITCHING
JOEHILL
JOSHING
KACHINA
KACHING
KOSHIBA
LASHING
LATHING
LITHIUM
LOTHIAN
LUCHINO
LUSHIER
LUTHIER
MACHINA
MACHINE
MASHIES
MASHING
MATHIAS
MATHIEU
MESHIER
MESHING
MISHIMA
MISHITS
MOSHING
MOTHIER
MRCHIPS
MUSHIER
MUSHILY
MUSHING
MYTHIFY
NEWHIRE
NICHING
NOBHILL
NONHITS
NOSHING
NOTHING
NOTHINS
ORCHIDS
OUTHIRE
OUTHISS
OUTHITS
PACHISI
PISHING
PITHIER
PITHILY
PITHING
PUSHIER
PUSHILY
PUSHING
PYTHIAN
PYTHIAS
RASHIDA
RAWHIDE
RESHIFT
RESHINE
RESHIPS
RETHINK
ROTHIRA
RUCHING
RUSHIER
RUSHING
SAMHILL
SASHIMI
SASHING
SAYHITO
SEPHIAS
SIGHING
SIKHISM
SKYHIGH
SOPHIES
SOPHISM
SOPHIST
SWAHILI
TAXHIKE
TECHIES
THEHILL
THWHITE
TITHING
TOOHIGH
TOSHIBA
TOSHIRO
TUSHIES
UNSHIER
UNSHIFT
UNSHINY
UNSHIPS
UNTHICK
UNTHINK
UNWHIPT
UNWHITE
UPSHIFT
UPWHIRL
URCHINS
WASHIER
WASHING
WICHITA
WISHING
WITHIES
YASHICA
YESHIVA

•••H•I•

ALLHAIL
ALSHAIN
ANAHEIM
ANTHEIL
ARCHAIC
BADHAIR
BATHOIL
BIGHAIR
BOTHNIA
BRAHMIN
BUSHPIG
BYAHAIR
CATHAIR
CICHLID
COCHAIR
DAPHNIA
DAPHNIS
DOGHAIR
ENCHAIN
FISHOIL
FUCHSIA
GUTHRIE
KASHMIR
LITHOID
LOTHAIR
MACHSIX
MANHEIM
MECHLIN
MIKHAIL
MOCHRIE
MOSHPIT
NEPHRIC
NIGHTIE
PETHAIR
PUSHKIN
PUSHPIN
REDHAIR
RUSHDIE
SECHZIG
TASHLIN
TOAHAIR
TYPHOID
UNCHAIN
UNCHAIR
XIPHOID
YACHTIE

•••H••I

AFGHANI
DASHIKI
LUTHULI
PACHISI
SASHIMI
SWAHILI

••••HI•

AIRSHIP
ALLTHIS
AWASHIN
BACCHIC
BASEHIT
BASRHIN
BIOCHIP
BOOTHIA
CHICHIS
COLCHIS
CYNTHIA
DAUPHIN
DEFGHIJ
DELPHIC
DOLPHIN
GEEWHIZ
GENGHIS
GETAHIT
GETSHIP
GETTHIS
GLYPHIC
GOTAHIT
GRAPHIC
GUNSHIP
HARDHIT
ITSAHIT
JOACHIM
KINSHIP
LAUGHIN
LEFTHIP
LITCHIS
MEGAHIT
MEMPHIS
MENUHIN
MIDSHIP
MISSHIP
MORPHIC
MORPHIN
MUNCHIE
MYRRHIC
NOWTHIS
NUNSHIP
NYMPHIC
ONAWHIM
ONECHIP
ONEWHIT
PERAHIA
PERCHIK
PITCHIN
POOCHIE
PRESHIP
PREWHIP
PSYCHIC
PUNCHIN
PYRRHIC
RALPHIE
REACHIN
REDCHIP
RITCHIE
ROSEHIP
ROUGHIT
SONSHIP
SYLPHIC
TEACHIN
TOPTHIS
TOUGHIE
VERYHIP
WARSHIP
WATCHIT
WEIGHIN
WELLHID
WELLHIT
WORSHIP
WORTHIT
XANTHIC

••••H•I

AMICHAI
BALIHAI
BOLSHOI
LAKSHMI

•••••HI

ACANTHI
ADELPHI
BELUSHI
BIANCHI
BRONCHI
CDEFGHI
FRANCHI
FRENCHI
GNOCCHI
HAMACHI
HIBACHI
HITACHI
JOSEPHI
KARACHI
KENICHI
MALACHI
MIZRAHI
NOGUCHI
SAATCHI
SCACCHI

HJ•••••

HJALMAR
HJHEINZ

H•J••••

HIJACKS
HIJINKS
HIJKLMN

H••J•••

HEYJUDE

H•••J••

HADAJOB
HOLYJOE

H•••••J

HEYMRDJ

•H•J•••

GHIJKLM
THEJERK
THEJETS

••H•J••

FGHIJKL
JOHNJAY

•••H•J•

EFGHIJK

••••H•J

DEFGHIJ

H•K••••

HIKEDUP
HIKEOUT
HIKESUP
HOKIEST

H••K•••

HACKERS
HACKETT
HACKIES
HACKING
HACKLED
HACKLER
HACKLES
HACKMAN
HACKNEY
HACKOFF
HACKSAW
HACKSIT
HACKSUP
HAIKAIS
HANKERS
HANKIBA
HANKIES
HAPKIDO
HARKENS
HARKING
HASKELL
HAWKERS
HAWKEYE
HAWKING
HAWKINS
HAWKISH
HAWKMAN
HECKART
HECKLED
HECKLER
HECKLES
HECKMAN
HECKUVA
HECKYES
HICKEYS
HICKMAN
HICKORY
HIJKLMN
HINKIER
HOCKERS
HOCKING
HONKERS
HONKING
HONKSAT
HOOKAHS
HOOKING
HOOKSON
HOOKSUP
HOOKUPS
HOPKINS
HOSKINS
HOTKEYS
HULKIER
HULKING
HUNKERS
HUNKIER
HUSKERS
HUSKIER
HUSKIES
HUSKILY
HUSKING

H•••K••
HAECKEL
HANUKAH
HEARKEN
HOBOKEN

H••••K•
HAGLIKE
HATLIKE
HENLIKE
HIJACKS
HIJINKS
HIPLIKE
HOECAKE
HOGLIKE
HOLYOKE
HOTCAKE
HUNLIKE
HUTLIKE

H•••••K
HADDOCK
HAMHOCK
HAMMOCK
HANCOCK
HARNICK
HARTACK
HASSOCK
HATRACK
HAYFORK
HAYRACK
HAYRICK
HEMLOCK
HENPECK
HERRICK
HEYLOOK
HILLOCK
HITBACK
HOGBACK
HOLMOAK
HOLYARK
HOTLICK
HOTLINK
HOTMILK
HOTPACK
HOTPINK
HOWARDK

•H•K•••
CHAKRAS
CHEKHOV
CHOKEON
CHOKERS
CHOKEUP
CHOKIER
CHOKING
CHUKKER
SHAKERS
SHAKEUP
SHAKIER
SHAKILY
SHAKING
SHAKIRA
SHAKOES
SHEKELS
SHIKOKU
THEKING
THEKISS
WHOKNEW

•H••K••
CHALKED
CHALKUP
CHECKED
CHECKER
CHECKIN
CHECKON
CHECKUP
CHEEKED
CHICKEN
CHILKAT
CHINKED
CHOCKED
CHUCKED
CHUCKIT
CHUCKLE
CHUKKER
CHUNKED
GHERKIN
GHIJKLM
KHARKOV
SHACKED
SHACKLE
SHANKAR
SHANKED
SHARKEY
SHEIKHS
SHIRKED
SHIRKER
SHOCKED
SHOCKER
SHOOKUP
SHOPKOS
SHRIKES
SHUCKED
SHUCKER
THANKED
THANKER
THICKEN
THICKER
THICKET
THICKLY
THINKER
THINKOF
THINKSO
THINKUP
THUNKED
WHACKED
WHACKER
WHISKAS
WHISKED
WHISKER
WHISKEY
WHIZKID

•H•••K•
CHACHKA
CHOMSKY
RHEBOKS
SHIKOKU
SHLOCKY
SHNOOKS
SHRIEKS
SHRINKS
SHTICKS
SHTICKY
THEDUKE
THELIKE
THWACKS

•H••••K
CHARPAK
CHINOOK
PHILIPK
SHYLOCK
THATSOK
THEHULK
THEJERK
THELARK
THELOOK
THEMASK
THEMICK
THERINK
THEROCK
THESACK

••HK•••
OSHKOSH

••H•K••
CAHOKIA

••H••K•
ASHCAKE
FGHIJKL
MOHAWKS
REHOOKS
SCHICKS
UNHOOKS
UNHUSKS

••H•••K
OKHOTSK
SCHLOCK
SCHNOOK
SCHTICK

•••HK••
BISHKEK
KISHKES
PUSHKIN

•••H•K•
DASHIKI
GOTHIKA
TAXHIKE
UNCHOKE

•••H••K
BETHINK
BISHKEK
EFGHIJK
EYEHOOK
FUTHARK
GOSHAWK
HAMHOCK
INCHECK
INSHOCK
POTHOOK
RECHALK
RECHECK
REDHAWK
RETHANK
RETHINK
SEAHAWK
SKYHOOK
THEHULK
UNCHECK
UNTHICK
UNTHINK
WARHAWK
YASHMAK

••••HK•
CHACHKA
ROETHKE

••••H•K
KAISHEK
PERCHIK
SAWCHUK
YITZHAK

H•L••••
HALALAS
HALAVAH
HALCYON
HALDANE
HALFBAD
HALFCUT
HALFDAY
HALFDUG
HALFFED
HALFIES
HALFMAD
HALFRAW
HALFROD
HALFSHY
HALFWAY
HALFWIT
HALFWON
HALIBUT
HALIDES
HALIFAX
HALITES
HALLEYS
HALLOOS
HALLOWS
HALLWAY
HALOGEN
HALOIDS
HALOING
HALSTON
HALTERS
HALTING
HALVAHS
HALVERS
HALVING
HALYARD
HELDOFF
HELDOUT
HELICAL
HELICES
HELICON
HELIPAD
HELIXES
HELLBOY
HELLCAT
HELLENE
HELLENO
HELLION
HELLISH
HELLMAN
HELLOED
HELLOES
HELLUVA
HELLYES
HELMETS
HELMING
HELMOND
HELOISE
HELOTRY
HELPERS
HELPFUL
HELPING
HELPOUT
HELPSIN
HELPSON
HELPSUP
HELSING
HILAIRE
HILBERT
HILLARY
HILLIER
HILLING
HILLMAN
HILLMEN
HILLOCK
HILLTOP
HILTING
HILTONS
HOLBEIN
HOLBERG
HOLDALL
HOLDERS
HOLDING
HOLDOFF
HOLDOUT
HOLDSIN
HOLDSIT
HOLDSON
HOLDSTO
HOLDSUP
HOLDUPS
HOLEDUP
HOLEOUT
HOLESUP
HOLIDAY
HOLIEST
HOLISTS
HOLLAND
HOLLERS
HOLLIES
HOLLOWS
HOLMIUM
HOLMOAK
HOLSTER
HOLYARK
HOLYCOW
HOLYDAY
HOLYJOE
HOLYMAN
HOLYMEN
HOLYOIL
HOLYOKE
HOLYONE
HOLYSEE
HOLYWAR
HOLZMAN
HULKIER
HULKING
HULLERS
HULLING
HULLOED

H••L•••
HAGLIKE
HAILERS
HAILING
HALLEYS
HALLOOS
HALLOWS
HALLWAY
HAMLETS
HAMLINE
HAPLESS
HAPLOID
HARLAND
HARLEYS
HARLINE
HARLOTS
HATLESS
HATLIKE
HAULAGE
HAULERS
HAULING
HAULOFF
HAULSIN
HAULSUP
HAYLOFT
HAZLITT
HEALALL
HEALERS
HEALING
HEALSUP
HEALTHY
HEELERS
HEELING
HEELPAD
HEELTAP
HELLBOY
HELLCAT
HELLENE
HELLENO
HELLION
HELLISH
HELLMAN
HELLOED
HELLOES
HELLUVA
HELLYES
HEMLINE
HEMLOCK
HENLIKE
HEWLETT
HEYLOOK
HIALEAH
HILLARY
HILLIER
HILLING
HILLMAN
HILLMEN
HILLOCK
HILLTOP
HIPLESS
HIPLIKE
HITLESS
HITLIST
HJALMAR
HOGLIKE
HOLLAND
HOLLERS
HOLLIES
HOLLOWS
HOPLITE
HOTLEAD
HOTLICK
HOTLINE
HOTLINK
HOTLIPS
HOVLANE
HOWLAME
HOWLERS
HOWLING
HOWLONG
HOWLSAT
HUELESS
HULLERS
HULLING
HULLOED
HUNLIKE
HURLERS
HURLING
HUTLIKE
HYALITE
HYALOID

H•••L••
HAARLEM
HABILIS
HACKLED
HACKLER
HACKLES
HAGGLED
HAGGLER
HAGGLES
HALALAS
HAMELIN
HAMULUS
HANDLED
HANDLER
HANDLES
HANDLIN
HAROLDI
HARTLEY
HASSLED
HASSLES
HECKLED
HECKLER
HECKLES
HEMSLEY
HENSLEY
HERALDS
HGWELLS
HIBBLER
HIDALGO
HIGGLED
HIGGLER
HIGGLES
HIGHLOW
HIJKLMN
HIMALIA
HINDLEG
HITPLAY
HOBBLED
HOBBLER
HOBBLES
HOMELAB
HONALEE
HOODLUM
HOOPLAS
HORSLEY
HOSTLER
HOTGLUE
HOWELLS
HOWELSE
HUDDLED
HUDDLER
HUDDLES
HUMBLED
HUMBLER
HUMBLES
HUNTLEY
HURDLED
HURDLER
HURDLES
HURTLED
HURTLES
HUSTLED
HUSTLER
HUSTLES
HYGELAC

H••••L•
HADPULL
HAMMILY
HANDILY
HANSOLO
HAPPILY
HARDILY
HARROLD
HARSHLY
HARWELL
HASKELL
HASPULL
HASTILY
HATABLE
HATFULS
HAYBALE
HEADILY
HEALALL
HEAVILY
HEFTILY
HERBALS
HERCULE
HERSELF
HGWELLS
HIDABLE
HIMSELF
HIRABLE
HITFILM
HOARILY
HOGCALL
HOGWILD
HOLDALL
HORSILY
HOSCALE
HOSTELS
HOSTILE
HOTMILK
HOTROLL
HOWDULL
HOWELLS
HUBBELL
HUFFILY
HUMANLY
HUMIDLY
HUMMELS
HUSKILY
HYMNALS

H•••••L
HADPULL
HAECKEL
HAIRGEL
HANDFUL
HANDSEL
HARMFUL
HARWELL
HASKELL
HASPULL
HATEFUL
HEADFUL
HEALALL
HEATFUL
HEEDFUL
HELICAL
HELPFUL
HOBNAIL
HOGCALL
HOLDALL
HOLYOIL
HOOTOWL
HOPEFUL
HOTCOAL
HOTMAIL
HOTMEAL
HOTROLL
HOWDULL
HRETHEL
HUBBELL
HUMERAL
HUMORAL
HURTFUL
HUSHFUL
HUSSERL

•HL••••
CHLORIC
NHLGAME
NHLTEAM
PHLEGMY
PHLOEMS
PHLOXES
SHLOCKY

•H•L•••
CHALCIS
CHALETS
CHALICE
CHALKED
CHALKUP
CHALLAH
CHALONS
CHALUPA
CHELATE
CHELSEA
CHILCAT
CHILEAN
CHILIAD
CHILIES
CHILKAT
CHILLED
CHILLER
CHILLIS
CHILLUM
CHOLERA
CHOLERS
CHOLINE
CHOLLAS
EHRLICH
FHALOAN
PHALANX
PHILBIN
PHILCOS
PHILEAS
PHILIPK
PHILIPS
PHILIPV
PHILLIE
PHILLIP
PHILOUS
PHILTER
PHILTRE
PHYLLIS
PHYLLOS
SHALALA
SHALIER
SHALLOT
SHALLOW
SHALLWE
SHALOMS
SHELDON
SHELLAC
SHELLED
SHELLER
SHELLEY
SHELTER
SHELTIE
SHELVED
SHELVER
SHELVES
SHILLED
SHULMAN
SHYLOCK
THALERS
THELAMB
THELARK
THELEFT
THELIKE
THELOOK
THELOOP
THULIUM
WHALERS
WHALING
WHALLEY
WHELMED
WHELPED
WHILING

•H••L••
CHABLIS
CHALLAH
CHAPLET
CHAPLIN
CHARLES
CHARLEY
CHARLIE
CHEMLAB
CHICLES
CHICLET
CHILLED
CHILLER
CHILLIS
CHILLUM
CHITLIN
CHOLLAS
OHANLON
OHMSLAW
PHARLAP
PHILLIE
PHILLIP
PHYLLIS
PHYLLOS
SHALLOT
SHALLOW
SHALLWE
SHAWLED
SHEILAE
SHEILAS
SHELLAC
SHELLED
SHELLER
SHELLEY
SHIELDS
SHILLED
SHIRLEY
SHOALED
SHOULDA
SHOULDI
SHRILLS
SHRILLY
THEALPS
THEBLOB
THEFLEA
THEFLOP
THRALLS
THRILLA
THRILLS
WHALLEY
WHEELED
WHEELER
WHEELIE
WHEELIN
WHIRLED
WHIRLER
WHORLED

•H•••L•
AHASSLE
CHAGALL
CHANELS
CHAPALA
CHAPELS
CHARILY
CHEADLE
CHEAPLY
CHIEFLY
CHISELS
CHORALE
CHORALS
CHORTLE
CHUCKLE
GHASTLY
GHIJKLM
GHOSTLY
PHENOLS
PHONILY
SHACKLE
SHADILY
SHAKILY
SHALALA
SHAMBLE
SHAPELY
SHARPLY
SHEERLY
SHEKELS
SHEWOLF
SHINGLE
SHINGLY
SHINILY
SHINOLA
SHOOFLY
SHORTLY
SHOVELS
SHOWILY
SHRILLS
SHRILLY
SHTETLS
SHUFFLE
SHUTTLE
THEBELL
THEDELL
THEDOLE
THEFALL
THEGOLD
THEHELP
THEHILL
THEHULK
THEMALL
THENILE
THERULE
THESELF
THEWALL
THICKLY
THIMBLE
THIRDLY
THISTLE
THISTLY
THRALLS
THRILLA
THRILLS
THYSELF
WHEEDLE
WHERELL
WHIFFLE
WHIPPLE
WHISTLE
WHITELY
WHITTLE

•H••••L
CHAGALL
CHANCEL
CHANNEL
CHASMAL
CHATTEL
CHERVIL
CHORDAL
CHUNNEL
OHCAROL
PHRASAL
SHIPFUL
SHOPFUL
SHRIVEL
THEBELL
THEDELL
THEFALL
THEFOOL
THEHILL
THEMALL
THERMAL
THEWALL
WHERELL

••HL•••
ASHLAND
ASHLARS
ASHLESS
ATHLETE
DAHLIAS
OOHLALA
PAHLAVI
SCHLEPP
SCHLEPS
SCHLITZ
SCHLOCK
SCHLUBS
SCHLUMP

••H•L••
ACHILLE
APHELIA
APHILIP
BEHOLDS
ECHELON
EXHALED
EXHALES
INHALED
INHALER
INHALES
JOHNLAW
JOHNLEE
MAHALIA
MCHALES
MRHULOT
OPHELIA
OTHELLO
SCHELDT
SCHOLAR
SCHOLES
SCHULTZ
TOHELEN
UNHELMS
UNHILLY
UNHULLS
UPHILLS
UPHOLDS

••H••L•
ACHILLE
ATHRILL
DEHMELT
OOHLALA
OTHELLO
REHAULS
REHEALS
REHEELS
SCHOOLS
UNHILLY
UNHULLS
UPHILLS
VEHICLE

••H•••L
ATHRILL
DUHAMEL
ETHANOL
ETHICAL
FGHIJKL
ISHMAEL
NAHUATL
SPHERAL

•••HL••
CICHLID
COCHLEA
COGHLAN
HIGHLOW
KOEHLER
MECHLIN
RICHLER
TASHLIN

•••H•L•
AIRHOLE
ANTHILL
ARMHOLE
ARSHILE
ASPHALT
BETHELS
BIGHALF
BOGHOLE
BUSHELS
BUSHILY
CEPHALO
CEPHALY
CUSHILY
DESHELL
DRYHOLE
EARHOLE
EYEHOLE
FISHILY
FOXHOLE
GETHELP
GOTHELP
GUSHILY
IANHOLM
ICEHOLE
INAHOLE
ISOHELS
JOEHILL
JONHALL
KEYHOLE
LIGHTLY
LITHELY
LUTHULI
MANHOLE
MUDHOLE
MUSHILY
NICHOLS
NIGHTLY
NOBHILL
OMPHALO
ONEHALF
PIEHOLE
PINHOLE
PITHILY
POTHOLE
PUSHILY
RATHOLE
RECHALK
RECHALL
RIGHTLY
SAMHILL
SIGHTLY
SPYHOLE
SUBHALL
SWAHILI
THEHELP
THEHILL
THEHULK
TIGHTLY
TIMHOLT
TOEHOLD
TOPHOLE
UNSHELL
UNSHYLY
UNWHOLE
VFWHALL
WILHELM

•••H••L
ALLHAIL
ALLHEAL
ANTHEIL
ANTHILL
BASHFUL
BATHOIL
BSCHOOL
DESHELL
DISHFUL
ENTHRAL
FISHOIL
HUSHFUL
ISCHIAL
JOEHILL
JONHALL
LOWHEEL
MICHAEL
MIKHAIL
NOBHILL
ONTHEDL
OUTHAUL
OUTHOWL
OUTHURL
PREHEAL
PUSHFUL
QSCHOOL
RACHAEL
RAPHAEL
RECHALL
RUTHFUL
SAMHILL
SIGHFUL
SUBHALL
TARHEEL
THEHILL
UNSHELL
UNWHEEL
UPWHIRL
VFWHALL
WISHFUL

••••HL•
APISHLY
BRASHLY
DASCHLE
EARTHLY
FIFTHLY
FLESHLY
FRESHLY
HARSHLY
LOATHLY
MONTHLY
NINTHLY
PLUSHLY
ROUGHLY
SIXTHLY
TENTHLY
TOUGHLY

••••H•L
ALCOHOL
EPOCHAL
GASOHOL
HRETHEL
MARSHAL
MENTHOL
NARWHAL
NYMPHAL
PASCHAL
SATCHEL

•••••HL
KENWAHL

H•M••••
HAMACHI
HAMBONE
HAMBURG
HAMELIN
HAMHOCK
HAMITES
HAMITIC
HAMITUP
HAMLETS
HAMLINE
HAMMERS
HAMMETT
HAMMIER
HAMMILY
HAMMING
HAMMOCK
HAMMOND
HAMPERS
HAMPTON
HAMSTER
HAMULUS
HEMATIC
HEMATIN
HEMLINE
HEMLOCK
HEMMERS
HEMMING
HEMPIER
HEMSLEY
HHMUNRO
HIMALIA
HIMSELF
HOMAGER
HOMAGES
HOMBRES
HOMBURG
HOMEBOY
HOMEDIN
HOMEICE
HOMEIER
HOMELAB
HOMERED
HOMERIC
HOMERUN
HOMESIN
HOMIEST
HOMINID
HOMONYM
HUMANLY
HUMANUM
HUMBARD
HUMBERT
HUMBLED
HUMBLER
HUMBLES
HUMBUGS
HUMDRUM
HUMERAL
HUMERUS
HUMIDEX
HUMIDLY
HUMIDOR
HUMMELS
HUMMERS
HUMMING
HUMORAL
HUMORED
HUMORME
HUMOURS
HUMPHED
HUMPHRY
HUMPIER
HUMUSES
HUMVEES
HYMNALS
HYMNARY
HYMNING
HYMNODY

H••M•••
HAIMISH
HAMMERS
HAMMETT
HAMMIER
HAMMILY
HAMMING
HAMMOCK
HAMMOND
HARMERS
HARMFUL
HARMING
HARMONY
HAYMOWS
HAZMATS
HELMETS
HELMING
HELMOND
HEMMERS
HEMMING
HERMANA
HERMANN
HERMANO
HERMANS
HERMITS
HERMOSA
HERMOSO
HEYMANS
HEYMRDJ
HOFMANN
HOLMIUM
HOLMOAK
HORMONE
HOTMAIL
HOTMEAL
HOTMILK
HOWMANY
HOWMUCH
HUMMELS
HUMMERS
HUMMING

H•••M••
HACKMAN
HALFMAD
HANGMAN
HANGMEN
HARTMAN
HARTMUT
HAWKMAN
HEADMAN
HEADMEN
HECKMAN
HEISMAN
HELLMAN
HICKMAN
HILLMAN
HILLMEN
HJALMAR
HOFFMAN
HOLYMAN
HOLYMEN
HOLZMAN
HOOPMAN
HOOPMEN
HOUSMAN
HUFFMAN

H••••M•
HADSOME
HADTIME
HANSOMS
HASTIME
HIJKLMN
HITHOME
HOTCOMB
HOTTIME
HOWCOME
HOWLAME
HUMORME

H•••••M
HAARLEM
HADROOM
HAFNIUM
HAHNIUM
HASIDIM
HASROOM
HASSIUM
HATBRIM
HAZANIM
HEIRDOM
HEREIAM
HEROISM
HITFILM
HOBOISM
HOLMIUM
HOMONYM
HOODLUM
HOTITEM
HUMANUM
HUMDRUM
HYPONYM

•HM••••
HHMUNRO
OHMAGES
OHMSLAW

•H•M•••
CHAMBER
CHAMBRE
CHAMFER
CHAMOIS
CHAMPED
CHAMPER
CHEMISE
CHEMIST
CHEMLAB
CHIMEIN
CHIMERA
CHIMERS
CHIMING
CHIMINH
CHIMNEY
CHOMPED
CHOMPON
CHOMSKY
CHUMASH
CHUMMED
CHUMPED
PHEMIUS
RHOMBIC
RHOMBUS
RHUMBAS
RHYMERS
RHYMING
RHYMIST
SHAMANS
SHAMBLE
SHAMING
SHAMMED
SHAMPOO
SHIMMER
THEMAGI
THEMALL
THEMASK
THEMAVS
THEMAYO
THEMETS
THEMICK
THEMOON
THEMOST
THIMBLE
THIMPHU
THOMSON
THUMBED
THUMPED
THUMPER
THYMINE
WHAMMED
WHIMPER
WHOMPED

•H••M••
CHAPMAN
CHAPMEN
CHARMAN
CHARMED
CHARMEN
CHARMER
CHARMIN
CHASMAL
CHASMIC
CHEXMIX
CHEZMOI
CHROMAT
CHROMED
CHROMES
CHROMIC
CHUMMED
DHARMAS
DHARMIC
RHEUMIC
SHAMMED
SHERMÀN
SHIMMER
SHIPMAN
SHIPMEN
SHOWMAN
SHOWMEN
SHRIMPS
SHRIMPY
SHULMAN
THEOMEN
THEOMNI
THERMAL
THERMIC
THERMOS
THIAMIN
THINMAN
THURMAN
WHAMMED
WHELMED
WHITMAN

•H•••M•
CHRISMS
KHATAMI
NHLGAME
PHENOMS
PHLEGMY
PHLOEMS
PHONEME
RHIZOME
RHYTHMS
SHALOMS
THEARMY
THEBOMB
THEGAME
THEISMS
THELAMB
THEPUMP
THERAMS
THESAME
THESIMS
WHATAMI

•H••••M
CHATHAM
CHETRUM
CHEWGUM
CHILLUM
CHRISOM
GHIJKLM
KHAYYAM
NHLTEAM
PHANTOM
RHENIUM
RHODIUM
SHAHDOM
SHYFROM
THEFIRM
THEOREM
THEROOM
THORIUM
THREEAM
THREEPM
THULIUM

••HM•••
DEHMELT
ETHMOID
ISHMAEL
LEHMANN
SCHMEAR
SCHMEER
SCHMIDT
SCHMITT
SCHMOES

••H•M••
ASHAMED
ATHOMES
BAHAMAS
BAHAMEN
BEHRMAN
BOHEMIA
DAHOMEY
DUHAMEL
EXHUMED
EXHUMER
EXHUMES
INHUMAN
INHUMED
INHUMER
INHUMES
OGHAMIC
SCHEMAS
SCHEMED
SCHEMER
SCHEMES
SCHUMER
TOHOMER
UNHUMAN
UNHUMID

••H••M•
ASHRAMS
MAHATMA
SCHISMS
SCHLUMP
UNHELMS

••H•••M
ATHEISM
BAHAISM
BOHRIUM
ECHOISM
EPHRAIM
HAHNIUM
LCHAYIM
MAHDISM

•••HM••
ASTHMAS
BACHMAN
BATHMAT
BRAHMAN
BRAHMAS
BRAHMIN
BUCHMAN
BUSHMAN
BUSHMEN
ISTHMUS
KASHMIR
RICHMAN
RICHMEN
TUCHMAN
YASHMAK
YEAHMAN

•••H•M•
ALCHEMY
ANTHEMS
DIRHAMS
DUCHAMP
FATHOMS
GRAHAME
GRAHAMS
HITHOME
MAYHEMS
MIAHAMM
MISHIMA
NONHOME
NOTHOME
RAMHOME
RANHOME
RUNHOME
SACHEMS
SASHIMI
SATHOME
SITHOME
UNRHYME

•••H••M
ANAHEIM
ARTHURM
BECHARM
EIGHTAM
EIGHTPM
IANHOLM
ISCHIUM
LITHIUM
MANHEIM
MIAHAMM
ORPHEUM
SHAHDOM
SIKHISM
SOPHISM
WILHELM

••••HM•
DRACHMA
LAKSHMI
MEGOHMS
PINCHME
RHYTHMS
SATCHMO

••••H•M
ABRAHAM
APOTHEM
BEACHAM
BECKHAM
BEECHAM
BENTHAM
BINGHAM
BRIGHAM
CHATHAM
DELIHAM
EASTHAM
FORDHAM
FULGHUM
GINGHAM
GRESHAM
GRISHAM
JOACHIM
KETCHAM
KETCHUM
LANGHAM
MARKHAM
MAUGHAM
MITCHUM
NEEDHAM
ONAWHIM
PINKHAM
SORGHUM
WALTHAM
WYNDHAM

•••••HM
TERAOHM

H•N••••
HANAPER
HANCOCK
HANDAXE
HANDBAG
HANDCAR
HANDERS
HANDEYE
HANDFED
HANDFUL
HANDGUN
HANDIER
HANDILY
HANDING
HANDLED
HANDLER
HANDLES
HANDLIN
HANDOFF
HANDOUT
HANDSAW
HANDSEL
HANDSET
HANDSIN
HANDSON
HANDSUP
HANDYTO
HANGARS
HANGBYS
HANGDOG
HANGERS
HANGING
HANGMAN
HANGMEN
HANGOFF
HANGOUT
HANGSBY
HANGSIN
HANGSON
HANGSUP
HANGTEN
HANGUPS
HANKERS
HANKIBA
HANKIES
HANOVER
HANSARP
HANSOLO
HANSOMS
HANUKAH
HENBANE
HENBITS
HENCOOP
HENDECA
HENDRIX
HENDRYX
HENLIKE
HENNAED
HENNERY
HENNISH
HENPECK
HENREID
HENRICH
HENRIES
HENRYII
HENRYIV
HENRYVI
HENSLEY
HENTOFF
HINDERS
HINDLEG
HINDPAW
HINGEON
HINGING
HINKIER
HINNIES
HINTERS
HINTING
HINTSAT
HONALEE
HONCHOS
HONEDIN
HONESIN
HONESTY
HONEYED
HONIARA
HONKERS
HONKING
HONKSAT
HONORED
HONOREE
HONORER
HONOURS
HUNCHED
HUNCHES
HUNDRED
HUNGARY
HUNGERS
HUNGOFF
HUNGOUT
HUNGTEN
HUNKERS
HUNKIER
HUNLIKE
HUNNISH
HUNNYBS
HUNTERS
HUNTFOR
HUNTING
HUNTLEY
HUNTSUP

H••N•••
HAFNIUM
HAHNIUM
HARNESS
HARNICK
HAUNTED
HAUNTER
HEINOUS
HENNAED
HENNERY
HENNISH
HERNANI
HERNDON
HERNIAE
HERNIAS
HERNIBS
HEXNUTS
HINNIES
HIPNESS
HISNIBS
HOBNAIL
HOBNOBS
HOGNOSE
HOGNUTS
HOHNERS
HORNETS
HORNIER
HORNING
HORNISH
HORNIST
HORNSBY
HORNSIN
HORNUNG
HOTNESS
HOUNDED
HOUNDER
HOWNICE
HUANGHE
HUANGTI
HUNNISH
HUNNYBS
HYANNIS
HYMNALS
HYMNARY
HYMNING
HYMNODY
HYPNOID
HYUNDAI

H•••N••
HACKNEY
HADANIP
HAIRNET
HAPENNY
HASANIP
HAVANAN
HAVANAS
HAVENER
HAVENOT
HAYINGS
HAZANIM
HAZINGS
HEDONIC
HERENOW
HERONRY
HEXANES
HHMUNRO
HIDINGS
HIJINKS
HITINTO
HOMINID
HOMONYM
HOPENOT
HOPINTO
HOSANNA
HOTONES
HRYVNIA
HUMANLY
HUMANUM
HYANNIS
HYGINUS
HYPONYM

H••••N•
HACKING
HADDONE
HADRONS
HAFTING
HAILING
HALDANE
HALOING
HALTING
HALVING
HAMBONE
HAMLINE
HAMMING
HAMMOND
HANDING
HANGING
HAPENNY
HAPPENS
HARDENS
HARDING
HARKENS
HARKING
HARLAND
HARLINE
HARMING
HARMONY
HARPING
HASDONE
HASHING
HASPING
HASTENS
HASTING
HATBAND
HATPINS
HATTING
HAULING
HAVEONE
HAWKING
HAWKINS
HEADEND
HEADING

HEALING
HEAPING
HEARING
HEATING
HEAVENS
HEAVING
HEDGING
HEEDING
HEELING
HEFTING
HELLENE
HELLENO
HELMING
HELMOND
HELPING
HELSING
HEMLINE
HEMMING
HENBANE
HERDING
HERMANA
HERMANN
HERMANO
HERMANS
HERNANI
HEROINE
HERRING
HEYMANS
HIBBING
HIBERNO
HIGGINS
HIGHEND
HILLING
HILTING
HILTONS
HINGING
HINTING
HIPBONE
HIRCINE
HISPANO
HISSING
HITSONG
HITTING
HITTUNE
HJHEINZ
HOAXING
HOBOING
HOBSONS
HOCKING
HODDING
HOFMANN
HOGGING
HOLDING
HOLLAND
HOLYONE
HONKING
HOODING
HOOFING
HOOKING
HOOPING
HOOTING
HOPKINS
HOPPING
HOPSING
HORDING
HORMONE
HORNING
HORNUNG
HORSING
HOSANNA
HOSKINS
HOSTING
HOTHAND
HOTLINE
HOTLINK
HOTPINK
HOTTUNA
HOTZONE
HOUDINI
HOUSING
HOVLANE
HOWLING
HOWLONG
HOWMANY
HOYDENS
HUFFING
HUGGING
HUGGINS
HULKING
HULLING
HUMMING
HUNTING
HURLING
HURTING
HUSBAND
HUSHING
HUSKING
HUTTING
HUYGENS
HYDRANT
HYGIENE
HYMNING
HYPHENS
HYPOING

H•••••N

HACKMAN
HADBEEN
HADRIAN
HAIRPIN
HAITIAN
HALCYON
HALFWON
HALOGEN
HALSTON
HAMELIN
HAMPTON
HANDGUN
HANDLIN
HANDSIN
HANDSON
HANGMAN
HANGMEN
HANGSIN
HANGSON
HANGTEN
HARDPAN
HARDTEN
HARDWON
HARPOON
HARPSON
HARSHEN
HARTMAN
HASBEEN
HAULSIN
HAVANAN
HAVEFUN
HAWKMAN
HEADMAN
HEADMEN
HEADPIN
HEADSIN
HEAPSON
HEARKEN
HEARTEN
HEATFAN
HEATHEN
HECKMAN
HEDISON
HEISMAN
HELICON
HELLION
HELLMAN
HELPSIN
HELPSON
HEMATIN
HEPARIN
HEPBURN
HERMANN
HERNDON
HESHVAN
HESSIAN
HEXAGON
HEXSIGN
HICKMAN
HIJKLMN
HILLMAN
HILLMEN
HINGEON
HIREDON
HIRESON
HITCHON
HITTOWN
HITUPON
HOARSEN
HOBOKEN
HOEDOWN
HOFFMAN
HOFMANN
HOLBEIN
HOLDSIN
HOLDSON
HOLYMAN
HOLYMEN
HOLZMAN
HOMEDIN
HOMERUN
HOMESIN
HONEDIN
HONESIN
HOOKSON
HOOPMAN
HOOPMEN
HORIZON
HORNSIN
HOUSMAN
HOUSTON
HOWTHEN
HUFFMAN
HUNGTEN
HURSTON
HUSSEIN
HYPERON

•HN••••

SHNOOKS

•H•N•••

CHANCED
CHANCEL
CHANCER
CHANCES
CHANELS
CHANGED
CHANGER
CHANGES
CHANNEL
CHANOYU
CHANSON
CHANTED
CHANTER
CHANTEY
CHANTRY
CHENIER
CHINESE
CHINKED
CHINNED
CHINOIS
CHINOOK
CHINTZY
CHINUPS
CHINWAG
CHUNKED
CHUNNEL
GHANIAN
KHANATE
OHANLON
PHANTOM
PHENOLS
PHENOMS
PHINEAS
PHONEIN
PHONEME
PHONENO
PHONERS
PHONEYS
PHONICS
PHONIER
PHONIES
PHONILY
PHONING
PHONYUP
RHENISH
RHENIUM
SHANANA
SHANGRI
SHANKAR
SHANKED
SHANNEN
SHANNON
SHANTER
SHINDIG
SHINEON
SHINERS
SHINEUP
SHINGLE
SHINGLY
SHINIER
SHINILY
SHINING
SHINNED
SHINOLA
SHINPAD
SHONUFF
SHUNNED
SHUNTED
SHUNTER
SHYNESS
THANDIE
THANKED
THANKER
THENETS
THENEWS
THENILE
THINAIR
THINICE
THINKER
THINKOF
THINKSO
THINKUP
THINMAN
THINNED
THINNER
THINOUT
THUNDER
THUNKED
WHANGED
WHINERS
WHINIER
WHINING

•H••N••

CHAINED
CHAINES
CHAINUP
CHANNEL
CHARNIN
CHIANTI
CHIGNON
CHIMNEY
CHINNED
CHRONIC
CHUNNEL
CHURNED
CHURNER
CHURNUP
CHUTNEY
HHMUNRO
PHOENIX
PHRENIC
SHANNEN
SHANNON
SHATNER
SHAWNEE
SHINNED
SHOPNBC
SHOWNIN
SHOWNUP
SHRINED
SHRINER
SHRINES
SHRINKS
SHUNNED
THINNED
THINNER
THORNED
THRONES
THRONGS
WHATNOT
WHATNOW
WHITNEY
WHOKNEW

•H•••N•

BHUTANI
CHAFING
CHALONS
CHARING
CHASING
CHAWING
CHAZANS
CHEFING
CHEVONS
CHEWING
CHICANA
CHICANE
CHICANO
CHIDING
CHIMING
CHIMINH
CHITONS
CHOKING
CHOLINE
CHOPINE
CHORINE
CHOWING
CHUTING
CHYRONS
LHASANS
OHIOANS
PHALANX
PHARYNX
PHASING
PHONENO
PHONING
PHOTONS
RHYMING
SHADING
SHAKING
SHAMANS
SHAMING
SHANANA
SHAPING
SHARING
SHARONA
SHAVING
SHEBANG
SHINING
SHOEING
SHOGUNS
SHOOING
SHOOINS
SHORING
SHOVING
SHOWING
SHUTINS
THATONE
THAWING
THEBAND
THEBANS
THEFONZ
THEGANG
THEKING
THEOMNI
THEPOND
THERENT
THERING
THERINK
THESUNS
THEWIND
THISONE
THREENO
THYMINE
WHALING
WHILING
WHINING
WHITENS
WHITING

•H••••N

CHAGRIN
CHANSON
CHAPLIN
CHAPMAN
CHAPMEN
CHARMAN
CHARMEN
CHARMIN
CHARNIN
CHASTEN
CHATWIN
CHAZZAN
CHEAPEN
CHEATIN
CHEATON
CHECHEN
CHECKIN
CHECKON
CHEERON
CHEVRON
CHEWSON
CHICHEN
CHICKEN
CHIDDEN
CHIFFON
CHIGNON
CHILEAN
CHIMEIN
CHIPSIN
CHITLIN
CHITOWN
CHOKEON
CHOMPON
FHALOAN
GHANIAN
GHERKIN
OHANLON
PHAETON
PHASEIN
PHILBIN
PHONEIN
RHODIAN
SHANNEN
SHANNON
SHAREIN
SHARPEN
SHAVIAN
SHEDSON
SHEEHAN
SHELDON
SHERMAN
SHERWIN
SHINEON
SHIPMAN
SHIPMEN
SHODDEN
SHOOSIN
SHORTEN
SHOTGUN
SHOVEIN
SHOWMAN
SHOWMEN
SHOWNIN
SHOWSIN
SHULMAN
SHUTSIN
THEMOON
THEOMEN
THEREIN
THEREON
THESWAN
THETURN
THIAMIN
THICKEN
THIGPEN
THINMAN
THOMSON
THORSON
THREWIN
THREWON
THRIVEN
THROWIN
THROWON
THURMAN
WHARTON
WHAUDEN
WHEATEN
WHEATON
WHEELIN
WHEREIN
WHEREON
WHIPSIN
WHITMAN
WHITSUN

••HN•••

ETHNICS
HAHNIUM
HOHNERS
JOHNBOY
JOHNDOE
JOHNGAY
JOHNIII
JOHNJAY
JOHNLAW
JOHNLEE
JOHNNIE
JOHNNYB
JOHNSON
JOHNVII
JOHNWOO
JOHNXII
JOHNXIV
JOHNXIX
JOHNXVI
JOHNXXI
SCHNAPS
SCHNOOK
SCHNOZZ

••H•N••

ACHENES
APHONIA
APHONIC
ASHANTI
BEHINDS
ENHANCE
ETHANES
ETHANOL
ETHENES
FTHENRY
GEHENNA
JOHANNA
JOHNNIE
JOHNNYB
KAHUNAS
MAHONEY
MCHENRY
MRHANEY
NOHANDS
OCHENTA
REHANGS
REHINGE
REHONED
REHONES
REHONOR
TAHINIS
UNHANDS
UNHANDY
UNHINGE
UNHONED
WAHINES
WCHANDY

••H••N•

ACHTUNG
ASHBINS
ASHCANS
ASHLAND
ASHPANS
BAHIANS
BEHRENS
BEHRING
DEHORNS
ECHIDNA
ECHOING
GEHENNA
HJHEINZ
JOHANNA
LAHAINA
LEHMANN
OAHUANS
SCHWANN
SCHWINN

••H•••N

ACHERON
ACHESON
ASHBURN
BAHAMEN
BAHRAIN
BAHREIN
BEHRMAN
DEHAVEN
ECHELON
GAHAGAN
ICHDIEN
INHUMAN
ITHACAN
JOHNSON
LEHMANN
MOHEGAN
MOHICAN
SAHARAN
SCHWANN
SCHWINN
TEHERAN
TOHELEN
UNHUMAN
USHERIN

•••HN••

BOCHNER
BOTHNIA
BUCHNER
DAPHNES
DAPHNIA
DAPHNIS
FECHNER
FISHNET
MISHNAH
TECHNOS

•••H•N•

AFGHANI
AFGHANS
ALTHING
ANTHONY
ARCHING
ARCHONS
BACHING
BADHAND
BASHING
BATHING
BETHANY
BETHINK
BETHUNE
BICHONS
BIGHAND
BUSHING
BYPHONE
CACHING
CASHING
CASHINS
COSHING
COWHAND
CUSHING
DABHAND
DASHING
DIAHANN
DISHING
EGGHUNT
ENCHANT
ETCHANT
ETCHING
EUPHONY
EYEHAND
FISHING
FOXHUNT
GASHING
GUSHING
HASHING
HIGHEND
HOTHAND
HUSHING
HYPHENS
INCHING
INTHING
ITCHING
JOBHUNT
JOSHING
KACHINA
KACHING
KUCHENS
LASHING
LATHING
LICHENS
LOWHAND
LUCHINO
MACHINA
MACHINE
MACHONE
MANHUNT
MASHING
MCSHANE
MESHING
METHANE
MIGHTNT
MOSHING
MUDHENS
MUSHING
NATHANS
NEWHAND
NICHING
NOSHING
NOTHING
NOTHINS
OFFHAND
OLDHAND
OMAHANE
OMAHANS
ONEHAND
ORPHANS
ORPHANT
OUGHTNT
OUTHUNT
PATHAND
PATHANS
PEAHENS
PISHING
PITHING
PUSHING
PYTHONS
REDHENS
REPHONE
RESHINE
RETHANK
RETHINK
RICHENS
RUCHING
RUSHING
RUTHANN
SASHING
SEAHUNT
SIGHING
SIPHONS
TERHUNE
TITHING
UNSHINY
UNTHINK
URCHINS
UTAHANS
WASHING
WISHING

•••H••N

AIRHORN
ALSHAIN
ALTHORN
AMPHION
BACHMAN
BIGHORN
BRAHMAN
BRAHMIN
BUCHMAN
BUSHMAN
BUSHMEN
CALHOUN
CARHORN
COCHRAN
COGHLAN
CUSHION
DIAHANN
DISHPAN
ENCHAIN
FASHION
FOGHORN
HESHVAN
IDAHOAN
INKHORN
KATHRYN
LEGHORN
LETHEAN
LIGHTEN
LIGHTON
LOTHIAN
MACHAON
MECHLIN
ORPHEAN
PUSHKIN
PUSHPIN
PYTHIAN
RESHOWN
RICHMAN
RICHMEN
RIGHTON
RUTHANN
SAXHORN
SOTHERN
TACHYON
TASHLIN
TIGHTEN
TINHORN
TUCHMAN
TYPHOON
UNCHAIN
UNCHURN
UNSHORN
UNSHOWN
VECHTEN
YEAHMAN

••••HN•

ARACHNE
ARACHNO
KRISHNA
STJOHNS

••••H•N

AGAKHAN
ALYKHAN
ANDTHEN
AWASHIN
BASRHIN
BEECHEN
BIRCHEN
BLUEHEN
BLUSHON
CATCHON
CAUTHEN
CHECHEN
CHICHEN
DAUPHIN
DIAPHAN
DOLPHIN
EARTHEN
EREWHON
FLASHON
FRESHEN
GERSHON
GREYHEN
GRYPHON
HARSHEN
HEATHEN
HITCHON
HOWTHEN
ISFAHAN
KEESHAN
KEOGHAN
KITCHEN
LARCHEN
LATCHON
LAUGHIN
LOWCHEN
MADCHEN
MARCHON
MCLUHAN
MCMAHON
MENUHIN
MOORHEN
MORPHIN
MUNCHEN
MUNCHON
NOWTHEN
PATCHEN
PITCHIN
PUNCHIN
PYNCHON
REACHIN
ROUGHEN
SAGEHEN
SAYWHEN
SHEEHAN
SIOBHAN
STEPHEN
TEACHIN
TOUCHON
TOUGHEN
VAUGHAN
WEIGHIN
WEIGHON
XANTHAN
YOUTHEN

•••••HN

BIGJOHN
IIIJOHN
ROYCOHN

HO•••••

HOAGIES
HOARDED
HOARDER
HOARIER

HOARILY
HOARSEN
HOARSER
HOAXERS
HOAXING
HOBBIES
HOBBITS
HOBBLED
HOBBLER
HOBBLES
HOBNAIL
HOBNOBS
HOBOING
HOBOISM
HOBOKEN
HOBSONS
HOCKERS
HOCKING
HOCUSED
HODADDY
HODDING
HOECAKE
HOEDOWN
HOFBRAU
HOFFMAN
HOFMANN
HOFSTRA
HOGARTH
HOGBACK
HOGCALL
HOGGERY
HOGGING
HOGGISH
HOGLIKE
HOGNOSE
HOGNUTS
HOGTIED
HOGTIES
HOGWASH
HOGWEED
HOGWILD
HOHNERS
HOISTED
HOISTER
HOISTUP
HOKIEST
HOLBEIN
HOLBERG
HOLDALL
HOLDERS
HOLDING
HOLDOFF
HOLDOUT
HOLDSIN
HOLDSIT
HOLDSON
HOLDSTO
HOLDSUP
HOLDUPS
HOLEDUP
HOLEOUT
HOLESUP
HOLIDAY
HOLIEST
HOLISTS
HOLLAND
HOLLERS
HOLLIES
HOLLOWS
HOLMIUM
HOLMOAK
HOLSTER
HOLYARK
HOLYCOW
HOLYDAY
HOLYJOE
HOLYMAN
HOLYMEN
HOLYOIL
HOLYOKE
HOLYONE
HOLYSEE
HOLYWAR
HOLZMAN
HOMAGER
HOMAGES
HOMBRES
HOMBURG
HOMEBOY
HOMEDIN
HOMEICE
HOMEIER
HOMELAB
HOMERED
HOMERIC
HOMERUN
HOMESIN
HOMIEST
HOMINID
HOMONYM
HONALEE
HONCHOS
HONEDIN
HONESIN
HONESTY
HONEYED
HONIARA
HONKERS
HONKING
HONKSAT
HONORED
HONOREE
HONORER
HONOURS
HOOCHES
HOODIES
HOODING
HOODLUM
HOODOOS
HOOFERS
HOOFING
HOOFSIT
HOOHAHS
HOOKAHS
HOOKING
HOOKSON
HOOKSUP
HOOKUPS
HOOPERS
HOOPING
HOOPLAS
HOOPMAN
HOOPMEN
HOOPOES
HOOPTOY
HOORAHS
HOORAYS
HOOSIER
HOOTERS
HOOTING
HOOTOWL
HOOTSAT
HOOVERS
HOPACAB
HOPEDSO
HOPEDTO
HOPEFOR
HOPEFUL
HOPENOT
HOPESSO
HOPESTO
HOPINTO
HOPKINS
HOPLITE
HOPOVER
HOPPERS
HOPPIER
HOPPING
HOPSING
HOPSOFF
HOPSOUT
HOPTOIT
HORATIO
HORDING
HORIZON
HORMONE
HORNETS
HORNIER
HORNING
HORNISH
HORNIST
HORNSBY
HORNSIN
HORNUNG
HORRIFY
HORRORS
HORSIER
HORSILY
HORSING
HORSLEY
HORVITZ
HOSANNA
HOSCALE
HOSIERS
HOSIERY
HOSKINS
HOSPICE
HOSTAGE
HOSTELS
HOSTESS
HOSTILE
HOSTING
HOSTLER
HOTBATH
HOTBEDS
HOTCAKE
HOTCAPS
HOTCARS
HOTCOAL
HOTCOMB
HOTCUPS
HOTDATE
HOTDAYS
HOTDOGS
HOTFOOT
HOTGLUE
HOTHAND
HOTHEAD
HOTITEM
HOTKEYS
HOTLEAD
HOTLICK
HOTLINE
HOTLINK
HOTLIPS
HOTMAIL
HOTMEAL
HOTMILK
HOTNESS
HOTONES
HOTOVER
HOTPACK
HOTPINK
HOTPOTS
HOTRODS
HOTROLL
HOTSEAT
HOTSHOT
HOTSOUP
HOTSPOT
HOTSPUR
HOTTEAS
HOTTEST
HOTTIES
HOTTIME
HOTTIPS
HOTTUBS
HOTTUNA
HOTWARS
HOTWIRE
HOTZONE
HOUDINI
HOUNDED
HOUNDER
HOUSING
HOUSMAN
HOUSSAY
HOUSTON
HOVERED
HOVERER
HOVLANE
HOWARDK
HOWARDS
HOWARDU
HOWBEIT
HOWCOME
HOWDAHS
HOWDEDO
HOWDULL
HOWDYDO
HOWELLS
HOWELSE
HOWEVER
HOWHIGH
HOWLAME
HOWLERS
HOWLING
HOWLONG
HOWLSAT
HOWMANY
HOWMUCH
HOWNICE
HOWTHEN
HOYDENS

H•O••••

HOOCHES
HOODIES
HOODING
HOODLUM
HOODOOS
HOOFERS
HOOFING
HOOFSIT
HOOHAHS
HOOKAHS
HOOKING
HOOKSON
HOOKSUP
HOOKUPS
HOOPERS
HOOPING
HOOPLAS
HOOPMAN
HOOPMEN
HOOPOES
HOOPTOY
HOORAHS
HOORAYS
HOOSIER
HOOTERS
HOOTING
HOOTOWL
HOOTSAT
HOOVERS

H••O•••

HADOVER
HALOGEN
HALOIDS
HALOING
HANOVER
HAROLDI
HASOVER
HAWORTH
HEDONIC
HELOISE
HELOTRY
HEROICS
HEROINE
HEROISM
HERONRY
HEXOSES
HOBOING
HOBOISM
HOBOKEN
HOMONYM
HONORED
HONOREE
HONORER
HONOURS
HOPOVER
HOTONES
HOTOVER
HUMORAL
HUMORED
HUMORME
HUMOURS
HYPOING
HYPONYM

H•••O••

HACKOFF
HADDOCK
HADDONE
HADRONS
HADROOM
HADSOME
HADTOBE
HALLOOS
HALLOWS
HAMBONE
HAMHOCK
HAMMOCK
HAMMOND
HANCOCK
HANDOFF
HANDOUT
HANGOFF
HANGOUT
HANSOLO
HANSOMS
HAPLOID
HARBORS
HARBOUR
HARLOTS
HARMONY
HARPOON
HARRODS
HARROLD
HARROWS
HASDONE
HASHOUT
HASROOM
HASSOCK
HASTOBE
HATSOFF
HAULOFF
HAVEONE
HAVEOUT
HAYFORK
HAYLOFT
HAYMOWS
HEADOFF
HEADOUT
HEAROUT
HECTORS
HEINOUS
HELDOFF
HELDOUT
HELLOED
HELLOES
HELMOND
HELPOUT
HEMLOCK
HENCOOP
HENTOFF
HERMOSA
HERMOSO
HEYLOOK
HEYWOOD
HICKORY
HIDEOUS
HIDEOUT
HIKEOUT
HILLOCK
HILTONS
HIPBONE
HIPBOOT
HIPROOF
HIREOUT
HISTORY
HITHOME
HITSOFF
HITSONG
HITSOUT
HITTOWN
HIVEOFF
HOBNOBS
HOBSONS
HOEDOWN
HOGNOSE
HOLDOFF
HOLDOUT
HOLEOUT
HOLLOWS
HOLMOAK
HOLYOIL
HOLYOKE
HOLYONE
HOODOOS
HOOPOES
HOOTOWL
HOPSOFF
HOPSOUT
HOPTOIT
HORMONE
HORRORS
HOTCOAL
HOTCOMB
HOTDOGS
HOTFOOT
HOTPOTS
HOTRODS
HOTROLL
HOTSOUP
HOTZONE
HOWCOME
HOWLONG
HULLOED
HUNGOFF
HUNGOUT
HYALOID
HYDROUS
HYMNODY
HYPNOID
HYSSOPS

H••••O•

HADACOW
HADAJOB
HADAROW
HADROOM
HAIRDOS
HALCYON
HALFROD
HALFWON
HALLOOS
HALSTON
HAMPTON
HANDSON
HANGDOG
HANGSON
HARDTOP
HARDWON
HARICOT
HARPOON
HARPSON
HASACOW
HASAROW
HASROOM
HAUTBOY
HAVENOT
HEADFOR
HEAPSOF
HEAPSON
HEARDOF
HEARSOF
HEDISON
HEIRDOM
HELICON
HELLBOY
HELLION
HELPSON
HENCOOP
HERENOW
HERITOR
HERNDON
HERRIOT
HEXAGON
HEXAPOD
HEYLOOK
HEYWOOD
HIGHBOY
HIGHLOW
HIGHTOP
HILLTOP
HINGEON
HIPBOOT
HIPROOF
HIREDON
HIRESON
HITCHON
HITSFOR
HITSHOW
HITUPON
HOLDSON
HOLYCOW
HOLYJOE
HOMEBOY
HONCHOS
HOODOOS
HOOKSON
HOOPTOY
HOPEFOR
HOPENOT
HORIZON
HOTFOOT
HOTSHOT
HOTSPOT
HOUSTON
HUMIDOR
HUNTFOR
HURSTON
HURTFOR
HYPERON

H•••••O

HANDYTO
HANSOLO
HAPKIDO
HAPPYTO
HAVEAGO
HEADSTO
HEAVEHO
HEAVETO
HEIGHHO
HELLENO
HERESTO
HERMANO
HERMOSO
HERPETO
HEWEDTO
HHMUNRO
HIBERNO
HIDALGO
HISPANO
HITINTO
HOLDSTO
HOPEDSO
HOPEDTO
HOPESSO
HOPESTO
HOPINTO
HORATIO
HOWDEDO
HOWDYDO

•HO••••

AHOSTOF
CHOCKED
CHOCTAW
CHOICER
CHOICES
CHOIRED
CHOKEON
CHOKERS
CHOKEUP
CHOKIER
CHOKING
CHOLERA
CHOLERS
CHOLINE
CHOLLAS
CHOMPED
CHOMPON
CHOMSKY
CHOOSER
CHOOSES
CHOOSEY
CHOPINE
CHOPOFF
CHOPPED
CHOPPER
CHOPSUP
CHORALE
CHORALS
CHORDAL
CHORDED
CHORINE
CHORIST
CHORIZO
CHORTLE
CHOSEUP
CHOUGHS
CHOWDER
CHOWING
GHOSTED
GHOSTLY
IHOPESO
PHOBIAS
PHOBICS
PHOEBES
PHOEBUS
PHOENIX
PHONEIN
PHONEME
PHONENO
PHONERS
PHONEYS
PHONICS
PHONIER
PHONIES
PHONILY
PHONING
PHONYUP
PHOTICS
PHOTOGS
PHOTOID
PHOTONS
PHOTOOP
RHODIAN
RHODIUM
RHOECUS
RHOMBIC
RHOMBUS
SHOALED
SHOCKED
SHOCKER
SHODDEN
SHOEBOX
SHOEING
SHOEPAC
SHOFARS
SHOGUNS
SHONUFF
SHOOFLY
SHOOING
SHOOINS
SHOOKUP
SHOOOFF
SHOOSIN
SHOOTAT
SHOOTBY
SHOOTER
SHOOTUP
SHOPFOR
SHOPFUL
SHOPKOS
SHOPNBC
SHOPPED
SHOPPER
SHOPPES
SHOPSAT
SHOREUP
SHORING
SHORTED
SHORTEN
SHORTER
SHORTIE
SHORTLY
SHORTOF
SHOTFOR
SHOTGUN
SHOTOUT
SHOTPAR
SHOTPUT
SHOULDA
SHOULDI
SHOUTAT
SHOUTED
SHOUTER
SHOVEIN
SHOVELS
SHOVERS
SHOVING
SHOWBIZ
SHOWCAT
SHOWDOG
SHOWERS
SHOWERY
SHOWHOW
SHOWIER
SHOWILY
SHOWING
SHOWMAN
SHOWMEN
SHOWNIN
SHOWNUP
SHOWOFF
SHOWOUT
SHOWSIN
SHOWSUP
THOMSON
THOREAU
THORIUM
THORNED
THORSON
THOUGHT
WHOEVER
WHOISIT
WHOKNEW
WHOMPED
WHOOPED
WHOOPEE
WHOOPER
WHOOPIE
WHOOSIS
WHOPPED
WHOPPER
WHORLED
WHOSAID
WHOSOUT
WHOSWHO

•H•O•••

CHAOTIC
CHLORIC
CHOOSER
CHOOSES
CHOOSEY
CHROMAT
CHROMED
CHROMES
CHROMIC
CHRONIC
OHIOANS
OHIOART
PHLOEMS
PHLOXES
SHLOCKY
SHNOOKS
SHOOFLY
SHOOING
SHOOINS
SHOOKUP
SHOOOFF
SHOOSIN
SHOOTAT
SHOOTBY
SHOOTER
SHOOTUP
SHROUDS
THEOATH
THEODOR
THEOMEN
THEOMNI
THEOREM
THROATS
THROATY
THRONES
THRONGS
THROUGH
THROWAT
THROWER
THROWIN
THROWON
THROWUP
WHOOPED
WHOOPEE
WHOOPER
WHOOPIE
WHOOSIS
WHWORDS

•H••O••

AHCHOOS
CHALONS
CHAMOIS
CHANOYU
CHAYOTE
CHEROOT
CHEVONS
CHEWOUT
CHICORY
CHIGOES
CHINOIS
CHINOOK
CHITONS
CHITOWN
CHOPOFF
CHYRONS
FHALOAN
PHENOLS
PHENOMS
PHILOUS
PHOTOGS
PHOTOID
PHOTONS
PHOTOOP
RHEBOKS
RHETORS
RHIZOME
SHADOWS
SHADOWY
SHAKOES
SHALOMS
SHARONA
SHEGOAT
SHEWOLF
SHIKOKU
SHINOLA
SHIPOUT
SHNOOKS
SHOOOFF
SHOTOUT
SHOWOFF
SHOWOUT
SHUTOFF
SHUTOUT
SHYLOCK
THATONE
THAWOUT
THEBOBO
THEBODY
THEBOMB
THEBOSS
THEBOYS
THEDOLE
THEFONZ
THEFOOL
THEGOLD
THEHOGS
THEHOOD
THEHOPE
THELOOK
THELOOP
THEMOON
THEMOST
THEPOND
THEPOOH
THEPOPE
THEPOST
THEROBE
THEROCK
THEROOM
THEROPE
THEROSE
THEROUX
THETOUR
THINOUT
THISONE
THYROID
WHOSOUT

•H•••O•

AHCHOOS
AHEADOF
AHOSTOF
CHANSON
CHARCOT
CHARIOT
CHARROS
CHEATON
CHECKON
CHEERON
CHEETOS
CHEKHOV
CHEROOT
CHEVIOT
CHEVRON
CHEWSON
CHEWTOY
CHEZMOI
CHIFFON
CHIGNON
CHINOOK
CHOKEON
CHOMPON
CHRISOM
CHURROS
GHETTOS
KHARKOV
OHANLON
OHCAROL

PHAETON
PHANTOM
PHARAOH
PHILCOS
PHOTOOP
PHYLLOS
SHADROE
SHAHDOM
SHALLOT
SHALLOW
SHAMPOO
SHANNON
SHAVUOT
SHEDSON
SHELDON
SHINEON
SHOEBOX
SHOPFOR
SHOPKOS
SHORTOF
SHOTFOR
SHOWDOG
SHOWHOW
SHYFROM
THATSOK
THEBLOB
THECROW
THEFLOP
THEFOOL
THEHOOD
THELOOK
THELOOP
THEMOON
THEODOR
THEPOOH
THEREOF
THEREON
THERMOS
THEROOM
THESHOW
THINKOF
THOMSON
THORSON
THREWON
THROWON
WHARTON
WHATFOR
WHATNOT
WHATNOW
WHEATON
WHEREOF
WHEREON

•H••••O

CHEERIO
CHICAGO
CHICANO
CHIRICO
CHORIZO
CHRISTO
HHMUNRO
IHOPESO
PHONENO
SHAMPOO
SHAPIRO
THEBOBO
THEHERO
THEMAYO
THERETO
THINKSO
THREENO
WHERETO
WHOSWHO
ZHIVAGO

••HO•••

APHONIA
APHONIC
ATHOMES
BEHOLDS
BEHOOVE
CAHOKIA
CAHOOTS
COHORTS
COHOSTS
DAHOMEY
DEHORNS
ECHOERS
ECHOING
ECHOISM
EXHORTS
IMHOTEP
INHOUSE
MAHONEY
MAHOUTS
MRHOBBS
MRHORSE
OKHOTSK
REHONED
REHONES
REHONOR
REHOOKS
REHOUSE
SCHOLAR
SCHOLES
SCHOOLS
TOHOMER
TOHORSE
UNHONED
UNHOODS
UNHOOKS
UNHOPED
UNHORSE
UNHOUSE
UPHOARD
UPHOLDS

••H•O••

ASHFORD
BEHOOVE
CAHOOTS
ETHMOID
MAHFOUZ
MAHZORS
OCHROID
OCHROUS
OSHKOSH
REHOOKS
SCHLOCK
SCHMOES
SCHNOOK
SCHNOZZ
SCHOOLS
UNHOODS
UNHOOKS

••H••O•

ACHEFOR
ACHERON
ACHESON
ECHELON
ETHANOL
ICHABOD
JOHNBOY
JOHNDOE
JOHNSON
JOHNWOO
MRHULOT
REHONOR
SCHNOOK

••H•••O

JOHNWOO
OTHELLO
SCHERZO
SUHARTO

•••HO••

AHCHOOS
AIRHOLE
AIRHORN
AIRHOSE
ALTHORN
AMPHORA
ANCHORS
ANCHOVY
ANTHONY
ANYHOPE
ARCHONS
ARMHOLE
AUTHORS
BARHOPS
BATHOIL
BBSHOTS
BICHONS
BIGHORN
BISHOPS
BOBHOPE
BOGHOLE
BOOHOOS
BOYHOOD
BSCHOOL
BYPHONE
CALHOUN
CARHOPS
CARHORN
CASHOUT
CATHODE
DASHOFF
DAYHOPS
DEGHOST
DISHOUT
DOSHOTS
DRYHOLE
EARHOLE
EUPHONY
EYEHOLE
EYEHOOK
FATHOMS
FISHOIL
FISHOUT
FOGHORN
FOXHOLE
GASHOGS
GODHOOD
GUSHOUT
HAMHOCK
HASHOUT
HITHOME
IANHOLM
ICEHOLE
IDAHOAN
IMAHOGG
INAHOLE
INKHORN
INSHOCK
INSHORE
INSHORT
JIMHOGG
JOBHOPS
KEYHOLE
LADHOOD
LASHOUT
LEGHORN
LEWHOAD
LITHOID
MACHONE
MANHOLE
MANHOOD
MANHOUR
METHODS
MILHOUS
MUDHOLE
NEWHOPE
NICHOLS
NONHOME
NOSHOWS
NOTHOME
NUNHOOD
OFFHOUR
OKSHOOT
ONEHOUR
ONSHORE
OUTHOWL
PIEHOLE
PINHOLE
POTHOLE
POTHOOK
PUSHOFF
PUSHOUT
PYTHONS
QSCHOOL
QUAHOGS
RAMHOME
RANHOME
RATHOLE
RECHOSE
REDHOTS
REPHONE
RESHOES
RESHOOT
RESHOWN
RESHOWS
RUNHOME
RUSHOFF
RUSHOUT
SATHOME
SAXHORN
SENHORA
SIPHONS
SITHOME
SKYHOOK
SPYHOLE
SYDHOFF
THEHOGS
THEHOOD
THEHOPE
TIMHOLT
TINHORN
TOEHOLD
TOPHOLE
TOYHOOP
TVSHOWS
TWOHOUR
TYPHOID
TYPHOON
UNCHOKE
UNSHOED
UNSHOES
UNSHORN
UNSHORT
UNSHOWN
UNSHOWY
UNWHOLE
UPSHOOT
UPSHOTS
WASHOFF
WASHOUT
WEEHOUR
WITHOUT
XIPHOID
YOOHOOS

•••H•O•

AHCHOOS
ALOHAOE
AMPHION
ARCHFOE
BOOHOOS
BOYHOOD
BSCHOOL
BUSHHOG
CASHBOX
CASHCOW
CUSHION
DASHDOT
DASHPOT
DRCHAOS
EYEHOOK
FASHION
FISHFOR
GODHOOD
HIGHBOY
HIGHLOW
HIGHTOP
ITCHFOR
LADHOOD
LIGHTON
LITHGOW
LOTHROP
MACHAON
MANHOOD
NUNHOOD
OKSHOOT
POTHOOK
PUSHFOR
PUSHROD
QSCHOOL
RESHOOT
RIGHTON
SHAHDOM
SIGHFOR
SKYHOOK
TACHYON
TECHNOS
THEHOOD
TOYHOOP
TYPHOON
UPSHOOT
UPTHROW
WISHFOR
YEAHYOU
YOOHOOS

•••H••O

AKIHITO
BEAHERO
BUSHIDO
CEPHALO
LUCHINO
MACHTWO
NONHERO
OMPHALO
ONTHEGO
OUGHTTO
SAYHITO
SEAHERO
THEHERO
TOSHIRO
WARHERO

••••HO•

AIRSHOW
ALCOHOL
ARTSHOP
ARTSHOW
BACKHOE
BADSHOT
BAGEHOT
BELLHOP
BENTHOS
BIGSHOT
BIGSHOW
BLUSHON
BOKCHOY
BOLSHOI
BOWSHOT
BUSHHOG
CAMPHOR
CARSHOW
CATCHON
CATCHOW
CATSHOW
CHEKHOV
CONCHOS
COPSHOP
DOGCHOW
DOGSHOW
DONOHOE
EARSHOT
EREWHON
EYESHOT
FLASHON
FLUSHOT
FORSHOW
GASOHOL
GAUCHOS
GERSHON
GETSHOT
GLASHOW
GRYPHON
GUMSHOE
GUNSHOT
GYMSHOE
HITCHON
HITSHOW
HONCHOS
HOTSHOT
ICESHOW
INASHOE
IVANHOE
JOBSHOP
KNEWHOW
KNOWHOW
LATCHON
MALEHOG
MARCHON
MCMAHON
MENTHOL
MTATHOS
MUGSHOT
MUNCHON
NAVAHOS
NORTHOF
ODDSHOE
OLDSHOE
ONESHOE
ONESHOT
OUTSHOT
OUTSHOW
OVERHOT
PETSHOP
PINCHOT
PONCHOS
PORTHOS
POSTHOC
POTSHOT
PRESHOW
PROSHOP
PRUDHOE
PSYCHOS
PYNCHON
RAGSHOP
RANCHOS
RIMSHOT
ROADHOG
RUMSHOP
SALCHOW
SANDHOG
SETSHOT
SHOWHOW
SKISHOP
SOCKHOP
SOMEHOW
SOUTHOF
TAPSHOE
TEASHOP
TEESHOT
THESHOW
TOESHOE
TOUCHON
TOYSHOP
TWOSHOT
USOSHOW
VERYHOT
VOSKHOD
WAPSHOT
WARTHOG
WEIGHON

••••H•O

ARACHNO
ERYTHRO
HEIGHHO
LOATHTO
PITCHTO
ROUGHGO
SATCHMO

•••••HO

ARAPAHO
BOWECHO
BRONCHO
CAMACHO
DERECHO
GROUCHO
HEAVEHO
HEIGHHO
JERICHO
LESOTHO
MRMACHO
ORNITHO
OUTECHO
SAYSWHO
SUBECHO
TALLYHO
UNMACHO
WHOSWHO

H•P••••

HAPENNY
HAPKIDO
HAPLESS
HAPLOID
HAPPENS
HAPPIER
HAPPIFY
HAPPILY
HAPPYTO
HAPTICS
HEPARIN
HEPATIC
HEPBURN
HEPCATS
HEPPEST
HEPTADS
HIPBATH
HIPBONE
HIPBOOT
HIPLESS
HIPLIKE
HIPNESS
HIPPEST
HIPPIER
HIPPIES
HIPPISH
HIPPITY
HIPROOF
HIPSTER
HOPACAB
HOPEDSO
HOPEDTO
HOPEFOR
HOPEFUL
HOPENOT
HOPESSO
HOPESTO
HOPINTO
HOPKINS
HOPLITE
HOPOVER
HOPPERS
HOPPIER
HOPPING
HOPSING
HOPSOFF
HOPSOUT
HOPTOIT
HUPPAHS
HUPPERT
HYPATIA
HYPEDUP
HYPERON
HYPESUP
HYPHENS
HYPNOID
HYPOING
HYPONYM

H••P•••

HADPULL
HAMPERS
HAMPTON
HAPPENS
HAPPIER
HAPPIFY
HAPPILY
HAPPYTO
HARPERS
HARPIES
HARPING
HARPIST
HARPOON
HARPSON
HASPING
HASPULL
HATPINS
HEAPERS
HEAPING
HEAPSOF
HEAPSON
HEAPSUP
HELPERS
HELPFUL
HELPING
HELPOUT
HELPSIN
HELPSON
HELPSUP
HEMPIER
HENPECK
HEPPEST
HERPETO
HIPPEST
HIPPIER
HIPPIES
HIPPISH
HIPPITY
HISPANO
HISPEED
HITPLAY
HOOPERS
HOOPING
HOOPLAS
HOOPMAN
HOOPMEN
HOOPOES
HOOPTOY
HOPPERS
HOPPIER
HOPPING
HOSPICE
HOTPACK
HOTPINK
HOTPOTS
HUMPHED
HUMPHRY
HUMPIER
HUPPAHS
HUPPERT

H•••P••

HAIRPIN
HANAPER
HARDPAN
HARDPUT
HEADPIN
HEELPAD
HELIPAD
HEXAPOD
HIGHPAY
HINDPAW
HITUPON
HOTSPOT
HOTSPUR

H••••P•

HANGUPS
HICCUPS
HOLDUPS
HOOKUPS
HOTCAPS
HOTCUPS
HOTLIPS
HOTTIPS
HUBCAPS
HYSSOPS

H•••••P

HACKSUP
HADANIP
HAMITUP
HANDSUP
HANGSUP
HANSARP
HARDTOP
HASANIP
HAULSUP
HEADSUP
HEALSUP
HEAPSUP
HEATSUP
HEELTAP
HELPSUP
HENCOOP
HIGHTOP
HIKEDUP
HIKESUP
HILLTOP
HITCHUP
HOISTUP
HOLDSUP
HOLEDUP
HOLESUP
HOOKSUP
HOTSOUP
HUNTSUP
HURRYUP
HYPEDUP
HYPESUP

•H•P•••

CHAPALA
CHAPATI
CHAPEAU
CHAPELS
CHAPLET
CHAPLIN
CHAPMAN
CHAPMEN
CHAPPED
CHAPPIE
CHAPTER
CHIPPED
CHIPPER
CHIPSIN
CHIPSUP
CHOPINE
CHOPOFF
CHOPPED
CHOPPER
CHOPSUP
CHUPPAH
CHUPPAS
IHOPESO
SHAPELY
SHAPERS
SHAPEUP
SHAPING
SHAPIRO
SHEPARD
SHIPFUL
SHIPMAN
SHIPMEN
SHIPOUT
SHIPPED
SHIPPER
SHIPWAY
SHOPFOR
SHOPFUL
SHOPKOS
SHOPNBC
SHOPPED
SHOPPER
SHOPPES
SHOPSAT
THEPIPS
THEPITS
THEPOND
THEPOOH
THEPOPE
THEPOST
THEPUMP
WHAPPED
WHIPPED
WHIPPER
WHIPPET
WHIPPLE
WHIPSAW
WHIPSIN
WHIPSUP
WHOPPED
WHOPPER
WHUPPED

•H••P••

CHAMPED
CHAMPER
CHAPPED
CHAPPIE
CHARPAK
CHEAPEN
CHEAPER
CHEAPIE
CHEAPLY
CHEEPED
CHEEPER
CHIAPAS
CHIAPET
CHIPPED
CHIPPER
CHIRPED
CHIRPER
CHOMPED
CHOMPON
CHOPPED
CHOPPER
CHUMPED
CHUPPAH
CHUPPAS
SHAMPOO
SHARPED
SHARPEI
SHARPEN
SHARPER
SHARPIE
SHARPLY
SHERPAS
SHINPAD
SHIPPED
SHIPPER
SHOEPAC
SHOPPED
SHOPPER
SHOPPES
SHOTPAR
SHOTPUT
THESPIS
THIGPEN
THIMPHU
THRUPUT
THUMPED
THUMPER
WHAPPED
WHELPED
WHIMPER
WHIPPED
WHIPPER
WHIPPET
WHIPPLE
WHISPER
WHOMPED
WHOOPED
WHOOPEE
WHOOPER
WHOOPIE
WHOPPED
WHOPPER
WHUPPED

•H•••P•

CHALUPA
CHINUPS
CHUTZPA
PHILIPK
PHILIPS
PHILIPV
SHRIMPS
SHRIMPY
THEALPS
THECAPE
THEHOPE
THEPIPS
THEPOPE
THERAPY
THEROPE
THEVIPS
THEYIPS
THREEPM

•H••••P

CHAINUP
CHALKUP
CHATSUP
CHECKUP
CHEERUP
CHEWSUP
CHIPSUP
CHIRRUP
CHOKEUP
CHOPSUP
CHOSEUP
CHURNUP
PHARLAP
PHILLIP
PHONYUP
PHOTOOP
SHAKEUP
SHAPEUP
SHINEUP
SHOOKUP
SHOOTUP
SHOREUP
SHOWNUP
SHOWSUP
SHUTSUP
THEDEEP
THEFLOP
THEHELP
THELOOP
THEPUMP
THINKUP
THREEUP
THREWUP
THROWUP
WHATSUP
WHIPSUP

••HP•••

ASHPANS
ASHPITS

••H•P••

BEHAPPY

ECHAPPE
IMHAPPY
LSHAPED
OSHAPED
SSHAPED
TSHAPED
TSHAPES
UNHAPPY
UNHOPED
USHAPED
USHAPES
VSHAPED
VSHAPES
YSHAPED
YSHAPES

••H••P•
BEHAPPY
ECHAPPE
IMHAPPY
SCHLEPP
SCHLEPS
SCHNAPS
UNHAPPY
UNHASPS
UPHEAPS

••H•••P
APHILIP
ASHHEAP
IMHOTEP
SCHLEPP
SCHLUMP

•••HP••
BUSHPIG
DASHPOT
DISHPAN
HIGHPAY
JODHPUR
MOSHPIT
PUSHPIN

•••H•P•
ANYHOPE
BARHOPS
BISHOPS
BOBHOPE
CARHOPS
DAYHOPS
EIGHTPM
INSHAPE
JOBHOPS
LASHUPS
MISHAPS
MRCHIPS
NEWHOPE
PERHAPS
PUSHUPS
RESHAPE
RESHIPS
THEHOPE
UNSHIPS
UNWHIPT
WASHUPS

•••H••P
ASHHEAP
ASSHARP
DUCHAMP
EIGHTUP
GETHELP
GOTHELP
HIGHTOP
INAHEAP
LIGHTUP
LOTHROP
THEHELP
TOYHOOP
UNSHARP

••••H•P
AIRSHIP
ARTSHOP
BELLHOP
BIOCHIP
BOTCHUP
BRUSHUP
BUNCHUP
CATCHUP
COPSHOP
COUGHUP
FROTHUP
GETSHEP
GETSHIP
GUNSHIP
HITCHUP
JOBSHOP
KETCHUP
KINSHIP
LEFTHIP
MATCHUP
MIDSHIP
MISSHIP
NUNSHIP
OLDCHAP
ONECHIP
PATCHUP
PETSHOP
PRESHIP
PREWHIP
PROSHOP
PSYCHUP
PUNCHUP
RAGSHOP
REACHUP
REDCHIP
ROSEHIP
ROUGHUP
RUMSHOP
SKISHOP
SMASHUP
SOCKHOP
SONSHIP
TEASHOP
TOUCHUP
TOYSHOP
VERYHIP
WARSHIP
WEIGHUP
WORSHIP

H••••Q•
HIGHIQS

•H•Q•••
CHEQUER
CHEQUES

•••H•Q•
HIGHIQS
ONTHEQT

HR•••••
HRETHEL
HRYVNIA

H•R••••
HARBACH
HARBORS
HARBOUR
HARBURG
HARDDAY
HARDEES
HARDENS
HARDEST
HARDHAT
HARDHIT
HARDIER
HARDILY
HARDING
HARDISH
HARDPAN
HARDPUT
HARDSET
HARDSIX
HARDTEN
HARDTOP
HARDWAY
HARDWON
HARHARS
HARICOT
HARKENS
HARKING
HARLAND
HARLEYS
HARLINE
HARLOTS
HARMERS
HARMFUL
HARMING
HARMONY
HARNESS
HARNICK
HAROLDI
HARPERS
HARPIES
HARPING
HARPIST
HARPOON
HARPSON
HARRAHS
HARRIED
HARRIER
HARRIES
HARRIET
HARRODS
HARROLD
HARROWS
HARSHEN
HARSHER
HARSHLY
HARTACK
HARTLEY
HARTMAN
HARTMUT
HARVARD
HARVEST
HARWELL
HERALDS
HERBAGE
HERBALS
HERBART
HERBAUT
HERBERT
HERBIER
HERBTEA
HERCULE
HERDERS
HERDING
HEREDIA
HEREIAM
HERENOW
HERESTO
HERETIC
HERITOR
HERMANA
HERMANN
HERMANO
HERMANS
HERMITS
HERMOSA
HERMOSO
HERNANI
HERNDON
HERNIAE
HERNIAS
HERNIBS
HEROICS
HEROINE
HEROISM
HERONRY
HERPETO
HERRICK
HERRING
HERRIOT
HERSELF
HERSHEY
HIRABLE
HIRCINE
HIREDON
HIREOUT
HIRESON
HIRSUTE
HORATIO
HORDING
HORIZON
HORMONE
HORNETS
HORNIER
HORNING
HORNISH
HORNIST
HORNSBY
HORNSIN
HORNUNG
HORRIFY
HORRORS
HORSIER
HORSILY
HORSING
HORSLEY
HORVITZ
HURDLED
HURDLER
HURDLES
HURLERS
HURLING
HURRAHS
HURRAYS
HURRIED
HURRIER
HURRIES
HURRYUP
HURSTON
HURTERS
HURTFOR
HURTFUL
HURTING
HURTLED
HURTLES
HYRACES
HYRAXES

H••R•••
HAARLEM
HADRIAN
HADRONS
HADROOM
HAIRCUT
HAIRDOS
HAIRDYE
HAIRGEL
HAIRIER
HAIRNET
HAIRPIN
HARRAHS
HARRIED
HARRIER
HARRIES
HARRIET
HARRODS
HARROLD
HARROWS
HASROOM
HATRACK
HATREDS
HAYRACK
HAYRICK
HAYRIDE
HEARDOF
HEARERS
HEARING
HEARKEN
HEAROUT
HEARSAY
HEARSES
HEARSOF
HEARTED
HEARTEN
HEARTHS
HEBRAIC
HEBREWS
HEIRDOM
HEIRESS
HENREID
HENRICH
HENRIES
HENRYII
HENRYIV
HENRYVI
HERRICK
HERRING
HERRIOT
HEURIGE
HEYRUBE
HIPROOF
HOARDED
HOARDER
HOARIER
HOARILY
HOARSEN
HOARSER
HOORAHS
HOORAYS
HORRIFY
HORRORS
HOTRODS
HOTROLL
HURRAHS
HURRAYS
HURRIED
HURRIER
HURRIES
HURRYUP
HYBRIDS
HYDRANT
HYDRATE
HYDRIDE
HYDROUS

H•••R••
HADAROW
HAGERTY
HALFRAW
HALFROD
HASAROW
HATBRIM
HAVARTI
HAWORTH
HAZARDS
HEATRAY
HEGIRAS
HENDRIX
HENDRYX
HEPARIN
HEYMRDJ
HIBERNO
HIGHRES
HOFBRAU
HOGARTH
HOMBRES
HOMERED
HOMERIC
HOMERUN
HONORED
HONOREE
HONORER
HOVERED
HOVERER
HOWARDK
HOWARDS
HOWARDU
HUMDRUM
HUMERAL
HUMERUS
HUMORAL
HUMORED
HUMORME
HUNDRED
HYPERON

H••••R•
HACKERS
HAGGARD
HAILERS
HALTERS
HALVERS
HALYARD
HAMBURG
HAMMERS
HAMPERS
HANDERS
HANGARS
HANGERS
HANKERS
HANSARP
HARBORS
HARBURG
HARHARS
HARMERS
HARPERS
HARVARD
HASTERT
HATTERS
HAULERS
HAWKERS
HAWSERS
HAYFORK
HAYWARD
HAYWIRE
HEADERS
HEALERS
HEAPERS
HEARERS
HEATERS
HEAVERS
HECKART
HECTARE
HECTORS
HEDGERS
HEEDERS
HEELERS
HEFTERS
HEIFERS
HELOTRY
HELPERS
HEMMERS
HENNERY
HEPBURN
HERBART
HERBERT
HERDERS
HERONRY
HEYWARD
HHMUNRO
HICKORY
HIGHART
HILAIRE
HILBERT
HILLARY
HINDERS
HINTERS
HISSERS
HISTORY
HITHERE
HITTERS
HOAXERS
HOCKERS
HOFSTRA
HOGGERY
HOHNERS
HOLBERG
HOLDERS
HOLLERS
HOLYARK
HOMBURG
HONIARA
HONKERS
HONOURS
HOOFERS
HOOPERS
HOOTERS
HOOVERS
HOPPERS
HORRORS
HOSIERS
HOSIERY
HOTCARS
HOTWARS
HOTWIRE
HOWLERS
HUBBARD
HUGGERS
HULLERS
HUMBARD
HUMBERT
HUMMERS
HUMOURS
HUMPHRY
HUNGARY
HUNGERS
HUNKERS
HUNTERS
HUPPERT
HURLERS
HURTERS
HUSKERS
HUSSARS
HUSSERL
HYMNARY

H•••••R
HACKLER
HADOVER
HAGGLER
HAIRIER
HAMMIER
HAMSTER
HANAPER
HANDCAR
HANDIER
HANDLER
HANOVER
HAPPIER
HARBOUR
HARDIER
HARRIER
HARSHER
HASOVER
HASTIER
HATCHER
HAUNTER
HAUTEUR
HAVENER
HEADFOR
HEADIER
HEATHER
HEATTER
HEAVIER
HECKLER
HEDGIER
HEFTIER
HEMPIER
HERBIER
HERITOR
HIBBLER
HIGGLER
HIGHBAR
HILLIER
HINKIER
HIPPIER
HIPSTER
HISSIER
HITCHER
HITSFOR
HJALMAR
HOARDER
HOARIER
HOARSER
HOBBLER
HOISTER
HOLSTER
HOLYWAR
HOMAGER
HOMEIER
HONORER
HOOSIER
HOPEFOR
HOPOVER
HOPPIER
HORNIER
HORSIER
HOSTLER
HOTOVER
HOTSPUR
HOUNDER
HOVERER
HOWEVER
HUDDLER
HUFFIER
HULKIER
HUMBLER
HUMIDOR
HUMPIER
HUNKIER
HUNTFOR
HURDLER
HURRIER
HURTFOR
HUSKIER
HUSTLER

•HR••••
CHRISMS
CHRISOM
CHRISTA
CHRISTI
CHRISTO
CHRISTY
CHROMAT
CHROMED
CHROMES
CHROMIC
CHRONIC
EHRLICH
PHRASAL
PHRASED
PHRASES
PHRENIC
PHRYGIA
SHRIEKS
SHRIKES
SHRILLS
SHRILLY
SHRIMPS
SHRIMPY
SHRINED
SHRINER
SHRINES
SHRINKS
SHRIVEL
SHRIVER
SHRIVES
SHROUDS
SHRUBBY
THRALLS
THREADS
THREADY
THREATS
THREEAD
THREEAM
THREEBC
THREEEE
THREENO
THREEPM
THREERS
THREEUP
THREWAT
THREWIN
THREWON
THREWUP
THRIFTS
THRIFTY
THRILLA
THRILLS
THRIVED
THRIVEN
THRIVER
THRIVES
THROATS
THROATY
THRONES
THRONGS
THROUGH
THROWAT
THROWER
THROWIN
THROWON
THROWUP
THRUPUT
THRUSTS
THRUWAY

•H•R•••
CHARADE
CHARCOT
CHARGED
CHARGER
CHARGES
CHARIER
CHARILY
CHARING
CHARIOT
CHARITY
CHARLES
CHARLEY
CHARLIE
CHARMAN
CHARMED
CHARMEN
CHARMER
CHARMIN
CHARNIN
CHARPAK
CHARRED
CHARRER
CHARROS
CHARTED
CHARTER
CHARVET
CHERISH
CHEROOT
CHERUBS
CHERVIL
CHIRICO
CHIRPED
CHIRPER
CHIRRED
CHIRRUP
CHORALE
CHORALS
CHORDAL
CHORDED
CHORINE
CHORIST
CHORIZO
CHORTLE
CHURCHY
CHURNED
CHURNER
CHURNUP
CHURROS
CHYRONS
DHARMAS
DHARMIC
DHURRIE
GHERKIN
KHARKOV
PHARAOH
PHARLAP
PHARYNX
SHAREIN
SHARERS
SHARING
SHARKEY
SHARONA
SHARPED
SHARPEI
SHARPEN
SHARPER
SHARPIE
SHARPLY
SHERBET
SHERIFF
SHERIFS
SHERMAN
SHERPAS
SHERWIN
SHIRKED
SHIRKER
SHIRLEY
SHIRRED
SHOREUP
SHORING
SHORTED
SHORTEN
SHORTER
SHORTIE
SHORTLY
SHORTOF
THERAMS
THERAPY
THEREAT
THEREBY
THEREDS
THEREIN
THERENT
THEREOF
THEREON
THERESA
THERETO
THERIAC
THERING
THERINK
THERITZ
THERMAL
THERMIC
THERMOS
THEROBE
THEROCK
THEROOM
THEROPE
THEROSE
THEROUX
THERULE
THIRDLY
THIRSTS
THIRSTY
THOREAU
THORIUM
THORNED
THORSON
THURBER
THURGAU
THURMAN
THYROID
WHARFED
WHARTON
WHARVES
WHEREAS
WHEREAT
WHEREBY
WHEREIN
WHERELL
WHEREOF
WHEREON
WHERERE
WHERETO
WHEREVE
WHIRLED
WHIRLER
WHIRRED
WHORLED

•H••R••
CHAGRIN
CHAIRED
CHAKRAS
CHARRED
CHARRER
CHARROS
CHEERED
CHEERER
CHEERIO
CHEERON
CHEERUP
CHETRUM
CHEVRES
CHEVRET
CHEVRON
CHIRRED
CHIRRUP
CHLORIC
CHOIRED
CHURROS
DHURRIE
IHEARYA
OHCAROL
SHADROE
SHAGRUG
SHEARED
SHEARER
SHECRAB
SHEERED
SHEERER
SHEERLY
SHIRRED
SHYFROM
THEARMY
THEARTS
THEBRAT
THECRAB
THECROW
THEFRUG
THEOREM
THETREE
THETRIB
THIERRY
THWARTS
WHIRRED
WHWORDS

•H•••R•
CHAFERS
CHAMBRE
CHANTRY
CHASERS
CHEDERS
CHEWERS
CHICORY
CHIDERS
CHIMERA
CHIMERS
CHOKERS
CHOLERA
CHOLERS
HHMUNRO
OHIOART
PHAEDRA
PHASERS
PHILTRE
PHONERS

RHETORS
RHUBARB
RHYMERS
SHADERS
SHAKERS
SHAKIRA
SHANGRI
SHAPERS
SHAPIRO
SHARERS
SHASTRI
SHAVERS
SHEPARD
SHINERS
SHIVERS
SHIVERY
SHOFARS
SHOVERS
SHOWERS
SHOWERY
SHUBERT
THALERS
THAWERS
THEATRE
THEBARD
THECARS
THEFIRM
THEHERO
THEJERK
THELARK
THETURN
THIERRY
THREERS
WHALERS
WHERERE
WHINERS

•H••••R

CHAFFER
CHAMBER
CHAMFER
CHAMPER
CHANCER
CHANGER
CHANTER
CHAPTER
CHARGER
CHARIER
CHARMER
CHARRER
CHARTER
CHASTER
CHATTER
CHAUCER
CHEAPER
CHEATER
CHECKER
CHEDDAR
CHEEPER
CHEERER
CHEEVER
CHENIER
CHEQUER
CHESTER
CHEWIER
CHIGGER
CHILLER
CHIPPER
CHIRPER
CHITTER
CHOICER
CHOKIER
CHOOSER
CHOPPER
CHOWDER
CHUGGER
CHUKKER
CHURNER
PHATTER
PHILTER
PHISHER
PHONIER
SHADIER
SHAFFER
SHAKIER
SHALIER
SHANKAR
SHANTER
SHARPER
SHATNER
SHATTER
SHEARER
SHEBEAR
SHEDDER
SHEERER
SHEFFER
SHELLER
SHELTER
SHELVER
SHIFTER
SHIMMER
SHINIER
SHIPPER
SHIRKER
SHOCKER
SHOOTER
SHOPFOR
SHOPPER
SHORTER
SHOTFOR
SHOTPAR
SHOUTER
SHOWIER
SHRINER
SHRIVER
SHUCKER
SHUDDER
SHUNTER
SHUSTER
SHUTTER
SHYSTER
THANKER
THEATER
THEBEAR
THEODOR
THESTAR
THETOUR
THEUSSR
THICKER
THINAIR
THINKER
THINNER
THITHER
THRIVER
THROWER
THUMPER
THUNDER
THURBER
THUSFAR
WHACKER
WHATFOR
WHEELER
WHEEZER
WHETHER
WHETTER
WHIFFER
WHIMPER
WHINIER
WHIPPER
WHIRLER
WHISKER
WHISPER
WHITHER
WHIZZER
WHOEVER
WHOOPER
WHOPPER
WHYEVER

••HR•••

ASHRAMS
ATHRILL
BAHRAIN
BAHREIN
BEHRENS
BEHRING
BEHRMAN
BOHRIUM
EPHRAIM
OCHROID
OCHROUS

••H•R••

ACHERON
ADHERED
ADHERER
ADHERES
AMHARIC
AMHERST
ASHTRAY
ASHTREE
ATHIRST
COHERED
COHERER
COHERES
COHORTS
DEHIRED
DEHIRES
DEHORNS
DOHERTY
ETHERIC
EXHORTS
INHERED
INHERES
INHERIT
ITHIRTY
MAHARIS
MRHORSE
REHIRED
REHIRES
SAHARAN
SCHERZI
SCHERZO
SCHIRRA
SPHERAL
SPHERED
SPHERES
SPHERIC
SUHARTO
TEHERAN
TOHORSE
TSHIRTS
UNHARDY
UNHARSH
UNHIRED
UNHIRES
UNHORSE
USHERED
USHERIN
VIHARAS

••H••R•

ASHBERY
ASHBURN
ASHBURY
ASHFORD
ASHLARS
ATHEART
ATHWART
BEHEARD
BYHEART
CAHIERS
COHEIRS
DEHAIRS
ECHOERS
EPHEDRA
EXHEDRA
FTHENRY
HOHNERS
LEHAVRE
MAHZORS
MCHENRY
MOHAIRS
OXHEART
REHEARD
REHEARS
SCHIRRA
TOHEART
UNHAIRS
UNHAIRY
UNHEARD
UPHOARD

••H•••R

ACHEFOR
ADHERER
ASHIVER
COHERER
EXHUMER
INHALER
INHUMER
REHONOR
SCHEMER
SCHMEAR
SCHMEER
SCHOLAR
SCHUMER
TOHOMER

•••HR••

ANTHRAX
ATTHREE
COCHRAN
DISHRAG
ENTHRAL
EUCHRED
EUCHRES
GUTHRIE
HIGHRES
INTHREE
KATHRYN
LOTHROP
MACHREE
MITHRAS
MOCHRIE
MPTHREE
NEPHRIC
ONTHREE
PUSHROD
UPTHROW
WASHRAG

•••H•R•

AIRHORN
ALLHERE
ALPHARD
ALTHORN
AMPHORA
ANCHORS
ANTHERS
ARCHERS
ARCHERY
ARTHURC
ARTHURM
ARTHURS
ASSHARP
ATTHIRD
AUTHORS
BASHERS
BATHERS
BEAHERO
BECHARM
BETHERE
BIGHORN
BOKHARA
BOTHERS
BUKHARA
BUSHERS
CARHORN
CIPHERS
COSHERS
COWHERD
CYPHERS
DASHERS
DIEHARD
DITHERS
DITHERY
EARHART
EATHERE
ECKHART
ELKHART
ESCHERS
ETCHERS
FATHERS
FISHERS
FISHERY
FISHFRY
FOGHORN
FORHIRE
FUTHARK
GATHERS
GETHURT
GOPHERS
GOTHURT
GUSHERS
HARHARS
HIGHART
HITHERE
IMTHERE
INCHERS
INKHORN
INSHORE
INSHORT
INTHERE
INTHIRD
ITSHERE
JOSHERS
KITHARA
KOSHERS
LASHERS
LATHERS
LATHERY
LECHERS
LEGHORN
MASHERS
MATHERS
MOSHERS
MOTHERS
MOTHERY
MULHARE
MUSHERS
NEWHART
NEWHIRE
NONHERO
NOSHERS
NOTHERE
NOWHERE
ONSHORE
ORCHARD
OUTHERE
OUTHIRE
OUTHURL
PETHARE
POTHERB
POTHERS
PUSHERS
RASHERS
RECHART
RESHARE
RICHARD
ROTHIRA
RUSHERS
SAXHORN
SEAHERO
SEEHERE
SENHORA
SIGHERS
SOTHERE
SOTHERN
TETHERS
THEHERO
TINHORN
TITHERS
TOOHARD
TOSHIRO
TRYHARD
TUSHERY
UNCHARY
UNCHURN
UNSHARP
UNSHORN
UNSHORT
UPTHERE
UPWHIRL
WARHERO
WASHERS
WISHERS
WITHERS
YOGHURT
YOTHERS
ZACHARY
ZEPHYRS
ZITHERS

•••H••R

BADHAIR
BIGHAIR
BOCHNER
BONHEUR
BUCHNER
BUSHIER
BYAHAIR
CASHBAR
CASHIER
CATHAIR
COCHAIR
CUSHIER
DASHIER
DICHTER
DISHIER
DOGHAIR
FECHNER
FIGHTER
FISHFOR
FISHIER
GUSHIER
HIGHBAR
ITCHFOR
ITCHIER
JODHPUR
KASHMIR
KOEHLER
LIGHTER
LOTHAIR
LUSHIER
LUTHIER
MANHOUR
MESHIER
MISHEAR
MOTHIER
MUSHIER
MYNHEER
NIGHTER
OFFHOUR
ONEHOUR
OUTHEAR
PETHAIR
PITHIER
PUSHFOR
PUSHIER
REDHAIR
RICHLER
RICHTER
RIGHTER
RUSHIER
SIGHFOR
SIGHTER
TIGHTER
TOAHAIR
TWOHOUR
UNCHAIR
UNSHEER
UNSHIER
UNSHYER
WASHIER
WEEHOUR
WISHFOR
YACHTER

••••HR•

ERYTHRO
HUMPHRY
SEETHRU

••••H•R

ANOTHER
BEECHER
BELCHER
BENCHER
BLATHER
BLITHER
BLUSHER
BOTCHER
BOUCHER
BRASHER
BROTHER
BRUSHER
BULGHUR
BURGHER
BUTCHER
CAMPHOR
CATCHER
CLASHER
CRASHER
CRUSHER
DITCHER
FARTHER
FEATHER
FETCHER
FILCHER
FISCHER
FLASHER
FLUSHER
FRESHER
FROTHER
FURTHER
GAUCHER
GNASHER
GUNTHER
HARSHER
HATCHER
HEATHER
HITCHER
IRISHER
KUTCHER
LAUGHER
LEACHER
LEATHER
LOATHER
LUNCHER
LURCHER
MARCHER
MATCHER
MOOCHER
MOUTHER
MUNCHER
NEITHER
NOOTHER
NORTHER
NOTCHER
PANTHER
PATCHER
PERCHER
PHISHER
PINCHER
PITCHER
PLUSHER
POACHER
PUNCHER
RANCHER
REACHER
REUTHER
ROUGHER
SLASHER
SLATHER
SLITHER
SMASHER
SMOTHER
SOOTHER
SULPHUR
TEACHER
TEETHER
TEICHER
THITHER
TORCHER
TOUCHER
TOUGHER
TRASHER
VOUCHER
WALTHER
WATCHER
WEATHER
WEIGHER
WERNHER
WERTHER
WHETHER
WHITHER
WINCHER
WRITHER

•••••HR

NIEBUHR

H•S••••

HASACOW
HASAFIT
HASAGAS
HASANIP
HASAROW
HASASAY
HASASET
HASATIT
HASBEEN
HASDONE
HASFITS
HASHING
HASHISH
HASHOUT
HASIDIC
HASIDIM
HASKELL
HASOVER
HASPING
HASPULL
HASROOM
HASSIUM
HASSLED
HASSLES
HASSOCK
HASTENS
HASTERT
HASTIER
HASTILY
HASTIME
HASTING
HASTOBE
HESHVAN
HESSAFE
HESSIAN
HISNIBS
HISPANO
HISPEED
HISSERS
HISSIER
HISSING
HISTORY
HOSANNA
HOSCALE
HOSIERS
HOSIERY
HOSKINS
HOSPICE
HOSTAGE
HOSTELS
HOSTESS
HOSTILE
HOSTING
HOSTLER
HUSBAND
HUSHABY
HUSHFUL
HUSHING
HUSKERS
HUSKIER
HUSKIES
HUSKILY
HUSKING
HUSSARS
HUSSEIN
HUSSERL
HUSSIES
HUSSITE
HUSTLED
HUSTLER
HUSTLES
HYSSOPS

H••S•••

HADSOME
HALSTON
HAMSTER
HANSARP
HANSOLO
HANSOMS
HARSHEN
HARSHER
HARSHLY
HASSIUM
HASSLED
HASSLES
HASSOCK
HATSIZE
HATSOFF
HAWSERS
HAYSEED
HEISMAN
HEISTED
HELSING
HEMSLEY
HENSLEY
HERSELF
HERSHEY
HESSAFE
HESSIAN
HEXSIGN
HIMSELF
HIPSTER
HIRSUTE
HISSERS
HISSIER
HISSING
HITSFOR
HITSHOW
HITSOFF
HITSONG
HITSOUT
HOBSONS
HOFSTRA
HOISTED
HOISTER
HOISTUP
HOLSTER
HOOSIER
HOPSING
HOPSOFF
HOPSOUT
HORSIER
HORSILY
HORSING
HORSLEY
HOTSEAT
HOTSHOT
HOTSOUP
HOTSPOT
HOTSPUR
HOUSING
HOUSMAN
HOUSSAY
HOUSTON
HURSTON
HUSSARS
HUSSEIN
HUSSERL
HUSSIES
HUSSITE
HYSSOPS

H•••S••

HACKSAW
HACKSIT
HACKSUP
HADASAY
HADASET
HALFSHY
HANDSAW
HANDSEL
HANDSET
HANDSIN
HANDSON
HANDSUP
HANGSBY
HANGSIN
HANGSON
HANGSUP
HARDSET
HARDSIX
HARPSON
HASASAY
HASASET
HATESIT
HAULSIN
HAULSUP
HAYESES
HDTVSET
HEADSAW
HEADSET
HEADSIN
HEADSTO
HEADSUP
HEALSUP
HEAPSOF
HEAPSON
HEAPSUP
HEARSAY
HEARSES
HEARSOF
HEATSUP
HEDISON
HELPSIN
HELPSON
HELPSUP
HERESTO
HEXOSES
HIGHSEA
HIKESUP
HINTSAT
HIRESON
HOARSEN
HOARSER
HOCUSED
HOLDSIN
HOLDSIT
HOLDSON
HOLDSTO
HOLDSUP
HOLESUP
HOLISTS
HOLYSEE
HOMESIN
HONESIN
HONESTY
HONKSAT
HOOFSIT
HOOKSON
HOOKSUP
HOOTSAT
HOPESSO
HOPESTO
HORNSBY
HORNSIN
HOUSSAY
HOWLSAT
HUMUSES
HUNTSUP
HYPESUP

H••••S•

HADBEST
HAGGISH
HAIMISH
HAPLESS
HARDEST
HARDISH
HARNESS
HARPIST
HARVEST
HASHISH
HATLESS
HAWKISH
HAZIEST
HEIRESS
HELLISH
HELOISE
HENNISH
HEPPEST
HERMOSA
HERMOSO
HEROISM
HIGHEST
HIGHISH
HIPLESS
HIPNESS
HIPPEST
HIPPISH
HITLESS
HITLIST
HOBOISM
HOGGISH
HOGNOSE
HOGWASH
HOKIEST
HOLIEST
HOMIEST
HOPEDSO
HOPESSO
HORNISH
HORNIST
HOSTESS
HOTNESS
HOTTEST
HOWELSE
HUELESS
HUFFISH
HUNNISH

H•••••S

HABILIS
HACKERS
HACKIES
HACKLES
HADAGAS
HADFITS
HADRONS
HAGGLES
HAIKAIS
HAILERS
HAIRDOS
HALALAS
HALFIES
HALIDES
HALITES
HALLEYS
HALLOOS
HALLOWS

HALOIDS
HALTERS
HALVAHS
HALVERS
HAMITES
HAMLETS
HAMMERS
HAMPERS
HAMULUS
HANDERS
HANDLES
HANGARS
HANGBYS
HANGERS
HANGUPS
HANKERS
HANKIES
HANSOMS
HAPLESS
HAPPENS
HAPTICS
HARBORS
HARDEES
HARDENS
HARHARS
HARKENS
HARLEYS
HARLOTS
HARMERS
HARNESS
HARPERS
HARPIES
HARRAHS
HARRIES
HARRODS
HARROWS
HASAGAS
HASFITS
HASSLES
HASTENS
HATCHES
HATFULS
HATLESS
HATPINS
HATREDS
HATTERS
HAULERS
HAVANAS
HAWHAWS
HAWKERS
HAWKINS
HAWSERS
HAYESES
HAYINGS
HAYMOWS
HAZARDS
HAZINGS
HAZMATS
HEADERS
HEALERS
HEAPERS
HEARERS
HEARSES
HEARTHS
HEATERS
HEAVENS
HEAVERS
HEAVIES

HEBREWS
HECKLES
HECKYES
HECTORS
HEDGERS
HEEDERS
HEEHAWS
HEELERS
HEFTERS
HEGIRAS
HEHHEHS
HEIFERS
HEIGHTS
HEINOUS
HEIRESS
HELICES
HELIXES
HELLOES
HELLYES
HELMETS
HELPERS
HEMMERS
HENBITS
HENRIES
HEPCATS
HEPTADS
HERALDS
HERBALS
HERDERS
HERMANS
HERMITS
HERNIAS
HERNIBS
HEROICS
HEXANES
HEXNUTS
HEXOSES
HEYDAYS
HEYMANS
HGWELLS
HICCUPS
HICKEYS
HIDEOUS
HIDINGS
HIGGINS
HIGGLES
HIGHIQS
HIGHRES
HIJACKS
HIJINKS
HILTONS
HINDERS
HINNIES
HINTERS
HIPLESS
HIPNESS
HIPPIES
HISNIBS
HISSERS
HITCHES
HITLESS
HITTERS
HOAGIES
HOAXERS
HOBBIES
HOBBITS
HOBBLES
HOBNOBS

HOBSONS
HOCKERS
HOGNUTS
HOGTIES
HOHNERS
HOLDERS
HOLDUPS
HOLISTS
HOLLERS
HOLLIES
HOLLOWS
HOMAGES
HOMBRES
HONCHOS
HONKERS
HONOURS
HOOCHES
HOODIES
HOODOOS
HOOFERS
HOOHAHS
HOOKAHS
HOOKUPS
HOOPERS
HOOPLAS
HOOPOES
HOORAHS
HOORAYS
HOOTERS
HOOVERS
HOPKINS
HOPPERS
HORNETS
HORRORS
HOSIERS
HOSKINS
HOSTELS
HOSTESS
HOTBEDS
HOTCAPS
HOTCARS
HOTCUPS
HOTDAYS
HOTDOGS
HOTKEYS
HOTLIPS
HOTNESS
HOTONES
HOTPOTS
HOTRODS
HOTTEAS
HOTTIES
HOTTIPS
HOTTUBS
HOTWARS
HOWARDS
HOWDAHS
HOWELLS
HOWLERS
HOYDENS
HUBBIES
HUBBUBS
HUBCAPS
HUDDLES
HUELESS
HUGGERS
HUGGIES
HUGGINS

HULLERS
HUMBLES
HUMBUGS
HUMERUS
HUMMELS
HUMMERS
HUMOURS
HUMUSES
HUMVEES
HUNCHES
HUNGERS
HUNKERS
HUNNYBS
HUNTERS
HUPPAHS
HURDLES
HURLERS
HURRAHS
HURRAYS
HURRIES
HURTERS
HURTLES
HUSKERS
HUSKIES
HUSSARS
HUSSIES
HUSTLES
HUTCHES
HUYGENS
HUZZAHS
HYANNIS
HYBRIDS
HYDROUS
HYGINUS
HYMNALS
HYPHENS
HYRACES
HYRAXES
HYSSOPS

•H•S•••

AHASSLE
AHOSTOF
CHASERS
CHASING
CHASMAL
CHASMIC
CHASSED
CHASSES
CHASSIS
CHASTEN
CHASTER
CHESTED
CHESTER
CHISELS
CHOSEUP
GHASTLY
GHOSTED
GHOSTLY
LHASANS
OHMSLAW
PHASEIN
PHASERS
PHASING
PHISHED
PHISHER
PHISHES
PHYSICS

SHASTRI
SHUSHED
SHUSHES
SHUSTER
SHYSTER
THESACK
THESAME
THESELF
THESEUS
THESHOW
THESIMS
THESPIS
THESTAR
THESUNS
THESWAN
THISDAY
THISONE
THISTLE
THISTLY
THISWAY
THUSFAR
THYSELF
WHISHED
WHISHES
WHISKAS
WHISKED
WHISKER
WHISKEY
WHISPER
WHISTLE
WHOSAID
WHOSOUT
WHOSWHO

•H••S••

AHASSLE
CHAISES
CHANSON
CHASSED
CHASSES
CHASSIS
CHATSUP
CHEESED
CHEESES
CHELSEA
CHEWSON
CHEWSUP
CHIPSIN
CHIPSUP
CHOMSKY
CHOOSER
CHOOSES
CHOOSEY
CHOPSUP
CHRISMS
CHRISOM
CHRISTA
CHRISTI
CHRISTO
CHRISTY
PHRASAL
PHRASED
PHRASES
SHEDSON
SHOOSIN
SHOPSAT
SHOWSIN
SHOWSUP

SHUTSIN
SHUTSUP
THATSIT
THATSOK
THEISMS
THEISTS
THEUSSR
THEYSAY
THIRSTS
THIRSTY
THOMSON
THORSON
THRUSTS
WHATSAY
WHATSIS
WHATSIT
WHATSUP
WHIPSAW
WHIPSIN
WHIPSUP
WHITSUN
WHOISIT
WHOOSIS
WHYISIT

•H•••S•

CHEMISE
CHEMIST
CHERISH
CHICEST
CHINESE
CHORIST
CHUMASH
CHUTIST
IHOPESO
RHENISH
RHYMIST
SHIATSU
SHYNESS
THEBEST
THEBOSS
THEBUSH
THEEAST
THEKISS
THEMASK
THEMOST
THEPOST
THERESA
THEROSE
THEUSSR
THINKSO
WHEYISH
WHITEST
WHITISH

•H••••S

AHCHOOS
CHABLIS
CHACHAS
CHAFERS
CHAINES
CHAISES
CHAKRAS
CHALCIS
CHALETS
CHALONS
CHAMOIS
CHANCES

CHANELS
CHANGES
CHAPELS
CHARGES
CHARLES
CHARROS
CHASERS
CHASSES
CHASSIS
CHAZANS
CHEDERS
CHEESES
CHEETAS
CHEETOS
CHEQUES
CHERUBS
CHEVETS
CHEVONS
CHEVRES
CHEWERS
CHIAPAS
CHICHAS
CHICHIS
CHICLES
CHIDERS
CHIGOES
CHILIES
CHILLIS
CHIMERS
CHINOIS
CHINUPS
CHISELS
CHITONS
CHIVIES
CHOICES
CHOKERS
CHOLERS
CHOLLAS
CHOOSES
CHORALS
CHOUGHS
CHRISMS
CHROMES
CHUPPAS
CHURROS
CHYRONS
DHARMAS
GHETTOS
LHASANS
OHIOANS
OHMAGES
PHASERS
PHEMIUS
PHENOLS
PHENOMS
PHIDIAS
PHILCOS
PHILEAS
PHILIPS
PHILOUS
PHINEAS
PHISHES
PHLOEMS
PHLOXES
PHOBIAS
PHOBICS
PHOEBES
PHOEBUS

PHONERS
PHONEYS
PHONICS
PHONIES
PHOTICS
PHOTOGS
PHOTONS
PHRASES
PHYLLIS
PHYLLOS
PHYSICS
RHEBOKS
RHETORS
RHOECUS
RHOMBUS
RHUMBAS
RHYMERS
RHYTHMS
SHADERS
SHADOWS
SHAKERS
SHAKOES
SHALOMS
SHAMANS
SHAPERS
SHARERS
SHAVERS
SHEATHS
SHEAVES
SHEIKHS
SHEILAS
SHEKELS
SHELVES
SHERIFS
SHERPAS
SHEVATS
SHIELDS
SHIITES
SHINERS
SHIVERS
SHNOOKS
SHOFARS
SHOGUNS
SHOOINS
SHOPKOS
SHOPPES
SHOVELS
SHOVERS
SHOWERS
SHRIEKS
SHRIKES
SHRILLS
SHRIMPS
SHRINES
SHRINKS
SHRIVES
SHROUDS
SHTETLS
SHTICKS
SHUSHES
SHUTINS
SHYNESS
THALERS
THAWERS
THEABCS
THEAGES
THEALPS
THEARTS

THEAXIS
THEBANS
THEBOSS
THEBOYS
THECARS
THECAVS
THECUBS
THEFEDS
THEHOGS
THEISMS
THEISTS
THEJETS
THEKISS
THEMAVS
THEMETS
THENETS
THENEWS
THEPIPS
THEPITS
THERAMS
THEREDS
THERMOS
THESEUS
THESIMS
THESPIS
THESUNS
THEVIPS
THEYIPS
THIEVES
THIRSTS
THRALLS
THREADS
THREATS
THREERS
THRIFTS
THRILLS
THRIVES
THROATS
THRONES
THRONGS
THRUSTS
THWACKS
THWARTS
WHALERS
WHARVES
WHATIFS
WHATSIS
WHEEZES
WHEREAS
WHINERS
WHISHES
WHISKAS
WHITENS
WHIZZES
WHOOSIS
WHWORDS

••H•S••

ACHESON
APHASIA
APHASIC
BEHESTS
COHOSTS
DEHISCE
EPHESUS
INHASTE
JOHNSON
SCHISMS

SCHISTS
UNHASPS
UNHASTY
UNHUSKS

••H••S•

ACHIEST
AMHERST
ASHIEST
ASHLESS
ATHEISM
ATHEIST
ATHIRST
BAHAISM
BAHAIST
ECHOISM
EXHAUST
INHOUSE
MAHDISM
MAHDIST
MRHORSE
OKHOTSK
OSHKOSH
REHOUSE
TOHORSE
UNHARSH
UNHORSE
UNHOUSE

••H•••S

ACHENES
ADHERES
APHIDES
ASHBINS
ASHCANS
ASHLARS
ASHLESS
ASHPANS
ASHPITS
ASHRAMS
ATHOMES
AXHEADS
BAHAMAS
BAHIANS
BEHAVES
BEHEADS
BEHESTS
BEHINDS
BEHOLDS
BEHRENS
CAHIERS
CAHOOTS
COHEIRS
COHERES
COHORTS
COHOSTS
DAHLIAS
DEHAIRS
DEHEXES
DEHIRES
DEHORNS
ECHOERS
EPHEBUS
EPHESUS
ETHANES
ETHENES
ETHNICS
EXHALES

EXHORTS
EXHUMES
HEHHEHS
HOHNERS
INHALES
INHERES
INHUMES
KAHUNAS
MAHARIS
MAHOUTS
MAHZORS
MCHALES
MOHAIRS
MOHAVES
MOHAWKS
MRHOBBS
NOHANDS
OAHUANS
OCHROUS
OXHIDES
REHANGS
REHAULS
REHEALS
REHEARS
REHEATS
REHEELS
REHIDES
REHIRES
REHONES
REHOOKS
SCHAYES
SCHEMAS
SCHEMES
SCHICKS
SCHISMS
SCHISTS
SCHLEPS
SCHLUBS
SCHMOES
SCHNAPS
SCHOLES
SCHOOLS
SPHERES
TAHINIS
TSHAPES
TSHIRTS
UNHAIRS
UNHANDS
UNHASPS
UNHEEDS
UNHELMS
UNHIRES
UNHOODS
UNHOOKS
UNHULLS
UNHUSKS
UPHEAPS
UPHILLS
UPHOLDS
USHAPES
VIHARAS
VSHAPES
WAHINES
WAHWAHS
YSHAPES

•••HS••

ARCHSEE

FUCHSIA
HIGHSEA
MACHSIX
SIGHSAT

•••H•S•

AIRHOSE
ARCHEST
BOOHISS
COCHISE
DEGHOST
DUCHESS
ENCHASE
ENTHUSE
HASHISH
HIGHEST
HIGHISH
INPHASE
LITHEST
LUSHEST
NIGHEST
OUTHISS
PACHISI
POSHEST
RASHEST
RECHOSE
REPHASE
RICHEST
SIKHISM
SOPHISM
SOPHIST
UPPHASE

•••H••S

AFGHANS
AHCHOOS
ANCHORS
ANTHEMS
ANTHERS
ARCHERS
ARCHIES
ARCHONS
ARTHURS
ASTHMAS
AUTHORS
BADHATS
BARHOPS
BASHERS
BATHERS
BAUHAUS
BBSHOTS
BETHELS
BICHONS
BIGHITS
BIGHUGS
BISHOPS
BOOHISS
BOOHOOS
BOTHERS
BRAHMAS
BUSHELS
BUSHERS
CACHETS
CARHOPS
CASHEWS
CASHINS
CEPHEUS
CIPHERS

COSHERS
CUSHAWS
CYPHERS
DAPHNES
DAPHNIS
DASHERS
DAYHOPS
DIRHAMS
DITHERS
DOSHOTS
DRCHAOS
DUCHESS
DUCHIES
EIGHTHS
ESCHERS
ESCHEWS
ETCHERS
EUCHRES
FATHERS
FATHOMS
FISHERS
GASHOGS
GATHERS
GOPHERS
GOTHICS
GRAHAMS
GUSHERS
HARHARS
HAWHAWS
HEEHAWS
HEHHEHS
HIGHIQS
HIGHRES
HOOHAHS
HYPHENS
INCHERS
ISOHELS
ISTHMUS
JOBHOPS
JOSHERS
KISHKES
KOSHERS
KUCHENS
LASHERS
LASHUPS
LATHERS
LECHERS
LICHEES
LICHENS
MARHAUS
MASHERS
MASHIES
MATHERS
MATHEWS
MATHIAS
MAYHEMS
METHODS
MILHOUS
MISHAPS
MISHITS
MITHRAS
MOSHERS
MOTHERS
MRCHIPS
MUDHENS
MUSHERS
NATHANS
NEPHEWS

NEWHATS
NICHOLS
NONHITS
NOSHERS
NOSHOWS
NOTHINS
OMAHANS
ORCHIDS
ORPHANS
ORPHEUS
OUTHISS
OUTHITS
PATHANS
PEAHENS
PERHAPS
POTHERS
PUSHERS
PUSHUPS
PYTHIAS
PYTHONS
QUAHOGS
RASHERS
RECHEWS
REDHATS
REDHENS
REDHOTS
RESHIPS
RESHOES
RESHOWS
RESHUTS
RETHAWS
RICHENS
ROCHETS
RUSHEES
RUSHERS
SACHEMS
SACHETS
SASHAYS
SEPHIAS
SIGHERS
SIPHONS
SKIHATS
SOPHIES
SUNHATS
TECHIES
TECHNOS
TEEHEES
TETHERS
THEHOGS
TINHATS
TITHERS
TOPHATS
TOWHEES
TOYHATS
TUSHIES
TVSHOWS
UNSHIPS
UNSHOES
UNTHAWS
UPSHOTS
URCHINS
UTAHANS
WASHERS
WASHUPS
WISHERS
WITHERS
WITHIES
YOOHOOS
YOTHERS
ZEPHYRS
ZITHERS

••••H•S

ABASHES
AGULHAS
AITCHES
ALIGHTS
ALLTHIS
APACHES
BACCHUS
BATCHES
BEACHES
BEECHES
BELCHES
BENCHES
BENTHOS
BERTHAS
BIRCHES
BLIGHTS
BLUSHES
BOTCHES
BOUCHES
BRASHES
BRIGHTS
BRUSHES
BUDDHAS
BUNCHES
BUQSHAS
BUTCHES
CANCHAS
CATCHES
CHACHAS
CHICHAS
CHICHIS
CINCHES
CLASHES
CLICHES
CLOCHES
CLOTHES
COACHES
COLCHIS
CONCHES
CONCHOS
COUCHES
CRASHES
CRECHES
CRUSHES
CULCHES
DITCHES
FETCHES
FILCHES
FINCHES
FLASHES
FLECHES
FLESHES
FLIGHTS
FLUSHES
FRESHES
FRIGHTS
GAUCHOS
GEISHAS
GENGHIS
GETTHIS
GNASHES
GOTCHAS
GULCHES
GURKHAS
HATCHES
HEIGHTS
HITCHES
HONCHOS
HOOCHES
HUNCHES
HUTCHES
KETCHES
KNIGHTS
KNISHES
KOOSHES
KWACHAS
LARCHES
LATCHES
LEACHES
LEASHES
LEECHES
LITCHIS
LOATHES
LUNCHES
LURCHES
MALTHUS
MARCHES
MARSHES
MATCHES
MEGOHMS
MEMPHIS
MERCHES
MOOCHES
MTATHOS
MULCHES
MUNCHES
MURPHYS
NAUGHTS
NAVAHOS
NOTCHES
NOUGHTS
NOWTHIS
NUDZHES
PARCHES
PATCHES
PEACHES
PERCHES
PHISHES
PINCHAS
PINCHES
PITCHES
PLASHES
PLIGHTS
PLUSHES
POACHES
PONCHOS
POOCHES
PORCHES
PORTHOS
POUCHES
PSYCHES
PSYCHOS
PUNCHES
PYRRHUS
QUASHES
QUICHES
RANCHES
RANCHOS
REACHES
RHYTHMS
ROACHES
SCATHES
SCYTHES
SEETHES
SHUSHES
SKOSHES
SLASHES
SLIGHTS
SLOSHES
SLUSHES
SMASHES
SMUSHES
SOOTHES
SPATHES
STASHES
STJOHNS
SWASHES
SWATHES
SWISHES
TEACHES
TEETHES
TENCHES
TOPTHIS
TORCHES
TOUCHES
TRASHES
TROCHES
VEIGHTS
VETCHES
VOUCHES
WATCHES
WEIGHTS
WENCHES
WHISHES
WINCHES
WITCHES
WOOSHES
WRIGHTS
WRITHES
YAMAHAS
ZILCHES

•••••HS

ALIYAHS
ANARCHS
BREATHS
BYPATHS
CALIPHS
CHOUGHS
DALETHS
DEARTHS
DEMOTHS
EIGHTHS
EMPATHS
EOLITHS
EPARCHS
EXARCHS
FELLAHS
FOURTHS
FRENCHS
GROWTHS
GULLAHS
HALVAHS
HARRAHS
HEARTHS
HEHHEHS
HOOHAHS
HOOKAHS
HOORAHS
HOWDAHS
HUPPAHS
HURRAHS
HUZZAHS
IOMOTHS
LENGTHS
LOOFAHS
MATZOHS
MULLAHS
OOMPAHS
PARAPHS
PARIAHS
PLINTHS
PLOUGHS
RUPIAHS
SAMEKHS
SERAPHS
SHEATHS
SHEIKHS
SLEIGHS
SLEUTHS
SLOUGHS
SMOOTHS
TEMPEHS
TROUGHS
VOTECHS
WAHWAHS
WEALTHS
WRAITHS
WREATHS
ZENITHS

H•T••••

HATABLE
HATBAND
HATBRIM
HATCHED
HATCHER
HATCHES
HATCHET
HATEDIT
HATEFUL
HATESIT
HATFULS
HATLESS
HATLIKE
HATPINS
HATRACK
HATREDS
HATSIZE
HATSOFF
HATTERS
HATTING
HDTVSET
HITACHI
HITBACK
HITCHED
HITCHER
HITCHES
HITCHON
HITCHUP
HITFILM
HITHERE
HITHOME
HITINTO
HITLESS
HITLIST
HITPLAY
HITSFOR
HITSHOW
HITSOFF
HITSONG
HITSOUT
HITTERS
HITTING
HITTITE
HITTOWN
HITTUNE
HITUPON
HOTBATH
HOTBEDS
HOTCAKE
HOTCAPS
HOTCARS
HOTCOAL
HOTCOMB
HOTCUPS
HOTDATE
HOTDAYS
HOTDOGS
HOTFOOT
HOTGLUE
HOTHAND
HOTHEAD
HOTITEM
HOTKEYS
HOTLEAD
HOTLICK
HOTLINE
HOTLINK
HOTLIPS
HOTMAIL
HOTMEAL
HOTMILK
HOTNESS
HOTONES
HOTOVER
HOTPACK
HOTPINK
HOTPOTS
HOTRODS
HOTROLL
HOTSEAT
HOTSHOT
HOTSOUP
HOTSPOT
HOTSPUR
HOTTEAS
HOTTEST
HOTTIES
HOTTIME
HOTTIPS
HOTTUBS
HOTTUNA
HOTWARS
HOTWIRE
HOTZONE
HUTCHES
HUTLIKE
HUTTING

H••T•••

HADTIME
HADTOBE
HAFTING
HAITIAN
HALTERS
HALTING
HAPTICS
HARTACK
HARTLEY
HARTMAN
HARTMUT
HASTENS
HASTERT
HASTIER
HASTILY
HASTIME
HASTING
HASTOBE
HATTERS
HATTING
HAUTBOY
HAUTEUR
HEATERS
HEATFAN
HEATFUL
HEATHEN
HEATHER
HEATING
HEATRAY
HEATSUP
HEATTER
HECTARE
HECTORS
HEFTERS
HEFTIER
HEFTILY
HEFTING
HENTOFF
HEPTADS
HILTING
HILTONS
HINTERS
HINTING
HINTSAT
HISTORY
HITTERS
HITTING
HITTITE
HITTOWN
HITTUNE
HOGTIED
HOGTIES
HOOTERS
HOOTING
HOOTOWL
HOOTSAT
HOPTOIT
HOSTAGE
HOSTELS
HOSTESS
HOSTILE
HOSTING
HOSTLER
HOTTEAS
HOTTEST
HOTTIES
HOTTIME
HOTTIPS
HOTTUBS
HOTTUNA
HOWTHEN
HRETHEL
HUNTERS
HUNTFOR
HUNTING
HUNTLEY
HUNTSUP
HURTERS
HURTFOR
HURTFUL
HURTING
HURTLED
HURTLES
HUSTLED
HUSTLER
HUSTLES
HUTTING

H•••T••

HABITAT
HABITED
HABITUE
HADATIT
HALITES
HALSTON
HAMITES
HAMITIC
HAMITUP
HAMPTON
HAMSTER
HANGTEN
HARDTEN
HARDTOP
HASATIT
HAUNTED
HAUNTER
HEALTHY
HEARTED
HEARTEN
HEARTHS
HEATTER
HEELTAP
HEISTED
HELOTRY
HEMATIC
HEMATIN
HEPATIC
HERBTEA
HERETIC
HERITOR
HIGHTEA
HIGHTOP
HILLTOP
HIPSTER
HOFSTRA
HOISTED
HOISTER
HOISTUP
HOLSTER
HOOPTOY
HORATIO
HOTITEM
HOUSTON
HUNGTEN
HURSTON
HYPATIA

H••••T•

HACKETT
HADFITS
HAGERTY
HAMLETS
HAMMETT
HANDYTO
HAPPYTO
HARLOTS
HASFITS
HAUGHTY
HAVARTI
HAWORTH
HAZLITT
HAZMATS
HEADSTO
HEAVETO
HEIFETZ
HEIGHTS
HELMETS
HENBITS
HEPCATS
HERESTO
HERMITS
HERPETO
HEWEDTO
HEWLETT
HEXNUTS
HIPBATH
HIPPITY
HIRSUTE
HITINTO
HITTITE
HOBBITS
HOGARTH
HOGNUTS
HOLDSTO
HOLISTS
HONESTY
HOPEDTO
HOPESTO
HOPINTO
HOPLITE
HORNETS
HORVITZ
HOTBATH
HOTDATE
HOTPOTS
HUANGTI
HUSSITE
HYALITE
HYDRATE

H•••••T

HABITAT
HACKETT
HACKSIT
HADAFIT
HADASET
HADATIT
HADBEST
HAIRCUT
HAIRNET
HALFCUT
HALFWIT
HALIBUT
HAMMETT
HANDOUT
HANDSET
HANGOUT
HARDEST
HARDHAT
HARDHIT
HARDPUT
HARDSET
HARICOT
HARPIST
HARRIET
HARTMUT
HARVEST
HASAFIT
HASASET
HASATIT
HASHOUT
HASTERT
HATCHET
HATEDIT
HATESIT
HAVENOT
HAVEOUT
HAYLOFT
HAZIEST
HAZLITT
HDTVSET
HEADOUT
HEADSET
HEAROUT
HECKART
HELDOUT
HELLCAT
HELPOUT
HEPPEST
HERBART
HERBAUT
HERBERT
HERRIOT
HEWLETT
HIDEOUT
HIGHART
HIGHEST
HIGHHAT
HIKEOUT
HILBERT
HINTSAT
HIPBOOT
HIPPEST
HIREOUT
HITLIST
HITSOUT
HOKIEST
HOLDOUT
HOLDSIT
HOLEOUT
HOLIEST
HOMIEST
HONKSAT
HOOFSIT
HOOTSAT
HOPENOT
HOPSOUT
HOPTOIT
HORNIST
HOTFOOT
HOTSEAT
HOTSHOT
HOTSPOT
HOTTEST
HOWBEIT
HOWLSAT
HUMBERT
HUNGOUT
HUPPERT
HYDRANT

•HT••••

SHTETLS
SHTICKS
SHTICKY

•H•T•••

BHUTANI
CHATEAU
CHATHAM
CHATSUP
CHATTED
CHATTEL
CHATTER
CHATWIN
CHETRUM
CHITLIN
CHITONS
CHITOWN
CHITTER
CHUTING
CHUTIST
CHUTNEY
CHUTZPA
GHETTOS
IHATEIT
KHATAMI
NHLTEAM
PHATTER
PHOTICS
PHOTOGS
PHOTOID
PHOTONS
PHOTOOP
RHETORS
RHYTHMS
SHATNER
SHATTER
SHOTFOR
SHOTGUN
SHOTOUT
SHOTPAR
SHOTPUT
SHUTEYE
SHUTINS
SHUTOFF
SHUTOUT
SHUTSIN
SHUTSUP
SHUTTER
SHUTTLE
THATCHY
THATONE
THATSIT
THATSOK
THATWAY
THETOUR
THETREE
THETRIB
THETUBE
THETURN
THITHER
WHATAMI
WHATFOR
WHATIFS
WHATNOT
WHATNOW
WHATSAY
WHATSIS
WHATSIT
WHATSUP
WHATTHE
WHETHER
WHETTED
WHETTER
WHITELY
WHITENS
WHITEST
WHITHER
WHITING
WHITISH
WHITMAN
WHITNEY
WHITSUN
WHITTLE

•H••T••

AHOSTOF
CHANTED
CHANTER
CHANTEY
CHANTRY
CHAOTIC
CHAPTER
CHARTED
CHARTER
CHASTEN
CHASTER
CHATTED
CHATTEL
CHATTER
CHEATED
CHEATER
CHEATIN
CHEATON
CHEETAH
CHEETAS
CHEETOS
CHESTED
CHESTER
CHEWTOY
CHINTZY
CHITTER
CHOCTAW
CHORTLE
GHASTLY
GHETTOS
GHOSTED
GHOSTLY
PHAETON
PHANTOM
PHATTER
PHILTER
PHILTRE
SHAFTED
SHANTER
SHASTRI
SHATTER
SHEATHE
SHEATHS
SHEETED
SHELTER
SHELTIE
SHIATSU
SHIFTED
SHIFTER
SHIHTZU
SHIITES
SHOOTAT
SHOOTBY
SHOOTER
SHOOTUP
SHORTED
SHORTEN
SHORTER
SHORTIE
SHORTLY
SHORTOF
SHOUTAT
SHOUTED
SHOUTER
SHTETLS
SHUNTED
SHUNTER
SHUSTER
SHUTTER
SHUTTLE
SHYSTER
THEATER
THEATRE
THESTAR
THISTLE
THISTLY
WHARTON
WHATTHE
WHEATEN
WHEATON
WHETTED
WHETTER
WHISTLE
WHITTLE

•H•••T•

CHALETS
CHAPATI
CHARITY
CHAYOTE
CHELATE
CHEVETS
CHIANTI
CHRISTA
CHRISTI
CHRISTO
CHRISTY
KHANATE
SHEVATS
THEARTS
THECITY
THEISTS
THEJETS
THEMETS
THENETS
THEOATH
THEPITS
THERETO
THERITZ
THIRSTS
THIRSTY
THREATS
THRIFTS

THRIFTY
THROATS
THROATY
THRUSTS
THWARTS
THWHITE
WHERETO

•H••••T
CHAPLET
CHARCOT
CHARIOT
CHARVET
CHEEZIT
CHEMIST
CHEROOT
CHEVIOT
CHEVRET
CHEWOUT
CHIAPET
CHICEST
CHICLET
CHILCAT
CHILKAT
CHORIST
CHROMAT
CHUCKIT
CHUTIST
IHATEIT
IHAVEIT
OHIOART
RHYMIST
SHABBAT
SHALLOT
SHAVUOT
SHEGOAT
SHERBET
SHIPOUT
SHOOTAT
SHOPSAT
SHOTOUT
SHOTPUT
SHOUTAT
SHOWCAT
SHOWOUT
SHUBERT
SHUTOUT
THATSIT
THAWOUT
THEBEST
THEBRAT
THEDIET
THEEAST
THEGIFT
THEHEAT
THELEFT
THEMOST
THEPOST
THEREAT
THERENT
THICKET
THINOUT
THOUGHT
THREWAT
THROWAT
THRUPUT
WHATNOT
WHATSIT
WHEREAT
WHIPPET
WHITEST
WHOISIT
WHOSOUT
WHYISIT
WHYWAIT

••HT•••
ACHTUNG
ASHTRAY
ASHTREE
SCHTICK
YAHTZEE

••H•T••
IMHOTEP
MAHATMA
OKHOTSK
REHITCH
UNHATED
UNHITCH

••H••T•
ASHANTI
ASHPITS
ATHLETE
BEHESTS
CAHOOTS
COHORTS
COHOSTS
DOHERTY
EXHORTS
INHASTE
ITHIRTY
MAHOUTS
NAHUATL
OCHENTA
REHEATS
SCHISTS
SCHLITZ
SCHMITT
SCHULTZ
SUHARTO
TSHIRTS
UNHASTY

••H•••T
ACHIEST
ADHIBIT
AMHERST
ASHIEST
ATHEART
ATHEIST
ATHIRST
ATHWART
BAHAIST
BYHEART
COHABIT
DEHMELT
EXHAUST
EXHIBIT
INHABIT
INHERIT
INHIBIT
MAHDIST
MRHULOT
OXHEART
SCHELDT
SCHMIDT
SCHMITT
TOHEART

•••HT••
BATHTUB
DICHTER
EIGHTAD
EIGHTAM
EIGHTBC
EIGHTEE
EIGHTHS
EIGHTPM
EIGHTUP
FIGHTER
HIGHTEA
HIGHTOP
JEPHTHA
LIGHTED
LIGHTEN
LIGHTER
LIGHTLY
LIGHTON
LIGHTUP
MACHTWO
MIGHTNT
NAPHTHA
NIGHTER
NIGHTIE
NIGHTLY
OUGHTNT
OUGHTTO
RICHTER
RIGHTED
RIGHTER
RIGHTLY
RIGHTON
SHIHTZU
SIGHTED
SIGHTER
SIGHTLY
TIGHTEN
TIGHTER
TIGHTLY
VECHTEN
WASHTUB
YACHTED
YACHTER
YACHTIE

•••H•T•
AKIHITO
BACHATA
BADHATS
BBSHOTS
BIGHITS
CACHETS
DOSHOTS
EBWHITE
ESTHETE
INWHITE
JAPHETH
MACHETE
MISHITS
NEWHATS
NONHITS
OUGHTTO
OUTHITS
REDHATS
REDHOTS
RESHUTS
ROCHETS
SACHETS
SAYHITO
SKIHATS
SUNHATS
THWHITE
TINHATS
TOPHATS
TOYHATS
UNWHITE
UPSHOTS
WICHITA

•••H••T
ARCHEST
ASPHALT
BATHMAT
CASHOUT
DASHDOT
DASHPOT
DEGHOST
DISHOUT
DRYHEAT
EARHART
ECKHART
EGGHUNT
ELKHART
ENCHANT
ESCHEAT
ETCHANT
FISHNET
FISHOUT
FOXHUNT
GASHEAT
GETHURT
GOTHURT
GUSHOUT
HASHOUT
HIGHART
HIGHEST
HIGHHAT
IDTHEFT
INSHORT
JOBHUNT
LASHOUT
LITHEST
LUSHEST
MANHUNT
MIGHTNT
MOSHPIT
NEWHART
NIGHEST
OILHEAT
OKSHOOT
ONTHEQT
ORPHANT
OUGHTNT
OUTHUNT
POSHEST
PREHEAT
PUSHOUT
RASHEST
RECHART
REDHEAT
RESHIFT
RESHOOT
RICHEST
RUSHOUT
SEAHUNT
SIGHSAT
SOPHIST
THEHEAT
TIMHOLT
UNSHIFT
UNSHORT
UNWHIPT
UPSHIFT
UPSHOOT
WASHOUT
WITHOUT
YEAHBUT
YOGHURT

••••HT•
ALIGHTS
BLIGHTS
BLIGHTY
BRIGHTS
DOUGHTY
DWIGHTD
FLIGHTS
FLIGHTY
FRIGHTS
HAUGHTY
HEIGHTS
IEIGHTY
KNIGHTS
LOATHTO
NAUGHTS
NAUGHTY
NOUGHTS
PITCHTO
PLIGHTS
SLIGHTS
TRASHTV
VEIGHTS
WATCHTV
WEIGHTS
WEIGHTY
WRIGHTS

••••H•T
ALLTHAT
BADSHOT
BAGEHOT
BASEHIT
BIGSHOT
BOWSHOT
CROCHET
EARSHOT
EPITHET
EYESHOT
FELTHAT
FIREHAT
FLATHAT
FLUSHOT
FRESHET
GETAHIT
GETSHOT
GOTAHIT
GUNSHOT
HARDHAT
HARDHIT
HATCHET
HIGHHAT
HOTSHOT
ITSAHIT
LAUGHAT
MEGAHIT
MUGSHOT
NOWWHAT
ONESHOT
ONEWHIT
OUTSHOT
OVERHOT
PINCHOT
POTSHOT
PROPHET
RAINHAT
RATCHET
RIMSHOT
ROUGHIT
SAYWHAT
SETSHOT
SILKHAT
SNOWHAT
TEESHOT
TWOSHOT
VERYHOT
WAPSHOT
WATCHIT
WELLHIT
WOOLHAT
WORTHIT

•••••HT
ALRIGHT
ATEIGHT
ATNIGHT
ATSIGHT
BORSCHT
BROUGHT
BYRIGHT
DELIGHT
DORIGHT
DRAUGHT
DROUGHT
ENRIGHT
FRAUGHT
FREIGHT
INSIGHT
MRRIGHT
ONSIGHT
REFIGHT
RELIGHT
RESIGHT
SLEIGHT
THOUGHT
TONIGHT
UNLIGHT
UNSIGHT
UPLIGHT
UPRIGHT
UPTIGHT
UTRECHT
WROUGHT

HU•••••
HUANGHE
HUANGTI
HUBBARD
HUBBELL
HUBBIES
HUBBUBS
HUBCAPS
HUDDLED
HUDDLER
HUDDLES
HUELESS
HUFFIER
HUFFILY
HUFFING
HUFFISH
HUFFMAN
HUGGERS
HUGGIES
HUGGING
HUGGINS
HULKIER
HULKING
HULLERS
HULLING
HULLOED
HUMANLY
HUMANUM
HUMBARD
HUMBERT
HUMBLED
HUMBLER
HUMBLES
HUMBUGS
HUMDRUM
HUMERAL
HUMERUS
HUMIDEX
HUMIDLY
HUMIDOR
HUMMELS
HUMMERS
HUMMING
HUMORAL
HUMORED
HUMORME
HUMOURS
HUMPHED
HUMPHRY
HUMPIER
HUMUSES
HUMVEES
HUNCHED
HUNCHES
HUNDRED
HUNGARY
HUNGERS
HUNGOFF
HUNGOUT
HUNGTEN
HUNKERS
HUNKIER
HUNLIKE
HUNNISH
HUNNYBS
HUNTERS
HUNTFOR
HUNTING
HUNTLEY
HUNTSUP
HUPPAHS
HUPPERT
HURDLED
HURDLER
HURDLES
HURLERS
HURLING
HURRAHS
HURRAYS
HURRIED
HURRIER
HURRIES
HURRYUP
HURSTON
HURTERS
HURTFOR
HURTFUL
HURTING
HURTLED
HURTLES
HUSBAND
HUSHABY
HUSHFUL
HUSHING
HUSKERS
HUSKIER
HUSKIES
HUSKILY
HUSKING
HUSSARS
HUSSEIN
HUSSERL
HUSSIES
HUSSITE
HUSTLED
HUSTLER
HUSTLES
HUTCHES
HUTLIKE
HUTTING
HUYGENS
HUZZAHS

H•U••••
HAUGHTY
HAULAGE
HAULERS
HAULING
HAULOFF
HAULSIN
HAULSUP
HAUNTED
HAUNTER
HAUTBOY
HAUTEUR
HEURIGE
HOUDINI
HOUNDED
HOUNDER
HOUSING
HOUSMAN
HOUSSAY
HOUSTON
HYUNDAI

H••U•••
HAMULUS
HANUKAH
HHMUNRO
HITUPON
HOCUSED
HUMUSES

H•••U••
HADPULL
HAMBURG
HANGUPS
HARBURG
HASPULL
HATFULS
HECKUVA
HELLUVA
HEPBURN
HERCULE
HEXNUTS
HEYJUDE
HEYRUBE
HICCUPS
HIRSUTE
HITTUNE
HOGNUTS
HOLDUPS
HOMBURG
HONOURS
HOOKUPS
HORNUNG
HOTCUPS
HOTTUBS
HOTTUNA
HOWDULL
HOWMUCH
HUBBUBS
HUMBUGS
HUMOURS

H••••U•
HABITUE
HACKSUP
HAFNIUM
HAHNIUM
HAIRCUT
HALFCUT
HALFDUG
HALIBUT
HAMITUP
HAMULUS
HANDFUL
HANDGUN
HANDOUT
HANDSUP
HANGOUT
HANGSUP
HARBOUR
HARDPUT
HARMFUL
HARTMUT
HASHOUT
HASSIUM
HATEFUL
HAULSUP
HAUTEUR
HAVEFUN
HAVEOUT
HEADFUL
HEADOUT
HEADSUP
HEALSUP
HEAPSUP
HEAROUT
HEATFUL
HEATSUP
HEEDFUL
HEINOUS
HELDOUT
HELPFUL
HELPOUT
HELPSUP
HERBAUT
HIDEOUS
HIDEOUT
HIKEDUP
HIKEOUT
HIKESUP
HIREOUT
HITCHUP
HITSOUT
HOISTUP
HOLDOUT
HOLDSUP
HOLEDUP
HOLEOUT
HOLESUP
HOLMIUM
HOMERUN
HOODLUM
HOOKSUP
HOPEFUL
HOPSOUT
HOTGLUE
HOTSOUP
HOTSPUR
HUMANUM
HUMDRUM
HUMERUS
HUNGOUT
HUNTSUP
HURRYUP
HURTFUL
HUSHFUL
HYDROUS
HYGINUS
HYPEDUP
HYPESUP

H•••••U
HOFBRAU
HOWARDU

•HU••••
BHUTANI
CHUCKED
CHUCKIT
CHUCKLE
CHUFFED
CHUGGED
CHUGGER
CHUKKER
CHUMASH
CHUMMED
CHUMPED
CHUNKED
CHUNNEL
CHUPPAH
CHUPPAS
CHURCHY
CHURNED
CHURNER
CHURNUP
CHURROS
CHUTING
CHUTIST
CHUTNEY
CHUTZPA
DHURRIE
RHUBARB
RHUMBAS
SHUBERT
SHUCKED
SHUCKER
SHUDDER
SHUFFLE
SHULMAN
SHUNNED
SHUNTED
SHUNTER
SHUSHED
SHUSHES
SHUSTER
SHUTEYE
SHUTINS
SHUTOFF
SHUTOUT
SHUTSIN
SHUTSUP
SHUTTER
SHUTTLE
THUDDED
THULIUM
THUMBED
THUMPED
THUMPER
THUNDER
THUNKED
THURBER
THURGAU
THURMAN
THUSFAR
WHUPPED

•H•U•••
CHAUCER
CHOUGHS
HHMUNRO
OHFUDGE
RHEUMIC
SHOULDA
SHOULDI
SHOUTAT
SHOUTED
SHOUTER
SHRUBBY
THEUSSR
THOUGHT
THRUPUT
THRUSTS
THRUWAY
WHAUDEN

•H••U••
CHALUPA
CHEQUER
CHEQUES
CHERUBS
CHINUPS
SHAVUOT
SHOGUNS
SHONUFF
SHROUDS
THEBUSH
THECUBS
THEDUKE
THEHULK
THEPUMP
THERULE
THESUNS
THETUBE
THETURN
THROUGH

•H•••U•
CHAINUP
CHALKUP
CHATSUP
CHECKUP
CHEERUP
CHETRUM
CHEVAUX
CHEWGUM
CHEWOUT
CHEWSUP
CHILLUM
CHIPSUP
CHIRRUP
CHOKEUP
CHOPSUP
CHOSEUP
CHURNUP
PHEMIUS
PHILOUS
PHOEBUS
PHONYUP
RHENIUM
RHODIUM
RHOECUS
RHOMBUS
SHAGRUG
SHAKEUP
SHAPEUP
SHINEUP
SHIPFUL
SHIPOUT
SHOOKUP
SHOOTUP
SHOPFUL
SHOREUP
SHOTGUN
SHOTOUT
SHOTPUT
SHOWNUP
SHOWOUT
SHOWSUP
SHUTOUT
SHUTSUP
THAWOUT
THEFRUG
THEROUX
THESEUS
THETOUR
THINKUP
THINOUT
THORIUM
THREEUP
THREWUP
THROWUP
THRUPUT
THULIUM
WHATSUP
WHIPSUP
WHITSUN
WHOSOUT

•H••••U
CHANOYU
CHAPEAU
CHATEAU
SHIATSU
SHIHTZU
SHIKOKU
THIMPHU
THOREAU
THURGAU

••HU•••
EXHUMED
EXHUMER
EXHUMES
INHUMAN
INHUMED
INHUMER
INHUMES
KAHUNAS
MRHULOT
NAHUATL
OAHUANS
SCHULTZ
SCHUMER
UNHULLS
UNHUMAN
UNHUMID
UNHUSKS

••H•U••
ACHTUNG
ASHBURN
ASHBURY
EXHAUST
INHOUSE
MAHOUTS
REHAULS
REHOUSE
SCHLUBS
SCHLUMP
UNHOUSE

••H••U•
BOHRIUM
EPHEBUS
EPHESUS
HAHNIUM
MAHFOUZ
OCHROUS

••H•••U
LEHIGHU

•••HU••
ARTHURC
ARTHURM
ARTHURS

BETHUNE
BIGHUGS
EGGHUNT
ENTHUSE
FOXHUNT
GETHURT
GOTHURT
INAHUFF
JOBHUNT
LASHUPS
LUTHULI
MANHUNT
MESHUGA
OUTHUNT
OUTHURL
PUSHUPS
RESHUTS
SAMHUFF
SEAHUNT
TERHUNE
THEHULK
UNCHURN
WASHUPS
YOGHURT

•••H•U•
BASHFUL
BATHTUB
BAUHAUS
BONHEUR
CALHOUN
CASHOUT
CEPHEUS
DISHFUL
DISHOUT
EIGHTUP
FISHOUT
GUSHOUT
HASHOUT
HUSHFUL
ISCHIUM
ISTHMUS
JODHPUR
JOUHAUX
LASHOUT
LIGHTUP
LITHIUM
MANHOUR
MARHAUS
MICHAUX
MILHAUD
MILHOUS
OFFHOUR
ONEHOUR
ORPHEUM
ORPHEUS
OUTHAUL
PUSHFUL
PUSHOUT
RUSHOUT
RUTHFUL
SIGHFUL
TWOHOUR
WASHOUT
WASHTUB
WEEHOUR
WISHFUL
WITHOUT
YEAHBUT

•••H••U
MATHIEU
SHIHTZU
YEAHYOU

••••HU•
BACCHUS
BEARHUG
BOTCHUP
BRUSHUP
BULGHUR
BUNCHUP
CATCHUP
COUGHUP
DONAHUE
FROTHUP
FULGHUM
HITCHUP
KETCHUM
KETCHUP
MALTHUS
MATCHUP
MITCHUM
PATCHUP
PSYCHUP
PUNCHUP
PYRRHUS
QUECHUA
REACHUP
ROUGHUP
SAWCHUK
SMASHUP
SORGHUM
SULPHUR
TOUCHUP
WEIGHUP

••••H•U
MATTHAU
SEETHRU

•••••HU
LEHIGHU
THIMPHU

H•V••••
HAVANAN
HAVANAS
HAVARTI
HAVEAGO
HAVEFUN
HAVENER
HAVENOT
HAVEONE
HAVEOUT
HIVEOFF
HOVERED
HOVERER
HOVLANE

H••V•••
HALVAHS
HALVERS
HALVING
HARVARD
HARVEST
HDTVSET
HEAVEHO
HEAVENS
HEAVERS
HEAVETO
HEAVIER
HEAVIES
HEAVILY
HEAVING
HOOVERS
HORVITZ
HRYVNIA
HUMVEES

H•••V••
HADOVER
HALAVAH
HANOVER
HASOVER
HESHVAN
HOPOVER
HOTOVER
HOWEVER

H••••V•
HECKUVA
HELLUVA
HENRYVI

H•••••V
HENRYIV

•H•V•••
CHEVAUX
CHEVETS
CHEVIOT
CHEVONS
CHEVRES
CHEVRET
CHEVRON
CHIVIED
CHIVIES
IHAVEIT
SHAVERS
SHAVIAN
SHAVING
SHAVUOT
SHEVATS
SHIVERS
SHIVERY
SHOVEIN
SHOVELS
SHOVERS
SHOVING
THEVIEW
THEVIPS
ZHIVAGO

•H••V••
CHARVET
CHEEVER
CHERVIL
SHEAVED
SHEAVES
SHELVED
SHELVER
SHELVES
SHRIVEL
SHRIVER
SHRIVES
THIEVED
THIEVES
THRIVED
THRIVEN
THRIVER
THRIVES
WHARVES
WHOEVER
WHYEVER

•H•••V•
KHEDIVE
THECAVS
THEFIVE
THEMAVS
THEWAVE
WHEREVE

•H••••V
CHEKHOV
KHARKOV
PHILIPV

••H•V••
ASHIVER
BEHAVED
BEHAVES
DEHAVEN
JOHNVII
LEHAVRE
MOHAVES
SOHAVEI

••H••V•
ACHIEVA
ACHIEVE
BEHOOVE
JOHNXVI
PAHLAVI
UNHEAVY
UPHEAVE

••H•••V
JOHNXIV

•••HV••
HESHVAN

•••H•V•
ANCHOVY
ARCHIVE
BEEHIVE
LETHAVE
RESHAVE
YESHIVA

••••H•V
CHEKHOV
TRASHTV
WATCHTV

H•W••••
HAWHAWS
HAWKERS
HAWKEYE
HAWKING
HAWKINS
HAWKISH
HAWKMAN
HAWORTH
HAWSERS
HEWEDTO
HEWLETT
HGWELLS
HOWARDK
HOWARDS
HOWARDU
HOWBEIT
HOWCOME
HOWDAHS
HOWDEDO
HOWDULL
HOWDYDO
HOWELLS
HOWELSE
HOWEVER
HOWHIGH
HOWLAME
HOWLERS
HOWLING
HOWLONG
HOWLSAT
HOWMANY
HOWMUCH
HOWNICE
HOWTHEN

H••W•••
HARWELL
HAYWARD
HAYWIRE
HEYWARD
HEYWOOD
HOGWASH
HOGWEED
HOGWILD
HOTWARS
HOTWIRE

H•••W••
HALFWAY
HALFWIT
HALFWON
HALLWAY
HARDWAY
HARDWON
HEADWAY
HIDAWAY
HIGHWAY
HOLYWAR

H••••W•
HALLOWS
HARROWS
HAWHAWS
HAYMOWS
HEBREWS
HEEHAWS
HITTOWN
HOEDOWN
HOLLOWS
HOOTOWL

H•••••W
HACKSAW
HADACOW
HADAROW
HALFRAW
HANDSAW
HASACOW
HASAROW
HEADSAW
HERENOW
HIGHLOW
HINDPAW
HITSHOW
HOLYCOW

•HW••••
THWACKS
THWARTS
THWHITE
WHWORDS

•H•W•••
CHAWING
CHEWERS
CHEWGUM
CHEWIER
CHEWING
CHEWOUT
CHEWSON
CHEWSUP
CHEWTOY
CHOWDER
CHOWING
SHAWLED
SHAWNEE
SHEWOLF
SHOWBIZ
SHOWCAT
SHOWDOG
SHOWERS
SHOWERY
SHOWHOW
SHOWIER
SHOWILY
SHOWING
SHOWMAN
SHOWMEN
SHOWNIN
SHOWNUP
SHOWOFF
SHOWOUT
SHOWSIN
SHOWSUP
THAWERS
THAWING
THAWOUT
THEWALL
THEWAVE
THEWIND
WHYWAIT

•H••W••
CHATWIN
CHINWAG
SHERWIN
SHIPWAY
SHYAWAY
THATWAY
THESWAN
THISWAY
THREWAT
THREWIN
THREWON
THREWUP
THROWAT
THROWER
THROWIN
THROWON
THROWUP
THRUWAY
WHOSWHO

•H•••W•
CHITOWN
SHADOWS
SHADOWY
SHALLWE
THENEWS

•H••••W
CHOCTAW
OHMSLAW
SHALLOW
SHOWHOW
THECROW
THESHOW
THEVIEW
WHATNOW
WHIPSAW
WHOKNEW

••HW•••
ATHWART
SCHWANN
SCHWINN
WAHWAHS

••H•W••
JOHNWOO
MOHAWKS
PSHAWED
UNHEWED

••H•••W
JOHNLAW

•••HW••
ARCHWAY
BUSHWAH
HIGHWAY
PATHWAY

•••H•W•
CASHEWS
CUSHAWS
ESCHEWS
GOSHAWK
HAWHAWS
HEEHAWS
MACHTWO
MATHEWS
NEPHEWS
NOSHOWS
OUTHOWL
RECHEWS
REDHAWK
RESHOWN
RESHOWS
RETHAWS
SEAHAWK
TVSHOWS
UNSHOWN
UNSHOWY
UNTHAWS
WARHAWK

•••H••W
CASHCOW
HIGHLOW
LITHGOW
UPTHROW

••••H•W
AIRSHOW
ARTSHOW
BIGSHOW
CAPSHAW
CARSHOW
CATCHOW
CATSHOW
CRASHAW
CUMSHAW
DOGCHEW
DOGCHOW
DOGSHOW
FORSHOW
GLASHOW
HITSHOW
ICESHOW
KERSHAW
KNEWHOW
KNOWHOW
MATTHEW
OUTSHOW
PETCHEW
PRESHOW
SALCHOW
SHOWHOW
SOMEHOW
THESHOW
USOSHOW

H•X••••
HEXADIC
HEXAGON
HEXANES
HEXAPOD
HEXNUTS
HEXOSES
HEXSIGN

H••X•••
HOAXERS
HOAXING

H•••X••
HELIXES
HYRAXES

H••••X•
HANDAXE

H•••••X
HALIFAX
HARDSIX
HENDRIX
HENDRYX
HUMIDEX

•H•X•••
CHEXMIX

•H••X••
PHLOXES
THEAXIS

•H••••X
CHEVAUX
CHEXMIX
PHALANX
PHARYNX
PHOENIX
SHOEBOX
THEROUX

••H•X••
DEHEXED
DEHEXES
JOHNXII
JOHNXIV
JOHNXIX
JOHNXVI
JOHNXXI

••H••X•
JOHNXXI

••H•••X
JOHNXIX

•••H••X
ANTHRAX
CASHBOX
JOUHAUX
MACHSIX
MICHAUX

••••H•X
NARTHEX
PANCHAX

HY•••••
HYALITE
HYALOID
HYANNIS
HYBRIDS
HYDRANT
HYDRATE
HYDRIDE
HYDROUS
HYGELAC
HYGIEIA
HYGIENE
HYGINUS
HYMNALS
HYMNARY
HYMNING
HYMNODY
HYPATIA
HYPEDUP
HYPERON
HYPESUP
HYPHENS
HYPNOID
HYPOING
HYPONYM
HYRACES
HYRAXES
HYSSOPS
HYUNDAI

H•Y••••
HAYBALE
HAYESES
HAYFORK
HAYINGS
HAYLOFT
HAYMOWS
HAYRACK
HAYRICK
HAYRIDE
HAYSEED
HAYWARD
HAYWIRE
HEYDAYS
HEYJUDE
HEYLOOK
HEYMANS
HEYMRDJ
HEYRUBE
HEYWARD
HEYWOOD
HOYDENS
HRYVNIA
HUYGENS

H••Y•••
HALYARD
HOLYARK
HOLYCOW
HOLYDAY
HOLYJOE
HOLYMAN
HOLYMEN
HOLYOIL
HOLYOKE
HOLYONE
HOLYSEE
HOLYWAR

H•••Y••
HALCYON
HANDYTO
HAPPYTO
HECKYES
HELLYES
HENRYII
HENRYIV
HENRYVI
HONEYED
HOWDYDO
HUNNYBS
HURRYUP

H••••Y•
HAIRDYE
HALLEYS
HANDEYE
HANGBYS
HARLEYS
HAWKEYE
HENDRYX
HEYDAYS
HICKEYS
HOMONYM
HOORAYS
HOTDAYS
HOTKEYS
HURRAYS
HYPONYM

H•••••Y
HACKNEY
HADASAY
HAGERTY
HALFDAY
HALFSHY
HALFWAY
HALLWAY
HAMMILY
HANDILY
HANGSBY
HAPENNY
HAPPIFY
HAPPILY
HARDDAY
HARDILY
HARDWAY
HARMONY
HARSHLY
HARTLEY
HASASAY
HASTILY
HAUGHTY
HAUTBOY
HEADILY
HEADWAY
HEALTHY
HEARSAY
HEATRAY
HEAVILY
HEFTILY
HELLBOY
HELOTRY
HEMSLEY
HENNERY
HENSLEY
HERONRY
HERSHEY
HICKORY
HIDAWAY
HIGHBOY
HIGHDAY
HIGHPAY
HIGHWAY
HILLARY
HIPPITY
HISTORY
HITPLAY
HOARILY
HODADDY
HOGGERY
HOLIDAY
HOLYDAY
HOMEBOY
HONESTY
HOOPTOY
HORNSBY
HORRIFY
HORSILY
HORSLEY
HOSIERY
HOUSSAY
HOWMANY
HUFFILY
HUMANLY
HUMIDLY
HUMPHRY
HUNGARY
HUNTLEY
HUSHABY
HUSKILY
HYMNARY
HYMNODY

•HY••••
CHYRONS
PHYLLIS
PHYLLOS
PHYSICS
RHYMERS
RHYMING
RHYMIST
RHYTHMS
SHYAWAY
SHYFROM
SHYLOCK
SHYNESS
SHYSTER
THYMINE
THYROID
THYSELF
WHYEVER
WHYISIT
WHYWAIT

•H•Y•••
CHAYOTE
KHAYYAM
PHRYGIA
THEYIPS
THEYSAY
WHEYISH

•H••Y••
KHAYYAM
PHARYNX
PHONYUP

•H•••Y•
CHANOYU
IHEARYA
PHONEYS
SHUTEYE
THEBOYS
THEMAYO

•H••••Y
CHANTEY
CHANTRY
CHARILY
CHARITY
CHARLEY
CHEAPLY
CHEWTOY
CHICORY
CHIEFLY
CHIMNEY
CHINTZY
CHOMSKY
CHOOSEY
CHRISTY
CHURCHY
CHUTNEY
GHASTLY
GHOSTLY
PHLEGMY
PHONILY
SHADILY
SHADOWY
SHAKILY
SHAPELY
SHARKEY
SHARPLY
SHEERLY
SHELLEY
SHINGLY
SHINILY
SHIPWAY
SHIRLEY
SHIVERY
SHLOCKY
SHOOFLY
SHOOTBY
SHORTLY
SHOWERY
SHOWILY
SHRILLY
SHRIMPY
SHRUBBY
SHTICKY
SHYAWAY
THATCHY
THATWAY
THEARMY
THEBABY
THEBODY
THECITY
THERAPY
THEREBY
THEYSAY
THICKLY
THIERRY
THIRDLY
THIRSTY
THISDAY
THISTLY
THISWAY
THREADY
THRIFTY
THROATY
THRUWAY
WHALLEY
WHATSAY
WHEREBY
WHISKEY
WHITELY
WHITNEY

••H•Y••
LCHAYIM
SCHAYES
UNHAYED

••H••Y•
JOHNNYB

••H•••Y
ASHBERY
ASHBURY
ASHTRAY
BEHAPPY
DAHOMEY
DOHERTY
FTHENRY
IMHAPPY
ITHIRTY
JOHNBOY
JOHNGAY
JOHNJAY
MAHONEY
MCHENRY
MRHANEY
UNHAIRY
UNHANDY
UNHAPPY
UNHARDY
UNHASTY
UNHEADY
UNHEAVY
UNHILLY
WCHANDY

•••HY••
TACHYON
UNRHYME
UNSHYER
UNSHYLY
YEAHYOU
ZEPHYRS

•••H•Y•
FISHEYE
KATHRYN
SASHAYS

•••H••Y
ALCHEMY
ANCHOVY
ANTHONY
ARCHERY
ARCHWAY
BETHANY
BUSHILY
BYTHEBY
CEPHALY
CUSHILY
DITHERY
EUPHONY
FISHERY
FISHFRY
FISHILY
GUSHILY
HIGHBOY
HIGHDAY
HIGHPAY
HIGHWAY
HUSHABY
LATHERY
LIGHTLY
LITHELY
MOTHERY
MUSHILY
MYTHIFY
NIGHTLY
PATHWAY
PITHILY
PUSHILY
RIGHTLY
SIGHTLY
SOTHEBY
TIGHTLY
TUSHERY
UNCHARY
UNSHADY
UNSHINY
UNSHOWY
UNSHYLY
WASHDAY
ZACHARY

••••HY•
MURPHYS

••••H•Y
AINTHAY
APISHLY
BLIGHTY
BOKCHOY
BRASHLY
DOUGHTY
EARTHLY
FIFTHLY
FLESHLY
FLIGHTY
FRESHLY
HARSHLY
HAUGHTY
HERSHEY
HUMPHRY
IEIGHTY
LOATHLY
MADEHAY
MAKEHAY
MONTHLY
NAUGHTY
NINTHLY
PLUSHLY
ROUGHLY
SIXTHLY
SOUTHEY
TENTHLY
TOUGHLY
WEIGHTY

•••••HY
ANARCHY
ATROPHY
BLOTCHY
BRANCHY
BREATHY
CHURCHY
CLUTCHY
CRUNCHY
DENNEHY
DOROTHY
EMPATHY
EPARCHY
GIRLSHY
GLITCHY
GROUCHY
HALFSHY
HEALTHY
KITSCHY
KVETCHY
LENGTHY
MENSCHY
MULCAHY
PAUNCHY
PREACHY
RAUNCHY
SKETCHY
SLOUCHY
SMOOTHY
SPLASHY
SQUASHY
SQUISHY
STARCHY
SWARTHY
THATCHY
TIMOTHY
TWITCHY
VERYSHY
WEALTHY
WORKSHY
WREATHY

H•Z••••
HAZANIM
HAZARDS
HAZIEST
HAZINGS
HAZLITT
HAZMATS
HUZZAHS

H••Z•••
HOLZMAN
HOTZONE
HUZZAHS

H•••Z••
HORIZON

H••••Z•
HATSIZE

H•••••Z
HEIFETZ
HJHEINZ
HORVITZ

•H•Z•••
CHAZANS
CHAZZAN
CHEZMOI
RHIZOME
WHIZKID
WHIZZED
WHIZZER
WHIZZES

•H••Z••
CHAZZAN
CHEEZIT
CHUTZPA
WHEEZED
WHEEZER
WHEEZES
WHIZZED
WHIZZER
WHIZZES

•H•••Z•
CHINTZY
CHORIZO
SHIHTZU

•H••••Z
SHOWBIZ
THEFONZ
THERITZ

••HZ•••
MAHZORS

••H•Z••
UNHAZED
YAHTZEE

••H••Z•
SCHERZI
SCHERZO
SCHNOZZ

••H•••Z
HJHEINZ
MAHFOUZ
SCHLITZ
SCHNOZZ
SCHULTZ

•••HZ••
SECHZIG

•••H•Z•
SHIHTZU

••••H•Z
GEEWHIZ
NATCHEZ

IA•••••
IACOCCA
IAMBICS
IAMBIST
IAMLOVE
IANHOLM
IAPETUS
IATRICS

I•A••••
ICANNOT
IDAHOAN
IDAREDS
IHATEIT
IHAVEIT
IMADEIT
IMAGERS
IMAGERY
IMAGINE
IMAGING
IMAGISM
IMAGIST
IMAGOES
IMAHOGG
IMAMATE
IMAMESS
IMARETS
INABALL
INABIND
INACAST
INADAZE
INAFUNK
INAFURY
INAHEAP
INAHOLE
INAHUFF
INAIDOF
INAJIFF
INAKNOT
INALINE
INAMESS
INAMOOD
INANELY
INANEST
INANITY
INAPILE
INAPOEM
INAPOKE
INAPRIL
INAPTER
INAPTLY
INARAGE
INARUSH
INASHOE
INASNAP
INASNIT
INASPIN
INASPOT
INASTEW
INASTIR
INASUIT
INATRAP
INAVALE
INAWEOF
INAWINK
INAWORD
IPANEMA
IRANIAN
IRATELY
IRATEST
ISABEAU
ISADORA
ISADORE
ISAHEAD
ISAIDNO
ITALIAN
ITALICS
IVANHOE
IVANIII
IVANOVO
IWANTIT
IWANTTO
IZATION

I••A•••
ICEAGES
ICEAXES
ICHABOD
IDBADGE
IDCARDS
IDEALLY
IDEAMAN
IDEAMEN
IDEATED
IDEATES
IDIAMIN
IDSAYSO
IGNARRO
IGNATOW
IGRAINE
IGUANAS
IGUANID
IGUASSU
IHEARYA
ILIADIC
ILIAMNA
IMEANIT
IMHAPPY
IMPACTS
IMPAIRS
IMPALAS
IMPALED
IMPALER
IMPALES
IMPANEL
IMPARTS
IMPASSE
IMPASTO
IMPAVID
INCANTS
INCASED
INCASES
INFAITH
INFANCY
INFANTA
INFANTE
INFANTS
INFAVOR
INGALLS
INGATES
INHABIT
INHALED
INHALER
INHALES
INHASTE
INLABOR
INLANDS
INLARGE
INLAYER
INMARCH
INMATES
INNAGES
INNARDS
INRANGE
INSALES
INSANER
INTAILS
INTAKES
INTASTE
INVACUO
INVADED
INVADER
INVADES
INVALID
INWARDS
IODATED
IODATES
ISFAHAN
ISLAMIC
ISLANDS
ISRAELI
ISRAFEL
ITHACAN
ITMAYBE
ITSABOY
ITSAHIT
ITSALIE
ITSALOT
ITSASIN
ITSATIE
IZZATSO

I•••A••
IBIZANS
IBNSAUD
ICEBAGS
ICEBATH
ICECAPS
ICECAVE
ICEDAMS
ICEFALL
ICELAND
ICEPACK
IKEBANA
ILLCALL
ILLEANA
ILLMADE
ILLPASS
ILOCANO
IMAMATE
IMITATE
IMPEACH
IMPLANT
IMREADY
INABALL
INACAST
INADAZE
INARAGE
INAVALE
INBLACK
INBOARD
INCLASS
INDIANA
INDIANS
INDRAFT
INDRAWN
INEXACT
INFLAME
INFLATE
INFRACT
INGOALS
INGRAFT
INGRAIN
INGRATE
INKMARK
INKPADS
INKSACS
INPEACE
INPHASE
INPLACE
INREACH
INROADS
INSCALE
INSEAMS
INSHAPE
INSPACE
INSPANS
INSTALL
INSTALS
INSTANT
INSTATE
INTEARS
INTRADE
INTRAYS
INULASE
INWEAVE
INYEARS
IONIANS
IRELAND
IRONAGE
ISHMAEL
ISITAGO
ISOBARS
ISOLATE
ISOLATO
ISSUANT
ITERANT
ITERATE
ITSEASY
ITSLATE

I••••A•
IBERIAN
ICEBOAT
ICETEAS
ICETRAY
IDAHOAN
IDEAMAN
IFWEMAY
IGUANAS
ILLCLAD
ILLEGAL
IMGREAT
IMMORAL
IMPALAS
IMPLEAD
INAHEAP
INASNAP
INATRAP
INDYCAR
INGEMAR
INHUMAN
INITIAL
INKYCAP
INNOWAY
INSOFAR
INSTEAD
INSULAR
INTOTAL
IONBEAM
IRANIAN
IREPEAT
IRONBAR
IRONMAN
ISABEAU
ISAHEAD
ISCHIAL
ISFAHAN
ISOGRAM
ISSUEAD
ISTRIAN
ISUREAM
ITALIAN
ITHACAN
ITSOKAY
IVORIAN

I•••••A
IACOCCA
ICEDTEA
IGOTCHA
IHEARYA
IKEBANA
ILIAMNA
ILLEANA
ILLYRIA
ILOVELA
IMPREZA
INDIANA
INDICIA
INEDITA
INERTIA
INFANTA
INGESTA
INOCULA
INSECTA
INTEGRA
INVICTA
IPANEMA
ISADORA
IWOJIMA

•IA••••
BIAFRAN
BIALIES
BIANCHI
BIASING
BIASPLY
BIASSED
BIASSES
BIAXIAL
DIABLES
DIABLOS
DIABOLO
DIADEMS
DIAGRAM
DIAHANN
DIALECT
DIALEDO
DIALERS
DIALING
DIALLED
DIALOGS
DIALOUT
DIALSIN
DIALSUP
DIALUPS
DIAMOND
DIAPERS
DIAPHAN
DIARIES
DIARIOS
DIARIST
DIATOMS
DIAVOLO
FIACRES
FIANCEE
FIANCES
FIASCOS
FIATLUX
GIACOMO
GIAUQUE
HIALEAH
KIARIOS
LIAISED
LIAISES
LIAISON
MIAHAMM
MIAMIAN
MIAMIFL
MIAOUED
MIAOWED
MIASARA
MIASMAL
MIASMAS
MIASMIC
NIAGARA
NIALONG
NIANTIC
PIAFFED
PIAFFES
PIANISM
PIANIST
PIANOLA
PIASTER
PIASTRE
PIAZZAS
RIALTOS
RIANTLY
SIAMESE
TIARAED
VIADENT
VIADUCT
VIALFUL
VIALING
VIALLED
VIATICA

•I•A•••
AIRACES
BICARBS
BIGAPES
BIVALVE
BIZARRE
BIZARRO
CICADAE
CICADAS
CIMABUE
CITABLE
CITADEL
DIDACTS
DIDASET
DIEAWAY
DILATED
DILATES
DILATOR
DIMAGES
DINADAM
DINARIC
DISABLE
DISARMS
DISAVOW
DIZAINS
FINABLE
FINAGLE
FINALES
FINALLY
FINANCE
FIXABLE
FIXATED
FIXATES
GIGABIT
GIGATON
GIRAFFE
GIRASOL
GITANOS
HIBACHI
HIDABLE
HIDALGO
HIDAWAY
HIJACKS
HILAIRE
HIMALIA
HIRABLE
HITACHI
JICAMAS
JIRASEK
KILAUEA
KIWANIS
LIEABED
LIEATOP
LIGANDS
LIGATED
LIGATES
LIKABLE
LILALEE
LIMACON
LINABLE
LINAGES
LIPARIS
LIPASES
LISAGAY
LIVABLE
LIZARDS
MICAELA
MIDASES
MIKADOS
MIKASAS
MILAGRO
MINABLE
MINARET
MIRABEL
MIRACLE
MIRADAS
MIRADOR
MIRAGES
MIRAMAR
MIRAMAX
MIRANDA
MISACTS
MISADDS
MISAIMS
MISALLY
MISAVER
MIXABLE
PICADOR
PICANTE
PICARAS
PICARDO
PICARDY
PICAROS
PICASSO
PILATES
PILATUS
PINATAS
PIPAGES
PIRAEUS
PIRANHA
PIRATED
PIRATES
PIRATIC
PISANIO
PISARRO
PITAPAT
PITAYAS
PIZARRO
RIBALDS
RIBANDS
RICARDO
RIDABLE
RINALDO
RITAGAM
RITALIN
RITAMAE
RITARDS
RIVALED
RIVALRY
SINATRA
SITATOP
SIZABLE
SIZABLY
TIDALLY
TINAFEY
TINAMOU
TIRADES
TISANES
TITANAE
TITANIA
TITANIC
VIDALIA
VIHARAS
VIRAGOS
VISAGED
VISAGES
VISAING
VISALIA
VISAVIS
VISAYAN
VITALIS
VITALLY
VITAMIN
VITARAS
VIVALDI
VIVANTS
VIVARIA
WIRABLE
WIZARDS
ZIMARRA

•I••A••
AIRBAGS
AIRBALL
AIRBASE
AIRDAMS
AIRDATE
AIRFARE
AIRLANE
AIRMADA
AIRMAIL
AIRMASS
AIRPACK
AIRPARK
AIRRACE
AIRRAGE
AIRRAID
AIRSACS
AIRTANK
AIRTAXI
AIRWARS
AIRWAVE
AIRWAYS
BIDFAIR
BIGBABY
BIGBAND
BIGBANG
BIGCARS
BIGCATS
BIGDAYS
BIGEARS
BIGEAST
BIGEASY
BIGFANS
BIGGAME
BIGHAIR
BIGHALF
BIGHAND
BIGJAKE
BIGMACS
BIGMAMA
BIGNAME
BIGSALE
BIGTALK
BIODATA
BIOLABS
BIOMASS
BIPLANE
BIRIANI
BIRMANS
BIRYANI
BISTATE
BITMAPS
BITPART
CILIARY
CILIATE
CINZANO
CIRRATE
CISEAUX
CITRATE
DIAHANN
DICTATE
DIDLAPS
DIECAST
DIEHARD
DIETARY
DIGRAMS
DIGRAPH
DIKTATS
DILLARD
DIORAMA
DIRHAMS
DISBAND
DISBARS
DISCARD
DISDAIN
DISEASE
DISMALS
DISMAST
DISMAYS
DISPART
DISRATE
DISTAFF
DISTANT
FIGBARS
FIJIANS
FINBACK
FINEART
FINGALS

FINIALS
FINIANS
FINLAND
FINNAIR
FIRBANK
FIREANT
FIREARM
FIVEAAA
GIGBAGS
GIMBALS
GINGAME
GISCARD
GIZZARD
HIGHART
HILLARY
HIPBATH
HISPANO
HITBACK
JIGSAWS
JIMDALE
JIMJAMS
JIMKAAT
KIDNAPS
KILDARE
KIMBALL
KINCAID
KINKAID
KIRMANS
KITBAGS
KITHARA
KITKATS
LIBRANS
LIBRARY
LIBYANS
LIEBACK
LIMEADE
LINEAGE
LINEARA
LINEARB
LINEATE
LINKAGE
LIPBALM
LIPMANN
LIQUATE
LIVEAID
MIAHAMM
MIASARA
MICHAEL
MICHAUX
MICMACS
MIDCAPS
MIDDAYS
MIDEAST
MIDLAND
MIDWAYS
MIGRANT
MIGRATE
MIKHAIL
MILEAGE
MILHAUD
MILLAGE
MILLAIS
MILLAND
MILLARD
MINOANS
MINTAGE
MINYANS
MISCALL

MISCAST
MISDATE
MISGAVE
MISHAPS
MISLAID
MISLAYS
MISMARK
MISMATE
MISNAME
MISPAGE
MISRATE
MISSAID
MISSALS
MISSAYS
MISTAKE
MIZRAHI
NIAGARA
NICCAGE
NICTATE
NIKEADS
NIRVANA
NISSANS
NISSANZ
NITRATE
NITTANY
OILBASE
OILCAKE
OILCANS
OILLAMP
OILPALM
OILPANS
OILSAND
OILTANK
OISEAUX
PICCARD
PICCATA
PICKAXE
PIEBALD
PIEPANS
PIESAFE
PIESALE
PIGTAIL
PILEATE
PILLAGE
PILLARS
PINBALL
PINNACE
PINNATE
PINOAKS
PINTAIL
PINWALE
PIPCARD
PIQUANT
PITFALL
PITSAWS
PIZZAZZ
QINTARS
RIBCAGE
RIBPADS
RICHARD
RICRACS
RIEMANN
RIMBAUD
RIOTACT
RIPRAPS
RIPSAWN
RIPSAWS
RITEAID

RITUALS
SIDEARM
SIGNAGE
SIGNALS
SIMIANS
SINKAGE
SINUATE
SIOUANS
SITBACK
SITUATE
SIXBALL
SIXLANE
SIXPACK
TIARAED
TICTACS
TIEBACK
TIEBARS
TIEGAME
TIERACK
TIETACK
TIETACS
TIFFANY
TIJUANA
TILLAGE
TIMBALE
TIMBALS
TIMPANI
TINCANS
TINEARS
TINHATS
TINWARE
TIPCART
TIPJARS
TITIANS
TITLARK
TITRATE
VIBRANT
VIBRATE
VIBRATO
VICDANA
VILLAGE
VILLAIN
VILLARD
VILLARI
VINLAND
VINTAGE
VIOLATE
VIRGATE
VISTAED
VISUALS
VITIATE
WICCANS
WIDMARK
WIELAND
WIGWAGS
WIGWAMS
WILLARD
WINBACK
WINDAGE
WINDAUS
ZIGZAGS

•I•••A•

AIMEDAT
AINTHAY
AIRBOAT
AIRHEAD
AIRPLAY

AIRTRAP
BIAFRAN
BIAXIAL
BIFOCAL
BIGBEAR
BIGBEAT
BIGDEAL
BIGHEAD
BIGLEAD
BIGMEAL
BIGSTAR
BIKEWAY
BIMETAL
BIMODAL
BINGHAM
BIPEDAL
BIPOLAR
BIRDMAN
BITONAL
BIVOUAC
CICADAE
CICADAS
CINEMAS
CINEMAX
CITYGAL
DIAGRAM
DIAPHAN
DIDTOAT
DIEAWAY
DIGICAM
DIGITAL
DILLMAN
DINADAM
DINEDAT
DINESAT
DINGBAT
DIPOLAR
DIRTBAG
DISCMAN
DISHPAN
DISHRAG
DISPLAY
DIURNAL
EIGHTAD
EIGHTAM
EIJKMAN
FIBULAE
FIBULAR
FIBULAS
FIESTAS
FIFTYAD
FIGLEAF
FIGURAL
FILOFAX
FINDLAY
FINICAL
FIREDAT
FIREHAT
FIREMAN
FIRESAT
FIVEAAA
FIVEDAY
FIVEMAN
FIVEWAY
GIBESAT
GIDDYAP
GIFTTAX
GILBLAS

GILLIAM
GILLIAN
GILLMAN
GINGHAM
GIVEEAR
GIVEWAY
HIALEAH
HICKMAN
HIDAWAY
HIGHBAR
HIGHDAY
HIGHHAT
HIGHPAY
HIGHWAY
HILLMAN
HINDPAW
HINTSAT
HITPLAY
JIBEDAT
JIBESAT
JICAMAS
JILLIAN
JIMBEAM
JIMDIAL
JIMKAAT
KIDSEAT
KILOBAR
KINGMAN
KINGRAT
KINNEAR
KINSMAN
LIBERAL
LIKEMAD
LILINAU
LILLIAN
LILYPAD
LIMINAL
LINBIAO
LINDSAY
LINEMAN
LINGUAE
LINGUAL
LINPIAO
LIPREAD
LISAGAY
LITERAL
LIVEOAK
LIVESAT
MIAMIAN
MIASMAL
MIASMAS
MIDYEAR
MIKASAS
MILKBAR
MILKCAN
MILKMAN
MILLDAM
MIMOSAS
MINERAL
MINIBAR
MINICAB
MINICAM
MINICAR
MINILAB
MINIMAL
MINIMAX
MINIVAC
MINIVAN

MIRADAS
MIRAMAR
MIRAMAX
MISDEAL
MISDIAL
MISDRAW
MISHEAR
MISHNAH
MISLEAD
MISPLAN
MISPLAY
MISREAD
MISSEAT
MISTRAL
MITHRAS
MITZVAH
MIZUNAS
NICEDAY
NICEMAN
NICOBAR
NICOLAS
NIKOLAI
NIKOLAY
OILHEAT
PIAZZAS
PICARAS
PICKSAT
PIERIAN
PIGMEAT
PINATAS
PINCHAS
PINESAP
PINETAR
PINHEAD
PINKHAM
PINSEAL
PISCEAN
PITAPAT
PITAYAS
PITHEAD
PITTMAN
PIVOTAL
RIBMEAT
RICHMAN
RICKMAN
RIDGWAY
RIESMAN
RIKSDAG
RINKRAT
RIORDAN
RITAGAM
RITAMAE
SICKBAY
SICKDAY
SICKPAY
SIDEBAR
SIDECAR
SIDEMAN
SIDEWAY
SIENNAS
SIERRAS
SIESTAS
SIGHSAT
SILICAS
SILKHAT
SIMILAC
SIMILAR
SINDBAD

SINUTAB
SIOBHAN
SITEMAP
SITSPAT
SIXTYAD
SIXYEAR
TIBETAN
TIEBEAM
TIENDAS
TILTSAT
TIMELAG
TIMEWAS
TINSTAR
TIREMAN
TITANAE
TITULAR
VICINAL
VICTUAL
VICUNAS
VIETNAM
VIHARAS
VIMINAL
VINEGAR
VIRGOAN
VIRTUAL
VISAYAN
VITARAS
VIVICAA
VIVITAR
VIZSLAS
WILDCAT
WILDMAN
WILLIAM
WINDBAG
WINEBAR
WINESAP
WINEVAT
WINGMAN
WINKSAT
WIREMAN
WIRETAP
WISEMAN
YITZHAK
ZINNIAS

•I••••A

AIRMADA
BIENNIA
BIGIDEA
BIGMAMA
BIODATA
BIRETTA
CINESIA
DILEMMA
DIORAMA
DIOTIMA
DIPLOMA
FIDELIA
FIORINA
FIRENZA
FIVEAAA
GINGIVA
HIGHSEA
HIGHTEA
HIMALIA
KILAUEA
KITHARA
LIBERIA

LIDWINA
LIGURIA
LINEARA
LINGULA
MIASARA
MICAELA
MILITIA
MINEOLA
MINERVA
MINOLTA
MINORCA
MINTTEA
MINUTIA
MIRANDA
MISHIMA
MISSUSA
NIAGARA
NICOSIA
NIGERIA
NIRVANA
PIANOLA
PICCATA
PINOTTA
PIRANHA
RICKSHA
RICOTTA
RIGVEDA
RIORITA
RIVIERA
SIBERIA
SICILIA
SIGNORA
SILENTA
SILESIA
SINATRA
TIJUANA
TITANIA
VIATICA
VICDANA
VICENZA
VIDALIA
VIGNOLA
VINCULA
VISALIA
VISCERA
VISTULA
VITORIA
VIVARIA
VIVICAA
WICHITA
ZIMARRA

••IA•••

ALIASES
AMIABLE
AMIABLY
ARIADNE
ARIANES
ASIAGOS
ASIATIC
AVIANCA
AVIATED
AVIATES
AVIATIC
AVIATOR
AXIALLY
BOIARDO
BRIARDS

CHIANTI
CHIAPAS
CHIAPET
ESIASON
FRIABLE
FRIARLY
IDIAMIN
ILIADIC
ILIAMNA
JAIALAI
NAIADES
OPIATES
PLIABLE
PLIABLY
PLIANCY
SCIATIC
SHIATSU
SKIABLE
SKIAREA
THIAMIN
TRIABLE
TRIADIC
TRIAGES
UNIATES

••I•A••

ABIGAIL
AGITATE
AGITATO
ALIBABA
ALIDADE
ALIYAHS
AMIDALA
AMILATE
ANIMACY
ANIMALS
ANIMATE
ANIMATO
ARIGATO
ARIKARA
ASISAID
BOITANO
BRIDALS
BRIGADE
BRIGAND
BRITAIN
CAIMANS
CHICAGO
CHICANA
CHICANE
CHICANO
CLIMATE
CLIMATS
CLIPART
COINAGE
CUIRASS
DOIDARE
EDINAMN
ELIYALE
EMIRATE
EPICARP
EPILADY
EPILATE
EPITAPH
FAISALI
FBICASE
FRIDAYS
FRIGATE

GRIMACE
GUITARS
HAIKAIS
IBIZANS
IMITATE
ISITAGO
MAITAIS
NAIPAUL
OCICATS
OHIOANS
OHIOART
OKINAWA
ORIGAMI
OVIPARA
OVISACS
OXIDANT
OXIDASE
OXIDATE
PAIDADS
PAISANO
PAISANS
PLICATE
PRIMACY
PRIMARY
PRIMATE
PRIVACY
PRIVATE
QUINARY
QUINATE
RAILAGE
REIMAGE
RUINATE
SAIDAAH
SAIDAYE
SKICAPS
SKIHATS
SKIMASK
SKIRACE
SKIRACK
SOILAGE
SPINACH
SPIRALS
SZILARD
THINAIR
TRINARY
UNIBALL
UNITARD
UNITARY
UNIVACS
UTICANS
UTICANY
WAIKATO
ZHIVAGO

••I••A•

ABIDJAN
AMICHAI
AMISTAD
ANITRAS
ARISTAE
ARISTAS
AVIDFAN
AVIVIAN
AXILLAE
AXILLAR
AXILLAS
BAITCAR
BLINKAT

BRIGHAM
CHIAPAS
CHICHAS
CHILCAT
CHILEAN
CHILIAD
CHILKAT
CHINWAG
CRIMEAN
CRITIAS
DRIPPAN
DRISTAN
DRIVEAT
EDICTAL
ENIGMAS
EPIGRAM
FAIRFAX
FAIRWAY
FLIESAT
FLINGAT
FRIEDAN
FRISIAN
GAINSAY
GEISHAS
GOINGAT
GRIDMAP
GRINSAT
GRISHAM
GUINEAN
GUINEAS
HAITIAN
HEISMAN
INITIAL
JAIALAI
MAILBAG
MAILCAR
MAILMAN
MAINMAN
MOISSAN
MRISCAN
OJIBWAS
OJIBWAY
OSIRIAN
OVIDIAN
PHIDIAS
PHILEAS
PHINEAS
POINTAT
PRINTAD
QUINLAN
QUINTAL
QUINTAS
RAILCAR
RAILMAN
RAILSAT
RAILWAY
RAINHAT
RAINMAN
REITMAN
SAIDAAH
SAIDNAY
SEISMAL
SHINPAD
SHIPMAN
SHIPWAY
SKIWEAR
SMILEAT
SMILLAS

SNIFFAT
SNIPEAT
SPIREAS
STIGMAS
SWINGAT
TAILWAG
THINMAN
THISDAY
THISWAY
TOILSAT
TRIGRAM
TRIMTAB
TRISTAN
TRISTAR
TRIVIAL
UNIDEAL
WEIDMAN
WEIRDAL
WHIPSAW
WHISKAS
WHITMAN
ZAIRIAN
ZWICKAU

••I•••A

ABINTRA
ALIBABA
AMIDALA
ARIETTA
ARIKARA
ARIZONA
AVIANCA
CHICANA
CHIMERA
ERIGENA
ERITREA
ILIAMNA
KRISHNA
OKINAWA
OVIPARA
PRIMERA
QUINELA
SCIORRA
SHINOLA
SKIAREA
SPINOZA
TRIBECA
TRIPLEA

•••IA••

ADRIANA
AERIALS
AFFIANT
ANDIAMO
ANTIART
BAHIANS
BIRIANI
BONIATO
BURIALS
CAVIARE
CAVIARS
CILIARY
CILIATE
DECIARE
DEFIANT
DENIALS
DEVIANT
DEVIATE

EQUIANO
ESPIALS
EXPIATE
FACIALS
FIJIANS
FINIALS
FINIANS
FOLIAGE
FOLIATE
GAVIALS
GOLIATH
HONIARA
INDIANA
INDIANS
IONIANS
JULIANA
KODIAKS
LABIALS
LABIATE
LARIATS
LUCIANA
LUCIANO
MALIANS
MANIACS
MARIANA
MARIANO
MEDIANS
MEDIANT
MEDIATE
MENIALS
MYGIANT
MYRIADS
NUBIANS
NYGIANT
OBVIATE
ORGIAST
OSTIARY
PARIAHS
PERIAPT
PONIARD
RADIALS
RADIANS
RADIANT
RADIATE
REDIALS
RELIANT
RETIARY
RUPIAHS
SATIATE
SERIALS
SERIATE
SIMIANS
SOCIALS
SORIANO
STRIATE
SYRIANA
SYRIANS
TAMIAMI
TATIANA
TITIANS
TOPIARY
UNCIALS
VALIANT
VARIANT
VARIATE
VITIATE
XENIAOH
ZODIACS

ZONIANS
ZUNIANS

•••I•A•

AALIYAH
ACTIVAS
ADMIRAL
AFRICAN
ALNILAM
ALNITAK
ALNIYAT
ALTIMAS
AMRITAS
ANTITAX
ANTIWAR
AQUINAS
ARNICAS
ARRIVAL
ARTISAN
BABIYAR
BALIHAI
BASINAL
BERIGAN
BKLIBAN
BOLIVAR
CALIBAN
CANIDAE
CAPITAL
CAPITAN
CARINAE
CARINAS
CASITAS
CAVILAT
CELICAS
COMICAL
CONICAL
CUBICAL
CUBITAL
CYNICAL
DECIMAL
DELIHAM
DELILAH
DELIMAN
DIGICAM
DIGITAL
DOMICAL
ENCINAS
EQUIFAX
ESTIVAL
ETHICAL
FADIMAN
FAJITAS
FARINAS
FINICAL
FLAILAT
FLUIDAL
FREITAG
FUJISAN
GAVILAN
HABITAT
HALIFAX
HEGIRAS
HELICAL
HELIPAD
HOLIDAY
KAPITAL
LADIDAS
LAMINAE
LAMINAL
LAMINAR
LAMINAS
LATIFAH
LATINAS
LEXICAL
LILINAU
LIMINAL
LOGICAL
LONIGAN
LUCIDAE
LUMINAS
LYRICAL
MADIGAN
MAGICAL
MANILAS
MARIDAS
MARINAS
MARITAL
MATINAL
MAXIMAL
MAXIMAS
MEDICAL
MEDIGAP
MEDIVAC
MEXICAN
MINIBAR
MINICAB
MINICAM
MINICAR
MINILAB
MINIMAL
MINIMAX
MINIVAC
MINIVAN
MOHICAN
MTSINAI
MUSICAL
NAVIDAD
NODICAL
NOMINAL
NOVISAD
NUBIRAS
OEDIPAL
OMNIMAX
ONEIDAS
OPTICAL
OPTIMAL
OPTIMAS
ORBITAL
ORDINAL
OVOIDAL
PATINAS
PEDICAB
PELICAN
PEPITAS
PURITAN
RADICAL
RADIOAD
RAPIDAN
RARITAN
RECITAL
REGINAL
REGINAS
RETINAE
RETINAL
RETINAS
REVISAL
REVIVAL
RUFIYAA
SAGINAW
SALINAS
SALIVAS
SEMINAL
SEMINAR
SEMIRAW
SEPIRAS
SERIPAK
SHEILAE
SHEILAS
SILICAS
SIMILAC
SIMILAR
STOICAL
SURINAM
TALIBAN
TAXICAB
TAXIMAN
TAXIWAY
TOPICAL
TROIKAS
TYPICAL
ULTIMAS
UNVITAL
VATICAL
VATICAN
VERITAS
VICINAL
VIMINAL
VIVICAA
VIVITAR
XENICAL
YAKIMAS
YESICAN
ZOOIDAL

•••I••A

ACHIEVA
ADRIANA
AGRIPPA
ALGIEBA
ANTIGUA
BADIDEA
BARISTA
BATISTA
BELINDA
BENICIA
BIGIDEA
BOLIVIA
BONILLA
CALISTA
CAMILLA
CARIOCA
CECILIA
CEDILLA
CHRISTA
CURIOSA
DANIELA
DASILVA
DELIRIA
DRYIDEA
ECHIDNA
ERMINIA
FAMILIA
FELICIA
GALICIA
GORILLA
HONIARA
HYGIEIA
INDIANA
INDICIA
INVICTA
JERITZA
JULIANA
KAPITSA
KATISHA
KOPIYKA
LAVINIA
LETITIA
LUCIANA
LUCINDA
MAGILLA
MARIANA
MARILLA
MARIMBA
MATILDA
MAXILLA
MEGILLA
MELINDA
MELISMA
MELISSA
MELITTA
MILITIA
MOZILLA
NAMIBIA
NERISSA
NEWIDEA
NORIEGA
ONEIOTA
PAPILLA
PERISSA
PREIDEA
RESIDUA
RIVIERA
RUFIYAA
RUZICKA
SCHIRRA
SEVILLA
SICILIA
SOYINKA
SUBIDEA
SYRIANA
TABITHA
TAPIOCA
TATIANA
THEIDEA
THRILLA
TREINTA
TUNISIA
TURISTA
VANILLA
VIVICAA

••••IA•

ACACIAS
ACADIAN
AEOLIAN
ANANIAS
ANEMIAS
APULIAN
ARABIAN
ASOCIAL
AVIVIAN
AZANIAN
AZORIAN
BELGIAN
BESTIAL
BIAXIAL
BORGIAS
BOSNIAN
CARDIAC
CARDIAL
CASPIAN
CASSIAS
CHILIAD
COAXIAL
CORDIAL
CORDIAS
CRANIAL
CRITIAS
CRUCIAL
CUMBIAS
CYPRIAN
DAHLIAS
DRUZIAN
EGERIAS
ELEGIAC
ELENIAK
ELUVIAL
ELYSIAN
ETESIAN
ETONIAN
FASCIAE
FASCIAL
FASCIAS
FLORIAN
FLUVIAL
FRISIAN
FUSTIAN
GAMBIAN
GENTIAN
GHANIAN
GILLIAM
GILLIAN
GLACIAL
GLORIAS
GORDIAN
GRACIAS
GRATIAS
GRECIAN
HADRIAN
HAITIAN
HEREIAM
HERNIAE
HERNIAS
HESSIAN
IBERIAN
INITIAL
IRANIAN
ISCHIAL
ISTRIAN
ITALIAN
IVORIAN
JILLIAN
JIMDIAL
JUNGIAN
KANTIAN
LANCIAS
LAOTIAN
LATVIAN
LILLIAN
LINBIAO
LINPIAO
LOGGIAS
LOTHIAN
MARDIAN
MARTIAL
MARTIAN
MARXIAN
MATHIAS
MAURIAC
MAURIAT
MERCIAN
MERRIAM
MESSIAH
MIAMIAN
MISDIAL
MONDIAL
MYOPIAS
NUPTIAL
NUTRIAS
OBADIAH
ONABIAS
ONTRIAL
OSIRIAN
OVIDIAN
OXONIAN
PARTIAL
PENZIAS
PEORIAN
PERMIAN
PERSIAN
PHIDIAS
PHOBIAS
PIERIAN
PLEBIAN
PLUVIAL
PONTIAC
PONTIAN
PREVIAS
PYTHIAN
PYTHIAS
RAFFIAS
RETRIAL
RHODIAN
RUFFIAN
RUSSIAN
SAURIAN
SCORIAS
SCOTIAN
SEPHIAS
SERBIAN
SHAVIAN
SPACIAL
SPATIAL
SPECIAL
STELIAS
STYGIAN
SUBBIAS
SUNDIAL
SUREIAM
THERIAC
TREDIAS
TRIVIAL
UMBRIAN
UTOPIAN
UTOPIAS
UXORIAL
VOSGIAN
WILLIAM
WOZNIAK
YTTRIAS
ZAIRIAN
ZAMBIAN
ZINNIAS
ZOYSIAS

••••I•A

ADELINA
ALUMINA
AMANITA
AMERICA
AMERIKA
ARABICA
AVENIDA
BAMBINA
BERNINA
BOBVILA
BURKINA
CANDIDA
CANTINA
CAPTIVA
CARMINA
COQUINA
CORRIDA
CORSICA
CORTINA
CORVINA
CZARINA
DERRIDA
DESPINA
DIOTIMA
EMERITA
EROTICA
ETVOILA
EXOTICA
FESTINA
FESTIVA
FIORINA
FLORIDA
FONTINA
FORMICA
GINGIVA
GORDITA
GOTHIKA
GRANITA
HANKIBA
INEDITA
IWOJIMA
JAMAICA
JESSICA
JUDAICA
KACHINA
KATRINA
KOSCINA
KOSHIBA
LAHAINA
LEMPIRA
LIDWINA
MACHINA
MADEIRA
MALLIKA
MALVINA
MARTINA
MESSINA
MISHIMA
MUSCIDA
NAUTICA
NORDICA
OCARINA
ONELIRA
OUGUIYA
PAPRIKA
PARAIBA
PARTITA
PASTINA
PAULINA
PERDITA
PODRIDA
POETICA
POPDIVA
PROXIMA
QUERIDA
RASHIDA
REPLICA
RETSINA
RIORITA
RORAIMA
ROTHIRA
SABRINA
SESTINA
SHAKIRA
STAMINA
TEQUILA
THEBIGA
TOSHIBA
TSARINA
TUTUILA
TZARINA
VAMPIRA
VIATICA
WICHITA
YASHICA
YESHIVA
YUCAIPA
ZOSSIMA

•••••IA

ALBANIA
ALEGRIA
ALGERIA
ALLUVIA
ALMERIA
ALSATIA
AMMONIA
AMNESIA
ANAEMIA
ANOSMIA
ANSONIA
ANTONIA
APHAGIA
APHASIA
APHELIA
APHONIA
AQUARIA
ARCADIA
ARMENIA
ASSYRIA
ASTORIA
AUSTRIA
AUTOPIA
BACTRIA
BATAVIA
BAVARIA
BEDELIA
BEGONIA
BENICIA
BIENNIA
BOHEMIA
BOLIVIA
BOOTHIA
BOTHNIA
BRESCIA
CAHOKIA
CAMBRIA
CARAMIA
CATANIA
CECILIA
CINESIA
CLAUDIA
COMEDIA
CROATIA
CUMBRIA
CYNTHIA
DAPHNIA
DELIRIA
EMPORIA
ENCOMIA
ERMINIA
ESTONIA
ETRURIA
EUGENIA
EUNOMIA
EURASIA
EXORDIA
EXURBIA
FAMILIA
FELICIA
FIDELIA
FREESIA
FUCHSIA
GALATIA
GALICIA
GANGLIA
GEORGIA
HEREDIA
HIMALIA
HRYVNIA
HYGIEIA
HYPATIA
ILLYRIA
INDICIA
INERTIA
LACONIA
LAVINIA
LETITIA
LIBERIA
LIGURIA
LUCANIA
LUTETIA
MAHALIA
MALARIA
MAMAMIA
MELANIA
MELODIA
MILITIA
MINUTIA
MORAVIA
MYALGIA
NAMIBIA
NATALIA
NICOSIA
NIGERIA
OCEANIA
OCTAVIA
ODONTIA
OLYMPIA
OPHELIA
OPUNTIA
OTALGIA
PERAHIA
PERUGIA
PETULIA
PETUNIA
PHRYGIA
POLONIA
POMPEIA
PRUSSIA
PYREXIA
RATAFIA
REGALIA
ROMANIA
ROSALIA
RUMANIA
SAMARIA
SANGRIA
SEDALIA
SEGOVIA
SEQUOIA
SIBERIA
SICILIA
SILESIA
SOLARIA
SOMALIA
STLUCIA
TALARIA
TITANIA
TOCELIA
TUNISIA
VENEZIA
VERONIA
VIDALIA
VISALIA
VITORIA
VIVARIA
ZENOBIA

IB•••••

IBEGYOU
IBERIAN
IBILITY
IBIZANS
IBNSAUD

I•B••••

IDBADGE
IMBIBED
IMBIBER
IMBIBES
IMBORED
IMBROKE
IMBRUED
IMBRUES
IMBUING
INBLACK
INBLOOM
INBOARD
INBOUND
INBOXES
INBREED
INBRIEF
INBROWN
INBUILT
IOBJECT

I••B•••

IAMBICS
IAMBIST
ICEBAGS
ICEBATH
ICEBEER
ICEBERG
ICEBLUE
ICEBOAT
IKEBANA
ILLBITE
ILLBRED
INABALL
INABIND
INKBLOT
IONBEAM
ISABEAU
ISOBARS
ITSBEST

I•••B••

ICHABOD
IGNOBLE
IGNOBLY
IMBIBED
IMBIBER
IMBIBES
INCUBUS
INHABIT
INHIBIT
INLABOR
INORBIT
IRONBAR
ITSABOY
IVTUBES

I••••B•

ICECUBE
INDOUBT
INLIMBO
ITMAYBE

•IB••••

BIBBERS
BIBBIDI
BIBBING
BIBCOCK
BIBELOT
BIBLESS
BIBLIKE
BIBLIOG
DIBBLED
DIBBLER
DIBBLES
FIBBERS
FIBBING
FIBERED
FIBIGER
FIBRINS
FIBROID
FIBROUS
FIBSTER
FIBULAE
FIBULAR
FIBULAS
GIBBERS
GIBBONS
GIBBOUS
GIBESAT
GIBLETS
GIBLUES
GIBSONS
GIBUSES
HIBACHI
HIBBING
HIBBLER
HIBERNO
JIBBOOM
JIBEDAT
JIBESAT
KIBBLED
KIBBLES
KIBBUTZ
LIBBERS
LIBBING
LIBELED
LIBELEE
LIBELER
LIBERAL
LIBERIA
LIBERTE
LIBERTY
LIBIDOS
LIBRANS
LIBRARY
LIBYANS
NIBBLED
NIBBLER
NIBBLES
NIBLETS
NIBLICK
NIBLIKE
RIBALDS
RIBANDS
RIBBERS
RIBBIER
RIBBIES
RIBBING
RIBBONS
RIBBONY
RIBCAGE
RIBCUTS
RIBEYES
RIBLESS
RIBLETS
RIBLIKE
RIBMEAT
RIBPADS
SIBERIA
SIBLING
SIBYLIC
TIBBETT
TIBETAN
TIBURON
VIBISTS
VIBRANT
VIBRATE
VIBRATO

•I•B•••

AIRBAGS
AIRBALL
AIRBASE
AIRBILL
AIRBOAT
BIBBERS
BIBBIDI
BIBBING
BIGBABY
BIGBAND
BIGBANG
BIGBEAR
BIGBEAT
BIGBEND
BIGBETS
BIGBIRD
BIGBLUE
BIGBOSS
BIGBOYS
BIMBOES
DIABLES
DIABLOS
DIABOLO
DIBBLED
DIBBLER
DIBBLES
DIEBOLD
DILBERT
DIMBULB
DISBAND
DISBARS
DISBUDS
FIBBERS
FIBBING
FIGBARS
FILBERT
FINBACK
FIRBANK
GIBBERS
GIBBONS
GIBBOUS
GIGBAGS
GILBERT
GILBLAS
GIMBALS
GIMBELS
HIBBING
HIBBLER
HILBERT
HIPBATH
HIPBONE
HIPBOOT
HITBACK
JIBBOOM
JIMBEAM
KIBBLED
KIBBLES
KIBBUTZ
KIMBALL
KITBAGS
LIBBERS
LIBBING
LIEBACK
LIMBERS
LIMBING
LIMBURG
LINBIAO
LIPBALM
LISBETH
MISBILL
MISBIND

MISBREW
NIBBLED
NIBBLER
NIBBLES
NIEBUHR
NIMBLER
NIOBITE
NIOBIUM
OILBASE
OILBIRD
PIEBALD
PINBALL
PINBOYS
PITBOSS
PITBULL
RIBBERS
RIBBIER
RIBBIES
RIBBING
RIBBONS
RIBBONY
RIMBAUD
SIEBZIG
SIOBHAN
SITBACK
SIXBALL
TIBBETT
TIDBITS
TIEBACK
TIEBARS
TIEBEAM
TIMBALE
TIMBALS
TIMBERS
TIMBERY
TIMBRES
WILBERT
WINBACK

•I••B••

BILOBED
CIMABUE
CITABLE
CITYBOY
DINGBAT
DIRTBAG
DISABLE
DISOBEY
FILIBEG
FINABLE
FIREBOX
FIREBUG
FIXABLE
GIFTBOX
GIGABIT
HIDABLE
HIGHBAR
HIGHBOY
HIRABLE
KICKBOX
KILOBAR
KILOBIT
LIEABED
LIKABLE
LINABLE
LIVABLE
MILKBAR
MINABLE
MINIBAR
MINIBUS
MIRABEL
MISTBOW
MIXABLE
NICEBOY
NICOBAR
PILLBOX
PILLBUG
RIDABLE
RIDEBYS
RISIBLE
RISIBLY
SICKBAY
SICKBED
SIDEBAR
SIDEBET
SINDBAD
SIZABLE
SIZABLY
TINYBIT
VISIBLE
VISIBLY
VITEBSK
WINDBAG
WINEBAR
WINSBIG
WIRABLE

•I•••B•

AIRTUBE
BICARBS
BIGBABY
BIOLABS
DISROBE
EIGHTBC
FIFTYBC
FILEDBY
FILESBY
GIVENBY
HISNIBS
MICROBE
MIDRIBS
OILRUBS
RIDESBY
RIOLOBO
SIXTYBC
TICKSBY

•I••••B

DIMBULB
DISTURB
LINEARB
LIONCUB
MINICAB
MINILAB
MINISUB
NICEJOB
SILENTB
SINUTAB

••IB•••

ALIBABA
ALIBIED
AMIBLUE
BRIBEES
BRIBERS
BRIBERY
BRIBING
CLIBURN
CRIBBED
CRIBBER
CUIBONO
DRIBBLE
DRIBLET
EDIBLES
FOIBLES
FRIBBLE
GLIBBER
LEIBNIZ
OJIBWAS
OJIBWAY
QUIBBLE
SKIBIBS
SKIBOBS
SKIBOOT
SKIBUMS
TRIBBLE
TRIBECA
TRIBORO
TRIBUNE
TRIBUTE
UNIBALL
UNIBODY

••I•B••

AMIABLE
AMIABLY
CLIMBED
CLIMBER
CLIMBIN
CLIMBON
CLIMBTO
CLIMBUP
COINBOX
CRIBBED
CRIBBER
DRIBBLE
FRIABLE
FRIBBLE
FRISBEE
GLIBBER
MAILBAG
MAILBIN
MAILBOX
PHILBIN
PLIABLE
PLIABLY
QUIBBLE
RAILBUS
RAINBOW
SAIDBOO
SKIABLE
THIMBLE
TRIABLE
TRIBBLE
TWINBED

••I••B•

ABIDEBY
ABITIBI
ALIBABA
DRIVEBY
EKINGBY
FLIESBY
FLITSBY
GLIDEBY
GOINGBY
GRIMSBY
LYINGBY
NAIROBI
SKIBIBS
SKIBOBS
SKIPSBY
SLIDEBY
SLIPSBY
STICKBY
SWINGBY

••I•••B

TRIMTAB

•••IB••

ADDIBLE
ADHIBIT
AGRIBIZ
ANTIBES
AUDIBLE
AUDIBLY
BKLIBAN
CALIBAN
CALIBER
CALIBRE
CARIBES
CARIBOO
CARIBOU
DECIBEL
DELIBES
EXHIBIT
FILIBEG
FUSIBLE
HALIBUT
IMBIBED
IMBIBER
IMBIBES
INHIBIT
KLEIBER
LEGIBLE
LEGIBLY
MINIBAR
MINIBUS
MRTIBBS
NAMIBIA
OMNIBUS
PARIBUS
RISIBLE
RISIBLY
SANIBEL
SCRIBED
SCRIBER
SCRIBES
TALIBAN
VISIBLE
VISIBLY

•••I•B•

ALGIEBA
CANITBE
INLIMBO
LETITBE
MARIMBA
MRTIBBS

•••I••B

MINICAB
MINILAB
MINISUB
PEDICAB
TAXICAB

••••IB•

ABITIBI
ARECIBO
ASCRIBE
BBQRIBS
ETALIBI
HANKIBA
HERNIBS
HISNIBS
KOSHIBA
MADLIBS
MIDRIBS
OUTRIBS
PARAIBA
SKIBIBS
TOSHIBA

••••I•B

RECLIMB
UPCLIMB

•••••IB

THETRIB
TRUERIB

IC•••••

ICANNOT
ICEAGES
ICEAXES
ICEBAGS
ICEBATH
ICEBEER
ICEBERG
ICEBLUE
ICEBOAT
ICECAPS
ICECAVE
ICECOLD
ICECUBE
ICEDAMS
ICEDOUT
ICEDOWN
ICEDTEA
ICEFALL
ICEFLOE
ICEFOGS
ICEFREE
ICEHOLE
ICELAND
ICELESS
ICELIKE
ICELINE
ICEMILK
ICEOUTS
ICEOVER
ICEPACK
ICEPICK
ICEPOPS
ICERINK
ICERUNS
ICESHOW
ICESOUT
ICETEAS
ICETRAY
ICEWINE
ICHABOD
ICHDIEN
ICICLES
ICINESS
ICINGIN
ICINGIT
ICINGUP
ICKIEST
ICKYPOO
ICONIFY
ICTERUS
ICTINUS
ICTUSES
ICYWIND

I•C••••

IACOCCA
IDCARDS
INCANTS
INCASED
INCASES
INCENSE
INCENTS
INCEPTS
INCHECK
INCHERS
INCHING
INCISED
INCISES
INCISOR
INCITED
INCITER
INCITES
INCIVIL
INCLASS
INCLINE
INCLOSE
INCLUDE
INCOLOR
INCOMER
INCOMES
INCOURT
INCROWD
INCRUST
INCUBUS
INCUDES
INCURVE
INCUSED
INCUSES
IPCRESS
ISCHIAL
ISCHIUM
ITCHFOR
ITCHIER
ITCHING

I••C•••

ICECAPS
ICECAVE
ICECOLD
ICECUBE
ICICLES
ILLCALL
ILLCLAD
ILOCANO
INACAST
INOCULA
INSCALE
IRECKON
ISECOND
ITSCOLD

I•••C••

IACOCCA
IGOTCHA
ILLICIT
IMPACTS
INDICES
INDICIA
INDICTS
INDUCED
INDUCER
INDUCES
INDUCTS
INDYCAR
INFECTS
INFOCUS
INJECTS
INKYCAP
INSECTA
INSECTS
INVACUO
INVICTA
ITHACAN

I••••C•

IACOCCA
IAMBICS
IATRICS
ICEPACK
ICEPICK
ILIESCU
ILLLUCK
IMPEACH
INBLACK
INCHECK
INDUTCH
INEXACT
INFANCY
INFLECT
INFLICT
INFORCE
INFRACT
INKSACS
INMARCH
INPEACE
INPLACE
INREACH
INSHOCK
INSPACE
INSPECT
INSTOCK
INSYNCH
INTOUCH
INVOICE
IOBJECT
IONESCO
IPSWICH
IRENICS
ITALICS

I•••••C

IDENTIC
IDIOTIC
IDYLLIC
ILIADIC
ILLOGIC
ISLAMIC

•IC••••

BICARBS
BICHONS
BICKERS
BICOLOR
BICORNE
BICORNS
BICYCLE
CICADAE
CICADAS
CICCONE
CICHLID
DICECUP
DICHTER
DICIEST
DICILLO
DICKENS
DICKERS
DICKEYS
DICKIES
DICKORY
DICKSON
DICTATE
DICTION
DICTUMS
FICKLER
FICTILE
FICTION
FICTIVE
FICUSES
HICCUPS
HICKEYS
HICKMAN
HICKORY
JICAMAS
KICKBOX
KICKERS
KICKIER
KICKING
KICKOFF
KICKOUT
KICKSIN
KICKSUP
KICKUPS
LICENCE
LICENSE
LICHEES
LICHENS
LICITLY
LICKERS
LICKETY
LICKING
LICKSUP
MICAELA
MICHAEL
MICHAUX
MICKEYS
MICMACS
MICROBE
MICRONS
NICCAGE
NICCOLO
NICEBOY
NICEDAY
NICEDOG
NICEGUY
NICEJOB
NICEKID
NICEMAN
NICEMEN
NICEONE
NICETRY
NICHING
NICHOLS
NICKELS
NICKERS
NICKING
NICKLES
NICOBAR
NICOISE
NICOLAS
NICOLET
NICOLLE
NICOSIA
NICTATE
PICADOR
PICANTE
PICARAS
PICARDO
PICARDY
PICAROS
PICASSO
PICCARD
PICCATA
PICCOLO
PICEOUS
PICKAXE
PICKENS
PICKERS
PICKETS
PICKETT
PICKIER
PICKING
PICKLED
PICKLES
PICKOFF
PICKOUT
PICKSAT
PICKSON
PICKSUP
PICKUPS
PICNICS
PICOTED
PICTISH
PICTURE
RICARDO
RICHARD
RICHENS
RICHEST
RICHLER
RICHMAN
RICHMEN
RICHTER
RICKETY
RICKEYS
RICKLES
RICKMAN
RICKSHA
RICOTTA
RICRACS
SICCING
SICILIA
SICKBAY
SICKBED
SICKDAY
SICKENS
SICKEST
SICKISH
SICKLES
SICKOUT
SICKPAY
TICCING
TICKERS
TICKETS
TICKING
TICKLED
TICKLER
TICKLES
TICKOFF
TICKSBY
TICOTIN
TICTACS
VICDANA
VICENTE
VICENZA
VICEROY
VICINAL
VICIOUS
VICKERS
VICKREY
VICOMTE
VICTIMS
VICTORS
VICTORY
VICTRIX
VICTUAL
VICUNAS
WICCANS
WICHITA
WICKERS
WICKETS
WICKING
WICKIUP
WICKLOW

•I•C•••

AIRCOOL
AIRCREW
AITCHES
BIBCOCK
BIGCARS
BIGCATS
BIGCITY
BIOCHIP
BIOCIDE
BIRCHED
BIRCHEN
BIRCHES
BISCUIT
CICCONE
CINCHED
CINCHES
CIRCLED
CIRCLER
CIRCLES
CIRCLET
CIRCUIT
CIRCUSY
CISCOES
DIECAST
DIECUTS
DIOCESE
DISCARD
DISCERN
DISCING
DISCMAN
DISCOED
DISCOID
DISCORD
DISCUSS
DITCHED
DITCHER
DITCHES
FIACRES
FILCHED
FILCHER
FILCHES
FINCHES
FISCHER
GIACOMO
GIOCOSO
GISCARD
HICCUPS
HIRCINE
HITCHED
HITCHER
HITCHES
HITCHON
HITCHUP
JIMCHEE
KIDCOMS
KIMCHEE
KINCAID
KITCHEN
LINCOLN
LITCHIS
LITCRIT
MIDCAPS
MINCERS
MINCING
MIOCENE
MISCALL
MISCAST
MISCITE
MISCODE
MISCOIN
MISCOPY
MISCUED
MISCUES
MISCUTS
MITCHUM
NICCAGE
NICCOLO
OILCAKE
OILCANS
OILCUPS
PICCARD
PICCATA
PICCOLO
PIECERS
PIECING
PILCROW
PINCERS
PINCHAS
PINCHED
PINCHER
PINCHES
PINCHME
PINCHOT
PINCURL
PIPCARD
PISCEAN
PISCINE
PISCOPO
PITCHED
PITCHER
PITCHES
PITCHIN
PITCHTO
PITCREW
RIBCAGE
RIBCUTS
RIPCORD
RITCHIE
SICCING
SIMCITY
SINCERE
SINCITY
SITCOMS
TICCING
TIECLIP
TINCANS
TINCTED
TIPCART
VINCENT
VINCULA
VISCERA
VISCOUS
VISCUSO
WICCANS
WINCERS
WINCHED
WINCHER
WINCHES
WINCING
WITCHED
WITCHES
ZILCHES
ZINCIFY
ZINCING
ZINCITE
ZINCKED
ZINCOUS
ZIPCODE
ZIPCUFF
ZIRCONS
ZITCOMS

•I••C••

AIRACES
BIANCHI
BICYCLE
BIFOCAL
BINOCHE
BISECTS
DICECUP
DIDACTS
DIGICAM
DIRECTS
DIRECTV
FIANCEE
FIANCES
FIASCOS
FIERCER
FINICAL
FINICKY
HIBACHI
HIJACKS
HITACHI
KITSCHY
LIMACON
LINECUT
LINGCOD
LIONCUB
MILKCAN
MILKCOW
MIMICRY
MINICAB
MINICAM
MINICAR
MIRACLE
MISACTS
PIERCED
PIERCER
PIERCES
SIDECAR
SILICAS
SILICON
SIROCCO
TIERCES
TIMECOP
VIDICON
VIVICAA
WILDCAT

•I•••C•

AIRDUCT
AIRLOCK
AIRPACK
AIRRACE
AIRSACS
AIRSICK
AIRSOCK
AIRWICK
BIBCOCK
BIGMACS
BIONICS
BIOPICS
BIOTECH
DIALECT
DIPTYCH
DISSECT
DISTICH
DIVORCE
FINANCE
FINBACK
FIREICE
GIMMICK
HILLOCK
HITBACK
JIMRICE
KIDROCK
LICENCE
LIEBACK
LIKEICE
MICMACS
MINORCA
MIRISCH
MIXTECS
NIBLICK

NIDETCH
NIPMUCK
NITPICK
OILRICH
PICNICS
PIMLICO
PINNACE
RICRACS
RIDDICK
RIMROCK
RIOTACT
SILENCE
SIROCCO
SITBACK
SIXPACK
TICTACS
TIEBACK
TIERACK
TIETACK
TIETACS
TIMRICE
TITMICE
VIADUCT
VIATICA
VITRICS
WINBACK
ZIPLOCK
ZIPLOCS

•I••••C

BIVOUAC
DINARIC
EIDETIC
EIDOLIC
EIGHTBC
FIFTYBC
KINESIC
KINETIC
LIPIDIC
LIPSYNC
MIASMIC
MIDDLEC
MIMETIC
MINIVAC
MISKOLC
MITOTIC
NIANTIC
PIRATIC
SIBYLIC
SILENTC
SIMILAC
SIXTYBC
TITANIC
VINYLIC

••IC•••

AMICHAI
BRICKED
BRICKLE
BRICKUP
CHICAGO
CHICANA
CHICANE
CHICANO
CHICEST
CHICHAS
CHICHEN
CHICHIS
CHICKEN
CHICLES
CHICLET
CHICORY
CLICHED
CLICHES
CLICKED
CLICKER
CLICKON
CRICKED
CRICKET
DEICERS
DEICING
EDICTAL
ELICITS
EPICARP
EPICENE
EPICURE
ERICSON
ETICKET
EVICTED
EVICTEE
EVICTOR
FBICASE
FLICKED
FLICKER
FRICKER
ICICLES
JUICERS
JUICEUP
JUICIER
JUICILY
JUICING
LAICIZE
OCICATS
OLICOOK
OMICRON
PLICATE
PRICERS
PRICIER
PRICILY
PRICING
PRICKED
PRICKLE
PRICKLY
PRICKUP
QUICHES
QUICKEN
QUICKER
QUICKIE
QUICKLY
REICING
SKICAPS
SLICERS
SLICEUP
SLICING
SLICKED
SLICKER
SLICKLY
SNICKER
SNICKET
SPICERS
SPICERY
SPICEUP
SPICIER
SPICILY
SPICING
STICKBY
STICKER
STICKIN
STICKON
STICKTO
STICKUM
STICKUP
TEICHER
THICKEN
THICKER
THICKET
THICKLY
TRICEPS
TRICKED
TRICKER
TRICKLE
TRICORN
TRICOTS
UNICODE
UNICORN
UTICANS
UTICANY
VOICERS
VOICING
ZWICKAU

••I•C••

BAITCAR
BRIOCHE
BRITCOM
CHILCAT
EVINCED
EVINCES
GLITCHY
HAIRCUT
MAILCAR
MRISCAN
PHILCOS
PRINCES
QUINCES
QUINCEY
RAILCAR
TWITCHY

••I••C•

ANIMACY
AVIANCA
CHIRICO
CLINICS
CRITICS
DRIESCH
EDIFICE
FAIENCE
GRIMACE
ILIESCU
ORIFICE
ORINOCO
OVIDUCT
OVISACS
PLIANCY
PRIMACY
PRIVACY
SCIENCE
SCITECH
SKIRACE
SKIRACK
SPINACH
THINICE
TRIBECA
TRISECT
UNIVACS

••I•••C

ABIOTIC
ANIONIC
ASIATIC
AVIATIC
AVIONIC
DEISTIC
EKISTIC
ERISTIC
IDIOTIC
ILIADIC
MEIOTIC
QUINTIC
SCIATIC
SEISMIC
TRIADIC

•••IC••

ADDICTS
ADVICES
AFRICAN
ALNICOS
APRICOT
ARNICAS
ARTICLE
ATTICUS
AURICLE
BENICIA
BENICIO
BODICES
CALICES
CALICOS
CELICAS
CEVICHE
CHOICER
CHOICES
CODICES
CODICIL
COLICKY
COMICAL
COMICES
CONICAL
CUBICAL
CUBICLE
CUBICLY
CUTICLE
CYNICAL
DEFICIT
DELICTI
DELICTO
DELICTS
DEPICTS
DEVICES
DIGICAM
DOMICAL
DOMICIL
ENTICED
ENTICER
ENTICES
ETHICAL
FAMICOM
FELICIA
FINICAL
FINICKY
FRAICHE
GALICIA
HARICOT
HELICAL
HELICES
HELICON
ILLICIT
INDICES
INDICIA
INDICTS
INVICTA
JERICHO
KENICHI
LATICES
LEXICAL
LEXICON
LOGICAL
LYRICAL
LYRICON
MAGICAL
MALICES
MEDICAL
MEDICOS
MEXICAN
MIMICRY
MINICAB
MINICAM
MINICAR
MODICUM
MOHICAN
MUSICAL
MUSICKS
NODICAL
NOTICED
NOTICER
NOTICES
NOVICES
OFFICER
OFFICES
OFFICIO
OPTICAL
OPTICKS
OSSICLE
PANICKY
PANICLE
PEDICAB
PELICAN
PLAICES
POLICED
POLICER
POLICES
PUMICED
PUMICES
RADICAL
RADICES
RADICLE
REKICKS
RELICTS
REPICKS
RETICLE
RUBICON
RUZICKA
SCHICKS
SHTICKS
SHTICKY
SILICAS
SILICON
SLUICED
SLUICES
SOLICIT
SPLICED
SPLICER
SPLICES
STOICAL
TAXICAB
TOPICAL
TUNICLE
TYPICAL
UNPICKS
UPTICKS
VATICAL
VATICAN
VEHICLE
VESICLE
VIDICON
VIVICAA
WAVICLE
XENICAL
YESICAN

•••I•C•

ANTIOCH
BADITCH
BEWITCH
CARIOCA
DAVINCI
DEHISCE
DENIECE
EXTINCT
JALISCO
MANIACS
MENISCI
MIRISCH
NABISCO
ONEINCH
POLISCI
REHITCH
SQUINCH
STRITCH
TAPIOCA
UNCINCH
UNHITCH
ZODIACS

•••I••C

BASILIC
DOMINIC
DRUIDIC
EMPIRIC
FATIDIC
FLUIDIC
HAMITIC
HASIDIC
JURIDIC
LEVITIC
LIPIDIC
MEDIVAC
MINIVAC
ONEIRIC
OOLITIC
OSSIFIC
PACIFIC
POLITIC
PYRITIC
SATIRIC
SEMITIC
SIMILAC
UNCIVIC
VERIDIC

••••IC•

AFFLICT
AGARICS
AIRSICK
AIRWICK
ALDRICH
AMERICA
ARABICA
ARABICS
ATOMICS
ATONICS
AUSPICE
AVARICE
BARLICK
BEQUICK
BERBICK
BERWICK
BIONICS
BIOPICS
BLUEICE
BURDICK
CANDICE
CAPRICE
CELTICS
CHALICE
CHIRICO
CLARICE
CLERICS
CLINICS
CONNICK
CONVICT
COPPICE
CORNICE
CORSICA
CORTICO
COWLICK
CREVICE
CRITICS
CYMRICS
DERRICK
DERRICO
DISTICH
DOGTICK
DORMICE
DOTRICE
EBONICS
EDIFICE
EHRLICH
ELDRICH
ELDRICK
EMETICS
ERDRICH
EROTICA
EROTICS
ETHNICS
ETONICS
EXOTICA
EXOTICS
FABRICS
FANFICS
FIREICE
FORMICA
FOSDICK
FROLICS
GALLICO
GARLICS
GARRICK
GATWICK
GEDRICK
GIMMICK
GOTHICS
HAPTICS
HARNICK
HAYRICK
HENRICH
HEROICS
HERRICK
HOMEICE
HOSPICE
HOTLICK
HOWNICE
IAMBICS
IATRICS
ICEPICK
INFLICT
INVOICE
IPSWICH
IRENICS
ITALICS
JAMAICA
JESSICA
JIMRICE
JUDAICA
JUSTICE
KUBRICK
LABMICE
LATTICE
LIKEICE
MANRICO
MASTICS
MAURICE
MEDWICK
MERRICK
MESSICK
METRICS
MORTICE
MOSAICS
MYSTICS
NATWICK
NAUTICA
NEWRICH
NIBLICK
NITPICK
NOETICS
NORDICA
NORDICS
NORWICH
NOTNICE
OILRICH
OLDNICK
ONAKICK
ORIFICE
OSTRICH
OUTKICK
OUTPICK
OVERICE
PACKICE
PAMLICO
PATRICE
PATRICK
PEPSICO
PEPTICS
PETMICE
PHOBICS
PHONICS
PHOTICS
PHYSICS
PICNICS
PIMLICO
POETICA
POETICS
PORTICO
PREDICT
PUBLICS
REEVICT
REJOICE
RENWICK
REPLICA
REPRICE
RESPICE
RESTICK
REVOICE
RIDDICK
RODDICK
ROLLICK
RUBRICS
RUSTICS
SCENICS
SCHTICK
SEASICK
SERPICO
SERVICE
STATICE
STATICS
SUFFICE
SYNDICS
TACTICS
TAMPICO
THEMICK
THINICE
TIMRICE
TITMICE
TOEPICK
TOPKICK
TROPICS
UNJUICY
UNQUICK
UNSLICK
UNSPICY
UNSTICK
UNTHICK
UNVOICE
VARRICK
VERDICT
VIATICA
VITRICS
WARWICK
YANNICK
YASHICA

••••I•C

CARDIAC
ELEGIAC
MAURIAC
PONTIAC
THERIAC

•••••IC

ABIOTIC
ACERBIC
ACRYLIC
ACYCLIC
AELFRIC
AEROBIC
AGNATIC
ALEMBIC
ALLELIC
AMHARIC
AMMONIC
AMNESIC
AMOEBIC
ANAEMIC
ANGELIC
ANIONIC
ANOSMIC
APHAGIC
APHASIC
APHONIC
AQUATIC
ARAMAIC
ARCHAIC
ARSENIC
ASCETIC
ASEPTIC
ASIATIC
AVIATIC
AVIONIC
BACCHIC
BALDRIC
BASILIC
BENEFIC
BORONIC
BOSONIC
BOTANIC
BUCOLIC
BYRONIC
CALORIC
CAMBRIC
CANONIC
CAUSTIC
CENTRIC
CERAMIC
CHAOTIC
CHASMIC
CHLORIC
CHROMIC
CHRONIC
CLASSIC
COMEDIC
CROSTIC
CRYPTIC
DEISTIC
DELPHIC
DELTAIC
DEMONIC
DEMOTIC
DHARMIC
DINARIC
DOMINIC
DRASTIC
DRUIDIC
DRYADIC
DYNAMIC
EIDETIC
EIDOLIC
EKISTIC
ELASTIC
EMPIRIC
ENDEMIC
ENTERIC
ENZYMIC
ERGOTIC
ERISTIC
ERRATIC
ETHERIC
EUGENIC
FANATIC
FATIDIC
FJORDIC
FLUIDIC
FRANTIC
FREDRIC
GASTRIC
GENERIC
GENETIC
GENOMIC
GEORGIC
GLYPHIC
GLYPTIC
GNOSTIC
GRAPHIC
HAMITIC
HASIDIC
HEBRAIC
HEDONIC
HEMATIC
HEPATIC
HERETIC
HEXADIC
HOMERIC
IDENTIC
IDIOTIC
IDYLLIC
ILIADIC
ILLOGIC
ISLAMIC
JURIDIC
KETONIC
KINESIC
KINETIC
KORANIC
LACONIC
LECTRIC
LEVITIC
LIPIDIC
LUNATIC
MALEFIC
MANTRIC
MASONIC
MEIOTIC
MELANIC
MELODIC
MESONIC
MIASMIC
MIMETIC
MITOTIC
MONADIC
MONODIC
MORONIC
MORPHIC
MRMUSIC
MYALGIC
MYRRHIC
NEPHRIC
NEPOTIC
NIANTIC
NOMADIC
NONEPIC
NUCLEIC
NUMERIC
NYMPHIC
OCEANIC
OCTADIC
OGHAMIC
OLYMPIC
ONEIRIC
ONTOPIC
OOLITIC
ORECTIC
ORGANIC
OSMATIC
OSMOTIC
OSSIFIC
OTALGIC
PACIFIC
PADRAIC
PARODIC
PASSAIC
PELAGIC
PHRENIC
PIRATIC
PLASMIC
PLASTIC
PLUMBIC
POLEMIC
POLITIC
PRACTIC
PROSAIC
PSALMIC
PSYCHIC
PYRETIC
PYRITIC
PYRRHIC
QUADRIC
QUARTIC
QUINTIC
RHEUMIC
RHOMBIC
ROBOTIC
ROMANIC
SATANIC
SATIRIC
SATYRIC
SCEPTIC
SCIATIC
SEISMIC
SELENIC
SEMITIC
SIBYLIC
SKEPTIC
SOMATIC
SPHERIC
STANNIC
STEARIC
STYPTIC
SYLPHIC
SYNODIC
TACONIC
TELEPIC
THERMIC
TITANIC
TOTEMIC
TRAFFIC
TRIADIC
UNCIVIC
UNCOMIC
UNCUBIC
UNLYRIC
UNSTOIC
UNTOXIC
VANADIC
VENATIC
VERIDIC
VINYLIC
VOCALIC
VOLTAIC
WAREPIC
XANTHIC
XEROTIC
ZEBRAIC

ID•••••

IDAHOAN
IDAREDS
IDBADGE
IDCARDS
IDEALLY
IDEAMAN
IDEAMEN
IDEATED
IDEATES
IDENTIC
IDIAMIN
IDIDTOO
IDIOTIC
IDLESSE
IDOLISE
IDOLIST
IDOLIZE
IDOODIT
IDOTTER
IDSAYSO
IDTHEFT
IDYLIST
IDYLLIC

I•D••••

INDEEDY
INDENTS
INDEPTH
INDEXED
INDEXER
INDEXES
INDIANA
INDIANS
INDICES
INDICIA
INDICTS
INDIGEN
INDIGOS
INDITED
INDITER
INDITES
INDOORS
INDORSE
INDOUBT
INDRAFT
INDRAWN
INDUCED
INDUCER
INDUCES
INDUCTS
INDULGE

INDUTCH
INDWELL
INDWELT
INDYCAR
IODATED
IODATES
IODIDES
IODISED
IODISES
IODIZED
IODIZER
IODIZES

I••D•••

ICEDAMS
ICEDOUT
ICEDOWN
ICEDTEA
ICHDIEN
IDIDTOO
ILLDOIT
ILLDONE
IMADEIT
INADAZE
INEDITA
IRIDIUM
ISADORA
ISADORE
ISIDORE
ITSDONE

I•••D••

IDBADGE
IDOODIT
IFITDIE
ILIADIC
ILLUDED
ILLUDES
IMPEDED
IMPEDER
IMPEDES
INAIDOF
INCUDES
INFIDEL
INKEDIN
INORDER
INSIDER
INSIDES
INVADED
INVADER
INVADES
IODIDES
IPLEDGE
ISAIDNO
IWONDER

I••••D•

IDAREDS
IDCARDS
ILLMADE
IMPENDS
IMPLODE
IMREADY
INCLUDE
INDEEDY
INFOLDS
INKPADS
INLANDS
INNARDS
INROADS
INTENDS
INTRADE
INTRUDE
INWARDS
ISLANDS
ISOPODS
ISUREDO

I•••••D

IBNSAUD
ICECOLD
ICELAND
ICHABOD
ICYWIND
IDEATED
IGNITED
IGNORED
IGOOFED
IGUANID
ILLBRED
ILLCLAD
ILLFOLD
ILLUDED
ILLUMED
ILLUSED
ILLWIND
IMBIBED
IMBORED
IMBRUED
IMMIXED
IMMURED
IMPALED
IMPAVID
IMPEDED
IMPLEAD
IMPLIED
IMPOSED
IMPOUND
IMPUTED
IMTIRED
INABIND
INAMOOD
INAWORD
INBOARD
INBOUND
INBREED
INCASED
INCISED
INCITED
INCROWD
INCUSED
INDEXED
INDITED
INDUCED
INFIELD
INFIXED
INFUSED
INHALED
INHERED
INHUMED
INJURED
INSIPID
INSTEAD
INSURED
INTHIRD
INTONED
INVADED
INVALID
INVITED
INVOKED
IODATED
IODISED
IODIZED
IONISED
IONIZED
IRELAND
ISAHEAD
ISECOND
ISLETED
ISSUEAD
ITSCOLD

•ID••••

AIDLESS
BIDDERS
BIDDIES
BIDDING
BIDFAIR
BIDSFOR
DIDACTS
DIDASET
DIDDLED
DIDDLER
DIDDLES
DIDDLEY
DIDEROT
DIDFINE
DIDGOOD
DIDLAPS
DIDLIKE
DIDOVER
DIDSUMS
DIDTIME
DIDTOAT
DIDWELL
EIDETIC
EIDOLIC
EIDOLON
FIDDLED
FIDDLER
FIDDLES
FIDELES
FIDELIA
FIDELIO
FIDELIS
FIDGETS
FIDGETY
GIDDIED
GIDDIER
GIDDIES
GIDDILY
GIDDYAP
GIDDYUP
GIDEONS
HIDABLE
HIDALGO
HIDAWAY
HIDEOUS
HIDEOUT
HIDINGS
KIDCOMS
KIDDERS
KIDDIES
KIDDING
KIDDISH
KIDLIKE
KIDNAPS
KIDNEYS
KIDROCK
KIDSEAT
KIDSKIN
KIDSRUS
KIDULTS
KIDVIDS
LIDLESS
LIDWINA
MIDASES
MIDCAPS
MIDDAYS
MIDDIES
MIDDLEC
MIDDLED
MIDDLER
MIDDLES
MIDEAST
MIDGETS
MIDIRON
MIDJULY
MIDJUNE
MIDLAND
MIDLEGS
MIDLIFE
MIDLINE
MIDLIST
MIDMORN
MIDMOST
MIDNOON
MIDOFFS
MIDRIBS
MIDRIFF
MIDRISE
MIDSHIP
MIDSIZE
MIDSOLE
MIDTEEN
MIDTERM
MIDTOWN
MIDWAYS
MIDWEEK
MIDWEST
MIDWIFE
MIDYEAR
NIDETCH
PIDDLED
PIDDLES
PIDGEON
PIDGINS
RIDABLE
RIDDERS
RIDDICK
RIDDING
RIDDLED
RIDDLER
RIDDLES
RIDEBYS
RIDEOFF
RIDEOUT
RIDESBY
RIDESIN
RIDESTO
RIDESUP
RIDGIER
RIDGING
RIDGWAY
RIDINGS
RIDOTTO
SIDDONS
SIDDURS
SIDEARM
SIDEBAR
SIDEBET
SIDECAR
SIDEMAN
SIDEMEN
SIDEONE
SIDETWO
SIDEWAY
SIDINGS
SIDIOUS
SIDLING
TIDALLY
TIDBITS
TIDERIP
TIDIEST
TIDINGS
TIDYING
TIDYSUM
VIDALIA
VIDEOED
VIDETTE
VIDICON
VIDIOTS
WIDENED
WIDENER
WIDGEON
WIDGETS
WIDMARK
WIDOWED
WIDOWER
YIDDISH

•I•D•••

AIRDAMS
AIRDATE
AIRDRIE
AIRDROP
AIRDUCT
BIDDERS
BIDDIES
BIDDING
BIGDAYS
BIGDEAL
BIGDIGS
BIGDOGS
BINDERS
BINDERY
BINDING
BINDLES
BINDOFF
BINDSTO
BINDSUP
BIODATA
BIRDDOG
BIRDERS
BIRDFLU
BIRDIED
BIRDIES
BIRDING
BIRDMAN
BIRDMEN
CINDERS
CINDERY
DIADEMS
DIDDLED
DIDDLER
DIDDLES
DIDDLEY
DIEDFOR
DIEDOFF
DIEDOUT
DIEDOWN
DIKDIKS
DINDINS
DISDAIN
FIDDLED
FIDDLER
FIDDLES
FIEDLER
FINDERS
FINDING
FINDLAY
FINDLEY
FINDOUT
GIDDIED
GIDDIER
GIDDIES
GIDDILY
GIDDYAP
GIDDYUP
GILDERS
GILDING
GIRDERS
GIRDING
GIRDLED
GIRDLER
GIRDLES
HINDERS
HINDLEG
HINDPAW
JIMDALE
JIMDIAL
KIDDERS
KIDDIES
KIDDING
KIDDISH
KILDARE
KINDEST
KINDLED
KINDLER
KINDLES
KINDRED
LIEDFOR
LIEDOWN
LINDENS
LINDIED
LINDIES
LINDNER
LINDORF
LINDROS
LINDSAY
LINDSEY
MIDDAYS
MIDDIES
MIDDLEC
MIDDLED
MIDDLER
MIDDLES
MILDEST
MILDEWS
MILDEWY
MILDRED
MINDERS
MINDFUL
MINDING
MINDORO
MINDSET
MISDATE
MISDEAL
MISDEED
MISDEEM
MISDIAL
MISDOER
MISDOES
MISDONE
MISDRAW
MISDREW
OILDRUM
PIDDLED
PIDDLES
PINDOWN
RIDDERS
RIDDICK
RIDDING
RIDDLED
RIDDLER
RIDDLES
RINDIER
RITDYES
SIDDONS
SIDDURS
SINDBAD
SIRDUKE
SITDOWN
TIEDOFF
TIEDOWN
TIEDYED
TIEDYES
TINDERS
TINDERY
TIPDOWN
VIADENT
VIADUCT
VICDANA
VIEDFOR
WILDCAT
WILDDOG
WILDEST
WILDING
WILDISH
WILDMAN
WILDMEN
WILDONE
WILDPIG
WINDAGE
WINDAUS
WINDBAG
WINDERS
WINDGOD
WINDIER
WINDIGO
WINDILY
WINDING
WINDOMS
WINDOWS
WINDOWY
WINDSOR
WINDSUP
WINDTEE
WINDUPS
WISDOMS
YIDDISH
ZIPDISK

•I••D••

AIKIDOS
AIMEDAT
AIREDUP
BIGIDEA
BIMODAL
BIPEDAL
BIRDDOG
CICADAE
CICADAS
CITADEL
DINADAM
DINEDAT
DINEDIN
DINEDON
DIRNDLS
DIVEDIN
DIVIDED
DIVIDER
DIVIDES
FIEFDOM
FIELDED
FIELDER
FILEDBY
FILEDIN
FILMDOM
FIREDAT
FIREDOG
FIREDON
FIREDUP
FIVEDAY
FIXEDLY
FIXEDON
FIXEDUP
HIGHDAY
HIKEDUP
HIREDON
JIBEDAT
KIKIDEE
KILNDRY
KINGDOM
LIBIDOS
LINEDRY
LINEDUP
LIPIDIC
LIVEDIN
LIVEDON
LIVIDLY
MIKADOS
MILKDUD
MILLDAM
MIRADAS
MIRADOR
MISADDS
MISEDIT
MIXEDIN
MIXEDLY
MIXEDUP
NICEDAY
NICEDOG
PICADOR
PILEDIN
PILEDON
PILEDUP
PIPEDIN
PIPEDUP
RIGIDLY
RIKSDAG
RILEDUP
RIORDAN
SICKDAY
SINEDIE
SIZEDUP
TIENDAS
TIMIDER
TIMIDLY
TIRADES
TIREDER
TIREDLY
TIREDOF
VIVIDER
VIVIDLY
WIELDED
WIELDER
WILDDOG
WIPEDUP
WIREDIN
WIREDUP
WISEDUP
YIELDED
YIELDER
YIELDTO

•I•••D•

AIRMADA
BIBBIDI
BIGENDS
BIGKIDS
BIOCIDE
DIALEDO
DIOMEDE
DIOXIDE
DISBUDS
GIRONDE
KIDVIDS
LIGANDS
LIMEADE
LIQUIDS
LIZARDS
MILORDS
MIRANDA
MISADDS
MISCODE
NIKEADS
NIMRODS
NITRIDE
PICARDO
PICARDY
RIBALDS
RIBANDS
RIBPADS
RICARDO
RIGVEDA
RINALDO
RIPTIDE
RITARDS
TIERODS
TINGODS
VIVALDI
VIVENDI
WIZARDS
ZIPCODE

•I••••D

AIRHEAD
AIRRAID
BIASSED
BIGBAND
BIGBEND
BIGBIRD
BIGEYED
BIGHAND
BIGHEAD
BIGLEAD
BIGOTED
BILOBED
BIRCHED
BIRDIED
BIRTHED
CICHLID
CINCHED
CIRCLED
DIALLED
DIAMOND
DIBBLED
DIDDLED
DIDGOOD
DIEBOLD
DIEHARD
DILATED
DILLARD
DILUTED
DIMPLED
DIPLOID
DIRTIED
DISBAND
DISCARD
DISCOED
DISCOID
DISCORD
DISTEND
DISUSED
DITCHED
DITTOED
DIVIDED
DIVINED
DIVVIED
DIZZIED
EIGHTAD
FIBERED
FIBROID
FIDDLED
FIELDED
FIFTYAD
FIGURED
FILCHED
FINISHD
FINLAND
FIXATED
FIZZLED
GIDDIED
GIELGUD
GIFFORD
GIGGLED
GILFORD
GINGOLD
GIRDLED
GIRTHED
GISCARD
GIZZARD
HIGGLED
HIGHEND
HISPEED
HITCHED
JIGGLED
JIMMIED
JINGLED
KIBBLED
KINCAID
KINDLED
KINDRED
KINKAID
LIAISED
LIBELED
LIEABED
LIGATED
LIGHTED
LIKEMAD
LIKENED
LILYPAD
LIMITED
LINDIED
LINGCOD
LINSEED
LIPREAD
LITHOID
LIVEAID
LIVENED
LIVERED
MIAOUED
MIAOWED
MIDDLED
MIDLAND
MILDRED
MILHAUD
MILKDUD
MILKFED
MILLAND
MILLARD
MILLEND
MIMEOED
MINGLED
MINORED
MINOTND
MINUEND
MINUTED
MISBIND
MISCUED
MISDEED
MISFEED
MISLAID
MISLEAD
MISREAD
MISSAID
MISSEND
MISTOLD
MISUSED
MISWORD
MITERED
MITFORD
MIZZLED
NIBBLED
NICEKID
NIGGLED
OILBIRD
OILSAND
OILSEED
PIAFFED
PICCARD
PICKLED
PICOTED
PIDDLED
PIEBALD
PIEEYED
PIERCED
PIFFLED
PIGEYED
PIGWEED
PILOTED
PIMPLED
PINCHED
PINFOLD
PINGUID
PINHEAD
PIPCARD
PIRATED
PITCHED
PITHEAD
PIVOTED
RICHARD
RIDDLED
RIFFLED
RIGHTED
RIMBAUD
RIMPLED
RIPCORD
RIPENED
RIPPLED
RITEAID
RIVALED
RIVETED
SICKBED
SIGHTED
SIGMOID
SIGMUND
SILENTD
SINDBAD
SINEWED
SINGLED
SIRENED
SIXFOLD
SIXTYAD
SIZZLED
TIARAED
TICKLED
TIEDYED
TIMREID
TINCTED
TINGLED
TINKLED
TIPPLED
TIPTOED
VIALLED
VIDEOED
VILLARD
VINLAND
VISAGED
VISITED
VISORED
VISTAED
VIZORED
WIDENED
WIDOWED
WIELAND
WIELDED
WIGGLED
WILFORD
WILFRED
WILLARD
WIMPLED
WINCHED
WINDGOD
WINERED
WINWOOD
WITCHED
WITSEND
WIZENED
XIPHOID
YIELDED
ZINCKED

••ID•••

ABIDEBY
ABIDERS
ABIDING
ABIDJAN
ACIDIFY
ACIDITY
ALIDADE
AMIDALA
AMIDOLS
ARIDEST
ARIDITY
AVIDEST
AVIDFAN
AVIDITY
BRIDALS
BRIDGED
BRIDGER
BRIDGES
BRIDGET
BRIDLED
BRIDLER
BRIDLES
CHIDDEN
CHIDERS
CHIDING
DOIDARE
ELIDERS
ELIDING
EPIDERM
EPIDOTE
EVIDENT
FRIDAYS
FRIDGES
FRIDLEY
GLIDEBY
GLIDEIN
GLIDERS
GLIDING
GRIDDED
GRIDDER
GRIDDLE
GRIDMAP
GUIDERS
GUIDING
IDIDTOO
IRIDIUM
ISIDORE
LAIDFOR
LAIDLOW

LAIDOFF
LAIDOUT
LOIDING
MAIDENS
MAIDISH
OVIDIAN
OVIDUCT
OXIDANT
OXIDASE
OXIDATE
OXIDISE
OXIDIZE
PAIDADS
PAIDFOR
PAIDOFF
PAIDOUT
PHIDIAS
PRIDING
RAIDERS
RAIDING
SAIDAAH
SAIDAYE
SAIDBOO
SAIDIDO
SAIDNAY
SKIDDED
SKIDDER
SKIDDOO
SKIDLID
SKIDOOS
SKIDROW
SLIDEBY
SLIDEIN
SLIDERS
SLIDING
SLIDOFF
SLIDOUT
SMIDGEN
SMIDGES
SNIDELY
SNIDEST
SPIDERS
SPIDERY
TRIDENT
TVIDOLS
TWIDDLE
UNIDEAL
VOIDERS
VOIDING
VOIDOUT
WEIDMAN

••I•D••
ARIADNE
BLINDED
BLINDER
BLINDLY
BLINDTO
BRINDLE
BUILDER
BUILDIN
BUILDON
BUILDUP
CHIDDEN
CRIEDUP
DEIRDRE
DRIEDUP
DRIPDRY
DWINDLE
FLIEDTO
FRIEDAN
FRIEDUP
GRIDDED
GRIDDER
GRIDDLE
GRINDER
GUILDER
HAIRDOS
HAIRDYE
HEIRDOM
IFITDIE
ILIADIC
JOINDER
NAIADES
REINDEX
SHINDIG
SKIDDED
SKIDDER
SKIDDOO
SPIEDON
SPINDLE
SPINDLY
SPINDRY
SWINDLE
THIRDLY
THISDAY
TRIADIC
TRIEDIT
TRIEDON
TRIEDTO
TRIODES
TWIDDLE
UVINDEX
WEIRDAL
WEIRDED
WEIRDER
WEIRDLY
WEIRDOS

••I••D•
ALIDADE
BOIARDO
BRIARDS
BRIGADE
EPILADY
EPISODE
FRIENDS
PAIDADS
SAIDIDO
SHIELDS
TRIPODS
UNIBODY
UNICODE
UNIPODS

••I•••D
ALIBIED
ALIGNED
AMISTAD
ANISEED
ASISAID
AVIATED
BLINDED
BLINKED
BLIPPED
BLISSED
BLITZED
BOISEID
BRICKED
BRIDGED
BRIDLED
BRIEFED
BRIGAND
BRIMMED
BRISKED
CAIRNED
CHILIAD
CHILLED
CHINKED
CHINNED
CHIPPED
CHIRPED
CHIRRED
CHIVIED
CLICHED
CLICKED
CLIMBED
CLINKED
CLIPPED
CLIQUED
COIFFED
COIGNED
CRIBBED
CRICKED
CRIMPED
CRINGED
CRISPED
DEIFIED
DEIGNED
DRIFTED
DRILLED
DRIPPED
DWIGHTD
EDIFIED
EMITTED
ENISLED
EVICTED
EVINCED
EXISTED
FAINTED
FEIGNED
FEINTED
FLICKED
FLIPPED
FLIRTED
FLITTED
FOISTED
FRILLED
FRINGED
FRISKED
FRITTED
FRIZZED
GLINTED
GLITZED
GRIDDED
GRIEVED
GRIFTED
GRILLED
GRINNED
GRIPPED
GRITTED
HEISTED
HOISTED
JOINTED
JOISTED
KNITTED
MAITRED
NEIGHED
OMITTED
OSIERED
PAINTED
PHISHED
PLINKED
POINTED
PRICKED
PRIMMED
PRIMPED
PRINKED
PRINTAD
PRINTED
QUIETED
QUILLED
QUILTED
QUIPPED
QUIRTED
QUITTED
QUIZZED
RAINGOD
REIFIED
REIGNED
REINKED
SAINTED
SHIFTED
SHILLED
SHINNED
SHINPAD
SHIPPED
SHIRKED
SHIRRED
SKIDDED
SKIDLID
SKIFFED
SKILLED
SKIMMED
SKIMPED
SKINNED
SKIPPED
SKIRLED
SKIRTED
SLICKED
SLIMMED
SLINKED
SLIPPED
SLITTED
SMIRKED
SMITHED
SNIFFED
SNIPPED
SPIELED
SPIFFED
SPILLED
STIFFED
STIFLED
STILLED
STILTED
STINTED
STIPEND
STIRRED
SWIGGED
SWILLED
SWIRLED
SWISHED
SZILARD
TAILEND
TAINTED
THIEVED
THINNED
TRICKED
TRIFFID
TRIFLED
TRIFOLD
TRILLED
TRIMMED
TRIPLED
TRIPPED
TWILLED
TWINBED
TWINGED
TWINNED
TWIRLED
TWISTED
TWITTED
UNIFIED
UNINKED
UNITARD
WAISTED
WEIGHED
WEIRDED
WHIFFED
WHIPPED
WHIRLED
WHIRRED
WHISHED
WHISKED
WHIZKID
WHIZZED
WRITHED

•••ID••
ABRIDGE
ACRIDLY
AIKIDOS
APHIDES
APSIDES
AVOIDED
AVOIDER
BADIDEA
BESIDES
BETIDED
BETIDES
BIGIDEA
BOLIDES
BORIDES
BRAIDED
BRAIDER
BROIDER
CANIDAE
CCRIDER
DECIDED
DECIDER
DECIDES
DERIDED
DERIDER
DERIDES
DIVIDED
DIVIDER
DIVIDES
DOSIDOS
DREIDEL
DRUIDIC
DRYIDEA
ECHIDNA
EXCIDED
EXCIDES
FATIDIC
FETIDLY
FLUIDAL
FLUIDIC
FLUIDLY
GELIDLY
HALIDES
HASIDIC
HASIDIM
HOLIDAY
HUMIDEX
HUMIDLY
HUMIDOR
INAIDOF
INFIDEL
INSIDER
INSIDES
IODIDES
ISAIDNO
JURIDIC
KEMIDOV
KIKIDEE
LADIDAS
LEPIDUS
LIBIDOS
LIPIDIC
LIVIDLY
LUCIDAE
LUCIDLY
LURIDLY
MARIDAS
MARIDOS
MERIDEN
NAVIDAD
NEWIDEA
ONEIDAS
ONSIDES
ONVIDEO
OVOIDAL
OXHIDES
PAVIDLY
PERIDOT
PREIDEA
RABIDLY
RAPIDAN
RAPIDER
RAPIDLY
REHIDES
RERIDES
RESIDED
RESIDER
RESIDES
RESIDUA
RESIDUE
REWIDEN
RIGIDLY
SEMIDRY
SODIDWE
SOLIDER
SOLIDLY
STAIDER
STAIDLY
STRIDER
STRIDES
SUBIDEA
TEPIDLY
THEIDEA
TIMIDER
TIMIDLY
UNAIDED
UNGIDDY
UNSIDED
UPSIDES
VALIDID
VALIDLY
VAPIDLY
VERIDIC
VIVIDER
VIVIDLY
WEDIDIT
YESIDID
ZOOIDAL

•••I•D•
BEGIRDS
BEHINDS
BELINDA
DEWILDE
ENGILDS
ENGIRDS
ENWINDS
LUCINDA
MATILDA
MELINDA
MYRIADS
PERIODS
RADIODJ
REBINDS
REFINDS
REGILDS
REGIRDS
REMINDS
REWINDS
UNBINDS
UNGIDDY
UNGIRDS
UNWINDS
UNWINDY
UPGIRDS
UPWINDS

•••I••D
ACTIFED
ADMIRED
ADMIXED
ADVISED
AFFINED
AFFIXED
ARRIVED
ASPIRED
ATTIRED
AUDITED
AVAILED
AVOIDED
AWAITED
BATIKED
BEMIRED
BETIDED
BRAIDED
BRAINED
BRAISED
BROILED
BRUISED
BRUITED
BYLINED
CAVILED
CHAINED
CHAIRED
CHOIRED
CLAIMED
CRUISED
DEAIRED
DEBITED
DECIDED
DEFILED
DEFINED
DEHIRED
DEMIGOD
DEMISED
DENIMED
DERIDED
DERIVED
DESIRED
DEVILED
DEVISED
DEWIRED
DIVIDED
DIVINED
DRAINED
EMAILED
ENFIELD
ENGINED
ENOILED
ENSILED
ENTICED
ERMINED
ETAILED
EXCIDED
EXCISED
EXCITED
EXPIRED
FINISHD
FLAILED
FOLIOED
FRUITED
GRAINED
GROINED
HABITED
HELIPAD
HOMINID
IGNITED
IMBIBED
IMMIXED
IMTIRED
INCISED
INCITED
INDITED
INFIELD
INFIXED
INSIPID
INVITED
IODISED
IODIZED
IONISED
IONIZED
LIAISED
LIMITED
MERITED
MOTIVED
NAVIDAD
NOTICED
NOVISAD
OBLIGED
ORBITED
PERILED
PLAITED
POLICED
PONIARD
POSITED
PRAISED
PUMICED
QUAILED
QUOINED
QUOITED
RADIOAD
RADIOED
RAVINED
REAIMED
REAIRED
RECITED
REFILED
REFINED
REFIRED
REFIXED
REHIRED
RELINED
RELIVED
REMINED
REMISED
REMIXED
REOILED
REPINED
RESIDED
RESILED
RESINED
RESITED
RESIZED
RETILED
RETIMED
RETIRED
REVILED
REVISED
REVIVED
REWIPED
REWIRED
ROSINED
SCRIBED
SHRINED
SLUICED
SPLICED
SPOILED
SQUIRED
STAINED
STAIRED
STRIPED
STRIVED
THRIVED
TRAILED
TRAINED
UMPIRED
UNAIDED
UNAIMED
UNAIRED
UNCITED
UNDIKED
UNFILED
UNFINED
UNFIRED
UNFIXED
UNHIRED
UNLIKED
UNLINED
UNLIVED
UNMIKED
UNMINED
UNMIRED
UNMIXED
UNOILED
UNPILED
UNPIPED
UNRIGID
UNRILED
UNRIMED
UNRIVED
UNSIDED
UNSIZED
UNTILED
UNTIMED
UNTIMID
UNTIRED
UNVIVID
UNWIPED
UNWIRED
UPDIVED
UPFIELD
UPPILED
UPSIZED
VALIDID
VISITED
YESIDID

••••ID•
ACARIDS
ALCAIDE
ALTOIDS
ARAMIDS
ASTRIDE
AVENIDA
BANDIDO
BEDSIDE
BIBBIDI
BIGKIDS
BIOCIDE
BOBBIDI
BROMIDE
BUSHIDO
BUSRIDE
CABRIDE
CANDIDA
CANDIDE
CANDIDS
CARBIDE
CASSIDY
CERVIDS
COLLIDE
CONFIDE
CONOIDS
CORRIDA
CORVIDS
COWHIDE
CUBOIDS
CUEBIDS
CUSPIDS
CYANIDE
CYANIDS
DAYSIDE
DERRIDA
DIOXIDE
DOASIDO
EBBTIDE
ECOCIDE
ELAPIDS
EYELIDS
FAKEIDS
FARSIDE
FLORIDA
FORBIDS
GAPKIDS
HALOIDS
HAPKIDO
HAYRIDE
HYBRIDS
HYDRIDE
JOEKIDD
JOYRIDE
KIDVIDS
LEETIDE
LEONIDS
LETRIDE
LIQUIDS
LOWBIDS
LOWSIDE
LOWTIDE
MCBRIDE
MUSCIDA
NAVAIDS
NEREIDS
NEWKIDS
NITRIDE
NUCLIDE
OFFSIDE
ORCHIDS
OUTBIDS
OUTRIDE
OUTSIDE
PEPCIDS
PEPTIDE
PERDIDO
PERFIDY
PLACIDO
PODRIDA
PONGIDS
POTLIDS
PREBIDS
PRESIDE
PROVIDE
QUERIDA
QUERIDO
RASHIDA
RAWHIDE
REDTIDE
REGUIDE
RIPTIDE
ROLAIDS
SAIDIDO
SAYSIDO
SCHMIDT
SEASIDE
SPYKIDS
STUPIDS
SUBLIDS
SUBSIDE
SUBSIDY
SULFIDE
SUREIDO
TOPBIDS
TOPSIDE
TOROIDS
TVGUIDE
USERIDS
VERBIDS
VESPIDS
WAYSIDE

••••I•D
ALIBIED
ALLTIED
AMERIND
ANTBIRD
ANYKIND
APPLIED
ATTHIRD
BANDIED
BELLIED
BERRIED
BIGBIRD
BIRDIED
BOOBIRD
BOOGIED
BUDDIED
BULLIED
CADDIED
CANDIED
CARRIED
CATBIRD
CHILIAD
CHIVIED
CONRIED
COWBIRD
CULLIED
CURRIED
DALLIED
DECRIED
DEIFIED
DIRTIED
DIVVIED
DIZZIED
DOLLIED
DUMMIED
EDIFIED
EMPTIED
ENSKIED
EPOXIED
EXSCIND
FANCIED
FERRIED
GIDDIED
GLORIED
GULLIED
GUSSIED
HARRIED
HOGTIED
HOGWILD
HURRIED
ICYWIND
ILLWIND
IMPLIED
INABIND
INTHIRD
JAYBIRD
JELLIED
JETTIED
JIMMIED
JOEKIDD
JOLLIED
LINDIED
LOBBIED
MANKIND
MARRIED
MISBIND
MUDDIED
NANNIED
OFAKIND
OFAMIND
OILBIRD
OUTFIND
OUTVIED
OUTWIND
PARRIED
PARTIED
PETBIRD
PREBIND
PUTTIED
QUERIED
RALLIED
RANWILD
READIED
REBUILD
REDBIRD
REDRIED
REFRIED
REGRIND
REIFIED
REPLIED
RESCIND
RETRIED
RUDDIED
RUNWILD
SALLIED
SAVVIED
SEABIRD
SORTIED
STORIED
STUDIED
STYMIED
SULLIED
SUNBIRD
TALLIED
TARRIED
THEWIND
TOADIED
UNBUILD
UNCRIED
UNDRIED
UNFRIED
UNIFIED
UNPLIED
UNSPIED
UNTRIED
UPBUILD
UPDRIED
WEARIED
WORRIED

•••••ID
ADENOID
AIRRAID
AMEBOID
ANDROID
ANEROID

ANNELID
ANTACID
ARANEID
ASISAID
BANDAID
BARMAID
BOISEID
CAMELID
CAROTID
CICHLID
COCCOID
COLLOID
CTENOID
CYCLOID
DELTOID
DENTOID
DIPLOID
DISCOID
ETHMOID
FACTOID
FARMAID
FIBROID
FLACCID
GETSRID
GLOBOID
GOODKID
HAPLOID
HENREID
HOMINID
HYALOID
HYPNOID
IGUANID
IMPAVID
INSIPID
INVALID
JUMPBID
KATYDID
KINCAID
KINKAID
KOOLAID
LACTAID
LANGUID
LITHOID
LIVEAID
LOWPAID
MASTOID
MERMAID
MISLAID
MISSAID
NAYSAID
NEWLAID
NICEKID
NONACID
NONPAID
NONSKID
NONVOID
OCEANID
OCHROID
OLDMAID
OSTEOID
OUTLAID
OUTPAID
OUTSAID
OVERBID
OVERDID
PAROTID
PERSEID
PHOTOID
PINGUID
PREACID
PREPAID
PREVOID
PROMBID
PYRAMID
RITEAID
SCARWID
SIGMOID
SKIDLID
SQUALID
STEROID
SUBARID
SUNMAID
TABLOID
TAXPAID
THYROID
TIMREID
TRIFFID
TYPHOID
UNBRAID
UNFLUID
UNHUMID
UNLUCID
UNRIGID
UNSOLID
UNSTAID
UNTIMID
UNVIVID
UPBRAID
VALIDID
WAYLAID
WELLHID
WHIZKID
WHOSAID
XIPHOID
YESIDID
ZEBROID

IE•••••

IEIGHTY

I•E••••

IBEGYOU
IBERIAN
ICEAGES
ICEAXES
ICEBAGS
ICEBATH
ICEBEER
ICEBERG
ICEBLUE
ICEBOAT
ICECAPS
ICECAVE
ICECOLD
ICECUBE
ICEDAMS
ICEDOUT
ICEDOWN
ICEDTEA
ICEFALL
ICEFLOE
ICEFOGS
ICEFREE
ICEHOLE
ICELAND
ICELESS
ICELIKE
ICELINE
ICEMILK
ICEOUTS
ICEOVER
ICEPACK
ICEPICK
ICEPOPS
ICERINK
ICERUNS
ICESHOW
ICESOUT
ICETEAS
ICETRAY
ICEWINE
IDEALLY
IDEAMAN
IDEAMEN
IDEATED
IDEATES
IDENTIC
IHEARYA
IKEBANA
IMEANIT
IMEMINE
INEDITA
INEPTLY
INERROR
INERTIA
INERTLY
INEXACT
INEXILE
IRECKON
IREFUSE
IRELAND
IRELESS
IRENICS
IREPEAT
IRESIGN
ISECOND
ISEENOW
ISEEYOU
ITEMING
ITEMISE
ITEMIZE
ITEMONE
ITERANT
ITERATE
IVERSON

I••E•••

IAPETUS
ICTERUS
IDLESSE
IFWEMAY
IGNEOUS
IIPETER
IKNEWIT
ILIESCU
ILLEANA
ILLEGAL
ILLEGIT
IMMENSE
IMMERGE
IMMERSE
IMPEACH
IMPEDED
IMPEDER
IMPEDES
IMPENDS
IMPERIL
IMPETUS
IMREADY
INCENSE
INCENTS
INCEPTS
INDEEDY
INDENTS
INDEPTH
INDEXED
INDEXER
INDEXES
INFECTS
INFERNO
INFESTS
INGEMAR
INGENUE
INGESTA
INGESTS
INHERED
INHERES
INHERIT
INJECTS
INKEDIN
INNERLY
INNERVE
INPEACE
INPERIL
INREACH
INSEAMS
INSECTA
INSECTS
INSERTS
INTEARS
INTEGER
INTEGRA
INTENDS
INTENSE
INTENTS
INTERIM
INTERNE
INTERNS
INTERSE
INVEIGH
INVENTS
INVERSE
INVERTS
INVESTS
INWEAVE
INYEARS
IONESCO
IOWEYOU
IPLEDGE
IQTESTS
ISEENOW
ISEEYOU
ISLETED
ITSEASY
ITWELVE
ITWENTY

I•••E••

ICEBEER
ICEBERG
ICELESS
ICETEAS
ICINESS
ICKIEST
IDAREDS
IDTHEFT
IFFIEST
IFIFELL
IGIVEUP
IHATEIT
IHAVEIT
IHOPESO
ILIKEIT
ILLNESS
ILLTELL
ILOVEIT
ILOVELA
IMADEIT
IMAGERS
IMAGERY
IMAMESS
IMARETS
IMGREAT
IMOGENE
IMPIETY
IMPLEAD
IMPRESS
IMPREST
IMPREZA
IMSWELL
IMTHERE
INAHEAP
INAMESS
INANELY
INANEST
INAWEOF
INBREED
INCHECK
INCHERS
INDEEDY
INDWELL
INDWELT
INFIELD
INFLECT
INGLESE
INGREEN
INGRESS
ININETY
INKIEST
INKJETS
INKLESS
INKWELL
INNLESS
INQUEST
INSPECT
INSTEAD
INSTEPS
INSWEPT
INTHERE
INUTERO
IOBJECT
IONBEAM
IPANEMA
IPCRESS
IRATELY
IRATEST
IRELESS
IREPEAT
IRONERS
ISABEAU
ISAHEAD
ISOHELS
ISOMERS
ISRAELI
ISSUEAD
ISSUERS
ISUREAM
ISUREDO
ITSBEST
ITSHERE

I••••E•

ICEAGES
ICEAXES
ICEBEER
ICEDTEA
ICEFREE
ICEOVER
ICHDIEN
ICICLES
ICTUSES
IDEAMEN
IDEATED
IDEATES
IDOTTER
IFORGET
IGNITED
IGNITER
IGNITES
IGNORED
IGNORER
IGNORES
IGOOFED
IIPETER
ILLBRED
ILLUDED
ILLUDES
ILLUMED
ILLUMES
ILLUSED
ILLUSES
IMAGOES
IMBIBED
IMBIBER
IMBIBES
IMBORED
IMBRUED
IMBRUES
IMHOTEP
IMMIXED
IMMIXES
IMMUNES
IMMURED
IMMURES
IMPALED
IMPALER
IMPALES
IMPANEL
IMPEDED
IMPEDER
IMPEDES
IMPLIED
IMPLIES
IMPOSED
IMPOSER
IMPOSES
IMPURER
IMPUTED
IMPUTER
IMPUTES
IMTIRED
INAPOEM
INAPTER
INASTEW
INBOXES
INBREED
INBRIEF
INCASED
INCASES
INCISED
INCISES
INCITED
INCITER
INCITES
INCOMER
INCOMES
INCUDES
INCUSED
INCUSES
INDEXED
INDEXER
INDEXES
INDICES
INDIGEN
INDITED
INDITER
INDITES
INDUCED
INDUCER
INDUCES
INFIDEL
INFIVES
INFIXED
INFIXES
INFUSED
INFUSER
INFUSES
INGATES
INGREEN
INHALED
INHALER
INHALES
INHERED
INHERES
INHUMED
INHUMER
INHUMES
INJOKES
INJURED
INJURER
INJURES
INKSTER
INLAYER
INLINES
INMATES
INNAGES
INORDER
INPOWER
INSALES
INSANER
INSIDER
INSIDES
INSOLES
INSURED
INSURER
INSURES
INTAKES
INTEGER
INTHREE
INTONED
INTONER
INTONES
INVADED
INVADER
INVADES
INVITED
INVITEE
INVITER
INVITES
INVOKED
INVOKER
INVOKES
INWOVEN
IODATED
IODATES
IODIDES
IODISED
IODISES
IODIZED
IODIZER
IODIZES
IONISED
IONISER
IONISES
IONIZED
IONIZER
IONIZES
IONONES
IRISHER
IRONIES
IRONMEN
ISHMAEL
ISLETED
ISRAFEL
ITCHIER
ITSOPEN
ITSOVER
IVORIES
IVTUBES
IWONDER

I•••••E

IAMLOVE
ICEBLUE
ICECAVE
ICECUBE
ICEFLOE
ICEFREE
ICEHOLE
ICELIKE
ICELINE
ICEWINE
IDBADGE
IDLESSE
IDOLISE
IDOLIZE
IFITDIE
IFORONE
IFSTONE
IGNOBLE
IGRAINE
ILLBITE
ILLDONE
ILLLIVE
ILLMADE
IMAGINE
IMAMATE
IMBROKE
IMEMINE
IMITATE
IMMENSE
IMMERGE
IMMERSE
IMOGENE
IMPASSE
IMPINGE
IMPLODE
IMPLORE
IMPROVE
IMPULSE
IMTHERE
INADAZE
INAHOLE
INALINE
INAPILE
INAPOKE
INARAGE
INASHOE
INAVALE
INCENSE
INCLINE
INCLOSE
INCLUDE
INCURVE
INDORSE
INDULGE
INEXILE
INFANTE
INFLAME
INFLATE
INFORCE
INGENUE
INGLESE
INGRATE
INHASTE
INHOUSE
INKLIKE
INLARGE
INNERVE
INPEACE
INPHASE
INPLACE
INQUIRE
INRANGE
INSCALE
INSHAPE
INSHORE
INSIGNE
INSPACE
INSPIRE
INSPITE
INSTATE
INSTONE
INSTORE
INSTYLE
INTASTE
INTENSE
INTERNE
INTERSE
INTHERE
INTHREE
INTRADE
INTRUDE
INULASE
INUTILE
INVERSE
INVITEE
INVOGUE
INVOICE
INVOLVE
INWEAVE
INWHITE
IPLEDGE
IREFUSE
IRKSOME
IRONAGE
IRONORE
ISADORE
ISIDORE
ISOLATE
ISOLINE
ISOTONE
ISOTOPE
ITEMISE
ITEMIZE
ITEMONE
ITERATE
ITMAYBE
ITSALIE
ITSATIE
ITSDONE
ITSFINE
ITSGONE
ITSHERE
ITSLATE
ITSLOVE
ITSONME
ITSTIME
ITSTRUE
ITWELVE
IVANHOE
IVORINE
IVYLIKE

•IE••••

BIENNIA
BIENTOT
DIEAWAY
DIEBOLD
DIECAST
DIECUTS
DIEDFOR
DIEDOFF
DIEDOUT
DIEDOWN
DIEHARD
DIEMENS
DIEOFFS
DIESELS
DIESFOR
DIESOFF
DIESOUT
DIETARY
DIETERS
DIETING
FIEDLER
FIEFDOM
FIELDED
FIELDER
FIENNES
FIERCER
FIERIER
FIERILY
FIESTAS
GIELGUD
KIEFFER
LIEABED
LIEATOP
LIEBACK
LIEDFOR
LIEDOWN
LIEFEST
LIENEES
LIENORS
LIEOVER
LIESFOR
LIESLOW
LIETEST
NIEBUHR
NIELSEN
PIEBALD
PIECERS
PIECING
PIEEYED
PIEHOLE
PIELIKE
PIEPANS
PIERCED
PIERCER
PIERCES
PIERIAN
PIERROT
PIESAFE
PIESALE
PIETIES
PIETINS
PIETOSO
PIETROS
RIEGERT
RIEMANN
RIESENS
RIESMAN
RIESSEN
SIEBZIG
SIEGING
SIEMENS
SIENESE
SIENNAS
SIERRAS
SIESTAS
SIEVING
TIEBACK
TIEBARS
TIEBEAM
TIECLIP
TIEDOFF
TIEDOWN
TIEDYED
TIEDYES
TIEGAME
TIEINTO
TIELESS
TIELINE
TIEMPOS
TIENDAS
TIEPINS
TIEPOLO
TIERACK
TIERCES
TIERING
TIERNEY
TIERODS
TIEROPE
TIESOFF
TIETACK
TIETACS
VIEDFOR
VIELLES
VIERNES
VIERZIG
VIESFOR
VIETNAM
VIEWERS
VIEWIER
VIEWING
VIEWITH
WIELAND
WIELDED
WIELDER
WIENERS
WIENIES
YIELDED
YIELDER
YIELDTO
ZIEGLER
ZIERING

•I•E•••

AILERON
AIMEDAT
AIREDUP
BIBELOT
BIGEARS
BIGEAST
BIGEASY
BIGELOW
BIGENDS
BIGEYED
BIGEYES
BIKEWAY
BILEVEL
BIMETAL
BIPEDAL
BIREMES
BIRETTA
BISECTS
BITEOFF
BITESIN
BITESON
BITESUP
CILENTO
CINEMAS
CINEMAX
CINEOLE
CINERGY
CINESIA
CISEAUX
DICECUP
DIDEROT
DIGESTS
DILEMMA
DIMETER
DINEDAT
DINEDIN
DINEDON
DINEOUT
DINESAT
DINESEN
DINESIN
DINESON
DINETTE
DIRECTS
DIRECTV
DIREFUL
DISEASE
DISEURS
DISEUSE
DIVEDIN
DIVERGE
DIVERSE
DIVERTS
DIVESIN
DIVESTS
EIDETIC
FIBERED
FIDELES
FIDELIA
FIDELIO
FIDELIS
FILEDBY
FILEDIN
FILENES
FILEOUT
FILESBY
FILESIN
FINEART
FINESSE
FIREANT
FIREARM
FIREBOX
FIREBUG
FIREDAT
FIREDOG
FIREDON
FIREDUP
FIREFLY
FIREFOX
FIREHAT
FIREICE
FIRELIT
FIREMAN
FIREMEN
FIRENZA
FIRENZE
FIREOFF
FIREPIT
FIRESAT
FIRESON
FIRESUP
FIVEAAA
FIVEDAY
FIVEEEE
FIVEMAN
FIVEONE
FIVEPIN
FIVESIX
FIVETEN
FIVETWO
FIVEWAY
FIXEDLY
FIXEDON
FIXEDUP
FIXESON
FIXESUP

GIBESAT
GIDEONS
GISELLE
GIVEEAR
GIVENBY
GIVENIN
GIVENOF
GIVENON
GIVENTO
GIVENUP
GIVEOFF
GIVEOUT
GIVESIN
GIVESOF
GIVESON
GIVESTO
GIVESUP
GIVEUPS
GIVEWAY
HIBERNO
HIDEOUS
HIDEOUT
HIKEDUP
HIKEOUT
HIKESUP
HIREDON
HIREOUT
HIRESON
HIVEOFF
IIPETER
JIBEDAT
JIBESAT
JIMENEZ
KINESES
KINESIC
KINESIS
KINETIC
LIBELED
LIBELEE
LIBELER
LIBERAL
LIBERIA
LIBERTE
LIBERTY
LICENCE
LICENSE
LIFEFUL
LIFENET
LIKEICE
LIKEMAD
LIKENED
LIKENEW
LIKENTO
LIKEWOW
LILETEE
LIMEADE
LIMEPIE
LINEAGE
LINEARA
LINEARB
LINEATE
LINECUT
LINEDRY
LINEDUP
LINEMAN
LINEMEN
LINEONE
LINEOUT
LINESUP
LINETWO
LINEUPS
LISENTE
LITERAL
LIVEAID
LIVEDIN
LIVEDON
LIVEFOR
LIVENED
LIVENER
LIVENUP
LIVEOAK
LIVEONE
LIVEOUT
LIVERED
LIVESAT
LIVESET
LIVESEY
LIVESIN
LIVESON
LIZETTE
MIDEAST
MIGENES
MILEAGE
MILERUN
MIMEOED
MIMESES
MIMESIS
MIMETIC
MINEOLA
MINEPIT
MINERAL
MINERVA
MISEDIT
MISERLY
MITERED
MIXEDIN
MIXEDLY
MIXEDUP
MIXESIN
MIXESUP
NICEBOY
NICEDAY
NICEDOG
NICEGUY
NICEJOB
NICEKID
NICEMAN
NICEMEN
NICEONE
NICETRY
NIDETCH
NIGERIA
NIKEADS
NILESOH
NINEEEE
NINEPIN
NINEVEH
NIVEOUS
OISEAUX
PICEOUS
PIEEYED
PIGEONS
PIGEYED
PILEATE
PILEDIN
PILEDON
PILEDUP
PILEGGI
PILEOUS
PILESIN
PILESOF
PILESON
PILESUP
PILEUPS
PIMENTO
PIMESON
PINEFOR
PINENUT
PINEOIL
PINESAP
PINESOL
PINETAR
PINETOP
PINETUM
PIPEDIN
PIPEDUP
PIPEFUL
PIPESIN
PIPESUP
PIPETTE
PIRELLI
PITEOUS
RIBEYES
RIDEBYS
RIDEOFF
RIDEOUT
RIDESBY
RIDESIN
RIDESTO
RIDESUP
RILEDUP
RILESUP
RIPENED
RIPENER
RISENTO
RISESTO
RISESUP
RITEAID
RIVERPO
RIVETED
RIVETER
SIBERIA
SIDEARM
SIDEBAR
SIDEBET
SIDECAR
SIDEMAN
SIDEMEN
SIDEONE
SIDETWO
SIDEWAY
SILENCE
SILENTA
SILENTB
SILENTC
SILENTD
SILENTE
SILENTF
SILENTG
SILENTH
SILENTI
SILENTJ
SILENTK
SILENTL
SILENTM
SILENTN
SILENTO
SILENTP
SILENTQ
SILENTR
SILENTS
SILENTT
SILENTU
SILENTV
SILENTW
SILENTX
SILENTY
SILENTZ
SILESIA
SIMENON
SINEDIE
SINEWED
SIRENED
SISENOR
SITEMAP
SIXEEEE
SIZEDUP
SIZEONE
SIZESIX
SIZESUP
SIZETEN
SIZETWO
TIBETAN
TIDERIP
TIMECOP
TIMELAG
TIMEOFF
TIMEOUT
TIMESUP
TIMEWAS
TIMEXES
TINEARS
TIREDER
TIREDLY
TIREDOF
TIREMAN
TIREMEN
TIREOUT
TIRESOF
VICENTE
VICENZA
VICEROY
VIDEOED
VIDETTE
VINEGAR
VITEBSK
VIVENDI
VIXENLY
WIDENED
WIDENER
WINEBAR
WINERED
WINESAP
WINEVAT
WIPEDUP
WIPEOFF
WIPEOUT
WIPESUP
WIREDIN
WIREDUP
WIREMAN
WIREMEN
WIRESIN
WIRESUP
WIRETAP
WISEDUP
WISEGUY
WISEMAN
WISEMEN
WISEONE
WISESUP
WITEOUT
WIZENED
XIMENES

•I••E••

AIDLESS
AIGLETS
AIGRETS
AILMENT
AIMLESS
AIRHEAD
AIRIEST
AIRLESS
AIRNESS
AIRVENT
BIBBERS
BIBLESS
BICKERS
BIDDERS
BIGBEAR
BIGBEAT
BIGBEND
BIGBETS
BIGDEAL
BIGFEET
BIGGERS
BIGGEST
BIGHEAD
BIGJERK
BIGLEAD
BIGMEAL
BIGMESS
BIGNESS
BIGNEWS
BIGTENT
BILKERS
BILLERS
BILLETS
BINDERS
BINDERY
BINGERS
BIOTECH
BIRDERS
BIRLERS
BISSELL
BITLESS
BITTERN
BITTERS
CINDERS
CINDERY
CIPHERS
CISTERN
DIADEMS
DIALECT
DIALEDO
DIALERS
DIAPERS
DICIEST
DICKENS
DICKERS
DICKEYS
DIDWELL
DIEMENS
DIESELS
DIETERS
DIFFERS
DIGGERS
DIGRESS
DILBERT
DILUENT
DIMMERS
DIMMEST
DIMNESS
DINGERS
DINNERS
DIOCESE
DIOMEDE
DIPNETS
DIPPERS
DISCERN
DISPELS
DISSECT
DISSENT
DISSERT
DISTEND
DITHERS
DITHERY
FIBBERS
FIDGETS
FIDGETY
FIFTEEN
FIGLEAF
FIGMENT
FILBERT
FILLERS
FILLETS
FILTERS
FINDERS
FINGERS
FINLESS
FIRMEST
FISHERS
FISHERY
FISHEYE
FITNESS
FITTERS
FITTEST
FITWELL
FIVEEEE
FIZZERS
GIBBERS
GIBLETS
GIFTEES
GILBERT
GILDERS
GIMBELS
GIMLETS
GINGERS
GINGERY
GINSENG
GIRDERS
GIVEEAR
HIALEAH
HICKEYS
HIGHEND
HIGHEST
HILBERT
HIMSELF
HINDERS
HINGEON
HINTERS
HIPLESS
HIPNESS
HIPPEST
HISPEED
HISSERS
HITHERE
HITLESS
HITTERS
JIGGERS
JIGGERY
JILTERS
JIMBEAM
JINXERS
JITNEYS
JITTERS
JITTERY
JIVIEST
KICKERS
KIDDERS
KIDNEYS
KIDSEAT
KILLEEN
KILLERS
KINDEST
KINLESS
KINNEAR
KINNELL
KIPPERS
KISLEVS
KISMETS
KISSELS
KISSERS
KITTENS
KITTERY
LIBBERS
LICHEES
LICHENS
LICKERS
LICKETY
LIDLESS
LIEFEST
LIENEES
LIETEST
LIFTERS
LIGGETT
LIMBERS
LIMIEST
LIMNERS
LIMPEST
LIMPETS
LINDENS
LINGERS
LINIEST
LINKERS
LINNETS
LINSEED
LINTELS
LINTERS
LIONELL
LIONELS
LIONESS
LIONETS
LIPLESS
LIPPERS
LIPREAD
LIQUEFY
LIQUEUR
LISBETH
LISPERS
LISTEES
LISTENS
LISTERS
LITHELY
LITHEST
LITTERS
LITTERY
MICAELA
MICKEYS
MIDGETS
MIDLEGS
MIDTEEN
MIDTERM
MIDWEEK
MIDWEST
MIDYEAR
MILDEST
MILDEWS
MILDEWY
MILIEUS
MILIEUX
MILKERS
MILLEND
MILLERS
MILLETS
MILLETT
MIMIEUX
MINCERS
MINDERS
MINTERS
MINUEND
MINUETS
MIOCENE
MIRIEST
MISDEAL
MISDEED
MISDEEM
MISFEED
MISHEAR
MISKEYS
MISLEAD
MISMESH
MISREAD
MISRELY
MISSEAT
MISSEND
MISSENT
MISSETS
MISTELL
MISTERM
MISTERS
MISTERX
MITTENS
MIXTECS
MIZZENS
NIBLETS
NICKELS
NICKERS
NIGHEST
NIMIETY
NINEEEE
NIPPERS
OILHEAT
OILIEST
OILLESS
OILSEED
OILWELL
OINKERS
PICKENS
PICKERS
PICKETS
PICKETT
PIDGEON
PIECERS
PIGGERY
PIGLETS
PIGMEAT
PIGMENT
PIGPENS
PIGWEED
PILFERS
PINCERS
PINGERS
PINHEAD
PINIEST
PINKENS
PINKEST
PINKETT
PINLESS
PINNERS
PINSEAL
PIOLETS
PIONEER
PIPIEST
PIPLESS
PIRAEUS
PISCEAN
PITHEAD
PITIERS
RIBBERS
RIBLESS
RIBLETS
RIBMEAT
RICHENS
RICHEST
RICKETY
RICKEYS
RIDDERS
RIEGERT
RIESENS
RIFLERS
RIFLERY
RIGGERS
RIGUEUR
RIGVEDA
RILIEVO
RILLETS
RIMIEST
RIMLESS
RINGERS
RINSERS
RIOTERS
RIPIENI
RIPIENO
RIPPERS
RISKERS
RIVIERA
RIVIERE
SIAMESE
SICKENS
SICKEST
SIEMENS
SIENESE
SIFTERS
SIGHERS
SIGNEES
SIGNERS
SIGNETS
SILVERS
SILVERY
SIMMERS
SIMPERS
SINCERE
SINGERS
SINKERS
SINLESS
SINNERS
SIPPERS
SISTERS
SITTERS
SITWELL
SIXEEEE
SIXFEET
SIXTEEN
SIXWEEK
SIXYEAR
TIBBETT
TICKERS
TICKETS
TIDIEST
TIEBEAM
TIELESS
TIGRESS
TILLERS
TILLETS
TILTERS
TIMBERS
TIMBERY
TIMREID
TINDERS
TINDERY
TINIEST
TINKERS
TINNERS
TINSELS
TINTERN
TINTERS
TIPLESS
TIPPEES
TIPPERS
TIPPETS
TITHERS
TITTERS
VIADENT
VICKERS
VIEWERS
VILLEIN
VINCENT
VINIEST
VIOLENT
VIOLETS
VISCERA
VISTEON
VIZIERS
WICKERS
WICKETS
WIDGEON
WIDGETS
WIENERS
WIGGERY
WIGLESS
WIGLETS
WILBERT
WILDEST
WILHELM
WILIEST
WILKENS
WILLERS
WINCERS
WINDERS
WINGERS
WINIEST
WINKERS
WINLESS
WINNERS
WINTERS
WINTERY
WIRIEST
WISHERS
WITHERS
WITLESS
WITNESS
WITSEND
ZINGERS
ZIPPERS
ZITHERS

•I•••E•

AIRACES
AIRCREW
AITCHES
BIALIES
BIASSED
BIASSES
BIDDIES
BIGAPES
BIGEYED
BIGEYES
BIGFEET
BIGGIES
BIGIDEA
BIGLIES
BIGONES
BIGOTED
BIGTOES
BILEVEL
BILGIER
BILLIES
BILOBED
BIMBOES
BINDLES
BINGLES
BINGOES
BIOFUEL
BIRCHED
BIRCHEN
BIRCHES
BIRDIED
BIRDIES
BIRDMEN
BIREMES
BIRTHED
BISHKEK
BISQUES
BITSIER
BITTIER
CINCHED
CINCHES
CINQUES
CIRCLED
CIRCLER
CIRCLES
CIRCLET
CIRQUES
CISCOES
CITADEL
CITIZEN
CITROEN
CIVVIES
DIABLES
DIALLED
DIARIES
DIBBLED
DIBBLER
DIBBLES
DICHTER
DICKIES
DIDASET
DIDDLED
DIDDLER
DIDDLES
DIDDLEY
DIDOVER
DIGIPET
DILATED
DILATES
DILLIES
DILUTED
DILUTER
DILUTES
DIMAGES
DIMETER
DIMPLED
DIMPLES
DIMVIEW
DINESEN
DINGIER
DINGLES
DINGOES
DINKIER
DIOPTER
DIPOLES
DIPPIER
DIRKSEN
DIRTIED
DIRTIER
DIRTIES
DISCOED
DISHIER
DISOBEY
DISUSED
DISUSES
DITCHED
DITCHER
DITCHES
DITSIER
DITTIES
DITTOED
DITZIER
DIVIDED
DIVIDER
DIVIDES
DIVINED
DIVINER
DIVINES
DIVVIED
DIVVIES
DIZZIED
DIZZIER
DIZZIES
EIGHTEE
FIACRES
FIANCEE
FIANCES
FIBERED
FIBIGER
FIBSTER
FICKLER
FICUSES
FIDDLED
FIDDLER
FIDDLES
FIDELES
FIEDLER
FIELDED
FIELDER
FIENNES
FIERCER
FIERIER
FIFTEEN
FIFTIES
FIGHTER
FIGTREE
FIGURED
FIGURER
FIGURES
FILCHED
FILCHER
FILCHES
FILENES
FILIBEG
FILLIES
FILMIER
FILMSET
FINALES
FINCHES
FINDLEY
FINITES
FINNIER
FIPPLES
FIREMEN
FIRRIER
FIRTREE
FISCHER
FISHIER
FISHNET
FIVEEEE
FIVETEN
FIXATED
FIXATES
FIZZIER
FIZZLED
FIZZLER
FIZZLES
GIBLUES
GIBUSES
GIDDIED
GIDDIER
GIDDIES
GIFTEES
GIFTSET
GIGGLED
GIGGLER

GIGGLES
GILLNET
GIPSIES
GIRDLED
GIRDLER
GIRDLES
GIRLIER
GIRLIES
GIRTHED
HIBBLER
HIGGLED
HIGGLER
HIGGLES
HIGHRES
HIGHSEA
HIGHTEA
HILLIER
HILLMEN
HINDLEG
HINKIER
HINNIES
HIPPIER
HIPPIES
HIPSTER
HISPEED
HISSIER
HITCHED
HITCHER
HITCHES
IIPETER
JIFFIES
JIGGIER
JIGGLED
JIGGLES
JIMCHEE
JIMENEZ
JIMINEZ
JIMMIED
JIMMIES
JINGLED
JINGLER
JINGLES
JINGOES
JIRASEK
KIBBLED
KIBBLES
KICKIER
KIDDIES
KIEFFER
KIKIDEE
KILAUEA
KILLEEN
KILLFEE
KILTIES
KIMCHEE
KINDLED
KINDLER
KINDLES
KINDRED
KINESES
KINGLET
KINKIER
KINSMEN
KIRSTEN
KISHKES
KITCHEN
KITTIES
LIAISED

LIAISES
LIBELED
LIBELEE
LIBELER
LICHEES
LIEABED
LIENEES
LIEOVER
LIFENET
LIGATED
LIGATES
LIGHTED
LIGHTEN
LIGHTER
LIKENED
LIKENEW
LILALEE
LILETEE
LIMITED
LIMITER
LIMOGES
LINAGES
LINDIED
LINDIES
LINDNER
LINDSEY
LINEMEN
LINGOES
LINSEED
LINTIER
LIPASES
LIPPIER
LISTEES
LITOTES
LITTLER
LITTLES
LIVENED
LIVENER
LIVERED
LIVESET
LIVESEY
LIZZIES
MIAOUED
MIAOWED
MICHAEL
MIDASES
MIDDIES
MIDDLEC
MIDDLED
MIDDLER
MIDDLES
MIDTEEN
MIDWEEK
MIFFIER
MIGENES
MILDRED
MILKFED
MILKIER
MILKMEN
MIMEOED
MIMESES
MINARET
MINDSET
MINGIER
MINGLED
MINGLER
MINGLES
MINIVER

MINORED
MINSTER
MINTIER
MINTTEA
MINUSES
MINUTED
MINUTER
MINUTES
MIRABEL
MIRAGES
MISAVER
MISBREW
MISCUED
MISCUES
MISDEED
MISDEEM
MISDOER
MISDOES
MISDREW
MISFEED
MISKNEW
MISSIES
MISSTEP
MISTIER
MISUSED
MISUSER
MISUSES
MITERED
MITOSES
MIZZLED
MIZZLES
NIBBLED
NIBBLER
NIBBLES
NICEMEN
NICKLES
NICOLET
NIELSEN
NIFTIER
NIFTIES
NIGGLED
NIGGLER
NIGGLES
NIGHTER
NIMBLER
NINEEEE
NINEVEH
NINNIES
NIPPIER
NIPPLES
NITTIER
OILSEED
PIAFFED
PIAFFES
PIASTER
PICKIER
PICKLED
PICKLES
PICOTED
PIDDLED
PIDDLES
PIEEYED
PIERCED
PIERCER
PIERCES
PIETIES
PIFFLED
PIFFLES

PIGEYED
PIGGIER
PIGGIES
PIGWEED
PILATES
PILOTED
PILSNER
PIMPLED
PIMPLES
PINCHED
PINCHER
PINCHES
PINKIES
PINKOES
PINONES
PIONEER
PIPAGES
PIRATED
PIRATES
PIROGEN
PITCHED
PITCHER
PITCHES
PITCREW
PITHIER
PIVOTED
PIVOTER
RIBBIER
RIBBIES
RIBEYES
RICHLER
RICHMEN
RICHTER
RICKLES
RIDDLED
RIDDLER
RIDDLES
RIDGIER
RIESSEN
RIFFLED
RIFFLER
RIFFLES
RIGHTED
RIGHTER
RIMPLED
RIMPLES
RINDIER
RINGLET
RIPENED
RIPENER
RIPOPEN
RIPPLED
RIPPLES
RIPPLET
RISKIER
RITDYES
RITZIER
RIVALED
RIVETED
RIVETER
RIVULET
SICKBED
SICKLES
SIDEBET
SIDEMEN
SIGHTED
SIGHTER
SIGNEES

SILKIER
SILLIER
SILLIES
SILTIER
SIMILES
SIMPLER
SIMPLES
SIMPLEX
SINEWED
SINGLED
SINGLES
SINGLET
SINUSES
SIRENED
SISSIER
SISSIES
SIXEEEE
SIXFEET
SIXTEEN
SIXTIES
SIXWEEK
SIZETEN
SIZZLED
SIZZLER
SIZZLES
TIARAED
TICKLED
TICKLER
TICKLES
TIEDYED
TIEDYES
TIERCES
TIERNEY
TIGHTEN
TIGHTER
TIMBRES
TIMEXES
TIMIDER
TINAFEY
TINCTED
TINGLED
TINGLER
TINGLES
TINKLED
TINKLER
TINKLES
TINNIER
TINORES
TIPOVER
TIPPEES
TIPPIER
TIPPLED
TIPPLER
TIPPLES
TIPSIER
TIPSTER
TIPTOED
TIPTOES
TIRADES
TIREDER
TIREMEN
TISANES
TISSUES
TISSUEY
TITTLES
TIZZIES
VIALLED
VICKREY

VIDEOED
VIELLES
VIERNES
VIEWIER
VINTNER
VIRTUES
VIRUSES
VISAGED
VISAGES
VISITED
VISORED
VISTAED
VITTLES
VIVIDER
VIZORED
WIDENED
WIDENER
WIDOWED
WIDOWER
WIELDED
WIELDER
WIENIES
WIGGIER
WIGGLED
WIGGLER
WIGGLES
WILDMEN
WILFRED
WILLIES
WIMOWEH
WIMPIER
WIMPLED
WIMPLES
WINCHED
WINCHER
WINCHES
WINDIER
WINDTEE
WINERED
WINFREY
WINGLET
WINGMEN
WINKLER
WINOVER
WINSLET
WIREMEN
WISEMEN
WISPIER
WITCHED
WITCHES
WITHIES
WITTIER
WIZENED
XIMENES
YIELDED
YIELDER
YIPPIES
ZIEGLER
ZILCHES
ZINCKED
ZINGIER
ZINKIER
ZIPPIER

•I••••E

AIRBASE
AIRDATE
AIRDRIE
AIRFARE
AIRFONE
AIRHOLE
AIRHOSE
AIRLANE
AIRLIKE
AIRLINE
AIRMILE
AIRRACE
AIRRAGE
AIRTIME
AIRTUBE
AIRWAVE
BIBLIKE
BICORNE
BICYCLE
BIGBLUE
BIGFIVE
BIGGAME
BIGJAKE
BIGLOVE
BIGNAME
BIGNOSE
BIGSALE
BIGTIME
BILLNYE
BINOCHE
BIOCIDE
BIOLITE
BIOTITE
BIOTYPE
BIPLANE
BISTATE
BITROLE
BIVALVE
BIZARRE
CICADAE
CICCONE
CILIATE
CIMABUE
CINEOLE
CIRRATE
CITABLE
CITRATE
CITRINE
DICTATE
DIDFINE
DIDLIKE
DIDTIME
DIFFUSE
DINETTE
DIOCESE
DIOMEDE
DIORITE
DIOXIDE
DISABLE
DISEASE
DISEUSE
DISLIKE
DISPOSE
DISPUTE
DISRATE
DISROBE
DIVERGE
DIVERSE
DIVORCE
DIVULGE
DIVULSE

EIGHTEE
FIANCEE
FIBULAE
FICTILE
FICTIVE
FIGTREE
FINABLE
FINAGLE
FINANCE
FINESSE
FINLIKE
FIREICE
FIRENZE
FIRTREE
FISHEYE
FISSILE
FISSURE
FIVEEEE
FIVEONE
FIXABLE
FIXTURE
GIAUQUE
GILMORE
GINGAME
GIRAFFE
GIROLLE
GIRONDE
GISELLE
HIDABLE
HILAIRE
HIPBONE
HIPLIKE
HIRABLE
HIRCINE
HIRSUTE
HITHERE
HITHOME
HITTITE
HITTUNE
JIGLIKE
JIGTIME
JIMCHEE
JIMDALE
JIMRICE
KIDLIKE
KIKIDEE
KILDARE
KILLFEE
KIMCHEE
KIRSTIE
LIBELEE
LIBERTE
LICENCE
LICENSE
LIGNITE
LIKABLE
LIKEICE
LILALEE
LILETEE
LIMEADE
LIMEPIE
LIMNITE
LINABLE
LINEAGE
LINEATE
LINEONE
LINGUAE
LINKAGE

LIONISE
LIONIZE
LIPLIKE
LIQUATE
LISENTE
LISSOME
LIVABLE
LIVEONE
LIZETTE
MICROBE
MIDJUNE
MIDLIFE
MIDLINE
MIDRISE
MIDSIZE
MIDSOLE
MIDWIFE
MIGRATE
MILEAGE
MILLAGE
MILLIME
MINABLE
MINOGUE
MINTAGE
MIOCENE
MIRACLE
MISCITE
MISCODE
MISDATE
MISDONE
MISFILE
MISFIRE
MISGAVE
MISGIVE
MISLIKE
MISMATE
MISMOVE
MISNAME
MISPAGE
MISRATE
MISRULE
MISSILE
MISSIVE
MISTAKE
MISTIME
MISTUNE
MISTYPE
MISWIRE
MISZONE
MIXABLE
MIXTURE
NIBLIKE
NICCAGE
NICEONE
NICOISE
NICOLLE
NICTATE
NIGHTIE
NINEEEE
NIOBITE
NITRATE
NITRIDE
NITRITE
OILBASE
OILCAKE
OILLIKE
OILLINE
PIASTRE

PICANTE
PICKAXE
PICTURE
PIEHOLE
PIELIKE
PIESAFE
PIESALE
PIGLIKE
PILEATE
PILLAGE
PINCHME
PINHOLE
PINNACE
PINNATE
PINWALE
PIPETTE
PIROGUE
PISCINE
PISMIRE
PISTOLE
RIBCAGE
RIBLIKE
RIDABLE
RIPOSTE
RIPSONE
RIPTIDE
RISIBLE
RISSOLE
RITAMAE
RITCHIE
RIVIERE
SIAMESE
SIDEONE
SIENESE
SIGNAGE
SIGNORE
SILENCE
SILENTE
SILKTIE
SILLYME
SINCERE
SINEDIE
SINKAGE
SINLIKE
SINUATE
SIRDUKE
SISTINE
SITHOME
SITUATE
SIXEEEE
SIXFIVE
SIXLANE
SIXNINE
SIZABLE
SIZEONE
TIEGAME
TIELINE
TIEROPE
TILLAGE
TIMBALE
TIMRICE
TINLIKE
TINMINE
TINTYPE
TINWARE
TIPLINE
TITANAE
TITMICE

TITRATE
VIBRATE
VICENTE
VICOMTE
VIDETTE
VILLAGE
VINROSE
VINTAGE
VIOLATE
VIOLONE
VIRGATE
VIRGULE
VISIBLE
VITIATE
VITRINE
WIGLIKE
WILDONE
WILLKIE
WIMPOLE
WINDAGE
WINDTEE
WINSOME
WIRABLE
WISEONE
ZINCITE
ZIPCODE

••IE•••

ALIENEE
ALIENOR
ALIENTO
ARIETTA
ARIETTE
BRIEFED
BRIEFER
BRIEFLY
CHIEFLY
CLIENTS
CRIEDUP
CRIESUP
DNIEPER
DRIEDUP
DRIESCH
DRIESUP
ELIEZER
ETIENNE
FAIENCE
FLIEDTO
FLIESAT
FLIESBY
FLIESIN
FLIESON
FLIESTO
FLIESUP
FRIEDAN
FRIEDUP
FRIENDS
FRIESUP
FRIEZES
GRIEVED
GRIEVER
GRIEVES
ILIESCU
KNIEVEL
MSIEURS
ORIENTE
ORIENTS
OSIERED

PRIESTS
QUIETED
QUIETEN
QUIETER
QUIETLY
QUIETUS
SCIENCE
SHIELDS
SPIEDON
SPIEGEL
SPIELED
SPIELER
SPIESON
THIERRY
THIEVED
THIEVES
TRIEDIT
TRIEDON
TRIEDTO
TRIESIT
TRIESON
TRIESTE
TRIESTO

••I•E••

ABIDEBY
ABIDERS
ABILENE
AGILELY
AGILEST
ALIMENT
ALINERS
ALIVETO
ANISEED
APILEOF
ARIDEST
AVIDEST
BAILEES
BAILERS
BAITERS
BOILERS
BOISEID
BRIBEES
BRIBERS
BRIBERY
BRINERS
CAIRENE
CHICEST
CHIDERS
CHILEAN
CHIMEIN
CHIMERA
CHIMERS
CHINESE
CHISELS
COILERS
COINERS
CRIMEAN
DEICERS
DRIVEAT
DRIVEBY
DRIVEIN
DRIVELS
DRIVERS
DRIVETO
DRIVEUP
ELIDERS
ELITEST
EMINENT
EPICENE
EPIDERM
ERIGENA
EVIDENT
EVILEST
EVILEYE
EXIGENT
EXILERS
FAINEST
FAIREST
FRISEUR
GAINERS
GAITERS
GLIDEBY
GLIDEIN
GLIDERS
GOITERS
GRIPERS
GUIDERS
GUINEAN
GUINEAS
HAILERS
HEIFERS
HEIFETZ
HEIRESS
ICINESS
IFIFELL
IGIVEUP
ILIKEIT
ININETY
JAILERS
JOINERS
JOINERY
JUICERS
JUICEUP
KAISERS
KNIFERS
LOITERS
MAIDENS
MAILERS
MAIMERS
MAINERS
MOILERS
NAILERS
NAIVELY
NAIVEST
NAIVETE
NAIVETY
OPINERS
PAIRERS
PHILEAS
PHINEAS
POISERS
PRICERS
PRIMELY
PRIMERA
PRIMERO
PRIMERS
PRIVETS
QUINELA
QUITESO
QUIVERS
QUIVERY
RAIDERS
RAILERS
RAIMENT
RAISERS

RAISEUP
RUINERS
SAILERS
SCITECH
SEINERS
SEIZEON
SEIZERS
SHINEON
SHINERS
SHINEUP
SHIVERS
SHIVERY
SKIVEST
SKIWEAR
SLICERS
SLICEUP
SLIDEBY
SLIDEIN
SLIDERS
SLIVERS
SMILEAT
SMILEON
SMILERS
SMILEYS
SMITERS
SNIDELY
SNIDEST
SNIPEAT
SNIPERS
SNIVELS
SOIREES
SPICERS
SPICERY
SPICEUP
SPIDERS
SPIDERY
SPIKERS
SPIKETV
SPIKEUP
SPINELS
SPINETS
SPIREAS
STIPEND
SWIGERT
SWINERY
SWIPERS
SWIVELS
SWIVETS
TAILEND
TAILERS
TOILERS
TOILETS
TRIBECA
TRICEPS
TRIDENT
TRIJETS
TRIREME
TRISECT
TRITELY
TRITEST
TRIVETS
TWINERS
UNIDEAL
UNINERT
UNITERS
VAINEST
VEILERS
VOICERS
VOIDERS
WAILERS
WAITERS
WAIVERS
WHINERS
WHITELY
WHITENS
WHITEST
WRITEIN
WRITEME
WRITEON
WRITERS
WRITETO
WRITEUP

••I••E•

ALIASES
ALIBIED
ALIENEE
ALIGNED
ALIGNER
AMITIES
ANISEED
ARIANES
ASIMMER
AVIATED
AVIATES
AZINGER
BAILEES
BAINTER
BEIGNES
BEIGNET
BLINDED
BLINDER
BLINKED
BLINKER
BLIPPED
BLISSED
BLISSES
BLISTER
BLITHER
BLITZED
BLITZEN
BLITZER
BLITZES
BRIBEES
BRICKED
BRIDGED
BRIDGER
BRIDGES
BRIDGET
BRIDLED
BRIDLER
BRIDLES
BRIEFED
BRIEFER
BRIMLEY
BRIMMED
BRIMMER
BRINGER
BRINIER
BRINKER
BRIQUET
BRISKED
BRISKER
BRISKET
BRITNEY
BRITTEN
BUILDER
CAIRNED
CHIAPET
CHICHEN
CHICKEN
CHICLES
CHICLET
CHIDDEN
CHIGGER
CHIGOES
CHILIES
CHILLED
CHILLER
CHIMNEY
CHINKED
CHINNED
CHIPPED
CHIPPER
CHIRPED
CHIRPER
CHIRRED
CHITTER
CHIVIED
CHIVIES
CLICHED
CLICHES
CLICKED
CLICKER
CLIMBED
CLIMBER
CLINGER
CLINKED
CLINKER
CLIPPED
CLIPPER
CLIQUED
CLIQUES
CLIQUEY
COIFFED
COIGNED
COIGNES
CRIBBED
CRIBBER
CRICKED
CRICKET
CRIMPED
CRIMPER
CRINGED
CRINGES
CRISPED
CRISPEN
CRISPER
CRITTER
DAILIES
DAIMLER
DAIRIES
DAIRYER
DAISIES
DEIFIED
DEIFIER
DEIFIES
DEIGNED
DEITIES
DNIEPER
DOILIES
DRIBLET
DRIFTED
DRIFTER
DRILLED
DRILLER
DRINKER
DRIPPED
DRIPPER
EDIBLES
EDIFIED
EDIFIER
EDIFIES
ELIEZER
EMIGREE
EMIGRES
EMITTED
EMITTER
ENISLED
ENISLES
EPITHET
ERINYES
ERITREA
ETICKET
EVICTED
EVICTEE
EVILLER
EVINCED
EVINCES
EXISTED
EXITFEE
FAILLES
FAINTED
FAINTER
FAIRIES
FAIRSEX
FEIFFER
FEIGNED
FEIGNER
FEINTED
FLICKED
FLICKER
FLINGER
FLIPPED
FLIPPEN
FLIPPER
FLIRTED
FLIRTER
FLITTED
FLITTER
FLIVVER
FOIBLES
FOISTED
FRICKER
FRIDGES
FRIDLEY
FRIEZES
FRILLED
FRINGED
FRINGES
FRISBEE
FRISKED
FRISKER
FRITTED
FRITTER
FRIZZED
FRIZZER
FRIZZES
GLIBBER
GLIMMER
GLINTED
GLISTEN
GLISTER
GLITTER
GLITZED
GLITZES
GRIDDED
GRIDDER
GRIEVED
GRIEVER
GRIEVES
GRIFFEY
GRIFTED
GRIFTER
GRILLED
GRILLER
GRILLES
GRIMIER
GRIMMER
GRINDER
GRINNED
GRINNER
GRIPPED
GRIPPER
GRIPPES
GRISLET
GRISNEZ
GRISTER
GRITTED
GRITTER
GUILDER
HAIRGEL
HAIRIER
HAIRNET
HEISTED
HOISTED
HOISTER
ICICLES
IRISHER
JOINDER
JOINTED
JOINTER
JOISTED
JUICIER
JUILLET
KAISHEK
KEISTER
KLINGER
KLINKER
KLISTER
KNIEVEL
KNISHES
KNITTED
KNITTER
LAISSEZ
LAITIES
LEISTER
MAIGRET
MAILMEN
MAINMEN
MAITRED
MAITRES
MEIOSES
MEISSEN
MEISTER
MEITNER
MOISTEN
MOISTER
NAIADES
NAILKEG
NAILSET
NEIGHED
NEITHER
NOISIER
OLIVIER
OMITTED
OMITTER
OPIATES
ORIOLES
OSIERED
PAINTED
PAINTER
PAISLEY
PAIUTES
PHILTER
PHISHED
PHISHER
PHISHES
PLINKED
PLISSES
POINTED
POINTER
POINTES
POITIER
POIVRES
PRICIER
PRICKED
PRIMMED
PRIMMER
PRIMPED
PRINCES
PRINKED
PRINKER
PRINTED
PRINTER
PRISSES
PRITHEE
PRIUSES
PRIVIER
PRIVIES
QUICHES
QUICKEN
QUICKER
QUIETED
QUIETEN
QUIETER
QUIGLEY
QUILLED
QUILLER
QUILTED
QUILTER
QUINCES
QUINCEY
QUINTES
QUINTET
QUINZES
QUIPPED
QUIPPER
QUIRTED
QUITTED
QUITTER
QUIZZED
QUIZZER
QUIZZES
RAILMEN
RAINIER
REIFIED
REIFIES
REIGNED
REINDEX
REINKED
ROILIER
ROISTER
SAINTED
SAINTES
SHIFTED
SHIFTER
SHIITES
SHILLED
SHIMMER
SHINIER
SHINNED
SHIPMEN
SHIPPED
SHIPPER
SHIRKED
SHIRKER
SHIRLEY
SHIRRED
SKIAREA
SKIDDED
SKIDDER
SKIFFED
SKILLED
SKILLET
SKIMMED
SKIMMER
SKIMPED
SKINNED
SKINNER
SKIPPED
SKIPPER
SKIRLED
SKIRTED
SKIRTER
SKITTER
SLICKED
SLICKER
SLIMIER
SLIMMED
SLIMMER
SLINGER
SLINKED
SLINKER
SLIPPED
SLIPPER
SLITHER
SLITTED
SLITTER
SMIDGEN
SMIDGES
SMIRKED
SMIRKER
SMITHED
SMITTEN
SNICKER
SNICKET
SNIFFED
SNIFFER
SNIFTER
SNIGLET
SNIPPED
SNIPPER
SNIPPET
SOIGNEE
SOIREES
SPICIER
SPIEGEL
SPIELED
SPIELER
SPIFFED
SPIKIER
SPILLED
SPILLER
SPINIER
SPINNER
SPINNEY
SPIRIER
SPITTER
SPITZES
STICKER
STIFFED
STIFFEL
STIFFEN
STIFFER
STIFLED
STIFLES
STILLED
STILLER
STILTED
STINGER
STINKER
STINTED
STINTER
STIRRED
STIRRER
SWIFTER
SWIGGED
SWILLED
SWILLER
SWIMMER
SWINGER
SWIRLED
SWISHED
SWISHES
SWITZER
TAINTED
TEICHER
THICKEN
THICKER
THICKET
THIEVED
THIEVES
THIGPEN
THINKER
THINNED
THINNER
THITHER
TRIAGES
TRICKED
TRICKER
TRIFLED
TRIFLER
TRIFLES
TRIGGER
TRILLED
TRILLER
TRIMMED
TRIMMER
TRINKET
TRIODES
TRIOLET
TRIPLEA
TRIPLED
TRIPLES
TRIPLET
TRIPLEX
TRIPPED
TRIPPER
TRIPPET
TUILLES
TWILLED
TWINBED
TWINGED
TWINGES
TWINIER
TWINJET
TWINNED
TWINSET
TWIRLED
TWIRLER
TWISTED
TWISTER
TWITTED
TWITTER
TZIMMES
UNIATES
UNIFIED
UNIFIER
UNIFIES
UNINKED
UNIPLEX
UNIQUES
UNITIES
UVINDEX
VEINIER
VEINLET
VEINTES
WAISTED
WEIGHED
WEIGHER
WEIRDED
WEIRDER
WHIFFED
WHIFFER
WHIMPER
WHINIER
WHIPPED
WHIPPER
WHIPPET
WHIRLED
WHIRLER
WHIRRED
WHISHED
WHISHES
WHISKED
WHISKER
WHISKEY
WHISPER
WHITHER
WHITNEY
WHIZZED
WHIZZER
WHIZZES
WRIGLEY
WRINGER
WRITHED
WRITHER
WRITHES
WRITTEN

••I•••E

ABILENE
ADIPOSE
AGITATE
ALIDADE
ALIENEE
ALIGOTE
ALITTLE
AMIABLE
AMIBLUE
AMILATE
AMINUTE
ANILINE
ANIMATE
ARIADNE
ARIETTE
ARISTAE
ASININE
ATINGLE
ATIPTOE
ATISSUE
AXILLAE
BLIMPIE
BLINTZE
BRICKLE
BRIGADE
BRINDLE
BRIOCHE
BRISTLE
BRITTLE
CAIRENE
CHICANE
CHINESE
CLIMATE
COINAGE
CRINKLE
CRIPPLE
CUISINE
DEIRDRE
DOIDARE
DRIBBLE
DRINKME
DRIZZLE
DWINDLE
EDIFICE
ELIYALE
EMIGREE
EMIRATE
EPICENE
EPICURE
EPIDOTE
EPIGONE
EPILATE
EPISODE
EPISTLE
EPITOME
ETIENNE
EVICTEE
EVILEYE
EVILONE
EXITFEE
FAIENCE
FAILURE
FAIRUSE
FBICASE
FBIFILE
FRIABLE
FRIBBLE
FRIGATE
FRIJOLE
FRISBEE
FRIZZLE
GLIMPSE
GRIDDLE
GRIMACE
GRISTLE
GRIZZLE
HAIRDYE
IFITDIE
IMITATE
ISIDORE
KRINGLE
LAICIZE
LEISURE
NAIVETE
NOISOME
OLIVINE
ORIENTE
ORIFICE
ORIGINE
OXIDASE
OXIDATE
OXIDISE
OXIDIZE
PHILLIE
PHILTRE
PLIABLE
PLICATE
PRICKLE
PRIMATE
PRINGLE
PRITHEE
PRIVATE
QUIBBLE
QUICKIE
QUINATE
QUININE
QUINQUE
QUIVIVE
QUIXOTE
RAILAGE
REIMAGE
REISSUE
RHIZOME
RUINATE
SAIDAYE
SCIENCE
SEIZURE
SHINGLE
SKIABLE
SKIFFLE
SKIPOLE
SKIRACE
SKITTLE
SNIFFLE
SOIGNEE
SOILAGE
SPINDLE
SPITTLE
STIPPLE
SUITSME
SWINDLE
SWIZZLE
THIMBLE
THINICE
THISONE
THISTLE
TRIABLE
TRIBBLE
TRIBUNE
TRIBUTE
TRICKLE
TRIESTE
TRIREME
TRITONE
TWIDDLE
TWINKIE
TWINKLE
UNICODE
UNISIZE
UNITISE
UNITIVE
UNITIZE
UTILISE
UTILIZE
VEINULE
VOITURE
WHIFFLE
WHIPPLE
WHISTLE
WHITTLE
WRIGGLE
WRINKLE
WRITEME

•••IE••

ACHIEST
ACHIEVA
ACHIEVE
AERIEST
AIRIEST
ALFIERI
ALGIEBA
ALGIERS
AMBIENS
AMBIENT
ANCIENT
ANXIETY
ARRIERE
ARTIEST
ASHIEST
BABIEST
BELIEFS
BELIERS
BELIEVE
BESIEGE
BEZIERS
BONIEST
BOXIEST
BURIERS
BUSIEST
CAGIEST
CAHIERS
CAKIEST
CANIEST
COKIEST
COPIERS
COSIEST
COWIEST
COZIEST
DANIELA
DANIELJ
DANIELS
DEFIERS
DENIECE
DENIERS
DEWIEST
DICIEST
DOPIEST
DOZIEST
DUBIETY
EASIEST
EDGIEST
EELIEST
EERIEST
EGGIEST
ELMIEST
ENFIELD
ENVIERS
FOXIEST
FUMIEST
GAMIEST
GLUIEST
GOOIEST
GORIEST
HAZIEST
HOKIEST
HOLIEST
HOMIEST
HOSIERS
HOSIERY
HYGIEIA
HYGIENE
ICKIEST
IFFIEST
IMPIETY
INFIELD
INKIEST
JIVIEST
JOKIEST
LACIEST
LAKIEST
LAZIEST
LEMIEUX
LENIENT
LEVIERS
LIMIEST
LINIEST
LOGIEST
LORIENT
LUMIERE
MAZIEST
METIERS
MILIEUS
MILIEUX
MIMIEUX
MIRIEST
MOLIERE
MOPIEST
MURIELS
NAPIERS
NIMIETY
NORIEGA
NOSIEST
OAKIEST
OILIEST
ONLIEST
OOZIEST
ORVIETO
OWLIEST
PACIEST
PANIERS

7 IE

PAPIERS
PATIENT
PINIEST
PIPIEST
PITIERS
POKIEST
PUNIEST
RACIEST
RAPIERS
RELIEFS
RELIERS
RELIEVE
REVIEWS
RILIEVO
RIMIEST
RIPIENI
RIPIENO
RIVIERA
RIVIERE
ROPIEST
ROSIEST
RULIEST
SAGIEST
SALIENT
SALIERI
SAPIENS
SAPIENT
SATIETY
SERIESE
SERIESF
SERIESG
SERIESH
SERIESI
SERIESJ
SERIESK
SEXIEST
SHRIEKS
SOCIETY
SOVIETS
SPRIEST
TIDIEST
TINIEST
TONIEST
UGLIEST
UNFIERY
UNPIETY
UNTIERS
UPFIELD
VARIERS
VARIETY
VERIEST
VINIEST
VIZIERS
WANIEST
WARIEST
WAVIEST
WAXIEST
WILIEST
WINIEST
WIRIEST
XAVIERU
ZANIEST
ZOOIEST

•••I•E•

ABRILES
ACTIFED
ACTIVES
ADMIRED
ADMIRER
ADMIRES
ADMIXED
ADMIXES
ADVICES
ADVISED
ADVISEE
ADVISER
ADVISES
AEDILES
AEGISES
AFFINED
AFFINES
AFFIXED
AFFIXER
AFFIXES
ALBIREO
ALPINER
ALPINES
ANTIBES
ANTIGEN
APHIDES
APLITES
APSIDES
AQUIFER
AQUIVER
ARBITER
ARRISES
ARRIVED
ARRIVER
ARRIVES
ASHIVER
ASPIRED
ASPIRER
ASPIRES
ASSIZES
ATTIMES
ATTIRED
ATTIRER
ATTIRES
AUDILES
AUDITED
AUDITEE
AUGITES
AVAILED
AVOIDED
AVOIDER
AWAITED
AWAITER
BADIDEA
BARITES
BATIKED
BEDIZEN
BEMIRED
BEMIRES
BESIDES
BETIDED
BETIDES
BETIMES
BIGIDEA
BODICES
BOLIDES
BORIDES
BOVINES
BRAIDED
BRAIDER
BRAINED
BRAINER
BRAISED
BRAISES
BROIDER
BROILED
BROILER
BRUISED
BRUISER
BRUISES
BRUITED
BYFIVES
BYLINED
BYLINER
BYLINES
CABINET
CALIBER
CALICES
CALIPER
CAMISES
CANINES
CARIBES
CAVILED
CAVILER
CCRIDER
CERISES
CHAINED
CHAINES
CHAIRED
CHAISES
CHOICER
CHOICES
CHOIRED
CITIZEN
CLAIMED
CLAIMER
CODICES
COMICES
CONIFER
COSINES
CRUISED
CRUISER
CRUISES
CUTISES
DANIKEN
DANITES
DATIVES
DEAIRED
DEBITED
DECIBEL
DECIDED
DECIDER
DECIDES
DECILES
DEFILED
DEFILER
DEFILES
DEFINED
DEFINER
DEFINES
DEHIRED
DEHIRES
DELIBES
DELIMEN
DELIVER
DEMISED
DEMISES
DENIMED
DENIZEN
DERIDED
DERIDER
DERIDES
DERIVED
DERIVER
DERIVES
DESIRED
DESIREE
DESIRER
DESIRES
DEVICES
DEVILED
DEVISED
DEVISEE
DEVISER
DEVISES
DEWIRED
DEWIRES
DIGIPET
DIVIDED
DIVIDER
DIVIDES
DIVINED
DIVINER
DIVINES
DRAINED
DRAINER
DREIDEL
DREISER
DRYIDEA
EGLISES
ELAINES
EMAILED
EMAILER
EMPIRES
ENDIVES
ENGINED
ENGINES
ENLIVEN
ENOILED
ENSILED
ENSILES
ENTICED
ENTICER
ENTICES
ENTIRES
EOSINES
EQUINES
ERMINED
ERMINES
ETAILED
ETAILER
ETOILES
EXCIDED
EXCIDES
EXCISED
EXCISES
EXCITED
EXCITER
EXCITES
EXOILER
EXPIRED
EXPIRES
EXWIVES
FAMINES
FELINES
FIBIGER
FILIBEG
FINITES
FLAILED
FOLIOED
FRAILER
FRAISES
FRUITED
FTRILEY
GALILEE
GALILEI
GALILEO
GAMINES
GRAINED
GRAINER
GROINED
GUNITES
HABITED
HALIDES
HALITES
HAMITES
HELICES
HELIXES
HOTITEM
HUMIDEX
IGNITED
IGNITER
IGNITES
IMBIBED
IMBIBER
IMBIBES
IMMIXED
IMMIXES
IMTIRED
INCISED
INCISES
INCITED
INCITER
INCITES
INDICES
INDIGEN
INDITED
INDITER
INDITES
INFIDEL
INFIVES
INFIXED
INFIXES
INLINES
INSIDER
INSIDES
INVITED
INVITEE
INVITER
INVITES
IODIDES
IODISED
IODISES
IODIZED
IODIZER
IODIZES
IONISED
IONISER
IONISES
IONIZED
IONIZER
IONIZES
JIMINEZ
JUBILEE
JUNIPER
JUPITER
KIKIDEE
KLEIBER
KLEISER
KURILES
LATICES
LATIMES
LEVITES
LEXISES
LIAISED
LIAISES
LIMITED
LIMITER
LORISES
LUCIFER
LUCITES
LUPINES
MALICES
MARINER
MARINES
MATINEE
MAVISES
MAXIXES
MERIDEN
MERIMEE
MERITED
MINIVER
MOBILES
MONIKER
MOTIVED
MOTIVES
MRTIGER
NATIVES
NETIZEN
NEWIDEA
NOMINEE
NORITES
NOSIREE
NOTICED
NOTICER
NOTICES
NOVICES
NOWISEE
NOWISER
NYTIMES
OBLIGED
OBLIGEE
OBLIGER
OBLIGES
OFFICER
OFFICES
ONSIDES
ONVIDEO
OOLITES
ORBITED
ORBITER
ORDINES
ORRISES
OSCINES
OSSIPEE
OXHIDES
PERIGEE
PERILED
PETITES
PLAICES
PLAINER
PLAINES
PLAITED
PLAITER
POLICED
POLICER
POLICES
POLITER
PORIVER
POSITED
PRAISED
PRAISER
PRAISES
PREIDEA
PUMICED
PUMICES
PYRITES
QUAILED
QUOINED
QUOITED
RADICES
RADIOED
RADIOER
RADIXES
RAMIREZ
RAPIDER
RAPINES
RATINES
RATITES
RAVINED
RAVINES
REAIMED
REAIRED
RECIPES
RECITED
RECITER
RECITES
REFILED
REFILES
REFINED
REFINER
REFINES
REFIRED
REFIRES
REFIXED
REFIXES
REGIMEN
REGIMES
REGIVEN
REGIVES
REHIDES
REHIRED
REHIRES
RELINED
RELINES
RELIVED
RELIVES
REMINED
REMINES
REMISED
REMISES
REMIXED
REMIXES
REOILED
REPINED
REPINER
REPINES
RERIDES
RERISEN
RERISES
RESIDED
RESIDER
RESIDES
RESILED
RESILES
RESINED
RESITED
RESIZED
RESIZER
RESIZES
RETILED
RETILES
RETIMED
RETIMES
RETIRED
RETIREE
RETIRES
REVILED
REVILER
REVILES
REVISED
REVISER
REVISES
REVIVED
REVIVER
REVIVES
REWIDEN
REWIPED
REWIPES
REWIRED
REWIRES
ROSINED
ROTIFER
RUTILES
SABINES
SALINES
SAMISEN
SANIBEL
SATINET
SATIRES
SCRIBED
SCRIBER
SCRIBES
SEMITES
SHIITES
SHRIKES
SHRINED
SHRINER
SHRINES
SHRIVEL
SHRIVER
SHRIVES
SIMILES
SLUICED
SLUICES
SOLIDER
SOMINEX
SPLICED
SPLICER
SPLICES
SPLINES
SPOILED
SPOILER
SPRITES
SQUIRED
SQUIRES
STAIDER
STAINED
STAINER
STAIRED
STEIGER
STEINEM
STEINER
STRIDER
STRIDES
STRIFES
STRIKER
STRIKES
STRIPED
STRIPER
STRIPES
STRIVED
STRIVEN
STRIVER
STRIVES
SUBIDEA
SUBITEM
TAXIMEN
THEIDEA
THRIVED
THRIVEN
THRIVER
THRIVES
TIMIDER
TRAILED
TRAILER
TRAINED
TRAINEE
TRAINER
TREIZES
UMPIRED
UMPIRES
UNAIDED
UNAIMED
UNAIRED
UNCITED
UNDIKED
UNDINES
UNFILED
UNFILES
UNFINED
UNFINES
UNFIRED
UNFIXED
UNFIXES
UNGIVEN
UNHIRED
UNHIRES
UNLIKED
UNLIKES
UNLINED
UNLIVED
UNLIVES
UNMIKED
UNMINED
UNMIRED
UNMITER
UNMIXED
UNMIXES
UNOILED
UNPILED
UNPILES
UNPIPED
UNRILED
UNRIMED
UNRIPER
UNRISEN
UNRIVED
UNRIVEN
UNSIDED
UNSIZED
UNTILED
UNTIMED
UNTIRED
UNWIPED
UNWIRED
UNWISER
UPDIVED
UPDIVES
UPPILED
UPPILES
UPRISEN
UPRISER
UPRISES
UPRIVER
UPSIDES
UPSIZED
UPSIZES
UPTIMES
VALINES
VALISES
VARITEK
VISITED
VIVIDER
VOTIVES
WAHINES
YESISEE

•••I••E

AAMILNE
ABRIDGE
ACHIEVE
ACHILLE
ADDIBLE
ADVISEE
ANTIQUE
ARRIERE
ARTICLE
ARTISTE
AUDIBLE
AUDITEE
AURICLE
BATISTE
BELIEVE
BESIEGE
BEZIQUE
BRAILLE
CACIQUE
CALIBRE
CAMILLE
CANIDAE
CANITBE
CARINAE
CARIOLE
CAVIARE
CEVICHE
CILIATE
COMIQUE
CORINNE
CRAIGIE
CUBICLE
CUTICLE
DECIARE
DEHISCE
DEMILLE
DENIECE
DESIREE
DEVIATE
DEVILLE
DEVISEE
DEWILDE
ECLIPSE
EGOISTE
ELLIPSE
ENRIQUE
ENTITLE
EXPIATE
FAMILLE
FATIGUE
FOLIAGE
FOLIATE
FOLIOSE
FRAICHE
FUSIBLE
GALILEE
GEFILTE
HABITUE
HYGIENE
IMPINGE
INSIGNE
INVITEE
JUBILEE
KIKIDEE
LABIATE
LAFITTE
LALIQUE
LAMINAE
LEGIBLE
LETITBE
LUCIDAE
LUCILLE
LUMIERE
MANIPLE
MATINEE
MATISSE
MEDIATE
MERIMEE
MODISTE
MOLIERE
NEVILLE
NOMINEE
NOSIREE
NOWISEE
OBLIGEE
OBLIQUE
OBVIATE
ORVILLE
OSSICLE
OSSIPEE
PANICLE
PELISSE
PERIGEE
PETIOLE
PRAIRIE
RADIATE
RADICLE
REHINGE
RELIEVE
RERINSE
RESIDUE
RETICLE
RETINAE
RETINGE
RETINUE
RETIREE
RETITLE
RISIBLE
RIVIERE
SATIATE
SERIATE
SERIESE
SEVILLE
SHEILAE
SODIDWE
STRIATE
SYRINGE
TRAINEE
TRAIPSE
TUNICLE
UNHINGE
UNMITRE
VARIATE
VEHICLE
VESICLE
VISIBLE
VITIATE
WAVICLE
WOEISME
YESISEE

••••IE•

ADELIES
AGONIES
ALIBIED
ALLTIED
AMBRIES
AMITIES
ANGRIER
ANOMIES
ANTSIER
APEDIET
APERIES
APPLIED
APPLIER
APPLIES
ARCHIES
ARTSIER
ASQUIET
ATELIER
ATOMIES
ATONIES
AUNTIES
AUSSIES
BADDIES
BADLIES
BAFFIES
BAGGIER
BAGGIES
BALDIES
BALKIER
BALMIER
BAMMIES
BANDIED
BANDIER
BANDIES
BARBIES
BARKIER
BARMIER
BARRIER
BASSIER
BATTIER
BAWDIER
BEADIER
BEAMIER
BEANIES
BEEFIER
BEERIER
BEETIER
BELLIED
BELLIES
BENDIER
BEQUIET
BERRIED
BERRIES
BIALIES
BIDDIES
BIGGIES
BIGLIES
BILGIER
BILLIES
BIRDIED
BIRDIES
BITSIER
BITTIER
BLOWIER
BMOVIES
BOBBIES
BOCCIES
BOGGIER
BONNIER
BOOBIES
BOOGIED
BOOGIES
BOOKIES
BOOMIER
BOONIES
BOOTIES
BOOZIER
BOSSIER
BOUVIER
BOWTIES
BRASIER
BRAZIER
BRINIER
BRODIES
BUDDIED
BUDDIES
BUDGIES
BUGGIER
BUGGIES
BULGIER
BULKIER
BULLIED
BULLIES
BUMPIER
BUNNIES
BURLIER
BURRIER
BUSBIES
BUSHIER
BUSTIER
BUZZIER
CABBIES
CADDIED
CADDIES
CAMMIES
CAMPIER
CANDIED
CANDIES

CANNIER
CARNIES
CARRIED
CARRIER
CARRIES
CARTIER
CASHIER
CATTIER
CHARIER
CHENIER
CHEWIER
CHILIES
CHIVIED
CHIVIES
CHOKIER
CIVVIES
CLAVIER
CLAYIER
COCKIER
COLLIER
COLLIES
COMBIEN
COMFIER
CONRIED
COOKIES
COOLIES
COOTIES
CORKIER
CORNIER
COURIER
COWRIES
CRAZIER
CRAZIES
CRONIES
CROSIER
CROZIER
CUBBIES
CUDDIES
CULLIED
CULLIES
CUPPIER
CURDIER
CURLIER
CURRIED
CURRIER
CURRIES
CURVIER
CUSHIER
DADDIES
DAFFIER
DAILIES
DAIRIES
DAISIES
DALLIED
DALLIER
DALLIES
DANDIER
DANDIES
DASHIER
DAUMIER
DEARIES
DEBRIEF
DECRIED
DECRIER
DECRIES
DEIFIED
DEIFIER
DEIFIES

DEITIES
DERBIES
DERNIER
DEVRIES
DIARIES
DICKIES
DILLIES
DIMVIEW
DINGIER
DINKIER
DIPPIER
DIRTIED
DIRTIER
DIRTIES
DISHIER
DITSIER
DITTIES
DITZIER
DIVVIED
DIVVIES
DIZZIED
DIZZIER
DIZZIES
DODGIER
DOGGIER
DOGGIES
DOILIES
DOLLIED
DOLLIES
DOOLIES
DOOMIER
DOOZIES
DORKIER
DOSSIER
DOTTIER
DOWDIER
DOWDIES
DOWNIER
DOWRIES
DROXIES
DUCHIES
DUCKIER
DUCKIES
DUMMIED
DUMMIES
DUMPIER
DUSKIER
DUSTIER
EARLIER
EARLIES
EBONIES
EDIFIED
EDIFIER
EDIFIES
ELEGIES
EMERIES
EMPTIED
EMPTIER
EMPTIES
ENEMIES
ENSKIED
ENSKIES
ENTRIES
EPOXIED
EPOXIES
EWERIES
EZEKIEL
FADDIER

FADDIET
FAERIES
FAIRIES
FANCIED
FANCIER
FANCIES
FARRIER
FATTIER
FENNIER
FERNIER
FERRIED
FERRIES
FEVRIER
FIERIER
FIFTIES
FILLIES
FILMIER
FINNIER
FIRRIER
FISHIER
FIZZIER
FLAKIER
FLAMIER
FLAWIER
FLAXIER
FLUKIER
FLUTIER
FLUTIES
FLYTIER
FOAMIER
FOGGIER
FOLKIER
FOLKIES
FOLLIES
FOODIES
FORKIER
FORTIES
FOURIER
FRASIER
FRAZIER
FUBSIER
FUDDIES
FUNKIER
FUNNIER
FUNNIES
FURRIER
FUSSIER
FUSTIER
FUZZIER
GABBIER
GABRIEL
GAMBIER
GASSIER
GAUDIER
GAUDIES
GAUTIER
GAUZIER
GAWKIER
GEEKIER
GEMMIER
GERMIER
GIDDIED
GIDDIER
GIDDIES
GIPSIES
GIRLIER
GIRLIES
GLACIER

GLAZIER
GLORIED
GLORIES
GOALIES
GODLIER
GOODIES
GOOFIER
GOONIER
GOONIES
GOOPIER
GOOSIER
GORSIER
GOUTIER
GRAPIER
GRAVIES
GRAZIER
GRIMIER
GRODIER
GROLIER
GUCKIER
GULLIED
GULLIES
GULPIER
GUMMIER
GUNKIER
GUNNIES
GUPPIES
GUSHIER
GUSSIED
GUSSIES
GUSTIER
GUTSIER
GUTTIER
GYPSIES
HACKIES
HAIRIER
HALFIES
HAMMIER
HANDIER
HANKIES
HAPPIER
HARDIER
HARPIES
HARRIED
HARRIER
HARRIES
HARRIET
HASTIER
HEADIER
HEAVIER
HEAVIES
HEDGIER
HEFTIER
HEMPIER
HENRIES
HERBIER
HILLIER
HINKIER
HINNIES
HIPPIER
HIPPIES
HISSIER
HOAGIES
HOARIER
HOBBIES
HOGTIED
HOGTIES
HOLLIES

HOMEIER
HOODIES
HOOSIER
HOPPIER
HORNIER
HORSIER
HOTTIES
HUBBIES
HUFFIER
HUGGIES
HULKIER
HUMPIER
HUNKIER
HURRIED
HURRIER
HURRIES
HUSKIER
HUSKIES
HUSSIES
ICHDIEN
IMPLIED
IMPLIES
INBRIEF
IRONIES
ITCHIER
IVORIES
JACKIEO
JAGGIER
JAGGIES
JAMMIER
JAMMIES
JANVIER
JAZZIER
JEEBIES
JELLIED
JELLIES
JERKIER
JERKIES
JETTIED
JETTIES
JIFFIES
JIGGIER
JIMMIED
JIMMIES
JOLLIED
JOLLIER
JOLLIES
JOLLIET
JOLTIER
JOWLIER
JUICIER
JUMPIER
JUNKIER
JUNKIES
KELPIES
KEWPIES
KICKIER
KIDDIES
KILTIES
KINKIER
KITTIES
KOOKIER
LADDIES
LAITIES
LANKIER
LARDIER
LARKIER
LASSIES

LEADIER
LEAFIER
LEAKIER
LEDGIER
LEERIER
LEFTIES
LEGGIER
LINDIED
LINDIES
LINTIER
LIPPIER
LIZZIES
LOAMIER
LOBBIED
LOBBIES
LOFTIER
LOLLIES
LONGIES
LOOBIES
LOONIER
LOONIES
LOOPIER
LOPPIER
LORRIES
LOUSIER
LOWLIER
LUCKIER
LUMPIER
LUSHIER
LUSTIER
LUTHIER
MAGPIES
MALTIER
MANGIER
MANLIER
MANNIES
MARLIER
MARNIER
MARRIED
MARRIES
MARVIER
MASHIES
MASSIER
MATHIEU
MEALIER
MEALIES
MEANIES
MEATIER
MEEMIES
MENZIES
MERCIES
MERRIER
MESHIER
MESSIER
MIDDIES
MIFFIER
MILKIER
MINGIER
MINTIER
MISSIES
MISTIER
MOLDIER
MOLLIES
MOMMIES
MONDIEU
MOODIER
MOONIER
MOONIES

MOORIER
MOSSIER
MOTHIER
MOUSIER
MUCKIER
MUDDIED
MUDDIER
MUDDIES
MUDPIES
MUGGIER
MUMMIES
MURKIER
MUSHIER
MUSKIER
MUSKIES
MUSSIER
MUSTIER
MUYBIEN
MUZZIER
NAGGIER
NANNIED
NANNIES
NAPPIER
NAPPIES
NASTIER
NASTIES
NATTIER
NEEDIER
NERDIER
NERVIER
NEWBIES
NEWSIER
NEWSIES
NIFTIER
NIFTIES
NINNIES
NIPPIER
NITTIER
NOBBIER
NODDIES
NOISIER
NONDIET
NOOGIES
NUBBIER
NUTSIER
NUTTIER
OLIVIER
OLOGIES
ONADIET
ORACIES
OTARIES
OUTLIER
OUTLIES
OUTVIED
OUTVIES
OVARIES
PADDIES
PALLIER
PALMIER
PANNIER
PANSIES
PANTIES
PAPPIES
PARRIED
PARRIER
PARRIES
PARTIED
PARTIER

PARTIES
PASTIER
PASTIES
PATRIES
PATSIES
PATTIES
PEAKIER
PEATIER
PENNIES
PEONIES
PEPPIER
PERDIEM
PERKIER
PERRIER
PESKIER
PETTIER
PHONIER
PHONIES
PICKIER
PIETIES
PIGGIER
PIGGIES
PINKIES
PITHIER
PLATIER
PLATIES
PLUMIER
POESIES
POITIER
POPPIES
PORGIES
PORKIER
POSTIES
POTPIES
POTTIER
POTTIES
POUTIER
PREDIET
PREMIER
PREMIES
PREVIEW
PREXIES
PRICIER
PRIVIER
PRIVIES
PROBIES
PROSIER
PROXIES
PUDGIER
PUFFIER
PULPIER
PUNKIER
PUNKIES
PUNNIER
PUPPIES
PURLIEU
PURSIER
PURTIER
PURVIEW
PUSHIER
PUSSIES
PUTTIED
PUTTIES
PYGMIES
QUAKIER
QUAKIES
QUERIED
QUERIER

QUERIES
RAGGIER
RAGGIES
RAINIER
RALLIED
RALLIER
RALLIES
RANDIER
RANGIER
RASPIER
RATTIER
RAZZIES
READIED
READIER
READIES
REDRIED
REDRIES
REDTIES
REEDIER
REEFIER
REEKIER
REFLIES
REFRIED
REFRIES
REGNIER
REIFIED
REIFIES
RENTIER
REPLIED
REPLIER
REPLIES
REQUIEM
RETRIED
RETRIES
RIBBIER
RIBBIES
RIDGIER
RINDIER
RISKIER
RITZIER
ROADIES
ROCKIER
ROCKIES
ROILIER
ROOKIER
ROOKIES
ROOMIER
ROOMIES
ROOTIER
ROWDIER
ROWDIES
RUDDIED
RUDDIER
RUMMIES
RUNNIER
RUNTIER
RUSHIER
RUSTIER
RUTTIER
SAGGIER
SALLIED
SALLIER
SALLIES
SALTIER
SANDIER
SAPPIER
SASSIER
SAUCIER

SAVVIED
SAVVIER
SAVVIES
SCALIER
SCARIER
SEAMIER
SEDGIER
SEEDIER
SEEPIER
SHADIER
SHAKIER
SHALIER
SHINIER
SHOWIER
SILKIER
SILLIER
SILLIES
SILTIER
SISSIER
SISSIES
SIXTIES
SLATIER
SLIMIER
SMOKIER
SMOKIES
SNAKIER
SNOWIER
SOAPIER
SODDIER
SOFTIES
SOGGIER
SOLDIER
SOOTIER
SOPHIES
SOPPIER
SORRIER
SORTIED
SORTIES
SOUPIER
SPACIER
SPANIEL
SPECIES
SPICIER
SPIKIER
SPINIER
SPIRIER
SPUMIER
STAGIER
STEWIER
STOGIES
STONIER
STORIED
STORIES
STUDIED
STUDIER
STUDIES
STYMIED
STYMIES
SUCKIER
SUDSIER
SULKIER
SULKIES
SULLIED
SULLIES
SUNNIER
SURFIER
SURLIER
TABBIES

TACKIER
TAFFIES
TALKIER
TALKIES
TALLIED
TALLIER
TALLIES
TANGIER
TANSIES
TARDIER
TARRIED
TARRIER
TARRIES
TARTIER
TASTIER
TATTIER
TAWNIER
TEARIER
TECHIES
TEDDIES
TEENIER
TEKKIES
TELLIES
TENNIEL
TENNIES
TERRIER
TERRIES
TESTIER
THEDIET
THEVIEW
TINNIER
TIPPIER
TIPSIER
TIZZIES
TOADIED
TOADIES
TODDIES
TOLKIEN
TOONIES
TOWNIES
TUBBIER
TUFTIER
TUMMIES
TURFIER
TUSHIES
TWINIER
UMBRIEL
UNBRIEF
UNCRIED
UNDRIED
UNFRIED
UNIFIED
UNIFIER
UNIFIES
UNITIES
UNPLIED
UNQUIET
UNSHIER
UNSLIER
UNSPIED
UNTRIED
UPDRIED
UPDRIES
USURIES
VAMPIER
VANDIEN
VASTIER
VEALIER

VEERIES
VEGGIES
VEINIER
VERNIER
VIEWIER
WACKIER
WARTIER
WASHIER
WASPIER
WEARIED
WEARIER
WEARIES
WEBBIER
WEDGIER
WEDGIES
WEEDIER
WEENIES
WEEPIER
WESTIES
WHINIER
WIENIES
WIGGIER
WILLIES
WIMPIER
WINDIER
WISPIER
WITHIES
WITTIER
WOODIER
WOODIES
WOOKIEE
WOOLIER
WOOLIES
WOOZIER
WORDIER
WORMIER
WORRIED
WORRIER
WORRIES
YAWNIER
YETTIES
YIPPIES
YORKIES
YUCKIER
YUMMIER
YUPPIES
ZAPPIER
ZESTIER
ZINGIER
ZINKIER
ZIPPIER
ZOMBIES

••••I•E

ABSCISE
ABUSIVE
ACONITE
ACQUIRE
ACTFIVE
ACTLIKE
ADAMITE
ADELINE
ADENINE
AFFAIRE
AGATINE
AGEFIVE
AGENINE
AGONISE
AGONIZE
AIRLIKE
AIRLINE
AIRMILE
AIRTIME
ALADINE
ALANINE
ALCAIDE
ALEWIFE
ALLMINE
ALLRISE
ALLTIME
ALLWISE
AMATIVE
ANILINE
ANODISE
ANODIZE
ANTLIKE
ANTOINE
ANYTIME
ANYWISE
APATITE
APELIKE
APPRISE
ARCHIVE
ARCSINE
ARMLIKE
ARMOIRE
ARSHILE
ASCRIBE
ASININE
ASSLIKE
ASTAIRE
ASTRIDE
ATATIME
ATOMISE
ATOMIZE
ATTRITE
AUSPICE
AVARICE
AXELIKE
AZURITE
BAALITE
BADTIME
BAGLIKE
BAGPIPE
BAPTISE
BAPTIZE
BATLIKE
BAUXITE
BEDLIKE
BEDSIDE
BEDTIME
BEEHIVE
BEELIKE
BEELINE
BEGRIME
BEGUILE
BEGUINE
BIBLIKE
BIGFIVE
BIGTIME
BIOCIDE
BIOLITE
BIOTITE
BLUEICE
BONAIRE
BONFIRE

BOWLIKE
BOWLINE
BOXKITE
BOXLIKE
BOYLIKE
BRASIZE
BROMIDE
BROMINE
BUDLIKE
BUDTIME
BUSLINE
BUSRIDE
BUYTIME
BYAMILE
CABRIDE
CALCITE
CANDICE
CANDIDE
CAPRICE
CAPRINE
CAPSIZE
CAPTIVE
CARBIDE
CARBINE
CARMINE
CARTIRE
CASTILE
CATLIKE
CENTIME
CERVINE
CESAIRE
CHALICE
CHEMISE
CHOLINE
CHOPINE
CHORINE
CITRINE
CLARICE
COCAINE
COCHISE
CODEINE
COGNIZE
COLLIDE
COLLINE
COMBINE
COMPILE
CONCISE
CONFIDE
CONFINE
CONNIVE
COPPICE
CORDITE
CORNICE
CORVINE
CORZINE
COSTIVE
COUSINE
COWHIDE
COWLIKE
COWRITE
CREVICE
CUISINE
CUPLIKE
CUPRITE
CURLIKE
CURSIVE
CUTTIME
CYANIDE
DAYSIDE
DAYTIME
DEBOITE
DECEIVE
DECLINE
DELUISE
DENTINE
DEPRIVE
DESPISE
DESPITE
DESTINE
DEWLINE
DIDFINE
DIDLIKE
DIDTIME
DIORITE
DIOXIDE
DISLIKE
DOGBITE
DOGLIKE
DOGPILE
DOMAINE
DORMICE
DOTLIKE
DOTRICE
DUALIZE
DUCTILE
EARLIKE
EBBTIDE
EBONITE
EBONIZE
EBWHITE
ECOCIDE
EDIFICE
EDOMITE
EELLIKE
EGALITE
EGGLIKE
ELAMITE
ELEGIZE
ELFLIKE
ELUSIVE
EMBOITE
EMOTIVE
EMPRISE
ENDLINE
ENDWISE
ENPRISE
ENQUIRE
ENSUITE
ENTWINE
EONLINE
EPONINE
EREMITE
EROSIVE
ERSKINE
ERUDITE
ESQUIRE
ETAMINE
EVASIVE
EXAMINE
EYELIKE
EYELINE
FADLIKE
FANLIKE
FANTINE
FANWISE
FANZINE
FARSIDE
FASCIAE
FATLIKE
FBIFILE
FEBRILE
FERRITE
FERTILE
FESTIVE
FICTILE
FICTIVE
FINLIKE
FIREICE
FISSILE
FLEXILE
FORGIVE
FORHIRE
FORLIFE
FORSIZE
FOXFIRE
FOXLIKE
FRAGILE
FUNTIME
FURTIVE
GAGLINE
GARPIKE
GASLINE
GASPIPE
GEMLIKE
GENOISE
GENTILE
GENUINE
GETWISE
GLAVINE
GLYCINE
GODLIKE
GOTWISE
GRACILE
GRANITE
GRECIZE
GUANINE
GUMLIKE
GUNFIRE
HADTIME
HAGLIKE
HAMLINE
HARLINE
HASTIME
HATLIKE
HATSIZE
HAYRIDE
HAYWIRE
HELOISE
HEMLINE
HENLIKE
HERNIAE
HEROINE
HEURIGE
HILAIRE
HIPLIKE
HIRCINE
HITTITE
HOGLIKE
HOMEICE
HOPLITE
HOSPICE
HOSTILE
HOTLINE
HOTTIME
HOTWIRE
HOWNICE
HUNLIKE
HUSSITE
HUTLIKE
HYALITE
HYDRIDE
ICELIKE
ICELINE
ICEWINE
IDOLISE
IDOLIZE
IGRAINE
ILLBITE
ILLLIVE
IMAGINE
IMEMINE
INALINE
INAPILE
INCLINE
INEXILE
INKLIKE
INQUIRE
INSPIRE
INSPITE
INUTILE
INVOICE
INWHITE
ISOLINE
ITEMISE
ITEMIZE
ITSFINE
ITSTIME
IVORINE
IVYLIKE
JADEITE
JAMLIKE
JARDINE
JASMINE
JAWLIKE
JAWLINE
JETFIRE
JIGLIKE
JIGTIME
JIMRICE
JOYRIDE
JUGWINE
JUSTICE
JUSTINE
KATRINE
KEYLIME
KHEDIVE
KIDLIKE
LABMICE
LAICIZE
LARAINE
LATRINE
LATTICE
LAVAINE
LAWLIKE
LEETIDE
LEGLIKE
LEONINE
LETLIVE
LETRIDE
LEUCINE
LIGNITE
LIKEICE
LIMNITE
LIONISE
LIONIZE
LIPLIKE
LOWDIVE
LOWLIFE
LOWRISE
LOWSIDE
LOWTIDE
LUDDITE
LYDDITE
MACHINE
MAGUIRE
MALAISE
MALDIVE
MANLIKE
MANSIZE
MASSINE
MASSIVE
MAURICE
MAYTIME
MAYWINE
MCBRIDE
MCGUIRE
MCGWIRE
MCSWINE
MEMOIRE
METLIFE
MIDLIFE
MIDLINE
MIDRISE
MIDSIZE
MIDWIFE
MILLIME
MISCITE
MISFILE
MISFIRE
MISGIVE
MISLIKE
MISSILE
MISSIVE
MISTIME
MISWIRE
MOABITE
MORAINE
MORTICE
MORTISE
NAPTIME
NBALIVE
NERVINE
NETLIKE
NEWHIRE
NEWLIFE
NEWLINE
NIBLIKE
NICOISE
NIOBITE
NITRIDE
NITRITE
NONLIFE
NONLIVE
NONOISE
NOTLIKE
NOTLIVE
NOTMINE
NOTNICE
NUCLIDE
NUNLIKE
NUTLIKE
NUTPINE
OAKLIKE
OARLIKE
OATLIKE
OBELISE
OBELIZE
ODORIZE
OFFLINE
OFFSIDE
OFFSITE
OILLIKE
OILLINE
OLDLINE
OLDTIME
OLIVINE
ONALINE
ONEDIME
ONEMILE
ONESIZE
ONETIME
OPALINE
ORBLIKE
ORIFICE
ORIGINE
OUTFIRE
OUTGIVE
OUTHIRE
OUTLINE
OUTLIVE
OUTPIPE
OUTRIDE
OUTSIDE
OUTSIZE
OUTTIRE
OUTWILE
OVERICE
OWLLIKE
OXIDISE
OXIDIZE
OZONISE
OZONIZE
PACKICE
PADSITE
PANPIPE
PANTILE
PARFIVE
PARTITE
PASSIVE
PASTIME
PATRICE
PAULINE
PEALIKE
PEGLIKE
PENLIKE
PENLITE
PENNINE
PENSIVE
PEPTIDE
PERLITE
PERRINE
PETMICE
PIELIKE
PIGLIKE
PISCINE
PISMIRE
PLOSIVE
PODLIKE
POETISE
POETIZE
POPWINE
PORCINE
PRALINE
PRECISE
PRECITE
PREDIVE
PREFILE
PRELIFE
PREMISE
PRESIDE
PRETIRE
PREWIRE
PROFILE
PROLIFE
PROMISE
PROVIDE
PROVINE
PUERILE
PVCPIPE
QUININE
QUIVIVE
RAGTIME
RAMLIKE
RANKINE
RATLIKE
RATLINE
RAWHIDE
RAYLIKE
REALINE
REALISE
REALIZE
REARISE
RECEIVE
RECLINE
REDFIVE
REDLINE
REDNINE
REDPINE
REDRIVE
REDTIDE
REDWINE
REGUIDE
REJOICE
REPRICE
REPRIME
REPRISE
REPTILE
REQUIRE
REQUITE
RERAISE
RESEIZE
RESHINE
RESPICE
RESPIRE
RESPITE
RESTIVE
RETWINE
REUNITE
REVOICE
REWRITE
RIBLIKE
RIPTIDE
RLSTINE
RODLIKE
ROGAINE
ROMAINE
ROUTINE
RUGLIKE
RUNTIME
SACLIKE
SALTINE
SAMWISE
SARDINE
SAWLIKE
SEALIFE
SEALIKE
SEAMILE
SEASIDE
SERVICE
SERVILE
SESSILE
SINLIKE
SISTINE
SIXFIVE
SIXNINE
SKYDIVE
SKYLIKE
SKYLINE
SONLIKE
SOUBISE
SOWLIKE
STABILE
STANINE
STATICE
STERILE
STYLISE
STYLIZE
SUASIVE
SUBFILE
SUBLIME
SUBSIDE
SUFFICE
SULFIDE
SULFITE
SUNFIRE
SUNLIKE
SUNRISE
SURMISE
SURVIVE
SUSPIRE
SVERIGE
TACTILE
TAGLIKE
TAGLINE
TANLINE
TAURINE
TAXHIKE
TEATIME
TEETIME
TENMILE
TENSILE
TENSIVE
TERMITE
TERRINE
TEXTILE
THEFIVE
THELIKE
THENILE
THINICE
THWHITE
THYMINE
TIELINE
TIMRICE
TINLIKE
TINMINE
TIPLINE
TITMICE
TMOBILE
TOELIKE
TOMKITE
TONTINE
TOPFIVE
TOPLINE
TOPSIDE
TOWLINE
TOYBIKE
TOYKITE
TOYLIKE
TUBLIKE
TURBINE
TUSSIVE
TVGUIDE
TWOTIME
UKRAINE
UNAGILE
UNALIKE
UNISIZE
UNITISE
UNITIVE
UNITIZE
UNNAIVE
UNTRITE
UNTWINE
UNVOICE
UNWHITE
UPRAISE
URANITE
URNLIKE
UTILISE
UTILIZE
VACCINE
VAMPIRE
VANDINE
VANLINE
VEREINE
VESTIGE
VITRINE
VULPINE
WARLIKE
WARTIME
WAXLIKE
WAYSIDE
WEBLIKE
WEBSITE
WEBZINE
WIGLIKE
WOOKIEE
WOOLITE
YASMINE
YESSIRE
ZADKINE
ZEBRINE
ZERNIKE
ZINCITE

•••••IE

AIRDRIE
BEASTIE
BEATTIE
BLACKIE
BLIMPIE
BLONDIE
BOLATIE
BOLOTIE
BOOPSIE
BRASSIE
BROWNIE
CALORIE
CAPAPIE
CHAPPIE
CHARLIE
CHEAPIE
COMEDIE
COTERIE
CRAIGIE
CRAPPIE
DHURRIE
DONTLIE
DOORDIE
EUGENIE
FLOSSIE
FOOTSIE
FRANKIE
FREDDIE
FREEBIE
GALAXIE
GEORGIE
GRANNIE
GROUPIE
GUTHRIE
IFITDIE
ITSALIE
ITSATIE
JEANNIE
JOHNNIE
KIRSTIE
LARAMIE
LIMEPIE
MALTBIE
MEATPIE
MELANIE
MOCHRIE
MOONPIE
MOUNTIE
MUNCHIE
NATALIE
NECKTIE
NIGHTIE
NOTALIE
OVERLIE
PHILLIE
PLUMPIE
POOCHIE
POOPSIE
PORKPIE
PRAIRIE
PREEMIE
PREPPIE
QUEENIE
QUICKIE
RALPHIE
REVERIE
RITCHIE
ROSALIE
RUSHDIE
SCOTTIE
SHARPIE
SHELTIE
SHORTIE
SILKTIE
SINEDIE
STEELIE
STOOLIE
SWEETIE
SWOOSIE
TEENSIE
THANDIE
TOOTSIE
TOUGHIE
TREKKIE
TVMOVIE
TWINKIE
TWOONIE
VALERIE
WHEELIE
WHOOPIE
WILLKIE
YACHTIE

IF•••••

IFFIEST
IFIFELL
IFITDIE
IFORGET
IFORGOT
IFORONE
IFSTONE
IFWEMAY
IFYOUGO

I•F••••

IFFIEST
IMFORIT
INFAITH
INFANCY
INFANTA
INFANTE
INFANTS
INFAVOR
INFECTS
INFERNO
INFESTS
INFIDEL
INFIELD
INFIRST
INFIVES
INFIXED
INFIXES
INFLAME
INFLATE
INFLECT
INFLICT
INFLOWS
INFOCUS
INFOLDS
INFORCE
INFORIT
INFORMS
INFRACT
INFRONT
INFUSED
INFUSER
INFUSES
ISFAHAN

I••F•••

ICEFALL
ICEFLOE
ICEFOGS
ICEFREE
IFIFELL
ILLFOLD
INAFUNK
INAFURY
IREFUSE
IRSFORM
ITSFINE

I•••F••

IGOOFED
INSOFAR
ISRAFEL
ITCHFOR

I••••F•

ICONIFY
IDTHEFT
INAHUFF
INAJIFF
INDRAFT
INGRAFT
INGULFS

I•••••F

INAHUFF
INAIDOF
INAJIFF
INAWEOF
INBRIEF

•IF••••

BIFFING
BIFOCAL
DIFFERS
DIFFUSE
FIFTEEN
FIFTHLY
FIFTIES
FIFTYAD
FIFTYBC
GIFFORD
GIFTBOX
GIFTEES
GIFTING
GIFTSET
GIFTTAX
JIFFIES
LIFEFUL
LIFENET
LIFTERS
LIFTING
LIFTOFF
LIFTSUP
MIFFIER
MIFFING
MIFFLIN
NIFTIER
NIFTIES
NIFTILY
PIFFLED
PIFFLES
RIFFING
RIFFLED
RIFFLER
RIFFLES
RIFLERS
RIFLERY
RIFLING
RIFTING
SIFTERS
SIFTING
TIFFANY
TIFFING
TIFFINS
WIFYING

•I•F•••

AIRFARE
AIRFLOW
AIRFOIL
AIRFONE
BIAFRAN
BIDFAIR
BIFFING
BIGFANS
BIGFEET
BIGFISH
BIGFIVE
BIGFOOT
BIGFOUR
BIOFUEL
DIDFINE
DIFFERS
DIFFUSE
FIEFDOM
GIFFORD
GILFORD
GINFIZZ
HITFILM
JIFFIES
JIMFIXX
KIEFFER
KINFOLK
LIEFEST
MIFFIER
MIFFING
MIFFLIN
MISFEED
MISFILE
MISFIRE
MISFITS
MISFORM
MITFORD
PIAFFED
PIAFFES
PIFFLED
PIFFLES
PIGFISH
PILFERS
PINFOLD
PITFALL
RIFFING
RIFFLED
RIFFLER
RIFFLES
SIXFEET
SIXFIVE
SIXFOLD
SIXFOOT
SIXFOUR
TIFFANY
TIFFING
TIFFINS
TINFISH

TINFOIL
WILFORD
WILFRED
WINFREY

•I••F••

AIMSFOR
BIDSFOR
BIRDFLU
DIEDFOR
DIEOFFS
DIESFOR
DIGSFOR
DIREFUL
DISHFUL
FILOFAX
FIREFLY
FIREFOX
FISHFOR
FISHFRY
FISTFUL
GIRAFFE
HITSFOR
KIEFFER
KILLFEE
LIEDFOR
LIESFOR
LIFEFUL
LIVEFOR
MIDOFFS
MILKFED
MINDFUL
PIAFFED
PIAFFES
PINEFOR
PIPEFUL
PITIFUL
RINGFOR
RIPOFFS
SIGHFOR
SIGHFUL
SIGNFOR
SITSFOR
TINAFEY
TIPOFFS
VIALFUL
VIEDFOR
VIESFOR
WILLFUL
WISHFOR
WISHFUL
WISTFUL

•I•••F•

AIRLIFT
BINDOFF
BITEOFF
DIEDOFF
DIEOFFS
DIESOFF
DIGNIFY
DISTAFF
FIREOFF
GIRAFFE
GIVEOFF
HITSOFF
HIVEOFF
KICKOFF
KISSOFF
LIFTOFF
LIGNIFY
LIPSOFF
LIQUEFY
MIAMIFL
MIDLIFE
MIDOFFS
MIDRIFF
MIDWIFE
NITRIFY
PICKOFF
PIESAFE
RIDEOFF
RINGOFF
RIPOFFS
RIPSOFF
SIGNIFY
SIGNOFF
TICKOFF
TIEDOFF
TIESOFF
TIMEOFF
TIPOFFS
TIPSOFF
VITRIFY
WIPEOFF
ZINCIFY
ZIPCUFF
ZIPSOFF

•I••••F

AIRWOLF
BIGHALF
BINDOFF
BITEOFF
DIEDOFF
DIESOFF
DISTAFF
FIGLEAF
FIREOFF
GIVENOF
GIVEOFF
GIVESOF
HIMSELF
HIPROOF
HITSOFF
HIVEOFF
KICKOFF
KISSOFF
LIFTOFF
LINDORF
LIPSOFF
MIDRIFF
PICKOFF
PILESOF
RIDEOFF
RINGOFF
RIPSOFF
SIGNOFF
SILENTF
TICKOFF
TIEDOFF
TIESOFF
TIMEOFF
TINROOF
TIPSOFF
TIREDOF
TIRESOF
WIPEOFF
ZIPCUFF
ZIPSOFF

••IF•••

ALIFORM
CHIFFON
CLIFTON
COIFFED
COIFING
DEIFIED
DEIFIER
DEIFIES
DRIFTED
DRIFTER
DRIFTIN
DRIFTUP
EDIFICE
EDIFIED
EDIFIER
EDIFIES
FBIFILE
FEIFFER
GRIFFEY
GRIFFIN
GRIFFON
GRIFTED
GRIFTER
HEIFERS
HEIFETZ
IFIFELL
KNIFERS
KNIFING
ORIFICE
OVIFORM
REIFIED
REIFIES
SHIFTED
SHIFTER
SKIFFED
SKIFFLE
SNIFFAT
SNIFFED
SNIFFER
SNIFFLE
SNIFFLY
SNIFFUP
SNIFTER
SPIFFED
SPIFFUP
STIFFED
STIFFEL
STIFFEN
STIFFER
STIFFLY
STIFLED
STIFLES
SWIFTER
SWIFTLY
TRIFFID
TRIFLED
TRIFLER
TRIFLES
TRIFOLD
TRIFORM
UNIFIED
UNIFIER
UNIFIES
UNIFORM
WAIFISH
WHIFFED
WHIFFER
WHIFFLE

••I•F••

AVIDFAN
BRIEFED
BRIEFER
BRIEFLY
BRIMFUL
CHIEFLY
CHIFFON
COIFFED
EXITFEE
FAIRFAX
FEIFFER
GAINFUL
GOINFOR
GRIFFEY
GRIFFIN
GRIFFON
LAIDFOR
PAIDFOR
PAILFUL
PAINFUL
SHIPFUL
SKIFFED
SKIFFLE
SKILFUL
SNIFFAT
SNIFFED
SNIFFER
SNIFFLE
SNIFFLY
SNIFFUP
SPIFFED
SPIFFUP
STIFFED
STIFFEL
STIFFEN
STIFFER
STIFFLY
STIRFRY
TAILFIN
TOILFUL
TRIFFID
WAILFUL
WAITFOR
WHIFFED
WHIFFER
WHIFFLE

••I••F•

ACIDIFY
BAILIFF
BOILOFF
CLIPOFF
FAIROFF
LAIDOFF
PAIDOFF
PAIROFF
SKILIFT
SLIDOFF
SLIPOFF
SNIPOFF
SPINOFF
TAILOFF
TRIMOFF

••I•••F

APILEOF
BAILIFF
BOILOFF
CLIPOFF
FAIROFF
LAIDOFF
PAIDOFF
PAIROFF
SLIDOFF
SLIPOFF
SNIPOFF
SPINOFF
TAILOFF
THINKOF
TRIMOFF

•••IF••

ACTIFED
ANTIFOG
AQUIFER
CONIFER
DUTIFUL
EQUIFAX
HALIFAX
LATIFAH
LUCIFER
NOGIFTS
OSSIFIC
PACIFIC
PITIFUL
REGIFTS
RESIFTS
ROTIFER
STRIFES
TARIFFS
THRIFTS
THRIFTY
UPLIFTS

•••I•F•

BELIEFS
RELIEFS
SATISFY
TARIFFS

•••I••F

APAIROF
INAIDOF
SERIESF
STRIPOF

••••IF•

ACETIFY
ACIDIFY
AIRLIFT
ALEWIFE
AMPLIFY
ASAGIFT
ASSTIFF
BAILIFF
BEATIFY
BRANIFF
CALCIFY
CARDIFF
CERTIFY
CLARIFY
CONNIFF
DANDIFY
DENSIFY
DIGNIFY
DULCIFY
EYELIFT
FALSIFY
FANCIFY
FORLIFE
FORTIFY
GLORIFY
GRATIFY
HAPPIFY
HORRIFY
ICONIFY
INAJIFF
JELLIFY
JOLLIFY
JUSTIFY
LIGNIFY
LOWLIFE
MAGNIFY
MASSIFS
MASTIFF
MCGRIFF
METLIFE
MIAMIFL
MIDLIFE
MIDRIFF
MIDWIFE
MOLLIFY
MORTIFY
MUMMIFY
MYSTIFY
MYTHIFY
NEWLIFE
NITRIFY
NONLIFE
NULLIFY
OUTSIFT
PETRIFY
PONTIFF
PRELIFE
PRESIFT
PROLIFE
PULPIFY
QUALIFY
RECTIFY
RESHIFT
REUNIFY
SCARIFY
SEALIFE
SEALIFT
SHERIFF
SHERIFS
SIGNIFY
SKILIFT
SPECIFY
TERRIFY
TESTIFY
THEGIFT
UNSHIFT
UNSTIFF
UPDRIFT
UPSHIFT
VERBIFY
VERSIFY
VITRIFY
WHATIFS
YUPPIFY
ZINCIFY
ZOMBIFY

••••I•F

ASSTIFF
BAILIFF
BRANIFF
CARDIFF
CONNIFF
DEBRIEF
INAJIFF
INBRIEF
MASTIFF
MCGRIFF
MIDRIFF
PONTIFF
SHERIFF
UNBRIEF
UNSTIFF

IG•••••

IGGYPOP
IGIVEUP
IGNARRO
IGNATOW
IGNEOUS
IGNITED
IGNITER
IGNITES
IGNITOR
IGNOBLE
IGNOBLY
IGNORED
IGNORER
IGNORES
IGOOFED
IGOROTS
IGOTCHA
IGOTYOU
IGRAINE
IGUANAS
IGUANID
IGUASSU

I•G••••

IGGYPOP
IMGOING
IMGREAT
INGALLS
INGATES
INGEMAR
INGENUE
INGESTA
INGESTS
INGLESE
INGOALS
INGOING
INGRAFT
INGRAIN
INGRATE
INGREEN
INGRESS
INGROUP
INGROWN
INGULFS
ITGIRLS

I••G•••

IBEGYOU
IEIGHTY
IMAGERS
IMAGERY
IMAGINE
IMAGING
IMAGISM
IMAGIST
IMAGOES
IMOGENE
ISOGONS
ISOGRAM
ITSGONE

I•••G••

ICEAGES
ICINGIN
ICINGIT
ICINGUP
IFORGET
IFORGOT
ILLEGAL
ILLEGIT
ILLOGIC
IMPUGNS
INDIGEN
INDIGOS
INNAGES
INSIGHT
INSIGNE
INTEGER
INTEGRA
INVOGUE

I••••G•

ICEBAGS
ICEFOGS
IDBADGE
IFYOUGO
IIKINGS
IMAHOGG
IMMERGE
IMPINGE
IMUSTGO
INARAGE
INDULGE
INKINGS
INLARGE
INNINGS
INRANGE
INVEIGH
IPLEDGE
IRESIGN
IRONAGE
ISITAGO

I•••••G

ICEBERG
IMAGING
IMAHOGG
IMBUING
IMGOING
INCHING
INGOING
INKLING
INLYING
INTHING
INURING
IRISING
IRONING
ISSUING
ITCHING
ITEMING

•IG••••

AIGLETS
AIGRETS
BIGAPES
BIGBABY
BIGBAND
BIGBANG
BIGBEAR
BIGBEAT
BIGBEND
BIGBETS
BIGBIRD
BIGBLUE
BIGBOSS
BIGBOYS
BIGCARS
BIGCATS
BIGCITY
BIGDAYS
BIGDEAL
BIGDIGS
BIGDOGS
BIGEARS
BIGEAST
BIGEASY
BIGELOW
BIGENDS
BIGEYED
BIGEYES
BIGFANS
BIGFEET
BIGFISH
BIGFIVE
BIGFOOT
BIGFOUR
BIGGAME
BIGGERS
BIGGEST
BIGGIES
BIGGIRL
BIGGISH
BIGGITY
BIGGULP
BIGGUNS
BIGHAIR
BIGHALF
BIGHAND
BIGHEAD
BIGHITS
BIGHORN
BIGHUGS
BIGIDEA
BIGJAKE
BIGJERK
BIGJOHN
BIGKIDS
BIGLEAD
BIGLIES
BIGLOTS
BIGLOVE
BIGMACS
BIGMAMA
BIGMEAL
BIGMESS
BIGNAME
BIGNESS
BIGNEWS
BIGNOSE
BIGONES
BIGOTED
BIGOTRY
BIGRIGS
BIGSALE
BIGSHOT
BIGSHOW
BIGSTAR
BIGTALK
BIGTENT
BIGTIME
BIGTOES
BIGTOPS
BIGTOWN
BIGUNIT
BIGWIGS
BIGWINS
DIGESTS
DIGGERS
DIGGING
DIGGITY
DIGGORY
DIGICAM
DIGINTO
DIGIPET
DIGITAL
DIGLOTS
DIGNIFY
DIGNITY
DIGRAMS
DIGRAPH
DIGRESS
DIGSFOR
DIGSOUT
EIGHTAD
EIGHTAM
EIGHTBC
EIGHTEE
EIGHTHS
EIGHTPM
EIGHTUP
FIGBARS
FIGHTER
FIGLEAF
FIGMENT
FIGTREE
FIGURAL
FIGURED
FIGURER
FIGURES
GIGABIT
GIGATON
GIGBAGS
GIGGING
GIGGLED
GIGGLER
GIGGLES
GIGOLOS
HIGGINS
HIGGLED
HIGGLER
HIGGLES
HIGHART
HIGHBAR
HIGHBOY
HIGHDAY
HIGHEND
HIGHEST
HIGHHAT
HIGHIQS
HIGHISH
HIGHLOW
HIGHPAY
HIGHRES
HIGHSEA
HIGHTEA
HIGHTOP
HIGHWAY
JIGGERS
JIGGERY
JIGGIER
JIGGING
JIGGISH
JIGGLED
JIGGLES
JIGLIKE
JIGSAWS
JIGTIME
LIGANDS
LIGATED
LIGATES
LIGGETT
LIGHTED
LIGHTEN
LIGHTER
LIGHTLY
LIGHTON
LIGHTUP
LIGNIFY
LIGNINS
LIGNITE
LIGURIA
MIGENES
MIGHTNT
MIGNONS
MIGRANT
MIGRATE
NIGERIA
NIGGLED
NIGGLER
NIGGLES
NIGHEST
NIGHTER
NIGHTIE
NIGHTLY
PIGEONS
PIGEYED
PIGFISH
PIGGERY
PIGGIER
PIGGIES
PIGGING
PIGGISH
PIGIRON
PIGLETS
PIGLIKE
PIGMEAT
PIGMENT
PIGNUTS
PIGOUTS
PIGPENS
PIGSKIN
PIGSOUT
PIGTAIL
PIGWEED
RIGGERS
RIGGING
RIGHTED
RIGHTER
RIGHTLY
RIGHTON
RIGIDLY
RIGOURS
RIGSOUT
RIGUEUR
RIGVEDA
SIGHERS
SIGHFOR
SIGHFUL
SIGHING
SIGHSAT
SIGHTED
SIGHTER
SIGHTLY
SIGMOID
SIGMUND
SIGNAGE
SIGNALS
SIGNEES
SIGNERS
SIGNETS
SIGNFOR
SIGNIFY
SIGNING
SIGNOFF
SIGNORA
SIGNORE
SIGNORS
SIGNOUT
SIGNSIN
SIGNSON
SIGNSUP
SIGNUPS
TIGHTEN
TIGHTER
TIGHTLY
TIGLONS
TIGRESS
VIGNOLA
VIGOURS
WIGGERY
WIGGIER
WIGGING
WIGGLED
WIGGLER
WIGGLES
WIGLESS
WIGLETS
WIGLIKE
WIGSOUT
WIGWAGS
WIGWAMS
ZIGGING
ZIGZAGS

•I•G•••

AIRGLOW
AIRGUNS
BIGGAME
BIGGERS
BIGGEST
BIGGIES
BIGGIRL
BIGGISH
BIGGITY
BIGGULP
BIGGUNS
BILGIER
BINGERS
BINGHAM
BINGING
BINGLES
BINGOES
DIAGRAM
DIDGOOD
DIGGERS
DIGGING
DIGGITY
DIGGORY
DINGBAT
DINGERS
DINGIER
DINGILY
DINGING
DINGLES
DINGOES
DISGUST
FIDGETS
FIDGETY
FINGALS
FINGERS
FIZGIGS
GIGGING
GIGGLED
GIGGLER
GIGGLES
GINGAME
GINGERS
GINGERY
GINGHAM
GINGIVA
GINGKOS
GINGOLD
HIGGINS
HIGGLED
HIGGLER
HIGGLES
HINGEON
HINGING
JIGGERS
JIGGERY
JIGGIER
JIGGING
JIGGISH
JIGGLED
JIGGLES
JINGLED
JINGLER
JINGLES
JINGOES
KINGDOM

KINGING
KINGLET
KINGMAN
KINGPIN
KINGRAT
KINGTUT
LIGGETT
LINGCOD
LINGERS
LINGOES
LINGUAE
LINGUAL
LINGULA
MIDGETS
MINGIER
MINGLED
MINGLER
MINGLES
MISGAVE
MISGIVE
NIAGARA
NIGGLED
NIGGLER
NIGGLES
PIDGEON
PIDGINS
PIGGERY
PIGGIER
PIGGIES
PIGGING
PIGGISH
PILGRIM
PINGERS
PINGING
PINGUID
RIDGIER
RIDGING
RIDGWAY
RIEGERT
RIGGERS
RIGGING
RINGERS
RINGFOR
RINGING
RINGLET
RINGOFF
RINGOUT
RINGSIN
RINGSUP
SIEGING
SINGERS
SINGING
SINGLED
SINGLES
SINGLET
SINGOUT
SINGSTO
SIXGUNS
TIEGAME
TINGING
TINGLED
TINGLER
TINGLES
TINGODS
VIRGATE
VIRGINS
VIRGOAN
VIRGULE
WIDGEON
WIDGETS
WIGGERY
WIGGIER
WIGGING
WIGGLED
WIGGLER
WIGGLES
WINGERS
WINGING
WINGLET
WINGMAN
WINGMEN
WINGNUT
WINGSIT
WINGTIP
XINGOUT
ZIEGLER
ZIGGING
ZINGERS
ZINGIER
ZINGING
ZIPGUNS

•I••G••

CITYGAL
DIMAGES
FIBIGER
FINAGLE
GIELGUD
GINKGOS
GIORGIO
GIORGOS
LIMOGES
LINAGES
LISAGAY
LITHGOW
MILAGRO
MINOGUE
MIRAGES
NICEGUY
NIPIGON
PILEGGI
PIPAGES
PIROGEN
PIROGUE
RIOTGUN
RITAGAM
VINEGAR
VIRAGOS
VISAGED
VISAGES
WINDGOD
WISEGUY

•I•••G•

AIMHIGH
AIRBAGS
AIRINGS
AIRLOGS
AIRRAGE
AIRSIGN
BIGDIGS
BIGDOGS
BIGHUGS
BIGRIGS
BIGWIGS
BIOLOGY
CINERGY
DIALOGS
DIVERGE
DIVULGE
FILINGS
FIRINGS
FIXINGS
FIZGIGS
GIGBAGS
HIDALGO
HIDINGS
IIKINGS
JIMHOGG
KITBAGS
LIKINGS
LINEAGE
LININGS
LINKAGE
LITURGY
LIVINGS
MIDLEGS
MILEAGE
MILLAGE
MININGS
MINTAGE
MISPAGE
NICCAGE
OILRIGS
PILEGGI
PILINGS
PILLAGE
PIPINGS
RIBCAGE
RIDINGS
RISINGS
SIDINGS
SIGNAGE
SINKAGE
TIDINGS
TILINGS
TILLAGE
TIMINGS
VIKINGS
VILLAGE
VINTAGE
WIGWAGS
WINDAGE
WINDIGO
WIRINGS
ZIGZAGS

•I••••G

BIASING
BIBBING
BIBLIOG
BIDDING
BIFFING
BIGBANG
BILKING
BILLING
BINDING
BINGING
BINNING
BIRDDOG
BIRDING
BIRLING
BIRRING
BITTING
DIALING
DIETING
DIGGING
DIMMING
DINGING
DINNING
DINTING
DIPPING
DIRKING
DIRTBAG
DISCING
DISHING
DISHRAG
DISKING
DISSING
FIBBING
FILIBEG
FILLING
FILMING
FINDING
FINKING
FIREBUG
FIREDOG
FIRMING
FISHING
FITTING
FIZZING
GIFTING
GIGGING
GILDING
GILLING
GIMPING
GINNING
GINSENG
GIRDING
GIRTING
GISSING
GITTING
HIBBING
HILLING
HILTING
HINDLEG
HINGING
HINTING
HISSING
HITSONG
HITTING
JIGGING
JILTING
JIMHOGG
JINXING
KICKING
KIDDING
KILLING
KILNING
KILTING
KINGING
KINKING
KIPLING
KIPPING
KISSING
KITTING
LIBBING
LICKING
LIFTING
LILTING
LIMBING
LIMBURG
LIMNING
LIMPING
LINKING
LINTING
LIPPING
LISPING
LISTING
MIFFING
MILKING
MILLING
MINCING
MINDING
MINTING
MISSING
MISTING
MITRING
NIALONG
NICEDOG
NICHING
NICKING
NIPPING
OILRING
OINKING
PICKING
PIECING
PIGGING
PILLBUG
PILLING
PINGING
PINKING
PINNING
PIQUING
PISHING
PITHING
PITTING
PITYING
RIBBING
RIDDING
RIDGING
RIFFING
RIFLING
RIFTING
RIGGING
RIKSDAG
RIMMING
RINGING
RINSING
RIOTING
RIPPING
RISKING
SIBLING
SICCING
SIDLING
SIEBZIG
SIEGING
SIEVING
SIFTING
SIGHING
SIGNING
SILENTG
SILOING
SILTING
SINGING
SINKING
SINNING
SIPPING
SITTING
TICCING
TICKING
TIDYING
TIERING
TIFFING
TILLING
TILTING
TIMELAG
TINGING
TINNING
TINTING
TIPPING
TITHING
TITLING
TITRING
VIALING
VIERZIG
VIEWING
VISAING
WICKING
WIFYING
WIGGING
WILDDOG
WILDING
WILDPIG
WILLING
WILTING
WIMPING
WINCING
WINDBAG
WINDING
WINGING
WINKING
WINNING
WINSBIG
WISHING
WISPING
WITLING
WITTING
YIPPING
ZIERING
ZIGGING
ZINCING
ZINGING
ZIPPING

••IG•••

ABIGAIL
ALIGHTS
ALIGNED
ALIGNER
ALIGOTE
ARIGATO
AVIGNON
BEIGNES
BEIGNET
BLIGHTS
BLIGHTY
BRIGADE
BRIGAND
BRIGHAM
BRIGHTS
CHIGGER
CHIGNON
CHIGOES
COIGNED
COIGNES
DEIGNED
DEIGNTO
DWIGHTD
ELIGIUS
EMIGREE
EMIGRES
ENIGMAS
EPIGONE
EPIGRAM
ERIGENA
EXIGENT
FEIGNED
FEIGNER
FLIGHTS
FLIGHTY
FRIGATE
FRIGHTS
GRIGRIS
GUIGNOL
HEIGHHO
HEIGHTS
IEIGHTY
KNIGHTS
MAIGRET
NEIGHED
OMIGOSH
ORIGAMI
ORIGINE
ORIGINS
PLIGHTS
QUIGLEY
REIGNED
SLIGHTS
SNIGLET
SOIGNEE
SPIGOTS
STIGMAS
SWIGERT
SWIGGED
THIGPEN
TRIGGER
TRIGONS
TRIGRAM
VEIGHTS
WEIGHED
WEIGHER
WEIGHIN
WEIGHON
WEIGHTS
WEIGHTY
WEIGHUP
WRIGGLE
WRIGGLY
WRIGHTS
WRIGLEY

••I•G••

ACINGIT
ASIAGOS
ATINGLE
AZINGER
BRIDGED
BRIDGER
BRIDGES
BRIDGET
BRINGER
BRINGIN
BRINGIT
BRINGON
BRINGTO
BRINGUP
CHIGGER
CLINGER
CLINGTO
CRINGED
CRINGES
CUINGIN
DOINGIN
DOINGOK
DOINGSO
DOINGTO
DOINGUP
EKINGBY
FLINGAT
FLINGER
FRIDGES
FRINGED
FRINGES
GOINGAT
GOINGBY
GOINGIN
GOINGON
GOINGTO
GOINGUP
GRINGOS
HAIRGEL
ICINGIN
ICINGIT
ICINGUP
KLINGER
KLINGON
KRINGLE
LYINGBY
LYINGON
LYINGTO
LYINGUP
NAILGUN
ODINGON
OWINGON
OWINGTO
PRINGLE
RAINGOD
SHINGLE
SHINGLY
SLINGER
SMIDGEN
SMIDGES
SPIEGEL
STINGER
SWIGGED
SWINGAT
SWINGBY
SWINGER
SWINGIT
TLINGIT
TRIAGES
TRIGGER
TWINGED
TWINGES
TYINGIN
TYINGON
TYINGTO
TYINGUP
USINGIN
USINGUP
WRIGGLE
WRIGGLY
WRINGER
ZWINGLI

••I••G•

CHICAGO
COINAGE
EPILOGS
ISITAGO
RAILAGE
REIMAGE
SOILAGE
TRILOGY
ZHIVAGO

••I•••G

ABIDING
ALINING
ARISING
BAILING
BAITING
BEIJING
BOILING
BRIBING
BRILLIG
BRINING
CEILING
CHIDING
CHIMING
CHINWAG
COIFING
COILING
COINING
DEICING
DRIVING
EDITING
ELIDING
EXILING
EXITING
FAILING
FAIRING
FOILING
GAINING
GAITING
GLIDING
GRIMING
GRIPING
GUIDING
GUILING
HAILING
IRISING
JAILING
JOINING
JUICING
KNIFING
LAIRING
LEIPZIG
LOIDING
MAILBAG
MAILING
MAIMING
MOILING
NAILING
NAILKEG
NOISING
OPINING
PAINING
PAIRING
PEIPING
POISING
PRICING
PRIDING
PRIMING
PRIZING
RAIDING
RAILING
RAINING
RAISING
REICING
REINING
ROILING
RUINING
SAILING
SEINING
SEIZING
SHINDIG
SHINING
SLICING
SLIDING
SLIMING
SMILING
SMITING
SNIPING
SOILING
SPICING
SPIKING
SPITING
SUITING
SWIPING
TAILING
TAILWAG
TOILING
TWINING
UNITING
VEILING
VEINING
VOICING
VOIDING
WAILING
WAITING
WAIVING
WHILING
WHINING
WHITING
WRITING
ZEITUNG

•••IG••

ALRIGHT
ANTIGEN
ANTIGUA
ANTIGUN
ASSIGNS
ATEIGHT
ATNIGHT
ATSIGHT
ATSIGNS
BENIGNI
BENIGNO
BERIGAN
BYRIGHT
COSIGNS
CRAIGIE
DELIGHT
DEMIGOD
DESIGNS
DORIGHT
ENRIGHT
ENSIGNS
FATIGUE
FIBIGER
FREIGHT
INDIGEN
INDIGOS
INSIGHT
INSIGNE
LATIGOS
LEHIGHU
LONIGAN
MADIGAN
MALIGNS
MEDIGAP
MRRIGHT
MRTIGER
MUSIGNY
NIPIGON
OBLIGED
OBLIGEE
OBLIGER
OBLIGES
OBLIGOR
ONSIGHT
PERIGEE
REFIGHT
RELIGHT
RESIGHT
RESIGNS
SEVIGNY
SLEIGHS
SLEIGHT
STEIGER
TONIGHT
UNLIGHT
UNRIGID
UNSIGHT
UPLIGHT
UPRIGHT
UPTIGHT

•••I•G•

ABRIDGE
AIRINGS
ARCINGS
AWNINGS
BESIEGE
BLUINGS
BODINGS
BOEINGS
BORINGS
BYJINGO
CANINGS
CASINGS
COMINGS
DATINGS
DOMINGO
EDGINGS
ENDINGS
FACINGS
FILINGS
FIRINGS
FIXINGS
FOLIAGE
GATINGS
HAYINGS
HAZINGS
HIDINGS
IIKINGS
IMPINGE
INKINGS
INNINGS
LACINGS
LADINGS
LETITGO
LIKINGS
LININGS
LIVINGS
LOSINGS
MAKINGS
MAYINGS
MININGS
MOWINGS
MUSINGS
NORIEGA
OFFINGS
OUTINGS
PAGINGS
PALINGS
PARINGS
PAVINGS
PILINGS
PIPINGS
RAGINGS
RATINGS
RAVINGS
REHINGE
RESINGS
RETINGE
RIDINGS
RISINGS
ROVINGS
RULINGS
SAVINGS
SAYINGS
SIDINGS
SPRINGS
SPRINGY
SPYINGS
STRINGS
STRINGY
SYRINGE
TAKINGS
TAPINGS
TIDINGS
TILINGS
TIMINGS
TOWINGS
UNHINGE
URGINGS
VIKINGS
WAKINGS
WAXINGS
WIRINGS

•••I••G

ANTIFOG
ANTILOG
FILIBEG
FREITAG
PERIWIG
SEMILOG
SERIESG
TAXIING
WYSIWYG

••••IG•

ACEHIGH
AIMHIGH
AIRSIGN
AMERIGO
ARRAIGN
BADSIGN
BAGWIGS
BIGDIGS
BIGRIGS
BIGWIGS
CATRIGS
CONDIGN
CONSIGN
EARWIGS
FIZGIGS
FLYHIGH
FOREIGN
HEURIGE
HEXSIGN
HOWHIGH
INVEIGH
IRESIGN
LENTIGO
OILRIGS
OUTRIGS
OUTSIGH
PETPIGS
PRODIGY
RALEIGH
REALIGN
REWEIGH
RODRIGO
SKYHIGH
SVERIGE
THEBIGA
TOOHIGH
VERTIGO
VESTIGE
WINDIGO

••••I•G

ABASING
ABATING
ABIDING
ABUSING
ADDLING
ADORING
ALAKING
ALAYING
ALINING
ALLYING
ALTHING
AMAZING
AMBLING
AMUSING
ANELING
ANGLING
ANTEING
APPLING
ARCHING
ARGUING
ARISING
ATONING
AUTOING
AVOWING
AWAKING
BABYING

BACHING
BACKING
BAFFING
BAGGING
BAILING
BAITING
BALDING
BALKING
BAMMING
BANDING
BANGING
BANKING
BANNING
BANTING
BARBING
BARGING
BARKING
BARNING
BARRING
BASHING
BASKING
BASTING
BATHING
BATTING
BATWING
BAWLING
BEADING
BEAMING
BEANING
BEARING
BEATING
BEDDING
BEEFING
BEEPING
BEGGING
BEHRING
BEIJING
BELLING
BELTING
BELYING
BENDING
BENNING
BERMING
BESTING
BETTING
BIASING
BIBBING
BIBLIOG
BIDDING
BIFFING
BILKING
BILLING
BINDING
BINGING
BINNING
BIRDING
BIRLING
BIRRING
BITTING
BLADING
BLAMING
BLARING
BLAZING
BLOWING
BLUEING
BOATING
BOBBING
BOFFING

BOGGING
BOILING
BOLLING
BOLTING
BOMBING
BONDING
BONGING
BONKING
BOOKING
BOOMING
BOOTING
BOOZING
BOPPING
BORKING
BOSSING
BOWLING
BRACING
BRAKING
BRAVING
BRAYING
BRAZING
BREWING
BRIBING
BRINING
BRUXING
BUCKING
BUDDING
BUDGING
BUFFING
BUGGING
BUGLING
BULGING
BULKING
BULLING
BUMMING
BUMPING
BUNGING
BUNKING
BUNNING
BUNTING
BUOYING
BURLING
BURNING
BURPING
BURRING
BURYING
BUSHING
BUSKING
BUSSING
BUSTING
BUSYING
BUTTING
BUZZING
CABBING
CABLING
CACHING
CADGING
CALKING
CALLING
CALMING
CALVING
CAMPING
CANNING
CANTING
CAPPING
CARDING
CARKING
CARLING

CARPING
CARTING
CARVING
CASHING
CASKING
CASTING
CAUSING
CEASING
CEILING
CENSING
CESSING
CHAFING
CHARING
CHASING
CHAWING
CHEFING
CHEWING
CHIDING
CHIMING
CHOKING
CHOWING
CHUTING
CLAWING
CLAYING
CLEWING
CLONING
CLOSING
CLOYING
CLUEING
COALING
COATING
COAXING
COCKING
COGGING
COIFING
COILING
COINING
COMBING
COMPING
CONKING
CONNING
COOKING
COOLING
COOPING
COPPING
COPYING
CORDING
CORKING
CORNING
COSHING
COSTING
COSYING
COUPING
COWLING
COZYING
CRANING
CRAPING
CRATING
CRAVING
CRAZING
CREPING
CREWING
CROWING
CUBBING
CUFFING
CULLING
CUNNING
CUPPING

CURBING
CURDING
CURLING
CURRING
CURSING
CURVING
CUSHING
CUSSING
CUTTING
CYCLING
DABBING
DADOING
DAMMING
DAMNING
DAMPING
DANCING
DANNING
DAPPING
DARLING
DARNING
DARTING
DASHING
DAUBING
DAWNING
DEALING
DECKING
DEEDING
DEEMING
DEFYING
DEICING
DEKEING
DELEING
DELVING
DEMOING
DENNING
DENTING
DENYING
DERRING
DEUCING
DIALING
DIETING
DIGGING
DIMMING
DINGING
DINNING
DINTING
DIPPING
DIRKING
DISCING
DISHING
DISKING
DISSING
DOCKING
DODGING
DOFFING
DOGGING
DOLLING
DONKING
DONNING
DOOMING
DOSSING
DOTTING
DOUSING
DOWLING
DOWNING
DOWSING
DRAPING
DRAWING

DRAYING
DRIVING
DRONING
DUBBING
DUCKING
DUCTING
DUELING
DUETING
DULLING
DUMBING
DUMPING
DUNKING
DUNNING
DURNING
DUSKING
DUSTING
EAGLING
EARNING
EARRING
EASTING
ECHOING
EDDYING
EDITING
EDUCING
ELATING
ELIDING
ELOPING
ELUDING
ELUTING
EMOTING
ENDUING
ENSUING
ENURING
ENVYING
ERASING
ERODING
ESPYING
ESTRING
ETCHING
EVADING
EVENING
EVOKING
EXILING
EXITING
EXUDING
FABLING
FAILING
FAIRING
FALLING
FANGING
FANNING
FARCING
FARMING
FASTING
FATLING
FATTING
FAWNING
FEARING
FEEDING
FEELING
FELLING
FELTING
FENCING
FENDING
FESSING
FEUDING
FIBBING
FILLING

FILMING
FINDING
FINKING
FIRMING
FISHING
FITTING
FIZZING
FLAKING
FLAMING
FLARING
FLAWING
FLAYING
FLEEING
FLEMING
FLEXING
FLOWING
FLUTING
FLUXING
FOALING
FOAMING
FOBBING
FOGGING
FOILING
FOLDING
FOOLING
FOOTING
FORCING
FORDING
FORGING
FORKING
FORMING
FOULING
FOWLING
FRAMING
FRAYING
FREEING
FRODING
FUDGING
FUELING
FUNDING
FUNKING
FUNNING
FURLING
FURRING
FUSSING
FUTZING
FUZZING
GABBING
GADDING
GAFFING
GAGGING
GAINING
GAITING
GALLING
GAMMING
GANGING
GAOLING
GAPPING
GARBING
GASHING
GASPING
GASSING
GATLING
GAUGING
GAWKING
GAWPING
GEARING
GELDING

GELLING
GETTING
GIFTING
GIGGING
GILDING
GILLING
GIMPING
GINNING
GIRDING
GIRTING
GISSING
GITTING
GLARING
GLAZING
GLIDING
GLOBING
GLOVING
GLOWING
GNAWING
GOADING
GODLING
GOLDING
GOLFING
GONGING
GOODING
GOOFING
GOOSING
GORGING
GORMING
GOSLING
GOUGING
GOWNING
GRACING
GRADING
GRATING
GRAVING
GRAYING
GRAZING
GREYING
GRIMING
GRIPING
GROPING
GROWING
GSTRING
GUIDING
GUILING
GULFING
GULLING
GULPING
GUMMING
GUNNING
GUSHING
GUSTING
GUTTING
GYPPING
HACKING
HAFTING
HAILING
HALOING
HALTING
HALVING
HAMMING
HANDING
HANGING
HARDING
HARKING
HARMING
HARPING

HASHING
HASPING
HASTING
HATTING
HAULING
HAWKING
HEADING
HEALING
HEAPING
HEARING
HEATING
HEAVING
HEDGING
HEEDING
HEELING
HEFTING
HELMING
HELPING
HELSING
HEMMING
HERDING
HERRING
HIBBING
HILLING
HILTING
HINGING
HINTING
HISSING
HITTING
HOAXING
HOBOING
HOCKING
HODDING
HOGGING
HOLDING
HONKING
HOODING
HOOFING
HOOKING
HOOPING
HOOTING
HOPPING
HOPSING
HORDING
HORNING
HORSING
HOSTING
HOUSING
HOWLING
HUFFING
HUGGING
HULKING
HULLING
HUMMING
HUNTING
HURLING
HURTING
HUSHING
HUSKING
HUTTING
HYMNING
HYPOING
IMAGING
IMBUING
IMGOING
INCHING
INGOING
INKLING

INLYING
INTHING
INURING
IRISING
IRONING
ISSUING
ITCHING
ITEMING
JABBING
JACKING
JAGGING
JAILING
JAMMING
JARRING
JAZZING
JEERING
JELLING
JERKING
JESTING
JETTING
JIGGING
JILTING
JINXING
JOBBING
JOGGING
JOINING
JOLTING
JOSHING
JOTTING
JREWING
JUDGING
JUGGING
JUICING
JUMPING
JUNKING
JURYING
JUTTING
KACHING
KAYOING
KEDGING
KEELING
KEENING
KEEPING
KEGGING
KENNING
KEYRING
KICKING
KIDDING
KILLING
KILNING
KILTING
KINGING
KINKING
KIPLING
KIPPING
KISSING
KITTING
KNEEING
KNIFING
KNOWING
KOONING
LACKING
LADLING
LAGGING
LAIRING
LALLING
LAMBING
LAMMING

LANCING
LANDING
LANSING
LAPPING
LAPSING
LAPWING
LARDING
LARKING
LASHING
LASTING
LATHING
LAUDING
LEADING
LEAFING
LEAKING
LEANING
LEAPING
LEASING
LEAVING
LEERING
LEGGING
LEMMING
LENDING
LESSING
LETTING
LEVYING
LIBBING
LICKING
LIFTING
LILTING
LIMBING
LIMNING
LIMPING
LINKING
LINTING
LIPPING
LISPING
LISTING
LOADING
LOAFING
LOAMING
LOANING
LOBBING
LOCKING
LODGING
LOFTING
LOGGING
LOIDING
LOLLING
LONGING
LOOKING
LOOMING
LOOPING
LOOSING
LOOTING
LOPPING
LORDING
LOTTING
LOURING
LOUSING
LOUTING
LUCKING
LUFFING
LUGGING
LULLING
LUMPING
LUNGING
LURKING

LUSTING
MADDING
MAILING
MAIMING
MALTING
MANNING
MAPPING
MARKING
MARRING
MASHING
MASKING
MASSING
MASTING
MATTING
MAULING
MEANING
MEETING
MELDING
MELTING
MEMLING
MENDING
MEOWING
MERGING
MESHING
MESSING
MEWLING
MIFFING
MILKING
MILLING
MINCING
MINDING
MINTING
MISSING
MISTING
MITRING
MOANING
MOBBING
MOCKING
MOILING
MOLDING
MOLTING
MOONING
MOORING
MOOTING
MOPPING
MORNING
MOSHING
MOSSING
MOUSING
MUCKING
MUDDING
MUFFING
MUGGING
MULLING
MUMMING
MUSHING
MUSSING
NABBING
NAGGING
NAILING
NANJING
NANKING
NAPPING
NEARING
NECKING
NEEDING
NERVING
NESTING

NETTING
NICHING
NICKING
NIPPING
NOCKING
NODDING
NOISING
NOONING
NOOSING
NOSHING
NOTHING
NOTTING
NUDGING
NULLING
NUMBING
NURSING
NUTTING
OBEYING
OILRING
OINKING
OKAYING
OMENING
ONGOING
OPENING
OPINING
ORATING
OUSTING
OUTKING
OUTRING
OUTSING
OUTWING
PACKING
PADDING
PAINING
PAIRING
PALLING
PALMING
PANNING
PANTING
PARGING
PARKING
PARRING
PARSING
PARTING
PASSING
PASTING
PATTING
PAULING
PAUSING
PAWNING
PEAKING
PEALING
PECKING
PEEKING
PEELING
PEENING
PEEPING
PEERING
PEEVING
PEGGING
PEIPING
PELTING
PENDING
PENNING
PEPPING
PERKING
PERMING
PETTING

PHASING
PHONING
PICKING
PIECING
PIGGING
PILLING
PINGING
PINKING
PINNING
PIQUING
PISHING
PITHING
PITTING
PITYING
PLACING
PLANING
PLATING
PLAYING
PLOWING
PLUMING
POISING
POLLING
PONDING
PONYING
POOLING
POOPING
POPPING
PORKING
PORTING
POSTING
POTTING
POURING
POUTING
PRATING
PRAYING
PREYING
PRICING
PRIDING
PRIMING
PRIZING
PROBING
PROSING
PROVING
PRUNING
PUDDING
PUFFING
PULLING
PULPING
PULSING
PUMPING
PUNNING
PUNTING
PURGING
PURLING
PURRING
PURSING
PUSHING
PUTTING
QUAKING
QUEUING
QUOTING
RACKING
RAFTING
RAGGING
RAIDING
RAILING
RAINING
RAISING

RAMMING
RAMPING
RANGING
RANKING
RANTING
RAPPING
RASPING
RATTING
RAZZING
RDLAING
READING
REAMING
REAPING
REARING
REAVING
REDDING
REDKING
REDOING
REDWING
REDYING
REEDING
REEFING
REEKING
REELING
REEVING
REFFING
REFYING
REICING
REINING
RELYING
RENDING
RENTING
REPPING
RESTING
RETTING
REUSING
REVVING
RHYMING
RIBBING
RIDDING
RIDGING
RIFFING
RIFLING
RIFTING
RIGGING
RIMMING
RINGING
RINSING
RIOTING
RIPPING
RISKING
ROAMING
ROARING
ROBBING
ROCKING
RODDING
ROGUING
ROILING
ROLFING
ROLLING
ROMPING
ROOFING
ROOKING
ROOMING
ROOTING
ROTTING
ROUGING
ROUSING
ROUTING
ROWLING
RRATING
RSVPING
RUBBING
RUCHING
RUCKING
RUFFING
RUINING
RUNNING
RUSHING
RUSTING
RUTTING
SACKING
SAGGING
SAILING
SALTING
SALVING
SANDING
SAPLING
SAPPING
SASHING
SASSING
SAUCING
SCALING
SCARING
SCOPING
SCORING
SEALING
SEAMING
SEARING
SEATING
SEBRING
SEEDING
SEEKING
SEEMING
SEEPING
SEINING
SEIZING
SELLING
SENDING
SENSING
SERLING
SERVING
SETTING
SHADING
SHAKING
SHAMING
SHAPING
SHARING
SHAVING
SHINING
SHOEING
SHOOING
SHORING
SHOVING
SHOWING
SIBLING
SICCING
SIDLING
SIEGING
SIEVING
SIFTING
SIGHING
SIGNING
SILOING
SILTING
SINGING
SINKING
SINNING
SIPPING
SITTING
SKATING
SKEWING
SLAKING
SLATING
SLAVING
SLAYING
SLEWING
SLICING
SLIDING
SLIMING
SLOPING
SLOWING
SMILING
SMITING
SMOKING
SNAKING
SNARING
SNIPING
SNORING
SNOWING
SOAKING
SOAPING
SOARING
SOBBING
SOCKING
SODDING
SOILING
SOLOING
SOLVING
SOPPING
SORTING
SOURING
SOUSING
SPACING
SPADING
SPARING
SPAYING
SPECING
SPEWING
SPICING
SPIKING
SPITING
SPOKING
SPUMING
SPYRING
STAGING
STAKING
STARING
STATING
STAVING
STAYING
STEWING
STOKING
STONING
STORING
STOWING
STUBING
STYLING
SUBBING
SUBKING
SUCKING
SUDSING
SUITING
SULKING
SUMMING
SUNNING
SUPPING
SURFING
SURGING
SUSSING
SWAYING
SWIPING
SYNCING
TABBING
TABLING
TABUING
TACKING
TAGGING
TAILING
TALKING
TAMPING
TANGING
TANKING
TANNING
TAPPING
TARRING
TARTING
TASKING
TASTING
TATTING
TAXIING
TEAMING
TEARING
TEASING
TEEMING
TELLING
TEMPING
TENDING
TENSING
TENTING
TENZING
TERMING
TESTING
TEXTING
THAWING
THEKING
THERING
TICCING
TICKING
TIDYING
TIERING
TIFFING
TILLING
TILTING
TINGING
TINNING
TINTING
TIPPING
TITHING
TITLING
TITRING
TOGGING
TOILING
TOLLING
TONGING
TOOLING
TOOTING
TOPPING
TOSSING
TOTTING
TOURING
TOUTING
TRACING
TRADING
TREEING
TROWING
TRUEING
TUBBING
TUCKING
TUFTING
TUGGING
TURFING
TURNING
TUSKING
TUTTING
TWINING
UNAGING
UNDOING
UNDYING
UNITING
UNLYING
UNOWING
UNSLING
UNTYING
UNVYING
UPFLING
UPGOING
UPSWING
VALUING
VAMPING
VANNING
VARYING
VATTING
VEERING
VEGGING
VEILING
VEINING
VENDING
VENTING
VERGING
VERSING
VESTING
VETOING
VETTING
VIALING
VIEWING
VISAING
VOGUING
VOICING
VOIDING
WADDING
WAFTING
WAGGING
WAILING
WAITING
WAIVING
WALKING
WALLING
WANNING
WANTING
WARDING
WARMING
WARNING
WARPING
WARRING
WASHING
WASTING
WAXWING
WEANING
WEARING
WEAVING
WEBBING
WEDDING
WEDGING
WEEDING
WEEPING
WELDING
WELLING
WELTING
WENDING
WETTING
WHALING
WHILING
WHINING
WHITING
WICKING
WIFYING
WIGGING
WILDING
WILLING
WILTING
WIMPING
WINCING
WINDING
WINGING
WINKING
WINNING
WISHING
WISPING
WITLING
WITTING
WOLFING
WONTING
WOODING
WOOFING
WORDING
WORKING
WORMING
WRITING
WYOMING
XRATING
XRAYING
YAKKING
YANKING
YAOMING
YAPPING
YARDING
YARNING
YAWNING
YAWPING
YEANING
YELLING
YELPING
YENNING
YESSING
YIPPING
YOWLING
YOYOING
YUKKING
ZAGGING
ZAPPING
ZEROING
ZESTING
ZIERING
ZIGGING
ZINCING
ZINGING
ZIPPING
ZONKING
ZOOMING

•••••IG

BRILLIG
BUSHPIG
FUNFZIG
GREWBIG
GROWBIG
JURYRIG
LEIPZIG
LOSEBIG
LOSTBIG
MALEPIG
OVERBIG
PERIWIG
PFENNIG
SECHZIG
SHINDIG
SIEBZIG
TALKBIG
VERYBIG
VIERZIG
WILDPIG
WINSBIG
ZAGAZIG
ZWANZIG

IH•••••

IHATEIT
IHAVEIT
IHEARYA
IHOPESO

I•H••••

ICHABOD
ICHDIEN
IMHAPPY
IMHOTEP
INHABIT
INHALED
INHALER
INHALES
INHASTE
INHERED
INHERES
INHERIT
INHIBIT
INHOUSE
INHUMAN
INHUMED
INHUMER
INHUMES
ISHMAEL
ITHACAN
ITHIRTY

I••H•••

IANHOLM
ICEHOLE
IDAHOAN
IDTHEFT
IMAHOGG
IMTHERE
INAHEAP
INAHOLE
INAHUFF
INCHECK
INCHERS
INCHING
INKHORN
INPHASE
INSHAPE
INSHOCK
INSHORE
INSHORT
INTHERE
INTHING
INTHIRD
INTHREE
INWHITE
ISAHEAD
ISCHIAL
ISCHIUM
ISOHELS
ISTHMUS
ITCHFOR
ITCHIER
ITCHING
ITSHERE

I•••H••

ICESHOW
IEIGHTY
INASHOE
IRISHER
ISFAHAN
ITSAHIT
IVANHOE

I••••H•

IGOTCHA
IIIJOHN
INSIGHT
IOMOTHS

I•••••H

ICEBATH
IMPEACH
INARUSH
INDEPTH
INDUTCH
INFAITH
INMARCH
INREACH
INSYNCH
INTOUCH
INTRUTH
INVEIGH
IPSWICH

•IH••••

VIHARAS

•I•H•••

AIMHIGH
AIRHEAD
AIRHOLE
AIRHORN
AIRHOSE
BICHONS
BIGHAIR
BIGHALF
BIGHAND
BIGHEAD
BIGHITS
BIGHORN
BIGHUGS
BISHKEK
BISHOPS
CICHLID
CIPHERS
DIAHANN
DICHTER
DIEHARD
DIRHAMS
DISHFUL
DISHIER
DISHING
DISHOUT
DISHPAN
DISHRAG
DITHERS
DITHERY
EIGHTAD
EIGHTAM
EIGHTBC
EIGHTEE
EIGHTHS
EIGHTPM
EIGHTUP
FIGHTER
FISHERS
FISHERY
FISHEYE
FISHFOR
FISHFRY
FISHIER
FISHILY
FISHING
FISHNET
FISHOIL
FISHOUT
HIGHART
HIGHBAR
HIGHBOY
HIGHDAY
HIGHEND
HIGHEST
HIGHHAT
HIGHIQS
HIGHISH
HIGHLOW
HIGHPAY
HIGHRES
HIGHSEA
HIGHTEA
HIGHTOP
HIGHWAY
HITHERE
HITHOME
JIMHOGG
KISHKES
KITHARA
LICHEES
LICHENS
LIGHTED
LIGHTEN
LIGHTER
LIGHTLY
LIGHTON
LIGHTUP
LITHELY
LITHEST
LITHGOW
LITHIUM
LITHOID
MIAHAMM
MICHAEL
MICHAUX
MIGHTNT
MIKHAIL
MILHAUD
MILHOUS
MISHAPS
MISHEAR
MISHIMA
MISHITS
MISHNAH
MITHRAS
NICHING
NICHOLS
NIGHEST
NIGHTER
NIGHTIE
NIGHTLY
OILHEAT
PIEHOLE
PINHEAD
PINHOLE
PISHING
PITHEAD
PITHIER
PITHILY
PITHING
RICHARD
RICHENS
RICHEST
RICHLER
RICHMAN
RICHMEN
RICHTER
RIGHTED
RIGHTER
RIGHTLY
RIGHTON
SIGHERS
SIGHFOR
SIGHFUL
SIGHING
SIGHSAT
SIGHTED
SIGHTER
SIGHTLY
SIKHISM
SIPHONS
SITHOME
TIGHTEN
TIGHTER
TIGHTLY
TIMHOLT
TINHATS
TINHORN
TITHERS
TITHING
WICHITA
WILHELM
WISHERS
WISHFOR
WISHFUL
WISHING
WITHERS
WITHIES
WITHOUT
XIPHOID
ZITHERS

•I••H••

AINTHAY
AIRSHIP
AIRSHOW
AITCHES
BIGSHOT
BIGSHOW
BINGHAM
BIOCHIP
BIRCHED
BIRCHEN
BIRCHES
BIRTHED
CINCHED
CINCHES
DIAPHAN
DITCHED
DITCHER
DITCHES
FIFTHLY
FILCHED
FILCHER
FILCHES
FINCHES
FIREHAT
FISCHER
GINGHAM
GIRTHED
HIGHHAT
HITCHED
HITCHER
HITCHES
HITCHON
HITCHUP
HITSHOW
JIMCHEE
KIMCHEE
KINSHIP
KITCHEN
LITCHIS
MIDSHIP
MISSHIP
MITCHUM
NINTHLY
PINCHAS
PINCHED
PINCHER
PINCHES
PINCHME
PINCHOT
PINKHAM
PITCHED
PITCHER
PITCHES
PITCHIN
PITCHTO
RIMSHOT
RITCHIE
SILKHAT
SIOBHAN
SIXTHLY
WINCHED
WINCHER
WINCHES
WITCHED
WITCHES
YITZHAK
ZILCHES

•I•••H•

BIANCHI
BIGJOHN
BINOCHE
EIGHTHS
FINISHD
GIRLSHY
HIBACHI
HITACHI
IIIJOHN
KITSCHY
MIZRAHI
NIEBUHR
PIRANHA
RICKSHA
TIMOTHY

•I••••H

AIMHIGH
BIGFISH
BIGGISH
BIOTECH
BISMUTH
DIGRAPH
DIPTYCH
DISTICH
FINNISH
GIRLISH
HIALEAH
HIGHISH
HIPBATH
HIPPISH
JIGGISH
KIDDISH
LISBETH
MINXISH
MIRISCH
MISHNAH
MISMESH
MISSISH
MITZVAH
NIDETCH
NILESOH
NINEVEH
OILRICH
PICTISH
PIGFISH
PIGGISH
PINKISH
PIXYISH
SICKISH
SILENTH
SITWITH
TIMROTH
TINFISH
VIEWITH
WILDISH
WIMOWEH
WIMPISH
YIDDISH

••IH•••

AKIHITO
SHIHTZU
SKIHATS

••I•H••

ALIGHTS
AMICHAI
APISHLY
BLIGHTS
BLIGHTY
BLITHER
BRIGHAM
BRIGHTS
CHICHAS
CHICHEN
CHICHIS
CLICHED
CLICHES
DWIGHTD
EPITHET
FLIGHTS
FLIGHTY
FRIGHTS
GEISHAS
GRISHAM
HEIGHHO
HEIGHTS
IEIGHTY
IRISHER
KAISHEK
KNIGHTS
KNISHES
KRISHNA
NEIGHED
NEITHER
PHISHED
PHISHER
PHISHES
PLIGHTS
PRITHEE
QUICHES
RAINHAT
SKISHOP
SLIGHTS
SLITHER
SMITHED
SWISHED
SWISHES
TEICHER
THITHER
VEIGHTS
WEIGHED
WEIGHER
WEIGHIN
WEIGHON
WEIGHTS
WEIGHTY
WEIGHUP
WHISHED
WHISHES
WHITHER
WRIGHTS
WRITHED
WRITHER
WRITHES

••I••H•
ALIYAHS
BRIOCHE
GLITCHY
HEIGHHO
IIIJOHN
PLINTHS
THIMPHU
TWITCHY

••I•••H
AZIMUTH
BRINISH
BRITISH
CHIMINH
DRIESCH
EPITAPH
FAIRISH
GOIRISH
HAIMISH
MAIDISH
OMIGOSH
SAIDAAH
SCITECH
SPINACH
SWINISH
TRIUMPH
WAIFISH
WHITISH

•••IH••
BALIHAI
DELIHAM

•••I•H•
ALRIGHT
ATEIGHT
ATNIGHT
ATSIGHT
BYRIGHT
CALIPHS
CEVICHE
DELIGHT
DORIGHT
ENRIGHT
EOLITHS
FINISHD
FRAICHE
FREIGHT
INSIGHT
JERICHO
KATISHA
KENICHI
LEHIGHU
MRRIGHT
ONSIGHT
ORNITHO
PARIAHS
REFIGHT
RELIGHT
RESIGHT
RUPIAHS
SHEIKHS
SLEIGHS
SLEIGHT
SQUISHY
TABITHA
TONIGHT
UNLIGHT
UNSIGHT
UPLIGHT
UPRIGHT
UPTIGHT
WRAITHS
ZENITHS

•••I••H
AALIYAH
ABSINTH
ANTIOCH
BADITCH
BEWITCH
BYBIRTH
CORINTH
DELILAH
GOLIATH
JACINTH
LATIFAH
MIRISCH
ONEINCH
REBIRTH
REHITCH
SERIESH
SQUINCH
STRITCH
UNCINCH
UNHITCH
XENIAOH

••••I•H
ABOLISH
ACEHIGH
AIMHIGH
ALDRICH
ALSMITH
ANGUISH
ANOUILH
ASQUITH
BAALISH
BABYISH
BADDISH
BALDISH
BEAMISH
BEARISH
BEAUISH
BIGFISH
BIGGISH
BLEMISH
BLUEISH
BOARISH
BOGGISH
BOOKISH
BOORISH
BRINISH
BRITISH
BRUTISH
BULLISH
BURNISH
CADDISH
CATFISH
CATTISH
CHERISH
CHIMINH
CLAYISH
COCKISH
CODFISH
COLDISH
COLTISH
COMMISH
COOLISH
CORNISH
COWFISH
CUBBISH
CULTISH
CURRISH
DAMPISH
DARKISH
DEEPISH
DERVISH
DISTICH
DOGFISH
DOGGISH
DOLLISH
DOLTISH
DONNISH
DRONISH
DULLISH
DUMPISH
DUNCISH
DUSKISH
EHRLICH
ELDRICH
ENGLISH
ERDRICH
EVANISH
FADDISH
FAIRISH
FATTISH
FINNISH
FLEMISH
FLYFISH
FLYHIGH
FOGYISH
FOLKISH
FOOLISH
FOPPISH
FURBISH
FURNISH
GARNISH
GAULISH
GAWKISH
GIRLISH
GNOMISH
GOATISH
GOIRISH
GOODISH
GOUTISH
GRAYISH
GREYISH
HAGGISH
HAIMISH
HARDISH
HASHISH
HAWKISH
HELLISH
HENNISH
HENRICH
HIGHISH
HIPPISH
HOGGISH
HORNISH
HOWHIGH
HUFFISH
HUNNISH
INFAITH
INVEIGH
IPSWICH
JAZZISH
JIGGISH
KADDISH
KENTISH
KIDDISH
KNAVISH
KURDISH
LADDISH
LADYISH
LAPPISH
LARGISH
LARKISH
LAZYISH
LEFTISH
LETTISH
LOGGISH
LONGISH
LOUDISH
LOUTISH
LUMPISH
MADDISH
MAIDISH
MANNISH
MAWKISH
MESSIAH
METWITH
MINXISH
MISSISH
MOBBISH
MONKISH
MOONISH
MOORISH
MRSMITH
MUDFISH
MUGGISH
MURKISH
NAGGISH
NEBBISH
NEOLITH
NERDISH
NESMITH
NEWRICH
NORRISH
NORWICH
NOTWITH
NOURISH
NUNNISH
OBADIAH
OGREISH
OILRICH
OPALISH
OSTRICH
OUTFISH
OUTSIGH
OUTWISH
OUTWITH
PANFISH
PARRISH
PEAKISH
PECKISH
PEEVISH
PELTISH
PERKISH
PETFISH
PETTISH
PICTISH
PIGFISH
PIGGISH
PINKISH
PIXYISH
PLANISH
PLENISH
POORISH
PORKISH
PRUDISH
PUBLISH
PUCKISH
PUGGISH
RAFFISH
RALEIGH
RAMMISH
RANKISH
RANWITH
RASPISH
RATTISH
RAWFISH
REDDISH
REDFISH
REWEIGH
RHENISH
ROGUISH
ROMPISH
ROOKISH
RUBBISH
RUNTISH
RUNWITH
RUTTISH
SALTISH
SATWITH
SAWFISH
SELFISH
SICKISH
SITWITH
SKYHIGH
SLAVISH
SLOWISH
SOFTISH
SOPWITH
SOTTISH
SOURISH
SPANISH
STYLISH
SUNFISH
SWEDISH
SWINISH
TALLISH
TALLITH
TANNISH
TARNISH
TARTISH
TINFISH
TOADISH
TOOHIGH
TORYISH
TOWNISH
TOYWITH
TURKISH
UNFAITH
VAMPISH
VARNISH
VIEWITH
VOGUISH
WAGGISH
WAIFISH
WANNISH
WARMISH
WASPISH
WEAKISH
WETTISH
WHEYISH
WHITISH
WILDISH
WIMPISH
WOLFISH
WORMISH
YERKISH
YIDDISH
YOBBISH
YOUWISH
ZANYISH

II•••••
IIIJOHN
IIKINGS
IINSIST
IIPETER

I•I••••
IBILITY
IBIZANS
ICICLES
ICINESS
ICINGIN
ICINGIT
ICINGUP
IDIAMIN
IDIDTOO
IDIOTIC
IEIGHTY
IFIFELL
IFITDIE
IGIVEUP
IIIJOHN
ILIADIC
ILIAMNA
ILIESCU
ILIKEIT
IMITATE
ININETY
INIRONS
INITIAL
IRIDIUM
IRISHER
IRISING
IRISOUT
ISIDORE
ISITAGO
ITISTOO

I••I•••
ICKIEST
ICTINUS
IFFIEST
IGNITED
IGNITER
IGNITES
IGNITOR
IIKINGS
ILLICIT
IMBIBED
IMBIBER
IMBIBES
IMMIXED
IMMIXES
IMPIETY
IMPINGE
IMPIOUS
IMTIRED
INAIDOF
INCISED
INCISES
INCISOR
INCITED
INCITER
INCITES
INCIVIL
INDIANA
INDIANS
INDICES
INDICIA
INDICTS
INDIGEN
INDIGOS
INDITED
INDITER
INDITES
INFIDEL
INFIELD
INFIRST
INFIVES
INFIXED
INFIXES
INHIBIT
INKIEST
INKINGS
INLIMBO
INLINES
INNINGS
INSIDER
INSIDES
INSIGHT
INSIGNE
INSIPID
INSISTS
INVICTA
INVITED
INVITEE
INVITER
INVITES
INVITRO
IODIDES
IODISED
IODISES
IODIZED
IODIZER
IODIZES
IONIANS
IONISED
IONISER
IONISES
IONIUMS
IONIZED
IONIZER
IONIZES
ISAIDNO
ITGIRLS
ITHIRTY

I•••I••
IAMBICS
IAMBIST
IATRICS
IBERIAN
IBILITY
ICELIKE
ICELINE
ICEMILK
ICEPICK
ICERINK
ICEWINE
ICHDIEN
ICONIFY
ICYWIND
IDOLISE
IDOLIST
IDOLIZE
IDYLIST
IGRAINE
IINSIST
ILLBITE
ILLLIVE
ILLWILL
ILLWIND
IMAGINE
IMAGING
IMAGISM
IMAGIST
IMBUING
IMEMINE
IMGOING
IMPAIRS
IMPLIED
IMPLIES
IMPRINT
INABIND
INAJIFF
INALINE
INANITY
INAPILE
INAWINK
INBRIEF
INBUILT
INCHING
INCLINE
INEDITA
INEXILE
INFAITH
INFLICT
INGOING
INITIAL
INKLIKE
INKLING
INLYING
INPOINT
INPRINT
INQUIRE
INQUIRY
INRUINS
INSPIRE
INSPITE
INSTILL
INSTILS
INTAILS
INTHING
INTHIRD
INTUITS
INURING
INUTILE
INVEIGH
INVOICE
INWHITE
IPSWICH
IRANIAN
IRENICS
IRESIGN
IRIDIUM
IRISING
IRONIES
IRONING
IRONIST
ISCHIAL
ISCHIUM
ISOLINE
ISSUING
ISTRIAN
ITALIAN
ITALICS
ITCHIER
ITCHING
ITEMING
ITEMISE
ITEMIZE
ITSFINE
ITSTIME
IVANIII
IVORIAN
IVORIES
IVORINE
IVYLIKE
IWOJIMA
IZATION

I••••I•
ICINGIN
ICINGIT
IDENTIC
IDIAMIN
IDIOTIC
IDOODIT
IDYLLIC
IFITDIE
IGUANID
IHATEIT
IHAVEIT
IKNEWIT
IKNOWIT
ILIADIC
ILIKEIT
ILLDOIT
ILLEGIT
ILLICIT
ILLOGIC
ILLYRIA
ILOSTIT
ILOVEIT
IMADEIT
IMEANIT
IMFORIT
IMPAVID
IMPERIL
INAPRIL
INASNIT
INASPIN
INASTIR
INASUIT
INCIVIL
INDICIA
INERTIA
INFORIT
INGRAIN
INHABIT
INHERIT
INHIBIT
INKEDIN
INORBIT
INPERIL
INSIPID
INSULIN
INTERIM
INTROIT
INVALID
ISLAMIC
ISTOMIN
ITSAHIT
ITSALIE
ITSASIN
ITSATIE
IVANIII
IWANTIT

I•••••I
ISRAELI
IVANIII

•II••••
IIIJOHN

•I•I•••
AIKIDOS
AIRIEST
AIRINGS
BIGIDEA
BIKINIS
BILIOUS
BIMINIS
BIRIANI
CILIARY
CILIATE
CITIZEN
CIVILLY
DICIEST
DICILLO
DIGICAM
DIGINTO
DIGIPET
DIGITAL
DIMITRI
DIPINTO
DIVIDED
DIVIDER
DIVIDES
DIVINED
DIVINER
DIVINES
DIVISOR
FIBIGER
FIJIANS
FILIBEG
FILINGS
FILIPPO
FINIALS
FINIANS
FINICAL
FINICKY
FINISHD
FINITES
FIRINGS
FITINTO
FIXINGS
HIDINGS
HIJINKS
HITINTO
IIKINGS
JIMINEZ
JIVIEST
KIKIDEE
KINISON
LIAISED
LIAISES
LIAISON
LIBIDOS
LICITLY
LIKINGS
LILINAU
LIMIEST
LIMINAL
LIMITED
LIMITER
LINIEST
LININGS
LIPIDIC
LITINTO
LIVIDLY
LIVINGS
MIDIRON
MILIEUS
MILIEUX
MILITIA
MIMICRY
MIMIEUX
MINIBAR
MINIBUS
MINICAB
MINICAM
MINICAR
MINIKIN
MINILAB
MINIMAL
MINIMAX
MINIMUM
MINIMUS
MININGS
MINIONS
MINISKI
MINISUB
MINITVS
MINIVAC
MINIVAN
MINIVER
MINIZOO
MIRIEST
MIRISCH
MIXITUP
NIMIETY
NIPIGON
OILIEST
PIGIRON
PILINGS
PINIEST
PINIONS
PIPIEST
PIPINGS
PITIERS
PITIFUL
PITILLO
RIDINGS
RIGIDLY
RILIEVO
RIMIEST
RIPIENI
RIPIENO
RIPINTO
RISIBLE
RISIBLY
RISINGS
RIVIERA
RIVIERE
SICILIA
SIDINGS
SIDIOUS
SILICAS
SILICON
SIMIANS
SIMILAC
SIMILAR
SIMILES
SITINON
SIXIRON
TIDIEST
TIDINGS
TIEINTO
TILINGS
TIMIDER
TIMIDLY
TIMINGS
TINIEST
TITIANS
VIBISTS
VICINAL
VICIOUS
VIDICON
VIDIOTS
VIKINGS
VIMINAL
VINIEST
VISIBLE
VISIBLY
VISIONS
VISITED
VISITOR
VITIATE
VIVICAA
VIVIDER
VIVIDLY
VIVITAR
VIZIERS
WILIEST
WINIEST
WIRIEST
WIRINGS

•I••I••
AIMHIGH
AIRBILL
AIRKISS
AIRLIFT
AIRLIKE
AIRLINE
AIRMILE
AIRSICK
AIRSIGN
AIRTIME
AIRWICK
BIALIES
BIASING
BIAXIAL
BIBBIDI
BIBBING
BIBLIKE
BIBLIOG
BIDDIES
BIDDING
BIFFING
BIGBIRD
BIGCITY
BIGDIGS
BIGFISH
BIGFIVE
BIGGIES
BIGGIRL
BIGGISH
BIGGITY
BIGHITS
BIGKIDS
BIGLIES
BIGRIGS
BIGTIME
BIGWIGS
BIGWINS
BILGIER
BILKING
BILLIES
BILLING
BILLION
BINDING
BINGING
BINNING
BIOCIDE
BIOLITE
BIONICS
BIOPICS
BIOTITE
BIRDIED
BIRDIES
BIRDING
BIRLING
BIRRING
BITSIER
BITTIER
BITTING
CITRINE
CIVVIES
DIALING
DIARIES
DIARIOS
DIARIST
DICKIES
DICTION
DIDFINE
DIDLIKE
DIDTIME
DIETING
DIGGING
DIGGITY
DIGNIFY
DIGNITY

DIKDIKS
DILLIES
DIMMING
DIMVIEW
DIMWITS
DINDINS
DINGIER
DINGILY
DINGING
DINKIER
DINNING
DINTING
DIORITE
DIOTIMA
DIOXIDE
DIOXINS
DIPPIER
DIPPING
DIRKING
DIRTIED
DIRTIER
DIRTIES
DIRTILY
DISCING
DISHIER
DISHING
DISKING
DISLIKE
DISMISS
DISSING
DISTICH
DISTILL
DISTILS
DITSIER
DITTIES
DITZIER
DIVVIED
DIVVIES
DIZAINS
DIZZIED
DIZZIER
DIZZIES
DIZZILY
FIBBING
FIBRINS
FICTILE
FICTION
FICTIVE
FIERIER
FIERILY
FIFTIES
FILLIES
FILLING
FILLINS
FILLIPS
FILMIER
FILMILY
FILMING
FINDING
FINKING
FINLIKE
FINNIER
FINNISH
FIORINA
FIREICE
FIRKINS
FIRMING
FIRRIER
FISHIER
FISHILY
FISHING
FISSILE
FISSION
FITTING
FIZGIGS
FIZZIER
FIZZING
GIDDIED
GIDDIER
GIDDIES
GIDDILY
GIFTING
GIGGING
GILDING
GILLIAM
GILLIAN
GILLING
GIMMICK
GIMPING
GINFIZZ
GINGIVA
GINMILL
GINNING
GIPSIES
GIRDING
GIRLIER
GIRLIES
GIRLISH
GIRTING
GISSING
GITTING
HIBBING
HIGGINS
HIGHIQS
HIGHISH
HILAIRE
HILLIER
HILLING
HILTING
HINGING
HINKIER
HINNIES
HINTING
HIPLIKE
HIPPIER
HIPPIES
HIPPISH
HIPPITY
HIRCINE
HISNIBS
HISSIER
HISSING
HITFILM
HITLIST
HITTING
HITTITE
IINSIST
JIFFIES
JIGGIER
JIGGING
JIGGISH
JIGLIKE
JIGTIME
JILLIAN
JILLION
JILTING
JIMDIAL
JIMFIXX
JIMMIED
JIMMIES
JIMRICE
JINXING
KIARIOS
KICKIER
KICKING
KIDDIES
KIDDING
KIDDISH
KIDLIKE
KIDVIDS
KILLING
KILNING
KILTIES
KILTING
KINGING
KINKIER
KINKILY
KINKING
KIPLING
KIPPING
KISSING
KITTIES
KITTING
LIBBING
LICKING
LIDWINA
LIFTING
LIGNIFY
LIGNINS
LIGNITE
LIKEICE
LILLIAN
LILTING
LIMBING
LIMNING
LIMNITE
LIMPING
LINBIAO
LINDIED
LINDIES
LINKING
LINPIAO
LINTIER
LINTING
LIONISE
LIONIZE
LIPLIKE
LIPPIER
LIPPING
LIQUIDS
LISPING
LISTING
LITHIUM
LIZZIES
MIAMIAN
MIAMIFL
MIDDIES
MIDLIFE
MIDLINE
MIDLIST
MIDRIBS
MIDRIFF
MIDRISE
MIDSIZE
MIDWIFE
MIFFIER
MIFFING
MILKIER
MILKILY
MILKING
MILLIME
MILLING
MILLION
MINCING
MINDING
MINGIER
MINTIER
MINTING
MINXISH
MISAIMS
MISBILL
MISBIND
MISCITE
MISDIAL
MISFILE
MISFIRE
MISFITS
MISGIVE
MISHIMA
MISHITS
MISLIKE
MISSIES
MISSILE
MISSING
MISSION
MISSISH
MISSIVE
MISTIER
MISTILY
MISTIME
MISTING
MISWIRE
MITRING
NIBLICK
NIBLIKE
NICHING
NICKING
NICOISE
NIFTIER
NIFTIES
NIFTILY
NINNIES
NIOBITE
NIOBIUM
NIPPIER
NIPPILY
NIPPING
NITPICK
NITRIDE
NITRIFY
NITRITE
NITTIER
NITWITS
OILBIRD
OILLIKE
OILLINE
OILRICH
OILRIGS
OILRING
OINKING
PIANISM
PIANIST
PICKIER
PICKING
PICNICS
PICTISH
PIDGINS
PIECING
PIELIKE
PIERIAN
PIETIES
PIETINS
PIGFISH
PIGGIER
PIGGIES
PIGGING
PIGGISH
PIGLIKE
PILLING
PILLION
PIMLICO
PINGING
PINKIES
PINKING
PINKISH
PINNING
PIOSITY
PIPPINS
PIQUING
PISCINE
PISHING
PISMIRE
PISTILS
PITHIER
PITHILY
PITHING
PITTING
PITYING
PIUSIII
PIXYISH
RIBBIER
RIBBIES
RIBBING
RIBLIKE
RIDDICK
RIDDING
RIDGIER
RIDGING
RIFFING
RIFLING
RIFTING
RIGGING
RIMMING
RINDIER
RINGING
RINSING
RIORITA
RIOTING
RIPPING
RIPTIDE
RISKIER
RISKILY
RISKING
RITZIER
RITZILY
SIBLING
SICCING
SICKISH
SIDLING
SIEGING
SIEVING
SIFTING
SIGHING
SIGNIFY
SIGNING
SIKHISM
SILKIER
SILKILY
SILLIER
SILLIES
SILOING
SILTIER
SILTING
SIMCITY
SINCITY
SINGING
SINKING
SINLIKE
SINNING
SIPPING
SISSIER
SISSIES
SISTINE
SITTING
SITWITH
SIXFIVE
SIXNINE
SIXTIES
TICCING
TICKING
TIDBITS
TIDYING
TIELINE
TIEPINS
TIERING
TIFFING
TIFFINS
TILLING
TILSITS
TILTING
TIMMINS
TIMRICE
TINFISH
TINGING
TINLIKE
TINMINE
TINNIER
TINNILY
TINNING
TINTING
TIPLINE
TIPPIER
TIPPING
TIPSIER
TIPSILY
TIRPITZ
TITHING
TITLING
TITLIST
TITMICE
TITOISM
TITOIST
TITRING
TIZZIES
VIALING
VIATICA
VICTIMS
VIEWIER
VIEWING
VIEWITH
VILNIUS
VIOLINS
VIOLIST
VIRGINS
VISAING
VITRICS
VITRIFY
VITRINE
VITRIOL
WICHITA
WICKING
WICKIUP
WIENIES
WIFYING
WIGGIER
WIGGING
WIGLIKE
WILDING
WILDISH
WILKINS
WILLIAM
WILLIES
WILLING
WILTING
WIMPIER
WIMPING
WIMPISH
WINCING
WINDIER
WINDIGO
WINDILY
WINDING
WINGING
WINKING
WINNING
WISHING
WISPIER
WISPILY
WISPING
WITHIES
WITLING
WITTIER
WITTILY
WITTING
YIDDISH
YIPPIES
YIPPING
ZIERING
ZIGGING
ZILLION
ZINCIFY
ZINCING
ZINCITE
ZINGIER
ZINGING
ZINKIER
ZINNIAS
ZIONISM
ZIONIST
ZIPDISK
ZIPPIER
ZIPPING

•|•••|•

AIRDRIE
AIRFOIL
AIRMAIL
AIRRAID
AIRSHIP
BIDFAIR
BIENNIA
BIGHAIR
BIGUNIT
BIKINIS
BIMINIS
BIOCHIP
BISCUIT
BITESIN
CICHLID
CINESIA
CIRCUIT
DIALSIN
DINARIC
DINEDIN
DINESIN
DIPLOID
DISCOID
DISDAIN
DISJOIN
DIVEDIN
DIVESIN
EIDETIC
EIDOLIC
FIBROID
FIDELIA
FIDELIO
FIDELIS
FILEDIN
FILESIN
FILLSIN
FINNAIR
FIRELIT
FIREPIT
FISHOIL
FIVEPIN
FIVESIX
GIGABIT
GIORGIO
GIVENIN
GIVESIN
HIMALIA
KICKSIN
KIDSKIN
KILOBIT
KINCAID
KINESIC
KINESIS
KINETIC
KINGPIN
KINKAID
KINSHIP
KIRSTIE
KIWANIS
LIBERIA
LIGURIA
LIMEPIE
LIPARIS
LIPIDIC
LITCHIS
LITCRIT
LITHOID
LIVEAID
LIVEDIN
LIVESIN
MIASMIC
MIDSHIP
MIFFLIN
MIKHAIL
MILITIA
MILLAIS
MIMESIS
MIMETIC
MINEPIT
MINIKIN
MINORIN
MINUTIA
MISCOIN
MISEDIT
MISJOIN
MISLAID
MISSAID
MISSHIP
MITOSIS
MITOTIC
MIXEDIN
MIXESIN
NIANTIC
NICEKID
NICOSIA
NIGERIA
NIGHTIE
NINEPIN
OILSKIN
PIGSKIN
PIGTAIL
PILEDIN
PILESIN
PILGRIM
PINEOIL
PINGUID
PINTAIL
PIPEDIN
PIPESIN
PIRATIC
PISANIO
PITCHIN
PIUSIII
PIUSVII
PIUSXII
RIDESIN
RINGSIN
RISKSIT
RITALIN
RITCHIE
RITEAID
SIBERIA
SIBYLIC
SICILIA
SIEBZIG
SIGMOID
SIGNSIN
SILESIA
SILKTIE
SIMONIZ
SINEDIE
SINKSIN
SIRLOIN
SITONIT
SIZESIX
TICOTIN
TIDERIP
TIECLIP
TIMREID
TINFOIL
TINYBIT
TINYTIM
TIOMKIN
TITANIA
TITANIC
VICTRIX
VIDALIA
VIERZIG
VILLAIN
VILLEIN
VINYLIC
VISALIA
VISAVIS
VITALIS
VITAMIN
VITORIA
VIVARIA
WILDPIG
WILLKIE
WINGSIT
WINGTIP
WINSBIG
WIREDIN
WIRESIN
XIPHOID

•|••••|

AIRTAXI
BIANCHI
BIBBIDI
BIRIANI
BIRYANI
DIMITRI
HIBACHI
HITACHI
MINISKI
MIZRAHI
NIKOLAI
PILEGGI
PIRELLI
PIUSIII
PIUSVII
PIUSXII
RIOMUNI
RIPIENI
SILENTI
TIMPANI
VILLARI
VIVALDI
VIVENDI

••||•••

SHIITES

••|•|••

ABIDING
ABILITY
ABITIBI
ACIDIFY
ACIDITY
AGILITY
AKIHITO
ALIBIED
ALINING
AMITIES
ANILINE
ANILITY
ANIMISM
ANIMIST
ARIDITY
ARISING
ASININE
AVIDITY
AVIVIAN
BAILIFF
BAILING
BAITING
BEIJING
BOILING
BRIBING
BRINIER
BRINING
BRINISH
BRITISH
CEILING
CHIDING
CHILIAD
CHILIES
CHIMING
CHIMINH
CHIRICO
CHIVIED
CHIVIES
CLINICS
COIFING
COILING
COINING
CRIMINY
CRITIAS
CRITICS
CUISINE
DAILIES
DAIRIES
DAISIES
DEICING
DEIFIED
DEIFIER
DEIFIES
DEITIES
DOILIES
DRIVING
EDIFICE
EDIFIED
EDIFIER
EDIFIES
EDITING
EDITION
ELICITS
ELIDING
ELIGIUS
ELISION
ELITISM
ELITIST
ELIXIRS
EXILING
EXITING
FAILING
FAIRIES
FAIRING
FAIRISH
FBIFILE
FOILING
FRISIAN
GAINING
GAITING
GLIDING
GOIRISH
GRIMIER
GRIMILY
GRIMING
GRIPING
GUIDING
GUILING
HAILING
HAIMISH
HAIRIER
HAITIAN
IBILITY
INITIAL
IRIDIUM
IRISING
JAILING
JAINISM
JAINIST
JOINING
JUICIER
JUICILY
JUICING
KNIFING
LAICIZE
LAIRING
LAITIES
LOIDING
MAIDISH
MAILING
MAILINS
MAIMING
MAIMITI
MOILING
NAILING
NOISIER
NOISILY
NOISING
OLIVIER
OLIVINE
OPINING
OPINION
ORIFICE
ORIGINE
ORIGINS
OSIRIAN
OVIDIAN
OXIDISE
OXIDIZE
PAINING
PAIRING
PEIPING
PHIDIAS
PHILIPK
PHILIPS
PHILIPV
POISING
POITIER
PRICIER
PRICILY
PRICING
PRIDING
PRIMING
PRIVIER
PRIVIES
PRIVILY
PRIVITY
PRIZING
QUININE
QUINION
QUIVIVE
RAIDING
RAILING
RAINIER
RAINILY
RAINING
RAISING
RAISINS
RAISINY
REICING
REIFIED
REIFIES
REINING
ROILIER
ROILING
RUINING
SAIDIDO
SAILING
SEINING
SEIZING
SHINIER
SHINILY
SHINING
SKIBIBS
SKILIFT
SLICING
SLIDING
SLIMIER
SLIMILY
SLIMING
SMILING
SMITING
SNIPING
SOILING
SPICIER
SPICILY
SPICING
SPIKIER
SPIKILY
SPIKING
SPINIER
SPIRIER
SPIRITS
SPITING
SUITING
SWINISH
SWIPING
TAILING
TBILISI
THINICE
TOILING
TRINITY
TRITIUM
TRIVIAL
TRIVIOT
TRIVIUM
TUITION
TWINIER
TWINING
UNIFIED
UNIFIER
UNIFIES
UNISIZE
UNITIES
UNITING

UNITISE
UNITIVE
UNITIZE
UTILISE
UTILITY
UTILIZE
VEILING
VEINIER
VEINING
VOICING
VOIDING
WAIFISH
WAIKIKI
WAILING
WAITING
WAIVING
WHILING
WHINIER
WHINING
WHITING
WHITISH
WRITING
ZAIRIAN

••I••I•
ABIGAIL
ABIOTIC
ACINGIT
ANIONIC
ASIATIC
ASISAID
AVIATIC
AVIONIC
BLIMPIE
BOISEID
BRILLIG
BRINGIN
BRINGIT
BRITAIN
BUILDIN
BUILTIN
CHICHIS
CHILLIS
CHIMEIN
CHINOIS
CHIPSIN
CHITLIN
CLIMBIN
CRISPIN
CRISPIX
CUINGIN
DEISTIC
DJINNIS
DOINGIN
DRIFTIN
DRINKIN
DRIVEIN
EDITRIX
EKISTIC
ERISTIC
FLIESIN
FLITSIN
GLIDEIN
GOINGIN
GRIFFIN
GRIGRIS
HAIKAIS
HAIRPIN
ICINGIN
ICINGIT
IDIAMIN
IDIOTIC
IFITDIE
ILIADIC
ILIKEIT
JOINSIN
KRISTIN
LEIBNIZ
LEIPZIG
LEITRIM
MAILBIN
MAILSIN
MAITAIS
MEIOSIS
MEIOTIC
NAILSIN
NAILSIT
NAILTIP
PHILBIN
PHILLIE
PHILLIP
PRIZZIS
QUICKIE
QUINTIC
QUITSIT
RAINSIN
REINSIN
SCIATIC
SEISMIC
SHINDIG
SKIDLID
SKISUIT
SKITRIP
SLIDEIN
SLIMJIM
SLINKIN
SLIPSIN
STICKIN
STIRSIN
SWINGIT
TAILFIN
TAILPIN
THIAMIN
THINAIR
TLINGIT
TRIADIC
TRIEDIT
TRIESIT
TRIFFID
TRILLIN
TWINKIE
TYINGIN
USINGIN
WEIGHIN
WHIPSIN
WHIZKID
WRITEIN

••I•••I
ABITIBI
AMICHAI
BUITONI
CHIANTI
FAISALI
FLINTMI
JAIALAI
MAIMITI
MAISOUI
NAIROBI
ORIGAMI
STIMULI
TBILISI
TRIPOLI
WAIKIKI
ZWINGLI

•••II••
TAXIING
YOGIISM

•••I•I•
ADHIBIT
AGRIBIZ
APHILIP
ASPIRIN
BASILIC
BASILIO
BENICIA
BENICIO
BIKINIS
BIMINIS
BOLIVIA
CASIMIR
CECILIA
CODICIL
CRAIGIE
CRAISIN
DEFICIT
DELIMIT
DELIRIA
DOMICIL
DOMINIC
DRUIDIC
EMPIRIC
EMPIRIN
ERMINIA
EXHIBIT
FAMILIA
FATIDIC
FELICIA
FLUIDIC
GALICIA
GEMINIS
HABILIS
HAMITIC
HASIDIC
HASIDIM
HOMINID
HYGIEIA
ILLICIT
INCIVIL
INDICIA
INHIBIT
INSIPID
JURIDIC
KALININ
LATINII
LAVINIA
LETITIA
LEVITIC
LIPIDIC
LOUISII
LOUISIV
LOUISIX
MANIKIN
MILITIA
MINIKIN
MRFIXIT
NAMIBIA
NOLIMIT
OFFICIO
ONEIRIC
OOLITIC
OSSIFIC
PACIFIC
PANINIS
PERIWIG
PLAISIR
POLITIC
PRAIRIE
PYRITIC
RADIOIN
RAPINIS
RELIMIT
REVISIT
RUBITIN
SATIRIC
SEMITIC
SICILIA
SOLICIT
SURIMIS
TAHINIS
TRAININ
TUNISIA
UNCIVIC
UNCIVIL
UNRIGID
UNTIMID
UNVIVID
VALIDID
VERIDIC
WAPITIS
WEDIDIT
WHOISIT
WHYISIT
YESIDID
YESITIS
YOGINIS

•••I••I
ALFIERI
APRIORI
BACILLI
BALIHAI
BENIGNI
BIRIANI
CHRISTI
DARIUSI
DAVINCI
DELICTI
DIMITRI
ELMISTI
FUSILLI
GALILEI
KENICHI
LATINII
LEVILLI
LOUISII
LOUISVI
LOUISXI
LUCIUSI
MAFIOSI
MENISCI
MINISKI
MTSINAI
POLISCI
RAVIOLI
RIPIENI
SALIERI
SERIESI
STPIUSI
TAMIAMI
VANILLI

••••II•
BAMBIII
BOOKIII
IVANIII
JOHNIII
LEOVIII
LEOXIII
MARKIII
OLAFIII
OLAVIII
OTTOIII
PARTIII
PAULIII
PIUSIII

••••I•I
ABITIBI
BAMBIII
BAMBINI
BELLINI
BERNINI
BIBBIDI
BOBBIDI
BOOKIII
CABRINI
CASSINI
CELLINI
CREMINI
DASHIKI
EMERITI
ETALIBI
FABRIZI
FELLINI
HOUDINI
IVANIII
JOHNIII
KONTIKI
KUWAITI
LANDINI
LEOVIII
LEOXIII
MAIMITI
MANCINI
MARKIII
MARTINI
MAZZINI
NAUTILI
OLAFIII
OLAVIII
OTTOIII
PACHISI
PARTIII
PAULIII
PIUSIII
PUCCINI
ROSSINI
SANTINI
SASHIMI
SORDINI
SWAHILI
TANKINI
TBILISI
TERMINI
VALMIKI
WAIKIKI

•••••II
BAMBIII
BOOKIII
BOOKVII
CAROLII
CYRUSII
DANTEII
DENARII
HENRYII
IVANIII
JAMESII
JOHNIII
JOHNVII
JOHNXII
LATINII
LEOVIII
LEOXIII
LOUISII
MARKIII
MARKVII
OLAFIII
OLAVIII
OTTOIII
PARTIII
PAULIII
PETERII
PIUSIII
PIUSVII
PIUSXII
POMPEII
ROCKYII
SCENEII
URBANII

IJ•••••
IJKLMNO

I•J••••
INJECTS
INJOKES
INJURED
INJURER
INJURES

I••J•••
IIIJOHN
INAJIFF
INKJETS
IOBJECT
IWOJIMA

•IJ••••
EIJKMAN
FIJIANS
HIJACKS
HIJINKS
HIJKLMN
TIJUANA

•I•J•••
BIGJAKE
BIGJERK
BIGJOHN
DISJOIN
IIIJOHN
JIMJAMS
MIDJULY
MIDJUNE
MISJOIN
TIPJARS

•I••J••
KILLJOY
NICEJOB

•I••••J
SILENTJ

••IJ•••
BEIJING
FRIJOLE
GHIJKLM
IIIJOHN
SKIJUMP
TRIJETS

••I•J••
ABIDJAN
SLIMJIM
TWINJET

•••IJ••
FGHIJKL

•••I••J
DANIELJ
FTDIXNJ
RADIODJ
SERIESJ

••••IJ•
EFGHIJK
VANRIJN

•••••IJ
DEFGHIJ

IK•••••
IKEBANA
IKNEWIT
IKNOWIT

I•K••••
ICKIEST
ICKYPOO
IIKINGS
IJKLMNO
INKBLOT
INKEDIN
INKHORN
INKIEST
INKINGS
INKJETS
INKLESS
INKLIKE
INKLING
INKMARK
INKNOTS
INKPADS
INKPOTS
INKSACS
INKSPOT
INKSTER
INKWELL
INKYCAP
IRKSOME
IRKUTSK

I••K•••
ILIKEIT
ILLKNOW
INAKNOT

I•••K••
INJOKES
INTAKES
INVOKED
INVOKER
INVOKES
IRECKON
ITSOKAY

I••••K•
ICELIKE
IMBROKE
INAPOKE
INKLIKE
IVYLIKE

I•••••K
ICEMILK
ICEPACK
ICEPICK
ICERINK
ILLLUCK
INAFUNK
INAWINK
INBLACK
INCHECK
INKMARK
INSHOCK
INSTOCK
IRKUTSK

•IK••••
AIKIDOS
BIKEWAY
BIKINIS
DIKDIKS
DIKTATS
HIKEDUP
HIKEOUT
HIKESUP
IIKINGS
KIKIDEE
KIKUYUS
LIKABLE
LIKEICE
LIKEMAD
LIKENED
LIKENEW
LIKENTO
LIKEWOW
LIKINGS
MIKADOS
MIKASAS
MIKHAIL
NIKEADS
NIKOLAI
NIKOLAY
RIKSDAG
SIKHISM
VIKINGS

•I•K•••
AIRKISS
BICKERS
BIGKIDS
BILKERS
BILKING
DICKENS
DICKERS
DICKEYS
DICKIES
DICKORY
DICKSON
DINKIER
DIRKING
DIRKSEN
DISKING
EIJKMAN
FICKLER
FINKING
FINKSON
FIRKINS
GINKGOS
HICKEYS
HICKMAN
HICKORY
HIJKLMN
HINKIER
JIMKAAT
KICKBOX
KICKERS
KICKIER
KICKING
KICKOFF
KICKOUT
KICKSIN
KICKSUP
KICKUPS
KINKAID
KINKIER
KINKILY
KINKING
KITKATS
LICKERS
LICKETY
LICKING
LICKSUP
LINKAGE
LINKERS
LINKING
LINKSUP
LINKUPS
MICKEYS
MILKBAR
MILKCAN
MILKCOW
MILKDUD
MILKERS
MILKFED
MILKIER
MILKILY
MILKING
MILKMAN
MILKMEN
MILKRUN
MILKSOP
MISKEYS
MISKNEW
MISKNOW
MISKOLC
NICKELS
NICKERS
NICKING
NICKLES
OINKERS
OINKING
PICKAXE
PICKENS
PICKERS
PICKETS
PICKETT
PICKIER
PICKING
PICKLED
PICKLES
PICKOFF
PICKOUT
PICKSAT
PICKSON
PICKSUP
PICKUPS
PINKENS
PINKEST
PINKETT
PINKHAM
PINKIES
PINKING
PINKISH
PINKOES
RICKETY
RICKEYS
RICKLES
RICKMAN
RICKSHA
RINKRAT
RISKERS
RISKIER
RISKILY
RISKING
RISKSIT
SICKBAY
SICKBED
SICKDAY
SICKENS
SICKEST
SICKISH
SICKLES
SICKOUT
SICKPAY
SILKHAT
SILKIER
SILKILY
SILKTIE
SINKAGE
SINKERS
SINKING
SINKSIN
TICKERS
TICKETS
TICKING
TICKLED
TICKLER
TICKLES
TICKOFF
TICKSBY
TINKERS
TINKLED
TINKLER
TINKLES
VICKERS
VICKREY
WICKERS
WICKETS
WICKING
WICKIUP
WICKLOW
WILKENS
WILKINS
WINKERS
WINKING
WINKLER
WINKOUT
WINKSAT
ZINKIER

•I••K••
BISHKEK
GINGKOS
KIDSKIN
KISHKES
MINIKIN
MINSKYS
NICEKID
OILSKIN
PIGSKIN
TIOMKIN
WILLKIE
ZINCKED

•I•••K•
AIRLIKE
BIBLIKE
BIGJAKE
DIDLIKE
DIKDIKS
DISLIKE
FINICKY
FINLIKE
HIJACKS
HIJINKS
HIPLIKE
JIGLIKE
KIDLIKE
LIPLIKE
MINISKI
MISLIKE
MISTAKE
NIBLIKE
OILCAKE
OILLIKE
PIELIKE
PIGLIKE
PINOAKS
RIBLIKE
SINLIKE
SIRDUKE
TINLIKE
WIGLIKE

•I••••K
AIRLOCK
AIRPACK
AIRPARK
AIRSICK
AIRSOCK
AIRTANK
AIRWICK
BIBCOCK
BIGJERK
BIGTALK
BISHKEK
FINBACK
FIRBANK
GIMMICK
HILLOCK
HITBACK
JIRASEK
KIDROCK
KINFOLK
LIEBACK
LITOVSK
LIVEOAK
MIDWEEK
MISMARK
MISTOOK
NIBLICK
NIPMUCK
NITPICK
OILTANK
RIDDICK
RIMROCK
SILENTK
SITBACK
SIXPACK
SIXWEEK
TIEBACK
TIERACK
TIETACK
TINWORK
TITLARK
VITEBSK
WIDMARK
WINBACK
YITZHAK
ZIPDISK
ZIPLOCK

••IK•••
ARIKARA
ERIKSON
HAIKAIS
ILIKEIT
SHIKOKU
SPIKERS
SPIKETV
SPIKEUP
SPIKIER
SPIKILY
SPIKING
WAIKATO
WAIKIKI

••I•K••
BLINKAT
BLINKED
BLINKER
BRICKED
BRICKLE
BRICKUP
BRINKER
BRISKED
BRISKER
BRISKET
BRISKLY
CHICKEN
CHILKAT
CHINKED
CLICKED
CLICKER
CLICKON
CLINKED
CLINKER
CRICKED
CRICKET
CRINKLE
CRINKLY
DRINKER
DRINKIN
DRINKME
DRINKTO
DRINKUP
ETICKET
FLICKED
FLICKER
FRICKER
FRISKED
FRISKER
GHIJKLM
GRINKOV
KLINKER
NAILKEG
PLINKED
PRICKED
PRICKLE
PRICKLY
PRICKUP
PRINKED
PRINKER
QUICKEN
QUICKER
QUICKIE
QUICKLY
REINKED
SHIRKED
SHIRKER
SLICKED
SLICKER
SLICKLY
SLINKED
SLINKER
SLINKIN
SLINKUP
SMIRKED
SMIRKER
SNICKER
SNICKET
STICKBY
STICKER
STICKIN
STICKON
STICKTO
STICKUM

STICKUP
STINKER
STINKUP
THICKEN
THICKER
THICKET
THICKLY
THINKER
THINKOF
THINKSO
THINKUP
TRICKED
TRICKER
TRICKLE
TRINKET
TWINKIE
TWINKLE
TWINKLY
UNINKED
WHISKAS
WHISKED
WHISKER
WHISKEY
WHIZKID
WRINKLE
WRINKLY
ZWICKAU

••I••K•
SHIKOKU
WAIKIKI

••I•••K
CHINOOK
DOINGOK
KAISHEK
OLICOOK
PHILIPK
SKIMASK
SKIRACK

•••IK••
BATIKED
DANIKEN
MANIKIN
MINIKIN
MONIKER
SHEIKHS
SHRIKES
STRIKER
STRIKES
TROIKAS
UNDIKED
UNLIKED
UNLIKES
UNMIKED

•••I•K•
COLICKY
ENLINKS
FGHIJKL
FINICKY
HIJINKS
KODIAKS
KOPIYKA
MINISKI
MUSICKS
OPTICKS
PANICKY
REKICKS
RELINKS
REPICKS
RESINKS
RUZICKA
SCHICKS
SHRIEKS
SHRINKS
SHTICKS
SHTICKY
SOYINKA
SOYINKS
UNKINKS
UNLINKS
UNPICKS
UNRISKY
UPLINKS
UPTICKS

•••I••K
ALNITAK
SERIESK
SERIPAK
VARITEK

••••IK•
ACTLIKE
AIRLIKE
AMERIKA
ANTLIKE
APELIKE
ARMLIKE
ASSLIKE
AXELIKE
BAGLIKE
BATLIKE
BEDLIKE
BEELIKE
BIBLIKE
BOWLIKE
BOXLIKE
BOYLIKE
BUDLIKE
CATLIKE
COWLIKE
CUPLIKE
CURLIKE
DASHIKI
DIDLIKE
DIKDIKS
DISLIKE
DOGLIKE
DOTLIKE
EARLIKE
EELLIKE
EGGLIKE
ELFLIKE
EYELIKE
FADLIKE
FANLIKE
FATLIKE
FINLIKE
FOXLIKE
GARPIKE
GEMLIKE
GODLIKE
GOTHIKA
GUMLIKE
HAGLIKE
HATLIKE
HENLIKE
HIPLIKE
HOGLIKE
HUNLIKE
HUTLIKE
ICELIKE
INKLIKE
IVYLIKE
JAMLIKE
JAWLIKE
JIGLIKE
KIDLIKE
KONTIKI
LAWLIKE
LEGLIKE
LIPLIKE
MALLIKA
MANLIKE
MISLIKE
NETLIKE
NIBLIKE
NOTLIKE
NUDNIKS
NUNLIKE
NUTLIKE
OAKLIKE
OARLIKE
OATLIKE
OILLIKE
ORBLIKE
OWLLIKE
PAPRIKA
PEALIKE
PEGLIKE
PENLIKE
PIELIKE
PIGLIKE
PODLIKE
RAMLIKE
RATLIKE
RAYLIKE
RIBLIKE
RODLIKE
RUGLIKE
SACLIKE
SAWLIKE
SEALIKE
SINLIKE
SKYLIKE
SONLIKE
SOWLIKE
SUNLIKE
TAGLIKE
TAXHIKE
THELIKE
TINLIKE
TOELIKE
TOYBIKE
TOYLIKE
TUBLIKE
TUGRIKS
UNALIKE
URNLIKE
VALMIKI
WAIKIKI
WARLIKE
WAXLIKE
WEBLIKE
WIGLIKE
ZERNIKE

••••I•K
AIRSICK
AIRWICK
BARLICK
BEQUICK
BERBICK
BERWICK
BETHINK
BURDICK
CONNICK
COWLICK
DERRICK
DOGTICK
DUNKIRK
EFGHIJK
ELDRICK
ELENIAK
EYEWINK
FALKIRK
FOSDICK
GARRICK
GATWICK
GEDRICK
GIMMICK
GOTMILK
HARNICK
HAYRICK
HERRICK
HOTLICK
HOTLINK
HOTMILK
HOTPINK
ICEMILK
ICEPICK
ICERINK
INAWINK
KUBRICK
LOWRISK
MEDWICK
MERRICK
MESSICK
NATWICK
NIBLICK
NITPICK
OBELISK
OLDNICK
ONAKICK
OUTKICK
OUTPICK
PATRICK
PHILIPK
RATFINK
RAWSILK
RENWICK
RESTICK
RETHINK
RIDDICK
RODDICK
ROLLICK
SCHTICK
SEASICK
SELKIRK
SOYMILK
THEMICK
THERINK
TOEPICK
TOPKICK
UNQUICK
UNSLICK
UNSTICK
UNTHICK
UNTHINK
VARRICK
WARWICK
WOZNIAK
YANNICK
ZIPDISK

•••••IK
BEATNIK
GOODNIK
JONERIK
KRAMNIK
KUBELIK
NEATNIK
NESQUIK
PERCHIK
SPUTNIK

IL•••••
ILIADIC
ILIAMNA
ILIESCU
ILIKEIT
ILLBITE
ILLBRED
ILLCALL
ILLCLAD
ILLDOIT
ILLDONE
ILLEANA
ILLEGAL
ILLEGIT
ILLFOLD
ILLICIT
ILLKNOW
ILLLIVE
ILLLUCK
ILLMADE
ILLNESS
ILLOGIC
ILLPASS
ILLTELL
ILLUDED
ILLUDES
ILLUMED
ILLUMES
ILLUSED
ILLUSES
ILLWILL
ILLWIND
ILLYRIA
ILOCANO
ILOSTIT
ILOVEIT
ILOVELA

I•L••••
IDLESSE
ILLBITE
ILLBRED
ILLCALL
ILLCLAD
ILLDOIT
ILLDONE
ILLEANA
ILLEGAL
ILLEGIT
ILLFOLD
ILLICIT
ILLKNOW
ILLLIVE
ILLLUCK
ILLMADE
ILLNESS
ILLOGIC
ILLPASS
ILLTELL
ILLUDED
ILLUDES
ILLUMED
ILLUMES
ILLUSED
ILLUSES
ILLWILL
ILLWIND
ILLYRIA
INLABOR
INLANDS
INLARGE
INLAYER
INLIMBO
INLINES
INLYING
IPLEDGE
ISLAMIC
ISLANDS
ISLETED

I••L•••
IAMLOVE
IBILITY
ICELAND
ICELESS
ICELIKE
ICELINE
IDOLISE
IDOLIST
IDOLIZE
IDYLIST
IDYLLIC
IJKLMNO
ILLLIVE
ILLLUCK
IMPLANT
IMPLEAD
IMPLIED
IMPLIES
IMPLODE
IMPLORE
INALINE
INBLACK
INBLOOM
INCLASS
INCLINE
INCLOSE
INCLUDE
INFLAME
INFLATE
INFLECT
INFLICT
INFLOWS
INGLESE
INKLESS
INKLIKE
INKLING
INNLESS
INPLACE
INULASE
IRELAND
IRELESS
ISOLATE
ISOLATO
ISOLINE
ITALIAN
ITALICS
ITSLATE
ITSLOVE
IVYLIKE

I•••L••
ICEBLUE
ICEFLOE
ICICLES
IDEALLY
IDYLLIC
ILLCLAD
IMPALAS
IMPALED
IMPALER
IMPALES
IMPULSE
INCOLOR
INDULGE
INFOLDS
INGALLS
INGULFS
INHALED
INHALER
INHALES
INKBLOT
INSALES
INSOLES
INSULAR
INSULIN
INSULTS
INVALID
INVOLVE
ITSALIE
ITSALOT
ITWELVE

I••••L•
IANHOLM
ICECOLD
ICEFALL
ICEHOLE
ICEMILK
IDEALLY
IFIFELL
IGNOBLE
IGNOBLY
ILLCALL
ILLFOLD
ILLTELL
ILLWILL
ILOVELA
IMSWELL
INABALL
INAHOLE
INANELY
INAPILE
INAPTLY
INAVALE
INBUILT
INDWELL
INDWELT
INEPTLY
INERTLY
INEXILE
INFIELD
INGALLS
INGOALS
INKWELL
INNERLY
INOCULA
INSCALE
INSTALL
INSTALS
INSTILL
INSTILS
INSTYLE
INTAILS
INUTILE
IRATELY
ISOHELS
ISRAELI
ITGIRLS
ITSCOLD

I•••••L
ICEFALL
IFIFELL
ILLCALL
ILLEGAL
ILLTELL
ILLWILL
IMMORAL
IMPANEL
IMPERIL
IMSWELL
INABALL
INAPRIL
INCIVIL
INDWELL
INFIDEL
INITIAL
INKWELL
INPERIL
INSTALL
INSTILL
INTOTAL
ISCHIAL
ISHMAEL
ISRAFEL

•IL••••
AILERON
AILMENT
BILEVEL
BILGIER
BILIOUS
BILKERS
BILKING
BILLERS
BILLETS
BILLIES
BILLING
BILLION
BILLNYE
BILLOWS
BILLOWY
BILOBED
CILENTO
CILIARY
CILIATE
DILATED
DILATES
DILATOR
DILBERT
DILEMMA
DILLARD
DILLIES
DILLMAN
DILUENT
DILUTED
DILUTER
DILUTES
DILUTOR
FILBERT
FILCHED
FILCHER
FILCHES
FILEDBY
FILEDIN
FILENES
FILEOUT
FILESBY
FILESIN
FILIBEG
FILINGS
FILIPPO
FILLERS
FILLETS
FILLIES
FILLING
FILLINS
FILLIPS
FILLOUT
FILLSIN
FILLSUP
FILLUPS
FILMDOM
FILMIER
FILMILY
FILMING
FILMSET
FILOFAX
FILTERS
GILBERT
GILBLAS
GILDERS
GILDING
GILFORD
GILLIAM
GILLIAN
GILLING
GILLMAN
GILLNET
GILMORE
HILAIRE
HILBERT
HILLARY
HILLIER
HILLING
HILLMAN
HILLMEN
HILLOCK
HILLTOP
HILTING
HILTONS
JILLIAN
JILLION
JILTERS
JILTING
KILAUEA
KILDARE
KILLEEN
KILLERS
KILLFEE
KILLING
KILLJOY
KILNDRY
KILNING
KILOBAR
KILOBIT
KILOTON
KILTIES
KILTING
LILALEE
LILETEE
LILINAU
LILLIAN
LILTING
LILYPAD
MILAGRO
MILDEST
MILDEWS
MILDEWY
MILDRED
MILEAGE
MILERUN
MILHAUD
MILHOUS
MILIEUS
MILIEUX
MILITIA
MILKBAR
MILKCAN
MILKCOW
MILKDUD
MILKERS
MILKFED
MILKIER
MILKILY
MILKING
MILKMAN
MILKMEN
MILKRUN
MILKSOP
MILLAGE
MILLAIS
MILLAND
MILLARD
MILLDAM
MILLEND
MILLERS
MILLETS
MILLETT
MILLIME
MILLING
MILLION
MILLRUN
MILORDS
NILESOH
NILSSON
OILBASE
OILBIRD
OILCAKE
OILCANS
OILCUPS
OILDRUM
OILHEAT
OILIEST
OILLAMP
OILLESS
OILLIKE
OILLINE
OILPALM
OILPANS
OILRICH
OILRIGS
OILRING
OILRUBS
OILSAND
OILSEED
OILSKIN
OILSPOT
OILTANK
OILWELL
PILATES
PILATUS
PILCROW
PILEATE
PILEDIN
PILEDON
PILEDUP
PILEGGI
PILEOUS
PILESIN
PILESOF
PILESON
PILESUP
PILEUPS
PILFERS
PILGRIM
PILINGS
PILLAGE
PILLARS
PILLBOX
PILLBUG
PILLING
PILLION
PILLORY
PILLOWS
PILLOWY
PILOTED
PILSNER
RILEDUP
RILESUP
RILIEVO
RILLETS
SILENCE
SILENTA
SILENTB
SILENTC
SILENTD
SILENTE
SILENTF
SILENTG
SILENTH
SILENTI
SILENTJ
SILENTK
SILENTL
SILENTM
SILENTN
SILENTO
SILENTP
SILENTQ
SILENTR
SILENTS
SILENTT
SILENTU
SILENTV
SILENTW
SILENTX
SILENTY
SILENTZ
SILESIA
SILICAS
SILICON
SILKHAT
SILKIER
SILKILY
SILKTIE
SILLIER
SILLIES
SILLYME
SILOING
SILTIER
SILTING
SILVERS
SILVERY
TILINGS
TILLAGE
TILLERS
TILLETS
TILLING
TILLNOW
TILSITS
TILTERS
TILTING
TILTSAT
TILTSUP
TILTTOP
VILLAGE
VILLAIN
VILLARD
VILLARI
VILLEIN
VILNIUS
WILBERT
WILDCAT
WILDDOG
WILDEST
WILDING
WILDISH
WILDMAN
WILDMEN
WILDONE
WILDPIG
WILFORD
WILFRED
WILHELM
WILIEST
WILKENS
WILKINS
WILLARD
WILLERS
WILLFUL
WILLIAM
WILLIES
WILLING
WILLKIE
WILLOWS
WILLOWY
WILLSON
WILLYOU
WILSONS
WILTING
ZILCHES
ZILLION

•I•L•••
AIDLESS
AIGLETS
AIMLESS
AIRLANE
AIRLESS
AIRLIFT
AIRLIKE
AIRLINE
AIRLOCK
AIRLOGS
BIALIES
BIBLESS
BIBLIKE
BIBLIOG
BIGLEAD
BIGLIES
BIGLOTS
BIGLOVE
BILLERS
BILLETS
BILLIES
BILLING
BILLION
BILLNYE
BILLOWS
BILLOWY
BIOLABS
BIOLITE
BIOLOGY
BIPLANE
BIRLERS
BIRLING
BITLESS
DIALECT
DIALEDO
DIALERS
DIALING
DIALLED
DIALOGS
DIALOUT
DIALSIN
DIALSUP
DIALUPS
DIDLAPS
DIDLIKE
DIGLOTS
DILLARD
DILLIES
DILLMAN

DIPLOID
DIPLOMA
DISLIKE
FIELDED
FIELDER
FIGLEAF
FILLERS
FILLETS
FILLIES
FILLING
FILLINS
FILLIPS
FILLOUT
FILLSIN
FILLSUP
FILLUPS
FINLAND
FINLESS
FINLIKE
GIBLETS
GIBLUES
GIELGUD
GILLIAM
GILLIAN
GILLING
GILLMAN
GILLNET
GIMLETS
GIRLIER
GIRLIES
GIRLISH
GIRLSHY
HIALEAH
HILLARY
HILLIER
HILLING
HILLMAN
HILLMEN
HILLOCK
HILLTOP
HIPLESS
HIPLIKE
HITLESS
HITLIST
JIGLIKE
JILLIAN
JILLION
KIDLIKE
KILLEEN
KILLERS
KILLFEE
KILLING
KILLJOY
KINLESS
KIPLING
KISLEVS
LIDLESS
LILLIAN
LIPLESS
LIPLIKE
MIDLAND
MIDLEGS
MIDLIFE
MIDLINE
MIDLIST
MILLAGE
MILLAIS
MILLAND
MILLARD
MILLDAM
MILLEND
MILLERS
MILLETS
MILLETT
MILLIME
MILLING
MILLION
MILLRUN
MISLAID
MISLAYS
MISLEAD
MISLIKE
NIALONG
NIBLETS
NIBLICK
NIBLIKE
NIELSEN
OILLAMP
OILLESS
OILLIKE
OILLINE
PIELIKE
PIGLETS
PIGLIKE
PILLAGE
PILLARS
PILLBOX
PILLBUG
PILLING
PILLION
PILLORY
PILLOWS
PILLOWY
PIMLICO
PINLESS
PIOLETS
PIPLESS
RIALTOS
RIBLESS
RIBLETS
RIBLIKE
RIFLERS
RIFLERY
RIFLING
RILLETS
RIMLESS
RIOLOBO
SIBLING
SIDLING
SILLIER
SILLIES
SILLYME
SINLESS
SINLIKE
SIRLOIN
SIXLANE
TIELESS
TIELINE
TIGLONS
TILLAGE
TILLERS
TILLETS
TILLING
TILLNOW
TINLIKE
TIPLESS
TIPLINE
TITLARK
TITLING
TITLIST
VIALFUL
VIALING
VIALLED
VIELLES
VILLAGE
VILLAIN
VILLARD
VILLARI
VILLEIN
VINLAND
VIOLATE
VIOLENT
VIOLETS
VIOLINS
VIOLIST
VIOLONE
WIELAND
WIELDED
WIELDER
WIGLESS
WIGLETS
WIGLIKE
WILLARD
WILLERS
WILLFUL
WILLIAM
WILLIES
WILLING
WILLKIE
WILLOWS
WILLOWY
WILLSON
WILLYOU
WINLESS
WITLESS
WITLING
YIELDED
YIELDER
YIELDTO
ZILLION
ZIPLOCK
ZIPLOCS

•I••L••

AIRFLOW
AIRGLOW
AIRPLAY
BIBELOT
BICOLOR
BIGBLUE
BIGELOW
BINDLES
BINGLES
BIPOLAR
BIVALVE
CICHLID
CIRCLED
CIRCLER
CIRCLES
CIRCLET
CIVILLY
DIABLES
DIABLOS
DIALLED
DIBBLED
DIBBLER
DIBBLES
DICILLO
DIDDLED
DIDDLER
DIDDLES
DIDDLEY
DIMPLED
DIMPLES
DINGLES
DIPOLAR
DIPOLES
DISPLAY
DIVULGE
DIVULSE
EIDOLIC
EIDOLON
FIATLUX
FIBULAE
FIBULAR
FIBULAS
FICKLER
FIDDLED
FIDDLER
FIDDLES
FIDELES
FIDELIA
FIDELIO
FIDELIS
FIEDLER
FINALES
FINALLY
FINDLAY
FINDLEY
FIPPLES
FIRELIT
FIZZLED
FIZZLER
FIZZLES
GIGGLED
GIGGLER
GIGGLES
GIGOLOS
GILBLAS
GIRDLED
GIRDLER
GIRDLES
GIROLLE
GISELLE
HIBBLER
HIDALGO
HIGGLED
HIGGLER
HIGGLES
HIGHLOW
HIJKLMN
HIMALIA
HINDLEG
HITPLAY
JIGGLED
JIGGLES
JINGLED
JINGLER
JINGLES
KIBBLED
KIBBLES
KIDULTS
KINDLED
KINDLER
KINDLES
KINGLET
LIBELED
LIBELEE
LIBELER
LIESLOW
LILALEE
LITTLER
LITTLES
MIDDLEC
MIDDLED
MIDDLER
MIDDLES
MIFFLIN
MINGLED
MINGLER
MINGLES
MINILAB
MINOLTA
MISALLY
MISPLAN
MISPLAY
MIZZLED
MIZZLES
NIBBLED
NIBBLER
NIBBLES
NICKLES
NICOLAS
NICOLET
NICOLLE
NIGGLED
NIGGLER
NIGGLES
NIKOLAI
NIKOLAY
NIMBLER
NIPPLES
PICKLED
PICKLES
PIDDLED
PIDDLES
PIFFLED
PIFFLES
PIMPLED
PIMPLES
PIRELLI
PITILLO
RIBALDS
RICHLER
RICKLES
RIDDLED
RIDDLER
RIDDLES
RIFFLED
RIFFLER
RIFFLES
RIMPLED
RIMPLES
RINALDO
RINGLET
RIPPLED
RIPPLES
RIPPLET
RITALIN
RIVALED
RIVALRY
RIVULET
SIBYLIC
SICILIA
SICKLES
SIMILAC
SIMILAR
SIMILES
SIMPLER
SIMPLES
SIMPLEX
SINGLED
SINGLES
SINGLET
SIZZLED
SIZZLER
SIZZLES
TICKLED
TICKLER
TICKLES
TIDALLY
TIECLIP
TIMELAG
TINGLED
TINGLER
TINGLES
TINKLED
TINKLER
TINKLES
TIPPLED
TIPPLER
TIPPLES
TITTLES
TITULAR
VIALLED
VIDALIA
VIELLES
VINYLIC
VISALIA
VITALIS
VITALLY
VITTLES
VIVALDI
VIZSLAS
WICKLOW
WIGGLED
WIGGLER
WIGGLES
WIMPLED
WIMPLES
WINGLET
WINKLER
WINSLET
WINSLOW
ZIEGLER

•I•••L•

AIRBALL
AIRBILL
AIRHOLE
AIRMILE
AIRWOLF
BIASPLY
BICYCLE
BIGGULP
BIGHALF
BIGSALE
BIGTALK
BIRDFLU
BISSELL
BITROLE
CINEOLE
CITABLE
CIVILLY
DIABOLO
DIAVOLO
DICILLO
DIDWELL
DIEBOLD
DIESELS
DIMBULB
DINGILY
DIRNDLS
DIRTILY
DISABLE
DISMALS
DISPELS
DISTILL
DISTILS
DIZZILY
FICTILE
FIERILY
FIFTHLY
FILMILY
FINABLE
FINAGLE
FINALLY
FINGALS
FINIALS
FIREFLY
FIRSTLY
FISHILY
FISSILE
FITWELL
FIXABLE
FIXEDLY
GIDDILY
GIMBALS
GIMBELS
GINGOLD
GINMILL
GIROLLE
GISELLE
HIDABLE
HIMSELF
HIRABLE
HITFILM
JIMDALE
KIMBALL
KINFOLK
KINKILY
KINNELL
KISSELS
LICITLY
LIGHTLY
LIKABLE
LINABLE
LINCOLN
LINGULA
LINTELS
LIONELL
LIONELS
LIPBALM
LITHELY
LIVABLE
LIVIDLY
MICAELA
MIDJULY
MIDSOLE
MILKILY
MINABLE
MINEOLA
MIRACLE
MISALLY
MISBILL
MISCALL
MISERLY
MISFILE
MISKOLC
MISRELY
MISRULE
MISSALS
MISSILE
MISTELL
MISTILY
MISTOLD
MIXABLE
MIXEDLY
NICCOLO
NICHOLS
NICKELS
NICOLLE
NIFTILY
NIGHTLY
NINTHLY
NIPPILY
OILPALM
OILWELL
PIANOLA
PICCOLO
PIEBALD
PIEHOLE
PIESALE
PINBALL
PINFOLD
PINHOLE
PINWALE
PIOUSLY
PIRELLI
PISTILS
PISTOLE
PISTOLS
PITBULL
PITFALL
PITHILY
PITILLO
RIANTLY
RIDABLE
RIGHTLY
RIGIDLY
RISIBLE
RISIBLY
RISKILY
RISSOLE
RITUALS
RITZILY
SIGHTLY
SIGNALS
SILKILY
SITWELL
SIXBALL
SIXFOLD
SIXTHLY
SIZABLE
SIZABLY
TIDALLY
TIEPOLO
TIGHTLY
TIMBALE
TIMBALS
TIMHOLT
TIMIDLY
TINNILY
TINSELS
TIPSILY
TIREDLY
VIGNOLA
VINCULA
VIRGULE
VISIBLE
VISIBLY
VISTULA
VISUALS
VITALLY
VIVIDLY
VIXENLY
WILHELM
WIMPOLE
WINDILY
WIRABLE
WISPILY
WITTILY

•I••••L

AIRBALL
AIRBILL
AIRCOOL
AIRFOIL
AIRMAIL
BIAXIAL
BIFOCAL
BIGDEAL
BIGGIRL
BIGMEAL
BILEVEL
BIMETAL
BIMODAL
BIOFUEL
BIPEDAL
BISSELL
BITONAL
CITADEL
CITYGAL
DIDWELL
DIGITAL
DIREFUL
DISHFUL
DISTILL
DIURNAL
FIGURAL
FINICAL
FISHOIL
FISTFUL
FITWELL
GINMILL
GIRASOL
JIMDIAL
KIMBALL
KINNELL
LIBERAL
LIFEFUL
LIMINAL
LINGUAL
LIONELL
LITERAL
MIAMIFL
MIASMAL
MICHAEL
MIKHAIL
MINDFUL
MINERAL
MINIMAL
MIRABEL
MISBILL
MISCALL
MISDEAL
MISDIAL
MISTELL
MISTRAL
OILWELL
PIGTAIL
PINBALL
PINCURL
PINEOIL
PINESOL
PINSEAL
PINTAIL
PIPEFUL
PITBULL
PITFALL
PITIFUL
PIVOTAL
SIGHFUL
SILENTL
SITWELL
SIXBALL
TINFOIL
VIALFUL
VICINAL
VICTUAL
VIMINAL
VIRTUAL
VITRIOL
WILLFUL
WISHFUL
WISTFUL

••IL•••

ABILENE
ABILITY
AGILELY
AGILEST
AGILITY
AMILATE
ANILINE
ANILITY
APILEOF
AXILLAE
AXILLAR
AXILLAS
BAILEES
BAILERS
BAILIFF
BAILING
BAILORS
BAILOUT
BAILSON
BOILERS
BOILING
BOILOFF
BOILOUT
BOILSUP
BRILLIG
BRILLOS
BUILDER
BUILDIN
BUILDON
BUILDUP
BUILTIN
BUILTON
BUILTUP
CAILLOU
CEILING
CHILCAT
CHILEAN
CHILIAD
CHILIES
CHILKAT
CHILLED
CHILLER
CHILLIS
CHILLUM
COILERS
COILING
COILSUP
DAILIES
DOILIES
DRILLED
DRILLER
EPILADY
EPILATE
EPILOGS
EVILEST
EVILEYE
EVILLER
EVILONE
EXILERS
EXILING
FAILING
FAILLES
FAILSTO
FAILURE
FOILING
FRILLED
GRILLED
GRILLER
GRILLES
GUILDER
GUILING
HAILERS
HAILING
IBILITY
JAILERS
JAILING
JAILORS
JUILLET
KEILLOR
MAILBAG
MAILBIN
MAILBOX
MAILCAR
MAILERS
MAILING
MAILINS
MAILLOL
MAILLOT
MAILMAN
MAILMEN
MAILOUT
MAILSIN
MOILERS
MOILING
NAILERS
NAILGUN
NAILING
NAILKEG
NAILSET
NAILSIN
NAILSIT
NAILSUP
NAILTIP
PAILFUL
PHILBIN
PHILCOS
PHILEAS
PHILIPK
PHILIPS
PHILIPV
PHILLIE
PHILLIP
PHILOUS
PHILTER
PHILTRE
QUILLED
QUILLER
QUILTED
QUILTER
RAILAGE
RAILBUS
RAILCAR
RAILERS
RAILING
RAILMAN
RAILMEN
RAILSAT
RAILSON
RAILWAY
ROILIER
ROILING
SAILERS
SAILING
SAILORS
SAILSON
SAILSTO
SHILLED
SKILFUL
SKILIFT
SKILLED
SKILLET
SMILEAT
SMILEON
SMILERS
SMILEYS
SMILING
SMILLAS
SOILAGE
SOILING
SPILLED
SPILLER
STILLED
STILLER
STILLUP
STILTED
STILTON
SWILLED
SWILLER
SZILARD
TAILEND
TAILERS
TAILFIN
TAILING
TAILOFF
TAILORS
TAILPIN
TAILWAG
TBILISI
TOILERS
TOILETS
TOILFUL
TOILING
TOILSAT
TRILLED
TRILLER
TRILLIN
TRILOGY
TUILLES
TWILLED
UTILISE
UTILITY
UTILIZE
VEILERS
VEILING
WAILERS
WAILFUL
WAILING
WHILING

••I•L••

AMIBLUE
AXIALLY
AXILLAE
AXILLAR
AXILLAS
BRIDLED
BRIDLER
BRIDLES
BRILLIG
BRILLOS
BRIMLEY
CAILLOU
CHICLES
CHICLET
CHILLED
CHILLER
CHILLIS
CHILLUM
CHITLIN
DAIMLER
DRIBLET
DRILLED
DRILLER
EDIBLES
ENISLED
ENISLES
EVILLER
FAILLES
FOIBLES
FRIDLEY
FRILLED
GRILLED
GRILLER
GRILLES
GRISLET
ICICLES

JAIALAI
JUILLET
KEILLOR
LAIDLOW
MAILLOL
MAILLOT
ORIOLES
PAISLEY
PHILLIE
PHILLIP
QUIGLEY
QUILLED
QUILLER
QUINLAN
SHIELDS
SHILLED
SHIRLEY
SKIDLID
SKILLED
SKILLET
SKIRLED
SMILLAS
SNIGLET
SPIELED
SPIELER
SPILLED
SPILLER
STIFLED
STIFLES
STILLED
STILLER
STILLUP
SWILLED
SWILLER
SWIRLED
TRIFLED
TRIFLER
TRIFLES
TRILLED
TRILLER
TRILLIN
TRIOLET
TRIPLEA
TRIPLED
TRIPLES
TRIPLET
TRIPLEX
TUILLES
TWILLED
TWIRLED
TWIRLER
UNIPLEX
VEINLET
WHIRLED
WHIRLER
WRIGLEY

••I••L•

AGILELY
ALITTLE
AMIABLE
AMIABLY
AMIDALA
AMIDOLS
ANIMALS
APISHLY
ATINGLE
AXIALLY
BLINDLY
BRICKLE
BRIDALS
BRIEFLY
BRINDLE
BRISKLY
BRISTLE
BRISTLY
BRITTLE
CHIEFLY
CHISELS
CRINKLE
CRINKLY
CRIPPLE
CRISPLY
DRIBBLE
DRIVELS
DRIZZLE
DRIZZLY
DWINDLE
ELIYALE
EPISTLE
FAINTLY
FAISALI
FBIFILE
FRIABLE
FRIARLY
FRIBBLE
FRIJOLE
FRIVOLS
FRIZZLE
FRIZZLY
GHIJKLM
GRIDDLE
GRIMILY
GRISTLE
GRISTLY
GRIZZLE
GRIZZLY
IFIFELL
JOINTLY
JUICILY
KRINGLE
MOISTLY
NAIVELY
NOISILY
PLIABLE
PLIABLY
PRICILY
PRICKLE
PRICKLY
PRIMELY
PRINGLE
PRIVILY
QUIBBLE
QUICKLY
QUIETLY
QUINELA
RAINILY
REIMPLY
SAINTLO
SAINTLY
SHINGLE
SHINGLY
SHINILY
SHINOLA
SKIABLE
SKIFFLE
SKIPOLE
SKITTLE
SLICKLY
SLIMILY
SNIDELY
SNIFFLE
SNIFFLY
SNIVELS
SPICILY
SPIKILY
SPINDLE
SPINDLY
SPINELS
SPIRALS
SPITTLE
STIFFLY
STIMULI
STIPPLE
SWIFTLY
SWINDLE
SWIVELS
SWIZZLE
THICKLY
THIMBLE
THIRDLY
THISTLE
THISTLY
TRIABLE
TRIBBLE
TRICKLE
TRIFOLD
TRIPOLI
TRITELY
TVIDOLS
TWIDDLE
TWINKLE
TWINKLY
UNIBALL
VEINULE
WEIRDLY
WHIFFLE
WHIPPLE
WHISTLE
WHITELY
WHITTLE
WRIGGLE
WRIGGLY
WRINKLE
WRINKLY
ZWINGLI

••I•••L

ABIGAIL
BRIMFUL
BRISTOL
EDICTAL
GAINFUL
GUIGNOL
HAIRGEL
IFIFELL
INITIAL
KNIEVEL
MAILLOL
NAIPAUL
PAILFUL
PAINFUL
QUINTAL
SEISMAL
SHIPFUL
SKILFUL
SPIEGEL
STIFFEL
TOILFUL
TRIVIAL
UNIBALL
UNIDEAL
WAILFUL
WEIRDAL

•••IL••

AAMILNE
ABRILES
ACHILLE
AEDILES
ALNILAM
ANTILOG
APHILIP
AUDILES
AVAILED
BACILLI
BASILIC
BASILIO
BONILLA
BRAILLE
BROILED
BROILER
CAMILLA
CAMILLE
CAVILAT
CAVILED
CAVILER
CECILIA
CEDILLA
CIVILLY
COPILOT
DASILVA
DECILES
DEFILED
DEFILER
DEFILES
DELILAH
DELILLO
DEMILLE
DESILTS
DEVILED
DEVILLE
DEVILRY
DEWILDE
DICILLO
EMAILED
EMAILER
ENGILDS
ENOILED
ENSILED
ENSILES
EPSILON
ETAILED
ETAILER
ETOILES
EXOILER
FAMILIA
FAMILLE
FLAILAT
FLAILED
FRAILER
FRAILLY
FRAILTY
FTRILEY
FURILLO
FUSILLI
GALILEE
GALILEI
GALILEO
GAVILAN
GEFILTE
GORILLA
HABILIS
JERILYN
JUBILEE
KURILES
LEVILLI
LUCILLE
MAGILLA
MANILAS
MANILOW
MARILLA
MARILYN
MATILDA
MAXILLA
MEGILLA
MINILAB
MOBILES
MOZILLA
MURILLO
NEUILLY
NEVILLE
OREILLY
ORVILLE
PAPILLA
PERILED
PITILLO
QUAILED
REBILLS
REFILED
REFILES
REFILLS
REFILMS
REGILDS
REMILLS
REOILED
RESILED
RESILES
RETILED
RETILES
RETILLS
REVILED
REVILER
REVILES
RUTILES
SEMILOG
SEVILLA
SEVILLE
SHEILAE
SHEILAS
SHRILLS
SHRILLY
SICILIA
SIMILAC
SIMILAR
SIMILES
SPOILED
SPOILER
THRILLA
THRILLS
TRAILED
TRAILER
TROILUS
UNFILED
UNFILES
UNHILLY
UNOILED
UNPILED
UNPILES
UNRILED
UNSILLY
UNTILED
UPHILLS
UPPILED
UPPILES
UPSILON
UPTILTS
UTRILLO
VANILLA
VANILLI
ZEDILLO

•••I•L•

ACHILLE
ACRIDLY
ADDIBLE
AERIALS
ARTICLE
AUDIBLE
AUDIBLY
AURICLE
BACILLI
BONILLA
BRAILLE
BURIALS
CAMILLA
CAMILLE
CARIOLE
CEDILLA
CIVILLY
CUBICLE
CUBICLY
CUTICLE
DANIELA
DANIELJ
DANIELS
DELILLO
DEMILLE
DENIALS
DEVILLE
DICILLO
ENFIELD
ENTITLE
ESPIALS
FACIALS
FAMILLE
FETIDLY
FINIALS
FLUIDLY
FRAILLY
FURILLO
FUSIBLE
FUSILLI
GAVIALS
GELIDLY
GOGIRLS
GORILLA
HUMIDLY
INFIELD
ITGIRLS
LABIALS
LEGIBLE
LEGIBLY
LEVILLI
LICITLY
LIVIDLY
LUCIDLY
LUCILLE
LURIDLY
MAGILLA
MANIPLE
MARILLA
MAXILLA
MEGILLA
MENIALS
MOZILLA
MURIELS
MURILLO
NEUILLY
NEVILLE
OREILLY
ORVILLE
OSSICLE
PANICLE
PAPILLA
PAVIDLY
PETIOLE
PITILLO
PLAINLY
RABIDLY
RADIALS
RADICLE
RAPIDLY
RAVIOLI
REBILLS
REDIALS
REFILLS
REMILLS
RETICLE
RETILLS
RETITLE
RIGIDLY
RISIBLE
RISIBLY
SERIALS
SEVILLA
SEVILLE
SHRILLS
SHRILLY
SOCIALS
SOLIDLY
STAIDLY
TACITLY
TEPIDLY
THRILLA
THRILLS
TIMIDLY
TUNICLE
UNCIALS
UNFITLY
UNHILLY
UNSILLY
UPFIELD
UPHILLS
UTRILLO
VALIDLY
VANILLA
VANILLI
VAPIDLY
VEHICLE
VESICLE
VISIBLE
VISIBLY
VIVIDLY
WAVICLE
ZEDILLO

•••I••L

ADMIRAL
ARRIVAL
BASINAL
CAPITAL
CAPITOL
CLAIROL
CODICIL
COMICAL
CONICAL
CUBICAL
CUBITAL
CYNICAL
DECIBEL
DECIMAL
DIGITAL
DOMICAL
DOMICIL
DREIDEL
DUTIFUL
ESTIVAL
ETHICAL
FGHIJKL
FINICAL
FLUIDAL
GERITOL
HELICAL
INCIVIL
INFIDEL
KAPITAL
LAMINAL
LEXICAL
LIMINAL
LOGICAL
LYRICAL
MAGICAL
MARITAL
MATINAL
MAXIMAL
MEDICAL
MINIMAL
MUSICAL
NODICAL
NOMINAL
OEDIPAL
OPTICAL
OPTIMAL
ORBITAL
ORDINAL
OVOIDAL
PITIFUL
RADICAL
RECITAL
REGINAL
RETINAL
RETINOL
REVISAL
REVIVAL
SANIBEL
SEMINAL
SHRIVEL
STOICAL
TOPICAL
TYPICAL
UNCIVIL
UNVITAL
VATICAL
VICINAL
VIMINAL
XENICAL
ZOOIDAL

••••IL•

AGNAILS
AIRBILL
AIRMILE
ANGRILY
ANOUILH
ANTHILL
ARSHILE
ARTFILM
ASSAILS
ATATILT
ATHRILL
AVERILL
BAGGILY
BALKILY
BALMILY
BARBILL
BAWDILY
BEADILY
BEEFILY
BEGUILE
BESTILL
BEWAILS
BOBVILA
BONNILY
BOOZILY
BOSSILY
BUMPILY
BUSHILY
BYAMILE
CAMPILY
CANNILY
CANTILY
CASTILE
CATTILY
CHARILY
COCKILY
COMPILE
CORNILY
CRAZILY
CUSHILY
DAFFILY
DANDILY
DATRILS
DAYLILY
DERAILS
DETAILS
DINGILY
DIRTILY
DISTILL
DISTILS
DIZZILY
DOGPILE
DOTTILY
DOWDILY
DUCTILE
DUMPILY
DUSKILY
DUSTILY
EADGILS
EMPTILY
ENTAILS
ENVEILS
ETVOILA
FANCILY
FATTILY
FBIFILE
FEBRILE
FEELILL
FELTILL
FERTILE
FICTILE
FIERILY
FILMILY
FISHILY
FISSILE
FLAKILY
FLEXILE
FLUKILY
FOAMILY
FOGGILY
FOSSILS
FRAGILE
FULFILL
FULFILS
FUNKILY
FUNNILY
FUSSILY
FUSTILY
FUZZILY
GAUDILY
GAUZILY
GAWKILY
GENTILE
GERBILS
GIDDILY
GINMILL
GLAZILY
GOOFILY
GOONILY
GOTMILK
GOUTILY
GRACILE
GRIMILY
GUSHILY
GUSTILY
GUTSILY
HAMMILY
HANDILY
HAPPILY
HARDILY
HASTILY
HEADILY
HEAVILY
HEFTILY
HITFILM
HOARILY
HOGWILD
HORSILY
HOSTILE
HOTMILK
HUFFILY
HUSKILY
ICEMILK
ILLWILL
INAPILE
INBUILT
INEXILE
INSTILL
INSTILS
INTAILS
INUTILE
JAZZILY
JERKILY
JOEHILL
JOLLILY
JUICILY
JUMPILY
KINKILY
LANKILY
LEERILY
LENTILS
LOFTILY
LOONILY
LOUSILY
LOWLILY
LUCKILY
LUMPILY
LUSTILY
MADEILL
MAKEILL
MCNEILL
MEATILY
MERRILL
MERRILY
MESSILY
MILKILY
MISBILL
MISFILE
MISSILE
MISTILY
MOODILY
MOONILY
MOUSILY
MRQUILP
MUDDILY
MURKILY
MUSHILY
MUSSILY
MUSTILY
MUZZILY
NASTILY
NATTILY
NAUTILI
NEEDILY
NERVILY
NIFTILY
NIPPILY
NOBHILL
NOISILY
NONOILY
NUTOILS
NUTTILY
OLDFILM
ONEKILO
ONEMILE
OUTKILL
OUTWILE
OUTWILL
OXTAILS
PANTILE
PENCILS
PEPPILL
PEPPILY
PERKILY
PESKILY
PETTILY
PHONILY
PISTILS
PITHILY
PREBILL
PREFILE
PRICILY
PRIVILY
PROFILE
PROSILY
PUDGILY
PUERILE
PUFFILY
PUNNILY
PUSHILY
QUAKILY
RAINILY
RANWILD
RAWSILK
READILY
REBOILS
REBUILD
REBUILT
RECOILS
REDRILL
REJAILS
REMAILS
RENAILS
REPTILE
RESOILS
RETAILS
RISKILY
RITZILY
ROCKILY
ROOMILY
ROWDILY
RUDDILY
RUNWILD
RUSTILY
SALTILY
SAMHILL
SAPPILY
SASSILY
SAUCILY
SAVVILY
SAWMILL
SCARILY
SEALILY
SEAMILE
SEEDILY
SERVILE
SESSILE
SHADILY
SHAKILY
SHINILY
SHOWILY
SILKILY
SLIMILY
SMOKILY
SNAKILY
SNOWILY
SOAPILY
SOGGILY
SOOTILY
SORRILY
SOYMILK
SPICILY
SPIKILY
STABILE
STAGILY
STERILE
STONILY
SUBFILE
SULKILY
SUNNILY
SURLILY
SWAHILI
TACKILY
TACTILE
TAKEILL
TARDILY
TAROILS
TARTILY
TASTILY
TATTILY
TAWNILY
TEARILY
TENMILE
TENSILE
TEQUILA
TESTILY
TEXTILE
THEHILL
THENILE
TINNILY
TIPSILY
TMOBILE
TONSILS
TOOKILL
TORVILL
TUTUILA
UNAGILE
UNBUILD
UNBUILT
UNCOILS
UNFRILL
UNNAILS
UNSPILT
UNVEILS
UPBUILD
UPCOILS
URACILS
VERYILL
WACKILY
WASPILY
WASSILY
WAYBILL
WEARILY
WEEDILY
WEEVILS
WINDILY
WISPILY
WITTILY
WOOZILY
WORDILY
ZESTILY

••••I•L

AIRBILL

ANTHILL
ASOCIAL
ATHRILL
AVERILL
BADGIRL
BAGGIRL
BALLIOL
BARBILL
BATGIRL
BESTIAL
BESTILL
BIAXIAL
BIGGIRL
BUSGIRL
CAMGIRL
CARDIAL
COAXIAL
CORDIAL
COWGIRL
CRANIAL
CRUCIAL
DISTILL
ELUVIAL
EZEKIEL
FASCIAL
FEELILL
FELTILL
FLUVIAL
FLYGIRL
FULFILL
GABRIEL
GINMILL
GLACIAL
ILLWILL
INITIAL
INSTILL
ISCHIAL
JIMDIAL
JOEHILL
MADEILL
MAKEILL
MARTIAL
MCNEILL
MERRILL
MIAMIFL
MISBILL
MISDIAL
MONDIAL
NOBHILL
NUPTIAL
OLDGIRL
ONTRIAL
OUTKILL
OUTWILL
PARTIAL
PEPPILL
PLUVIAL
PREBILL
REDRILL
RETRIAL
SAMHILL
SAWMILL
SPACIAL
SPANIEL
SPATIAL
SPECIAL
SUNDIAL
TAKEILL

TENNIEL
THEHILL
TOOKILL
TORVILL
TRIVIAL
UMBRIEL
UNFRILL
UPWHIRL
UXORIAL
VERYILL
VITRIOL
WAYBILL

•••••IL

ABIGAIL
AIRFOIL
AIRMAIL
ALLHAIL
ANTHEIL
ATABOIL
BABYOIL
BATHOIL
BEANOIL
BEDEVIL
BEDRAIL
BOBTAIL
CATTAIL
CHERVIL
COALOIL
CODICIL
CORNOIL
COUNCIL
CURTAIL
DAYQUIL
DAYSAIL
DESPOIL
DOGTAIL
DOMICIL
DWEEZIL
EMBROIL
ESTORIL
FANEUIL
FANMAIL
FANTAIL
FISHOIL
FOXTAIL
FUELOIL
GELUSIL
GODEVIL
GONERIL
GULFOIL
HOBNAIL
HOLYOIL
HOTMAIL
IMPERIL
INAPRIL
INCIVIL
INPERIL
JETFOIL
JONQUIL
LAMPOIL
LESTOIL
LUGSAIL
MACNEIL
MIKHAIL
NONEVIL
NOSTRIL
OLEOOIL

OUTRAIL
OUTSAIL
PALMOIL
PARBOIL
PIGTAIL
PINEOIL
PINTAIL
POTBOIL
PREBOIL
PRECOIL
PREVAIL
RATTAIL
REAVAIL
REDTAIL
ROCKOIL
ROSEOIL
SETBAIL
SETSAIL
STBASIL
STENCIL
SUBSOIL
SURVEIL
TENDRIL
TINFOIL
TOENAIL
TOPSAIL
TOPSOIL
TOYPAIL
TRAVAIL
TREFOIL
TRYSAIL
TUNAOIL
TUNGOIL
TURMOIL
UNCIVIL
UNFRAIL
UTENSIL
VERMEIL
WASSAIL
WEBMAIL

IM•••••

IMADEIT
IMAGERS
IMAGERY
IMAGINE
IMAGING
IMAGISM
IMAGIST
IMAGOES
IMAHOGG
IMAMATE
IMAMESS
IMARETS
IMBIBED
IMBIBER
IMBIBES
IMBORED
IMBROKE
IMBRUED
IMBRUES
IMBUING
IMEANIT
IMEMINE
IMFORIT
IMGOING
IMGREAT
IMHAPPY

IMHOTEP
IMITATE
IMMENSE
IMMERGE
IMMERSE
IMMIXED
IMMIXES
IMMORAL
IMMUNES
IMMURED
IMMURES
IMOGENE
IMPACTS
IMPAIRS
IMPALAS
IMPALED
IMPALER
IMPALES
IMPANEL
IMPARTS
IMPASSE
IMPASTO
IMPAVID
IMPEACH
IMPEDED
IMPEDER
IMPEDES
IMPENDS
IMPERIL
IMPETUS
IMPIETY
IMPINGE
IMPIOUS
IMPLANT
IMPLEAD
IMPLIED
IMPLIES
IMPLODE
IMPLORE
IMPORTS
IMPOSED
IMPOSER
IMPOSES
IMPOSTS
IMPOUND
IMPRESS
IMPREST
IMPREZA
IMPRINT
IMPROVE
IMPUGNS
IMPULSE
IMPURER
IMPUTED
IMPUTER
IMPUTES
IMREADY
IMSORRY
IMSWELL
IMTHERE
IMTIRED
IMUSTGO
IMYOURS

I•M••••

IAMBICS
IAMBIST
IAMLOVE

IMMENSE
IMMERGE
IMMERSE
IMMIXED
IMMIXES
IMMORAL
IMMUNES
IMMURED
IMMURES
INMARCH
INMATES
IOMOTHS
ITMAYBE

I••M•••

ICEMILK
ILLMADE
IMAMATE
IMAMESS
IMEMINE
INAMESS
INAMOOD
INKMARK
ISHMAEL
ISOMERS
ITEMING
ITEMISE
ITEMIZE
ITEMONE

I•••M••

IDEAMAN
IDEAMEN
IDIAMIN
IFWEMAY
IJKLMNO
ILIAMNA
ILLUMED
ILLUMES
INCOMER
INCOMES
INGEMAR
INHUMAN
INHUMED
INHUMER
INHUMES
INLIMBO
IRONMAN
IRONMEN
ISLAMIC
ISTHMUS
ISTOMIN

I••••M•

ICEDAMS
INFLAME
INFORMS
INSEAMS
IONIUMS
IPANEMA
IRKSOME
ISONOMY
ITSONME
ITSTIME
IWOJIMA

I•••••M

IANHOLM

IMAGISM
INAPOEM
INBLOOM
INTERIM
IONBEAM
IRIDIUM
IRSFORM
ISCHIUM
ISOGRAM
ISUREAM

•IM••••

AIMEDAT
AIMHIGH
AIMLESS
AIMSFOR
BIMBOES
BIMETAL
BIMINIS
BIMODAL
CIMABUE
DIMAGES
DIMBULB
DIMETER
DIMITRI
DIMMERS
DIMMEST
DIMMING
DIMNESS
DIMOUTS
DIMPLED
DIMPLES
DIMSOUT
DIMVIEW
DIMWITS
GIMBALS
GIMBELS
GIMLETS
GIMMICK
GIMPING
HIMALIA
HIMSELF
JIMBEAM
JIMCHEE
JIMDALE
JIMDIAL
JIMENEZ
JIMFIXX
JIMHOGG
JIMINEZ
JIMJAMS
JIMKAAT
JIMMIED
JIMMIES
JIMRICE
JIMRYUN
JIMSONS
KIMBALL
KIMCHEE
KIMONOS
LIMACON
LIMBERS
LIMBING
LIMBURG
LIMEADE
LIMEPIE
LIMIEST
LIMINAL

LIMITED
LIMITER
LIMNERS
LIMNING
LIMNITE
LIMOGES
LIMPEST
LIMPETS
LIMPING
LIMPOPO
MIMEOED
MIMESES
MIMESIS
MIMETIC
MIMICRY
MIMIEUX
MIMOSAS
NIMBLER
NIMIETY
NIMRODS
PIMENTO
PIMESON
PIMLICO
PIMPLED
PIMPLES
RIMBAUD
RIMIEST
RIMLESS
RIMMING
RIMPLED
RIMPLES
RIMROCK
RIMSHOT
SIMCITY
SIMENON
SIMIANS
SIMILAC
SIMILAR
SIMILES
SIMMERS
SIMMONS
SIMONIZ
SIMPERS
SIMPLER
SIMPLES
SIMPLEX
SIMPSON
TIMBALE
TIMBALS
TIMBERS
TIMBERY
TIMBRES
TIMECOP
TIMELAG
TIMEOFF
TIMEOUT
TIMESUP
TIMEWAS
TIMEXES
TIMHOLT
TIMIDER
TIMIDLY
TIMINGS
TIMMINS
TIMOTHY
TIMPANI
TIMREID
TIMRICE

TIMROTH
VIMINAL
WIMOWEH
WIMPIER
WIMPING
WIMPISH
WIMPLED
WIMPLES
WIMPOLE
WIMPOUT
XIMENES
ZIMARRA

•I•M•••

AILMENT
AIRMADA
AIRMAIL
AIRMASS
AIRMILE
BIGMACS
BIGMAMA
BIGMEAL
BIGMESS
BIOMASS
BIRMANS
BISMUTH
BITMAPS
DIAMOND
DIEMENS
DIMMERS
DIMMEST
DIMMING
DINMONT
DIOMEDE
DISMALS
DISMAST
DISMAYS
DISMISS
FIGMENT
FILMDOM
FILMIER
FILMILY
FILMING
FILMSET
FIRMEST
FIRMING
FIRMSUP
GILMORE
GIMMICK
GINMILL
JIMMIED
JIMMIES
KINMONT
KIRMANS
KISMETS
LIPMANN
MIAMIAN
MIAMIFL
MICMACS
MIDMORN
MIDMOST
MISMARK
MISMATE
MISMESH
MISMOVE
NIPMUCK
PIGMEAT
PIGMENT

PISMIRE
RIBMEAT
RIEMANN
RIMMING
RIOMUNI
SIAMESE
SIEMENS
SIGMOID
SIGMUND
SIMMERS
SIMMONS
TIEMPOS
TIMMINS
TINMINE
TIOMKIN
TITMICE
WIDMARK

•I••M••

BIRDMAN
BIRDMEN
BIREMES
CINEMAS
CINEMAX
DILEMMA
DILLMAN
DISCMAN
EIJKMAN
FIREMAN
FIREMEN
FIVEMAN
GILLMAN
HICKMAN
HILLMAN
HILLMEN
JICAMAS
KINGMAN
KINSMAN
KINSMEN
LIKEMAD
LINEMAN
LINEMEN
MIASMAL
MIASMAS
MIASMIC
MILKMAN
MILKMEN
MINIMAL
MINIMAX
MINIMUM
MINIMUS
MIRAMAR
MIRAMAX
NICEMAN
NICEMEN
PITTMAN
RICHMAN
RICHMEN
RICKMAN
RIESMAN
RITAMAE
SIDEMAN
SIDEMEN
SITEMAP
TINAMOU
TIREMAN
TIREMEN
VICOMTE

VITAMIN
WILDMAN
WILDMEN
WINGMAN
WINGMEN
WIREMAN
WIREMEN
WISEMAN
WISEMEN

•I•••M•

AIRDAMS
AIRPUMP
AIRTIME
BIGGAME
BIGMAMA
BIGNAME
BIGTIME
DIADEMS
DIATOMS
DICTUMS
DIDSUMS
DIDTIME
DIGRAMS
DILEMMA
DIORAMA
DIOTIMA
DIPLOMA
DIRHAMS
DISARMS
GIACOMO
GINGAME
HIJKLMN
HITHOME
JIGTIME
JIMJAMS
KIDCOMS
LISSOME
MIAHAMM
MILLIME
MISAIMS
MISHIMA
MISNAME
MISTIME
OILLAMP
PINCHME
SILLYME
SITCOMS
SITHOME
TIEGAME
VICTIMS
WIGWAMS
WINDOMS
WINSOME
WISDOMS
ZITCOMS

•I••••M

BINGHAM
DIAGRAM
DIGICAM
DINADAM
EIGHTAM
EIGHTPM
FIEFDOM
FILMDOM
FIREARM
GILLIAM

GINGHAM
HITFILM
JIBBOOM
JIMBEAM
KINGDOM
LIPBALM
LITHIUM
MIAHAMM
MIDTERM
MILLDAM
MINICAM
MINIMUM
MISDEEM
MISFORM
MISTERM
MITCHUM
NIOBIUM
OILDRUM
OILPALM
PIANISM
PILGRIM
PINETUM
PINKHAM
RITAGAM
SIDEARM
SIKHISM
SILENTM
TIDYSUM
TIEBEAM
TINYTIM
TITOISM
VIETNAM
WILHELM
WILLIAM
ZIONISM

••IM•••

ALIMENT
ALIMONY
ANIMACY
ANIMALS
ANIMATE
ANIMATO
ANIMISM
ANIMIST
ASIMMER
AZIMUTH
BLIMPIE
BRIMFUL
BRIMLEY
BRIMMED
BRIMMER
CAIMANS
CHIMEIN
CHIMERA
CHIMERS
CHIMING
CHIMINH
CHIMNEY
CLIMATE
CLIMATS
CLIMBED
CLIMBER
CLIMBIN
CLIMBON
CLIMBTO
CLIMBUP
CRIMEAN

CRIMINY
CRIMPED
CRIMPER
CRIMSON
DAIMLER
GLIMMER
GLIMPSE
GRIMACE
GRIMIER
GRIMILY
GRIMING
GRIMMER
GRIMSBY
HAIMISH
MAIMERS
MAIMING
MAIMITI
PRIMACY
PRIMARY
PRIMATE
PRIMELY
PRIMERA
PRIMERO
PRIMERS
PRIMING
PRIMMED
PRIMMER
PRIMPED
RAIMENT
REIMAGE
REIMPLY
SHIMMER
SKIMASK
SKIMMED
SKIMMER
SKIMPED
SKIMPON
SLIMIER
SLIMILY
SLIMING
SLIMJIM
SLIMMED
SLIMMER
STIMSON
STIMULI
SWIMMER
SWIMSUP
THIMBLE
THIMPHU
TRIMMED
TRIMMER
TRIMOFF
TRIMTAB
TZIMMES
WHIMPER

••I•M••

ASIMMER
BRIMMED
BRIMMER
ENIGMAS
GLIMMER
GRIDMAP
GRIMMER
HEISMAN
IDIAMIN
ILIAMNA
MAILMAN

MAILMEN
MAINMAN
MAINMEN
PRIMMED
PRIMMER
RAILMAN
RAILMEN
RAINMAN
REITMAN
SEISMAL
SEISMIC
SHIMMER
SHIPMAN
SHIPMEN
SKIMMED
SKIMMER
SLIMMED
SLIMMER
STIGMAS
SWIMMER
THIAMIN
THINMAN
TRIMMED
TRIMMER
TRIUMPH
TZIMMES
WEIDMAN
WHITMAN

••I••M•

DRINKME
EDINAMN
EPITOME
FLINTMI
NOISOME
ORIGAMI
RHIZOME
SKIBUMS
SKIJUMP
SUITSME
TRIREME
UNISOMS
WRITEME

••I•••M

ALIFORM
ANIMISM
BRIGHAM
BRITCOM
CHILLUM
ELITISM
EPIDERM
EPIGRAM
GHIJKLM
GRISHAM
GRISSOM
HEIRDOM
IRIDIUM
JAINISM
LEITRIM
OVIFORM
SLIMJIM
STICKUM
TRIFORM
TRIGRAM
TRITIUM
TRIVIUM
UNIFORM

•••IM••
AJSIMON
ALTIMAS
ATTIMES
BETIMES
CASIMIR
CLAIMED
CLAIMER
DECIMAL
DELIMAN
DELIMEN
DELIMIT
DENIMED
DONIMUS
ESKIMOS
FADIMAN
INLIMBO
LATIMES
MARIMBA
MAXIMAL
MAXIMAS
MAXIMUM
MAXIMUS
MERIMEE
MINIMAL
MINIMAX
MINIMUM
MINIMUS
NOLIMIT
NYTIMES
OMNIMAX
OPTIMAL
OPTIMAS
OPTIMUM
REAIMED
REGIMEN
REGIMES
RELIMIT
RETIMED
RETIMES
SCRIMPS
SCRIMPY
SHRIMPS
SHRIMPY
STSIMON
SURIMIS
TAXIMAN
TAXIMEN
ULTIMAS
UNAIMED
UNRIMED
UNTIMED
UNTIMID
UPTIMES
YAKIMAS
ZOSIMUS

•••I•M•
AFFIRMS
ALLIUMS
ANDIAMO
ATRIUMS
CHRISMS
IONIUMS
MEDIUMS
MELISMA
PODIUMS
PRFIRMS
REFILMS
SCHISMS
SQUIRMS
SQUIRMY
TAMIAMI
TEDIUMS
THEISMS
TRUISMS
TURISMO
VERISMO
WOEISME

•••I••M
ALNILAM
CHRISOM
DELIHAM
DIGICAM
FAMICOM
FEMINUM
HASIDIM
HOTITEM
MAXIMUM
MINICAM
MINIMUM
MODICUM
OPTIMUM
STEINEM
SUBITEM
SURINAM
YOGIISM

••••IM•
AIRTIME
ALLTIME
ANYTIME
ATATIME
BADTIME
BEDTIME
BEGRIME
BIGTIME
BUDTIME
BUYTIME
CENTIME
CENTIMO
CUTTIME
DAYTIME
DIDTIME
DIOTIMA
EXANIMO
FUNTIME
HADTIME
HASTIME
HOTTIME
ITSTIME
IWOJIMA
JIGTIME
KEYLIME
LACRIMO
MAYTIME
MEGRIMS
MILLIME
MISAIMS
MISHIMA
MISTIME
MUSLIMS
NANAIMO
NAPTIME
OLDTIME
ONEDIME
ONETIME
OUTLIMN
PASTIME
PRELIMS
PROXIMA
PROXIMO
RAGTIME
RECLIMB
REPRIME
RESWIMS
RETRIMS
RORAIMA
RUNTIME
SASHIMI
SUBLIME
TEATIME
TEETIME
THESIMS
TWOTIME
UPCLIMB
VICTIMS
WARTIME
ZOSSIMA

••••I•M
AGONISM
ANIMISM
ARTFILM
ATAVISM
ATHEISM
ATOMISM
BAALISM
BAHAISM
BAPTISM
BELGIUM
BOHRIUM
BOSSISM
BRUXISM
CADMIUM
CALCIUM
CARDIUM
COMTISM
CONFIRM
CRANIUM
CULTISM
CZARISM
DADAISM
DUALISM
DUBNIUM
ECHOISM
EGOTISM
ELITISM
ELUVIUM
ELYSIUM
EXOTISM
FADDISM
FASCISM
FAUVISM
FERMIUM
FOGYISM
GALLIUM
GILLIAM
GRECISM
HAFNIUM
HAHNIUM
HASSIUM
HEREIAM
HEROISM
HITFILM
HOBOISM
HOLMIUM
IMAGISM
IRIDIUM
ISCHIUM
JAINISM
JUDAISM
LAMAISM
LEFTISM
LITHIUM
LOOKISM
LUDDISM
MAHDISM
MARXISM
MERRIAM
MOBBISM
NATRIUM
NIOBIUM
OLDFILM
ORARIUM
PENTIUM
PERDIEM
PIANISM
PREMIUM
REALISM
REQUIEM
RHENIUM
RHODIUM
SIKHISM
SOPHISM
STADIUM
STATISM
SUREIAM
TERBIUM
THEFIRM
THORIUM
THULIUM
TITOISM
TORYISM
TOURISM
TRITIUM
TRIVIUM
TROPISM
TSARISM
URANIUM
UTOPISM
WILLIAM
YOGIISM
YTTRIUM
ZANYISM
ZIONISM

•••••IM
ACCLAIM
ANAHEIM
DECLAIM
EPHRAIM
EXCLAIM
GOODAIM
GREWDIM
GROWDIM
HASIDIM
HATBRIM
HAZANIM
INTERIM
JOACHIM
LCHAYIM
LEITRIM
LORDJIM
MANHEIM
ONAWHIM
OUTSWIM
PILGRIM
PRETRIM
RECLAIM
SLIMJIM
TAKEAIM
TINYTIM
TOOKAIM

IN•••••
INABALL
INABIND
INACAST
INADAZE
INAFUNK
INAFURY
INAHEAP
INAHOLE
INAHUFF
INAIDOF
INAJIFF
INAKNOT
INALINE
INAMESS
INAMOOD
INANELY
INANEST
INANITY
INAPILE
INAPOEM
INAPOKE
INAPRIL
INAPTER
INAPTLY
INARAGE
INARUSH
INASHOE
INASNAP
INASNIT
INASPIN
INASPOT
INASTEW
INASTIR
INASUIT
INATRAP
INAVALE
INAWEOF
INAWINK
INAWORD
INBLACK
INBLOOM
INBOARD
INBOUND
INBOXES
INBREED
INBRIEF
INBROWN
INBUILT
INCANTS
INCASED
INCASES
INCENSE
INCENTS
INCEPTS
INCHECK
INCHERS
INCHING
INCISED
INCISES
INCISOR
INCITED
INCITER
INCITES
INCIVIL
INCLASS
INCLINE
INCLOSE
INCLUDE
INCOLOR
INCOMER
INCOMES
INCOURT
INCROWD
INCRUST
INCUBUS
INCUDES
INCURVE
INCUSED
INCUSES
INDEEDY
INDENTS
INDEPTH
INDEXED
INDEXER
INDEXES
INDIANA
INDIANS
INDICES
INDICIA
INDICTS
INDIGEN
INDIGOS
INDITED
INDITER
INDITES
INDOORS
INDORSE
INDOUBT
INDRAFT
INDRAWN
INDUCED
INDUCER
INDUCES
INDUCTS
INDULGE
INDUTCH
INDWELL
INDWELT
INDYCAR
INEDITA
INEPTLY
INERROR
INERTIA
INERTLY
INEXACT
INEXILE
INFAITH
INFANCY
INFANTA
INFANTE
INFANTS
INFAVOR
INFECTS
INFERNO
INFESTS
INFIDEL
INFIELD
INFIRST
INFIVES
INFIXED
INFIXES
INFLAME
INFLATE
INFLECT
INFLICT
INFLOWS
INFOCUS
INFOLDS
INFORCE
INFORIT
INFORMS
INFRACT
INFRONT
INFUSED
INFUSER
INFUSES
INGALLS
INGATES
INGEMAR
INGENUE
INGESTA
INGESTS
INGLESE
INGOALS
INGOING
INGRAFT
INGRAIN
INGRATE
INGREEN
INGRESS
INGROUP
INGROWN
INGULFS
INHABIT
INHALED
INHALER
INHALES
INHASTE
INHERED
INHERES
INHERIT
INHIBIT
INHOUSE
INHUMAN
INHUMED
INHUMER
INHUMES
ININETY
INIRONS
INITIAL
INJECTS
INJOKES
INJURED
INJURER
INJURES
INKBLOT
INKEDIN
INKHORN
INKIEST
INKINGS
INKJETS
INKLESS
INKLIKE
INKLING
INKMARK
INKNOTS
INKPADS
INKPOTS
INKSACS
INKSPOT
INKSTER
INKWELL
INKYCAP
INLABOR
INLANDS
INLARGE
INLAYER
INLIMBO
INLINES
INLYING
INMARCH
INMATES
INNAGES
INNARDS
INNERLY
INNERVE
INNINGS
INNLESS
INNOWAY
INOCULA
INORBIT
INORDER
INPEACE
INPERIL
INPHASE
INPLACE
INPOINT
INPOURS
INPOWER
INPRINT
INQUEST
INQUIRE
INQUIRY
INRANGE
INREACH
INROADS
INRUINS
INSALES
INSANER
INSCALE
INSEAMS
INSECTA
INSECTS
INSERTS
INSHAPE
INSHOCK
INSHORE
INSHORT
INSIDER
INSIDES
INSIGHT
INSIGNE
INSIPID
INSISTS
INSOFAR
INSOLES
INSPACE
INSPANS
INSPECT
INSPIRE
INSPITE
INSPOTS
INSTALL
INSTALS
INSTANT
INSTATE
INSTEAD
INSTEPS
INSTILL
INSTILS
INSTOCK
INSTONE
INSTORE
INSTYLE
INSULAR
INSULIN
INSULTS
INSURED
INSURER
INSURES
INSWEPT
INSYNCH
INTAILS
INTAKES
INTASTE
INTEARS
INTEGER
INTEGRA
INTENDS
INTENSE
INTENTS
INTERIM
INTERNE
INTERNS
INTERSE
INTHERE
INTHING
INTHIRD
INTHREE
INTONED
INTONER
INTONES
INTOTAL
INTOUCH
INTRADE
INTRAYS
INTROIT
INTRUDE
INTRUST
INTRUTH
INTUITS
INTURNS
INULASE
INURING
INUTERO
INUTILE
INVACUO
INVADED
INVADER
INVADES
INVALID
INVEIGH
INVENTS
INVERSE
INVERTS
INVESTS
INVICTA
INVITED
INVITEE
INVITER
INVITES
INVITRO
INVOGUE
INVOICE
INVOKED
INVOKER
INVOKES
INVOLVE
INWARDS
INWEAVE
INWHITE
INWOVEN
INYEARS

I•N••••
IANHOLM
IBNSAUD
IGNARRO
IGNATOW
IGNEOUS
IGNITED
IGNITER
IGNITES
IGNITOR
IGNOBLE
IGNOBLY
IGNORED
IGNORER
IGNORES
IINSIST
IKNEWIT
IKNOWIT
INNAGES
INNARDS
INNERLY
INNERVE
INNINGS
INNLESS
INNOWAY
IONBEAM
IONESCO
IONIANS
IONISED
IONISER
IONISES
IONIUMS
IONIZED
IONIZER
IONIZES
IONONES

I••N•••
ICANNOT
ICINESS
ICINGIN
ICINGIT
ICINGUP
ICONIFY
IDENTIC
ILLNESS
INANELY
INANEST
INANITY
ININETY
INKNOTS
IPANEMA
IRANIAN
IRENICS
IRONAGE
IRONBAR
IRONERS
IRONIES
IRONING
IRONIST
IRONMAN
IRONMEN
IRONONS
IRONORE
IRONOUT
IRONSON
ISONOMY
IVANHOE
IVANIII
IVANOVO
IWANTIT
IWANTTO
IWONDER

I•••N••
ICANNOT
ICTINUS
IGUANAS
IGUANID
IIKINGS
ILLKNOW
IMEANIT
IMMENSE
IMMUNES
IMPANEL
IMPENDS
IMPINGE
INAKNOT
INASNAP
INASNIT
INCANTS
INCENSE
INCENTS
INDENTS
INFANCY
INFANTA
INFANTE
INFANTS
INGENUE
INKINGS
INLANDS
INLINES
INNINGS
INRANGE
INSANER
INSYNCH
INTENDS
INTENSE
INTENTS
INTONED
INTONER
INTONES
INVENTS
IONONES
ISEENOW
ISLANDS
ITSONME
ITWENTY

I••••N•
IBIZANS
ICELAND
ICELINE
ICERINK
ICERUNS
ICEWINE
ICYWIND
IFORONE
IFSTONE
IGRAINE
IJKLMNO
IKEBANA
ILIAMNA
ILLDONE
ILLEANA
ILLWIND
ILOCANO
IMAGINE
IMAGING
IMBUING
IMEMINE
IMGOING
IMOGENE
IMPLANT
IMPOUND
IMPRINT
IMPUGNS
INABIND
INAFUNK
INALINE
INAWINK
INBOUND
INCHING
INCLINE
INDIANA
INDIANS
INFERNO
INFRONT
INGOING
INIRONS
INKLING
INLYING
INPOINT
INPRINT
INRUINS
INSIGNE
INSPANS
INSTANT
INSTONE
INTERNE
INTERNS
INTHING
INTURNS
INURING
IONIANS
IRELAND
IRISING
IRONING
IRONONS
ISAIDNO
ISECOND
ISOGONS
ISOLINE
ISOTONE
ISSUANT
ISSUING
ITCHING
ITEMING
ITEMONE
ITERANT
ITSDONE
ITSFINE
ITSGONE
IVORINE

I•••••N
IBERIAN
ICEDOWN
ICHDIEN
ICINGIN
IDAHOAN
IDEAMAN
IDEAMEN
IDIAMIN
IIIJOHN
INASPIN
INBROWN
INDIGEN
INDRAWN
INGRAIN
INGREEN
INGROWN
INHUMAN
INKEDIN
INKHORN
INSULIN
INWOVEN
IRANIAN
IRECKON
IRESIGN
IRONMAN
IRONMEN
IRONSON
ISFAHAN
ISTOMIN
ISTRIAN
ITALIAN
ITHACAN
ITSASIN
ITSOPEN
IVERSON
IVORIAN
IZATION

•IN••••
AINTHAY
BINDERS
BINDERY
BINDING
BINDLES
BINDOFF
BINDSTO
BINDSUP
BINGERS
BINGHAM
BINGING
BINGLES
BINGOES
BINNING
BINOCHE
CINCHED
CINCHES
CINDERS

CINDERY
CINEMAS
CINEMAX
CINEOLE
CINERGY
CINESIA
CINQUES
CINZANO
DINADAM
DINARIC
DINDINS
DINEDAT
DINEDIN
DINEDON
DINEOUT
DINESAT
DINESEN
DINESIN
DINESON
DINETTE
DINGBAT
DINGERS
DINGIER
DINGILY
DINGING
DINGLES
DINGOES
DINKIER
DINMONT
DINNERS
DINNING
DINTING
FINABLE
FINAGLE
FINALES
FINALLY
FINANCE
FINBACK
FINCHES
FINDERS
FINDING
FINDLAY
FINDLEY
FINDOUT
FINEART
FINESSE
FINGALS
FINGERS
FINIALS
FINIANS
FINICAL
FINICKY
FINISHD
FINITES
FINKING
FINKSON
FINLAND
FINLESS
FINLIKE
FINNAIR
FINNIER
FINNISH
GINFIZZ
GINGAME
GINGERS
GINGERY
GINGHAM
GINGIVA

GINGKOS
GINGOLD
GINKGOS
GINMILL
GINNING
GINSENG
HINDERS
HINDLEG
HINDPAW
HINGEON
HINGING
HINKIER
HINNIES
HINTERS
HINTING
HINTSAT
IINSIST
JINGLED
JINGLER
JINGLES
JINGOES
JINXERS
JINXING
KINCAID
KINDEST
KINDLED
KINDLER
KINDLES
KINDRED
KINESES
KINESIC
KINESIS
KINETIC
KINFOLK
KINGDOM
KINGING
KINGLET
KINGMAN
KINGPIN
KINGRAT
KINGTUT
KINISON
KINKAID
KINKIER
KINKILY
KINKING
KINLESS
KINMONT
KINNEAR
KINNELL
KINSHIP
KINSMAN
KINSMEN
LINABLE
LINAGES
LINBIAO
LINCOLN
LINDENS
LINDIED
LINDIES
LINDNER
LINDORF
LINDROS
LINDSAY
LINDSEY
LINEAGE
LINEARA
LINEARB

LINEATE
LINECUT
LINEDRY
LINEDUP
LINEMAN
LINEMEN
LINEONE
LINEOUT
LINESUP
LINETWO
LINEUPS
LINGCOD
LINGERS
LINGOES
LINGUAE
LINGUAL
LINGULA
LINIEST
LININGS
LINKAGE
LINKERS
LINKING
LINKSUP
LINKUPS
LINNETS
LINPIAO
LINSEED
LINTELS
LINTERS
LINTIER
LINTING
MINABLE
MINARET
MINCERS
MINCING
MINDERS
MINDFUL
MINDING
MINDORO
MINDSET
MINEOLA
MINEPIT
MINERAL
MINERVA
MINGIER
MINGLED
MINGLER
MINGLES
MINIBAR
MINIBUS
MINICAB
MINICAM
MINICAR
MINIKIN
MINILAB
MINIMAL
MINIMAX
MINIMUM
MINIMUS
MININGS
MINIONS
MINISKI
MINISUB
MINITVS
MINIVAC
MINIVAN
MINIVER
MINIZOO

MINNOWS
MINOANS
MINOGUE
MINOLTA
MINORCA
MINORED
MINORIN
MINOTND
MINSKYS
MINSTER
MINTAGE
MINTERS
MINTIER
MINTING
MINTTEA
MINUEND
MINUETS
MINUSES
MINUTED
MINUTER
MINUTES
MINUTIA
MINXISH
MINYANS
NINEEEE
NINEPIN
NINEVEH
NINNIES
NINTHLY
OINKERS
OINKING
PINATAS
PINBALL
PINBOYS
PINCERS
PINCHAS
PINCHED
PINCHER
PINCHES
PINCHME
PINCHOT
PINCURL
PINDOWN
PINEFOR
PINENUT
PINEOIL
PINESAP
PINESOL
PINETAR
PINETOP
PINETUM
PINFOLD
PINGERS
PINGING
PINGUID
PINHEAD
PINHOLE
PINIEST
PINIONS
PINKENS
PINKEST
PINKETT
PINKHAM
PINKIES
PINKING
PINKISH
PINKOES
PINLESS

PINNACE
PINNATE
PINNERS
PINNING
PINOAKS
PINONES
PINOTTA
PINSEAL
PINTAIL
PINWALE
QINTARS
RINALDO
RINDIER
RINGERS
RINGFOR
RINGING
RINGLET
RINGOFF
RINGOUT
RINGSIN
RINGSUP
RINKRAT
RINSERS
RINSING
SINATRA
SINCERE
SINCITY
SINDBAD
SINEDIE
SINEWED
SINGERS
SINGING
SINGLED
SINGLES
SINGLET
SINGOUT
SINGSTO
SINKAGE
SINKERS
SINKING
SINKSIN
SINLESS
SINLIKE
SINNERS
SINNING
SINUATE
SINUOUS
SINUSES
SINUTAB
TINAFEY
TINAMOU
TINCANS
TINCTED
TINDERS
TINDERY
TINEARS
TINFISH
TINFOIL
TINGING
TINGLED
TINGLER
TINGLES
TINGODS
TINHATS
TINHORN
TINIEST
TINKERS
TINKLED

TINKLER
TINKLES
TINLIKE
TINMINE
TINNERS
TINNIER
TINNILY
TINNING
TINORES
TINROOF
TINSELS
TINSTAR
TINTERN
TINTERS
TINTING
TINTYPE
TINWARE
TINWORK
TINYBIT
TINYTIM
TINYTOT
VINCENT
VINCULA
VINEGAR
VINIEST
VINLAND
VINROSE
VINTAGE
VINTNER
VINYLIC
WINBACK
WINCERS
WINCHED
WINCHER
WINCHES
WINCING
WINDAGE
WINDAUS
WINDBAG
WINDERS
WINDGOD
WINDIER
WINDIGO
WINDILY
WINDING
WINDOMS
WINDOWS
WINDOWY
WINDSOR
WINDSUP
WINDTEE
WINDUPS
WINEBAR
WINERED
WINESAP
WINEVAT
WINFREY
WINGERS
WINGING
WINGLET
WINGMAN
WINGMEN
WINGNUT
WINGSIT
WINGTIP
WINIEST
WINKERS
WINKING

WINKLER
WINKOUT
WINKSAT
WINLESS
WINNERS
WINNING
WINNOWS
WINOVER
WINSBIG
WINSLET
WINSLOW
WINSOME
WINSOUT
WINSTON
WINTERS
WINTERY
WINWOOD
XINGOUT
ZINCIFY
ZINCING
ZINCITE
ZINCKED
ZINCOUS
ZINGERS
ZINGIER
ZINGING
ZINKIER
ZINNIAS

•I•N•••

AIRNESS
BIANCHI
BIENNIA
BIENTOT
BIGNAME
BIGNESS
BIGNEWS
BIGNOSE
BINNING
BIONICS
DIGNIFY
DIGNITY
DIMNESS
DINNERS
DINNING
DIPNETS
DIRNDLS
FIANCEE
FIANCES
FIENNES
FINNAIR
FINNIER
FINNISH
FITNESS
GINNING
HINNIES
HIPNESS
HISNIBS
JITNEYS
KIDNAPS
KIDNEYS
KILNDRY
KILNING
KINNEAR
KINNELL
LIENEES
LIENORS
LIGNIFY
LIGNINS
LIGNITE
LIMNERS
LIMNING
LIMNITE
LINNETS
LIONCUB
LIONELL
LIONELS
LIONESS
LIONETS
LIONISE
LIONIZE
MIDNOON
MIGNONS
MINNOWS
MISNAME
NIANTIC
NINNIES
PIANISM
PIANIST
PIANOLA
PICNICS
PIGNUTS
PINNACE
PINNATE
PINNERS
PINNING
PIONEER
RIANTLY
SIENESE
SIENNAS
SIGNAGE
SIGNALS
SIGNEES
SIGNERS
SIGNETS
SIGNFOR
SIGNIFY
SIGNING
SIGNOFF
SIGNORA
SIGNORE
SIGNORS
SIGNOUT
SIGNSIN
SIGNSON
SIGNSUP
SIGNUPS
SINNERS
SINNING
SIXNINE
TIENDAS
TINNERS
TINNIER
TINNILY
TINNING
VIGNOLA
VILNIUS
WIENERS
WIENIES
WINNERS
WINNING
WINNOWS
WITNESS
ZINNIAS
ZIONISM
ZIONIST

•I••N••

AIRINGS
BIENNIA
BIGENDS
BIGONES
BIGUNIT
BIKINIS
BILLNYE
BIMINIS
BITONAL
CILENTO
DIGINTO
DIPINTO
DIURNAL
DIVINED
DIVINER
DIVINES
FIENNES
FILENES
FILINGS
FINANCE
FIRENZA
FIRENZE
FIRINGS
FISHNET
FITINTO
FIXINGS
GILLNET
GIRONDE
GITANOS
GIVENBY
GIVENIN
GIVENOF
GIVENON
GIVENTO
GIVENUP
HIDINGS
HIJINKS
HITINTO
IIKINGS
JIMENEZ
JIMINEZ
KIMONOS
KIWANIS
LICENCE
LICENSE
LIFENET
LIGANDS
LIKENED
LIKENEW
LIKENTO
LIKINGS
LILINAU
LIMINAL
LINDNER
LININGS
LISENTE
LITINTO
LIVENED
LIVENER
LIVENUP
LIVINGS
MIGENES
MININGS
MIRANDA
MISHNAH
MISKNEW
MISKNOW
MIZUNAS
PICANTE
PILINGS
PILSNER
PIMENTO
PINENUT
PINONES
PIPINGS
PIRANHA
PISANIO
RIBANDS
RIDINGS
RIPENED
RIPENER
RIPINTO
RISENTO
RISINGS
SIDINGS
SIENNAS
SILENCE
SILENTA
SILENTB
SILENTC
SILENTD
SILENTE
SILENTF
SILENTG
SILENTH
SILENTI
SILENTJ
SILENTK
SILENTL
SILENTM
SILENTN
SILENTO
SILENTP
SILENTQ
SILENTR
SILENTS
SILENTT
SILENTU
SILENTV
SILENTW
SILENTX
SILENTY
SILENTZ
SIMENON
SIMONIZ
SIRENED
SISENOR
SITINON
SITONIT
TIDINGS
TIEINTO
TIERNEY
TILINGS
TILLNOW
TIMINGS
TISANES
TITANAE
TITANIA
TITANIC
VICENTE
VICENZA
VICINAL
VICUNAS
VIERNES
VIETNAM
VIKINGS
VIMINAL
VINTNER
VIVANTS
VIVENDI
VIXENLY
WIDENED
WIDENER
WINGNUT
WIRINGS
WIZENED
XIMENES

•I•••N•

AILMENT
AIRFONE
AIRGUNS
AIRLANE
AIRLINE
AIRTANK
AIRVENT
BIASING
BIBBING
BICHONS
BICORNE
BICORNS
BIDDING
BIFFING
BIGBAND
BIGBANG
BIGBEND
BIGFANS
BIGGUNS
BIGHAND
BIGTENT
BIGWINS
BILKING
BILLING
BINDING
BINGING
BINNING
BIPLANE
BIRDING
BIRIANI
BIRLING
BIRMANS
BIRRING
BIRYANI
BITTING
CICCONE
CINZANO
CITRINE
CITRONS
DIAHANN
DIALING
DIAMOND
DICKENS
DIDFINE
DIEMENS
DIETING
DIGGING
DILUENT
DIMMING
DINDINS
DINGING
DINMONT
DINNING
DINTING
DIOXINS
DIPPING
DIRKING
DISBAND
DISCING
DISHING
DISKING
DISOWNS
DISSENT
DISSING
DISTANT
DISTEND
DIZAINS
FIBBING
FIBRINS
FIGMENT
FIJIANS
FILLING
FILLINS
FILMING
FINDING
FINIANS
FINKING
FINLAND
FIORINA
FIRBANK
FIREANT
FIRKINS
FIRMING
FISHING
FITTING
FIVEONE
FIZZING
GIBBONS
GIBSONS
GIDEONS
GIFTING
GIGGING
GILDING
GILLING
GIMPING
GINNING
GINSENG
GIRDING
GIRTING
GISSING
GITTING
HIBBING
HIBERNO
HIGGINS
HIGHEND
HILLING
HILTING
HILTONS
HINGING
HINTING
HIPBONE
HIRCINE
HISPANO
HISSING
HITSONG
HITTING
HITTUNE
JIGGING
JILTING
JIMSONS
JINXING
KICKING
KIDDING
KILLING
KILNING
KILTING
KINGING
KINKING
KINMONT
KIPLING
KIPPING
KIRMANS
KISSING
KITTENS
KITTING
LIBBING
LIBRANS
LIBYANS
LICHENS
LICKING
LIDWINA
LIFTING
LIGNINS
LILTING
LIMBING
LIMNING
LIMPING
LINDENS
LINEONE
LINKING
LINTING
LIPMANN
LIPPING
LIPSYNC
LISPING
LISTENS
LISTING
LIVEONE
LIVORNO
MICRONS
MIDJUNE
MIDLAND
MIDLINE
MIFFING
MIGHTNT
MIGNONS
MIGRANT
MILKING
MILLAND
MILLEND
MILLING
MINCING
MINDING
MINIONS
MINOANS
MINOTND
MINTING
MINUEND
MINYANS
MIOCENE
MISBIND
MISDONE
MISSEND
MISSENT
MISSING
MISTING
MISTUNE
MISZONE
MITRING
MITTENS

MIZZENS
NIALONG
NICEONE
NICHING
NICKING
NIPPING
NIRVANA
NISSANS
NISSANZ
NITTANY
OILCANS
OILLINE
OILPANS
OILRING
OILSAND
OILTANK
OINKING
PICKENS
PICKING
PIDGINS
PIECING
PIEPANS
PIETINS
PIGEONS
PIGGING
PIGMENT
PIGPENS
PILLING
PINGING
PINIONS
PINKENS
PINKING
PINNING
PIPPINS
PIQUANT
PIQUING
PISCINE
PISHING
PISTONS
PITHING
PITTING
PITYING
RIBBING
RIBBONS
RIBBONY
RICHENS
RIDDING
RIDGING
RIEMANN
RIESENS
RIFFING
RIFLING
RIFTING
RIGGING
RIMMING
RINGING
RINSING
RIOMUNI
RIOTING
RIPIENI
RIPIENO
RIPPING
RIPSONE
RISKING
SIBLING
SICCING
SICKENS
SIDDONS
SIDEONE
SIDLING
SIEGING
SIEMENS
SIEVING
SIFTING
SIGHING
SIGMUND
SIGNING
SILOING
SILTING
SIMIANS
SIMMONS
SINGING
SINKING
SINNING
SIOUANS
SIPHONS
SIPPING
SISTINE
SITTING
SIXGUNS
SIXLANE
SIXNINE
SIZEONE
TICCING
TICKING
TIDYING
TIELINE
TIEPINS
TIERING
TIFFANY
TIFFING
TIFFINS
TIGLONS
TIJUANA
TILLING
TILTING
TIMMINS
TIMPANI
TINCANS
TINGING
TINMINE
TINNING
TINTING
TIPLINE
TIPPING
TITHING
TITIANS
TITLING
TITRING
VIADENT
VIALING
VIBRANT
VICDANA
VIEWING
VINCENT
VINLAND
VIOLENT
VIOLINS
VIOLONE
VIRGINS
VISAING
VISIONS
VITRINE
WICCANS
WICKING
WIELAND
WIFYING
WIGGING
WILDING
WILDONE
WILKENS
WILKINS
WILLING
WILSONS
WILTING
WIMPING
WINCING
WINDING
WINGING
WINKING
WINNING
WISEONE
WISHING
WISPING
WITLING
WITSEND
WITTING
YIPPING
ZIERING
ZIGGING
ZINCING
ZINGING
ZIPGUNS
ZIPPING
ZIRCONS

•I••••N

AILERON
AIRHORN
AIRSIGN
BIAFRAN
BIGHORN
BIGJOHN
BIGTOWN
BILLION
BIRCHEN
BIRDMAN
BIRDMEN
BITESIN
BITESON
BITTERN
CISTERN
CITIZEN
CITROEN
DIAHANN
DIALSIN
DIAPHAN
DICKSON
DICTION
DIEDOWN
DILLMAN
DINEDIN
DINEDON
DINESEN
DINESIN
DINESON
DIRKSEN
DISCERN
DISCMAN
DISDAIN
DISHPAN
DISJOIN
DIVEDIN
DIVESIN
EIDOLON
EIJKMAN
FICTION
FIFTEEN
FILEDIN
FILESIN
FILLSIN
FINKSON
FIREDON
FIREMAN
FIREMEN
FIRESON
FISSION
FIVEMAN
FIVEPIN
FIVETEN
FIXEDON
FIXESON
FIXUPON
GIGATON
GILLIAN
GILLMAN
GIVENIN
GIVENON
GIVESIN
GIVESON
HICKMAN
HIJKLMN
HILLMAN
HILLMEN
HINGEON
HIREDON
HIRESON
HITCHON
HITTOWN
HITUPON
IIIJOHN
JILLIAN
JILLION
JIMRYUN
KICKSIN
KIDSKIN
KILLEEN
KILOTON
KINGMAN
KINGPIN
KINISON
KINSMAN
KINSMEN
KIRSTEN
KITCHEN
LIAISON
LIEDOWN
LIGHTEN
LIGHTON
LILLIAN
LIMACON
LINCOLN
LINEMAN
LINEMEN
LIPMANN
LIVEDIN
LIVEDON
LIVESIN
LIVESON
MIAMIAN
MIDIRON
MIDMORN
MIDNOON
MIDTEEN
MIDTOWN
MIFFLIN
MILERUN
MILKCAN
MILKMAN
MILKMEN
MILKRUN
MILLION
MILLRUN
MINIKIN
MINIVAN
MINORIN
MISCOIN
MISJOIN
MISPLAN
MISSION
MIXEDIN
MIXESIN
NICEMAN
NICEMEN
NIELSEN
NILSSON
NINEPIN
NIPIGON
OILSKIN
PICKSON
PIDGEON
PIERIAN
PIGIRON
PIGSKIN
PILEDIN
PILEDON
PILESIN
PILESON
PILLION
PIMESON
PINDOWN
PIPEDIN
PIPESIN
PIROGEN
PISCEAN
PITCHIN
PITTMAN
RICHMAN
RICHMEN
RICKMAN
RIDESIN
RIEMANN
RIESMAN
RIESSEN
RIGHTON
RINGSIN
RIORDAN
RIOTGUN
RIPOPEN
RIPSAWN
RIPTORN
RITALIN
SIDEMAN
SIDEMEN
SIGNSIN
SIGNSON
SILENTN
SILICON
SIMENON
SIMPSON
SINKSIN
SIOBHAN
SIRLOIN
SITDOWN
SITINON
SITUPON
SIXIRON
SIXTEEN
SIZETEN
TIBETAN
TIBURON
TICOTIN
TIEDOWN
TIGHTEN
TINHORN
TINTERN
TIOMKIN
TIPDOWN
TIREMAN
TIREMEN
VIDICON
VILLAIN
VILLEIN
VIRGOAN
VISAYAN
VISTEON
VITAMIN
WIDGEON
WILDMAN
WILDMEN
WILLSON
WINGMAN
WINGMEN
WINSTON
WIREDIN
WIREMAN
WIREMEN
WIRESIN
WISEMAN
WISEMEN
ZILLION

••IN•••

ABINTRA
ACINGIT
ALINERS
ALINING
AMINUTE
ASININE
ATINGLE
AZINGER
BAINTER
BLINDED
BLINDER
BLINDLY
BLINDTO
BLINKAT
BLINKED
BLINKER
BLINTZE
BRINDLE
BRINERS
BRINGER
BRINGIN
BRINGIT
BRINGON
BRINGTO
BRINGUP
BRINIER
BRINING
BRINISH
BRINKER
CHINESE
CHINKED
CHINNED
CHINOIS
CHINOOK
CHINTZY
CHINUPS
CHINWAG
CLINGER
CLINGTO
CLINICS
CLINKED
CLINKER
CLINTON
COINAGE
COINBOX
COINERS
COINING
COINOPS
CRINGED
CRINGES
CRINKLE
CRINKLY
CUINGIN
DJINNIS
DOINGIN
DOINGOK
DOINGSO
DOINGTO
DOINGUP
DRINKER
DRINKIN
DRINKME
DRINKTO
DRINKUP
DWINDLE
EDINAMN
EKINGBY
EMINENT
ERINYES
EVINCED
EVINCES
FAINEST
FAINTED
FAINTER
FAINTLY
FEINTED
FLINGAT
FLINGER
FLINTMI
FRINGED
FRINGES
GAINERS
GAINFUL
GAINING
GAINSAY
GAINSON
GLINTED
GOINFOR
GOINGAT
GOINGBY
GOINGIN
GOINGON
GOINGTO
GOINGUP
GRINDER
GRINGOS
GRINKOV
GRINNED
GRINNER
GRINSAT
GUINEAN
GUINEAS
HEINOUS
ICINESS
ICINGIN
ICINGIT
ICINGUP
ININETY
JAINISM
JAINIST
JOINDER
JOINERS
JOINERY
JOINING
JOINSIN
JOINSUP
JOINTED
JOINTER
JOINTLY
KLINGER
KLINGON
KLINKER
KRINGLE
LYINGBY
LYINGON
LYINGTO
LYINGUP
MAINERS
MAINMAN
MAINMEN
MAINTOP
ODINGON
OKINAWA
OMINOUS
OPINERS
OPINING
OPINION
ORINOCO
OWINGON
OWINGTO
PAINFUL
PAINING
PAINTED
PAINTER
PHINEAS
PLINKED
PLINTHS
POINTAT
POINTED
POINTER
POINTES
POINTTO
POINTUP
PRINCES
PRINGLE
PRINKED
PRINKER
PRINTAD
PRINTED
PRINTER
PRINTUP
QUINARY
QUINATE
QUINCES
QUINCEY
QUINELA
QUININE
QUINION
QUINLAN
QUINQUE
QUINTAL
QUINTAS
QUINTES
QUINTET
QUINTIC
QUINTON
QUINTUS
QUINZES
RAINBOW
RAINGOD
RAINHAT
RAINIER
RAINILY
RAINING
RAINMAN
RAINOUT
RAINSIN
RAINSON
REINDEX
REINING
REINKED
REINSIN
RUINATE
RUINERS
RUINING
RUINOUS
SAINTED
SAINTES
SAINTLO
SAINTLY
SEINERS
SEINING
SHINDIG
SHINEON
SHINERS
SHINEUP
SHINGLE
SHINGLY
SHINIER
SHINILY
SHINING
SHINNED
SHINOLA
SHINPAD
SKINNED
SKINNER
SLINGER
SLINKED
SLINKER
SLINKIN
SLINKUP
SPINACH
SPINDLE
SPINDLY
SPINDRY
SPINELS
SPINETS
SPINIER
SPINNER
SPINNEY
SPINOFF
SPINOUT
SPINOZA
STINGER
STINKER
STINKUP
STINTED
STINTER
SWINDLE
SWINERY
SWINGAT
SWINGBY
SWINGER
SWINGIT
SWINISH
SWINTON
TAINTED
THINAIR
THINICE
THINKER
THINKOF
THINKSO
THINKUP
THINMAN
THINNED
THINNER
THINOUT
TLINGIT
TRINARY
TRINITY
TRINKET
TWINBED
TWINERS
TWINGED
TWINGES
TWINIER
TWINING
TWINJET
TWINKIE
TWINKLE
TWINKLY
TWINNED
TWINSET
TYINGIN
TYINGON
TYINGTO
TYINGUP
UNINERT
UNINKED
USINGIN
USINGUP
UVINDEX
VAINEST
VEINIER
VEINING
VEINLET
VEINTES
VEINULE
WHINERS
WHINIER
WHINING
WRINGER
WRINKLE
WRINKLY
ZWINGLI

••I•N••

ALIENEE
ALIENOR
ALIENTO
ALIGNED
ALIGNER
ANIONIC
ARIANES
AVIANCA
AVIGNON
AVIONIC
BEIGNES
BEIGNET
BRITNEY
CAIRNED
CHIANTI
CHIGNON
CHIMNEY
CHINNED
CLIENTS
COIGNED
COIGNES
DEIGNED
DEIGNTO
DJINNIS
DOITNOW
ETIENNE
EXITNOW
FAIENCE
FEIGNED
FEIGNER
FRIENDS
GRINNED
GRINNER
GRISNEZ
GUIGNOL
HAIRNET
LEIBNIZ
MEITNER
ORIENTE
ORIENTS
PLIANCY
QUIZNOS
REIGNED
SAIDNAY
SCIENCE
SHINNED
SKINNED
SKINNER
SMIRNOV
SOIGNEE
SPINNER
SPINNEY
THINNED
THINNER
TWINNED
WHITNEY

••I••N•

ABIDING
ABILENE
ALIMENT
ALIMONY
ALINING
ANILINE
ARIADNE
ARISING
ARIZONA
ASININE
BAILING
BAITING
BEIJING
BOILING
BOITANO
BRIBING
BRIGAND
BRINING
BRITONS
BUITONI
CAIMANS
CAIRENE
CEILING
CHICANA
CHICANE
CHICANO
CHIDING
CHIMING
CHIMINH
CHITONS
CLIPONS
COIFING
COILING
COINING
CRIMINY
CUIBONO
CUISINE
DEICING
DRIVING
EDITING
ELIDING
EMINENT
EPICENE
EPIGONE
ERIGENA
ETIENNE
EVIDENT
EVILONE
EXIGENT
EXILING
EXITING
FAILING
FAIRING
FOILING
GAINING
GAITING
GLIDING
GRIMING
GRIPING
GUIDING
GUILING
HAILING
IBIZANS
ILIAMNA
INIRONS
IRISING
JAILING
JOINING
JUICING
KNIFING
KRISHNA
LAIRING
LOIDING
MAIDENS
MAILING
MAILINS
MAIMING
MAISONS
MOILING
NAILING
NOISING
OHIOANS
OLIVINE
OPINING
ORIGINE
ORIGINS
ORISONS
OXIDANT
PAINING
PAIRING
PAISANO
PAISANS
PEIPING
POISING
POISONS
PRICING
PRIDING
PRIMING
PRISONS
PRIZING
QUININE
RAIDING
RAILING
RAIMENT
RAINING
RAISING
RAISINS
RAISINY
RAISONS
REICING
REINING
ROILING
RUINING
SAILING
SAISONS
SEINING
SEIZING
SHINING
SKIRUNS
SLICING
SLIDING
SLIMING
SLIPONS
SMILING
SMITING
SNIPING
SOILING
SPICING
SPIKING
SPITING
STIPEND
SUITING
SWIPING
TAILEND
TAILING
THISONE
TOILING
TRIBUNE
TRIDENT
TRIGONS
TRITONE
TRITONS
TWINING
UNISONS
UNITING

UTICANS
UTICANY
VEILING
VEINING
VOICING
VOIDING
WAILING
WAITING
WAIVING
WHILING
WHINING
WHITENS
WHITING
WRITING
ZEITUNG

••I•••N

ABIDJAN
ANISTON
AVIDFAN
AVIGNON
AVIVIAN
BAILSON
BLITZEN
BRINGIN
BRINGON
BRITAIN
BRITTEN
BRITTON
BUILDIN
BUILDON
BUILTIN
BUILTON
BUISSON
CAISSON
CHICHEN
CHICKEN
CHIDDEN
CHIFFON
CHIGNON
CHILEAN
CHIMEIN
CHIPSIN
CHITLIN
CHITOWN
CLIBURN
CLICKON
CLIFTON
CLIMBIN
CLIMBON
CLINTON
CLIPSON
CRIMEAN
CRIMSON
CRISPEN
CRISPIN
CUINGIN
DOINGIN
DRIFTIN
DRINKIN
DRIPPAN
DRIPSON
DRISTAN
DRIVEIN
EDINAMN
EDITION
ELISION
ERICSON
ERIKSON
ESIASON
FLIESIN
FLIESON
FLIPPEN
FLITSIN
FOISTON
FRIEDAN
FRISIAN
FRISSON
GAINSON
GLIDEIN
GLISTEN
GOINGIN
GOINGON
GRIFFIN
GRIFFON
GUINEAN
HAIRPIN
HAITIAN
HEISMAN
ICINGIN
IDIAMIN
IIIJOHN
JOINSIN
KLINGON
KRISTIN
LYINGON
MAILBIN
MAILMAN
MAILMEN
MAILSIN
MAINMAN
MAINMEN
MEISSEN
MOISSAN
MOISTEN
MRISCAN
NAILGUN
NAILSIN
ODINGON
OMICRON
OPINION
OSIRIAN
OVIDIAN
OWINGON
PHILBIN
POISSON
QUICKEN
QUIETEN
QUINION
QUINLAN
QUINTON
RAILMAN
RAILMEN
RAILSON
RAINMAN
RAINSIN
RAINSON
REINSIN
REITMAN
SAILSON
SEIZEON
SHINEON
SHIPMAN
SHIPMEN
SKIMPON
SLIDEIN
SLINKIN
SLIPSIN
SLIPSON
SMIDGEN
SMILEON
SMITTEN
SPIEDON
SPIESON
SPITSON
STICKIN
STICKON
STIFFEN
STILTON
STIMSON
STIRSIN
SWINTON
TAILFIN
TAILPIN
THIAMIN
THICKEN
THIGPEN
THINMAN
TRICORN
TRIEDON
TRIESON
TRILLIN
TRIPSON
TRISTAN
TUITION
TWISTON
TYINGIN
TYINGON
UNICORN
USINGIN
VUITTON
WAITRON
WAITSON
WEIDMAN
WEIGHIN
WEIGHON
WEIRTON
WHIPSIN
WHITMAN
WHITSUN
WRITEIN
WRITEON
WRITTEN
ZAIRIAN

•••IN••

ABSINTH
ACTINON
AFFINED
AFFINES
AGAINST
AIRINGS
ALBINOS
ALPINER
ALPINES
ANOINTS
AQUINAS
ARCINGS
ATEINTO
AWNINGS
BASINAL
BEHINDS
BELINDA
BIKINIS
BIMINIS
BLUINGS
BODINGS
BOEINGS
BORINGS
BOVINES
BRAINED
BRAINER
BUYINTO
BYJINGO
BYLINED
BYLINER
BYLINES
CABINET
CAMINOS
CANINES
CANINGS
CARINAE
CARINAS
CASINGS
CASINOS
CHAINED
CHAINES
CHAINUP
COMINGS
CORINNE
CORINTH
COSINES
CUTINON
CUTINTO
DATINGS
DAVINCI
DEFINED
DEFINER
DEFINES
DELINTS
DIGINTO
DIPINTO
DIVINED
DIVINER
DIVINES
DOMINGO
DOMINIC
DOMINOS
DOMINUS
DRAINED
DRAINER
DUGINTO
EATINTO
EDGINGS
ELAINES
ELNINOS
ENCINAS
ENDINGS
ENGINED
ENGINES
ENLINKS
ENWINDS
EOSINES
EQUINES
EQUINOX
ERMINED
ERMINES
ERMINIA
EXTINCT
FACINGS
FAMINES
FARINAS
FEDINTO
FELINES
FEMINUM
FILINGS
FIRINGS
FITINTO
FIXINGS
FLYINTO
FORINTS
GAMINES
GATINGS
GEMINIS
GETINON
GETINTO
GOTINON
GOTINTO
GRAINED
GRAINER
GROINED
HAYINGS
HAZINGS
HIDINGS
HIJINKS
HITINTO
HOMINID
HOPINTO
HYGINUS
ICTINUS
IIKINGS
IMPINGE
INKINGS
INLINES
INNINGS
JACINTH
JACINTO
JIMINEZ
KALININ
KEYINON
LACINGS
LADINGS
LADINOS
LAMINAE
LAMINAL
LAMINAR
LAMINAS
LAMINTO
LATINAS
LATINII
LATINOS
LATINUS
LAVINIA
LAYINTO
LEDINTO
LETINON
LIKINGS
LILINAU
LIMINAL
LININGS
LITINTO
LIVINGS
LOSINGS
LUCINDA
LUMINAS
LUPINES
MAGINOT
MAKINGS
MARINAS
MARINER
MARINES
MATINAL
MATINEE
MAYINGS
MELINDA
MERINOS
MININGS
MOWINGS
MTSINAI
MUSINGS
NOMINAL
NOMINEE
OFFINGS
ONEINCH
ORDINAL
ORDINES
OSCINES
OUTINGS
PAGINGS
PALINGS
PANINIS
PARINGS
PATINAS
PAVINGS
PAXINOU
PAYINTO
PILINGS
PIPINGS
PLAINER
PLAINES
PLAINLY
PLAINTS
PRYINTO
QUOINED
RACINOS
RAGINGS
RAMINTO
RANINTO
RAPINES
RAPINIS
RATINES
RATINGS
RAVINED
RAVINES
RAVINGS
REBINDS
REFINDS
REFINED
REFINER
REFINES
REGINAL
REGINAS
REHINGE
RELINED
RELINES
RELINKS
REMINDS
REMINED
REMINES
REMINTS
REPINED
REPINER
REPINES
RERINSE
RESINED
RESINGS
RESINKS
RETINAE
RETINAL
RETINAS
RETINGE
RETINOL
RETINTS
RETINUE
REWINDS
RIDINGS
RIPINTO
RISINGS
ROSINED
ROVINGS
RULINGS
RUNINTO
SABINES
SAGINAW
SALINAS
SALINES
SATINET
SATINON
SAVINGS
SAWINTO
SAYINGS
SEEINTO
SEMINAL
SEMINAR
SETINTO
SHRINED
SHRINER
SHRINES
SHRINKS
SIDINGS
SITINON
SOMINEX
SOYINKA
SOYINKS
SPLINES
SPLINTS
SPRINGS
SPRINGY
SPRINTS
SPYINGS
SQUINCH
SQUINTS
SQUINTY
STAINED
STAINER
STEINEM
STEINER
STRINGS
STRINGY
SURINAM
SYRINGE
TAHINIS
TAKINGS
TAPINGS
TAPINTO
TIDINGS
TIEINTO
TILINGS
TIMINGS
TORINOS
TOTINOS
TOWINGS
TRAINED
TRAINEE
TRAINER
TRAININ
TREINTA
UNBINDS
UNCINCH
UNDINES
UNFINED
UNFINES
UNHINGE
UNKINKS
UNLINED
UNLINKS
UNMINED
UNWINDS
UNWINDY
UPLINKS
UPWINDS
URGINGS
URSINUS
USTINOV
VALINES
VICINAL
VIKINGS
VIMINAL
WAHINES
WAKINGS
WAXINGS
WIRINGS
YOGINIS

•••I•N•

AAMILNE
ACTIONS
ADRIANA
AFFIANT
AMBIENS
AMBIENT
AMNIONS
ANCIENT
ASSIGNS
ATSIGNS
BAHIANS
BCLIONS
BENIGNI
BENIGNO
BIRIANI
BUNIONS
CAMIONS
CATIONS
CORINNE
COSIGNS
DEFIANT
DESIGNS
DEVIANT
ECHIDNA
ENSIGNS
EQUIANO
FANIONS
FIJIANS
FINIANS
FTDIXNJ
FUSIONS
HYGIENE
INDIANA
INDIANS
INSIGNE
IONIANS
ISAIDNO
JULIANA
LEGIONS
LENIENT
LESIONS
LORIENT
LOTIONS
LUCIANA
LUCIANO
MALIANS
MALIGNS
MARIANA
MARIANO
MEDIANS
MEDIANT
MINIONS
MOTIONS
MUSIGNY
MYGIANT
NATIONS
NOTIONS
NUBIANS
NYGIANT
OPTIONS
PATIENT
PINIONS
POTIONS
RADIANS
RADIANT
RATIONS
REGIONS
RELIANT
RESIGNS
RIPIENI
RIPIENO
SALIENT
SAPIENS
SAPIENT
SEVIGNY
SIMIANS
SORIANO
SYRIANA
SYRIANS
TATIANA
TAXIING
TITIANS
VALIANT
VARIANT
VISIONS
ZONIANS
ZUNIANS

•••I••N

ACTINON
ADDISON
AFRICAN
AJSIMON
ALLISON
ANDIRON
ANTIGEN
ANTIGUN
ARTISAN
ASPIRIN
BEDIZEN
BENISON
BERIGAN
BKLIBAN
CALIBAN
CAPITAN
CITIZEN
CRAISIN
CUTINON
DANIKEN
DAVISON
DELIMAN
DELIMEN
DENISON
DENIZEN
ELEISON
ELLISON
EMPIRIN
ENLIVEN
ENVIRON
EPSILON
FADIMAN
FUJISAN
GAVILAN
GETINON
GETITON
GOTINON
GOTITON
HEDISON
HELICON
HORIZON
INDIGEN
JAMISON
JEMISON
JERILYN
JEWISON
KALININ
KEYINON
KINISON
LAYITON
LEGIRON
LETINON
LEXICON
LIAISON
LONIGAN
LYRICON
MADIGAN
MADISON
MANIKIN
MARILYN
MERIDEN
MEXICAN
MIDIRON
MINIKIN
MINIVAN
MOHICAN
NETIZEN
NIPIGON
NONIRON
ONEIRON
ORBISON
PELICAN
PIGIRON
PURITAN
RADIOIN
RAPIDAN
RARITAN
REGIMEN
REGIVEN
RERISEN
REWIDEN
RUBICON
RUBITIN
SAMISEN
SATINON
SILICON
SITINON
SIXIRON
STRIVEN
STSIMON
TALIBAN
TAXIMAN
TAXIMEN
THRIVEN
TRAININ
TRYITON
TWOIRON
UNGIVEN
UNRISEN
UNRIVEN
UPRISEN
UPSILON
VATICAN
VENISON
VERIZON
VIDICON
YESICAN

••••IN•

ABASING
ABATING
ABIDING
ABUSING
ADDLING
ADELINA
ADELINE
ADENINE
ADJOINS
ADORING
AGATINE
AGENINE
AIRLINE
ALADINE
ALAKING
ALANINE
ALAYING
ALINING
ALLMINE
ALLYING
ALTHING
ALUMINA
AMAZING
AMBLING
AMERIND
AMUSING
ANACINS
ANELING
ANGLING
ANILINE
ANTEING
ANTOINE
ANYKIND
APPLING
APPOINT
ARCHING
ARCSINE
ARETINO
ARGUING
ARISING
ASHBINS
ASININE
ASQUINT
ATONING
ATTAINS
ATTAINT
AUSTINS
AUTOING
AVOWING
AWAKING
BABYING
BACHING
BACKING
BAFFING
BAGGING
BAGGINS
BAILING
BAITING
BALDING
BALKING
BAMBINA
BAMBINI
BAMBINO
BAMMING
BANDING
BANGING
BANKING
BANNING
BANTING
BARBING
BARGING
BARKING
BARNING
BARRING
BASHING
BASKING
BASTING
BATHING
BATTING
BATWING
BAWLING
BEADING
BEAMING
BEANING
BEARING
BEATING
BEDDING
BEEFING
BEELINE
BEEPING
BEGGING
BEGUINE
BEHRING
BEIJING
BELLING
BELLINI
BELTING
BELYING
BENDING
BENNING
BERMING
BERNINA
BERNINI
BESTING
BETHINK
BETTING
BIASING
BIBBING
BIDDING
BIFFING
BIGWINS
BILKING
BILLING
BINDING
BINGING
BINNING
BIRDING
BIRLING
BIRRING
BITTING
BLADING
BLAMING
BLARING
BLAZING
BLOWING
BLUEING
BOATING
BOBBING
BOBBINS
BODKINS
BOFFING
BOFFINS
BOGGING
BOILING
BOLLING
BOLTING
BOMBING
BONDING
BONGING
BONKING
BOOKING
BOOMING
BOOTING
BOOZING
BOPPING
BORKING
BOSSING
BOUDINS
BOWFINS
BOWLINE
BOWLING
BRACING
BRAKING
BRAVING
BRAYING
BRAZING
BREWING
BRIBING
BRINING
BROMINE
BRUXING
BUCKING
BUDDING
BUDGING
BUFFING
BUGGING
BUGLING
BULGING
BULKING
BULLING
BULLINS
BUMMING
BUMPING
BUNGING
BUNKING
BUNNING
BUNTING
BUOYING
BURKINA
BURLING
BURNING

BURPING	CHORINE	CUPPING	DISSING	ESTRING	FOILING	GLOBING	HEALING	ICERINK	JUTTING	LEONINE	MARKING	MUSLINS
BURRING	CHOWING	CURBING	DIZAINS	ETAMINE	FOLDING	GLOBINS	HEAPING	ICEWINE	KACHINA	LESSING	MARLINS	MUSSING
BURYING	CHUTING	CURDING	DOBBINS	ETCHING	FONTINA	GLOVING	HEARING	ICYWIND	KACHING	LETTING	MARRING	NABBING
BUSHING	CITRINE	CURLING	DOCKING	EVADING	FOOLING	GLOWING	HEATING	IGRAINE	KATRINA	LEUCINE	MARTINA	NAGGING
BUSKING	CLAWING	CURRING	DODGING	EVENING	FOOTING	GLYCINE	HEAVING	ILLWIND	KATRINE	LEVYING	MARTINI	NAILING
BUSLINE	CLAYING	CURSING	DOFFING	EVOKING	FORCING	GNAWING	HEDGING	IMAGINE	KAYOING	LIBBING	MARTINO	NANJING
BUSSING	CLEWING	CURVING	DOGGING	EXAMINE	FORDING	GOADING	HEEDING	IMAGING	KEDGING	LICKING	MARTINS	NANKING
BUSTING	CLONING	CUSHING	DOLLING	EXILING	FORGING	GOBLINS	HEELING	IMBUING	KEELING	LIDWINA	MARTINU	NAPKINS
BUSYING	CLOSING	CUSSING	DOMAINE	EXITING	FORKING	GODLING	HEFTING	IMEMINE	KEENING	LIFTING	MARTINV	NAPPING
BUTTING	CLOYING	CUTTING	DOMAINS	EXSCIND	FORMING	GOLDING	HELMING	IMGOING	KEEPING	LIGNINS	MASHING	NEARING
BUZZING	CLUEING	CYCLING	DONKING	EXUDING	FOULING	GOLFING	HELPING	IMPRINT	KEGGING	LILTING	MASKING	NECKING
CABBING	COALING	CZARINA	DONNING	EYELINE	FOWLING	GONGING	HELSING	INABIND	KELVINS	LIMBING	MASSINE	NEEDING
CABLING	COATING	DABBING	DOOMING	EYEWINK	FRAMING	GOODING	HEMLINE	INALINE	KENNING	LIMNING	MASSING	NERVINE
CABRINI	COAXING	DADOING	DOSSING	FABLING	FRAYING	GOOFING	HEMMING	INAWINK	KEYRING	LIMPING	MASTING	NERVING
CACHING	COCAINE	DAMMING	DOTTING	FADEINS	FREEING	GOOSING	HERDING	INCHING	KICKING	LINKING	MATTING	NESTING
CADGING	COCKING	DAMNING	DOUSING	FAILING	FRODING	GORGING	HEROINE	INCLINE	KIDDING	LINTING	MAULING	NETTING
CALKING	CODEINE	DAMPING	DOWLING	FAIRING	FUDGING	GORMING	HERRING	INGOING	KILLING	LIPPING	MAYWINE	NEWLINE
CALKINS	COFFINS	DANCING	DOWNING	FALLING	FUELING	GOSLING	HIBBING	INKLING	KILNING	LISPING	MAZZINI	NEWMINT
CALLING	COGGING	DANNING	DOWSING	FANGING	FUNDING	GOUGING	HIGGINS	INLYING	KILTING	LISTING	MCSWINE	NICHING
CALLINS	COIFING	DAPPING	DRAPING	FANNING	FUNKING	GOWNING	HILLING	INPOINT	KINGING	LOADING	MEANING	NICKING
CALMING	COILING	DARLING	DRAWING	FANTINE	FUNNING	GRACING	HILTING	INPRINT	KINKING	LOAFING	MEETING	NIPPING
CALVING	COINING	DARNING	DRAYING	FANZINE	FURLING	GRADING	HINGING	INRUINS	KIPLING	LOAMING	MELDING	NOCKING
CALVINO	COLLINE	DARTING	DRIVING	FARCING	FURRING	GRATING	HINTING	INTHING	KIPPING	LOANING	MELTING	NODDING
CAMPING	COLLINS	DASHING	DRONING	FARMING	FUSSING	GRAVING	HIRCINE	INURING	KISSING	LOBBING	MEMLING	NOGGINS
CANNING	COMBINE	DAUBING	DROPINS	FASTING	FUTZING	GRAYING	HISSING	IRISING	KITTING	LOCKING	MENDING	NOISING
CANTINA	COMBING	DAWKINS	DRQUINN	FATLING	FUZZING	GRAZING	HITTING	IRONING	KNEEING	LOCKINS	MEOWING	NOONING
CANTING	COMPING	DAWNING	DUBBING	FATTING	GABBING	GREYING	HJHEINZ	ISOLINE	KNIFING	LODGING	MERGING	NOOSING
CANTINO	CONFINE	DAYSINN	DUCKING	FAWNING	GADDING	GRIMING	HOAXING	ISSUING	KNOWING	LOFTING	MERLINS	NOSHING
CAPPING	CONKING	DEALING	DUCTING	FEARING	GAFFING	GRIPING	HOBOING	ITCHING	KOONING	LOGGING	MESHING	NOTHING
CAPRINE	CONNING	DECKING	DUELING	FEEDING	GAGGING	GROPING	HOCKING	ITEMING	KOSCINA	LOGGINS	MESSINA	NOTHINS
CARBINE	COOKING	DECLINE	DUETING	FEELING	GAGLINE	GROWING	HODDING	ITSFINE	LACKING	LOIDING	MESSING	NOTMINE
CARDING	COOLING	DEEDING	DULLING	FELLING	GAINING	GSTRING	HOGGING	IVORINE	LADLING	LOLLING	MEWLING	NOTTING
CARKING	COOPING	DEEMING	DUMBING	FELLINI	GAITING	GUANINE	HOLDING	JABBING	LAGGING	LONGING	MIDLINE	NUBBINS
CARLING	COPPING	DEFYING	DUMPING	FELTING	GALLING	GUIDING	HONKING	JACKING	LAHAINA	LOOKING	MIFFING	NUDGING
CARMINA	COPYING	DEICING	DUNKING	FENCING	GAMMING	GUILING	HOODING	JAGGING	LAIRING	LOOKINS	MILKING	NULLING
CARMINE	COQUINA	DEKEING	DUNLINS	FENDING	GANGING	GULFING	HOOFING	JAILING	LALLING	LOOMING	MILLING	NUMBING
CARPING	CORDING	DELEING	DUNNING	FESSING	GAOLING	GULLING	HOOKING	JAMMING	LAMBING	LOOPING	MINCING	NURSING
CARTING	CORKING	DELVING	DURNING	FESTINA	GAPPING	GULPING	HOOPING	JARDINE	LAMMING	LOOSING	MINDING	NUTPINE
CARVING	CORNING	DEMOING	DUSKING	FEUDING	GARBING	GUMMING	HOOTING	JARDINS	LANCING	LOOTING	MINTING	NUTTING
CASEINS	CORTINA	DENNING	DUSTING	FIBBING	GASHING	GUNNING	HOPKINS	JARRING	LANDING	LOPPING	MISBIND	OBEYING
CASHING	CORVINA	DENTINE	EAGLING	FIBRINS	GASLINE	GUSHING	HOPPING	JASMINE	LANDINI	LORDING	MISSING	OBTAINS
CASHINS	CORVINE	DENTING	EARNING	FILLING	GASPING	GUSTING	HOPSING	JAWLINE	LANSING	LOTTING	MISTING	OCARINA
CASKING	CORZINE	DENTINS	EARRING	FILLINS	GASSING	GUTTING	HORDING	JAZZING	LANVINS	LOURING	MITRING	OFAKIND
CASSINI	COSHING	DENYING	EASTING	FILMING	GATLING	GYPPING	HORNING	JEERING	LAPPING	LOUSING	MOANING	OFAMIND
CASSINO	COSTING	DERRING	ECHOING	FINDING	GATLINS	HACKING	HORSING	JELLING	LAPSING	LOUTING	MOBBING	OFFLINE
CASTING	COSYING	DESPINA	EDDYING	FINKING	GAUGING	HAFTING	HOSKINS	JENKINS	LAPWING	LOVEINS	MOCKING	OILLINE
CATKINS	COUPING	DESTINE	EDITING	FIORINA	GAWKING	HAILING	HOSTING	JERKING	LARAINE	LUCHINO	MOILING	OILRING
CATMINT	COUSINE	DESTINO	EDUCING	FIRKINS	GAWPING	HALOING	HOTLINE	JERKINS	LARDING	LUCKING	MOLDING	OINKING
CAUSING	COUSINS	DESTINY	ELATING	FIRMING	GEARING	HALTING	HOTLINK	JESTING	LARKING	LUFFING	MOLTING	OKAYING
CAVEINS	COWLING	DETAINS	ELIDING	FISHING	GELDING	HALVING	HOTPINK	JETTING	LARKINS	LUGGING	MOONING	OLDLINE
CEASING	COZYING	DEUCING	ELOPING	FITTING	GELLING	HAMLINE	HOUDINI	JIGGING	LASHING	LULLING	MOORING	OLEFINS
CEILING	CRANING	DEVEINS	ELUDING	FIZZING	GENUINE	HAMMING	HOUSING	JILTING	LASTING	LUMPING	MOOTING	OLIVINE
CELLINI	CRAPING	DEWLINE	ELUTING	FLAKING	GERAINT	HANDING	HOWLING	JINXING	LATHING	LUNGING	MOPPING	OMENING
CENSING	CRATING	DIALING	EMOTING	FLAMING	GETTING	HANGING	HUFFING	JOBBING	LATRINE	LURKING	MORAINE	ONALINE
CERVINE	CRAVING	DIDFINE	ENDLINE	FLARING	GIFTING	HARDING	HUGGING	JOGGING	LAUDING	LUSTING	MORNING	ONEPINT
CESSING	CRAZING	DIETING	ENDPINS	FLAWING	GIGGING	HARKING	HUGGINS	JOINING	LAVAINE	MACHINA	MOSHING	ONGOING
CHAFING	CREMINI	DIGGING	ENDUING	FLAYING	GILDING	HARLINE	HULKING	JOLTING	LEADING	MACHINE	MOSSING	ONPOINT
CHARING	CREPING	DIMMING	ENJOINS	FLEEING	GILLING	HARMING	HULLING	JOSHING	LEADINS	MADDING	MOTRINS	OPALINE
CHASING	CRETINS	DINDINS	ENSUING	FLEMING	GIMPING	HARPING	HUMMING	JOTTING	LEAFING	MAILING	MOUSING	OPENING
CHAWING	CREWING	DINGING	ENTWINE	FLEXING	GINNING	HASHING	HUNTING	JREWING	LEAKING	MAILINS	MUCKING	OPINING
CHEFING	CRIMINY	DINNING	ENURING	FLORINS	GIRDING	HASPING	HURLING	JUDGING	LEANING	MAIMING	MUDDING	ORATING
CHEWING	CROWING	DINTING	ENVYING	FLOWING	GIRTING	HASTING	HURTING	JUGGING	LEAPING	MALTING	MUFFING	ORDAINS
CHIDING	CUBBING	DIOXINS	EONLINE	FLUTING	GISSING	HATPINS	HUSHING	JUGWINE	LEASING	MALVINA	MUFFINS	ORIGINE
CHIMING	CUBBINS	DIPPING	EPONINE	FLUXING	GITTING	HATTING	HUSKING	JUICING	LEAVING	MANCINI	MUGGING	ORIGINS
CHIMINH	CUFFING	DIRKING	ERASING	FOALING	GLARING	HAULING	HUTTING	JUMPING	LEERING	MANKIND	MULLING	OUSTING
CHOKING	CUISINE	DISCING	ERODING	FOAMING	GLAVINE	HAWKING	HYMNING	JUNKING	LEGGING	MANNING	MULLINS	OUTFIND
CHOLINE	CULLING	DISHING	ERSKINE	FOBBING	GLAZING	HAWKINS	HYPOING	JURYING	LEMMING	MAPPING	MUMMING	OUTJINX
CHOPINE	CUNNING	DISKING	ESPYING	FOGGING	GLIDING	HEADING	ICELINE	JUSTINE	LENDING	MARGINS	MUSHING	OUTKING

OUTLINE
OUTRING
OUTSING
OUTSINS
OUTWIND
OUTWING
PACKING
PADDING
PAINING
PAIRING
PALLING
PALMING
PANNING
PANTING
PARGING
PARKING
PARKINS
PARRING
PARSING
PARTING
PASSING
PASTINA
PASTING
PATTING
PAULINA
PAULINE
PAULING
PAUSING
PAWNING
PEAKING
PEALING
PECKING
PECTINS
PEEKING
PEELING
PEENING
PEEPING
PEERING
PEEVING
PEGGING
PEIPING
PELTING
PENDING
PENNINE
PENNING
PEPPING
PEPPINO
PEPSINS
PERKING
PERKINS
PERMING
PERRINE
PERRINS
PETTING
PHASING
PHONING
PICKING
PIDGINS
PIECING
PIETINS
PIGGING
PILLING
PINGING
PINKING
PINNING
PIPPINS
PIQUING
PISCINE
PISHING
PITHING
PITTING
PITYING
PLACING
PLANING
PLATING
PLAYING
PLOWING
PLUGINS
PLUMING
POISING
POLLING
PONDING
PONYING
POOLING
POOPING
POPLINS
POPPING
POPPINS
POPWINE
PORCINE
PORKING
PORTING
POSTING
POTTING
POURING
POUTING
PRALINE
PRATING
PRAYING
PREBIND
PREYING
PRICING
PRIDING
PRIMING
PRIZING
PROBING
PROSING
PROVINE
PROVING
PRUNING
PUCCINI
PUDDING
PUFFING
PUFFINS
PULLING
PULLINS
PULPING
PULSING
PUMPING
PUNNING
PUNTING
PURGING
PURLING
PURRING
PURSING
PUSHING
PUTTING
QUAKING
QUEUING
QUININE
QUOTING
RACKING
RAFTING
RAGGING
RAIDING
RAILING
RAINING
RAISING
RAISINS
RAISINY
RAMMING
RAMPING
RANGING
RANKINE
RANKING
RANTING
RAPPING
RASPING
RATFINK
RATLINE
RATLINS
RATTING
RAWLINS
RAZZING
RDLAING
READING
REALINE
REAMING
REAPING
REARING
REAVING
RECLINE
RECOINS
REDDING
REDFINS
REDKING
REDLINE
REDNINE
REDOING
REDPINE
REDWINE
REDWING
REDYING
REEDING
REEFING
REEKING
REELING
REEVING
REFFING
REFYING
REGAINS
REGRIND
REICING
REINING
REJOINS
RELYING
REMAINS
RENDING
RENNINS
RENTING
REPAINT
REPOINT
REPPING
REPRINT
RESCIND
RESHINE
RESPINS
RESTING
RETAINS
RETHINK
RETSINA
RETTING
RETWINE
REUSING
REVVING
RHYMING
RIBBING
RIDDING
RIDGING
RIFFING
RIFLING
RIFTING
RIGGING
RIMMING
RINGING
RINSING
RIOTING
RIPPING
RISKING
RLSTINE
ROAMING
ROARING
ROBBING
ROBBINS
ROCKING
RODDING
ROGAINE
ROGUING
ROILING
ROLFING
ROLLING
ROLLINS
ROMAINE
ROMAINS
ROMPING
ROOFING
ROOKING
ROOMING
ROOTING
ROSSINI
ROTTING
ROUGING
ROUSING
ROUTINE
ROUTING
ROWLING
RRATING
RSVPING
RUBBING
RUCHING
RUCKING
RUFFING
RUINING
RUNNING
RUSHING
RUSTING
RUTTING
SABRINA
SACKING
SAGGING
SAILING
SALTINE
SALTING
SALVING
SANDING
SANTINI
SAPLING
SAPPING
SARDINE
SASHING
SASSING
SAUCING
SCALING
SCARING
SCHWINN
SCOPING
SCORING
SEALING
SEAMING
SEARING
SEATING
SEBRING
SEEDING
SEEKING
SEEMING
SEEPING
SEINING
SEIZING
SELLING
SENDING
SENSING
SEQUINS
SERLING
SERVING
SESTINA
SETTING
SHADING
SHAKING
SHAMING
SHAPING
SHARING
SHAVING
SHINING
SHOEING
SHOOING
SHOOINS
SHORING
SHOVING
SHOWING
SHUTINS
SIBLING
SICCING
SIDLING
SIEGING
SIEVING
SIFTING
SIGHING
SIGNING
SILOING
SILTING
SINGING
SINKING
SINNING
SIPPING
SISTINE
SITTING
SIXNINE
SKATING
SKEWING
SKYLINE
SLAKING
SLATING
SLAVING
SLAYING
SLEWING
SLICING
SLIDING
SLIMING
SLOPING
SLOWING
SMILING
SMITING
SMOKING
SNAKING
SNARING
SNIPING
SNORING
SNOWING
SOAKING
SOAPING
SOARING
SOBBING
SOCKING
SODDING
SOILING
SOLOING
SOLVING
SOPPING
SORDINI
SORDINO
SORTING
SORVINO
SOURING
SOUSING
SPACING
SPADING
SPARING
SPAYING
SPECING
SPEWING
SPICING
SPIKING
SPITING
SPOKING
SPRAINS
SPUMING
SPYRING
STAGING
STAKING
STAMINA
STANINE
STARING
STATING
STATINS
STAVING
STAYING
STEPINS
STEWING
STOKING
STONING
STORING
STOTINS
STOWING
STRAINS
STUBING
STYLING
SUBBING
SUBKING
SUCKING
SUDSING
SUITING
SULKING
SUMMING
SUNNING
SUPPING
SURFING
SURGING
SUSSING
SWAYING
SWIPING
SYNCING
TABBING
TABLING
TABUING
TACKING
TAGGING
TAGLINE
TAILING
TAKEINS
TALKING
TALLINN
TAMPING
TANGING
TANKING
TANKINI
TANLINE
TANNING
TANNINS
TAPPING
TARRING
TARTING
TASKING
TASTING
TATTING
TAURINE
TAXIING
TEAMING
TEARING
TEASING
TEEMING
TELLING
TEMPING
TENDING
TENPINS
TENSING
TENTING
TENZING
TERMING
TERMINI
TERRINE
TESTING
TEXTING
THAWING
THEKING
THERING
THERINK
THEWIND
THYMINE
TICCING
TICKING
TIDYING
TIELINE
TIEPINS
TIERING
TIFFING
TIFFINS
TILLING
TILTING
TIMMINS
TINGING
TINMINE
TINNING
TINTING
TIPLINE
TIPPING
TITHING
TITLING
TITRING
TOCSINS
TOGGING
TOILING
TOLLING
TONGING
TONTINE
TOOLING
TOOTING
TOPLINE
TOPPING
TOSSING
TOTTING
TOURING
TOUTING
TOWLINE
TRACING
TRADING
TREEING
TREVINO
TROWING
TRUEING
TSARINA
TUBBING
TUCKING
TUFTING
TUGGING
TURBINE
TURFING
TURNING
TUSKING
TUTTING
TWINING
TZARINA
UGOLINO
UKRAINE
UNAGING
UNDOING
UNDYING
UNITING
UNJOINS
UNJOINT
UNLYING
UNOWING
UNRAINY
UNSHINY
UNSLING
UNTHINK
UNTWINE
UNTYING
UNVYING
UPFLING
UPGOING
UPSPINS
UPSWING
URCHINS
VACCINE
VALUING
VAMPING
VANDINE
VANLINE
VANNING
VARMINT
VARYING
VATTING
VEERING
VEGGING
VEILING
VEINING
VENDING
VENTING
VERDINS
VEREINE
VERGING
VERMINY
VERSING
VESTING
VETOING
VETTING
VIALING
VIEWING
VIOLINS
VIRGINS
VISAING
VITRINE
VOGUING
VOICING
VOIDING
VULPINE
WADDING
WADKINS
WAFTING
WAGGING
WAILING
WAITING
WAIVING
WALKING
WALKINS
WALLING
WANNING
WANTING
WARDING
WARMING
WARNING
WARPING
WARRING
WASHING
WASTING
WATKINS
WAXWING
WEANING
WEARING
WEAVING
WEBBING
WEBZINE
WEDDING
WEDGING
WEEDING
WEEPING
WELDING
WELLING
WELTING
WENDING
WESTINS
WETTING
WHALING
WHILING
WHINING
WHITING
WICKING
WIFYING
WIGGING
WILDING
WILKINS
WILLING
WILTING
WIMPING
WINCING
WINDING
WINGING
WINKING
WINNING
WISHING
WISPING
WITLING
WITTING
WOLFING
WONTING
WOODING
WOOFING
WORDING
WORKING
WORMING
WRITING
WYOMING
XRATING
XRAYING
YAKKING
YANKING
YAOMING
YAPPING
YARDING
YARNING
YASMINE
YAWNING
YAWPING
YEANING
YELLING
YELPING
YENNING
YESSING
YIPPING
YOWLING
YOYOING
YUKKING
ZADKINE
ZAGGING
ZAPPING
ZEBRINE
ZEROING
ZESTING
ZIERING
ZIGGING
ZINCING
ZINGING
ZIPPING
ZONKING
ZOOMING

••••I•N

ACADIAN
AEOLIAN
AIRSIGN
AMPHION
ANTLION
APULIAN
ARABIAN
ARRAIGN
AUCTION
AVIVIAN
AZANIAN
AZORIAN
BADSIGN
BASTION
BEALION
BELGIAN
BILLION
BOSNIAN
BULLION
CAMPION
CAPTION
CASPIAN
CAUTION
CESSION
CLARION
COMBIEN
CONDIGN
CONSIGN
CRATION
CUSHION
CYPRIAN
DAYSINN
DICTION
DREGION
DRQUINN
DRUZIAN
EDITION
ELAAIUN
ELATION
ELISION
ELUTION
ELYSIAN
EMOTION
EROSION
ETESIAN
ETONIAN
EVASION
FACTION
FASHION
FERMION
FICTION
FISSION
FLEXION
FLORIAN
FLUXION
FOREIGN
FRISIAN
FUSTIAN
GAMBIAN
GENTIAN
GHANIAN
GILLIAN
GORDIAN
GRECIAN
GRUNION
HADRIAN
HAITIAN
HELLION
HESSIAN
HEXSIGN
IBERIAN
ICHDIEN
IRANIAN
IRESIGN
ISTRIAN
ITALIAN
IVORIAN
IZATION
JILLIAN
JILLION
JUNGIAN
KANTIAN
KRATION
LAOTIAN
LATVIAN
LILLIAN
LOTHIAN
MANSION
MARDIAN
MARMION
MARTIAN
MARXIAN
MENTION
MERCIAN
MGMLION
MIAMIAN
MILLION
MISSION
MUYBIEN
OPINION
ORARION
ORATION
OSIRIAN
OUTLIMN
OVATION
OVIDIAN
OXONIAN
PASSION
PENSION
PEORIAN
PERMIAN
PERSIAN
PETLION
PIERIAN
PILLION
PLEBIAN
PLOSION
PONTIAN
PORTION
PYTHIAN
QUINION
REALIGN
REUNION
RHODIAN
RUCTION
RUFFIAN
RUSSIAN
SAURIAN
SCHWINN
SCOTIAN
SEALION
SECTION
SERBIAN
SESSION
SHAVIAN
STARION
STATION
STYGIAN
SUASION
SUCTION
TALLINN
TENSION
TOLKIEN
TORSION
TUITION
UMBRIAN
UNCTION
UTOPIAN
VANDIEN
VANRIJN
VERSION
VOSGIAN
ZAIRIAN
ZAMBIAN
ZILLION

•••••IN

ABSTAIN
ACTEDIN
ADDEDIN
ALADDIN
ALAMEIN
ALBUMIN
ALDUBIN
ALLOWIN
ALSHAIN
ANNAKIN
ANTONIN
ASKEDIN
ASPIRIN
AWASHIN
BACKSIN
BAHRAIN
BAHREIN
BALDWIN
BALMAIN
BARGAIN
BARGEIN
BASRHIN
BEDOUIN
BITESIN
BLENDIN
BLENTIN
BLOWNIN
BLOWSIN
BLUEFIN
BORODIN
BOWDOIN
BOXEDIN
BOXESIN
BRAHMIN
BREAKIN
BRESLIN
BRINGIN
BRITAIN
BROKEIN
BUILDIN
BUILTIN
BUMPKIN
BURNSIN
BURNTIN
BURSTIN
BUSTSIN
BUTTSIN
BYTRAIN
CAGEDIN
CAKETIN
CALLSIN
CAPTAIN
CAROTIN
CARRYIN
CARTSIN
CAVEDIN
CAVESIN
CERTAIN
CHAGRIN
CHAPLIN

CHARMIN
CHARNIN
CHATWIN
CHEATIN
CHECKIN
CHIMEIN
CHIPSIN
CHITLIN
CLIMBIN
CLOCKIN
CLOSEIN
CLUEDIN
CLUESIN
COALBIN
COMESIN
COMPLIN
CONJOIN
CONKLIN
CONTAIN
CORNBIN
COSTAIN
COUNTIN
COWSKIN
CRAISIN
CRAMSIN
CREEPIN
CREPTIN
CRESPIN
CRISPIN
CROWDIN
CUINGIN
CURLSIN
CURTAIN
DAUPHIN
DEALSIN
DEALTIN
DESTAIN
DETRAIN
DEXTRIN
DIALSIN
DINEDIN
DINESIN
DISDAIN
DISJOIN
DIVEDIN
DIVESIN
DOAGAIN
DOESKIN
DOINGIN
DOLPHIN
DOONEIN
DRAGSIN
DRANKIN
DRAWNIN
DRAWSIN
DREAMIN
DRESSIN
DRIFTIN
DRINKIN
DRIVEIN
DROPSIN
DROVEIN
DRUMLIN
DUCKPIN
DUNEDIN
DUSTBIN
DWELLIN
EASEDIN

EASESIN
ECOTRIN
EDGEDIN
EDGESIN
EELSKIN
ELASTIN
ELTRAIN
EMPIRIN
ENCHAIN
ENDEDIN
ENGRAIN
ENTERIN
ENTRAIN
EPSTEIN
ESTAMIN
EUCERIN
EXCELIN
EXPLAIN
FADEDIN
FADESIN
FALLSIN
FEEDBIN
FEEDSIN
FENCEIN
FILEDIN
FILESIN
FILLSIN
FIVEPIN
FLIESIN
FLITSIN
FLOWNIN
FLOWSIN
FOLDSIN
FORCEIN
FOURPIN
GAGARIN
GASMAIN
GAUGUIN
GELATIN
GERMAIN
GHERKIN
GIVENIN
GIVESIN
GLIDEIN
GLOAMIN
GOBELIN
GOINGIN
GOODWIN
GREMLIN
GRIFFIN
GROOVIN
HAIRPIN
HAMELIN
HANDLIN
HANDSIN
HANGSIN
HAULSIN
HEADPIN
HEADSIN
HELPSIN
HEMATIN
HEPARIN
HOLBEIN
HOLDSIN
HOMEDIN
HOMESIN
HONEDIN
HONESIN

HORNSIN
HUSSEIN
ICINGIN
IDIAMIN
INASPIN
INGRAIN
INKEDIN
INSULIN
ISTOMIN
ITSASIN
JACOBIN
JAVELIN
JOAQUIN
JOINSIN
JUMPSIN
KALININ
KEEPSIN
KENOLIN
KERATIN
KEYEDIN
KICKSIN
KIDSKIN
KINGPIN
KJELLIN
KOSYGIN
KREMLIN
KRESKIN
KRISTIN
KTOSLIN
LADYKIN
LAMBKIN
LANOLIN
LAUGHIN
LEADSIN
LEAKSIN
LEANSIN
LEAPSIN
LEAPTIN
LEAVEIN
LETEMIN
LETMEIN
LIVEDIN
LIVESIN
LOADSIN
LOCKLIN
LOCKSIN
LODGEIN
LOOKSIN
LUMPSIN
LUREDIN
LURESIN
MAILBIN
MAILSIN
MAJORIN
MANIKIN
MANOLIN
MARRYIN
MATALIN
MAUDLIN
MAULDIN
MAYALIN
MAZARIN
MCGAVIN
MECHLIN
MELANIN
MENUHIN
MIFFLIN
MINIKIN

MINORIN
MISCOIN
MISJOIN
MIXEDIN
MIXESIN
MORPHIN
MOVEDIN
MOVESIN
MUEZZIN
NAILSIN
NESTSIN
NETGAIN
NINEPIN
NOSEDIN
NOSESIN
NOSTAIN
OBERLIN
OILSKIN
OPTEDIN
ORDERIN
OUTGAIN
OUTGRIN
OUTLAIN
OUTSPIN
PACKSIN
PACQUIN
PALADIN
PASTEIN
PEEKSIN
PEERSIN
PENGUIN
PERTAIN
PHASEIN
PHILBIN
PHONEIN
PIGSKIN
PILEDIN
PILESIN
PIPEDIN
PIPESIN
PITCHIN
PLUGSIN
POURSIN
POUSSIN
PREGAIN
PROTEIN
PULLPIN
PULLSIN
PUMPKIN
PUNCHIN
PURLOIN
PUSHKIN
PUSHPIN
QUENTIN
RACEDIN
RADIOIN
RAINSIN
RAKEDIN
RAKESIN
RAMBLIN
RAMEKIN
RANONIN
REACHIN
READSIN
REBEGIN
REDSKIN
REELSIN
REFRAIN

REINSIN
RESTAIN
RESTSIN
RETRAIN
REVELIN
RIDESIN
RINGSIN
RITALIN
ROLLSIN
ROPEDIN
ROPESIN
RUBITIN
RUNONIN
SALADIN
SAVARIN
SEALSIN
SEEPSIN
SENDSIN
SHAREIN
SHERWIN
SHOOSIN
SHOVEIN
SHOWNIN
SHOWSIN
SHUTSIN
SIGNSIN
SINKSIN
SIRLOIN
SLATKIN
SLEEPIN
SLEPTIN
SLIDEIN
SLINKIN
SLIPSIN
SLOEGIN
SLUNKIN
SNEAKIN
SNOWSIN
SOAKSIN
SOCKSIN
SPORTIN
STANDIN
STARSIN
STARTIN
STAYSIN
STEALIN
STEARIN
STEEPIN
STEPSIN
STICKIN
STIRSIN
STOLEIN
STOMPIN
STOODIN
STOPSIN
STORMIN
STRAPIN
STUCKIN
STUFFIN
SUBJOIN
SUCKSIN
SUSTAIN
SWEARIN
SWOOPIN
SWOREIN
TAILFIN
TAILPIN
TAKENIN

TAKESIN
TASHLIN
TEACHIN
TERRAIN
THEREIN
THIAMIN
THREWIN
THROWIN
TICOTIN
TIOMKIN
TOPSPIN
TOWEDIN
TRADEIN
TRAININ
TRILLIN
TROMPIN
TROOPIN
TRUSTIN
TUCKSIN
TUNEDIN
TUNESIN
TURNSIN
TYINGIN
TYPEDIN
TYPESIN
UNCHAIN
UNSLAIN
UPANDIN
USHERIN
USINGIN
VILLAIN
VILLEIN
VITAMIN
VOTEDIN
VOTESIN
WADEDIN
WADESIN
WALLSIN
WANTSIN
WAVEDIN
WAVESIN
WEDGEIN
WEIGHIN
WHEELIN
WHEREIN
WHIPSIN
WIREDIN
WIRESIN
WOODBIN
WORKSIN
WRITEIN
WROTEIN
YELTSIN
ZEROSIN
ZOOMSIN

IO•••••

IOBJECT
IODATED
IODATES
IODIDES
IODISED
IODISES
IODIZED
IODIZER
IODIZES
IOMOTHS
IONBEAM
IONESCO
IONIANS
IONISED
IONISER
IONISES
IONIUMS
IONIZED
IONIZER
IONIZES
IONONES
IOWEYOU

I•O••••

ICONIFY
IDOLISE
IDOLIST
IDOLIZE
IDOODIT
IDOTTER
IFORGET
IFORGOT
IFORONE
IGOOFED
IGOROTS
IGOTCHA
IGOTYOU
IHOPESO
ILOCANO
ILOSTIT
ILOVEIT
ILOVELA
IMOGENE
INOCULA
INORBIT
INORDER
IRONAGE
IRONBAR
IRONERS
IRONIES
IRONING
IRONIST
IRONMAN
IRONMEN
IRONONS
IRONORE
IRONOUT
IRONSON
ISOBARS
ISOGONS
ISOGRAM
ISOHELS
ISOLATE
ISOLATO
ISOLINE
ISOMERS
ISONOMY
ISOPODS
ISOTONE
ISOTOPE
ISOTOPY
IVORIAN
IVORIES
IVORINE
IWOJIMA
IWONDER

I••O•••

IACOCCA
ICEOUTS
ICEOVER
IDIOTIC
IDOODIT
IFYOUGO
IGNOBLE
IGNOBLY
IGNORED
IGNORER
IGNORES
IGOOFED
IKNOWIT
ILLOGIC
IMBORED
IMFORIT
IMGOING
IMHOTEP
IMMORAL
IMPORTS
IMPOSED
IMPOSER
IMPOSES
IMPOSTS
IMPOUND
IMSORRY
IMYOURS
INBOARD
INBOUND
INBOXES
INCOLOR
INCOMER
INCOMES
INCOURT
INDOORS
INDORSE
INDOUBT
INFOCUS
INFOLDS
INFORCE
INFORIT
INFORMS
INGOALS
INGOING
INHOUSE
INJOKES
INNOWAY
INPOINT
INPOURS
INPOWER
INROADS
INSOFAR
INSOLES
INTONED
INTONER
INTONES
INTOTAL
INTOUCH
INVOGUE
INVOICE
INVOKED
INVOKER
INVOKES
INVOLVE
INWOVEN
IOMOTHS
IONONES
ISTOMIN
ITSOKAY
ITSONME
ITSOPEN
ITSOVER

I•••O••

IAMLOVE
IANHOLM
ICEBOAT
ICECOLD
ICEDOUT
ICEDOWN
ICEFOGS
ICEHOLE
ICEPOPS
ICESOUT
IDAHOAN
IFORONE
IFSTONE
IGNEOUS
IGOROTS
IIIJOHN
ILLDOIT
ILLDONE
ILLFOLD
IMAGOES
IMAHOGG
IMBROKE
IMPIOUS
IMPLODE
IMPLORE
IMPROVE
INAHOLE
INAMOOD
INAPOEM
INAPOKE
INAWORD
INBLOOM
INBROWN
INCLOSE
INCROWD
INDOORS
INFLOWS
INFRONT
INGROUP
INGROWN
INIRONS
INKHORN
INKNOTS
INKPOTS
INSHOCK
INSHORE
INSHORT
INSPOTS
INSTOCK
INSTONE
INSTORE
INTROIT
IRISOUT
IRKSOME
IRONONS
IRONORE
IRONOUT
IRSFORM
ISADORA
ISADORE
ISECOND
ISIDORE
ISOGONS
ISONOMY
ISOPODS
ISOTONE
ISOTOPE
ISOTOPY
ITEMONE
ITSCOLD
ITSDONE
ITSGONE
ITSLOVE
IVANOVO

I••••O•

IBEGYOU
ICANNOT
ICEFLOE
ICESHOW
ICHABOD
ICKYPOO
IDIDTOO
IFORGOT
IGGYPOP
IGNATOW
IGNITOR
IGOTYOU
ILLKNOW
INAIDOF
INAKNOT
INAMOOD
INASHOE
INASPOT
INAWEOF
INBLOOM
INCISOR
INCOLOR
INDIGOS
INERROR
INFAVOR
INKBLOT
INKSPOT
INLABOR
IOWEYOU
IRECKON
IRONSON
ISEENOW
ISEEYOU
ITCHFOR
ITISTOO
ITSABOY
ITSALOT
IVANHOE
IVERSON
IZATION

I•••••O

ICKYPOO
IDIDTOO
IDSAYSO
IFYOUGO
IGNARRO
IHOPESO
IJKLMNO
ILOCANO
IMPASTO
IMUSTGO
INFERNO
INLIMBO
INUTERO
INVACUO
INVITRO
IONESCO
ISAIDNO
ISITAGO
ISOLATO
ISUREDO
ITISTOO
IVANOVO
IWANTTO
IZZATSO

•IO••••

BIOCHIP
BIOCIDE
BIODATA
BIOFUEL
BIOLABS
BIOLITE
BIOLOGY
BIOMASS
BIONICS
BIOPICS
BIOTECH
BIOTITE
BIOTYPE
DIOCESE
DIOMEDE
DIOPTER
DIORAMA
DIORITE
DIOTIMA
DIOXIDE
DIOXINS
FIORINA
GIOCOSO
GIORGIO
GIORGOS
LIONCUB
LIONELL
LIONELS
LIONESS
LIONETS
LIONISE
LIONIZE
MIOCENE
NIOBITE
NIOBIUM
PIOLETS
PIONEER
PIOSITY
PIOUSLY
RIOLOBO
RIOMUNI
RIORDAN
RIORITA
RIOTACT
RIOTERS
RIOTGUN
RIOTING
RIOTOUS
SIOBHAN
SIOUANS
TIOMKIN
VIOLATE
VIOLENT
VIOLETS
VIOLINS
VIOLIST
VIOLONE
ZIONISM
ZIONIST

•I•O•••

BICOLOR
BICORNE
BICORNS
BIFOCAL
BIGONES
BIGOTED
BIGOTRY
BILOBED
BIMODAL
BINOCHE
BIPOLAR
BITONAL
BIVOUAC
DIDOVER
DIEOFFS
DIMOUTS
DIPOLAR
DIPOLES
DISOBEY
DISOWNS
DIVORCE
EIDOLIC
EIDOLON
FILOFAX
GIGOLOS
GIROLLE
GIRONDE
KILOBAR
KILOBIT
KILOTON
KIMONOS
LIEOVER
LIMOGES
LITOTES
LITOVSK
LIVORNO
MIAOUED
MIAOWED
MIDOFFS
MILORDS
MIMOSAS
MINOANS
MINOGUE
MINOLTA
MINORCA
MINORED
MINORIN
MINOTND
MITOSES
MITOSIS
MITOTIC
NICOBAR
NICOISE
NICOLAS
NICOLET
NICOLLE
NICOSIA
NIKOLAI
NIKOLAY
PICOTED
PIGOUTS
PILOTED
PINOAKS
PINONES
PINOTTA
PIROGEN
PIROGUE
PIVOTAL
PIVOTED
PIVOTER
RICOTTA
RIDOTTO
RIGOURS
RIPOFFS
RIPOPEN
RIPOSTE
RIPOSTS
RISOTTO
SILOING
SIMONIZ
SIROCCO
SITONIT
TICOTIN
TIMOTHY
TINORES
TIPOFFS
TIPOVER
TITOISM
TITOIST
VICOMTE
VIGOURS
VISORED
VITORIA
VIZORED
WIDOWED
WIDOWER
WIMOWEH
WINOVER

•I••O••

AIRBOAT
AIRCOOL
AIRFOIL
AIRFONE
AIRHOLE
AIRHORN
AIRHOSE
AIRLOCK
AIRLOGS
AIRPOPS
AIRPORT
AIRPOTS
AIRSOCK
AIRSOUT
AIRWOLF
BIBCOCK
BICHONS
BIGBOSS
BIGBOYS
BIGDOGS
BIGFOOT
BIGFOUR
BIGHORN
BIGJOHN
BIGLOTS
BIGLOVE
BIGNOSE
BIGTOES
BIGTOPS
BIGTOWN

BILIOUS BILLOWS BILLOWY BIMBOES BINDOFF BINGOES BIOLOGY BISHOPS BITEOFF BITROLE CICCONE CINEOLE CISCOES CITROEN CITRONS CITROUS DIABOLO DIALOGS DIALOUT DIAMOND DIATOMS DIAVOLO DICKORY DIDGOOD DIDTOAT DIEBOLD DIEDOFF DIEDOUT DIEDOWN DIESOFF DIESOUT DIGGORY DIGLOTS DIGSOUT DIMSOUT DINEOUT DINGOES DINMONT DIPLOID DIPLOMA DISCOED DISCOID DISCORD DISHOUT DISJOIN DISPORT DISPOSE DISROBE DISTORT DITTOED FIBROID FIBROUS FILEOUT FILLOUT FINDOUT FIREOFF FISHOIL FISHOUT FIVEONE GIACOMO GIBBONS GIBBOUS GIBSONS GIDEONS GIFFORD GILFORD GILMORE GINGOLD

GIOCOSO GIVEOFF GIVEOUT HICKORY HIDEOUS HIDEOUT HIKEOUT HILLOCK HILTONS HIPBONE HIPBOOT HIPROOF HIREOUT HISTORY HITHOME HITSOFF HITSONG HITSOUT HITTOWN HIVEOFF IIIJOHN JIBBOOM JIMHOGG JIMSONS JINGOES KICKOFF KICKOUT KIDCOMS KIDROCK KINFOLK KINMONT KISSOFF LIEDOWN LIENORS LIFTOFF LIMPOPO LINCOLN LINDORF LINEONE LINEOUT LINGOES LIPSOFF LIPSOUT LIQUORS LISSOME LITHOID LIVEOAK LIVEONE LIVEOUT MICROBE MICRONS MIDMORN MIDMOST MIDNOON MIDSOLE MIDTOWN MIGNONS MILHOUS MIMEOED MINDORO MINEOLA MINIONS MINNOWS MIRRORS MISCODE MISCOIN MISCOPY MISDOER

MISDOES MISDONE MISFORM MISJOIN MISKOLC MISMOVE MISSORT MISSOUT MISTOLD MISTOOK MISWORD MISZONE MITFORD NIALONG NICCOLO NICEONE NICHOLS NIMRODS NITROUS NIVEOUS PIANOLA PICCOLO PICEOUS PICKOFF PICKOUT PIEHOLE PIETOSO PIGEONS PIGSOUT PILEOUS PILLORY PILLOWS PILLOWY PINBOYS PINDOWN PINEOIL PINFOLD PINHOLE PINIONS PINKOES PISCOPO PISTOLE PISTOLS PISTONS PISTOUS PITBOSS PITEOUS PITROWS RIBBONS RIBBONY RIDEOFF RIDEOUT RIGSOUT RIMROCK RINGOFF RINGOUT RIOLOBO RIOTOUS RIPCORD RIPSOFF RIPSONE RIPSOUT RIPTORN RISSOLE SICKOUT SIDDONS SIDEONE SIDIOUS

SIGMOID SIGNOFF SIGNORA SIGNORE SIGNORS SIGNOUT SIMMONS SINGOUT SINUOUS SIPHONS SIRLOIN SITCOMS SITDOWN SITHOME SITSOUT SIXFOLD SIXFOOT SIXFOUR SIZEONE TICKOFF TIEDOFF TIEDOWN TIEPOLO TIERODS TIEROPE TIESOFF TIGLONS TIMEOFF TIMEOUT TIMHOLT TIMROTH TINFOIL TINGODS TINHORN TINROOF TINWORK TIPDOWN TIPSOFF TIPTOED TIPTOES TIPTOPS TIREOUT TISSOTS VICIOUS VICTORS VICTORY VIDEOED VIDIOTS VIGNOLA VINROSE VIOLONE VIRGOAN VISCOUS VISIONS WIGSOUT WILDONE WILFORD WILLOWS WILLOWY WILSONS WIMPOLE WIMPOUT WINDOMS WINDOWS WINDOWY WINKOUT WINNOWS WINSOME

WINSOUT WINWOOD WIPEOFF WIPEOUT WISDOMS WISEONE WITEOUT WITHOUT XINGOUT XIPHOID ZINCOUS ZIPCODE ZIPLOCK ZIPLOCS ZIPSOFF ZIPTOPS ZIRCONS ZITCOMS

•I•••O•

AIKIDOS AILERON AIMSFOR AIRCOOL AIRDROP AIRFLOW AIRGLOW AIRSHOW BIBELOT BIBLIOG BICOLOR BIDSFOR BIENTOT BIGELOW BIGFOOT BIGSHOT BIGSHOW BILLION BIRDDOG BISTROS BITESON CITYBOY DIABLOS DIARIOS DICKSON DICTION DIDEROT DIDGOOD DIEDFOR DIESFOR DIGSFOR DILATOR DILUTOR DINEDON DINESON DISAVOW DISTROS DIVISOR EIDOLON FIASCOS FICTION FIEFDOM FILMDOM FINKSON FIREBOX FIREDOG FIREDON FIREFOX

FIRESON FISHFOR FISSION FITZROY FIXEDON FIXESON FIXUPON GIFTBOX GIGATON GIGOLOS GINGKOS GINKGOS GIORGOS GIRASOL GITANOS GIVENOF GIVENON GIVESOF GIVESON HIGHBOY HIGHLOW HIGHTOP HILLTOP HINGEON HIPBOOT HIPROOF HIREDON HIRESON HITCHON HITSFOR HITSHOW HITUPON JIBBOOM JILLION KIARIOS KICKBOX KILLJOY KILOTON KIMONOS KINGDOM KINISON LIAISON LIBIDOS LIEATOP LIEDFOR LIESFOR LIESLOW LIGHTON LIKEWOW LIMACON LINDROS LINGCOD LITHGOW LIVEDON LIVEFOR LIVESON MIDIRON MIDNOON MIKADOS MILKCOW MILKSOP MILLION MINIZOO MIRADOR MISKNOW MISSION MISSYOU MISTBOW

MISTOOK NICEBOY NICEDOG NICEJOB NILESOH NILSSON NIPIGON OILSPOT PICADOR PICAROS PICKSON PIDGEON PIERROT PIETROS PIGIRON PILCROW PILEDON PILESOF PILESON PILLBOX PILLION PIMESON PINCHOT PINEFOR PINESOL PINETOP PITSTOP RIALTOS RIGHTON RIMSHOT RINGFOR RIPSTOP SIGHFOR SIGNFOR SIGNSON SILICON SIMENON SIMPSON SISENOR SITATOP SITINON SITSFOR SITUPON SIXFOOT SIXIRON TIBURON TIEMPOS TILLNOW TILTTOP TIMECOP TINAMOU TINROOF TINYTOT TIREDOF TIRESOF VICEROY VIDICON VIEDFOR VIESFOR VIRAGOS VISITOR VISTEON VITRIOL WICKLOW WIDGEON WILDDOG WILLSON WILLYOU

WINDGOD WINDSOR WINSLOW WINSTON WINWOOD WISHFOR ZILLION

•I••••O

BINDSTO BIZARRO CILENTO CINZANO DIABOLO DIALEDO DIAVOLO DICILLO DIGINTO DIPINTO FIDELIO FILIPPO FITINTO FIVETWO GIACOMO GIOCOSO GIORGIO GIVENTO GIVESTO HIBERNO HIDALGO HISPANO HITINTO LIKENTO LIMPOPO LINBIAO LINETWO LINPIAO LITINTO LIVORNO MILAGRO MINDORO MINIZOO NICCOLO PICARDO PICASSO PICCOLO PIETOSO PIMENTO PIMLICO PISANIO PISARRO PISCOPO PITCHTO PITILLO PIZARRO RICARDO RIDESTO RIDOTTO RILIEVO RINALDO RIOLOBO RIPIENO RIPINTO RISENTO RISESTO RISOTTO RIVERPO RIZZUTO

SIDETWO SILENTO SINGSTO SIROCCO SIZETWO TIEINTO TIEPOLO VIBRATO VISCUSO WINDIGO YIELDTO

••IO•••

ABIOTIC ANIONIC ARIOSOS ARIOSTO AVIONIC BRIOCHE IDIOTIC MEIOSES MEIOSIS MEIOTIC OHIOANS OHIOART ORIOLES PRIORTO SCIORRA TRIODES TRIOLET

••I•O••

ADIPOSE ALIFORM ALIGOTE ALIMONY AMIDOLS ARIZONA BAILORS BAILOUT BOILOFF BOILOUT BRITONS BUITONI CHICORY CHIGOES CHINOIS CHINOOK CHITONS CHITOWN CLIPOFF CLIPONS CLIPOUT COINOPS CUIBONO EDITORS EDITOUT EPIDOTE EPIGONE EPILOGS EPISODE EPITOME EVILONE FAIROFF FLIPOUT FRIJOLE FRIVOLS HEINOUS

IIIJOHN INIRONS IRISOUT ISIDORE JAILORS LAIDOFF LAIDOUT MAILOUT MAISONS MAISOUI NAIROBI NOISOME OLICOOK OMIGOSH OMINOUS ORINOCO ORISONS OVIFORM PAIDOFF PAIDOUT PAIROFF PHILOUS POISONS PRISONS QUIXOTE RAINOUT RAISONS RHIZOME RUINOUS SAILORS SAISONS SEIZORS SHIKOKU SHINOLA SHIPOUT SKIBOBS SKIBOOT SKIDOOS SKIPOLE SKIPOUT SKITOWS SLIDOFF SLIDOUT SLIPOFF SLIPONS SLIPOUT SNIPOFF SPIGOTS SPINOFF SPINOUT SPINOZA SPITOUT SUITORS TAILOFF TAILORS THINOUT THISONE TRIBORO TRICORN TRICOTS TRIFOLD TRIFORM TRIGONS TRILOGY TRIMOFF TRIPODS TRIPOLI TRITONE

TRITONS TVIDOLS UNIBODY UNICODE UNICORN UNIFORM UNIPODS UNISOMS UNISONS VOIDOUT WAITOUT

••I••O•

ALIENOR ANISTON APILEOF ARIOSOS ARISTOS ASIAGOS ATIPTOE AVIATOR AVIGNON BAILSON BRILLOS BRINGON BRISTOL BRITCOM BRITPOP BRITTON BUILDON BUILTON BUISSON CAILLOU CAISSON CHIFFON CHIGNON CHINOOK CLICKON CLIFTON CLIMBON CLINTON CLIPSON COINBOX CRIMSON DOINGOK DOITNOW DRIPSON EDITION ELISION ERICSON ERIKSON ESIASON EVICTOR EXITNOW FLIESON FLIPTOP FOISTON FRISSON GAINSON GOINFOR GOINGON GRIFFON GRINGOS GRINKOV GRISSOM GUIGNOL HAIRDOS HEIRDOM

IDIDTOO ITISTOO KEILLOR KLINGON LAIDFOR LAIDLOW LYINGON MAILBOX MAILLOL MAILLOT MAINTOP ODINGON OLICOOK OMICRON OPINION OWINGON PAIDFOR PHILCOS POISSON QUINION QUINTON QUIZNOS RAILSON RAINBOW RAINGOD RAINSON SAIDBOO SAILSON SCISSOR SEIZEON SHINEON SKIBOOT SKIDDOO SKIDOOS SKIDROW SKIMPON SKISHOP SLIPSON SMILEON SMIRNOV SPIEDON SPIESON SPITSON STICKON STILTON STIMSON SWINTON THINKOF TRIEDON TRIESON TRIPSON TRIVIOT TUITION TWISTON TYINGON VUITTON WAITFOR WAITRON WAITSON WEIGHON WEIRDOS WEIRTON WRITEON

••I•••O

AGITATO AKIHITO ALIENTO

ALIVETO ANIMATO ARIGATO ARIOSTO BLINDTO BOIARDO BOITANO BRINGTO CHICAGO CHICANO CHIRICO CLIMBTO CLINGTO CUIBONO DEIGNTO DOINGSO DOINGTO DRINKTO DRIVETO FAILSTO FLIEDTO FLIESTO GOINGTO HEIGHHO IDIDTOO ISITAGO ITISTOO LYINGTO ORINOCO OWINGTO PAISANO POINTTO PRIMERO PRIORTO PRIVYTO QUITESO SAIDBOO SAIDIDO SAILSTO SAINTLO SKIDDOO STICKTO THINKSO TRIBORO TRIEDTO TRIESTO TYINGTO WAIKATO WRITETO ZHIVAGO

•••IO••

ACTIONS AMNIONS ANTIOCH ANXIOUS APRIORI BCLIONS BILIOUS BUNIONS CAMIONS CARIOCA CARIOLE CARIOUS CATIONS COPIOUS CURIOSA CURIOUS

DEVIOUS
DUBIOUS
ELLIOTT
ENVIOUS
FANIONS
FOLIOED
FOLIOSE
FURIOSO
FURIOUS
FUSIONS
IMPIOUS
JUNIORS
LEGIONS
LESIONS
LOTIONS
MAFIOSI
MAFIOSO
MINJONS
MOTIONS
NATIONS
NOTIONS
NOXIOUS
OBVIOUS
ONEIOTA
OPTIONS
PAVIORS
PAVIOUR
PERIODS
PETIOLE
PINIONS
POTIONS
RADIOAD
RADIODJ
RADIOED
RADIOER
RADIOIN
RATIONS
RAVIOLI
REGIONS
RUBIOUS
SAVIORS
SAVIOUR
SENIORS
SERIOUS
SIDIOUS
TAPIOCA
TEDIOUS
UNPIOUS
VARIOUS
VICIOUS
VIDIOTS
VISIONS

•••I•O•

ACTINON
ADDISON
ADVISOR
AIKIDOS
AJSIMON
ALBINOS
ALLISON
ALNICOS
ANDIRON
ANTIFOG
ANTILOG
APAIROF
APRICOT
AUDITOR
BENISON
BONITOS
CALICOS
CAMINOS
CAPITOL
CARIBOO
CARIBOU
CASINOS
CHRISOM
CLAIROL
COPILOT
CUTINON
DAVISON
DEMIGOD
DENISON
DEVISOR
DIVISOR
DOMINOS
DORITOS
DOSIDOS
ELEISON
ELLISON
ELNINOS
ENVIRON
ENVIROS
EPSILON
EQUINOX
ESKIMOS
EXCITOR
FAMICOM
GENITOR
GERITOL
GETINON
GETITON
GOTINON
GOTITON
HARICOT
HEDISON
HELICON
HERITOR
HORIZON
HUMIDOR
IGNITOR
INAIDOF
INCISOR
INDIGOS
JAMISON
JANITOR
JEMISON
JEWISON
KEMIDOV
KEYINON
KINISON
LADINOS
LATIGOS
LATINOS
LAYITON
LEGIRON
LETINON
LEXICON
LIAISON
LIBIDOS
LYRICON
MADISON
MAGINOT
MANILOW
MARIDOS
MEDICOS
MERINOS
MIDIRON
MINIZOO
MOJITOS
MOLITOR
MONITOR
MORISOT
NIPIGON
NONIRON
OBLIGOR
ONEIRON
ORBISON
PAXINOU
PERIDOT
PIGIRON
QUEIROS
RACINOS
RETINOL
REVISOR
RUBICON
SATINON
SEMILOG
SILICON
SITINON
SIXIRON
STRIPOF
STSIMON
TORINOS
TOTINOS
TRAITOR
TRYITON
TWOIRON
UPSILON
USTINOV
VENISON
VERIZON
VIDICON
VISITOR
XENIAOH

•••I••O

ADMITTO
ALBIREO
ANDIAMO
ATEINTO
BASILIO
BENICIO
BENIGNO
BONIATO
BUYINTO
BYJINGO
CARIBOO
CHRISTO
CUTINTO
DELICTO
DELILLO
DICILLO
DIGINTO
DIPINTO
DOMINGO
DUGINTO
EATINTO
EQUIANO
FEDINTO
FILIPPO
FITINTO
FLYINTO
FURILLO
FURIOSO
GALILEO
GETINTO
GOTINTO
HITINTO
HOPINTO
INLIMBO
INVITRO
ISAIDNO
JACINTO
JALISCO
JERICHO
LAMINTO
LAYINTO
LEDINTO
LETITGO
LITINTO
LUCIANO
MAFIOSO
MARIANO
MINIZOO
MURILLO
NABISCO
OFFICIO
ONVIDEO
ORNITHO
ORVIETO
PAYINTO
PITILLO
PRYINTO
PUTITTO
RAMINTO
RANINTO
RILIEVO
RIPIENO
RIPINTO
RUNINTO
SAWINTO
SEEINTO
SEMIPRO
SETINTO
SORIANO
TAPINTO
TIEINTO
TURISMO
UTRILLO
VERISMO
ZEDILLO

••••IO•

ADAGIOS
AMPHION
ANTLION
AUCTION
BAGNIOS
BALLIOL
BARRIOS
BASTION
BEALION
BERLIOZ
BIBLIOG
BILLION
BLERIOT
BULLION
CABRIOS
CAMPION
CAPTION
CAUTION
CESSION
CHARIOT
CHEVIOT
CLARION
CRATION
CUSHION
CYPRIOT
DIARIOS
DICTION
DREGION
EDITION
ELATION
ELISION
ELUTION
EMOTION
EROSION
EVASION
FACTION
FASHION
FERMION
FICTION
FISSION
FLEXION
FLUXION
GRUNION
HELLION
HERRIOT
IZATION
JILLION
KIARIOS
KRATION
MANSION
MARMION
MENTION
MGMLION
MILLION
MISSION
NUNCIOS
OPINION
ORARION
ORATION
OVATION
PASSION
PATRIOT
PENSION
PETLION
PILLION
PLOSION
PORTION
PRERIOT
QRATIOS
QUINION
RANRIOT
REUNION
RUCTION
RUNRIOT
SEALION
SECTION
SESSION
STARION
STATION
STUDIOS
SUASION
SUCTION
TENSION
TORSION
TRIVIOT
TSELIOT
TUITION
UNCTION
VERSION
VITRIOL
WARRIOR
ZILLION

••••I•O

AKIHITO
AMERIGO
ARECIBO
ARETINO
BAMBINO
BANDIDO
BANDITO
BURRITO
BUSHIDO
CALVINO
CANTINO
CASSINO
CENTIMO
CHIRICO
CHORIZO
CORTICO
DERRICO
DESTINO
DOASIDO
EXANIMO
GALLICO
HAPKIDO
JACKIEO
JANEIRO
LACRIMO
LENTIGO
LINBIAO
LINPIAO
LUCHINO
MANRICO
MARTINO
NANAIMO
ONEKILO
PAMLICO
PEPPINO
PEPSICO
PERDIDO
PIMLICO
PLACIDO
PORTICO
PROVISO
PROXIMO
QUERIDO
RODRIGO
SAIDIDO
SAYHITO
SAYSIDO
SERPICO
SHAPIRO
SORDINO
SORVINO
SUREIDO
TAMPICO
TOSHIRO
TREVINO
UGOLINO
VERTIGO
WINDIGO

•••••IO

AJACCIO
AMRADIO
ANTONIO
ARSENIO
ARTERIO
AUTOBIO
BASILIO
BENICIO
BONARIO
CBRADIO
CHEERIO
CLAUDIO
CONBRIO
DRMARIO
FIDELIO
FMRADIO
GENNAIO
GIORGIO
HORATIO
OCTAVIO
OFFICIO
ONTARIO
OTTAVIO
PERATIO
PISANIO
ROSARIO
SCORPIO
XMRADIO

IP•••••

IPANEMA
IPCRESS
IPLEDGE
IPSWICH

I•P••••

IAPETUS
IIPETER
IMPACTS
IMPAIRS
IMPALAS
IMPALED
IMPALER
IMPALES
IMPANEL
IMPARTS
IMPASSE
IMPASTO
IMPAVID
IMPEACH
IMPEDED
IMPEDER
IMPEDES
IMPENDS
IMPERIL
IMPETUS
IMPIETY
IMPINGE
IMPIOUS
IMPLANT
IMPLEAD
IMPLIED
IMPLIES
IMPLODE
IMPLORE
IMPORTS
IMPOSED
IMPOSER
IMPOSES
IMPOSTS
IMPOUND
IMPRESS
IMPREST
IMPREZA
IMPRINT
IMPROVE
IMPUGNS
IMPULSE
IMPURER
IMPUTED
IMPUTER
IMPUTES
INPEACE
INPERIL
INPHASE
INPLACE
INPOINT
INPOURS
INPOWER
INPRINT

I••P•••

ICEPACK
ICEPICK
ICEPOPS
IHOPESO
ILLPASS
INAPILE
INAPOEM
INAPOKE
INAPRIL
INAPTER
INAPTLY
INEPTLY
INKPADS
INKPOTS
INSPACE
INSPANS
INSPECT
INSPIRE
INSPITE
INSPOTS
IREPEAT
ISOPODS

I•••P••

ICKYPOO
IGGYPOP
IMHAPPY
INASPIN
INASPOT
INCEPTS
INDEPTH
INKSPOT
INSIPID
IRRUPTS
ITSOPEN

I••••P•

ICECAPS
ICEPOPS
IMHAPPY
INSHAPE
INSTEPS
INSWEPT
ISOTOPE
ISOTOPY

I•••••P

ICINGUP
IGGYPOP
IGIVEUP
IMHOTEP
INAHEAP
INASNAP
INATRAP
INGROUP
INKYCAP

•IP••••

BIPEDAL
BIPLANE
BIPOLAR
CIPHERS
DIPINTO
DIPLOID
DIPLOMA
DIPNETS
DIPOLAR
DIPOLES
DIPPERS
DIPPIER
DIPPING
DIPTYCH
FIPPLES
GIPSIES
HIPBATH
HIPBONE
HIPBOOT
HIPLESS
HIPLIKE
HIPNESS
HIPPEST
HIPPIER
HIPPIES
HIPPISH
HIPPITY
HIPROOF
HIPSTER
IIPETER
KIPLING
KIPPERS
KIPPING
LIPARIS
LIPASES
LIPBALM
LIPIDIC
LIPLESS
LIPLIKE
LIPMANN
LIPPERS
LIPPIER
LIPPING
LIPREAD
LIPSOFF
LIPSOUT
LIPSYNC
NIPIGON
NIPMUCK
NIPPERS
NIPPIER
NIPPILY
NIPPING
NIPPLES
PIPAGES
PIPCARD
PIPEDIN
PIPEDUP
PIPEFUL
PIPESIN
PIPESUP
PIPETTE
PIPIEST
PIPINGS
PIPLESS
PIPPINS
RIPCORD
RIPENED
RIPENER
RIPIENI
RIPIENO
RIPINTO
RIPOFFS
RIPOPEN
RIPOSTE
RIPOSTS
RIPPERS
RIPPING
RIPPLED
RIPPLES
RIPPLET
RIPRAPS
RIPSAWN
RIPSAWS
RIPSOFF
RIPSONE
RIPSOUT
RIPSTOP
RIPTIDE
RIPTORN
SIPHONS
SIPPERS
SIPPING
TIPCART
TIPDOWN
TIPJARS
TIPLESS
TIPLINE
TIPOFFS
TIPOVER
TIPPEES
TIPPERS
TIPPETS
TIPPIER
TIPPING
TIPPLED
TIPPLER
TIPPLES
TIPSIER
TIPSILY
TIPSOFF
TIPSTER
TIPTOED
TIPTOES
TIPTOPS
WIPEDUP
WIPEOFF
WIPEOUT
WIPESUP
XIPHOID
YIPPIES
YIPPING
ZIPCODE
ZIPCUFF
ZIPDISK
ZIPGUNS
ZIPLOCK
ZIPLOCS
ZIPPERS
ZIPPIER
ZIPPING
ZIPSOFF
ZIPTOPS

•I•P•••

AIRPACK
AIRPARK
AIRPLAY
AIRPOPS
AIRPORT
AIRPOTS
AIRPUMP
BIOPICS
BITPART
DIAPERS
DIAPHAN
DIMPLED
DIMPLES
DIOPTER
DIPPERS
DIPPIER
DIPPING
DISPART
DISPELS
DISPLAY
DISPORT
DISPOSE
DISPUTE
FIPPLES
GIMPING
HIPPEST
HIPPIER
HIPPIES
HIPPISH
HIPPITY
HISPANO
HISPEED
HITPLAY
KIPPERS
KIPPING
LIMPEST
LIMPETS
LIMPING
LIMPOPO
LINPIAO
LIPPERS
LIPPIER
LIPPING
LISPERS
LISPING
MISPAGE
MISPLAN
MISPLAY
NIPPERS
NIPPIER
NIPPILY
NIPPING
NIPPLES
NITPICK
OILPALM
OILPANS
PIEPANS
PIGPENS
PIMPLED
PIMPLES
PIPPINS
RIBPADS
RIMPLED
RIMPLES
RIPPERS
RIPPING
RIPPLED
RIPPLES
RIPPLET
SIMPERS
SIMPLER
SIMPLES
SIMPLEX
SIMPSON
SIPPERS
SIPPING
SIXPACK
TIEPINS
TIEPOLO
TIMPANI
TIPPEES
TIPPERS
TIPPETS
TIPPIER
TIPPING
TIPPLED
TIPPLER
TIPPLES
TIRPITZ
WIMPIER
WIMPING
WIMPISH
WIMPLED
WIMPLES
WIMPOLE
WIMPOUT
WISPIER
WISPILY
WISPING
YIPPIES
YIPPING
ZIPPERS
ZIPPIER
ZIPPING

•I••P••

BIASPLY
BIGAPES
DIGIPET
DISHPAN
FILIPPO
FIREPIT
FIVEPIN
FIXUPON
HIGHPAY
HINDPAW
HITUPON
KINGPIN
LILYPAD
LIMEPIE
MINEPIT
NINEPIN
OILSPOT
PITAPAT
RIPOPEN
SICKPAY
SITSPAT
SITUPON
TIEMPOS
WILDPIG

•I•••P•

AIRPOPS
BIGTOPS
BIOTYPE
BISHOPS
BITMAPS
DIALUPS
DIDLAPS
DIGRAPH
DISRUPT
EIGHTPM
FILIPPO
FILLIPS
FILLUPS
GIVEUPS
HICCUPS
KICKUPS
KIDNAPS
LIMPOPO
LINEUPS
LINKUPS
MIDCAPS
MISCOPY
MISHAPS
MISTYPE
OILCUPS
PICKUPS
PILEUPS
PISCOPO
RIPRAPS
RIVERPO
SIGNUPS
TIEROPE
TINTYPE
TIPTOPS
WINDUPS
ZIPTOPS

•I••••P

AIRDROP
AIREDUP
AIRPUMP
AIRSHIP
AIRTRAP
BIGGULP
BINDSUP
BIOCHIP
BITESUP
DIALSUP
DICECUP
DIVVYUP
EIGHTUP
FILLSUP
FIREDUP
FIRESUP
FIRMSUP
FIRSTUP
FIXEDUP
FIXESUP

GIDDYAP
GIDDYUP
GIVENUP
GIVESUP
HIGHTOP
HIKEDUP
HIKESUP
HILLTOP
HITCHUP
KICKSUP
KINSHIP
LICKSUP
LIEATOP
LIFTSUP
LIGHTUP
LINEDUP
LINESUP
LINKSUP
LIVENUP
MIDSHIP
MILKSOP
MISSHIP
MISSTEP
MISTSUP
MIXEDUP
MIXESUP
MIXITUP
OILLAMP
PICKSUP
PILEDUP
PILESUP
PINESAP
PINETOP
PIPEDUP
PIPESUP
PITSTOP
RIDESUP
RILEDUP
RILESUP
RINGSUP
RIPSTOP
RISESUP
SIGNSUP
SILENTP
SITATOP
SITEMAP
SIZEDUP
SIZESUP
TIDERIP
TIECLIP
TILTSUP
TILTTOP
TIMECOP
TIMESUP
WICKIUP
WINDSUP
WINESAP
WINGTIP
WIPEDUP
WIPESUP
WIREDUP
WIRESUP
WIRETAP
WISEDUP
WISESUP

••IP•••

ADIPOSE
ATIPTOE
BLIPPED
CHIPPED
CHIPPER
CHIPSIN
CHIPSUP
CLIPART
CLIPOFF
CLIPONS
CLIPOUT
CLIPPED
CLIPPER
CLIPSON
CRIPPLE
DRIPDRY
DRIPPAN
DRIPPED
DRIPPER
DRIPSON
FLIPOUT
FLIPPED
FLIPPEN
FLIPPER
FLIPTOP
FLIPUPS
GRIPERS
GRIPING
GRIPPED
GRIPPER
GRIPPES
LEIPZIG
NAIPAUL
OVIPARA
PEIPING
QUIPPED
QUIPPER
SHIPFUL
SHIPMAN
SHIPMEN
SHIPOUT
SHIPPED
SHIPPER
SHIPWAY
SKIPOLE
SKIPOUT
SKIPPED
SKIPPER
SKIPSBY
SLIPOFF
SLIPONS
SLIPOUT
SLIPPED
SLIPPER
SLIPSBY
SLIPSIN
SLIPSON
SLIPSUP
SLIPUPS
SNIPEAT
SNIPERS
SNIPING
SNIPOFF
SNIPPED
SNIPPER
SNIPPET
STIPEND
STIPPLE
SWIPERS
SWIPING
TRIPLEA
TRIPLED
TRIPLES
TRIPLET
TRIPLEX
TRIPODS
TRIPOLI
TRIPPED
TRIPPER
TRIPPET
TRIPSON
TRIPSUP
UNIPLEX
UNIPODS
WHIPPED
WHIPPER
WHIPPET
WHIPPLE
WHIPSAW
WHIPSIN
WHIPSUP

••I•P••

BLIMPIE
BLIPPED
BRITPOP
CHIAPAS
CHIAPET
CHIPPED
CHIPPER
CHIRPED
CHIRPER
CLIPPED
CLIPPER
CRIMPED
CRIMPER
CRIPPLE
CRISPED
CRISPEN
CRISPER
CRISPIN
CRISPIX
CRISPLY
CRISPUS
DNIEPER
DRIPPAN
DRIPPED
DRIPPER
FLIPPED
FLIPPEN
FLIPPER
GLIMPSE
GRIPPED
GRIPPER
GRIPPES
HAIRPIN
PRIMPED
QUIPPED
QUIPPER
REIMPLY
SHINPAD
SHIPPED
SHIPPER
SKIMPED
SKIMPON
SKIPPED
SKIPPER
SLIPPED
SLIPPER
SNIPPED
SNIPPER
SNIPPET
STIPPLE
TAILPIN
THIGPEN
THIMPHU
TRIPPED
TRIPPER
TRIPPET
WHIMPER
WHIPPED
WHIPPER
WHIPPET
WHIPPLE
WHISPER

••I••P•

CHINUPS
COINOPS
EPITAPH
FLIPUPS
PHILIPK
PHILIPS
PHILIPV
SKICAPS
SLIPUPS
TRICEPS
TRIUMPH

••I•••P

BOILSUP
BRICKUP
BRINGUP
BRITPOP
BUILDUP
BUILTUP
CHIPSUP
CHIRRUP
CLIMBUP
COILSUP
CRIEDUP
CRIESUP
DOINGUP
DRIEDUP
DRIESUP
DRIFTUP
DRINKUP
DRIVEUP
EPICARP
FAIRSUP
FLIESUP
FLIPTOP
FRIEDUP
FRIESUP
GOINGUP
GRIDMAP
HOISTUP
ICINGUP
IGIVEUP
JOINSUP
JUICEUP
LYINGUP
MAINTOP
NAILSUP
NAILTIP
PAIRSUP
PHILLIP
POINTUP
PRICKUP
PRINTUP
RAISEUP
SHINEUP
SKIJUMP
SKISHOP
SKITRIP
SLICEUP
SLINKUP
SLIPSUP
SNIFFUP
SPICEUP
SPIFFUP
SPIKEUP
STICKUP
STILLUP
STINKUP
STIRRUP
STIRSUP
SUITSUP
SWIMSUP
THINKUP
TRIPSUP
TWISTUP
TYINGUP
USINGUP
WAITSUP
WEIGHUP
WHIPSUP
WRITEUP

•••IP••

AGRIPPA
CALIPER
CALIPHS
DIGIPET
ECLIPSE
ELLIPSE
FILIPPO
HELIPAD
INSIPID
JUNIPER
MANIPLE
MANIPUR
OCCIPUT
OEDIPAL
OEDIPUS
OSSIPEE
RECIPES
REWIPED
REWIPES
SCRIPPS
SCRIPTS
SEMIPRO
SERIPAK
STRIPED
STRIPER
STRIPES
STRIPOF
TRAIPSE
UNPIPED
UNRIPER
UNWIPED

•••I•P•

AGRIPPA
FILIPPO
PERIAPT
SCRIMPS
SCRIMPY
SCRIPPS
SHRIMPS
SHRIMPY

•••I••P

APHILIP
ATEITUP
CHAINUP
EATITUP
HAMITUP
MEDIGAP
MIXITUP
RANITUP
REVITUP
RUNITUP
SPLITUP
SUMITUP
TEEITUP

••••IP•

BAGPIPE
CATNIPS
CUETIPS
FATLIPS
FILLIPS
GASPIPE
GOSSIPS
GOSSIPY
HOTLIPS
HOTTIPS
MRCHIPS
OUTLIPS
OUTPIPE
PANPIPE
PHILIPK
PHILIPS
PHILIPV
PVCPIPE
RECEIPT
REFLIPS
REGRIPS
RESHIPS
THEPIPS
THEVIPS
THEYIPS
TURNIPS
UNCLIPS
UNCLIPT
UNGRIPS
UNSHIPS
UNWHIPT
YUCAIPA

••••I•P

MRQUILP
WICKIUP

•••••IP

AIRSHIP
APHILIP
ATACLIP
BADTRIP
BEANDIP
BIOCHIP
BUSTRIP
CANTRIP
CARTRIP
CLAMDIP
COWSLIP
DAYTRIP
EARCLIP
EGOTRIP
FELTTIP
FLEADIP
FOULTIP
GETATIP
GETSHIP
GOLDTIP
GOTATIP
GUNSHIP
HADANIP
HASANIP
KEYGRIP
KINSHIP
LEFTHIP
LETSLIP
LETSRIP
MIDSHIP
MISSHIP
NAILTIP
NONDRIP
NONSLIP
NUNSHIP
ONATRIP
ONECHIP
OUTSKIP
OVERTIP
PARSNIP
PAYSLIP
PHILLIP
PRESHIP
PREWHIP
REDCHIP
REEQUIP
RESTRIP
ROSEHIP
SEATRIP
SKITRIP
SONSHIP
TIDERIP
TIECLIP
VERYHIP
WARSHIP
WINGTIP
WORSHIP

IQ•••••

IQTESTS

I•Q••••

INQUEST
INQUIRE
INQUIRY

•IQ••••

LIQUATE
LIQUEFY
LIQUEUR
LIQUIDS
LIQUORS
PIQUANT
PIQUING

•I•Q•••

BISQUES
CINQUES
CIRQUES

•I••Q••

GIAUQUE

•I•••Q•

HIGHIQS

•I••••Q

SILENTQ

••IQ•••

BRIQUET
CLIQUED
CLIQUES
CLIQUEY
UNIQUES

••I•Q••

QUINQUE

•••IQ••

ANTIQUE
BEZIQUE
CACIQUE
COMIQUE
ENRIQUE
LALIQUE
OBLIQUE

••••IQ•

HIGHIQS

IR•••••

IRANIAN
IRATELY
IRATEST
IRECKON
IREFUSE
IRELAND
IRELESS
IRENICS
IREPEAT
IRESIGN
IRIDIUM
IRISHER
IRISING
IRISOUT
IRKSOME
IRKUTSK
IRONAGE
IRONBAR
IRONERS
IRONIES
IRONING
IRONIST
IRONMAN
IRONMEN
IRONONS
IRONORE
IRONOUT
IRONSON
IRRUPTS
IRSFORM

I•R••••

IGRAINE
IMREADY
INRANGE
INREACH
INROADS
INRUINS
IRRUPTS
ISRAELI
ISRAFEL

I••R•••

IATRICS
IBERIAN
ICERINK
ICERUNS
IDAREDS
IFORGET
IFORGOT
IFORONE
IGOROTS
IMARETS
IMBROKE
IMBRUED
IMBRUES
IMGREAT
IMPRESS
IMPREST
IMPREZA
IMPRINT
IMPROVE
INARAGE
INARUSH
INBREED
INBRIEF
INBROWN
INCROWD
INCRUST
INDRAFT
INDRAWN
INERROR
INERTIA
INERTLY
INFRACT
INFRONT
INGRAFT
INGRAIN
INGRATE
INGREEN
INGRESS
INGROUP
INGROWN
INIRONS
INORBIT
INORDER
INPRINT
INTRADE
INTRAYS
INTROIT
INTRUDE
INTRUST
INTRUTH
INURING
IPCRESS
ISTRIAN
ISUREAM
ISUREDO
ITERANT
ITERATE
IVERSON
IVORIAN
IVORIES
IVORINE

I•••R••

ICEFREE
ICETRAY
ICTERUS
IDCARDS
IGNARRO
IGNORED
IGNORER
IGNORES
IHEARYA
ILLBRED
ILLYRIA
IMBORED
IMFORIT
IMMERGE
IMMERSE
IMMORAL
IMMURED
IMMURES
IMPARTS
IMPERIL
IMPORTS
IMPURER
IMSORRY
IMTIRED
INAPRIL
INATRAP
INCURVE
INDORSE
INERROR
INFERNO
INFIRST
INFORCE
INFORIT
INFORMS
INHERED
INHERES
INHERIT
INJURED
INJURER
INJURES
INLARGE
INMARCH
INNARDS
INNERLY
INNERVE
INPERIL
INSERTS
INSURED
INSURER
INSURES
INTERIM
INTERNE
INTERNS
INTERSE
INTHREE
INTURNS
INVERSE
INVERTS
INWARDS
ISOGRAM
ITGIRLS
ITHIRTY
ITSTRUE

I••••R•

ICEBERG
IGNARRO
IMAGERS
IMAGERY
IMPAIRS
IMPLORE
IMSORRY
IMTHERE
IMYOURS
INAFURY
INAWORD
INBOARD
INCHERS
INCOURT
INDOORS
INKHORN
INKMARK
INPOURS
INQUIRE
INQUIRY
INSHORE
INSHORT
INSPIRE
INSTORE
INTEARS
INTEGRA
INTHERE
INTHIRD
INUTERO
INVITRO
INYEARS
IRONERS
IRONORE
IRSFORM
ISADORA
ISADORE
ISIDORE
ISOBARS
ISOMERS
ISSUERS
ITSHERE

I•••••R

ICEBEER
ICEOVER
IDOTTER
IGNITER
IGNITOR
IGNORER
IIPETER
IMBIBER
IMPALER
IMPEDER
IMPOSER
IMPURER
IMPUTER
INAPTER
INASTIR
INCISOR
INCITER
INCOLOR
INCOMER
INDEXER
INDITER
INDUCER
INDYCAR
INERROR
INFAVOR
INFUSER
INGEMAR
INHALER
INHUMER
INJURER
INKSTER
INLABOR
INLAYER
INORDER
INPOWER
INSANER
INSIDER
INSOFAR
INSULAR
INSURER
INTEGER
INTONER
INVADER
INVITER
INVOKER
IODIZER
IONISER
IONIZER
IRISHER
IRONBAR
ITCHFOR
ITCHIER
ITSOVER
IWONDER

•IR••••

AIRACES
AIRBAGS
AIRBALL
AIRBASE
AIRBILL
AIRBOAT
AIRCOOL
AIRCREW
AIRDAMS
AIRDATE
AIRDRIE
AIRDROP
AIRDUCT
AIREDUP
AIRFARE
AIRFLOW
AIRFOIL
AIRFONE
AIRGLOW
AIRGUNS
AIRHEAD
AIRHOLE
AIRHORN
AIRHOSE
AIRIEST
AIRINGS
AIRKISS
AIRLANE
AIRLESS
AIRLIFT
AIRLIKE
AIRLINE
AIRLOCK
AIRLOGS
AIRMADA
AIRMAIL
AIRMASS
AIRMILE
AIRNESS
AIRPACK
AIRPARK
AIRPLAY
AIRPOPS
AIRPORT
AIRPOTS
AIRPUMP
AIRRACE
AIRRAGE
AIRRAID
AIRSACS
AIRSHIP
AIRSHOW
AIRSICK
AIRSIGN
AIRSOCK
AIRSOUT
AIRTANK
AIRTAXI
AIRTIME
AIRTRAP
AIRTUBE
AIRVENT
AIRWARS
AIRWAVE
AIRWAYS
AIRWICK
AIRWOLF
BIRCHED
BIRCHEN
BIRCHES
BIRDDOG
BIRDERS
BIRDFLU
BIRDIED
BIRDIES
BIRDING
BIRDMAN
BIRDMEN
BIREMES
BIRETTA
BIRIANI
BIRLERS
BIRLING
BIRMANS
BIRRING
BIRTHED
BIRYANI
CIRCLED
CIRCLER
CIRCLES
CIRCLET
CIRCUIT
CIRCUSY
CIRQUES
CIRRATE
DIRECTS
DIRECTV
DIREFUL

DIRHAMS
DIRKING
DIRKSEN
DIRNDLS
DIRTBAG
DIRTIED
DIRTIER
DIRTIES
DIRTILY
FIRBANK
FIREANT
FIREARM
FIREBOX
FIREBUG
FIREDAT
FIREDOG
FIREDON
FIREDUP
FIREFLY
FIREFOX
FIREHAT
FIREICE
FIRELIT
FIREMAN
FIREMEN
FIRENZA
FIRENZE
FIREOFF
FIREPIT
FIRESAT
FIRESON
FIRESUP
FIRINGS
FIRKINS
FIRMEST
FIRMING
FIRMSUP
FIRRIER
FIRSTLY
FIRSTUP
FIRTREE
GIRAFFE
GIRASOL
GIRDERS
GIRDING
GIRDLED
GIRDLER
GIRDLES
GIRLIER
GIRLIES
GIRLISH
GIRLSHY
GIROLLE
GIRONDE
GIRTHED
GIRTING
HIRABLE
HIRCINE
HIREDON
HIREOUT
HIRESON
HIRSUTE
JIRASEK
KIRMANS
KIRSTEN
KIRSTIE
MIRABEL
MIRACLE
MIRADAS
MIRADOR
MIRAGES
MIRAMAR
MIRAMAX
MIRANDA
MIRIEST
MIRISCH
MIRRORS
NIRVANA
PIRAEUS
PIRANHA
PIRATED
PIRATES
PIRATIC
PIRELLI
PIROGEN
PIROGUE
SIRDUKE
SIRENED
SIRLOIN
SIROCCO
TIRADES
TIREDER
TIREDLY
TIREDOF
TIREMAN
TIREMEN
TIREOUT
TIRESOF
TIRPITZ
VIRAGOS
VIRGATE
VIRGINS
VIRGOAN
VIRGULE
VIRTUAL
VIRTUES
VIRUSES
WIRABLE
WIREDIN
WIREDUP
WIREMAN
WIREMEN
WIRESIN
WIRESUP
WIRETAP
WIRIEST
WIRINGS
ZIRCONS

•I•R•••

AIGRETS
AIRRACE
AIRRAGE
AIRRAID
BIGRIGS
BIRRING
BITROLE
CIRRATE
CITRATE
CITRINE
CITROEN
CITRONS
CITROUS
DIARIES
DIARIOS
DIARIST
DIGRAMS
DIGRAPH
DIGRESS
DIORAMA
DIORITE
DISRATE
DISROBE
DISRUPT
DIURNAL
FIBRINS
FIBROID
FIBROUS
FIERCER
FIERIER
FIERILY
FIORINA
FIRRIER
GIORGIO
GIORGOS
HIPROOF
JIMRICE
JIMRYUN
KIARIOS
KIDROCK
LIBRANS
LIBRARY
LIPREAD
MICROBE
MICRONS
MIDRIBS
MIDRIFF
MIDRISE
MIGRANT
MIGRATE
MIRRORS
MISRATE
MISREAD
MISRELY
MISRULE
MITRING
MIZRAHI
NIMRODS
NITRATE
NITRIDE
NITRIFY
NITRITE
NITROUS
OILRICH
OILRIGS
OILRING
OILRUBS
PIERCED
PIERCER
PIERCES
PIERIAN
PIERROT
PITROWS
RICRACS
RIMROCK
RIORDAN
RIORITA
RIPRAPS
SIERRAS
TIARAED
TIERACK
TIERCES
TIERING
TIERNEY
TIERODS
TIEROPE
TIGRESS
TIMREID
TIMRICE
TIMROTH
TINROOF
TITRATE
TITRING
VIBRANT
VIBRATE
VIBRATO
VIERNES
VIERZIG
VINROSE
VITRICS
VITRIFY
VITRINE
VITRIOL
ZIERING

•I••R••

AILERON
AIRCREW
AIRDRIE
AIRDROP
AIRTRAP
BIAFRAN
BICARBS
BICORNE
BICORNS
BISTROS
BIZARRE
BIZARRO
CINERGY
DIAGRAM
DIDEROT
DINARIC
DISARMS
DISHRAG
DISTROS
DIVERGE
DIVERSE
DIVERTS
DIVORCE
FIACRES
FIBERED
FIGTREE
FIGURAL
FIGURED
FIGURER
FIGURES
FIRTREE
FITZROY
HIBERNO
HIGHRES
KIDSRUS
KINDRED
KINGRAT
LIBERAL
LIBERIA
LIBERTE
LIBERTY
LIGURIA
LINDROS
LIPARIS
LITCRIT
LITERAL
LITURGY
LIVERED
LIVORNO
LIZARDS
MIDIRON
MILDRED
MILERUN
MILKRUN
MILLRUN
MILORDS
MINARET
MINERAL
MINERVA
MINORCA
MINORED
MINORIN
MISBREW
MISDRAW
MISDREW
MISERLY
MISTRAL
MITERED
MITHRAS
NIGERIA
OILDRUM
PICARAS
PICARDO
PICARDY
PICAROS
PIERROT
PIETROS
PIGIRON
PILCROW
PILGRIM
PISARRO
PITCREW
PIZARRO
RICARDO
RINKRAT
RITARDS
RIVERPO
SIBERIA
SIERRAS
SIXIRON
TIBURON
TIDERIP
TIMBRES
TINORES
VICEROY
VICKREY
VICTRIX
VIHARAS
VISORED
VITARAS
VITORIA
VIVARIA
VIZORED
WILFRED
WINERED
WINFREY
WIZARDS
ZIMARRA

•I•••R•

AIRFARE
AIRHORN
AIRPARK
AIRPORT
AIRWARS
BIBBERS
BICKERS
BIDDERS
BIGBIRD
BIGCARS
BIGEARS
BIGGERS
BIGGIRL
BIGHORN
BIGJERK
BIGOTRY
BILKERS
BILLERS
BINDERS
BINDERY
BINGERS
BIRDERS
BIRLERS
BITPART
BITTERN
BITTERS
BIZARRE
BIZARRO
CILIARY
CINDERS
CINDERY
CIPHERS
CISTERN
DIALERS
DIAPERS
DICKERS
DICKORY
DIEHARD
DIETARY
DIETERS
DIFFERS
DIGGERS
DIGGORY
DILBERT
DILLARD
DIMITRI
DIMMERS
DINGERS
DINNERS
DIPPERS
DISBARS
DISCARD
DISCERN
DISCORD
DISEURS
DISPART
DISPORT
DISSERT
DISTORT
DISTURB
DITHERS
DITHERY
FIBBERS
FIGBARS
FILBERT
FILLERS
FILTERS
FINDERS
FINEART
FINGERS
FIREARM
FISHERS
FISHERY
FISHFRY
FISSURE
FITTERS
FIXTURE
FIZZERS
GIBBERS
GIFFORD
GILBERT
GILDERS
GILFORD
GILMORE
GINGERS
GINGERY
GIRDERS
GISCARD
GIZZARD
HICKORY
HIGHART
HILAIRE
HILBERT
HILLARY
HINDERS
HINTERS
HISSERS
HISTORY
HITHERE
HITTERS
JIGGERS
JIGGERY
JILTERS
JINXERS
JITTERS
JITTERY
KICKERS
KIDDERS
KILDARE
KILLERS
KILNDRY
KIPPERS
KISSERS
KITHARA
KITTERY
LIBBERS
LIBRARY
LICKERS
LIENORS
LIFTERS
LIMBERS
LIMBURG
LIMNERS
LINDORF
LINEARA
LINEARB
LINEDRY
LINGERS
LINKERS
LINTERS
LIPPERS
LIQUORS
LISPERS
LISTERS
LITTERS
LITTERY
MIASARA
MIDMORN
MIDTERM
MILAGRO
MILKERS
MILLARD
MILLERS
MIMICRY
MINCERS
MINDERS
MINDORO
MINTERS
MIRRORS
MISFIRE
MISFORM
MISMARK
MISSORT
MISTERM
MISTERS
MISTERX
MISWIRE
MISWORD
MITFORD
MIXTURE
NIAGARA
NICETRY
NICKERS
NIPPERS
OILBIRD
OINKERS
PIASTRE
PICCARD
PICKERS
PICTURE
PIECERS
PIGGERY
PILFERS
PILLARS
PILLORY
PINCERS
PINCURL
PINGERS
PINNERS
PIPCARD
PISARRO
PISMIRE
PITIERS
PIZARRO
QINTARS
RIBBERS
RICHARD
RIDDERS
RIEGERT
RIFLERS
RIFLERY
RIGGERS
RIGOURS
RINGERS
RINSERS
RIOTERS
RIPCORD
RIPPERS
RIPTORN
RISKERS
RIVALRY
RIVIERA
RIVIERE
SIDDURS
SIDEARM
SIFTERS
SIGHERS
SIGNERS
SIGNORA
SIGNORE
SIGNORS
SILVERS
SILVERY
SIMMERS
SIMPERS
SINATRA
SINCERE
SINGERS
SINKERS
SINNERS
SIPPERS
SISTERS
SITTERS
TICKERS
TIEBARS
TILLERS
TILTERS
TIMBERS
TIMBERY
TINDERS
TINDERY
TINEARS
TINHORN
TINKERS
TINNERS
TINTERN
TINTERS
TINWARE
TINWORK
TIPCART
TIPJARS
TIPPERS
TITHERS
TITLARK
TITTERS
VICKERS
VICTORS
VICTORY
VIEWERS
VIGOURS
VILLARD
VILLARI
VISCERA
VIZIERS
WICKERS
WIDMARK
WIENERS
WIGGERY
WILBERT
WILFORD
WILLARD
WILLERS
WINCERS
WINDERS
WINGERS
WINKERS
WINNERS
WINTERS
WINTERY
WISHERS
WITHERS
ZIMARRA
ZINGERS
ZIPPERS
ZITHERS

•I••••R

AIMSFOR
BICOLOR
BIDFAIR
BIDSFOR
BIGBEAR
BIGFOUR
BIGHAIR
BIGSTAR
BILGIER
BIPOLAR
BITSIER
BITTIER
CIRCLER
DIBBLER
DICHTER
DIDDLER
DIDOVER
DIEDFOR
DIESFOR
DIGSFOR
DILATOR
DILUTER
DILUTOR
DIMETER
DINGIER
DINKIER
DIOPTER
DIPOLAR
DIPPIER
DIRTIER
DISHIER
DITCHER
DITSIER
DITZIER
DIVIDER
DIVINER
DIVISOR
DIZZIER
FIBIGER
FIBSTER
FIBULAR
FICKLER
FIDDLER
FIEDLER
FIELDER
FIERCER
FIERIER
FIGHTER
FIGURER
FILCHER
FILMIER
FINNAIR
FINNIER
FIRRIER
FISCHER
FISHFOR
FISHIER
FIZZIER
FIZZLER
GIDDIER
GIGGLER
GIRDLER
GIRLIER
GIVEEAR
HIBBLER
HIGGLER
HIGHBAR
HILLIER
HINKIER
HIPPIER
HIPSTER
HISSIER
HITCHER
HITSFOR
IIPETER
JIGGIER
JINGLER
KICKIER
KIEFFER
KILOBAR
KINDLER
KINKIER
KINNEAR
LIBELER
LIEDFOR
LIEOVER
LIESFOR
LIGHTER
LIMITER
LINDNER
LINTIER
LIPPIER
LIQUEUR
LITTLER
LIVEFOR
LIVENER
MIDDLER
MIDYEAR
MIFFIER
MILKBAR
MILKIER
MINGIER
MINGLER
MINIBAR
MINICAR
MINIVER
MINSTER
MINTIER
MINUTER
MIRADOR
MIRAMAR
MISAVER
MISDOER
MISHEAR
MISTIER
MISUSER
NIBBLER
NICOBAR
NIEBUHR
NIFTIER
NIGGLER
NIGHTER
NIMBLER
NIPPIER
NITTIER
PIASTER
PICADOR
PICKIER
PIERCER
PIGGIER
PILSNER
PINCHER
PINEFOR
PINETAR
PIONEER
PITCHER
PITHIER
PIVOTER
RIBBIER
RICHLER
RICHTER
RIDDLER
RIDGIER
RIFFLER
RIGHTER
RIGUEUR
RINDIER
RINGFOR
RIPENER
RISKIER
RITZIER
RIVETER
SIDEBAR
SIDECAR
SIGHFOR
SIGHTER
SIGNFOR
SILENTR
SILKIER
SILLIER
SILTIER
SIMILAR
SIMPLER
SISENOR
SISSIER
SITSFOR
SIXFOUR
SIXYEAR
SIZZLER
TICKLER
TIGHTER
TIMIDER
TINGLER
TINKLER
TINNIER
TINSTAR
TIPOVER
TIPPIER
TIPPLER
TIPSIER
TIPSTER
TIREDER
TITULAR
VIEDFOR
VIESFOR
VIEWIER
VINEGAR
VINTNER
VISITOR
VIVIDER
VIVITAR
WIDENER
WIDOWER
WIELDER
WIGGIER
WIGGLER
WIMPIER
WINCHER
WINDIER
WINDSOR
WINEBAR
WINKLER
WINOVER
WISHFOR
WISPIER
WITTIER
YIELDER
ZIEGLER
ZINGIER
ZINKIER
ZIPPIER

••IR•••

CAIRENE
CAIRNED
CHIRICO
CHIRPED
CHIRPER
CHIRRED
CHIRRUP
CUIRASS
DAIRIES
DAIRYER
DEIRDRE
EMIRATE
FAIREST
FAIRFAX
FAIRIES
FAIRING
FAIRISH
FAIROFF
FAIRSEX
FAIRSUP
FAIRUSE
FAIRWAY
FLIRTED
FLIRTER
GOIRISH
HAIRCUT
HAIRDOS
HAIRDYE
HAIRGEL
HAIRIER
HAIRNET
HAIRPIN
HEIRDOM
HEIRESS
INIRONS
LAIRING
NAIROBI
OSIRIAN
PAIRERS
PAIRING
PAIROFF
PAIRSUP
QUIRTED
SHIRKED
SHIRKER
SHIRLEY
SHIRRED
SKIRACE
SKIRACK
SKIRLED
SKIRTED
SKIRTER
SKIRUNS
SMIRKED
SMIRKER
SMIRNOV
SOIREES
SPIRALS

SPIREAS
SPIRIER
SPIRITS
STIRFRY
STIRRED
STIRRER
STIRRUP
STIRSIN
STIRSUP
SWIRLED
THIRDLY
THIRSTS
THIRSTY
TRIREME
TWIRLED
TWIRLER
WEIRDAL
WEIRDED
WEIRDER
WEIRDLY
WEIRDOS
WEIRTON
WHIRLED
WHIRLER
WHIRRED
ZAIRIAN

••I•R••

ANITRAS
BOIARDO
BRIARDS
CHIRRED
CHIRRUP
EDITRIX
EMIGREE
EMIGRES
EPIGRAM
ERITREA
FRIARLY
GRIGRIS
LEITRIM
MAIGRET
MAITRED
MAITRES
OMICRON
OSIERED
POIVRES
PRIORTO
SCIORRA
SHIRRED
SKIAREA
SKIDROW
SKITRIP
STIRRED
STIRRER
STIRRUP
THIERRY
TRIGRAM
WAITRON
WHIRRED

••I••R•

ABIDERS
ABINTRA
ALIFORM
ALINERS
ARIKARA
BAILERS
BAILORS
BAITERS
BOILERS
BRIBERS
BRIBERY
BRINERS
CHICORY
CHIDERS
CHIMERA
CHIMERS
CLIBURN
CLIPART
COILERS
COINERS
DEICERS
DEIRDRE
DOIDARE
DRIPDRY
DRIVERS
EDITORS
ELIDERS
ELIXIRS
EPICARP
EPICURE
EPIDERM
EXILERS
FAILURE
GAINERS
GAITERS
GLIDERS
GOITERS
GRIPERS
GUIDERS
GUITARS
HAILERS
HEIFERS
ISIDORE
JAILERS
JAILORS
JOINERS
JOINERY
JUICERS
KAISERS
KNIFERS
LEISURE
LOITERS
MAILERS
MAIMERS
MAINERS
MOILERS
MSIEURS
NAILERS
OHIOART
OPINERS
OVIFORM
OVIPARA
PAIRERS
PHILTRE
POISERS
PRICERS
PRIMARY
PRIMERA
PRIMERO
PRIMERS
QUINARY
QUIVERS
QUIVERY
RAIDERS
RAILERS
RAISERS
RUINERS
SAILERS
SAILORS
SCIORRA
SEINERS
SEIZERS
SEIZORS
SEIZURE
SHINERS
SHIVERS
SHIVERY
SLICERS
SLIDERS
SLIVERS
SMILERS
SMITERS
SNIPERS
SPICERS
SPICERY
SPIDERS
SPIDERY
SPIKERS
SPINDRY
STIRFRY
SUITORS
SWIGERT
SWINERY
SWIPERS
SZILARD
TAILERS
TAILORS
THIERRY
TOILERS
TRIBORO
TRICORN
TRIFORM
TRINARY
TWINERS
UNICORN
UNIFORM
UNINERT
UNITARD
UNITARY
UNITERS
VEILERS
VOICERS
VOIDERS
VOITURE
WAILERS
WAITERS
WAIVERS
WHINERS
WRITERS

••I•••R

ALIENOR
ALIGNER
ASIMMER
AVIATOR
AXILLAR
AZINGER
BAINTER
BAITCAR
BLINDER
BLINKER
BLISTER
BLITHER
BLITZER
BRIDGER
BRIDLER
BRIEFER
BRIMMER
BRINGER
BRINIER
BRINKER
BRISKER
BUILDER
CHIGGER
CHILLER
CHIPPER
CHIRPER
CHITTER
CLICKER
CLIMBER
CLINGER
CLINKER
CLIPPER
CRIBBER
CRIMPER
CRISPER
CRITTER
CRITTUR
DAIMLER
DAIRYER
DEIFIER
DNIEPER
DRIFTER
DRILLER
DRINKER
DRIPPER
EDIFIER
ELIEZER
EMITTER
EVICTOR
EVILLER
FAINTER
FEIFFER
FEIGNER
FLICKER
FLINGER
FLIPPER
FLIRTER
FLITTER
FLIVVER
FRICKER
FRISEUR
FRISKER
FRITTER
FRIZZER
GLIBBER
GLIMMER
GLISTER
GLITTER
GOINFOR
GRIDDER
GRIEVER
GRIFTER
GRILLER
GRIMIER
GRIMMER
GRINDER
GRINNER
GRIPPER
GRISTER
GRITTER
GUILDER
HAIRIER
HOISTER
IRISHER
JOINDER
JOINTER
JUICIER
KEILLOR
KEISTER
KLINGER
KLINKER
KLISTER
KNITTER
LAIDFOR
LEISTER
MAILCAR
MEISTER
MEITNER
MOISTER
NEITHER
NOISIER
OLIVIER
OMITTER
PAIDFOR
PAINTER
PHILTER
PHISHER
POINTER
POITIER
PRICIER
PRIMMER
PRINKER
PRINTER
PRIVIER
QUICKER
QUIETER
QUILLER
QUILTER
QUIPPER
QUITTER
QUIZZER
RAILCAR
RAINIER
ROILIER
ROISTER
SCISSOR
SHIFTER
SHIMMER
SHINIER
SHIPPER
SHIRKER
SKIDDER
SKIMMER
SKINNER
SKIPPER
SKIRTER
SKITTER
SKIWEAR
SLICKER
SLIMIER
SLIMMER
SLINGER
SLINKER
SLIPPER
SLITHER
SLITTER
SMIRKER
SNICKER
SNIFFER
SNIFTER
SNIPPER
SPICIER
SPIELER
SPIKIER
SPILLER
SPINIER
SPINNER
SPIRIER
SPITTER
STICKER
STIFFER
STILLER
STINGER
STINKER
STINTER
STIRRER
SWIFTER
SWILLER
SWIMMER
SWINGER
SWITZER
TEICHER
THICKER
THINAIR
THINKER
THINNER
THITHER
TRICKER
TRIFLER
TRIGGER
TRILLER
TRIMMER
TRIPPER
TRISTAR
TWINIER
TWIRLER
TWISTER
TWITTER
UNIFIER
VEINIER
WAITFOR
WEIGHER
WEIRDER
WHIFFER
WHIMPER
WHINIER
WHIPPER
WHIRLER
WHISKER
WHISPER
WHITHER
WHIZZER
WRINGER
WRITHER

•••IR••

ADMIRAL
ADMIRED
ADMIRER
ADMIRES
AFFIRMS
ALBIREO
ANDIRON
APAIROF
ASPIRED
ASPIRER
ASPIRES
ASPIRIN
ATFIRST
ATHIRST
ATTIRED
ATTIRER
ATTIRES
BEGIRDS
BEMIRED
BEMIRES
BYBIRTH
CHAIRED
CHOIRED
CLAIROL
DEAIRED
DEHIRED
DEHIRES
DELIRIA
DESIRED
DESIREE
DESIRER
DESIRES
DEWIRED
DEWIRES
EMPIRES
EMPIRIC
EMPIRIN
ENGIRDS
ENTIRES
ENVIRON
ENVIROS
EXPIRED
EXPIRES
GOFIRST
GOGIRLS
HEGIRAS
IMTIRED
INFIRST
ITGIRLS
ITHIRTY
LEGIRON
MEFIRST
MIDIRON
NONIRON
NOSIREE
NUBIRAS
ONEIRIC
ONEIRON
ONFIRST
PIGIRON
PRAIRIE
PRFIRMS
QUEIROS
RAMIREZ
REAIRED
REBIRTH
REFIRED
REFIRES
REGIRDS
REHIRED
REHIRES
RETIRED
RETIREE
RETIRES
REWIRED
REWIRES
SATIRES
SATIRIC
SCHIRRA
SEMIRAW
SEPIRAS
SIXIRON
SQUIRED
SQUIRES
SQUIRMS
SQUIRMY
SQUIRTS
STAIRED
TSHIRTS
TWOIRON
UMPIRED
UMPIRES
UNAIRED
UNFIRED
UNGIRDS
UNHIRED
UNHIRES
UNMIRED
UNTIRED
UNWIRED
UPFIRST
UPGIRDS

•••I•R•

ALFIERI
ALGIERS
ANTIART
APRIORI
ARRIERE
BELIERS
BEZIERS
BURIERS
CAHIERS
CALIBRE
CAVIARE
CAVIARS
CILIARY
COPIERS
DECIARE
DEFIERS
DENIERS
DEVILRY
DIMITRI
ENVIERS
HONIARA
HOSIERS
HOSIERY
INVITRO
JUNIORS
LEVIERS
LUMIERE
METIERS
MIMICRY
MOLIERE
NAPIERS
OSTIARY
PANIERS
PAPIERS
PAVIORS
PITIERS
PONIARD
RAPIERS
RELIERS
RETIARY
RIVIERA
RIVIERE
SALIERI
SAVIORS
SCHIRRA
SEMIDRY
SEMIPRO
SENIORS
TOPIARY
UNFIERY
UNMITRE
UNTIERS
VARIERS
VIZIERS
XAVIERU

•••I••R

ADMIRER
ADVISER
ADVISOR
AFFIXER
ALPINER
ANTIWAR
AQUIFER
AQUIVER
ARBITER
ARRIVER
ASHIVER
ASPIRER
ATTIRER
AUDITOR
AVOIDER
AWAITER
BABIYAR
BOLIVAR
BRAIDER
BRAINER
BROIDER
BROILER
BRUISER
BYLINER
CALIBER
CALIPER
CASIMIR
CAVILER
CCRIDER
CHOICER
CLAIMER
CONIFER
CRUISER
DECIDER
DEFILER
DEFINER
DELIVER
DERIDER
DERIVER
DESIRER
DEVISER
DEVISOR
DIVIDER
DIVINER
DIVISOR
DRAINER
DREISER
EMAILER
ENTICER
ETAILER
EXCITER
EXCITOR
EXOILER
FIBIGER
FRAILER
GENITOR
GRAINER
HERITOR
HUMIDOR
IGNITER
IGNITOR
IMBIBER
INCISOR
INCITER
INDITER
INSIDER
INVITER
IODIZER
IONISER
IONIZER
JANITOR
JUNIPER
JUPITER
KLEIBER
KLEISER
LAMINAR
LIMITER
LUCIFER
MANIPUR
MARINER
MINIBAR
MINICAR
MINIVER
MOLITOR
MONIKER
MONITOR
MRTIGER
NOTICER
NOWISER
OBLIGER
OBLIGOR
OFFICER
ORBITER
PAVIOUR
PLAINER
PLAISIR
PLAITER
POLICER
POLITER
PORIVER
PRAISER
RADIOER
RAPIDER
RECITER
REFINER
REPINER
RESIDER
RESIZER
REVILER
REVISER
REVISOR
REVIVER
ROTIFER
SAVIOUR
SCRIBER
SEMINAR
SHRINER
SHRIVER
SIMILAR
SOLIDER
SPLICER
SPOILER
STAIDER
STAINER
STEIGER
STEINER
STRIDER
STRIKER
STRIPER
STRIVER
THRIVER
TIMIDER
TRAILER
TRAINER
TRAITOR
UNMITER
UNRIPER
UNWISER
UPRISER
UPRIVER
VISITOR
VIVIDER
VIVITAR

••••IR•

ACQUIRE
AFFAIRE
AFFAIRS
ANTBIRD
ARMOIRE
ASTAIRE
ATEDIRT
ATTHIRD
AUPAIRS
BADGIRL
BAGGIRL
BATGIRL
BELAIRS
BESTIRS
BIGBIRD
BIGGIRL
BONAIRE
BONFIRE
BOOBIRD
BUSGIRL
CAMGIRL
CARTIRE
CATBIRD
CESAIRE
COHEIRS
CONFIRM
COWBIRD
COWGIRL
DEHAIRS
DEVOIRS
DUNKIRK
EATDIRT
ECLAIRS
ELIXIRS
ENQUIRE
ENQUIRY
ESQUIRE
FALKIRK
FLYGIRL
FORHIRE
FOXFIRE
GUNFIRE
HAYWIRE
HILAIRE
HOTWIRE
IMPAIRS
INQUIRE
INQUIRY
INSPIRE
INTHIRD
JANEIRO
JAYBIRD
JETFIRE
LEMPIRA
MADEIRA
MAGUIRE
MCGUIRE
MCGWIRE
MEMOIRE
MEMOIRS
MISFIRE
MISWIRE
MOHAIRS
NEWHIRE
OILBIRD
OLDGIRL
ONELIRA
OUTFIRE
OUTHIRE
OUTTIRE
PAYDIRT
PETBIRD
PISMIRE
PRETIRE
PREWIRE
REDBIRD
REDFIRS
RENOIRS
REPAIRS
REQUIRE
RESPIRE
RESTIRS
ROTHIRA
SEABIRD
SEAGIRT
SELKIRK
SHAKIRA
SHAPIRO
SUNBIRD
SUNFIRE
SUSPIRE
THEFIRM
TOSHIRO
UNHAIRS
UNHAIRY
UPSTIRS
UPWHIRL
VAMPIRA
VAMPIRE
YESSIRE

••••I•R

ANGRIER
ANTSIER
APPLIER
ARTSIER
ATELIER
BAGGIER
BALKIER
BALMIER
BANDIER
BARKIER
BARMIER
BARRIER
BASSIER
BATTIER
BAWDIER
BEADIER
BEAMIER
BEEFIER
BEERIER
BEETIER
BENDIER
BILGIER
BITSIER
BITTIER
BLOWIER
BOGGIER
BONNIER
BOOMIER
BOOZIER
BOSSIER
BOUVIER
BRASIER
BRAZIER
BRINIER
BUGGIER
BULGIER
BULKIER
BUMPIER
BURLIER
BURRIER
BUSHIER
BUSTIER
BUZZIER
CAMPIER
CANNIER
CARRIER
CARTIER
CASHIER
CATTIER
CHARIER
CHENIER
CHEWIER
CHOKIER
CLAVIER
CLAYIER
COCKIER
COLLIER
COMFIER
CORKIER
CORNIER
COURIER
CRAZIER
CROSIER
CROZIER
CUPPIER
CURDIER
CURLIER
CURRIER
CURVIER
CUSHIER
DAFFIER
DALLIER
DANDIER
DASHIER
DAUMIER
DECRIER
DEIFIER

DERNIER
DINGIER
DINKIER
DIPPIER
DIRTIER
DISHIER
DITSIER
DITZIER
DIZZIER
DODGIER
DOGGIER
DOOMIER
DORKIER
DOSSIER
DOTTIER
DOWDIER
DOWNIER
DUCKIER
DUMPIER
DUSKIER
DUSTIER
EARLIER
EDIFIER
EMPTIER
FADDIER
FANCIER
FARRIER
FATTIER
FENNIER
FERNIER
FEVRIER
FIERIER
FILMIER
FINNIER
FIRRIER
FISHIER
FIZZIER
FLAKIER
FLAMIER
FLAWIER
FLAXIER
FLUKIER
FLUTIER
FLYTIER
FOAMIER
FOGGIER
FOLKIER
FORKIER
FOURIER
FRASIER
FRAZIER
FUBSIER
FUNKIER
FUNNIER
FURRIER
FUSSIER
FUSTIER
FUZZIER
GABBIER
GAMBIER
GASSIER
GAUDIER
GAUTIER
GAUZIER
GAWKIER
GEEKIER
GEMMIER
GERMIER
GIDDIER
GIRLIER
GLACIER
GLAZIER
GODLIER
GOOFIER
GOONIER
GOOPIER
GOOSIER
GORSIER
GOUTIER
GRAPIER
GRAZIER
GRIMIER
GRODIER
GROLIER
GUCKIER
GULPIER
GUMMIER
GUNKIER
GUSHIER
GUSTIER
GUTSIER
GUTTIER
HAIRIER
HAMMIER
HANDIER
HAPPIER
HARDIER
HARRIER
HASTIER
HEADIER
HEAVIER
HEDGIER
HEFTIER
HEMPIER
HERBIER
HILLIER
HINKIER
HIPPIER
HISSIER
HOARIER
HOMEIER
HOOSIER
HOPPIER
HORNIER
HORSIER
HUFFIER
HULKIER
HUMPIER
HUNKIER
HURRIER
HUSKIER
ITCHIER
JAGGIER
JAMMIER
JANVIER
JAZZIER
JERKIER
JIGGIER
JOLLIER
JOLTIER
JOWLIER
JUICIER
JUMPIER
JUNKIER
KICKIER
KINKIER
KOOKIER
LANKIER
LARDIER
LARKIER
LEADIER
LEAFIER
LEAKIER
LEDGIER
LEERIER
LEGGIER
LINTIER
LIPPIER
LOAMIER
LOFTIER
LOONIER
LOOPIER
LOPPIER
LOUSIER
LOWLIER
LUCKIER
LUMPIER
LUSHIER
LUSTIER
LUTHIER
MALTIER
MANGIER
MANLIER
MARLIER
MARNIER
MARVIER
MASSIER
MEALIER
MEATIER
MERRIER
MESHIER
MESSIER
MIFFIER
MILKIER
MINGIER
MINTIER
MISTIER
MOLDIER
MOODIER
MOONIER
MOORIER
MOSSIER
MOTHIER
MOUSIER
MUCKIER
MUDDIER
MUGGIER
MURKIER
MUSHIER
MUSKIER
MUSSIER
MUSTIER
MUZZIER
NAGGIER
NAPPIER
NASTIER
NATTIER
NEEDIER
NERDIER
NERVIER
NEWSIER
NIFTIER
NIPPIER
NITTIER
NOBBIER
NOISIER
NUBBIER
NUTSIER
NUTTIER
OLIVIER
OUTLIER
PALLIER
PALMIER
PANNIER
PARRIER
PARTIER
PASTIER
PEAKIER
PEATIER
PEPPIER
PERKIER
PERRIER
PESKIER
PETTIER
PHONIER
PICKIER
PIGGIER
PITHIER
PLATIER
PLUMIER
POITIER
PORKIER
POTTIER
POUTIER
PREMIER
PRICIER
PRIVIER
PROSIER
PUDGIER
PUFFIER
PULPIER
PUNKIER
PUNNIER
PURSIER
PURTIER
PUSHIER
QUAKIER
QUERIER
RAGGIER
RAINIER
RALLIER
RANDIER
RANGIER
RASPIER
RATTIER
READIER
REEDIER
REEFIER
REEKIER
REGNIER
RENTIER
REPLIER
RIBBIER
RIDGIER
RINDIER
RISKIER
RITZIER
ROCKIER
ROILIER
ROOKIER
ROOMIER
ROOTIER
ROWDIER
RUDDIER
RUNNIER
RUNTIER
RUSHIER
RUSTIER
RUTTIER
SAGGIER
SALLIER
SALTIER
SANDIER
SAPPIER
SASSIER
SAUCIER
SAVVIER
SCALIER
SCARIER
SEAMIER
SEDGIER
SEEDIER
SEEPIER
SHADIER
SHAKIER
SHALIER
SHINIER
SHOWIER
SILKIER
SILLIER
SILTIER
SISSIER
SLATIER
SLIMIER
SMOKIER
SNAKIER
SNOWIER
SOAPIER
SODDIER
SOGGIER
SOLDIER
SOOTIER
SOPPIER
SORRIER
SOUPIER
SPACIER
SPICIER
SPIKIER
SPINIER
SPIRIER
SPUMIER
STAGIER
STEWIER
STONIER
STUDIER
SUCKIER
SUDSIER
SULKIER
SUNNIER
SURFIER
SURLIER
TACKIER
TALKIER
TALLIER
TANGIER
TARDIER
TARRIER
TARTIER
TASTIER
TATTIER
TAWNIER
TEARIER
TEENIER
TERRIER
TESTIER
TINNIER
TIPPIER
TIPSIER
TUBBIER
TUFTIER
TURFIER
TWINIER
UNIFIER
UNSHIER
UNSLIER
VAMPIER
VASTIER
VEALIER
VEINIER
VERNIER
VIEWIER
WACKIER
WARRIOR
WARTIER
WASHIER
WASPIER
WEARIER
WEBBIER
WEDGIER
WEEDIER
WEEPIER
WHINIER
WIGGIER
WIMPIER
WINDIER
WISPIER
WITTIER
WOODIER
WOOLIER
WOOZIER
WORDIER
WORMIER
WORRIER
YAWNIER
YUCKIER
YUMMIER
ZAPPIER
ZESTIER
ZINGIER
ZINKIER
ZIPPIER

••••••IR

ARTFAIR
BADHAIR
BELVOIR
BENAZIR
BIDFAIR
BIGHAIR
BOBWEIR
BONSOIR
BOROMIR
BOUDOIR
BYAHAIR
CASIMIR
CATHAIR
COCHAIR
COOLAIR
CORSAIR
CORVAIR
DEADAIR
DEARSIR
DESPAIR
DOGHAIR
DUUMVIR
FINNAIR
FREEAIR
FUNFAIR
GOBYAIR
INASTIR
JAROMIR
JOBFAIR
KASHMIR
LOTHAIR
LOWPAIR
MAYFAIR
MRSMUIR
NOTFAIR
ONEPAIR
OPENAIR
PETHAIR
PLAISIR
REDHAIR
SPANAIR
TERROIR
THINAIR
TOAHAIR
TOYFAIR
TWOPAIR
UNCHAIR
UPSTAIR
WASFAIR

IS•••••

ISABEAU
ISADORA
ISADORE
ISAHEAD
ISAIDNO
ISCHIAL
ISCHIUM
ISECOND
ISEENOW
ISEEYOU
ISFAHAN
ISHMAEL
ISIDORE
ISITAGO
ISLAMIC
ISLANDS
ISLETED
ISOBARS
ISOGONS
ISOGRAM
ISOHELS
ISOLATE
ISOLATO
ISOLINE
ISOMERS
ISONOMY
ISOPODS
ISOTONE
ISOTOPE
ISOTOPY
ISRAELI
ISRAFEL
ISSUANT
ISSUEAD
ISSUERS
ISSUING
ISTHMUS
ISTOMIN
ISTRIAN
ISUREAM
ISUREDO

I•S••••

IDSAYSO
IFSTONE
IMSORRY
IMSWELL
INSALES
INSANER
INSCALE
INSEAMS
INSECTA
INSECTS
INSERTS
INSHAPE
INSHOCK
INSHORE
INSHORT
INSIDER
INSIDES
INSIGHT
INSIGNE
INSIPID
INSISTS
INSOFAR
INSOLES
INSPACE
INSPANS
INSPECT
INSPIRE
INSPITE
INSPOTS
INSTALL
INSTALS
INSTANT
INSTATE
INSTEAD
INSTEPS
INSTILL
INSTILS
INSTOCK
INSTONE
INSTORE
INSTYLE
INSULAR
INSULIN
INSULTS
INSURED
INSURER
INSURES
INSWEPT
INSYNCH
IPSWICH
IRSFORM
ISSUANT
ISSUEAD
ISSUERS
ISSUING
ITSABOY
ITSAHIT
ITSALIE
ITSALOT
ITSASIN
ITSATIE
ITSBEST
ITSCOLD
ITSDONE
ITSEASY
ITSFINE
ITSGONE
ITSHERE
ITSLATE
ITSLOVE
ITSOKAY
ITSONME
ITSOPEN
ITSOVER
ITSTIME
ITSTRUE

I••S•••

IBNSAUD
ICESHOW
ICESOUT
IINSIST
ILOSTIT
IMUSTGO
INASHOE
INASNAP
INASNIT
INASPIN
INASPOT
INASTEW
INASTIR
INASUIT
INKSACS
INKSPOT
INKSTER
IRESIGN
IRISHER
IRISING
IRISOUT
IRKSOME
ITISTOO

I•••S••

ICTUSES
IDLESSE
IGUASSU
ILIESCU
ILLUSED
ILLUSES
IMPASSE
IMPASTO
IMPOSED
IMPOSER
IMPOSES
IMPOSTS
INCASED
INCASES
INCISED
INCISES
INCISOR
INCUSED
INCUSES
INFESTS
INFUSED
INFUSER
INFUSES
INGESTA
INGESTS
INHASTE
INSISTS
INTASTE
INVESTS
IODISED
IODISES
IONESCO
IONISED
IONISER
IONISES
IQTESTS
IRONSON
ITSASIN
IVERSON

I••••S•

IAMBIST
ICELESS
ICINESS
ICKIEST
IDLESSE
IDOLISE
IDOLIST
IDSAYSO
IDYLIST
IFFIEST
IGUASSU
IHOPESO
IINSIST
ILLNESS
ILLPASS
IMAGISM
IMAGIST
IMAMESS
IMMENSE
IMMERSE
IMPASSE
IMPRESS
IMPREST
IMPULSE
INACAST
INAMESS
INANEST
INARUSH
INCENSE
INCLASS
INCLOSE
INCRUST
INDORSE
INFIRST
INGLESE
INGRESS
INHOUSE
INKIEST
INKLESS
INNLESS
INPHASE
INQUEST
INTENSE
INTERSE
INTRUST
INULASE
INVERSE
IPCRESS
IRATEST
IREFUSE
IRELESS
IRKUTSK
IRONIST
ITEMISE
ITSBEST
ITSEASY
IZZATSO

I•••••S

IAMBICS
IAPETUS
IATRICS
IBIZANS
ICEAGES
ICEAXES
ICEBAGS
ICECAPS
ICEDAMS
ICEFOGS
ICELESS
ICEOUTS
ICEPOPS
ICERUNS
ICETEAS
ICICLES
ICINESS
ICTERUS
ICTINUS
ICTUSES
IDAREDS
IDCARDS
IDEATES
IGNEOUS
IGNITES
IGNORES
IGOROTS
IGUANAS
IIKINGS
ILLNESS
ILLPASS
ILLUDES
ILLUMES
ILLUSES
IMAGERS
IMAGOES
IMAMESS
IMARETS
IMBIBES
IMBRUES
IMMIXES
IMMUNES
IMMURES
IMPACTS
IMPAIRS
IMPALAS
IMPALES
IMPARTS
IMPEDES
IMPENDS
IMPETUS
IMPIOUS
IMPLIES
IMPORTS
IMPOSES
IMPOSTS
IMPRESS
IMPUGNS
IMPUTES
IMYOURS
INAMESS
INBOXES
INCANTS
INCASES
INCENTS
INCEPTS
INCHERS
INCISES
INCITES
INCLASS
INCOMES
INCUBUS
INCUDES
INCUSES
INDENTS
INDEXES
INDIANS
INDICES
INDICTS
INDIGOS
INDITES
INDOORS
INDUCES
INDUCTS
INFANTS
INFECTS
INFESTS
INFIVES
INFIXES
INFLOWS
INFOCUS
INFOLDS
INFORMS
INFUSES
INGALLS
INGATES
INGESTS
INGOALS
INGRESS
INGULFS
INHALES
INHERES
INHUMES
INIRONS
INJECTS
INJOKES
INJURES
INKINGS
INKJETS
INKLESS
INKNOTS
INKPADS
INKPOTS
INKSACS
INLANDS
INLINES
INMATES
INNAGES
INNARDS
INNINGS
INNLESS
INPOURS
INROADS
INRUINS
INSALES
INSEAMS
INSECTS
INSERTS
INSIDES
INSISTS
INSOLES
INSPANS
INSPOTS
INSTALS
INSTEPS
INSTILS
INSULTS
INSURES
INTAILS
INTAKES
INTEARS
INTENDS
INTENTS
INTERNS
INTONES
INTRAYS
INTUITS
INTURNS
INVADES
INVENTS
INVERTS
INVESTS
INVITES
INVOKES
INWARDS
INYEARS
IODATES
IODIDES
IODISES
IODIZES
IOMOTHS
IONIANS
IONISES
IONIUMS
IONIZES
IONONES
IPCRESS
IQTESTS
IRELESS
IRENICS
IRONERS
IRONIES
IRONONS
IRRUPTS
ISLANDS
ISOBARS
ISOGONS
ISOHELS
ISOMERS
ISOPODS
ISSUERS
ISTHMUS
ITALICS
ITGIRLS
IVORIES
IVTUBES

•IS••••

BISCUIT
BISECTS
BISHKEK
BISHOPS
BISMUTH
BISQUES

BISSELL
BISTATE
BISTROS
CISCOES
CISEAUX
CISTERN
DISABLE
DISARMS
DISAVOW
DISBAND
DISBARS
DISBUDS
DISCARD
DISCERN
DISCING
DISCMAN
DISCOED
DISCOID
DISCORD
DISCUSS
DISDAIN
DISEASE
DISEURS
DISEUSE
DISGUST
DISHFUL
DISHIER
DISHING
DISHOUT
DISHPAN
DISHRAG
DISJOIN
DISKING
DISLIKE
DISMALS
DISMAST
DISMAYS
DISMISS
DISOBEY
DISOWNS
DISPART
DISPELS
DISPLAY
DISPORT
DISPOSE
DISPUTE
DISRATE
DISROBE
DISRUPT
DISSECT
DISSENT
DISSERT
DISSING
DISTAFF
DISTANT
DISTEND
DISTICH
DISTILL
DISTILS
DISTORT
DISTROS
DISTURB
DISUSED
DISUSES
FISCHER
FISHERS
FISHERY
FISHEYE
FISHFOR
FISHFRY
FISHIER
FISHILY
FISHING
FISHNET
FISHOIL
FISHOUT
FISSILE
FISSION
FISSURE
FISTFUL
GISCARD
GISELLE
GISSING
HISNIBS
HISPANO
HISPEED
HISSERS
HISSIER
HISSING
HISTORY
KISHKES
KISLEVS
KISMETS
KISSELS
KISSERS
KISSING
KISSOFF
LISAGAY
LISBETH
LISENTE
LISPERS
LISPING
LISSOME
LISTEES
LISTENS
LISTERS
LISTING
MISACTS
MISADDS
MISAIMS
MISALLY
MISAVER
MISBILL
MISBIND
MISBREW
MISCALL
MISCAST
MISCITE
MISCODE
MISCOIN
MISCOPY
MISCUED
MISCUES
MISCUTS
MISDATE
MISDEAL
MISDEED
MISDEEM
MISDIAL
MISDOER
MISDOES
MISDONE
MISDRAW
MISDREW
MISEDIT
MISERLY
MISFEED
MISFILE
MISFIRE
MISFITS
MISFORM
MISGAVE
MISGIVE
MISHAPS
MISHEAR
MISHIMA
MISHITS
MISHNAH
MISJOIN
MISKEYS
MISKNEW
MISKNOW
MISKOLC
MISLAID
MISLAYS
MISLEAD
MISLIKE
MISMARK
MISMATE
MISMESH
MISMOVE
MISNAME
MISPAGE
MISPLAN
MISPLAY
MISRATE
MISREAD
MISRELY
MISRULE
MISSAID
MISSALS
MISSAYS
MISSEAT
MISSEND
MISSENT
MISSETS
MISSHIP
MISSIES
MISSILE
MISSING
MISSION
MISSISH
MISSIVE
MISSORT
MISSOUT
MISSTEP
MISSUSA
MISSYOU
MISTAKE
MISTBOW
MISTELL
MISTERM
MISTERS
MISTERX
MISTIER
MISTILY
MISTIME
MISTING
MISTOLD
MISTOOK
MISTRAL
MISTSUP
MISTUNE
MISTYPE
MISUSED
MISUSER
MISUSES
MISWIRE
MISWORD
MISZONE
NISSANS
NISSANZ
OISEAUX
PISANIO
PISARRO
PISCEAN
PISCINE
PISCOPO
PISHING
PISMIRE
PISTILS
PISTOLE
PISTOLS
PISTONS
PISTOUS
RISENTO
RISESTO
RISESUP
RISIBLE
RISIBLY
RISINGS
RISKERS
RISKIER
RISKILY
RISKING
RISKSIT
RISOTTO
RISSOLE
SISENOR
SISSIER
SISSIES
SISTERS
SISTINE
TISANES
TISSOTS
TISSUES
TISSUEY
VISAGED
VISAGES
VISAING
VISALIA
VISAVIS
VISAYAN
VISCERA
VISCOUS
VISCUSO
VISIBLE
VISIBLY
VISIONS
VISITED
VISITOR
VISORED
VISTAED
VISTEON
VISTULA
VISUALS
WISDOMS
WISEDUP
WISEGUY
WISEMAN
WISEMEN
WISEONE
WISESUP
WISHERS
WISHFOR
WISHFUL
WISHING
WISPIER
WISPILY
WISPING
WISTFUL

•I•S•••

AIMSFOR
AIRSACS
AIRSHIP
AIRSHOW
AIRSICK
AIRSIGN
AIRSOCK
AIRSOUT
BIASING
BIASPLY
BIASSED
BIASSES
BIDSFOR
BIGSALE
BIGSHOT
BIGSHOW
BIGSTAR
BISSELL
BITSIER
DIDSUMS
DIESELS
DIESFOR
DIESOFF
DIESOUT
DIGSFOR
DIGSOUT
DIMSOUT
DISSECT
DISSENT
DISSERT
DISSING
DITSIER
FIASCOS
FIBSTER
FIESTAS
FIRSTLY
FIRSTUP
FISSILE
FISSION
FISSURE
GIBSONS
GINSENG
GIPSIES
GISSING
HIMSELF
HIPSTER
HIRSUTE
HISSERS
HISSIER
HISSING
HITSFOR
HITSHOW
HITSOFF
HITSONG
HITSOUT
IINSIST
JIGSAWS
JIMSONS
KIDSEAT
KIDSKIN
KIDSRUS
KINSHIP
KINSMAN
KINSMEN
KIRSTEN
KIRSTIE
KISSELS
KISSERS
KISSING
KISSOFF
KITSCHY
LIESFOR
LIESLOW
LINSEED
LIPSOFF
LIPSOUT
LIPSYNC
LISSOME
MIASARA
MIASMAL
MIASMAS
MIASMIC
MIDSHIP
MIDSIZE
MIDSOLE
MINSKYS
MINSTER
MISSAID
MISSALS
MISSAYS
MISSEAT
MISSEND
MISSENT
MISSETS
MISSHIP
MISSIES
MISSILE
MISSING
MISSION
MISSISH
MISSIVE
MISSORT
MISSOUT
MISSTEP
MISSUSA
MISSYOU
NILSSON
NISSANS
NISSANZ
OILSAND
OILSEED
OILSKIN
OILSPOT
PIASTER
PIASTRE
PIESAFE
PIESALE
PIGSKIN
PIGSOUT
PILSNER
PINSEAL
PIOSITY
PITSAWS
PITSTOP
PIUSIII
PIUSVII
PIUSXII
RIESENS
RIESMAN
RIESSEN
RIGSOUT
RIKSDAG
RIMSHOT
RINSERS
RINSING
RIPSAWN
RIPSAWS
RIPSOFF
RIPSONE
RIPSOUT
RIPSTOP
RISSOLE
SIESTAS
SISSIER
SISSIES
SITSFOR
SITSOUT
SITSPAT
TIESOFF
TILSITS
TINSELS
TINSTAR
TIPSIER
TIPSILY
TIPSOFF
TIPSTER
TISSOTS
TISSUES
TISSUEY
VIESFOR
VIZSLAS
WIGSOUT
WILSONS
WINSBIG
WINSLET
WINSLOW
WINSOME
WINSOUT
WINSTON
WITSEND
ZIPSOFF

•I••S••

BIASSED
BIASSES
BINDSTO
BINDSUP
BITESIN
BITESON
BITESUP
CINESIA
DIALSIN
DIALSUP
DICKSON
DIDASET
DIGESTS
DINESAT
DINESEN
DINESIN
DINESON
DIRKSEN
DISUSED
DISUSES
DIVESIN
DIVESTS
DIVISOR
FICUSES
FILESBY
FILESIN
FILLSIN
FILLSUP
FILMSET
FINESSE
FINISHD
FINKSON
FIRESAT
FIRESON
FIRESUP
FIRMSUP
FIVESIX
FIXESON
FIXESUP
GIBESAT
GIBUSES
GIFTSET
GIRASOL
GIRLSHY
GIVESIN
GIVESOF
GIVESON
GIVESTO
GIVESUP
HIGHSEA
HIKESUP
HINTSAT
HIRESON
JIBESAT
JIRASEK
KICKSIN
KICKSUP
KINESES
KINESIC
KINESIS
KINISON
LIAISED
LIAISES
LIAISON
LICKSUP
LIFTSUP
LINDSAY
LINDSEY
LINESUP
LINKSUP
LIPASES
LIVESAT
LIVESET
LIVESEY
LIVESIN
LIVESON
MIDASES
MIKASAS
MILKSOP
MIMESES
MIMESIS
MIMOSAS
MINDSET
MINISKI
MINISUB
MINUSES
MIRISCH
MISTSUP
MISUSED
MISUSER
MISUSES
MITOSES
MITOSIS
MIXESIN
MIXESUP
NICOSIA
NIELSEN
NILESOH
NILSSON
PICASSO
PICKSAT
PICKSON
PICKSUP
PILESIN
PILESOF
PILESON
PILESUP
PIMESON
PINESAP
PINESOL
PIOUSLY
PIPESIN
PIPESUP
RICKSHA
RIDESBY
RIDESIN
RIDESTO
RIDESUP
RIESSEN
RILESUP
RINGSIN
RINGSUP
RIPOSTE
RIPOSTS
RISESTO
RISESUP
RISKSIT
SIGHSAT
SIGNSIN
SIGNSON
SIGNSUP
SILESIA
SIMPSON
SINGSTO
SINKSIN
SINUSES
SIZESIX
SIZESUP
TICKSBY
TIDYSUM
TILTSAT
TILTSUP
TIMESUP
TIRESOF
VIBISTS
VIRUSES
WILLSON
WINDSOR
WINDSUP
WINESAP
WINGSIT
WINKSAT
WIPESUP
WIRESIN
WIRESUP
WISESUP

•I•••S•

AIDLESS
AIMLESS
AIRBASE
AIRHOSE
AIRIEST
AIRKISS
AIRLESS
AIRMASS
AIRNESS
BIBLESS
BIGBOSS
BIGEAST
BIGEASY
BIGFISH
BIGGEST
BIGGISH
BIGMESS
BIGNESS
BIGNOSE
BIOMASS
BITLESS
CIRCUSY
DIARIST
DICIEST
DIECAST
DIFFUSE
DIGRESS
DIMMEST
DIMNESS
DIOCESE
DISCUSS
DISEASE
DISEUSE
DISGUST
DISMAST
DISMISS
DISPOSE
DIVERSE
DIVULSE
FINESSE
FINLESS
FINNISH
FIRMEST
FITNESS
FITTEST
GIOCOSO
GIRLISH
HIGHEST
HIGHISH
HIPLESS
HIPNESS
HIPPEST
HIPPISH
HITLESS
HITLIST
IINSIST
JIGGISH
JIVIEST
KIDDISH
KINDEST
KINLESS
LICENSE
LIDLESS
LIEFEST
LIETEST
LIMIEST
LIMPEST
LINIEST
LIONESS
LIONISE
LIPLESS
LITHEST
LITOVSK
MIDEAST
MIDLIST
MIDMOST
MIDRISE
MIDWEST
MILDEST
MINXISH
MIRIEST
MISCAST
MISMESH
MISSISH
MISSUSA
NICOISE
NIGHEST
OILBASE
OILIEST
OILLESS
PIANISM
PIANIST
PICASSO
PICTISH
PIETOSO
PIGFISH
PIGGISH
PINIEST
PINKEST
PINKISH
PINLESS
PIPIEST
PIPLESS
PITBOSS
PIXYISH
RIBLESS
RICHEST
RIMIEST
RIMLESS
SIAMESE
SICKEST
SICKISH
SIENESE
SIKHISM
SINLESS
TIDIEST
TIELESS
TIGRESS
TINFISH
TINIEST
TIPLESS
TITLIST
TITOISM
TITOIST
VINIEST
VINROSE
VIOLIST
VISCUSO
VITEBSK
WIGLESS
WILDEST
WILDISH
WILIEST
WIMPISH
WINIEST
WINLESS
WIRIEST
WITLESS
WITNESS
YIDDISH
ZIONISM
ZIONIST
ZIPDISK

•I••••S

AIDLESS
AIGLETS
AIGRETS
AIKIDOS
AIMLESS
AIRACES
AIRBAGS
AIRDAMS
AIRGUNS
AIRINGS
AIRKISS
AIRLESS
AIRLOGS
AIRMASS
AIRNESS
AIRPOPS
AIRPOTS
AIRSACS
AIRWARS
AIRWAYS
AITCHES
BIALIES
BIASSES
BIBBERS
BIBLESS
BICARBS
BICHONS
BICKERS
BICORNS
BIDDERS
BIDDIES
BIGAPES
BIGBETS
BIGBOSS
BIGBOYS
BIGCARS
BIGCATS
BIGDAYS
BIGDIGS
BIGDOGS
BIGEARS
BIGENDS
BIGEYES
BIGFANS
BIGGERS
BIGGIES
BIGGUNS
BIGHITS
BIGHUGS
BIGKIDS
BIGLIES
BIGLOTS
BIGMACS
BIGMESS
BIGNESS
BIGNEWS
BIGONES
BIGRIGS
BIGTOES
BIGTOPS
BIGWIGS
BIGWINS
BIKINIS
BILIOUS
BILKERS
BILLERS
BILLETS
BILLIES
BILLOWS
BIMBOES
BIMINIS
BINDERS
BINDLES
BINGERS
BINGLES
BINGOES
BIOLABS
BIOMASS
BIONICS
BIOPICS
BIRCHES
BIRDERS
BIRDIES
BIREMES
BIRLERS
BIRMANS
BISECTS
BISHOPS
BISQUES
BISTROS
BITLESS
BITMAPS
BITTERS
CICADAS
CINCHES
CINDERS
CINEMAS
CINQUES
CIPHERS
CIRCLES
CIRQUES
CISCOES
CITRONS
CITROUS
CIVVIES
DIABLES
DIABLOS
DIADEMS
DIALERS
DIALOGS
DIALUPS
DIAPERS
DIARIES
DIARIOS
DIATOMS
DIBBLES
DICKENS
DICKERS
DICKEYS
DICKIES
DICTUMS
DIDACTS
DIDDLES
DIDLAPS
DIDSUMS
DIECUTS

DIEMENS
DIEOFFS
DIESELS
DIETERS
DIFFERS
DIGESTS
DIGGERS
DIGLOTS
DIGRAMS
DIGRESS
DIKDIKS
DIKTATS
DILATES
DILLIES
DILUTES
DIMAGES
DIMMERS
DIMNESS
DIMOUTS
DIMPLES
DIMWITS
DINDINS
DINGERS
DINGLES
DINGOES
DINNERS
DIOXINS
DIPNETS
DIPOLES
DIPPERS
DIRECTS
DIRHAMS
DIRNDLS
DIRTIES
DISARMS
DISBARS
DISBUDS
DISCUSS
DISEURS
DISMALS
DISMAYS
DISMISS
DISOWNS
DISPELS
DISTILS
DISTROS
DISUSES
DITCHES
DITHERS
DITTIES
DIVERTS
DIVESTS
DIVIDES
DIVINES
DIVVIES
DIZAINS
DIZZIES
EIGHTHS
FIACRES
FIANCES
FIASCOS
FIBBERS
FIBRINS
FIBROUS
FIBULAS
FICUSES
FIDDLES
FIDELES

FIDELIS
FIDGETS
FIENNES
FIESTAS
FIFTIES
FIGBARS
FIGURES
FIJIANS
FILCHES
FILENES
FILINGS
FILLERS
FILLETS
FILLIES
FILLINS
FILLIPS
FILLUPS
FILTERS
FINALES
FINCHES
FINDERS
FINGALS
FINGERS
FINIALS
FINIANS
FINITES
FINLESS
FIPPLES
FIRINGS
FIRKINS
FISHERS
FITNESS
FITTERS
FIXATES
FIXINGS
FIZGIGS
FIZZERS
FIZZLES
GIBBERS
GIBBONS
GIBBOUS
GIBLETS
GIBLUES
GIBSONS
GIBUSES
GIDDIES
GIDEONS
GIFTEES
GIGBAGS
GIGGLES
GIGOLOS
GILBLAS
GILDERS
GIMBALS
GIMBELS
GIMLETS
GINGERS
GINGKOS
GINKGOS
GIORGOS
GIPSIES
GIRDERS
GIRDLES
GIRLIES
GITANOS
GIVEUPS
HICCUPS
HICKEYS

HIDEOUS
HIDINGS
HIGGINS
HIGGLES
HIGHIQS
HIGHRES
HIJACKS
HIJINKS
HILTONS
HINDERS
HINNIES
HINTERS
HIPLESS
HIPNESS
HIPPIES
HISNIBS
HISSERS
HITCHES
HITLESS
HITTERS
IIKINGS
JICAMAS
JIFFIES
JIGGERS
JIGGLES
JIGSAWS
JILTERS
JIMJAMS
JIMMIES
JIMSONS
JINGLES
JINGOES
JINXERS
JITNEYS
JITTERS
KIARIOS
KIBBLES
KICKERS
KICKUPS
KIDCOMS
KIDDERS
KIDDIES
KIDNAPS
KIDNEYS
KIDSRUS
KIDULTS
KIDVIDS
KIKUYUS
KILLERS
KILTIES
KIMONOS
KINDLES
KINESES
KINESIS
KINLESS
KIPPERS
KIRMANS
KISHKES
KISLEVS
KISMETS
KISSELS
KISSERS
KITBAGS
KITKATS
KITTENS
KITTIES
KIWANIS
LIAISES

LIBBERS
LIBIDOS
LIBRANS
LIBYANS
LICHEES
LICHENS
LICKERS
LIDLESS
LIENEES
LIENORS
LIFTERS
LIGANDS
LIGATES
LIGNINS
LIKINGS
LIMBERS
LIMNERS
LIMOGES
LIMPETS
LINAGES
LINDENS
LINDIES
LINDROS
LINEUPS
LINGERS
LINGOES
LININGS
LINKERS
LINKUPS
LINNETS
LINTELS
LINTERS
LIONELS
LIONESS
LIONETS
LIPARIS
LIPASES
LIPLESS
LIPPERS
LIQUIDS
LIQUORS
LISPERS
LISTEES
LISTENS
LISTERS
LITCHIS
LITOTES
LITTERS
LITTLES
LIVINGS
LIZARDS
LIZZIES
MIASMAS
MICKEYS
MICMACS
MICRONS
MIDASES
MIDCAPS
MIDDAYS
MIDDIES
MIDDLES
MIDGETS
MIDLEGS
MIDOFFS
MIDRIBS
MIDWAYS
MIGENES
MIGNONS

MIKADOS
MIKASAS
MILDEWS
MILHOUS
MILIEUS
MILKERS
MILLAIS
MILLERS
MILLETS
MILORDS
MIMESES
MIMESIS
MIMOSAS
MINCERS
MINDERS
MINGLES
MINIBUS
MINIMUS
MININGS
MINIONS
MINITVS
MINNOWS
MINOANS
MINSKYS
MINTERS
MINUETS
MINUSES
MINUTES
MINYANS
MIRADAS
MIRAGES
MIRRORS
MISACTS
MISADDS
MISAIMS
MISCUES
MISCUTS
MISDOES
MISFITS
MISHAPS
MISHITS
MISKEYS
MISLAYS
MISSALS
MISSAYS
MISSETS
MISSIES
MISTERS
MISUSES
MITHRAS
MITOSES
MITOSIS
MITTENS
MIXTECS
MIZUNAS
MIZZENS
MIZZLES
NIBBLES
NIBLETS
NICHOLS
NICKELS
NICKERS
NICKLES
NICOLAS
NIFTIES
NIGGLES
NIKEADS
NIMRODS

NINNIES
NIPPERS
NIPPLES
NISSANS
NITROUS
NITWITS
NIVEOUS
OILCANS
OILCUPS
OILLESS
OILPANS
OILRIGS
OILRUBS
OINKERS
PIAFFES
PIAZZAS
PICARAS
PICAROS
PICEOUS
PICKENS
PICKERS
PICKETS
PICKLES
PICKUPS
PICNICS
PIDDLES
PIDGINS
PIECERS
PIEPANS
PIERCES
PIETIES
PIETINS
PIETROS
PIFFLES
PIGEONS
PIGGIES
PIGLETS
PIGNUTS
PIGOUTS
PIGPENS
PILATES
PILATUS
PILEOUS
PILEUPS
PILFERS
PILINGS
PILLARS
PILLOWS
PIMPLES
PINATAS
PINBOYS
PINCERS
PINCHAS
PINCHES
PINGERS
PINIONS
PINKENS
PINKIES
PINKOES
PINLESS
PINNERS
PINOAKS
PINONES
PIOLETS
PIPAGES
PIPINGS
PIPLESS
PIPPINS

PIRAEUS
PIRATES
PISTILS
PISTOLS
PISTONS
PISTOUS
PITAYAS
PITBOSS
PITCHES
PITEOUS
PITIERS
PITROWS
PITSAWS
QINTARS
RIALTOS
RIBALDS
RIBANDS
RIBBERS
RIBBIES
RIBBONS
RIBCUTS
RIBEYES
RIBLESS
RIBLETS
RIBPADS
RICHENS
RICKEYS
RICKLES
RICRACS
RIDDERS
RIDDLES
RIDEBYS
RIDINGS
RIESENS
RIFFLES
RIFLERS
RIGGERS
RIGOURS
RILLETS
RIMLESS
RIMPLES
RINGERS
RINSERS
RIOTERS
RIOTOUS
RIPOFFS
RIPOSTS
RIPPERS
RIPPLES
RIPRAPS
RIPSAWS
RISINGS
RISKERS
RITARDS
RITDYES
RITUALS
SICKENS
SICKLES
SIDDONS
SIDDURS
SIDINGS
SIDIOUS
SIEMENS
SIENNAS
SIERRAS
SIESTAS
SIFTERS
SIGHERS

SIGNALS
SIGNEES
SIGNERS
SIGNETS
SIGNORS
SIGNUPS
SILENTS
SILICAS
SILLIES
SILVERS
SIMIANS
SIMILES
SIMMERS
SIMMONS
SIMPERS
SIMPLES
SINGERS
SINGLES
SINKERS
SINLESS
SINNERS
SINUOUS
SINUSES
SIOUANS
SIPHONS
SIPPERS
SISSIES
SISTERS
SITCOMS
SITTERS
SIXGUNS
SIXTIES
SIZZLES
TICKERS
TICKETS
TICKLES
TICTACS
TIDBITS
TIDINGS
TIEBARS
TIEDYES
TIELESS
TIEMPOS
TIENDAS
TIEPINS
TIERCES
TIERODS
TIETACS
TIFFINS
TIGLONS
TIGRESS
TILINGS
TILLERS
TILLETS
TILSITS
TILTERS
TIMBALS
TIMBERS
TIMBRES
TIMEWAS
TIMEXES
TIMINGS
TIMMINS
TINCANS
TINDERS
TINEARS
TINGLES
TINGODS

TINHATS
TINKERS
TINKLES
TINNERS
TINORES
TINSELS
TINTERS
TIPJARS
TIPLESS
TIPOFFS
TIPPEES
TIPPERS
TIPPETS
TIPPLES
TIPTOES
TIPTOPS
TIRADES
TISANES
TISSOTS
TISSUES
TITHERS
TITIANS
TITTERS
TITTLES
TIZZIES
VIBISTS
VICIOUS
VICKERS
VICTIMS
VICTORS
VICUNAS
VIDIOTS
VIELLES
VIERNES
VIEWERS
VIGOURS
VIHARAS
VIKINGS
VILNIUS
VIOLETS
VIOLINS
VIRAGOS
VIRGINS
VIRTUES
VIRUSES
VISAGES
VISAVIS
VISCOUS
VISIONS
VISUALS
VITALIS
VITARAS
VITRICS
VITTLES
VIVANTS
VIZIERS
VIZSLAS
WICCANS
WICKERS
WICKETS
WIDGETS
WIENERS
WIENIES
WIGGLES
WIGLESS
WIGLETS
WIGWAGS
WIGWAMS

WILKENS
WILKINS
WILLERS
WILLIES
WILLOWS
WILSONS
WIMPLES
WINCERS
WINCHES
WINDAUS
WINDERS
WINDOMS
WINDOWS
WINDUPS
WINGERS
WINKERS
WINLESS
WINNERS
WINNOWS
WINTERS
WIRINGS
WISDOMS
WISHERS
WITCHES
WITHERS
WITHIES
WITLESS
WITNESS
WIZARDS
XIMENES
YIPPIES
ZIGZAGS
ZILCHES
ZINCOUS
ZINGERS
ZINNIAS
ZIPGUNS
ZIPLOCS
ZIPPERS
ZIPTOPS
ZIRCONS
ZITCOMS
ZITHERS

••IS•••

AMISTAD
ANISEED
ANISTON
APISHLY
ARISING
ARISTAE
ARISTAS
ARISTOS
ASISAID
ATISSUE
BLISSED
BLISSES
BLISTER
BOISEID
BRISKED
BRISKER
BRISKET
BRISKLY
BRISTLE
BRISTLY
BRISTOL
BUISSON
CAISSON

CHISELS
CRISPED
CRISPEN
CRISPER
CRISPIN
CRISPIX
CRISPLY
CRISPUS
CUISINE
DAISIES
DEISTIC
DRISTAN
EKISTIC
ELISION
ENISLED
ENISLES
EPISODE
EPISTLE
ERISTIC
EXISTED
FAISALI
FOISTED
FOISTON
FRISBEE
FRISEUR
FRISIAN
FRISKED
FRISKER
FRISSON
GEISHAS
GLISTEN
GLISTER
GRISHAM
GRISLET
GRISNEZ
GRISSOM
GRISTER
GRISTLE
GRISTLY
HEISMAN
HEISTED
HOISTED
HOISTER
HOISTUP
IRISHER
IRISING
IRISOUT
ITISTOO
JOISTED
KAISERS
KAISHEK
KEISTER
KLISTER
KNISHES
KRISHNA
KRISTIN
LAISSEZ
LEISTER
LEISURE
MAISONS
MAISOUI
MEISSEN
MEISTER
MOISSAN
MOISTEN
MOISTER
MOISTLY
MRISCAN

NOISIER
NOISILY
NOISING
NOISOME
ORISONS
OVISACS
PAISANO
PAISANS
PAISLEY
PHISHED
PHISHER
PHISHES
PLISSES
POISERS
POISING
POISONS
POISSON
PRISONS
PRISSES
RAISERS
RAISEUP
RAISING
RAISINS
RAISINY
RAISONS
REISSUE
ROISTER
SAISONS
SCISSOR
SEISMAL
SEISMIC
SKISHOP
SKISUIT
SWISHED
SWISHES
THISDAY
THISONE
THISTLE
THISTLY
THISWAY
TRISECT
TRISTAN
TRISTAR
TWISTED
TWISTER
TWISTON
TWISTUP
UNISIZE
UNISOMS
UNISONS
WAISTED
WHISHED
WHISHES
WHISKAS
WHISKED
WHISKER
WHISKEY
WHISPER
WHISTLE

••I•S••

ALIASES
ARIOSOS
ARIOSTO
ATISSUE
BAILSON
BLISSED
BLISSES
BOILSUP
BUISSON
CAISSON
CHIPSIN
CHIPSUP
CLIPSON
COILSUP
CRIESUP
CRIMSON
DRIESCH
DRIESUP
DRIPSON
ERICSON
ERIKSON
ESIASON
FAILSTO
FAIRSEX
FAIRSUP
FLIESAT
FLIESBY
FLIESIN
FLIESON
FLIESTO
FLIESUP
FLITSBY
FLITSIN
FRIESUP
FRISSON
GAINSAY
GAINSON
GRIMSBY
GRINSAT
GRISSOM
ILIESCU
JOINSIN
JOINSUP
LAISSEZ
MAILSIN
MEIOSES
MEIOSIS
MEISSEN
MOISSAN
NAILSET
NAILSIN
NAILSIT
NAILSUP
PAIRSUP
PLISSES
POISSON
PRIESTS
PRISSES
PRIUSES
QUITSIT
RAILSAT
RAILSON
RAINSIN
RAINSON
REINSIN
REISSUE
SAILSON
SAILSTO
SCISSOR
SKIPSBY
SLIPSBY
SLIPSIN
SLIPSON
SLIPSUP
SPIESON

SPITSON
STIMSON
STIRSIN
STIRSUP
SUITSME
SUITSUP
SWIMSUP
THIRSTS
THIRSTY
TOILSAT
TRIESIT
TRIESON
TRIESTE
TRIESTO
TRIPSON
TRIPSUP
TWINSET
WAITSON
WAITSUP
WHIPSAW
WHIPSIN
WHIPSUP
WHITSUN

••I••S•

ADIPOSE
AGILEST
ANIMISM
ANIMIST
ARIDEST
AVIDEST
BRINISH
BRITISH
CHICEST
CHINESE
CUIRASS
DOINGSO
ELITEST
ELITISM
ELITIST
EVILEST
FAINEST
FAIREST
FAIRISH
FAIRUSE
FBICASE
GLIMPSE
GOIRISH
HAIMISH
HEIRESS
ICINESS
JAINISM
JAINIST
MAIDISH
NAIVEST
OMIGOSH
OXIDASE
OXIDISE
QUITESO
SHIATSU
SKIMASK
SKIVEST
SNIDEST
SWINISH
TBILISI
THINKSO
TRITEST
UNITISE
UTILISE
VAINEST
WAIFISH
WHITEST
WHITISH

••I•••S

ABIDERS
ALIASES
ALIGHTS
ALINERS
ALIYAHS
AMIDOLS
AMITIES
ANIMALS
ANITRAS
ARIANES
ARIOSOS
ARISTAS
ARISTOS
ASIAGOS
AVIATES
AXILLAS
BAILEES
BAILERS
BAILORS
BAITERS
BEIGNES
BLIGHTS
BLISSES
BLITZES
BOILERS
BRIARDS
BRIBEES
BRIBERS
BRIDALS
BRIDGES
BRIDLES
BRIGHTS
BRILLOS
BRINERS
BRITONS
CAIMANS
CHIAPAS
CHICHAS
CHICHIS
CHICLES
CHIDERS
CHIGOES
CHILIES
CHILLIS
CHIMERS
CHINOIS
CHINUPS
CHISELS
CHITONS
CHIVIES
CLICHES
CLIENTS
CLIMATS
CLINICS
CLIPONS
CLIQUES
COIGNES
COILERS
COINERS
COINOPS
CRINGES
CRISPUS
CRITIAS
CRITICS
CUIRASS
DAILIES
DAIRIES
DAISIES
DEICERS
DEIFIES
DEITIES
DJINNIS
DOILIES
DRIVELS
DRIVERS
EDIBLES
EDIFIES
EDITORS
ELICITS
ELIDERS
ELIGIUS
ELIXIRS
EMIGRES
ENIGMAS
ENISLES
EPILOGS
ERINYES
EVINCES
EXILERS
FAILLES
FAIRIES
FLIGHTS
FLIPUPS
FOIBLES
FRIDAYS
FRIDGES
FRIENDS
FRIEZES
FRIGHTS
FRINGES
FRIVOLS
FRIZZES
GAINERS
GAITERS
GEISHAS
GLIDERS
GLITZES
GOITERS
GRIEVES
GRIGRIS
GRILLES
GRINGOS
GRIPERS
GRIPPES
GUIDERS
GUINEAS
GUITARS
HAIKAIS
HAILERS
HAIRDOS
HEIFERS
HEIGHTS
HEINOUS
HEIRESS
IBIZANS
ICICLES
ICINESS
INIRONS
JAILERS
JAILORS
JOINERS
JUICERS
KAISERS
KNIFERS
KNIGHTS
KNISHES
LAITIES
LOITERS
MAIDENS
MAILERS
MAILINS
MAIMERS
MAINERS
MAISONS
MAITAIS
MAITRES
MEIOSES
MEIOSIS
MOILERS
MSIEURS
NAIADES
NAILERS
OCICATS
OHIOANS
OJIBWAS
OMINOUS
OPIATES
OPINERS
ORIENTS
ORIGINS
ORIOLES
ORISONS
OVISACS
PAIDADS
PAIRERS
PAISANS
PAIUTES
PHIDIAS
PHILCOS
PHILEAS
PHILIPS
PHILOUS
PHINEAS
PHISHES
PLIGHTS
PLINTHS
PLISSES
POINTES
POISERS
POISONS
POIVRES
PRICERS
PRIESTS
PRIMERS
PRINCES
PRISONS
PRISSES
PRIUSES
PRIVETS
PRIVIES
PRIZZIS
QUICHES
QUIETUS
QUINCES
QUINTAS
QUINTES
QUINTUS
QUINZES
QUIVERS
QUIZNOS
QUIZZES
RAIDERS
RAILBUS
RAILERS
RAISERS
RAISINS
RAISONS
REIFIES
RUINERS
RUINOUS
SAILERS
SAILORS
SAINTES
SAISONS
SEINERS
SEIZERS
SEIZORS
SHIELDS
SHIITES
SHINERS
SHIVERS
SKIBIBS
SKIBOBS
SKIBUMS
SKICAPS
SKIDOOS
SKIHATS
SKIRUNS
SKITOWS
SLICERS
SLIDERS
SLIGHTS
SLIPONS
SLIPUPS
SLIVERS
SMIDGES
SMILERS
SMILEYS
SMILLAS
SMITERS
SNIPERS
SNIVELS
SOIREES
SPICERS
SPIDERS
SPIGOTS
SPIKERS
SPINELS
SPINETS
SPIRALS
SPIREAS
SPIRITS
SPITZES
STIFLES
STIGMAS
SUITORS
SWIPERS
SWISHES
SWIVELS
SWIVETS
TAILERS
TAILORS
THIEVES
THIRSTS
TOILERS
TOILETS
TRIAGES
TRICEPS
TRICOTS
TRIFLES
TRIGONS
TRIJETS
TRIODES
TRIPLES
TRIPODS
TRITONS
TRIVETS
TUILLES
TVIDOLS
TWINERS
TWINGES
TZIMMES
UNIATES
UNIFIES
UNIPODS
UNIQUES
UNISOMS
UNISONS
UNITERS
UNITIES
UNIVACS
UTICANS
VEIGHTS
VEILERS
VEINTES
VOICERS
VOIDERS
WAILERS
WAITERS
WAIVERS
WEIGHTS
WEIRDOS
WHINERS
WHISHES
WHISKAS
WHITENS
WHIZZES
WRIGHTS
WRITERS
WRITHES

•••IS••

ADDISON
ADVISED
ADVISEE
ADVISER
ADVISES
ADVISOR
AEGISES
AGEISTS
ALLISON
ARRISES
ARTISAN
ARTISTE
ARTISTS
ASSISTS
AURISTS
AUTISTS
BARISTA
BATISTA
BATISTE
BENISON
BRAISED
BRAISES
BRUISED
BRUISER
BRUISES
CALISTA
CAMISES
CERISES
CHAISES
CHRISMS
CHRISOM
CHRISTA
CHRISTI
CHRISTO
CHRISTY
CRAISIN
CRUISED
CRUISER
CRUISES
CUBISTS
CUTISES
DAVISON
DEHISCE
DELISTS
DEMISED
DEMISES
DEMISTS
DENISON
DESISTS
DEVISED
DEVISEE
DEVISER
DEVISES
DEVISOR
DIVISOR
DREISER
EGLISES
EGOISTE
EGOISTS
ELEISON
ELLISON
ELMISTI
ENLISTS
EXCISED
EXCISES
FINISHD
FRAISES
FUJISAN
HEDISON
HOLISTS
INCISED
INCISES
INCISOR
INSISTS
IODISED
IODISES
IONISED
IONISER
IONISES
JALISCO
JAMISON
JEMISON
JEWISON
JURISTS
KATISHA
KINISON
KLEISER
LAKISTS
LEGISTS
LEXISES
LIAISED
LIAISES
LIAISON
LORISES
LOUISII
LOUISIV
LOUISIX
LOUISVI
LOUISXI
LOUISXV
LUTISTS
LYRISTS
MADISON
MAOISTS
MATISSE
MAVISES
MELISMA
MELISSA
MENISCI
MINISKI
MINISUB
MIRISCH
MODISTE
MORISOT
NABISCO
NERISSA
NOVISAD
NOWISEE
NOWISER
NUDISTS
OBOISTS
ORBISON
ORRISES
PAPISTS
PELISSE
PERISSA
PLAISIR
POLISCI
PRAISED
PRAISER
PRAISES
PURISTS
RACISTS
RAWISTS
RELISTS
REMISED
REMISES
RERISEN
RERISES
RESISTS
REVISAL
REVISED
REVISER
REVISES
REVISIT
REVISOR
SADISTS
SAMISEN
SATISFY
SCHISMS
SCHISTS
SEWISTS
SEXISTS
SQUISHY
TAOISTS
THEISMS
THEISTS
TRUISMS
TUBISTS
TUNISIA
TURISMO
TURISTA
TYPISTS
UNRISEN
UNRISKY
UNWISER
UPRISEN
UPRISER
UPRISES
VALISES
VEDISTS
VENISON
VERISMO
VERISTS
VIBISTS
WHOISIT
WHYISIT
WOEISME
YESISEE
ZENISTS

•••I•S•

ACHIEST
AERIEST
AGAINST
AIRIEST
ARTIEST
ASHIEST
ATFIRST
ATHIRST
BABIEST
BONIEST
BOXIEST
BUSIEST
CAGIEST
CAKIEST
CANIEST
COKIEST
COSIEST
COWIEST
COZIEST
CURIOSA
DARIUSI
DEWIEST
DICIEST
DOPIEST
DOZIEST
EASIEST
ECLIPSE
EDGIEST
EELIEST
EERIEST
EGGIEST
ELLIPSE
ELMIEST
FOLIOSE
FOXIEST
FUJITSU
FUMIEST
FURIOSO
GAMIEST
GLUIEST
GOFIRST
GOOIEST
GORIEST
HAZIEST
HOKIEST
HOLIEST
HOMIEST
ICKIEST
IFFIEST
INFIRST
INKIEST
JIVIEST
JOKIEST
JUJITSU
KAPITSA
LACIEST
LAKIEST
LAZIEST
LIMIEST
LINIEST
LOGIEST
LUCIUSI
MAFIOSI
MAFIOSO
MATISSE
MAZIEST
MEFIRST
MELISSA
MIRIEST
MOPIEST
NERISSA
NOSIEST
OAKIEST
OILIEST
ONFIRST
ONLIEST
OOZIEST
ORGIAST
OWLIEST
PACIEST
PELISSE
PERISSA
PINIEST
PIPIEST
POKIEST
PUNIEST
RACIEST
RERINSE
RIMIEST
ROPIEST
ROSIEST
RULIEST
SAGIEST
SERIESE
SERIESF
SERIESG
SERIESH
SERIESI
SERIESJ
SERIESK
SEXIEST
SPRIEST
STPIUSI
STPIUSV
STPIUSX
TIDIEST
TINIEST
TONIEST
TRAIPSE
UGLIEST
UPFIRST
VERIEST
VINIEST
WANIEST
WARIEST
WAVIEST
WAXIEST
WILIEST
WINIEST
WIRIEST
YOGIISM
ZANIEST
ZOOIEST

•••I••S

ABRILES
ACTIONS
ACTIVAS
ACTIVES
ADDICTS
ADMIRES
ADMIXES
ADVICES
ADVISES
AEDILES
AEGISES
AERIALS
AFFINES
AFFIRMS
AFFIXES
AGEISTS
AIKIDOS
AIRINGS
ALBINOS
ALGIERS
ALLIUMS
ALNICOS
ALPINES
ALTIMAS
AMBIENS
AMNIONS
AMRITAS
ANOINTS
ANTIBES
ANXIOUS
APHIDES
APLITES
APSIDES
AQUINAS
ARCINGS
ARNICAS
ARRISES
ARRIVES
ARTISTS
ASPIRES
ASSIGNS
ASSISTS
ASSIZES
ATRIUMS
ATSIGNS
ATTICUS
ATTIMES
ATTIRES
AUDILES
AUGITES
AURISTS
AUTISTS
AWNINGS
BAHIANS
BARITES
BCLIONS
BEGIRDS
BEHINDS
BELIEFS
BELIERS
BEMIRES
BESIDES
BETIDES
BETIMES
BEZIERS
BIKINIS
BILIOUS
BIMINIS
BLUINGS
BODICES
BODINGS
BOEINGS
BOLIDES
BONITOS
BORIDES
BORINGS
BOVINES
BRAISES
BRUISES
BUNIONS
BURIALS
BURIERS
BYFIVES
BYLINES
CAHIERS
CALICES
CALICOS
CALIPHS
CAMINOS
CAMIONS
CAMISES
CANINES
CANINGS
CARIBES
CARINAS
CARIOUS
CASINGS
CASINOS
CASITAS
CATIONS
CAVIARS
CELICAS
CERISES
CHAINES
CHAISES
CHOICES
CHRISMS
CODICES
COMICES
COMINGS
COPIERS
COPIOUS
COSIGNS
COSINES
CRUISES
CUBISTS
CUBITUS
CURIOUS
CUTISES
DANIELS
DANITES
DATINGS
DATIVES
DECIDES
DECILES
DEFIERS
DEFILES
DEFINES
DEHIRES
DELIBES
DELICTS
DELINTS
DELISTS
DEMISES
DEMISTS
DENIALS
DENIERS
DEPICTS
DERIDES
DERIVES
DESIGNS
DESILTS
DESIRES
DESISTS
DEVICES
DEVIOUS
DEVISES
DEWIRES
DIVIDES
DIVINES
DOMINOS
DOMINUS
DONIMUS
DORITOS
DOSIDOS
DUBIOUS
EDGINGS
EGLISES
EGOISTS
ELAINES
ELNINOS
EMPIRES
ENCINAS
ENDINGS
ENDIVES
ENGILDS
ENGINES
ENGIRDS
ENLINKS
ENLISTS
ENSIGNS
ENSILES
ENTICES
ENTIRES
ENVIERS
ENVIOUS
ENVIROS
ENWINDS
EOLITHS
EOSINES
EQUINES
ERMINES
ESKIMOS
ESPIALS
ETOILES
EXCIDES
EXCISES
EXCITES
EXPIRES
EXWIVES

FACIALS
FACINGS
FAJITAS
FAMINES
FANIONS
FARINAS
FELINES
FIJIANS
FILINGS
FINIALS
FINIANS
FINITES
FIRINGS
FIXINGS
FORINTS
FRAISES
FURIOUS
FUSIONS
GAMINES
GATINGS
GAVIALS
GEMINIS
GOGIRLS
GUNITES
HABILIS
HALIDES
HALITES
HAMITES
HAYINGS
HAZINGS
HEGIRAS
HELICES
HELIXES
HIDINGS
HIJINKS
HOLISTS
HOSIERS
HYGINUS
ICTINUS
IGNITES
IIKINGS
IMBIBES
IMMIXES
IMPIOUS
INCISES
INCITES
INDIANS
INDICES
INDICTS
INDIGOS
INDITES
INFIVES
INFIXES
INKINGS
INLINES
INNINGS
INSIDES
INSISTS
INVITES
IODIDES
IODISES
IODIZES
IONIANS
IONISES
IONIUMS
IONIZES
ITGIRLS
JUNIORS
JURISTS
KODIAKS
KURILES
LABIALS
LACINGS
LADIDAS
LADINGS
LADINOS
LAKISTS
LAMINAS
LARIATS
LATICES
LATIGOS
LATIMES
LATINAS
LATINOS
LATINUS
LEGIONS
LEGISTS
LEPIDUS
LESIONS
LEVIERS
LEVITES
LEXISES
LIAISES
LIBIDOS
LIKINGS
LININGS
LIVINGS
LORISES
LOSINGS
LOTIONS
LUCITES
LUMINAS
LUPINES
LUTISTS
LYRISTS
MAKINGS
MALIANS
MALICES
MALIGNS
MANIACS
MANILAS
MAOISTS
MARIDAS
MARIDOS
MARINAS
MARINES
MAVISES
MAXIMAS
MAXIMUS
MAXIXES
MAYINGS
MEDIANS
MEDICOS
MEDIUMS
MENIALS
MERINOS
METIERS
MILIEUS
MINIBUS
MINIMUS
MININGS
MINIONS
MINITVS
MOBILES
MOJITOS
MOTIONS
MOTIVES
MOWINGS
MRTIBBS
MURIELS
MUSICKS
MUSINGS
MYRIADS
NAPIERS
NATIONS
NATIVES
NOGIFTS
NORITES
NOTICES
NOTIONS
NOVICES
NOXIOUS
NUBIANS
NUBIRAS
NUDISTS
NYTIMES
OBLIGES
OBOISTS
OBVIOUS
OEDIPUS
OFFICES
OFFINGS
OMNIBUS
ONEIDAS
ONSIDES
OOLITES
OPTICKS
OPTIMAS
OPTIONS
ORDINES
ORRISES
OSCINES
OUTINGS
OXHIDES
PAGINGS
PALINGS
PANIERS
PANINIS
PAPIERS
PAPISTS
PARIAHS
PARIBUS
PARINGS
PATINAS
PAVINGS
PAVIORS
PEPITAS
PERIODS
PERITUS
PETITES
PILINGS
PINIONS
PIPINGS
PITIERS
PLAICES
PLAINES
PLAINTS
PODIUMS
POLICES
POTIONS
PRAISES
PRFIRMS
PUMICES
PURISTS
PYRITES
QUEIROS
RACINOS
RACISTS
RADIALS
RADIANS
RADICES
RADIXES
RAGINGS
RAPIERS
RAPINES
RAPINIS
RATINES
RATINGS
RATIONS
RATITES
RAVINES
RAVINGS
RAWISTS
REBILLS
REBINDS
RECIPES
RECITES
REDIALS
REFILES
REFILLS
REFILMS
REFINDS
REFINES
REFIRES
REFIXES
REGIFTS
REGILDS
REGIMES
REGINAS
REGIONS
REGIRDS
REGIVES
REHIDES
REHIRES
REKICKS
RELICTS
RELIEFS
RELIERS
RELINES
RELINKS
RELISTS
RELIVES
REMILLS
REMINDS
REMINES
REMINTS
REMISES
REMIXES
REPICKS
REPINES
RERIDES
RERISES
RESIDES
RESIFTS
RESIGNS
RESILES
RESINGS
RESINKS
RESISTS
RESIZES
RETILES
RETILLS
RETIMES
RETINAS
RETINTS
RETIRES
REVIEWS
REVILES
REVISES
REVIVES
REWINDS
REWIPES
REWIRES
RIDINGS
RISINGS
ROVINGS
RUBIOUS
RULINGS
RUPIAHS
RUTILES
SABINES
SADISTS
SALINAS
SALINES
SALIVAS
SAPIENS
SATIRES
SAVINGS
SAVIORS
SAYINGS
SCHICKS
SCHISMS
SCHISTS
SCRIBES
SCRIMPS
SCRIPPS
SCRIPTS
SEMITES
SENIORS
SEPIRAS
SERIALS
SERIOUS
SEWISTS
SEXISTS
SHEIKHS
SHEILAS
SHIITES
SHRIEKS
SHRIKES
SHRILLS
SHRIMPS
SHRINES
SHRINKS
SHRIVES
SHTICKS
SIDINGS
SIDIOUS
SILICAS
SIMIANS
SIMILES
SLEIGHS
SLUICES
SOCIALS
SOVIETS
SOYINKS
SPLICES
SPLINES
SPLINTS
SPRINGS
SPRINTS
SPRITES
SPYINGS
SQUINTS
SQUIRES
SQUIRMS
SQUIRTS
STKITTS
STRIDES
STRIFES
STRIKES
STRINGS
STRIPES
STRIVES
SURIMIS
SYRIANS
TACITUS
TAHINIS
TAKINGS
TAOISTS
TAPINGS
TARIFFS
TEDIOUS
TEDIUMS
THEISMS
THEISTS
THRIFTS
THRILLS
THRIVES
TIDINGS
TILINGS
TIMINGS
TITIANS
TORINOS
TOTINOS
TOWINGS
TREIZES
TROIKAS
TROILUS
TRUISMS
TSHIRTS
TUBISTS
TYPISTS
ULTIMAS
UMPIRES
UNBINDS
UNCIALS
UNDINES
UNFILES
UNFINES
UNFIXES
UNGIRDS
UNHIRES
UNKINKS
UNLIKES
UNLINKS
UNLIVES
UNMIXES
UNPICKS
UNPILES
UNPIOUS
UNTIERS
UNWINDS
UPDIVES
UPGIRDS
UPHILLS
UPLIFTS
UPLINKS
UPPILES
UPRISES
UPSIDES
UPSIZES
UPTICKS
UPTILTS
UPTIMES
UPWINDS
URGINGS
URSINUS
VALINES
VALISES
VARIERS
VARIOUS
VEDISTS
VERISTS
VERITAS
VIBISTS
VICIOUS
VIDIOTS
VIKINGS
VISIONS
VIZIERS
VOTIVES
WAHINES
WAKINGS
WAPITIS
WAXINGS
WIRINGS
WRAITHS
YAKIMAS
YESITIS
YOGINIS
ZENISTS
ZENITHS
ZODIACS
ZONIANS
ZOSIMUS
ZUNIANS

••••IS•

ABOLISH
ABSCISE
AGONISE
AGONISM
AGONIST
AIRKISS
ALLRISE
ALLWISE
ALQUIST
ALTOIST
AMORIST
ANGUISH
ANIMISM
ANIMIST
ANODISE
ANYWISE
APPRISE
ARABIST
ATAVISM
ATAVIST
ATHEISM
ATHEIST
ATOMISE
ATOMISM
ATOMIST
BAALISH
BAALISM
BAALIST
BABYISH
BADDISH
BAHAISM
BAHAIST
BALDISH
BAPTISE
BAPTISM
BAPTIST
BASSIST
BEAMISH
BEARISH
BEAUISH
BIGFISH
BIGGISH
BLEMISH
BLUEISH
BOARISH
BOGGISH
BOOHISS
BOOKISH
BOORISH
BOSSISM
BRINISH
BRITISH
BRUTISH
BRUXISM
BULLISH
BURNISH
CADDISH
CASUIST
CATFISH
CATTISH
CELLIST
CHEMISE
CHEMIST
CHERISH
CHORIST
CHUTIST
CLAYISH
CLERISY
COCHISE
COCKISH
CODFISH
COEXIST
COLDISH
COLTISH
COMMISH
COMTISM
COMTIST
CONCISE
CONSIST
COOLISH
COPYIST
CORNISH
COWFISH
CUBBISH
CULTISH
CULTISM
CULTIST
CURRISH
CURTISS
CYCLIST
CZARISM
CZARIST
DADAISM
DADAIST
DAMPISH
DARKISH
DEEPISH
DELUISE
DENTIST
DERVISH
DESPISE
DIARIST
DISMISS
DOGFISH
DOGGISH
DOLLISH
DOLTISH
DONNISH
DRFRIST
DRONISH
DUALISM
DUALIST
DUELIST
DULLISH
DUMPISH
DUNCISH
DUSKISH
ECHOISM
EGOTISM
EGOTIST
ELEGIST
ELITISM
ELITIST
EMPRISE
ENDWISE
ENGLISH
ENPRISE
ENTWIST
EPEEIST
EVANISH
EXOTISM
FADDISH
FADDISM
FADDIST
FAIRISH
FANWISE
FASCISM
FASCIST
FATTISH
FAUVISM
FAUVIST
FEUDIST
FINNISH
FLEMISH
FLORIST
FLUTIST
FLYFISH
FOGYISH
FOGYISM
FOLKISH
FOOLISH
FOPPISH
FTBLISS
FURBISH
FURNISH
GARNISH
GAULISH
GAWKISH
GENOISE
GETWISE
GIRLISH
GNOMISH
GNOMIST
GOAMISS
GOATISH
GOIRISH
GOODISH
GOTWISE
GOUTISH
GRAYISH
GRECISM
GREYISH
HAGGISH
HAIMISH
HARDISH
HARPIST
HASHISH
HAWKISH
HELLISH
HELOISE
HENNISH
HEROISM
HIGHISH
HIPPISH
HITLIST
HOBOISM
HOGGISH
HORNISH
HORNIST
HUFFISH
HUNNISH
IAMBIST
IDOLISE
IDOLIST
IDYLIST
IINSIST
IMAGISM
IMAGIST
IRONIST
ITEMISE
JAINISM
JAINIST
JAZZISH
JIGGISH
JUDAISM
JUDOIST
KADDISH
KENTISH
KIDDISH
KNAVISH
KURDISH
LADDISH
LADYISH
LAMAISM
LAMAIST
LAPPISH
LARGISH
LARKISH
LAZYISH
LEFTISH
LEFTISM
LEFTIST
LETTISH
LIONISE
LOGGISH
LONGISH
LOOKISM
LOOKIST
LOUDISH
LOUTISH
LOWRISE
LOWRISK
LUDDISM
LUMPISH
MADDISH
MAHDISM
MAHDIST
MAIDISH
MALAISE
MANNISH
MARXISM
MARXIST
MAWKISH
METRIST
MIDLIST
MIDRISE
MINXISH
MISSISH
MOBBISH
MOBBISM
MOBBIST
MONKISH
MOONISH
MOORISH
MORTISE
MRBLISS
MUDFISH
MUGGISH
MURKISH
NAGGISH
NEBBISH
NERDISH
NICOISE
NONOISE
NORRISH
NOURISH
NUNNISH
OBELISE
OBELISK
OCULIST
OGREISH
OLEMISS
OPALISH
ORALIST
OUTFISH
OUTHISS
OUTKISS
OUTWISH
OXIDISE
OZONISE
PACHISI
PALMIST
PANFISH
PARRISH
PAULIST
PEAKISH
PECKISH
PEEVISH
PELTISH
PERKISH
PERSIST
PETFISH
PETTISH
PIANISM
PIANIST
PICTISH
PIGFISH
PIGGISH
PINKISH
PIXYISH
PLANISH
PLENISH
POETISE
POLOIST
POORISH
PORKISH
PRECISE
PREMISE
PREMISS
PROMISE
PROTIST
PROVISO
PRUDISH
PUBLISH
PUCKISH
PUGGISH
QUERIST
RAFFISH
RAMMISH
RANKISH
RASPISH
RATTISH
RAWFISH
REALISE
REALISM
REALIST
REARISE
REDDISH
REDFISH
REPRISE
RERAISE
RETWIST
RHENISH
RHYMIST
ROGUISH
ROMPISH
ROOKISH
RUBBISH
RUNTISH
RUTTISH
SALTISH
SAMWISE
SAWFISH
SEAMIST
SELFISH
SICKISH
SIKHISM
SLAVISH
SLOWISH
SOFTISH
SOLOIST
SOPHISM
SOPHIST
SOTTISH
SOUBISE
SOURISH
SPANISH
STATISM
STATIST
STYLISE
STYLISH
STYLIST
SUBSIST
SUMOIST
SUNFISH
SUNKIST
SUNRISE
SURMISE
SWEDISH
SWINISH
TALLISH
TANNISH
TARNISH
TARTISH
TBILISI
THEKISS
TINFISH
TITLIST
TITOISM
TITOIST
TOADISH
TORYISH
TORYISM
TOURISM
TOURIST
TOWNISH
TROPISM
TSARISM
TSARIST
TUBAIST
TURKISH
UNITISE
UNMOIST
UNNOISY
UNTWIST
UPRAISE
UTILISE
UTOPISM
UTOPIST
VAMPISH
VARNISH
VIOLIST
VOGUISH
WAGGISH
WAIFISH
WANNISH
WARMISH
WASPISH
WEAKISH
WETKISS
WETTISH
WHEYISH
WHITISH
WILDISH
WIMPISH
WOLFISH
WORMISH
YERKISH
YIDDISH
YOBBISH
YOGIISM
YORKIST
YOUWISH
ZANYISH
ZANYISM
ZIONISM
ZIONIST
ZIPDISK

••••I•S

ACACIAS
ACARIDS
ACQUITS
ADAGIOS
ADELIES
ADJOINS

AFFAIRS
AGARICS
AGNAILS
AGONIES
AIRKISS
ALTOIDS
AMBRIES
AMITIES
ANACINS
ANANIAS
ANEMIAS
ANOMIES
APERIES
APPLIES
ARABICS
ARAMIDS
ARCHIES
ARMPITS
ASHBINS
ASHPITS
ASSAILS
ATOMICS
ATOMIES
ATONICS
ATONIES
ATTAINS
ATTRITS
AUNTIES
AUPAIRS
AUSSIES
AUSTINS
BADDIES
BADFITS
BADLIES
BAFFIES
BAGGIES
BAGGINS
BAGNIOS
BAGWIGS
BALDIES
BAMMIES
BANDIES
BANDITS
BANKITS
BARBIES
BARRIOS
BBQPITS
BBQRIBS
BEANIES
BEDSITS
BELAIRS
BELLIES
BERGIUS
BERRIES
BESTIRS
BEWAILS
BIALIES
BIDDIES
BIGDIGS
BIGGIES
BIGHITS
BIGKIDS
BIGLIES
BIGRIGS
BIGWIGS
BIGWINS
BILLIES
BIONICS

BIOPICS
BIRDIES
BMOVIES
BOBBIES
BOBBINS
BOCCIES
BODKINS
BOFFINS
BOOBIES
BOOGIES
BOOHISS
BOOKIES
BOONIES
BOOTIES
BORGIAS
BOUDINS
BOWFINS
BOWTIES
BRODIES
BUDDIES
BUDGIES
BUGGIES
BULLIES
BULLINS
BUNNIES
BUSBIES
CABBIES
CABRIOS
CADDIES
CALKINS
CALLINS
CAMMIES
CANDIDS
CANDIES
CARNIES
CARRIES
CASEINS
CASHINS
CASSIAS
CASSIUS
CATFITS
CATKINS
CATNIPS
CATRIGS
CATSITS
CAVEINS
CELSIUS
CELTICS
CERVIDS
CHILIES
CHIVIES
CIVVIES
CLERICS
CLINICS
COEDITS
COFFINS
COHEIRS
COLLIES
COLLINS
COMFITS
COMMITS
CONFITS
CONOIDS
COOKIES
COOLIES
COOTIES
CORDIAS
CORVIDS

COUSINS
COWRIES
CRAZIES
CREDITS
CRETINS
CRITIAS
CRITICS
CRONIES
CUBBIES
CUBBINS
CUBOIDS
CUDDIES
CUEBIDS
CUETIPS
CULLIES
CUMBIAS
CURRIES
CURTISS
CUSPIDS
CYANIDS
CYMRICS
DADDIES
DAHLIAS
DAILIES
DAIRIES
DAISIES
DALLIES
DANDIES
DATRILS
DAWKINS
DEARIES
DECEITS
DECRIES
DEHAIRS
DEIFIES
DEITIES
DENTINS
DERAILS
DERBIES
DETAILS
DETAINS
DEVEINS
DEVOIRS
DEVRIES
DIARIES
DIARIOS
DICKIES
DIKDIKS
DILLIES
DIMWITS
DINDINS
DIOXINS
DIRTIES
DISMISS
DISTILS
DITTIES
DIVVIES
DIZAINS
DIZZIES
DOBBINS
DOGGIES
DOGSITS
DOILIES
DOLLIES
DOMAINS
DOOLIES
DOOZIES
DOWDIES

DOWRIES
DROPINS
DROXIES
DUCHIES
DUCKIES
DUMMIES
DUNLINS
EADGILS
EARLIES
EARWIGS
EBONICS
EBONIES
ECLAIRS
EDIFIES
EGERIAS
ELAPIDS
ELEGIES
ELEGITS
ELICITS
ELIGIUS
ELIXIRS
EMERIES
EMETICS
EMPTIES
ENDPINS
ENEMIES
ENJOINS
ENSKIES
ENTAILS
ENTRIES
ENVEILS
EPOXIES
EROTICS
ESPRITS
ETHNICS
ETONICS
EWERIES
EXOTICS
EYELIDS
EYEPITS
FABRICS
FADEINS
FAERIES
FAIRIES
FAKEIDS
FANCIES
FANFICS
FASCIAS
FATLIPS
FERRIES
FIBRINS
FIFTIES
FILLIES
FILLINS
FILLIPS
FIRKINS
FIZGIGS
FLAVIUS
FLORINS
FLUTIES
FOLKIES
FOLLIES
FOODIES
FORBIDS
FORTIES
FORTIUS
FOSSILS
FROLICS

FTBLISS
FUDDIES
FULFILS
FUNNIES
GAMBITS
GAPKIDS
GARLICS
GARLITS
GATLINS
GAUDIES
GERBILS
GIDDIES
GIPSIES
GIRLIES
GLOBINS
GLORIAS
GLORIES
GOALIES
GOAMISS
GOBLINS
GODWITS
GOODIES
GOONIES
GORDIUS
GOSSIPS
GOTHICS
GRACIAS
GRATIAS
GRAVIES
GROPIUS
GROTIUS
GULLIES
GUNNIES
GUPPIES
GUSSIES
GYPSIES
HACKIES
HADFITS
HALFIES
HALOIDS
HANKIES
HAPTICS
HARPIES
HARRIES
HASFITS
HATPINS
HAWKINS
HEAVIES
HENBITS
HENRIES
HERMITS
HERNIAS
HERNIBS
HEROICS
HIGGINS
HIGHIQS
HINNIES
HIPPIES
HISNIBS
HOAGIES
HOBBIES
HOBBITS
HOGTIES
HOLLIES
HOODIES
HOPKINS
HOSKINS
HOTLIPS

HOTTIES
HOTTIPS
HUBBIES
HUGGIES
HUGGINS
HURRIES
HUSKIES
HUSSIES
HYBRIDS
IAMBICS
IATRICS
IMPAIRS
IMPLIES
INRUINS
INSTILS
INTAILS
INTUITS
IRENICS
IRONIES
ITALICS
IVORIES
JAGGIES
JAMMIES
JARDINS
JEEBIES
JELLIES
JENKINS
JERKIES
JERKINS
JESUITS
JETTIES
JIFFIES
JIMMIES
JOLLIES
JUNKIES
KELPIES
KELVINS
KEWPIES
KIARIOS
KIDDIES
KIDVIDS
KILTIES
KITTIES
LADDIES
LAITIES
LANCIAS
LANVINS
LARKINS
LASSIES
LEADINS
LEFTIES
LENTILS
LEONIDS
LIGNINS
LINDIES
LIQUIDS
LIZZIES
LOBBIES
LOCKINS
LOGGIAS
LOGGINS
LOLLIES
LONGIES
LOOBIES
LOOKINS
LOONIES
LORRIES
LOVEINS

LOWBIDS
MADLIBS
MAGPIES
MAILINS
MANNIES
MARGINS
MARLINS
MARRIES
MARTINS
MARTIUS
MASHIES
MASSIFS
MASTICS
MATHIAS
MEALIES
MEANIES
MEEMIES
MEGRIMS
MEMOIRS
MENCIUS
MENZIES
MERCIES
MERLINS
METRICS
MIDDIES
MIDRIBS
MISAIMS
MISFITS
MISHITS
MISSIES
MOHAIRS
MOLLIES
MOMMIES
MOONIES
MOSAICS
MOTRINS
MRBLISS
MRCHIPS
MUDDIES
MUDPIES
MUFFINS
MULLINS
MUMMIES
MUSKIES
MUSLIMS
MUSLINS
MYOPIAS
MYSTICS
NANNIES
NAPKINS
NAPPIES
NASTIES
NAVAIDS
NENNIUS
NEREIDS
NEWBIES
NEWKIDS
NEWSIES
NIFTIES
NINNIES
NITWITS
NODDIES
NOETICS
NOGGINS
NONHITS
NOOGIES
NORDICS
NOTHINS

NUBBINS
NUDNIKS
NUNCIOS
NUTOILS
NUTRIAS
OBTAINS
OILRIGS
OLEFINS
OLEMISS
OLOGIES
ONABIAS
ORACIES
ORCHIDS
ORDAINS
ORIGINS
OTARIES
OUTBIDS
OUTFITS
OUTHISS
OUTHITS
OUTKISS
OUTLIES
OUTLIPS
OUTRIBS
OUTRIGS
OUTSINS
OUTSITS
OUTVIES
OUTWITS
OVARIES
OXTAILS
PADDIES
PANDITS
PANSIES
PANTIES
PAPPIES
PARKINS
PARRIES
PARTIES
PASTIES
PATRIES
PATSIES
PATTIES
PECTINS
PENCILS
PENNIES
PENZIAS
PEONIES
PEPCIDS
PEPSINS
PEPTICS
PERKINS
PERMITS
PERRINS
PERSIUS
PETPIGS
PETSITS
PHEMIUS
PHIDIAS
PHILIPS
PHOBIAS
PHOBICS
PHONICS
PHONIES
PHOTICS
PHYSICS
PICNICS
PIDGINS

PIETIES
PIETINS
PIGGIES
PINKIES
PIPPINS
PISTILS
PLATIES
PLUGINS
POESIES
POETICS
PONGIDS
PONTIUS
POPLINS
POPPIES
POPPINS
PORGIES
POSTIES
POSTITS
POTLIDS
POTPIES
POTTIES
PREBIDS
PRELIMS
PREMIES
PREMISS
PREVIAS
PREXIES
PRIVIES
PROBIES
PROFITS
PROXIES
PUBLICS
PUBLIUS
PUFFINS
PULLINS
PULPITS
PUNDITS
PUNKIES
PUPPIES
PUSSIES
PUTTIES
PYGMIES
PYTHIAS
QRATIOS
QUAKIES
QUERIES
RABBITS
RAFFIAS
RAGGIES
RAISINS
RALLIES
RATLINS
RAWLINS
RAZZIES
READIES
REBAITS
REBOILS
RECOILS
RECOINS
REDFINS
REDFIRS
REDRIES
REDTIES
REEDITS
REEMITS
REFLIES
REFLIPS
REFRIES

REGAINS
REGRIPS
REIFIES
REJAILS
REJOINS
REKNITS
REMAILS
REMAINS
RENAILS
RENNINS
RENOIRS
REPAIRS
REPLIES
RESHIPS
RESOILS
RESPINS
RESTIRS
RESUITS
RESWIMS
RETAILS
RETAINS
RETRIES
RETRIMS
RIBBIES
ROADIES
ROBBINS
ROCKIES
ROLAIDS
ROLLINS
ROMAINS
ROOKIES
ROOMIES
ROWDIES
RUBRICS
RUMMIES
RUSTICS
SALLIES
SAVVIES
SAWPITS
SCENICS
SCORIAS
SEPHIAS
SEQUINS
SHERIFS
SHOOINS
SHUTINS
SILLIES
SISSIES
SIXTIES
SKIBIBS
SMOKIES
SOFFITS
SOFTIES
SOPHIES
SORTIES
SPECIES
SPIRITS
SPRAINS
SPYKIDS
STATICS
STATINS
STELIAS
STEPINS
STOGIES
STORIES
STOTINS
STRAINS
STRAITS

STUDIES
STUDIOS
STUPIDS
STYMIES
SUBBIAS
SUBLIDS
SUBMITS
SULKIES
SULLIES
SUMMITS
SYNDICS
TABBIES
TACTICS
TAFFIES
TAKEINS
TALKIES
TALLIES
TANNINS
TANSIES
TAROILS
TARPITS
TARRIES
TECHIES
TEDDIES
TEKKIES
TELLIES
TENNIES
TENPINS
TERRIES
THEKISS
THEPIPS
THEPITS
THESIMS
THEVIPS
THEYIPS
TIDBITS
TIEPINS
TIFFINS
TILSITS
TIMMINS
TIZZIES
TOADIES
TOCSINS
TODDIES
TOMTITS
TONSILS
TOONIES
TOPBIDS
TOROIDS
TOWNIES
TREDIAS
TROPICS
TUGRIKS
TUMMIES
TURNIPS
TUSHIES
TWOBITS
UNBAITS
UNCLIPS
UNCOILS
UNGRIPS
UNHAIRS
UNIFIES
UNITIES
UNJOINS
UNKNITS
UNNAILS
UNSHIPS

UNVEILS
UPCOILS
UPDRIES
UPSPINS
UPSTIRS
URACILS
URCHINS
USERIDS
USURIES
UTOPIAS
VEERIES
VEGGIES
VERBIDS
VERDINS
VESPIDS
VICTIMS
VILNIUS
VIOLINS
VIRGINS
VITRICS
WABBITS
WADKINS
WALKINS
WATKINS
WEARIES
WEDGIES
WEEBITS
WEENIES
WEEVILS
WESKITS
WESTIES
WESTINS
WETKISS
WHATIFS
WIENIES
WILKINS
WILLIES
WITHIES
WOODIES
WOOLIES
WORRIES
YETTIES
YIPPIES
YORKIES
YTTRIAS
YUPPIES
ZINNIAS
ZOMBIES
ZOYSIAS

•••••IS

ADONAIS
ADZUKIS
AGOUTIS
ALDAVIS
ALKALIS
ALLEWIS
ALLTHIS
AMANTIS
AMNERIS
ANGLAIS
ARGALIS
ARTEMIS
ASEPSIS
AVANTIS
BANZAIS
BIKINIS
BIMINIS

BONACIS
BORZOIS
CETERIS
CHABLIS
CHALCIS
CHAMOIS
CHASSIS
CHICHIS
CHILLIS
CHINOIS
COEPTIS
COLCHIS
CROQUIS
CSLEWIS
DALASIS
DAPHNIS
DELORIS
DJINNIS
DUKAKIS
ECDYSIS
FEMORIS
FIDELIS
FRANCIS
GELATIS
GEMINIS
GENERIS
GENESIS
GENGHIS
GERVAIS
GETTHIS
GLOTTIS
GLYNNIS
GRIGRIS
HABILIS
HAIKAIS
HYANNIS
JETSKIS
KABUKIS
KINESIS
KIWANIS
LAVORIS
LEXUSIS
LIPARIS
LITCHIS
MAHARIS
MAITAIS
MARQUIS
MAUROIS
MAUVAIS
MEIOSIS
MEMPHIS
MESAMIS
MILLAIS
MIMESIS
MITOSIS
MORANIS
MUESLIS
NEMESIS
NEPALIS
NOKOMIS
NOVALIS
NOWTHIS
OCTROIS
ONASSIS
OSMOSIS
OSTOSIS
PANINIS
PHYLLIS

POLARIS
PRIZZIS
QATARIS
RAPINIS
RENVOIS
RESNAIS
ROLLEIS
ROMAJIS
ROMANIS
RUMAKIS
SAFARIS
SALAMIS
SALUKIS
SAMEDIS
SANSEIS
SATORIS
SEFERIS
SENSEIS
SERAPIS
SNUGLIS
SOMALIS
STDENIS
STENNIS
STLOUIS
STREGIS
STYPSIS
SURIMIS
SUZUKIS
TAHINIS
TATAMIS
THEAXIS
THESPIS
TOPTHIS
TRELLIS
TSOURIS
VAUDOIS
VENTRIS
VISAVIS
VITALIS
WAPITIS
WASABIS
WATUSIS
WHATSIS
WHOOSIS
XEROSIS
YANQUIS
YEMENIS
YESITIS
YOGINIS
YUKOLIS

IT•••••

ITALIAN
ITALICS
ITCHFOR
ITCHIER
ITCHING
ITEMING
ITEMISE
ITEMIZE
ITEMONE
ITERANT
ITERATE
ITGIRLS
ITHACAN
ITHIRTY
ITISTOO
ITMAYBE
ITSABOY
ITSAHIT
ITSALIE
ITSALOT
ITSASIN
ITSATIE
ITSBEST
ITSCOLD
ITSDONE
ITSEASY
ITSFINE
ITSGONE
ITSHERE
ITSLATE
ITSLOVE
ITSOKAY
ITSONME
ITSOPEN
ITSOVER
ITSTIME
ITSTRUE
ITWELVE
ITWENTY

I•T••••

IATRICS
ICTERUS
ICTINUS
ICTUSES
IDTHEFT
IMTHERE
IMTIRED
INTAILS
INTAKES
INTASTE
INTEARS
INTEGER
INTEGRA
INTENDS
INTENSE
INTENTS
INTERIM
INTERNE
INTERNS
INTERSE
INTHERE
INTHING
INTHIRD
INTHREE
INTONED
INTONER
INTONES
INTOTAL
INTOUCH
INTRADE
INTRAYS
INTROIT
INTRUDE
INTRUST
INTRUTH
INTUITS
INTURNS
IQTESTS
ISTHMUS
ISTOMIN
ISTRIAN
IVTUBES

I••T•••

ICETEAS
ICETRAY
IDOTTER
IFITDIE
IFSTONE
IGOTCHA
IGOTYOU
IHATEIT
ILLTELL
IMITATE
INATRAP
INITIAL
INSTALL
INSTALS
INSTANT
INSTATE
INSTEAD
INSTEPS
INSTILL
INSTILS
INSTOCK
INSTONE
INSTORE
INSTYLE
INUTERO
INUTILE
IRATELY
IRATEST
ISITAGO
ISOTONE
ISOTOPE
ISOTOPY
ITSTIME
ITSTRUE
IZATION

I•••T••

IAPETUS
ICEDTEA
IDEATED
IDEATES
IDENTIC
IDIDTOO
IDIOTIC
IDOTTER
IGNATOW
IGNITED
IGNITER
IGNITES
IGNITOR
IIPETER
ILOSTIT
IMHOTEP
IMPETUS
IMPUTED
IMPUTER
IMPUTES
IMUSTGO
INAPTER
INAPTLY
INASTEW
INASTIR
INCITED
INCITER
INCITES
INDITED
INDITER
INDITES
INDUTCH
INEPTLY
INERTIA
INERTLY
INGATES
INKSTER
INMATES
INTOTAL
INVITED
INVITEE
INVITER
INVITES
INVITRO
IODATED
IODATES
IOMOTHS
IRKUTSK
ISLETED
ITISTOO
ITSATIE
IWANTIT
IWANTTO
IZZATSO

I••••T•

IBILITY
ICEBATH
ICEOUTS
IEIGHTY
IGOROTS
ILLBITE
IMAMATE
IMARETS
IMITATE
IMPACTS
IMPARTS
IMPASTO
IMPIETY
IMPORTS
IMPOSTS
INANITY
INCANTS
INCENTS
INCEPTS
INDENTS
INDEPTH
INDICTS
INDUCTS
INEDITA
INFAITH
INFANTA
INFANTE
INFANTS
INFECTS
INFESTS
INFLATE
INGESTA
INGESTS
INGRATE
INHASTE
ININETY
INJECTS
INKJETS
INKNOTS
INKPOTS
INSECTA
INSECTS
INSERTS
INSISTS
INSPITE
INSPOTS
INSTATE
INSULTS
INTASTE
INTENTS
INTRUTH
INTUITS
INVENTS
INVERTS
INVESTS
INVICTA
INWHITE
IQTESTS
IRRUPTS
ISOLATE
ISOLATO
ITERATE
ITHIRTY
ITSLATE
ITWENTY
IWANTTO

I•••••T

IAMBIST
ICANNOT
ICEBOAT
ICEDOUT
ICESOUT
ICINGIT
ICKIEST
IDOLIST
IDOODIT
IDTHEFT
IDYLIST
IFFIEST
IFORGET
IFORGOT
IHATEIT
IHAVEIT
IINSIST
IKNEWIT
IKNOWIT
ILIKEIT
ILLDOIT
ILLEGIT
ILLICIT
ILOSTIT
ILOVEIT
IMADEIT
IMAGIST
IMEANIT
IMFORIT
IMGREAT
IMPLANT
IMPREST
IMPRINT
INACAST
INAKNOT
INANEST
INASNIT
INASPOT
INASUIT
INBUILT
INCOURT
INCRUST
INDOUBT
INDRAFT
INDWELT
INEXACT
INFIRST
INFLECT
INFLICT
INFORIT
INFRACT
INFRONT
INGRAFT
INHABIT
INHERIT
INHIBIT
INKBLOT
INKIEST
INKSPOT
INORBIT
INPOINT
INPRINT
INQUEST
INSHORT
INSIGHT
INSPECT
INSTANT
INSWEPT
INTROIT
INTRUST
IOBJECT
IRATEST
IREPEAT
IRISOUT
IRONIST
IRONOUT
ISSUANT
ITERANT
ITSAHIT
ITSALOT
ITSBEST
IWANTIT

•IT••••

AITCHES
BITEOFF
BITESIN
BITESON
BITESUP
BITLESS
BITMAPS
BITONAL
BITPART
BITROLE
BITSIER
BITTERN
BITTERS
BITTIER
BITTING
CITABLE
CITADEL
CITIZEN
CITRATE
CITRINE
CITROEN
CITRONS
CITROUS
CITYBOY
CITYGAL
DITCHED
DITCHER
DITCHES
DITHERS
DITHERY
DITSIER
DITTIES
DITTOED
DITZIER
FITINTO
FITNESS
FITTERS
FITTEST
FITTING
FITWELL
FITZROY
GITANOS
GITTING
HITACHI
HITBACK
HITCHED
HITCHER
HITCHES
HITCHON
HITCHUP
HITFILM
HITHERE
HITHOME
HITINTO
HITLESS
HITLIST
HITPLAY
HITSFOR
HITSHOW
HITSOFF
HITSONG
HITSOUT
HITTERS
HITTING
HITTITE
HITTOWN
HITTUNE
HITUPON
JITNEYS
JITTERS
JITTERY
KITBAGS
KITCHEN
KITHARA
KITKATS
KITSCHY
KITTENS
KITTERY
KITTIES
KITTING
LITCHIS
LITCRIT
LITERAL
LITHELY
LITHEST
LITHGOW
LITHIUM
LITHOID
LITINTO
LITOTES
LITOVSK
LITTERS
LITTERY
LITTLER
LITTLES
LITURGY
MITCHUM
MITERED
MITFORD
MITHRAS
MITOSES
MITOSIS
MITOTIC
MITRING
MITTENS
MITZVAH
NITPICK
NITRATE
NITRIDE
NITRIFY
NITRITE
NITROUS
NITTANY
NITTIER
NITWITS
PITAPAT
PITAYAS
PITBOSS
PITBULL
PITCHED
PITCHER
PITCHES
PITCHIN
PITCHTO
PITCREW
PITEOUS
PITFALL
PITHEAD
PITHIER
PITHILY
PITHING
PITIERS
PITIFUL
PITILLO
PITROWS
PITSAWS
PITSTOP
PITTING
PITTMAN
PITYING
RITAGAM
RITALIN
RITAMAE
RITARDS
RITCHIE
RITDYES
RITEAID
RITUALS
RITZIER
RITZILY
SITATOP
SITBACK
SITCOMS
SITDOWN
SITEMAP
SITHOME
SITINON
SITONIT
SITSFOR
SITSOUT
SITSPAT
SITTERS
SITTING
SITUATE
SITUPON
SITWELL
SITWITH
TITANAE
TITANIA
TITANIC
TITHERS
TITHING
TITIANS
TITLARK
TITLING
TITLIST
TITMICE
TITOISM
TITOIST
TITRATE
TITRING
TITTERS
TITTLES
TITULAR
VITALIS
VITALLY
VITAMIN
VITARAS
VITEBSK
VITIATE
VITORIA
VITRICS
VITRIFY
VITRINE
VITRIOL
VITTLES
WITCHED
WITCHES
WITEOUT
WITHERS
WITHIES
WITHOUT
WITLESS
WITLING
WITNESS
WITSEND
WITTIER
WITTILY
WITTING
YITZHAK
ZITCOMS
ZITHERS

•I•T•••

AINTHAY
AIRTANK
AIRTAXI
AIRTIME
AIRTRAP
AIRTUBE
BIGTALK
BIGTENT
BIGTIME
BIGTOES
BIGTOPS
BIGTOWN
BIOTECH
BIOTITE
BIOTYPE
BIRTHED
BISTATE
BISTROS
BITTERN
BITTERS
BITTIER
BITTING
CISTERN
DIATOMS
DICTATE
DICTION
DICTUMS
DIDTIME
DIDTOAT
DIETARY
DIETERS
DIETING
DIKTATS
DINTING
DIOTIMA
DIPTYCH
DIRTBAG
DIRTIED
DIRTIER
DIRTIES
DIRTILY
DISTAFF
DISTANT
DISTEND
DISTICH
DISTILL
DISTILS
DISTORT
DISTROS
DISTURB
DITTIES
DITTOED
FIATLUX
FICTILE
FICTION
FICTIVE
FIFTEEN
FIFTHLY
FIFTIES
FIFTYAD
FIFTYBC
FIGTREE
FILTERS
FIRTREE
FISTFUL
FITTERS
FITTEST
FITTING
FIXTURE
GIFTBOX
GIFTEES
GIFTING
GIFTSET
GIFTTAX
GIRTHED
GIRTING
GITTING
HILTING
HILTONS
HINTERS
HINTING
HINTSAT
HISTORY
HITTERS
HITTING
HITTITE
HITTOWN
HITTUNE
JIGTIME
JILTERS
JILTING
JITTERS
JITTERY
KILTIES
KILTING
KITTENS
KITTERY
KITTIES
KITTING
LIETEST
LIFTERS
LIFTING
LIFTOFF
LIFTSUP
LILTING
LINTELS
LINTERS
LINTIER
LINTING
LISTEES
LISTENS
LISTERS
LISTING
LITTERS
LITTERY
LITTLER
LITTLES
MIDTEEN
MIDTERM
MIDTOWN
MINTAGE
MINTERS
MINTIER
MINTING
MINTTEA
MISTAKE
MISTBOW
MISTELL
MISTERM
MISTERS
MISTERX
MISTIER
MISTILY
MISTIME
MISTING
MISTOLD
MISTOOK
MISTRAL
MISTSUP
MISTUNE
MISTYPE
MITTENS
MIXTECS
MIXTURE
NICTATE
NIFTIER
NIFTIES
NIFTILY
NINTHLY
NITTANY
NITTIER
OILTANK
PICTISH
PICTURE
PIETIES
PIETINS
PIETOSO
PIETROS
PIGTAIL
PINTAIL
PISTILS
PISTOLE
PISTOLS
PISTONS
PISTOUS
PITTING
PITTMAN
QINTARS
RIFTING
RIOTACT
RIOTERS
RIOTGUN
RIOTING
RIOTOUS
RIPTIDE
RIPTORN
SIFTERS
SIFTING
SILTIER
SILTING
SISTERS
SISTINE
SITTERS
SITTING
SIXTEEN
SIXTHLY
SIXTIES
SIXTYAD
SIXTYBC
TICTACS
TIETACK
TIETACS
TILTERS
TILTING
TILTSAT
TILTSUP
TILTTOP
TINTERN
TINTERS
TINTING
TINTYPE
TIPTOED
TIPTOES
TIPTOPS
TITTERS
TITTLES
VIATICA
VICTIMS
VICTORS
VICTORY
VICTRIX
VICTUAL
VIETNAM
VINTAGE
VINTNER
VIRTUAL
VIRTUES
VISTAED
VISTEON
VISTULA
VITTLES
WILTING
WINTERS
WINTERY
WISTFUL
WITTIER
WITTILY
WITTING
ZIPTOPS

•I••T••

BIENTOT
BIGOTED
BIGOTRY
BIGSTAR
BIMETAL
BIRETTA
DICHTER
DIGITAL
DILATED
DILATES
DILATOR
DILUTED
DILUTER
DILUTES
DILUTOR
DIMETER
DIMITRI
DINETTE
DIOPTER
EIDETIC
EIGHTAD
EIGHTAM
EIGHTBC
EIGHTEE
EIGHTHS
EIGHTPM
EIGHTUP
FIBSTER
FIESTAS
FIGHTER
FINITES
FIRSTLY
FIRSTUP
FIVETEN
FIVETWO
FIXATED
FIXATES
GIFTTAX
GIGATON
HIGHTEA
HIGHTOP
HILLTOP
HIPSTER
IIPETER
KILOTON
KINETIC
KINGTUT
KIRSTEN
KIRSTIE
LICITLY
LIEATOP
LIGATED
LIGATES
LIGHTED
LIGHTEN
LIGHTER
LIGHTLY

LIGHTON
LIGHTUP
LILETEE
LIMITED
LIMITER
LINETWO
LITOTES
LIZETTE
MIGHTNT
MILITIA
MIMETIC
MINITVS
MINOTND
MINSTER
MINTTEA
MINUTED
MINUTER
MINUTES
MINUTIA
MISSTEP
MITOTIC
MIXITUP
NIANTIC
NICETRY
NIDETCH
NIGHTER
NIGHTIE
NIGHTLY
PIASTER
PIASTRE
PICOTED
PILATES
PILATUS
PILOTED
PINATAS
PINETAR
PINETOP
PINETUM
PINOTTA
PIPETTE
PIRATED
PIRATES
PIRATIC
PITSTOP
PIVOTAL
PIVOTED
PIVOTER
RIALTOS
RIANTLY
RICHTER
RICOTTA
RIDOTTO
RIGHTED
RIGHTER
RIGHTLY
RIGHTON
RIPSTOP
RISOTTO
RIVETED
RIVETER
SIDETWO
SIESTAS
SIGHTED
SIGHTER
SIGHTLY
SILKTIE
SINATRA
SINUTAB

SITATOP
SIZETEN
SIZETWO
TIBETAN
TICOTIN
TIGHTEN
TIGHTER
TIGHTLY
TILTTOP
TIMOTHY
TINCTED
TINSTAR
TINYTIM
TINYTOT
TIPSTER
VIDETTE
VISITED
VISITOR
VIVITAR
WINDTEE
WINGTIP
WINSTON
WIRETAP

•I•••T•

AIGLETS
AIGRETS
AIRDATE
AIRPOTS
BIGBETS
BIGCATS
BIGCITY
BIGGITY
BIGHITS
BIGLOTS
BILLETS
BINDSTO
BIODATA
BIOLITE
BIOTITE
BIRETTA
BISECTS
BISMUTH
BISTATE
CILENTO
CILIATE
CIRRATE
CITRATE
DICTATE
DIDACTS
DIECUTS
DIGESTS
DIGGITY
DIGINTO
DIGLOTS
DIGNITY
DIKTATS
DIMOUTS
DIMWITS
DINETTE
DIORITE
DIPINTO
DIPNETS
DIRECTS
DIRECTV
DISPUTE
DISRATE
DIVERTS

DIVESTS
FIDGETS
FIDGETY
FILLETS
FITINTO
GIBLETS
GIMLETS
GIVENTO
GIVESTO
HIPBATH
HIPPITY
HIRSUTE
HITINTO
HITTITE
KIBBUTZ
KIDULTS
KISMETS
KITKATS
LIBERTE
LIBERTY
LICKETY
LIGGETT
LIGNITE
LIKENTO
LIMNITE
LIMPETS
LINEATE
LINNETS
LIONETS
LIQUATE
LISBETH
LISENTE
LITINTO
LIZETTE
MIDGETS
MIGRATE
MILLETS
MILLETT
MINOLTA
MINUETS
MISACTS
MISCITE
MISCUTS
MISDATE
MISFITS
MISHITS
MISMATE
MISRATE
MISSETS
NIBLETS
NICTATE
NIMIETY
NIOBITE
NITRATE
NITRITE
NITWITS
PICANTE
PICCATA
PICKETS
PICKETT
PIGLETS
PIGNUTS
PIGOUTS
PILEATE
PIMENTO
PINKETT
PINNATE
PINOTTA

PIOLETS
PIOSITY
PIPETTE
PITCHTO
RIBCUTS
RIBLETS
RICKETY
RICOTTA
RIDESTO
RIDOTTO
RILLETS
RIORITA
RIPINTO
RIPOSTE
RIPOSTS
RISENTO
RISESTO
RISOTTO
RIZZUTO
SIGNETS
SILENTA
SILENTB
SILENTC
SILENTD
SILENTE
SILENTF
SILENTG
SILENTH
SILENTI
SILENTJ
SILENTK
SILENTL
SILENTM
SILENTN
SILENTO
SILENTP
SILENTQ
SILENTR
SILENTS
SILENTT
SILENTU
SILENTV
SILENTW
SILENTX
SILENTY
SILENTZ
SIMCITY
SINCITY
SINGSTO
SINUATE
SITUATE
SITWITH
TIBBETT
TICKETS
TIDBITS
TIEINTO
TILLETS
TILSITS
TIMROTH
TINHATS
TIPPETS
TIRPITZ
TISSOTS
TITRATE
VIBISTS
VIBRATE
VIBRATO
VICENTE

VICOMTE
VIDETTE
VIDIOTS
VIEWITH
VIOLATE
VIOLETS
VIRGATE
VITIATE
VIVANTS
WICHITA
WICKETS
WIDGETS
WIGLETS
YIELDTO
ZINCITE

•I••••T

AILMENT
AIMEDAT
AIRBOAT
AIRDUCT
AIRIEST
AIRLIFT
AIRPORT
AIRSOUT
AIRVENT
BIBELOT
BIENTOT
BIGBEAT
BIGEAST
BIGFEET
BIGFOOT
BIGGEST
BIGSHOT
BIGTENT
BIGUNIT
BISCUIT
BITPART
CIRCLET
CIRCUIT
DIALECT
DIALOUT
DIARIST
DICIEST
DIDASET
DIDEROT
DIDTOAT
DIECAST
DIEDOUT
DIESOUT
DIGIPET
DIGSOUT
DILBERT
DILUENT
DIMMEST
DIMSOUT
DINEDAT
DINEOUT
DINESAT
DINGBAT
DINMONT
DISGUST
DISHOUT
DISMAST
DISPART
DISPORT
DISRUPT
DISSECT

DISSENT
DISSERT
DISTANT
DISTORT
FIGMENT
FILBERT
FILEOUT
FILLOUT
FILMSET
FINDOUT
FINEART
FIREANT
FIREDAT
FIREHAT
FIRELIT
FIREPIT
FIRESAT
FIRMEST
FISHNET
FISHOUT
FITTEST
GIBESAT
GIFTSET
GIGABIT
GILBERT
GILLNET
GIVEOUT
HIDEOUT
HIGHART
HIGHEST
HIGHHAT
HIKEOUT
HILBERT
HINTSAT
HIPBOOT
HIPPEST
HIREOUT
HITLIST
HITSOUT
IINSIST
JIBEDAT
JIBESAT
JIMKAAT
JIVIEST
KICKOUT
KIDSEAT
KILOBIT
KINDEST
KINGLET
KINGRAT
KINGTUT
KINMONT
LIEFEST
LIETEST
LIFENET
LIGGETT
LIMIEST
LIMPEST
LINECUT
LINEOUT
LINIEST
LIPSOUT
LITCRIT
LITHEST
LIVEOUT
LIVESAT
LIVESET
MIDEAST

MIDLIST
MIDMOST
MIDWEST
MIGHTNT
MIGRANT
MILDEST
MILLETT
MINARET
MINDSET
MINEPIT
MIRIEST
MISCAST
MISEDIT
MISSEAT
MISSENT
MISSORT
MISSOUT
NICOLET
NIGHEST
OILHEAT
OILIEST
OILSPOT
PIANIST
PICKETT
PICKOUT
PICKSAT
PIERROT
PIGMEAT
PIGMENT
PIGSOUT
PINCHOT
PINENUT
PINIEST
PINKEST
PINKETT
PIPIEST
PIQUANT
PITAPAT
RIBMEAT
RICHEST
RIDEOUT
RIEGERT
RIGSOUT
RIMIEST
RIMSHOT
RINGLET
RINGOUT
RINKRAT
RIOTACT
RIPPLET
RIPSOUT
RISKSIT
RIVULET
SICKEST
SICKOUT
SIDEBET
SIGHSAT
SIGNOUT
SILENTT
SILKHAT
SINGLET
SINGOUT
SITONIT
SITSOUT
SITSPAT
SIXFEET
SIXFOOT
TIBBETT

TIDIEST
TILTSAT
TIMEOUT
TIMHOLT
TINIEST
TINYBIT
TINYTOT
TIPCART
TIREOUT
TITLIST
TITOIST
VIADENT
VIADUCT
VIBRANT
VINCENT
VINIEST
VIOLENT
VIOLIST
WIGSOUT
WILBERT
WILDCAT
WILDEST
WILIEST
WIMPOUT
WINEVAT
WINGLET
WINGNUT
WINGSIT
WINIEST
WINKOUT
WINKSAT
WINSLET
WINSOUT
WIPEOUT
WIRIEST
WITEOUT
WITHOUT
XINGOUT
ZIONIST

••IT•••

ABITIBI
AGITATE
AGITATO
ALITTLE
AMITIES
ANITRAS
BAITCAR
BAITERS
BAITING
BLITHER
BLITZED
BLITZEN
BLITZER
BLITZES
BOITANO
BRITAIN
BRITCOM
BRITISH
BRITNEY
BRITONS
BRITPOP
BRITTEN
BRITTLE
BRITTON
BUITONI
CHITLIN
CHITONS

CHITOWN
CHITTER
CRITIAS
CRITICS
CRITTER
CRITTUR
DEITIES
DOITNOW
EDITING
EDITION
EDITORS
EDITOUT
EDITRIX
ELITEST
ELITISM
ELITIST
EMITTED
EMITTER
EPITAPH
EPITHET
EPITOME
ERITREA
EXITFEE
EXITING
EXITNOW
FLITSBY
FLITSIN
FLITTED
FLITTER
FRITTED
FRITTER
GAITERS
GAITING
GLITCHY
GLITTER
GLITZED
GLITZES
GOITERS
GRITTED
GRITTER
GUITARS
HAITIAN
IFITDIE
IMITATE
INITIAL
ISITAGO
KNITTED
KNITTER
LAITIES
LEITRIM
LOITERS
MAITAIS
MAITRED
MAITRES
MEITNER
NEITHER
OMITTED
OMITTER
POITIER
PRITHEE
QUITESO
QUITSIT
QUITTED
QUITTER
REITMAN
SCITECH
SKITOWS
SKITRIP

SKITTER
SKITTLE
SLITHER
SLITTED
SLITTER
SMITERS
SMITHED
SMITING
SMITTEN
SPITING
SPITOUT
SPITSON
SPITTER
SPITTLE
SPITZES
SUITING
SUITORS
SUITSME
SUITSUP
SWITZER
THITHER
TRITELY
TRITEST
TRITIUM
TRITONE
TRITONS
TUITION
TWITCHY
TWITTED
TWITTER
UNITARD
UNITARY
UNITERS
UNITIES
UNITING
UNITISE
UNITIVE
UNITIZE
VOITURE
VUITTON
WAITERS
WAITFOR
WAITING
WAITOUT
WAITRON
WAITSON
WAITSUP
WHITELY
WHITENS
WHITEST
WHITHER
WHITING
WHITISH
WHITMAN
WHITNEY
WHITSUN
WHITTLE
WRITEIN
WRITEME
WRITEON
WRITERS
WRITETO
WRITEUP
WRITHED
WRITHER
WRITHES
WRITING
WRITTEN

ZEITUNG

••I•T••

ABINTRA
ABIOTIC
ALITTLE
AMISTAD
ANISTON
ARIETTA
ARIETTE
ARISTAE
ARISTAS
ARISTOS
ASIATIC
ATIPTOE
AVIATED
AVIATES
AVIATIC
AVIATOR
BAINTER
BLINTZE
BLISTER
BRISTLE
BRISTLY
BRISTOL
BRITTEN
BRITTLE
BRITTON
BUILTIN
BUILTON
BUILTUP
CHINTZY
CHITTER
CLIFTON
CLINTON
CRITTER
CRITTUR
DEISTIC
DRIFTED
DRIFTER
DRIFTIN
DRIFTUP
DRISTAN
EDICTAL
EKISTIC
EMITTED
EMITTER
EPISTLE
ERISTIC
EVICTED
EVICTEE
EVICTOR
EXISTED
FAINTED
FAINTER
FAINTLY
FEINTED
FLINTMI
FLIPTOP
FLIRTED
FLIRTER
FLITTED
FLITTER
FOISTED
FOISTON
FRITTED
FRITTER
GLINTED

GLISTEN
GLISTER
GLITTER
GRIFTED
GRIFTER
GRISTER
GRISTLE
GRISTLY
GRITTED
GRITTER
HEISTED
HOISTED
HOISTER
HOISTUP
IDIDTOO
IDIOTIC
ITISTOO
JOINTED
JOINTER
JOINTLY
JOISTED
KEISTER
KLISTER
KNITTED
KNITTER
KRISTIN
LEISTER
MAINTOP
MEIOTIC
MEISTER
MOISTEN
MOISTER
MOISTLY
NAILTIP
OMITTED
OMITTER
OPIATES
PAINTED
PAINTER
PAIUTES
PHILTER
PHILTRE
PLINTHS
POINTAT
POINTED
POINTER
POINTES
POINTTO
POINTUP
PRINTAD
PRINTED
PRINTER
PRINTUP
QUIETED
QUIETEN
QUIETER
QUIETLY
QUIETUS
QUILTED
QUILTER
QUINTAL
QUINTAS
QUINTES
QUINTET
QUINTIC
QUINTON
QUINTUS
QUIRTED

QUITTED
QUITTER
ROISTER
SAINTED
SAINTES
SAINTLO
SAINTLY
SCIATIC
SHIATSU
SHIFTED
SHIFTER
SHIHTZU
SHIITES
SKIRTED
SKIRTER
SKITTER
SKITTLE
SLITTED
SLITTER
SMITTEN
SNIFTER
SPITTER
SPITTLE
STILTED
STILTON
STINTED
STINTER
SWIFTER
SWIFTLY
SWINTON
TAINTED
THISTLE
THISTLY
TRIMTAB
TRISTAN
TRISTAR
TWISTED
TWISTER
TWISTON
TWISTUP
TWITTED
TWITTER
UNIATES
VEINTES
VUITTON
WAISTED
WEIRTON
WHISTLE
WHITTLE
WRITTEN

••I••T•

ABILITY
ACIDITY
AGILITY
AGITATE
AGITATO
AKIHITO
ALIENTO
ALIGHTS
ALIGOTE
ALIVETO
AMILATE
AMINUTE
ANILITY
ANIMATE
ANIMATO
ARIDITY

ARIETTA
ARIETTE
ARIGATO
ARIOSTO
AVIDITY
AZIMUTH
BLIGHTS
BLIGHTY
BLINDTO
BRIGHTS
BRINGTO
CHIANTI
CLIENTS
CLIMATE
CLIMATS
CLIMBTO
CLINGTO
DEIGNTO
DOINGTO
DRINKTO
DRIVETO
DWIGHTD
ELICITS
EMIRATE
EPIDOTE
EPILATE
FAILSTO
FLIEDTO
FLIESTO
FLIGHTS
FLIGHTY
FRIGATE
FRIGHTS
GOINGTO
HEIFETZ
HEIGHTS
IBILITY
IEIGHTY
IMITATE
ININETY
KNIGHTS
LYINGTO
MAIMITI
NAIVETE
NAIVETY
OCICATS
ORIENTE
ORIENTS
OWINGTO
OXIDATE
PLICATE
PLIGHTS
POINTTO
PRIESTS
PRIMATE
PRIORTO
PRIVATE
PRIVETS
PRIVITY
PRIVYTO
QUINATE
QUIXOTE
RUINATE
SAILSTO
SKIHATS
SLIGHTS
SPIGOTS
SPIKETV
SPINETS
SPIRITS
STICKTO
SWIVETS
THIRSTS
THIRSTY
TOILETS
TRIBUTE
TRICOTS
TRIEDTO
TRIESTE
TRIESTO
TRIJETS
TRINITY
TRIVETS
TYINGTO
UTILITY
VEIGHTS
WAIKATO
WEIGHTS
WEIGHTY
WRIGHTS
WRITETO

7 IT

••I•••T

ACINGIT
AGILEST
ALIMENT
ANIMIST
ARIDEST
AVIDEST
BAILOUT
BEIGNET
BLINKAT
BOILOUT
BRIDGET
BRINGIT
BRIQUET
BRISKET
CHIAPET
CHICEST
CHICLET
CHILCAT
CHILKAT
CLIPART
CLIPOUT
CRICKET
DRIBLET
DRIVEAT
EDITOUT
ELITEST
ELITIST
EMINENT
EPITHET
ETICKET
EVIDENT
EVILEST
EXIGENT
FAINEST
FAIREST
FLIESAT
FLINGAT
FLIPOUT
GOINGAT
GRINSAT
GRISLET
HAIRCUT
HAIRNET
ICINGIT
ILIKEIT
IRISOUT
JAINIST
JUILLET
LAIDOUT
MAIGRET
MAILLOT
MAILOUT
NAILSET
NAILSIT
NAIVEST
OHIOART
OVIDUCT
OXIDANT
PAIDOUT
POINTAT
QUINTET
QUITSIT
RAILSAT
RAIMENT
RAINHAT
RAINOUT
SHIPOUT
SKIBOOT
SKILIFT
SKILLET
SKIPOUT
SKISUIT
SKIVEST
SLIDOUT
SLIPOUT
SMILEAT
SNICKET
SNIDEST
SNIFFAT
SNIGLET
SNIPEAT
SNIPPET
SPINOUT
SPITOUT
SWIGERT
SWINGAT
SWINGIT
THICKET
THINOUT
TLINGIT
TOILSAT
TRIDENT
TRIEDIT
TRIESIT
TRINKET
TRIOLET
TRIPLET
TRIPPET
TRISECT
TRITEST
TRIVIOT
TWINJET
TWINSET
UNINERT
VAINEST
VEINLET
VOIDOUT
WAITOUT
WHIPPET
WHITEST

•••IT••

ADMITTO
ALNITAK
AMRITAS
ANTITAX
APLITES
ARBITER
ATEITUP
AUDITED
AUDITEE
AUDITOR
AUGITES
AWAITED
AWAITER
BADITCH
BARITES
BEWITCH
BONITOS
BRUITED
CANITBE
CAPITAL
CAPITAN
CAPITOL
CASITAS
CUBITAL
CUBITUS
DANITES
DEBITED
DIGITAL
DIMITRI
DORITOS
EATITUP
ENTITLE
EOLITHS
EXCITED
EXCITER
EXCITES
EXCITOR
FAJITAS
FINITES
FREITAG
FRUITED
FUJITSU
GENITOR
GERITOL
GETITON
GOTITON
GUNITES
HABITAT
HABITED
HABITUE
HALITES
HAMITES
HAMITIC
HAMITUP
HERITOR
HOTITEM
IGNITED
IGNITER
IGNITES
IGNITOR
INCITED
INCITER
INCITES
INDITED
INDITER
INDITES
INVITED
INVITEE
INVITER
INVITES
INVITRO
JANITOR
JERITZA
JUJITSU
JUPITER
KAPITAL
KAPITSA
LAFITTE
LAYITON
LETITBE
LETITGO
LETITIA
LEVITES
LEVITIC
LICITLY
LIMITED
LIMITER
LUCITES
MARITAL
MELITTA
MERITED
MILITIA
MINITVS
MIXITUP
MOJITOS
MOLITOR
MONITOR
NORITES
OOLITES
OOLITIC
ORBITAL
ORBITED
ORBITER
ORNITHO
PEPITAS
PERITUS
PETITES
PLAITED
PLAITER
POLITER
POLITIC
POSITED
PURITAN
PUTITTO
PYRITES
PYRITIC
QUOITED
RANITUP
RARITAN
RATITES
RECITAL
RECITED
RECITER
RECITES
REHITCH
RESITED
RETITLE
REVITUP
RUBITIN
RUNITUP
SEMITES
SEMITIC
SHIITES
SPLITUP
SPRITES
STKITTS
STRITCH
SUBITEM
SUMITUP
TABITHA
TACITLY
TACITUS
TEEITUP
TRAITOR
TRYITON
UNCITED
UNFITLY
UNHITCH
UNMITER
UNMITRE
UNVITAL
UNWITTY
VARITEK
VERITAS
VISITED
VISITOR
VIVITAR
WAPITIS
WRAITHS
YESITIS
ZENITHS

•••I•T•

ABSINTH
ADDICTS
ADMITTO
AGEISTS
ANOINTS
ANXIETY
ARTISTE
ARTISTS
ASSISTS
ATEINTO
AURISTS
AUTISTS
BARISTA
BATISTA
BATISTE
BONIATO
BUYINTO
BYBIRTH
CALISTA
CHRISTA
CHRISTI
CHRISTO
CHRISTY
CILIATE
CORINTH
CUBISTS
CUTINTO
DELICTI
DELICTO
DELICTS
DELINTS
DELISTS
DEMISTS
DEPICTS
DESILTS
DESISTS
DEVIATE
DIGINTO
DIPINTO
DUBIETY
DUGINTO
EATINTO
EGOISTE
EGOISTS
ELLIOTT
ELMISTI
ENLISTS
EXPIATE
FEDINTO
FITINTO
FLYINTO
FOLIATE
FORINTS
FRAILTY
GEFILTE
GETINTO
GOLIATH
GOTINTO
HITINTO
HOLISTS
HOPINTO
IMPIETY
INDICTS
INSISTS
INVICTA
ITHIRTY
JACINTH
JACINTO
JURISTS
LABIATE
LAFITTE
LAKISTS
LAMINTO
LARIATS
LAYINTO
LEDINTO
LEGISTS
LITINTO
LUTISTS
LYRISTS
MAOISTS
MEDIATE
MELITTA
MODISTE
NIMIETY
NOGIFTS
NUDISTS
OBOISTS
OBVIATE
ONEIOTA
ORVIETO
PAPISTS
PAYINTO
PLAINTS
PRYINTO
PURISTS
PUTITTO
RACISTS
RADIATE
RAMINTO
RANINTO
RAWISTS
REBIRTH
REGIFTS
RELICTS
RELISTS
REMINTS
RESIFTS
RESISTS
RETINTS
RIPINTO
RUNINTO
SADISTS
SATIATE
SATIETY
SAWINTO
SCHISTS
SCRIPTS
SEEINTO
SERIATE
SETINTO
SEWISTS
SEXISTS
SOCIETY
SOVIETS
SPLINTS
SPRINTS
SQUINTS
SQUINTY
SQUIRTS
STKITTS
STRIATE
TAOISTS
TAPINTO
THEISTS
THRIFTS
THRIFTY
TIEINTO
TREINTA
TSHIRTS
TUBISTS
TURISTA
TYPISTS
UNPIETY
UNWITTY
UPLIFTS
UPTILTS
VARIATE
VARIETY
VEDISTS
VERISTS
VIBISTS
VIDIOTS
VITIATE
ZENISTS

•••I••T

ACHIEST
ADHIBIT
AERIEST
AFFIANT
AGAINST
AIRIEST
ALNIYAT
ALRIGHT
AMBIENT
ANCIENT
ANTIART
APRICOT
ARTIEST
ASHIEST
ATEIGHT
ATFIRST
ATHIRST
ATNIGHT
ATSIGHT
BABIEST
BONIEST
BOXIEST
BUSIEST
BYRIGHT
CABINET
CAGIEST
CAKIEST
CANIEST
CAVILAT
COKIEST
COPILOT
COSIEST
COWIEST
COZIEST
DEFIANT
DEFICIT
DELIGHT
DELIMIT
DEVIANT
DEWIEST
DICIEST
DIGIPET
DOPIEST
DORIGHT
DOZIEST
EASIEST
EDGIEST
EELIEST
EERIEST
EGGIEST
ELLIOTT
ELMIEST
ENRIGHT
EXHIBIT
EXTINCT
FLAILAT
FOXIEST
FREIGHT
FUMIEST
GAMIEST
GLUIEST
GOFIRST
GOOIEST
GORIEST
HABITAT
HALIBUT
HARICOT
HAZIEST
HOKIEST
HOLIEST
HOMIEST
ICKIEST
IFFIEST
ILLICIT
INFIRST
INHIBIT
INKIEST
INSIGHT
JIVIEST
JOKIEST
LACIEST
LAKIEST
LAZIEST
LENIENT
LIMIEST
LINIEST
LOGIEST
LORIENT
MAGINOT
MAZIEST
MEDIANT
MEFIRST
MIRIEST
MOPIEST
MORISOT
MRFIXIT
MRRIGHT
MYGIANT
NOLIMIT
NOSIEST
NYGIANT
OAKIEST
OCCIPUT
OILIEST
ONFIRST
ONLIEST
ONSIGHT
OOZIEST
ORGIAST
OWLIEST
PACIEST
PATIENT
PERIAPT
PERIDOT
PINIEST
PIPIEST
POKIEST
PUNIEST
RACIEST
RADIANT
REFIGHT
RELIANT
RELIGHT
RELIMIT
RESIGHT
REVISIT
RIMIEST
ROPIEST
ROSIEST
RULIEST
SAGIEST
SALIENT
SAPIENT
SATINET
SEXIEST
SLEIGHT
SOLICIT
SPRIEST
TIDIEST
TINIEST
TONIEST
TONIGHT
UGLIEST
UNLIGHT
UNSIGHT
UPFIRST
UPLIGHT
UPRIGHT
UPTIGHT
VALIANT
VARIANT
VERIEST
VINIEST
WANIEST
WARIEST
WAVIEST
WAXIEST
WEDIDIT
WHOISIT
WHYISIT
WILIEST
WINIEST
WIRIEST
ZANIEST
ZOOIEST

••••IT•

ABILITY
ACIDITY
ACONITE
ACQUITS
ADAMITE
AGILITY
AKIHITO
ALSMITH
AMANITA
AMENITY
ANILITY
ANNUITY
APATITE
ARIDITY
ARMPITS
ASHPITS
ASQUITH
ATTRITE
ATTRITS
AVIDITY
AZURITE
BAALITE
BABBITT
BADFITS
BANDITO
BANDITS
BANKITS
BAUXITE
BAYCITY
BBQPITS
BEDSITS
BERLITZ
BIGCITY
BIGGITY
BIGHITS
BIOLITE
BIOTITE
BOXKITE
BREVITY
BULLITT
BURRITO
CALCITE
CATFITS
CATSITS
CHARITY
CLARITY
COEDITS
COMFITS
COMMITS
CONFITS
CORDITE
COWRITE
CREDITS
CRUDITY
CUPRITE
DEBOITE
DECEITS
DELCITY
DENSITY
DESPITE
DIGGITY
DIGNITY
DIMWITS
DIORITE
DOGBITE
DOGSITS
DUALITY
EBONITE
EBWHITE
EDACITY
EDOMITE
EGALITE
ELAMITE
ELEGITS
ELICITS
ELMCITY
EMBOITE
EMERITA
EMERITI
ENSUITE
EREMITE
ERUDITE
ESPRITS
EYEPITS
FALSITY
FATCITY
FATUITY
FERRITE
FOGCITY
GAMBITS
GARLITS
GASEITY
GODWITS
GORDITA
GRANITA
GRANITE
GRAVITY
HADFITS
HASFITS
HAZLITT
HENBITS
HERMITS
HIPPITY
HITTITE
HOBBITS
HOPLITE
HORVITZ
HUSSITE
HYALITE
IBILITY
ILLBITE
INANITY
INEDITA
INFAITH
INSPITE
INTUITS
INWHITE
JADEITE
JESUITS
JOLLITY
KUWAITI
LAURITZ
LIGNITE
LIMNITE
LUDDITE
LYDDITE
MAIMITI
METWITH
MISCITE
MISFITS
MISHITS
MOABITE
MRSMITH
NEOLITH
NESBITT
NESMITH
NIOBITE
NITRITE
NITWITS
NONHITS
NOTWITH
NULLITY
OBESITY
OFFSITE
OLDCITY
OPACITY
OUTCITY
OUTFITS
OUTHITS
OUTPITY
OUTSITS
OUTWITH
OUTWITS
PADSITE
PANDITS
PARTITA
PARTITE
PAUCITY
PENLITE
PERDITA
PERLITE
PERMITS
PETSITS
PIOSITY
POSTITS
PRECITE
PREWITT
PRIVITY
PROBITY
PROCITY
PROFITS
PULPITS
PUNDITS
QUALITY
RABBITS
RABBITT
RABBITY
RANWITH
REALITY
REBAITS
REEDITS
REEMITS
REKNITS
REQUITE
RESPITE
RESUITS
REUNITE
REWRITE
RIORITA
RUNWITH
SATWITH
SAWPITS

SAYHITO
SCHLITZ
SCHMITT
SIMCITY
SINCITY
SITWITH
SOFFITS
SOPWITH
SPIRITS
STRAITS
SUAVITY
SUBMITS
SULFITE
SUMMITS
SUNCITY
TALLITH
TARPITS
TENSITY
TENUITY
TERMITE
THECITY
THEPITS
THERITZ
THWHITE
TIDBITS
TILSITS
TIRPITZ
TOMKITE
TOMTITS
TOYKITE
TOYWITH
TRINITY
TWOBITS
UNBAITS
UNFAITH
UNKNITS
UNTRITE
UNWHITE
URANITE
UTILITY
VACUITY
VARSITY
VASTITY
VIEWITH
WABBITS
WEBSITE
WEEBITS
WESKITS
WICHITA
WOOLITE
ZINCITE

••••I•T

AFFLICT
AGONIST
AIRLIFT
ALQUIST
ALTOIST
AMORIST
ANIMIST
APEDIET
APPOINT
ARABIST
ASAGIFT
ASQUIET
ASQUINT
ATATILT
ATAVIST
ATEDIRT
ATHEIST
ATOMIST
ATTAINT
BAALIST
BABBITT
BAHAIST
BAPTIST
BASSIST
BEQUIET
BETWIXT
BLERIOT
BULLITT
CASUIST
CATMINT
CELLIST
CHARIOT
CHEMIST
CHEVIOT
CHORIST
CHUTIST
COEXIST
COMTIST
CONSIST
CONVICT
COPYIST
CULTIST
CYCLIST
CYPRIOT
CZARIST
DADAIST
DENTIST
DIARIST
DRFRIST
DUALIST
DUELIST
EATDIRT
EGOTIST
ELEGIST
ELITIST
ENTWIST
EPEEIST
EYELIFT
FADDIET
FADDIST
FASCIST
FAUVIST
FEUDIST
FLORIST
FLUTIST
GERAINT
GNOMIST
HARPIST
HARRIET
HAZLITT
HERRIOT
HITLIST
HORNIST
IAMBIST
IDOLIST
IDYLIST
IINSIST
IMAGIST
IMPRINT
INBUILT
INFLICT
INPOINT
INPRINT
IRONIST
JAINIST
JOLLIET
JUDOIST
LAMAIST
LEFTIST
LOOKIST
MAHDIST
MARXIST
MAURIAT
METRIST
MIDLIST
MOBBIST
NESBITT
NEWMINT
NONDIET
OCULIST
ONADIET
ONEPINT
ONPOINT
ORALIST
OUTSIFT
PALMIST
PATRIOT
PAULIST
PAYDIRT
PERSIST
PIANIST
POLOIST
PREDICT
PREDIET
PRERIOT
PRESIFT
PREWITT
PROTIST
QUERIST
RABBITT
RANRIOT
REALIST
REBUILT
RECEIPT
REEVICT
REPAINT
REPOINT
REPRINT
RESHIFT
RETWIST
RHYMIST
RUNRIOT
SCHMIDT
SCHMITT
SEAGIRT
SEALIFT
SEAMIST
SKILIFT
SOLOIST
SOPHIST
STATIST
STYLIST
SUBSIST
SUMOIST
SUNKIST
THEDIET
THEGIFT
TITLIST
TITOIST
TOURIST
TRIVIOT
TSARIST
TSELIOT
TUBAIST
UNBUILT
UNCLIPT
UNJOINT
UNMOIST
UNQUIET
UNSHIFT
UNSPILT
UNTWIST
UNWHIPT
UPDRIFT
UPSHIFT
UTOPIST
VARMINT
VERDICT
VIOLIST
YORKIST
ZIONIST

•••••IT

ABOUTIT
ACINGIT
ADHIBIT
ALLOFIT
APESUIT
APPETIT
AQUAVIT
ATEABIT
AWEEBIT
BABYSIT
BACKBIT
BACKLIT
BASEHIT
BATSUIT
BEARPIT
BEATSIT
BENEFIT
BIGUNIT
BISCUIT
BLOWSIT
BLUETIT
BODYKIT
BOOTSIT
BRINGIT
CALLSIT
CATSUIT
CESSPIT
CHEEZIT
CHUCKIT
CIRCUIT
CLAYPIT
COALPIT
COCKPIT
COHABIT
CONCEIT
CONDUIT
COOLSIT
CULPRIT
DEFICIT
DELIMIT
DEMERIT
DEORBIT
DEPOSIT
DETROIT
DOUBTIT
DROPSIT
DRYSUIT
EARNSIT
EATABIT
ENDEDIT
EXHIBIT
EXPLOIT
EXPOSIT
FACEDIT
FACESIT
FAKEDIT
FAKESIT
FIRELIT
FIREPIT
FLEAPIT
FLOORIT
FOOTSIT
FORABIT
FORFEIT
GETAHIT
GETONIT
GETSFIT
GETTOIT
GIGABIT
GOFORIT
GOTAHIT
GOTONIT
GOTTOIT
GYMSUIT
HACKSIT
HADAFIT
HADATIT
HALFWIT
HARDHIT
HASAFIT
HASATIT
HATEDIT
HATESIT
HOLDSIT
HOOFSIT
HOPTOIT
HOWBEIT
ICINGIT
IDOODIT
IHATEIT
IHAVEIT
IKNEWIT
IKNOWIT
ILIKEIT
ILLDOIT
ILLEGIT
ILLICIT
ILOSTIT
ILOVEIT
IMADEIT
IMEANIT
IMFORIT
INASNIT
INASUIT
INFORIT
INHABIT
INHERIT
INHIBIT
INORBIT
INTROIT
ITSAHIT
IWANTIT
KEEPFIT
KEPTFIT
KILOBIT
LACKWIT
LAMPLIT
LAWSUIT
LEAVEIT
LITCRIT
LORDSIT
LOSESIT
LOVEDIT
LOVESIT
LUMPSIT
MADEFIT
MAKEFIT
MAKESIT
MANUMIT
MAOSUIT
MEANSIT
MEANTIT
MEGABIT
MEGAHIT
MESSKIT
MINEPIT
MISEDIT
MOONLIT
MOSHPIT
MOVEDIT
MOVESIT
MRFIXIT
NAILSIT
NAYARIT
NOLIMIT
NOTABIT
ONEUNIT
ONEWHIT
OPENPIT
OUTOFIT
OUTSPIT
OUTWAIT
OVERFIT
OVERLIT
PARFAIT
PARKSIT
PLAUDIT
POLESIT
PREEDIT
PREOMIT
PROVEIT
PURSUIT
QUEENIT
QUITSIT
RAREBIT
READMIT
REARLIT
REAUDIT
RECRUIT
REDEBIT
REDSUIT
RELIMIT
RENUZIT
REPOSIT
RESPLIT
REVISIT
RISKSIT
ROUGHIT
SALTPIT
SANDPIT
SAWTOIT
SAYWAIT
SEENFIT
SEESFIT
SEETOIT
SELLSIT
SITONIT
SKISUIT
SNUGFIT
SOLICIT
SOLVEIT
SPOTLIT
STARLIT
STOPSIT
STOWSIT
SUBUNIT
SUNSUIT
SURFEIT
SWEATIT
SWINGIT
SWUNGIT
TAKESIT
TASTEIT
TEARSIT
TELLSIT
TESTKIT
THATSIT
TINYBIT
TLINGIT
TOOLKIT
TRANSIT
TRIEDIT
TRIESIT
TWOUNIT
UNPLAIT
UNSPLIT
UPFORIT
VERYFIT
WATCHIT
WEDIDIT
WELLHIT
WELLLIT
WETSUIT
WHATSIT
WHOISIT
WHYISIT
WHYWAIT
WINGSIT
WORTHIT
YOPLAIT
YOUREIT

I•U••••

IGUANAS
IGUANID
IGUASSU
IMUSTGO
INULASE
INURING
INUTERO
INUTILE
ISUREAM
ISUREDO

I••U•••

ICTUSES
ILLUDED
ILLUDES
ILLUMED
ILLUMES
ILLUSED
ILLUSES
IMBUING
IMMUNES
IMMURED
IMMURES
IMPUGNS
IMPULSE
IMPURER
IMPUTED
IMPUTER
IMPUTES
INBUILT
INCUBUS
INCUDES
INCURVE
INCUSED
INCUSES
INDUCED
INDUCER
INDUCES
INDUCTS
INDULGE
INDUTCH
INFUSED
INFUSER
INFUSES
INGULFS
INHUMAN
INHUMED
INHUMER
INHUMES
INJURED
INJURER
INJURES
INQUEST
INQUIRE
INQUIRY
INRUINS
INSULAR
INSULIN
INSULTS
INSURED
INSURER
INSURES
INTUITS
INTURNS
IRKUTSK
IRRUPTS
ISSUANT
ISSUEAD
ISSUERS
ISSUING
IVTUBES

I•••U••

ICECUBE
ICEOUTS
ICERUNS
IFYOUGO
ILLLUCK
IMBRUED
IMBRUES
IMPOUND
IMYOURS
INAFUNK
INAFURY
INAHUFF
INARUSH
INASUIT
INBOUND
INCLUDE
INCOURT
INCRUST
INDOUBT
INHOUSE
INOCULA
INPOURS
INTOUCH
INTRUDE
INTRUST
INTRUTH
IONIUMS
IREFUSE

I••••U•

IAPETUS
IBNSAUD
ICEBLUE
ICEDOUT
ICESOUT
ICINGUP
ICTERUS
ICTINUS
IGIVEUP
IGNEOUS
IMPETUS
IMPIOUS
INCUBUS
INFOCUS
INGENUE
INGROUP
INVACUO
INVOGUE
IRIDIUM
IRISOUT
IRONOUT
ISCHIUM
ISTHMUS
ITSTRUE

I•••••U

IBEGYOU
IGOTYOU
IGUASSU
ILIESCU
IOWEYOU
ISABEAU
ISEEYOU

•IU••••

DIURNAL
PIUSIII
PIUSVII
PIUSXII

•I•U•••

BIGUNIT
DILUENT
DILUTED
DILUTER
DILUTES
DILUTOR
DISUSED
DISUSES
DIVULGE
DIVULSE
FIBULAE
FIBULAR
FIBULAS
FICUSES
FIGURAL
FIGURED
FIGURER
FIGURES
FIXUPON
GIAUQUE
GIBUSES
HITUPON
KIDULTS
KIKUYUS
LIGURIA
LIQUATE
LIQUEFY
LIQUEUR
LIQUIDS
LIQUORS
LITURGY
MINUEND
MINUETS
MINUSES
MINUTED
MINUTER
MINUTES
MINUTIA
MISUSED
MISUSER
MISUSES
MIZUNAS
PIOUSLY
PIQUANT
PIQUING
RIGUEUR
RITUALS
RIVULET
SINUATE
SINUOUS
SINUSES
SINUTAB
SIOUANS
SITUATE
SITUPON
TIBURON
TIJUANA
TITULAR
VICUNAS
VIRUSES
VISUALS

•I••U••

AIRDUCT
AIRGUNS
AIRPUMP
AIRTUBE
BIGGULP
BIGGUNS
BIGHUGS
BIOFUEL
BISCUIT
BISMUTH
BISQUES
BIVOUAC
CINQUES
CIRCUIT
CIRCUSY
CIRQUES
DIALUPS
DICTUMS
DIDSUMS
DIECUTS
DIFFUSE
DIMBULB
DIMOUTS
DISBUDS
DISCUSS
DISEURS
DISEUSE
DISGUST
DISPUTE
DISRUPT
DISTURB
FILLUPS
FISSURE
FIXTURE
GIBLUES
GIVEUPS
HICCUPS
HIRSUTE
HITTUNE
KIBBUTZ
KICKUPS
KILAUEA
LIMBURG
LINEUPS
LINGUAE
LINGUAL
LINGULA
LINKUPS
MIAOUED
MIDJULY
MIDJUNE
MISCUED
MISCUES
MISCUTS
MISRULE
MISSUSA
MISTUNE
MIXTURE
NIEBUHR
NIPMUCK
OILCUPS
OILRUBS
PICKUPS
PICTURE
PIGNUTS
PIGOUTS
PILEUPS
PINCURL
PINGUID
PITBULL
RIBCUTS
RIGOURS
RIOMUNI
RIZZUTO
SIDDURS
SIGMUND
SIGNUPS
SIRDUKE
SIXGUNS
TISSUES
TISSUEY
VIADUCT
VICTUAL
VIGOURS
VINCULA
VIRGULE
VIRTUAL
VIRTUES
VISCUSO
VISTULA
WINDUPS
ZIPCUFF
ZIPGUNS

•I•••U•

AIREDUP
AIRSOUT
BIGBLUE
BIGFOUR
BILIOUS
BINDSUP
BITESUP
CIMABUE
CISEAUX
CITROUS
DIALOUT
DIALSUP
DICECUP
DIEDOUT
DIESOUT
DIGSOUT
DIMSOUT
DINEOUT
DIREFUL
DISHFUL
DISHOUT
DIVVYUP
EIGHTUP
FIATLUX
FIBROUS
FILEOUT
FILLOUT
FILLSUP
FINDOUT
FIREBUG
FIREDUP
FIRESUP
FIRMSUP
FIRSTUP
FISHOUT
FISTFUL
FIXEDUP
FIXESUP
GIAUQUE
GIBBOUS
GIDDYUP
GIELGUD
GIVENUP
GIVEOUT
GIVESUP
HIDEOUS
HIDEOUT
HIKEDUP
HIKEOUT
HIKESUP
HIREOUT
HITCHUP
HITSOUT
JIMRYUN
KICKOUT
KICKSUP
KIDSRUS
KIKUYUS
KINGTUT
LICKSUP
LIFEFUL
LIFTSUP
LIGHTUP
LINECUT
LINEDUP
LINEOUT
LINESUP
LINKSUP
LIONCUB
LIPSOUT
LIQUEUR
LITHIUM
LIVENUP
LIVEOUT
MICHAUX
MILERUN
MILHAUD
MILHOUS
MILIEUS
MILIEUX
MILKDUD
MILKRUN
MILLRUN
MIMIEUX
MINDFUL
MINIBUS
MINIMUM
MINIMUS
MINISUB
MINOGUE
MISSOUT
MISTSUP
MITCHUM
MIXEDUP
MIXESUP
MIXITUP
NICEGUY
NIOBIUM
NITROUS
NIVEOUS
OILDRUM
OISEAUX
PICEOUS
PICKOUT
PICKSUP
PIGSOUT
PILATUS
PILEDUP
PILEOUS
PILESUP
PILLBUG
PINENUT
PINETUM
PIPEDUP
PIPEFUL
PIPESUP
PIRAEUS
PIROGUE
PISTOUS
PITEOUS
PITIFUL
RIDEOUT
RIDESUP

RIGSOUT
RIGUEUR
RILEDUP
RILESUP
RIMBAUD
RINGOUT
RINGSUP
RIOTGUN
RIOTOUS
RIPSOUT
RISESUP
SICKOUT
SIDIOUS
SIGHFUL
SIGNOUT
SIGNSUP
SINGOUT
SINUOUS
SITSOUT
SIXFOUR
SIZEDUP
SIZESUP
TIDYSUM
TILTSUP
TIMEOUT
TIMESUP
TIREOUT
VIALFUL
VICIOUS
VILNIUS
VISCOUS
WICKIUP
WIGSOUT
WILLFUL
WIMPOUT
WINDAUS
WINDSUP
WINGNUT
WINKOUT
WINSOUT
WIPEDUP
WIPEOUT
WIPESUP
WIREDUP
WIRESUP
WISEDUP
WISEGUY
WISESUP
WISHFUL
WISTFUL
WITEOUT
WITHOUT
XINGOUT
ZINCOUS

•I••••U

BIRDFLU
LILINAU
MISSYOU
SILENTU
TINAMOU
WILLYOU

••IU•••

PAIUTES
PRIUSES
TRIUMPH

••I•U••

AMINUTE
AZIMUTH
BRIQUET
CHINUPS
CLIBURN
CLIQUED
CLIQUES
CLIQUEY
EPICURE
FAILURE
FAIRUSE
FLIPUPS
LEISURE
MSIEURS
OVIDUCT
SEIZURE
SKIBUMS
SKIJUMP
SKIRUNS
SKISUIT
SLIPUPS
STIMULI
TRIBUNE
TRIBUTE
UNIQUES
VEINULE
VOITURE
ZEITUNG

••I••U•

AMIBLUE
ATISSUE
BAILOUT
BOILOUT
BOILSUP
BRICKUP
BRIMFUL
BRINGUP
BUILDUP
BUILTUP
CHILLUM
CHIPSUP
CHIRRUP
CLIMBUP
CLIPOUT
COILSUP
CRIEDUP
CRIESUP
CRISPUS
CRITTUR
DOINGUP
DRIEDUP
DRIESUP
DRIFTUP
DRINKUP
DRIVEUP
EDITOUT
ELIGIUS
FAIRSUP
FLIESUP
FLIPOUT
FRIEDUP
FRIESUP
FRISEUR
GAINFUL
GOINGUP
HAIRCUT
HEINOUS
HOISTUP
ICINGUP
IGIVEUP
IRIDIUM
IRISOUT
JOINSUP
JUICEUP
LAIDOUT
LYINGUP
MAILOUT
MAISOUI
NAILGUN
NAILSUP
NAIPAUL
OMINOUS
PAIDOUT
PAILFUL
PAINFUL
PAIRSUP
PHILOUS
POINTUP
PRICKUP
PRINTUP
QUIETUS
QUINQUE
QUINTUS
RAILBUS
RAINOUT
RAISEUP
REISSUE
RUINOUS
SHINEUP
SHIPFUL
SHIPOUT
SKILFUL
SKIPOUT
SLICEUP
SLIDOUT
SLINKUP
SLIPOUT
SLIPSUP
SNIFFUP
SPICEUP
SPIFFUP
SPIKEUP
SPINOUT
SPITOUT
STICKUM
STICKUP
STILLUP
STINKUP
STIRRUP
STIRSUP
SUITSUP
SWIMSUP
THINKUP
THINOUT
TOILFUL
TRIPSUP
TRITIUM
TRIVIUM
TWISTUP
TYINGUP
USINGUP
VOIDOUT
WAILFUL
WAITOUT
WAITSUP
WEIGHUP
WHIPSUP
WHITSUN
WRITEUP

••I•••U

CAILLOU
ILIESCU
SHIATSU
SHIHTZU
SHIKOKU
THIMPHU
ZWICKAU

•••IU••

ALLIUMS
ATRIUMS
DARIUSI
IONIUMS
LUCIUSI
MEDIUMS
PODIUMS
STPIUSI
STPIUSV
STPIUSX
TEDIUMS

•••I•U•

ANTIGUA
ANTIGUN
ANTIQUE
ANXIOUS
ATEITUP
ATTICUS
BEZIQUE
BILIOUS
CACIQUE
CARIOUS
CHAINUP
COMIQUE
COPIOUS
CUBITUS
CURIOUS
DEVIOUS
DOMINUS
DONIMUS
DUBIOUS
DUTIFUL
EATITUP
ENRIQUE
ENVIOUS
FATIGUE
FEMINUM
FURIOUS
HABITUE
HALIBUT
HAMITUP
HYGINUS
ICTINUS
IMPIOUS
LALIQUE
LATINUS
LEMIEUX
LEPIDUS
MANIPUR
MAXIMUM
MAXIMUS
MILIEUS
MILIEUX
MIMIEUX
MINIBUS
MINIMUM
MINIMUS
MINISUB
MIXITUP
MODICUM
NOXIOUS
OBLIQUE
OBVIOUS
OCCIPUT
OEDIPUS
OMNIBUS
OPTIMUM
PARIBUS
PAVIOUR
PERITUS
PITIFUL
RANITUP
RESIDUA
RESIDUE
RETINUE
REVITUP
RUBIOUS
RUNITUP
SAVIOUR
SERIOUS
SIDIOUS
SPLITUP
SUMITUP
TACITUS
TEDIOUS
TEEITUP
TROILUS
UNPIOUS
URSINUS
VARIOUS
VICIOUS
ZOSIMUS

•••I••U

CARIBOU
FUJITSU
JUJITSU
LEHIGHU
LILINAU
PAXINOU
XAVIERU

••••IU•

BELGIUM
BERGIUS
BOHRIUM
CADMIUM
CALCIUM
CARDIUM
CASSIUS
CELSIUS
CRANIUM
DUBNIUM
ELAAIUN
ELIGIUS
ELUVIUM
ELYSIUM
FERMIUM
FLAVIUS
FORTIUS
GALLIUM
GORDIUS
GROPIUS
GROTIUS
HAFNIUM
HAHNIUM
HASSIUM
HOLMIUM
IRIDIUM
ISCHIUM
LITHIUM
MARTIUS
MENCIUS
NATRIUM
NENNIUS
NIOBIUM
ORARIUM
PENTIUM
PERSIUS
PHEMIUS
PONTIUS
PREMIUM
PUBLIUS
RHENIUM
RHODIUM
STADIUM
TERBIUM
THORIUM
THULIUM
TRITIUM
TRIVIUM
URANIUM
VILNIUS
WICKIUP
YTTRIUM

••••I•U

MARTINU
MATHIEU
MONDIEU
PURLIEU

•••••IU

LUCYLIU

IV•••••

IVANHOE
IVANIII
IVANOVO
IVERSON
IVORIAN
IVORIES
IVORINE
IVTUBES
IVYLIKE

I•V••••

INVACUO
INVADED
INVADER
INVADES
INVALID
INVEIGH
INVENTS
INVERSE
INVERTS
INVESTS
INVICTA
INVITED
INVITEE
INVITER
INVITES
INVITRO
INVOGUE
INVOICE
INVOKED
INVOKER
INVOKES
INVOLVE

I••V•••

IGIVEUP
IHAVEIT
ILOVEIT
ILOVELA
INAVALE

I•••V••

ICEOVER
IMPAVID
INCIVIL
INFAVOR
INFIVES
INWOVEN
ITSOVER

I••••V•

IAMLOVE
ICECAVE
ILLLIVE
IMPROVE
INCURVE
INNERVE
INVOLVE
INWEAVE
ITSLOVE
ITWELVE
IVANOVO

•IV••••

BIVALVE
BIVOUAC
CIVILLY
CIVVIES
DIVEDIN
DIVERGE
DIVERSE
DIVERTS
DIVESIN
DIVESTS
DIVIDED
DIVIDER
DIVIDES
DIVINED
DIVINER
DIVINES
DIVISOR
DIVORCE
DIVULGE
DIVULSE
DIVVIED
DIVVIES
DIVVYUP
FIVEAAA
FIVEDAY
FIVEEEE
FIVEMAN
FIVEONE
FIVEPIN
FIVESIX
FIVETEN
FIVETWO
FIVEWAY
GIVEEAR
GIVENBY
GIVENIN
GIVENOF
GIVENON
GIVENTO
GIVENUP
GIVEOFF
GIVEOUT
GIVESIN
GIVESOF
GIVESON
GIVESTO
GIVESUP
GIVEUPS
GIVEWAY
HIVEOFF
JIVIEST
LIVABLE
LIVEAID
LIVEDIN
LIVEDON
LIVEFOR
LIVENED
LIVENER
LIVENUP
LIVEOAK
LIVEONE
LIVEOUT
LIVERED
LIVESAT
LIVESET
LIVESEY
LIVESIN
LIVESON
LIVIDLY
LIVINGS
LIVORNO
NIVEOUS
PIVOTAL
PIVOTED
PIVOTER
RIVALED
RIVALRY
RIVERPO
RIVETED
RIVETER
RIVIERA
RIVIERE
RIVULET
VIVALDI
VIVANTS
VIVARIA
VIVENDI
VIVICAA
VIVIDER
VIVIDLY
VIVITAR

•I•V•••

AIRVENT
CIVVIES
DIAVOLO
DIMVIEW
DIVVIED
DIVVIES
DIVVYUP
KIDVIDS
NIRVANA
RIGVEDA
SIEVING
SILVERS
SILVERY

•I••V••

BILEVEL
DIDOVER
DISAVOW
LIEOVER
LITOVSK
MINIVAC
MINIVAN
MINIVER
MISAVER
MITZVAH
NINEVEH
PIUSVII
TIPOVER
VISAVIS
WINEVAT
WINOVER

•I•••V•

AIRWAVE
BIGFIVE
BIGLOVE
BIVALVE
FICTIVE
GINGIVA
KISLEVS
MINERVA
MINITVS
MISGAVE
MISGIVE
MISMOVE
MISSIVE
RILIEVO
SIXFIVE

•I••••V

DIRECTV
SILENTV

••IV•••

ALIVETO
AVIVIAN
CHIVIED
CHIVIES
DRIVEAT
DRIVEBY
DRIVEIN
DRIVELS
DRIVERS
DRIVETO
DRIVEUP
DRIVING
FLIVVER
FRIVOLS
IGIVEUP
NAIVELY
NAIVEST
NAIVETE
NAIVETY
OLIVIER
OLIVINE
POIVRES
PRIVACY
PRIVATE
PRIVETS
PRIVIER
PRIVIES
PRIVILY
PRIVITY
PRIVYTO
QUIVERS
QUIVERY
QUIVIVE
SHIVERS
SHIVERY
SKIVEST
SLIVERS
SNIVELS
SWIVELS
SWIVETS
TRIVETS
TRIVIAL
TRIVIOT
TRIVIUM
UNIVACS
WAIVERS
WAIVING
ZHIVAGO

••I•V••

FLIVVER
GRIEVED
GRIEVER
GRIEVES
KNIEVEL
THIEVED
THIEVES

••I••V•

QUIVIVE
UNITIVE

••I•••V

GRINKOV
PHILIPV
SMIRNOV
SPIKETV

•••IV••

ACTIVAS
ACTIVES
AQUIVER
ARRIVAL
ARRIVED
ARRIVER
ARRIVES
ASHIVER
BOLIVAR
BOLIVIA
BYFIVES
DATIVES
DELIVER
DERIVED
DERIVER
DERIVES
ENDIVES
ENLIVEN
ESTIVAL
EXWIVES
INCIVIL
INFIVES
MEDIVAC
MINIVAC
MINIVAN
MINIVER
MOTIVED
MOTIVES
NATIVES
PORIVER
REGIVEN
REGIVES
RELIVED
RELIVES
REVIVAL
REVIVED
REVIVER
REVIVES
SALIVAS
SHRIVEL
SHRIVER
SHRIVES
STRIVED
STRIVEN
STRIVER
STRIVES
THRIVED
THRIVEN
THRIVER
THRIVES
UNCIVIC
UNCIVIL
UNGIVEN
UNLIVED
UNLIVES
UNRIVED
UNRIVEN
UNVIVID
UPDIVED
UPDIVES
UPRIVER
VOTIVES

•••I•V•

ACHIEVA
ACHIEVE
BELIEVE
DASILVA
LOUISVI
MINITVS
RELIEVE
RILIEVO

•••I••V

KEMIDOV
LOUISIV
LOUISXV
STPIUSV
USTINOV

••••IV•

ABUSIVE
ACTFIVE
AGEFIVE
AMATIVE
ARCHIVE
BEEHIVE
BIGFIVE
CAPTIVA
CAPTIVE
CONNIVE
COSTIVE
CURSIVE
DECEIVE
DEPRIVE
ELUSIVE
EMOTIVE
EROSIVE
EVASIVE
FESTIVA
FESTIVE
FICTIVE
FORGIVE
FURTIVE
GINGIVA
ILLLIVE
KHEDIVE
LETLIVE
LOWDIVE
MALDIVE
MASSIVE
MISGIVE
MISSIVE
NBALIVE
NONLIVE
NOTLIVE
OUTGIVE
OUTLIVE
PARFIVE
PASSIVE
PENSIVE
PLOSIVE
POPDIVA
PREDIVE
QUIVIVE
RECEIVE
REDFIVE
REDRIVE
RESTIVE
SIXFIVE
SKYDIVE
SUASIVE
SURVIVE
TANTIVY
TENSIVE
THEFIVE
TOPFIVE
TUSSIVE
UNITIVE
UNNAIVE
YESHIVA

••••I•V

MARTINV
PHILIPV

•••••IV

HENRYIV
JAMESIV
JOHNXIV
LOUISIV
PLOVDIV
ROCKYIV
ROYGBIV
SCENEIV
TELAVIV
URBANIV

IW•••••

IWANTIT
IWANTTO
IWOJIMA
IWONDER

I•W••••

IFWEMAY
INWARDS
INWEAVE
INWHITE
INWOVEN
IOWEYOU
ITWELVE
ITWENTY

I••W•••

ICEWINE
ICYWIND
ILLWILL
ILLWIND
IMSWELL
INAWEOF
INAWINK
INAWORD
INDWELL
INDWELT
INKWELL
INSWEPT
IPSWICH

I•••W••

IKNEWIT
IKNOWIT
INNOWAY
INPOWER

I••••W•

ICEDOWN
INBROWN
INCROWD
INDRAWN
INFLOWS
INGROWN

I•••••W

ICESHOW
IGNATOW
ILLKNOW
INASTEW
ISEENOW

•IW••••

KIWANIS

•I•W•••

AIRWARS
AIRWAVE

AIRWAYS
AIRWICK
AIRWOLF
BIGWIGS
BIGWINS
DIDWELL
DIMWITS
FITWELL
LIDWINA
MIDWAYS
MIDWEEK
MIDWEST
MIDWIFE
MISWIRE
MISWORD
NITWITS
OILWELL
PIGWEED
PINWALE
SITWELL
SITWITH
SIXWEEK
TINWARE
TINWORK
VIEWERS
VIEWIER
VIEWING
VIEWITH
WIGWAGS
WIGWAMS
WINWOOD

•I••W••

BIKEWAY
DIEAWAY
DISOWNS
FIVEWAY
GIVEWAY
HIDAWAY
HIGHWAY
LIKEWOW
MIAOWED
RIDGWAY
SIDEWAY
SINEWED
TIMEWAS
WIDOWED
WIDOWER
WIMOWEH

•I•••W•

BIGNEWS
BIGTOWN
BILLOWS
BILLOWY
DIEDOWN
FIVETWO
HITTOWN
JIGSAWS
LIEDOWN
LINETWO
MIDTOWN
MILDEWS
MILDEWY
MINNOWS
PILLOWS
PILLOWY
PINDOWN
PITROWS
PITSAWS
RIPSAWN
RIPSAWS
SIDETWO
SITDOWN
SIZETWO
TIEDOWN
TIPDOWN
WILLOWS
WILLOWY
WINDOWS
WINDOWY
WINNOWS

•I••••W

AIRCREW
AIRFLOW
AIRGLOW
AIRSHOW
BIGELOW
BIGSHOW
DIMVIEW
DISAVOW
HIGHLOW
HINDPAW
HITSHOW
LIESLOW
LIKENEW
LIKEWOW
LITHGOW
MILKCOW
MISBREW
MISDRAW
MISDREW
MISKNEW
MISKNOW
MISTBOW
PILCROW
PITCREW
SILENTW
TILLNOW
WICKLOW
WINSLOW

••IW•••

SKIWEAR

••I•W••

CHINWAG
FAIRWAY
OJIBWAS
OJIBWAY
RAILWAY
SHIPWAY
TAILWAG
THISWAY

••I••W•

CHITOWN
OKINAWA
SKITOWS

••I•••W

DOITNOW
EXITNOW
LAIDLOW
RAINBOW
SKIDROW
WHIPSAW

•••IW••

ANTIWAR
PERIWIG
TAXIWAY
WYSIWYG

•••I•W•

REVIEWS
SODIDWE

•••I••W

MANILOW
SAGINAW
SEMIRAW

••••I•W

DIMVIEW
PREVIEW
PURVIEW
THEVIEW

I••X•••

INEXACT
INEXILE

I•••X••

ICEAXES
IMMIXED
IMMIXES
INBOXES
INDEXED
INDEXER
INDEXES
INFIXED
INFIXES

•IX••••

FIXABLE
FIXATED
FIXATES
FIXEDLY
FIXEDON
FIXEDUP
FIXESON
FIXESUP
FIXINGS
FIXTURE
FIXUPON
MIXABLE
MIXEDIN
MIXEDLY
MIXEDUP
MIXESIN
MIXESUP
MIXITUP
MIXTECS
MIXTURE
PIXYISH
SIXBALL
SIXEEEE
SIXFEET
SIXFIVE
SIXFOLD
SIXFOOT
SIXFOUR
SIXGUNS
SIXIRON
SIXLANE
SIXNINE
SIXPACK
SIXTEEN
SIXTHLY
SIXTIES
SIXTYAD
SIXTYBC
SIXWEEK
SIXYEAR
VIXENLY

•I•X•••

BIAXIAL
DIOXIDE
DIOXINS
JINXERS
JINXING
MINXISH

•I••X••

PIUSXII
TIMEXES

•I•••X•

AIRTAXI
JIMFIXX
PICKAXE

•I••••X

CINEMAX
CISEAUX
FIATLUX
FILOFAX
FIREBOX
FIREFOX
FIVESIX
GIFTBOX
GIFTTAX
JIMFIXX
KICKBOX
MICHAUX
MILIEUX
MIMIEUX
MINIMAX
MIRAMAX
MISTERX
OISEAUX
PILLBOX
SILENTX
SIMPLEX
SIZESIX
VICTRIX

••IX•••

ELIXIRS
QUIXOTE

••I•••X

COINBOX
CRISPIX
EDITRIX
FAIRFAX
FAIRSEX
MAILBOX
REINDEX
TRIPLEX
UNIPLEX
UVINDEX

•••IX••

ADMIXED
ADMIXES
AFFIXED
AFFIXER
AFFIXES
FTDIXNJ
HELIXES
IMMIXED
IMMIXES
INFIXED
INFIXES
MAXIXES
MRFIXIT
RADIXES
REFIXED
REFIXES
REMIXED
REMIXES
UNFIXED
UNFIXES
UNMIXED
UNMIXES

•••I•X•

LOUISXI
LOUISXV

•••I••X

ANTITAX
EQUIFAX
EQUINOX
HALIFAX
HUMIDEX
LEMIEUX
LOUISIX
MILIEUX
MIMIEUX
MINIMAX
OMNIMAX
SOMINEX
STPIUSX

••••IX•

BETWIXT
JIMFIXX

••••I•X

JIMFIXX
OUTJINX

•••••IX

ASTERIX
BASESIX
BEATRIX
BERVOIX
CAKEMIX
CHEXMIX
COOLPIX
CRISPIX
DEEPSIX
EDITRIX
FIVESIX
FORTDIX
HARDSIX
HENDRIX
JOHNXIX
LOUISIX
MACHSIX
MEOWMIX
MUESLIX
NETFLIX
ORATRIX
OVERFIX
OVERMIX
PAGESIX
PHOENIX
POSTFIX
REAFFIX
ROUBAIX
SIZESIX
SKEEZIX
SOUPMIX
STCROIX
TELEPIX
VICTRIX

I•Y••••

ICYWIND
IDYLIST
IDYLLIC
IFYOUGO
IMYOURS
INYEARS
IVYLIKE

I••Y•••

ICKYPOO
IGGYPOP
ILLYRIA
INDYCAR
INKYCAP
INLYING
INSYNCH

I•••Y••

IBEGYOU
IDSAYSO
IGOTYOU
INLAYER
INSTYLE
IOWEYOU
ISEEYOU
ITMAYBE

I••••Y•

IHEARYA
INTRAYS

I•••••Y

IBILITY
ICETRAY
ICONIFY
IDEALLY
IEIGHTY
IFWEMAY
IGNOBLY
IMAGERY
IMHAPPY
IMPIETY
IMREADY
IMSORRY
INAFURY
INANELY
INANITY
INAPTLY
INDEEDY
INEPTLY
INERTLY
INFANCY
ININETY
INNERLY
INNOWAY
INQUIRY
IRATELY
ISONOMY
ISOTOPY
ITHIRTY
ITSABOY
ITSEASY
ITSOKAY
ITWENTY

•I•Y•••

BICYCLE
BIRYANI
CITYBOY
CITYGAL
LIBYANS
LILYPAD
MIDYEAR
MINYANS
PITYING
PIXYISH
SIBYLIC
SIXYEAR
TIDYING
TIDYSUM
TINYBIT
TINYTIM
TINYTOT
VINYLIC
WIFYING

•I••Y••

BIGEYED
BIGEYES
BIOTYPE
DIPTYCH
DIVVYUP
FIFTYAD
FIFTYBC
GIDDYAP
GIDDYUP
JIMRYUN
KIKUYUS
LIPSYNC
MISSYOU
MISTYPE
PIEEYED
PIGEYED
PITAYAS
RIBEYES
RITDYES
SILLYME
SIXTYAD
SIXTYBC
TIEDYED
TIEDYES
TINTYPE
VISAYAN
WILLYOU

•I•••Y•

AIRWAYS
BIGBOYS
BIGDAYS
BILLNYE
DICKEYS
DISMAYS
FISHEYE
HICKEYS
JITNEYS
KIDNEYS
MICKEYS
MIDDAYS
MIDWAYS
MINSKYS
MISKEYS
MISLAYS
MISSAYS
PINBOYS
RICKEYS
RIDEBYS

•I••••Y

AINTHAY
AIRPLAY
BIASPLY
BIGBABY
BIGCITY
BIGEASY
BIGGITY
BIGOTRY
BIKEWAY
BILLOWY
BINDERY
BIOLOGY
CILIARY
CINDERY
CINERGY
CIRCUSY
CITYBOY
CIVILLY
DICKORY
DIDDLEY
DIEAWAY
DIETARY
DIGGITY
DIGGORY
DIGNIFY
DIGNITY
DINGILY
DIRTILY
DISOBEY
DISPLAY
DITHERY
DIZZILY
FIDGETY
FIERILY
FIFTHLY
FILEDBY
FILESBY
FILMILY
FINALLY
FINDLAY
FINDLEY
FINICKY
FIREFLY
FIRSTLY
FISHERY
FISHFRY
FISHILY
FITZROY
FIVEDAY
FIVEWAY
FIXEDLY
GIDDILY
GINGERY
GIRLSHY
GIVENBY
GIVEWAY
HICKORY
HIDAWAY
HIGHBOY
HIGHDAY
HIGHPAY
HIGHWAY
HILLARY
HIPPITY
HISTORY
HITPLAY
JIGGERY
JITTERY
KILLJOY
KILNDRY
KINKILY
KITSCHY
KITTERY
LIBERTY
LIBRARY
LICITLY
LICKETY
LIGHTLY
LIGNIFY
LINDSAY
LINDSEY
LINEDRY
LIQUEFY
LISAGAY
LITHELY
LITTERY
LITURGY
LIVESEY
LIVIDLY
MIDJULY
MILDEWY
MILKILY
MIMICRY
MISALLY
MISCOPY
MISERLY
MISPLAY
MISRELY
MISTILY
MIXEDLY
NICEBOY
NICEDAY
NICEGUY
NICETRY
NIFTILY
NIGHTLY
NIKOLAY
NIMIETY
NINTHLY
NIPPILY
NITRIFY
NITTANY
PICARDY
PIGGERY
PILLORY
PILLOWY
PIOSITY
PIOUSLY
PITHILY
RIANTLY
RIBBONY
RICKETY
RIDESBY
RIDGWAY
RIFLERY
RIGHTLY
RIGIDLY
RISIBLY
RISKILY
RITZILY
RIVALRY
SICKBAY
SICKDAY
SICKPAY
SIDEWAY
SIGHTLY
SIGNIFY
SILENTY
SILKILY
SILVERY
SIMCITY
SINCITY
SIXTHLY
SIZABLY
TICKSBY
TIDALLY
TIERNEY
TIFFANY
TIGHTLY
TIMBERY
TIMIDLY
TIMOTHY
TINAFEY
TINDERY
TINNILY
TIPSILY
TIREDLY
TISSUEY
VICEROY
VICKREY
VICTORY
VISIBLY
VITALLY
VITRIFY
VIVIDLY
VIXENLY
WIGGERY
WILLOWY
WINDILY
WINDOWY
WINFREY
WINTERY
WISEGUY
WISPILY
WITTILY
ZINCIFY

••IY•••

ALIYAHS
ELIYALE

••I•Y••

DAIRYER
ERINYES
PRIVYTO

••I••Y•

EVILEYE
FRIDAYS
HAIRDYE
SAIDAYE
SMILEYS

••I•••Y

ABIDEBY
ABILITY
ACIDIFY
ACIDITY
AGILELY
AGILITY
ALIMONY
AMIABLY
ANILITY
ANIMACY
APISHLY
ARIDITY
AVIDITY
AXIALLY
BLIGHTY
BLINDLY
BRIBERY
BRIEFLY
BRIMLEY
BRISKLY
BRISTLY
BRITNEY
CHICORY
CHIEFLY
CHIMNEY
CHINTZY
CLIQUEY
CRIMINY
CRINKLY
CRISPLY
DRIPDRY
DRIVEBY
DRIZZLY
EKINGBY
EPILADY
FAINTLY
FAIRWAY
FLIESBY
FLIGHTY
FLITSBY
FRIARLY
FRIDLEY
FRIZZLY
GAINSAY
GLIDEBY
GLITCHY
GOINGBY
GRIFFEY
GRIMILY
GRIMSBY
GRISTLY
GRIZZLY
IBILITY
IEIGHTY
ININETY
JOINERY
JOINTLY
JUICILY
LYINGBY
MOISTLY
NAIVELY
NAIVETY
NOISILY
OJIBWAY
PAISLEY
PLIABLY
PLIANCY
PRICILY
PRICKLY
PRIMACY
PRIMARY
PRIMELY
PRIVACY
PRIVILY
PRIVITY
QUICKLY
QUIETLY
QUIGLEY
QUINARY
QUINCEY
QUIVERY
RAILWAY
RAINILY
RAISINY
REIMPLY
SAIDNAY
SAINTLY
SHINGLY
SHINILY
SHIPWAY
SHIRLEY
SHIVERY
SKIPSBY
SLICKLY
SLIDEBY
SLIMILY
SLIPSBY
SNIDELY
SNIFFLY
SPICERY
SPICILY
SPIDERY
SPIKILY
SPINDLY
SPINDRY
SPINNEY
STICKBY
STIFFLY
STIRFRY
SWIFTLY
SWINERY
SWINGBY
THICKLY
THIERRY
THIRDLY
THIRSTY
THISDAY
THISTLY
THISWAY
TRILOGY
TRINARY
TRINITY
TRITELY
TWINKLY
TWITCHY
UNIBODY
UNITARY
UTICANY
UTILITY
WEIGHTY
WEIRDLY
WHISKEY
WHITELY
WHITNEY
WRIGGLY
WRIGLEY
WRINKLY

•••IY••

AALIYAH
ALNIYAT
BABIYAR
KOPIYKA
RUFIYAA

•••I•Y•

JERILYN
MARILYN
WYSIWYG

•••I••Y

ACRIDLY
ANXIETY
AUDIBLY
CHRISTY
CILIARY
CIVILLY
COLICKY
CUBICLY
DEVILRY
DUBIETY
FETIDLY
FINICKY
FLUIDLY
FRAILLY
FRAILTY
FTRILEY
GELIDLY
HOLIDAY
HOSIERY
HUMIDLY
IMPIETY
ITHIRTY
LEGIBLY
LICITLY
LIVIDLY
LUCIDLY
LURIDLY
MIMICRY
MUSIGNY
NEUILLY
NIMIETY
OREILLY
OSTIARY
PANICKY
PAVIDLY
PLAINLY

RABIDLY
RAPIDLY
RETIARY
RIGIDLY
RISIBLY
SATIETY
SATISFY
SCRIMPY
SEMIDRY
SEVIGNY
SHRILLY
SHRIMPY
SHTICKY
SOCIETY
SOLIDLY
SPRINGY
SQUINTY
SQUIRMY
SQUISHY
STAIDLY
STRINGY
TACITLY
TAXIWAY
TEPIDLY
THRIFTY
TIMIDLY
TOPIARY
UNFIERY
UNFITLY
UNGIDDY
UNHILLY
UNPIETY
UNRISKY
UNSILLY
UNWINDY
UNWITTY
VALIDLY
VAPIDLY
VARIETY
VISIBLY
VIVIDLY

••••IY•

OUGUIYA

••••I•Y

ABILITY
ACETIFY
ACIDIFY
ACIDITY
AGILITY
AMENITY
AMPLIFY
ANGRILY
ANILITY
ANNUITY
ARIDITY
AVIDITY
BAGGILY
BALKILY
BALMILY
BAWDILY
BAYCITY
BEADILY
BEATIFY
BEEFILY
BIGCITY
BIGGITY
BONNILY
BOOZILY
BOSSILY
BREVITY
BUMPILY
BUSHILY
CALCIFY
CAMPILY
CANNILY
CANTILY
CASSIDY
CATTILY
CERTIFY
CHARILY
CHARITY
CLARIFY
CLARITY
CLERISY
COCKILY
CORNILY
CRAZILY
CRIMINY
CRUDITY
CUSHILY
DAFFILY
DANDIFY
DANDILY
DAYLILY
DELCITY
DENSIFY
DENSITY
DESTINY
DIGGITY
DIGNIFY
DIGNITY
DINGILY
DIRTILY
DIZZILY
DOTTILY
DOWDILY
DUALITY
DULCIFY
DUMPILY
DUSKILY
DUSTILY
EDACITY
ELMCITY
EMPTILY
ENQUIRY
FALSIFY
FALSITY
FANCIFY
FANCILY
FATCITY
FATTILY
FATUITY
FIERILY
FILMILY
FISHILY
FLAKILY
FLUKILY
FOAMILY
FOGCITY
FOGGILY
FORTIFY
FUNKILY
FUNNILY
FUSSILY
FUSTILY
FUZZILY
GASEITY
GAUDILY
GAUZILY
GAWKILY
GIDDILY
GLAZILY
GLORIFY
GOOFILY
GOONILY
GOSSIPY
GOUTILY
GRATIFY
GRAVITY
GRIMILY
GUSHILY
GUSTILY
GUTSILY
HAMMILY
HANDILY
HAPPIFY
HAPPILY
HARDILY
HASTILY
HEADILY
HEAVILY
HEFTILY
HIPPITY
HOARILY
HORRIFY
HORSILY
HUFFILY
HUSKILY
IBILITY
ICONIFY
INANITY
INQUIRY
JAZZILY
JELLIFY
JERKILY
JOLLIFY
JOLLILY
JOLLITY
JUICILY
JUMPILY
JUSTIFY
KINKILY
LANKILY
LEERILY
LIGNIFY
LOFTILY
LOONILY
LOUSILY
LOWLILY
LUCKILY
LUMPILY
LUSTILY
MAGNIFY
MEATILY
MERRILY
MESSILY
MILKILY
MISTILY
MOLLIFY
MOODILY
MOONILY
MORTIFY
MOUSILY
MUDDILY
MUMMIFY
MURKILY
MUSHILY
MUSSILY
MUSTILY
MUZZILY
MYSTIFY
MYTHIFY
NASTILY
NATTILY
NEEDILY
NERVILY
NIFTILY
NIPPILY
NITRIFY
NOISILY
NONOILY
NULLIFY
NULLITY
NUTTILY
OBESITY
OLDCITY
OPACITY
OUTCITY
OUTPITY
PAUCITY
PEPPILY
PERFIDY
PERKILY
PESKILY
PETRIFY
PETTILY
PHONILY
PIOSITY
PITHILY
PRICILY
PRIVILY
PRIVITY
PROBITY
PROCITY
PRODIGY
PROSILY
PUDGILY
PUFFILY
PULPIFY
PUNNILY
PUSHILY
QUAKILY
QUALIFY
QUALITY
RABBITY
RAINILY
RAISINY
READILY
REALITY
RECTIFY
REUNIFY
RISKILY
RITZILY
ROCKILY
ROOMILY
ROWDILY
RUDDILY
RUSTILY
SALTILY
SAPPILY
SASSILY
SAUCILY
SAVVILY
SCARIFY
SCARILY
SEALILY
SEEDILY
SHADILY
SHAKILY
SHINILY
SHOWILY
SIGNIFY
SILKILY
SIMCITY
SINCITY
SLIMILY
SMOKILY
SNAKILY
SNOWILY
SOAPILY
SOGGILY
SOOTILY
SORRILY
SPECIFY
SPICILY
SPIKILY
STAGILY
STONILY
SUAVITY
SUBSIDY
SULKILY
SUNCITY
SUNNILY
SURLILY
TACKILY
TANTIVY
TARDILY
TARTILY
TASTILY
TATTILY
TAWNILY
TEARILY
TENSITY
TENUITY
TERRIFY
TESTIFY
TESTILY
THECITY
TINNILY
TIPSILY
TRINITY
UNHAIRY
UNJUICY
UNNOISY
UNRAINY
UNSHINY
UNSPICY
UTILITY
VACUITY
VARSITY
VASTITY
VERBIFY
VERMINY
VERSIFY
VITRIFY
WACKILY
WASPILY
WASSILY
WEARILY
WEEDILY
WINDILY
WISPILY
WITTILY
WOOZILY
WORDILY
YUPPIFY
ZESTILY
ZINCIFY
ZOMBIFY

IZ•••••

IZATION
IZZATSO

I•Z••••

IZZATSO

I••Z•••

IBIZANS

I•••Z••

IODIZED
IODIZER
IODIZES
IONIZED
IONIZER
IONIZES

I••••Z•

IDOLIZE
IMPREZA
INADAZE
ITEMIZE

•IZ••••

BIZARRE
BIZARRO
DIZAINS
DIZZIED
DIZZIER
DIZZIES
DIZZILY
FIZGIGS
FIZZERS
FIZZIER
FIZZING
FIZZLED
FIZZLER
FIZZLES
GIZZARD
LIZARDS
LIZETTE
LIZZIES
MIZRAHI
MIZUNAS
MIZZENS
MIZZLED
MIZZLES
PIZARRO
PIZZAZZ
RIZZUTO
SIZABLE
SIZABLY
SIZEDUP
SIZEONE
SIZESIX
SIZESUP
SIZETEN
SIZETWO
SIZZLED
SIZZLER
SIZZLES
TIZZIES
VIZIERS
VIZORED
VIZSLAS
WIZARDS
WIZENED

•I•Z•••

CINZANO
DITZIER
DIZZIED
DIZZIER
DIZZIES
DIZZILY
FITZROY
FIZZERS
FIZZIER
FIZZING
FIZZLED
FIZZLER
FIZZLES
GIZZARD
LIZZIES
MISZONE
MITZVAH
MIZZENS
MIZZLED
MIZZLES
PIAZZAS
PIZZAZZ
RITZIER
RITZILY
RIZZUTO
SIZZLED
SIZZLER
SIZZLES
TIZZIES
YITZHAK
ZIGZAGS

•I••Z••

CITIZEN
MINIZOO
PIAZZAS
SIEBZIG
VIERZIG

•I•••Z•

FIRENZA
FIRENZE
GINFIZZ
LIONIZE
MIDSIZE
PIZZAZZ
VICENZA

•I••••Z

GINFIZZ
JIMENEZ
JIMINEZ
KIBBUTZ
NISSANZ
PIZZAZZ
SILENTZ
SIMONIZ
TIRPITZ

••IZ•••

ARIZONA
DRIZZLE
DRIZZLY
FRIZZED
FRIZZER
FRIZZES
FRIZZLE
FRIZZLY
GRIZZLE
GRIZZLY
IBIZANS
PRIZING
PRIZZIS
QUIZNOS
QUIZZED
QUIZZER
QUIZZES
RHIZOME
SEIZEON
SEIZERS
SEIZING
SEIZORS
SEIZURE
SWIZZLE
WHIZKID
WHIZZED
WHIZZER
WHIZZES

••I•Z••

BLITZED
BLITZEN
BLITZER
BLITZES
DRIZZLE
DRIZZLY
ELIEZER
FRIEZES
FRIZZED
FRIZZER
FRIZZES
FRIZZLE
FRIZZLY
GLITZED
GLITZES
GRIZZLE
GRIZZLY
LEIPZIG
PRIZZIS
QUINZES
QUIZZED
QUIZZER
QUIZZES
SPITZES
SWITZER
SWIZZLE
WHIZZED
WHIZZER
WHIZZES

••I••Z•

BLINTZE
CHINTZY
LAICIZE
OXIDIZE
SHIHTZU
SPINOZA
UNISIZE
UNITIZE
UTILIZE

••I•••Z

GRISNEZ
HEIFETZ
LAISSEZ
LEIBNIZ

•••IZ••

ASSIZES
BEDIZEN
CITIZEN
DENIZEN
HORIZON
IODIZED
IODIZER
IODIZES
IONIZED
IONIZER
IONIZES
MINIZOO
NETIZEN
RESIZED
RESIZER
RESIZES
TREIZES
UNSIZED
UPSIZED
UPSIZES
VERIZON

•••I•Z•

JERITZA

•••I••Z

AGRIBIZ
JIMINEZ
RAMIREZ

••••IZ•

AGONIZE
ANODIZE
ATOMIZE
BAPTIZE
BRASIZE
CAPSIZE
CHORIZO
COGNIZE
DUALIZE
EBONIZE
ELEGIZE
FABRIZI
FORSIZE
GINFIZZ
GRECIZE
HATSIZE
IDOLIZE
ITEMIZE
LAICIZE
LIONIZE
MANSIZE
MIDSIZE
OBELIZE
ODORIZE
ONESIZE
OUTSIZE
OXIDIZE
OZONIZE
POETIZE
REALIZE
RESEIZE
STYLIZE
UNISIZE
UNITIZE
UTILIZE

••••I•Z

BERLIOZ
BERLITZ
GINFIZZ
HJHEINZ
HORVITZ
LAURITZ
SCHLITZ
THERITZ
TIRPITZ

•••••IZ

AGASSIZ
AGRIBIZ
ALBENIZ
GEEWHIZ
LEIBNIZ
POPQUIZ
SHOWBIZ
SIMONIZ

JA•••••

JABBERS
JABBING
JACALES
JACAMAR
JACCUSE
JACINTH
JACINTO
JACKALS
JACKASS
JACKDAW
JACKETS
JACKIEO
JACKING
JACKPOT
JACKSON
JACKSOO
JACKSUP
JACKTAR
JACOBIN
JACONET
JACQUES
JACUZZI
JADEDLY
JADEITE
JAECKEL
JAEGERS
JAGGIER
JAGGIES
JAGGING
JAGLESS
JAGUARS
JAIALAI
JAILERS
JAILING
JAILORS
JAINISM
JAINIST
JAKARTA
JALISCO
JAMAICA
JAMBAND
JAMBEAU
JAMCAMS
JAMESII
JAMESIV
JAMESON
JAMESVI
JAMISON
JAMLIKE
JAMMERS
JAMMIER
JAMMIES
JAMMING
JAMPACK
JANACEK
JANEANE
JANEDOE
JANEIRO
JANEWAY
JANGLED
JANGLER
JANGLES
JANITOR
JANKLOW
JANSSEN
JANSSON
JANUARY
JANVIER
JAPHETH
JARDINE
JARDINS
JARFULS
JARGONS
JARGONY
JARLESS
JAROMIR
JARRELL
JARRETT
JARRING
JARROTT
JASMINE
JASPERS
JASPERY
JAUNTED
JAVAMAN
JAVELIN
JAWBONE
JAWEDAT
JAWLESS
JAWLIKE
JAWLINE
JAYBIRD
JAYCEES
JAYLENO
JAYVEES
JAYWALK
JAYWARD
JAZZAGE
JAZZBOS
JAZZERS
JAZZIER
JAZZILY
JAZZING
JAZZISH
JAZZMAN
JAZZMEN

J•A••••

JCARROL
JEALOUS
JEANARP
JEANLUC
JEANNIE
JEANNOT
JOACHIM
JOAQUIN

J••A•••

JACALES
JACAMAR
JAIALAI
JAKARTA
JAMAICA
JANACEK
JAVAMAN
JICAMAS
JIRASEK
JOCASTA
JOHANNA
JOMARCH
JUDAICA
JUDAISM
JUDASES
JUMADAS
JUMANJI

J•••A••

JACKALS
JACKASS
JAGUARS
JAMBAND
JAMCAMS
JAMPACK
JANEANE
JANUARY
JAYWALK
JAYWARD
JAZZAGE
JEANARP
JETFANS
JETLAGS
JETPACK
JETWASH
JETWAYS
JIGSAWS
JIMDALE
JIMJAMS
JIMKAAT
JOBBANK
JOBFAIR
JOBJARS
JOECAMP
JONHALL
JORDANA
JOUHAUX
JOYPADS
JUDEANS
JUGBAND
JULIANA
JUNKART
JUTLAND

J••••A•

JACAMAR
JACKDAW
JACKTAR
JAIALAI
JAMBEAU
JANEWAY
JAVAMAN
JAWEDAT
JAZZMAN
JEERSAT
JERBOAS
JETBOAT
JETSFAN
JETSTAR
JIBEDAT
JIBESAT
JICAMAS
JILLIAN
JIMBEAM
JIMDIAL
JIMKAAT
JOCULAR
JOGBRAS
JOHNGAY
JOHNJAY
JOHNLAW
JOJOBAS
JOURDAN
JOURNAL
JOYCEAN
JUDELAW
JUDOKAS
JUGHEAD
JUGULAR
JULYDAY
JUMADAS
JUMPSAT
JUNEDAY
JUNGIAN
JUNKCAR
JUNKFAX
JUNKMAN
JURYMAN
JUVENAL

J•••••A

JAKARTA
JAMAICA
JEPHTHA
JERITZA
JESSICA
JOCASTA
JOHANNA
JORDANA
JOSEPHA
JUDAICA
JULIANA
JUNKDNA

•JA••••

AJACCIO
HJALMAR

•J••A••
AJOWANS

•J•••A•
HJALMAR
OJIBWAS
OJIBWAY

••JA•••
GUJARAT
HIJACKS
MOJAVES
PAJAMAS
PDJAMES
RAJARAO
REJAILS
STJAMES
TEJANAS
TEJANOS
UNJADED

••J•A••
FIJIANS
TIJUANA

••J••A•
EIJKMAN
FAJITAS
FUJISAN
GUJARAT
JOJOBAS
PAJAMAS
RAJARAO
TEJANAS

••J•••A
LAJOLLA
MAJORCA
TIJUANA
WOJTYLA

•••JA••
BIGJAKE
CARJACK
DEEJAYS
JIMJAMS
JOBJARS
LOGJAMS
PUNJABI
REDJACK
SKYJACK
TIPJARS
TROJANS
VEEJAYS

•••J•A•
DONJUAN
SANJUAN
TOMJOAD
VALJEAN

•••J••A
IWOJIMA

••••JA•
ABIDJAN
ALANJAY
BELLJAR
BLUEJAY
CULTJAM
GRAYJAY
JOHNJAY
KARAJAN
KELLJAN
LEFTJAB
LOCKJAW
LTKOJAK

•••••JA
ALFORJA
MARUSJA

J•B••••
JABBERS
JABBING
JEBBUSH
JIBBOOM
JIBEDAT
JIBESAT
JOBBANK
JOBBERS
JOBBERY
JOBBING
JOBCUTS
JOBFAIR
JOBHOPS
JOBHUNT
JOBJARS
JOBLESS
JOBLOCK
JOBLOTS
JOBSHOP
JUBILEE

J••B•••
JABBERS
JABBING
JAMBAND
JAMBEAU
JAWBONE
JAYBIRD
JEBBUSH
JEEBIES
JERBOAS
JETBOAT
JIBBOOM
JIMBEAM
JOBBANK
JOBBERS
JOBBERY
JOBBING
JOEBLOW
JOEBUCK
JOGBRAS
JOSBOYS
JROBERT
JUGBAND
JUMBLED
JUMBLER
JUMBLES
JUMBUCK

J•••B••
JACOBIN
JAZZBOS
JEZEBEL
JOHNBOY
JOJOBAS
JUJUBES
JUKEBOX
JUMPBID
JUNEBUG
JURYBOX

J•••••B
JOHNNYB

•J•B•••
OJIBWAS
OJIBWAY

••J•B••
JOJOBAS
JUJUBES

••J••B•
AAJUMBO

•••J•B•
BAGJOBS
CONJOBS
DAYJOBS
DYEJOBS
NEWJOBS
ODDJOBS
PUNJABI

••••J•B
BANKJOB
EASYJOB
GETAJOB
GOODJOB
GOTAJOB
HADAJOB
LEFTJAB
LUBEJOB
NICEJOB
NOSEJOB
SNOWJOB
TEMPJOB

JC•••••
JCARROL
JCPOWYS

J•C••••
JACALES
JACAMAR
JACCUSE
JACINTH
JACINTO
JACKALS
JACKASS
JACKDAW
JACKETS
JACKIEO
JACKING
JACKPOT
JACKSON
JACKSOO
JACKSUP
JACKTAR
JACOBIN
JACONET
JACQUES
JACUZZI
JICAMAS
JOCASTA
JOCELYN
JOCKEYS
JOCULAR

J••C•••
JACCUSE
JAECKEL
JAMCAMS
JAYCEES
JIMCHEE
JOACHIM
JOBCUTS
JOECAMP
JOECOOL
JOYCEAN
JUICERS
JUICEUP
JUICIER
JUICILY
JUICING
JUNCOES

J•••C••
JANACEK
JERICHO
JOUNCED
JOUNCES
JUMPCUT
JUNKCAR

J••••C•
JALISCO
JAMAICA
JAMPACK
JESSICA
JETPACK
JIMRICE
JOBLOCK
JOEBUCK
JOMARCH
JUDAICA
JUMBUCK
JUSTICE

J•••••C
JEANLUC
JURIDIC

•J•C•••
AJACCIO
EJECTED
EJECTOR

•J••C••
AJACCIO

•J••••C
FJORDIC

••J•C••
DEJECTS
HIJACKS
INJECTS
OBJECTS
REJECTS

••J••C•
ADJUNCT
MAJORCA
REJOICE
UNJUICY

•••J•C•
CARJACK
IOBJECT
PROJECT
REDJACK
REEJECT
SKYJACK
SUBJECT

JD•••••
JDPOWER

J•D••••
JADEDLY
JADEITE
JODHPUR
JODRELL
JUDAICA
JUDAISM
JUDASES
JUDEANS
JUDELAW
JUDGERS
JUDGING
JUDOIST
JUDOKAS

J••D•••
JARDINE
JARDINS
JIMDALE
JIMDIAL
JORDANA
JOTDOWN

J•••D••
JACKDAW
JADEDLY
JANEDOE
JAWEDAT
JIBEDAT
JOEYDEE
JOHNDOE
JOINDER
JOURDAN
JULYDAY
JUMADAS
JUNEDAY
JUNKDNA
JURIDIC

J••••D•
JOEKIDD
JOYPADS
JOYRIDE

J•••••D
JAMBAND
JANGLED
JAUNTED
JAYBIRD
JAYWARD
JELLIED
JETTIED
JEWELED
JIGGLED
JIMMIED
JINGLED
JOEKIDD
JOGGLED
JOINTED
JOISTED
JOLLIED
JONESED
JOSTLED
JOUNCED
JOUSTED
JUGBAND
JUGGLED
JUGHEAD
JUMBLED
JUMPBID
JUTLAND

•J••D••
FJORDIC

•J••••D
EJECTED

••J•D••
ADJUDGE
REJUDGE
UNJADED

••J•••D
ABJURED
ADJURED
CAJOLED
ENJOYED
INJURED
MAJORED
UNJADED
UNJOYED

•••J•D•
HEYJUDE

••••J•D
TOMJOAD

JE•••••
JEALOUS
JEANARP
JEANLUC
JEANNIE
JEANNOT
JEBBUSH
JEEBIES
JEEPERS
JEERERS
JEERING
JEERSAT
JEFFERS
JEFFREY
JEJUNUM
JELLIED
JELLIES
JELLIFY
JELLING
JEMISON
JENKINS
JENNETS
JEPHTHA
JERBOAS
JERGENS
JERICHO
JERILYN
JERITZA
JERKERS
JERKIER
JERKIES
JERKILY
JERKING
JERKINS
JERKOUT
JERKSUP
JERSEYS
JESSICA
JESTERS
JESTING
JESUITS
JETBOAT
JETFANS
JETFIRE
JETFOIL
JETGUNS
JETLAGS
JETPACK
JETPORT
JETSETS
JETSFAN
JETSKIS
JETSONS
JETSTAR
JETTIED
JETTIES
JETTING
JETWASH
JETWAYS
JEWELED
JEWELER
JEWELRY
JEWISON
JEZEBEL

J•E••••
JAECKEL
JAEGERS
JEEBIES
JEEPERS
JEERERS
JEERING
JEERSAT
JOEBLOW
JOEBUCK
JOECAMP
JOECOOL
JOEHILL
JOEKIDD
JOEROTH
JOEYDEE
JREWING

J••E•••
JADEDLY
JADEITE
JAMESII
JAMESIV
JAMESON
JAMESVI
JANEANE
JANEDOE
JANEIRO
JANEWAY
JAVELIN
JAWEDAT
JEWELED
JEWELER
JEWELRY
JEZEBEL
JIBEDAT
JIBESAT
JIMENEZ
JOCELYN
JONERIK
JONESED
JONESES
JOSEPHA
JOSEPHI
JUDEANS
JUDELAW
JUKEBOX
JUNEBUG
JUNEDAY
JUVENAL

J•••E••
JABBERS
JACKETS
JAEGERS
JAGLESS
JAILERS
JAMBEAU
JAMMERS
JAPHETH
JARLESS
JARRELL
JARRETT
JASPERS
JASPERY
JAWLESS
JAYCEES
JAYLENO
JAYVEES
JAZZERS
JEEPERS
JEERERS
JEFFERS
JENNETS
JERGENS
JERKERS
JERSEYS
JESTERS
JETSETS
JIGGERS
JIGGERY
JILTERS
JIMBEAM
JINXERS
JITNEYS
JITTERS
JITTERY
JIVIEST
JOBBERS
JOBBERY
JOBLESS
JOCKEYS
JODRELL
JOGGERS
JOINERS
JOINERY
JOKIEST
JOLTERS
JOSHERS
JOTTERS
JOYCEAN
JOYLESS
JROBERT
JUDGERS
JUGHEAD
JUICERS
JUICEUP
JUMPERS
JUNKERS
JUNKETS
JURGENS
JUSTEST

J••••E•
JACALES
JACKIEO
JACONET
JACQUES
JAECKEL
JAGGIER
JAGGIES
JAMMIER
JAMMIES
JANACEK
JANGLED
JANGLER
JANGLES
JANSSEN
JANVIER
JAUNTED
JAYCEES
JAYVEES
JAZZIER
JAZZMEN
JDPOWER
JEEBIES
JEFFREY
JELLIED
JELLIES
JERKIER
JERKIES
JETTIED
JETTIES
JEWELED
JEWELER
JEZEBEL
JIFFIES
JIGGIER
JIGGLED
JIGGLES
JIMCHEE
JIMENEZ
JIMINEZ
JIMMIED
JIMMIES
JINGLED
JINGLER
JINGLES
JINGOES
JIRASEK
JOEYDEE
JOFFREY
JOGGLED
JOGGLER
JOGGLES
JOHNLEE
JOINDER
JOINTED
JOINTER
JOISTED
JOLLIED
JOLLIER
JOLLIES
JOLLIET
JOLTIER
JONESED
JONESES
JOSTLED
JOSTLER
JOSTLES
JOUNCED
JOUNCES
JOURNEE
JOURNEY
JOUSTED
JOUSTER
JOWLIER
JTMONEY
JUBILEE
JUDASES
JUGGLED
JUGGLER
JUGGLES
JUICIER
JUILLET
JUJUBES
JUMBLED
JUMBLER
JUMBLES
JUMPIER
JUNCOES
JUNGLES
JUNIPER
JUNKIER
JUNKIES
JUNKMEN
JUPITER
JURYMEN

J•••••E
JACCUSE
JADEITE
JAMLIKE
JANEANE
JANEDOE
JARDINE
JASMINE
JAWBONE
JAWLIKE
JAWLINE
JAZZAGE
JEANNIE
JETFIRE
JIGLIKE
JIGTIME
JIMCHEE
JIMDALE
JIMRICE
JOEYDEE
JOHNDOE
JOHNLEE
JOHNNIE
JOURNEE
JOYRIDE
JSTROKE
JUBILEE
JUGWINE
JUSTICE
JUSTINE
JUSTONE

•JE••••
EJECTED
EJECTOR
EJEMPLO
GJETOST
KJELLIN

•J•E•••
HJHEINZ

•J•••E•
EJECTED

••JE•••
BEJEWEL
DEJECTS
INJECTS
LEJEUNE
MAJESTE
MAJESTY
MAJEURE
MUJERES
OBJECTS
REJECTS

••J•E••
MAJGENS

••J••E•
ABJURED
ABJURER
ABJURES
ADJURED
ADJURER
ADJURES
BEJEWEL
BUJONES
CAJOLED
CAJOLER
CAJOLES
ENJOYED
ENJOYER
INJOKES
INJURED
INJURER
INJURES
JUJUBES
KCJONES
MAJORED
MOJAVES
MRJONES
MUJERES
PDJAMES
STJAMES
UNJADED
UNJOYED

••J•••E
ADJUDGE
LEJEUNE
MAJESTE
MAJEURE
REJOICE
REJUDGE

•••JE••
BIGJERK
FANJETS
GASJETS
INKJETS
IOBJECT
NONJEWS
OUTJEST
OUTJETS
PROJECT
PROJETS
RAMJETS
REEJECT
SUBJECT
THEJERK
THEJETS
TRIJETS
VALJEAN

•••J•E•
BANJOES
PALJOEY

•••J••E
ASAJOKE
BADJOKE
BIGJAKE
CONJURE
DONJOSE
FRIJOLE
HEYJUDE
MIDJUNE
OLDJOKE
PERJURE
SANJOSE

••••JE•
LEARJET
PROPJET
RESOJET
TWINJET

••••J•E
GOODJOE
HOLYJOE
MEANJOE

J•F••••
JEFFERS
JEFFREY
JIFFIES
JOFFREY

J••F•••
JARFULS
JEFFERS
JEFFREY
JETFANS
JETFIRE
JETFOIL
JIFFIES
JIMFIXX
JOBFAIR
JOFFREY
JUGFULS

J•••F••
JETSFAN
JUNKFAX

J••••F•
JELLIFY
JOLLIFY
JUMPOFF
JUSTIFY

J•••••F
JUMPOFF

•••J•F•
INAJIFF

•••J••F
INAJIFF

J•G••••
JAGGIER
JAGGIES
JAGGING
JAGLESS
JAGUARS
JIGGERS
JIGGERY
JIGGIER
JIGGING
JIGGISH
JIGGLED
JIGGLES
JIGLIKE
JIGSAWS
JIGTIME
JOGBRAS
JOGGERS
JOGGING
JOGGLED
JOGGLER
JOGGLES
JOGTROT
JUGBAND
JUGFULS
JUGGING
JUGGLED
JUGGLER
JUGGLES
JUGHEAD
JUGULAR
JUGWINE

J••G•••
JAEGERS
JAGGIER

JAGGIES
JAGGING
JANGLED
JANGLER
JANGLES
JARGONS
JARGONY
JERGENS
JETGUNS
JIGGERS
JIGGERY
JIGGIER
JIGGING
JIGGISH
JIGGLED
JIGGLES
JINGLED
JINGLER
JINGLES
JINGOES
JOGGERS
JOGGING
JOGGLED
JOGGLER
JOGGLES
JUDGERS
JUDGING
JUGGING
JUGGLED
JUGGLER
JUGGLES
JUNGIAN
JUNGLES
JURGENS

J•••G••
JOHNGAY

J••••G•
JAZZAGE
JETLAGS
JIMHOGG

J•••••G
JABBING
JACKING
JAGGING
JAILING
JAMMING
JARRING
JAZZING
JEERING
JELLING
JERKING
JESTING
JETTING
JIGGING
JILTING
JIMHOGG
JINXING
JOBBING
JOGGING
JOINING
JOLTING
JOSHING
JOTTING
JREWING
JUDGING
JUGGING
JUICING
JUMPING
JUNEBUG
JUNKING
JURYING
JURYRIG
JUTTING

••JG•••
MAJGENS

••J••G•
ADJUDGE
BYJINGO
REJUDGE

•••J••G
BEIJING
NANJING

J•H••••
JOHANNA
JOHNBOY
JOHNDOE
JOHNGAY
JOHNIII
JOHNJAY
JOHNLAW
JOHNLEE
JOHNNIE
JOHNNYB
JOHNSON
JOHNVII
JOHNWOO
JOHNXII
JOHNXIV
JOHNXIX
JOHNXVI
JOHNXXI

J••H•••
JAPHETH
JEPHTHA
JIMHOGG
JOBHOPS
JOBHUNT
JODHPUR
JOEHILL
JONHALL
JOSHERS
JOSHING
JOUHAUX
JUGHEAD

J•••H••
JIMCHEE
JOACHIM
JOBSHOP

J••••H•
JEPHTHA
JERICHO
JOSEPHA
JOSEPHI

J•••••H
JACINTH
JAPHETH
JAZZISH
JEBBUSH
JETWASH
JIGGISH
JOEROTH
JOMARCH

•JH••••
HJHEINZ

••J•H••
STJOHNS

•••J•H•
BIGJOHN
IIIJOHN

JI•••••
JIBBOOM
JIBEDAT
JIBESAT
JICAMAS
JIFFIES
JIGGERS
JIGGERY
JIGGIER
JIGGING
JIGGISH
JIGGLED
JIGGLES
JIGLIKE
JIGSAWS
JIGTIME
JILLIAN
JILLION
JILTERS
JILTING
JIMBEAM
JIMCHEE
JIMDALE
JIMDIAL
JIMENEZ
JIMFIXX
JIMHOGG
JIMINEZ
JIMJAMS
JIMKAAT
JIMMIED
JIMMIES
JIMRICE
JIMRYUN
JIMSONS
JINGLED
JINGLER
JINGLES
JINGOES
JINXERS
JINXING
JIRASEK
JITNEYS
JITTERS
JITTERY
JIVIEST

J•I••••
JAIALAI
JAILERS
JAILING
JAILORS
JAINISM
JAINIST
JOINDER
JOINERS
JOINERY
JOINING
JOINSIN
JOINSUP
JOINTED
JOINTER
JOINTLY
JOISTED
JUICERS
JUICEUP
JUICIER
JUICILY
JUICING
JUILLET

J••I•••
JACINTH
JACINTO
JALISCO
JAMISON
JANITOR
JEMISON
JERICHO
JERILYN
JERITZA
JEWISON
JIMINEZ
JIVIEST
JOKIEST
JUBILEE
JUJITSU
JULIANA
JUNIORS
JUNIPER
JUPITER
JURIDIC
JURISTS

J•••I••
JABBING
JACKIEO
JACKING
JADEITE
JAGGIER
JAGGIES
JAGGING
JAILING
JAINISM
JAINIST
JAMAICA
JAMLIKE
JAMMIER
JAMMIES
JAMMING
JANEIRO
JANVIER
JARDINE
JARDINS
JARRING
JASMINE
JAWLIKE
JAWLINE
JAYBIRD
JAZZIER
JAZZILY
JAZZING
JAZZISH
JEEBIES
JEERING
JELLIED
JELLIES
JELLIFY
JELLING
JENKINS
JERKIER
JERKIES
JERKILY
JERKING
JERKINS
JESSICA
JESTING
JESUITS
JETFIRE
JETTIED
JETTIES
JETTING
JIFFIES
JIGGIER
JIGGING
JIGGISH
JIGLIKE
JIGTIME
JILLIAN
JILLION
JILTING
JIMDIAL
JIMFIXX
JIMMIED
JIMMIES
JIMRICE
JINXING
JOBBING
JOEHILL
JOEKIDD
JOGGING
JOHNIII
JOINING
JOLLIED
JOLLIER
JOLLIES
JOLLIET
JOLLIFY
JOLLILY
JOLLITY
JOLTIER
JOLTING
JOSHING
JOTTING
JOWLIER
JOYRIDE
JREWING
JUDAICA
JUDAISM
JUDGING
JUDOIST
JUGGING
JUGWINE
JUICIER
JUICILY
JUICING
JUMPIER
JUMPILY
JUMPING
JUNGIAN
JUNKIER
JUNKIES
JUNKING
JURYING
JUSTICE
JUSTIFY
JUSTINE
JUTTING

J••••I•
JACOBIN
JAMESII
JAMESIV
JAROMIR
JAVELIN
JEANNIE
JETFOIL
JETSKIS
JOACHIM
JOAQUIN
JOBFAIR
JOHNIII
JOHNNIE
JOHNVII
JOHNXII
JOHNXIV
JOHNXIX
JOINSIN
JONERIK
JONQUIL
JUMPBID
JUMPSIN
JURIDIC
JURYRIG

J•••••I
JACUZZI
JAIALAI
JAMESII
JAMESVI
JOHNIII
JOHNVII
JOHNXII
JOHNXVI
JOHNXXI
JOSEPHI
JUMANJI

•JI••••
DJINNIS
OJIBWAS
OJIBWAY

•J•I•••
AJSIMON

•J••I••
HJHEINZ

•J•••I•
AJACCIO
DJINNIS
FJORDIC
KJELLIN

••JI•••
BYJINGO
FAJITAS
FIJIANS
FUJISAN
FUJITSU
HIJINKS
JUJITSU
MOJITOS

••J•I••
ADJOINS
ENJOINS
REJAILS
REJOICE
REJOINS
UNJOINS
UNJOINT
UNJUICY

••J••I•
MAJORIN

•••JI••
BEIJING
INAJIFF
IWOJIMA
NANJING
OUTJINX

•••J•I•
CONJOIN
DISJOIN
MISJOIN
SUBJOIN

•••J••I
BONJOVI
PUNJABI

••••JI•
LORDJIM
ROMAJIS
SLIMJIM

•••••JI
BASENJI
JUMANJI

J•J••••
JEJUNUM
JOJOBAS
JUJITSU
JUJUBES

J••J•••
JIMJAMS
JOBJARS

J•••J••
JOHNJAY

J••••J•
JUMANJI

JK•••••
JKLMNOP

J•K••••
JAKARTA
JOKIEST
JUKEBOX

J••K•••
JACKALS
JACKASS
JACKDAW
JACKETS
JACKIEO
JACKING
JACKPOT
JACKSON
JACKSOO
JACKSUP
JACKTAR
JANKLOW
JENKINS
JERKERS
JERKIER
JERKIES
JERKILY
JERKING
JERKINS
JERKOUT
JERKSUP
JIMKAAT
JOCKEYS
JOEKIDD
JUNKART
JUNKCAR
JUNKDNA
JUNKERS
JUNKETS
JUNKFAX
JUNKIER
JUNKIES
JUNKING
JUNKMAN
JUNKMEN

J•••K••
JAECKEL
JETSKIS
JUDOKAS

J••••K•
JAMLIKE
JAWLIKE
JIGLIKE
JSTROKE

J•••••K
JAMPACK
JANACEK
JAYWALK
JETPACK
JIRASEK
JOBBANK
JOBLOCK
JOEBUCK
JONERIK
JUMBUCK

•JK••••
IJKLMNO

••JK•••
EIJKMAN
HIJKLMN

••J•K••
INJOKES

••J••K•
DEJUNKS
HIJACKS
HIJINKS

•••JK••
GHIJKLM

•••J•K•
ASAJOKE
BADJOKE
BIGJAKE
OLDJOKE

•••J••K
BIGJERK
CARJACK
REDJACK
SKYJACK
THEJERK

••••JK•
FGHIJKL

•••••JK
EFGHIJK

J•L••••
JALISCO
JELLIED
JELLIES
JELLIFY
JELLING
JILLIAN
JILLION
JILTERS
JILTING
JKLMNOP
JOLLIED
JOLLIER
JOLLIES
JOLLIET
JOLLIFY
JOLLILY
JOLLITY
JOLTERS
JOLTIER
JOLTING
JULIANA
JULYDAY

J••L•••
JAGLESS
JAILERS
JAILING
JAILORS
JAMLIKE
JARLESS
JAWLESS
JAWLIKE
JAWLINE
JAYLENO
JEALOUS
JELLIED
JELLIES
JELLIFY
JELLING
JETLAGS
JIGLIKE
JILLIAN
JILLION
JOBLESS
JOBLOCK
JOBLOTS
JOLLIED
JOLLIER
JOLLIES
JOLLIET
JOLLIFY
JOLLILY
JOLLITY
JOWLIER
JOYLESS
JUILLET
JUTLAND

J•••L••
JACALES
JAIALAI
JANGLED
JANGLER
JANGLES
JANKLOW
JAVELIN
JEANLUC
JERILYN
JEWELED
JEWELER
JEWELRY
JIGGLED
JIGGLES
JINGLED
JINGLER
JINGLES
JOCELYN
JOCULAR
JOEBLOW
JOGGLED
JOGGLER
JOGGLES
JOHNLAW
JOHNLEE
JOSTLED
JOSTLER
JOSTLES
JUBILEE
JUDELAW
JUGGLED
JUGGLER
JUGGLES
JUGULAR
JUILLET
JUMBLED
JUMBLER
JUMBLES
JUNGLES

J••••L•
JACKALS
JADEDLY
JARFULS
JARRELL
JAYWALK
JAZZILY
JERKILY
JIMDALE
JODRELL
JOEHILL
JOINTLY
JOLLILY
JONHALL
JOPPOLO
JUGFULS
JUICILY
JUMPILY

J•••••L
JAECKEL
JARRELL
JCARROL
JETFOIL
JEZEBEL
JIMDIAL
JODRELL
JOECOOL
JOEHILL
JONHALL
JONQUIL
JOURNAL
JUVENAL

•J•L•••
HJALMAR
IJKLMNO
KJELLIN

•J••L••
KJELLIN

•J•••L•
EJEMPLO

••J•L••
CAJOLED
CAJOLER
CAJOLES
HIJKLMN
LAJOLLA
UNJOLLY

••J••L•
LAJOLLA
REJAILS
UNJOLLY
WOJTYLA

••J•••L
BEJEWEL

•••J•L•
FRIJOLE
GHIJKLM
MIDJULY

••••J•L
FGHIJKL

J•M••••
JAMAICA
JAMBAND
JAMBEAU
JAMCAMS
JAMESII
JAMESIV
JAMESON
JAMESVI
JAMISON
JAMLIKE
JAMMERS
JAMMIER
JAMMIES
JAMMING
JAMPACK
JEMISON
JIMBEAM
JIMCHEE
JIMDALE
JIMDIAL
JIMENEZ
JIMFIXX
JIMHOGG
JIMINEZ
JIMJAMS
JIMKAAT
JIMMIED
JIMMIES
JIMRICE
JIMRYUN
JIMSONS
JOMARCH
JTMONEY
JUMADAS
JUMANJI
JUMBLED
JUMBLER
JUMBLES
JUMBUCK
JUMPBID
JUMPCUT
JUMPERS
JUMPIER
JUMPILY
JUMPING
JUMPOFF
JUMPSAT
JUMPSIN
JUMPSON
JUMPSUP

J••M•••
JAMMERS
JAMMIER
JAMMIES
JAMMING
JASMINE
JIMMIED
JIMMIES
JKLMNOP

J•••M••
JACAMAR
JAROMIR
JAVAMAN
JAZZMAN
JAZZMEN
JICAMAS
JUNKMAN
JUNKMEN
JURYMAN
JURYMEN

J••••M•
JAMCAMS
JIGTIME
JIMJAMS
JOECAMP

J•••••M
JAINISM
JEJUNUM
JIBBOOM
JIMBEAM
JOACHIM
JUDAISM

•J•M•••
EJEMPLO

•J••M••
AJSIMON
HJALMAR
IJKLMNO

••J•M••
AAJUMBO
EIJKMAN
PAJAMAS
PDJAMES
STJAMES

••J••M•
HIJKLMN

••J•••M
JEJUNUM

•••J•M•
IWOJIMA
JIMJAMS
LOGJAMS
OUTJUMP
SKIJUMP

•••J••M
GHIJKLM

••••J•M
CULTJAM
LORDJIM
SLIMJIM

J•N••••
JANACEK
JANEANE
JANEDOE
JANEIRO
JANEWAY
JANGLED
JANGLER
JANGLES

7
JG

JANITOR
JANKLOW
JANSSEN
JANSSON
JANUARY
JANVIER
JENKINS
JENNETS
JINGLED
JINGLER
JINGLES
JINGOES
JINXERS
JINXING
JONERIK
JONESED
JONESES
JONHALL
JONQUIL
JUNCOES
JUNEBUG
JUNEDAY
JUNGIAN
JUNGLES
JUNIORS
JUNIPER
JUNKART
JUNKCAR
JUNKDNA
JUNKERS
JUNKETS
JUNKFAX
JUNKIER
JUNKIES
JUNKING
JUNKMAN
JUNKMEN

J••N•••

JAINISM
JAINIST
JAUNTED
JEANARP
JEANLUC
JEANNIE
JEANNOT
JENNETS
JITNEYS
JOHNBOY
JOHNDOE
JOHNGAY
JOHNIII
JOHNJAY
JOHNLAW
JOHNLEE
JOHNNIE
JOHNNYB
JOHNSON
JOHNVII
JOHNWOO
JOHNXII
JOHNXIV
JOHNXIX
JOHNXVI
JOHNXXI
JOINDER
JOINERS
JOINERY
JOINING
JOINSIN
JOINSUP
JOINTED
JOINTER
JOINTLY
JOUNCED
JOUNCES

J•••N••

JACINTH
JACINTO
JACONET
JEANNIE
JEANNOT
JEJUNUM
JIMENEZ
JIMINEZ
JKLMNOP
JOHANNA
JOHNNIE
JOHNNYB
JOURNAL
JOURNEE
JOURNEY
JOURNOS
JTMONEY
JUMANJI
JUSTNOW
JUVENAL

J••••N•

JABBING
JACKING
JAGGING
JAILING
JAMBAND
JAMMING
JANEANE
JARDINE
JARDINS
JARGONS
JARGONY
JARRING
JASMINE
JAWBONE
JAWLINE
JAYLENO
JAZZING
JEERING
JELLING
JENKINS
JERGENS
JERKING
JERKINS
JESTING
JETFANS
JETGUNS
JETSONS
JETTING
JIGGING
JILTING
JIMSONS
JINXING
JOBBANK
JOBBING
JOBHUNT
JOGGING
JOHANNA
JOINING
JOLTING
JORDANA
JOSHING
JOTTING
JREWING
JUDEANS
JUDGING
JUGBAND
JUGGING
JUGWINE
JUICING
JULIANA
JUMPING
JUNKDNA
JUNKING
JURGENS
JURYING
JUSTINE
JUSTONE
JUTLAND
JUTTING

J••••••N

JACKSON
JACOBIN
JAMESON
JAMISON
JANSSEN
JANSSON
JAVAMAN
JAVELIN
JAZZMAN
JAZZMEN
JEMISON
JERILYN
JETSFAN
JEWISON
JILLIAN
JILLION
JIMRYUN
JOAQUIN
JOCELYN
JOHNSON
JOINSIN
JOTDOWN
JOURDAN
JOYCEAN
JUMPSIN
JUMPSON
JUNGIAN
JUNKMAN
JUNKMEN
JURYMAN
JURYMEN

•J•N•••

DJINNIS

•J••N••

DJINNIS

•J•••N•

AJOWANS
HJHEINZ
IJKLMNO

•J••••N

AJSIMON
KJELLIN

••J•N••

ADJUNCT
BUJONES
BYJINGO
DEJUNKS
HIJINKS
JEJUNUM
KCJONES
MRJONES
TEJANAS
TEJANOS

••J••N•

ADJOINS
ENJOINS
FIJIANS
LEJEUNE
MAJGENS
REJOINS
STJOHNS
TIJUANA
UNJOINS
UNJOINT

••J•••N

ADJOURN
EIJKMAN
FUJISAN
HIJKLMN
MAJORIN
SOJOURN

•••J•N•

BEIJING
DONJONS
MIDJUNE
NANJING
OUTJINX
TROJANS

•••J••N

BIGJOHN
CONJOIN
DISJOIN
DONJUAN
IIIJOHN
MISJOIN
SANJUAN
SUBJOIN
VALJEAN

••••J•N

ABIDJAN
ELCAJON
KARAJAN
KELLJAN

•••••JN

VANRIJN

JO•••••

JOACHIM
JOAQUIN
JOBBANK
JOBBERS
JOBBERY
JOBBING
JOBCUTS
JOBFAIR
JOBHOPS
JOBHUNT
JOBJARS
JOBLESS
JOBLOCK
JOBLOTS
JOBSHOP
JOCASTA
JOCELYN
JOCKEYS
JOCULAR
JODHPUR
JODRELL
JOEBLOW
JOEBUCK
JOECAMP
JOECOOL
JOEHILL
JOEKIDD
JOEROTH
JOEYDEE
JOFFREY
JOGBRAS
JOGGERS
JOGGING
JOGGLED
JOGGLER
JOGGLES
JOGTROT
JOHANNA
JOHNBOY
JOHNDOE
JOHNGAY
JOHNIII
JOHNJAY
JOHNLAW
JOHNLEE
JOHNNIE
JOHNNYB
JOHNSON
JOHNVII
JOHNWOO
JOHNXII
JOHNXIV
JOHNXIX
JOHNXVI
JOHNXXI
JOINDER
JOINERS
JOINERY
JOINING
JOINSIN
JOINSUP
JOINTED
JOINTER
JOINTLY
JOISTED
JOJOBAS
JOKIEST
JOLLIED
JOLLIER
JOLLIES
JOLLIET
JOLLIFY
JOLLILY
JOLLITY
JOLTERS
JOLTIER
JOLTING
JOMARCH
JONERIK
JONESED
JONESES
JONHALL
JONQUIL
JOPPOLO
JORDANA
JOSBOYS
JOSEPHA
JOSEPHI
JOSHERS
JOSHING
JOSTLED
JOSTLER
JOSTLES
JOTDOWN
JOTTERS
JOTTING
JOUHAUX
JOUNCED
JOUNCES
JOURDAN
JOURNAL
JOURNEE
JOURNEY
JOURNOS
JOUSTED
JOUSTER
JOWLIER
JOYCEAN
JOYLESS
JOYPADS
JOYRIDE

J•O••••

JROBERT

J••O•••

JACOBIN
JACONET
JAROMIR
JCPOWYS
JDPOWER
JOJOBAS
JTMONEY
JUDOIST
JUDOKAS

J•••O••

JAILORS
JARGONS
JARGONY
JARROTT
JAWBONE
JEALOUS
JERBOAS
JERKOUT
JETBOAT
JETFOIL
JETPORT
JETSONS
JIBBOOM
JIMHOGG
JIMSONS
JINGOES
JOBHOPS
JOBLOCK
JOBLOTS
JOECOOL
JOEROTH
JOPPOLO
JOSBOYS
JOTDOWN
JSTROKE
JUMPOFF
JUNCOES
JUNIORS
JUSTONE
JUSTOUT

J••••O•

JACKPOT
JACKSON
JACKSOO
JAMESON
JAMISON
JANEDOE
JANITOR
JANKLOW
JANSSON
JAZZBOS
JCARROL
JEANNOT
JEMISON
JEWISON
JIBBOOM
JILLION
JKLMNOP
JOBSHOP
JOEBLOW
JOECOOL
JOGTROT
JOHNBOY
JOHNDOE
JOHNSON
JOHNWOO
JOURNOS
JUKEBOX
JUMPSON
JURYBOX
JUSTNOW

J•••••O

JACINTO
JACKIEO
JACKSOO
JALISCO
JANEIRO
JAYLENO
JERICHO
JOHNWOO
JOPPOLO

•JO••••

AJOWANS
FJORDIC

•J••O••

GJETOST

•J•••O•

AJSIMON
EJECTOR

•J••••O

AJACCIO
EJEMPLO
IJKLMNO

••JO•••

ADJOINS
ADJOURN
BUJONES
CAJOLED
CAJOLER
CAJOLES
ENJOINS
ENJOYED
ENJOYER
INJOKES
JOJOBAS
KCJONES
LAJOLLA
MAJORCA
MAJORED
MAJORIN
MRJONES
REJOICE
REJOINS
SOJOURN
STJOHNS
UNJOINS
UNJOINT
UNJOLLY
UNJOYED

••J••O•

ADJUROR
COJUROR
MOJITOS
TEJANOS

••J•••O

AAJUMBO
BYJINGO
RAJARAO

•••JO••

ASAJOKE
BADJOKE
BAGJOBS
BANJOES
BIGJOHN
BONJOUR
BONJOVI
CONJOBS
CONJOIN
DAYJOBS
DISJOIN
DONJONS
DONJOSE
DYEJOBS
FRIJOLE
IIIJOHN
MISJOIN
NEWJOBS
ODDJOBS
OLDJOKE
PALJOEY
SANJOSE
SUBJOIN
TOMJOAD

••••JO•

BANKJOB
EASYJOB
ELCAJON
GETAJOB
GOODJOB
GOODJOE
GOTAJOB
HADAJOB
HOLYJOE
KILLJOY
LOVEJOY
LUBEJOB
MEANJOE
NAVAJOS
NICEJOB
NOSEJOB
OVERJOY
REENJOY
SNOWJOB
TEMPJOB

•••••JO

AZULEJO
SAMMYJO
VALLEJO

J•P••••

JAPHETH
JCPOWYS
JDPOWER
JEPHTHA
JOPPOLO
JUPITER

J••P•••

JAMPACK
JASPERS
JASPERY
JEEPERS
JETPACK
JETPORT
JOPPOLO
JOYPADS
JUMPBID
JUMPCUT
JUMPERS
JUMPIER
JUMPILY
JUMPING
JUMPOFF
JUMPSAT
JUMPSIN
JUMPSON
JUMPSUP

J•••P••

JACKPOT
JODHPUR
JOSEPHA
JOSEPHI
JUNIPER

J••••P•

JOBHOPS

J•••••P

JACKSUP
JEANARP
JERKSUP
JKLMNOP
JOBSHOP
JOECAMP
JOINSUP
JUICEUP
JUMPSUP

•J•P•••

EJEMPLO

•••J••P

OUTJUMP
SKIJUMP

J••Q•••

JACQUES
JOAQUIN
JONQUIL

JR•••••

JREWING
JROBERT

J•R••••

JARDINE
JARDINS
JARFULS
JARGONS
JARGONY
JARLESS
JAROMIR
JARRELL
JARRETT
JARRING
JARROTT
JERBOAS
JERGENS
JERICHO
JERILYN
JERITZA
JERKERS
JERKIER
JERKIES
JERKILY
JERKING
JERKINS
JERKOUT
JERKSUP
JERSEYS
JIRASEK
JORDANA
JURGENS
JURIDIC
JURISTS
JURYBOX
JURYING
JURYMAN
JURYMEN
JURYRIG

J••R•••

JARRELL
JARRETT
JARRING
JARROTT
JCARROL
JEERERS
JEERING
JEERSAT
JIMRICE
JIMRYUN
JODRELL
JOEROTH
JOURDAN
JOURNAL
JOURNEE
JOURNEY
JOURNOS
JOYRIDE
JSTROKE

J•••R••

JAKARTA
JCARROL
JEFFREY
JOFFREY
JOGBRAS
JOGTROT
JOMARCH
JONERIK
JURYRIG

J••••R•

JABBERS
JAEGERS
JAGUARS
JAILERS
JAILORS
JAMMERS
JANEIRO
JANUARY
JASPERS
JASPERY
JAYBIRD
JAYWARD
JAZZERS
JEANARP
JEEPERS
JEERERS
JEFFERS
JERKERS
JESTERS
JETFIRE
JETPORT
JEWELRY
JIGGERS
JIGGERY
JILTERS
JINXERS
JITTERS
JITTERY
JOBBERS
JOBBERY
JOBJARS
JOGGERS
JOINERS
JOINERY
JOLTERS
JOSHERS
JOTTERS
JROBERT
JUDGERS
JUICERS
JUMPERS
JUNIORS
JUNKART
JUNKERS

J•••••R

JACAMAR
JACKTAR
JAGGIER
JAMMIER
JANGLER
JANITOR
JANVIER
JAROMIR
JAZZIER
JDPOWER
JERKIER
JETSTAR
JEWELER
JIGGIER
JINGLER
JOBFAIR
JOCULAR
JODHPUR
JOGGLER
JOINDER
JOINTER
JOLLIER
JOLTIER
JOSTLER
JOUSTER
JOWLIER
JUGGLER
JUGULAR
JUICIER
JUMBLER
JUMPIER
JUNIPER
JUNKCAR
JUNKIER
JUPITER

•J•R•••

FJORDIC

•J••••R

EJECTOR
HJALMAR

••J•R••

ABJURED
ABJURER
ABJURES
ADJURED
ADJURER
ADJURES
ADJUROR
COJUROR
GUJARAT
INJURED
INJURER
INJURES
MAJORCA
MAJORED
MAJORIN
MUJERES
RAJARAO

••J••R•

ADJOURN
MAJEURE
SOJOURN

••J•••R

ABJURER
ADJURER
ADJUROR
CAJOLER
COJUROR
ENJOYER
INJURER

•••J•R•

BIGJERK
CONJURE
CONJURY
JOBJARS
NONJURY
ONAJURY
PERJURE
PERJURY
THEJERK
TIPJARS

•••J••R

BONJOUR

••••J•R

BELLJAR

JS•••••

JSTROKE

J•S••••

JASMINE
JASPERS
JASPERY
JESSICA
JESTERS
JESTING
JESUITS
JOSBOYS
JOSEPHA
JOSEPHI
JOSHERS
JOSHING
JOSTLED
JOSTLER
JOSTLES
JUSTEST
JUSTICE
JUSTIFY
JUSTINE
JUSTNOW
JUSTONE
JUSTOUT

J••S•••

JANSSEN
JANSSON
JERSEYS

JESSICA
JETSETS
JETSFAN
JETSKIS
JETSONS
JETSTAR
JIGSAWS
JIMSONS
JOBSHOP
JOISTED
JOUSTED
JOUSTER

J•••S••
JACKSON
JACKSOO
JACKSUP
JALISCO
JAMESII
JAMESIV
JAMESON
JAMESVI
JAMISON
JANSSEN
JANSSON
JEERSAT
JEMISON
JERKSUP
JEWISON
JIBESAT
JIRASEK
JOCASTA
JOHNSON
JOINSIN
JOINSUP
JONESED
JONESES
JUDASES
JUMPSAT
JUMPSIN
JUMPSON
JUMPSUP
JURISTS

J••••S•
JACCUSE
JACKASS
JAGLESS
JAINISM
JAINIST
JARLESS
JAWLESS
JAZZISH
JEBBUSH
JETWASH
JIGGISH
JIVIEST
JOBLESS
JOKIEST
JOYLESS
JUDAISM
JUDOIST
JUJITSU
JUSTEST

J•••••S
JABBERS
JACALES
JACKALS
JACKASS
JACKETS
JACQUES
JAEGERS
JAGGIES
JAGLESS
JAGUARS
JAILERS
JAILORS
JAMCAMS
JAMMERS
JAMMIES
JANGLES
JARDINS
JARFULS
JARGONS
JARLESS
JASPERS
JAWLESS
JAYCEES
JAYVEES
JAZZBOS
JAZZERS
JCPOWYS
JEALOUS
JEEBIES
JEEPERS
JEERERS
JEFFERS
JELLIES
JENKINS
JENNETS
JERBOAS
JERGENS
JERKERS
JERKIES
JERKINS
JERSEYS
JESTERS
JESUITS
JETFANS
JETGUNS
JETLAGS
JETSETS
JETSKIS
JETSONS
JETTIES
JETWAYS
JICAMAS
JIFFIES
JIGGERS
JIGGLES
JIGSAWS
JILTERS
JIMJAMS
JIMMIES
JIMSONS
JINGLES
JINGOES
JINXERS
JITNEYS
JITTERS
JOBBERS
JOBCUTS
JOBHOPS
JOBJARS
JOBLESS
JOBLOTS
JOCKEYS
JOGBRAS
JOGGERS
JOGGLES
JOINERS
JOJOBAS
JOLLIES
JOLTERS
JONESES
JOSBOYS
JOSHERS
JOSTLES
JOTTERS
JOUNCES
JOURNOS
JOYLESS
JOYPADS
JUDASES
JUDEANS
JUDGERS
JUDOKAS
JUGFULS
JUGGLES
JUICERS
JUJUBES
JUMADAS
JUMBLES
JUMPERS
JUNCOES
JUNGLES
JUNIORS
JUNKERS
JUNKETS
JUNKIES
JURGENS
JURISTS

•JS••••
AJSIMON

•J•••S•
GJETOST

•J••••S
AJOWANS
DJINNIS
OJIBWAS

••J•S••
ADJUSTS
FUJISAN
MAJESTE
MAJESTY

••J••S•
FUJITSU
JUJITSU

••J•••S
ABJURES
ADJOINS
ADJURES
ADJUSTS
BUJONES
CAJOLES
DEJECTS
DEJUNKS
ENJOINS
FAJITAS
FIJIANS
HIJACKS
HIJINKS
INJECTS
INJOKES
INJURES
JOJOBAS
JUJUBES
KCJONES
MAJGENS
MOJAVES
MOJITOS
MRJONES
MUJERES
OBJECTS
PAJAMAS
PDJAMES
REJAILS
REJECTS
REJOINS
STJAMES
STJOHNS
TEJANAS
TEJANOS
UNJOINS

•••J•S•
DONJOSE
OUTJEST
SANJOSE

•••J••S
BAGJOBS
BANJOES
CONJOBS
DAYJOBS
DEEJAYS
DONJONS
DYEJOBS
FANJETS
GASJETS
INKJETS
JIMJAMS
JOBJARS
LOGJAMS
NEWJOBS
NONJEWS
ODDJOBS
OUTJETS
OUTJUTS
PROJETS
RAMJETS
THEJETS
TIPJARS
TRIJETS
TROJANS
VEEJAYS

••••J•S
NAVAJOS
ROMAJIS

•••••JS
PBANDJS

JT•••••
JTMONEY

J•T••••
JETBOAT
JETFANS
JETFIRE
JETFOIL
JETGUNS
JETLAGS
JETPACK
JETPORT
JETSETS
JETSFAN
JETSKIS
JETSONS
JETSTAR
JETTIED
JETTIES
JETTING
JETWASH
JETWAYS
JITNEYS
JITTERS
JITTERY
JOTDOWN
JOTTERS
JOTTING
JSTROKE
JUTLAND
JUTTING

J••T•••
JESTERS
JESTING
JETTIED
JETTIES
JETTING
JIGTIME
JILTERS
JILTING
JITTERS
JITTERY
JOGTROT
JOLTERS
JOLTIER
JOLTING
JOSTLED
JOSTLER
JOSTLES
JOTTERS
JOTTING
JUSTEST
JUSTICE
JUSTIFY
JUSTINE
JUSTNOW
JUSTONE
JUSTOUT
JUTTING

J•••T••
JACKTAR
JANITOR
JAUNTED
JEPHTHA
JERITZA
JETSTAR
JOINTED
JOINTER
JOINTLY
JOISTED
JOUSTED
JOUSTER
JUJITSU
JUPITER

J••••T•
JACINTH
JACINTO
JACKETS
JADEITE
JAKARTA
JAPHETH
JARRETT
JARROTT
JENNETS
JESUITS
JETSETS
JOBCUTS
JOBLOTS
JOCASTA
JOEROTH
JOLLITY
JUNKETS
JURISTS

J•••••T
JACKPOT
JACONET
JAINIST
JARRETT
JARROTT
JAWEDAT
JEANNOT
JEERSAT
JERKOUT
JETBOAT
JETPORT
JIBEDAT
JIBESAT
JIMKAAT
JIVIEST
JOBHUNT
JOGTROT
JOKIEST
JOLLIET
JROBERT
JUDOIST
JUILLET
JUMPCUT
JUMPSAT
JUNKART
JUSTEST
JUSTOUT

•J•T•••
GJETOST

•J••T••
EJECTED
EJECTOR

•J••••T
GJETOST

••JT•••
WOJTYLA

••J•T••
FAJITAS
FUJITSU
JUJITSU
MOJITOS

••J••T•
ADJUSTS
DEJECTS
INJECTS
MAJESTE
MAJESTY
OBJECTS
REJECTS

••J•••T
ADJUNCT
GUJARAT
UNJOINT

•••J•T•
FANJETS
GASJETS
INKJETS
OUTJETS
OUTJUTS
PROJETS
RAMJETS
THEJETS
TRIJETS

•••J••T
IOBJECT
OUTJEST
PROJECT
REEJECT
SUBJECT

••••J•T
LEARJET
PROPJET
RESOJET
TWINJET

JU•••••
JUBILEE
JUDAICA
JUDAISM
JUDASES
JUDEANS
JUDELAW
JUDGERS
JUDGING
JUDOIST
JUDOKAS
JUGBAND
JUGFULS
JUGGING
JUGGLED
JUGGLER
JUGGLES
JUGHEAD
JUGULAR
JUGWINE
JUICERS
JUICEUP
JUICIER
JUICILY
JUICING
JUILLET
JUJITSU
JUJUBES
JUKEBOX
JULIANA
JULYDAY
JUMADAS
JUMANJI
JUMBLED
JUMBLER
JUMBLES
JUMBUCK
JUMPBID
JUMPCUT
JUMPERS
JUMPIER
JUMPILY
JUMPING
JUMPOFF
JUMPSAT
JUMPSIN
JUMPSON
JUMPSUP
JUNCOES
JUNEBUG
JUNEDAY
JUNGIAN
JUNGLES
JUNIORS
JUNIPER
JUNKART
JUNKCAR
JUNKDNA
JUNKERS
JUNKETS
JUNKFAX
JUNKIER
JUNKIES
JUNKING
JUNKMAN
JUNKMEN
JUPITER
JURGENS
JURIDIC
JURISTS
JURYBOX
JURYING
JURYMAN
JURYMEN
JURYRIG
JUSTEST
JUSTICE
JUSTIFY
JUSTINE
JUSTNOW
JUSTONE
JUSTOUT
JUTLAND
JUTTING
JUVENAL

J•U••••
JAUNTED
JOUHAUX
JOUNCED
JOUNCES
JOURDAN
JOURNAL
JOURNEE
JOURNEY
JOURNOS
JOUSTED
JOUSTER

J••U•••
JACUZZI
JAGUARS
JANUARY
JEJUNUM
JESUITS
JOCULAR
JUGULAR
JUJUBES

J•••U••
JACCUSE
JACQUES
JARFULS
JEBBUSH
JETGUNS
JOAQUIN
JOBCUTS
JOBHUNT
JOEBUCK
JONQUIL
JUGFULS
JUMBUCK

J••••U•
JACKSUP
JEALOUS
JEANLUC
JEJUNUM
JERKOUT
JERKSUP
JIMRYUN
JODHPUR
JOINSUP
JOUHAUX
JUICEUP
JUMPCUT
JUMPSUP
JUNEBUG
JUSTOUT

J•••••U
JAMBEAU
JUJITSU

••JU•••
AAJUMBO
ABJURED
ABJURER
ABJURES
ADJUDGE
ADJUNCT
ADJURED
ADJURER
ADJURES
ADJUROR
ADJUSTS
COJUROR
DEJUNKS
INJURED
INJURER
INJURES
JEJUNUM
JUJUBES
REJUDGE
TIJUANA
UNJUICY

••J•U••
ADJOURN
LEJEUNE
MAJEURE
SOJOURN

••J••U•
JEJUNUM

••J•••U
FUJITSU
JUJITSU

•••JU••
CONJURE
CONJURY
DONJUAN
HEYJUDE
MIDJULY
MIDJUNE
NONJURY
ONAJURY
OUTJUMP
OUTJUTS
PERJURE
PERJURY
SANJUAN
SKIJUMP

•••J•U•
BONJOUR

J•V••••
JAVAMAN
JAVELIN
JIVIEST
JUVENAL

J••V•••
JANVIER
JAYVEES

J•••V••
JOHNVII

J••••V•
JAMESVI
JOHNXVI

J•••••V
JAMESIV
JOHNXIV

••J•V••
MOJAVES

•••J•V•
BONJOVI

J•W••••
JAWBONE
JAWEDAT
JAWLESS
JAWLIKE
JAWLINE
JEWELED
JEWELER
JEWELRY
JEWISON
JOWLIER

J••W•••
JAYWALK
JAYWARD
JETWASH
JETWAYS
JREWING
JUGWINE

J•••W••
JANEWAY
JCPOWYS
JDPOWER
JOHNWOO

J••••W•
JIGSAWS
JOTDOWN

J•••••W
JACKDAW
JANKLOW
JOEBLOW
JOHNLAW
JUDELAW
JUSTNOW

•J•W•••
AJOWANS

•J••W••
OJIBWAS
OJIBWAY

••J•W••
BEJEWEL

•••J•W•
NONJEWS

••••J•W
LOCKJAW

J••X•••
JINXERS
JINXING

J•••X••
JOHNXII
JOHNXIV
JOHNXIX
JOHNXVI
JOHNXXI

J••••X•
JIMFIXX
JOHNXXI

J•••••X
JIMFIXX
JOHNXIX
JOUHAUX
JUKEBOX
JUNKFAX
JURYBOX

•••J••X
OUTJINX

J•Y••••
JAYBIRD
JAYCEES
JAYLENO
JAYVEES
JAYWALK
JAYWARD
JOYCEAN
JOYLESS
JOYPADS
JOYRIDE

J••Y•••
JOEYDEE
JULYDAY
JURYBOX
JURYING
JURYMAN
JURYMEN
JURYRIG

J•••Y••
JIMRYUN

J••••Y•
JCPOWYS
JERILYN
JERSEYS
JETWAYS
JITNEYS
JOCELYN
JOCKEYS
JOHNNYB
JOSBOYS

J•••••Y
JADEDLY
JANEWAY
JANUARY
JARGONY
JASPERY
JAZZILY
JEFFREY
JELLIFY
JERKILY
JEWELRY
JIGGERY
JITTERY
JOBBERY
JOFFREY
JOHNBOY
JOHNGAY
JOHNJAY
JOINERY
JOINTLY
JOLLIFY
JOLLILY
JOLLITY
JOURNEY
JTMONEY
JUICILY
JULYDAY
JUMPILY
JUNEDAY
JUSTIFY

•J••••Y
OJIBWAY

••J•Y••
ENJOYED
ENJOYER
UNJOYED
WOJTYLA

••J•••Y
MAJESTY
UNJOLLY
UNJUICY

•••J•Y•
DEEJAYS
VEEJAYS

•••J••Y
CONJURY
MIDJULY
NONJURY
ONAJURY
PALJOEY
PERJURY

••••J•Y
ALANJAY
BLUEJAY
GRAYJAY
JOHNJAY
KILLJOY
LOVEJOY
OVERJOY
REENJOY

J•Z••••
JAZZAGE
JAZZBOS
JAZZERS
JAZZIER
JAZZILY
JAZZING
JAZZISH
JAZZMAN
JAZZMEN
JEZEBEL

J••Z•••
JAZZAGE
JAZZBOS
JAZZERS
JAZZIER
JAZZILY
JAZZING
JAZZISH
JAZZMAN
JAZZMEN

J•••Z••
JACUZZI

J••••Z•
JACUZZI
JERITZA

J•••••Z
JIMENEZ
JIMINEZ

•J••••Z
HJHEINZ

KA•••••
KABBALA
KABUKIS
KACHINA
KACHING
KADDISH
KADETTS
KAHUNAS
KAISERS
KAISHEK
KAKAPOS
KAKUROS
KALININ
KAMERAD
KAMFONG
KAMPALA
KANAKAS
KANEOHE
KANSANS
KANTIAN
KAPITAL
KAPITSA
KAPTURE
KARACHI
KARAJAN
KARAKUM
KARAOKE
KARASEA
KARATES
KARLOFF
KARLOVY
KARLSON
KAROLYI
KASHMIR
KASTLER
KATAYEV
KATHRYN
KATISHA
KATRINA
KATRINE
KATYDID
KAUFMAN
KAYAKED
KAYAKER
KAYLENZ
KAYOING

K•A••••
KEARNEY
KHANATE
KHARKOV
KHATAMI
KHAYYAM
KIARIOS
KLAMATH
KLAMMER
KLATSCH
KLAXONS
KNARRED
KNAVERY
KNAVISH
KRACKEL
KRAKENS
KRAMDEN
KRAMNIK
KRASNER
KRATION
KVASSES
KWACHAS
KWANZAA
KWANZAS

K••A•••
KAKAPOS
KANAKAS
KARACHI
KARAJAN
KARAKUM
KARAOKE
KARASEA
KARATES
KATAYEV
KAYAKED
KAYAKER
KERATIN
KILAUEA
KIWANIS
KNEADED
KNEADER
KOLANUT
KOMATSU
KORANIC
KOWADLO
KUWAITI

K•••A••
KABBALA
KAMPALA
KANSANS
KENDALL
KENWAHL
KENYANS
KEYBANK
KEYCARD
KEYCASE
KEYPADS
KEYPALS
KEYWAYS
KHANATE
KHATAMI
KIDNAPS
KILDARE
KIMBALL
KINCAID
KINKAID
KIRMANS
KITBAGS
KITHARA
KITKATS
KKKKATY
KLAMATH
KNOWALL
KODIAKS
KOLKATA
KOOLAID
KOREANS

K••••A•
KAHUNAS
KAMERAD
KANAKAS
KANTIAN
KAPITAL
KARAJAN
KAUFMAN
KEEPSAT
KEESHAN
KEESLAR
KELLJAN
KEOGHAN
KEROUAC
KERSHAW
KETCHAM
KEYSPAN
KHAYYAM
KIDSEAT
KILOBAR
KINGMAN
KINGRAT
KINNEAR
KINSMAN
KLUGMAN
KNEECAP
KNEEPAD
KORUNAS
KOSOVAR
KUMQUAT
KWACHAS
KWANZAA
KWANZAS

K•••••A
KABBALA
KACHINA
KAMPALA
KAPITSA
KARASEA
KATISHA
KATRINA
KEDROVA
KELOWNA
KENOSHA
KILAUEA
KITHARA
KOLKATA
KOPIYKA
KOSCINA
KOSHIBA
KRISHNA
KUNDERA
KWANZAA

•KA••••
OKAYGUY
OKAYING
SKAGWAY
SKATERS
SKATING

•K•A•••
AKSAKOV
SKIABLE
SKIAREA
UKRAINE

•K••A••
IKEBANA
KKKKATY
OKINAWA
SKICAPS
SKIHATS
SKIMASK
SKIRACE
SKIRACK
SKYCAMS
SKYCAPS
SKYJACK
SKYLARK
SKYMAPS
SKYWALK
SKYWARD
SKYWAYS

•K•••A•
BKLIBAN
NKRUMAH
SKAGWAY
SKIWEAR

•K••••A
IKEBANA
OKINAWA
SKIAREA

••KA•••
ACKACKS
ALKALIS
ANKARAN
ASKANCE
ASKAWAY
AZKABAN
DUKAKIS
GOKAPUT
GOKARTS
JAKARTA
KAKAPOS
LIKABLE
MAKABLE
MIKADOS
MIKASAS
RAKABLE
SUKARNO
TAKABLE
WAKAMES
YUKATAS

••K•A••
AWKWARD
BAKLAVA
BOKHARA
BUKHARA
DAKTARI
DIKTATS
ECKHART
ELKHART
INKMARK
INKPADS
INKSACS
KKKKATY
KKKKATY
MIKHAIL
NIKEADS
OAKCASK
OAKLAND
OAKLAWN
OAKPARK
OAKTAGS
TAKEAIM

••K••A•
ANKARAN
ASKAWAY
AZKABAN
BAKEPAN
BIKEWAY
CAKEPAN
DAKOTAN
DAKOTAS
INKYCAP
LAKOTAS
LIKEMAD
LTKOJAK
MAKEHAY
MAKEMAD
MAKEPAR
MAKEWAR
MAKEWAY
MIKASAS
NIKOLAI
NIKOLAY
OAKLEAF
POKEDAT
POKESAT
REKNEAD
RIKSDAG
WAKSMAN
YAKIMAS
YUKATAS

••K•••A
BAKLAVA
BOKHARA
BUKHARA
DYKSTRA
JAKARTA
MCKENNA
MTKENYA
TAKETEA
ZAKUSKA

•••KA••
ARIKARA
BALKANS
BOBKANE
COCKADE
CORKAGE
DARKAGE
DOCKAGE
FOLKART
HAIKAIS
HECKART
HOOKAHS
JACKALS
JACKASS
JIMKAAT
JUNKART
KINKAID
KITKATS
KOLKATA
LEAKAGE
LINKAGE
LOCKAGE
MANKATO
OSAKANS
OUTKAST
PACKAGE
PACKARD
PARKADE
PARKAVE
PICKAXE
PLAKATS
POLKAED
ROCKABY
RYOKANS
SINKAGE
SPOKANE
TANKAGE
TANKARD
TOOKAIM
TOPKAPI
WAIKATO

•••K•A•
AGAKHAN
ALYKHAN
BACKBAR
BACKBAY
BACKPAY
BACKSAW
BACKWAY
BALKSAT
BARKSAT
BECKHAM
BOOKBAG
BOOKMAN
BUCKRAM
BUCKSAW
CHAKRAS
CORKOAK
DARKMAN
DARKTAN
EIJKMAN
FOLKWAY
GAWKSAT
GURKHAS
HACKMAN
HACKSAW
HAWKMAN
HECKMAN
HICKMAN
HONKSAT
JACKDAW
JACKTAR
JIMKAAT
JUNKCAR
JUNKFAX
JUNKMAN
LOCKEAN
LOCKJAW
LOOKSAD
LOOKSAT
LUCKMAN
MARKHAM
MARKKAA
MILKBAR
MILKCAN
MILKMAN
MUSKRAT
ONTKEAN
PACKRAT
PARKMAN
PARKWAY
PECKSAT
PEEKSAT
PICKSAT
PINKHAM
RICKMAN
RINKRAT
SICKBAY
SICKDAY
SICKPAY
SILKHAT
TALKSAT
TANKCAR
TASKBAR
WALKMAN
WALKWAY
WEEKDAY
WINKSAT
WORKDAY
WORKMAN
WORKSAT
YANKSAT

•••K••A
ARIKARA
BURKINA
ELEKTRA
HANKIBA
HECKUVA
JUNKDNA
KOLKATA
MARKKAA
MARKOVA
NDAKOTA
RICKSHA
SDAKOTA
SHAKIRA

••••KA•
ALASKAN
ALASKAS
BLINKAT
CHILKAT
EUREKAS
HANUKAH
ITSOKAY
JUDOKAS
KANAKAS
MARKKAA
MARYKAY
MEDAKAS
MEERKAT
MOLOKAI
NOOTKAS
REBEKAH
SHANKAR
TOPEKAN
TROIKAS
WHISKAS
ZWICKAU

••••K•A
CAHOKIA
MARKKAA

•••••KA
AMERIKA
BAZOOKA
CHACHKA
EMMUSKA
GOTHIKA
KOPIYKA
MALLIKA
MAZURKA
PALOOKA
PAPRIKA
RUZICKA
SOYINKA
ZAKUSKA

K•B••••
KABBALA
KABUKIS
KIBBLED
KIBBLES
KIBBUTZ
KOBLENZ
KOBOLDS
KUBELIK
KUBRICK

K••B•••
KABBALA
KEEBLER
KEYBANK
KIBBLED
KIBBLES
KIBBUTZ
KIMBALL
KITBAGS
KNOBBED

K•••B••
KICKBOX
KILOBAR
KILOBIT
KLEIBER
KNOBBED

K••••B•
KOSHIBA

K•••••B
KEYCLUB

•K•B•••
AKEBONO
IKEBANA
SKIBIBS
SKIBOBS
SKIBOOT
SKIBUMS
SKYBLUE

•K••B••
BKLIBAN
OKTOBER
SKIABLE

•K•••B•
EKINGBY
SKIBIBS
SKIBOBS
SKIPSBY

••KB•••
INKBLOT

••K•B••
AZKABAN
JUKEBOX
LAKEBED
LIKABLE
MAKABLE
RAKABLE
TAKABLE

••K••B•
TAKENBY

•••KB••
BACKBAR
BACKBAY
BACKBIT
BOOKBAG
BUNKBED
KICKBOX
LOCKBOX
MILKBAR
SICKBAY
SICKBED
TALKBIG
TASKBAR
WORKBOX

•••K•B•
HANKIBA
ROCKABY
TICKSBY
WALKSBY

•••K••B
BACKRUB
BANKJOB

••••KB•
SNEAKBY
STICKBY
STUCKBY

KC•••••
KCJONES

K•C••••
KACHINA
KACHING
KICKBOX
KICKERS
KICKIER
KICKING
KICKOFF
KICKOUT
KICKSIN
KICKSUP
KICKUPS
KUCHENS

K••C•••
KETCHAM
KETCHES
KETCHUM
KETCHUP
KEYCARD
KEYCASE
KEYCLUB
KIDCOMS
KIMCHEE
KINCAID
KITCHEN
KNOCKED
KNOCKER
KNOCKON
KNUCKLE
KNUCKLY
KOSCINA
KRACKEL
KUTCHER
KWACHAS

K•••C••
KARACHI
KENICHI
KITSCHY
KNEECAP
KOPECKS
KVETCHY

K••••C•
KEYLOCK
KIDROCK
KLATSCH
KLENSCH
KUBRICK

K•••••C
KEROUAC
KETONIC
KINESIC
KINETIC
KORANIC

•K•C•••
SKICAPS
SKYCAMS
SKYCAPS

•K••C••
SKETCHY

•K•••C•
SKIRACE
SKIRACK
SKYJACK

•K••••C
EKISTIC
SKEPTIC

••KC•••
BOKCHOY
OAKCASK

••K•C••
ACKACKS
INKYCAP
REKICKS

••K••C•
ASKANCE
INKSACS
LIKEICE
NOKNOCK
REKNOCK

•••KC••
JUNKCAR
MILKCAN
MILKCOW
ROCKCOD
TANKCAR

•••K•C•
ONAKICK
OUTKICK
PACKICE
TOPKICK

•••K••C
MISKOLC
RAYKROC

K•D••••
KADDISH
KADETTS
KEDGERS
KEDGING
KEDROVA
KIDCOMS
KIDDERS
KIDDIES
KIDDING
KIDDISH
KIDLIKE
KIDNAPS
KIDNEYS
KIDROCK
KIDSEAT
KIDSKIN
KIDSRUS
KIDULTS
KIDVIDS
KODIAKS

K••D•••
KADDISH
KENDALL
KENDOLL
KENDREW
KEYDETS
KHEDIVE
KIDDERS
KIDDIES
KIDDING
KIDDISH
KILDARE
KINDEST
KINDLED
KINDLER
KINDLES
KINDRED
KLUDGED
KLUDGES
KORDELL
KUNDERA
KURDISH

K•••D••
KATYDID
KEMIDOV
KEYEDIN
KEYEDON
KEYEDUP
KIKIDEE
KILNDRY
KINGDOM
KNEADED
KNEADER
KOWADLO
KRAMDEN
KYOODLE

K••••D•
KENNEDY
KEYPADS
KIDVIDS
KOBOLDS

K•••••D
KAMERAD
KATYDID
KAYAKED
KEYCARD
KEYWORD
KIBBLED
KINCAID
KINDLED
KINDRED
KINKAID
KLUDGED
KNARRED
KNEADED
KNEELED
KNEEPAD
KNELLED
KNITTED
KNOBBED
KNOCKED
KNOTTED
KNOUTED
KNURLED
KOOLAID
KVELLED

•K•D•••
EKEDOUT
SKIDDED
SKIDDER
SKIDDOO
SKIDLID
SKIDOOS
SKIDROW
SKYDIVE
SKYDOME

•K••D••
SKIDDED
SKIDDER
SKIDDOO

•K••••D
SKIDDED
SKIDLID
SKIFFED
SKILLED
SKIMMED
SKIMPED
SKINNED
SKIPPED
SKIRLED
SKIRTED
SKULKED
SKULLED
SKUNKED
SKYNYRD
SKYWARD

••KD•••
DIKDIKS
OAKDESK

••K•D••
AIKIDOS
ASKEDIN
ASKEDOF
ASKEDUP
CAKEDUP
DUKEDOM
FAKEDIT
HIKEDUP
INKEDIN
KIKIDEE
MAKEDOS
MIKADOS
NAKEDLY
POKEDAT
RAKEDIN
RAKEDUP
RIKSDAG
WAKEDUP

••K••D•
FAKEIDS
INKPADS
MAKESDO
NIKEADS

••K•••D
AWKWARD
AYKROYD
LAKEBED
LIKEMAD
LIKENED
MAKEMAD
OAKLAND
OAKWOOD
REKEYED
REKNEAD
TOKENED
UNKEYED
WAKENED

•••KD••
GEEKDOM
JACKDAW
JUNKDNA
MILKDUD
SICKDAY
SUCKDRY
WEEKDAY

WORKDAY

•••K•D•
BIGKIDS
COCKADE
GAPKIDS
HAPKIDO
JOEKIDD
NEWKIDS
PARKADE
PROKEDS
SPYKIDS

•••K••D
ANYKIND
BACKEND
BOOKEND
BUCKLED
BUNKBED
BUNKOED
CACKLED
COCKLED
DARKLED
DARKRED
DECKLED
ENSKIED
GROKKED
HACKLED
HECKLED
JOEKIDD
KINKAID
LOOKSAD
MANKIND
MILKDUD
MILKFED
OFAKIND
PACKARD
PICKLED
POLKAED
RANKLED
ROCKCOD
SICKBED
TACKLED
TANKARD
TICKLED
TINKLED
TREKKED
VOSKHOD
WEEKEND

••••K•D
BATIKED
BAULKED
BLACKED
BLANKED
BLINKED
BLOCKED
BRICKED
BRISKED
BROOKED
CAULKED
CHALKED
CHECKED
CHEEKED
CHINKED
CHOCKED
CHUCKED
CHUNKED
CLACKED
CLANKED
CLERKED
CLICKED
CLINKED
CLOAKED
CLOCKED
CLONKED
CLUCKED
CLUNKED
CRACKED
CRANKED
CREAKED
CRICKED
CROAKED
CROCKED
CROOKED
EBANKED
FLACKED
FLANKED
FLECKED
FLICKED
FLOCKED
FLUNKED
FRANKED
FREAKED
FRISKED
FROCKED
GOODKID
GROKKED
INVOKED
KAYAKED
KNOCKED
NICEKID
NONSKED
NONSKID
PLANKED
PLINKED
PLONKED
PLUCKED
PLUNKED
PRICKED
PRINKED
QUACKED
REASKED
REBAKED
REBUKED
REINKED
RERAKED
REVOKED
REWAKED
REYOKED
SHACKED
SHANKED
SHIRKED
SHOCKED
SHUCKED
SKULKED
SKUNKED
SLACKED
SLEEKED
SLICKED
SLINKED
SMACKED
SMIRKED
SNACKED
SNEAKED
SPANKED
SPARKED
SPECKED
SPOOKED
STACKED
STALKED
STOCKED
STROKED
SWANKED
TALCKED
THANKED
THUNKED
TRACKED
TREKKED
TRICKED
TRUCKED
TWEAKED
UNASKED
UNBAKED
UNCAKED
UNDIKED
UNFAKED
UNINKED
UNLIKED
UNMIKED
UNRAKED
UNWAKED
UNYOKED
VNECKED
WHACKED
WHISKED
WHIZKID
WRACKED
WREAKED
WRECKED
ZINCKED

KE•••••
KEARNEY
KEDGERS
KEDGING
KEDROVA
KEEBLER
KEELING
KEENENH
KEENERS
KEENEST
KEENING
KEEPERS
KEEPFIT
KEEPING
KEEPMUM
KEEPOFF
KEEPOUT
KEEPSAT
KEEPSIN
KEEPSON
KEEPSTO
KEEPSUP
KEESHAN
KEESLAR
KEESLER
KEGGERS
KEGGING
KEGLERS
KEILLOR
KEISTER
KELLJAN
KELLOGG
KELOWNA
KELPIES
KELVINS
KEMIDOV
KEMPTON
KENDALL
KENDOLL
KENDREW
KENICHI
KENMORE
KENNEDY
KENNELS
KENNETH
KENNING
KENOLIN
KENOSHA
KENTISH
KENWAHL
KENYANS
KEOGHAN
KEPTFIT
KEPTMUM
KEPTOFF
KEPTOUT
KERATIN
KERFLOP
KERNELS
KEROUAC
KERPLOP
KERSHAW
KERTESZ
KESTREL
KETCHAM
KETCHES
KETCHUM
KETCHUP
KETONES
KETONIC
KETTLES
KEWPIES
KEYBANK
KEYCARD
KEYCASE
KEYCLUB
KEYDETS
KEYEDIN
KEYEDON
KEYEDUP
KEYGRIP
KEYHOLE
KEYINON
KEYLESS
KEYLIME
KEYLOCK
KEYNOTE
KEYPADS
KEYPALS
KEYRING
KEYSPAN
KEYWAYS
KEYWEST
KEYWORD

K•E••••
KEEBLER
KEELING
KEENENH
KEENERS
KEENEST
KEENING
KEEPERS
KEEPFIT
KEEPING
KEEPMUM
KEEPOFF
KEEPOUT
KEEPSAT
KEEPSIN
KEEPSON
KEEPSTO
KEEPSUP
KEESHAN
KEESLAR
KEESLER
KHEDIVE
KIEFFER
KJELLIN
KLEENEX
KLEIBER
KLEISER
KLENSCH
KLEPTOS
KLEZMER
KMESONS
KNEADED
KNEADER
KNEECAP
KNEEING
KNEELED
KNEELER
KNEEPAD
KNEESUP
KNELLED
KNESSET
KNEWHOW
KOEHLER
KREMLIN
KRESKIN
KVELLED
KVETCHY

K••E•••
KADETTS
KAMERAD
KANEOHE
KEYEDIN
KEYEDON
KEYEDUP
KINESES
KINESIC
KINESIS
KINETIC
KLEENEX
KNEECAP
KNEEING
KNEELED
KNEELER
KNEEPAD
KNEESUP
KNIEVEL
KOPECKS
KOREANS
KROEMER
KRUEGER
KUBELIK

K•••E••
KAISERS
KAYLENZ
KEDGERS
KEENENH
KEENERS
KEENEST
KEEPERS
KEGGERS
KEGLERS
KENNEDY
KENNELS
KENNETH
KERNELS
KERTESZ
KEYDETS
KEYLESS
KEYWEST
KICKERS
KIDDERS
KIDNEYS
KIDSEAT
KILLEEN
KILLERS
KINDEST
KINLESS
KINNEAR
KINNELL
KIPPERS
KISLEVS
KISMETS
KISSELS
KISSERS
KITTENS
KITTERY
KNAVERY
KNIFERS
KNOWERS
KNOWETH
KOBLENZ
KORDELL
KOSHERS
KRAKENS
KUCHENS
KUMMELS
KUNDERA
KURRENT
KUZNETS

K••••E•
KAISHEK
KARASEA
KARATES
KASTLER
KATAYEV
KAYAKED
KAYAKER
KCJONES
KEARNEY
KEEBLER
KEESLER
KEISTER
KELPIES
KENDREW
KESTREL
KETCHES
KETONES
KETTLES
KEWPIES
KIBBLED
KIBBLES
KICKIER
KIDDIES
KIEFFER
KIKIDEE
KILAUEA
KILLEEN
KILLFEE
KILTIES
KIMCHEE
KINDLED
KINDLER
KINDLES
KINDRED
KINESES
KINGLET
KINKIER
KINSMEN
KIRSTEN
KISHKES
KITCHEN
KITTIES
KLAMMER
KLEENEX
KLEIBER
KLEISER
KLEZMER
KLINGER
KLINKER
KLISTER
KLUDGED
KLUDGES
KLUTZES
KNARRED
KNEADED
KNEADER
KNEELED
KNEELER
KNELLED
KNESSET
KNIEVEL
KNISHES
KNITTED
KNITTER
KNOBBED
KNOCKED
KNOCKER
KNOTTED
KNOTTER
KNOUTED
KNOWLES
KNURLED
KOEHLER
KOOKIER
KOOSHES
KRACKEL
KRAMDEN
KRASNER
KROEMER
KRUEGER
KURILES
KUTCHER
KVASSES
KVELLED

K•••••E
KANEOHE
KAPTURE
KARAOKE
KATRINE
KENMORE
KEYCASE
KEYHOLE
KEYLIME
KEYNOTE
KHANATE
KHEDIVE
KIDLIKE
KIKIDEE
KILDARE
KILLFEE
KIMCHEE
KIRSTIE
KNUCKLE
KRINGLE
KRYSTLE
KYOODLE

•KE••••
AKEBONO
AKERLOF
EKEDOUT
EKESOUT
IKEBANA
OKEEFFE
OKELLEY
SKEETER
SKEEZIX
SKELTER
SKELTON
SKEPTIC
SKETCHY
SKEWERS
SKEWING
UKELELE

•K•E•••
EKUELES
EKWENSI
IKNEWIT
OKEEFFE
SKEETER
SKEEZIX

•K••E••
SKATERS
SKEWERS
SKIVEST
SKIWEAR
SKYLESS
UKELELE
UKULELE

•K•••E•
EKUELES
OKELLEY
OKTOBER
SKEETER
SKELTER
SKIAREA
SKIDDED
SKIDDER
SKIFFED
SKILLED
SKILLET
SKIMMED
SKIMMER
SKIMPED
SKINNED
SKINNER
SKIPPED
SKIPPER
SKIRLED
SKIRTED
SKIRTER
SKITTER
SKOSHES
SKULKED
SKULKER
SKULLED
SKUNKED

•K••••E
OKEEFFE
SKIABLE
SKIFFLE
SKIPOLE
SKIRACE
SKITTLE
SKYBLUE
SKYDIVE
SKYDOME
SKYLIKE
SKYLINE
UKELELE
UKRAINE
UKULELE

••KE•••
ALKENES
ASKEDIN
ASKEDOF
ASKEDUP
BAKEOFF
BAKEPAN
BAKERST
BIKEWAY
CAKEDUP
CAKEMIX
CAKEPAN
CAKESUP
CAKETIN
DEKEING
DUKEDOM
FAKEDIT
FAKEFUR
FAKEIDS
FAKEOUT
FAKESIT
HIKEDUP
HIKEOUT
HIKESUP
INKEDIN
JUKEBOX
LAKEBED
LIKEICE
LIKEMAD
LIKENED
LIKENEW
LIKENTO
LIKEWOW
MAKEDOS
MAKEFIT
MAKEFOR
MAKEFUN
MAKEHAY
MAKEILL
MAKEMAD
MAKEOFF
MAKEONE
MAKEOUT
MAKEPAR
MAKERUN
MAKESDO
MAKESGO
MAKESIT
MAKESUP
MAKEUPS
MAKEWAR
MAKEWAY
MCKENNA
MTKENYA
NAKEDLY
NIKEADS
PEKEPOO
POKEDAT
POKEFUN
POKEMON
POKEOUT
POKESAT
RAKEDIN
RAKEDUP
RAKEOFF
RAKESIN
RAKESUP
REKEYED
TAKEAIM
TAKEFOR
TAKEILL
TAKEINS
TAKENBY
TAKENIN
TAKENON
TAKENTO
TAKENUP
TAKEOFF
TAKEONE
TAKEOUT
TAKESIN
TAKESIT
TAKESON
TAKESTO
TAKESUP
TAKETEA
TAKETEN
TOKENED
UNKEMPT
UNKEYED
UPKEEPS
WAKEDUP
WAKEFUL
WAKENED
WAKENER
WAKESUP
WAKEUPS
WOKENUP

••K•E••
ANKLERS
ANKLETS
AUKLETS
BOKKENS
CAKIEST
COKIEST
DEKLERK
FOKKERS
HOKIEST
ICKIEST
INKIEST
INKJETS
INKLESS
INKWELL
JOKIEST
LAKIEST
OAKDESK
OAKFERN
OAKIEST
OAKLEAF
ORKNEYS
POKIEST
REKNEAD
UPKEEPS
YAKKERS

••K••E•
ALKENES
ASKOVER
INKSTER
KIKIDEE
LAKEBED
LIKENED
LIKENEW
OAKTREE
REKEYED
TAKETEA
TAKETEN
TEKKIES
TOKENED
UNKEYED
WAKAMES
WAKENED
WAKENER

••K•••E
ASKANCE
INKLIKE
IRKSOME
KIKIDEE
LIKABLE
LIKEICE
MAKABLE
MAKEONE
OAKLIKE
OAKTREE
RAKABLE
TAKABLE
TAKEONE

•••KE••
ALEKEGS
ALTKEYS
AWAKENS
AWAKERS
BACKEND
BACKERS
BALKERS
BANKERS
BARKEEP
BARKERS
BASKETS
BASKETT
BEAKERS
BECKETT
BICKERS
BILKERS
BLAKELY
BOKKENS
BONKERS
BOOKEND
BOOKERS
BOOKERT
BROKEIN
BROKERS
BROKEUP
BUCKERS
BUCKETS
BUCKEYE
BUNKERS
BUSKERS
CALKERS
CANKERS
CARKEYS
CASKETS
CHOKEON
CHOKERS
CHOKEUP
COCKERS
CONKERS
COOKERS
COOKERY
CORKERS
DANKEST
DARKENS
DARKEST
DECKERS
DELKEYS
DICKENS
DICKERS
DICKEYS
DOCKERS
DOCKETS
DONKEYS
DUCKERS
DUNKERS
EVOKERS
FLAKERS
FOKKERS
FORKERS
GASKELL
GASKETS
GAWKERS
HACKERS
HACKETT
HANKERS
HARKENS
HASKELL
HAWKERS
HAWKEYE
HICKEYS
HOCKERS
HONKERS
HOTKEYS
HUNKERS
HUSKERS
ILIKEIT
JACKETS
JERKERS
JOCKEYS
JUNKERS
JUNKETS
KICKERS
KRAKENS
LACKEYS
LANKEST
LARKERS
LEAKERS
LEAKEYS
LICKERS
LICKETY
LINKERS
LOCKEAN
LOCKERS
LOCKETS
LOOKERS
LUNKERS
LURKERS
MARKERS
MARKETS
MASKERS
MEEKEST
MICKEYS
MILKERS
MISKEYS
MOCKERS
MOCKERY
MONKEES
MONKEYS
MUCKERS
MUSKEGO
MUSKETS
NECKERS
NICKELS
NICKERS
OINKERS
ONTKEAN
OUTKEEP
OUTKEPT
PACKERS
PACKETS
PARKERS
PEEKERS
PICKENS
PICKERS
PICKETS
PICKETT
PINKENS
PINKEST
PINKETT
POCKETS
PORKERS
PROKEDS
PUCKERS
PUCKERY
PUCKETT
PUNKERS
QUAKERS
RACKERS
RACKETS
RACKETY
RANKERS
RANKEST
REEKERS
RICKETY

RICKEYS
RISKERS
ROCKERS
ROCKERY
ROCKETS
ROOKERY
RUCKERT
SACKERS
SECKELS
SEEKERS
SHAKERS
SHAKEUP
SHEKELS
SICKENS
SICKEST
SINKERS
SLAKERS
SMOKERS
SMOKEUP
SMOKEYS
SNAKERS
SOAKERS
SOCKETS
SOCKEYE
SPIKERS
SPIKETV
SPIKEUP
SPOKEOF
SPOKETO
SPOKEUP
STOKELY
STOKERS
STOKEUP
SUCKERS
SULKERS
TABKEYS
TACKERS
TALKERS
TANKERS
TICKERS
TICKETS
TINKERS
TUCKERS
TURKEYS
TUSKERS
UNSKEWS
VICKERS
WACKEST
WALKERS
WANKELS
WEAKENS
WEAKEST
WEEKEND
WICKERS
WICKETS
WILKENS
WINKERS
WORKERS
YAKKERS
YANKEES
YANKERS
YONKERS
YORKERS

•••K•E•
ALEKSEI
BALKIER
BANKFEE
BARKEEP
BARKIER
BARKLEY
BERKLEY
BERKNER
BLAKLEY
BOOKIES
BOOKLET
BOOKMEN
BUCKLED
BUCKLES
BUCKLEY
BUCKNER
BUCKOES
BULKIER
BUNKBED
BUNKOED
CACKLED
CACKLER
CACKLES
CHOKIER
CHUKKER
COCKIER
COCKLED
COCKLES
COCKNEY
COOKIES
CORKIER
DARKLED
DARKLES
DARKRED
DECKLED
DECKLES
DESKSET
DICKIES
DINKIER
DIRKSEN
DORKIER
DUCKIER
DUCKIES
DUSKIER
ENSKIED
ENSKIES
EZEKIEL
FICKLER
FLAKIER
FLUKIER
FOLKIER
FOLKIES
FORKIER
FUNKIER
GAWKIER
GECKOES
GEEKIER
GROKKED
GUCKIER
GUNKIER
HACKIES
HACKLED
HACKLER
HACKLES
HACKNEY
HANKIES
HECKLED
HECKLER
HECKLES
HECKYES
HINKIER
HULKIER
HUNKIER
HUSKIER
HUSKIES
JACKIEO
JERKIER
JERKIES
JUNKIER
JUNKIES
JUNKMEN
KICKIER
KINKIER
KOOKIER
LANKIER
LARKIER
LEAKIER
LOCKLET
LOCKSET
LOOKSEE
LUCKIER
MILKFED
MILKIER
MILKMEN
MISKNEW
MONKEES
MUCKIER
MURKIER
MUSKIER
MUSKIES
NECKLET
NICKLES
OUTKEEP
PEAKIER
PERKIER
PESKIER
PICKIER
PICKLED
PICKLES
PINKIES
PINKOES
POLKAED
PORKIER
PUNKIER
PUNKIES
QUAKIER
QUAKIES
RANKLED
RANKLES
REEKIER
RICKLES
RISKIER
ROCKIER
ROCKIES
ROOKIER
ROOKIES
SHAKIER
SHAKOES
SICKBED
SICKLES
SILKIER
SMOKIER
SMOKIES
SNAKIER
SPIKIER
SUCKIER
SULKIER
SULKIES
TACKIER
TACKLED
TACKLER
TACKLES
TALKIER
TALKIES
TEKKIES
TICKLED
TICKLER
TICKLES
TINKLED
TINKLER
TINKLES
TOLKIEN
TOOKTEN
TREKKED
TREKKER
VICKREY
WACKIER
WHOKNEW
WINKLER
WOOKIEE
WORKMEN
YANKEES
YORKIES
YUCKIER
ZINKIER

•••K••E
BACKHOE
BANKFEE
BANKONE
BOBKANE
BOXKITE
BUCKEYE
COCKADE
CORKAGE
DARKAGE
DOCKAGE
ERSKINE
HAWKEYE
LEAKAGE
LINKAGE
LOCKAGE
LOOKSEE
NECKTIE
PACKAGE
PACKICE
PARKADE
PARKAVE
PICKAXE
PORKPIE
RANKINE
SILKTIE
SINKAGE
SOCKEYE
SPOKANE
TANKAGE
TOMKITE
TOYKITE
TREKKIE
WALKURE
WOOKIEE
ZADKINE

••••KE•
ALROKER
BATIKED
BAULKED
BAULKER
BEERKEG
BETAKEN
BETAKES
BETOKEN
BISHKEK
BLACKED
BLACKEN
BLACKER
BLANKED
BLANKER
BLANKET
BLEAKER
BLINKED
BLINKER
BLOCKED
BLOCKER
BLYNKEN
BRACKEN
BRACKET
BREAKER
BRICKED
BRINKER
BRISKED
BRISKER
BRISKET
BRODKEY
BROOKED
CARDKEY
CAULKED
CAULKER
CHALKED
CHECKED
CHECKER
CHEEKED
CHICKEN
CHINKED
CHOCKED
CHUCKED
CHUKKER
CHUNKED
CLACKED
CLACKER
CLANKED
CLERKED
CLICKED
CLICKER
CLINKED
CLINKER
CLOAKED
CLOCKED
CLOCKER
CLONKED
CLUCKED
CLUCKER
CLUNKED
CLUNKER
COMAKER
CRACKED
CRACKER
CRANKED
CREAKED
CRICKED
CRICKET
CROAKED
CROAKER
CROCKED
CROCKER
CROCKET
CROOKED
CROOKES
DANIKEN
DEBAKEY
DRINKER
DRUCKER
DRUNKEN
DRUNKER
EBANKED
ETICKET
FLACKED
FLANKED
FLANKEN
FLANKER
FLECKED
FLICKED
FLICKER
FLOCKED
FLUNKED
FLUNKER
FRANKED
FRANKEN
FRANKER
FREAKED
FRICKER
FRISKED
FRISKER
FROCKED
GROKKED
HAECKEL
HEARKEN
HOBOKEN
INJOKES
INTAKES
INVOKED
INVOKER
INVOKES
JAECKEL
KAYAKED
KAYAKER
KISHKES
KLINKER
KNOCKED
KNOCKER
KRACKEL
LALAKER
MENCKEN
MONIKER
NAILKEG
NONSKED
NONUKES
PASSKEY
PERUKES
PLACKET
PLANKED
PLINKED
PLONKED
PLUCKED
PLUNKED
PLUNKER
PONYKEG
PRICKED
PRINKED
PRINKER
QUACKED
QUACKER
QUICKEN
QUICKER
REASKED
REBAKED
REBAKES
REBUKED
REBUKER
REBUKES
REINKED
REMAKES
RERAKED
RERAKES
RETAKEN
RETAKER
RETAKES
REVOKED
REVOKER
REVOKES
REWAKED
REWAKEN
REWAKES
REWOKEN
REYOKED
REYOKES
SHACKED
SHANKED
SHARKEY
SHIRKED
SHIRKER
SHOCKED
SHOCKER
SHRIKES
SHUCKED
SHUCKER
SKULKED
SKULKER
SKUNKED
SLACKED
SLACKEN
SLACKER
SLEEKED
SLEEKEN
SLEEKER
SLICKED
SLICKER
SLINKED
SLINKER
SMACKED
SMACKER
SMIRKED
SMIRKER
SMUCKER
SNACKED
SNACKER
SNEAKED
SNEAKER
SNICKER
SNICKET
SNOOKER
SNORKEL
SPANKED
SPANKER
SPARKED
SPEAKER
SPECKED
SPOOKED
STACKED
STACKER
STALKED
STALKER
STARKER
STARKEY
STICKER
STINKER
STLUKES
STOCKED
STOCKER
STOOKEY
STRIKER
STRIKES
STROKED
STROKER
STROKES
SWANKED
SWANKER
TALCKED
THANKED
THANKER
THICKEN
THICKER
THICKET
THINKER
THUNKED
TRACKED
TRACKER
TREKKED
TREKKER
TRICKED
TRICKER
TRINKET
TRUCKED
TRUCKEE
TRUCKER
TURNKEY
TWEAKED
UNASKED
UNBAKED
UNCAKED
UNCAKES
UNDIKED
UNFAKED
UNINKED
UNLIKED
UNLIKES
UNMAKER
UNMAKES
UNMIKED
UNRAKED
UNTAKEN
UNWAKED
UNYOKED
UNYOKES
UPTAKES
VNECKED
VOLCKER
WHACKED
WHACKER
WHISKED
WHISKER
WHISKEY
WRACKED
WREAKED
WREAKER
WRECKED
WRECKER
ZINCKED

••••K•E
BLACKIE
BRICKLE
CHUCKLE
CRACKLE
CRINKLE
DRINKME
FRANKIE
FRECKLE
GRACKLE
KNUCKLE
PRICKLE
QUICKIE
SHACKLE
SPACKLE
SPARKLE
SPECKLE
TREKKIE
TRICKLE
TRUCKEE
TRUCKLE
TWINKIE
TWINKLE
WILLKIE
WRINKLE

•••••KE
ACTLIKE
AIRLIKE
ANTLIKE
APELIKE
ARMLIKE
ASAJOKE
ASHCAKE
ASSLIKE
ATSTAKE
AXELIKE
BADJOKE
BAGLIKE
BATLIKE
BEDLIKE
BEELIKE
BESPOKE
BIBLIKE
BIGJAKE
BOWLIKE
BOXLIKE
BOYLIKE
BUDLIKE
CATLIKE
CODCAKE
CONVOKE
COWLIKE
COWPOKE
CUPCAKE
CUPLIKE
CURLIKE
DIDLIKE
DISLIKE
DOGLIKE
DOTLIKE
EARLIKE
EATCAKE
EELLIKE
EGGLIKE
ELFLIKE
EYELIKE
FADLIKE
FANLIKE
FATLIKE
FINLIKE
FORSAKE
FOXLIKE
GARPIKE
GEMLIKE
GOBROKE
GODLIKE
GUMLIKE
HAGLIKE
HATLIKE
HENLIKE
HIPLIKE
HOECAKE
HOGLIKE
HOLYOKE
HOTCAKE
HUNLIKE
HUTLIKE
ICELIKE
IMBROKE
INAPOKE
INKLIKE
IVYLIKE
JAMLIKE
JAWLIKE
JIGLIKE
JSTROKE
KARAOKE
KIDLIKE
LAWLIKE
LEGLIKE
LIPLIKE
MANLIKE
MISLIKE
MISTAKE
NETLIKE
NETSUKE
NIBLIKE
NOTLIKE
NUNLIKE
NUTLIKE
OAKLIKE
OARLIKE
OATCAKE
OATLIKE
OILCAKE
OILLIKE
OLDJOKE
ORBLIKE
OROURKE
OUTBAKE
OUTTAKE
OWLLIKE
PANCAKE
PARBAKE
PARTAKE
PEALIKE
PEGLIKE
PENLIKE
PIELIKE
PIGLIKE
PODLIKE
PREBAKE
PREMAKE
PROVOKE
RAMLIKE
RATLIKE
RAYLIKE
REAWAKE
REAWOKE
REBROKE
REEVOKE
RESPOKE
RESTOKE
RIBLIKE
ROANOKE
RODLIKE
ROETHKE
RUGLIKE
RUMCAKE
SACLIKE
SAWLIKE
SEALIKE
SINLIKE
SIRDUKE
SKYLIKE
SONLIKE
SOWLIKE
SUNLIKE
TAGLIKE
TAXHIKE
TEACAKE
THEDUKE
THELIKE
TINLIKE
TOELIKE
TOYBIKE
TOYLIKE
TUBLIKE
UNALIKE
UNAWAKE
UNBRAKE
UNBROKE
UNCHOKE
UNSPOKE
URNLIKE
VANDYKE
WARLIKE
WAXLIKE
WEBLIKE
WIGLIKE
ZERNIKE

K••F•••
KAMFONG
KAUFMAN
KERFLOP
KIEFFER
KINFOLK
KNIFERS
KNIFING

K•••F••
KEEPFIT
KEPTFIT
KIEFFER
KILLFEE

K••••F•
KARLOFF
KEEPOFF
KEPTOFF
KICKOFF
KISSOFF

K•••••F
KARLOFF
KEEPOFF
KEPTOFF
KICKOFF
KISSOFF
KNOWSOF

•K•F•••
SKIFFED
SKIFFLE

•K••F••
OKEEFFE
SKIFFED
SKIFFLE
SKILFUL

•K•••F•
OKEEFFE
SKILIFT

•K••••F
AKERLOF
SKYSURF

••KF•••
OAKFERN

••K•F••
ASKSFOR
FAKEFUR
MAKEFIT
MAKEFOR
MAKEFUN
POKEFUN
TAKEFOR
WAKEFUL

••K••F•
BAKEOFF
MAKEOFF
RAKEOFF
TAKEOFF

••K•••F
ASKEDOF
BAKEOFF
MAKEOFF
OAKLEAF
RAKEOFF
TAKEOFF

•••KF••
BANKFEE
BUCKFOR
DESKFUL
FORKFUL
JUNKFAX
LOOKFOR
MILKFED
SACKFUL
TANKFUL
TOOKFOR
WORKFOR

•••K•F•
BACKOFF
CONKOFF
COOKOFF
HACKOFF
KICKOFF
MARKOFF
PACKOFF
PICKOFF
TICKOFF
TOOKOFF
WALKOFF
WORKOFF
YANKOFF

•••K••F
BACKOFF
CONKOFF
COOKOFF
HACKOFF
KICKOFF
MARKOFF
PACKOFF
PICKOFF
REEKSOF
SPOKEOF
TALKSOF
TICKOFF
TOOKOFF
WALKOFF
WORKOFF
YANKOFF

••••K•F
ALACKOF
APECKOF
SMACKOF
SPEAKOF
THINKOF

K•G••••
KEGGERS
KEGGING
KEGLERS

K••G•••
KEDGERS
KEDGING
KEGGERS
KEGGING
KEOGHAN
KEYGRIP
KINGDOM
KINGING
KINGLET
KINGMAN
KINGPIN
KINGRAT
KINGTUT
KLUGMAN
KNIGHTS

K•••G••
KLINGER
KLINGON
KLUDGED
KLUDGES
KOSYGIN
KRINGLE
KRUEGER

K••••G•
KELLOGG
KITBAGS

K•••••G
KACHING
KAMFONG
KAYOING
KEDGING
KEELING
KEENING
KEEPING
KEGGING
KELLOGG
KENNING
KEYRING
KICKING
KIDDING
KILLING
KILNING
KILTING
KINGING
KINKING
KIPLING
KIPPING
KISSING
KITTING
KNEEING
KNIFING
KNOWING
KOONING

•K•G•••
SKAGWAY

•K••G••
EKINGBY
OKAYGUY

•K•••G•
SKYHIGH

•K••••G
OKAYING
SKATING
SKEWING

••K••G•
IIKINGS
INKINGS
LIKINGS
MAKESGO
MAKINGS
OAKTAGS
TAKINGS
VIKINGS
WAKINGS

••K•••G
DEKEING
INKLING
RIKSDAG
YAKKING
YUKKING

•••KG••
GINKGOS

•••K•G•
ALEKEGS
CORKAGE
DARKAGE
DOCKAGE
LEAKAGE
LINKAGE
LOCKAGE
MUSKEGO
PACKAGE
SINKAGE
TANKAGE

•••K••G
ALAKING
AWAKING
BACKING
BACKLOG
BALKING
BANKING
BARKING
BASKING
BILKING
BONKING
BOOKBAG
BOOKING
BORKING
BRAKING
BUCKING
BULKING
BUNKING
BUSKING
CALKING
CARKING
CASKING
CHOKING
COCKING
CONKING
COOKING
CORKING
DECKING
DIRKING
DISKING
DOCKING
DONKING
DUCKING
DUNKING
DUSKING
EVOKING
FINKING
FLAKING
FORKING
FUNKING
GAWKING
HACKING
HARKING
HAWKING
HOCKING
HONKING
HOOKING
HULKING
HUSKING
JACKING
JERKING
JUNKING
KICKING
KINKING
LACKING
LARKING
LEAKING
LICKING
LINKING
LOCKING
LOOKING
LUCKING
LURKING
MARKING
MASKING
MILKING
MOCKING
MUCKING
NANKING
NECKING
NICKING
NOCKING
OINKING
OUTKING
PACKING
PARKING
PEAKING
PECKING
PEEKING
PERKING
PICKING
PINKING
PORKING
QUAKING
RACKING
RANKING
REDKING
REEKING
RISKING
ROCKING
ROOKING
RUCKING
SACKING
SEEKING
SHAKING
SINKING
SLAKING
SMOKING
SNAKING
SOAKING
SOCKING
SPIKING
SPOKING
STAKING
STOKING
SUBKING
SUCKING
SULKING
TACKING
TALKBIG
TALKING
TANKING
TASKING
THEKING
TICKING
TUCKING
TUSKING
WALKING
WICKING
WINKING
WORKING
YAKKING
YANKING
YUKKING
ZONKING

••••K•G
BEERKEG
NAILKEG
PONYKEG

KH•••••
KHANATE
KHARKOV
KHATAMI
KHAYYAM
KHEDIVE

K•H••••
KAHUNAS

K••H•••
KACHINA
KACHING
KASHMIR
KATHRYN
KEYHOLE
KISHKES
KITHARA
KOEHLER
KOSHERS
KOSHIBA
KUCHENS

K•••H••
KAISHEK
KEESHAN
KEOGHAN
KERSHAW
KETCHAM
KETCHES
KETCHUM
KETCHUP
KIMCHEE
KINSHIP
KITCHEN
KNEWHOW
KNIGHTS
KNISHES
KNOWHOW
KOOSHES
KRISHNA
KUTCHER
KWACHAS

K••••H•
KANEOHE
KARACHI
KATISHA
KENICHI
KENOSHA
KENWAHL
KITSCHY
KVETCHY

K•••••H
KADDISH
KEENENH
KENNETH
KENTISH
KIDDISH
KLAMATH
KLATSCH
KLENSCH
KNAVISH
KNOWETH
KOSSUTH
KURDISH

•KH••••
OKHOTSK

•K•H•••
AKIHITO
OKSHOOT
SKIHATS
SKYHIGH
SKYHOOK

•K••H••
SKISHOP
SKOSHES

•K•••H•
SKETCHY

•K••••H
AKRONOH
NKRUMAH
SKYHIGH

••KH•••
BOKHARA
BUKHARA
ECKHART
ELKHART
INKHORN
MIKHAIL
SIKHISM

••K•H••
BOKCHOY
LAKSHMI
MAKEHAY

••K••H
SUKKOTH

•••KH••
AGAKHAN
ALYKHAN
BACKHOE
BECKHAM
CHEKHOV
GURKHAS
MARKHAM
PINKHAM
SILKHAT
SOCKHOP
VOSKHOD

•••K•H•
HOOKAHS
RICKSHA
WORKSHY

•••K••H
BOOKISH
COCKISH
DARKISH
DUSKISH
FOLKISH
GAWKISH
HAWKISH
LARKISH
MAWKISH
MONKISH
MURKISH
OSHKOSH
PEAKISH
PECKISH
PERKISH
PINKISH
PORKISH
PUCKISH
RANKISH
ROOKISH
SICKISH
SUKKOTH
TURKISH
WEAKISH
YERKISH

••••KH•
SAMEKHS
SHEIKHS

••••K•H
HANUKAH
REBEKAH

KI•••••
KIARIOS
KIBBLED
KIBBLES
KIBBUTZ
KICKBOX
KICKERS
KICKIER
KICKING
KICKOFF
KICKOUT
KICKSIN
KICKSUP
KICKUPS
KIDCOMS
KIDDERS
KIDDIES
KIDDING
KIDDISH
KIDLIKE
KIDNAPS
KIDNEYS
KIDROCK
KIDSEAT
KIDSKIN
KIDSRUS
KIDULTS
KIDVIDS
KIEFFER
KIKIDEE
KIKUYUS
KILAUEA
KILDARE
KILLEEN
KILLERS
KILLFEE
KILLING
KILLJOY
KILNDRY
KILNING
KILOBAR
KILOBIT
KILOTON
KILTIES
KILTING
KIMBALL
KIMCHEE
KIMONOS
KINCAID
KINDEST
KINDLED
KINDLER
KINDLES
KINDRED
KINESES
KINESIC
KINESIS
KINETIC
KINFOLK
KINGDOM
KINGING
KINGLET
KINGMAN
KINGPIN
KINGRAT
KINGTUT
KINISON
KINKAID
KINKIER
KINKILY
KINKING
KINLESS
KINMONT
KINNEAR
KINNELL
KINSHIP
KINSMAN
KINSMEN
KIPLING
KIPPERS
KIPPING
KIRMANS
KIRSTEN
KIRSTIE
KISHKES
KISLEVS
KISMETS
KISSELS
KISSERS
KISSING
KISSOFF
KITBAGS
KITCHEN
KITHARA
KITKATS
KITSCHY
KITTENS
KITTERY
KITTIES
KITTING
KIWANIS

K•I••••
KAISERS
KAISHEK
KEILLOR
KEISTER
KLINGER
KLINGON
KLINKER
KLISTER
KNIEVEL
KNIFERS
KNIFING
KNIGHTS
KNISHES
KNITTED
KNITTER
KRINGLE
KRISHNA
KRISTIN

K••I•••
KALININ
KAPITAL
KAPITSA
KATISHA
KEMIDOV
KENICHI
KEYINON
KIKIDEE
KINISON
KLEIBER
KLEISER
KODIAKS
KOPIYKA
KURILES

K•••I••
KACHINA
KACHING
KADDISH
KANTIAN
KATRINA
KATRINE
KAYOING
KEDGING
KEELING
KEENING
KEEPING
KEGGING
KELPIES
KELVINS
KENNING
KENTISH
KEWPIES
KEYLIME
KEYRING
KHEDIVE
KIARIOS
KICKIER
KICKING
KIDDIES
KIDDING
KIDDISH
KIDLIKE
KIDVIDS
KILLING
KILNING
KILTIES
KILTING
KINGING
KINKIER
KINKILY
KINKING
KIPLING
KIPPING
KISSING
KITTIES
KITTING
KNAVISH
KNEEING
KNIFING
KNOWING
KONTIKI
KOOKIER
KOONING
KOSCINA
KOSHIBA
KRATION
KUBRICK
KURDISH
KUWAITI

K••••I•
KABUKIS
KALININ
KASHMIR
KATYDID
KEEPFIT
KEEPSIN
KENOLIN
KEPTFIT
KERATIN
KETONIC
KEYEDIN
KEYGRIP
KICKSIN
KIDSKIN
KILOBIT
KINCAID
KINESIC
KINESIS
KINETIC
KINGPIN
KINKAID
KINSHIP
KIRSTIE
KIWANIS
KJELLIN
KOOLAID
KORANIC
KOSYGIN
KRAMNIK
KREMLIN
KRESKIN
KRISTIN
KTOSLIN
KUBELIK

K•••••I
KARACHI
KAROLYI
KENICHI
KHATAMI
KONTIKI
KUWAITI

•KI••••
AKIHITO
EKINGBY
EKISTIC
OKINAWA
SKIABLE
SKIAREA
SKIBIBS
SKIBOBS
SKIBOOT
SKIBUMS
SKICAPS
SKIDDED
SKIDDER
SKIDDOO
SKIDLID
SKIDOOS
SKIDROW
SKIFFED
SKIFFLE
SKIHATS
SKIJUMP
SKILFUL
SKILIFT
SKILLED
SKILLET
SKIMASK
SKIMMED
SKIMMER
SKIMPED
SKIMPON
SKINNED
SKINNER
SKIPOLE
SKIPOUT
SKIPPED
SKIPPER
SKIPSBY
SKIRACE
SKIRACK
SKIRLED
SKIRTED
SKIRTER
SKIRUNS
SKISHOP
SKISUIT
SKITOWS
SKITRIP
SKITTER
SKITTLE
SKIVEST
SKIWEAR

•K•I•••
BKLIBAN

•K••I••
AKIHITO
OKAYING
SKATING
SKEWING
SKIBIBS
SKILIFT
SKYDIVE
SKYHIGH
SKYLIKE
SKYLINE
UKRAINE

•K•••I•
EKISTIC
IKNEWIT
IKNOWIT
SKEEZIX
SKEPTIC
SKIDLID
SKISUIT
SKITRIP

•K••••I
EKWENSI

••KI•••
AIKIDOS
BIKINIS
CAKIEST
COKIEST
ESKIMOS
HOKIEST
ICKIEST
IIKINGS
INKIEST
INKINGS
JOKIEST
KIKIDEE
LAKIEST
LAKISTS
LIKINGS
MAKINGS
OAKIEST
POKIEST
REKICKS
STKITTS
TAKINGS
UNKINKS
VIKINGS
WAKINGS
YAKIMAS

••K•I••
DEKEING
DIKDIKS
FAKEIDS
INKLIKE
INKLING
LIKEICE
MAKEILL
OAKLIKE
REKNITS
SIKHISM
TAKEILL
TAKEINS
TEKKIES
UNKNITS
YAKKING
YUKKING

••K••I•
ALKALIS
ASKEDIN
BIKINIS
CAKEMIX
CAKETIN
DUKAKIS
FAKEDIT
FAKESIT
INKEDIN
MAKEFIT
MAKESIT
MIKHAIL
NOKOMIS
RAKEDIN
RAKESIN
TAKEAIM
TAKENIN
TAKESIN
TAKESIT
YUKOLIS

••K•••I
DAKTARI
LAKSHMI
NIKOLAI

•••KI••
AIRKISS
ALAKING
ANYKIND
AWAKING
BACKING
BALKIER
BALKILY
BALKING
BANKING
BANKITS
BARKIER
BARKING
BASKING
BIGKIDS
BILKING
BODKINS
BONKING
BOOKIES
BOOKIII
BOOKING
BOOKISH
BORKING
BOXKITE
BRAKING
BUCKING
BULKIER
BULKING
BUNKING
BURKINA
BUSKING
CALKING
CALKINS
CARKING
CASKING
CATKINS
CHOKIER
CHOKING
COCKIER
COCKILY
COCKING
COCKISH
CONKING
COOKIES
COOKING
CORKIER
CORKING
DARKISH
DAWKINS
DECKING
DICKIES
DINKIER
DIRKING
DISKING
DOCKING
DONKING
DORKIER
DUCKIER
DUCKIES
DUCKING
DUNKING
DUNKIRK
DUSKIER
DUSKILY
DUSKING
DUSKISH
ENSKIED
ENSKIES
ERSKINE
EVOKING
EZEKIEL
FALKIRK
FINKING
FIRKINS
FLAKIER
FLAKILY
FLAKING
FLUKIER
FLUKILY
FOLKIER
FOLKIES
FOLKISH
FORKIER
FORKING
FUNKIER
FUNKILY
FUNKING
GAPKIDS
GAWKIER
GAWKILY
GAWKING
GAWKISH
GEEKIER
GUCKIER
GUNKIER
HACKIES
HACKING
HANKIBA
HANKIES
HAPKIDO
HARKING
HAWKING
HAWKINS
HAWKISH
HINKIER
HOCKING
HONKING
HOOKING
HOPKINS
HOSKINS
HULKIER
HULKING
HUNKIER
HUSKIER
HUSKIES
HUSKILY
HUSKING
JACKIEO
JACKING

JENKINS
JERKIER
JERKIES
JERKILY
JERKING
JERKINS
JOEKIDD
JUNKIER
JUNKIES
JUNKING
KICKIER
KICKING
KINKIER
KINKILY
KINKING
KOOKIER
LACKING
LANKIER
LANKILY
LARKIER
LARKING
LARKINS
LARKISH
LEAKIER
LEAKING
LICKING
LINKING
LOCKING
LOCKINS
LOOKING
LOOKINS
LOOKISM
LOOKIST
LUCKIER
LUCKILY
LUCKING
LURKING
MANKIND
MARKIII
MARKING
MASKING
MAWKISH
MILKIER
MILKILY
MILKING
MOCKING
MONKISH
MUCKIER
MUCKING
MURKIER
MURKILY
MURKISH
MUSKIER
MUSKIES
NANKING
NAPKINS
NECKING
NEWKIDS
NICKING
NOCKING
OFAKIND
OINKING
ONAKICK
ONEKILO
OUTKICK
OUTKILL
OUTKING
OUTKISS
PACKICE
PACKING
PARKING
PARKINS
PEAKIER
PEAKING
PEAKISH
PECKING
PECKISH
PEEKING
PERKIER
PERKILY
PERKING
PERKINS
PERKISH
PESKIER
PESKILY
PICKIER
PICKING
PINKIES
PINKING
PINKISH
PORKIER
PORKING
PORKISH
PUCKISH
PUNKIER
PUNKIES
QUAKIER
QUAKIES
QUAKILY
QUAKING
RACKING
RANKINE
RANKING
RANKISH
REDKING
REEKIER
REEKING
RISKIER
RISKILY
RISKING
ROCKIER
ROCKIES
ROCKILY
ROCKING
ROOKIER
ROOKIES
ROOKING
ROOKISH
RUCKING
SACKING
SEEKING
SELKIRK
SHAKIER
SHAKILY
SHAKING
SHAKIRA
SICKISH
SILKIER
SILKILY
SINKING
SLAKING
SMOKIER
SMOKIES
SMOKILY
SMOKING
SNAKIER
SNAKILY
SNAKING
SOAKING
SOCKING
SPIKIER
SPIKILY
SPIKING
SPOKING
SPYKIDS
STAKING
STOKING
SUBKING
SUCKIER
SUCKING
SULKIER
SULKIES
SULKILY
SULKING
SUNKIST
TACKIER
TACKILY
TACKING
TALKIER
TALKIES
TALKING
TANKING
TANKINI
TASKING
TEKKIES
THEKING
THEKISS
TICKING
TOLKIEN
TOMKITE
TOOKILL
TOPKICK
TOYKITE
TUCKING
TURKISH
TUSKING
WACKIER
WACKILY
WADKINS
WAIKIKI
WALKING
WALKINS
WATKINS
WEAKISH
WESKITS
WETKISS
WICKING
WICKIUP
WILKINS
WINKING
WOOKIEE
WORKING
YAKKING
YANKING
YERKISH
YORKIES
YORKIST
YUCKIER
YUKKING
ZADKINE
ZINKIER
ZONKING

•••K•I•

BACKBIT
BACKLIT
BACKSIN
BOOKIII
BOOKVII
BROKEIN
COCKPIT
CONKLIN
DUCKPIN
HACKSIT
HAIKAIS
ILIKEIT
KICKSIN
KINKAID
LACKWIT
LEAKSIN
LOCKLIN
LOCKSIN
LOOKSIN
MARKIII
MARKVII
NECKTIE
PACKSIN
PARKSIT
PEEKSIN
PORKPIE
RISKSIT
ROCKOIL
ROCKYII
ROCKYIV
SILKTIE
SINKSIN
SOAKSIN
SOCKSIN
SUCKSIN
TALKBIG
TOOKAIM
TREKKIE
TUCKSIN
WORKSIN

•••K••I

ALEKSEI
BOOKIII
BOOKVII
MARKIII
MARKVII
ROCKYII
TANKINI
TOPKAPI
WAIKIKI

••••KI•

ADZUKIS
ANNAKIN
BLACKIE
BODYKIT
BREAKIN
BUMPKIN
CAHOKIA
CHECKIN
CHUCKIT
CLOCKIN
COWSKIN
DOESKIN
DRANKIN
DRINKIN
DUKAKIS
EELSKIN
FRANKIE
GHERKIN
GOODKID
JETSKIS
KABUKIS
KIDSKIN
KRESKIN
LADYKIN
LAMBKIN
MANIKIN
MESSKIT
MINIKIN
NICEKID
NONSKID
OILSKIN
OUTSKIP
PIGSKIN
PUMPKIN
PUSHKIN
QUICKIE
RAMEKIN
REDSKIN
RUMAKIS
SALUKIS
SLATKIN
SLINKIN
SLUNKIN
SNEAKIN
STICKIN
STUCKIN
SUZUKIS
TESTKIT
TIOMKIN
TOOLKIT
TREKKIE
TWINKIE
WHIZKID
WILLKIE

••••K•I

MOLOKAI

•••••KI

BREWSKI
DASHIKI
FAROUKI
KONTIKI
MANDOKI
MINISKI
MONOSKI
PARASKI
PULASKI
SNOWSKI
TURFSKI
VALMIKI
WAIKIKI

KJ•••••

KJELLIN

K•J••••

KCJONES

K•••J••

KARAJAN
KELLJAN
KILLJOY

•K•J•••

SKIJUMP
SKYJACK

••KJ•••

INKJETS

••K•J••

LTKOJAK

•••KJ••

BANKJOB
LOCKJAW

KK•••••

KKKKATY

K•K••••

KAKAPOS
KAKUROS
KIKIDEE
KIKUYUS
KKKKATY

K••K•••

KICKBOX
KICKERS
KICKIER
KICKING
KICKOFF
KICKOUT
KICKSIN
KICKSUP
KICKUPS
KINKAID
KINKIER
KINKILY
KINKING
KITKATS
KKKKATY
KOLKATA
KOOKIER
KRAKENS

K•••K••

KABUKIS
KANAKAS
KARAKUM
KAYAKED
KAYAKER
KHARKOV
KIDSKIN
KISHKES
KLINKER
KNOCKED
KNOCKER
KNOCKON
KNUCKLE
KNUCKLY
KRACKEL
KRESKIN

K••••K•

KARAOKE
KIDLIKE
KODIAKS
KONTIKI
KOPECKS
KOPIYKA

K•••••K

KAISHEK
KEYBANK
KEYLOCK
KIDROCK
KINFOLK
KRAMNIK
KUBELIK
KUBRICK

•KK••••

KKKKATY

•K•K•••

KKKKATY

•K••K••

AKSAKOV
SKULKED
SKULKER
SKUNKED

•K•••K•

SKYLIKE

•K••••K

OKHOTSK
SKIMASK
SKIRACK
SKYHOOK
SKYJACK
SKYLARK
SKYWALK

••KK•••

BOKKENS
FOKKERS
KKKKATY
SUKKOTH
TEKKIES
YAKKERS
YAKKING
YUKKING

••K•K••

DUKAKIS

••K••K•

ACKACKS
DIKDIKS
INKLIKE
MUKLUKS
OAKLIKE
REKICKS
TSKTSKS
UNKINKS
ZAKUSKA

••K•••K

DEKLERK
INKMARK
IRKUTSK
LTKOJAK
NOKNOCK
OAKCASK
OAKDESK
OAKPARK
REKNOCK
YAKUTSK

•••KK••

CHUKKER
GROKKED
MARKKAA
TREKKED
TREKKER
TREKKIE

•••K•K•

SHIKOKU
WAIKIKI

•••K••K

CORKOAK
DUNKIRK
FALKIRK
ONAKICK
OUTKICK
SELKIRK
TOPKICK

••••K•K

BANGKOK
BISHKEK

KL•••••

KLAMATH
KLAMMER
KLATSCH
KLAXONS
KLEENEX
KLEIBER
KLEISER
KLENSCH
KLEPTOS
KLEZMER
KLINGER
KLINGON
KLINKER
KLISTER
KLMNOPQ
KLUDGED
KLUDGES
KLUGMAN
KLUTZES

K•L••••

KALININ
KELLJAN
KELLOGG
KELOWNA
KELPIES
KELVINS
KILAUEA
KILDARE
KILLEEN
KILLERS
KILLFEE
KILLING
KILLJOY
KILNDRY
KILNING
KILOBAR
KILOBIT
KILOTON
KILTIES
KILTING
KOLANUT
KOLKATA

K••L•••

KARLOFF
KARLOVY
KARLSON
KAYLENZ
KEELING
KEGLERS
KEILLOR
KELLJAN
KELLOGG
KEYLESS
KEYLIME
KEYLOCK
KIDLIKE
KILLEEN
KILLERS
KILLFEE
KILLING
KILLJOY
KINLESS
KIPLING
KISLEVS
KJELLIN
KNELLED
KOBLENZ
KOOLAID
KOWLOON
KVELLED

K•••L••

KAROLYI
KASTLER
KEEBLER
KEESLAR
KEESLER
KEILLOR
KENOLIN
KERFLOP
KERPLOP
KETTLES
KEYCLUB
KIBBLED
KIBBLES
KIDULTS
KINDLED
KINDLER
KINDLES
KINGLET
KJELLIN
KNEELED
KNEELER
KNELLED
KNOWLES
KNURLED
KOBOLDS
KOEHLER
KREMLIN
KTOSLIN
KUBELIK
KURILES
KVELLED

K••••L•

KABBALA
KAMPALA
KENDALL
KENDOLL
KENNELS
KERNELS
KEYHOLE
KEYPALS
KIMBALL
KINFOLK
KINKILY
KINNELL
KISSELS
KNOWALL
KNUCKLE
KNUCKLY
KORDELL
KOWADLO
KRINGLE
KRYSTLE
KUMMELS
KYOODLE

K•••••L

KAPITAL
KENDALL
KENDOLL
KENWAHL
KESTREL
KIMBALL
KINNELL
KNIEVEL
KNOWALL
KORDELL
KRACKEL

•KL••••

BKLIBAN
JKLMNOP

•K•L•••

OKELLEY
SKELTER
SKELTON
SKILFUL
SKILIFT
SKILLED
SKILLET
SKULKED
SKULKER
SKULLED
SKYLARK
SKYLESS
SKYLIKE
SKYLINE
UKELELE
UKULELE

•K••L••

AKERLOF
EKUELES
OKELLEY
SKIDLID
SKILLED
SKILLET
SKIRLED
SKULLED
SKYBLUE

•K•••L•

SKIABLE
SKIFFLE
SKIPOLE
SKITTLE
SKYWALK
UKELELE
UKULELE

•K••••L

SKILFUL

••KL•••

ANKLERS
ANKLETS
AUKLETS
BAKLAVA
DEKLERK
IJKLMNO
INKLESS
INKLIKE
INKLING
MUKLUKS
OAKLAND
OAKLAWN
OAKLEAF
OAKLIKE

••K•L••

ALKALIS
INKBLOT
NIKOLAI
NIKOLAY
YUKOLIS

••K••L•

INKWELL
LIKABLE
MAKABLE
MAKEILL
NAKEDLY
RAKABLE
TAKABLE
TAKEILL

••K•••L

INKWELL
MAKEILL
MIKHAIL
TAKEILL
WAKEFUL

•••KL••

BACKLIT
BACKLOG
BACKLOT
BARKLEY
BERKLEY
BLAKLEY
BOOKLET
BUCKLED
BUCKLES
BUCKLEY
CACKLED
CACKLER
CACKLES
COCKLED
COCKLES
CONKLIN
DARKLED
DARKLES
DECKLED
DECKLES
FICKLER
HACKLED
HACKLER
HACKLES
HECKLED
HECKLER
HECKLES
HIJKLMN
JANKLOW
LOCKLET
LOCKLIN
NECKLET
NICKLES
PICKLED
PICKLES
RANKLED
RANKLES
RICKLES
SICKLES
TACKLED
TACKLER
TACKLES
TICKLED
TICKLER
TICKLES
TINKLED
TINKLER
TINKLES
WICKLOW
WINKLER

•••K•L•

BALKILY
BLAKELY
COCKILY
DUSKILY
FLAKILY
FLUKILY
FUNKILY
GASKELL
GAWKILY
HASKELL
HUSKILY
JACKALS
JERKILY
KINKILY
LANKILY
LUCKILY
MILKILY
MISKOLC
MURKILY
NICKELS
ONEKILO
OUTKILL
PERKILY
PESKILY
QUAKILY
RISKILY
ROCKILY
SECKELS
SHAKILY
SHEKELS
SILKILY
SMOKILY
SNAKILY
SPIKILY
STOKELY
SULKILY
TACKILY
TOOKILL
WACKILY
WANKELS

•••K••L

DESKFUL
EZEKIEL
FORKFUL
GASKELL
HASKELL
OUTKILL
ROCKOIL
SACKFUL
TANKFUL
TOOKILL

••••KL•

BLACKLY
BLANKLY
BLEAKLY
BRICKLE
BRISKLY
CHUCKLE
CLERKLY
CRACKLE
CRACKLY
CRINKLE
CRINKLY
FRANKLY
FRECKLE
FRECKLY
GHIJKLM
GRACKLE
KNUCKLE
KNUCKLY
PRICKLE
PRICKLY
QUICKLY
SHACKLE
SLACKLY
SLEEKLY
SLICKLY
SPACKLE
SPARKLE
SPARKLY
SPECKLE
STARKLY
THICKLY
TRICKLE
TRUCKLE
TWINKLE
TWINKLY
WRINKLE
WRINKLY

••••K•L

HAECKEL
JAECKEL

KRACKEL
SNORKEL

•••••KL
FGHIJKL

KM•••••
KMESONS

K•M••••
KAMERAD
KAMFONG
KAMPALA
KEMIDOV
KEMPTON
KIMBALL
KIMCHEE
KIMONOS
KLMNOPQ
KOMATSU
KUMMELS
KUMQUAT

K••M•••
KENMORE
KINMONT
KIRMANS
KISMETS
KLAMATH
KLAMMER
KRAMDEN
KRAMNIK
KREMLIN
KUMMELS

K•••M••
KASHMIR
KAUFMAN
KEEPMUM
KEPTMUM
KINGMAN
KINSMAN
KINSMEN
KLAMMER
KLEZMER
KLUGMAN
KROEMER

K••••M•
KEYLIME
KHATAMI
KIDCOMS

K•••••M
KARAKUM
KEEPMUM
KEPTMUM
KETCHAM
KETCHUM
KHAYYAM
KINGDOM

•K•M•••
JKLMNOP
SKIMASK
SKIMMED
SKIMMER
SKIMPED
SKIMPON
SKYMAPS

•K••M••
NKRUMAH
SKIMMED
SKIMMER

•K•••M•
SKIBUMS
SKIJUMP
SKYCAMS
SKYDOME

••KM•••
INKMARK
OAKMOSS

••K•M••
CAKEMIX
ESKIMOS
IJKLMNO
LIKEMAD
MAKEMAD
NOKOMIS
POKEMON
UNKEMPT
WAKAMES
WAKSMAN
YAKIMAS

••K••M•
IRKSOME
LAKSHMI

••K•••M
DUKEDOM
SIKHISM
TAKEAIM

•••KM••
BOOKMAN
BOOKMEN
DARKMAN
EIJKMAN
HACKMAN
HAWKMAN
HECKMAN
HICKMAN
JUNKMAN
JUNKMEN
LUCKMAN
MILKMAN
MILKMEN
PARKMAN
RICKMAN
WALKMAN
WORKMAN
WORKMEN

•••K•M•
BUNKUMS
HIJKLMN

•••K••M
BECKHAM
BUCKRAM
GEEKDOM
LOOKISM
MARKHAM
PINKHAM
TOOKAIM

••••KM•
DRINKME

••••K•M
GHIJKLM
KARAKUM
STICKUM

KN•••••
KNARRED
KNAVERY
KNAVISH
KNEADED
KNEADER
KNEECAP
KNEEING
KNEELED
KNEELER
KNEEPAD
KNEESUP
KNELLED
KNESSET
KNEWHOW
KNIEVEL
KNIFERS
KNIFING
KNIGHTS
KNISHES
KNITTED
KNITTER
KNOBBED
KNOCKED
KNOCKER
KNOCKON
KNOSSOS
KNOTSUP
KNOTTED
KNOTTER
KNOUTED
KNOWALL
KNOWERS
KNOWETH
KNOWHOW
KNOWING
KNOWLES
KNOWSOF
KNUCKLE
KNUCKLY
KNURLED

K•N••••
KANAKAS
KANEOHE
KANSANS
KANTIAN
KENDALL
KENDOLL
KENDREW
KENICHI
KENMORE
KENNEDY
KENNELS
KENNETH
KENNING
KENOLIN
KENOSHA
KENTISH
KENWAHL
KENYANS
KINCAID
KINDEST
KINDLED
KINDLER
KINDLES
KINDRED
KINESES
KINESIC
KINESIS
KINETIC
KINFOLK
KINGDOM
KINGING
KINGLET
KINGMAN
KINGPIN
KINGRAT
KINGTUT
KINISON
KINKAID
KINKIER
KINKILY
KINKING
KINLESS
KINMONT
KINNEAR
KINNELL
KINSHIP
KINSMAN
KINSMEN
KONTIKI
KUNDERA

K••N•••
KEENENH
KEENERS
KEENEST
KEENING
KENNEDY
KENNELS
KENNETH
KENNING
KERNELS
KEYNOTE
KHANATE
KIDNAPS
KIDNEYS
KILNDRY
KILNING
KINNEAR
KINNELL
KLENSCH
KLINGER
KLINGON
KLINKER
KLMNOPQ
KOONING
KRINGLE
KUZNETS
KWANZAA
KWANZAS

K•••N••
KAHUNAS
KALININ
KCJONES
KEARNEY
KETONES
KETONIC
KEYINON
KIMONOS
KIWANIS
KLEENEX
KOLANUT
KORANIC
KORUNAS
KRAMNIK
KRASNER

K••••N•
KACHINA
KACHING
KAMFONG
KANSANS
KATRINA
KATRINE
KAYLENZ
KAYOING
KEDGING
KEELING
KEENENH
KEENING
KEEPING
KEGGING
KELOWNA
KELVINS
KENNING
KENYANS
KEYBANK
KEYRING
KICKING
KIDDING
KILLING
KILNING
KILTING
KINGING
KINKING
KINMONT
KIPLING
KIPPING
KIRMANS
KISSING
KITTENS
KITTING
KLAXONS
KMESONS
KNEEING
KNIFING
KNOWING
KOBLENZ
KOONING
KOREANS
KOSCINA
KRAKENS
KRISHNA
KUCHENS
KURRENT

K•••••N
KALININ
KANTIAN
KARAJAN
KARLSON
KATHRYN
KAUFMAN
KEEPSIN
KEEPSON
KEESHAN
KELLJAN
KEMPTON
KENOLIN
KEOGHAN
KERATIN
KEYEDIN
KEYEDON
KEYINON
KEYSPAN
KICKSIN
KIDSKIN
KILLEEN
KILOTON
KINGMAN
KINGPIN
KINISON
KINSMAN
KINSMEN
KIRSTEN
KITCHEN
KJELLIN
KLINGON
KLUGMAN
KNOCKON
KOSYGIN
KOWLOON
KRAMDEN
KRATION
KREMLIN
KRESKIN
KRISTIN
KRYPTON
KTOSLIN

•KN••••
IKNEWIT
IKNOWIT

•K•N•••
EKINGBY
OKINAWA
SKINNED
SKINNER
SKUNKED
SKYNYRD

•K••N••
AKRONOH
EKWENSI
JKLMNOP
SKINNED
SKINNER

•K•••N•
AKEBONO
IKEBANA
OKAYING
SKATING
SKEWING
SKIRUNS
SKYLINE
UKRAINE

•K••••N
BKLIBAN
SKELTON
SKIMPON

••KN•••
INKNOTS
NOKNOCK
ORKNEYS
REKNEAD
REKNITS
REKNOCK
REKNOTS
UNKNITS
UNKNOTS
UNKNOWN

••K•N••
ALKENES
ASKANCE
BIKINIS
IIKINGS
INKINGS
LIKENED
LIKENEW
LIKENTO
LIKINGS
MAKINGS
MCKENNA
MTKENYA
MYKONOS
TAKENBY
TAKENIN
TAKENON
TAKENTO
TAKENUP
TAKINGS
TOKENED
UNKINKS
VIKINGS
WAKENED
WAKENER
WAKINGS
WOKENUP

••K••N•
BOKKENS
DEKEING
IJKLMNO
INKLING
MAKEONE
MCKENNA
OAKLAND
SUKARNO
TAKEINS
TAKEONE
YAKKING
YOKOONO
YUKKING

••K•••N
ANKARAN
ASKEDIN
AZKABAN
BAKEPAN
CAKEPAN
CAKETIN
DAKOTAN
INKEDIN
INKHORN
MAKEFUN
MAKERUN
OAKFERN
OAKLAWN
POKEFUN
POKEMON
RAKEDIN
RAKESIN
TAKENIN
TAKENON
TAKESIN
TAKESON
TAKETEN
UNKNOWN
WAKSMAN

•••KN••
BERKNER
BOWKNOT
BUCKNER
COCKNEY
HACKNEY
ILLKNOW
INAKNOT
LETKNOW
LOCKNUT
LUCKNOW
MISKNEW
MISKNOW
TOPKNOT
WHOKNEW
YOUKNOW

•••K•N•
ALAKING
ANYKIND
AWAKENS
AWAKING
BACKEND
BACKING
BALKANS
BALKING
BANKING
BANKONE
BARKING
BASKING
BECKONS
BILKING
BOBKANE
BODKINS
BOKKENS
BONKING
BOOKEND
BOOKING
BORKING
BRAKING
BUCKING
BULKING
BUNKING
BURKINA
BUSKING
CALKING
CALKINS
CARKING
CASKING
CATKINS
CHOKING
COCKING
CONKING
COOKING
CORKING
DARKENS
DAWKINS
DECKING
DICKENS
DIRKING
DISKING
DOCKING
DONKING
DUCKING
DUNKING
DUSKING
ERSKINE
EVOKING
FINKING
FIRKINS
FLAKING
FORKING
FUNKING
GAWKING
HACKING
HARKENS
HARKING
HAWKING
HAWKINS
HOCKING
HONKING
HOOKING
HOPKINS
HOSKINS
HULKING
HUSKING
JACKING
JENKINS
JERKING
JERKINS
JUNKDNA
JUNKING
KICKING
KINKING
KRAKENS
LACKING
LARKING
LARKINS
LEAKING
LICKING
LINKING
LOCKING
LOCKINS
LOOKING
LOOKINS
LUCKING
LURKING
MANKIND
MARKING
MASKING
MILKING
MOCKING
MUCKING
NANKING
NAPKINS
NECKING
NICKING
NOCKING
OFAKIND
OINKING
OSAKANS
OUTKING
PACKING
PARKING
PARKINS
PEAKING
PECKING
PEEKING
PERKING
PERKINS
PICKENS
PICKING
PINKENS
PINKING
PORKING
QUAKING
RACKING
RANKINE
RANKING
RECKONS
REDKING
REEKING
RISKING
ROCKING
ROOKING
RUCKING
RYOKANS
SACKING
SEEKING
SHAKING
SICKENS
SINKING
SLAKING
SMOKING
SNAKING
SOAKING
SOCKING
SPIKING
SPOKANE
SPOKING
STAKING
STOKING
SUBKING
SUCKING
SULKING
TACKING
TALKING
TANKING
TANKINI
TASKING
THEKING
TICKING
TUCKING
TUSKING
WADKINS
WALKING
WALKINS
WALKONS
WATKINS
WEAKENS
WEAKONS
WEEKEND
WICKING
WILKENS
WILKINS
WINKING
WORKING
YAKKING
YANKING
YUKKING
ZADKINE
ZONKING

•••K••N
AGAKHAN
ALYKHAN
BACKSIN
BANKSON
BOOKMAN
BOOKMEN
BROKEIN
CHOKEON
CONKLIN
DARKMAN
DARKTAN
DICKSON
DIRKSEN
DUCKPIN
EIJKMAN
ERIKSON
FINKSON
HACKMAN
HAWKMAN
HECKMAN
HICKMAN
HIJKLMN
HOOKSON
JACKSON
JUNKMAN
JUNKMEN
KICKSIN
LEAKSIN
LOCKEAN
LOCKLIN
LOCKSIN
LOCKSON
LOOKSIN
LOOKSON
LUCKMAN
MILKCAN
MILKMAN
MILKMEN
MILKRUN
ONTKEAN
PACKSIN
PACKSON
PARKMAN
PEEKSIN
PICKSON
RICKMAN
ROCKOON
SINKSIN
SOAKSIN
SOCKSIN
SUCKSIN
TACKSON
TALKSON
TENKRUN
TOLKIEN
TOOKTEN
TUCKSIN
WALKMAN
WALKSON
WORKMAN
WORKMEN
WORKSIN
WORKSON
YANKSON
YANKTON
YORKTON

••••K•N
ALASKAN
ANNAKIN
BETAKEN
BETOKEN
BLACKEN
BLYNKEN
BRACKEN
BREAKIN
BUMPKIN
CHECKIN
CHECKON
CHICKEN
CLICKON
CLOCKIN
COWSKIN
DANIKEN
DOESKIN
DRANKIN
DRINKIN
DRUNKEN
EELSKIN
FLANKEN
FRANKEN
GHERKIN
HEARKEN
HOBOKEN
IRECKON
KIDSKIN
KNOCKON
KRESKIN
LADYKIN
LAMBKIN
MANIKIN
MENCKEN
MINIKIN
OILSKIN
PIGSKIN
PUMPKIN
PUSHKIN
QUICKEN
RAMEKIN
REDSKIN
RETAKEN
REWAKEN
REWOKEN
SLACKEN
SLATKIN
SLEEKEN
SLINKIN
SLUNKIN
SNACKON
SNEAKIN
STICKIN
STICKON
STUCKIN
STUCKON
THICKEN
TIOMKIN
TOPEKAN
UNTAKEN

KO•••••
KOBLENZ
KOBOLDS
KODIAKS
KOEHLER
KOLANUT
KOLKATA
KOMATSU
KONTIKI
KOOKIER
KOOLAID
KOONING
KOOSHES
KOPECKS
KOPIYKA
KORANIC
KORDELL
KOREANS
KORUNAS
KOSCINA
KOSHERS
KOSHIBA
KOSOVAR
KOSSUTH
KOSYGIN
KOWADLO
KOWLOON
KOWTOWS

K•O••••
KEOGHAN
KNOBBED
KNOCKED
KNOCKER
KNOCKON
KNOSSOS
KNOTSUP
KNOTTED
KNOTTER
KNOUTED
KNOWALL
KNOWERS
KNOWETH
KNOWHOW
KNOWING
KNOWLES
KNOWSOF
KOOKIER
KOOLAID
KOONING
KOOSHES
KROEMER
KTOSLIN
KYOODLE

K••O•••
KAROLYI
KAYOING
KCJONES
KELOWNA
KENOLIN
KENOSHA
KEROUAC
KETONES

KETONIC
KILOBAR
KILOBIT
KILOTON
KIMONOS
KOBOLDS
KOSOVAR
KYOODLE

K•••O••
KAMFONG
KANEOHE
KARAOKE
KARLOFF
KARLOVY
KEDROVA
KEEPOFF
KEEPOUT
KELLOGG
KENDOLL
KENMORE
KEPTOFF
KEPTOUT
KEYHOLE
KEYLOCK
KEYNOTE
KEYWORD
KICKOFF
KICKOUT
KIDCOMS
KIDROCK
KINFOLK
KINMONT
KISSOFF
KLAXONS
KLMNOPQ
KMESONS
KOWLOON
KOWTOWS

K••••O•
KAKAPOS
KAKUROS
KARLSON
KEEPSON
KEILLOR
KEMIDOV
KEMPTON
KERFLOP
KERPLOP
KEYEDON
KEYINON
KHARKOV
KIARIOS
KICKBOX
KILLJOY
KILOTON
KIMONOS
KINGDOM
KINISON
KLEPTOS
KLINGON
KNEWHOW
KNOCKON
KNOSSOS
KNOWHOW
KNOWSOF
KOWLOON
KRATION
KRYPTON
KUTUZOV

K•••••O
KEEPSTO
KOWADLO

•KO••••
SKOSHES

•K•O•••
AKRONOH
IKNOWIT
OKHOTSK
OKTOBER

•K••O••
AKEBONO
EKEDOUT
EKESOUT
OKSHOOT
SKIBOBS
SKIBOOT
SKIDOOS
SKIPOLE
SKIPOUT
SKITOWS
SKYDOME
SKYHOOK

•K•••O•
AKERLOF
AKRONOH
AKSAKOV
JKLMNOP
OKSHOOT
SKELTON
SKIBOOT
SKIDDOO
SKIDOOS
SKIDROW
SKIMPON
SKISHOP
SKYHOOK

•K••••O
AKEBONO
AKIHITO
SKIDDOO

••KO•••
ASKOVER
DAKOTAN
DAKOTAS
LAKOTAS
LTKOJAK
MYKONOS
NIKOLAI
NIKOLAY
NOKOMIS
YOKOONO
YUKOLIS

••K•O••
ASKSOUT
AYKROYD
BAKEOFF
FAKEOUT
HIKEOUT
INKHORN
INKNOTS
INKPOTS
IRKSOME
MAKEOFF
MAKEONE
MAKEOUT
NOKNOCK
OAKMOSS
OAKWOOD
POKEOUT
RAKEOFF
REKNOCK
REKNOTS
SUKKOTH
TAKEOFF
TAKEONE
TAKEOUT
UNKNOTS
UNKNOWN
YOKOONO

••K••O•
AIKIDOS
ASKEDOF
ASKSFOR
BOKCHOY
DUKEDOM
ESKIMOS
ICKYPOO
INKBLOT
INKSPOT
JUKEBOX
KAKAPOS
KAKUROS
LIKEWOW
MAKEDOS
MAKEFOR
MIKADOS
MYKONOS
OAKWOOD
PEKEPOO
POKEMON
TAKEFOR
TAKENON
TAKESON

••K•••O
ICKYPOO
IJKLMNO
LIKENTO
MAKESDO
MAKESGO
PEKEPOO
SUKARNO
TAKENTO
TAKESTO
YOKOONO

•••KO••
BACKOFF
BACKOUT
BANKONE
BECKONS
BUCKOES
BUNKOED
CONKOFF
CONKOUT
COOKOFF
COOKOUT
CORKOAK
CUCKOOS
DECKOUT
DICKORY
DUCKOUT
FORKOUT
GECKOES
HACKOFF
HICKORY
JERKOUT
KICKOFF
KICKOUT
LOCKOUT
LOOKOUT
LUCKOUT
MARKOFF
MARKOUT
MARKOVA
MISKOLC
NDAKOTA
OSHKOSH
PACKOFF
PEEKOUT
PICKOFF
PICKOUT
PINKOES
RACKOUT
RANKOUT
RECKONS
ROCKOIL
ROCKOON
SACKOUT
SDAKOTA
SEEKOUT
SHAKOES
SHIKOKU
SICKOUT
SUKKOTH
TALKOUT
TICKOFF
TOOKOFF
TOOKOUT
WALKOFF
WALKONS
WALKOUT
WEAKONS
WINKOUT
WORKOFF
WORKOUT
YANKOFF
YANKOUT
ZONKOUT

•••K•O•
BACKHOE
BACKLOG
BACKLOT
BACKROW
BANKJOB
BANKSON
BOWKNOT
BUCKFOR
CHEKHOV
CHOKEON
COOKPOT
COOKTOP
CUCKOOS
DESKTOP
DICKSON
ERIKSON
FINKSON
GEEKDOM
GINKGOS
HOOKSON
ILLKNOW
INAKNOT
JACKPOT
JACKSON
JACKSOO
JANKLOW
KICKBOX
LETKNOW
LOCKBOX
LOCKSON
LOOKFOR
LOOKSON
LOOKYOU
LUCKNOW
MILKCOW
MILKSOP
MISKNOW
PACKSON
PICKSON
RAYKROC
REEKSOF
ROCKCOD
ROCKOON
SOCKHOP
SPOKEOF
TACKSON
TALKSOF
TALKSON
TANKTOP
TOOKFOR
TOPKNOT
VOSKHOD
WALKSON
WICKLOW
WORKBOX
WORKFOR
WORKSON
YANKSON
YANKTON
YORKTON
YOUKNOW

•••K••O
HAPKIDO
JACKIEO
JACKSOO
LOOKSTO
MANKATO
MUSKEGO
ONEKILO
SPOKETO
TALKSTO
WAIKATO
WALKSTO

••••KO•
AKSAKOV
ALACKOF
APECKOF
BANGKOK
CHECKON
CLICKON
DAVEKOZ
FRANKOZ
GINGKOS
GRINKOV
IRECKON
KHARKOV
KNOCKON
NABOKOV
SHOPKOS
SMACKOF
SNACKON
SPEAKOF
STICKON
STUCKON
THINKOF
WENDKOS

••••K•O
DRANKTO
DRINKTO
FLOCKTO
SPEAKTO
STICKTO
STUCKTO
THINKSO

•••••KO
DANEYKO
FEDERKO
GROMYKO
LYSENKO

K•P••••
KAPITAL
KAPITSA
KAPTURE
KEPTFIT
KEPTMUM
KEPTOFF
KEPTOUT
KIPLING
KIPPERS
KIPPING
KOPECKS
KOPIYKA

K••P•••
KAMPALA
KEEPERS
KEEPFIT
KEEPING
KEEPMUM
KEEPOFF
KEEPOUT
KEEPSAT
KEEPSIN
KEEPSON
KEEPSTO
KEEPSUP
KELPIES
KEMPTON
KERPLOP
KEWPIES
KEYPADS
KEYPALS
KIPPERS
KIPPING
KLEPTOS
KRYPTON

K•••P••
KAKAPOS
KEYSPAN
KINGPIN
KNEEPAD

K••••P•
KICKUPS
KIDNAPS
KLMNOPQ

K•••••P
KEEPSUP
KERFLOP
KERPLOP
KETCHUP
KEYEDUP
KEYGRIP
KICKSUP
KINSHIP
KNEECAP
KNEESUP
KNOTSUP

•K•P•••
SKEPTIC
SKIPOLE
SKIPOUT
SKIPPED
SKIPPER
SKIPSBY

•K••P••
SKIMPED
SKIMPON
SKIPPED
SKIPPER

•K•••P•
SKICAPS
SKYCAPS
SKYMAPS

•K••••P
JKLMNOP
SKIJUMP
SKISHOP
SKITRIP

••KP•••
INKPADS
INKPOTS
OAKPARK

••K•P••
BAKEPAN
CAKEPAN
GOKAPUT
ICKYPOO
INKSPOT
KAKAPOS
MAKEPAR
PEKEPOO

••K••P•
MAKEUPS
UNKEMPT
UPKEEPS
WAKEUPS

••K•••P
ASKEDUP
CAKEDUP
CAKESUP
HIKEDUP
HIKESUP
INKYCAP
MAKESUP
RAKEDUP
RAKESUP
TAKENUP
TAKESUP
WAKEDUP
WAKESUP
WOKENUP

•••KP••
BACKPAY
COCKPIT
COOKPOT
DUCKPIN
JACKPOT
PORKPIE
SICKPAY

•••K•P•
BACKUPS
HOOKUPS
KICKUPS
LINKUPS
LOCKUPS
LOOKUPS
MARKUPS
MOCKUPS
OUTKEPT
PICKUPS
TOPKAPI
WALKUPS
WORKUPS

•••K••P
BACKSUP
BANKSUP
BARKEEP
BROKEUP
BUCKSUP
BULKSUP
CHOKEUP
COOKSUP
COOKTOP
CORKSUP
DESKTOP
FORKSUP
HACKSUP
HOOKSUP
JACKSUP
JERKSUP
KICKSUP
LICKSUP
LINKSUP
LOCKSUP
LOOKSUP
MARKSUP
MILKSOP
MOCKSUP
MUCKSUP
OUTKEEP
PACKSUP
PERKSUP
PICKSUP
RACKSUP
RUCKSUP
SACKSUP
SHAKEUP
SMOKEUP
SOAKSUP
SOCKHOP
SPIKEUP
SPOKEUP
STOKEUP
SUCKSUP
TACKSUP
TALKSUP
TANKSUP
TANKTOP
WICKIUP
WORKSUP

••••K•P
BLOCKUP
BREAKUP
BRICKUP
CHALKUP
CHECKUP
CRACKUP
CRANKUP
DRANKUP
DRINKUP
OUTSKIP
PRICKUP
SHOOKUP
SLACKUP
SLINKUP
SLUNKUP
SMACKUP
SNEAKUP
SNUCKUP
SPEAKUP
STACKUP
STANKUP
STICKUP
STINKUP
STOCKUP
STUCKUP
SWANKUP
THINKUP
WRACKUP

K••Q•••
KUMQUAT

K•••••Q
KLMNOPQ

KR•••••
KRACKEL
KRAKENS
KRAMDEN
KRAMNIK
KRASNER
KRATION
KREMLIN
KRESKIN
KRINGLE
KRISHNA
KRISTIN
KROEMER
KRUEGER
KRYPTON
KRYSTLE

K•R••••
KARACHI
KARAJAN
KARAKUM
KARAOKE
KARASEA
KARATES
KARLOFF
KARLOVY
KARLSON
KAROLYI
KERATIN
KERFLOP
KERNELS
KEROUAC
KERPLOP
KERSHAW
KERTESZ
KIRMANS
KIRSTEN
KIRSTIE
KORANIC
KORDELL
KOREANS
KORUNAS
KURDISH
KURILES
KURRENT

K••R•••
KATRINA
KATRINE
KEARNEY
KEDROVA
KEYRING
KHARKOV
KIARIOS
KIDROCK
KNARRED
KNURLED
KUBRICK
KURRENT

K•••R••
KAKUROS
KAMERAD
KATHRYN
KENDREW
KESTREL
KEYGRIP
KIDSRUS
KINDRED
KINGRAT
KNARRED

K••••R•
KAISERS
KAPTURE
KEDGERS
KEENERS
KEEPERS
KEGGERS
KEGLERS
KENMORE
KEYCARD
KEYWORD
KICKERS
KIDDERS
KILDARE
KILLERS
KILNDRY
KIPPERS
KISSERS
KITHARA
KITTERY
KNAVERY
KNIFERS
KNOWERS
KOSHERS
KUNDERA

K•••••R
KASHMIR
KASTLER
KAYAKER
KEEBLER
KEESLAR
KEESLER
KEILLOR
KEISTER
KICKIER
KIEFFER
KILOBAR
KINDLER
KINKIER
KINNEAR
KLAMMER
KLEIBER
KLEISER
KLEZMER
KLINGER
KLINKER
KLISTER
KNEADER
KNEELER
KNITTER
KNOCKER
KNOTTER
KOEHLER
KOOKIER
KOSOVAR
KRASNER
KROEMER
KRUEGER
KUTCHER

•KR••••
AKRONOH
NKRUMAH
UKRAINE

•K•R•••
AKERLOF
SKIRACE
SKIRACK
SKIRLED
SKIRTED
SKIRTER
SKIRUNS

•K••R••
SKIAREA
SKIDROW
SKITRIP

•K•••R•
SKATERS
SKEWERS
SKYLARK
SKYNYRD
SKYSURF
SKYWARD

•K••••R
OKTOBER
SKEETER
SKELTER
SKIDDER
SKIMMER
SKINNER
SKIPPER
SKIRTER
SKITTER
SKIWEAR
SKULKER

••KR•••
AYKROYD

••K•R••
ANKARAN
BAKERST
GOKARTS
JAKARTA
KAKUROS
MAKERUN
OAKTREE
SUKARNO

••K••R•
ANKLERS
AWKWARD
BOKHARA
BUKHARA
DAKTARI
DEKLERK
DYKSTRA
ECKHART
ELKHART
FOKKERS
INKHORN
INKMARK
OAKFERN
OAKPARK
YAKKERS

••K•••R
ASKOVER
ASKSFOR
FAKEFUR
INKSTER
MAKEFOR
MAKEPAR
MAKEWAR
TAKEFOR
WAKENER

•••KR••
BACKROW
BACKRUB
BUCKRAM
CHAKRAS
DARKRED
MILKRUN
MUSKRAT
PACKRAT
RAYKROC
RINKRAT
TENKRUN
VICKREY

•••K•R•
ARIKARA
AWAKERS
BACKERS
BALKERS
BANKERS
BARKERS
BEAKERS
BICKERS
BILKERS
BONKERS
BOOKERS
BOOKERT
BROKERS
BUCKERS
BUNKERS
BUSKERS
CALKERS
CANKERS
CHOKERS
COCKERS
CONKERS
COOKERS
COOKERY
CORKERS
DECKERS
DICKERS
DICKORY
DOCKERS
DUCKERS
DUNKERS
DUNKIRK
ELEKTRA
EVOKERS
FALKIRK
FLAKERS
FOKKERS
FOLKART
FORKERS
GAWKERS
HACKERS
HANKERS
HAWKERS
HECKART
HICKORY
HOCKERS
HONKERS
HUNKERS

HUSKERS
JERKERS
JUNKART
JUNKERS
KICKERS
LARKERS
LEAKERS
LICKERS
LINKERS
LOCKERS
LOOKERS
LUNKERS
LURKERS
MARKERS
MASKERS
MILKERS
MOCKERS
MOCKERY
MUCKERS
NECKERS
NICKERS
OINKERS
PACKARD
PACKERS
PARKERS
PEEKERS
PICKERS
PORKERS
PUCKERS
PUCKERY
PUNKERS
QUAKERS
RACKERS
RANKERS
REEKERS
RISKERS
ROCKERS
ROCKERY
ROOKERY
RUCKERT
SACKERS
SEEKERS
SELKIRK
SHAKERS
SHAKIRA
SINKERS
SLAKERS
SMOKERS
SNAKERS
SOAKERS
SPIKERS
STOKERS
SUCKDRY
SUCKERS
SULKERS
TACKERS
TALKERS
TANKARD
TANKERS
TICKERS
TINKERS
TUCKERS
TUSKERS
VICKERS
WALKERS
WALKURE
WICKERS
WINKERS
WORKERS
YAKKERS
YANKERS
YONKERS
YORKERS

•••K••R

BACKBAR
BALKIER
BARKIER
BERKNER
BUCKFOR
BUCKNER
BULKIER
CACKLER
CHOKIER
CHUKKER
COCKIER
CORKIER
DINKIER
DORKIER
DUCKIER
DUSKIER
FICKLER
FLAKIER
FLUKIER
FOLKIER
FORKIER
FUNKIER
GAWKIER
GEEKIER
GUCKIER
GUNKIER
HACKLER
HECKLER
HINKIER
HULKIER
HUNKIER
HUSKIER
JACKTAR
JERKIER
JUNKCAR
JUNKIER
KICKIER
KINKIER
KOOKIER
LANKIER
LARKIER
LEAKIER
LOOKFOR
LUCKIER
MILKBAR
MILKIER
MUCKIER
MURKIER
MUSKIER
PEAKIER
PERKIER
PESKIER
PICKIER
PORKIER
PUNKIER
QUAKIER
REEKIER
RISKIER
ROCKIER
ROOKIER
SHAKIER
SILKIER
SMOKIER
SNAKIER
SPIKIER
SUCKIER
SULKIER
TACKIER
TACKLER
TALKIER
TANKCAR
TASKBAR
TICKLER
TINKLER
TOOKFOR
TREKKER
WACKIER
WINKLER
WORKFOR
YUCKIER
ZINKIER

••••KR•

CONAKRY

••••K•R

ALROKER
BAULKER
BLACKER
BLANKER
BLEAKER
BLINKER
BLOCKER
BREAKER
BRINKER
BRISKER
CAULKER
CHECKER
CHUKKER
CLACKER
CLICKER
CLINKER
CLOCKER
CLUCKER
CLUNKER
COMAKER
CRACKER
CROAKER
CROCKER
DRINKER
DRUCKER
DRUNKER
FLANKER
FLICKER
FLUNKER
FRANKER
FRICKER
FRISKER
INVOKER
KAYAKER
KLINKER
KNOCKER
LALAKER
MONIKER
PLUNKER
PRINKER
QUACKER
QUICKER
REBUKER
RETAKER
REVOKER
SHANKAR
SHIRKER
SHOCKER
SHUCKER
SKULKER
SLACKER
SLEEKER
SLICKER
SLINKER
SMACKER
SMIRKER
SMUCKER
SNACKER
SNEAKER
SNICKER
SNOOKER
SPANKER
SPEAKER
STACKER
STALKER
STARKER
STICKER
STINKER
STOCKER
STRIKER
STROKER
SWANKER
THANKER
THICKER
THINKER
TRACKER
TREKKER
TRICKER
TRUCKER
UNMAKER
VOLCKER
WHACKER
WHISKER
WREAKER
WRECKER

K•S••••

KASHMIR
KASTLER
KESTREL
KISHKES
KISLEVS
KISMETS
KISSELS
KISSERS
KISSING
KISSOFF
KOSCINA
KOSHERS
KOSHIBA
KOSOVAR
KOSSUTH
KOSYGIN

K••S•••

KAISERS
KAISHEK
KANSANS
KEESHAN
KEESLAR
KEESLER
KEISTER
KERSHAW
KEYSPAN
KIDSEAT
KIDSKIN
KIDSRUS
KINSHIP
KINSMAN
KINSMEN
KIRSTEN
KIRSTIE
KISSELS
KISSERS
KISSING
KISSOFF
KITSCHY
KLISTER
KMESONS
KNESSET
KNISHES
KNOSSOS
KOOSHES
KOSSUTH
KRASNER
KRESKIN
KRISHNA
KRISTIN
KRYSTLE
KTOSLIN
KVASSES

K•••S••

KARASEA
KARLSON
KATISHA
KEEPSAT
KEEPSIN
KEEPSON
KEEPSTO
KEEPSUP
KENOSHA
KICKSIN
KICKSUP
KINESES
KINESIC
KINESIS
KINISON
KLATSCH
KLEISER
KLENSCH
KNEESUP
KNESSET
KNOSSOS
KNOTSUP
KNOWSOF
KVASSES

K••••S•

KADDISH
KAPITSA
KEENEST
KENTISH
KERTESZ
KEYCASE
KEYLESS
KEYWEST
KIDDISH
KINDEST
KINLESS
KNAVISH
KOMATSU
KURDISH

K•••••S

KABUKIS
KADETTS
KAHUNAS
KAISERS
KAKAPOS
KAKUROS
KANAKAS
KANSANS
KARATES
KCJONES
KEDGERS
KEENERS
KEEPERS
KEGGERS
KEGLERS
KELPIES
KELVINS
KENNELS
KENYANS
KERNELS
KETCHES
KETONES
KETTLES
KEWPIES
KEYDETS
KEYLESS
KEYPADS
KEYPALS
KEYWAYS
KIARIOS
KIBBLES
KICKERS
KICKUPS
KIDCOMS
KIDDERS
KIDDIES
KIDNAPS
KIDNEYS
KIDSRUS
KIDULTS
KIDVIDS
KIKUYUS
KILLERS
KILTIES
KIMONOS
KINDLES
KINESES
KINESIS
KINLESS
KIPPERS
KIRMANS
KISHKES
KISLEVS
KISMETS
KISSELS
KISSERS
KITBAGS
KITKATS
KITTENS
KITTIES
KIWANIS
KLAXONS
KLEPTOS
KLUDGES
KLUTZES
KMESONS
KNIFERS
KNIGHTS
KNISHES
KNOSSOS
KNOWERS
KNOWLES
KOBOLDS
KODIAKS
KOOSHES
KOPECKS
KOREANS
KORUNAS
KOSHERS
KOWTOWS
KRAKENS
KUCHENS
KUMMELS
KURILES
KUZNETS
KVASSES
KWACHAS
KWANZAS

•KS••••

AKSAKOV
OKSHOOT

•K•S•••

EKESOUT
EKISTIC
SKISHOP
SKISUIT
SKOSHES
SKYSURF

•K••S••

SKIPSBY

•K•••S•

EKWENSI
OKHOTSK
SKIMASK
SKIVEST
SKYLESS

•K••••S

EKUELES
SKATERS
SKEWERS
SKIBIBS
SKIBOBS
SKIBUMS
SKICAPS
SKIDOOS
SKIHATS
SKIRUNS
SKITOWS
SKOSHES
SKYCAMS
SKYCAPS
SKYLESS
SKYMAPS
SKYWAYS

••KS•••

ASKSFOR
ASKSOUT
DYKSTRA
INKSACS
INKSPOT
INKSTER
IRKSOME
LAKSHMI
RIKSDAG
WAKSMAN

••K•S••

CAKESUP
FAKESIT
HIKESUP
LAKISTS
MAKESDO
MAKESGO
MAKESIT
MAKESUP
MIKASAS
POKESAT
RAKESIN
RAKESUP
TAKESIN
TAKESIT
TAKESON
TAKESTO
TAKESUP
TSKTSKS
WAKESUP
ZAKUSKA

••K••S•

BAKERST
CAKIEST
COKIEST
HOKIEST
ICKIEST
INKIEST
INKLESS
IRKUTSK
JOKIEST
LAKIEST
OAKCASK
OAKDESK
OAKIEST
OAKMOSS
POKIEST
SIKHISM
YAKUTSK

••K•••S

ACKACKS
AIKIDOS
ALKALIS
ALKENES
ANKLERS
ANKLETS
AUKLETS
BIKINIS
BOKKENS
DAKOTAS
DIKDIKS
DIKTATS
DUKAKIS
ESKIMOS
FAKEIDS
FOKKERS
GOKARTS
IIKINGS
INKINGS
INKJETS
INKLESS
INKNOTS
INKPADS
INKPOTS
INKSACS
KAKAPOS
KAKUROS
KIKUYUS
LAKISTS
LAKOTAS
LIKINGS
MAKEDOS
MAKEUPS
MAKINGS
MIKADOS
MIKASAS
MUKLUKS
MYKONOS
NIKEADS
NOKOMIS
OAKMOSS
OAKTAGS
ORKNEYS
REKICKS
REKNITS
REKNOTS
STKITTS
TAKEINS
TAKINGS
TEKKIES
TSKTSKS
UNKINKS
UNKNITS
UNKNOTS
UPKEEPS
VIKINGS
WAKAMES
WAKEUPS
WAKINGS
YAKIMAS
YAKKERS
YUKATAS
YUKOLIS

•••KS••

ALEKSEI
BACKSAW
BACKSIN
BACKSUP
BALKSAT
BANKSON
BANKSUP
BARKSAT
BUCKSAW
BUCKSUP
BULKSUP
COOKSUP
CORKSUP
DESKSET
DICKSON
DIRKSEN
ERIKSON
FINKSON
FORKSUP
GAWKSAT
HACKSAW
HACKSIT
HACKSUP
HONKSAT
HOOKSON
HOOKSUP
JACKSON
JACKSOO
JACKSUP
JERKSUP
KICKSIN
KICKSUP
LEAKSIN
LICKSUP
LINKSUP
LOCKSET
LOCKSIN
LOCKSON
LOCKSUP
LOOKSAD
LOOKSAT
LOOKSEE
LOOKSIN
LOOKSON
LOOKSTO
LOOKSUP
MARKSUP
MILKSOP
MOCKSUP
MUCKSUP
PACKSIN
PACKSON
PACKSUP
PARKSIT
PECKSAT
PEEKSAT
PEEKSIN
PERKSUP
PICKSAT
PICKSON
PICKSUP
RACKSUP
REEKSOF
RICKSHA
RISKSIT
RUCKSUP
SACKSUP
SINKSIN
SOAKSIN
SOAKSUP
SOCKSIN
SUCKSIN
SUCKSUP
TACKSON
TACKSUP
TALKSAT
TALKSOF
TALKSON
TALKSTO
TALKSUP
TANKSUP
TICKSBY
TUCKSIN
WALKSBY
WALKSON
WALKSTO
WINKSAT
WORKSAT
WORKSHY
WORKSIN
WORKSON
WORKSUP
YANKSAT
YANKSON

•••K•S•

AIRKISS
BOOKISH
COCKISH
DANKEST
DARKEST
DARKISH
DUSKISH
FOLKISH
GAWKISH
HAWKISH
JACKASS
LANKEST
LARKISH
LOOKISM
LOOKIST
MAWKISH
MEEKEST
MONKISH
MURKISH
OSHKOSH
OUTKAST
OUTKISS
PEAKISH
PECKISH
PERKISH
PINKEST
PINKISH
PORKISH
PUCKISH
RANKEST
RANKISH
ROOKISH
SICKEST
SICKISH
SUNKIST
THEKISS
TURKISH
WACKEST
WEAKEST
WEAKISH
WETKISS
YERKISH
YORKIST

•••K••S

AIRKISS
ALEKEGS
ALTKEYS
AWAKENS
AWAKERS
BACKERS
BACKUPS
BALKANS
BALKERS
BANKERS
BANKITS
BARKERS
BASKETS
BEAKERS
BECKONS
BICKERS
BIGKIDS
BILKERS
BODKINS
BOKKENS
BONKERS
BOOKERS
BOOKIES
BROKERS
BUCKERS
BUCKETS
BUCKLES
BUCKOES
BUNKERS
BUNKUMS
BUSKERS
CACKLES
CALKERS
CALKINS
CANKERS
CARKEYS
CASKETS
CATKINS
CHAKRAS
CHOKERS
COCKERS
COCKLES
CONKERS
COOKERS
COOKIES
CORKERS
CUCKOOS
DARKENS
DARKLES
DAWKINS
DECKERS
DECKLES
DELKEYS
DICKENS
DICKERS
DICKEYS
DICKIES
DOCKERS
DOCKETS
DONKEYS
DUCKERS
DUCKIES
DUNKERS
ENSKIES
EVOKERS
FIRKINS
FLAKERS
FOKKERS
FOLKIES
FORKERS
GAPKIDS
GASKETS
GAWKERS
GECKOES
GINKGOS
GURKHAS
HACKERS
HACKIES
HACKLES
HAIKAIS
HANKERS
HANKIES
HARKENS
HAWKERS
HAWKINS
HECKLES
HECKYES
HICKEYS
HOCKERS
HONKERS
HOOKAHS
HOOKUPS
HOPKINS
HOSKINS
HOTKEYS
HUNKERS
HUSKERS
HUSKIES
JACKALS
JACKASS
JACKETS
JENKINS
JERKERS
JERKIES
JERKINS
JOCKEYS
JUNKERS
JUNKETS
JUNKIES
KICKERS
KICKUPS
KITKATS
KRAKENS
LACKEYS
LARKERS
LARKINS
LEAKERS
LEAKEYS
LICKERS
LINKERS
LINKUPS
LOCKERS
LOCKETS
LOCKINS
LOCKUPS
LOOKERS
LOOKINS
LOOKUPS
LUNKERS
LURKERS
MARKERS
MARKETS
MARKUPS
MASKERS
MICKEYS
MILKERS
MISKEYS
MOCKERS
MOCKUPS
MONKEES
MONKEYS
MUCKERS
MUSKETS
MUSKIES
NAPKINS
NECKERS
NEWKIDS
NICKELS

NICKERS
NICKLES
OINKERS
OSAKANS
OUTKISS
PACKERS
PACKETS
PARKERS
PARKINS
PEEKERS
PERKINS
PICKENS
PICKERS
PICKETS
PICKLES
PICKUPS
PINKENS
PINKIES
PINKOES
PLAKATS
POCKETS
PORKERS
PROKEDS
PUCKERS
PUNKERS
PUNKIES
QUAKERS
QUAKIES
RACKERS
RACKETS
RANKERS
RANKLES
RECKONS
REEKERS
RICKEYS
RICKLES
RISKERS
ROCKERS
ROCKETS
ROCKIES
ROOKIES
RYOKANS
RYUKYUS
SACKERS
SECKELS
SEEKERS
SHAKERS
SHAKOES
SHEKELS
SICKENS
SICKLES
SINKERS
SLAKERS
SMOKERS
SMOKEYS
SMOKIES
SNAKERS
SOAKERS
SOCKETS
SPIKERS
SPYKIDS
STOKERS
SUCKERS
SULKERS
SULKIES
TABKEYS
TACKERS
TACKLES
TALKERS
TALKIES
TANKERS
TEKKIES
THEKISS
TICKERS
TICKETS
TICKLES
TINKERS
TINKLES
TUCKERS
TURKEYS
TUSKERS
UNSKEWS
VICKERS
WADKINS
WALKERS
WALKINS
WALKONS
WALKUPS
WANKELS
WATKINS
WEAKENS
WEAKONS
WESKITS
WETKISS
WICKERS
WICKETS
WILKENS
WILKINS
WINKERS
WORKERS
WORKUPS
YAKKERS
YANKEES
YANKERS
YONKERS
YORKERS
YORKIES

••••KS•
THINKSO

••••K•S
ADZUKIS
ALASKAS
BETAKES
CROOKES
DUKAKIS
EUREKAS
GINGKOS
INJOKES
INTAKES
INVOKES
JETSKIS
JUDOKAS
KABUKIS
KANAKAS
KISHKES
MEDAKAS
MINSKYS
NONUKES
NOOTKAS
PERUKES
REBAKES
REBUKES
REMAKES
RERAKES
RETAKES
REVOKES
REWAKES
REYOKES
RUMAKIS
SALUKIS
SAMEKHS
SHEIKHS
SHOPKOS
SHRIKES
STLUKES
STRIKES
STROKES
SUDOKUS
SUZUKIS
TROIKAS
UNCAKES
UNLIKES
UNMAKES
UNYOKES
UPTAKES
WENDKOS
WHISKAS

•••••KS
ACKACKS
ANORAKS
ARRACKS
ATTACKS
ATTUCKS
BEDECKS
BUROAKS
BYTALKS
CANUCKS
CDRACKS
DAMASKS
DEBARKS
DEBUNKS
DEJUNKS
DEMARKS
DIKDIKS
DYBBUKS
EMBANKS
EMBARKS
ENLINKS
ENRANKS
EUBANKS
EXWORKS
EXYANKS
HIJACKS
HIJINKS
KODIAKS
KOPECKS
MOHAWKS
MUKLUKS
MUSICKS
NUDNIKS
NYYANKS
OPTICKS
OUTASKS
PINOAKS
REBANKS
REBOOKS
RECOCKS
RECOOKS
RECORKS
REDOAKS
REDOCKS
REEBOKS
REHOOKS
REKICKS
RELINKS
RELOCKS
RELOOKS
REMARKS
REPACKS
REPARKS
REPERKS
REPICKS
RERACKS
RERANKS
RESEEKS
RESINKS
RESOAKS
RETACKS
REWORKS
RHEBOKS
RVPARKS
SCHICKS
SCREAKS
SHNOOKS
SHRIEKS
SHRINKS
SHTICKS
SLOVAKS
SOYINKS
SQUAWKS
SQUEAKS
STMARKS
STREAKS
TANOAKS
THWACKS
TSKTSKS
TUGRIKS
UNCASKS
UNCORKS
UNDOCKS
UNFORKS
UNHOOKS
UNHUSKS
UNKINKS
UNLINKS
UNLOCKS
UNMASKS
UNPACKS
UNPICKS
UNRACKS
UNTACKS
UNTUCKS
UPLINKS
UPTALKS
UPTICKS
UQUARKS
ZEDONKS

KT•••••
KTOSLIN

K•T••••
KATAYEV
KATHRYN
KATISHA
KATRINA
KATRINE
KATYDID
KETCHAM
KETCHES
KETCHUM
KETCHUP
KETONES
KETONIC
KETTLES
KITBAGS
KITCHEN
KITHARA
KITKATS
KITSCHY
KITTENS
KITTERY
KITTIES
KITTING
KUTCHER
KUTUZOV

K••T•••
KANTIAN
KAPTURE
KASTLER
KENTISH
KEPTFIT
KEPTMUM
KEPTOFF
KEPTOUT
KERTESZ
KESTREL
KETTLES
KHATAMI
KILTIES
KILTING
KITTENS
KITTERY
KITTIES
KITTING
KLATSCH
KLUTZES
KNITTED
KNITTER
KNOTSUP
KNOTTED
KNOTTER
KONTIKI
KOWTOWS
KRATION
KVETCHY

K•••T••
KADETTS
KAPITAL
KAPITSA
KARATES
KEISTER
KEMPTON
KERATIN
KILOTON
KINETIC
KINGTUT
KIRSTEN
KIRSTIE
KLEPTOS
KLISTER
KNITTED
KNITTER
KNOTTED
KNOTTER
KNOUTED
KOMATSU
KRISTIN
KRYPTON
KRYSTLE

K••••T•
KADETTS
KEEPSTO
KENNETH
KEYDETS
KEYNOTE
KHANATE
KIBBUTZ
KIDULTS
KISMETS
KITKATS
KKKKATY
KLAMATH
KNIGHTS
KNOWETH
KOLKATA
KOSSUTH
KUWAITI
KUZNETS

K•••••T
KEENEST
KEEPFIT
KEEPOUT
KEEPSAT
KEPTFIT
KEPTOUT
KEYWEST
KICKOUT
KIDSEAT
KILOBIT
KINDEST
KINGLET
KINGRAT
KINGTUT
KINMONT
KNESSET
KOLANUT
KUMQUAT
KURRENT

•KT••••
OKTOBER

•K•T•••
SKATERS
SKATING
SKETCHY
SKITOWS
SKITRIP
SKITTER
SKITTLE

•K••T••
EKISTIC
OKHOTSK
SKEETER
SKELTER
SKELTON
SKEPTIC
SKIRTED
SKIRTER
SKITTER
SKITTLE

•K•••T•
AKIHITO
KKKKATY
SKIHATS

•K••••T
EKEDOUT
EKESOUT
IKNEWIT
IKNOWIT
OKSHOOT
SKIBOOT
SKILIFT
SKILLET
SKIPOUT
SKISUIT
SKIVEST

••KT•••
DAKTARI
DIKTATS
OAKTAGS
OAKTREE
TSKTSKS

••K•T••
CAKETIN
DAKOTAN
DAKOTAS
DYKSTRA
INKSTER
IRKUTSK
LAKOTAS
STKITTS
TAKETEA
TAKETEN
YAKUTSK
YUKATAS

••K••T•
ANKLETS
AUKLETS
DIKTATS
GOKARTS
INKJETS
INKNOTS
INKPOTS
JAKARTA
KKKKATY
LAKISTS
LIKENTO
REKNITS
REKNOTS
STKITTS
SUKKOTH
TAKENTO
TAKESTO
UNKNITS
UNKNOTS

••K•••T
ASKSOUT
BAKERST
CAKIEST
COKIEST
ECKHART
ELKHART
FAKEDIT
FAKEOUT
FAKESIT
GOKAPUT
HIKEOUT
HOKIEST
ICKIEST
INKBLOT
INKIEST
INKSPOT
JOKIEST
LAKIEST
MAKEFIT
MAKEOUT
MAKESIT
OAKIEST
POKEDAT
POKEOUT
POKESAT
POKIEST
TAKEOUT
TAKESIT
UNKEMPT

•••KT••
COOKTOP
DARKTAN
DESKTOP
ELEKTRA
JACKTAR
NECKTIE
SILKTIE
TANKTOP
TOOKTEN
YANKTON
YORKTON

•••K•T•
BANKITS
BASKETS
BASKETT
BECKETT
BOXKITE
BUCKETS
CASKETS
DOCKETS
GASKETS
HACKETT
JACKETS
JUNKETS
KITKATS
KKKKATY
KOLKATA
LICKETY
LOCKETS
LOOKSTO
MANKATO
MARKETS
MUSKETS
NDAKOTA
PACKETS
PICKETS
PICKETT
PINKETT
PLAKATS
POCKETS
PUCKETT
RACKETS
RACKETY
RICKETY
ROCKETS
SDAKOTA
SOCKETS
SPIKETV
SPOKETO
SUKKOTH
TALKSTO
TICKETS
TOMKITE
TOYKITE
WAIKATO
WALKSTO
WESKITS
WICKETS

•••K••T
BACKBIT
BACKLIT
BACKLOT
BACKOUT
BALKSAT
BARKSAT
BASKETT
BECKETT
BOOKERT
BOOKLET
BOWKNOT
COCKPIT
CONKOUT
COOKOUT
COOKPOT
DANKEST
DARKEST
DECKOUT
DESKSET
DUCKOUT
FOLKART
FORKOUT
GAWKSAT
HACKETT
HACKSIT
HECKART
HONKSAT
ILIKEIT
INAKNOT
JACKPOT
JERKOUT
JIMKAAT
JUNKART
KICKOUT
LACKWIT
LANKEST
LOCKLET
LOCKNUT
LOCKOUT
LOCKSET
LOOKIST
LOOKOUT
LOOKSAT
LUCKOUT
MARKOUT
MEEKEST
MUSKRAT
NECKLET
OUTKAST
OUTKEPT
PACKRAT
PARKSIT
PECKSAT
PEEKOUT
PEEKSAT
PICKETT
PICKOUT
PICKSAT
PINKEST
PINKETT
PUCKETT
RACKOUT
RANKEST
RANKOUT
RINKRAT
RISKSIT
RUCKERT
SACKOUT
SEEKOUT
SICKEST
SICKOUT
SILKHAT
SUNKIST
TALKOUT
TALKSAT
TOOKOUT
TOPKNOT
WACKEST
WALKOUT
WEAKEST
WINKOUT
WINKSAT
WORKOUT
WORKSAT
YANKOUT
YANKSAT
YORKIST
ZONKOUT

••••KT•
DRANKTO
DRINKTO
FLOCKTO
SPEAKTO
STICKTO
STUCKTO

••••K•T
BLANKET
BLINKAT
BODYKIT
BRACKET
BRISKET
CHILKAT
CHUCKIT
CRICKET
CROCKET
ETICKET
MEERKAT
MESSKIT
MONGKUT
PLACKET
SNICKET
TESTKIT
THICKET
TOOLKIT
TRINKET

KU•••••
KUBELIK
KUBRICK
KUCHENS
KUMMELS
KUMQUAT
KUNDERA
KURDISH
KURILES
KURRENT
KUTCHER
KUTUZOV
KUWAITI
KUZNETS

K•U••••
KAUFMAN
KLUDGED
KLUDGES
KLUGMAN
KLUTZES
KNUCKLE
KNUCKLY
KNURLED
KRÜEGER

K••U•••
KABUKIS
KAHUNAS
KAKUROS
KIDULTS
KIKUYUS
KNOUTED
KORUNAS
KUTUZOV

K•••U••
KAPTURE
KEROUAC
KIBBUTZ
KICKUPS
KILAUEA
KOSSUTH
KUMQUAT

K••••U•
KARAKUM
KEEPMUM
KEEPOUT
KEEPSUP
KEPTMUM
KEPTOUT
KETCHUM
KETCHUP
KEYCLUB
KEYEDUP
KICKOUT
KICKSUP
KIDSRUS
KIKUYUS
KINGTUT
KNEESUP
KNOTSUP
KOLANUT

K•••••U
KOMATSU

•KU••••
EKUELES
SKULKED
SKULKER
SKULLED
SKUNKED
UKULELE

•K•U•••
NKRUMAH

•K••U••
SKIBUMS
SKIJUMP
SKIRUNS
SKISUIT
SKYSURF

•K•••U•
EKEDOUT
EKESOUT
OKAYGUY
SKILFUL
SKIPOUT
SKYBLUE

••KU•••
IRKUTSK
KAKUROS
KIKUYUS
YAKUTSK
ZAKUSKA

••K•U••
MAKEUPS
MUKLUKS
WAKEUPS

••K••U•
ASKEDUP
ASKSOUT
CAKEDUP
CAKESUP
FAKEFUR
FAKEOUT
GOKAPUT
HIKEDUP
HIKEOUT
HIKESUP
KIKUYUS
MAKEFUN
MAKEOUT
MAKERUN
MAKESUP
POKEFUN
POKEOUT
RAKEDUP
RAKESUP
TAKENUP
TAKEOUT
TAKESUP
WAKEDUP
WAKEFUL
WAKESUP
WOKENUP

•••KU••
BACKUPS
BUNKUMS
HECKUVA
HOOKUPS
KICKUPS
LINKUPS
LOCKUPS
LOOKUPS
MARKUPS
MOCKUPS
PICKUPS
WALKUPS
WALKURE
WORKUPS

•••K•U•
BACKOUT
BACKRUB
BACKSUP
BANKSUP
BROKEUP
BUCKSUP
BULKSUP
CHOKEUP
CONKOUT
COOKOUT
COOKSUP
CORKSUP
DECKOUT
DESKFUL
DUCKOUT
FORKFUL
FORKOUT
FORKSUP
HACKSUP
HOOKSUP
JACKSUP
JERKOUT
JERKSUP
KICKOUT
KICKSUP
LICKSUP
LINKSUP
LOCKNUT
LOCKOUT
LOCKSUP
LOOKOUT
LOOKSUP
LUCKOUT
MARKOUT
MARKSUP
MILKDUD
MILKRUN
MOCKSUP
MUCKSUP
PACKSUP
PEEKOUT
PERKSUP
PICKOUT
PICKSUP
RACKOUT
RACKSUP
RANKOUT
RUCKSUP
RYUKYUS
SACKFUL
SACKOUT

SACKSUP
SEEKOUT
SHAKEUP
SICKOUT
SMOKEUP
SOAKSUP
SPIKEUP
SPOKEUP
STOKEUP
SUCKSUP
TACKSUP
TALKOUT
TALKSUP
TANKFUL
TANKSUP
TENKRUN
TOOKOUT
WALKOUT
WICKIUP
WINKOUT
WORKOUT
WORKSUP
YANKOUT
ZONKOUT

•••K••U
LOOKYOU
SHIKOKU

••••KU•
BLOCKUP
BREAKUP
BRICKUP
CHALKUP
CHECKUP
CRACKUP
CRANKUP
DRANKUP
DRINKUP
KARAKUM
MONGKUT
PRICKUP
SHOOKUP
SLACKUP
SLINKUP
SLUNKUP
SMACKUP
SNEAKUP
SNUCKUP
SPEAKUP
STACKUP
STANKUP
STICKUM
STICKUP
STINKUP
STOCKUP
STUCKUP
SUDOKUS
SWANKUP
THINKUP
WRACKUP

••••K•U
ZWICKAU

•••••KU
BUNRAKU
SHIKOKU

KV•••••
KVASSES
KVELLED
KVETCHY

K••V•••
KELVINS
KIDVIDS
KNAVERY
KNAVISH

K•••V••
KNIEVEL
KOSOVAR

K••••V•
KARLOVY
KEDROVA
KHEDIVE
KISLEVS

K•••••V
KATAYEV
KEMIDOV
KHARKOV
KUTUZOV

•K•V•••
SKIVEST

•K•••V•
SKYDIVE

•K••••V
AKSAKOV

••K•V••
ASKOVER

••K••V•
BAKLAVA

•••KV••
BOOKVII
MARKVII

•••K•V•
HECKUVA
MARKOVA
PARKAVE

•••K••V
CHEKHOV
ROCKYIV
SPIKETV

••••K•V
AKSAKOV
GRINKOV
KHARKOV
NABOKOV

KW•••••
KWACHAS
KWANZAA
KWANZAS

K•W••••
KEWPIES
KIWANIS
KOWADLO
KOWLOON
KOWTOWS
KUWAITI

K••W•••
KENWAHL
KEYWAYS
KEYWEST
KEYWORD
KNEWHOW
KNOWALL
KNOWERS
KNOWETH
KNOWHOW
KNOWING
KNOWLES
KNOWSOF

K•••W••
KELOWNA

K••••W•
KOWTOWS

K•••••W
KENDREW
KERSHAW
KNEWHOW
KNOWHOW

•KW••••
EKWENSI

•K•W•••
SKEWERS
SKEWING
SKIWEAR
SKYWALK
SKYWARD
SKYWAYS

•K••W••
IKNEWIT
IKNOWIT
SKAGWAY

•K•••W•
OKINAWA
SKITOWS

•K••••W
SKIDROW

••KW•••
AWKWARD
INKWELL
OAKWOOD

••K•W••
ASKAWAY
BIKEWAY
LIKEWOW
MAKEWAR
MAKEWAY

••K••W•
OAKLAWN
UNKNOWN

••K•••W
LIKENEW
LIKEWOW

•••KW••
BACKWAY
FOLKWAY
LACKWIT
PARKWAY
WALKWAY

•••K•W•
UNSKEWS

•••K••W
BACKROW
BACKSAW
BUCKSAW
HACKSAW
ILLKNOW
JACKDAW
JANKLOW
LETKNOW
LOCKJAW
LUCKNOW
MILKCOW
MISKNEW
MISKNOW
WHOKNEW
WICKLOW
YOUKNOW

K••X•••
KLAXONS

K•••••X
KICKBOX
KLEENEX

•K••••X
SKEEZIX

••K•••X
CAKEMIX
JUKEBOX

•••K•X•
PICKAXE

•••K••X
JUNKFAX
KICKBOX
LOCKBOX
WORKBOX

KY•••••
KYOODLE

K•Y••••
KAYAKED
KAYAKER
KAYLENZ
KAYOING
KEYBANK
KEYCARD
KEYCASE
KEYCLUB
KEYDETS
KEYEDIN
KEYEDON
KEYEDUP
KEYGRIP
KEYHOLE
KEYINON
KEYLESS
KEYLIME
KEYLOCK
KEYNOTE
KEYPADS
KEYPALS
KEYRING
KEYSPAN
KEYWAYS
KEYWEST
KEYWORD
KRYPTON
KRYSTLE

K••Y•••
KATYDID
KENYANS
KHAYYAM
KOSYGIN

K•••Y••
KATAYEV
KHAYYAM
KIKUYUS
KOPIYKA

K••••Y•
KAROLYI
KATHRYN
KEYWAYS
KIDNEYS

K•••••Y
KARLOVY
KEARNEY
KENNEDY
KILLJOY
KILNDRY
KINKILY
KITSCHY
KITTERY
KKKKATY
KNAVERY
KNUCKLY
KVETCHY

•KY••••
SKYBLUE
SKYCAMS
SKYCAPS
SKYDIVE
SKYDOME
SKYHIGH
SKYHOOK
SKYJACK
SKYLARK
SKYLESS
SKYLIKE
SKYLINE
SKYMAPS
SKYNYRD
SKYSURF
SKYWALK
SKYWARD
SKYWAYS

•K•Y•••
OKAYGUY
OKAYING

•K••Y••
SKYNYRD

•K•••Y•
SKYWAYS

•K••••Y
EKINGBY
KKKKATY
OKAYGUY
OKELLEY
SKAGWAY
SKETCHY
SKIPSBY

••KY•••
ICKYPOO
INKYCAP

••K•Y••
KIKUYUS
REKEYED
UNKEYED

••K••Y•
AYKROYD
MTKENYA
ORKNEYS

••K•••Y
ASKAWAY
BIKEWAY
BOKCHOY
KKKKATY
MAKEHAY
MAKEWAY
NAKEDLY
NIKOLAY
TAKENBY

•••KY••
HECKYES
LOOKYOU
ROCKYII
ROCKYIV
RYUKYUS

•••K•Y•
ALTKEYS
BUCKEYE
CARKEYS
DELKEYS
DICKEYS
DONKEYS
HAWKEYE
HICKEYS
HOTKEYS
JOCKEYS
LACKEYS
LEAKEYS
MICKEYS
MISKEYS
MONKEYS
RICKEYS
SMOKEYS
SOCKEYE
TABKEYS
TURKEYS

•••K••Y
BACKBAY
BACKPAY
BACKWAY
BALKILY
BARKLEY
BERKLEY
BLAKELY
BLAKLEY
BUCKLEY
COCKILY
COCKNEY
COOKERY
DICKORY
DUSKILY
FLAKILY
FLUKILY
FOLKWAY
FUNKILY
GAWKILY
HACKNEY
HICKORY
HUSKILY
JERKILY
KINKILY
KKKKATY
LANKILY
LICKETY
LUCKILY
MILKILY
MOCKERY
MURKILY
PARKWAY
PERKILY
PESKILY
PUCKERY
QUAKILY
RACKETY
RICKETY
RISKILY
ROCKABY
ROCKERY
ROCKILY
ROOKERY
SHAKILY
SICKBAY
SICKDAY
SICKPAY
SILKILY
SMOKILY
SNAKILY
SPIKILY
STOKELY
SUCKDRY
SULKILY
TACKILY
TICKSBY
VICKREY
WACKILY
WALKSBY
WALKWAY
WEEKDAY
WORKDAY
WORKSHY

••••KY•
MINSKYS

••••K•Y
BLACKLY
BLANKLY
BLEAKLY
BRISKLY
BRODKEY
CARDKEY
CLERKLY
CONAKRY
CRACKLY
CRINKLY
DEBAKEY
FRANKLY
FRECKLY
ITSOKAY
KNUCKLY
MARYKAY
PASSKEY
PRICKLY
QUICKLY
SHARKEY
SLACKLY
SLEEKLY
SLICKLY
SNEAKBY
SPARKLY
STARKEY
STARKLY
STICKBY
STOOKEY
STUCKBY
THICKLY
TURNKEY
TWINKLY
WHISKEY
WRINKLY

•••••KY
ARENSKY
AUTARKY
BLUESKY
BRODSKY
CHOMSKY
COLICKY
DEEPSKY
FINICKY
GRETZKY
MALARKY
MRLUCKY
PANICKY
SHLOCKY
SHTICKY
SPASSKY
SQUAWKY
SQUEAKY
STARSKY
STREAKY
TROTSKY
UNBULKY
UNFLAKY
UNLEAKY
UNLUCKY
UNRISKY
UNROCKY
UNSMOKY
UNSNAKY
UNSULKY
VRONSKY

K•Z••••
KUZNETS

K••Z•••
KLEZMER

K•••Z••
KLUTZES
KUTUZOV
KWANZAA
KWANZAS

K•••••Z
KAYLENZ
KERTESZ
KIBBUTZ
KOBLENZ

•K••Z••
SKEEZIX

••••K•Z
DAVEKOZ
FRANKOZ

LA•••••
LABAMBA
LABATTS
LABCOAT
LABELED
LABELER
LABELLE
LABFEES
LABIALS
LABIATE
LABMICE
LABORAT
LABORED
LABORER
LABOURS
LABRATS
LABTECH
LABTEST
LABTUBE
LACEDUP
LACERTA
LACESON
LACESUP
LACEUPS
LACIEST
LACINGS
LACKEYS
LACKING
LACKWIT
LACONIA
LACONIC
LACOSTE
LACQUER
LACRIMO
LACTAID
LACTASE
LACTATE
LACTEAL
LACTOSE
LACUNAE
LACUNAL
LACUNAR
LACUNAS
LACUREE
LADADOG
LADDERS
LADDIES
LADDISH
LADHOOD
LADIDAS
LADINGS
LADINOS
LADLERS
LADLING
LADOUCE
LADRONE
LADYBUG
LADYDAY
LADYISH
LADYKIN
LADYNAS
LAEMMLE
LAENNEC
LAERTES
LAFARGE
LAFEMME
LAFITTE
LAFLEUR
LAGASSE
LAGGARD
LAGGERS
LAGGING
LAGOONS
LAGUNAS
LAHAINA
LAICIZE
LAIDFOR
LAIDLOW
LAIDOFF
LAIDOUT
LAIRING
LAISSEZ
LAITIES
LAJOLLA
LAKEBED
LAKIEST
LAKISTS
LAKOTAS
LAKSHMI
LALAKER
LALANNE
LALIQUE
LALLING
LALOOSH
LAMAISM
LAMAIST
LAMARCK
LAMBADA
LAMBDAS
LAMBEAU
LAMBENT
LAMBERT
LAMBETH
LAMBING
LAMBKIN
LAMENTS
LAMINAE
LAMINAL
LAMINAR
LAMINAS
LAMINTO
LAMMING
LAMOTTA
LAMOTTE
LAMPERT
LAMPLIT
LAMPOIL
LAMPOON
LAMPREY
LANCERS
LANCETS
LANCIAS
LANCING
LANCOME
LANDAUS
LANDERS
LANDING
LANDINI
LANDLER
LANDMAN
LANDMEN
LANDSAT
LANDSUP
LANDTAG
LANDTAX
LANEONE
LANETWO
LANFORD
LANGDON
LANGHAM
LANGLEY
LANGTON
LANGTRY
LANGUID
LANGUOR
LANGWAY
LANKEST
LANKIER
LANKILY
LANOLIN
LANOTTE
LANSING
LANTANA
LANTERN
LANVINS
LANYARD
LAOCOON
LAOTIAN
LAPALMA
LAPBELT
LAPCATS
LAPDOGS
LAPELED
LAPERMS
LAPFULS
LAPLACA
LAPLACE
LAPLAND
LAPLATA
LAPORTE
LAPPERS
LAPPETS
LAPPING
LAPPISH
LAPROBE
LAPSANG
LAPSERS
LAPSING
LAPTOPS
LAPUTAN
LAPWARE
LAPWING
LARAINE
LARAMIE
LARCENY
LARCHEN
LARCHES
LARDERS
LARDIER
LARDING
LARDNER
LARDONS
LAREDOS
LARGELY
LARGENT
LARGEOJ
LARGESS
LARGEST
LARGISH
LARIATS
LARKERS
LARKIER
LARKING
LARKINS
LARKISH
LAROCHE
LARRUPS
LARUSSA
LASAGNA
LASAGNE
LASALLE
LASCALA
LASCARS
LASCAUX
LASHERS
LASHING
LASHOUT
LASHUPS
LASORDA
LASSIES
LASSOED
LASSOER
LASSOES
LASTACT
LASTDON
LASTGAS
LASTING
LASTLAP
LASTLEG
LASTMAY
LASTONE
LASTORY
LASTROW
LATCHED
LATCHES
LATCHON
LATEENS
LATEFEE
LATENCY
LATENED
LATENTS
LATERAL
LATERAN
LATERON
LATETAG
LATEXES
LATHERS
LATHERY
LATHING
LATICES
LATIFAH
LATIGOS
LATIMES
LATINAS
LATINII
LATINOS
LATINUS
LATOSCA
LATRELL
LATRINE
LATROBE
LATTICE
LATVIAN
LAUDERS
LAUDING
LAUGHAT
LAUGHED
LAUGHER
LAUGHIN
LAULAUS
LAUNDER
LAUNDRY
LAURELS
LAURENT
LAURITZ
LAUTREC
LAVABOS
LAVACHE
LAVAGES
LAVAINE
LAVALSE
LAVELLI
LAVERAN
LAVERNE
LAVINIA
LAVORIS
LAWANDA
LAWBOOK
LAWCASE
LAWFORD
LAWLESS
LAWLIKE
LAWSUIT
LAWYERS
LAXNESS
LAYAWAY
LAYBACK
LAYBARE
LAYDOWN
LAYERED
LAYETTE

LAYINTO
LAYITON
LAYODDS
LAYOFFS
LAYOPEN
LAYOUTS
LAYOVER
LAYSFOR
LAYSLOW
LAYSOFF
LAYSOUT
LAYUPON
LAZARUS
LAZBOYS
LAZENBY
LAZIEST
LAZONGA
LAZYISH
LAZZERI

L•A••••

LEACHED
LEACHER
LEACHES
LEACOCK
LEADDOG
LEADENS
LEADERS
LEADETH
LEADIER
LEADING
LEADINS
LEADMAN
LEADMEN
LEADOFF
LEADORE
LEADOUT
LEADSIN
LEADSON
LEADSTO
LEADSUP
LEADUPS
LEAFAGE
LEAFIER
LEAFING
LEAFLET
LEAFOUT
LEAGUED
LEAGUER
LEAGUES
LEAKAGE
LEAKERS
LEAKEYS
LEAKIER
LEAKING
LEAKSIN
LEANCUT
LEANDER
LEANERS
LEANEST
LEANING
LEANSIN
LEANSON
LEANSTO
LEANTOS
LEAPDAY
LEAPERS
LEAPFOR
LEAPING
LEAPSAT
LEAPSIN
LEAPSON
LEAPSUP
LEAPTAT
LEAPTIN
LEAPTON
LEAPTUP
LEARJET
LEARNED
LEARNER
LEARNOF
LEARNTO
LEASERS
LEASETO
LEASHED
LEASHES
LEASING
LEATHER
LEAVEBE
LEAVEIN
LEAVEIT
LEAVENS
LEAVEON
LEAVING
LEAWOOD
LHASANS
LIAISED
LIAISES
LIAISON
LLADROS
LLANERO
LOADERS
LOADING
LOADSIN
LOADSOF
LOADSUP
LOAFERS
LOAFING
LOAFPAN
LOAMIER
LOAMING
LOANERS
LOANING
LOANOUT
LOATHED
LOATHER
LOATHES
LOATHLY
LOATHTO

L••A•••

LABAMBA
LABATTS
LADADOG
LAFARGE
LAGASSE
LAHAINA
LALAKER
LALANNE
LAMAISM
LAMAIST
LAMARCK
LAPALMA
LARAINE
LARAMIE
LASAGNA
LASAGNE
LASALLE
LAVABOS
LAVACHE
LAVAGES
LAVAINE
LAVALSE
LAWANDA
LAYAWAY
LAZARUS
LCHAYIM
LEBANON
LEBARON
LECARRE
LEDAWAY
LEGALLY
LEGANZA
LEGATEE
LEGATES
LEGATOR
LEGATOS
LEHAVRE
LEPANTO
LESABRE
LEVADES
LEVATOR
LIEABED
LIEATOP
LIGANDS
LIGATED
LIGATES
LIKABLE
LILALEE
LIMACON
LINABLE
LINAGES
LIPARIS
LIPASES
LISAGAY
LIVABLE
LIZARDS
LOBATED
LOCALES
LOCALLY
LOCARNO
LOCATED
LOCATER
LOCATES
LOCATOR
LOGANUT
LORANGE
LOSABLE
LOVABLE
LOVABLY
LOVAGES
LOYALER
LOYALES
LOYALLY
LOYALTO
LOYALTY
LSHAPED
LUCANIA
LUCARNE
LUNATED
LUNATES
LUNATIC
LUXATED
LUXATES

L•••A••

LABIALS
LABIATE
LABRATS
LACTAID
LACTASE
LACTATE
LAGGARD
LAMBADA
LANDAUS
LANTANA
LANYARD
LAPCATS
LAPLACA
LAPLACE
LAPLAND
LAPLATA
LAPSANG
LAPWARE
LARIATS
LASCALA
LASCARS
LASCAUX
LASTACT
LAULAUS
LAWCASE
LAYBACK
LAYBARE
LEAFAGE
LEAKAGE
LEBLANC
LEEWARD
LEEWAYS
LEFTARM
LEGRAND
LEHMANN
LEMMATA
LENFANT
LEONARD
LEONATO
LEOPARD
LEOTARD
LEPPARD
LESCAUT
LESPAUL
LETFALL
LETHAVE
LETPASS
LEXMARK
LHASANS
LIBRANS
LIBRARY
LIBYANS
LIEBACK
LIMEADE
LINEAGE
LINEARA
LINEARB
LINEATE
LINKAGE
LIPBALM
LIPMANN
LIQUATE
LIVEAID
LOCKAGE
LOGJAMS
LOLLARD
LOMBARD
LONGAGO
LONGARM
LOOFAHS
LOQUATS
LOSTART
LOTHAIR
LOWBALL
LOWCARB
LOWCARD
LOWHAND
LOWLAND
LOWMASS
LOWPAID
LOWPAIR
LUCIANA
LUCIANO
LUGGAGE
LUGSAIL
LULLABY
LUMBAGO
LUMBARS

L••••A•

LABCOAT
LABORAT
LACTEAL
LACUNAE
LACUNAL
LACUNAR
LACUNAS
LADIDAS
LADYDAY
LADYNAS
LAGUNAS
LAKOTAS
LAMBDAS
LAMBEAU
LAMINAE
LAMINAL
LAMINAR
LAMINAS
LANCIAS
LANDMAN
LANDSAT
LANDTAG
LANDTAX
LANGHAM
LANGWAY
LAOTIAN
LAPUTAN
LASTGAS
LASTLAP
LASTMAY
LATERAL
LATERAN
LATETAG
LATIFAH
LATINAS
LATVIAN
LAUGHAT
LAVERAN
LAYAWAY
LEADMAN
LEAPDAY
LEAPSAT
LEAPTAT
LEDAWAY
LEERSAT
LEFREAK
LEFTEAR
LEFTJAB
LEGOLAS
LEGTRAP
LEGWEAR
LENGUAS
LENSCAP
LENSMAN
LEONDAY
LESSFAT
LESSTAR
LETHEAN
LETSEAT
LEWHOAD
LEXICAL
LIBERAL
LIKEMAD
LILINAU
LILLIAN
LILYPAD
LIMINAL
LINBIAO
LINDSAY
LINEMAN
LINGUAE
LINGUAL
LINPIAO
LIPREAD
LISAGAY
LITERAL
LIVEOAK
LIVESAT
LOAFPAN
LOCKEAN
LOCKJAW
LOGGIAS
LOGICAL
LONGDAY
LONGWAY
LONIGAN
LOOKSAD
LOOKSAT
LOOMPAS
LORELAI
LOSTCAT
LOTHIAN
LOVETAP
LOWBEAM
LOWGEAR
LOWROAD
LOYOLAU
LTKOJAK
LUCIDAE
LUCKMAN
LUMINAS
LUNGEAT
LUNULAE
LUNULAR
LUSTRAL
LYESOAP
LYRICAL

L•••••A

LABAMBA
LACERTA
LACONIA
LAHAINA
LAJOLLA
LAMBADA
LAMOTTA
LANTANA
LAPALMA
LAPLACA
LAPLATA
LARUSSA
LASAGNA
LASCALA
LASORDA
LATOSCA
LAVINIA
LAWANDA
LAZONGA
LECUONA
LEGANZA
LEMMATA
LEMPIRA
LEONORA
LETITIA
LETTERA
LIBERIA
LIDWINA
LIGURIA
LINEARA
LINGULA
LORETTA
LOUELLA
LUCANIA
LUCETTA
LUCIANA
LUCINDA
LUNESTA
LUTETIA

•LA••••

ALABAMA
ALABAMY
ALACKOF
ALADDIN
ALADINE
ALAKING
ALAMEDA
ALAMEIN
ALAMODE
ALAMOSA
ALANINE
ALANJAY
ALANNAH
ALARBUS
ALARCON
ALARMED
ALARMER
ALARUMS
ALASKAN
ALASKAS
ALASSAD
ALATEEN
ALAYING
BLABBED
BLABBER
BLACKED
BLACKEN
BLACKER
BLACKIE
BLACKLY
BLACULA
BLADDER
BLADERS
BLADING
BLAKELY
BLAKLEY
BLALOCK
BLAMEON
BLAMERS
BLAMING
BLANCHE
BLANDER
BLANDLY
BLANKED
BLANKER
BLANKET
BLANKLY
BLANTON
BLARING
BLARNEY
BLASTED
BLASTER
BLATANT
BLATHER
BLATTED
BLAUBOK
BLAZERS
BLAZEUP
BLAZING
BLAZONS
CLABBER
CLACKED
CLACKER
CLACTON
CLADDED
CLAIMED
CLAIMER
CLAIROL
CLAMANT
CLAMATO
CLAMBAR
CLAMBER
CLAMDIP
CLAMMED
CLAMMER
CLAMORS
CLAMOUR
CLAMPED
CLAMPER
CLAMPON
CLAMSUP
CLANGED
CLANGER
CLANGOR
CLANKED
CLANTON
CLAPFOR
CLAPPED
CLAPPER
CLAPTON
CLAQUES
CLARETS
CLARICE
CLARIFY
CLARION
CLARITY
CLASHED
CLASHER
CLASHES
CLASPED
CLASPER
CLASSED
CLASSER
CLASSES
CLASSIC
CLASSON
CLATTER
CLAUDEL
CLAUDIA
CLAUDIO
CLAUSAL
CLAUSES
CLAVATE
CLAVELL
CLAVIER
CLAWERS
CLAWING
CLAWSAT
CLAYIER
CLAYING
CLAYISH
CLAYPIT
CLAYTON
ELAAIUN
ELAINES
ELAMITE
ELANCES
ELANETS
ELANTRA
ELAPIDS
ELAPSED
ELAPSES
ELASTIC
ELASTIN
ELATERS
ELATING
ELATION
FLACCID
FLACKED
FLACONS
FLAGDAY
FLAGGED
FLAGGER
FLAGMAN
FLAGMEN
FLAGONS
FLAILAT
FLAILED
FLAKERS
FLAKIER
FLAKILY
FLAKING
FLAMBED
FLAMBES
FLAMERS
FLAMEUP
FLAMIER
FLAMING
FLAMMED
FLANEUR
FLANGES
FLANKED
FLANKEN
FLANKER
FLANNEL
FLAPPED
FLAPPER
FLAREUP
FLARING
FLASHED
FLASHER
FLASHES
FLASHON
FLATBED
FLATCAR
FLATHAT
FLATLET
FLATOUT
FLATTAX
FLATTED
FLATTEN
FLATTER
FLATTOP
FLATTVS
FLAUNTS
FLAUNTY
FLAUTAS
FLAVIUS
FLAVORS
FLAVORY
FLAVOUR
FLAWIER
FLAWING
FLAXIER
FLAYERS
FLAYING
GLACEED
GLACIAL
GLACIER
GLADDEN
GLADDER
GLADEYE
GLAMORS
GLAMOUR
GLAMSUP
GLANCED
GLANCES
GLAREAT
GLARING
GLASGOW
GLASHOW
GLASSED
GLASSES
GLAVINE
GLAZERS
GLAZIER
GLAZILY
GLAZING
KLAMATH
KLAMMER
KLATSCH
KLAXONS
LLADROS
LLANERO
OLAFIII
OLAVIII
PLACARD
PLACATE
PLACEBO
PLACERS
PLACIDO
PLACING
PLACKET
PLAGUED
PLAGUES
PLAICES
PLAINER
PLAINES
PLAINLY
PLAINTS
PLAISIR
PLAITED
PLAITER
PLAKATS
PLANATE
PLANERS
PLANETS
PLANFOR
PLANING
PLANISH
PLANKED
PLANNED
PLANNER
PLANOUT
PLANSON
PLANSTO
PLANTAR
PLANTED
PLANTER
PLAQUES
PLASHED
PLASHES
PLASMAS
PLASMIC
PLASTER
PLASTIC
PLATEAU
PLATENS
PLATERS
PLATIER
PLATIES
PLATING
PLATOON
PLATTED
PLATTER
PLATYPI
PLAUDIT
PLAUTUS
PLAYACT
PLAYBOY
PLAYDOH
PLAYERS
PLAYFUL
PLAYING
PLAYLET
PLAYOFF
PLAYOUT
PLAYPEN
PLAYSAT
PLAYSBY
PLAYSON
PLAYSTO
PLAYSUP
PLAYTEX
SLABBED
SLACKED
SLACKEN
SLACKER
SLACKLY
SLACKUP
SLAKERS
SLAKING
SLALOMS
SLAMMED
SLAMMER
SLAMSON
SLANDER
SLANTED
SLANTLY
SLANTUP
SLAPPED
SLAPPER
SLAPSON
SLASHED
SLASHER
SLASHES
SLATERS
SLATHER
SLATIER
SLATING
SLATKIN
SLATTED
SLAVERS
SLAVERY
SLAVING
SLAVISH
SLAYERS
SLAYING
SLAYTON
ULALUME
ULANOVA
ULANUDE

•L•A•••

ALBANIA
ALCAIDE
ALCALDE
ALCAZAR
ALDAVIS
ALEARDI
ALFALFA
ALGARVE
ALIASES
ALKALIS
ALLAGES
ALLANTE
ALLAYED
ALLAYER
ALMAATA
ALMADEN
ALMANAC
ALOADOF
ALPACAS
ALSATIA
ALVAREZ
BLEAKER
BLEAKLY
BLEARED
BLEATED
BLEATER
BLOATED
CLEANED
CLEANER
CLEANLY
CLEANSE
CLEANTE
CLEANUP
CLEARED
CLEARER
CLEARLY
CLEAROF
CLEARUP
CLEATED
CLEAVED
CLEAVER
CLEAVES
CLEAVON
CLOAKED
ELAAIUN
ELCAJON
ELCAMPO
ELEANOR
ELEAZAR
ELGALLO
ELLAMAE
ELUANTS
ELUATES
FLEABAG
FLEADIP
FLEANCE
FLEAPIT
FLOATBY
FLOATED
FLOATER
FLOATUP
FLYABLE
FLYAWAY
GLEAMED
GLEANED
GLEANER
GLEASON
GLOAMIN
GLOATED
GLOATER
ILIADIC
ILIAMNA
OLEANNA
OLEANNY
OLEATES
PLEADED
PLEADER
PLEADTO
PLEASED
PLEASER
PLEASES
PLEATED
PLIABLE
PLIABLY
PLIANCY
SLEAZES
ULLAGES
ULYANOV
ULZANAS

•L••A••

ALABAMA
ALABAMY
ALEGARS
ALETAPS
ALEYARD
ALIBABA
ALIDADE
ALIYAHS
ALLCAPS
ALLCASH
ALLEARS
ALLHAIL
ALLMALE
ALMAATA

ALOHAOE
ALPHARD
ALREADY
ALSHAIN
ALTTABS
BLATANT
CLAMANT
CLAMATO
CLAVATE
CLIMATE
CLIMATS
CLIPART
ELEGANT
ELEVATE
ELIYALE
ELKHART
ELLMANN
ELPRADO
ELTRAIN
FLOTAGE
FLOWAGE
FLYBALL
FLYCAST
FLYPAST
FLYWAYS
GLOBATE
ILLCALL
ILLEANA
ILLMADE
ILLPASS
ILOCANO
KLAMATH
OLDBATS
OLDCARS
OLDDAYS
OLDGAGS
OLDHAND
OLDLADY
OLDMAID
OLDNAVY
OLDPALS
OLDSALT
OLDSAWS
OLDWAYS
PLACARD
PLACATE
PLAKATS
PLANATE
PLAYACT
PLENARY
PLICATE
PLUMAGE
PLURALS
SLOGANS
SLOVAKS
ULLMANN
ULULANT
ULULATE

•L•••A•

ALANJAY
ALANNAH
ALASKAN
ALASKAS
ALASSAD
ALBORAK
ALCAZAR
ALDORAY
ALLBRAN
ALLCLAD
ALLHEAL
ALLOWAY
ALLSTAR
ALLTHAT
ALMANAC
ALMSMAN
ALNILAM
ALNITAK
ALNIYAT
ALPACAS
ALSORAN
ALTIMAS
ALTOSAX
ALUMNAE
ALUMNAL
ALYKHAN
BLINKAT
BLUEJAY
BLUELAW
CLAMBAR
CLAUSAL
CLAWSAT
CLUBCAR
ELEAZAR
ELEGIAC
ELENIAK
ELLAMAE
ELLYMAY
ELUVIAL
ELYSIAN
FLAGDAY
FLAGMAN
FLAILAT
FLATCAR
FLATHAT
FLATTAX
FLAUTAS
FLEABAG
FLIESAT
FLINGAT
FLOREAL
FLORIAN
FLOTSAM
FLOWNAT
FLUIDAL
FLUNGAT
FLUVIAL
FLYAWAY
FLYLEAF
FLYTRAP
GLACIAL
GLAREAT
GLEEMAN
GLORIAS
GLOSSAE
GLOSSAL
GLOSSAS
GLOTTAL
GLUTEAL
ILLCLAD
ILLEGAL
KLUGMAN
OLDBEAN
OLDCHAP
OLDUVAI
PLANTAR
PLASMAS
PLATEAU
PLAYSAT
PLEBIAN
PLEURAE
PLEURAL
PLOWMAN
PLUSTAX
PLUVIAL
SLOTCAR
SLOWDAY
ULTIMAS
ULZANAS

•L••••A

ALABAMA
ALAMEDA
ALAMOSA
ALBANIA
ALBERTA
ALEGRIA
ALFALFA
ALFORJA
ALFREDA
ALGEBRA
ALGERIA
ALGIEBA
ALIBABA
ALLEGRA
ALLUVIA
ALMAATA
ALMERIA
ALSATIA
ALTOONA
ALUMINA
ALYOSHA
BLACULA
CLAUDIA
ELANTRA
ELBERTA
ELECTRA
ELEKTRA
ELEVENA
FLORIDA
ILIAMNA
ILLEANA
ILLYRIA
ILOVELA
OLEANNA
OLESTRA
OLYMPIA
PLECTRA
PLUGOLA
ULANOVA

••LA•••

AALARGE
ABLATED
ABLATES
ALLAGES
ALLANTE
ALLAYED
ALLAYER
ATLANTA
ATLARGE
ATLASES
BALABAN
BALANCE
BALASES
BALATAS
BALATON
BELABOR
BELAIRS
BELARUS
BELASCO
BELATED
BELAYED
BELAYER
BOLATIE
CALABRO
CALAMAR
CALANDO
CCLAMPS
CELADON
CELAENO
COLADAS
DALASIS
DELANEY
DELARUE
DELAYED
DELAYER
DILATED
DILATES
DILATOR
DRLAURA
ECLAIRS
ELLAMAE
ENLACED
ENLACES
ENLARGE
ERLANGS
EULABUS
FALAFEL
FOLATES
GALAHAD
GALANOS
GALANTS
GALATEA
GALATIA
GALAXES
GALAXIE
GELATED
GELATES
GELATIN
GELATIS
GELATOS
HALALAS
HALAVAH
HILAIRE
INLABOR
INLANDS
INLARGE
INLAYER
ISLAMIC
ISLANDS
KILAUEA
KOLANUT
LALAKER
LALANNE
LILALEE
MALABAR
MALACCA
MALACHI
MALAGAN
MALAGAS
MALAISE
MALAMUD
MALARIA
MALARKY
MALAYAN
MELAMED
MELANGE
MELANIA
MELANIC
MELANIE
MELANIN
MILAGRO
MULATTO
MYLANTA
OBLASTS
OBLATES
OGLALAS
ORLANDO
PALABRA
PALACES
PALADIN
PALAMAS
PALANCE
PALATAL
PALATES
PALAVER
PALAZZI
PALAZZO
PELAGES
PELAGIC
PILATES
PILATUS
POLANER
POLANYI
POLARAS
POLARIS
PULASKI
RDLAING
RELABEL
RELACED
RELACES
RELANCE
RELANDS
RELANES
RELAPSE
RELATCH
RELATED
RELATER
RELATES
RELATOR
RELAXED
RELAXER
RELAXES
RELAYED
RELAYER
ROLAIDS
SALAAMS
SALABLE
SALADES
SALADIN
SALAMIS
SALAZAR
SCLAFFS
SOLACED
SOLACER
SOLACES
SOLARAS
SOLARIA
SPLASHY
SPLAYED
TALARIA
TELAVIV
TULANEU
ULLAGES
UMLAUTS
UNLACED
UNLACES
UNLADED
UNLADEN
UNLADES
UNLARGE
UNLATCH
UNLAVED
UNLAXED
UNLAXES
UPLANDS
VALADON
VALANCE
VOLANTE
YOLANDA
ZELAZNY

••L•A••

ALLCAPS
ALLCASH
ALLEARS
ALLHAIL
ALLMALE
ATLEAST
BALKANS
BALLADE
BALLADS
BALLARD
BALLAST
BALMAIN
BALSAMS
BALSAMY
BELDAME
BELDAMS
BELFAST
BELLAMY
BELTANE
BULGARI
BULGARS
BULWARK
CALGARY
CALVARY
CELLARS
CILIARY
CILIATE
COLGATE
COLLAGE
COLLARD
COLLARS
COLLATE
DELEADS
DELRAYS
DELTAIC
DILLARD
DOLLARS
DOLMANS
DULLARD
ELLMANN
FALCATE
FALLACY
FALLALS
FELLAHS
FOLIAGE
FOLIATE
FOLKART
FULMARS
GALEATE
GALLANT
GALPALS
GALVANI
GALVANO
GELCAPS
GOLDARN
GOLIATH
GULLAHS
HALDANE
HALVAHS
HALYARD
HILLARY
HOLDALL
HOLLAND
HOLYARK
ILLCALL
ILLEANA
ILLMADE
ILLPASS
JULIANA
KILDARE
KOLKATA
LOLLARD
LULLABY
MALEANT
MALIANS
MALLARD
MALPASO
MALRAUX
MALTASE
MALWARE
MELTAGE
MILEAGE
MILHAUD
MILLAGE
MILLAIS
MILLAND
MILLARD
MULCAHY
MULDAUR
MULHARE
MULLAHS
NFLGAME
NHLGAME
NOLOADS
OILBASE
OILCAKE
OILCANS
OILLAMP
OILPALM
OILPANS
OILSAND
OILTANK
ONLEASE
ONLEASH
ONLEAVE
ONLOADS
ORLEANS
PALEALE
PALMARY
PALMATE
PALPATE
PELTATE
PILEATE
PILLAGE
PILLARS
POLEAXE
POLKAED
POLLACK
POLLARD
POLTAVA
PULSARS
PULSATE
RELEADS
RELEAPS
RELEARN
RELEASE
RELIANT
RELOADS
RELOANS
ROLLAND
ROLVAAG
SALAAMS
SALTANT
SALVAGE
SELMAAL
SELVAGE
SOLLATI
SOLOACT
SULFATE
SULTANA
SULTANS
SYLLABI
TELLALL
TILLAGE
TOLDALL
TOLEASE
TOLLAGE
TULSANS
TULSAOK
ULLMANN
UNLEADS
UNLEAFS
UNLEAKY
UNLEARN
UNLEASH
UNLOADS
UNLOATH
UPLEAPS
UPLEAPT
UPLOADS
VALIANT
VALUATE
VALVATE
VILLAGE
VILLAIN
VILLARD
VILLARI
VOLCANO
VOLTAGE
VOLTAIC
VULCANS
VULGATE
WALLABY
WALLACE
WALLACH
WALMART
WELFARE
WELLAND
WILLARD

••L••A•

AALIYAH
ALLBRAN
ALLCLAD
ALLHEAL
ALLOWAY
ALLSTAR
ALLTHAT
BALABAN
BALATAS
BALBOAS
BALIHAI
BALKSAT
BELGIAN
BELLEAU
BELLJAR
BELLLAP
BELLMAN
BELTBAG
BELTRAN
BELTSAW
BELTWAY
BELUGAS
BKLIBAN
BOLIVAR
BULOVAS
CALAMAR
CALIBAN
CELICAS
COLADAS
COLDDAY
COLDWAR
COLEMAN
CULTJAM
DELIHAM
DELILAH
DELIMAN
DILLMAN
ELLAMAE
ELLYMAY
FELDMAN
FELTBAD
FELTHAT
FILOFAX
FOLKWAY
FULLDAY
GALAHAD
GALENAS
GILBLAS
GILLIAM
GILLIAN
GILLMAN
GOLDMAN
GOLFBAG
GOLFCAR
GULFWAR
HALALAS
HALAVAH
HALFBAD
HALFDAY
HALFMAD
HALFRAW
HALFWAY
HALIFAX
HALLWAY
HELICAL
HELIPAD
HELLCAT
HELLMAN
HILLMAN
HOLIDAY
HOLMOAK
HOLYDAY
HOLYMAN
HOLYWAR
HOLZMAN
ILLCLAD
ILLEGAL
JILLIAN
JULYDAY
KELLJAN
KILOBAR
LILINAU
LILLIAN
LILYPAD
MALABAR
MALAGAN
MALAGAS
MALAYAN
MALECAT
MALLRAT
MCLUHAN
MILKBAR
MILKCAN
MILKMAN
MILLDAM
MOLERAT
MOLOKAI
MTLOGAN
MULETAS
NFLTEAM
NHLTEAM
OGLALAS
OILHEAT
PALAMAS
PALATAL
PALOMAR
PALOMAS
PALUDAL
PELICAN
PELLEAS
PELOTAS
POLARAS
POLECAR
POLECAT
POLEMAN
POLESAT
POLLTAX
PULLMAN
PULLTAB
ROLLBAR
ROLLWAY
ROLVAAG
SALAZAR
SALINAS
SALIVAS
SCLERAE
SCLERAL
SCLERAS
SELMAAL
SILICAS
SILKHAT
SOLARAS
SOLEDAD
TALIBAN
TALKSAT
TELEFAX
TELERAN
TELSTAR
TILTSAT
TOLEDAN
TOLLBAR
TOLLMAN
TOLLWAY
UNLEGAL
UNLOCAL
UNLOYAL
VALJEAN
VELTMAN
WALKMAN
WALKWAY
WALLMAP
WALTHAM
WELLMAN
WILDCAT
WILDMAN
WILLIAM
WOLFGAL
WOLFMAN
WOLFRAM
YALELAW
YALEMAN
YELLSAT

••L•••A

ALLEGRA
ALLUVIA
ATLANTA
AULETTA
BELINDA
BOLIVIA
BOLOGNA
CALDERA
CALISTA
CALMSEA
CELESTA
COLONNA
COLUMBA
DELEDDA
DELIRIA
DELTONA
DILEMMA
DRLAURA
FELICIA
GALATEA
GALATIA
GALICIA
HELLUVA
ILLEANA
ILLYRIA
JULIANA
KELOWNA
KILAUEA
KOLKATA
MALACCA
MALARIA
MALLIKA
MALVINA
MELANIA
MELINDA
MELISMA
MELISSA
MELITTA
MELODIA
MILITIA
MOLDOVA
MOLUCCA
MYLANTA
PALABRA
PALMYRA
PALOOKA
POLENTA
POLLERA
POLONIA
POLTAVA
ROLONDA
SALONGA
SALSODA
SALTSEA
SILENTA
SILESIA
SOLARIA
SPLENDA
STLUCIA
SULTANA
SULUSEA
TALARIA
VALVULA
YOLANDA

•••LA••

ABELARD
ACCLAIM
ADULATE
AIRLANE
AMILATE
AMYLASE
ANGLAIS
APPLAUD
ARCLAMP
ASALARK
ASHLAND
ASHLARS
ATELATE
BADLAND
BAGLADY
BAKLAVA
BALLADE
BALLADS
BALLARD
BALLAST
BEDLAMP
BEDLAMS
BELLAMY
BIOLABS
BIPLANE
BORLAUG
BURLAPS
BUSLANE
BYPLAYS
CELLARS
CHELATE
COLLAGE
COLLARD
COLLARS
COLLATE
COOLAIR
COOLANT
COPLAND
CUTLASS
DECLAIM
DECLARE
DECLASS
DECLAWS
DEFLATE
DEGLAZE
DEPLANE
DEWLAPS
DIDLAPS
DILLARD
DNALABS
DOLLARS
DULLARD
EARLAPS
EATLATE
EMBLAZE
EMPLACE
EMPLANE
EMULATE
ENCLASP
ENCLAVE
ENDLATE
ENFLAME
ENGLAND
ENPLANE
ENSLAVE
EPILADY
EPILATE
EWELAMB
EXCLAIM
EXCLAVE
EXPLAIN
EYELASH
FALLACY
FALLALS
FELLAHS
FINLAND
FOGLAMP
FORLANI
FOULARD
GAGLAWS
GALLANT
GARLAND
GASLAMP
GOBLANK
GOULASH
GULLAHS
GUNLAPS
GUNLAWS
HARLAND
HAULAGE
HEALALL
HILLARY
HOLLAND
HOVLANE
HOWLAME
ICELAND
IMPLANT
INBLACK
INCLASS
INFLAME
INFLATE
INPLACE
INULASE
IRELAND
ISOLATE
ISOLATO
ITSLATE
JETLAGS
JUTLAND

KOOLAID
LAPLACA
LAPLACE
LAPLAND
LAPLATA
LAULAUS
LEBLANC
LOLLARD
LOWLAND
LULLABY
MALLARD
MIDLAND
MILLAGE
MILLAIS
MILLAND
MILLARD
MISLAID
MISLAYS
MOULAGE
MRSLATE
MTBLANC
MUDLARK
MULLAHS
NEDLAND
NEWLAID
NOCLASS
NOPLACE
OAKLAND
OAKLAWN
OCALAFL
OCULARS
OILLAMP
OLDLADY
ONALARK
ONELANE
OOHLALA
OUTLAID
OUTLAIN
OUTLAND
OUTLASH
OUTLAST
OUTLAWS
OUTLAYS
OXALATE
PAHLAVI
PARLAYS
PETLAMB
PHALANX
PILLAGE
PILLARS
POBLANO
POLLACK
POLLARD
POPLARS
PRELACY
PRELATE
PROLATE
RAGLANS
RAILAGE
RANLAPS
RANLATE
RECLADS
RECLAIM
RECLAME
RECLASP
RECLASS
REFLAGS
REFLATE
REGLAZE
REPLACE
REPLANE
REPLANS
REPLANT
REPLATE
REPLAYS
RESLATE
ROLLAND
ROULADE
ROWLAND
RUNLAPS
RUNLATE
RUTLAND
SCALAGE
SCALARS
SCOLARI
SEALABS
SEALANE
SEALANT
SHALALA
SIXLANE
SKYLARK
SOILAGE
SOLLATI
STALAGS
SUNLAMP
SYLLABI
SZILARD
TAXLAWS
TELLALL
THELAMB
THELARK
TILLAGE
TITLARK
TOBLAME
TOLLAGE
TOOLATE
TOYLAND
TRALALA
TWOLANE
ULULANT
ULULATE
UNBLADE
UNCLAMP
UNCLASP
UNFLAKY
UNPLAIT
UNPLANS
UNSLACK
UNSLAIN
USFLAGS
VARLAAM
VILLAGE
VILLAIN
VILLARD
VILLARI
VINLAND
VIOLATE
VONLAUE
VORLAGE
WALLABY
WALLACE
WALLACH
WASLATE
WAYLAID
WAYLAND
WAYLAYS
WELLAND
WETLAND
WIELAND
WILLARD
YOPLAIT
ZEALAND
ZEELAND

•••L•A•

ABOLLAE
ADOLLAR
AEOLIAN
AGULHAS
AMALGAM
APULIAN
ARMLOAD
AXILLAE
AXILLAR
AXILLAS
AZALEAS
BAYLEAF
BELLEAU
BELLJAR
BELLLAP
BELLMAN
BIGLEAD
BOOLEAN
BUSLOAD
CARLOAD
CARLOAN
CHALLAH
CHILCAT
CHILEAN
CHILIAD
CHILKAT
CHOLLAS
COALCAR
COALGAS
COALTAR
COOLCAT
COOLMAX
DAHLIAS
DEFLEAS
DILLMAN
DRSLOAN
DWELLAT
ENDLEAF
FEELBAD
FHALOAN
FIGLEAF
FLYLEAF
FULLDAY
GASLEAK
GILLIAM
GILLIAN
GILLMAN
HALLWAY
HEELPAD
HEELTAP
HELLCAT
HELLMAN
HIALEAH
HILLMAN
HJALMAR
HOTLEAD
HOWLSAT
IMPLEAD
ITALIAN
JILLIAN
KELLJAN
LILLIAN
MACLEAN
MAILBAG
MAILCAR
MAILMAN
MALLRAT
MILLDAM
MISLEAD
MRCLEAN
NEWLEAF
NUCLEAR
OAKLEAF
OCELLAR
OFFLOAD
ONALEAD
OUTLEAD
OUTLEAP
PAELLAS
PAYLOAD
PELLEAS
PERLMAN
PHILEAS
POLLTAX
POOLMAN
PRELOAD
PRELOAN
PULLMAN
PULLTAB
RAILCAR
RAILMAN
RAILSAT
RAILWAY
REALMAN
RECLEAN
REFLOAT
REPLEAD
ROLLBAR
ROLLWAY
ROULEAU
RYELOAF
SHELLAC
SHULMAN
SMALLAD
SMILEAT
SMILLAS
SOULMAN
STELIAS
STELLAR
TABLEAU
TAILWAG
TEALEAF
TOILSAT
TOLLBAR
TOLLMAN
TOLLWAY
TOOLBAR
UNCLEAN
UNCLEAR
UNCLOAK
VANLOAD
VARLAAM
WALLMAP
WELLMAN
WILLIAM
WOOLFAT
WOOLHAT
YELLSAT

•••L••A

ADELINA
ARALSEA
BAKLAVA
CARLOTA
CHALUPA
CHELSEA
CHOLERA
DIPLOMA
EUGLENA
EVALUNA
HELLUVA
LAPLACA
LAPLATA
MALLIKA
MYALGIA
ONELIRA
OOHLALA
OTALGIA
PAULINA
PAVLOVA
POLLERA
REPLICA
SHALALA
TRALALA
TWELVEA

••••LA•

ABOLLAE
ADOLLAR
AIRPLAY
ALLCLAD
ALNILAM
AMESLAN
ANGELAS
ANGOLAN
ANGULAR
ANNULAR
AREOLAE
AREOLAR
AREOLAS
ASTOLAT
AXILLAE
AXILLAR
AXILLAS
BARCLAY
BELLLAP
BIPOLAR
BLUELAW
BURGLAR
CABALAS
CANOLAS
CANULAE
CANULAS
CASELAW
CATALAN
CATFLAP
CAVILAT
CHALLAH
CHEMLAB
CHOLLAS
COGHLAN
COPULAE
COPULAR
COPULAS
CUPOLAS
CUPULAR
DANELAW
DELILAH
DEMOLAY
DEWCLAW
DIPOLAR
DISPLAY
DOUGLAS
DWELLAT
EARFLAP
ENDPLAY
EXCELAT
FACULAE
FIBULAE
FIBULAR
FIBULAS
FINDLAY
FLAILAT
GAMELAN
GAMELAW
GAVILAN
GILBLAS
GRAVLAX
GRAYLAG
GREYLAG
GUNPLAY
HALALAS
HITPLAY
HOMELAB
HOOPLAS
HYGELAC
ILLCLAD
IMPALAS
INSULAR
JAIALAI
JOCULAR
JOHNLAW
JUDELAW
JUGULAR
KEESLAR
LASTLAP
LEGOLAS
LORELAI
LOYOLAU
LUNULAE
LUNULAR
MACULAE
MACULAR
MANILAS
MINILAB
MISPLAN
MISPLAY
MODELAS
MODULAR
MUDFLAP
MUDFLAT
NEBULAE
NEBULAR
NEBULAS
NICOLAS
NIKOLAI
NIKOLAY
NODULAR
NONPLAY
NOVELAS
OCELLAR
OGLALAS
OHMSLAW
ONECLAM
ORTOLAN
OSCULAR
OUTPLAN
OUTPLAY
OVERLAP
OVERLAX
OVERLAY
PACELAP
PAELLAS
PAYOLAS
PHARLAP
POORLAW
POPULAR
PREPLAN
QABALAH
QABALAS
QUINLAN
RCCOLAS
REDCLAY
REDFLAG
REGULAR
ROMULAN
ROTBLAT
RUSSLAN
RUYBLAS
SANBLAS
SAVALAS
SCHOLAR
SECULAR
SETPLAY
SHEILAE
SHEILAS
SHELLAC
SIMILAC
SIMILAR
SMALLAD
SMILLAS
SNARLAT
STELLAR
SUBCLAN
SZYSLAK
TABULAR
TEMPLAR
TESTLAB
TIMELAG
TITULAR
TORTLAW
TUBULAR
TUTELAR
UNDULAR
UNGULAE
UNGULAR
URSULAK
VIZSLAS
WROCLAW
XRAYLAB
YALELAW
ZONULAR

••••L•A

ALFALFA
APHELIA
AVONLEA
BEDELIA
BONILLA
CAMILLA
CAPELLA
CASELLA
CATALPA
CATFLEA
CECILIA
CEDILLA
COCHLEA
COROLLA
CRUELLA
DASILVA
DEFALLA
DEPALMA
DESYLVA
DOGFLEA
DOUBLEA
ESTELLA
FAMILIA
FIDELIA
GANGLIA
GORILLA
HIMALIA
LAJOLLA
LAPALMA
LOUELLA
MAGILLA
MAHALIA
MARILLA
MATILDA
MAXILLA
MEDULLA
MEGILLA
MINOLTA
MORELLA
MOZILLA
NATALIA
NOVELLA
OPHELIA
PAPILLA
PATELLA
PETULIA
REDALGA
REGALIA
ROSALIA
ROSELLA
RUBELLA
SEDALIA
SEVILLA
SHOULDA
SICILIA
SOMALIA
THEFLEA
THRILLA
TOCELIA
TRIPLEA
VANILLA
VIDALIA
VISALIA

•••••LA

ACEROLA
AMAPOLA
AMIDALA
ARUGULA
AUREOLA
BLACULA
BOBVILA
BOFFOLA
BONILLA
CABBALA
CAMILLA
CANDELA
CANNULA
CAPELLA
CARMELA
CASELLA
CASSOLA
CEDILLA
CHAPALA
COPPOLA
COROLLA
CRAPOLA
CRAYOLA
CRUELLA
DANIELA
DEFALLA
DRACULA
ESCUELA
ESTELLA
ETVOILA
EXEMPLA
FORMULA
GONDOLA
GORILLA
GRANOLA
ILOVELA
INOCULA
KABBALA
KAMPALA
LAJOLLA
LASCALA
LINGULA
LOUELLA
MAGILLA
MANDALA
MANDELA
MARILLA
MARSALA
MAXILLA
MEDULLA
MEGILLA
MESSALA
MICAELA
MINEOLA
MORELLA
MOZILLA
NONCOLA
NOVELLA
OOHLALA
OSCEOLA
PAPILLA
PATELLA
PERGOLA
PIANOLA
PLUGOLA
QUINELA
ROSELLA
ROSEOLA
RUBELLA
RUBEOLA
SCAPULA
SEVILLA
SHALALA
SHINOLA
SPATULA
TAMBALA
TEQUILA
THRILLA
TOMGOLA
TORTOLA
TRALALA
TUTUILA
UPPSALA
VALVULA
VANILLA
VIGNOLA
VINCULA
VISTULA
WOJTYLA

L•B••••

LABAMBA
LABATTS
LABCOAT
LABELED
LABELER
LABELLE
LABFEES
LABIALS
LABIATE
LABMICE
LABORAT
LABORED
LABORER
LABOURS
LABRATS
LABTECH
LABTEST
LABTUBE
LEBANON
LEBARON
LEBLANC
LEBROCK
LIBBERS
LIBBING
LIBELED
LIBELEE
LIBELER
LIBERAL
LIBERIA
LIBERTE
LIBERTY
LIBIDOS
LIBRANS
LIBRARY
LIBYANS
LOBATED
LOBBERS
LOBBIED
LOBBIES
LOBBING
LOBBYER
LOBSTER
LOBULES
LUBBERS
LUBBOCK
LUBEJOB

L••B•••

LAMBADA
LAMBDAS
LAMBEAU
LAMBENT
LAMBERT
LAMBETH
LAMBING
LAMBKIN
LAPBELT
LAWBOOK
LAYBACK
LAYBARE
LAZBOYS
LEGBONE
LEIBNIZ
LIBBERS
LIBBING
LIEBACK
LIMBERS
LIMBING
LIMBURG
LINBIAO
LIPBALM
LISBETH
LOBBERS
LOBBIED
LOBBIES
LOBBING
LOBBYER
LOGBOOK
LOMBARD
LONBORG
LOOBIES
LOWBALL
LOWBEAM
LOWBIDS
LOWBLOW
LOWBORN
LOWBOYS
LOWBRED
LOWBROW
LUBBERS
LUBBOCK
LUMBAGO
LUMBARS
LUMBERS

L•••B••

LADYBUG
LAKEBED
LAVABOS
LEGIBLE
LEGIBLY
LESABRE
LIEABED
LIKABLE
LINABLE
LIVABLE
LOCKBOX
LOFTBED
LONGBED
LONGBOW
LOSABLE
LOSEBIG
LOSTBIG
LOVABLE
LOVABLY
LOVEBUG

L••••B•

LABAMBA
LABTUBE
LAPROBE
LATROBE
LAZENBY
LEAVEBE
LETGOBY
LETITBE
LETMEBE
LULLABY
LYINGBY

L•••••B

LEFTJAB
LETTERB
LINEARB
LIONCUB
LOWCARB
LUBEJOB
LYNDONB

•LB••••

ALBANIA
ALBEDOS
ALBENIZ
ALBERTA
ALBERTI
ALBERTO
ALBINOS
ALBIREO
ALBORAK
ALBSURE
ALBUMEN
ALBUMIN
ALBUNDY
ELBERTA
ELBOWED
ELBOWER

•L•B•••

ALABAMA
ALABAMY
ALIBABA
ALIBIED
ALLBRAN
BLABBED
BLABBER
BLOBBED
BLUBBER
CLABBER
CLIBURN
CLOBBER
CLUBBED
CLUBBER
CLUBCAR
CLUBMED
CLUBSUP
FLUBBED
FLUBBER
FLUBDUB
FLUBUGS
FLYBALL
FLYBOYS
GLIBBER
GLOBATE
GLOBING
GLOBINS
GLOBOID
GLOBOSE
GLOBOUS
GLOBULE
ILLBITE
ILLBRED
OLDBATS
OLDBEAN
OLDBLUE
OLDBOYS
OLEBULL
PLEBIAN
SLABBED
SLOBBER

•L••B••

ALARBUS
ALDUBIN
ALEMBIC
ALGEBRA
BLABBED
BLABBER
BLAUBOK
BLOBBED
BLUBBER
BLUEBOY
BLURBER
CLABBER
CLAMBAR
CLAMBER
CLIMBED
CLIMBER
CLIMBIN
CLIMBON
CLIMBTO
CLIMBUP
CLOBBER
CLUBBED
CLUBBER
FLAMBED
FLAMBES
FLATBED
FLEABAG
FLUBBED
FLUBBER
FLYABLE
GLIBBER
KLEIBER
PLAYBOY
PLIABLE
PLIABLY
PLOWBOY
PLUMBED
PLUMBER
PLUMBIC
PLUMBUM
SLABBED
SLOBBER
SLUMBER

•L•••B•

ALGIEBA
ALIBABA
ALLENBY
ALTTABS
CLOSEBY
FLIESBY
FLITSBY
FLOATBY
FLOWNBY
GLIDEBY
GLORYBE
PLACEBO
PLAYSBY

SLIDEBY
SLIPSBY

•L••••B
ELEVENB
FLUBDUB

••LB•••
ALLBRAN
ARLBERG
BALBOAS
BULBLET
BULBOUS
COLBERT
DELBERT
DILBERT
FILBERT
GILBERT
GILBLAS
HILBERT
HOLBEIN
HOLBERG
ILLBITE
ILLBRED
OILBASE
OILBIRD
WILBERT

••L•B••
BALABAN
BALLBOY
BELABOR
BELLBOY
BELTBAG
BILOBED
BKLIBAN
CALABRO
CALIBAN
CALIBER
CALIBRE
CALLBOX
CALLBOY
CELEBES
CELEBRE
DELIBES
EULABUS
FELTBAD
FILIBEG
GOLDBUG
GOLFBAG
HALFBAD
HALIBUT
HELLBOY
INLABOR
KILOBAR
KILOBIT
MALABAR
MALEBEE
MALTBIE
MILKBAR
PALABRA
PILLBOX
PILLBUG
RELABEL
ROLLBAR
SALABLE
SALTBOX
SOLUBLE
TALIBAN
TALKBIG
TOLLBAR
UNLOBED
VOLUBLE
VOLUBLY

••L••B•
ALLENBY
COLOMBO
COLUMBA
COLUMBO
FILEDBY
FILESBY
INLIMBO
LULLABY
OILRUBS
ROLLSBY
RULEDBY
SYLLABI
WALKSBY
WALLABY

••L•••B
PULLTAB
SILENTB
WOLFCUB

•••LB••
BALLBOY
BELLBOY
CALLBOX
CALLBOY
CDALBUM
COALBIN
FEELBAD
HELLBOY
MAILBAG
MAILBIN
MAILBOX
PHILBIN
PILLBOX
PILLBUG
RAILBUS
ROLLBAR
TOLLBAR
TOOLBAR
TOOLBOX

•••L•B•
BIOLABS
COULDBE
DNALABS
EARLOBE
ETALIBI
LULLABY
MADLIBS
RIOLOBO
ROLLSBY
SCHLUBS
SEALABS
SYLLABI
WALLABY
WOULDBE

•••L••B
COULOMB
EWELAMB
PETLAMB
PULLTAB
RECLIMB
REPLUMB
THELAMB
TWELVEB
UNPLUMB
UPCLIMB

••••LB•
DRWELBY
MODELBS

••••L•B
CARCLUB
CHEMLAB
DOUBLEB
FANCLUB
GYMCLUB
HOMELAB
KEYCLUB
MINILAB
ONECLUB
TESTLAB
THEBLOB
WARCLUB
XRAYLAB

•••••LB
DIMBULB
DRYBULB
WETBULB

LC•••••
LCHAYIM

L•C••••
LACEDUP
LACERTA
LACESON
LACESUP
LACEUPS
LACIEST
LACINGS
LACKEYS
LACKING
LACKWIT
LACONIA
LACONIC
LACOSTE
LACQUER
LACRIMO
LACTAID
LACTASE
LACTATE
LACTEAL
LACTOSE
LACUNAE
LACUNAL
LACUNAR
LACUNAS
LACUREE
LECARRE
LECHERS
LECONTE
LECTERN
LECTORS
LECTRIC
LECTURE
LECUONA
LICENCE
LICENSE
LICHEES
LICHENS
LICITLY
LICKERS
LICKETY
LICKING
LICKSUP
LLCOOLJ
LOCALES
LOCALLY
LOCARNO
LOCATED
LOCATER
LOCATES
LOCATOR
LOCKAGE
LOCKBOX
LOCKEAN
LOCKERS
LOCKETS
LOCKING
LOCKINS
LOCKJAW
LOCKLET
LOCKLIN
LOCKNUT
LOCKOUT
LOCKSET
LOCKSIN
LOCKSON
LOCKSUP
LOCKUPS
LOCULUS
LOCUSTS
LUCANIA
LUCARNE
LUCENCY
LUCERNE
LUCETTA
LUCHINO
LUCIANA
LUCIANO
LUCIDAE
LUCIDLY
LUCIFER
LUCILLE
LUCINDA
LUCITES
LUCIUSI
LUCKIER
LUCKILY
LUCKING
LUCKMAN
LUCKNOW
LUCKOUT
LUCYLIU
LYCEUMS

L••C•••
LABCOAT
LAICIZE
LANCERS
LANCETS
LANCIAS
LANCING
LANCOME
LAOCOON
LAPCATS
LARCENY
LARCHEN
LARCHES
LASCALA
LASCARS
LASCAUX
LATCHED
LATCHES
LATCHON
LAWCASE
LEACHED
LEACHER
LEACHES
LEACOCK
LEECHED
LEECHEE
LEECHES
LESCAUT
LEUCINE
LINCOLN
LITCHIS
LITCRIT
LOWCARB
LOWCARD
LOWCHEN
LOWCOST
LUNCHED
LUNCHER
LUNCHES
LURCHED
LURCHER
LURCHES
LYOCELL

L•••C••
LAROCHE
LATICES
LAVACHE
LEANCUT
LENSCAP
LEXICAL
LEXICON
LIMACON
LINECUT
LINGCOD
LIONCUB
LOGICAL
LOSTCAT
LYRICAL
LYRICON

L••••C•
LABMICE
LABTECH
LADOUCE
LAMARCK
LAPLACA
LAPLACE
LASTACT
LATENCY
LATOSCA
LATTICE
LAYBACK
LEACOCK
LEBROCK
LELOUCH
LETTUCE
LICENCE
LIEBACK
LIKEICE
LOWNECK
LOWTECH
LUBBOCK
LUCENCY

L•••••C
LACONIC
LAENNEC
LAUTREC
LEBLANC
LECTRIC
LETTERC
LEVITIC
LEXUSSC
LIPIDIC
LIPSYNC
LUNATIC

•LC••••
ALCAIDE
ALCALDE
ALCAZAR
ALCESTE
ALCHEMY
ALCOHOL
ALCOPOP
ALCOVES
ALCYONE
ELCAJON
ELCAMPO
LLCOOLJ

•L•C•••
ALACKOF
ALLCAPS
ALLCASH
ALLCLAD
BLACKED
BLACKEN
BLACKER
BLACKIE
BLACKLY
BLACULA
BLOCKED
BLOCKER
BLOCKUP
CLACKED
CLACKER
CLACTON
CLICHED
CLICHES
CLICKED
CLICKER
CLICKON
CLOCHES
CLOCKED
CLOCKER
CLOCKIN
CLUCKED
CLUCKER
ELECTED
ELECTEE
ELECTME
ELECTOR
ELECTRA
ELECTRO
ELICITS
ELMCITY
ELOCUTE
FLACCID
FLACKED
FLACONS
FLECHES
FLECKED
FLICKED
FLICKER
FLOCKED
FLOCKTO
FLYCAST
GLACEED
GLACIAL
GLACIER
GLUCOSE
GLYCINE
GLYCOLS
ILLCALL
ILLCLAD
ILOCANO
OLDCARS
OLDCHAP
OLDCITY
OLICOOK
PLACARD
PLACATE
PLACEBO
PLACERS
PLACIDO
PLACING
PLACKET
PLECTRA
PLICATE
PLUCKED
SLACKED
SLACKEN
SLACKER
SLACKLY
SLACKUP
SLICERS
SLICEUP
SLICING
SLICKED
SLICKER
SLICKLY

•L••C••
ALARCON
ALENCON
ALNICOS
ALPACAS
BLANCHE
BLOTCHY
CLUBCAR
CLUTCHY
ELANCES
FLACCID
FLATCAR
FLEECED
FLEECER
FLEECES
GLANCED
GLANCES
GLENCOE
GLITCHY
ILLICIT
PLAICES
PLUMCOT
SLOTCAR
SLOUCHY
SLUICED
SLUICES

•L•••C•
ALDRICH
BLALOCK
BLUEICE
CLARICE
CLERICS
CLINICS
ELDRICH
ELDRICK
ELFLOCK
ELGRECO
FLEANCE
FLOUNCE
FLOUNCY
FLUENCY
ILIESCU
ILLLUCK
KLATSCH
KLENSCH
OLDNICK
PLAYACT
PLIANCY

•L••••C
ALEMBIC
ALLELIC
ALMANAC
CLASSIC
ELASTIC
ELEGIAC
ELEVENC
FLUIDIC
GLYPHIC
GLYPTIC
ILIADIC
ILLOGIC
OLYMPIC
PLASMIC
PLASTIC
PLUMBIC

••LC•••
ALLCAPS
ALLCASH
ALLCLAD
BALCONY
BELCHED
BELCHER
BELCHES
CALCIFY
CALCITE
CALCIUM
CALCULI
COLCHIS
CULCHES
DELCITY
DULCIFY
FALCATE
FALCONS
FILCHED
FILCHER
FILCHES
FULCRUM
GELCAPS
GULCHES
HALCYON
ILLCALL
ILLCLAD
MALCOLM
MULCAHY
MULCHED
MULCHES
MULCTED
OILCAKE
OILCANS
OILCUPS
PILCROW
SALCHOW
TALCKED
TALCUMS
VELCROS
VOLCANO
VOLCKER
VULCANS
WALCOTT
WELCOME
ZILCHES

••L•C••
CALICES
CALICOS
CALYCES
CELICAS
COLDCUP
COLDCUT
COLICKY
DELICTI
DELICTO
DELICTS
ENLACED
ENLACES
FELICIA
GALICIA
GOLFCAR
HALFCUT
HELICAL
HELICES
HELICON
HELLCAT
HOLYCOW
ILLICIT
MALACCA
MALACHI
MALECAT
MALICES
MILKCAN
MILKCOW
MOLUCCA
MRLUCKY
PALACES
PELICAN
POLECAR
POLECAT
POLICED
POLICER
POLICES
RELACED
RELACES
RELICTS
RELOCKS
RELUCTS
SELECTS
SHLOCKY
SILICAS
SILICON
SOLACED
SOLACER
SOLACES
SOLICIT
SPLICED
SPLICER
SPLICES
STLUCIA
TELECOM
UNLACED
UNLACES
UNLOCAL
UNLOCKS
UNLUCID
UNLUCKY
WELLCUT
WILDCAT
WOLFCUB

••L••C•
ATLUNCH
BALANCE
BELASCO
BULLOCK
CALTECH
CELTICS
COLLECT
DOLUNCH
FALLACY
GALLICO
HILLOCK
ILLLUCK
JALISCO
LELOUCH
MALACCA
MOLUCCA
OILRICH
PALANCE
POLISCI
POLLACK
POLLOCK
POLYSCI
RELANCE
RELATCH
ROLLICK
SELLECK
SILENCE
SOLOACT
SPLOTCH
TOLTECS
UNLATCH
VALANCE
VALENCE
WALLACE
WALLACH

••L•••C
AELFRIC
ALLELIC
BALDRIC
CALORIC
CHLORIC
DELPHIC
DELTAIC
ILLOGIC
ISLAMIC
MALEFIC
MELANIC
MELODIC
MOLLUSC
OOLITIC
PELAGIC
POLEMIC
POLITIC
SELENIC
SILENTC
SYLPHIC
TELEPIC
UNLYRIC
VOLTAIC

•••LC••
CHALCIS
CHILCAT
COALCAR
COOLCAT
HELLCAT
MAILCAR
PHILCOS
POOLCUE
RAILCAR
WELLCUT

•••L•C•
AFFLECK
AFFLICT
AIRLOCK
ANYLUCK
ARMLOCK
BADLUCK
BARLICK
BLALOCK
BULLOCK
CHALICE
COLLECT
COWLICK
DEFLECT
DIALECT
EARLOCK
EHRLICH
ELFLOCK
EMPLACE
FALLACY
FETLOCK
FROLICS
GALLICO
GARLICS
GENLOCK
GUNLOCK
HEMLOCK
HILLOCK
HOTLICK
ILLLUCK
INBLACK
INFLECT
INFLICT
INPLACE
ITALICS
JOBLOCK
KEYLOCK
LAPLACA
LAPLACE
MADLOCK
MATLOCK
MORLOCK
NEGLECT
NIBLICK
NOPLACE
NUMLOCK
OARLOCK
OOBLECK
PADLOCK
PAMLICO
PIMLICO
POLLACK
POLLOCK
POTLUCK
PRELACY
PUBLICS
REBLOCK
REELECT
REFLECT
REPLACE
REPLICA
ROLLICK
SCHLOCK
SELLECK
SHYLOCK
UNBLOCK
UNSLACK
UNSLICK
WALLACE
WALLACH
WARLOCK
WEDLOCK
ZIPLOCK
ZIPLOCS

•••L••C
IDYLLIC
LEBLANC
MOLLUSC
MTBLANC
MYALGIC
NUCLEIC
OTALGIC
POULENC
PSALMIC
SHELLAC
TWELVEC

••••LC•
ACDELCO
NORELCO
SQUELCH

••••L•C
ACRYLIC
ACYCLIC
ALLELIC
ANGELIC
BASILIC
BUCOLIC
DOUBLEC
EIDOLIC
HYGELAC
IDYLLIC
JEANLUC
MIDDLEC
SHELLAC
SIBYLIC
SIMILAC
TONELOC
VINYLIC
VOCALIC

•••••LC
MISKOLC

L•D••••
LADADOG
LADDERS
LADDIES
LADDISH
LADHOOD
LADIDAS
LADINGS
LADINOS
LADLERS
LADLING
LADOUCE
LADRONE
LADYBUG
LADYDAY
LADYISH
LADYKIN
LADYNAS
LEDAWAY
LEDERER
LEDGERS
LEDGIER
LEDINTO
LEDUPTO
LIDLESS
LIDWINA
LODGEIN
LODGERS
LODGING
LUDDISM
LUDDITE
LYDDITE

L••D•••
LADDERS
LADDIES
LADDISH
LAIDFOR
LAIDLOW
LAIDOFF
LAIDOUT
LANDAUS
LANDERS
LANDING
LANDINI
LANDLER
LANDMAN
LANDMEN
LANDSAT
LANDSUP
LANDTAG
LANDTAX
LAPDOGS

LARDERS
LARDIER
LARDING
LARDNER
LARDONS
LAUDERS
LAUDING
LAYDOWN
LEADDOG
LEADENS
LEADERS
LEADETH
LEADIER
LEADING
LEADINS
LEADMAN
LEADMEN
LEADOFF
LEADORE
LEADOUT
LEADSIN
LEADSON
LEADSTO
LEADSUP
LEADUPS
LENDERS
LENDING
LENDOUT
LETDOWN
LETDROP
LEWDEST
LIEDFOR
LIEDOWN
LINDENS
LINDIED
LINDIES
LINDNER
LINDORF
LINDROS
LINDSAY
LINDSEY
LLADROS
LOADERS
LOADING
LOADSIN
LOADSOF
LOADSUP
LOIDING
LONDRES
LORDING
LORDJIM
LORDSIT
LOUDENS
LOUDEST
LOUDISH
LOWDIVE
LOWDOWN
LUDDISM
LUDDITE
LYDDITE
LYNDONB

L•••D••

LACEDUP
LADADOG
LADIDAS
LADYDAY
LAMBDAS
LANGDON
LAREDOS
LASTDON
LAUNDER
LAUNDRY
LAYODDS
LEADDOG
LEANDER
LEAPDAY
LEONDAY
LEPIDUS
LEVADES
LIBIDOS
LINEDRY
LINEDUP
LIPIDIC
LIVEDIN
LIVEDON
LIVIDLY
LONGDAY
LONGDEN
LOSTDOG
LOURDES
LOVEDIT
LOVEDTO
LUCIDAE
LUCIDLY
LUREDIN
LURIDLY

L••••D•

LAMBADA
LASORDA
LAWANDA
LAYODDS
LEETIDE
LEGENDS
LEMONDE
LEONIDS
LETRIDE
LIGANDS
LIMEADE
LIQUIDS
LIZARDS
LOWBIDS
LOWSIDE
LOWTIDE
LUCINDA

L•••••D

LABELED
LABORED
LACTAID
LADHOOD
LAGGARD
LAKEBED
LANFORD
LANGUID
LANYARD
LAPELED
LAPLAND
LASSOED
LATCHED
LATENED
LAUGHED
LAWFORD
LAYERED
LEACHED
LEAGUED
LEARNED
LEASHED
LEAWOOD
LEECHED
LEEFORD
LEEWARD
LEFTEND
LEGRAND
LEONARD
LEOPARD
LEOPOLD
LEOTARD
LEPPARD
LETTERD
LEVELED
LEVERED
LEWHOAD
LIAISED
LIBELED
LIEABED
LIGATED
LIGHTED
LIKEMAD
LIKENED
LILYPAD
LIMITED
LINDIED
LINGCOD
LINSEED
LIPREAD
LITHOID
LIVEAID
LIVENED
LIVERED
LOATHED
LOBATED
LOBBIED
LOCATED
LOFTBED
LOLLARD
LOMBARD
LONGBED
LOOKSAD
LOUNGED
LOUREED
LOUVRED
LOWBRED
LOWCARD
LOWERED
LOWHAND
LOWLAND
LOWPAID
LOWROAD
LSHAPED
LUNATED
LUNCHED
LURCHED
LUSTRED
LUXATED

•LD••••

ALDAVIS
ALDENTE
ALDORAY
ALDRICH
ALDUBIN
ELDERLY
ELDRICH
ELDRICK
OLDBATS
OLDBEAN
OLDBLUE
OLDBOYS
OLDCARS
OLDCHAP
OLDCITY
OLDDAYS
OLDDOGS
OLDFILM
OLDFOGY
OLDGAGS
OLDGIRL
OLDGOLD
OLDHAND
OLDJOKE
OLDLADY
OLDLINE
OLDLYME
OLDMAID
OLDMOON
OLDNAVY
OLDNESS
OLDNEWS
OLDNICK
OLDPALS
OLDPROS
OLDROSE
OLDSALT
OLDSAWS
OLDSHOE
OLDSONG
OLDSTER
OLDTIME
OLDTOWN
OLDUVAI
OLDWAYS
OLDWEST

•L•D•••

ALADDIN
ALADINE
ALIDADE
ALLDONE
ALTDORF
ALUDELS
BLADDER
BLADERS
BLADING
BLEDSOE
BLUDGED
BLUDGER
BLUDGES
CLADDED
ELIDERS
ELIDING
ELUDERS
ELUDING
FLEDGED
FLEDGES
GLADDEN
GLADDER
GLADEYE
GLIDEBY
GLIDEIN
GLIDERS
GLIDING
ILLDOIT
ILLDONE
KLUDGED
KLUDGES
LLADROS
OLDDAYS
OLDDOGS
PLEDGED
PLEDGEE
PLEDGER
PLEDGES
PLODDED
PLODDER
SLEDDED
SLEDDER
SLEDDOG
SLEDFUL
SLEDGED
SLEDGES
SLIDEBY
SLIDEIN
SLIDERS
SLIDING
SLIDOFF
SLIDOUT
SLUDGES

•L••D••

ALADDIN
ALBEDOS
ALLUDED
ALLUDES
ALMADEN
ALOADOF
BLADDER
BLANDER
BLANDLY
BLEEDER
BLENDED
BLENDER
BLENDES
BLENDIN
BLINDED
BLINDER
BLINDLY
BLINDTO
BLONDER
BLONDES
BLONDIE
BLOODED
BLOWDRY
BLUNDEN
BLUNDER
CLADDED
CLAMDIP
CLAUDEL
CLAUDIA
CLAUDIO
CLOUDED
CLOUDUP
CLOWDER
CLUEDIN
ELFUDGE
FLAGDAY
FLEADIP
FLIEDTO
FLOODED
FLUBDUB
FLUIDAL
FLUIDIC
FLUIDLY
GLADDEN
GLADDER
GLUEDON
GLUEDTO
ILIADIC
ILLUDED
ILLUDES
PLAUDIT
PLAYDOH
PLEADED
PLEADER
PLEADTO
PLODDED
PLODDER
PLOVDIV
PLUNDER
SLANDER
SLEDDED
SLEDDER
SLEDDOG
SLENDER
SLOWDAY

•L•••D•

ALAMEDA
ALAMODE
ALBUNDY
ALCAIDE
ALCALDE
ALEARDI
ALFREDA
ALFREDE
ALFREDO
ALFREDU
ALIDADE
ALLENDE
ALMONDS
ALMONDY
ALREADY
ALTOIDS
ELAPIDS
ELMUNDO
ELPRADO
FLORIDA
FLYRODS
ILLMADE
OLDLADY
PLACIDO
ULANUDE

•L••••D

ALARMED
ALASSAD
ALERTED
ALEYARD
ALIBIED
ALIGNED
ALLAYED
ALLCLAD
ALLEGED
ALLGOOD
ALLOWED
ALLOYED
ALLTIED
ALLTOLD
ALLUDED
ALLURED
ALPHARD
ALTERED
BLABBED
BLACKED
BLANKED
BLASTED
BLATTED
BLEARED
BLEATED
BLEEPED
BLENDED
BLESSED
BLINDED
BLINKED
BLIPPED
BLISSED
BLITZED
BLOATED
BLOBBED
BLOCKED
BLOGGED
BLOODED
BLOOMED
BLOOPED
BLOTTED
BLOUSED
BLOWZED
BLUDGED
BLUERED
BLUFFED
BLUNTED
BLURRED
BLURTED
BLUSHED
CLACKED
CLADDED
CLAIMED
CLAMMED
CLAMPED
CLANGED
CLANKED
CLAPPED
CLASHED
CLASPED
CLASSED
CLEANED
CLEARED
CLEATED
CLEAVED
CLERKED
CLICHED
CLICKED
CLIMBED
CLINKED
CLIPPED
CLIQUED
CLOAKED
CLOCKED
CLOGGED
CLOMPED
CLONKED
CLOPPED
CLOTHED
CLOTTED
CLOUDED
CLOUTED
CLOWNED
CLUBBED
CLUBMED
CLUCKED
CLUMPED
CLUNKED
ELAPSED
ELBOWED
ELECTED
ELEVEND
ELMWOOD
FLACCID
FLACKED
FLAGGED
FLAILED
FLAMBED
FLAMMED
FLANKED
FLAPPED
FLASHED
FLATBED
FLATTED
FLECKED
FLEDGED
FLEECED
FLEERED
FLEETED
FLENSED
FLESHED
FLICKED
FLIPPED
FLIRTED
FLITTED
FLOATED
FLOCKED
FLOGGED
FLOODED
FLOORED
FLOPPED
FLOSSED
FLOURED
FLOUTED
FLUBBED
FLUFFED
FLUNKED
FLUSHED
GLACEED
GLANCED
GLASSED
GLEAMED
GLEANED
GLINTED
GLITZED
GLOATED
GLOBOID
GLOMMED
GLOOMED
GLORIED
GLOSSED
GLUGGED
GLUMMED
GLUTTED
ILLBRED
ILLCLAD
ILLFOLD
ILLUDED
ILLUMED
ILLUSED
ILLWIND
KLUDGED
OLDGOLD
OLDHAND
OLDMAID
OLMSTED
PLACARD
PLAGUED
PLAITED
PLANKED
PLANNED
PLANTED
PLASHED
PLATTED
PLEADED
PLEASED
PLEATED
PLEDGED
PLINKED
PLODDED
PLONKED
PLOPPED
PLOTTED
PLOTZED
PLUCKED
PLUGGED
PLUMBED
PLUMPED
PLUNGED
PLUNKED
PLYWOOD
SLABBED
SLACKED
SLAMMED
SLANTED
SLAPPED
SLASHED
SLATTED
SLEDDED
SLEDGED
SLEEKED
SLEETED
SLEEVED
SLICKED
SLIMMED
SLINKED
SLIPPED
SLITTED
SLOGGED
SLOPPED
SLOSHED
SLOTTED
SLUGGED
SLUICED
SLUMMED
SLUMPED
SLURPED
SLURRED
SLUSHED

••LD•••

ALLDONE
AULDSOD
BALDEST
BALDIES
BALDING
BALDISH
BALDRIC
BALDWIN
BELDAME
BELDAMS
BOLDEST
CALDERA
CALDERS
CALDRON
COLDCUP
COLDCUT
COLDDAY
COLDEST
COLDISH
COLDONE
COLDWAR
FELDMAN
FOLDERS
FOLDING
FOLDOUT
FOLDSIN
FOLDSUP
FOLDUPS
GELDING
GILDERS
GILDING
GOLDARN
GOLDBUG
GOLDING
GOLDMAN
GOLDONI
GOLDTIP
GOLDWYN
GULDENS
HALDANE
HELDOFF
HELDOUT
HOLDALL
HOLDERS
HOLDING
HOLDOFF
HOLDOUT
HOLDSIN
HOLDSIT
HOLDSON
HOLDSTO
HOLDSUP
HOLDUPS
ILLDOIT
ILLDONE
KILDARE
MALDIVE
MELDERS
MELDING
MILDEST
MILDEWS
MILDEWY
MILDRED
MOLDERS
MOLDIER
MOLDING
MOLDOVA
MULDAUR
MULDOON
OILDRUM
SOLDERS
SOLDFOR
SOLDIER
SOLDOFF
SOLDOUT
TOLDALL
TOLDOFF
WALDORF
WELDERS
WELDING
WILDCAT
WILDDOG
WILDEST
WILDING
WILDISH
WILDMAN
WILDMEN
WILDONE
WILDPIG

••L•D••

ALLUDED
ALLUDES
ARLEDGE
BOLIDES
BULLDOG
CELADON
COLADAS
COLDDAY
DELEDDA
DELUDED
DELUDER
DELUDES
FALLDUE
FELLDUE
FILEDBY
FILEDIN
FILMDOM
FULLDAY
GELIDLY
HALFDAY
HALFDUG
HALIDES
HOLEDUP
HOLIDAY
HOLYDAY
ILLUDED
ILLUDES
IPLEDGE
JULYDAY
KILNDRY
MALEDOG
MALODOR
MELODIA
MELODIC
MILKDUD
MILLDAM
PALADIN
PALEDRY
PALUDAL
PILEDIN
PILEDON
PILEDUP
RILEDUP
ROLODEX
RULEDBY
RULEDON
SALADES
SALADIN
SOLEDAD
SOLIDER
SOLIDLY
TOLEDAN
TOLEDOS
UNLADED
UNLADEN
UNLADES
VALADON
VALIDID
VALIDLY
WILDDOG
WOLFDOG

••L••D•

ALLENDE
BALLADE
BALLADS
BELINDA
CALANDO
CALENDS
COLLIDE
COLLODI
COLLUDE
DELEADS
DELEDDA
HALOIDS
ILLMADE
INLANDS
ISLANDS
MALTEDS
MELINDA
MILORDS
NOLOADS
ONLOADS
ORLANDO
RELANDS
RELEADS
RELENDS
RELOADS
ROLAIDS
ROLONDA
SALSODA
SPLENDA
SULFIDE
UNLEADS
UNLOADS
UPLANDS
UPLOADS
YOLANDA

••L•••D

ABLATED
ALLAYED
ALLCLAD
ALLEGED
ALLGOOD
ALLOWED
ALLOYED
ALLTIED
ALLTOLD
ALLUDED
ALLURED
AULDSOD
BALLARD
BELATED
BELAYED
BELCHED
BELLIED
BELOVED
BILOBED
BULLIED
BYLINED
COLLARD
COLLOID
COLORED
CULLIED
DALLIED
DELAYED
DELETED
DELTOID
DELUDED
DELUGED
DILATED
DILLARD
DILUTED
DOLLIED
DULLARD
ENLACED
FELTBAD
FILCHED
FOLIOED
GALAHAD
GALOPED
GELATED
GILFORD
GULLIED
HALFBAD
HALFFED
HALFMAD
HALFROD
HALYARD
HELIPAD
HELLOED
HELMOND
HOLLAND
HULLOED
ILLBRED
ILLCLAD
ILLFOLD
ILLUDED
ILLUMED
ILLUSED
ILLWIND
ISLETED
JELLIED
JOLLIED
LILYPAD
LOLLARD
MALAMUD
MALLARD
MELAMED
MILDRED
MILHAUD
MILKDUD
MILKFED
MILLAND
MILLARD
MILLEND
MULCHED
MULCTED
OBLIGED
OILBIRD
OILSAND
OILSEED
OWLEYED
PILOTED
POLICED
POLKAED

POLLARD
POLYPED
POLYPOD
RALLIED
RELACED
RELATED
RELAXED
RELAYED
RELINED
RELIVED
RELUMED
ROLLAND
SALLIED
SALUTED
SILENTD
SOLACED
SOLEDAD
SPLAYED
SPLICED
SULLIED
TALCKED
TALLIED
TALONED
TELEXED
UNLACED
UNLADED
UNLAVED
UNLAXED
UNLIKED
UNLINED
UNLIVED
UNLOBED
UNLOVED
UNLUCID
UNLURED
VALETED
VALIDID
VILLARD
VOLUMED
VOLUTED
WALTZED
WELLAND
WELLFED
WELLHID
WELLLED
WILFORD
WILFRED
WILLARD

•••LD••
BOULDER
BUILDER
BUILDIN
BUILDON
BUILDUP
BULLDOG
COULDBE
COULDNT
EARLDOM
FALLDUE
FELLDUE
FIELDED
FIELDER
FULLDAY
GUILDER
MAULDIN
MILLDAM
MOULDED
MOULDER
SCALDED
SCALDER
SCOLDED
SCOLDER
SHELDON
SMOLDER
WIELDED
WIELDER
WORLDLY
WOULDBE
WOULDNT
WOULDST
YIELDED
YIELDER
YIELDTO

•••L•D•
BAGLADY
BALLADE
BALLADS
COLLIDE
COLLODI
COLLUDE
DIALEDO
EPILADY
EXCLUDE
EXPLODE
EYELIDS
IMPLODE
INCLUDE
NUCLIDE
OCCLUDE
OLDLADY
POTLIDS
PRELUDE
RECLADS
ROULADE
SECLUDE
SUBLIDS
UNBLADE

•••L••D
ABELARD
APPLAUD
APPLIED
ARMLOAD
ASHLAND
AVULSED
AXELROD
BADLAND
BALLARD
BAULKED
BECLOUD
BELLIED
BIGLEAD
BULLIED
BUSLOAD
CARLOAD
CAULKED
CHALKED
CHILIAD
CHILLED
COLLARD
COLLOID
COPLAND
CULLIED
CYCLOID
DALLIED
DIALLED
DILLARD
DIPLOID
DOLLIED
DRILLED
DUELLED
DULLARD
DWELLED
ENGLAND
ENGLUND
EVOLVED
EVULSED
EXALTED
EXULTED
FAULTED
FEELBAD
FIELDED
FINLAND
FOULARD
FRILLED
FUELLED
FUELROD
GARLAND
GAYLORD
GIELGUD
GRILLED
GULLIED
HAPLOID
HARLAND
HEELPAD
HELLOED
HOLLAND
HOTLEAD
HULLOED
HYALOID
ICELAND
IMPLEAD
IMPLIED
IRELAND
JELLIED
JOLLIED
JUTLAND
KNELLED
KOOLAID
KVELLED
LAPLAND
LOLLARD
LOWLAND
MACLEOD
MALLARD
MCCLOUD
MIDLAND
MILLAND
MILLARD
MILLEND
MISLAID
MISLEAD
MOULDED
MOULTED
NEDLAND
NEWLAID
OAKLAND
OFFLOAD
ONALEAD
OUTLAID
OUTLAND
OUTLEAD
OUTLOUD
OXBLOOD
PAYLOAD
POLLARD
PRELOAD
QUELLED
QUILLED
QUILTED
RALLIED
REFLOOD
REGLUED
REPLEAD
REPLIED
ROLLAND
ROWLAND
RUTLAND
SALLIED
SAMLOYD
SCALDED
SCALPED
SCOLDED
SCULLED
SCULPED
SHELLED
SHELVED
SHILLED
SKILLED
SKULKED
SKULLED
SMALLAD
SMELLED
SMELTED
SPELLED
SPILLED
STALKED
STALLED
STCLOUD
STILLED
STILTED
SULLIED
SWELLED
SWILLED
SZILARD
TABLOID
TAILEND
TALLIED
TOYLAND
TRILLED
TROLLED
TWELVED
TWILLED
UNBLUED
UNCLOUD
UNFLUID
UNGLUED
UNPLIED
VANLOAD
VAULTED
VIALLED
VILLARD
VINLAND
WARLORD
WAYLAID
WAYLAND
WELLAND
WELLFED
WELLHID
WELLLED
WETLAND
WHELMED
WHELPED
WIELAND
WIELDED
WILLARD
YIELDED
ZEALAND
ZEELAND

••••LD•
ALCALDE
ARNOLDS
BEHOLDS
DEWILDE
ENFOLDS
ENGILDS
GERALDO
HAROLDI
HERALDS
INFOLDS
KOBOLDS
MATILDA
MTBALDY
REFOLDS
REGILDS
REMOLDS
RENALDO
REWELDS
RIBALDS
RINALDO
SCHELDT
SHIELDS
SHOULDA
SHOULDI
TEBALDI
UNBELDI
UNFOLDS
UNMOLDS
UNMOLDY
UPFOLDS
UPHOLDS
VIVALDI

••••L•D
ALLCLAD
ANNELID
AVAILED
BABBLED
BAFFLED
BANGLED
BATTLED
BEVELED
BOBBLED
BOBSLED
BOGGLED
BOTTLED
BRAWLED
BRIDLED
BROILED
BUBBLED
BUCKLED
BUMBLED
BUNDLED
BUNGLED
BURBLED
BURGLED
BUSTLED
CACKLED
CAJOLED
CAMELID
CANALED
CANDLED
CAROLED
CASTLED
CAVILED
CHILLED
CICHLID
CIRCLED
COBBLED
COCKLED
CODDLED
COUPLED
CRADLED
CRAWLED
CUDDLED
CUPELED
CURDLED
DABBLED
DANDLED
DANGLED
DAPPLED
DARKLED
DARTLED
DAWDLED
DAZZLED
DECKLED
DEFILED
DEVILED
DIALLED
DIBBLED
DIDDLED
DIMPLED
DOGSLED
DOODLED
DOUBLED
DRAWLED
DRILLED
DROOLED
DUELLED
DWELLED
EASELED
EMAILED
EMPALED
ENABLED
ENISLED
ENOILED
ENSILED
EQUALED
ETAILED
EXHALED
FIDDLED
FIZZLED
FLAILED
FONDLED
FOOTLED
FOOZLED
FORDLTD
FRILLED
FUDDLED
FUELLED
FUMBLED
GABBLED
GAMBLED
GARBLED
GARGLED
GAVELED
GENTLED
GIGGLED
GIRDLED
GNARLED
GOBBLED
GOGGLED
GOOGLED
GRILLED
GROWLED
GURGLED
GUZZLED
HACKLED
HAGGLED
HANDLED
HASSLED
HECKLED
HIGGLED
HOBBLED
HUDDLED
HUMBLED
HURDLED
HURTLED
HUSTLED
ILLCLAD
IMPALED
INHALED
INVALID
JANGLED
JEWELED
JIGGLED
JINGLED
JOGGLED
JOSTLED
JUGGLED
JUMBLED
KIBBLED
KINDLED
KNEELED
KNELLED
KNURLED
KVELLED
LABELED
LAPELED
LEVELED
LIBELED
MANGLED
MANTLED
MARBLED
MEDALED
MEDDLED
METALED
MIDDLED
MINGLED
MIZZLED
MODELED
MOTTLED
MUDDLED
MUFFLED
MUMBLED
MURALED
MUSCLED
MUZZLED
NEEDLED
NESTLED
NETTLED
NIBBLED
NIGGLED
NODULED
NOODLED
NUZZLED
OUTPLOD
PADDLED
PANELED
PAROLED
PEARLED
PEBBLED
PEDALED
PEDDLED
PEOPLED
PERILED
PESTLED
PETALED
PICKLED
PIDDLED
PIFFLED
PIMPLED
POPPLED
PROWLED
PUDDLED
PURFLED
PURPLED
PUZZLED
QUAILED
QUELLED
QUILLED
RABBLED
RAFFLED
RAMBLED
RANKLED
RASSLED
RATTLED
RAVELED
REBALED
REFILED
REGALED
REOILED
RESILED
RESOLED
RETILED
REVELED
REVILED
RIDDLED
RIFFLED
RIMPLED
RIPPLED
RIVALED
ROOTLED
ROWELED
RUFFLED
RUMBLED
RUMPLED
RUSTLED
SADDLED
SAMPLED
SCOWLED
SCULLED
SEPALED
SETTLED
SHAWLED
SHELLED
SHILLED
SHOALED
SINGLED
SIZZLED
SKIDLID
SKILLED
SKIRLED
SKULLED
SMALLAD
SMELLED
SNARLED
SPELLED
SPIELED
SPILLED
SPOILED
SPOOLED
SQUALID
STABLED
STALLED
STAPLED
STEELED
STIFLED
STILLED
STOOLED
SUPPLED
SWELLED
SWILLED
SWIRLED
TACKLED
TANGLED
TATTLED
TEMPLED
TICKLED
TINGLED
TINKLED
TIPPLED
TODDLED
TOGGLED
TOOTLED
TOPPLED
TOTALED
TOUSLED
TOWELED
TOYSLED
TRAILED
TRAWLED
TREBLED
TRIFLED
TRILLED
TRIPLED
TROLLED
TUMBLED
TURTLED
TUSSLED
TWILLED
TWIRLED
UNAXLED
UNBALED
UNFILED
UNOGLED
UNOILED
UNPALED
UNPILED
UNPOLED
UNRILED
UNRULED
UNSOLED
UNSOLID
UNTILED
UPPILED
VIALLED
WADDLED
WAFFLED
WAGGLED
WAMBLED
WANGLED
WARBLED
WATTLED
WEDELED
WELLLED
WHEELED
WHIRLED
WHORLED
WIGGLED
WIMPLED
WOBBLED
YODELED

•••••LD
ALLTOLD
ARCWELD
BADCOLD
BAGNOLD
DIEBOLD
EMERALD
ENFIELD
EYEFOLD
FANFOLD
GETCOLD
GETSOLD
GINGOLD
GOTCOLD
GREWOLD
GROWOLD
HARROLD
HOGWILD
ICECOLD
ILLFOLD
INFIELD
ITSCOLD
LEOPOLD
MISTOLD
MYWORLD
NONGOLD
OLDGOLD
ONEFOLD
OSTWALD
OUTCOLD
OUTSOLD
OUTTOLD
PCWORLD
PIEBALD
PINFOLD
PRESOLD
PRETOLD
RANWILD
REBUILD
RUNWILD
SAMEOLD
SIXFOLD
TENFOLD
THEGOLD
TOEHOLD
TORVALD
TRIFOLD
TWOFOLD
UNBUILD
UNMOULD
UPBUILD
UPFIELD
VERYOLD

LE•••••
LEACHED
LEACHER
LEACHES
LEACOCK
LEADDOG
LEADENS
LEADERS
LEADETH
LEADIER
LEADING
LEADINS
LEADMAN
LEADMEN
LEADOFF
LEADORE
LEADOUT
LEADSIN
LEADSON
LEADSTO
LEADSUP
LEADUPS
LEAFAGE
LEAFIER
LEAFING
LEAFLET
LEAFOUT
LEAGUED
LEAGUER
LEAGUES
LEAKAGE
LEAKERS
LEAKEYS
LEAKIER
LEAKING
LEAKSIN
LEANCUT
LEANDER
LEANERS
LEANEST
LEANING
LEANSIN
LEANSON
LEANSTO
LEANTOS
LEAPDAY
LEAPERS
LEAPFOR
LEAPING
LEAPSAT
LEAPSIN
LEAPSON
LEAPSUP
LEAPTAT
LEAPTIN
LEAPTON
LEAPTUP
LEARJET
LEARNED
LEARNER
LEARNOF
LEARNTO
LEASERS
LEASETO
LEASHED
LEASHES
LEASING
LEATHER
LEAVEBE
LEAVEIN
LEAVEIT
LEAVENS
LEAVEON
LEAVING
LEAWOOD
LEBANON
LEBARON
LEBLANC
LEBROCK
LECARRE
LECHERS
LECONTE
LECTERN
LECTORS
LECTRIC
LECTURE
LECUONA
LEDAWAY
LEDERER
LEDGERS
LEDGIER
LEDINTO
LEDUPTO
LEECHED
LEECHEE
LEECHES
LEEFORD
LEERERS
LEERIER
LEERILY
LEERING
LEERSAT
LEETIDE
LEEWARD
LEEWAYS
LEFREAK
LEFTARM
LEFTEAR
LEFTEND
LEFTEST
LEFTEYE
LEFTFOR
LEFTHIP
LEFTIES
LEFTISH
LEFTISM
LEFTIST
LEFTJAB
LEFTLEG
LEFTOFF
LEFTOUT
LEGALLY
LEGANZA
LEGATEE
LEGATES
LEGATOR
LEGATOS
LEGBONE
LEGENDS
LEGGIER
LEGGING
LEGHORN
LEGIBLE
LEGIBLY
LEGIONS
LEGIRON
LEGISTS
LEGLESS
LEGLIKE
LEGOLAS
LEGOSET
LEGPULL
LEGRAND
LEGREST
LEGROOM
LEGROPE
LEGTRAP
LEGUMES
LEGWEAR
LEGWORK
LEHAVRE
LEHIGHU
LEHMANN
LEIBNIZ
LEIPZIG
LEISTER
LEISURE
LEITRIM
LEJEUNE
LELOUCH
LEMIEUX
LEMMATA
LEMMING
LEMONDE
LEMOYNE
LEMPIRA
LENDERS
LENDING
LENDOUT
LENFANT
LENGTHS
LENGTHY
LENGUAS
LENIENT
LENNONS
LENOVOS
LENSCAP
LENSMAN
LENSMEN
LENTIGO
LENTILS
LEOGENN
LEONARD
LEONATO
LEONDAY
LEONIDS
LEONINE
LEONORA
LEONORE
LEOPARD
LEOPOLD
LEOTARD
LEOVIII
LEOXIII
LEPANTO
LEPIDUS
LEPPARD
LEPTONS
LESABRE
LESCAUT
LESIONS
LESOTHO
LESPAUL
LESSEES

LESSENS
LESSEPS
LESSFAT
LESSING
LESSONS
LESSORS
LESSTAR
LESTOIL
LETDOWN
LETDROP
LETEMIN
LETFALL
LETGOBY
LETGOOF
LETHAVE
LETHEAN
LETINON
LETITBE
LETITGO
LETITIA
LETKNOW
LETLIVE
LETMEBE
LETMEGO
LETMEIN
LETPASS
LETRIDE
LETROLL
LETSEAT
LETSFLY
LETSLIP
LETSNOT
LETSOFF
LETSOUT
LETSRIP
LETSSEE
LETSUSE
LETTERA
LETTERB
LETTERC
LETTERD
LETTERE
LETTERF
LETTERG
LETTERH
LETTERI
LETTERJ
LETTERK
LETTERL
LETTERM
LETTERN
LETTERO
LETTERP
LETTERQ
LETTERR
LETTERS
LETTERT
LETTERU
LETTERV
LETTERW
LETTERX
LETTERY
LETTERZ
LETTING
LETTISH
LETTRES
LETTUCE
LETUPON
LEUCINE
LEVADES
LEVATOR
LEVELED
LEVELER
LEVELLY
LEVERED
LEVERET
LEVIERS
LEVILLI
LEVITES
LEVITIC
LEVYING
LEWDEST
LEWHOAD
LEXICAL
LEXICON
LEXISES
LEXMARK
LEXUSES
LEXUSGS
LEXUSGX
LEXUSIS
LEXUSLS
LEXUSLX
LEXUSRX
LEXUSSC

L•E••••

LAEMMLE
LAENNEC
LAERTES
LEECHED
LEECHEE
LEECHES
LEEFORD
LEERERS
LEERIER
LEERILY
LEERING
LEERSAT
LEETIDE
LEEWARD
LEEWAYS
LIEABED
LIEATOP
LIEBACK
LIEDFOR
LIEDOWN
LIEFEST
LIENEES
LIENORS
LIEOVER
LIESFOR
LIESLOW
LIETEST
LLEYTON
LOESSER
LOESSES
LYESOAP

L••E•••

LABELED
LABELER
LABELLE
LACEDUP
LACERTA
LACESON
LACESUP
LACEUPS
LAFEMME
LAKEBED
LAMENTS
LANEONE
LANETWO
LAPELED
LAPERMS
LAREDOS
LATEENS
LATEFEE
LATENCY
LATENED
LATENTS
LATERAL
LATERAN
LATERON
LATETAG
LATEXES
LAVELLI
LAVERAN
LAVERNE
LAYERED
LAYETTE
LAZENBY
LEDERER
LEGENDS
LEJEUNE
LETEMIN
LEVELED
LEVELER
LEVELLY
LEVERED
LEVERET
LIBELED
LIBELEE
LIBELER
LIBERAL
LIBERIA
LIBERTE
LIBERTY
LICENCE
LICENSE
LIFEFUL
LIFENET
LIKEICE
LIKEMAD
LIKENED
LIKENEW
LIKENTO
LIKEWOW
LILETEE
LIMEADE
LIMEPIE
LINEAGE
LINEARA
LINEARB
LINEATE
LINECUT
LINEDRY
LINEDUP
LINEMAN
LINEMEN
LINEONE
LINEOUT
LINESUP
LINETWO
LINEUPS
LISENTE
LITERAL
LIVEAID
LIVEDIN
LIVEDON
LIVEFOR
LIVENED
LIVENER
LIVENUP
LIVEOAK
LIVEONE
LIVEOUT
LIVERED
LIVESAT
LIVESET
LIVESEY
LIVESIN
LIVESON
LIZETTE
LONETTE
LORELAI
LORELEI
LORENTZ
LORENZO
LORETTA
LOSEBIG
LOSEOUT
LOSESIT
LOSESTO
LOUELLA
LOVEBUG
LOVEDIT
LOVEDTO
LOVEINS
LOVEJOY
LOVERLY
LOVESET
LOVESIT
LOVESTO
LOVETAP
LOVEYOU
LOWEEZY
LOWERED
LOZENGE
LUBEJOB
LUCENCY
LUCERNE
LUCETTA
LUNESTA
LUNETTE
LUREDIN
LURESIN
LUREXES
LUTETIA
LYCEUMS
LYNETTE
LYSENKO

L•••E••

LABFEES
LABTECH
LABTEST
LACIEST
LACKEYS
LACTEAL
LADDERS
LADLERS
LAFLEUR
LAGGERS
LAKIEST
LAMBEAU
LAMBENT
LAMBERT
LAMBETH
LAMPERT
LANCERS
LANCETS
LANDERS
LANKEST
LANTERN
LAPBELT
LAPPERS
LAPPETS
LAPSERS
LARCENY
LARDERS
LARGELY
LARGENT
LARGEOJ
LARGESS
LARGEST
LARKERS
LASHERS
LATEENS
LATHERS
LATHERY
LATRELL
LAUDERS
LAURELS
LAURENT
LAWLESS
LAWYERS
LAXNESS
LAZIEST
LAZZERI
LEADENS
LEADERS
LEADETH
LEAKERS
LEAKEYS
LEANERS
LEANEST
LEAPERS
LEASERS
LEASETO
LEAVEBE
LEAVEIN
LEAVEIT
LEAVENS
LEAVEON
LECHERS
LECTERN
LEDGERS
LEERERS
LEFREAK
LEFTEAR
LEFTEND
LEFTEST
LEFTEYE
LEGLESS
LEGREST
LEGWEAR
LEMIEUX
LENDERS
LENIENT
LEOGENN
LESSEES
LESSENS
LESSEPS
LETHEAN
LETMEBE
LETMEGO
LETMEIN
LETSEAT
LETTERA
LETTERB
LETTERC
LETTERD
LETTERE
LETTERF
LETTERG
LETTERH
LETTERI
LETTERJ
LETTERK
LETTERL
LETTERM
LETTERN
LETTERO
LETTERP
LETTERQ
LETTERR
LETTERS
LETTERT
LETTERU
LETTERV
LETTERW
LETTERX
LETTERY
LETTERZ
LEVIERS
LEWDEST
LIBBERS
LICHEES
LICHENS
LICKERS
LICKETY
LIDLESS
LIEFEST
LIENEES
LIETEST
LIFTERS
LIGGETT
LIMBERS
LIMIEST
LIMNERS
LIMPEST
LIMPETS
LINDENS
LINGERS
LINIEST
LINKERS
LINNETS
LINSEED
LINTELS
LINTERS
LIONELL
LIONELS
LIONESS
LIONETS
LIPLESS
LIPPERS
LIPREAD
LIQUEFY
LIQUEUR
LISBETH
LISPERS
LISTEES
LISTENS
LISTERS
LITHELY
LITHEST
LITTERS
LITTERY
LLANERO
LOADERS
LOAFERS
LOANERS
LOBBERS
LOCKEAN
LOCKERS
LOCKETS
LODGEIN
LODGERS
LOFTERS
LOGGERS
LOGIEST
LOITERS
LOLLERS
LONGEST
LOOKERS
LOOPERS
LOOSELY
LOOSENS
LOOSEST
LOOTERS
LOPPERS
LORIENT
LOTTERS
LOTTERY
LOUDENS
LOUDEST
LOUREED
LOUSEUP
LOUVERS
LOWBEAM
LOWEEZY
LOWGEAR
LOWHEEL
LOWNECK
LOWNESS
LOWRENT
LOWTECH
LUBBERS
LUGGERS
LULLERS
LUMBERS
LUMIERE
LUMPERS
LUNGEAT
LUNGERS
LUNKERS
LURKERS
LURLEEN
LUSHEST
LUSTERS
LYOCELL
LYONELL

L••••E•

LABELED
LABELER
LABFEES
LABORED
LABORER
LACQUER
LACUREE
LADDIES
LAENNEC
LAERTES
LAISSEZ
LAITIES
LAKEBED
LALAKER
LAMPREY
LANDLER
LANDMEN
LANGLEY
LANKIER
LAPELED
LARCHEN
LARCHES
LARDIER
LARDNER
LARKIER
LASSIES
LASSOED
LASSOER
LASSOES
LASTLEG
LATCHED
LATCHES
LATEFEE
LATENED
LATEXES
LATICES
LATIMES
LAUGHED
LAUGHER
LAUNDER
LAUTREC
LAVAGES
LAYERED
LAYOPEN
LAYOVER
LEACHED
LEACHER
LEACHES
LEADIER
LEADMEN
LEAFIER
LEAFLET
LEAGUED
LEAGUER
LEAGUES
LEAKIER
LEANDER
LEARJET
LEARNED
LEARNER
LEASHED
LEASHES
LEATHER
LEDERER
LEDGIER
LEECHED
LEECHEE
LEECHES
LEERIER
LEFTIES
LEFTLEG
LEGATEE
LEGATES
LEGGIER
LEGOSET
LEGUMES
LEISTER
LENSMEN
LESSEES
LETSSEE
LETTRES
LEVADES
LEVELED
LEVELER
LEVERED
LEVERET
LEVITES
LEXISES
LEXUSES
LIAISED
LIAISES
LIBELED
LIBELEE
LIBELER
LICHEES
LIEABED
LIENEES
LIEOVER
LIFENET
LIGATED
LIGATES
LIGHTED
LIGHTEN
LIGHTER
LIKENED
LIKENEW
LILALEE
LILETEE
LIMITED
LIMITER
LIMOGES
LINAGES
LINDIED
LINDIES
LINDNER
LINDSEY
LINEMEN
LINGOES
LINSEED
LINTIER
LIPASES
LIPPIER
LISTEES
LITOTES
LITTLER
LITTLES
LIVENED
LIVENER
LIVERED
LIVESET
LIVESEY
LIZZIES
LOAMIER
LOATHED
LOATHER
LOATHES
LOBATED
LOBBIED
LOBBIES
LOBBYER
LOBSTER
LOBULES
LOCALES
LOCATED
LOCATER
LOCATES
LOCKLET
LOCKSET
LOESSER
LOESSES
LOFTBED
LOFTIER
LOLLIES
LONDRES
LONGBED
LONGDEN
LONGIES
LONGUES
LOOBIES
LOOKSEE
LOONIER
LOONIES
LOOPIER
LOPPIER
LORELEI
LORISES
LORRIES
LORUSES
LOSTPET
LOTUSES
LOUNGED
LOUNGER
LOUNGES
LOURDES
LOUREED
LOUSIER
LOUVRED
LOUVRES
LOVAGES
LOVESET
LOWBRED
LOWCHEN
LOWERED
LOWHEEL
LOWLIER
LOYALER
LOYALES
LSHAPED
LUCIFER
LUCITES
LUCKIER
LUMPIER
LUNATED
LUNATES
LUNCHED
LUNCHER
LUNCHES
LUPINES
LURCHED
LURCHER
LURCHES
LUREXES
LURLEEN
LUSHIER
LUSTIER
LUSTRED
LUSTRES
LUTHIER
LUXATED
LUXATES

L•••••E

LABELLE
LABIATE
LABMICE
LABTUBE
LACOSTE
LACTASE
LACTATE
LACTOSE
LACUNAE
LACUREE
LADOUCE
LADRONE
LAEMMLE
LAFARGE
LAFEMME
LAFITTE
LAGASSE
LAICIZE
LALANNE
LALIQUE
LAMINAE
LAMOTTE
LANCOME
LANEONE
LANOTTE
LAPLACE
LAPORTE
LAPROBE
LAPWARE
LARAINE
LARAMIE
LAROCHE
LASAGNE
LASALLE
LASTONE
LATEFEE
LATRINE
LATROBE
LATTICE
LAVACHE
LAVAINE
LAVALSE
LAVERNE
LAWCASE
LAWLIKE
LAYBARE
LAYETTE
LEADORE
LEAFAGE
LEAKAGE
LEAVEBE
LECARRE
LECONTE
LECTURE
LEECHEE
LEETIDE
LEFTEYE
LEGATEE
LEGBONE
LEGIBLE
LEGLIKE
LEGROPE
LEHAVRE
LEISURE
LEJEUNE
LEMONDE
LEMOYNE
LEONINE
LEONORE
LESABRE
LETHAVE
LETITBE
LETLIVE
LETMEBE
LETRIDE
LETSSEE
LETSUSE
LETTERE
LETTUCE
LEUCINE
LIBELEE
LIBERTE
LICENCE
LICENSE
LIGNITE
LIKABLE
LIKEICE
LILALEE
LILETEE
LIMEADE
LIMEPIE
LIMNITE
LINABLE
LINEAGE
LINEATE
LINEONE
LINGUAE
LINKAGE
LIONISE
LIONIZE
LIPLIKE
LIQUATE
LISENTE
LISSOME
LIVABLE
LIVEONE
LIZETTE
LOCKAGE
LONETTE
LOOKSEE
LORANGE
LOSABLE
LOVABLE
LOWDIVE
LOWLIFE
LOWRISE
LOWSIDE
LOWTIDE
LOZENGE
LUCARNE
LUCERNE
LUCIDAE
LUCILLE
LUDDITE
LUGGAGE
LUMIERE
LUNETTE
LUNULAE
LYDDITE
LYNETTE

•LE••••

ALEARDI
ALEGARS
ALEGRIA
ALEKEGS
ALEKSEI
ALEMBIC
ALENCON
ALERTED
ALERTER
ALERTLY
ALERTTO
ALETAPS
ALETTES
ALEVELS
ALEWIFE
ALEYARD
BLEAKER
BLEAKLY
BLEARED
BLEATED
BLEATER
BLEDSOE
BLEEDER
BLEEPED
BLEEPER
BLEMISH
BLENDED
BLENDER
BLENDES
BLENDIN
BLENTIN
BLERIOT
BLESSED
BLESSER
BLESSES
BLEWOFF
BLEWOUT
CLEANED
CLEANER
CLEANLY
CLEANSE
CLEANTE
CLEANUP
CLEARED
CLEARER
CLEARLY
CLEAROF
CLEARUP
CLEATED
CLEAVED
CLEAVER
CLEAVES
CLEAVON
CLEMENS
CLEMENT
CLEMSON
CLERICS
CLERISY
CLERKED
CLERKLY
CLEWING
ELEANOR
ELEAZAR
ELECTED
ELECTEE

ELECTME
ELECTOR
ELECTRA
ELECTRO
ELEGANT
ELEGIAC
ELEGIES
ELEGIST
ELEGITS
ELEGIZE
ELEISON
ELEKTRA
ELEMENT
ELENIAK
ELEVATE
ELEVENA
ELEVENB
ELEVENC
ELEVEND
ELEVENE
ELEVENS
ELEVONS
FLEABAG
FLEADIP
FLEANCE
FLEAPIT
FLECHES
FLECKED
FLEDGED
FLEDGES
FLEECED
FLEECER
FLEECES
FLEEGLE
FLEEING
FLEERED
FLEETED
FLEETER
FLEETLY
FLEMING
FLEMISH
FLENSED
FLENSER
FLENSES
FLESHED
FLESHES
FLESHLY
FLEURON
FLEXILE
FLEXING
FLEXION
FLEXNER
FLEXORS
FLEXURE
GLEAMED
GLEANED
GLEANER
GLEASON
GLEEFUL
GLEEMAN
GLEEMEN
GLENCOE
KLEENEX
KLEIBER
KLEISER
KLENSCH
KLEPTOS
KLEZMER
LLEYTON
OLEANNA
OLEANNY
OLEATES
OLEBULL
OLEFINS
OLEMISS
OLEOOIL
OLESTRA
OLEVELS
PLEADED
PLEADER
PLEADTO
PLEASED
PLEASER
PLEASES
PLEATED
PLEBIAN
PLECTRA
PLEDGED
PLEDGEE
PLEDGER
PLEDGES
PLENARY
PLENISH
PLENUMS
PLEURAE
PLEURAL
PLEXORS
SLEAZES
SLEDDED
SLEDDER
SLEDDOG
SLEDFUL
SLEDGED
SLEDGES
SLEEKED
SLEEKEN
SLEEKER
SLEEKLY
SLEEPER
SLEEPIN
SLEEPON
SLEETED
SLEEVED
SLEEVES
SLEIGHS
SLEIGHT
SLENDER
SLEPTIN
SLEPTON
SLEUTHS
SLEWING

•L•E•••

ALBEDOS
ALBENIZ
ALBERTA
ALBERTI
ALBERTO
ALCESTE
ALDENTE
ALFEROV
ALGEBRA
ALGERIA
ALIENEE
ALIENOR
ALIENTO
ALKENES
ALLEARS
ALLEGED
ALLEGER
ALLEGES
ALLEGRA
ALLEGRO
ALLELES
ALLELIC
ALLELSE
ALLENBY
ALLENDE
ALLERGY
ALLEWIS
ALLEYES
ALMERIA
ALREADY
ALTERED
ALTERER
ALVEOLI
BLEEDER
BLEEPED
BLEEPER
BLUEBOY
BLUEFIN
BLUEFLU
BLUEFOX
BLUEHEN
BLUEICE
BLUEING
BLUEISH
BLUEJAY
BLUELAW
BLUERED
BLUESKY
BLUESUN
BLUETIT
CLIENTS
CLUEDIN
CLUEFUL
CLUEING
CLUESIN
ELBERTA
ELDERLY
ELIEZER
FLEECED
FLEECER
FLEECES
FLEEGLE
FLEEING
FLEERED
FLEETED
FLEETER
FLEETLY
FLIEDTO
FLIESAT
FLIESBY
FLIESIN
FLIESON
FLIESTO
FLIESUP
FLUENCY
GLEEFUL
GLEEMAN
GLEEMEN
GLUEDON
GLUEDTO
GLUEGUN
GLUESON
GLUESTO
ILIESCU
ILLEANA
ILLEGAL
ILLEGIT
KLEENEX
PLOESTI
SLEEKED
SLEEKEN
SLEEKER
SLEEKLY
SLEEPER
SLEEPIN
SLEEPON
SLEETED
SLEEVED
SLEEVES
SLOEGIN

•L••E••

ALAMEDA
ALAMEIN
ALATEEN
ALCHEMY
ALEKEGS
ALEVELS
ALFIERI
ALFREDA
ALFREDE
ALFREDO
ALFREDU
ALGIEBA
ALGIERS
ALGREEN
ALIMENT
ALINERS
ALIVETO
ALLHEAL
ALLHERE
ALLNESS
ALLNEWS
ALTKEYS
ALUDELS
BLADERS
BLAKELY
BLAMEON
BLAMERS
BLAZERS
BLAZEUP
BLOWERS
CLARETS
CLAVELL
CLAWERS
CLEMENS
CLEMENT
CLONERS
CLORETS
CLOSEBY
CLOSEIN
CLOSELY
CLOSERS
CLOSEST
CLOSETO
CLOSETS
CLOSEUP
CLOVERS
CLOVERY
ELANETS
ELATERS
ELEMENT
ELEVENA
ELEVENB
ELEVENC
ELEVEND
ELEVENE
ELEVENS
ELGRECO
ELIDERS
ELITEST
ELMIEST
ELOPERS
ELUDERS
ELYSEES
FLAKERS
FLAMERS
FLAMEUP
FLANEUR
FLAREUP
FLAYERS
FLOREAL
FLORENZ
FLORETS
FLOWERS
FLOWERY
FLUTERS
FLYLEAF
FLYLESS
FLYNETS
GLACEED
GLADEYE
GLAREAT
GLAZERS
GLIDEBY
GLIDEIN
GLIDERS
GLOWERS
GLUIEST
GLUTEAL
GLUTENS
GLUTEUS
ILIKEIT
ILLNESS
ILLTELL
ILOVEIT
ILOVELA
LLANERO
OLDBEAN
OLDNESS
OLDNEWS
OLDWEST
OLEVELS
PLACEBO
PLACERS
PLANERS
PLANETS
PLATEAU
PLATENS
PLATERS
PLAYERS
PLOVERS
PLOWERS
SLAKERS
SLATERS
SLAVERS
SLAVERY
SLAYERS
SLICERS
SLICEUP
SLIDEBY
SLIDEIN
SLIDERS
SLIVERS
SLOPERS
SLOVENE
SLOVENS
SLOWEST
SLYNESS
ULSTERS

•L•••E•

ALARMED
ALARMER
ALATEEN
ALBIREO
ALBUMEN
ALCOVES
ALEKSEI
ALERTED
ALERTER
ALETTES
ALGREEN
ALIASES
ALIBIED
ALIENEE
ALIGNED
ALIGNER
ALKENES
ALLAGES
ALLAYED
ALLAYER
ALLEGED
ALLEGER
ALLEGES
ALLELES
ALLEYES
ALLOPEZ
ALLOVER
ALLOWED
ALLOYED
ALLTIED
ALLUDED
ALLUDES
ALLURED
ALLURER
ALLURES
ALMADEN
ALMONER
ALMSMEN
ALPINER
ALPINES
ALROKER
ALROSEN
ALTERED
ALTERER
ALUNSER
ALVAREZ
BLABBED
BLABBER
BLACKED
BLACKEN
BLACKER
BLADDER
BLAKLEY
BLANDER
BLANKED
BLANKER
BLANKET
BLARNEY
BLASTED
BLASTER
BLATHER
BLATTED
BLEAKER
BLEARED
BLEATED
BLEATER
BLEEDER
BLEEPED
BLEEPER
BLENDED
BLENDER
BLENDES
BLESSED
BLESSER
BLESSES
BLINDED
BLINDER
BLINKED
BLINKER
BLIPPED
BLISSED
BLISSES
BLISTER
BLITHER
BLITZED
BLITZEN
BLITZER
BLITZES
BLOATED
BLOBBED
BLOCKED
BLOCKER
BLOGGED
BLOGGER
BLONDER
BLONDES
BLOODED
BLOOMED
BLOOMER
BLOOPED
BLOOPER
BLOTTED
BLOTTER
BLOUSED
BLOUSES
BLOWIER
BLOWZED
BLUBBER
BLUDGED
BLUDGER
BLUDGES
BLUEHEN
BLUERED
BLUFFED
BLUFFER
BLUNDEN
BLUNDER
BLUNTED
BLUNTER
BLURBER
BLURRED
BLURTED
BLURTER
BLUSHED
BLUSHER
BLUSHES
BLUSTER
BLYNKEN
CLABBER
CLACKED
CLACKER
CLADDED
CLAIMED
CLAIMER
CLAMBER
CLAMMED
CLAMMER
CLAMPED
CLAMPER
CLANGED
CLANGER
CLANKED
CLAPPED
CLAPPER
CLAQUES
CLASHED
CLASHER
CLASHES
CLASPED
CLASPER
CLASSED
CLASSER
CLASSES
CLATTER
CLAUDEL
CLAUSES
CLAVIER
CLAYIER
CLEANED
CLEANER
CLEARED
CLEARER
CLEATED
CLEAVED
CLEAVER
CLEAVES
CLERKED
CLICHED
CLICHES
CLICKED
CLICKER
CLIMBED
CLIMBER
CLINGER
CLINKED
CLINKER
CLIPPED
CLIPPER
CLIQUED
CLIQUES
CLIQUEY
CLOAKED
CLOBBER
CLOCHES
CLOCKED
CLOCKER
CLOGGED
CLOMPED
CLONKED
CLOONEY
CLOPPED
CLOTHED
CLOTHES
CLOTTED
CLOUDED
CLOUTED
CLOUTER
CLOWDER
CLOWNED
CLUBBED
CLUBBER
CLUBMED
CLUCKED
CLUCKER
CLUMPED
CLUNKED
CLUNKER
CLUSTER
CLUTTER
ELAINES
ELANCES
ELAPSED
ELAPSES
ELBOWED
ELBOWER
ELECTED
ELECTEE
ELEGIES
ELIEZER
ELMTREE
ELUATES
ELYSEES
FLACKED
FLAGGED
FLAGGER
FLAGMEN
FLAILED
FLAKIER
FLAMBED
FLAMBES
FLAMIER
FLAMMED
FLANGES
FLANKED
FLANKEN
FLANKER
FLANNEL
FLAPPED
FLAPPER
FLASHED
FLASHER
FLASHES
FLATBED
FLATLET
FLATTED
FLATTEN
FLATTER
FLAWIER
FLAXIER
FLECHES
FLECKED
FLEDGED
FLEDGES
FLEECED
FLEECER
FLEECES
FLEERED
FLEETED
FLEETER
FLENSED
FLENSER
FLENSES
FLESHED
FLESHES
FLEXNER
FLICKED
FLICKER
FLINGER
FLIPPED
FLIPPEN
FLIPPER
FLIRTED
FLIRTER
FLITTED
FLITTER
FLIVVER
FLOATED
FLOATER
FLOCKED
FLOGGED
FLOGGER
FLOODED
FLOORED
FLOORER
FLOPPED
FLOPPER
FLOSSED
FLOSSER
FLOSSES
FLOURED
FLOUTED
FLOUTER
FLUBBED
FLUBBER
FLUFFED
FLUFFER
FLUKIER
FLUNKED
FLUNKER
FLUSHED
FLUSHER
FLUSHES
FLUSTER
FLUTIER
FLUTIES
FLUTTER
FLYOPEN
FLYOVER
FLYTIER
GLACEED
GLACIER
GLADDEN
GLADDER
GLANCED
GLANCES
GLASSED
GLASSES
GLAZIER
GLEAMED
GLEANED
GLEANER
GLEEMEN
GLIBBER
GLIMMER
GLINTED
GLISTEN
GLISTER
GLITTER
GLITZED
GLITZES
GLOATED
GLOATER
GLOMMED
GLOOMED
GLORIED
GLORIES
GLOSSED
GLOSSER
GLOSSES
GLUGGED
GLUMMED
GLUMMER
GLURGES
GLUTTED
ILLBRED
ILLUDED
ILLUDES
ILLUMED
ILLUMES
ILLUSED
ILLUSES
KLAMMER
KLEENEX
KLEIBER
KLEISER
KLEZMER
KLINGER
KLINKER
KLISTER
KLUDGED
KLUDGES
KLUTZES
OLDSTER
OLEATES
OLIVIER
OLMSTED
OLOGIES
PLACKET
PLAGUED
PLAGUES
PLAICES
PLAINER
PLAINES
PLAITED
PLAITER
PLANKED
PLANNED
PLANNER
PLANTED
PLANTER
PLAQUES
PLASHED
PLASHES
PLASTER
PLATIER
PLATIES
PLATTED
PLATTER
PLAYLET
PLAYPEN
PLAYTEX
PLEADED
PLEADER
PLEASED
PLEASER
PLEASES
PLEATED
PLEDGED
PLEDGEE
PLEDGER
PLEDGES
PLINKED
PLISSES
PLODDED
PLODDER
PLONKED
PLOPPED
PLOTTED
PLOTTER
PLOTZED
PLOTZES
PLOWMEN
PLUCKED
PLUGGED
PLUGGER
PLUMBED
PLUMBER
PLUMIER
PLUMMER
PLUMMET
PLUMPED
PLUMPER
PLUNDER
PLUNGED
PLUNGER
PLUNGES
PLUNKED
PLUNKER
PLUSHER
PLUSHES
PLUSSES
SLABBED
SLACKED
SLACKEN
SLACKER
SLAMMED
SLAMMER
SLANDER
SLANTED
SLAPPED
SLAPPER
SLASHED
SLASHER
SLASHES
SLATHER
SLATIER
SLATTED
SLEAZES
SLEDDED
SLEDDER
SLEDGED
SLEDGES
SLEEKED
SLEEKEN
SLEEKER
SLEEPER
SLEETED
SLEEVED
SLEEVES
SLENDER
SLICKED
SLICKER
SLIMIER
SLIMMED
SLIMMER
SLINGER
SLINKED
SLINKER
SLIPPED
SLIPPER
SLITHER
SLITTED
SLITTER
SLOBBER
SLOGGED
SLOGGER
SLOPPED
SLOSHED
SLOSHES
SLOTTED
SLOTTER
SLUDGES
SLUGGED
SLUGGER
SLUICED
SLUICES
SLUMBER
SLUMMED
SLUMMER
SLUMPED
SLURPED
SLURPEE
SLURPER
SLURRED
SLUSHED
SLUSHES
ULLAGES
ULYSSES

•L••••E

ALADINE
ALAMODE
ALANINE
ALBSURE
ALCAIDE
ALCALDE
ALCESTE
ALCYONE
ALDENTE
ALEWIFE
ALFONSE
ALFREDE
ALGARVE
ALIDADE
ALIENEE
ALIGOTE
ALITTLE
ALLANTE
ALLDONE
ALLELSE
ALLENDE
ALLGONE
ALLHERE
ALLMALE
ALLMINE
ALLOFME
ALLONGE
ALLOWME
ALLRISE

ALLTIME
ALLWISE
ALOHAOE
ALUMNAE
BLACKIE
BLANCHE
BLEDSOE
BLIMPIE
BLINTZE
BLONDIE
BLUEICE
CLARICE
CLAVATE
CLEANSE
CLEANTE
CLIMATE
CLOSURE
CLOTURE
ELAMITE
ELECTEE
ELECTME
ELEGIZE
ELEVATE
ELEVENE
ELFLIKE
ELFUDGE
ELIYALE
ELLAMAE
ELLIPSE
ELMONTE
ELMTREE
ELNORTE
ELOCUTE
ELUSIVE
FLEANCE
FLEEGLE
FLEXILE
FLEXURE
FLOSSIE
FLOTAGE
FLOUNCE
FLOWAGE
FLYABLE
GLADEYE
GLAVINE
GLENCOE
GLIMPSE
GLOBATE
GLOBOSE
GLOBULE
GLORYBE
GLOSSAE
GLUCOSE
GLYCINE
ILLBITE
ILLDONE
ILLLIVE
ILLMADE
OLDBLUE
OLDJOKE
OLDLINE
OLDLYME
OLDROSE
OLDSHOE
OLDTIME
OLIVINE
PLACATE
PLANATE
PLEDGEE
PLEURAE
PLIABLE
PLICATE
PLOSIVE
PLUMAGE
PLUMOSE
PLUMPIE
PLUMULE
PLUSONE
RLSTINE
SLOVENE
SLURPEE
ULALUME
ULANUDE
ULULATE

••LE•••

AILERON
ALLEARS
ALLEGED
ALLEGER
ALLEGES
ALLEGRA
ALLEGRO
ALLELES
ALLELIC
ALLELSE
ALLENBY
ALLENDE
ALLERGY
ALLEWIS
ALLEYES
APLENTY
ARLEDGE
ASLEWOF
ATLEAST
AULETTA
BALEENS
BALEFUL
BELEVEN
BILEVEL
BOLEROS
CALENDS
CELEBES
CELEBRE
CELESTA
CELESTE
CILENTO
COLEMAN
COLETTE
CSLEWIS
CULEXES
DALETHS
DELEADS
DELEDDA
DELEING
DELETED
DELETES
DILEMMA
DOLEFUL
DOLEOUT
FILEDBY
FILEDIN
FILENES
FILEOUT
FILESBY
FILESIN
FOLENGO
GALEATE
GALENAS
GALENTO
GALETTE
HOLEDUP
HOLEOUT
HOLESUP
IDLESSE
ILLEANA
ILLEGAL
ILLEGIT
IPLEDGE
ISLETED
LILETEE
MALEANT
MALEBEE
MALECAT
MALEDOG
MALEFIC
MALEHOG
MALEPIG
MILEAGE
MILERUN
MOLERAT
MOLESTS
MULETAS
NILESOH
ONLEASE
ONLEASH
ONLEAVE
ORLEANS
OWLEGGS
OWLEYED
PALEALE
PALEDRY
PALEMON
PALERMO
PALETTE
PHLEGMY
PILEATE
PILEDIN
PILEDON
PILEDUP
PILEGGI
PILEOUS
PILESIN
PILESOF
PILESON
PILESUP
PILEUPS
POLEAXE
POLECAR
POLECAT
POLEMAN
POLEMEN
POLEMIC
POLENTA
POLESAT
POLESIT
RALEIGH
RELEADS
RELEAPS
RELEARN
RELEASE
RELENDS
RELENTS
RELEVEL
RELEVER
RELEVES
RILEDUP
RILESUP
ROLEXES
RULEDBY
RULEDON
RULEONE
RULEOUT
RULESON
SALEMOR
SALERNO
SCLERAE
SCLERAL
SCLERAS
SELECTS
SELENIC
SILENCE
SILENTA
SILENTB
SILENTC
SILENTD
SILENTE
SILENTF
SILENTG
SILENTH
SILENTI
SILENTJ
SILENTK
SILENTL
SILENTM
SILENTN
SILENTO
SILENTP
SILENTQ
SILENTR
SILENTS
SILENTT
SILENTU
SILENTV
SILENTW
SILENTX
SILENTY
SILENTZ
SILESIA
SOLEDAD
SPLEENS
SPLEENY
SPLENDA
TALENTS
TELECOM
TELEFAX
TELEPIC
TELEPIX
TELERAN
TELESTO
TELEXED
TELEXES
TOLEASE
TOLEDAN
TOLEDOS
TYLENOL
UNLEADS
UNLEAFS
UNLEAKY
UNLEARN
UNLEASH
UNLEGAL
UNLEVEL
UPLEAPS
UPLEAPT
VALENCE
VALENTE
VALENTI
VALERIE
VALETED
VOLENTE
YALELAW
YALEMAN
YALEMEN
YULELOG

••L•E••

AILMENT
ALLHEAL
ALLHERE
ALLNESS
ALLNEWS
ARLBERG
BALDEST
BALEENS
BALKERS
BALLETS
BELIEFS
BELIERS
BELIEVE
BELLEAU
BELLEEK
BELTERS
BILKERS
BILLERS
BILLETS
BOLDEST
BOLTERS
BULLETS
CALDERA
CALDERS
CALKERS
CALLEES
CALLERS
CALMEST
CALTECH
CALVERT
CELAENO
COLBERT
COLDEST
COLLECT
COLLEEN
COLLEGE
COLLETS
CULLERS
CULLETS
CULVERT
DELBERT
DELKEYS
DELVERS
DILBERT
DILUENT
DULLEST
EELIEST
FALLERS
FALSELY
FALSEST
FALTERS
FALWELL
FELLERS
FILBERT
FILLERS
FILLETS
FILTERS
FOLDERS
FOLGERS
FOLLETT
FULGENT
FULLEST
FULNESS
GALLEON
GALLERY
GALLEYS
GELPENS
GILBERT
GILDERS
GOLFERS
GULDENS
GULLETS
GULPERS
HALLEYS
HALTERS
HALVERS
HELLENE
HELLENO
HELMETS
HELPERS
HILBERT
HOLBEIN
HOLBERG
HOLDERS
HOLIEST
HOLLERS
HULLERS
ILLNESS
ILLTELL
JILTERS
JOLTERS
KILLEEN
KILLERS
LOLLERS
LULLERS
MALLETS
MALLEUS
MALTEDS
MALTESE
MELDERS
MELTERS
MILDEST
MILDEWS
MILDEWY
MILIEUS
MILIEUX
MILKERS
MILLEND
MILLERS
MILLETS
MILLETT
MOLDERS
MOLIERE
MOLTERS
MULLERS
MULLETS
NFLTEAM
NHLTEAM
OILHEAT
OILIEST
OILLESS
OILSEED
OILWELL
ONLIEST
OWLIEST
PALLETS
PALMERS
PALTERS
PELLEAS
PELLETS
PELTERS
PHLOEMS
PILFERS
POLLEES
POLLENS
POLLERA
POLLERS
PULLERS
PULLETS
PULLEYS
PULPERS
RELIEFS
RELIERS
RELIEVE
RELLENO
RILIEVO
RILLETS
ROLFERS
ROLLEIS
ROLLERS
RULIEST
SALIENT
SALIERI
SALTERS
SALVERS
SELLECK
SELLERS
SILVERS
SILVERY
SOLDERS
SOLFEGE
SOLNESS
SOLVEIT
SOLVENT
SOLVERS
SPLEENS
SPLEENY
SULKERS
TALKERS
TALLEST
TELLERS
TILLERS
TILLETS
TILTERS
TOLLERS
TOLTECS
TOLUENE
UGLIEST
VALJEAN
VALLEJO
VALLEYS
VALUERS
VELVETS
VELVETY
VILLEIN
VOLLEYS
WALKERS
WALLETS
WALLEYE
WALTERS
WELDERS
WELTERS
WILBERT
WILDEST
WILHELM
WILIEST
WILKENS
WILLERS
YELLERS
YELPERS

••L••E•

ABLATED
ABLATES
ALLAGES
ALLAYED
ALLAYER
ALLEGED
ALLEGER
ALLEGES
ALLELES
ALLEYES
ALLOPEZ
ALLOVER
ALLOWED
ALLOYED
ALLTIED
ALLUDED
ALLUDES
ALLURED
ALLURER
ALLURES
APLITES
APLUSES
ATLASES
BALASES
BALDIES
BALKIER
BALLMER
BALLUET
BALMIER
BALONEY
BELATED
BELAYED
BELAYER
BELCHED
BELCHER
BELCHES
BELEVEN
BELLEEK
BELLIED
BELLIES
BELLMEN
BELOVED
BILEVEL
BILGIER
BILLIES
BILOBED
BOLIDES
BOLSTER
BOLUSES
BPLUSES
BULBLET
BULGIER
BULKIER
BULLIED
BULLIES
BULLPEN
BYLINED
BYLINER
BYLINES
CALIBER
CALICES
CALIPER
CALLEES
CALMSEA
CALUMET
CALYCES
CALYXES
CELEBES
CELOTEX
COLLEEN
COLLIER
COLLIES
COLLYER
COLONEL
COLONES
COLORED
COLORER
CPLUSES
CULCHES
CULEXES
CULLIED
CULLIES
DALLIED
DALLIER
DALLIES
DALTREY
DELANEY
DELAYED
DELAYER
DELETED
DELETES
DELIBES
DELIMEN
DELIVER
DELUDED
DELUDER
DELUDES
DELUGED
DELUGES
DILATED
DILATES
DILLIES
DILUTED
DILUTER
DILUTES
DOLLIED
DOLLIES
DOLORES
DPLUSES
EGLISES
ENLACED
ENLACES
ENLIVEN
FALAFEL
FELINES
FELTPEN
FILCHED
FILCHER
FILCHES
FILENES
FILIBEG
FILLIES
FILMIER
FILMSET
FOLATES
FOLIOED
FOLKIER
FOLKIES
FOLLIES
GALATEA
GALAXES
GALILEE
GALILEI
GALILEO
GALOPED
GELATED
GELATES
GILLNET
GOLFTEE
GULCHES
GULLIED
GULLIES
GULPIER
HALFFED
HALFIES
HALIDES
HALITES
HALOGEN
HELICES
HELIXES
HELLOED
HELLOES
HELLYES
HILLIER
HILLMEN
HOLLIES
HOLSTER
HOLYMEN
HOLYSEE
HULKIER
HULLOED
ILLBRED
ILLUDED
ILLUDES
ILLUMED
ILLUMES
ILLUSED
ILLUSES
INLAYER
INLINES
ISLETED
JELLIED
JELLIES
JOLLIED
JOLLIER
JOLLIES
JOLLIET
JOLTIER
KELPIES
KILAUEA
KILLEEN
KILLFEE
KILTIES
LALAKER
LILALEE
LILETEE
LOLLIES
MALEBEE
MALICES
MALMSEY
MALTIER
MELAMED
MILDRED
MILKFED
MILKIER
MILKMEN
MOLDIER
MOLLIES
MULCHED
MULCHES
MULCTED
MULGREW
NULLSET
OBLATES
OBLIGED
OBLIGEE
OBLIGER
OBLIGES
OILSEED
OOLITES
OWLEYED
PALACES
PALATES
PALAVER
PALFREY
PALJOEY
PALLIER
PALMIER
PELAGES
PHLOXES
PILATES
PILOTED
PILSNER
POLANER
POLEMEN
POLICED
POLICER
POLICES
POLITER
POLKAED
POLLEES
POLYMER
POLYPED
PULPIER
RALLIED
RALLIER
RALLIES
RALLYES
RELABEL
RELACED
RELACES
RELANES
RELATED
RELATER
RELATES
RELAXED
RELAXER
RELAXES
RELAYED
RELAYER
RELEVEL
RELEVER
RELEVES
RELINED
RELINES
RELIVED
RELIVES
RELOSES
RELUMED
RELUMES
ROLEXES
ROLODEX
SALADES
SALINES
SALLIED
SALLIER
SALLIES
SALTIER
SALTSEA
SALUTED
SALUTER
SALUTES
SALVOES
SELTZER
SILKIER
SILLIER
SILLIES
SILTIER
SOLACED
SOLACER
SOLACES
SOLDIER
SOLIDER
SOLUTES
SPLAYED
SPLICED
SPLICER
SPLICES
SPLINES
STLUKES
SULKIER
SULKIES
SULLIED
SULLIES
SULUSEA
TALCKED
TALKIER
TALKIES
TALLIED
TALLIER
TALLIES
TALONED
TALUSES
TELEXED
TELEXES
TELLIES
TOLKIEN
TOLLMEN
TULANEU
ULLAGES
UNLACED
UNLACES
UNLADED
UNLADEN
UNLADES
UNLAVED
UNLAXED
UNLAXES
UNLEVEL
UNLIKED
UNLIKES
UNLINED
UNLIVED
UNLIVES
UNLOBED
UNLOVED
UNLURED
VALETED
VALINES
VALISES
VALOREM
VELOXES
VELURES
VOLCKER
VOLUMED
VOLUMES
VOLUTED
VOLUTES
WALTHER
WALTZED
WALTZER
WALTZES
WELLFED
WELLLED
WELLSEE
WELLSET
WELLYES
WILDMEN
WILFRED
WILLIES
WOLFMEN
XYLOSES
YALEMEN
ZILCHES

••L•••E

AALARGE
ALLANTE
ALLDONE
ALLELSE
ALLENDE
ALLGONE
ALLHERE
ALLMALE
ALLMINE
ALLOFME
ALLONGE
ALLOWME
ALLRISE
ALLTIME
ALLWISE
ARLEDGE
ATLARGE
AXLROSE
BALANCE
BALLADE
BALLONE
BELDAME
BELIEVE
BELTANE
BILLNYE
BOLATIE
BOLOTIE
CALCITE
CALIBRE
CALORIE
CALOTTE
CALZONE
CELEBRE
CELESTE
CELLULE
CILIATE
COLDONE
COLETTE
COLGATE

COLLAGE
COLLATE
COLLEGE
COLLIDE
COLLINE
COLLUDE
COLOGNE
CULOTTE
CULTURE
DELARUE
DELMORE
DELORME
DELOUSE
DELUISE
ECLIPSE
ECLOGUE
EELLIKE
ELLAMAE
ELLIPSE
ENLARGE
FALCATE
FALLDUE
FELLDUE
FOLIAGE
FOLIATE
FOLIOSE
FULSOME
GALAXIE
GALEATE
GALETTE
GALILEE
GILMORE
GOLFTEE
HALDANE
HELLENE
HELOISE
HILAIRE
HOLYJOE
HOLYOKE
HOLYONE
HOLYSEE
IDLESSE
ILLBITE
ILLDONE
ILLLIVE
ILLMADE
INLARGE
IPLEDGE
KILDARE
KILLFEE
LALANNE
LALIQUE
LILALEE
LILETEE
MALAISE
MALDIVE
MALEBEE
MALTASE
MALTBIE
MALTESE
MALTOSE
MALWARE
MELANGE
MELANIE
MELROSE
MELTAGE
MILEAGE
MILLAGE
MILLIME
MOLIERE
MULHARE
NFLGAME
NHLGAME
OBLIGEE
OBLIQUE
OILBASE
OILCAKE
OILLIKE
OILLINE
ONLEASE
ONLEAVE
OWLLIKE
PALANCE
PALEALE
PALETTE
PALMATE
PALPATE
PELISSE
PELTATE
PILEATE
PILLAGE
POLEAXE
POLLUTE
PULSATE
RALPHIE
RELANCE
RELAPSE
RELEASE
RELIEVE
RULEONE
SALABLE
SALTINE
SALVAGE
SCLERAE
SELVAGE
SILENCE
SILENTE
SILKTIE
SILLYME
SOLFEGE
SOLUBLE
SPLURGE
SULFATE
SULFIDE
SULFITE
TALLONE
TILLAGE
TOLEASE
TOLLAGE
TOLUENE
UNLARGE
UNLOOSE
VALANCE
VALENCE
VALENTE
VALERIE
VALLONE
VALOTTE
VALUATE
VALVATE
VALVULE
VBLOUSE
VELOUTE
VILLAGE
VOLANTE
VOLENTE
VOLPONE
VOLTAGE
VOLTORE
VOLUBLE
VULGATE
VULPINE
VULTURE
WALKURE
WALLACE
WALLEYE
WALPOLE
WELCOME
WELFARE
WELLSEE
WILDONE
WILLKIE

•••LE••

ABILENE
AFFLECK
AGELESS
AGILELY
AGILEST
AIDLESS
AIGLETS
AIMLESS
AIRLESS
AMBLERS
AMPLEST
AMULETS
ANGLERS
ANKLERS
ANKLETS
ANTLERS
APELETS
APILEOF
APPLETS
ARMLESS
ARMLETS
ARTLESS
ASHLESS
ATELESS
ATHLETE
AUKLETS
AUSLESE
AWELESS
AWNLESS
AZALEAS
AZULEJO
BAILEES
BAILERS
BALLETS
BARLESS
BARLEYS
BAWLERS
BAYLEAF
BEDLESS
BELLEAU
BELLEEK
BIBLESS
BIGLEAD
BILLERS
BILLETS
BIRLERS
BITLESS
BOILERS
BOOLEAN
BOWLERS
BOWLESS
BRALESS
BUDLESS
BUGLERS
BULLETS
BUMLEGS
BURLERS
BUTLERS
CABLERS
CABLETS
CABLETV
CALLEES
CALLERS
CAPLESS
CAPLETS
CARLENE
CARLESS
CHALETS
CHILEAN
CHOLERA
CHOLERS
COALERS
COBLENZ
COILERS
COLLECT
COLLEEN
COLLEGE
COLLETS
COOLERS
COOLEST
COULEES
COXLESS
CULLERS
CULLETS
CURLERS
CURLEWS
CUTLERS
CUTLERY
CUTLETS
CYCLERS
DARLEEN
DARLENE
DEALERS
DEFLEAS
DEFLECT
DEKLERK
DEPLETE
DEWLESS
DIALECT
DIALEDO
DIALERS
DOGLEGS
DOGLESS
DONLEVY
DUELERS
DULLEST
EAGLETS
EARLESS
EARLETS
EATLESS
ECCLESI
EGGLERS
EGGLESS
EMBLEMS
ENDLEAF
ENDLESS
EUGLENA
EVILEST
EVILEYE
EXILERS
EYELESS
EYELETS
FABLERS
FALLERS
FARLEFT
FATLESS
FEELERS
FEELESS
FELLERS
FIGLEAF
FILLERS
FILLETS
FINLESS
FLYLEAF
FLYLESS
FOELESS
FOGLESS
FOLLETT
FOOLERS
FOOLERY
FOULEST
FOWLERS
FRELENG
FUELERS
FULLEST
FURLERS
FURLESS
GALLEON
GALLERY
GALLEYS
GAOLERS
GAPLESS
GASLEAK
GASLESS
GEMLESS
GIBLETS
GIMLETS
GOBLETS
GODLESS
GULLETS
GUMLESS
GUNLESS
GUTLESS
HAILERS
HALLEYS
HAMLETS
HAPLESS
HARLEYS
HATLESS
HAULERS
HEALERS
HEELERS
HELLENE
HELLENO
HEWLETT
HIALEAH
HIPLESS
HITLESS
HOLLERS
HOTLEAD
HOWLERS
HUELESS
HULLERS
HURLERS
ICELESS
IMPLEAD
INFLECT
INGLESE
INKLESS
INNLESS
IRELESS
JAGLESS
JAILERS
JARLESS
JAWLESS
JAYLENO
JOBLESS
JOYLESS
KAYLENZ
KEGLERS
KEYLESS
KILLEEN
KILLERS
KINLESS
KISLEVS
KOBLENZ
LADLERS
LAFLEUR
LAWLESS
LEGLESS
LIDLESS
LIPLESS
LOLLERS
LULLERS
LURLEEN
MACLEAN
MACLEOD
MAGLEVS
MAILERS
MALLETS
MALLEUS
MANLESS
MARLENE
MATLESS
MAULERS
MEDLEYS
MEWLERS
MIDLEGS
MILLEND
MILLERS
MILLETS
MILLETT
MISLEAD
MOILERS
MOSLEMS
MOTLEYS
MRCLEAN
MULLERS
MULLETS
NAILERS
NAPLESS
NEGLECT
NETLESS
NEWLEAF
NEWLEFT
NIBLETS
NOBLEST
NUCLEAR
NUCLEIC
NUCLEON
NUCLEUS
NUTLETS
OAKLEAF
OARLESS
ODELETS
OILLESS
OMELETS
ONALEAD
ONALERT
OOBLECK
OPULENT
ORBLESS
ORELESS
OSTLERS
OUTLEAD
OUTLEAP
OUTLETS
PALLETS
PARLEYS
PAYLESS
PEELERS
PEGLEGS
PEGLESS
PELLEAS
PELLETS
PHILEAS
PIGLETS
PINLESS
PIOLETS
PIPLESS
POLLEES
POLLENS
POLLERA
POLLERS
POOLERS
POULENC
PTOLEMY
PULLERS
PULLETS
PULLEYS
PUNLESS
RAILERS
RAYLESS
REALEST
RECLEAN
REDLEGS
REELECT
REELERS
REFLECT
RELLENO
REPLEAD
REPLETE
RIBLESS
RIBLETS
RIFLERS
RIFLERY
RILLETS
RIMLESS
RODLESS
ROLLEIS
ROLLERS
ROULEAU
RUMLESS
RUNLESS
RUNLETS
SAILERS
SAMLETS
SAPLESS
SCALENE
SCALERS
SCALEUP
SCHLEPP
SCHLEPS
SEALEGS
SEALERS
SEALERY
SELLECK
SELLERS
SEXLESS
SINLESS
SKYLESS
SMILEAT
SMILEON
SMILERS
SMILEYS
SODLESS
SONLESS
SOYLENT
STALELY
STALEST
STOLEIN
STYLERS
STYLETS
SUBLETS
SUMLESS
SUNLESS
TABLEAU
TABLETS
TAILEND
TAILERS
TALLEST
TAXLESS
TAXLEVY
TEALEAF
TEALESS
TELLERS
THALERS
THELEFT
TIELESS
TILLERS
TILLETS
TIPLESS
TOELESS
TOILERS
TOILETS
TOLLERS
TOOLERS
TOPLESS
TOYLESS
TUGLESS
UKELELE
UKULELE
UNALERT
UNBLENT
UNBLEST
UNCLEAN
UNCLEAR
UNCLEFT
UNSLEEK
USELESS
VALLEJO
VALLEYS
VARLETS
VEILERS
VILLEIN
VIOLENT
VIOLETS
VOLLEYS
VOWLESS
WAILERS
WALLETS
WALLEYE
WARLESS
WAYLESS
WEBLESS
WHALERS
WIGLESS
WIGLETS
WILLERS
WINLESS
WITLESS
WOOLENS
WOOLERY
YELLERS
YESLETS
YOWLERS

•••L•E•

ADELIES
APPLIED
APPLIER
APPLIES
ARALSEA
ATELIER
AVULSED
AVULSES
BADLIES
BAILEES
BALLMER
BALLUET
BAULKED
BAULKER
BEDLOES
BELLEEK
BELLIED
BELLIES
BELLMEN
BIALIES
BIGLIES
BILLIES
BOULDER
BUELLER
BUILDER
BULLIED
BULLIES
BULLPEN
BURLIER
CALLEES
CAULKED
CAULKER
CHALKED
CHELSEA
CHILIES
CHILLED
CHILLER
COLLEEN
COLLIER
COLLIES
COLLYER
COOLIES
COULEES
COULTER
CRULLER
CULLIED
CULLIES
CURLIER
DAILIES
DALLIED
DALLIER
DALLIES
DARLEEN
DIALLED
DILLIES
DOILIES
DOLLIED
DOLLIES
DOOLIES
DRILLED
DRILLER
DROLLER
DUELLED
DWELLED
DWELLER
EARLIER
EARLIES
EVILLER
EVOLVED
EVOLVER
EVOLVES
EVULSED
EVULSES
EXALTED
EXALTER
EXULTED
FAILLES
FAULTED
FIELDED
FIELDER
FILLIES
FOLLIES
FRILLED
FUELLED
GIBLUES
GILLNET
GIRLIER
GIRLIES
GOALIES
GODLIER
GRILLED
GRILLER
GRILLES
GROLIER
GUILDER
GULLIED
GULLIES
HELLOED
HELLOES
HELLYES
HILLIER
HILLMEN
HOLLIES
HULLOED
IMPLIED
IMPLIES
JELLIED
JELLIES
JOLLIED
JOLLIER
JOLLIES
JOLLIET
JOWLIER
JUILLET
KILLEEN
KILLFEE
KNELLED
KVELLED
LOLLIES
LOWLIER
LURLEEN
MAILMEN
MANLIER
MARLIER
MCALLEN
MEALIER
MEALIES
MOLLIES
MOULDED
MOULDER
MOULTED
MUELLER
NAILKEG
NAILSET
NIELSEN
NULLSET
OKELLEY
OMALLEY
OUTLIER
OUTLIES
PALLIER
PAULSEN
PHILTER
POLLEES
POOLMEN
PSALTER
PURLIEU
QUELLED
QUELLER
QUILLED
QUILLER
QUILTED
QUILTER
RAILMEN
RALLIED
RALLIER
RALLIES
RALLYES
REALMEN
REALTER
REFLIES
REGLUED
REGLUES
REPLIED
REPLIER
REPLIES
ROILIER
RVALUES
SALLIED
SALLIER
SALLIES
SCALDED
SCALDER
SCALIER
SCALPED
SCALPEL
SCALPER
SCOLDED
SCOLDER
SCULLED
SCULLER
SCULPED
SHALIER
SHELLED
SHELLER
SHELLEY
SHELTER
SHELVED
SHELVER
SHELVES
SHILLED
SILLIER
SILLIES
SKELTER
SKILLED
SKILLET
SKULKED
SKULKER
SKULLED
SMALLER
SMELLED
SMELLER
SMELTED
SMELTER
SMOLDER
SNELLEN
SPELLED
SPELLER
SPILLED
SPILLER
STALKED
STALKER
STALLED
STALLER
STILLED
STILLER
STILTED
STOLLEN
SUELLEN
SULLIED
SULLIES
SURLIER
SVELTER
SWELLED
SWELLER
SWELTER
SWILLED
SWILLER
SWOLLEN
TALLIED
TALLIER
TALLIES
TELLIES
TOLLMEN
TOOLSET
TRILLED
TRILLER
TROLLED
TROLLER
TROLLEY
TUILLES
TWELVEA
TWELVEB
TWELVEC
TWELVED
TWELVEE
TWELVES
TWILLED
UNBLUED
UNGLUED
UNGLUES
UNPLIED
UNSLEEK
UNSLIER
UNSLYER
UVALUES
VAULTED
VAULTER
VEALIER
VIALLED
VIELLES
WELLFED
WELLLED
WELLSEE
WELLSET
WELLYES
WHALLEY
WHELMED
WHELPED
WIELDED
WIELDER
WILLIES
WOOLIER
WOOLIES
WOOLLEN
WOOLLEY
WOOLSEY
YIELDED
YIELDER
ZOELLER

•••L••E

ABALONE
ABILENE
ABOLLAE
ACOLYTE
ACTLIKE
ADELINE
ADOLPHE
ADULATE
AIRLANE
AIRLIKE
AIRLINE
AMILATE
AMYLASE
ANALYSE
ANALYTE
ANALYZE
ANILINE
ANTLIKE
APELIKE
ARMLIKE
ASSLIKE
ATELATE
ATHLETE
AUSLESE
AXELIKE
AXILLAE
BAALITE
BADLOVE
BAGLIKE
BALLADE
BALLONE
BATLIKE
BEDLIKE
BEELIKE
BEELINE
BIBLIKE
BIGLOVE
BILLNYE
BIOLITE
BIPLANE

BOWLIKE
BOWLINE
BOXLIKE
BOYLIKE
BUDLIKE
BUSLANE
BUSLINE
CARLENE
CARLYLE
CATLIKE
CELLULE
CHALICE
CHELATE
CHOLINE
COLLAGE
COLLATE
COLLEGE
COLLIDE
COLLINE
COLLUDE
COULDBE
COWLIKE
CUPLIKE
CURLIKE
CYCLONE
DARLENE
DECLARE
DECLINE
DEFLATE
DEGLAZE
DEPLANE
DEPLETE
DEPLORE
DEWLINE
DIDLIKE
DISLIKE
DOGLIKE
DOTLIKE
DUALIZE
EARLIKE
EARLOBE
EATLATE
EELLIKE
EGALITE
EGGLIKE
ELFLIKE
EMBLAZE
EMPLACE
EMPLANE
EMULATE
ENCLAVE
ENCLOSE
ENDLATE
ENDLINE
ENFLAME
ENPLANE
ENSLAVE
EONLINE
EPILATE
EVILEYE
EVILONE
EVOLUTE
EXCLAVE
EXCLUDE
EXPLODE
EXPLORE
EYELIKE
EYELINE

FADLIKE
FAILURE
FALLDUE
FANLIKE
FATLIKE
FAXLORE
FELLDUE
FINLIKE
FORLIFE
FORLOVE
FOXLIKE
GAGLINE
GASLINE
GEMLIKE
GODLIKE
GUMLIKE
HAGLIKE
HAMLINE
HARLINE
HATLIKE
HAULAGE
HELLENE
HEMLINE
HENLIKE
HIPLIKE
HOGLIKE
HOPLITE
HOTLINE
HOVLANE
HOWLAME
HUNLIKE
HUTLIKE
HYALITE
IAMLOVE
ICELIKE
ICELINE
IDOLISE
IDOLIZE
ILLLIVE
IMPLODE
IMPLORE
INALINE
INCLINE
INCLOSE
INCLUDE
INFLAME
INFLATE
INGLESE
INKLIKE
INPLACE
INULASE
ISOLATE
ISOLINE
ITSLATE
ITSLOVE
IVYLIKE
JAMLIKE
JAWLIKE
JAWLINE
JIGLIKE
KEYLIME
KIDLIKE
KILLFEE
LAPLACE
LAWLIKE
LEGLIKE
LETLIVE
LIPLIKE

LOWLIFE
MANLIKE
MARLENE
MARLOWE
MCCLURE
METLIFE
MIDLIFE
MIDLINE
MILLAGE
MILLIME
MISLIKE
MOULAGE
MRSLATE
NBALIVE
NEOLYTE
NETLIKE
NEWLIFE
NEWLINE
NEWLOVE
NIBLIKE
NONLIFE
NONLIVE
NOPLACE
NOTLIKE
NOTLIVE
NUCLIDE
NUNLIKE
NUTLIKE
OAKLIKE
OARLIKE
OATLIKE
OBELISE
OBELIZE
OCCLUDE
OFFLINE
OILLIKE
OILLINE
OLDLINE
OLDLYME
ONALINE
ONELANE
ONELOVE
OPALINE
ORBLIKE
OUTLINE
OUTLIVE
OUTLOVE
OWLLIKE
OXALATE
PAULINE
PCCLONE
PEALIKE
PEGLIKE
PENLIKE
PENLITE
PERLITE
PHILLIE
PHILTRE
PIELIKE
PIGLIKE
PILLAGE
PODLIKE
POLLUTE
POOLCUE
PRALINE
PRELATE
PRELIFE
PRELUDE

PROLATE
PROLIFE
QUELQUE
RAILAGE
RAMLIKE
RANLATE
RATLIKE
RATLINE
RAYLIKE
REALINE
REALISE
REALIZE
RECLAME
RECLINE
RECLUSE
REDLINE
REFLATE
REGLAZE
REPLACE
REPLANE
REPLATE
REPLETE
REPLUME
RESLATE
RIBLIKE
ROBLOWE
RODLIKE
ROULADE
RUGLIKE
RUNLATE
SACLIKE
SAWLIKE
SCALAGE
SCALENE
SEALANE
SEALIFE
SEALIKE
SECLUDE
SHALLWE
SHELTIE
SILLYME
SINLIKE
SIXLANE
SKYLIKE
SKYLINE
SOILAGE
SONLIKE
SOWLIKE
STYLISE
STYLIZE
SUBLIME
SUNLIKE
TAGLIKE
TAGLINE
TALLONE
TANLINE
THELIKE
TIELINE
TILLAGE
TINLIKE
TIPLINE
TOBLAME
TOELIKE
TOLLAGE
TOOLATE
TOPLINE
TOWLINE
TOYLIKE

TUBLIKE
TWELVEE
TWOLANE
UKELELE
UKULELE
ULALUME
ULULATE
UNALIKE
UNALONE
UNBLADE
UNCLOSE
UNGLOVE
UPCLOSE
UPSLOPE
URNLIKE
UTILISE
UTILIZE
VALLONE
VANLINE
VILLAGE
VIOLATE
VIOLONE
VONLAUE
VORLAGE
WALLACE
WALLEYE
WARLIKE
WASLATE
WAXLIKE
WEBLIKE
WELLSEE
WIGLIKE
WILLKIE
WOOLITE
WOULDBE
YOULOSE

••••LE•

ABRILES
AEDILES
ALLELES
AMPULES
ANGELES
ANNALEE
ANNALES
ANNULET
ARABLES
ARBOLES
AREOLES
ARGYLES
AUDILES
AURALEE
AVAILED
AVONLEA
BABBLED
BABBLER
BABBLES
BAFFLED
BAFFLER
BAFFLES
BANALER
BANDLET
BANGLED
BANGLES
BARKLEY
BARTLES
BARTLET
BATTLED

BATTLER
BATTLES
BAUBLES
BEADLES
BEAGLES
BEASLEY
BEATLES
BEETLES
BENTLEY
BERKLEY
BEVELED
BEVELER
BINDLES
BINGLES
BLAKLEY
BOBBLED
BOBBLER
BOBBLES
BOBSLED
BOGGLED
BOGGLER
BOGGLES
BOMBLET
BONELET
BOODLES
BOOKLET
BOOMLET
BOOSLER
BOOTLEG
BOTTLED
BOTTLER
BOTTLES
BOWDLER
BRADLEE
BRADLEY
BRAMLEY
BRAWLED
BRAWLER
BRAWLEY
BRIDLED
BRIDLER
BRIDLES
BRIMLEY
BROILED
BROILER
BUBBLED
BUBBLES
BUCKLED
BUCKLES
BUCKLEY
BUELLER
BUGGLES
BULBLET
BUMBLED
BUMBLER
BUMBLES
BUNDLED
BUNDLER
BUNDLES
BUNGLED
BUNGLER
BUNGLES
BURBLED
BURBLER
BURBLES
BURGLED
BURGLES
BURNLEY

BUSTLED
BUSTLER
BUSTLES
CACKLED
CACKLER
CACKLES
CAJOLED
CAJOLER
CAJOLES
CANALED
CANDLED
CANDLER
CANDLES
CANTLES
CAPELET
CAPULET
CAROLED
CAROLER
CASTLED
CASTLES
CATFLEA
CAVILED
CAVILER
CHAPLET
CHARLES
CHARLEY
CHICLES
CHICLET
CHILLED
CHILLER
CIRCLED
CIRCLER
CIRCLES
CIRCLET
COBBLED
COBBLER
COBBLES
COCHLEA
COCKLED
COCKLES
CODDLED
CODDLER
CODDLES
COGGLES
COMPLEX
CONELET
COUPLED
COUPLER
COUPLES
COUPLET
CRADLED
CRADLER
CRADLES
CRAWLED
CRAWLER
CRAWLEY
CREELEY
CREOLES
CROWLEY
CRUELER
CRULLER
CUDDLED
CUDDLES
CUPELED
CUPELER
CUPULES
CURDLED
CURDLER

CURDLES
CUSSLER
DABBLED
DABBLER
DABBLES
DAIMLER
DANDLED
DANDLER
DANDLES
DANGLED
DANGLER
DANGLES
DAPPLED
DAPPLES
DARKLED
DARKLES
DARTLED
DARTLES
DAWDLED
DAWDLER
DAWDLES
DAZZLED
DAZZLER
DAZZLES
DECILES
DECKLED
DECKLES
DEFILED
DEFILER
DEFILES
DEVILED
DIABLES
DIALLED
DIBBLED
DIBBLER
DIBBLES
DIDDLED
DIDDLER
DIDDLES
DIDDLEY
DIMPLED
DIMPLES
DINGLES
DIPOLES
DOGFLEA
DOGSLED
DONGLES
DOODLED
DOODLER
DOODLES
DOPPLER
DOTTLES
DOUBLEA
DOUBLEB
DOUBLEC
DOUBLED
DOUBLEE
DOUBLEF
DOUBLEG
DOUBLEH
DOUBLEI
DOUBLEJ
DOUBLEK
DOUBLEL
DOUBLEM
DOUBLEN
DOUBLEO
DOUBLEP

DOUBLEQ
DOUBLER
DOUBLES
DOUBLET
DOUBLEU
DOUBLEV
DOUBLEW
DOUBLEX
DOUBLEY
DOUBLEZ
DOVELET
DRAWLED
DRAWLER
DREXLER
DRIBLET
DRILLED
DRILLER
DROLLER
DROOLED
DROOLER
DROPLET
DUELLED
DUFFLES
DWELLED
DWELLER
EASELED
EDIBLES
EKUELES
EMAILED
EMAILER
EMPALED
EMPALES
ENABLED
ENABLER
ENABLES
ENISLED
ENISLES
ENOILED
ENSILED
ENSILES
EPAULET
EQUALED
ETAILED
ETAILER
ETOILES
EVILLER
EXHALED
EXHALES
EXOILER
FAILLES
FANSLER
FARTLEK
FATALES
FEEBLER
FEMALES
FERULES
FETTLES
FICKLER
FIDDLED
FIDDLER
FIDDLES
FIDELES
FIEDLER
FINALES
FINDLEY
FIPPLES
FIZZLED
FIZZLER

FIZZLES
FLAILED
FLATLET
FOCSLES
FOIBLES
FONDLED
FONDLER
FONDLES
FOOTLED
FOOTLER
FOOTLES
FOOTLET
FOOZLED
FOOZLER
FOOZLES
FORELEG
FORTLEE
FRAILER
FRAWLEY
FRIDLEY
FRILLED
FROGLEG
FROGLET
FTRILEY
FUDDLED
FUDDLES
FUELLED
FUMBLED
FUMBLER
FUMBLES
FUNPLEX
GABBLED
GABBLES
GAGGLES
GALILEE
GALILEI
GALILEO
GAMBLED
GAMBLER
GAMBLES
GAMELEG
GANTLET
GARBLED
GARBLER
GARBLES
GARGLED
GARGLER
GARGLES
GATELEG
GAVELED
GENTLED
GENTLER
GENTLES
GIGGLED
GIGGLER
GIGGLES
GIRDLED
GIRDLER
GIRDLES
GNARLED
GOBBLED
GOBBLER
GOBBLES
GOGGLED
GOGGLER
GOGGLES
GOOGLED
GOOGLER

GOOGLES
GREELEY
GRILLED
GRILLER
GRILLES
GRISLET
GROWLED
GROWLER
GURGLED
GURGLES
GUZZLED
GUZZLER
GUZZLES
HAARLEM
HACKLED
HACKLER
HACKLES
HAGGLED
HAGGLER
HAGGLES
HANDLED
HANDLER
HANDLES
HARTLEY
HASSLED
HASSLES
HECKLED
HECKLER
HECKLES
HEMSLEY
HENSLEY
HIBBLER
HIGGLED
HIGGLER
HIGGLES
HINDLEG
HOBBLED
HOBBLER
HOBBLES
HONALEE
HORSLEY
HOSTLER
HUDDLED
HUDDLER
HUDDLES
HUMBLED
HUMBLER
HUMBLES
HUNTLEY
HURDLED
HURDLER
HURDLES
HURTLED
HURTLES
HUSTLED
HUSTLER
HUSTLES
ICICLES
IMPALED
IMPALER
IMPALES
INHALED
INHALER
INHALES
INSALES
INSOLES
JACALES
JANGLED

JANGLER
JANGLES
JEWELED
JEWELER
JIGGLED
JIGGLES
JINGLED
JINGLER
JINGLES
JOGGLED
JOGGLER
JOGGLES
JOHNLEE
JOSTLED
JOSTLER
JOSTLES
JUBILEE
JUGGLED
JUGGLER
JUGGLES
JUILLET
JUMBLED
JUMBLER
JUMBLES
JUNGLES
KASTLER
KEEBLER
KEESLER
KETTLES
KIBBLED
KIBBLES
KINDLED
KINDLER
KINDLES
KINGLET
KNEELED
KNEELER
KNELLED
KNOWLES
KNURLED
KOEHLER
KURILES
KVELLED
LABELED
LABELER
LANDLER
LANGLEY
LAPELED
LASTLEG
LEAFLET
LEFTLEG
LEVELED
LEVELER
LIBELED
LIBELEE
LIBELER
LILALEE
LITTLER
LITTLES
LOBULES
LOCALES
LOCKLET
LORELEI
LOYALER
LOYALES
MANGLED
MANGLER
MANGLES

MANTLED
MANTLES
MANTLET
MARBLED
MARBLER
MARBLES
MCALLEN
MCHALES
MEAGLES
MEASLES
MEDALED
MEDDLED
MEDDLER
MEDDLES
MEDELES
METALED
METTLER
METTLES
MIDDLEC
MIDDLED
MIDDLER
MIDDLES
MINGLED
MINGLER
MINGLES
MIZZLED
MIZZLES
MOBILES
MODELED
MODELER
MODULES
MOONLET
MORALES
MOTTLED
MOTTLES
MTPELEE
MUDDLED
MUDDLER
MUDDLES
MUELLER
MUFFLED
MUFFLER
MUFFLES
MUGGLES
MUMBLED
MUMBLER
MUMBLES
MURALED
MUSCLED
MUSCLES
MUZZLED
MUZZLER
MUZZLES
MYRTLES
NECKLET
NEEDLED
NEEDLER
NEEDLES
NESTLED
NESTLER
NESTLES
NETTLED
NETTLES
NIBBLED
NIBBLER
NIBBLES
NICKLES
NICOLET

NIGGLED
NIGGLER
NIGGLES
NIMBLER
NIPPLES
NODULED
NODULES
NOGALES
NOODLED
NOODLES
NOPALES
NOZZLES
NTUPLES
NUBBLES
NUZZLED
NUZZLER
NUZZLES
OKELLEY
OMALLEY
ORACLES
ORIOLES
OSCULES
OUTFLEE
OVERLET
PADDLED
PADDLER
PADDLES
PAISLEY
PANELED
PANTLEG
PAPELES
PAROLED
PAROLEE
PAROLES
PARSLEY
PEARLED
PEARLER
PEBBLED
PEBBLES
PEDALED
PEDALER
PEDDLED
PEDDLER
PEDDLES
PEEBLES
PEEPLES
PEOPLED
PEOPLES
PERILED
PERPLEX
PESTLED
PESTLES
PETALED
PETALES
PICKLED
PICKLES
PIDDLED
PIDDLES
PIFFLED
PIFFLES
PIMPLED
PIMPLES
PLAYLET
POODLES
POPELEO
POPPLED
POPPLES
POSOLES
POZOLES
PRESLEY
PROBLEM
PROWLED
PROWLER
PUDDLED
PUDDLES
PUGGLES
PUGSLEY
PURFLED
PURFLER
PURFLES
PURPLED
PURPLES
PUZZLED
PUZZLER
PUZZLES
QUAILED
QUARLES
QUELLED
QUELLER
QUIGLEY
QUILLED
QUILLER
RABBLED
RABBLES
RAFFLED
RAFFLER
RAFFLES
RAMBLED
RAMBLER
RAMBLES
RANKLED
RANKLES
RASSLED
RASSLER
RASSLES
RATTLED
RATTLER
RATTLES
RAVELED
REBALED
REBALES
REFILED
REFILES
REGALED
REGALER
REGALES
REOILED
RESALES
RESILED
RESILES
RESOLED
RESOLER
RESOLES
RETILED
RETILES
REVELED
REVELER
REVILED
REVILER
REVILES
RICHLER
RICKLES
RIDDLED
RIDDLER
RIDDLES
RIFFLED
RIFFLER
RIFFLES
RIMPLED
RIMPLES
RINGLET
RIPPLED
RIPPLES
RIPPLET
RIVALED
RIVULET
ROOTLED
ROOTLES
ROOTLET
ROWELED
ROYALES
RUBBLES
RUFFLED
RUFFLER
RUFFLES
RUGGLES
RUMBLED
RUMBLER
RUMBLES
RUMPLED
RUMPLES
RUNDLES
RUSTLED
RUSTLER
RUSTLES
RUTALEE
RUTILES
SADDLED
SADDLER
SADDLES
SAMPLED
SAMPLER
SAMPLES
SANDLER
SARALEE
SCARLET
SCHOLES
SCOWLED
SCOWLER
SCULLED
SCULLER
SEEDLET
SEPALED
SETTLED
SETTLER
SETTLES
SHAWLED
SHELLED
SHELLER
SHELLEY
SHILLED
SHIRLEY
SHOALED
SICKLES
SIMILES
SIMPLER
SIMPLES
SIMPLEX
SINGLED
SINGLES
SINGLET
SIZZLED
SIZZLER
SIZZLES
SKILLED
SKILLET
SKIRLED
SKULLED
SMALLER
SMELLED
SMELLER
SNARLED
SNARLER
SNELLEN
SNIGLET
SPELLED
SPELLER
SPIELED
SPIELER
SPILLED
SPILLER
SPOILED
SPOILER
SPOOLED
SPOOLER
STABLED
STABLER
STABLES
STADLER
STALLED
STALLER
STANLEE
STANLEY
STAPLED
STAPLER
STAPLES
STARLET
STATLER
STEALER
STEELED
STEELER
STIFLED
STIFLES
STILLED
STILLER
STOLLEN
STOOLED
SUBTLER
SUELLEN
SUPPLED
SUPPLER
SUPPLES
SWELLED
SWELLER
SWILLED
SWILLER
SWIRLED
SWOLLEN
TACKLED
TACKLER
TACKLES
TAMALES
TAMGLEN
TANGLED
TANGLER
TANGLES
TARTLET
TATTLED
TATTLER
TATTLES
TEMPLED
TEMPLES
THEFLEA
TICKLED
TICKLER
TICKLES
TINGLED
TINGLER
TINGLES
TINKLED
TINKLER
TINKLES
TIPPLED
TIPPLER
TIPPLES
TITTLES
TODDLED
TODDLER
TODDLES
TOFFLER
TOGGLED
TOGGLER
TOGGLES
TOHELEN
TOODLES
TOOTLED
TOOTLER
TOOTLES
TOPPLED
TOPPLES
TOTALED
TOTALER
TOUSLED
TOUSLES
TOWELED
TOWNLET
TOYSLED
TRAILED
TRAILER
TRAWLED
TRAWLER
TREBLED
TREBLES
TREELET
TRIFLED
TRIFLER
TRIFLES
TRILLED
TRILLER
TRIOLET
TRIPLEA
TRIPLED
TRIPLES
TRIPLET
TRIPLEX
TROLLED
TROLLER
TROLLEY
TUBULES
TUILLES
TUMBLED
TUMBLER
TUMBLES
TUMMLER
TUPOLEV
TURTLED
TURTLES
TUSSLED
TUSSLES
TWILLED
TWIRLED
TWIRLER
UNAXLED
UNBALED
UNBALES
UNFILED
UNFILES
UNIPLEX
UNOGLED
UNOILED
UNPALED
UNPILED
UNPILES
UNPOLED
UNRILED
UNRULED
UNSOLED
UNSOLES
UNTILED
UPPILED
UPPILES
USABLES
VEINLET
VENULES
VIALLED
VIELLES
VITTLES
WADDLED
WADDLER
WADDLES
WAFFLED
WAFFLER
WAFFLES
WAGGLED
WAGGLER
WAGGLES
WAMBLED
WAMBLES
WANGLED
WANGLER
WANGLES
WARBLED
WARBLER
WARBLES
WATTLED
WATTLES
WAVELET
WEDELED
WELLLED
WEMBLEY
WHALLEY
WHEELED
WHEELER
WHIRLED
WHIRLER
WHORLED
WIGGLED
WIGGLER
WIGGLES
WIMPLED
WIMPLES
WINGLET
WINKLER
WINSLET
WOBBLED
WOBBLER
WOBBLES
WOODLEY
WOOLLEN
WOOLLEY
WORSLEY
WRIGLEY
YODELED
YODELER
ZIEGLER
ZOELLER
ZONULES

••••L•E

AAMILNE
ABOLLAE
ABSOLVE
ACHILLE
ALCALDE
ALLELSE
AMIBLUE
ANNALEE
AREOLAE
AURALEE
AXILLAE
BENBLUE
BIGBLUE
BIVALVE
BRADLEE
BRAILLE
BTWELVE
CABALLE
CAMILLE
CANULAE
CHARLIE
COPULAE
DEMILLE
DERALTE
DEVALUE
DEVILLE
DEVOLVE
DEWILDE
DIVULGE
DIVULSE
DONTLIE
DOUBLEE
ECUELLE
ESTELLE
FACULAE
FAMILLE
FIBULAE
FORTLEE
GALILEE
GAZELLE
GEFILTE
GIROLLE
GISELLE
HONALEE
HOTGLUE
HOWELSE
ICEBLUE
ICEFLOE
IMPULSE
INDULGE
INVOLVE
ITSALIE
ITWELVE
JOHNLEE
JUBILEE
LABELLE
LASALLE
LAVALSE
LIBELEE
LILALEE
LUCILLE
LUNULAE
MACULAE
MOSELLE
MTPELEE
NACELLE
NATALIE
NBCBLUE
NEBULAE
NEVILLE
NICOLLE
NOTALIE
NOVELLE
OFVALUE
OLDBLUE
ORVILLE
OUTFLEE
OVERLIE
PAROLEE
PASALLE
PHILLIE
RAVELOE
REPULSE
RESOLVE
REVALUE
REVOLVE
ROSALIE
ROSELLE
ROTELLE
ROYALWE
ROZELLE
RUTALEE
SARALEE
SEABLUE
SEVILLE
SHALLWE
SHEILAE
SKYBLUE
STANLEE
STEELIE
STOOLIE
UNGULAE
UPVALUE
WHEELIE

•••••LE

ACHILLE
ACOUPLE
ACTABLE
ADDABLE
ADDIBLE
AFFABLE
AHASSLE
AIRHOLE
AIRMILE
ALITTLE
ALLMALE
AMIABLE
AMPOULE
ANATOLE
APOSTLE
ARMHOLE
ARSHILE
ARTICLE
ARTSALE
ASARULE
ATINGLE
AUDIBLE
AUREOLE
AURICLE
AUSABLE
BARBULE
BASSALE
BEGUILE
BICYCLE
BIGSALE
BITROLE
BOBDOLE
BOGHOLE
BRAILLE
BRAMBLE
BRATTLE
BRICKLE
BRINDLE
BRISTLE
BRITTLE
BUYABLE
BYAMILE
CABALLE
CAMILLE
CAMRYLE
CAPABLE
CAPSULE
CARIOLE
CARLYLE
CARSALE
CASTILE
CELLULE
CENACLE
CHEADLE
CHORALE
CHORTLE
CHUCKLE
CINEOLE
CITABLE
COMPILE
CONDOLE
CONSOLE
CORACLE
CRACKLE
CRINKLE
CRIPPLE
CRUMBLE
CRUMPLE
CUBICLE
CURABLE
CUTICLE
DASCHLE
DATABLE
DEBACLE
DEBOULE
DECUPLE
DEMILLE
DEVILLE
DISABLE
DOGPILE
DRABBLE
DRAGGLE
DRIBBLE
DRIZZLE
DRYABLE
DRYHOLE
DUCTILE
DURABLE
DWINDLE
EARHOLE
EATABLE
ECUELLE
EFFABLE
ELIYALE
ENDABLE
ENNOBLE
ENTITLE
EPISTLE
EQUABLE
ERRABLE
ESTELLE
EXAMPLE
EYEHOLE
FAMILLE
FBIFILE
FEBRILE
FERRULE
FERTILE
FICTILE
FINABLE
FINAGLE
FISSILE
FIXABLE
FLEEGLE
FLEXILE
FLYABLE
FORSALE
FOXHOLE
FRAGGLE
FRAGILE
FRAZZLE
FRECKLE
FRIABLE
FRIBBLE
FRIJOLE
FRIZZLE
FROOGLE
FRYABLE
FUSIBLE
GAGRULE
GAZELLE
GENTILE
GETABLE
GIROLLE
GISELLE
GLOBULE
GOSTALE
GRACILE
GRACKLE
GRANULE
GRAPPLE
GRASSLE
GRIDDLE
GRISTLE
GRIZZLE
GRUMBLE
GUNWALE
HATABLE
HAYBALE
HERCULE
HIDABLE
HIRABLE
HOSCALE
HOSTILE
ICEHOLE
IGNOBLE
INAHOLE
INAPILE
INAVALE
INEXILE
INSCALE
INSTYLE
INUTILE
JIMDALE
KEYHOLE
KNUCKLE
KRINGLE
KRYSTLE
KYOODLE
LABELLE
LAEMMLE
LASALLE
LEGIBLE
LIKABLE
LINABLE
LIVABLE
LOSABLE
LOVABLE
LUCILLE
MAKABLE
MANACLE
MANHOLE
MANIPLE
MAYPOLE
MCARDLE
MIDSOLE
MINABLE
MIRACLE
MISFILE
MISRULE
MISSILE
MIXABLE
MOBRULE
MONDALE
MONOCLE
MONTALE
MOSELLE
MOVABLE
MUDHOLE
MUTABLE
NACELLE
NAMABLE
NERVULE
NEVILLE
NICOLLE
NONSALE
NONUPLE
NOTABLE
NOVELLE
OCTUPLE
ONEMILE
ORVILLE
OSSICLE
OUTSOLE
OUTWILE
PALEALE
PANICLE
PANTILE
PARABLE
PASALLE
PAYABLE
PERCALE
PETIOLE
PETMULE
PIEHOLE
PIESALE
PINHOLE
PINWALE
PISTOLE
PLIABLE
PLUMULE
POSABLE
POTABLE
POTHOLE
PRATTLE
PREFILE
PRESALE
PRICKLE
PRINGLE
PROFILE
PUERILE
QUIBBLE
RADICLE
RAKABLE
RATABLE
RATHOLE
RECABLE
RECYCLE
REPTILE
RESCALE
RESTYLE
RETABLE
RETICLE
RETITLE
RIDABLE
RISIBLE
RISSOLE
ROSELLE
ROTELLE
ROZELLE
RUMPOLE
SALABLE
SAVABLE
SAYABLE
SCRUPLE
SCUFFLE
SCUTTLE
SEAMILE
SEATTLE
SEEABLE
SERVILE
SESSILE
SEVILLE
SHACKLE
SHAMBLE
SHINGLE
SHUFFLE
SHUTTLE
SIZABLE
SKIABLE
SKIFFLE
SKIPOLE
SKITTLE
SMUGGLE
SNAPPLE
SNIFFLE
SNUFFLE
SNUGGLE
SOLUBLE
SOUFFLE
SOURALE
SPACKLE
SPANGLE
SPARKLE
SPECKLE
SPINDLE
SPITTLE
SPYHOLE
STABILE
STARTLE
STEEPLE
STERILE
STIPPLE
STOPPLE
STUBBLE
STUMBLE
SUBFILE
SWADDLE
SWINDLE
SWIZZLE
SYSTOLE
TACTILE
TADPOLE
TAGSALE
TAKABLE
TAMABLE
TAXABLE
TAXSALE
TENABLE
TENMILE
TENSILE
TEXTILE
THEDOLE
THENILE
THERULE
THIMBLE
THISTLE
TIMBALE
TMOBILE
TOPHOLE
TOSCALE
TOTABLE
TOWABLE
TRAMPLE
TREACLE
TREADLE
TREMBLE
TRESTLE
TRIABLE
TRIBBLE
TRICKLE
TROUBLE
TRUCKLE
TRUFFLE
TRUNDLE
TUNABLE
TUNICLE
TVTABLE
TWADDLE
TWEEDLE
TWIDDLE
TWINKLE
UKELELE
UKULELE
UNAGILE
UNWHOLE
UPSCALE
VACUOLE
VALVULE

VEHICLE
VEINULE
VENABLE
VESICLE
VIRGULE
VISIBLE
VOCABLE
VOLUBLE
VOTABLE
WALPOLE
WAVICLE
WAXABLE
WHEEDLE
WHIFFLE
WHIPPLE
WHISTLE
WHITTLE
WIMPOLE
WIRABLE
WRANGLE
WRESTLE
WRIGGLE
WRINKLE
ZEPPOLE

L•F••••

LAFARGE
LAFEMME
LAFITTE
LAFLEUR
LEFREAK
LEFTARM
LEFTEAR
LEFTEND
LEFTEST
LEFTEYE
LEFTFOR
LEFTHIP
LEFTIES
LEFTISH
LEFTISM
LEFTIST
LEFTJAB
LEFTLEG
LEFTOFF
LEFTOUT
LIFEFUL
LIFENET
LIFTERS
LIFTING
LIFTOFF
LIFTSUP
LOFTBED
LOFTERS
LOFTIER
LOFTILY
LOFTING
LUFFING

L••F•••

LABFEES
LANFORD
LAPFULS
LAWFORD
LEAFAGE
LEAFIER
LEAFING
LEAFLET
LEAFOUT
LEEFORD
LENFANT
LETFALL
LIEFEST
LOAFERS
LOAFING
LOAFPAN
LOOFAHS
LUFFING

L•••F••

LAIDFOR
LATEFEE
LATIFAH
LAYOFFS
LAYSFOR
LEAPFOR
LEFTFOR
LESSFAT
LETSFLY
LIEDFOR
LIESFOR
LIFEFUL
LIVEFOR
LOGOFFS
LONGFOR
LOOKFOR
LUCIFER
LUSTFUL

L••••F•

LAIDOFF
LAYOFFS
LAYSOFF
LEADOFF
LEFTOFF
LETSOFF
LIFTOFF
LIGNIFY
LIPSOFF
LIQUEFY
LOGOFFS
LOGSOFF
LOPSOFF
LOWLIFE

L•••••F

LAIDOFF
LAYSOFF
LEADOFF
LEARNOF
LEFTOFF
LETGOOF
LETSOFF
LETTERF
LIFTOFF
LINDORF
LIPSOFF
LOADSOF
LOGSOFF
LOPSOFF

•LF••••

ALFALFA
ALFEROV
ALFIERI
ALFONSE
ALFONSO
ALFORJA
ALFREDA
ALFREDE
ALFREDO
ALFREDU
ELFLIKE
ELFLOCK
ELFOWLS
ELFUDGE

•L•F•••

ALIFORM
BLUFFED
BLUFFER
BLUFFLY
CLIFTON
FLUFFED
FLUFFER
FLUFFUP
FLYFISH
ILLFOLD
OLAFIII
OLDFILM
OLDFOGY
OLEFINS

•L••F••

ALLOFIT
ALLOFME
ALLOFUS
ALOOFLY
BLOWFLY
BLUEFIN
BLUEFLU
BLUEFOX
BLUFFED
BLUFFER
BLUFFLY
CLAPFOR
CLUEFUL
FLUFFED
FLUFFER
FLUFFUP
GLEEFUL
PLANFOR
PLAYFUL
PLOTFUL
SLEDFUL

•L•••F•

ALEWIFE
ALFALFA
BLEWOFF
BLOWOFF
CLARIFY
CLIPOFF
GLORIFY
PLAYOFF
SLIDOFF
SLIPOFF

•L••••F

ALACKOF
ALOADOF
ALTDORF
BLEWOFF
BLOWOFF
CLEAROF
CLIPOFF
FLYLEAF
PLAYOFF
SLIDOFF
SLIPOFF

••LF•••

AELFRIC
BALFOUR
BELFAST
BELFORT
FULFILL
FULFILS
GILFORD
GOLFBAG
GOLFCAR
GOLFERS
GOLFING
GOLFPRO
GOLFTEE
GULFING
GULFOIL
GULFWAR
HALFBAD
HALFCUT
HALFDAY
HALFDUG
HALFFED
HALFIES
HALFMAD
HALFRAW
HALFROD
HALFSHY
HALFWAY
HALFWIT
HALFWON
ILLFOLD
PALFREY
PILFERS
ROLFERS
ROLFING
SELFISH
SOLFEGE
SULFATE
SULFIDE
SULFITE
WELFARE
WILFORD
WILFRED
WOLFCUB
WOLFDOG
WOLFGAL
WOLFING
WOLFISH
WOLFMAN
WOLFMEN
WOLFRAM

••L•F••

ALLOFIT
ALLOFME
ALLOFUS
BALEFUL
CALLFOR
DOLEFUL
FALAFEL
FALLFOR
FELLFOR
FELTFOR
FILOFAX
HALFFED
HALIFAX
HELPFUL
KILLFEE
MALEFIC
MILKFED
PALMFUL
PULLFOR
SCLAFFS
SELLFOR
SOLDFOR
TELEFAX
UNLOFTY
UPLIFTS
WELLFED
WILLFUL
YELLFOR

••L••F•

BELIEFS
CALCIFY
CALLOFF
DULCIFY
FALLOFF
FALSIFY
FELLOFF
FELTOFF
HELDOFF
HOLDOFF
JELLIFY
JOLLIFY
MOLLIFY
NULLIFY
PALMOFF
PULLOFF
PULPIFY
RELIEFS
ROLLOFF
SCLAFFS
SELLOFF
SOLDOFF
TELLOFF
TOLDOFF
UNLEAFS
WALKOFF
WALLOFF
WELLOFF

••L•••F

ASLEWOF
CALLOFF
FALLOFF
FELLOFF
FELTOFF
HELDOFF
HOLDOFF
PALMOFF
PILESOF
PULLOFF
ROLLOFF
SELLOFF
SILENTF
SOLDOFF
TALKSOF
TELLOFF
TELLSOF
TOLDOFF
WALDORF
WALKOFF
WALLOFF
WELLOFF

•••LF••

BOWLFUL
CALLFOR
FALLFOR
FEELFOR
FELLFOR
KILLFEE
PAILFUL
PULLFOR
SELLFOR
SKILFUL
SOULFUL
TAILFIN
TOILFUL
TWELFTH
VIALFUL
WAILFUL
WELLFED
WILLFUL
WOOLFAT
YELLFOR

•••L•F•

AIRLIFT
AMPLIFY
BAILIFF
BOILOFF
CALLOFF
EYELIFT
FALLOFF
FARLEFT
FEELOFF
FELLOFF
FORLIFE
HAULOFF
HAYLOFT
JELLIFY
JOLLIFY
KARLOFF
LOWLIFE
METLIFE
MIDLIFE
MOLLIFY
NEWLEFT
NEWLIFE
NONLIFE
NULLIFY
OCALAFL
PEELOFF
PRELIFE
PROLIFE
PULLOFF
QUALIFY
REELOFF
ROLLOFF
SEALIFE
SEALIFT
SEALOFF
SELLOFF
SKILIFT
TAILOFF
TELLOFF
THELEFT
UNCLEFT
WALLOFF
WELLOFF

•••L••F

APILEOF
BAILIFF
BAYLEAF
BOILOFF
CALLOFF
ENDLEAF
FALLOFF
FEELOFF
FELLOFF
FIGLEAF
FLYLEAF
HAULOFF
KARLOFF
NEWLEAF
OAKLEAF
PEELOFF
PULLOFF
REELOFF
ROLLOFF
RYELOAF
SEALOFF
SELLOFF
TAILOFF
TEALEAF
TELLOFF
TELLSOF
WALLOFF
WELLOFF

••••LF•

ALFALFA
DRMELFI
ENGULFS
INGULFS
RODOLFO
RUDOLFI

••••L•F

AFOULOF
AKERLOF
DOUBLEF

•••••LF

AIRWOLF
BEOWULF
BIGHALF
CRYWOLF
DARRYLF
GANDALF
HERSELF
HIMSELF
METCALF
NONSELF
ONEHALF
ONESELF
OURSELF
PETCALF
REDWOLF
SEAWOLF
SHEWOLF
THESELF
THYSELF

L•G••••

LAGASSE
LAGGARD
LAGGERS
LAGGING
LAGOONS
LAGUNAS
LEGALLY
LEGANZA
LEGATEE
LEGATES
LEGATOR
LEGATOS
LEGBONE
LEGENDS
LEGGIER
LEGGING
LEGHORN
LEGIBLE
LEGIBLY
LEGIONS
LEGIRON
LEGISTS
LEGLESS
LEGLIKE
LEGOLAS
LEGOSET
LEGPULL
LEGRAND
LEGREST
LEGROOM
LEGROPE
LEGTRAP
LEGUMES
LEGWEAR
LEGWORK
LIGANDS
LIGATED
LIGATES
LIGGETT
LIGHTED
LIGHTEN
LIGHTER
LIGHTLY
LIGHTON
LIGHTUP
LIGNIFY
LIGNINS
LIGNITE
LIGURIA
LOGANUT
LOGBOOK
LOGGERS
LOGGIAS
LOGGING
LOGGINS
LOGGISH
LOGICAL
LOGIEST
LOGJAMS
LOGOFFS
LOGONTO
LOGOUTS
LOGROLL
LOGSOFF
LOGSOUT
LUGGAGE
LUGGERS
LUGGING
LUGNUTS
LUGSAIL
LUGSOUT
LUGWORM

L••G•••

LAGGARD
LAGGERS
LAGGING
LANGDON
LANGHAM
LANGLEY
LANGTON
LANGTRY
LANGUID
LANGUOR
LANGWAY
LARGELY
LARGENT
LARGEOJ
LARGESS
LARGEST
LARGISH
LAUGHAT
LAUGHED
LAUGHER
LAUGHIN
LEAGUED
LEAGUER
LEAGUES
LEDGERS
LEDGIER
LEGGIER
LEGGING
LENGTHS
LENGTHY
LENGUAS
LEOGENN
LETGOBY
LETGOOF
LIGGETT
LINGCOD
LINGERS
LINGOES
LINGUAE
LINGUAL
LINGULA
LODGEIN
LODGERS
LODGING
LOGGERS
LOGGIAS
LOGGING
LOGGINS
LOGGISH
LONGAGO
LONGARM
LONGBED
LONGBOW
LONGDAY
LONGDEN
LONGEST
LONGFOR
LONGIES
LONGING
LONGISH
LONGRUN
LONGTOM
LONGTON
LONGUES
LONGWAY
LORGNON
LOWGEAR
LUGGAGE
LUGGERS
LUGGING
LUNGEAT
LUNGERS
LUNGING

L•••G••

LASAGNA
LASAGNE
LASTGAS
LATIGOS
LAVAGES
LEHIGHU
LIMOGES
LINAGES
LISAGAY
LITHGOW
LONIGAN
LOUNGED
LOUNGER
LOUNGES
LOVAGES
LYINGBY
LYINGON
LYINGTO
LYINGUP

L••••G•

LACINGS
LADINGS
LAFARGE
LAPDOGS
LAZONGA
LEAFAGE
LEAKAGE
LENTIGO
LETITGO
LETMEGO
LEXUSGS
LEXUSGX
LIKINGS
LINEAGE
LININGS
LINKAGE
LITURGY
LIVINGS
LOCKAGE
LONGAGO
LORANGE
LOSINGS
LOZENGE
LUGGAGE
LUMBAGO

L•••••G

LACKING
LADADOG
LADLING
LADYBUG
LAGGING
LAIRING
LALLING
LAMBING
LAMMING
LANCING
LANDING
LANDTAG
LANSING
LAPPING
LAPSANG
LAPSING
LAPWING
LARDING
LARKING
LASHING
LASTING
LASTLEG
LATETAG
LATHING
LAUDING
LEADDOG
LEADING
LEAFING
LEAKING
LEANING
LEAPING
LEASING
LEAVING
LEERING
LEFTLEG
LEGGING
LEIPZIG
LEMMING
LENDING
LESSING
LETTERG
LETTING
LEVYING
LIBBING
LICKING
LIFTING
LILTING
LIMBING
LIMBURG
LIMNING
LIMPING
LINKING
LINTING
LIPPING
LISPING
LISTING
LOADING
LOAFING
LOAMING
LOANING
LOBBING
LOCKING
LODGING
LOFTING
LOGGING
LOIDING
LOLLING
LONBORG
LONGING
LOOKING
LOOMING
LOOPING
LOOSING
LOOTING
LOPPING
LORDING
LOSEBIG
LOSTBIG
LOSTDOG
LOTTING
LOURING
LOUSING
LOUTING
LOVEBUG
LUCKING
LUFFING
LUGGING
LULLING
LUMPING
LUNGING
LURKING
LUSTING

•LG••••

ALGARVE
ALGEBRA
ALGERIA
ALGIEBA
ALGIERS
ALGREEN
ELGALLO
ELGRECO

•L•G•••

ALEGARS
ALEGRIA
ALIGHTS
ALIGNED
ALIGNER
ALIGOTE
ALLGONE
ALLGOOD
BLIGHTS
BLIGHTY
BLOGGED
BLOGGER
CLOGGED
CLOGSUP
ELEGANT
ELEGIAC
ELEGIES
ELEGIST
ELEGITS
ELEGIZE
ELIGIUS
FLAGDAY
FLAGGED
FLAGGER
FLAGMAN
FLAGMEN
FLAGONS
FLIGHTS
FLIGHTY
FLOGGED
FLOGGER
FLYGIRL
GLUGGED
KLUGMAN
OLDGAGS
OLDGIRL
OLDGOLD
OLOGIES
PLAGUED
PLAGUES
PLIGHTS
PLUGGED
PLUGGER
PLUGINS
PLUGOLA
PLUGSIN
PLUGSUP
SLIGHTS
SLOGANS
SLOGGED
SLOGGER
SLUGGED
SLUGGER

•L••G••

ALLAGES
ALLEGED
ALLEGER
ALLEGES
ALLEGRA
ALLEGRO
ALRIGHT
BLOGGED
BLOGGER
BLOWGUN
BLUDGED
BLUDGER
BLUDGES
CLANGED
CLANGER
CLANGOR
CLINGER
CLINGTO
CLOGGED
CLUNGTO
FLAGGED
FLAGGER
FLANGES
FLEDGED
FLEDGES
FLEEGLE
FLINGAT
FLINGER
FLOGGED
FLOGGER
FLUNGAT
GLASGOW
GLUEGUN
GLUGGED
GLURGES
ILLEGAL
ILLEGIT
ILLOGIC
KLINGER
KLINGON
KLUDGED
KLUDGES
PLEDGED
PLEDGEE
PLEDGER
PLEDGES
PLOUGHS
PLUGGED
PLUGGER

PLUNGED
PLUNGER
PLUNGES
SLEDGED
SLEDGES
SLEIGHS
SLEIGHT
SLINGER
SLOEGIN
SLOGGED
SLOGGER
SLOUGHS
SLUDGES
SLUGGED
SLUGGER
TLINGIT
ULLAGES

•L•••G•

ALEKEGS
ALLERGY
ALLONGE
BLTTOGO
BLUINGS
ELFUDGE
FLOTAGE
FLOWAGE
FLUBUGS
FLYHIGH
OLDDOGS
OLDFOGY
OLDGAGS
PLUMAGE

•L••••G

ALAKING
ALAYING
ALINING
ALLYING
ALTHING
BLADING
BLAMING
BLARING
BLAZING
BLOWING
BLUEING
CLAWING
CLAYING
CLEWING
CLONING
CLOSING
CLOYING
CLUEING
ELATING
ELIDING
ELOPING
ELUDING
ELUTING
FLAKING
FLAMING
FLARING
FLAWING
FLAYING
FLEABAG
FLEEING
FLEMING
FLEXING
FLOWING
FLUTING
FLUXING
GLARING
GLAZING
GLIDING
GLOBING
GLOVING
GLOWING
OLDSONG
PLACING
PLANING
PLATING
PLAYING
PLOWING
PLUMING
SLAKING
SLATING
SLAVING
SLAYING
SLEDDOG
SLEWING
SLICING
SLIDING
SLIMING
SLOPING
SLOWING

••LG•••

ALLGONE
ALLGOOD
BELGIAN
BELGIUM
BILGIER
BULGARI
BULGARS
BULGHUR
BULGIER
BULGING
BULGURS
CALGARY
COLGATE
FOLGERS
FULGENT
FULGHUM
MULGREW
NFLGAME
NHLGAME
PILGRIM
VULGATE

••L•G••

ALLAGES
ALLEGED
ALLEGER
ALLEGES
ALLEGRA
ALLEGRO
BELUGAS
BOLOGNA
COLOGNE
DELIGHT
DELUGED
DELUGES
ECLOGUE
FALLGUY
HALOGEN
ILLEGAL
ILLEGIT
ILLOGIC
MALAGAN
MALAGAS
MALIGNS
MILAGRO
MTLOGAN
OBLIGED
OBLIGEE
OBLIGER
OBLIGES
OBLIGOR
OWLEGGS
PELAGES
PELAGIC
PHLEGMY
PILEGGI
POLYGON
RELIGHT
ULLAGES
UNLEGAL
UNLIGHT
UPLIGHT
WOLFGAL

••L••G•

AALARGE
ALLERGY
ALLONGE
ARLEDGE
ATLARGE
BELONGS
COLLAGE
COLLEGE
ENLARGE
ERLANGS
FILINGS
FOLENGO
FOLIAGE
INLARGE
IPLEDGE
KELLOGG
MELANGE
MELTAGE
MILEAGE
MILLAGE
OBLONGS
OILRIGS
OOLONGS
OWLEGGS
PALINGS
PILEGGI
PILINGS
PILLAGE
RALEIGH
RULINGS
SALONGA
SALVAGE
SELVAGE
SOLFEGE
SPLURGE
TILINGS
TILLAGE
TOLLAGE
UNLARGE
VILLAGE
VOLTAGE

••L•••G

ALLYING
ARLBERG
BALDING
BALKING
BELLING
BELTBAG
BELTING
BELYING
BILKING
BILLING
BOLLING
BOLTING
BULGING
BULKING
BULLDOG
BULLING
CALKING
CALLING
CALMING
CALVING
CULLING
DELEING
DELVING
DOLLING
DULLING
FALLING
FELLING
FELTING
FILIBEG
FILLING
FILMING
FOLDING
GALLING
GELDING
GELLING
GILDING
GILLING
GOLDBUG
GOLDING
GOLFBAG
GOLFING
GULFING
GULLING
GULPING
HALFDUG
HALOING
HALTING
HALVING
HELMING
HELPING
HELSING
HILLING
HILTING
HOLBERG
HOLDING
HULKING
HULLING
INLYING
JELLING
JILTING
JOLTING
KELLOGG
KILLING
KILNING
KILTING
LALLING
LILTING
LOLLING
LULLING
MALEDOG
MALEHOG
MALEPIG
MALTING
MELDING
MELTING
MILKING
MILLING
MOLDING
MOLTING
MULLING
NULLING
OILRING
PALLING
PALMING
PELTING
PILLBUG
PILLING
POLLING
PULLING
PULPING
PULSING
RDLAING
RELYING
ROLFING
ROLLING
ROLVAAG
SALTING
SALVING
SELLING
SILENTG
SILOING
SILTING
SOLOING
SOLVING
SULKING
TALKBIG
TALKING
TELLING
TILLING
TILTING
TOLLING
UNLYING
VALUING
WALKING
WALLING
WELDING
WELLING
WELTING
WILDDOG
WILDING
WILDPIG
WILLING
WILTING
WOLFDOG
WOLFING
YELLING
YELPING
YULELOG

•••LG••

AMALGAM
COALGAS
FALLGUY
GIELGUD
MYALGIA
MYALGIC
NAILGUN
OTALGIA
OTALGIC

•••L•G•

AIRLOGS
ANALOGS
ANALOGY
APOLOGY
BIOLOGY
BUMLEGS
COLLAGE
COLLEGE
DIALOGS
DOGLEGS
ECOLOGY
ENOLOGY
EPILOGS
GASLOGS
GEOLOGY
HAULAGE
JETLAGS
KELLOGG
MIDLEGS
MILLAGE
MOULAGE
MYOLOGY
NEOLOGY
OROLOGY
OTOLOGY
PEGLEGS
PILLAGE
PROLOGS
RAILAGE
REALIGN
REDLEGS
REFLAGS
SAWLOGS
SCALAGE
SEALEGS
SOILAGE
STALAGS
TILLAGE
TOLLAGE
TRILOGY
UFOLOGY
UNCLOGS
UNPLUGS
UROLOGY
USFLAGS
VILLAGE
VORLAGE
WEBLOGS
ZOOLOGY

•••L••G

ADDLING
AGELONG
AMBLING
ANELING
ANGLING
APPLING
BAILING
BAWLING
BELLING
BIBLIOG
BILLING
BIRLING
BOILING
BOLLING
BORLAUG
BOWLING
BRILLIG
BUGLING
BULLDOG
BULLING
BURLING
CABLING
CALLING
CARLING
CEILING
COALING
COILING
COOLING
COWLING
CULLING
CURLING
CYCLING
DARLING
DAYLONG
DEALING
DIALING
DOLLING
DOWLING
DUELING
DULLING
EAGLING
ENDLONG
ERELONG
EVELONG
EXILING
FABLING
FAILING
FALLING
FATLING
FEELING
FELLING
FILLING
FOALING
FOILING
FOOLING
FOULING
FOWLING
FRELENG
FUELING
FURLING
FURLONG
GALLING
GAOLING
GATLING
GELLING
GILLING
GOALONG
GODLING
GOSLING
GUILING
GULLING
HAILING
HAULING
HEALING
HEELING
HILLING
HOWLING
HOWLONG
HULLING
HURLING
INKLING
JAILING
JELLING
KEELING
KELLOGG
KILLING
KIPLING
LADLING
LALLING
LOLLING
LULLING
MAILBAG
MAILING
MAULING
MCCLURG
MEMLING
MEWLING
MILLING
MOILING
MULLING
NAILING
NAILKEG
NIALONG
NULLING
PALLING
PAULING
PEALING
PEELING
PILLBUG
PILLING
POLLING
POOLING
PROLONG
PULLING
PURLING
RAILING
REELING
RIFLING
ROILING
ROLLING
ROWLING
SAILING
SAPLING
SCALING
SEALING
SELLING
SERLING
SIBLING
SIDLING
SMILING
SOILING
STYLING
SUBLONG
TABLING
TAILING
TAILWAG
TELLING
TILLING
TITLING
TOILING
TOLLING
TOOLING
TOOLONG
UNSLING
UNSLUNG
UPFLING
VEILING
VIALING
WAILING
WALLING
WELLING
WHALING
WHILING
WILLING
WITLING
YELLING
YOWLING

••••LG•

DIVULGE
HIDALGO
INDULGE
REDALGA

••••L•G

ANTILOG
BACKLOG
BOOTLEG
BRILLIG
CATALOG
DECALOG
DOUBLEG
EARPLUG
FORELEG
FROGLEG
GAMELEG
GATELEG
GRAYLAG
GREYLAG
HINDLEG
LASTLEG
LEFTLEG
MAGALOG
MONOLOG
PANTLEG
REDFLAG
SEASLUG
SEMILOG
STARLOG
TAGALOG
TIMELAG
YULELOG

LH•••••

LHASANS

L•H••••

LAHAINA
LCHAYIM
LEHAVRE
LEHIGHU
LEHMANN
LSHAPED

L••H•••

LADHOOD
LASHERS
LASHING
LASHOUT
LASHUPS
LATHERS
LATHERY
LATHING
LECHERS
LEGHORN
LETHAVE
LETHEAN
LEWHOAD
LICHEES
LICHENS
LIGHTED
LIGHTEN
LIGHTER
LIGHTLY
LIGHTON
LIGHTUP
LITHELY
LITHEST
LITHGOW
LITHIUM
LITHOID
LOTHAIR
LOTHIAN
LOTHROP
LOWHAND
LOWHEEL
LUCHINO
LUSHEST
LUSHIER
LUTHIER
LUTHULI

L•••H••

LAKSHMI
LANGHAM
LARCHEN
LARCHES
LATCHED
LATCHES
LATCHON
LAUGHAT
LAUGHED
LAUGHER
LAUGHIN
LEACHED
LEACHER
LEACHES
LEASHED
LEASHES
LEATHER
LEECHED
LEECHEE
LEECHES
LEFTHIP
LITCHIS
LOATHED
LOATHER
LOATHES
LOATHLY
LOATHTO
LOWCHEN
LUNCHED
LUNCHER
LUNCHES
LURCHED
LURCHER
LURCHES

L••••H•

LAROCHE
LAVACHE
LEHIGHU
LENGTHS
LENGTHY
LESOTHO
LOOFAHS

L•••••H

LABTECH
LADDISH
LADYISH
LALOOSH
LAMBETH
LAPPISH
LARGISH
LARKISH
LATIFAH
LAZYISH
LEADETH
LEFTISH
LELOUCH
LETTERH
LETTISH
LISBETH
LOGGISH
LONGISH
LOUDISH
LOUTISH
LOWTECH
LUMPISH

•L•H•••

ALCHEMY
ALLHAIL
ALLHEAL
ALLHERE
ALOHAOE
ALPHARD
ALSHAIN
ALTHING
ALTHORN
ELKHART
FLYHIGH
OLDHAND

•L••H••

ALCOHOL
ALIGHTS
ALLTHAT
ALLTHIS
ALYKHAN
BLATHER
BLIGHTS
BLIGHTY
BLITHER
BLUEHEN
BLUSHED
BLUSHER
BLUSHES
BLUSHON
CLASHED
CLASHER
CLASHES
CLICHED
CLICHES
CLOCHES
CLOTHED
CLOTHES
FLASHED
FLASHER
FLASHES
FLASHON
FLATHAT
FLECHES
FLESHED
FLESHES
FLESHLY
FLIGHTS
FLIGHTY
FLUSHED
FLUSHER
FLUSHES
FLUSHOT
GLASHOW
GLYPHIC
OLDCHAP
OLDSHOE
PLASHED
PLASHES
PLIGHTS
PLUSHER
PLUSHES
PLUSHLY
SLASHED
SLASHER
SLASHES
SLATHER
SLIGHTS
SLITHER
SLOSHED
SLOSHES
SLUSHED
SLUSHES

•L•••H•

ALIYAHS
ALRIGHT
ALYOSHA
BLANCHE
BLOTCHY
CLUTCHY
GLITCHY
PLINTHS
PLOUGHS
SLEIGHS
SLEIGHT
SLEUTHS
SLOUCHY
SLOUGHS

•L••••H

ALANNAH
ALDRICH
ALLCASH
ALSMITH
ALWORTH
BLEMISH
BLUEISH
CLAYISH
ELDRICH
FLEMISH
FLYFISH
FLYHIGH
KLAMATH
KLATSCH
KLENSCH
PLANISH
PLAYDOH
PLENISH
SLAVISH
SLOWISH

••LH•••

ALLHAIL
ALLHEAL
ALLHERE
CALHOUN
MILHAUD
MILHOUS
MULHARE
OILHEAT
WILHELM

••L•H••

ALLTHAT
ALLTHIS
BALIHAI
BELCHED
BELCHER
BELCHES
BELLHOP
BOLSHOI
BULGHUR
COLCHIS
CULCHES
DELIHAM
DELPHIC
DOLPHIN
FELTHAT
FILCHED
FILCHER
FILCHES
FULGHUM
GALAHAD
GULCHES
MALEHOG
MALTHUS
MCLUHAN
MULCHED
MULCHES
RALPHIE
SALCHOW
SILKHAT
SULPHUR
SYLPHIC
WALTHAM
WALTHER
WELLHID
WELLHIT
ZILCHES

••L••H•

BELUSHI
CALIPHS
DALETHS
DELIGHT
EOLITHS
FELLAHS
GULLAHS
HALFSHY
HALVAHS
MALACHI
MULCAHY
MULLAHS
RELIGHT
SPLASHY
TALLYHO

UNLIGHT
UPLIGHT

••L•••H
AALIYAH
ALLCASH
ATLUNCH
BALDISH
BULLISH
BULRUSH
CALTECH
COLDISH
COLTISH
CULTISH
DELILAH
DELRUTH
DOLLISH
DOLTISH
DOLUNCH
DULLISH
FOLKISH
GALUMPH
GOLIATH
HALAVAH
HELLISH
LALOOSH
LELOUCH
NILESOH
OILRICH
ONLEASH
PELTISH
RALEIGH
RELATCH
SALTISH
SELFISH
SILENTH
SPLOTCH
TALLISH
TALLITH
UNLATCH
UNLEASH
UNLOATH
WALLACH
WILDISH
WOLFISH

•••LH••
AGULHAS
BELLHOP
WELLHID
WELLHIT
WOOLHAT

•••L•H•
ADELPHI
ADOLPHE
FELLAHS
GIRLSHY
GULLAHS
HEALTHY
MULLAHS
TALLYHO
WEALTHS
WEALTHY

•••L••H
ABOLISH
BAALISH
BULLISH
CHALLAH
COOLISH
DOLLISH
DULLISH
EHRLICH
ENGLISH
EYELASH
FOOLISH
GAULISH
GIRLISH
GOULASH
HELLISH
HIALEAH
NEOLITH
OPALISH
OUTLASH
PUBLISH
STYLISH
TALLISH
TALLITH
TWELFTH
WALLACH

••••L•H
CHALLAH
DELILAH
DOUBLEH
QABALAH
RUDOLPH
SQUELCH
STEALTH

•••••LH
ANOUILH

LI•••••
LIAISED
LIAISES
LIAISON
LIBBERS
LIBBING
LIBELED
LIBELEE
LIBELER
LIBERAL
LIBERIA
LIBERTE
LIBERTY
LIBIDOS
LIBRANS
LIBRARY
LIBYANS
LICENCE
LICENSE
LICHEES
LICHENS
LICITLY
LICKERS
LICKETY
LICKING
LICKSUP
LIDLESS
LIDWINA
LIEABED
LIEATOP
LIEBACK
LIEDFOR
LIEDOWN
LIEFEST
LIENEES
LIENORS
LIEOVER
LIESFOR
LIESLOW
LIETEST
LIFEFUL
LIFENET
LIFTERS
LIFTING
LIFTOFF
LIFTSUP
LIGANDS
LIGATED
LIGATES
LIGGETT
LIGHTED
LIGHTEN
LIGHTER
LIGHTLY
LIGHTON
LIGHTUP
LIGNIFY
LIGNINS
LIGNITE
LIGURIA
LIKABLE
LIKEICE
LIKEMAD
LIKENED
LIKENEW
LIKENTO
LIKEWOW
LIKINGS
LILALEE
LILETEE
LILINAU
LILLIAN
LILTING
LILYPAD
LIMACON
LIMBERS
LIMBING
LIMBURG
LIMEADE
LIMEPIE
LIMIEST
LIMINAL
LIMITED
LIMITER
LIMNERS
LIMNING
LIMNITE
LIMOGES
LIMPEST
LIMPETS
LIMPING
LIMPOPO
LINABLE
LINAGES
LINBIAO
LINCOLN
LINDENS
LINDIED
LINDIES
LINDNER
LINDORF
LINDROS
LINDSAY
LINDSEY
LINEAGE
LINEARA
LINEARB
LINEATE
LINECUT
LINEDRY
LINEDUP
LINEMAN
LINEMEN
LINEONE
LINEOUT
LINESUP
LINETWO
LINEUPS
LINGCOD
LINGERS
LINGOES
LINGUAE
LINGUAL
LINGULA
LINIEST
LININGS
LINKAGE
LINKERS
LINKING
LINKSUP
LINKUPS
LINNETS
LINPIAO
LINSEED
LINTELS
LINTERS
LINTIER
LINTING
LIONCUB
LIONELL
LIONELS
LIONESS
LIONETS
LIONISE
LIONIZE
LIPARIS
LIPASES
LIPBALM
LIPIDIC
LIPLESS
LIPLIKE
LIPMANN
LIPPERS
LIPPIER
LIPPING
LIPREAD
LIPSOFF
LIPSOUT
LIPSYNC
LIQUATE
LIQUEFY
LIQUEUR
LIQUIDS
LIQUORS
LISAGAY
LISBETH
LISENTE
LISPERS
LISPING
LISSOME
LISTEES
LISTENS
LISTERS
LISTING
LITCHIS
LITCRIT
LITERAL
LITHELY
LITHEST
LITHGOW
LITHIUM
LITHOID
LITINTO
LITOTES
LITOVSK
LITTERS
LITTERY
LITTLER
LITTLES
LITURGY
LIVABLE
LIVEAID
LIVEDIN
LIVEDON
LIVEFOR
LIVENED
LIVENER
LIVENUP
LIVEOAK
LIVEONE
LIVEOUT
LIVERED
LIVESAT
LIVESET
LIVESEY
LIVESIN
LIVESON
LIVIDLY
LIVINGS
LIVORNO
LIZARDS
LIZETTE
LIZZIES

L•I••••
LAICIZE
LAIDFOR
LAIDLOW
LAIDOFF
LAIDOUT
LAIRING
LAISSEZ
LAITIES
LEIBNIZ
LEIPZIG
LEISTER
LEISURE
LEITRIM
LOIDING
LOITERS
LYINGBY
LYINGON
LYINGTO
LYINGUP

L••I•••
LABIALS
LABIATE
LACIEST
LACINGS
LADIDAS
LADINGS
LADINOS
LAFITTE
LAKIEST
LAKISTS
LALIQUE
LAMINAE
LAMINAL
LAMINAR
LAMINAS
LAMINTO
LARIATS
LATICES
LATIFAH
LATIGOS
LATIMES
LATINAS
LATINII
LATINOS
LATINUS
LAVINIA
LAYINTO
LAYITON
LAZIEST
LEDINTO
LEGIBLE
LEGIBLY
LEGIONS
LEGIRON
LEGISTS
LEHIGHU
LEMIEUX
LENIENT
LEPIDUS
LESIONS
LETINON
LETITBE
LETITGO
LETITIA
LEVIERS
LEVILLI
LEVITES
LEVITIC
LEXICAL
LEXICON
LEXISES
LIAISED
LIAISES
LIAISON
LIBIDOS
LICITLY
LIKINGS
LILINAU
LIMIEST
LIMINAL
LIMITED
LIMITER
LINIEST
LININGS
LIPIDIC
LITINTO
LIVIDLY
LIVINGS
LOGICAL
LOGIEST
LONIGAN
LORIENT
LORISES
LOSINGS
LOTIONS
LOUISII
LOUISIV
LOUISIX
LOUISVI
LOUISXI
LOUISXV
LUCIANA
LUCIANO
LUCIDAE
LUCIDLY
LUCIFER
LUCILLE
LUCINDA
LUCITES
LUCIUSI
LUMIERE
LUMINAS
LUPINES
LURIDLY
LUTISTS
LYRICAL
LYRICON
LYRISTS

L•••I••
LABMICE
LACKING
LACRIMO
LADDIES
LADDISH
LADLING
LADYISH
LAGGING
LAHAINA
LAICIZE
LAIRING
LAITIES
LALLING
LAMAISM
LAMAIST
LAMBING
LAMMING
LANCIAS
LANCING
LANDING
LANDINI
LANKIER
LANKILY
LANSING
LANVINS
LAOTIAN
LAPPING
LAPPISH
LAPSING
LAPWING
LARAINE
LARDIER
LARDING
LARGISH
LARKIER
LARKING
LARKINS
LARKISH
LASHING
LASSIES
LASTING
LATHING
LATRINE
LATTICE
LATVIAN
LAUDING
LAURITZ
LAVAINE
LAWLIKE
LAZYISH
LEADIER
LEADING
LEADINS
LEAFIER
LEAFING
LEAKIER
LEAKING
LEANING
LEAPING
LEASING
LEAVING
LEDGIER
LEERIER
LEERILY
LEERING
LEETIDE
LEFTIES
LEFTISH
LEFTISM
LEFTIST
LEGGIER
LEGGING
LEGLIKE
LEMMING
LEMPIRA
LENDING
LENTIGO
LENTILS
LEONIDS
LEONINE
LEOVIII
LEOXIII
LESSING
LETLIVE
LETRIDE
LETTING
LETTISH
LEUCINE
LEVYING
LIBBING
LICKING
LIDWINA
LIFTING
LIGNIFY
LIGNINS
LIGNITE
LIKEICE
LILLIAN
LILTING
LIMBING
LIMNING
LIMNITE
LIMPING
LINBIAO
LINDIED
LINDIES
LINKING
LINPIAO
LINTIER
LINTING
LIONISE
LIONIZE
LIPLIKE
LIPPIER
LIPPING
LIQUIDS
LISPING
LISTING
LITHIUM
LIZZIES
LOADING
LOAFING
LOAMIER
LOAMING
LOANING
LOBBIED
LOBBIES
LOBBING
LOCKING
LOCKINS
LODGING
LOFTIER
LOFTILY
LOFTING
LOGGIAS
LOGGING
LOGGINS
LOGGISH
LOIDING
LOLLIES
LOLLING
LONGIES
LONGING
LONGISH
LOOBIES
LOOKING
LOOKINS
LOOKISM
LOOKIST
LOOMING
LOONIER
LOONIES
LOONILY
LOOPIER
LOOPING
LOOSING
LOOTING
LOPPIER
LOPPING
LORDING
LORRIES
LOTHIAN
LOTTING
LOUDISH
LOURING
LOUSIER
LOUSILY
LOUSING
LOUTING
LOUTISH
LOVEINS
LOWBIDS
LOWDIVE
LOWLIER
LOWLIFE
LOWLILY
LOWRISE
LOWRISK
LOWSIDE
LOWTIDE
LUCHINO
LUCKIER
LUCKILY
LUCKING
LUDDISM
LUDDITE
LUFFING
LUGGING
LULLING
LUMPIER
LUMPILY
LUMPING
LUMPISH
LUNGING
LURKING
LUSHIER
LUSTIER
LUSTILY
LUSTING
LUTHIER
LYDDITE

L••••I•
LACKWIT
LACONIA
LACONIC
LACTAID
LADYKIN
LAMBKIN
LAMPLIT
LAMPOIL
LANGUID
LANOLIN
LARAMIE
LATINII
LAUGHIN
LAVINIA
LAVORIS
LAWSUIT
LCHAYIM
LEADSIN
LEAKSIN
LEANSIN
LEAPSIN
LEAPTIN
LEAVEIN
LEAVEIT
LECTRIC
LEFTHIP
LEIBNIZ
LEIPZIG
LEITRIM
LEOVIII
LEOXIII
LESTOIL
LETEMIN
LETITIA
LETMEIN
LETSLIP
LETSRIP
LEVITIC
LEXUSIS
LIBERIA
LIGURIA
LIMEPIE
LIPARIS
LIPIDIC
LITCHIS
LITCRIT
LITHOID
LIVEAID
LIVEDIN
LIVESIN
LOADSIN
LOCKLIN
LOCKSIN
LODGEIN
LOOKSIN
LORDJIM
LORDSIT
LOSEBIG
LOSESIT
LOSTBIG
LOTHAIR
LOUISII
LOUISIV
LOUISIX
LOVEDIT
LOVESIT
LOWPAID
LOWPAIR
LUCANIA
LUCYLIU
LUGSAIL
LUMPSIN
LUMPSIT
LUNATIC
LUREDIN
LURESIN
LUTETIA

L•••••I
LAKSHMI
LANDINI
LATINII
LAVELLI
LAZZERI
LEOVIII
LEOXIII
LETTERI
LEVILLI
LORELAI
LORELEI
LOUISII
LOUISVI
LOUISXI
LUCIUSI
LUTHULI

•LI••••
ALIASES
ALIBABA
ALIBIED
ALIDADE
ALIENEE
ALIENOR
ALIENTO
ALIFORM
ALIGHTS
ALIGNED
ALIGNER
ALIGOTE
ALIMENT
ALIMONY
ALINERS
ALINING
ALITTLE
ALIVETO
ALIYAHS
BLIGHTS
BLIGHTY
BLIMPIE
BLINDED
BLINDER
BLINDLY
BLINDTO
BLINKAT
BLINKED
BLINKER
BLINTZE
BLIPPED
BLISSED
BLISSES
BLISTER
BLITHER
BLITZED
BLITZEN
BLITZER
BLITZES
CLIBURN
CLICHED
CLICHES
CLICKED
CLICKER
CLICKON
CLIENTS
CLIFTON
CLIMATE
CLIMATS
CLIMBED
CLIMBER
CLIMBIN
CLIMBON
CLIMBTO
CLIMBUP
CLINGER
CLINGTO
CLINICS
CLINKED
CLINKER
CLINTON
CLIPART
CLIPOFF
CLIPONS
CLIPOUT
CLIPPED
CLIPPER
CLIPSON
CLIQUED
CLIQUES
CLIQUEY
ELICITS
ELIDERS
ELIDING
ELIEZER
ELIGIUS
ELISION
ELITEST
ELITISM
ELITIST
ELIXIRS
ELIYALE
FLICKED
FLICKER
FLIEDTO
FLIESAT
FLIESBY
FLIESIN
FLIESON
FLIESTO
FLIESUP
FLIGHTS
FLIGHTY
FLINGAT
FLINGER
FLINTMI
FLIPOUT
FLIPPED
FLIPPEN
FLIPPER
FLIPTOP
FLIPUPS
FLIRTED
FLIRTER
FLITSBY
FLITSIN
FLITTED
FLITTER
FLIVVER
GLIBBER
GLIDEBY
GLIDEIN
GLIDERS
GLIDING
GLIMMER
GLIMPSE
GLINTED
GLISTEN
GLISTER
GLITCHY
GLITTER
GLITZED
GLITZES
ILIADIC
ILIAMNA
ILIESCU
ILIKEIT
KLINGER
KLINGON
KLINKER
KLISTER
OLICOOK
OLIVIER
OLIVINE
PLIABLE
PLIABLY
PLIANCY
PLICATE
PLIGHTS
PLINKED
PLINTHS
PLISSES
SLICERS

SLICEUP
SLICING
SLICKED
SLICKER
SLICKLY
SLIDEBY
SLIDEIN
SLIDERS
SLIDING
SLIDOFF
SLIDOUT
SLIGHTS
SLIMIER
SLIMILY
SLIMING
SLIMJIM
SLIMMED
SLIMMER
SLINGER
SLINKED
SLINKER
SLINKIN
SLINKUP
SLIPOFF
SLIPONS
SLIPOUT
SLIPPED
SLIPPER
SLIPSBY
SLIPSIN
SLIPSON
SLIPSUP
SLIPUPS
SLITHER
SLITTED
SLITTER
SLIVERS
TLINGIT

•L•I•••

ALBINOS
ALBIREO
ALFIERI
ALGIEBA
ALGIERS
ALLISON
ALLIUMS
ALNICOS
ALNILAM
ALNITAK
ALNIYAT
ALPINER
ALPINES
ALRIGHT
ALTIMAS
BLUINGS
CLAIMED
CLAIMER
CLAIROL
ELAINES
ELEISON
ELLIOTT
ELLIPSE
ELLISON
ELMIEST
ELMISTI
ELNINOS
FLAILAT
FLAILED
FLUIDAL
FLUIDIC
FLUIDLY
FLYINTO
GLUIEST
ILLICIT
KLEIBER
KLEISER
PLAICES
PLAINER
PLAINES
PLAINLY
PLAINTS
PLAISIR
PLAITED
PLAITER
SLEIGHS
SLEIGHT
SLUICED
SLUICES
ULTIMAS

•L••I••

ALADINE
ALAKING
ALANINE
ALAYING
ALCAIDE
ALDRICH
ALEWIFE
ALIBIED
ALINING
ALLMINE
ALLRISE
ALLTIED
ALLTIME
ALLWISE
ALLYING
ALQUIST
ALSMITH
ALTHING
ALTOIDS
ALTOIST
ALUMINA
BLADING
BLAMING
BLARING
BLAZING
BLEMISH
BLERIOT
BLOWIER
BLOWING
BLUEICE
BLUEING
BLUEISH
CLARICE
CLARIFY
CLARION
CLARITY
CLAVIER
CLAWING
CLAYIER
CLAYING
CLAYISH
CLERICS
CLERISY
CLEWING
CLINICS
CLONING
CLOSING
CLOYING
CLUEING
ELAAIUN
ELAMITE
ELAPIDS
ELATING
ELATION
ELDRICH
ELDRICK
ELEGIAC
ELEGIES
ELEGIST
ELEGITS
ELEGIZE
ELENIAK
ELFLIKE
ELICITS
ELIDING
ELIGIUS
ELISION
ELITISM
ELITIST
ELIXIRS
ELMCITY
ELOPING
ELUDING
ELUSIVE
ELUTING
ELUTION
ELUVIAL
ELUVIUM
ELYSIAN
ELYSIUM
FLAKIER
FLAKILY
FLAKING
FLAMIER
FLAMING
FLARING
FLAVIUS
FLAWIER
FLAWING
FLAXIER
FLAYING
FLEEING
FLEMING
FLEMISH
FLEXILE
FLEXING
FLEXION
FLORIAN
FLORIDA
FLORINS
FLORIST
FLOWING
FLUKIER
FLUKILY
FLUTIER
FLUTIES
FLUTING
FLUTIST
FLUVIAL
FLUXING
FLUXION
FLYFISH
FLYGIRL
FLYHIGH
FLYTIER
GLACIAL
GLACIER
GLARING
GLAVINE
GLAZIER
GLAZILY
GLAZING
GLIDING
GLOBING
GLOBINS
GLORIAS
GLORIED
GLORIES
GLORIFY
GLOVING
GLOWING
GLYCINE
ILLBITE
ILLLIVE
ILLWILL
ILLWIND
OLAFIII
OLAVIII
OLDCITY
OLDFILM
OLDGIRL
OLDLINE
OLDNICK
OLDTIME
OLEFINS
OLEMISS
OLIVIER
OLIVINE
OLOGIES
PLACIDO
PLACING
PLANING
PLANISH
PLATIER
PLATIES
PLATING
PLAYING
PLEBIAN
PLENISH
PLOSION
PLOSIVE
PLOWING
PLUGINS
PLUMIER
PLUMING
PLUVIAL
RLSTINE
SLAKING
SLATIER
SLATING
SLAVING
SLAVISH
SLAYING
SLEWING
SLICING
SLIDING
SLIMIER
SLIMILY
SLIMING
SLOPING
SLOWING
SLOWISH

•L•••I•

ALADDIN
ALAMEIN
ALBANIA
ALBENIZ
ALBUMIN
ALDAVIS
ALDUBIN
ALEGRIA
ALEMBIC
ALGERIA
ALKALIS
ALLELIC
ALLEWIS
ALLHAIL
ALLOFIT
ALLOWIN
ALLTHIS
ALLUVIA
ALMERIA
ALSATIA
ALSHAIN
BLACKIE
BLENDIN
BLENTIN
BLIMPIE
BLONDIE
BLOWNIN
BLOWSIN
BLOWSIT
BLUEFIN
BLUETIT
CLAMDIP
CLASSIC
CLAUDIA
CLAUDIO
CLAYPIT
CLIMBIN
CLOCKIN
CLOSEIN
CLUEDIN
CLUESIN
ELASTIC
ELASTIN
ELTRAIN
FLACCID
FLEADIP
FLEAPIT
FLIESIN
FLITSIN
FLOORIT
FLOSSIE
FLOWNIN
FLOWSIN
FLUIDIC
GLIDEIN
GLOAMIN
GLOBOID
GLOTTIS
GLYNNIS
GLYPHIC
GLYPTIC
ILIADIC
ILIKEIT
ILLDOIT
ILLEGIT
ILLICIT
ILLOGIC
ILLYRIA
ILOSTIT
ILOVEIT
OLAFIII
OLAVIII
OLDMAID
OLEOOIL
OLYMPIA
OLYMPIC
PLAISIR
PLASMIC
PLASTIC
PLAUDIT
PLOVDIV
PLUGSIN
PLUMBIC
PLUMPIE
SLATKIN
SLEEPIN
SLEPTIN
SLIDEIN
SLIMJIM
SLINKIN
SLIPSIN
SLOEGIN
SLUNKIN
TLINGIT

•L••••I

ALBERTI
ALEARDI
ALEKSEI
ALFIERI
ALVEOLI
ELMISTI
FLINTMI
OLAFIII
OLAVIII
OLDUVAI
PLATYPI
PLOESTI

••LI•••

AALIYAH
ALLISON
ALLIUMS
APLITES
BALIHAI
BCLIONS
BELIEFS
BELIERS
BELIEVE
BELINDA
BILIOUS
BKLIBAN
BOLIDES
BOLIVAR
BOLIVIA
BYLINED
BYLINER
BYLINES
CALIBAN
CALIBER
CALIBRE
CALICES
CALICOS
CALIPER
CALIPHS
CALISTA
CELICAS
CILIARY
CILIATE
COLICKY
DELIBES
DELICTI
DELICTO
DELICTS
DELIGHT
DELIHAM
DELILAH
DELILLO
DELIMAN
DELIMEN
DELIMIT
DELINTS
DELIRIA
DELISTS
DELIVER
ECLIPSE
EELIEST
EGLISES
ELLIOTT
ELLIPSE
ELLISON
ENLINKS
ENLISTS
ENLIVEN
EOLITHS
FELICIA
FELINES
FILIBEG
FILINGS
FILIPPO
FOLIAGE
FOLIATE
FOLIOED
FOLIOSE
GALICIA
GALILEE
GALILEI
GALILEO
GELIDLY
GOLIATH
HALIBUT
HALIDES
HALIFAX
HALITES
HELICAL
HELICES
HELICON
HELIPAD
HELIXES
HOLIDAY
HOLIEST
HOLISTS
ILLICIT
INLIMBO
INLINES
JALISCO
JULIANA
KALININ
LALIQUE
LILINAU
MALIANS
MALICES
MALIGNS
MELINDA
MELISMA
MELISSA
MELITTA
MILIEUS
MILIEUX
MILITIA
MOLIERE
MOLITOR
NOLIMIT
OBLIGED
OBLIGEE
OBLIGER
OBLIGES
OBLIGOR
OBLIQUE
OILIEST
ONLIEST
OOLITES
OOLITIC
OWLIEST
PALINGS
PELICAN
PELISSE
PILINGS
POLICED
POLICER
POLICES
POLISCI
POLITER
POLITIC
RELIANT
RELICTS
RELIEFS
RELIERS
RELIEVE
RELIGHT
RELIMIT
RELINED
RELINES
RELINKS
RELISTS
RELIVED
RELIVES
RILIEVO
RULIEST
RULINGS
SALIENT
SALIERI
SALINAS
SALINES
SALIVAS
SILICAS
SILICON
SOLICIT
SOLIDER
SOLIDLY
SPLICED
SPLICER
SPLICES
SPLINES
SPLINTS
SPLITUP
TALIBAN
TILINGS
UGLIEST
UNLIGHT
UNLIKED
UNLIKES
UNLINED
UNLINKS
UNLIVED
UNLIVES
UPLIFTS
UPLIGHT
UPLINKS
VALIANT
VALIDID
VALIDLY
VALINES
VALISES
WILIEST

••L•I••

ALLMINE
ALLRISE
ALLTIED
ALLTIME
ALLWISE
ALLYING
BALDIES
BALDING
BALDISH
BALKIER
BALKILY
BALKING
BALLIOL
BALMIER
BALMILY
BELAIRS
BELGIAN
BELGIUM
BELLIED
BELLIES
BELLING
BELLINI
BELTING
BELYING
BILGIER
BILKING
BILLIES
BILLING
BILLION
BOLLING
BOLTING
BULGIER
BULGING
BULKIER
BULKING
BULLIED
BULLIES
BULLING
BULLINS
BULLION
BULLISH
BULLITT
CALCIFY
CALCITE
CALCIUM
CALKING
CALKINS
CALLING
CALLINS
CALMING
CALVING
CALVINO
CELLINI
CELLIST
CELSIUS
CELTICS
COLDISH
COLLIDE
COLLIER
COLLIES
COLLINE
COLLINS
COLTISH
CULLIED
CULLIES
CULLING
CULTISH
CULTISM
CULTIST
DALLIED
DALLIER
DALLIES
DELCITY
DELEING
DELUISE
DELVING
DILLIES
DOLLIED
DOLLIES
DOLLING
DOLLISH
DOLTISH
DULCIFY
DULLING
DULLISH
ECLAIRS
EELLIKE
FALKIRK
FALLING
FALSIFY
FALSITY
FELLING
FELLINI
FELTILL
FELTING
FILLIES
FILLING
FILLINS
FILLIPS
FILMIER
FILMILY
FILMING
FOLDING
FOLKIER
FOLKIES
FOLKISH
FOLLIES
FULFILL
FULFILS
GALLICO
GALLING
GALLIUM
GELDING
GELLING
GILDING
GILLIAM
GILLIAN
GILLING
GOLDING
GOLFING
GULFING
GULLIED
GULLIES
GULLING
GULPIER
GULPING
HALFIES
HALOIDS
HALOING
HALTING
HALVING
HELLION
HELLISH
HELMING
HELOISE
HELPING
HELSING
HILAIRE
HILLIER
HILLING
HILTING
HOLDING
HOLLIES
HOLMIUM
HULKIER
HULKING
HULLING
ILLBITE
ILLLIVE
ILLWILL
ILLWIND
INLYING
JELLIED
JELLIES
JELLIFY
JELLING
JILLIAN
JILLION
JILTING
JOLLIED
JOLLIER
JOLLIES
JOLLIET
JOLLIFY
JOLLILY
JOLLITY
JOLTIER
JOLTING
KELPIES
KELVINS
KILLING
KILNING
KILTIES
KILTING
LALLING
LILLIAN
LILTING
LOLLIES
LOLLING
LULLING
MALAISE
MALDIVE
MALLIKA
MALTIER
MALTING
MALVINA
MELDING
MELTING
MILKIER
MILKILY
MILKING
MILLIME
MILLING
MILLION
MOLDIER
MOLDING
MOLLIES
MOLLIFY
MOLTING
MULLING
MULLINS
NULLIFY
NULLING
NULLITY
OILBIRD
OILLIKE
OILLINE
OILRICH
OILRIGS
OILRING
OWLLIKE
PALLIER
PALLING
PALMIER
PALMING
PALMIST
PELTING
PELTISH
PILLING
PILLION
POLLING
POLOIST
PULLING
PULLINS
PULPIER
PULPIFY
PULPING
PULPITS
PULSING
RALEIGH
RALLIED
RALLIER
RALLIES
RDLAING
RELYING
ROLAIDS
ROLFING
ROLLICK
ROLLING
ROLLINS
SALLIED
SALLIER
SALLIES
SALTIER
SALTILY
SALTINE
SALTING
SALTISH
SALVING
SELFISH
SELKIRK
SELLING
SILKIER
SILKILY
SILLIER
SILLIES
SILOING
SILTIER
SILTING
SOLDIER
SOLOING
SOLOIST
SOLVING
SULFIDE
SULFITE
SULKIER
SULKIES
SULKILY
SULKING
SULLIED
SULLIES
TALKIER
TALKIES
TALKING
TALLIED
TALLIER
TALLIES
TALLINN
TALLISH
TALLITH
TELLIES
TELLING
TILLING
TILSITS
TILTING
TOLKIEN
TOLLING
UNLYING
VALMIKI
VALUING
VILNIUS
VULPINE
WALKING
WALKINS
WALLING
WELDING
WELLING
WELTING
WILDING
WILDISH
WILKINS
WILLIAM
WILLIES
WILLING
WILTING
WOLFING
WOLFISH
YELLING
YELPING
ZILLION

••L••I•

AELFRIC
ALLELIC
ALLEWIS
ALLHAIL
ALLOFIT
ALLOWIN
ALLTHIS
ALLUVIA
BALDRIC

BALDWIN BALMAIN BELVOIR BOLATIE BOLIVIA BOLOTIE CALLSIN CALLSIT CALORIC CALORIE CHLORIC COLCHIS COLLOID CSLEWIS CULPRIT DALASIS DELIMIT DELIRIA DELORIS DELPHIC DELTAIC DELTOID DOLPHIN EELSKIN FALLSIN FELICIA FELTTIP FILEDIN FILESIN FILLSIN FOLDSIN GALATIA GALAXIE GALICIA GELATIN GELATIS GELUSIL GOLDTIP GULFOIL HALFWIT HELPSIN HOLBEIN HOLDSIN HOLDSIT HOLYOIL ILLDOIT ILLEGIT ILLICIT ILLOGIC ILLYRIA ISLAMIC KALININ KILOBIT MALARIA MALEFIC MALEPIG MALTBIE MELANIA MELANIC MELANIE MELANIN MELODIA MELODIC MILITIA MILLAIS NOLIMIT OILSKIN OOLITIC

PALADIN PALMOIL PELAGIC PILEDIN PILESIN PILGRIM POLARIS POLEMIC POLESIT POLITIC POLONIA PULLPIN PULLSIN RALPHIE RELIMIT ROLLEIS ROLLSIN SALADIN SALAMIS SALTPIT SALUKIS SELENIC SELLSIT SILESIA SILKTIE SOLARIA SOLICIT SOLVEIT STLOUIS STLUCIA SYLPHIC TALARIA TALKBIG TELAVIV TELEPIC TELEPIX TELLSIT UNLUCID UNLYRIC VALERIE VALIDID VILLAIN VILLEIN VOLTAIC WALLSIN WELLHID WELLHIT WELLLIT WILDPIG WILLKIE YELTSIN

••L•••I

BALIHAI BELLINI BELUSHI BELZONI BOLSHOI BULGARI CALCULI CELLINI COLLODI COLOSSI DELICTI FELLINI GALILEI GALVANI GOLDONI

MALACHI MOLOKAI PALAZZI PILEGGI POLANYI POLISCI POLYSCI PULASKI PULMONI SALIERI SILENTI SOLLATI SYLLABI TOLSTOI VALENTI VALMIKI VILLARI

•••LI••

ABILITY ABOLISH ACTLIKE ADDLING ADELIES ADELINA ADELINE AEOLIAN AFFLICT AGILITY AIRLIFT AIRLIKE AIRLINE AMBLING AMPLIFY ANELING ANGLING ANILINE ANILITY ANTLIKE ANTLION APELIKE APPLIED APPLIER APPLIES APPLING APULIAN ARMLIKE ASSLIKE ATELIER AXELIKE BAALISH BAALISM BAALIST BAALITE BADLIES BAGLIKE BAILIFF BAILING BALLIOL BARLICK BATLIKE BAWLING BEALION BEDLIKE BEELIKE BEELINE BELLIED BELLIES

BELLING BELLINI BERLIOZ BERLITZ BIALIES BIBLIKE BIBLIOG BIGLIES BILLIES BILLING BILLION BIOLITE BIRLING BOILING BOLLING BOWLIKE BOWLINE BOWLING BOXLIKE BOYLIKE BUDLIKE BUGLING BULLIED BULLIES BULLING BULLINS BULLION BULLISH BULLITT BURLIER BURLING BUSLINE CABLING CALLING CALLINS CARLING CATLIKE CEILING CELLINI CELLIST CHALICE CHILIAD CHILIES CHOLINE COALING COILING COLLIDE COLLIER COLLIES COLLINE COLLINS COOLIES COOLING COOLISH COWLICK COWLIKE COWLING CULLIED CULLIES CULLING CUPLIKE CURLIER CURLIKE CURLING CYCLING CYCLIST DAHLIAS DAILIES

DALLIED DALLIER DALLIES DARLING DAYLILY DEALING DECLINE DEWLINE DIALING DIDLIKE DILLIES DISLIKE DOGLIKE DOILIES DOLLIED DOLLIES DOLLING DOLLISH DOOLIES DOTLIKE DOWLING DUALISM DUALIST DUALITY DUALIZE DUELING DUELIST DULLING DULLISH DUNLINS EAGLING EARLIER EARLIES EARLIKE EELLIKE EGALITE EGGLIKE EHRLICH ELFLIKE ENDLINE ENGLISH EONLINE ETALIBI EXILING EYELIDS EYELIFT EYELIKE EYELINE FABLING FADLIKE FAILING FALLING FANLIKE FATLIKE FATLING FATLIPS FEELILL FEELING FELLING FELLINI FILLIES FILLING FILLINS FILLIPS FINLIKE FOALING FOILING FOLLIES

FOOLING FOOLISH FORLIFE FOULING FOWLING FOXLIKE FROLICS FTBLISS FUELING FURLING GAGLINE GALLICO GALLING GALLIUM GAOLING GARLICS GARLITS GASLINE GATLING GATLINS GAULISH GELLING GEMLIKE GILLIAM GILLIAN GILLING GIRLIER GIRLIES GIRLISH GOALIES GOBLINS GODLIER GODLIKE GODLING GOSLING GROLIER GUILING GULLIED GULLIES GULLING GUMLIKE HAGLIKE HAILING HAMLINE HARLINE HATLIKE HAULING HAZLITT HEALING HEELING HELLION HELLISH HEMLINE HENLIKE HILLIER HILLING HIPLIKE HITLIST HOGLIKE HOLLIES HOPLITE HOTLICK HOTLINE HOTLINK HOTLIPS HOWLING HULLING HUNLIKE

HURLING HUTLIKE HYALITE IBILITY ICELIKE ICELINE IDOLISE IDOLIST IDOLIZE IDYLIST ILLLIVE IMPLIED IMPLIES INALINE INCLINE INFLICT INKLIKE INKLING ISOLINE ITALIAN ITALICS IVYLIKE JAILING JAMLIKE JAWLIKE JAWLINE JELLIED JELLIES JELLIFY JELLING JIGLIKE JILLIAN JILLION JOLLIED JOLLIER JOLLIES JOLLIET JOLLIFY JOLLILY JOLLITY JOWLIER KEELING KEYLIME KIDLIKE KILLING KIPLING LADLING LALLING LAWLIKE LEGLIKE LETLIVE LILLIAN LIPLIKE LOLLIES LOLLING LOWLIER LOWLIFE LOWLILY LULLING MADLIBS MAILING MAILINS MALLIKA MANLIER MANLIKE MARLIER MARLINS MAULING

MEALIER MEALIES MEMLING MERLINS METLIFE MEWLING MGMLION MIDLIFE MIDLINE MIDLIST MILLIME MILLING MILLION MISLIKE MOILING MOLLIES MOLLIFY MRBLISS MULLING MULLINS MUSLIMS MUSLINS NAILING NBALIVE NEOLITH NETLIKE NEWLIFE NEWLINE NIBLICK NIBLIKE NONLIFE NONLIVE NOTLIKE NOTLIVE NUCLIDE NULLIFY NULLING NULLITY NUNLIKE NUTLIKE OAKLIKE OARLIKE OATLIKE OBELISE OBELISK OBELIZE OCULIST OFFLINE OILLIKE OILLINE OLDLINE ONALINE ONELIRA OPALINE OPALISH ORALIST ORBLIKE OUTLIER OUTLIES OUTLIMN OUTLINE OUTLIPS OUTLIVE OWLLIKE PALLIER PALLING PAMLICO PAULIII

PAULINA PAULINE PAULING PAULIST PEALIKE PEALING PEELING PEGLIKE PENLIKE PENLITE PERLITE PETLION PHILIPK PHILIPS PHILIPV PIELIKE PIGLIKE PILLING PILLION PIMLICO PODLIKE POLLING POOLING POPLINS POTLIDS PRALINE PRELIFE PRELIMS PROLIFE PUBLICS PUBLISH PUBLIUS PULLING PULLINS PURLIEU PURLING QUALIFY QUALITY RAILING RALLIED RALLIER RALLIES RAMLIKE RATLIKE RATLINE RATLINS RAWLINS RAYLIKE REALIGN REALINE REALISE REALISM REALIST REALITY REALIZE RECLIMB RECLINE REDLINE REELING REFLIES REFLIPS REPLICA REPLIED REPLIER REPLIES RIBLIKE RIFLING RODLIKE

ROILIER ROILING ROLLICK ROLLING ROLLINS ROWLING RUGLIKE SACLIKE SAILING SALLIED SALLIER SALLIES SAPLING SAWLIKE SCALIER SCALING SCHLITZ SEALIFE SEALIFT SEALIKE SEALILY SEALING SEALION SELLING SERLING SHALIER SIBLING SIDLING SILLIER SILLIES SINLIKE SKILIFT SKYLIKE SKYLINE SMILING SOILING SONLIKE SOWLIKE STELIAS STYLING STYLISE STYLISH STYLIST STYLIZE SUBLIDS SUBLIME SULLIED SULLIES SUNLIKE SURLIER SURLILY TABLING TAGLIKE TAGLINE TAILING TALLIED TALLIER TALLIES TALLINN TALLISH TALLITH TANLINE TBILISI TELLIES TELLING THELIKE THULIUM TIELINE

TILLING TINLIKE TIPLINE TITLING TITLIST TOELIKE TOILING TOLLING TOOLING TOPLINE TOWLINE TOYLIKE TSELIOT TUBLIKE UGOLINO UNALIKE UNCLIPS UNCLIPT UNPLIED UNSLICK UNSLIER UNSLING UPCLIMB UPFLING URNLIKE UTILISE UTILITY UTILIZE VANLINE VEALIER VEILING VIALING VIOLINS VIOLIST WAILING WALLING WARLIKE WAXLIKE WEBLIKE WELLING WHALING WHILING WIGLIKE WILLIAM WILLIES WILLING WITLING WOOLIER WOOLIES WOOLITE YELLING YOWLING ZILLION

•••L•I•

ACCLAIM ANGLAIS BRILLIG BUILDIN BUILTIN CALLSIN CALLSIT CHALCIS CHILLIS COALBIN COALOIL COALPIT COLLOID

COOLAIR COOLPIX COOLSIT CURLSIN CYCLOID DEALSIN DEALTIN DECLAIM DIALSIN DIPLOID DWELLIN EXCLAIM EXPLAIN EXPLOIT FALLSIN FILLSIN FOULTIP FUELOIL HAPLOID HAULSIN HYALOID IDYLLIC KJELLIN KOOLAID MAILBIN MAILSIN MAULDIN MILLAIS MISLAID MYALGIA MYALGIC NAILSIN NAILSIT NAILTIP NEWLAID NUCLEIC OTALGIA OTALGIC OUTLAID OUTLAIN PAULIII PHILBIN PHILLIE PHILLIP PHYLLIS PSALMIC PULLPIN PULLSIN PURLOIN RECLAIM REELSIN ROLLEIS ROLLSIN SEALSIN SELLSIT SHELTIE SIRLOIN STOLEIN TABLOID TAILFIN TAILPIN TELLSIT TOOLKIT TRELLIS TRILLIN UNFLUID UNPLAIT UNSLAIN

VILLAIN VILLEIN WALLSIN WAYLAID WELLHID WELLHIT WELLLIT WILLKIE YOPLAIT

•••L••I

ADELPHI BELLINI CELLINI COLLODI ECCLESI ETALIBI FELLINI FORLANI PAHLAVI PAULIII SCOLARI SOLLATI SYLLABI TBILISI VILLARI

••••LI•

ACRYLIC ACYCLIC ALKALIS ALLELIC ANGELIC ANNELID APHELIA APHILIP ARGALIS ATACLIP BACKLIT BASILIC BASILIO BEDELIA BRESLIN BRILLIG BUCOLIC CAMELID CAROLII CECILIA CHABLIS CHAPLIN CHARLIE CHILLIS CHITLIN CICHLID COMPLIN CONKLIN COWSLIP DONTLIE DRUMLIN DWELLIN EARCLIP EIDOLIC EXCELIN FAMILIA FIDELIA FIDELIO FIDELIS FIRELIT

GANGLIA GOBELIN GREMLIN HABILIS HAMELIN HANDLIN HIMALIA IDYLLIC INSULIN INVALID ITSALIE JAVELIN KENOLIN KJELLIN KREMLIN KTOSLIN KUBELIK LAMPLIT LANOLIN LETSLIP LOCKLIN LUCYLIU MAHALIA MANOLIN MATALIN MAUDLIN MAYALIN MECHLIN MIFFLIN MOONLIT MUESLIS MUESLIX NATALIA NATALIE NEPALIS NETFLIX NONSLIP NOTALIE NOVALIS OBERLIN OPHELIA OVERLIE OVERLIT PAYSLIP PETULIA PHILLIE PHILLIP PHYLLIS RAMBLIN REARLIT REGALIA RESPLIT REVELIN RITALIN ROSALIA ROSALIE SEDALIA SIBYLIC SICILIA SKIDLID SNUGLIS SOMALIA SOMALIS SPOTLIT SQUALID STARLIT STEALIN STEELIE STOOLIE TASHLIN TIECLIP TOCELIA TRELLIS TRILLIN UNSOLID UNSPLIT VIDALIA VINYLIC VISALIA VITALIS VOCALIC WELLLIT WHEELIE WHEELIN YUKOLIS

••••L•I

BACILLI BOCELLI CAROLII CORELLI DOUBLEI DRMELFI FUSILLI GALILEI GEMELLI HAROLDI JAIALAI KAROLYI LAVELLI LEVILLI LORELAI LORELEI NIKOLAI PIRELLI RUDOLFI SHOULDI TEBALDI UNBELDI VANILLI VIVALDI

•••••LI

ALVEOLI BACILLI BENGALI BENZALI BOCELLI CALCULI CANNOLI CORELLI FAISALI FUSILLI GEMELLI ISRAELI LAVELLI LEVILLI LUTHULI NAUTILI PASCOLI PIRELLI RAVIOLI STIMULI SWAHILI TABOULI TRIPOLI VANILLI ZEPPOLI ZWINGLI

L•J••••

LAJOLLA LEJEUNE

L••J•••

LOGJAMS

L•••J••

LEARJET LEFTJAB LOCKJAW LORDJIM LOVEJOY LTKOJAK LUBEJOB

L•••••J

LARGEOJ LETTERJ LLCOOLJ

•L•J•••

OLDJOKE

•L••J••

ALANJAY BLUEJAY ELCAJON SLIMJIM

•L•••J•

ALFORJA

•L••••J

LLCOOLJ

••LJ•••

PALJOEY VALJEAN

••L•J••

BELLJAR CULTJAM HOLYJOE KELLJAN KILLJOY

••L••J•

VALLEJO

••L•••J

SILENTJ

•••LJ••

BELLJAR KELLJAN KILLJOY

•••L•J•

AZULEJO VALLEJO

•••L••J

SMALLOJ

••••L•J

DOUBLEJ SMALLOJ

•••••LJ

DANIELJ LLCOOLJ

L•K••••

LAKEBED LAKIEST LAKISTS LAKOTAS LAKSHMI LIKABLE LIKEICE LIKEMAD LIKENED LIKENEW LIKENTO LIKEWOW LIKINGS LTKOJAK

L••K•••

LACKEYS LACKING LACKWIT LANKEST LANKIER LANKILY LARKERS LARKIER LARKING LARKINS LARKISH LEAKAGE LEAKERS LEAKEYS LEAKIER LEAKING LEAKSIN LETKNOW LICKERS LICKETY LICKING LICKSUP LINKAGE LINKERS LINKING LINKSUP LINKUPS LOCKAGE LOCKBOX LOCKEAN LOCKERS LOCKETS LOCKING LOCKINS LOCKJAW LOCKLET LOCKLIN LOCKNUT LOCKOUT LOCKSET LOCKSIN LOCKSON LOCKSUP LOCKUPS LOOKERS LOOKFOR LOOKING LOOKINS LOOKISM LOOKIST LOOKOUT LOOKSAD LOOKSAT LOOKSEE LOOKSIN LOOKSON LOOKSTO LOOKSUP LOOKUPS LOOKYOU LUCKIER LUCKILY LUCKING LUCKMAN LUCKNOW LUCKOUT LUNKERS LURKERS LURKING

L•••K••

LADYKIN LALAKER LAMBKIN

L••••K•

LAWLIKE LEGLIKE LIPLIKE LYSENKO

L•••••K

LAMARCK LAWBOOK LAYBACK LEACOCK LEBROCK LEFREAK LEGWORK LETTERK LEXMARK LIEBACK LITOVSK LIVEOAK LOGBOOK LOWNECK LOWRISK LTKOJAK LUBBOCK

•LK••••

ALKALIS ALKENES ELKHART

•L•K•••

ALAKING ALEKEGS ALEKSEI ALTKEYS ALYKHAN BLAKELY BLAKLEY ELEKTRA FLAKERS FLAKIER FLAKILY FLAKING FLUKIER FLUKILY ILIKEIT ILLKNOW PLAKATS SLAKERS SLAKING

•L••K••

ALACKOF ALASKAN ALASKAS ALROKER BLACKED BLACKEN BLACKER BLACKIE BLACKLY BLANKED BLANKER BLANKET BLANKLY BLEAKER BLEAKLY BLINKAT BLINKED BLINKER BLOCKED BLOCKER BLOCKUP BLYNKEN CLACKED CLACKER CLANKED CLERKED CLERKLY CLICKED CLICKER CLICKON CLINKED CLINKER CLOAKED CLOCKED CLOCKER CLOCKIN CLONKED CLUCKED CLUCKER CLUNKED CLUNKER FLACKED FLANKED FLANKEN FLANKER FLECKED FLICKED FLICKER FLOCKED FLOCKTO FLUNKED FLUNKER KLINKER PLACKET PLANKED PLINKED PLONKED PLUCKED PLUNKED PLUNKER SLACKED SLACKEN SLACKER SLACKLY SLACKUP SLATKIN SLEEKED SLEEKEN SLEEKER SLEEKLY SLICKED SLICKER SLICKLY SLINKED SLINKER SLINKIN SLINKUP SLUNKIN SLUNKUP

•L•••K•

BLUESKY ELFLIKE OLDJOKE SLOVAKS

•L••••K

ALBORAK ALNITAK BLALOCK BLAUBOK ELDRICK ELENIAK ELFLOCK ILLLUCK OLDNICK OLICOOK SLYLOOK

••LK•••

BALKANS BALKERS BALKIER BALKILY BALKING BALKSAT BILKERS BILKING BULKIER BULKING BULKSUP CALKERS CALKING CALKINS DELKEYS FALKIRK FOLKART FOLKIER FOLKIES FOLKISH FOLKWAY HULKIER HULKING ILLKNOW KOLKATA MILKBAR MILKCAN MILKCOW MILKDUD MILKERS MILKFED MILKIER MILKILY MILKING MILKMAN MILKMEN MILKRUN MILKSOP POLKAED SELKIRK SILKHAT SILKIER SILKILY SILKTIE SULKERS SULKIER SULKIES SULKILY SULKING TALKBIG TALKERS TALKIER TALKIES TALKING TALKOUT TALKSAT TALKSOF TALKSON TALKSTO TALKSUP TOLKIEN WALKERS WALKING WALKINS WALKMAN WALKOFF WALKONS WALKOUT WALKSBY WALKSON WALKSTO WALKUPS WALKURE WALKWAY WILKENS WILKINS

••L•K••

EELSKIN LALAKER MOLOKAI OILSKIN SALUKIS STLUKES TALCKED UNLIKED UNLIKES VOLCKER WILLKIE

••L••K•

COLICKY EELLIKE ENLINKS HOLYOKE MALARKY MALLIKA MRLUCKY OILCAKE OILLIKE OWLLIKE PALOOKA PULASKI RELINKS RELOCKS RELOOKS SHLOCKY UNLEAKY UNLINKS UNLOCKS UNLUCKY UPLINKS VALMIKI

••L•••K

BELLEEK BULLOCK BULWARK FALKIRK HILLOCK HOLMOAK HOLYARK ILLLUCK MOLLUSK OILTANK POLLACK POLLOCK ROLLICK SELKIRK SELLECK SILENTK TULSAOK

•••LK••

BAULKED BAULKER CAULKED CAULKER CHALKED CHALKUP CHILKAT NAILKEG SKULKED SKULKER STALKED STALKER TOOLKIT WILLKIE

•••L•K•

ACTLIKE AIRLIKE ANTLIKE APELIKE ARMLIKE ASSLIKE AXELIKE BAGLIKE BATLIKE BEDLIKE BEELIKE BIBLIKE BOWLIKE BOXLIKE BOYLIKE BUDLIKE CATLIKE COWLIKE CUPLIKE CURLIKE DIDLIKE DISLIKE DOGLIKE DOTLIKE EARLIKE EELLIKE EGGLIKE ELFLIKE EYELIKE FADLIKE FANLIKE FATLIKE FINLIKE FOXLIKE GEMLIKE GODLIKE GUMLIKE HAGLIKE HATLIKE HENLIKE HIPLIKE HOGLIKE HUNLIKE HUTLIKE ICELIKE INKLIKE IVYLIKE JAMLIKE JAWLIKE JIGLIKE KIDLIKE LAWLIKE LEGLIKE LIPLIKE MALLIKA MANLIKE MISLIKE MUKLUKS NETLIKE NIBLIKE NOTLIKE NUNLIKE NUTLIKE OAKLIKE OARLIKE OATLIKE OILLIKE ORBLIKE OWLLIKE PEALIKE PEGLIKE PENLIKE PIELIKE PIGLIKE PODLIKE RAMLIKE RATLIKE RAYLIKE RIBLIKE RODLIKE RUGLIKE SACLIKE SAWLIKE SEALIKE SINLIKE SKYLIKE SONLIKE SOWLIKE SUNLIKE TAGLIKE THELIKE TINLIKE TOELIKE TOYLIKE TUBLIKE UNALIKE UNFLAKY URNLIKE WARLIKE WAXLIKE WEBLIKE WIGLIKE

•••L••K

AFFLECK AIRLOCK ANYLUCK ARMLOCK ASALARK BADLUCK BARLICK BELLEEK BLALOCK BULLOCK COWLICK DEKLERK EARLOCK ELFLOCK FEELSOK FETLOCK GASLEAK GENLOCK GOBLANK GUNLOCK HEMLOCK HEYLOOK HILLOCK HOTLICK HOTLINK ILLLUCK INBLACK JOBLOCK KEYLOCK MADLOCK MATLOCK MOLLUSK MORLOCK MUDLARK NEWLOOK NIBLICK NOWLOOK NUMLOCK OARLOCK OBELISK ONALARK ONELOOK OOBLECK OUTLOOK PADLOCK PHILIPK POLLACK POLLOCK POTLUCK REBLOCK ROLLICK SCHLOCK SELLECK SHYLOCK SKYLARK SLYLOOK SPELUNK THELARK THELOOK TITLARK UNBLOCK UNCLOAK UNSLACK UNSLEEK UNSLICK WARLOCK WEDLOCK WETLOOK ZIPLOCK

••••LK•

BYTALKS UNBULKY UNSULKY UPTALKS

••••L•K

DOUBLEK FARTLEK KUBELIK SZYSLAK URSULAK

•••••LK

BIGTALK BTFSPLK CARTALK CATWALK DUNDALK GOTMILK HOTMILK ICEMILK JAYWALK KINFOLK MENFOLK NORFOLK NORWALK OUTBULK OUTSULK OUTTALK OUTWALK PEPTALK RAWSILK RECHALK SKYWALK SOYMILK SUFFOLK THEHULK WEEFOLK

LL•••••

LLADROS LLANERO LLCOOLJ LLEYTON

L•L••••

LALAKER LALANNE LALIQUE LALLING LALOOSH LELOUCH LILALEE LILETEE LILINAU LILLIAN LILTING LILYPAD LOLLARD LOLLERS LOLLIES LOLLING LULLABY LULLERS LULLING

L••L•••

LADLERS LADLING LAFLEUR LALLING LAPLACA LAPLACE LAPLAND LAPLATA LAULAUS LAWLESS LAWLIKE LEBLANC LEGLESS LEGLIKE LETLIVE LIDLESS LILLIAN LIPLESS LIPLIKE LOLLARD LOLLERS LOLLIES LOLLING LOWLAND LOWLIER LOWLIFE LOWLILY LULLABY LULLERS LULLING LURLEEN

L•••L••

LABELED LABELER LABELLE

LAIDLOW LAJOLLA LAMPLIT LANDLER LANGLEY LANOLIN LAPALMA LAPELED LASALLE LASTLAP LASTLEG LAVALSE LAVELLI LAYSLOW LEAFLET LEFTLEG LEGALLY LEGOLAS LETSLIP LEVELED LEVELER LEVELLY LEVILLI LIBELED LIBELEE LIBELER LIESLOW LILALEE LITTLER LITTLES LOBULES LOCALES LOCALLY LOCKLET LOCKLIN LOCULUS LORELAI LORELEI LOUELLA LOWBLOW LOYALER LOYALES LOYALLY LOYALTO LOYALTY LOYOLAU LUCILLE LUCYLIU LUNULAE LUNULAR

L••••L•

LABELLE LABIALS LAEMMLE LAJOLLA LANKILY LAPBELT LAPFULS LARGELY LASALLE LASCALA LATRELL LAURELS LAVELLI LEERILY LEGALLY LEGIBLE LEGIBLY LEGPULL LENTILS LEOPOLD LETFALL LETROLL LETSFLY LEVELLY LEVILLI LEXUSLS LEXUSLX LICITLY LIGHTLY LIKABLE LINABLE LINCOLN LINGULA LINTELS LIONELL LIONELS LIPBALM LITHELY LIVABLE LIVIDLY LLCOOLJ LOATHLY LOCALLY LOFTILY LOGROLL LOONILY LOOSELY LOSABLE LOUELLA LOUSILY LOVABLE LOVABLY LOVERLY LOWBALL LOWLILY LOYALLY LUCIDLY LUCILLE LUCKILY LUMPILY LURIDLY LUSTILY LUTHULI LYOCELL LYONELL

L•••••L

LACTEAL LACUNAL LAMINAL LAMPOIL LATERAL LATRELL LEGPULL LESPAUL LESTOIL LETFALL LETROLL LETTERL LEXICAL LIBERAL LIFEFUL LIMINAL LINGUAL LIONELL LITERAL LOGICAL LOGROLL LOWBALL LOWHEEL LUGSAIL LUSTFUL LUSTRAL LYOCELL LYONELL LYRICAL

•LL••••

ALLAGES ALLANTE ALLAYED ALLAYER ALLBRAN ALLCAPS ALLCASH ALLCLAD ALLDONE ALLEARS ALLEGED ALLEGER ALLEGES ALLEGRA ALLEGRO ALLELES ALLELIC ALLELSE ALLENBY ALLENDE ALLERGY ALLEWIS ALLEYES ALLGONE ALLGOOD ALLHAIL ALLHEAL ALLHERE ALLISON ALLIUMS ALLMALE ALLMINE ALLNESS ALLNEWS ALLOFIT ALLOFME ALLOFUS ALLONGE ALLONYM ALLOPEZ ALLOVER ALLOWAY ALLOWED ALLOWIN ALLOWME ALLOYED ALLRISE ALLSTAR ALLSTON ALLTHAT ALLTHIS ALLTIED ALLTIME ALLTOLD ALLUDED ALLUDES ALLURED ALLURER ALLURES ALLUVIA ALLWISE ALLYING ALLYSON ELLAMAE ELLIOTT ELLIPSE ELLISON ELLMANN ELLYMAY ILLBITE ILLBRED ILLCALL ILLCLAD ILLDOIT ILLDONE ILLEANA ILLEGAL ILLEGIT ILLFOLD ILLICIT ILLKNOW ILLLIVE ILLLUCK ILLMADE ILLNESS ILLOGIC ILLPASS ILLTELL ILLUDED ILLUDES ILLUMED ILLUMES ILLUSED ILLUSES ILLWILL ILLWIND ILLYRIA ULLAGES ULLMANN

•L•L•••

BLALOCK ELFLIKE ELFLOCK FLYLEAF FLYLESS ILLLIVE ILLLUCK OLDLADY OLDLINE OLDLYME SLALOMS SLYLOOK ULALUME ULULANT ULULATE

•L••L••

ALCALDE ALFALFA ALKALIS ALLCLAD ALLELES ALLELIC ALLELSE ALNILAM BLAKLEY BLUELAW ELGALLO FLAILAT FLAILED FLATLET ILLCLAD OLDBLUE PLAYLET

•L•••L•

ALERTLY ALEVELS ALITTLE ALLMALE ALLTOLD ALOOFLY ALUDELS ALVEOLI BLACKLY BLACULA BLAKELY BLANDLY BLANKLY BLEAKLY BLINDLY BLOWFLY BLUEFLU BLUFFLY BLUNTLY CLAVELL CLEANLY CLEARLY CLERKLY CLOSELY ELDERLY ELFOWLS ELGALLO ELIYALE FLAKILY FLEEGLE FLEETLY FLESHLY FLEXILE FLUIDLY FLUKILY FLYABLE FLYBALL FLYSOLO GLAZILY GLOBULE GLYCOLS ILLCALL ILLFOLD ILLTELL ILLWILL ILOVELA LLCOOLJ OLDFILM OLDGOLD OLDPALS OLDSALT OLEBULL OLEVELS PLAINLY PLIABLE PLIABLY PLUGOLA PLUMPLY PLUMULE PLURALS PLUSHLY SLACKLY SLANTLY SLEEKLY SLICKLY SLIMILY

•L••••L

ALCOHOL ALLHAIL ALLHEAL ALUMNAL CLAIROL CLAUDEL CLAUSAL CLAVELL CLUEFUL ELUVIAL FLANNEL FLOREAL FLUIDAL FLUVIAL FLYBALL FLYGIRL GLACIAL GLEEFUL GLOSSAL GLOTTAL GLUTEAL ILLCALL ILLEGAL ILLTELL ILLWILL OLDGIRL OLEBULL OLEOOIL PLAYFUL PLEURAL PLOTFUL PLUVIAL SLEDFUL

••LL•••

BALLADE BALLADS BALLARD BALLAST BALLBOY BALLETS BALLIOL BALLMER BALLONE BALLOON BALLOTS BALLSUP BALLTWO BALLUET BELLAMY BELLBOY BELLEAU BELLEEK BELLHOP BELLIED BELLIES BELLING BELLINI BELLJAR BELLLAP BELLMAN BELLMEN BELLOWS BELLSON BELLYUP BILLERS BILLETS BILLIES BILLING BILLION BILLNYE BILLOWS BILLOWY BOLLING BULLDOG BULLETS BULLIED BULLIES BULLING BULLINS BULLION BULLISH BULLITT BULLOCK BULLPEN BULLRUN CALLBOX CALLBOY CALLEES CALLERS CALLFOR CALLING CALLINS CALLNOW CALLOFF CALLOUS CALLOUT CALLSIN CALLSIT CALLSON CALLSTO CALLSUP CALLUPS CELLARS CELLINI CELLIST CELLULE COLLAGE COLLARD COLLARS COLLATE COLLECT COLLEEN COLLEGE COLLETS COLLIDE COLLIER COLLIES COLLINE COLLINS COLLODI COLLOID COLLOPS COLLUDE COLLYER CULLERS CULLETS CULLIED CULLIES CULLING DALLIED DALLIER DALLIES DILLARD DILLIES DILLMAN DOLLARS DOLLIED DOLLIES DOLLING DOLLISH DOLLOPS DOLLSUP DULLARD DULLEST DULLING DULLISH EELLIKE FALLACY FALLALS FALLDUE FALLERS FALLFOR FALLGUY FALLING FALLOFF FALLOUT FALLOWS FALLSIN FALLSON FALLSTO FELLAHS FELLDUE FELLERS FELLFOR FELLING FELLINI FELLOFF FELLOUT FELLOWS FILLERS FILLETS FILLIES FILLING FILLINS FILLIPS FILLOUT FILLSIN FILLSUP FILLUPS FOLLETT FOLLIES FOLLOWS FULLDAY FULLEST FULLLOT FULLOUT GALLANT GALLEON GALLERY GALLEYS GALLICO GALLING GALLIUM GALLONS GALLOPS GALLOWS GELLING GILLIAM GILLIAN GILLING GILLMAN GILLNET GULLAHS GULLETS GULLIED GULLIES GULLING HALLEYS HALLOOS HALLOWS HALLWAY HELLBOY HELLCAT HELLENE HELLENO HELLION HELLISH HELLMAN HELLOED HELLOES HELLUVA HELLYES HILLARY HILLIER HILLING HILLMAN HILLMEN HILLOCK HILLTOP HOLLAND HOLLERS HOLLIES HOLLOWS HULLERS HULLING HULLOED ILLLIVE ILLLUCK JELLIED JELLIES JELLIFY JELLING JILLIAN JILLION JOLLIED JOLLIER JOLLIES JOLLIET JOLLIFY JOLLILY JOLLITY KELLJAN KELLOGG KILLEEN KILLERS KILLFEE KILLING KILLJOY LALLING LILLIAN LOLLARD LOLLERS LOLLIES LOLLING LULLABY LULLERS LULLING MALLARD MALLETS MALLEUS MALLIKA MALLOWS MALLRAT MELLOWS MILLAGE MILLAIS MILLAND MILLARD MILLDAM MILLEND MILLERS MILLETS MILLETT MILLIME MILLING MILLION MILLRUN MOLLIES MOLLIFY MOLLUSC MOLLUSK MULLAHS MULLERS MULLETS MULLING MULLINS NULLIFY NULLING NULLITY NULLSET OILLAMP OILLESS OILLIKE OILLINE OWLLIKE PALLETS PALLIER PALLING PALLORS PELLEAS PELLETS PILLAGE PILLARS PILLBOX PILLBUG PILLING PILLION PILLORY PILLOWS PILLOWY POLLACK POLLARD POLLEES POLLENS POLLERA POLLERS POLLING POLLOCK POLLTAX POLLUTE PULLERS PULLETS PULLEYS PULLFOR PULLING PULLINS PULLMAN PULLOFF PULLONS PULLOUT PULLPIN PULLSIN PULLSON PULLSUP PULLTAB PULLTOY PULLUPS RALLIED RALLIER RALLIES RALLYES RALLYTO RELLENO RILLETS ROLLAND ROLLBAR ROLLEIS ROLLERS ROLLICK ROLLING ROLLINS ROLLMOP ROLLOFF ROLLONS ROLLOUT ROLLSBY ROLLSIN ROLLSON ROLLSUP ROLLTOP ROLLUPS ROLLWAY SALLIED SALLIER SALLIES SELLECK SELLERS SELLFOR SELLING SELLOFF SELLOUT SELLSIT SELLSTO SILLIER SILLIES SILLYME SOLLATI SULLIED SULLIES SYLLABI TALLEST TALLIED TALLIER TALLIES TALLINN TALLISH TALLITH TALLONE TALLOWS TALLOWY TALLYHO TALLYUP TELLALL TELLERS TELLIES TELLING TELLOFF TELLSIT TELLSOF TELLSON TILLAGE TILLERS TILLETS TILLING TILLNOW TOLLAGE TOLLBAR TOLLERS TOLLING TOLLMAN TOLLMEN TOLLWAY VALLEJO VALLEYS VALLONE VELLUMS VILLAGE VILLAIN VILLARD VILLARI VILLEIN VOLLEYS WALLABY WALLACE WALLACH WALLETS WALLEYE WALLING WALLMAP WALLOFF WALLOON WALLOPS WALLOWS WALLSIN WALLSUP WELLAND WELLCUT WELLFED WELLHID WELLHIT WELLING WELLLED WELLLIT WELLMAN WELLOFF WELLPUT WELLRUN WELLSEE WELLSET WELLSUP WELLWON WELLYES WILLARD WILLERS WILLFUL WILLIAM WILLIES WILLING WILLKIE WILLOWS WILLOWY WILLSON WILLYOU YELLERS YELLFOR YELLING YELLOUT YELLOWS YELLOWY YELLSAT ZILLION

••L•L••

ALLCLAD ALLELES ALLELIC ALLELSE BELLLAP BULBLET DELILAH DELILLO FULLLOT GALILEE GALILEI GALILEO GILBLAS HALALAS ILLCLAD LILALEE OGLALAS WELLLED WELLLIT YALELAW YULELOG

••L••L•

ALLMALE ALLTOLD BALKILY BALMILY CALCULI CALPOLY CELLULE DELILLO DELSOLS FALLALS FALSELY FALWELL FELTILL FILMILY FULFILL FULFILS GALPALS GELIDLY HOLDALL ILLCALL ILLFOLD ILLTELL

ILLWILL
JOLLILY
MALCOLM
MILKILY
OILPALM
OILWELL
PALEALE
SALABLE
SALTILY
SILKILY
SOLIDLY
SOLUBLE
SULKILY
TELLALL
TOLDALL
UNLOWLY
VALIDLY
VALVULA
VALVULE
VOLUBLE
VOLUBLY
WALPOLE
WILHELM

••L•••L

ALLHAIL
ALLHEAL
BALEFUL
BALLIOL
BILEVEL
COLONEL
DOLEFUL
FALAFEL
FALWELL
FELTILL
FULFILL
GELUSIL
GULFOIL
HELICAL
HELPFUL
HOLDALL
HOLYOIL
ILLCALL
ILLEGAL
ILLTELL
ILLWILL
OILWELL
PALATAL
PALMFUL
PALMOIL
PALUDAL
RELABEL
RELEVEL
SCLERAL
SELMAAL
SILENTL
TELLALL
TOLDALL
TYLENOL
UNLEGAL
UNLEVEL
UNLOCAL
UNLOYAL
WILLFUL
WOLFGAL

•••LL••

ABOLLAE
ADOLLAR
AGALLOP
APOLLOS
AXILLAE
AXILLAR
AXILLAS
BELLLAP
BRILLIG
BRILLOS
BUELLER
CAILLOU
CHALLAH
CHILLED
CHILLER
CHILLIS
CHILLUM
CHOLLAS
CRULLER
DIALLED
DRILLED
DRILLER
DROLLER
DUELLED
DWELLAT
DWELLED
DWELLER
DWELLIN
DWELLON
EVILLER
FAILLES
FRILLED
FUELLED
FULLLOT
GRILLED
GRILLER
GRILLES
IDYLLIC
JUILLET
KEILLOR
KJELLIN
KNELLED
KVELLED
MAILLOL
MAILLOT
MCALLEN
MUELLER
OCELLAR
OCELLUS
OKELLEY
OMALLEY
PAELLAS
PHILLIE
PHILLIP
PHYLLIS
PHYLLOS
QUELLED
QUELLER
QUILLED
QUILLER
REALLOT
SCALLOP
SCULLED
SCULLER
SHALLOT
SHALLOW
SHALLWE
SHELLAC
SHELLED
SHELLER
SHELLEY
SHILLED
SKILLED
SKILLET
SKULLED
SMALLAD
SMALLER
SMALLOJ
SMELLED
SMELLER
SMILLAS
SNELLEN
SPELLED
SPELLER
SPILLED
SPILLER
STALLED
STALLER
STELLAR
STILLED
STILLER
STILLUP
STOLLEN
SUELLEN
SWALLOW
SWELLED
SWELLER
SWELLUP
SWILLED
SWILLER
SWOLLEN
TRELLIS
TRILLED
TRILLER
TRILLIN
TROLLED
TROLLER
TROLLEY
TROLLOP
TUILLES
TWILLED
VIALLED
VIELLES
WELLLED
WELLLIT
WHALLEY
WOOLLEN
WOOLLEY
ZOELLER

•••L•L•

ADULTLY
AGILELY
CARLYLE
CELLULE
DAYLILY
FALLALS
FEELILL
HEALALL
JOLLILY
LOWLILY
OOHLALA
SEALILY
SHALALA
STALELY
SURLILY
TELLALL
TRALALA
UKELELE
UKULELE
UNSLYLY
WORLDLY

•••L••L

AXOLOTL
BALLIOL
BOWLFUL
COALOIL
FEELILL
FUELOIL
HEALALL
MAILLOL
OCALAFL
PAILFUL
SCALPEL
SKILFUL
SOULFUL
TELLALL
TOILFUL
VIALFUL
WAILFUL
WILLFUL

••••LL•

AACELLS
ACHILLE
APPALLS
AURALLY
AWFULLY
AXIALLY
BACILLI
BANALLY
BASALLY
BEFALLS
BOCELLI
BONILLA
BRAILLE
BYGOLLY
CABALLE
CAMILLA
CAMILLE
CAPELLA
CASELLA
CEDILLA
CIVILLY
CORELLI
COROLLA
CRUELLA
CRUELLY
DEFALLA
DELILLO
DEMILLE
DEVILLE
DICILLO
DUCALLY
ECUELLE
ELGALLO
ENDALLS
ENROLLS
EQUALLY
ESTELLA
ESTELLE
EXTOLLS
FAMILLE
FATALLY
FINALLY
FRAILLY
FUGALLY
FURILLO
FUSILLI
GAZELLE
GEMELLI
GIROLLE
GISELLE
GORILLA
GYRALLY
HGWELLS
HOWELLS
IDEALLY
INGALLS
LABELLE
LAJOLLA
LASALLE
LAVELLI
LEGALLY
LEVELLY
LEVILLI
LOCALLY
LOUELLA
LOYALLY
LUCILLE
MAGILLA
MARILLA
MARULLO
MAXILLA
MCCALLS
MCNALLY
MEDULLA
MEGILLA
MISALLY
MORALLY
MORELLA
MORELLO
MOSELLE
MOZILLA
MURILLO
NACELLE
NASALLY
NEUILLY
NEVILLE
NICOLLE
NOVELLA
NOVELLE
NOVELLO
OREILLY
ORVILLE
OTHELLO
PAPILLA
PASALLE
PATELLA
PIRELLI
PITILLO
PREALLY
RAPALLO
RAVELLY
REBILLS
RECALLS
REFALLS
REFILLS
REGALLY
REMILLS
RENALLY
REPOLLS
REROLLS
RESELLS
RETALLY
RETELLS
RETILLS
ROSELLA
ROSELLE
ROTELLE
ROYALLY
ROZELLE
RUBELLA
RURALLY
SCROLLS
SEVILLA
SEVILLE
SHRILLS
SHRILLY
SQUALLS
SQUALLY
STROLLS
THRALLS
THRILLA
THRILLS
TIDALLY
TONALLY
TOTALLY
UCCELLO
UNFULLY
UNHILLY
UNHULLS
UNJOLLY
UNROLLS
UNSELLS
UNSILLY
UNWALLS
UPHILLS
UPWELLS
USUALLY
UTRILLO
VANILLA
VANILLI
VENALLY
VITALLY
VOCALLY
VOWELLY
ZEDILLO
ZONALLY

••••L•L

DOUBLEL
MAILLOL

•••••LL

AAACELL
AIRBALL
AIRBILL
ANTHILL
ARTWALL
ATHRILL
AVERELL
AVERILL
BADCALL
BAGWELL
BARBELL
BARBILL
BEATALL
BEDROLL
BENZELL
BESSELL
BESTILL
BISSELL
BOSWELL
BOXBALL
BUZZELL
CANNELL
CARROLL
CATCALL
CHAGALL
CLAVELL
CORDELL
CORNELL
CORYELL
COWBELL
CROWELL
CUEBALL
CUREALL
DARNELL
DARWELL
DESHELL
DEWFALL
DIDWELL
DISTILL
DONNALL
DRYCELL
DRYWALL
DRYWELL
DURRELL
EGGROLL
EYEBALL
EYEROLL
EYEWALL
FALWELL
FARRELL
FATCELL
FEELILL
FELTILL
FITWELL
FLYBALL
FULFILL
FURBALL
GASKELL
GETWELL
GINMILL
GOODALL
GOTWELL
GUMBALL
GUNMOLL
GYMBALL
HADPULL
HARWELL
HASKELL
HASPULL
HEALALL
HOGCALL
HOLDALL
HOTROLL
HOWDULL
HUBBELL
ICEFALL
IFIFELL
ILLCALL
ILLTELL
ILLWILL
IMSWELL
INABALL
INDWELL
INKWELL
INSTALL
INSTILL
JARRELL
JODRELL
JOEHILL
JONHALL
KENDALL
KENDOLL
KIMBALL
KINNELL
KNOWALL
KORDELL
LATRELL
LEGPULL
LETFALL
LETROLL
LIONELL
LOGROLL
LOWBALL
LYOCELL
LYONELL
MADEILL
MAKEILL
MARVELL
MAXWELL
MCNEILL
MERRILL
MEYNELL
MISBILL
MISCALL
MISTELL
NETBALL
NOBHILL
NOTWELL
ODDBALL
OILWELL
OLEBULL
ONAROLL
ONEBALL
ONEBELL
ONECALL
ONECELL
OUTCALL
OUTCULL
OUTKILL
OUTPOLL
OUTPULL
OUTROLL
OUTSELL
OUTTELL
OUTTOLL
OUTWELL
OUTWILL
OUTYELL
OVERALL
PACBELL
PAYROLL
PAYWELL
PEPPILL
PINBALL
PITBULL
PITFALL
PREBILL
PRESELL
PRETELL
PROBALL
PURCELL
RAGDOLL
RANDALL
RAYNELL
RECHALL
REDCELL
REDPOLL
REDRILL
RENDELL
RESPELL
ROSWELL
RUSSELL
SAMHILL
SAMUELL
SATWELL
SAWMILL
SEAGULL
SEAWALL
SEENALL
SEESALL
SITWELL
SIXBALL
SNOBALL
SORRELL
SUBCELL
SUBHALL
TAKEILL
TARBELL
TEABALL
TELLALL
TENBALL
TERRELL
THEBELL
THEDELL
THEFALL
THEHILL
THEMALL
THEWALL
TOLDALL
TOOKILL
TOOTALL
TORVILL
TOYBALL
TOYDOLL
TWOBALL
TYNDALL
UNFRILL
UNIBALL
UNSHELL
UPSWELL
VERDELL
VERYILL
VFWHALL
VONZELL
WADDELL
WAYBILL
WEDDELL
WENDELL
WETCELL
WHERELL
WORRELL
YARNELL

LM•••••

LMNOPQR

L•M••••

LAMAISM
LAMAIST
LAMARCK
LAMBADA
LAMBDAS
LAMBEAU
LAMBENT
LAMBERT
LAMBETH
LAMBING
LAMBKIN
LAMENTS
LAMINAE
LAMINAL
LAMINAR
LAMINAS
LAMINTO
LAMMING
LAMOTTA
LAMOTTE
LAMPERT
LAMPLIT
LAMPOIL
LAMPOON
LAMPREY
LEMIEUX
LEMMATA
LEMMING
LEMONDE
LEMOYNE
LEMPIRA
LIMACON
LIMBERS
LIMBING
LIMBURG
LIMEADE
LIMEPIE
LIMIEST
LIMINAL
LIMITED
LIMITER
LIMNERS
LIMNING
LIMNITE
LIMOGES
LIMPEST
LIMPETS
LIMPING
LIMPOPO
LOMBARD
LUMBAGO
LUMBARS
LUMBERS
LUMIERE
LUMINAS
LUMPERS
LUMPIER
LUMPILY
LUMPING
LUMPISH
LUMPSIN
LUMPSIT
LUMPSUM

L••M•••

LABMICE
LAEMMLE
LAMMING
LEHMANN
LEMMATA
LEMMING
LETMEBE
LETMEGO
LETMEIN
LEXMARK
LIPMANN
LOAMIER
LOAMING
LOOMING
LOOMPAS
LOWMASS

L•••M••

LABAMBA
LAEMMLE
LAFEMME
LANDMAN
LANDMEN
LARAMIE
LASTMAY
LATIMES
LEADMAN
LEADMEN
LEGUMES
LENSMAN
LENSMEN
LETEMIN
LIKEMAD
LINEMAN
LINEMEN
LUCKMAN

L••••M•

LACRIMO
LAFEMME
LAKSHMI
LANCOME
LAPALMA
LAPERMS
LISSOME
LOGJAMS
LYCEUMS

L•••••M

LAMAISM
LANGHAM
LCHAYIM
LEFTARM
LEFTISM
LEGROOM
LEITRIM
LETTERM
LIPBALM
LITHIUM
LONGARM
LONGTOM
LOOKISM
LORDJIM
LOWBEAM
LUDDISM
LUGWORM
LUMPSUM
LUSTRUM

•LM••••

ALMAATA
ALMADEN
ALMANAC
ALMERIA
ALMONDS
ALMONDY
ALMONER
ALMONRY
ALMSMAN
ALMSMEN
ELMCITY
ELMIEST
ELMISTI
ELMONTE
ELMTREE
ELMUNDO
ELMWOOD
KLMNOPQ
OLMSTED

•L•M•••

ALAMEDA
ALAMEIN
ALAMODE
ALAMOSA
ALEMBIC
ALIMENT
ALIMONY
ALLMALE
ALLMINE
ALSMITH
ALUMINA
ALUMNAE
ALUMNAL
ALUMNUS
BLAMEON
BLAMERS
BLAMING
BLEMISH
BLIMPIE
CLAMANT
CLAMATO
CLAMBAR
CLAMBER
CLAMDIP
CLAMMED
CLAMMER
CLAMORS
CLAMOUR
CLAMPED
CLAMPER
CLAMPON
CLAMSUP
CLEMENS
CLEMENT
CLEMSON
CLIMATE
CLIMATS
CLIMBED
CLIMBER
CLIMBIN
CLIMBON
CLIMBTO
CLIMBUP
CLOMPED
CLUMPED
ELAMITE
ELEMENT
ELLMANN
FLAMBED
FLAMBES
FLAMERS
FLAMEUP
FLAMIER
FLAMING
FLAMMED
FLEMING
FLEMISH
FLUMMOX
GLAMORS
GLAMOUR
GLAMSUP
GLIMMER
GLIMPSE
GLOMMED
GLUMMED
GLUMMER
ILLMADE
KLAMATH
KLAMMER
OLDMAID
OLDMOON
OLEMISS
OLYMPIA
OLYMPIC
OLYMPUS
PLUMAGE
PLUMBED
PLUMBER
PLUMBIC
PLUMBUM
PLUMCOT
PLUMIER
PLUMING
PLUMMER
PLUMMET
PLUMOSE
PLUMPED
PLUMPER
PLUMPIE
PLUMPLY
PLUMULE
SLAMMED
SLAMMER
SLAMSON
SLIMIER
SLIMILY
SLIMING
SLIMJIM
SLIMMED
SLIMMER
SLUMBER
SLUMMED
SLUMMER
SLUMPED
ULLMANN

•L••M••

ALARMED
ALARMER
ALBUMEN
ALBUMIN
ALMSMAN
ALMSMEN
ALTIMAS
BLOOMED
BLOOMER
CLAIMED
CLAIMER

CLAMMED
CLAMMER
CLUBMED
ELCAMPO
ELLAMAE
ELLYMAY
FLAGMAN
FLAGMEN
FLAMMED
FLUMMOX
GLEAMED
GLEEMAN
GLEEMEN
GLIMMER
GLOAMIN
GLOMMED
GLOOMED
GLUMMED
GLUMMER
ILIAMNA
ILLUMED
ILLUMES
KLAMMER
KLEZMER
KLUGMAN
PLASMAS
PLASMIC
PLOWMAN
PLOWMEN
PLUMMER
PLUMMET
SLAMMED
SLAMMER
SLIMMED
SLIMMER
SLUMMED
SLUMMER
ULTIMAS

•L•••M•

ALABAMA
ALABAMY
ALARUMS
ALCHEMY
ALLIUMS
ALLOFME
ALLOWME
ALLTIME
ELECTME
FLINTMI
OLDLYME
OLDTIME
PLENUMS
SLALOMS
ULALUME

•L••••M

ALIFORM
ALLONYM
ALNILAM
ALYSSUM
BLOSSOM
ELITISM
ELUVIUM
ELYSIUM
FLOTSAM
OLDFILM
PLUMBUM
SLIMJIM

••LM•••

AILMENT
ALLMALE
ALLMINE
BALMAIN
BALMIER
BALMILY
BELMONT
CALMEST
CALMING
CALMSEA
DELMONT
DELMORE
DOLMANS
ELLMANN
FILMDOM
FILMIER
FILMILY
FILMING
FILMSET
FULMARS
GILMORE
HELMETS
HELMING
HELMOND
HOLMIUM
HOLMOAK
ILLMADE
JKLMNOP
MALMSEY
PALMARY
PALMATE
PALMERS
PALMFUL
PALMIER
PALMING
PALMIST
PALMOFF
PALMOIL
PALMTOP
PALMYRA
PULMONI
PULMONO
SALMONP
SALMONS
SELMAAL
ULLMANN
VALMIKI
WALMART

••L•M••

BALLMER
BELLMAN
BELLMEN
CALAMAR
CALUMET
CALUMNY
CCLAMPS
COLEMAN
COLOMBO
COLUMBA
COLUMBO
COLUMNS
DELIMAN
DELIMEN
DELIMIT
DILEMMA
DILLMAN
ELLAMAE
ELLYMAY
FELDMAN
GALUMPH
GILLMAN
GOLDMAN
HALFMAD
HELLMAN
HILLMAN
HILLMEN
HOLYMAN
HOLYMEN
HOLZMAN
ILLUMED
ILLUMES
INLIMBO
ISLAMIC
MALAMUD
MELAMED
MILKMAN
MILKMEN
NOLIMIT
PALAMAS
PALEMON
PALOMAR
PALOMAS
POLEMAN
POLEMEN
POLEMIC
POLYMER
PULLMAN
RELIMIT
RELUMED
RELUMES
ROLLMOP
SALAMIS
SALEMOR
SALOMON
SOLOMON
TOLLMAN
TOLLMEN
UNLUMPY
VELTMAN
VOLUMED
VOLUMES
WALKMAN
WALLMAP
WELLMAN
WILDMAN
WILDMEN
WOLFMAN
WOLFMEN
YALEMAN
YALEMEN

••L•M•

ALLIUMS
ALLOFME
ALLOWME
ALLTIME
BALSAMS
BALSAMY
BELDAME
BELDAMS
BELLAMY
DELORME
DILEMMA
FULSOME
MELISMA
MILLIME
NFLGAME
NHLGAME
OILLAMP
PALERMO
PHLEGMY
PHLOEMS
SALAAMS
SILLYME
TALCUMS
VELLUMS
WELCOME

••L•••M

ALLONYM
BELGIUM
CALCIUM
CULTISM
CULTJAM
DELIHAM
EELWORM
FILMDOM
FULCRUM
FULGHUM
GALLIUM
GILLIAM
HOLMIUM
MALCOLM
MILLDAM
NFLTEAM
NHLTEAM
OILDRUM
OILPALM
PILGRIM
SILENTM
TELECOM
VALOREM
WALTHAM
WILHELM
WILLIAM
WOLFRAM

•••LM••

BALLMER
BELLMAN
BELLMEN
COOLMAX
DILLMAN
GILLMAN
HELLMAN
HILLMAN
HILLMEN
HJALMAR
IJKLMNO
MAILMAN
MAILMEN
PERLMAN
POOLMAN
POOLMEN
PSALMIC
PULLMAN
RAILMAN
RAILMEN
REALMAN
REALMEN
ROLLMOP
SHULMAN
SOULMAN
TOLLMAN
TOLLMEN
WALLMAP
WELLMAN
WHELMED

•••L•M•

ARCLAMP
ASYLUMS
BEDLAMP
BEDLAMS
BELLAMY
COULOMB
DESLUMS
DIPLOMA
EMBLEMS
ENFLAME
EWELAMB
FOGLAMP
GASLAMP
HOWLAME
INFLAME
KEYLIME
MILLIME
MOSLEMS
MUSLIMS
OILLAMP
OLDLYME
ONELUMP
OUTLIMN
PABLUMS
PEPLUMS
PETLAMB
PRELIMS
PTOLEMY
RECLAME
RECLIMB
REPLUMB
REPLUME
SCHLUMP
SHALOMS
SILLYME
SLALOMS
SUBLIME
SUNLAMP
THELAMB
TOBLAME
ULALUME
UNCLAMP
UNPLUMB
UPCLIMB
VELLUMS

•••L••M

ACCLAIM
AMALGAM
BAALISM
CDALBUM
CHILLUM
DECLAIM
DUALISM
EARLDOM
EXCLAIM
GALLIUM
GILLIAM
INBLOOM
MILLDAM
REALISM
REBLOOM
RECLAIM
THULIUM
VARLAAM
WILLIAM

••••LM•

ANSELMO
BECALMS
DEPALMA
EMBALMS
HIJKLMN
LAPALMA
NAPALMS
REFILMS
UNHELMS

••••L•M

ABSALOM
ALNILAM
BORGLUM
CHILLUM
DOUBLEM
HAARLEM
HOODLUM
ONECLAM
PABULUM
PROBLEM

•••••LM

ARTFILM
FANPALM
GHIJKLM
HITFILM
IANHOLM
LIPBALM
MALCOLM
OILPALM
OLDFILM
SEACALM
WILHELM

L•N••••

LANCERS
LANCETS
LANCIAS
LANCING
LANCOME
LANDAUS
LANDERS
LANDING
LANDINI
LANDLER
LANDMAN
LANDMEN
LANDSAT
LANDSUP
LANDTAG
LANDTAX
LANEONE
LANETWO
LANFORD
LANGDON
LANGHAM
LANGLEY
LANGTON
LANGTRY
LANGUID
LANGUOR
LANGWAY
LANKEST
LANKIER
LANKILY
LANOLIN
LANOTTE
LANSING
LANTANA
LANTERN
LANVINS
LANYARD
LENDERS
LENDING
LENDOUT
LENFANT
LENGTHS
LENGTHY
LENGUAS
LENIENT
LENNONS
LENOVOS
LENSCAP
LENSMAN
LENSMEN
LENTIGO
LENTILS
LINABLE
LINAGES
LINBIAO
LINCOLN
LINDENS
LINDIED
LINDIES
LINDNER
LINDORF
LINDROS
LINDSAY
LINDSEY
LINEAGE
LINEARA
LINEARB
LINEATE
LINECUT
LINEDRY
LINEDUP
LINEMAN
LINEMEN
LINEONE
LINEOUT
LINESUP
LINETWO
LINEUPS
LINGCOD
LINGERS
LINGOES
LINGUAE
LINGUAL
LINGULA
LINIEST
LININGS
LINKAGE
LINKERS
LINKING
LINKSUP
LINKUPS
LINNETS
LINPIAO
LINSEED
LINTELS
LINTERS
LINTIER
LINTING
LMNOPQR
LONBORG
LONDRES
LONETTE
LONGAGO
LONGARM
LONGBED
LONGBOW
LONGDAY
LONGDEN
LONGEST
LONGFOR
LONGIES
LONGING
LONGISH
LONGRUN
LONGTOM
LONGTON
LONGUES
LONGWAY
LONIGAN
LUNATED
LUNATES
LUNATIC
LUNCHED
LUNCHER
LUNCHES
LUNESTA
LUNETTE
LUNGEAT
LUNGERS
LUNGING
LUNKERS
LUNULAE
LUNULAR
LYNDONB
LYNETTE

L••N•••

LAENNEC
LAUNDER
LAUNDRY
LAXNESS
LEANCUT
LEANDER
LEANERS
LEANEST
LEANING
LEANSIN
LEANSON
LEANSTO
LEANTOS
LENNONS
LEONARD
LEONATO
LEONDAY
LEONIDS
LEONINE
LEONORA
LEONORE
LIENEES
LIENORS
LIGNIFY
LIGNINS
LIGNITE
LIMNERS
LIMNING
LIMNITE
LINNETS
LIONCUB
LIONELL
LIONELS
LIONESS
LIONETS
LIONISE
LIONIZE
LLANERO
LOANERS
LOANING
LOANOUT
LOONIER
LOONIES
LOONILY
LOUNGED
LOUNGER
LOUNGES
LOWNECK
LOWNESS
LUGNUTS
LYINGBY
LYINGON
LYINGTO
LYINGUP
LYONELL

L•••N••

LACINGS
LACONIA
LACONIC
LACUNAE
LACUNAL
LACUNAR
LACUNAS
LADINGS
LADINOS
LADYNAS
LAENNEC
LAGUNAS
LALANNE
LAMENTS
LAMINAE
LAMINAL
LAMINAR
LAMINAS
LAMINTO
LARDNER
LATENCY
LATENED
LATENTS
LATINAS
LATINII
LATINOS
LATINUS
LAVINIA
LAWANDA
LAYINTO
LAZENBY
LAZONGA
LEARNED
LEARNER
LEARNOF
LEARNTO
LEBANON
LECONTE
LEDINTO
LEGANZA
LEGENDS
LEIBNIZ
LEMONDE
LEPANTO
LETINON
LETKNOW
LETSNOT
LICENCE
LICENSE
LIFENET
LIGANDS
LIKENED
LIKENEW
LIKENTO
LIKINGS
LILINAU
LIMINAL
LINDNER
LININGS
LISENTE
LITINTO
LIVENED
LIVENER
LIVENUP
LIVINGS
LOCKNUT
LOGANUT
LOGONTO
LORANGE
LORENTZ
LORENZO
LORGNON
LOSINGS
LOZENGE
LUCANIA
LUCENCY
LUCINDA
LUCKNOW
LUMINAS
LUPINES
LYSENKO

L••••N•

LACKING
LADLING
LADRONE
LAGGING
LAGOONS
LAHAINA
LAIRING
LALANNE
LALLING
LAMBENT
LAMBING
LAMMING
LANCING
LANDING
LANDINI
LANEONE
LANSING
LANTANA
LANVINS
LAPLAND
LAPPING
LAPSANG
LAPSING
LAPWING
LARAINE
LARCENY
LARDING
LARDONS
LARGENT
LARKING
LARKINS
LASAGNA
LASAGNE
LASHING
LASTING
LASTONE
LATEENS
LATHING
LATRINE
LAUDING
LAURENT
LAVAINE
LAVERNE
LEADENS
LEADING
LEADINS
LEAFING
LEAKING
LEANING
LEAPING
LEASING
LEAVENS
LEAVING
LEBLANC
LECUONA
LEERING
LEFTEND
LEGBONE
LEGGING
LEGIONS
LEGRAND
LEHMANN
LEJEUNE
LEMMING
LEMOYNE
LENDING
LENFANT
LENIENT
LENNONS
LEOGENN
LEONINE
LEPTONS
LESIONS
LESSENS
LESSING
LESSONS
LETTING
LEUCINE
LEVYING
LHASANS
LIBBING
LIBRANS
LIBYANS
LICHENS
LICKING
LIDWINA
LIFTING
LIGNINS
LILTING
LIMBING
LIMNING
LIMPING
LINDENS
LINEONE
LINKING
LINTING
LIPMANN
LIPPING
LIPSYNC
LISPING
LISTENS
LISTING
LIVEONE
LIVORNO
LOADING
LOAFING
LOAMING
LOANING
LOBBING
LOCARNO
LOCKING
LOCKINS
LODGING
LOFTING
LOGGING
LOGGINS
LOIDING
LOLLING
LONGING
LOOKING
LOOKINS
LOOMING
LOOPING
LOOSENS
LOOSING
LOOTING
LOPPING
LORDING
LORIENT
LOTIONS
LOTTING
LOUDENS
LOURING
LOUSING
LOUTING
LOVEINS
LOWHAND
LOWLAND
LOWRENT
LUCARNE
LUCERNE
LUCHINO
LUCIANA
LUCIANO
LUCKING
LUFFING
LUGGING
LULLING
LUMPING
LUNGING
LURKING
LUSTING
LYNDONB

L•••••N

LACESON
LADYKIN
LAMBKIN
LAMPOON
LANDMAN
LANDMEN
LANGDON
LANGTON
LANOLIN
LANTERN
LAOCOON
LAOTIAN
LAPUTAN
LARCHEN
LASTDON
LATCHON
LATERAN
LATERON
LATVIAN
LAUGHIN
LAVERAN
LAYDOWN
LAYITON
LAYOPEN
LAYUPON
LEADMAN
LEADMEN
LEADSIN
LEADSON
LEAKSIN
LEANSIN
LEANSON
LEAPSIN
LEAPSON
LEAPTIN
LEAPTON
LEAVEIN
LEAVEON
LEBANON
LEBARON
LECTERN
LEGHORN
LEGIRON
LEHMANN
LENSMAN
LENSMEN
LEOGENN
LETDOWN
LETEMIN
LETHEAN
LETINON
LETMEIN
LETTERN
LETUPON
LEXICON
LIAISON
LIEDOWN
LIGHTEN
LIGHTON
LILLIAN
LIMACON
LINCOLN
LINEMAN
LINEMEN
LIPMANN
LIVEDIN
LIVEDON

LIVESIN
LIVESON
LLEYTON
LOADSIN
LOAFPAN
LOCKEAN
LOCKLIN
LOCKSIN
LOCKSON
LODGEIN
LONGDEN
LONGRUN
LONGTON
LONIGAN
LOOKSIN
LOOKSON
LORGNON
LOTHIAN
LOWBORN
LOWCHEN
LOWDOWN
LUCKMAN
LUMPSIN
LUREDIN
LURESIN
LURLEEN
LYINGON
LYRICON

•LN••••

ALNICOS
ALNILAM
ALNITAK
ALNIYAT
ELNINOS
ELNORTE

•L•N•••

ALANINE
ALANJAY
ALANNAH
ALENCON
ALINERS
ALINING
ALLNESS
ALLNEWS
ALUNSER
BLANCHE
BLANDER
BLANDLY
BLANKED
BLANKER
BLANKET
BLANKLY
BLANTON
BLENDED
BLENDER
BLENDES
BLENDIN
BLENTIN
BLINDED
BLINDER
BLINDLY
BLINDTO
BLINKAT
BLINKED
BLINKER
BLINTZE
BLONDER
BLONDES
BLONDIE
BLUNDEN
BLUNDER
BLUNTED
BLUNTER
BLUNTLY
BLYNKEN
CLANGED
CLANGER
CLANGOR
CLANKED
CLANTON
CLINGER
CLINGTO
CLINICS
CLINKED
CLINKER
CLINTON
CLONERS
CLONING
CLONKED
CLUNGTO
CLUNKED
CLUNKER
ELANCES
ELANETS
ELANTRA
ELENIAK
FLANEUR
FLANGES
FLANKED
FLANKEN
FLANKER
FLANNEL
FLENSED
FLENSER
FLENSES
FLINGAT
FLINGER
FLINTMI
FLUNGAT
FLUNKED
FLUNKER
FLYNETS
GLANCED
GLANCES
GLENCOE
GLINTED
GLYNNIS
ILLNESS
KLENSCH
KLINGER
KLINGON
KLINKER
KLMNOPQ
LLANERO
OLDNAVY
OLDNESS
OLDNEWS
OLDNICK
PLANATE
PLANERS
PLANETS
PLANFOR
PLANING
PLANISH
PLANKED
PLANNED
PLANNER
PLANOUT
PLANSON
PLANSTO
PLANTAR
PLANTED
PLANTER
PLENARY
PLENISH
PLENUMS
PLINKED
PLINTHS
PLONKED
PLUNDER
PLUNGED
PLUNGER
PLUNGES
PLUNKED
PLUNKER
SLANDER
SLANTED
SLANTLY
SLANTUP
SLENDER
SLINGER
SLINKED
SLINKER
SLINKIN
SLINKUP
SLUNKIN
SLUNKUP
SLYNESS
TLINGIT
ULANOVA
ULANUDE

•L••N••

ALANNAH
ALBANIA
ALBENIZ
ALBINOS
ALBUNDY
ALDENTE
ALFONSE
ALFONSO
ALIENEE
ALIENOR
ALIENTO
ALIGNED
ALIGNER
ALKENES
ALLANTE
ALLENBY
ALLENDE
ALLONGE
ALLONYM
ALMANAC
ALMONDS
ALMONDY
ALMONER
ALMONRY
ALPINER
ALPINES
ALUMNAE
ALUMNAL
ALUMNUS
BLARNEY
BLOWNIN
BLOWNUP
BLUINGS
CLEANED
CLEANER
CLEANLY
CLEANSE
CLEANTE
CLEANUP
CLIENTS
CLOONEY
CLOWNED
ELAINES
ELEANOR
ELMONTE
ELMUNDO
ELNINOS
ELUANTS
FLANNEL
FLAUNTS
FLAUNTY
FLEANCE
FLEXNER
FLOUNCE
FLOUNCY
FLOWNAT
FLOWNBY
FLOWNIN
FLOWNON
FLOWNTO
FLOWNUP
FLUENCY
FLYINTO
GLEANED
GLEANER
GLYNNIS
ILLKNOW
KLEENEX
OLEANNA
OLEANNY
PLAINER
PLAINES
PLAINLY
PLAINTS
PLANNED
PLANNER
PLIANCY
ULYANOV
ULZANAS

•L•••N•

ALADINE
ALAKING
ALANINE
ALAYING
ALCYONE
ALIMENT
ALIMONY
ALINING
ALLDONE
ALLGONE
ALLMINE
ALLYING
ALTHING
ALTOONA
ALUMINA
BLADING
BLAMING
BLARING
BLATANT
BLAZING
BLAZONS
BLOWING
BLUEING
CLAMANT
CLAWING
CLAYING
CLEMENS
CLEMENT
CLEWING
CLIPONS
CLONING
CLOSING
CLOYING
CLUEING
ELATING
ELEGANT
ELEMENT
ELEVENA
ELEVENB
ELEVENC
ELEVEND
ELEVENE
ELEVENS
ELEVONS
ELIDING
ELLMANN
ELOPING
ELUDING
ELUTING
FLACONS
FLAGONS
FLAKING
FLAMING
FLARING
FLAWING
FLAYING
FLEEING
FLEMING
FLEXING
FLORENZ
FLORINS
FLOWING
FLUTING
FLUXING
GLARING
GLAVINE
GLAZING
GLIDING
GLOBING
GLOBINS
GLOVING
GLOWING
GLUTENS
GLYCINE
ILIAMNA
ILLDONE
ILLEANA
ILLWIND
ILOCANO
KLAXONS
OLDHAND
OLDLINE
OLDSONG
OLEANNA
OLEANNY
OLEFINS
OLIVINE
PLACING
PLANING
PLATENS
PLATING
PLAYING
PLOWING
PLUGINS
PLUMING
PLUSONE
PLUTONS
RLSTINE
SLAKING
SLATING
SLAVING
SLAYING
SLEWING
SLICING
SLIDING
SLIMING
SLIPONS
SLOGANS
SLOPING
SLOVENE
SLOVENS
SLOWING
ULLMANN
ULULANT

•L••••N

ALADDIN
ALAMEIN
ALARCON
ALASKAN
ALATEEN
ALBUMEN
ALBUMIN
ALDUBIN
ALENCON
ALGREEN
ALLBRAN
ALLISON
ALLOWIN
ALLSTON
ALLYSON
ALMADEN
ALMSMAN
ALMSMEN
ALROSEN
ALSHAIN
ALSORAN
ALTHORN
ALYKHAN
BLACKEN
BLAMEON
BLANTON
BLENDIN
BLENTIN
BLITZEN
BLOUSON
BLOWGUN
BLOWNIN
BLOWSIN
BLOWSON
BLUEFIN
BLUEHEN
BLUESUN
BLUNDEN
BLUSHON
BLYNKEN
CLACTON
CLAMPON
CLANTON
CLAPTON
CLARION
CLASSON
CLAYTON
CLEAVON
CLEMSON
CLIBURN
CLICKON
CLIFTON
CLIMBIN
CLIMBON
CLINTON
CLIPSON
CLOCKIN
CLOSEIN
CLUEDIN
CLUESIN
ELAAIUN
ELASTIN
ELATION
ELCAJON
ELEISON
ELISION
ELLISON
ELLMANN
ELTRAIN
ELUTION
ELYSIAN
FLAGMAN
FLAGMEN
FLANKEN
FLASHON
FLATTEN
FLEURON
FLEXION
FLIESIN
FLIESON
FLIPPEN
FLITSIN
FLORIAN
FLOWNIN
FLOWNON
FLOWSIN
FLUXION
FLYOPEN
GLADDEN
GLEASON
GLEEMAN
GLEEMEN
GLIDEIN
GLISTEN
GLOAMIN
GLUEDON
GLUEGUN
GLUESON
GLUTTON
KLINGON
KLUGMAN
LLEYTON
OLDBEAN
OLDMOON
OLDTOWN
PLANSON
PLATOON
PLAYPEN
PLAYSON
PLEBIAN
PLOSION
PLOWMAN
PLOWMEN
PLOWSON
PLUGSIN
SLACKEN
SLAMSON
SLAPSON
SLATKIN
SLAYTON
SLEEKEN
SLEEPIN
SLEEPON
SLEPTIN
SLEPTON
SLIDEIN
SLINKIN
SLIPSIN
SLIPSON
SLOEGIN
SLOPSON
SLUNKIN
ULLMANN

••LN•••

ALLNESS
ALLNEWS
FULNESS
ILLNESS
KILNDRY
KILNING
SOLNESS
VILNIUS
WALNUTS

••L•N••

ALLANTE
ALLENBY
ALLENDE
ALLONGE
ALLONYM
APLENTY
ATLANTA
ATLUNCH
BALANCE
BALONEY
BELINDA
BELONGS
BILLNYE
BYLINED
BYLINER
BYLINES
CALANDO
CALENDS
CALLNOW
CILENTO
COLONEL
COLONES
COLONNA
COLONUS
DELANEY
DELINTS
DOLUNCH
ENLINKS
ERLANGS
FELINES
FELONRY
FILENES
FILINGS
FOLENGO
GALANOS
GALANTS
GALENAS
GALENTO
GILLNET
ILLKNOW
INLANDS
INLINES
ISLANDS
JKLMNOP
KALININ
KOLANUT
LALANNE
LILINAU
MELANGE
MELANIA
MELANIC
MELANIE
MELANIN
MELINDA
MYLANTA
OBLONGS
OOLONGS
ORLANDO
PALANCE
PALINGS
PILINGS
PILSNER
POLANER
POLANYI
POLENTA
POLONIA
RELANCE
RELANDS
RELANES
RELENDS
RELENTS
RELINED
RELINES
RELINKS
ROLONDA
RULINGS
SALINAS
SALINES
SALONGA
SELENIC
SILENCE
SILENTA
SILENTB
SILENTC
SILENTD
SILENTE
SILENTF
SILENTG
SILENTH
SILENTI
SILENTJ
SILENTK
SILENTL
SILENTM
SILENTN
SILENTO
SILENTP
SILENTQ
SILENTR
SILENTS
SILENTT
SILENTU
SILENTV
SILENTW
SILENTX
SILENTY
SILENTZ
SPLENDA
SPLINES
SPLINTS
TALENTS
TALONED
TILINGS
TILLNOW
TULANEU
TYLENOL
UNLINED
UNLINKS
UPLANDS
UPLINKS
VALANCE
VALENCE
VALENTE
VALENTI
VALINES
VOLANTE
VOLENTE
YOLANDA

••L••N•

AILMENT
ALLDONE
ALLGONE
ALLMINE
ALLYING
BALCONY
BALDING
BALEENS
BALKANS
BALKING
BALLONE
BCLIONS
BELLING
BELLINI
BELMONT
BELTANE
BELTING
BELYING
BELZONI
BILKING
BILLING
BOLLING
BOLOGNA
BOLTING
BULGING
BULKING
BULLING
BULLINS
CALKING
CALKINS
CALLING
CALLINS
CALMING
CALUMNY
CALVING
CALVINO
CALZONE
CELAENO
CELLINI
COLDONE
COLLINE
COLLINS
COLOGNE
COLONNA
COLUMNS
CULLING
DALTONS
DELEING
DELMONT
DELTONA
DELVING
DILUENT
DOLLING
DOLMANS
DULLING
ELLMANN
FALCONS
FALLING
FELLING
FELLINI
FELTING
FILLING
FILLINS
FILMING
FOLDING
FULGENT
GALLANT
GALLING
GALLONS
GALVANI
GALVANO
GELDING
GELLING
GELPENS
GILDING
GILLING
GOLDING
GOLDONI
GOLFING
GULDENS
GULFING
GULLING
GULPING
HALDANE
HALOING
HALTING
HALVING
HELLENE
HELLENO
HELMING
HELMOND
HELPING
HELSING
HILLING
HILTING
HILTONS
HOLDING
HOLLAND
HOLYONE
HULKING
HULLING
ILLDONE
ILLEANA
ILLWIND
INLYING
JELLING
JILTING
JOLTING
JULIANA
KELOWNA
KELVINS
KILLING
KILNING
KILTING
LALANNE
LALLING
LILTING
LOLLING
LULLING
MALEANT
MALIANS
MALIGNS
MALTING
MALVINA
MELDING
MELTING
MILKING
MILLAND
MILLEND
MILLING
MOLDING
MOLSONS
MOLTING
MULLING
MULLINS
NELSONS
NULLING
OILCANS
OILLINE
OILPANS
OILRING
OILSAND
OILTANK
ORLEANS
PALLING
PALMING
PELTING
PILLING
POLLENS
POLLING
PULLING
PULLINS
PULLONS
PULMONI
PULMONO
PULPING
PULSING
RDLAING
RELIANT
RELLENO
RELOANS
RELYING
ROLFING
ROLLAND
ROLLING
ROLLINS
ROLLONS
RULEONE
SALERNO
SALIENT
SALMONP
SALMONS
SALOONS
SALTANT
SALTINE
SALTING
SALVING
SELLING
SILOING
SILTING
SOLOING
SOLVENT
SOLVING
SPLEENS
SPLEENY
SULKING
SULTANA
SULTANS
TALKING
TALLINN
TALLONE
TELLING
TILLING
TILTING
TOLLING
TOLUENE
TULSANS
ULLMANN
UNLYING
VALIANT
VALLONE
VALUING
VOLCANO
VOLPONE
VULCANS
VULPINE
WALKING
WALKINS
WALKONS
WALLING
WALTONS
WELDING
WELLAND
WELLING
WELTING
WILDING
WILDONE
WILKENS
WILKINS
WILLING
WILSONS
WILTING
WOLFING
YELLING
YELPING
ZELAZNY

••L•••N

AILERON
ALLBRAN
ALLISON
ALLOWIN
ALLSTON
ALLYSON
BALABAN
BALATON

BALDWIN
BALLOON
BALMAIN
BELEVEN
BELGIAN
BELLMAN
BELLMEN
BELLSON
BELTRAN
BILLION
BKLIBAN
BULLION
BULLPEN
BULLRUN
CALDRON
CALHOUN
CALIBAN
CALLSIN
CALLSON
CELADON
COLEMAN
COLLEEN
DELIMAN
DELIMEN
DILLMAN
DOLPHIN
EELSKIN
ELLISON
ELLMANN
ENLIVEN
FALLSIN
FALLSON
FELDMAN
FELTPEN
FILEDIN
FILESIN
FILLSIN
FOLDSIN
GALLEON
GELATIN
GILLIAN
GILLMAN
GOLDARN
GOLDMAN
GOLDWYN
HALCYON
HALFWON
HALOGEN
HALSTON
HELICON
HELLION
HELLMAN
HELPSIN
HELPSON
HILLMAN
HILLMEN
HOLBEIN
HOLDSIN
HOLDSON
HOLYMAN
HOLYMEN
HOLZMAN
JILLIAN
JILLION
KALININ
KELLJAN
KILLEEN
KILOTON
LILLIAN
MALAGAN
MALAYAN
MCLUHAN
MELANIN
MILERUN
MILKCAN
MILKMAN
MILKMEN
MILKRUN
MILLION
MILLRUN
MTLOGAN
MULDOON
NILSSON
OILSKIN
PALADIN
PALEMON
PELICAN
PELOTON
PILEDIN
PILEDON
PILESIN
PILESON
PILLION
POLEMAN
POLEMEN
POLYGON
PULLMAN
PULLPIN
PULLSIN
PULLSON
RALSTON
RELEARN
ROLLSIN
ROLLSON
RULEDON
RULESON
SALADIN
SALOMON
SILENTN
SILICON
SOLOMON
TALIBAN
TALKSON
TALLINN
TELERAN
TELLSON
TOLEDAN
TOLKIEN
TOLLMAN
TOLLMEN
ULLMANN
UNLADEN
UNLEARN
VALADON
VALJEAN
VELTMAN
VILLAIN
VILLEIN
WALKMAN
WALKSON
WALLOON
WALLSIN
WALSTON
WELLMAN
WELLRUN
WELLWON
WILDMAN
WILDMEN
WILLSON
WOLFMAN
WOLFMEN
YALEMAN
YALEMEN
YELTSIN
ZILLION

•••LN••

BILLNYE
CALLNOW
GILLNET
TILLNOW

•••L•N•

ABALONE
ABILENE
ADDLING
ADELINA
ADELINE
AGELONG
AIRLANE
AIRLINE
AMBLING
ANELING
ANGLING
ANILINE
APPLING
ASHLAND
AVALONS
BADLAND
BAILING
BALLONE
BAWLING
BAYLYNX
BEELINE
BELLING
BELLINI
BILLING
BIPLANE
BIRLING
BOILING
BOLLING
BOWLINE
BOWLING
BUGLING
BULLING
BULLINS
BURLING
BUSLANE
BUSLINE
CABLING
CALLING
CALLINS
CARLENE
CARLING
CEILING
CELLINI
CHALONS
CHOLINE
COALING
COBLENZ
COILING
COLLINE
COLLINS
COOLANT
COOLING
COPLAND
COULDNT
COWLING
CULLING
CURLING
CYCLING
CYCLONE
DARLENE
DARLING
DAYLONG
DEALING
DECLINE
DEPLANE
DEWLINE
DIALING
DOLLING
DOWLING
DUELING
DULLING
DUNLINS
EAGLING
EMPLANE
ENDLINE
ENDLONG
ENGLAND
ENGLUND
ENPLANE
EONLINE
ERELONG
EUGLENA
EVALUNA
EVELONG
EVILONE
EXILING
EYELINE
FABLING
FAILING
FALLING
FATLING
FEELING
FELLING
FELLINI
FILLING
FILLINS
FINLAND
FOALING
FOILING
FOOLING
FORLANI
FOULING
FOWLING
FRELENG
FUELING
FURLING
FURLONG
GAGLINE
GALLANT
GALLING
GALLONS
GAOLING
GARLAND
GASLINE
GATLING
GATLINS
GELLING
GILLING
GOALONG
GOBLANK
GOBLINS
GODLING
GOSLING
GUILING
GULLING
HAILING
HAMLINE
HARLAND
HARLINE
HAULING
HEALING
HEELING
HELLENE
HELLENO
HEMLINE
HILLING
HOLLAND
HOTLINE
HOTLINK
HOVLANE
HOWLING
HOWLONG
HULLING
HURLING
ICELAND
ICELINE
IJKLMNO
IMPLANT
INALINE
INCLINE
INKLING
IRELAND
ISOLINE
JAILING
JAWLINE
JAYLENO
JELLING
JUTLAND
KAYLENZ
KEELING
KILLING
KIPLING
KOBLENZ
LADLING
LALLING
LAPLAND
LEBLANC
LOLLING
LOWLAND
LULLING
MAILING
MAILINS
MARLENE
MARLINS
MAULING
MEMLING
MERLINS
MEWLING
MIDLAND
MIDLINE
MILLAND
MILLEND
MILLING
MOILING
MTBLANC
MULLING
MULLINS
MUSLINS
NAILING
NEDLAND
NEWLINE
NIALONG
NULLING
OAKLAND
OFFLINE
OILLINE
OLDLINE
ONALINE
ONELANE
OPALINE
OPULENT
OUTLAND
OUTLINE
PALLING
PAULINA
PAULINE
PAULING
PCCLONE
PEALING
PEELING
PHALANX
PILLING
POBLANO
POLLENS
POLLING
POOLING
POPLINS
POULENC
PRALINE
PROLONG
PULLING
PULLINS
PULLONS
PURLING
RAGLANS
RAILING
RATLINE
RATLINS
RAWLINS
REALINE
RECLINE
REDLINE
REELING
RELLENO
REPLANE
REPLANS
REPLANT
RIFLING
ROILING
ROLLAND
ROLLING
ROLLINS
ROLLONS
ROWLAND
ROWLING
RUTLAND
SAILING
SAPLING
SCALENE
SCALING
SEALANE
SEALANT
SEALING
SELLING
SERLING
SIBLING
SIDLING
SIXLANE
SKYLINE
SMILING
SOILING
SOYLENT
SPELUNK
STOLONS
STYLING
SUBLONG
TABLING
TAGLINE
TAILEND
TAILING
TALLINN
TALLONE
TANLINE
TEFLONS
TELLING
TIELINE
TIGLONS
TILLING
TIPLINE
TITLING
TOILING
TOLLING
TOOLING
TOOLONG
TOPLINE
TOWLINE
TOYLAND
TWOLANE
UGOLINO
ULULANT
UNALONE
UNBLENT
UNPLANS
UNSLING
UNSLUNG
UPFLING
VALLONE
VANLINE
VEILING
VIALING
VINLAND
VIOLENT
VIOLINS
VIOLONE
WAILING
WALLING
WAYLAND
WELLAND
WELLING
WETLAND
WHALING
WHILING
WIELAND
WILLING
WITLING
WOOLENS
WOULDNT
YELLING
YOWLING
ZEALAND
ZEELAND

•••L••N

AEOLIAN
ANTLION
APULIAN
BAILSON
BALLOON
BDALTON
BEALION
BELLMAN
BELLMEN
BELLSON
BILLION
BOOLEAN
BUILDIN
BUILDON
BUILTIN
BUILTON
BULLION
BULLPEN
BULLRUN
CALLSIN
CALLSON
CARLOAN
CARLSON
CARLTON
CHILEAN
COALBIN
COLLEEN
CURLSIN
DARLEEN
DEALSIN
DEALTIN
DIALSIN
DILLMAN
DRSLOAN
DWELLIN
DWELLON
DWELTON
EARLYON
EXPLAIN
FALLSIN
FALLSON
FHALOAN
FILLSIN
FORLORN
GALLEON
GILLIAN
GILLMAN
HAULSIN
HELLION
HELLMAN
HILLMAN
HILLMEN
ITALIAN
JILLIAN
JILLION
KARLSON
KELLJAN
KILLEEN
KJELLIN
KOWLOON
LILLIAN
LURLEEN
MACLEAN
MAILBIN
MAILMAN
MAILMEN
MAILSIN
MAULDIN
MCALLEN
MGMLION
MILLION
MILLRUN
MRCLEAN
NAILGUN
NAILSIN
NIELSEN
NUCLEON
OAKLAWN
OUTLAIN
OUTLIMN
PAULSEN
PERLMAN
PETLION
PHILBIN
PILLION
POOLMAN
POOLMEN
PRELOAN
PULLMAN
PULLPIN
PULLSIN
PULLSON
PURLOIN
RAILMAN
RAILMEN
RAILSON
REALIGN
REALMAN
REALMEN
REBLOWN
RECLEAN
REELSIN
REFLOWN
ROLLSIN
ROLLSON
SAILSON
SEALION
SEALSIN
SHELDON
SHULMAN
SIRLOIN
SKELTON
SMILEON
SNELLEN
SOULMAN
STILTON
STOLEIN
STOLLEN
SUELLEN
SUELYON
SWOLLEN
TAILFIN
TAILPIN
TALLINN
TELLSON
TOLLMAN
TOLLMEN
TRILLIN
UNBLOWN
UNCLEAN
UNFLOWN
UNSLAIN
VILLAIN
VILLEIN
WALLOON
WALLSIN
WELLMAN
WELLRUN
WELLWON
WILLSON
WOOLLEN
ZILLION

••••LN•

AAMILNE
WEDELNS

••••L•N

AMESLAN
ANGOLAN
BABYLON
BRESLIN
CAROLYN
CATALAN
CHAPLIN
CHITLIN
COGHLAN
COMPLIN
CONKLIN
DOUBLEN
DRUMLIN
DWELLIN
DWELLON
ECHELON
EIDOLON
EPSILON
EXCELIN
FENELON
GAMELAN
GAVILAN
GOBELIN
GREMLIN
HAMELIN
HANDLIN
HIJKLMN
INSULIN
JAVELIN
JERILYN
JOCELYN
KENOLIN
KJELLIN
KREMLIN
KTOSLIN
LANOLIN
LOCKLIN
MADALYN
MADELON
MANOLIN
MARILYN
MATALIN
MAUDLIN
MAYALIN
MCALLEN
MECHLIN
MEGALON
MIFFLIN
MISPLAN
OBERLIN
OHANLON
ORTOLAN
OUTPLAN
PREPLAN
QUINLAN
RAMBLIN
REVELIN
RITALIN
ROMULAN
ROSALYN
RUSSLAN
SNELLEN
STEALIN
STOLLEN
SUBCLAN
SUELLEN
SWOLLEN
TAMBLYN
TAMGLEN
TASHLIN
TOHELEN
TRILLIN
UPSILON
WHEELIN
WOOLLEN
ZEBULON
ZEBULUN

•••••LN

LINCOLN

LO•••••

LOADERS
LOADING
LOADSIN
LOADSOF
LOADSUP
LOAFERS
LOAFING
LOAFPAN
LOAMIER
LOAMING
LOANERS
LOANING
LOANOUT
LOATHED
LOATHER
LOATHES
LOATHLY
LOATHTO
LOBATED
LOBBERS
LOBBIED
LOBBIES
LOBBING
LOBBYER
LOBSTER
LOBULES
LOCALES
LOCALLY
LOCARNO
LOCATED
LOCATER
LOCATES
LOCATOR
LOCKAGE
LOCKBOX
LOCKEAN
LOCKERS
LOCKETS
LOCKING
LOCKINS
LOCKJAW
LOCKLET
LOCKLIN
LOCKNUT
LOCKOUT
LOCKSET
LOCKSIN
LOCKSON
LOCKSUP
LOCKUPS
LOCULUS
LOCUSTS
LODGEIN
LODGERS
LODGING
LOESSER
LOESSES
LOFTBED
LOFTERS
LOFTIER
LOFTILY
LOFTING
LOGANUT
LOGBOOK
LOGGERS
LOGGIAS
LOGGING
LOGGINS
LOGGISH
LOGICAL
LOGIEST
LOGJAMS
LOGOFFS
LOGONTO
LOGOUTS
LOGROLL
LOGSOFF
LOGSOUT
LOIDING
LOITERS
LOLLARD
LOLLERS
LOLLIES
LOLLING
LOMBARD
LONBORG
LONDRES
LONETTE
LONGAGO
LONGARM
LONGBED
LONGBOW
LONGDAY
LONGDEN
LONGEST
LONGFOR
LONGIES
LONGING
LONGISH
LONGRUN
LONGTOM
LONGTON
LONGUES
LONGWAY
LONIGAN
LOOBIES
LOOFAHS
LOOKERS
LOOKFOR
LOOKING
LOOKINS
LOOKISM
LOOKIST
LOOKOUT
LOOKSAD
LOOKSAT
LOOKSEE
LOOKSIN
LOOKSON
LOOKSTO
LOOKSUP
LOOKUPS
LOOKYOU
LOOMING
LOOMPAS
LOONIER
LOONIES
LOONILY
LOOPERS
LOOPIER
LOOPING
LOOSELY
LOOSENS
LOOSEST
LOOSING
LOOTERS
LOOTING
LOPPERS
LOPPIER
LOPPING
LOPSOFF
LOQUATS
LORANGE
LORDING
LORDJIM
LORDSIT
LORELAI
LORELEI
LORENTZ
LORENZO
LORETTA
LORGNON
LORIENT
LORISES
LORRIES
LORUSES
LOSABLE
LOSEBIG
LOSEOUT
LOSESIT
LOSESTO
LOSINGS
LOSTART
LOSTBIG
LOSTCAT
LOSTDOG
LOSTOUT
LOSTPET
LOTHAIR
LOTHIAN
LOTHROP
LOTIONS
LOTTERS
LOTTERY
LOTTING
LOTUSES
LOUDENS

LOUDEST
LOUDISH
LOUELLA
LOUISII
LOUISIV
LOUISIX
LOUISVI
LOUISXI
LOUISXV
LOUNGED
LOUNGER
LOUNGES
LOURDES
LOUREED
LOURING
LOUSEUP
LOUSIER
LOUSILY
LOUSING
LOUTING
LOUTISH
LOUVERS
LOUVRED
LOUVRES
LOVABLE
LOVABLY
LOVAGES
LOVEBUG
LOVEDIT
LOVEDTO
LOVEINS
LOVEJOY
LOVERLY
LOVESET
LOVESIT
LOVESTO
LOVETAP
LOVEYOU
LOWBALL
LOWBEAM
LOWBIDS
LOWBLOW
LOWBORN
LOWBOYS
LOWBRED
LOWBROW
LOWCARB
LOWCARD
LOWCHEN
LOWCOST
LOWDIVE
LOWDOWN
LOWEEZY
LOWERED
LOWGEAR
LOWHAND
LOWHEEL
LOWLAND
LOWLIER
LOWLIFE
LOWLILY
LOWMASS
LOWNECK
LOWNESS
LOWPAID
LOWPAIR
LOWPOST
LOWRENT
LOWRISE
LOWRISK
LOWROAD
LOWSIDE
LOWTECH
LOWTIDE
LOWTOPS
LOYALER
LOYALES
LOYALLY
LOYALTO
LOYALTY
LOYOLAU
LOZENGE

L•O••••

LAOCOON
LAOTIAN
LEOGENN
LEONARD
LEONATO
LEONDAY
LEONIDS
LEONINE
LEONORA
LEONORE
LEOPARD
LEOPOLD
LEOTARD
LEOVIII
LEOXIII
LIONCUB
LIONELL
LIONELS
LIONESS
LIONETS
LIONISE
LIONIZE
LOOBIES
LOOFAHS
LOOKERS
LOOKFOR
LOOKING
LOOKINS
LOOKISM
LOOKIST
LOOKOUT
LOOKSAD
LOOKSAT
LOOKSEE
LOOKSIN
LOOKSON
LOOKSTO
LOOKSUP
LOOKUPS
LOOKYOU
LOOMING
LOOMPAS
LOONIER
LOONIES
LOONILY
LOOPERS
LOOPIER
LOOPING
LOOSELY
LOOSENS
LOOSEST
LOOSING
LOOTERS
LOOTING
LYOCELL
LYONELL

L••O•••

LABORAT
LABORED
LABORER
LABOURS
LACONIA
LACONIC
LACOSTE
LADOUCE
LAGOONS
LAJOLLA
LAKOTAS
LALOOSH
LAMOTTA
LAMOTTE
LANOLIN
LANOTTE
LAPORTE
LAROCHE
LASORDA
LATOSCA
LAVORIS
LAYODDS
LAYOFFS
LAYOPEN
LAYOUTS
LAYOVER
LAZONGA
LECONTE
LEGOLAS
LEGOSET
LELOUCH
LEMONDE
LEMOYNE
LENOVOS
LESOTHO
LIEOVER
LIMOGES
LITOTES
LITOVSK
LIVORNO
LLCOOLJ
LMNOPQR
LOGOFFS
LOGONTO
LOGOUTS
LOYOLAU
LTKOJAK

L•••O••

LABCOAT
LACTOSE
LADHOOD
LADRONE
LAGOONS
LAIDOFF
LAIDOUT
LALOOSH
LAMPOIL
LAMPOON
LANCOME
LANEONE
LANFORD
LAOCOON
LAPDOGS
LAPROBE
LAPTOPS
LARDONS
LASHOUT
LASSOED
LASSOER
LASSOES
LASTONE
LASTORY
LATROBE
LAWBOOK
LAWFORD
LAYDOWN
LAYSOFF
LAYSOUT
LAZBOYS
LEACOCK
LEADOFF
LEADORE
LEADOUT
LEAFOUT
LEAWOOD
LEBROCK
LECTORS
LECUONA
LEEFORD
LEFTOFF
LEFTOUT
LEGBONE
LEGHORN
LEGIONS
LEGROOM
LEGROPE
LEGWORK
LENDOUT
LENNONS
LEONORA
LEONORE
LEOPOLD
LEPTONS
LESIONS
LESSONS
LESSORS
LESTOIL
LETDOWN
LETGOBY
LETGOOF
LETROLL
LETSOFF
LETSOUT
LEWHOAD
LIEDOWN
LIENORS
LIFTOFF
LIMPOPO
LINCOLN
LINDORF
LINEONE
LINEOUT
LINGOES
LIPSOFF
LIPSOUT
LIQUORS
LISSOME
LITHOID
LIVEOAK
LIVEONE
LIVEOUT
LLCOOLJ
LOANOUT
LOCKOUT
LOGBOOK
LOGROLL
LOGSOFF
LOGSOUT
LONBORG
LOOKOUT
LOPSOFF
LOSEOUT
LOSTOUT
LOTIONS
LOWBORN
LOWBOYS
LOWCOST
LOWDOWN
LOWPOST
LOWROAD
LOWTOPS
LUBBOCK
LUCKOUT
LUGSOUT
LUGWORM
LYESOAP
LYNDONB

L••••O•

LACESON
LADADOG
LADHOOD
LADINOS
LAIDFOR
LAIDLOW
LAMPOON
LANGDON
LANGTON
LANGUOR
LAOCOON
LAREDOS
LARGEOJ
LASTDON
LASTROW
LATCHON
LATERON
LATIGOS
LATINOS
LAVABOS
LAWBOOK
LAYITON
LAYSFOR
LAYSLOW
LAYUPON
LEADDOG
LEADSON
LEANSON
LEANTOS
LEAPFOR
LEAPSON
LEAPTON
LEARNOF
LEAVEON
LEAWOOD
LEBANON
LEBARON
LEFTFOR
LEGATOR
LEGATOS
LEGIRON
LEGROOM
LENOVOS
LETDROP
LETGOOF
LETINON
LETKNOW
LETSNOT
LETUPON
LEVATOR
LEXICON
LIAISON
LIBIDOS
LIEATOP
LIEDFOR
LIESFOR
LIESLOW
LIGHTON
LIKEWOW
LIMACON
LINDROS
LINGCOD
LITHGOW
LIVEDON
LIVEFOR
LIVESON
LLADROS
LLEYTON
LOADSOF
LOCATOR
LOCKBOX
LOCKSON
LOGBOOK
LONGBOW
LONGFOR
LONGTOM
LONGTON
LOOKFOR
LOOKSON
LOOKYOU
LORGNON
LOSTDOG
LOTHROP
LOVEJOY
LOVEYOU
LOWBLOW
LOWBROW
LUBEJOB
LUCKNOW
LYINGON
LYRICON

L•••••O

LACRIMO
LAMINTO
LANETWO
LAYINTO
LEADSTO
LEANSTO
LEARNTO
LEASETO
LEDINTO
LEDUPTO
LENTIGO
LEONATO
LEPANTO
LESOTHO
LETITGO
LETMEGO
LETTERO
LIKENTO
LIMPOPO
LINBIAO
LINETWO
LINPIAO
LITINTO
LIVORNO
LLANERO
LOATHTO
LOCARNO
LOGONTO
LONGAGO
LOOKSTO
LORENZO
LOSESTO
LOVEDTO
LOVESTO
LOYALTO
LUCHINO
LUCIANO
LUMBAGO
LYINGTO
LYSENKO

•LO••••

ALOADOF
ALOHAOE
ALOOFLY
BLOATED
BLOBBED
BLOCKED
BLOCKER
BLOCKUP
BLOGGED
BLOGGER
BLONDER
BLONDES
BLONDIE
BLOODED
BLOOMED
BLOOMER
BLOOPED
BLOOPER
BLOSSOM
BLOTCHY
BLOTOUT
BLOTSUP
BLOTTED
BLOTTER
BLOUSED
BLOUSES
BLOUSON
BLOWDRY
BLOWERS
BLOWFLY
BLOWGUN
BLOWIER
BLOWING
BLOWNIN
BLOWNUP
BLOWOFF
BLOWOUT
BLOWPOP
BLOWSIN
BLOWSIT
BLOWSON
BLOWSUP
BLOWUPS
BLOWZED
CLOAKED
CLOBBER
CLOCHES
CLOCKED
CLOCKER
CLOCKIN
CLOGGED
CLOGSUP
CLOMPED
CLONERS
CLONING
CLONKED
CLOONEY
CLOPPED
CLORETS
CLOSEBY
CLOSEIN
CLOSELY
CLOSERS
CLOSEST
CLOSETO
CLOSETS
CLOSEUP
CLOSING
CLOSURE
CLOTHED
CLOTHES
CLOTSUP
CLOTTED
CLOTURE
CLOUDED
CLOUDUP
CLOUTED
CLOUTER
CLOVERS
CLOVERY
CLOWDER
CLOWNED
CLOYING
ELOCUTE
ELOPERS
ELOPING
FLOATBY
FLOATED
FLOATER
FLOATUP
FLOCKED
FLOCKTO
FLOGGED
FLOGGER
FLOODED
FLOORED
FLOORER
FLOORIT
FLOPPED
FLOPPER
FLOREAL
FLORENZ
FLORETS
FLORIAN
FLORIDA
FLORINS
FLORIST
FLOSSED
FLOSSER
FLOSSES
FLOSSIE
FLOTAGE
FLOTSAM
FLOUNCE
FLOUNCY
FLOURED
FLOUTED
FLOUTER
FLOWAGE
FLOWERS
FLOWERY
FLOWING
FLOWNAT
FLOWNBY
FLOWNIN
FLOWNON
FLOWNTO
FLOWNUP
FLOWOUT
FLOWSIN
GLOAMIN
GLOATED
GLOATER
GLOBATE
GLOBING
GLOBINS
GLOBOID
GLOBOSE
GLOBOUS
GLOBULE
GLOMMED
GLOOMED
GLORIAS
GLORIED
GLORIES
GLORIFY
GLORYBE
GLOSSAE
GLOSSAL
GLOSSAS
GLOSSED
GLOSSER
GLOSSES
GLOTTAL
GLOTTIS
GLOVING
GLOWERS
GLOWING
ILOCANO
ILOSTIT
ILOVEIT
ILOVELA
OLOGIES
OLOROSO
PLODDED
PLODDER
PLOESTI
PLONKED
PLOPPED
PLOSION
PLOSIVE
PLOTFUL
PLOTTED
PLOTTER
PLOTZED
PLOTZES
PLOUGHS
PLOVDIV
PLOVERS
PLOWBOY
PLOWERS
PLOWING
PLOWMAN
PLOWMEN
PLOWSON
PLOWSUP
SLOBBER
SLOEGIN
SLOGANS
SLOGGED
SLOGGER
SLOPERS
SLOPING
SLOPPED
SLOPSON
SLOSHED
SLOSHES
SLOTCAR
SLOTTED
SLOTTER
SLOUCHY
SLOUGHS
SLOVAKS
SLOVENE
SLOVENS
SLOWDAY
SLOWEST
SLOWING
SLOWISH
SLOWSUP
SLOWUPS

•L•O•••

ALBORAK
ALCOHOL
ALCOPOP
ALCOVES
ALDORAY
ALFONSE
ALFONSO
ALFORJA
ALLOFIT
ALLOFME
ALLOFUS
ALLONGE
ALLONYM
ALLOPEZ
ALLOVER
ALLOWAY
ALLOWED
ALLOWIN
ALLOWME
ALLOYED
ALMONDS
ALMONDY
ALMONER
ALMONRY
ALOOFLY
ALROKER
ALROSEN
ALSORAN
ALTOIDS
ALTOIST
ALTOONA
ALTOSAX
ALWORTH
ALYOSHA
BLOODED
BLOOMED
BLOOMER
BLOOPED
BLOOPER
CLOONEY
ELBOWED
ELBOWER
ELFOWLS
ELMONTE
ELNORTE
FLOODED
FLOORED
FLOORER
FLOORIT
FLYOPEN
FLYOVER
GLOOMED
ILLOGIC
LLCOOLJ
OLEOOIL

•L••O••

ALAMODE
ALAMOSA
ALCYONE
ALIFORM
ALIGOTE
ALIMONY
ALLDONE
ALLGONE
ALLGOOD
ALLTOLD
ALTDORF
ALTHORN
ALTOONA
ALVEOLI
BLALOCK
BLAZONS
BLEWOFF
BLEWOUT
BLOTOUT
BLOWOFF
BLOWOUT
BLTTOGO
CLAMORS
CLAMOUR
CLIPOFF
CLIPONS
CLIPOUT
ELEVONS
ELFLOCK
ELLIOTT
ELMWOOD
ELUSORY
FLACONS
FLAGONS
FLATOUT
FLAVORS
FLAVORY
FLAVOUR
FLEXORS
FLIPOUT
FLOWOUT
FLYBOYS
FLYRODS
FLYSOLO
GLAMORS
GLAMOUR
GLOBOID
GLOBOSE
GLOBOUS
GLUCOSE
GLYCOLS
ILLDOIT
ILLDONE
ILLFOLD
KLAXONS
KLMNOPQ
LLCOOLJ
OLDBOYS
OLDDOGS
OLDFOGY
OLDGOLD
OLDJOKE
OLDMOON
OLDROSE
OLDSONG
OLDTOWN
OLEOOIL
OLICOOK
OLOROSO
PLANOUT
PLATOON
PLAYOFF
PLAYOUT
PLEXORS
PLUGOLA
PLUMOSE
PLUSONE
PLUTONS
PLYWOOD
SLALOMS
SLIDOFF
SLIDOUT
SLIPOFF
SLIPONS
SLIPOUT
SLYLOOK
ULANOVA

•L•••O•

ALACKOF
ALARCON
ALBEDOS
ALBINOS
ALCOHOL
ALCOPOP
ALENCON
ALFEROV
ALIENOR
ALLGOOD
ALLISON
ALLSTON
ALLYSON
ALNICOS
ALOADOF
ALOHAOE
BLAMEON
BLANTON
BLAUBOK
BLEDSOE
BLERIOT
BLOSSOM
BLOUSON
BLOWPOP
BLOWSON
BLUEBOY
BLUEFOX
BLUSHON
CLACTON
CLAIROL
CLAMPON
CLANGOR
CLANTON
CLAPFOR
CLAPTON
CLARION
CLASSON
CLAYTON
CLEAROF
CLEAVON
CLEMSON
CLICKON
CLIFTON
CLIMBON
CLINTON
CLIPSON
ELATION
ELCAJON
ELEANOR
ELECTOR
ELEISON
ELISION
ELLISON
ELMWOOD
ELNINOS
ELUTION
FLASHON
FLATTOP
FLEURON
FLEXION
FLIESON
FLIPTOP
FLOWNON
FLUMMOX
FLUSHOT
FLUXION
GLASGOW
GLASHOW
GLEASON
GLENCOE
GLUEDON
GLUESON
GLUTTON
ILLKNOW
KLEPTOS
KLINGON
LLADROS
LLEYTON
OLDMOON
OLDPROS
OLDSHOE
OLICOOK
PLANFOR
PLANSON
PLATOON
PLAYBOY
PLAYDOH
PLAYSON

PLOSION
PLOWBOY
PLOWSON
PLUMCOT
PLYWOOD
SLAMSON
SLAPSON
SLAYTON
SLEDDOG
SLEEPON
SLEPTON
SLIPSON
SLOPSON
SLYLOOK
ULYANOV

•L••••O

ALBERTO
ALBIREO
ALERTTO
ALFONSO
ALFREDO
ALIENTO
ALIVETO
ALLEGRO
BLINDTO
BLTTOGO
CLAMATO
CLAUDIO
CLIMBTO
CLINGTO
CLOSETO
CLUNGTO
ELCAMPO
ELECTRO
ELGALLO
ELGRECO
ELMUNDO
ELPRADO
FLIEDTO
FLIESTO
FLOCKTO
FLOWNTO
FLYINTO
FLYSOLO
GLUEDTO
GLUESTO
ILOCANO
LLANERO
OLOROSO
PLACEBO
PLACIDO
PLANSTO
PLAYSTO
PLEADTO
PLUSTWO

••LO•••

ALLOFIT
ALLOFME
ALLOFUS
ALLONGE
ALLONYM
ALLOPEZ
ALLOVER
ALLOWAY
ALLOWED
ALLOWIN
ALLOWME
ALLOYED
BALONEY
BELONGS
BELOVED
BILOBED
BOLOGNA
BOLOTIE
BULOVAS
CALORIC
CALORIE
CALOTTE
CELOTEX
CHLORIC
COLOGNE
COLOMBO
COLONEL
COLONES
COLONNA
COLONUS
COLORED
COLORER
COLORTV
COLOSSI
COLOURS
CULOTTE
DELORIS
DELORME
DELOUSE
DOLORES
DOLOURS
ECLOGUE
FELONRY
FILOFAX
GALOOTS
GALOPED
HALOGEN
HALOIDS
HALOING
HELOISE
HELOTRY
ILLOGIC
KELOWNA
KILOBAR
KILOBIT
KILOTON
LALOOSH
LELOUCH
MALODOR
MELODIA
MELODIC
MILORDS
MOLOKAI
MOLOTOV
MTLOGAN
NOLOADS
OBLONGS
OBLOQUY
ONLOADS
OOLONGS
PALOMAR
PALOMAS
PALOOKA
PELOTAS
PELOTON
PHLOEMS
PHLOXES
PILOTED
POLOIST
POLONIA
RELOADS
RELOANS
RELOCKS
RELOOKS
RELOSES
ROLODEX
ROLONDA
SALOMON
SALONGA
SALOONS
SHLOCKY
SILOING
SOLOACT
SOLOING
SOLOIST
SOLOMON
SPLOTCH
STLOUIS
TALONED
UNLOADS
UNLOATH
UNLOBED
UNLOCAL
UNLOCKS
UNLOFTY
UNLOOPS
UNLOOSE
UNLOVED
UNLOWLY
UNLOYAL
UPLOADS
VALOREM
VALOTTE
VALOURS
VBLOUSE
VELOURS
VELOUTE
VELOXES
XYLOSES

••L•O••

ALLDONE
ALLGONE
ALLGOOD
ALLTOLD
AXLROSE
BALBOAS
BALCONY
BALFOUR
BALLONE
BALLOON
BALLOTS
BCLIONS
BELFORT
BELLOWS
BELMONT
BELTOUT
BELVOIR
BELVOUR
BELZONI
BILIOUS
BILLOWS
BILLOWY
BULBOUS
BULLOCK
CALHOUN
CALLOFF
CALLOUS
CALLOUT
CALPOLY
CALZONE
COLDONE
COLLODI
COLLOID
COLLOPS
DALTONS
DELMONT
DELMORE
DELSOLS
DELTOID
DELTONA
DELTORO
DOLEOUT
DOLLOPS
EELPOTS
EELPOUT
EELWORM
ELLIOTT
FALCONS
FALLOFF
FALLOUT
FALLOWS
FELLOFF
FELLOUT
FELLOWS
FELTOFF
FELTOUT
FILEOUT
FILLOUT
FOLDOUT
FOLIOED
FOLIOSE
FOLLOWS
FULLOUT
FULSOME
GALLONS
GALLOPS
GALLOWS
GALOOTS
GILFORD
GILMORE
GOLDONI
GULFOIL
HALLOOS
HALLOWS
HELDOFF
HELDOUT
HELLOED
HELLOES
HELMOND
HELPOUT
HILLOCK
HILTONS
HOLDOFF
HOLDOUT
HOLEOUT
HOLLOWS
HOLMOAK
HOLYOIL
HOLYOKE
HOLYONE
HULLOED
ILLDOIT
ILLDONE
ILLFOLD
KELLOGG
LALOOSH
MALCOLM
MALLOWS
MALTOSE
MELLOWS
MELROSE
MILHOUS
MOLDOVA
MOLSONS
MULDOON
NELSONS
PALJOEY
PALLORS
PALMOFF
PALMOIL
PALOOKA
PILEOUS
PILLORY
PILLOWS
PILLOWY
POLLOCK
PULLOFF
PULLONS
PULLOUT
PULMONI
PULMONO
RELOOKS
ROLLOFF
ROLLONS
ROLLOUT
RULEONE
RULEOUT
SALMONP
SALMONS
SALOONS
SALSODA
SALVOES
SALVORS
SELLOFF
SELLOUT
SOLDOFF
SOLDOUT
TALKOUT
TALLONE
TALLOWS
TALLOWY
TELLOFF
TOLDOFF
UNLOOPS
UNLOOSE
VALLONE
VOLPONE
VOLTORE
WALCOTT
WALDORF
WALKOFF
WALKONS
WALKOUT
WALLOFF
WALLOON
WALLOPS
WALLOWS
WALPOLE
WALTONS
WELCOME
WELLOFF
WILDONE
WILFORD
WILLOWS
WILLOWY
WILSONS
YELLOUT
YELLOWS
YELLOWY

••L••O•

AILERON
ALLGOOD
ALLISON
ALLSTON
ALLYSON
ASLEWOF
AULDSOD
BALATON
BALLBOY
BALLIOL
BALLOON
BELABOR
BELLBOY
BELLHOP
BELLSON
BILLION
BOLEROS
BOLSHOI
BULLDOG
BULLION
CALDRON
CALICOS
CALLBOX
CALLBOY
CALLFOR
CALLNOW
CALLSON
CELADON
DILATOR
DILUTOR
ELLISON
FALLFOR
FALLSON
FELLFOR
FELTFOR
FILMDOM
FULLLOT
GALANOS
GALLEON
GELATOS
HALCYON
HALFROD
HALFWON
HALLOOS
HALSTON
HELICON
HELLBOY
HELLION
HELPSON
HILLTOP
HOLDSON
HOLYCOW
HOLYJOE
ILLKNOW
INLABOR
JILLION
JKLMNOP
KILLJOY
KILOTON
MALEDOG
MALEHOG
MALODOR
MILKCOW
MILKSOP
MILLION
MOLITOR
MOLOTOV
MULDOON
NILESOH
NILSSON
OBLIGOR
OILSPOT
ONLYTOO
ONLYYOU
PALEMON
PALMTOP
PALTROW
PELOTON
PILCROW
PILEDON
PILESOF
PILESON
PILLBOX
PILLION
POLYGON
POLYPOD
PULLFOR
PULLSON
PULLTOY
RALSTON
RELATOR
ROLLMOP
ROLLSON
ROLLTOP
RULEDON
RULESON
SALCHOW
SALEMOR
SALOMON
SALTBOX
SELLFOR
SILICON
SOLDFOR
SOLOMON
TALKSOF
TALKSON
TELECOM
TELLSOF
TELLSON
TILLNOW
TILTTOP
TOLEDOS
TOLSTOI
TOLSTOY
TULSAOK
TYLENOL
VALADON
VELCROS
WALKSON
WALLOON
WALSTON
WELLWON
WILDDOG
WILLSON
WILLYOU
WOLFDOG
YELLFOR
YULELOG
ZILLION

••L•••O

ALLEGRO
BALLTWO
BELASCO
CALABRO
CALANDO
CALLSTO
CALVINO
CALYPSO
CELAENO
CILENTO
COLOMBO
COLUMBO
DELICTO
DELILLO
DELTORO
FALLSTO
FILIPPO
FOLENGO
GALENTO
GALILEO
GALLICO
GALVANO
GOLFPRO
HELLENO
HOLDSTO
INLIMBO
JALISCO
MALPASO
MILAGRO
MULATTO
ONLYTOO
ORLANDO
PALAZZO
PALERMO
PULMONO
RALLYTO
RELLENO
RILIEVO
SALERNO
SELLSTO
SILENTO
TALKSTO
TALLYHO
TELESTO
VALLEJO
VOLCANO
WALKSTO

•••LO••

ABALONE
AGELONG
AIRLOCK
AIRLOGS
ANALOGS
ANALOGY
APOLOGY
ARMLOAD
ARMLOCK
ATALOSS
AVALONS
AXOLOTL
BADLOTS
BADLOVE
BAILORS
BAILOUT
BALLONE
BALLOON
BALLOTS
BAWLOUT
BAYLORU
BECLOUD
BEDLOES
BELLOWS
BIGLOTS
BIGLOVE
BILLOWS
BILLOWY
BIOLOGY
BLALOCK
BOILOFF
BOILOUT
BULLOCK
BUSLOAD
CALLOFF
CALLOUS
CALLOUT
CARLOAD
CARLOAN
CARLOTA
CARLOTS
CHALONS
COALOIL
COLLODI
COLLOID
COLLOPS
COOLOUT
COULOMB
CYCLOID
CYCLONE
CYCLOPS
DAYLONG
DEALOUT
DECLOTS
DEPLORE
DEPLOYS
DIALOGS
DIALOUT
DIGLOTS
DIPLOID
DIPLOMA
DOLLOPS
DRSLOAN
DUNLOPS
DYELOTS
EARLOBE
EARLOCK
ECOLOGY
ELFLOCK
EMPLOYS
EMULOUS
ENCLOSE
ENDLONG
ENOLOGY
EPILOGS
ERELONG
EVELONG
EVILONE
EXPLODE
EXPLOIT
EXPLORE
FALLOFF
FALLOUT
FALLOWS
FAXLORE
FEELOFF
FEELOUT
FELLOFF
FELLOUT
FELLOWS
FETLOCK
FHALOAN
FILLOUT
FOLLOWS
FORLORN
FORLOVE
FOULOUT
FUELOIL
FULLOUT
FURLONG
GALLONS
GALLOPS
GALLOWS
GASLOGS
GAYLORD
GENLOCK
GEOLOGY
GETLOST
GOALONG
GOTLOST
GUNLOCK
HALLOOS
HALLOWS
HAPLOID
HARLOTS
HAULOFF
HAYLOFT
HELLOED
HELLOES
HEMLOCK
HEYLOOK
HILLOCK
HOLLOWS
HOWLONG
HULLOED
HYALOID
IAMLOVE
IMPLODE
IMPLORE
INBLOOM
INCLOSE
INFLOWS
ITSLOVE
JAILORS
JEALOUS
JOBLOCK
JOBLOTS
KARLOFF
KARLOVY
KELLOGG
KEYLOCK
KOWLOON
MADLOCK
MAILOUT
MALLOWS
MARLOWE
MATLOCK
MCCLOUD
MELLOWS
MERLOTS
MORLOCK
MYOLOGY
NEOLOGY
NETLOSS
NEWLOOK
NEWLOVE
NIALONG
NOWLOOK
NUMLOCK
OARLOCK
OCELOTS
ODDLOTS
OFFLOAD
ONELOOK
ONELOVE
OROLOGY
OTOLOGY
OUTLOOK
OUTLOUD
OUTLOVE
OXBLOOD
PADLOCK
PALLORS
PARLORS
PARLOUR
PARLOUS
PAVLOVA
PAYLOAD
PCCLONE
PEELOFF
PEELOUT
PHILOUS
PILLORY
PILLOWS
PILLOWY
POLLOCK
PRELOAD
PRELOAN
PRELOSS
PROLOGS
PROLONG
PULLOFF
PULLONS
PULLOUT
PURLOIN
REBLOCK
REBLOOM
REBLOWN
REELOFF
REELOUT
REFLOAT
REFLOOD
REFLOWN
REFLOWS
REGLOSS
REGLOWS
REPLOTS
REPLOWS
RIOLOBO
ROBLOWE
ROLLOFF
ROLLONS
ROLLOUT
RYELOAF
SAILORS
SAMLOYD
SAWLOGS
SCHLOCK
SEALOFF
SELLOFF
SELLOUT
SHALOMS
SHYLOCK
SIRLOIN
SLALOMS
SLYLOOK
STCLOUD
STOLONS
SUBLONG
SUBLOTS
TABLOID
TAILOFF
TAILORS
TALLONE
TALLOWS
TALLOWY
TAYLORS
TEFLONS
TELLOFF
THELOOK
THELOOP
TIGLONS
TOELOOP
TOOLONG
TRILOGY
UFOLOGY
UNALONE
UNBLOCK
UNBLOWN
UNCLOAK
UNCLOGS
UNCLOSE
UNCLOUD
UNFLOOR
UNFLOWN
UNGLOVE
UPCLOSE
UPFLOWS
UPSLOPE
UROLOGY
VALLONE
VANLOAD
VIOLONE
WALLOFF
WALLOON
WALLOPS
WALLOWS
WARLOCK
WARLORD
WEBLOGS
WEDLOCK
WELLOFF
WETLOOK
WILLOWS
WILLOWY
YELLOUT
YELLOWS
YELLOWY
YOULOSE
ZEALOTS
ZEALOUS
ZIPLOCK
ZIPLOCS
ZOOLOGY

•••L•O•

AGALLOP
ANTLION
APILEOF
APOLLOS
AXELROD
BAILSON
BALLBOY
BALLIOL
BALLOON
BDALTON
BEALION
BELLBOY
BELLHOP
BELLSON
BERLIOZ
BIBLIOG
BILLION
BRILLOS
BUILDON
BUILTON
BULLDOG
BULLION
CAILLOU
CALLBOX
CALLBOY
CALLFOR
CALLNOW
CALLSON
CARLSON
CARLTON
DWELLON
DWELTON
EARLDOM
EARLYON
FALLFOR
FALLSON
FEELFOR
FEELSOK
FELLFOR
FUELROD
FULLLOT
GALLEON
HALLOOS
HELLBOY
HELLION
HEYLOOK
HILLTOP
INBLOOM
JILLION
KARLSON
KEILLOR
KILLJOY
KOWLOON
MACLEOD
MAILBOX
MAILLOL
MAILLOT
MGMLION
MILLION
NEWLOOK
NOWLOOK
NUCLEON
ONELOOK
OUTLOOK
OXBLOOD
PETLION
PHILCOS

PHYLLOS
PILLBOX
PILLION
PULLFOR
PULLSON
PULLTOY
RAILSON
REALLOT
REALTOR
REBLOOM
REFLOOD
RIALTOS
ROLLMOP
ROLLSON
ROLLTOP
SAILSON
SCALLOP
SEALION
SELLFOR
SHALLOT
SHALLOW
SHELDON
SKELTON
SLYLOOK
SMALLOJ
SMILEON
STILTON
SUELYON
SWALLOW
TELLSOF
TELLSON
THELOOK
THELOOP
TILLNOW
TOELOOP
TOOLBOX
TROLLOP
TSELIOT
UNFLOOR
WALLOON
WELLWON
WETLOOK
WILLSON
WILLYOU
YELLFOR
ZILLION

•••L••O

APPLYTO
AZULEJO
BALLTWO
CALLSTO
DEALSTO
DEALTTO
DIALEDO
FAILSTO
FALLSTO
GALLICO
HELLENO
IJKLMNO
ISOLATO
JAYLENO
PAMLICO
PIMLICO
POBLANO
RALLYTO
RELLENO
REPLYTO
RIOLOBO
SAILSTO
SELLSTO
TALLYHO
UGOLINO
VALLEJO
YIELDTO

••••LO•

ABSALOM
AFATLOT
AFOULOF
AGALLOP
AIRFLOW
AIRGLOW
AKERLOF
ANGELOU
ANTILOG
APOLLOS
ATEALOT
BABYLON
BACKLOG
BACKLOT
BAROLOS
BIBELOT
BICOLOR
BIGELOW
BRILLOS
BUGALOO
CAILLOU
CAMELOT
CASELOT
CATALOG
CATALOS
COPILOT
DECALOG
DECOLOR
DEVELOP
DIABLOS
DWELLON
EATALOT
ECHELON
EIDOLON
EMMYLOU
ENVELOP
EPSILON
ESCALOP
FEEDLOT
FENELON
FULLLOT
GIGOLOS
GOBELOW
HIGHLOW
ICEFLOE
INCOLOR
INKBLOT
ITSALOT
JANKLOW
JOEBLOW
KEILLOR
KERFLOP
KERPLOP
LAIDLOW
LAYSLOW
LIESLOW
LOWBLOW
MADELON
MAGALOG
MAILLOL
MAILLOT
MANILOW
MARYLOU
MEGALON
MONOLOG
MORELOS
MRHULOT
MUDFLOW
NOTALOT
OHANLON
OUTBLOT
OUTBLOW
OUTFLOW
OUTGLOW
OUTPLOD
OUTPLOT
PHYLLOS
POMELOS
PREPLOT
PUEBLOS
RAVELOE
REALLOT
RECOLOR
RUNSLOW
SANDLOT
SCALLOP
SEMILOG
SETTLOR
SHALLOT
SHALLOW
SMALLOJ
SQUALOR
STARLOG
SUBPLOT
SUNGLOW
SWALLOW
TAGALOG
TEMBLOR
THEBLOB
THEFLOP
TONELOC
TOOSLOW
TROLLOP
TUPELOS
UPSILON
VERYLOW
WICKLOW
WINSLOW
WOODLOT
YULELOG
ZEBULON
ZOCALOS

••••L•O

ACDELCO
ANSELMO
BASILIO
BUGALOO
DELILLO
DICILLO
DOUBLEO
ELGALLO
EQUALTO
FIDELIO
FURILLO
GALILEO
GERALDO
HIDALGO
LOYALTO
MARULLO
MORELLO
MURILLO
NORELCO
NOVELLO
OTHELLO
PITILLO
POPELEO
RAPALLO
RENALDO
RINALDO
RODOLFO
SEEALSO
UCCELLO
UTRILLO
ZEDILLO

•••••LO

BARTOLO
BEEFALO
BUFFALO
BUNUELO
CATTALO
CEMBALO
CEPHALO
DANGELO
DECARLO
DELILLO
DIABOLO
DIAVOLO
DICILLO
EJEMPLO
ELGALLO
FLYSOLO
FOSCOLO
FURILLO
HANSOLO
JOPPOLO
KOWADLO
MARULLO
MORELLO
MURILLO
NICCOLO
NOVELLO
OMPHALO
ONEKILO
OTHELLO
PICCOLO
PITILLO
RAPALLO
RUFFALO
SAINTLO
TANGELO
TIEPOLO
TREMOLO
UCCELLO
UTRILLO
ZEDILLO

L•P••••

LAPALMA
LAPBELT
LAPCATS
LAPDOGS
LAPELED
LAPERMS
LAPFULS
LAPLACA
LAPLACE
LAPLAND
LAPLATA
LAPORTE
LAPPERS
LAPPETS
LAPPING
LAPPISH
LAPROBE
LAPSANG
LAPSERS
LAPSING
LAPTOPS
LAPUTAN
LAPWARE
LAPWING
LEPANTO
LEPIDUS
LEPPARD
LEPTONS
LIPARIS
LIPASES
LIPBALM
LIPIDIC
LIPLESS
LIPLIKE
LIPMANN
LIPPERS
LIPPIER
LIPPING
LIPREAD
LIPSOFF
LIPSOUT
LIPSYNC
LOPPERS
LOPPIER
LOPPING
LOPSOFF
LUPINES

L••P•••

LAMPERT
LAMPLIT
LAMPOIL
LAMPOON
LAMPREY
LAPPERS
LAPPETS
LAPPING
LAPPISH
LEAPDAY
LEAPERS
LEAPFOR
LEAPING
LEAPSAT
LEAPSIN
LEAPSON
LEAPSUP
LEAPTAT
LEAPTIN
LEAPTON
LEAPTUP
LEGPULL
LEIPZIG
LEMPIRA
LEOPARD
LEOPOLD
LEPPARD
LESPAUL
LETPASS
LIMPEST
LIMPETS
LIMPING
LIMPOPO
LINPIAO
LIPPERS
LIPPIER
LIPPING
LISPERS
LISPING
LOOPERS
LOOPIER
LOOPING
LOPPERS
LOPPIER
LOPPING
LOWPAID
LOWPAIR
LOWPOST
LUMPERS
LUMPIER
LUMPILY
LUMPING
LUMPISH
LUMPSIN
LUMPSIT
LUMPSUM

L•••P••

LAYOPEN
LAYUPON
LEDUPTO
LETUPON
LILYPAD
LIMEPIE
LMNOPQR
LOAFPAN
LOOMPAS
LOSTPET
LSHAPED

L••••P•

LACEUPS
LAPTOPS
LARRUPS
LASHUPS
LEADUPS
LEGROPE
LESSEPS
LIMPOPO
LINEUPS
LINKUPS
LOCKUPS
LOOKUPS
LOWTOPS

L•••••P

LACEDUP
LACESUP
LANDSUP
LASTLAP
LEADSUP
LEAPSUP
LEAPTUP
LEFTHIP
LEGTRAP
LENSCAP
LETDROP
LETSLIP
LETSRIP
LETTERP
LICKSUP
LIEATOP
LIFTSUP
LIGHTUP
LINEDUP
LINESUP
LINKSUP
LIVENUP
LOADSUP
LOCKSUP
LOOKSUP
LOTHROP
LOUSEUP
LOVETAP
LYESOAP
LYINGUP

•LP••••

ALPACAS
ALPHARD
ALPINER
ALPINES
ELPRADO

•L•P•••

BLIPPED
CLAPFOR
CLAPPED
CLAPPER
CLAPTON
CLIPART
CLIPOFF
CLIPONS
CLIPOUT
CLIPPED
CLIPPER
CLIPSON
CLOPPED
ELAPIDS
ELAPSED
ELAPSES
ELOPERS
ELOPING
FLAPPED
FLAPPER
FLIPOUT
FLIPPED
FLIPPEN
FLIPPER
FLIPTOP
FLIPUPS
FLOPPED
FLOPPER
FLYPAST
GLYPHIC
GLYPTIC
ILLPASS
KLEPTOS
OLDPALS
OLDPROS
PLOPPED
SLAPPED
SLAPPER
SLAPSON
SLEPTIN
SLEPTON
SLIPOFF
SLIPONS
SLIPOUT
SLIPPED
SLIPPER
SLIPSBY
SLIPSIN
SLIPSON
SLIPSUP
SLIPUPS
SLOPERS
SLOPING
SLOPPED
SLOPSON

•L••P••

ALCOPOP
ALLOPEZ
BLEEPED
BLEEPER
BLIMPIE
BLIPPED
BLOOPED
BLOOPER
BLOWPOP
CLAMPED
CLAMPER
CLAMPON
CLAPPED
CLAPPER
CLASPED
CLASPER
CLAYPIT
CLIPPED
CLIPPER
CLOMPED
CLOPPED
CLUMPED
ELLIPSE
FLAPPED
FLAPPER
FLEAPIT
FLIPPED
FLIPPEN
FLIPPER
FLOPPED
FLOPPER
FLYOPEN
GLIMPSE
OLYMPIA
OLYMPIC
OLYMPUS
PLAYPEN
PLOPPED
PLUMPED
PLUMPER
PLUMPIE
PLUMPLY
SLAPPED
SLAPPER
SLEEPER
SLEEPIN
SLEEPON
SLIPPED
SLIPPER
SLOPPED
SLUMPED
SLURPED
SLURPEE
SLURPER

•L•••P•

ALETAPS
ALLCAPS
BLOWUPS
ELCAMPO
FLIPUPS
KLMNOPQ
PLATYPI
SLIPUPS
SLOWUPS

•L••••P

ALCOPOP
BLAZEUP
BLOCKUP
BLOTSUP
BLOWNUP
BLOWPOP
BLOWSUP
CLAMDIP
CLAMSUP
CLEANUP
CLEARUP
CLIMBUP
CLOGSUP
CLOSEUP
CLOTSUP
CLOUDUP
CLUBSUP
FLAMEUP
FLAREUP
FLATTOP
FLEADIP
FLIESUP
FLIPTOP
FLOATUP
FLOWNUP
FLUFFUP
FLYTRAP
GLAMSUP
OLDCHAP
PLAYSUP
PLOWSUP
PLUGSUP
SLACKUP
SLANTUP
SLICEUP
SLINKUP
SLIPSUP
SLOWSUP
SLUNKUP

••LP•••

CALPOLY
CULPRIT
DELPHIC
DOLPHIN
EELPOTS
EELPOUT
GALPALS
GELPENS
GULPERS
GULPIER
GULPING
HELPERS
HELPFUL
HELPING
HELPOUT
HELPSIN
HELPSON
HELPSUP
ILLPASS
KELPIES
MALPASO
OILPALM
OILPANS
PALPATE
PULPERS
PULPIER
PULPIFY
PULPING
PULPITS
RALPHIE
SULPHUR
SYLPHIC
VOLPONE
VULPINE
WALPOLE
YELPERS
YELPING

••L•P••

ALLOPEZ
BULLPEN
CALIPER
CALIPHS
CALYPSO
ECLIPSE
ELLIPSE
FELTPEN
FILIPPO
GALOPED
GOLFPRO
HELIPAD
LILYPAD
MALEPIG
OILSPOT
POLYPED
POLYPOD
PULLPIN
RELAPSE
SALTPIT
TELEPIC
TELEPIX
WELLPUT
WILDPIG

••L••P•

ALLCAPS
CALLUPS
CCLAMPS
COLLOPS
DOLLOPS
FILIPPO
FILLIPS
FILLUPS
FOLDUPS
GALLOPS
GALUMPH
GELCAPS
HOLDUPS
OILCUPS
PILEUPS
PULLUPS
RELEAPS
ROLLUPS
UNLOOPS
UNLUMPY
UPLEAPS
UPLEAPT
WALKUPS
WALLOPS

••L•••P

BALLSUP
BELLHOP
BELLLAP
BELLYUP
BELTSUP
BOLTSUP
BULKSUP
CALLSUP
COLDCUP
DOLLSUP
FELTTIP
FILLSUP
FOLDSUP
GOLDTIP
HELPSUP
HILLTOP
HOLDSUP
HOLEDUP
HOLESUP
JKLMNOP
MILKSOP
OILLAMP
PALMTOP
PILEDUP
PILESUP
PULLSUP
RILEDUP
RILESUP
ROLLMOP
ROLLSUP
ROLLTOP
SALMONP
SILENTP
SPLITUP
TALKSUP
TALLYUP
TILTSUP
TILTTOP
WALLMAP
WALLSUP
WELLSUP

•••LP••

ADELPHI
ADOLPHE
BULLPEN
COALPIT
COOLPIX
HEELPAD
PAULPRY
PULLPIN
SCALPED
SCALPEL
SCALPER
SCULPED
SCULPTS
TAILPIN
WELLPUT
WHELPED

•••L•P•

BURLAPS
CALLUPS
CHALUPA
COLLOPS
CYCLOPS
DEWLAPS
DIALUPS
DIDLAPS
DOLLOPS
DUNLOPS
EARLAPS
FATLIPS
FILLIPS
FILLUPS
FOULUPS
GALLOPS
GUNLAPS
HOTLIPS
OUTLIPS
PHILIPK
PHILIPS
PHILIPV
PULLUPS
RANLAPS
REFLIPS
ROLLUPS
RUNLAPS
SCHLEPP
SCHLEPS
UNCLIPS
UNCLIPT
UPSLOPE
WALLOPS

•••L••P

AGALLOP
ARCLAMP
BALLSUP
BEDLAMP
BELLHOP
BELLLAP
BELLYUP
BOILSUP
BUILDUP
BUILTUP
CALLSUP
CHALKUP
COILSUP
CURLSUP
DEALSUP
DEALTUP
DIALSUP
DOLLSUP
ENCLASP
FILLSUP
FOGLAMP
FOULSUP
FOULTIP
FUELSUP
GASLAMP
HAULSUP
HEALSUP
HEELTAP
HILLTOP
NAILSUP
NAILTIP
OILLAMP
ONELUMP
OUTLEAP
PHILLIP
PULLSUP
RECLASP
REELSUP
ROLLMOP
ROLLSUP
ROLLTOP
SCALEUP
SCALLOP
SCHLEPP
SCHLUMP
SEALSUP
STILLUP
SUNLAMP
SWELLUP
TALLYUP
THELOOP
TOELOOP
TOOLSUP
TROLLOP
UNCLAMP
UNCLASP
WALLMAP
WALLSUP
WELLSUP

••••LP•

CATALPA
DEPULPS
RUDOLPH
THEALPS

••••L•P

AGALLOP
APHILIP
ATACLIP
BELLLAP
CATFLAP
COWSLIP
DEVELOP
DOUBLEP
EARCLIP
EARFLAP
ENVELOP
ESCALOP
KERFLOP
KERPLOP
LASTLAP
LETSLIP
MUDFLAP
NONSLIP
OVERLAP
PACELAP
PAYSLIP
PHARLAP
PHILLIP
SCALLOP
SNARLUP

STILLUP
SWELLUP
THEFLOP
TIECLIP
TOTALUP
TROLLOP

•••••LP
BIGGULP
GETHELP
GOTHELP
MRQUILP
OUTYELP
THEHELP

L•Q••••
LIQUATE
LIQUEFY
LIQUEUR
LIQUIDS
LIQUORS
LOQUATS

L••Q•••
LACQUER

L•••Q••
LALIQUE

L••••Q•
LMNOPQR

L•••••Q
LETTERQ

•LQ••••
ALQUIST

•L•Q•••
CLAQUES
CLIQUED
CLIQUES
CLIQUEY
PLAQUES

•L••••Q
KLMNOPQ

••L•Q••
LALIQUE
OBLIQUE
OBLOQUY

••L•••Q
SILENTQ

•••LQ••
QUELQUE

••••LQ•
POSSLQS

••••L•Q
DOUBLEQ

L•R••••
LARAINE
LARAMIE
LARCENY
LARCHEN
LARCHES
LARDERS
LARDIER
LARDING
LARDNER
LARDONS
LAREDOS
LARGELY
LARGENT
LARGEOJ
LARGESS
LARGEST
LARGISH
LARIATS
LARKERS
LARKIER
LARKING
LARKINS
LARKISH
LAROCHE
LARRUPS
LARUSSA
LORANGE
LORDING
LORDJIM
LORDSIT
LORELAI
LORELEI
LORENTZ
LORENZO
LORETTA
LORGNON
LORIENT
LORISES
LORRIES
LORUSES
LURCHED
LURCHER
LURCHES
LUREDIN
LURESIN
LUREXES
LURIDLY
LURKERS
LURKING
LURLEEN
LYRICAL
LYRICON
LYRISTS

L••R•••
LABRATS
LACRIMO
LADRONE
LAERTES
LAIRING
LAPROBE
LARRUPS
LATRELL
LATRINE
LATROBE
LAURELS
LAURENT
LAURITZ
LEARJET
LEARNED
LEARNER
LEARNOF
LEARNTO
LEBROCK
LEERERS
LEERIER
LEERILY
LEERING
LEERSAT
LEFREAK
LEGRAND
LEGREST
LEGROOM
LEGROPE
LETRIDE
LETROLL
LIBRANS
LIBRARY
LIPREAD
LOGROLL
LORRIES
LOURDES
LOUREED
LOURING
LOWRENT
LOWRISE
LOWRISK
LOWROAD

L•••R••
LABORAT
LABORED
LABORER
LACERTA
LACUREE
LAFARGE
LAMARCK
LAMPREY
LAPERMS
LAPORTE
LASORDA
LASTROW
LATERAL
LATERAN
LATERON
LAUTREC
LAVERAN
LAVERNE
LAVORIS
LAYERED
LAZARUS
LEBARON
LECARRE
LECTRIC
LEDERER
LEGIRON
LEGTRAP
LEITRIM
LETDROP
LETSRIP
LETTRES
LEVERED
LEVERET
LIBERAL
LIBERIA
LIBERTE
LIBERTY
LIGURIA
LINDROS
LIPARIS
LITCRIT
LITERAL
LITURGY
LIVERED
LIVORNO
LIZARDS
LLADROS
LOCARNO
LONDRES
LONGRUN
LOTHROP
LOUVRED
LOUVRES
LOVERLY
LOWBRED
LOWBROW
LOWERED
LUCARNE
LUCERNE
LUSTRAL
LUSTRED
LUSTRES
LUSTRUM

L••••R•
LABOURS
LADDERS
LADLERS
LAGGARD
LAGGERS
LAMBERT
LAMPERT
LANCERS
LANDERS
LANFORD
LANGTRY
LANTERN
LANYARD
LAPPERS
LAPSERS
LAPWARE
LARDERS
LARKERS
LASCARS
LASHERS
LASTORY
LATHERS
LATHERY
LAUDERS
LAUNDRY
LAWFORD
LAWYERS
LAYBARE
LAZZERI
LEADERS
LEADORE
LEAKERS
LEANERS
LEAPERS
LEASERS
LECARRE
LECHERS
LECTERN
LECTORS
LECTURE
LEDGERS
LEEFORD
LEERERS
LEEWARD
LEFTARM
LEGHORN
LEGWORK
LEHAVRE
LEISURE
LEMPIRA
LENDERS
LEONARD
LEONORA
LEONORE
LEOPARD
LEOTARD
LEPPARD
LESABRE
LESSORS
LETTERA
LETTERB
LETTERC
LETTERD
LETTERE
LETTERF
LETTERG
LETTERH
LETTERI
LETTERJ
LETTERK
LETTERL
LETTERM
LETTERN
LETTERO
LETTERP
LETTERQ
LETTERR
LETTERS
LETTERT
LETTERU
LETTERV
LETTERW
LETTERX
LETTERY
LETTERZ
LEVIERS
LEXMARK
LEXUSRX
LIBBERS
LIBRARY
LICKERS
LIENORS
LIFTERS
LIMBERS
LIMBURG
LIMNERS
LINDORF
LINEARA
LINEARB
LINEDRY
LINGERS
LINKERS
LINTERS
LIPPERS
LIQUORS
LISPERS
LISTERS
LITTERS
LITTERY
LLANERO
LOADERS
LOAFERS
LOANERS
LOBBERS
LOCKERS
LODGERS
LOFTERS
LOGGERS
LOITERS
LOLLARD
LOLLERS
LOMBARD
LONBORG
LONGARM
LOOKERS
LOOPERS
LOOTERS
LOPPERS
LOSTART
LOTTERS
LOTTERY
LOUVERS
LOWBORN
LOWCARB
LOWCARD
LUBBERS
LUGGERS
LUGWORM
LULLERS
LUMBARS
LUMBERS
LUMIERE
LUMPERS
LUNGERS
LUNKERS
LURKERS
LUSTERS

L•••••R
LABELER
LABORER
LACQUER
LACUNAR
LAFLEUR
LAIDFOR
LALAKER
LAMINAR
LANDLER
LANGUOR
LANKIER
LARDIER
LARDNER
LARKIER
LASSOER
LAUGHER
LAUNDER
LAYOVER
LAYSFOR
LEACHER
LEADIER
LEAFIER
LEAGUER
LEAKIER
LEANDER
LEAPFOR
LEARNER
LEATHER
LEDERER
LEDGIER
LEERIER
LEFTEAR
LEFTFOR
LEGATOR
LEGGIER
LEGWEAR
LEISTER
LESSTAR
LETTERR
LEVATOR
LEVELER
LIBELER
LIEDFOR
LIEOVER
LIESFOR
LIGHTER
LIMITER
LINDNER
LINTIER
LIPPIER
LIQUEUR
LITTLER
LIVEFOR
LIVENER
LMNOPQR
LOAMIER
LOATHER
LOBBYER
LOBSTER
LOCATER
LOCATOR
LOESSER
LOFTIER
LONGFOR
LOOKFOR
LOONIER
LOOPIER
LOPPIER
LOTHAIR
LOUNGER
LOUSIER
LOWGEAR
LOWLIER
LOWPAIR
LOYALER
LUCIFER
LUCKIER
LUMPIER
LUNCHER
LUNULAR
LURCHER
LUSHIER
LUSTIER
LUTHIER

•LR••••
ALREADY
ALRIGHT
ALROKER
ALROSEN

•L•R•••
ALARBUS
ALARCON
ALARMED
ALARMER
ALARUMS
ALDRICH
ALERTED
ALERTER
ALERTLY
ALERTTO
ALFREDA
ALFREDE
ALFREDO
ALFREDU
ALGREEN
ALLRISE
BLARING
BLARNEY
BLERIOT
BLURBER
BLURRED
BLURTED
BLURTER
CLARETS
CLARICE
CLARIFY
CLARION
CLARITY
CLERICS
CLERISY
CLERKED
CLERKLY
CLORETS
ELDRICH
ELDRICK
ELGRECO
ELPRADO
ELTRAIN
FLAREUP
FLARING
FLIRTED
FLIRTER
FLOREAL
FLORENZ
FLORETS
FLORIAN
FLORIDA
FLORINS
FLORIST
FLYRODS
GLAREAT
GLARING
GLORIAS
GLORIED
GLORIES
GLORIFY
GLORYBE
GLURGES
OLDROSE
OLOROSO
PLURALS
SLURPED
SLURPEE
SLURPER
SLURRED

•L••R••
ALBERTA
ALBERTI
ALBERTO
ALBIREO
ALBORAK
ALDORAY
ALEARDI
ALEGRIA
ALFEROV
ALFORJA
ALGARVE
ALGERIA
ALLBRAN
ALLERGY
ALLURED
ALLURER
ALLURES
ALMERIA
ALSORAN
ALTERED
ALTERER
ALVAREZ
ALWORTH
BLEARED
BLUERED
BLURRED
CLAIROL
CLEARED
CLEARER
CLEARLY
CLEAROF
CLEARUP
ELBERTA
ELDERLY
ELMTREE
ELNORTE
FLEERED
FLEURON
FLOORED
FLOORER
FLOORIT
FLOURED
FLYTRAP
ILLBRED
ILLYRIA
LLADROS
OLDPROS
PLEURAE
PLEURAL
SLURRED

•L•••R•
ALBSURE
ALEGARS
ALEYARD
ALFIERI
ALGEBRA
ALGIERS
ALIFORM
ALINERS
ALLEARS
ALLEGRA
ALLEGRO
ALLHERE
ALMONRY
ALPHARD
ALTDORF
ALTHORN
BLADERS
BLAMERS
BLAZERS
BLOWDRY
BLOWERS
CLAMORS
CLAWERS
CLIBURN
CLIPART
CLONERS
CLOSERS
CLOSURE
CLOTURE
CLOVERS
CLOVERY
ELANTRA
ELATERS
ELECTRA
ELECTRO
ELEKTRA
ELIDERS
ELIXIRS
ELKHART
ELOPERS
ELUDERS
ELUSORY
FLAKERS
FLAMERS
FLAVORS
FLAVORY
FLAYERS
FLEXORS
FLEXURE
FLOWERS
FLOWERY
FLUTERS
FLYGIRL
GLAMORS
GLAZERS
GLIDERS
GLOWERS
LLANERO
OLDCARS
OLDGIRL
OLESTRA
PLACARD
PLACERS
PLANERS
PLATERS
PLAYERS
PLECTRA
PLENARY
PLEXORS
PLOVERS
PLOWERS
SLAKERS
SLATERS
SLAVERS
SLAVERY
SLAYERS
SLICERS
SLIDERS
SLIVERS
SLOPERS
ULSTERS

•L••••R
ALARMER
ALCAZAR
ALERTER
ALIENOR
ALIGNER
ALLAYER
ALLEGER
ALLOVER
ALLSTAR
ALLURER
ALMONER
ALPINER
ALROKER
ALTERER
ALUNSER
BLABBER
BLACKER
BLADDER
BLANDER
BLANKER
BLASTER
BLATHER
BLEAKER
BLEATER
BLEEDER
BLEEPER
BLENDER
BLESSER
BLINDER
BLINKER
BLISTER
BLITHER
BLITZER
BLOCKER
BLOGGER
BLONDER
BLOOMER
BLOOPER
BLOTTER
BLOWIER
BLUBBER
BLUDGER
BLUFFER
BLUNDER
BLUNTER
BLURBER
BLURTER
BLUSHER
BLUSTER
CLABBER
CLACKER
CLAIMER
CLAMBAR
CLAMBER
CLAMMER
CLAMOUR
CLAMPER
CLANGER
CLANGOR
CLAPFOR
CLAPPER
CLASHER
CLASPER
CLASSER
CLATTER
CLAVIER
CLAYIER
CLEANER
CLEARER
CLEAVER
CLICKER
CLIMBER
CLINGER
CLINKER
CLIPPER
CLOBBER
CLOCKER
CLOUTER
CLOWDER
CLUBBER
CLUBCAR
CLUCKER
CLUNKER
CLUSTER
CLUTTER
ELBOWER
ELEANOR
ELEAZAR
ELECTOR
ELIEZER
FLAGGER
FLAKIER
FLAMIER
FLANEUR
FLANKER
FLAPPER
FLASHER
FLATCAR
FLATTER
FLAVOUR
FLAWIER
FLAXIER
FLEECER
FLEETER
FLENSER
FLEXNER
FLICKER
FLINGER
FLIPPER
FLIRTER
FLITTER
FLIVVER
FLOATER
FLOGGER
FLOORER
FLOPPER
FLOSSER
FLOUTER
FLUBBER
FLUFFER
FLUKIER
FLUNKER
FLUSHER
FLUSTER
FLUTIER
FLUTTER
FLYOVER
FLYTIER
GLACIER
GLADDER
GLAMOUR
GLAZIER
GLEANER
GLIBBER
GLIMMER
GLISTER
GLITTER
GLOATER
GLOSSER
GLUMMER
KLAMMER
KLEIBER
KLEISER
KLEZMER
KLINGER
KLINKER
KLISTER
OLDSTER
OLIVIER
PLAINER
PLAISIR
PLAITER
PLANFOR
PLANNER
PLANTAR
PLANTER
PLASTER
PLATIER
PLATTER
PLEADER
PLEASER
PLEDGER
PLODDER
PLOTTER
PLUGGER
PLUMBER
PLUMIER
PLUMMER
PLUMPER
PLUNDER
PLUNGER
PLUNKER
PLUSHER
SLACKER
SLAMMER
SLANDER
SLAPPER
SLASHER
SLATHER
SLATIER
SLEDDER
SLEEKER
SLEEPER
SLENDER
SLICKER
SLIMIER
SLIMMER
SLINGER
SLINKER
SLIPPER
SLITHER
SLITTER
SLOBBER
SLOGGER
SLOTCAR
SLOTTER
SLUGGER
SLUMBER
SLUMMER
SLURPER

••LR•••
ALLRISE
AXLROSE
BULRUSH
DELRAYS
DELRUTH
MALRAUX
MELROSE
OILRICH

OILRIGS
OILRING
OILRUBS

••L•R••

AALARGE
AELFRIC
AILERON
ALLBRAN
ALLERGY
ALLURED
ALLURER
ALLURES
ATLARGE
BALDRIC
BELARUS
BELTRAN
BOLEROS
BULLRUN
CALDRON
CALORIC
CALORIE
CHLORIC
COLORED
COLORER
COLORTV
CULPRIT
DALTREY
DELARUE
DELIRIA
DELORIS
DELORME
DOLORES
ENLARGE
FULCRUM
HALFRAW
HALFROD
ILLBRED
ILLYRIA
INLARGE
MALARIA
MALARKY
MALLRAT
MILDRED
MILERUN
MILKRUN
MILLRUN
MILORDS
MOLERAT
MULGREW
OILDRUM
PALERMO
PALFREY
PALTROW
PILCROW
PILGRIM
POLARAS
POLARIS
SALERNO
SCLERAE
SCLERAL
SCLERAS
SOLARAS
SOLARIA
SPLURGE
TALARIA
TELERAN
UNLARGE
UNLURED
UNLYRIC
VALERIE
VALOREM
VELCROS
VELURES
WELLRUN
WILFRED
WOLFRAM

••L••R•

ALLEARS
ALLEGRA
ALLEGRO
ALLHERE
ARLBERG
BALKERS
BALLARD
BELAIRS
BELFORT
BELIERS
BELTERS
BILKERS
BILLERS
BOLTERS
BULGARI
BULGARS
BULGURS
BULWARK
CALABRO
CALDERA
CALDERS
CALGARY
CALIBRE
CALKERS
CALLERS
CALVARY
CALVERT
CELEBRE
CELLARS
CILIARY
COLBERT
COLLARD
COLLARS
COLOURS
CULLERS
CULTURE
CULVERT
DELBERT
DELMORE
DELTORO
DELVERS
DILBERT
DILLARD
DOLLARS
DOLOURS
DRLAURA
DULLARD
ECLAIRS
EELWORM
FALKIRK
FALLERS
FALTERS
FELLERS
FELONRY
FILBERT
FILLERS
FILTERS
FOLDERS
FOLGERS
FOLKART
FULMARS
GALLERY
GILBERT
GILDERS
GILFORD
GILMORE
GOLDARN
GOLFERS
GOLFPRO
GULPERS
HALTERS
HALVERS
HALYARD
HELOTRY
HELPERS
HILAIRE
HILBERT
HILLARY
HOLBERG
HOLDERS
HOLLERS
HOLYARK
HULLERS
JILTERS
JOLTERS
KILDARE
KILLERS
KILNDRY
LOLLARD
LOLLERS
LULLERS
MALLARD
MALWARE
MELDERS
MELTERS
MILAGRO
MILKERS
MILLARD
MILLERS
MOLDERS
MOLIERE
MOLTERS
MULHARE
MULLERS
OILBIRD
PALABRA
PALEDRY
PALLORS
PALMARY
PALMERS
PALMYRA
PALTERS
PELTERS
PILFERS
PILLARS
PILLORY
POLLARD
POLLERA
POLLERS
PULLERS
PULPERS
PULSARS
RELEARN
RELIERS
ROLFERS
ROLLERS
SALIERI
SALTERS
SALVERS
SALVORS
SELKIRK
SELLERS
SILVERS
SILVERY
SOLDERS
SOLVERS
SULKERS
TALKERS
TELLERS
TILLERS
TILTERS
TOLLERS
UNLEARN
VALOURS
VALUERS
VELOURS
VILLARD
VILLARI
VOLTORE
VULTURE
WALDORF
WALKERS
WALKURE
WALMART
WALTERS
WELDERS
WELFARE
WELTERS
WILBERT
WILFORD
WILLARD
WILLERS
YELLERS
YELPERS

••L•••R

ALLAYER
ALLEGER
ALLOVER
ALLSTAR
ALLURER
BALFOUR
BALKIER
BALLMER
BALMIER
BELABOR
BELAYER
BELCHER
BELLJAR
BELVOIR
BELVOUR
BILGIER
BOLIVAR
BOLSTER
BULGHUR
BULGIER
BULKIER
BYLINER
CALAMAR
CALIBER
CALIPER
CALLFOR
COLDWAR
COLLIER
COLLYER
COLORER
DALLIER
DELAYER
DELIVER
DELUDER
DILATOR
DILUTER
DILUTOR
FALLFOR
FELLFOR
FELTFOR
FILCHER
FILMIER
FOLKIER
GOLFCAR
GULFWAR
GULPIER
HILLIER
HOLSTER
HOLYWAR
HULKIER
INLABOR
INLAYER
JOLLIER
JOLTIER
KILOBAR
LALAKER
MALABAR
MALODOR
MALTIER
MILKBAR
MILKIER
MOLDIER
MOLITOR
MULDAUR
OBLIGER
OBLIGOR
PALAVER
PALLIER
PALMIER
PALOMAR
PILSNER
POLANER
POLECAR
POLICER
POLITER
POLYMER
PULLFOR
PULPIER
RALLIER
RELATER
RELATOR
RELAXER
RELAYER
RELEVER
ROLLBAR
SALAZAR
SALEMOR
SALLIER
SALTIER
SALUTER
SELLFOR
SELTZER
SILENTR
SILKIER
SILLIER
SILTIER
SOLACER
SOLDFOR
SOLDIER
SOLIDER
SPLICER
SULKIER
SULPHUR
TALKIER
TALLIER
TELSTAR
TOLLBAR
VOLCKER
WALTHER
WALTZER
YELLFOR

•••LR••

AXELROD
BULLRUN
FUELROD
MALLRAT
MILLRUN
WELLRUN

•••L•R•

ABELARD
AMBLERS
ANGLERS
ANKLERS
ANTLERS
ASALARK
ASHLARS
BAILERS
BAILORS
BALLARD
BAWLERS
BAYLORU
BILLERS
BIRLERS
BOILERS
BOWLERS
BUGLERS
BURLERS
BUTLERS
CABLERS
CALLERS
CELLARS
CHOLERA
CHOLERS
COALERS
COILERS
COLLARD
COLLARS
COOLERS
CULLERS
CURLERS
CUTLERS
CUTLERY
CYCLERS
DEALERS
DEBLURS
DECLARE
DEKLERK
DEPLORE
DIALERS
DILLARD
DOLLARS
DUELERS
DULLARD
EGGLERS
EXILERS
EXPLORE
FABLERS
FAILURE
FALLERS
FAXLORE
FEELERS
FELLERS
FILLERS
FOOLERS
FOOLERY
FORLORN
FOULARD
FOWLERS
FUELERS
FURLERS
GALLERY
GAOLERS
GAYLORD
HAILERS
HAULERS
HEALERS
HEELERS
HILLARY
HOLLERS
HOWLERS
HULLERS
HURLERS
IMPLORE
JAILERS
JAILORS
KEGLERS
KILLERS
LADLERS
LOLLARD
LOLLERS
LULLERS
MAILERS
MALLARD
MAULERS
MCCLURE
MCCLURG
MEWLERS
MILLARD
MILLERS
MOILERS
MUDLARK
MULLERS
NAILERS
OCULARS
ONALARK
ONALERT
ONELIRA
OSTLERS
PALLORS
PARLORS
PAULPRY
PEELERS
PHILTRE
PILLARS
PILLORY
POLLARD
POLLERA
POLLERS
POOLERS
POPLARS
POULTRY
PULLERS
RAILERS
REELERS
RIFLERS
RIFLERY
ROLLERS
SAILERS
SAILORS
SCALARS
SCALERS
SCOLARI
SEALERS
SEALERY
SELLERS
SKYLARK
SMILERS
STYLERS
SWELTRY
SZILARD
TAILERS
TAILORS
TAYLORS
TELLERS
THALERS
THELARK
TILLERS
TITLARK
TOILERS
TOLLERS
TOOLERS
UNALERT
VEILERS
VILLARD
VILLARI
WAILERS
WARLORD
WHALERS
WILLARD
WILLERS
WOOLERY
YELLERS
YOWLERS

•••L••R

ADOLLAR
APPLIER
ATELIER
AXILLAR
BALLMER
BAULKER
BELLJAR
BOULDER
BUELLER
BUILDER
BURLIER
CALLFOR
CAULKER
CHILLER
COALCAR
COALTAR
COLLIER
COLLYER
COOLAIR
COULTER
CRULLER
CURLIER
DALLIER
DRILLER
DROLLER
DWELLER
EARLIER
EVILLER
EVOLVER
EXALTER
FALLFOR
FEELFOR
FELLFOR
FIELDER
GIRLIER
GODLIER
GRILLER
GROLIER
GUILDER
HILLIER
HJALMAR
JOLLIER
JOWLIER
KEILLOR
LAFLEUR
LOWLIER
MAILCAR
MANLIER
MARLIER
MEALIER
MOULDER
MUELLER
NUCLEAR
OCELLAR
OUTLIER
PALLIER
PARLOUR
PHILTER
PSALTER
PULLFOR
QUELLER
QUILLER
QUILTER
RAILCAR
RALLIER
REALTER
REALTOR
REPLIER
ROILIER
ROLLBAR
SALLIER
SCALDER
SCALIER
SCALPER
SCOLDER
SCULLER
SELLFOR
SHALIER
SHELLER
SHELTER
SHELVER
SILLIER
SKELTER
SKULKER
SMALLER
SMELLER
SMELTER
SMOLDER
SPELLER
SPILLER
STALKER
STALLER
STELLAR
STILLER
SURLIER
SVELTER
SWELLER
SWELTER
SWILLER
TALLIER
TOLLBAR
TOOLBAR
TRILLER
TROLLER
UNCLEAR
UNFLOOR
UNSLIER
UNSLYER
VAULTER
VEALIER
WIELDER
WOOLIER
YELLFOR
YIELDER
ZOELLER

••••LR•

CAVALRY
DEVILRY
JEWELRY
REVELRY
RIVALRY

••••L•R

ADOLLAR
ANGULAR
ANNULAR
AREOLAR
AXILLAR
BABBLER
BAFFLER
BANALER
BATTLER
BEVELER
BICOLOR
BIPOLAR
BOBBLER
BOGGLER
BOOSLER
BOTTLER
BOWDLER
BRAWLER
BRIDLER
BROILER
BUELLER
BUMBLER
BUNDLER
BUNGLER
BURBLER
BURGLAR
BUSTLER
CACKLER
CAJOLER
CANDLER
CAROLER
CAVILER
CHILLER
CIRCLER
COBBLER
CODDLER
COPULAR
COUPLER
CRADLER
CRAWLER
CRUELER
CRULLER
CUPELER
CUPULAR
CURDLER
CUSSLER
DABBLER
DAIMLER
DANDLER
DANGLER
DAWDLER
DAZZLER
DECOLOR
DEFILER
DIBBLER
DIDDLER
DIPOLAR
DOODLER
DOPPLER
DOUBLER
DRAWLER
DREXLER
DRILLER
DROLLER
DROOLER
DWELLER
EMAILER
ENABLER
ETAILER
EVILLER
EXOILER
FANSLER
FEEBLER
FIBULAR
FICKLER
FIDDLER
FIEDLER
FIZZLER
FONDLER
FOOTLER
FOOZLER
FRAILER
FUMBLER
GAMBLER
GARBLER
GARGLER
GENTLER
GIGGLER
GIRDLER
GOBBLER
GOGGLER
GOOGLER
GRILLER
GROWLER
GUZZLER
HACKLER
HAGGLER
HANDLER
HECKLER
HIBBLER
HIGGLER
HOBBLER
HOSTLER
HUDDLER
HUMBLER
HURDLER
HUSTLER
IMPALER
INCOLOR
INHALER
INSULAR
JANGLER
JEWELER
JINGLER
JOCULAR
JOGGLER
JOSTLER
JUGGLER
JUGULAR
JUMBLER
KASTLER
KEEBLER
KEESLAR
KEESLER
KEILLOR
KINDLER
KNEELER
KOEHLER
LABELER
LANDLER
LEVELER
LIBELER
LITTLER
LOYALER
LUNULAR
MACULAR
MANGLER
MARBLER
MEDDLER
METTLER
MIDDLER
MINGLER
MODELER
MODULAR
MUDDLER
MUELLER
MUFFLER
MUMBLER
MUZZLER
NEBULAR
NEEDLER
NESTLER
NIBBLER
NIGGLER
NIMBLER
NODULAR
NUZZLER
OCELLAR
OSCULAR
PADDLER
PEARLER
PEDALER
PEDDLER
POPULAR
PROWLER
PURFLER
PUZZLER
QUELLER
QUILLER
RAFFLER
RAMBLER
RASSLER
RATTLER
RECOLOR
REGALER
REGULAR
RESOLER
REVELER
REVILER
RICHLER
RIDDLER
RIFFLER
RUFFLER
RUMBLER
RUSTLER
SADDLER
SAMPLER
SANDLER
SCHOLAR
SCOWLER
SCULLER
SECULAR
SETTLER
SETTLOR
SHELLER
SIMILAR
SIMPLER
SIZZLER
SMALLER
SMELLER
SNARLER
SPELLER
SPIELER
SPILLER
SPOILER
SPOOLER
SQUALOR
STABLER
STADLER
STALLER
STAPLER
STATLER
STEALER
STEELER
STELLAR
STILLER
SUBTLER
SUPPLER
SWELLER
SWILLER
TABULAR
TACKLER
TANGLER
TATTLER
TEMBLOR
TEMPLAR
TICKLER
TINGLER
TINKLER
TIPPLER
TITULAR
TODDLER
TOFFLER
TOGGLER
TOOTLER
TOTALER
TRAILER
TRAWLER

TRIFLER
TRILLER
TROLLER
TUBULAR
TUMBLER
TUMMLER
TUTELAR
TWIRLER
UNDULAR
UNGULAR
WADDLER
WAFFLER
WAGGLER
WANGLER
WARBLER
WHEELER
WHIRLER
WIGGLER
WINKLER
WOBBLER
YODELER
ZIEGLER
ZOELLER
ZONULAR

LS•••••

LSHAPED

L•S••••

LASAGNA
LASAGNE
LASALLE
LÂSCALA
LASCARS
LASCAUX
LASHERS
LASHING
LASHOUT
LASHUPS
LASORDA
LASSIES
LASSOED
LASSOER
LASSOES
LASTACT
LASTDON
LASTGAS
LASTING
LASTLAP
LASTLEG
LASTMAY
LASTONE
LASTORY
LASTROW
LESABRE
LESCAUT
LESIONS
LESOTHO
LESPAUL
LESSEES
LESSENS
LESSEPS
LESSFAT
LESSING
LESSONS
LESSORS
LESSTAR
LESTOIL
LISAGAY
LISBETH
LISENTE
LISPERS
LISPING
LISSOME
LISTEES
LISTENS
LISTERS
LISTING
LOSABLE
LOSEBIG
LOSEOUT
LOSESIT
LOSESTO
LOSINGS
LOSTART
LOSTBIG
LOSTCAT
LOSTDOG
LOSTOUT
LOSTPET
LUSHEST
LUSHIER
LUSTERS
LUSTFUL
LUSTIER
LUSTILY
LUSTING
LUSTRAL
LUSTRED
LUSTRES
LUSTRUM
LYSENKO

L••S•••

LAISSEZ
LAKSHMI
LANSING
LAPSANG
LAPSERS
LAPSING
LASSIES
LASSOED
LASSOER
LASSOES
LAWSUIT
LAYSFOR
LAYSLOW
LAYSOFF
LAYSOUT
LEASERS
LEASETO
LEASHED
LEASHES
LEASING
LEISTER
LEISURE
LENSCAP
LENSMAN
LENSMEN
LESSEES
LESSENS
LESSEPS
LESSFAT
LESSING
LESSONS
LESSORS
LESSTAR
LETSEAT
LETSFLY
LETSLIP
LETSNOT
LETSOFF
LETSOUT
LETSRIP
LETSSEE
LETSUSE
LHASANS
LIESFOR
LIESLOW
LINSEED
LIPSOFF
LIPSOUT
LIPSYNC
LISSOME
LOBSTER
LOESSER
LOESSES
LOGSOFF
LOGSOUT
LOOSELY
LOOSENS
LOOSEST
LOOSING
LOPSOFF
LOUSEUP
LOUSIER
LOUSILY
LOUSING
LOWSIDE
LUGSAIL
LUGSOUT
LYESOAP

L•••S••

LACESON
LACESUP
LACOSTE
LAGASSE
LAISSEZ
LAKISTS
LANDSAT
LANDSUP
LARUSSA
LATOSCA
LEADSIN
LEADSON
LEADSTO
LEADSUP
LEAKSIN
LEANSIN
LEANSON
LEANSTO
LEAPSAT
LEAPSIN
LEAPSON
LEAPSUP
LEERSAT
LEGISTS
LEGOSET
LETSSEE
LEXISES
LEXUSES
LEXUSGS
LEXUSGX
LEXUSIS
LEXUSLS
LEXUSLX
LEXUSRX
LEXUSSC
LIAISED
LIAISES
LIAISON
LICKSUP
LIFTSUP
LINDSAY
LINDSEY
LINESUP
LINKSUP
LIPASES
LIVESAT
LIVESET
LIVESEY
LIVESIN
LIVESON
LOADSIN
LOADSOF
LOADSUP
LOCKSET
LOCKSIN
LOCKSON
LOCKSUP
LOCUSTS
LOESSER
LOESSES
LOOKSAD
LOOKSAT
LOOKSEE
LOOKSIN
LOOKSON
LOOKSTO
LOOKSUP
LORDSIT
LORISES
LORUSES
LOSESIT
LOSESTO
LOTUSES
LOUISII
LOUISIV
LOUISIX
LOUISVI
LOUISXI
LOUISXV
LOVESET
LOVESIT
LOVESTO
LUMPSIN
LUMPSIT
LUMPSUM
LUNESTA
LURESIN
LUTISTS
LYRISTS

L••••S•

LABTEST
LACIEST
LACTASE
LACTOSE
LADDISH
LADYISH
LAGASSE
LAKIEST
LALOOSH
LAMAISM
LAMAIST
LANKEST
LAPPISH
LARGESS
LARGEST
LARGISH
LARKISH
LARUSSA
LAVALSE
LAWCASE
LAWLESS
LAXNESS
LAZIEST
LAZYISH
LEANEST
LEFTEST
LEFTISH
LEFTISM
LEFTIST
LEGLESS
LEGREST
LETPASS
LETSUSE
LETTISH
LEWDEST
LEXUSSC
LICENSE
LIDLESS
LIEFEST
LIETEST
LIMIEST
LIMPEST
LINIEST
LIONESS
LIONISE
LIPLESS
LITHEST
LITOVSK
LOGGISH
LOGIEST
LONGEST
LONGISH
LOOKISM
LOOKIST
LOOSEST
LOUDEST
LOUDISH
LOUTISH
LOWCOST
LOWMASS
LOWNESS
LOWPOST
LOWRISE
LOWRISK
LUCIUSI
LUDDISM
LUMPISH
LUSHEST

L•••••S

LABATTS
LABFEES
LABIALS
LABOURS
LABRATS
LACEUPS
LACINGS
LACKEYS
LACUNAS
LADDERS
LADDIES
LADIDAS
LADINGS
LADINOS
LADLERS
LADYNAS
LAERTES
LAGGERS
LAGOONS
LAGUNAS
LAITIES
LAKISTS
LAKOTAS
LAMBDAS
LAMENTS
LAMINAS
LANCERS
LANCETS
LANCIAS
LANDAUS
LANDERS
LANVINS
LAPCATS
LAPDOGS
LAPERMS
LAPFULS
LAPPERS
LAPPETS
LAPSERS
LAPTOPS
LARCHES
LARDERS
LARDONS
LAREDOS
LARGESS
LARIATS
LARKERS
LARKINS
LARRUPS
LASCARS
LASHERS
LASHUPS
LASSIES
LASSOES
LASTGAS
LATCHES
LATEENS
LATENTS
LATEXES
LATHERS
LATICES
LATIGOS
LATIMES
LATINAS
LATINOS
LATINUS
LAUDERS
LAULAUS
LAURELS
LAVABOS
LAVAGES
LAVORIS
LAWLESS
LAWYERS
LAXNESS
LAYODDS
LAYOFFS
LAYOUTS
LAZARUS
LAZBOYS
LEACHES
LEADENS
LEADERS
LEADINS
LEADUPS
LEAGUES
LEAKERS
LEAKEYS
LEANERS
LEANTOS
LEAPERS
LEASERS
LEASHES
LEAVENS
LECHERS
LECTORS
LEDGERS
LEECHES
LEERERS
LEEWAYS
LEFTIES
LEGATES
LEGATOS
LEGENDS
LEGIONS
LEGISTS
LEGLESS
LEGOLAS
LEGUMES
LENDERS
LENGTHS
LENGUAS
LENNONS
LENOVOS
LENTILS
LEONIDS
LEPIDUS
LEPTONS
LESIONS
LESSEES
LESSENS
LESSEPS
LESSONS
LESSORS
LETPASS
LETTERS
LETTRES
LEVADES
LEVIERS
LEVITES
LEXISES
LEXUSES
LEXUSGS
LEXUSIS
LEXUSLS
LHASANS
LIAISES
LIBBERS
LIBIDOS
LIBRANS
LIBYANS
LICHEES
LICHENS
LICKERS
LIDLESS
LIENEES
LIENORS
LIFTERS
LIGANDS
LIGATES
LIGNINS
LIKINGS
LIMBERS
LIMNERS
LIMOGES
LIMPETS
LINAGES
LINDENS
LINDIES
LINDROS
LINEUPS
LINGERS
LINGOES
LININGS
LINKERS
LINKUPS
LINNETS
LINTELS
LINTERS
LIONELS
LIONESS
LIONETS
LIPARIS
LIPASES
LIPLESS
LIPPERS
LIQUIDS
LIQUORS
LISPERS
LISTEES
LISTENS
LISTERS
LITCHIS
LITOTES
LITTERS
LITTLES
LIVINGS
LIZARDS
LIZZIES
LLADROS
LOADERS
LOAFERS
LOANERS
LOATHES
LOBBERS
LOBBIES
LOBULES
LOCALES
LOCATES
LOCKERS
LOCKETS
LOCKINS
LOCKUPS
LOCULUS
LOCUSTS
LODGERS
LOESSES
LOFTERS
LOGGERS
LOGGIAS
LOGGINS
LOGJAMS
LOGOFFS
LOGOUTS
LOITERS
LOLLERS
LOLLIES
LONDRES
LONGIES
LONGUES
LOOBIES
LOOFAHS
LOOKERS
LOOKINS
LOOKUPS
LOOMPAS
LOONIES
LOOPERS
LOOSENS
LOOTERS
LOPPERS
LOQUATS
LORISES
LORRIES
LORUSES
LOSINGS
LOTIONS
LOTTERS
LOTUSES
LOUDENS
LOUNGES
LOURDES
LOUVERS
LOUVRES
LOVAGES
LOVEINS
LOWBIDS
LOWBOYS
LOWMASS
LOWNESS
LOWTOPS
LOYALES
LUBBERS
LUCITES
LUGGERS
LUGNUTS
LULLERS
LUMBARS
LUMBERS
LUMINAS
LUMPERS
LUNATES
LUNCHES
LUNGERS
LUNKERS
LUPINES
LURCHES
LUREXES
LURKERS
LUSTERS
LUSTRES
LUTISTS
LUXATES
LYCEUMS
LYRISTS

•LS••••

ALSATIA
ALSHAIN
ALSMITH
ALSORAN
RLSTINE
ULSTERS

•L•S•••

ALASKAN
ALASKAS
ALASSAD
ALBSURE
ALLSTAR
ALLSTON
ALMSMAN
ALMSMEN
ALYSSUM
BLASTED
BLASTER
BLESSED
BLESSER
BLESSES
BLISSED
BLISSES
BLISTER
BLOSSOM
BLUSHED
BLUSHER
BLUSHES
BLUSHON
BLUSTER
CLASHED
CLASHER
CLASHES
CLASPED
CLASPER
CLASSED
CLASSER
CLASSES
CLASSIC
CLASSON
CLOSEBY
CLOSEIN
CLOSELY
CLOSERS
CLOSEST
CLOSETO
CLOSETS
CLOSEUP
CLOSING
CLOSURE
CLUSTER
ELASTIC
ELASTIN
ELISION
ELUSIVE
ELUSORY
ELYSEES
ELYSIAN
ELYSIUM
FLASHED
FLASHER
FLASHES
FLASHON
FLESHED
FLESHES
FLESHLY
FLOSSED
FLOSSER
FLOSSES
FLOSSIE
FLUSHED
FLUSHER
FLUSHES
FLUSHOT
FLUSTER
FLYSOLO
GLASGOW
GLASHOW
GLASSED
GLASSES
GLISTEN
GLISTER
GLOSSAE
GLOSSAL
GLOSSAS
GLOSSED
GLOSSER
GLOSSES
ILOSTIT
KLISTER
OLDSALT
OLDSAWS
OLDSHOE
OLDSONG
OLDSTER
OLESTRA
OLMSTED
PLASHED
PLASHES
PLASMAS
PLASMIC
PLASTER
PLASTIC
PLISSES
PLOSION
PLOSIVE
PLUSHER
PLUSHES
PLUSHLY
PLUSONE
PLUSSES
PLUSTAX
PLUSTWO
SLASHED
SLASHER
SLASHES
SLOSHED
SLOSHES
SLUSHED
SLUSHES
ULYSSES

•L••S••

ALASSAD
ALCESTE
ALEKSEI
ALIASES
ALLISON
ALLYSON
ALROSEN
ALTOSAX
ALUNSER
ALYOSHA
ALYSSUM
BLEDSOE
BLESSED
BLESSER
BLESSES
BLISSED
BLISSES
BLOSSOM
BLOTSUP
BLOUSED
BLOUSES
BLOUSON
BLOWSIN
BLOWSIT
BLOWSON
BLOWSUP
BLUESKY
BLUESUN
CLAMSUP
CLASSED
CLASSER
CLASSES
CLASSIC
CLASSON
CLAUSAL
CLAUSES
CLAWSAT
CLEMSON
CLIPSON
CLOGSUP
CLOTSUP
CLUBSUP
CLUESIN
ELAPSED
ELAPSES
ELEISON
ELLISON
ELMISTI
FLENSED
FLENSER
FLENSES
FLIESAT
FLIESBY
FLIESIN
FLIESON
FLIESTO
FLIESUP
FLITSBY
FLITSIN
FLOSSED
FLOSSER
FLOSSES
FLOSSIE
FLOTSAM
FLOWSIN
GLAMSUP
GLASSED
GLASSES
GLEASON
GLOSSAE
GLOSSAL
GLOSSAS
GLOSSED
GLOSSER
GLOSSES
GLUESON
GLUESTO
ILIESCU
ILLUSED
ILLUSES
KLATSCH
KLEISER
KLENSCH
PLAISIR
PLANSON
PLANSTO
PLAYSAT
PLAYSBY
PLAYSON
PLAYSTO
PLAYSUP
PLEASED
PLEASER
PLEASES
PLISSES
PLOESTI
PLOWSON
PLOWSUP
PLUGSIN
PLUGSUP
PLUSSES
SLAMSON
SLAPSON
SLIPSBY
SLIPSIN
SLIPSON
SLIPSUP
SLOPSON
SLOWSUP
ULYSSES

•L•••S•

ALAMOSA
ALFONSE
ALFONSO
ALLCASH
ALLELSE
ALLNESS
ALLRISE
ALLWISE
ALQUIST
ALTOIST
BLEMISH
BLUEISH
CLAYISH
CLEANSE
CLERISY
CLOSEST
ELEGIST
ELITEST
ELITISM
ELITIST
ELLIPSE
ELMIEST
FLEMISH
FLORIST
FLUTIST
FLYCAST
FLYFISH
FLYLESS
FLYPAST
GLIMPSE
GLOBOSE
GLUCOSE
GLUIEST
ILLNESS
ILLPASS

OLDNESS
OLDROSE
OLDWEST
OLEMISS
OLOROSO
PLANISH
PLENISH
PLUMOSE
SLAVISH
SLOWEST
SLOWISH
SLYNESS

•L••••S

ALARBUS
ALARUMS
ALASKAS
ALBEDOS
ALBINOS
ALCOVES
ALDAVIS
ALEGARS
ALEKEGS
ALETAPS
ALETTES
ALEVELS
ALGIERS
ALIASES
ALIGHTS
ALINERS
ALIYAHS
ALKALIS
ALKENES
ALLAGES
ALLCAPS
ALLEARS
ALLEGES
ALLELES
ALLEWIS
ALLEYES
ALLIUMS
ALLNESS
ALLNEWS
ALLOFUS
ALLTHIS
ALLUDES
ALLURES
ALMONDS
ALNICOS
ALPACAS
ALPINES
ALTIMAS
ALTKEYS
ALTOIDS
ALTTABS
ALUDELS
ALUMNUS
BLADERS
BLAMERS
BLAZERS
BLAZONS
BLENDES
BLESSES
BLIGHTS
BLISSES
BLITZES
BLONDES
BLOUSES
BLOWERS
BLOWUPS
BLUDGES
BLUINGS
BLUSHES
CLAMORS
CLAQUES
CLARETS
CLASHES
CLASSES
CLAUSES
CLAWERS
CLEAVES
CLEMENS
CLERICS
CLICHES
CLIENTS
CLIMATS
CLINICS
CLIPONS
CLIQUES
CLOCHES
CLONERS
CLORETS
CLOSERS
CLOSETS
CLOTHES
CLOVERS
ELAINES
ELANCES
ELANETS
ELAPIDS
ELAPSES
ELATERS
ELEGIES
ELEGITS
ELEVENS
ELEVONS
ELFOWLS
ELICITS
ELIDERS
ELIGIUS
ELIXIRS
ELNINOS
ELOPERS
ELUANTS
ELUATES
ELUDERS
ELYSEES
FLACONS
FLAGONS
FLAKERS
FLAMBES
FLAMERS
FLANGES
FLASHES
FLATTVS
FLAUNTS
FLAUTAS
FLAVIUS
FLAVORS
FLAYERS
FLECHES
FLEDGES
FLEECES
FLENSES
FLESHES
FLEXORS
FLIGHTS
FLIPUPS
FLORETS
FLORINS
FLOSSES
FLOWERS
FLUBUGS
FLUSHES
FLUTERS
FLUTIES
FLYBOYS
FLYLESS
FLYNETS
FLYRODS
FLYWAYS
GLAMORS
GLANCES
GLASSES
GLAZERS
GLIDERS
GLITZES
GLOBINS
GLOBOUS
GLORIAS
GLORIES
GLOSSAS
GLOSSES
GLOTTIS
GLOWERS
GLURGES
GLUTENS
GLUTEUS
GLYCOLS
GLYNNIS
ILLNESS
ILLPASS
ILLUDES
ILLUMES
ILLUSES
KLAXONS
KLEPTOS
KLUDGES
KLUTZES
LLADROS
OLDBATS
OLDBOYS
OLDCARS
OLDDAYS
OLDDOGS
OLDGAGS
OLDNESS
OLDNEWS
OLDPALS
OLDPROS
OLDSAWS
OLDWAYS
OLEATES
OLEFINS
OLEMISS
OLEVELS
OLOGIES
OLYMPUS
PLACERS
PLAGUES
PLAICES
PLAINES
PLAINTS
PLAKATS
PLANERS
PLANETS
PLAQUES
PLASHES
PLASMAS
PLATENS
PLATERS
PLATIES
PLAUTUS
PLAYERS
PLEASES
PLEDGES
PLENUMS
PLEXORS
PLIGHTS
PLINTHS
PLISSES
PLOTZES
PLOUGHS
PLOVERS
PLOWERS
PLUGINS
PLUNGES
PLURALS
PLUSHES
PLUSSES
PLUTONS
SLAKERS
SLALOMS
SLASHES
SLATERS
SLAVERS
SLAYERS
SLEAZES
SLEDGES
SLEEVES
SLEIGHS
SLEUTHS
SLICERS
SLIDERS
SLIGHTS
SLIPONS
SLIPUPS
SLIVERS
SLOGANS
SLOPERS
SLOSHES
SLOUGHS
SLOVAKS
SLOVENS
SLOWUPS
SLUDGES
SLUICES
SLUSHES
SLYNESS
ULLAGES
ULSTERS
ULTIMAS
ULYSSES
ULZANAS

••LS•••

ALLSTAR
ALLSTON
BALSAMS
BALSAMY
BOLSHOI
BOLSTER
CELSIUS
DELSOLS
EELSKIN
FALSELY
FALSEST
FALSIFY
FALSITY
FULSOME
HALSTON
HELSING
HOLSTER
MOLSONS
NELSONS
NILSSON
OILSAND
OILSEED
OILSKIN
OILSPOT
PILSNER
PULSARS
PULSATE
PULSING
RALSTON
SALSODA
TELSTAR
TILSITS
TOLSTOI
TOLSTOY
TULSANS
TULSAOK
WALSTON
WILSONS

••L•S••

ALLISON
ALLYSON
APLUSES
ATLASES
AULDSOD
BALASES
BALKSAT
BALLSUP
BELASCO
BELLSON
BELTSAW
BELTSUP
BELUSHI
BOLTSUP
BOLUSES
BPLUSES
BULKSUP
CALISTA
CALLSIN
CALLSIT
CALLSON
CALLSTO
CALLSUP
CALMSEA
CELESTA
CELESTE
COLOSSI
CPLUSES
DALASIS
DELISTS
DOLLSUP
DPLUSES
EGLISES
ELLISON
ENLISTS
FALLSIN
FALLSON
FALLSTO
FILESBY
FILESIN
FILLSIN
FILLSUP
FILMSET
FOLDSIN
FOLDSUP
GELUSIL
HALFSHY
HELPSIN
HELPSON
HELPSUP
HOLDSIN
HOLDSIT
HOLDSON
HOLDSTO
HOLDSUP
HOLESUP
HOLISTS
HOLYSEE
IDLESSE
ILLUSED
ILLUSES
JALISCO
MALMSEY
MELISMA
MELISSA
MILKSOP
MOLESTS
NILESOH
NILSSON
NULLSET
OBLASTS
PELISSE
PILESIN
PILESOF
PILESON
PILESUP
POLESAT
POLESIT
POLISCI
POLYSCI
PULASKI
PULLSIN
PULLSON
PULLSUP
RELISTS
RELOSES
RILESUP
ROLLSBY
ROLLSIN
ROLLSON
ROLLSUP
RULESON
SALTSEA
SELLSIT
SELLSTO
SILESIA
SPLASHY
SULUSEA
TALKSAT
TALKSOF
TALKSON
TALKSTO
TALKSUP
TALUSES
TELESTO
TELLSIT
TELLSOF
TELLSON
TILTSAT
TILTSUP
UNLUSTY
VALISES
WALKSBY
WALKSON
WALKSTO
WALLSIN
WALLSUP
WELLSEE
WELLSET
WELLSUP
WILLSON
XYLOSES
YELLSAT
YELTSIN

••L••S•

ALLCASH
ALLELSE
ALLNESS
ALLRISE
ALLWISE
ATLEAST
AXLROSE
BALDEST
BALDISH
BALLAST
BELFAST
BOLDEST
BULLISH
BULRUSH
CALMEST
CALYPSO
CELLIST
COLDEST
COLDISH
COLOSSI
COLTISH
CULTISH
CULTISM
CULTIST
DELOUSE
DELUISE
DOLLISH
DOLTISH
DULLEST
DULLISH
ECLIPSE
EELIEST
ELLIPSE
FALSEST
FOLIOSE
FOLKISH
FULLEST
FULNESS
HELLISH
HELOISE
HOLIEST
IDLESSE
ILLNESS
ILLPASS
LALOOSH
MALAISE
MALPASO
MALTASE
MALTESE
MALTOSE
MELISSA
MELROSE
MILDEST
MOLLUSC
MOLLUSK
OILBASE
OILIEST
OILLESS
ONLEASE
ONLEASH
ONLIEST
OWLIEST
PALMIST
PELISSE
PELTISH
POLOIST
RELAPSE
RELEASE
RULIEST
SALTISH
SELFISH
SOLNESS
SOLOIST
TALLEST
TALLISH
TOLEASE
UGLIEST
UNLEASH
UNLOOSE
VBLOUSE
WILDEST
WILDISH
WILIEST
WOLFISH

••L•••S

ABLATES
ALLAGES
ALLCAPS
ALLEARS
ALLEGES
ALLELES
ALLEWIS
ALLEYES
ALLIUMS
ALLNESS
ALLNEWS
ALLOFUS
ALLTHIS
ALLUDES
ALLURES
APLITES
APLUSES
ATLASES
BALASES
BALATAS
BALBOAS
BALDIES
BALEENS
BALKANS
BALKERS
BALLADS
BALLETS
BALLOTS
BALSAMS
BCLIONS
BELAIRS
BELARUS
BELCHES
BELDAMS
BELIEFS
BELIERS
BELLIES
BELLOWS
BELONGS
BELTERS
BELUGAS
BILIOUS
BILKERS
BILLERS
BILLETS
BILLIES
BILLOWS
BOLEROS
BOLIDES
BOLTERS
BOLUSES
BPLUSES
BULBOUS
BULGARS
BULGURS
BULLETS
BULLIES
BULLINS
BULOVAS
BYLINES
CALDERS
CALENDS
CALICES
CALICOS
CALIPHS
CALKERS
CALKINS
CALLEES
CALLERS
CALLINS
CALLOUS
CALLUPS
CALYCES
CALYXES
CCLAMPS
CELEBES
CELICAS
CELLARS
CELSIUS
CELTICS
COLADAS
COLCHIS
COLLARS
COLLETS
COLLIES
COLLINS
COLLOPS
COLONES
COLONUS
COLOURS
COLUMNS
CPLUSES
CSLEWIS
CULCHES
CULEXES
CULLERS
CULLETS
CULLIES
DALASIS
DALETHS
DALLIES
DALTONS
DELEADS
DELETES
DELIBES
DELICTS
DELINTS
DELISTS
DELKEYS
DELORIS
DELRAYS
DELSOLS
DELUDES
DELUGES
DELVERS
DILATES
DILLIES
DILUTES
DOLLARS
DOLLIES
DOLLOPS
DOLMANS
DOLORES
DOLOURS
DPLUSES
ECLAIRS
EELPOTS
EGLISES
ENLACES
ENLINKS
ENLISTS
EOLITHS
ERLANGS
EULABUS
FALCONS
FALLALS
FALLERS
FALLOWS
FALTERS
FELINES
FELLAHS
FELLERS
FELLOWS
FILCHES
FILENES
FILINGS
FILLERS
FILLETS
FILLIES
FILLINS
FILLIPS
FILLUPS
FILTERS
FOLATES
FOLDERS
FOLDUPS
FOLGERS
FOLKIES
FOLLIES
FOLLOWS
FULFILS
FULMARS
FULNESS
GALANOS
GALANTS
GALAXES
GALENAS
GALLEYS
GALLONS
GALLOPS
GALLOWS
GALOOTS
GALPALS
GELATES
GELATIS
GELATOS
GELCAPS
GELPENS
GILBLAS
GILDERS
GOLFERS
GULCHES
GULDENS
GULLAHS
GULLETS
GULLIES
GULPERS
HALALAS
HALFIES
HALIDES
HALITES
HALLEYS
HALLOOS
HALLOWS
HALOIDS
HALTERS
HALVAHS
HALVERS
HELICES
HELIXES
HELLOES
HELLYES
HELMETS
HELPERS
HILTONS
HOLDERS
HOLDUPS
HOLISTS
HOLLERS
HOLLIES
HOLLOWS
HULLERS
ILLNESS
ILLPASS
ILLUDES
ILLUMES
ILLUSES
INLANDS
INLINES
ISLANDS
JELLIES
JILTERS
JOLLIES
JOLTERS
KELPIES
KELVINS
KILLERS
KILTIES
LOLLERS
LOLLIES
LULLERS
MALAGAS
MALIANS
MALICES
MALIGNS
MALLETS
MALLEUS
MALLOWS
MALTEDS
MALTHUS
MELDERS
MELLOWS
MELTERS
MILDEWS
MILHOUS
MILIEUS
MILKERS
MILLAIS
MILLERS
MILLETS
MILORDS
MOLDERS
MOLESTS
MOLLIES
MOLSONS
MOLTERS
MULCHES
MULETAS
MULLAHS
MULLERS
MULLETS
MULLINS
NELSONS
NOLOADS
OBLASTS
OBLATES
OBLIGES
OBLONGS
OGLALAS
OILCANS
OILCUPS
OILLESS
OILPANS
OILRIGS
OILRUBS
ONLOADS
OOLITES
OOLONGS
ORLEANS
OWLEGGS
PALACES
PALAMAS
PALATES
PALINGS
PALLETS
PALLORS
PALMERS
PALOMAS
PALTERS
PELAGES
PELLEAS
PELLETS
PELOTAS
PELTERS
PHLOEMS
PHLOXES
PILATES
PILATUS
PILEOUS
PILEUPS
PILFERS
PILINGS
PILLARS
PILLOWS
POLARAS
POLARIS
POLICES
POLLEES
POLLENS
POLLERS
PULLERS
PULLETS
PULLEYS
PULLINS
PULLONS
PULLUPS
PULPERS
PULPITS
PULSARS
RALLIES
RALLYES
RELACES
RELANDS
RELANES
RELATES
RELAXES
RELEADS
RELEAPS
RELENDS
RELENTS
RELEVES
RELICTS
RELIEFS
RELIERS
RELINES
RELINKS
RELISTS
RELIVES
RELOADS
RELOANS
RELOCKS
RELOOKS
RELOSES
RELUCTS
RELUMES
RILLETS
ROLAIDS
ROLEXES
ROLFERS
ROLLEIS
ROLLERS
ROLLINS
ROLLONS
ROLLUPS
RULINGS
SALAAMS
SALADES
SALAMIS
SALINAS
SALINES
SALIVAS
SALLIES
SALMONS
SALOONS
SALTERS
SALUKIS

SALUTES
SALVERS
SALVOES
SALVORS
SCLAFFS
SCLERAS
SELECTS
SELLERS
SILENTS
SILICAS
SILLIES
SILVERS
SOLACES
SOLARAS
SOLDERS
SOLNESS
SOLUTES
SOLVERS
SPLEENS
SPLICES
SPLINES
SPLINTS
STLOUIS
STLUKES
SULKERS
SULKIES
SULLIES
SULTANS
TALCUMS
TALENTS
TALKERS
TALKIES
TALLIES
TALLOWS
TALUSES
TELEXES
TELLERS
TELLIES
TILINGS
TILLERS
TILLETS
TILSITS
TILTERS
TOLEDOS
TOLLERS
TOLTECS
TULSANS
ULLAGES
UMLAUTS
UNLACES
UNLADES
UNLAXES
UNLEADS
UNLEAFS
UNLIKES
UNLINKS
UNLIVES
UNLOADS
UNLOCKS
UNLOOPS
UPLANDS
UPLEAPS
UPLIFTS
UPLINKS
UPLOADS
VALINES
VALISES
VALLEYS
VALOURS
VALUERS
VELCROS
VELLUMS
VELOURS
VELOXES
VELURES
VELVETS
VILNIUS
VOLLEYS
VOLUMES
VOLUTES
VULCANS
WALKERS
WALKINS
WALKONS
WALKUPS
WALLETS
WALLOPS
WALLOWS
WALNUTS
WALTERS
WALTONS
WALTZES
WELDERS
WELLYES
WELTERS
WILKENS
WILKINS
WILLERS
WILLIES
WILLOWS
WILSONS
XYLOSES
YELLERS
YELLOWS
YELPERS
ZILCHES

•••LS••

ARALSEA
AVULSED
AVULSES
BAILSON
BALLSUP
BELLSON
BOILSUP
CALLSIN
CALLSIT
CALLSON
CALLSTO
CALLSUP
CARLSON
CHELSEA
COILSUP
COOLSIT
CURLSIN
CURLSUP
DEALSIN
DEALSTO
DEALSUP
DIALSIN
DIALSUP
DOLLSUP
EVULSED
EVULSES
FAILSTO
FALLSIN
FALLSON
FALLSTO
FEELSOK
FILLSIN
FILLSUP
FOULSUP
FUELSUP
GIRLSHY
HAULSIN
HAULSUP
HEALSUP
HOWLSAT
KARLSON
MAILSIN
NAILSET
NAILSIN
NAILSIT
NAILSUP
NIELSEN
NULLSET
PAULSEN
PULLSIN
PULLSON
PULLSUP
RAILSAT
RAILSON
REELSIN
REELSUP
ROLLSBY
ROLLSIN
ROLLSON
ROLLSUP
SAILSON
SAILSTO
SEALSIN
SEALSUP
SELLSIT
SELLSTO
TELLSIT
TELLSOF
TELLSON
TOILSAT
TOOLSET
TOOLSUP
WALLSIN
WALLSUP
WELLSEE
WELLSET
WELLSUP
WILLSON
WOOLSEY
YELLSAT

•••L•S•

ABOLISH
AGELESS
AGILEST
AIDLESS
AIMLESS
AIRLESS
AMPLEST
AMYLASE
ANALYSE
ANALYST
ARMLESS
ARTLESS
ASHLESS
ATALOSS
ATELESS
AUSLESE
AWELESS
AWNLESS
BAALISH
BAALISM
BAALIST
BALLAST
BARLESS
BEDLESS
BIBLESS
BITLESS
BOWLESS
BRALESS
BUDLESS
BULLISH
CAPLESS
CARLESS
CELLIST
COOLEST
COOLISH
COXLESS
CUTLASS
CYCLIST
DECLASS
DEWLESS
DOGLESS
DOLLISH
DUALISM
DUALIST
DUELIST
DULLEST
DULLISH
EARLESS
EATLESS
ECCLESI
EGGLESS
ENCLASP
ENCLOSE
ENDLESS
ENGLISH
EVILEST
EYELASH
EYELESS
FATLESS
FEELESS
FINLESS
FLYLESS
FOELESS
FOGLESS
FOOLISH
FOULEST
FTBLISS
FULLEST
FURLESS
GAPLESS
GASLESS
GAULISH
GEMLESS
GETLOST
GIRLISH
GODLESS
GOTLOST
GOULASH
GUMLESS
GUNLESS
GUTLESS
HAPLESS
HATLESS
HELLISH
HIPLESS
HITLESS
HITLIST
HUELESS
ICELESS
IDOLISE
IDOLIST
IDYLIST
INCLASS
INCLOSE
INGLESE
INKLESS
INNLESS
INULASE
IRELESS
JAGLESS
JARLESS
JAWLESS
JOBLESS
JOYLESS
KEYLESS
KINLESS
LAWLESS
LEGLESS
LIDLESS
LIPLESS
MANLESS
MATLESS
MIDLIST
MOLLUSC
MOLLUSK
MRBLISS
NAPLESS
NETLESS
NETLOSS
NOBLEST
NOCLASS
OARLESS
OBELISE
OBELISK
OCULIST
OILLESS
OPALISH
ORALIST
ORBLESS
ORELESS
OUTLASH
OUTLAST
PAULIST
PAYLESS
PEGLESS
PINLESS
PIPLESS
PRELOSS
PUBLISH
PUNLESS
RAYLESS
REALEST
REALISE
REALISM
REALIST
RECLASP
RECLASS
RECLUSE
REGLOSS
RIBLESS
RIMLESS
RODLESS
RUMLESS
RUNLESS
SAPLESS
SEXLESS
SINLESS
SKYLESS
SODLESS
SONLESS
STALEST
STYLISE
STYLISH
STYLIST
SUMLESS
SUNLESS
TALLEST
TALLISH
TAXLESS
TBILISI
TEALESS
TIELESS
TIPLESS
TITLIST
TOELESS
TOPLESS
TOYLESS
TUGLESS
UNBLEST
UNCLASP
UNCLOSE
UPCLOSE
USELESS
UTILISE
VIOLIST
VOWLESS
WARLESS
WAYLESS
WEBLESS
WIGLESS
WINLESS
WITLESS
WOULDST
YOULOSE

•••L••S

ADELIES
AGELESS
AGULHAS
AIDLESS
AIGLETS
AIMLESS
AIRLESS
AIRLOGS
AMBLERS
AMULETS
ANALOGS
ANGLAIS
ANGLERS
ANKLERS
ANKLETS
ANTLERS
APELETS
APOLLOS
APPLETS
APPLIES
ARMLESS
ARMLETS
ARTLESS
ASHLARS
ASHLESS
ASYLUMS
ATALOSS
ATELESS
AUKLETS
AVALONS
AVULSES
AWELESS
AWNLESS
AXILLAS
AZALEAS
BADLIES
BADLOTS
BAILEES
BAILERS
BAILORS
BALLADS
BALLETS
BALLOTS
BARLESS
BARLEYS
BAWLERS
BEDLAMS
BEDLESS
BEDLOES
BELLIES
BELLOWS
BIALIES
BIBLESS
BIGLIES
BIGLOTS
BILLERS
BILLETS
BILLIES
BILLOWS
BIOLABS
BIRLERS
BITLESS
BOILERS
BOWLERS
BOWLESS
BRALESS
BRILLOS
BUDLESS
BUGLERS
BULLETS
BULLIES
BULLINS
BUMLEGS
BURLAPS
BURLERS
BUTLERS
BYPLAYS
CABLERS
CABLETS
CALLEES
CALLERS
CALLINS
CALLOUS
CALLUPS
CAPLESS
CAPLETS
CARLESS
CARLOTS
CELLARS
CHALCIS
CHALETS
CHALONS
CHILIES
CHILLIS
CHOLERS
CHOLLAS
COALERS
COALGAS
COILERS
COLLARS
COLLETS
COLLIES
COLLINS
COLLOPS
COOLERS
COOLIES
COULEES
COXLESS
CULLERS
CULLETS
CULLIES
CURLERS
CURLEWS
CUTLASS
CUTLERS
CUTLETS
CYCLERS
CYCLOPS
DAHLIAS
DAILIES
DALLIES
DEALERS
DEBLURS
DECLASS
DECLAWS
DECLOTS
DEFLEAS
DEPLOYS
DESLUMS
DEWLAPS
DEWLESS
DIALERS
DIALOGS
DIALUPS
DIDLAPS
DIGLOTS
DILLIES
DNALABS
DOGLEGS
DOGLESS
DOILIES
DOLLARS
DOLLIES
DOLLOPS
DOOLIES
DUELERS
DUNLINS
DUNLOPS
DYELOTS
EAGLETS
EARLAPS
EARLESS
EARLETS
EARLIES
EATLESS
EGGLERS
EGGLESS
EMBLEMS
EMPLOYS
EMULOUS
ENDLESS
ENGLUTS
EPILOGS
EVOLVES
EVULSES
EXILERS
EYELESS
EYELETS
EYELIDS
FABLERS
FAILLES
FALLALS
FALLERS
FALLOWS
FATLESS
FATLIPS
FEELERS
FEELESS
FELLAHS
FELLERS
FELLOWS
FILLERS
FILLETS
FILLIES
FILLINS
FILLIPS
FILLUPS
FINLESS
FLYLESS
FOELESS
FOGLESS
FOLLIES
FOLLOWS
FOOLERS
FOULUPS
FOWLERS
FROLICS
FTBLISS
FUELERS
FURLERS
FURLESS
GAGLAWS
GALLEYS
GALLONS
GALLOPS
GALLOWS
GAOLERS
GAPLESS
GARLICS
GARLITS
GASLESS
GASLOGS
GATLINS
GEMLESS
GIBLETS
GIBLUES
GIMLETS
GIRLIES
GOALIES
GOBLETS
GOBLINS
GODLESS
GRILLES
GULLAHS
GULLETS
GULLIES
GUMLESS
GUNLAPS
GUNLAWS
GUNLESS
GUTLESS
HAILERS
HALLEYS
HALLOOS
HALLOWS
HAMLETS
HAPLESS
HARLEYS
HARLOTS
HATLESS
HAULERS
HEALERS
HEELERS
HELLOES
HELLYES
HIPLESS
HITLESS
HOLLERS
HOLLIES
HOLLOWS
HOTLIPS
HOWLERS
HUELESS
HULLERS
HURLERS
ICELESS
IMPLIES
INCLASS
INFLOWS
INKLESS
INNLESS
IRELESS
ITALICS
JAGLESS
JAILERS
JAILORS
JARLESS
JAWLESS
JEALOUS
JELLIES
JETLAGS
JOBLESS
JOBLOTS
JOLLIES
JOYLESS
KEGLERS
KEYLESS
KILLERS
KINLESS
KISLEVS
LADLERS
LAULAUS
LAWLESS
LEGLESS
LIDLESS
LIPLESS
LOLLERS
LOLLIES
LULLERS
MADLIBS
MAGLEVS
MAILERS
MAILINS
MALLETS
MALLEUS
MALLOWS
MANLESS
MARLINS
MATLESS
MAULERS
MEALIES
MEDLEYS
MELLOWS
MERLINS
MERLOTS
MEWLERS
MIDLEGS
MILLAIS
MILLERS
MILLETS
MISLAYS
MOILERS
MOLLIES
MOSLEMS
MOTLEYS
MRBLISS
MUKLUKS
MULLAHS
MULLERS
MULLETS
MULLINS
MUSLIMS
MUSLINS
NAILERS
NAPLESS
NETLESS
NETLOSS
NIBLETS
NOCLASS
NUCLEUS
NUTLETS
OARLESS
OCELLUS
OCELOTS
OCULARS
ODDLOTS
ODELETS
OILLESS
OMELETS
ORBLESS
ORELESS
OSTLERS
OUTLAWS
OUTLAYS
OUTLETS
OUTLIES
OUTLIPS
PABLUMS
PAELLAS
PALLETS
PALLORS
PARLAYS
PARLEYS
PARLORS
PARLOUS
PAYLESS
PEELERS
PEGLEGS
PEGLESS
PELLEAS
PELLETS
PEPLUMS
PHILCOS
PHILEAS
PHILIPS
PHILOUS
PHYLLIS
PHYLLOS
PIGLETS
PILLARS
PILLOWS
PINLESS
PIOLETS
PIPLESS
POLLEES
POLLENS
POLLERS
POOLERS
POPLARS
POPLINS
POTLIDS
PRELIMS
PRELOSS
PROLOGS
PUBLICS
PUBLIUS
PULLERS
PULLETS
PULLEYS
PULLINS
PULLONS
PULLUPS
PUNLESS
RAGLANS
RAILBUS
RAILERS
RALLIES
RALLYES
RANLAPS
RATLINS
RAWLINS
RAYLESS
RECLADS
RECLASS
REDLEGS
REELERS
REFLAGS
REFLIES
REFLIPS
REFLOWS
REGLOSS
REGLOWS
REGLUES
REPLANS
REPLAYS
REPLIES
REPLOTS
REPLOWS
RIALTOS
RIBLESS
RIBLETS
RIFLERS
RILLETS
RIMLESS
RODLESS
ROLLEIS
ROLLERS
ROLLINS
ROLLONS
ROLLUPS
RUMLESS
RUNLAPS
RUNLESS
RUNLETS
RVALUES
SAILERS
SAILORS
SALLIES
SAMLETS
SAPLESS
SAWLOGS
SCALARS
SCALERS
SCHLEPS
SCHLUBS
SCULPTS
SEALABS
SEALEGS
SEALERS
SELLERS
SEXLESS
SHALOMS
SHELVES
SILLIES
SINLESS
SKYLESS
SLALOMS
SMILERS
SMILEYS
SMILLAS
SODLESS
SONLESS
STALAGS
STELIAS
STOLONS
STYLERS
STYLETS
SUBLETS
SUBLIDS
SUBLOTS
SULLIES
SUMLESS
SUNLESS
TABLETS
TAILERS
TAILORS
TALLIES
TALLOWS
TAXLAWS
TAXLESS
TAYLORS
TEALESS
TEFLONS
TELLERS
TELLIES
THALERS
TIELESS
TIGLONS
TILLERS
TILLETS
TIPLESS
TOELESS
TOILERS
TOILETS
TOLLERS
TOOLERS
TOPLESS
TOYLESS

TRELLIS
TUGLESS
TUILLES
TWELVES
UNCLIPS
UNCLOGS
UNGLUES
UNPLANS
UNPLUGS
UPFLOWS
USELESS
USFLAGS
UVALUES
VALLEYS
VARLETS
VEILERS
VELLUMS
VIELLES
VIOLETS
VIOLINS
VOLLEYS
VOWLESS
WAILERS
WALLETS
WALLOPS
WALLOWS
WARLESS
WAYLAYS
WAYLESS
WEALTHS
WEBLESS
WEBLOGS
WELLYES
WHALERS
WIGLESS
WIGLETS
WILLERS
WILLIES
WILLOWS
WINLESS
WITLESS
WOOLENS
WOOLIES
YELLERS
YELLOWS
YESLETS
YOWLERS
ZEALOTS
ZEALOUS
ZIPLOCS

••••LS•

ALLELSE
DIVULSE
HOWELSE
IMPULSE
LAVALSE
REPULSE
SEEALSO

••••L•S

AACELLS
ABRILES
AEDILES
ALKALIS
ALLELES
AMPULES
ANGELAS
ANGELES
ANGELUS
ANNALES
ANNULUS
APOLLOS
APPALLS
ARABLES
ARBOLES
AREOLAS
AREOLES
ARGALIS
ARGYLES
ARNOLDS
AUDILES
AXILLAS
BABBLES
BAFFLES
BANGLES
BAROLOS
BARTLES
BASALTS
BATTLES
BAUBLES
BEADLES
BEAGLES
BEATLES
BECALMS
BEETLES
BEFALLS
BEHOLDS
BINDLES
BINGLES
BOBBLES
BOGGLES
BOODLES
BOTTLES
BRIDLES
BRILLOS
BUBBLES
BUCKLES
BUGGLES
BUMBLES
BUNDLES
BUNGLES
BURBLES
BURGLES
BUSTLES
BYTALKS
CABALAS
CACKLES
CAJOLES
CANDLES
CANOLAS
CANTLES
CANULAS
CASTLES
CATALOS
CHABLIS
CHARLES
CHICLES
CHILLIS
CHOLLAS
CIRCLES
COBALTS
COBBLES
COCKLES
CODDLES
COGGLES
COPULAS
COUPLES
CRADLES
CREOLES
CUDDLES
CUMULUS
CUPOLAS
CUPULES
CURDLES
DABBLES
DANDLES
DANGLES
DAPPLES
DARKLES
DARTLES
DAWDLES
DAZZLES
DECILES
DECKLES
DEDALUS
DEFILES
DEPULPS
DESALTS
DESILTS
DIABLES
DIABLOS
DIBBLES
DIDDLES
DIMPLES
DINGLES
DIPOLES
DONGLES
DOODLES
DOTTLES
DOUBLES
DOUGLAS
DUFFLES
EDIBLES
EKUELES
EMBALMS
EMPALES
ENABLES
ENDALLS
ENFOLDS
ENGILDS
ENGULFS
ENISLES
ENROLLS
ENSILES
ESCALUS
ETOILES
EVERLYS
EXHALES
EXTOLLS
FAILLES
FAMULUS
FATALES
FEMALES
FERULES
FETTLES
FIBULAS
FIDDLES
FIDELES
FIDELIS
FINALES
FIPPLES
FIZZLES
FOCSLES
FOIBLES
FONDLES
FOOTLES
FOOZLES
FUDDLES
FUMBLES
GABBLES
GAGGLES
GAMBLES
GARBLES
GARGLES
GENTLES
GIGGLES
GIGOLOS
GILBLAS
GIRDLES
GOBBLES
GOGGLES
GOOGLES
GRILLES
GURGLES
GUZZLES
HABILIS
HACKLES
HAGGLES
HALALAS
HAMULUS
HANDLES
HASSLES
HECKLES
HERALDS
HGWELLS
HIGGLES
HOBBLES
HOOPLAS
HOWELLS
HUDDLES
HUMBLES
HURDLES
HURTLES
HUSTLES
ICICLES
IMPALAS
IMPALES
INFOLDS
INGALLS
INGULFS
INHALES
INSALES
INSOLES
INSULTS
JACALES
JANGLES
JIGGLES
JINGLES
JOGGLES
JOSTLES
JUGGLES
JUMBLES
JUNGLES
KETTLES
KIBBLES
KIDULTS
KINDLES
KNOWLES
KOBOLDS
KURILES
LEGOLAS
LITTLES
LOBULES
LOCALES
LOCULUS
LOYALES
MANGLES
MANILAS
MANTLES
MARBLES
MCCALLS
MCHALES
MEAGLES
MEASLES
MEDDLES
MEDELES
METTLES
MIDDLES
MINGLES
MIZZLES
MOBILES
MODELAS
MODELBS
MODELTS
MODULES
MODULUS
MORALES
MORELOS
MOTTLES
MUDDLES
MUESLIS
MUFFLES
MUGGLES
MUMBLES
MUSCLES
MUZZLES
MYRTLES
NAPALMS
NEBULAS
NEEDLES
NEPALIS
NESTLES
NETTLES
NIBBLES
NICKLES
NICOLAS
NIGGLES
NIPPLES
NODULES
NOGALES
NONPLUS
NOODLES
NOPALES
NOVALIS
NOVELAS
NOZZLES
NTUPLES
NUBBLES
NUZZLES
OCCULTS
OCELLUS
OGLALAS
ORACLES
ORIOLES
ORMOLUS
OSCULES
PADDLES
PAELLAS
PAPELES
PAROLES
PAYOLAS
PEBBLES
PEDDLES
PEEBLES
PEEPLES
PENULTS
PEOPLES
PESTLES
PETALES
PHYLLIS
PHYLLOS
PICKLES
PIDDLES
PIFFLES
PIMPLES
POMELOS
POODLES
POPPLES
POSOLES
POSSLQS
POZOLES
PROCLUS
PUDDLES
PUEBLOS
PUGGLES
PURFLES
PURPLES
PUZZLES
QABALAS
QUARLES
RABBLES
RAFFLES
RAMBLES
RANKLES
RASSLES
RATTLES
RCCOLAS
REBALES
REBILLS
REBOLTS
RECALLS
REFALLS
REFILES
REFILLS
REFILMS
REFOLDS
REGALES
REGILDS
REGULUS
REMELTS
REMILLS
REMOLDS
REPOLLS
REROLLS
RESALES
RESALTS
RESELLS
RESILES
RESOLES
RESULTS
RETELLS
RETILES
RETILLS
REVILES
REVOLTS
REWELDS
RIBALDS
RICKLES
RIDDLES
RIFFLES
RIMPLES
RIPPLES
ROMULUS
ROOTLES
ROYALES
RUBBLES
RUFFLES
RUGGLES
RUMBLES
RUMPLES
RUNDLES
RUSTLES
RUTILES
RUYBLAS
SADDLES
SAMPLES
SANBLAS
SAVALAS
SCHOLES
SCROLLS
SETTLES
SHEILAS
SHIELDS
SHRILLS
SICKLES
SIMILES
SIMPLES
SINGLES
SIZZLES
SMILLAS
SNUGLIS
SOMALIS
SQUALLS
STABLES
STAPLES
STIFLES
STROLLS
SUPPLES
SURPLUS
TACKLES
TAMALES
TANGLES
TATTLES
TEMPLES
THEALPS
THRALLS
THRILLS
TICKLES
TINGLES
TINKLES
TIPPLES
TITTLES
TODDLES
TOGGLES
TOODLES
TOOTLES
TOPPLES
TOUSLES
TREBLES
TRELLIS
TRIFLES
TRIPLES
TROILUS
TUBULES
TUILLES
TUMBLES
TUMULTS
TUPELOS
TURTLES
TUSSLES
UNBALES
UNBELTS
UNBOLTS
UNFILES
UNFOLDS
UNHELMS
UNHULLS
UNMOLDS
UNPILES
UNROLLS
UNSELLS
UNSOLES
UNWALLS
UPFOLDS
UPHILLS
UPHOLDS
UPPILES
UPTALKS
UPTILTS
UPWELLS
USABLES
VENULES
VIELLES
VITALIS
VITTLES
VIZSLAS
WADDLES
WAFFLES
WAGGLES
WAMBLES
WANGLES
WARBLES
WATTLES
WEDELNS
WIGGLES
WIMPLES
WOBBLES
YUKOLIS
ZOCALOS
ZONULES

•••••LS

AACELLS
ACETALS
AERIALS
AGNAILS
ALEVELS
ALUDELS
AMATOLS
AMIDOLS
AMSTELS
ANIMALS
ANNEALS
ANNUALS
APPALLS
APPEALS
ARMFULS
ASSAILS
AVOWALS
BAGFULS
BARRELS
BEFALLS
BEFOOLS
BEFOULS
BENGALS
BETHELS
BEWAILS
BOATELS
BOXFULS
BRIDALS
BURIALS
BUSHELS
CANCELS
CANFULS
CANNELS
CANTALS
CAPFULS
CARFULS
CARPALS
CARPELS
CARRELS
CARTELS
CARVELS
CASUALS
CENTALS
CEREALS
CHANELS
CHAPELS
CHISELS
CHORALS
COEVALS
COMPELS
CONSULS
CORBELS
CORRALS
CRENELS
CREWELS
CUDGELS
CUPFULS
CYMBALS
DACTYLS
DAMSELS
DANIELS
DATRILS
DEFUELS
DELSOLS
DENIALS
DENTALS
DERAILS
DETAILS
DIESELS
DIRNDLS
DISMALS
DISPELS
DISTILS
DORSALS
DOSSALS
DRIVELS
DUFFELS
EADGILS
EARFULS
ELFOWLS
ENAMELS
ENDALLS
ENROLLS
ENSEALS
ENSOULS
ENTAILS
ENVEILS
ESPIALS
EXTOLLS
EYEFULS
FACIALS
FALLALS
FARFELS
FENNELS
FINGALS
FINIALS
FORMALS
FOSSILS
FRIVOLS
FULFILS
FUNNELS
GALPALS
GAMBOLS
GAVIALS
GERBILS
GIMBALS
GIMBELS
GLYCOLS
GOGIRLS
GOOGOLS
GOSPELS
GRAVELS
GROVELS
GUNSELS
HATFULS
HERBALS
HGWELLS
HOSTELS
HOWELLS
HUMMELS
HYMNALS
INGALLS
INGOALS
INSTALS
INSTILS
INTAILS
ISOHELS
ITGIRLS
JACKALS
JARFULS
JUGFULS
KENNELS
KERNELS
KEYPALS
KISSELS
KUMMELS
LABIALS
LAPFULS
LAURELS
LENTILS
LEXUSLS
LINTELS
LIONELS
MAMMALS
MANTELS
MANUALS
MARCELS
MARVELS
MCCALLS
MENDELS
MENIALS
MESCALS
MISSALS
MONGOLS
MORSELS
MORTALS
MUDEELS
MUGFULS
MURIELS
MUSSELS
MUTUALS
NETFULS
NICHOLS
NICKELS
NORMALS
NUTOILS
OLDPALS
OLEVELS
ORDEALS
OXTAILS
PANFULS
PARCELS
PASSELS
PASTELS
PATROLS
PENCILS
PENPALS
PENTELS
PETRELS
PETROLS
PHENOLS
PISTILS
PISTOLS
PLURALS
POMMELS
PORTALS
POTFULS
PROPELS
PUMMELS
RADIALS
RAPPELS
RASCALS
REBILLS
REBOILS
RECALLS
RECOALS
RECOILS
RECOOLS
RECURLS
REDEALS
REDIALS
REFALLS
REFILLS
REFUELS
REHAULS
REHEALS
REHEELS
REJAILS
REMAILS
REMILLS
RENAILS
RENTALS
REPEALS
REPOLLS
REREELS
REROLLS
RESEALS
RESELLS
RESOILS
RETAILS
RETELLS
RETILLS
RETOOLS
REVEALS
RITUALS
RONDELS
RUNNELS
SANDALS
SCHOOLS
SCRAWLS
SCROLLS
SEAEELS
SECKELS
SEQUELS
SERIALS
SHEKELS
SHOVELS
SHRILLS
SHTETLS
SIGNALS
SNIVELS
SOCIALS
SORRELS
SPINELS
SPIRALS
SPRAWLS
SQUALLS
SQUEALS
STEROLS
STPAULS
STROLLS
SWIVELS
SYMBOLS
TAROILS
TARSALS
TASSELS
TEASELS
TERCELS
THRALLS
THRILLS
TIMBALS
TINSELS
TONSILS
TRAVELS
TROWELS
TUBFULS
TUNNELS
TVIDOLS
UNCIALS
UNCOILS
UNCURLS
UNFURLS
UNHULLS
UNNAILS
UNPEELS
UNREELS
UNROLLS
UNSEALS
UNSELLS
UNVEILS
UNWALLS
UPCOILS
UPCURLS
UPHILLS
UPWELLS
URACILS
URNFULS
VANDALS
VASSALS
VATFULS
VERBALS
VESSELS
VESTALS
VISUALS
WANKELS
WEASELS
WEEVILS

LT•••••

LTKOJAK

L•T••••

LATCHED
LATCHES
LATCHON
LATEENS
LATEFEE
LATENCY
LATENED
LATENTS
LATERAL
LATERAN
LATERON
LATETAG
LATEXES
LATHERS
LATHERY
LATHING
LATICES
LATIFAH
LATIGOS
LATIMES
LATINAS
LATINII
LATINOS
LATINUS
LATOSCA
LATRELL
LATRINE
LATROBE
LATTICE
LATVIAN
LETDOWN
LETDROP
LETEMIN
LETFALL
LETGOBY
LETGOOF
LETHAVE
LETHEAN
LETINON
LETITBE
LETITGO
LETITIA
LETKNOW
LETLIVE
LETMEBE
LETMEGO
LETMEIN
LETPASS
LETRIDE
LETROLL
LETSEAT
LETSFLY
LETSLIP
LETSNOT
LETSOFF
LETSOUT
LETSRIP
LETSSEE
LETSUSE

LETTERA
LETTERB
LETTERC
LETTERD
LETTERE
LETTERF
LETTERG
LETTERH
LETTERI
LETTERJ
LETTERK
LETTERL
LETTERM
LETTERN
LETTERO
LETTERP
LETTERQ
LETTERR
LETTERS
LETTERT
LETTERU
LETTERV
LETTERW
LETTERX
LETTERY
LETTERZ
LETTING
LETTISH
LETTRES
LETTUCE
LETUPON
LITCHIS
LITCRIT
LITERAL
LITHELY
LITHEST
LITHGOW
LITHIUM
LITHOID
LITINTO
LITOTES
LITOVSK
LITTERS
LITTERY
LITTLER
LITTLES
LITURGY
LOTHAIR
LOTHIAN
LOTHROP
LOTIONS
LOTTERS
LOTTERY
LOTTING
LOTUSES
LUTETIA
LUTHIER
LUTHULI
LUTISTS

L••T•••

LABTECH
LABTEST
LABTUBE
LACTAID
LACTASE
LACTATE
LACTEAL
LACTOSE
LAITIES
LANTANA
LANTERN
LAOTIAN
LAPTOPS
LASTACT
LASTDON
LASTGAS
LASTING
LASTLAP
LASTLEG
LASTMAY
LASTONE
LASTORY
LASTROW
LATTICE
LAUTREC
LEATHER
LECTERN
LECTORS
LECTRIC
LECTURE
LEETIDE
LEFTARM
LEFTEAR
LEFTEND
LEFTEST
LEFTEYE
LEFTFOR
LEFTHIP
LEFTIES
LEFTISH
LEFTISM
LEFTIST
LEFTJAB
LEFTLEG
LEFTOFF
LEFTOUT
LEGTRAP
LEITRIM
LENTIGO
LENTILS
LEOTARD
LEPTONS
LESTOIL
LETTERA
LETTERB
LETTERC
LETTERD
LETTERE
LETTERF
LETTERG
LETTERH
LETTERI
LETTERJ
LETTERK
LETTERL
LETTERM
LETTERN
LETTERO
LETTERP
LETTERQ
LETTERR
LETTERS
LETTERT
LETTERU
LETTERV
LETTERW
LETTERX
LETTERY
LETTERZ
LETTING
LETTISH
LETTRES
LETTUCE
LIETEST
LIFTERS
LIFTING
LIFTOFF
LIFTSUP
LILTING
LINTELS
LINTERS
LINTIER
LINTING
LISTEES
LISTENS
LISTERS
LISTING
LITTERS
LITTERY
LITTLER
LITTLES
LOATHED
LOATHER
LOATHES
LOATHLY
LOATHTO
LOFTBED
LOFTERS
LOFTIER
LOFTILY
LOFTING
LOITERS
LOOTERS
LOOTING
LOSTART
LOSTBIG
LOSTCAT
LOSTDOG
LOSTOUT
LOSTPET
LOTTERS
LOTTERY
LOTTING
LOUTING
LOUTISH
LOWTECH
LOWTIDE
LOWTOPS
LUSTERS
LUSTFUL
LUSTIER
LUSTILY
LUSTING
LUSTRAL
LUSTRED
LUSTRES
LUSTRUM

L•••T••

LABATTS
LAERTES
LAFITTE
LAKOTAS
LAMOTTA
LAMOTTE
LANDTAG
LANDTAX
LANETWO
LANGTON
LANGTRY
LANOTTE
LAPUTAN
LATETAG
LAYETTE
LAYITON
LEANTOS
LEAPTAT
LEAPTIN
LEAPTON
LEAPTUP
LEGATEE
LEGATES
LEGATOR
LEGATOS
LEISTER
LENGTHS
LENGTHY
LESOTHO
LESSTAR
LETITBE
LETITGO
LETITIA
LEVATOR
LEVITES
LEVITIC
LICITLY
LIEATOP
LIGATED
LIGATES
LIGHTED
LIGHTEN
LIGHTER
LIGHTLY
LIGHTON
LIGHTUP
LILETEE
LIMITED
LIMITER
LINETWO
LITOTES
LIZETTE
LLEYTON
LOBATED
LOBSTER
LOCATED
LOCATER
LOCATES
LOCATOR
LONETTE
LONGTOM
LONGTON
LORETTA
LOVETAP
LUCETTA
LUCITES
LUNATED
LUNATES
LUNATIC
LUNETTE
LUTETIA
LUXATED
LUXATES
LYNETTE

L••••T•

LABATTS
LABIATE
LABRATS
LACERTA
LACOSTE
LACTATE
LAFITTE
LAKISTS
LAMBETH
LAMENTS
LAMINTO
LAMOTTA
LAMOTTE
LANCETS
LANOTTE
LAPCATS
LAPLATA
LAPORTE
LAPPETS
LARIATS
LATENTS
LAURITZ
LAYETTE
LAYINTO
LAYOUTS
LEADETH
LEADSTO
LEANSTO
LEARNTO
LEASETO
LECONTE
LEDINTO
LEDUPTO
LEGISTS
LEMMATA
LEONATO
LEPANTO
LIBERTE
LIBERTY
LICKETY
LIGGETT
LIGNITE
LIKENTO
LIMNITE
LIMPETS
LINEATE
LINNETS
LIONETS
LIQUATE
LISBETH
LISENTE
LITINTO
LIZETTE
LOATHTO
LOCKETS
LOCUSTS
LOGONTO
LOGOUTS
LONETTE
LOOKSTO
LOQUATS
LORENTZ
LORETTA
LOSESTO
LOVEDTO
LOVESTO
LOYALTO
LOYALTY
LUCETTA
LUDDITE
LUGNUTS
LUNESTA
LUNETTE
LUTISTS
LYDDITE
LYINGTO
LYNETTE
LYRISTS

L•••••T

LABCOAT
LABORAT
LABTEST
LACIEST
LACKWIT
LAIDOUT
LAKIEST
LAMAIST
LAMBENT
LAMBERT
LAMPERT
LAMPLIT
LANDSAT
LANKEST
LAPBELT
LARGENT
LARGEST
LASHOUT
LASTACT
LAUGHAT
LAURENT
LAWSUIT
LAYSOUT
LAZIEST
LEADOUT
LEAFLET
LEAFOUT
LEANCUT
LEANEST
LEAPSAT
LEAPTAT
LEARJET
LEAVEIT
LEERSAT
LEFTEST
LEFTIST
LEFTOUT
LEGOSET
LEGREST
LENDOUT
LENFANT
LENIENT
LESCAUT
LESSFAT
LETSEAT
LETSNOT
LETSOUT
LETTERT
LEVERET
LEWDEST
LIEFEST
LIETEST
LIFENET
LIGGETT
LIMIEST
LIMPEST
LINECUT
LINEOUT
LINIEST
LIPSOUT
LITCRIT
LITHEST
LIVEOUT
LIVESAT
LIVESET
LOANOUT
LOCKLET
LOCKNUT
LOCKOUT
LOCKSET
LOGANUT
LOGIEST
LOGSOUT
LONGEST
LOOKIST
LOOKOUT
LOOKSAT
LOOSEST
LORDSIT
LORIENT
LOSEOUT
LOSESIT
LOSTART
LOSTCAT
LOSTOUT
LOSTPET
LOUDEST
LOVEDIT
LOVESET
LOVESIT
LOWCOST
LOWPOST
LOWRENT
LUCKOUT
LUGSOUT
LUMPSIT
LUNGEAT
LUSHEST

•LT••••

ALTDORF
ALTERED
ALTERER
ALTHING
ALTHORN
ALTIMAS
ALTKEYS
ALTOIDS
ALTOIST
ALTOONA
ALTOSAX
ALTTABS
BLTTOGO
ELTRAIN
ULTIMAS

•L•T•••

ALATEEN
ALETAPS
ALETTES
ALITTLE
ALLTHAT
ALLTHIS
ALLTIED
ALLTIME
ALLTOLD
ALTTABS
BLATANT
BLATHER
BLATTED
BLITHER
BLITZED
BLITZEN
BLITZER
BLITZES
BLOTCHY
BLOTOUT
BLOTSUP
BLOTTED
BLOTTER
BLTTOGO
CLATTER
CLOTHED
CLOTHES
CLOTSUP
CLOTTED
CLOTURE
CLUTCHY
CLUTTER
ELATERS
ELATING
ELATION
ELITEST
ELITISM
ELITIST
ELMTREE
ELUTING
ELUTION
FLATBED
FLATCAR
FLATHAT
FLATLET
FLATOUT
FLATTAX
FLATTED
FLATTEN
FLATTER
FLATTOP
FLATTVS
FLITSBY
FLITSIN
FLITTED
FLITTER
FLOTAGE
FLOTSAM
FLUTERS
FLUTIER
FLUTIES
FLUTING
FLUTIST
FLUTTER
FLYTIER
FLYTRAP
GLITCHY
GLITTER
GLITZED
GLITZES
GLOTTAL
GLOTTIS
GLUTEAL
GLUTENS
GLUTEUS
GLUTTED
GLUTTON
ILLTELL
KLATSCH
KLUTZES
OLDTIME
OLDTOWN
PLATEAU
PLATENS
PLATERS
PLATIER
PLATIES
PLATING
PLATOON
PLATTED
PLATTER
PLATYPI
PLOTFUL
PLOTTED
PLOTTER
PLOTZED
PLOTZES
PLUTONS
RLSTINE
SLATERS
SLATHER
SLATIER
SLATING
SLATKIN
SLATTED
SLITHER
SLITTED
SLITTER
SLOTCAR
SLOTTED
SLOTTER
ULSTERS

•L••T••

ALERTED
ALERTER
ALERTLY
ALERTTO
ALETTES
ALITTLE
ALLSTAR
ALLSTON
ALNITAK
ALSATIA
BLANTON
BLASTED
BLASTER
BLATTED
BLEATED
BLEATER
BLENTIN
BLINTZE
BLISTER
BLOATED
BLOTTED
BLOTTER
BLUETIT
BLUNTED
BLUNTER
BLUNTLY
BLURTED
BLURTER
BLUSTER
CLACTON
CLANTON
CLAPTON
CLATTER
CLAYTON
CLEATED
CLIFTON
CLINTON
CLOTTED
CLOUTED
CLOUTER
CLUSTER
CLUTTER
ELANTRA
ELASTIC
ELASTIN
ELECTED
ELECTEE
ELECTME
ELECTOR
ELECTRA
ELECTRO
ELEKTRA
ELUATES
FLATTAX
FLATTED
FLATTEN
FLATTER
FLATTOP
FLATTVS
FLAUTAS
FLEETED
FLEETER
FLEETLY
FLINTMI
FLIPTOP
FLIRTED
FLIRTER
FLITTED
FLITTER
FLOATBY
FLOATED
FLOATER
FLOATUP
FLOUTED
FLOUTER
FLUSTER
FLUTTER
GLINTED
GLISTEN
GLISTER
GLITTER
GLOATED
GLOATER
GLOTTAL
GLOTTIS
GLUTTED
GLUTTON
GLYPTIC
ILOSTIT
KLEPTOS
KLISTER
LLEYTON
OLDSTER
OLEATES
OLESTRA
OLMSTED
PLAITED
PLAITER
PLANTAR
PLANTED
PLANTER
PLASTER
PLASTIC
PLATTED
PLATTER
PLAUTUS
PLAYTEX
PLEATED
PLECTRA
PLINTHS
PLOTTED
PLOTTER
PLUSTAX
PLUSTWO
SLANTED
SLANTLY
SLANTUP
SLATTED
SLAYTON
SLEETED
SLEPTIN
SLEPTON
SLEUTHS
SLITTED
SLITTER
SLOTTED
SLOTTER

•L•••T•

ALBERTA
ALBERTI
ALBERTO
ALCESTE
ALDENTE
ALERTTO
ALIENTO
ALIGHTS
ALIGOTE
ALIVETO
ALLANTE
ALMAATA
ALSMITH
ALWORTH
BLIGHTS
BLIGHTY
BLINDTO
CLAMATO
CLARETS
CLARITY
CLAVATE
CLEANTE
CLIENTS
CLIMATE
CLIMATS
CLIMBTO
CLINGTO
CLORETS
CLOSETO
CLOSETS
CLUNGTO
ELAMITE
ELANETS
ELBERTA
ELEGITS
ELEVATE
ELICITS
ELLIOTT
ELMCITY
ELMISTI
ELMONTE
ELNORTE
ELOCUTE
ELUANTS
FLAUNTS
FLAUNTY
FLIEDTO
FLIESTO
FLIGHTS
FLIGHTY
FLOCKTO
FLORETS
FLOWNTO
FLYINTO
FLYNETS
GLOBATE
GLUEDTO
GLUESTO
ILLBITE
KLAMATH
OLDBATS
OLDCITY
PLACATE
PLAINTS
PLAKATS
PLANATE
PLANETS
PLANSTO
PLAYSTO
PLEADTO
PLICATE
PLIGHTS
PLOESTI
SLIGHTS
ULULATE

•L••••T

ALIMENT
ALLOFIT
ALLTHAT
ALNIYAT
ALQUIST
ALRIGHT
ALTOIST
BLANKET
BLATANT
BLERIOT
BLEWOUT
BLINKAT
BLOTOUT
BLOWOUT
BLOWSIT
BLUETIT
CLAMANT
CLAWSAT
CLAYPIT
CLEMENT
CLIPART
CLIPOUT
CLOSEST
ELEGANT
ELEGIST
ELEMENT
ELITEST
ELITIST
ELKHART
ELLIOTT
ELMIEST
FLAILAT
FLATHAT
FLATLET
FLATOUT
FLEAPIT
FLIESAT
FLINGAT
FLIPOUT
FLOORIT
FLORIST
FLOWNAT
FLOWOUT
FLUNGAT
FLUSHOT
FLUTIST
FLYCAST
FLYPAST
GLAREAT
GLUIEST
ILIKEIT
ILLDOIT
ILLEGIT
ILLICIT
ILOSTIT
ILOVEIT
OLDSALT
OLDWEST
PLACKET
PLANOUT
PLAUDIT
PLAYACT
PLAYLET
PLAYOUT
PLAYSAT
PLUMCOT
PLUMMET
SLEIGHT
SLIDOUT
SLIPOUT
SLOWEST
TLINGIT
ULULANT

••LT•••

ALLTHAT
ALLTHIS
ALLTIED
ALLTIME
ALLTOLD
BELTANE
BELTBAG
BELTERS
BELTING
BELTOUT
BELTRAN
BELTSAW
BELTSUP
BELTWAY
BOLTERS
BOLTING

BOLTSUP
CALTECH
CELTICS
COLTISH
CULTISH
CULTISM
CULTIST
CULTJAM
CULTURE
DALTONS
DALTREY
DELTAIC
DELTOID
DELTONA
DELTORO
DOLTISH
FALTERS
FELTBAD
FELTFOR
FELTHAT
FELTILL
FELTING
FELTOFF
FELTOUT
FELTPEN
FELTTIP
FILTERS
HALTERS
HALTING
HILTING
HILTONS
ILLTELL
JILTERS
JILTING
JOLTERS
JOLTIER
JOLTING
KILTIES
KILTING
LILTING
MALTASE
MALTBIE
MALTEDS
MALTESE
MALTHUS
MALTIER
MALTING
MALTOSE
MELTAGE
MELTERS
MELTING
MOLTERS
MOLTING
NFLTEAM
NHLTEAM
OILTANK
PALTERS
PALTROW
PELTATE
PELTERS
PELTING
PELTISH
POLTAVA
SALTANT
SALTBOX
SALTERS
SALTIER
SALTILY
SALTINE
SALTING
SALTISH
SALTPIT
SALTSEA
SELTZER
SILTIER
SILTING
SULTANA
SULTANS
TILTERS
TILTING
TILTSAT
TILTSUP
TILTTOP
TOLTECS
VELTMAN
VOLTAGE
VOLTAIC
VOLTORE
VULTURE
WALTERS
WALTHAM
WALTHER
WALTONS
WALTZED
WALTZER
WALTZES
WELTERS
WELTING
WILTING
YELTSIN

••L•T••

ABLATED
ABLATES
ALLSTAR
ALLSTON
APLITES
AULETTA
BALATAS
BALATON
BALLTWO
BELATED
BOLATIE
BOLOTIE
BOLSTER
CALOTTE
CELOTEX
COLETTE
CULOTTE
DALETHS
DELETED
DELETES
DILATED
DILATES
DILATOR
DILUTED
DILUTER
DILUTES
DILUTOR
EOLITHS
FELTTIP
FOLATES
GALATEA
GALATIA
GALETTE
GELATED
GELATES
GELATIN
GELATIS
GELATOS
GOLDTIP
GOLFTEE
HALITES
HALSTON
HELOTRY
HILLTOP
HOLSTER
ISLETED
KILOTON
LILETEE
MELITTA
MILITIA
MOLITOR
MOLOTOV
MULATTO
MULCTED
MULETAS
OBLATES
ONLYTOO
OOLITES
OOLITIC
PALATAL
PALATES
PALETTE
PALMTOP
PELOTAS
PELOTON
PILATES
PILATUS
PILOTED
POLITER
POLITIC
POLLTAX
PULLTAB
PULLTOY
RALSTON
RELATCH
RELATED
RELATER
RELATES
RELATOR
ROLLTOP
SALUTED
SALUTER
SALUTES
SILKTIE
SOLUTES
SPLITUP
SPLOTCH
TELSTAR
TILTTOP
TOLSTOI
TOLSTOY
UNLATCH
VALETED
VALOTTE
VOLUTED
VOLUTES
WALSTON

••L••T•

ALLANTE
APLENTY
ATLANTA
AULETTA
BALLETS
BALLOTS
BILLETS
BULLETS
BULLITT
CALCITE
CALISTA
CALLSTO
CALOTTE
CELESTA
CELESTE
CILENTO
CILIATE
COLETTE
COLGATE
COLLATE
COLLETS
COLORTV
CULLETS
CULOTTE
DELCITY
DELICTI
DELICTO
DELICTS
DELINTS
DELISTS
DELRUTH
EELPOTS
ELLIOTT
ENLISTS
FALCATE
FALLSTO
FALSITY
FILLETS
FOLIATE
FOLLETT
GALANTS
GALEATE
GALENTO
GALETTE
GALOOTS
GOLIATH
GULLETS
HELMETS
HOLDSTO
HOLISTS
ILLBITE
JOLLITY
KOLKATA
MALLETS
MELITTA
MILLETS
MILLETT
MOLESTS
MULATTO
MULLETS
MYLANTA
NULLITY
OBLASTS
PALETTE
PALLETS
PALMATE
PALPATE
PELLETS
PELTATE
PILEATE
POLENTA
POLLUTE
PULLETS
PULPITS
PULSATE
RALLYTO
RELENTS
RELICTS
RELISTS
RELUCTS
RILLETS
SELECTS
SELLSTO
SILENTA
SILENTB
SILENTC
SILENTD
SILENTE
SILENTF
SILENTG
SILENTH
SILENTI
SILENTJ
SILENTK
SILENTL
SILENTM
SILENTN
SILENTO
SILENTP
SILENTQ
SILENTR
SILENTS
SILENTT
SILENTU
SILENTV
SILENTW
SILENTX
SILENTY
SILENTZ
SOLLATI
SPLINTS
SULFATE
SULFITE
TALENTS
TALKSTO
TALLITH
TELESTO
TILLETS
TILSITS
UMLAUTS
UNLOATH
UNLOFTY
UNLUSTY
UPLIFTS
VALENTE
VALENTI
VALOTTE
VALUATE
VALVATE
VELOUTE
VELVETS
VELVETY
VOLANTE
VOLENTE
VULGATE
WALCOTT
WALKSTO
WALLETS
WALNUTS

••L•••T

AILMENT
ALLOFIT
ALLTHAT
ATLEAST
BALDEST
BALKSAT
BALLAST
BALLUET
BELFAST
BELFORT
BELMONT
BELTOUT
BOLDEST
BULBLET
BULLITT
CALLOUT
CALLSIT
CALMEST
CALUMET
CALVERT
CELLIST
COLBERT
COLDCUT
COLDEST
COLLECT
CULPRIT
CULTIST
CULVERT
DELBERT
DELIGHT
DELIMIT
DELMONT
DILBERT
DILUENT
DOLEOUT
DULLEST
EELIEST
EELPOUT
ELLIOTT
FALLOUT
FALSEST
FELLOUT
FELTHAT
FELTOUT
FILBERT
FILEOUT
FILLOUT
FILMSET
FOLDOUT
FOLKART
FOLLETT
FULGENT
FULLEST
FULLLOT
FULLOUT
GALLANT
GILBERT
GILLNET
HALFCUT
HALFWIT
HALIBUT
HELDOUT
HELLCAT
HELPOUT
HILBERT
HOLDOUT
HOLDSIT
HOLEOUT
HOLIEST
ILLDOIT
ILLEGIT
ILLICIT
JOLLIET
KILOBIT
KOLANUT
MALEANT
MALECAT
MALLRAT
MILDEST
MILLETT
MOLERAT
NOLIMIT
NULLSET
OILHEAT
OILIEST
OILSPOT
ONLIEST
OWLIEST
PALMIST
POLECAT
POLESAT
POLESIT
POLOIST
PULLOUT
RELIANT
RELIGHT
RELIMIT
ROLLOUT
RULEOUT
RULIEST
SALIENT
SALTANT
SALTPIT
SELLOUT
SELLSIT
SILENTT
SILKHAT
SOLDOUT
SOLICIT
SOLOACT
SOLOIST
SOLVEIT
SOLVENT
TALKOUT
TALKSAT
TALLEST
TELLSIT
TILTSAT
UGLIEST
UNLIGHT
UPLEAPT
UPLIGHT
VALIANT
WALCOTT
WALKOUT
WALMART
WELLCUT
WELLHIT
WELLLIT
WELLPUT
WELLSET
WILBERT
WILDCAT
WILDEST
WILIEST
YELLOUT
YELLSAT

•••LT••

ADULTLY
BALLTWO
BDALTON
BUILTIN
BUILTON
BUILTUP
CARLTON
COALTAR
COULTER
DEALTIN
DEALTTO
DEALTUP
DWELTON
EXALTED
EXALTER
EXULTED
FAULTED
FOULTIP
HEALTHY
HEELTAP
HILLTOP
MOULTED
NAILTIP
PHILTER
PHILTRE
POLLTAX
POULTRY
PSALTER
PULLTAB
PULLTOY
QUILTED
QUILTER
REALTER
REALTOR
RIALTOS
ROLLTOP
SHELTER
SHELTIE
SKELTER
SKELTON
SMELTED
SMELTER
STILTED
STILTON
SVELTER
SWELTER
SWELTRY
VAULTED
VAULTER
WEALTHS
WEALTHY

•••L•T•

ABILITY
ACOLYTE
ADULATE
AGILITY
AIGLETS
AMILATE
AMULETS
ANALYTE
ANILITY
ANKLETS
APELETS
APPLETS
APPLYTO
ARMLETS
ATELATE
ATHLETE
AUKLETS
AXOLOTL
BAALITE
BADLOTS
BALLETS
BALLOTS
BERLITZ
BIGLOTS
BILLETS
BIOLITE
BULLETS
BULLITT
CABLETS
CABLETV
CALLSTO
CAPLETS
CARLOTA
CARLOTS
CHALETS
CHELATE
COLLATE
COLLETS
CULLETS
CUTLETS
DEALSTO
DEALTTO
DECLOTS
DEFLATE
DEPLETE
DIGLOTS
DUALITY
DYELOTS
EAGLETS
EARLETS
EATLATE
EGALITE
EMULATE
ENDLATE
ENGLUTS
EPILATE
EVOLUTE
EYELETS
FAILSTO
FALLSTO
FILLETS
FOLLETT
GARLITS
GIBLETS
GIMLETS
GOBLETS
GULLETS
HAMLETS
HARLOTS
HAZLITT
HEWLETT
HOPLITE
HYALITE
IBILITY
INFLATE
ISOLATE
ISOLATO
ITSLATE
JOBLOTS
JOLLITY
LAPLATA
MALLETS
MERLOTS
MILLETS
MILLETT
MRSLATE
MULLETS
NEOLITH
NEOLYTE
NIBLETS
NULLITY
NUTLETS
OCELOTS
ODDLOTS
ODELETS
OMELETS
OUTLETS
OXALATE
PALLETS
PELLETS
PENLITE
PERLITE
PIGLETS
PIOLETS
POLLUTE
PRELATE
PROLATE
PULLETS
QUALITY
RALLYTO
RANLATE
REALITY
REFLATE
REPLATE
REPLETE
REPLOTS
REPLYTO
RESLATE
RIBLETS
RILLETS
RUNLATE
RUNLETS
SAILSTO
SAMLETS
SCHLITZ
SCULPTS
SELLSTO
SOLLATI
STYLETS
SUBLETS
SUBLOTS
TABLETS
TALLITH
TILLETS
TOILETS
TOOLATE
TWELFTH
ULULATE
UTILITY
VARLETS
VIOLATE
VIOLETS
WALLETS
WASLATE
WIGLETS
WOOLITE
YESLETS
YIELDTO
ZEALOTS

•••L••T

AFFLICT
AGILEST
AIRLIFT
AMPLEST
ANALYST
BAALIST
BAILOUT
BALLAST
BALLUET
BAWLOUT
BOILOUT
BULLITT
CALLOUT
CALLSIT
CELLIST
CHILCAT
CHILKAT
COALPIT
COLLECT
COOLANT
COOLCAT
COOLEST
COOLOUT
COOLSIT
COULDNT
CYCLIST
DEALOUT
DEFLECT
DIALECT
DIALOUT
DUALIST
DUELIST
DULLEST
DWELLAT
EVILEST
EXPLOIT
EYELIFT
FALLOUT
FARLEFT
FEELOUT
FELLOUT
FILLOUT
FOLLETT
FOULEST
FOULOUT
FULLEST
FULLLOT
FULLOUT
GALLANT
GETLOST
GILLNET
GOTLOST
HAYLOFT
HAZLITT
HELLCAT
HEWLETT
HITLIST
HOWLSAT
IDOLIST
IDYLIST
IMPLANT
INFLECT
INFLICT
JOLLIET
JUILLET
MAILLOT
MAILOUT
MALLRAT
MIDLIST
MILLETT
NAILSET
NAILSIT
NEGLECT
NEWLEFT
NOBLEST
NULLSET
OCULIST
ONALERT
OPULENT
ORALIST
OUTLAST
PAULIST
PEELOUT
PULLOUT
RAILSAT
REALEST
REALIST
REALLOT
REELECT
REELOUT
REFLECT
REFLOAT
REPLANT
ROLLOUT
SEALANT
SEALIFT
SELLOUT
SELLSIT
SHALLOT
SKILIFT
SKILLET
SMILEAT
SOYLENT
STALEST
STYLIST
TALLEST
TELLSIT
THELEFT
TITLIST
TOILSAT
TOOLKIT
TOOLSET
TSELIOT
ULULANT
UNALERT
UNBLENT
UNBLEST
UNCLEFT
UNCLIPT
UNPLAIT
VIOLENT
VIOLIST
WELLCUT
WELLHIT
WELLLIT
WELLPUT
WELLSET
WOOLFAT
WOOLHAT
WOULDNT
WOULDST
YELLOUT
YELLSAT
YOPLAIT

••••LT•

BASALTS
COBALTS
CRUELTY
DERALTE
DESALTS
DESILTS
EQUALTO
FACULTY
FORDLTD
FRAILTY
GEFILTE
INSULTS
KIDULTS
LOYALTO
LOYALTY
MINOLTA
MODELTS
NOVELTY
OCCULTS
PENALTY
PENULTS
REBOLTS
REMELTS
RESALTS
RESULTS
REVOLTS
ROYALTY
SCHULTZ
STEALTH
TUMULTS
UNBELTS
UNBOLTS
UNSALTY
UPTILTS

••••L•T

ABSOLUT
AFATLOT
ANNULET
ASTOLAT
ATEALOT
BACKLIT
BACKLOT
BANDLET
BARTLET
BIBELOT
BOMBLET
BONELET
BOOKLET
BOOMLET
BULBLET
CAMELOT
CAPELET
CAPULET
CASELOT
CAVILAT
CHAPLET
CHICLET
CIRCLET
CONELET
COPILOT
COUPLET
DOUBLET
DOVELET

DRIBLET
DROPLET
DWELLAT
EATALOT
EPAULET
EXCELAT
FEEDLOT
FIRELIT
FLAILAT
FLATLET
FOOTLET
FROGLET
FULLLOT
GANTLET
GRISLET
INKBLOT
ITSALOT
JUILLET
KINGLET
LAMPLIT
LEAFLET
LOCKLET
MAILLOT
MANTLET
MOONLET
MOONLIT
MRHULOT
MUDFLAT
NECKLET
NICOLET
NOTALOT
OUTBLOT
OUTPLOT
OVERLET
OVERLIT
PLAYLET
PREPLOT
REALLOT
REARLIT
RESPLIT
RINGLET
RIPPLET
RIVULET
ROOTLET
ROTBLAT
SANDLOT
SCARLET
SCHELDT
SEEDLET
SHALLOT
SINGLET
SKILLET
SNARLAT
SNIGLET
SPOTLIT
STARLET
STARLIT
SUBPLOT
TARTLET
TOWNLET
TREELET
TRIOLET
TRIPLET
UNSPLIT
VEINLET
WAVELET
WELLLIT
WINGLET
WINSLET
WOODLOT

•••••LT

ADDSALT
ASPHALT
ASSAULT
ATATILT
ATFAULT
BERTOLT
CONSULT
DEFAULT
DEHMELT
EYEBOLT
FANBELT
GESTALT
GUNBELT
INBUILT
INDWELT
LAPBELT
MYFAULT
NEWBOLT
NOFAULT
OLDSALT
PRESALT
REBUILT
REDEALT
RENAULT
RESMELT
RESPELT
ROUAULT
SEASALT
SUNBELT
TIMHOLT
UNADULT
UNBUILT
UNDEALT
UNSPELT
UNSPILT
VANPELT
ZUMWALT

LU•••••

LUBBERS
LUBBOCK
LUBEJOB
LUCANIA
LUCARNE
LUCENCY
LUCERNE
LUCETTA
LUCHINO
LUCIANA
LUCIANO
LUCIDAE
LUCIDLY
LUCIFER
LUCILLE
LUCINDA
LUCITES
LUCIUSI
LUCKIER
LUCKILY
LUCKING
LUCKMAN
LUCKNOW
LUCKOUT
LUCYLIU
LUDDISM
LUDDITE
LUFFING
LUGGAGE
LUGGERS
LUGGING
LUGNUTS
LUGSAIL
LUGSOUT
LUGWORM
LULLABY
LULLERS
LULLING
LUMBAGO
LUMBARS
LUMBERS
LUMIERE
LUMINAS
LUMPERS
LUMPIER
LUMPILY
LUMPING
LUMPISH
LUMPSIN
LUMPSIT
LUMPSUM
LUNATED
LUNATES
LUNATIC
LUNCHED
LUNCHER
LUNCHES
LUNESTA
LUNETTE
LUNGEAT
LUNGERS
LUNGING
LUNKERS
LUNULAE
LUNULAR
LUPINES
LURCHED
LURCHER
LURCHES
LUREDIN
LURESIN
LUREXES
LURIDLY
LURKERS
LURKING
LURLEEN
LUSHEST
LUSHIER
LUSTERS
LUSTFUL
LUSTIER
LUSTILY
LUSTING
LUSTRAL
LUSTRED
LUSTRES
LUSTRUM
LUTETIA
LUTHIER
LUTHULI
LUTISTS
LUXATED
LUXATES

L•U••••

LAUDERS
LAUDING
LAUGHAT
LAUGHED
LAUGHER
LAUGHIN
LAULAUS
LAUNDER
LAUNDRY
LAURELS
LAURENT
LAURITZ
LAUTREC
LEUCINE
LOUDENS
LOUDEST
LOUDISH
LOUELLA
LOUISII
LOUISIV
LOUISIX
LOUISVI
LOUISXI
LOUISXV
LOUNGED
LOUNGER
LOUNGES
LOURDES
LOUREED
LOURING
LOUSEUP
LOUSIER
LOUSILY
LOUSING
LOUTING
LOUTISH
LOUVERS
LOUVRED
LOUVRES

L••U•••

LACUNAE
LACUNAL
LACUNAR
LACUNAS
LACUREE
LAGUNAS
LAPUTAN
LARUSSA
LAYUPON
LECUONA
LEDUPTO
LEGUMES
LETUPON
LEXUSES
LEXUSGS
LEXUSGX
LEXUSIS
LEXUSLS
LEXUSLX
LEXUSRX
LEXUSSC
LIGURIA
LIQUATE
LIQUEFY
LIQUEUR
LIQUIDS
LIQUORS
LITURGY
LOBULES
LOCULUS
LOCUSTS
LOQUATS
LORUSES
LOTUSES
LUNULAE
LUNULAR

L•••U••

LABOURS
LABTUBE
LACEUPS
LACQUER
LADOUCE
LANGUID
LANGUOR
LAPFULS
LARRUPS
LASHUPS
LAWSUIT
LAYOUTS
LEADUPS
LEAGUED
LEAGUER
LEAGUES
LECTURE
LEGPULL
LEISURE
LEJEUNE
LELOUCH
LENGUAS
LETSUSE
LETTUCE
LIMBURG
LINEUPS
LINGUAE
LINGUAL
LINGULA
LINKUPS
LOCKUPS
LOGOUTS
LONGUES
LOOKUPS
LUCIUSI
LUGNUTS
LUTHULI
LYCEUMS

L••••U•

LACEDUP
LACESUP
LADYBUG
LAFLEUR
LAIDOUT
LALIQUE
LANDAUS
LANDSUP
LASCAUX
LASHOUT
LATINUS
LAULAUS
LAYSOUT
LAZARUS
LEADOUT
LEADSUP
LEAFOUT
LEANCUT
LEAPSUP
LEAPTUP
LEFTOUT
LEMIEUX
LENDOUT
LEPIDUS
LESCAUT
LESPAUL
LETSOUT
LICKSUP
LIFEFUL
LIFTSUP
LIGHTUP
LINECUT
LINEDUP
LINEOUT
LINESUP
LINKSUP
LIONCUB
LIPSOUT
LIQUEUR
LITHIUM
LIVENUP
LIVEOUT
LOADSUP
LOANOUT
LOCKNUT
LOCKOUT
LOCKSUP
LOCULUS
LOGANUT
LOGSOUT
LONGRUN
LOOKOUT
LOOKSUP
LOSEOUT
LOSTOUT
LOUSEUP
LOVEBUG
LUCKOUT
LUGSOUT
LUMPSUM
LUSTFUL
LUSTRUM
LYINGUP

L•••••U

LAMBEAU
LEHIGHU
LETTERU
LILINAU
LOOKYOU
LOVEYOU
LOYOLAU
LUCYLIU

•LU••••

ALUDELS
ALUMINA
ALUMNAE
ALUMNAL
ALUMNUS
ALUNSER
BLUBBER
BLUDGED
BLUDGER
BLUDGES
BLUEBOY
BLUEFIN
BLUEFLU
BLUEFOX
BLUEHEN
BLUEICE
BLUEING
BLUEISH
BLUEJAY
BLUELAW
BLUERED
BLUESKY
BLUESUN
BLUETIT
BLUFFED
BLUFFER
BLUFFLY
BLUINGS
BLUNDEN
BLUNDER
BLUNTED
BLUNTER
BLUNTLY
BLURBER
BLURRED
BLURTED
BLURTER
BLUSHED
BLUSHER
BLUSHES
BLUSHON
BLUSTER
CLUBBED
CLUBBER
CLUBCAR
CLUBMED
CLUBSUP
CLUCKED
CLUCKER
CLUEDIN
CLUEFUL
CLUEING
CLUESIN
CLUMPED
CLUNGTO
CLUNKED
CLUNKER
CLUSTER
CLUTCHY
CLUTTER
ELUANTS
ELUATES
ELUDERS
ELUDING
ELUSIVE
ELUSORY
ELUTING
ELUTION
ELUVIAL
ELUVIUM
FLUBBED
FLUBBER
FLUBDUB
FLUBUGS
FLUENCY
FLUFFED
FLUFFER
FLUFFUP
FLUIDAL
FLUIDIC
FLUIDLY
FLUKIER
FLUKILY
FLUMMOX
FLUNGAT
FLUNKED
FLUNKER
FLUSHED
FLUSHER
FLUSHES
FLUSHOT
FLUSTER
FLUTERS
FLUTIER
FLUTIES
FLUTING
FLUTIST
FLUTTER
FLUVIAL
FLUXING
FLUXION
GLUCOSE
GLUEDON
GLUEDTO
GLUEGUN
GLUESON
GLUESTO
GLUGGED
GLUIEST
GLUMMED
GLUMMER
GLURGES
GLUTEAL
GLUTENS
GLUTEUS
GLUTTED
GLUTTON
KLUDGED
KLUDGES
KLUGMAN
KLUTZES
PLUCKED
PLUGGED
PLUGGER
PLUGINS
PLUGOLA
PLUGSIN
PLUGSUP
PLUMAGE
PLUMBED
PLUMBER
PLUMBIC
PLUMBUM
PLUMCOT
PLUMIER
PLUMING
PLUMMER
PLUMMET
PLUMOSE
PLUMPED
PLUMPER
PLUMPIE
PLUMPLY
PLUMULE
PLUNDER
PLUNGED
PLUNGER
PLUNGES
PLUNKED
PLUNKER
PLURALS
PLUSHER
PLUSHES
PLUSHLY
PLUSONE
PLUSSES
PLUSTAX
PLUSTWO
PLUTONS
PLUVIAL
SLUDGES
SLUGGED
SLUGGER
SLUICED
SLUICES
SLUMBER
SLUMMED
SLUMMER
SLUMPED
SLUNKIN
SLUNKUP
SLURPED
SLURPEE
SLURPER
SLURRED
SLUSHED
SLUSHES
ULULANT
ULULATE

•L•U•••

ALBUMEN
ALBUMIN
ALBUNDY
ALDUBIN
ALLUDED
ALLUDES
ALLURED
ALLURER
ALLURES
ALLUVIA
ALQUIST
BLAUBOK
BLOUSED
BLOUSES
BLOUSON
CLAUDEL
CLAUDIA
CLAUDIO
CLAUSAL
CLAUSES
CLOUDED
CLOUDUP
CLOUTED
CLOUTER
ELFUDGE
ELMUNDO
FLAUNTS
FLAUNTY
FLAUTAS
FLEURON
FLOUNCE
FLOUNCY
FLOURED
FLOUTED
FLOUTER
ILLUDED
ILLUDES
ILLUMED
ILLUMES
ILLUSED
ILLUSES
OLDUVAI
PLAUDIT
PLAUTUS
PLEURAE
PLEURAL
PLOUGHS
SLEUTHS
SLOUCHY
SLOUGHS

•L••U••

ALARUMS
ALBSURE
ALLIUMS
BLACULA
BLOWUPS
CLAQUES
CLIBURN
CLIQUED
CLIQUES
CLIQUEY
CLOSURE
CLOTURE
ELOCUTE
FLEXURE
FLIPUPS
FLUBUGS
GLOBULE
ILLLUCK
OLEBULL
PLAGUED
PLAGUES
PLAQUES
PLENUMS
PLUMULE
SLIPUPS
SLOWUPS
ULALUME
ULANUDE

•L•••U•

ALARBUS
ALLOFUS
ALUMNUS
ALYSSUM
BLAZEUP
BLEWOUT
BLOCKUP
BLOTOUT
BLOTSUP
BLOWGUN
BLOWNUP
BLOWOUT
BLOWSUP
BLUESUN
CLAMOUR
CLAMSUP
CLEANUP
CLEARUP
CLIMBUP
CLIPOUT
CLOGSUP
CLOSEUP
CLOTSUP
CLOUDUP
CLUBSUP
CLUEFUL
ELAAIUN
ELIGIUS
ELUVIUM
ELYSIUM
FLAMEUP
FLANEUR
FLAREUP
FLATOUT
FLAVIUS
FLAVOUR
FLIESUP
FLIPOUT
FLOATUP
FLOWNUP
FLOWOUT
FLUBDUB
FLUFFUP
GLAMOUR
GLAMSUP
GLEEFUL
GLOBOUS
GLUEGUN
GLUTEUS
OLDBLUE
OLYMPUS
PLANOUT
PLAUTUS
PLAYFUL
PLAYOUT
PLAYSUP
PLOTFUL
PLOWSUP
PLUGSUP
PLUMBUM
SLACKUP
SLANTUP
SLEDFUL
SLICEUP
SLIDOUT
SLINKUP
SLIPOUT
SLIPSUP
SLOWSUP
SLUNKUP

•L••••U

ALFREDU
BLUEFLU
ILIESCU
PLATEAU

••LU•••

ALLUDED
ALLUDES
ALLURED
ALLURER
ALLURES
ALLUVIA
APLUSES
ATLUNCH
BELUGAS
BELUSHI
BOLUSES
BPLUSES
CALUMET
CALUMNY
COLUMBA
COLUMBO
COLUMNS
CPLUSES
DELUDED
DELUDER
DELUDES
DELUGED
DELUGES
DELUISE
DILUENT
DILUTED
DILUTER
DILUTES
DILUTOR
DOLUNCH
DPLUSES
GALUMPH
GELUSIL
ILLUDED
ILLUDES
ILLUMED
ILLUMES
ILLUSED
ILLUSES
MCLUHAN
MOLUCCA
MRLUCKY
PALUDAL
RELUCTS
RELUMED
RELUMES
SALUKIS
SALUTED
SALUTER
SALUTES
SOLUBLE
SOLUTES
SPLURGE
STLUCIA
STLUKES
SULUSEA
TALUSES
TOLUENE
UNLUCID
UNLUCKY
UNLUMPY
UNLURED
UNLUSTY
VALUATE
VALUERS
VALUING
VELURES
VOLUBLE
VOLUBLY
VOLUMED
VOLUMES
VOLUTED
VOLUTES

••L•U••

ALLIUMS
BALLUET
BULGURS
BULRUSH
CALCULI
CALLUPS
CELLULE
COLLUDE
COLOURS
CULTURE
DELOUSE
DELRUTH
DOLOURS
DRLAURA
FILLUPS
FOLDUPS
HELLUVA
HOLDUPS
ILLLUCK
KILAUEA
LELOUCH
MOLLUSC
MOLLUSK
OILCUPS
OILRUBS
PILEUPS
POLLUTE
PULLUPS
ROLLUPS
STLOUIS
TALCUMS
UMLAUTS
VALOURS
VALVULA
VALVULE
VBLOUSE
VELLUMS
VELOURS
VELOUTE
VULTURE
WALKUPS
WALKURE
WALNUTS

••L••U•

ALLOFUS
BALEFUL
BALFOUR
BALLSUP
BELARUS
BELGIUM
BELLYUP
BELTOUT
BELTSUP
BELVOUR
BILIOUS
BOLTSUP
BULBOUS
BULGHUR
BULKSUP
BULLRUN
CALCIUM
CALHOUN
CALLOUS
CALLOUT
CALLSUP
CELSIUS
COLDCUP
COLDCUT

COLONUS
DELARUE
DOLEFUL
DOLEOUT
DOLLSUP
ECLOGUE
EELPOUT
EULABUS
FALLDUE
FALLGUY
FALLOUT
FELLDUE
FELLOUT
FELTOUT
FILEOUT
FILLOUT
FILLSUP
FOLDOUT
FOLDSUP
FULCRUM
FULGHUM
FULLOUT
GALLIUM
GOLDBUG
HALFCUT
HALFDUG
HALIBUT
HELDOUT
HELPFUL
HELPOUT
HELPSUP
HOLDOUT
HOLDSUP
HOLEDUP
HOLEOUT
HOLESUP
HOLMIUM
KOLANUT
LALIQUE
MALAMUD
MALLEUS
MALRAUX
MALTHUS
MILERUN
MILHAUD
MILHOUS
MILIEUS
MILIEUX
MILKDUD
MILKRUN
MILLRUN
MULDAUR
OBLIQUE
OBLOQUY
OILDRUM
PALMFUL
PILATUS
PILEDUP
PILEOUS
PILESUP
PILLBUG
PULLOUT
PULLSUP
RILEDUP
RILESUP
ROLLOUT
ROLLSUP
RULEOUT
SELLOUT
SOLDOUT
SPLITUP
SULPHUR
TALKOUT
TALKSUP
TALLYUP
TILTSUP
VILNIUS
WALKOUT
WALLSUP
WELLCUT
WELLPUT
WELLRUN
WELLSUP
WILLFUL
WOLFCUB
YELLOUT

••L•••U

BELLEAU
LILINAU
ONLYYOU
SILENTU
TULANEU
WILLYOU

•••LU••

ANYLUCK
ASYLUMS
BADLUCK
BALLUET
CALLUPS
CELLULE
CHALUPA
COLLUDE
DEBLURS
DESLUMS
DIALUPS
ENGLUND
ENGLUTS
EVALUNA
EVOLUTE
EXCLUDE
FAILURE
FILLUPS
FOULUPS
GIBLUES
HELLUVA
ILLLUCK
INCLUDE
MCCLURE
MCCLURG
MOLLUSC
MOLLUSK
MUKLUKS
OCCLUDE
ONELUMP
PABLUMS
PEPLUMS
POLLUTE
POTLUCK
PRELUDE
PULLUPS
RECLUSE
REGLUED
REGLUES
REPLUMB
REPLUME
ROLLUPS
RVALUES
SCHLUBS
SCHLUMP
SECLUDE
SPELUNK
ULALUME
UNBLUED
UNFLUID
UNGLUED
UNGLUES
UNPLUGS
UNPLUMB
UNSLUNG
UVALUES
VELLUMS

•••L•U•

APPLAUD
BAILOUT
BALLSUP
BAWLOUT
BECLOUD
BELLYUP
BOILOUT
BOILSUP
BORLAUG
BOWLFUL
BUILDUP
BUILTUP
BULLRUN
CALLOUS
CALLOUT
CALLSUP
CDALBUM
CHALKUP
CHILLUM
COILSUP
COOLOUT
CURLSUP
DEALOUT
DEALSUP
DEALTUP
DIALOUT
DIALSUP
DOLLSUP
EMULOUS
FALLDUE
FALLGUY
FALLOUT
FEELOUT
FELLDUE
FELLOUT
FILLOUT
FILLSUP
FOULOUT
FOULSUP
FUELSUP
FULLOUT
GALLIUM
GIELGUD
HAULSUP
HEALSUP
JEALOUS
LAFLEUR
LAULAUS
MAILOUT
MALLEUS
MCCLOUD
MILLRUN
NAILGUN
NAILSUP
NUCLEUS
OCELLUS
OUTLOUD
PAILFUL
PARLOUR
PARLOUS
PEELOUT
PHILOUS
PILLBUG
POOLCUE
PUBLIUS
PULLOUT
PULLSUP
QUELQUE
RAILBUS
REELOUT
REELSUP
ROLLOUT
ROLLSUP
SCALEUP
SEALSUP
SELLOUT
SKILFUL
SOULFUL
STCLOUD
STILLUP
SWELLUP
TALLYUP
THULIUM
TOILFUL
TOOLSUP
UNCLOUD
VIALFUL
VONLAUE
WAILFUL
WALLSUP
WELLCUT
WELLPUT
WELLRUN
WELLSUP
WILLFUL
YELLOUT
ZEALOUS

•••L••U

BAYLORU
BELLEAU
CAILLOU
PURLIEU
ROULEAU
TABLEAU
WILLYOU

••••LU•

ABSOLUT
AMIBLUE
ANGELUS
ANNULUS
BENBLUE
BENELUX
BIGBLUE
BORGLUM
CARCLUB
CHILLUM
CUMULUS
DEDALUS
DEVALUE
EARPLUG
ESCALUS
FAMULUS
FANCLUB
FIATLUX
GYMCLUB
HAMULUS
HOODLUM
HOTGLUE
ICEBLUE
JEANLUC
KEYCLUB
LOCULUS
MODULUS
NBCBLUE
NONFLUX
NONPLUS
OCELLUS
OFVALUE
OLDBLUE
ONECLUB
ORMOLUS
OUTFLUX
PABULUM
PROCLUS
REGULUS
REVALUE
ROMULUS
SEABLUE
SEASLUG
SKYBLUE
SNARLUP
STILLUP
SURPLUS
SWELLUP
TOTALUP
TROILUS
UPVALUE
WARCLUB
ZEBULUN

••••L•U

ANGELOU
CAILLOU
DOUBLEU
EMMYLOU
LOYOLAU
LUCYLIU
MARYLOU

•••••LU

BIRDFLU
BLUEFLU
DEPAULU
DREXELU

L•V••••

LAVABOS
LAVACHE
LAVAGES
LAVAINE
LAVALSE
LAVELLI
LAVERAN
LAVERNE
LAVINIA
LAVORIS
LEVADES
LEVATOR
LEVELED
LEVELER
LEVELLY
LEVERED
LEVERET
LEVIERS
LEVILLI
LEVITES
LEVITIC
LEVYING
LIVABLE
LIVEAID
LIVEDIN
LIVEDON
LIVEFOR
LIVENED
LIVENER
LIVENUP
LIVEOAK
LIVEONE
LIVEOUT
LIVERED
LIVESAT
LIVESET
LIVESEY
LIVESIN
LIVESON
LIVIDLY
LIVINGS
LIVORNO
LOVABLE
LOVABLY
LOVAGES
LOVEBUG
LOVEDIT
LOVEDTO
LOVEINS
LOVEJOY
LOVERLY
LOVESET
LOVESIT
LOVESTO
LOVETAP
LOVEYOU

L••V•••

LANVINS
LATVIAN
LEAVEBE
LEAVEIN
LEAVEIT
LEAVENS
LEAVEON
LEAVING
LEOVIII
LOUVERS
LOUVRED
LOUVRES

L•••V••

LAYOVER
LEHAVRE
LENOVOS
LIEOVER
LITOVSK

L••••V•

LETHAVE
LETLIVE
LOUISVI
LOWDIVE

L•••••V

LETTERV
LOUISIV
LOUISXV

•LV••••

ALVAREZ
ALVEOLI

•L•V•••

ALEVELS
ALIVETO
CLAVATE
CLAVELL
CLAVIER
CLOVERS
CLOVERY
ELEVATE
ELEVENA
ELEVENB
ELEVENC
ELEVEND
ELEVENE
ELEVENS
ELEVONS
ELUVIAL
ELUVIUM
FLAVIUS
FLAVORS
FLAVORY
FLAVOUR
FLIVVER
FLUVIAL
GLAVINE
GLOVING
ILOVEIT
ILOVELA
OLAVIII
OLEVELS
OLIVIER
OLIVINE
PLOVDIV
PLOVERS
PLUVIAL
SLAVERS
SLAVERY
SLAVING
SLAVISH
SLIVERS
SLOVAKS
SLOVENE
SLOVENS

•L••V••

ALCOVES
ALDAVIS
ALLOVER
ALLUVIA
CLEAVED
CLEAVER
CLEAVES
CLEAVON
FLIVVER
FLYOVER
OLDUVAI
SLEEVED
SLEEVES

•L•••V•

ALGARVE
ELUSIVE
FLATTVS
ILLLIVE
OLDNAVY
PLOSIVE
ULANOVA

•L••••V

ALFEROV
PLOVDIV
ULYANOV

••LV•••

BELVOIR
BELVOUR
CALVARY
CALVERT
CALVING
CALVINO
CULVERT
DELVERS
DELVING
GALVANI
GALVANO
HALVAHS
HALVERS
HALVING
KELVINS
MALVINA
ROLVAAG
SALVAGE
SALVERS
SALVING
SALVOES
SALVORS
SELVAGE
SILVERS
SILVERY
SOLVEIT
SOLVENT
SOLVERS
SOLVING
VALVATE
VALVULA
VALVULE
VELVETS
VELVETY

••L•V••

ALLOVER
ALLUVIA
BELEVEN
BELOVED
BILEVEL
BOLIVAR
BOLIVIA
BULOVAS
DELIVER
ENLIVEN
HALAVAH
PALAVER
RELEVEL
RELEVER
RELEVES
RELIVED
RELIVES
SALIVAS
TELAVIV
UNLAVED
UNLEVEL
UNLIVED
UNLIVES
UNLOVED

••L••V•

BELIEVE
HELLUVA
ILLLIVE
MALDIVE
MOLDOVA
ONLEAVE
POLTAVA
RELIEVE
RILIEVO

••L•••V

COLORTV
MOLOTOV
SILENTV
TELAVIV

•••LV••

EVOLVED
EVOLVER
EVOLVES
SHELVED
SHELVER
SHELVES
TWELVEA
TWELVEB
TWELVEC
TWELVED
TWELVEE
TWELVES

•••L•V•

BADLOVE
BAKLAVA
BIGLOVE
DONLEVY
ENCLAVE
ENSLAVE
EXCLAVE
FORLOVE
HELLUVA
IAMLOVE
ILLLIVE
ITSLOVE
KARLOVY
KISLEVS
LETLIVE
MAGLEVS
NBALIVE
NEWLOVE
NONLIVE
NOTLIVE
ONELOVE
OUTLIVE
OUTLOVE
PAHLAVI
PAVLOVA
TAXLEVY
UNGLOVE

•••L••V

CABLETV
PHILIPV

••••LV•

ABSOLVE
BIVALVE
BTWELVE
DASILVA
DESYLVA
DEVOLVE
INVOLVE
ITWELVE
RESOLVE
REVOLVE

••••L•V

DOUBLEV
TUPOLEV

L•W••••

LAWANDA
LAWBOOK
LAWCASE
LAWFORD
LAWLESS
LAWLIKE
LAWSUIT
LAWYERS
LEWDEST
LEWHOAD
LOWBALL
LOWBEAM
LOWBIDS
LOWBLOW
LOWBORN
LOWBOYS
LOWBRED
LOWBROW
LOWCARB
LOWCARD
LOWCHEN
LOWCOST
LOWDIVE
LOWDOWN
LOWEEZY
LOWERED
LOWGEAR
LOWHAND
LOWHEEL
LOWLAND
LOWLIER
LOWLIFE
LOWLILY
LOWMASS
LOWNECK
LOWNESS
LOWPAID
LOWPAIR
LOWPOST
LOWRENT
LOWRISE
LOWRISK
LOWROAD
LOWSIDE
LOWTECH
LOWTIDE
LOWTOPS

L••W•••

LAPWARE
LAPWING
LEAWOOD
LEEWARD
LEEWAYS
LEGWEAR
LEGWORK
LIDWINA
LUGWORM

L•••W••

LACKWIT
LANGWAY
LAYAWAY
LEDAWAY
LIKEWOW
LONGWAY

L••••W•

LANETWO
LAYDOWN
LETDOWN
LIEDOWN
LINETWO
LOWDOWN

L•••••W

LAIDLOW
LASTROW
LAYSLOW
LETKNOW
LETTERW
LIESLOW
LIKENEW
LIKEWOW
LITHGOW
LOCKJAW
LONGBOW
LOWBLOW
LOWBROW
LUCKNOW

•LW••••

ALWORTH

•L•W•••

ALEWIFE
ALLWISE
BLEWOFF
BLEWOUT
BLOWDRY
BLOWERS
BLOWFLY
BLOWGUN
BLOWIER
BLOWING
BLOWNIN
BLOWNUP
BLOWOFF
BLOWOUT
BLOWPOP
BLOWSIN
BLOWSIT
BLOWSON
BLOWSUP
BLOWUPS
BLOWZED
CLAWERS
CLAWING
CLAWSAT
CLEWING
CLOWDER
CLOWNED
ELMWOOD
FLAWIER
FLAWING
FLOWAGE
FLOWERS
FLOWERY
FLOWING
FLOWNAT
FLOWNBY
FLOWNIN
FLOWNON
FLOWNTO
FLOWNUP
FLOWOUT
FLOWSIN
FLYWAYS
GLOWERS
GLOWING
ILLWILL
ILLWIND
OLDWAYS
OLDWEST
PLOWBOY
PLOWERS
PLOWING
PLOWMAN
PLOWMEN
PLOWSON
PLOWSUP
PLYWOOD
SLEWING
SLOWDAY
SLOWEST
SLOWING
SLOWISH
SLOWSUP
SLOWUPS

•L••W••

ALLEWIS
ALLOWAY
ALLOWED
ALLOWIN
ALLOWME
ELBOWED
ELBOWER
ELFOWLS
FLYAWAY

•L•••W•

ALLNEWS
OLDNEWS
OLDSAWS
OLDTOWN
PLUSTWO

•L••••W

BLUELAW
GLASGOW
GLASHOW
ILLKNOW

••LW•••

ALLWISE
BULWARK
EELWORM
FALWELL
ILLWILL
ILLWIND
MALWARE
OILWELL

••L•W••

ALLEWIS
ALLOWAY
ALLOWED
ALLOWIN
ALLOWME
ASLEWOF
BALDWIN
BELTWAY
COLDWAR
CSLEWIS
FOLKWAY
GOLDWYN
GULFWAR
HALFWAY
HALFWIT
HALFWON
HALLWAY
HOLYWAR
KELOWNA
ROLLWAY
TOLLWAY
UNLOWLY
WALKWAY
WELLWON

••L••W•

ALLNEWS
BALLTWO
BELLOWS
BILLOWS
BILLOWY
FALLOWS
FELLOWS
FOLLOWS
GALLOWS
HALLOWS
HOLLOWS
MALLOWS
MELLOWS
MILDEWS
MILDEWY
PILLOWS
PILLOWY
TALLOWS
TALLOWY
WALLOWS
WILLOWS

WILLOWY
YELLOWS
YELLOWY

••L•••W
BELTSAW
CALLNOW
HALFRAW
HOLYCOW
ILLKNOW
MILKCOW
MULGREW
PALTROW
PILCROW
SALCHOW
SILENTW
TILLNOW
YALELAW

•••LW••
HALLWAY
RAILWAY
ROLLWAY
TAILWAG
TOLLWAY
WELLWON

•••L•W•
BALLTWO
BELLOWS
BILLOWS
BILLOWY
CURLEWS
DECLAWS
FALLOWS
FELLOWS
FOLLOWS
GAGLAWS
GALLOWS
GUNLAWS
HALLOWS
HOLLOWS
INFLOWS
MALLOWS
MARLOWE
MELLOWS
OAKLAWN
OUTLAWS
PILLOWS
PILLOWY
REBLOWN
REFLOWN
REFLOWS
REGLOWS
REPLOWS
ROBLOWE
SHALLWE
TALLOWS
TALLOWY
TAXLAWS
UNBLOWN
UNFLOWN
UPFLOWS
WALLOWS
WILLOWS
WILLOWY
YELLOWS
YELLOWY

•••L••W
CALLNOW
SHALLOW
SWALLOW
TILLNOW

••••LW•
ROYALWE
SHALLWE

••••L•W
AIRFLOW
AIRGLOW
BIGELOW
BLUELAW
CASELAW
DANELAW
DEWCLAW
DOUBLEW
GAMELAW
GOBELOW
HIGHLOW
JANKLOW
JOEBLOW
JOHNLAW
JUDELAW
LAIDLOW
LAYSLOW
LIESLOW
LOWBLOW
MANILOW
MUDFLOW
OHMSLAW
OUTBLOW
OUTFLOW
OUTGLOW
POORLAW
RUNSLOW
SHALLOW
SUNGLOW
SWALLOW
TOOSLOW
TORTLAW
VERYLOW
WICKLOW
WINSLOW
WROCLAW
YALELAW

L•X••••
LAXNESS
LEXICAL
LEXICON
LEXISES
LEXMARK
LEXUSES
LEXUSGS
LEXUSGX
LEXUSIS
LEXUSLS
LEXUSLX
LEXUSRX
LEXUSSC
LUXATED
LUXATES

L••X•••
LEOXIII

L•••X••
LATEXES
LUREXES

L••••X•
LOUISXI
LOUISXV

L•••••X
LANDTAX
LASCAUX
LEMIEUX
LETTERX
LEXUSGX
LEXUSLX
LEXUSRX
LOCKBOX
LOUISIX

•L•X•••
ELIXIRS
FLAXIER
FLEXILE
FLEXING
FLEXION
FLEXNER
FLEXORS
FLEXURE
FLUXING
FLUXION
KLAXONS
PLEXORS

•L••••X
ALTOSAX
BLUEFOX
FLATTAX
FLUMMOX
KLEENEX
PLAYTEX
PLUSTAX

••L•X••
CALYXES
CULEXES
GALAXES
GALAXIE
HELIXES
PHLOXES
RELAXED
RELAXER
RELAXES
ROLEXES
TELEXED
TELEXES
UNLAXED
UNLAXES
VELOXES

••L••X•
POLEAXE

••L•••X
CALLBOX
CELOTEX
FILOFAX
HALIFAX
MALRAUX
MILIEUX
PILLBOX
POLLTAX
ROLODEX
SALTBOX
SILENTX
TELEFAX
TELEPIX

•••L••X
BAYLYNX
CALLBOX
COOLMAX
COOLPIX
MAILBOX
PHALANX
PILLBOX
POLLTAX
TOOLBOX

••••L•X
BENELUX
COMPLEX
DOUBLEX
FIATLUX
FUNPLEX
GRAVLAX
MUESLIX
NETFLIX
NONFLUX
OUTFLUX
OVERLAX
PERPLEX
SIMPLEX
TRIPLEX
UNIPLEX

•••••LX
LEXUSLX

LY•••••
LYCEUMS
LYDDITE
LYESOAP
LYINGBY
LYINGON
LYINGTO
LYINGUP
LYNDONB
LYNETTE
LYOCELL
LYONELL
LYRICAL
LYRICON
LYRISTS
LYSENKO

L•Y••••
LAYAWAY
LAYBACK
LAYBARE
LAYDOWN
LAYERED
LAYETTE
LAYINTO
LAYITON
LAYODDS
LAYOFFS
LAYOPEN
LAYOUTS
LAYOVER
LAYSFOR
LAYSLOW
LAYSOFF
LAYSOUT
LAYUPON
LOYALER
LOYALES
LOYALLY
LOYALTO
LOYALTY
LOYOLAU

L••Y•••
LADYBUG
LADYDAY
LADYISH
LADYKIN
LADYNAS
LANYARD
LAWYERS
LAZYISH
LEVYING
LIBYANS
LILYPAD
LLEYTON
LUCYLIU

L•••Y••
LCHAYIM
LEMOYNE
LIPSYNC
LOBBYER
LOOKYOU
LOVEYOU

L••••Y•
LACKEYS
LAZBOYS
LEAKEYS
LEEWAYS
LEFTEYE
LOWBOYS

L•••••Y
LADYDAY
LAMPREY
LANGLEY
LANGTRY
LANGWAY
LANKILY
LARCENY
LARGELY
LASTMAY
LASTORY
LATENCY
LATHERY
LAUNDRY
LAYAWAY
LAZENBY
LEAPDAY
LEDAWAY
LEERILY
LEGALLY
LEGIBLY
LENGTHY
LEONDAY
LETGOBY
LETSFLY
LETTERY
LEVELLY
LIBERTY
LIBRARY
LICITLY
LICKETY
LIGHTLY
LIGNIFY
LINDSAY
LINDSEY
LINEDRY
LIQUEFY
LISAGAY
LITHELY
LITTERY
LITURGY
LIVESEY
LIVIDLY
LOATHLY
LOCALLY
LOFTILY
LONGDAY
LONGWAY
LOONILY
LOOSELY
LOTTERY
LOUSILY
LOVABLY
LOVEJOY
LOVERLY
LOWEEZY
LOWLILY
LOYALLY
LOYALTY
LUCENCY
LUCIDLY
LUCKILY
LULLABY
LUMPILY
LURIDLY
LUSTILY
LYINGBY

•LY••••
ALYKHAN
ALYOSHA
ALYSSUM
BLYNKEN
ELYSEES
ELYSIAN
ELYSIUM
FLYABLE
FLYAWAY
FLYBALL
FLYBOYS
FLYCAST
FLYFISH
FLYGIRL
FLYHIGH
FLYINTO
FLYLEAF
FLYLESS
FLYNETS
FLYOPEN
FLYOVER
FLYPAST
FLYRODS
FLYSOLO
FLYTIER
FLYTRAP
FLYWAYS
GLYCINE
GLYCOLS
GLYNNIS
GLYPHIC
GLYPTIC
OLYMPIA
OLYMPIC
OLYMPUS
PLYWOOD
SLYLOOK
SLYNESS
ULYANOV
ULYSSES

•L•Y•••
ALAYING
ALCYONE
ALEYARD
ALIYAHS
ALLYING
ALLYSON
CLAYIER
CLAYING
CLAYISH
CLAYPIT
CLAYTON
CLOYING
ELIYALE
ELLYMAY
FLAYERS
FLAYING
ILLYRIA
LLEYTON
PLAYACT
PLAYBOY
PLAYDOH
PLAYERS
PLAYFUL
PLAYING
PLAYLET
PLAYOFF
PLAYOUT
PLAYPEN
PLAYSAT
PLAYSBY
PLAYSON
PLAYSTO
PLAYSUP
PLAYTEX
SLAYERS
SLAYING
SLAYTON

•L••Y••
ALLAYED
ALLAYER
ALLEYES
ALLOYED
ALNIYAT
GLORYBE
OLDLYME
PLATYPI

•L•••Y•
ALLONYM
ALTKEYS
FLYBOYS
FLYWAYS
GLADEYE
OLDBOYS
OLDDAYS
OLDWAYS

•L••••Y
ALABAMY
ALANJAY
ALBUNDY
ALCHEMY
ALDORAY
ALERTLY
ALIMONY
ALLENBY
ALLERGY
ALLOWAY
ALMONDY
ALMONRY
ALOOFLY
ALREADY
BLACKLY
BLAKELY
BLAKLEY
BLANDLY
BLANKLY
BLARNEY
BLEAKLY
BLIGHTY
BLINDLY
BLOTCHY
BLOWDRY
BLOWFLY
BLUEBOY
BLUEJAY
BLUESKY
BLUFFLY
BLUNTLY
CLARIFY
CLARITY
CLEANLY
CLEARLY
CLERISY
CLERKLY
CLIQUEY
CLOONEY
CLOSEBY
CLOSELY
CLOVERY
CLUTCHY
ELDERLY
ELLYMAY
ELMCITY
ELUSORY
FLAGDAY
FLAKILY
FLAUNTY
FLAVORY
FLEETLY
FLESHLY
FLIESBY
FLIGHTY
FLITSBY
FLOATBY
FLOUNCY
FLOWERY
FLOWNBY
FLUENCY
FLUIDLY
FLUKILY
FLYAWAY
GLAZILY
GLIDEBY
GLITCHY
GLORIFY
OLDCITY
OLDFOGY
OLDLADY
OLDNAVY
OLEANNY
PLAINLY
PLAYBOY
PLAYSBY
PLENARY
PLIABLY
PLIANCY
PLOWBOY
PLUMPLY
PLUSHLY
SLACKLY
SLANTLY
SLAVERY
SLEEKLY
SLICKLY
SLIDEBY
SLIMILY
SLIPSBY
SLOUCHY
SLOWDAY

••LY•••
ALLYING
ALLYSON
BELYING
CALYCES
CALYPSO
CALYXES
ELLYMAY
HALYARD
HOLYARK
HOLYCOW
HOLYDAY
HOLYJOE
HOLYMAN
HOLYMEN
HOLYOIL
HOLYOKE
HOLYONE
HOLYSEE
HOLYWAR
ILLYRIA
INLYING
JULYDAY
LILYPAD
ONLYTOO
ONLYYOU
POLYGON
POLYMER
POLYPED
POLYPOD
POLYSCI
RELYING
UNLYING
UNLYRIC

••L•Y••
AALIYAH
ALLAYED
ALLAYER
ALLEYES
ALLOYED
BELAYED
BELAYER
BELLYUP
COLLYER
DELAYED
DELAYER
HALCYON
HELLYES
INLAYER
MALAYAN
ONLYYOU
OWLEYED
PALMYRA
RALLYES
RALLYTO
RELAYED
RELAYER
SILLYME
SPLAYED
TALLYHO
TALLYUP
UNLOYAL
WELLYES
WILLYOU

••L••Y•
ALLONYM
BILLNYE
DELKEYS
DELRAYS
GALLEYS
GOLDWYN
HALLEYS
POLANYI
PULLEYS
VALLEYS
VOLLEYS
WALLEYE

••L•••Y
ALLENBY
ALLERGY
ALLOWAY
APLENTY
BALCONY
BALKILY
BALLBOY
BALMILY
BALONEY
BALSAMY
BELLAMY
BELLBOY
BELTWAY
BILLOWY
CALCIFY
CALGARY
CALLBOY
CALPOLY
CALUMNY
CALVARY
CILIARY
COLDDAY
COLICKY
DALTREY
DELANEY
DELCITY
DULCIFY
ELLYMAY
FALLACY
FALLGUY
FALSELY
FALSIFY
FALSITY
FELONRY
FILEDBY
FILESBY
FILMILY
FOLKWAY
FULLDAY
GALLERY
GELIDLY
HALFDAY
HALFSHY
HALFWAY
HALLWAY
HELLBOY
HELOTRY
HILLARY
HOLIDAY
HOLYDAY
JELLIFY
JOLLIFY
JOLLILY
JOLLITY
JULYDAY
KILLJOY
KILNDRY
LULLABY
MALARKY
MALMSEY
MILDEWY
MILKILY
MOLLIFY
MRLUCKY
MULCAHY
NULLIFY
NULLITY
OBLOQUY
PALEDRY
PALFREY
PALJOEY
PALMARY
PHLEGMY
PILLORY
PILLOWY
PULLTOY
PULPIFY
ROLLSBY
ROLLWAY
RULEDBY
SALTILY
SHLOCKY
SILENTY
SILKILY
SILVERY
SOLIDLY
SPLASHY
SPLEENY
SULKILY
TALLOWY
TOLLWAY
TOLSTOY
UNLEAKY
UNLOFTY
UNLOWLY
UNLUCKY
UNLUMPY
UNLUSTY
VALIDLY
VELVETY
VOLUBLY
WALKSBY
WALKWAY
WALLABY
WILLOWY
YELLOWY
ZELAZNY

•••LY••
ACOLYTE
ANALYSE
ANALYST
ANALYTE
ANALYZE
APPLYTO
BAYLYNX
BELLYUP
CARLYLE
COLLYER
EARLYON
HELLYES
NEOLYTE
OLDLYME
RALLYES
RALLYTO
REPLYTO
SILLYME
SUELYON
TALLYHO
TALLYUP
UNSLYER
UNSLYLY
WELLYES
WILLYOU

•••L•Y•
BARLEYS
BILLNYE
BYPLAYS
DEPLOYS
EMPLOYS
EVILEYE
GALLEYS
HALLEYS
HARLEYS
MEDLEYS
MISLAYS
MOTLEYS
OUTLAYS
PARLAYS
PARLEYS
PULLEYS
REPLAYS
SAMLOYD
SMILEYS
VALLEYS
VOLLEYS
WALLEYE
WAYLAYS

•••L••Y
ABILITY
ADULTLY
AGILELY
AGILITY
AMPLIFY
ANALOGY
ANILITY
APOLOGY
BAGLADY
BALLBOY
BELLAMY
BELLBOY
BILLOWY
BIOLOGY
CALLBOY
CUTLERY
DAYLILY
DONLEVY
DUALITY
ECOLOGY
ENOLOGY
EPILADY
FALLACY
FALLGUY
FOOLERY
FULLDAY
GALLERY
GEOLOGY
GIRLSHY
HALLWAY
HEALTHY
HELLBOY
HILLARY
IBILITY
JELLIFY
JOLLIFY
JOLLILY
JOLLITY
KARLOVY
KILLJOY
LOWLILY
LULLABY
MOLLIFY
MYOLOGY
NEOLOGY
NULLIFY
NULLITY
OKELLEY
OLDLADY
OMALLEY
OROLOGY
OTOLOGY
PAULPRY
PILLORY
PILLOWY
POULTRY
PRELACY
PTOLEMY
PULLTOY
QUALIFY
QUALITY
RAILWAY

REALITY
RIFLERY
ROLLSBY
ROLLWAY
SEALERY
SEALILY
SHELLEY
STALELY
SURLILY
SWELTRY
TALLOWY
TAXLEVY
TOLLWAY
TRILOGY
TROLLEY
UFOLOGY
UNFLAKY
UNSLYLY
UROLOGY
UTILITY
WALLABY
WEALTHY
WHALLEY
WILLOWY
WOOLERY
WOOLLEY
WOOLSEY
WORLDLY
YELLOWY
ZOOLOGY

••••LY•

CAROLYN
EVERLYS
JERILYN
JOCELYN
KAROLYI
MADALYN
MARILYN
ROSALYN
TAMBLYN

••••L•Y

AIRPLAY
AURALLY
AWFULLY
AXIALLY
BANALLY
BARCLAY
BARKLEY
BASALLY
BEASLEY
BENTLEY
BERKLEY
BLAKLEY
BRADLEY
BRAMLEY
BRAWLEY
BRIMLEY
BUCKLEY
BURNLEY
BYGOLLY
CAVALRY
CHARLEY
CIVILLY
CRAWLEY
CREELEY
CROWLEY
CRUELLY
CRUELTY
DEMOLAY
DEVILRY
DIDDLEY
DISPLAY
DOUBLEY
DRWELBY
DUCALLY
ENDPLAY
EQUALLY
FACULTY
FATALLY
FINALLY
FINDLAY
FINDLEY
FRAILLY
FRAILTY
FRAWLEY
FRIDLEY
FTRILEY
FUGALLY
GREELEY
GUNPLAY
GYRALLY
HARTLEY
HEMSLEY
HENSLEY
HITPLAY
HORSLEY
HUNTLEY
IDEALLY
JEWELRY
LANGLEY
LEGALLY
LEVELLY
LOCALLY
LOYALLY
LOYALTY
MCNALLY
MISALLY
MISPLAY
MORALLY
MTBALDY
NASALLY
NEUILLY
NIKOLAY
NONPLAY
NOVELTY
OKELLEY
OMALLEY
OREILLY
OUTPLAY
OVERLAY
PAISLEY
PARSLEY
PENALTY
PREALLY
PRESLEY
PUGSLEY
QUIGLEY
RAVELLY
REDCLAY
REGALLY
RENALLY
RETALLY
REVELRY
RIVALRY
ROYALLY
ROYALTY
RURALLY
SETPLAY
SHELLEY
SHIRLEY
SHRILLY
SQUALLY
STANLEY
TIDALLY
TONALLY
TOTALLY
TROLLEY
UNBULKY
UNFULLY
UNHILLY
UNJOLLY
UNMOLDY
UNSALTY
UNSILLY
UNSULKY
USUALLY
VENALLY
VITALLY
VOCALLY
VOWELLY
WEMBLEY
WHALLEY
WOODLEY
WOOLLEY
WORSLEY
WRIGLEY
ZONALLY

•••••LY

ACRIDLY
ACTORLY
ACUTELY
ADDEDLY
ADEPTLY
ADULTLY
AFFABLY
AGILELY
ALERTLY
ALOOFLY
AMIABLY
ANATOLY
ANGRILY
ANOMALY
APISHLY
AUDIBLY
AURALLY
AWFULLY
AXIALLY
BAGGILY
BALKILY
BALMILY
BANALLY
BASALLY
BAWDILY
BEADILY
BEASTLY
BEEFILY
BEVERLY
BIASPLY
BLACKLY
BLAKELY
BLANDLY
BLANKLY
BLEAKLY
BLINDLY
BLOWFLY
BLUFFLY
BLUNTLY
BOGUSLY
BONNILY
BOOZILY
BOSSILY
BRAMBLY
BRASHLY
BRAVELY
BRIEFLY
BRISKLY
BRISTLY
BROADLY
BRUTELY
BUMPILY
BUSHILY
BUXOMLY
BYGOLLY
CALPOLY
CAMPILY
CANNILY
CANTILY
CAPABLY
CATTILY
CEPHALY
CHARILY
CHEAPLY
CHIEFLY
CIVILLY
CLEANLY
CLEARLY
CLERKLY
CLOSELY
COCKILY
CORNILY
COURTLY
CRACKLY
CRASSLY
CRAZILY
CRINKLY
CRISPLY
CROSSLY
CRUDELY
CRUELLY
CRUMBLY
CRUMPLY
CUBICLY
CURABLY
CUSHILY
DAFFILY
DANDILY
DATEDLY
DAYLILY
DAZEDLY
DEERFLY
DENSELY
DINGILY
DIRTILY
DIZZILY
DOTTILY
DOWDILY
DRIZZLY
DUCALLY
DUMPILY
DUOPOLY
DURABLY
DUSKILY
DUSTILY
EAGERLY
EARTHLY
EFFABLY
ELDERLY
EMPTILY
EPPERLY
EQUABLY
EQUALLY
ERECTLY
EROSELY
EXACTLY
FADEDLY
FAINTLY
FALSELY
FANCILY
FATALLY
FATTILY
FETIDLY
FIERILY
FIFTHLY
FILMILY
FINALLY
FIREFLY
FIRSTLY
FISHILY
FIXEDLY
FLAKILY
FLEETLY
FLESHLY
FLUIDLY
FLUKILY
FOAMILY
FOGGILY
FRAILLY
FRANKLY
FRECKLY
FRESHLY
FRIARLY
FRIZZLY
FUGALLY
FUNKILY
FUNNILY
FUSSILY
FUSTILY
FUZZILY
GAUDILY
GAUNTLY
GAUZILY
GAWKILY
GELIDLY
GHASTLY
GHOSTLY
GIDDILY
GLAZILY
GOOFILY
GOONILY
GOUTILY
GRANDLY
GRAVELY
GREATLY
GREENLY
GRIMILY
GRISTLY
GRIZZLY
GROSSLY
GRUFFLY
GRUMBLY
GUSHILY
GUSTILY
GUTSILY
GYRALLY
HAMMILY
HANDILY
HAPPILY
HARDILY
HARSHLY
HASTILY
HEADILY
HEAVILY
HEFTILY
HOARILY
HORSILY
HUFFILY
HUMANLY
HUMIDLY
HUSKILY
IDEALLY
IGNOBLY
INANELY
INAPTLY
INEPTLY
INERTLY
INNERLY
IRATELY
JADEDLY
JAZZILY
JERKILY
JOINTLY
JOLLILY
JUICILY
JUMPILY
KINKILY
KNUCKLY
LANKILY
LARGELY
LEERILY
LEGALLY
LEGIBLY
LETSFLY
LEVELLY
LICITLY
LIGHTLY
LITHELY
LIVIDLY
LOATHLY
LOCALLY
LOFTILY
LOONILY
LOOSELY
LOUSILY
LOVABLY
LOVERLY
LOWLILY
LOYALLY
LUCIDLY
LUCKILY
LUMPILY
LURIDLY
LUSTILY
MCNALLY
MEATILY
MERRILY
MESSILY
MIDJULY
MILKILY
MISALLY
MISERLY
MISRELY
MISTILY
MIXEDLY
MOISTLY
MONTHLY
MOODILY
MOONILY
MORALLY
MOUSILY
MOVABLY
MUDDILY
MURKILY
MUSHILY
MUSSILY
MUSTILY
MUTABLY
MUTEDLY
MUZZILY
NAIVELY
NAKEDLY
NAMABLY
NASALLY
NASTILY
NATTILY
NEEDILY
NERVILY
NEUILLY
NIFTILY
NIGHTLY
NINTHLY
NIPPILY
NOISILY
NONOILY
NOTABLY
NOTEDLY
NUTTILY
OBESELY
OCTUPLY
ORDERLY
OREILLY
OVERFLY
OVERPLY
OVERTLY
PANOPLY
PAVIDLY
PEPPILY
PERKILY
PESKILY
PETTILY
PHONILY
PIOUSLY
PITHILY
PLAINLY
PLIABLY
PLUMPLY
PLUSHLY
PREALLY
PRICILY
PRICKLY
PRIMELY
PRIVILY
PRONELY
PROSILY
PROUDLY
PUDGILY
PUFFILY
PUNNILY
PUSHILY
QUAKILY
QUEENLY
QUEERLY
QUICKLY
QUIETLY
RABIDLY
RAINILY
RAPIDLY
RAVELLY
READILY
REAPPLY
REGALLY
REIMPLY
RENALLY
RETALLY
RIANTLY
RIGHTLY
RIGIDLY
RISIBLY
RISKILY
RITZILY
ROCKILY
ROOMILY
ROUGHLY
ROUNDLY
ROWDILY
ROYALLY
RUDDILY
RURALLY
RUSTILY
SAINTLY
SALTILY
SANDFLY
SAPPILY
SASSILY
SAUCILY
SAVVILY
SCANTLY
SCARILY
SCRAWLY
SEALILY
SEEDILY
SHADILY
SHAKILY
SHAPELY
SHARPLY
SHEERLY
SHINGLY
SHINILY
SHOOFLY
SHORTLY
SHOWILY
SHRILLY
SIGHTLY
SILKILY
SIXTHLY
SIZABLY
SLACKLY
SLANTLY
SLEEKLY
SLICKLY
SLIMILY
SMARTLY
SMOKILY
SNAKILY
SNIDELY
SNIFFLY
SNOWILY
SNUGGLY
SOAPILY
SOBERLY
SOGGILY
SOLIDLY
SOOTILY
SORRILY
SOUNDLY
SPACELY
SPANGLY
SPARELY
SPARKLY
SPICILY
SPIKILY
SPINDLY
SPRAWLY
SQUALLY
SQUATLY
STAGILY
STAIDLY
STALELY
STARKLY
STATELY
STEEPLY
STERNLY
STIFFLY
STOKELY
STONILY
STOUTLY
STUBBLY
SUAVELY
SULKILY
SUNNILY
SURLILY
SWEETLY
SWIFTLY
TACITLY
TACKILY
TARDILY
TARTILY
TASTILY
TATTILY
TAWNILY
TEARILY
TENABLY
TENSELY
TENTHLY
TEPIDLY
TERSELY
TESTFLY
TESTILY
THICKLY
THIRDLY
THISTLY
TIDALLY
TIGHTLY
TIMIDLY
TINNILY
TIPSILY
TIREDLY
TONALLY
TOTALLY
TOUGHLY
TREACLY
TREMBLY
TRITELY
TWINKLY
UNAPTLY
UNBURLY
UNCOYLY
UNFITLY
UNFULLY
UNGODLY
UNHILLY
UNJOLLY
UNLOWLY
UNMADLY
UNMANLY
UNSADLY
UNSCALY
UNSHYLY
UNSILLY
UNSLYLY
UNSURLY
UNTRULY
UPEARLY
USUALLY
UTTERLY
VAGUELY
VALIDLY
VAPIDLY
VENALLY
VEXEDLY
VISIBLY
VITALLY
VIVIDLY
VIXENLY
VOCABLY
VOCALLY
VOLUBLY
VOWELLY
WACKILY
WASPILY
WASSILY
WEARILY
WEEDILY
WEIRDLY
WHITELY
WINDILY
WISPILY
WITTILY
WOMANLY
WOOZILY
WORDILY
WORLDLY
WRIGGLY
WRINKLY
WRONGLY
ZESTILY
ZONALLY

L•Z••••

LAZARUS
LAZBOYS
LAZENBY
LAZIEST
LAZONGA
LAZYISH
LAZZERI
LIZARDS
LIZETTE
LIZZIES
LOZENGE

L••Z•••

LAZZERI
LIZZIES

L•••Z••

LEIPZIG

L••••Z•

LAICIZE
LEGANZA
LIONIZE
LORENZO
LOWEEZY

L•••••Z

LAISSEZ
LAURITZ
LEIBNIZ
LETTERZ
LORENTZ

•LZ••••

ULZANAS

•L•Z•••

BLAZERS
BLAZEUP
BLAZING
BLAZONS
GLAZERS
GLAZIER
GLAZILY
GLAZING
KLEZMER

•L••Z••

ALCAZAR
BLITZED
BLITZEN
BLITZER
BLITZES
BLOWZED
ELEAZAR
ELIEZER
GLITZED
GLITZES
KLUTZES
PLOTZED
PLOTZES
SLEAZES

•L•••Z•

BLINTZE
ELEGIZE

•L••••Z

ALBENIZ
ALLOPEZ
ALVAREZ
FLORENZ

••LZ•••

BELZONI
CALZONE
HOLZMAN

••L•Z••

PALAZZI
PALAZZO
SALAZAR
SELTZER
WALTZED
WALTZER
WALTZES
ZELAZNY

••L••Z•

PALAZZI
PALAZZO

••L•••Z

ALLOPEZ
SILENTZ

•••L•Z•

ANALYZE
DEGLAZE
DUALIZE
EMBLAZE
IDOLIZE
OBELIZE
REALIZE
REGLAZE
STYLIZE
UTILIZE

•••L••Z

BERLIOZ
BERLITZ
COBLENZ
KAYLENZ
KOBLENZ
SCHLITZ

••••L•Z

DOUBLEZ
SCHULTZ

MA•••••

MAANDPA
MAARTEN
MACABRE
MACACOS
MACADAM
MACAQUE
MACBETH
MACDUFF
MACEDON
MACGRAW
MACHAON
MACHETE
MACHINA
MACHINE
MACHONE
MACHREE
MACHSIX
MACHTWO
MACLEAN
MACLEOD
MACNEIL
MACONGA
MACOUNS
MACRAME
MACRONS
MACULAE
MACULAR
MACUSER
MADALYN
MADAMES
MADAMEX
MADCAPS
MADCHEN
MADDASH
MADDENS
MADDERS
MADDEST
MADDING
MADDISH
MADDOGS
MADEFIT
MADEFOR
MADEFUN
MADEHAY
MADEILL
MADEIRA
MADELON
MADEMAD
MADEOFF
MADEONE
MADEOUT
MADEPAR
MADERUN
MADEWAR
MADEWAY
MADIGAN
MADISON
MADLIBS
MADLOCK
MADNESS
MADONNA
MADRUSH
MADUROS
MAENADS
MAESTRO
MAEWEST
MAFIOSI
MAFIOSO
MAGALOG
MAGENTA
MAGGOTS
MAGICAL
MAGILLA
MAGINOT
MAGLEVS
MAGNANI
MAGNATE
MAGNETO
MAGNETS
MAGNIFY
MAGNUMS
MAGPIES
MAGUIRE
MAGYARS
MAHALIA
MAHARIS
MAHATMA
MAHDISM
MAHDIST
MAHFOUZ
MAHONEY
MAHOUTS
MAHZORS

MAIDENS
MAIDISH
MAIGRET
MAILBAG
MAILBIN
MAILBOX
MAILCAR
MAILERS
MAILING
MAILINS
MAILLOL
MAILLOT
MAILMAN
MAILMEN
MAILOUT
MAILSIN
MAIMERS
MAIMING
MAIMITI
MAINERS
MAINMAN
MAINMEN
MAINTOP
MAISONS
MAISOUI
MAITAIS
MAITRED
MAITRES
MAJESTE
MAJESTY
MAJEURE
MAJGENS
MAJORCA
MAJORED
MAJORIN
MAKABLE
MAKEDOS
MAKEFIT
MAKEFOR
MAKEFUN
MAKEHAY
MAKEILL
MAKEMAD
MAKEOFF
MAKEONE
MAKEOUT
MAKEPAR
MAKERUN
MAKESDO
MAKESGO
MAKESIT
MAKESUP
MAKEUPS
MAKEWAR
MAKEWAY
MAKINGS
MALABAR
MALACCA
MALACHI
MALAGAN
MALAGAS
MALAISE
MALAMUD
MALARIA
MALARKY
MALAYAN
MALCOLM
MALDIVE
MALEANT
MALEBEE
MALECAT
MALEDOG
MALEFIC
MALEHOG
MALEPIG
MALIANS
MALICES
MALIGNS
MALLARD
MALLETS
MALLEUS
MALLIKA
MALLOWS
MALLRAT
MALMSEY
MALODOR
MALPASO
MALRAUX
MALTASE
MALTBIE
MALTEDS
MALTESE
MALTHUS
MALTIER
MALTING
MALTOSE
MALVINA
MALWARE
MAMAMIA
MAMBOED
MAMMALS
MAMMOTH
MANACLE
MANAGED
MANAGER
MANAGES
MANAGUA
MANANAS
MANATEE
MANCINI
MANCUSO
MANDALA
MANDANS
MANDATE
MANDAYS
MANDELA
MANDOKI
MANDREL
MANEGES
MANETTE
MANFRED
MANGANO
MANGERS
MANGIER
MANGLED
MANGLER
MANGLES
MANGOES
MANHEIM
MANHOLE
MANHOOD
MANHOUR
MANHUNT
MANIACS
MANIKIN
MANILAS
MANILOW
MANIPLE
MANIPUR
MANKATO
MANKIND
MANLESS
MANLIER
MANLIKE
MANMADE
MANNERS
MANNIES
MANNING
MANNISH
MANOLIN
MANOWAR
MANRICO
MANROPE
MANSARD
MANSION
MANSIZE
MANSMAN
MANTECA
MANTELS
MANTLED
MANTLES
MANTLET
MANTRAP
MANTRAS
MANTRIC
MANTUAN
MANUALS
MANUMIT
MANURED
MANURES
MANXCAT
MANXMAN
MANXMEN
MANYEAR
MAOISTS
MAOSUIT
MAPPERS
MAPPING
MAPSOUT
MARACAS
MARANTZ
MARAUDS
MARBLED
MARBLER
MARBLES
MARCATO
MARCEAU
MARCELS
MARCHED
MARCHER
MARCHES
MARCHON
MARCONI
MARCUSE
MARDIAN
MARENGO
MARGATE
MARGAUX
MARGERY
MARGINS
MARGRET
MARHAUS
MARIANA
MARIANO
MARIDAS
MARIDOS
MARILLA
MARILYN
MARIMBA
MARINAS
MARINER
MARINES
MARITAL
MARKERS
MARKETS
MARKHAM
MARKIII
MARKING
MARKKAA
MARKOFF
MARKOUT
MARKOVA
MARKSUP
MARKUPS
MARKVII
MARLENE
MARLIER
MARLINS
MARLOWE
MARMARA
MARMION
MARMOTS
MARNIER
MAROONS
MARQUEE
MARQUES
MARQUEZ
MARQUIS
MARRERS
MARRIED
MARRIES
MARRING
MARRONS
MARROWS
MARRYAT
MARRYIN
MARRYME
MARSALA
MARSBAR
MARSDEN
MARSHAL
MARSHES
MARSRED
MARSTON
MARTENS
MARTIAL
MARTIAN
MARTINA
MARTINI
MARTINO
MARTINS
MARTINU
MARTINV
MARTIUS
MARTYRS
MARULLO
MARUSJA
MARVELL
MARVELS
MARVIER
MARXIAN
MARXISM
MARXIST
MARYANN
MARYKAY
MARYLOU
MARYURE
MASARYK
MASCARA
MASCOTS
MASHERS
MASHIES
MASHING
MASKERS
MASKING
MASONED
MASONIC
MASONRY
MASQUER
MASQUES
MASSAGE
MASSEUR
MASSIER
MASSIFS
MASSINE
MASSING
MASSIVE
MASTERP
MASTERS
MASTERY
MASTICS
MASTIFF
MASTING
MASTOID
MATADOR
MATALIN
MATCHED
MATCHER
MATCHES
MATCHUP
MATEWAN
MATHERS
MATHEWS
MATHIAS
MATHIEU
MATILDA
MATINAL
MATINEE
MATISSE
MATLESS
MATLOCK
MATRONS
MATTERS
MATTHAU
MATTHEW
MATTING
MATTOCK
MATURED
MATURER
MATURES
MATZOHS
MATZOTH
MAUDLIN
MAUGHAM
MAULDIN
MAULERS
MAULING
MAUMAUS
MAUNDER
MAUPRAT
MAUREEN
MAURIAC
MAURIAT
MAURICE
MAUROIS
MAUSERS
MAUVAIS
MAVISES
MAWKISH
MAXBAER
MAXBORN
MAXILLA
MAXIMAL
MAXIMAS
MAXIMUM
MAXIMUS
MAXIXES
MAXWELL
MAYALIN
MAYBESO
MAYDAYS
MAYFAIR
MAYHEMS
MAYINGS
MAYNARD
MAYORAL
MAYPOLE
MAYTAGS
MAYTIME
MAYWINE
MAZARIN
MAZEPPA
MAZIEST
MAZURKA
MAZZINI

M•A••••

MAANDPA
MAARTEN
MBABANE
MCADAMS
MCALLEN
MCARDLE
MEADOWS
MEADOWY
MEAGLES
MEALIER
MEALIES
MEANAGE
MEANDER
MEANEST
MEANIES
MEANING
MEANJOE
MEANSIT
MEANSTO
MEANTIT
MEANTTO
MEASLES
MEASURE
MEATAXE
MEATIER
MEATILY
MEATMAN
MEATMEN
MEATPIE
MIAHAMM
MIAMIAN
MIAMIFL
MIAOUED
MIAOWED
MIASARA
MIASMAL
MIASMAS
MIASMIC
MOABITE
MOANERS
MOANFUL
MOANING
MTADAMS
MTATHOS
MUAMMAR
MYALGIA
MYALGIC
MYANMAR

M••A•••

MACABRE
MACACOS
MACADAM
MACAQUE
MADALYN
MADAMES
MADAMEX
MAGALOG
MAHALIA
MAHARIS
MAHATMA
MAKABLE
MALABAR
MALACCA
MALACHI
MALAGAN
MALAGAS
MALAISE
MALAMUD
MALARIA
MALARKY
MALAYAN
MAMAMIA
MANACLE
MANAGED
MANAGER
MANAGES
MANAGUA
MANANAS
MANATEE
MARACAS
MARANTZ
MARAUDS
MASARYK
MATADOR
MATALIN
MAYALIN
MAZARIN
MCCALLS
MCCAREY
MCGAVIN
MCHALES
MCMAHON
MCNALLY
MCPAPER
MCRANEY
MEDAKAS
MEDALED
MEDAWAR
MEGABIT
MEGAERA
MEGAERG
MEGAHIT
MEGALON
MEGANES
MEGATON
MELAMED
MELANGE
MELANIA
MELANIC
MELANIE
MELANIN
MENACED
MENACER
MENACES
MENAGES
MESAMIS
METALED
METATES
MICAELA
MIDASES
MIKADOS
MIKASAS
MILAGRO
MINABLE
MINARET
MIRABEL
MIRACLE
MIRADAS
MIRADOR
MIRAGES
MIRAMAR
MIRAMAX
MIRANDA
MISACTS
MISADDS
MISAIMS
MISALLY
MISAVER
MIXABLE
MOGADOR
MOGAMBO
MOHAIRS
MOHAVES
MOHAWKS
MOJAVES
MONACAN
MONADAL
MONADIC
MONARCH
MORAINE
MORALES
MORALLY
MORANIS
MORANTE
MORAVIA
MOSAICS
MOVABLE
MOVABLY
MOVADOS
MRDARCY
MRHANEY
MRMACHO
MRMAGOO
MRMARCH
MRNANNY
MRPADRE
MTBALDY
MTMARCY
MUBARAK
MULATTO
MURALED
MURANOS
MUSANTE
MUTABLE
MUTABLY
MUTAGEN
MUTANTS
MUTATED
MUTATES
MYFAULT
MYLANTA
MYMAMMY

M•••A••

MACHAON
MACRAME
MADCAPS
MADDASH
MAENADS
MAGNANI
MAGNATE
MAGYARS
MAITAIS
MALEANT
MALIANS
MALLARD
MALPASO
MALRAUX
MALTASE
MALWARE
MAMMALS
MANDALA
MANDANS
MANDATE
MANDAYS
MANGANO
MANIACS
MANKATO
MANMADE
MANSARD
MANUALS
MARCATO
MARGATE
MARGAUX
MARHAUS
MARIANA
MARIANO
MARMARA
MARSALA
MARYANN
MASCARA
MASSAGE
MAUMAUS
MAUVAIS
MAXBAER
MAYDAYS
MAYFAIR
MAYNARD
MAYTAGS
MBABANE
MCADAMS
MCCRARY
MCSHANE
MEANAGE
MEATAXE
MECCANS
MEDIANS
MEDIANT
MEDIATE
MELTAGE
MENIALS
MENSANS
MERCADO
MERMAID
MESCALS
MESHACH
MESSAGE
MESSALA
METCALF
METFANS
METHANE
MIAHAMM
MIASARA
MICHAEL
MICHAUX
MICMACS
MIDCAPS
MIDDAYS
MIDEAST
MIDLAND
MIDWAYS
MIGRANT
MIGRATE
MIKHAIL
MILEAGE
MILHAUD
MILLAGE
MILLAIS
MILLAND
MILLARD
MINOANS
MINTAGE
MINYANS
MISCALL
MISCAST
MISDATE
MISGAVE
MISHAPS
MISLAID
MISLAYS
MISMARK
MISMATE
MISNAME
MISPAGE
MISRATE
MISSAID
MISSALS
MISSAYS
MISTAKE
MIZRAHI
MOMBASA
MONDALE
MONDAVI
MONDAYS
MONTAGE
MONTAGU
MONTALE
MONTANA
MONTAND
MONTANO
MONTAUK
MOORAGE
MORDANT
MORGANA
MORGANS
MORTALS
MORTARS
MOSCATO
MOULAGE
MRSBASS
MRSLATE
MRSPAUL
MTADAMS
MTBLANC
MTEVANS
MUDBATH
MUDCATS
MUDLARK
MUDPACK
MUDWASP
MULCAHY
MULDAUR
MULHARE
MULLAHS
MUNDANE
MUSCATS
MUSTAFA
MUSTANG
MUSTARD
MUTUALS
MYGIANT
MYRIADS
MYSPACE
MYSTARS

M••••A•

MACADAM
MACGRAW
MACLEAN
MACULAE
MACULAR
MADEHAY
MADEMAD
MADEPAR
MADEWAR
MADEWAY
MADIGAN
MAGICAL
MAILBAG
MAILCAR
MAILMAN
MAINMAN
MAKEHAY
MAKEMAD
MAKEPAR
MAKEWAR
MAKEWAY
MALABAR
MALAGAN
MALAGAS
MALAYAN
MALECAT
MALLRAT
MANANAS
MANILAS
MANOWAR
MANSMAN
MANTRAP
MANTRAS
MANTUAN
MANXCAT
MANXMAN
MANYEAR
MARACAS
MARCEAU
MARDIAN
MARIDAS
MARINAS
MARITAL
MARKHAM
MARKKAA
MARRYAT
MARSBAR
MARSHAL
MARTIAL
MARTIAN
MARXIAN
MARYKAY
MATEWAN
MATHIAS
MATINAL
MATTHAU
MAUGHAM
MAUPRAT
MAURIAC
MAURIAT
MAXIMAL
MAXIMAS
MAYORAL
MCLUHAN
MEATMAN
MEDAKAS
MEDAWAR
MEDEVAC
MEDICAL
MEDIGAP
MEDIVAC
MEDUSAE
MEDUSAN
MEDUSAS
MEERKAT
MEGRYAN
MEMOPAD
MENORAH
MENUBAR
MERCIAN
MERRIAM
MESSIAH
METSFAN
MEXICAN
MEZUZAH
MEZUZAS
MIAMIAN
MIASMAL
MIASMAS
MIDYEAR
MIKASAS
MILKBAR
MILKCAN
MILKMAN
MILLDAM
MIMOSAS
MINERAL
MINIBAR
MINICAB
MINICAM
MINICAR
MINILAB
MINIMAL
MINIMAX
MINIVAC
MINIVAN
MIRADAS
MIRAMAR
MIRAMAX
MISDEAL
MISDIAL
MISDRAW
MISHEAR
MISHNAH
MISLEAD
MISPLAN
MISPLAY
MISREAD
MISSEAT
MISTRAL
MITHRAS
MITZVAH
MIZUNAS
MODELAS
MODULAR
MOHEGAN
MOHICAN
MOISSAN
MOLERAT
MOLOKAI
MONACAN
MONADAL
MONDIAL
MOPHEAD
MOREPAY
MOWBRAY
MRCLEAN
MRISCAN
MRNOVAK
MTLOGAN
MTSINAI
MUAMMAR
MUBARAK
MUDFLAP
MUDFLAT
MULETAS
MUSICAL
MUSKRAT
MYANMAR
MYCENAE
MYOPIAS
MYTREAT

M•••••A

MAANDPA
MACHINA
MACONGA
MADEIRA
MADONNA
MAGENTA
MAGILLA
MAHALIA
MAHATMA
MAJORCA
MALACCA
MALARIA
MALLIKA
MALVINA
MAMAMIA
MANAGUA

MANDALA
MANDELA
MANTECA
MARIANA
MARILLA
MARIMBA
MARKKAA
MARKOVA
MARMARA
MARSALA
MARTINA
MARUSJA
MASCARA
MATILDA
MAXILLA
MAZEPPA
MAZURKA
MCKENNA
MEDULLA
MEGAERA
MEGILLA
MELANIA
MELINDA
MELISMA
MELISSA
MELITTA
MELODIA
MENORCA
MESHUGA
MESSALA
MESSINA
MIASARA
MICAELA
MILITIA
MINEOLA
MINERVA
MINOLTA
MINORCA
MINTTEA
MINUTIA
MIRANDA
MISHIMA
MISSUSA
MOLDOVA
MOLUCCA
MOMBASA
MOMENTA
MONTANA
MONTOYA
MORAVIA
MORELLA
MORGANA
MOZETTA
MOZILLA
MTKENYA
MUSCIDA
MUSETTA
MUSTAFA
MYALGIA
MYLANTA

•MA••••

AMADEUS
AMALGAM
AMANITA
AMANTIS
AMAPOLA
AMARONE
AMASSED
AMASSER
AMASSES
AMATEUR
AMATIVE
AMATOLS
AMATORY
AMAZING
AMAZONS
EMAILED
EMAILER
EMANANT
EMANATE
EMANUEL
IMADEIT
IMAGERS
IMAGERY
IMAGINE
IMAGING
IMAGISM
IMAGIST
IMAGOES
IMAHOGG
IMAMATE
IMAMESS
IMARETS
OMAHANE
OMAHANS
OMALLEY
SMACKED
SMACKER
SMACKOF
SMACKUP
SMALLAD
SMALLER
SMALLOJ
SMARTED
SMARTEN
SMARTER
SMARTLY
SMASHED
SMASHER
SMASHES
SMASHUP
SMATTER

•M•A•••

AMHARIC
AMIABLE
AMIABLY
AMRADIO
EMBALMS
EMBANKS
EMBARGO
EMBARKS
EMBASSY
EMBAYED
EMPALED
EMPALES
EMPANEL
EMPATHS
EMPATHY
FMBANDS
FMRADIO
IMEANIT
IMHAPPY
IMPACTS
IMPAIRS
IMPALAS
IMPALED
IMPALER
IMPALES
IMPANEL
IMPARTS
IMPASSE
IMPASTO
IMPAVID
SMEAGOL
SMEARED
SMEARER
SMEARON
UMLAUTS
XMRADIO

•M••A••

AMERADA
AMIDALA
AMILATE
AMTRACK
AMTRACS
AMYLASE
EMANANT
EMANATE
EMBLAZE
EMBRACE
EMERALD
EMIRATE
EMPLACE
EMPLANE
EMQUADS
EMULATE
IMAMATE
IMITATE
IMPEACH
IMPLANT
IMREADY
OMAHANE
OMAHANS
OMPHALO
SMETANA
UMBRAGE

•M•••A•

AMALGAM
AMESLAN
AMICHAI
AMISTAD
AMOEBAE
AMOEBAS
AMRITAS
AMSCRAY
FMURRAY
IMGREAT
IMMORAL
IMPALAS
IMPLEAD
OMNIMAX
SMALLAD
SMILEAT
SMILLAS
UMBRIAN

•M••••A

AMANITA
AMAPOLA
AMERADA
AMERICA
AMERIKA
AMIDALA
AMMONIA
AMNESIA
AMPHORA
AMREETA
EMERITA
EMMUSKA
EMPORIA
IMPREZA
SMETANA

••MA•••

ALMAATA
ALMADEN
ALMANAC
ARMADAS
ASMARAN
CAMACHO
CAMAROS
CIMABUE
COMAKER
DAMAGED
DAMAGES
DAMASKS
DAMASUS
DEMAGOG
DEMANDS
DEMARCO
DEMARET
DEMARKS
DEMASTS
DIMAGES
DOMAINE
DOMAINS
DRMARIO
ENMASSE
EXMATES
EXMAYOR
FEMALES
GEMAYEL
HAMACHI
HEMATIC
HEMATIN
HIMALIA
HOMAGER
HOMAGES
HUMANLY
HUMANUM
INMARCH
INMATES
ITMAYBE
JAMAICA
JOMARCH
JUMADAS
JUMANJI
KOMATSU
LAMAISM
LAMAIST
LAMARCK
LIMACON
MAMAMIA
MCMAHON
MRMACHO
MRMAGOO
MRMARCH
MTMARCY
MYMAMMY
NAMABLE
NAMABLY
NOMADIC
OHMAGES
ORMANDY
OSMATIC
POMADED
POMADES
RAMADAN
RAMADAS
REMAILS
REMAINS
REMAKES
REMANDS
REMARKS
REMARRY
REMATCH
REMATED
REMATES
ROMAINE
ROMAINS
ROMAJIS
ROMANCE
ROMANIA
ROMANIC
ROMANIS
ROMANOS
ROMANOV
ROMANSH
ROMANUS
RUMAKIS
RUMANIA
SAMARAS
SAMARIA
SEMANAS
SOMALIA
SOMALIS
SOMATIC
STMARKS
STMARYS
SUMATRA
TAMABLE
TAMALES
TAMARAC
UNMACHO
UNMADLY
UNMAKER
UNMAKES
UNMANED
UNMANLY
UNMASKS
UNMASTS
UNMATED
UNMATES
WOMANLY
YAMAHAS
ZIMARRA

••M•A••

ALMAATA
ARMBAND
ARMYANT
ATMCARD
BEMOANS
BOMBARD
BOMBAST
BUMRAPS
CAMPARI
CEMBALO
COMBATS
COMCAST
COMMAND
COMPACT
COMPANY
COMPAQS
COMPARE
COMPART
COMPASS
COMRADE
COMSATS
CYMBALS
DEMEANS
FTMEADE
GAMBADO
GEMMATE
GIMBALS
GUMBALL
GYMBAGS
GYMBALL
GYMNAST
GYMRATS
HUMBARD
HYMNALS
HYMNARY
JAMBAND
JAMCAMS
JAMPACK
JIMDALE
JIMJAMS
JIMKAAT
KAMPALA
KIMBALL
LAMBADA
LEMMATA
LIMEADE
LOMBARD
LUMBAGO
LUMBARS
MAMMALS
MOMBASA
NUMBATS
OOMPAHS
POMMARD
POMPANO
RAMFANS
RAMPAGE
RAMPANT
RAMPART
REMNANT
RIMBAUD
RUMBAED
RUMCAKE
RUMMAGE
SAMBAED
SAMBASS
SAMOANS
SAMPANS
SIMIANS
SUMMAND
SUMMARY
SUMMATE
TAMBALA
TAMIAMI
TAMMANY
TAMPAFL
TAMTAMS
TIMBALE
TIMBALS
TIMPANI
TOMCATS
TYMPANA
TYMPANI
UNMEANT
WOMBATS
ZUMWALT

••M••A•

ADMIRAL
AIMEDAT
ALMANAC
ALMSMAN
ARMADAS
ARMLOAD
ASMARAN
BIMETAL
BIMODAL
BUMDEAL
CAMERAE
CAMERAL
CAMERAS
COMESAS
COMESAT
COMICAL
COMORAN
CUMBIAS
CUMSHAW
DEMOLAY
DOMECAR
DOMICAL
FEMORAL
FUMEDAT
FUMESAT
GAMBIAN
GAMEBAG
GAMELAN
GAMELAW
GAMETAL
HOMELAB
HUMERAL
HUMORAL
IMMORAL
JAMBEAU
JIMBEAM
JIMDIAL
JIMKAAT
JUMADAS
JUMPSAT
KAMERAD
KUMQUAT
LAMBDAS
LAMBEAU
LAMINAE
LAMINAL
LAMINAR
LAMINAS
LIMINAL
LUMINAS
MEMOPAD
MIMOSAS
NAMEDAY
NAMETAG
NOMINAL
NUMERAL
NYMPHAL
OHMSLAW
RAMADAN
RAMADAS
RAMSFAN
REMORAS
REMOVAL
ROMULAN
SAMARAS
SAMEDAY
SAMOSAS
SAMOVAR
SAMPRAS
SAMURAI
SEMANAS
SEMINAL
SEMINAR
SEMIRAW
SIMILAC
SIMILAR
SOMEDAY
SOMESAY
SOMEWAY
TAMARAC
TEMPEAZ
TEMPLAR
TIMELAG
TIMEWAS
TOMJOAD
VIMINAL
YAMAHAS
ZAMBIAN

••M•••A

ALMAATA
ALMERIA
AMMONIA
ARMENIA
BAMBINA
CAMBRIA
CAMILLA
COMEDIA
CUMBRIA
EMMUSKA
ERMINIA
FAMILIA
HIMALIA
JAMAICA
KAMPALA
LAMBADA
LAMOTTA
LEMMATA
LEMPIRA
MAMAMIA
MOMBASA
MOMENTA
NAMIBIA
POMPEIA
ROMANIA
RUMANIA
SAMARIA
SAMBORA
SAMBUCA
SOMALIA
SUMATRA
TAMBALA
TEMPERA
TEMPURA
TOMGOLA
TYMPANA
VAMPIRA
ZIMARRA

•••MA••

AAAMAPS
ADAMANT
AGEMATE
AIRMADA
AIRMAIL
AIRMASS
ALLMALE
ANIMACY
ANIMALS
ANIMATE
ANIMATO
ANOMALY
ARAMAIC
ARAMARK
ATAMANS
BALMAIN
BARMAID
BASMATI
BEDMATE
BIGMACS
BIGMAMA
BIOMASS
BIRMANS
BITMAPS
BROMATE
BURMANS
BUSMANS
CAIMANS
CAYMANS
CHUMASH
CLAMANT
CLAMATO
CLIMATE
CLIMATS
COMMAND
CORMACK
CREMATE
DAYMARE
DENMARK
DERMATO
DISMALS
DISMAST
DISMAYS
DOGMATA
DOLMANS
DORMANT
DRAMADY
EARMARK
EDEMATA
ELLMANN
EYEMASK
FANMAIL
FARMAID
FERMATA
FERMATE
FERMATS
FORMALS
FORMATS
FROMAGE
FULMARS
GASMAIN
GASMASK
GEMMATE
GERMAIN
GERMANE
GERMANS
GERMANY
GODMAMA
GRIMACE
HAZMATS
HERMANA
HERMANN
HERMANO
HERMANS
HEYMANS
HOFMANN
HOTMAIL
HOWMANY
ILLMADE
IMAMATE
INKMARK
ISHMAEL
KIRMANS
KLAMATH
LEHMANN
LEMMATA
LEXMARK
LIPMANN
LOWMASS
MAMMALS
MANMADE
MARMARA
MAUMAUS
MERMAID
MICMACS
MISMARK
MISMATE
NEUMANN
NEWMADE
NEWMANS
NEWMATH
NORMALS
NORMAND
NORMANS
NOTMANY
OLDMAID
OSTMARK
OUTMANS
OUTMATE
PALMARY
PALMATE
PLUMAGE
POMMARD
PREMADE
PREMAKE
PREMATE
PRIMACY
PRIMARY
PRIMATE
RAGMANS
REAMASS
REIMAGE
RIEMANN
RUMMAGE
SAYMASS
SEAMAPS
SELMAAL
SHAMANS
SKIMASK
SKYMAPS
STOMACH
STOMATA
SUMMAND
SUMMARY
SUMMATE
SUNMAID
TAMMANY
TARMACS
TEDMACK
THEMAGI
THEMALL
THEMASK
THEMAVS
THEMAYO
TOOMANY
TOPMAST
TRUMANS
ULLMANN
UNSMART
WALMART
WEBMAIL
WIDMARK
YEOMANS
YESMAAM
YOUMANS
ZERMATT

•••M•A•

ALUMNAE
ALUMNAL
ANEMIAS
ARAMEAN
BESMEAR
BIGMEAL
BOOMCAR
CHEMLAB
CLAMBAR
CRIMEAN
FARMGAL
GOOMBAH
GOOMBAY
GRAMMAR
GRAMPAS
GRUMMAN
HOLMOAK
HOTMEAL
LOOMPAS
MIAMIAN
MUAMMAR
NONMEAT
NUTMEAT
OATMEAL
PERMIAN
PIGMEAT
RAWMEAT
REDMEAT
RHUMBAS
RIBMEAT
ROOMBAS
SCHMEAR
SELMAAL
SOYMEAL
TRAMCAR
TRAMPAS
TRAMWAY
TRIMTAB
YESMAAM

•••M••A

AIRMADA
ALAMEDA
ALAMOSA
ALUMINA
BERMUDA
BIGMAMA
CALMSEA
CARMELA
CARMINA
CHIMERA
CREMONA
CREMORA
DOGMATA
EDEMATA
EXEMPLA
FERMATA
FORMICA
FORMOSA
FORMULA
GODMAMA
HERMANA
HERMOSA
LEMMATA
MARMARA
OLYMPIA
OXYMORA
PALMYRA
PRIMERA
STAMINA
STOMATA
TEAMUSA

••••MA•

ABYSMAL
ADWOMAN
ALMSMAN
ALTIMAS
ANDAMAN
ANNAMAY
AQUAMAN
AREAMAP
ASTHMAS
AUTOMAT
BACHMAN
BAHAMAS
BASEMAN
BATEMAN
BATHMAT
BATSMAN
BEHRMAN
BELLMAN
BERGMAN
BESTMAN
BETAMAX
BIRDMAN
BOATMAN
BOGYMAN
BONDMAN
BOOKMAN
BOORMAN
BOSSMAN
BOZEMAN
BRAHMAN
BRAHMAS
BUCHMAN
BUSHMAN
CALAMAR
CAPEMAY
CAVEMAN
CHAPMAN
CHARMAN
CHASMAL
CHROMAT
CINEMAS
CINEMAX
COLEMAN
COOLMAX
COPYMAN
CREWMAN
DARKMAN
DECIMAL
DELIMAN
DHARMAS
DILLMAN
DISCMAN
DOORMAN
DOORMAT
DORFMAN
DRAWMAN
DRAYMAN
DUSTMAN
EASTMAN
ECZEMAS
EDNAMAY
EIJKMAN
ELLAMAE
ELLYMAY
ENIGMAS
FADIMAN
FELDMAN
FEYNMAN
FIREMAN
FIVEMAN
FLAGMAN
FOOTMAN
FOREMAN
FOTOMAT
FOURMAN
FREEMAN
FROGMAN
FUSUMAS
GASSMAN
GATEMAN
GETSMAD
GILLMAN
GLEEMAN
GOESMAD
GOLDMAN
GONEMAD
GOODMAN
GRAMMAR
GRAUMAN
GRIDMAP
GRUMMAN
HACKMAN
HALFMAD
HANGMAN
HARTMAN
HAWKMAN
HEADMAN
HECKMAN
HEISMAN
HELLMAN
HICKMAN
HILLMAN

HJALMAR
HOFFMAN
HOLYMAN
HOLZMAN
HOOPMAN
HOUSMAN
HUFFMAN
IDEAMAN
IFWEMAY
INGEMAR
INHUMAN
IRONMAN
JACAMAR
JAVAMAN
JAZZMAN
JICAMAS
JUNKMAN
JURYMAN
KAUFMAN
KINGMAN
KINSMAN
KLUGMAN
LANDMAN
LASTMAY
LEADMAN
LENSMAN
LIKEMAD
LINEMAN
LUCKMAN
MADEMAD
MAILMAN
MAINMAN
MAKEMAD
MANSMAN
MANXMAN
MAXIMAL
MAXIMAS
MEATMAN
MIASMAL
MIASMAS
MILKMAN
MINIMAL
MINIMAX
MIRAMAR
MIRAMAX
MUAMMAR
MYANMAR
NAVYMAN
NESSMAN
NEWSMAN
NICEMAN
NKRUMAH
OARSMAN
OMNIMAX
OPTIMAL
OPTIMAS
OTTOMAN
OVERMAN
PAJAMAS
PALAMAS
PALOMAR
PALOMAS
PANAMAS
PARKMAN
PERLMAN
PETEMAN
PITTMAN
PLASMAS
PLOWMAN
PNEUMAS
PNEUMAT
POLEMAN
POOLMAN
POORMAN
PORTMAN
POSTMAN
POTOMAC
PROPMAN
PULLMAN
RAILMAN
RAINMAN
REALMAN
REEDMAN
REITMAN
REPOMAN
RICHMAN
RICKMAN
RIESMAN
RITAMAE
ROADMAP
SANDMAN
SARUMAN
SCATMAN
SCHEMAS
SEISMAL
SHERMAN
SHIPMAN
SHOWMAN
SHULMAN
SIDEMAN
SITEMAP
SNOWMAN
SOULMAN
STARMAN
STARMAP
STIGMAS
SURFMAN
SWAGMAN
SYNGMAN
TACOMAS
TAPEMAN
TAXIMAN
THERMAL
THINMAN
THURMAN
TIREMAN
TOLLMAN
TRAUMAS
TUCHMAN
TURFMAN
ULTIMAS
UNHUMAN
VELTMAN
VENEMAN
VERYMAD
WAKSMAN
WALKMAN
WALLMAP
WEIDMAN
WELLMAN
WENTMAD
WHITMAN
WILDMAN
WINGMAN
WIREMAN
WISEMAN
WOLFMAN
WORKMAN
YAKIMAS
YALEMAN
YARDMAN
YASHMAK
YEAHMAN
YOGAMAT
YZERMAN

••••M•A
ANAEMIA
ANOSMIA
BOHEMIA
CARAMBA
CARAMIA
COLUMBA
DILEMMA
ENCOMIA
EUNOMIA
ILIAMNA
LABAMBA
MAMAMIA
MARIMBA
OTTUMWA

•••••MA
ALABAMA
ATACAMA
BIGMAMA
DEPALMA
DILEMMA
DIORAMA
DIOTIMA
DIPLOMA
DRACHMA
GAUTAMA
GODMAMA
GRANDMA
IPANEMA
IWOJIMA
LAPALMA
MAHATMA
MELISMA
MISHIMA
NOXZEMA
PROXIMA
RORAIMA
SATSUMA
ZOSSIMA

MB•••••
MBABANE

M•B••••
MCBRIDE
MOBBERS
MOBBING
MOBBISH
MOBBISM
MOBBIST
MOBILES
MOBRULE
MOBSTER
MRBLISS
MRBODDY
MRBONES
MRBROWN
MRBURNS
MRBUTTS
MTBALDY
MTBLANC
MUBARAK
MYBUDDY

M••B•••
MACBETH
MAMBOED
MARBLED
MARBLER
MARBLES
MAXBAER
MAXBORN
MAYBESO
MBABANE
MEMBERS
MISBILL
MISBIND
MISBREW
MOABITE
MOBBERS
MOBBING
MOBBISH
MOBBISM
MOBBIST
MOEBERG
MOMBASA
MOWBRAY
MRSBASS
MUDBATH
MUMBLED
MUMBLER
MUMBLES
MUYBIEN

M•••B••
MACABRE
MAILBAG
MAILBIN
MAILBOX
MAKABLE
MALABAR
MALEBEE
MALTBIE
MARSBAR
MEGABIT
MENUBAR
MILKBAR
MINABLE
MINIBAR
MINIBUS
MIRABEL
MISTBOW
MIXABLE
MOONBOW
MOVABLE
MOVABLY
MRHOBBS
MRTIBBS
MUTABLE
MUTABLY

M••••B•
MADLIBS
MARIMBA
MICROBE
MIDRIBS
MODELBS
MOGAMBO
MORESBY
MRHOBBS
MRTIBBS

M•••••B
MCCRUMB
MINICAB
MINILAB
MINISUB

•MB••••
AMBIENS
AMBIENT
AMBLERS
AMBLING
AMBRIES
AMBROSE
EMBALMS
EMBANKS
EMBARGO
EMBARKS
EMBASSY
EMBAYED
EMBLAZE
EMBLEMS
EMBOITE
EMBOSOM
EMBOWER
EMBRACE
EMBROIL
EMBROWN
EMBRUED
EMBRUES
EMBRYOS
FMBANDS
IMBIBED
IMBIBER
IMBIBES
IMBORED
IMBROKE
IMBRUED
IMBRUES
IMBUING
UMBERED
UMBERTO
UMBRAGE
UMBRIAN
UMBRIEL

•M•B•••
AMEBOID
AMIBLUE
TMOBILE

•M••B••
AMIABLE
AMIABLY
AMOEBAE
AMOEBAS
AMOEBIC
IMBIBED
IMBIBER
IMBIBES
OMNIBUS

••MB•••
ARMBAND
ARMBONE
BAMBIII
BAMBINA
BAMBINI
BAMBINO
BAMBOOS
BIMBOES
BOMBARD
BOMBAST
BOMBECK
BOMBERS
BOMBING
BOMBLET
BUMBLED
BUMBLER
BUMBLES
CAMBERS
CAMBOYS
CAMBRIA
CAMBRIC
CEMBALO
COMBATS
COMBERS
COMBIEN
COMBINE
COMBING
COMBUST
CUMBERS
CUMBIAS
CUMBRIA
CYMBALS
DEMBUMS
DIMBULB
DUMBEST
DUMBING
FEMBOTS
FUMBLED
FUMBLER
FUMBLES
GAMBADO
GAMBIAN
GAMBIER
GAMBITS
GAMBLED
GAMBLER
GAMBLES
GAMBOLS
GIMBALS
GIMBELS
GUMBALL
GUMBOOT
GYMBAGS
GYMBALL
HAMBONE
HAMBURG
HOMBRES
HOMBURG
HUMBARD
HUMBERT
HUMBLED
HUMBLER
HUMBLES
HUMBUGS
IAMBICS
IAMBIST
JAMBAND
JAMBEAU
JIMBEAM
JUMBLED
JUMBLER
JUMBLES
JUMBUCK
KIMBALL
LAMBADA
LAMBDAS
LAMBEAU
LAMBENT
LAMBERT
LAMBETH
LAMBING
LAMBKIN
LIMBERS
LIMBING
LIMBURG
LOMBARD
LUMBAGO
LUMBARS
LUMBERS
MAMBOED
MEMBERS
MOMBASA
MUMBLED
MUMBLER
MUMBLES
NIMBLER
NOMBRES
NUMBATS
NUMBERS
NUMBEST
NUMBING
RAMBLED
RAMBLER
RAMBLES
RAMBLIN
RIMBAUD
ROMBERG
RUMBAED
RUMBLED
RUMBLER
RUMBLES
SAMBAED
SAMBASS
SAMBORA
SAMBUCA
SYMBOLS
TAMBALA
TAMBLYN
TEMBLOR
TIMBALE
TIMBALS
TIMBERS
TIMBERY
TIMBRES
TOMBOYS
TUMBLED
TUMBLER
TUMBLES
TUMBREL
WAMBLED
WAMBLES
WEMBLEY
WOMBATS
ZAMBEZI
ZAMBIAN
ZAMBONI
ZOMBIES
ZOMBIFY

••M•B••
CAMPBED
CIMABUE
GAMEBAG
GAMEBOY
GEMSBOK
HOMEBOY
JUMPBID
NAMABLE
NAMABLY
NAMIBIA
TAMABLE

••M••B•
COMESBY
ITMAYBE

••M•••B
DIMBULB
GYMCLUB
HOMELAB
TEMPJOB

•••MB••
ALEMBIC
BOOMBOX
BRAMBLE
BRAMBLY
CHAMBER
CHAMBRE
CLAMBAR
CLAMBER
CLIMBED
CLIMBER
CLIMBIN
CLIMBON
CLIMBTO
CLIMBUP
CRUMBED
CRUMBLE
CRUMBLY
CRUMBUM
FARMBOY
FLAMBED
FLAMBES
FNUMBER
GOOMBAH
GOOMBAY
GRUMBLE
GRUMBLY
PLUMBED
PLUMBER
PLUMBIC
PLUMBUM
PROMBID
RHOMBIC
RHOMBUS
RHUMBAS
ROOMBAS
SHAMBLE
SLUMBER
SPAMBOT
STUMBLE
THIMBLE
THUMBED
TREMBLE
TREMBLY

•••M•B•
GRIMSBY
LETMEBE

•••M••B
CHEMLAB
TRIMTAB

••••MB•
AAJUMBO
BENUMBS
CARAMBA
COLOMBO
COLUMBA
COLUMBO
ENTOMBS
INLIMBO
LABAMBA
MARIMBA
MOGAMBO
RECOMBS

•••••MB
CATCOMB
COULOMB
COXCOMB
DECRUMB
DOGCOMB
DOTBOMB
EWELAMB
HOTCOMB
MCCRUMB
PETCOMB
PETLAMB
RECLIMB
REPLUMB
SUCCUMB
THEBOMB
THELAMB
UNPLUMB
UPCLIMB

MC•••••
MCADAMS
MCALLEN
MCARDLE
MCBRIDE
MCCALLS
MCCAREY
MCCLOUD
MCCLURE
MCCLURG
MCCOURT
MCCOVEY
MCCOWEN
MCCRARY
MCCRUMB
MCENROE
MCGAVIN
MCGRIFF
MCGRORY
MCGRUFF
MCGUIRE
MCGWIRE
MCHALES
MCHENRY
MCKENNA
MCLUHAN
MCMAHON
MCMURDO
MCNALLY
MCNEILL
MCPAPER
MCQUEEN
MCRANEY
MCSHANE
MCSWINE

M•C••••
MACABRE
MACACOS
MACADAM
MACAQUE
MACBETH
MACDUFF
MACEDON
MACGRAW
MACHAON
MACHETE
MACHINA
MACHINE
MACHONE
MACHREE
MACHSIX
MACHTWO
MACLEAN
MACLEOD
MACNEIL
MACONGA
MACOUNS
MACRAME
MACRONS
MACULAE
MACULAR
MACUSER
MCCALLS
MCCAREY
MCCLOUD
MCCLURE
MCCLURG
MCCOURT
MCCOVEY
MCCOWEN
MCCRARY
MCCRUMB
MECCANS
MECHLIN
MICAELA
MICHAEL
MICHAUX
MICKEYS
MICMACS
MICROBE
MICRONS
MOCHRIE
MOCKERS
MOCKERY
MOCKING
MOCKSUP
MOCKUPS
MRCHIPS
MRCLEAN
MUCKERS
MUCKIER
MUCKING
MUCKSUP
MYCENAE
MYCROFT

M••C•••
MADCAPS
MADCHEN
MALCOLM
MANCINI
MANCUSO
MARCATO
MARCEAU
MARCELS
MARCHED
MARCHER
MARCHES
MARCHON
MARCONI
MARCUSE
MASCARA
MASCOTS
MATCHED
MATCHER
MATCHES
MATCHUP
MECCANS
MENCIUS
MENCKEN
MERCADO
MERCERS
MERCERY
MERCHES
MERCIAN
MERCIES
MERCURE
MERCURY
MESCALS
METCALF
MIDCAPS
MINCERS
MINCING
MIOCENE
MISCALL
MISCAST
MISCITE
MISCODE
MISCOIN
MISCOPY
MISCUED
MISCUES
MISCUTS
MITCHUM
MONCTON
MOOCHED
MOOCHER
MOOCHES
MOOCOWS
MORCERF
MOSCATO
MOSCONI
MRSCOTT
MUDCATS
MULCAHY
MULCHED
MULCHES
MULCTED
MUNCHED
MUNCHEN
MUNCHER
MUNCHES
MUNCHIE
MUNCHON
MUSCATS
MUSCIDA
MUSCLED
MUSCLES

M•••C••
MACACOS
MAGICAL
MAILCAR
MALACCA
MALACHI
MALECAT
MALICES
MANACLE
MANXCAT
MARACAS
MEDICAL
MEDICOS
MENACED
MENACER
MENACES
MENSCHY
MEXICAN
MILKCAN
MILKCOW
MIMICRY
MINICAB
MINICAM
MINICAR
MIRACLE
MISACTS
MODICUM
MOHICAN
MOLUCCA
MONACAN
MONOCLE
MOROCCO
MRISCAN
MRLUCKY
MRMACHO
MUSICAL
MUSICKS

M••••C•
MADLOCK
MAJORCA
MALACCA
MANIACS
MANRICO
MANTECA
MASTICS
MATLOCK
MATTOCK
MAURICE
MEDWICK
MENISCI
MENORCA
MERRICK
MESHACH
MESSICK
METRICS
MICMACS
MINORCA
MIRISCH
MIXTECS
MOLUCCA
MONARCH
MORLOCK
MOROCCO
MORTICE
MOSAICS
MRDARCY
MRMARCH
MRSPOCK
MTMARCY
MUDPACK
MURDOCH
MYSPACE
MYSTICS

M•••••C
MALEFIC
MANTRIC
MASONIC
MAURIAC
MEDEVAC
MEDIVAC
MEIOTIC
MELANIC
MELODIC
MESONIC
MIASMIC
MIDDLEC
MIMETIC
MINIVAC
MISKOLC
MITOTIC
MOLLUSC
MONADIC
MONODIC
MORONIC
MORPHIC
MRMUSIC
MTBLANC
MYALGIC
MYRRHIC

•M•C•••
AMICHAI
AMSCRAY
OMICRON
SMACKED
SMACKER
SMACKOF
SMACKUP
SMUCKER

•M••C••
AMERCED
AMERCER
AMERCES
IMPACTS

•M•••C•
AMERICA
AMTRACK
AMTRACS
EMBRACE
EMETICS

EMPLACE
IMPEACH

•M••••C
AMHARIC
AMMONIC
AMNESIC
AMOEBIC
EMPIRIC

••MC•••
ATMCARD
COMCAST
DRMCCOY
ELMCITY
GYMCLUB
JAMCAMS
JIMCHEE
KIMCHEE
ROMCOMS
RUMCAKE
SIMCITY
TOMCATS

••M•C••
CAMACHO
COMICAL
COMICES
DOMECAR
DOMICAL
DOMICIL
DRMCCOY
FAMICOM
HAMACHI
JUMPCUT
LIMACON
MIMICRY
MRMACHO
PUMICED
PUMICES
TIMECOP
UNMACHO

••M••C•
ARMLOCK
BOMBECK
COMPACT
CYMRICS
DEMARCO
GIMMICK
GYMSOCK
HAMHOCK
HAMMOCK
HEMLOCK
HOMEICE
IAMBICS
INMARCH
JAMAICA
JAMPACK
JIMRICE
JOMARCH
JUMBUCK
LAMARCK
MRMARCH
MTMARCY
NOMERCY
NUMLOCK
PAMLICO
PIMLICO
REMATCH
RIMROCK
ROMANCE
SAMBUCA
TAMPICO
TIMRICE
TUMESCE

••M•••C
ALMANAC
AMMONIC
CAMBRIC
COMEDIC
DEMONIC
DEMOTIC
DOMINIC
HAMITIC
HEMATIC
HOMERIC
MIMETIC
MRMUSIC
NOMADIC
NUMERIC
NYMPHIC
OSMATIC
OSMOTIC
ROMANIC
SEMITIC
SIMILAC
SOMATIC
TAMARAC

•••MC••
BOOMCAR
PLUMCOT
TRAMCAR

•••M•C•
ANIMACY
ATOMICS
BIGMACS
CORMACK
DORMICE
FORMICA
GIMMICK
GRIMACE
HAMMOCK
HOWMUCH
LABMICE
MICMACS
NIPMUCK
NOTMUCH
PETMICE
PRIMACY
STOMACH
TARMACS
TEDMACK
THEMICK
TITMICE
TOOMUCH

•••M••C
ALEMBIC
ARAMAIC
OLYMPIC
PLUMBIC
RHOMBIC

••••M•C
ANAEMIC
ANOSMIC
CERAMIC
CHASMIC
CHROMIC
DHARMIC
DYNAMIC
ENDEMIC
ENZYMIC
GENOMIC
ISLAMIC
MIASMIC
OGHAMIC
PLASMIC
POLEMIC
POTOMAC
PSALMIC
RHEUMIC
SEISMIC
THERMIC
TOTEMIC
UNCOMIC

•••••MC
YOUNGMC

M•D••••
MADALYN
MADAMES
MADAMEX
MADCAPS
MADCHEN
MADDASH
MADDENS
MADDERS
MADDEST
MADDING
MADDISH
MADDOGS
MADEFIT
MADEFOR
MADEFUN
MADEHAY
MADEILL
MADEIRA
MADELON
MADEMAD
MADEOFF
MADEONE
MADEOUT
MADEPAR
MADERUN
MADEWAR
MADEWAY
MADIGAN
MADISON
MADLIBS
MADLOCK
MADNESS
MADONNA
MADRUSH
MADUROS
MEDAKAS
MEDALED
MEDAWAR
MEDDLED
MEDDLER
MEDDLES
MEDELES
MEDEVAC
MEDFORD
MEDIANS
MEDIANT
MEDIATE
MEDICAL
MEDICOS
MEDIGAP
MEDIUMS
MEDIVAC
MEDLEYS
MEDULLA
MEDUSAE
MEDUSAN
MEDUSAS
MEDWICK
MIDASES
MIDCAPS
MIDDAYS
MIDDIES
MIDDLEC
MIDDLED
MIDDLER
MIDDLES
MIDEAST
MIDGETS
MIDIRON
MIDJULY
MIDJUNE
MIDLAND
MIDLEGS
MIDLIFE
MIDLINE
MIDLIST
MIDMORN
MIDMOST
MIDNOON
MIDOFFS
MIDRIBS
MIDRIFF
MIDRISE
MIDSHIP
MIDSIZE
MIDSOLE
MIDTEEN
MIDTERM
MIDTOWN
MIDWAYS
MIDWEEK
MIDWEST
MIDWIFE
MIDYEAR
MODELAS
MODELBS
MODELED
MODELER
MODELTS
MODEMED
MODERNE
MODERNS
MODESTO
MODESTY
MODICUM
MODISTE
MODULAR
MODULES
MODULUS
MRDARCY
MRDEEDS
MUDBATH
MUDCATS
MUDDERS
MUDDIED
MUDDIER
MUDDIES
MUDDILY
MUDDING
MUDDLED
MUDDLER
MUDDLES
MUDEELS
MUDFISH
MUDFLAP
MUDFLAT
MUDFLOW
MUDHENS
MUDHOLE
MUDLARK
MUDPACK
MUDPIES
MUDROOM
MUDWASP

M••D•••
MACDUFF
MADDASH
MADDENS
MADDERS
MADDEST
MADDING
MADDISH
MADDOGS
MAHDISM
MAHDIST
MAIDENS
MAIDISH
MALDIVE
MANDALA
MANDANS
MANDATE
MANDAYS
MANDELA
MANDOKI
MANDREL
MARDIAN
MAUDLIN
MAYDAYS
MCADAMS
MEADOWS
MEADOWY
MEDDLED
MEDDLER
MEDDLES
MELDERS
MELDING
MENDELS
MENDERS
MENDING
MIDDAYS
MIDDIES
MIDDLEC
MIDDLED
MIDDLER
MIDDLES
MILDEST
MILDEWS
MILDEWY
MILDRED
MINDERS
MINDFUL
MINDING
MINDORO
MINDSET
MISDATE
MISDEAL
MISDEED
MISDEEM
MISDIAL
MISDOER
MISDOES
MISDONE
MISDRAW
MISDREW
MOLDERS
MOLDIER
MOLDING
MOLDOVA
MONDALE
MONDAVI
MONDAYS
MONDESI
MONDIAL
MONDIEU
MOODIER
MOODILY
MORDANT
MORDENT
MORDRED
MOWDOWN
MTADAMS
MUDDERS
MUDDIED
MUDDIER
MUDDIES
MUDDILY
MUDDING
MUDDLED
MUDDLER
MUDDLES
MULDAUR
MULDOON
MUNDANE
MURDERS
MURDOCH

M•••D••
MAANDPA
MACADAM
MACEDON
MAKEDOS
MALEDOG
MALODOR
MARIDAS
MARIDOS
MARSDEN
MATADOR
MAULDIN
MAUNDER
MCARDLE
MEANDER
MELODIA
MELODIC
MENUDOS
MERIDEN
MIKADOS
MILKDUD
MILLDAM
MIRADAS
MIRADOR
MISADDS
MISEDIT
MIXEDIN
MIXEDLY
MIXEDUP
MOGADOR
MONADAL
MONADIC
MONODIC
MOONDOG
MOULDED
MOULDER
MOUNDED
MOVADOS
MOVEDIN
MOVEDIT
MOVEDON
MOVEDTO
MOVEDUP
MRBODDY
MRPADRE
MUSEDON
MUSTDOS
MUTEDLY
MYBUDDY

M••••D•
MAENADS
MAKESDO
MALTEDS
MANMADE
MARAUDS
MATILDA
MCBRIDE
MCMURDO
MELINDA
MERCADO
METHODS
MILORDS
MIRANDA
MISADDS
MISCODE
MRBODDY
MRDEEDS
MRWORDS
MTBALDY
MUSCIDA
MYBUDDY
MYRIADS

M•••••D
MACLEOD
MADEMAD
MAITRED
MAJORED
MAKEMAD
MALAMUD
MALLARD
MAMBOED
MANAGED
MANFRED
MANGLED
MANHOOD
MANKIND
MANSARD
MANTLED
MANURED
MARBLED
MARCHED
MARRIED
MARSRED
MASONED
MASTOID
MATCHED
MATURED
MAYNARD
MCCLOUD
MEDALED
MEDDLED
MEDFORD
MELAMED
MEMOPAD
MENACED
MERITED
MERMAID
METALED
METERED
MIAOUED
MIAOWED
MIDDLED
MIDLAND
MILDRED
MILHAUD
MILKDUD
MILKFED
MILLAND
MILLARD
MILLEND
MIMEOED
MINGLED
MINORED
MINOTND
MINUEND
MINUTED
MISBIND
MISCUED
MISDEED
MISFEED
MISLAID
MISLEAD
MISREAD
MISSAID
MISSEND
MISTOLD
MISUSED
MISWORD
MITERED
MITFORD
MIZZLED
MODELED
MODEMED
MONEYED
MONOPOD
MONTAND
MOOCHED
MOONGOD
MOPHEAD
MORDRED
MORPHED
MOSEYED
MOTIVED
MOTORED
MOTTLED
MOULDED
MOULTED
MOUNDED
MOUNTED
MOURNED
MOUSSED
MOUTHED
MUDDIED
MUDDLED
MUFFLED
MULCHED
MULCTED
MUMBLED
MUMFORD
MUNCHED
MURALED
MUSCLED
MUSTARD
MUTATED
MUZZLED
MYRRHED
MYWORLD

•M•D•••
AMADEUS
AMIDALA
AMIDOLS
IMADEIT
SMIDGEN
SMIDGES
SMUDGED
SMUDGES

•M••D••
AMENDED
AMENDER
AMPEDUP
AMRADIO
EMENDED
EMENDER
FMRADIO
IMPEDED
IMPEDER
IMPEDES
SMOLDER
XMRADIO

•M•••D•
AMERADA
EMQUADS
FMBANDS
IMPENDS
IMPLODE
IMREADY

•M••••D
AMASSED
AMEBOID
AMENDED
AMERCED
AMERIND
AMISTAD
EMAILED
EMBAYED
EMBRUED
EMENDED
EMERALD
EMERGED
EMERSED
EMITTED
EMPALED
EMPTIED
IMBIBED
IMBORED
IMBRUED
IMMIXED
IMMURED
IMPALED
IMPAVID
IMPEDED
IMPLEAD
IMPLIED
IMPOSED
IMPOUND
IMPUTED
IMTIRED
OMITTED
SMACKED
SMALLAD
SMARTED
SMASHED
SMEARED
SMELLED
SMELTED
SMIRKED
SMITHED
SMUDGED
SMUSHED
UMBERED
UMPIRED

••MD•••
BUMDEAL
DUMDUMS
GUMDROP
HUMDRUM
JIMDALE
JIMDIAL
RAMDOWN

••M•D••
AIMEDAT
ALMADEN
ARMADAS
BIMODAL
CAMEDUE
COMEDIA
COMEDIC
COMEDIE
COMEDUE
DAMPDRY
FUMEDAT
GQMODEL
HOMEDIN
HUMIDEX
HUMIDLY
HUMIDOR
JUMADAS
KEMIDOV
LAMBDAS
NAMEDAY
NOMADIC
POMADED
POMADES
RAMADAN
RAMADAS
REMODEL
SAMEDAY
SAMEDIS
SEMIDRY
SOMEDAY
TIMIDER
TIMIDLY
UNMADLY
UNMUDDY

••M••D•
ALMONDS
ALMONDY
COMMODE
COMRADE
DEMANDS
EDMONDS
EDMUNDI
EDMUNDS
ELMUNDO
FTMEADE
GAMBADO
HYMNODY
LAMBADA
LEMONDE
LIMEADE
MCMURDO
NIMRODS
ORMANDY
OSMONDS
OSMUNDS
RAMRODS
REMANDS
REMENDS
REMINDS
REMOLDS
UNMOLDS
UNMOLDY
UNMOODY
UNMUDDY

••M•••D
ADMIRED
ADMIXED
ARMBAND
ARMLOAD
ARMORED
ATMCARD
BEMIRED
BEMUSED
BOMBARD
BUMBLED
CAMELID
CAMEOED
CAMPBED
COMMAND
COMMEND
COMPEND
DAMAGED
DEMIGOD
DEMISED
DEMOTED
DIMPLED
DUMMIED
ELMWOOD
ERMINED
FUMBLED
GAMBLED
GUMWOOD
HAMMOND
HOMERED
HOMINID
HUMBARD
HUMBLED
HUMORED
HUMPHED
IMMIXED
IMMURED
JAMBAND
JIMMIED
JUMBLED
JUMPBID
KAMERAD
LIMITED
LOMBARD
MAMBOED
MEMOPAD
MIMEOED
MUMBLED
MUMFORD
OLMSTED
OSMOSED
PIMPLED
POMADED
POMMARD
PUMICED
RAMBLED
REMATED
REMINED
REMISED
REMIXED
REMOVED
REMOWED
RIMBAUD
RIMPLED
RUMBAED
RUMBLED
RUMFORD
RUMORED
RUMPEND
RUMPLED
SAMBAED
SAMEOLD
SAMLOYD
SAMOYED
SAMPLED
SUMMAND
TEMPLED
TEMPTED
TIMREID
TOMJOAD
TUMBLED
UNMANED
UNMATED
UNMEWED
UNMIKED
UNMINED
UNMIRED
UNMIXED
UNMOULD
UNMOVED
UNMOWED
UNMUTED
WAMBLED
WIMPLED

•••MD••
CLAMDIP
FILMDOM
KRAMDEN

•••M•D•
AIRMADA
ALAMEDA
ALAMODE
ARAMIDS
BERMUDA
BROMIDE
COMMODE
DIOMEDE
DRAMADY
DRAMEDY
HEYMRDJ
ILLMADE
MANMADE
NEWMADE
OUTMODE
PREMADE
PREMEDS
SCHMIDT

•••M••D
BADMOOD
BARMAID
BRIMMED
CHAMPED
CHOMPED
CHUMMED
CHUMPED
CLAMMED
CLAMPED
CLIMBED
CLOMPED
CLUMPED
COMMAND
COMMEND
CRAMMED
CRAMPED
CRIMPED
CRUMBED
CRUMPED
DESMOND
DIAMOND
DRUMMED
DUMMIED
EANMUND
ETHMOID
FARMAID
FLAMBED
FLAMMED
GLOMMED
GLUMMED
GRUMPED
HAMMOND
HELMOND
INAMOOD
JIMMIED
MERMAID
NORMAND
OFAMIND

OLDMAID
PLUMBED
PLUMPED
POMMARD
PRIMMED
PRIMPED
PROMBID
PROMOED
RAYMOND
REAMEND
REDMOND
SCAMMED
SCAMPED
SHAMMED
SIGMOID
SIGMUND
SKIMMED
SKIMPED
SLAMMED
SLIMMED
SLUMMED
SLUMPED
SPAMMED
STAMPED
STEMMED
STOMPED
STUMPED
STYMIED
SUMMAND
SUNMAID
SWAMPED
THUMBED
THUMPED
TRAMMED
TRAMPED
TRIMMED
TROMPED
TRUMPED
WHAMMED
WHOMPED

••••M•D

ALARMED
ASHAMED
ASSUMED
BLOOMED
BOSOMED
BRIMMED
BROOMED
CAROMED
CHARMED
CHROMED
CHUMMED
CLAIMED
CLAMMED
CLUBMED
CRAMMED
CREAMED
DEFAMED
DENIMED
DREAMED
DRUMMED
ENARMED
EXHUMED
FLAMMED
GETSMAD
GLEAMED
GLOMMED
GLOOMED
GLUMMED
GOESMAD
GONEMAD
GROOMED
HALFMAD
ILLUMED
INHUMED
LIKEMAD
MADEMAD
MAKEMAD
MALAMUD
MELAMED
MODEMED
PRIMMED
PYRAMID
REAIMED
REARMED
RELUMED
RENAMED
RESUMED
RETAMED
RETIMED
SCAMMED
SCHEMED
SHAMMED
SKIMMED
SLAMMED
SLIMMED
SLUMMED
SPAMMED
STEAMED
STEMMED
STORMED
SWARMED
TRAMMED
TRIMMED
UNAIMED
UNARMED
UNDOMED
UNFAMED
UNHUMID
UNNAMED
UNRIMED
UNTAMED
UNTIMED
UNTIMID
VERYMAD
VOLUMED
VROOMED
WENTMAD
WHAMMED
WHELMED

ME•••••

MEADOWS
MEADOWY
MEAGLES
MEALIER
MEALIES
MEANAGE
MEANDER
MEANEST
MEANIES
MEANING
MEANJOE
MEANSIT
MEANSTO
MEANTIT
MEANTTO
MEASLES
MEASURE
MEATAXE
MEATIER
MEATILY
MEATMAN
MEATMEN
MEATPIE
MECCANS
MECHLIN
MEDAKAS
MEDALED
MEDAWAR
MEDDLED
MEDDLER
MEDDLES
MEDELES
MEDEVAC
MEDFORD
MEDIANS
MEDIANT
MEDIATE
MEDICAL
MEDICOS
MEDIGAP
MEDIUMS
MEDIVAC
MEDLEYS
MEDULLA
MEDUSAE
MEDUSAN
MEDUSAS
MEDWICK
MEEKEST
MEEMIES
MEERKAT
MEETERS
MEETING
MEETSUP
MEFIRST
MEGABIT
MEGAERA
MEGAERG
MEGAHIT
MEGALON
MEGANES
MEGATON
MEGILLA
MEGOHMS
MEGRIMS
MEGRYAN
MEIOSES
MEIOSIS
MEIOTIC
MEISSEN
MEISTER
MEITNER
MELAMED
MELANGE
MELANIA
MELANIC
MELANIE
MELANIN
MELDERS
MELDING
MELINDA
MELISMA
MELISSA
MELITTA
MELLOWS
MELODIA
MELODIC
MELROSE
MELTAGE
MELTERS
MELTING
MEMBERS
MEMENTO
MEMLING
MEMOIRE
MEMOIRS
MEMOPAD
MEMOREX
MEMPHIS
MENACED
MENACER
MENACES
MENAGES
MENCIUS
MENCKEN
MENDELS
MENDERS
MENDING
MENFOLK
MENIALS
MENISCI
MENORAH
MENORCA
MENOTTI
MENSANS
MENSCHY
MENTEES
MENTHOL
MENTION
MENTORS
MENUBAR
MENUDOS
MENUHIN
MENZIES
MEOWERS
MEOWING
MEOWMIX
MERCADO
MERCERS
MERCERY
MERCHES
MERCIAN
MERCIES
MERCURE
MERCURY
MERGEES
MERGERS
MERGING
MERIDEN
MERIMEE
MERINOS
MERITED
MERLINS
MERLOTS
MERMAID
MERRIAM
MERRICK
MERRIER
MERRILL
MERRILY
MESAMIS
MESCALS
MESEEMS
MESHACH
MESHIER
MESHING
MESHUGA
MESONIC
MESSAGE
MESSALA
MESSIAH
MESSICK
MESSIER
MESSILY
MESSINA
MESSING
MESSKIT
MESSUPS
METALED
METATES
METCALF
METEORS
METEOUT
METERED
METFANS
METHANE
METHODS
METIERS
METLIFE
METOOER
METRICS
METRIST
METSFAN
METTLER
METTLES
METWITH
MEWLERS
MEWLING
MEXICAN
MEYNELL
MEZUZAH
MEZUZAS

M•E••••

MAENADS
MAESTRO
MAEWEST
MCENROE
MEEKEST
MEEMIES
MEERKAT
MEETERS
MEETING
MEETSUP
MOEBERG
MTEVANS
MUELLER
MUESLIS
MUESLIX
MUEZZIN
MYERSON

M••E•••

MACEDON
MADEFIT
MADEFOR
MADEFUN
MADEHAY
MADEILL
MADEIRA
MADELON
MADEMAD
MADEOFF
MADEONE
MADEOUT
MADEPAR
MADERUN
MADEWAR
MADEWAY
MAGENTA
MAJESTE
MAJESTY
MAJEURE
MAKEDOS
MAKEFIT
MAKEFOR
MAKEFUN
MAKEHAY
MAKEILL
MAKEMAD
MAKEOFF
MAKEONE
MAKEOUT
MAKEPAR
MAKERUN
MAKESDO
MAKESGO
MAKESIT
MAKESUP
MAKEUPS
MAKEWAR
MAKEWAY
MALEANT
MALEBEE
MALECAT
MALEDOG
MALEFIC
MALEHOG
MALEPIG
MANEGES
MANETTE
MARENGO
MATEWAN
MAZEPPA
MCHENRY
MCKENNA
MCNEILL
MEDELES
MEDEVAC
MEMENTO
MESEEMS
METEORS
METEOUT
METERED
MIDEAST
MIGENES
MILEAGE
MILERUN
MIMEOED
MIMESES
MIMESIS
MIMETIC
MINEOLA
MINEPIT
MINERAL
MINERVA
MISEDIT
MISERLY
MITERED
MIXEDIN
MIXEDLY
MIXEDUP
MIXESIN
MIXESUP
MODELAS
MODELBS
MODELED
MODELER
MODELTS
MODEMED
MODERNE
MODERNS
MODESTO
MODESTY
MOHEGAN
MOLERAT
MOLESTS
MOMENTA
MOMENTS
MONEYED
MOREENS
MORELLA
MORELLO
MORELOS
MOREPAY
MORESBY
MORETTI
MOSELLE
MOSEYED
MOVEDIN
MOVEDIT
MOVEDON
MOVEDTO
MOVEDUP
MOVEOFF
MOVEOUT
MOVESIN
MOVESIT
MOVESON
MOVESTO
MOVESUP
MOZETTA
MRDEEDS
MSIEURS
MTKENYA
MTPELEE
MUDEELS
MUJERES
MULETAS
MUMESON
MUSEDON
MUSEFUL
MUSESON
MUSETTA
MUSETTE
MUSEUMS
MUTEDLY
MYCENAE

M•••E••

MACBETH
MACHETE
MACLEAN
MACLEOD
MACNEIL
MADDENS
MADDERS
MADDEST
MADNESS
MAEWEST
MAGLEVS
MAGNETO
MAGNETS
MAIDENS
MAILERS
MAIMERS
MAINERS
MAJGENS
MALLETS
MALLEUS
MALTEDS
MALTESE
MANDELA
MANGERS
MANHEIM
MANLESS
MANNERS
MANTECA
MANTELS
MANYEAR
MAPPERS
MARCEAU
MARCELS
MARGERY
MARKERS
MARKETS
MARLENE
MARRERS
MARTENS
MARVELL
MARVELS
MASHERS
MASKERS
MASSEUR
MASTERP
MASTERS
MASTERY
MATHERS
MATHEWS
MATLESS
MATTERS
MAULERS
MAUREEN
MAUSERS
MAXWELL
MAYBESO
MAYHEMS
MAZIEST
MCQUEEN
MEANEST
MEDLEYS
MEEKEST
MEETERS
MEGAERA
MEGAERG
MELDERS
MELTERS
MEMBERS
MENDELS
MENDERS
MENTEES
MEOWERS
MERCERS
MERCERY
MERGEES
MERGERS
MESEEMS
METIERS
MEWLERS
MEYNELL
MICAELA
MICKEYS
MIDGETS
MIDLEGS
MIDTEEN
MIDTERM
MIDWEEK
MIDWEST
MIDYEAR
MILDEST
MILDEWS
MILDEWY
MILIEUS
MILIEUX
MILKERS
MILLEND
MILLERS
MILLETS
MILLETT
MIMIEUX
MINCERS
MINDERS
MINTERS
MINUEND
MINUETS
MIOCENE
MIRIEST
MISDEAL
MISDEED
MISDEEM
MISFEED
MISHEAR
MISKEYS
MISLEAD
MISMESH
MISREAD
MISRELY
MISSEAT
MISSEND
MISSENT
MISSETS
MISTELL
MISTERM
MISTERS
MISTERX
MITTENS
MIXTECS
MIZZENS
MOANERS
MOBBERS
MOCKERS
MOCKERY
MOEBERG
MOILERS
MOLDERS
MOLIERE
MOLTERS
MONDESI
MONGERS
MONKEES
MONKEYS
MONTEGO
MONTERO
MONTEUX
MOONERS
MOONEYE
MOOTERS
MOPHEAD
MOPIEST
MOPPERS
MOPPETS
MORCERF
MORDENT
MOREENS
MORSELS
MOSHERS
MOSLEMS
MOTHERS
MOTHERY
MOTLEYS
MOUSERS
MRCLEAN
MRDEEDS
MRGREEN
MRSPEEL
MUCKERS
MUDDERS
MUDEELS
MUDHENS
MUGGERS
MULLERS
MULLETS
MUMMERS
MUMMERY
MUPPETS
MURDERS
MURIELS
MUSHERS
MUSKEGO
MUSKETS
MUSSELS
MUSTERS
MUTTERS
MYNHEER
MYSTERY
MYTREAT

M••••E•

MAARTEN
MACHREE
MACUSER
MADAMES
MADAMEX
MADCHEN
MAGPIES
MAHONEY
MAIGRET
MAILMEN
MAINMEN
MAITRED
MAITRES
MAJORED
MALEBEE
MALICES
MALMSEY
MALTIER
MAMBOED
MANAGED
MANAGER
MANAGES
MANATEE
MANDREL
MANEGES
MANFRED
MANGIER
MANGLED
MANGLER
MANGLES
MANGOES
MANLIER
MANNIES
MANTLED
MANTLES
MANTLET
MANURED
MANURES
MANXMEN
MARBLED
MARBLER
MARBLES
MARCHED
MARCHER
MARCHES
MARGRET
MARINER
MARINES
MARLIER
MARNIER
MARQUEE
MARQUES
MARQUEZ
MARRIED
MARRIES
MARSDEN
MARSHES
MARSRED
MARVIER
MASHIES
MASONED
MASQUER
MASQUES
MASSIER
MATCHED
MATCHER
MATCHES
MATHIEU
MATINEE
MATTHEW
MATURED
MATURER
MATURES
MAUNDER
MAUREEN
MAVISES
MAXBAER
MAXIXES
MCALLEN
MCCAREY
MCCOVEY
MCCOWEN
MCHALES
MCPAPER
MCQUEEN
MCRANEY
MEAGLES
MEALIER
MEALIES
MEANDER
MEANIES
MEASLES
MEATIER
MEATMEN
MEDALED
MEDDLED
MEDDLER
MEDDLES
MEDELES
MEEMIES
MEGANES
MEIOSES
MEISSEN
MEISTER
MEITNER
MELAMED
MEMOREX
MENACED
MENACER
MENACES
MENAGES
MENCKEN
MENTEES
MENZIES
MERCHES
MERCIES
MERGEES
MERIDEN
MERIMEE
MERITED
MERRIER
MESHIER
MESSIER
METALED
METATES
METERED
METOOER
METTLER
METTLES
MIAOUED
MIAOWED
MICHAEL
MIDASES
MIDDIES
MIDDLEC
MIDDLED
MIDDLER
MIDDLES
MIDTEEN
MIDWEEK
MIFFIER
MIGENES
MILDRED
MILKFED
MILKIER
MILKMEN
MIMEOED
MIMESES
MINARET
MINDSET
MINGIER
MINGLED
MINGLER
MINGLES
MINIVER
MINORED
MINSTER
MINTIER
MINTTEA
MINUSES
MINUTED
MINUTER
MINUTES
MIRABEL
MIRAGES
MISAVER
MISBREW
MISCUED
MISCUES
MISDEED
MISDEEM
MISDOER
MISDOES
MISDREW
MISFEED
MISKNEW
MISSIES
MISSTEP
MISTIER
MISUSED
MISUSER
MISUSES
MITERED
MITOSES
MIZZLED
MIZZLES
MOBILES
MOBSTER
MODELED
MODELER
MODEMED
MODULES
MOHAVES
MOISTEN
MOISTER
MOJAVES
MOLDIER
MOLLIES
MOMMIES
MOMMSEN
MOMONEY
MOMUSES
MONDIEU
MONEYED
MONGREL
MONIKER
MONKEES
MONOMER
MONROES
MONSTER
MOOCHED
MOOCHER
MOOCHES
MOODIER
MOONIER
MOONIES
MOONLET
MOONSET
MOORHEN
MOORIER
MORALES
MORDRED
MORGUES

7 ME

MORPHED
MOSEYED
MOSQUES
MOSSIER
MOTHIER
MOTIVED
MOTIVES
MOTORED
MOTTLED
MOTTLES
MOTTOES
MOULDED
MOULDER
MOULTED
MOUNDED
MOUNTED
MOUNTER
MOURNED
MOURNER
MOUSIER
MOUSSED
MOUSSES
MOUTHED
MOUTHER
MPTHREE
MRBONES
MRGREEN
MRHANEY
MRJONES
MRSPEEL
MRTIGER
MTPELEE
MUCKIER
MUDDIED
MUDDIER
MUDDIES
MUDDLED
MUDDLER
MUDDLES
MUDPIES
MUELLER
MUFFLED
MUFFLER
MUFFLES
MUGGIER
MUGGLES
MUJERES
MULCHED
MULCHES
MULCTED
MULGREW
MUMBLED
MUMBLER
MUMBLES
MUMMIES
MUNCHED
MUNCHEN
MUNCHER
MUNCHES
MUNSTER
MURALED
MURKIER
MUSCLED
MUSCLES
MUSHIER
MUSKIER
MUSKIES
MUSSIER
MUSTIER
MUSTSEE
MUTAGEN
MUTATED
MUTATES
MUYBIEN
MUZZIER
MUZZLED
MUZZLER
MUZZLES
MYNHEER
MYRRHED
MYRTLES

M•••••E

MACABRE
MACAQUE
MACHETE
MACHINE
MACHONE
MACHREE
MACRAME
MACULAE
MADEONE
MAGNATE
MAGUIRE
MAJESTE
MAJEURE
MAKABLE
MAKEONE
MALAISE
MALDIVE
MALEBEE
MALTASE
MALTBIE
MALTESE
MALTOSE
MALWARE
MANACLE
MANATEE
MANDATE
MANETTE
MANHOLE
MANIPLE
MANLIKE
MANMADE
MANROPE
MANSIZE
MARCUSE
MARGATE
MARLENE
MARLOWE
MARQUEE
MARRYME
MARYURE
MASSAGE
MASSINE
MASSIVE
MATINEE
MATISSE
MAURICE
MAYPOLE
MAYTIME
MAYWINE
MBABANE
MCARDLE
MCBRIDE
MCCLURE
MCENROE
MCGUIRE
MCGWIRE
MCSHANE
MCSWINE
MEANAGE
MEANJOE
MEASURE
MEATAXE
MEATPIE
MEDIATE
MEDUSAE
MELANGE
MELANIE
MELROSE
MELTAGE
MEMOIRE
MERCURE
MERIMEE
MESSAGE
METHANE
METLIFE
MICROBE
MIDJUNE
MIDLIFE
MIDLINE
MIDRISE
MIDSIZE
MIDSOLE
MIDWIFE
MIGRATE
MILEAGE
MILLAGE
MILLIME
MINABLE
MINOGUE
MINTAGE
MIOCENE
MIRACLE
MISCITE
MISCODE
MISDATE
MISDONE
MISFILE
MISFIRE
MISGAVE
MISGIVE
MISLIKE
MISMATE
MISMOVE
MISNAME
MISPAGE
MISRATE
MISRULE
MISSILE
MISSIVE
MISTAKE
MISTIME
MISTUNE
MISTYPE
MISWIRE
MISZONE
MIXABLE
MIXTURE
MOABITE
MOBRULE
MOCHRIE
MODERNE
MODISTE
MOLIERE
MONDALE
MONOCLE
MONTAGE
MONTALE
MOONEYE
MOONPIE
MOORAGE
MORAINE
MORANTE
MORTICE
MORTISE
MOSELLE
MOULAGE
MOUNTIE
MOVABLE
MPTHREE
MRHORSE
MRMOOSE
MRPADRE
MRSLATE
MTPELEE
MUDHOLE
MULHARE
MUNCHIE
MUNDANE
MUSANTE
MUSETTE
MUSTSEE
MUTABLE
MYCENAE
MYSPACE

•ME••••

AMEBOID
AMENDED
AMENDER
AMENITY
AMERADA
AMERCED
AMERCER
AMERCES
AMERICA
AMERIGO
AMERIKA
AMERIND
AMESLAN
EMENDED
EMENDER
EMERALD
EMERGED
EMERGES
EMERIES
EMERITA
EMERITI
EMERSED
EMERSON
EMETICS
IMEANIT
IMEMINE
KMESONS
OMELETS
OMENING
SMEAGOL
SMEARED
SMEARER
SMEARON
SMELLED
SMELLER
SMELTED
SMELTER
SMETANA

•M•E•••

AMHERST
AMMETER
AMNERIS
AMNESIA
AMNESIC
AMNESTY
AMOEBAE
AMOEBAS
AMOEBIC
AMPEDUP
AMPERES
AMREETA
EMPEROR
IMMENSE
IMMERGE
IMMERSE
IMPEACH
IMPEDED
IMPEDER
IMPEDES
IMPENDS
IMPERIL
IMPETUS
IMREADY
UMBERED
UMBERTO

•M••E••

AMADEUS
AMATEUR
AMBIENS
AMBIENT
AMBLERS
AMPLEST
AMREETA
AMSTELS
AMULETS
AMUSEME
AMUSERS
EMBLEMS
EMINENT
EMOTERS
EMPRESS
IMADEIT
IMAGERS
IMAGERY
IMAMESS
IMARETS
IMGREAT
IMOGENE
IMPIETY
IMPLEAD
IMPRESS
IMPREST
IMPREZA
IMSWELL
IMTHERE
OMELETS
SMILEAT
SMILEON
SMILERS
SMILEYS
SMITERS
SMOKERS
SMOKEUP
SMOKEYS
UMPTEEN

•M•••E•

AMASSED
AMASSER
AMASSES
AMBRIES
AMENDED
AMENDER
AMERCED
AMERCER
AMERCES
AMITIES
AMMETER
AMPERES
AMPULES
BMOVIES
EMAILED
EMAILER
EMANUEL
EMBAYED
EMBOWER
EMBRUED
EMBRUES
EMENDED
EMENDER
EMERGED
EMERGES
EMERIES
EMERSED
EMIGREE
EMIGRES
EMITTED
EMITTER
EMPALED
EMPALES
EMPANEL
EMPIRES
EMPOWER
EMPTIED
EMPTIER
EMPTIES
IMAGOES
IMBIBED
IMBIBER
IMBIBES
IMBORED
IMBRUED
IMBRUES
IMHOTEP
IMMIXED
IMMIXES
IMMUNES
IMMURED
IMMURES
IMPALED
IMPALER
IMPALES
IMPANEL
IMPEDED
IMPEDER
IMPEDES
IMPLIED
IMPLIES
IMPOSED
IMPOSER
IMPOSES
IMPURER
IMPUTED
IMPUTER
IMPUTES
IMTIRED
OMALLEY
OMITTED
OMITTER
SMACKED
SMACKER
SMALLER
SMARTED
SMARTEN
SMARTER
SMASHED
SMASHER
SMASHES
SMATTER
SMEARED
SMEARER
SMELLED
SMELLER
SMELTED
SMELTER
SMIDGEN
SMIDGES
SMIRKED
SMIRKER
SMITHED
SMITTEN
SMOKIER
SMOKIES
SMOLDER
SMOTHER
SMUCKER
SMUDGED
SMUDGES
SMUGGER
SMUSHED
SMUSHES
UMBERED
UMBRIEL
UMPIRED
UMPIRES
UMPTEEN

•M••••E

AMARONE
AMATIVE
AMBROSE
AMIABLE
AMIBLUE
AMILATE
AMINUTE
AMOEBAE
AMPOULE
AMUSEME
AMYLASE
EMANATE
EMBLAZE
EMBOITE
EMBRACE
EMIGREE
EMIRATE
EMOTIVE
EMPLACE
EMPLANE
EMPRISE
EMULATE
IMAGINE
IMAMATE
IMBROKE
IMEMINE
IMITATE
IMMENSE
IMMERGE
IMMERSE
IMOGENE
IMPASSE
IMPINGE
IMPLODE
IMPLORE
IMPROVE
IMPULSE
IMTHERE
OMAHANE
SMUGGLE
TMOBILE
UMBRAGE

••ME•••

AIMEDAT
ALMERIA
AMMETER
ARMENIA
BIMETAL
CAMEDUE
CAMELID
CAMELOT
CAMEOED
CAMEOFF
CAMEOUT
CAMERAE
CAMERAL
CAMERAS
CAMERON
CEMENTS
COMEDIA
COMEDIC
COMEDIE
COMEDUE
COMENOW
COMEOFF
COMEONS
COMEOUT
COMESAS
COMESAT
COMESBY
COMESIN
COMESON
COMESTO
COMESUP
DEMEANS
DEMENTO
DEMERGE
DEMERIT
DEMEROL
DEMESNE
DEMETER
DIMETER
DOMECAR
DRMELFI
EDMEESE
FOMENTS
FTMEADE
FUMEDAT
FUMESAT
GAMEBAG
GAMEBOY
GAMELAN
GAMELAW
GAMELEG
GAMETAL
GAMETES
GEMELLI
HAMELIN
HOMEBOY
HOMEDIN
HOMEICE
HOMEIER
HOMELAB
HOMERED
HOMERIC
HOMERUN
HOMESIN
HUMERAL
HUMERUS
IMMENSE
IMMERGE
IMMERSE
JAMESII
JAMESIV
JAMESON
JAMESVI
JIMENEZ
KAMERAD
LAMENTS
LIMEADE
LIMEPIE
MEMENTO
MIMEOED
MIMESES
MIMESIS
MIMETIC
MOMENTA
MOMENTS
MUMESON
NAMEDAY
NAMEONE
NAMETAG
NEMEROV
NEMESES
NEMESIS
NOMERCY
NOMERGE
NUMERAL
NUMERIC
NUMEROS
PIMENTO
PIMESON
POMELOS
RAMEKIN
RAMESES
REMEETS
REMELTS
REMENDS
REMERGE
SAMEDAY
SAMEDIS
SAMEKHS
SAMEOLD
SIMENON
SOMEDAY
SOMEHOW
SOMEONE
SOMESAY
SOMEWAY
TIMECOP
TIMELAG
TIMEOFF
TIMEOUT
TIMESUP
TIMEWAS
TIMEXES
TUMESCE
UNMEANT
UNMERGE
UNMERRY
UNMEWED
VUMETER
XIMENES
YEMENIS

••M•E••

AIMLESS
ARMLESS
ARMLETS
ARMREST
ATMFEES
BOMBECK
BOMBERS
BUMDEAL
BUMLEGS
BUMMERS
BUMPERS
CAMBERS
CAMPERS
COMBERS
COMMEND
COMMENT
COMPEER
COMPELS
COMPEND
COMPERE
COMPETE
CUMBERS
DAMMERS
DAMNERS
DAMPENS
DAMPERS
DAMPEST
DAMSELS
DIMMERS
DIMMEST
DIMNESS
DUMBEST
DUMPERS
EDMEESE
ELMIEST
FTMYERS
FUMIEST
GAMIEST
GAMMERS
GEMLESS
GIMBELS
GIMLETS
GOMPERS
GUMLESS
HAMLETS
HAMMERS
HAMMETT
HAMPERS
HEMMERS
HIMSELF
HOMIEST
HUMBERT
HUMMELS
HUMMERS
HUMVEES
JAMBEAU
JAMMERS
JIMBEAM
JUMPERS
KUMMELS
LAMBEAU
LAMBENT
LAMBERT
LAMBETH
LAMPERT
LEMIEUX
LIMBERS
LIMIEST
LIMNERS
LIMPEST
LIMPETS
LUMBERS
LUMIERE
LUMPERS
MEMBERS
MIMIEUX
MUMMERS
MUMMERY
NIMIETY
NUMBERS
NUMBEST
PAMPERS
POMMELS
POMPEIA
POMPEII
PUMMELS
PUMPERS
RAMJETS
RAMMERS
RAMSESI
REMEETS
RIMIEST
RIMLESS
ROMBERG
ROMNEYS
ROMPERS
RUMLESS
RUMMERS
RUMPEND
SAMLETS
SAMUELL
SIMMERS
SIMPERS
SUMLESS
SUMMERS
SUMMERY
TAMPERS
TEMPEAZ
TEMPEHS
TEMPERA
TEMPERS
TEMPEST
TIMBERS
TIMBERY
TIMREID
VAMPERS
YAMMERS
ZAMBEZI

••M••E•

ADMIRED
ADMIRER
ADMIRES
ADMIXED
ADMIXES
ALMADEN
ALMONER
ALMSMEN
AMMETER
ARMORED
ARMORER
ATMFEES
BAMMIES
BEMIRED
BEMIRES
BEMUSED
BEMUSES
BIMBOES
BOMBLET
BUMBLED
BUMBLER
BUMBLES
BUMPIER
CAMEOED
CAMISES
CAMMIES
CAMPBED
CAMPIER
COMAKER
COMBIEN
COMFIER
COMICES
COMPEER
COMPLEX
COMTREX
DAMAGED
DAMAGES
DAMOSEL
DEMARET
DEMETER
DEMISED
DEMISES
DEMOTED
DEMOTES
DEMPSEY
DEMURER
DIMAGES
DIMETER
DIMPLED
DIMPLES
DIMVIEW
DUMMIED
DUMMIES
DUMPIER
ELMTREE
ERMINED
ERMINES
EXMATES
FAMINES
FEMALES
FUMBLED
FUMBLER
FUMBLES
GAMBIER
GAMBLED
GAMBLER
GAMBLES
GAMELEG
GAMETES
GAMINES
GEMAYEL
GEMMIER
GOMODEL
GUMMIER
GUMTREE
HAMITES
HAMMIER
HAMSTER
HEMPIER
HEMSLEY
HOMAGER
HOMAGES
HOMBRES
HOMEIER
HOMERED
HUMBLED
HUMBLER
HUMBLES
HUMIDEX
HUMORED
HUMPHED
HUMPIER
HUMUSES
HUMVEES
IMMIXED
IMMIXES
IMMUNES
IMMURED
IMMURES
INMATES
JAMMIER
JAMMIES
JIMCHEE
JIMENEZ
JIMINEZ
JIMMIED
JIMMIES
JTMONEY
JUMBLED
JUMBLER
JUMBLES
JUMPIER
KIMCHEE
LAMPREY
LIMITED
LIMITER
LIMOGES
LUMPIER
MAMBOED
MEMOREX
MIMEOED
MIMESES
MOMMIES
MOMMSEN
MOMONEY
MOMUSES
MUMBLED
MUMBLER

MUMBLES
MUMMIES
NEMESES
NIMBLER
NOMBRES
NOMINEE
OHMAGES
OLMSTED
OSMOSED
OSMOSES
PIMPLED
PIMPLES
POMADED
POMADES
PUMICED
PUMICES
RAMBLED
RAMBLER
RAMBLES
RAMESES
RAMIREZ
RAMONES
REMAKES
REMATED
REMATES
REMINED
REMINES
REMISED
REMISES
REMIXED
REMIXES
REMODEL
REMOTER
REMOTES
REMOVED
REMOVER
REMOVES
REMOWED
RIMPLED
RIMPLES
RUMBAED
RUMBLED
RUMBLER
RUMBLES
RUMMIES
RUMORED
RUMPLED
RUMPLES
SAMBAED
SAMISEN
SAMOSET
SAMOYED
SAMPLED
SAMPLER
SAMPLES
SEMITES
SIMILES
SIMPLER
SIMPLES
SIMPLEX
SOMINEX
TAMALES
TAMGLEN
TEMPLED
TEMPLES
TEMPTED
TEMPTER
TIMBRES

TIMEXES
TIMIDER
TUMBLED
TUMBLER
TUMBLES
TUMBREL
TUMMIES
TUMMLER
UNMAKER
UNMAKES
UNMANED
UNMATED
UNMATES
UNMEWED
UNMIKED
UNMINED
UNMIRED
UNMITER
UNMIXED
UNMIXES
UNMOVED
UNMOWED
UNMUTED
VAMPIER
VUMETER
WAMBLED
WAMBLES
WEMBLEY
WIMOWEH
WIMPIER
WIMPLED
WIMPLES
XIMENES
YUMMIER
ZOMBIES

••M•••E

AAMILNE
ARMBONE
ARMHOLE
ARMLIKE
ARMOIRE
CAMEDUE
CAMERAE
CAMILLE
CAMRYLE
CIMABUE
COMBINE
COMEDIE
COMEDUE
COMIQUE
COMMODE
COMMOVE
COMMUNE
COMMUTE
COMPARE
COMPERE
COMPETE
COMPILE
COMPOSE
COMPOTE
COMPUTE
COMRADE
DEMERGE
DEMESNE
DEMILLE
DOMAINE
EDMEESE

ELMONTE
ELMTREE
ENMASSE
FAMILLE
FTMEADE
GEMLIKE
GEMMATE
GUMLIKE
GUMSHOE
GUMTREE
GYMSHOE
HAMBONE
HAMLINE
HEMLINE
HOMEICE
HUMORME
IAMLOVE
IMMENSE
IMMERGE
IMMERSE
ITMAYBE
JAMLIKE
JIMCHEE
JIMDALE
JIMRICE
KIMCHEE
LAMINAE
LAMOTTE
LEMONDE
LEMOYNE
LIMEADE
LIMEPIE
LIMNITE
LUMIERE
MEMOIRE
MRMOOSE
NAMABLE
NAMEONE
NOMERGE
NOMINEE
RAMHOME
RAMLIKE
RAMPAGE
REMERGE
REMORSE
ROMAINE
ROMANCE
RUMCAKE
RUMMAGE
RUMPOLE
SAMWISE
SOMEONE
SUMMATE
TAMABLE
TEMPORE
TIMBALE
TIMRICE
TOMKITE
TUMESCE
TVMOVIE
UNMERGE
UNMITRE
VAMOOSE
VAMPIRE
WIMPOLE

•••ME••

ACUMENS

AILMENT
ALAMEDA
ALAMEIN
ALIMENT
ARAMEAN
AUGMENT
BEAMERS
BEEMERS
BESMEAR
BIGMEAL
BIGMESS
BLAMEON
BLAMERS
BOOMERS
BUMMERS
BURMESE
CALMEST
CARMELA
CHIMEIN
CHIMERA
CHIMERS
CLEMENS
CLEMENT
COMMEND
COMMENT
CRIMEAN
DAMMERS
DEHMELT
DIEMENS
DIMMERS
DIMMEST
DIOMEDE
DORMERS
DRAMEDY
ELEMENT
ENAMELS
FARMERS
FARMERY
FERMENT
FIGMENT
FIRMEST
FLAMERS
FLAMEUP
FOAMERS
FORMERS
FRAMERS
FRAMEUP
GAMMERS
GARMENT
HAMMERS
HAMMETT
HARMERS
HELMETS
HEMMERS
HOTMEAL
HUMMELS
HUMMERS
IMAMESS
INAMESS
ISOMERS
JAMMERS
KISMETS
KUMMELS
LETMEBE
LETMEGO
LETMEIN
MAIMERS
MISMESH

MUMMERS
MUMMERY
NONMEAT
NUTMEAT
NUTMEGS
OATMEAL
ODDMENT
PALMERS
PAYMENT
PIGMEAT
PIGMENT
POMMELS
PREMEDS
PREMEET
PRIMELY
PRIMERA
PRIMERO
PRIMERS
PUMMELS
RAIMENT
RAMMERS
RAWMEAT
REAMEND
REAMERS
REDMEAT
RESMELT
RHYMERS
RIBMEAT
ROAMERS
ROOMERS
RUMMERS
SCHMEAR
SCHMEER
SEAMERS
SEGMENT
SIAMESE
SIEMENS
SIMMERS
SOYMEAL
STAMENS
SUMMERS
SUMMERY
THEMETS
TORMENT
VERMEER
VERMEIL
WARMERS
WARMEST
WORMERS
YAMMERS

•••M•E•

ADAMSES
ANOMIES
ASIMMER
ATOMIES
BALMIER
BAMMIES
BARMIER
BEAMIER
BOOMIER
BOOMLET
BRAMLEY
BRIMLEY
BRIMMED
BRIMMER
BRUMMEL
CALMSEA

CAMMIES
CHAMBER
CHAMFER
CHAMPED
CHAMPER
CHIMNEY
CHOMPED
CHUMMED
CHUMPED
CLAMBER
CLAMMED
CLAMMER
CLAMPED
CLAMPER
CLIMBED
CLIMBER
CLOMPED
CLUMPED
CRAMMED
CRAMMER
CRAMPED
CRIMPED
CRIMPER
CRUMBED
CRUMPED
CRUMPET
DAIMLER
DAUMIER
DOOMIER
DRUMMED
DRUMMER
DRUMSET
DUMMIED
DUMMIES
ENEMIES
FILMIER
FILMSET
FLAMBED
FLAMBES
FLAMIER
FLAMMED
FNUMBER
FOAMIER
FROMMER
GEMMIER
GERMIER
GLIMMER
GLOMMED
GLUMMED
GLUMMER
GRAMMER
GRAMMES
GRIMIER
GRIMMER
GROMMET
GRUMPED
GUMMIER
HAMMIER
ISHMAEL
JAMMIER
JAMMIES
JIMMIED
JIMMIES
KLAMMER
KRAMDEN
LOAMIER
MALMSEY
MEEMIES

MOMMIES
MOMMSEN
MUMMIES
PALMIER
PLUMBED
PLUMBER
PLUMIER
PLUMMER
PLUMMET
PLUMPED
PLUMPER
PREMEET
PREMIER
PREMIES
PRIMMED
PRIMMER
PRIMPED
PROMOED
PYGMIES
ROOMIER
ROOMIES
RUMMIES
SCAMMED
SCAMMER
SCAMPED
SCAMPER
SCHMEER
SCHMOES
SEAMIER
SHAMMED
SHIMMER
SKIMMED
SKIMMER
SKIMPED
SLAMMED
SLAMMER
SLIMIER
SLIMMED
SLIMMER
SLUMBER
SLUMMED
SLUMMER
SLUMPED
SPAMMED
SPAMMER
SPUMIER
STAMMER
STAMPED
STAMPER
STEMMED
STEMPEL
STOMPED
STUMPED
STUMPER
STYMIED
STYMIES
SWAMPED
SWIMMER
THUMBED
THUMPED
THUMPER
TRAMMED
TRAMMEL
TRAMPED
TRAMPER
TRIMMED
TRIMMER
TROMPED

TRUMPED
TRUMPET
TUMMIES
TUMMLER
TZIMMES
VERMEER
WHAMMED
WHIMPER
WHOMPED
WORMIER
YUMMIER

•••M••E

ADAMITE
AGEMATE
AIRMILE
ALAMODE
ALLMALE
ALLMINE
ALUMNAE
ANDMORE
ANEMONE
ANIMATE
ANYMORE
ARDMORE
ATEMORE
ATOMISE
ATOMIZE
BADMOVE
BEDMATE
BLIMPIE
BRAMBLE
BROMATE
BROMIDE
BROMINE
BURMESE
BYAMILE
CARMINE
CHAMBRE
CHEMISE
CLIMATE
COMMODE
COMMOVE
COMMUNE
COMMUTE
CREMATE
CRUMBLE
CRUMPLE
DAYMARE
DELMORE
DIOMEDE
DORMICE
EATMORE
EDOMITE
ELAMITE
EREMITE
ETAMINE
EXAMINE
EXAMPLE
FARMORE
FERMATE
FROMAGE
GEMMATE
GERMANE
GILMORE
GLIMPSE
GRIMACE
GRUMBLE

HORMONE
ILLMADE
IMAMATE
IMEMINE
ITEMISE
ITEMIZE
ITEMONE
JASMINE
KENMORE
LABMICE
LAEMMLE
LETMEBE
MANMADE
MISMATE
MISMOVE
NEWMADE
NOTMINE
ONEMILE
ONEMORE
OUTMATE
OUTMODE
OUTMOVE
PALMATE
PAYMORE
PERMUTE
PETMICE
PETMULE
PISMIRE
PLUMAGE
PLUMOSE
PLUMPIE
PLUMULE
PREMADE
PREMAKE
PREMATE
PREMISE
PRIMATE
PROMISE
PROMOTE
REIMAGE
RUMMAGE
SAYMORE
SEAMILE
SHAMBLE
SIAMESE
SPUMONE
STUMBLE
SUMMATE
SURMISE
TENMILE
TERMITE
THIMBLE
THYMINE
TINMINE
TITMICE
TRAMPLE
TREMBLE
TWOMORE
YASMINE

••••ME•

ABDOMEN
ADWOMEN
AFRAMES
AGNOMEN
ALARMED
ALARMER
ALBUMEN

ALMSMEN
ASHAMED
ASIMMER
ASSUMED
ASSUMER
ASSUMES
ATHOMES
ATTIMES
BADOMEN
BAHAMEN
BALLMER
BASEMEN
BATSMEN
BECOMES
BELLMEN
BESTMEN
BETIMES
BIRDMEN
BIREMES
BLOOMED
BLOOMER
BOATMEN
BOGYMEN
BONDMEN
BOOKMEN
BOSOMED
BOSSMEN
BRIMMED
BRIMMER
BROOMED
BRUMMEL
BUSHMEN
BYNAMES
CALUMET
CARAMEL
CAROMED
CAVEMEN
CERUMEN
CHAPMEN
CHARMED
CHARMEN
CHARMER
CHROMED
CHROMES
CHUMMED
CLAIMED
CLAIMER
CLAMMED
CLAMMER
CLUBMED
COPYMEN
COZUMEL
CRAMMED
CRAMMER
CRANMER
CREAMED
CREAMER
CREWMEN
DAHOMEY
DEFAMED
DEFAMER
DEFAMES
DELIMEN
DENIMED
DOORMEN
DRAWMEN
DRAYMEN
DREAMED

DREAMER
DRUMMED
DRUMMER
DUHAMEL
DUSTMEN
ENARMED
ENZYMES
EXHUMED
EXHUMER
EXHUMES
FIREMEN
FLAGMEN
FLAMMED
FOOTMEN
FOREMEN
FREEMEN
FROGMEN
FROMMER
GATEMEN
GENOMES
GLEAMED
GLEEMEN
GLIMMER
GLOMMED
GLOOMED
GLUMMED
GLUMMER
GOODMEN
GOURMET
GRAMMER
GRAMMES
GRIMMER
GROMMET
GROOMED
GROOMER
HANGMEN
HEADMEN
HILLMEN
HOLYMEN
HOOPMEN
IDEAMEN
ILLUMED
ILLUMES
INCOMER
INCOMES
INHUMED
INHUMER
INHUMES
IRONMEN
JAZZMEN
JUNKMEN
JURYMEN
KINSMEN
KLAMMER
KLEZMER
KROEMER
LANDMEN
LATIMES
LEADMEN
LEGUMES
LENSMEN
LINEMEN
MADAMES
MADAMEX
MAILMEN
MAINMEN
MANXMEN
MEATMEN

MELAMED
MERIMEE
MILKMEN
MODEMED
MONOMER
NAVYMEN
NEWSMEN
NICEMEN
NONAMES
NYTIMES
OARSMEN
PDJAMES
PETEMEN
PLOWMEN
PLUMMER
PLUMMET
POLEMEN
POLYMER
POOLMEN
POORMEN
POSTMEN
PRIMMED
PRIMMER
PROPMEN
RACEMES
RADAMES
RADOMES
RAILMEN
REAIMED
REALMEN
REARMED
REEDMEN
REGIMEN
REGIMES
RELUMED
RELUMES
RENAMED
RENAMES
RESUMED
RESUMES
RETAMED
RETAMES
RETIMED
RETIMES
RICHMEN
SANDMEN
SAYAMEN
SCAMMED
SCAMMER
SCHEMED
SCHEMER
SCHEMES
SCHUMER
SESAMES
SHAMMED
SHIMMER
SHIPMEN
SHOWMEN
SIDEMEN
SKIMMED
SKIMMER
SLAMMED
SLAMMER
SLIMMED
SLIMMER
SLUMMED
SLUMMER
SNOWMEN

SPAMMED
SPAMMER
STAMMER
STEAMED
STEAMER
STEMMED
STJAMES
STORMED
SURFMEN
SWAGMEN
SWARMED
SWARMER
SWIMMER
TAGAMET
TAPEMEN
TAXIMEN
THEOMEN
TIREMEN
TOHOMER
TOLLMEN
TONEMES
TRAMMED
TRAMMEL
TRIMMED
TRIMMER
TURFMEN
TVGAMES
TZIMMES
UNAIMED
UNARMED
UNDOMED
UNFAMED
UNNAMED
UNRIMED
UNTAMED
UNTAMES
UNTIMED
UPTIMES
VOLUMED
VOLUMES
VROOMED
WAKAMES
WHAMMED
WHELMED
WILDMEN
WINGMEN
WIREMEN
WISEMEN
WOLFMEN
WORKMEN
YALEMEN
YARDMEN

••••M•E

AUTOMNE
ELLAMAE
LAEMMLE
LAFEMME
LARAMIE
MERIMEE
PREEMIE
RITAMAE
VICOMTE

•••••ME

ACADEME
AIRTIME
ALLOFME

7 ME

ALLOWME
ALLTIME
AMUSEME
ANYTIME
ATATIME
AWESOME
BADNAME
BADTIME
BEATSME
BEDTIME
BEGRIME
BELDAME
BIGGAME
BIGNAME
BIGTIME
BUDTIME
BUYTIME
CENTIME
CONGAME
CONSUME
COSTUME
COVERME
CUTTIME
DAYGAME
DAYTIME
DEFRAME
DELORME
DIDTIME
DRINKME
ELECTME
ENDGAME
ENFLAME
ENFRAME
EPITOME
EXTREME
FULSOME
FUNTIME
GENZYME
GINGAME
GRAHAME
HADSOME
HADTIME
HASTIME
HITHOME
HOTTIME
HOWCOME
HOWLAME
HUMORME
INFLAME
IRKSOME
ITSONME
ITSTIME
JIGTIME
KEYLIME
LAFEMME
LANCOME
LISSOME
MACRAME
MARRYME
MAYTIME
MILLIME
MISNAME
MISTIME
NAPTIME
NATSUME
NBAGAME
NETGAME
NEWNAME
NEWSOME
NFLGAME
NHLGAME
NOISOME
NONHOME
NOTHOME
OLDLYME
OLDTIME
ONEDIME
ONENAME
ONETIME
OUTCOME
OUTGAME
PASTIME
PENNAME
PERFUME
PETNAME
PHONEME
PINCHME
PREGAME
PRENAME
PRESUME
PUBGAME
RAGTIME
RAMHOME
RANHOME
RCADOME
RECLAME
REFRAME
REPLUME
REPRIME
RHIZOME
RUNHOME
RUNTIME
SAOTOME
SATHOME
SCUSEME
SILLYME
SITHOME
SKYDOME
SOSUEME
SPAREME
SUBLIME
SUBSUME
SUITSME
SUPREME
SURNAME
TEATIME
TEETIME
THEGAME
THESAME
TIEGAME
TOBLAME
TOPNAME
TRIREME
TRUSTME
TWOSOME
TWOTIME
ULALUME
UNRHYME
VENDOME
WARGAME
WARTIME
WELCOME
WINSOME
WOEISME
WRITEME

M•F••••
MAFIOSI
MAFIOSO
MEFIRST
MIFFIER
MIFFING
MIFFLIN
MRFIXIT
MUFFING
MUFFINS
MUFFLED
MUFFLER
MUFFLES
MYFAULT

M••F•••
MAHFOUZ
MANFRED
MAYFAIR
MEDFORD
MENFOLK
METFANS
MIFFIER
MIFFING
MIFFLIN
MISFEED
MISFILE
MISFIRE
MISFITS
MISFORM
MITFORD
MUDFISH
MUDFLAP
MUDFLAT
MUDFLOW
MUFFING
MUFFINS
MUFFLED
MUFFLER
MUFFLES
MUGFULS
MUMFORD

M•••F••
MADEFIT
MADEFOR
MADEFUN
MAKEFIT
MAKEFOR
MAKEFUN
MALEFIC
METSFAN
MIDOFFS
MILKFED
MINDFUL
MOANFUL
MUSEFUL

M••••F•
MACDUFF
MADEOFF
MAGNIFY
MAKEOFF
MARKOFF
MASSIFS
MASTIFF
MCGRIFF
MCGRUFF
METLIFE
MIAMIFL
MIDLIFE
MIDOFFS
MIDRIFF
MIDWIFE
MOLLIFY
MORTIFY
MOVEOFF
MUMMIFY
MUSTAFA
MYCROFT
MYSTIFY
MYTHIFY

M•••••F
MACDUFF
MADEOFF
MAKEOFF
MARKOFF
MASTIFF
MCGRIFF
MCGRUFF
METCALF
MIDRIFF
MORCERF
MOVEOFF

•MF••••
IMFORIT

•M•••F•
AMPLIFY

•M••••F
SMACKOF

••MF•••
ARMFULS
ATMFEES
COMFIER
COMFITS
COMFORT
JIMFIXX
KAMFONG
MUMFORD
RAMFANS
RUMFORD
TOMFOOL

••M•F••
AIMSFOR
RAMSFAN

••M••F•
CAMEOFF
COMEOFF
DAMPOFF
DRMELFI
JUMPOFF
MUMMIFY
SAMHUFF
TAMPAFL
TIMEOFF
ZOMBIFY

••M•••F
CAMEOFF
COMEOFF
DAMPOFF
HIMSELF
JUMPOFF
SAMHUFF
TIMEOFF

•••MF••
BRIMFUL
CHAMFER
DOOMFUL
FORMFUL
HARMFUL
PALMFUL
ROOMFUL

•••M•F•
EARMUFF
MIAMIFL
MUMMIFY
PALMOFF
TRIMOFF

•••M••F
EARMUFF
PALMOFF
TRIMOFF

••••M•F
DREAMOF

MG•••••
MGMLION

M•G••••
MAGALOG
MAGENTA
MAGGOTS
MAGICAL
MAGILLA
MAGINOT
MAGLEVS
MAGNANI
MAGNATE
MAGNETO
MAGNETS
MAGNIFY
MAGNUMS
MAGPIES
MAGUIRE
MAGYARS
MCGAVIN
MCGRIFF
MCGRORY
MCGRUFF
MCGUIRE
MCGWIRE
MEGABIT
MEGAERA
MEGAERG
MEGAHIT
MEGALON
MEGANES
MEGATON
MEGILLA
MEGOHMS
MEGRIMS
MEGRYAN
MIGENES
MIGHTNT
MIGNONS
MIGRANT
MIGRATE
MOGADOR
MOGAMBO
MRGREEN
MUGFULS
MUGGERS
MUGGIER
MUGGING
MUGGISH
MUGGLES
MUGSHOT
MUGWUMP
MYGIANT

M••G•••
MACGRAW
MAGGOTS
MAIGRET
MAJGENS
MANGANO
MANGERS
MANGIER
MANGLED
MANGLER
MANGLES
MANGOES
MARGATE
MARGAUX
MARGERY
MARGINS
MARGRET
MAUGHAM
MEAGLES
MERGEES
MERGERS
MERGING
MIDGETS
MINGIER
MINGLED
MINGLER
MINGLES
MISGAVE
MISGIVE
MONGERS
MONGKUT
MONGOLS
MONGREL
MORGANA
MORGANS
MORGUES
MUGGERS
MUGGIER
MUGGING
MUGGISH
MUGGLES
MULGREW

M•••G••
MADIGAN
MALAGAN
MALAGAS
MALIGNS
MANAGED
MANAGER
MANAGES
MANAGUA
MANEGES
MEDIGAP
MENAGES
MILAGRO
MINOGUE
MIRAGES
MOHEGAN
MOONGOD
MRMAGOO
MRRIGHT
MRTIGER
MTLOGAN
MUSIGNY
MUTAGEN
MYALGIA
MYALGIC

M••••G•
MACONGA
MADDOGS
MAKESGO
MAKINGS
MARENGO
MASSAGE
MAYINGS
MAYTAGS
MEANAGE
MELANGE
MELTAGE
MESHUGA
MESSAGE
MIDLEGS
MILEAGE
MILLAGE
MININGS
MINTAGE
MISPAGE
MONTAGE
MONTAGU
MONTEGO
MOORAGE
MOULAGE
MOWINGS
MUSINGS
MUSKEGO
MYOLOGY

M•••••G
MADDING
MAGALOG
MAILBAG
MAILING
MAIMING
MALEDOG
MALEHOG
MALEPIG
MALTING
MANNING
MAPPING
MARKING
MARRING
MASHING
MASKING
MASSING
MASTING
MATTING
MAULING
MCCLURG
MEANING
MEETING
MEGAERG
MELDING
MELTING
MEMLING
MENDING
MEOWING
MERGING
MESHING
MESSING
MEWLING
MIFFING
MILKING
MILLING
MINCING
MINDING
MINTING
MISSING
MISTING
MITRING
MOANING
MOBBING
MOCKING
MOEBERG
MOILING
MOLDING
MOLTING
MONOLOG
MOONDOG
MOONING
MOORING
MOOTING
MOPPING
MORNING
MOSHING
MOSSING
MOUSING
MRWRONG
MUCKING
MUDDING
MUFFING
MUGGING
MULLING
MUMMING
MUSHING
MUSSING
MUSTANG

•MG••••
IMGOING
IMGREAT

•M•G•••
EMIGREE
EMIGRES
IMAGERS
IMAGERY
IMAGINE
IMAGING
IMAGISM
IMAGIST
IMAGOES
IMOGENE
OMIGOSH
SMUGGER
SMUGGLE

•M••G••
AMALGAM
AMONGST
EMERGED
EMERGES
IMPUGNS
SMEAGOL
SMIDGEN
SMIDGES
SMUDGED
SMUDGES
SMUGGER
SMUGGLE

•M•••G•
AMERIGO
EMBARGO
IMAHOGG
IMMERGE
IMPINGE
IMUSTGO
UMBRAGE

•M••••G
AMAZING
AMBLING
AMUSING
EMOTING
IMAGING
IMAHOGG
IMBUING
IMGOING
OMENING
SMILING
SMITING
SMOKING

••MG•••
CAMGIRL
TAMGLEN
TOMGOLA

••M•G••
DAMAGED
DAMAGES
DEMAGOG
DEMIGOD
DIMAGES
HOMAGER
HOMAGES
LIMOGES
MRMAGOO
OHMAGES

••M••G•
AIMHIGH
BUMLEGS
COMINGS
DEMERGE
DOMINGO
GYMBAGS
HUMBUGS
IMMERGE
JIMHOGG
LUMBAGO
NOMERGE
RAMPAGE
REMERGE
RUMMAGE
TIMINGS
UNMERGE
ZYMURGY

••M•••G
BAMMING
BOMBING
BUMMING
BUMPING
CAMPING
COMBING
COMPING
DAMMING
DAMNING
DAMPING
DEMAGOG
DEMOING
DIMMING
DUMBING
DUMPING
GAMEBAG
GAMELEG
GAMMING
GIMPING
GUMMING
HAMBURG
HAMMING
HEMMING
HOMBURG
HUMMING
HYMNING
JAMMING
JIMHOGG
JUMPING
KAMFONG
LAMBING
LAMMING
LEMMING
LIMBING
LIMBURG
LIMNING
LIMPING
LUMPING
MEMLING
MUMMING
NAMETAG
NUMBING
PUMPING
RAMMING
RAMPING
RIMMING
ROMBERG
ROMPING
SAMSUNG
SEMILOG
SUMMING
TAMPING
TEMPING
TIMELAG
VAMPING
WIMPING

•••MG••
FARMGAL

•••M•G•
DESMOGS
FROMAGE
LETMEGO
NUTMEGS
PLUMAGE
REIMAGE
RUMMAGE
THEMAGI

•••M••G
BAMMING
BEAMING
BERMING
BLAMING
BOOMING
BUMMING
CALMING
CHIMING
DAMMING
DEEMING
DIMMING
DOOMING
FARMING
FILMING
FIRMING
FLAMING
FLEMING
FOAMING
FORMING
FRAMING
GAMMING
GORMING
GRIMING
GUMMING
HAMMING
HARMING
HELMING
HEMMING
HUMMING
ITEMING
JAMMING
LAMMING
LEMMING
LOAMING
LOOMING
MAIMING
MUMMING
PALMING
PERMING
PLUMING
PRIMING
RAMMING
REAMING
RHYMING
RIMMING
ROAMING
ROOMING
SEAMING
SEEMING
SHAMING
SLIMING
SPUMING
SUMMING
TEAMING
TEEMING
TERMING
WARMING
WORMING
WYOMING
YAOMING
ZOOMING

••••M•G
BEERMUG

M•H••••
MAHALIA
MAHARIS
MAHATMA
MAHDISM
MAHDIST
MAHFOUZ
MAHONEY
MAHOUTS
MAHZORS
MCHALES
MCHENRY
MOHAIRS
MOHAVES
MOHAWKS
MOHEGAN
MOHICAN
MRHANEY
MRHOBBS
MRHORSE
MRHULOT

M••H•••
MACHAON
MACHETE
MACHINA
MACHINE
MACHONE
MACHREE
MACHSIX
MACHTWO
MANHEIM
MANHOLE
MANHOOD
MANHOUR
MANHUNT
MARHAUS
MASHERS
MASHIES
MASHING
MATHERS
MATHEWS
MATHIAS
MATHIEU
MAYHEMS
MCSHANE
MECHLIN
MESHACH
MESHIER
MESHING
MESHUGA
METHANE
METHODS
MIAHAMM
MICHAEL
MICHAUX
MIGHTNT
MIKHAIL
MILHAUD
MILHOUS
MISHAPS
MISHEAR
MISHIMA
MISHITS
MISHNAH
MITHRAS
MOCHRIE
MOPHEAD
MOSHERS
MOSHING
MOSHPIT
MOTHERS
MOTHERY
MOTHIER
MPTHREE
MRCHIPS
MUDHENS
MUDHOLE
MULHARE
MUSHERS
MUSHIER
MUSHILY
MUSHING
MYNHEER
MYTHIFY

M•••H••
MADCHEN
MADEHAY
MAKEHAY
MALEHOG
MALTHUS
MARCHED
MARCHER
MARCHES
MARCHON
MARKHAM
MARSHAL
MARSHES
MATCHED
MATCHER
MATCHES
MATCHUP
MATTHAU
MATTHEW
MAUGHAM
MCLUHAN
MCMAHON
MEGAHIT
MEGOHMS
MEMPHIS
MENTHOL
MENUHIN
MERCHES
MIDSHIP
MISSHIP
MITCHUM
MONTHLY
MOOCHED
MOOCHER
MOOCHES
MOORHEN
MORPHED
MORPHIC
MORPHIN
MOUTHED
MOUTHER
MTATHOS

7 MF

MUGSHOT
MULCHED
MULCHES
MUNCHED
MUNCHEN
MUNCHER
MUNCHES
MUNCHIE
MUNCHON
MURPHYS
MYRRHED
MYRRHIC

M••••H•
MALACHI
MATZOHS
MENSCHY
MIZRAHI
MRMACHO
MRRIGHT
MULCAHY
MULLAHS

M•••••H
MACBETH
MADDASH
MADDISH
MADRUSH
MAIDISH
MAMMOTH
MANNISH
MATZOTH
MAWKISH
MENORAH
MESHACH
MESSIAH
METWITH
MEZUZAH
MINXISH
MIRISCH
MISHNAH
MISMESH
MISSISH
MITZVAH
MOBBISH
MONARCH
MONKISH
MOONISH
MOORISH
MRMARCH
MRNORTH
MRSMITH
MUDBATH
MUDFISH
MUGGISH
MURDOCH
MURKISH

•MH••••
AMHARIC
AMHERST
IMHAPPY
IMHOTEP

•M•H•••
AMPHION
AMPHORA
IMAHOGG
IMTHERE
OMAHANE
OMAHANS
OMPHALO

•M••H••
AMICHAI
SMASHED
SMASHER
SMASHES
SMASHUP
SMITHED
SMOTHER
SMUSHED
SMUSHES

•M•••H•
EMPATHS
EMPATHY
SMOOTHS
SMOOTHY

•M••••H
IMPEACH
OMIGOSH

••MH•••
AIMHIGH
ARMHOLE
HAMHOCK
JIMHOGG
RAMHOME
SAMHILL
SAMHUFF
TIMHOLT

••M•H••
CAMPHOR
CUMSHAW
GUMSHOE
GYMSHOE
HUMPHED
HUMPHRY
JIMCHEE
KIMCHEE
MCMAHON
MEMPHIS
NYMPHAL
NYMPHIC
RIMSHOT
RUMSHOP
SOMEHOW
YAMAHAS

••M••H•
CAMACHO
DEMOTHS
HAMACHI
IOMOTHS
MRMACHO
OOMPAHS
SAMEKHS
TEMPEHS
TIMOTHY
UNMACHO

••M•••H
AIMHIGH
BUMRUSH
BYMOUTH
COMMISH
DAMPISH
DUMPISH
INMARCH
JOMARCH
LAMBETH
LUMPISH
MAMMOTH
MRMARCH
RAMMISH
REMATCH
ROMANSH
ROMPISH
TIMROTH
VAMPISH
WIMOWEH
WIMPISH

•••M•H•
THIMPHU

•••M••H
ALSMITH
AZIMUTH
BEAMISH
BISMUTH
BLEMISH
CHIMINH
CHUMASH
COMMISH
FLEMISH
GNOMISH
GOOMBAH
HAIMISH
HOWMUCH
KLAMATH
MAMMOTH
MISMESH
MRSMITH
NESMITH
NEWMATH
NOTMUCH
RAMMISH
STOMACH
TOOMUCH
WARMISH
WORMISH

••••M•H
GALUMPH
NKRUMAH
TRIUMPH

MI•••••
MIAHAMM
MIAMIAN
MIAMIFL
MIAOUED
MIAOWED
MIASARA
MIASMAL
MIASMAS
MIASMIC
MICAELA
MICHAEL
MICHAUX
MICKEYS
MICMACS
MICROBE
MICRONS
MIDASES
MIDCAPS
MIDDAYS
MIDDIES
MIDDLEC
MIDDLED
MIDDLER
MIDDLES
MIDEAST
MIDGETS
MIDIRON
MIDJULY
MIDJUNE
MIDLAND
MIDLEGS
MIDLIFE
MIDLINE
MIDLIST
MIDMORN
MIDMOST
MIDNOON
MIDOFFS
MIDRIBS
MIDRIFF
MIDRISE
MIDSHIP
MIDSIZE
MIDSOLE
MIDTEEN
MIDTERM
MIDTOWN
MIDWAYS
MIDWEEK
MIDWEST
MIDWIFE
MIDYEAR
MIFFIER
MIFFING
MIFFLIN
MIGENES
MIGHTNT
MIGNONS
MIGRANT
MIGRATE
MIKADOS
MIKASAS
MIKHAIL
MILAGRO
MILDEST
MILDEWS
MILDEWY
MILDRED
MILEAGE
MILERUN
MILHAUD
MILHOUS
MILIEUS
MILIEUX
MILITIA
MILKBAR
MILKCAN
MILKCOW
MILKDUD
MILKERS
MILKFED
MILKIER
MILKILY
MILKING
MILKMAN
MILKMEN
MILKRUN
MILKSOP
MILLAGE
MILLAIS
MILLAND
MILLARD
MILLDAM
MILLEND
MILLERS
MILLETS
MILLETT
MILLIME
MILLING
MILLION
MILLRUN
MILORDS
MIMEOED
MIMESES
MIMESIS
MIMETIC
MIMICRY
MIMIEUX
MIMOSAS
MINABLE
MINARET
MINCERS
MINCING
MINDERS
MINDFUL
MINDING
MINDORO
MINDSET
MINEOLA
MINEPIT
MINERAL
MINERVA
MINGIER
MINGLED
MINGLER
MINGLES
MINIBAR
MINIBUS
MINICAB
MINICAM
MINICAR
MINIKIN
MINILAB
MINIMAL
MINIMAX
MINIMUM
MINIMUS
MININGS
MINIONS
MINISKI
MINISUB
MINITVS
MINIVAC
MINIVAN
MINIVER
MINIZOO
MINNOWS
MINOANS
MINOGUE
MINOLTA
MINORCA
MINORED
MINORIN
MINOTND
MINSKYS
MINSTER
MINTAGE
MINTERS
MINTIER
MINTING
MINTTEA
MINUEND
MINUETS
MINUSES
MINUTED
MINUTER
MINUTES
MINUTIA
MINXISH
MINYANS
MIOCENE
MIRABEL
MIRACLE
MIRADAS
MIRADOR
MIRAGES
MIRAMAR
MIRAMAX
MIRANDA
MIRIEST
MIRISCH
MIRRORS
MISACTS
MISADDS
MISAIMS
MISALLY
MISAVER
MISBILL
MISBIND
MISBREW
MISCALL
MISCAST
MISCITE
MISCODE
MISCOIN
MISCOPY
MISCUED
MISCUES
MISCUTS
MISDATE
MISDEAL
MISDEED
MISDEEM
MISDIAL
MISDOER
MISDOES
MISDONE
MISDRAW
MISDREW
MISEDIT
MISERLY
MISFEED
MISFILE
MISFIRE
MISFITS
MISFORM
MISGAVE
MISGIVE
MISHAPS
MISHEAR
MISHIMA
MISHITS
MISHNAH
MISJOIN
MISKEYS
MISKNEW
MISKNOW
MISKOLC
MISLAID
MISLAYS
MISLEAD
MISLIKE
MISMARK
MISMATE
MISMESH
MISMOVE
MISNAME
MISPAGE
MISPLAN
MISPLAY
MISRATE
MISREAD
MISRELY
MISRULE
MISSAID
MISSALS
MISSAYS
MISSEAT
MISSEND
MISSENT
MISSETS
MISSHIP
MISSIES
MISSILE
MISSING
MISSION
MISSISH
MISSIVE
MISSORT
MISSOUT
MISSTEP
MISSUSA
MISSYOU
MISTAKE
MISTBOW
MISTELL
MISTERM
MISTERS
MISTERX
MISTIER
MISTILY
MISTIME
MISTING
MISTOLD
MISTOOK
MISTRAL
MISTSUP
MISTUNE
MISTYPE
MISUSED
MISUSER
MISUSES
MISWIRE
MISWORD
MISZONE
MITCHUM
MITERED
MITFORD
MITHRAS
MITOSES
MITOSIS
MITOTIC
MITRING
MITTENS
MITZVAH
MIXABLE
MIXEDIN
MIXEDLY
MIXEDUP
MIXESIN
MIXESUP
MIXITUP
MIXTECS
MIXTURE
MIZRAHI
MIZUNAS
MIZZENS
MIZZLED
MIZZLES

M•I••••
MAIDENS
MAIDISH
MAIGRET
MAILBAG
MAILBIN
MAILBOX
MAILCAR
MAILERS
MAILING
MAILINS
MAILLOL
MAILLOT
MAILMAN
MAILMEN
MAILOUT
MAILSIN
MAIMERS
MAIMING
MAIMITI
MAINERS
MAINMAN
MAINMEN
MAINTOP
MAISONS
MAISOUI
MAITAIS
MAITRED
MAITRES
MEIOSES
MEIOSIS
MEIOTIC
MEISSEN
MEISTER
MEITNER
MOILERS
MOILING
MOISSAN
MOISTEN
MOISTER
MOISTLY
MRISCAN
MSIEURS

M••I•••
MADIGAN
MADISON
MAFIOSI
MAFIOSO
MAGICAL
MAGILLA
MAGINOT
MAKINGS
MALIANS
MALICES
MALIGNS
MANIACS
MANIKIN
MANILAS
MANILOW
MANIPLE
MANIPUR
MAOISTS
MARIANA
MARIANO
MARIDAS
MARIDOS
MARILLA
MARILYN
MARIMBA
MARINAS
MARINER
MARINES
MARITAL
MATILDA
MATINAL
MATINEE
MATISSE
MAVISES
MAXILLA
MAXIMAL
MAXIMAS
MAXIMUM
MAXIMUS
MAXIXES
MAYINGS
MAZIEST
MEDIANS
MEDIANT
MEDIATE
MEDICAL
MEDICOS
MEDIGAP
MEDIUMS
MEDIVAC
MEFIRST
MEGILLA
MELINDA
MELISMA
MELISSA
MELITTA
MENIALS
MENISCI
MERIDEN
MERIMEE
MERINOS
MERITED
METIERS
MEXICAN
MIDIRON
MILIEUS
MILIEUX
MILITIA
MIMICRY
MIMIEUX
MINIBAR
MINIBUS
MINICAB
MINICAM
MINICAR
MINIKIN
MINILAB
MINIMAL
MINIMAX
MINIMUM
MINIMUS
MININGS
MINIONS
MINISKI
MINISUB
MINITVS
MINIVAC
MINIVAN
MINIVER
MINIZOO
MIRIEST
MIRISCH
MIXITUP
MOBILES
MODICUM
MODISTE
MOHICAN
MOJITOS
MOLIERE
MOLITOR
MONIKER
MONITOR
MOPIEST
MORISOT
MOTIONS
MOTIVED
MOTIVES
MOWINGS
MOZILLA
MRFIXIT
MRRIGHT
MRTIBBS
MRTIGER
MTSINAI
MURIELS
MURILLO
MUSICAL
MUSICKS
MUSIGNY
MUSINGS
MYGIANT
MYRIADS

M•••I••
MACHINA
MACHINE
MADDING
MADDISH
MADEILL
MADEIRA
MADLIBS
MAGNIFY
MAGPIES
MAGUIRE
MAHDISM
MAHDIST
MAIDISH
MAILING
MAILINS
MAIMING
MAIMITI
MAKEILL
MALAISE
MALDIVE
MALLIKA
MALTIER
MALTING
MALVINA
MANCINI
MANGIER
MANKIND
MANLIER
MANLIKE
MANNIES
MANNING
MANNISH
MANRICO
MANSION
MANSIZE
MAPPING
MARDIAN
MARGINS
MARKIII
MARKING
MARLIER
MARLINS
MARMION
MARNIER
MARRIED
MARRIES
MARRING
MARTIAL
MARTIAN
MARTINA
MARTINI
MARTINO
MARTINS
MARTINU
MARTINV
MARTIUS
MARVIER
MARXIAN
MARXISM
MARXIST
MASHIES
MASHING
MASKING
MASSIER
MASSIFS
MASSINE
MASSING
MASSIVE
MASTICS
MASTIFF
MASTING
MATHIAS
MATHIEU
MATTING
MAULING
MAURIAC
MAURIAT
MAURICE
MAWKISH
MAYTIME
MAYWINE
MAZZINI
MCBRIDE
MCGRIFF
MCGUIRE
MCGWIRE
MCNEILL
MCSWINE
MEALIER
MEALIES
MEANIES
MEANING
MEATIER
MEATILY
MEDWICK
MEEMIES
MEETING
MEGRIMS
MELDING
MELTING
MEMLING
MEMOIRE
MEMOIRS
MENCIUS
MENDING
MENTION
MENZIES
MEOWING
MERCIAN
MERCIES
MERGING
MERLINS
MERRIAM
MERRICK
MERRIER
MERRILL
MERRILY
MESHIER
MESHING
MESSIAH
MESSICK
MESSIER
MESSILY
MESSINA
MESSING
METLIFE
METRICS
METRIST
METWITH
MEWLING
MGMLION
MIAMIAN
MIAMIFL
MIDDIES
MIDLIFE
MIDLINE
MIDLIST
MIDRIBS
MIDRIFF
MIDRISE
MIDSIZE
MIDWIFE
MIFFIER
MIFFING
MILKIER
MILKILY
MILKING
MILLIME
MILLING
MILLION
MINCING
MINDING
MINGIER
MINTIER
MINTING
MINXISH
MISAIMS
MISBILL
MISBIND
MISCITE
MISDIAL
MISFILE
MISFIRE
MISFITS
MISGIVE
MISHIMA
MISHITS
MISLIKE
MISSIES
MISSILE
MISSING
MISSION
MISSISH
MISSIVE
MISTIER
MISTILY
MISTIME
MISTING
MISWIRE
MITRING
MOABITE
MOANING
MOBBING
MOBBISH
MOBBISM
MOBBIST
MOCKING
MOHAIRS
MOILING
MOLDIER
MOLDING
MOLLIES
MOLLIFY
MOLTING
MOMMIES
MONDIAL
MONDIEU
MONKISH
MOODIER
MOODILY
MOONIER
MOONIES
MOONILY
MOONING
MOONISH
MOORIER
MOORING
MOORISH
MOOTING
MOPPING
MORAINE
MORNING
MORTICE

MORTIFY
MORTISE
MOSAICS
MOSHING
MOSSIER
MOSSING
MOTHIER
MOTRINS
MOUSIER
MOUSILY
MOUSING
MRBLISS
MRCHIPS
MRQUILP
MRSMITH
MUCKIER
MUCKING
MUDDIED
MUDDIER
MUDDIES
MUDDILY
MUDDING
MUDFISH
MUDPIES
MUFFING
MUFFINS
MUGGIER
MUGGING
MUGGISH
MULLING
MULLINS
MUMMIES
MUMMIFY
MUMMING
MURKIER
MURKILY
MURKISH
MUSCIDA
MUSHIER
MUSHILY
MUSHING
MUSKIER
MUSKIES
MUSLIMS
MUSLINS
MUSSIER
MUSSILY
MUSSING
MUSTIER
MUSTILY
MUYBIEN
MUZZIER
MUZZILY
MYOPIAS
MYSTICS
MYSTIFY
MYTHIFY

M••••I•

MACHSIX
MACNEIL
MADEFIT
MAHALIA
MAHARIS
MAILBIN
MAILSIN
MAITAIS
MAJORIN
MAKEFIT
MAKESIT
MALARIA
MALEFIC
MALEPIG
MALTBIE
MAMAMIA
MANHEIM
MANIKIN
MANOLIN
MANTRIC
MANUMIT
MAOSUIT
MARKIII
MARKVII
MARQUIS
MARRYIN
MASONIC
MASTOID
MATALIN
MAUDLIN
MAULDIN
MAUROIS
MAUVAIS
MAYALIN
MAYFAIR
MAZARIN
MCGAVIN
MEANSIT
MEANTIT
MEATPIE
MECHLIN
MEGABIT
MEGAHIT
MEIOSIS
MEIOTIC
MELANIA
MELANIC
MELANIE
MELANIN
MELODIA
MELODIC
MEMPHIS
MENUHIN
MEOWMIX
MERMAID
MESAMIS
MESONIC
MESSKIT
MIASMIC
MIDSHIP
MIFFLIN
MIKHAIL
MILITIA
MILLAIS
MIMESIS
MIMETIC
MINEPIT
MINIKIN
MINORIN
MINUTIA
MISCOIN
MISEDIT
MISJOIN
MISLAID
MISSAID
MISSHIP
MITOSIS
MITOTIC
MIXEDIN
MIXESIN
MOCHRIE
MONADIC
MONODIC
MOONLIT
MOONPIE
MORANIS
MORAVIA
MORONIC
MORPHIC
MORPHIN
MOSHPIT
MOUNTIE
MOVEDIN
MOVEDIT
MOVESIN
MOVESIT
MRFIXIT
MRMUSIC
MRSMUIR
MUESLIS
MUESLIX
MUEZZIN
MUNCHIE
MYALGIA
MYALGIC
MYRRHIC

M•••••I

MAFIOSI
MAGNANI
MAIMITI
MAISOUI
MALACHI
MANCINI
MANDOKI
MARCONI
MARKIII
MARKVII
MARTINI
MAZZINI
MENISCI
MENOTTI
MINISKI
MIZRAHI
MOLOKAI
MONDAVI
MONDESI
MONOSKI
MORETTI
MOSCONI
MTSINAI

•MI••••

AMIABLE
AMIABLY
AMIBLUE
AMICHAI
AMIDALA
AMIDOLS
AMILATE
AMINUTE
AMISTAD
AMITIES
EMIGREE
EMIGRES
EMINENT
EMIRATE
EMITTED
EMITTER
IMITATE
OMICRON
OMIGOSH
OMINOUS
OMITTED
OMITTER
SMIDGEN
SMIDGES
SMILEAT
SMILEON
SMILERS
SMILEYS
SMILING
SMILLAS
SMIRKED
SMIRKER
SMIRNOV
SMITERS
SMITHED
SMITING
SMITTEN

•M•I•••

AMBIENS
AMBIENT
AMNIONS
AMRITAS
EMAILED
EMAILER
EMPIRES
EMPIRIC
EMPIRIN
IMBIBED
IMBIBER
IMBIBES
IMMIXED
IMMIXES
IMPIETY
IMPINGE
IMPIOUS
IMTIRED
OMNIBUS
OMNIMAX
UMPIRED
UMPIRES

•M••I••

AMANITA
AMATIVE
AMAZING
AMBLING
AMBRIES
AMENITY
AMERICA
AMERIGO
AMERIKA
AMERIND
AMITIES
AMORIST
AMPHION
AMPLIFY
AMUSING
BMOVIES
EMBOITE
EMERIES
EMERITA
EMERITI
EMETICS
EMOTING
EMOTION
EMOTIVE
EMPRISE
EMPTIED
EMPTIER
EMPTIES
EMPTILY
IMAGINE
IMAGING
IMAGISM
IMAGIST
IMBUING
IMEMINE
IMGOING
IMPAIRS
IMPLIED
IMPLIES
IMPRINT
OMENING
SMILING
SMITING
SMOKIER
SMOKIES
SMOKILY
SMOKING
TMOBILE
UMBRIAN
UMBRIEL

•M•••I•

AMANTIS
AMEBOID
AMHARIC
AMMONIA
AMMONIC
AMNERIS
AMNESIA
AMNESIC
AMOEBIC
AMRADIO
EMBROIL
EMPIRIC
EMPIRIN
EMPORIA
FMRADIO
IMADEIT
IMEANIT
IMFORIT
IMPAVID
IMPERIL
XMRADIO

•M••••I

AMICHAI
EMERITI

••MI•••

AAMILNE
ADMIRAL
ADMIRED
ADMIRER
ADMIRES
ADMITTO
ADMIXED
ADMIXES
BEMIRED
BEMIRES
BIMINIS
CAMILLA
CAMILLE
CAMINOS
CAMIONS
CAMISES
COMICAL
COMICES
COMINGS
COMIQUE
DEMIGOD
DEMILLE
DEMISED
DEMISES
DEMISTS
DIMITRI
DOMICAL
DOMICIL
DOMINGO
DOMINIC
DOMINOS
DOMINUS
ELMIEST
ELMISTI
ERMINED
ERMINES
ERMINIA
FAMICOM
FAMILIA
FAMILLE
FAMINES
FEMINUM
FUMIEST
GAMIEST
GAMINES
GEMINIS
HAMITES
HAMITIC
HAMITUP
HOMIEST
HOMINID
HUMIDEX
HUMIDLY
HUMIDOR
IMMIXED
IMMIXES
JAMISON
JEMISON
JIMINEZ
KEMIDOV
LAMINAE
LAMINAL
LAMINAR
LAMINAS
LAMINTO
LEMIEUX
LIMIEST
LIMINAL
LIMITED
LIMITER
LUMIERE
LUMINAS
MIMICRY
MIMIEUX
NAMIBIA
NIMIETY
NOMINAL
NOMINEE
PUMICED
PUMICES
RAMINTO
RAMIREZ
REMILLS
REMINDS
REMINED
REMINES
REMINTS
REMISED
REMISES
REMIXED
REMIXES
RIMIEST
SAMISEN
SEMIDRY
SEMILOG
SEMINAL
SEMINAR
SEMIPRO
SEMIRAW
SEMITES
SEMITIC
SIMIANS
SIMILAC
SIMILAR
SIMILES
SOMINEX
SUMITUP
TAMIAMI
TIMIDER
TIMIDLY
TIMINGS
UNMIKED
UNMINED
UNMIRED
UNMITER
UNMITRE
UNMIXED
UNMIXES
VIMINAL

••M•I••

AIMHIGH
ARMLIKE
ARMOIRE
ARMPITS
BAMBIII
BAMBINA
BAMBINI
BAMBINO
BAMMIES
BAMMING
BOMBING
BUMMING
BUMPIER
BUMPILY
BUMPING
CAMGIRL
CAMMIES
CAMPIER
CAMPILY
CAMPING
CAMPION
COMBIEN
COMBINE
COMBING
COMFIER
COMFITS
COMMISH
COMMITS
COMPILE
COMPING
COMTISM
COMTIST
CUMBIAS
CYMRICS
DAMMING
DAMNING
DAMPING
DAMPISH
DEMOING
DIMMING
DIMVIEW
DIMWITS
DOMAINE
DOMAINS
DUMBING
DUMMIED
DUMMIES
DUMPIER
DUMPILY
DUMPING
DUMPISH
ELMCITY
GAMBIAN
GAMBIER
GAMBITS
GAMMING
GEMLIKE
GEMMIER
GIMMICK
GIMPING
GUMLIKE
GUMMIER
GUMMING
HAMLINE
HAMMIER
HAMMILY
HAMMING
HEMLINE
HEMMING
HEMPIER
HOMEICE
HOMEIER
HUMMING
HUMPIER
HYMNING
IAMBICS
IAMBIST
JAMAICA
JAMLIKE
JAMMIER
JAMMIES
JAMMING
JIMDIAL
JIMFIXX
JIMMIED
JIMMIES
JIMRICE
JUMPIER
JUMPILY
JUMPING
LAMAISM
LAMAIST
LAMBING
LAMMING
LEMMING
LEMPIRA
LIMBING
LIMNING
LIMNITE
LIMPING
LUMPIER
LUMPILY
LUMPING
LUMPISH
MEMLING
MEMOIRE
MEMOIRS
MGMLION
MOMMIES
MUMMIES
MUMMIFY
MUMMING
NUMBING
PAMLICO
PIMLICO
PUMPING
RAMLIKE
RAMMING
RAMMISH
RAMPING
REMAILS
REMAINS
RIMMING
ROMAINE
ROMAINS
ROMPING
ROMPISH
RUMMIES
SAMHILL
SAMWISE
SIMCITY
SUMMING
SUMMITS
SUMOIST
TAMPICO
TAMPING
TEMPING
TIMMINS
TIMRICE
TOMKITE
TOMTITS
TUMMIES
UNMOIST
VAMPIER
VAMPING
VAMPIRA
VAMPIRE
VAMPISH
WIMPIER
WIMPING
WIMPISH
YUMMIER
ZAMBIAN
ZOMBIES
ZOMBIFY

••M••I•

ALMERIA
AMMONIA
AMMONIC
ARMENIA
BAMBIII
BIMINIS
BUMPKIN
CAMBRIA
CAMBRIC
CAMELID
COMEDIA
COMEDIC
COMEDIE
COMESIN
COMPLIN
CUMBRIA
DEMERIT
DEMONIC
DEMOTIC
DOMICIL
DOMINIC
DRMARIO
ERMINIA
FAMILIA
FEMORIS
GEMINIS
GYMSUIT
HAMELIN
HAMITIC
HEMATIC
HEMATIN
HIMALIA
HOMEDIN
HOMERIC
HOMESIN
HOMINID
JAMESII
JAMESIV
JUMPBID
JUMPSIN
LAMBKIN
LAMPLIT
LAMPOIL
LIMEPIE
LUMPSIN
LUMPSIT
MAMAMIA
MEMPHIS
MIMESIS
MIMETIC
MRMUSIC
NAMIBIA
NEMESIS
NOMADIC
NUMERIC
NYMPHIC
OSMATIC
OSMOSIS
OSMOTIC
POMPEIA
POMPEII
PUMPKIN
RAMBLIN
RAMEKIN
ROMAJIS
ROMANIA
ROMANIC
ROMANIS
RUMAKIS
RUMANIA
SAMARIA
SAMEDIS
SEMITIC
SIMONIZ
SOMALIA
SOMALIS
SOMATIC
TIMREID
TVMOVIE
YEMENIS

••M•••I

BAMBIII
BAMBINI
CAMPARI
DIMITRI
DRMELFI
EDMUNDI
ELMISTI
GEMELLI
HAMACHI
JAMESII
JAMESVI
JUMANJI
POMPEII
RAMSESI
SAMURAI
TAMIAMI
TIMPANI
TYMPANI
ZAMBEZI
ZAMBONI

•••MI••

ADAMITE
AIRMILE
ALLMINE
ALSMITH
ALUMINA
ANEMIAS
ANIMISM
ANIMIST
ANOMIES
ARAMIDS
ATOMICS
ATOMIES
ATOMISE
ATOMISM
ATOMIST
ATOMIZE
BALMIER
BALMILY
BAMMIES
BAMMING
BARMIER
BEAMIER
BEAMING
BEAMISH
BERMING
BLAMING
BLEMISH
BOOMIER
BOOMING
BROMIDE
BROMINE
BUMMING
BYAMILE
CADMIUM
CALMING
CAMMIES
CARMINA
CARMINE
CATMINT
CHEMISE
CHEMIST
CHIMING
CHIMINH
COMMISH
COMMITS
CREMINI
CRIMINY
DAMMING
DAUMIER
DEEMING
DIMMING
DISMISS
DOOMIER
DOOMING
DORMICE
DUMMIED
DUMMIES
EDOMITE
ELAMITE
ENEMIES
EREMITE
ETAMINE
EXAMINE
FARMING
FERMION
FERMIUM
FILMIER
FILMILY
FILMING
FIRMING
FLAMIER
FLAMING
FLEMING
FLEMISH
FOAMIER
FOAMILY
FOAMING
FORMICA
FORMING
FRAMING
GAMMING
GEMMIER
GERMIER
GIMMICK
GINMILL
GNOMISH
GNOMIST
GOAMISS
GORMING
GOTMILK
GRIMIER
GRIMILY
GRIMING
GUMMIER
GUMMING
HAIMISH
HAMMIER
HAMMILY
HAMMING
HARMING
HELMING
HEMMING
HERMITS
HOLMIUM
HOTMILK
HUMMING
ICEMILK
IMEMINE
ITEMING
ITEMISE
ITEMIZE
JAMMIER
JAMMIES
JAMMING
JASMINE
JIMMIED
JIMMIES
LABMICE
LAMMING
LEMMING
LOAMIER
LOAMING
LOOMING
MAIMING
MAIMITI
MARMION
MEEMIES
MIAMIAN
MIAMIFL
MOMMIES
MRSMITH
MUMMIES
MUMMIFY
MUMMING
NESMITH
NEWMINT
NOTMINE
OFAMIND
OLEMISS
ONEMILE
PALMIER
PALMING
PALMIST
PERMIAN
PERMING
PERMITS
PETMICE
PHEMIUS
PISMIRE
PLUMIER
PLUMING
PREMIER
PREMIES
PREMISE
PREMISS
PREMIUM
PRIMING
PROMISE
PYGMIES
RAMMING
RAMMISH
REAMING
REEMITS
RHYMING
RHYMIST
RIMMING
ROAMING

ROOMIER
ROOMIES
ROOMILY
ROOMING
RUMMIES
SAWMILL
SCHMIDT
SCHMITT
SEAMIER
SEAMILE
SEAMING
SEAMIST
SEEMING
SHAMING
SLIMIER
SLIMILY
SLIMING
SOYMILK
SPUMIER
SPUMING
STAMINA
STYMIED
STYMIES
SUBMITS
SUMMING
SUMMITS
SURMISE
TEAMING
TEEMING
TENMILE
TERMING
TERMINI
TERMITE
THEMICK
THYMINE
TIMMINS
TINMINE
TITMICE
TUMMIES
VALMIKI
VARMINT
VERMINY
WARMING
WARMISH
WORMIER
WORMING
WORMISH
WYOMING
YAOMING
YASMINE
YUMMIER
ZOOMING

•••M•I•
AIRMAIL
ALAMEIN
ALEMBIC
ARAMAIC
BALMAIN
BARMAID
BLIMPIE
CHAMOIS
CHIMEIN
CLAMDIP
CLIMBIN
CRAMSIN
DRUMLIN
DUUMVIR
ETHMOID
FANMAIL
FARMAID
GASMAIN
GERMAIN
GREMLIN
HOTMAIL
KRAMNIK
KREMLIN
LETMEIN
MERMAID
MRSMUIR
OLDMAID
OLYMPIA
OLYMPIC
PALMOIL
PLUMBIC
PLUMPIE
PROMBID
RHOMBIC
SIGMOID
SLIMJIM
STOMPIN
SUNMAID
TIOMKIN
TROMPIN
TURMOIL
VERMEIL
WEBMAIL
ZOOMSIN

•••M••I
BASMATI
CREMINI
MAIMITI
PULMONI
RIOMUNI
SPUMONI
STIMULI
TERMINI
THEMAGI
VALMIKI

••••MI•
ALBUMIN
ANAEMIA
ANAEMIC
ANOSMIA
ANOSMIC
ARTEMIS
BOHEMIA
BOROMIR
BRAHMIN
CAKEMIX
CARAMIA
CASIMIR
CERAMIC
CHARMIN
CHASMIC
CHEXMIX
CHROMIC
DELIMIT
DHARMIC
DREAMIN
DYNAMIC
ENCOMIA
ENDEMIC
ENZYMIC
ESTAMIN
EUNOMIA
GENOMIC
GLOAMIN
IDIAMIN
ISLAMIC
ISTOMIN
JAROMIR
KASHMIR
LARAMIE
LETEMIN
MAMAMIA
MANUMIT
MEOWMIX
MESAMIS
MIASMIC
NOKOMIS
NOLIMIT
OGHAMIC
OVERMIX
PLASMIC
POLEMIC
PREEMIE
PREOMIT
PSALMIC
PYRAMID
READMIT
RELIMIT
RHEUMIC
SALAMIS
SEISMIC
SOUPMIX
STORMIN
SURIMIS
TATAMIS
THERMIC
THIAMIN
TOTEMIC
UNCOMIC
UNHUMID
UNTIMID
VITAMIN

••••M•I
CESTMOI
CHEZMOI
THEOMNI

•••••MI
BUSCEMI
FLINTMI
GOURAMI
KHATAMI
LAKSHMI
ORIGAMI
SASHIMI
TAMIAMI
TSUNAMI
WHATAMI

M•J••••
MAJESTE
MAJESTY
MAJEURE
MAJGENS
MAJORCA
MAJORED
MAJORIN
MOJAVES
MOJITOS
MRJONES
MUJERES

M••J•••
MIDJULY
MIDJUNE
MISJOIN

M•••J••
MEANJOE

M••••J•
MARUSJA

•M••••J
SMALLOJ

••MJ•••
JIMJAMS
RAMJETS
TOMJOAD

••M•J••
ROMAJIS
TEMPJOB

••M••J•
JUMANJI
SAMMYJO

•••MJ••
SLIMJIM

•••M•J•
SAMMYJO

•••M••J
HEYMRDJ

M•K••••
MAKABLE
MAKEDOS
MAKEFIT
MAKEFOR
MAKEFUN
MAKEHAY
MAKEILL
MAKEMAD
MAKEOFF
MAKEONE
MAKEOUT
MAKEPAR
MAKERUN
MAKESDO
MAKESGO
MAKESIT
MAKESUP
MAKEUPS
MAKEWAR
MAKEWAY
MAKINGS
MCKENNA
MIKADOS
MIKASAS
MIKHAIL
MTKENYA
MUKLUKS
MYKONOS

M••K•••
MANKATO
MANKIND
MARKERS
MARKETS
MARKHAM
MARKIII
MARKING
MARKKAA
MARKOFF
MARKOUT
MARKOVA
MARKSUP
MARKUPS
MARKVII
MASKERS
MASKING
MAWKISH
MEEKEST
MICKEYS
MILKBAR
MILKCAN
MILKCOW
MILKDUD
MILKERS
MILKFED
MILKIER
MILKILY
MILKING
MILKMAN
MILKMEN
MILKRUN
MILKSOP
MISKEYS
MISKNEW
MISKNOW
MISKOLC
MOCKERS
MOCKERY
MOCKING
MOCKSUP
MOCKUPS
MONKEES
MONKEYS
MONKISH
MUCKERS
MUCKIER
MUCKING
MUCKSUP
MURKIER
MURKILY
MURKISH
MUSKEGO
MUSKETS
MUSKIER
MUSKIES
MUSKRAT

M•••K••
MANIKIN
MARKKAA
MARYKAY
MEDAKAS
MEERKAT
MENCKEN
MESSKIT
MINIKIN
MINSKYS
MOLOKAI
MONGKUT
MONIKER

M••••K•
MALARKY
MALLIKA
MANDOKI
MANLIKE
MAZURKA
MINISKI
MISLIKE
MISTAKE
MOHAWKS
MONOSKI
MRLUCKY
MUKLUKS
MUSICKS

M•••••K
MADLOCK
MASARYK
MATLOCK
MATTOCK
MEDWICK
MENFOLK
MERRICK
MESSICK
MIDWEEK
MISMARK
MISTOOK
MOLLUSK
MONTAUK
MORLOCK
MRNOVAK
MRSPOCK
MUBARAK
MUDLARK
MUDPACK

•M•K•••
SMOKERS
SMOKEUP
SMOKEYS
SMOKIER
SMOKIES
SMOKILY
SMOKING

•M••K••
SMACKED
SMACKER
SMACKOF
SMACKUP
SMIRKED
SMIRKER
SMUCKER

•M•••K•
AMERIKA
EMBANKS
EMBARKS
EMMUSKA
IMBROKE

•M••••K
AMTRACK
DMYTRYK

••MK•••
JIMKAAT
TOMKITE

••M•K••
BUMPKIN
COMAKER
LAMBKIN
PUMPKIN
RAMEKIN
REMAKES
RUMAKIS
SAMEKHS
UNMAKER
UNMAKES
UNMIKED

••M••K•
ARMLIKE
DAMASKS
DEMARKS
EMMUSKA
GEMLIKE
GUMLIKE
JAMLIKE
RAMLIKE
REMARKS
RUMCAKE
STMARKS
UNMASKS

••M•••K
ARMLOCK
BOMBECK
GEMSBOK
GIMMICK
GYMSOCK
HAMHOCK
HAMMOCK
HEMLOCK
JAMPACK
JUMBUCK
LAMARCK
NUMLOCK
RIMROCK

•••MK••
TIOMKIN

•••M•K•
CHOMSKY
GROMYKO
PREMAKE
UNSMOKY
VALMIKI

•••M••K
ARAMARK
CORMACK
DENMARK
EARMARK
EYEMASK
GASMASK
GIMMICK
GOTMILK
HAMMOCK
HOLMOAK
HOTMILK
ICEMILK
INKMARK
KRAMNIK
LEXMARK
MISMARK
NIPMUCK
OSTMARK
SKIMASK
SOYMILK
TEDMACK
THEMASK
THEMICK
WIDMARK

••••M•K
RANAMOK
RUNAMOK
YASHMAK

M•L••••
MALABAR
MALACCA
MALACHI
MALAGAN
MALAGAS
MALAISE
MALAMUD
MALARIA
MALARKY
MALAYAN
MALCOLM
MALDIVE
MALEANT
MALEBEE
MALECAT
MALEDOG
MALEFIC
MALEHOG
MALEPIG
MALIANS
MALICES
MALIGNS
MALLARD
MALLETS
MALLEUS
MALLIKA
MALLOWS
MALLRAT
MALMSEY
MALODOR
MALPASO
MALRAUX
MALTASE
MALTBIE
MALTEDS
MALTESE
MALTHUS
MALTIER
MALTING
MALTOSE
MALVINA
MALWARE
MCLUHAN
MELAMED
MELANGE
MELANIA
MELANIC
MELANIE
MELANIN
MELDERS
MELDING
MELINDA
MELISMA
MELISSA
MELITTA
MELLOWS
MELODIA
MELODIC
MELROSE
MELTAGE
MELTERS
MELTING
MILAGRO
MILDEST
MILDEWS
MILDEWY
MILDRED
MILEAGE
MILERUN
MILHAUD
MILHOUS
MILIEUS
MILIEUX
MILITIA
MILKBAR
MILKCAN
MILKCOW
MILKDUD
MILKERS
MILKFED
MILKIER
MILKILY
MILKING
MILKMAN
MILKMEN
MILKRUN
MILKSOP
MILLAGE
MILLAIS
MILLAND
MILLARD
MILLDAM
MILLEND
MILLERS
MILLETS
MILLETT
MILLIME
MILLING
MILLION
MILLRUN
MILORDS
MOLDERS
MOLDIER
MOLDING
MOLDOVA
MOLERAT
MOLESTS
MOLIERE
MOLITOR
MOLLIES
MOLLIFY
MOLLUSC
MOLLUSK
MOLOKAI
MOLOTOV
MOLSONS
MOLTERS
MOLTING
MOLUCCA
MRLUCKY
MTLOGAN
MULATTO
MULCAHY
MULCHED
MULCHES
MULCTED
MULDAUR
MULDOON
MULETAS
MULGREW
MULHARE
MULLAHS
MULLERS
MULLETS
MULLING
MULLINS
MYLANTA

M••L•••
MACLEAN
MACLEOD
MADLIBS
MADLOCK
MAGLEVS
MAILBAG
MAILBIN
MAILBOX
MAILCAR
MAILERS
MAILING
MAILINS
MAILLOL
MAILLOT
MAILMAN
MAILMEN
MAILOUT
MAILSIN
MALLARD
MALLETS
MALLEUS
MALLIKA
MALLOWS
MALLRAT
MANLESS
MANLIER
MANLIKE
MARLENE
MARLIER
MARLINS
MARLOWE
MATLESS
MATLOCK
MAULDIN
MAULERS
MAULING
MCALLEN
MCCLOUD
MCCLURE
MCCLURG
MEALIER
MEALIES
MEDLEYS
MELLOWS
MEMLING
MERLINS
MERLOTS
METLIFE
MEWLERS
MEWLING
MGMLION
MIDLAND
MIDLEGS
MIDLIFE
MIDLINE
MIDLIST
MILLAGE
MILLAIS
MILLAND
MILLARD
MILLDAM
MILLEND
MILLERS
MILLETS
MILLETT
MILLIME
MILLING
MILLION
MILLRUN
MISLAID
MISLAYS
MISLEAD
MISLIKE
MOILERS
MOILING
MOLLIES
MOLLIFY
MOLLUSC
MOLLUSK
MORLOCK
MOSLEMS
MOTLEYS
MOULAGE
MOULDED
MOULDER
MOULTED
MRBLISS
MRCLEAN
MRSLATE
MTBLANC
MUDLARK
MUELLER
MUKLUKS
MULLAHS
MULLERS
MULLETS
MULLING
MULLINS
MUSLIMS
MUSLINS
MYALGIA
MYALGIC
MYOLOGY

M•••L••
MACULAE
MACULAR
MADALYN
MADELON
MAGALOG
MAGILLA
MAHALIA
MAILLOL
MAILLOT
MANGLED
MANGLER
MANGLES
MANILAS
MANILOW
MANOLIN
MANTLED
MANTLES
MANTLET
MARBLED
MARBLER
MARBLES
MARILLA
MARILYN
MARULLO
MARYLOU
MATALIN
MATILDA
MAUDLIN
MAXILLA
MAYALIN
MCALLEN
MCCALLS
MCHALES
MCNALLY
MEAGLES
MEASLES
MECHLIN
MEDALED
MEDDLED
MEDDLER
MEDDLES
MEDELES
MEDULLA
MEGALON
MEGILLA
METALED
METTLER
METTLES
MIDDLEC
MIDDLED
MIDDLER
MIDDLES
MIFFLIN
MINGLED
MINGLER
MINGLES
MINILAB
MINOLTA
MISALLY
MISPLAN
MISPLAY
MIZZLED
MIZZLES
MOBILES
MODELAS
MODELBS
MODELED
MODELER
MODELTS
MODULAR
MODULES
MODULUS
MONOLOG
MOONLET
MOONLIT
MORALES
MORALLY
MORELLA
MORELLO
MORELOS
MOSELLE
MOTTLED
MOTTLES
MOZILLA
MRHULOT
MTBALDY
MTPELEE
MUDDLED
MUDDLER
MUDDLES
MUDFLAP
MUDFLAT
MUDFLOW
MUELLER
MUESLIS
MUESLIX
MUFFLED
MUFFLER
MUFFLES
MUGGLES
MUMBLED
MUMBLER
MUMBLES
MURALED
MURILLO
MUSCLED
MUSCLES
MUZZLED
MUZZLER
MUZZLES
MYRTLES

M••••L•
MADEILL
MAGILLA
MAKABLE
MAKEILL
MALCOLM
MAMMALS
MANACLE
MANDALA
MANDELA
MANHOLE
MANIPLE
MANTELS
MANUALS
MARCELS
MARILLA
MARSALA
MARULLO
MARVELL
MARVELS
MAXILLA
MAXWELL
MAYPOLE
MCARDLE
MCCALLS
MCNALLY
MCNEILL
MEATILY

MEDULLA MEGILLA MENDELS MENFOLK MENIALS MERRILL MERRILY MESCALS MESSALA MESSILY METCALF MEYNELL MICAELA MIDJULY MIDSOLE MILKILY MINABLE MINEOLA MIRACLE MISALLY MISBILL MISCALL MISERLY MISFILE MISKOLC MISRELY MISRULE MISSALS MISSILE MISTELL MISTILY MISTOLD MIXABLE MIXEDLY MOBRULE MOISTLY MONDALE MONGOLS MONOCLE MONTALE MONTHLY MOODILY MOONILY MORALLY MORELLA MORELLO MORSELS MORTALS MOSELLE MOUSILY MOVABLE MOVABLY MOZILLA MRQUILP MUDDILY MUDEELS MUDHOLE MUGFULS MURIELS MURILLO MURKILY MUSHILY MUSSELS MUSSILY MUSTILY MUTABLE MUTABLY MUTEDLY MUTUALS MUZZILY MYFAULT MYWORLD

M•••••L

MACNEIL MADEILL MAGICAL MAILLOL MAKEILL MANDREL MARITAL MARSHAL MARTIAL MARVELL MATINAL MAXIMAL MAXWELL MAYORAL MCNEILL MEDICAL MENTHOL MERRILL MEYNELL MIAMIFL MIASMAL MICHAEL MIKHAIL MINDFUL MINERAL MINIMAL MIRABEL MISBILL MISCALL MISDEAL MISDIAL MISTELL MISTRAL MOANFUL MONADAL MONDIAL MONGREL MRSPAUL MRSPEEL MUSEFUL MUSICAL

•ML••••

UMLAUTS

•M•L•••

AMALGAM AMBLERS AMBLING AMILATE AMPLEST AMPLIFY AMULETS AMYLASE EMBLAZE EMBLEMS EMPLACE EMPLANE EMPLOYS EMULATE EMULOUS IMPLANT IMPLEAD IMPLIED IMPLIES IMPLODE IMPLORE OMALLEY OMELETS SMALLAD SMALLER SMALLOJ SMELLED SMELLER SMELTED SMELTER SMILEAT SMILEON SMILERS SMILEYS SMILING SMILLAS SMOLDER

•M••L••

AMESLAN AMIBLUE AMPULES EMAILED EMAILER EMBALMS EMMYLOU EMPALED EMPALES IMPALAS IMPALED IMPALER IMPALES IMPULSE OMALLEY SMALLAD SMALLER SMALLOJ SMELLED SMELLER SMILLAS

•M•••L•

AMAPOLA AMATOLS AMIABLE AMIABLY AMIDALA AMIDOLS AMPOULE AMSTELS EMERALD EMPTILY IMSWELL OMPHALO SMARTLY SMOKILY SMUGGLE TMOBILE

•M••••L

EMANUEL EMBROIL EMPANEL IMMORAL IMPANEL IMPERIL IMSWELL SMEAGOL UMBRIEL

••ML•••

AIMLESS ARMLESS ARMLETS ARMLIKE ARMLOAD ARMLOCK BUMLEGS GEMLESS GEMLIKE GIMLETS GUMLESS GUMLIKE HAMLETS HAMLINE HEMLINE HEMLOCK IAMLOVE JAMLIKE MEMLING MGMLION NUMLOCK PAMLICO PIMLICO RAMLIKE RIMLESS RUMLESS SAMLETS SAMLOYD SUMLESS

••M•L••

AAMILNE BOMBLET BUMBLED BUMBLER BUMBLES CAMELID CAMELOT CAMILLA CAMILLE COMPLEX COMPLIN CUMULUS DEMILLE DEMOLAY DIMPLED DIMPLES DRMELFI EMMYLOU FAMILIA FAMILLE FAMULUS FEMALES FUMBLED FUMBLER FUMBLES GAMBLED GAMBLER GAMBLES GAMELAN GAMELAW GAMELEG GEMELLI GYMCLUB HAMELIN HAMULUS HEMSLEY HIMALIA HOMELAB HUMBLED HUMBLER HUMBLES JUMBLED JUMBLER JUMBLES LAMPLIT MUMBLED MUMBLER MUMBLES NIMBLER OHMSLAW ORMOLUS PIMPLED PIMPLES POMELOS RAMBLED RAMBLER RAMBLES RAMBLIN REMELTS REMILLS REMOLDS RIMPLED RIMPLES ROMULAN ROMULUS RUMBLED RUMBLER RUMBLES RUMPLED RUMPLES SAMPLED SAMPLER SAMPLES SEMILOG SIMILAC SIMILAR SIMILES SIMPLER SIMPLES SIMPLEX SOMALIA SOMALIS TAMALES TAMBLYN TAMGLEN TEMBLOR TEMPLAR TEMPLED TEMPLES TIMELAG TUMBLED TUMBLER TUMBLES TUMMLER TUMULTS UNMOLDS UNMOLDY WAMBLED WAMBLES WEMBLEY WIMPLED WIMPLES

••M••L•

ARMFULS ARMHOLE BUMPILY CAMILLA CAMILLE CAMPILY CAMRYLE CEMBALO COMPELS COMPILE CYMBALS DAMSELS DEMILLE DIMBULB DUMPILY FAMILLE GAMBOLS GEMELLI GIMBALS GIMBELS GUMBALL GYMBALL HAMMILY HIMSELF HUMANLY HUMIDLY HUMMELS HYMNALS JIMDALE JUMPILY KAMPALA KIMBALL KUMMELS LUMPILY MAMMALS NAMABLE NAMABLY POMMELS PUMMELS REMAILS REMILLS RUMPOLE SAMEOLD SAMHILL SAMUELL SYMBOLS TAMABLE TAMBALA TIMBALE TIMBALS TIMHOLT TIMIDLY TOMGOLA UNMADLY UNMANLY UNMOULD WIMPOLE WOMANLY ZUMWALT

••M•••L

ADMIRAL BIMETAL BIMODAL BUMDEAL CAMERAL CAMGIRL COMICAL DAMOSEL DEMEROL DOMICAL DOMICIL FEMORAL GAMETAL GEMAYEL GQMODEL GUMBALL GYMBALL HUMERAL HUMORAL IMMORAL JIMDIAL KIMBALL LAMINAL LAMPOIL LIMINAL NOMINAL NUMERAL NYMPHAL REMODEL REMOVAL SAMHILL SAMUELL SEMINAL TAMPAFL TOMFOOL TUMBREL VIMINAL

•••ML••

BOOMLET BRAMLEY BRIMLEY CHEMLAB DAIMLER DRUMLIN GREMLIN KREMLIN TUMMLER

•••M•L•

AIRMILE ALLMALE ANIMALS ANOMALY BALMILY BRAMBLE BRAMBLY BYAMILE CARMELA CRUMBLE CRUMBLY CRUMPLE CRUMPLY DEHMELT DISMALS EJEMPLO ENAMELS EXAMPLE EXEMPLA FILMILY FOAMILY FORMALS FORMULA GINMILL GOTMILK GRIMILY GRUMBLE GRUMBLY GUNMOLL HAMMILY HOTMILK HUMMELS ICEMILK KUMMELS LAEMMLE MAMMALS NORMALS ONEMILE PETMULE PLUMPLY PLUMULE POMMELS PRIMELY PUMMELS REIMPLY RESMELT ROOMILY SAWMILL SEAMILE SHAMBLE SLIMILY SOYMILK STIMULI STUMBLE TENMILE THEMALL THIMBLE TRAMPLE TREMBLE TREMBLY TREMOLO

•••M••L

AIRMAIL ALUMNAL BIGMEAL BRIMFUL BRUMMEL DOOMFUL FANMAIL FARMGAL FORMFUL GINMILL GUNMOLL HARMFUL HOTMAIL HOTMEAL ISHMAEL MIAMIFL OATMEAL PALMFUL PALMOIL ROOMFUL SAWMILL SELMAAL SOYMEAL STEMPEL THEMALL TRAMMEL TURMOIL VERMEIL WEBMAIL

••••ML•

BUXOMLY LAEMMLE

••••M•L

ABYSMAL BRUMMEL CARAMEL CHASMAL COZUMEL DECIMAL DUHAMEL MAXIMAL MIASMAL MINIMAL OPTIMAL SEISMAL THERMAL TRAMMEL

M•M••••

MAMAMIA MAMBOED MAMMALS MAMMOTH MCMAHON MCMURDO MEMBERS MEMENTO MEMLING MEMOIRE MEMOIRS MEMOPAD MEMOREX MEMPHIS MGMLION MIMEOED MIMESES MIMESIS MIMETIC MIMICRY MIMIEUX MIMOSAS MOMBASA MOMENTA MOMENTS MOMMIES MOMMSEN MOMONEY MOMUSES MRMACHO MRMAGOO MRMARCH MRMOOSE MRMUSIC MTMARCY MUMBLED MUMBLER MUMBLES MUMESON MUMFORD MUMMERS MUMMERY MUMMIES MUMMIFY MUMMING MYMAMMY

M••M•••

MAIMERS MAIMING MAIMITI MALMSEY MAMMALS MAMMOTH MANMADE MARMARA MARMION MARMOTS MAUMAUS MEEMIES MERMAID MIAMIAN MIAMIFL MICMACS MIDMORN MIDMOST MISMARK MISMATE MISMESH MISMOVE MOMMIES MOMMSEN MORMONS MRSMITH MRSMUIR MUAMMAR MUMMERS MUMMERY MUMMIES MUMMIFY MUMMING MURMURS MUUMUUS

M•••M••

MADAMES MADAMEX MADEMAD MAILMAN MAILMEN MAINMAN MAINMEN MAKEMAD MALAMUD MAMAMIA MANSMAN MANUMIT MANXMAN MANXMEN MARIMBA MAXIMAL MAXIMAS MAXIMUM MAXIMUS MEATMAN MEATMEN MELAMED MEOWMIX MERIMEE MESAMIS MIASMAL MIASMAS MIASMIC MILKMAN MILKMEN MINIMAL MINIMAX MINIMUM MINIMUS MIRAMAR MIRAMAX MODEMED MOGAMBO MONOMER MUAMMAR MYANMAR MYMAMMY

M••••M•

MACRAME MAGNUMS MAHATMA MARRYME MAYHEMS MAYTIME MCADAMS MCCRUMB MEDIUMS MEGOHMS MEGRIMS MELISMA MESEEMS MIAHAMM MILLIME MISAIMS MISHIMA MISNAME MISTIME MOSLEMS MTADAMS MUGWUMP MUSEUMS MUSLIMS MYMAMMY

M•••••M

MACADAM MAHDISM MALCOLM MANHEIM MARKHAM MARXISM MAUGHAM MAXIMUM MERRIAM MIAHAMM MIDTERM MILLDAM MINICAM MINIMUM MISDEEM MISFORM MISTERM MITCHUM MOBBISM MODICUM MUDROOM

•MM••••

AMMETER AMMONIA AMMONIC EMMUSKA EMMYLOU IMMENSE IMMERGE IMMERSE IMMIXED IMMIXES IMMORAL IMMUNES IMMURED IMMURES

•M•M•••

IMAMATE IMAMESS IMEMINE

•M••M••

OMNIMAX

•M•••M•

AMUSEME EMBALMS EMBLEMS

•M••••M

AMALGAM EMBOSOM IMAGISM

••MM•••

BAMMIES BAMMING BUMMERS BUMMING CAMMIES COMMAND COMMEND COMMENT COMMISH COMMITS COMMODE COMMONS COMMOVE COMMUNE COMMUTE DAMMERS DAMMING DIMMERS DIMMEST DIMMING DUMMIED DUMMIES DUMMYUP GAMMERS GAMMING GAMMONS GEMMATE GEMMIER GIMMICK GUMMIER GUMMING HAMMERS HAMMETT HAMMIER HAMMILY HAMMING HAMMOCK HAMMOND HEMMERS HEMMING HUMMELS HUMMERS HUMMING JAMMERS JAMMIER JAMMIES JAMMING JIMMIED JIMMIES KUMMELS LAMMING LEMMATA LEMMING MAMMALS MAMMOTH MOMMIES MOMMSEN MUMMERS MUMMERY MUMMIES MUMMIFY MUMMING POMMARD POMMELS PUMMELS RAMMERS RAMMING RAMMISH RIMMING RUMMAGE RUMMERS RUMMIES SAMMYJO SIMMERS SIMMONS SUMMAND SUMMARY SUMMATE SUMMERS SUMMERY SUMMING SUMMITS SUMMONS TAMMANY TIMMINS TUMMIES TUMMLER YAMMERS YUMMIER

••M•M••

ALMSMAN ALMSMEN DAMPMOP MAMAMIA MYMAMMY

••M••M•

DEMBUMS DUMDUMS HUMORME

JAMCAMS
JIMJAMS
MYMAMMY
POMPOMS
RAMHOME
ROMCOMS
TAMIAMI
TAMTAMS
TOMTOMS
WAMPUMS

••M•••M

COMTISM
DEMONYM
FAMICOM
FEMINUM
HOMONYM
HUMANUM
HUMDRUM
JIMBEAM
LAMAISM
LUMPSUM
SYMPTOM

•••MM••

ASIMMER
BRIMMED
BRIMMER
BRUMMEL
CHUMMED
CLAMMED
CLAMMER
CRAMMED
CRAMMER
DRUMMED
DRUMMER
FLAMMED
FLUMMOX
FROMMER
GLIMMER
GLOMMED
GLUMMED
GLUMMER
GRAMMAR
GRAMMER
GRAMMES
GRAMMYS
GRIMMER
GROMMET
GRUMMAN
KLAMMER
LAEMMLE
MUAMMAR
PLUMMER
PLUMMET
PRIMMED
PRIMMER
SCAMMED
SCAMMER
SHAMMED
SHIMMER
SKIMMED
SKIMMER
SLAMMED
SLAMMER
SLIMMED
SLIMMER
SLUMMED
SLUMMER
SPAMMED
SPAMMER
STAMMER
STEMMED
SWIMMER
TRAMMED
TRAMMEL
TRIMMED
TRIMMER
TZIMMES
WHAMMED

•••M•M•

BIGMAMA
DENMOMS
GODMAMA

•••M••M

ANIMISM
ATOMISM
CADMIUM
CRUMBUM
FERMIUM
FILMDOM
HOLMIUM
PLUMBUM
PREMIUM
SLIMJIM
YESMAAM

••••MM•

DILEMMA
LAFEMME
MYMAMMY

••••M•M

KEEPMUM
KEPTMUM
MAXIMUM
MINIMUM
OPTIMUM
STEPMOM

•••••MM

MIAHAMM

MN•••••

MNOPQRS

M•N••••

MANACLE
MANAGED
MANAGER
MANAGES
MANAGUA
MANANAS
MANATEE
MANCINI
MANCUSO
MANDALA
MANDANS
MANDATE
MANDAYS
MANDELA
MANDOKI
MANDREL
MANEGES
MANETTE
MANFRED
MANGANO
MANGERS
MANGIER
MANGLED
MANGLER
MANGLES
MANGOES
MANHEIM
MANHOLE
MANHOOD
MANHOUR
MANHUNT
MANIACS
MANIKIN
MANILAS
MANILOW
MANIPLE
MANIPUR
MANKATO
MANKIND
MANLESS
MANLIER
MANLIKE
MANMADE
MANNERS
MANNIES
MANNING
MANNISH
MANOLIN
MANOWAR
MANRICO
MANROPE
MANSARD
MANSION
MANSIZE
MANSMAN
MANTECA
MANTELS
MANTLED
MANTLES
MANTLET
MANTRAP
MANTRAS
MANTRIC
MANTUAN
MANUALS
MANUMIT
MANURED
MANURES
MANXCAT
MANXMAN
MANXMEN
MANYEAR
MCNALLY
MCNEILL
MENACED
MENACER
MENACES
MENAGES
MENCIUS
MENCKEN
MENDELS
MENDERS
MENDING
MENFOLK
MENIALS
MENISCI
MENORAH
MENORCA
MENOTTI
MENSANS
MENSCHY
MENTEES
MENTHOL
MENTION
MENTORS
MENUBAR
MENUDOS
MENUHIN
MENZIES
MINABLE
MINARET
MINCERS
MINCING
MINDERS
MINDFUL
MINDING
MINDORO
MINDSET
MINEOLA
MINEPIT
MINERAL
MINERVA
MINGIER
MINGLED
MINGLER
MINGLES
MINIBAR
MINIBUS
MINICAB
MINICAM
MINICAR
MINIKIN
MINILAB
MINIMAL
MINIMAX
MINIMUM
MINIMUS
MININGS
MINIONS
MINISKI
MINISUB
MINITVS
MINIVAC
MINIVAN
MINIVER
MINIZOO
MINNOWS
MINOANS
MINOGUE
MINOLTA
MINORCA
MINORED
MINORIN
MINOTND
MINSKYS
MINSTER
MINTAGE
MINTERS
MINTIER
MINTING
MINTTEA
MINUEND
MINUETS
MINUSES
MINUTED
MINUTER
MINUTES
MINUTIA
MINXISH
MINYANS
MONACAN
MONADAL
MONADIC
MONARCH
MONCTON
MONDALE
MONDAVI
MONDAYS
MONDESI
MONDIAL
MONDIEU
MONEYED
MONGERS
MONGKUT
MONGOLS
MONGREL
MONIKER
MONITOR
MONKEES
MONKEYS
MONKISH
MONOCLE
MONODIC
MONOLOG
MONOMER
MONOPOD
MONOSKI
MONROES
MONSOON
MONSTER
MONSTRO
MONTAGE
MONTAGU
MONTALE
MONTANA
MONTAND
MONTANO
MONTAUK
MONTEGO
MONTERO
MONTEUX
MONTHLY
MONTOYA
MONTUNO
MRNANNY
MRNORTH
MRNOVAK
MUNCHED
MUNCHEN
MUNCHER
MUNCHES
MUNCHIE
MUNCHON
MUNDANE
MUNSTER
MYNHEER

M••N•••

MAANDPA
MACNEIL
MADNESS
MAENADS
MAGNANI
MAGNATE
MAGNETO
MAGNETS
MAGNIFY
MAGNUMS
MAINERS
MAINMAN
MAINMEN
MAINTOP
MANNERS
MANNIES
MANNING
MANNISH
MARNIER
MAUNDER
MAYNARD
MCENROE
MEANAGE
MEANDER
MEANEST
MEANIES
MEANING
MEANJOE
MEANSIT
MEANSTO
MEANTIT
MEANTTO
MEYNELL
MIDNOON
MIGNONS
MINNOWS
MISNAME
MOANERS
MOANFUL
MOANING
MOONBOW
MOONDOG
MOONERS
MOONEYE
MOONGOD
MOONIER
MOONIES
MOONILY
MOONING
MOONISH
MOONLET
MOONLIT
MOONPIE
MOONSET
MORNING
MOUNDED
MOUNTED
MOUNTER
MOUNTIE
MOUNTUP
MYANMAR

M•••N••

MACONGA
MADONNA
MAGENTA
MAGINOT
MAHONEY
MAKINGS
MANANAS
MARANTZ
MARENGO
MARINAS
MARINER
MARINES
MASONED
MASONIC
MASONRY
MATINAL
MATINEE
MAYINGS
MCHENRY
MCKENNA
MCRANEY
MEGANES
MEITNER
MELANGE
MELANIA
MELANIC
MELANIE
MELANIN
MELINDA
MEMENTO
MERINOS
MESONIC
MIGENES
MININGS
MIRANDA
MISHNAH
MISKNEW
MISKNOW
MIZUNAS
MOMENTA
MOMENTS
MOMONEY
MORANIS
MORANTE
MORONIC
MOURNED
MOURNER
MOWINGS
MRBONES
MRHANEY
MRJONES
MRNANNY
MTKENYA
MTSINAI
MURANOS
MUSANTE
MUSINGS
MUTANTS
MYCENAE
MYKONOS
MYLANTA

M••••N•

MACHINA
MACHINE
MACHONE
MACOUNS
MACRONS
MADDENS
MADDING
MADEONE
MADONNA
MAGNANI
MAIDENS
MAILING
MAILINS
MAIMING
MAISONS
MAJGENS
MAKEONE
MALEANT
MALIANS
MALIGNS
MALTING
MALVINA
MANCINI
MANDANS
MANGANO
MANHUNT
MANKIND
MANNING
MAPPING
MARCONI
MARGINS
MARIANA
MARIANO
MARKING
MARLENE
MARLINS
MAROONS
MARRING
MARRONS
MARTENS
MARTINA
MARTINI
MARTINO
MARTINS
MARTINU
MARTINV
MARYANN
MASHING
MASKING
MASSINE
MASSING
MASTING
MATRONS
MATTING
MAULING
MAYWINE
MAZZINI
MBABANE
MCKENNA
MCSHANE
MCSWINE
MEANING
MECCANS
MEDIANS
MEDIANT
MEETING
MELDING
MELTING
MEMLING
MENDING
MENSANS
MEOWING
MERGING
MERLINS
MESHING
MESSINA
MESSING
METFANS
METHANE
MEWLING
MICRONS
MIDJUNE
MIDLAND
MIDLINE
MIFFING
MIGHTNT
MIGNONS
MIGRANT
MILKING
MILLAND
MILLEND
MILLING
MINCING
MINDING
MINIONS
MINOANS
MINOTND
MINTING
MINUEND
MINYANS
MIOCENE
MISBIND
MISDONE
MISSEND
MISSENT
MISSING
MISTING
MISTUNE
MISZONE
MITRING
MITTENS
MIZZENS
MOANING
MOBBING
MOCKING
MODERNE
MODERNS
MOILING
MOLDING
MOLSONS
MOLTING
MONTANA
MONTAND
MONTANO
MONTUNO
MOONING
MOORING
MOOTING
MOPPING
MORAINE
MORDANT
MORDENT
MOREENS
MORGANA
MORGANS
MORMONS
MORNING
MORTONS
MOSCONI
MOSHING
MOSSING
MOTIONS
MOTRINS
MOUSING
MRBURNS
MRNANNY
MRWRONG
MTBLANC
MTEVANS
MUCKING
MUDDING
MUDHENS
MUFFING
MUFFINS
MUGGING
MULLING
MULLINS
MUMMING
MUNDANE
MUSHING
MUSIGNY
MUSLINS
MUSSING
MUSTANG
MUTTONS
MYGIANT

M•••••N

MAARTEN
MACEDON
MACHAON
MACLEAN
MADALYN
MADCHEN
MADEFUN
MADELON
MADERUN
MADIGAN
MADISON
MAILBIN
MAILMAN
MAILMEN
MAILSIN
MAINMAN
MAINMEN
MAJORIN
MAKEFUN
MAKERUN
MALAGAN
MALAYAN
MANIKIN
MANOLIN
MANSION
MANSMAN
MANTUAN
MANXMAN
MANXMEN
MARCHON
MARDIAN
MARILYN
MARMION
MARRYIN
MARSDEN
MARSTON
MARTIAN
MARXIAN
MARYANN
MATALIN
MATEWAN
MAUDLIN
MAULDIN
MAUREEN
MAXBORN
MAYALIN
MAZARIN
MCALLEN
MCCOWEN
MCGAVIN
MCLUHAN
MCMAHON
MCQUEEN
MEATMAN
MEATMEN
MECHLIN
MEDUSAN
MEGALON
MEGATON
MEGRYAN
MEISSEN
MELANIN
MENCKEN
MENTION
MENUHIN
MERCIAN
MERIDEN
METSFAN
MEXICAN
MGMLION
MIAMIAN
MIDIRON
MIDMORN
MIDNOON
MIDTEEN
MIDTOWN
MIFFLIN
MILERUN
MILKCAN
MILKMAN
MILKMEN
MILKRUN
MILLION
MILLRUN
MINIKIN
MINIVAN
MINORIN
MISCOIN
MISJOIN
MISPLAN
MISSION
MIXEDIN
MIXESIN
MOHEGAN
MOHICAN
MOISSAN
MOISTEN
MOMMSEN
MONACAN
MONCTON
MONSOON
MOORHEN
MORPHIN
MOVEDIN
MOVEDON
MOVESIN
MOVESON
MOWDOWN
MRBROWN
MRCLEAN
MRGREEN
MRISCAN
MTLOGAN
MUEZZIN
MULDOON
MUMESON
MUNCHEN
MUNCHON
MUSEDON
MUSESON
MUTAGEN
MUYBIEN
MYERSON

•MN••••

AMNERIS
AMNESIA
AMNESIC
AMNESTY
AMNIONS
LMNOPQR
OMNIBUS
OMNIMAX

•M•N•••

AMANITA
AMANTIS
AMENDED
AMENDER
AMENITY
AMINUTE
AMONGST
EMANANT
EMANATE
EMANUEL
EMENDED
EMENDER
EMINENT
OMENING
OMINOUS

•M••N••

AMMONIA
AMMONIC
AMOUNTS
EMBANKS
EMPANEL
FMBANDS
IMEANIT
IMMENSE
IMMUNES
IMPANEL
IMPENDS
IMPINGE
SMIRNOV

•M•••N•

AMARONE
AMAZING
AMAZONS
AMBIENS
AMBIENT
AMBLING
AMERIND
AMNIONS
AMUSING
EMANANT
EMINENT
EMOTING
EMPLANE
IMAGINE
IMAGING
IMBUING
IMEMINE
IMGOING
IMOGENE
IMPLANT
IMPOUND
IMPRINT
IMPUGNS
KMESONS
OMAHANE
OMAHANS
OMENING
SMETANA
SMILING
SMITING
SMOKING

•M••••N

AMESLAN
AMPHION
EMBROWN
EMERSON
EMOTION
EMPIRIN
OMICRON
SMARTEN
SMEARON
SMIDGEN
SMILEON
SMITTEN
UMBRIAN
UMPTEEN

••MN•••

DAMNERS
DAMNING
DIMNESS
GYMNAST
HYMNALS
HYMNARY
HYMNING
HYMNODY
KLMNOPQ
LIMNERS
LIMNING
LIMNITE
REMNANT
ROMNEYS
SAMNUNN

••M•N••

ALMANAC
ALMONDS
ALMONDY
ALMONER
ALMONRY
AMMONIA
AMMONIC
ARMENIA
BIMINIS
CAMINOS
CEMENTS
COMENOW
COMINGS
DEMANDS
DEMENTO
DEMONIC
DEMONYM
DOMINGO
DOMINIC
DOMINOS

DOMINUS
EDMONDS
EDMUNDI
EDMUNDS
ELMONTE
ELMUNDO
ERMINED
ERMINES
ERMINIA
FAMINES
FEMINUM
FOMENTS
GAMINES
GEMINIS
HHMUNRO
HOMINID
HOMONYM
HUMANLY
HUMANUM
IMMENSE
IMMUNES
JIMENEZ
JIMINEZ
JTMONEY
JUMANJI
KIMONOS
LAMENTS
LAMINAE
LAMINAL
LAMINAR
LAMINAS
LAMINTO
LEMONDE
LIMINAL
LUMINAS
MEMENTO
MOMENTA
MOMENTS
MOMONEY
NOMINAL
NOMINEE
ORMANDY
OSMONDS
OSMUNDS
PIMENTO
RAMINTO
RAMONES
REMANDS
REMENDS
REMINDS
REMINED
REMINES
REMINTS
ROMANCE
ROMANIA
ROMANIC
ROMANIS
ROMANOS
ROMANOV
ROMANSH
ROMANUS
RUMANIA
SEMANAS
SEMINAL
SEMINAR
SIMENON
SIMONIZ
SOMINEX
TIMINGS
UNMANED
UNMANLY
UNMINED
VIMINAL
WOMANLY
XIMENES
YEMENIS

••M••N•

AAMILNE
ARMBAND
ARMBONE
ARMYANT
BAMBINA
BAMBINI
BAMBINO
BAMMING
BEMOANS
BOMBING
BUMMING
BUMPING
CAMIONS
CAMPING
COMBINE
COMBING
COMEONS
COMMAND
COMMEND
COMMENT
COMMONS
COMMUNE
COMPANY
COMPEND
COMPING
DAMMING
DAMNING
DAMPENS
DAMPING
DAMSONS
DEMEANS
DEMESNE
DEMOING
DEMOUNT
DIMMING
DOMAINE
DOMAINS
DUMBING
DUMPING
GAMMING
GAMMONS
GIMPING
GUMMING
HAMBONE
HAMLINE
HAMMING
HAMMOND
HEMLINE
HEMMING
HUMMING
HYMNING
JAMBAND
JAMMING
JIMSONS
JUMPING
KAMFONG
LAMBENT
LAMBING
LAMMING
LEMMING
LEMOYNE
LIMBING
LIMNING
LIMPING
LUMPING
MEMLING
MUMMING
NAMEONE
NUMBING
POMPANO
POMPONS
PUMPING
RAMFANS
RAMMING
RAMPANT
RAMPING
RAMSONS
REMAINS
REMNANT
REMOUNT
RIMMING
ROMAINE
ROMAINS
ROMPING
RUMPEND
SAMNUNN
SAMOANS
SAMPANS
SAMSONS
SAMSUNG
SIMIANS
SIMMONS
SOMEONE
SUMMAND
SUMMING
SUMMONS
TAMMANY
TAMPING
TEMPING
TIMMINS
TIMPANI
TYMPANA
TYMPANI
UNMEANT
VAMPING
WIMPING
XAMOUNT
ZAMBONI

••M•••N

ALMADEN
ALMSMAN
ALMSMEN
ASMARAN
BUMPKIN
CAMERON
CAMPION
COMBIEN
COMESIN
COMESON
COMORAN
COMPLIN
COMPTON
DUMPSON
GAMBIAN
GAMELAN
HAMELIN
HAMPTON
HEMATIN
HOMEDIN
HOMERUN
HOMESIN
JAMESON
JAMISON
JEMISON
JIMRYUN
JUMPSIN
JUMPSON
KEMPTON
LAMBKIN
LAMPOON
LIMACON
LUMPSIN
MCMAHON
MGMLION
MOMMSEN
MUMESON
ONMYOWN
PIMESON
PUMPKIN
RAMADAN
RAMBLIN
RAMDOWN
RAMEKIN
RAMSFAN
ROMULAN
SAMISEN
SAMNUNN
SAMPSON
SIMENON
SIMPSON
TAMBLYN
TAMGLEN
ZAMBIAN

•••MN••

ALUMNAE
ALUMNAL
ALUMNUS
CHIMNEY
JKLMNOP
KRAMNIK

•••M•N•

ACUMENS
ADAMANT
AILMENT
ALIMENT
ALIMONY
ALLMINE
ALUMINA
ANEMONE
ATAMANS
AUGMENT
BAMMING
BEAMING
BELMONT
BERMING
BIRMANS
BLAMING
BOOMING
BROMINE
BUMMING
BURMANS
BUSMANS
CAIMANS
CALMING
CARMINA
CARMINE
CATMINT
CAYMANS
CHIMING
CHIMINH
CLAMANT
CLEMENS
CLEMENT
COMMAND
COMMEND
COMMENT
COMMONS
COMMUNE
CREMINI
CREMONA
CRIMINY
DAEMONS
DAMMING
DEEMING
DELMONT
DESMOND
DIAMOND
DIEMENS
DIMMING
DINMONT
DOLMANS
DOOMING
DORMANT
EANMUND
ELEMENT
ELLMANN
ETAMINE
ETYMONS
EXAMINE
FARMING
FERMENT
FIGMENT
FILMING
FIRMING
FLAMING
FLEMING
FOAMING
FORMING
FRAMING
FREMONT
GAMMING
GAMMONS
GARMENT
GERMANE
GERMANS
GERMANY
GNOMONS
GORMING
GRIMING
GUMMING
HAMMING
HAMMOND
HARMING
HARMONY
HELMING
HELMOND
HEMMING
HERMANA
HERMANN
HERMANO
HERMANS
HEYMANS
HOFMANN
HORMONE
HOWMANY
HUMMING
IMEMINE
ITEMING
ITEMONE
JAMMING
JASMINE
KINMONT
KIRMANS
LAMMING
LEHMANN
LEMMING
LIPMANN
LOAMING
LOOMING
MAIMING
MORMONS
MUMMING
NEUMANN
NEWMANS
NEWMINT
NEWMONT
NORMAND
NORMANS
NOTMANY
NOTMINE
ODDMENT
OFAMIND
OUTMANS
PALMING
PAYMENT
PERMING
PIGMENT
PLUMING
PRIMING
PULMONI
PULMONO
RAGMANS
RAIMENT
RAMMING
RAYMOND
REAMEND
REAMING
REDMOND
REYMONT
RHYMING
RIEMANN
RIMMING
RIOMUNI
ROAMING
ROOMING
SALMONP
SALMONS
SEAMING
SEEMING
SEGMENT
SERMONS
SHAMANS
SHAMING
SIEMENS
SIGMUND
SIMMONS
SLIMING
SPUMING
SPUMONE
SPUMONI
STAMENS
STAMINA
SUMMAND
SUMMING
SUMMONS
TAMMANY
TEAMING
TEEMING
TERMING
TERMINI
THYMINE
TIMMINS
TINMINE
TOOMANY
TORMENT
TRUMANS
ULLMANN
UNAMUNO
VARMINT
VERMINY
VERMONT
WARMING
WORMING
WYOMING
YAOMING
YASMINE
YEOMANS
YOUMANS
ZOOMING

•••M••N

ADAMSON
ALAMEIN
ARAMEAN
BALMAIN
BLAMEON
CHIMEIN
CHOMPON
CLAMPON
CLEMSON
CLIMBIN
CLIMBON
CRAMPON
CRAMSIN
CRIMEAN
CRIMSON
DRUMLIN
ELLMANN
FERMION
GASMAIN
GERMAIN
GREMLIN
GRUMMAN
HERMANN
HOFMANN
KRAMDEN
KREMLIN
LEHMANN
LETMEIN
LIPMANN
MARMION
MIAMIAN
MIDMORN
MOMMSEN
NEUMANN
NEWMOON
NEWMOWN
OLDMOON
PERMIAN
RIEMANN
SKIMPON
SLAMSON
STIMSON
STOMPIN
STOMPON
THEMOON
THOMSON
TIOMKIN
TROMPIN
ULLMANN
ZOOMSIN

••••MN•

AUTOMNE
AUTUMNS
CALUMNY
COLUMNS
IJKLMNO
ILIAMNA
THEOMNI

••••M•N

ABDOMEN
ADWOMAN
ADWOMEN
AGNOMEN
AJSIMON
ALBUMEN
ALBUMIN
ALMSMAN
ALMSMEN
ANDAMAN
AQUAMAN
BACHMAN
BADOMEN
BAHAMEN
BASEMAN
BASEMEN
BATEMAN
BATSMAN
BATSMEN
BEHRMAN
BELLMAN
BELLMEN
BERGMAN
BESTMAN
BESTMEN
BIRDMAN
BIRDMEN
BOATMAN
BOATMEN
BOGYMAN
BOGYMEN
BONDMAN
BONDMEN
BOOKMAN
BOOKMEN
BOORMAN
BOSSMAN
BOSSMEN
BOZEMAN
BRAHMAN
BRAHMIN
BUCHMAN
BUSHMAN
BUSHMEN
CAVEMAN
CAVEMEN
CERUMEN
CHAPMAN
CHAPMEN
CHARMAN
CHARMEN
CHARMIN
COLEMAN
COPYMAN
COPYMEN
CREWMAN
CREWMEN
DARKMAN
DELIMAN
DELIMEN
DILLMAN
DISCMAN
DOORMAN
DOORMEN
DORFMAN
DRAWMAN
DRAWMEN
DRAYMAN
DRAYMEN
DREAMIN
DREAMON
DUSTMAN
DUSTMEN
EASTMAN
EIJKMAN
ESTAMIN
EUDEMON
FADIMAN
FELDMAN
FEYNMAN
FIREMAN
FIREMEN
FIVEMAN
FLAGMAN
FLAGMEN
FOOTMAN
FOOTMEN
FOREMAN
FOREMEN
FOURMAN
FREEMAN
FREEMEN
FROGMAN
FROGMEN
GASSMAN
GATEMAN
GATEMEN
GILLMAN
GLEEMAN
GLEEMEN
GLOAMIN
GOLDMAN
GOODMAN
GOODMEN
GRAUMAN
GRUMMAN
HACKMAN
HANGMAN
HANGMEN
HARTMAN
HAWKMAN
HEADMAN
HEADMEN
HECKMAN
HEISMAN
HELLMAN
HICKMAN
HILLMAN
HILLMEN
HOFFMAN
HOLYMAN
HOLYMEN
HOLZMAN
HOOPMAN
HOOPMEN
HOUSMAN
HUFFMAN
IDEAMAN
IDEAMEN
IDIAMIN
INHUMAN
IRONMAN
IRONMEN
ISTOMIN
JAVAMAN
JAZZMAN
JAZZMEN
JUNKMAN
JUNKMEN
JURYMAN
JURYMEN
KAUFMAN
KINGMAN
KINSMAN
KINSMEN
KLUGMAN
LANDMAN
LANDMEN
LEADMAN
LEADMEN
LENSMAN
LENSMEN
LETEMIN
LINEMAN
LINEMEN
LUCKMAN
MAILMAN
MAILMEN
MAINMAN
MAINMEN
MANSMAN
MANXMAN
MANXMEN
MEATMAN
MEATMEN
MILKMAN
MILKMEN
NAVYMAN
NAVYMEN
NESSMAN
NEWSMAN
NEWSMEN
NICEMAN
NICEMEN
OARSMAN
OARSMEN
OTTOMAN
OVERMAN
PALEMON
PARKMAN
PERLMAN
PETEMAN
PETEMEN
PITTMAN
PLOWMAN
PLOWMEN
PNEUMON
POKEMON
POLEMAN
POLEMEN
POOLMAN
POOLMEN
POORMAN
POORMEN
PORTMAN
POSTMAN
POSTMEN
PROPMAN
PROPMEN
PULLMAN
RAILMAN
RAILMEN
RAINMAN
REALMAN
REALMEN
REEDMAN
REEDMEN
REGIMEN
REITMAN
REPOMAN
RICHMAN
RICHMEN
RICKMAN
RIESMAN
SALOMON
SANDMAN
SANDMEN
SARUMAN
SAYAMEN
SCATMAN
SHERMAN
SHIPMAN
SHIPMEN
SHOWMAN
SHOWMEN
SHULMAN
SIDEMAN
SIDEMEN
SNOWMAN
SNOWMEN
SOLOMON
SOULMAN
STARMAN
STORMIN
STSIMON
SURFMAN
SURFMEN
SWAGMAN
SWAGMEN
SYNGMAN
TAPEMAN
TAPEMEN
TAXIMAN
TAXIMEN
THEOMEN
THIAMIN
THINMAN
THURMAN
TIREMAN
TIREMEN
TOLLMAN
TOLLMEN
TUCHMAN
TURFMAN
TURFMEN
UNHUMAN
VELTMAN
VENEMAN
VITAMIN
WAKSMAN
WALKMAN
WEIDMAN
WELLMAN
WHITMAN
WILDMAN
WILDMEN
WINGMAN
WINGMEN
WIREMAN
WIREMEN
WISEMAN
WISEMEN
WOLFMAN
WOLFMEN
WORKMAN
WORKMEN
YALEMAN
YALEMEN
YARDMAN
YARDMEN
YEAHMAN
YZERMAN

•••••MN

CONDEMN
CONTEMN
EDINAMN
HIJKLMN
OUTLIMN

MO•••••

MOABITE
MOANERS
MOANFUL
MOANING
MOBBERS
MOBBING
MOBBISH
MOBBISM
MOBBIST
MOBILES
MOBRULE
MOBSTER
MOCHRIE
MOCKERS
MOCKERY
MOCKING
MOCKSUP
MOCKUPS
MODELAS
MODELBS
MODELED
MODELER
MODELTS
MODEMED
MODERNE
MODERNS
MODESTO
MODESTY
MODICUM
MODISTE
MODULAR
MODULES
MODULUS
MOEBERG
MOGADOR
MOGAMBO
MOHAIRS
MOHAVES
MOHAWKS
MOHEGAN
MOHICAN
MOILERS
MOILING
MOISSAN
MOISTEN
MOISTER
MOISTLY
MOJAVES
MOJITOS
MOLDERS
MOLDIER
MOLDING
MOLDOVA
MOLERAT
MOLESTS
MOLIERE
MOLITOR
MOLLIES
MOLLIFY
MOLLUSC
MOLLUSK
MOLOKAI
MOLOTOV
MOLSONS
MOLTERS
MOLTING
MOLUCCA
MOMBASA
MOMENTA
MOMENTS
MOMMIES
MOMMSEN
MOMONEY
MOMUSES
MONACAN
MONADAL
MONADIC
MONARCH
MONCTON
MONDALE
MONDAVI
MONDAYS
MONDESI
MONDIAL
MONDIEU
MONEYED
MONGERS
MONGKUT
MONGOLS
MONGREL

MONIKER
MONITOR
MONKEES
MONKEYS
MONKISH
MONOCLE
MONODIC
MONOLOG
MONOMER
MONOPOD
MONOSKI
MONROES
MONSOON
MONSTER
MONSTRO
MONTAGE
MONTAGU
MONTALE
MONTANA
MONTAND
MONTANO
MONTAUK
MONTEGO
MONTERO
MONTEUX
MONTHLY
MONTOYA
MONTUNO
MOOCHED
MOOCHER
MOOCHES
MOOCOWS
MOODIER
MOODILY
MOONBOW
MOONDOG
MOONERS
MOONEYE
MOONGOD
MOONIER
MOONIES
MOONILY
MOONING
MOONISH
MOONLET
MOONLIT
MOONPIE
MOONSET
MOORAGE
MOORHEN
MOORIER
MOORING
MOORISH
MOOTERS
MOOTING
MOPHEAD
MOPIEST
MOPPERS
MOPPETS
MOPPING
MOPTOPS
MORAINE
MORALES
MORALLY
MORANIS
MORANTE
MORAVIA
MORCERF
MORDANT
MORDENT
MORDRED
MOREENS
MORELLA
MORELLO
MORELOS
MOREPAY
MORESBY
MORETTI
MORGANA
MORGANS
MORGUES
MORISOT
MORLOCK
MORMONS
MORNING
MOROCCO
MORONIC
MORPHED
MORPHIC
MORPHIN
MORROWS
MORSELS
MORTALS
MORTARS
MORTICE
MORTIFY
MORTISE
MORTONS
MOSAICS
MOSCATO
MOSCONI
MOSELLE
MOSEYED
MOSHERS
MOSHING
MOSHPIT
MOSLEMS
MOSQUES
MOSSIER
MOSSING
MOTHERS
MOTHERY
MOTHIER
MOTIONS
MOTIVED
MOTIVES
MOTLEYS
MOTORED
MOTRINS
MOTTLED
MOTTLES
MOTTOES
MOULAGE
MOULDED
MOULDER
MOULTED
MOUNDED
MOUNTED
MOUNTER
MOUNTIE
MOUNTUP
MOURNED
MOURNER
MOUSERS
MOUSIER
MOUSILY
MOUSING
MOUSSED
MOUSSES
MOUTHED
MOUTHER
MOVABLE
MOVABLY
MOVADOS
MOVEDIN
MOVEDIT
MOVEDON
MOVEDTO
MOVEDUP
MOVEOFF
MOVEOUT
MOVESIN
MOVESIT
MOVESON
MOVESTO
MOVESUP
MOWBRAY
MOWDOWN
MOWINGS
MOZETTA
MOZILLA

M•O••••

MAOISTS
MAOSUIT
MEOWERS
MEOWING
MEOWMIX
MIOCENE
MNOPQRS
MOOCHED
MOOCHER
MOOCHES
MOOCOWS
MOODIER
MOODILY
MOONBOW
MOONDOG
MOONERS
MOONEYE
MOONGOD
MOONIER
MOONIES
MOONILY
MOONING
MOONISH
MOONLET
MOONLIT
MOONPIE
MOONSET
MOORAGE
MOORHEN
MOORIER
MOORING
MOORISH
MOOTERS
MOOTING
MYOLOGY
MYOPIAS

M••O•••

MACONGA
MACOUNS
MADONNA
MAHONEY
MAHOUTS
MAJORCA
MAJORED
MAJORIN
MALODOR
MANOLIN
MANOWAR
MAROONS
MASONED
MASONIC
MASONRY
MAYORAL
MCCOURT
MCCOVEY
MCCOWEN
MEGOHMS
MEIOSES
MEIOSIS
MEIOTIC
MELODIA
MELODIC
MEMOIRE
MEMOIRS
MEMOPAD
MEMOREX
MENORAH
MENORCA
MENOTTI
MESONIC
METOOER
MIAOUED
MIAOWED
MIDOFFS
MILORDS
MIMOSAS
MINOANS
MINOGUE
MINOLTA
MINORCA
MINORED
MINORIN
MINOTND
MITOSES
MITOSIS
MITOTIC
MOLOKAI
MOLOTOV
MOMONEY
MONOCLE
MONODIC
MONOLOG
MONOMER
MONOPOD
MONOSKI
MOROCCO
MORONIC
MOTORED
MRBODDY
MRBONES
MRHOBBS
MRHORSE
MRJONES
MRMOOSE
MRNORTH
MRNOVAK
MRWORDS
MTLOGAN
MYKONOS
MYWORLD

M•••O••

MACHONE
MACRONS
MADDOGS
MADEOFF
MADEONE
MADEOUT
MADLOCK
MAFIOSI
MAFIOSO
MAGGOTS
MAHFOUZ
MAHZORS
MAILOUT
MAISONS
MAISOUI
MAKEOFF
MAKEONE
MAKEOUT
MALCOLM
MALLOWS
MALTOSE
MAMBOED
MAMMOTH
MANDOKI
MANGOES
MANHOLE
MANHOOD
MANHOUR
MANROPE
MAPSOUT
MARCONI
MARKOFF
MARKOUT
MARKOVA
MARLOWE
MARMOTS
MAROONS
MARRONS
MARROWS
MASCOTS
MASTOID
MATLOCK
MATRONS
MATTOCK
MATZOHS
MATZOTH
MAUROIS
MAXBORN
MAYPOLE
MCCLOUD
MCGRORY
MEADOWS
MEADOWY
MEDFORD
MELLOWS
MELROSE
MENFOLK
MENTORS
MERLOTS
METEORS
METEOUT
METHODS
METOOER
MICROBE
MICRONS
MIDMORN
MIDMOST
MIDNOON
MIDSOLE
MIDTOWN
MIGNONS
MILHOUS
MIMEOED
MINDORO
MINEOLA
MINIONS
MINNOWS
MIRRORS
MISCODE
MISCOIN
MISCOPY
MISDOER
MISDOES
MISDONE
MISFORM
MISJOIN
MISKOLC
MISMOVE
MISSORT
MISSOUT
MISTOLD
MISTOOK
MISWORD
MISZONE
MITFORD
MOLDOVA
MOLSONS
MONGOLS
MONROES
MONSOON
MONTOYA
MOOCOWS
MOPTOPS
MORLOCK
MORMONS
MORROWS
MORTONS
MOSCONI
MOTIONS
MOTTOES
MOVEOFF
MOVEOUT
MOWDOWN
MRBROWN
MRMOOSE
MRSCOTT
MRSPOCK
MRWRONG
MUDHOLE
MUDROOM
MULDOON
MUMFORD
MURDOCH
MUTTONS
MYCROFT
MYOLOGY

M••••O•

MACACOS
MACEDON
MACHAON
MACLEOD
MADEFOR
MADELON
MADISON
MADUROS
MAGALOG
MAGINOT
MAILBOX
MAILLOL
MAILLOT
MAINTOP
MAKEDOS
MAKEFOR
MALEDOG
MALEHOG
MALODOR
MANHOOD
MANILOW
MANSION
MARCHON
MARIDOS
MARMION
MARSTON
MARYLOU
MATADOR
MCENROE
MCMAHON
MEANJOE
MEDICOS
MEGALON
MEGATON
MENTHOL
MENTION
MENUDOS
MERINOS
MGMLION
MIDIRON
MIDNOON
MIKADOS
MILKCOW
MILKSOP
MILLION
MINIZOO
MIRADOR
MISKNOW
MISSION
MISSYOU
MISTBOW
MISTOOK
MOGADOR
MOJITOS
MOLITOR
MOLOTOV
MONCTON
MONITOR
MONOLOG
MONOPOD
MONSOON
MOONBOW
MOONDOG
MOONGOD
MORELOS
MORISOT
MOVADOS
MOVEDON
MOVESON
MRHULOT
MRMAGOO
MTATHOS
MUDFLOW
MUDROOM
MUGSHOT
MULDOON
MUMESON
MUNCHON
MURANOS
MUSEDON
MUSESON
MUSTDOS
MYERSON
MYKONOS

M•••••O

MACHTWO
MAESTRO
MAFIOSO
MAGNETO
MAKESDO
MAKESGO
MALPASO
MANCUSO
MANGANO
MANKATO
MANRICO
MARCATO
MARENGO
MARIANO
MARTINO
MARULLO
MAYBESO
MCMURDO
MEANSTO
MEANTTO
MEMENTO
MERCADO
MILAGRO
MINDORO
MINIZOO
MODESTO
MOGAMBO
MONSTRO
MONTANO
MONTEGO
MONTERO
MONTUNO
MORELLO
MOROCCO
MOSCATO
MOVEDTO
MOVESTO
MRMACHO
MRMAGOO
MULATTO
MURILLO
MUSKEGO

•MO••••

AMOEBAE
AMOEBAS
AMOEBIC
AMONGST
AMORIST
AMOROSO
AMOROUS
AMOUNTS
BMOVIES
EMOTERS
EMOTING
EMOTION
EMOTIVE
IMOGENE
SMOKERS
SMOKEUP
SMOKEYS
SMOKIER
SMOKIES
SMOKILY
SMOKING
SMOLDER
SMOOTHS
SMOOTHY
SMOTHER
TMOBILE

•M•O•••

AMMONIA
AMMONIC
AMPOULE
EMBOITE
EMBOSOM
EMBOWER
EMPORIA
EMPOWER
IMBORED
IMFORIT
IMGOING
IMHOTEP
IMMORAL
IMPORTS
IMPOSED
IMPOSER
IMPOSES
IMPOSTS
IMPOUND
IMSORRY
IMYOURS
LMNOPQR
SMOOTHS
SMOOTHY

•M••O••

AMAPOLA
AMARONE
AMATOLS
AMATORY
AMAZONS
AMBROSE
AMEBOID
AMIDOLS
AMNIONS
AMOROSO
AMOROUS
AMPHORA
EMBROIL
EMBROWN
EMPLOYS
EMULOUS
IMAGOES
IMAHOGG
IMBROKE
IMPIOUS
IMPLODE
IMPLORE
IMPROVE
KMESONS
OMIGOSH
OMINOUS

•M•••O•

AMPHION
EMBOSOM
EMBRYOS
EMERSON
EMMYLOU
EMOTION
EMPEROR
OMICRON
SMACKOF
SMALLOJ
SMEAGOL
SMEARON
SMILEON
SMIRNOV

•M••••O

AMERIGO
AMOROSO
AMRADIO
EMBARGO
FMRADIO
IMPASTO
IMUSTGO
OMPHALO
UMBERTO
XMRADIO

••MO•••

ALMONDS
ALMONDY
ALMONER
ALMONRY
AMMONIA
AMMONIC
ARMOIRE
ARMORED
ARMORER
ARMOURS
ARMOURY
BEMOANS
BIMODAL
BYMOUTH
COMORAN
COMOROS
DAMOSEL
DEMOING
DEMOLAY
DEMONIC
DEMONYM
DEMOTED
DEMOTES
DEMOTHS
DEMOTIC
DEMOUNT
DIMOUTS
EDMONDS
ELMONTE
FEMORAL
FEMORIS
GQMODEL
HOMONYM
HUMORAL
HUMORED
HUMORME
HUMOURS
IMMORAL
IOMOTHS
JTMONEY
KIMONOS
LAMOTTA
LAMOTTE
LEMONDE
LEMOYNE
LIMOGES
MEMOIRE
MEMOIRS
MEMOPAD
MEMOREX
MIMOSAS
MOMONEY
MRMOOSE
ORMOLUS
OSMONDS
OSMOSED
OSMOSES
OSMOSIS
OSMOTIC
RAMONES
REMODEL
REMOLDS
REMORAS
REMORSE
REMOTER
REMOTES
REMOUNT
REMOVAL
REMOVED
REMOVER
REMOVES
REMOWED
RUMORED
RUMOURS
SAMOANS
SAMOSAS
SAMOSET
SAMOVAR
SAMOYED
SIMONIZ
SUMOIST
TIMOTHY
TVMOVIE
UNMOIST
UNMOLDS
UNMOLDY
UNMOODY
UNMOORS
UNMOSSY
UNMOULD
UNMOVED
UNMOWED
UTMOSTS
VAMOOSE
WIMOWEH
XAMOUNT

••M•O••

ARMBONE
ARMHOLE
ARMLOAD
ARMLOCK
BAMBOOS
BIMBOES
BUMSOUT
CAMBOYS
CAMEOED
CAMEOFF
CAMEOUT
CAMIONS
CAMPOUT
COMEOFF
COMEONS
COMEOUT
COMFORT
COMMODE
COMMONS
COMMOVE
COMPORT
COMPOSE
COMPOST
COMPOTE
DAMPOFF
DAMSONS
DIMSOUT
DUMPOUT
ELMWOOD
FEMBOTS
GAMBOLS
GAMMONS
GUMBOOT
GUMWOOD
GYMSOCK
HAMBONE
HAMHOCK
HAMMOCK
HAMMOND
HEMLOCK
HYMNODY
IAMLOVE
JIMHOGG
JIMSONS
JUMPOFF
KAMFONG
KLMNOPQ
LAMPOIL
LAMPOON
LIMPOPO
MAMBOED
MAMMOTH
MIMEOED
MRMOOSE
MUMFORD
NAMEONE
NIMRODS
NUMLOCK
ONMYOWN
POMPOMS
POMPONS
POMPOUS
PUMPOUT
RAMDOWN
RAMHOME
RAMRODS
RAMSONS
RIMROCK
ROMCOMS
RUMFORD
RUMPOLE
SAMBORA
SAMEOLD
SAMLOYD
SAMSONS
SIMMONS
SOMEONE
SUMMONS
SYMBOLS
TEMPORE
TIMEOFF
TIMEOUT
TIMHOLT
TIMROTH
TOMBOYS
TOMFOOL
TOMGOLA
TOMJOAD
TOMTOMS
UNMOODY
UNMOORS
VAMOOSE
WIMPOLE
WIMPOUT
YOMTOVS
ZAMBONI

••M••O•

AIMSFOR
BAMBOOS
CAMAROS
CAMELOT
CAMERON
CAMINOS
CAMPHOR
CAMPION
COMENOW
COMESON
COMOROS
COMPTON
DAMPMOP
DEMAGOG
DEMEROL
DEMIGOD
DOMINOS
DRMCCOY
DUMPSON
ELMWOOD
EMMYLOU
EXMAYOR
FAMICOM
GAMEBOY
GEMSBOK
GUMBOOT
GUMDROP
GUMSHOE
GUMWOOD
GYMSHOE
HAMPTON
HOMEBOY
HUMIDOR
JAMESON
JAMISON
JEMISON
JUMPSON
KEMIDOV
KEMPTON
KIMONOS
LAMPOON
LIMACON
MCMAHON
MGMLION

MRMAGOO
MUMESON
NEMEROV
NUMEROS
PIMESON
POMELOS
RIMSHOT
ROMANOS
ROMANOV
RUMSHOP
SAMPSON
SEMILOG
SIMENON
SIMPSON
SOMEHOW
SYMPTOM
TEMBLOR
TEMPJOB
TIMECOP
TOMFOOL

••M•••O

ADMITTO
BAMBINO
CAMACHO
CEMBALO
COMESTO
DEMARCO
DEMENTO
DOMINGO
DRMARIO
ELMUNDO
GAMBADO
HHMUNRO
LAMINTO
LIMPOPO
LUMBAGO
MCMURDO
MEMENTO
MRMACHO
MRMAGOO
PAMLICO
PIMENTO
PIMLICO
POMPANO
RAMINTO
SAMMYJO
SEMIPRO
SUMUPTO
TAMPICO
UNMACHO
ZEMSTVO

•••MO••

AFTMOST
ALAMODE
ALAMOSA
ALIMONY
ANDMORE
ANEMONE
ANYMORE
ARDMORE
ATEMORE
BADMOOD
BADMOVE
BELMONT
BONMOTS
BRUMOUS
CHAMOIS
CLAMORS
CLAMOUR
COMMODE
COMMONS
COMMOVE
CONMOTO
CREMONA
CREMORA
DAEMONS
DELMONT
DELMORE
DENMOMS
DESMOGS
DESMOND
DIAMOND
DINMONT
DRUMOUT
DRYMOPS
EATMORE
ENAMORS
ENAMOUR
ENDMOST
ETHMOID
ETYMONS
FARMORE
FARMOUT
FORMOSA
FREMONT
GAMMONS
GILMORE
GLAMORS
GLAMOUR
GNOMONS
GUNMOLL
HAMMOCK
HAMMOND
HARMONY
HAYMOWS
HELMOND
HERMOSA
HERMOSO
HOLMOAK
HORMONE
INAMOOD
ITEMONE
KENMORE
KINMONT
MAMMOTH
MARMOTS
MIDMORN
MIDMOST
MISMOVE
MORMONS
NEWMONT
NEWMOON
NEWMOWN
OAKMOSS
OLDMOON
ONEMORE
OUTMODE
OUTMOST
OUTMOVE
OXYMORA
PALMOFF
PALMOIL
PAYMORE
PLUMOSE
PROMOED
PROMOTE
PULMONI
PULMONO
RAGMOPS
RAYMOND
REAMOUT
REDMOND
REYMONT
SALMONP
SALMONS
SAYMORE
SCHMOES
SEAMOSS
SERMONS
SEYMOUR
SIGMOID
SIMMONS
SPUMONE
SPUMONI
SUMMONS
THEMOON
THEMOST
TOPMOST
TREMOLO
TREMORS
TRIMOFF
TURMOIL
TWOMORE
UNSMOKY
VERMONT
WETMOPS
ZOOMOUT

•••M•O•

ADAMSON
BADMOOD
BLAMEON
BOOMBOX
CHOMPON
CLAMPON
CLEMSON
CLIMBON
CRAMPON
CRIMSON
FARMBOY
FERMION
FILMDOM
FLUMMOX
INAMOOD
JKLMNOP
MARMION
NEWMOON
OLDMOON
PALMTOP
PLUMCOT
SHAMPOO
SKIMPON
SLAMSON
SPAMBOT
STIMSON
STOMPON
THEMOON
THOMSON
TIEMPOS

•••M••O

ANIMATO
CLAMATO
CLIMBTO
CONMOTO
DERMATO
DOOMSTO
EJEMPLO
GROMYKO
HERMANO
HERMOSO
LETMEGO
PRIMERO
PULMONO
SAMMYJO
SEEMSTO
SHAMPOO
THEMAYO
TREMOLO
UNAMUNO
WARMSTO

••••MO•

AJSIMON
CESTMOI
CHEZMOI
DAMPMOP
DREAMOF
DREAMON
DUSTMOP
DYNAMOS
ESKIMOS
EUDEMON
FLUMMOX
PALEMON
PNEUMON
POKEMON
RANAMOK
ROLLMOP
RUNAMOK
SALEMOR
SALOMON
SOLOMON
STEPMOM
STSIMON
THERMOS
TINAMOU

••••M•O

AAJUMBO
COLOMBO
COLUMBO
ELCAMPO
IJKLMNO
INLIMBO
MOGAMBO
UPTEMPO

•••••MO

ANDIAMO
ANSELMO
BERGAMO
CENTIMO
EXANIMO
GIACOMO
LACRIMO
NANAIMO
PALERMO
PROXIMO
SANREMO
SATCHMO
TURISMO
VERISMO
YOTEAMO

MP•••••

MPTHREE

M•P••••

MAPPERS
MAPPING
MAPSOUT
MCPAPER
MOPHEAD
MOPIEST
MOPPERS
MOPPETS
MOPPING
MOPTOPS
MRPADRE
MTPELEE
MUPPETS

M••P•••

MAGPIES
MALPASO
MAPPERS
MAPPING
MAUPRAT
MAYPOLE
MEMPHIS
MISPAGE
MISPLAN
MISPLAY
MNOPQRS
MOPPERS
MOPPETS
MOPPING
MORPHED
MORPHIC
MORPHIN
MRSPAUL
MRSPEEL
MRSPOCK
MUDPACK
MUDPIES
MUPPETS
MURPHYS
MYOPIAS
MYSPACE

M•••P••

MADEPAR
MAKEPAR
MALEPIG
MANIPLE
MANIPUR
MAZEPPA
MCPAPER
MEATPIE
MEMOPAD
MINEPIT
MONOPOD
MOONPIE
MOREPAY
MOSHPIT

M••••P•

MAANDPA
MADCAPS
MAKEUPS
MANROPE
MARKUPS
MAZEPPA
MESSUPS
MIDCAPS
MISCOPY
MISHAPS
MISTYPE
MOCKUPS
MOPTOPS
MRCHIPS

M•••••P

MAINTOP
MAKESUP
MANTRAP
MARKSUP
MASTERP
MATCHUP
MEDIGAP
MEETSUP
MIDSHIP
MILKSOP
MISSHIP
MISSTEP
MISTSUP
MIXEDUP
MIXESUP
MIXITUP
MOCKSUP
MOUNTUP
MOVEDUP
MOVESUP
MRQUILP
MUCKSUP
MUDFLAP
MUDWASP
MUGWUMP

•MP••••

AMPEDUP
AMPERES
AMPHION
AMPHORA
AMPLEST
AMPLIFY
AMPOULE
AMPULES
EMPALED
EMPALES
EMPANEL
EMPATHS
EMPATHY
EMPEROR
EMPIRES
EMPIRIC
EMPIRIN
EMPLACE
EMPLANE
EMPLOYS
EMPORIA
EMPOWER
EMPRESS
EMPRISE
EMPTIED
EMPTIER
EMPTIES
EMPTILY
IMPACTS
IMPAIRS
IMPALAS
IMPALED
IMPALER
IMPALES
IMPANEL
IMPARTS
IMPASSE
IMPASTO
IMPAVID
IMPEACH
IMPEDED
IMPEDER
IMPEDES
IMPENDS
IMPERIL
IMPETUS
IMPIETY
IMPINGE
IMPIOUS
IMPLANT
IMPLEAD
IMPLIED
IMPLIES
IMPLODE
IMPLORE
IMPORTS
IMPOSED
IMPOSER
IMPOSES
IMPOSTS
IMPOUND
IMPRESS
IMPREST
IMPREZA
IMPRINT
IMPROVE
IMPUGNS
IMPULSE
IMPURER
IMPUTED
IMPUTER
IMPUTES
OMPHALO
UMPIRED
UMPIRES
UMPTEEN

•M•P•••

AMAPOLA

•M••P••

IMHAPPY
LMNOPQR

•M•••P•

IMHAPPY

•M••••P

AMPEDUP
IMHOTEP
SMACKUP
SMASHUP
SMOKEUP

••MP•••

ARMPITS
BUMPERS
BUMPIER
BUMPILY
BUMPING
BUMPKIN
BUMPSUP
CAMPARI
CAMPBED
CAMPERS
CAMPHOR
CAMPIER
CAMPILY
CAMPING
CAMPION
CAMPOUT
CAMPSUP
COMPACT
COMPANY
COMPAQS
COMPARE
COMPART
COMPASS
COMPEER
COMPELS
COMPEND
COMPERE
COMPETE
COMPILE
COMPING
COMPLEX
COMPLIN
COMPORT
COMPOSE
COMPOST
COMPOTE
COMPTON
COMPUTE
DAMPDRY
DAMPENS
DAMPERS
DAMPEST
DAMPING
DAMPISH
DAMPMOP
DAMPOFF
DEMPSEY
DIMPLED
DIMPLES
DUMPERS
DUMPIER
DUMPILY
DUMPING
DUMPISH
DUMPOUT
DUMPSON
GIMPING
GOMPERS
HAMPERS
HAMPTON
HEMPIER
HUMPHED
HUMPHRY
HUMPIER
JAMPACK
JUMPBID
JUMPCUT
JUMPERS
JUMPIER
JUMPILY
JUMPING
JUMPOFF
JUMPSAT
JUMPSIN
JUMPSON
JUMPSUP
KAMPALA
KEMPTON
LAMPERT
LAMPLIT
LAMPOIL
LAMPOON
LAMPREY
LEMPIRA
LIMPEST
LIMPETS
LIMPING
LIMPOPO
LUMPERS
LUMPIER
LUMPILY
LUMPING
LUMPISH
LUMPSIN
LUMPSIT
LUMPSUM
MEMPHIS
NYMPHAL
NYMPHIC
OOMPAHS
PAMPERS
PIMPLED
PIMPLES
POMPANO
POMPEIA
POMPEII
POMPOMS
POMPONS
POMPOUS
PUMPERS
PUMPING
PUMPKIN
PUMPOUT
PUMPSUP
RAMPAGE
RAMPANT
RAMPART
RAMPING
RAMPSUP
RIMPLED
RIMPLES
ROMPERS
ROMPING
ROMPISH
RUMPEND
RUMPLED
RUMPLES
RUMPOLE
SAMPANS
SAMPLED
SAMPLER
SAMPLES
SAMPRAS
SAMPSON
SIMPERS
SIMPLER
SIMPLES
SIMPLEX
SIMPSON
SYMPTOM
TAMPAFL
TAMPERS
TAMPICO
TAMPING
TEMPEAZ
TEMPEHS
TEMPERA
TEMPERS
TEMPEST
TEMPING
TEMPJOB
TEMPLAR
TEMPLED
TEMPLES
TEMPORE
TEMPTED
TEMPTER
TEMPURA
TIMPANI
TYMPANA
TYMPANI
VAMPERS
VAMPIER
VAMPING
VAMPIRA
VAMPIRE
VAMPISH
WAMPUMS
WIMPIER
WIMPING
WIMPISH
WIMPLED
WIMPLES
WIMPOLE
WIMPOUT

••M•P••

LIMEPIE
MEMOPAD
SEMIPRO
SUMUPTO

••M••P•

BUMRAPS
KLMNOPQ
LIMPOPO

••M•••P

BUMPSUP
CAMPSUP
COMESUP
DAMPMOP
DUMMYUP
GUMDROP
HAMITUP
JUMPSUP
PUMPSUP
RAMPSUP
RUMSHOP
SUMITUP
TIMECOP
TIMESUP

•••MP••

BLIMPIE
CHAMPED
CHAMPER
CHOMPED
CHOMPON
CHUMPED
CLAMPED
CLAMPER
CLAMPON
CLOMPED
CLUMPED
CRAMPED
CRAMPON
CRIMPED
CRIMPER
CRUMPED
CRUMPET
CRUMPLE
CRUMPLY
EJEMPLO
EXAMPLE
EXEMPLA
EXEMPTS
GLIMPSE
GRAMPAS
GRAMPUS
GRUMPED
LOOMPAS
OLYMPIA
OLYMPIC
OLYMPUS
ONEMPTY
PLUMPED
PLUMPER
PLUMPIE
PLUMPLY
PRIMPED
PROMPTS
REIMPLY
SCAMPED
SCAMPER
SHAMPOO
SKIMPED
SKIMPON
SLUMPED
STAMPED
STAMPER
STEMPEL
STOMPED
STOMPIN
STOMPON
STUMPED
STUMPER
SWAMPED
THIMPHU
THUMPED
THUMPER
TIEMPOS
TRAMPAS
TRAMPED
TRAMPER
TRAMPLE
TROMPED
TROMPIN
TRUMPED
TRUMPET
TRUMPUP
UNEMPTY
WHIMPER
WHOMPED

•••M•P•

AAAMAPS
BITMAPS
DRYMOPS
RAGMOPS
SEAMAPS
SKYMAPS
WARMUPS
WETMOPS

•••M••P

BEAMSUP
CLAMDIP
CLAMSUP
CLIMBUP
DRUMSUP
DUMMYUP
FIRMSUP
FLAMEUP
FRAMEUP
GLAMSUP
JKLMNOP
PALMTOP
SALMONP
SWIMSUP
TEAMSUP
TRUMPUP
WARMSUP

••••MP•

ATTEMPT
CCLAMPS
DECAMPS
ELCAMPO
ENCAMPS
GALUMPH
ONRAMPS
PREAMPS
PREEMPT
REPUMPS
REVAMPS
SCRIMPS
SCRIMPY
SHRIMPS
SHRIMPY
TRIUMPH
UNKEMPT
UNLUMPY
UPTEMPO

••••M•P

AREAMAP
DAMPMOP
DREAMUP
DUSTMOP
GRIDMAP
PUTEMUP
ROADMAP
ROLLMOP
SITEMAP
STARMAP
STEAMUP
WALLMAP

•••••MP

AIRPUMP
ARCLAMP
BEDLAMP
DAYCAMP
DUCHAMP
FOGLAMP
GASLAMP
GASPUMP
JOECAMP
MUGWUMP
NOTRUMP
OFFRAMP
OILLAMP
ONELUMP
OUTJUMP
RESTAMP
SCHLUMP
SKIJUMP
SUNLAMP
THEPUMP
UNCLAMP
UNCRAMP
VANCAMP

M•Q••••

MCQUEEN
MRQUILP

M••Q•••

MARQUEE
MARQUES
MARQUEZ
MARQUIS
MASQUER
MASQUES
MOSQUES

M•••Q••

MACAQUE
MNOPQRS

•MQ••••

EMQUADS

•M•••Q•

LMNOPQR

••MQ•••

KUMQUAT

••M•Q••

COMIQUE

••M••Q•

COMPAQS

••M•••Q

KLMNOPQ

MR•••••

MRBLISS
MRBODDY
MRBONES
MRBROWN
MRBURNS

MRBUTTS
MRCHIPS
MRCLEAN
MRDARCY
MRDEEDS
MRFIXIT
MRGREEN
MRHANEY
MRHOBBS
MRHORSE
MRHULOT
MRISCAN
MRJONES
MRLUCKY
MRMACHO
MRMAGOO
MRMARCH
MRMOOSE
MRMUSIC
MRNANNY
MRNORTH
MRNOVAK
MRPADRE
MRQUILP
MRRIGHT
MRSBASS
MRSCOTT
MRSLATE
MRSMITH
MRSMUIR
MRSPAUL
MRSPEEL
MRSPOCK
MRTIBBS
MRTIGER
MRWORDS
MRWRONG

M•R••••

MARACAS
MARANTZ
MARAUDS
MARBLED
MARBLER
MARBLES
MARCATO
MARCEAU
MARCELS
MARCHED
MARCHER
MARCHES
MARCHON
MARCONI
MARCUSE
MARDIAN
MARENGO
MARGATE
MARGAUX
MARGERY
MARGINS
MARGRET
MARHAUS
MARIANA
MARIANO
MARIDAS
MARIDOS
MARILLA
MARILYN
MARIMBA
MARINAS
MARINER
MARINES
MARITAL
MARKERS
MARKETS
MARKHAM
MARKIII
MARKING
MARKKAA
MARKOFF
MARKOUT
MARKOVA
MARKSUP
MARKUPS
MARKVII
MARLENE
MARLIER
MARLINS
MARLOWE
MARMARA
MARMION
MARMOTS
MARNIER
MAROONS
MARQUEE
MARQUES
MARQUEZ
MARQUIS
MARRERS
MARRIED
MARRIES
MARRING
MARRONS
MARROWS
MARRYAT
MARRYIN
MARRYME
MARSALA
MARSBAR
MARSDEN
MARSHAL
MARSHES
MARSRED
MARSTON
MARTENS
MARTIAL
MARTIAN
MARTINA
MARTINI
MARTINO
MARTINS
MARTINU
MARTINV
MARTIUS
MARTYRS
MARULLO
MARUSJA
MARVELL
MARVELS
MARVIER
MARXIAN
MARXISM
MARXIST
MARYANN
MARYKAY
MARYLOU
MARYURE
MCRANEY
MERCADO
MERCERS
MERCERY
MERCHES
MERCIAN
MERCIES
MERCURE
MERCURY
MERGEES
MERGERS
MERGING
MERIDEN
MERIMEE
MERINOS
MERITED
MERLINS
MERLOTS
MERMAID
MERRIAM
MERRICK
MERRIER
MERRILL
MERRILY
MIRABEL
MIRACLE
MIRADAS
MIRADOR
MIRAGES
MIRAMAR
MIRAMAX
MIRANDA
MIRIEST
MIRISCH
MIRRORS
MORAINE
MORALES
MORALLY
MORANIS
MORANTE
MORAVIA
MORCERF
MORDANT
MORDENT
MORDRED
MOREENS
MORELLA
MORELLO
MORELOS
MOREPAY
MORESBY
MORETTI
MORGANA
MORGANS
MORGUES
MORISOT
MORLOCK
MORMONS
MORNING
MOROCCO
MORONIC
MORPHED
MORPHIC
MORPHIN
MORROWS
MORSELS
MORTALS
MORTARS
MORTICE
MORTIFY
MORTISE
MORTONS
MRRIGHT
MURALED
MURANOS
MURDERS
MURDOCH
MURIELS
MURILLO
MURKIER
MURKILY
MURKISH
MURMURS
MURPHYS
MYRIADS
MYRRHED
MYRRHIC
MYRTLES

M••R•••

MAARTEN
MACRAME
MACRONS
MADRUSH
MALRAUX
MANRICO
MANROPE
MARRERS
MARRIED
MARRIES
MARRING
MARRONS
MARROWS
MARRYAT
MARRYIN
MARRYME
MATRONS
MAUREEN
MAURIAC
MAURIAT
MAURICE
MAUROIS
MCARDLE
MCBRIDE
MCCRARY
MCCRUMB
MCGRIFF
MCGRORY
MCGRUFF
MEERKAT
MEGRIMS
MEGRYAN
MELROSE
MERRIAM
MERRICK
MERRIER
MERRILL
MERRILY
METRICS
METRIST
MICROBE
MICRONS
MIDRIBS
MIDRIFF
MIDRISE
MIGRANT
MIGRATE
MIRRORS
MISRATE
MISREAD
MISRELY
MISRULE
MITRING
MIZRAHI
MOBRULE
MONROES
MOORAGE
MOORHEN
MOORIER
MOORING
MOORISH
MORROWS
MOTRINS
MOURNED
MOURNER
MRBROWN
MRGREEN
MRWRONG
MUDROOM
MYCROFT
MYERSON
MYRRHED
MYRRHIC
MYTREAT

M•••R••

MACGRAW
MACHREE
MADERUN
MADUROS
MAHARIS
MAIGRET
MAITRED
MAITRES
MAJORCA
MAJORED
MAJORIN
MAKERUN
MALARIA
MALARKY
MALLRAT
MANDREL
MANFRED
MANTRAP
MANTRAS
MANTRIC
MANURED
MANURES
MARGRET
MARSRED
MASARYK
MATURED
MATURER
MATURES
MAUPRAT
MAYORAL
MAZARIN
MAZURKA
MCCAREY
MCENROE
MCMURDO
MEFIRST
MEMOREX
MENORAH
MENORCA
METERED
MIDIRON
MILDRED
MILERUN
MILKRUN
MILLRUN
MILORDS
MINARET
MINERAL
MINERVA
MINORCA
MINORED
MINORIN
MISBREW
MISDRAW
MISDREW
MISERLY
MISTRAL
MITERED
MITHRAS
MOCHRIE
MODERNE
MODERNS
MOLERAT
MONARCH
MONGREL
MORDRED
MOTORED
MOWBRAY
MPTHREE
MRBURNS
MRDARCY
MRHORSE
MRMARCH
MRNORTH
MRWORDS
MTMARCY
MUBARAK
MUJERES
MULGREW
MUSKRAT
MYWORLD

M••••R•

MACABRE
MADDERS
MADEIRA
MAESTRO
MAGUIRE
MAGYARS
MAHZORS
MAILERS
MAIMERS
MAINERS
MAJEURE
MALLARD
MALWARE
MANGERS
MANNERS
MANSARD
MAPPERS
MARGERY
MARKERS
MARMARA
MARRERS
MARTYRS
MARYURE
MASCARA
MASHERS
MASKERS
MASONRY
MASTERP
MASTERS
MASTERY
MATHERS
MATTERS
MAULERS
MAUSERS
MAXBORN
MAYNARD
MCCLURE
MCCLURG
MCCOURT
MCCRARY
MCGRORY
MCGUIRE
MCGWIRE
MCHENRY
MEASURE
MEDFORD
MEETERS
MEGAERA
MEGAERG
MELDERS
MELTERS
MEMBERS
MEMOIRE
MEMOIRS
MENDERS
MENTORS
MEOWERS
MERCERS
MERCERY
MERCURE
MERCURY
MERGERS
METEORS
METIERS
MEWLERS
MIASARA
MIDMORN
MIDTERM
MILAGRO
MILKERS
MILLARD
MILLERS
MIMICRY
MINCERS
MINDERS
MINDORO
MINTERS
MIRRORS
MISFIRE
MISFORM
MISMARK
MISSORT
MISTERM
MISTERS
MISTERX
MISWIRE
MISWORD
MITFORD
MIXTURE
MNOPQRS
MOANERS
MOBBERS
MOCKERS
MOCKERY
MOEBERG
MOHAIRS
MOILERS
MOLDERS
MOLIERE
MOLTERS
MONGERS
MONSTRO
MONTERO
MOONERS
MOOTERS
MOPPERS
MORCERF
MORTARS
MOSHERS
MOTHERS
MOTHERY
MOUSERS
MRPADRE
MSIEURS
MUCKERS
MUDDERS
MUDLARK
MUGGERS
MULHARE
MULLERS
MUMFORD
MUMMERS
MUMMERY
MURDERS
MURMURS
MUSHERS
MUSTARD
MUSTERS
MUTTERS
MYSTARS
MYSTERY

M•••••R

MACULAR
MACUSER
MADEFOR
MADEPAR
MADEWAR
MAILCAR
MAKEFOR
MAKEPAR
MAKEWAR
MALABAR
MALODOR
MALTIER
MANAGER
MANGIER
MANGLER
MANHOUR
MANIPUR
MANLIER
MANOWAR
MANYEAR
MARBLER
MARCHER
MARINER
MARLIER
MARNIER
MARSBAR
MARVIER
MASQUER
MASSEUR
MASSIER
MATADOR
MATCHER
MATURER
MAUNDER
MAXBAER
MAYFAIR
MCPAPER
MEALIER
MEANDER
MEATIER
MEDAWAR
MEDDLER
MEISTER
MEITNER
MENACER
MENUBAR
MERRIER
MESHIER
MESSIER
METOOER
METTLER
MIDDLER
MIDYEAR
MIFFIER
MILKBAR
MILKIER
MINGIER
MINGLER
MINIBAR
MINICAR
MINIVER
MINSTER
MINTIER
MINUTER
MIRADOR
MIRAMAR
MISAVER
MISDOER
MISHEAR
MISTIER
MISUSER
MOBSTER
MODELER
MODULAR
MOGADOR
MOISTER
MOLDIER
MOLITOR
MONIKER
MONITOR
MONOMER
MONSTER
MOOCHER
MOODIER
MOONIER
MOORIER
MOSSIER
MOTHIER
MOULDER
MOUNTER
MOURNER
MOUSIER
MOUTHER
MRSMUIR
MRTIGER
MUAMMAR
MUCKIER
MUDDIER
MUDDLER
MUELLER
MUFFLER
MUGGIER
MULDAUR
MUMBLER
MUNCHER
MUNSTER
MURKIER
MUSHIER
MUSKIER
MUSSIER
MUSTIER
MUZZIER
MUZZLER
MYANMAR
MYNHEER

•MR••••

AMRADIO
AMREETA
AMRITAS
FMRADIO
IMREADY
XMRADIO

•M•R•••

AMARONE
AMBRIES
AMBROSE
AMERADA
AMERCED
AMERCER
AMERCES
AMERICA
AMERIGO
AMERIKA
AMERIND
AMORIST
AMOROSO
AMOROUS
AMTRACK
AMTRACS
EMBRACE
EMBROIL
EMBROWN
EMBRUED
EMBRUES
EMBRYOS
EMERALD
EMERGED
EMERGES
EMERIES
EMERITA
EMERITI
EMERSED
EMERSON
EMIRATE
EMPRESS
EMPRISE
FMURRAY
IMARETS
IMBROKE
IMBRUED
IMBRUES
IMGREAT
IMPRESS
IMPREST
IMPREZA
IMPRINT
IMPROVE
SMARTED
SMARTEN
SMARTER
SMARTLY
SMIRKED
SMIRKER
SMIRNOV
UMBRAGE
UMBRIAN
UMBRIEL

•M••R••

AMHARIC
AMHERST
AMNERIS
AMPERES
AMSCRAY
DMYTRYK
EMBARGO
EMBARKS
EMIGREE
EMIGRES
EMPEROR
EMPIRES
EMPIRIC
EMPIRIN
EMPORIA
FMURRAY
IMBORED
IMFORIT
IMMERGE
IMMERSE
IMMORAL
IMMURED
IMMURES
IMPARTS
IMPERIL
IMPORTS
IMPURER
IMSORRY
IMTIRED
OMICRON
SMEARED
SMEARER
SMEARON
UMBERED
UMBERTO
UMPIRED
UMPIRES

•M•••R•

AMATORY
AMBLERS
AMPHORA
AMUSERS
EMOTERS
IMAGERS
IMAGERY
IMPAIRS
IMPLORE
IMSORRY
IMTHERE
IMYOURS
SMILERS
SMITERS
SMOKERS

•M••••R

AMASSER
AMATEUR
AMENDER
AMERCER
AMMETER
EMAILER
EMBOWER
EMENDER
EMITTER
EMPEROR
EMPOWER
EMPTIER
IMBIBER
IMPALER
IMPEDER
IMPOSER
IMPURER
IMPUTER
LMNOPQR
OMITTER
SMACKER
SMALLER
SMARTER
SMASHER
SMATTER
SMEARER
SMELLER
SMELTER
SMIRKER
SMOKIER
SMOLDER
SMOTHER
SMUCKER
SMUGGER

••MR•••

ARMREST
BUMRAPS
BUMRUSH
CAMRYLE
COMRADE
CYMRICS
GYMRATS
JIMRICE
JIMRYUN
NIMRODS
RAMRODS
RIMROCK
TIMREID
TIMRICE
TIMROTH

••M•R••

ADMIRAL
ADMIRED
ADMIRER
ADMIRES
ALMERIA
ARMORED
ARMORER
ASMARAN
BEMIRED
BEMIRES
CAMAROS
CAMBRIA
CAMBRIC
CAMERAE
CAMERAL
CAMERAS
CAMERON
COMORAN
COMOROS
COMTREX
CUMBRIA
DEMARCO
DEMARET
DEMARKS
DEMERGE
DEMERIT
DEMEROL
DEMURER
DRMARIO
ELMTREE
FEMORAL
FEMORIS
GUMDROP
GUMTREE
HOMBRES
HOMERED
HOMERIC
HOMERUN
HUMDRUM
HUMERAL
HUMERUS
HUMORAL
HUMORED
HUMORME
IMMERGE
IMMERSE
IMMORAL
IMMURED
IMMURES
INMARCH
JOMARCH
KAMERAD
LAMARCK
LAMPREY
MCMURDO
MEMOREX
MRMARCH
MTMARCY
NEMEROV
NOMBRES
NOMERCY
NOMERGE
NUMERAL
NUMERIC
NUMEROS
RAMIREZ
REMARKS
REMARRY
REMERGE
REMORAS
REMORSE
RUMORED
SAMARAS
SAMARIA
SAMPRAS

SAMURAI
SEMIRAW
STMARKS
STMARYS
TAMARAC
TIMBRES
TUMBREL
UNMERGE
UNMERRY
UNMIRED
ZIMARRA
ZYMURGY

••M••R•

ALMONRY
ARMOIRE
ARMOURS
ARMOURY
ATMCARD
BOMBARD
BOMBERS
BUMMERS
BUMPERS
CAMBERS
CAMGIRL
CAMPARI
CAMPERS
COMBERS
COMFORT
COMPARE
COMPART
COMPERE
COMPORT
CUMBERS
DAMMERS
DAMNERS
DAMPDRY
DAMPERS
DIMITRI
DIMMERS
DUMPERS
FTMYERS
GAMMERS
GOMPERS
HAMBURG
HAMMERS
HAMPERS
HEMMERS
HHMUNRO
HOMBURG
HUMBARD
HUMBERT
HUMMERS
HUMOURS
HUMPHRY
HYMNARY
JAMMERS
JUMPERS
LAMBERT
LAMPERT
LEMPIRA
LIMBERS
LIMBURG
LIMNERS
LOMBARD
LUMBARS
LUMBERS
LUMIERE
LUMPERS
MEMBERS
MEMOIRE
MEMOIRS
MIMICRY
MUMFORD
MUMMERS
MUMMERY
NUMBERS
PAMPERS
POMMARD
PUMPERS
RAMMERS
RAMPART
REMARRY
ROMBERG
ROMPERS
RUMFORD
RUMMERS
RUMOURS
SAMBORA
SEMIDRY
SEMIPRO
SIMMERS
SIMPERS
SUMATRA
SUMMARY
SUMMERS
SUMMERY
TAMPERS
TEMPERA
TEMPERS
TEMPORE
TEMPURA
TIMBERS
TIMBERY
UNMERRY
UNMITRE
UNMOORS
VAMPERS
VAMPIRA
VAMPIRE
YAMMERS
ZIMARRA

••M•••R

ADMIRER
AIMSFOR
ALMONER
AMMETER
ARMORER
BUMBLER
BUMPIER
CAMPHOR
CAMPIER
COMAKER
COMFIER
COMPEER
DEMETER
DEMURER
DIMETER
DOMECAR
DUMPIER
EXMAYOR
FUMBLER
GAMBIER
GAMBLER
GEMMIER
GUMMIER
HAMMIER
HAMSTER
HEMPIER
HOMAGER
HOMEIER
HUMBLER
HUMIDOR
HUMPIER
JAMMIER
JUMBLER
JUMPIER
LAMINAR
LIMITER
LUMPIER
MUMBLER
NIMBLER
RAMBLER
REMOTER
REMOVER
RUMBLER
SAMOVAR
SAMPLER
SEMINAR
SIMILAR
SIMPLER
TEMBLOR
TEMPLAR
TEMPTER
TIMIDER
TUMBLER
TUMMLER
UNMAKER
UNMITER
VAMPIER
VUMETER
WIMPIER
YUMMIER

•••MR••

HEYMRDJ

•••M•R•

ANDMORE
ANYMORE
ARAMARK
ARDMORE
ATEMORE
BEAMERS
BEEMERS
BLAMERS
BOOMERS
BUMMERS
CHAMBRE
CHIMERA
CHIMERS
CLAMORS
CREMORA
DAMMERS
DAYMARE
DELMORE
DENMARK
DIMMERS
DORMERS
EARMARK
EATMORE
ENAMORS
FARMERS
FARMERY
FARMORE
FLAMERS
FOAMERS
FORMERS
FRAMERS
FULMARS
GAMMERS
GILMORE
GLAMORS
HAMMERS
HARMERS
HEMMERS
HUMMERS
INKMARK
ISOMERS
JAMMERS
KENMORE
LEXMARK
MAIMERS
MARMARA
MIDMORN
MISMARK
MUMMERS
MUMMERY
MURMURS
ONEMORE
OSTMARK
OXYMORA
PALMARY
PALMERS
PALMYRA
PAYMORE
PISMIRE
POMMARD
PRIMARY
PRIMERA
PRIMERO
PRIMERS
RAMMERS
REAMERS
RHYMERS
ROAMERS
ROOMERS
RUMMERS
SAYMORE
SEAMERS
SIMMERS
SUMMARY
SUMMERS
SUMMERY
TREMORS
TWOMORE
UNSMART
WALMART
WARMERS
WIDMARK
WORMERS
YAMMERS

•••M••R

ASIMMER
BALMIER
BARMIER
BEAMIER
BESMEAR
BOOMCAR
BOOMIER
BRIMMER
CHAMBER
CHAMFER
CHAMPER
CLAMBAR
CLAMBER
CLAMMER
CLAMOUR
CLAMPER
CLIMBER
CRAMMER
CRIMPER
DAIMLER
DAUMIER
DOOMIER
DRUMMER
DUUMVIR
ENAMOUR
FILMIER
FLAMIER
FNUMBER
FOAMIER
FROMMER
GEMMIER
GERMIER
GLAMOUR
GLIMMER
GLUMMER
GRAMMAR
GRAMMER
GRIMIER
GRIMMER
GUMMIER
HAMMIER
JAMMIER
KLAMMER
LOAMIER
MRSMUIR
MUAMMAR
PALMIER
PLUMBER
PLUMIER
PLUMMER
PLUMPER
PREMIER
PRIMMER
ROOMIER
SCAMMER
SCAMPER
SCHMEAR
SCHMEER
SEAMIER
SEYMOUR
SHIMMER
SKIMMER
SLAMMER
SLIMIER
SLIMMER
SLUMBER
SLUMMER
SPAMMER
SPUMIER
STAMMER
STAMPER
STUMPER
SWIMMER
THUMPER
TRAMCAR
TRAMPER
TRIMMER
TUMMLER
VERMEER
WHIMPER
WORMIER
YUMMIER

••••M•R

ALARMER
ASIMMER
ASSUMER
BALLMER
BLOOMER
BOROMIR
BRIMMER
CALAMAR
CASIMIR
CHARMER
CLAIMER
CLAMMER
CRAMMER
CRANMER
CREAMER
DEFAMER
DREAMER
DRUMMER
EXHUMER
FROMMER
GLIMMER
GLUMMER
GRAMMAR
GRAMMER
GRIMMER
GROOMER
HJALMAR
INCOMER
INGEMAR
INHUMER
JACAMAR
JAROMIR
KASHMIR
KLAMMER
KLEZMER
KROEMER
MIRAMAR
MONOMER
MUAMMAR
MYANMAR
PALOMAR
PLUMMER
POLYMER
PRIMMER
REAUMUR
SALEMOR
SCAMMER
SCHEMER
SCHUMER
SHIMMER
SKIMMER
SLAMMER
SLIMMER
SLUMMER
SPAMMER
STAMMER
STEAMER
SWARMER
SWIMMER
TOHOMER
TRIMMER

MS•••••

MSIEURS

M•S••••

MASARYK
MASCARA
MASCOTS
MASHERS
MASHIES
MASHING
MASKERS
MASKING
MASONED
MASONIC
MASONRY
MASQUER
MASQUES
MASSAGE
MASSEUR
MASSIER
MASSIFS
MASSINE
MASSING
MASSIVE
MASTERP
MASTERS
MASTERY
MASTICS
MASTIFF
MASTING
MASTOID
MCSHANE
MCSWINE
MESAMIS
MESCALS
MESEEMS
MESHACH
MESHIER
MESHING
MESHUGA
MESONIC
MESSAGE
MESSALA
MESSIAH
MESSICK
MESSIER
MESSILY
MESSINA
MESSING
MESSKIT
MESSUPS
MISACTS
MISADDS
MISAIMS
MISALLY
MISAVER
MISBILL
MISBIND
MISBREW
MISCALL
MISCAST
MISCITE
MISCODE
MISCOIN
MISCOPY
MISCUED
MISCUES
MISCUTS
MISDATE
MISDEAL
MISDEED
MISDEEM
MISDIAL
MISDOER
MISDOES
MISDONE
MISDRAW
MISDREW
MISEDIT
MISERLY
MISFEED
MISFILE
MISFIRE
MISFITS
MISFORM
MISGAVE
MISGIVE
MISHAPS
MISHEAR
MISHIMA
MISHITS
MISHNAH
MISJOIN
MISKEYS
MISKNEW
MISKNOW
MISKOLC
MISLAID
MISLAYS
MISLEAD
MISLIKE
MISMARK
MISMATE
MISMESH
MISMOVE
MISNAME
MISPAGE
MISPLAN
MISPLAY
MISRATE
MISREAD
MISRELY
MISRULE
MISSAID
MISSALS
MISSAYS
MISSEAT
MISSEND
MISSENT
MISSETS
MISSHIP
MISSIES
MISSILE
MISSING
MISSION
MISSISH
MISSIVE
MISSORT
MISSOUT
MISSTEP
MISSUSA
MISSYOU
MISTAKE
MISTBOW
MISTELL
MISTERM
MISTERS
MISTERX
MISTIER
MISTILY
MISTIME
MISTING
MISTOLD
MISTOOK
MISTRAL
MISTSUP
MISTUNE
MISTYPE
MISUSED
MISUSER
MISUSES
MISWIRE
MISWORD
MISZONE
MOSAICS
MOSCATO
MOSCONI
MOSELLE
MOSEYED
MOSHERS
MOSHING
MOSHPIT
MOSLEMS
MOSQUES
MOSSIER
MOSSING
MRSBASS
MRSCOTT
MRSLATE
MRSMITH
MRSMUIR
MRSPAUL
MRSPEEL
MRSPOCK
MTSINAI
MUSANTE
MUSCATS
MUSCIDA
MUSCLED
MUSCLES
MUSEDON
MUSEFUL
MUSESON
MUSETTA
MUSETTE
MUSEUMS
MUSHERS
MUSHIER
MUSHILY
MUSHING
MUSICAL
MUSICKS
MUSIGNY
MUSINGS
MUSKEGO
MUSKETS
MUSKIER
MUSKIES
MUSKRAT
MUSLIMS
MUSLINS
MUSSELS
MUSSIER
MUSSILY
MUSSING
MUSTAFA
MUSTANG
MUSTARD
MUSTDOS
MUSTERS
MUSTIER
MUSTILY
MUSTSEE
MYSPACE
MYSTARS
MYSTERY
MYSTICS
MYSTIFY

M••S•••

MAESTRO
MAISONS
MAISOUI
MANSARD
MANSION
MANSIZE
MANSMAN
MAOSUIT
MAPSOUT
MARSALA
MARSBAR
MARSDEN
MARSHAL
MARSHES
MARSRED
MARSTON
MASSAGE
MASSEUR
MASSIER
MASSIFS
MASSINE
MASSING
MASSIVE
MAUSERS
MEASLES
MEASURE
MEISSEN
MEISTER
MENSANS
MENSCHY
MESSAGE
MESSALA
MESSIAH
MESSICK
MESSIER
MESSILY
MESSINA
MESSING
MESSKIT
MESSUPS
METSFAN
MIASARA
MIASMAL
MIASMAS
MIASMIC
MIDSHIP
MIDSIZE
MIDSOLE
MINSKYS
MINSTER
MISSAID
MISSALS
MISSAYS
MISSEAT
MISSEND
MISSENT
MISSETS
MISSHIP
MISSIES
MISSILE
MISSING
MISSION
MISSISH
MISSIVE
MISSORT
MISSOUT
MISSTEP
MISSUSA
MISSYOU
MOBSTER
MOISSAN
MOISTEN
MOISTER
MOISTLY
MOLSONS
MONSOON
MONSTER
MONSTRO
MORSELS
MOSSIER
MOSSING
MOUSERS
MOUSIER
MOUSILY
MOUSING
MOUSSED
MOUSSES
MRISCAN
MUESLIS
MUESLIX
MUGSHOT
MUNSTER
MUSSELS
MUSSIER
MUSSILY
MUSSING

M•••S••

MACHSIX
MACUSER
MADISON
MAILSIN
MAJESTE
MAJESTY
MAKESDO
MAKESGO
MAKESIT
MAKESUP
MALMSEY
MAOISTS
MARKSUP
MARUSJA
MATISSE
MAVISES
MEANSIT
MEANSTO
MEDUSAE
MEDUSAN
MEDUSAS
MEETSUP
MEIOSES
MEIOSIS
MEISSEN
MELISMA
MELISSA
MENISCI
MIDASES
MIKASAS
MILKSOP
MIMESES
MIMESIS
MIMOSAS
MINDSET
MINISKI
MINISUB
MINUSES
MIRISCH
MISTSUP
MISUSED
MISUSER
MISUSES
MITOSES
MITOSIS
MIXESIN
MIXESUP
MOCKSUP
MODESTO
MODESTY
MODISTE
MOISSAN
MOLESTS
MOMMSEN
MOMUSES
MONOSKI
MOONSET
MORESBY
MORISOT
MOUSSED
MOUSSES
MOVESIN
MOVESIT
MOVESON
MOVESTO
MOVESUP
MRMUSIC
MUCKSUP
MUMESON
MUSESON
MUSTSEE
MYERSON

M••••S•

MADDASH
MADDEST
MADDISH
MADNESS
MADRUSH
MAEWEST
MAFIOSI
MAFIOSO
MAHDISM
MAHDIST
MAIDISH
MALAISE
MALPASO
MALTASE
MALTESE
MALTOSE
MANCUSO
MANLESS
MANNISH
MARCUSE
MARXISM
MARXIST
MATISSE
MATLESS
MAWKISH
MAYBESO
MAZIEST
MEANEST
MEEKEST
MEFIRST
MELISSA
MELROSE
METRIST
MIDEAST
MIDLIST
MIDMOST
MIDRISE
MIDWEST
MILDEST
MINXISH
MIRIEST
MISCAST
MISMESH
MISSISH
MISSUSA
MOBBISH
MOBBISM
MOBBIST
MOLLUSC
MOLLUSK
MOMBASA
MONDESI
MONKISH
MOONISH
MOORISH
MOPIEST
MORTISE
MRBLISS
MRHORSE
MRMOOSE
MRSBASS
MUDFISH
MUDWASP
MUGGISH
MURKISH

M•••••S

MACACOS
MACOUNS
MACRONS
MADAMES
MADCAPS
MADDENS
MADDERS
MADDOGS
MADLIBS
MADNESS
MADUROS
MAENADS
MAGGOTS
MAGLEVS

MAGNETS
MAGNUMS
MAGPIES
MAGYARS
MAHARIS
MAHOUTS
MAHZORS
MAIDENS
MAILERS
MAILINS
MAIMERS
MAINERS
MAISONS
MAITAIS
MAITRES
MAJGENS
MAKEDOS
MAKEUPS
MAKINGS
MALAGAS
MALIANS
MALICES
MALIGNS
MALLETS
MALLEUS
MALLOWS
MALTEDS
MALTHUS
MAMMALS
MANAGES
MANANAS
MANDANS
MANDAYS
MANEGES
MANGERS
MANGLES
MANGOES
MANIACS
MANILAS
MANLESS
MANNERS
MANNIES
MANTELS
MANTLES
MANTRAS
MANUALS
MANURES
MAOISTS
MAPPERS
MARACAS
MARAUDS
MARBLES
MARCELS
MARCHES
MARGINS
MARHAUS
MARIDAS
MARIDOS
MARINAS
MARINES
MARKERS
MARKETS
MARKUPS
MARLINS
MARMOTS
MAROONS
MARQUES
MARQUIS
MARRERS
MARRIES
MARRONS
MARROWS
MARSHES
MARTENS
MARTINS
MARTIUS
MARTYRS
MARVELS
MASCOTS
MASHERS
MASHIES
MASKERS
MASQUES
MASSIFS
MASTERS
MASTICS
MATCHES
MATHERS
MATHEWS
MATHIAS
MATLESS
MATRONS
MATTERS
MATURES
MATZOHS
MAULERS
MAUMAUS
MAUROIS
MAUSERS
MAUVAIS
MAVISES
MAXIMAS
MAXIMUS
MAXIXES
MAYDAYS
MAYHEMS
MAYINGS
MAYTAGS
MCADAMS
MCCALLS
MCHALES
MEADOWS
MEAGLES
MEALIES
MEANIES
MEASLES
MECCANS
MEDAKAS
MEDDLES
MEDELES
MEDIANS
MEDICOS
MEDIUMS
MEDLEYS
MEDUSAS
MEEMIES
MEETERS
MEGANES
MEGOHMS
MEGRIMS
MEIOSES
MEIOSIS
MELDERS
MELLOWS
MELTERS
MEMBERS
MEMOIRS
MEMPHIS
MENACES
MENAGES
MENCIUS
MENDELS
MENDERS
MENIALS
MENSANS
MENTEES
MENTORS
MENUDOS
MENZIES
MEOWERS
MERCERS
MERCHES
MERCIES
MERGEES
MERGERS
MERINOS
MERLINS
MERLOTS
MESAMIS
MESCALS
MESEEMS
MESSUPS
METATES
METEORS
METFANS
METHODS
METIERS
METRICS
METTLES
MEWLERS
MEZUZAS
MIASMAS
MICKEYS
MICMACS
MICRONS
MIDASES
MIDCAPS
MIDDAYS
MIDDIES
MIDDLES
MIDGETS
MIDLEGS
MIDOFFS
MIDRIBS
MIDWAYS
MIGENES
MIGNONS
MIKADOS
MIKASAS
MILDEWS
MILHOUS
MILIEUS
MILKERS
MILLAIS
MILLERS
MILLETS
MILORDS
MIMESES
MIMESIS
MIMOSAS
MINCERS
MINDERS
MINGLES
MINIBUS
MINIMUS
MININGS
MINIONS
MINITVS
MINNOWS
MINOANS
MINSKYS
MINTERS
MINUETS
MINUSES
MINUTES
MINYANS
MIRADAS
MIRAGES
MIRRORS
MISACTS
MISADDS
MISAIMS
MISCUES
MISCUTS
MISDOES
MISFITS
MISHAPS
MISHITS
MISKEYS
MISLAYS
MISSALS
MISSAYS
MISSETS
MISSIES
MISTERS
MISUSES
MITHRAS
MITOSES
MITOSIS
MITTENS
MIXTECS
MIZUNAS
MIZZENS
MIZZLES
MNOPQRS
MOANERS
MOBBERS
MOBILES
MOCKERS
MOCKUPS
MODELAS
MODELBS
MODELTS
MODERNS
MODULES
MODULUS
MOHAIRS
MOHAVES
MOHAWKS
MOILERS
MOJAVES
MOJITOS
MOLDERS
MOLESTS
MOLLIES
MOLSONS
MOLTERS
MOMENTS
MOMMIES
MOMUSES
MONDAYS
MONGERS
MONGOLS
MONKEES
MONKEYS
MONROES
MOOCHES
MOOCOWS
MOONERS
MOONIES
MOOTERS
MOPPERS
MOPPETS
MOPTOPS
MORALES
MORANIS
MOREENS
MORELOS
MORGANS
MORGUES
MORMONS
MORROWS
MORSELS
MORTALS
MORTARS
MORTONS
MOSAICS
MOSHERS
MOSLEMS
MOSQUES
MOTHERS
MOTIONS
MOTIVES
MOTLEYS
MOTRINS
MOTTLES
MOTTOES
MOUSERS
MOUSSES
MOVADOS
MOWINGS
MRBLISS
MRBONES
MRBURNS
MRBUTTS
MRCHIPS
MRDEEDS
MRHOBBS
MRJONES
MRSBASS
MRTIBBS
MRWORDS
MSIEURS
MTADAMS
MTATHOS
MTEVANS
MUCKERS
MUDCATS
MUDDERS
MUDDIES
MUDDLES
MUDEELS
MUDHENS
MUDPIES
MUESLIS
MUFFINS
MUFFLES
MUGFULS
MUGGERS
MUGGLES
MUJERES
MUKLUKS
MULCHES
MULETAS
MULLAHS
MULLERS
MULLETS
MULLINS
MUMBLES
MUMMERS
MUMMIES
MUNCHES
MUPPETS
MURANOS
MURDERS
MURIELS
MURMURS
MURPHYS
MUSCATS
MUSCLES
MUSEUMS
MUSHERS
MUSICKS
MUSINGS
MUSKETS
MUSKIES
MUSLIMS
MUSLINS
MUSSELS
MUSTDOS
MUSTERS
MUTANTS
MUTATES
MUTTERS
MUTTONS
MUTUALS
MUUMUUS
MUZZLES
MYKONOS
MYOPIAS
MYRIADS
MYRTLES
MYSTARS
MYSTICS

•MS••••

AMSCRAY
AMSTELS
IMSORRY
IMSWELL

•M•S•••

AMASSED
AMASSER
AMASSES
AMESLAN
AMISTAD
AMUSEME
AMUSERS
AMUSING
IMUSTGO
KMESONS
SMASHED
SMASHER
SMASHES
SMASHUP
SMUSHED
SMUSHES

•M••S••

AMASSED
AMASSER
AMASSES
AMNESIA
AMNESIC
AMNESTY
EMBASSY
EMBOSOM
EMERSED
EMERSON
EMMUSKA
IMPASSE
IMPASTO
IMPOSED
IMPOSER
IMPOSES
IMPOSTS

•M•••S•

AMBROSE
AMHERST
AMONGST
AMORIST
AMOROSO
AMPLEST
AMYLASE
EMBASSY
EMPRESS
EMPRISE
IMAGISM
IMAGIST
IMAMESS
IMMENSE
IMMERSE
IMPASSE
IMPRESS
IMPREST
IMPULSE
OMIGOSH

•M••••S

AMADEUS
AMANTIS
AMASSES
AMATOLS
AMAZONS
AMBIENS
AMBLERS
AMBRIES
AMERCES
AMIDOLS
AMITIES
AMNERIS
AMNIONS
AMOEBAS
AMOROUS
AMOUNTS
AMPERES
AMPULES
AMRITAS
AMSTELS
AMTRACS
AMULETS
AMUSERS
BMOVIES
EMBALMS
EMBANKS
EMBARKS
EMBLEMS
EMBRUES
EMBRYOS
EMERGES
EMERIES
EMETICS
EMIGRES
EMOTERS
EMPALES
EMPATHS
EMPIRES
EMPLOYS
EMPRESS
EMPTIES
EMQUADS
EMULOUS
FMBANDS
IMAGERS
IMAGOES
IMAMESS
IMARETS
IMBIBES
IMBRUES
IMMIXES
IMMUNES
IMMURES
IMPACTS
IMPAIRS
IMPALAS
IMPALES
IMPARTS
IMPEDES
IMPENDS
IMPETUS
IMPIOUS
IMPLIES
IMPORTS
IMPOSES
IMPOSTS
IMPRESS
IMPUGNS
IMPUTES
IMYOURS
KMESONS
OMAHANS
OMELETS
OMINOUS
OMNIBUS
SMASHES
SMIDGES
SMILERS
SMILEYS
SMILLAS
SMITERS
SMOKERS
SMOKEYS
SMOKIES
SMOOTHS
SMUDGES
SMUSHES
UMLAUTS
UMPIRES

••MS•••

AIMSFOR
ALMSMAN
ALMSMEN
BUMSOUT
COMSATS
CUMSHAW
DAMSELS
DAMSONS
DIMSOUT
GEMSBOK
GUMSHOE
GYMSHOE
GYMSOCK
GYMSUIT
HAMSTER
HEMSLEY
HIMSELF
JIMSONS
OHMSLAW
OLMSTED
RAMSESI
RAMSFAN
RAMSONS
RIMSHOT
RUMSHOP
SAMSONS
SAMSUNG
ZEMSTVO

••M•S••

BEMUSED
BEMUSES
BUMPSUP
CAMISES
CAMPSUP
COMESAS
COMESAT
COMESBY
COMESIN
COMESON
COMESTO
COMESUP
DAMASKS
DAMASUS
DAMOSEL
DEMASTS
DEMESNE
DEMISED
DEMISES
DEMISTS
DEMPSEY
DUMPSON
ELMISTI
EMMUSKA
ENMASSE
FUMESAT
HOMESIN
HUMUSES
JAMESII
JAMESIV
JAMESON
JAMESVI
JAMISON
JEMISON
JUMPSAT
JUMPSIN
JUMPSON
JUMPSUP
LUMPSIN
LUMPSIT
LUMPSUM
MIMESES
MIMESIS
MIMOSAS
MOMMSEN
MOMUSES
MRMUSIC
MUMESON
NEMESES
NEMESIS
OSMOSED
OSMOSES
OSMOSIS
PIMESON
PUMPSUP
RAMESES
RAMPSUP
REMISED
REMISES
SAMISEN
SAMOSAS
SAMOSET
SAMPSON
SIMPSON
SOMESAY
TIMESUP
TUMESCE
UNMASKS
UNMASTS
UNMOSSY
UTMOSTS

••M••S•

AIMLESS
ARMLESS
ARMREST
BOMBAST
BUMRUSH
COMBUST
COMCAST
COMMISH
COMPASS
COMPOSE
COMPOST
COMTISM
COMTIST
DAMPEST
DAMPISH
DIMMEST
DIMNESS
DUMBEST
DUMPISH
EDMEESE
ELMIEST
ENMASSE
FUMIEST
GAMIEST
GEMLESS
GUMLESS
GYMNAST
HOMIEST
IAMBIST
IMMENSE
IMMERSE
KOMATSU
LAMAISM
LAMAIST
LIMIEST
LIMPEST
LUMPISH
MOMBASA
MRMOOSE
NUMBEST
RAMMISH
RAMSESI
REMORSE
RIMIEST
RIMLESS
ROMANSH
ROMPISH
RUMLESS
SAMBASS
SAMWISE
SUMLESS
SUMOIST
TEMPEST
UNMOIST
UNMOSSY
VAMOOSE
VAMPISH
WIMPISH

••M•••S

ADMIRES
ADMIXES
AIMLESS
ALMONDS
ARMADAS
ARMFULS
ARMLESS
ARMLETS
ARMOURS
ARMPITS
ATMFEES
BAMBOOS
BAMMIES
BEMIRES
BEMOANS
BEMUSES
BIMBOES
BIMINIS
BOMBERS
BUMBLES
BUMLEGS
BUMMERS
BUMPERS
BUMRAPS
CAMAROS
CAMBERS
CAMBOYS
CAMERAS
CAMINOS
CAMIONS
CAMISES
CAMMIES
CAMPERS
CEMENTS
COMBATS
COMBERS
COMEONS
COMESAS
COMFITS
COMICES
COMINGS
COMMITS
COMMONS
COMOROS
COMPAQS
COMPASS
COMPELS
COMSATS
CUMBERS
CUMBIAS
CUMULUS
CYMBALS
CYMRICS
DAMAGES
DAMASKS
DAMASUS
DAMMERS
DAMNERS
DAMPENS
DAMPERS
DAMSELS
DAMSONS
DEMANDS
DEMARKS
DEMASTS
DEMBUMS
DEMEANS
DEMISES
DEMISTS
DEMOTES
DEMOTHS
DIMAGES
DIMMERS
DIMNESS
DIMOUTS
DIMPLES
DIMWITS
DOMAINS
DOMINOS
DOMINUS
DUMDUMS
DUMMIES
DUMPERS
EDMONDS
EDMUNDS
ERMINES
EXMATES
FAMINES
FAMULUS
FEMALES
FEMBOTS
FEMORIS
FOMENTS
FTMYERS
FUMBLES
GAMBITS
GAMBLES
GAMBOLS
GAMETES
GAMINES
GAMMERS
GAMMONS
GEMINIS
GEMLESS
GIMBALS
GIMBELS
GIMLETS
GOMPERS
GUMLESS
GYMBAGS
GYMRATS
HAMITES
HAMLETS
HAMMERS
HAMPERS
HAMULUS
HEMMERS
HOMAGES
HOMBRES
HUMBLES
HUMBUGS
HUMERUS
HUMMELS
HUMMERS
HUMOURS
HUMUSES
HUMVEES
HYMNALS
IAMBICS
IMMIXES
IMMUNES
IMMURES
INMATES
IOMOTHS
JAMCAMS
JAMMERS
JAMMIES
JIMJAMS
JIMMIES
JIMSONS
JUMADAS
JUMBLES
JUMPERS
KIMONOS
KUMMELS
LAMBDAS
LAMENTS
LAMINAS
LIMBERS
LIMNERS
LIMOGES
LIMPETS
LUMBARS
LUMBERS
LUMINAS
LUMPERS
MAMMALS
MEMBERS
MEMOIRS
MEMPHIS
MIMESES
MIMESIS
MIMOSAS
MOMENTS
MOMMIES
MOMUSES
MUMBLES
MUMMERS
MUMMIES
NEMESES
NEMESIS
NIMRODS
NOMBRES
NUMBATS
NUMBERS
NUMEROS
OHMAGES
OOMPAHS
ORMOLUS
OSMONDS

OSMOSES
OSMOSIS
OSMUNDS
PAMPERS
PIMPLES
POMADES
POMELOS
POMMELS
POMPOMS
POMPONS
POMPOUS
PUMICES
PUMMELS
PUMPERS
RAMADAS
RAMBLES
RAMESES
RAMFANS
RAMJETS
RAMMERS
RAMONES
RAMRODS
RAMSONS
REMAILS
REMAINS
REMAKES
REMANDS
REMARKS
REMATES
REMEETS
REMELTS
REMENDS
REMILLS
REMINDS
REMINES
REMINTS
REMISES
REMIXES
REMOLDS
REMORAS
REMOTES
REMOVES
RIMLESS
RIMPLES
ROMAINS
ROMAJIS
ROMANIS
ROMANOS
ROMANUS
ROMCOMS
ROMNEYS
ROMPERS
ROMULUS
RUMAKIS
RUMBLES
RUMLESS
RUMMERS
RUMMIES
RUMOURS
RUMPLES
SAMARAS
SAMBASS
SAMEDIS
SAMEKHS
SAMLETS
SAMOANS
SAMOSAS
SAMPANS
SAMPLES
SAMPRAS
SAMSONS
SEMANAS
SEMITES
SIMIANS
SIMILES
SIMMERS
SIMMONS
SIMPERS
SIMPLES
SOMALIS
STMARKS
STMARYS
SUMLESS
SUMMERS
SUMMITS
SUMMONS
SYMBOLS
TAMALES
TAMPERS
TAMTAMS
TEMPEHS
TEMPERS
TEMPLES
TIMBALS
TIMBERS
TIMBRES
TIMEWAS
TIMEXES
TIMINGS
TIMMINS
TOMBOYS
TOMCATS
TOMTITS
TOMTOMS
TUMBLES
TUMMIES
TUMULTS
UNMAKES
UNMASKS
UNMASTS
UNMATES
UNMIXES
UNMOLDS
UNMOORS
UTMOSTS
VAMPERS
WAMBLES
WAMPUMS
WIMPLES
WOMBATS
XIMENES
YAMAHAS
YAMMERS
YEMENIS
YOMTOVS
ZOMBIES

•••MS••

ADAMSES
ADAMSON
BEAMSUP
CALMSEA
CHOMSKY
CLAMSUP
CLEMSON
CRAMSIN
CRIMSON
DOOMSTO
DRUMSET
DRUMSUP
FILMSET
FIRMSUP
GLAMSUP
GRIMSBY
MALMSEY
MOMMSEN
SEEMSTO
SLAMSON
STIMSON
SWIMSUP
TEAMSUP
THOMSON
WARMSTO
WARMSUP
ZOOMSIN

•••M•S•

AFTMOST
AIRMASS
ALAMOSA
ANIMISM
ANIMIST
ATOMISE
ATOMISM
ATOMIST
BEAMISH
BIGMESS
BIOMASS
BLEMISH
BURMESE
CALMEST
CHEMISE
CHEMIST
CHUMASH
COMMISH
DIMMEST
DISMAST
DISMISS
ENDMOST
EYEMASK
FIRMEST
FLEMISH
FORMOSA
GASMASK
GLIMPSE
GNOMISH
GNOMIST
GOAMISS
HAIMISH
HERMOSA
HERMOSO
IMAMESS
INAMESS
ITEMISE
LOWMASS
MIDMOST
MISMESH
OAKMOSS
OLEMISS
OUTMOST
PALMIST
PLUMOSE
PREMISE
PREMISS
PROMISE
RAMMISH
REAMASS
RHYMIST
SAYMASS
SEAMIST
SEAMOSS
SIAMESE
SKIMASK
SURMISE
TEAMUSA
THEMASK
THEMOST
TOPMAST
TOPMOST
WARMEST
WARMISH
WORMISH

•••M••S

AAAMAPS
ACUMENS
ADAMSES
AIRMASS
ALUMNUS
ANEMIAS
ANIMALS
ANOMIES
ARAMIDS
ATAMANS
ATOMICS
ATOMIES
BAMMIES
BEAMERS
BEEMERS
BIGMACS
BIGMESS
BIOMASS
BIRMANS
BITMAPS
BLAMERS
BONMOTS
BOOMERS
BRUMOUS
BUMMERS
BURMANS
BUSMANS
CAIMANS
CAMMIES
CAYMANS
CHAMOIS
CHIMERS
CLAMORS
CLEMENS
CLIMATS
COMMITS
COMMONS
DAEMONS
DAMMERS
DENMOMS
DESMOGS
DIEMENS
DIMMERS
DISMALS
DISMAYS
DISMISS
DOLMANS
DORMERS
DRYMOPS
DUMMIES
ENAMELS
ENAMORS
ENEMIES
ETYMONS
EXEMPTS
FARMERS
FERMATS
FLAMBES
FLAMERS
FOAMERS
FORMALS
FORMATS
FORMERS
FRAMERS
FULMARS
GAMMERS
GAMMONS
GERMANS
GLAMORS
GNOMONS
GOAMISS
GRAMMES
GRAMMYS
GRAMPAS
GRAMPUS
HAMMERS
HARMERS
HAYMOWS
HAZMATS
HELMETS
HEMMERS
HERMANS
HERMITS
HEYMANS
HUMMELS
HUMMERS
IMAMESS
INAMESS
ISOMERS
JAMMERS
JAMMIES
JIMMIES
KIRMANS
KISMETS
KUMMELS
LOOMPAS
LOWMASS
MAIMERS
MAMMALS
MARMOTS
MAUMAUS
MEEMIES
MICMACS
MOMMIES
MORMONS
MUMMERS
MUMMIES
MURMURS
MUUMUUS
NEWMANS
NORMALS
NORMANS
NUTMEGS
OAKMOSS
OLEMISS
OLYMPUS
OUTMANS
PALMERS
PERMITS
PHEMIUS
POMMELS
PREMEDS
PREMIES
PREMISS
PRIMERS
PROMPTS
PUMMELS
PYGMIES
RAGMANS
RAGMOPS
RAMMERS
REAMASS
REAMERS
REEMITS
RHOMBUS
RHUMBAS
RHYMERS
ROAMERS
ROOMBAS
ROOMERS
ROOMIES
RUMMERS
RUMMIES
SALMONS
SAYMASS
SCHMOES
SEAMAPS
SEAMERS
SEAMOSS
SERMONS
SHAMANS
SIEMENS
SIMMERS
SIMMONS
SKYMAPS
STAMENS
STYMIES
SUBMITS
SUMMERS
SUMMITS
SUMMONS
TARMACS
THEMAVS
THEMETS
TIEMPOS
TIMMINS
TRAMPAS
TREMORS
TRUMANS
TUMMIES
TZIMMES
WARMERS
WARMUPS
WETMOPS
WORMERS
YAMMERS
YEOMANS
YOUMANS

••••M•S

AFRAMES
ALTIMAS
ARTEMIS
ARTEMUS
ASSUMES
ASTHMAS
ATHOMES
ATTIMES
AUTUMNS
BAHAMAS
BECOMES
BENUMBS
BETIMES
BIREMES
BRAHMAS
BYNAMES
CCLAMPS
CHROMES
CINEMAS
COLUMNS
DECAMPS
DEFAMES
DHARMAS
DONIMUS
DYNAMOS
ECZEMAS
ENCAMPS
ENIGMAS
ENTOMBS
ENZYMES
ERASMUS
ESKIMOS
EXHUMES
FUSUMAS
GENOMES
GRAMMES
GRAMMYS
ILLUMES
INCOMES
INHUMES
ISTHMUS
JICAMAS
LATIMES
LEGUMES
MADAMES
MAXIMAS
MAXIMUS
MESAMIS
MIASMAS
MINIMUS
NOKOMIS
NONAMES
NYTIMES
ONRAMPS
OPTIMAS
PAJAMAS
PALAMAS
PALOMAS
PANAMAS
PARAMUS
PDJAMES
PLASMAS
PNEUMAS
POTAMUS
PREAMPS
PYRAMUS
RACEMES
RADAMES
RADOMES
RECOMBS
REGIMES
RELUMES
RENAMES
REPUMPS
RESUMES
RETAMES
RETIMES
REVAMPS
SALAMIS
SCHEMAS
SCHEMES
SCRIMPS
SESAMES
SHRIMPS
STIGMAS
STJAMES
SURIMIS
TACOMAS
TATAMIS
THERMOS
TONEMES
TRAUMAS
TVGAMES
TZIMMES
ULTIMAS
UNTAMES
UPTIMES
VOLUMES
WAKAMES
YAKIMAS
ZOSIMUS

•••••MS

AFFIRMS
AIRDAMS
ALARUMS
ALLIUMS
ANADEMS
ANONYMS
ANTHEMS
ASHRAMS
ASYLUMS
ATRIUMS
BALSAMS
BANTAMS
BARNUMS
BAYRUMS
BECALMS
BEDLAMS
BELDAMS
BOTTOMS
BUNKUMS
BYFORMS
CHRISMS
CORFAMS
CUSTOMS
DEFOAMS
DEFORMS
DEGERMS
DEMBUMS
DENMOMS
DESLUMS
DESTEMS
DEWORMS
DIADEMS
DIATOMS
DICTUMS
DIDSUMS
DIGRAMS
DIRHAMS
DISARMS
DODGEMS
DOTCOMS
DUMDUMS
EMBALMS
EMBLEMS
ENGRAMS
EPONYMS
ESTEEMS
EUONYMS
EXONYMS
FANDOMS
FATHOMS
GRAHAMS
GYPSUMS
HANSOMS
ICEDAMS
INFORMS
INSEAMS
IONIUMS
JAMCAMS
JIMJAMS
KIDCOMS
LAPERMS
LOGJAMS
LYCEUMS
MAGNUMS
MAYHEMS
MCADAMS
MEDIUMS
MEGOHMS
MEGRIMS
MESEEMS
MISAIMS
MOSLEMS
MTADAMS
MUSEUMS
MUSLIMS
NAPALMS
NONCOMS
OUTSUMS
PABLUMS
PARFUMS
PEPLUMS
PHENOMS
PHLOEMS
PLENUMS
PODIUMS
POMPOMS
POSSUMS
PREARMS
PRELIMS
PRFIRMS
QUORUMS
RANSOMS
REDEEMS
REFILMS
REFORMS
RESEAMS
RESWIMS
RETRIMS
REWARMS
RHYTHMS
ROMCOMS
SACHEMS
SALAAMS
SATCOMS
SCHISMS
SCREAMS
SEAARMS
SHALOMS
SITCOMS
SKIBUMS
SKYCAMS
SLALOMS
SPYCAMS
SQUIRMS
STREAMS
SYSTEMS
TALCUMS
TAMTAMS
TANDEMS
TEDEUMS
TEDIUMS
THEISMS
THERAMS
THESIMS
TOMTOMS
TRUISMS
TVROOMS
UNHELMS
UNISOMS
UNSEAMS
VACUUMS
VELLUMS
VICTIMS
WAMPUMS
WEBCAMS
WIGWAMS
WINDOMS
WISDOMS
ZITCOMS

MT•••••

MTADAMS
MTATHOS
MTBALDY
MTBLANC
MTEVANS
MTKENYA
MTLOGAN
MTMARCY
MTPELEE
MTSINAI

M•T••••

MATADOR
MATALIN
MATCHED
MATCHER
MATCHES
MATCHUP
MATEWAN
MATHERS
MATHEWS
MATHIAS
MATHIEU
MATILDA
MATINAL
MATINEE
MATISSE
MATLESS
MATLOCK
MATRONS
MATTERS
MATTHAU
MATTHEW
MATTING
MATTOCK
MATURED
MATURER
MATURES
MATZOHS
MATZOTH
METALED
METATES
METCALF
METEORS
METEOUT
METERED
METFANS
METHANE
METHODS
METIERS
METLIFE
METOOER
METRICS
METRIST
METSFAN
METTLER
METTLES
METWITH
MITCHUM
MITERED
MITFORD
MITHRAS
MITOSES
MITOSIS
MITOTIC
MITRING
MITTENS
MITZVAH
MOTHERS
MOTHERY
MOTHIER
MOTIONS
MOTIVED
MOTIVES
MOTLEYS
MOTORED
MOTRINS
MOTTLED
MOTTLES
MOTTOES
MPTHREE
MRTIBBS
MRTIGER
MUTABLE
MUTABLY
MUTAGEN
MUTANTS
MUTATED
MUTATES
MUTEDLY
MUTTERS
MUTTONS
MUTUALS
MYTHIFY
MYTREAT

M••T•••

MAITAIS
MAITRED
MAITRES
MALTASE
MALTBIE
MALTEDS
MALTESE
MALTHUS
MALTIER
MALTING
MALTOSE
MANTECA
MANTELS
MANTLED
MANTLES
MANTLET
MANTRAP
MANTRAS
MANTRIC
MANTUAN
MARTENS
MARTIAL
MARTIAN
MARTINA
MARTINI
MARTINO
MARTINS
MARTINU
MARTINV
MARTIUS
MARTYRS
MASTERP
MASTERS
MASTERY
MASTICS
MASTIFF
MASTING
MASTOID
MATTERS
MATTHAU
MATTHEW
MATTING
MATTOCK
MAYTAGS
MAYTIME
MEATAXE
MEATIER
MEATILY
MEATMAN
MEATMEN
MEATPIE
MEETERS
MEETING
MEETSUP
MEITNER
MELTAGE
MELTERS
MELTING
MENTEES
MENTHOL
MENTION
MENTORS
METTLER
METTLES
MIDTEEN
MIDTERM
MIDTOWN
MINTAGE
MINTERS
MINTIER
MINTING
MINTTEA
MISTAKE
MISTBOW
MISTELL
MISTERM
MISTERS
MISTERX
MISTIER
MISTILY
MISTIME
MISTING
MISTOLD
MISTOOK
MISTRAL
MISTSUP
MISTUNE
MISTYPE
MITTENS
MIXTECS
MIXTURE
MOLTERS
MOLTING
MONTAGE
MONTAGU
MONTALE
MONTANA
MONTAND
MONTANO
MONTAUK
MONTEGO
MONTERO
MONTEUX
MONTHLY
MONTOYA
MONTUNO
MOOTERS
MOOTING
MOPTOPS
MORTALS
MORTARS
MORTICE
MORTIFY
MORTISE
MORTONS
MOTTLED
MOTTLES
MOTTOES
MOUTHED
MOUTHER
MTATHOS
MUSTAFA
MUSTANG
MUSTARD
MUSTDOS
MUSTERS
MUSTIER
MUSTILY
MUSTSEE
MUTTERS
MUTTONS
MYRTLES
MYSTARS
MYSTERY
MYSTICS
MYSTIFY

M•••T••

MAARTEN

MACHTWO
MAESTRO
MAHATMA
MAINTOP
MANATEE
MANETTE
MARITAL
MARSTON
MEANTIT
MEANTTO
MEGATON
MEIOTIC
MEISTER
MELITTA
MENOTTI
MERITED
METATES
MIGHTNT
MILITIA
MIMETIC
MINITVS
MINOTND
MINSTER
MINTTEA
MINUTED
MINUTER
MINUTES
MINUTIA
MISSTEP
MITOTIC
MIXITUP
MOBSTER
MOISTEN
MOISTER
MOISTLY
MOJITOS
MOLITOR
MOLOTOV
MONCTON
MONITOR
MONSTER
MONSTRO
MORETTI
MOULTED
MOUNTED
MOUNTER
MOUNTIE
MOUNTUP
MOZETTA
MRBUTTS
MULATTO
MULCTED
MULETAS
MUNSTER
MUSETTA
MUSETTE
MUTATED
MUTATES

M•••T••

MACBETH
MACHETE
MAGENTA
MAGGOTS
MAGNATE
MAGNETO
MAGNETS
MAHOUTS
MAIMITI
MAJESTE
MAJESTY
MALLETS
MAMMOTH
MANDATE
MANETTE
MANKATO
MAOISTS
MARANTZ
MARCATO
MARGATE
MARKETS
MARMOTS
MASCOTS
MATZOTH
MEANSTO
MEANTTO
MEDIATE
MELITTA
MEMENTO
MENOTTI
MERLOTS
METWITH
MIDGETS
MIGRATE
MILLETS
MILLETT
MINOLTA
MINUETS
MISACTS
MISCITE
MISCUTS
MISDATE
MISFITS
MISHITS
MISMATE
MISRATE
MISSETS
MOABITE
MODELTS
MODESTO
MODESTY
MODISTE
MOLESTS
MOMENTA
MOMENTS
MOPPETS
MORANTE
MORETTI
MOSCATO
MOVEDTO
MOVESTO
MOZETTA
MRBUTTS
MRNORTH
MRSCOTT
MRSLATE
MRSMITH
MUDBATH
MUDCATS
MULATTO
MULLETS
MUPPETS
MUSANTE
MUSCATS
MUSETTA
MUSETTE
MUSKETS
MUTANTS
MYLANTA

M•••••T

MADDEST
MADEFIT
MADEOUT
MAEWEST
MAGINOT
MAHDIST
MAIGRET
MAILLOT
MAILOUT
MAKEFIT
MAKEOUT
MAKESIT
MALEANT
MALECAT
MALLRAT
MANHUNT
MANTLET
MANUMIT
MANXCAT
MAOSUIT
MAPSOUT
MARGRET
MARKOUT
MARRYAT
MARXIST
MAUPRAT
MAURIAT
MAZIEST
MCCOURT
MEANEST
MEANSIT
MEANTIT
MEDIANT
MEEKEST
MEERKAT
MEFIRST
MEGABIT
MEGAHIT
MESSKIT
METEOUT
METRIST
MIDEAST
MIDLIST
MIDMOST
MIDWEST
MIGHTNT
MIGRANT
MILDEST
MILLETT
MINARET
MINDSET
MINEPIT
MIRIEST
MISCAST
MISEDIT
MISSEAT
MISSENT
MISSORT
MISSOUT
MOBBIST
MOLERAT
MONGKUT
MOONLET
MOONLIT
MOONSET
MOPIEST
MORDANT
MORDENT
MORISOT
MOSHPIT
MOVEDIT
MOVEOUT
MOVESIT
MRFIXIT
MRHULOT
MRRIGHT
MRSCOTT
MUDFLAT
MUGSHOT
MUSKRAT
MYCROFT
MYFAULT
MYGIANT
MYTREAT

•MT••••

AMTRACK
AMTRACS
IMTHERE
IMTIRED

•M•T•••

AMATEUR
AMATIVE
AMATOLS
AMATORY
AMITIES
AMSTELS
DMYTRYK
EMETICS
EMITTED
EMITTER
EMOTERS
EMOTING
EMOTION
EMOTIVE
EMPTIED
EMPTIER
EMPTIES
EMPTILY
IMITATE
OMITTED
OMITTER
SMATTER
SMETANA
SMITERS
SMITHED
SMITING
SMITTEN
SMOTHER
UMPTEEN

•M••T••

AMANTIS
AMISTAD
AMMETER
AMRITAS
EMITTED
EMITTER
EMPATHS
EMPATHY
IMHOTEP
IMPETUS
IMPUTED
IMPUTER
IMPUTES
IMUSTGO
OMITTED
OMITTER
SMARTED
SMARTEN
SMARTER
SMARTLY
SMATTER
SMELTED
SMELTER
SMITTEN
SMOOTHS
SMOOTHY

•M•••T•

AMANITA
AMENITY
AMILATE
AMINUTE
AMNESTY
AMOUNTS
AMREETA
AMULETS
EMANATE
EMBOITE
EMERITA
EMERITI
EMIRATE
EMULATE
IMAMATE
IMARETS
IMITATE
IMPACTS
IMPARTS
IMPASTO
IMPIETY
IMPORTS
IMPOSTS
OMELETS
UMBERTO
UMLAUTS

•M••••T

AMBIENT
AMHERST
AMONGST
AMORIST
AMPLEST
EMANANT
EMINENT
IMADEIT
IMAGIST
IMEANIT
IMFORIT
IMGREAT
IMPLANT
IMPREST
IMPRINT
SMILEAT

••MT•••

COMTISM
COMTIST
COMTREX
ELMTREE
GUMTREE
TAMTAMS
TOMTITS
TOMTOMS
YOMTOVS

••M•T••

ADMITTO
AMMETER
BIMETAL
COMPTON
DEMETER
DEMOTED
DEMOTES
DEMOTHS
DEMOTIC
DIMETER
DIMITRI
EXMATES
GAMETAL
GAMETES
HAMITES
HAMITIC
HAMITUP
HAMPTON
HAMSTER
HEMATIC
HEMATIN
INMATES
IOMOTHS
KEMPTON
KOMATSU
LAMOTTA
LAMOTTE
LIMITED
LIMITER
MIMETIC
NAMETAG
OLMSTED
OSMATIC
OSMOTIC
REMATCH
REMATED
REMATES
REMOTER
REMOTES
SEMITES
SEMITIC
SOMATIC
SUMATRA
SUMITUP
SYMPTOM
TEMPTED
TEMPTER
TIMOTHY
UNMATED
UNMATES
UNMITER
UNMITRE
UNMUTED
VUMETER
ZEMSTVO

••M••T•

ADMITTO
ALMAATA
ARMLETS
ARMPITS
BYMOUTH
CEMENTS
COMBATS
COMESTO
COMFITS
COMMITS
COMMUTE
COMPETE
COMPOTE
COMPUTE
COMSATS
DEMASTS
DEMENTO
DEMISTS
DIMOUTS
DIMWITS
ELMCITY
ELMISTI
ELMONTE
FEMBOTS
FOMENTS
GAMBITS
GEMMATE
GIMLETS
GYMRATS
HAMLETS
HAMMETT
LAMBETH
LAMENTS
LAMINTO
LAMOTTA
LAMOTTE
LEMMATA
LIMNITE
LIMPETS
MAMMOTH
MEMENTO
MOMENTA
MOMENTS
NIMIETY
NUMBATS
PIMENTO
RAMINTO
RAMJETS
REMEETS
REMELTS
REMINTS
SAMLETS
SIMCITY
SUMMATE
SUMMITS
SUMUPTO
TIMROTH
TOMCATS
TOMKITE
TOMTITS
TUMULTS
UNMASTS
UTMOSTS
WOMBATS

••M•••T

AIMEDAT
ARMREST
ARMYANT
BOMBAST
BOMBLET
BUMSOUT
CAMELOT
CAMEOUT
CAMPOUT
COMBUST
COMCAST
COMEOUT
COMESAT
COMFORT
COMMENT
COMPACT
COMPART
COMPORT
COMPOST
COMTIST
DAMPEST
DEMARET
DEMERIT
DEMOUNT
DIMMEST
DIMSOUT
DUMBEST
DUMPOUT
ELMIEST
FUMEDAT
FUMESAT
FUMIEST
GAMIEST
GUMBOOT
GYMNAST
GYMSUIT
HAMMETT
HOMIEST
HUMBERT
IAMBIST
JIMKAAT
JUMPCUT
JUMPSAT
KUMQUAT
LAMAIST
LAMBENT
LAMBERT
LAMPERT
LAMPLIT
LIMIEST
LIMPEST
LUMPSIT
NUMBEST
PUMPOUT
RAMPANT
RAMPART
REMNANT
REMOUNT
RIMIEST
RIMSHOT
SAMOSET
SUMOIST
TEMPEST
TIMEOUT
TIMHOLT
UNMEANT
UNMOIST
WIMPOUT
XAMOUNT
ZUMWALT

•••MT••

PALMTOP
TRIMTAB

•••M•T•

ADAMITE
AGEMATE
ALSMITH
ANIMATE
ANIMATO
AZIMUTH
BASMATI
BEDMATE
BISMUTH
BONMOTS
BROMATE
CLAMATO
CLIMATE
CLIMATS
CLIMBTO
COMMITS
COMMUTE
CONMOTO
CREMATE
DERMATO
DOGMATA
DOOMSTO
EDEMATA
EDOMITE
ELAMITE
EREMITE
EXEMPTS
FERMATA
FERMATE
FERMATS
FORMATS
GEMMATE
HAMMETT
HAZMATS
HELMETS
HERMITS
IMAMATE
KISMETS
KLAMATH
LEMMATA
MAIMITI
MAMMOTH
MARMOTS
MISMATE
MRSMITH
NESMITH
NEWMATH
ONEMPTY
OUTMATE
PALMATE
PERMITS
PERMUTE
PREMATE
PRIMATE
PROMOTE
PROMPTS
REEMITS
SCHMITT
SEEMSTO
STOMATA
SUBMITS
SUMMATE
SUMMITS
TERMITE
THEMETS
UNEMPTY
WARMSTO
ZERMATT

•••M••T

ADAMANT
AFTMOST
AILMENT
ALIMENT
ANIMIST
ATOMIST
AUGMENT
BELMONT
BOOMLET
CALMEST
CATMINT
CHEMIST
CLAMANT
CLEMENT
COMMENT
CRUMPET
DEHMELT
DELMONT
DIMMEST
DINMONT
DISMAST
DORMANT
DRUMOUT
DRUMSET
ELEMENT
ENDMOST
FARMOUT
FERMENT
FIGMENT
FILMSET
FIRMEST
FREMONT
GARMENT
GNOMIST
GROMMET
HAMMETT
KINMONT
MIDMOST
NEWMINT
NEWMONT
NONMEAT
NUTMEAT
ODDMENT
OUTMOST
PALMIST
PAYMENT
PIGMEAT
PIGMENT
PLUMCOT
PLUMMET
PREMEET
RAIMENT
RAWMEAT
REAMOUT
REDMEAT
RESMELT
REYMONT
RHYMIST
RIBMEAT
SCHMIDT
SCHMITT
SEAMIST
SEGMENT
SPAMBOT
THEMOST
TOPMAST
TOPMOST
TORMENT
TRUMPET
UNSMART
VARMINT
VERMONT
WALMART
WARMEST
ZERMATT
ZOOMOUT

••••MT•

VICOMTE

••••M•T

ATTEMPT
AUTOMAT
BATHMAT
CALUMET
CHROMAT
DELIMIT
DOORMAT
FOTOMAT
GOURMET
GROMMET
HARTMUT
MANUMIT
NOLIMIT
PLUMMET
PNEUMAT
PREEMPT
PREOMIT
READMIT
RELIMIT
TAGAMET
UNKEMPT
YOGAMAT

•••••MT

BUTTEMT

MU•••••

MUAMMAR
MUBARAK
MUCKERS
MUCKIER
MUCKING
MUCKSUP
MUDBATH
MUDCATS
MUDDERS
MUDDIED
MUDDIER
MUDDIES
MUDDILY
MUDDING
MUDDLED
MUDDLER
MUDDLES
MUDEELS
MUDFISH
MUDFLAP
MUDFLAT
MUDFLOW
MUDHENS
MUDHOLE
MUDLARK
MUDPACK
MUDPIES
MUDROOM
MUDWASP
MUELLER
MUESLIS
MUESLIX
MUEZZIN
MUFFING
MUFFINS
MUFFLED
MUFFLER
MUFFLES
MUGFULS
MUGGERS
MUGGIER
MUGGING
MUGGISH
MUGGLES
MUGSHOT
MUGWUMP
MUJERES
MUKLUKS
MULATTO
MULCAHY
MULCHED
MULCHES
MULCTED
MULDAUR
MULDOON
MULETAS
MULGREW
MULHARE
MULLAHS
MULLERS
MULLETS
MULLING
MULLINS
MUMBLED
MUMBLER
MUMBLES
MUMESON
MUMFORD
MUMMERS
MUMMERY
MUMMIES
MUMMIFY
MUMMING
MUNCHED
MUNCHEN
MUNCHER
MUNCHES
MUNCHIE
MUNCHON
MUNDANE
MUNSTER
MUPPETS
MURALED
MURANOS
MURDERS
MURDOCH
MURIELS
MURILLO
MURKIER
MURKILY
MURKISH
MURMURS
MURPHYS
MUSANTE
MUSCATS
MUSCIDA
MUSCLED
MUSCLES
MUSEDON
MUSEFUL
MUSESON
MUSETTA
MUSETTE
MUSEUMS
MUSHERS
MUSHIER
MUSHILY
MUSHING
MUSICAL
MUSICKS
MUSIGNY
MUSINGS
MUSKEGO
MUSKETS
MUSKIER
MUSKIES
MUSKRAT
MUSLIMS
MUSLINS
MUSSELS
MUSSIER
MUSSILY
MUSSING
MUSTAFA
MUSTANG
MUSTARD
MUSTDOS
MUSTERS
MUSTIER
MUSTILY
MUSTSEE
MUTABLE
MUTABLY
MUTAGEN
MUTANTS
MUTATED
MUTATES
MUTEDLY
MUTTERS
MUTTONS
MUTUALS
MUUMUUS
MUYBIEN
MUZZIER
MUZZILY
MUZZLED
MUZZLER
MUZZLES

M•U••••

MAUDLIN
MAUGHAM
MAULDIN
MAULERS
MAULING
MAUMAUS
MAUNDER

MAUPRAT
MAUREEN
MAURIAC
MAURIAT
MAURICE
MAUROIS
MAUSERS
MAUVAIS
MOULAGE
MOULDED
MOULDER
MOULTED
MOUNDED
MOUNTED
MOUNTER
MOUNTIE
MOUNTUP
MOURNED
MOURNER
MOUSERS
MOUSIER
MOUSILY
MOUSING
MOUSSED
MOUSSES
MOUTHED
MOUTHER
MUUMUUS

M••U•••
MACULAE
MACULAR
MACUSER
MADUROS
MAGUIRE
MANUALS
MANUMIT
MANURED
MANURES
MARULLO
MARUSJA
MATURED
MATURER
MATURES
MAZURKA
MCGUIRE
MCLUHAN
MCMURDO
MCQUEEN
MEDULLA
MEDUSAE
MEDUSAN
MEDUSAS
MENUBAR
MENUDOS
MENUHIN
MEZUZAH
MEZUZAS
MINUEND
MINUETS
MINUSES
MINUTED
MINUTER
MINUTES
MINUTIA
MISUSED
MISUSER
MISUSES
MIZUNAS
MODULAR
MODULES
MODULUS
MOLUCCA
MOMUSES
MRBURNS
MRBUTTS
MRHULOT
MRLUCKY
MRMUSIC
MRQUILP
MUTUALS
MYBUDDY

M•••U••
MACDUFF
MACOUNS
MADRUSH
MAGNUMS
MAHOUTS
MAJEURE
MAKEUPS
MANCUSO
MANHUNT
MANTUAN
MAOSUIT
MARAUDS
MARCUSE
MARKUPS
MARQUEE
MARQUES
MARQUEZ
MARQUIS
MARYURE
MASQUER
MASQUES
MCCLURE
MCCLURG
MCCOURT
MCCRUMB
MCGRUFF
MEASURE
MEDIUMS
MERCURE
MERCURY
MESHUGA
MESSUPS
MIAOUED
MIDJULY
MIDJUNE
MISCUED
MISCUES
MISCUTS
MISRULE
MISSUSA
MISTUNE
MIXTURE
MOBRULE
MOCKUPS
MOLLUSC
MOLLUSK
MONTUNO
MORGUES
MOSQUES
MRSMUIR
MSIEURS
MUGFULS
MUGWUMP
MUKLUKS
MURMURS
MUSEUMS
MUUMUUS
MYFAULT

M••••U•
MACAQUE
MADEFUN
MADEOUT
MADERUN
MAHFOUZ
MAILOUT
MAISOUI
MAKEFUN
MAKEOUT
MAKERUN
MAKESUP
MALAMUD
MALLEUS
MALRAUX
MALTHUS
MANAGUA
MANHOUR
MANIPUR
MAPSOUT
MARGAUX
MARHAUS
MARKOUT
MARKSUP
MARTIUS
MASSEUR
MATCHUP
MAUMAUS
MAXIMUM
MAXIMUS
MCCLOUD
MEETSUP
MENCIUS
METEOUT
MICHAUX
MILERUN
MILHAUD
MILHOUS
MILIEUS
MILIEUX
MILKDUD
MILKRUN
MILLRUN
MIMIEUX
MINDFUL
MINIBUS
MINIMUM
MINIMUS
MINISUB
MINOGUE
MISSOUT
MISTSUP
MITCHUM
MIXEDUP
MIXESUP
MIXITUP
MOANFUL
MOCKSUP
MODICUM
MODULUS
MONGKUT
MONTAUK
MONTEUX
MOUNTUP
MOVEDUP
MOVEOUT
MOVESUP
MRSPAUL
MUCKSUP
MULDAUR
MUSEFUL
MUUMUUS

M•••••U
MARCEAU
MARTINU
MARYLOU
MATHIEU
MATTHAU
MISSYOU
MONDIEU
MONTAGU

•MU••••
AMULETS
AMUSEME
AMUSERS
AMUSING
EMULATE
EMULOUS
FMURRAY
IMUSTGO
SMUCKER
SMUDGED
SMUDGES
SMUGGER
SMUGGLE
SMUSHED
SMUSHES

•M•U•••
AMOUNTS
AMPULES
EMMUSKA
EMQUADS
IMBUING
IMMUNES
IMMURED
IMMURES
IMPUGNS
IMPULSE
IMPURER
IMPUTED
IMPUTER
IMPUTES

•M••U••
AMINUTE
AMPOULE
EMANUEL
EMBRUED
EMBRUES
IMBRUED
IMBRUES
IMPOUND
IMYOURS
UMLAUTS

•M•••U•
AMADEUS
AMATEUR
AMIBLUE
AMOROUS
AMPEDUP
EMULOUS
IMPETUS
IMPIOUS
OMINOUS
OMNIBUS
SMACKUP
SMASHUP
SMOKEUP

•M••••U
EMMYLOU

••MU•••
BEMUSED
BEMUSES
CUMULUS
DEMURER
EDMUNDI
EDMUNDS
ELMUNDO
EMMUSKA
FAMULUS
HAMULUS
HHMUNRO
HUMUSES
IMMUNES
IMMURED
IMMURES
MCMURDO
MOMUSES
MRMUSIC
OSMUNDS
ROMULAN
ROMULUS
SAMUELL
SAMURAI
SUMUPTO
TUMULTS
UNMUDDY
UNMUTED
ZYMURGY

••M•U••
ARMFULS
ARMOURS
ARMOURY
BUMRUSH
BYMOUTH
COMBUST
COMMUNE
COMMUTE
COMPUTE
DEMBUMS
DEMOUNT
DIMBULB
DIMOUTS
DUMDUMS
GYMSUIT
HAMBURG
HOMBURG
HUMBUGS
HUMOURS
JUMBUCK
KUMQUAT
LIMBURG
REMOUNT
RUMOURS
SAMBUCA
SAMHUFF
SAMNUNN
SAMSUNG
TEMPURA
UNMOULD
WAMPUMS
XAMOUNT

••M••U•
BUMPSUP
BUMSOUT
CAMEDUE
CAMEOUT
CAMPOUT
CAMPSUP
CIMABUE
COMEDUE
COMEOUT
COMESUP
COMIQUE
CUMULUS
DAMASUS
DIMSOUT
DOMINUS
DUMMYUP
DUMPOUT
FAMULUS
FEMINUM
GYMCLUB
HAMITUP
HAMULUS
HOMERUN
HUMANUM
HUMDRUM
HUMERUS
JIMRYUN
JUMPCUT
JUMPSUP
LEMIEUX
LUMPSUM
MIMIEUX
ORMOLUS
POMPOUS
PUMPOUT
PUMPSUP
RAMPSUP
RIMBAUD
ROMANUS
ROMULUS
SUMITUP
TIMEOUT
TIMESUP
WIMPOUT

••M•••U
EMMYLOU
JAMBEAU
KOMATSU
LAMBEAU

•••MU••
AZIMUTH
BERMUDA
BISMUTH
COMMUNE
COMMUTE
EANMUND
EARMUFF
FORMULA
HOWMUCH
MRSMUIR
MURMURS
MUUMUUS
NIPMUCK
NOTMUCH
PERMUTE
PETMULE
PLUMULE
RIOMUNI
SIGMUND
STIMULI
TEAMUSA
TOOMUCH
UNAMUNO
WARMUPS

•••M•U•
ALUMNUS
BEAMSUP
BRIMFUL
BRUMOUS
CADMIUM
CLAMOUR
CLAMSUP
CLIMBUP
CRUMBUM
DOOMFUL
DRUMOUT
DRUMSUP
DUMMYUP
ENAMOUR
FARMOUT
FERMIUM
FIRMSUP
FLAMEUP
FORMFUL
FRAMEUP
GLAMOUR
GLAMSUP
GRAMPUS
HARMFUL
HOLMIUM
MAUMAUS
MUUMUUS
OLYMPUS
PALMFUL
PHEMIUS
PLUMBUM
PREMIUM
REAMOUT
RHOMBUS
ROOMFUL
SEYMOUR
SWIMSUP
TEAMSUP
TRUMPUP
WARMSUP
ZOOMOUT

•••M••U
THIMPHU

••••MU•
ARTEMUS
BEERMUG
DONIMUS
DREAMUP
ERASMUS
HARTMUT
ISTHMUS
KEEPMUM
KEPTMUM
MALAMUD
MAXIMUM
MAXIMUS
MINIMUM
MINIMUS
OPTIMUM
PARAMUS
POTAMUS
PUTEMUP
PYRAMUS
REAUMUR
STEAMUP
ZOSIMUS

••••M•U
TINAMOU

M•V••••
MAVISES
MOVABLE
MOVABLY
MOVADOS
MOVEDIN
MOVEDIT
MOVEDON
MOVEDTO
MOVEDUP
MOVEOFF
MOVEOUT
MOVESIN
MOVESIT
MOVESON
MOVESTO
MOVESUP

M••V•••
MALVINA
MARVELL
MARVELS
MARVIER
MAUVAIS
MTEVANS

M•••V••
MARKVII
MCCOVEY
MCGAVIN
MEDEVAC
MEDIVAC
MINIVAC
MINIVAN
MINIVER
MISAVER
MITZVAH
MOHAVES
MOJAVES
MORAVIA
MOTIVED
MOTIVES
MRNOVAK

M••••V•
MAGLEVS
MALDIVE
MARKOVA
MASSIVE
MINERVA
MINITVS
MISGAVE
MISGIVE
MISMOVE
MISSIVE
MOLDOVA
MONDAVI

M•••••V
MARTINV
MOLOTOV

•M•V•••
BMOVIES

•M••V••
IMPAVID

•M•••V•
AMATIVE
EMOTIVE
IMPROVE

•M••••V
SMIRNOV

••MV•••
DIMVIEW
HUMVEES

••M•V••
REMOVAL
REMOVED
REMOVER
REMOVES
SAMOVAR
TVMOVIE
UNMOVED

••M••V•
COMMOVE
IAMLOVE
JAMESVI
YOMTOVS
ZEMSTVO

••M•••V
JAMESIV
KEMIDOV
NEMEROV
ROMANOV

•••MV••
DUUMVIR

•••M•V•
BADMOVE
COMMOVE
MISMOVE
OUTMOVE
THEMAVS

M•W••••
MAWKISH
MEWLERS
MEWLING
MOWBRAY
MOWDOWN
MOWINGS
MRWORDS
MRWRONG
MYWORLD

M••W•••
MAEWEST
MALWARE
MAXWELL
MAYWINE
MCGWIRE
MCSWINE
MEDWICK
MEOWERS
MEOWING
MEOWMIX
METWITH
MIDWAYS
MIDWEEK
MIDWEST
MIDWIFE
MISWIRE
MISWORD
MUDWASP
MUGWUMP

M•••W••
MADEWAR
MADEWAY
MAKEWAR
MAKEWAY
MANOWAR
MATEWAN
MCCOWEN
MEDAWAR
MIAOWED
MOHAWKS

M••••W•
MACHTWO
MALLOWS
MARLOWE
MARROWS
MATHEWS
MEADOWS
MEADOWY
MELLOWS
MIDTOWN
MILDEWS
MILDEWY
MINNOWS
MOOCOWS
MORROWS
MOWDOWN
MRBROWN

M•••••W
MACGRAW
MANILOW
MATTHEW
MILKCOW
MISBREW
MISDRAW
MISDREW
MISKNEW
MISKNOW
MISTBOW
MOONBOW
MUDFLOW
MULGREW

•M•W•••
IMSWELL

•M••W••
EMBOWER
EMPOWER

•M•••W•
EMBROWN

••MW•••
DIMWITS
ELMWOOD
GUMWOOD
SAMWISE
ZUMWALT

••M•W••
REMOWED
SOMEWAY
TIMEWAS
UNMEWED
UNMOWED
WIMOWEH

••M••W•
ONMYOWN
RAMDOWN

••M•••W
COMENOW
CUMSHAW
DIMVIEW
GAMELAW
OHMSLAW
SEMIRAW
SOMEHOW

•••MW••
TRAMWAY

•••M•W•
HAYMOWS
NEWMOWN

••••MW•
OTTUMWA

M•X••••
MAXBAER
MAXBORN
MAXILLA
MAXIMAL
MAXIMAS
MAXIMUM
MAXIMUS
MAXIXES
MAXWELL
MEXICAN
MIXABLE
MIXEDIN
MIXEDLY
MIXEDUP
MIXESIN
MIXESUP
MIXITUP
MIXTECS
MIXTURE

M••X•••
MANXCAT
MANXMAN
MANXMEN
MARXIAN
MARXISM
MARXIST
MINXISH

M•••X••
MAXIXES
MRFIXIT

M••••X•
MEATAXE

M•••••X
MACHSIX
MADAMEX
MAILBOX
MALRAUX
MARGAUX
MEMOREX
MEOWMIX
MICHAUX
MILIEUX
MIMIEUX
MINIMAX
MIRAMAX
MISTERX
MONTEUX
MUESLIX

•M••X••
IMMIXED
IMMIXES

•M••••X
OMNIMAX

••M•X••
ADMIXED
ADMIXES
IMMIXED
IMMIXES
REMIXED
REMIXES
TIMEXES
UNMIXED
UNMIXES

••M••X•
JIMFIXX

••M•••X
COMPLEX
COMTREX
HUMIDEX
JIMFIXX
LEMIEUX
MEMOREX
MIMIEUX
SIMPLEX
SOMINEX

•••M••X
BOOMBOX
FLUMMOX

••••M•X
BETAMAX
CAKEMIX
CHEXMIX
CINEMAX
COOLMAX
FLUMMOX
MADAMEX
MEOWMIX
MINIMAX
MIRAMAX
OMNIMAX
OVERMIX
SOUPMIX

MY•••••
MYALGIA
MYALGIC
MYANMAR
MYBUDDY
MYCENAE
MYCROFT
MYERSON
MYFAULT
MYGIANT
MYKONOS
MYLANTA
MYMAMMY
MYNHEER
MYOLOGY
MYOPIAS
MYRIADS
MYRRHED
MYRRHIC
MYRTLES
MYSPACE
MYSTARS
MYSTERY
MYSTICS
MYSTIFY
MYTHIFY
MYTREAT
MYWORLD

M•Y••••
MAYALIN
MAYBESO
MAYDAYS
MAYFAIR
MAYHEMS

MAYINGS
MAYNARD
MAYORAL
MAYPOLE
MAYTAGS
MAYTIME
MAYWINE
MEYNELL
MUYBIEN

M••Y•••
MAGYARS
MANYEAR
MARYANN
MARYKAY
MARYLOU
MARYURE
MIDYEAR
MINYANS

M•••Y••
MALAYAN
MARRYAT
MARRYIN
MARRYME
MARTYRS
MEGRYAN
MISSYOU
MISTYPE
MONEYED
MOSEYED

M••••Y•
MADALYN
MANDAYS
MARILYN
MASARYK
MAYDAYS
MEDLEYS
MICKEYS
MIDDAYS
MIDWAYS
MINSKYS
MISKEYS
MISLAYS
MISSAYS
MONDAYS
MONKEYS
MONTOYA
MOONEYE
MOTLEYS
MTKENYA
MURPHYS

M•••••Y
MADEHAY
MADEWAY
MAGNIFY
MAHONEY
MAJESTY
MAKEHAY
MAKEWAY
MALARKY
MALMSEY
MARGERY
MARYKAY
MASONRY
MASTERY
MCCAREY
MCCOVEY
MCCRARY
MCGRORY
MCHENRY
MCNALLY
MCRANEY
MEADOWY
MEATILY
MENSCHY
MERCERY
MERCURY
MERRILY
MESSILY
MIDJULY
MILDEWY
MILKILY
MIMICRY
MISALLY
MISCOPY
MISERLY
MISPLAY
MISRELY
MISTILY
MIXEDLY
MOCKERY
MODESTY
MOISTLY
MOLLIFY
MOMONEY
MONTHLY
MOODILY
MOONILY
MORALLY
MOREPAY
MORESBY
MORTIFY
MOTHERY
MOUSILY
MOVABLY
MOWBRAY
MRBODDY
MRDARCY
MRHANEY
MRLUCKY
MRNANNY
MTBALDY
MTMARCY
MUDDILY
MULCAHY
MUMMERY
MUMMIFY
MURKILY
MUSHILY
MUSIGNY
MUSSILY
MUSTILY
MUTABLY
MUTEDLY
MUZZILY
MYBUDDY
MYMAMMY
MYOLOGY
MYSTERY
MYSTIFY
MYTHIFY

•MY••••
AMYLASE
DMYTRYK
IMYOURS

•M•Y•••
EMMYLOU

•M••Y••
EMBAYED
EMBRYOS

•M•••Y•
DMYTRYK
EMPLOYS
SMILEYS
SMOKEYS

•M••••Y
AMATORY
AMENITY
AMIABLY
AMNESTY
AMPLIFY
AMSCRAY
EMBASSY
EMPATHY
EMPTILY
FMURRAY
IMAGERY
IMHAPPY
IMPIETY
IMREADY
IMSORRY
OMALLEY
SMARTLY
SMOKILY
SMOOTHY

••MY•••
ARMYANT
EMMYLOU
FTMYERS
ONMYOWN

••M•Y••
CAMRYLE
DUMMYUP
EXMAYOR
GEMAYEL
ITMAYBE
JIMRYUN
LEMOYNE
SAMMYJO
SAMOYED

••M••Y•
CAMBOYS
DEMONYM
HOMONYM
ROMNEYS
SAMLOYD
STMARYS
TAMBLYN
TOMBOYS

••M•••Y
ALMONDY
ALMONRY
ARMOURY
BUMPILY
CAMPILY
COMESBY
COMPANY
DAMPDRY
DEMOLAY
DEMPSEY
DRMCCOY
DUMPILY
ELMCITY
GAMEBOY
HAMMILY
HEMSLEY
HOMEBOY
HUMANLY
HUMIDLY
HUMPHRY
HYMNARY
HYMNODY
JTMONEY
JUMPILY
LAMPREY
LUMPILY
MIMICRY
MOMONEY
MTMARCY
MUMMERY
MUMMIFY
MYMAMMY
NAMABLY
NAMEDAY
NIMIETY
NOMERCY
ORMANDY
REMARRY
SAMEDAY
SEMIDRY
SIMCITY
SOMEDAY
SOMESAY
SOMEWAY
SUMMARY
SUMMERY
TAMMANY
TIMBERY
TIMIDLY
TIMOTHY
UNMADLY
UNMANLY
UNMERRY
UNMOLDY
UNMOODY
UNMOSSY
UNMUDDY
WEMBLEY
WOMANLY
ZOMBIFY
ZYMURGY

•••MY••
DUMMYUP
GROMYKO
PALMYRA
SAMMYJO

•••M•Y•
DISMAYS
GRAMMYS
THEMAYO

•••M••Y
ALIMONY
ANIMACY
ANOMALY
BALMILY
BRAMBLY
BRAMLEY
BRIMLEY
CHIMNEY
CHOMSKY
CRIMINY
CRUMBLY
CRUMPLY
DRAMADY
DRAMEDY
FARMBOY
FARMERY
FILMILY
FOAMILY
GERMANY
GOOMBAY
GRIMILY
GRIMSBY
GRUMBLY
HAMMILY
HARMONY
HOWMANY
MALMSEY
MUMMERY
MUMMIFY
NOTMANY
ONEMPTY
PALMARY
PLUMPLY
PRIMACY
PRIMARY
PRIMELY
REIMPLY
ROOMILY
SLIMILY
SUMMARY
SUMMERY
TAMMANY
TOOMANY
TRAMWAY
TREMBLY
UNEMPTY
UNSMOKY
VERMINY

••••MY•
GRAMMYS

••••M•Y
ANNAMAY
BUXOMLY
CALUMNY
CAPEMAY
DAHOMEY
EDNAMAY
ELLYMAY
IFWEMAY
LASTMAY
MYMAMMY
SCRIMPY
SHRIMPY
UNLUMPY

•••••MY
ACADEMY
ALABAMY
ALCHEMY
ANATOMY
BALSAMY
BELLAMY
ECONOMY
EPONYMY
EXENEMY
EXOGAMY
FRENEMY
ISONOMY
MYMAMMY
PERFUMY
PHLEGMY
PTOLEMY
REDARMY
SQUIRMY
THEARMY
UNROOMY
UNWORMY

M•Z••••
MAZARIN
MAZEPPA
MAZIEST
MAZURKA
MAZZINI
MEZUZAH
MEZUZAS
MIZRAHI
MIZUNAS
MIZZENS
MIZZLED
MIZZLES
MOZETTA
MOZILLA
MUZZIER
MUZZILY
MUZZLED
MUZZLER
MUZZLES

M••Z•••
MAHZORS
MATZOHS
MATZOTH
MAZZINI
MENZIES
MISZONE
MITZVAH
MIZZENS
MIZZLED
MIZZLES
MUEZZIN
MUZZIER
MUZZILY
MUZZLED
MUZZLER
MUZZLES

M•••Z••
MEZUZAH
MEZUZAS
MINIZOO
MUEZZIN

M••••Z•
MANSIZE
MIDSIZE

M•••••Z
MAHFOUZ
MARANTZ
MARQUEZ

•M•Z•••
AMAZING
AMAZONS

•M•••Z•
EMBLAZE
IMPREZA

••M••Z•
ZAMBEZI

••M•••Z
JIMENEZ
JIMINEZ
RAMIREZ
SIMONIZ
TEMPEAZ

•••M•Z•
ATOMIZE
ITEMIZE

NA•••••
NABBERS
NABBING
NABISCO
NABOKOV
NABUCCO
NACELLE
NAGGERS
NAGGIER
NAGGING
NAGGISH
NAHUATL
NAIADES
NAILERS
NAILGUN
NAILING
NAILKEG
NAILSET
NAILSIN
NAILSIT
NAILSUP
NAILTIP
NAIPAUL
NAIROBI
NAIVELY
NAIVEST
NAIVETE
NAIVETY
NAKEDLY
NAMABLE
NAMABLY
NAMEDAY
NAMEONE
NAMETAG
NAMIBIA
NANAIMO
NANETTE
NANJING
NANKING
NANNIED
NANNIES
NAPALMS
NAPHTHA
NAPIERS
NAPKINS
NAPLESS
NAPPERS
NAPPIER
NAPPIES
NAPPING
NAPSTER
NAPTIME
NARAYAN
NARRATE
NARROWS
NARTHEX
NARVAEZ
NARWHAL
NASALLY
NASCENT
NASTASE
NASTIER
NASTIES
NASTILY
NATALIA
NATALIE
NATASHA
NATATOR
NATCHEZ
NATHANS
NATIONS
NATIVES
NATRIUM
NATSUME
NATTERS
NATTIER
NATTILY
NATURAL
NATURED
NATUREL
NATURES
NATWICK
NAUGHTS
NAUGHTY
NAUSEAM
NAUTICA
NAUTILI
NAVAHOS
NAVAIDS
NAVAJOS
NAVARRE
NAVIDAD
NAVYMAN
NAVYMEN
NAYARIT
NAYSAID
NAYSAYS

N•A••••
NBAGAME
NBALIVE
NBATEAM
NDAKOTA
NEAREST
NEARING
NEARPAR
NEARYOU
NEATENS
NEATEST
NEATNIK
NIAGARA
NIALONG
NIANTIC
NOANGEL
NUANCED
NUANCES

N••A•••
NAIADES
NAMABLE
NAMABLY
NANAIMO
NAPALMS
NARAYAN
NASALLY
NATALIA
NATALIE
NATASHA
NATATOR
NAVAHOS
NAVAIDS
NAVAJOS
NAVARRE
NAYARIT
NEGATED
NEGATER
NEGATES
NEGATOR
NEPALIS
NEVADAN
NEWAGER
NEWAGEY
NOCANDO
NOCARBS
NOCATCH
NOFAULT
NOGALES
NOHANDS
NOMADIC
NONACID
NONAGES
NONAGON
NONAMES
NONARAB
NONARTS
NOPALES
NOTABIT
NOTABLE
NOTABLY
NOTALIE
NOTALOT
NOTAONE
NOTASTE
NOTATED
NOTATES
NOVALIS
NOVARRO
NUNAVUT
NUTATED
NUTATES
NYYANKS

N•••A••
NAHUATL
NAIPAUL
NARRATE
NARVAEZ
NASTASE
NATHANS
NAYSAID
NAYSAYS
NBAGAME
NECTARS
NECTARY
NEDLAND
NEONATE
NESCAFE
NETBALL
NETCAFE
NETGAIN
NETGAME
NETWARE
NEUMANN
NEWCARS
NEWFACE
NEWGATE
NEWHAND
NEWHART
NEWHATS
NEWLAID
NEWMADE
NEWMANS
NEWMATH
NEWNAME
NEWWAVE
NEXRADS
NFLGAME
NHLGAME
NIAGARA
NICCAGE
NICTATE
NIKEADS
NIRVANA
NISSANS
NISSANZ
NITRATE
NITTANY
NOCLASS
NOLOADS
NONBANK
NONBASE
NONCASH
NONDARK
NONFACT
NONFANS
NONFARM
NONPAID
NONPARS
NONPAST
NONSALE
NONSANE
NONWAGE
NONWARS
NOPLACE
NORMALS
NORMAND
NORMANS
NORWALK
NOSEATS
NOSTAIN
NOSTARS
NOTEASY
NOTFAIR
NOTMANY
NOTRADE
NOTRARE
NOTSAFE
NOUGATS
NUBIANS
NUMBATS
NYGIANT

N••••A•
NAMEDAY
NAMETAG
NARAYAN
NARWHAL
NATURAL
NAUSEAM
NAVIDAD
NAVYMAN
NBATEAM
NEARPAR
NEBULAE
NEBULAR
NEBULAS
NEEDHAM
NEONGAS
NESSMAN
NEUTRAL
NEVADAN
NEWDEAL
NEWLEAF
NEWSDAY
NEWSMAN
NEWYEAR
NEXTDAY
NFCTEAM
NFLTEAM
NHLTEAM
NICEDAY
NICEMAN
NICOBAR
NICOLAS
NIKOLAI
NIKOLAY
NKRUMAH
NODICAL
NODULAR
NOMINAL
NONARAB
NONDEAF
NONMEAT
NONORAL
NONPEAK
NONPLAY
NOONDAY
NOOTKAS
NOSEBAG
NOSEGAY
NOSUGAR
NOSWEAT
NOTEPAD
NOTNEAR
NOTREAL
NOUVEAU
NOVELAS
NOVENAS
NOVISAD
NOWWHAT
NUBIRAS
NUCLEAR
NUMERAL
NUPTIAL
NUTMEAT
NUTRIAS
NYMPHAL

N•••••A
NAMIBIA
NAPHTHA
NATALIA
NATASHA
NAUTICA
NDAKOTA
NERISSA
NEWIDEA
NIAGARA
NICOSIA
NIGERIA
NIRVANA
NONCOLA
NORDICA
NORIEGA
NOSEBRA
NOVELLA
NOXZEMA
NUESTRA

•NA••••
ANACINS
ANADEMS
ANAEMIA
ANAEMIC
ANAGRAM
ANAHEIM
ANALOGS
ANALOGY
ANALYSE
ANALYST
ANALYTE
ANALYZE
ANANIAS
ANAPEST
ANARCHS
ANARCHY
ANASAZI
ANATASE
ANATOLE
ANATOLY
ANATOMY
DNAASES
DNACODE
DNALABS
DNATEST
ENABLED
ENABLER
ENABLES
ENACTED
ENACTOR
ENAMELS
ENAMORS
ENAMOUR
ENARBOR
ENARMED
GNARLED
GNARRED
GNASHED
GNASHER
GNASHES
GNAWERS
GNAWING
GNAWSAT
GNAWSON
INABALL
INABIND
INACAST
INADAZE
INAFUNK
INAFURY
INAHEAP
INAHOLE
INAHUFF
INAIDOF
INAJIFF
INAKNOT
INALINE
INAMESS
INAMOOD
INANELY
INANEST
INANITY
INAPILE
INAPOEM
INAPOKE
INAPRIL
INAPTER
INAPTLY
INARAGE
INARUSH
INASHOE
INASNAP
INASNIT
INASPIN
INASPOT
INASTEW
INASTIR
INASUIT
INATRAP
INAVALE
INAWEOF
INAWINK
INAWORD
KNARRED
KNAVERY
KNAVISH
ONABIAS
ONADARE
ONADATE
ONADIET
ONAGERS
ONAJURY
ONAKICK
ONALARK
ONALEAD
ONALERT
ONALINE
ONANDON

ONAROLL
ONASSIS
ONATEAR
ONATOOT
ONATRIP
ONAWHIM
SNACKED
SNACKER
SNACKON
SNAFUED
SNAGGED
SNAGGER
SNAGSUP
SNAKERS
SNAKIER
SNAKILY
SNAKING
SNAPONS
SNAPPEA
SNAPPED
SNAPPER
SNAPPLE
SNAPSAT
SNAPSON
SNAPSTO
SNAPSUP
SNARERS
SNARFED
SNARING
SNARLAT
SNARLED
SNARLER
SNARLUP
SNAZZUP
UNACTED
UNADDED
UNADEPT
UNADULT
UNAGILE
UNAGING
UNAIDED
UNAIMED
UNAIRED
UNALERT
UNALIKE
UNALONE
UNAMUNO
UNANGRY
UNAPTLY
UNARMED
UNASKED
UNAWAKE
UNAWARE
UNAWFUL
UNAXLED

•N•A•••

ANDAMAN
ANDANTE
ANKARAN
ANNABEL
ANNAKIN
ANNALEE
ANNALES
ANNAMAY
ANNATTO
ANTACID
ANTARES
DNAASES
ENCAGED
ENCAGES
ENCAMPS
ENCARRE
ENCARTA
ENCASED
ENCASES
ENDABLE
ENDALLS
ENFACED
ENFACES
ENFANTS
ENGAGED
ENGAGER
ENGAGES
ENGARDE
ENHANCE
ENLACED
ENLACES
ENLARGE
ENMASSE
ENRAGED
ENRAGES
ENRANKS
ENTAILS
INCANTS
INCASED
INCASES
INFAITH
INFANCY
INFANTA
INFANTE
INFANTS
INFAVOR
INGALLS
INGATES
INHABIT
INHALED
INHALER
INHALES
INHASTE
INLABOR
INLANDS
INLARGE
INLAYER
INMARCH
INMATES
INNAGES
INNARDS
INRANGE
INSALES
INSANER
INTAILS
INTAKES
INTASTE
INVACUO
INVADED
INVADER
INVADES
INVALID
INWARDS
KNEADED
KNEADER
ONEACAT
ONEACRE
ONEACTS
ONEADAY
ONEARTH
ONPAPER
ONRAMPS
ONSAGER
ONTARIO
ONWARDS
ONWATER
SNEAKBY
SNEAKED
SNEAKER
SNEAKIN
SNEAKUP
UNBAITS
UNBAKED
UNBALED
UNBALES
UNBARED
UNBARES
UNBASED
UNBATED
UNCAGED
UNCAGES
UNCAKED
UNCAKES
UNCANED
UNCANNY
UNCAPED
UNCASED
UNCASES
UNCASKS
UNDARED
UNDATED
UNDAZED
UNEAGER
UNEARTH
UNEASES
UNEATEN
UNEAVED
UNFACED
UNFACTS
UNFADED
UNFAITH
UNFAKED
UNFAMED
UNFANCY
UNFATED
UNFATTY
UNFAZED
UNGATED
UNGAUDY
UNHAIRS
UNHAIRY
UNHANDS
UNHANDY
UNHAPPY
UNHARDY
UNHARSH
UNHASPS
UNHASTY
UNHATED
UNHAYED
UNHAZED
UNIATES
UNJADED
UNLACED
UNLACES
UNLADED
UNLADEN
UNLADES
UNLARGE
UNLATCH
UNLAVED
UNLAXED
UNLAXES
UNMACHO
UNMADLY
UNMAKER
UNMAKES
UNMANED
UNMANLY
UNMASKS
UNMASTS
UNMATED
UNMATES
UNNAILS
UNNAIVE
UNNAMED
UNNASAL
UNPACED
UNPACKS
UNPAGAN
UNPAGED
UNPALED
UNPARED
UNPASTE
UNPAVED
UNPAWED
UNPAWNS
UNRACKS
UNRAINY
UNRAKED
UNRASPY
UNRATED
UNRAVEL
UNRAYED
UNRAZED
UNSADLY
UNSAFER
UNSALTY
UNSATED
UNSAVED
UNSAVVY
UNSAWED
UNTACKS
UNTAKEN
UNTAMED
UNTAMES
UNTAPED
UNTAPES
UNTASTY
UNTAXED
UNTAXES
UNVAGUE
UNWADED
UNWAGED
UNWAKED
UNWALLS
UNWANED
UNWAVED
UNWAXED

•N••A••

ANASAZI
ANATASE
ANDEANS
ANDIAMO
ANDRADE
ANGLAIS
ANIMACY
ANIMALS
ANIMATE
ANIMATO
ANNEALS
ANNUALS
ANOMALY
ANORAKS
ANSPACH
ANTFARM
ANTIART
ANYWAYS
DNALABS
ENCHAIN
ENCHANT
ENCHASE
ENCLASP
ENCLAVE
ENDEARS
ENDGAME
ENDLATE
ENDWAYS
ENFLAME
ENFRAME
ENGLAND
ENGRAFT
ENGRAIN
ENGRAMS
ENGRAVE
ENNEADS
ENPLANE
ENQUADS
ENSEALS
ENSEATS
ENSLAVE
ENSNARE
ENSNARL
ENTRADA
ENTRAIN
ENTRANT
ENTRAPS
ENWRAPS
INABALL
INACAST
INADAZE
INARAGE
INAVALE
INBLACK
INBOARD
INCLASS
INDIANA
INDIANS
INDRAFT
INDRAWN
INEXACT
INFLAME
INFLATE
INFRACT
INGOALS
INGRAFT
INGRAIN
INGRATE
INKMARK
INKPADS
INKSACS
INPEACE
INPHASE
INPLACE
INREACH
INROADS
INSCALE
INSEAMS
INSHAPE
INSPACE
INSPANS
INSTALL
INSTALS
INSTANT
INSTATE
INTEARS
INTRADE
INTRAYS
INULASE
INWEAVE
INYEARS
KNOWALL
ONADARE
ONADATE
ONALARK
ONBOARD
ONEBALL
ONEBASE
ONECALL
ONEHALF
ONEHAND
ONELANE
ONENAME
ONEPAGE
ONEPAIR
ONEPART
ONEYARD
ONGUARD
ONLEASE
ONLEASH
ONLEAVE
ONLOADS
ONORATI
ONSTAFF
ONSTAGE
ONTOAST
ONTRACK
SNOBALL
SNOCAPS
SNOCATS
UNAWAKE
UNAWARE
UNBEARD
UNBLADE
UNBRACE
UNBRAID
UNBRAKE
UNBRAVE
UNCHAIN
UNCHAIR
UNCHARY
UNCIALS
UNCLAMP
UNCLASP
UNCRAMP
UNCRATE
UNCRAZY
UNDEALT
UNDRAPE
UNDRAWN
UNDRAWS
UNFLAKY
UNFRAIL
UNFRANK
UNGRAND
UNGUARD
UNHEADY
UNHEARD
UNHEAVY
UNIBALL
UNITARD
UNITARY
UNIVACS
UNLEADS
UNLEAFS
UNLEAKY
UNLEARN
UNLEASH
UNLOADS
UNLOATH
UNMEANT
UNPLAIT
UNPLANS
UNREADY
UNSCALY
UNSEALS
UNSEAMS
UNSEATS
UNSHADE
UNSHADY
UNSHARP
UNSLACK
UNSLAIN
UNSMART
UNSNAGS
UNSNAKY
UNSNAPS
UNSNARL
UNSPANS
UNSTACK
UNSTAGY
UNSTAID
UNSTATE
UNTEACH
UNTHAWS
UNTRACK
UNTRAPS
UNWEARY
UNWEAVE
UNWRAPS

•N•••A•

ANAGRAM
ANANIAS
ANDAMAN
ANDREAS
ANEMIAS
ANGELAS
ANGOLAN
ANGORAS
ANGRYAT
ANGULAR
ANITRAS
ANKARAN
ANNAMAY
ANNULAR
ANTBEAR
ANTHRAX
ANTITAX
ANTIWAR
ANYROAD
ENCINAS
ENDEDAT
ENDLEAF
ENDPLAY
ENDUPAT
ENIGMAS
ENTHRAL
ENTREAT
GNAWSAT
INAHEAP
INASNAP
INATRAP
INDYCAR
INGEMAR
INHUMAN
INITIAL
INKYCAP
INNOWAY
INSOFAR
INSTEAD
INSULAR
INTOTAL
KNEECAP
KNEEPAD
ONABIAS
ONALEAD
ONATEAR
ONBREAK
ONEACAT
ONEADAY
ONECLAM
ONEGRAM
ONEIDAS
ONEOCAT
ONESTAR
ONEYEAR
ONTKEAN
ONTRIAL
PNEUMAS
PNEUMAT
SNAPSAT
SNARLAT
SNEERAT
SNIFFAT
SNIPEAT
SNORTAT
SNOWCAP
SNOWCAT
SNOWDAY
SNOWHAT
SNOWMAN
UNCLEAN
UNCLEAR
UNCLOAK
UNDULAR
UNEQUAL
UNGULAE
UNGULAR
UNHUMAN
UNIDEAL
UNLEGAL
UNLOCAL
UNLOYAL
UNNASAL
UNPAGAN
UNREGAL
UNRURAL
UNSPEAK
UNSTRAP
UNSWEAR
UNTREAD
UNURBAN
UNUSUAL
UNVENAL
UNVITAL
UNVOCAL

•N••••A

ANAEMIA
ANDORRA
ANOSMIA
ANSONIA
ANTENNA
ANTIGUA
ANTONIA
ENCARTA
ENCOMIA
ENTRADA
INDIANA
INDICIA
INEDITA
INERTIA
INFANTA
INGESTA
INOCULA
INSECTA
INTEGRA
INVICTA
ONEIOTA
ONELIRA
ONEONTA
SNAPPEA
SNOWPEA

••NA•••

AGNAILS
AGNATES
AGNATIC
ANNABEL
ANNAKIN
ANNALEE
ANNALES
ANNAMAY
ANNATTO
BANACEK
BANALER
BANALLY
BANANAS
BANANES
BENARES
BENATAR
BENAZIR
BONACIS
BONAIRE
BONANZA
BONARIO
BYNAMES
CANALED
CANAPES
CANARDS
CANASTA
CENACLE
CONAGRA
CONAKRY
DANANAS
DENARII
DINADAM
DINARIC
DONAHUE
DONATED
DONATEE
DONATES
DONATOR
DONATUS
DUNAWAY
DYNAMIC
DYNAMOS
DYNASTS
DYNASTY
EDNAMAY
FANATIC
FINABLE
FINAGLE
FINALES
FINALLY
FINANCE
HANAPER
HONALEE
IGNARRO
IGNATOW
INNAGES
INNARDS
JANACEK
KANAKAS
LINABLE
LINAGES
LUNATED
LUNATES
LUNATIC
MANACLE
MANAGED
MANAGER
MANAGES
MANAGUA
MANANAS
MANATEE
MCNALLY
MENACED
MENACER
MENACES
MENAGES
MINABLE
MINARET
MONACAN
MONADAL
MONADIC
MONARCH
MRNANNY
NANAIMO
NONACID
NONAGES
NONAGON
NONAMES
NONARAB
NONARTS
NUNAVUT
PANACEA
PANACHE
PANADAS
PANAMAS
PANARAB
PENALTY
PENANCE
PENATES
PINATAS
RANAMOK
RANATAB
RANAWAY
RENAILS
RENALDO
RENALLY
RENAMED
RENAMES
RENAULT
RINALDO
RUNAMOK
RUNATAB
RUNAWAY
SENATES
SENATOR
SINATRA
SONANCE
SONATAS
SYNAPSE
TANAGER
TENABLE
TENABLY
TENACES
TENACRE
TENANCY
TENANTS
TINAFEY
TINAMOU
TONALLY
TUNABLE
TUNAOIL
TUNASUB
UNNAILS
UNNAIVE
UNNAMED
UNNASAL
VANADIC
VENABLE
VENALLY
VENATIC
XANADUS
ZENANAS
ZONALLY

••N•A••

ANNEALS
ANNUALS
AYNRAND
BANDAGE
BANDAID
BANDANA
BANTAMS
BANYANS
BANZAIS
BENDAYS
BENEATH
BENGALI
BENGALS
BENZALI
BONDAGE
BONEASH
BONIATO
BONNARD
BUNRAKU
CANCANS
CANDACE
CANTABS
CANTALS
CANTATA
CANVASS
CENTALS
CENTARE
CENTAUR
CENTAVO
CINZANO
CONCAVE
CONFABS
CONGAED
CONGAME
CONNATE
CONRACK
CONTACS
CONTACT
CONTAIN
CUNEATE
DENHAAG
DENIALS
DENMARK
DENTALS
DENTATE
DONNALL
DONTASK
DUNDALK
DUNNAGE
ENNEADS
FANBASE
FANFARE
FANMAIL
FANPALM
FANTAIL
FANTANS
FANTASM
FANTAST
FANTASY
FINBACK
FINEART
FINGALS
FINIALS
FINIANS
FINLAND
FINNAIR
FONDANT
FONTANA
FONTANE
FUNFAIR
GANDALF
GENNAIO
GENNARO
GINGAME
GONEAFT
GONEAPE
GONZAGA
GUNCASE
GUNLAPS
GUNLAWS
GUNWALE
HANDAXE
HANGARS
HANSARP
HENBANE
HENNAED
HONIARA
HUNGARY
IBNSAUD
IONIANS
JANEANE
JANUARY
JONHALL
JUNKART
KANSANS
KENDALL
KENWAHL
KENYANS
KINCAID
KINKAID
LANDAUS
LANTANA
LANYARD
LENFANT
LINEAGE
LINEARA
LINEARB
LINEATE
LINKAGE
LONGAGO
LONGARM
MANDALA
MANDANS
MANDATE
MANDAYS
MANGANO
MANIACS
MANKATO
MANMADE
MANSARD
MANUALS
MENIALS
MENSANS
MINOANS
MINTAGE
MINYANS
MONDALE
MONDAVI
MONDAYS
MONTAGE
MONTAGU
MONTALE
MONTANA
MONTAND
MONTANO
MONTAUK
MUNDANE
NONBANK
NONBASE
NONCASH
NONDARK
NONFACT
NONFANS
NONFARM
NONPAID
NONPARS
NONPAST
NONSALE
NONSANE
NONWAGE
NONWARS
PANCAKE
PANGAEA
PENCASE
PENDANT

PENNAME
PENNANT
PENNATE
PENPALS
PENTADS
PENTANE
PINBALL
PINNACE
PINNATE
PINOAKS
PINTAIL
PINWALE
PONIARD
PONTANO
PUNJABI
QINTARS
RANBACK
RANDALL
RANLAPS
RANLATE
RANPAST
RANSACK
RENTALS
RONSARD
RUNBACK
RUNLAPS
RUNLATE
RUNPAST
RUNWAYS
SANDALS
SANTAFE
SANTANA
SENSATE
SINKAGE
SINUATE
SUNBATH
SUNDAES
SUNDAYS
SUNFANS
SUNFAST
SUNHATS
SUNLAMP
SUNMAID
SUNRAYS
SUNTANS
SUNWARD
TANBARK
TANKAGE
TANKARD
TANOAKS
TANTARA
TENBALL
TENDAYS
TENNANT
TENPAST
TINCANS
TINEARS
TINHATS
TINWARE
TONEARM
TONGANS
TONNAGE
TYNDALL
VANCAMP
VANDALS
VANSANT
VANTAGE
VANUATU
VANWARD
VANZANT
VENTAGE
VINLAND
VINTAGE
VONBAER
VONLAUE
WANNABE
WANTADS
WANTAGH
WENTAFT
WENTAPE
WINBACK
WINDAGE
WINDAUS
XENIAOH
ZONIANS
ZUNIANS

••N••A•

AINTHAY
ALNILAM
ALNITAK
ALNIYAT
ANNAMAY
ANNULAR
ARNICAS
BANANAS
BANDEAU
BANDSAW
BENATAR
BENTHAM
BINGHAM
BONDMAN
CANCHAS
CANIDAE
CANOLAS
CANTSAY
CANULAE
CANULAS
CENTRAL
CINEMAS
CINEMAX
CONCEAL
CONCHAE
CONGEAL
CONICAL
CONTRAS
CYNICAL
DANANAS
DANELAW
DANTEAN
DENHAAG
DINADAM
DINEDAT
DINESAT
DINGBAT
DONEBAD
DONEGAL
DONEGAN
DONJUAN
DONOVAN
DUNAWAY
DUNSTAN
EDNAMAY
FINDLAY
FINICAL
GANGSAW
GANGWAY
GENERAL
GENEVAN
GENTIAN
GINGHAM
GONEBAD
GONEFAR
GONEMAD
GUNBOAT
GUNPLAY
HANDBAG
HANDCAR
HANDSAW
HANGMAN
HANUKAH
HINDPAW
HINTSAT
HONKSAT
INNOWAY
IONBEAM
JANEWAY
JUNEDAY
JUNGIAN
JUNKCAR
JUNKFAX
JUNKMAN
KANAKAS
KANTIAN
KINGMAN
KINGRAT
KINNEAR
KINSMAN
LANCIAS
LANDMAN
LANDSAT
LANDTAG
LANDTAX
LANGHAM
LANGWAY
LENGUAS
LENSCAP
LENSMAN
LINBIAO
LINDSAY
LINEMAN
LINGUAE
LINGUAL
LINPIAO
LONGDAY
LONGWAY
LONIGAN
LUNGEAT
LUNULAE
LUNULAR
MANANAS
MANILAS
MANOWAR
MANSMAN
MANTRAP
MANTRAS
MANTUAN
MANXCAT
MANXMAN
MANYEAR
MENORAH
MENUBAR
MINERAL
MINIBAR
MINICAB
MINICAM
MINICAR
MINILAB
MINIMAL
MINIMAX
MINIVAC
MINIVAN
MONACAN
MONADAL
MONDIAL
MRNOVAK
NONARAB
NONDEAF
NONMEAT
NONORAL
NONPEAK
NONPLAY
OMNIMAX
OWNGOAL
PANADAS
PANAMAS
PANARAB
PANCHAX
PANGRAM
PENZIAS
PINATAS
PINCHAS
PINESAP
PINETAR
PINHEAD
PINKHAM
PINSEAL
PONTIAC
PONTIAN
RANATAB
RANAWAY
RANTSAT
RENEWAL
RINKRAT
RONDEAU
RUNATAB
RUNAWAY
SANBLAS
SANDBAG
SANDBAR
SANDDAB
SANDMAN
SANJUAN
SENECAN
SENECAS
SENEGAL
SENORAS
SENSUAL
SENTRAS
SINDBAD
SINUTAB
SONATAS
SONORAN
SUNBEAM
SUNDIAL
SUNSFAN
SYNGMAN
SYNODAL
TANGRAM
TANKCAR
TENYEAR
TINSTAR
TONNEAU
TUNDRAS
UNNASAL
VANLOAD
VENEMAN
VENTRAD
VENTRAL
VINEGAR
WENTBAD
WENTFAR
WENTMAD
WINDBAG
WINEBAR
WINESAP
WINEVAT
WINGMAN
WINKSAT
WYNDHAM
XANTHAN
XENICAL
YANKSAT
ZENANAS
ZINNIAS
ZONULAR

••N•••A

AMNESIA
BANDANA
BANDERA
BENBOVA
BENICIA
BONANZA
BONILLA
CANASTA
CANDELA
CANDIDA
CANNULA
CANTATA
CANTINA
CANZONA
CINESIA
CONAGRA
CYNTHIA
DANIELA
ERNESTA
EUNOMIA
FONTANA
FONTINA
GANGLIA
GANGSTA
GINGIVA
GONDOLA
GONGORA
GONZAGA
HANKIBA
HENDECA
HONIARA
JUNKDNA
KENOSHA
KUNDERA
LANTANA
LINEARA
LINGULA
LUNESTA
MANAGUA
MANDALA
MANDELA
MANTECA
MENORCA
MINEOLA
MINERVA
MINOLTA
MINORCA
MINTTEA
MINUTIA
MONTANA
MONTOYA
NONCOLA
PANACEA
PANDORA
PANETTA
PANGAEA
PANTERA
PINOTTA
SANGRIA
SANTANA
SENHORA
SINATRA
TANTARA
TUNISIA
VANDURA
VANESSA
VANILLA
VENEZIA
VENTURA
VINCULA
WYNONNA
ZENOBIA

•••NA••

ADONAIS
ASONANT
BADNAME
BARNABY
BARNARD
BERNARD
BERNAYS
BIGNAME
BONNARD
BRANAGH
BURNABY
CARNABY
CARNAGE
CATNAPS
COGNACS
COGNATE
COINAGE
CONNATE
CRENATE
DOGNAPS
DONNALL
DUNNAGE
EDINAMN
EMANANT
EMANATE
ENSNARE
ENSNARL
FERNAND
FINNAIR
FURNACE
GENNAIO
GENNARO
GRANADA
GRANARY
GRENADA
GRENADE
GUANACO
GYMNAST
HENNAED
HERNANI
HOBNAIL
HYMNALS
HYMNARY
IRONAGE
JEANARP
KHANATE
KIDNAPS
LEONARD
LEONATO
MAENADS
MAGNANI
MAGNATE
MAYNARD
MEANAGE
MISNAME
NEONATE
NEWNAME
OCANADA
OFANAGE
OKINAWA
OLDNAVY
ONENAME
OPENAIR
PENNAME
PENNANT
PENNATE
PEONAGE
PETNAME
PETNAPS
PINNACE
PINNATE
PLANATE
PLENARY
PRENAME
PRONATE
PRONAVY
QUINARY
QUINATE
REENACT
REGNANT
REGNARD
REMNANT
RESNAIS
RESNAPS
REYNARD
REYNAUD
RUINATE
SAUNAED
SCHNAPS
SEENALL
SHANANA
SIGNAGE
SIGNALS
SPANAIR
SPINACH
SURNAME
TEENAGE
TENNANT
TERNARY
TERNATE
THINAIR
TOENAIL
TONNAGE
TOPNAME
TORNADO
TRENARY
TRINARY
TSUNAMI
UNSNAGS
UNSNAKY
UNSNAPS
UNSNARL
WANNABE
WETNAPS

•••N•A•

AGENDAS
ALANJAY
ALANNAH
ANANIAS
ARONNAX
AZANIAN
BEANBAG
BLINKAT
BORNEAN
BOSNIAN
BRENDAN
BRENNAN
CHINWAG
COONCAN
COONCAT
CORNEAL
CORNEAS
CRANIAL
DOWNPAT
DUENNAS
ELENIAK
ETONIAN
EVENPAR
FERNBAR
FEYNMAN
FLINGAT
FLUNGAT
FRENEAU
FRONTAL
GAINSAY
GARNEAU
GHANIAN
GOINGAT
GRANDAM
GRANPAS
GRINSAT
GUINEAN
GUINEAS
HERNIAE
HERNIAS
HYUNDAI
IRANIAN
IRONBAR
IRONMAN
JOHNGAY
JOHNJAY
JOHNLAW
KINNEAR
KWANZAA
KWANZAS
LEONDAY
MAINMAN
MYANMAR
NEONGAS
NOONDAY
NOTNEAR
OPENBAR
OPENTAP
OXONIAN
PAANGAS
PHINEAS
PLANTAR
POINTAT
PRINTAD
QBSNEAK
QUENEAU
QUINLAN
QUINTAL
QUINTAS
QUONDAM
RAINHAT
RAINMAN
REKNEAD
RUANDAS
RWANDAN
SCANDAL
SHANKAR
SHINPAD
SIENNAS
STANZAS
STONEAX
SWINGAT
SWUNGAT
THINMAN
TIENDAS
TONNEAU
TOWNCAR
TRANSAM
TSONGAS
TURNBAD
UGANDAN
WOZNIAK
ZINNIAS

•••N••A

ABINTRA
AMANITA
ARANTXA
AVENIDA
AVONLEA
BERNINA
BIENNIA
CANNULA
CARNERA
ELANTRA
GRANADA
GRANDMA
GRANDPA
GRANITA
GRANOLA
GRENADA
IPANEMA
KWANZAA
LEONORA
MAANDPA
OCANADA
ODONTIA
OKINAWA
OPENSEA
OPUNTIA
PIANOLA
QUINELA
REYNOSA
SHANANA
SHINOLA
SIGNORA
SPINOZA
SWANSEA
ULANOVA
VIGNOLA

••••NA•

ADRENAL
ALANNAH
ALMANAC
ALUMNAE
ALUMNAL
AQUINAS
ARONNAX
ARSENAL
AVERNAL
BANANAS
BASINAL
BITONAL
BRENNAN
BROSNAN
CABANAS
CARINAE
CARINAS
CATENAE
CATENAS
CESSNAS
CORONAE
CORONAL
CORONAS
DANANAS
DIURNAL
DUENNAS
EATENAT
ENCINAS
EPERNAY
ETERNAL
FARINAS
FLOWNAT
FROWNAT
GALENAS
HAVANAN
HAVANAS
IGUANAS
INASNAP
JOURNAL
JUVENAL
KAHUNAS
KORUNAS
LACUNAE
LACUNAL
LACUNAR
LACUNAS
LADYNAS
LAGUNAS
LAMINAE
LAMINAL
LAMINAR
LAMINAS
LATINAS
LILINAU
LIMINAL
LUMINAS
MANANAS
MARINAS
MATINAL
MISHNAH
MIZUNAS
MTSINAI
MYCENAE
NOMINAL
NOVENAS
ORDINAL
OUTGNAW
PATINAS
QUESNAY
RAVENAL
REGINAL
REGINAS
RETINAE
RETINAL
RETINAS
SAGINAW
SAIDNAY
SALINAS
SARANAC
SAVANAS
SAYSNAY
SEDONAS
SEMANAS
SEMINAL
SEMINAR
SEVENAD
SEVENAM
SIENNAS
STERNAL
SURINAM
TEJANAS
TITANAE
ULZANAS
UNVENAL
VICINAL
VICUNAS
VIETNAM
VIMINAL
VOTENAY
WOOSNAM
ZENANAS

••••N•A

ADDENDA
ALBANIA
AMMONIA
ANSONIA
ANTENNA
ANTONIA
APHONIA
ARMENIA
ASSUNTA
ATLANTA
AVIANCA
BEGONIA
BELINDA
BIENNIA
BONANZA
BOTHNIA
CADENZA
CATANIA
COLONNA
DAPHNIA
DERONDA
ERMINIA
ESTONIA
EUGENIA
FIRENZA
FORENZA
GEHENNA
HOSANNA
HRYVNIA
INFANTA
JOHANNA
LACONIA
LAVINIA
LAWANDA
LAZONGA
LEGANZA
LUCANIA
LUCINDA
MACONGA
MADONNA
MAGENTA
MCKENNA
MELANIA
MELINDA
MIRANDA
MOMENTA
MTKENYA
MYLANTA
OCEANIA
OCHENTA
OLEANNA
ONEONTA
ORGANZA
PETUNIA
PIRANHA
POLENTA
POLONIA
RAVENNA
ROLONDA
ROMANIA
ROSANNA
ROTUNDA
RUMANIA
SALONGA
SAVANNA
SETENTA
SILENTA
SOYINKA
SPLENDA
SUSANNA
TITANIA
TREINTA
VERANDA
VERONIA
VICENZA
WYNONNA
YOLANDA

•••••NA

ADELINA
ADRIANA
ALTOONA
ALUMINA
ANTENNA
ARIZONA
BAMBINA
BANDANA
BERNINA
BOLOGNA
BURKINA
CANTINA
CANZONA
CAPUANA
CARMINA
CHICANA
COLONNA
COQUINA
CORTINA
CORVINA
CREMONA
CZARINA
DAYTONA
DELTONA
DESPINA
DUODENA
ECHIDNA
ELEVENA
ERIGENA
EUGLENA
EVALUNA
FESTINA
FIORINA
FONTANA
FONTINA
FORTUNA
GABBANA
GARDENA
GEHENNA
GETSANA
HERMANA
HOSANNA
HOTTUNA
IKEBANA
ILIAMNA
ILLEANA
INDIANA
JOHANNA
JORDANA
JULIANA
JUNKDNA
KACHINA
KATRINA
KELOWNA
KOSCINA
KRISHNA
LAHAINA
LANTANA
LASAGNA
LECUONA
LIDWINA
LUCIANA
MACHINA
MADONNA
MALVINA
MARIANA
MARTINA
MCKENNA
MESSINA
MONTANA
MORGANA
NIRVANA
OCARINA
OLEANNA
PASTINA
PAULINA
PERSONA
PORSENA
RAVENNA
RETSINA
ROSANNA
SABRINA

SANTANA
SAVANNA
SESTINA
SHANANA
SHARONA
SMETANA
STAMINA
SULTANA
SUSANNA
SYRIANA
TARZANA
TATIANA
TAVERNA
TIJUANA
TSARINA
TYMPANA
TZARINA
VERBENA
VICDANA
WYNONNA
WYOTANA

NB•••••
NBAGAME
NBALIVE
NBATEAM
NBCBLUE
NBCNEWS

N•B••••
NABBERS
NABBING
NABISCO
NABOKOV
NABUCCO
NEBBISH
NEBULAE
NEBULAR
NEBULAS
NIBBLED
NIBBLER
NIBBLES
NIBLETS
NIBLICK
NIBLIKE
NOBBIER
NOBHILL
NOBLEST
NOBODYS
NUBBERS
NUBBIER
NUBBINS
NUBBLES
NUBIANS
NUBIRAS

N••B•••
NABBERS
NABBING
NBCBLUE
NEBBISH
NESBITT
NETBALL
NEWBERN
NEWBERY
NEWBIES
NEWBOLT
NEWBORN
NEWBURG
NIBBLED
NIBBLER
NIBBLES
NIEBUHR
NIMBLER
NIOBITE
NIOBIUM
NOBBIER
NOMBRES
NONBANK
NONBASE
NONBODY
NONBOOK
NONBUSY
NORBERT
NOTBEEN
NUBBERS
NUBBIER
NUBBINS
NUBBLES
NUMBATS
NUMBERS
NUMBEST
NUMBING

N•••B••
NAMABLE
NAMABLY
NAMIBIA
NEWSBOY
NICEBOY
NICOBAR
NOSEBAG
NOSEBRA
NOTABIT
NOTABLE
NOTABLY

N••••B•
NAIROBI
NEWJOBS
NOCARBS
NODOUBT
NOTTOBE

N•••••B
NICEJOB
NONARAB
NOSEJOB

•NB••••
ANBESOL
INBLACK
INBLOOM
INBOARD
INBOUND
INBOXES
INBREED
INBRIEF
INBROWN
INBUILT
ONBOARD
ONBREAK
UNBAITS
UNBAKED
UNBALED
UNBALES
UNBARED
UNBARES
UNBASED
UNBATED
UNBEARD
UNBELDI
UNBELTS
UNBENCH
UNBENDS
UNBERTH
UNBESET
UNBINDS
UNBLADE
UNBLENT
UNBLEST
UNBLOCK
UNBLOWN
UNBLUED
UNBOGGY
UNBOLTS
UNBONED
UNBORED
UNBORNE
UNBOSOM
UNBOUND
UNBOWED
UNBOXED
UNBOXES
UNBRACE
UNBRAID
UNBRAKE
UNBRAVE
UNBRIEF
UNBROKE
UNBUILD
UNBUILT
UNBULKY
UNBURLY
UNBURNT
UNBURST

•N•B•••
ANTBEAR
ANTBIRD
ANYBODY
ENABLED
ENABLER
ENABLES
INABALL
INABIND
INKBLOT
KNOBBED
ONABIAS
ONEBALL
ONEBASE
ONEBELL
ONEBYTE
SNOBALL
SNUBBED
SNUBBER
UNEBBED
UNIBALL
UNIBODY
UNOBESE

•N••B••
ANNABEL
ANTIBES
ENARBOR
ENDABLE
ENNOBLE
ENROBED
ENROBES
ENTEBBE
FNUMBER
INCUBUS
INHABIT
INHIBIT
INLABOR
INORBIT
KNOBBED
SNUBBED
SNUBBER
UNCUBIC
UNEBBED
UNLOBED
UNORBED
UNROBED
UNROBES
UNSOBER
UNURBAN

•N•••B•
DNALABS
ENDERBY
ENTEBBE
ENTOMBS
INDOUBT
INLIMBO
SNEAKBY
UNCURBS

•N••••B
ONECLUB
SNOWJOB
UNPLUMB

••NB•••
BANBURY
BENBLUE
BENBOVA
BONBONS
CONBRIO
DANBURY
FANBASE
FANBELT
FINBACK
GUNBELT
GUNBOAT
HENBANE
HENBITS
IONBEAM
LINBIAO
LONBORG
NONBANK
NONBASE
NONBODY
NONBOOK
NONBUSY
PINBALL
PINBOYS
RANBACK
RUNBACK
SANBLAS
SANBORN
SUNBATH
SUNBEAM
SUNBELT
SUNBIRD
SUNBOWL
SUNBOWS
SUNBURN
TANBARK
TENBALL
VONBAER
WINBACK

••N•B••
ANNABEL
AUNTBEE
BANDBOX
BUNKBED
DINGBAT
DONEBAD
DONTBEE
ENNOBLE
FINABLE
GONEBAD
HANDBAG
HANGBYS
IGNOBLE
IGNOBLY
JUNEBUG
LINABLE
LONGBED
LONGBOW
MENUBAR
MINABLE
MINIBAR
MINIBUS
OMNIBUS
SANDBAG
SANDBAR
SANDBOX
SANDBUR
SANIBEL
SINDBAD
TENABLE
TENABLY
TENTBED
TINYBIT
TUNABLE
VENABLE
WENTBAD
WINDBAG
WINEBAR
WINSBIG
ZENOBIA

••N••B•
BENUMBS
CANITBE
CANTABS
CONFABS
CONJOBS
HANGSBY
HANKIBA
HUNNYBS
PUNJABI
SENDSBY
WANNABE

••N•••B
BANKJOB
FANCLUB
LINEARB
LYNDONB
MINICAB
MINILAB
MINISUB
NONARAB
PANARAB
RANATAB
RUNATAB
SANDDAB
SINUTAB
TUNASUB

•••NB••
BEANBAG
COINBOX
CORNBIN
DOWNBOW
EVENBET
FERNBAR
IRONBAR
JOHNBOY
MOONBOW
OPENBAR
RAINBOW
TOYNBEE
TURNBAD
TWINBED

•••N•B•
BARNABY
BURNABY
BYANDBY
CARNABY
EKINGBY
GOINGBY
HERNIBS
HISNIBS
HOBNOBS
HORNSBY
HUNNYBS
LYINGBY
STANDBY
SWINGBY
SWUNGBY
WANNABE

•••N••B
CORNCOB
JOHNNYB
LIONCUB

••••NB•
ALLENBY
FLOWNBY
GIVENBY
LAZENBY
SEVENBC
SHOPNBC
TAKENBY

••••N•B
JOHNNYB
SILENTB

•••••NB
ELEVENB
LYNDONB

NC•••••
NCWYETH

N•C••••
NACELLE
NBCBLUE
NBCNEWS
NECKERS
NECKING
NECKLET
NECKTIE
NECTARS
NECTARY
NFCTEAM
NICCAGE
NICCOLO
NICEBOY
NICEDAY
NICEDOG
NICEGUY
NICEJOB
NICEKID
NICEMAN
NICEMEN
NICEONE
NICETRY
NICHING
NICHOLS
NICKELS
NICKERS
NICKING
NICKLES
NICOBAR
NICOISE
NICOLAS
NICOLET
NICOLLE
NICOSIA
NICTATE
NOCANDO
NOCARBS
NOCATCH
NOCKING
NOCLASS
NOCOUNT
NOCUOUS
NUCLEAR
NUCLEIC
NUCLEON
NUCLEUS
NUCLIDE

N••C•••
NASCENT
NATCHEZ
NEOCENE
NEOCONS
NESCAFE
NETCAFE
NETCOST
NEWCARS
NICCAGE
NICCOLO
NONCASH
NONCOLA
NONCOMS
NONCORE
NONCROP
NOSCORE
NOTCHED
NOTCHER
NOTCHES
NUNCIOS

N•••C••
NABUCCO
NODICAL
NOGUCHI
NONACID
NOTICED
NOTICER
NOTICES
NOVICES
NUANCED
NUANCES

N••••C•
NABISCO
NABUCCO
NATWICK
NAUTICA
NEGLECT
NEWFACE
NEWRICH
NIBLICK
NIDETCH
NIPMUCK
NITPICK
NOCATCH
NOETICS
NOKNOCK
NOMERCY
NONFACT
NONSUCH
NOPLACE
NORDICA
NORDICS
NORELCO
NORWICH
NOTMUCH
NOTNICE
NOTONCE
NUMLOCK

N•••••C
NEPHRIC
NEPOTIC
NIANTIC
NOMADIC
NONEPIC
NUCLEIC
NUMERIC
NYMPHIC

•NC••••
ANCHORS
ANCHOVY
ANCIENT
ENCAGED
ENCAGES
ENCAMPS
ENCARRE
ENCARTA
ENCASED
ENCASES
ENCHAIN
ENCHANT
ENCHASE
ENCINAS
ENCLASP
ENCLAVE
ENCLOSE
ENCODED
ENCODER
ENCODES
ENCOMIA
ENCORED
ENCORES
ENCRUST
ENCRYPT
INCANTS
INCASED
INCASES
INCENSE
INCENTS
INCEPTS
INCHECK
INCHERS
INCHING
INCISED
INCISES
INCISOR
INCITED
INCITER
INCITES
INCIVIL
INCLASS
INCLINE
INCLOSE
INCLUDE
INCOLOR
INCOMER
INCOMES
INCOURT
INCROWD
INCRUST
INCUBUS
INCUDES
INCURVE
INCUSED
INCUSES
UNCAGED
UNCAGES
UNCAKED
UNCAKES
UNCANED
UNCANNY
UNCAPED
UNCASED
UNCASES
UNCASKS
UNCEDED
UNCHAIN
UNCHAIR
UNCHARY
UNCHECK
UNCHOKE
UNCHURN
UNCIALS
UNCINCH
UNCITED
UNCIVIC
UNCIVIL
UNCLAMP
UNCLASP
UNCLEAN
UNCLEAR
UNCLEFT
UNCLIPS
UNCLIPT
UNCLOAK
UNCLOGS
UNCLOSE
UNCLOUD
UNCODED
UNCOILS
UNCOMIC
UNCOOPS
UNCORED
UNCORES
UNCORKS
UNCOUTH
UNCOVER
UNCOWED
UNCOYER
UNCOYLY
UNCRAMP
UNCRATE
UNCRAZY
UNCRIED
UNCROSS
UNCROWN
UNCRUDE
UNCRUEL
UNCTION
UNCUBIC
UNCUFFS
UNCURBS
UNCURED
UNCURLS

•N•C•••
ANACINS
ANTCOWS
DNACODE
ENACTED
ENACTOR
ENDCUTS
GNOCCHI
INACAST
INOCULA
INSCALE
KNOCKED
KNOCKER
KNOCKON
KNUCKLE
KNUCKLY
ONECALL
ONECELL
ONECENT
ONECHIP
ONECLAM
ONECLUB
SNACKED
SNACKER
SNACKON
SNICKER
SNICKET
SNOCAPS
SNOCATS
SNOCONE
SNUCKUP
UNACTED
UNICODE
UNICORN
UNSCALY
UNSCREW
VNECKED

•N••C••
ANARCHS
ANARCHY
ANTACID
ENFACED
ENFACES
ENLACED
ENLACES
ENTICED
ENTICER
ENTICES
GNOCCHI
INDICES
INDICIA
INDICTS
INDUCED
INDUCER
INDUCES
INDUCTS
INDYCAR
INFECTS
INFOCUS
INJECTS
INKYCAP
INSECTA
INSECTS
INVACUO
INVICTA
KNEECAP
ONEACAT
ONEACRE
ONEACTS
ONEOCAT
SNOWCAP
SNOWCAT
UNDOCKS
UNFACED
UNFACTS
UNLACED
UNLACES
UNLOCAL
UNLOCKS
UNLUCID
UNLUCKY
UNMACHO
UNPACED
UNPACKS
UNPICKS
UNRACKS
UNROCKY
UNTACKS
UNTUCKS
UNVOCAL

•N•••C•
ANDSUCH
ANIMACY
ANSPACH
ANTIOCH
ANYLUCK
ENFORCE
ENHANCE
ENOUNCE
INBLACK
INCHECK
INDUTCH
INEXACT
INFANCY
INFLECT
INFLICT
INFORCE
INFRACT
INKSACS
INMARCH
INPEACE
INPLACE
INREACH
INSHOCK
INSPACE
INSPECT
INSTOCK
INSYNCH
INTOUCH
INVOICE
ONAKICK
ONEINCH
ONESOCK
ONTRACK
SNEETCH
UNBENCH
UNBLOCK
UNBRACE
UNCHECK
UNCINCH
UNERECT
UNFANCY
UNFENCE
UNFROCK
UNHITCH
UNIVACS
UNJUICY
UNLATCH
UNQUICK
UNSLACK
UNSLICK
UNSPICY
UNSTACK
UNSTICK
UNSTUCK
UNTEACH
UNTHICK
UNTRACK
UNVOICE

•N••••C
ANAEMIC
ANGELIC
ANIONIC
ANOSMIC
ENDEMIC
ENTERIC
ENZYMIC
GNOSTIC
ONEIRIC
ONTOPIC
UNCIVIC
UNCOMIC
UNCUBIC
UNLYRIC
UNSTOIC
UNTOXIC

••NC•••
BENCHED
BENCHER
BENCHES
BUNCHED
BUNCHES
BUNCHUP
BUNCOED
CANCANS
CANCELS
CANCERS
CANCHAS
CINCHED
CINCHES
CONCAVE
CONCEAL
CONCEDE
CONCEIT
CONCEPT
CONCERN
CONCERT
CONCHAE
CONCHES
CONCHOS
CONCISE
CONCOCT
CONCORD
CONCURS
CONCUSS
DANCERS
DANCING
DUNCISH
FANCIED
FANCIER
FANCIES
FANCIFY
FANCILY
FANCLUB
FANCYUP
FENCEIN
FENCERS
FENCEUP
FENCING
FINCHES
GUNCASE
HANCOCK
HENCOOP
HONCHOS
HUNCHED
HUNCHES
JUNCOES
KINCAID
LANCERS
LANCETS
LANCIAS
LANCING
LANCOME
LINCOLN
LUNCHED
LUNCHER
LUNCHES
MANCINI
MANCUSO

MENCIUS
MENCKEN
MINCERS
MINCING
MONCTON
MUNCHED
MUNCHEN
MUNCHER
MUNCHES
MUNCHIE
MUNCHON
NONCASH
NONCOLA
NONCOMS
NONCORE
NONCROP
NUNCIOS
PANCAKE
PANCHAX
PENCASE
PENCILS
PINCERS
PINCHAS
PINCHED
PINCHER
PINCHES
PINCHME
PINCHOT
PINCURL
PONCHOS
PUNCHED
PUNCHER
PUNCHES
PUNCHIN
PUNCHUP
PYNCHON
RANCHED
RANCHER
RANCHES
RANCHOS
RANCORS
RANCOUR
SANCTUM
SANCTUS
SINCERE
SINCITY
SUNCITY
SYNCHED
SYNCING
SYNCOPE
TENCENT
TENCHES
TENCODE
TINCANS
TINCTED
VANCAMP
VINCENT
VINCULA
WENCHES
WINCERS
WINCHED
WINCHER
WINCHES
WINCING
ZINCIFY
ZINCING
ZINCITE
ZINCKED
ZINCOUS

••N•C••

ALNICOS
ARNICAS
BANACEK
BENICIA
BENICIO
BINOCHE
BONACIS
CANUCKS
CENACLE
CONICAL
CYNICAL
DONTCRY
FINICAL
FINICKY
HANDCAR
JANACEK
JUNKCAR
KENICHI
LENSCAP
LINECUT
LINGCOD
MANACLE
MANXCAT
MENACED
MENACER
MENACES
MENSCHY
MINICAB
MINICAM
MINICAR
MONACAN
MONOCLE
NONACID
PANACEA
PANACHE
PANICKY
PANICLE
PENUCHE
SENECAN
SENECAS
TANKCAR
TENACES
TENACRE
TUNICLE
VANOCUR
XENICAL

••N•C•

CANDACE
CANDICE
CANNOCK
CANSECO
CONCOCT
CONDUCE
CONDUCT
CONFECT
CONNECT
CONNICK
CONRACK
CONTACS
CONTACT
CONVECT
CONVICT
DENIECE
FANFICS
FINANCE
FINBACK
GENLOCK
GUNLOCK
HANCOCK
HENDECA
HENPECK
HENRICH
IONESCO
MANIACS
MANRICO
MANTECA
MENISCI
MENORCA
MINORCA
MONARCH
NONFACT
NONSUCH
PENANCE
PENNOCK
PINNACE
RANBACK
RANSACK
RENWICK
RUNBACK
SENESCE
SONANCE
SUNDECK
SYNDICS
TENANCY
TENNECO
VANDYCK
VANEYCK
VANWYCK
WINBACK
YANNICK

••N•••C

AGNATIC
AMNESIC
BENEFIC
CANONIC
CENTRIC
DINARIC
DYNAMIC
FANATIC
GENERIC
GENETIC
GENOMIC
KINESIC
KINETIC
LUNATIC
MANTRIC
MINIVAC
MONADIC
MONODIC
NONEPIC
PONTIAC
SYNODIC
TONELOC
VANADIC
VENATIC
VINYLIC
XANTHIC

•••NC••

AGENCES
ALENCON
BIANCHI
BLANCHE
BOUNCED
BOUNCER
BOUNCES
BRANCHY
BRONCHI
BRONCHO
BRONCOS
CHANCED
CHANCEL
CHANCER
CHANCES
COONCAN
COONCAT
CORNCOB
COUNCIL
CRUNCHY
ELANCES
EVINCED
EVINCES
FIANCEE
FIANCES
FRANCES
FRANCHI
FRANCIS
FRENCHI
FRENCHS
GLANCED
GLANCES
GLENCOE
JOUNCED
JOUNCES
LEANCUT
LIONCUB
NUANCED
NUANCES
PAUNCHY
POUNCED
POUNCER
POUNCES
PRANCED
PRANCER
PRANCES
PRINCES
QUINCES
QUINCEY
RAUNCHY
SCONCES
SEANCES
SPENCER
STANCES
STENCIL
TOWNCAR
TRANCED
TRANCES
USANCES

•••N•C•

ATONICS
BIONICS
BYANECK
CANNOCK
CLINICS
COGNACS
CONNECT
CONNICK
CORNICE
EBONICS
ETHNICS
ETONICS
EWENECK
FURNACE
GUANACO
HARNICK
HOWNICE
IRENICS
KLENSCH
LOWNECK
NOKNOCK
NOTNICE
OLDNICK
ORINOCO
PENNOCK
PHONICS
PICNICS
PINNACE
REDNECK
REENACT
REKNOCK
SCENICS
SPINACH
TEANECK
TENNECO
THINICE
VEENECK
YANNICK

•••N••C

FRANTIC
IDENTIC
JEANLUC
LAENNEC
NIANTIC
QUINTIC
STANNIC
YOUNGMC

••••NC•

ABSENCE
ADJUNCT
ADVANCE
ARDENCY
ASKANCE
ASPENCO
ATLUNCH
AVIANCA
BABENCO
BALANCE
BEYONCE
CADENCE
CADENCY
COGENCY
DAVINCI
DECENCY
DEFENCE
DEFUNCT
DOLUNCH
DURANCE
ENHANCE
ENOUNCE
ERRANCY
ESCENCE
ESSENCE
EXTINCT
FAIENCE
FINANCE
FLEANCE
FLOUNCE
FLOUNCY
FLUENCY
FORONCE
INFANCY
INSYNCH
LATENCY
LICENCE
LUCENCY
NOTONCE
OFFENCE
ONEINCH
PALANCE
PATENCY
PENANCE
PLIANCY
POTENCE
POTENCY
PUDENCY
RECENCY
REFENCE
REGENCY
RELANCE
ROMANCE
SCIENCE
SCRUNCH
SILENCE
SONANCE
SQUINCH
STAUNCH
TENANCY
TERENCE
TROUNCE
TRUANCY
UNBENCH
UNCINCH
UNFANCY
UNFENCE
URGENCY
VACANCY
VALANCE
VALENCE

••••N•C

ALMANAC
AMMONIC
ANIONIC
APHONIC
ARSENIC
AVIONIC
BORONIC
BOSONIC
BOTANIC
BYRONIC
CANONIC
CHRONIC
DEMONIC
DOMINIC
EUGENIC
HEDONIC
KETONIC
KORANIC
LACONIC
LAENNEC
MASONIC
MELANIC
MESONIC
MORONIC
OCEANIC
ORGANIC
PHRENIC
ROMANIC
SARANAC
SATANIC
SELENIC
SEVENBC
SHOPNBC
SILENTC
STANNIC
TACONIC
TITANIC

•••••NC

ELEVENC
LEBLANC
LIPSYNC
MTBLANC
POULENC

ND•••••

NDAKOTA

N•D••••

NEDLAND
NIDETCH
NODDERS
NODDIES
NODDING
NODICAL
NODOUBT
NODSOFF
NODULAR
NODULED
NODULES
NUDGERS
NUDGING
NUDISTS
NUDNIKS
NUDZHED
NUDZHES

N••D•••

NEEDERS
NEEDFUL
NEEDHAM
NEEDIER
NEEDILY
NEEDING
NEEDLED
NEEDLER
NEEDLES
NEEDNOT
NEEDSTO
NERDIER
NERDISH
NEWDEAL
NODDERS
NODDIES
NODDING
NONDARK
NONDEAF
NONDEEP
NONDIET
NONDRIP
NONDRUG
NOODGED
NOODGES
NOODLED
NOODLES
NORDICA
NORDICS
NORDOFF
NORDOWE
NOTDONE

N•••D••

NAIADES
NAKEDLY
NAMEDAY
NAVIDAD
NEVADAN
NEWIDEA
NEWSDAY
NEXTDAY
NICEDAY
NICEDOG
NOBODYS
NOENDOF
NOENDTO
NOMADIC
NOONDAY
NOSEDIN
NOSEDUP
NOTEDLY

N••••D•

NAVAIDS
NEREIDS
NEWKIDS
NEWMADE
NEXRADS
NIKEADS
NIMRODS
NITRIDE
NOCANDO
NOGOODS
NOHANDS
NOLOADS
NONBODY
NOTRADE
NUCLIDE

N•••••D

NANNIED
NATURED
NAVIDAD
NAYSAID
NEDLAND
NEEDLED
NEGATED
NEIGHED
NESTLED
NETTLED
NEWHAND
NEWLAID
NEWWORD
NIBBLED
NICEKID
NIGGLED
NODULED
NONACID
NONFOOD
NONGOLD
NONPAID
NONSKED
NONSKID
NONVOID
NONWORD
NOODGED
NOODLED
NORMAND
NORWOOD
NOTATED
NOTCHED
NOTEPAD
NOTGOOD
NOTICED
NOTUSED
NOVISAD
NUANCED
NUDZHED
NUNHOOD
NUTATED
NUTWOOD
NUZZLED

•ND••••

ANDAMAN
ANDANTE
ANDEANS
ANDIAMO
ANDIRON
ANDMORE
ANDORRA
ANDOVER
ANDRADE
ANDREAS
ANDRESS
ANDREWS
ANDROID
ANDROUS
ANDSOON
ANDSUCH
ANDTHEN
ENDABLE
ENDALLS
ENDCUTS
ENDEARS
ENDEDAT
ENDEDIN
ENDEDIT
ENDEDON
ENDEDUP
ENDEMIC
ENDERBY
ENDGAME
ENDINGS
ENDIVES
ENDLATE
ENDLEAF
ENDLESS
ENDLINE
ENDLONG
ENDMOST
ENDNOTE
ENDORSE
ENDOWED
ENDOWER
ENDPINS
ENDPLAY
ENDRUNS
ENDUING
ENDUPAT
ENDURED
ENDURER
ENDURES
ENDUROS
ENDUSER
ENDUSES
ENDWAYS
ENDWISE
ENDZONE
INDEEDY
INDENTS
INDEPTH
INDEXED
INDEXER
INDEXES
INDIANA
INDIANS
INDICES
INDICIA
INDICTS
INDIGEN
INDIGOS
INDITED
INDITER
INDITES
INDOORS
INDORSE
INDOUBT
INDRAFT
INDRAWN
INDUCED
INDUCER
INDUCES
INDUCTS
INDULGE
INDUTCH
INDWELL
INDWELT
INDYCAR
UNDARED
UNDATED
UNDAZED
UNDEALT
UNDERDO
UNDERGO
UNDEWED
UNDIKED
UNDINES
UNDOCKS
UNDOERS
UNDOING
UNDOMED
UNDRAPE
UNDRAWN
UNDRAWS
UNDRESS
UNDRIED
UNDRUNK
UNDULAR
UNDUPED
UNDUSTY
UNDYING

•N•D•••

ANADEMS
ANODISE
ANODIZE
ANODYNE
INADAZE
INEDITA
ONADARE
ONADATE
ONADIET
ONEDIME
ONEDOWN
SNIDELY
SNIDEST
UNADDED
UNADEPT
UNADULT
UNEDGED
UNEDGES
UNIDEAL

•N••D••

ANTEDUP
ENCODED
ENCODER
ENCODES
ENDEDAT
ENDEDIN
ENDEDIT
ENDEDON
ENDEDUP
INAIDOF
INCUDES
INFIDEL
INKEDIN
INORDER
INSIDER
INSIDES
INVADED
INVADER
INVADES
KNEADED
KNEADER
ONANDON
ONEADAY
ONEIDAS
ONORDER
ONSIDES
ONVIDEO
SNOWDAY
SNOWDON
UNADDED
UNAIDED
UNCEDED
UNCODED
UNENDED
UNFADED
UNGIDDY
UNGODLY
UNJADED
UNLADED
UNLADEN
UNLADES
UNMADLY
UNMUDDY
UNSADLY
UNSIDED
UNWADED
UNWEDGE

•N•••D•

ANDRADE
ANYBODY
DNACODE
ENFOLDS
ENGARDE
ENGILDS
ENGIRDS
ENNEADS
ENQUADS
ENTRADA
ENWINDS
INCLUDE
INDEEDY
INFOLDS
INKPADS
INLANDS
INNARDS
INROADS
INTENDS
INTRADE
INTRUDE
INWARDS
ONLOADS
ONTHEDL
ONWARDS
UNBELDI
UNBENDS
UNBINDS
UNBLADE
UNCRUDE
UNDERDO
UNFOLDS
UNGAUDY
UNGIDDY
UNGIRDS
UNHANDS
UNHANDY
UNHARDY
UNHEADY
UNHEEDS
UNHOODS
UNIBODY
UNICODE
UNIPODS
UNLEADS
UNLOADS
UNMOLDS
UNMOLDY
UNMOODY
UNMUDDY
UNNEEDY
UNREADY
UNROWDY
UNSHADE
UNSHADY
UNWINDS
UNWINDY

•N••••D

ANDROID
ANEROID
ANGERED
ANISEED
ANNELID
ANNEXED
ANNOYED
ANTACID
ANTBIRD
ANYKIND
ANYROAD
ENABLED
ENACTED
ENARMED
ENCAGED
ENCASED
ENCODED
ENCORED
ENDOWED
ENDURED
ENFACED
ENFIELD
ENGAGED
ENGINED
ENGLAND
ENGLUND
ENISLED
ENJOYED
ENLACED
ENOILED
ENRAGED
ENROBED
ENSILED
ENSKIED
ENSURED
ENTERED
ENTICED
ENWOUND
GNARLED
GNARRED
GNASHED
INABIND
INAMOOD
INAWORD
INBOARD
INBOUND
INBREED
INCASED
INCISED
INCITED
INCROWD
INCUSED
INDEXED
INDITED
INDUCED
INFIELD
INFIXED
INFUSED
INHALED
INHERED
INHUMED
INJURED
INSIPID
INSTEAD
INSURED
INTHIRD
INTONED
INVADED
INVALID
INVITED
INVOKED
KNARRED
KNEADED
KNEELED
KNEEPAD
KNELLED

KNITTED KNOBBED KNOCKED KNOTTED KNOUTED KNURLED ONALEAD ONBOARD ONEEYED ONEFOLD ONEHAND ONEWOOD ONEYARD ONGUARD SNACKED SNAFUED SNAGGED SNAPPED SNARFED SNARLED SNEAKED SNEERED SNEEZED SNIFFED SNIPPED SNOOPED SNOOTED SNOOZED SNORTED SNOUTED SNUBBED SNUFFED SNUGGED UNACTED UNADDED UNAIDED UNAIMED UNAIRED UNARMED UNASKED UNAXLED UNBAKED UNBALED UNBARED UNBASED UNBATED UNBEARD UNBLUED UNBONED UNBORED UNBOUND UNBOWED UNBOXED UNBRAID UNBUILD UNCAGED UNCAKED UNCANED UNCAPED UNCASED UNCEDED UNCITED UNCLOUD UNCODED UNCORED UNCOWED UNCRIED UNCURED

UNDARED UNDATED UNDAZED UNDEWED UNDIKED UNDOMED UNDRIED UNDUPED UNEAVED UNEBBED UNEDGED UNENDED UNFACED UNFADED UNFAKED UNFAMED UNFATED UNFAZED UNFETED UNFILED UNFINED UNFIRED UNFIXED UNFLUID UNFOUND UNFOXED UNFREED UNFRIED UNFUSED UNGATED UNGLUED UNGORED UNGRAND UNGUARD UNGUYED UNGYVED UNHATED UNHAYED UNHAZED UNHEARD UNHEWED UNHIRED UNHONED UNHOPED UNHUMID UNIFIED UNINKED UNITARD UNJADED UNJOYED UNKEYED UNLACED UNLADED UNLAVED UNLAXED UNLIKED UNLINED UNLIVED UNLOBED UNLOVED UNLUCID UNLURED UNMANED UNMATED UNMEWED UNMIKED UNMINED UNMIRED

UNMIXED UNMOULD UNMOVED UNMOWED UNMUTED UNNAMED UNNOSED UNNOTED UNOGLED UNOILED UNOPTED UNORBED UNOWNED UNPACED UNPAGED UNPALED UNPARED UNPAVED UNPAWED UNPILED UNPIPED UNPLIED UNPOLED UNPOSED UNPROUD UNRAKED UNRATED UNRAYED UNRAZED UNRIGID UNRILED UNRIMED UNRIVED UNROBED UNROPED UNROUND UNRULED UNSATED UNSAVED UNSAWED UNSEWED UNSHOED UNSIDED UNSIZED UNSOLED UNSOLID UNSOUND UNSOWED UNSPIED UNSTAID UNTAMED UNTAPED UNTAXED UNTILED UNTIMED UNTIMID UNTIRED UNTONED UNTREAD UNTREED UNTRIED UNTUNED UNTYPED UNURGED UNVEXED UNVIVID UNVOTED UNVOWED

UNWADED UNWAGED UNWAKED UNWANED UNWAVED UNWAXED UNWIPED UNWIRED UNWOOED UNWOUND UNYOKED UNZONED VNECKED

••ND•••

BANDAGE BANDAID BANDANA BANDBOX BANDEAU BANDERA BANDERS BANDIDO BANDIED BANDIER BANDIES BANDING BANDITO BANDITS BANDLET BANDSAW BENDAYS BENDERS BENDIER BENDING BINDERS BINDERY BINDING BINDLES BINDOFF BINDSTO BINDSUP BONDAGE BONDERS BONDING BONDMAN BONDMEN BUNDLED BUNDLER BUNDLES CANDACE CANDELA CANDENT CANDICE CANDIDA CANDIDE CANDIDS CANDIED CANDIES CANDLED CANDLER CANDLES CANDOUR CINDERS CINDERY CONDEMN CONDIGN CONDOLE

CONDONE CONDORS CONDUCE CONDUCT CONDUIT DANDERS DANDIER DANDIES DANDIFY DANDILY DANDLED DANDLER DANDLES DENDRON DINDINS DUNDALK FANDOMS FENDERS FENDING FENDOFF FINDERS FINDING FINDLAY FINDLEY FINDOUT FONDANT FONDEST FONDLED FONDLER FONDLES FONDUED FONDUES FUNDERS FUNDING GANDALF GANDERS GENDERS GONDOLA GUNDOGS HANDAXE HANDBAG HANDCAR HANDERS HANDEYE HANDFED HANDFUL HANDGUN HANDIER HANDILY HANDING HANDLED HANDLER HANDLES HANDLIN HANDOFF HANDOUT HANDSAW HANDSEL HANDSET HANDSIN HANDSON HANDSUP HANDYTO HENDECA HENDRIX HENDRYX HINDERS HINDLEG

HINDPAW HUNDRED KENDALL KENDOLL KENDREW KINDEST KINDLED KINDLER KINDLES KINDRED KUNDERA LANDAUS LANDERS LANDING LANDINI LANDLER LANDMAN LANDMEN LANDSAT LANDSUP LANDTAG LANDTAX LENDERS LENDING LENDOUT LINDENS LINDIED LINDIES LINDNER LINDORF LINDROS LINDSAY LINDSEY LONDRES LYNDONB MANDALA MANDANS MANDATE MANDAYS MANDELA MANDOKI MANDREL MENDELS MENDERS MENDING MINDERS MINDFUL MINDING MINDORO MINDSET MONDALE MONDAVI MONDAYS MONDESI MONDIAL MONDIEU MUNDANE NONDARK NONDEAF NONDEEP NONDIET NONDRIP NONDRUG PANDERS PANDITS PANDORA PENDANT PENDENT

PENDING PINDOWN PONDERS PONDING PUNDITS RANDALL RANDEEP RANDIER RANDOWN RENDELL RENDERS RENDING RINDIER RONDEAU RONDELS RONDURE RUNDEEP RUNDLES RUNDOWN SANDALS SANDBAG SANDBAR SANDBOX SANDBUR SANDDAB SANDERS SANDFLY SANDHOG SANDIER SANDING SANDLER SANDLOT SANDMAN SANDMEN SANDPIT SENDEES SENDERS SENDFOR SENDING SENDOFF SENDOUT SENDSBY SENDSIN SENDSON SENDSTO SENDSUP SENDUPS SINDBAD SUNDAES SUNDAYS SUNDECK SUNDERS SUNDIAL SUNDOGS SUNDOWN SYNDICS TANDEMS TANDOOR TENDAYS TENDERS TENDING TENDONS TENDRIL TENDSTO TINDERS TINDERY TUNDRAS TYNDALL

VANDALS VANDIEN VANDINE VANDURA VANDUYN VANDYCK VANDYKE VENDEES VENDERS VENDING VENDOME VENDORS VENDUES WANDERS WENDELL WENDERS WENDING WENDKOS WINDAGE WINDAUS WINDBAG WINDERS WINDGOD WINDIER WINDIGO WINDILY WINDING WINDOMS WINDOWS WINDOWY WINDSOR WINDSUP WINDTEE WINDUPS WONDERS WYNDHAM

••N•D••

BONEDRY BONEDUP CANIDAE DENUDED DENUDER DENUDES DINADAM DINEDAT DINEDIN DINEDON DUNEDIN DYNODES HANGDOG HONEDIN JANEDOE JUNEDAY JUNKDNA KINGDOM LANGDON LINEDRY LINEDUP LONGDAY LONGDEN MENUDOS MONADAL MONADIC MONODIC OWNEDUP PANADAS RUNSDRY

SANDDAB SINEDIE SYNODAL SYNODIC TONEDUP TONYDOW TUNEDIN TUNEDTO TUNEDUP VANADIC XANADUS

••N••D•

ARNOLDS BANDIDO CANARDS CANDIDA CANDIDE CANDIDS CONCEDE CONFIDE CONOIDS ENNEADS FANTODS INNARDS KENNEDY MANMADE NONBODY PENTADS PONGIDS RENALDO RINALDO SUNGODS TENCODE TINGODS UNNEEDY WANTADS

••N•••D

ANNELID ANNEXED ANNOYED AYNRAND BANDAID BANDIED BANGLED BENCHED BENOTED BONNARD BUNCHED BUNCOED BUNDLED BUNGLED BUNKBED BUNKOED CANALED CANDIED CANDLED CENTRED CINCHED CONCORD CONGAED CONRIED CONTEND DANDLED DANGLED DENIMED DENOTED

DENTOID DENUDED DONATED DONEBAD EANMUND FANCIED FANFOLD FINISHD FINLAND FONDLED FONDUED GENTLED GINGOLD GONEBAD GONEMAD HANDFED HANDLED HENNAED HENREID HONEYED HONORED HUNCHED HUNDRED IBNSAUD IGNITED IGNORED IONISED IONIZED JANGLED JINGLED JONESED KINCAID KINDLED KINDRED KINKAID LANFORD LANGUID LANYARD LINDIED LINGCOD LINSEED LONGBED LUNATED LUNCHED MANAGED MANFRED MANGLED MANHOOD MANKIND MANSARD MANTLED MANURED MENACED MINGLED MINORED MINOTND MINUEND MINUTED MONEYED MONOPOD MONTAND MUNCHED NANNIED NONACID NONFOOD NONGOLD NONPAID NONSKED

NONSKID NONVOID NONWORD NUNHOOD PANELED PINCHED PINFOLD PINGUID PINHEAD PONIARD PUNCHED RANCHED RANKLED RANWILD RENAMED RENEGED RENEWED RENOTED RONSARD RONWOOD RUNWILD SANFORD SINDBAD SINEWED SINGLED SUNBIRD SUNMAID SUNWARD SYNCHED TANGLED TANGOED TANKARD TENFOLD TENONED TENTBED TENURED TINCTED TINGLED TINKLED UNNAMED UNNOSED UNNOTED VANLOAD VANWARD VENTRAD VINLAND WANGLED WENTBAD WENTMAD WINCHED WINDGOD WINERED WINWOOD ZINCKED

•••ND••

ABANDON AGENDAS AGENDUM AMENDED AMENDER ARUNDEL ASUNDER BEANDIP BLANDER BLANDLY BLENDED BLENDER

BLENDES BLENDIN BLINDED BLINDER BLINDLY BLINDTO BLONDER BLONDES BLONDIE BLUNDEN BLUNDER BOUNDED BOUNDER BOUNDTO BOUNDUP BRANDED BRANDER BRANDON BRENDAN BRENDEL BRENDON BRINDLE BYANDBY COONDOG CORNDOG DIRNDLS DWINDLE EMENDED EMENDER EVANDER FOUNDED FOUNDER FOUNDRY GOUNDER GRANDAM GRANDEE GRANDER GRANDLY GRANDMA GRANDPA GRENDEL GRINDER HERNDON HOUNDED HOUNDER HYUNDAI IWONDER JOHNDOE JOINDER KILNDRY LAUNDER LAUNDRY LEANDER LEONDAY MAANDPA MAUNDER MEANDER MOONDOG MOUNDED NOENDOF NOENDTO NOONDAY ONANDON PBANDJS PLUNDER POUNDED POUNDER PSANDQS

QUONDAM REENDOW REINDEX ROUNDED ROUNDEL ROUNDER ROUNDLY ROUNDON ROUNDUP RUANDAS RWANDAN SCANDAL SHINDIG SLANDER SLENDER SOANDSO SOUNDED SOUNDER SOUNDLY SPANDEX SPENDER SPENDON SPINDLE SPINDLY SPINDRY SPONDEE STANDBY STANDEE STANDER STANDIN STANDON STANDTO STANDUP SWINDLE THANDIE THUNDER TIENDAS TRENDED TRUNDLE UGANDAN UNENDED UPANDIN UPENDED UVINDEX WOUNDED WOUNDUP XSANDOS

•••N•D•

AVENIDA CYANIDE CYANIDS GRANADA GRENADA GRENADE HYMNODY KENNEDY LEONIDS MAENADS OCANADA TORNADO ULANUDE

•••N••D

ADENOID AGENTED AMENDED ARANEID

ATANEND
AVENGED
BAGNOLD
BARNARD
BARNRED
BERNARD
BLANKED
BLENDED
BLINDED
BLINKED
BLUNTED
BONNARD
BOUNCED
BOUNDED
BRANDED
BRONZED
CHANCED
CHANGED
CHANTED
CHINKED
CHINNED
CHUNKED
CLANGED
CLANKED
CLINKED
CLONKED
CLUNKED
CORNFED
COUNTED
CRANKED
CRINGED
CTENOID
DAUNTED
EBANKED
EMENDED
EVINCED
FAINTED
FEINTED
FERNAND
FLANKED
FLENSED
FLUNKED
FOUNDED
FRANKED
FRINGED
FRONTED
GLANCED
GLINTED
GRANTED
GRINNED
GRUNTED
HAUNTED
HENNAED
HOUNDED
HYPNOID
JAUNTED
JOINTED
JOUNCED
LEONARD
LOUNGED
MAYNARD
MOONGOD
MOUNDED
MOUNTED
NANNIED
NUANCED
OPENEND
PAINTED

PLANKED
PLANNED
PLANTED
PLINKED
PLONKED
PLUNGED
PLUNKED
POINTED
POUNCED
POUNDED
PRANCED
PRINKED
PRINTAD
PRINTED
PRONGED
RAINGOD
REGNARD
REINKED
REKNEAD
REYNARD
REYNAUD
ROUNDED
SAINTED
SAUNAED
SCANNED
SCANTED
SCENTED
SHANKED
SHINNED
SHINPAD
SHUNNED
SHUNTED
SKINNED
SKUNKED
SKYNYRD
SLANTED
SLINKED
SOUNDED
SPANKED
SPANNED
SPONGED
STINTED
STUNNED
STUNTED
SWANKED
TAINTED
TAUNTED
THANKED
THINNED
THUNKED
TRANCED
TRENDED
TURNBAD
TURNRED
TWANGED
TWINBED
TWINGED
TWINNED
UNENDED
UNINKED
UPENDED
VAUNTED
WHANGED
WOUNDED
WRONGED

••••ND•

ABOUNDS
ADDENDA
ADDENDS
ALBUNDY
ALLENDE
ALMONDS
ALMONDY
APPENDS
ASCENDS
ATTENDS
AUGENDS
BADENDS
BEHINDS
BELINDA
BERENDT
BIGENDS
BURUNDI
CALANDO
CALENDS
DEFENDS
DEFUNDS
DEMANDS
DEPENDS
DERONDA
EDMONDS
EDMUNDI
EDMUNDS
EFFENDI
ELMUNDO
ENWINDS
ERRANDS
EXPANDS
EXPENDS
EXTENDS
FAGENDS
FMBANDS
FRIENDS
GERUNDS
GIRONDE
GROUNDS
IMPENDS
INLANDS
INTENDS
ISLANDS
LAWANDA
LEGENDS
LEMONDE
LIGANDS
LUCINDA
MELINDA
MIRANDA
NOCANDO
NOHANDS
OBTUNDS
OFFENDS
ORGANDY
ORLANDO
ORMANDY
OSMONDS
OSMUNDS
REBENDS
REBINDS
REDONDO
REFINDS
REFUNDS
RELANDS
RELENDS
REMANDS
REMENDS

REMINDS
RESANDS
RESENDS
REVENDS
REWINDS
RIBANDS
ROLONDA
ROTUNDA
SECONDI
SECONDO
SECONDR
SECONDS
SPLENDA
STRANDS
TAGENDS
UNBENDS
UNBINDS
UNHANDS
UNHANDY
UNWINDS
UNWINDY
UPLANDS
UPSENDS
UPWINDS
VERANDA
VIVENDI
WCHANDY
YAOUNDE
YOLANDA
YOUANDI

••••N•D

ACORNED
ADORNED
AFFINED
ALIGNED
APRONED
ATTUNED
BRAINED
BROWNED
BYLINED
CAIRNED
CHAINED
CHINNED
CHURNED
CLEANED
CLOWNED
COIGNED
COOWNED
COZENED
CROONED
CROWNED
DEBONED
DEFINED
DEIGNED
DEPONED
DETUNED
DIVINED
DRAINED
DROWNED
ENGINED
ERMINED
FEIGNED
FROWNED
GLEANED
GRAINED
GREENED
GRINNED

GROANED
GROINED
HOMINID
IGUANID
INTONED
LATENED
LEARNED
LIKENED
LIVENED
MASONED
MOURNED
OCEANID
PLANNED
PRAWNED
PREENED
QUEENED
QUOINED
RAVENED
RAVINED
RECANED
REFINED
REHONED
REIGNED
RELINED
REMINED
REOWNED
REPINED
RESINED
RETONED
RETUNED
REZONED
RIPENED
ROSINED
SCANNED
SCORNED
SEVENAD
SHINNED
SHRINED
SHUNNED
SILENTD
SIRENED
SKINNED
SPANNED
SPAWNED
SPOONED
SPURNED
STAINED
STUNNED
SWOONED
TALONED
TENONED
THINNED
THORNED
TOKENED
TRAINED
TWINNED
UNBONED
UNCANED
UNFINED
UNHONED
UNLINED
UNMANED
UNMINED
UNOWNED
UNTONED
UNTUNED
UNWANED
UNZONED

WAGONED
WAKENED
WIDENED
WIZENED
YEARNED

•••••ND

ABSCOND
AGROUND
AMERIND
ANYKIND
ARMBAND
ASHLAND
ASTOUND
ATANEND
AYNRAND
BACKEND
BADHAND
BADLAND
BARTEND
BIGBAND
BIGBEND
BIGHAND
BOOKEND
BOYBAND
BRIGAND
COBRAND
COFOUND
COMMAND
COMMEND
COMPEND
CONTEND
COPLAND
COWHAND
DABHAND
DAYSEND
DEADEND
DEEPEND
DESCEND
DESMOND
DESPOND
DIAMOND
DISBAND
DISTEND
EANMUND
EASTEND
ELEVEND
ENGLAND
ENGLUND
ENWOUND
EXPOUND
EXSCIND
EYEHAND
FARGOND
FERNAND
FINLAND
FORFEND
GARLAND
GODSEND
GOROUND
HAMMOND
HARLAND
HATBAND
HEADEND
HELMOND
HIGHEND
HOLLAND
HOTHAND

HUSBAND
ICELAND
ICYWIND
ILLWIND
IMPOUND
INABIND
INBOUND
IRELAND
ISECOND
JAMBAND
JUGBAND
JUTLAND
LAPLAND
LEFTEND
LEGRAND
LOWHAND
LOWLAND
MANKIND
MIDLAND
MILLAND
MILLEND
MINOTND
MINUEND
MISBIND
MISSEND
MONTAND
NEDLAND
NEWHAND
NORMAND
OAKLAND
OFAKIND
OFAMIND
OFFHAND
OILSAND
OLDHAND
ONEHAND
OPENEND
OPERAND
OROTUND
OUTBEND
OUTFIND
OUTLAND
OUTWIND
PATHAND
PEPBAND
PORTEND
PREBIND
PREFUND
PRETEND
RAYMOND
REAMEND
REAREND
REBOUND
REBRAND
REDMOND
REDOUND
REFOUND
REGRIND
RESCIND
RESOUND
RESPOND
REWOUND
ROLLAND
ROSTAND
ROWLAND
RUMPEND
RUTLAND
SIGMUND

STIPEND
SUBBAND
SUBTEND
SUMMAND
SUSPEND
TAILEND
THEBAND
THEPOND
THEWIND
TOYLAND
UNBOUND
UNFOUND
UNGRAND
UNROUND
UNSOUND
UNWOUND
UPBOUND
UPSTAND
UPTREND
VINLAND
WARBOND
WAYLAND
WEEKEND
WELLAND
WESTEND
WETLAND
WIELAND
WITSEND
YEAREND
ZEALAND
ZEELAND

NE•••••

NEAREST
NEARING
NEARPAR
NEARYOU
NEATENS
NEATEST
NEATNIK
NEBBISH
NEBULAE
NEBULAR
NEBULAS
NECKERS
NECKING
NECKLET
NECKTIE
NECTARS
NECTARY
NEDLAND
NEEDERS
NEEDFUL
NEEDHAM
NEEDIER
NEEDILY
NEEDING
NEEDLED
NEEDLER
NEEDLES
NEEDNOT
NEEDSTO
NEGATED
NEGATER
NEGATES
NEGATOR
NEGLECT
NEGRONI

NEGUSES
NEIGHED
NEITHER
NELSONS
NEMEROV
NEMESES
NEMESIS
NENNIUS
NEOCENE
NEOCONS
NEOGENE
NEOLITH
NEOLOGY
NEOLYTE
NEONATE
NEONGAS
NEPALIS
NEPHEWS
NEPHRIC
NEPOTIC
NEPTUNE
NERDIER
NERDISH
NEREIDS
NERISSA
NERVIER
NERVILY
NERVINE
NERVING
NERVOUS
NERVULE
NESBITT
NESCAFE
NESMITH
NESQUIK
NESSMAN
NESTEGG
NESTERS
NESTFUL
NESTING
NESTLED
NESTLER
NESTLES
NESTORS
NESTSIN
NETBALL
NETCAFE
NETCOST
NETFLIX
NETFULS
NETGAIN
NETGAME
NETIZEN
NETLESS
NETLIKE
NETLOSS
NETSTER
NETSUKE
NETSURF
NETTERS
NETTING
NETTLED
NETTLES
NETTONS
NETWARE
NETWORK
NETZERO
NEUILLY

NEUMANN
NEURONE
NEURONS
NEUTERS
NEUTRAL
NEUTRON
NEVADAN
NEVILLE
NEWAGER
NEWAGEY
NEWBERN
NEWBERY
NEWBIES
NEWBOLT
NEWBORN
NEWBURG
NEWCARS
NEWDEAL
NEWFACE
NEWGATE
NEWHAND
NEWHART
NEWHATS
NEWHIRE
NEWHOPE
NEWIDEA
NEWJOBS
NEWKIDS
NEWLAID
NEWLEAF
NEWLEFT
NEWLIFE
NEWLINE
NEWLOOK
NEWLOVE
NEWMADE
NEWMANS
NEWMATH
NEWMINT
NEWMONT
NEWMOON
NEWMOWN
NEWNAME
NEWNESS
NEWPORT
NEWRICH
NEWSBOY
NEWSDAY
NEWSIER
NEWSIES
NEWSMAN
NEWSMEN
NEWSOME
NEWSPEG
NEWTONS
NEWTOWN
NEWTOYS
NEWWAVE
NEWWEEK
NEWWORD
NEWYEAR
NEWYORK
NEXRADS
NEXTDAY
NEXUSES

N•E••••

NEEDERS
NEEDFUL
NEEDHAM
NEEDIER
NEEDILY
NEEDING
NEEDLED
NEEDLER
NEEDLES
NEEDNOT
NEEDSTO
NIEBUHR
NIELSEN
NOENDOF
NOENDTO
NOENTRY
NOETICS
NUESTRA
NUESTRO

N••E•••

NACELLE
NAKEDLY
NAMEDAY
NAMEONE
NAMETAG
NANETTE
NEMEROV
NEMESES
NEMESIS
NEREIDS
NICEBOY
NICEDAY
NICEDOG
NICEGUY
NICEJOB
NICEKID
NICEMAN
NICEMEN
NICEONE
NICETRY
NIDETCH
NIGERIA
NIKEADS
NILESOH
NINEEEE
NINEPIN
NINEVEH
NIVEOUS
NOMERCY
NOMERGE
NONEPIC
NONETTE
NONEVER
NONEVIL
NORELCO
NOSEATS
NOSEBAG
NOSEBRA
NOSEDIN
NOSEDUP
NOSEEUM
NOSEGAY
NOSEJOB
NOSEOUT
NOSESIN
NOSESUP
NOTEASY
NOTEDLY
NOTEPAD
NOTEVEN
NOTEVER
NOVELAS
NOVELLA
NOVELLE
NOVELLO
NOVELTY
NOVENAS
NUMERAL
NUMERIC
NUMEROS
NUREYEV

N•••E••

NABBERS
NAGGERS
NAILERS
NAIVELY
NAIVEST
NAIVETE
NAIVETY
NAPIERS
NAPLESS
NAPPERS
NASCENT
NATTERS
NAUSEAM
NBATEAM
NBCNEWS
NCWYETH
NEAREST
NEATENS
NEATEST
NECKERS
NEEDERS
NEGLECT
NEOCENE
NEOGENE
NEPHEWS
NESTEGG
NESTERS
NETLESS
NETTERS
NETZERO
NEUTERS
NEWBERN
NEWBERY
NEWDEAL
NEWLEAF
NEWLEFT
NEWNESS
NEWWEEK
NEWYEAR
NFCTEAM
NFLTEAM
NHLTEAM
NIBLETS
NICKELS
NICKERS
NIGHEST
NIMIETY
NINEEEE
NIPPERS
NOBLEST
NODDERS
NONDEAF
NONDEEP
NONHERO
NONJEWS
NONMEAT
NONNEWS
NONPEAK
NONSELF
NONZERO
NOONERS
NOOSERS
NORBERT
NORIEGA
NOSEEUM
NOSHERS
NOSIEST
NOSWEAT
NOTBEEN
NOTHERE
NOTNEAR
NOTREAL
NOTWELL
NOUVEAU
NOWHERE
NOWNESS
NOXZEMA
NUBBERS
NUCLEAR
NUCLEIC
NUCLEON
NUCLEUS
NUDGERS
NUGGETS
NUGGETY
NUMBERS
NUMBEST
NUNNERY
NURSERS
NURSERY
NUTLETS
NUTMEAT
NUTMEGS
NUTTERS

N••••E•

NAGGIER
NAIADES
NAILKEG
NAILSET
NANNIED
NANNIES
NAPPIER
NAPPIES
NAPSTER
NARTHEX
NARVAEZ
NASTIER
NASTIES
NATCHEZ
NATIVES
NATTIER
NATURED
NATUREL
NATURES
NAVYMEN
NECKLET
NEEDIER
NEEDLED
NEEDLER
NEEDLES

NEGATED
NEGATER
NEGATES
NEGUSES
NEIGHED
NEITHER
NEMESES
NERDIER
NERVIER
NESTLED
NESTLER
NESTLES
NETIZEN
NETSTER
NETTLED
NETTLES
NEWAGER
NEWAGEY
NEWBIES
NEWIDEA
NEWSIER
NEWSIES
NEWSMEN
NEWSPEG
NEWWEEK
NEXUSES
NIBBLED
NIBBLER
NIBBLES
NICEMEN
NICKLES
NICOLET
NIELSEN
NIFTIER
NIFTIES
NIGGLED
NIGGLER
NIGGLES
NIGHTER
NIMBLER
NINEEEE
NINEVEH
NINNIES
NIPPIER
NIPPLES
NITTIER
NOANGEL
NOBBIER
NODDIES
NODULED
NODULES
NOGALES
NOISIER
NOMBRES
NOMINEE
NONAGES
NONAMES
NONDEEP
NONDIET
NONEVER
NONFUEL
NONPOET
NONSKED
NONUKES
NONUSER
NOODGED
NOODGES
NOODLED
NOODLES
NOOGIES
NOOTHER
NOPALES
NORITES
NORTHER
NOSIREE
NOTATED
NOTATES
NOTBEEN
NOTCHED
NOTCHER
NOTCHES
NOTEVEN
NOTEVER
NOTICED
NOTICER
NOTICES
NOTOPEN
NOTOVER
NOTUSED
NOVICES
NOVOTES
NOWISEE
NOWISER
NOWTHEN
NOZZLES
NTUPLES
NUANCED
NUANCES
NUBBIER
NUBBLES
NUDZHED
NUDZHES
NULLSET
NUNGWEN
NUREYEV
NUTATED
NUTATES
NUTSIER
NUTTIER
NUTTREE
NUZZLED
NUZZLER
NUZZLES
NYTIMES

N•••••E

NACELLE
NAIVETE
NAMABLE
NAMEONE
NANETTE
NAPTIME
NARRATE
NASTASE
NATALIE
NATSUME
NAVARRE
NBAGAME
NBALIVE
NBCBLUE
NEBULAE
NECKTIE
NEOCENE
NEOGENE
NEOLYTE
NEONATE
NEPTUNE
NERVINE
NERVULE
NESCAFE
NETCAFE
NETGAME
NETLIKE
NETSUKE
NETWARE
NEURONE
NEVILLE
NEWFACE
NEWGATE
NEWHIRE
NEWHOPE
NEWLIFE
NEWLINE
NEWLOVE
NEWMADE
NEWNAME
NEWSOME
NEWWAVE
NFLGAME
NHLGAME
NIBLIKE
NICCAGE
NICEONE
NICOISE
NICOLLE
NICTATE
NIGHTIE
NINEEEE
NIOBITE
NITRATE
NITRIDE
NITRITE
NOISOME
NOMERGE
NOMINEE
NONBASE
NONCORE
NONETTE
NONHOME
NONLIFE
NONLIVE
NONOISE
NONSALE
NONSANE
NONUPLE
NONWAGE
NOPLACE
NORDOWE
NOSCORE
NOSIREE
NOTABLE
NOTALIE
NOTAONE
NOTASTE
NOTDONE
NOTHERE
NOTHOME
NOTLIKE
NOTLIVE
NOTMINE
NOTNICE
NOTONCE
NOTRADE
NOTRARE
NOTSAFE
NOTSURE
NOTTOBE
NOTTRUE
NOVELLE
NOWHERE
NOWISEE
NOWORSE
NUCLIDE
NUNLIKE
NURTURE
NUTLIKE
NUTPINE
NUTTREE

•NE••••

ANELING
ANEMIAS
ANEMONE
ANEROID
ENEMIES
INEDITA
INEPTLY
INERROR
INERTIA
INERTLY
INEXACT
INEXILE
KNEADED
KNEADER
KNEECAP
KNEEING
KNEELED
KNEELER
KNEEPAD
KNEESUP
KNELLED
KNESSET
KNEWHOW
ONEACAT
ONEACRE
ONEACTS
ONEADAY
ONEARTH
ONEBALL
ONEBASE
ONEBELL
ONEBYTE
ONECALL
ONECELL
ONECENT
ONECHIP
ONECLAM
ONECLUB
ONEDIME
ONEDOWN
ONEEEEE
ONEEYED
ONEFOLD
ONEFOOT
ONEGRAM
ONEHALF
ONEHAND
ONEHOUR
ONEIDAS
ONEINCH
ONEIOTA
ONEIRIC
ONEIRON
ONEKILO
ONELANE
ONELIRA
ONELOOK
ONELOVE
ONELUMP
ONEMILE
ONEMORE
ONEMPTY
ONENAME
ONENESS
ONENOTE
ONEOCAT
ONEOFFS
ONEOFUS
ONEONTA
ONEOVER
ONEPAGE
ONEPAIR
ONEPART
ONEPINT
ONEREEL
ONEROOM
ONEROUS
ONESELF
ONESHOE
ONESHOT
ONESIZE
ONESOCK
ONESPOT
ONESTAR
ONESTEP
ONESTOP
ONETERM
ONETIME
ONETOGO
ONETWOS
ONEUNIT
ONEVOTE
ONEWEEK
ONEWHIT
ONEWOOD
ONEYARD
ONEYEAR
PNEUMAS
PNEUMAT
PNEUMON
SNEAKBY
SNEAKED
SNEAKER
SNEAKIN
SNEAKUP
SNEERAT
SNEERED
SNEERER
SNEETCH
SNEEZED
SNEEZER
SNEEZES
SNELLEN
UNEAGER
UNEARTH
UNEASES
UNEATEN
UNEAVED
UNEBBED
UNEDGED
UNEDGES
UNEMPTY
UNENDED
UNEQUAL
UNERECT
VNECKED

•N•E•••

ANAEMIA
ANAEMIC
ANBESOL
ANDEANS
ANGELAS
ANGELES
ANGELIC
ANGELOU
ANGELUS
ANGERED
ANNEALS
ANNELID
ANNETTE
ANNEXED
ANNEXES
ANSELMO
ANTEDUP
ANTEING
ANTENNA
ANTERUS
ANTESUP
DNIEPER
ENDEARS
ENDEDAT
ENDEDIN
ENDEDIT
ENDEDON
ENDEDUP
ENDEMIC
ENDERBY
ENNEADS
ENSEALS
ENSEATS
ENTEBBE
ENTENTE
ENTERED
ENTERER
ENTERIC
ENTERIN
ENTERON
ENVEILS
ENVELOP
ENVENOM
INCENSE
INCENTS
INCEPTS
INDEEDY
INDENTS
INDEPTH
INDEXED
INDEXER
INDEXES
INFECTS
INFERNO
INFESTS
INGEMAR
INGENUE
INGESTA
INGESTS
INHERED
INHERES
INHERIT
INJECTS
INKEDIN
INNERLY
INNERVE
INPEACE
INPERIL
INREACH
INSEAMS
INSECTA
INSECTS
INSERTS
INTEARS
INTEGER
INTEGRA
INTENDS
INTENSE
INTENTS
INTERIM
INTERNE
INTERNS
INTERSE
INVEIGH
INVENTS
INVERSE
INVERTS
INVESTS
INWEAVE
INYEARS
KNEECAP
KNEEING
KNEELED
KNEELER
KNEEPAD
KNEESUP
KNIEVEL
ONEEEEE
ONEEYED
ONLEASE
ONLEASH
ONLEAVE
ONSERVE
SNEERAT
SNEERED
SNEERER
SNEETCH
SNEEZED
SNEEZER
SNEEZES
UNBEARD
UNBELDI
UNBELTS
UNBENCH
UNBENDS
UNBERTH
UNBESET
UNCEDED
UNDEALT
UNDERDO
UNDERGO
UNDEWED
UNFENCE
UNFERTH
UNFETED
UNHEADY
UNHEARD
UNHEAVY
UNHEEDS
UNHELMS
UNHEWED
UNKEMPT
UNKEYED
UNLEADS
UNLEAFS
UNLEAKY
UNLEARN
UNLEASH
UNLEGAL
UNLEVEL
UNMEANT
UNMERGE
UNMERRY
UNMEWED
UNNEEDY
UNNERVE
UNPEELS
UNREADY
UNREELS
UNREGAL
UNRESTS
UNSEALS
UNSEAMS
UNSEATS
UNSELLS
UNSEWED
UNTEACH
UNTENSE
UNTERSE
UNVEILS
UNVENAL
UNVEXED
UNWEARY
UNWEAVE
UNWEDGE

•N••E••

ANADEMS
ANAHEIM
ANAPEST
ANCIENT
ANDREAS
ANDRESS
ANDREWS
ANGLERS
ANISEED
ANKLERS
ANKLETS
ANSWERS
ANTBEAR
ANTHEIL
ANTHEMS
ANTHERS
ANTLERS
ANTWERP
ANXIETY
ANYNEWS
DNATEST
ENAMELS
ENDLEAF
ENDLESS
ENFIELD
ENQUEUE
ENTREAT
ENTREES
ENVIERS
GNAWERS
INAHEAP
INAMESS
INANELY
INANEST
INAWEOF
INBREED
INCHECK
INCHERS
INDEEDY
INDWELL
INDWELT
INFIELD
INFLECT
INGLESE
INGREEN
INGRESS
ININETY
INKIEST
INKJETS
INKLESS
INKWELL
INNLESS
INQUEST
INSPECT
INSTEAD
INSTEPS
INSWEPT
INTHERE
INUTERO
KNAVERY
KNIFERS
KNOWERS
KNOWETH
ONAGERS
ONALEAD
ONALERT
ONATEAR
ONBREAK
ONEBELL
ONECELL
ONECENT
ONEEEEE
ONENESS
ONEREEL
ONESELF
ONETERM
ONEWEEK
ONEYEAR
ONLIEST
ONTHEDL
ONTHEGO
ONTHEQT
ONTKEAN
SNAKERS
SNARERS
SNIDELY
SNIDEST
SNIPEAT
SNIPERS
SNIVELS
SNORERS
UNADEPT
UNALERT
UNBLENT
UNBLEST
UNCHECK
UNCLEAN
UNCLEAR
UNCLEFT
UNDOERS
UNDRESS
UNERECT
UNFIERY
UNFREED
UNFREES
UNGREEN
UNGUENT
UNHEEDS
UNIDEAL
UNINERT
UNITERS
UNNEEDY
UNOBESE
UNOVERT
UNPEELS
UNPIETY
UNREELS
UNSHEER
UNSHELL
UNSKEWS
UNSLEEK
UNSPEAK
UNSPELT
UNSPENT
UNSTEEL
UNSTEPS
UNSTERN
UNSWEAR
UNSWEET
UNSWEPT
UNTIERS
UNTREAD
UNTREED
UNWHEEL

•N•••E•

ANDOVER
ANDTHEN
ANGELES
ANGERED
ANGRIER
ANISEED
ANNABEL
ANNALEE
ANNALES
ANNEXED
ANNEXES
ANNOYED
ANNOYER
ANNULET
ANOMIES
ANOTHER
ANTARES
ANTIBES
ANTIGEN
ANTSIER
ANYONES
CNTOWER
DNAASES
DNIEPER
ENABLED
ENABLER
ENABLES
ENACTED
ENARMED
ENCAGED
ENCAGES
ENCASED
ENCASES
ENCODED
ENCODER
ENCODES
ENCORED
ENCORES
ENDIVES
ENDOWED
ENDOWER
ENDURED
ENDURER
ENDURES
ENDUSER
ENDUSES
ENEMIES
ENFACED
ENFACES
ENGAGED
ENGAGER
ENGAGES
ENGINED
ENGINES
ENISLED
ENISLES
ENJOYED
ENJOYER
ENLACED
ENLACES
ENLIVEN
ENOILED
ENRAGED
ENRAGES
ENROBED
ENROBES
ENSILED
ENSILES
ENSKIED
ENSKIES
ENSURED
ENSURER
ENSURES
ENTERED
ENTERER
ENTICED
ENTICER
ENTICES
ENTIRES
ENTREES
ENTRIES
ENZYMES
FNUMBER
GNARLED
GNARRED
GNASHED
GNASHER
GNASHES
INAPOEM
INAPTER
INASTEW
INBOXES
INBREED
INBRIEF
INCASED
INCASES
INCISED
INCISES
INCITED
INCITER
INCITES
INCOMER
INCOMES
INCUDES
INCUSED
INCUSES
INDEXED
INDEXER
INDEXES
INDICES
INDIGEN
INDITED
INDITER
INDITES
INDUCED
INDUCER
INDUCES
INFIDEL
INFIVES
INFIXED
INFIXES
INFUSED
INFUSER
INFUSES
INGATES
INGREEN
INHALED
INHALER
INHALES
INHERED
INHERES
INHUMED
INHUMER
INHUMES
INJOKES
INJURED
INJURER
INJURES
INKSTER
INLAYER
INLINES
INMATES
INNAGES
INORDER
INPOWER
INSALES
INSANER
INSIDER
INSIDES
INSOLES
INSURED
INSURER
INSURES
INTAKES
INTEGER
INTHREE
INTONED
INTONER
INTONES
INVADED
INVADER
INVADES
INVITED
INVITEE
INVITER
INVITES
INVOKED
INVOKER
INVOKES
INWOVEN
KNARRED
KNEADED
KNEADER
KNEELED
KNEELER
KNELLED
KNESSET
KNIEVEL
KNISHES
KNITTED
KNITTER
KNOBBED
KNOCKED
KNOCKER
KNOTTED
KNOTTER
KNOUTED
KNOWLES
KNURLED
ONADIET
ONEEEEE
ONEEYED
ONEOVER
ONEREEL
ONESTEP
ONEWEEK
ONORDER
ONPAPER
ONSAGER
ONSIDES
ONTHREE
ONVIDEO
ONWATER
SNACKED
SNACKER
SNAFUED
SNAGGED
SNAGGER
SNAKIER
SNAPPEA
SNAPPED
SNAPPER
SNARFED
SNARLED
SNARLER
SNEAKED
SNEAKER
SNEERED
SNEERER
SNEEZED
SNEEZER
SNEEZES
SNELLEN
SNICKER
SNICKET
SNIFFED
SNIFFER
SNIFTER
SNIGLET
SNIPPED
SNIPPER
SNIPPET
SNOOKER

SNOOPED
SNOOPER
SNOOTED
SNOOZED
SNOOZER
SNOOZES
SNORKEL
SNORTED
SNORTER
SNOUTED
SNOWIER
SNOWMEN
SNOWPEA
SNUBBED
SNUBBER
SNUFFED
SNUFFER
SNUGGED
SNUGGER
UNACTED
UNADDED
UNAIDED
UNAIMED
UNAIRED
UNARMED
UNASKED
UNAXLED
UNBAKED
UNBALED
UNBALES
UNBARED
UNBARES
UNBASED
UNBATED
UNBESET
UNBLUED
UNBONED
UNBORED
UNBOWED
UNBOXED
UNBOXES
UNBRIEF
UNCAGED
UNCAGES
UNCAKED
UNCAKES
UNCANED
UNCAPED
UNCASED
UNCASES
UNCEDED
UNCITED
UNCODED
UNCORED
UNCORES
UNCOVER
UNCOWED
UNCOYER
UNCRIED
UNCRUEL
UNCURED
UNDARED
UNDATED
UNDAZED
UNDEWED
UNDIKED
UNDINES
UNDOMED
UNDRIED
UNDUPED
UNEAGER
UNEASES
UNEATEN
UNEAVED
UNEBBED
UNEDGED
UNEDGES
UNENDED
UNFACED
UNFADED
UNFAKED
UNFAMED
UNFATED
UNFAZED
UNFETED
UNFILED
UNFILES
UNFINED
UNFINES
UNFIRED
UNFIXED
UNFIXES
UNFOXED
UNFREED
UNFREES
UNFRIED
UNFUSED
UNGATED
UNGIVEN
UNGLUED
UNGLUES
UNGORED
UNGREEN
UNGUYED
UNGYVED
UNHATED
UNHAYED
UNHAZED
UNHEWED
UNHIRED
UNHIRES
UNHONED
UNHOPED
UNIATES
UNIFIED
UNIFIER
UNIFIES
UNINKED
UNIPLEX
UNIQUES
UNITIES
UNJADED
UNJOYED
UNKEYED
UNLACED
UNLACES
UNLADED
UNLADEN
UNLADES
UNLAVED
UNLAXED
UNLAXES
UNLEVEL
UNLIKED
UNLIKES
UNLINED
UNLIVED
UNLIVES
UNLOBED
UNLOVED
UNLURED
UNMAKER
UNMAKES
UNMANED
UNMATED
UNMATES
UNMEWED
UNMIKED
UNMINED
UNMIRED
UNMITER
UNMIXED
UNMIXES
UNMOVED
UNMOWED
UNMUTED
UNNAMED
UNNOSED
UNNOTED
UNNOVEL
UNOFTEN
UNOGLED
UNOILED
UNOPTED
UNORBED
UNOWNED
UNPACED
UNPAGED
UNPALED
UNPARED
UNPAVED
UNPAWED
UNPILED
UNPILES
UNPIPED
UNPLIED
UNPOLED
UNPOSED
UNQUIET
UNRAKED
UNRATED
UNRAVEL
UNRAYED
UNRAZED
UNRILED
UNRIMED
UNRIPER
UNRISEN
UNRIVED
UNRIVEN
UNROBED
UNROBES
UNROPED
UNROPES
UNRULED
UNSAFER
UNSATED
UNSAVED
UNSAWED
UNSCREW
UNSEWED
UNSHEER
UNSHIER
UNSHOED
UNSHOES
UNSHYER
UNSIDED
UNSIZED
UNSLEEK
UNSLIER
UNSLYER
UNSOBER
UNSOLED
UNSOLES
UNSOWED
UNSPIED
UNSTEEL
UNSWEET
UNTAKEN
UNTAMED
UNTAMES
UNTAPED
UNTAPES
UNTAXED
UNTAXES
UNTILED
UNTIMED
UNTIRED
UNTONED
UNTREED
UNTRIED
UNTRUER
UNTUNED
UNTUNES
UNTYPED
UNURGED
UNVEXED
UNVOTED
UNVOWED
UNWADED
UNWAGED
UNWAKED
UNWANED
UNWAVED
UNWAXED
UNWHEEL
UNWIPED
UNWIRED
UNWISER
UNWOOED
UNWOVEN
UNYOKED
UNYOKES
UNZONED
UNZONES
VNECKED

•N••••E

ANALYSE
ANALYTE
ANALYZE
ANATASE
ANATOLE
ANDANTE
ANDMORE
ANDRADE
ANEMONE
ANILINE
ANIMATE
ANNALEE
ANNETTE
ANODISE
ANODIZE
ANODYNE
ANTIQUE
ANTLIKE
ANTOINE
ANYHOPE
ANYMORE
ANYTIME
ANYWISE
DNACODE
ENCARRE
ENCHASE
ENCLAVE
ENCLOSE
ENDABLE
ENDGAME
ENDLATE
ENDLINE
ENDNOTE
ENDORSE
ENDWISE
ENDZONE
ENFLAME
ENFORCE
ENFRAME
ENGARDE
ENGORGE
ENGRAVE
ENHANCE
ENLARGE
ENMASSE
ENNOBLE
ENOUNCE
ENPLANE
ENPRISE
ENQUEUE
ENQUIRE
ENRIQUE
ENROUTE
ENSLAVE
ENSNARE
ENSUITE
ENTEBBE
ENTENTE
ENTHUSE
ENTITLE
ENTWINE
ENVOGUE
INADAZE
INAHOLE
INALINE
INAPILE
INAPOKE
INARAGE
INASHOE
INAVALE
INCENSE
INCLINE
INCLOSE
INCLUDE
INCURVE
INDORSE
INDULGE
INEXILE
INFANTE
INFLAME
INFLATE
INFORCE
INGENUE
INGLESE
INGRATE
INHASTE
INHOUSE
INKLIKE
INLARGE
INNERVE
INPEACE
INPHASE
INPLACE
INQUIRE
INRANGE
INSCALE
INSHAPE
INSHORE
INSIGNE
INSPACE
INSPIRE
INSPITE
INSTATE
INSTONE
INSTORE
INSTYLE
INTASTE
INTENSE
INTERNE
INTERSE
INTHERE
INTHREE
INTRADE
INTRUDE
INULASE
INUTILE
INVERSE
INVITEE
INVOGUE
INVOICE
INVOLVE
INWEAVE
INWHITE
KNUCKLE
ONADARE
ONADATE
ONALINE
ONEACRE
ONEBASE
ONEBYTE
ONEDIME
ONEEEEE
ONELANE
ONELOVE
ONEMILE
ONEMORE
ONENAME
ONENOTE
ONEPAGE
ONESHOE
ONESIZE
ONETIME
ONEVOTE
ONLEASE
ONLEAVE
ONSERVE
ONSHORE
ONSTAGE
ONTHREE
SNAPPLE
SNIFFLE
SNOCONE
SNUFFLE
SNUGGLE
UNAGILE
UNALIKE
UNALONE
UNAWAKE
UNAWARE
UNBLADE
UNBORNE
UNBRACE
UNBRAKE
UNBRAVE
UNBROKE
UNCHOKE
UNCLOSE
UNCRATE
UNCRUDE
UNDRAPE
UNFENCE
UNFROZE
UNGLOVE
UNGULAE
UNHINGE
UNHORSE
UNHOUSE
UNICODE
UNISIZE
UNITISE
UNITIVE
UNITIZE
UNLARGE
UNLOOSE
UNMERGE
UNMITRE
UNNAIVE
UNNERVE
UNOBESE
UNPASTE
UNQUOTE
UNRHYME
UNSHADE
UNSPOKE
UNSTATE
UNSWORE
UNTENSE
UNTERSE
UNTRITE
UNTWINE
UNVAGUE
UNVOICE
UNWEAVE
UNWEDGE
UNWHITE
UNWHOLE

••NE•••

AMNERIS
AMNESIA
AMNESIC
AMNESTY
ANNEALS
ANNELID
ANNETTE
ANNEXED
ANNEXES
BANEFUL
BENEATH
BENEFIC
BENEFIT
BENELUX
BONEASH
BONEDRY
BONEDUP
BONELET
BONESET
BONESUP
BONEYER
CANETTI
CINEMAS
CINEMAX
CINEOLE
CINERGY
CINESIA
CONELET
CUNEATE
DANELAW
DANEYKO
DENEUVE
DINEDAT
DINEDIN
DINEDON
DINEOUT
DINESAT
DINESEN
DINESIN
DINESON
DINETTE
DONEBAD
DONEFOR
DONEGAL
DONEGAN
DONETSK
DUNEDIN
ENNEADS
ERNESTA
ERNESTO
FANEUIL
FENELON
FENETRE
FINEART
FINESSE
GENERAL
GENERIC
GENERIS
GENESEE
GENESES
GENESET
GENESIS
GENETIC
GENEVAN
GONEAFT
GONEAPE
GONEBAD
GONEFAR
GONEFOR
GONEMAD
GONEOFF
GONEOUT
GONEPRO
GONERIL
HONEDIN
HONESIN
HONESTY
HONEYED
IGNEOUS
IKNEWIT
INNERLY
INNERVE
IONESCO
JANEANE
JANEDOE
JANEIRO
JANEWAY
JONERIK
JONESED
JONESES
JUNEBUG
JUNEDAY
KANEOHE
KINESES
KINESIC
KINESIS
KINETIC
LANEONE
LANETWO
LINEAGE
LINEARA
LINEARB
LINEATE
LINECUT
LINEDRY
LINEDUP
LINEMAN
LINEMEN
LINEONE
LINEOUT
LINESUP
LINETWO
LINEUPS
LONETTE
LUNESTA
LUNETTE
LYNETTE
MANEGES
MANETTE
MCNEILL
MINEOLA
MINEPIT
MINERAL
MINERVA
MONEYED
NANETTE
NINEEEE
NINEPIN
NINEVEH
NONEPIC
NONETTE
NONEVER
NONEVIL
ORNETTE
OWNEDUP
PANELED
PANETTA
PINEFOR
PINENUT
PINEOIL
PINESAP
PINESOL
PINETAR
PINETOP
PINETUM
RENEGED
RENEGER
RENEGES
RENESTS
RENEWAL
RENEWED
RENEWER
RONETTE
SENECAN
SENECAS
SENEGAL
SENESCE
SINEDIE
SINEWED
SYNERGY
TENEEEE
TINEARS
TONEARM
TONEDUP
TONELOC
TONEMES
TONEROW
TONESUP
TONETTE
TUNEDIN
TUNEDTO
TUNEDUP
TUNEFUL
TUNEOUT
TUNESIN
TUNESTO
TUNESUP
TUNEUPS
UNNEEDY
UNNERVE
VANESSA
VANEXEL
VANEYCK
VENEERS
VENEMAN
VENEZIA
VINEGAR
WINEBAR
WINERED
WINESAP
WINEVAT
WYNETTE
ZANETTO
ZONEOUT

••N•E••

AWNLESS
BANDEAU
BANDERA
BANDERS
BANGERS
BANKERS
BANNERS
BANTERS
BENDERS
BENNETT
BENZELL
BENZENE
BINDERS
BINDERY
BINGERS
BONDERS
BONHEUR
BONIEST
BONKERS
BONNETS
BUNGEES
BUNKERS
BUNTERS
BUNUELO
CANCELS
CANCERS
CANDELA
CANDENT
CANIEST
CANKERS
CANNELL
CANNELS
CANNERS
CANNERY
CANOERS
CANSECO
CANTEEN
CANTERS
CENSERS
CENTERS
CINDERS
CINDERY
CONCEAL
CONCEDE
CONCEIT
CONCEPT
CONCERN
CONCERT
CONDEMN
CONFECT
CONFERS
CONFESS
CONGEAL
CONGERS
CONGEST
CONKERS
CONNECT
CONNERY
CONSENT
CONTEMN
CONTEND
CONTENT
CONTEST
CONTEXT
CONVECT
CONVENE
CONVENT
CONVERT
CONVEYS
DANCERS
DANDERS
DANGELO
DANGERS
DANIELA
DANIELJ
DANIELS
DANKEST
DANSEUR
DANTEAN
DANTEII
DANVERS
DENIECE
DENIERS
DENNEHY
DENSELY
DENSEST
DINGERS
DINNERS
DONKEYS
DONLEVY
DUNGEON
DUNKERS
DUNNERS
FANBELT
FANFEST
FANJETS
FANNERS
FENCEIN
FENCERS
FENCEUP
FENDERS
FENNELS
FINDERS
FINGERS
FINLESS
FONDEST
FONTEYN
FUNDERS
FUNFEST
FUNNELS
GANDERS
GANGERS
GANNETS
GANNETT
GENDERS
GENOESE
GENTEEL
GENXERS
GINGERS
GINGERY
GINSENG
GUNBELT
GUNLESS
GUNNERS
GUNNERY
GUNSELS
HANDERS
HANDEYE
HANGERS
HANKERS
HENDECA
HENNERY
HENPECK
HENREID
HINDERS
HINGEON
HINTERS
HONKERS
HUNGERS
HUNKERS
HUNTERS
INNLESS
IONBEAM
JENNETS
JINXERS
JUNKERS
JUNKETS
KENNEDY
KENNELS
KENNETH
KINDEST
KINLESS
KINNEAR
KINNELL
KUNDERA
LANCERS
LANCETS
LANDERS
LANKEST
LANTERN
LENDERS
LENIENT
LINDENS
LINGERS
LINIEST
LINKERS
LINNETS
LINSEED
LINTELS
LINTERS
LONGEST
LUNGEAT
LUNGERS
LUNKERS
MANDELA
MANGERS
MANHEIM
MANLESS
MANNERS
MANTECA
MANTELS
MANYEAR
MENDELS
MENDERS
MENTEES
MINCERS
MINDERS
MINTERS
MINUEND
MINUETS
MONDESI
MONGERS
MONKEES
MONKEYS
MONTEGO
MONTERO
MONTEUX
MYNHEER
NINEEEE
NONDEAF
NONDEEP
NONHERO
NONJEWS
NONMEAT
NONNEWS
NONPEAK
NONSELF
NONZERO
NUNNERY
OINKERS
PANDERS
PANIERS
PANNERS
PANTENE
PANTERA
PANTERS
PANZERS
PENDENT
PENNERS
PENNEYS
PENSEES
PENTELS

PINCERS
PINGERS
PINHEAD
PINIEST
PINKENS
PINKEST
PINKETT
PINLESS
PINNERS
PINSEAL
PONDERS
PONGEES
PUNGENT
PUNIEST
PUNKERS
PUNLESS
PUNNERS
PUNTERS
RANDEEP
RANGERS
RANKERS
RANKEST
RANTERS
RENDELL
RENDERS
RENNETS
RENTEES
RENTERS
RINGERS
RINSERS
RONDEAU
RONDELS
RUNDEEP
RUNLESS
RUNLETS
RUNNELS
RUNNERS
RUNNETH
SANDERS
SANREMO
SANSEIS
SENDEES
SENDERS
SENNETT
SENSEIS
SENSENS
SINCERE
SINGERS
SINKERS
SINLESS
SINNERS
SONLESS
SONNETS
SUNBEAM
SUNBELT
SUNDECK
SUNDERS
SUNLESS
SUNSETS
TANDEMS
TANGELO
TANGENT
TANKERS
TANNERS
TANNERY
TANNEST
TENCENT
TENDERS
TENEEEE
TENFEET
TENNECO
TENNERS
TENSELY
TENSEST
TENSEUP
TENTERS
TENWEEK
TENYEAR
TINDERS
TINDERY
TINIEST
TINKERS
TINNERS
TINSELS
TINTERN
TINTERS
TONIEST
TONNEAU
TUNNELS
UNNEEDY
VANPELT
VENDEES
VENDERS
VENEERS
VENTERS
VINCENT
VINIEST
VONZELL
WANDERS
WANIEST
WANKELS
WANNESS
WANNEST
WANTERS
WENDELL
WENDERS
WINCERS
WINDERS
WINGERS
WINIEST
WINKERS
WINLESS
WINNERS
WINTERS
WINTERY
WONDERS
YANKEES
YANKERS
YONKERS
ZANIEST
ZINGERS

••N••E•

AGNATES
AGNOMEN
ANNABEL
ANNALEE
ANNALES
ANNEXED
ANNEXES
ANNOYED
ANNOYER
ANNULET
AUNTBEE
AUNTIES
BANACEK
BANALER
BANANES
BANDIED
BANDIER
BANDIES
BANDLET
BANGLED
BANGLES
BANJOES
BANKFEE
BANQUES
BANQUET
BANSHEE
BENARES
BENCHED
BENCHER
BENCHES
BENDIER
BENOTED
BENOTES
BENTLEY
BENTSEN
BINDLES
BINGLES
BINGOES
BONDMEN
BONELET
BONESET
BONEYER
BONGOES
BONNIER
BONUSES
BUNCHED
BUNCHES
BUNCOED
BUNDLED
BUNDLER
BUNDLES
BUNGEES
BUNGLED
BUNGLER
BUNGLES
BUNKBED
BUNKOED
BUNNIES
BYNAMES
CANALED
CANAPES
CANDIED
CANDIES
CANDLED
CANDLER
CANDLES
CANINES
CANNIER
CANTEEN
CANTLES
CENTRED
CENTRES
CINCHED
CINCHES
CINQUES
CONCHES
CONELET
CONFREY
CONGAED
CONIFER
CONQUER
CONRIED
CONURES
DANDIER
DANDIES
DANDLED
DANDLER
DANDLES
DANGLED
DANGLER
DANGLES
DANIKEN
DANITES
DENIMED
DENIZEN
DENOTED
DENOTES
DENUDED
DENUDER
DENUDES
DINESEN
DINGIER
DINGLES
DINGOES
DINKIER
DONATED
DONATEE
DONATES
DONGLES
DONTBEE
DYNODES
FANCIED
FANCIER
FANCIES
FANSLER
FENNIER
FINALES
FINCHES
FINDLEY
FINITES
FINNIER
FONDLED
FONDLER
FONDLES
FONDUED
FONDUES
FUNGOES
FUNKIER
FUNNIER
FUNNIES
FUNPLEX
FUNSTER
GANTLET
GENESEE
GENESES
GENESET
GENOMES
GENTEEL
GENTLED
GENTLER
GENTLES
GENUSES
GUNITES
GUNKIER
GUNNIES
GUNTHER
GUNUSER
HANAPER
HANDFED
HANDIER
HANDLED
HANDLER
HANDLES
HANDSEL
HANDSET
HANGMEN
HANGTEN
HANKIES
HANOVER
HENNAED
HENRIES
HENSLEY
HINDLEG
HINKIER
HINNIES
HONALEE
HONEYED
HONORED
HONOREE
HONORER
HUNCHED
HUNCHES
HUNDRED
HUNGTEN
HUNKIER
HUNTLEY
IGNITED
IGNITER
IGNITES
IGNORED
IGNORER
IGNORES
INNAGES
IONISED
IONISER
IONISES
IONIZED
IONIZER
IONIZES
IONONES
JANACEK
JANGLED
JANGLER
JANGLES
JANSSEN
JANVIER
JINGLED
JINGLER
JINGLES
JINGOES
JONESED
JONESES
JUNCOES
JUNGLES
JUNIPER
JUNKIER
JUNKIES
JUNKMEN
KENDREW
KINDLED
KINDLER
KINDLES
KINDRED
KINESES
KINGLET
KINKIER
KINSMEN
LANDLER
LANDMEN
LANGLEY
LANKIER
LENSMEN
LINAGES
LINDIED
LINDIES
LINDNER
LINDSEY
LINEMEN
LINGOES
LINSEED
LINTIER
LONDRES
LONGBED
LONGDEN
LONGIES
LONGUES
LUNATED
LUNATES
LUNCHED
LUNCHER
LUNCHES
MANAGED
MANAGER
MANAGES
MANATEE
MANDREL
MANEGES
MANFRED
MANGIER
MANGLED
MANGLER
MANGLES
MANGOES
MANLIER
MANNIES
MANTLED
MANTLES
MANTLET
MANURED
MANURES
MANXMEN
MENACED
MENACER
MENACES
MENAGES
MENCKEN
MENTEES
MENZIES
MINARET
MINDSET
MINGIER
MINGLED
MINGLER
MINGLES
MINIVER
MINORED
MINSTER
MINTIER
MINTTEA
MINUSES
MINUTED
MINUTER
MINUTES
MONDIEU
MONEYED
MONGREL
MONIKER
MONKEES
MONOMER
MONROES
MONSTER
MUNCHED
MUNCHEN
MUNCHER
MUNCHES
MUNSTER
MYNHEER
NANNIED
NANNIES
NINEEEE
NINEVEH
NINNIES
NONAGES
NONAMES
NONDEEP
NONDIET
NONEVER
NONFUEL
NONPOET
NONSKED
NONUKES
NONUSER
NUNGWEN
PANACEA
PANELED
PANGAEA
PANNIER
PANSIES
PANTHER
PANTIES
PANTLEG
PENATES
PENNIES
PENSEES
PINCHED
PINCHER
PINCHES
PINKIES
PINKOES
PINONES
PONGEES
PONYKEG
PUNCHED
PUNCHER
PUNCHES
PUNKIER
PUNKIES
PUNNIER
PUNSTER
RANCHED
RANCHER
RANCHES
RANDEEP
RANDIER
RANFREE
RANGIER
RANKLED
RANKLES
RANOVER
RENAMED
RENAMES
RENEGED
RENEGER
RENEGES
RENEWED
RENEWER
RENFREW
RENOTED
RENOTES
RENTEES
RENTIER
RINDIER
RINGLET
RONTGEN
RUNDEEP
RUNDLES
RUNFREE
RUNNIER
RUNOVER
RUNTIER
SANDIER
SANDLER
SANDMEN
SANIBEL
SENATES
SENDEES
SENORES
SINEWED
SINGLED
SINGLES
SINGLET
SINUSES
SUNDAES
SUNNIER
SYNCHED
SYNFUEL
TANAGER
TANGIER
TANGLED
TANGLER
TANGLES
TANGOED
TANGOER
TANSIES
TENACES
TENCHES
TENEEEE
TENFEET
TENNIEL
TENNIES
TENONED
TENONER
TENTBED
TENTPEG
TENURED
TENURES
TENWEEK
TINAFEY
TINCTED
TINGLED
TINGLER
TINGLES
TINKLED
TINKLER
TINKLES
TINNIER
TINORES
TONEMES
TONGUES
TONUSES
UNNAMED
UNNOSED
UNNOTED
UNNOVEL
VANDIEN
VANEXEL
VANOWEN
VENDEES
VENDUES
VENULES
VENUSES
VINTNER
VONBAER
VONOPEL
WANGLED
WANGLER
WANGLES
WENCHES
WINCHED
WINCHER
WINCHES
WINDIER
WINDTEE
WINERED
WINFREY
WINGLET
WINGMEN
WINKLER
WINOVER
WINSLET
WONOVER
YANKEES
ZINCKED
ZINGIER
ZINKIER
ZONULES

••N•••E

ANNALEE
ANNETTE
AUNTBEE
BANDAGE
BANKFEE
BANKONE
BANSHEE
BENBLUE
BENZENE
BINOCHE
BONAIRE
BONDAGE
BONFIRE
CANDACE
CANDICE
CANDIDE
CANIDAE
CANITBE
CANULAE
CANZONE
CENACLE
CENSURE
CENTARE
CENTIME
CINEOLE
CONCAVE
CONCEDE
CONCHAE
CONCISE
CONDOLE
CONDONE
CONDUCE
CONFIDE
CONFINE
CONFUSE
CONFUTE
CONGAME
CONJURE
CONNATE
CONNIVE
CONNOTE
CONSOLE
CONSUME
CONTUSE
CONVENE
CONVOKE
CUNEATE
DENEUVE
DENIECE
DENTATE
DENTINE
DENTURE
DENTYNE
DINETTE
DONAHUE
DONATEE
DONJOSE
DONOHOE
DONTBEE
DONTLIE
DUNNAGE
ELNORTE
ENNOBLE
EONLINE
FANBASE
FANFARE
FANLIKE
FANTINE
FANWISE
FANZINE
FENETRE
FINABLE
FINAGLE
FINANCE
FINESSE
FINLIKE
FONTANE
FUNTIME
GENESEE
GENOESE
GENOISE
GENTILE
GENUINE
GENZYME
GINGAME
GONEAPE
GUNCASE
GUNFIRE
GUNWALE
HANDAXE
HANDEYE
HENBANE
HENLIKE
HONALEE
HONOREE
HUNLIKE
IGNOBLE
INNERVE
JANEANE
JANEDOE
KANEOHE
KENMORE
LANCOME
LANEONE
LANOTTE
LINABLE
LINEAGE
LINEATE
LINEONE
LINGUAE
LINKAGE
LONETTE
LUNETTE
LUNULAE
LYNETTE
MANACLE
MANATEE
MANDATE
MANETTE
MANHOLE
MANIPLE
MANLIKE
MANMADE
MANROPE
MANSIZE
MINABLE
MINOGUE
MINTAGE
MONDALE
MONOCLE
MONTAGE
MONTALE
MUNCHIE
MUNDANE
NANETTE
NINEEEE
NONBASE
NONCORE
NONETTE
NONHOME
NONLIFE
NONLIVE
NONOISE
NONSALE
NONSANE
NONUPLE
NONWAGE
NUNLIKE
OFNOUSE
ORNETTE
PANACHE
PANCAKE
PANICLE
PANPIPE
PANTENE
PANTILE
PANTONE
PANURGE
PENANCE
PENCASE
PENLIKE
PENLITE
PENNAME
PENNATE
PENNINE
PENROSE
PENSIVE
PENTANE
PENUCHE
PINCHME
PINHOLE
PINNACE
PINNATE
PINWALE
RANFREE
RANHOME
RANKINE
RANLATE
RONDURE
RONETTE
RUNFREE
RUNHOME
RUNLATE
RUNTIME
SANJOSE
SANTAFE
SENESCE
SENSATE
SINCERE
SINEDIE
SINKAGE
SINLIKE
SINUATE
SONANCE
SONLIKE
SUNFIRE
SUNLIKE
SUNRISE
SYNAPSE
SYNCOPE
TANKAGE
TANLINE
TENABLE
TENACRE
TENCODE
TENEEEE
TENMILE
TENSILE
TENSIVE
TINLIKE
TINMINE
TINTYPE
TINWARE
TONETTE
TONNAGE
TONSURE
TONTINE
TUNABLE
TUNICLE
UNNAIVE
UNNERVE
URNLIKE
VANDINE
VANDYKE
VANLINE
VANTAGE
VENABLE
VENDOME
VENTAGE
VENTURE
VINROSE
VINTAGE
VONLAUE
WANNABE
WENTAPE
WINDAGE
WINDTEE
WINSOME
WYNETTE
YANGTZE
ZINCITE

•••NE••

ABCNEWS
AIRNESS
ALINERS
ALLNESS
ALLNEWS
ANYNEWS
APTNESS
ARANEID
ATANEND
ATONERS
BADNESS
BADNEWS
BANNERS
BARNEYS
BATNEXT
BEANERY
BENNETT
BERNESE
BIGNESS
BIGNEWS
BONNETS
BORNEAN
BORNEUP
BRINERS
BRUNETS
BURNERS
BURNETT
BYANECK
CANNELL
CANNELS
CANNERS
CANNERY
CARNERA
CARNETS
CBSNEWS
CHANELS
CHINESE
CLONERS
COINERS
CONNECT
CONNERY
CORNEAL
CORNEAS
CORNELL
CORNERS
CORNETS
COYNESS
CRENELS
CYGNETS
DAMNERS
DARNELL
DARNERS
DEANERY
DENNEHY
DIMNESS
DINNERS
DIPNETS
DOONEIN
DOWNERS
DRONEON

DRONERS
DRYNESS
DUNNERS
EARNERS
EARNEST
ELANETS
EMINENT
ESPNEWS
EVENERS
EVENEST
EWENECK
EXENEMY
FAINEST
FANNERS
FARNESS
FATNESS
FAWNERS
FENNELS
FERNERY
FEWNESS
FEYNESS
FITNESS
FLANEUR
FLYNETS
FOXNEWS
FRENEAU
FRENEMY
FRENESI
FULNESS
FUNNELS
FURNESS
GAINERS
GANNETS
GANNETT
GARNEAU
GARNERS
GARNETS
GARNETT
GAYNESS
GOONEYS
GUINEAN
GUINEAS
GUNNERS
GUNNERY
GURNEYS
GWYNETH
HARNESS
HENNERY
HIPNESS
HOHNERS
HORNETS
HOTNESS
ICINESS
ILLNESS
INANELY
INANEST
ININETY
IPANEMA
IRONERS
JENNETS
JITNEYS
JOINERS
JOINERY
KEENENH
KEENERS
KEENEST
KENNEDY
KENNELS
KENNETH
KERNELS
KIDNEYS
KINNEAR
KINNELL
KUZNETS
LAXNESS
LEANERS
LEANEST
LIENEES
LIMNERS
LINNETS
LIONELL
LIONELS
LIONESS
LIONETS
LLANERO
LOANERS
LOWNECK
LOWNESS
LYONELL
MACNEIL
MADNESS
MAGNETO
MAGNETS
MAINERS
MANNERS
MEANEST
MEYNELL
MOANERS
MOONERS
MOONEYE
NBCNEWS
NEWNESS
NONNEWS
NOONERS
NOTNEAR
NOWNESS
NUNNERY
ODDNESS
OLDNESS
OLDNEWS
ONENESS
OPENEND
OPENERS
OPINERS
ORKNEYS
PANNERS
PATNESS
PAWNEES
PAWNERS
PENNERS
PENNEYS
PHINEAS
PHONEIN
PHONEME
PHONENO
PHONERS
PHONEYS
PINNERS
PIONEER
PLANERS
PLANETS
PRONELY
PRONETO
PRUNERS
PUNNERS
QBSNEAK
QUENEAU
QUINELA
RAWNESS
RAYNELL
REDNECK
REDNESS
REKNEAD
RENNETS
REUNERS
ROMNEYS
RUINERS
RUNNELS
RUNNERS
RUNNETH
SADNESS
SCENEII
SCENEIV
SCENERY
SCENEVI
SEINERS
SENNETT
SHINEON
SHINERS
SHINEUP
SHYNESS
SIENESE
SIGNEES
SIGNERS
SIGNETS
SINNERS
SLYNESS
SOLNESS
SONNETS
SOONERS
SOONEST
SPINELS
SPINETS
STONEAX
STONERS
SUBNETS
SWINERY
TANNERS
TANNERY
TANNEST
TEANECK
TEENERS
TENNECO
TENNERS
THENETS
THENEWS
TINNERS
TONNEAU
TOWNERS
TUNNELS
TURNERS
TURNERY
TWINERS
UNINERT
VAINEST
VEENECK
WANNESS
WANNEST
WEANERS
WEENESS
WETNESS
WHINERS
WIENERS
WINNERS
WITNESS
WRYNESS
YARNELL
YAWNERS

•••N•E•

AGENCES
AGENTED
AGONIES
ALUNSER
AMENDED
AMENDER
ARUNDEL
ASANTES
ASUNDER
ATONIES
AVENGED
AVENGER
AVENGES
AVENUEQ
AVENUES
AVONLEA
AZINGER
BAINTER
BARNRED
BEANIES
BERNSEN
BLANDER
BLANKED
BLANKER
BLANKET
BLENDED
BLENDER
BLENDES
BLINDED
BLINDER
BLINKED
BLINKER
BLONDER
BLONDES
BLUNDEN
BLUNDER
BLUNTED
BLUNTER
BLYNKEN
BONNIER
BOONIES
BOUNCED
BOUNCER
BOUNCES
BOUNDED
BOUNDER
BRANDED
BRANDER
BRENDEL
BRENNER
BRINGER
BRINIER
BRINKER
BRONTES
BRONWEN
BRONZED
BRONZER
BRONZES
BRYNNER
BUNNIES
BURNLEY
CANNIER
CARNIES
CHANCED
CHANCEL
CHANCER
CHANCES
CHANGED
CHANGER
CHANGES
CHANNEL
CHANTED
CHANTER
CHANTEY
CHENIER
CHINKED
CHINNED
CHUNKED
CHUNNEL
CLANGED
CLANGER
CLANKED
CLINGER
CLINKED
CLINKER
CLONKED
CLUNKED
CLUNKER
CORNFED
CORNIER
COUNSEL
COUNTED
COUNTEE
COUNTEM
COUNTER
CRANKED
CRANMER
CRINGED
CRINGES
CRONIES
DAUNTED
DAUNTER
DERNIER
DOWNIER
DRINKER
DRUNKEN
DRUNKER
EBANKED
EBONIES
ELANCES
EMANUEL
EMENDED
EMENDER
ERINYES
EVANDER
EVANGEL
EVENBET
EVINCED
EVINCES
FAINTED
FAINTER
FEINTED
FENNIER
FERNIER
FIANCEE
FIANCES
FIENNES
FINNIER
FLANGES
FLANKED
FLANKEN
FLANKER
FLANNEL
FLENSED
FLENSER
FLENSES
FLINGER
FLUNKED
FLUNKER
FOUNDED
FOUNDER
FRANCES
FRANKED
FRANKEN
FRANKER
FRINGED
FRINGES
FRONTED
FUENTES
FUNNIER
FUNNIES
GAUNTER
GLANCED
GLANCES
GLINTED
GOONIER
GOONIES
GOUNDER
GRANDEE
GRANDER
GRANGER
GRANGES
GRANTED
GRANTEE
GRANTER
GRENDEL
GRINDER
GRINNED
GRINNER
GRUNGER
GRUNGES
GRUNTED
GRUNTER
GUNNIES
HAUNTED
HAUNTER
HENNAED
HINNIES
HORNIER
HOUNDED
HOUNDER
IRONIES
IRONMEN
IWONDER
JAUNTED
JOHNLEE
JOINDER
JOINTED
JOINTER
JOUNCED
JOUNCES
KLINGER
KLINKER
LAENNEC
LAUNDER
LEANDER
LIENEES
LOONIER
LOONIES
LOUNGED
LOUNGER
LOUNGES
MAINMEN
MANNIES
MARNIER
MAUNDER
MEANDER
MEANIES
MOONIER
MOONIES
MOONLET
MOONSET
MOUNDED
MOUNTED
MOUNTER
NANNIED
NANNIES
NINNIES
NOANGEL
NUANCED
NUANCES
OPENNET
OPENSEA
ORANGES
ORANGEY
ORANTES
PAINTED
PAINTER
PANNIER
PAWNEES
PENNIES
PEONIES
PHONIER
PHONIES
PIONEER
PLANKED
PLANNED
PLANNER
PLANTED
PLANTER
PLINKED
PLONKED
PLUNDER
PLUNGED
PLUNGER
PLUNGES
PLUNKED
PLUNKER
POINTED
POINTER
POINTES
POUNCED
POUNCER
POUNCES
POUNDED
POUNDER
PRANCED
PRANCER
PRANCES
PRINCES
PRINKED
PRINKER
PRINTED
PRINTER
PRONGED
PUNNIER
QUINCES
QUINCEY
QUINTES
QUINTET
QUINZES
QUONSET
RAINIER
REANNEX
REENTER
REGNIER
REINDEX
REINKED
ROUNDED
ROUNDEL
ROUNDER
RUNNIER
SAINTED
SAINTES
SAUNAED
SAUNTER
SCANNED
SCANNER
SCANTED
SCANTER
SCENTED
SCENTER
SCONCES
SEANCES
SHANKED
SHANNEN
SHANTER
SHINIER
SHINNED
SHUNNED
SHUNTED
SHUNTER
SIGNEES
SKINNED
SKINNER
SKUNKED
SLANDER
SLANTED
SLENDER
SLINGER
SLINKED
SLINKER
SOUNDED
SOUNDER
SPANDEX
SPANIEL
SPANKED
SPANKER
SPANNED
SPANNER
SPENCER
SPENDER
SPENSER
SPINIER
SPINNER
SPINNEY
SPONDEE
SPONGED
SPONGER
SPONGES
STANCES
STANDEE
STANDER
STANLEE
STANLEY
STENGEL
STINGER
STINKER
STINTED
STINTER
STONIER
STUNNED
STUNNER
STUNTED
SUNNIER
SWANKED
SWANKER
SWANSEA
SWINGER
TAINTED
TAUNTED
TAUNTER
TAWNIER
TEENIER
TENNIEL
TENNIES
THANKED
THANKER
THINKER
THINNED
THINNER
THUNDER
THUNKED
TINNIER
TOONIES
TOWNIES
TOWNLET
TOYNBEE
TRANCED
TRANCES
TRENDED
TRINKET
TURNKEY
TURNRED
TWANGED
TWANGER
TWINBED
TWINGED
TWINGES
TWINIER
TWINJET
TWINNED
TWINSET
UNENDED
UNINKED
UPENDED
USANCES
UVINDEX
VAUNTED
VAUNTER
VEINIER
VEINLET
VEINTES
VERNIER
WEENIES
WERNHER
WHANGED
WHINIER
WIENIES
WOUNDED
WRANGEL
WRINGER
WRONGED
WRONGER
YAWNIER
YOUNGER

•••N••E

ACONITE
ADENINE
AGENINE
AGONISE
AGONIZE
ALANINE
AMINUTE
ARENOSE
ASININE
ATINGLE
BADNAME
BARNONE
BERNESE
BIGNAME
BIGNOSE
BLANCHE
BLINTZE
BLONDIE
BRINDLE
BYANOSE
CARNAGE
CHINESE
COGNATE
COGNIZE
COINAGE
CONNATE
CONNIVE
CONNOTE
CORNICE
CORNUTE
COUNTEE
CRENATE
CRINKLE
CYANIDE
DRINKME
DUNNAGE
DWINDLE
EBONITE
EBONIZE
EMANATE
ENDNOTE
ENSNARE
EPONINE
FIANCEE
FRANKIE
FURNACE
GLENCOE
GRANDEE
GRANITE
GRANNIE
GRANTEE
GRANULE
GRENADE
GUANINE
HERNIAE
HOGNOSE
HOWNICE
HUANGHE
IRONAGE
IRONORE
IVANHOE
JEANNIE
JOHNDOE
JOHNLEE
JOHNNIE
KEYNOTE
KHANATE
KRINGLE
LEONINE
LEONORE
LIGNITE
LIMNITE
LIONISE
LIONIZE
MAGNATE
MCENROE
MEANAGE
MEANJOE
MISNAME
MOONEYE
MOONPIE
MOUNTIE
NEONATE
NEWNAME
NOTNICE
OFANAGE
ONENAME
ONENOTE
OPENTOE
OZONISE
OZONIZE
PENNAME
PENNATE
PENNINE
PEONAGE
PETNAME
PHONEME
PINNACE
PINNATE
PLANATE
PRENAME
PRINGLE
PRONATE
PUGNOSE
QUINATE
QUININE
QUINQUE
REDNINE
REDNOSE
REUNITE
ROANOKE
RUINATE
SHINGLE
SIENESE
SIGNAGE
SIGNORE
SIXNINE
SPANGLE
SPINDLE
SPONDEE
STANDEE
STANINE
STANLEE
SURNAME
SWINDLE
TEENAGE
TEENSIE
TERNATE
THANDIE
THENILE
THINICE
TONNAGE
TOPNAME
TOYNBEE
TRUNDLE
TWINKIE
TWINKLE
ULANUDE
URANITE
VEINULE
WANNABE
WRANGLE
WRINKLE
ZERNIKE

••••NE•

ACHENES
ACORNED
ADORNED
ADORNER
AFFINED
AFFINES
ALIENEE
ALIGNED
ALIGNER
ALKENES
ALMONER
ALPINER
ALPINES
ANYONES
APRONED
ARIANES
ATTUNED
ATTUNES
BALONEY
BANANES
BARONET
BAYONET
BEIGNES
BEIGNET
BERKNER
BIGONES
BLARNEY
BOCHNER
BOVINES
BRAINED
BRAINER
BRENNER
BRITNEY
BROWNED
BROWNER
BRYNNER
BUCHNER
BUCKNER
BUJONES
BUTANES
BUTENES
BYGONES
BYLINED
BYLINER
BYLINES
CABINET
CAIRNED
CANINES
CETANES
CHAINED
CHAINES
CHANNEL
CHIMNEY
CHINNED
CHUNNEL
CHURNED
CHURNER
CHUTNEY
CLEANED
CLEANER
CLOONEY
CLOWNED
COCKNEY
COIGNED
COIGNES
COLONEL
COLONES
COOWNED
CORONER
CORONET
COSINES
COSTNER
COZENED
COZENER
CROONED
CROONER
CROWNED
CROWNER
DAPHNES
DEBONED
DEBONES
DEFINED
DEFINER
DEFINES
DEIGNED
DELANEY
DEPONED
DEPONER
DEPONES
DETUNED
DETUNES
DIVINED
DIVINER
DIVINES
DOUANES
DRAGNET
DRAINED
DRAINER
DROPNET
DROWNED
EDASNER
ELAINES
EMPANEL
ENGINED
ENGINES
EOSINES
EQUINES
ERMINED
ERMINES
ESSENES
ETHANES
ETHENES
FAMINES
FASTNET
FATONES
FECHNER
FEIGNED
FEIGNER
FELINES
FIENNES

FILENES
FISHNET
FLANNEL
FLEXNER
FRESNEL
FROWNED
FROWNER
GAMINES
GARDNER
GILLNET
GLEANED
GLEANER
GORTNER
GRAINED
GRAINER
GRAPNEL
GREENED
GREENER
GRINNED
GRINNER
GRISNEZ
GROANED
GROANER
GROINED
GYRENES
HACKNEY
HAIRNET
HAVENER
HEXANES
HOTONES
IMMUNES
IMPANEL
INLINES
INSANER
INTONED
INTONER
INTONES
IONONES
JACONET
JIMENEZ
JIMINEZ
JOURNEE
JOURNEY
JTMONEY
KCJONES
KEARNEY
KETONES
KLEENEX
KRASNER
LAENNEC
LARDNER
LATENED
LEARNED
LEARNER
LIFENET
LIKENED
LIKENEW
LINDNER
LIVENED
LIVENER
LUPINES
MAHONEY
MARINER
MARINES
MASONED
MATINEE
MCRANEY
MEGANES

MEITNER
MIGENES
MISKNEW
MOMONEY
MOURNED
MOURNER
MRBONES
MRHANEY
MRJONES
NOMINEE
OCTANES
OFTENER
OPENNET
ORDINES
ORDONEZ
OSCINES
OVERNEW
PARDNER
PARTNER
PAVANES
PILSNER
PINONES
PLAINER
PLAINES
PLANNED
PLANNER
POLANER
PRAWNED
PREENED
PREENER
QUEENED
QUOINED
RAMONES
RAPINES
RATINES
RAVENED
RAVINED
RAVINES
REANNEX
RECANED
RECANES
REFINED
REFINER
REFINES
REHONED
REHONES
REIGNED
RELANES
RELINED
RELINES
REMINED
REMINES
REOWNED
REPANEL
REPINED
REPINER
REPINES
RESINED
RETONED
RETONES
RETUNED
RETUNES
REZONED
REZONES
RIPENED
RIPENER
ROBBNEN
ROSINED

ROSSNER
SABINES
SALINES
SATINET
SCANNED
SCANNER
SCORNED
SCORNER
SERENER
SEVENEE
SHANNEN
SHATNER
SHAWNEE
SHINNED
SHRINED
SHRINER
SHRINES
SHUNNED
SIRENED
SKINNED
SKINNER
SOAPNET
SOIGNEE
SOMINEX
SPANNED
SPANNER
SPAWNED
SPAWNER
SPINNER
SPINNEY
SPLINES
SPOONED
SPOONER
SPURNED
SPURNER
STAGNES
STAINED
STAINER
STEINEM
STEINER
STERNER
STUNNED
STUNNER
SWEENEY
SWOONED
SWOONER
TALONED
TENONED
TENONER
THINNED
THINNER
THORNED
THRONES
TIERNEY
TISANES
TOKENED
TOURNEY
TRAINED
TRAINEE
TRAINER
TULANEU
TWEENER
TWINNED
UNBONED
UNCANED
UNDINES
UNFINED
UNFINES

UNHONED
UNLINED
UNMANED
UNMINED
UNOWNED
UNTONED
UNTUNED
UNTUNES
UNWANED
UNZONED
UNZONES
URBANER
VALINES
VERYNEW
VIERNES
VINTNER
WAGONED
WAGONER
WAHINES
WAKENED
WAKENER
WEEONES
WEGENER
WETONES
WHITNEY
WHOKNEW
WIDENED
WIDENER
WIZENED
XIMENES
YEARNED
YEARNER

••••N•E

ABSENCE
ADVANCE
ALDENTE
ALFONSE
ALIENEE
ALLANTE
ALLENDE
ALLONGE
ALUMNAE
ANDANTE
ARGANTE
ARGONNE
ARRANGE
ASKANCE
ASSANTE
BALANCE
BAYONNE
BEYONCE
BILLNYE
BROWNIE
CADENCE
CARINAE
CATENAE
CAYENNE
CEZANNE
CLEANSE
CLEANTE
CORINNE
CORONAE
DEFENCE
DEFENSE
DERANGE
DETENTE
DOYENNE

DURANCE
DURANTE
ELMONTE
ENHANCE
ENOUNCE
ENTENTE
ESCENCE
ESSENCE
ETIENNE
EUGENIE
EXPANSE
EXPENSE
EXPUNGE
FACONNE
FAIENCE
FINANCE
FIRENZE
FLEANCE
FLOUNCE
FORONCE
GARONNE
GIRONDE
GRANNIE
IMMENSE
IMPINGE
INCENSE
INFANTE
INGENUE
INRANGE
INTENSE
ITSONME
JEANNIE
JOHNNIE
JOURNEE
LACUNAE
LALANNE
LAMINAE
LECONTE
LEMONDE
LICENCE
LICENSE
LISENTE
LORANGE
LOZENGE
MATINEE
MELANGE
MELANIE
MORANTE
MUSANTE
MYCENAE
NOMINEE
NOTONCE
OFFENCE
OFFENSE
ORIENTE
PALANCE
PENANCE
PESANTE
PICANTE
POTENCE
QUEENIE
REFENCE
REHINGE
RELANCE
RERINSE
RETINAE
RETINGE
RETINUE

REVENGE
REVENUE
ROMANCE
ROSANNE
ROXANNE
SCIENCE
SEVENEE
SHAWNEE
SILENCE
SILENTE
SOIGNEE
SONANCE
STEANNE
STRANGE
SUSANNE
SUZANNE
SYRINGE
TERENCE
TITANAE
TRAINEE
TROUNCE
TWOONIE
UNFENCE
UNHINGE
UNTENSE
VALANCE
VALENCE
VALENTE
VICENTE
VOLANTE
VOLENTE
YAOUNDE

•••••NE

AAMILNE
ABALONE
ABILENE
ACETONE
ADELINE
ADENINE
AGATINE
AGENINE
AIRFONE
AIRLANE
AIRLINE
ALADINE
ALANINE
ALCYONE
ALLDONE
ALLGONE
ALLMINE
AMARONE
ANEMONE
ANILINE
ANODYNE
ANTOINE
ARACHNE
ARCSINE
ARGONNE
ARIADNE
ARMBONE
ASININE
AUTOMNE
BALLONE
BANKONE
BARNONE
BAYONNE
BEELINE

BEGUINE
BELTANE
BENZENE
BEROWNE
BESTONE
BETHUNE
BICORNE
BIPLANE
BOBKANE
BOWLINE
BROMINE
BUSLANE
BUSLINE
BYPHONE
CAIRENE
CALZONE
CANZONE
CAPRINE
CARBINE
CARLENE
CARMINE
CASERNE
CAYENNE
CERVINE
CEZANNE
CHICANE
CHOLINE
CHOPINE
CHORINE
CICCONE
CITRINE
COCAINE
CODEINE
COLDONE
COLLINE
COLOGNE
COMBINE
COMMUNE
CONDONE
CONFINE
CONVENE
CORINNE
CORVINE
CORZINE
COUSINE
COWBANE
CUISINE
CYCLONE
DARLENE
DEARONE
DECLINE
DEMESNE
DENTINE
DENTYNE
DEPLANE
DESTINE
DEWLINE
DIDFINE
DOGBANE
DOGBONE
DOGGONE
DOMAINE
DOYENNE
DUOTONE
EARBONE
EASYONE
ELEVENE
EMPLANE

ENDLINE
ENDZONE
ENPLANE
ENTWINE
EONLINE
EPERGNE
EPICENE
EPIGONE
EPONINE
ERSKINE
ETAMINE
ETIENNE
EVILONE
EXAMINE
EXTERNE
EYELINE
FACONNE
FANTINE
FANZINE
FARGONE
FASTONE
FIVEONE
FONTANE
FORDONE
FORGONE
FORTUNE
FROZONE
FTWAYNE
GAGLINE
GARONNE
GASLINE
GASTONE
GENUINE
GERMANE
GETDONE
GLAVINE
GLYCINE
GOODONE
GOTDONE
GUANINE
HADDONE
HALDANE
HAMBONE
HAMLINE
HARLINE
HASDONE
HAVEONE
HELLENE
HEMLINE
HENBANE
HEROINE
HIPBONE
HIRCINE
HITTUNE
HOLYONE
HORMONE
HOTLINE
HOTZONE
HOVLANE
HYGIENE
ICELINE
ICEWINE
IFORONE
IFSTONE
IGRAINE
ILLDONE
IMAGINE
IMEMINE

IMOGENE
INALINE
INCLINE
INSIGNE
INSTONE
INTERNE
ISOLINE
ISOTONE
ITEMONE
ITSDONE
ITSFINE
ITSGONE
IVORINE
JANEANE
JARDINE
JASMINE
JAWBONE
JAWLINE
JUGWINE
JUSTINE
JUSTONE
KATRINE
LADRONE
LALANNE
LANEONE
LARAINE
LASAGNE
LASTONE
LATRINE
LAVAINE
LAVERNE
LEGBONE
LEJEUNE
LEMOYNE
LEONINE
LEUCINE
LINEONE
LIVEONE
LUCARNE
LUCERNE
MACHINE
MACHONE
MADEONE
MAKEONE
MARLENE
MASSINE
MAYWINE
MBABANE
MCSHANE
MCSWINE
METHANE
MIDJUNE
MIDLINE
MIOCENE
MISDONE
MISTUNE
MISZONE
MODERNE
MORAINE
MUNDANE
NAMEONE
NEOCENE
NEOGENE
NEPTUNE
NERVINE
NEURONE
NEWLINE
NICEONE

NONSANE
NOTAONE
NOTDONE
NOTMINE
NUTPINE
OBSCENE
OFFLINE
OILLINE
OLDLINE
OLIVINE
OMAHANE
ONALINE
ONELANE
OPALINE
OPUSONE
ORIGINE
OSBORNE
OUTDONE
OUTLINE
PADRONE
PAGEONE
PANTENE
PANTONE
PARTONE
PAULINE
PCCLONE
PENNINE
PENTANE
PEPTONE
PERRINE
PISCINE
PLUSONE
POPTUNE
POPWINE
PORCINE
PRALINE
PROFANE
PROPANE
PROPONE
PROVINE
QUININE
RANKINE
RAPTUNE
RATLINE
REALINE
RECLINE
REDBONE
REDLINE
REDNINE
REDPINE
REDWINE
REDZONE
REPHONE
REPLANE
REPRUNE
RESHINE
RETWINE
RIPSONE
RLSTINE
ROGAINE
ROMAINE
ROSANNE
ROUTINE
ROXANNE
RULEONE
SALTINE
SARDINE
SCALENE

SEALANE
SIDEONE
SISTINE
SIXLANE
SIXNINE
SIZEONE
SKYLINE
SLOVENE
SNOCONE
SOMEONE
SPOKANE
SPUMONE
STANINE
STEANNE
STEPONE
STYRENE
SUBTONE
SUBVENE
SUBZONE
SUSANNE
SUZANNE
TAGLINE
TAKEONE
TALLONE
TANLINE
TAURINE
TERHUNE
TERRENE
TERRINE
THATONE
THISONE
THYMINE
TIELINE
TINMINE
TIPLINE
TOLUENE
TONTINE
TOPLINE
TOWLINE
TRIBUNE
TRITONE
TURBINE
TWOLANE
TWOTONE
UKRAINE
UNALONE
UNBORNE
UNTWINE
UPBORNE
VACCINE
VALLONE
VANDINE
VANLINE
VEREINE
VIOLONE
VITRINE
VOLPONE
VULPINE
WARZONE
WEBZINE
WILDONE
WISEONE
WORDONE
YASMINE
YEARONE
ZADKINE
ZEBRINE

NF•••••

NFCTEAM
NFLGAME
NFLTEAM

N•F••••

NIFTIER
NIFTIES
NIFTILY
NOFAULT

N••F•••

NETFLIX
NETFULS
NEWFACE
NONFACT
NONFANS
NONFARM
NONFLUX
NONFOOD
NONFORM
NONFUEL
NORFOLK
NOTFAIR

N•••F••

NEEDFUL
NESTFUL
NOGIFTS

N••••F•

NESCAFE
NETCAFE
NEWLEFT
NEWLIFE
NITRIFY
NODSOFF
NONLIFE
NORDOFF
NOTSAFE
NULLIFY

N•••••F

NETSURF
NEWLEAF
NODSOFF
NOENDOF
NONDEAF
NONSELF
NORDOFF
NORTHOF

•NF••••

ENFACED
ENFACES
ENFANTS
ENFIELD
ENFLAME
ENFOLDS
ENFORCE
ENFRAME
INFAITH
INFANCY
INFANTA
INFANTE
INFANTS
INFAVOR
INFECTS

INFERNO
INFESTS
INFIDEL
INFIELD
INFIRST
INFIVES
INFIXED
INFIXES
INFLAME
INFLATE
INFLECT
INFLICT
INFLOWS
INFOCUS
INFOLDS
INFORCE
INFORIT
INFORMS
INFRACT
INFRONT
INFUSED
INFUSER
INFUSES
ONFIRST
UNFACED
UNFACTS
UNFADED
UNFAITH
UNFAKED
UNFAMED
UNFANCY
UNFATED
UNFATTY
UNFAZED
UNFENCE
UNFERTH
UNFETED
UNFIERY
UNFILED
UNFILES
UNFINED
UNFINES
UNFIRED
UNFITLY
UNFIXED
UNFIXES
UNFLAKY
UNFLOOR
UNFLOWN
UNFLUID
UNFOGGY
UNFOLDS
UNFORKS
UNFOUND
UNFOXED
UNFRAIL
UNFRANK
UNFREED
UNFREES
UNFRIED
UNFRILL
UNFROCK
UNFROST
UNFROZE
UNFULLY
UNFUNNY
UNFURLS
UNFUSED

UNFUSSY

•N•F•••
ANTFARM
INAFUNK
INAFURY
KNIFERS
KNIFING
ONEFOLD
ONEFOOT
SNAFUED
SNIFFAT
SNIFFED
SNIFFER
SNIFFLE
SNIFFLY
SNIFFUP
SNIFTER
SNUFFED
SNUFFER
SNUFFLE
UNIFIED
UNIFIER
UNIFIES
UNIFORM
UNOFTEN

•N••F••
ANTIFOG
INSOFAR
ONEOFFS
ONEOFUS
SNARFED
SNIFFAT
SNIFFED
SNIFFER
SNIFFLE
SNIFFLY
SNIFFUP
SNUFFED
SNUFFER
SNUFFLE
SNUGFIT
UNAWFUL
UNCUFFS
UNLOFTY
UNSAFER

•N•••F•
ENGRAFT
ENGULFS
INAHUFF
INAJIFF
INDRAFT
INGRAFT
INGULFS
ONEOFFS
ONSTAFF
SNIPOFF
UNCLEFT
UNCUFFS
UNGRUFF
UNLEAFS
UNROOFS
UNSHIFT
UNSTIFF

•N••••F
ENDLEAF
INAHUFF
INAIDOF
INAJIFF
INAWEOF
INBRIEF
KNOWSOF
ONEHALF
ONESELF
ONSTAFF
ONTOPOF
SNIPOFF
UNBRIEF
UNGRUFF
UNSTIFF

••NF•••
BONFIRE
CANFULS
CONFABS
CONFECT
CONFERS
CONFESS
CONFIDE
CONFINE
CONFIRM
CONFITS
CONFORM
CONFREY
CONFUSE
CONFUTE
FANFARE
FANFEST
FANFICS
FANFOLD
FUNFAIR
FUNFEST
FUNFURS
FUNFZIG
GINFIZZ
GUNFIRE
KINFOLK
LANFORD
LENFANT
MANFRED
MENFOLK
NONFACT
NONFANS
NONFARM
NONFLUX
NONFOOD
NONFORM
NONFUEL
PANFISH
PANFULS
PINFOLD
RANFREE
RENFREW
RUNFREE
SANFORD
SUNFANS
SUNFAST
SUNFIRE
SUNFISH
SYNFUEL
TENFEET
TENFOLD
TENFOOT
TENFOUR
TINFISH
TINFOIL
URNFULS
WINFREY

••N•F••
BANEFUL
BANKFEE
BENEFIC
BENEFIT
CONIFER
DONEFOR
GONEFAR
GONEFOR
GUNSFOR
HANDFED
HANDFUL
HUNTFOR
JUNKFAX
LONGFOR
MINDFUL
PINEFOR
RANGFOR
RINGFOR
RUNGFOR
RUNOFFS
RUNSFOR
SANDFLY
SENDFOR
SENTFOR
SONGFUL
SUNSFAN
TANKFUL
TENTFUL
TINAFEY
TUNEFUL
WENTFAR
WENTFOR
YENSFOR

••N••F•
BINDOFF
CONKOFF
CONNIFF
DANDIFY
DENSIFY
FANCIFY
FENDOFF
GONEAFT
GONEOFF
HANDOFF
HANGOFF
HENTOFF
HUNGOFF
NONLIFE
PONTIFF
RANGOFF
RINGOFF
RUNGOFF
RUNOFFS
RUNSOFF
SANTAFE
SENDOFF
SENTOFF
WENTAFT
WENTOFF
YANKOFF
ZINCIFY

••N•••F
BINDOFF
CONKOFF
CONNIFF
FENDOFF
GANDALF
GONEOFF
HANDOFF
HANGOFF
HENTOFF
HUNGOFF
LINDORF
NONDEAF
NONSELF
PONTIFF
RANGOFF
RINGOFF
RUNGOFF
RUNSOFF
SENDOFF
SENTOFF
SUNROOF
TINROOF
WENTOFF
YANKOFF

•••NF••
BURNFOR
CORNFED
GAINFUL
GOINFOR
MOANFUL
PAINFUL
PLANFOR
SEENFIT
SIGNFOR
YAWNFUL

•••N•F•
BRANIFF
BURNOFF
DIGNIFY
EVENOFF
ICONIFY
LIGNIFY
MAGNIFY
PAWNOFF
REUNIFY
SARNOFF
SAWNOFF
SEENOFF
SHONUFF
SIGNIFY
SIGNOFF
SPINOFF
SPUNOFF
TORNOFF
TURNOFF
WARNOFF
WORNOFF

•••N••F
BRANIFF
BURNOFF
CONNIFF
EVENOFF
NOENDOF
PAWNOFF
SARNOFF
SAWNOFF
SEENOFF
SHONUFF
SIGNOFF
SPINOFF
SPUNOFF
THINKOF
TORNOFF
TURNOFF
WARNOFF
WARNSOF
WORNOFF

••••N•F
BARANOF
GIVENOF
LEARNOF
SILENTF

•••••NF
GETSANF

N•G••••
NAGGERS
NAGGIER
NAGGING
NAGGISH
NEGATED
NEGATER
NEGATES
NEGATOR
NEGLECT
NEGRONI
NEGUSES
NIGERIA
NIGGLED
NIGGLER
NIGGLES
NIGHEST
NIGHTER
NIGHTIE
NIGHTLY
NOGALES
NOGGINS
NOGIFTS
NOGOODS
NOGUCHI
NUGGETS
NUGGETY
NYGIANT

N••G•••
NAGGERS
NAGGIER
NAGGING
NAGGISH
NAUGHTS
NAUGHTY
NBAGAME
NEIGHED
NEOGENE
NETGAIN
NETGAME
NEWGATE
NFLGAME
NHLGAME
NIAGARA
NIGGLED
NIGGLER
NIGGLES
NOGGINS
NONGOGO
NONGOLD
NOOGIES
NOTGOOD
NOUGATS
NOUGHTS
NUDGERS
NUDGING
NUGGETS
NUGGETY
NUNGWEN

N•••G••
NAILGUN
NEONGAS
NEWAGER
NEWAGEY
NICEGUY
NIPIGON
NOANGEL
NONAGES
NONAGON
NOODGED
NOODGES
NOSEGAY
NOSUGAR

N••••G•
NEOLOGY
NESTEGG
NICCAGE
NOMERGE
NONGOGO
NONWAGE
NORIEGA
NUTMEGS

N•••••G
NABBING
NAGGING
NAILING
NAILKEG
NAMETAG
NANJING
NANKING
NAPPING
NEARING
NECKING
NEEDING
NERVING
NESTEGG
NESTING
NETTING
NEWBURG
NEWSPEG
NIALONG
NICEDOG
NICHING
NICKING
NIPPING
NOCKING
NODDING
NOISING
NONDRUG
NOONING
NOOSING
NOSEBAG
NOSHING
NOTHING
NOTTING
NUDGING
NULLING
NUMBING
NURSING
NUTTING

•NG••••
ANGELAS
ANGELES
ANGELIC
ANGELOU
ANGELUS
ANGERED
ANGLAIS
ANGLERS
ANGLING
ANGOLAN
ANGORAS
ANGRIER
ANGRILY
ANGRYAT
ANGUISH
ANGULAR
ENGAGED
ENGAGER
ENGAGES
ENGARDE
ENGILDS
ENGINED
ENGINES
ENGIRDS
ENGLAND
ENGLISH
ENGLUND
ENGLUTS
ENGORGE
ENGRAFT
ENGRAIN
ENGRAMS
ENGRAVE
ENGROSS
ENGULFS
INGALLS
INGATES
INGEMAR
INGENUE
INGESTA
INGESTS
INGLESE
INGOALS
INGOING
INGRAFT
INGRAIN
INGRATE
INGREEN
INGRESS
INGROUP
INGROWN
INGULFS
ONGOING
ONGUARD
UNGATED
UNGAUDY
UNGIDDY
UNGIRDS
UNGIVEN
UNGLOVE
UNGLUED
UNGLUES
UNGODLY
UNGORED
UNGRAND
UNGREEN
UNGRIPS
UNGROSS
UNGROWN
UNGRUFF
UNGUARD
UNGUENT
UNGULAE
UNGULAR
UNGUYED
UNGYVED

•N•G•••
ANAGRAM
ENDGAME
ENIGMAS
KNIGHTS
ONAGERS
ONEGRAM
SNAGGED
SNAGGER
SNAGSUP
SNIGLET
SNUGFIT
SNUGGED
SNUGGER
SNUGGLE
SNUGGLY
SNUGLIS
UNAGILE
UNAGING
UNOGLED

•N••G••
ANTIGEN
ANTIGUA
ANTIGUN
ENCAGED
ENCAGES
ENGAGED
ENGAGER
ENGAGES
ENRAGED
ENRAGES
ENRIGHT
ENSIGNS
ENVOGUE
INDIGEN
INDIGOS
INNAGES
INSIGHT
INSIGNE
INTEGER
INTEGRA
INVOGUE
ONSAGER
ONSIGHT
SNAGGED
SNAGGER
SNUGGED
SNUGGER
SNUGGLE
SNUGGLY
UNANGRY
UNBOGGY
UNCAGED
UNCAGES
UNEAGER
UNEDGED
UNEDGES
UNFOGGY
UNLEGAL
UNLIGHT
UNPAGAN
UNPAGED
UNREGAL
UNRIGID
UNSIGHT
UNSOGGY
UNURGED
UNVAGUE
UNWAGED

•N•••G•
ANALOGS
ANALOGY
ENDINGS
ENGORGE
ENLARGE
ENOLOGY
INARAGE
INDULGE
INKINGS
INLARGE
INNINGS
INRANGE
INVEIGH
ONEPAGE
ONETOGO
ONSTAGE
ONTHEGO
UNBOGGY
UNCLOGS
UNDERGO
UNFOGGY
UNHINGE
UNLARGE
UNMERGE
UNPLUGS
UNSNAGS
UNSOGGY
UNSTAGY
UNTOUGH
UNWEDGE

•N••••G
ANELING
ANGLING
ANTEING
ANTIFOG
ANTILOG
ENDLONG
ENDUING
ENSUING
ENURING
ENVYING
GNAWING
INCHING
INGOING
INKLING
INLYING
INTHING
INURING
KNEEING
KNIFING
KNOWING
ONGOING
SNAKING
SNARING
SNIPING
SNORING
SNOWING
UNAGING
UNDOING
UNDYING
UNITING
UNLYING
UNOWING
UNSLING
UNSLUNG
UNSTUNG
UNSWUNG
UNTYING
UNVYING
UNWRUNG
UNYOUNG

••NG•••
BANGERS
BANGING
BANGKOK
BANGLED
BANGLES
BANGOUT
BANGSON
BANGSUP
BENGALI
BENGALS
BENGUNN
BINGERS
BINGHAM
BINGING
BINGLES
BINGOES
BONGING
BONGOES
BUNGEES
BUNGING
BUNGLED
BUNGLER
BUNGLES
CONGAED
CONGAME
CONGEAL
CONGERS
CONGEST
CONGOUS
DANGELO
DANGERS
DANGLED
DANGLER
DANGLES
DINGBAT
DINGERS
DINGIER
DINGILY
DINGING
DINGLES
DINGOES
DONGLES
DUNGEON
FANGING
FINGALS
FINGERS
FUNGOES
GANGERS
GANGING
GANGLIA
GANGSAW
GANGSTA
GANGSUP
GANGTOK
GANGWAY
GENGHIS
GINGAME
GINGERS
GINGERY
GINGHAM
GINGIVA
GINGKOS
GINGOLD
GONGING
GONGORA
HANGARS
HANGBYS
HANGDOG
HANGERS
HANGING
HANGMAN
HANGMEN
HANGOFF
HANGOUT
HANGSBY
HANGSIN
HANGSON
HANGSUP
HANGTEN
HANGUPS
HINGEON
HINGING
HUNGARY
HUNGERS
HUNGOFF
HUNGOUT
HUNGTEN
JANGLED
JANGLER
JANGLES
JINGLED
JINGLER
JINGLES
JINGOES
JUNGIAN
JUNGLES
KINGDOM
KINGING
KINGLET
KINGMAN
KINGPIN
KINGRAT
KINGTUT
LANGDON
LANGHAM
LANGLEY
LANGTON
LANGTRY
LANGUID
LANGUOR
LANGWAY
LENGTHS
LENGTHY
LENGUAS
LINGCOD
LINGERS
LINGOES
LINGUAE
LINGUAL
LINGULA
LONGAGO
LONGARM
LONGBED
LONGBOW
LONGDAY
LONGDEN
LONGEST
LONGFOR
LONGIES
LONGING
LONGISH
LONGRUN
LONGTOM
LONGTON
LONGUES
LONGWAY
LUNGEAT
LUNGERS
LUNGING
MANGANO
MANGERS
MANGIER
MANGLED
MANGLER
MANGLES
MANGOES
MINGIER
MINGLED
MINGLER
MINGLES
MONGERS
MONGKUT
MONGOLS
MONGREL
NONGOGO
NONGOLD
NUNGWEN
OWNGOAL
PANGAEA
PANGRAM
PENGUIN
PINGERS
PINGING
PINGUID
PONGEES
PONGIDS
PUNGENT
RANGERS
RANGFOR
RANGIER
RANGING
RANGOFF
RANGOON
RANGOUT
RINGERS
RINGFOR
RINGING
RINGLET
RINGOFF
RINGOUT
RINGSIN
RINGSUP
RUNGFOR
RUNGOFF
RUNGOUT
SANGOUT
SANGRIA
SINGERS
SINGING
SINGLED
SINGLES
SINGLET
SINGOUT
SINGSTO
SONGFUL
SUNGLOW
SUNGODS
SYNGMAN
TANGELO
TANGENT
TANGIER
TANGING
TANGLED
TANGLER
TANGLES
TANGOED
TANGOER
TANGRAM
TINGING
TINGLED
TINGLER
TINGLES
TINGODS
TONGANS
TONGING
TONGUES
TUNGOIL
VANGOGH
WANGLED
WANGLER
WANGLES
WINGERS
WINGING
WINGLET
WINGMAN
WINGMEN
WINGNUT
WINGSIT
WINGTIP
XINGOUT
YANGTZE
ZINGERS
ZINGIER
ZINGING

••N•G••
ATNIGHT
BENIGNI
BENIGNO
CONAGRA
DONEGAL
DONEGAN
FINAGLE
GINKGOS
HANDGUN
INNAGES
LINAGES
LONIGAN
MANAGED
MANAGER
MANAGES
MANAGUA
MANEGES
MENAGES
MINOGUE
NONAGES
NONAGON
RENEGED
RENEGER
RENEGES
RONTGEN
SENEGAL
TANAGER
TONIGHT
VINEGAR
WINDGOD

••N••G•
AWNINGS
BANDAGE
BONDAGE
CANINGS
CINERGY
CONDIGN
CONSIGN
DONOTGO
DUNNAGE
GONZAGA
GUNDOGS
INNINGS
LENTIGO
LINEAGE
LININGS
LINKAGE
LONGAGO
MININGS
MINTAGE
MONTAGE
MONTAGU
MONTEGO
NONGOGO
NONWAGE
PANURGE
SINKAGE
SUNDOGS
SYNERGY
TANKAGE
TONNAGE
VANGOGH
VANTAGE
VANVOGT
VENTAGE
VINTAGE
WANTAGH
WINDAGE
WINDIGO

••N•••G
BANDING
BANGING
BANKING
BANNING
BANTING
BENDING
BENNING
BINDING
BINGING
BINNING
BONDING
BONGING
BONKING
BUNGING
BUNKING
BUNNING
BUNTING
CANNING
CANTING
CENSING
CONKING
CONNING
CUNNING
DANCING
DANNING
DENHAAG
DENNING
DENTING
DENYING
DINGING
DINNING
DINTING
DONKING
DONNING
DUNKING
DUNNING
FANGING
FANNING
FENCING
FENDING
FINDING
FINKING
FUNDING
FUNFZIG
FUNKING
FUNNING
GANGING
GINNING
GINSENG
GONGING
GUNNING
HANDBAG
HANDING
HANGDOG
HANGING
HINDLEG
HINGING
HINTING
HONKING
HUNTING
JINXING
JUNEBUG
JUNKING
KENNING
KINGING
KINKING
LANCING
LANDING
LANDTAG
LANSING
LENDING
LINKING
LINTING
LONBORG
LONGING
LUNGING
MANNING
MENDING
MINCING
MINDING
MINTING
MONOLOG
NANJING
NANKING
NONDRUG
OINKING
PANNING
PANTING
PANTLEG
PENDING
PENNING
PINGING
PINKING
PINNING
PONDING
PONYING
PONYKEG
PUNNING
PUNTING
RANGING
RANKING
RANTING
RENDING
RENTING
RINGING
RINSING
RUNNING
SANDBAG
SANDHOG
SANDING
SENDING
SENSING
SINGING
SINKING
SINNING
SUNNING
SYNCING
TANGING
TANKING
TANNING
TENDING
TENSING
TENTING
TENTPEG
TENZING
TINGING
TINNING
TINTING
TONGING
VANNING
VENDING
VENTING
WANNING
WANTING
WENDING
WINCING
WINDBAG
WINDING
WINGING
WINKING
WINNING
WINSBIG
WONTING
YANKING
YENNING
ZINCING
ZINGING
ZONKING

•••NG••
ACINGIT
AMONGST
ATINGLE
AVENGED
AVENGER
AVENGES
AZINGER
BRENGUN
BRINGER
BRINGIN
BRINGIT
BRINGON
BRINGTO
BRINGUP
CHANGED
CHANGER
CHANGES
CLANGED
CLANGER
CLANGOR
CLINGER
CLINGTO
CLUNGTO
CRINGED
CRINGES
CUINGIN
DOINGIN
DOINGOK
DOINGSO
DOINGTO
DOINGUP
EKINGBY
ERYNGOS
EVANGEL
FLANGES
FLINGAT
FLINGER
FLUNGAT
FRINGED
FRINGES
GOINGAT
GOINGBY
GOINGIN
GOINGON
GOINGTO
GOINGUP
GRANGER
GRANGES
GRINGOS
GRUNGER
GRUNGES
HUANGHE
HUANGTI
ICINGIN
ICINGIT
ICINGUP
JOHNGAY
KLINGER
KLINGON
KRINGLE
LOUNGED
LOUNGER
LOUNGES
LYINGBY
LYINGON
LYINGTO
LYINGUP
MOONGOD
NEONGAS
NOANGEL
ODINGON
ORANGES
ORANGEY
OWINGON
OWINGTO
PAANGAS
PLUNGED
PLUNGER
PLUNGES
PRINGLE
PRONGED
RAINGOD
SHANGRI
SHINGLE
SHINGLY
SLINGER
SPANGLE
SPANGLY
SPONGED
SPONGER
SPONGES
STENGEL
STENGUN
STINGER
STUNGUN
SWINGAT
SWINGBY
SWINGER
SWINGIT
SWUNGAT
SWUNGBY
SWUNGIT
TLINGIT
TSONGAS
TWANGED
TWANGER
TWINGED
TWINGES
TYINGIN
TYINGON
TYINGTO
TYINGUP
UNANGRY
USINGIN
USINGUP
WHANGED
WRANGEL
WRANGLE
WRINGER
WRONGED
WRONGER
WRONGLY
YOUNGER
YOUNGMC
YOUNGUN
ZWINGLI

•••N•G•
BRANAGH
CARNAGE
COINAGE
DUNNAGE
EGGNOGS
IRONAGE
MEANAGE
OFANAGE
PEONAGE
SIGNAGE
TEENAGE
TONNAGE
UNSNAGS

•••N••G
ALINING
ATONING
BANNING
BARNING
BEANBAG
BEANING
BENNING
BINNING
BRINING
BUNNING
BURNING
CANNING
CHINWAG
CLONING
COINING
CONNING
COONDOG
CORNDOG
CORNING
CRANING
CUNNING
DAMNING
DANNING
DARNING
DAWNING
DENNING
DINNING
DONNING
DOWNING
DRONING
DUNNING
DURNING
EARNING
EVENING
FANNING
FAWNING
FUNNING
GAINING
GINNING
GOWNING
GUNNING
HORNING
HORNUNG
HYMNING
IRONING
JOINING
KEENING
KENNING
KILNING
KOONING
LEANING
LIMNING
LOANING
MANNING
MEANING
MOANING
MOONDOG
MOONING
MORNING
NOONING
OMENING
OPENING
OPINING
PAINING
PANNING
PAWNING
PEENING
PENNING
PFENNIG
PHONING
PINNING
PLANING
PRUNING
PUNNING
RAINING
REINING
RUINING
RUNNING
SEINING
SHINDIG
SHINING
SIGNING
SINNING
STONING
SUNNING
TANNING
TINNING
TURNING
TWINING
VANNING
VEINING
WANNING
WARNING
WEANING
WHINING
WINNING
YARNING
YAWNING
YEANING
YENNING
ZWANZIG

••••NG•
AIRINGS
ALLONGE
ARCINGS
ARRANGE
AWNINGS
BELONGS
BLUINGS
BODINGS
BOEINGS
BORINGS
BYJINGO
CANINGS
CASINGS
COMINGS
DATINGS
DEFANGS
DERANGE
DOMINGO
DUGONGS
DURANGO
EDGINGS
ENDINGS
ERLANGS
EXPUNGE
FACINGS
FILINGS
FIRINGS
FIXINGS
FOLENGO
GATINGS
HAYINGS
HAZINGS
HIDINGS
IIKINGS
IMPINGE
INKINGS
INNINGS
INRANGE
LACINGS
LADINGS
LAZONGA
LIKINGS
LININGS
LIVINGS
LORANGE
LOSINGS
LOZENGE
MACONGA
MAKINGS
MARENGO
MAYINGS
MELANGE
MININGS
MOWINGS
MUSINGS
OBLONGS
OFFINGS
OOLONGS
OUTINGS
PAGINGS
PALINGS
PARINGS
PAVINGS
PILINGS
PIPINGS
RAGINGS
RATINGS
RAVINGS
REHANGS
REHINGE
RESINGS
RETINGE
REVENGE
RIDINGS
RISINGS
ROVINGS
RULINGS
SALONGA
SARONGS
SAVINGS
SAYINGS
SIDINGS
SPRINGS
SPRINGY
SPYINGS
STRANGE
STRINGS
STRINGY
SYRINGE
TAKINGS
TAPINGS
THRONGS
TIDINGS
TILINGS
TIMINGS
TOWINGS
UNHINGE
URGINGS
VIKINGS
WAKINGS
WAXINGS
WIRINGS

••••N•G
PFENNIG
SILENTG

•••••NG
ABASING
ABATING
ABIDING
ABUSING
ACHTUNG
ADDLING
ADORING
AGELONG
ALAKING
ALAYING
ALINING
ALLYING
ALTHING
AMAZING
AMBLING
AMUSING
ANELING
ANGLING
ANTEING
APPLING
ARCHING
ARGUING
ARISING
ARTSONG
ATONING
AUTOING
AVOWING
AWAKING
BABYING
BACHING
BACKING
BAFFING
BAGGING
BAILING
BAITING
BALDING
BALKING
BAMMING
BANDING
BANGING
BANKING
BANNING
BANTING
BARBING
BARGING
BARKING
BARNING
BARRING
BASHING
BASKING
BASTING
BATHING
BATTING
BATWING
BAWLING
BEADING
BEAMING
BEANING
BEARING
BEATING
BEDDING
BEEFING
BEEPING
BEGGING
BEHRING
BEIJING
BELLING
BELTING
BELYING
BENDING
BENNING
BERMING
BESTING
BETTING
BIASING
BIBBING
BIDDING
BIFFING
BIGBANG
BILKING
BILLING
BINDING
BINGING
BINNING
BIRDING
BIRLING
BIRRING
BITTING
BLADING
BLAMING
BLARING
BLAZING
BLOWING
BLUEING
BOATING
BOBBING
BOFFING
BOGGING
BOILING
BOLLING
BOLTING
BOMBING
BONDING
BONGING
BONKING
BOOKING
BOOMING
BOOTING
BOOZING
BOPPING
BORKING
BOSSING
BOWLING
BRACING
BRAKING
BRAVING
BRAYING
BRAZING
BREWING
BRIBING
BRINING
BRUXING
BUCKING
BUDDING
BUDGING
BUFFING
BUGGING
BUGLING
BULGING
BULKING
BULLING
BUMMING
BUMPING
BUNGING
BUNKING
BUNNING
BUNTING
BUOYING
BURLING
BURNING
BURPING
BURRING
BURYING
BUSHING
BUSKING
BUSSING
BUSTING
BUSYING
BUTTING
BUZZING
CABBING
CABLING
CACHING
CADGING
CALKING
CALLING
CALMING
CALVING
CAMPING
CANNING
CANTING
CAPPING
CARDING
CARKING
CARLING
CARPING
CARTING
CARVING
CASHING
CASKING
CASTING
CAUSING
CEASING
CEILING
CENSING
CESSING
CHAFING
CHARING
CHASING
CHAWING
CHEFING
CHEWING
CHIDING
CHIMING
CHOKING
CHOWING
CHUTING
CLAWING
CLAYING
CLEWING
CLONING
CLOSING
CLOYING
CLUEING
COALING
COATING
COAXING
COCKING
COGGING
COIFING
COILING
COINING
COMBING
COMPING
CONKING
CONNING
COOKING
COOLING
COOPING
COPPING
COPYING
CORDING
CORKING
CORNING
COSHING
COSTING
COSYING
COUPING
COWLING
COZYING
CRANING
CRAPING
CRATING
CRAVING
CRAZING
CREPING
CREWING
CROWING
CUBBING
CUFFING
CULLING
CUNNING
CUPPING
CURBING
CURDING
CURLING
CURRING
CURSING
CURVING
CUSHING
CUSSING
CUTTING
CYCLING
CYYOUNG
DABBING
DADOING
DAMMING
DAMNING
DAMPING
DANCING
DANNING
DAPPING
DARLING
DARNING
DARTING
DASHING
DAUBING
DAWNING
DAYLONG
DEALING
DECKING
DEEDING
DEEMING
DEFYING
DEICING
DEKEING
DELEING
DELVING
DEMOING
DENNING
DENTING
DENYING
DERRING
DEUCING
DEYOUNG
DIALING
DIETING
DIGGING
DIMMING
DINGING
DINNING
DINTING
DIPPING
DIRKING
DISCING
DISHING
DISKING
DISSING
DOCKING
DODGING
DOFFING
DOGGING
DOLLING
DONKING
DONNING
DOOMING
DOSSING
DOTTING
DOUSING
DOWLING
DOWNING
DOWRONG
DOWSING
DRAPING
DRAWING
DRAYING
DRIVING

DRONING	FILLING	GAWPING	HANDING	HUTTING	KNIFING	LOTTING	MUSSING	PAUSING	PUFFING	RIGGING	SERLING	SPECING
DUBBING	FILMING	GEARING	HANGING	HYMNING	KNOWING	LOURING	MUSTANG	PAWNING	PULLING	RIMMING	SERVING	SPEWING
DUCKING	FINDING	GELDING	HARDING	HYPOING	KOONING	LOUSING	NABBING	PEAKING	PULPING	RINGING	SETTING	SPICING
DUCTING	FINKING	GELLING	HARKING	IMAGING	LACKING	LOUTING	NAGGING	PEALING	PULSING	RINSING	SHADING	SPIKING
DUELING	FIRMING	GETTING	HARMING	IMBUING	LADLING	LUCKING	NAILING	PECKING	PUMPING	RIOTING	SHAKING	SPITING
DUETING	FISHING	GIFTING	HARPING	IMGOING	LAGGING	LUFFING	NANJING	PEEKING	PUNNING	RIPPING	SHAMING	SPOKING
DULLING	FITTING	GIGGING	HASHING	INCHING	LAIRING	LUGGING	NANKING	PEELING	PUNTING	RISKING	SHAPING	SPUMING
DUMBING	FIZZING	GILDING	HASPING	INGOING	LALLING	LULLING	NAPPING	PEENING	PURGING	ROAMING	SHARING	SPYRING
DUMPING	FLAKING	GILLING	HASTING	INKLING	LAMBING	LUMPING	NEARING	PEEPING	PURLING	ROARING	SHAVING	STAGING
DUNKING	FLAMING	GIMPING	HATTING	INLYING	LAMMING	LUNGING	NECKING	PEERING	PURRING	ROBBING	SHEBANG	STAKING
DUNNING	FLARING	GINNING	HAULING	INTHING	LANCING	LURKING	NEEDING	PEEVING	PURSING	ROCKING	SHINING	STARING
DURNING	FLAWING	GINSENG	HAWKING	INURING	LANDING	LUSTING	NERVING	PEGGING	PUSHING	RODDING	SHOEING	STATING
DUSKING	FLAYING	GIRDING	HEADING	IRISING	LANSING	MADDING	NESTING	PEIPING	PUTTING	ROGUING	SHOOING	STAVING
DUSTING	FLEEING	GIRTING	HEALING	IRONING	LAPPING	MAILING	NETTING	PELTING	QUAKING	ROILING	SHORING	STAYING
EAGLING	FLEMING	GISSING	HEAPING	ISSUING	LAPSANG	MAIMING	NIALONG	PENDING	QUEUING	ROLFING	SHOVING	STEWING
EARNING	FLEXING	GITTING	HEARING	ITCHING	LAPSING	MALTING	NICHING	PENNING	QUOTING	ROLLING	SHOWING	STOKING
EARRING	FLOWING	GLARING	HEATING	ITEMING	LAPWING	MANNING	NICKING	PEPPING	RACKING	ROMPING	SIBLING	STONING
EASTING	FLUTING	GLAZING	HEAVING	JABBING	LARDING	MAPPING	NIPPING	PERKING	RAFTING	ROOFING	SICCING	STORING
ECHOING	FLUXING	GLIDING	HEDGING	JACKING	LARKING	MARKING	NOCKING	PERMING	RAGGING	ROOKING	SIDLING	STOWING
EDDYING	FOALING	GLOBING	HEEDING	JAGGING	LASHING	MARRING	NODDING	PETTING	RAIDING	ROOMING	SIEGING	STUBING
EDITING	FOAMING	GLOVING	HEELING	JAILING	LASTING	MASHING	NOISING	PHASING	RAILING	ROOTING	SIEVING	STYLING
EDUCING	FOBBING	GLOWING	HEFTING	JAMMING	LATHING	MASKING	NOONING	PHONING	RAINING	ROTTING	SIFTING	SUBBING
ELATING	FOGGING	GNAWING	HELMING	JARRING	LAUDING	MASSING	NOOSING	PICKING	RAISING	ROUGING	SIGHING	SUBKING
ELIDING	FOILING	GOADING	HELPING	JAZZING	LEADING	MASTING	NOSHING	PIECING	RAMMING	ROUSING	SIGNING	SUBLONG
ELOPING	FOLDING	GOALONG	HELSING	JEERING	LEAFING	MATTING	NOTHING	PIGGING	RAMPING	ROUTING	SILOING	SUCKING
ELUDING	FOOLING	GODLING	HEMMING	JELLING	LEAKING	MAULING	NOTTING	PILLING	RANGING	ROWLING	SILTING	SUDSING
ELUTING	FOOTING	GOLDING	HERDING	JERKING	LEANING	MEANING	NUDGING	PINGING	RANKING	RRATING	SINGING	SUITING
EMOTING	FORCING	GOLFING	HERRING	JESTING	LEAPING	MEETING	NULLING	PINKING	RANTING	RSVPING	SINKING	SULKING
ENDLONG	FORDING	GONGING	HIBBING	JETTING	LEASING	MELDING	NUMBING	PINNING	RAPPING	RUBBING	SINNING	SUMMING
ENDUING	FORGING	GOODING	HILLING	JIGGING	LEAVING	MELTING	NURSING	PIQUING	RAPSONG	RUCHING	SIPPING	SUNNING
ENSUING	FORKING	GOOFING	HILTING	JILTING	LEERING	MEMLING	NUTTING	PISHING	RASPING	RUCKING	SITTING	SUPPING
ENURING	FORMING	GOOSING	HINGING	JINXING	LEGGING	MENDING	OBEYING	PITHING	RATTING	RUFFING	SKATING	SURFING
ENVYING	FOULING	GORGING	HINTING	JOBBING	LEMMING	MEOWING	OILRING	PITTING	RAZZING	RUINING	SKEWING	SURGING
ERASING	FOWLING	GORMING	HISSING	JOGGING	LENDING	MERGING	OINKING	PITYING	RDLAING	RUNNING	SLAKING	SUSSING
ERELONG	FRAMING	GOSLING	HITSONG	JOINING	LESSING	MESHING	OKAYING	PLACING	READING	RUSHING	SLATING	SWAYING
ERODING	FRAYING	GOUGING	HITTING	JOLTING	LETTING	MESSING	OLDSONG	PLANING	REAMING	RUSTING	SLAVING	SWIPING
ESPYING	FREEING	GOWNING	HOAXING	JOSHING	LEVYING	MEWLING	OMENING	PLATING	REAPING	RUTTING	SLAYING	SYNCING
ESTRING	FRELENG	GOWRONG	HOBOING	JOTTING	LIBBING	MIFFING	ONGOING	PLAYING	REARING	SACKING	SLEWING	TABBING
ETCHING	FRODING	GRACING	HOCKING	JREWING	LICKING	MILKING	OPENING	PLOWING	REAVING	SADSONG	SLICING	TABLING
EVADING	FUDGING	GRADING	HODDING	JUDGING	LIFTING	MILLING	OPINING	PLUMING	REDDING	SAGGING	SLIDING	TABUING
EVELONG	FUELING	GRATING	HOGGING	JUGGING	LILTING	MINCING	ORATING	POISING	REDKING	SAILING	SLIMING	TACKING
EVENING	FUNDING	GRAVING	HOLDING	JUICING	LIMBING	MINDING	OURGANG	POLLING	REDOING	SALTING	SLOPING	TAGGING
EVOKING	FUNKING	GRAYING	HONKING	JUMPING	LIMNING	MINTING	OURSONG	PONDING	REDWING	SALVING	SLOWING	TAILING
EXILING	FUNNING	GRAZING	HOODING	JUNKING	LIMPING	MISSING	OUSTING	PONYING	REDYING	SAMSUNG	SMILING	TALKING
EXITING	FURLING	GREYING	HOOFING	JURYING	LINKING	MISTING	OUTKING	POOLING	REEDING	SANDING	SMITING	TAMPING
EXUDING	FURLONG	GRIMING	HOOKING	JUTTING	LINTING	MITRING	OUTRANG	POOPING	REEFING	SAPLING	SMOKING	TANGING
FABLING	FURRING	GRIPING	HOOPING	KACHING	LIPPING	MOANING	OUTRING	POPPING	REEKING	SAPPING	SNAKING	TANKING
FAILING	FUSSING	GROPING	HOOTING	KAMFONG	LISPING	MOBBING	OUTSANG	POPSONG	REELING	SASHING	SNARING	TANNING
FAIRING	FUTZING	GROWING	HOPPING	KAYOING	LISTING	MOCKING	OUTSING	PORKING	REEVING	SASSING	SNIPING	TAPPING
FALLING	FUZZING	GSTRING	HOPSING	KEDGING	LOADING	MOILING	OUTSUNG	PORTING	REFFING	SAUCING	SNORING	TARRING
FANGING	GABBING	GUIDING	HORDING	KEELING	LOAFING	MOLDING	OUTWING	POSTING	REFYING	SCALING	SNOWING	TARTING
FANNING	GADDING	GUILING	HORNING	KEENING	LOAMING	MOLTING	PACKING	POTTING	REICING	SCARING	SOAKING	TASKING
FARCING	GAFFING	GULFING	HORNUNG	KEEPING	LOANING	MOONING	PADDING	POURING	REINING	SCOPING	SOAPING	TASTING
FARMING	GAGGING	GULLING	HORSING	KEGGING	LOBBING	MOORING	PAINING	POUTING	RELYING	SCORING	SOARING	TATTING
FASTING	GAINING	GULPING	HOSTING	KENNING	LOCKING	MOOTING	PAIRING	PRATING	RENDING	SEALING	SOBBING	TAXIING
FATLING	GAITING	GUMMING	HOUSING	KEYRING	LODGING	MOPPING	PALLING	PRAYING	RENTING	SEAMING	SOCKING	TEAMING
FATTING	GALLING	GUNNING	HOWLING	KICKING	LOFTING	MORNING	PALMING	PRESONG	REPPING	SEARING	SODDING	TEARING
FAWNING	GAMMING	GUSHING	HOWLONG	KIDDING	LOGGING	MOSHING	PANNING	PREYING	RESTING	SEATING	SOILING	TEASING
FEARING	GANGING	GUSTING	HUFFING	KILLING	LOIDING	MOSSING	PANTING	PRICING	RETTING	SEBRING	SOLOING	TEEMING
FEEDING	GAOLING	GUTTING	HUGGING	KILNING	LOLLING	MOUSING	PARGING	PRIDING	REUSING	SEEDING	SOLVING	TELLING
FEELING	GAPPING	GYPPING	HULKING	KILTING	LONGING	MRWRONG	PARKING	PRIMING	REVVING	SEEKING	SOPPING	TEMPING
FELLING	GARBING	HACKING	HULLING	KINGING	LOOKING	MUCKING	PARRING	PRIZING	RHYMING	SEEMING	SORTING	TENDING
FELTING	GASHING	HAFTING	HUMMING	KINKING	LOOMING	MUDDING	PARSING	PROBING	RIBBING	SEEPING	SOURING	TENSING
FENCING	GASPING	HAILING	HUNTING	KIPLING	LOOPING	MUFFING	PARTING	PROLONG	RIDDING	SEINING	SOUSING	TENTING
FENDING	GASSING	HALOING	HURLING	KIPPING	LOOSING	MUGGING	PASSING	PROSING	RIDGING	SEIZING	SPACING	TENZING
FESSING	GATLING	HALTING	HURTING	KISSING	LOOTING	MULLING	PASTING	PROVING	RIFFING	SELLING	SPADING	TERMING
FEUDING	GAUGING	HALVING	HUSHING	KITTING	LOPPING	MUMMING	PATTING	PRUNING	RIFLING	SENDING	SPARING	TESTING
FIBBING	GAWKING	HAMMING	HUSKING	KNEEING	LORDING	MUSHING	PAULING	PUDDING	RIFTING	SENSING	SPAYING	TEXTING

THAWING
THEGANG
THEKING
THERING
TICCING
TICKING
TIDYING
TIERING
TIFFING
TILLING
TILTING
TINGING
TINNING
TINTING
TIPPING
TITHING
TITLING
TITRING
TOGGING
TOILING
TOLLING
TONGING
TOOLING
TOOLONG
TOOTING
TOPPING
TOSSING
TOTTING
TOURING
TOUTING
TRACING
TRADING
TREEING
TROWING
TRUEING
TSETUNG
TUBBING
TUCKING
TUFTING
TUGGING
TURFING
TURNING
TUSKING
TUTTING
TWINING
UNAGING
UNDOING
UNDYING
UNITING
UNLYING
UNOWING
UNSLING
UNSLUNG
UNSTUNG
UNSWUNG
UNTYING
UNVYING
UNWRUNG
UNYOUNG
UPFLING
UPGOING
UPSWING
VALUING
VAMPING
VANNING
VARYING
VATTING
VEERING

VEGGING
VEILING
VEINING
VENDING
VENTING
VERGING
VERSING
VESTING
VETOING
VETTING
VIALING
VIEWING
VISAING
VOGUING
VOICING
VOIDING
WADDING
WAFTING
WAGGING
WAILING
WAITING
WAIVING
WALKING
WALLING
WANNING
WANTING
WARDING
WARMING
WARNING
WARPING
WARRENG
WARRING
WASHING
WASTING
WAXWING
WEANING
WEARING
WEAVING
WEBBING
WEDDING
WEDGING
WEEDING
WEEPING
WELDING
WELLING
WELTING
WENDING
WETTING
WHALING
WHILING
WHINING
WHITING
WICKING
WIFYING
WIGGING
WILDING
WILLING
WILTING
WIMPING
WINCING
WINDING
WINGING
WINKING
WINNING
WISHING
WISPING
WITLING
WITTING

WOLFING
WONTING
WOODING
WOOFING
WORDING
WORKING
WORMING
WRITING
WYOMING
XRATING
XRAYING
YAKKING
YANKING
YAOMING
YAPPING
YARDING
YARNING
YAWNING
YAWPING
YEANING
YELLING
YELPING
YENNING
YESSING
YIPPING
YOURANG
YOWLING
YOYOING
YUKKING
ZAGGING
ZAPPING
ZEITUNG
ZEROING
ZESTING
ZIERING
ZIGGING
ZINCING
ZINGING
ZIPPING
ZONKING
ZOOMING

NH•••••
NHLGAME
NHLTEAM

N•H••••
NAHUATL
NOHANDS

N••H•••
NAPHTHA
NATHANS
NEPHEWS
NEPHRIC
NEWHAND
NEWHART
NEWHATS
NEWHIRE
NEWHOPE
NICHING
NICHOLS
NIGHEST
NIGHTER
NIGHTIE
NIGHTLY
NOBHILL
NONHERO

NONHITS
NONHOME
NOSHERS
NOSHING
NOSHOWS
NOTHERE
NOTHING
NOTHINS
NOTHOME
NOWHERE
NUNHOOD

N•••H••
NARTHEX
NARWHAL
NATCHEZ
NAUGHTS
NAUGHTY
NAVAHOS
NEEDHAM
NEIGHED
NEITHER
NINTHLY
NOOTHER
NORTHER
NORTHOF
NOTCHED
NOTCHER
NOTCHES
NOUGHTS
NOWTHEN
NOWTHIS
NOWWHAT
NUDZHED
NUDZHES
NUNSHIP
NYMPHAL
NYMPHIC

N••••H•
NAPHTHA
NATASHA
NIEBUHR
NOGUCHI

N•••••H
NAGGISH
NCWYETH
NEBBISH
NEOLITH
NERDISH
NESMITH
NEWMATH
NEWRICH
NIDETCH
NILESOH
NINEVEH
NKRUMAH
NOCATCH
NONCASH
NONSUCH
NORRISH
NORWICH
NOTMUCH
NOTWITH
NOURISH
NUNNISH

•NH••••
ENHANCE
INHABIT
INHALED
INHALER
INHALES
INHASTE
INHERED
INHERES
INHERIT
INHIBIT
INHOUSE
INHUMAN
INHUMED
INHUMER
INHUMES
UNHAIRS
UNHAIRY
UNHANDS
UNHANDY
UNHAPPY
UNHARDY
UNHARSH
UNHASPS
UNHASTY
UNHATED
UNHAYED
UNHAZED
UNHEADY
UNHEARD
UNHEAVY
UNHEEDS
UNHELMS
UNHEWED
UNHILLY
UNHINGE
UNHIRED
UNHIRES
UNHITCH
UNHONED
UNHOODS
UNHOOKS
UNHOPED
UNHORSE
UNHOUSE
UNHULLS
UNHUMAN
UNHUMID
UNHUSKS

•N•H•••
ANAHEIM
ANCHORS
ANCHOVY
ANTHEIL
ANTHEMS
ANTHERS
ANTHILL
ANTHONY
ANTHRAX
ANYHOPE
ENCHAIN
ENCHANT
ENCHASE
ENTHRAL
ENTHUSE
INAHEAP
INAHOLE

INAHUFF
INCHECK
INCHERS
INCHING
INKHORN
INPHASE
INSHAPE
INSHOCK
INSHORE
INSHORT
INTHERE
INTHING
INTHIRD
INTHREE
INWHITE
ONEHALF
ONEHAND
ONEHOUR
ONSHORE
ONTHEDL
ONTHEGO
ONTHEQT
ONTHREE
UNCHAIN
UNCHAIR
UNCHARY
UNCHECK
UNCHOKE
UNCHURN
UNRHYME
UNSHADE
UNSHADY
UNSHARP
UNSHEER
UNSHELL
UNSHIER
UNSHIFT
UNSHINY
UNSHIPS
UNSHOED
UNSHOES
UNSHORN
UNSHORT
UNSHOWN
UNSHOWY
UNSHYER
UNSHYLY
UNTHAWS
UNTHICK
UNTHINK
UNWHEEL
UNWHIPT
UNWHITE
UNWHOLE

•N••H••
ANDTHEN
ANOTHER
GNASHED
GNASHER
GNASHES
INASHOE
KNEWHOW
KNIGHTS
KNISHES
KNOWHOW
ONAWHIM
ONECHIP

ONESHOE
ONESHOT
ONEWHIT
SNOWHAT-

•N•••H•
ANARCHS
ANARCHY
ENRIGHT
GNOCCHI
INSIGHT
ONSIGHT
UNLIGHT
UNMACHO
UNSIGHT

•N••••H
ANDSUCH
ANGUISH
ANOUILH
ANSPACH
ANTIOCH
ENGLISH
GNOMISH
INARUSH
INDEPTH
INDUTCH
INFAITH
INMARCH
INREACH
INSYNCH
INTOUCH
INTRUTH
INVEIGH
KNAVISH
KNOWETH
ONEARTH
ONEINCH
ONLEASH
SNEETCH
UNBENCH
UNBERTH
UNCINCH
UNCOUTH
UNEARTH
UNFAITH
UNFERTH
UNHARSH
UNHITCH
UNLATCH
UNLEASH
UNLOATH
UNTEACH
UNTOUGH
UNTRUTH

••NH•••
BONHEUR
DENHAAG
IANHOLM
JONHALL
MANHEIM
MANHOLE
MANHOOD
MANHOUR
MANHUNT
MYNHEER
NONHERO

NONHITS
NONHOME
NUNHOOD
PINHEAD
PINHOLE
RANHOME
RUNHOME
SENHORA
SUNHATS
TINHATS
TINHORN

••N•H••
AINTHAY
BANSHEE
BENCHED
BENCHER
BENCHES
BENTHAM
BENTHOS
BINGHAM
BUNCHED
BUNCHES
BUNCHUP
CANCHAS
CINCHED
CINCHES
CONCHAE
CONCHES
CONCHOS
CYNTHIA
DONAHUE
DONOHOE
FINCHES
GENGHIS
GINGHAM
GUNSHIP
GUNSHOT
GUNTHER
HONCHOS
HUNCHED
HUNCHES
KINSHIP
LANGHAM
LUNCHED
LUNCHER
LUNCHES
MENTHOL
MENUHIN
MONTHLY
MUNCHED
MUNCHEN
MUNCHER
MUNCHES
MUNCHIE
MUNCHON
NINTHLY
NUNSHIP
PANCHAX
PANTHER
PINCHAS
PINCHED
PINCHER
PINCHES
PINCHME
PINCHOT
PINKHAM
PONCHOS

PUNCHED
PUNCHER
PUNCHES
PUNCHIN
PUNCHUP
PYNCHON
RANCHED
RANCHER
RANCHES
RANCHOS
SANDHOG
SONSHIP
SYNCHED
TENCHES
TENTHLY
WENCHES
WINCHED
WINCHER
WINCHES
WYNDHAM
XANTHAN
XANTHIC

••N••H•
ATNIGHT
BINOCHE
DENNEHY
FINISHD
KANEOHE
KENICHI
KENOSHA
KENWAHL
LENGTHS
LENGTHY
MENSCHY
ORNITHO
PANACHE
PENUCHE
TONIGHT
ZENITHS

••N•••H
BENEATH
BONEASH
DONNISH
DUNCISH
FINNISH
HANUKAH
HENNISH
HENRICH
HUNNISH
KENNETH
KENTISH
LONGISH
MANNISH
MENORAH
MINXISH
MONARCH
MONKISH
MRNORTH
NINEVEH
NONCASH
NONSUCH
NUNNISH
PANFISH
PINKISH
RANKISH
RANWITH

RUNNETH
RUNTISH
RUNWITH
SUNBATH
SUNFISH
TANNISH
TINFISH
UPNORTH
VANGOGH
WANNISH
WANTAGH
XENIAOH
ZANYISH

•••NH••
IVANHOE
RAINHAT
WERNHER

•••N•H•
ACANTHI
BIANCHI
BLANCHE
BRANCHY
BRONCHI
BRONCHO
CRUNCHY
DENNEHY
FRANCHI
FRENCHI
FRENCHS
HUANGHE
PAUNCHY
PLINTHS
RAUNCHY

•••N••H
ALANNAH
BRANAGH
BRINISH
BURNISH
CORNISH
DONNISH
DRONISH
EVANISH
FURNISH
GARNISH
GWYNETH
HENNISH
HORNISH
HUNNISH
KEENENH
KENNETH
KLENSCH
MANNISH
MOONISH
NUNNISH
PLANISH
PLENISH
RHENISH
RUNNETH
SPANISH
SPINACH
SWINISH
TANNISH
TARNISH
TOWNISH

VARNISH
WANNISH

••••NH•
PIRANHA

••••N•H
ABSINTH
AKRONOH
ALANNAH
ATLUNCH
CORINTH
DOLUNCH
DOZENTH
INSYNCH
JACINTH
MISHNAH
ONEINCH
ROMANSH
SCRUNCH
SEVENTH
SILENTH
SQUINCH
STAUNCH
UNBENCH
UNCINCH

•••••NH
CHIMINH
KEENENH

NI•••••
NIAGARA
NIALONG
NIANTIC
NIBBLED
NIBBLER
NIBBLES
NIBLETS
NIBLICK
NIBLIKE
NICCAGE
NICCOLO
NICEBOY
NICEDAY
NICEDOG
NICEGUY
NICEJOB
NICEKID
NICEMAN
NICEMEN
NICEONE
NICETRY
NICHING
NICHOLS
NICKELS
NICKERS
NICKING
NICKLES
NICOBAR
NICOISE
NICOLAS
NICOLET
NICOLLE
NICOSIA
NICTATE
NIDETCH
NIEBUHR

NIELSEN
NIFTIER
NIFTIES
NIFTILY
NIGERIA
NIGGLED
NIGGLER
NIGGLES
NIGHEST
NIGHTER
NIGHTIE
NIGHTLY
NIKEADS
NIKOLAI
NIKOLAY
NILESOH
NILSSON
NIMBLER
NIMIETY
NIMRODS
NINEEEE
NINEPIN
NINEVEH
NINNIES
NINTHLY
NIOBITE
NIOBIUM
NIPIGON
NIPMUCK
NIPPERS
NIPPIER
NIPPILY
NIPPING
NIPPLES
NIRVANA
NISSANS
NISSANZ
NITPICK
NITRATE
NITRIDE
NITRIFY
NITRITE
NITROUS
NITTANY
NITTIER
NITWITS
NIVEOUS

N•I••••
NAIADES
NAILERS
NAILGUN
NAILING
NAILKEG
NAILSET
NAILSIN
NAILSIT
NAILSUP
NAILTIP
NAIPAUL
NAIROBI
NAIVELY
NAIVEST
NAIVETE
NAIVETY
NEIGHED
NEITHER
NOISIER

NOISILY
NOISING
NOISOME

N••I•••
NABISCO
NAMIBIA
NAPIERS
NATIONS
NATIVES
NAVIDAD
NERISSA
NETIZEN
NEUILLY
NEVILLE
NEWIDEA
NIMIETY
NIPIGON
NODICAL
NOGIFTS
NOLIMIT
NOMINAL
NOMINEE
NONIRON
NORIEGA
NORITES
NOSIEST
NOSIREE
NOTICED
NOTICER
NOTICES
NOTIONS
NOVICES
NOVISAD
NOWISEE
NOWISER
NOXIOUS
NUBIANS
NUBIRAS
NUDISTS
NYGIANT
NYTIMES

N•••I••
NABBING
NAGGIER
NAGGING
NAGGISH
NAILING
NANAIMO
NANJING
NANKING
NANNIED
NANNIES
NAPKINS
NAPPIER
NAPPIES
NAPPING
NAPTIME
NASTIER
NASTIES
NASTILY
NATRIUM
NATTIER
NATTILY
NATWICK
NAUTICA
NAUTILI

NAVAIDS NBALIVE NEARING NEBBISH NECKING NEEDIER NEEDILY NEEDING NENNIUS NEOLITH NERDIER NERDISH NEREIDS NERVIER NERVILY NERVINE NERVING NESBITT NESMITH NESTING NETLIKE NETTING NEWBIES NEWHIRE NEWKIDS NEWLIFE NEWLINE NEWMINT NEWRICH NEWSIER NEWSIES NIBLICK NIBLIKE NICHING NICKING NICOISE NIFTIER NIFTIES NIFTILY NINNIES NIOBITE NIOBIUM NIPPIER NIPPILY NIPPING NITPICK NITRIDE NITRIFY NITRITE NITTIER NITWITS NOBBIER NOBHILL NOCKING NODDIES NODDING NOETICS NOGGINS NOISIER NOISILY NOISING NONDIET NONHITS NONLIFE NONLIVE NONOILY NONOISE NOOGIES NOONING NOOSING NORDICA NORDICS NORRISH NORWICH NOSHING NOTHING NOTHINS NOTLIKE NOTLIVE NOTMINE NOTNICE NOTTING NOTWITH NOURISH NUBBIER NUBBINS NUCLIDE NUDGING NUDNIKS NULLIFY NULLING NULLITY NUMBING NUNCIOS NUNLIKE NUNNISH NUPTIAL NURSING NUTLIKE NUTOILS NUTPINE NUTRIAS NUTSIER NUTTIER NUTTILY NUTTING

N••••I•

NAILSIN NAILSIT NAILTIP NAMIBIA NATALIA NATALIE NAYARIT NAYSAID NEATNIK NECKTIE NEMESIS NEPALIS NEPHRIC NEPOTIC NESQUIK NESTSIN NETFLIX NETGAIN NEWLAID NIANTIC NICEKID NICOSIA NIGERIA NIGHTIE NINEPIN NOKOMIS NOLIMIT NOMADIC NONACID NONDRIP NONEPIC NONEVIL NONPAID NONSKID NONSLIP NONVOID NOSEDIN NOSESIN NOSTAIN NOSTRIL NOTABIT NOTALIE NOTFAIR NOVALIS NOWTHIS NUCLEIC NUMERIC NUNSHIP NYMPHIC

N•••••I

NAIROBI NAUTILI NEGRONI NIKOLAI NOGUCHI

•NI••••

ANILINE ANILITY ANIMACY ANIMALS ANIMATE ANIMATO ANIMISM ANIMIST ANIONIC ANISEED ANISTON ANITRAS DNIEPER ENIGMAS ENISLED ENISLES ININETY INIRONS INITIAL KNIEVEL KNIFERS KNIFING KNIGHTS KNISHES KNITTED KNITTER SNICKER SNICKET SNIDELY SNIDEST SNIFFAT SNIFFED SNIFFER SNIFFLE SNIFFLY SNIFFUP SNIFTER SNIGLET SNIPEAT SNIPERS SNIPING SNIPOFF SNIPPED SNIPPER SNIPPET SNIVELS UNIATES UNIBALL UNIBODY UNICODE UNICORN UNIDEAL UNIFIED UNIFIER UNIFIES UNIFORM UNINERT UNINKED UNIPLEX UNIPODS UNIQUES UNISIZE UNISOMS UNISONS UNITARD UNITARY UNITERS UNITIES UNITING UNITISE UNITIVE UNITIZE UNIVACS

•N•I•••

ANCIENT ANDIAMO ANDIRON ANOINTS ANTIART ANTIBES ANTIFOG ANTIGEN ANTIGUA ANTIGUN ANTILOG ANTIOCH ANTIQUE ANTITAX ANTIWAR ANXIETY ANXIOUS ENCINAS ENDINGS ENDIVES ENFIELD ENGILDS ENGINED ENGINES ENGIRDS ENLINKS ENLISTS ENLIVEN ENOILED ENRIGHT ENRIQUE ENSIGNS ENSILED ENSILES ENTICED ENTICER ENTICES ENTIRES ENTITLE ENVIERS ENVIOUS ENVIRON ENVIROS ENWINDS INAIDOF INCISED INCISES INCISOR INCITED INCITER INCITES INCIVIL INDIANA INDIANS INDICES INDICIA INDICTS INDIGEN INDIGOS INDITED INDITER INDITES INFIDEL INFIELD INFIRST INFIVES INFIXED INFIXES INHIBIT INKIEST INKINGS INLIMBO INLINES INNINGS INSIDER INSIDES INSIGHT INSIGNE INSIPID INSISTS INVICTA INVITED INVITEE INVITER INVITES INVITRO ONEIDAS ONEINCH ONEIOTA ONEIRIC ONEIRON ONFIRST ONLIEST ONSIDES ONSIGHT ONVIDEO UNAIDED UNAIMED UNAIRED UNBINDS UNCIALS UNCINCH UNCITED UNCIVIC UNCIVIL UNDIKED UNDINES UNFIERY UNFILED UNFILES UNFINED UNFINES UNFIRED UNFITLY UNFIXED UNFIXES UNGIDDY UNGIRDS UNGIVEN UNHILLY UNHINGE UNHIRED UNHIRES UNHITCH UNKINKS UNLIGHT UNLIKED UNLIKES UNLINED UNLINKS UNLIVED UNLIVES UNMIKED UNMINED UNMIRED UNMITER UNMITRE UNMIXED UNMIXES UNOILED UNPICKS UNPIETY UNPILED UNPILES UNPIOUS UNPIPED UNRIGID UNRILED UNRIMED UNRIPER UNRISEN UNRISKY UNRIVED UNRIVEN UNSIDED UNSIGHT UNSILLY UNSIZED UNTIERS UNTILED UNTIMED UNTIMID UNTIRED UNVITAL UNVIVID UNWINDS UNWINDY UNWIPED UNWIRED UNWISER UNWITTY

•N••I••

ANACINS ANANIAS ANELING ANEMIAS ANGLING ANGRIER ANGRILY ANGUISH ANILINE ANILITY ANIMISM ANIMIST ANNUITY ANODISE ANODIZE ANOMIES ANOUILH ANTBIRD ANTEING ANTHILL ANTLIKE ANTLION ANTOINE ANTSIER ANYKIND ANYTIME ANYWISE ENDLINE ENDPINS ENDUING ENDWISE ENEMIES ENGLISH ENJOINS ENPRISE ENQUIRE ENQUIRY ENSKIED ENSKIES ENSUING ENSUITE ENTAILS ENTRIES ENTWINE ENTWIST ENURING ENVEILS ENVYING GNAWING GNOMISH GNOMIST INABIND INAJIFF INALINE INANITY INAPILE INAWINK INBRIEF INBUILT INCHING INCLINE INEDITA INEXILE INFAITH INFLICT INGOING INITIAL INKLIKE INKLING INLYING INPOINT INPRINT INQUIRE INQUIRY INRUINS INSPIRE INSPITE INSTILL INSTILS INTAILS INTHING INTHIRD INTUITS INURING INUTILE INVEIGH INVOICE INWHITE KNAVISH KNEEING KNIFING KNOWING ONABIAS ONADIET ONAKICK ONALINE ONEDIME ONEKILO ONELIRA ONEMILE ONEPINT ONESIZE ONETIME ONGOING ONPOINT ONTRIAL SNAKIER SNAKILY SNAKING SNARING SNIPING SNORING SNOWIER SNOWILY SNOWING UNAGILE UNAGING UNALIKE UNBAITS UNBRIEF UNBUILD UNBUILT UNCLIPS UNCLIPT UNCOILS UNCRIED UNCTION UNDOING UNDRIED UNDYING UNFAITH UNFRIED UNFRILL UNGRIPS UNHAIRS UNHAIRY UNIFIED UNIFIER UNIFIES UNISIZE UNITIES UNITING UNITISE UNITIVE UNITIZE UNJOINS UNJOINT UNJUICY UNKNITS UNLYING UNMOIST UNNAILS UNNAIVE UNNOISY UNOWING UNPLIED UNQUICK UNQUIET UNRAINY UNSHIER UNSHIFT UNSHINY UNSHIPS UNSLICK UNSLIER UNSLING UNSPICY UNSPIED UNSPILT UNSTICK UNSTIFF UNTHICK UNTHINK UNTRIED UNTRITE UNTWINE UNTWIST UNTYING UNVEILS UNVOICE UNVYING UNWHIPT UNWHITE

•N•••I•

ANAEMIA ANAEMIC ANAHEIM ANDROID ANEROID ANGELIC ANGLAIS ANIONIC ANNAKIN ANNELID ANOSMIA ANOSMIC ANSONIA ANTACID ANTHEIL ANTONIA ANTONIN ANTONIO ENCHAIN ENCOMIA ENDEDIN ENDEDIT ENDEMIC ENGRAIN ENTERIC ENTERIN ENTRAIN ENZYMIC GNOSTIC INAPRIL INASNIT INASPIN INASTIR INASUIT INCIVIL INDICIA INERTIA INFORIT INGRAIN INHABIT INHERIT INHIBIT INKEDIN INORBIT INPERIL INSIPID INSULIN INTERIM INTROIT INVALID ONASSIS ONATRIP ONAWHIM ONECHIP ONEIRIC ONEPAIR ONEUNIT ONEWHIT ONTARIO ONTOPIC SNEAKIN SNOWSIN SNUGFIT SNUGLIS UNBRAID UNCHAIN UNCHAIR UNCIVIC UNCIVIL UNCOMIC UNCUBIC UNFLUID UNFRAIL UNHUMID UNLUCID UNLYRIC UNPLAIT UNRIGID UNSLAIN UNSOLID UNSPLIT UNSTAID UNSTOIC UNTIMID UNTOXIC UNVIVID

•N••••I

ANASAZI GNOCCHI ONORATI SNOWSKI UNBELDI

••NI•••

ALNICOS ALNILAM ALNITAK ALNIYAT AMNIONS ARNICAS ATNIGHT AWNINGS BENICIA BENICIO BENIGNI BENIGNO BENISON BONIATO BONIEST BONILLA BONITOS BUNIONS CANIDAE CANIEST CANINES CANINGS CANITBE CONICAL CONIFER CYNICAL DANIELA DANIELJ DANIELS DANIKEN DANITES DENIALS DENIECE DENIERS DENIMED DENISON DENIZEN DONIMUS ELNINOS FANIONS FINIALS FINIANS FINICAL FINICKY FINISHD FINITES GENITOR GUNITES HONIARA IGNITED IGNITER IGNITES IGNITOR INNINGS IONIANS IONISED IONISER IONISES IONIUMS IONIZED IONIZER IONIZES JANITOR JUNIORS JUNIPER KENICHI KINISON LENIENT LINIEST LININGS LONIGAN MANIACS MANIKIN MANILAS MANILOW MANIPLE MANIPUR MENIALS MENISCI MINIBAR MINIBUS MINICAB MINICAM MINICAR MINIKIN MINILAB MINIMAL MINIMAX MINIMUM MINIMUS MININGS MINIONS MINISKI MINISUB MINITVS MINIVAC MINIVAN MINIVER MINIZOO MONIKER MONITOR NONIRON OMNIBUS OMNIMAX ORNITHO PANICKY PANICLE PANIERS PANINIS PINIEST PINIONS PONIARD PUNIEST RANINTO RANITUP RUNINTO RUNITUP SANIBEL SENIORS TINIEST TONIEST TONIGHT TUNICLE TUNISIA VANILLA VANILLI VENISON VINIEST WANIEST WINIEST XENIAOH XENICAL ZANIEST ZENISTS ZENITHS ZONIANS ZUNIANS

••N•I••

AGNAILS ANNUITY AUNTIES BANDIDO BANDIED BANDIER BANDIES BANDING BANDITO BANDITS BANGING BANKING BANKITS BANNING BANTING BENDIER BENDING BENNING BINDING BINGING BINNING BONAIRE BONDING BONFIRE BONGING BONKING BONNIER BONNILY BUNGING BUNKING BUNNIES BUNNING BUNTING CANDICE CANDIDA CANDIDE CANDIDS CANDIED CANDIES CANNIER CANNILY CANNING CANTILY CANTINA CANTING CANTINO CENSING CENTIME CENTIMO CONCISE CONDIGN

CONFIDE
CONFINE
CONFIRM
CONFITS
CONKING
CONNICK
CONNIFF
CONNING
CONNIVE
CONOIDS
CONRIED
CONSIGN
CONSIST
CONVICT
CUNNING
DANCING
DANDIER
DANDIES
DANDIFY
DANDILY
DANNING
DENNING
DENSIFY
DENSITY
DENTINE
DENTING
DENTINS
DENTIST
DENYING
DINDINS
DINGIER
DINGILY
DINGING
DINKIER
DINNING
DINTING
DONKING
DONNING
DONNISH
DUNCISH
DUNKING
DUNKIRK
DUNLINS
DUNNING
EONLINE
FANCIED
FANCIER
FANCIES
FANCIFY
FANCILY
FANFICS
FANGING
FANLIKE
FANNING
FANTINE
FANWISE
FANZINE
FENCING
FENDING
FENNIER
FINDING
FINKING
FINLIKE
FINNIER
FINNISH
FONTINA
FUNDING
FUNKIER
FUNKILY
FUNKING
FUNNIER
FUNNIES
FUNNILY
FUNNING
FUNTIME
GANGING
GENOISE
GENTIAN
GENTILE
GENUINE
GINFIZZ
GINGIVA
GINMILL
GINNING
GONGING
GUNFIRE
GUNKIER
GUNNIES
GUNNING
HANDIER
HANDILY
HANDING
HANGING
HANKIBA
HANKIES
HENBITS
HENLIKE
HENNISH
HENRICH
HENRIES
HINGING
HINKIER
HINNIES
HINTING
HONKING
HUNKIER
HUNLIKE
HUNNISH
HUNTING
IINSIST
JANEIRO
JANVIER
JENKINS
JINXING
JUNGIAN
JUNKIER
JUNKIES
JUNKING
KANTIAN
KENNING
KENTISH
KINGING
KINKIER
KINKILY
KINKING
KONTIKI
LANCIAS
LANCING
LANDING
LANDINI
LANKIER
LANKILY
LANSING
LANVINS
LENDING
LENTIGO
LENTILS
LINBIAO
LINDIED
LINDIES
LINKING
LINPIAO
LINTIER
LINTING
LONGIES
LONGING
LONGISH
LUNGING
MANCINI
MANGIER
MANKIND
MANLIER
MANLIKE
MANNIES
MANNING
MANNISH
MANRICO
MANSION
MANSIZE
MCNEILL
MENCIUS
MENDING
MENTION
MENZIES
MINCING
MINDING
MINGIER
MINTIER
MINTING
MINXISH
MONDIAL
MONDIEU
MONKISH
NANAIMO
NANJING
NANKING
NANNIED
NANNIES
NENNIUS
NINNIES
NONDIET
NONHITS
NONLIFE
NONLIVE
NONOILY
NONOISE
NUNCIOS
NUNLIKE
NUNNISH
OINKING
PANDITS
PANFISH
PANNIER
PANNING
PANPIPE
PANSIES
PANTIES
PANTILE
PANTING
PENCILS
PENDING
PENLIKE
PENLITE
PENNIES
PENNINE
PENNING
PENSION
PENSIVE
PENTIUM
PENZIAS
PINGING
PINKIES
PINKING
PINKISH
PINNING
PONDING
PONGIDS
PONTIAC
PONTIAN
PONTIFF
PONTIUS
PONYING
PUNDITS
PUNKIER
PUNKIES
PUNNIER
PUNNILY
PUNNING
PUNTING
RANDIER
RANGIER
RANGING
RANKINE
RANKING
RANKISH
RANRIOT
RANTING
RANWILD
RANWITH
RENAILS
RENDING
RENNINS
RENOIRS
RENTIER
RENTING
RENWICK
RINDIER
RINGING
RINSING
RUNNIER
RUNNING
RUNRIOT
RUNTIER
RUNTIME
RUNTISH
RUNWILD
RUNWITH
SANDIER
SANDING
SANTINI
SENDING
SENSING
SINCITY
SINGING
SINKING
SINLIKE
SINNING
SONLIKE
SUNBIRD
SUNCITY
SUNDIAL
SUNFIRE
SUNFISH
SUNKIST
SUNLIKE
SUNNIER
SUNNILY
SUNNING
SUNRISE
SYNCING
SYNDICS
TANGIER
TANGING
TANKING
TANKINI
TANLINE
TANNING
TANNINS
TANNISH
TANSIES
TANTIVY
TENDING
TENMILE
TENNIEL
TENNIES
TENPINS
TENSILE
TENSING
TENSION
TENSITY
TENSIVE
TENTING
TENUITY
TENZING
TINFISH
TINGING
TINLIKE
TINMINE
TINNIER
TINNILY
TINNING
TINTING
TONGING
TONSILS
TONTINE
UNNAILS
UNNAIVE
UNNOISY
URNLIKE
VANDIEN
VANDINE
VANLINE
VANNING
VANRIJN
VENDING
VENTING
WANNING
WANNISH
WANTING
WENDING
WINCING
WINDIER
WINDIGO
WINDILY
WINDING
WINGING
WINKING
WINNING
WONTING
YANKING
YANNICK
YENNING
ZANYISH
ZANYISM
ZINCIFY
ZINCING
ZINCITE
ZINGIER
ZINGING
ZINKIER
ZINNIAS
ZONKING

••N••I•

AGNATIC
AMNERIS
AMNESIA
AMNESIC
ANNAKIN
ANNELID
BANDAID
BANZAIS
BENAZIR
BENEFIC
BENEFIT
BENICIA
BENICIO
BONACIS
BONARIO
BONSOIR
CANONIC
CANTRIP
CENTRIC
CINESIA
CONBRIO
CONCEIT
CONDUIT
CONJOIN
CONKLIN
CONTAIN
CYNTHIA
DANTEII
DENARII
DENTOID
DINARIC
DINEDIN
DINESIN
DONTLIE
DUNEDIN
DYNAMIC
EUNOMIA
FANATIC
FANEUIL
FANMAIL
FANTAIL
FENCEIN
FINNAIR
FUNFAIR
FUNFZIG
GANGLIA
GENERIC
GENERIS
GENESIS
GENETIC
GENGHIS
GENNAIO
GENOMIC
GONERIL
GUNSHIP
HANDLIN
HANDSIN
HANGSIN
HENDRIX
HENREID
HENRYII
HENRYIV
HONEDIN
HONESIN
IKNEWIT
IKNOWIT
JONERIK
JONQUIL
KENOLIN
KINCAID
KINESIC
KINESIS
KINETIC
KINGPIN
KINKAID
KINSHIP
LANGUID
LANOLIN
LUNATIC
MANHEIM
MANIKIN
MANOLIN
MANTRIC
MANUMIT
MENUHIN
MINEPIT
MINIKIN
MINORIN
MINUTIA
MONADIC
MONODIC
MUNCHIE
NINEPIN
NONACID
NONDRIP
NONEPIC
NONEVIL
NONPAID
NONSKID
NONSLIP
NONVOID
NUNSHIP
PANINIS
PENGUIN
PINEOIL
PINGUID
PINTAIL
PUNCHIN
RANONIN
RENUZIT
RENVOIS
RINGSIN
RUNONIN
SANDPIT
SANGRIA
SANSEIS
SENDSIN
SENSEIS
SINEDIE
SINKSIN
SONSHIP
SUNMAID
SUNSUIT
SYNODIC
TENDRIL
TINFOIL
TINYBIT
TINYTIM
TUNAOIL
TUNEDIN
TUNESIN
TUNGOIL
TUNISIA
VANADIC
VENATIC
VENEZIA
VENTRIS
VINYLIC
WANTSIN
WINGSIT
WINGTIP
WINSBIG
XANTHIC
YANQUIS
ZENOBIA

••N•••I

BENGALI
BENIGNI
BENZALI
BONJOVI
CANETTI
CANNOLI
CANZONI
DANTEII
DENARII
HENRYII
HENRYVI
KENICHI
KONTIKI
LANDINI
MANCINI
MANDOKI
MENISCI
MENOTTI
MINISKI
MONDAVI
MONDESI
MONOSKI
PUNJABI
RONZONI
SANTINI
TANKINI
VANILLI
VENTURI

•••NI••

ACONITE
ADENINE
AGENINE
AGONIES
AGONISE
AGONISM
AGONIST
AGONIZE
ALANINE
ALINING
AMANITA
AMENITY
ANANIAS
ASININE
ATONICS
ATONIES
ATONING
AVENIDA
AZANIAN
BAGNIOS
BANNING
BARNING
BEANIES
BEANING
BENNING
BERNINA
BERNINI
BINNING
BIONICS
BONNIER
BONNILY
BOONIES
BOSNIAN
BRANIFF
BRINIER
BRINING
BRINISH
BUNNIES
BUNNING
BURNING
BURNISH
CANNIER
CANNILY
CANNING
CARNIES
CATNIPS
CHENIER
CLINICS
CLONING
COGNIZE
COINING
CONNICK
CONNIFF
CONNING
CONNIVE
CORNICE
CORNIER
CORNILY
CORNING
CORNISH
CRANIAL
CRANING
CRANIUM
CRONIES
CUNNING
CYANIDE
CYANIDS
DAMNING
DANNING
DARNING
DAWNING
DENNING
DERNIER
DIGNIFY
DIGNITY
DINNING
DONNING
DONNISH
DOWNIER
DOWNING
DRONING
DRONISH
DUBNIUM
DUNNING
DURNING
EARNING
EBONICS
EBONIES
EBONITE
EBONIZE
ELENIAK
EPONINE
ETHNICS
ETONIAN
ETONICS
EVANISH
EVENING
EXANIMO
FANNING
FAWNING
FENNIER
FERNIER
FINNIER
FINNISH
FUNNIER
FUNNIES
FUNNILY
FUNNING
FURNISH
GAINING
GARNISH
GHANIAN
GINNING
GOONIER
GOONIES
GOONILY
GOWNING
GRANITA
GRANITE
GRUNION
GUANINE
GUNNIES
GUNNING
HAFNIUM
HAHNIUM
HARNICK
HENNISH
HERNIAE
HERNIAS
HERNIBS
HINNIES
HISNIBS
HORNIER
HORNING
HORNISH
HORNIST
HOWNICE
HUNNISH
HYMNING
ICONIFY
INANITY
IRANIAN
IRENICS
IRONIES
IRONING
IRONIST
IVANIII
JAINISM
JAINIST
JOHNIII
JOINING
KEENING
KENNING
KILNING
KOONING
LEANING
LEONIDS
LEONINE
LIGNIFY
LIGNINS
LIGNITE
LIMNING
LIMNITE
LIONISE
LIONIZE
LOANING
LOONIER
LOONIES
LOONILY
MAGNIFY
MANNIES
MANNING
MANNISH
MARNIER
MEANIES
MEANING
MOANING
MOONIER
MOONIES
MOONILY
MOONING
MOONISH
MORNING
NANNIED
NANNIES
NENNIUS
NINNIES
NOONING
NOTNICE
NUDNIKS
NUNNISH
OLDNICK
OMENING
OPENING
OPINING
OPINION
OXONIAN
OZONISE
OZONIZE
PAINING
PANNIER
PANNING
PAWNING
PEENING
PENNIES
PENNINE
PENNING
PEONIES
PHONICS
PHONIER
PHONIES
PHONILY
PHONING
PIANISM
PIANIST
PICNICS
PINNING
PLANING
PLANISH
PLENISH
PRUNING
PUNNIER
PUNNILY
PUNNING
QUININE
QUINION
RAINIER
RAINILY
RAINING
REDNINE
REGNIER
REINING
REKNITS
RENNINS
REUNIFY
REUNION
REUNITE
RHENISH
RHENIUM
RUINING
RUNNIER
RUNNING
SCENICS
SEINING
SHINIER
SHINILY
SHINING
SIGNIFY
SIGNING
SINNING
SIXNINE
SPANIEL
SPANISH
SPINIER
STANINE
STONIER
STONILY
STONING
SUNNIER
SUNNILY
SUNNING
SWINISH
TANNING
TANNINS
TANNISH
TARNISH
TAWNIER
TAWNILY
TEENIER
TENNIEL
TENNIES
THENILE
THINICE
TINNIER
TINNILY
TINNING
TOONIES
TOWNIES
TOWNISH
TRINITY
TURNING
TURNIPS
TWINIER
TWINING
UNKNITS
URANITE
URANIUM
VANNING
VARNISH
VEINIER
VEINING
VERNIER
VILNIUS
WANNING
WANNISH
WARNING
WEANING
WEENIES
WHINIER
WHINING
WIENIES
WINNING
WOZNIAK
YANNICK
YARNING
YAWNIER
YAWNING
YEANING
YENNING
ZERNIKE
ZINNIAS
ZIONISM
ZIONIST

•••N•I•

ACINGIT
ADENOID
ADONAIS
AMANTIS
ARANEID
AVANTIS
BEANDIP
BEANOIL
BIENNIA
BLENDIN
BLENTIN
BLONDIE
BRINGIN
BRINGIT
BURNSIN
BURNTIN
CHINOIS
CORNBIN
CORNOIL
COUNCIL
COUNTIN
CTENOID
CUINGIN
DJINNIS
DOINGIN
DOONEIN
DRANKIN
DRINKIN
EARNSIT
FINNAIR
FRANCIS
FRANKIE
FRANTIC
GENNAIO
GLYNNIS
GOINGIN
GRANNIE
HOBNAIL

HORNSIN
HYANNIS
HYPNOID
ICINGIN
ICINGIT
IDENTIC
IVANIII
IWANTIT
JEANNIE
JOHNIII
JOHNNIE
JOHNVII
JOHNXII
JOHNXIV
JOHNXIX
JOINSIN
LEANSIN
MACNEIL
MEANSIT
MEANTIT
MOONLIT
MOONPIE
MOUNTIE
NIANTIC
ODONTIA
OPENAIR
OPENPIT
OPUNTIA
PFENNIG
PHONEIN
QUENTIN
QUINTIC
RAINSIN
REINSIN
RESNAIS
SCENEII
SCENEIV
SEENFIT
SHINDIG
SIGNSIN
SLINKIN
SLUNKIN
SPANAIR
STANDIN
STANNIC
STENCIL
STENNIS
SWINGIT
SWUNGIT
TEENSIE
THANDIE
THINAIR
TLINGIT
TOENAIL
TRANSIT
TURNSIN
TWINKIE
TYINGIN
UPANDIN
USINGIN
UTENSIL
ZWANZIG

•••N••I
ACANTHI
BERNINI
BIANCHI
BRONCHI
CANNOLI
FLINTMI
FRANCHI
FRENCHI
FRENESI
HERNANI
HUANGTI
HYUNDAI
IVANIII
JOHNIII
JOHNVII
JOHNXII
JOHNXVI
JOHNXXI
MAGNANI
SCENEII
SCENEVI
SHANGRI
TSUNAMI
ZWINGLI

••••NI•
ALBANIA
ALBENIZ
AMMONIA
AMMONIC
ANIONIC
ANSONIA
ANTONIA
ANTONIN
ANTONIO
APHONIA
APHONIC
ARMENIA
ARSENIC
ARSENIO
AVIONIC
BEATNIK
BEGONIA
BIENNIA
BIGUNIT
BIKINIS
BIMINIS
BLOWNIN
BORONIC
BOSONIC
BOTANIC
BOTHNIA
BROWNIE
BYRONIC
CANONIC
CATANIA
CHARNIN
CHRONIC
DAPHNIA
DAPHNIS
DEMONIC
DJINNIS
DOMINIC
DRAWNIN
ERMINIA
ESTONIA
EUGENIA
EUGENIC
EUGENIE
FLOWNIN
GEMINIS
GETONIT
GIVENIN
GLYNNIS
GOODNIK
GOTONIT
GRANNIE
HADANIP
HASANIP
HAZANIM
HEDONIC
HOMINID
HRYVNIA
HYANNIS
IGUANID
IMEANIT
INASNIT
JEANNIE
JOHNNIE
KALININ
KETONIC
KIWANIS
KORANIC
KRAMNIK
LACONIA
LACONIC
LATINII
LAVINIA
LEIBNIZ
LUCANIA
MASONIC
MELANIA
MELANIC
MELANIE
MELANIN
MESONIC
MORANIS
MORONIC
NEATNIK
OCEANIA
OCEANIC
OCEANID
ONEUNIT
ORGANIC
PANINIS
PARSNIP
PETUNIA
PFENNIG
PHOENIX
PHRENIC
PISANIO
POLONIA
QUEENIE
QUEENIT
RANONIN
RAPINIS
ROMANIA
ROMANIC
ROMANIS
RUMANIA
RUNONIN
SATANIC
SELENIC
SHOWNIN
SIMONIZ
SITONIT
SPUTNIK
STANNIC
STDENIS
STENNIS
SUBUNIT
TACONIC
TAHINIS
TAKENIN
TITANIA
TITANIC
TRAININ
TWOONIE
TWOUNIT
URBANII
URBANIV
VERONIA
YEMENIS
YOGINIS

•••••N•I
ARGENTI
ASHANTI
BASENJI
BURUNDI
CHIANTI
DAVINCI
EDMUNDI
EFFENDI
EKWENSI
JUMANJI
LATINII
MTSINAI
POLANYI
RAPANUI
SECONDI
SILENTI
URBANII
URBANVI
VALENTI
VIVENDI
YOUANDI

•••••NI
AFGHANI
BAMBINI
BASSANI
BELLINI
BELZONI
BENIGNI
BERNINI
BHUTANI
BIRIANI
BIRYANI
BORDONI
BUITONI
CABRINI
CANZONI
CASSINI
CELLINI
CREMINI
FELLINI
FORLANI
GALVANI
GOLDONI
GUARANI
HERNANI
HOUDINI
LANDINI
MAGNANI
MANCINI
MARCONI
MARTINI
MAZZINI
MOSCONI
NEGRONI
PUCCINI
PULMONI
RIOMUNI
RIPIENI
RONZONI
ROSSINI
SANTINI
SOPRANI
SORDINI
SPUMONI
STEFANI
TANKINI
TERMINI
THEOMNI
TIMPANI
TORTONI
TYMPANI
ZAMBONI

N••J•••
NANJING
NEWJOBS
NONJEWS
NONJURY

N•••J••
NAVAJOS
NICEJOB
NOSEJOB

•NJ••••
ENJOINS
ENJOYED
ENJOYER
INJECTS
INJOKES
INJURED
INJURER
INJURES
UNJADED
UNJOINS
UNJOINT
UNJOLLY
UNJOYED
UNJUICY

•N•J•••
INAJIFF
INKJETS
ONAJURY

•N••J••
SNOWJOB

••NJ•••
BANJOES
BONJOUR
BONJOVI
CONJOBS
CONJOIN
CONJURE
CONJURY
DONJONS
DONJOSE
DONJUAN
FANJETS
NANJING
NONJEWS
NONJURY
PUNJABI
SANJOSE
SANJUAN

••N•J••
BANKJOB

••N••J•
VANRIJN

••N•••J
DANIELJ

•••NJ••
ALANJAY
JOHNJAY
MEANJOE
REENJOY
TWINJET

•••N•J•
PBANDJS

••••NJ•
BASENJI
JUMANJI

••••N•J
SILENTJ

•••••NJ
FTDIXNJ

NK•••••
NKRUMAH

N•K••••
NAKEDLY
NIKEADS
NIKOLAI
NIKOLAY
NOKNOCK
NOKOMIS

N••K•••
NANKING
NAPKINS
NDAKOTA
NECKERS
NECKING
NECKLET
NECKTIE
NEWKIDS
NICKELS
NICKERS
NICKING
NICKLES
NOCKING

N•••K••
NABOKOV
NAILKEG
NICEKID
NONSKED
NONSKID
NONUKES
NOOTKAS

N••••K•
NETLIKE
NETSUKE
NIBLIKE
NOTLIKE
NUDNIKS
NUNLIKE
NUTLIKE
NYYANKS

N•••••K
NATWICK
NEATNIK
NESQUIK
NETWORK
NEWLOOK
NEWWEEK
NEWYORK
NIBLICK
NIPMUCK
NITPICK
NOKNOCK
NONBANK
NONBOOK
NONDARK
NONPEAK
NONWORK
NORFOLK
NORWALK
NOWLOOK
NUMLOCK

•NK••••
ANKARAN
ANKLERS
ANKLETS
INKBLOT
INKEDIN
INKHORN
INKIEST
INKINGS
INKJETS
INKLESS
INKLIKE
INKLING
INKMARK
INKNOTS
INKPADS
INKPOTS
INKSACS
INKSPOT
INKSTER
INKWELL
INKYCAP
UNKEMPT
UNKEYED
UNKINKS
UNKNITS
UNKNOTS
UNKNOWN

•N•K•••
ANYKIND
ENSKIED
ENSKIES
INAKNOT
ONAKICK
ONEKILO
ONTKEAN
SNAKERS
SNAKIER
SNAKILY
SNAKING
UNSKEWS

•N••K••
ANNAKIN
INJOKES
INTAKES
INVOKED
INVOKER
INVOKES
KNOCKED
KNOCKER
KNOCKON
KNUCKLE
KNUCKLY
SNACKED
SNACKER
SNACKON
SNEAKBY
SNEAKED
SNEAKER
SNEAKIN
SNEAKUP
SNICKER
SNICKET
SNOOKER
SNORKEL
SNUCKUP
UNASKED
UNBAKED
UNCAKED
UNCAKES
UNDIKED
UNFAKED
UNINKED
UNLIKED
UNLIKES
UNMAKER
UNMAKES
UNMIKED
UNRAKED
UNTAKEN
UNWAKED
UNYOKED
UNYOKES
VNECKED

•N•••K•
ANORAKS
ANTLIKE
ENLINKS
ENRANKS
INAPOKE
INKLIKE
SNOWSKI
UNALIKE
UNAWAKE
UNBRAKE
UNBROKE
UNBULKY
UNCASKS
UNCHOKE
UNCORKS
UNDOCKS
UNFLAKY
UNFORKS
UNHOOKS
UNHUSKS
UNKINKS
UNLEAKY
UNLINKS
UNLOCKS
UNLUCKY
UNMASKS
UNPACKS
UNPICKS
UNRACKS
UNRISKY
UNROCKY
UNSMOKY
UNSNAKY
UNSPOKE
UNSULKY
UNTACKS
UNTUCKS

•N••••K
ANYLUCK
INAFUNK
INAWINK
INBLACK
INCHECK
INKMARK
INSHOCK
INSTOCK
ONAKICK
ONALARK
ONBREAK
ONELOOK
ONESOCK
ONEWEEK
ONTRACK
UNBLOCK
UNCHECK
UNCLOAK
UNDRUNK
UNFRANK
UNFROCK
UNQUICK
UNSLACK
UNSLEEK
UNSLICK
UNSPEAK
UNSTACK
UNSTICK
UNSTUCK
UNTHICK
UNTHINK
UNTRACK

••NK•••
BANKERS
BANKFEE
BANKING
BANKITS
BANKJOB
BANKONE
BANKSON
BANKSUP
BONKERS
BONKING
BUNKBED
BUNKERS
BUNKING
BUNKOED
BUNKUMS
CANKERS
CONKERS
CONKING
CONKLIN
CONKOFF
CONKOUT
DANKEST
DINKIER
DONKEYS
DONKING
DUNKERS
DUNKING
DUNKIRK
FINKING
FINKSON
FUNKIER
FUNKILY
FUNKING
GINKGOS
GUNKIER
HANKERS
HANKIBA
HANKIES
HINKIER
HONKERS
HONKING
HONKSAT
HUNKERS
HUNKIER
JANKLOW
JENKINS
JUNKART
JUNKCAR
JUNKDNA
JUNKERS
JUNKETS
JUNKFAX
JUNKIER
JUNKIES
JUNKING
JUNKMAN
JUNKMEN
KINKAID
KINKIER
KINKILY
KINKING
LANKEST
LANKIER
LANKILY
LINKAGE
LINKERS
LINKING
LINKSUP
LINKUPS
LUNKERS
MANKATO
MANKIND
MONKEES
MONKEYS
MONKISH
NANKING
OINKERS
OINKING
PINKENS
PINKEST
PINKETT
PINKHAM
PINKIES
PINKING
PINKISH
PINKOES
PUNKERS
PUNKIER
PUNKIES
RANKERS
RANKEST
RANKINE
RANKING
RANKISH
RANKLED
RANKLES
RANKOUT
RINKRAT
SINKAGE
SINKERS
SINKING
SINKSIN
SUNKIST
TANKAGE
TANKARD
TANKCAR
TANKERS
TANKFUL
TANKING
TANKINI
TANKSUP
TANKTOP
TENKRUN
TINKERS
TINKLED
TINKLER
TINKLES
WANKELS
WINKERS
WINKING
WINKLER
WINKOUT
WINKSAT
YANKEES
YANKERS
YANKING
YANKOFF
YANKOUT
YANKSAT
YANKSON
YANKTON
YONKERS
ZINKIER
ZONKING
ZONKOUT

••N•K••
ANNAKIN
BANGKOK
CONAKRY
DANIKEN
GINGKOS
HANUKAH
KANAKAS
MANIKIN
MENCKEN
MINIKIN
MINSKYS
MONGKUT
MONIKER
NONSKED
NONSKID
NONUKES
PONYKEG
WENDKOS
ZINCKED

••N••K•
BUNRAKU
CANUCKS
CONVOKE
DANEYKO
FANLIKE
FINICKY
FINLIKE
HENLIKE
HUNLIKE
KONTIKI
MANDOKI
MANLIKE
MINISKI
MONOSKI
NUNLIKE
PANCAKE
PANICKY
PENLIKE
PINOAKS
SHNOOKS
SINLIKE
SONLIKE
SUNLIKE
TANOAKS
TINLIKE
URNLIKE
VANDYKE

••N•••K
ALNITAK
BANACEK
BANGKOK
CANNOCK
CONNICK
CONRACK
DENMARK
DONETSK
DONTASK
DUNDALK
DUNKIRK
FINBACK
GANGTOK
GENLOCK
GUNLOCK
HANCOCK
HENPECK
JANACEK
JONERIK
KINFOLK
MENFOLK
MONTAUK
MRNOVAK
NONBANK
NONBOOK
NONDARK
NONPEAK
NONWORK
PENNOCK
RANAMOK
RANBACK
RANSACK
RENWICK
RUNAMOK
RUNBACK
SUNDECK
TANBARK
TENWEEK
TINWORK
VANDYCK
VANEYCK
VANWYCK
WINBACK
YANNICK

•••NK••
BLANKED
BLANKER
BLANKET
BLANKLY
BLINKAT
BLINKED
BLINKER
BLYNKEN
BRINKER
CHINKED
CHUNKED
CLANKED
CLINKED
CLINKER
CLONKED
CLUNKED
CLUNKER
CRANKED
CRANKUP
CRINKLE
CRINKLY
DRANKIN
DRANKTO
DRANKUP
DRINKER
DRINKIN
DRINKME
DRINKTO
DRINKUP
DRUNKEN
DRUNKER
EBANKED
FLANKED
FLANKEN
FLANKER
FLUNKED
FLUNKER
FRANKED
FRANKEN
FRANKER
FRANKIE
FRANKLY
FRANKOZ
GRINKOV
KLINKER
PLANKED

PLINKED
PLONKED
PLUNKED
PLUNKER
PRINKED
PRINKER
REINKED
SHANKAR
SHANKED
SKUNKED
SLINKED
SLINKER
SLINKIN
SLINKUP
SLUNKIN
SLUNKUP
SPANKED
SPANKER
STANKUP
STINKER
STINKUP
SWANKED
SWANKER
SWANKUP
THANKED
THANKER
THINKER
THINKOF
THINKSO
THINKUP
THUNKED
TRINKET
TURNKEY
TWINKIE
TWINKLE
TWINKLY
UNINKED
WRINKLE
WRINKLY

•••N•K•

ARENSKY
NUDNIKS
ROANOKE
UNSNAKY
VRONSKY
ZERNIKE

•••N••K

BYANECK
CANNOCK
CHINOOK
CONNICK
DOINGOK
ELENIAK
EWENECK
HARNICK
LOWNECK
NOKNOCK
OLDNICK
PENNOCK
QBSNEAK
REDNECK
REKNOCK
SCHNOOK
TEANECK
VEENECK
WOZNIAK
YANNICK

••••NK•

DEBUNKS
DEJUNKS
EMBANKS
ENLINKS
ENRANKS
EUBANKS
EXYANKS
HIJINKS
LYSENKO
NYYANKS
REBANKS
RELINKS
RERANKS
RESINKS
SHRINKS
SOYINKA
SOYINKS
UNKINKS
UNLINKS
UPLINKS
ZEDONKS

••••N•K

BEATNIK
GOODNIK
KRAMNIK
NEATNIK
SILENTK
SPUTNIK

•••••NK

AIRTANK
BETHINK
BURBANK
EYEBANK
EYEWINK
FIRBANK
FOGBANK
GASTANK
GOBLANK
HOTLINK
HOTPINK
ICERINK
INAFUNK
INAWINK
JOBBANK
KEYBANK
NONBANK
OILTANK
OUTRANK
RATFINK
RECRANK
RETHANK
RETHINK
SPELUNK
SUBBANK
THERINK
TOPRANK
UNDRUNK
UNFRANK
UNTHINK

N•L••••

NELSONS
NFLGAME
NFLTEAM
NHLGAME
NHLTEAM
NILESOH
NILSSON
NOLIMIT
NOLOADS
NULLIFY
NULLING
NULLITY
NULLSET

N••L•••

NAILERS
NAILGUN
NAILING
NAILKEG
NAILSET
NAILSIN
NAILSIT
NAILSUP
NAILTIP
NAPLESS
NBALIVE
NEDLAND
NEGLECT
NEOLITH
NEOLOGY
NEOLYTE
NETLESS
NETLIKE
NETLOSS
NEWLAID
NEWLEAF
NEWLEFT
NEWLIFE
NEWLINE
NEWLOOK
NEWLOVE
NIALONG
NIBLETS
NIBLICK
NIBLIKE
NIELSEN
NOBLEST
NOCLASS
NONLIFE
NONLIVE
NOPLACE
NOTLIKE
NOTLIVE
NOWLOOK
NUCLEAR
NUCLEIC
NUCLEON
NUCLEUS
NUCLIDE
NULLIFY
NULLING
NULLITY
NULLSET
NUMLOCK
NUNLIKE
NUTLETS
NUTLIKE

N•••L••

NACELLE
NAPALMS
NASALLY
NATALIA
NATALIE
NBCBLUE
NEBULAE
NEBULAR
NEBULAS
NECKLET
NEEDLED
NEEDLER
NEEDLES
NEPALIS
NESTLED
NESTLER
NESTLES
NETFLIX
NETTLED
NETTLES
NEUILLY
NEVILLE
NIBBLED
NIBBLER
NIBBLES
NICKLES
NICOLAS
NICOLET
NICOLLE
NIGGLED
NIGGLER
NIGGLES
NIKOLAI
NIKOLAY
NIMBLER
NIPPLES
NODULAR
NODULED
NODULES
NOGALES
NONFLUX
NONPLAY
NONPLUS
NONSLIP
NOODLED
NOODLES
NOPALES
NORELCO
NOTALIE
NOTALOT
NOVALIS
NOVELAS
NOVELLA
NOVELLE
NOVELLO
NOVELTY
NOZZLES
NTUPLES
NUBBLES
NUZZLED
NUZZLER
NUZZLES

N••••L•

NACELLE
NAIVELY
NAKEDLY
NAMABLE
NAMABLY
NASALLY
NASTILY
NATTILY
NAUTILI
NEEDILY
NERVILY
NERVULE
NETBALL
NETFULS
NEUILLY
NEVILLE
NEWBOLT
NICCOLO
NICHOLS
NICKELS
NICOLLE
NIFTILY
NIGHTLY
NINTHLY
NIPPILY
NOBHILL
NOFAULT
NOISILY
NONCOLA
NONGOLD
NONOILY
NONSALE
NONSELF
NONUPLE
NORFOLK
NORMALS
NORWALK
NOTABLE
NOTABLY
NOTEDLY
NOTWELL
NOVELLA
NOVELLE
NOVELLO
NUTOILS
NUTTILY

N•••••L

NAHUATL
NAIPAUL
NARWHAL
NATURAL
NATUREL
NEEDFUL
NESTFUL
NETBALL
NEUTRAL
NEWDEAL
NOANGEL
NOBHILL
NODICAL
NOMINAL
NONEVIL
NONFUEL
NONORAL
NONWOOL
NOSTRIL
NOTREAL
NOTWELL
NUMERAL
NUPTIAL
NYMPHAL

•NL••••

ENLACED
ENLACES
ENLARGE
ENLINKS
ENLISTS
ENLIVEN
INLABOR
INLANDS
INLARGE
INLAYER
INLIMBO
INLINES
INLYING
ONLEASE
ONLEASH
ONLEAVE
ONLIEST
ONLOADS
ONLYTOO
ONLYYOU
UNLACED
UNLACES
UNLADED
UNLADEN
UNLADES
UNLARGE
UNLATCH
UNLAVED
UNLAXED
UNLAXES
UNLEADS
UNLEAFS
UNLEAKY
UNLEARN
UNLEASH
UNLEGAL
UNLEVEL
UNLIGHT
UNLIKED
UNLIKES
UNLINED
UNLINKS
UNLIVED
UNLIVES
UNLOADS
UNLOATH
UNLOBED
UNLOCAL
UNLOCKS
UNLOFTY
UNLOOPS
UNLOOSE
UNLOVED
UNLOWLY
UNLOYAL
UNLUCID
UNLUCKY
UNLUMPY
UNLURED
UNLUSTY
UNLYING
UNLYRIC

•N•L•••

ANALOGS
ANALOGY
ANALYSE
ANALYST
ANALYTE
ANALYZE
ANELING
ANGLAIS
ANGLERS
ANGLING
ANILINE
ANILITY
ANKLERS
ANKLETS
ANTLERS
ANTLIKE
ANTLION
ANYLUCK
DNALABS
ENCLASP
ENCLAVE
ENCLOSE
ENDLATE
ENDLEAF
ENDLESS
ENDLINE
ENDLONG
ENFLAME
ENGLAND
ENGLISH
ENGLUND
ENGLUTS
ENOLOGY
ENPLANE
ENSLAVE
INALINE
INBLACK
INBLOOM
INCLASS
INCLINE
INCLOSE
INCLUDE
INFLAME
INFLATE
INFLECT
INFLICT
INFLOWS
INGLESE
INKLESS
INKLIKE
INKLING
INNLESS
INPLACE
INULASE
KNELLED
ONALARK
ONALEAD
ONALERT
ONALINE
ONELANE
ONELIRA
ONELOOK
ONELOVE
ONELUMP
SNELLEN
UNALERT
UNALIKE
UNALONE
UNBLADE
UNBLENT
UNBLEST
UNBLOCK
UNBLOWN
UNBLUED
UNCLAMP
UNCLASP
UNCLEAN
UNCLEAR
UNCLEFT
UNCLIPS
UNCLIPT
UNCLOAK
UNCLOGS
UNCLOSE
UNCLOUD
UNFLAKY
UNFLOOR
UNFLOWN
UNFLUID
UNGLOVE
UNGLUED
UNGLUES
UNPLAIT
UNPLANS
UNPLIED
UNPLUGS
UNPLUMB
UNSLACK
UNSLAIN
UNSLEEK
UNSLICK
UNSLIER
UNSLING
UNSLUNG
UNSLYER
UNSLYLY

•N••L••

ANGELAS
ANGELES
ANGELIC
ANGELOU
ANGELUS
ANGOLAN
ANGULAR
ANNALEE
ANNALES
ANNELID
ANNULAR
ANNULET
ANNULUS
ANSELMO
ANTILOG
ENABLED
ENABLER
ENABLES
ENDALLS
ENDPLAY
ENFOLDS
ENGILDS
ENGULFS
ENISLED
ENISLES
ENOILED
ENROLLS
ENSILED
ENSILES
ENVELOP
GNARLED
INCOLOR
INDULGE
INFOLDS
INGALLS
INGULFS
INHALED
INHALER
INHALES
INKBLOT
INSALES
INSOLES
INSULAR
INSULIN
INSULTS
INVALID
INVOLVE
KNEELED
KNEELER
KNELLED
KNOWLES
KNURLED
ONECLAM
ONECLUB
SNARLAT
SNARLED
SNARLER
SNARLUP
SNELLEN
SNIGLET
SNUGLIS
UNAXLED
UNBALED
UNBALES
UNBELDI
UNBELTS
UNBOLTS
UNBULKY
UNDULAR
UNFILED
UNFILES
UNFOLDS
UNFULLY
UNGULAE
UNGULAR
UNHELMS
UNHILLY
UNHULLS
UNIPLEX
UNJOLLY
UNMOLDS
UNMOLDY
UNOGLED
UNOILED
UNPALED
UNPILED
UNPILES
UNPOLED
UNRILED
UNROLLS
UNRULED
UNSALTY
UNSELLS
UNSILLY
UNSOLED
UNSOLES
UNSOLID
UNSPLIT
UNSULKY
UNTILED
UNWALLS

•N•••L•

ANATOLE
ANATOLY
ANGRILY
ANIMALS
ANNEALS
ANNUALS
ANOMALY
ANOUILH
ANTHILL
ENAMELS
ENDABLE
ENDALLS
ENFIELD
ENNOBLE
ENROLLS
ENSEALS
ENSOULS
ENTAILS
ENTITLE
ENVEILS
INABALL
INAHOLE
INANELY
INAPILE
INAPTLY
INAVALE
INBUILT
INDWELL
INDWELT
INEPTLY
INERTLY
INEXILE
INFIELD
INGALLS
INGOALS
INKWELL
INNERLY
INOCULA
INSCALE
INSTALL
INSTALS
INSTILL
INSTILS
INSTYLE
INTAILS
INUTILE
KNOWALL
KNUCKLE
KNUCKLY
ONAROLL
ONEBALL
ONEBELL
ONECALL
ONECELL
ONEFOLD
ONEHALF
ONEKILO
ONEMILE
ONESELF
SNAKILY
SNAPPLE
SNIDELY
SNIFFLE
SNIFFLY
SNIVELS
SNOBALL
SNOWILY
SNUFFLE
SNUGGLE
SNUGGLY
UNADULT
UNAGILE
UNAPTLY
UNBUILD
UNBUILT
UNBURLY
UNCIALS
UNCOILS
UNCOYLY
UNCURLS
UNDEALT
UNFITLY
UNFRILL
UNFULLY
UNFURLS
UNGODLY
UNHILLY
UNHULLS
UNIBALL
UNJOLLY
UNLOWLY
UNMADLY
UNMANLY
UNMOULD
UNNAILS
UNPEELS
UNREELS
UNROLLS
UNSADLY
UNSCALY
UNSEALS
UNSELLS
UNSHELL
UNSHYLY
UNSILLY
UNSLYLY
UNSPELT
UNSPILT
UNSURLY
UNTRULY
UNVEILS
UNWALLS
UNWHOLE

•N••••L

ANBESOL
ANNABEL
ANTHEIL
ANTHILL
ENSNARL
ENTHRAL
INABALL
INAPRIL
INCIVIL
INDWELL
INFIDEL
INITIAL
INKWELL
INPERIL
INSTALL
INSTILL
INTOTAL
KNIEVEL
KNOWALL
ONAROLL
ONEBALL
ONEBELL
ONECALL
ONECELL
ONEREEL
ONTHEDL
ONTRIAL
SNOBALL
SNORKEL
UNAWFUL
UNCIVIL
UNCRUEL
UNEQUAL
UNFRAIL
UNFRILL
UNIBALL
UNIDEAL
UNLEGAL
UNLEVEL
UNLOCAL
UNLOYAL
UNNASAL
UNNOVEL
UNRAVEL
UNREGAL
UNRURAL
UNSHELL
UNSNARL
UNSPOOL
UNSTEEL
UNUSUAL
UNVENAL
UNVITAL
UNVOCAL
UNWHEEL

••NL•••

AWNLESS
DONLEVY
DUNLINS
DUNLOPS
EONLINE
FANLIKE
FINLAND
FINLESS
FINLIKE
GENLOCK
GUNLAPS
GUNLAWS
GUNLESS
GUNLOCK
HENLIKE
HUNLIKE
INNLESS
KINLESS
MANLESS
MANLIER
MANLIKE
NONLIFE
NONLIVE
NUNLIKE
PENLIKE
PENLITE
PINLESS
PUNLESS
RANLAPS
RANLATE
RUNLAPS
RUNLATE
RUNLESS
RUNLETS
SINLESS
SINLIKE
SONLESS
SONLIKE
SUNLAMP
SUNLESS
SUNLIKE
TANLINE
TINLIKE
URNLIKE
VANLINE
VANLOAD
VINLAND
VONLAUE
WINLESS

••N•L••

ALNILAM
ANNALEE
ANNALES
ANNELID
ANNULAR
ANNULET
ANNULUS
ARNOLDS
BANALER
BANALLY
BANDLET
BANGLED
BANGLES
BENBLUE
BENELUX
BENTLEY
BINDLES
BINGLES
BONELET
BONILLA
BUNDLED
BUNDLER
BUNDLES
BUNGLED
BUNGLER
BUNGLES
CANALED
CANDLED
CANDLER
CANDLES
CANOLAS
CANTLES
CANULAE
CANULAS
CONELET
CONKLIN
DANDLED
DANDLER
DANDLES
DANELAW
DANGLED
DANGLER
DANGLES
DINGLES
DONGLES

DONTLIE
FANCLUB
FANSLER
FENELON
FINALES
FINALLY
FINDLAY
FINDLEY
FONDLED
FONDLER
FONDLES
FUNPLEX
GANGLIA
GANTLET
GENTLED
GENTLER
GENTLES
GUNPLAY
HANDLED
HANDLER
HANDLES
HANDLIN
HENSLEY
HINDLEG
HONALEE
HUNTLEY
JANGLED
JANGLER
JANGLES
JANKLOW
JINGLED
JINGLER
JINGLES
JUNGLES
KENOLIN
KINDLED
KINDLER
KINDLES
KINGLET
LANDLER
LANGLEY
LANOLIN
LUNULAE
LUNULAR
MANGLED
MANGLER
MANGLES
MANILAS
MANILOW
MANOLIN
MANTLED
MANTLES
MANTLET
MCNALLY
MINGLED
MINGLER
MINGLES
MINILAB
MINOLTA
MONOLOG
NONFLUX
NONPLAY
NONPLUS
NONSLIP
PANELED
PANTLEG
PENALTY
PENULTS
RANKLED
RANKLES
RENALDO
RENALLY
RINALDO
RINGLET
RUNDLES
RUNSLOW
SANBLAS
SANDLER
SANDLOT
SINGLED
SINGLES
SINGLET
SUNGLOW
TANGLED
TANGLER
TANGLES
TINGLED
TINGLER
TINGLES
TINKLED
TINKLER
TINKLES
TONALLY
TONELOC
VANILLA
VANILLI
VENALLY
VENULES
VINYLIC
WANGLED
WANGLER
WANGLES
WINGLET
WINKLER
WINSLET
WINSLOW
ZONALLY
ZONULAR
ZONULES

••N••L•

AGNAILS
ANNEALS
ANNUALS
BANALLY
BENGALI
BENGALS
BENZALI
BENZELL
BONILLA
BONNILY
BUNUELO
CANCELS
CANDELA
CANFULS
CANNELL
CANNELS
CANNILY
CANNOLI
CANNULA
CANTALS
CANTILY
CENACLE
CENTALS
CINEOLE
CONDOLE
CONSOLE
CONSULS
CONSULT
DANDILY
DANGELO
DANIELA
DANIELJ
DANIELS
DENIALS
DENSELY
DENTALS
DINGILY
DONNALL
DUNDALK
ENNOBLE
FANBELT
FANCILY
FANFOLD
FANPALM
FENNELS
FINABLE
FINAGLE
FINALLY
FINGALS
FINIALS
FUNKILY
FUNNELS
FUNNILY
GANDALF
GENTILE
GINGOLD
GINMILL
GONDOLA
GUNBELT
GUNMOLL
GUNSELS
GUNWALE
HANDILY
HANSOLO
IANHOLM
IGNOBLE
IGNOBLY
INNERLY
JONHALL
KENDALL
KENDOLL
KENNELS
KINFOLK
KINKILY
KINNELL
LANKILY
LENTILS
LINABLE
LINCOLN
LINGULA
LINTELS
MANACLE
MANDALA
MANDELA
MANHOLE
MANIPLE
MANTELS
MANUALS
MCNALLY
MCNEILL
MENDELS
MENFOLK
MENIALS
MINABLE
MINEOLA
MONDALE
MONGOLS
MONOCLE
MONTALE
MONTHLY
NINTHLY
NONCOLA
NONGOLD
NONOILY
NONSALE
NONSELF
NONUPLE
PANFULS
PANICLE
PANOPLY
PANTILE
PENCILS
PENPALS
PENTELS
PINBALL
PINFOLD
PINHOLE
PINWALE
PUNNILY
RANDALL
RANWILD
RENAILS
RENALLY
RENAULT
RENDELL
RENTALS
RONDELS
RUNNELS
RUNWILD
SANDALS
SANDFLY
SUNBELT
SUNNILY
TANGELO
TENABLE
TENABLY
TENBALL
TENFOLD
TENMILE
TENSELY
TENSILE
TENTHLY
TINNILY
TINSELS
TONALLY
TONSILS
TUNABLE
TUNICLE
TUNNELS
TYNDALL
UNNAILS
URNFULS
VANDALS
VANILLA
VANILLI
VANPELT
VENABLE
VENALLY
VINCULA
VONZELL
WANKELS
WENDELL
WINDILY
ZONALLY

••N•••L

ANNABEL
BANEFUL
BENZELL
CANNELL
CENTRAL
CONCEAL
CONGEAL
CONICAL
CONTROL
CYNICAL
DONEGAL
DONNALL
FANEUIL
FANMAIL
FANTAIL
FINICAL
GENERAL
GENTEEL
GINMILL
GONERIL
GUNMOLL
HANDFUL
HANDSEL
JONHALL
JONQUIL
KENDALL
KENDOLL
KENWAHL
KINNELL
LINGUAL
MANDREL
MCNEILL
MENTHOL
MINDFUL
MINERAL
MINIMAL
MONADAL
MONDIAL
MONGREL
NONEVIL
NONFUEL
NONORAL
NONWOOL
OWNGOAL
PINBALL
PINCURL
PINEOIL
PINESOL
PINSEAL
PINTAIL
RANDALL
RENDELL
RENEWAL
SANIBEL
SENEGAL
SENSUAL
SONGFUL
SUNBOWL
SUNDIAL
SYNFUEL
SYNODAL
TANKFUL
TENBALL
TENDRIL
TENNIEL
TENTFUL
TINFOIL
TUNAOIL
TUNEFUL
TUNGOIL
TYNDALL
UNNASAL
UNNOVEL
VANEXEL
VANPOOL
VENTRAL
VONOPEL
VONZELL
WENDELL
XENICAL

•••NL••

AVONLEA
BURNLEY
JEANLUC
JOHNLAW
JOHNLEE
MOONLET
MOONLIT
OHANLON
QUINLAN
STANLEE
STANLEY
TOWNLET
VEINLET

•••N•L•

ATINGLE
BAGNOLD
BLANDLY
BLANKLY
BLINDLY
BLUNTLY
BONNILY
BRINDLE
CANNELL
CANNELS
CANNILY
CANNOLI
CANNULA
CHANELS
CORNELL
CORNILY
CRENELS
CRINKLE
CRINKLY
DARNELL
DIRNDLS
DONNALL
DWINDLE
FAINTLY
FENNELS
FRANKLY
FUNNELS
FUNNILY
GAUNTLY
GOONILY
GRANDLY
GRANOLA
GRANULE
HYMNALS
INANELY
JOINTLY
KENNELS
KERNELS
KINNELL
KRINGLE
LIONELL
LIONELS
LOONILY
LYONELL
MEYNELL
MOONILY
PHENOLS
PHONILY
PIANOLA
PRINGLE
PRONELY
PUNNILY
QUINELA
RAINILY
RAYNELL
RIANTLY
ROUNDLY
RUNNELS
SAINTLO
SAINTLY
SCANTLY
SEENALL
SHINGLE
SHINGLY
SHINILY
SHINOLA
SIGNALS
SLANTLY
SOUNDLY
SPANGLE
SPANGLY
SPINDLE
SPINDLY
SPINELS
STONILY
SUNNILY
SWINDLE
TAWNILY
THENILE
TINNILY
TRUNDLE
TUNNELS
TWINKLE
TWINKLY
VEINULE
VIGNOLA
WRANGLE
WRINKLE
WRINKLY
WRONGLY
YARNELL
ZWINGLI

•••N••L

ARUNDEL
BARNOWL
BEANOIL
BRENDEL
CANNELL
CHANCEL
CHANNEL
CHUNNEL
CORNEAL
CORNELL
CORNOIL
COUNCIL
COUNSEL
CRANIAL
DARNELL
DONNALL
EMANUEL
ENSNARL
EVANGEL
FLANNEL
FRONTAL
GAINFUL
GRENDEL
HOBNAIL
KINNELL
LIONELL
LYONELL
MACNEIL
MEYNELL
MOANFUL
NOANGEL
PAINFUL
QUINTAL
RAYNELL
ROUNDEL
SCANDAL
SEENALL
SPANIEL
STENCIL
STENGEL
TENNIEL
TOENAIL
UNSNARL
UTENSIL
WRANGEL
YARNELL
YAWNFUL

••••NL•

CLEANLY
GREENLY
HUMANLY
PLAINLY
QUEENLY
STERNLY
UNMANLY
VIXENLY
WOMANLY

••••N•L

ADRENAL
ALUMNAL
ARSENAL
AVERNAL
BASINAL
BITONAL
CHANNEL
CHUNNEL
COLONEL
CORONAL
DIURNAL
EMPANEL
ESPANOL
ETERNAL
ETHANOL
FLANNEL
FRESNEL
GRAPNEL
GUIGNOL
IMPANEL
JOURNAL
JUVENAL
LACUNAL
LAMINAL
LIMINAL
MATINAL
NOMINAL
ORDINAL
RAVENAL
REGINAL
REPANEL
RETINAL
RETINOL
SEMINAL
SILENTL
STERNAL
TYLENOL
UNVENAL
VICINAL
VIMINAL

N•M••••

NAMABLE
NAMABLY
NAMEDAY
NAMEONE
NAMETAG
NAMIBIA
NEMEROV
NEMESES
NEMESIS
NIMBLER
NIMIETY
NIMRODS
NOMADIC
NOMBRES
NOMERCY
NOMERGE
NOMINAL
NOMINEE
NUMBATS
NUMBERS
NUMBEST
NUMBING
NUMERAL
NUMERIC
NUMEROS
NUMLOCK
NYMPHAL
NYMPHIC

N••M•••

NESMITH
NEUMANN
NEWMADE
NEWMANS
NEWMATH
NEWMINT
NEWMONT
NEWMOON
NEWMOWN
NIPMUCK
NONMEAT
NORMALS
NORMAND
NORMANS
NOTMANY
NOTMINE
NOTMUCH
NUTMEAT
NUTMEGS

N•••M••

NAVYMAN
NAVYMEN
NESSMAN
NEWSMAN
NEWSMEN
NICEMAN
NICEMEN
NKRUMAH
NOKOMIS
NOLIMIT
NONAMES
NYTIMES

N••••M•

NANAIMO
NAPALMS
NAPTIME
NATSUME
NBAGAME
NETGAME
NEWNAME
NEWSOME
NFLGAME
NHLGAME
NOISOME
NONCOMS
NONHOME
NOTHOME
NOTRUMP
NOXZEMA

N•••••M

NATRIUM
NAUSEAM
NBATEAM
NEEDHAM
NFCTEAM
NFLTEAM
NHLTEAM
NIOBIUM
NONFARM
NONFORM
NOSEEUM
NOSTRUM

•NM••••

ENMASSE
INMARCH
INMATES
ONMYOWN
UNMACHO
UNMADLY
UNMAKER
UNMAKES
UNMANED
UNMANLY
UNMASKS
UNMASTS
UNMATED
UNMATES
UNMEANT
UNMERGE
UNMERRY
UNMEWED
UNMIKED
UNMINED
UNMIRED
UNMITER
UNMITRE
UNMIXED
UNMIXES
UNMOIST
UNMOLDS
UNMOLDY
UNMOODY
UNMOORS
UNMOSSY
UNMOULD
UNMOVED
UNMOWED
UNMUDDY
UNMUTED

•N•M•••

ANDMORE
ANEMIAS
ANEMONE
ANIMACY
ANIMALS
ANIMATE
ANIMATO
ANIMISM
ANIMIST
ANOMALY
ANOMIES
ANYMORE
ENAMELS
ENAMORS
ENAMOUR
ENDMOST
ENEMIES
FNUMBER
GNOMISH
GNOMIST
GNOMONS
INAMESS
INAMOOD
INKMARK
ONEMILE
ONEMORE
ONEMPTY
UNAMUNO
UNEMPTY
UNSMART
UNSMOKY

•N••M••

ANAEMIA
ANAEMIC
ANDAMAN
ANNAMAY
ANOSMIA
ANOSMIC
ENARMED
ENCAMPS
ENCOMIA
ENDEMIC
ENIGMAS
ENTOMBS
ENZYMES
ENZYMIC
INCOMER
INCOMES
INGEMAR
INHUMAN
INHUMED
INHUMER
INHUMES
INLIMBO
ONRAMPS
PNEUMAS
PNEUMAT
PNEUMON
SNOWMAN
SNOWMEN
UNAIMED
UNARMED
UNCOMIC
UNDOMED
UNFAMED
UNHUMAN
UNHUMID
UNKEMPT
UNLUMPY
UNNAMED
UNRIMED
UNTAMED
UNTAMES
UNTIMED
UNTIMID

•N•••M•

ANADEMS
ANATOMY
ANDIAMO
ANONYMS
ANSELMO
ANTHEMS
ANYTIME
ENDGAME
ENFLAME
ENFRAME
ENGRAMS
INFLAME
INFORMS
INSEAMS
ONEDIME
ONELUMP
ONENAME
ONETIME
UNCLAMP
UNCRAMP
UNHELMS
UNISOMS
UNPLUMB
UNRHYME
UNROOMY
UNSEAMS
UNWORMY

•N••••M

ANAGRAM
ANAHEIM
ANIMISM
ANTFARM
ANTONYM
ENVENOM
INAPOEM
INBLOOM
INTERIM
ONAWHIM
ONECLAM
ONEGRAM
ONEROOM
ONETERM
UNBOSOM
UNIFORM

••NM•••

BONMOTS
CONMOTO
DENMARK
DENMOMS
DINMONT
EANMUND
FANMAIL
GINMILL
GUNMOLL
KENMORE
KINMONT
MANMADE
NONMEAT
SUNMAID
TENMILE
TINMINE

••N•M••

AGNOMEN
ANNAMAY
BENUMBS
BONDMAN
BONDMEN
BYNAMES
CINEMAS
CINEMAX
DENIMED
DONIMUS
DYNAMIC
DYNAMOS
EDNAMAY
EUNOMIA
GENOMES
GENOMIC
GONEMAD
HANGMAN
HANGMEN
JUNKMAN
JUNKMEN
KINGMAN
KINSMAN
KINSMEN
LANDMAN
LANDMEN
LENSMAN
LENSMEN
LINEMAN
LINEMEN
MANSMAN
MANUMIT
MANXMAN
MANXMEN
MINIMAL
MINIMAX

MINIMUM
MINIMUS
MONOMER
NONAMES
OMNIMAX
PANAMAS
RANAMOK
RENAMED
RENAMES
RUNAMOK
SANDMAN
SANDMEN
SYNGMAN
TINAMOU
TONEMES
UNNAMED
VENEMAN
WENTMAD
WINGMAN
WINGMEN

••N••M•

BANTAMS
BUNKUMS
CENTIME
CENTIMO
CONDEMN
CONGAME
CONSUME
CONTEMN
DENMOMS
FANDOMS
FUNTIME
GENZYME
GINGAME
HANSOMS
IONIUMS
LANCOME
NANAIMO
NONCOMS
NONHOME
PENNAME
PINCHME
RANHOME
RANSOMS
RUNHOME
RUNTIME
SANREMO
SUNLAMP
TANDEMS
VANCAMP
VENDOME
WINDOMS
WINSOME

••N•••M

ALNILAM
BENTHAM
BINGHAM
CENTRUM
CONFIRM
CONFORM
DINADAM
FANPALM
FANTASM
GINGHAM
GUNROOM
IANHOLM
IONBEAM
KINGDOM
LANGHAM
LONGARM
LONGTOM
MANHEIM
MINICAM
MINIMUM
NONFARM
NONFORM
PANGRAM
PENTIUM
PINETUM
PINKHAM
SANCTUM
SUNBEAM
SUNROOM
SYNONYM
TANGRAM
TANTRUM
TINYTIM
TONEARM
WYNDHAM
ZANYISM

•••NM••

CRANMER
FEYNMAN
IRONMAN
IRONMEN
MAINMAN
MAINMEN
MYANMAR
RAINMAN
THINMAN

•••N•M•

ANONYMS
BADNAME
BARNUMS
BIGNAME
DRINKME
ECONOMY
EDINAMN
EPONYMS
EPONYMY
EUONYMS
EXANIMO
EXENEMY
EXONYMS
FLINTMI
FRENEMY
GRANDMA
IPANEMA
ISONOMY
MAGNUMS
MISNAME
NEWNAME
ONENAME
PENNAME
PETNAME
PHENOMS
PHONEME
PLENUMS
PRENAME
SURNAME
TOPNAME
TSUNAMI
YOUNGMC

•••N••M

AGENDUM
AGONISM
COUNTEM
CRANIUM
DUBNIUM
GRANDAM
HAFNIUM
HAHNIUM
JAINISM
PHANTOM
PIANISM
QUANTUM
QUONDAM
RHENIUM
STANNUM
TRANSAM
TRANSOM
URANIUM
ZIONISM

••••NM•

ITSONME

••••N•M

ACRONYM
ALLONYM
ANTONYM
ARCANUM
AUTONYM
CACONYM
DEMONYM
ENVENOM
FEMINUM
HAZANIM
HOMONYM
HUMANUM
HYPONYM
JEJUNUM
PARONYM
SEVENAM
SEVENPM
SILENTM
STANNUM
STEINEM
STERNUM
SURINAM
SYNONYM
TOPONYM
VIETNAM
WOOSNAM

N•N••••

NANAIMO
NANETTE
NANJING
NANKING
NANNIED
NANNIES
NENNIUS
NINEEEE
NINEPIN
NINEVEH
NINNIES
NINTHLY
NONACID
NONAGES
NONAGON
NONAMES
NONARAB
NONARTS
NONBANK
NONBASE
NONBODY
NONBOOK
NONBUSY
NONCASH
NONCOLA
NONCOMS
NONCORE
NONCROP
NONDARK
NONDEAF
NONDEEP
NONDIET
NONDRIP
NONDRUG
NONEPIC
NONETTE
NONEVER
NONEVIL
NONFACT
NONFANS
NONFARM
NONFLUX
NONFOOD
NONFORM
NONFUEL
NONGOGO
NONGOLD
NONHERO
NONHITS
NONHOME
NONIRON
NONJEWS
NONJURY
NONLIFE
NONLIVE
NONMEAT
NONNEWS
NONOILY
NONOISE
NONORAL
NONPAID
NONPARS
NONPAST
NONPEAK
NONPLAY
NONPLUS
NONPOET
NONPOOR
NONPROS
NONSALE
NONSANE
NONSELF
NONSKED
NONSKID
NONSLIP
NONSTOP
NONSUCH
NONUKES
NONUPLE
NONUSER
NONVOID
NONWAGE
NONWARS
NONWOOL
NONWORD
NONWORK
NONZERO
NUNAVUT
NUNCIOS
NUNGWEN
NUNHOOD
NUNLIKE
NUNNERY
NUNNISH
NUNSHIP

N••N•••

NANNIED
NANNIES
NBCNEWS
NENNIUS
NEONATE
NEONGAS
NEWNAME
NEWNESS
NIANTIC
NINNIES
NOANGEL
NOENDOF
NOENDTO
NOENTRY
NOKNOCK
NONNEWS
NOONDAY
NOONERS
NOONING
NOTNEAR
NOTNICE
NOWNESS
NUANCED
NUANCES
NUDNIKS
NUNNERY
NUNNISH

N•••N••

NEATNIK
NEEDNOT
NOCANDO
NOHANDS
NOMINAL
NOMINEE
NOTONCE
NOVENAS
NYYANKS

N••••N•

NABBING
NAGGING
NAILING
NAMEONE
NANJING
NANKING
NAPKINS
NAPPING
NASCENT
NATHANS
NATIONS
NEARING
NEATENS
NECKING
NEDLAND
NEEDING
NEGRONI
NELSONS
NEOCENE
NEOCONS
NEOGENE
NEPTUNE
NERVINE
NERVING
NESTING
NETTING
NETTONS
NEUMANN
NEURONE
NEURONS
NEWHAND
NEWLINE
NEWMANS
NEWMINT
NEWMONT
NEWTONS
NIALONG
NICEONE
NICHING
NICKING
NIPPING
NIRVANA
NISSANS
NISSANZ
NITTANY
NOCKING
NOCOUNT
NODDING
NOGGINS
NOISING
NONBANK
NONFANS
NONSANE
NOONING
NOOSING
NORMAND
NORMANS
NORTONS
NOSHING
NOTAONE
NOTDONE
NOTHING
NOTHINS
NOTIONS
NOTMANY
NOTMINE
NOTTING
NOTURNS
NOVOTNY
NUBBINS
NUBIANS
NUDGING
NULLING
NUMBING
NURSING
NUTPINE
NUTTING
NYGIANT

N•••••N

NAILGUN
NAILSIN
NARAYAN
NAVYMAN
NAVYMEN
NESSMAN
NESTSIN
NETGAIN
NETIZEN
NEUMANN
NEUTRON
NEVADAN
NEWBERN
NEWBORN
NEWMOON
NEWMOWN
NEWSMAN
NEWSMEN
NEWTOWN
NICEMAN
NICEMEN
NIELSEN
NILSSON
NINEPIN
NIPIGON
NONAGON
NONIRON
NOSEDIN
NOSESIN
NOSTAIN
NOTBEEN
NOTEVEN
NOTOPEN
NOUTURN
NOWTHEN
NUCLEON
NUNGWEN

•NN••••

ANNABEL
ANNAKIN
ANNALEE
ANNALES
ANNAMAY
ANNATTO
ANNEALS
ANNELID
ANNETTE
ANNEXED
ANNEXES
ANNOYED
ANNOYER
ANNUALS
ANNUITY
ANNULAR
ANNULET
ANNULUS
ENNEADS
ENNOBLE
INNAGES
INNARDS
INNERLY
INNERVE
INNINGS
INNLESS
INNOWAY
UNNAILS
UNNAIVE
UNNAMED
UNNASAL
UNNEEDY
UNNERVE
UNNOISY
UNNOSED
UNNOTED
UNNOVEL

•N•N•••

ANANIAS
ANONYMS
ANYNEWS
ENDNOTE
ENSNARE
ENSNARL
INANELY
INANEST
INANITY
ININETY
INKNOTS
ONANDON
ONENAME
ONENESS
ONENOTE
UNANGRY
UNENDED
UNINERT
UNINKED
UNKNITS
UNKNOTS
UNKNOWN
UNSNAGS
UNSNAKY
UNSNAPS
UNSNARL

•N••N••

ANDANTE
ANIONIC
ANOINTS
ANSONIA
ANTENNA
ANTONIA
ANTONIN
ANTONIO
ANTONYM
ANYONES
ENCINAS
ENDINGS
ENFANTS
ENGINED
ENGINES
ENHANCE
ENLINKS
ENOUNCE
ENRANKS
ENTENTE
ENVENOM
ENWINDS
INAKNOT
INASNAP
INASNIT
INCANTS
INCENSE
INCENTS
INDENTS
INFANCY
INFANTA
INFANTE
INFANTS
INGENUE
INKINGS
INLANDS
INLINES
INNINGS
INRANGE
INSANER
INSYNCH
INTENDS
INTENSE
INTENTS
INTONED
INTONER
INTONES
INVENTS
ONEINCH
ONEONTA
ONEUNIT
UNBENCH
UNBENDS
UNBINDS
UNBONED
UNCANED
UNCANNY
UNCINCH
UNDINES
UNFANCY
UNFENCE
UNFINED
UNFINES
UNFUNNY
UNHANDS
UNHANDY
UNHINGE
UNHONED
UNKINKS
UNLINED
UNLINKS
UNMANED
UNMANLY
UNMINED
UNOWNED
UNSUNNY
UNTENSE
UNTONED
UNTUNED
UNTUNES
UNVENAL
UNWANED
UNWINDS
UNWINDY
UNZONED
UNZONES

•N•••N•

ANACINS
ANCIENT
ANDEANS
ANELING
ANEMONE
ANGLING
ANILINE
ANODYNE
ANTEING
ANTENNA
ANTHONY
ANTOINE
ANYKIND
ENCHANT
ENDLINE
ENDLONG
ENDPINS
ENDRUNS
ENDUING
ENDZONE
ENGLAND
ENGLUND
ENJOINS
ENPLANE
ENSIGNS
ENSUING
ENTRANT
ENTWINE
ENURING
ENVYING
ENWOUND
GNAWING
GNOMONS
INABIND
INAFUNK
INALINE
INAWINK
INBOUND
INCHING
INCLINE
INDIANA
INDIANS
INFERNO
INFRONT
INGOING
INIRONS
INKLING
INLYING
INPOINT
INPRINT
INRUINS
INSIGNE
INSPANS
INSTANT
INSTONE
INTERNE
INTERNS
INTHING
INTURNS
INURING
KNEEING
KNIFING
KNOWING
ONALINE
ONECENT
ONEHAND
ONELANE
ONEPINT
ONGOING
ONPOINT
SNAKING
SNAPONS
SNARING
SNIPING
SNOCONE
SNORING
SNOWING
UNAGING
UNALONE
UNAMUNO
UNBLENT
UNBORNE
UNBOUND
UNBURNT
UNCANNY
UNDOING
UNDRUNK
UNDYING
UNFOUND
UNFRANK
UNFUNNY
UNGRAND
UNGUENT
UNISONS
UNITING
UNJOINS
UNJOINT
UNLYING
UNMEANT
UNOWING
UNPAWNS
UNPLANS
UNRAINY
UNROUND
UNSHINY
UNSLING
UNSLUNG
UNSOUND
UNSPANS
UNSPENT
UNSTONY
UNSTUNG
UNSUNNY
UNSWUNG
UNTHINK
UNTWINE
UNTYING
UNVYING
UNWOUND
UNWRUNG
UNYOUNG

•N••••N

ANDAMAN
ANDIRON
ANDSOON
ANDTHEN
ANGOLAN
ANISTON
ANKARAN
ANNAKIN
ANTIGEN
ANTIGUN
ANTLION
ANTONIN
ANYTOWN
ENCHAIN
ENDEDIN
ENDEDON
ENGRAIN
ENLIVEN
ENTERIN
ENTERON
ENTRAIN
ENVIRON
GNAWSON
INASPIN
INBROWN
INDIGEN
INDRAWN
INGRAIN
INGREEN
INGROWN
INHUMAN
INKEDIN
INKHORN
INSULIN
INWOVEN
KNOCKON
ONANDON
ONEDOWN
ONEIRON
ONMYOWN
ONTKEAN
PNEUMON
SNACKON
SNAPSON
SNEAKIN
SNELLEN
SNOWDON
SNOWMAN
SNOWMEN
SNOWSIN
UNBLOWN
UNCHAIN
UNCHURN
UNCLEAN
UNCROWN
UNCTION
UNDRAWN
UNEATEN
UNFLOWN
UNGIVEN
UNGREEN
UNGROWN
UNHUMAN
UNICORN
UNKNOWN
UNLADEN
UNLEARN
UNOFTEN
UNPAGAN
UNRISEN
UNRIVEN
UNSHORN
UNSHOWN
UNSLAIN
UNSTERN
UNSWORN
UNTAKEN
UNURBAN
UNWOVEN

••NN•••

BANNERS
BANNING
BENNETT
BENNING
BINNING
BONNARD
BONNETS
BONNIER
BONNILY
BUNNIES
BUNNING
CANNELL
CANNELS
CANNERS
CANNERY
CANNIER
CANNILY
CANNING
CANNOCK
CANNOLI
CANNONS
CANNULA
CONNATE
CONNECT
CONNERY
CONNICK
CONNIFF
CONNING
CONNIVE
CONNORS
CONNOTE
CUNNING
DANNING
DENNEHY
DENNING
DINNERS
DINNING
DONNALL
DONNING
DONNISH
DUNNAGE
DUNNERS
DUNNING
FANNERS
FANNING
FENNELS
FENNIER
FINNAIR
FINNIER
FINNISH
FUNNELS
FUNNIER
FUNNIES
FUNNILY
FUNNING
GANNETS
GANNETT
GENNAIO
GENNARO
GINNING
GUNNERS
GUNNERY
GUNNIES
GUNNING
HENNAED
HENNERY
HENNISH
HINNIES
HUNNISH
HUNNYBS
JENNETS
KENNEDY
KENNELS
KENNETH
KENNING
KINNEAR
KINNELL

LENNONS
LINNETS
MANNERS
MANNIES
MANNING
MANNISH
MINNOWS
NANNIED
NANNIES
NENNIUS
NINNIES
NONNEWS
NUNNERY
NUNNISH
PANNERS
PANNIER
PANNING
PENNAME
PENNANT
PENNATE
PENNERS
PENNEYS
PENNIES
PENNINE
PENNING
PENNOCK
PENNONS
PINNACE
PINNATE
PINNERS
PINNING
PUNNERS
PUNNIER
PUNNILY
PUNNING
RENNETS
RENNINS
RUNNELS
RUNNERS
RUNNETH
RUNNIER
RUNNING
SENNETT
SINNERS
SINNING
SONNETS
SUNNIER
SUNNILY
SUNNING
TANNERS
TANNERY
TANNEST
TANNING
TANNINS
TANNISH
TENNANT
TENNECO
TENNERS
TENNIEL
TENNIES
TINNERS
TINNIER
TINNILY
TINNING
TONNAGE
TONNEAU
TUNNELS
VANNING
WANNABE
WANNESS
WANNEST
WANNING
WANNISH
WINNERS
WINNING
WINNOWS
YANNICK
YENNING
ZINNIAS

••N•N••

AWNINGS
BANANAS
BANANES
BONANZA
CANINES
CANINGS
CANONIC
CANONRY
DANANAS
ELNINOS
FINANCE
INNINGS
IONONES
LINDNER
LININGS
MANANAS
MININGS
MRNANNY
PANINIS
PENANCE
PINENUT
PINONES
RANINTO
RANONIN
RUNINTO
RUNONIN
SONANCE
SYNONYM
TENANCY
TENANTS
TENONED
TENONER
VENTNOR
VINTNER
WINGNUT
WYNONNA
ZENANAS

••N••N•

ADNOUNS
AMNIONS
AYNRAND
BANDANA
BANDING
BANGING
BANKING
BANKONE
BANNING
BANTING
BANYANS
BENDING
BENGUNN
BENIGNI
BENIGNO
BENNING
BENZENE
BINDING
BINGING
BINNING
BONBONS
BONDING
BONGING
BONKING
BUNGING
BUNIONS
BUNKING
BUNNING
BUNTING
CANCANS
CANDENT
CANNING
CANNONS
CANTINA
CANTING
CANTINO
CANTONS
CANYONS
CANZONA
CANZONE
CANZONI
CENSING
CINZANO
CONDONE
CONFINE
CONKING
CONNING
CONSENT
CONTEND
CONTENT
CONVENE
CONVENT
CUNNING
DANCING
DANNING
DENNING
DENTINE
DENTING
DENTINS
DENTONS
DENTYNE
DENYING
DINDINS
DINGING
DINMONT
DINNING
DINTING
DONJONS
DONKING
DONNING
DUNKING
DUNLINS
DUNNING
EANMUND
EONLINE
FANGING
FANIONS
FANNING
FANTANS
FANTINE
FANZINE
FENCING
FENDING
FINDING
FINIANS
FINKING
FINLAND
FONDANT
FONTANA
FONTANE
FONTINA
FUNDING
FUNKING
FUNNING
FUNRUNS
GANGING
GENUINE
GINNING
GINSENG
GONGING
GUNNING
HANDING
HANGING
HENBANE
HINGING
HINTING
HONKING
HUNTING
IONIANS
JANEANE
JENKINS
JINXING
JUNKDNA
JUNKING
KANSANS
KENNING
KENYANS
KINGING
KINKING
KINMONT
LANCING
LANDING
LANDINI
LANEONE
LANSING
LANTANA
LANVINS
LENDING
LENFANT
LENIENT
LENNONS
LINDENS
LINEONE
LINKING
LINTING
LONGING
LUNGING
LYNDONB
MANCINI
MANDANS
MANGANO
MANHUNT
MANKIND
MANNING
MENDING
MENSANS
MINCING
MINDING
MINIONS
MINOANS
MINOTND
MINTING
MINUEND
MINYANS
MONTANA
MONTAND
MONTANO
MONTUNO
MRNANNY
MUNDANE
NANJING
NANKING
NONBANK
NONFANS
NONSANE
OINKING
PANNING
PANTENE
PANTING
PANTONE
PENDANT
PENDENT
PENDING
PENNANT
PENNINE
PENNING
PENNONS
PENTANE
PINGING
PINIONS
PINKENS
PINKING
PINNING
PONDING
PONTANO
PONYING
PUNGENT
PUNNING
PUNTING
RANGING
RANKINE
RANKING
RANTING
RENDING
RENNINS
RENOWNS
RENTING
RINGING
RINSING
RONSONS
RONZONI
RUNNING
SANDING
SANTANA
SANTINI
SENDING
SENSENS
SENSING
SINGING
SINKING
SINNING
SUNFANS
SUNNING
SUNTANS
SYNCING
TANGENT
TANGING
TANKING
TANKINI
TANLINE
TANNING
TANNINS
TENCENT
TENDING
TENDONS
TENNANT
TENPINS
TENSING
TENTING
TENTONS
TENZING
TINCANS
TINGING
TINMINE
TINNING
TINTING
TONGANS
TONGING
TONTINE
VANDINE
VANLINE
VANNING
VANSANT
VANZANT
VENDING
VENTING
VINCENT
VINLAND
WANNING
WANTING
WANTONS
WENDING
WINCING
WINDING
WINGING
WINKING
WINNING
WONTING
WONTONS
WYNONNA
YANKING
YENNING
ZINCING
ZINGING
ZONIANS
ZONKING
ZUNIANS

••N•••N

AGNOMEN
ANNAKIN
BANGSON
BANKSON
BENGUNN
BENISON
BENTSEN
BONDMAN
BONDMEN
CANTEEN
CONCERN
CONDEMN
CONDIGN
CONJOIN
CONKLIN
CONSIGN
CONTAIN
CONTEMN
DANIKEN
DANTEAN
DENDRON
DENISON
DENIZEN
DINEDIN
DINEDON
DINESEN
DINESIN
DINESON
DONEGAN
DONJUAN
DONOVAN
DUNEDIN
DUNGEON
DUNSTAN
FENCEIN
FENELON
FINKSON
FONTEYN
GENEVAN
GENTIAN
HANDGUN
HANDLIN
HANDSIN
HANDSON
HANGMAN
HANGMEN
HANGSIN
HANGSON
HANGTEN
HINGEON
HONEDIN
HONESIN
HUNGTEN
JANSSEN
JANSSON
JUNGIAN
JUNKMAN
JUNKMEN
KANTIAN
KENOLIN
KINGMAN
KINGPIN
KINISON
KINSMAN
KINSMEN
LANDMAN
LANDMEN
LANGDON
LANGTON
LANOLIN
LANTERN
LENSMAN
LENSMEN
LINCOLN
LINEMAN
LINEMEN
LONGDEN
LONGRUN
LONGTON
LONIGAN
MANIKIN
MANOLIN
MANSION
MANSMAN
MANTUAN
MANXMAN
MANXMEN
MENCKEN
MENTION
MENUHIN
MINIKIN
MINIVAN
MINORIN
MONACAN
MONCTON
MONSOON
MUNCHEN
MUNCHON
NINEPIN
NONAGON
NONIRON
NUNGWEN
PENGUIN
PENSION
PINDOWN
PONTIAN
PONTOON
PUNCHIN
PYNCHON
RANDOWN
RANGOON
RANONIN
RINGSIN
RONTGEN
RUNDOWN
RUNONIN
SANBORN
SANDMAN
SANDMEN
SANJUAN
SENDSIN
SENDSON
SENECAN
SINKSIN
SONORAN
SUNBURN
SUNDOWN
SUNSFAN
SYNGMAN
TENKRUN
TENSION
TINHORN
TINTERN
TUNEDIN
TUNESIN
VANDIEN
VANDUYN
VANOWEN
VANRIJN
VENEMAN
VENISON
WANTSIN
WINGMAN
WINGMEN
WINSTON
XANTHAN
YANKSON
YANKTON

•••NN••

ALANNAH
ARONNAX
BIENNIA
BRENNAN
BRENNER
BRYNNER
CHANNEL
CHINNED
CHUNNEL
DJINNIS
DUENNAS
EVENNOW
FIENNES
FLANNEL
GLYNNIS
GRANNIE
GRINNED
GRINNER
HYANNIS
ICANNOT
JEANNIE
JEANNOT
JOHNNIE
JOHNNYB
LAENNEC
OCONNOR
OPENNET
PFENNIG
PLANNED
PLANNER
REANNEX
SCANNED
SCANNER
SHANNEN
SHANNON
SHINNED
SHUNNED
SIENNAS
SKINNED
SKINNER
SPANNED
SPANNER
SPINNER
SPINNEY
STANNIC
STANNUM
STENNIS
STUNNED
STUNNER
THINNED
THINNER
TWINNED

•••N•N•

ADENINE
AGENINE
ALANINE
ALINING
ASININE
ASONANT
ATANEND
ATONING
BANNING
BARNING
BARNONE
BEANING
BENNING
BERNINA
BERNINI
BINNING
BRINING
BUNNING
BURNING
CANNING
CANNONS
CLONING
COINING
CONNING
CORNING
CRANING
CUNNING
DAMNING
DANNING
DARNING
DAWNING
DENNING
DINNING
DONNING
DOWNING
DRONING
DUNNING
DURNING
EARNING
EMANANT
EMINENT
EPONINE
EVENING
FANNING
FAWNING
FERNAND
FUNNING
GAINING
GINNING
GOWNING
GUANINE
GUNNING
HERNANI
HORNING
HORNUNG
HYMNING
IRONING
IRONONS
JOINING
KEENENH
KEENING
KENNING
KILNING
KOONING
LEANING
LENNONS
LEONINE
LIGNINS
LIMNING
LOANING
MAGNANI
MANNING
MEANING
MIGNONS
MOANING
MOONING
MORNING
NOONING
OMENING
OPENEND
OPENING
OPINING
PAINING
PANNING
PAWNING
PEENING
PENNANT
PENNINE
PENNING
PENNONS
PHONENO
PHONING
PINNING
PLANING
PRUNING
PUNNING
QUININE
RAINING
REDNINE
REGNANT
REINING
REMNANT
RENNINS
RUINING
RUNNING
SAMNUNN
SEINING
SHANANA
SHINING
SIGNING
SINNING
SIXNINE
STANINE
STONING
SUNNING
TANNING
TANNINS
TENNANT
TINNING
TURNING
TURNONS
TWINING
VANNING
VEINING
WANNING
WARNING
WEANING
WHINING
WINNING
YARNING
YAWNING
YEANING
YENNING

•••N••N

ABANDON
ALENCON
AZANIAN
BERNSEN
BLANTON
BLENDIN
BLENTIN
BLUNDEN
BLYNKEN
BORNEAN
BOSNIAN
BRANDON
BRANSON
BRENDAN
BRENDON
BRENGUN
BRENNAN
BRINGIN
BRINGON
BRONSON
BRONWEN
BURNSIN
BURNTIN
CHANSON
CLANTON
CLINTON
COONCAN
CORNBIN
COUNTIN
COUNTON
CUINGIN
DAWNSON
DOINGIN
DOONEIN
DRANKIN
DRINKIN
DRONEON
DRUNKEN
EDINAMN
ETONIAN
FAWNSON
FEYNMAN
FLANKEN
FRANKEN
FRONTON
GAINSON
GHANIAN
GOINGIN
GOINGON
GRUNION
GUINEAN
HERNDON
HORNSIN
ICINGIN
IRANIAN
IRONMAN
IRONMEN
IRONSON
JOHNSON
JOINSIN
KLINGON
LEANSIN
LEANSON
LYINGON
MAINMAN
MAINMEN
MIDNOON
ODINGON
OHANLON
ONANDON
OPINION
OWINGON
OXONIAN
PHONEIN
PLANSON
PRENOON
PRONOUN
QUENTIN
QUINION
QUINLAN
QUINTON
RAINMAN
RAINSIN
RAINSON
REINSIN
REUNION
ROUNDON
RWANDAN
SAMNUNN
SHANNEN
SHANNON
SHINEON
SIGNSIN
SIGNSON
SLINKIN
SLUNKIN
SPENDON
SPENTON
STANDIN
STANDON
STANTON
STENGUN
STUNGUN
SWANSON
SWENSON
SWINTON
TAUNTON
THINMAN
TRENTON
TURNSIN
TURNSON
TYINGIN
TYINGON
UGANDAN
UNKNOWN
UPANDIN
USINGIN
YOUNGUN

••••NN•

ANTENNA
ARGONNE
BAYONNE
CAYENNE
CEZANNE
COLONNA
CORINNE
DOYENNE
ETIENNE
FACONNE
GARONNE
GEHENNA
HAPENNY
HOSANNA
JOHANNA
LALANNE
MADONNA
MCKENNA
MRNANNY
OLEANNA
OLEANNY
RAVENNA
ROSANNA
ROSANNE
ROXANNE
SAVANNA
SEVENNO
STEANNE
SUSANNA
SUSANNE
SUZANNE
TYRANNY
UNCANNY
UNFUNNY
UNSUNNY
WYNONNA

••••N•N
ACTINON
ANTONIN
AVIGNON
BLOWNIN
BRENNAN
BROSNAN
CHARNIN
CHIGNON
CUTINON
DRAWNIN
DRAWNON
FLOWNIN
FLOWNON
FROWNON
GETINON
GIVENIN
GIVENON
GOTINON
GROWNON
HAVANAN
KALININ
KEYINON
LEBANON
LETINON
LORGNON
MELANIN
RANONIN
ROBBNEN
RUNONIN
SATINON
SHANNEN
SHANNON
SHOWNIN
SILENTN
SIMENON
SITINON
TAKENIN
TAKENON
TRAININ

•••••NN
BENGUNN
CAPEANN
DAYSINN
DIAHANN
DRQUINN
ELLMANN
HERMANN
HOFMANN
LEHMANN
LEOGENN
LIPMANN
MARYANN
NEUMANN
RIEMANN
RUTHANN
SAMNUNN
SCHWANN
SCHWINN
TALLINN
ULLMANN

NO•••••
NOANGEL
NOBBIER
NOBHILL
NOBLEST
NOBODYS
NOCANDO
NOCARBS
NOCATCH
NOCKING
NOCLASS
NOCOUNT
NOCUOUS
NODDERS
NODDIES
NODDING
NODICAL
NODOUBT
NODSOFF
NODULAR
NODULED
NODULES
NOENDOF
NOENDTO
NOENTRY
NOETICS
NOFAULT
NOGALES
NOGGINS
NOGIFTS
NOGOODS
NOGUCHI
NOHANDS
NOISIER
NOISILY
NOISING
NOISOME
NOKNOCK
NOKOMIS
NOLIMIT
NOLOADS
NOMADIC
NOMBRES
NOMERCY
NOMERGE
NOMINAL
NOMINEE
NONACID
NONAGES
NONAGON
NONAMES
NONARAB
NONARTS
NONBANK
NONBASE
NONBODY
NONBOOK
NONBUSY
NONCASH
NONCOLA
NONCOMS
NONCORE
NONCROP
NONDARK
NONDEAF
NONDEEP
NONDIET
NONDRIP
NONDRUG
NONEPIC
NONETTE
NONEVER
NONEVIL
NONFACT
NONFANS
NONFARM
NONFLUX
NONFOOD
NONFORM
NONFUEL
NONGOGO
NONGOLD
NONHERO
NONHITS
NONHOME
NONIRON
NONJEWS
NONJURY
NONLIFE
NONLIVE
NONMEAT
NONNEWS
NONOILY
NONOISE
NONORAL
NONPAID
NONPARS
NONPAST
NONPEAK
NONPLAY
NONPLUS
NONPOET
NONPOOR
NONPROS
NONSALE
NONSANE
NONSELF
NONSKED
NONSKID
NONSLIP
NONSTOP
NONSUCH
NONUKES
NONUPLE
NONUSER
NONVOID
NONWAGE
NONWARS
NONWOOL
NONWORD
NONWORK
NONZERO
NOODGED
NOODGES
NOODLED
NOODLES
NOOGIES
NOONDAY
NOONERS
NOONING
NOOSERS
NOOSING
NOOTHER
NOOTKAS
NOPALES
NOPLACE
NOPQRST
NORBERT
NORDICA
NORDICS
NORDOFF
NORDOWE
NORELCO
NORFOLK
NORIEGA
NORITES
NORMALS
NORMAND
NORMANS
NORRISH
NORTHER
NORTHOF
NORTONS
NORWALK
NORWICH
NORWOOD
NOSCORE
NOSEATS
NOSEBAG
NOSEBRA
NOSEDIN
NOSEDUP
NOSEEUM
NOSEGAY
NOSEJOB
NOSEOUT
NOSESIN
NOSESUP
NOSHERS
NOSHING
NOSHOWS
NOSIEST
NOSIREE
NOSTAIN
NOSTARS
NOSTRIL
NOSTRUM
NOSUGAR
NOSWEAT
NOTABIT
NOTABLE
NOTABLY
NOTALIE
NOTALOT
NOTAONE
NOTASTE
NOTATED
NOTATES
NOTBEEN
NOTCHED
NOTCHER
NOTCHES
NOTDONE
NOTEASY
NOTEDLY
NOTEPAD
NOTEVEN
NOTEVER
NOTFAIR
NOTGOOD
NOTHERE
NOTHING
NOTHINS
NOTHOME
NOTICED
NOTICER
NOTICES
NOTIONS
NOTLIKE
NOTLIVE
NOTMANY
NOTMINE
NOTMUCH
NOTNEAR
NOTNICE
NOTONCE
NOTOPEN
NOTOVER
NOTRADE
NOTRARE
NOTREAL
NOTRUMP
NOTSAFE
NOTSURE
NOTTING
NOTTOBE
NOTTRUE
NOTUPTO
NOTURNS
NOTUSED
NOTWELL
NOTWITH
NOUGATS
NOUGHTS
NOURISH
NOUTURN
NOUVEAU
NOVALIS
NOVARRO
NOVELAS
NOVELLA
NOVELLE
NOVELLO
NOVELTY
NOVENAS
NOVICES
NOVISAD
NOVOTES
NOVOTNY
NOWHERE
NOWISEE
NOWISER
NOWLOOK
NOWNESS
NOWORSE
NOWTHEN
NOWTHIS
NOWWHAT
NOXIOUS
NOXZEMA
NOZZLES

N•O••••
NEOCENE
NEOCONS
NEOGENE
NEOLITH
NEOLOGY
NEOLYTE
NEONATE
NEONGAS
NIOBITE
NIOBIUM
NOODGED
NOODGES
NOODLED
NOODLES
NOOGIES
NOONDAY
NOONERS
NOONING
NOOSERS
NOOSING
NOOTHER
NOOTKAS

N••O•••
NABOKOV
NEPOTIC
NICOBAR
NICOISE
NICOLAS
NICOLET
NICOLLE
NICOSIA
NIKOLAI
NIKOLAY
NOBODYS
NOCOUNT
NODOUBT
NOGOODS
NOKOMIS
NOLOADS
NONOILY
NONOISE
NONORAL
NOTONCE
NOTOPEN
NOTOVER
NOVOTES
NOVOTNY
NOWORSE
NUTOILS

N•••O••
NAIROBI
NAMEONE
NARROWS
NATIONS
NDAKOTA
NEGRONI
NELSONS
NEOCONS
NEOLOGY
NERVOUS
NESTORS
NETCOST
NETLOSS
NETTONS
NETWORK
NEURONE
NEURONS
NEWBOLT
NEWBORN
NEWHOPE
NEWJOBS
NEWLOOK
NEWLOVE
NEWMONT
NEWMOON
NEWMOWN
NEWPORT
NEWSOME
NEWTONS
NEWTOWN
NEWTOYS
NEWWORD
NEWYORK
NIALONG
NICCOLO
NICEONE
NICHOLS
NIMRODS
NITROUS
NIVEOUS
NOCUOUS
NODSOFF
NOGOODS
NOISOME
NOKNOCK
NONBODY
NONBOOK
NONCOLA
NONCOMS
NONCORE
NONFOOD
NONFORM
NONGOGO
NONGOLD
NONHOME
NONPOET
NONPOOR
NONVOID
NONWOOL
NONWORD
NONWORK
NORDOFF
NORDOWE
NORFOLK
NORTONS
NORWOOD
NOSCORE
NOSEOUT
NOSHOWS
NOTAONE
NOTDONE
NOTGOOD
NOTHOME
NOTIONS
NOTTOBE
NOWLOOK
NOXIOUS
NUMLOCK
NUNHOOD
NUTWOOD

N••••O•
NABOKOV
NATATOR
NAVAHOS
NAVAJOS
NEARYOU
NEEDNOT
NEGATOR
NEMEROV
NEUTRON
NEWLOOK
NEWMOON
NEWSBOY
NICEBOY
NICEDOG
NICEJOB
NILESOH
NILSSON
NIPIGON
NOENDOF
NONAGON
NONBOOK
NONCROP
NONFOOD
NONIRON
NONPOOR
NONPROS
NONSTOP
NONWOOL
NORTHOF
NORWOOD
NOSEJOB
NOTALOT
NOTGOOD
NOWLOOK
NUCLEON
NUMEROS
NUNCIOS
NUNHOOD
NUTWOOD

N•••••O
NABISCO
NABUCCO
NANAIMO
NEEDSTO
NETZERO
NICCOLO
NOCANDO
NOENDTO
NONGOGO
NONHERO
NONZERO
NORELCO
NOTUPTO
NOVARRO
NOVELLO
NUESTRO

•NO••••
ANODISE
ANODIZE
ANODYNE
ANOINTS
ANOMALY
ANOMIES
ANONYMS
ANORAKS
ANOSMIA
ANOSMIC
ANOTHER
ANOUILH
CNOSSUS
ENOILED
ENOLOGY
ENOUNCE
GNOCCHI
GNOMISH
GNOMIST
GNOMONS
GNOSSUS
GNOSTIC
INOCULA
INORBIT
INORDER
KNOBBED
KNOCKED
KNOCKER
KNOCKON
KNOSSOS
KNOTSUP
KNOTTED
KNOTTER
KNOUTED
KNOWALL
KNOWERS
KNOWETH
KNOWHOW
KNOWING
KNOWLES
KNOWSOF
MNOPQRS
ONORATI
ONORDER
SNOBALL
SNOCAPS
SNOCATS
SNOCONE
SNOOKER
SNOOPED
SNOOPER
SNOOTED
SNOOZED
SNOOZER
SNOOZES
SNORERS
SNORING
SNORKEL
SNORTAT
SNORTED
SNORTER
SNOUTED
SNOWCAP
SNOWCAT
SNOWDAY
SNOWDON
SNOWHAT
SNOWIER
SNOWILY
SNOWING
SNOWJOB
SNOWMAN
SNOWMEN
SNOWPEA
SNOWSIN
SNOWSKI
UNOBESE
UNOFTEN
UNOGLED
UNOILED
UNOPTED
UNORBED
UNOVERT
UNOWING
UNOWNED

•N•O•••
ANDORRA
ANDOVER
ANGOLAN
ANGORAS
ANIONIC
ANNOYED
ANNOYER
ANSONIA
ANTOINE
ANTONIA
ANTONIN
ANTONIO
ANTONYM
ANYONES
CNTOWER
ENCODED
ENCODER
ENCODES
ENCOMIA
ENCORED
ENCORES
ENDORSE
ENDOWED
ENDOWER
ENFOLDS
ENFORCE
ENGORGE
ENJOINS
ENJOYED
ENJOYER
ENNOBLE
ENROBED
ENROBES
ENROLLS
ENROOTS
ENROUTE
ENSOULS
ENTOMBS
ENVOGUE
ENWOUND
INBOARD
INBOUND
INBOXES
INCOLOR
INCOMER
INCOMES
INCOURT
INDOORS
INDORSE
INDOUBT
INFOCUS
INFOLDS
INFORCE
INFORIT
INFORMS
INGOALS
INGOING
INHOUSE
INJOKES
INNOWAY
INPOINT
INPOURS
INPOWER
INROADS
INSOFAR
INSOLES
INTONED
INTONER
INTONES
INTOTAL
INTOUCH
INVOGUE
INVOICE
INVOKED
INVOKER
INVOKES
INVOLVE
INWOVEN
ONBOARD
ONEOCAT
ONEOFFS
ONEOFUS
ONEONTA
ONEOVER
ONGOING
ONLOADS
ONPOINT
ONTOAST
ONTOPIC
ONTOPOF
SNOOKER
SNOOPED
SNOOPER
SNOOTED
SNOOZED
SNOOZER
SNOOZES
UNBOGGY
UNBOLTS
UNBONED
UNBORED
UNBORNE
UNBOSOM
UNBOUND
UNBOWED
UNBOXED
UNBOXES
UNCODED
UNCOILS
UNCOMIC
UNCOOPS
UNCORED
UNCORES
UNCORKS
UNCOUTH
UNCOVER
UNCOWED
UNCOYER
UNCOYLY
UNDOCKS
UNDOERS
UNDOING
UNDOMED
UNFOGGY
UNFOLDS
UNFORKS
UNFOUND
UNFOXED
UNGODLY
UNGORED
UNHONED
UNHOODS
UNHOOKS
UNHOPED
UNHORSE
UNHOUSE
UNJOINS
UNJOINT
UNJOLLY
UNJOYED
UNLOADS
UNLOATH
UNLOBED
UNLOCAL
UNLOCKS
UNLOFTY
UNLOOPS
UNLOOSE
UNLOVED
UNLOWLY
UNLOYAL
UNMOIST
UNMOLDS
UNMOLDY
UNMOODY
UNMOORS
UNMOSSY
UNMOULD
UNMOVED
UNMOWED
UNNOISY
UNNOSED
UNNOTED
UNNOVEL
UNPOLED
UNPOSED
UNROBED
UNROBES
UNROCKY
UNROLLS
UNROOFS
UNROOMY
UNROOTS
UNROPED
UNROPES
UNROUND
UNROWDY
UNSOBER
UNSOGGY
UNSOLED
UNSOLES
UNSOLID
UNSOOTY
UNSORRY
UNSORTS
UNSOUND
UNSOWED
UNTONED
UNTOUGH
UNTOXIC
UNVOCAL
UNVOICE
UNVOTED
UNVOWED
UNWOOED
UNWORMY
UNWOUND
UNWOVEN
UNYOKED
UNYOKES
UNYOUNG
UNZONED
UNZONES

•N••O••
ANALOGS
ANALOGY
ANATOLE
ANATOLY
ANATOMY
ANCHORS
ANCHOVY
ANDMORE
ANDROID
ANDROUS
ANDSOON
ANEMONE
ANEROID
ANTCOWS
ANTHONY
ANTIOCH
ANXIOUS
ANYBODY
ANYHOPE
ANYMORE
ANYROAD
ANYTOWN
DNACODE
ENAMORS
ENAMOUR
ENCLOSE
ENDLONG
ENDMOST
ENDNOTE
ENDZONE
ENGROSS
ENOLOGY
ENROOTS
ENTROPY
ENVIOUS
GNOMONS
INAHOLE
INAMOOD
INAPOEM
INAPOKE
INAWORD
INBLOOM
INBROWN
INCLOSE
INCROWD
INDOORS
INFLOWS
INFRONT
INGROUP
INGROWN
INIRONS
INKHORN
INKNOTS
INKPOTS
INSHOCK
INSHORE
INSHORT
INSPOTS
INSTOCK
INSTONE
INSTORE
INTROIT
ONAROLL
ONATOOT
ONEDOWN
ONEFOLD
ONEFOOT
ONEHOUR
ONEIOTA
ONELOOK
ONELOVE
ONEMORE
ONENOTE

ONEROOM
ONEROUS
ONESOCK
ONETOGO
ONEVOTE
ONEWOOD
ONMYOWN
ONSHORE
SNAPONS
SNIPOFF
SNOCONE
UNALONE
UNBLOCK
UNBLOWN
UNBROKE
UNCHOKE
UNCLOAK
UNCLOGS
UNCLOSE
UNCLOUD
UNCOOPS
UNCROSS
UNCROWN
UNFLOOR
UNFLOWN
UNFROCK
UNFROST
UNFROZE
UNGLOVE
UNGROSS
UNGROWN
UNHOODS
UNHOOKS
UNIBODY
UNICODE
UNICORN
UNIFORM
UNIPODS
UNISOMS
UNISONS
UNKNOTS
UNKNOWN
UNLOOPS
UNLOOSE
UNMOODY
UNMOORS
UNPIOUS
UNPROUD
UNQUOTE
UNROOFS
UNROOMY
UNROOTS
UNSHOED
UNSHOES
UNSHORN
UNSHORT
UNSHOWN
UNSHOWY
UNSMOKY
UNSOOTY
UNSPOKE
UNSPOOL
UNSTOIC
UNSTONY
UNSTOPS
UNSTOUT
UNSTOWS
UNSWORE
UNSWORN
UNWHOLE
UNWOOED

•N•••O•

ANBESOL
ANDIRON
ANDSOON
ANGELOU
ANISTON
ANTIFOG
ANTILOG
ANTLION
ENACTOR
ENARBOR
ENDEDON
ENDUROS
ENTERON
ENVELOP
ENVENOM
ENVIRON
ENVIROS
GNAWSON
INAIDOF
INAKNOT
INAMOOD
INASHOE
INASPOT
INAWEOF
INBLOOM
INCISOR
INCOLOR
INDIGOS
INERROR
INFAVOR
INKBLOT
INKSPOT
INLABOR
KNEWHOW
KNOCKON
KNOSSOS
KNOWHOW
KNOWSOF
ONANDON
ONATOOT
ONEFOOT
ONEIRON
ONELOOK
ONEROOM
ONESHOE
ONESHOT
ONESPOT
ONESTOP
ONETWOS
ONEWOOD
ONLYTOO
ONLYYOU
ONTOPOF
PNEUMON
SNACKON
SNAPSON
SNOWDON
SNOWJOB
UNBOSOM
UNCTION
UNFLOOR
UNSPOOL

•N••••O

ANDIAMO
ANIMATO
ANNATTO
ANSELMO
ANTONIO
INFERNO
INLIMBO
INUTERO
INVACUO
INVITRO
ONEKILO
ONETOGO
ONLYTOO
ONTARIO
ONTHEGO
ONVIDEO
SNAPSTO
UNAMUNO
UNDERDO
UNDERGO
UNMACHO

••NO•••

ADNOUNS
AGNOMEN
ANNOYED
ANNOYER
ARNOLDS
BENOTED
BENOTES
BINOCHE
CANOERS
CANOLAS
CANONIC
CANONRY
CANOPUS
CONOIDS
DENOTED
DENOTES
DONOHOE
DONOTGO
DONOVAN
DYNODES
ELNORTE
ENNOBLE
EUNOMIA
FANOUTS
GENOESE
GENOISE
GENOMES
GENOMIC
HANOVER
HONORED
HONOREE
HONORER
HONOURS
IGNOBLE
IGNOBLY
IGNORED
IGNORER
IGNORES
IKNOWIT
INNOWAY
IONONES
KENOLIN
KENOSHA
LANOLIN
LANOTTE
LENOVOS
LMNOPQR
MANOLIN
MANOWAR
MENORAH
MENORCA
MENOTTI
MINOANS
MINOGUE
MINOLTA
MINORCA
MINORED
MINORIN
MINOTND
MONOCLE
MONODIC
MONOLOG
MONOMER
MONOPOD
MONOSKI
MRNORTH
MRNOVAK
NONOILY
NONOISE
NONORAL
OFNOUSE
PANOPLY
PINOAKS
PINONES
PINOTTA
RANONIN
RANOVER
RENOIRS
RENOTED
RENOTES
RENOWNS
RUNOFFS
RUNONIN
RUNOUTS
RUNOVER
SENORAS
SENORES
SHNOOKS
SONORAN
SYNODAL
SYNODIC
SYNONYM
TANOAKS
TENONED
TENONER
TINORES
UNNOISY
UNNOSED
UNNOTED
UNNOVEL
UPNORTH
VANOCUR
VANOWEN
VONOPEL
WINOVER
WONOVER
WYNONNA
ZENOBIA

••N•O••

AMNIONS
BANGOUT
BANJOES
BANKONE
BENBOVA
BINDOFF
BINGOES
BONBONS
BONGOES
BONJOUR
BONJOVI
BONMOTS
BONSOIR
BUNCOED
BUNIONS
BUNKOED
CANDOUR
CANNOCK
CANNOLI
CANNONS
CANTONS
CANTORS
CANYONS
CANZONA
CANZONE
CANZONI
CENSORS
CINEOLE
CONCOCT
CONCORD
CONDOLE
CONDONE
CONDORS
CONFORM
CONGOUS
CONJOBS
CONJOIN
CONKOFF
CONKOUT
CONMOTO
CONNORS
CONNOTE
CONSOLE
CONSORT
CONTORT
CONTOUR
CONVOKE
CONVOYS
DENMOMS
DENTOID
DENTONS
DINEOUT
DINGOES
DINMONT
DONJONS
DONJOSE
DUNLOPS
FANDOMS
FANFOLD
FANIONS
FANSOUT
FANTODS
FENDOFF
FINDOUT
FUNGOES
GENLOCK
GINGOLD
GONDOLA
GONEOFF
GONEOUT
GONGORA
GUNBOAT
GUNDOGS
GUNLOCK
GUNMOLL
GUNROOM
HANCOCK
HANDOFF
HANDOUT
HANGOFF
HANGOUT
HANSOLO
HANSOMS
HENCOOP
HENTOFF
HUNGOFF
HUNGOUT
IANHOLM
IGNEOUS
JINGOES
JUNCOES
JUNIORS
KANEOHE
KENDOLL
KENMORE
KINFOLK
KINMONT
LANCOME
LANEONE
LANFORD
LENDOUT
LENNONS
LINCOLN
LINDORF
LINEONE
LINEOUT
LINGOES
LONBORG
LYNDONB
MANDOKI
MANGOES
MANHOLE
MANHOOD
MANHOUR
MANROPE
MENFOLK
MENTORS
MINDORO
MINEOLA
MINIONS
MINNOWS
MONGOLS
MONROES
MONSOON
MONTOYA
NONBODY
NONBOOK
NONCOLA
NONCOMS
NONCORE
NONFOOD
NONFORM
NONGOGO
NONGOLD
NONHOME
NONPOET
NONPOOR
NONVOID
NONWOOL
NONWORD
NONWORK
NUNHOOD
OWNGOAL
PANDORA
PANSOUT
PANTONE
PENNOCK
PENNONS
PENROSE
PINBOYS
PINDOWN
PINEOIL
PINFOLD
PINHOLE
PINIONS
PINKOES
PONTOON
RANCORS
RANCOUR
RANDOWN
RANGOFF
RANGOON
RANGOUT
RANHOME
RANKOUT
RANSOMS
RENTOUT
RENVOIS
RINGOFF
RINGOUT
RONSONS
RONWOOD
RONZONI
RUNDOWN
RUNGOFF
RUNGOUT
RUNHOME
RUNSOFF
RUNSOUT
SANBORN
SANFORD
SANGOUT
SANJOSE
SENDOFF
SENDOUT
SENHORA
SENIORS
SENSORS
SENSORY
SENTOFF
SENTOUT
SHNOOKS
SINGOUT
SINUOUS
SUNBOWL
SUNBOWS
SUNDOGS
SUNDOWN
SUNGODS
SUNROOF
SUNROOM
SYNCOPE
TANDOOR
TANGOED
TANGOER
TENCODE
TENDONS
TENFOLD
TENFOOT
TENFOUR
TENSORS
TENTONS
TENUOUS
TINFOIL
TINGODS
TINHORN
TINROOF
TINWORK
TUNAOIL
TUNEOUT
TUNGOIL
VANGOGH
VANLOAD
VANPOOL
VANVOGT
VENDOME
VENDORS
VINROSE
WANTONS
WANTOUT
WENTOFF
WENTOUT
WINDOMS
WINDOWS
WINDOWY
WINKOUT
WINNOWS
WINSOME
WINSOUT
WINWOOD
WONTONS
XINGOUT
YANKOFF
YANKOUT
ZINCOUS
ZONEOUT
ZONKOUT

••N••O•

ALNICOS
BANDBOX
BANGKOK
BANGSON
BANKJOB
BANKSON
BENISON
BENTHOS
BONITOS
CONCHOS
CONTROL
DENDRON
DENISON
DINEDON
DINESON
DONATOR
DONEFOR
DONOHOE
DUNGEON
DYNAMOS
ELNINOS
FENELON
FINKSON
GANGTOK
GENITOR
GINGKOS
GINKGOS
GONEFOR
GUNROOM
GUNSFOR
GUNSHOT
HANDSON
HANGDOG
HANGSON
HENCOOP
HINGEON
HONCHOS
HUNTFOR
IGNATOW
IGNITOR
JANEDOE
JANITOR
JANKLOW
JANSSON
KINGDOM
KINISON
LANGDON
LANGTON
LANGUOR
LENOVOS
LINDROS
LINGCOD
LONGBOW
LONGFOR
LONGTOM
LONGTON
MANHOOD
MANILOW
MANSION
MENTHOL
MENTION
MENUDOS
MINIZOO
MONCTON
MONITOR
MONOLOG
MONOPOD
MONSOON
MUNCHON
NONAGON
NONBOOK
NONCROP
NONFOOD
NONIRON
NONPOOR
NONPROS
NONSTOP
NONWOOL
NUNCIOS
NUNHOOD
PENSION
PINCHOT
PINEFOR
PINESOL
PINETOP
PONCHOS
PONTOON
PYNCHON
RANAMOK
RANCHOS
RANGFOR
RANGOON
RANRIOT
RINGFOR
RONWOOD
RUNAMOK
RUNGFOR
RUNRIOT
RUNSFOR
RUNSLOW
SANDBOX
SANDHOG
SANDLOT
SENATOR
SENDFOR
SENDSON
SENTFOR
SUNGLOW
SUNROOF
SUNROOM
SUNSPOT
TANDOOR
TANKTOP
TENFOOT
TENSION
TENSPOT
TINAMOU
TINROOF
TINYTOT
TONELOC
TONEROW
TONYDOW
VANPOOL
VENISON
VENTNOR
WENDKOS
WENTFOR
WINDGOD
WINDSOR
WINSLOW
WINSTON
WINWOOD
XENIAOH
YANKSON
YANKTON
YENSFOR

••N•••O

ANNATTO
BANDIDO
BANDITO
BENICIO
BENIGNO
BONARIO
BONIATO
BUNUELO
CANSECO
CANTINO
CENTAVO
CENTIMO
CINZANO
CONBRIO
CONMOTO
DANEYKO
DANGELO
DONOTGO
ERNESTO
GENNAIO
GENNARO
GONEPRO
HANDYTO
HANSOLO
IGNARRO
IONESCO
JANEIRO
LANETWO
LENTIGO
LINBIAO
LINETWO
LINPIAO
LONGAGO
MANCUSO
MANGANO
MANKATO
MANRICO
MINDORO
MINIZOO
MONSTRO
MONTANO
MONTEGO
MONTERO
MONTUNO
NANAIMO
NONGOGO
NONHERO
NONZERO
ORNITHO
OWNUPTO
PONTANO
RANINTO
RANUPTO
RENALDO
RENTSTO
RINALDO
RUNINTO
RUNUPTO
SANREMO
SENDSTO
SINGSTO
TANGELO
TENDSTO
TENNECO
TUNEDTO
TUNESTO
WANTSTO
WENTPRO
WINDIGO
ZANETTO

•••NO••

ADENOID
ARENOSE
BAGNOLD
BARNONE
BARNOWL
BEANOIL
BEDNORZ
BIGNOSE
BURNOFF
BURNOUT
BYANOSE
CANNOCK
CANNOLI
CANNONS
CHANOYU
CHINOIS
CHINOOK
COINOPS
CONNORS
CONNOTE
CORNOIL
CTENOID
ECONOMY
EGGNOGS
ENDNOTE
EVENOFF
EVENOUT
GRANOLA
GUVNORS
HEINOUS
HOBNOBS
HOGNOSE
HYMNODY
HYPNOID
INKNOTS
IRONONS
IRONORE
IRONOUT
ISONOMY
IVANOVO
KEYNOTE
KLMNOPQ
LENNONS
LEONORA
LEONORE
LIENORS
LOANOUT
MIDNOON
MIGNONS
MINNOWS
NOKNOCK
OMINOUS
ONENOTE
OPENOUT
ORINOCO
OZONOUS
PAWNOFF
PENNOCK
PENNONS
PHENOLS
PHENOMS
PIANOLA
PLANOUT
PRENOON
PRONOUN
PUGNOSE
RAINOUT
REDNOSE
REKNOCK
REKNOTS
REYNOSA
ROANOKE
RUINOUS
SARNOFF
SAWNOFF
SAYNOTO
SCHNOOK
SCHNOZZ
SEENOFF
SEENOUT
SHINOLA
SIGNOFF
SIGNORA
SIGNORE
SIGNORS
SIGNOUT
SPINOFF
SPINOUT
SPINOZA
SPUNOFF
SPUNOUT
THINOUT
TORNOFF
TORNOUT
TURNOFF
TURNONS
TURNOUT
ULANOVA
UNKNOTS
UNKNOWN
VIGNOLA
WARNOFF
WINNOWS
WORNOFF
WORNOUT

•••N•O•

ABANDON
ALENCON
BAGNIOS
BIENTOT
BLANTON
BRANDON
BRANSON
BRENDON
BRINGON
BRONCOS
BRONSON
BURNFOR
CHANSON
CHINOOK
CLANGOR
CLANTON
CLINTON
COINBOX
COONDOG
CORNCOB
CORNDOG
CORNROW
COUNTON
DAWNSON
DOINGOK
DOWNBOW
DRONEON
ERYNGOS
EVENNOW
FAWNSON
FRANKOZ
FRONTON
GAINSON
GLENCOE
GOINFOR
GOINGON
GRANTOR
GRINGOS
GRINKOV
GRUNION
HERNDON
ICANNOT
IRONSON
IVANHOE
JEANNOT
JOHNBOY
JOHNDOE

JOHNSON
JOHNWOO
KLINGON
LEANSON
LEANTOS
LYINGON
MAINTOP
MCENROE
MEANJOE
MIDNOON
MOONBOW
MOONDOG
MOONGOD
NOENDOF
OBENTOS
OCONNOR
ODINGON
OHANLON
ONANDON
OPENTOE
OPENTOP
OPINION
OWINGON
PHANTOM
PLANFOR
PLANSON
PRENOON
QUINION
QUINTON
RAINBOW
RAINGOD
RAINSON
REENDOW
REENJOY
REUNION
ROUNDON
SCHNOOK
SHANNON
SHINEON
SIGNFOR
SIGNSON
SPENDON
SPENTON
SPONSOR
STANDON
STANTON
STENTOR
SWANSON
SWENSON
SWINTON
TAUNTON
THINKOF
TRANSOM
TRENTON
TURNSON
TYINGON
WARNSOF
XSANDOS

•••N••O

BLINDTO
BOUNDTO
BRINGTO
BRONCHO
CLINGTO
CLUNGTO
DOINGSO
DOINGTO
DRANKTO
DRINKTO
EXANIMO
GENNAIO
GENNARO
GOINGTO
GUANACO
IVANOVO
IWANTTO
JOHNWOO
LEANSTO
LEONATO
LLANERO
LYINGTO
MAGNETO
MEANSTO
MEANTTO
NOENDTO
ORINOCO
OWINGTO
PHONENO
PLANSTO
POINTTO
PRONETO
SAINTLO
SAYNOTO
SOANDSO
STANDTO
TENNECO
THINKSO
TORNADO
TURNPRO
TURNSTO
TYINGTO

••••NO•

ACCTNOS
ACTINON
AKRONOH
ALBINOS
ALIENOR
ASOFNOW
AVIGNON
AWOONOR
BADENOV
BARANOF
BOWKNOT
CALLNOW
CAMINOS
CASINOS
CHIGNON
COMENOW
CUTINON
DARENOT
DOESNOT
DOITNOW
DOMINOS
DRAWNON
ELEANOR
ELNINOS
ENVENOM
EQUINOX
ESPANOL
ETHANOL
EVENNOW
EXITNOW
FEARNOT
FLOWNON
FROWNON
GALANOS
GETINON
GITANOS
GIVENOF
GIVENON
GODUNOV
GOTINON
GROWNON
GUIGNOL
HAVENOT
HERENOW
HOPENOT
ICANNOT
ILLKNOW
INAKNOT
ISEENOW
JEANNOT
JKLMNOP
JOURNOS
JUSTNOW
KEYINON
KIMONOS
LADINOS
LATINOS
LEARNOF
LEBANON
LETINON
LETKNOW
LETSNOT
LORGNON
LUCKNOW
MAGINOT
MERINOS
MISKNOW
MURANOS
MYKONOS
NEEDNOT
OCONNOR
PAXINOU
PAYSNOW
POCONOS
PORTNOY
QUIZNOS
RACINOS
REHONOR
RETINOL
ROMANOS
ROMANOV
ROZANOV
SATINON
SHANNON
SIMENON
SISENOR
SITINON
SMIRNOV
STERNOS
TAKENON
TECHNOS
TEJANOS
TILLNOW
TOPKNOT
TORINOS
TOTINOS
TRAYNOR
TYLENOL
ULYANOV
UPTONOW
USTINOV
VENTNOR
WHATNOT
WHATNOW
YOUKNOW

••••N•O

ADDONTO
ALFONSO
ALIENTO
ANTONIO
ARGENTO
ARSENIO
ASPENCO
ATEINTO
BABENCO
BEGANTO
BUYINTO
BYJINGO
CALANDO
CILENTO
CUTINTO
DEIGNTO
DEMENTO
DIGINTO
DIPINTO
DOMINGO
DRAWNTO
DUGINTO
DURANGO
EATINTO
ELMUNDO
EXTENSO
FEDINTO
FITINTO
FLOWNTO
FLYINTO
FOLENGO
GALENTO
GETINTO
GETONTO
GIVENTO
GOTINTO
GOTONTO
HHMUNRO
HITINTO
HOPINTO
JACINTO
LAMINTO
LAYINTO
LEARNTO
LEDINTO
LEPANTO
LIKENTO
LITINTO
LOGONTO
LORENZO
LYSENKO
MARENGO
MEMENTO
NOCANDO
ORLANDO
OTRANTO
PAYINTO
PIMENTO
PISANIO
PRYINTO
RAMINTO
RANINTO
REDONDO
RIPINTO
RISENTO
RUNINTO
SAWINTO
SECONDO
SEEINTO
SETINTO
SEVENNO
SILENTO
SORENTO
SQUANTO
TAKENTO
TAPINTO
TARANTO
TIEINTO
TORONTO
WASONTO
YEARNTO

•••••NO

AKEBONO
ARACHNO
ARETINO
BAMBINO
BASSANO
BENIGNO
BOITANO
BOUSONO
CALVINO
CANTINO
CASSINO
CELAENO
CHICANO
CINZANO
CUIBONO
DESTINO
EQUIANO
GAETANO
GALVANO
HELLENO
HERMANO
HIBERNO
HISPANO
IJKLMNO
ILOCANO
INFERNO
ISAIDNO
JAYLENO
LIVORNO
LOCARNO
LUCHINO
LUCIANO
MANGANO
MARIANO
MARTINO
MONTANO
MONTUNO
OREGANO
PAISANO
PATERNO
PEPPINO
PHONENO
POBLANO
POMPANO
PONTANO
PROBONO
PULMONO
RELLENO
RIPIENO
ROSSANO
SALERNO
SEVENNO
SOPRANO
SORDINO
SORIANO
SORVINO
SUKARNO
THREENO
TREVINO
UGOLINO
UNAMUNO
VOLCANO
VOTEDNO
VOTESNO
YESORNO
YOKOONO

N•P••••

NAPALMS
NAPHTHA
NAPIERS
NAPKINS
NAPLESS
NAPPERS
NAPPIER
NAPPIES
NAPPING
NAPSTER
NAPTIME
NEPALIS
NEPHEWS
NEPHRIC
NEPOTIC
NEPTUNE
NIPIGON
NIPMUCK
NIPPERS
NIPPIER
NIPPILY
NIPPING
NIPPLES
NOPALES
NOPLACE
NOPQRST
NUPTIAL

N••P•••

NAIPAUL
NAPPERS
NAPPIER
NAPPIES
NAPPING
NEWPORT
NIPPERS
NIPPIER
NIPPILY
NIPPING
NIPPLES
NITPICK
NONPAID
NONPARS
NONPAST
NONPEAK
NONPLAY
NONPLUS
NONPOET
NONPOOR
NONPROS
NTUPLES
NUTPINE
NYMPHAL
NYMPHIC

N•••P••

NEARPAR
NEWSPEG
NINEPIN
NONEPIC
NONUPLE
NOTEPAD
NOTOPEN
NOTUPTO

N••••P•

NEWHOPE

N•••••P

NAILSUP
NAILTIP
NONCROP
NONDEEP
NONDRIP
NONSLIP
NONSTOP
NOSEDUP
NOSESUP
NOTRUMP
NUNSHIP

•NP••••

ENPLANE
ENPRISE
INPEACE
INPERIL
INPHASE
INPLACE
INPOINT
INPOURS
INPOWER
INPRINT
ONPAPER
ONPOINT
UNPACED
UNPACKS
UNPAGAN
UNPAGED
UNPALED
UNPARED
UNPASTE
UNPAVED
UNPAWED
UNPAWNS
UNPEELS
UNPICKS
UNPIETY
UNPILED
UNPILES
UNPIOUS
UNPIPED
UNPLAIT
UNPLANS
UNPLIED
UNPLUGS
UNPLUMB
UNPOLED
UNPOSED
UNPROUD

•N•P•••

ANAPEST
ANSPACH
ENDPINS
ENDPLAY
INAPILE
INAPOEM
INAPOKE
INAPRIL
INAPTER
INAPTLY
INEPTLY
INKPADS
INKPOTS
INSPACE
INSPANS
INSPECT
INSPIRE
INSPITE
INSPOTS
MNOPQRS
ONEPAGE
ONEPAIR
ONEPART
ONEPINT
SNAPONS
SNAPPEA
SNAPPED
SNAPPER
SNAPPLE
SNAPSAT
SNAPSON
SNAPSTO
SNAPSUP
SNIPEAT
SNIPERS
SNIPING
SNIPOFF
SNIPPED
SNIPPER
SNIPPET
UNAPTLY
UNIPLEX
UNIPODS
UNOPTED
UNSPANS
UNSPEAK
UNSPELT
UNSPENT
UNSPICY
UNSPIED
UNSPILT
UNSPLIT
UNSPOKE
UNSPOOL

•N••P••

DNIEPER
ENDUPAT
INASPIN
INASPOT
INCEPTS
INDEPTH
INKSPOT
INSIPID
KNEEPAD
ONEMPTY
ONESPOT
ONPAPER
ONTOPIC
ONTOPOF
SNAPPEA
SNAPPED
SNAPPER
SNAPPLE
SNIPPED
SNIPPER
SNIPPET
SNOOPED
SNOOPER
SNOWPEA
UNCAPED
UNDUPED
UNEMPTY
UNHAPPY
UNHOPED
UNPIPED
UNRIPER
UNROPED
UNROPES
UNTAPED
UNTAPES
UNTYPED
UNWIPED

•N•••P•

ANYHOPE
ENCAMPS
ENCRYPT
ENTRAPS
ENTROPY
ENWRAPS
INSHAPE
INSTEPS
INSWEPT
ONRAMPS
SNOCAPS
UNADEPT
UNCLIPS
UNCLIPT
UNCOOPS
UNDRAPE
UNGRIPS
UNHAPPY
UNHASPS
UNKEMPT
UNLOOPS
UNLUMPY
UNRASPY
UNSHIPS
UNSNAPS
UNSTEPS
UNSTOPS
UNSWEPT
UNTRAPS
UNWHIPT
UNWRAPS

•N••••P

ANTEDUP
ANTESUP
ANTWERP
ENCLASP
ENDEDUP
ENVELOP
INAHEAP
INASNAP
INATRAP
INGROUP
INKYCAP
KNEECAP
KNEESUP
KNOTSUP
ONATRIP
ONECHIP
ONELUMP
ONESTEP
ONESTOP
SNAGSUP
SNAPSUP
SNARLUP
SNAZZUP
SNEAKUP
SNIFFUP
SNOWCAP
SNUCKUP
UNCLAMP
UNCLASP
UNCRAMP
UNSHARP
UNSTRAP

••NP•••

FANPALM
FUNPLEX
GUNPLAY
HENPECK
LINPIAO
NONPAID
NONPARS
NONPAST
NONPEAK
NONPLAY
NONPLUS
NONPOET
NONPOOR
NONPROS
PANPIPE
PENPALS
RANPAST
RUNPAST
TENPAST
TENPINS
VANPELT
VANPOOL

••N•P••

CANAPES
CANOPUS
GONEPRO
HANAPER
HINDPAW
JUNIPER
KINGPIN
LMNOPQR
MANIPLE
MANIPUR
MINEPIT
MONOPOD
NINEPIN
NONEPIC
NONUPLE
OWNUPTO
PANOPLY
RANUPTO
RUNUPTO
SANDPIT
SUNSPOT
SYNAPSE
TENSPOT
TENTPEG
VONOPEL
WENTPRO

••N••P•

CONCEPT
DUNLOPS
GONEAPE
GUNLAPS
HANGUPS
LINEUPS
LINKUPS
MANROPE
PANPIPE
RANLAPS
RUNLAPS
SENDUPS
SYNCOPE
TINTYPE
TUNEUPS
WENTAPE
WINDUPS

••N•••P

BANGSUP
BANKSUP
BINDSUP
BONEDUP
BONESUP
BUNCHUP
CANTRIP
FANCYUP
FENCEUP
GANGSUP
GUNSHIP
HANDSUP
HANGSUP
HANSARP
HENCOOP
HUNTSUP
KINSHIP
LANDSUP
LENSCAP
LINEDUP
LINESUP
LINKSUP
MANTRAP
NONCROP
NONDEEP
NONDRIP
NONSLIP
NONSTOP
NUNSHIP
OWNEDUP
PINESAP
PINETOP
PUNCHUP
RANDEEP
RANITUP
RINGSUP
RUNDEEP
RUNITUP
SENDSUP
SONSHIP
SUNLAMP
TANKSUP
TANKTOP
TENSEUP
TONEDUP
TONESUP
TUNEDUP
TUNESUP
VANCAMP
WINDSUP
WINESAP
WINGTIP

•••NP••

DOWNPAT
EVENPAR
GRANPAS
MOONPIE
OPENPIT
SHINPAD
TURNPRO

•••N•P•

CATNAPS
CATNIPS
CHINUPS
COINOPS
DOGNAPS
GRANDPA
KIDNAPS
KLMNOPQ
MAANDPA
PETNAPS
PRENUPS
RESNAPS
SCHNAPS
SIGNUPS
TURNIPS
TURNUPS
UNSNAPS
WETNAPS

•••N••P

BEANDIP
BORNEUP
BOUNDUP
BRINGUP
BURNSUP
BURNTUP
COUNTUP
CRANKUP
DOINGUP
DRANKUP
DRINKUP
EVENSUP
GOINGUP
ICINGUP
JEANARP
JOINSUP
LYINGUP
MAINTOP
MOUNTUP
OPENSUP
OPENTAP
OPENTOP
PHONYUP
POINTUP
PRINTUP
ROUNDUP
SHINEUP
SIGNSUP
SLANTUP
SLINKUP
SLUNKUP
STANDUP
STANKUP
STINKUP
SWANKUP
THINKUP
TURNSUP
TYINGUP
USINGUP
WOUNDUP

••••NP•

SEVENPM

••••N•P

BLOWNUP
CHAINUP
CHURNUP
CLEANUP
DRAWNUP
EATENUP
FLOWNUP
GIVENUP
GROWNUP
HADANIP
HASANIP
INASNAP
JKLMNOP
LIVENUP
PARSNIP
SEVENUP
SHOWNUP
SILENTP
TAKENUP
WOKENUP

•••••NP

SALMONP

N••Q•••

NESQUIK
NOPQRST

•NQ••••

ENQUADS
ENQUEUE
ENQUIRE
ENQUIRY
INQUEST
INQUIRE
INQUIRY
UNQUICK
UNQUIET
UNQUOTE

•N•Q•••
UNEQUAL
UNIQUES

•N••Q••
ANTIQUE
ENRIQUE
MNOPQRS

•N•••Q•
ONTHEQT

••NQ•••
BANQUES
BANQUET
CINQUES
CONQUER
JONQUIL
YANQUIS

••N••Q•
LMNOPQR

•••NQ••
QUINQUE

•••N•Q•
PSANDQS

•••N••Q
AVENUEQ
KLMNOPQ

••••N•Q
SILENTQ

N•R••••
NARAYAN
NARRATE
NARROWS
NARTHEX
NARVAEZ
NARWHAL
NERDIER
NERDISH
NEREIDS
NERISSA
NERVIER
NERVILY
NERVINE
NERVING
NERVOUS
NERVULE
NIRVANA
NKRUMAH
NORBERT
NORDICA
NORDICS
NORDOFF
NORDOWE
NORELCO
NORFOLK
NORIEGA
NORITES
NORMALS
NORMAND
NORMANS
NORRISH
NORTHER
NORTHOF
NORTONS
NORWALK
NORWICH
NORWOOD
NUREYEV
NURSERS
NURSERY
NURSING
NURTURE

N••R•••
NAIROBI
NARRATE
NARROWS
NATRIUM
NEAREST
NEARING
NEARPAR
NEARYOU
NEGRONI
NEURONE
NEURONS
NEWRICH
NEXRADS
NIMRODS
NITRATE
NITRIDE
NITRIFY
NITRITE
NITROUS
NORRISH
NOTRADE
NOTRARE
NOTREAL
NOTRUMP
NOURISH
NUTRIAS

N•••R••
NATURAL
NATURED
NATUREL
NATURES
NAVARRE
NAYARIT
NEMEROV
NEPHRIC
NEUTRAL
NEUTRON
NIGERIA
NOCARBS
NOMBRES
NOMERCY
NOMERGE
NONARAB
NONARTS
NONCROP
NONDRIP
NONDRUG
NONIRON
NONORAL
NONPROS
NOPQRST
NOSIREE
NOSTRIL
NOSTRUM
NOTTRUE
NOTURNS
NOVARRO
NOWORSE
NUBIRAS
NUMERAL
NUMERIC
NUMEROS
NUTTREE

N••••R•
NABBERS
NAGGERS
NAILERS
NAPIERS
NAPPERS
NATTERS
NAVARRE
NECKERS
NECTARS
NECTARY
NEEDERS
NESTERS
NESTORS
NETSURF
NETTERS
NETWARE
NETWORK
NETZERO
NEUTERS
NEWBERN
NEWBERY
NEWBORN
NEWBURG
NEWCARS
NEWHART
NEWHIRE
NEWPORT
NEWWORD
NEWYORK
NIAGARA
NICETRY
NICKERS
NIPPERS
NODDERS
NOENTRY
NONCORE
NONDARK
NONFARM
NONFORM
NONHERO
NONJURY
NONPARS
NONWARS
NONWORD
NONWORK
NONZERO
NOONERS
NOOSERS
NORBERT
NOSCORE
NOSEBRA
NOSHERS
NOSTARS
NOTHERE
NOTRARE
NOTSURE
NOUTURN
NOVARRO
NOWHERE
NUBBERS
NUDGERS
NUESTRA
NUESTRO
NUMBERS
NUNNERY
NURSERS
NURSERY
NURTURE
NUTTERS

N•••••R
NAGGIER
NAPPIER
NAPSTER
NASTIER
NATATOR
NATTIER
NEARPAR
NEBULAR
NEEDIER
NEEDLER
NEGATER
NEGATOR
NEITHER
NERDIER
NERVIER
NESTLER
NETSTER
NEWAGER
NEWSIER
NEWYEAR
NIBBLER
NICOBAR
NIEBUHR
NIFTIER
NIGGLER
NIGHTER
NIMBLER
NIPPIER
NITTIER
NOBBIER
NODULAR
NOISIER
NONEVER
NONPOOR
NONUSER
NOOTHER
NORTHER
NOSUGAR
NOTCHER
NOTEVER
NOTFAIR
NOTICER
NOTNEAR
NOTOVER
NOWISER
NUBBIER
NUCLEAR
NUTSIER
NUTTIER
NUZZLER

•NR••••
ENRAGED
ENRAGES
ENRANKS
ENRIGHT
ENRIQUE
ENROBED
ENROBES
ENROLLS
ENROOTS
ENROUTE
INRANGE
INREACH
INROADS
INRUINS
ONRAMPS
UNRACKS
UNRAINY
UNRAKED
UNRASPY
UNRATED
UNRAVEL
UNRAYED
UNRAZED
UNREADY
UNREELS
UNREGAL
UNRESTS
UNRHYME
UNRIGID
UNRILED
UNRIMED
UNRIPER
UNRISEN
UNRISKY
UNRIVED
UNRIVEN
UNROBED
UNROBES
UNROCKY
UNROLLS
UNROOFS
UNROOMY
UNROOTS
UNROPED
UNROPES
UNROUND
UNROWDY
UNRULED
UNRURAL

•N•R•••
ANARCHS
ANARCHY
ANDRADE
ANDREAS
ANDRESS
ANDREWS
ANDROID
ANDROUS
ANEROID
ANGRIER
ANGRILY
ANGRYAT
ANORAKS
ANYROAD
ENARBOR
ENARMED
ENCRUST
ENCRYPT
ENDRUNS
ENFRAME
ENGRAFT
ENGRAIN
ENGRAMS
ENGRAVE
ENGROSS
ENPRISE
ENTRADA
ENTRAIN
ENTRANT
ENTRAPS
ENTREAT
ENTREES
ENTRIES
ENTROPY
ENTRUST
ENURING
ENWRAPS
GNARLED
GNARRED
INARAGE
INARUSH
INBREED
INBRIEF
INBROWN
INCROWD
INCRUST
INDRAFT
INDRAWN
INERROR
INERTIA
INERTLY
INFRACT
INFRONT
INGRAFT
INGRAIN
INGRATE
INGREEN
INGRESS
INGROUP
INGROWN
INIRONS
INORBIT
INORDER
INPRINT
INTRADE
INTRAYS
INTROIT
INTRUDE
INTRUST
INTRUTH
INURING
KNARRED
KNURLED
ONAROLL
ONBREAK
ONEREEL
ONEROOM
ONEROUS
ONORATI
ONORDER
ONTRACK
ONTRIAL
SNARERS
SNARFED
SNARING
SNARLAT
SNARLED
SNARLER
SNARLUP
SNORERS
SNORING
SNORKEL
SNORTAT
SNORTED
SNORTER
UNARMED
UNBRACE
UNBRAID
UNBRAKE
UNBRAVE
UNBRIEF
UNBROKE
UNCRAMP
UNCRATE
UNCRAZY
UNCRIED
UNCROSS
UNCROWN
UNCRUDE
UNCRUEL
UNDRAPE
UNDRAWN
UNDRAWS
UNDRESS
UNDRIED
UNDRUNK
UNERECT
UNFRAIL
UNFRANK
UNFREED
UNFREES
UNFRIED
UNFRILL
UNFROCK
UNFROST
UNFROZE
UNGRAND
UNGREEN
UNGRIPS
UNGROSS
UNGROWN
UNGRUFF
UNORBED
UNPROUD
UNTRACK
UNTRAPS
UNTREAD
UNTREED
UNTRIED
UNTRITE
UNTRUER
UNTRULY
UNTRUSS
UNTRUTH
UNURBAN
UNURGED
UNWRAPS
UNWRUNG

•N••R••
ANAGRAM
ANDIRON
ANDORRA
ANGERED
ANGORAS
ANITRAS
ANKARAN
ANTARES
ANTERUS
ANTHRAX
ENCARRE
ENCARTA
ENCORED
ENCORES
ENDERBY
ENDORSE
ENDURED
ENDURER
ENDURES
ENDUROS
ENFORCE
ENGARDE
ENGIRDS
ENGORGE
ENLARGE
ENSURED
ENSURER
ENSURES
ENTERED
ENTERER
ENTERIC
ENTERIN
ENTERON
ENTHRAL
ENTIRES
ENVIRON
ENVIROS
GNARRED
INAPRIL
INATRAP
INCURVE
INDORSE
INERROR
INFERNO
INFIRST
INFORCE
INFORIT
INFORMS
INHERED
INHERES
INHERIT
INJURED
INJURER
INJURES
INLARGE
INMARCH
INNARDS
INNERLY
INNERVE
INPERIL
INSERTS
INSURED
INSURER
INSURES
INTERIM
INTERNE
INTERNS
INTERSE
INTHREE
INTURNS
INVERSE
INVERTS
INWARDS
KNARRED
ONATRIP
ONEARTH
ONEGRAM
ONEIRIC
ONEIRON
ONFIRST
ONSERVE
ONTARIO
ONTHREE
ONWARDS
SNEERAT
SNEERED
SNEERER
UNAIRED
UNBARED
UNBARES
UNBERTH
UNBORED
UNBORNE
UNBURLY
UNBURNT
UNBURST
UNCORED
UNCORES
UNCORKS
UNCURBS
UNCURED
UNCURLS
UNDARED
UNDERDO
UNDERGO
UNEARTH
UNFERTH
UNFIRED
UNFORKS
UNFURLS
UNGIRDS
UNGORED
UNHARDY
UNHARSH
UNHIRED
UNHIRES
UNHORSE
UNLARGE
UNLURED
UNLYRIC
UNMERGE
UNMERRY
UNMIRED
UNNERVE
UNPARED
UNRURAL
UNSCREW
UNSORRY
UNSORTS
UNSTRAP
UNSURLY
UNTERSE
UNTIRED
UNWIRED
UNWORMY

•N•••R•
ANCHORS
ANDMORE
ANDORRA
ANGLERS
ANKLERS
ANSWERS
ANTBIRD
ANTFARM
ANTHERS
ANTIART
ANTLERS
ANTWERP
ANYMORE
ENAMORS
ENCARRE
ENDEARS
ENQUIRE
ENQUIRY
ENSNARE
ENSNARL
ENVIERS
GNAWERS
INAFURY
INAWORD
INBOARD
INCHERS
INCOURT
INDOORS
INKHORN
INKMARK
INPOURS
INQUIRE
INQUIRY
INSHORE
INSHORT
INSPIRE
INSTORE
INTEARS
INTEGRA
INTHERE
INTHIRD
INUTERO
INVITRO
INYEARS
KNAVERY
KNIFERS
KNOWERS
MNOPQRS
ONADARE
ONAGERS
ONAJURY
ONALARK
ONALERT
ONBOARD
ONEACRE
ONELIRA
ONEMORE
ONEPART
ONETERM
ONEYARD
ONGUARD
ONSHORE
SNAKERS
SNARERS
SNIPERS
SNORERS
UNALERT
UNANGRY
UNAWARE
UNBEARD
UNCHARY
UNCHURN
UNDOERS
UNFIERY
UNGUARD
UNHAIRS
UNHAIRY
UNHEARD
UNICORN
UNIFORM
UNINERT
UNITARD
UNITARY
UNITERS
UNLEARN
UNMERRY
UNMITRE
UNMOORS
UNOVERT
UNSHARP
UNSHORN
UNSHORT
UNSMART
UNSNARL
UNSORRY
UNSTERN
UNSWORE
UNSWORN
UNTIERS
UNWEARY

•N••••R
ANDOVER
ANGRIER
ANGULAR
ANNOYER
ANNULAR
ANOTHER
ANTBEAR
ANTIWAR
ANTSIER
CNTOWER
DNIEPER
ENABLER
ENACTOR
ENAMOUR
ENARBOR
ENCODER
ENDOWER
ENDURER
ENDUSER
ENGAGER
ENJOYER
ENSURER
ENTERER
ENTICER
FNUMBER
GNASHER
INAPTER
INASTIR
INCISOR
INCITER
INCOLOR
INCOMER
INDEXER
INDITER
INDUCER
INDYCAR
INERROR
INFAVOR
INFUSER
INGEMAR
INHALER
INHUMER
INJURER
INKSTER
INLABOR
INLAYER
INORDER
INPOWER
INSANER
INSIDER
INSOFAR
INSULAR
INSURER
INTEGER
INTONER
INVADER
INVITER
INVOKER
KNEADER
KNEELER
KNITTER
KNOCKER
KNOTTER
ONATEAR
ONEHOUR
ONEOVER
ONEPAIR
ONESTAR
ONEYEAR
ONORDER
ONPAPER
ONSAGER
ONWATER
SNACKER
SNAGGER
SNAKIER
SNAPPER
SNARLER
SNEAKER
SNEERER
SNEEZER
SNICKER
SNIFFER
SNIFTER
SNIPPER
SNOOKER
SNOOPER
SNOOZER
SNORTER
SNOWIER
SNUBBER
SNUFFER
SNUGGER
UNCHAIR
UNCLEAR
UNCOVER
UNCOYER
UNDULAR
UNEAGER
UNFLOOR
UNGULAR
UNIFIER
UNMAKER
UNMITER
UNRIPER
UNSAFER
UNSHEER
UNSHIER
UNSHYER
UNSLIER
UNSLYER
UNSOBER
UNSWEAR
UNTRUER
UNWISER

••NR•••
AYNRAND
BUNRAKU
CONRACK
CONRIED
DONRUSS
FUNRUNS
GUNROOM
HENREID
HENRICH
HENRIES
HENRYII
HENRYIV
HENRYVI
MANRICO
MANROPE
MONROES
PENROSE
RANRIOT
RUNRIOT
SANREMO
SUNRAYS
SUNRISE
SUNROOF
SUNROOM
TINROOF
VANRIJN
VINROSE

••N•R••
AMNERIS
BENARES
BONARIO
CANARDS
CANTRIP
CENTRAL
CENTRED
CENTRES
CENTRIC
CENTRUM
CINERGY
CONBRIO
CONFREY
CONTRAS
CONTROL
CONURES
DENARII
DENDRON
DINARIC
ELNORTE
GENERAL
GENERIC
GENERIS
GONERIL
HENDRIX
HENDRYX
HONORED
HONOREE

HONORER
HUNDRED
IGNARRO
IGNORED
IGNORER
IGNORES
INNARDS
INNERLY
INNERVE
JONERIK
KENDREW
KINDRED
KINGRAT
LINDROS
LONDRES
LONGRUN
MANDREL
MANFRED
MANTRAP
MANTRAS
MANTRIC
MANURED
MANURES
MENORAH
MENORCA
MINARET
MINERAL
MINERVA
MINORCA
MINORED
MINORIN
MONARCH
MONGREL
MRNORTH
NONARAB
NONARTS
NONCROP
NONDRIP
NONDRUG
NONIRON
NONORAL
NONPROS
PANARAB
PANGRAM
PANURGE
RANFREE
RENFREW
RINKRAT
RUNFREE
SANGRIA
SENORAS
SENORES
SENTRAS
SONORAN
SYNERGY
TANGRAM
TANTRUM
TENDRIL
TENKRUN
TENURED
TENURES
TINORES
TONEROW
TUNDRAS
UNNERVE
UPNORTH
VENTRAD
VENTRAL
VENTRIS
WINERED
WINFREY

••N••R•

BANBURY
BANDERA
BANDERS
BANGERS
BANKERS
BANNERS
BANTERS
BENDERS
BINDERS
BINDERY
BINGERS
BONAIRE
BONDERS
BONEDRY
BONFIRE
BONKERS
BONNARD
BUNKERS
BUNTERS
CANCERS
CANKERS
CANNERS
CANNERY
CANOERS
CANONRY
CANTERS
CANTORS
CENSERS
CENSORS
CENSURE
CENTARE
CENTERS
CENTURY
CINDERS
CINDERY
CONAGRA
CONAKRY
CONCERN
CONCERT
CONCORD
CONCURS
CONDORS
CONFERS
CONFIRM
CONFORM
CONGERS
CONJURE
CONJURY
CONKERS
CONNERY
CONNORS
CONSORT
CONTORT
CONVERT
DANBURY
DANCERS
DANDERS
DANGERS
DANVERS
DENIERS
DENMARK
DENTURE
DINGERS
DINNERS
DONTCRY
DUNKERS
DUNKIRK
DUNNERS
FANFARE
FANNERS
FENCERS
FENDERS
FENETRE
FINDERS
FINEART
FINGERS
FUNDERS
FUNFURS
GANDERS
GANGERS
GENDERS
GENNARO
GENXERS
GINGERS
GINGERY
GONEPRO
GONGORA
GUNFIRE
GUNNERS
GUNNERY
HANDERS
HANGARS
HANGERS
HANKERS
HANSARP
HENNERY
HINDERS
HINTERS
HONIARA
HONKERS
HONOURS
HUNGARY
HUNGERS
HUNKERS
HUNTERS
IGNARRO
JANEIRO
JANUARY
JINXERS
JUNIORS
JUNKART
JUNKERS
KENMORE
KUNDERA
LANCERS
LANDERS
LANFORD
LANGTRY
LANTERN
LANYARD
LENDERS
LINDORF
LINEARA
LINEARB
LINEDRY
LINGERS
LINKERS
LINTERS
LONBORG
LONGARM
LUNGERS
LUNKERS
MANGERS
MANNERS
MANSARD
MENDERS
MENTORS
MINCERS
MINDERS
MINDORO
MINTERS
MONGERS
MONSTRO
MONTERO
NONCORE
NONDARK
NONFARM
NONFORM
NONHERO
NONJURY
NONPARS
NONWARS
NONWORD
NONWORK
NONZERO
NUNNERY
OINKERS
PANDERS
PANDORA
PANIERS
PANNERS
PANTERA
PANTERS
PANZERS
PENNERS
PINCERS
PINCURL
PINGERS
PINNERS
PONDERS
PONIARD
PUNKERS
PUNNERS
PUNTERS
QINTARS
RANCORS
RANGERS
RANKERS
RANTERS
RENDERS
RENOIRS
RENTERS
RINGERS
RINSERS
RONDURE
RONSARD
RUNNERS
RUNSDRY
SANBORN
SANDERS
SANFORD
SENDERS
SENHORA
SENIORS
SENSORS
SENSORY
SINATRA
SINCERE
SINGERS
SINKERS
SINNERS
SUNBIRD
SUNBURN
SUNDERS
SUNFIRE
SUNWARD
TANBARK
TANKARD
TANKERS
TANNERS
TANNERY
TANTARA
TENACRE
TENDERS
TENNERS
TENSORS
TENTERS
TINDERS
TINDERY
TINEARS
TINHORN
TINKERS
TINNERS
TINTERN
TINTERS
TINWARE
TINWORK
TONEARM
TONSURE
VANDURA
VANWARD
VENDERS
VENDORS
VENEERS
VENTERS
VENTURA
VENTURE
VENTURI
WANDERS
WANTERS
WENDERS
WENTPRO
WINCERS
WINDERS
WINGERS
WINKERS
WINNERS
WINTERS
WINTERY
WONDERS
YANKERS
YONKERS
ZINGERS

••N•••R

ANNOYER
ANNULAR
BANALER
BANDIER
BENATAR
BENAZIR
BENCHER
BENDIER
BONEYER
BONHEUR
BONJOUR
BONNIER
BONSOIR
BUNDLER
BUNGLER
CANDLER
CANDOUR
CANNIER
CENTAUR
CONIFER
CONQUER
CONTOUR
DANDIER
DANDLER
DANGLER
DANSEUR
DENUDER
DINGIER
DINKIER
DONATOR
DONEFOR
FANCIER
FANSLER
FENNIER
FINNAIR
FINNIER
FONDLER
FUNFAIR
FUNKIER
FUNNIER
FUNSTER
GENITOR
GENTLER
GONEFAR
GONEFOR
GUNKIER
GUNSFOR
GUNTHER
GUNUSER
HANAPER
HANDCAR
HANDIER
HANDLER
HANOVER
HINKIER
HONORER
HUNKIER
HUNTFOR
IGNITER
IGNITOR
IGNORER
IONISER
IONIZER
JANGLER
JANITOR
JANVIER
JINGLER
JUNIPER
JUNKCAR
JUNKIER
KINDLER
KINKIER
KINNEAR
LANDLER
LANGUOR
LANKIER
LINDNER
LINTIER
LMNOPQR
LONGFOR
LUNCHER
LUNULAR
MANAGER
MANGIER
MANGLER
MANHOUR
MANIPUR
MANLIER
MANOWAR
MANYEAR
MENACER
MENUBAR
MINGIER
MINGLER
MINIBAR
MINICAR
MINIVER
MINSTER
MINTIER
MINUTER
MONIKER
MONITOR
MONOMER
MONSTER
MUNCHER
MUNSTER
MYNHEER
NONEVER
NONPOOR
NONUSER
PANNIER
PANTHER
PINCHER
PINEFOR
PINETAR
PUNCHER
PUNKIER
PUNNIER
PUNSTER
RANCHER
RANCOUR
RANDIER
RANGFOR
RANGIER
RANOVER
RENEGER
RENEWER
RENTIER
RINDIER
RINGFOR
RUNGFOR
RUNNIER
RUNOVER
RUNSFOR
RUNTIER
SANDBAR
SANDBUR
SANDIER
SANDLER
SENATOR
SENDFOR
SENTFOR
SUNNIER
TANAGER
TANDOOR
TANGIER
TANGLER
TANGOER
TANKCAR
TENFOUR
TENONER
TENYEAR
TINGLER
TINKLER
TINNIER
TINSTAR
VANOCUR
VENTNOR
VINEGAR
VINTNER
VONBAER
WANGLER
WENTFAR
WENTFOR
WINCHER
WINDIER
WINDSOR
WINEBAR
WINKLER
WINOVER
WONOVER
YENSFOR
ZINGIER
ZINKIER
ZONULAR

•••NR••

BARNRED
CORNROW
MCENROE
TURNRED

•••N•R•

ABINTRA
AGENTRY
ALINERS
ATONERS
BANNERS
BARNARD
BEANERY
BEDNORZ
BERNARD
BONNARD
BRINERS
BURNERS
CANNERS
CANNERY
CARNERA
CHANTRY
CLONERS
COINERS
CONNERY
CONNORS
CORNERS
COUNTRY
DAMNERS
DARNERS
DEANERY
DINNERS
DOWNERS
DRONERS
DUNNERS
EARNERS
ELANTRA
ENSNARE
ENSNARL
EVENERS
FANNERS
FAWNERS
FERNERY
FOUNDRY
GAINERS
GARNERS
GENNARO
GRANARY
GUNNERS
GUNNERY
GUVNORS
HENNERY
HOHNERS
HYMNARY
IRONERS
IRONORE
JEANARP
JOINERS
JOINERY
KEENERS
KILNDRY
LAUNDRY
LEANERS
LEONARD
LEONORA
LEONORE
LIENORS
LIMNERS
LLANERO
LOANERS
MAINERS
MANNERS
MAYNARD
MOANERS
MOONERS
NOENTRY
NOONERS
NUNNERY
OPENERS
OPINERS
PANNERS
PAWNERS
PENNERS
PHONERS
PINNERS
PLANERS
PLENARY
PRUNERS
PUNNERS
QUINARY
REENTRY
REGNARD
REUNERS
REYNARD
RUINERS
RUNNERS
SCENERY
SEINERS
SHANGRI
SHINERS
SIGNERS
SIGNORA
SIGNORE
SIGNORS
SINNERS
SKYNYRD
SOONERS
SPINDRY
STONERS
SWINERY
TANNERS
TANNERY
TEENERS
TENNERS
TERNARY
TINNERS
TOWNERS
TRENARY
TRINARY
TURNERS
TURNERY
TURNPRO
TWINERS
UNANGRY
UNINERT
UNSNARL
WEANERS
WHINERS
WIENERS
WINNERS
YAWNERS

•••N••R

ALUNSER
AMENDER
ASUNDER
AVENGER
AZINGER
BAINTER
BLANDER
BLANKER
BLENDER
BLINDER
BLINKER
BLONDER
BLUNDER
BLUNTER
BONNIER
BOUNCER
BOUNDER
BRANDER
BRENNER
BRINGER
BRINIER
BRINKER
BRONZER
BRYNNER
BURNFOR
CANNIER
CHANCER
CHANGER
CHANTER
CHENIER
CLANGER
CLANGOR
CLINGER
CLINKER
CLUNKER
CORNIER
COUNTER
CRANMER
DAUNTER
DERNIER
DOWNIER
DRINKER
DRUNKER
EMENDER
EVANDER
EVENPAR
FAINTER
FENNIER
FERNBAR
FERNIER
FINNAIR
FINNIER
FLANEUR
FLANKER
FLENSER
FLINGER
FLUNKER
FOUNDER
FRANKER
FUNNIER
GAUNTER
GOINFOR
GOONIER
GOUNDER
GRANDER
GRANGER
GRANTER
GRANTOR
GRINDER
GRINNER
GRUNGER
GRUNTER
HAUNTER
HORNIER
HOUNDER
IRONBAR
IWONDER
JOINDER
JOINTER
KINNEAR
KLINGER
KLINKER
LAUNDER
LEANDER
LOONIER
LOUNGER
MARNIER
MAUNDER
MEANDER
MOONIER
MOUNTER
MYANMAR
NOTNEAR
OCONNOR
OPENAIR
OPENBAR
PAINTER
PANNIER
PHONIER
PIONEER
PLANFOR
PLANNER
PLANTAR
PLANTER
PLUNDER
PLUNGER
PLUNKER
POINTER
POUNCER
POUNDER
PRANCER
PRINKER
PRINTER
PUNNIER
RAINIER
REENTER
REGNIER
ROUNDER
RUNNIER
SAUNTER
SCANNER
SCANTER
SCENTER
SHANKAR
SHANTER
SHINIER
SHUNTER
SIGNFOR
SKINNER
SLANDER
SLENDER
SLINGER
SLINKER
SOUNDER
SPANAIR
SPANKER
SPANNER
SPENCER
SPENDER
SPENSER
SPINIER
SPINNER
SPONGER
SPONSOR
STANDER
STENTOR
STINGER
STINKER
STINTER
STONIER
STUNNER
SUNNIER
SWANKER
SWINGER
TAUNTER
TAWNIER
TEENIER
THANKER
THINAIR
THINKER
THINNER
THUNDER
TINNIER
TOWNCAR
TWANGER
TWINIER
VAUNTER
VEINIER
VERNIER
WERNHER
WHINIER
WRINGER
WRONGER
YAWNIER
YOUNGER

••••NR•

ALMONRY
CANONRY
FELONRY
FTHENRY
HERONRY
HHMUNRO
MASONRY
MCHENRY

••••N•R

ADORNER
ALIENOR
ALIGNER
ALMONER
ALPINER
AWOONOR
BERKNER
BOCHNER
BRAINER
BRENNER
BROWNER
BRYNNER
BUCHNER
BUCKNER
BYLINER
CHURNER
CLEANER
CORONER
COSTNER
COZENER
CROONER
CROWNER
DEFINER
DEPONER
DIVINER
DRAINER
EDASNER
ELEANOR
FECHNER
FEIGNER
FLEXNER
FROWNER
GARDNER
GLEANER
GORTNER
GRAINER
GREENER
GRINNER
GROANER
HAVENER
INSANER
INTONER
KRASNER
LACUNAR
LAMINAR
LARDNER
LEARNER
LINDNER
LIVENER
MARINER
MEITNER
MOURNER
OCONNOR
OFTENER
PARDNER
PARTNER
PILSNER
PLAINER
PLANNER

POLANER
PREENER
REFINER
REHONOR
REPINER
RIPENER
ROSSNER
SCANNER
SCORNER
SECONDR
SEMINAR
SERENER
SHATNER
SHRINER
SILENTR
SISENOR
SKINNER
SPANNER
SPAWNER
SPINNER
SPOONER
SPURNER
STAINER
STEINER
STERNER
STUNNER
SWOONER
TENONER
THINNER
TRAINER
TRAYNOR
TWEENER
URBANER
VENTNOR
VINTNER
WAGONER
WAKENER
WEGENER
WIDENER
YEARNER

N•S••••

NASALLY
NASCENT
NASTASE
NASTIER
NASTIES
NASTILY
NESBITT
NESCAFE
NESMITH
NESQUIK
NESSMAN
NESTEGG
NESTERS
NESTFUL
NESTING
NESTLED
NESTLER
NESTLES
NESTORS
NESTSIN
NISSANS
NISSANZ
NOSCORE
NOSEATS
NOSEBAG
NOSEBRA
NOSEDIN
NOSEDUP
NOSEEUM
NOSEGAY
NOSEJOB
NOSEOUT
NOSESIN
NOSESUP
NOSHERS
NOSHING
NOSHOWS
NOSIEST
NOSIREE
NOSTAIN
NOSTARS
NOSTRIL
NOSTRUM
NOSUGAR
NOSWEAT

N••S•••

NAPSTER
NATSUME
NAUSEAM
NAYSAID
NAYSAYS
NELSONS
NESSMAN
NETSTER
NETSUKE
NETSURF
NEWSBOY
NEWSDAY
NEWSIER
NEWSIES
NEWSMAN
NEWSMEN
NEWSOME
NEWSPEG
NILSSON
NISSANS
NISSANZ
NODSOFF
NOISIER
NOISILY
NOISING
NOISOME
NONSALE
NONSANE
NONSELF
NONSKED
NONSKID
NONSLIP
NONSTOP
NONSUCH
NOOSERS
NOOSING
NOTSAFE
NOTSURE
NUESTRA
NUESTRO
NUNSHIP
NURSERS
NURSERY
NURSING
NUTSIER

N•••S••

NABISCO
NAILSET
NAILSIN
NAILSIT
NAILSUP
NATASHA
NEEDSTO
NEGUSES
NEMESES
NEMESIS
NERISSA
NESTSIN
NEXUSES
NICOSIA
NIELSEN
NILESOH
NILSSON
NONUSER
NOSESIN
NOSESUP
NOTASTE
NOTUSED
NOVISAD
NOWISEE
NOWISER
NUDISTS
NULLSET

N••••S•

NAGGISH
NAIVEST
NAPLESS
NASTASE
NEAREST
NEATEST
NEBBISH
NERDISH
NERISSA
NETCOST
NETLESS
NETLOSS
NEWNESS
NICOISE
NIGHEST
NOBLEST
NOCLASS
NONBASE
NONBUSY
NONCASH
NONOISE
NONPAST
NOPQRST
NORRISH
NOSIEST
NOTEASY
NOURISH
NOWNESS
NOWORSE
NUMBEST
NUNNISH

N•••••S

NABBERS
NAGGERS
NAIADES
NAILERS
NANNIES
NAPALMS
NAPIERS
NAPKINS
NAPLESS
NAPPERS
NAPPIES
NARROWS
NASTIES
NATHANS
NATIONS
NATIVES
NATTERS
NATURES
NAUGHTS
NAVAHOS
NAVAIDS
NAVAJOS
NAYSAYS
NBCNEWS
NEATENS
NEBULAS
NECKERS
NECTARS
NEEDERS
NEEDLES
NEGATES
NEGUSES
NELSONS
NEMESES
NEMESIS
NENNIUS
NEOCONS
NEONGAS
NEPALIS
NEPHEWS
NEREIDS
NERVOUS
NESTERS
NESTLES
NESTORS
NETFULS
NETLESS
NETLOSS
NETTERS
NETTLES
NETTONS
NEURONS
NEUTERS
NEWBIES
NEWCARS
NEWHATS
NEWJOBS
NEWKIDS
NEWMANS
NEWNESS
NEWSIES
NEWTONS
NEWTOYS
NEXRADS
NEXUSES
NIBBLES
NIBLETS
NICHOLS
NICKELS
NICKERS
NICKLES
NICOLAS
NIFTIES
NIGGLES
NIKEADS
NIMRODS
NINNIES
NIPPERS
NIPPLES
NISSANS
NITROUS
NITWITS
NIVEOUS
NOBODYS
NOCARBS
NOCLASS
NOCUOUS
NODDERS
NODDIES
NODULES
NOETICS
NOGALES
NOGGINS
NOGIFTS
NOGOODS
NOHANDS
NOKOMIS
NOLOADS
NOMBRES
NONAGES
NONAMES
NONARTS
NONCOMS
NONFANS
NONHITS
NONJEWS
NONNEWS
NONPARS
NONPLUS
NONPROS
NONUKES
NONWARS
NOODGES
NOODLES
NOOGIES
NOONERS
NOOSERS
NOOTKAS
NOPALES
NORDICS
NORITES
NORMALS
NORMANS
NORTONS
NOSEATS
NOSHERS
NOSHOWS
NOSTARS
NOTATES
NOTCHES
NOTHINS
NOTICES
NOTIONS
NOTURNS
NOUGATS
NOUGHTS
NOVALIS
NOVELAS
NOVENAS
NOVICES
NOVOTES
NOWNESS
NOWTHIS
NOXIOUS
NOZZLES
NTUPLES
NUANCES
NUBBERS
NUBBINS
NUBBLES
NUBIANS
NUBIRAS
NUCLEUS
NUDGERS
NUDISTS
NUDNIKS
NUDZHES
NUGGETS
NUMBATS
NUMBERS
NUMEROS
NUNCIOS
NURSERS
NUTATES
NUTLETS
NUTMEGS
NUTOILS
NUTRIAS
NUTTERS
NUZZLES
NYTIMES
NYYANKS

•NS••••

ANSELMO
ANSONIA
ANSPACH
ANSWERS
ENSEALS
ENSEATS
ENSIGNS
ENSILED
ENSILES
ENSKIED
ENSKIES
ENSLAVE
ENSNARE
ENSNARL
ENSOULS
ENSUING
ENSUITE
ENSURED
ENSURER
ENSURES
INSALES
INSANER
INSCALE
INSEAMS
INSECTA
INSECTS
INSERTS
INSHAPE
INSHOCK
INSHORE
INSHORT
INSIDER
INSIDES
INSIGHT
INSIGNE
INSIPID
INSISTS
INSOFAR
INSOLES
INSPACE
INSPANS
INSPECT
INSPIRE
INSPITE
INSPOTS
INSTALL
INSTALS
INSTANT
INSTATE
INSTEAD
INSTEPS
INSTILL
INSTILS
INSTOCK
INSTONE
INSTORE
INSTYLE
INSULAR
INSULIN
INSULTS
INSURED
INSURER
INSURES
INSWEPT
INSYNCH
ONSAGER
ONSERVE
ONSHORE
ONSIDES
ONSIGHT
ONSTAFF
ONSTAGE
UNSADLY
UNSAFER
UNSALTY
UNSATED
UNSAVED
UNSAVVY
UNSAWED
UNSCALY
UNSCREW
UNSEALS
UNSEAMS
UNSEATS
UNSELLS
UNSEWED
UNSHADE
UNSHADY
UNSHARP
UNSHEER
UNSHELL
UNSHIER
UNSHIFT
UNSHINY
UNSHIPS
UNSHOED
UNSHOES
UNSHORN
UNSHORT
UNSHOWN
UNSHOWY
UNSHYER
UNSHYLY
UNSIDED
UNSIGHT
UNSILLY
UNSIZED
UNSKEWS
UNSLACK
UNSLAIN
UNSLEEK
UNSLICK
UNSLIER
UNSLING
UNSLUNG
UNSLYER
UNSLYLY
UNSMART
UNSMOKY
UNSNAGS
UNSNAKY
UNSNAPS
UNSNARL
UNSOBER
UNSOGGY
UNSOLED
UNSOLES
UNSOLID
UNSOOTY
UNSORRY
UNSORTS
UNSOUND
UNSOWED
UNSPANS
UNSPEAK
UNSPELT
UNSPENT
UNSPICY
UNSPIED
UNSPILT
UNSPLIT
UNSPOKE
UNSPOOL
UNSTACK
UNSTAGY
UNSTAID
UNSTATE
UNSTEEL
UNSTEPS
UNSTERN
UNSTICK
UNSTIFF
UNSTOIC
UNSTONY
UNSTOPS
UNSTOUT
UNSTOWS
UNSTRAP
UNSTUCK
UNSTUNG
UNSULKY
UNSUNNY
UNSURLY
UNSWEAR
UNSWEET
UNSWEPT
UNSWORE
UNSWORN
UNSWUNG

•N•S•••

ANASAZI
ANDSOON
ANDSUCH
ANISEED
ANISTON
ANOSMIA
ANOSMIC
ANTSIER
CNOSSUS
ENISLED
ENISLES
GNASHED
GNASHER
GNASHES
GNOSSUS
GNOSTIC
INASHOE
INASNAP
INASNIT
INASPIN
INASPOT
INASTEW
INASTIR
INASUIT
INKSACS
INKSPOT
INKSTER
KNESSET
KNISHES
KNOSSOS
ONASSIS
ONESELF
ONESHOE
ONESHOT
ONESIZE
ONESOCK
ONESPOT
ONESTAR
ONESTEP
ONESTOP
UNASKED
UNISIZE
UNISOMS
UNISONS
UNUSUAL

•N••S••

ANBESOL
ANTESUP
CNOSSUS
DNAASES
ENCASED
ENCASES
ENDUSER
ENDUSES
ENLISTS
ENMASSE
GNAWSAT
GNAWSON
GNOSSUS
INCASED
INCASES
INCISED
INCISES
INCISOR
INCUSED
INCUSES
INFESTS
INFUSED
INFUSER
INFUSES
INGESTA
INGESTS
INHASTE
INSISTS
INTASTE
INVESTS
KNEESUP
KNESSET
KNOSSOS
KNOTSUP
KNOWSOF
ONASSIS
SNAGSUP
SNAPSAT
SNAPSON
SNAPSTO
SNAPSUP
SNOWSIN
SNOWSKI
UNBASED
UNBESET
UNBOSOM
UNCASED
UNCASES
UNCASKS
UNDUSTY
UNEASES
UNFUSED
UNFUSSY
UNHASPS
UNHASTY
UNHUSKS
UNLUSTY
UNMASKS
UNMASTS
UNMOSSY
UNNASAL
UNNOSED
UNPASTE
UNPOSED
UNRASPY
UNRESTS
UNRISEN
UNRISKY
UNTASTY
UNWISER

•N•••S•

ANALYSE
ANALYST
ANAPEST
ANATASE
ANDRESS
ANGUISH
ANIMISM
ANIMIST
ANODISE
ANYWISE
DNATEST
ENCHASE
ENCLASP
ENCLOSE
ENCRUST
ENDLESS
ENDMOST
ENDORSE
ENDWISE
ENGLISH
ENGROSS
ENMASSE
ENPRISE
ENTHUSE
ENTRUST
ENTWIST
GNOMISH
GNOMIST
INACAST
INAMESS
INANEST
INARUSH
INCENSE
INCLASS
INCLOSE
INCRUST
INDORSE
INFIRST
INGLESE
INGRESS
INHOUSE
INKIEST
INKLESS
INNLESS
INPHASE
INQUEST
INTENSE
INTERSE
INTRUST
INULASE
INVERSE
KNAVISH
ONEBASE
ONENESS
ONFIRST
ONLEASE
ONLEASH
ONLIEST
ONTOAST
SNIDEST
UNBLEST
UNBURST
UNCLASP
UNCLOSE
UNCROSS
UNDRESS
UNFROST
UNFUSSY
UNGROSS
UNHARSH
UNHORSE
UNHOUSE
UNITISE
UNLEASH
UNLOOSE
UNMOIST
UNMOSSY
UNNOISY
UNOBESE
UNTENSE
UNTERSE
UNTRUSS
UNTWIST

•N••••S

ANACINS
ANADEMS
ANALOGS
ANANIAS
ANARCHS
ANCHORS
ANDEANS
ANDREAS
ANDRESS
ANDREWS
ANDROUS
ANEMIAS
ANGELAS
ANGELES
ANGELUS
ANGLAIS
ANGLERS
ANGORAS
ANIMALS
ANITRAS
ANKLERS
ANKLETS
ANNALES
ANNEALS
ANNEXES
ANNUALS
ANNULUS
ANOINTS
ANOMIES
ANONYMS
ANORAKS
ANSWERS
ANTARES
ANTCOWS
ANTERUS
ANTHEMS
ANTHERS
ANTIBES
ANTLERS
ANXIOUS
ANYNEWS
ANYONES
ANYWAYS
CNOSSUS
DNAASES
DNALABS
ENABLES
ENAMELS
ENAMORS
ENCAGES
ENCAMPS
ENCASES
ENCINAS
ENCODES
ENCORES
ENDALLS
ENDCUTS
ENDEARS
ENDINGS
ENDIVES
ENDLESS
ENDPINS
ENDRUNS
ENDURES
ENDUROS
ENDUSES
ENDWAYS
ENEMIES
ENFACES
ENFANTS
ENFOLDS
ENGAGES
ENGILDS
ENGINES
ENGIRDS
ENGLUTS
ENGRAMS
ENGROSS
ENGULFS
ENIGMAS
ENISLES
ENJOINS
ENLACES
ENLINKS
ENLISTS
ENNEADS
ENQUADS
ENRAGES
ENRANKS
ENROBES
ENROLLS
ENROOTS
ENSEALS
ENSEATS
ENSIGNS
ENSILES
ENSKIES
ENSOULS
ENSURES
ENTAILS
ENTICES
ENTIRES
ENTOMBS
ENTRAPS
ENTREES
ENTRIES
ENVEILS
ENVIERS
ENVIOUS
ENVIROS
ENWINDS
ENWRAPS
ENZYMES
GNASHES
GNAWERS
GNOMONS
GNOSSUS
INAMESS
INBOXES
INCANTS
INCASES
INCENTS
INCEPTS
INCHERS
INCISES
INCITES
INCLASS
INCOMES
INCUBUS
INCUDES
INCUSES
INDENTS
INDEXES
INDIANS
INDICES

7 NS

INDICTS
INDIGOS
INDITES
INDOORS
INDUCES
INDUCTS
INFANTS
INFECTS
INFESTS
INFIVES
INFIXES
INFLOWS
INFOCUS
INFOLDS
INFORMS
INFUSES
INGALLS
INGATES
INGESTS
INGOALS
INGRESS
INGULFS
INHALES
INHERES
INHUMES
INIRONS
INJECTS
INJOKES
INJURES
INKINGS
INKJETS
INKLESS
INKNOTS
INKPADS
INKPOTS
INKSACS
INLANDS
INLINES
INMATES
INNAGES
INNARDS
INNINGS
INNLESS
INPOURS
INROADS
INRUINS
INSALES
INSEAMS
INSECTS
INSERTS
INSIDES
INSISTS
INSOLES
INSPANS
INSPOTS
INSTALS
INSTEPS
INSTILS
INSULTS
INSURES
INTAILS
INTAKES
INTEARS
INTENDS
INTENTS
INTERNS
INTONES
INTRAYS
INTUITS
INTURNS
INVADES
INVENTS
INVERTS
INVESTS
INVITES
INVOKES
INWARDS
INYEARS
KNIFERS
KNIGHTS
KNISHES
KNOSSOS
KNOWERS
KNOWLES
MNOPQRS
ONABIAS
ONAGERS
ONASSIS
ONEACTS
ONEIDAS
ONENESS
ONEOFFS
ONEOFUS
ONEROUS
ONETWOS
ONLOADS
ONRAMPS
ONSIDES
ONWARDS
PNEUMAS
SNAKERS
SNAPONS
SNARERS
SNEEZES
SNIPERS
SNIVELS
SNOCAPS
SNOCATS
SNOOZES
SNORERS
SNUGLIS
UNBAITS
UNBALES
UNBARES
UNBELTS
UNBENDS
UNBINDS
UNBOLTS
UNBOXES
UNCAGES
UNCAKES
UNCASES
UNCASKS
UNCIALS
UNCLIPS
UNCLOGS
UNCOILS
UNCOOPS
UNCORES
UNCORKS
UNCROSS
UNCUFFS
UNCURBS
UNCURLS
UNDINES
UNDOCKS
UNDOERS
UNDRAWS
UNDRESS
UNEASES
UNEDGES
UNFACTS
UNFILES
UNFINES
UNFIXES
UNFOLDS
UNFORKS
UNFREES
UNFURLS
UNGIRDS
UNGLUES
UNGRIPS
UNGROSS
UNHAIRS
UNHANDS
UNHASPS
UNHEEDS
UNHELMS
UNHIRES
UNHOODS
UNHOOKS
UNHULLS
UNHUSKS
UNIATES
UNIFIES
UNIPODS
UNIQUES
UNISOMS
UNISONS
UNITERS
UNITIES
UNIVACS
UNJOINS
UNKINKS
UNKNITS
UNKNOTS
UNLACES
UNLADES
UNLAXES
UNLEADS
UNLEAFS
UNLIKES
UNLINKS
UNLIVES
UNLOADS
UNLOCKS
UNLOOPS
UNMAKES
UNMASKS
UNMASTS
UNMATES
UNMIXES
UNMOLDS
UNMOORS
UNNAILS
UNPACKS
UNPAWNS
UNPEELS
UNPICKS
UNPILES
UNPIOUS
UNPLANS
UNPLUGS
UNRACKS
UNREELS
UNRESTS
UNROBES
UNROLLS
UNROOFS
UNROOTS
UNROPES
UNSEALS
UNSEAMS
UNSEATS
UNSELLS
UNSHIPS
UNSHOES
UNSKEWS
UNSNAGS
UNSNAPS
UNSOLES
UNSORTS
UNSPANS
UNSTEPS
UNSTOPS
UNSTOWS
UNTACKS
UNTAMES
UNTAPES
UNTAXES
UNTHAWS
UNTIERS
UNTRAPS
UNTRUSS
UNTUCKS
UNTUNES
UNVEILS
UNWALLS
UNWINDS
UNWRAPS
UNYOKES
UNZONES

••NS•••

BANSHEE
BONSOIR
CANSECO
CENSERS
CENSING
CENSORS
CENSURE
CONSENT
CONSIGN
CONSIST
CONSOLE
CONSORT
CONSULS
CONSULT
CONSUME
DANSEUR
DENSELY
DENSEST
DENSIFY
DENSITY
DUNSTAN
FANSLER
FANSOUT
FUNSTER
GINSENG
GUNSELS
GUNSFOR
GUNSHIP
GUNSHOT
HANSARP
HANSOLO
HANSOMS
HENSLEY
IBNSAUD
IINSIST
JANSSEN
JANSSON
KANSANS
KINSHIP
KINSMAN
KINSMEN
LANSING
LENSCAP
LENSMAN
LENSMEN
LINSEED
MANSARD
MANSION
MANSIZE
MANSMAN
MENSANS
MENSCHY
MINSKYS
MINSTER
MONSOON
MONSTER
MONSTRO
MUNSTER
NONSALE
NONSANE
NONSELF
NONSKED
NONSKID
NONSLIP
NONSTOP
NONSUCH
NUNSHIP
PANSIES
PANSOUT
PENSEES
PENSION
PENSIVE
PINSEAL
PUNSTER
RANSACK
RANSOMS
RINSERS
RINSING
RONSARD
RONSONS
RUNSDRY
RUNSFOR
RUNSLOW
RUNSOFF
RUNSOUT
SANSEIS
SENSATE
SENSEIS
SENSENS
SENSING
SENSORS
SENSORY
SENSUAL
SONSHIP
SUNSETS
SUNSFAN
SUNSPOT
SUNSUIT
TANSIES
TENSELY
TENSEST
TENSEUP
TENSILE
TENSING
TENSION
TENSITY
TENSIVE
TENSORS
TENSPOT
TINSELS
TINSTAR
TONSILS
TONSURE
VANSANT
WINSBIG
WINSLET
WINSLOW
WINSOME
WINSOUT
WINSTON
YENSFOR

••N•S••

AMNESIA
AMNESIC
AMNESTY
BANDSAW
BANGSON
BANGSUP
BANKSON
BANKSUP
BENISON
BENTSEN
BINDSTO
BINDSUP
BONESET
BONESUP
BONUSES
CANASTA
CANTSAY
CINESIA
DENISON
DINESAT
DINESEN
DINESIN
DINESON
DYNASTS
DYNASTY
ERNESTA
ERNESTO
FINESSE
FINISHD
FINKSON
GANGSAW
GANGSTA
GANGSUP
GENESEE
GENESES
GENESET
GENESIS
GENUSES
GUNUSER
HANDSAW
HANDSEL
HANDSET
HANDSIN
HANDSON
HANDSUP
HANGSBY
HANGSIN
HANGSON
HANGSUP
HINTSAT
HONESIN
HONESTY
HONKSAT
HUNTSUP
IONESCO
IONISED
IONISER
IONISES
JANSSEN
JANSSON
JONESED
JONESES
KENOSHA
KINESES
KINESIC
KINESIS
KINISON
LANDSAT
LANDSUP
LINDSAY
LINDSEY
LINESUP
LINKSUP
LUNESTA
MENISCI
MINDSET
MINISKI
MINISUB
MINUSES
MONOSKI
NONUSER
PINESAP
PINESOL
RANTSAT
RENESTS
RENTSTO
RINGSIN
RINGSUP
SENDSBY
SENDSIN
SENDSON
SENDSTO
SENDSUP
SENESCE
SINGSTO
SINKSIN
SINUSES
TANKSUP
TENDSTO
TONESUP
TONUSES
TUNASUB
TUNESIN
TUNESTO
TUNESUP
TUNISIA
UNNASAL
UNNOSED
VANESSA
VENISON
VENUSES
WANTSIN
WANTSTO
WINDSOR
WINDSUP
WINESAP
WINGSIT
WINKSAT
YANKSAT
YANKSON
ZENISTS

••N••S•

AWNLESS
BONEASH
BONIEST
CANIEST
CANVASS
CONCISE
CONCUSS
CONFESS
CONFUSE
CONGEST
CONSIST
CONTEST
CONTUSE
DANKEST
DENSEST
DENTIST
DONETSK
DONJOSE
DONNISH
DONRUSS
DONTASK
DUNCISH
FANBASE
FANFEST
FANTASM
FANTAST
FANTASY
FANWISE
FINESSE
FINLESS
FINNISH
FONDEST
FUNFEST
GENOESE
GENOISE
GUNCASE
GUNLESS
HENNISH
HUNNISH
IINSIST
INNLESS
KENTISH
KINDEST
KINLESS
LANKEST
LINIEST
LONGEST
LONGISH
MANCUSO
MANLESS
MANNISH
MINXISH
MONDESI
MONKISH
NONBASE
NONBUSY
NONCASH
NONOISE
NONPAST
NUNNISH
OFNOUSE
PANFISH
PENCASE
PENROSE
PINIEST
PINKEST
PINKISH
PINLESS
PUNIEST
PUNLESS
RANKEST
RANKISH
RANPAST
RUNLESS
RUNPAST
RUNTISH
SANJOSE
SINLESS
SONLESS
SUNFAST
SUNFISH
SUNKIST
SUNLESS
SUNRISE
SYNAPSE
TANNEST
TANNISH
TENPAST
TENSEST
TINFISH
TINIEST
TONIEST
UNNOISY
VANESSA
VINIEST
VINROSE
WANIEST
WANNESS
WANNEST
WANNISH
WINIEST
WINLESS
ZANIEST
ZANYISH
ZANYISM

••N•••S

ADNOUNS
AGNAILS
AGNATES
ALNICOS
AMNERIS
AMNIONS
ANNALES
ANNEALS
ANNEXES
ANNUALS
ANNULUS
ARNICAS
ARNOLDS
AUNTIES
AWNINGS
AWNLESS
BANANAS
BANANES
BANDERS
BANDIES
BANDITS
BANGERS
BANGLES
BANJOES
BANKERS
BANKITS
BANNERS
BANQUES
BANTAMS
BANTERS
BANYANS
BANZAIS
BENARES
BENCHES
BENDAYS
BENDERS
BENGALS
BENOTES
BENTHOS
BENUMBS
BINDERS
BINDLES
BINGERS
BINGLES
BINGOES
BONACIS
BONBONS
BONDERS
BONGOES
BONITOS
BONKERS
BONMOTS
BONNETS
BONUSES
BUNCHES
BUNDLES
BUNGEES
BUNGLES
BUNIONS
BUNKERS
BUNKUMS
BUNNIES
BUNTERS
BYNAMES
CANAPES
CANARDS
CANCANS
CANCELS
CANCERS
CANCHAS
CANDIDS
CANDIES
CANDLES
CANFULS
CANINES
CANINGS
CANKERS
CANNELS
CANNERS
CANNONS
CANOERS
CANOLAS
CANOPUS
CANTABS
CANTALS
CANTERS
CANTLES
CANTONS
CANTORS
CANUCKS
CANULAS
CANVASS
CANYONS
CENSERS
CENSORS
CENTALS
CENTERS
CENTRES
CINCHES
CINDERS
CINEMAS
CINQUES
CONCHES
CONCHOS
CONCURS
CONCUSS
CONDORS
CONFABS
CONFERS
CONFESS
CONFITS
CONGERS
CONGOUS
CONJOBS
CONKERS
CONNORS
CONOIDS
CONSULS
CONTACS
CONTRAS
CONURES
CONVEYS
CONVOYS
DANANAS
DANCERS
DANDERS
DANDIES
DANDLES
DANGERS
DANGLES
DANIELS
DANITES
DANVERS
DENIALS
DENIERS
DENMOMS
DENOTES
DENTALS
DENTINS
DENTONS
DENUDES
DINDINS
DINGERS
DINGLES
DINGOES
DINNERS
DONATES
DONATUS
DONGLES
DONIMUS
DONJONS
DONKEYS
DONRUSS
DUNKERS
DUNLINS
DUNLOPS
DUNNERS
DYNAMOS
DYNASTS
DYNODES
ELNINOS
ENNEADS
FANCIES
FANDOMS
FANFICS
FANIONS
FANJETS
FANNERS
FANOUTS
FANTANS
FANTODS
FENCERS
FENDERS
FENNELS
FINALES
FINCHES
FINDERS
FINGALS
FINGERS
FINIALS
FINIANS
FINITES
FINLESS
FONDLES
FONDUES
FUNDERS
FUNFURS
FUNGOES
FUNNELS
FUNNIES
FUNRUNS
GANDERS
GANGERS
GANNETS
GENDERS
GENERIS
GENESES
GENESIS
GENGHIS
GENOMES
GENTLES
GENUSES
GENXERS
GINGERS
GINGKOS
GINKGOS
GUNDOGS
GUNITES
GUNLAPS
GUNLAWS
GUNLESS
GUNNERS
GUNNIES
GUNSELS
HANDERS
HANDLES
HANGARS
HANGBYS
HANGERS
HANGUPS
HANKERS
HANKIES
HANSOMS
HENBITS
HENRIES
HINDERS
HINNIES
HINTERS
HONCHOS
HONKERS
HONOURS
HUNCHES
HUNGERS
HUNKERS
HUNNYBS
HUNTERS
IGNEOUS
IGNITES
IGNORES
INNAGES
INNARDS
INNINGS
INNLESS
IONIANS
IONISES
IONIUMS
IONIZES
IONONES
JANGLES
JENKINS
JENNETS
JINGLES
JINGOES
JINXERS
JONESES
JUNCOES
JUNGLES
JUNIORS
JUNKERS
JUNKETS
JUNKIES
KANAKAS
KANSANS
KENNELS
KENYANS
KINDLES
KINESES
KINESIS
KINLESS
LANCERS
LANCETS
LANCIAS
LANDAUS
LANDERS
LANVINS
LENDERS
LENGTHS
LENGUAS
LENNONS
LENOVOS
LENTILS
LINAGES
LINDENS
LINDIES
LINDROS
LINEUPS
LINGERS

LINGOES
LININGS
LINKERS
LINKUPS
LINNETS
LINTELS
LINTERS
LONDRES
LONGIES
LONGUES
LUNATES
LUNCHES
LUNGERS
LUNKERS
MANAGES
MANANAS
MANDANS
MANDAYS
MANEGES
MANGERS
MANGLES
MANGOES
MANIACS
MANILAS
MANLESS
MANNERS
MANNIES
MANTELS
MANTLES
MANTRAS
MANUALS
MANURES
MENACES
MENAGES
MENCIUS
MENDELS
MENDERS
MENIALS
MENSANS
MENTEES
MENTORS
MENUDOS
MENZIES
MINCERS
MINDERS
MINGLES
MINIBUS
MINIMUS
MININGS
MINIONS
MINITVS
MINNOWS
MINOANS
MINSKYS
MINTERS
MINUETS
MINUSES
MINUTES
MINYANS
MONDAYS
MONGERS
MONGOLS
MONKEES
MONKEYS
MONROES
MUNCHES
NANNIES
NENNIUS
NINNIES
NONAGES
NONAMES
NONARTS
NONCOMS
NONFANS
NONHITS
NONJEWS
NONNEWS
NONPARS
NONPLUS
NONPROS
NONUKES
NONWARS
NUNCIOS
OINKERS
OMNIBUS
PANADAS
PANAMAS
PANDERS
PANDITS
PANFULS
PANIERS
PANINIS
PANNERS
PANSIES
PANTERS
PANTIES
PANZERS
PENATES
PENCILS
PENNERS
PENNEYS
PENNIES
PENNONS
PENPALS
PENSEES
PENTADS
PENTELS
PENULTS
PENZIAS
PINATAS
PINBOYS
PINCERS
PINCHAS
PINCHES
PINGERS
PINIONS
PINKENS
PINKIES
PINKOES
PINLESS
PINNERS
PINOAKS
PINONES
PONCHOS
PONDERS
PONGEES
PONGIDS
PONTIUS
PUNCHES
PUNDITS
PUNKERS
PUNKIES
PUNLESS
PUNNERS
PUNTERS
QINTARS
RANCHES
RANCHOS
RANCORS
RANGERS
RANKERS
RANKLES
RANLAPS
RANSOMS
RANTERS
RENAILS
RENAMES
RENDERS
RENEGES
RENESTS
RENNETS
RENNINS
RENOIRS
RENOTES
RENOWNS
RENTALS
RENTEES
RENTERS
RENVOIS
RINGERS
RINSERS
RONDELS
RONSONS
RUNDLES
RUNLAPS
RUNLESS
RUNLETS
RUNNELS
RUNNERS
RUNOFFS
RUNOUTS
RUNWAYS
SANBLAS
SANCTUS
SANDALS
SANDERS
SANSEIS
SENATES
SENDEES
SENDERS
SENDUPS
SENECAS
SENIORS
SENORAS
SENORES
SENSEIS
SENSENS
SENSORS
SENTRAS
SHNOOKS
SINGERS
SINGLES
SINKERS
SINLESS
SINNERS
SINUOUS
SINUSES
SONATAS
SONLESS
SONNETS
SUNBOWS
SUNDAES
SUNDAYS
SUNDERS
SUNDOGS
SUNFANS
SUNGODS
SUNHATS
SUNLESS
SUNRAYS
SUNSETS
SUNTANS
SYNDICS
TANDEMS
TANGLES
TANKERS
TANNERS
TANNINS
TANOAKS
TANSIES
TENACES
TENANTS
TENCHES
TENDAYS
TENDERS
TENDONS
TENNERS
TENNIES
TENPINS
TENSORS
TENTERS
TENTONS
TENUOUS
TENURES
TINCANS
TINDERS
TINEARS
TINGLES
TINGODS
TINHATS
TINKERS
TINKLES
TINNERS
TINORES
TINSELS
TINTERS
TONEMES
TONGANS
TONGUES
TONSILS
TONUSES
TUNDRAS
TUNEUPS
TUNNELS
UNNAILS
URNFULS
VANDALS
VENDEES
VENDERS
VENDORS
VENDUES
VENEERS
VENTERS
VENTRIS
VENULES
VENUSES
WANDERS
WANGLES
WANKELS
WANNESS
WANTADS
WANTERS
WANTONS
WENCHES
WENDERS
WENDKOS
WINCERS
WINCHES
WINDAUS
WINDERS
WINDOMS
WINDOWS
WINDUPS
WINGERS
WINKERS
WINLESS
WINNERS
WINNOWS
WINTERS
WONDERS
WONTONS
XANADUS
YANKEES
YANKERS
YANQUIS
YONKERS
ZENANAS
ZENISTS
ZENITHS
ZINCOUS
ZINGERS
ZINNIAS
ZONIANS
ZONULES
ZUNIANS

•••NS••

ALUNSER
ARENSKY
BERNSEN
BRANSON
BRONSON
BURNSIN
BURNSUP
CHANSON
COUNSEL
DAWNSON
EARNSIT
EVENSUP
FAWNSON
FLENSED
FLENSER
FLENSES
GAINSAY
GAINSON
GRINSAT
HORNSBY
HORNSIN
IRONSON
JOHNSON
JOINSIN
JOINSUP
KLENSCH
LEANSIN
LEANSON
LEANSTO
MEANSIT
MEANSTO
MOONSET
OPENSEA
OPENSUP
PLANSON
PLANSTO
QUONSET
RAINSIN
RAINSON
REINSIN
SIGNSIN
SIGNSON
SIGNSUP
SPENSER
SPONSOR
SWANSEA
SWANSON
SWENSON
TEENSIE
TRANSAM
TRANSIT
TRANSOM
TURNSIN
TURNSON
TURNSTO
TURNSUP
TWINSET
UTENSIL
VRONSKY
WARNSOF

•••N•S•

AGONISE
AGONISM
AGONIST
AIRNESS
ALLNESS
AMONGST
APTNESS
ARENOSE
BADNESS
BERNESE
BIGNESS
BIGNOSE
BRINISH
BURNISH
BYANOSE
CHINESE
CORNISH
COYNESS
DIMNESS
DOINGSO
DONNISH
DRONISH
DRYNESS
EARNEST
EVANISH
EVENEST
FAINEST
FARNESS
FATNESS
FEWNESS
FEYNESS
FINNISH
FITNESS
FRENESI
FULNESS
FURNESS
FURNISH
GARNISH
GAYNESS
GYMNAST
HARNESS
HENNISH
HIPNESS
HOGNOSE
HORNISH
HORNIST
HOTNESS
HUNNISH
ICINESS
ILLNESS
INANEST
IRONIST
JAINISM
JAINIST
KEENEST
LAXNESS
LEANEST
LIONESS
LIONISE
LOWNESS
MADNESS
MANNISH
MEANEST
MOONISH
NEWNESS
NOWNESS
NUNNISH
ODDNESS
OLDNESS
ONENESS
OZONISE
PATNESS
PIANISM
PIANIST
PLANISH
PLENISH
PUGNOSE
RAWNESS
REDNESS
REDNOSE
REYNOSA
RHENISH
SADNESS
SHYNESS
SIENESE
SLYNESS
SOANDSO
SOLNESS
SOONEST
SPANISH
SWINISH
TANNEST
TANNISH
TARNISH
THINKSO
TOWNISH
VAINEST
VARNISH
WANNESS
WANNEST
WANNISH
WEENESS
WETNESS
WITNESS
WRYNESS
ZIONISM
ZIONIST

•••N••S

ABCNEWS
ADONAIS
AGENCES
AGENDAS
AGONIES
AIRNESS
ALINERS
ALLNESS
ALLNEWS
AMANTIS
ANANIAS
ANONYMS
ANYNEWS
APTNESS
ASANTES
ATONERS
ATONICS
ATONIES
AVANTIS
AVENGES
AVENUES
BADNESS
BADNEWS
BAGNIOS
BANNERS
BARNEYS
BARNUMS
BEANIES
BERNAYS
BIGNESS
BIGNEWS
BIONICS
BLENDES
BLONDES
BONNETS
BOONIES
BOUNCES
BRINERS
BRONCOS
BRONTES
BRONZES
BRUNETS
BUNNIES
BURNERS
CANNELS
CANNERS
CANNONS
CAPNUTS
CARNETS
CARNIES
CATNAPS
CATNIPS
CBSNEWS
CHANCES
CHANELS
CHANGES
CHINOIS
CHINUPS
CLINICS
CLONERS
COBNUTS
COGNACS
COINERS
COINOPS
CONNORS
CORNEAS
CORNERS
CORNETS
COYNESS
CRENELS
CRINGES
CRONIES
CYANIDS
CYGNETS
DAMNERS
DARNERS
DIMNESS
DINNERS
DIPNETS
DIRNDLS
DJINNIS
DOGNAPS
DOWNERS
DRONERS
DRYNESS
DUENNAS
DUNNERS
EARNERS
EBONICS
EBONIES
EGGNOGS
ELANCES
ELANETS
EPONYMS
ERINYES
ERYNGOS
ESPNEWS
ETHNICS
ETONICS
EUONYMS
EVENERS
EVINCES
EXONYMS
FANNERS
FARNESS
FATNESS
FAWNERS
FENNELS
FEWNESS
FEYNESS
FIANCES
FIENNES
FITNESS
FLANGES
FLENSES
FLYNETS
FOXNEWS
FRANCES
FRANCIS
FRENCHS
FRINGES
FUENTES
FULNESS
FUNNELS
FUNNIES
FURNESS
GAINERS
GANNETS
GARNERS
GARNETS
GAYNESS
GLANCES
GLYNNIS
GOONEYS
GOONIES
GRANGES
GRANPAS
GRINGOS
GRUNGES
GUINEAS
GUNNERS
GUNNIES
GURNEYS
GUVNORS
HARNESS
HEINOUS
HERNIAS
HERNIBS
HEXNUTS
HINNIES
HIPNESS
HISNIBS
HOBNOBS
HOGNUTS
HOHNERS
HORNETS
HOTNESS
HUNNYBS
HYANNIS
HYMNALS
ICINESS
ILLNESS
INKNOTS
IRENICS
IRONERS
IRONIES
IRONONS
JENNETS
JITNEYS
JOINERS
JOUNCES
KEENERS
KENNELS
KERNELS
KIDNAPS
KIDNEYS
KUZNETS
KWANZAS
LAXNESS
LEANERS
LEANTOS
LENNONS
LEONIDS
LIENEES
LIENORS
LIGNINS
LIMNERS
LINNETS
LIONELS
LIONESS
LIONETS
LOANERS
LOONIES
LOUNGES
LOWNESS
LUGNUTS
MADNESS
MAENADS
MAGNETS
MAGNUMS
MAINERS
MANNERS
MANNIES
MEANIES
MIGNONS
MINNOWS
MOANERS
MOONERS
MOONIES
NANNIES
NBCNEWS
NENNIUS
NEONGAS
NEWNESS
NINNIES
NONNEWS
NOONERS
NOWNESS
NUANCES
NUDNIKS
OBENTOS
ODDNESS
OLDNESS
OLDNEWS
OMINOUS
ONENESS
OPENERS
OPINERS
ORANGES
ORANTES
ORKNEYS
OZONOUS
PAANGAS
PANNERS
PATNESS
PAWNEES
PAWNERS
PBANDJS
PEANUTS
PENNERS
PENNEYS
PENNIES
PENNONS
PEONIES
PETNAPS
PHENOLS
PHENOMS
PHINEAS
PHONERS
PHONEYS
PHONICS
PHONIES
PICNICS
PIGNUTS
PINNERS
PLANERS
PLANETS
PLENUMS
PLINTHS
PLUNGES
POINTES
POUNCES
PRANCES
PRENUPS
PRINCES
PRUNERS
PSANDQS
PUNNERS
QUINCES
QUINTAS
QUINTES
QUINTUS
QUINZES
RAWNESS
REDNESS
REKNITS
REKNOTS
RENNETS
RENNINS
RESNAIS
RESNAPS
REUNERS
ROMNEYS
RUANDAS
RUINERS
RUINOUS
RUNNELS
RUNNERS
SADNESS
SAINTES
SCENICS
SCHNAPS
SCONCES
SEANCES
SEINERS
SHINERS
SHYNESS
SIENNAS
SIGNALS
SIGNEES
SIGNERS
SIGNETS
SIGNORS
SIGNUPS
SINNERS
SLYNESS
SOLNESS
SONNETS
SOONERS
SPINELS
SPINETS
SPONGES
STANCES
STANZAS
STENNIS
STONERS
SUBNETS
TANNERS
TANNINS
TEENERS
TENNERS
TENNIES
THENETS
THENEWS
TIENDAS
TINNERS
TOONIES
TOWNERS
TOWNIES
TRANCES
TSONGAS
TUNNELS
TURNERS
TURNIPS
TURNONS
TURNUPS
TWINERS
TWINGES
UNKNITS
UNKNOTS
UNSNAGS
UNSNAPS
USANCES
VEINTES
VILNIUS
WALNUTS
WANNESS
WEANERS
WEENESS
WEENIES
WETNAPS
WETNESS
WHINERS
WIENERS
WIENIES
WINNERS
WINNOWS
WITNESS
WRYNESS
XSANDOS
YAWNERS
ZAGNUTS
ZINNIAS

••••NS•

AGAINST
ALFONSE
ALFONSO
CLEANSE
DEFENSE
EKWENSI
EXPANSE
EXPENSE
EXTENSO
IMMENSE
INCENSE
INTENSE
LICENSE
OFFENSE
RERINSE
ROMANSH
UNTENSE

••••N•S

ABOUNDS
ABSENTS
ACCENTS
ACCTNOS
ACHENES
ADDENDS
ADVENTS
AFFINES
AIRINGS
ALBINOS
ALKENES
ALMONDS
ALPINES
ALUMNUS
AMOUNTS
ANOINTS
ANYONES
APPENDS
AQUINAS
ARCINGS
ARGENTS
ARIANES
ASCENDS

ASCENTS	DOCENTS	HIJINKS	MYKONOS	REPENTS	TILINGS	AWAKENS	CITRONS	FALCONS	JARDINS	MENSANS	PARDONS	RENNINS
ASSENTS	DOMINOS	HOTONES	NOHANDS	REPINES	TIMINGS	BABOONS	CLEMENS	FANIONS	JARGONS	MERLINS	PARKINS	RENOWNS
ATTENDS	DOMINUS	HYANNIS	NOVENAS	RERANKS	TISANES	BAGGINS	CLIPONS	FANTANS	JENKINS	METFANS	PARSONS	REOPENS
ATTUNES	DOUANES	HYGINUS	NYYANKS	RERENTS	TORINOS	BAHIANS	COCOONS	FASTENS	JERGENS	MICRONS	PATHANS	REPLANS
AUGENDS	DUENNAS	ICTINUS	OBLONGS	RESANDS	TOTINOS	BALEENS	COFFINS	FATTENS	JERKINS	MIGNONS	PATRONS	REPUGNS
AVERNUS	DUGONGS	IGUANAS	OBTUNDS	RESENDS	TOWINGS	BALKANS	COLLINS	FIBRINS	JETFANS	MINIONS	PEAHENS	RESCANS
AWNINGS	EDGINGS	IIKINGS	OCEANUS	RESENTS	TRUANTS	BANYANS	COLUMNS	FIJIANS	JETGUNS	MINOANS	PECTINS	RESIGNS
BADENDS	EDMONDS	IMMUNES	OCTANES	RESINGS	TYRANTS	BARRENS	COMEONS	FILLINS	JETSONS	MINYANS	PENNONS	RESPANS
BANANAS	EDMUNDS	IMPENDS	OCTANTS	RESINKS	ULZANAS	BARRONS	COMMONS	FINIANS	JIMSONS	MITTENS	PEPSINS	RESPINS
BANANES	ELAINES	INCANTS	OFFENDS	RETINAS	UNBENDS	BARYONS	CORDONS	FIRKINS	JUDEANS	MIZZENS	PERKINS	RETAINS
BARENTS	ELNINOS	INCENTS	OFFINGS	RETINTS	UNBINDS	BATTENS	COSIGNS	FLACONS	JURGENS	MODERNS	PERRINS	RETURNS
BEHINDS	ELUANTS	INDENTS	OOLONGS	RETONES	UNDINES	BCLIONS	COTTONS	FLAGONS	KANSANS	MOLSONS	PERSONS	REUBENS
BEIGNES	EMBANKS	INFANTS	ORDINES	RETUNES	UNFINES	BEACONS	COUPONS	FLORINS	KELVINS	MOREENS	PHOTONS	REWARNS
BELONGS	ENCINAS	INKINGS	ORIENTS	REVENDS	UNHANDS	BECKONS	COUSINS	FRYPANS	KENYANS	MORGANS	PICKENS	RIBBONS
BIGENDS	ENDINGS	INLANDS	OSCINES	REWINDS	UNKINKS	BEHRENS	COZZENS	FUNRUNS	KIRMANS	MORMONS	PIDGINS	RICHENS
BIGONES	ENFANTS	INLINES	OSMONDS	REZONES	UNLINKS	BEMOANS	CRAVENS	FUSIONS	KITTENS	MORTONS	PIEPANS	RIESENS
BIKINIS	ENGINES	INNINGS	OSMUNDS	RIBANDS	UNTUNES	BICHONS	CRAYONS	GALLONS	KLAXONS	MOTIONS	PIETINS	ROBBINS
BIMINIS	ENLINKS	INTENDS	OUTINGS	RIDINGS	UNWINDS	BICORNS	CRETANS	GAMMONS	KMESONS	MOTRINS	PIGEONS	ROLLINS
BLUINGS	ENRANKS	INTENTS	PAGINGS	RISINGS	UNZONES	BIGFANS	CRETINS	GARCONS	KOREANS	MRBURNS	PIGPENS	ROLLONS
BODINGS	ENWINDS	INTONES	PALINGS	RODENTS	UPLANDS	BIGGUNS	CROTONS	GARDENS	KRAKENS	MTEVANS	PINIONS	ROMAINS
BOEINGS	EOSINES	INVENTS	PANINIS	ROMANIS	UPLINKS	BIGWINS	CRUZANS	GASCANS	KUCHENS	MUDHENS	PINKENS	RONSONS
BORINGS	EQUINES	IONONES	PARENTS	ROMANOS	UPSENDS	BIRMANS	CTSCANS	GASCONS	LAGOONS	MUFFINS	PIPPINS	RYOKANS
BOVINES	ERLANGS	ISLANDS	PARINGS	ROMANUS	UPWINDS	BLAZONS	CUBBINS	GATLINS	LANVINS	MULLINS	PISTONS	SADDENS
BUJONES	ERMINES	JOURNOS	PATENTS	ROVINGS	URGINGS	BOBBINS	CUBFANS	GAUDENS	LARDONS	MUSLINS	PLATENS	SAISONS
BUTANES	ERRANDS	KAHUNAS	PATINAS	RULINGS	URSINUS	BODKINS	DACRONS	GELPENS	LARKINS	MUTTONS	PLUGINS	SALMONS
BUTENES	ESSENES	KCJONES	PAVANES	SABINES	VALINES	BOFFINS	DAEMONS	GERMANS	LATEENS	NAPKINS	PLUTONS	SALOONS
BYGONES	ETHANES	KETONES	PAVINGS	SALINAS	VICUNAS	BOKKENS	DALTONS	GIBBONS	LEADENS	NATHANS	POISONS	SAMOANS
BYLINES	ETHENES	KIMONOS	PEDANTS	SALINES	VIERNES	BONBONS	DAMPENS	GIBSONS	LEADINS	NATIONS	POLLENS	SAMPANS
CABANAS	EUBANKS	KIWANIS	PILINGS	SARONGS	VIKINGS	BOSTONS	DAMSONS	GIDEONS	LEAVENS	NEATENS	POMPONS	SAMSONS
CALENDS	EXEUNTS	KORUNAS	PINONES	SAVANAS	VIVANTS	BOUDINS	DARKENS	GLOBINS	LEGIONS	NELSONS	POPGUNS	SAPIENS
CAMINOS	EXPANDS	LACINGS	PIPINGS	SAVANTS	WAHINES	BOWFINS	DATSUNS	GLUTENS	LENNONS	NEOCONS	POPLINS	SATEENS
CANINES	EXPENDS	LACUNAS	PLAINES	SAVINGS	WAKINGS	BRAZENS	DAWKINS	GNOMONS	LEPTONS	NETTONS	POPPINS	SATURNS
CANINGS	EXTENDS	LADINGS	PLAINTS	SAYINGS	WAXINGS	BRETONS	DEACONS	GOBLINS	LESIONS	NEURONS	POTEENS	SCREENS
CARINAS	EXTENTS	LADINOS	POCONOS	SECANTS	WEEONES	BRITONS	DEADENS	GODSONS	LESSENS	NEWMANS	POTIONS	SEASONS
CASINGS	EXYANKS	LADYNAS	QUIZNOS	SECONDS	WETONES	BROGANS	DEAFENS	GORGONS	LESSONS	NEWTONS	PRISONS	SENSENS
CASINOS	FACINGS	LAGUNAS	RACINOS	SEDONAS	WIRINGS	BULLINS	DEEPENS	GOVERNS	LHASANS	NISSANS	PROTONS	SEQUINS
CATENAS	FAGENDS	LAMENTS	RAGINGS	SEMANAS	XIMENES	BUNIONS	DEFCONS	GULDENS	LIBRANS	NOGGINS	PUFFINS	SERMONS
CEMENTS	FAMINES	LAMINAS	RAMONES	SHRINES	YEMENIS	BURDENS	DEHORNS	HADRONS	LIBYANS	NONFANS	PULLINS	SERPENS
CESSNAS	FARINAS	LATENTS	RAPINES	SHRINKS	YOGINIS	BURMANS	DEMEANS	HAPPENS	LICHENS	NORMANS	PULLONS	SEXTANS
CETANES	FATONES	LATINAS	RAPINIS	SIDINGS	ZEDONKS	BUSMANS	DENTINS	HARDENS	LIGNINS	NORTONS	PYTHONS	SEXTONS
CHAINES	FELINES	LATINOS	RATINES	SIENNAS	ZENANAS	BUTTONS	DENTONS	HARKENS	LINDENS	NOTHINS	RADIANS	SHAMANS
CLIENTS	FIENNES	LATINUS	RATINGS	SILENTS		BYTURNS	DESIGNS	HASTENS	LISTENS	NOTIONS	RAGLANS	SHOGUNS
COIGNES	FILENES	LEGENDS	RAVINES	SOYINKS	•••••NS	CAFTANS	DETAINS	HATPINS	LOCKINS	NOTURNS	RAGMANS	SHOOINS
COLONES	FILINGS	LIGANDS	RAVINGS	SPLINES	ACTIONS	CAIMANS	DEVEINS	HAWKINS	LOGGINS	NUBBINS	RAISINS	SHUTINS
COLONUS	FIRINGS	LIKINGS	REBANKS	SPLINTS	ACUMENS	CALKINS	DICKENS	HEAVENS	LOOKINS	NUBIANS	RAISONS	SICKENS
COMINGS	FIXINGS	LININGS	REBENDS	SPRINGS	ADJOINS	CALLINS	DIEMENS	HERMANS	LOOSENS	OAHUANS	RAMFANS	SIDDONS
CORONAS	FLAUNTS	LIVINGS	REBINDS	SPRINTS	ADNOUNS	CAMIONS	DINDINS	HEYMANS	LOTIONS	OBTAINS	RAMSONS	SIEMENS
COSINES	FMBANDS	LOSINGS	RECANES	SPYINGS	AFGHANS	CANCANS	DIOXINS	HIGGINS	LOUDENS	OHIOANS	RATIONS	SIMIANS
DANANAS	FOMENTS	LUMINAS	RECANTS	SQUINTS	AIRGUNS	CANNONS	DISOWNS	HILTONS	LOVEINS	OILCANS	RATLINS	SIMMONS
DAPHNES	FORINTS	LUPINES	REDANTS	STAGNES	AJOWANS	CANTONS	DIZAINS	HOBSONS	MACOUNS	OILPANS	RATTANS	SIOUANS
DAPHNIS	FRIENDS	MAKINGS	REFINDS	STDENIS	AMAZONS	CANYONS	DOBBINS	HOPKINS	MACRONS	OLEFINS	RAWLINS	SIPHONS
DATINGS	GALANOS	MANANAS	REFINES	STENNIS	AMBIENS	CAPGUNS	DOGRUNS	HOSKINS	MADDENS	OMAHANS	RAYBANS	SIXGUNS
DEBONES	GALANTS	MARINAS	REFUNDS	STERNOS	AMNIONS	CARBONS	DOLMANS	HOYDENS	MAIDENS	OPPUGNS	RAYGUNS	SKIRUNS
DEBUNKS	GALENAS	MARINES	REGENTS	STRANDS	ANACINS	CAREENS	DOMAINS	HUGGINS	MAILINS	OPTIONS	REAGANS	SLIPONS
DECANTS	GAMINES	MAYINGS	REGINAS	STRINGS	ANDEANS	CARTONS	DONJONS	HUYGENS	MAISONS	ORDAINS	REASONS	SLOGANS
DEFANGS	GATINGS	MEGANES	REHANGS	TAGENDS	ARCHONS	CASEINS	DRAGONS	HYPHENS	MAJGENS	ORIGINS	RECKONS	SLOVENS
DEFENDS	GEMINIS	MERINOS	REHONES	TAHINIS	ARUBANS	CASERNS	DROPINS	IBIZANS	MALIANS	ORISONS	RECOINS	SNAPONS
DEFINES	GERENTS	MIGENES	RELANDS	TAKINGS	ASHBINS	CASHINS	DRYRUNS	ICERUNS	MALIGNS	ORLEANS	REDARNS	SOFTENS
DEFUNDS	GERUNDS	MININGS	RELANES	TALENTS	ASHCANS	CATIONS	DUNLINS	IMPUGNS	MANDANS	ORPHANS	REDDENS	SOXFANS
DEJUNKS	GITANOS	MIZUNAS	RELENDS	TAPINGS	ASHPANS	CATKINS	ELEVENS	INDIANS	MARGINS	OSAKANS	REDFINS	SPLEENS
DELINTS	GLYNNIS	MOMENTS	RELENTS	TECHNOS	ASSIGNS	CAVEINS	ELEVONS	INIRONS	MARLINS	OUTBANS	REDHENS	SPRAINS
DEMANDS	GROUNDS	MORANIS	RELINES	TEJANAS	ATAMANS	CAVERNS	ENDPINS	INRUINS	MAROONS	OUTGUNS	REDSUNS	STAMENS
DEPENDS	GYRENES	MOWINGS	RELINKS	TEJANOS	ATSIGNS	CAYMANS	ENDRUNS	INSPANS	MARRONS	OUTMANS	REEARNS	STATINS
DEPONES	HAVANAS	MRBONES	REMANDS	TENANTS	ATTAINS	CHALONS	ENJOINS	INTERNS	MARTENS	OUTRUNS	REGAINS	STEARNS
DETENTS	HAYINGS	MRJONES	REMENDS	TETANUS	AUBURNS	CHAZANS	ENSIGNS	INTURNS	MARTINS	OUTSINS	REGIONS	STEPINS
DETUNES	HAZINGS	MURANOS	REMINDS	THRONES	AUSTINS	CHEVONS	ETYMONS	IONIANS	MATRONS	PADUANS	REJOINS	STEVENS
DIVINES	HEXANES	MUSINGS	REMINES	THRONGS	AUTUMNS	CHITONS	EXTERNS	IRONONS	MECCANS	PAISANS	RELOANS	STJOHNS
DJINNIS	HIDINGS	MUTANTS	REMINTS	TIDINGS	AVALONS	CHYRONS	FADEINS	ISOGONS	MEDIANS	PAPUANS	REMAINS	STOLONS

STOTINS
STRAINS
SUBORNS
SULTANS
SUMMONS
SUNFANS
SUNTANS
SYRIANS
TAKEINS
TANNINS
TAPPANS
TARPONS
TARTANS
TARZANS
TAUTENS
TAVERNS
TEAURNS
TEFLONS
TENDONS
TENPINS
TENTONS
TERRANS
TEUTONS
THEBANS
THESUNS
TIEPINS
TIFFINS
TIGLONS
TIMMINS
TINCANS
TITIANS
TOCSINS
TONGANS
TOPGUNS
TOPTENS
TOUCANS
TOYGUNS
TREPANS
TRIGONS
TRITONS
TROJANS
TRUMANS
TUCSONS
TULSANS
TURBANS
TUREENS
TURNONS
TUSCANS
TWOTONS
TYCOONS
UNISONS
UNJOINS
UNPAWNS
UNPLANS
UNSPANS
UPSPINS
UPTOWNS
UPTURNS
URCHINS
USOPENS
UTAHANS
UTICANS
VERDINS
VIOLINS
VIRGINS
VISIONS
VULCANS
WADKINS
WALKINS
WALKONS
WALTONS
WANTONS
WARDENS
WARRENS
WATKINS
WEAKENS
WEAKONS
WEAPONS
WEDELNS
WESTINS
WHITENS
WICCANS
WILKENS
WILKINS
WILSONS
WONTONS
WOOLENS
WORSENS
WYVERNS
YEOMANS
YOUMANS
ZIPGUNS
ZIRCONS
ZONIANS
ZUNIANS

NT•••••

NTUPLES

N•T••••

NATALIA
NATALIE
NATASHA
NATATOR
NATCHEZ
NATHANS
NATIONS
NATIVES
NATRIUM
NATSUME
NATTERS
NATTIER
NATTILY
NATURAL
NATURED
NATUREL
NATURES
NATWICK
NETBALL
NETCAFE
NETCOST
NETFLIX
NETFULS
NETGAIN
NETGAME
NETIZEN
NETLESS
NETLIKE
NETLOSS
NETSTER
NETSUKE
NETSURF
NETTERS
NETTING
NETTLED
NETTLES
NETTONS
NETWARE
NETWORK
NETZERO
NITPICK
NITRATE
NITRIDE
NITRIFY
NITRITE
NITROUS
NITTANY
NITTIER
NITWITS
NOTABIT
NOTABLE
NOTABLY
NOTALIE
NOTALOT
NOTAONE
NOTASTE
NOTATED
NOTATES
NOTBEEN
NOTCHED
NOTCHER
NOTCHES
NOTDONE
NOTEASY
NOTEDLY
NOTEPAD
NOTEVEN
NOTEVER
NOTFAIR
NOTGOOD
NOTHERE
NOTHING
NOTHINS
NOTHOME
NOTICED
NOTICER
NOTICES
NOTIONS
NOTLIKE
NOTLIVE
NOTMANY
NOTMINE
NOTMUCH
NOTNEAR
NOTNICE
NOTONCE
NOTOPEN
NOTOVER
NOTRADE
NOTRARE
NOTREAL
NOTRUMP
NOTSAFE
NOTSURE
NOTTING
NOTTOBE
NOTTRUE
NOTUPTO
NOTURNS
NOTUSED
NOTWELL
NOTWITH
NUTATED
NUTATES
NUTLETS
NUTLIKE
NUTMEAT
NUTMEGS
NUTOILS
NUTPINE
NUTRIAS
NUTSIER
NUTTERS
NUTTIER
NUTTILY
NUTTING
NUTTREE
NUTWOOD
NYTIMES

N••T•••

NAPTIME
NARTHEX
NASTASE
NASTIER
NASTIES
NASTILY
NATTERS
NATTIER
NATTILY
NAUTICA
NAUTILI
NBATEAM
NEATENS
NEATEST
NEATNIK
NECTARS
NECTARY
NEITHER
NEPTUNE
NESTEGG
NESTERS
NESTFUL
NESTING
NESTLED
NESTLER
NESTLES
NESTORS
NESTSIN
NETTERS
NETTING
NETTLED
NETTLES
NETTONS
NEUTERS
NEUTRAL
NEUTRON
NEWTONS
NEWTOWN
NEWTOYS
NEXTDAY
NFCTEAM
NFLTEAM
NHLTEAM
NICTATE
NIFTIER
NIFTIES
NIFTILY
NINTHLY
NITTANY
NITTIER
NOETICS
NOOTHER
NOOTKAS
NORTHER
NORTHOF
NORTONS
NOSTAIN
NOSTARS
NOSTRIL
NOSTRUM
NOTTING
NOTTOBE
NOTTRUE
NOUTURN
NOWTHEN
NOWTHIS
NUPTIAL
NURTURE
NUTTERS
NUTTIER
NUTTILY
NUTTING
NUTTREE

N•••T••

NAILTIP
NAMETAG
NANETTE
NAPHTHA
NAPSTER
NATATOR
NECKTIE
NEGATED
NEGATER
NEGATES
NEGATOR
NEPOTIC
NETSTER
NIANTIC
NICETRY
NIDETCH
NIGHTER
NIGHTIE
NIGHTLY
NOCATCH
NOENTRY
NONETTE
NONSTOP
NORITES
NOTATED
NOTATES
NOVOTES
NOVOTNY
NUESTRA
NUESTRO
NUTATED
NUTATES

N••••T•

NAHUATL
NAIVETE
NAIVETY
NANETTE
NARRATE
NAUGHTS
NAUGHTY
NCWYETH
NDAKOTA
NEEDSTO
NEOLITH
NEOLYTE
NEONATE
NESBITT
NESMITH
NEWGATE
NEWHATS
NEWMATH
NIBLETS
NICTATE
NIMIETY
NIOBITE
NITRATE
NITRITE
NITWITS
NOENDTO
NOGIFTS
NONARTS
NONETTE
NONHITS
NOSEATS
NOTASTE
NOTUPTO
NOTWITH
NOUGATS
NOUGHTS
NOVELTY
NUDISTS
NUGGETS
NUGGETY
NULLITY
NUMBATS
NUTLETS

N•••••T

NAILSET
NAILSIT
NAIVEST
NASCENT
NAYARIT
NEAREST
NEATEST
NECKLET
NEEDNOT
NEGLECT
NESBITT
NETCOST
NEWBOLT
NEWHART
NEWLEFT
NEWMINT
NEWMONT
NEWPORT
NICOLET
NIGHEST
NOBLEST
NOCOUNT
NODOUBT
NOFAULT
NOLIMIT
NONDIET
NONFACT
NONMEAT
NONPAST
NONPOET
NOPQRST
NORBERT
NOSEOUT
NOSIEST
NOSWEAT
NOTABIT
NOTALOT
NOWWHAT
NULLSET
NUMBEST
NUNAVUT
NUTMEAT
NYGIANT

•NT••••

ANTACID
ANTARES
ANTBEAR
ANTBIRD
ANTCOWS
ANTEDUP
ANTEING
ANTENNA
ANTERUS
ANTESUP
ANTFARM
ANTHEIL
ANTHEMS
ANTHERS
ANTHILL
ANTHONY
ANTHRAX
ANTIART
ANTIBES
ANTIFOG
ANTIGEN
ANTIGUA
ANTIGUN
ANTILOG
ANTIOCH
ANTIQUE
ANTITAX
ANTIWAR
ANTLERS
ANTLIKE
ANTLION
ANTOINE
ANTONIA
ANTONIN
ANTONIO
ANTONYM
ANTSIER
ANTWERP
CNTOWER
ENTAILS
ENTEBBE
ENTENTE
ENTERED
ENTERER
ENTERIC
ENTERIN
ENTERON
ENTHRAL
ENTHUSE
ENTICED
ENTICER
ENTICES
ENTIRES
ENTITLE
ENTOMBS
ENTRADA
ENTRAIN
ENTRANT
ENTRAPS
ENTREAT
ENTREES
ENTRIES
ENTROPY
ENTRUST
ENTWINE
ENTWIST
INTAILS
INTAKES
INTASTE
INTEARS
INTEGER
INTEGRA
INTENDS
INTENSE
INTENTS
INTERIM
INTERNE
INTERNS
INTERSE
INTHERE
INTHING
INTHIRD
INTHREE
INTONED
INTONER
INTONES
INTOTAL
INTOUCH
INTRADE
INTRAYS
INTROIT
INTRUDE
INTRUST
INTRUTH
INTUITS
INTURNS
ONTARIO
ONTHEDL
ONTHEGO
ONTHEQT
ONTHREE
ONTKEAN
ONTOAST
ONTOPIC
ONTOPOF
ONTRACK
ONTRIAL
UNTACKS
UNTAKEN
UNTAMED
UNTAMES
UNTAPED
UNTAPES
UNTASTY
UNTAXED
UNTAXES
UNTEACH
UNTENSE
UNTERSE
UNTHAWS
UNTHICK
UNTHINK
UNTIERS
UNTILED
UNTIMED
UNTIMID
UNTIRED
UNTONED
UNTOUGH
UNTOXIC
UNTRACK
UNTRAPS
UNTREAD
UNTREED
UNTRIED
UNTRITE
UNTRUER
UNTRULY
UNTRUSS
UNTRUTH
UNTUCKS
UNTUNED
UNTUNES
UNTWINE
UNTWIST
UNTYING
UNTYPED

•N•T•••

ANATASE
ANATOLE
ANATOLY
ANATOMY
ANDTHEN
ANITRAS
ANOTHER
ANYTIME
ANYTOWN
DNATEST
INATRAP
INITIAL
INSTALL
INSTALS
INSTANT
INSTATE
INSTEAD
INSTEPS
INSTILL
INSTILS
INSTOCK
INSTONE
INSTORE
INSTYLE
INUTERO
INUTILE
KNITTED
KNITTER
KNOTSUP
KNOTTED
KNOTTER
ONATEAR
ONATOOT
ONATRIP
ONETERM
ONETIME
ONETOGO
ONETWOS
ONSTAFF
ONSTAGE
UNCTION
UNITARD
UNITARY
UNITERS
UNITIES
UNITING
UNITISE
UNITIVE
UNITIZE
UNSTACK
UNSTAGY
UNSTAID
UNSTATE
UNSTEEL
UNSTEPS
UNSTERN
UNSTICK
UNSTIFF
UNSTOIC
UNSTONY
UNSTOPS
UNSTOUT
UNSTOWS
UNSTRAP
UNSTUCK
UNSTUNG

•N••T••

ANISTON
ANNATTO
ANNETTE
ANTITAX
ENACTED
ENACTOR
ENTITLE
GNOSTIC
INAPTER
INAPTLY
INASTEW
INASTIR
INCITED
INCITER
INCITES
INDITED
INDITER
INDITES
INDUTCH
INEPTLY
INERTIA
INERTLY
INGATES
INKSTER
INMATES
INTOTAL
INVITED
INVITEE
INVITER
INVITES
INVITRO
KNITTED
KNITTER
KNOTTED
KNOTTER
KNOUTED
ONESTAR
ONESTEP
ONESTOP
ONLYTOO
ONWATER
SNEETCH
SNIFTER
SNOOTED
SNORTAT
SNORTED
SNORTER
SNOUTED
UNACTED
UNAPTLY
UNBATED
UNCITED
UNDATED
UNEATEN
UNFATED
UNFATTY
UNFETED
UNFITLY
UNGATED
UNHATED
UNHITCH
UNIATES
UNLATCH
UNMATED
UNMATES
UNMITER
UNMITRE
UNMUTED
UNNOTED
UNOFTEN
UNOPTED
UNRATED
UNSATED
UNVITAL
UNVOTED
UNWITTY

•N•••T•

ANALYTE
ANDANTE
ANILITY
ANIMATE
ANIMATO
ANKLETS
ANNATTO
ANNETTE
ANNUITY
ANOINTS
ANXIETY
ENCARTA
ENDCUTS
ENDLATE
ENDNOTE
ENFANTS
ENGLUTS
ENLISTS
ENROOTS
ENROUTE
ENSEATS
ENSUITE
ENTENTE
INANITY
INCANTS
INCENTS
INCEPTS
INDENTS
INDEPTH
INDICTS
INDUCTS
INEDITA
INFAITH
INFANTA
INFANTE
INFANTS
INFECTS
INFESTS
INFLATE
INGESTA
INGESTS
INGRATE
INHASTE
ININETY
INJECTS
INKJETS
INKNOTS
INKPOTS
INSECTA
INSECTS
INSERTS
INSISTS
INSPITE
INSPOTS
INSTATE
INSULTS
INTASTE
INTENTS
INTRUTH
INTUITS
INVENTS
INVERTS
INVESTS
INVICTA
INWHITE
KNIGHTS
KNOWETH
ONADATE
ONEACTS
ONEARTH
ONEBYTE
ONEIOTA
ONEMPTY
ONENOTE
ONEONTA
ONEVOTE
ONORATI
SNAPSTO
SNOCATS
UNBAITS
UNBELTS
UNBERTH
UNBOLTS
UNCOUTH
UNCRATE
UNDUSTY
UNEARTH
UNEMPTY
UNFACTS
UNFAITH
UNFATTY
UNFERTH
UNHASTY
UNKNITS
UNKNOTS
UNLOATH
UNLOFTY
UNLUSTY
UNMASTS
UNPASTE
UNPIETY
UNQUOTE
UNRESTS
UNROOTS
UNSALTY
UNSEATS
UNSOOTY
UNSORTS
UNSTATE
UNTASTY
UNTRITE
UNTRUTH
UNWHITE
UNWITTY

•N••••T

ANALYST
ANAPEST
ANCIENT
ANGRYAT
ANIMIST
ANNULET
ANTIART
DNATEST
ENCHANT
ENCRUST
ENCRYPT
ENDEDAT
ENDEDIT
ENDMOST
ENDUPAT
ENGRAFT
ENRIGHT
ENTRANT
ENTREAT
ENTRUST
ENTWIST
GNAWSAT
GNOMIST
INACAST
INAKNOT
INANEST
INASNIT
INASPOT
INASUIT
INBUILT
INCOURT
INCRUST
INDOUBT
INDRAFT
INDWELT
INEXACT
INFIRST
INFLECT
INFLICT
INFORIT
INFRACT
INFRONT
INGRAFT
INHABIT
INHERIT
INHIBIT
INKBLOT
INKIEST
INKSPOT
INORBIT
INPOINT
INPRINT
INQUEST

INSHORT
INSIGHT
INSPECT
INSTANT
INSWEPT
INTROIT
INTRUST
KNESSET
ONADIET
ONALERT
ONATOOT
ONEACAT
ONECENT
ONEFOOT
ONEOCAT
ONEPART
ONEPINT
ONESHOT
ONESPOT
ONEUNIT
ONEWHIT
ONFIRST
ONLIEST
ONPOINT
ONSIGHT
ONTHEQT
ONTOAST
PNEUMAT
SNAPSAT
SNARLAT
SNEERAT
SNICKET
SNIDEST
SNIFFAT
SNIGLET
SNIPEAT
SNIPPET
SNORTAT
SNOWCAT
SNOWHAT
SNUGFIT
UNADEPT
UNADULT
UNALERT
UNBESET
UNBLENT
UNBLEST
UNBUILT
UNBURNT
UNBURST
UNCLEFT
UNCLIPT
UNDEALT
UNERECT
UNFROST
UNGUENT
UNINERT
UNJOINT
UNKEMPT
UNLIGHT
UNMEANT
UNMOIST
UNOVERT
UNPLAIT
UNQUIET
UNSHIFT
UNSHORT
UNSIGHT
UNSMART
UNSPELT
UNSPENT
UNSPILT
UNSPLIT
UNSTOUT
UNSWEET
UNSWEPT
UNTWIST
UNWHIPT

••NT•••

AINTHAY
AUNTBEE
AUNTIES
BANTAMS
BANTERS
BANTING
BENTHAM
BENTHOS
BENTLEY
BENTSEN
BUNTERS
BUNTING
CANTABS
CANTALS
CANTATA
CANTEEN
CANTERS
CANTILY
CANTINA
CANTING
CANTINO
CANTLES
CANTONS
CANTORS
CANTRIP
CANTSAY
CENTALS
CENTARE
CENTAUR
CENTAVO
CENTERS
CENTIME
CENTIMO
CENTRAL
CENTRED
CENTRES
CENTRIC
CENTRUM
CENTURY
CONTACS
CONTACT
CONTAIN
CONTEMN
CONTEND
CONTENT
CONTEST
CONTEXT
CONTORT
CONTOUR
CONTRAS
CONTROL
CONTUSE
CYNTHIA
DANTEAN
DANTEII
DENTALS
DENTATE
DENTINE
DENTING
DENTINS
DENTIST
DENTOID
DENTONS
DENTURE
DENTYNE
DINTING
DONTASK
DONTBEE
DONTCRY
DONTLIE
FANTAIL
FANTANS
FANTASM
FANTAST
FANTASY
FANTINE
FANTODS
FONTANA
FONTANE
FONTEYN
FONTINA
FUNTIME
GANTLET
GENTEEL
GENTIAN
GENTILE
GENTLED
GENTLER
GENTLES
GUNTHER
HENTOFF
HINTERS
HINTING
HINTSAT
HUNTERS
HUNTFOR
HUNTING
HUNTLEY
HUNTSUP
KANTIAN
KENTISH
KONTIKI
LANTANA
LANTERN
LENTIGO
LENTILS
LINTELS
LINTERS
LINTIER
LINTING
MANTECA
MANTELS
MANTLED
MANTLES
MANTLET
MANTRAP
MANTRAS
MANTRIC
MANTUAN
MENTEES
MENTHOL
MENTION
MENTORS
MINTAGE
MINTERS
MINTIER
MINTING
MINTTEA
MONTAGE
MONTAGU
MONTALE
MONTANA
MONTAND
MONTANO
MONTAUK
MONTEGO
MONTERO
MONTEUX
MONTHLY
MONTOYA
MONTUNO
NINTHLY
PANTENE
PANTERA
PANTERS
PANTHER
PANTIES
PANTILE
PANTING
PANTLEG
PANTONE
PENTADS
PENTANE
PENTELS
PENTIUM
PINTAIL
PONTANO
PONTIAC
PONTIAN
PONTIFF
PONTIUS
PONTOON
PUNTERS
PUNTING
QINTARS
RANTERS
RANTING
RANTSAT
RENTALS
RENTEES
RENTERS
RENTIER
RENTING
RENTOUT
RENTSTO
RONTGEN
RUNTIER
RUNTIME
RUNTISH
SANTAFE
SANTANA
SANTINI
SENTFOR
SENTOFF
SENTOUT
SENTRAS
SUNTANS
TANTARA
TANTIVY
TANTRUM
TENTBED
TENTERS
TENTFUL
TENTHLY
TENTING
TENTONS
TENTPEG
TINTERN
TINTERS
TINTING
TINTYPE
TONTINE
VANTAGE
VENTAGE
VENTERS
VENTING
VENTNOR
VENTRAD
VENTRAL
VENTRIS
VENTURA
VENTURE
VENTURI
VINTAGE
VINTNER
WANTADS
WANTAGH
WANTERS
WANTING
WANTONS
WANTOUT
WANTSIN
WANTSTO
WENTAFT
WENTAPE
WENTBAD
WENTFAR
WENTFOR
WENTMAD
WENTOFF
WENTOUT
WENTPRO
WINTERS
WINTERY
WONTING
WONTONS
XANTHAN
XANTHIC

••N•T••

AGNATES
AGNATIC
ALNITAK
ANNATTO
ANNETTE
BENATAR
BENOTED
BENOTES
BONITOS
CANETTI
CANITBE
DANITES
DENOTED
DENOTES
DINETTE
DONATED
DONATEE
DONATES
DONATOR
DONATUS
DONETSK
DONOTGO
DUNSTAN
FANATIC
FENETRE
FINITES
FUNSTER
GANGTOK
GENETIC
GENITOR
GUNITES
HANGTEN
HUNGTEN
IGNATOW
IGNITED
IGNITER
IGNITES
IGNITOR
JANITOR
KINETIC
KINGTUT
LANDTAG
LANDTAX
LANETWO
LANGTON
LANGTRY
LANOTTE
LENGTHS
LENGTHY
LINETWO
LONETTE
LONGTOM
LONGTON
LUNATED
LUNATES
LUNATIC
LUNETTE
LYNETTE
MANATEE
MANETTE
MENOTTI
MINITVS
MINOTND
MINSTER
MINTTEA
MINUTED
MINUTER
MINUTES
MINUTIA
MONCTON
MONITOR
MONSTER
MONSTRO
MUNSTER
NANETTE
NONETTE
NONSTOP
ORNETTE
ORNITHO
PANETTA
PENATES
PINATAS
PINETAR
PINETOP
PINETUM
PINOTTA
PUNSTER
RANATAB
RANITUP
RENOTED
RENOTES
RONETTE
RUNATAB
RUNITUP
SANCTUM
SANCTUS
SENATES
SENATOR
SINATRA
SINUTAB
SONATAS
TANKTOP
TINCTED
TINSTAR
TINYTIM
TINYTOT
TONETTE
UNNOTED
VENATIC
WINDTEE
WINGTIP
WINSTON
WYNETTE
YANGTZE
YANKTON
ZANETTO
ZENITHS

••N••T•

AMNESTY
ANNATTO
ANNETTE
ANNUITY
BANDITO
BANDITS
BANKITS
BENEATH
BENNETT
BINDSTO
BONIATO
BONMOTS
BONNETS
CANASTA
CANETTI
CANTATA
CONFITS
CONFUTE
CONMOTO
CONNATE
CONNOTE
CUNEATE
DENSITY
DENTATE
DINETTE
DYNASTS
DYNASTY
ELNORTE
ERNESTA
ERNESTO
FANJETS
FANOUTS
GANGSTA
GANNETS
GANNETT
HANDYTO
HENBITS
HONESTY
JENNETS
JUNKETS
KENNETH
LANCETS
LANOTTE
LINEATE
LINNETS
LONETTE
LUNESTA
LUNETTE
LYNETTE
MANDATE
MANETTE
MANKATO
MENOTTI
MINOLTA
MINUETS
MRNORTH
NANETTE
NONARTS
NONETTE
NONHITS
ORNETTE
OWNUPTO
PANDITS
PANETTA
PENALTY
PENLITE
PENNATE
PENULTS
PINKETT
PINNATE
PINOTTA
PUNDITS
RANINTO
RANLATE
RANUPTO
RANWITH
RENESTS
RENNETS
RENTSTO
RONETTE
RUNINTO
RUNLATE
RUNLETS
RUNNETH
RUNOUTS
RUNUPTO
RUNWITH
SENDSTO
SENNETT
SENSATE
SINCITY
SINGSTO
SINUATE
SONNETS
SUNBATH
SUNCITY
SUNHATS
SUNSETS
TENANTS
TENDSTO
TENSITY
TENUITY
TINHATS
TONETTE
TUNEDTO
TUNESTO
UPNORTH
VANUATU
WANTSTO
WYNETTE
ZANETTO
ZENISTS
ZINCITE

••N•••T

ALNIYAT
ANNULET
ATNIGHT
BANDLET
BANGOUT
BANQUET
BENEFIT
BENNETT
BONELET
BONESET
BONIEST
CANDENT
CANIEST
CONCEIT
CONCEPT
CONCERT
CONCOCT
CONDUCT
CONDUIT
CONELET
CONFECT
CONGEST
CONKOUT
CONNECT
CONSENT
CONSIST
CONSORT
CONSULT
CONTACT
CONTENT
CONTEST
CONTEXT
CONTORT
CONVECT
CONVENT
CONVERT
CONVICT
DANKEST
DENSEST
DENTIST
DINEDAT
DINEOUT
DINESAT
DINGBAT
DINMONT
FANBELT
FANFEST
FANSOUT
FANTAST
FINDOUT
FINEART
FONDANT
FONDEST
FUNFEST
GANNETT
GANTLET
GENESET
GONEAFT
GONEOUT
GUNBELT
GUNBOAT
GUNSHOT
HANDOUT
HANDSET
HANGOUT
HINTSAT
HONKSAT
HUNGOUT
IINSIST
IKNEWIT
IKNOWIT
JUNKART
KINDEST
KINGLET
KINGRAT
KINGTUT
KINMONT
LANDSAT
LANKEST
LENDOUT
LENFANT
LENIENT
LINECUT
LINEOUT
LINIEST
LONGEST
LUNGEAT
MANHUNT
MANTLET
MANUMIT
MANXCAT
MINARET
MINDSET
MINEPIT
MONGKUT
NONDIET
NONFACT
NONMEAT
NONPAST
NONPOET
NUNAVUT
PANSOUT
PENDANT
PENDENT
PENNANT
PINCHOT
PINENUT
PINIEST
PINKEST
PINKETT
PUNGENT
PUNIEST
RANGOUT
RANKEST
RANKOUT
RANPAST
RANRIOT
RANTSAT
RENAULT
RENTOUT
RENUZIT
RINGLET
RINGOUT
RINKRAT
RUNGOUT
RUNPAST
RUNRIOT
RUNSOUT
SANDLOT
SANDPIT
SANGOUT
SENDOUT
SENNETT
SENTOUT
SINGLET
SINGOUT
SUNBELT
SUNFAST
SUNKIST
SUNSPOT
SUNSUIT
TANGENT
TANNEST
TENCENT
TENFEET
TENFOOT
TENNANT
TENPAST
TENSEST
TENSPOT
TINIEST
TINYBIT
TINYTOT
TONIEST
TONIGHT
TUNEOUT
VANPELT
VANSANT
VANVOGT
VANZANT
VINCENT
VINIEST
WANIEST
WANNEST
WANTOUT
WENTAFT
WENTOUT
WINEVAT
WINGLET
WINGNUT
WINGSIT
WINIEST
WINKOUT
WINKSAT
WINSLET
WINSOUT
XINGOUT
YANKOUT
YANKSAT
ZANIEST
ZONEOUT
ZONKOUT

•••NT••

ABINTRA
ACANTHI
AGENTED
AGENTRY
AMANTIS
ARANTXA
ASANTES
AVANTIS
BAINTER
BIENTOT
BLANTON
BLENTIN
BLINTZE
BLUNTED
BLUNTER
BLUNTLY
BRONTES
BURNTIN
BURNTUP
CHANTED
CHANTER
CHANTEY
CHANTRY
CHINTZY
CLANTON
CLINTON
COUNTED
COUNTEE
COUNTEM
COUNTER
COUNTIN
COUNTON
COUNTRY
COUNTUP
DAUNTED
DAUNTER
ELANTRA
FAINTED
FAINTER
FAINTLY
FEINTED
FLINTMI
FRANTIC
FRONTAL
FRONTED
FRONTON
FUENTES
GAUNTER
GAUNTLY
GLINTED
GRANTED
GRANTEE
GRANTER
GRANTOR
GRUNTED
GRUNTER
HAUNTED
HAUNTER
IDENTIC
IWANTIT
IWANTTO
JAUNTED
JOINTED
JOINTER
JOINTLY
LEANTOS
MAINTOP
MEANTIT
MEANTTO
MOUNTED
MOUNTER
MOUNTIE
MOUNTUP
NIANTIC
NOENTRY
OBENTOS
ODONTIA
OPENTAP
OPENTOE
OPENTOP
OPUNTIA
ORANTES
PAINTED
PAINTER
PHANTOM
PLANTAR
PLANTED
PLANTER
PLINTHS
POINTAT
POINTED
POINTER
POINTES
POINTTO
POINTUP
PRINTAD
PRINTED
PRINTER
PRINTUP
QUANTUM
QUENTIN
QUINTAL
QUINTAS
QUINTES
QUINTET
QUINTIC
QUINTON
QUINTUS
REENTER
REENTRY
RIANTLY
SAINTED
SAINTES
SAINTLO
SAINTLY
SAUNTER
SCANTED
SCANTER
SCANTLY
SCENTED
SCENTER
SHANTER
SHUNTED
SHUNTER
SLANTED
SLANTLY
SLANTUP
SPENTON
STANTON
STENTOR
STINTED
STINTER
STUNTED
SWINTON
TAINTED
TAUNTED
TAUNTER
TAUNTON
TRENTON
VAUNTED
VAUNTER
VEINTES

•••N•T•

ACONITE
AMANITA

AMENITY
AMINUTE
BENNETT
BLINDTO
BONNETS
BOUNDTO
BRINGTO
BRUNETS
BURNETT
CAPNUTS
CARNETS
CLINGTO
CLUNGTO
COBNUTS
COGNATE
CONNATE
CONNOTE
CORNETS
CORNUTE
CRENATE
CYGNETS
DIGNITY
DIPNETS
DOINGTO
DRANKTO
DRINKTO
EBONITE
ELANETS
EMANATE
ENDNOTE
FLYNETS
GANNETS
GANNETT
GARNETS
GARNETT
GOINGTO
GRANITA
GRANITE
GWYNETH
HEXNUTS
HOGNUTS
HORNETS
HUANGTI
INANITY
ININETY
INKNOTS
IWANTTO
JENNETS
KENNETH
KEYNOTE
KHANATE
KUZNETS
LEANSTO
LEONATO
LIGNITE
LIMNITE
LINNETS
LIONETS
LUGNUTS
LYINGTO
MAGNATE
MAGNETO
MAGNETS
MEANSTO
MEANTTO
NEONATE
NOENDTO
ONENOTE
OWINGTO
PEANUTS
PENNATE
PIGNUTS
PINNATE
PLANATE
PLANETS
PLANSTO
POINTTO
PRONATE
PRONETO
QUINATE
REKNITS
REKNOTS
RENNETS
REUNITE
RUINATE
RUNNETH
SAYNOTO
SENNETT
SIGNETS
SONNETS
SPINETS
STANDTO
SUBNETS
TERNATE
THENETS
TRINITY
TURNSTO
TYINGTO
UNKNITS
UNKNOTS
URANITE
WALNUTS
ZAGNUTS

•••N••T

ACINGIT
AGONIST
AMONGST
ASONANT
BATNEXT
BENNETT
BIENTOT
BLANKET
BLINKAT
BRINGIT
BURNETT
BURNOUT
CONNECT
COONCAT
DOWNPAT
EARNEST
EARNSIT
EMANANT
EMINENT
EVENBET
EVENEST
EVENOUT
FAINEST
FLINGAT
FLUNGAT
GANNETT
GARNETT
GOINGAT
GRINSAT
GYMNAST
HORNIST
ICANNOT
ICINGIT
INANEST
IRONIST
IRONOUT
IWANTIT
JAINIST
JEANNOT
KEENEST
LEANCUT
LEANEST
LOANOUT
MEANEST
MEANSIT
MEANTIT
MOONLET
MOONLIT
MOONSET
OPENNET
OPENOUT
OPENPIT
PENNANT
PIANIST
PLANOUT
POINTAT
QUINTET
QUONSET
RAINHAT
RAINOUT
REENACT
REGNANT
REMNANT
SEENFIT
SEENOUT
SENNETT
SIGNOUT
SOONEST
SPINOUT
SPUNOUT
SWINGAT
SWINGIT
SWUNGAT
SWUNGIT
TANNEST
TENNANT
THINOUT
TLINGIT
TORNOUT
TOWNLET
TRANSIT
TRINKET
TURNOUT
TWINJET
TWINSET
UNINERT
VAINEST
VEINLET
WANNEST
WORNOUT
ZIONIST

••••NT•

ABSENTS
ABSINTH
ACCENTS
ADDONTO
ADVENTS
ALDENTE
ALIENTO
ALLANTE
AMOUNTS
ANDANTE
ANOINTS
APLENTY
ARGANTE
ARGENTI
ARGENTO
ARGENTS
ASCENTS
ASHANTI
ASSANTE
ASSENTS
ASSUNTA
ATEINTO
ATLANTA
BARENTS
BEGANTO
BUYINTO
CEMENTS
CHIANTI
CILENTO
CLEANTE
CLIENTS
CORINTH
CUTINTO
DECANTS
DEIGNTO
DELINTS
DEMENTO
DETENTE
DETENTS
DIGINTO
DIPINTO
DOCENTS
DOZENTH
DRAWNTO
DUGINTO
DURANTE
EATINTO
ELMONTE
ELUANTS
ENFANTS
ENTENTE
EXEUNTS
EXTENTS
FEDINTO
FITINTO
FLAUNTS
FLAUNTY
FLOWNTO
FLYINTO
FOMENTS
FORINTS
GALANTS
GALENTO
GERENTS
GETINTO
GETONTO
GIVENTO
GOTINTO
GOTONTO
HITINTO
HOPINTO
INCANTS
INCENTS
INDENTS
INFANTA
INFANTE
INFANTS
INTENTS
INVENTS
ITWENTY
JACINTH
JACINTO
LAMENTS
LAMINTO
LATENTS
LAYINTO
LEARNTO
LECONTE
LEDINTO
LEPANTO
LIKENTO
LISENTE
LITINTO
LOGONTO
LORENTZ
MAGENTA
MARANTZ
MEMENTO
MOMENTA
MOMENTS
MORANTE
MUSANTE
MUTANTS
MYLANTA
OCHENTA
OCTANTS
ONEONTA
ORIENTE
ORIENTS
OTRANTO
PARENTS
PATENTS
PAYINTO
PEDANTS
PESANTE
PICANTE
PIMENTO
PLAINTS
POLENTA
PRYINTO
RAMINTO
RANINTO
RECANTS
REDANTS
REGENTS
RELENTS
REMINTS
REPENTS
RERENTS
RESENTS
RETINTS
RIPINTO
RISENTO
RODENTS
RUNINTO
SAVANTS
SAWINTO
SECANTS
SEEINTO
SETENTA
SETINTO
SEVENTH
SEVENTY
SILENTA
SILENTB
SILENTC
SILENTD
SILENTE
SILENTF
SILENTG
SILENTH
SILENTI
SILENTJ
SILENTK
SILENTL
SILENTM
SILENTN
SILENTO
SILENTP
SILENTQ
SILENTR
SILENTS
SILENTT
SILENTU
SILENTV
SILENTW
SILENTX
SILENTY
SILENTZ
SORENTO
SPLINTS
SPRINTS
SQUANTO
SQUINTS
SQUINTY
TAKENTO
TALENTS
TAPINTO
TARANTO
TENANTS
TIEINTO
TORONTO
TREINTA
TRUANTS
TYRANTS
VALENTE
VALENTI
VICENTE
VIVANTS
VOLANTE
VOLENTE
WASONTO
YEARNTO

••••N•T

ADJUNCT
AGAINST
BARONET
BAYONET
BEIGNET
BERENDT
BIGUNIT
BOWKNOT
CABINET
COCONUT
CORONET
DARENOT
DEFUNCT
DOESNOT
DRAGNET
DROPNET
EATENAT
EXTINCT
FASTNET
FEARNOT
FISHNET
FLOWNAT
FROWNAT
GETONIT
GILLNET
GOTONIT
HAIRNET
HAVENOT
HOPENOT
ICANNOT
IMEANIT
INAKNOT
INASNIT
JACONET
JEANNOT
KOLANUT
LETSNOT
LIFENET
LOCKNUT
LOGANUT
MAGINOT
NEEDNOT
OGDENUT
ONEUNIT
OPENNET
PINENUT
QUEENIT
SATINET
SILENTT
SITONIT
SOAPNET
SUBUNIT
TOPKNOT
TWOUNIT
WHATNOT
WINGNUT

•••••NT

ABEYANT
ACCOUNT
ADAMANT
AFFIANT
AFFRONT
AILMENT
AIRVENT
ALIMENT
AMBIENT
ANCIENT
APPOINT
ARMYANT
ASONANT
ASQUINT
ATTAINT
AUGMENT
BELMONT
BERSUNT
BIGTENT
BLATANT
BUOYANT
CANDENT
CATMINT
CLAMANT
CLEMENT
COAGENT
COMMENT
CONSENT
CONTENT
CONVENT
COOLANT
COULDNT
COURANT
CURRANT
CURRENT
DEFIANT
DELMONT
DEMOUNT
DERWENT
DESCANT
DESCENT
DEVIANT
DILUENT
DINMONT
DISSENT
DISTANT
DORMANT
DURWENT
EGGHUNT
ELEGANT
ELEMENT
EMANANT
EMINENT
ENCHANT
ENTRANT
ERODENT
ETCHANT
EVIDENT
EXIGENT
FERMENT
FERVENT
FIGMENT
FIREANT
FONDANT
FORRENT
FORWENT
FOXHUNT
FREMONT
FULGENT
GALLANT
GARMENT
GERAINT
GETBENT
GODSENT
HYDRANT
IMPLANT
IMPRINT
INFRONT
INPOINT
INPRINT
INSTANT
ISSUANT
ITERANT
JOBHUNT
KINMONT
KURRENT
LAMBENT
LARGENT
LAURENT
LENFANT
LENIENT
LORIENT
LOWRENT
MALEANT
MANHUNT
MEDIANT
MIGHTNT
MIGRANT
MISSENT
MORDANT
MORDENT
MYGIANT
NASCENT
NEWMINT
NEWMONT
NOCOUNT
NYGIANT
ODDMENT
ODORANT
ONECENT
ONEPINT
ONPOINT
OPERANT
OPULENT
ORPHANT
OUGHTNT
OUTCANT
OUTHUNT
OUTRANT
OUTWENT
OXIDANT
PAGEANT
PASSANT
PATIENT
PAYMENT
PEASANT
PECCANT
PENDANT
PENDENT
PENNANT
PERCENT
PIGMENT
PIQUANT
PORTENT
PRERENT
PRESENT
PREVENT
PRUDENT
PUNGENT
PUPTENT
RADIANT
RAIMENT
RAMPANT
REAGENT
REBOANT
RECOUNT
REDCENT
REFRONT
REGNANT
REGRANT
RELIANT
REMNANT
REMOUNT
REPAINT
REPLANT
REPOINT
REPRINT
REYMONT
SALIENT
SALTANT
SAPIENT
SARGENT
SEAHUNT
SEALANT
SEGMENT
SERPENT
SERVANT
SEXTANT
SOLVENT
SOYLENT
STUDENT
TAGGANT
TANGENT
TENCENT
TENNANT
THERENT
TORMENT
TORRENT
TRIDENT
TWERENT
ULULANT
UNBLENT
UNBURNT
UNGUENT
UNJOINT
UNMEANT
UNSPENT
UPFRONT
USGRANT
VAGRANT
VALIANT
VANSANT
VANZANT
VARIANT
VARMINT
VERDANT
VERMONT
VERSANT
VIADENT
VIBRANT
VINCENT
VIOLENT
WARRANT
WOULDNT
XAMOUNT

NU•••••

NUANCED
NUANCES
NUBBERS
NUBBIER
NUBBINS
NUBBLES
NUBIANS
NUBIRAS
NUCLEAR
NUCLEIC
NUCLEON
NUCLEUS
NUCLIDE
NUDGERS
NUDGING
NUDISTS
NUDNIKS
NUDZHED
NUDZHES
NUESTRA
NUESTRO
NUGGETS
NUGGETY
NULLIFY
NULLING
NULLITY
NULLSET
NUMBATS
NUMBERS
NUMBEST
NUMBING
NUMERAL
NUMERIC
NUMEROS
NUMLOCK
NUNAVUT
NUNCIOS
NUNGWEN
NUNHOOD
NUNLIKE
NUNNERY
NUNNISH
NUNSHIP
NUPTIAL
NUREYEV
NURSERS
NURSERY
NURSING
NURTURE
NUTATED
NUTATES
NUTLETS
NUTLIKE
NUTMEAT
NUTMEGS
NUTOILS
NUTPINE
NUTRIAS
NUTSIER
NUTTERS
NUTTIER
NUTTILY
NUTTING
NUTTREE
NUTWOOD
NUZZLED
NUZZLER
NUZZLES

N•U••••

NAUGHTS
NAUGHTY
NAUSEAM
NAUTICA
NAUTILI
NEUILLY
NEUMANN
NEURONE
NEURONS
NEUTERS
NEUTRAL
NEUTRON
NOUGATS
NOUGHTS
NOURISH
NOUTURN
NOUVEAU
NTUPLES

N••U•••

NABUCCO
NAHUATL
NATURAL
NATURED
NATUREL
NATURES
NEBULAE
NEBULAR
NEBULAS
NEGUSES
NEXUSES
NKRUMAH
NOCUOUS
NODULAR
NODULED
NODULES
NOGUCHI
NONUKES
NONUPLE
NONUSER
NOSUGAR
NOTUPTO
NOTURNS
NOTUSED

N•••U••

NATSUME
NEPTUNE
NERVULE
NESQUIK
NETFULS
NETSUKE
NETSURF
NEWBURG
NIEBUHR
NIPMUCK
NOCOUNT
NODOUBT
NOFAULT
NONBUSY
NONFUEL
NONJURY
NONSUCH
NOTMUCH
NOTRUMP
NOTSURE
NOUTURN
NURTURE

N••••U•

NAILGUN
NAILSUP
NAIPAUL
NATRIUM
NBCBLUE
NEEDFUL
NENNIUS
NERVOUS
NESTFUL
NICEGUY
NIOBIUM
NITROUS
NIVEOUS
NOCUOUS
NONDRUG
NONFLUX
NONPLUS
NOSEDUP
NOSEEUM
NOSEOUT
NOSESUP
NOSTRUM
NOTTRUE
NOXIOUS
NUCLEUS
NUNAVUT

N•••••U

NEARYOU
NOUVEAU

•NU••••

ENURING
FNUMBER
INULASE
INURING
INUTERO
INUTILE
KNUCKLE
KNUCKLY
KNURLED
SNUBBED
SNUBBER
SNUCKUP
SNUFFED
SNUFFER
SNUFFLE
SNUGFIT
SNUGGED
SNUGGER
SNUGGLE
SNUGGLY
SNUGLIS
UNURBAN
UNURGED
UNUSUAL

•N•U•••

ANGUISH
ANGULAR
ANNUALS
ANNUITY
ANNULAR
ANNULET
ANNULUS
ANOUILH
ENDUING
ENDUPAT
ENDURED
ENDURER
ENDURES
ENDUROS
ENDUSER
ENDUSES
ENGULFS
ENOUNCE
ENQUADS
ENQUEUE
ENQUIRE
ENQUIRY
ENSUING
ENSUITE
ENSURED
ENSURER
ENSURES

INBUILT
INCUBUS
INCUDES
INCURVE
INCUSED
INCUSES
INDUCED
INDUCER
INDUCES
INDUCTS
INDULGE
INDUTCH
INFUSED
INFUSER
INFUSES
INGULFS
INHUMAN
INHUMED
INHUMER
INHUMES
INJURED
INJURER
INJURES
INQUEST
INQUIRE
INQUIRY
INRUINS
INSULAR
INSULIN
INSULTS
INSURED
INSURER
INSURES
INTUITS
INTURNS
KNOUTED
ONEUNIT
ONGUARD
PNEUMAS
PNEUMAT
PNEUMON
SNOUTED
UNBUILD
UNBUILT
UNBULKY
UNBURLY
UNBURNT
UNBURST
UNCUBIC
UNCUFFS
UNCURBS
UNCURED
UNCURLS
UNDULAR
UNDUPED
UNDUSTY
UNFULLY
UNFUNNY
UNFURLS
UNFUSED
UNFUSSY
UNGUARD
UNGUENT
UNGULAE
UNGULAR
UNGUYED
UNHULLS
UNHUMAN
UNHUMID
UNHUSKS
UNJUICY
UNLUCID
UNLUCKY
UNLUMPY
UNLURED
UNLUSTY
UNMUDDY
UNMUTED
UNQUICK
UNQUIET
UNQUOTE
UNRULED
UNRURAL
UNSULKY
UNSUNNY
UNSURLY
UNTUCKS
UNTUNED
UNTUNES

•N••U••

ANDSUCH
ANYLUCK
ENCRUST
ENDCUTS
ENDRUNS
ENGLUND
ENGLUTS
ENROUTE
ENSOULS
ENTHUSE
ENTRUST
ENWOUND
INAFUNK
INAFURY
INAHUFF
INARUSH
INASUIT
INBOUND
INCLUDE
INCOURT
INCRUST
INDOUBT
INHOUSE
INOCULA
INPOURS
INTOUCH
INTRUDE
INTRUST
INTRUTH
ONAJURY
ONELUMP
SNAFUED
UNADULT
UNAMUNO
UNBLUED
UNBOUND
UNCHURN
UNCOUTH
UNCRUDE
UNCRUEL
UNDRUNK
UNEQUAL
UNFLUID
UNFOUND
UNGAUDY
UNGLUED
UNGLUES
UNGRUFF
UNHOUSE
UNIQUES
UNMOULD
UNPLUGS
UNPLUMB
UNROUND
UNSLUNG
UNSOUND
UNSTUCK
UNSTUNG
UNSWUNG
UNTOUGH
UNTRUER
UNTRULY
UNTRUSS
UNTRUTH
UNUSUAL
UNWOUND
UNWRUNG
UNYOUNG

•N•••U•

ANDROUS
ANGELUS
ANNULUS
ANTEDUP
ANTERUS
ANTESUP
ANTIGUA
ANTIGUN
ANTIQUE
ANXIOUS
CNOSSUS
ENAMOUR
ENDEDUP
ENQUEUE
ENRIQUE
ENVIOUS
ENVOGUE
GNOSSUS
INCUBUS
INFOCUS
INGENUE
INGROUP
INVACUO
INVOGUE
KNEESUP
KNOTSUP
ONECLUB
ONEHOUR
ONEOFUS
ONEROUS
SNAGSUP
SNAPSUP
SNARLUP
SNAZZUP
SNEAKUP
SNIFFUP
SNUCKUP
UNAWFUL
UNCLOUD
UNPIOUS
UNPROUD
UNSTOUT
UNVAGUE

•N••••U

ANGELOU
ONLYYOU

••NU•••

ANNUALS
ANNUITY
ANNULAR
ANNULET
ANNULUS
BENUMBS
BONUSES
BUNUELO
CANUCKS
CANULAE
CANULAS
CONURES
DENUDED
DENUDER
DENUDES
GENUINE
GENUSES
GUNUSER
HANUKAH
JANUARY
LUNULAE
LUNULAR
MANUALS
MANUMIT
MANURED
MANURES
MENUBAR
MENUDOS
MENUHIN
MINUEND
MINUETS
MINUSES
MINUTED
MINUTER
MINUTES
MINUTIA
NONUKES
NONUPLE
NONUSER
OWNUPTO
PANURGE
PENUCHE
PENULTS
RANUPTO
RENUZIT
RUNUPTO
SINUATE
SINUOUS
SINUSES
SINUTAB
TENUITY
TENUOUS
TENURED
TENURES
TONUSES
VANUATU
VENULES
VENUSES
ZONULAR
ZONULES

••N•U••

ADNOUNS
BANBURY
BANQUES
BANQUET
BENGUNN
BUNKUMS
CANFULS
CANNULA
CENSURE
CENTURY
CINQUES
CONCURS
CONCUSS
CONDUCE
CONDUCT
CONDUIT
CONFUSE
CONFUTE
CONJURE
CONJURY
CONQUER
CONSULS
CONSULT
CONSUME
CONTUSE
DANBURY
DENEUVE
DENTURE
DONJUAN
DONRUSS
EANMUND
FANEUIL
FANOUTS
FONDUED
FONDUES
FUNFURS
FUNRUNS
HANGUPS
HONOURS
IONIUMS
JONQUIL
LANGUID
LANGUOR
LENGUAS
LINEUPS
LINGUAE
LINGUAL
LINGULA
LINKUPS
LONGUES
MANCUSO
MANHUNT
MANTUAN
MONTUNO
NONBUSY
NONFUEL
NONJURY
NONSUCH
OFNOUSE
PANFULS
PENGUIN
PINCURL
PINGUID
RENAULT
RONDURE
RUNOUTS
SANJUAN
SENDUPS
SENSUAL
SUNBURN
SUNSUIT
SYNFUEL
TONGUES
TONSURE
TUNEUPS
URNFULS
VANDURA
VANDUYN
VENDUES
VENTURA
VENTURE
VENTURI
VINCULA
WINDUPS
YANQUIS

••N••U•

ANNULUS
BANEFUL
BANGOUT
BANGSUP
BANKSUP
BENBLUE
BENELUX
BINDSUP
BONEDUP
BONESUP
BONHEUR
BONJOUR
BUNCHUP
CANDOUR
CANOPUS
CENTAUR
CENTRUM
CONGOUS
CONKOUT
CONTOUR
DANSEUR
DINEOUT
DONAHUE
DONATUS
DONIMUS
FANCLUB
FANCYUP
FANSOUT
FENCEUP
FINDOUT
GANGSUP
GONEOUT
HANDFUL
HANDGUN
HANDOUT
HANDSUP
HANGOUT
HANGSUP
HUNGOUT
HUNTSUP
IBNSAUD
IGNEOUS
JUNEBUG
KINGTUT
LANDAUS
LANDSUP
LENDOUT
LINECUT
LINEDUP
LINEOUT
LINESUP
LINKSUP
LONGRUN
MANAGUA
MANHOUR
MANIPUR
MENCIUS
MINDFUL
MINIBUS
MINIMUM
MINIMUS
MINISUB
MINOGUE
MONGKUT
MONTAUK
MONTEUX
NENNIUS
NONDRUG
NONFLUX
NONPLUS
NUNAVUT
OMNIBUS
OWNEDUP
PANSOUT
PENTIUM
PINENUT
PINETUM
PONTIUS
PUNCHUP
RANCOUR
RANGOUT
RANITUP
RANKOUT
RENTOUT
RINGOUT
RINGSUP
RUNGOUT
RUNITUP
RUNSOUT
SANCTUM
SANCTUS
SANDBUR
SANGOUT
SENDOUT
SENDSUP
SENTOUT
SINGOUT
SINUOUS
SONGFUL
TANKFUL
TANKSUP
TANTRUM
TENFOUR
TENKRUN
TENSEUP
TENTFUL
TENUOUS
TONEDUP
TONESUP
TUNASUB
TUNEDUP
TUNEFUL
TUNEOUT
TUNESUP
VANOCUR
VONLAUE
WANTOUT
WENTOUT
WINDAUS
WINDSUP
WINGNUT
WINKOUT
WINSOUT
XANADUS
XINGOUT
YANKOUT
ZINCOUS
ZONEOUT
ZONKOUT

••N•••U

BANDEAU
BUNRAKU
MONDIEU
MONTAGU
RONDEAU
TINAMOU
TONNEAU
VANUATU

•••NU••

AMINUTE
AVENUEQ
AVENUES
BARNUMS
CANNULA
CAPNUTS
CHINUPS
COBNUTS
CORNUTE
EMANUEL
GRANULE
HEXNUTS
HOGNUTS
HORNUNG
LUGNUTS
MAGNUMS
PEANUTS
PIGNUTS
PLENUMS
PRENUPS
SAMNUNN
SHONUFF
SIGNUPS
TURNUPS
ULANUDE
VEINULE
WALNUTS
ZAGNUTS

•••N•U•

AGENDUM
BORNEUP
BOUNDUP
BRENGUN
BRINGUP
BURNOUT
BURNSUP
BURNTUP
COUNTUP
CRANIUM
CRANKUP
DOINGUP
DRANKUP
DRINKUP
DUBNIUM
EVENOUT
EVENSUP
FLANEUR
GAINFUL
GOINGUP
HAFNIUM
HAHNIUM
HEINOUS
ICINGUP
IRONOUT
JEANLUC
JOINSUP
LEANCUT
LIONCUB
LOANOUT
LYINGUP
MOANFUL
MOUNTUP
NENNIUS
OMINOUS
OPENOUT
OPENSUP
OZONOUS
PAINFUL
PHONYUP
PLANOUT
POINTUP
PRINTUP
PRONOUN
QUANTUM
QUINQUE
QUINTUS
RAINOUT
REYNAUD
RHENIUM
ROUNDUP
RUINOUS
SEENOUT
SHINEUP
SIGNOUT
SIGNSUP
SLANTUP
SLINKUP
SLUNKUP
SPINOUT
SPUNOUT
STANDUP
STANKUP
STANNUM
STENGUN
STINKUP
STUNGUN
SWANKUP
THINKUP
THINOUT
TORNOUT
TURNOUT
TURNSUP
TYINGUP
URANIUM
USINGUP
VILNIUS
WORNOUT
WOUNDUP
YAWNFUL
YOUNGUN

•••N••U

CHANOYU
FRENEAU
GARNEAU
QUENEAU
TONNEAU

••••NU•

ALUMNUS
ARCANUM
AVERNUS
BLOWNUP
CHAINUP
CHURNUP
CLEANUP
COCONUT
COLONUS
DOMINUS
DRAWNUP
EATENUP
FEMINUM
FLOWNUP
GIVENUP
GROWNUP
HUMANUM
HYGINUS
ICTINUS
INGENUE
JEJUNUM
KOLANUT
LATINUS
LIVENUP
LOCKNUT
LOGANUT
OCEANUS
OGDENUT
PINENUT
RAPANUI
RETINUE
REVENUE
ROMANUS
SEVENUP
SHOWNUP
STANNUM
STERNUM
TAKENUP
TETANUS
URSINUS
WINGNUT
WOKENUP

••••N•U

LILINAU
PAXINOU
SILENTU
TULANEU

•••••NU

AUBURNU
BOSTONU
MARTINU
PARVENU

N•V••••

NAVAHOS
NAVAIDS
NAVAJOS
NAVARRE
NAVIDAD
NAVYMAN
NAVYMEN
NEVADAN
NEVILLE
NIVEOUS
NOVALIS
NOVARRO
NOVELAS
NOVELLA
NOVELLE
NOVELLO
NOVELTY
NOVENAS
NOVICES
NOVISAD
NOVOTES
NOVOTNY

N••V•••

NAIVELY
NAIVEST
NAIVETE
NAIVETY
NARVAEZ
NERVIER
NERVILY
NERVINE
NERVING
NERVOUS
NERVULE
NIRVANA
NONVOID
NOUVEAU

N•••V••

NATIVES
NINEVEH
NONEVER
NONEVIL
NOTEVEN
NOTEVER
NOTOVER
NUNAVUT

N••••V•

NBALIVE
NEWLOVE
NEWWAVE
NONLIVE
NOTLIVE

N•••••V

NABOKOV
NEMEROV
NUREYEV

•NV••••

ENVEILS
ENVELOP
ENVENOM
ENVIERS
ENVIOUS
ENVIRON
ENVIROS
ENVOGUE
ENVYING
INVACUO
INVADED
INVADER
INVADES
INVALID
INVEIGH
INVENTS
INVERSE
INVERTS
INVESTS
INVICTA
INVITED
INVITEE
INVITER
INVITES
INVITRO
INVOGUE
INVOICE
INVOKED
INVOKER
INVOKES
INVOLVE
ONVIDEO
UNVAGUE
UNVEILS
UNVENAL
UNVEXED
UNVITAL
UNVIVID
UNVOCAL
UNVOICE
UNVOTED
UNVOWED
UNVYING

•N•V•••

INAVALE
KNAVERY
KNAVISH
ONEVOTE
SNIVELS
UNIVACS
UNOVERT

•N••V••

ANDOVER
ENDIVES
ENLIVEN
INCIVIL
INFAVOR
INFIVES
INWOVEN
KNIEVEL
ONEOVER
UNCIVIC
UNCIVIL
UNCOVER
UNEAVED
UNGIVEN
UNGYVED
UNLAVED
UNLEVEL
UNLIVED
UNLIVES
UNLOVED
UNMOVED
UNNOVEL
UNPAVED
UNRAVEL
UNRIVED
UNRIVEN
UNSAVED
UNSAVVY
UNVIVID
UNWAVED
UNWOVEN

•N•••V•

ANCHOVY
ENCLAVE
ENGRAVE
ENSLAVE
INCURVE
INNERVE
INVOLVE
INWEAVE
ONELOVE
ONLEAVE
ONSERVE
UNBRAVE
UNGLOVE
UNHEAVY
UNITIVE
UNNAIVE
UNNERVE
UNSAVVY
UNWEAVE

••NV•••

CANVASS
CONVECT
CONVENE
CONVENT
CONVERT
CONVEYS
CONVICT
CONVOKE
CONVOYS
DANVERS
JANVIER
LANVINS
NONVOID
RENVOIS
VANVOGT

••N•V••

DONOVAN
GENEVAN
HANOVER
LENOVOS
MINIVAC
MINIVAN
MINIVER
MRNOVAK
NINEVEH
NONEVER
NONEVIL
NUNAVUT
RANOVER
RUNOVER
UNNOVEL
WINEVAT
WINOVER
WONOVER

••N••V•

BENBOVA

BONJOVI
CENTAVO
CONCAVE
CONNIVE
DENEUVE
DONLEVY
GINGIVA
HENRYVI
INNERVE
MINERVA
MINITVS
MONDAVI
NONLIVE
PENSIVE
TANTIVY
TENSIVE
UNNAIVE
UNNERVE

••N•••V
HENRYIV

•••NV••
JOHNVII

•••N•V•
CONNIVE
IVANOVO
JOHNXVI
OLDNAVY
PRONAVY
SCENEVI
ULANOVA

•••N••V
GRINKOV
JOHNXIV
SCENEIV

••••NV•
URBANVI

••••N•V
BADENOV
GODUNOV
ROMANOV
ROZANOV
SILENTV
SMIRNOV
ULYANOV
URBANIV
USTINOV

•••••NV
MARTINV

N•W••••
NCWYETH
NEWAGER
NEWAGEY
NEWBERN
NEWBERY
NEWBIES
NEWBOLT
NEWBORN
NEWBURG
NEWCARS
NEWDEAL
NEWFACE
NEWGATE
NEWHAND
NEWHART
NEWHATS
NEWHIRE
NEWHOPE
NEWIDEA
NEWJOBS
NEWKIDS
NEWLAID
NEWLEAF
NEWLEFT
NEWLIFE
NEWLINE
NEWLOOK
NEWLOVE
NEWMADE
NEWMANS
NEWMATH
NEWMINT
NEWMONT
NEWMOON
NEWMOWN
NEWNAME
NEWNESS
NEWPORT
NEWRICH
NEWSBOY
NEWSDAY
NEWSIER
NEWSIES
NEWSMAN
NEWSMEN
NEWSOME
NEWSPEG
NEWTONS
NEWTOWN
NEWTOYS
NEWWAVE
NEWWEEK
NEWWORD
NEWYEAR
NEWYORK
NOWHERE
NOWISEE
NOWISER
NOWLOOK
NOWNESS
NOWORSE
NOWTHEN
NOWTHIS
NOWWHAT

N••W•••
NARWHAL
NATWICK
NETWARE
NETWORK
NEWWAVE
NEWWEEK
NEWWORD
NITWITS
NONWAGE
NONWARS
NONWOOL
NONWORD
NONWORK
NORWALK
NORWICH
NORWOOD
NOSWEAT
NOTWELL
NOTWITH
NOWWHAT
NUTWOOD

N•••W••
NUNGWEN

N••••W•
NARROWS
NBCNEWS
NEPHEWS
NEWMOWN
NEWTOWN
NONJEWS
NONNEWS
NORDOWE
NOSHOWS

•NW••••
ENWINDS
ENWOUND
ENWRAPS
INWARDS
INWEAVE
INWHITE
INWOVEN
ONWARDS
ONWATER
UNWADED
UNWAGED
UNWAKED
UNWALLS
UNWANED
UNWAVED
UNWAXED
UNWEARY
UNWEAVE
UNWEDGE
UNWHEEL
UNWHIPT
UNWHITE
UNWHOLE
UNWINDS
UNWINDY
UNWIPED
UNWIRED
UNWISER
UNWITTY
UNWOOED
UNWORMY
UNWOUND
UNWOVEN
UNWRAPS
UNWRUNG

•N•W•••
ANSWERS
ANTWERP
ANYWAYS
ANYWISE
ENDWAYS
ENDWISE
ENTWINE
ENTWIST
GNAWERS
GNAWING
GNAWSAT
GNAWSON
INAWEOF
INAWINK
INAWORD
INDWELL
INDWELT
INKWELL
INSWEPT
KNEWHOW
KNOWALL
KNOWERS
KNOWETH
KNOWHOW
KNOWING
KNOWLES
KNOWSOF
ONAWHIM
ONEWEEK
ONEWHIT
ONEWOOD
SNOWCAP
SNOWCAT
SNOWDAY
SNOWDON
SNOWHAT
SNOWIER
SNOWILY
SNOWING
SNOWJOB
SNOWMAN
SNOWMEN
SNOWPEA
SNOWSIN
SNOWSKI
UNAWAKE
UNAWARE
UNAWFUL
UNOWING
UNOWNED
UNSWEAR
UNSWEET
UNSWEPT
UNSWORE
UNSWORN
UNSWUNG
UNTWINE
UNTWIST

•N••W••
ANTIWAR
CNTOWER
ENDOWED
ENDOWER
INNOWAY
INPOWER
ONETWOS
UNBOWED
UNCOWED
UNDEWED
UNHEWED
UNLOWLY
UNMEWED
UNMOWED
UNPAWED
UNPAWNS
UNROWDY
UNSAWED
UNSEWED
UNSOWED
UNVOWED

•N•••W•
ANDREWS
ANTCOWS
ANYNEWS
ANYTOWN
INBROWN
INCROWD
INDRAWN
INFLOWS
INGROWN
ONEDOWN
ONMYOWN
UNBLOWN
UNCROWN
UNDRAWN
UNDRAWS
UNFLOWN
UNGROWN
UNKNOWN
UNSHOWN
UNSHOWY
UNSKEWS
UNSTOWS
UNTHAWS

•N••••W
INASTEW
KNEWHOW
KNOWHOW
UNSCREW

••NW•••
FANWISE
GUNWALE
KENWAHL
NONWAGE
NONWARS
NONWOOL
NONWORD
NONWORK
PINWALE
RANWILD
RANWITH
RENWICK
RONWOOD
RUNWAYS
RUNWILD
RUNWITH
SUNWARD
TENWEEK
TINWARE
TINWORK
VANWARD
VANWYCK
WINWOOD

••N•W••
DUNAWAY
GANGWAY
IKNEWIT
IKNOWIT
INNOWAY
JANEWAY
LANGWAY
LONGWAY
MANOWAR
NUNGWEN
RANAWAY
RENEWAL
RENEWED
RENEWER
RENOWNS
RUNAWAY
SINEWED
VANOWEN

••N••W•
GUNLAWS
LANETWO
LINETWO
MINNOWS
NONJEWS
NONNEWS
PINDOWN
RANDOWN
RUNDOWN
SUNBOWL
SUNBOWS
SUNDOWN
WINDOWS
WINDOWY
WINNOWS

••N•••W
BANDSAW
DANELAW
GANGSAW
HANDSAW
HINDPAW
IGNATOW
JANKLOW
KENDREW
LONGBOW
MANILOW
RENFREW
RUNSLOW
SUNGLOW
TONEROW
TONYDOW
WINSLOW

•••NW••
BRONWEN
CHINWAG
JOHNWOO

•••N•W•
ABCNEWS
ALLNEWS
ANYNEWS
BADNEWS
BARNOWL
BIGNEWS
CBSNEWS
ESPNEWS
FOXNEWS
MINNOWS
NBCNEWS
NONNEWS
OKINAWA
OLDNEWS
THENEWS
UNKNOWN
WINNOWS

•••N••W
CORNROW
DOWNBOW
EVENNOW
JOHNLAW
MOONBOW
RAINBOW
REENDOW

••••N•W
ASOFNOW
CALLNOW
COMENOW
DOITNOW
EVENNOW
EXITNOW
HERENOW
ILLKNOW
ISEENOW
JUSTNOW
LETKNOW
LIKENEW
LUCKNOW
MISKNEW
MISKNOW
OUTGNAW
OVERNEW
PAYSNOW
SAGINAW
SILENTW
TILLNOW
UPTONOW
VERYNEW
WHATNOW
WHOKNEW
YOUKNOW

N•X••••
NEXRADS
NEXTDAY
NEXUSES
NOXIOUS
NOXZEMA

N•••••X
NARTHEX
NETFLIX
NONFLUX

•NX••••
ANXIETY
ANXIOUS

•N•X•••
INEXACT
INEXILE
UNAXLED

•N••X••
ANNEXED
ANNEXES
INBOXES
INDEXED
INDEXER
INDEXES
INFIXED
INFIXES
UNBOXED
UNBOXES
UNFIXED
UNFIXES
UNFOXED
UNLAXED
UNLAXES
UNMIXED
UNMIXES
UNTAXED
UNTAXES
UNTOXIC
UNVEXED
UNWAXED

•N••••X
ANTHRAX
ANTITAX
UNIPLEX

••NX•••
GENXERS
JINXERS
JINXING
MANXCAT
MANXMAN
MANXMEN
MINXISH

••N•X••
ANNEXED
ANNEXES
VANEXEL

••N••X•
CONTEXT
HANDAXE

••N•••X
BANDBOX
BENELUX
CINEMAX
FUNPLEX
HENDRIX
HENDRYX
JUNKFAX
LANDTAX
MINIMAX
MONTEUX
NONFLUX
OMNIMAX
PANCHAX
SANDBOX

•••NX••
JOHNXII
JOHNXIV
JOHNXIX
JOHNXVI
JOHNXXI

•••N•X•
ARANTXA
BATNEXT
JOHNXXI

•••N••X
ARONNAX
COINBOX
JOHNXIX
REANNEX
REINDEX
SPANDEX
STONEAX
UVINDEX

••••N•X
ARONNAX
EQUINOX
KLEENEX
PHOENIX
REANNEX
SILENTX
SOMINEX

•••••NX
BAYLYNX
OUTJINX
PHALANX
PHARYNX

NY•••••
NYGIANT
NYMPHAL
NYMPHIC
NYTIMES
NYYANKS

N•Y••••
NAYARIT
NAYSAID
NAYSAYS
NYYANKS

N••Y•••
NAVYMAN
NAVYMEN
NCWYETH
NEWYEAR
NEWYORK

N•••Y••
NARAYAN
NEARYOU
NEOLYTE
NUREYEV

N••••Y•
NAYSAYS
NEWTOYS
NOBODYS

N•••••Y
NAIVELY
NAIVETY
NAKEDLY
NAMABLY
NAMEDAY
NASALLY
NASTILY
NATTILY
NAUGHTY
NECTARY
NEEDILY
NEOLOGY
NERVILY
NEUILLY
NEWAGEY
NEWBERY
NEWSBOY
NEWSDAY
NEXTDAY
NICEBOY
NICEDAY
NICEGUY
NICETRY
NIFTILY
NIGHTLY
NIKOLAY
NIMIETY
NINTHLY
NIPPILY
NITRIFY
NITTANY
NOENTRY
NOISILY
NOMERCY
NONBODY
NONBUSY
NONJURY
NONOILY
NONPLAY
NOONDAY
NOSEGAY
NOTABLY
NOTEASY
NOTEDLY
NOTMANY
NOVELTY
NOVOTNY
NUGGETY
NULLIFY
NULLITY
NUNNERY
NURSERY
NUTTILY

•NY••••
ANYBODY
ANYHOPE
ANYKIND
ANYLUCK
ANYMORE
ANYNEWS
ANYONES
ANYROAD
ANYTIME
ANYTOWN
ANYWAYS
ANYWISE
INYEARS
UNYOKED
UNYOKES
UNYOUNG

•N•Y•••
ENVYING
ENZYMES
ENZYMIC
INDYCAR
INKYCAP
INLYING
INSYNCH
ONEYARD
ONEYEAR
ONLYTOO
ONLYYOU
ONMYOWN
UNDYING
UNGYVED
UNLYING
UNLYRIC
UNTYING
UNTYPED
UNVYING

•N••Y••
ANALYSE
ANALYST
ANALYTE
ANALYZE
ANGRYAT
ANNOYED
ANNOYER
ANODYNE
ANONYMS
ENCRYPT
ENJOYED
ENJOYER
INLAYER
INSTYLE
ONEBYTE
ONEEYED
ONLYYOU
UNCOYER
UNCOYLY
UNGUYED
UNHAYED
UNJOYED
UNKEYED
UNLOYAL
UNRAYED
UNRHYME
UNSHYER
UNSHYLY
UNSLYER
UNSLYLY

•N•••Y•
ANTONYM
ANYWAYS
ENDWAYS
INTRAYS

•N••••Y
ANALOGY
ANARCHY
ANATOLY
ANATOMY
ANCHOVY
ANGRILY
ANILITY
ANIMACY
ANNAMAY
ANNUITY
ANOMALY
ANTHONY
ANXIETY
ANYBODY
ENDERBY
ENDPLAY
ENOLOGY
ENQUIRY
ENTROPY
INAFURY
INANELY
INANITY
INAPTLY
INDEEDY
INEPTLY
INERTLY
INFANCY
ININETY
INNERLY
INNOWAY
INQUIRY
KNAVERY
KNUCKLY
ONAJURY
ONEADAY
ONEMPTY
SNAKILY
SNEAKBY
SNIDELY
SNIFFLY
SNOWDAY
SNOWILY
SNUGGLY
UNANGRY
UNAPTLY
UNBOGGY
UNBULKY
UNBURLY
UNCANNY
UNCHARY
UNCOYLY
UNCRAZY
UNDUSTY
UNEMPTY
UNFANCY
UNFATTY
UNFIERY
UNFITLY
UNFLAKY
UNFOGGY
UNFULLY
UNFUNNY
UNFUSSY
UNGAUDY
UNGIDDY
UNGODLY
UNHAIRY
UNHANDY
UNHAPPY
UNHARDY
UNHASTY
UNHEADY
UNHEAVY
UNHILLY
UNIBODY
UNITARY
UNJOLLY
UNJUICY
UNLEAKY
UNLOFTY
UNLOWLY
UNLUCKY
UNLUMPY
UNLUSTY
UNMADLY
UNMANLY
UNMERRY
UNMOLDY
UNMOODY
UNMOSSY
UNMUDDY
UNNEEDY
UNNOISY
UNPIETY
UNRAINY
UNRASPY
UNREADY
UNRISKY
UNROCKY
UNROOMY
UNROWDY
UNSADLY
UNSALTY
UNSAVVY
UNSCALY
UNSHADY
UNSHINY
UNSHOWY
UNSHYLY
UNSILLY
UNSLYLY
UNSMOKY
UNSNAKY
UNSOGGY
UNSOOTY
UNSORRY
UNSPICY
UNSTAGY
UNSTONY
UNSULKY
UNSUNNY
UNSURLY
UNTASTY
UNTRULY
UNWEARY
UNWINDY
UNWITTY
UNWORMY

••NY•••
BANYANS
CANYONS
DENYING
KENYANS
LANYARD
MANYEAR
MINYANS
PONYING
PONYKEG
TENYEAR
TINYBIT
TINYTIM
TINYTOT
TONYDOW
VINYLIC
ZANYISH
ZANYISM

••N•Y••
ALNIYAT
ANNOYED
ANNOYER
BONEYER
DANEYKO
DENTYNE
FANCYUP
GENZYME
HANDYTO
HENRYII
HENRYIV
HENRYVI
HONEYED
HUNNYBS
MONEYED
TINTYPE
VANDYCK
VANDYKE
VANEYCK
VANWYCK

••N••Y•
BENDAYS
CONVEYS
CONVOYS
DONKEYS
FONTEYN
HANDEYE
HANGBYS
HENDRYX
MANDAYS
MINSKYS
MONDAYS
MONKEYS
MONTOYA
PENNEYS
PINBOYS
RUNWAYS
SUNDAYS
SUNRAYS
SYNONYM
TENDAYS
VANDUYN

••N•••Y
AINTHAY
AMNESTY
ANNAMAY
ANNUITY
BANALLY
BANBURY
BENTLEY
BINDERY
BONEDRY
BONNILY
CANNERY
CANNILY
CANONRY
CANTILY
CANTSAY
CENTURY
CINDERY
CINERGY
CONAKRY
CONFREY
CONJURY
CONNERY
DANBURY
DANDIFY
DANDILY
DENNEHY
DENSELY
DENSIFY
DENSITY
DINGILY
DONLEVY
DONTCRY
DUNAWAY
DYNASTY
EDNAMAY
FANCIFY
FANCILY
FANTASY
FINALLY
FINDLAY
FINDLEY
FINICKY
FUNKILY
FUNNILY
GANGWAY
GINGERY
GUNNERY
GUNPLAY
HANDILY
HANGSBY
HENNERY
HENSLEY
HONESTY
HUNGARY
HUNTLEY
IGNOBLY
INNERLY
INNOWAY
JANEWAY
JANUARY
JUNEDAY
KENNEDY
KINKILY
LANGLEY
LANGTRY
LANGWAY
LANKILY
LENGTHY
LINDSAY
LINDSEY
LINEDRY
LONGDAY
LONGWAY
MCNALLY
MENSCHY
MONTHLY
MRNANNY
NINTHLY
NONBODY
NONBUSY
NONJURY
NONOILY
NONPLAY
NUNNERY
PANICKY
PANOPLY
PENALTY
PUNNILY
RANAWAY
RENALLY
RUNAWAY
RUNSDRY
SANDFLY
SENDSBY
SENSORY
SINCITY
SUNCITY
SUNNILY
SYNERGY
TANNERY
TANTIVY
TENABLY
TENANCY
TENSELY
TENSITY
TENTHLY
TENUITY
TINAFEY
TINDERY
TINNILY
TONALLY
UNNEEDY
UNNOISY
VENALLY
WINDILY
WINDOWY
WINFREY
WINTERY
ZINCIFY
ZONALLY

•••NY••
ANONYMS
EPONYMS
EPONYMY
ERINYES
EUONYMS
EXONYMS
HUNNYBS
PHONYUP
SKYNYRD

•••N•Y•
BARNEYS
BERNAYS
CHANOYU
GOONEYS
GURNEYS
JITNEYS
JOHNNYB
KIDNEYS
MOONEYE
ORKNEYS
PENNEYS
PHONEYS
ROMNEYS

•••N••Y
AGENTRY
ALANJAY
AMENITY
ARENSKY
BARNABY
BEANERY
BLANDLY
BLANKLY
BLINDLY
BLUNTLY
BONNILY
BRANCHY
BURNABY
BURNLEY
BYANDBY
CANNERY
CANNILY
CARNABY
CHANTEY
CHANTRY
CHINTZY
CONNERY
CORNILY
COUNTRY
CRINKLY
CRUNCHY
DEANERY
DENNEHY
DIGNIFY
DIGNITY
ECONOMY
EKINGBY
EPONYMY
EXENEMY
FAINTLY
FERNERY
FOUNDRY
FRANKLY
FRENEMY
FUNNILY
GAINSAY
GAUNTLY
GOINGBY
GOONILY
GRANARY
GRANDLY
GUNNERY
HENNERY
HORNSBY
HYMNARY
HYMNODY
ICONIFY
INANELY
INANITY
ININETY
ISONOMY
JOHNBOY
JOHNGAY
JOHNJAY
JOINERY
JOINTLY
KENNEDY
KILNDRY
LAUNDRY
LEONDAY
LIGNIFY
LOONILY
LYINGBY
MAGNIFY
MOONILY
NOENTRY
NOONDAY
NUNNERY
OLDNAVY
ORANGEY
PAUNCHY
PHONILY
PLENARY
PRONAVY
PRONELY
PUNNILY
QUINARY
QUINCEY
RAINILY
RAUNCHY
REENJOY
REENTRY
REUNIFY
RIANTLY
ROUNDLY
SAINTLY
SCANTLY
SCENERY
SHINGLY
SHINILY
SIGNIFY
SLANTLY
SOUNDLY
SPANGLY
SPINDLY
SPINDRY
SPINNEY
STANDBY
STANLEY
STONILY
SUNNILY
SWINERY
SWINGBY
SWUNGBY
TANNERY
TAWNILY
TERNARY
TINNILY
TRENARY
TRINARY
TRINITY
TURNERY
TURNKEY
TWINKLY
UNANGRY
UNSNAKY
VRONSKY
WRINKLY
WRONGLY

••••NY•
ACRONYM
ALLONYM
ANTONYM
AUTONYM
BILLNYE
CACONYM
DEMONYM
HOMONYM
HYPONYM
JOHNNYB
MTKENYA
PARONYM
POLANYI
SYNONYM
TOPONYM

••••N•Y
ALBUNDY
ALLENBY
ALMONDY
ALMONRY
APLENTY
ARDENCY
BALONEY
BLARNEY
BRITNEY
CADENCY
CANONRY
CHIMNEY
CHUTNEY
CLEANLY
CLOONEY
COCKNEY
COGENCY
DECENCY
DELANEY
EPERNAY
ERRANCY
FELONRY
FLAUNTY
FLOUNCY
FLOWNBY
FLUENCY
FTHENRY
GIVENBY
GREENLY
HACKNEY
HAPENNY
HERONRY
HUMANLY
INFANCY
ITWENTY
JOURNEY
JTMONEY
KEARNEY
LATENCY
LAZENBY
LUCENCY
MAHONEY
MASONRY
MCHENRY
MCRANEY
MOMONEY
MRHANEY
MRNANNY
OLEANNY
ORGANDY
ORMANDY
PATENCY
PLAINLY
PLIANCY
PORTNOY
POTENCY
PUDENCY
QUEENLY
QUESNAY
RECENCY
REGENCY
SAIDNAY
SAYSNAY
SEVENTY
SILENTY
SPINNEY
SPRINGY
SQUINTY
STERNLY
STRINGY
SWEENEY
TAKENBY
TENANCY
TIERNEY
TOURNEY
TRUANCY
TYRANNY
UNCANNY
UNFANCY
UNFUNNY
UNHANDY
UNMANLY
UNSUNNY
UNWINDY
URGENCY
VACANCY
VIXENLY
VOTENAY
WCHANDY
WHITNEY
WOMANLY

•••••NY
ALIMONY
ANTHONY
BALCONY
BETHANY
BETTANY
BUTTONY
CALUMNY
COMPANY
COTTONY
COWPONY
CRIMINY
DESTINY
EUPHONY
GASCONY
GERMANY
HAPENNY
HARMONY
HOWMANY
JARGONY
LARCENY
MRNANNY
MUSIGNY
NITTANY
NOTMANY
NOVOTNY
OLEANNY
OROGENY
PETPONY
PREDENY
PROGENY
RAISINY
REDPONY
RIBBONY
SAUCONY
SCRAWNY
SEVIGNY
SPLEENY
TAMMANY
TIFFANY
TOOMANY
TUSCANY
TYRANNY
UNCANNY
UNFUNNY
UNRAINY
UNSHINY
UNSTONY
UNSUNNY
UTICANY
VERMINY
YEVGENY
ZELAZNY

N•Z••••
NOZZLES
NUZZLED
NUZZLER
NUZZLES

N••Z•••
NETZERO
NONZERO
NOXZEMA
NOZZLES
NUDZHED
NUDZHES
NUZZLED
NUZZLER
NUZZLES

N•••Z••
NETIZEN

N•••••Z
NARVAEZ
NATCHEZ
NISSANZ

•NZ••••
ENZYMES
ENZYMIC
UNZONED
UNZONES

•N•Z•••
ENDZONE
SNAZZUP

•N••Z••
SNAZZUP
SNEEZED
SNEEZER
SNEEZES
SNOOZED
SNOOZER
SNOOZES
UNDAZED
UNFAZED
UNHAZED
UNRAZED
UNSIZED

•N•••Z•
ANALYZE
ANASAZI
ANODIZE
INADAZE
ONESIZE
UNCRAZY
UNFROZE
UNISIZE
UNITIZE

••NZ•••
BANZAIS
BENZALI
BENZELL
BENZENE
CANZONA
CANZONE
CANZONI
CINZANO
FANZINE
GENZYME
GONZAGA
MENZIES
NONZERO
PANZERS
PENZIAS
RONZONI
TENZING
VANZANT
VONZELL

••N•Z••
BENAZIR
DENIZEN
FUNFZIG
IONIZED
IONIZER
IONIZES
MINIZOO
RENUZIT
VENEZIA

••N••Z•
BONANZA
GINFIZZ
MANSIZE
YANGTZE

••N•••Z
GINFIZZ

•••NZ••
BRONZED
BRONZER
BRONZES
KWANZAA
KWANZAS
QUINZES
STANZAS
ZWANZIG

•••N•Z•
AGONIZE
BLINTZE
CHINTZY
COGNIZE
EBONIZE
LIONIZE
OZONIZE
SCHNOZZ
SPINOZA

•••N••Z
BEDNORZ
FRANKOZ
SCHNOZZ

••••NZ•
BONANZA
CADENZA
FIRENZA
FIRENZE
FORENZA
LEGANZA
LORENZO
ORGANZA
VICENZA

••••N•Z
ALBENIZ
GRISNEZ
JIMENEZ
JIMINEZ
LEIBNIZ
LORENTZ
MARANTZ
ORDONEZ
SILENTZ
SIMONIZ

•••••NZ
COBLENZ
FLORENZ
HJHEINZ
KAYLENZ
KOBLENZ
NISSANZ
THEFONZ

OA•••••
OAHUANS
OAKCASK
OAKDESK
OAKFERN
OAKIEST
OAKLAND
OAKLAWN
OAKLEAF
OAKLIKE
OAKMOSS
OAKPARK
OAKTAGS
OAKTREE
OAKWOOD
OARLESS
OARLIKE
OARLOCK
OARSMAN
OARSMEN
OATBRAN
OATCAKE
OATLIKE
OATMEAL
OAXACAN

O•A••••
OBADIAH
OCALAFL
OCANADA
OCARINA
OFAKIND
OFAMIND
OFANAGE
OFASORT
OHANLON
OKAYGUY
OKAYING
OLAFIII
OLAVIII
OMAHANE
OMAHANS
OMALLEY
ONABIAS
ONADARE
ONADATE
ONADIET
ONAGERS
ONAJURY
ONAKICK
ONALARK
ONALEAD
ONALERT
ONALINE
ONANDON
ONAROLL
ONASSIS
ONATEAR
ONATOOT
ONATRIP
ONAWHIM
OPACITY
OPALINE
OPALISH
OPAQUES
ORACIES
ORACLES
ORALIST
ORANGES
ORANGEY
ORANTES
ORARION
ORARIUM
ORATING
ORATION
ORATORS
ORATORY
ORATRIX
OSAKANS
OTALGIA
OTALGIC
OTARIES
OVARIES
OVATION
OXALATE

O••A•••
OAXACAN
OBLASTS
OBLATES
OBTAINS
OCEANIA
OCEANIC
OCEANID
OCEANUS
OCTADIC
OCTAGON
OCTANES
OCTANTS
OCTAVAL
OCTAVES
OCTAVIA
OCTAVIO
OCTAVOS
OFVALUE
OGHAMIC
OGLALAS
OHCAROL
OHMAGES
OLEANNA
OLEANNY
OLEATES
ONEACAT
ONEACRE
ONEACTS
ONEADAY
ONEARTH
ONPAPER
ONRAMPS
ONSAGER
ONTARIO
ONWARDS
ONWATER
OPIATES
ORDAINS
ORGANDY
ORGANIC
ORGANZA
ORLANDO
ORMANDY
OSHAPED
OSMATIC
OTRANTO
OTTAVIO
OTTAWAN
OTTAWAS
OUTACTS
OUTADDS
OUTAGES
OUTASKS
OUTAWED
OUTAWES
OXCARTS
OXTAILS

O•••A••
OAHUANS
OAKCASK
OAKLAND
OAKLAWN
OAKPARK
OAKTAGS
OATCAKE
OBVIATE
OCALAFL
OCANADA
OCICATS
OCULARS
ODDBALL
ODDSARE
ODORANT
OFANAGE
OFFBASE
OFFCAST
OFFDAYS
OFFHAND
OFFRAMP
OGDOADS
OHIOANS
OHIOART
OILBASE
OILCAKE
OILCANS
OILLAMP
OILPALM
OILPANS
OILSAND
OILTANK
OISEAUX
OKINAWA
OLDBATS
OLDCARS
OLDDAYS
OLDGAGS
OLDHAND
OLDLADY
OLDMAID
OLDNAVY
OLDPALS
OLDSALT
OLDSAWS
OLDWAYS
OMAHANE
OMAHANS
OMPHALO
ONADARE
ONADATE
ONALARK
ONBOARD
ONEBALL
ONEBASE
ONECALL
ONEHALF
ONEHAND
ONELANE
ONENAME
ONEPAGE
ONEPAIR
ONEPART
ONEYARD
ONGUARD
ONLEASE
ONLEASH
ONLEAVE
ONLOADS
ONORATI
ONSTAFF
ONSTAGE
ONTOAST
ONTRACK
OOHLALA
OOMPAHS
OPENAIR
OPERAND
OPERANT
OPERATE
ORCHARD
ORDEALS
OREGANO
ORGEATS
ORGIAST
ORIGAMI
ORLEANS
ORPHANS
ORPHANT
OSAKANS
OSSUARY
OSTIARY
OSTMARK
OSTRAVA

OSTWALD
OURGANG
OUTBACK
OUTBAKE
OUTBANS
OUTBARK
OUTBATS
OUTBAWL
OUTCALL
OUTCANT
OUTCAST
OUTDARE
OUTDATE
OUTEARN
OUTEATS
OUTFACE
OUTFAST
OUTFAWN
OUTGAIN
OUTGAME
OUTGAVE
OUTGAZE
OUTHAUL
OUTKAST
OUTLAID
OUTLAIN
OUTLAND
OUTLASH
OUTLAST
OUTLAWS
OUTLAYS
OUTMANS
OUTMATE
OUTPACE
OUTPAID
OUTPASS
OUTPATH
OUTPAYS
OUTRACE
OUTRAGE
OUTRAIL
OUTRANG
OUTRANK
OUTRANT
OUTRAPS
OUTRATE
OUTRAVE
OUTSAID
OUTSAIL
OUTSANG
OUTSAYS
OUTTAKE
OUTTALK
OUTWAIT
OUTWALK
OUTWARD
OUTWARS
OUTWASH
OUTWAVE
OVERACT
OVERAGE
OVERALL
OVERARM
OVERATE
OVERAWE
OVIPARA
OVISACS
OXALATE
OXHEART
OXIDANT
OXIDASE
OXIDATE

O••••A•

OAKLEAF
OARSMAN
OATBRAN
OATMEAL
OAXACAN
OBADIAH
OCELLAR
OCTAVAL
ODESSAN
OEDIPAL
OFFBEAT
OFFLOAD
OFFPEAK
OFFROAD
OFFYEAR
OGLALAS
OHMSLAW
OILHEAT
OJIBWAS
OJIBWAY
OLDBEAN
OLDCHAP
OLDUVAI
OMNIMAX
ONABIAS
ONALEAD
ONATEAR
ONBREAK
ONEACAT
ONEADAY
ONECLAM
ONEGRAM
ONEIDAS
ONEOCAT
ONESTAR
ONEYEAR
ONTKEAN
ONTRIAL
OPENBAR
OPENTAP
OPTICAL
OPTIMAL
OPTIMAS
ORBITAL
ORDINAL
ORPHEAN
ORTEGAL
ORTOLAN
OSCULAR
OSETRAS
OSIRIAN
OTTAWAN
OTTAWAS
OTTOMAN
OUTBEAM
OUTBRAG
OUTBRAY
OUTDRAG
OUTDRAW
OUTGNAW
OUTHEAR
OUTLEAD
OUTLEAP
OUTPLAN
OUTPLAY
OUTPRAY
OUTREAD
OUTROAR
OUTSOAR
OUTSTAY
OUTSWAM
OUTTEAR
OUTTRAY
OUTWEAR
OVEREAT
OVERFAR
OVERFAT
OVERLAP
OVERLAX
OVERLAY
OVERMAN
OVERPAR
OVERPAY
OVERRAN
OVERSAD
OVERSAW
OVERTAX
OVIDIAN
OVOIDAL
OWNGOAL
OXONIAN

O•••••A

OBSCURA
OCANADA
OCARINA
OCEANIA
OCHENTA
OCTAVIA
ODONTIA
OKINAWA
OLEANNA
OLESTRA
OLYMPIA
ONEIOTA
ONELIRA
ONEONTA
OOHLALA
OPENSEA
OPHELIA
OPUNTIA
ORGANZA
OSCEOLA
OSSETRA
OSTRAVA
OTALGIA
OTTUMWA
OUGUIYA
OVERSEA
OVIPARA
OXYMORA

•OA••••

BOARDED
BOARDER
BOARDUP
BOARISH
BOASTED
BOASTER
BOASTOF
BOATELS
BOATERS
BOATFUL
BOATING
BOATMAN
BOATMEN
COACHED
COACHES
COACTED
COAGENT
COALBIN
COALCAR
COALERS
COALGAS
COALING
COALOIL
COALPIT
COALTAR
COAPTED
COARSEN
COARSER
COASTAL
COASTED
COASTER
COATEES
COATERS
COATING
COAXERS
COAXIAL
COAXING
DOADEAL
DOAGAIN
DOASIDO
FOALING
FOAMERS
FOAMIER
FOAMILY
FOAMING
GOABOUT
GOADING
GOAFTER
GOAHEAD
GOALIES
GOALONG
GOAMISS
GOATEED
GOATEES
GOATISH
HOAGIES
HOARDED
HOARDER
HOARIER
HOARILY
HOARSEN
HOARSER
HOAXERS
HOAXING
JOACHIM
JOAQUIN
LOADERS
LOADING
LOADSIN
LOADSOF
LOADSUP
LOAFERS
LOAFING
LOAFPAN
LOAMIER
LOAMING
LOANERS
LOANING
LOANOUT
LOATHED
LOATHER
LOATHES
LOATHLY
LOATHTO
MOABITE
MOANERS
MOANFUL
MOANING
NOANGEL
POACHED
POACHER
POACHES
ROACHES
ROADBED
ROADEOS
ROADERS
ROADHOG
ROADIES
ROADMAP
ROADTAR
ROADTAX
ROADWAY
ROAMERS
ROAMING
ROANOKE
ROARERS
ROARING
ROARSAT
ROASTED
ROASTER
SOAKERS
SOAKING
SOAKSIN
SOAKSUP
SOANDSO
SOAPBOX
SOAPERS
SOAPIER
SOAPILY
SOAPING
SOAPNET
SOAPPAD
SOAPSUP
SOARERS
SOAREWE
SOARING
TOADIED
TOADIES
TOADISH
TOAHAIR
TOASTED
TOASTEE
TOASTER
TOATURN

•O•A•••

BOBATEA
BOGARDE
BOGARTS
BOIARDO
BOLATIE
BONACIS
BONAIRE
BONANZA
BONARIO
BORATES
BOTANIC
COBALTS
COCAINE
COHABIT
COLADAS
COMAKER
CONAGRA
CONAKRY
CORACLE
CORAZON
COWARDS
DOGAPES
DOMAINE
DOMAINS
DONAHUE
DONATED
DONATEE
DONATES
DONATOR
DONATUS
DOSADOS
DOSAGES
DOTAGES
DOTARDS
DOUANES
DOWAGER
FOLATES
FORABIT
FORADAY
FORAGED
FORAGER
FORAGES
FORASEC
FORAYED
GOCARTS
GOKAPUT
GOKARTS
GOTAHIT
GOTAJOB
GOTATIP
GOTAWAY
GOUACHE
HODADDY
HOGARTH
HOMAGER
HOMAGES
HONALEE
HOPACAB
HORATIO
HOSANNA
HOWARDK
HOWARDS
HOWARDU
IODATED
IODATES
JOCASTA
JOHANNA
JOMARCH
KOLANUT
KOMATSU
KORANIC
KOWADLO
LOBATED
LOCALES
LOCALLY
LOCARNO
LOCATED
LOCATER
LOCATES
LOCATOR
LOGANUT
LORANGE
LOSABLE
LOVABLE
LOVABLY
LOVAGES
LOYALER
LOYALES
LOYALLY
LOYALTO
LOYALTY
MOGADOR
MOGAMBO
MOHAIRS
MOHAVES
MOHAWKS
MOJAVES
MONACAN
MONADAL
MONADIC
MONARCH
MORAINE
MORALES
MORALLY
MORANIS
MORANTE
MORAVIA
MOSAICS
MOVABLE
MOVABLY
MOVADOS
NOCANDO
NOCARBS
NOCATCH
NOFAULT
NOGALES
NOHANDS
NOMADIC
NONACID
NONAGES
NONAGON
NONAMES
NONARAB
NONARTS
NOPALES
NOTABIT
NOTABLE
NOTABLY
NOTALIE
NOTALOT
NOTAONE
NOTASTE
NOTATED
NOTATES
NOVALIS
NOVARRO
POLANER
POLANYI
POLARAS
POLARIS
POMADED
POMADES
POSABLE
POSADAS
POTABLE
POTAGES
POTAMUS
ROBARDS
ROGAINE
ROLAIDS
ROMAINE
ROMAINS
ROMAJIS
ROMANCE
ROMANIA
ROMANIC
ROMANIS
ROMANOS
ROMANOV
ROMANSH
ROMANUS
RORAIMA
ROSABUD
ROSALIA
ROSALIE
ROSALYN
ROSANNA
ROSANNE
ROSARIO
ROTATED
ROTATES
ROTATOR
ROTAWAY
ROUAULT
ROXANNE
ROYALES
ROYALLY
ROYALTY
ROYALWE
ROZANOV
SODACAN
SODAPOP
SOFABED
SOFARAS
SOHAVEI
SOLACED
SOLACER
SOLACES
SOLARAS
SOLARIA
SOMALIA
SOMALIS
SOMATIC
SONANCE
SONATAS
TOBACCO
TONALLY
TOPAZES
TOTABLE
TOTALED
TOTALER
TOTALLY
TOTALUP
TOTASTE
TOUAREG
TOWABLE
TOWAGES
TOWARDS
TOWAWAY
VOCABLE
VOCABLY
VOCALIC
VOCALLY
VOLANTE
VOTABLE
VOYAGED
VOYAGER
VOYAGES
WOMANLY
YOGAMAT
YOLANDA
YOUANDI
ZOCALOS
ZONALLY

•O••A••

AOUDADS
BOBCATS
BOBKANE
BOBTAIL
BODYART
BOITANO
BOKHARA
BOMBARD
BOMBAST
BONDAGE
BONEASH
BONIATO
BONNARD
BORLAUG
BORZAGE
BOSCAGE
BOWOARS
BOWSAWS
BOXBALL
BOXCARS
BOYBAND
COBRAND
COCHAIR
COCKADE
CODCAKE
COEVALS
COGNACS
COGNATE
COINAGE
COLGATE
COLLAGE
COLLARD
COLLARS
COLLATE
COMBATS
COMCAST
COMMAND
COMPACT
COMPANY
COMPAQS
COMPARE
COMPART
COMPASS
COMRADE
COMSATS
CONCAVE
CONFABS
CONGAED
CONGAME
CONNATE
CONRACK
CONTACS
CONTACT
CONTAIN
COOLAIR
COOLANT
COPCARS
COPLAND
CORDAGE
CORDATE
CORFAMS
CORKAGE
CORMACK
CORRADE
CORRALS
CORSAGE
CORSAIR
CORVAIR
COSSACK
COSTAIN
COSTARD
COSTARS
COSTATE
COTEACH
COTTAGE
COUGARS
COURAGE
COURANT
COWBANE
COWHAND
DOAGAIN
DOCKAGE
DOGBANE
DOGCART
DOGDAYS
DOGEARS
DOGFACE
DOGGATE
DOGHAIR
DOGMATA
DOGNAPS
DOGRACE
DOGSAGE
DOGTAGS
DOGTAIL
DOIDARE
DOLLARS
DOLMANS
DONNALL
DONTASK
DOODADS
DORMANT
DORSALS
DOSSALS
DOTDASH
FOGBANK
FOGLAMP
FOLIAGE
FOLIATE
FOLKART
FONDANT
FONTANA
FONTANE
FOOTAGE
FORBADE
FOREACH
FOREARM
FORGAVE
FORLANI
FORMALS
FORMATS
FORSAKE
FORSALE
FORWARD
FOULARD
FOURAAA
FOXTAIL
GOBLANK
GOBYAIR
GOCRAZY
GODDARD
GODMAMA
GODPAPA
GOESAFT
GOESAPE
GOLDARN
GOLIATH
GONEAFT
GONEAPE
GONZAGA
GOODAIM
GOODALL
GOSHAWK
GOSSAGE
GOSTALE
GOTBACK
GOTCASH
GOTPAST
GOTTAGO
GOTWARM
GOULASH
GOURAMI
HOBNAIL
HOECAKE
HOFMANN
HOGBACK
HOGCALL
HOGWASH
HOLDALL
HOLLAND
HOLYARK
HONIARA
HOOHAHS
HOOKAHS
HOORAHS
HOORAYS
HOSCALE
HOSTAGE
HOTBATH
HOTCAKE
HOTCAPS
HOTCARS
HOTDATE
HOTDAYS
HOTHAND
HOTMAIL
HOTPACK
HOTWARS
HOVLANE
HOWDAHS
HOWLAME
HOWMANY
IONIANS
JOBBANK
JOBFAIR
JOBJARS
JOECAMP
JONHALL
JORDANA
JOUHAUX
JOYPADS
KODIAKS
KOLKATA
KOOLAID
KOREANS
LOCKAGE
LOGJAMS
LOLLARD
LOMBARD
LONGAGO
LONGARM
LOOFAHS
LOQUATS
LOSTART
LOTHAIR
LOWBALL
LOWCARB
LOWCARD
LOWHAND
LOWLAND
LOWMASS
LOWPAID
LOWPAIR
MOMBASA
MONDALE
MONDAVI
MONDAYS
MONTAGE
MONTAGU
MONTALE
MONTANA
MONTAND
MONTANO
MONTAUK
MOORAGE
MORDANT
MORGANA
MORGANS
MORTALS
MORTARS
MOSCATO
MOULAGE
NOCLASS
NOLOADS
NONBANK
NONBASE
NONCASH
NONDARK
NONFACT
NONFANS
NONFARM
NONPAID
NONPARS
NONPAST
NONSALE
NONSANE
NONWAGE
NONWARS
NOPLACE
NORMALS
NORMAND
NORMANS
NORWALK
NOSEATS
NOSTAIN
NOSTARS
NOTEASY
NOTFAIR
NOTMANY
NOTRADE
NOTRARE
NOTSAFE
NOUGATS
OOHLALA
OOMPAHS
POBLANO
PODCAST
POLEAXE
POLKAED
POLLACK
POLLARD
POLTAVA
POMMARD
POMPANO
PONIARD
PONTANO
POPEAFB
POPLARS
POPTART
PORTAGE
PORTALS
POSTAGE
POTTAGE
ROBSART
ROCKABY
ROLLAND
ROLVAAG
RONSARD
ROOFAGE
ROOTAGE
ROSEATE
ROSSANO
ROSTAND
ROUBAIX
ROULADE
ROWLAND
SOCIALS
SOILAGE
SOLLATI
SOLOACT
SOPRANI
SOPRANO
SORBATE
SORIANO
SOSPADS
SOURALE
SOXFANS
TOAHAIR
TOBLAME
TOCCATA
TOECAPS
TOENAIL
TOETAPS
TOHEART
TOLDALL
TOLEASE
TOLLAGE
TOMCATS
TONEARM
TONGANS
TONNAGE
TOOEASY
TOOHARD
TOOKAIM
TOOLATE

TOOMANY
TOOTALL
TOPHATS
TOPIARY
TOPKAPI
TOPMAST
TOPNAME
TOPRANK
TOPRATE
TOPSAIL
TORNADO
TORVALD
TOSCALE
TOSPARE
TOSTADA
TOSTART
TOUCANS
TOWBARS
TOWCARS
TOWPATH
TOYBALL
TOYCARS
TOYCART
TOYFAIR
TOYHATS
TOYLAND
TOYPAIL
VOLCANO
VOLTAGE
VOLTAIC
VONBAER
VONLAUE
VORLAGE
VOTEAYE
WOMBATS
WOODARD
WORDAGE
YOPLAIT
YOTEAMO
YOUMANS
YOURANG
ZODIACS
ZONIANS

•O•••A•

BOATMAN
BOBTWAY
BODEGAS
BODYBAR
BODYFAT
BOERWAR
BOGYMAN
BOLIVAR
BONDMAN
BOOEDAT
BOOHBAH
BOOKBAG
BOOKMAN
BOOLEAN
BOOMCAR
BOORMAN
BORGIAS
BORNEAN
BORSTAL
BOSNIAN
BOSSMAN
BOWHEAD
BOXCOAT
BOXSEAT
BOZEMAN
COALCAR
COALGAS
COALTAR
COASTAL
COAXIAL
COBCOAL
COCHRAN
COCTEAU
COEQUAL
COGHLAN
COLADAS
COLDDAY
COLDWAR
COLEMAN
COMESAS
COMESAT
COMICAL
COMORAN
CONCEAL
CONCHAE
CONGEAL
CONICAL
CONTRAS
COOLCAT
COOLMAX
COONCAN
COONCAT
COPULAE
COPULAR
COPULAS
COPYCAT
COPYMAN
CORDIAL
CORDIAS
CORKOAK
CORNEAL
CORNEAS
CORONAE
CORONAL
CORONAS
CORYZAS
COWERAT
COWPEAS
DOADEAL
DOESBAD
DOGCOAT
DOGREAT
DOGSEAR
DOGSTAR
DOMECAR
DOMICAL
DONEBAD
DONEGAL
DONEGAN
DONJUAN
DONOVAN
DOORMAN
DOORMAT
DOORWAY
DORFMAN
DOUGLAS
DOVEBAR
DOWNPAT
FOLKWAY
FOOTBAG
FOOTMAN
FOOTPAD
FOOTWAY
FORADAY
FORBEAR
FORDHAM
FOREBAY
FOREMAN
FOREPAW
FORERAN
FORESAW
FORREAL
FORTRAN
FORTYAD
FOTOMAT
FOURAAA
FOURDAY
FOURMAN
FOURWAY
GOAHEAD
GOBYCAB
GOBYCAR
GODHEAD
GODTHAB
GOESBAD
GOESFAR
GOESMAD
GOINGAT
GOLDMAN
GOLFBAG
GOLFCAR
GONEBAD
GONEFAR
GONEMAD
GOODBAR
GOODDAY
GOODMAN
GOODPAY
GOOMBAH
GOOMBAY
GORDIAN
GOTAWAY
GOTBEAT
GOTCHAS
GOTOGAL
GOTOWAR
GOTREAL
HOFBRAU
HOFFMAN
HOLIDAY
HOLMOAK
HOLYDAY
HOLYMAN
HOLYWAR
HOLZMAN
HOMELAB
HONKSAT
HOOPLAS
HOOPMAN
HOOTSAT
HOPACAB
HOTCOAL
HOTHEAD
HOTLEAD
HOTMEAL
HOTSEAT
HOTTEAS
HOUSMAN
HOUSSAY
HOWLSAT
IONBEAM
JOCULAR
JOGBRAS
JOHNGAY
JOHNJAY
JOHNLAW
JOJOBAS
JOURDAN
JOURNAL
JOYCEAN
KORUNAS
KOSOVAR
LOAFPAN
LOCKEAN
LOCKJAW
LOGGIAS
LOGICAL
LONGDAY
LONGWAY
LONIGAN
LOOKSAD
LOOKSAT
LOOMPAS
LORELAI
LOSTCAT
LOTHIAN
LOVETAP
LOWBEAM
LOWGEAR
LOWROAD
LOYOLAU
MODELAS
MODULAR
MOHEGAN
MOHICAN
MOISSAN
MOLERAT
MOLOKAI
MONACAN
MONADAL
MONDIAL
MOPHEAD
MOREPAY
MOWBRAY
NODICAL
NODULAR
NOMINAL
NONARAB
NONDEAF
NONMEAT
NONORAL
NONPEAK
NONPLAY
NOONDAY
NOOTKAS
NOSEBAG
NOSEGAY
NOSUGAR
NOSWEAT
NOTEPAD
NOTNEAR
NOTREAL
NOUVEAU
NOVELAS
NOVENAS
NOVISAD
NOWWHAT
POINTAT
POKEDAT
POKESAT
POLARAS
POLECAR
POLECAT
POLEMAN
POLESAT
POLLTAX
PONTIAC
PONTIAN
POOHBAH
POOLMAN
POORLAW
POORMAN
POORTAX
POPSTAR
POPULAR
POPUPAD
PORTMAN
PORTRAY
POSADAS
POSEDAS
POSESAS
POSTBAG
POSTMAN
POSTWAR
POTOMAC
POTSDAM
ROADMAP
ROADTAR
ROADTAX
ROADWAY
ROARSAT
ROLLBAR
ROLLWAY
ROLVAAG
ROMULAN
RONDEAU
ROOFRAT
ROOMBAS
ROOTCAP
RORQUAL
ROSEBAY
ROSTRAL
ROTAWAY
ROTBLAT
ROULEAU
ROWBOAT
ROYBEAN
SOAPPAD
SODACAN
SOFARAS
SOLARAS
SOLEDAD
SOMEDAY
SOMESAY
SOMEWAY
SONATAS
SONORAN
SORORAL
SOULMAN
SOUPCAN
SOWSEAR
SOYBEAN
SOYMEAL
TOBEHAD
TOILSAT
TOLEDAN
TOLLBAR
TOLLMAN
TOLLWAY
TOMJOAD
TONNEAU
TOOLBAR
TOOTSAT
TOPCOAT
TOPDRAW
TOPEKAN
TOPICAL
TORTLAW
TOTEBAG
TOWAWAY
TOWBOAT
TOWHEAD
TOWNCAR
TOYBOAT
TOYOTAS
VOSGIAN
VOTENAY
VOUVRAY
WOLFGAL
WOLFMAN
WOLFRAM
WOODSAW
WOODTAR
WOOLFAT
WOOLHAT
WOOSNAM
WORKDAY
WORKMAN
WORKSAT
WOZNIAK
YOGAMAT
ZONULAR
ZOOIDAL
ZOYSIAS

•O••••A

BOBATEA
BOBVILA
BOFFOLA
BOHEMIA
BOKHARA
BOLIVIA
BOLOGNA
BONANZA
BONILLA
BOOTHIA
BOTHNIA
BOTTEGA
COCHLEA
COLONNA
COLUMBA
COMEDIA
CONAGRA
COPPOLA
COQUINA
CORDOBA
CORETTA
COROLLA
CORPORA
CORRIDA
CORSICA
CORTINA
CORVINA
DOGFLEA
DOGMATA
DOUBLEA
FONTANA
FONTINA
FORENZA
FORMICA
FORMOSA
FORMULA
FORTUNA
FOURAAA
GOBYSEA
GODMAMA
GODPAPA
GONDOLA
GONGORA
GONZAGA
GORDITA
GORILLA
GOTHIKA
GOTOSEA
HOFSTRA
HONIARA
HOSANNA
HOTTUNA
JOCASTA
JOHANNA
JORDANA
JOSEPHA
KOLKATA
KOPIYKA
KOSCINA
KOSHIBA
LORETTA
LOUELLA
MOLDOVA
MOLUCCA
MOMBASA
MOMENTA
MONTANA
MONTOYA
MORAVIA
MORELLA
MORGANA
MOZETTA
MOZILLA
NONCOLA
NORDICA
NORIEGA
NOSEBRA
NOVELLA
NOXZEMA
OOHLALA
PODRIDA
POETICA
POLENTA
POLLERA
POLONIA
POLTAVA
POMPEIA
POPDIVA
PORSENA
ROBERTA
ROBUSTA
ROLONDA
ROMANIA
RORAIMA
ROSALIA
ROSANNA
ROSELLA
ROSEOLA
ROSETEA
ROSETTA
ROSSSEA
ROTHIRA
ROTUNDA
ROVETTA
SOLARIA
SOMALIA
SOYINKA
TOCCATA
TOCELIA
TOMGOLA
TORTOLA
TORTUGA
TOSHIBA
TOSTADA
VOTEYEA
WOJTYLA
YOLANDA
ZOSSIMA

••OA•••

ALOADOF
BLOATED
BROADAS
BROADAX
BROADEN
BROADER
BROADLY
BROASTS
CLOAKED
CROAKED
CROAKER
CROATIA
FLOATBY
FLOATED
FLOATER
FLOATUP
GLOAMIN
GLOATED
GLOATER
GROANED
GROANER
PROARAB
SHOALED
TWOACRE
TWOACTS

••O•A••

ADONAIS
AJOWANS
ALOHAOE
ANOMALY
ANORAKS
ASONANT
AVOCADO
AVOWALS
BAOBABS
BIODATA
BIOLABS
BIOMASS
BROCADE
BROGANS
BROMATE
BROWARD
BUOYANT
CHORALE
CHORALS
COOLAIR
COOLANT
DEODARS
DEODATO
DIORAMA
DOODADS
ECOTAGE
EDOUARD
EXOCARP
EXOGAMY
FLOTAGE
FLOWAGE
FOOTAGE
FROMAGE
FROWARD
GLOBATE
GOODAIM
GOODALL
HOOHAHS
HOOKAHS
HOORAHS
HOORAYS
ILOCANO
IRONAGE
ISOBARS
ISOLATE
ISOLATO
KNOWALL
KOOLAID
LEONARD
LEONATO
LEOPARD
LEOTARD
LOOFAHS
MOORAGE
NEONATE
ODORANT
ONORATI
PEONAGE
PROBALL
PROBATE
PROEAST
PROFANE
PROFARM
PROLATE
PRONATE
PRONAVY
PROPANE
PRORATA
PRORATE
PROSAIC
RIOTACT
ROOFAGE
ROOTAGE
RYOKANS
SCOLARI
SHOFARS
SIOUANS
SLOGANS
SLOVAKS
SNOBALL
SNOCAPS
SNOCATS
SPOKANE
STOMACH
STOMATA
STORAGE
STOWAGE
TOOEASY
TOOHARD
TOOKAIM
TOOLATE
TOOMANY
TOOTALL
TROJANS
TWOBALL
TWOBASE
TWODAYS
TWOFACE
TWOLANE
TWOPAIR
TWOPART
VIOLATE
WHOSAID
WOODARD
WYOTANA
YEOMANS

••O••A•

ABOLLAE
ADOLLAR
AEOLIAN
AMOEBAE
AMOEBAS
APOGEAL
APOGEAN
ARONNAX
AROUSAL
ASOCIAL
AZOREAN
AZORIAN
BEOGRAD
BOOEDAT
BOOHBAH
BOOKBAG
BOOKMAN
BOOLEAN
BOOMCAR
BOORMAN
BROADAS
BROADAX
BROSNAN
BROWWAX
CHOCTAW
CHOLLAS
CHORDAL
COOLCAT
COOLMAX
COONCAN
COONCAT
CROSSAT
CROWBAR
DOORMAN
DOORMAT
DOORWAY
DROPCAP
DROVEAT
EPOCHAL
ETONIAN
FLOREAL
FLORIAN
FLOTSAM
FLOWNAT
FOOTBAG
FOOTMAN
FOOTPAD
FOOTWAY
FROGMAN
FRONTAL
FROWNAT
GLORIAS
GLOSSAE
GLOSSAL
GLOSSAS
GLOTTAL
GOODBAR
GOODDAY
GOODMAN
GOODPAY
GOOMBAH
GOOMBAY
GROWFAT
HOOPLAS
HOOPMAN
HOOTSAT
IRONBAR
IRONMAN
ISOGRAM
IVORIAN
KEOGHAN
LAOTIAN
LEONDAY
LOOKSAD
LOOKSAT
LOOMPAS
MYOPIAS
NEONGAS
NOONDAY
NOOTKAS
OVOIDAL
OXONIAN
PEORIAN
PHOBIAS
PLOWMAN
POOHBAH
POOLMAN
POORLAW
POORMAN
POORTAX
PROARAB
PROGRAM
PROPMAN
PROSCAN
PROTEAM
PROTEAN
QUONDAM
RHODIAN
RIORDAN
ROOFRAT
ROOMBAS
ROOTCAP
SCOFFAT
SCOOBAS
SCORIAS
SCOTIAN
SHOEPAC
SHOOTAT
SHOPSAT
SHOTPAR
SHOUTAT
SHOWCAT
SHOWMAN
SIOBHAN
SLOTCAR
SLOWDAY
SNORTAT
SNOWCAP
SNOWCAT
SNOWDAY
SNOWHAT
SNOWMAN
SPORRAN
SPOUSAL
STOICAL
STONEAX
STOPGAP
STOPSAT
SWOREAT
THOREAU
TOOLBAR
TOOTSAT
TROIKAS
TSONGAS
TWOSTAR
TWOYEAR
UTOPIAN
UTOPIAS
UXORIAL
WOODSAW
WOODTAR
WOOLFAT
WOOLHAT
WOOSNAM
WROCLAW
ZOOIDAL

••O•••A

ANOSMIA
AVONLEA
BIODATA
BOOTHIA
CHOLERA
CROATIA
DIORAMA
DIOTIMA
DUODENA
EROTICA
EXORDIA
EXOTICA
FIORINA
FLORIDA
GEORGIA
IGOTCHA
ILOVELA
INOCULA
IWOJIMA
LEONORA
ODONTIA
PRORATA
PROXIMA
RIORITA
SHOULDA
SNOWPEA
STOMATA
WYOTANA

•••OA••

ABROACH
BEMOANS
BOWOARS
BUROAKS
BYROADS
DEFOAMS
INBOARD
INGOALS
INROADS
MINOANS
NOLOADS
OGDOADS
OHIOANS
OHIOART
ONBOARD
ONLOADS
ONTOAST
PINOAKS
PTBOATS
REBOANT
REBOARD
RECOALS
RECOATS
REDOAKS
RELOADS
RELOANS
RESOAKS
RESOAPS
RETOAST
SAMOANS
SOLOACT
TANOAKS
THEOATH
THROATS
THROATY
UNLOADS
UNLOATH
UPCOAST
UPHOARD
UPLOADS
UPROARS
UPSOARS

•••O•A•

ACROBAT
ADWOMAN
AEROBAT
ALBORAK
ALDORAY
ALLOWAY
ALSORAN
ALTOSAX
ANGOLAN
ANGORAS
AREOLAE
AREOLAR
AREOLAS
ASTOLAT
AURORAE
AURORAL
AURORAS
AUTOMAT
BIFOCAL
BIMODAL
BIPOLAR
BITONAL
BIVOUAC
BULOVAS
CANOLAS
CHROMAT

COMORAN
CORONAE
CORONAL
CORONAS
CUPOLAS
DAKOTAN
DAKOTAS
DEBORAH
DEMOLAY
DEPOSAL
DIPOLAR
DONOVAN
ESPOSAS
EUROVAN
FEDORAS
FEMORAL
FILOFAX
FOTOMAT
GOTOGAL
GOTOWAR
GYROCAR
HUMORAL
IMMORAL
INNOWAY
INSOFAR
INTOTAL
ITSOKAY
JOJOBAS
JUDOKAS
KEROUAC
KILOBAR
KOSOVAR
LABORAT
LAKOTAS
LEGOLAS
LOYOLAU
LTKOJAK
MANOWAR
MAYORAL
MEMOPAD
MENORAH
MIMOSAS
MOLOKAI
MRNOVAK
MTLOGAN
NICOBAR
NICOLAS
NIKOLAI
NIKOLAY
NONORAL
ONEOCAT
ORTOLAN
OTTOMAN
PAGODAS
PALOMAR
PALOMAS
PAYOLAS
PELOTAS
PERORAL
PIVOTAL
POTOMAC
PREORAL
RAYOVAC
RCCOLAS
REMORAS
REMOVAL
REPOMAN
RETOTAL

SAMOSAS
SAMOVAR
SAROYAN
SCHOLAR
SCOOBAS
SEDONAS
SENORAS
SHOOTAT
SONORAN
SORORAL
SYNODAL
TACOMAS
THROWAT
TOYOTAS
UNLOCAL
UNLOYAL
UNVOCAL
UPTOPAR

•••O••A

ALFORJA
ALTOONA
ALYOSHA
AMMONIA
ANDORRA
ANSONIA
ANTONIA
APHONIA
ASTORIA
AUTOPIA
BAZOOKA
BEGONIA
BEGORRA
BOLOGNA
CAHOKIA
COLONNA
COROLLA
DACOSTA
DERONDA
EMPORIA
ENCOMIA
ESTONIA
ETVOILA
EUNOMIA
GOTOSEA
IACOCCA
KELOWNA
KENOSHA
LACONIA
LAJOLLA
LAMOTTA
LASORDA
LATOSCA
LAZONGA
MACONGA
MADONNA
MAJORCA
MELODIA
MENORCA
MINOLTA
MINORCA
NICOSIA
ONEONTA
PALOOKA
PINOTTA
POLONIA
PWBOTHA
RICOTTA

ROLONDA
SALONGA
SCIORRA
SEGOVIA
VERONIA
VITORIA
WYNONNA
ZENOBIA

••••OA•

AIRBOAT
ANYROAD
ARMLOAD
BALBOAS
BARSOAP
BOXCOAT
BUSLOAD
CARCOAT
CARLOAD
CARLOAN
CATBOAT
COBCOAL
CORKOAK
DIDTOAT
DOGCOAT
DRSLOAN
FHALOAN
FURCOAT
GUNBOAT
HOLMOAK
HOTCOAL
ICEBOAT
IDAHOAN
JERBOAS
JETBOAT
LABCOAT
LEWHOAD
LIVEOAK
LOWROAD
LYESOAP
OFFLOAD
OFFROAD
OUTROAR
OUTSOAR
OWNGOAL
PAYLOAD
PEACOAT
PETBOAS
PETGOAT
PRELOAD
PRELOAN
PRESOAK
RADIOAD
REDCOAT
REFLOAT
ROWBOAT
RYELOAF
SEABOAT
SEAFOAM
SHEGOAT
SUBGOAL
TOMJOAD
TOPCOAT
TOWBOAT
TOYBOAT
TUGBOAT
UNCLOAK
VANLOAD

VIRGOAN

••••O•A

ACEROLA
ALAMOSA
ALTOONA
AMAPOLA
AMPHORA
ARIZONA
AUREOLA
BAZOOKA
BENBOVA
BOFFOLA
CANZONA
CARIOCA
CARLOTA
CASSOLA
COPPOLA
CORDOBA
CORPORA
CRAPOLA
CRAYOLA
CREMONA
CREMORA
CURIOSA
DAYTONA
DELTONA
DIPLOMA
FORMOSA
GONDOLA
GONGORA
GRANOLA
HERMOSA
ISADORA
KEDROVA
LECUONA
LEONORA
MARKOVA
MINEOLA
MOLDOVA
MONTOYA
NDAKOTA
NONCOLA
ONEIOTA
OSCEOLA
OXYMORA
PALOOKA
PANDORA
PAVLOVA
PERGOLA
PERSONA
PIANOLA
PLUGOLA
RASBORA
REYNOSA
ROSEOLA
RUBEOLA
SALSODA
SAMBORA
SDAKOTA
SENHORA
SEQUOIA
SEQUOYA
SHARONA
SHINOLA
SIGNORA
SPINOZA
SUBROSA

TAPIOCA
TOMGOLA
TORTOLA
ULANOVA
VIGNOLA

OB•••••

OBADIAH
OBELISE
OBELISK
OBELIZE
OBENTOS
OBERLIN
OBESELY
OBESITY
OBEYERS
OBEYING
OBJECTS
OBLASTS
OBLATES
OBLIGED
OBLIGEE
OBLIGER
OBLIGES
OBLIGOR
OBLIQUE
OBLONGS
OBLOQUY
OBOISTS
OBSCENE
OBSCURA
OBSCURE
OBSERVE
OBTAINS
OBTESTS
OBTRUDE
OBTUNDS
OBTUSER
OBVERSE
OBVERTS
OBVIATE
OBVIOUS

O•B••••

ONBOARD
ONBREAK
OOBLECK
ORBISON
ORBITAL
ORBITED
ORBITER
ORBLESS
ORBLIKE
OSBORNE
OXBLOOD

O••B•••

OATBRAN
ODDBALL
OFFBASE
OFFBEAT
OILBASE
OILBIRD
OJIBWAS
OJIBWAY
OLDBATS
OLDBEAN
OLDBLUE
OLDBOYS
OLEBULL
ONABIAS
ONEBALL
ONEBASE
ONEBELL
ONEBYTE
OREBODY
OUTBACK
OUTBAKE
OUTBANS
OUTBARK
OUTBATS
OUTBAWL
OUTBEAM
OUTBEGS
OUTBEND
OUTBIDS
OUTBLOT
OUTBLOW
OUTBOWL
OUTBOWS
OUTBRAG
OUTBRAY
OUTBRED
OUTBUDS
OUTBULK
OUTBURN
OUTBUYS
OUTBUZZ

O•••B••

OCTOBER
OCTOBRE
OCTUBRE
OKTOBER
OMNIBUS
OPENBAR
OVERBED
OVERBET
OVERBID
OVERBIG
OVERBUY

O••••B•

ODDJOBS
OILRUBS
OUTRIBS

O•••••B

ONECLUB
OVERDUB

•OB••••

BOBATEA
BOBBERS
BOBBIDI
BOBBIES
BOBBING
BOBBINS
BOBBLED
BOBBLER
BOBBLES
BOBBSEY
BOBCATS
BOBDOLE
BOBGOEN
BOBHOPE
BOBKANE
BOBSLED
BOBTAIL
BOBTWAY
BOBVILA
BOBWEIR
COBALTS
COBBLED
COBBLER
COBBLES
COBCOAL
COBLENZ
COBNUTS
COBRAND
COBUYER
COBWEBS
DOBBINS
FOBBING
FOBSOFF
GOBBLED
GOBBLER
GOBBLES
GOBELIN
GOBELOW
GOBLANK
GOBLETS
GOBLINS
GOBROKE
GOBYAIR
GOBYBUS
GOBYCAB
GOBYCAR
GOBYSEA
HOBBIES
HOBBITS
HOBBLED
HOBBLER
HOBBLES
HOBNAIL
HOBNOBS
HOBOING
HOBOISM
HOBOKEN
HOBSONS
IOBJECT
JOBBANK
JOBBERS
JOBBERY
JOBBING
JOBCUTS
JOBFAIR
JOBHOPS
JOBHUNT
JOBJARS
JOBLESS
JOBLOCK
JOBLOTS
JOBSHOP
KOBLENZ
KOBOLDS
LOBATED
LOBBERS
LOBBIED
LOBBIES
LOBBING
LOBBYER
LOBSTER
LOBULES
MOBBERS
MOBBING
MOBBISH
MOBBISM
MOBBIST
MOBILES
MOBRULE
MOBSTER
NOBBIER
NOBHILL
NOBLEST
NOBODYS
OOBLECK
POBLANO
POBOXES
ROBARDS
ROBBERS
ROBBERY
ROBBING
ROBBINS
ROBBNEN
ROBERTA
ROBERTE
ROBERTF
ROBERTH
ROBERTI
ROBERTO
ROBERTS
ROBESON
ROBLOWE
ROBOCOP
ROBOTIC
ROBOTRY
ROBROYS
ROBSART
ROBUSTA
ROBUSTO
SOBBERS
SOBBING
SOBERED
SOBERER
SOBERLY
TOBACCO
TOBEHAD
TOBLAME
WOBBLED
WOBBLER
WOBBLES
WOBEGON
YOBBISH

•O•B•••

BOBBERS
BOBBIDI
BOBBIES
BOBBING
BOBBINS
BOBBLED
BOBBLER
BOBBLES
BOBBSEY
BOMBARD
BOMBAST
BOMBECK
BOMBERS
BOMBING
BOMBLET
BONBONS
BOOBIES
BOOBIRD
BOOBOOS
BOXBALL
BOXBEDS
BOXBOYS
BOYBAND
COBBLED
COBBLER
COBBLES
COGBURN
COLBERT
COMBATS
COMBERS
COMBIEN
COMBINE
COMBING
COMBUST
CONBRIO
CORBELS
CORBETT
COWBANE
COWBELL
COWBIRD
COWBOYS
DOBBINS
DOGBANE
DOGBEDS
DOGBERT
DOGBITE
DOGBONE
DOGBOOT
DOGBOWL
DOTBOMB
DOUBLEA
DOUBLEB
DOUBLEC
DOUBLED
DOUBLEE
DOUBLEF
DOUBLEG
DOUBLEH
DOUBLEI
DOUBLEJ
DOUBLEK
DOUBLEL
DOUBLEM
DOUBLEN
DOUBLEO
DOUBLEP
DOUBLEQ
DOUBLER
DOUBLES
DOUBLET
DOUBLEU
DOUBLEV
DOUBLEW
DOUBLEX
DOUBLEY
DOUBLEZ
DOUBTED
DOUBTER
DOUBTIT
FOBBING
FOGBANK
FOGBOWS
FOIBLES
FORBADE
FORBEAR
FORBIDS
FORBORE
FORBUSH
FOXBORO
GOABOUT
GOBBLED
GOBBLER
GOBBLES
GOOBERS
GOTBACK
GOTBEAT
GOTBUSY
HOBBIES
HOBBITS
HOBBLED
HOBBLER
HOBBLES
HOFBRAU
HOGBACK
HOLBEIN
HOLBERG
HOMBRES
HOMBURG
HOTBATH
HOTBEDS
HOWBEIT
IONBEAM
JOBBANK
JOBBERS
JOBBERY
JOBBING
JOEBLOW
JOEBUCK
JOGBRAS
JOSBOYS
LOBBERS
LOBBIED
LOBBIES
LOBBING
LOBBYER
LOGBOOK
LOMBARD
LONBORG
LOOBIES
LOWBALL
LOWBEAM
LOWBIDS
LOWBLOW
LOWBORN
LOWBOYS
LOWBRED
LOWBROW
MOABITE
MOBBERS
MOBBING
MOBBISH
MOBBISM
MOBBIST
MOEBERG
MOMBASA
MOWBRAY
NOBBIER
NOMBRES
NONBANK
NONBASE
NONBODY
NONBOOK
NONBUSY
NORBERT
NOTBEEN
POTBOIL
ROBBERS
ROBBERY
ROBBING
ROBBINS
ROBBNEN
ROEBUCK
ROMBERG
ROTBLAT
ROUBAIX
ROWBOAT
ROXBURY
ROYBEAN
SOBBERS
SOBBING
SORBATE
SORBETS
SOUBISE
SOYBEAN
TOMBOYS
TOPBIDS
TOPBOOT
TOWBARS
TOWBOAT
TOYBALL
TOYBIKE
TOYBOAT
TOYBOOK
VONBAER
WOBBLED
WOBBLER
WOBBLES
WOMBATS
YOBBISH
ZOMBIES
ZOMBIFY

•O••B••

BODYBAR
BOOHBAH
BOOKBAG
BOOMBOX
BOURBON
COALBIN
COHABIT
COINBOX
COPYBOY
CORNBIN
COURBET
DOESBAD
DONEBAD
DONTBEE
DOVEBAR
DOWNBOW
FOOTBAG
FORABIT
FOREBAY
GOBYBUS
GOESBAD
GOLDBUG
GOLFBAG
GONEBAD
GOODBAR
GOODBUY
GOODBYE
GOODBYS
GOOMBAH
GOOMBAY
GOTOBED
HOMEBOY
JOHNBOY
JOJOBAS
LOCKBOX
LOFTBED
LONGBED
LONGBOW
LOSABLE
LOSEBIG
LOSTBIG
LOVABLE
LOVABLY
LOVEBUG
MOONBOW
MOVABLE
MOVABLY
NOSEBAG
NOSEBRA
NOTABIT
NOTABLE
NOTABLY
POOHBAH
POORBOX
POORBOY
POSABLE
POSTBAG
POSTBOX
POTABLE
ROADBED
ROLLBAR
ROOMBAS
ROSABUD
ROSEBAY
ROSEBUD
ROYGBIV
SOAPBOX
SOFABED
SOLUBLE
TOLLBAR
TOOLBAR
TOOLBOX
TOTABLE
TOTEBAG
TOURBUS
TOWABLE
TOYNBEE
VOCABLE
VOCABLY
VOLUBLE
VOLUBLY
VOTABLE
WOODBIN
WOODBOX
WORKBOX

•O•••B•

COBWEBS
COLOMBO
COLUMBA
COLUMBO
COMESBY
CONFABS
CONJOBS
CORDOBA
COULDBE
FORTYBC
GOINGBY
GOTOBED
HOBNOBS
HORNSBY
HOTTUBS
KOSHIBA
LOCKBOX
MODELBS
MOGAMBO
MORESBY
NOCARBS
NODOUBT
NOTTOBE
ROCKABY
ROLLSBY
SOTHEBY
TOSHIBA
WOULDBE

•O••••B

BODYRUB
CORNCOB
COULOMB
COXCOMB
DOGCOMB
DOTBOMB
DOUBLEB
FOODWEB
FOOTRUB
GOBYCAB
GODTHAB
GOODJOB
GOTAJOB
HOMELAB
HOPACAB
HOTCOMB
JOHNNYB
LOWCARB
NONARAB
NOSEJOB
POPEAFB
POTHERB
WOLFCUB

••OB•••

BAOBABS
BLOBBED
BOOBIES
BOOBIRD
BOOBOOS
CLOBBER
ESOBESO
GLOBATE
GLOBING
GLOBINS
GLOBOID
GLOBOSE
GLOBOUS
GLOBULE
GOOBERS
ISOBARS
JROBERT
KNOBBED
LOOBIES
NIOBITE
NIOBIUM
PHOBIAS
PHOBICS

PROBALL
PROBATE
PROBERS
PROBIES
PROBING
PROBITY
PROBLEM
PROBONO
PROBOWL
SIOBHAN
SLOBBER
SNOBALL
TMOBILE
TWOBALL
TWOBASE
TWOBITS
UNOBESE

••O•B••
AMOEBAE
AMOEBAS
AMOEBIC
BLOBBED
BOOHBAH
BOOKBAG
BOOMBOX
CLOBBER
CROWBAR
DEORBIT
DROPBOX
FOOTBAG
FROEBEL
GOODBAR
GOODBUY
GOODBYE
GOODBYS
GOOMBAH
GOOMBAY
GROWBIG
INORBIT
IRONBAR
KNOBBED
MOONBOW
PHOEBES
PHOEBUS
PLOWBOY
POOHBAH
POORBOX
POORBOY
PROMBID
RHOMBIC
RHOMBUS
ROOMBAS
SCOOBAS
SHOEBOX
SHOWBIZ
SLOBBER
TOOLBAR
TOOLBOX
TROUBLE
UNORBED
WOODBIN
WOODBOX

••O••B•
BAOBABS
BIOLABS
CLOSEBY
DROPSBY
DROVEBY
FLOATBY
FLOWNBY
GLORYBE
RIOLOBO
SHOOTBY
SHOPNBC
STOODBY
STOPSBY
SWOREBY

••O•••B
FOODWEB
FOOTRUB
GOODJOB
LIONCUB
PROARAB
PROVERB
SNOWJOB

•••OB••
ACROBAT
AEROBAT
AEROBES
AEROBIC
AUTOBIO
AUTOBUS
BILOBED
DISOBEY
ENNOBLE
ENROBED
ENROBES
GOTOBED
IGNOBLE
IGNOBLY
JACOBIN
JOJOBAS
KILOBAR
KILOBIT
MRHOBBS
NICOBAR
OCTOBER
OCTOBRE
OKTOBER
SCOOBAS
STROBES
UNLOBED
UNROBED
UNROBES
UNSOBER
ZENOBIA

•••O•B•
ABSORBS
ADSORBS
COLOMBO
ENTOMBS
INDOUBT
MRHOBBS
NODOUBT
RECOMBS
REDOUBT
RESORBS
SHOOTBY
STOODBY

•••O••B
VAPORUB

••••OB•
BAGJOBS
CONJOBS
CORDOBA
DAYJOBS
DISROBE
DYEJOBS
EARLOBE
HADTOBE
HASTOBE
HOBNOBS
LAPROBE
LATROBE
LETGOBY
MICROBE
NAIROBI
NEWJOBS
NOTTOBE
ODDJOBS
REDROBE
REPROBE
RIOLOBO
SKIBOBS
THEBOBO
THEROBE

••••O•B
CATCOMB
COULOMB
COXCOMB
DOGCOMB
DOTBOMB
HOTCOMB
LYNDONB
PETCOMB
THEBOMB

•••••OB
BANKJOB
CORNCOB
EASYJOB
GETAJOB
GOODJOB
GOTAJOB
HADAJOB
LUBEJOB
NICEJOB
NOSEJOB
SNOWJOB
TEMPJOB
THEBLOB

OC•••••
OCALAFL
OCANADA
OCARINA
OCCIPUT
OCCLUDE
OCCULTS
OCCURTO
OCEANIA
OCEANIC
OCEANID
OCEANUS
OCELLAR
OCELLUS
OCELOTS
OCHENTA
OCHROID
OCHROUS
OCICATS
OCONNOR
OCTADIC
OCTAGON
OCTANES
OCTANTS
OCTAVAL
OCTAVES
OCTAVIA
OCTAVIO
OCTAVOS
OCTETTE
OCTOBER
OCTOBRE
OCTOPOD
OCTOPUS
OCTROIS
OCTUBRE
OCTUPLE
OCTUPLY
OCULARS
OCULIST

O•C••••
OCCIPUT
OCCLUDE
OCCULTS
OCCURTO
OHCAROL
OOCYTES
ORCHARD
ORCHIDS
OSCEOLA
OSCINES
OSCULAR
OSCULES
OXCARTS

O••C•••
OAKCASK
OATCAKE
OBSCENE
OBSCURA
OBSCURE
OCICATS
OFFCAST
OILCAKE
OILCANS
OILCUPS
OLDCARS
OLDCHAP
OLDCITY
OLICOOK
OMICRON
ONECALL
ONECELL
ONECENT
ONECHIP
ONECLAM
ONECLUB
OPACITY
ORACIES
ORACLES
ORECTIC
OUTCALL
OUTCANT
OUTCAST
OUTCITY
OUTCOLD
OUTCOME
OUTCOOK
OUTCROP
OUTCROW
OUTCULL
OUTCURE
OUTCUTS

O•••C••
OAXACAN
OBJECTS
OFFICER
OFFICES
OFFICIO
ONEACAT
ONEACRE
ONEACTS
ONEOCAT
OPTICAL
OPTICKS
OSSICLE
OUTACTS
OUTECHO
OVERCOY
OVERCUT

O••••C•
OARLOCK
ODDDUCK
ODDSOCK
OFFENCE
OILRICH
OLDNICK
ONAKICK
ONEINCH
ONESOCK
ONTRACK
OOBLECK
ORIFICE
ORINOCO
OSTRICH
OUTBACK
OUTFACE
OUTKICK
OUTPACE
OUTPICK
OUTRACE
OUTROCK
OVERACT
OVERICE
OVIDUCT
OVISACS

O•••••C
OCEANIC
OCTADIC
OGHAMIC
OLYMPIC
ONEIRIC
ONTOPIC
OOLITIC
ORECTIC
ORGANIC
OSMATIC
OSMOTIC
OSSIFIC
OTALGIC

•OC••••
BOCCIES
BOCELLI
BOCHNER
COCAINE
COCCOID
COCHAIR
COCHISE
COCHLEA
COCHRAN
COCKADE
COCKERS
COCKIER
COCKILY
COCKING
COCKISH
COCKLED
COCKLES
COCKNEY
COCKPIT
COCONUT
COCOONS
COCTEAU
DOCENTS
DOCKAGE
DOCKERS
DOCKETS
DOCKING
DOCTORS
FOCSLES
FOCUSED
FOCUSER
FOCUSES
FOCUSON
GOCARTS
GOCRAZY
HOCKERS
HOCKING
HOCUSED
JOCASTA
JOCELYN
JOCKEYS
JOCULAR
LOCALES
LOCALLY
LOCARNO
LOCATED
LOCATER
LOCATES
LOCATOR
LOCKAGE
LOCKBOX
LOCKEAN
LOCKERS
LOCKETS
LOCKING
LOCKINS
LOCKJAW
LOCKLET
LOCKLIN
LOCKNUT
LOCKOUT
LOCKSET
LOCKSIN
LOCKSON
LOCKSUP
LOCKUPS
LOCULUS
LOCUSTS
MOCHRIE
MOCKERS
MOCKERY
MOCKING
MOCKSUP
MOCKUPS
NOCANDO
NOCARBS
NOCATCH
NOCKING
NOCLASS
NOCOUNT
NOCUOUS
OOCYTES
POCKETS
POCONOS
ROCHETS
ROCKABY
ROCKCOD
ROCKERS
ROCKERY
ROCKETS
ROCKIER
ROCKIES
ROCKILY
ROCKING
ROCKOIL
ROCKOON
ROCKYII
ROCKYIV
ROCOCOS
SOCIALS
SOCIETY
SOCKETS
SOCKEYE
SOCKHOP
SOCKING
SOCKSIN
TOCCATA
TOCELIA
TOCSINS
VOCABLE
VOCABLY
VOCALIC
VOCALLY
VOCODER
ZOCALOS

•O•C•••
BOBCATS
BOCCIES
BOKCHOY
BOOCOOS
BOSCAGE
BOTCHED
BOTCHER
BOTCHES
BOTCHUP
BOUCHER
BOUCHES
BOXCARS
BOXCOAT
BOYCOTT
COACHED
COACHES
COACTED
COBCOAL
COCCOID
CODCAKE
COLCHIS
COMCAST
CONCAVE
CONCEAL
CONCEDE
CONCEIT
CONCEPT
CONCERN
CONCERT
CONCHAE
CONCHES
CONCHOS
CONCISE
CONCOCT
CONCORD
CONCURS
CONCUSS
COPCARS
COUCHED
COUCHES
COXCOMB
DOGCART
DOGCHEW
DOGCHOW
DOGCOAT
DOGCOMB
DOTCOMS
DOUCEUR
FOGCITY
FORCEIN
FORCEON
FORCEPS
FORCERS
FORCEUP
FORCING
FOSCOLO
GOTCASH
GOTCHAS
GOTCOLD
GOTCUTE
HOECAKE
HOGCALL
HONCHOS
HOOCHES
HOSCALE
HOTCAKE
HOTCAPS
HOTCARS
HOTCOAL
HOTCOMB
HOTCUPS
HOWCOME
JOACHIM
JOBCUTS
JOECAMP
JOECOOL
JOYCEAN
KOSCINA
LOWCARB
LOWCARD
LOWCHEN
LOWCOST
MONCTON
MOOCHED
MOOCHER
MOOCHES
MOOCOWS
MORCERF
MOSCATO
MOSCONI
NONCASH
NONCOLA
NONCOMS
NONCORE
NONCROP
NOSCORE
NOTCHED
NOTCHER
NOTCHES
POACHED
POACHER
POACHES
PODCAST
PONCHOS
POOCHES
POOCHIE
POPCORN
PORCHES
PORCINE
POUCHED
POUCHES
ROACHES
ROMCOMS
ROSCOES
ROYCOHN
SORCERY
TOCCATA
TOECAPS
TOMCATS
TOPCOAT
TORCHED
TORCHER
TORCHES
TOSCALE
TOUCANS
TOUCHED
TOUCHER
TOUCHES
TOUCHON
TOUCHUP
TOWCARS
TOYCARS
TOYCART
VOICERS
VOICING
VOLCANO
VOLCKER
VOUCHED
VOUCHER
VOUCHES

•O••C••
BODICES
BONACIS
BOOMCAR
BOOTCUT
BORSCHT
BOUNCED
BOUNCER
BOUNCES
BOWECHO
COALCAR
CODICES
CODICIL
COERCED
COERCER
COERCES
COLDCUP
COLDCUT
COLICKY
COMICAL
COMICES
CONICAL
COOLCAT
COONCAN
COONCAT
COPYCAT
CORACLE
CORNCOB
COUNCIL
DOMECAR
DOMICAL
DOMICIL
DONTCRY
DOVECOT
GOBYCAB
GOBYCAR
GOLFCAR
GOUACHE
HOLYCOW
HOPACAB
JOUNCED
JOUNCES
KOPECKS
LOGICAL
LOSTCAT
MODICUM
MOHICAN
MOLUCCA
MONACAN
MONOCLE
MOROCCO
NODICAL
NOGUCHI
NONACID
NOTICED
NOTICER
NOTICES
NOVICES
POLECAR
POLECAT
POLICED
POLICER
POLICES
POOLCUE
PORSCHE
POUNCED
POUNCER
POUNCES
ROBOCOP
ROCKCOD
ROCOCOS
ROOTCAP
SODACAN
SOLACED
SOLACER
SOLACES
SOLICIT
SOUPCAN
SOUPCON
SOURCED
SOURCES
TOBACCO
TOPICAL
TOWNCAR
VOTECHS
WOLFCUB
WOODCUT

•O•••C•
BOMBECK
COGENCY
COGNACS
COLLECT
COMPACT
CONCOCT
CONDUCE
CONDUCT
CONFECT
CONNECT
CONNICK
CONRACK
CONTACS
CONTACT
CONVECT
CONVICT
COPPICE
CORMACK
CORNICE
CORRECT
CORSICA
CORTICO
COSSACK
COTEACH
COWLICK
DOGFACE
DOGRACE
DOGTICK
DOLUNCH
DORMICE
DOTRICE
FOREACH
FORMICA
FORONCE
FOSDICK
GODUTCH
GOTBACK
GOTHICS
HOGBACK
HOMEICE
HOSPICE
HOTLICK
HOTPACK
HOWMUCH
HOWNICE
IOBJECT
IONESCO
JOBLOCK
JOEBUCK
JOMARCH
LOWNECK
LOWTECH
MOLUCCA
MONARCH
MORLOCK
MOROCCO
MORTICE
MOSAICS
NOCATCH
NOETICS
NOKNOCK
NOMERCY
NONFACT
NONSUCH
NOPLACE
NORDICA
NORDICS
NORELCO
NORWICH
NOTMUCH
NOTNICE
NOTONCE
OOBLECK
POETICA
POETICS
POLISCI
POLLACK
POLLOCK
POLYSCI
POPROCK
PORTICO
POTENCE
POTENCY
POTLUCK
RODDICK
ROEBUCK
ROLLICK
ROMANCE
ROSTOCK
SOLOACT
SONANCE
TOBACCO
TOEPICK
TOLTECS
TOOMUCH
TOPKICK
WOZZECK
ZODIACS

•O••••C
BORONIC
BOSONIC
BOTANIC
COMEDIC
DOMINIC
DOUBLEC
FORASEC
FORTYBC
HOMERIC
KORANIC
MOLLUSC
MONADIC
MONODIC
MORONIC
MORPHIC
NOMADIC
NONEPIC
OOLITIC
POLEMIC
POLITIC
PONTIAC
POSTDOC
POSTHOC
POTOMAC
POULENC
ROBOTIC
ROMANIC
SOMATIC
TONELOC
TOTEMIC
VOCALIC
VOLTAIC
YOUNGMC

••OC•••
ASOCIAL
AVOCADO
AVOCETS
BIOCHIP
BIOCIDE
BLOCKED
BLOCKER
BLOCKUP
BOOCOOS
BROCADE
CHOCKED
CHOCTAW
CLOCHES
CLOCKED
CLOCKER
CLOCKIN
CROCHET
CROCKED
CROCKER
CROCKET
DIOCESE
ECOCIDE
ELOCUTE
EPOCHAL
EXOCARP
EXOCETS
FLOCKED
FLOCKTO
FROCKED
GEOCODE
GIOCOSO
GNOCCHI
GROCERS
GROCERY
HOOCHES
ILOCANO
INOCULA
KNOCKED
KNOCKER
KNOCKON
LAOCOON
LYOCELL
MIOCENE
MOOCHED
MOOCHER
MOOCHES
MOOCOWS
NEOCENE
NEOCONS
POOCHES
POOCHIE
PROCEED
PROCESS
PROCITY
PROCLUS

PROCTER
PROCTOR
PROCURE
PROCYON
REOCCUR
SHOCKED
SHOCKER
SNOCAPS
SNOCATS
SNOCONE
STOCKED
STOCKER
STOCKUP
TROCHEE
TROCHES
WROCLAW

••O•C••

BLOTCHY
BOOMCAR
BOOTCUT
BRONCHI
BRONCHO
BRONCOS
CHOICER
CHOICES
COOLCAT
COONCAN
COONCAT
DROPCAP
GFORCES
GNOCCHI
GROUCHO
GROUCHY
IGOTCHA
LIONCUB
POOLCUE
PROSCAN
REOCCUR
RHOECUS
ROOTCAP
SCONCES
SHOWCAT
SLOTCAR
SLOUCHY
SNOWCAP
SNOWCAT
STOICAL
TWOACRE
TWOACTS
WOODCUT

••O••C•

ATOMICS
ATONICS
BIONICS
BIOPICS
BIOTECH
EBONICS
ENOUNCE
EROTICA
EROTICS
ETONICS
EXOTICA
EXOTICS
FLOUNCE
FLOUNCY
FROLICS
GEODUCK
PHOBICS
PHONICS
PHOTICS
PRODUCE
PRODUCT
PROJECT
PROTECT
RIOTACT
SCOOTCH
STOMACH
TOOMUCH
TROPICS
TROUNCE
TWOFACE

••O•••C

AMOEBIC
ANOSMIC
CROSTIC
FJORDIC
GEORGEC
GEORGIC
GNOSTIC
PROSAIC
RHOMBIC
SHOEPAC
SHOPNBC

•••OC••

BIFOCAL
BINOCHE
BRIOCHE
DECOCTS
DEFOCUS
GYROCAR
IACOCCA
INFOCUS
LAROCHE
MONOCLE
MOROCCO
ONEOCAT
RECOCKS
REDOCKS
REFOCUS
RELOCKS
ROBOCOP
ROCOCOS
SHLOCKY
SIROCCO
UNDOCKS
UNLOCAL
UNLOCKS
UNROCKY
UNVOCAL
VANOCUR

•••O•C•

ABBOTCY
ABROACH
BEYONCE
BYFORCE
CATORCE
DIVORCE
ENFORCE
FORONCE
HEROICS
IACOCCA
INFORCE
INTOUCH
INVOICE
LADOUCE
LATOSCA
LELOUCH
MAJORCA
MENORCA
MINORCA
MOROCCO
NOTONCE
REJOICE
RETOUCH
REVOICE
SCOOTCH
SIROCCO
SOLOACT
SPLOTCH
UNVOICE

•••O••C

ABIOTIC
AEROBIC
AMMONIC
ANIONIC
APHONIC
AVIONIC
BIVOUAC
BORONIC
BOSONIC
BUCOLIC
BYRONIC
CALORIC
CANONIC
CHAOTIC
CHLORIC
CHROMIC
CHRONIC
DEMONIC
DEMOTIC
EIDOLIC
ERGOTIC
GENOMIC
HEDONIC
IDIOTIC
ILLOGIC
KEROUAC
KETONIC
LACONIC
MASONIC
MEIOTIC
MELODIC
MESONIC
MITOTIC
MONODIC
MORONIC
NEPOTIC
ONTOPIC
OSMOTIC
PARODIC
POTOMAC
RAYOVAC
ROBOTIC
SYNODIC
TACONIC
UNCOMIC
UNTOXIC
XEROTIC
ZAPOTEC

••••OC•

AIRLOCK
AIRSOCK
ANTIOCH
ARMLOCK
ARTROCK
BABCOCK
BEDROCK
BIBCOCK
BLALOCK
BULLOCK
CANNOCK
CARIOCA
CASSOCK
CONCOCT
DEFROCK
DESTOCK
DRSPOCK
DRYDOCK
EARLOCK
ELFLOCK
FETLOCK
GENLOCK
GUNLOCK
GYMSOCK
HADDOCK
HAMHOCK
HAMMOCK
HANCOCK
HASSOCK
HEMLOCK
HILLOCK
INSHOCK
INSTOCK
JOBLOCK
KEYLOCK
KIDROCK
LEACOCK
LEBROCK
LUBBOCK
MADLOCK
MATLOCK
MATTOCK
MORLOCK
MRSPOCK
MURDOCH
NOKNOCK
NUMLOCK
OARLOCK
ODDSOCK
ONESOCK
ORINOCO
OUTROCK
PADDOCK
PADLOCK
PEACOCK
PENNOCK
PETCOCK
PETROCK
POLLOCK
POPROCK
PREROCK
REBLOCK
REKNOCK
RESTOCK
RIMROCK
ROSTOCK
SCHLOCK
SHYLOCK
TAPIOCA
THEROCK
TUSSOCK
UNBLOCK
UNFROCK
WARLOCK
WEDLOCK
ZIPLOCK
ZIPLOCS

••••O•C

MISKOLC
UNSTOIC

•••••OC

PAPADOC
POSTDOC
POSTHOC
RAYKROC
TONELOC

OD•••••

ODDBALL
ODDDUCK
ODDJOBS
ODDLOTS
ODDMENT
ODDNESS
ODDSARE
ODDSHOE
ODDSOCK
ODELETS
ODESSAN
ODINGON
ODONTIA
ODORANT
ODORFUL
ODORIZE
ODOROUS
ODYSSEY

O•D••••

ODDBALL
ODDDUCK
ODDJOBS
ODDLOTS
ODDMENT
ODDNESS
ODDSARE
ODDSHOE
ODDSOCK
OEDIPAL
OEDIPUS
OGDENUT
OGDOADS
OLDBATS
OLDBEAN
OLDBLUE
OLDBOYS
OLDCARS
OLDCHAP
OLDCITY
OLDDAYS
OLDDOGS
OLDFILM
OLDFOGY
OLDGAGS
OLDGIRL
OLDGOLD
OLDHAND
OLDJOKE
OLDLADY
OLDLINE
OLDLYME
OLDMAID
OLDMOON
OLDNAVY
OLDNESS
OLDNEWS
OLDNICK
OLDPALS
OLDPROS
OLDROSE
OLDSALT
OLDSAWS
OLDSHOE
OLDSONG
OLDSTER
OLDTIME
OLDTOWN
OLDUVAI
OLDWAYS
OLDWEST
ORDAINS
ORDEALS
ORDERED
ORDERER
ORDERIN
ORDERLY
ORDERUP
ORDINAL
ORDINES
ORDONEZ

O••D•••

OAKDESK
OBADIAH
ODDDUCK
OFFDAYS
OFFDUTY
OILDRUM
OLDDAYS
OLDDOGS
ONADARE
ONADATE
ONADIET
ONEDIME
ONEDOWN
OUTDARE
OUTDATE
OUTDOER
OUTDOES
OUTDONE
OUTDOOR
OUTDRAG
OUTDRAW
OUTDREW
OUTDROP
OUTDUEL
OVIDIAN
OVIDUCT
OXIDANT
OXIDASE
OXIDATE
OXIDISE
OXIDIZE

O•••D••

OCTADIC
OHFUDGE
ONANDON
ONEADAY
ONEIDAS
ONORDER
ONSIDES
ONVIDEO
OPTEDIN
OPTEDTO
OUTADDS
OUTEDGE
OVERDID
OVERDOG
OVERDRY
OVERDUB
OVERDUE
OVERDYE
OVOIDAL
OWNEDUP
OXHIDES

O••••D•

OBTRUDE
OBTUNDS
OCANADA
OCCLUDE
OFFENDS
OFFSIDE
OGDOADS
OLDLADY
ONLOADS
ONTHEDL
ONWARDS
ORCHIDS
OREBODY
ORGANDY
ORLANDO
ORMANDY
OSMONDS
OSMUNDS
OUTADDS
OUTBIDS
OUTBUDS
OUTMODE
OUTRIDE
OUTRODE
OUTSIDE
OXFORDS

O•••••D

OAKLAND
OAKWOOD
OBLIGED
OCEANID
OCHROID
OCTOPOD
OERSTED
OFAKIND
OFAMIND
OFFERED
OFFHAND
OFFLOAD
OFFROAD
OILBIRD
OILSAND
OILSEED
OLDGOLD
OLDHAND
OLDMAID
OLMSTED
OMITTED
ONALEAD
ONBOARD
ONEEYED
ONEFOLD
ONEHAND
ONEWOOD
ONEYARD
ONGUARD
OPENEND
OPERAND
OPPOSED
ORBITED
ORCHARD
ORDERED
OROTUND
OSHAPED
OSIERED
OSMOSED
OSTEOID
OSTWALD
OUTAWED
OUTBEND
OUTBRED
OUTCOLD
OUTFEED
OUTFIND
OUTLAID
OUTLAND
OUTLEAD
OUTLOUD
OUTPAID
OUTPLOD
OUTREAD
OUTSAID
OUTSOLD
OUTSPED
OUTTOLD
OUTVIED
OUTWARD
OUTWEED
OUTWIND
OUTWORD
OVERBED
OVERBID
OVERDID
OVERFED
OVERSAD
OWLEYED
OXBLOOD

•OD••••

BODEFUL
BODEGAS
BODEREK
BODICES
BODINGS
BODKINS
BODYART
BODYBAR
BODYFAT
BODYKIT
BODYRUB
CODCAKE
CODDLED
CODDLER
CODDLES
CODEINE
CODERED
CODFISH
CODGERS
CODICES
CODICIL
DODDERS
DODDERY
DODGEMS
DODGERS
DODGIER
DODGING
DODGSON
FODDERS
GODDARD
GODDESS
GODEVIL
GODFREY
GODHEAD
GODHOOD
GODLESS
GODLIER
GODLIKE
GODLING
GODMAMA
GODPAPA
GODSEND
GODSENT
GODSONS
GODTHAB
GODUNOV
GODUTCH
GODWITS
HODADDY
HODDING
IODATED
IODATES
IODIDES
IODISED
IODISES
IODIZED
IODIZER
IODIZES
JODHPUR
JODRELL
KODIAKS
LODGEIN
LODGERS
LODGING
MODELAS
MODELBS
MODELED
MODELER
MODELTS
MODEMED
MODERNE
MODERNS
MODESTO
MODESTY
MODICUM
MODISTE
MODULAR
MODULES
MODULUS
NODDERS
NODDIES
NODDING
NODICAL
NODOUBT
NODSOFF
NODULAR
NODULED
NODULES
PODCAST
PODIUMS
PODLIKE
PODRIDA
RODDICK
RODDING
RODENTS
RODEOFF
RODEOUT
RODGERS
RODLESS
RODLIKE
RODOLFO
RODRIGO
SODACAN
SODAPOP
SODDIER
SODDING
SODIDWE
SODLESS
TODDIES
TODDLED
TODDLER
TODDLES
YODELED
YODELER
ZODIACS

•O•D•••

AOUDADS
BOBDOLE
BOGDOWN
BOLDEST
BONDAGE
BONDERS
BONDING
BONDMAN
BONDMEN
BOODLES
BORDERS
BORDONI
BOUDINS
BOUDOIR
BOWDLER
BOWDOIN
BOWDOWN
CODDLED
CODDLER
CODDLES
COEDITS
COLDCUP
COLDCUT
COLDDAY
COLDEST
COLDISH
COLDONE
COLDWAR
CONDEMN
CONDIGN
CONDOLE
CONDONE
CONDORS
CONDUCE
CONDUCT
CONDUIT
CORDAGE
CORDATE
CORDELL
CORDERO
CORDERS
CORDIAL
CORDIAS
CORDING
CORDITE
CORDOBA
CORDONS
COYDOGS
DOADEAL
DODDERS
DODDERY
DOGDAYS
DOGDOOR
DOIDARE
DOODADS
DOODLED
DOODLER
DOODLES
DOTDASH
DOWDIER
DOWDIES
DOWDILY
FODDERS
FOGDOGS
FOLDERS
FOLDING
FOLDOUT
FOLDSIN
FOLDSUP
FOLDUPS
FONDANT
FONDEST
FONDLED
FONDLER
FONDLES
FONDUED
FONDUES
FOODIES
FOODWEB
FORDGTS
FORDHAM
FORDING
FORDLTD
FORDOES
FORDONE
FOSDICK
FOUDRES
GOADING
GODDARD
GODDESS
GOLDARN
GOLDBUG
GOLDING
GOLDMAN
GOLDONI
GOLDTIP
GOLDWYN
GONDOLA
GOODAIM
GOODALL
GOODBAR
GOODBUY
GOODBYE
GOODBYS
GOODDAY
GOODDOG
GOODEGG
GOODERS
GOODFOR
GOODGUY
GOODIES
GOODING
GOODISH
GOODJOB
GOODJOE
GOODKID
GOODMAN
GOODMEN
GOODNIK
GOODONE
GOODPAY
GOODSON
GOODTRY
GOODUSE
GOODWIN
GORDIAN
GORDITA
GORDIUS
GOTDONE
GOTDOWN
HODDING
HOEDOWN
HOLDALL
HOLDERS
HOLDING
HOLDOFF
HOLDOUT
HOLDSIN
HOLDSIT
HOLDSON
HOLDSTO
HOLDSUP
HOLDUPS
HOODIES
HOODING
HOODLUM
HOODOOS
HORDING
HOTDATE
HOTDAYS
HOTDOGS
HOUDINI
HOWDAHS
HOWDEDO
HOWDULL
HOWDYDO
HOYDENS
JORDANA
JOTDOWN
KORDELL
LOADERS
LOADING
LOADSIN
LOADSOF
LOADSUP
LOIDING
LONDRES
LORDING
LORDJIM
LORDSIT
LOUDENS
LOUDEST
LOUDISH
LOWDIVE
LOWDOWN
MOLDERS
MOLDIER
MOLDING
MOLDOVA
MONDALE
MONDAVI
MONDAYS
MONDESI
MONDIAL
MONDIEU
MOODIER
MOODILY
MORDANT
MORDENT
MORDRED
MOWDOWN
NODDERS
NODDIES
NODDING
NONDARK
NONDEAF
NONDEEP
NONDIET
NONDRIP
NONDRUG
NOODGED
NOODGES
NOODLED
NOODLES
NORDICA
NORDICS
NORDOFF
NORDOWE
NOTDONE
PONDERS
PONDING
POODLES
POPDIVA
POUDRES
POWDERS
POWDERY
ROADBED
ROADEOS
ROADERS
ROADHOG
ROADIES
ROADMAP
ROADTAR
ROADTAX
ROADWAY
RODDICK
RODDING
ROEDEER
RONDEAU
RONDELS
RONDURE

ROWDIER
ROWDIES
ROWDILY
SODDIER
SODDING
SOLDERS
SOLDFOR
SOLDIER
SOLDOFF
SOLDOUT
SORDINI
SORDINO
TOADIED
TOADIES
TOADISH
TODDIES
TODDLED
TODDLER
TODDLES
TOLDALL
TOLDOFF
TOODLES
TOPDOGS
TOPDOWN
TOPDRAW
TOYDOGS
TOYDOLL
VOIDERS
VOIDING
VOIDOUT
VOODOOS
WONDERS
WOODARD
WOODBIN
WOODBOX
WOODCUT
WOODIER
WOODIES
WOODING
WOODLEY
WOODLOT
WOODROW
WOODSAW
WOODSON
WOODTAR
WORDAGE
WORDIER
WORDILY
WORDING
WORDONE

•O••D••

BOARDED
BOARDER
BOARDUP
BOLIDES
BONEDRY
BONEDUP
BOOEDAT
BOREDOM
BORIDES
BORODIN
BOULDER
BOUNDED
BOUNDER
BOUNDTO
BOUNDUP
BOWEDTO
BOXEDIN
BOXEDUP
COLADAS
COLDDAY
COMEDIA
COMEDIC
COMEDIE
COMEDUE
COONDOG
CORNDOG
COTEDOR
COULDBE
COULDNT
DOORDIE
DOSADOS
DOSIDOS
DOTEDON
FORADAY
FORTDIX
FOUNDED
FOUNDER
FOUNDRY
FOURDAY
GOODDAY
GOODDOG
GOUNDER
GOURDES
HOARDED
HOARDER
HODADDY
HOLEDUP
HOLIDAY
HOLYDAY
HOMEDIN
HONEDIN
HOPEDSO
HOPEDTO
HOUNDED
HOUNDER
IODIDES
JOEYDEE
JOHNDOE
JOINDER
JOURDAN
KOWADLO
LONGDAY
LONGDEN
LOSTDOG
LOURDES
LOVEDIT
LOVEDTO
MOGADOR
MONADAL
MONADIC
MONODIC
MOONDOG
MOULDED
MOULDER
MOUNDED
MOVADOS
MOVEDIN
MOVEDIT
MOVEDON
MOVEDTO
MOVEDUP
NOBODYS
NOENDOF
NOENDTO
NOMADIC
NOONDAY
NOSEDIN
NOSEDUP
NOTEDLY
POKEDAT
POMADED
POMADES
POPEDOM
POSADAS
POSEDAS
POSTDOC
POTSDAM
POUNDED
POUNDER
ROLODEX
ROPEDIN
ROPEDUP
ROUNDED
ROUNDEL
ROUNDER
ROUNDLY
ROUNDON
ROUNDUP
SOANDSO
SODIDWE
SOLEDAD
SOLIDER
SOLIDLY
SOMEDAY
SOUNDED
SOUNDER
SOUNDLY
TOLEDAN
TOLEDOS
TONEDUP
TONYDOW
TOORDER
TOWEDIN
VOCODER
VOTEDIN
VOTEDNO
VOTEDON
WOLFDOG
WORKDAY
WORLDLY
WOULDBE
WOULDNT
WOULDST
WOUNDED
WOUNDUP
WOWEDEM
ZOOIDAL

•O•••D•

AOUDADS
BOBBIDI
BOGARDE
BOIARDO
BOXBEDS
COCKADE
COLLIDE
COLLODI
COLLUDE
COMMODE
COMRADE
CONCEDE
CONFIDE
CONOIDS
CORRADE
CORRIDA
CORRODE
CORVIDS
COWARDS
COWHIDE
DOASIDO
DOGBEDS
DOODADS
DOTARDS
DOVERDE
FORBADE
FORBIDS
HODADDY
HOTBEDS
HOTRODS
HOWARDK
HOWARDS
HOWARDU
HOWDEDO
HOWDYDO
JOEKIDD
JOYPADS
JOYRIDE
KOBOLDS
LOWBIDS
LOWSIDE
LOWTIDE
NOCANDO
NOGOODS
NOHANDS
NOLOADS
NONBODY
NOTRADE
PODRIDA
PONGIDS
POTLIDS
ROBARDS
ROLAIDS
ROLONDA
ROTUNDA
ROULADE
SOSPADS
TOPBIDS
TOPSIDE
TORNADO
TOROIDS
TORPEDO
TOSTADA
TOWARDS
YOLANDA
YOUANDI

•O••••D

BOARDED
BOASTED
BOBBLED
BOBSLED
BOGEYED
BOGGLED
BOISEID
BOMBARD
BONNARD
BOOBIRD
BOOGIED
BOOKEND
BOOSTED
BOSOMED
BOTCHED
BOTTLED
BOUGHED
BOUNCED
BOUNDED
BOWERED
BOWHEAD
BOYBAND
BOYHOOD
COACHED
COACTED
COAPTED
COASTED
COBBLED
COBRAND
COCCOID
COCKLED
CODDLED
CODERED
COERCED
COFOUND
COHERED
COIFFED
COIGNED
COLLARD
COLLOID
COLORED
COMMAND
COMMEND
COMPEND
CONCORD
CONGAED
CONRIED
CONTEND
COOPTED
COOWNED
COPLAND
CORNFED
COSTARD
COUCHED
COUGHED
COUNTED
COUPLED
COURSED
COURTED
COVERED
COVETED
COWBIRD
COWERED
COWHAND
COWHERD
COWSHED
COZENED
DOEEYED
DOESBAD
DOGFOOD
DOGSLED
DOGWOOD
DOLLIED
DONATED
DONEBAD
DOODLED
DOUBLED
DOUBTED
DOWERED
FOCUSED
FOISTED
FOLIOED
FONDLED
FONDUED
FOOTLED
FOOTPAD
FOOZLED
FORAGED
FORAYED
FORDLTD
FORFEND
FORGOOD
FORTORD
FORTYAD
FORWARD
FOULARD
FOUNDED
GOAHEAD
GOATEED
GOBBLED
GODDARD
GODHEAD
GODHOOD
GODSEND
GOESBAD
GOESMAD
GOGGLED
GONEBAD
GONEMAD
GOODKID
GOOGLED
GOROUND
GOSFORD
GOTCOLD
GOTGOOD
GOTOBED
GOTWORD
HOARDED
HOBBLED
HOCUSED
HOGTIED
HOGWEED
HOGWILD
HOISTED
HOLLAND
HOMERED
HOMINID
HONEYED
HONORED
HOTHAND
HOTHEAD
HOTLEAD
HOUNDED
HOVERED
IODATED
IODISED
IODIZED
IONISED
IONIZED
JOEKIDD
JOGGLED
JOINTED
JOISTED
JOLLIED
JONESED
JOSTLED
JOUNCED
JOUSTED
KOOLAID
LOATHED
LOBATED
LOBBIED
LOCATED
LOFTBED
LOLLARD
LOMBARD
LONGBED
LOOKSAD
LOUNGED
LOUREED
LOUVRED
LOWBRED
LOWCARD
LOWERED
LOWHAND
LOWLAND
LOWPAID
LOWROAD
MODELED
MODEMED
MONEYED
MONOPOD
MONTAND
MOOCHED
MOONGOD
MOPHEAD
MORDRED
MORPHED
MOSEYED
MOTIVED
MOTORED
MOTTLED
MOULDED
MOULTED
MOUNDED
MOUNTED
MOURNED
MOUSSED
MOUTHED
NODULED
NONACID
NONFOOD
NONGOLD
NONPAID
NONSKED
NONSKID
NONVOID
NONWORD
NOODGED
NOODLED
NORMAND
NORWOOD
NOTATED
NOTCHED
NOTEPAD
NOTGOOD
NOTICED
NOTUSED
NOVISAD
POACHED
POINTED
POLICED
POLKAED
POLLARD
POLYPED
POLYPOD
POMADED
POMMARD
PONIARD
POPEYED
POPPLED
POPUPAD
PORTEND
POSITED
POUCHED
POUNCED
POUNDED
POWERED
ROADBED
ROASTED
ROCKCOD
ROGERED
ROLLAND
RONSARD
RONWOOD
ROOSTED
ROOTLED
ROSABUD
ROSEBUD
ROSERED
ROSINED
ROSTAND
ROTATED
ROUGHED
ROUNDED
ROUSTED
ROWELED
ROWLAND
SOAPPAD
SOBERED
SOFABED
SOLACED
SOLEDAD
SOOTHED
SORTIED
SOTWEED
SOUNDED
SOURCED
TOADIED
TOASTED
TOBEHAD
TODDLED
TOEHOLD
TOGGLED
TOKENED
TOMJOAD
TOOHARD
TOOTHED
TOOTLED
TOPPLED
TOPSEED
TORCHED
TORQUED
TORVALD
TOTALED
TOUCHED
TOUSLED
TOWELED
TOWERED
TOWHEAD
TOYLAND
TOYSLED
VOLUMED
VOLUTED
VOSKHOD
VOUCHED
VOYAGED
WOBBLED
WOODARD
WOOSHED
WORRIED
WORSTED
WOUNDED
YODELED

••OD•••

ANODISE
ANODIZE
ANODYNE
APODOUS
AZODYES
BIODATA
BOODLES
BRODIES
BRODKEY
BRODSKY
DEODARS
DEODATO
DOODADS
DOODLED
DOODLER
DOODLES
DUODENA
ERODENT
ERODERS
ERODING
FEODORI
FOODIES
FOODWEB
FRODING
GEODESY
GEODUCK
GOODAIM
GOODALL
GOODBAR
GOODBUY
GOODBYE
GOODBYS
GOODDAY
GOODDOG
GOODEGG
GOODERS
GOODFOR
GOODGUY
GOODIES
GOODING
GOODISH
GOODJOB
GOODJOE
GOODKID
GOODMAN
GOODMEN
GOODNIK
GOODONE
GOODPAY
GOODSON
GOODTRY
GOODUSE
GOODWIN
GRODIER
HOODIES
HOODING
HOODLUM
HOODOOS
MOODIER
MOODILY
NOODGED
NOODGES
NOODLED
NOODLES
PLODDED
PLODDER
POODLES
PRODDED
PRODDER
PRODIGY
PRODSON
PRODUCE
PRODUCT
RHODIAN
RHODIUM
SHODDEN
STODGED
STODGES
TOODLES
TRODDEN
TWODAYS
TWODEEP
TWODOOR
VOODOOS
WOODARD
WOODBIN
WOODBOX
WOODCUT
WOODIER
WOODIES
WOODING
WOODLEY
WOODLOT
WOODROW
WOODSAW
WOODSON
WOODTAR

••O•D••

ALOADOF
AVOIDED
AVOIDER
BLONDER
BLONDES
BLONDIE
BLOODED
BLOWDRY
BOOEDAT
BROADAS
BROADAX
BROADEN
BROADER
BROADLY
BROIDER
BROODED
BROODER
CHORDAL
CHORDED
CHOWDER
CLOUDED
CLOUDUP
CLOWDER
COONDOG
CROWDED
CROWDER
CROWDIN
DOORDIE
EXORDIA
FJORDIC
FLOODED
GGORDON
GOODDAY
GOODDOG
GROWDIM
IDOODIT
INORDER
IWONDER
KYOODLE
LEONDAY
MOONDOG
NOONDAY
ONORDER
OVOIDAL
PLODDED
PLODDER
PLOVDIV
PRODDED
PRODDER
PROUDER
PROUDLY
PROUDOF
QUONDAM
REORDER
RIORDAN
SCOLDED
SCOLDER
SHODDEN
SHOWDOG
SLOWDAY
SMOLDER
SNOWDAY
SNOWDON
SPONDEE
STOODBY
STOODIN
STOODON
STOODTO
STOODUP
TOORDER
TRODDEN
ZOOIDAL

••O••D•

ABOUNDS
AVOCADO
BIOCIDE
BROCADE
BROMIDE
DIOMEDE
DIOXIDE
DOODADS
ECOCIDE
FLORIDA
GEOCODE
GROUNDS
ISOPODS
LEONIDS
PROKEDS
PROSODY
PROVIDE
SHOULDA
SHOULDI
YAOUNDE

••O•••D

ABORTED
ACORNED
ADOPTED
ADORNED
AROUSED
AVOIDED
BEOGRAD
BLOATED
BLOBBED
BLOCKED
BLOGGED
BLOODED
BLOOMED
BLOOPED
BLOTTED
BLOUSED
BLOWZED
BOOBIRD
BOOGIED
BOOKEND
BOOSTED
BROILED
BRONZED
BROODED
BROOKED
BROOMED
BROWARD
BROWNED
BROWSED
CHOCKED
CHOIRED
CHOMPED
CHOPPED
CHORDED
CLOAKED
CLOCKED
CLOGGED
CLOMPED
CLONKED
CLOPPED
CLOTHED
CLOTTED
CLOUDED
CLOUTED
CLOWNED
COOPTED
COOWNED
CROAKED
CROCKED
CROOKED
CROONED
CROPPED
CROSSED
CROWDED
CROWNED
DOODLED
DROOLED
DROOPED
DROPPED
DROWNED
DROWSED
EDOUARD
ENOILED
EPOXIED
EVOLVED
FEOFFED
FLOATED
FLOCKED
FLOGGED
FLOODED
FLOORED
FLOPPED
FLOSSED
FLOURED
FLOUTED
FOOTLED
FOOTPAD
FOOZLED
FROCKED
FRONTED
FROSTED
FROTHED
FROWARD
FROWNED
GHOSTED
GLOATED
GLOBOID
GLOMMED
GLOOMED
GLORIED
GLOSSED
GOODKID
GOOGLED
GROANED
GROINED
GROKKED
GROOMED
GROOVED
GROSSED
GROUPED
GROUSED
GROUTED
GROWLED
GROWOLD
IGOOFED
KNOBBED
KNOCKED
KNOTTED
KNOUTED
KOOLAID
LEONARD
LEOPARD
LEOPOLD
LEOTARD
LOOKSAD
MOOCHED
MOONGOD
NOODGED
NOODLED
OROTUND
PEOPLED
PHOTOID
PLODDED
PLONKED
PLOPPED
PLOTTED
PLOTZED
PROCEED
PRODDED
PROMBID
PROMOED
PRONGED
PROOFED
PROPPED
PROWLED

QUOINED
QUOITED
REOILED
REOWNED
ROOSTED
ROOTLED
SCOFFED
SCOLDED
SCOOPED
SCOOTED
SCORNED
SCOURED
SCOUTED
SCOWLED
SHOALED
SHOCKED
SHOPPED
SHORTED
SHOUTED
SLOGGED
SLOPPED
SLOSHED
SLOTTED
SNOOPED
SNOOTED
SNOOZED
SNORTED
SNOUTED
SOOTHED
SPOILED
SPONGED
SPOOFED
SPOOKED
SPOOLED
SPOONED
SPORTED
SPOTTED
SPOUTED
STOCKED
STODGED
STOMPED
STOOGED
STOOLED
STOOPED
STOPPED
STORIED
STORMED
SWOONED
SWOOPED
THORNED
TOOHARD
TOOTHED
TOOTLED
TROLLED
TROMPED
TROOPED
TROTHED
TROTTED
TROUPED
TWOFOLD
TWOTOED
UNOGLED
UNOILED
UNOPTED
UNORBED
UNOWNED
VROOMED
WHOMPED

WHOOPED
WHOPPED
WHORLED
WHOSAID
WOODARD
WOOSHED
WRONGED

•••OD••

BIMODAL
BLOODED
BORODIN
BROODED
BROODER
DECODED
DECODER
DECODES
DYNODES
ENCODED
ENCODER
ENCODES
FLOODED
FTDODGE
GQMODEL
IDOODIT
KYOODLE
LAYODDS
MALODOR
MELODIA
MELODIC
MONODIC
MRBODDY
NOBODYS
PAGODAS
PARODIC
RECODED
RECODES
REMODEL
ROLODEX
STOODBY
STOODIN
STOODON
STOODTO
STOODUP
SYNODAL
SYNODIC
THEODOR
TRIODES
UNCODED
UNGODLY
VOCODER

•••O•D•

ACCORDS
AFFORDS
ALMONDS
ALMONDY
ALTOIDS
ARNOLDS
BEHOLDS
BYROADS
BYWORDS
CONOIDS
CUBOIDS
DERONDA
EDMONDS
ENFOLDS
GIRONDE

HALOIDS
HAROLDI
INFOLDS
INROADS
KOBOLDS
LASORDA
LAYODDS
LEMONDE
MILORDS
MRBODDY
MRWORDS
NOGOODS
NOLOADS
OGDOADS
ONLOADS
OSMONDS
OXFORDS
RECORDS
REDONDO
REFOLDS
RELOADS
REMOLDS
REWORDS
ROLONDA
SECONDI
SECONDO
SECONDR
SECONDS
SHROUDS
TOROIDS
UNFOLDS
UNHOODS
UNLOADS
UNMOLDS
UNMOLDY
UNMOODY
UNROWDY
UPFOLDS
UPHOLDS
UPLOADS
WHWORDS

•••O••D

AGROUND
ALLOWED
ALLOYED
ANNOYED
APPOSED
APRONED
ARBORED
ARMORED
ASTOUND
BELOVED
BENOTED
BIGOTED
BILOBED
BLOODED
BLOOMED
BLOOPED
BOSOMED
BROODED
BROOKED
BROOMED
CAJOLED
CAROLED
CAROMED
CAROTID
CHROMED

COFOUND
COLORED
CROOKED
CROONED
DEBONED
DECODED
DECOYED
DEMOTED
DENOTED
DEPONED
DEPOSED
DETOXED
DEVOTED
DROOLED
DROOPED
ELBOWED
ENCODED
ENCORED
ENDOWED
ENJOYED
ENROBED
ENWOUND
EXPOSED
EXPOUND
FAGOTED
FAVORED
FLOODED
FLOORED
GALOPED
GLOOMED
GOROUND
GOTOBED
GROOMED
GROOVED
HONORED
HUMORED
IGNORED
IGOOFED
IMBORED
IMPOSED
IMPOUND
INBOARD
INBOUND
INTONED
INVOKED
LABORED
MAJORED
MASONED
MEMOPAD
MIAOUED
MIAOWED
MINORED
MINOTND
MONOPOD
MOTORED
MYWORLD
OCTOPOD
ONBOARD
OPPOSED
OSMOSED
PAROLED
PAROTID
PCWORLD
PICOTED
PILOTED
PIVOTED
PROOFED
RAZORED

REBOARD
REBORED
REBOUND
REBOXED
RECODED
REDOSED
REDOUND
REFOUND
REHONED
REMOVED
REMOWED
RENOTED
REPOSED
RESOLED
RESOUND
RESOWED
RETONED
RETOWED
REVOKED
REVOTED
REWOUND
REYOKED
REZONED
RUMORED
SAMOYED
SAVORED
SCOOPED
SCOOTED
SNOOPED
SNOOTED
SNOOZED
SPOOFED
SPOOKED
SPOOLED
SPOONED
STOOGED
STOOLED
STOOPED
STROKED
SWOONED
SWOOPED
TABOOED
TALONED
TENONED
TROOPED
TUTORED
UNBONED
UNBORED
UNBOUND
UNBOWED
UNBOXED
UNCODED
UNCORED
UNCOWED
UNDOMED
UNFOUND
UNFOXED
UNGORED
UNHONED
UNHOPED
UNJOYED
UNLOBED
UNLOVED
UNMOULD
UNMOVED
UNMOWED
UNNOSED
UNNOTED

UNPOLED
UNPOSED
UNROBED
UNROPED
UNROUND
UNSOLED
UNSOLID
UNSOUND
UNSOWED
UNTONED
UNVOTED
UNVOWED
UNWOOED
UNWOUND
UNYOKED
UNZONED
UPBOUND
UPHOARD
VAPORED
VISORED
VIZORED
VROOMED
WAGONED
WHOOPED
WIDOWED
XEROXED

••••OD•

ALAMODE
ANYBODY
ASABODY
BARCODE
CATHODE
COLLODI
COMMODE
CORRODE
CUSTODY
DNACODE
EPISODE
EXPLODE
FANTODS
FLYRODS
GEOCODE
HARRODS
HOTRODS
HYMNODY
IMPLODE
ISOPODS
METHODS
MISCODE
NIMRODS
NOGOODS
NONBODY
OREBODY
OUTMODE
OUTRODE
PEABODY
PEAPODS
PERIODS
PRECODE
PROSODY
RADIODJ
RAMRODS
REDCODS
SALSODA
SEAGODS
SUBCODE
SUBGODS

SUNGODS
TAXCODE
TENCODE
TETRODE
THEBODY
TIERODS
TINGODS
TRIPODS
UNHOODS
UNIBODY
UNICODE
UNIPODS
UNMOODY
UPCCODE
VERYODD
WARGODS
ZIPCODE

••••O•D

ABSCOND
ADENOID
ALLGOOD
ALLTOLD
AMEBOID
ANDROID
ANEROID
ANYROAD
ARMLOAD
ASHFORD
AYKROYD
BADCOLD
BADMOOD
BADWORD
BAGNOLD
BECLOUD
BEDFORD
BOYHOOD
BRAVOED
BUNCOED
BUNKOED
BUSLOAD
BUTGOOD
CAMEOED
CARLOAD
CATFOOD
COCCOID
COLLOID
CONCORD
CTENOID
CYCLOID
DAGWOOD
DELTOID
DENTOID
DESMOND
DESPOND
DIAMOND
DIDGOOD
DIEBOLD
DIPLOID
DISCOED
DISCOID
DISCORD
DITTOED
DOGFOOD
DOGWOOD
DYEWOOD
ELMWOOD
ETHMOID

EYEFOLD
FACTOID
FANFOLD
FARGOND
FIBROID
FOLIOED
FORGOOD
FORTORD
GAYLORD
GESSOED
GETCOLD
GETGOOD
GETSOLD
GETWORD
GIFFORD
GILFORD
GINGOLD
GLOBOID
GODHOOD
GOSFORD
GOTCOLD
GOTGOOD
GOTWORD
GREWOLD
GROWOLD
GUMWOOD
HAMMOND
HAPLOID
HARROLD
HELLOED
HELMOND
HEYWOOD
HULLOED
HYALOID
HYPNOID
ICECOLD
ILLFOLD
INAMOOD
INAWORD
INCROWD
ISECOND
ITSCOLD
KEYWORD
LADHOOD
LANFORD
LASSOED
LAWFORD
LEAWOOD
LEEFORD
LEOPOLD
LEWHOAD
LITHOID
LOWROAD
MAMBOED
MANHOOD
MASTOID
MCCLOUD
MEDFORD
MIMEOED
MISTOLD
MISWORD
MITFORD
MUMFORD
NEWWORD
NONFOOD
NONGOLD
NONVOID
NONWORD

NORWOOD
NOTGOOD
NUNHOOD
NUTWOOD
OAKWOOD
OCHROID
OFFLOAD
OFFROAD
OLDGOLD
ONEFOLD
ONEWOOD
OSTEOID
OUTCOLD
OUTLOUD
OUTSOLD
OUTTOLD
OUTWORD
OXBLOOD
PAYLOAD
PHOTOID
PINFOLD
PLYWOOD
PRELOAD
PRESOLD
PRETOLD
PREVOID
PROMOED
RADFORD
RADIOAD
RADIOED
RAWFOOD
RAYMOND
REDFORD
REDMOND
REDWOOD
REFLOOD
RESPOND
RIPCORD
RONWOOD
RUMFORD
SAMEOLD
SAMLOYD
SANFORD
SAWWOOD
SEAFOOD
SIGMOID
SIXFOLD
STCLOUD
STEROID
TABLOID
TABOOED
TANGOED
TENFOLD
THEGOLD
THEHOOD
THEPOND
THYROID
TIPTOED
TOEHOLD
TOMJOAD
TRIFOLD
TWOFOLD
TWOTOED
TYPHOID
UNCLOUD
UNPROUD
UNSHOED
UNWOOED

UPSTOOD
VANLOAD
VERYODD
VERYOLD
VIDEOED
WARBOND
WARLORD
WATFORD
WEBTOED
WEXFORD
WILFORD
WINWOOD
XIPHOID
ZEBROID

•••••OD

ALLGOOD
AULDSOD
AXELROD
BADMOOD
BOYHOOD
BUTGOOD
CAPECOD
CATFOOD
DAGWOOD
DEARGOD
DECAPOD
DEMIGOD
DIDGOOD
DOGFOOD
DOGWOOD
DYEWOOD
ELMWOOD
FORGOOD
FUELROD
GETGOOD
GODHOOD
GOTGOOD
GUMWOOD
HALFROD
HEXAPOD
HEYWOOD
ICHABOD
INAMOOD
LADHOOD
LEAWOOD
LINGCOD
MACLEOD
MANHOOD
MONOPOD
MOONGOD
NONFOOD
NORWOOD
NOTGOOD
NUNHOOD
NUTWOOD
OAKWOOD
OCTOPOD
ONEWOOD
OUTPLOD
OXBLOOD
PLYWOOD
POLYPOD
PUSHROD
RAINGOD
RAWFOOD
REDWOOD
REFLOOD

ROCKCOD
RONWOOD
SAWWOOD
SEAFOOD
SEEDPOD
THEHOOD
UPSTOOD
VOSKHOD
WINDGOD
WINWOOD

OE•••••

OEDIPAL
OEDIPUS
OERSTED
OEUVRES

O•E••••

OBELISE
OBELISK
OBELIZE
OBENTOS
OBERLIN
OBESELY
OBESITY
OBEYERS
OBEYING
OCEANIA
OCEANIC
OCEANID
OCEANUS
OCELLAR
OCELLUS
OCELOTS
ODELETS
ODESSAN
OKEEFFE
OKELLEY
OLEANNA
OLEANNY
OLEATES
OLEBULL
OLEFINS
OLEMISS
OLEOOIL
OLESTRA
OLEVELS
OMELETS
OMENING
ONEACAT
ONEACRE
ONEACTS
ONEADAY
ONEARTH
ONEBALL
ONEBASE
ONEBELL
ONEBYTE
ONECALL
ONECELL
ONECENT
ONECHIP
ONECLAM
ONECLUB
ONEDIME
ONEDOWN
ONEEEEE
ONEEYED

ONEFOLD
ONEFOOT
ONEGRAM
ONEHALF
ONEHAND
ONEHOUR
ONEIDAS
ONEINCH
ONEIOTA
ONEIRIC
ONEIRON
ONEKILO
ONELANE
ONELIRA
ONELOOK
ONELOVE
ONELUMP
ONEMILE
ONEMORE
ONEMPTY
ONENAME
ONENESS
ONENOTE
ONEOCAT
ONEOFFS
ONEOFUS
ONEONTA
ONEOVER
ONEPAGE
ONEPAIR
ONEPART
ONEPINT
ONEREEL
ONEROOM
ONEROUS
ONESELF
ONESHOE
ONESHOT
ONESIZE
ONESOCK
ONESPOT
ONESTAR
ONESTEP
ONESTOP
ONETERM
ONETIME
ONETOGO
ONETWOS
ONEUNIT
ONEVOTE
ONEWEEK
ONEWHIT
ONEWOOD
ONEYARD
ONEYEAR
OPENAIR
OPENBAR
OPENEND
OPENERS
OPENING
OPENNET
OPENOUT
OPENPIT
OPENSEA
OPENSUP
OPENTAP
OPENTOE
OPENTOP

OPERAND
OPERANT
OPERATE
OPEROSE
OREBODY
ORECTIC
OREGANO
OREILLY
ORELESS
ORESTES
OSETRAS
OVERACT
OVERAGE
OVERALL
OVERARM
OVERATE
OVERAWE
OVERBED
OVERBET
OVERBID
OVERBIG
OVERBUY
OVERCOY
OVERCUT
OVERDID
OVERDOG
OVERDRY
OVERDUB
OVERDUE
OVERDYE
OVEREAT
OVERFAR
OVERFAT
OVERFED
OVERFEE
OVERFEW
OVERFIT
OVERFIX
OVERFLY
OVERHOT
OVERICE
OVERJOY
OVERLAP
OVERLAX
OVERLAY
OVERLET
OVERLIE
OVERLIT
OVERMAN
OVERMIX
OVERNEW
OVERPAR
OVERPAY
OVERPLY
OVERRAN
OVERRUN
OVERSAD
OVERSAW
OVERSEA
OVERSEE
OVERSET
OVERSEW
OVERSUP
OVERTAX
OVERTIP
OVERTLY
OVERTOP
OVERUSE

OVERWET

O••E•••

OBJECTS
OBSERVE
OBTESTS
OBVERSE
OBVERTS
OCHENTA
OCTETTE
OFFENCE
OFFENDS
OFFENSE
OFFERED
OFFEREE
OFFERER
OFFEROR
OFFERUP
OFTENER
OGDENUT
OGREISH
OISEAUX
OKEEFFE
ONEEEEE
ONEEYED
ONLEASE
ONLEASH
ONLEAVE
ONSERVE
OOZEOUT
OPHELIA
OPTEDIN
OPTEDTO
ORDEALS
ORDERED
ORDERER
ORDERIN
ORDERLY
ORDERUP
ORGEATS
ORIENTE
ORIENTS
ORLEANS
ORNETTE
ORTEGAL
OSCEOLA
OSIERED
OSSEOUS
OSSETRA
OSTEOID
OTHELLO
OUTEARN
OUTEATS
OUTECHO
OUTEDGE
OWLEGGS
OWLEYED
OWNEDUP
OXHEART

O•••E••

OAKDESK
OAKFERN
OAKIEST
OAKLEAF
OARLESS
OATMEAL
OBESELY
OBEYERS
OBSCENE
ODDMENT
ODDNESS
ODELETS
OFFBEAT
OFFPEAK
OFFSETS
OFFWEGO
OFFYEAR
OILHEAT
OILIEST
OILLESS
OILSEED
OILWELL
OINKERS
OLDBEAN
OLDNESS
OLDNEWS
OLDWEST
OLEVELS
OMELETS
ONAGERS
ONALEAD
ONALERT
ONATEAR
ONBREAK
ONEBELL
ONECELL
ONECENT
ONEEEEE
ONENESS
ONEREEL
ONESELF
ONETERM
ONEWEEK
ONEYEAR
ONLIEST
ONTHEDL
ONTHEGO
ONTHEQT
ONTKEAN
OOBLECK
OOZIEST
OPENEND
OPENERS
OPINERS
OPPRESS
OPULENT
ORBLESS
ORELESS
ORKNEYS
OROGENY
ORPHEAN
ORPHEUM
ORPHEUS
ORVIETO
OSPREYS
OSTLERS
OURSELF
OUSTERS
OUTBEAM
OUTBEGS
OUTBEND
OUTFEED
OUTFEEL
OUTHEAR
OUTHERE
OUTJEST
OUTJETS
OUTKEEP
OUTKEPT
OUTLEAD
OUTLEAP
OUTLETS
OUTPEEP
OUTREAD
OUTSEEK
OUTSEEN
OUTSEES
OUTSELL
OUTSERT
OUTSETS
OUTTEAR
OUTTELL
OUTWEAR
OUTWEED
OUTWEEP
OUTWELL
OUTWENT
OUTWEPT
OUTWEST
OUTYELL
OUTYELP
OVEREAT
OWLIEST
OYSTERS
OZZFEST

O••••E•

OAKTREE
OARSMEN
OBLATES
OBLIGED
OBLIGEE
OBLIGER
OBLIGES
OBTUSER
OCTANES
OCTAVES
OCTOBER
ODYSSEY
OERSTED
OEUVRES
OFFERED
OFFEREE
OFFERER
OFFICER
OFFICES
OFTENER
OHMAGES
OILSEED
OKELLEY
OKTOBER
OLDSTER
OLEATES
OLIVIER
OLMSTED
OLOGIES
OMALLEY
OMITTED
OMITTER
ONADIET
ONEEEEE
ONEEYED
ONEOVER
ONEREEL
ONESTEP
ONEWEEK
ONORDER
ONPAPER
ONSAGER
ONSIDES
ONTHREE
ONVIDEO
ONWATER
OOCYTES
OOLITES
OPAQUES
OPENNET
OPENSEA
OPIATES
OPPOSED
OPPOSER
OPPOSES
ORACIES
ORACLES
ORANGES
ORANGEY
ORANTES
ORBITED
ORBITER
ORDERED
ORDERER
ORDINES
ORDONEZ
ORESTES
ORIOLES
ORRISES
OSCINES
OSCULES
OSHAPED
OSIERED
OSMOSED
OSMOSES
OSSIPEE
OTARIES
OUTAGES
OUTAWED
OUTAWES
OUTBRED
OUTDOER
OUTDOES
OUTDREW
OUTDUEL
OUTFEED
OUTFEEL
OUTFLEE
OUTGOES
OUTGREW
OUTKEEP
OUTLIER
OUTLIES
OUTPEEP
OUTSEEK
OUTSEEN
OUTSEES
OUTSPED
OUTSTEP
OUTVIED
OUTVIES
OUTWEED
OUTWEEP
OVARIES
OVERBED
OVERBET
OVERFED
OVERFEE
OVERFEW
OVERLET
OVERNEW
OVERSEA
OVERSEE
OVERSET
OVERSEW
OVERWET
OWLEYED
OXHIDES

O•••••E

OAKLIKE
OAKTREE
OARLIKE
OATCAKE
OATLIKE
OBELISE
OBELIZE
OBLIGEE
OBLIQUE
OBSCENE
OBSCURE
OBSERVE
OBTRUDE
OBVERSE
OBVIATE
OCCLUDE
OCTETTE
OCTOBRE
OCTUBRE
OCTUPLE
ODDSARE
ODDSHOE
ODORIZE
OFANAGE
OFFBASE
OFFENCE
OFFENSE
OFFEREE
OFFLINE
OFFSIDE
OFFSITE
OFNOUSE
OFVALUE
OHFUDGE
OILBASE
OILCAKE
OILLIKE
OILLINE
OKEEFFE
OLDBLUE
OLDJOKE
OLDLINE
OLDLYME
OLDROSE
OLDSHOE
OLDTIME
OLIVINE
OMAHANE
ONADARE
ONADATE
ONALINE
ONEACRE
ONEBASE
ONEBYTE
ONEDIME
ONEEEEE
ONELANE
ONELOVE
ONEMILE
ONEMORE
ONENAME
ONENOTE
ONEPAGE
ONESHOE
ONESIZE
ONETIME
ONEVOTE
ONLEASE
ONLEAVE
ONSERVE
ONSHORE
ONSTAGE
ONTHREE
OPALINE
OPENTOE
OPERATE
OPEROSE
OPUSONE
ORBLIKE
ORIENTE
ORIFICE
ORIGINE
ORNETTE
OROURKE
ORVILLE
OSBORNE
OSSICLE
OSSIPEE
OUTBAKE
OUTCOME
OUTCURE
OUTDARE
OUTDATE
OUTDONE
OUTEDGE
OUTFACE
OUTFIRE
OUTFLEE
OUTGAME
OUTGAVE
OUTGAZE
OUTGIVE
OUTHERE
OUTHIRE
OUTLINE
OUTLIVE
OUTLOVE
OUTMATE
OUTMODE
OUTMOVE
OUTPACE
OUTPIPE
OUTRACE
OUTRAGE
OUTRATE
OUTRAVE
OUTRIDE
OUTRODE
OUTROVE
OUTSIDE
OUTSIZE
OUTSOLE
OUTTAKE
OUTTIRE
OUTTORE
OUTVOTE
OUTWAVE
OUTWILE
OUTWORE
OVERAGE
OVERATE
OVERAWE
OVERDUE
OVERDYE
OVERFEE
OVERICE
OVERLIE
OVERSEE
OVERUSE
OWLLIKE
OXALATE
OXIDASE
OXIDATE
OXIDISE
OXIDIZE
OZONISE
OZONIZE

•OE••••

BOEINGS
BOERWAR
COEDITS
COEPTIS
COEQUAL
COERCED
COERCER
COERCES
COETZEE
COEVALS
COEXIST
DOEEYED
DOESBAD
DOESFOR
DOESKIN
DOESNOT
DOESTOO
DOEUVRE
FOELESS
GOESAFT
GOESAPE
GOESBAD
GOESFAR
GOESFOR
GOESMAD
GOESOFF
GOESOUT
GOESPRO
HOECAKE
HOEDOWN
JOEBLOW
JOEBUCK
JOECAMP
JOECOOL
JOEHILL
JOEKIDD
JOEROTH
JOEYDEE
KOEHLER
LOESSER
LOESSES
MOEBERG
NOENDOF
NOENDTO
NOENTRY
NOETICS
POESIES
POETESS
POETICA
POETICS
POETISE
POETIZE
ROEBUCK
ROEDEER
ROETHKE
TOECAPS
TOEHOLD
TOELESS
TOELIKE
TOELOOP
TOENAIL
TOEPICK
TOESHOE
TOETAPS
WOEISME
ZOELLER

•O•E•••

BOCELLI
BODEFUL
BODEGAS
BODEREK
BOGEYED
BOHEMIA
BOLEROS
BONEASH
BONEDRY
BONEDUP
BONELET
BONESET
BONESUP
BONEYER
BOOEDAT
BOREDOM
BOREOUT
BOWECHO
BOWEDTO
BOWERED
BOXEDIN
BOXEDUP
BOXESIN
BOXESUP
BOZEMAN
CODEINE
CODERED
COGENCY
COHEIRS
COHERED
COHERER
COHERES
COLEMAN
COLETTE
COMEDIA
COMEDIC
COMEDIE
COMEDUE
COMENOW
COMEOFF
COMEONS
COMEOUT
COMESAS
COMESAT
COMESBY
COMESIN
COMESON
COMESTO
COMESUP
CONELET
CORELLI
CORETTA
COSETTE
COTEACH
COTEDOR
COTERIE
COVERED
COVERER
COVERME
COVERTS
COVERUP
COVETED
COVETER
COWERAT
COWERED
COZENED
COZENER
DOCENTS
DOEEYED
DOGEARS
DOHERTY
DOLEFUL
DOLEOUT
DOMECAR
DONEBAD
DONEFOR
DONEGAL
DONEGAN
DONETSK
DOPEOUT
DOTEDON
DOTESON
DOVEBAR
DOVECOT
DOVELET
DOVERDE
DOWERED
DOYENNE
DOZENTH
DOZEOFF
FOGERTY
FOLENGO
FOMENTS
FOREACH
FOREARM
FOREBAY
FOREIGN
FORELEG
FOREMAN
FOREMEN
FORENZA
FOREPAW
FORERAN
FORERUN
FORESAW
FORESEE
FORESTS
FORETOP
FOREVER
FOUETTE
GOBELIN
GOBELOW
GODEVIL
GOGETEM
GONEAFT
GONEAPE
GONEBAD
GONEFAR
GONEFOR
GONEMAD
GONEOFF
GONEOUT
GONEPRO
GONERIL
GORETEX
GOTEVEN
GOVERNS
HOLEDUP
HOLEOUT
HOLESUP
HOMEBOY
HOMEDIN
HOMEICE
HOMEIER
HOMELAB
HOMERED
HOMERIC
HOMERUN
HOMESIN
HONEDIN
HONESIN
HONESTY
HONEYED
HOPEDSO
HOPEDTO
HOPEFOR
HOPEFUL
HOPENOT
HOPESSO
HOPESTO
HOVERED
HOVERER
HOWELLS
HOWELSE
HOWEVER
IONESCO
IOWEYOU
JOCELYN
JONERIK
JONESED
JONESES
JOSEPHA
JOSEPHI
KOPECKS
KOREANS
LONETTE
LORELAI
LORELEI
LORENTZ
LORENZO
LORETTA
LOSEBIG
LOSEOUT
LOSESIT
LOSESTO
LOUELLA
LOVEBUG
LOVEDIT
LOVEDTO
LOVEINS
LOVEJOY
LOVERLY
LOVESET
LOVESIT
LOVESTO
LOVETAP
LOVEYOU
LOWEEZY
LOWERED
LOZENGE
MODELAS
MODELBS
MODELED
MODELER
MODELTS
MODEMED
MODERNE
MODERNS
MODESTO
MODESTY
MOHEGAN
MOLERAT
MOLESTS
MOMENTA
MOMENTS
MONEYED
MOREENS
MORELLA
MORELLO
MORELOS
MOREPAY
MORESBY
MORETTI
MOSELLE
MOSEYED
MOVEDIN
MOVEDIT
MOVEDON
MOVEDTO
MOVEDUP
MOVEOFF
MOVEOUT
MOVESIN
MOVESIT
MOVESON
MOVESTO
MOVESUP
MOZETTA
NOMERCY
NOMERGE
NONEPIC
NONETTE
NONEVER
NONEVIL
NORELCO
NOSEATS
NOSEBAG
NOSEBRA
NOSEDIN
NOSEDUP
NOSEEUM
NOSEGAY
NOSEJOB
NOSEOUT
NOSESIN
NOSESUP
NOTEASY
NOTEDLY
NOTEPAD
NOTEVEN
NOTEVER
NOVELAS
NOVELLA
NOVELLE
NOVELLO
NOVELTY
NOVENAS
OOZEOUT
POKEDAT
POKEFUN
POKEMON
POKEOUT
POKESAT
POLEAXE
POLECAR
POLECAT
POLEMAN
POLEMEN
POLEMIC
POLENTA
POLESAT
POLESIT
POMELOS
POPEAFB
POPEDOM
POPELEO
POPEYED
POPEYES
POSEDAS
POSESAS
POSEURS
POSEUSE
POTEENS
POTENCE
POTENCY
POVERTY
POWERED
POWERUP
ROBERTA
ROBERTE
ROBERTF
ROBERTH
ROBERTI
ROBERTO
ROBERTS
ROBESON
RODENTS
RODEOFF
RODEOUT
ROGERED
ROLEXES
RONETTE
ROPEDIN
ROPEDUP
ROPEOFF
ROPESIN
ROPESUP
ROPETOW
ROSEATE
ROSEBAY
ROSEBUD
ROSEHIP
ROSELLA
ROSELLE
ROSEOIL
ROSEOLA
ROSERED
ROSETEA
ROSETTA
ROSETTE
ROTELLE
ROVETTA
ROWELED
ROZELLE
SOBERED
SOBERER
SOBERLY
SOLEDAD
SOMEDAY
SOMEHOW
SOMEONE
SOMESAY
SOMEWAY
SORENTO
TOBEHAD
TOCELIA
TOHEART
TOHELEN
TOKENED
TOLEASE
TOLEDAN
TOLEDOS
TONEARM
TONEDUP
TONELOC
TONEMES
TONEROW
TONESUP
TONETTE
TOOEASY
TOPEKAN
TOREOFF
TOREOUT
TOREROS
TOTEBAG
TOTEMIC
TOTESUP
TOWEDIN
TOWELED
TOWERED
VOLENTE
VOTEAYE
VOTECHS
VOTEDIN
VOTEDNO
VOTEDON
VOTEFOR
VOTENAY
VOTEOUT
VOTESIN
VOTESNO
VOTESON
VOTEYEA
VOTEYES
VOWELLY
WOBEGON
WOKENUP
WOREOFF
WOREOUT

WOWEDEM
YODELED
YODELER
YOTEAMO
ZONEOUT

•O••E••

BOATELS
BOATERS
BOBBERS
BOBWEIR
BOILERS
BOISEID
BOKKENS
BOLDEST
BOLTERS
BOMBECK
BOMBERS
BONDERS
BONHEUR
BONIEST
BONKERS
BONNETS
BOOKEND
BOOKERS
BOOKERT
BOOLEAN
BOOMERS
BOOTEES
BOOTERS
BOOTERY
BOOZERS
BOPPERS
BORDERS
BORNEAN
BORNEUP
BOSWELL
BOTHERS
BOTREES
BOTTEGA
BOWHEAD
BOWLERS
BOWLESS
BOWYERS
BOXBEDS
BOXIEST
BOXSEAT
BOXSETS
COAGENT
COALERS
COATEES
COATERS
COAXERS
COBLENZ
COBWEBS
COCKERS
COCTEAU
CODGERS
COFFEES
COFFERS
COILERS
COINERS
COKIEST
COLBERT
COLDEST
COLLECT
COLLEEN
COLLEGE
COLLETS
COMBERS
COMMEND
COMMENT
COMPEER
COMPELS
COMPEND
COMPERE
COMPETE
CONCEAL
CONCEDE
CONCEIT
CONCEPT
CONCERN
CONCERT
CONDEMN
CONFECT
CONFERS
CONFESS
CONGEAL
CONGERS
CONGEST
CONKERS
CONNECT
CONNERY
CONSENT
CONTEMN
CONTEND
CONTENT
CONTEST
CONTEXT
CONVECT
CONVENE
CONVENT
CONVERT
CONVEYS
COOKERS
COOKERY
COOLERS
COOLEST
COOPERS
COOPERY
COOTERS
COPIERS
COPPERS
COPPERY
COPTERS
CORBELS
CORBETT
CORDELL
CORDERO
CORDERS
CORKERS
CORNEAL
CORNEAS
CORNELL
CORNERS
CORNETS
CORRECT
CORSETS
CORTEGE
CORVEES
CORYELL
COSHERS
COSIEST
COSSETS
COTTERS
COULEES
COUTERS
COWBELL
COWHERD
COWIEST
COWPEAS
COXLESS
COYNESS
COZIEST
COZZENS
DOADEAL
DOCKERS
DOCKETS
DODDERS
DODDERY
DODGEMS
DODGERS
DOFFERS
DOGBEDS
DOGBERT
DOGGETT
DOGLEGS
DOGLESS
DOGREAT
DOGSEAR
DOGVEST
DONKEYS
DONLEVY
DOONEIN
DOOVERS
DOOZERS
DOPIEST
DORMERS
DORSETT
DORSEYS
DOTTERS
DOUCEUR
DOUREST
DOUSERS
DOWNERS
DOWSERS
DOZIEST
FOAMERS
FODDERS
FOELESS
FOGGERS
FOGLESS
FOKKERS
FOLDERS
FOLGERS
FOLLETT
FONDEST
FONTEYN
FOOLERS
FOOLERY
FOOTERS
FOPPERY
FORBEAR
FORCEIN
FORCEON
FORCEPS
FORCERS
FORCEUP
FORFEIT
FORFEND
FORGERS
FORGERY
FORGETS
FORKERS
FORMERS
FORREAL
FORRENT
FORREST
FORWENT
FOSTERS
FOULEST
FOUREEE
FOWLERS
FOXIEST
FOXNEWS
GOAHEAD
GOATEED
GOATEES
GOBLETS
GODDESS
GODHEAD
GODLESS
GODSEND
GODSENT
GOITERS
GOLFERS
GOMPERS
GOOBERS
GOODEGG
GOODERS
GOOIEST
GOONEYS
GOPHERS
GORGERS
GORIEST
GOSPELS
GOSSETT
GOTBEAT
GOTHELP
GOTREAL
GOTWELL
GOUGERS
HOAXERS
HOCKERS
HOGGERY
HOGWEED
HOHNERS
HOKIEST
HOLBEIN
HOLBERG
HOLDERS
HOLIEST
HOLLERS
HOMIEST
HONKERS
HOOFERS
HOOPERS
HOOTERS
HOOVERS
HOPPERS
HORNETS
HOSIERS
HOSIERY
HOSTELS
HOSTESS
HOTBEDS
HOTHEAD
HOTKEYS
HOTLEAD
HOTMEAL
HOTNESS
HOTSEAT
HOTTEAS
HOTTEST
HOWBEIT
HOWDEDO
HOWLERS
HOYDENS
IOBJECT
IONBEAM
JOBBERS
JOBBERY
JOBLESS
JOCKEYS
JODRELL
JOGGERS
JOINERS
JOINERY
JOKIEST
JOLTERS
JOSHERS
JOTTERS
JOYCEAN
JOYLESS
KOBLENZ
KORDELL
KOSHERS
LOADERS
LOAFERS
LOANERS
LOBBERS
LOCKEAN
LOCKERS
LOCKETS
LODGEIN
LODGERS
LOFTERS
LOGGERS
LOGIEST
LOITERS
LOLLERS
LONGEST
LOOKERS
LOOPERS
LOOSELY
LOOSENS
LOOSEST
LOOTERS
LOPPERS
LORIENT
LOTTERS
LOTTERY
LOUDENS
LOUDEST
LOUREED
LOUSEUP
LOUVERS
LOWBEAM
LOWEEZY
LOWGEAR
LOWHEEL
LOWNECK
LOWNESS
LOWRENT
LOWTECH
MOANERS
MOBBERS
MOCKERS
MOCKERY
MOEBERG
MOILERS
MOLDERS
MOLIERE
MOLTERS
MONDESI
MONGERS
MONKEES
MONKEYS
MONTEGO
MONTERO
MONTEUX
MOONERS
MOONEYE
MOOTERS
MOPHEAD
MOPIEST
MOPPERS
MOPPETS
MORCERF
MORDENT
MOREENS
MORSELS
MOSHERS
MOSLEMS
MOTHERS
MOTHERY
MOTLEYS
MOUSERS
NOBLEST
NODDERS
NONDEAF
NONDEEP
NONHERO
NONJEWS
NONMEAT
NONNEWS
NONPEAK
NONSELF
NONZERO
NOONERS
NOOSERS
NORBERT
NORIEGA
NOSEEUM
NOSHERS
NOSIEST
NOSWEAT
NOTBEEN
NOTHERE
NOTNEAR
NOTREAL
NOTWELL
NOUVEAU
NOWHERE
NOWNESS
NOXZEMA
OOBLECK
OOZIEST
POCKETS
POETESS
POISERS
POKIEST
POLLEES
POLLENS
POLLERA
POLLERS
POMMELS
POMPEIA
POMPEII
PONDERS
PONGEES
POOLERS
POOREST
POPPERS
PORKERS
PORSENA
PORTEND
PORTENT
PORTERS
POSHEST
POSSESS
POSTERN
POSTERS
POTEENS
POTHERB
POTHERS
POTTERS
POTTERY
POULENC
POURERS
POUTERS
POWDERS
POWDERY
ROADEOS
ROADERS
ROAMERS
ROARERS
ROBBERS
ROBBERY
ROCHETS
ROCKERS
ROCKERY
ROCKETS
RODGERS
RODLESS
ROEDEER
ROGUERY
ROLFERS
ROLLEIS
ROLLERS
ROMBERG
ROMNEYS
ROMPERS
RONDEAU
RONDELS
ROOFERS
ROOKERY
ROOMERS
ROOTERS
ROPIEST
ROSIEST
ROSTERS
ROSWELL
ROTTERS
ROULEAU
ROUSERS
ROUTERS
ROYBEAN
SOAKERS
SOAPERS
SOARERS
SOAREWE
SOBBERS
SOCIETY
SOCKETS
SOCKEYE
SODLESS
SOFTENS
SOFTEST
SOIREES
SOLDERS
SOLFEGE
SOLNESS
SOLVEIT
SOLVENT
SOLVERS
SONLESS
SONNETS
SOONERS
SOONEST
SORBETS
SORCERY
SORRELL
SORRELS
SORTERS
SOSUEME
SOTHEBY
SOTHERE
SOTHERN
SOTWEED
SOUPERS
SOUREST
SOVIETS
SOWSEAR
SOYBEAN
SOYLENT
SOYMEAL
TOELESS
TOFFEES
TOGGERY
TOILERS
TOILETS
TOLLERS
TOLTECS
TOLUENE
TONIEST
TONNEAU
TOOLERS
TOOTERS
TOPLESS
TOPPERS
TOPSEED
TOPTENS
TORMENT
TORPEDO
TORREFY
TORRENT
TOSSERS
TOTTERS
TOTTERY
TOUPEES
TOURERS
TOUTERS
TOWHEAD
TOWHEES
TOWNERS
TOYLESS
VOGUERS
VOICERS
VOIDERS
VOLLEYS
VONZELL
VOWLESS
WONDERS
WOOFERS
WOOLENS
WOOLERY
WORKERS
WORMERS
WORRELL
WORSENS
WOZZECK
YONKERS
YORKERS
YOTHERS
YOUREIT
YOUREON
YOWLERS
ZOOIEST

•O•••E•

BOARDED
BOARDER
BOASTED
BOASTER
BOATMEN
BOBATEA
BOBBIES
BOBBLED
BOBBLER
BOBBLES
BOBBSEY
BOBGOEN
BOBSLED
BOCCIES
BOCHNER
BODEREK
BODICES
BOGEYED
BOGGIER
BOGGLED
BOGGLER
BOGGLES
BOGYMEN
BOLIDES
BOLSTER
BOLUSES
BOMBLET
BONDMEN
BONELET
BONESET
BONEYER
BONGOES
BONNIER
BONUSES
BOOBIES
BOODLES
BOOGIED
BOOGIES
BOOKIES
BOOKLET
BOOKMEN
BOOMIER
BOOMLET
BOONIES
BOOSLER
BOOSTED
BOOSTER
BOOTEES
BOOTIES
BOOTLEG
BOOZIER
BORATES
BORIDES
BOSOMED
BOSSIER
BOSSMEN
BOTCHED
BOTCHER
BOTCHES
BOTREES
BOTTLED
BOTTLER
BOTTLES
BOUCHER
BOUCHES
BOUFFES
BOUGHED
BOULDER
BOUNCED
BOUNCER
BOUNCES
BOUNDED
BOUNDER
BOUQUET
BOURGET
BOURSES
BOUVIER
BOVINES
BOWDLER
BOWERED
BOWTIES
BOXSTEP
BOXSTER
COACHED
COACHES
COACTED
COAPTED
COARSEN
COARSER
COASTED
COASTER
COATEES
COBBLED
COBBLER
COBBLES
COBUYER
COCHLEA
COCKIER
COCKLED
COCKLES
COCKNEY
CODDLED
CODDLER
CODDLES
CODERED
CODICES
COERCED
COERCER
COERCES
COETZEE
COFFEES
COGGLES
COHERED
COHERER
COHERES
COIFFED
COIGNED
COIGNES
COLLEEN
COLLIER
COLLIES
COLLYER
COLONEL
COLONES
COLORED
COLORER
COMAKER
COMBIEN
COMFIER
COMICES
COMPEER
COMPLEX
COMTREX
CONCHES
CONELET
CONFREY
CONGAED
CONIFER
CONQUER
CONRIED
CONURES
COOKIES
COOLIES
COOPTED
COOTIES
COOWNED
COPYMEN
CORKIER
CORNFED
CORNIER
CORONER
CORONET
CORPSES
CORVEES
COSINES
COSTNER
COUCHED
COUCHES
COUGHED
COULEES
COULTER
COUNSEL
COUNTED
COUNTEE
COUNTEM
COUNTER
COUPLED
COUPLER
COUPLES
COUPLET
COURBET
COURIER
COURSED
COURSER
COURSES
COURTED
COVERED
COVERER
COVETED
COVETER
COWERED
COWRIES
COWSHED
COYOTES
COZENED
COZENER
COZUMEL
DODGIER
DOEEYED
DOGAPES
DOGCHEW
DOGFLEA
DOGGIER
DOGGIES
DOGSLED
DOILIES
DOLLIED
DOLLIES
DOLORES
DONATED
DONATEE
DONATES
DONGLES
DONTBEE
DOODLED
DOODLER
DOODLES
DOOLIES
DOOMIER
DOORMEN
DOOZIES
DOPPLER
DORKIER
DOSAGES
DOSSIER
DOTAGES
DOTTIER
DOTTLES
DOUANES
DOUBLEA
DOUBLEB
DOUBLEC
DOUBLED
DOUBLEE
DOUBLEF
DOUBLEG
DOUBLEH
DOUBLEI
DOUBLEJ
DOUBLEK
DOUBLEL
DOUBLEM
DOUBLEN
DOUBLEO
DOUBLEP
DOUBLEQ
DOUBLER
DOUBLES
DOUBLET
DOUBLEU
DOUBLEV
DOUBLEW
DOUBLEX
DOUBLEY
DOUBLEZ
DOUBTED
DOUBTER
DOVELET
DOWAGER
DOWDIER
DOWDIES
DOWERED
DOWNIER
DOWRIES
EOSINES
FOAMIER
FOCSLES
FOCUSED
FOCUSER
FOCUSES
FOGGIER
FOIBLES
FOISTED
FOLATES
FOLIOED
FOLKIER
FOLKIES
FOLLIES
FONDLED
FONDLER
FONDLES
FONDUED
FONDUES
FOODIES
FOODWEB
FOOTLED
FOOTLER
FOOTLES
FOOTLET
FOOTMEN
FOOZLED
FOOZLER
FOOZLES
FORAGED
FORAGER
FORAGES
FORASEC
FORAYED
FORDOES
FORELEG
FOREMEN
FORESEE
FOREVER
FORFREE
FORGOER
FORGOES
FORKIER
FORSTER
FORTIES
FORTLEE
FOUDRES
FOUNDED
FOUNDER
FOUREEE
FOURIER
GOAFTER
GOALIES
GOATEED
GOATEES
GOBBLED
GOBBLER
GOBBLES
GOBYSEA
GODFREY
GODLIER
GOGETEM
GOGGLED
GOGGLER
GOGGLES
GOLFTEE
GOODIES
GOODMEN
GOOFIER

GOOGLED	HOVERED	LOFTIER	MOORHEN	NOTICES	POWERED	SOOTHER	TOWELED	BOLATIE	CONVOKE	FONTANE	HOVLANE	NOTHOME
GOOGLER	HOVERER	LOLLIES	MOORIER	NOTOPEN	POZOLES	SOOTHES	TOWERED	BOLOTIE	COPPICE	FOOTAGE	HOWCOME	NOTLIKE
GOOGLES	HOWEVER	LONDRES	MORALES	NOTOVER	ROACHES	SOOTIER	TOWHEES	BONAIRE	COPULAE	FOOTSIE	HOWELSE	NOTLIVE
GOONIER	HOWTHEN	LONGBED	MORDRED	NOTUSED	ROADBED	SOPHIES	TOWNIES	BONDAGE	CORACLE	FORBADE	HOWLAME	NOTMINE
GOONIES	IODATED	LONGDEN	MORGUES	NOVICES	ROADIES	SOPPIER	TOWNLET	BONFIRE	CORDAGE	FORBORE	HOWNICE	NOTNICE
GOOPIER	IODATES	LONGIES	MORPHED	NOVOTES	ROASTED	SORRIER	TOYNBEE	BOOPSIE	CORDATE	FORDONE	JOEYDEE	NOTONCE
GOOSIER	IODIDES	LONGUES	MOSEYED	NOWISEE	ROASTER	SORTIED	TOYSLED	BORZAGE	CORDITE	FORESEE	JOHNDOE	NOTRADE
GORETEX	IODISED	LOOBIES	MOSQUES	NOWISER	ROBBNEN	SORTIES	VOCODER	BOSCAGE	CORINNE	FORFREE	JOHNLEE	NOTRARE
GORSIER	IODISES	LOOKSEE	MOSSIER	NOWTHEN	ROCKIER	SOTWEED	VOLCKER	BOWLIKE	CORKAGE	FORGAVE	JOHNNIE	NOTSAFE
GORTNER	IODIZED	LOONIER	MOTHIER	NOZZLES	ROCKIES	SOUNDED	VOLUMED	BOWLINE	CORNICE	FORGIVE	JOURNEE	NOTSURE
GOTEVEN	IODIZER	LOONIES	MOTIVED	OOCYTES	ROEDEER	SOUNDER	VOLUMES	BOXKITE	CORNUTE	FORGONE	JOYRIDE	NOTTOBE
GOTFREE	IODIZES	LOOPIER	MOTIVES	OOLITES	ROGERED	SOUPIER	VOLUTED	BOXLIKE	CORONAE	FORHIRE	LOCKAGE	NOTTRUE
GOTOBED	IONISED	LOPPIER	MOTORED	POACHED	ROILIER	SOURCED	VOLUTES	BOYLIKE	CORRADE	FORLIFE	LONETTE	NOVELLE
GOTOSEA	IONISER	LORELEI	MOTTLED	POACHER	ROISTER	SOURCES	VONBAER	COCAINE	CORRODE	FORLOVE	LOOKSEE	NOWHERE
GOTOSEE	IONISES	LORISES	MOTTLES	POACHES	ROLEXES	SOUTHEY	VONOPEL	COCHISE	CORSAGE	FORONCE	LORANGE	NOWISEE
GOTOVER	IONIZED	LORRIES	MOTTOES	POBOXES	ROLODEX	TOADIED	VORSTER	COCKADE	CORTEGE	FORSAKE	LOSABLE	NOWORSE
GOUNDER	IONIZER	LORUSES	MOULDED	POESIES	RONTGEN	TOADIES	VOTEYEA	CODCAKE	CORVINE	FORSALE	LOVABLE	PODLIKE
GOURDES	IONIZES	LOSTPET	MOULDER	POINTED	ROOKIER	TOASTED	VOTEYES	CODEINE	CORZINE	FORSIZE	LOWDIVE	POETISE
GOURMET	IONONES	LOTUSES	MOULTED	POINTER	ROOKIES	TOASTEE	VOTIVES	COETZEE	COSETTE	FORSURE	LOWLIFE	POETIZE
GOUTIER	JOEYDEE	LOUNGED	MOUNDED	POINTES	ROOMIER	TOASTER	VOUCHED	COGNATE	COSTATE	FORSYTE	LOWRISE	POLEAXE
HOAGIES	JOFFREY	LOUNGER	MOUNTED	POITIER	ROOMIES	TODDIES	VOUCHER	COGNIZE	COSTIVE	FORTLEE	LOWSIDE	POLLUTE
HOARDED	JOGGLED	LOUNGES	MOUNTER	POIVRES	ROOSTED	TODDLED	VOUCHES	COINAGE	COSTUME	FORTUNE	LOWTIDE	POOCHIE
HOARDER	JOGGLER	LOURDES	MOURNED	POLANER	ROOSTER	TODDLER	VOYAGED	COLDONE	COTERIE	FOUETTE	LOZENGE	POOLCUE
HOARIER	JOGGLES	LOUREED	MOURNER	POLEMEN	ROOTIER	TODDLES	VOYAGER	COLETTE	COTTAGE	FOUREEE	MOABITE	POOPSIE
HOARSEN	JOHNLEE	LOUSIER	MOUSIER	POLICED	ROOTLED	TOFFEES	VOYAGES	COLGATE	COULDBE	FOXFIRE	MOBRULE	POPTUNE
HOARSER	JOINDER	LOUVRED	MOUSSED	POLICER	ROOTLES	TOFFLER	WOBBLED	COLLAGE	COUNTEE	FOXHOLE	MOCHRIE	POPWINE
HOBBIES	JOINTED	LOUVRES	MOUSSES	POLICES	ROOTLET	TOGGLED	WOBBLER	COLLATE	COURAGE	FOXLIKE	MODERNE	PORCINE
HOBBLED	JOINTER	LOVAGES	MOUTHED	POLITER	ROSCOES	TOGGLER	WOBBLES	COLLEGE	COUSINE	GOBROKE	MODISTE	PORKPIE
HOBBLER	JOISTED	LOVESET	MOUTHER	POLKAED	ROSERED	TOGGLES	WOLFMEN	COLLIDE	COUTURE	GODLIKE	MOLIERE	PORSCHE
HOBBLES	JOLLIED	LOWBRED	NOANGEL	POLLEES	ROSETEA	TOHELEN	WONOVER	COLLINE	COVERME	GOESAPE	MONDALE	PORTAGE
HOBOKEN	JOLLIER	LOWCHEN	NOBBIER	POLYMER	ROSINED	TOHOMER	WOODIER	COLLUDE	COWBANE	GOLFTEE	MONOCLE	POSABLE
HOCUSED	JOLLIES	LOWERED	NODDIES	POLYPED	ROSSNER	TOKENED	WOODIES	COLOGNE	COWHIDE	GONEAPE	MONTAGE	POSEUSE
HOGTIED	JOLLIET	LOWHEEL	NODULED	POMADED	ROSSSEA	TOLKIEN	WOODLEY	COMBINE	COWLIKE	GOODBYE	MONTALE	POSTAGE
HOGTIES	JOLTIER	LOWLIER	NODULES	POMADES	ROTATED	TOLLMEN	WOOKIEE	COMEDIE	COWPOKE	GOODJOE	MOONEYE	POSTURE
HOGWEED	JONESED	LOYALER	NOGALES	PONGEES	ROTATES	TONEMES	WOOLIER	COMEDUE	COWRITE	GOODONE	MOONPIE	POTABLE
HOISTED	JONESES	LOYALES	NOISIER	PONYKEG	ROTIFER	TONGUES	WOOLIES	COMIQUE	COWROTE	GOODUSE	MOORAGE	POTENCE
HOISTER	JOSTLED	MOBILES	NOMBRES	POOCHES	ROUGHED	TONUSES	WOOLLEN	COMMODE	DOCKAGE	GOSSAGE	MORAINE	POTHOLE
HOLLIES	JOSTLER	MOBSTER	NOMINEE	POODLES	ROUGHEN	TOODLES	WOOLLEY	COMMOVE	DOEUVRE	GOSTALE	MORANTE	POTTAGE
HOLSTER	JOSTLES	MODELED	NONAGES	POOLMEN	ROUGHER	TOOKTEN	WOOLSEY	COMMUNE	DOGBANE	GOTCUTE	MORTICE	ROANOKE
HOLYMEN	JOUNCED	MODELER	NONAMES	POORMEN	ROUNDED	TOOLSET	WOOSHED	COMMUTE	DOGBITE	GOTDONE	MORTISE	ROBERTE
HOLYSEE	JOUNCES	MODEMED	NONDEEP	POPELEO	ROUNDEL	TOONIES	WOOSHES	COMPARE	DOGBONE	GOTFREE	MOSELLE	ROBLOWE
HOMAGER	JOURNEE	MODULES	NONDIET	POPEYED	ROUNDER	TOORDER	WOOSTER	COMPERE	DOGFACE	GOTOSEE	MOULAGE	RODLIKE
HOMAGES	JOURNEY	MOHAVES	NONEVER	POPEYES	ROUSTED	TOOTHED	WOOZIER	COMPETE	DOGGATE	GOTSORE	MOUNTIE	ROETHKE
HOMBRES	JOUSTED	MOISTEN	NONFUEL	POPOVER	ROUSTER	TOOTLED	WORDIER	COMPILE	DOGGONE	GOTWISE	MOVABLE	ROGAINE
HOMEIER	JOUSTER	MOISTER	NONPOET	POPPIES	ROWDIER	TOOTLER	WORKMEN	COMPOSE	DOGLIKE	GOUACHE	NOISOME	ROMAINE
HOMERED	JOWLIER	MOJAVES	NONSKED	POPPLED	ROWDIES	TOOTLES	WORMIER	COMPOTE	DOGPILE	HOECAKE	NOMERGE	ROMANCE
HONALEE	KOEHLER	MOLDIER	NONUKES	POPPLES	ROWELED	TOPAZES	WORRIED	COMPUTE	DOGRACE	HOGLIKE	NOMINEE	RONDURE
HONEYED	KOOKIER	MOLLIES	NONUSER	PORCHES	ROYALES	TOPPLED	WORRIER	COMRADE	DOGROSE	HOGNOSE	NONBASE	RONETTE
HONORED	KOOSHES	MOMMIES	NOODGED	PORGIES	SOAPIER	TOPPLES	WORRIES	CONCAVE	DOGSAGE	HOLYJOE	NONCORE	ROOFAGE
HONOREE	LOAMIER	MOMMSEN	NOODGES	PORIVER	SOAPNET	TOPSEED	WORSLEY	CONCEDE	DOIDARE	HOLYOKE	NONETTE	ROOTAGE
HONORER	LOATHED	MOMONEY	NOODLED	PORKIER	SOBERED	TORCHED	WORSTED	CONCHAE	DOMAINE	HOLYONE	NONHOME	ROSALIE
HOOCHES	LOATHER	MOMUSES	NOODLES	POSITED	SOBERER	TORCHER	WOUNDED	CONCISE	DONAHUE	HOLYSEE	NONLIFE	ROSANNE
HOODIES	LOATHES	MONDIEU	NOOGIES	POSOLES	SODDIER	TORCHES	WOWEDEM	CONDOLE	DONATEE	HOMEICE	NONLIVE	ROSEATE
HOOPMEN	LOBATED	MONEYED	NOOTHER	POSTIES	SOFABED	TORQUED	YODELED	CONDONE	DONJOSE	HONALEE	NONOISE	ROSELLE
HOOPOES	LOBBIED	MONGREL	NOPALES	POSTMEN	SOFTGEL	TORQUES	YODELER	CONDUCE	DONOHOE	HONOREE	NONSALE	ROSETTE
HOOSIER	LOBBIES	MONIKER	NORITES	POTAGES	SOFTIES	TOTALED	YORKIES	CONFIDE	DONTBEE	HOPLITE	NONSANE	ROTELLE
HOPOVER	LOBBYER	MONKEES	NORTHER	POTPIES	SOGGIER	TOTALER	YOUNGER	CONFINE	DONTLIE	HORMONE	NONUPLE	ROULADE
HOPPIER	LOBSTER	MONOMER	NOSIREE	POTTIER	SOHAVEI	TOUAREG	YOUTHEN	CONFUSE	DOORDIE	HOSCALE	NONWAGE	ROUTINE
HORNIER	LOBULES	MONROES	NOTATED	POTTIES	SOIGNEE	TOUCHED	ZOELLER	CONFUTE	DORMICE	HOSPICE	NOPLACE	ROXANNE
HORSIER	LOCALES	MONSTER	NOTATES	POUCHED	SOIREES	TOUCHER	ZOMBIES	CONGAME	DOTLIKE	HOSTAGE	NORDOWE	ROYALWE
HORSLEY	LOCATED	MOOCHED	NOTBEEN	POUCHES	SOLACED	TOUCHES	ZONULES	CONJURE	DOTRICE	HOSTILE	NOSCORE	ROZELLE
HOSTLER	LOCATER	MOOCHER	NOTCHED	POUDRES	SOLACER	TOUGHEN		CONNATE	DOUBLEE	HOTCAKE	NOSIREE	SOAREWE
HOTITEM	LOCATES	MOOCHES	NOTCHER	POUNCED	SOLACES	TOUGHER	**•O••••E**	CONNIVE	DOVERDE	HOTDATE	NOTABLE	SOCKEYE
HOTONES	LOCKLET	MOODIER	NOTCHES	POUNCER	SOLDIER	TOUPEES	BOBDOLE	CONNOTE	DOYENNE	HOTGLUE	NOTALIE	SODIDWE
HOTOVER	LOCKSET	MOONIER	NOTEVEN	POUNCES	SOLIDER	TOURNEY	BOBHOPE	CONSOLE	EONLINE	HOTLINE	NOTAONE	SOIGNEE
HOTTIES	LOESSER	MOONIES	NOTEVER	POUNDED	SOLUTES	TOUSLED	BOBKANE	CONSUME	FOLIAGE	HOTTIME	NOTASTE	SOILAGE
HOUNDED	LOESSES	MOONLET	NOTICED	POUNDER	SOMINEX	TOUSLES	BOGARDE	CONTUSE	FOLIATE	HOTWIRE	NOTDONE	SOLFEGE
HOUNDER	LOFTBED	MOONSET	NOTICER	POUTIER	SOOTHED	TOWAGES	BOGHOLE	CONVENE	FOLIOSE	HOTZONE	NOTHERE	SOLUBLE

SOMEONE
SONANCE
SONLIKE
SORBATE
SOSUEME
SOTHERE
SOUBISE
SOUFFLE
SOURALE
SOWLIKE
TOASTEE
TOBLAME
TOELIKE
TOESHOE
TOHORSE
TOLEASE
TOLLAGE
TOLUENE
TOMKITE
TONETTE
TONNAGE
TONSURE
TONTINE
TOOLATE
TOOTSIE
TOPFIVE
TOPHOLE
TOPLINE
TOPNAME
TOPRATE
TOPSIDE
TORTURE
TOSCALE
TOSPARE
TOTABLE
TOTASTE
TOUGHIE
TOWABLE
TOWLINE
TOWROPE
TOYBIKE
TOYKITE
TOYLIKE
TOYNBEE
VOCABLE
VOITURE
VOLANTE
VOLENTE
VOLPONE
VOLTAGE
VOLTORE
VOLUBLE
VONLAUE
VORLAGE
VOTABLE
VOTEAYE
WOEISME
WOOKIEE
WOOLITE
WORDAGE
WORDONE
WOULDBE
YOULOSE

••OE•••

AMOEBAE
AMOEBAS
AMOEBIC
BOOEDAT
CROESUS
FROEBEL
KROEMER
PHOEBES
PHOEBUS
PHOENIX
PLOESTI
PROEAST
RHOECUS
SHOEBOX
SHOEING
SHOEPAC
SLOEGIN
TOOEASY
TWOEEEE
TWOEGGS
WHOEVER

••O•E••

ADORERS
APOGEAL
APOGEAN
APOGEES
ATONERS
AVOCETS
AVOWERS
AZOREAN
BIOTECH
BLOWERS
BOOKEND
BOOKERS
BOOKERT
BOOLEAN
BOOMERS
BOOTEES
BOOTERS
BOOTERY
BOOZERS
BROKEIN
BROKERS
BROKEUP
CHOKEON
CHOKERS
CHOKEUP
CHOLERA
CHOLERS
CHOSEUP
CLONERS
CLORETS
CLOSEBY
CLOSEIN
CLOSELY
CLOSERS
CLOSEST
CLOSETO
CLOSETS
CLOSEUP
CLOVERS
CLOVERY
COOKERS
COOKERY
COOLERS
COOLEST
COOPERS
COOPERY
COOTERS
CROWELL
CROWERS
DIOCESE
DIOMEDE
DOONEIN
DOOVERS
DOOZERS
DRONEON
DRONERS
DROVEAT
DROVEBY
DROVEIN
DROVERS
DROVETO
DROVEUP
DUODENA
ECOTEUR
ELOPERS
EMOTERS
EPOPEES
ERODENT
ERODERS
EROSELY
ESOBESO
ESOTERY
EVOKERS
EXOCETS
FLOREAL
FLORENZ
FLORETS
FLOWERS
FLOWERY
FOOLERS
FOOLERY
FOOTERS
FROZEUP
GAOLERS
GEODESY
GLOWERS
GOOBERS
GOODEGG
GOODERS
GOOIEST
GOONEYS
GROCERS
GROCERY
GROPERS
GROVELS
GROVERS
GROWERS
HOOFERS
HOOPERS
HOOTERS
HOOVERS
IHOPESO
ILOVEIT
ILOVELA
IMOGENE
IRONERS
ISOHELS
ISOMERS
JROBERT
KNOWERS
KNOWETH
LEOGENN
LIONELL
LIONELS
LIONESS
LIONETS
LOOKERS
LOOPERS
LOOSELY
LOOSENS
LOOSEST
LOOTERS
LYOCELL
LYONELL
MEOWERS
MIOCENE
MOONERS
MOONEYE
MOOTERS
NEOCENE
NEOGENE
NOONERS
NOOSERS
OROGENY
PHONEIN
PHONEME
PHONENO
PHONERS
PHONEYS
PIOLETS
PIONEER
PLOVERS
PLOWERS
POOLERS
POOREST
PROBERS
PROCEED
PROCESS
PROFESS
PROGENY
PROJECT
PROJETS
PROKEDS
PRONELY
PRONETO
PROPELS
PROSERS
PROTEAM
PROTEAN
PROTECT
PROTEGE
PROTEIN
PROTEST
PROTEUS
PROVEIT
PROVERB
PROVERS
PROWESS
PROWEST
PTOLEMY
QUOTEES
QUOTERS
REOPENS
RIOTERS
ROOFERS
ROOKERY
ROOMERS
ROOTERS
SCORERS
SCOTERS
SHOREUP
SHOVEIN
SHOVELS
SHOVERS
SHOWERS
SHOWERY
SLOPERS
SLOVENE
SLOVENS
SLOWEST
SMOKERS
SMOKEUP
SMOKEYS
SNORERS
SOONERS
SOONEST
SPOKEOF
SPOKETO
SPOKEUP
STOKELY
STOKERS
STOKEUP
STOLEIN
STONEAX
STONERS
STORERS
STOREUP
STOWERS
SWOREAT
SWOREBY
SWOREIN
SWORETO
THOREAU
TOOLERS
TOOTERS
TROWELS
TWODEEP
TWOEEEE
TWOFEET
TWOFERS
TWOTERM
TWOWEEK
TWOYEAR
UNOBESE
UNOVERT
USOPENS
VIOLENT
VIOLETS
WOOFERS
WOOLENS
WOOLERY
WROTEIN
WROTEON
WROTETO
WROTEUP
ZOOIEST

••O••E•

ABORTED
ACORNED
ADOPTED
ADOPTEE
ADOPTER
ADORNED
ADORNER
AGONIES
ANOMIES
ANOTHER
APOGEES
APOTHEM
AROUSED
AROUSER
AROUSES
ATOMIES
ATONIES
AVOIDED
AVOIDER
AVONLEA
AZODYES
BIOFUEL
BLOATED
BLOBBED
BLOCKED
BLOCKER
BLOGGED
BLOGGER
BLONDER
BLONDES
BLOODED
BLOOMED
BLOOMER
BLOOPED
BLOOPER
BLOTTED
BLOTTER
BLOUSED
BLOUSES
BLOWIER
BLOWZED
BMOVIES
BOOBIES
BOODLES
BOOGIED
BOOGIES
BOOKIES
BOOKLET
BOOKMEN
BOOMIER
BOOMLET
BOONIES
BOOSLER
BOOSTED
BOOSTER
BOOTEES
BOOTIES
BOOTLEG
BOOZIER
BROADEN
BROADER
BRODIES
BRODKEY
BROGUES
BROIDER
BROILED
BROILER
BRONTES
BRONWEN
BRONZED
BRONZER
BRONZES
BROODED
BROODER
BROOKED
BROOMED
BROSSES
BROTHER
BROWNED
BROWNER
BROWSED
BROWSER
BROWSES
CHOCKED
CHOICER
CHOICES
CHOIRED
CHOKIER
CHOMPED
CHOOSER
CHOOSES
CHOOSEY
CHOPPED
CHOPPER
CHORDED
CHOWDER
CLOAKED
CLOBBER
CLOCHES
CLOCKED
CLOCKER
CLOGGED
CLOMPED
CLONKED
CLOONEY
CLOPPED
CLOTHED
CLOTHES
CLOTTED
CLOUDED
CLOUTED
CLOUTER
CLOWDER
CLOWNED
COOKIES
COOLIES
COOPTED
COOTIES
COOWNED
CROAKED
CROAKER
CROCHET
CROCKED
CROCKER
CROCKET
CROFTER
CRONIES
CROOKED
CROOKES
CROONED
CROONER
CROPPED
CROPPER
CROQUET
CROSIER
CROSSED
CROSSER
CROSSES
CROUTES
CROWDED
CROWDER
CROWLEY
CROWNED
CROWNER
CROZIER
DIOPTER
DOODLED
DOODLER
DOODLES
DOOLIES
DOOMIER
DOORMEN
DOOZIES
DROGUES
DROLLER
DROOLED
DROOLER
DROOPED
DROPLET
DROPNET
DROPPED
DROPPER
DROSSES
DROWNED
DROWSED
DROWSES
DROXIES
EBONIES
ENOILED
EPOPEES
EPOQUES
EPOXIED
EPOXIES
ETOILES
EVOLVED
EVOLVER
EVOLVES
EXOILER
FEOFFED
FLOATED
FLOATER
FLOCKED
FLOGGED
FLOGGER
FLOODED
FLOORED
FLOORER
FLOPPED
FLOPPER
FLOSSED
FLOSSER
FLOSSES
FLOURED
FLOUTED
FLOUTER
FOODIES
FOODWEB
FOOTLED
FOOTLER
FOOTLES
FOOTLET
FOOTMEN
FOOZLED
FOOZLER
FOOZLES
FROCKED
FROEBEL
FROGGER
FROGLEG
FROGLET
FROGMEN
FROMMER
FRONTED
FROSTED
FROSTER
FROTHED
FROTHER
FROWNED
FROWNER
GEORGEC
GEORGEI
GEORGEM
GEORGES
GEORGEV
GEORGEW
GFORCES
GHOSTED
GLOATED
GLOATER
GLOMMED
GLOOMED
GLORIED
GLORIES
GLOSSED
GLOSSER
GLOSSES
GOODIES
GOODMEN
GOOFIER
GOOGLED
GOOGLER
GOOGLES
GOONIER
GOONIES
GOOPIER
GOOSIER
GROANED
GROANER
GRODIER
GROINED
GROKKED
GROLIER
GROMMET
GROOMED
GROOMER
GROOVED
GROOVES
GROSSED
GROSSER
GROSSES
GROUPED
GROUPER
GROUSED
GROUSER
GROUSES
GROUTED
GROUTER
GROWLED
GROWLER
HOOCHES
HOODIES
HOOPMEN
HOOPOES
HOOSIER
IDOTTER
IFORGET
IGOOFED
INORDER
IRONIES
IRONMEN
IVORIES
IWONDER
KNOBBED
KNOCKED
KNOCKER
KNOTTED
KNOTTER
KNOUTED
KNOWLES
KOOKIER
KOOSHES
KROEMER
LOOBIES
LOOKSEE
LOONIER
LOONIES
LOOPIER
MOOCHED
MOOCHER
MOOCHES
MOODIER
MOONIER
MOONIES
MOONLET
MOONSET
MOORHEN
MOORIER
NOODGED
NOODGES
NOODLED
NOODLES
NOOGIES
NOOTHER
OLOGIES
ONORDER
PEONIES
PEOPLED
PEOPLES
PHOEBES
PHONIER
PHONIES
PIONEER
PLODDED
PLODDER
PLONKED
PLOPPED
PLOTTED
PLOTTER
PLOTZED
PLOTZES
PLOWMEN
POOCHES
POODLES
POOLMEN
POORMEN
PROBIES
PROBLEM
PROCEED
PROCTER
PRODDED
PRODDER
PROFFER
PROMOED
PRONGED
PROOFED
PROOFER
PROPHET
PROPJET
PROPMEN
PROPPED
PROSIER
PROSPER
PROUDER
PROWLED
PROWLER
PROXIES
QUOINED
QUOITED
QUONSET
QUOTEES
REOFFER
REOILED
REORDER
REOWNED
ROOKIER
ROOKIES
ROOMIER
ROOMIES
ROOSTED
ROOSTER
ROOTIER
ROOTLED
ROOTLES
ROOTLET
SCOFFED
SCOFFER
SCOLDED
SCOLDER
SCONCES
SCOOPED
SCOOPER
SCOOTED
SCOOTER
SCORNED
SCORNER
SCOUPES
SCOURED
SCOURER
SCOUTED
SCOUTER
SCOWLED
SCOWLER
SHOALED
SHOCKED
SHOCKER
SHODDEN
SHOOTER
SHOPPED
SHOPPER
SHOPPES
SHORTED
SHORTEN
SHORTER
SHOUTED
SHOUTER
SHOWIER
SHOWMEN
SKOSHES
SLOBBER
SLOGGED
SLOGGER
SLOPPED
SLOSHED
SLOSHES
SLOTTED
SLOTTER
SMOKIER
SMOKIES
SMOLDER
SMOTHER
SNOOKER
SNOOPED
SNOOPER
SNOOTED
SNOOZED
SNOOZER
SNOOZES
SNORKEL
SNORTED
SNORTER
SNOUTED
SNOWIER
SNOWMEN
SNOWPEA
SOOTHED
SOOTHER
SOOTHES
SOOTIER
SPOILED
SPOILER
SPONDEE
SPONGED
SPONGER
SPONGES
SPOOFED
SPOOFER
SPOOKED
SPOOLED
SPOOLER
SPOONED
SPOONER
SPORTED
SPOTTED
SPOTTER
SPOUSES
SPOUTED
SPOUTER
STOCKED
STOCKER
STODGED
STODGES
STOGIES
STOLLEN
STOMPED
STONIER
STOOGED
STOOGES
STOOKEY
STOOLED
STOOPED
STOOPER
STOPPED
STOPPER
STORIED
STORIES
STORMED
STOUTEN
STOUTER
SWOLLEN
SWOONED
SWOONER
SWOOPED
SWOOPER
THORNED
TOODLES
TOOKTEN
TOOLSET
TOONIES
TOORDER
TOOTHED
TOOTLED
TOOTLER
TOOTLES
TROCHEE
TROCHES
TRODDEN
TROLLED
TROLLER
TROLLEY
TROMPED
TROOPED
TROOPER
TROTHED
TROTTED
TROTTER
TROUPED
TROUPER
TROUPES
TROUSER
TWODEEP
TWOEEEE
TWOFEET
TWOSTEP
TWOTOED
TWOWEEK
UNOFTEN
UNOGLED
UNOILED
UNOPTED
UNORBED
UNOWNED
VROOMED
WHOEVER
WHOKNEW
WHOMPED
WHOOPED
WHOOPEE
WHOOPER
WHOPPED
WHOPPER
WHORLED
WOODIER
WOODIES
WOODLEY
WOOKIEE
WOOLIER
WOOLIES
WOOLLEN
WOOLLEY
WOOLSEY
WOOSHED
WOOSHES
WOOSTER
WOOZIER
WRONGED
WRONGER

••O•••E

ABOLLAE
ACOLYTE
ACONITE
ACOUPLE
ADOLPHE
ADOPTEE
AGONISE
AGONIZE
ALOHAOE
AMOEBAE

ANODISE
ANODIZE
ANODYNE
APOSTLE
ATOMISE
ATOMIZE
BIOCIDE
BIOLITE
BIOTITE
BIOTYPE
BLONDIE
BOOPSIE
BROCADE
BROMATE
BROMIDE
BROMINE
BROWNIE
CHOLINE
CHOPINE
CHORALE
CHORINE
CHORTLE
CLOSURE
CLOTURE
DIOCESE
DIOMEDE
DIORITE
DIOXIDE
DOORDIE
DUOTONE
EBONITE
EBONIZE
ECOCIDE
ECOTAGE
ECOTYPE
EDOMITE
EGOISTE
ELOCUTE
EMOTIVE
ENOUNCE
EPONINE
EROSIVE
EVOLUTE
FLOSSIE
FLOTAGE
FLOUNCE
FLOWAGE
FOOTAGE
FOOTSIE
FROMAGE
FROOGLE
FROZONE
GEOCODE
GEORGIE
GLOBATE
GLOBOSE
GLOBULE
GLORYBE
GLOSSAE
GOODBYE
GOODJOE
GOODONE
GOODUSE
GROUPIE
IDOLISE
IDOLIZE
IFORONE
IMOGENE
IRONAGE
IRONORE
ISOLATE
ISOLINE
ISOTONE
ISOTOPE
IVORINE
KYOODLE
LEONINE
LEONORE
LIONISE
LIONIZE
LOOKSEE
MIOCENE
MOONEYE
MOONPIE
MOORAGE
NEOCENE
NEOGENE
NEOLYTE
NEONATE
NIOBITE
ODORIZE
OROURKE
OZONISE
OZONIZE
PEONAGE
PHONEME
PLOSIVE
POOCHIE
POOLCUE
POOPSIE
PROBATE
PROCURE
PRODUCE
PROFANE
PROFILE
PROFUSE
PROLATE
PROLIFE
PROMISE
PROMOTE
PRONATE
PROPANE
PROPONE
PROPOSE
PRORATE
PROTEGE
PROVIDE
PROVINE
PROVOKE
ROOFAGE
ROOTAGE
SAOTOME
SCOTTIE
SCOURGE
SHORTIE
SLOVENE
SNOCONE
SPOKANE
SPONDEE
STOOLIE
STOPPLE
STORAGE
STOWAGE
SWOOSIE
TMOBILE
TOOLATE
TOOTSIE
TROCHEE
TROUBLE
TROUNCE
TWOACRE
TWOBASE
TWOEEEE
TWOFACE
TWOLANE
TWOMORE
TWOONIE
TWOSOME
TWOTIME
TWOTONE
UNOBESE
VIOLATE
VIOLONE
WHOOPEE
WHOOPIE
WOOKIEE
WOOLITE
YAOUNDE

•••OE••

CANOERS
ECHOERS
FAROESE
GENOESE
PHLOEMS
UNDOERS
VETOERS

•••O•E•

ABDOMEN
ADWOMEN
AEROBES
AGNOMEN
ALCOVES
ALLOPEZ
ALLOVER
ALLOWED
ALLOYED
ALMONER
ALROKER
ALROSEN
ANDOVER
ANNOYED
ANNOYER
ANYONES
APPOSED
APPOSES
APRONED
ARBOLES
ARBORED
AREOLES
ARMORED
ARMORER
ASKOVER
ATEOVER
ATHOMES
AUTOPEN
BADOMEN
BALONEY
BARONET
BAYONET
BECOMES
BELOVED
BENOTED
BENOTES
BETOKEN
BIGONES
BIGOTED
BILOBED
BLOODED
BLOOMED
BLOOMER
BLOOPED
BLOOPER
BOSOMED
BROODED
BROODER
BROOKED
BROOMED
BUJONES
BYGONES
CAJOLED
CAJOLER
CAJOLES
CAPOTES
CAROLED
CAROLER
CAROMED
CDTOWER
CELOTEX
CHOOSER
CHOOSES
CHOOSEY
CHROMED
CHROMES
CLOONEY
CNTOWER
COLONEL
COLONES
COLORED
COLORER
CORONER
CORONET
COYOTES
CREOLES
CROOKED
CROOKES
CROONED
CROONER
CRYOGEN
CRYOVER
CUTOPEN
CUTOVER
DAHOMEY
DAMOSEL
DEBONED
DEBONES
DECODED
DECODER
DECODES
DECOYED
DECOYER
DEMOTED
DEMOTES
DENOTED
DENOTES
DEPONED
DEPONER
DEPONES
DEPOSED
DEPOSER
DEPOSES
DEPOWER
DETOXED
DETOXES
DEVORES
DEVOTED
DEVOTEE
DEVOTES
DIDOVER
DIPOLES
DISOBEY
DOLORES
DROOLED
DROOLER
DROOPED
DYNODES
EATOVER
ELBOWED
ELBOWER
EMBOWER
EMPOWER
ENCODED
ENCODER
ENCODES
ENCORED
ENCORES
ENDOWED
ENDOWER
ENJOYED
ENJOYER
ENROBED
ENROBES
EXPOSED
EXPOSER
EXPOSES
FAGOTED
FATONES
FAVORED
FAVORER
FLOODED
FLOORED
FLOORER
FLYOPEN
FLYOVER
FURORES
GALOPED
GASOVEN
GENOMES
GETOVER
GLOOMED
GOTOBED
GOTOSEA
GOTOSEE
GOTOVER
GOMODEL
GROOMED
GROOMER
GROOVED
GROOVES
HADOVER
HALOGEN
HANOVER
HASOVER
HEXOSES
HOBOKEN
HONORED
HONOREE
HONORER
HOPOVER
HOTONES
HOTOVER
HUMORED
ICEOVER
IGNORED
IGNORER
IGNORES
IGOOFED
IMBORED
IMHOTEP
IMPOSED
IMPOSER
IMPOSES
INBOXES
INCOMER
INCOMES
INJOKES
INPOWER
INSOLES
INTONED
INTONER
INTONES
INVOKED
INVOKER
INVOKES
INWOVEN
IONONES
ITSOPEN
ITSOVER
JACONET
JDPOWER
JTMONEY
KCJONES
KETONES
LABORED
LABORER
LAYOPEN
LAYOVER
LEGOSET
LIEOVER
LIMOGES
LITOTES
MAHONEY
MAJORED
MASONED
MCCOVEY
MCCOWEN
MEIOSES
MEMOREX
METOOER
MIAOUED
MIAOWED
MINORED
MITOSES
MOMONEY
MONOMER
MOTORED
MRBONES
MRJONES
NICOLET
NOTOPEN
NOTOVER
NOVOTES
OCTOBER
OKTOBER
ONEOVER
OPPOSED
OPPOSER
OPPOSES
ORDONEZ
ORIOLES
OSMOSED
OSMOSES
PAROLED
PAROLEE
PAROLES
PEYOTES
PHLOXES
PICOTED
PILOTED
PINONES
PIROGEN
PIVOTED
PIVOTER
POBOXES
POPOVER
POSOLES
POZOLES
PREOPEN
PROOFED
PROOFER
PRYOPEN
PUTOVER
RADOMES
RAMONES
RANOVER
RAZORED
REBORED
REBORES
REBOTES
REBOXED
REBOXES
RECODED
RECODES
RECOVER
REDOSED
REDOSES
REDOXES
REHONED
REHONES
RELOSES
REMODEL
REMOTER
REMOTES
REMOVED
REMOVER
REMOVES
REMOWED
RENOTED
RENOTES
REPOSED
REPOSER
REPOSES
REPOWER
RESOJET
RESOLED
RESOLER
RESOLES
RESOWED
RETONED
RETONES
RETOWED
REVOKED
REVOKER
REVOKES
REVOTED
REVOTES
REWOKEN
REWOVEN
REYOKED
REYOKES
REZONED
REZONES
RIPOPEN
ROLODEX
RUMORED
RUNOVER
SAMOSET
SAMOYED
SAVORED
SAVORER
SAYOVER
SCHOLES
SCOOPED
SCOOPER
SCOOTED
SCOOTER
SENORES
SHOOTER
SNOOKER
SNOOPED
SNOOPER
SNOOTED
SNOOZED
SNOOZER
SNOOZES
SPOOFED
SPOOFER
SPOOKED
SPOOLED
SPOOLER
SPOONED
SPOONER
STOOGED
STOOGES
STOOKEY
STOOLED
STOOPED
STOOPER
STROBES
STROKED
STROKER
STROKES
SWOONED
SWOONER
SWOOPED
SWOOPER
TABOOED
TABORET
TALONED
TENONED
TENONER
THEOMEN
THEOREM
THRONES
THROWER
TINORES
TIPOVER
TOHOMER
TRIODES
TRIOLET
TROOPED
TROOPER
TUPOLEV
TUTORED
UNBONED
UNBORED
UNBOWED
UNBOXED
UNBOXES
UNCODED
UNCORED
UNCORES
UNCOVER
UNCOWED
UNCOYER
UNDOMED
UNFOXED
UNGORED
UNHONED
UNHOPED
UNJOYED
UNLOBED
UNLOVED
UNMOVED
UNMOWED
UNNOSED
UNNOTED
UNNOVEL
UNPOLED
UNPOSED
UNROBED
UNROBES
UNROPED
UNROPES
UNSOBER
UNSOLED
UNSOLES
UNSOWED
UNTONED
UNVOTED
UNVOWED
UNWOOED
UNWOVEN
UNYOKED
UNYOKES
UNZONED
UNZONES
VALOREM
VANOWEN
VAPORED
VAPORER
VELOXES
VISORED
VIZORED
VOCODER
VONOPEL
VROOMED
WAGONED
WAGONER
WEEONES
WETONES
WHOOPED
WHOOPEE
WHOOPER
WIDOWED
WIDOWER
WIMOWEH
WINOVER
WONOVER
XEROSES
XEROXED
XEROXES
XYLOSES
ZAPOTEC
ZATOPEK
ZYGOTES

•••O••E

ABSOLVE
ALFONSE
ALLOFME
ALLONGE
ALLOWME
AMPOULE
ANTOINE
AREOLAE
ARGONNE
ARMOIRE
AURORAE
AUTOMNE
BAROQUE
BAYONNE
BEHOOVE
BEROWNE
BEYONCE
BICORNE
BINOCHE
BOLOTIE
BRIOCHE
BYFORCE
CABOOSE
CALORIE
CALOTTE
CAROUSE
CATORCE
COLOGNE
CORONAE
CULOTTE
DEBOITE
DEBOULE
DELORME
DELOUSE
DEVOLVE
DEVOTEE
DIVORCE
DONOHOE
ECLOGUE
ELMONTE
ELNORTE
EMBOITE
ENDORSE
ENFORCE
ENGORGE
ENNOBLE
ENROUTE
ENVOGUE
ESPOUSE
FACONNE
FAROESE
FORONCE
FROOGLE
FTDODGE
GARONNE
GAROTTE
GAVOTTE
GENOESE
GENOISE
GIROLLE
GIRONDE
GOTOSEE
HELOISE
HEROINE
HONOREE
HUMORME
IGNOBLE
INDORSE
INFORCE
INHOUSE
INVOGUE
INVOICE
INVOLVE
ITSONME
KYOODLE
LACOSTE
LADOUCE
LAMOTTE
LANOTTE
LAPORTE
LAROCHE
LECONTE
LEMONDE
LEMOYNE
MEMOIRE
MINOGUE
MONOCLE
MRHORSE
MRMOOSE
NICOISE
NICOLLE
NONOISE
NOTONCE
NOWORSE
OCTOBRE
OFNOUSE
OSBORNE
PAPOOSE
PAROLEE
PIROGUE
REFORGE
REHOUSE
REJOICE
REMORSE
REROUTE
RESOLVE
REVOICE
REVOLVE
RIPOSTE
SCROOGE
STOOLIE
STROPHE
STROUSE
SWOOSIE
TOHORSE
TVMOVIE
TWOONIE
UNBORNE
UNHORSE
UNHOUSE
UNLOOSE
UNVOICE
UPBORNE
UPROUSE
VALOTTE
VAMOOSE
VBLOUSE
VELOUTE
VICOMTE
WHOOPEE
WHOOPIE

••••OE•

BANJOES
BEDLOES
BIGTOES
BIMBOES
BINGOES
BOBGOEN
BONGOES
BRAVOED
BRAVOES
BUCKOES
BUNCOED
BUNKOED
CAMEOED
CARGOES
CHIGOES
CISCOES
CITROEN
DINGOES
DISCOED
DITTOED
FAEROES
FOLIOED
FORDOES
FORGOER
FORGOES
FUNGOES
GECKOES
GESSOED
GESSOES
GUSTOES
HELLOED
HELLOES
HOOPOES
HULLOED
IMAGOES
INAPOEM
JINGOES
JUNCOES
LASSOED
LASSOER
LASSOES
LINGOES
MAMBOED
MANGOES
METOOER
MIMEOED
MISDOER
MISDOES
MONROES
MOTTOES
NONPOET
OUTDOER
OUTDOES
OUTGOES
PALJOEY
PINKOES
PROMOED
RADIOED
RADIOER
RESHOES
ROSCOES
SALVOES
SCHMOES
SHAKOES
TABOOED
TANGOED
TANGOER
TIPTOED
TIPTOES
TWOTOED
UNSHOED
UNSHOES
UNWOOED
VIDEOED
WEBTOED

••••O•E

ABALONE
ACEROSE
ACETONE
ADIPOSE
AIRFONE
AIRHOLE
AIRHOSE
ALAMODE
ALCYONE
ALIGOTE
ALLDONE
ALLGONE
AMARONE
AMBROSE
ANATOLE
ANDMORE
ANEMONE
ANYHOPE
ANYMORE
APPROVE
ARDMORE
ARENOSE
ARMBONE
ARMHOLE
ASAJOKE
ATEMORE
AUREOLE
AWESOME
AXLROSE
BADJOKE
BADLOVE
BADMOVE
BALLONE
BANKONE
BARCODE
BARNONE
BEHOOVE
BESPOKE
BESTONE
BIGLOVE
BIGNOSE
BITROLE
BOBDOLE
BOBHOPE
BOGHOLE
BYANOSE
BYPHONE
CABOOSE
CALZONE
CANZONE
CARIOLE
CATHODE
CDSTORE
CHAYOTE
CICCONE

CINEOLE
COLDONE
COMMODE
COMMOVE
COMPOSE
COMPOTE
CONDOLE
CONDONE
CONNOTE
CONSOLE
CONVOKE
CORRODE
COWPOKE
COWROTE
CYCLONE
DEARONE
DELMORE
DEPLORE
DISPOSE
DISROBE
DNACODE
DOGBONE
DOGGONE
DOGROSE
DONJOSE
DRYHOLE
DUOTONE
EARBONE
EARHOLE
EARLOBE
EASYONE
EATMORE
ENCLOSE
ENDNOTE
ENDZONE
EPIDOTE
EPIGONE
EPISODE
EPITOME
EVILONE
EXPLODE
EXPLORE
EYEHOLE
EYESORE
FARGONE
FARMORE
FASTONE
FAXLORE
FIVEONE
FOLIOSE
FORBORE
FORDONE
FORGONE
FORLOVE
FOXHOLE
FRIJOLE
FROZONE
FULSOME
GARROTE
GASTONE
GEOCODE
GETDONE
GETSORE
GILMORE
GLOBOSE
GLUCOSE
GOBROKE
GOODONE
GOTDONE
GOTSORE
GUYROPE
HADDONE
HADSOME
HADTOBE
HAMBONE
HASDONE
HASTOBE
HAVEONE
HIPBONE
HITHOME
HOGNOSE
HOLYOKE
HOLYONE
HORMONE
HOTZONE
HOWCOME
IAMLOVE
ICEHOLE
IFORONE
IFSTONE
ILLDONE
IMBROKE
IMPLODE
IMPLORE
IMPROVE
INAHOLE
INAPOKE
INCLOSE
INSHORE
INSTONE
INSTORE
IRKSOME
IRONORE
ISADORE
ISIDORE
ISOTONE
ISOTOPE
ITEMONE
ITSDONE
ITSGONE
ITSLOVE
JAWBONE
JSTROKE
JUSTONE
KANEOHE
KARAOKE
KENMORE
KEYHOLE
KEYNOTE
LACTOSE
LADRONE
LANCOME
LANEONE
LAPROBE
LASTONE
LATROBE
LEADORE
LEGBONE
LEGROPE
LEONORE
LINEONE
LISSOME
LIVEONE
MACHONE
MADEONE
MAKEONE
MALTOSE
MANHOLE
MANROPE
MARLOWE
MAYPOLE
MELROSE
MICROBE
MIDSOLE
MISCODE
MISDONE
MISMOVE
MISZONE
MRMOOSE
MUDHOLE
NAMEONE
NEURONE
NEWHOPE
NEWLOVE
NEWSOME
NICEONE
NOISOME
NONCORE
NONHOME
NORDOWE
NOSCORE
NOTAONE
NOTDONE
NOTHOME
NOTTOBE
OLDJOKE
OLDROSE
ONELOVE
ONEMORE
ONENOTE
ONEVOTE
ONSHORE
OPEROSE
OPUSONE
OUTCOME
OUTDONE
OUTLOVE
OUTMODE
OUTMOVE
OUTRODE
OUTROVE
OUTSOLE
OUTTORE
OUTVOTE
OUTWORE
PADRONE
PAGEONE
PANTONE
PAPOOSE
PARTONE
PAYMORE
PCCLONE
PENROSE
PEPTONE
PETDOVE
PETIOLE
PIEHOLE
PINHOLE
PISTOLE
PLUMOSE
PLUSONE
POTHOLE
PRECODE
PROMOTE
PROPONE
PROPOSE
PROVOKE
PUGNOSE
PURPOSE
QUIXOTE
RAMHOME
RANHOME
RATHOLE
RCADOME
REAROSE
REAWOKE
REBROKE
RECHOSE
REDBONE
REDNOSE
REDROBE
REDROSE
REDZONE
REEVOKE
REPHONE
REPROBE
REPROVE
REQUOTE
RESCORE
RESPOKE
RESTOKE
RESTORE
RESWORE
REWROTE
RHIZOME
RIPSONE
RISSOLE
ROANOKE
ROBLOWE
RULEONE
RUMPOLE
RUNHOME
SANJOSE
SAOTOME
SATHOME
SAYMORE
SCROOGE
SIDEONE
SIGNORE
SITHOME
SIZEONE
SKIPOLE
SKYDOME
SNOCONE
SOMEONE
SPUMONE
SPYHOLE
STEPONE
SUBCODE
SUBTONE
SUBZONE
SUCROSE
SUPPOSE
SYNCOPE
SYSTOLE
TADPOLE
TAKEONE
TALLONE
TAXCODE
TEAROSE
TEMPORE
TENCODE
TETRODE
THATONE
THEDOLE
THEHOPE
THEPOPE
THEROBE
THEROPE
THEROSE
THISONE
TIEROPE
TOPHOLE
TOWROPE
TRITONE
TWOMORE
TWOSOME
TWOTONE
UNALONE
UNBROKE
UNCHOKE
UNCLOSE
UNFROZE
UNGLOVE
UNICODE
UNLOOSE
UNQUOTE
UNSPOKE
UNSWORE
UNWHOLE
UPABOVE
UPCCODE
UPCLOSE
UPSLOPE
VACUOLE
VALLONE
VAMOOSE
VENDOME
VERBOSE
VINROSE
VIOLONE
VOLPONE
VOLTORE
WALPOLE
WARZONE
WELCOME
WILDONE
WIMPOLE
WINSOME
WISEONE
WORDONE
YEARONE
YESVOTE
YOULOSE
ZEPPOLE
ZIPCODE

•••••OE

ALOHAOE
ARCHFOE
ATIPTOE
BACKHOE
BLEDSOE
DONOHOE
GLENCOE
GOODJOE
GUMSHOE
GYMSHOE
HOLYJOE
ICEFLOE
INASHOE
IVANHOE
JANEDOE
JOHNDOE
MCENROE
MEANJOE
ODDSHOE
OLDSHOE
ONESHOE
OPENTOE
PRUDHOE
RAVELOE
SHADROE
TAPSHOE
TOESHOE
TURFTOE

OF•••••

OFAKIND
OFAMIND
OFANAGE
OFASORT
OFFBASE
OFFBEAT
OFFCAST
OFFDAYS
OFFDUTY
OFFENCE
OFFENDS
OFFENSE
OFFERED
OFFEREE
OFFERER
OFFEROR
OFFERUP
OFFHAND
OFFHOUR
OFFICER
OFFICES
OFFICIO
OFFINGS
OFFLINE
OFFLOAD
OFFPEAK
OFFRAMP
OFFROAD
OFFSETS
OFFSIDE
OFFSITE
OFFWEGO
OFFYEAR
OFNOUSE
OFSORTS
OFTENER
OFVALUE

O•F••••

OFFBASE
OFFBEAT
OFFCAST
OFFDAYS
OFFDUTY
OFFENCE
OFFENDS
OFFENSE
OFFERED
OFFEREE
OFFERER
OFFEROR
OFFERUP
OFFHAND
OFFHOUR
OFFICER
OFFICES
OFFICIO
OFFINGS
OFFLINE
OFFLOAD
OFFPEAK
OFFRAMP
OFFROAD
OFFSETS
OFFSIDE
OFFSITE
OFFWEGO
OFFYEAR
OHFUDGE
ONFIRST
OXFORDS

O••F•••

OAKFERN
OLAFIII
OLDFILM
OLDFOGY
OLEFINS
ONEFOLD
ONEFOOT
ORIFICE
OUTFACE
OUTFAST
OUTFAWN
OUTFEED
OUTFEEL
OUTFIND
OUTFIRE
OUTFISH
OUTFITS
OUTFLEE
OUTFLOW
OUTFLUX
OUTFOOL
OUTFOOT
OVIFORM
OZZFEST

O•••F••

ODORFUL
OKEEFFE
ONEOFFS
ONEOFUS
OPTSFOR
OSSIFIC
OUTOFIT
OVERFAR
OVERFAT
OVERFED
OVERFEE
OVERFEW
OVERFIT
OVERFIX
OVERFLY

O••••F•

OCALAFL
OKEEFFE
ONEOFFS
ONSTAFF
OUTSIFT

O•••••F

OAKLEAF
ONEHALF
ONESELF
ONSTAFF
ONTOPOF
OURSELF

•OF••••

BOFFING
BOFFINS
BOFFOLA
COFFEES
COFFERS
COFFINS
COFOUND
DOFFERS
DOFFING
GOFIRST
GOFORIT
GOFORTH
HOFBRAU
HOFFMAN
HOFMANN
HOFSTRA
JOFFREY
LOFTBED
LOFTERS
LOFTIER
LOFTILY
LOFTING
NOFAULT
SOFABED
SOFARAS
SOFFITS
SOFTENS
SOFTEST
SOFTGEL
SOFTIES
SOFTISH
SOFTTOP
TOFFEES
TOFFLER
TOFUTTI

•O•F•••

BOFFING
BOFFINS
BOFFOLA
BONFIRE
BOUFFES
BOWFINS
BOXFULS
CODFISH
COFFEES
COFFERS
COFFINS
COIFFED
COIFING
COMFIER
COMFITS
COMFORT
CONFABS
CONFECT
CONFERS
CONFESS
CONFIDE
CONFINE
CONFIRM
CONFITS
CONFORM
CONFREY
CONFUSE
CONFUTE
CORFAMS
COWFISH
DOFFERS
DOFFING
DOGFACE
DOGFISH
DOGFLEA
DOGFOOD
DORFMAN
FORFEIT
FORFEND
FORFREE
FOXFIRE
GOAFTER
GODFREY
GOLFBAG
GOLFCAR
GOLFERS
GOLFING
GOLFPRO
GOLFTEE
GOOFIER
GOOFILY
GOOFING
GOOFOFF
GOOFSUP
GOOFUPS
GOSFORD
GOTFREE
HOFFMAN
HOOFERS
HOOFING
HOOFSIT
HOTFOOT
JOBFAIR
JOFFREY
LOAFERS
LOAFING
LOAFPAN
LOOFAHS
NONFACT
NONFANS
NONFARM
NONFLUX
NONFOOD
NONFORM
NONFUEL
NORFOLK
NOTFAIR
POTFULS
ROLFERS
ROLFING
ROOFAGE
ROOFERS
ROOFING
ROOFRAT
ROOFTOP
SOFFITS
SOLFEGE
SOUFFLE
SOXFANS
TOFFEES
TOFFLER
TOMFOOL
TOPFIVE
TOPFORM
TOYFAIR
WOLFCUB
WOLFDOG
WOLFGAL
WOLFING
WOLFISH
WOLFMAN
WOLFMEN
WOLFRAM
WOOFERS
WOOFING

•O••F••

BOATFUL
BODEFUL
BODYFAT
BOUFFES
BOWLFUL
COIFFED
CONIFER
CORNFED
DOESFOR
DOLEFUL
DONEFOR
DOOMFUL
FORKFUL
FORMFUL
GOESFAR
GOESFOR
GOINFOR
GONEFAR
GONEFOR
GOODFOR
HOPEFOR
HOPEFUL
LOGOFFS
LONGFOR
LOOKFOR
MOANFUL
NOGIFTS
POKEFUN
POPOFFS
POSTFIX
POUTFUL
ROOMFUL
ROOTFOR
ROTIFER
SOLDFOR
SONGFUL
SOUFFLE
SOULFUL
TOILFUL
TOOKFOR
VOTEFOR
WOOLFAT
WORKFOR

•O•••F•

BOILOFF
COMEOFF
CONKOFF
CONNIFF
COOKOFF
DOZEOFF
FOBSOFF
FORLIFE
FORTIFY
GOESAFT
GOESOFF
GONEAFT
GONEOFF
GOOFOFF
GOTSOFT
HOLDOFF
HOPSOFF
HORRIFY
JOLLIFY
LOGOFFS
LOGSOFF
LOPSOFF
LOWLIFE
MOLLIFY
MORTIFY
MOVEOFF
NODSOFF
NONLIFE
NORDOFF
NOTSAFE
PONTIFF
POPEAFB
POPOFFS
POPSOFF
RODEOFF
RODOLFO
ROLLOFF
ROPEOFF
SOLDOFF
TOLDOFF
TOOKOFF
TOPSOFF
TOREOFF
TORNOFF
TORREFY
TOSSOFF
WOREOFF
WORKOFF
WORNOFF
ZOMBIFY

•O••••F

BOASTOF
BOILOFF
COMEOFF
CONKOFF
CONNIFF
COOKOFF
DOOUTOF
DOUBLEF
DOZEOFF
FOBSOFF
GOESOFF
GONEOFF
GOOFOFF
HOLDOFF
HOPSOFF
LOADSOF
LOGSOFF
LOPSOFF
MORCERF
MOVEOFF
NODSOFF
NOENDOF
NONDEAF
NONSELF
NORDOFF
NORTHOF
PONTIFF
POPSOFF
ROBERTF
RODEOFF
ROLLOFF
ROPEOFF
SOLDOFF
SOUTHOF
TOLDOFF
TOOKOFF
TOPSOFF
TOREOFF
TORNOFF
TOSSOFF
WOREOFF
WORKOFF
WORNOFF

••OF•••

ASOFNOW
BIOFUEL
CROFTER
FEOFFED
GOOFIER
GOOFILY
GOOFING
GOOFOFF
GOOFSUP
GOOFUPS
HOOFERS
HOOFING
HOOFSIT
LOOFAHS
PROFANE
PROFARM
PROFESS
PROFFER
PROFILE
PROFITS
PROFUSE
REOFFER
ROOFAGE
ROOFERS
ROOFING
ROOFRAT
ROOFTOP
SCOFFAT
SCOFFED
SCOFFER
SHOFARS
TWOFACE
TWOFEET
TWOFERS
TWOFOLD
TWOFOOT
UNOFTEN
WOOFERS
WOOFING

••O•F••

ALOOFLY
BLOWFLY
DOOMFUL
FEOFFED
GOODFOR
GROWFAT
IGOOFED
LOOKFOR
ODORFUL
PLOTFUL
PROFFER
PROOFED
PROOFER
REOFFER
ROOMFUL
ROOTFOR
SCOFFAT
SCOFFED
SCOFFER
SHOOFLY
SHOPFOR
SHOPFUL
SHOTFOR
SPOOFED
SPOOFER
STOPFOR
TOOKFOR
WOOLFAT

••O••F•

BLOWOFF
CHOPOFF
COOKOFF
DROPOFF
GLORIFY
GOOFOFF
ICONIFY
PROLIFE
SHONUFF
SHOOOFF
SHOWOFF
STOPOFF
TOOKOFF
TROTOFF

••O•••F

AFOULOF
AHOSTOF
ALOADOF
BEOWULF
BLOWOFF
CHOPOFF
COOKOFF
DOOUTOF
DROPOFF
EGOSURF
GOOFOFF
KNOWSOF
PROUDOF
SHONUFF
SHOOOFF
SHORTOF
SHOWOFF
SPOKEOF
STOPOFF
TOOKOFF
TROTOFF

•••OF••
ALLOFIT
ALLOFME
ALLOFUS
ALOOFLY
BUYOFFS
CUTOFFS
DIEOFFS
FILOFAX
IGOOFED
INSOFAR
LAYOFFS
LOGOFFS
MIDOFFS
ONEOFFS
ONEOFUS
OUTOFIT
PAYOFFS
POPOFFS
PROOFED
PROOFER
PUTOFFS
RIPOFFS
RUNOFFS
SETOFFS
SHOOFLY
SPOOFED
SPOOFER
TEEOFFS
TIPOFFS
UNLOFTY

•••O•F•
BUYOFFS
CUTOFFS
DIEOFFS
LAYOFFS
LOGOFFS
MIDOFFS
ONEOFFS
PAYOFFS
POPOFFS
PUTOFFS
REROOFS
RIPOFFS
RODOLFO
RUDOLFI
RUNOFFS
SETOFFS
SHOOOFF
TEEOFFS
TIPOFFS
UNROOFS

•••O••F
ONTOPOF
SHOOOFF

••••OF•
BACKOFF
BAKEOFF
BEAROFF
BEATOFF
BEGSOFF
BESTOFF
BINDOFF
BITEOFF
BLEWOFF
BLOWOFF
BOILOFF
BUGSOFF
BURNOFF
BUYSOFF
BUZZOFF
CALLOFF
CAMEOFF
CARTOFF
CASTOFF
CHOPOFF
CLIPOFF
COMEOFF
CONKOFF
COOKOFF
CUTSOFF
DAMPOFF
DARTOFF
DASHOFF
DAYSOFF
DIEDOFF
DIESOFF
DOZEOFF
DRAGOFF
DRAWOFF
DREWOFF
DROPOFF
DUSTOFF
EASEOFF
EASYOFF
EVENOFF
FACEOFF
FAIROFF
FALLOFF
FEELOFF
FELLOFF
FELTOFF
FENDOFF
FIREOFF
FOBSOFF
GAVEOFF
GETSOFF
GETSOFT
GIVEOFF
GOESOFF
GONEOFF
GOOFOFF
GOTSOFT
HACKOFF
HANDOFF
HANGOFF
HATSOFF
HAULOFF
HAYLOFT
HEADOFF
HELDOFF
HENTOFF
HITSOFF
HIVEOFF
HOLDOFF
HOPSOFF
HUNGOFF
JUMPOFF
KARLOFF
KEEPOFF
KEPTOFF
KICKOFF
KISSOFF
LAIDOFF
LAYSOFF
LEADOFF
LEFTOFF
LETSOFF
LIFTOFF
LIPSOFF
LOGSOFF
LOPSOFF
MADEOFF
MAKEOFF
MARKOFF
MOVEOFF
MYCROFT
NODSOFF
NORDOFF
PACEOFF
PACKOFF
PAIDOFF
PAIROFF
PALMOFF
PASSOFF
PAWNOFF
PAYSOFF
PEELOFF
PERSOFF
PICKOFF
PLAYOFF
POPSOFF
PULLOFF
PUSHOFF
PUTSOFF
RAKEOFF
RANGOFF
READOFF
REELOFF
REROOFS
RIDEOFF
RINGOFF
RIPSOFF
RODEOFF
ROLLOFF
ROPEOFF
RUBSOFF
RUNGOFF
RUNSOFF
RUSHOFF
SARNOFF
SAWNOFF
SAWSOFF
SEALOFF
SEENOFF
SEESOFF
SELLOFF
SENDOFF
SENTOFF
SETSOFF
SHOOOFF
SHOWOFF
SHUTOFF
SIGNOFF
SLIDOFF
SLIPOFF
SNIPOFF
SOLDOFF
SPEDOFF
SPINOFF
SPUNOFF
STAYOFF
STEPOFF
STOPOFF
SYDHOFF
TAILOFF
TAKEOFF
TAPSOFF
TEAROFF
TEEDOFF
TEESOFF
TELLOFF
TICKOFF
TIEDOFF
TIESOFF
TIMEOFF
TIPSOFF
TOLDOFF
TOOKOFF
TOPSOFF
TOREOFF
TORNOFF
TOSSOFF
TRIMOFF
TROTOFF
TURNOFF
UNROOFS
VEEROFF
WALKOFF
WALLOFF
WARDOFF
WARNOFF
WASHOFF
WAVEOFF
WEAROFF
WELLOFF
WENTOFF
WIPEOFF
WOREOFF
WORKOFF
WORNOFF
YANKOFF
ZIPSOFF

••••O•F
AIRWOLF
ALTDORF
BACKOFF
BAKEOFF
BEAROFF
BEATOFF
BEGSOFF
BESTOFF
BINDOFF
BITEOFF
BLEWOFF
BLOWOFF
BOILOFF
BUGSOFF
BURNOFF
BUYSOFF
BUZZOFF
CALLOFF
CAMEOFF
CARTOFF
CASTOFF
CHOPOFF
CLIPOFF
COMEOFF
CONKOFF
COOKOFF
CRYWOLF
CUTSOFF
DAMPOFF
DARTOFF
DASHOFF
DAYSOFF
DIEDOFF
DIESOFF
DOZEOFF
DRAGOFF
DRAWOFF
DREWOFF
DROPOFF
DUSTOFF
EASEOFF
EASYOFF
EVENOFF
FACEOFF
FAIROFF
FALLOFF
FEELOFF
FELLOFF
FELTOFF
FENDOFF
FIREOFF
FOBSOFF
GAVEOFF
GETSOFF
GIVEOFF
GOESOFF
GONEOFF
GOOFOFF
HACKOFF
HANDOFF
HANGOFF
HATSOFF
HAULOFF
HEADOFF
HELDOFF
HENTOFF
HIPROOF
HITSOFF
HIVEOFF
HOLDOFF
HOPSOFF
HUNGOFF
JUMPOFF
KARLOFF
KEEPOFF
KEPTOFF
KICKOFF
KISSOFF
LAIDOFF
LAYSOFF
LEADOFF
LEFTOFF
LETGOOF
LETSOFF
LIFTOFF
LINDORF
LIPSOFF
LOGSOFF
LOPSOFF
MADEOFF
MAKEOFF
MARKOFF
MOVEOFF
NODSOFF
NORDOFF
PACEOFF
PACKOFF
PAIDOFF
PAIROFF
PALMOFF
PASSOFF
PAWNOFF
PAYSOFF
PEELOFF
PERSOFF
PICKOFF
PLAYOFF
POPSOFF
PULLOFF
PUSHOFF
PUTSOFF
RAKEOFF
RANGOFF
READOFF
REDWOLF
REELOFF
REPROOF
RIDEOFF
RINGOFF
RIPSOFF
RODEOFF
ROLLOFF
ROPEOFF
RUBSOFF
RUNGOFF
RUNSOFF
RUSHOFF
RYELOAF
SARNOFF
SAWNOFF
SAWSOFF
SEALOFF
SEAWOLF
SEENOFF
SEESOFF
SELLOFF
SENDOFF
SENTOFF
SETSOFF
SHEWOLF
SHOOOFF
SHOWOFF
SHUTOFF
SIGNOFF
SLIDOFF
SLIPOFF
SNIPOFF
SOLDOFF
SPEDOFF
SPINOFF
SPUNOFF
STAYOFF
STEPOFF
STOPOFF
SUNROOF
SYDHOFF
TAILOFF
TAKEOFF
TAPSOFF
TEAROFF
TEEDOFF
TEESOFF
TELLOFF
TICKOFF
TIEDOFF
TIESOFF
TIMEOFF
TINROOF
TIPSOFF
TOLDOFF
TOOKOFF
TOPSOFF
TOREOFF
TORNOFF
TOSSOFF
TRIMOFF
TROTOFF
TURNOFF
VEEROFF
WALDORF
WALKOFF
WALLOFF
WARDOFF
WARNOFF
WASHOFF
WAVEOFF
WEAROFF
WELLOFF
WENTOFF
WIPEOFF
WOREOFF
WORKOFF
WORNOFF
YANKOFF
ZIPSOFF

•••••OF
AFOULOF
AHEADOF
AHOSTOF
AKERLOF
ALACKOF
ALOADOF
APAIROF
APECKOF
APILEOF
ARAFTOF
ASKEDOF
ASLEWOF
AWAREOF
BARANOF
BOASTOF
BYWAYOF
CLEAROF
DOOUTOF
DREAMOF
FREEDOF
FREESOF
GIVENOF
GIVESOF
HEAPSOF
HEARDOF
HEARSOF
HIPROOF
INAIDOF
INAWEOF
KNOWSOF
LEARNOF
LETGOOF
LOADSOF
NOENDOF
NORTHOF
ONTOPOF
PILESOF
PROUDOF
REEKSOF
REPROOF
SCADSOF
SHORTOF
SMACKOF
SOUTHOF
SPEAKOF
SPOKEOF
STRIPOF
SUNROOF
SUREROF
TALKSOF
TELLSOF
THEREOF
THINKOF
TINROOF
TIREDOF
TIRESOF
WARNSOF
WHEREOF

OG•••••
OGDENUT
OGDOADS
OGHAMIC
OGLALAS
OGREISH

O•G••••
ONGOING
ONGUARD
ORGANDY
ORGANIC
ORGANZA
ORGEATS
ORGIAST
OUGHTNT
OUGHTTO
OUGUIYA

O••G•••
OLDGAGS
OLDGIRL
OLDGOLD
OLOGIES
OMIGOSH
ONAGERS
ONEGRAM
OREGANO
ORIGAMI
ORIGINE
ORIGINS
OROGENY
OURGANG
OUTGAIN
OUTGAME
OUTGAVE
OUTGAZE
OUTGIVE
OUTGLOW
OUTGNAW
OUTGOES
OUTGREW
OUTGRIN
OUTGROW
OUTGUNS
OUTGUSH
OWNGOAL

O•••G••
OBLIGED
OBLIGEE
OBLIGER
OBLIGES
OBLIGOR
OCTAGON
ODINGON
OHMAGES
OKAYGUY
ONSAGER
ONSIGHT
OPPUGNS
ORANGES
ORANGEY
ORTEGAL
OTALGIA
OTALGIC
OUTAGES
OWINGON
OWINGTO
OWLEGGS

O••••G•
OAKTAGS
OBLONGS
OFANAGE
OFFINGS
OFFWEGO
OHFUDGE
OILRIGS
OLDDOGS
OLDFOGY
OLDGAGS
ONEPAGE
ONETOGO
ONSTAGE
ONTHEGO
OOLONGS
OROLOGY
OTOLOGY
OUTBEGS
OUTEDGE
OUTINGS
OUTRAGE
OUTRIGS
OUTSIGH
OVERAGE
OWLEGGS

O•••••G
OBEYING
OILRING
OINKING
OKAYING
OLDSONG
OMENING
ONGOING
OPENING
OPINING
ORATING
OURGANG
OURSONG
OUSTING
OUTBRAG
OUTDRAG
OUTKING
OUTRANG
OUTRING
OUTSANG
OUTSING
OUTSUNG
OUTWING
OVERBIG
OVERDOG

•OG••••
BOGARDE
BOGARTS
BOGDOWN
BOGEYED
BOGGIER
BOGGING
BOGGISH
BOGGLED
BOGGLER
BOGGLES
BOGGUSS
BOGHOLE
BOGUSLY
BOGYMAN
BOGYMEN
COGBURN
COGENCY
COGGING
COGGLES
COGHLAN
COGNACS
COGNATE
COGNIZE
DOGAPES
DOGBANE
DOGBEDS
DOGBERT
DOGBITE
DOGBONE
DOGBOOT
DOGBOWL
DOGCART
DOGCHEW
DOGCHOW
DOGCOAT
DOGCOMB
DOGDAYS
DOGDOOR
DOGEARS
DOGFACE
DOGFISH
DOGFLEA
DOGFOOD
DOGGATE
DOGGETT
DOGGIER
DOGGIES
DOGGING
DOGGISH
DOGGONE
DOGHAIR
DOGLEGS
DOGLESS
DOGLIKE
DOGMATA
DOGNAPS
DOGPILE
DOGRACE
DOGREAT
DOGROSE
DOGRUNS
DOGSAGE
DOGSEAR
DOGSHOW
DOGSITS
DOGSLED
DOGSTAR
DOGTAGS
DOGTAIL
DOGTICK
DOGTOYS
DOGTROT
DOGVEST
DOGWOOD
FOGBANK
FOGBOWS
FOGCITY
FOGDOGS
FOGERTY
FOGGERS
FOGGIER
FOGGILY
FOGGING
FOGHORN
FOGLAMP
FOGLESS
FOGYISH
FOGYISM
GOGETEM
GOGGLED
GOGGLER
GOGGLES
GOGIRLS
HOGARTH
HOGBACK
HOGCALL
HOGGERY
HOGGING
HOGGISH
HOGLIKE
HOGNOSE
HOGNUTS
HOGTIED
HOGTIES
HOGWASH
HOGWEED
HOGWILD
JOGBRAS
JOGGERS
JOGGING
JOGGLED
JOGGLER
JOGGLES
JOGTROT
LOGANUT
LOGBOOK
LOGGERS
LOGGIAS
LOGGING
LOGGINS
LOGGISH
LOGICAL
LOGIEST
LOGJAMS
LOGOFFS
LOGONTO
LOGOUTS
LOGROLL
LOGSOFF
LOGSOUT
MOGADOR
MOGAMBO
NOGALES
NOGGINS
NOGIFTS
NOGOODS
NOGUCHI
ROGAINE
ROGERED
ROGUERY
ROGUING
ROGUISH
SOGGIER
SOGGILY
TOGGERY
TOGGING
TOGGLED
TOGGLER
TOGGLES
TOGSOUT
VOGUERS
VOGUING
VOGUISH
YOGAMAT
YOGHURT
YOGIISM
YOGINIS
YOGURTS

•O•G•••
BOBGOEN
BOGGIER
BOGGING
BOGGISH
BOGGLED
BOGGLER
BOGGLES
BOGGUSS
BONGING
BONGOES
BOOGIED
BOOGIES
BORGIAS
BORGLUM
BOUGHED
COAGENT
CODGERS
COGGING
COGGLES
COIGNED
COIGNES
COLGATE
CONGAED
CONGAME
CONGEAL
CONGERS
CONGEST
CONGOUS
COUGARS
COUGHED
COUGHUP
COWGIRL
DOAGAIN
DODGEMS
DODGERS
DODGIER
DODGING
DODGSON
DOGGATE
DOGGETT
DOGGIER
DOGGIES
DOGGING
DOGGISH
DOGGONE
DONGLES
DOUGHTY
DOUGLAS
FOGGERS
FOGGIER
FOGGILY
FOGGING
FOLGERS
FORGAVE
FORGERS
FORGERY
FORGETS
FORGING
FORGIVE
FORGOER
FORGOES
FORGONE
FORGOOD
GOGGLED
GOGGLER
GOGGLES
GONGING
GONGORA
GOOGLED
GOOGLER
GOOGLES
GOOGOLS
GORGERS
GORGING
GORGONS
GOTGOOD
GOUGERS
GOUGING
HOAGIES
HOGGERY
HOGGING
HOGGISH
HOTGLUE
JOGGERS
JOGGING
JOGGLED
JOGGLER
JOGGLES
LODGEIN
LODGERS
LODGING
LOGGERS
LOGGIAS
LOGGING
LOGGINS

LOGGISH
LONGAGO
LONGARM
LONGBED
LONGBOW
LONGDAY
LONGDEN
LONGEST
LONGFOR
LONGIES
LONGING
LONGISH
LONGRUN
LONGTOM
LONGTON
LONGUES
LONGWAY
LORGNON
LOWGEAR
MONGERS
MONGKUT
MONGOLS
MONGREL
MORGANA
MORGANS
MORGUES
NOGGINS
NONGOGO
NONGOLD
NOOGIES
NOTGOOD
NOUGATS
NOUGHTS
PONGEES
PONGIDS
POPGUNS
PORGIES
RODGERS
ROTGUTS
ROUGHED
ROUGHEN
ROUGHER
ROUGHGO
ROUGHIT
ROUGHLY
ROUGHUP
ROUGING
ROYGBIV
SOGGIER
SOGGILY
SOIGNEE
SONGFUL
SORGHUM
TOGGERY
TOGGING
TOGGLED
TOGGLER
TOGGLES
TOMGOLA
TONGANS
TONGING
TONGUES
TOPGUNS
TOUGHEN
TOUGHER
TOUGHIE
TOUGHLY
TOYGUNS
VOSGIAN

•O••G••

BODEGAS
BOLOGNA
BOURGET
COALGAS
COLOGNE
CONAGRA
COSIGNS
DOINGIN
DOINGOK
DOINGSO
DOINGTO
DOINGUP
DONEGAL
DONEGAN
DORIGHT
DOSAGES
DOTAGES
DOWAGER
FORAGED
FORAGER
FORAGES
FORDGTS
GOINGAT
GOINGBY
GOINGIN
GOINGON
GOINGTO
GOINGUP
GOODGUY
GOTOGAL
GOTOGUY
HOMAGER
HOMAGES
JOHNGAY
KOSYGIN
LONIGAN
LOUNGED
LOUNGER
LOUNGES
LOVAGES
MOHEGAN
MOONGOD
NOANGEL
NONAGES
NONAGON
NOODGED
NOODGES
NOSEGAY
NOSUGAR
POLYGON
POTAGES
RONTGEN
SOFTGEL
TONIGHT
TOWAGES
VOYAGED
VOYAGER
VOYAGES
WOBEGON
WOLFGAL
YOUNGER
YOUNGMC
YOUNGUN

•O•••G•

BODINGS
BOEINGS
BONDAGE
BORINGS
BOROUGH
BORZAGE
BOSCAGE
BOTTEGA
COINAGE
COLLAGE
COLLEGE
COMINGS
CONDIGN
CONSIGN
CORDAGE
CORKAGE
CORSAGE
CORTEGE
COTTAGE
COURAGE
COYDOGS
DOCKAGE
DOGLEGS
DOGSAGE
DOGTAGS
DOMINGO
DONOTGO
FOGDOGS
FOLENGO
FOLIAGE
FOOTAGE
FOREIGN
GONZAGA
GOODEGG
GOSSAGE
GOTTAGO
HOSTAGE
HOTDOGS
HOWHIGH
LOCKAGE
LONGAGO
LORANGE
LOSINGS
LOZENGE
MONTAGE
MONTAGU
MONTEGO
MOORAGE
MOULAGE
MOWINGS
NOMERGE
NONGOGO
NONWAGE
NORIEGA
OOLONGS
PORTAGE
POSTAGE
POTTAGE
RODRIGO
ROOFAGE
ROOTAGE
ROUGHGO
ROVINGS
SOILAGE
SOLFEGE
TOLLAGE
TONNAGE
TOOHIGH
TOPDOGS
TORTUGA
TOWINGS
TOYDOGS
VOLTAGE
VORLAGE
WORDAGE
ZOOLOGY

•O••••G

BOATING
BOBBING
BOFFING
BOGGING
BOILING
BOLLING
BOLTING
BOMBING
BONDING
BONGING
BONKING
BOOKBAG
BOOKING
BOOMING
BOOTING
BOOTLEG
BOOZING
BOPPING
BORKING
BORLAUG
BOSSING
BOWLING
COALING
COATING
COAXING
COCKING
COGGING
COIFING
COILING
COINING
COMBING
COMPING
CONKING
CONNING
COOKING
COOLING
COONDOG
COOPING
COPPING
COPYING
CORDING
CORKING
CORNDOG
CORNING
COSHING
COSTING
COSYING
COUPING
COWLING
COZYING
DOCKING
DODGING
DOFFING
DOGGING
DOLLING
DONKING
DONNING
DOOMING
DOSSING
DOTTING
DOUBLEG
DOUSING
DOWLING
DOWNING
DOWRONG
DOWSING
FOALING
FOAMING
FOBBING
FOGGING
FOILING
FOLDING
FOOLING
FOOTBAG
FOOTING
FORCING
FORDING
FORELEG
FORGING
FORKING
FORMING
FOULING
FOWLING
GOADING
GOALONG
GODLING
GOLDBUG
GOLDING
GOLFBAG
GOLFING
GONGING
GOODDOG
GOODEGG
GOODING
GOOFING
GOOSING
GORGING
GORMING
GOSLING
GOUGING
GOWNING
GOWRONG
HOAXING
HOBOING
HOCKING
HODDING
HOGGING
HOLBERG
HOLDING
HOMBURG
HONKING
HOODING
HOOFING
HOOKING
HOOPING
HOOTING
HOPPING
HOPSING
HORDING
HORNING
HORNUNG
HORSING
HOSTING
HOUSING
HOWLING
HOWLONG
JOBBING
JOGGING
JOINING
JOLTING
JOSHING
JOTTING
KOONING
LOADING
LOAFING
LOAMING
LOANING
LOBBING
LOCKING
LODGING
LOFTING
LOGGING
LOIDING
LOLLING
LONBORG
LONGING
LOOKING
LOOMING
LOOPING
LOOSING
LOOTING
LOPPING
LORDING
LOSEBIG
LOSTBIG
LOSTDOG
LOTTING
LOURING
LOUSING
LOUTING
LOVEBUG
MOANING
MOBBING
MOCKING
MOEBERG
MOILING
MOLDING
MOLTING
MONOLOG
MOONDOG
MOONING
MOORING
MOOTING
MOPPING
MORNING
MOSHING
MOSSING
MOUSING
NOCKING
NODDING
NOISING
NONDRUG
NOONING
NOOSING
NOSEBAG
NOSHING
NOTHING
NOTTING
POISING
POLLING
PONDING
PONYING
PONYKEG
POOLING
POOPING
POPPING
POPSONG
PORKING
PORTING
POSTBAG
POSTING
POTTING
POURING
POUTING
ROADHOG
ROAMING
ROARING
ROBBING
ROCKING
RODDING
ROGUING
ROILING
ROLFING
ROLLING
ROLVAAG
ROMBERG
ROMPING
ROOFING
ROOKING
ROOMING
ROOTING
ROTTING
ROUGING
ROUSING
ROUTING
ROWLING
SOAKING
SOAPING
SOARING
SOBBING
SOCKING
SODDING
SOILING
SOLOING
SOLVING
SOPPING
SORTING
SOURING
SOUSING
TOGGING
TOILING
TOLLING
TONGING
TOOLING
TOOLONG
TOOTING
TOPPING
TOSSING
TOTEBAG
TOTTING
TOUAREG
TOURING
TOUTING
VOGUING
VOICING
VOIDING
WOLFDOG
WOLFING
WONTING
WOODING
WOOFING
WORDING
WORKING
WORMING
YOURANG
YOWLING
YOYOING
ZONKING
ZOOMING

••OG•••

APOGEAL
APOGEAN
APOGEES
BEOGRAD
BLOGGED
BLOGGER
BOOGIED
BOOGIES
BROGANS
BROGUES
CLOGGED
CLOGSUP
DROGUES
EXOGAMY
FLOGGED
FLOGGER
FROGGER
FROGLEG
FROGLET
FROGMAN
FROGMEN
GOOGLED
GOOGLER
GOOGLES
GOOGOLS
IMOGENE
ISOGONS
ISOGRAM
KEOGHAN
LEOGENN
NEOGENE
NOOGIES
OLOGIES
OROGENY
PROGENY
PROGRAM
SHOGUNS
SLOGANS
SLOGGED
SLOGGER
STOGIES
UNOGLED

••O•G••

AMONGST
BLOGGED
BLOGGER
BLOWGUN
BROUGHT
CHOUGHS
CLOGGED
DROUGHT
FLOGGED
FLOGGER
FROGGER
FROOGLE
GEORGEC
GEORGEI
GEORGEM
GEORGES
GEORGEV
GEORGEW
GEORGIA
GEORGIC
GEORGIE
GIORGIO
GIORGOS
GOODGUY
IFORGET
IFORGOT
MOONGOD
NEONGAS
NOODGED
NOODGES
PLOUGHS
PRONGED
RIOTGUN
SHOTGUN
SLOEGIN
SLOGGED
SLOGGER
SLOUGHS
SPONGED
SPONGER
SPONGES
STODGED
STODGES
STOOGED
STOOGES
STOPGAP
THOUGHT
TROUGHS
TSONGAS
TWOEGGS
WRONGED
WRONGER
WRONGLY
WROUGHT

••O••G•

APOLOGY
BIOLOGY
ECOLOGY
ECOTAGE
ENOLOGY
FLOTAGE
FLOWAGE
FOOTAGE
FROMAGE
GEOLOGY
GOODEGG
IRONAGE
MOORAGE
MYOLOGY
NEOLOGY
OROLOGY
OTOLOGY
PEONAGE
PHOTOGS
PRODIGY
PROLOGS
PROTEGE
ROOFAGE
ROOTAGE
SCOURGE
STORAGE
STOWAGE
TOOHIGH
TWOEGGS
UFOLOGY
UROLOGY
ZOOLOGY

••O•••G

ADORING
ATONING
AVOWING
BLOWING
BOOKBAG
BOOKING
BOOMING
BOOTING
BOOTLEG
BOOZING
BUOYING
CHOKING
CHOWING
CLONING
CLOSING
CLOYING
COOKING
COOLING
COONDOG
COOPING
CROWING
DOOMING
DRONING
ELOPING
EMOTING
ERODING
EVOKING
FLOWING
FOOLING
FOOTBAG
FOOTING
FRODING
FROGLEG
GAOLING
GLOBING
GLOVING
GLOWING
GOODDOG
GOODEGG
GOODING
GOOFING
GOOSING
GROPING
GROWBIG
GROWING
HOODING
HOOFING
HOOKING
HOOPING
HOOTING
IRONING
KNOWING
KOONING
LOOKING
LOOMING
LOOPING
LOOSING
LOOTING
MEOWING
MOONDOG
MOONING
MOORING
MOOTING
NOONING
NOOSING
PHONING
PLOWING
POOLING
POOPING
PROBING
PROLONG
PROSING
PROVING
QUOTING
RIOTING
ROOFING
ROOKING
ROOMING
ROOTING
SCOPING
SCORING
SHOEING
SHOOING
SHORING
SHOVING
SHOWDOG
SHOWING
SLOPING
SLOWING
SMOKING
SNORING
SNOWING
SPOKING
STOKING
STONING
STORING
STOWING
TOOLING
TOOLONG
TOOTING
TROWING
UNOWING
WOODING
WOOFING
WYOMING
YAOMING
ZOOMING

•••OG••

BOLOGNA
COLOGNE
CRYOGEN
ECLOGUE
ENVOGUE
FROOGLE
GOTOGAL
GOTOGUY
HALOGEN
ILLOGIC
INVOGUE
LIMOGES
MINOGUE
MTLOGAN
PIROGEN
PIROGUE
STOOGED
STOOGES
UNBOGGY
UNFOGGY
UNSOGGY

•••O•G•

ALLONGE
BELONGS
BOROUGH
CYBORGS
DONOTGO
DUGONGS
ENGORGE
FTDODGE
IFYOUGO
LAZONGA
MACONGA
OBLONGS
OOLONGS
REFORGE
SALONGA
SARONGS
SCROOGE
THRONGS
THROUGH
UNBOGGY
UNFOGGY
UNSOGGY
UNTOUGH

•••O••G

AUTOING
CYYOUNG
DADOING
DEMOING
DEYOUNG
ECHOING
HALOING
HOBOING
HYPOING
IMGOING
INGOING
KAYOING
MONOLOG
ONGOING
REDOING
SHOOING
SILOING
SOLOING
UNDOING
UNYOUNG
UPGOING
VETOING
YOYOING
ZEROING

••••OG•

AIRLOGS
ANALOGS
ANALOGY
APOLOGY
BADDOGS
BIGDOGS
BIOLOGY
BLTTOGO
COYDOGS
DESMOGS
DIALOGS
DRYFOGS
ECOLOGY
EGGNOGS
ENOLOGY
EPILOGS
FOGDOGS
GASHOGS
GASLOGS
GEOLOGY
GUNDOGS
HOTDOGS
ICEFOGS
IMAHOGG
JIMHOGG
KELLOGG
LAPDOGS
MADDOGS
MYOLOGY
NEOLOGY
NONGOGO
OLDDOGS
OLDFOGY
ONETOGO
OROLOGY
OTOLOGY
PETDOGS
PHOTOGS
PROLOGS
PYEDOGS
QUAHOGS
REDDOGS
SAWLOGS
SCROOGE
SEADOGS
SUNDOGS
THEHOGS
TOPDOGS
TOYDOGS
TRILOGY
UFOLOGY
UNCLOGS
UROLOGY
VANGOGH
VANVOGT
WAYTOGO
WEBLOGS
ZOOLOGY

••••O•G

AGELONG
ARTSONG
DAYLONG
DOWRONG
ENDLONG
ERELONG
EVELONG
FURLONG
GOALONG
GOWRONG
HITSONG
HOWLONG
IMAHOGG
JIMHOGG
KAMFONG
KELLOGG
LONBORG
MRWRONG
NIALONG
OLDSONG
OURSONG

POPSONG
PRESONG
PROLONG
RAPSONG
SADSONG
SEABORG
SUBLONG
TOOLONG

•••••OG
ANTIFOG
ANTILOG
BACKLOG
BIBLIOG
BIRDDOG
BULLDOG
BUSHHOG
CATALOG
COONDOG
CORNDOG
DECALOG
DEMAGOG
FIREDOG
GOODDOG
HANGDOG
LADADOG
LEADDOG
LOSTDOG
MAGALOG
MALEDOG
MALEHOG
MONOLOG
MOONDOG
NICEDOG
OVERDOG
PEATBOG
PETFROG
ROADHOG
SANDHOG
SEMILOG
SHOWDOG
SLEDDOG
STARLOG
TAGALOG
WARTHOG
WILDDOG
WOLFDOG
YULELOG

OH•••••
OHANLON
OHCAROL
OHFUDGE
OHIOANS
OHIOART
OHMAGES
OHMSLAW

O•H••••
OAHUANS
OCHENTA
OCHROID
OCHROUS
OGHAMIC
OKHOTSK
OOHLALA
OPHELIA
OSHAPED
OSHKOSH
OTHELLO
OXHEART
OXHIDES

O••H•••
OFFHAND
OFFHOUR
OILHEAT
OKSHOOT
OLDHAND
OMAHANE
OMAHANS
OMPHALO
ONEHALF
ONEHAND
ONEHOUR
ONSHORE
ONTHEDL
ONTHEGO
ONTHEQT
ONTHREE
ORCHARD
ORCHIDS
ORPHANS
ORPHANT
ORPHEAN
ORPHEUM
ORPHEUS
OUGHTNT
OUGHTTO
OUTHAUL
OUTHEAR
OUTHERE
OUTHIRE
OUTHISS
OUTHITS
OUTHOWL
OUTHUNT
OUTHURL

O•••H••
ODDSHOE
OLDCHAP
OLDSHOE
ONAWHIM
ONECHIP
ONESHOE
ONESHOT
ONEWHIT
OUTSHOT
OUTSHOW
OVERHOT

O••••H•
ONSIGHT
OOMPAHS
ORNITHO
OUTECHO

O•••••H
OBADIAH
OGREISH
OILRICH
OMIGOSH
ONEARTH
ONEINCH
ONLEASH
OPALISH
OSHKOSH
OSTRICH
OUTFISH
OUTGUSH
OUTLASH
OUTPATH
OUTPUSH
OUTRUSH
OUTSIGH
OUTWASH
OUTWISH
OUTWITH

•OH••••
BOHEMIA
BOHRIUM
COHABIT
COHEIRS
COHERED
COHERER
COHERES
COHORTS
COHOSTS
DOHERTY
HOHNERS
JOHANNA
JOHNBOY
JOHNDOE
JOHNGAY
JOHNIII
JOHNJAY
JOHNLAW
JOHNLEE
JOHNNIE
JOHNNYB
JOHNSON
JOHNVII
JOHNWOO
JOHNXII
JOHNXIV
JOHNXIX
JOHNXVI
JOHNXXI
MOHAIRS
MOHAVES
MOHAWKS
MOHEGAN
MOHICAN
NOHANDS
OOHLALA
SOHAVEI
TOHEART
TOHELEN
TOHOMER
TOHORSE

•O•H•••
BOBHOPE
BOCHNER
BOGHOLE
BOKHARA
BONHEUR
BOOHBAH
BOOHISS
BOOHOOS
BOTHERS
BOTHNIA
BOWHEAD
BOYHOOD
COCHAIR
COCHISE
COCHLEA
COCHRAN
COGHLAN
COSHERS
COSHING
COWHAND
COWHERD
COWHIDE
DOGHAIR
DOSHOTS
FOGHORN
FORHIRE
FOXHOLE
FOXHUNT
GOAHEAD
GODHEAD
GODHOOD
GOPHERS
GOSHAWK
GOTHELP
GOTHICS
GOTHIKA
GOTHURT
HOOHAHS
HOTHAND
HOTHEAD
HOWHIGH
JOBHOPS
JOBHUNT
JODHPUR
JOEHILL
JONHALL
JOSHERS
JOSHING
JOUHAUX
KOEHLER
KOSHERS
KOSHIBA
LOTHAIR
LOTHIAN
LOTHROP
LOWHAND
LOWHEEL
MOCHRIE
MOPHEAD
MOSHERS
MOSHING
MOSHPIT
MOTHERS
MOTHERY
MOTHIER
NOBHILL
NONHERO
NONHITS
NONHOME
NOSHERS
NOSHING
NOSHOWS
NOTHERE
NOTHING
NOTHINS
NOTHOME
NOWHERE
POOHBAH
POSHEST
POTHERB
POTHERS
POTHOLE
POTHOOK
ROCHETS
ROTHIRA
SOPHIES
SOPHISM
SOPHIST
SOTHEBY
SOTHERE
SOTHERN
TOAHAIR
TOEHOLD
TOOHARD
TOOHIGH
TOPHATS
TOPHOLE
TOSHIBA
TOSHIRO
TOWHEAD
TOWHEES
TOYHATS
TOYHOOP
YOGHURT
YOOHOOS
YOTHERS

•O••H••
BOKCHOY
BOLSHOI
BOOTHIA
BOTCHED
BOTCHER
BOTCHES
BOTCHUP
BOUCHER
BOUCHES
BOUGHED
BOWSHOT
COACHED
COACHES
COLCHIS
CONCHAE
CONCHES
CONCHOS
COPSHOP
COUCHED
COUCHES
COUGHED
COUGHUP
COWSHED
DOGCHEW
DOGCHOW
DOGSHOW
DOLPHIN
DONAHUE
DONOHOE
DOUGHTY
FORDHAM
FORSHOW
GODTHAB
GOTAHIT
GOTCHAS
HONCHOS
HOOCHES
HOTSHOT
HOWTHEN
JOACHIM
JOBSHOP
KOOSHES
LOATHED
LOATHER
LOATHES
LOATHLY
LOATHTO
LOWCHEN
MONTHLY
MOOCHED
MOOCHER
MOOCHES
MOORHEN
MORPHED
MORPHIC
MORPHIN
MOUTHED
MOUTHER
NOOTHER
NORTHER
NORTHOF
NOTCHED
NOTCHER
NOTCHES
NOUGHTS
NOWTHEN
NOWTHIS
NOWWHAT
POACHED
POACHER
POACHES
PONCHOS
POOCHES
POOCHIE
PORCHES
PORTHOS
POSTHOC
POTSHOT
POUCHED
POUCHES
ROACHES
ROADHOG
ROETHKE
ROSEHIP
ROUGHED
ROUGHEN
ROUGHER
ROUGHGO
ROUGHIT
ROUGHLY
ROUGHUP
SOCKHOP
SOMEHOW
SONSHIP
SOOTHED
SOOTHER
SOOTHES
SORGHUM
SOUTHEY
SOUTHOF
TOBEHAD
TOESHOE
TOOTHED
TOPTHIS
TORCHED
TORCHER
TORCHES
TOUCHED
TOUCHER
TOUCHES
TOUCHON
TOUCHUP
TOUGHEN
TOUGHER
TOUGHIE
TOUGHLY
TOYSHOP
VOSKHOD
VOUCHED
VOUCHER
VOUCHES
WOOLHAT
WOOSHED
WOOSHES
WORSHIP
WORTHIT
YOUTHEN

•O•••H•
BORSCHT
BOWECHO
DORIGHT
DOROTHY
EOLITHS
FOURTHS
GOUACHE
HOOHAHS
HOOKAHS
HOORAHS
HOWDAHS
IOMOTHS
JOSEPHA
JOSEPHI
LOOFAHS
NOGUCHI
OOMPAHS
PORSCHE
ROYCOHN
TONIGHT
VOTECHS
WORKSHY

•O••••H
BOARISH
BOGGISH
BONEASH
BOOHBAH
BOOKISH
BOORISH
BOROUGH
COCKISH
CODFISH
COLDISH
COLTISH
COMMISH
COOLISH
CORINTH
CORNISH
COTEACH
COWFISH
DOGFISH
DOGGISH
DOLLISH
DOLTISH
DOLUNCH
DONNISH
DOTDASH
DOUBLEH
DOZENTH
FOGYISH
FOLKISH
FOOLISH
FOPPISH
FORBUSH
FOREACH
FORSYTH
GOATISH
GODUTCH
GOFORTH
GOIRISH
GOLIATH
GOODISH
GOOMBAH
GOSOUTH
GOTCASH
GOULASH
GOUTISH
HOGARTH
HOGGISH
HOGWASH
HORNISH
HOTBATH
HOWHIGH
HOWMUCH
JOEROTH
JOMARCH
KOSSUTH
LOGGISH
LONGISH
LOUDISH
LOUTISH
LOWTECH
MOBBISH
MONARCH
MONKISH
MOONISH
MOORISH
NOCATCH
NONCASH
NONSUCH
NORRISH
NORWICH
NOTMUCH
NOTWITH
NOURISH
POOHBAH
POORISH
PORKISH
ROBERTH
ROGUISH
ROMANSH
ROMPISH
ROOKISH
SOFTISH
SOPWITH
SOTTISH
SOURISH
TOADISH
TOOHIGH
TOOMUCH
TORYISH
TOWNISH
TOWPATH
TOYWITH
VOGUISH
WOLFISH
WORMISH
YOBBISH
YOUWISH

••OH•••
ALOHAOE
BOOHBAH
BOOHISS
BOOHOOS
HOOHAHS
ISOHELS
POOHBAH
TOOHARD
TOOHIGH
TWOHOUR
YOOHOOS

••O•H••
ANOTHER
APOTHEM
BIOCHIP
BOOTHIA
BROTHER
CLOCHES
CLOTHED
CLOTHES
CROCHET
EPOCHAL
FROTHED
FROTHER
FROTHUP
HOOCHES
KEOGHAN
KNOWHOW
KOOSHES
MOOCHED
MOOCHER
MOOCHES
MOORHEN
NOOTHER
POOCHES
POOCHIE
PROPHET
PROSHOP
SHOWHOW
SIOBHAN
SKOSHES
SLOSHED
SLOSHES
SMOTHER
SNOWHAT
SOOTHED
SOOTHER
SOOTHES
TOOTHED
TROCHEE
TROCHES
TROTHED
TWOSHOT
USOSHOW
WOOLHAT
WOOSHED
WOOSHES

••O••H•
ADOLPHE
BLOTCHY
BRONCHI
BRONCHO
BROUGHT
CHOUGHS
DROUGHT
GNOCCHI
GROUCHO
GROUCHY
GROWTHS
HOOHAHS
HOOKAHS
HOORAHS
IGOTCHA
LOOFAHS
PLOUGHS
SLOUCHY
SLOUGHS
SMOOTHS
SMOOTHY
THOUGHT
TROUGHS
WHOSWHO
WROUGHT

••O•••H
ABOLISH
ANOUILH
BIOTECH
BOOHBAH
BOOKISH
BOORISH
COOLISH
DRONISH
FOOLISH
GNOMISH
GOODISH
GOOMBAH
KNOWETH
MOONISH
MOORISH
NEOLITH
POOHBAH
POORISH
ROOKISH
SCOOTCH
SLOWISH
STOMACH
TOOHIGH
TOOMUCH

•••OH••
ALCOHOL
DONOHOE
GASOHOL
MEGOHMS
STJOHNS

•••O•H•
ALYOSHA
ATROPHY
BINOCHE
BRIOCHE
DEMOTHS
DOROTHY
IOMOTHS
KENOSHA
LAROCHE
LESOTHO
PWBOTHA
SMOOTHS
SMOOTHY
STROPHE
TIMOTHY

•••O••H
ABROACH
AKRONOH
ALWORTH
BOROUGH
BYMOUTH
DEBORAH
FATOUSH
FTWORTH
GOFORTH
GOSOUTH
HAWORTH
INTOUCH
LALOOSH
LELOUCH
MENORAH
MRNORTH
RETOUCH
RUDOLPH
SCOOTCH
SPLOTCH
THEOATH
THROUGH
UNCOUTH
UNLOATH
UNTOUGH
UPNORTH
WIMOWEH

••••OH•
BIGJOHN
IIIJOHN
KANEOHE
MATZOHS
ROYCOHN
TERAOHM

••••O•H
ANTIOCH
BETROTH
JOEROTH
LALOOSH
MAMMOTH
MATZOTH
MURDOCH
OMIGOSH
OSHKOSH
REXROTH
SUCCOTH
SUKKOTH
THEPOOH
TIMROTH
VANGOGH

•••••OH
AKRONOH
NILESOH
PHARAOH
PLAYDOH
THEPOOH
XENIAOH

OI•••••
OILBASE
OILBIRD
OILCAKE
OILCANS
OILCUPS
OILDRUM
OILHEAT
OILIEST
OILLAMP
OILLESS
OILLIKE
OILLINE
OILPALM
OILPANS
OILRICH
OILRIGS
OILRING
OILRUBS
OILSAND
OILSEED
OILSKIN
OILSPOT
OILTANK
OILWELL
OINKERS
OINKING
OISEAUX

O•I••••
OCICATS
ODINGON
OHIOANS
OHIOART
OJIBWAS
OJIBWAY
OKINAWA
OLICOOK
OLIVIER
OLIVINE
OMICRON
OMIGOSH
OMINOUS
OMITTED
OMITTER
OPIATES
OPINERS
OPINING
OPINION
ORIENTE
ORIENTS
ORIFICE
ORIGAMI
ORIGINE
ORIGINS
ORINOCO
ORIOLES
ORISONS
OSIERED
OSIRIAN
OVIDIAN
OVIDUCT
OVIFORM
OVIPARA
OVISACS
OWINGON
OWINGTO
OXIDANT
OXIDASE
OXIDATE
OXIDISE
OXIDIZE

O••I•••
OAKIEST
OBLIGED
OBLIGEE
OBLIGER
OBLIGES
OBLIGOR
OBLIQUE
OBOISTS
OBVIATE
OBVIOUS
OCCIPUT
OEDIPAL
OEDIPUS
OFFICER
OFFICES
OFFICIO
OFFINGS
OILIEST
OMNIBUS
OMNIMAX
ONEIDAS
ONEINCH
ONEIOTA
ONEIRIC
ONEIRON
ONFIRST
ONLIEST
ONSIDES
ONSIGHT
ONVIDEO
OOLITES
OOLITIC
OOZIEST
OPTICAL
OPTICKS
OPTIMAL
OPTIMAS
OPTIMUM
OPTIONS
ORBISON
ORBITAL
ORBITED
ORBITER
ORDINAL
ORDINES
OREILLY
ORGIAST
ORNITHO
ORRISES
ORVIETO
ORVILLE
OSCINES
OSSICLE
OSSIFIC
OSSIPEE
OSTIARY
OUTINGS
OVOIDAL
OWLIEST

OXHIDES

O•••I••

OAKLIKE
OARLIKE
OATLIKE
OBADIAH
OBELISE
OBELISK
OBELIZE
OBESITY
OBEYING
OBTAINS
OCARINA
OCULIST
ODORIZE
OFAKIND
OFAMIND
OFFLINE
OFFSIDE
OFFSITE
OGREISH
OILBIRD
OILLIKE
OILLINE
OILRICH
OILRIGS
OILRING
OINKING
OKAYING
OLAFIII
OLAVIII
OLDCITY
OLDFILM
OLDGIRL
OLDLINE
OLDNICK
OLDTIME
OLEFINS
OLEMISS
OLIVIER
OLIVINE
OLOGIES
OMENING
ONABIAS
ONADIET
ONAKICK
ONALINE
ONEDIME
ONEKILO
ONELIRA
ONEMILE
ONEPINT
ONESIZE
ONETIME
ONGOING
ONPOINT
ONTRIAL
OPACITY
OPALINE
OPALISH
OPENING
OPINING
OPINION
ORACIES
ORALIST
ORARION
ORARIUM
ORATING
ORATION
ORBLIKE
ORCHIDS
ORDAINS
ORIFICE
ORIGINE
ORIGINS
OSIRIAN
OSTRICH
OTARIES
OTTOIII
OUGUIYA
OUSTING
OUTBIDS
OUTCITY
OUTFIND
OUTFIRE
OUTFISH
OUTFITS
OUTGIVE
OUTHIRE
OUTHISS
OUTHITS
OUTJINX
OUTKICK
OUTKILL
OUTKING
OUTKISS
OUTLIER
OUTLIES
OUTLIMN
OUTLINE
OUTLIPS
OUTLIVE
OUTPICK
OUTPIPE
OUTPITY
OUTRIBS
OUTRIDE
OUTRIGS
OUTRING
OUTSIDE
OUTSIFT
OUTSIGH
OUTSING
OUTSINS
OUTSITS
OUTSIZE
OUTTIRE
OUTVIED
OUTVIES
OUTWILE
OUTWILL
OUTWIND
OUTWING
OUTWISH
OUTWITH
OUTWITS
OVARIES
OVATION
OVERICE
OVIDIAN
OWLLIKE
OXIDISE
OXIDIZE
OXONIAN
OXTAILS
OZONISE
OZONIZE

O••••I•

OBERLIN
OCEANIA
OCEANIC
OCEANID
OCHROID
OCTADIC
OCTAVIA
OCTAVIO
OCTROIS
ODONTIA
OFFICIO
OGHAMIC
OILSKIN
OLAFIII
OLAVIII
OLDMAID
OLEOOIL
OLYMPIA
OLYMPIC
ONASSIS
ONATRIP
ONAWHIM
ONECHIP
ONEIRIC
ONEPAIR
ONEUNIT
ONEWHIT
ONTARIO
ONTOPIC
OOLITIC
OPENAIR
OPENPIT
OPHELIA
OPTEDIN
OPUNTIA
ORATRIX
ORDERIN
ORECTIC
ORGANIC
OSMATIC
OSMOSIS
OSMOTIC
OSSIFIC
OSTEOID
OSTOSIS
OTALGIA
OTALGIC
OTTAVIO
OTTOIII
OUTGAIN
OUTGRIN
OUTLAID
OUTLAIN
OUTOFIT
OUTPAID
OUTRAIL
OUTSAID
OUTSAIL
OUTSKIP
OUTSPIN
OUTSPIT
OUTSWIM
OUTWAIT
OVERBID
OVERBIG
OVERDID
OVERFIT
OVERFIX
OVERLIE
OVERLIT
OVERMIX
OVERTIP

O•••••I

OLAFIII
OLAVIII
OLDUVAI
ONORATI
ORIGAMI
OTTOIII

•OI••••

BOIARDO
BOILERS
BOILING
BOILOFF
BOILOUT
BOILSUP
BOISEID
BOITANO
COIFFED
COIFING
COIGNED
COIGNES
COILERS
COILING
COILSUP
COINAGE
COINBOX
COINERS
COINING
COINOPS
DOIDARE
DOILIES
DOINGIN
DOINGOK
DOINGSO
DOINGTO
DOINGUP
DOITNOW
FOIBLES
FOILING
FOISTED
FOISTON
GOINFOR
GOINGAT
GOINGBY
GOINGIN
GOINGON
GOINGTO
GOINGUP
GOIRISH
GOITERS
HOISTED
HOISTER
HOISTUP
JOINDER
JOINERS
JOINERY
JOINING
JOINSIN
JOINSUP
JOINTED
JOINTER
JOINTLY
JOISTED
LOIDING
LOITERS
MOILERS
MOILING
MOISSAN
MOISTEN
MOISTER
MOISTLY
NOISIER
NOISILY
NOISING
NOISOME
POINTAT
POINTED
POINTER
POINTES
POINTTO
POINTUP
POISERS
POISING
POISONS
POISSON
POITIER
POIVRES
ROILIER
ROILING
ROISTER
SOIGNEE
SOILAGE
SOILING
SOIREES
TOILERS
TOILETS
TOILFUL
TOILING
TOILSAT
VOICERS
VOICING
VOIDERS
VOIDING
VOIDOUT
VOITURE

•O•I•••

BODICES
BODINGS
BOEINGS
BOLIDES
BOLIVAR
BOLIVIA
BONIATO
BONIEST
BONILLA
BONITOS
BORIDES
BORINGS
BOVINES
BOXIEST
CODICES
CODICIL
COKIEST
COLICKY
COMICAL
COMICES
COMINGS
COMIQUE
CONICAL
CONIFER
COPIERS
COPILOT
COPIOUS
CORINNE
CORINTH
COSIEST
COSIGNS
COSINES
COWIEST
COZIEST
DOMICAL
DOMICIL
DOMINGO
DOMINIC
DOMINOS
DOMINUS
DONIMUS
DOPIEST
DORIGHT
DORITOS
DOSIDOS
DOZIEST
EOLITHS
EOSINES
FOLIAGE
FOLIATE
FOLIOED
FOLIOSE
FORINTS
FOXIEST
GOFIRST
GOGIRLS
GOLIATH
GOOIEST
GORIEST
GORILLA
GOTINON
GOTINTO
GOTITON
HOKIEST
HOLIDAY
HOLIEST
HOLISTS
HOMIEST
HOMINID
HONIARA
HOPINTO
HORIZON
HOSIERS
HOSIERY
HOTITEM
IODIDES
IODISED
IODISES
IODIZED
IODIZER
IODIZES
IONIANS
IONISED
IONISER
IONISES
IONIUMS
IONIZED
IONIZER
IONIZES
JOKIEST
KODIAKS
KOPIYKA
LOGICAL
LOGIEST
LONIGAN
LORIENT
LORISES
LOSINGS
LOTIONS
LOUISII
LOUISIV
LOUISIX
LOUISVI
LOUISXI
LOUISXV
MOBILES
MODICUM
MODISTE
MOHICAN
MOJITOS
MOLIERE
MOLITOR
MONIKER
MONITOR
MOPIEST
MORISOT
MOTIONS
MOTIVED
MOTIVES
MOWINGS
MOZILLA
NODICAL
NOGIFTS
NOLIMIT
NOMINAL
NOMINEE
NONIRON
NORIEGA
NORITES
NOSIEST
NOSIREE
NOTICED
NOTICER
NOTICES
NOTIONS
NOVICES
NOVISAD
NOWISEE
NOWISER
NOXIOUS
OOLITES
OOLITIC
OOZIEST
PODIUMS
POKIEST
POLICED
POLICER
POLICES
POLISCI
POLITER
POLITIC
PONIARD
PORIVER
POSITED
POTIONS
ROPIEST
ROSIEST
ROSINED
ROTIFER
ROVINGS
SOCIALS
SOCIETY
SODIDWE
SOLICIT
SOLIDER
SOLIDLY
SOMINEX
SORIANO
SOVIETS
SOYINKA
SOYINKS
TONIEST
TONIGHT
TOPIARY
TOPICAL
TORINOS
TOTINOS
TOWINGS
VOTIVES
WOEISME
YOGIISM
YOGINIS
ZODIACS
ZONIANS
ZOOIDAL
ZOOIEST
ZOSIMUS

•O••I••

BOARISH
BOATING
BOBBIDI
BOBBIES
BOBBING
BOBBINS
BOBVILA
BOCCIES
BODKINS
BOFFING
BOFFINS
BOGGIER
BOGGING
BOGGISH
BOHRIUM
BOILING
BOLLING
BOLTING
BOMBING
BONAIRE
BONDING
BONFIRE
BONGING
BONKING
BONNIER
BONNILY
BOOBIES
BOOBIRD
BOOGIED
BOOGIES
BOOHISS
BOOKIES
BOOKIII
BOOKING
BOOKISH
BOOMIER
BOOMING
BOONIES
BOORISH
BOOTIES
BOOTING
BOOZIER
BOOZILY
BOOZING
BOPPING
BORGIAS
BORKING
BOSNIAN
BOSSIER
BOSSILY
BOSSING
BOSSISM
BOUDINS
BOUVIER
BOWFINS
BOWLIKE
BOWLINE
BOWLING
BOWTIES
BOXKITE
BOXLIKE
BOYLIKE
COALING
COATING
COAXIAL
COAXING
COCAINE
COCHISE
COCKIER
COCKILY
COCKING
COCKISH
CODEINE
CODFISH
COEDITS
COEXIST
COFFINS
COGGING
COGNIZE
COHEIRS
COIFING
COILING
COINING
COLDISH
COLLIDE
COLLIER
COLLIES
COLLINE
COLLINS
COLTISH
COMBIEN
COMBINE
COMBING
COMFIER
COMFITS
COMMISH
COMMITS
COMPILE
COMPING
COMTISM
COMTIST
CONCISE
CONDIGN
CONFIDE
CONFINE
CONFIRM
CONFITS
CONKING
CONNICK
CONNIFF
CONNING
CONNIVE
CONOIDS
CONRIED
CONSIGN
CONSIST
CONVICT
COOKIES
COOKING
COOLIES
COOLING
COOLISH
COOPING
COOTIES
COPPICE
COPPING
COPYING
COPYIST
COQUINA
CORDIAL
CORDIAS
CORDING
CORDITE
CORKIER
CORKING
CORNICE
CORNIER
CORNILY
CORNING
CORNISH
CORRIDA
CORSICA
CORTICO
CORTINA
CORVIDS
CORVINA
CORVINE
CORZINE
COSHING
COSTING
COSTIVE
COSYING
COUPING
COURIER
COUSINE
COUSINS
COWBIRD
COWFISH
COWGIRL
COWHIDE
COWLICK
COWLIKE
COWLING
COWRIES
COWRITE
COZYING
DOASIDO
DOBBINS
DOCKING
DODGIER
DODGING
DOFFING
DOGBITE
DOGFISH
DOGGIER
DOGGIES
DOGGING
DOGGISH
DOGLIKE
DOGPILE
DOGSITS
DOGTICK
DOILIES
DOLLIED
DOLLIES
DOLLING
DOLLISH
DOLTISH
DOMAINE
DOMAINS
DONKING
DONNING
DONNISH
DOOLIES
DOOMIER
DOOMING
DOOZIES
DORKIER
DORMICE
DOSSIER
DOSSING
DOTLIKE
DOTRICE
DOTTIER
DOTTILY
DOTTING
DOUSING
DOWDIER
DOWDIES
DOWDILY
DOWLING
DOWNIER
DOWNING
DOWRIES
DOWSING
EONLINE
FOALING
FOAMIER
FOAMILY
FOAMING
FOBBING
FOGCITY
FOGGIER
FOGGILY
FOGGING
FOGYISH
FOGYISM
FOILING
FOLDING
FOLKIER
FOLKIES
FOLKISH
FOLLIES
FONTINA
FOODIES
FOOLING
FOOLISH
FOOTING
FOPPISH
FORBIDS
FORCING
FORDING
FOREIGN
FORGING
FORGIVE
FORHIRE
FORKIER
FORKING
FORLIFE
FORMICA
FORMING
FORSIZE
FORTIES
FORTIFY
FORTIUS
FOSDICK
FOSSILS
FOULING
FOURIER
FOWLING
FOXFIRE
FOXLIKE
GOADING
GOALIES
GOAMISS
GOATISH
GOBLINS
GODLIER
GODLIKE
GODLING
GODWITS
GOIRISH
GOLDING
GOLFING
GONGING
GOODIES
GOODING
GOODISH
GOOFIER
GOOFILY
GOOFING
GOONIER
GOONIES
GOONILY
GOOPIER
GOOSIER
GOOSING
GORDIAN
GORDITA
GORDIUS
GORGING
GORMING
GORSIER
GOSLING
GOSSIPS
GOSSIPY
GOTHICS
GOTHIKA
GOTMILK
GOTWISE
GOUGING
GOUTIER
GOUTILY
GOUTISH
GOWNING
HOAGIES
HOARIER
HOARILY
HOAXING
HOBBIES
HOBBITS
HOBOING
HOBOISM
HOCKING
HODDING
HOGGING
HOGGISH
HOGLIKE
HOGTIED
HOGTIES
HOGWILD
HOLDING
HOLLIES
HOLMIUM
HOMEICE
HOMEIER
HONKING
HOODIES
HOODING
HOOFING
HOOKING
HOOPING
HOOSIER
HOOTING
HOPKINS
HOPLITE
HOPPIER
HOPPING
HOPSING
HORDING
HORNIER
HORNING
HORNISH
HORNIST
HORRIFY
HORSIER
HORSILY
HORSING
HORVITZ
HOSKINS
HOSPICE
HOSTILE
HOSTING
HOTLICK
HOTLINE
HOTLINK
HOTLIPS
HOTMILK
HOTPINK
HOTTIES
HOTTIME
HOTTIPS
HOTWIRE
HOUDINI
HOUSING
HOWHIGH
HOWLING
HOWNICE
JOBBING
JOEHILL
JOEKIDD
JOGGING
JOHNIII
JOINING
JOLLIED

JOLLIER
JOLLIES
JOLLIET
JOLLIFY
JOLLILY
JOLLITY
JOLTIER
JOLTING
JOSHING
JOTTING
JOWLIER
JOYRIDE
KONTIKI
KOOKIER
KOONING
KOSCINA
KOSHIBA
LOADING
LOAFING
LOAMIER
LOAMING
LOANING
LOBBIED
LOBBIES
LOBBING
LOCKING
LOCKINS
LODGING
LOFTIER
LOFTILY
LOFTING
LOGGIAS
LOGGING
LOGGINS
LOGGISH
LOIDING
LOLLIES
LOLLING
LONGIES
LONGING
LONGISH
LOOBIES
LOOKING
LOOKINS
LOOKISM
LOOKIST
LOOMING
LOONIER
LOONIES
LOONILY
LOOPIER
LOOPING
LOOSING
LOOTING
LOPPIER
LOPPING
LORDING
LORRIES
LOTHIAN
LOTTING
LOUDISH
LOURING
LOUSIER
LOUSILY
LOUSING
LOUTING
LOUTISH
LOVEINS

LOWBIDS
LOWDIVE
LOWLIER
LOWLIFE
LOWLILY
LOWRISE
LOWRISK
LOWSIDE
LOWTIDE
MOABITE
MOANING
MOBBING
MOBBISH
MOBBISM
MOBBIST
MOCKING
MOHAIRS
MOILING
MOLDIER
MOLDING
MOLLIES
MOLLIFY
MOLTING
MOMMIES
MONDIAL
MONDIEU
MONKISH
MOODIER
MOODILY
MOONIER
MOONIES
MOONILY
MOONING
MOONISH
MOORIER
MOORING
MOORISH
MOOTING
MOPPING
MORAINE
MORNING
MORTICE
MORTIFY
MORTISE
MOSAICS
MOSHING
MOSSIER
MOSSING
MOTHIER
MOTRINS
MOUSIER
MOUSILY
MOUSING
NOBBIER
NOBHILL
NOCKING
NODDIES
NODDING
NOETICS
NOGGINS
NOISIER
NOISILY
NOISING
NONDIET
NONHITS
NONLIFE
NONLIVE
NONOILY

NONOISE
NOOGIES
NOONING
NOOSING
NORDICA
NORDICS
NORRISH
NORWICH
NOSHING
NOTHING
NOTHINS
NOTLIKE
NOTLIVE
NOTMINE
NOTNICE
NOTTING
NOTWITH
NOURISH
PODLIKE
PODRIDA
POESIES
POETICA
POETICS
POETISE
POETIZE
POISING
POITIER
POLLING
POLOIST
PONDING
PONGIDS
PONTIAC
PONTIAN
PONTIFF
PONTIUS
PONYING
POOLING
POOPING
POORISH
POPDIVA
POPLINS
POPPIES
POPPING
POPPINS
POPWINE
PORCINE
PORGIES
PORKIER
PORKING
PORKISH
PORTICO
PORTING
PORTION
POSTIES
POSTING
POSTITS
POTLIDS
POTPIES
POTTIER
POTTIES
POTTING
POURING
POUTIER
POUTING
ROADIES
ROAMING
ROARING
ROBBING

ROBBINS
ROCKIER
ROCKIES
ROCKILY
ROCKING
RODDICK
RODDING
RODLIKE
RODRIGO
ROGAINE
ROGUING
ROGUISH
ROILIER
ROILING
ROLAIDS
ROLFING
ROLLICK
ROLLING
ROLLINS
ROMAINE
ROMAINS
ROMPING
ROMPISH
ROOFING
ROOKIER
ROOKIES
ROOKING
ROOKISH
ROOMIER
ROOMIES
ROOMILY
ROOMING
ROOTIER
ROOTING
RORAIMA
ROSSINI
ROTHIRA
ROTTING
ROUGING
ROUSING
ROUTINE
ROUTING
ROWDIER
ROWDIES
ROWDILY
ROWLING
SOAKING
SOAPIER
SOAPILY
SOAPING
SOARING
SOBBING
SOCKING
SODDIER
SODDING
SOFFITS
SOFTIES
SOFTISH
SOGGIER
SOGGILY
SOILING
SOLDIER
SOLOING
SOLOIST
SOLVING
SONLIKE
SOOTIER
SOOTILY

SOPHIES
SOPHISM
SOPHIST
SOPPIER
SOPPING
SOPWITH
SORDINI
SORDINO
SORRIER
SORRILY
SORTIED
SORTIES
SORTING
SORVINO
SOTTISH
SOUBISE
SOUPIER
SOURING
SOURISH
SOUSING
SOWLIKE
SOYMILK
TOADIED
TOADIES
TOADISH
TOCSINS
TODDIES
TOELIKE
TOEPICK
TOGGING
TOILING
TOLKIEN
TOLLING
TOMKITE
TOMTITS
TONGING
TONSILS
TONTINE
TOOHIGH
TOOKILL
TOOLING
TOONIES
TOOTING
TOPBIDS
TOPFIVE
TOPKICK
TOPLINE
TOPPING
TOPSIDE
TOROIDS
TORSION
TORVILL
TORYISH
TORYISM
TOSHIBA
TOSHIRO
TOSSING
TOTTING
TOURING
TOURISM
TOURIST
TOUTING
TOWLINE
TOWNIES
TOWNISH
TOYBIKE
TOYKITE
TOYLIKE

TOYWITH
VOGUING
VOGUISH
VOICING
VOIDING
VOSGIAN
WOLFING
WOLFISH
WONTING
WOODIER
WOODIES
WOODING
WOOFING
WOOKIEE
WOOLIER
WOOLIES
WOOLITE
WOOZIER
WOOZILY
WORDIER
WORDILY
WORDING
WORKING
WORMIER
WORMING
WORMISH
WORRIED
WORRIER
WORRIES
WOZNIAK
YOBBISH
YOGIISM
YORKIES
YORKIST
YOUWISH
YOWLING
YOYOING
ZOMBIES
ZOMBIFY
ZONKING
ZOOMING
ZOSSIMA
ZOYSIAS

•O•••I•

BOBTAIL
BOBWEIR
BODYKIT
BOHEMIA
BOISEID
BOLATIE
BOLIVIA
BOLOTIE
BONACIS
BONARIO
BONSOIR
BOOKIII
BOOKVII
BOOPSIE
BOOTHIA
BOOTSIT
BORODIN
BOROMIR
BORONIC
BORZOIS
BOSONIC
BOTANIC
BOTHNIA

BOUDOIR
BOWDOIN
BOXEDIN
BOXESIN
COALBIN
COALOIL
COALPIT
COCCOID
COCHAIR
COCKPIT
CODICIL
COEPTIS
COHABIT
COLCHIS
COLLOID
COMEDIA
COMEDIC
COMEDIE
COMESIN
COMPLIN
CONBRIO
CONCEIT
CONDUIT
CONJOIN
CONKLIN
CONTAIN
COOLAIR
COOLPIX
COOLSIT
CORNBIN
CORNOIL
CORSAIR
CORVAIR
COSTAIN
COTERIE
COUNCIL
COUNTIN
COWSKIN
COWSLIP
DOAGAIN
DOESKIN
DOGHAIR
DOGTAIL
DOINGIN
DOLPHIN
DOMICIL
DOMINIC
DONTLIE
DOONEIN
DOORDIE
DOUBTIT
FOLDSIN
FOOTSIE
FOOTSIT
FORABIT
FORCEIN
FORFEIT
FORTDIX
FOULTIP
FOURPIN
FOXTAIL
GOBELIN
GOBYAIR
GODEVIL
GOFORIT
GOINGIN
GOLDTIP
GONERIL

GOODAIM
GOODKID
GOODNIK
GOODWIN
GOTAHIT
GOTATIP
GOTONIT
GOTTOIT
HOBNAIL
HOLBEIN
HOLDSIN
HOLDSIT
HOLYOIL
HOMEDIN
HOMERIC
HOMESIN
HOMINID
HONEDIN
HONESIN
HOOFSIT
HOPTOIT
HORATIO
HORNSIN
HOTMAIL
HOWBEIT
JOACHIM
JOAQUIN
JOBFAIR
JOHNIII
JOHNNIE
JOHNVII
JOHNXII
JOHNXIV
JOHNXIX
JOINSIN
JONERIK
JONQUIL
KOOLAID
KORANIC
KOSYGIN
LOADSIN
LOCKLIN
LOCKSIN
LODGEIN
LOOKSIN
LORDJIM
LORDSIT
LOSEBIG
LOSESIT
LOSTBIG
LOTHAIR
LOUISII
LOUISIV
LOUISIX
LOVEDIT
LOVESIT
LOWPAID
LOWPAIR
MOCHRIE
MONADIC
MONODIC
MOONLIT
MOONPIE
MORANIS
MORAVIA
MORONIC
MORPHIC
MORPHIN

MOSHPIT
MOUNTIE
MOVEDIN
MOVEDIT
MOVESIN
MOVESIT
NOKOMIS
NOLIMIT
NOMADIC
NONACID
NONDRIP
NONEPIC
NONEVIL
NONPAID
NONSKID
NONSLIP
NONVOID
NOSEDIN
NOSESIN
NOSTAIN
NOSTRIL
NOTABIT
NOTALIE
NOTFAIR
NOVALIS
NOWTHIS
OOLITIC
POLARIS
POLEMIC
POLESIT
POLITIC
POLONIA
POMPEIA
POMPEII
POOCHIE
POOPSIE
POPQUIZ
PORKPIE
POSTFIX
POTBOIL
POURSIN
POUSSIN
ROBOTIC
ROCKOIL
ROCKYII
ROCKYIV
ROLLEIS
ROLLSIN
ROMAJIS
ROMANIA
ROMANIC
ROMANIS
ROPEDIN
ROPESIN
ROSALIA
ROSALIE
ROSARIO
ROSEHIP
ROSEOIL
ROUBAIX
ROUGHIT
ROYGBIV
SOAKSIN
SOCKSIN
SOLARIA
SOLICIT
SOLVEIT
SOMALIA

SOMALIS
SOMATIC
SONSHIP
SOUPMIX
TOAHAIR
TOCELIA
TOENAIL
TOOKAIM
TOOLKIT
TOOTSIE
TOPSAIL
TOPSOIL
TOPSPIN
TOPTHIS
TOTEMIC
TOUGHIE
TOWEDIN
TOYFAIR
TOYPAIL
VOCALIC
VOLTAIC
VOTEDIN
VOTESIN
WOODBIN
WORKSIN
WORSHIP
WORTHIT
YOGINIS
YOPLAIT
YOUREIT
ZOOMSIN

•O••••I

BOBBIDI
BOCELLI
BOLSHOI
BONJOVI
BOOKIII
BOOKVII
BORDONI
COLLODI
COLOSSI
CORELLI
DOUBLEI
FORLANI
GOLDONI
GOURAMI
HOUDINI
JOHNIII
JOHNVII
JOHNXII
JOHNXVI
JOHNXXI
JOSEPHI
KONTIKI
LORELAI
LORELEI
LOUISII
LOUISVI
LOUISXI
MOLOKAI
MONDAVI
MONDESI
MONOSKI
MORETTI
MOSCONI
NOGUCHI
POLANYI

POLISCI
POLYSCI
POMPEII
ROBERTI
ROCKYII
RONZONI
ROSSINI
SOHAVEI
SOLLATI
SOPRANI
SORDINI
TOFUTTI
TOLSTOI
TOPKAPI
TORTONI
YOUANDI

••OI•••

ANOINTS
AVOIDED
AVOIDER
BROIDER
BROILED
BROILER
CHOICER
CHOICES
CHOIRED
EGOISTE
EGOISTS
ENOILED
ETOILES
EXOILER
GOOIEST
GROINED
MAOISTS
OBOISTS
OVOIDAL
QUOINED
QUOITED
REOILED
SPOILED
SPOILER
STOICAL
TAOISTS
TROIKAS
TROILUS
TWOIRON
UNOILED
WHOISIT
ZOOIDAL
ZOOIEST

••O•I••

ABOLISH
ACONITE
ADORING
AEOLIAN
AGONIES
AGONISE
AGONISM
AGONIST
AGONIZE
AMORIST
ANODISE
ANODIZE
ANOMIES
ANOUILH
ASOCIAL

ATOMICS
ATOMIES
ATOMISE
ATOMISM
ATOMIST
ATOMIZE
ATONICS
ATONIES
ATONING
AVOWING
AZORIAN
BIOCIDE
BIOLITE
BIONICS
BIOPICS
BIOTITE
BLOWIER
BLOWING
BMOVIES
BOOBIES
BOOBIRD
BOOGIED
BOOGIES
BOOHISS
BOOKIES
BOOKIII
BOOKING
BOOKISH
BOOMIER
BOOMING
BOONIES
BOORISH
BOOTIES
BOOTING
BOOZIER
BOOZILY
BOOZING
BRODIES
BROMIDE
BROMINE
BUOYING
CHOKIER
CHOKING
CHOLINE
CHOPINE
CHORINE
CHORIST
CHORIZO
CHOWING
CLONING
CLOSING
CLOYING
COOKIES
COOKING
COOLIES
COOLING
COOLISH
COOPING
COOTIES
CRONIES
CROSIER
CROWING
CROZIER
DIORITE
DIOTIMA
DIOXIDE
DIOXINS
DOOLIES

DOOMIER
DOOMING
DOOZIES
DRONING
DRONISH
DROPINS
DROXIES
EBONICS
EBONIES
EBONITE
EBONIZE
ECOCIDE
EDOMITE
EGOTISM
EGOTIST
ELOPING
EMOTING
EMOTION
EMOTIVE
EPONINE
EPOXIED
EPOXIES
ERODING
EROSION
EROSIVE
EROTICA
EROTICS
ETONIAN
ETONICS
EVOKING
EXOTICA
EXOTICS
EXOTISM
FIORINA
FLORIAN
FLORIDA
FLORINS
FLORIST
FLOWING
FOODIES
FOOLING
FOOLISH
FOOTING
FRODING
FROLICS
GAOLING
GLOBING
GLOBINS
GLORIAS
GLORIED
GLORIES
GLORIFY
GLOVING
GLOWING
GNOMISH
GNOMIST
GOODIES
GOODING
GOODISH
GOOFIER
GOOFILY
GOOFING
GOONIER
GOONIES
GOONILY
GOOPIER
GOOSIER
GOOSING

GRODIER
GROLIER
GROPING
GROPIUS
GROTIUS
GROWING
HOODIES
HOODING
HOOFING
HOOKING
HOOPING
HOOSIER
HOOTING
ICONIFY
IDOLISE
IDOLIST
IDOLIZE
IRONIES
IRONING
IRONIST
ISOLINE
IVORIAN
IVORIES
IVORINE
IWOJIMA
KNOWING
KOOKIER
KOONING
LAOTIAN
LEONIDS
LEONINE
LEOVIII
LEOXIII
LIONISE
LIONIZE
LOOBIES
LOOKING
LOOKINS
LOOKISM
LOOKIST
LOOMING
LOONIER
LOONIES
LOONILY
LOOPIER
LOOPING
LOOSING
LOOTING
MEOWING
MOODIER
MOODILY
MOONIER
MOONIES
MOONILY
MOONING
MOONISH
MOORIER
MOORING
MOORISH
MOOTING
MYOPIAS
NEOLITH
NIOBITE
NIOBIUM
NOOGIES
NOONING
NOOSING
ODORIZE

OLOGIES
OXONIAN
OZONISE
OZONIZE
PEONIES
PEORIAN
PHOBIAS
PHOBICS
PHONICS
PHONIER
PHONIES
PHONILY
PHONING
PHOTICS
PIOSITY
PLOSION
PLOSIVE
PLOWING
POOLING
POOPING
POORISH
PROBIES
PROBING
PROBITY
PROCITY
PRODIGY
PROFILE
PROFITS
PROLIFE
PROMISE
PROSIER
PROSILY
PROSING
PROTIST
PROVIDE
PROVINE
PROVING
PROVISO
PROXIES
PROXIMA
PROXIMO
QUOTING
RHODIAN
RHODIUM
RIORITA
RIOTING
ROOFING
ROOKIER
ROOKIES
ROOKING
ROOKISH
ROOMIER
ROOMIES
ROOMILY
ROOMING
ROOTIER
ROOTING
SCOPING
SCORIAS
SCORING
SCOTIAN
SHOEING
SHOOING
SHOOINS
SHORING
SHOVING
SHOWIER
SHOWILY

SHOWING
SLOPING
SLOWING
SLOWISH
SMOKIER
SMOKIES
SMOKILY
SMOKING
SNORING
SNOWIER
SNOWILY
SNOWING
SOOTIER
SOOTILY
SPOKING
STOGIES
STOKING
STONIER
STONILY
STONING
STORIED
STORIES
STORING
STOTINS
STOWING
THORIUM
TMOBILE
TOOHIGH
TOOKILL
TOOLING
TOONIES
TOOTING
TROPICS
TROPISM
TROWING
TWOBITS
TWOTIME
UGOLINO
UNOWING
UTOPIAN
UTOPIAS
UTOPISM
UTOPIST
UXORIAL
VIOLINS
VIOLIST
WOODIER
WOODIES
WOODING
WOOFING
WOOKIEE
WOOLIER
WOOLIES
WOOLITE
WOOZIER
WOOZILY
WYOMING
YAOMING
ZIONISM
ZIONIST
ZOOMING

••O••I•
ABOUTIT
ADONAIS
AGOUTIS
AMOEBIC
ANOSMIA

ANOSMIC
BIOCHIP
BLONDIE
BLOWNIN
BLOWSIN
BLOWSIT
BOOKIII
BOOKVII
BOOPSIE
BOOTHIA
BOOTSIT
BROKEIN
BROWNIE
CLOCKIN
CLOSEIN
COOLAIR
COOLPIX
COOLSIT
CROATIA
CROQUIS
CROSTIC
CROWDIN
DEORBIT
DOONEIN
DOORDIE
DROPSIN
DROPSIT
DROVEIN
ECOTRIN
EGOTRIP
EXORDIA
FJORDIC
FLOORIT
FLOSSIE
FLOWNIN
FLOWSIN
FOOTSIE
FOOTSIT
GEORGIA
GEORGIC
GEORGIE
GIORGIO
GLOAMIN
GLOBOID
GLOTTIS
GNOSTIC
GOODAIM
GOODKID
GOODNIK
GOODWIN
GROOVIN
GROUPIE
GROWBIG
GROWDIM
HOOFSIT
IDOODIT
ILOSTIT
ILOVEIT
INORBIT
KOOLAID
KTOSLIN
LEOVIII
LEOXIII
LOOKSIN
MAOSUIT
MEOWMIX
MOONLIT
MOONPIE

ODONTIA
PHOENIX
PHONEIN
PHOTOID
PLOVDIV
POOCHIE
POOPSIE
PROMBID
PROSAIC
PROTEIN
PROVEIT
RHOMBIC
SCORPIO
SCOTTIE
SHOOSIN
SHORTIE
SHOVEIN
SHOWBIZ
SHOWNIN
SHOWSIN
SLOEGIN
SNOWSIN
SPORTIN
SPOTLIT
STOLEIN
STOMPIN
STOODIN
STOOLIE
STOPSIN
STOPSIT
STORMIN
STOWSIT
SWOOPIN
SWOOSIE
SWOREIN
TIOMKIN
TOOKAIM
TOOLKIT
TOOTSIE
TROMPIN
TROOPIN
TSOURIS
TWOONIE
TWOPAIR
TWOUNIT
WHOISIT
WHOOPIE
WHOOSIS
WHOSAID
WOODBIN
WROTEIN
ZOOMSIN

••O•••I
BOOKIII
BOOKVII
BRONCHI
FEODORI
GEORGEI
GNOCCHI
LEOVIII
LEOXIII
ONORATI
PLOESTI
RIOMUNI
SCOLARI
SHOULDI
SNOWSKI

•••OI••
ADJOINS
ALTOIDS
ALTOIST
ANTOINE
APPOINT
ARMOIRE
AUTOING
CONOIDS
CUBOIDS
DADOING
DEBOITE
DEMOING
DEVOIRS
ECHOING
ECHOISM
EMBOITE
ENJOINS
ETVOILA
GENOISE
HALOIDS
HALOING
HELOISE
HEROICS
HEROINE
HEROISM
HOBOING
HOBOISM
HYPOING
IMGOING
INGOING
INPOINT
INVOICE
JUDOIST
KAYOING
MEMOIRE
MEMOIRS
NICOISE
NONOILY
NONOISE
NUTOILS
ONGOING
ONPOINT
OTTOIII
POLOIST
REBOILS
RECOILS
RECOINS
REDOING
REJOICE
REJOINS
RENOIRS
REPOINT
RESOILS
REVOICE
SHOOING
SHOOINS
SILOING
SOLOING
SOLOIST
SUMOIST
TAROILS
TITOISM
TITOIST
TOROIDS
UNCOILS
UNDOING
UNJOINS
UNJOINT
UNMOIST
UNNOISY
UNVOICE
UPCOILS
UPGOING
VETOING
YOYOING
ZEROING

•••O•I•
ABIOTIC
AEROBIC
ALLOFIT
ALLOWIN
AMMONIA
AMMONIC
ANIONIC
ANSONIA
ANTONIA
ANTONIN
ANTONIO
APHONIA
APHONIC
ASTORIA
AUTOBIO
AUTOPIA
AVIONIC
BEDOUIN
BEGONIA
BOLOTIE
BORODIN
BOROMIR
BORONIC
BOSONIC
BUCOLIC
BYRONIC
CAHOKIA
CALORIC
CALORIE
CANONIC
CAROLII
CAROTID
CAROTIN
CHAOTIC
CHLORIC
CHROMIC
CHRONIC
DELORIS
DEMONIC
DEMOTIC
DEPOSIT
EIDOLIC
EMPORIA
ENCOMIA
ERGOTIC
ESTONIA
ESTORIL
EUNOMIA
EXPOSIT
FEMORIS
FLOORIT
GENOMIC
GETONIT
GOFORIT
GOTONIT
GROOVIN
HEDONIC
IDIOTIC
IDOODIT
IKNOWIT
ILLOGIC
IMFORIT
INFORIT
ISTOMIN
JACOBIN
JAROMIR
KENOLIN
KETONIC
KILOBIT
LACONIA
LACONIC
LANOLIN
LAVORIS
MAJORIN
MANOLIN
MASONIC
MEIOSIS
MEIOTIC
MELODIA
MELODIC
MESONIC
MINORIN
MITOSIS
MITOTIC
MONODIC
MORONIC
NEPOTIC
NICOSIA
NOKOMIS
OLEOOIL
ONTOPIC
OSMOSIS
OSMOTIC
OSTOSIS
OTTOIII
OUTOFIT
PARODIC
PAROTID
POLONIA
PREOMIT
RANONIN
REPOSIT
ROBOTIC
RUNONIN
SATORIS
SEGOVIA
SHOOSIN
SIMONIZ
SITONIT
STLOUIS
STOODIN
STOOLIE
SWOOPIN
SWOOSIE
SYNODIC
TACONIC
THROWIN
TICOTIN
TROOPIN
TVMOVIE
TWOONIE
UNCOMIC
UNSOLID
UNTOXIC
UPFORIT
VERONIA
VITORIA
WHOOPIE
WHOOSIS
XEROSIS
XEROTIC
YUKOLIS
ZENOBIA
ZEROSIN

•••O••I
CAROLII
COLOSSI
FAROUKI
HAROLDI
KAROLYI
MENOTTI
MOLOKAI
MONOSKI
NIKOLAI
OTTOIII
RUDOLFI
SECONDI
TABOULI
THEOMNI

••••OI•
ADENOID
AIRFOIL
AMEBOID
ANDROID
ANEROID
ATABOIL
BABYOIL
BATHOIL
BEANOIL
BELVOIR
BERVOIX
BONSOIR
BORZOIS
BOUDOIR
BOWDOIN
CHAMOIS
CHINOIS
COALOIL
COCCOID
COLLOID
CONJOIN
CORNOIL
CTENOID
CYCLOID
DELTOID
DENTOID
DESPOIL
DETROIT
DIPLOID
DISCOID
DISJOIN
EMBROIL
ETHMOID
EXPLOIT
FACTOID
FIBROID
FISHOIL
FUELOIL
GETTOIT
GLOBOID
GOTTOIT
GULFOIL
HAPLOID
HOLYOIL
HOPTOIT
HYALOID
HYPNOID
ILLDOIT
INTROIT
JETFOIL
LAMPOIL
LESTOIL
LITHOID
MASTOID
MAUROIS
MISCOIN
MISJOIN
NONVOID
OCHROID
OCTROIS
OLEOOIL
OSTEOID
PALMOIL
PARBOIL
PHOTOID
PINEOIL
POTBOIL
PREBOIL
PRECOIL
PREVOID
PURLOIN
RADIOIN
RENVOIS
ROCKOIL
ROSEOIL
SAWTOIT
SEETOIT
SEQUOIA
SIGMOID
SIRLOIN
STCROIX
STEROID
SUBJOIN
SUBSOIL
TABLOID
TERROIR
THYROID
TINFOIL
TOPSOIL
TREFOIL
TUNAOIL
TUNGOIL
TURMOIL
TYPHOID
UNSTOIC
VAUDOIS
XIPHOID
ZEBROID

••••O•I
ALVEOLI
APRIORI
BELZONI
BONJOVI
BORDONI
BUITONI
CANNOLI
CANZONI
COLLODI
DRAGOTI
FEODORI
GOLDONI
MAFIOSI
MAISOUI
MANDOKI
MARCONI
MOSCONI
NAIROBI
NEGRONI
PASCOLI
PULMONI
RAVIOLI
RONZONI
SPUMONI
TORTONI
TRIPOLI
ZAMBONI
ZEPPOLI

•••••OI
BOLSHOI
CESTMOI
CHEZMOI
TOLSTOI

OJ•••••
OJIBWAS
OJIBWAY

O•J••••
OBJECTS

O••J•••
ODDJOBS
OLDJOKE
ONAJURY
OUTJEST
OUTJETS
OUTJINX
OUTJUMP
OUTJUTS

O•••J••
OVERJOY

•OJ••••
COJUROR
JOJOBAS
MOJAVES
MOJITOS
SOJOURN
WOJTYLA

•O•J•••
BONJOUR
BONJOVI
CONJOBS
CONJOIN
CONJURE
CONJURY
DONJONS
DONJOSE
DONJUAN
IOBJECT
JOBJARS
LOGJAMS
NONJEWS
NONJURY
TOMJOAD

•O••J••
GOODJOB
GOODJOE
GOTAJOB
HOLYJOE
JOHNJAY
LOCKJAW
LORDJIM
LOVEJOY
NOSEJOB
ROMAJIS

•O••••J
DOUBLEJ

••OJ•••
IWOJIMA
PROJECT
PROJETS
TROJANS

••O•J••
GOODJOB
GOODJOE
PROPJET
SNOWJOB

•••OJ••
LTKOJAK
RESOJET

•••O•J•
ALFORJA

•••O••J
LLCOOLJ

••••O•J
LLCOOLJ
RADIODJ

•••••OJ
LARGEOJ
SMALLOJ

OK•••••
OKAYGUY
OKAYING
OKEEFFE
OKELLEY
OKHOTSK
OKINAWA
OKSHOOT
OKTOBER

O•K••••
OAKCASK
OAKDESK
OAKFERN
OAKIEST
OAKLAND
OAKLAWN
OAKLEAF
OAKLIKE
OAKMOSS
OAKPARK
OAKTAGS
OAKTREE
OAKWOOD
ORKNEYS

O••K•••
OFAKIND
OINKERS
OINKING
ONAKICK
ONEKILO
ONTKEAN
OSAKANS
OSHKOSH
OUTKAST
OUTKEEP
OUTKEPT
OUTKICK
OUTKILL
OUTKING
OUTKISS

O•••K••
OILSKIN
OUTSKIP

O••••K•
OAKLIKE
OARLIKE
OATCAKE
OATLIKE
OILCAKE
OILLIKE
OLDJOKE
OPTICKS
ORBLIKE
OROURKE
OUTASKS
OUTBAKE
OUTTAKE
OWLLIKE

O•••••K
OAKCASK
OAKDESK
OAKPARK
OARLOCK
OBELISK
ODDDUCK
ODDSOCK
OFFPEAK
OILTANK
OKHOTSK
OLDNICK
OLICOOK
ONAKICK
ONALARK
ONBREAK
ONELOOK
ONESOCK
ONEWEEK
ONTRACK
OOBLECK
OSTMARK
OUTBACK
OUTBARK
OUTBULK

OUTCOOK
OUTKICK
OUTLOOK
OUTPICK
OUTRANK
OUTROCK
OUTSEEK
OUTSULK
OUTTALK
OUTWALK
OUTWORK

•OK••••

BOKCHOY
BOKHARA
BOKKENS
COKIEST
FOKKERS
GOKAPUT
GOKARTS
HOKIEST
JOKIEST
NOKNOCK
NOKOMIS
POKEDAT
POKEFUN
POKEMON
POKEOUT
POKESAT
POKIEST
TOKENED
WOKENUP
YOKOONO

•O•K•••

BOBKANE
BODKINS
BOKKENS
BONKERS
BONKING
BOOKBAG
BOOKEND
BOOKERS
BOOKERT
BOOKIES
BOOKIII
BOOKING
BOOKISH
BOOKLET
BOOKMAN
BOOKMEN
BOOKVII
BORKING
BOWKNOT
BOXKITE
COCKADE
COCKERS
COCKIER
COCKILY
COCKING
COCKISH
COCKLED
COCKLES
COCKNEY
COCKPIT
CONKERS
CONKING
CONKLIN
CONKOFF
CONKOUT
COOKERS
COOKERY
COOKIES
COOKING
COOKOFF
COOKOUT
COOKPOT
COOKSUP
COOKTOP
CORKAGE
CORKERS
CORKIER
CORKING
CORKOAK
CORKSUP
DOCKAGE
DOCKERS
DOCKETS
DOCKING
DONKEYS
DONKING
DORKIER
FOKKERS
FOLKART
FOLKIER
FOLKIES
FOLKISH
FOLKWAY
FORKERS
FORKFUL
FORKIER
FORKING
FORKOUT
FORKSUP
HOCKERS
HOCKING
HONKERS
HONKING
HONKSAT
HOOKAHS
HOOKING
HOOKSON
HOOKSUP
HOOKUPS
HOPKINS
HOSKINS
HOTKEYS
JOCKEYS
JOEKIDD
KOLKATA
KOOKIER
LOCKAGE
LOCKBOX
LOCKEAN
LOCKERS
LOCKETS
LOCKING
LOCKINS
LOCKJAW
LOCKLET
LOCKLIN
LOCKNUT
LOCKOUT
LOCKSET
LOCKSIN
LOCKSON
LOCKSUP
LOCKUPS
LOOKERS
LOOKFOR
LOOKING
LOOKINS
LOOKISM
LOOKIST
LOOKOUT
LOOKSAD
LOOKSAT
LOOKSEE
LOOKSIN
LOOKSON
LOOKSTO
LOOKSUP
LOOKUPS
LOOKYOU
MOCKERS
MOCKERY
MOCKING
MOCKSUP
MOCKUPS
MONKEES
MONKEYS
MONKISH
NOCKING
POCKETS
POLKAED
PORKERS
PORKIER
PORKING
PORKISH
PORKPIE
ROCKABY
ROCKCOD
ROCKERS
ROCKERY
ROCKETS
ROCKIER
ROCKIES
ROCKILY
ROCKING
ROCKOIL
ROCKOON
ROCKYII
ROCKYIV
ROOKERY
ROOKIER
ROOKIES
ROOKING
ROOKISH
SOAKERS
SOAKING
SOAKSIN
SOAKSUP
SOCKETS
SOCKEYE
SOCKHOP
SOCKING
SOCKSIN
TOLKIEN
TOMKITE
TOOKAIM
TOOKFOR
TOOKILL
TOOKOFF
TOOKOUT
TOOKTEN
TOPKAPI
TOPKICK
TOPKNOT
TOYKITE
VOSKHOD
WOOKIEE
WORKBOX
WORKDAY
WORKERS
WORKFOR
WORKING
WORKMAN
WORKMEN
WORKOFF
WORKOUT
WORKSAT
WORKSHY
WORKSIN
WORKSON
WORKSUP
WORKUPS
YONKERS
YORKERS
YORKIES
YORKIST
YORKTON
YOUKNOW
ZONKING
ZONKOUT

•O••K••

BODYKIT
COMAKER
CONAKRY
COWSKIN
DOESKIN
GOODKID
HOBOKEN
MOLOKAI
MONGKUT
MONIKER
NONSKED
NONSKID
NONUKES
NOOTKAS
PONYKEG
TOOLKIT
TOPEKAN
VOLCKER

•O•••K•

BOWLIKE
BOXLIKE
BOYLIKE
CODCAKE
COLICKY
CONVOKE
COWLIKE
COWPOKE
DOGLIKE
DOTLIKE
FORSAKE
FOXLIKE
GOBROKE
GODLIKE
GOTHIKA
HOECAKE
HOGLIKE
HOLYOKE
HOTCAKE
KODIAKS
KONTIKI
KOPECKS
KOPIYKA
MOHAWKS
MONOSKI
NOTLIKE
PODLIKE
ROANOKE
RODLIKE
ROETHKE
SONLIKE
SOWLIKE
SOYINKA
SOYINKS
TOELIKE
TOYBIKE
TOYLIKE

•O••••K

BODEREK
BOMBECK
CONNICK
CONRACK
CORKOAK
CORMACK
COSSACK
COWLICK
DOGTICK
DOINGOK
DONETSK
DONTASK
DOUBLEK
FOGBANK
FORSOOK
FOSDICK
GOBLANK
GOODNIK
GOSHAWK
GOTBACK
GOTMILK
HOGBACK
HOLMOAK
HOLYARK
HOTLICK
HOTLINK
HOTMILK
HOTPACK
HOTPINK
HOWARDK
JOBBANK
JOBLOCK
JOEBUCK
JONERIK
LOGBOOK
LOWNECK
LOWRISK
MOLLUSK
MONTAUK
MORLOCK
NOKNOCK
NONBANK
NONBOOK
NONDARK
NONPEAK
NONWORK
NORFOLK
NORWALK
NOWLOOK
OOBLECK
POLLACK
POLLOCK
POPROCK
POTHOOK
POTLUCK
RODDICK
ROEBUCK
ROLLICK
ROSTOCK
SOYMILK
TOEPICK
TOPKICK
TOPRANK
TOYBOOK
WOZNIAK
WOZZECK

••OK•••

BOOKBAG
BOOKEND
BOOKERS
BOOKERT
BOOKIES
BOOKIII
BOOKING
BOOKISH
BOOKLET
BOOKMAN
BOOKMEN
BOOKVII
BROKEIN
BROKERS
BROKEUP
CHOKEON
CHOKERS
CHOKEUP
CHOKIER
CHOKING
COOKERS
COOKERY
COOKIES
COOKING
COOKOFF
COOKOUT
COOKPOT
COOKSUP
COOKTOP
EVOKERS
EVOKING
GROKKED
HOOKAHS
HOOKING
HOOKSON
HOOKSUP
HOOKUPS
KOOKIER
LOOKERS
LOOKFOR
LOOKING
LOOKINS
LOOKISM
LOOKIST
LOOKOUT
LOOKSAD
LOOKSAT
LOOKSEE
LOOKSIN
LOOKSON
LOOKSTO
LOOKSUP
LOOKUPS
LOOKYOU
PROKEDS
ROOKERY
ROOKIER
ROOKIES
ROOKING
ROOKISH
RYOKANS
SMOKERS
SMOKEUP
SMOKEYS
SMOKIER
SMOKIES
SMOKILY
SMOKING
SPOKANE
SPOKEOF
SPOKETO
SPOKEUP
SPOKING
STOKELY
STOKERS
STOKEUP
STOKING
TOOKAIM
TOOKFOR
TOOKILL
TOOKOFF
TOOKOUT
TOOKTEN
WHOKNEW
WOOKIEE

••O•K••

BLOCKED
BLOCKER
BLOCKUP
BRODKEY
BROOKED
CHOCKED
CLOAKED
CLOCKED
CLOCKER
CLOCKIN
CLONKED
CROAKED
CROAKER
CROCKED
CROCKER
CROCKET
CROOKED
CROOKES
FLOCKED
FLOCKTO
FROCKED
GOODKID
GROKKED
KNOCKED
KNOCKER
KNOCKON
NOOTKAS
PLONKED
SHOCKED
SHOCKER
SHOOKUP
SHOPKOS
SNOOKER
SNORKEL
SPOOKED
STOCKED
STOCKER
STOCKUP
STOOKEY
TIOMKIN
TOOLKIT
TROIKAS

••O••K•

ANORAKS
BRODSKY
CHOMSKY
GROMYKO
OROURKE
PROVOKE
SLOVAKS
SNOWSKI
TROTSKY
VRONSKY

••O•••K

GEODUCK
GOODNIK
TWOWEEK

•••OK••

ALROKER
BETOKEN
BROOKED
CAHOKIA
CROOKED
CROOKES
HOBOKEN
INJOKES
INVOKED
INVOKER
INVOKES
ITSOKAY
JUDOKAS
MOLOKAI
NABOKOV
REVOKED
REVOKER
REVOKES
REWOKEN
REYOKED
REYOKES
SHOOKUP
SNOOKER
SPOOKED
STOOKEY
STROKED
STROKER
STROKES
SUDOKUS
UNYOKED
UNYOKES

•••O•K•

BAZOOKA
BUROAKS
EXWORKS
FAROUKI
MONOSKI
PALOOKA
PINOAKS
REBOOKS
RECOCKS
RECOOKS
RECORKS
REDOAKS
REDOCKS
REHOOKS
RELOCKS
RELOOKS
RESOAKS
REWORKS
SHLOCKY
SHNOOKS
TANOAKS
UNCORKS
UNDOCKS
UNFORKS
UNHOOKS
UNLOCKS
UNROCKY
ZEDONKS

•••O••K

ALBORAK
LITOVSK
LTKOJAK
MRNOVAK
OKHOTSK
ZATOPEK

••••OK•

ASAJOKE
BADJOKE
BAZOOKA
BESPOKE
CONVOKE
COWPOKE
GOBROKE
HOLYOKE
IMBROKE
INAPOKE
JSTROKE
KARAOKE
MANDOKI
OLDJOKE
PALOOKA
PROVOKE
REAWOKE
REBOOKS
REBROKE
RECOOKS
REEBOKS
REEVOKE
REHOOKS
RELOOKS
RESPOKE
RESTOKE
RHEBOKS
ROANOKE
SHIKOKU
SHNOOKS
UNBROKE
UNCHOKE
UNHOOKS
UNSMOKY
UNSPOKE

••••O•K

AIRLOCK
AIRSOCK
ARMLOCK
ARTBOOK
ARTROCK
ARTWORK
BABCOCK
BBQPORK
BEDROCK
BIBCOCK
BLALOCK
BULLOCK
CANNOCK
CASSOCK
CHINOOK
CORKOAK
CUTWORK
DAYBOOK
DEFROCK
DESTOCK
DRSPOCK
DRYDOCK
EARLOCK
ELFLOCK
EYEHOOK
FETLOCK
FORSOOK
FRYCOOK
GENLOCK
GUNLOCK
GYMSOCK
HADDOCK
HAMHOCK
HAMMOCK
HANCOCK
HASSOCK
HAYFORK
HEMLOCK
HEYLOOK
HILLOCK
HOLMOAK
INSHOCK
INSTOCK
JOBLOCK
KEYLOCK
KIDROCK
KINFOLK
LAWBOOK
LEACOCK
LEBROCK
LEGWORK
LIVEOAK
LOGBOOK
LUBBOCK
MADLOCK
MATLOCK
MATTOCK
MENFOLK
MISTOOK
MORLOCK
MRSPOCK
NETWORK
NEWLOOK
NEWYORK
NOKNOCK
NONBOOK
NONWORK
NORFOLK
NOWLOOK
NUMLOCK
OARLOCK
ODDSOCK
OLICOOK
ONELOOK
ONESOCK
OUTCOOK
OUTLOOK
OUTROCK
OUTWORK
PADDOCK
PADLOCK
PARTOOK
PEACOCK
PENNOCK
PETCOCK
PETROCK
POLLOCK
POPROCK
POTHOOK
PREBOOK
PRECOOK
PREROCK
PRESOAK
PREWORK
REBLOCK
REDBOOK
REKNOCK
RESTOCK
RIMROCK
ROSTOCK
SCHLOCK
SCHNOOK
SHYLOCK
SKYHOOK
SLYLOOK
SUFFOLK
THELOOK
THEROCK
TINWORK
TOYBOOK
TUSSOCK
UNBLOCK
UNCLOAK
UNFROCK
WARLOCK
WAXWORK
WEDLOCK
WEEFOLK
WETLOOK
ZIPLOCK

•••••OK

ARTBOOK
BANGKOK
BLAUBOK
CHINOOK
DAYBOOK
DOINGOK
EYEHOOK
FEELSOK
FORSOOK
FRYCOOK
GANGTOK
GEMSBOK
HEYLOOK
LAWBOOK
LOGBOOK
MISTOOK
NEWLOOK
NONBOOK
NOWLOOK
OLICOOK
ONELOOK
OUTCOOK
OUTLOOK
PARTOOK
POTHOOK
PREBOOK
PRECOOK
RANAMOK
REDBOOK
RUNAMOK
SCHNOOK
SKYHOOK
SLYLOOK
THATSOK
THELOOK
TOYBOOK
TULSAOK
WETLOOK

OL•••••

OLAFIII
OLAVIII
OLDBATS
OLDBEAN
OLDBLUE
OLDBOYS
OLDCARS
OLDCHAP
OLDCITY
OLDDAYS
OLDDOGS
OLDFILM
OLDFOGY
OLDGAGS
OLDGIRL
OLDGOLD
OLDHAND
OLDJOKE
OLDLADY
OLDLINE
OLDLYME
OLDMAID
OLDMOON
OLDNAVY
OLDNESS
OLDNEWS
OLDNICK
OLDPALS
OLDPROS
OLDROSE
OLDSALT
OLDSAWS
OLDSHOE
OLDSONG
OLDSTER
OLDTIME
OLDTOWN
OLDUVAI
OLDWAYS
OLDWEST
OLEANNA
OLEANNY
OLEATES
OLEBULL
OLEFINS
OLEMISS
OLEOOIL
OLESTRA
OLEVELS
OLICOOK
OLIVIER
OLIVINE
OLMSTED
OLOGIES
OLOROSO
OLYMPIA
OLYMPIC
OLYMPUS

O•L••••

OBLASTS
OBLATES
OBLIGED
OBLIGEE
OBLIGER
OBLIGES
OBLIGOR
OBLIQUE
OBLONGS
OBLOQUY
OGLALAS
OILBASE
OILBIRD
OILCAKE
OILCANS
OILCUPS
OILDRUM
OILHEAT
OILIEST
OILLAMP
OILLESS
OILLIKE
OILLINE
OILPALM
OILPANS
OILRICH
OILRIGS
OILRING
OILRUBS
OILSAND
OILSEED
OILSKIN
OILSPOT
OILTANK
OILWELL
ONLEASE
ONLEASH
ONLEAVE
ONLIEST
ONLOADS
ONLYTOO
ONLYYOU

OOLITES
OOLITIC
OOLONGS
ORLANDO
ORLEANS
OWLEGGS
OWLEYED
OWLIEST
OWLLIKE

O••L•••

OAKLAND
OAKLAWN
OAKLEAF
OAKLIKE
OARLESS
OARLIKE
OARLOCK
OATLIKE
OBELISE
OBELISK
OBELIZE
OCALAFL
OCCLUDE
OCELLAR
OCELLUS
OCELOTS
OCULARS
OCULIST
ODDLOTS
ODELETS
OFFLINE
OFFLOAD
OILLAMP
OILLESS
OILLIKE
OILLINE
OKELLEY
OLDLADY
OLDLINE
OLDLYME
OMALLEY
OMELETS
ONALARK
ONALEAD
ONALERT
ONALINE
ONELANE
ONELIRA
ONELOOK
ONELOVE
ONELUMP
OOBLECK
OOHLALA
OPALINE
OPALISH
OPULENT
ORALIST
ORBLESS
ORBLIKE
ORELESS
OROLOGY
OSTLERS
OTALGIA
OTALGIC
OTOLOGY
OUTLAID
OUTLAIN
OUTLAND
OUTLASH
OUTLAST
OUTLAWS
OUTLAYS
OUTLEAD
OUTLEAP
OUTLETS
OUTLIER
OUTLIES
OUTLIMN
OUTLINE
OUTLIPS
OUTLIVE
OUTLOOK
OUTLOUD
OUTLOVE
OWLLIKE
OXALATE
OXBLOOD

O•••L••

OBERLIN
OCCULTS
OCELLAR
OCELLUS
OFVALUE
OGLALAS
OHANLON
OHMSLAW
OKELLEY
OLDBLUE
OMALLEY
ONECLAM
ONECLUB
OPHELIA
ORACLES
OREILLY
ORIOLES
ORMOLUS
ORTOLAN
ORVILLE
OSCULAR
OSCULES
OTHELLO
OUTBLOT
OUTBLOW
OUTFLEE
OUTFLOW
OUTFLUX
OUTGLOW
OUTPLAN
OUTPLAY
OUTPLOD
OUTPLOT
OVERLAP
OVERLAX
OVERLAY
OVERLET
OVERLIE
OVERLIT

O••••L•

OBESELY
OCTUPLE
OCTUPLY
ODDBALL
OILPALM
OILWELL
OLDFILM
OLDGOLD
OLDPALS
OLDSALT
OLEBULL
OLEVELS
OMPHALO
ONAROLL
ONEBALL
ONEBELL
ONECALL
ONECELL
ONEFOLD
ONEHALF
ONEKILO
ONEMILE
ONESELF
OOHLALA
ORDEALS
ORDERLY
OREILLY
ORVILLE
OSCEOLA
OSSICLE
OSTWALD
OTHELLO
OURSELF
OUTBULK
OUTCALL
OUTCOLD
OUTCULL
OUTKILL
OUTPOLL
OUTPULL
OUTROLL
OUTSELL
OUTSOLD
OUTSOLE
OUTSULK
OUTTALK
OUTTELL
OUTTOLD
OUTTOLL
OUTWALK
OUTWELL
OUTWILE
OUTWILL
OUTYELL
OUTYELP
OVERALL
OVERFLY
OVERPLY
OVERTLY
OXTAILS

O•••••L

OATMEAL
OCALAFL
OCTAVAL
ODDBALL
ODORFUL
OEDIPAL
OHCAROL
OILWELL
OLDGIRL
OLEBULL
OLEOOIL
ONAROLL
ONEBALL
ONEBELL
ONECALL
ONECELL
ONEREEL
ONTHEDL
ONTRIAL
OPTICAL
OPTIMAL
ORBITAL
ORDINAL
ORTEGAL
OUTBAWL
OUTBOWL
OUTCALL
OUTCULL
OUTDUEL
OUTFEEL
OUTFOOL
OUTHAUL
OUTHOWL
OUTHURL
OUTKILL
OUTPOLL
OUTPULL
OUTPURL
OUTRAIL
OUTROLL
OUTSAIL
OUTSELL
OUTTELL
OUTTOLL
OUTWELL
OUTWILL
OUTYELL
OVERALL
OVOIDAL
OWNGOAL

•OL••••

BOLATIE
BOLDEST
BOLEROS
BOLIDES
BOLIVAR
BOLIVIA
BOLLING
BOLOGNA
BOLOTIE
BOLSHOI
BOLSTER
BOLTERS
BOLTING
BOLTSUP
BOLUSES
COLADAS
COLBERT
COLCHIS
COLDCUP
COLDCUT
COLDDAY
COLDEST
COLDISH
COLDONE
COLDWAR
COLEMAN
COLETTE
COLGATE
COLICKY
COLLAGE
COLLARD
COLLARS
COLLATE
COLLECT
COLLEEN
COLLEGE
COLLETS
COLLIDE
COLLIER
COLLIES
COLLINE
COLLINS
COLLODI
COLLOID
COLLOPS
COLLUDE
COLLYER
COLOGNE
COLOMBO
COLONEL
COLONES
COLONNA
COLONUS
COLORED
COLORER
COLORTV
COLOSSI
COLOURS
COLTISH
COLUMBA
COLUMBO
COLUMNS
DOLEFUL
DOLEOUT
DOLLARS
DOLLIED
DOLLIES
DOLLING
DOLLISH
DOLLOPS
DOLLSUP
DOLMANS
DOLORES
DOLOURS
DOLPHIN
DOLTISH
DOLUNCH
EOLITHS
FOLATES
FOLDERS
FOLDING
FOLDOUT
FOLDSIN
FOLDSUP
FOLDUPS
FOLENGO
FOLGERS
FOLIAGE
FOLIATE
FOLIOED
FOLIOSE
FOLKART
FOLKIER
FOLKIES
FOLKISH
FOLKWAY
FOLLETT
FOLLIES
FOLLOWS
GOLDARN
GOLDBUG
GOLDING
GOLDMAN
GOLDONI
GOLDTIP
GOLDWYN
GOLFBAG
GOLFCAR
GOLFERS
GOLFING
GOLFPRO
GOLFTEE
GOLIATH
HOLBEIN
HOLBERG
HOLDALL
HOLDERS
HOLDING
HOLDOFF
HOLDOUT
HOLDSIN
HOLDSIT
HOLDSON
HOLDSTO
HOLDSUP
HOLDUPS
HOLEDUP
HOLEOUT
HOLESUP
HOLIDAY
HOLIEST
HOLISTS
HOLLAND
HOLLERS
HOLLIES
HOLLOWS
HOLMIUM
HOLMOAK
HOLSTER
HOLYARK
HOLYCOW
HOLYDAY
HOLYJOE
HOLYMAN
HOLYMEN
HOLYOIL
HOLYOKE
HOLYONE
HOLYSEE
HOLYWAR
HOLZMAN
JOLLIED
JOLLIER
JOLLIES
JOLLIET
JOLLIFY
JOLLILY
JOLLITY
JOLTERS
JOLTIER
JOLTING
KOLANUT
KOLKATA
LOLLARD
LOLLERS
LOLLIES
LOLLING
MOLDERS
MOLDIER
MOLDING
MOLDOVA
MOLERAT
MOLESTS
MOLIERE
MOLITOR
MOLLIES
MOLLIFY
MOLLUSC
MOLLUSK
MOLOKAI
MOLOTOV
MOLSONS
MOLTERS
MOLTING
MOLUCCA
NOLIMIT
NOLOADS
OOLITES
OOLITIC
OOLONGS
POLANER
POLANYI
POLARAS
POLARIS
POLEAXE
POLECAR
POLECAT
POLEMAN
POLEMEN
POLEMIC
POLENTA
POLESAT
POLESIT
POLICED
POLICER
POLICES
POLISCI
POLITER
POLITIC
POLKAED
POLLACK
POLLARD
POLLEES
POLLENS
POLLERA
POLLERS
POLLING
POLLOCK
POLLTAX
POLLUTE
POLOIST
POLONIA
POLTAVA
POLYGON
POLYMER
POLYPED
POLYPOD
POLYSCI
ROLAIDS
ROLEXES
ROLFERS
ROLFING
ROLLAND
ROLLBAR
ROLLEIS
ROLLERS
ROLLICK
ROLLING
ROLLINS
ROLLMOP
ROLLOFF
ROLLONS
ROLLOUT
ROLLSBY
ROLLSIN
ROLLSON
ROLLSUP
ROLLTOP
ROLLUPS
ROLLWAY
ROLODEX
ROLONDA
ROLVAAG
SOLACED
SOLACER
SOLACES
SOLARAS
SOLARIA
SOLDERS
SOLDFOR
SOLDIER
SOLDOFF
SOLDOUT
SOLEDAD
SOLFEGE
SOLICIT
SOLIDER
SOLIDLY
SOLLATI
SOLNESS
SOLOACT
SOLOING
SOLOIST
SOLOMON
SOLUBLE
SOLUTES
SOLVEIT
SOLVENT
SOLVERS
SOLVING
TOLDALL
TOLDOFF
TOLEASE
TOLEDAN
TOLEDOS
TOLKIEN
TOLLAGE
TOLLBAR
TOLLERS
TOLLING
TOLLMAN
TOLLMEN
TOLLWAY
TOLSTOI
TOLSTOY
TOLTECS
TOLUENE
VOLANTE
VOLCANO
VOLCKER
VOLENTE
VOLLEYS
VOLPONE
VOLTAGE
VOLTAIC
VOLTORE
VOLUBLE
VOLUBLY
VOLUMED
VOLUMES
VOLUTED
VOLUTES
WOLFCUB
WOLFDOG
WOLFGAL
WOLFING
WOLFISH
WOLFMAN
WOLFMEN
WOLFRAM
YOLANDA

•O•L•••

BOILERS
BOILING
BOILOFF
BOILOUT
BOILSUP
BOLLING
BOOLEAN
BORLAUG
BOULDER
BOWLERS
BOWLESS
BOWLFUL
BOWLIKE
BOWLINE
BOWLING
BOXLIKE
BOYLIKE
COALBIN
COALCAR
COALERS
COALGAS
COALING
COALOIL
COALPIT
COALTAR
COBLENZ
COILERS
COILING
COILSUP
COLLAGE
COLLARD
COLLARS
COLLATE
COLLECT
COLLEEN
COLLEGE
COLLETS
COLLIDE
COLLIER
COLLIES
COLLINE
COLLINS
COLLODI
COLLOID
COLLOPS
COLLUDE
COLLYER
COOLAIR
COOLANT
COOLCAT
COOLERS
COOLEST
COOLIES
COOLING
COOLISH
COOLMAX
COOLOUT
COOLPIX
COOLSIT
COPLAND
COULDBE
COULDNT
COULEES
COULOMB
COULTER
COWLICK
COWLIKE
COWLING
COXLESS
DOGLEGS
DOGLESS
DOGLIKE
DOILIES
DOLLARS
DOLLIED
DOLLIES
DOLLING
DOLLISH
DOLLOPS
DOLLSUP
DONLEVY
DOOLIES
DOTLIKE
DOWLING
EONLINE
FOALING
FOELESS
FOGLAMP
FOGLESS
FOILING
FOLLETT
FOLLIES
FOLLOWS
FOOLERS
FOOLERY
FOOLING
FOOLISH
FORLANI
FORLIFE
FORLORN
FORLOVE
FOULARD
FOULEST
FOULING
FOULOUT
FOULSUP
FOULTIP
FOULUPS
FOWLERS
FOWLING
FOXLIKE
GOALIES
GOALONG
GOBLANK
GOBLETS
GOBLINS
GODLESS
GODLIER
GODLIKE
GODLING
GOSLING
GOTLOST
GOULASH
HOGLIKE
HOLLAND
HOLLERS
HOLLIES
HOLLOWS
HOPLITE
HOTLEAD
HOTLICK
HOTLINE
HOTLINK
HOTLIPS
HOVLANE
HOWLAME
HOWLERS
HOWLING
HOWLONG
HOWLSAT
JOBLESS
JOBLOCK
JOBLOTS
JOLLIED
JOLLIER
JOLLIES
JOLLIET
JOLLIFY
JOLLILY
JOLLITY
JOWLIER
JOYLESS
KOBLENZ
KOOLAID
KOWLOON
LOLLARD
LOLLERS
LOLLIES
LOLLING
LOWLAND
LOWLIER
LOWLIFE
LOWLILY
MOILERS
MOILING
MOLLIES
MOLLIFY
MOLLUSC
MOLLUSK
MORLOCK
MOSLEMS
MOTLEYS
MOULAGE
MOULDED
MOULDER
MOULTED
NOBLEST
NOCLASS
NONLIFE
NONLIVE
NOPLACE
NOTLIKE
NOTLIVE
NOWLOOK
OOBLECK
OOHLALA
POBLANO
PODLIKE
POLLACK
POLLARD
POLLEES
POLLENS
POLLERA
POLLERS
POLLING
POLLOCK
POLLTAX
POLLUTE
POOLCUE
POOLERS
POOLING
POOLMAN
POOLMEN
POPLARS
POPLINS
POTLIDS
POTLUCK
POULENC
POULTRY
ROBLOWE
RODLESS
RODLIKE
ROILIER
ROILING
ROLLAND
ROLLBAR
ROLLEIS
ROLLERS
ROLLICK
ROLLING
ROLLINS
ROLLMOP
ROLLOFF
ROLLONS
ROLLOUT
ROLLSBY
ROLLSIN
ROLLSON
ROLLSUP
ROLLTOP
ROLLUPS
ROLLWAY
ROULADE
ROULEAU
ROWLAND
ROWLING
SODLESS
SOILAGE
SOILING
SOLLATI
SONLESS
SONLIKE
SOULFUL
SOULMAN
SOWLIKE
SOYLENT
TOBLAME
TOELESS
TOELIKE
TOELOOP
TOILERS
TOILETS
TOILFUL
TOILING
TOILSAT
TOLLAGE
TOLLBAR
TOLLERS
TOLLING
TOLLMAN
TOLLMEN
TOLLWAY
TOOLATE
TOOLBAR
TOOLBOX
TOOLERS
TOOLING
TOOLKIT
TOOLONG
TOOLSET
TOOLSUP
TOPLESS
TOPLINE
TOWLINE
TOYLAND
TOYLESS
TOYLIKE
VOLLEYS
VONLAUE
VORLAGE
VOWLESS
WOOLENS
WOOLERY
WOOLFAT
WOOLHAT
WOOLIER
WOOLIES
WOOLITE
WOOLLEN
WOOLLEY
WOOLSEY
WORLDLY
WOULDBE
WOULDNT
WOULDST
YOPLAIT
YOULOSE
YOWLERS
YOWLING
ZOELLER
ZOOLOGY

•O••L••

BOBBLED
BOBBLER
BOBBLES
BOBSLED
BOCELLI
BOGGLED
BOGGLER
BOGGLES
BOMBLET
BONELET
BONILLA
BOODLES
BOOKLET

BOOMLET
BOOSLER
BOOTLEG
BORGLUM
BOTTLED
BOTTLER
BOTTLES
BOWDLER
COBALTS
COBBLED
COBBLER
COBBLES
COCHLEA
COCKLED
COCKLES
CODDLED
CODDLER
CODDLES
COGGLES
COGHLAN
COMPLEX
COMPLIN
CONELET
CONKLIN
COPILOT
COPULAE
COPULAR
COPULAS
CORELLI
COROLLA
COUPLED
COUPLER
COUPLES
COUPLET
COWSLIP
DOGFLEA
DOGSLED
DONGLES
DONTLIE
DOODLED
DOODLER
DOODLES
DOPPLER
DOTTLES
DOUBLEA
DOUBLEB
DOUBLEC
DOUBLED
DOUBLEE
DOUBLEF
DOUBLEG
DOUBLEH
DOUBLEI
DOUBLEJ
DOUBLEK
DOUBLEL
DOUBLEM
DOUBLEN
DOUBLEO
DOUBLEP
DOUBLEQ
DOUBLER
DOUBLES
DOUBLET
DOUBLEU
DOUBLEV
DOUBLEW
DOUBLEX
DOUBLEY
DOUBLEZ
DOUGLAS
DOVELET
FOCSLES
FOIBLES
FONDLED
FONDLER
FONDLES
FOOTLED
FOOTLER
FOOTLES
FOOTLET
FOOZLED
FOOZLER
FOOZLES
FORDLTD
FORELEG
FORTLEE
GOBBLED
GOBBLER
GOBBLES
GOBELIN
GOBELOW
GOGGLED
GOGGLER
GOGGLES
GOOGLED
GOOGLER
GOOGLES
GORILLA
HOBBLED
HOBBLER
HOBBLES
HOMELAB
HONALEE
HOODLUM
HOOPLAS
HORSLEY
HOSTLER
HOTGLUE
HOWELLS
HOWELSE
JOCELYN
JOCULAR
JOEBLOW
JOGGLED
JOGGLER
JOGGLES
JOHNLAW
JOHNLEE
JOSTLED
JOSTLER
JOSTLES
KOBOLDS
KOEHLER
LOBULES
LOCALES
LOCALLY
LOCKLET
LOCKLIN
LOCULUS
LORELAI
LORELEI
LOUELLA
LOWBLOW
LOYALER
LOYALES
LOYALLY
LOYALTO
LOYALTY
LOYOLAU
MOBILES
MODELAS
MODELBS
MODELED
MODELER
MODELTS
MODULAR
MODULES
MODULUS
MONOLOG
MOONLET
MOONLIT
MORALES
MORALLY
MORELLA
MORELLO
MORELOS
MOSELLE
MOTTLED
MOTTLES
MOZILLA
NODULAR
NODULED
NODULES
NOGALES
NONFLUX
NONPLAY
NONPLUS
NONSLIP
NOODLED
NOODLES
NOPALES
NORELCO
NOTALIE
NOTALOT
NOVALIS
NOVELAS
NOVELLA
NOVELLE
NOVELLO
NOVELTY
NOZZLES
POMELOS
POODLES
POORLAW
POPELEO
POPPLED
POPPLES
POPULAR
POSOLES
POSSLQS
POZOLES
RODOLFO
ROMULAN
ROMULUS
ROOTLED
ROOTLES
ROOTLET
ROSALIA
ROSALIE
ROSALYN
ROSELLA
ROSELLE
ROTBLAT
ROTELLE
ROWELED
ROYALES
ROYALLY
ROYALTY
ROYALWE
ROZELLE
SOMALIA
SOMALIS
TOCELIA
TODDLED
TODDLER
TODDLES
TOFFLER
TOGGLED
TOGGLER
TOGGLES
TOHELEN
TONALLY
TONELOC
TOODLES
TOOSLOW
TOOTLED
TOOTLER
TOOTLES
TOPPLED
TOPPLES
TORTLAW
TOTALED
TOTALER
TOTALLY
TOTALUP
TOUSLED
TOUSLES
TOWELED
TOWNLET
TOYSLED
VOCALIC
VOCALLY
VOWELLY
WOBBLED
WOBBLER
WOBBLES
WOODLEY
WOODLOT
WOOLLEN
WOOLLEY
WORSLEY
YODELED
YODELER
ZOCALOS
ZOELLER
ZONALLY
ZONULAR
ZONULES

•O••L•

BOATELS
BOBDOLE
BOBVILA
BOCELLI
BOFFOLA
BOGHOLE
BOGUSLY
BONILLA
BONNILY
BOOZILY
BOSSILY
BOSWELL
BOXBALL
BOXFULS
COCKILY
COEVALS
COMPELS
COMPILE
CONDOLE
CONSOLE
CONSULS
CONSULT
COPPOLA
CORACLE
CORBELS
CORDELL
CORELLI
CORNELL
CORNILY
COROLLA
CORRALS
CORYELL
COURTLY
COWBELL
DOGPILE
DONNALL
DORSALS
DOSSALS
DOTTILY
DOWDILY
FOAMILY
FOGGILY
FORMALS
FORMULA
FORSALE
FOSCOLO
FOSSILS
FOXHOLE
GOGIRLS
GONDOLA
GOODALL
GOOFILY
GOOGOLS
GOONILY
GORILLA
GOSPELS
GOSTALE
GOTCOLD
GOTHELP
GOTMILK
GOTWELL
GOUTILY
HOARILY
HOGCALL
HOGWILD
HOLDALL
HORSILY
HOSCALE
HOSTELS
HOSTILE
HOTMILK
HOTROLL
HOWDULL
HOWELLS
JODRELL
JOEHILL
JOINTLY
JOLLILY
JONHALL
JOPPOLO
KORDELL
KOWADLO
LOATHLY
LOCALLY
LOFTILY
LOGROLL
LOONILY
LOOSELY
LOSABLE
LOUELLA
LOUSILY
LOVABLE
LOVABLY
LOVERLY
LOWBALL
LOWLILY
LOYALLY
MOBRULE
MOISTLY
MONDALE
MONGOLS
MONOCLE
MONTALE
MONTHLY
MOODILY
MOONILY
MORALLY
MORELLA
MORELLO
MORSELS
MORTALS
MOSELLE
MOUSILY
MOVABLE
MOVABLY
MOZILLA
NOBHILL
NOFAULT
NOISILY
NONCOLA
NONGOLD
NONOILY
NONSALE
NONSELF
NONUPLE
NORFOLK
NORMALS
NORWALK
NOTABLE
NOTABLY
NOTEDLY
NOTWELL
NOVELLA
NOVELLE
NOVELLO
OOHLALA
POMMELS
PORTALS
POSABLE
POTABLE
POTFULS
POTHOLE
ROCKILY
RONDELS
ROOMILY
ROSELLA
ROSELLE
ROSEOLA
ROSWELL
ROTELLE
ROUAULT
ROUGHLY
ROUNDLY
ROWDILY
ROYALLY
ROZELLE
SOAPILY
SOBERLY
SOCIALS
SOGGILY
SOLIDLY
SOLUBLE
SOOTILY
SORRELL
SORRELS
SORRILY
SOUFFLE
SOUNDLY
SOURALE
SOYMILK
TOEHOLD
TOLDALL
TOMGOLA
TONALLY
TONSILS
TOOKILL
TOOTALL
TOPHOLE
TORTOLA
TORVALD
TORVILL
TOSCALE
TOTABLE
TOTALLY
TOUGHLY
TOWABLE
TOYBALL
TOYDOLL
VOCABLE
VOCABLY
VOCALLY
VOLUBLE
VOLUBLY
VONZELL
VOTABLE
VOWELLY
WOJTYLA
WOMANLY
WOOZILY
WORDILY
WORLDLY
WORRELL
ZONALLY

•O••••L

BOATFUL
BOBTAIL
BODEFUL
BORSTAL
BOSWELL
BOWLFUL
BOXBALL
COALOIL
COASTAL
COAXIAL
COBCOAL
CODICIL
COEQUAL
COLONEL
COMICAL
CONCEAL
CONGEAL
CONICAL
CONTROL
CORDELL
CORDIAL
CORNEAL
CORNELL
CORNOIL
CORONAL
CORYELL
COUNCIL
COUNSEL
COWBELL
COWGIRL
COZUMEL
DOADEAL
DOGBOWL
DOGTAIL
DOLEFUL
DOMICAL
DOMICIL
DONEGAL
DONNALL
DOOMFUL
DOUBLEL
FORKFUL
FORMFUL
FORREAL
FOXTAIL
GODEVIL
GONERIL
GOODALL
GOTOGAL
GOTREAL
GOTWELL
HOBNAIL
HOGCALL
HOLDALL
HOLYOIL
HOOTOWL
HOPEFUL
HOTCOAL
HOTMAIL
HOTMEAL
HOTROLL
HOWDULL
JODRELL
JOECOOL
JOEHILL
JONHALL
JONQUIL
JOURNAL
KORDELL
LOGICAL
LOGROLL
LOWBALL
LOWHEEL
MOANFUL
MONADAL
MONDIAL
MONGREL
NOANGEL
NOBHILL
NODICAL
NOMINAL
NONEVIL
NONFUEL
NONORAL
NONWOOL
NOSTRIL
NOTREAL
NOTWELL
POTBOIL
POUTFUL
ROCKOIL
ROOMFUL
RORQUAL
ROSEOIL
ROSTRAL
ROSWELL
ROUNDEL
SOFTGEL
SONGFUL
SORORAL
SORRELL
SOULFUL
SOYMEAL
TOENAIL
TOILFUL
TOLDALL
TOMFOOL
TOOKILL
TOOTALL
TOPICAL
TOPSAIL
TOPSOIL
TORVILL
TOYBALL
TOYDOLL
TOYPAIL
VONOPEL
VONZELL
WOLFGAL
WORRELL
ZOOIDAL

••OL•••

ABOLISH
ABOLLAE
ACOLYTE
ADOLLAR
ADOLPHE
AEOLIAN
APOLLOS
APOLOGY
AXOLOTL
BIOLABS
BIOLITE
BIOLOGY
BOOLEAN
CHOLERA
CHOLERS
CHOLINE
CHOLLAS
COOLAIR
COOLANT
COOLCAT
COOLERS
COOLEST
COOLIES
COOLING
COOLISH
COOLMAX
COOLOUT
COOLPIX
COOLSIT
DOOLIES
DROLLER
ECOLOGY
ENOLOGY
EVOLUTE
EVOLVED
EVOLVER
EVOLVES
FOOLERS
FOOLERY
FOOLING
FOOLISH
FROLICS
GAOLERS
GAOLING
GEOLOGY
GROLIER
IDOLISE
IDOLIST
IDOLIZE
ISOLATE
ISOLATO
ISOLINE
KOOLAID
MYOLOGY
NEOLITH
NEOLOGY
NEOLYTE
OROLOGY
OTOLOGY
PIOLETS
POOLCUE
POOLERS
POOLING
POOLMAN
POOLMEN
PROLATE
PROLIFE
PROLOGS
PROLONG
PTOLEMY
RIOLOBO
SCOLARI
SCOLDED
SCOLDER
SMOLDER
STOLEIN
STOLLEN
STOLONS
SWOLLEN
TOOLATE
TOOLBAR
TOOLBOX
TOOLERS
TOOLING
TOOLKIT
TOOLONG
TOOLSET
TOOLSUP
TROLLED
TROLLER
TROLLEY
TROLLOP
TWOLANE
UFOLOGY
UGOLINO
UROLOGY
VIOLATE
VIOLENT
VIOLETS
VIOLINS
VIOLIST
VIOLONE
WOOLENS
WOOLERY
WOOLFAT
WOOLHAT
WOOLIER
WOOLIES
WOOLITE
WOOLLEN
WOOLLEY
WOOLSEY
ZOOLOGY

••O•L••

ABOLLAE
ADOLLAR
AFOULOF
APOLLOS
AVONLEA
BOODLES
BOOKLET
BOOMLET
BOOSLER
BOOTLEG
BROILED
BROILER
CHOLLAS
CROWLEY
DOODLED
DOODLER
DOODLES
DROLLER
DROOLED
DROOLER
DROPLET
ENOILED
ETOILES
EXOILER
FOOTLED
FOOTLER
FOOTLES
FOOTLET
FOOZLED
FOOZLER
FOOZLES
FROGLEG
FROGLET
GOOGLED
GOOGLER
GOOGLES
GROWLED
GROWLER
HOODLUM
HOOPLAS
KNOWLES
KTOSLIN
MOONLET
MOONLIT
NOODLED
NOODLES
PEOPLED
PEOPLES
POODLES
POORLAW
PROBLEM
PROCLUS
PROWLED
PROWLER
REOILED
ROOTLED
ROOTLES
ROOTLET
SCOWLED
SCOWLER
SHOALED
SHOULDA
SHOULDI
SPOILED
SPOILER
SPOOLED
SPOOLER
SPOTLIT
STOLLEN
STOOLED
STOOLIE
SWOLLEN
TOODLES
TOOSLOW
TOOTLED
TOOTLER
TOOTLES
TROILUS
TROLLED
TROLLER
TROLLEY
TROLLOP
UNOGLED
UNOILED
WHORLED
WOODLEY
WOODLOT
WOOLLEN
WOOLLEY
WROCLAW

••O••L•

ACOUPLE
ALOOFLY
ANOMALY
ANOUILH
APOSTLE
AVOWALS
BEOWULF
BLOWFLY
BOOZILY
BROADLY
CHORALE
CHORALS
CHORTLE
CLOSELY
CROSSLY
CROWELL
DUOPOLY
EROSELY
FROOGLE
GHOSTLY
GLOBULE
GOODALL
GOOFILY
GOOGOLS
GOONILY
GROSSLY
GROVELS
GROWOLD
ILOVELA
INOCULA
ISOHELS
KNOWALL
KYOODLE
LEOPOLD
LIONELL
LIONELS
LOONILY
LOOSELY
LYOCELL
LYONELL
MOODILY
MOONILY
PHONILY
PIOUSLY
PROBALL
PROFILE
PRONELY
PROPELS
PROSILY
PROUDLY
ROOMILY
SHOOFLY
SHORTLY
SHOVELS
SHOWILY
SMOKILY
SNOBALL
SNOWILY
SOOTILY
STOKELY
STONILY
STOPPLE
STOUTLY
TMOBILE
TOOKILL
TOOTALL
TROUBLE
TROWELS
TWOBALL
TWOFOLD
WOOZILY
WRONGLY

••O•••L

APOGEAL
AROUSAL
ASOCIAL
AXOLOTL
BIOFUEL
CHORDAL
CROWELL
DOOMFUL
EPOCHAL
FLOREAL
FROEBEL
FRONTAL
GLOSSAL
GLOTTAL

GOODALL
HOOTOWL
KNOWALL
LIONELL
LYOCELL
LYONELL
ODORFUL
OVOIDAL
PLOTFUL
PROBALL
PROBOWL
ROOMFUL
SHOPFUL
SNOBALL
SNORKEL
SPOUSAL
STOICAL
TOOKILL
TOOTALL
TWOBALL
UXORIAL
ZOOIDAL

•••OL••

ABSOLUT
ABSOLVE
ANGOLAN
ARBOLES
AREOLAE
AREOLAR
AREOLAS
AREOLES
ARNOLDS
ASTOLAT
BAROLOS
BEHOLDS
BICOLOR
BIPOLAR
BUCOLIC
BYGOLLY
CAJOLED
CAJOLER
CAJOLES
CANOLAS
CAROLED
CAROLER
CAROLII
CAROLYN
COROLLA
CREOLES
CUPOLAS
DECOLOR
DEMOLAY
DEVOLVE
DIPOLAR
DIPOLES
DROOLED
DROOLER
EIDOLIC
EIDOLON
ENFOLDS
ENROLLS
EXTOLLS
GIGOLOS
GIROLLE
HAROLDI
INCOLOR
INFOLDS
INSOLES
INVOLVE
KAROLYI
KENOLIN
KOBOLDS
LAJOLLA
LANOLIN
LEGOLAS
LOYOLAU
MANOLIN
MINOLTA
MONOLOG
NICOLAS
NICOLET
NICOLLE
NIKOLAI
NIKOLAY
ORIOLES
ORMOLUS
ORTOLAN
PAROLED
PAROLEE
PAROLES
PAYOLAS
POSOLES
POZOLES
RCCOLAS
REBOLTS
RECOLOR
REFOLDS
REMOLDS
REPOLLS
REROLLS
RESOLED
RESOLER
RESOLES
RESOLVE
REVOLTS
REVOLVE
RODOLFO
RUDOLFI
RUDOLPH
SCHOLAR
SCHOLES
SCROLLS
SPOOLED
SPOOLER
STOOLED
STOOLIE
STROLLS
TRIOLET
TUPOLEV
UNBOLTS
UNFOLDS
UNJOLLY
UNMOLDS
UNMOLDY
UNPOLED
UNROLLS
UNSOLED
UNSOLES
UNSOLID
UPFOLDS
UPHOLDS
YUKOLIS

•••O•L•

ACTORLY
ALOOFLY
AMPOULE
BEFOOLS
BEFOULS
BUXOMLY
BYGOLLY
COROLLA
DEBOULE
ELFOWLS
ENNOBLE
ENROLLS
ENSOULS
ETVOILA
EXTOLLS
FROOGLE
GIROLLE
IGNOBLE
IGNOBLY
INGOALS
KYOODLE
LAJOLLA
LLCOOLJ
MONOCLE
MYWORLD
NICOLLE
NONOILY
NUTOILS
PANOPLY
PCWORLD
REBOILS
RECOALS
RECOILS
RECOOLS
REPOLLS
REROLLS
RESOILS
RETOOLS
SCHOOLS
SCROLLS
SHOOFLY
STROLLS
TABOULI
TAROILS
UNCOILS
UNCOYLY
UNGODLY
UNJOLLY
UNLOWLY
UNMOULD
UNROLLS
UPCOILS

•••O••L

AEROSOL
ALCOHOL
AURORAL
BIFOCAL
BIMODAL
BITONAL
COLONEL
CORONAL
CREOSOL
DAMOSEL
DEPOSAL
ESTORIL
FEMORAL
GASOHOL
GOTOGAL
GQMODEL
HUMORAL
IMMORAL
INTOTAL
MAYORAL
NONORAL
OLEOOIL
PERORAL
PIVOTAL
PREORAL
REMODEL
REMOVAL
RETOTAL
SORORAL
SYNODAL
UNLOCAL
UNLOYAL
UNNOVEL
UNVOCAL
VONOPEL

••••OL•

ACEROLA
AIRHOLE
AIRWOLF
ALLTOLD
ALVEOLI
AMAPOLA
AMATOLS
AMIDOLS
ANATOLE
ANATOLY
ARMHOLE
AUREOLA
AUREOLE
BADCOLD
BAGNOLD
BARTOLO
BEDROLL
BEFOOLS
BERTOLT
BITROLE
BOBDOLE
BOFFOLA
BOGHOLE
CALPOLY
CANNOLI
CARIOLE
CARROLL
CASSOLA
CINEOLE
CONDOLE
CONSOLE
COPPOLA
CRAPOLA
CRAYOLA
CRYWOLF
DELSOLS
DIABOLO
DIAVOLO
DIEBOLD
DRYHOLE
DUOPOLY
EARHOLE
EGGROLL
EYEBOLT
EYEFOLD
EYEHOLE
EYEROLL
FANFOLD
FLYSOLO
FOSCOLO
FOXHOLE
FRIJOLE
FRIVOLS
GAMBOLS
GETCOLD
GETSOLD
GINGOLD
GLYCOLS
GONDOLA
GOOGOLS
GOTCOLD
GRANOLA
GREWOLD
GROWOLD
GUNMOLL
HANSOLO
HARROLD
HOTROLL
IANHOLM
ICECOLD
ICEHOLE
ILLFOLD
INAHOLE
ITSCOLD
JOPPOLO
KENDOLL
KEYHOLE
KINFOLK
LEOPOLD
LETROLL
LINCOLN
LLCOOLJ
LOGROLL
MALCOLM
MANHOLE
MAYPOLE
MENFOLK
MIDSOLE
MINEOLA
MISKOLC
MISTOLD
MONGOLS
MUDHOLE
NEWBOLT
NICCOLO
NICHOLS
NONCOLA
NONGOLD
NORFOLK
OLDGOLD
ONAROLL
ONEFOLD
OSCEOLA
OUTCOLD
OUTPOLL
OUTROLL
OUTSOLD
OUTSOLE
OUTTOLD
OUTTOLL
PASCOLI
PATROLS
PAYROLL
PERGOLA
PETIOLE
PETROLS
PHENOLS
PIANOLA
PICCOLO
PIEHOLE
PINFOLD
PINHOLE
PISTOLE
PISTOLS
PLUGOLA
POTHOLE
PRESOLD
PRETOLD
RAGDOLL
RATHOLE
RAVIOLI
RECOOLS
REDPOLL
REDWOLF
RETOOLS
RISSOLE
ROSEOLA
RUBEOLA
RUMPOLE
SAMEOLD
SCHOOLS
SEAWOLF
SHEWOLF
SHINOLA
SIXFOLD
SKIPOLE
SPYHOLE
STEROLS
SUFFOLK
SYMBOLS
SYSTOLE
TADPOLE
TENFOLD
THEDOLE
THEGOLD
TIEPOLO
TIMHOLT
TOEHOLD
TOMGOLA
TOPHOLE
TORTOLA
TOYDOLL
TREMOLO
TRIFOLD
TRIPOLI
TVIDOLS
TWOFOLD
UNWHOLE
VACUOLE
VERYOLD
VIGNOLA
WALPOLE
WEEFOLK
WIMPOLE
ZEPPOLE
ZEPPOLI

••••O•L

AIRCOOL
AIRFOIL
ATABOIL
AXOLOTL
BABYOIL
BARNOWL
BATHOIL
BEANOIL
BEDROLL
BSCHOOL
CARPOOL
CARROLL
CATBOWL
COALOIL
COBCOAL
CORNOIL
DESPOIL
DOGBOWL
EGGROLL
EMBROIL
EYEROLL
FISHOIL
FUELOIL
GULFOIL
GUNMOLL
HOLYOIL
HOOTOWL
HOTCOAL
HOTROLL
JETFOIL
JOECOOL
KENDOLL
LAMPOIL
LESTOIL
LETROLL
LOGROLL
NONWOOL
OLEOOIL
ONAROLL
OUTBOWL
OUTFOOL
OUTHOWL
OUTPOLL
OUTROLL
OUTTOLL
OWNGOAL
PALMOIL
PARBOIL
PAYROLL
PEAFOWL
PINEOIL
POTBOIL
PREBOIL
PRECOIL
PRECOOL
PROBOWL
QSCHOOL
RAGDOLL
REDPOLL
RESPOOL
ROCKOIL
ROSEOIL
SEAFOWL
SUBCOOL
SUBGOAL
SUBSOIL
SUNBOWL
THEFOOL
TINFOIL
TOMFOOL
TOPSOIL
TOYDOLL
TREFOIL
TUNAOIL
TUNGOIL
TURMOIL
UNSPOOL
VANPOOL
WAYCOOL

•••••OL

AEROSOL
AIRCOOL
ALCOHOL
ANBESOL
BALLIOL
BRISTOL
BSCHOOL
CAPITOL
CARPOOL
CASTROL
CLAIROL
CONTROL
CREOSOL
DEMEROL
ESPANOL
ETHANOL
GASOHOL
GERITOL
GIRASOL
GUIGNOL
JCARROL
JOECOOL
MAILLOL
MENTHOL
NONWOOL
OHCAROL
OUTFOOL
PARASOL
PINESOL
PRECOOL
QSCHOOL
RESPOOL
RETINOL
SMEAGOL
SUBCOOL
THEFOOL
TOMFOOL
TYLENOL
UNSPOOL
VANPOOL
VITRIOL
WAYCOOL

OM•••••

OMAHANE
OMAHANS
OMALLEY
OMELETS
OMENING
OMICRON
OMIGOSH
OMINOUS
OMITTED
OMITTER
OMNIBUS
OMNIMAX
OMPHALO

O•M••••

OHMAGES
OHMSLAW
OLMSTED
ONMYOWN
OOMPAHS
ORMANDY
ORMOLUS
OSMATIC
OSMONDS
OSMOSED
OSMOSES
OSMOSIS
OSMOTIC
OSMUNDS

O••M•••

OAKMOSS
OATMEAL
ODDMENT
OFAMIND
OLDMAID
OLDMOON
OLEMISS
OLYMPIA
OLYMPIC
OLYMPUS
ONEMILE
ONEMORE
ONEMPTY
OSTMARK
OUTMANS
OUTMATE
OUTMODE
OUTMOST
OUTMOVE
OXYMORA

O•••M••

OARSMAN
OARSMEN
OGHAMIC
OMNIMAX
ONRAMPS
OPTIMAL
OPTIMAS
OPTIMUM
OTTOMAN
OTTUMWA
OVERMAN
OVERMIX

O••••M•

OFFRAMP
OILLAMP
OLDLYME
OLDTIME
ONEDIME
ONELUMP
ONENAME
ONETIME
ORIGAMI
OUTCOME
OUTGAME
OUTJUMP
OUTLIMN
OUTSUMS

O•••••M

OILDRUM
OILPALM
OLDFILM
ONAWHIM
ONECLAM
ONEGRAM
ONEROOM
ONETERM
OPOSSUM
OPTIMUM
ORARIUM
ORPHEUM
OUTBEAM
OUTSWAM
OUTSWIM
OUTSWUM
OVERARM
OVIFORM

•OM••••

BOMBARD
BOMBAST
BOMBECK
BOMBERS
BOMBING
BOMBLET
COMAKER
COMBATS
COMBERS
COMBIEN
COMBINE
COMBING
COMBUST
COMCAST
COMEDIA
COMEDIC
COMEDIE
COMEDUE
COMENOW
COMEOFF
COMEONS
COMEOUT
COMESAS
COMESAT
COMESBY
COMESIN
COMESON
COMESTO
COMESUP
COMFIER
COMFITS
COMFORT
COMICAL
COMICES
COMINGS
COMIQUE
COMMAND
COMMEND
COMMENT
COMMISH
COMMITS
COMMODE
COMMONS
COMMOVE
COMMUNE
COMMUTE
COMORAN
COMOROS
COMPACT
COMPANY
COMPAQS
COMPARE
COMPART
COMPASS
COMPEER
COMPELS
COMPEND
COMPERE
COMPETE
COMPILE
COMPING
COMPLEX
COMPLIN
COMPORT
COMPOSE
COMPOST
COMPOTE
COMPTON
COMPUTE
COMRADE
COMSATS
COMTISM
COMTIST
COMTREX
DOMAINE
DOMAINS
DOMECAR
DOMICAL
DOMICIL
DOMINGO
DOMINIC
DOMINOS
DOMINUS
FOMENTS
GOMPERS
HOMAGER
HOMAGES
HOMBRES
HOMBURG
HOMEBOY
HOMEDIN
HOMEICE
HOMEIER
HOMELAB
HOMERED
HOMERIC
HOMERUN
HOMESIN
HOMIEST
HOMINID
HOMONYM
IOMOTHS
JOMARCH
KOMATSU
LOMBARD
MOMBASA
MOMENTA
MOMENTS
MOMMIES
MOMMSEN
MOMONEY
MOMUSES
NOMADIC
NOMBRES
NOMERCY
NOMERGE
NOMINAL
NOMINEE
OOMPAHS
POMADED
POMADES
POMELOS
POMMARD
POMMELS
POMPANO
POMPEIA
POMPEII
POMPOMS
POMPONS
POMPOUS
ROMAINE
ROMAINS
ROMAJIS
ROMANCE
ROMANIA
ROMANIC
ROMANIS
ROMANOS
ROMANOV
ROMANSH
ROMANUS
ROMBERG
ROMCOMS
ROMNEYS
ROMPERS
ROMPING
ROMPISH
ROMULAN
ROMULUS
SOMALIA
SOMALIS
SOMATIC
SOMEDAY
SOMEHOW
SOMEONE
SOMESAY
SOMEWAY
SOMINEX
TOMBOYS
TOMCATS
TOMFOOL
TOMGOLA
TOMJOAD
TOMKITE
TOMTITS
TOMTOMS
WOMANLY
WOMBATS
YOMTOVS
ZOMBIES
ZOMBIFY

•O•M•••

BONMOTS
BOOMBOX
BOOMCAR
BOOMERS
BOOMIER
BOOMING
BOOMLET
COMMAND
COMMEND
COMMENT
COMMISH
COMMITS
COMMODE
COMMONS
COMMOVE
COMMUNE
COMMUTE
CONMOTO
CORMACK
DOGMATA
DOLMANS
DOOMFUL
DOOMIER
DOOMING
DOOMSTO
DORMANT
DORMERS
DORMICE
FOAMERS
FOAMIER
FOAMILY
FOAMING
FORMALS
FORMATS
FORMERS
FORMFUL
FORMICA
FORMING
FORMOSA
FORMULA
GOAMISS
GODMAMA
GOOMBAH
GOOMBAY
GORMING
GOTMILK
HOFMANN
HOLMIUM
HOLMOAK
HORMONE
HOTMAIL
HOTMEAL
HOTMILK
HOWMANY
HOWMUCH
LOAMIER
LOAMING
LOOMING
LOOMPAS
LOWMASS
MOMMIES
MOMMSEN
MORMONS
NONMEAT
NORMALS
NORMAND
NORMANS
NOTMANY
NOTMINE
NOTMUCH
POMMARD
POMMELS
ROAMERS
ROAMING
ROOMBAS
ROOMERS
ROOMFUL
ROOMIER

ROOMIES
ROOMILY
ROOMING
SOYMEAL
SOYMILK
TOOMANY
TOOMUCH
TOPMAST
TOPMOST
TORMENT
WORMERS
WORMIER
WORMING
WORMISH
YOUMANS
ZOOMING
ZOOMOUT
ZOOMSIN

•O••M••

BOATMAN
BOATMEN
BOGYMAN
BOGYMEN
BOHEMIA
BONDMAN
BONDMEN
BOOKMAN
BOOKMEN
BOORMAN
BOROMIR
BOSOMED
BOSSMAN
BOSSMEN
BOZEMAN
COLEMAN
COLOMBO
COLUMBA
COLUMBO
COLUMNS
COOLMAX
COPYMAN
COPYMEN
COZUMEL
DONIMUS
DOORMAN
DOORMAT
DOORMEN
DORFMAN
FOOTMAN
FOOTMEN
FOREMAN
FOREMEN
FOTOMAT
FOURMAN
GOESMAD
GOLDMAN
GONEMAD
GOODMAN
GOODMEN
GOURMET
HOFFMAN
HOLYMAN
HOLYMEN
HOLZMAN
HOOPMAN
HOOPMEN
HOUSMAN
MODEMED
MOGAMBO
MONOMER
NOKOMIS
NOLIMIT
NONAMES
POKEMON
POLEMAN
POLEMEN
POLEMIC
POLYMER
POOLMAN
POOLMEN
POORMAN
POORMEN
PORTMAN
POSTMAN
POSTMEN
POTAMUS
POTOMAC
ROADMAP
ROLLMOP
SOLOMON
SOULMAN
SOUPMIX
TOHOMER
TOLLMAN
TOLLMEN
TONEMES
TOTEMIC
VOLUMED
VOLUMES
WOLFMAN
WOLFMEN
WORKMAN
WORKMEN
YOGAMAT
ZOSIMUS

•O•••M•

BOTTOMS
CONDEMN
CONGAME
CONSUME
CONTEMN
CORFAMS
COSTUME
COULOMB
COVERME
COXCOMB
DODGEMS
DOGCOMB
DOTBOMB
DOTCOMS
FOGLAMP
GODMAMA
GOURAMI
HOTCOMB
HOTTIME
HOWCOME
HOWLAME
IONIUMS
JOECAMP
LOGJAMS
MOSLEMS
NOISOME
NONCOMS
NONHOME
NOTHOME
NOTRUMP
NOXZEMA
PODIUMS
POMPOMS
POSSUMS
ROMCOMS
RORAIMA
SOSUEME
TOBLAME
TOMTOMS
TOPNAME
WOEISME
YOTEAMO
YOUNGMC
ZOSSIMA

•O••••M

BOHRIUM
BOREDOM
BORGLUM
BOSSISM
COMTISM
CONFIRM
CONFORM
COUNTEM
DOUBLEM
FOGYISM
FORDHAM
FOREARM
GOGETEM
GOODAIM
GOTWARM
HOBOISM
HOLMIUM
HOMONYM
HOODLUM
HOTITEM
IONBEAM
JOACHIM
LONGARM
LONGTOM
LOOKISM
LORDJIM
LOWBEAM
MOBBISM
MODICUM
NONFARM
NONFORM
NOSEEUM
NOSTRUM
POPEDOM
POTSDAM
ROSTRUM
SOPHISM
SORGHUM
TONEARM
TOOKAIM
TOPFORM
TOPONYM
TORYISM
TOURISM
WOLFRAM
WOOSNAM
WOWEDEM
YOGIISM

••OM•••

ANOMALY
ANOMIES
ATOMICS
ATOMIES
ATOMISE
ATOMISM
ATOMIST
ATOMIZE
BIOMASS
BOOMBOX
BOOMCAR
BOOMERS
BOOMIER
BOOMING
BOOMLET
BROMATE
BROMIDE
BROMINE
CHOMPED
CHOMPON
CHOMSKY
CLOMPED
DIOMEDE
DOOMFUL
DOOMIER
DOOMING
DOOMSTO
EDOMITE
FROMAGE
FROMMER
GLOMMED
GNOMISH
GNOMIST
GNOMONS
GOOMBAH
GOOMBAY
GROMMET
GROMYKO
ISOMERS
LOOMING
LOOMPAS
PROMBID
PROMISE
PROMOED
PROMOTE
PROMPTS
RHOMBIC
RHOMBUS
RIOMUNI
ROOMBAS
ROOMERS
ROOMFUL
ROOMIER
ROOMIES
ROOMILY
ROOMING
STOMACH
STOMATA
STOMPED
STOMPIN
STOMPON
THOMSON
TIOMKIN
TOOMANY
TOOMUCH
TROMPED
TROMPIN
TWOMORE
WHOMPED
WYOMING
YAOMING
YEOMANS
ZOOMING
ZOOMOUT
ZOOMSIN

••O•M••

ANOSMIA
ANOSMIC
BLOOMED
BLOOMER
BOOKMAN
BOOKMEN
BOORMAN
BROOMED
COOLMAX
DOORMAN
DOORMAT
DOORMEN
FOOTMAN
FOOTMEN
FROGMAN
FROGMEN
FROMMER
GLOAMIN
GLOMMED
GLOOMED
GOODMAN
GOODMEN
GROMMET
GROOMED
GROOMER
HOOPMAN
HOOPMEN
IRONMAN
IRONMEN
KROEMER
MEOWMIX
PLOWMAN
PLOWMEN
POOLMAN
POOLMEN
POORMAN
POORMEN
PROPMAN
PROPMEN
SHOWMAN
SHOWMEN
SNOWMAN
SNOWMEN
STORMED
STORMIN
VROOMED

••O••M•

ANONYMS
DIORAMA
DIOTIMA
ECONOMY
EPONYMS
EPONYMY
EUONYMS
EXOGAMY
EXONYMS
ISONOMY
IWOJIMA
PHONEME
PROXIMA
PROXIMO
PTOLEMY
QUORUMS
SAOTOME
TWOSOME
TWOTIME

••O•••M

AGONISM
APOTHEM
ATOMISM
BLOSSOM
EGOTISM
EXOTISM
FLOTSAM
GEORGEM
GOODAIM
GROWDIM
HOODLUM
ISOGRAM
LOOKISM
NIOBIUM
OPOSSUM
PROBLEM
PROFARM
PROGRAM
PROTEAM
QUONDAM
RHODIUM
THORIUM
TOOKAIM
TROPISM
TWOROOM
TWOTERM
UTOPISM
WOOSNAM
ZIONISM

•••OM••

ABDOMEN
ADWOMAN
ADWOMEN
AGNOMEN
ATHOMES
AUTOMAT
AUTOMNE
BADOMEN
BECOMES
BLOOMED
BLOOMER
BOROMIR
BOSOMED
BROOMED
BUXOMLY
CAROMED
CHROMAT
CHROMED
CHROMES
CHROMIC
COLOMBO
DAHOMEY
ENCOMIA
ENTOMBS
EUNOMIA
FOTOMAT
GENOMES
GENOMIC
GLOOMED
GROOMED
GROOMER
INCOMER
INCOMES
ISTOMIN
JAROMIR
MONOMER
NOKOMIS
OTTOMAN
PALOMAR
PALOMAS
POTOMAC
PREOMIT
RADOMES
RECOMBS
REPOMAN
SALOMON
SOLOMON
TACOMAS
THEOMEN
THEOMNI
TOHOMER
UNCOMIC
UNDOMED
VICOMTE
VROOMED

•••O•M•

ALLOFME
ALLOWME
BYFORMS
DEFOAMS
DEFORMS
DELORME
DEWORMS
HUMORME
INFORMS
ITSONME
MEGOHMS
PHLOEMS
REFORMS
TVROOMS
UNROOMY
UNWORMY

•••O••M

ACRONYM
ALLONYM
ANTONYM
AUTONYM
CACONYM
DECORUM
DEMONYM
ECHOISM
EMBOSOM
HEROISM
HOBOISM
HOMONYM
HYPONYM
PARONYM
SYNONYM
THEOREM
TITOISM
TOPONYM
UNBOSOM
VALOREM
ZEROSUM

••••OM•

ANATOMY
AWESOME
BOTTOMS
CATCOMB
COULOMB
COXCOMB
CUSTOMS
DENMOMS
DIATOMS
DIPLOMA
DOGCOMB
DOTBOMB
DOTCOMS
ECONOMY
EPITOME
FANDOMS
FATHOMS
FULSOME
GIACOMO
HADSOME
HANSOMS
HITHOME
HOTCOMB
HOWCOME
IRKSOME
ISONOMY
KIDCOMS
LANCOME
LISSOME
NEWSOME
NOISOME
NONCOMS
NONHOME
NOTHOME
OUTCOME
PETCOMB
PHENOMS
POMPOMS
RAMHOME
RANHOME
RANSOMS
RCADOME
RHIZOME
ROMCOMS
RUNHOME
SAOTOME
SATCOMS
SATHOME
SHALOMS
SITCOMS
SITHOME
SKYDOME
SLALOMS
THEBOMB
TOMTOMS
TVROOMS
TWOSOME
UNISOMS
UNROOMY
VENDOME
WELCOME
WINDOMS
WINSOME
WISDOMS
ZITCOMS

••••O•M

ALIFORM
ARTFORM
BADFORM
BARROOM
BEDROOM
BUDWORM
CONFORM
CUTWORM
DAYROOM
EELWORM
GUNROOM
HADROOM
HASROOM
IANHOLM
INAPOEM
INBLOOM
IRSFORM
JIBBOOM
LEGROOM
LUGWORM
MALCOLM
MISFORM
MUDROOM
NONFORM
ONEROOM
OVIFORM
PERFORM
PREBOOM
PREDOOM
PREFORM
REBLOOM
RECROOM
REDWORM
REGROOM
SEAFOAM
SUBFORM
SUNROOM
TAPROOM
TEAROOM
TERAOHM
THEROOM
TOPFORM
TRIFORM
TWOROOM
UNIFORM
WARROOM

•••••OM

ABSALOM
BARROOM
BEDROOM
BLOSSOM
BOREDOM
BRITCOM
CHRISOM
CZARDOM
DAYROOM
DUKEDOM
EARLDOM
EATFROM
EMBOSOM
ENVENOM
FAMICOM
FIEFDOM
FILMDOM
FREEDOM
GEEKDOM
GETFROM
GRISSOM
GUNROOM
HADROOM
HASROOM
HEIRDOM
INBLOOM
JIBBOOM
KINGDOM
LEGROOM
LONGTOM
MUDROOM
ONEROOM
PHANTOM
POPEDOM
PREBOOM
PREDOOM
REBLOOM
RECROOM
REGROOM
SERFDOM
SHAHDOM
SHYFROM
STARDOM
STEPMOM
SUNROOM
SYMPTOM
TAPROOM
TEAROOM
TELECOM
THEROOM
TRANSOM
TSARDOM
TWOROOM
UNBOSOM
WARROOM

ON•••••

ONABIAS
ONADARE
ONADATE
ONADIET
ONAGERS
ONAJURY
ONAKICK
ONALARK
ONALEAD
ONALERT
ONALINE
ONANDON
ONAROLL
ONASSIS
ONATEAR
ONATOOT
ONATRIP
ONAWHIM
ONBOARD
ONBREAK
ONEACAT
ONEACRE
ONEACTS
ONEADAY
ONEARTH
ONEBALL
ONEBASE
ONEBELL
ONEBYTE
ONECALL
ONECELL
ONECENT
ONECHIP
ONECLAM
ONECLUB
ONEDIME
ONEDOWN
ONEEEEE
ONEEYED
ONEFOLD
ONEFOOT
ONEGRAM
ONEHALF
ONEHAND
ONEHOUR
ONEIDAS
ONEINCH
ONEIOTA
ONEIRIC
ONEIRON
ONEKILO
ONELANE
ONELIRA
ONELOOK
ONELOVE
ONELUMP
ONEMILE
ONEMORE
ONEMPTY
ONENAME
ONENESS
ONENOTE
ONEOCAT
ONEOFFS
ONEOFUS
ONEONTA
ONEOVER
ONEPAGE
ONEPAIR
ONEPART
ONEPINT
ONEREEL
ONEROOM
ONEROUS
ONESELF
ONESHOE
ONESHOT
ONESIZE
ONESOCK
ONESPOT
ONESTAR
ONESTEP
ONESTOP
ONETERM
ONETIME
ONETOGO
ONETWOS
ONEUNIT
ONEVOTE
ONEWEEK
ONEWHIT
ONEWOOD
ONEYARD
ONEYEAR
ONFIRST
ONGOING
ONGUARD
ONLEASE
ONLEASH
ONLEAVE
ONLIEST
ONLOADS
ONLYTOO
ONLYYOU
ONMYOWN
ONORATI
ONORDER
ONPAPER
ONPOINT
ONRAMPS
ONSAGER
ONSERVE
ONSHORE
ONSIDES
ONSIGHT
ONSTAFF
ONSTAGE
ONTARIO
ONTHEDL
ONTHEGO
ONTHEQT
ONTHREE
ONTKEAN
ONTOAST
ONTOPIC
ONTOPOF
ONTRACK
ONTRIAL
ONVIDEO
ONWARDS
ONWATER

O•N••••

OFNOUSE
OINKERS
OINKING
OMNIBUS
OMNIMAX
ORNETTE
ORNITHO
OWNEDUP
OWNGOAL
OWNUPTO

O••N•••

OBENTOS
OCANADA
OCONNOR
ODDNESS
ODINGON
ODONTIA
OFANAGE
OHANLON
OKINAWA
OLDNAVY
OLDNESS
OLDNEWS
OLDNICK
OMENING
OMINOUS
ONANDON
ONENAME
ONENESS
ONENOTE
OPENAIR
OPENBAR
OPENEND
OPENERS
OPENING
OPENNET
OPENOUT
OPENPIT
OPENSEA
OPENSUP
OPENTAP
OPENTOE
OPENTOP
OPINERS
OPINING
OPINION
OPUNTIA
ORANGES
ORANGEY
ORANTES
ORINOCO
ORKNEYS
OWINGON
OWINGTO
OXONIAN
OZONISE
OZONIZE
OZONOUS

O•••N••

OBLONGS
OBTUNDS
OCEANIA
OCEANIC
OCEANID
OCEANUS
OCHENTA
OCONNOR
OCTANES
OCTANTS
OFFENCE
OFFENDS
OFFENSE
OFFINGS
OFTENER
OGDENUT
OLEANNA
OLEANNY
ONEINCH
ONEONTA
ONEUNIT
OOLONGS
OPENNET
ORDINAL
ORDINES
ORDONEZ
ORGANDY
ORGANIC
ORGANZA
ORIENTE
ORIENTS
ORLANDO
ORMANDY
OSCINES
OSMONDS
OSMUNDS
OTRANTO
OUTGNAW

OUTINGS
OVERNEW

O••••N•

OAHUANS
OAKLAND
OBEYING
OBSCENE
OBTAINS
OCARINA
ODDMENT
ODORANT
OFAKIND
OFAMIND
OFFHAND
OFFLINE
OHIOANS
OILCANS
OILLINE
OILPANS
OILRING
OILSAND
OILTANK
OINKING
OKAYING
OLDHAND
OLDLINE
OLDSONG
OLEANNA
OLEANNY
OLEFINS
OLIVINE
OMAHANE
OMAHANS
OMENING
ONALINE
ONECENT
ONEHAND
ONELANE
ONEPINT
ONGOING
ONPOINT
OPALINE
OPENEND
OPENING
OPERAND
OPERANT
OPINING
OPPUGNS
OPTIONS
OPULENT
OPUSONE
ORATING
ORDAINS
OREGANO
ORIGINE
ORIGINS
ORISONS
ORLEANS
OROGENY
OROTUND
ORPHANS
ORPHANT
OSAKANS
OSBORNE
OUGHTNT
OURGANG
OURSONG
OUSTING
OUTBANS
OUTBEND
OUTCANT
OUTDONE
OUTFIND
OUTGUNS
OUTHUNT
OUTJINX
OUTKING
OUTLAND
OUTLINE
OUTMANS
OUTRANG
OUTRANK
OUTRANT
OUTRING
OUTRUNS
OUTSANG
OUTSING
OUTSINS
OUTSUNG
OUTWENT
OUTWIND
OUTWING
OXIDANT

O•••••N

OAKFERN
OAKLAWN
OARSMAN
OARSMEN
OATBRAN
OAXACAN
OBERLIN
OCTAGON
ODESSAN
ODINGON
OHANLON
OILSKIN
OLDBEAN
OLDMOON
OLDTOWN
OMICRON
ONANDON
ONEDOWN
ONEIRON
ONMYOWN
ONTKEAN
OPINION
OPTEDIN
ORARION
ORATION
ORBISON
ORDERIN
ORPHEAN
ORTOLAN
OSIRIAN
OTTAWAN
OTTOMAN
OURTOWN
OUTBURN
OUTEARN
OUTFAWN
OUTGAIN
OUTGRIN
OUTLAIN
OUTLIMN
OUTPLAN
OUTSEEN
OUTSPIN
OUTTORN
OUTTURN
OUTWORN
OVATION
OVERMAN
OVERRAN
OVERRUN
OVIDIAN
OWINGON
OXONIAN

•ON••••

BONACIS
BONAIRE
BONANZA
BONARIO
BONBONS
BONDAGE
BONDERS
BONDING
BONDMAN
BONDMEN
BONEASH
BONEDRY
BONEDUP
BONELET
BONESET
BONESUP
BONEYER
BONFIRE
BONGING
BONGOES
BONHEUR
BONIATO
BONIEST
BONILLA
BONITOS
BONJOUR
BONJOVI
BONKERS
BONKING
BONMOTS
BONNARD
BONNETS
BONNIER
BONNILY
BONSOIR
BONUSES
CONAGRA
CONAKRY
CONBRIO
CONCAVE
CONCEAL
CONCEDE
CONCEIT
CONCEPT
CONCERN
CONCERT
CONCHAE
CONCHES
CONCHOS
CONCISE
CONCOCT
CONCORD
CONCURS
CONCUSS
CONDEMN
CONDIGN
CONDOLE
CONDONE
CONDORS
CONDUCE
CONDUCT
CONDUIT
CONELET
CONFABS
CONFECT
CONFERS
CONFESS
CONFIDE
CONFINE
CONFIRM
CONFITS
CONFORM
CONFREY
CONFUSE
CONFUTE
CONGAED
CONGAME
CONGEAL
CONGERS
CONGEST
CONGOUS
CONICAL
CONIFER
CONJOBS
CONJOIN
CONJURE
CONJURY
CONKERS
CONKING
CONKLIN
CONKOFF
CONKOUT
CONMOTO
CONNATE
CONNECT
CONNERY
CONNICK
CONNIFF
CONNING
CONNIVE
CONNORS
CONNOTE
CONOIDS
CONQUER
CONRACK
CONRIED
CONSENT
CONSIGN
CONSIST
CONSOLE
CONSORT
CONSULS
CONSULT
CONSUME
CONTACS
CONTACT
CONTAIN
CONTEMN
CONTEND
CONTENT
CONTEST
CONTEXT
CONTORT
CONTOUR
CONTRAS
CONTROL
CONTUSE
CONURES
CONVECT
CONVENE
CONVENT
CONVERT
CONVEYS
CONVICT
CONVOKE
CONVOYS
DONAHUE
DONATED
DONATEE
DONATES
DONATOR
DONATUS
DONEBAD
DONEFOR
DONEGAL
DONEGAN
DONETSK
DONGLES
DONIMUS
DONJONS
DONJOSE
DONJUAN
DONKEYS
DONKING
DONLEVY
DONNALL
DONNING
DONNISH
DONOHOE
DONOTGO
DONOVAN
DONRUSS
DONTASK
DONTBEE
DONTCRY
DONTLIE
EONLINE
FONDANT
FONDEST
FONDLED
FONDLER
FONDLES
FONDUED
FONDUES
FONTANA
FONTANE
FONTEYN
FONTINA
GONDOLA
GONEAFT
GONEAPE
GONEBAD
GONEFAR
GONEFOR
GONEMAD
GONEOFF
GONEOUT
GONEPRO
GONERIL
GONGING
GONGORA
GONZAGA
HONALEE
HONCHOS
HONEDIN
HONESIN
HONESTY
HONEYED
HONIARA
HONKERS
HONKING
HONKSAT
HONORED
HONOREE
HONORER
HONOURS
IONBEAM
IONESCO
IONIANS
IONISED
IONISER
IONISES
IONIUMS
IONIZED
IONIZER
IONIZES
IONONES
JONERIK
JONESED
JONESES
JONHALL
JONQUIL
KONTIKI
LONBORG
LONDRES
LONETTE
LONGAGO
LONGARM
LONGBED
LONGBOW
LONGDAY
LONGDEN
LONGEST
LONGFOR
LONGIES
LONGING
LONGISH
LONGRUN
LONGTOM
LONGTON
LONGUES
LONGWAY
LONIGAN
MONACAN
MONADAL
MONADIC
MONARCH
MONCTON
MONDALE
MONDAVI
MONDAYS
MONDESI
MONDIAL
MONDIEU
MONEYED
MONGERS
MONGKUT
MONGOLS
MONGREL
MONIKER
MONITOR
MONKEES
MONKEYS
MONKISH
MONOCLE
MONODIC
MONOLOG
MONOMER
MONOPOD
MONOSKI
MONROES
MONSOON
MONSTER
MONSTRO
MONTAGE
MONTAGU
MONTALE
MONTANA
MONTAND
MONTANO
MONTAUK
MONTEGO
MONTERO
MONTEUX
MONTHLY
MONTOYA
MONTUNO
NONACID
NONAGES
NONAGON
NONAMES
NONARAB
NONARTS
NONBANK
NONBASE
NONBODY
NONBOOK
NONBUSY
NONCASH
NONCOLA
NONCOMS
NONCORE
NONCROP
NONDARK
NONDEAF
NONDEEP
NONDIET
NONDRIP
NONDRUG
NONEPIC
NONETTE
NONEVER
NONEVIL
NONFACT
NONFANS
NONFARM
NONFLUX
NONFOOD
NONFORM
NONFUEL
NONGOGO
NONGOLD
NONHERO
NONHITS
NONHOME
NONIRON
NONJEWS
NONJURY
NONLIFE
NONLIVE
NONMEAT
NONNEWS
NONOILY
NONOISE
NONORAL
NONPAID
NONPARS
NONPAST
NONPEAK
NONPLAY
NONPLUS
NONPOET
NONPOOR
NONPROS
NONSALE
NONSANE
NONSELF
NONSKED
NONSKID
NONSLIP
NONSTOP
NONSUCH
NONUKES
NONUPLE
NONUSER
NONVOID
NONWAGE
NONWARS
NONWOOL
NONWORD
NONWORK
NONZERO
PONCHOS
PONDERS
PONDING
PONGEES
PONGIDS
PONIARD
PONTANO
PONTIAC
PONTIAN
PONTIFF
PONTIUS
PONTOON
PONYING
PONYKEG
RONDEAU
RONDELS
RONDURE
RONETTE
RONSARD
RONSONS
RONTGEN
RONWOOD
RONZONI
SONANCE
SONATAS
SONGFUL
SONLESS
SONLIKE
SONNETS
SONORAN
SONSHIP
TONALLY
TONEARM
TONEDUP
TONELOC
TONEMES
TONEROW
TONESUP
TONETTE
TONGANS
TONGING
TONGUES
TONIEST
TONIGHT
TONNAGE
TONNEAU
TONSILS
TONSURE
TONTINE
TONUSES
TONYDOW
VONBAER
VONLAUE
VONOPEL
VONZELL
WONDERS
WONOVER
WONTING
WONTONS
YONKERS
ZONALLY
ZONEOUT
ZONIANS
ZONKING
ZONKOUT
ZONULAR
ZONULES

•O•N•••

BONNARD
BONNETS
BONNIER
BONNILY
BOONIES
BORNEAN
BORNEUP
BOSNIAN
BOUNCED
BOUNCER
BOUNCES
BOUNDED
BOUNDER
BOUNDTO
BOUNDUP
COBNUTS
COGNACS
COGNATE
COGNIZE
COINAGE
COINBOX
COINERS
COINING
COINOPS
CONNATE
CONNECT
CONNERY
CONNICK
CONNIFF
CONNING
CONNIVE
CONNORS
CONNOTE
COONCAN
COONCAT
COONDOG
CORNBIN
CORNCOB
CORNDOG
CORNEAL
CORNEAS
CORNELL
CORNERS
CORNETS
CORNFED
CORNICE
CORNIER
CORNILY
CORNING
CORNISH
CORNOIL
CORNROW
CORNUTE
COUNCIL
COUNSEL
COUNTED
COUNTEE
COUNTEM
COUNTER
COUNTIN
COUNTON
COUNTRY
COUNTUP
COYNESS
DOGNAPS
DOINGIN
DOINGOK
DOINGSO
DOINGTO
DOINGUP
DONNALL
DONNING
DONNISH
DOONEIN
DOWNBOW
DOWNERS
DOWNIER
DOWNING
DOWNPAT
FOUNDED
FOUNDER
FOUNDRY
FOXNEWS
GOINFOR
GOINGAT
GOINGBY
GOINGIN
GOINGON
GOINGTO
GOINGUP
GOONEYS
GOONIER
GOONIES
GOONILY
GOUNDER
GOWNING
HOBNAIL
HOBNOBS
HOGNOSE
HOGNUTS
HOHNERS
HORNETS
HORNIER
HORNING
HORNISH
HORNIST
HORNSBY
HORNSIN
HORNUNG
HOTNESS
HOUNDED
HOUNDER
HOWNICE
JOHNBOY
JOHNDOE
JOHNGAY
JOHNIII
JOHNJAY
JOHNLAW
JOHNLEE
JOHNNIE
JOHNNYB
JOHNSON
JOHNVII
JOHNWOO
JOHNXII
JOHNXIV
JOHNXIX
JOHNXVI
JOHNXXI
JOINDER
JOINERS
JOINERY
JOINING
JOINSIN
JOINSUP
JOINTED
JOINTER
JOINTLY
JOUNCED
JOUNCES
KOONING
LOANERS
LOANING
LOANOUT
LOONIER
LOONIES
LOONILY
LOUNGED
LOUNGER
LOUNGES
LOWNECK
LOWNESS
MOANERS
MOANFUL
MOANING
MOONBOW
MOONDOG
MOONERS
MOONEYE
MOONGOD
MOONIER
MOONIES
MOONILY
MOONING
MOONISH
MOONLET
MOONLIT
MOONPIE
MOONSET
MORNING
MOUNDED
MOUNTED
MOUNTER
MOUNTIE
MOUNTUP
NOANGEL
NOENDOF
NOENDTO
NOENTRY
NOKNOCK
NONNEWS
NOONDAY
NOONERS
NOONING
NOTNEAR
NOTNICE
NOWNESS
POINTAT
POINTED
POINTER
POINTES
POINTTO
POINTUP
POUNCED
POUNCER
POUNCES
POUNDED
POUNDER
ROANOKE
ROMNEYS
ROUNDED
ROUNDEL
ROUNDER
ROUNDLY
ROUNDON
ROUNDUP
SOANDSO
SOLNESS
SONNETS
SOONERS
SOONEST
SOUNDED
SOUNDER
SOUNDLY
TOENAIL
TONNAGE
TONNEAU
TOONIES
TOPNAME
TORNADO
TORNOFF
TORNOUT
TOWNCAR
TOWNERS
TOWNIES
TOWNISH
TOWNLET
TOYNBEE
WORNOFF
WORNOUT
WOUNDED
WOUNDUP
WOZNIAK
YOUNGER
YOUNGMC
YOUNGUN

•O••N••

BOCHNER
BODINGS
BOEINGS
BONANZA
BORINGS
BORONIC
BOSONIC
BOTANIC
BOTHNIA
BOVINES
BOWKNOT
COCKNEY
COCONUT
COGENCY
COIGNED
COIGNES
COLONEL
COLONES
COLONNA
COLONUS
COMENOW
COMINGS
COOWNED
CORINNE
CORINTH
CORONAE
CORONAL
CORONAS
CORONER
CORONET
COSINES
COSTNER
COZENED
COZENER
DOCENTS
DOESNOT
DOITNOW
DOLUNCH
DOMINGO
DOMINIC
DOMINOS
DOMINUS
DOUANES
DOYENNE
DOZENTH
EOSINES
FOLENGO
FOMENTS
FORENZA
FORINTS
FORONCE
GODUNOV
GOODNIK
GORTNER
GOTINON
GOTINTO
GOTONIT
GOTONTO
HOMINID
HOMONYM
HOPENOT
HOPINTO
HOSANNA

HOTONES
IONONES
JOHANNA
JOHNNIE
JOHNNYB
JOURNAL
JOURNEE
JOURNEY
JOURNOS
KOLANUT
KORANIC
KORUNAS
LOCKNUT
LOGANUT
LOGONTO
LORANGE
LORENTZ
LORENZO
LORGNON
LOSINGS
LOZENGE
MOMENTA
MOMENTS
MOMONEY
MORANIS
MORANTE
MORONIC
MOURNED
MOURNER
MOWINGS
NOCANDO
NOHANDS
NOMINAL
NOMINEE
NOTONCE
NOVENAS
OOLONGS
POCONOS
POLANER
POLANYI
POLENTA
POLONIA
PORTNOY
POTENCE
POTENCY
ROBBNEN
RODENTS
ROLONDA
ROMANCE
ROMANIA
ROMANIC
ROMANIS
ROMANOS
ROMANOV
ROMANSH
ROMANUS
ROSANNA
ROSANNE
ROSINED
ROSSNER
ROTUNDA
ROVINGS
ROXANNE
ROZANOV
SOAPNET
SOIGNEE
SOMINEX
SONANCE
SORENTO
SOYINKA
SOYINKS
TOKENED
TOPKNOT
TOPONYM
TORINOS
TORONTO
TOTINOS
TOURNEY
TOWINGS
VOLANTE
VOLENTE
VOTENAY
WOKENUP
WOMANLY
WOOSNAM
YOGINIS
YOLANDA
YOUANDI
YOUKNOW

•O•••N•

BOATING
BOBBING
BOBBINS
BOBKANE
BODKINS
BOFFING
BOFFINS
BOGGING
BOILING
BOITANO
BOKKENS
BOLLING
BOLOGNA
BOLTING
BOMBING
BONBONS
BONDING
BONGING
BONKING
BOOKEND
BOOKING
BOOMING
BOOTING
BOOZING
BOPPING
BORDONI
BORKING
BOSSING
BOSTONS
BOSTONU
BOUDINS
BOUSONO
BOWFINS
BOWLINE
BOWLING
BOYBAND
COAGENT
COALING
COATING
COAXING
COBLENZ
COBRAND
COCAINE
COCKING
COCOONS
CODEINE
COFFINS
COFOUND
COGGING
COIFING
COILING
COINING
COLDONE
COLLINE
COLLINS
COLOGNE
COLONNA
COLUMNS
COMBINE
COMBING
COMEONS
COMMAND
COMMEND
COMMENT
COMMONS
COMMUNE
COMPANY
COMPEND
COMPING
CONDONE
CONFINE
CONKING
CONNING
CONSENT
CONTEND
CONTENT
CONVENE
CONVENT
COOKING
COOLANT
COOLING
COOPING
COPLAND
COPPING
COPYING
COQUINA
CORDING
CORDONS
CORINNE
CORKING
CORNING
CORTINA
CORVINA
CORVINE
CORZINE
COSHING
COSIGNS
COSTING
COSYING
COTTONS
COTTONY
COULDNT
COUPING
COUPONS
COURANT
COUSINE
COUSINS
COWBANE
COWHAND
COWLING
COWPONY
COZYING
COZZENS
DOBBINS
DOCKING
DODGING
DOFFING
DOGBANE
DOGBONE
DOGGING
DOGGONE
DOGRUNS
DOLLING
DOLMANS
DOMAINE
DOMAINS
DONJONS
DONKING
DONNING
DOOMING
DORMANT
DOSSING
DOTTING
DOUSING
DOWLING
DOWNING
DOWRONG
DOWSING
DOYENNE
EONLINE
FOALING
FOAMING
FOBBING
FOGBANK
FOGGING
FOILING
FOLDING
FONDANT
FONTANA
FONTANE
FONTINA
FOOLING
FOOTING
FORCING
FORDING
FORDONE
FORFEND
FORGING
FORGONE
FORKING
FORLANI
FORMING
FORRENT
FORTUNA
FORTUNE
FORWENT
FOULING
FOWLING
FOXHUNT
GOADING
GOALONG
GOBLANK
GOBLINS
GODLING
GODSEND
GODSENT
GODSONS
GOLDING
GOLDONI
GOLFING
GONGING
GOODING
GOODONE
GOOFING
GOOSING
GORGING
GORGONS
GORMING
GOROUND
GOSLING
GOTDONE
GOUGING
GOVERNS
GOWNING
GOWRONG
HOAXING
HOBOING
HOBSONS
HOCKING
HODDING
HOFMANN
HOGGING
HOLDING
HOLLAND
HOLYONE
HONKING
HOODING
HOOFING
HOOKING
HOOPING
HOOTING
HOPKINS
HOPPING
HOPSING
HORDING
HORMONE
HORNING
HORNUNG
HORSING
HOSANNA
HOSKINS
HOSTING
HOTHAND
HOTLINE
HOTLINK
HOTPINK
HOTTUNA
HOTZONE
HOUDINI
HOUSING
HOVLANE
HOWLING
HOWLONG
HOWMANY
HOYDENS
IONIANS
JOBBANK
JOBBING
JOBHUNT
JOGGING
JOHANNA
JOINING
JOLTING
JORDANA
JOSHING
JOTTING
KOBLENZ
KOONING
KOREANS
KOSCINA
LOADING
LOAFING
LOAMING
LOANING
LOBBING
LOCARNO
LOCKING
LOCKINS
LODGING
LOFTING
LOGGING
LOGGINS
LOIDING
LOLLING
LONGING
LOOKING
LOOKINS
LOOMING
LOOPING
LOOSENS
LOOSING
LOOTING
LOPPING
LORDING
LORIENT
LOTIONS
LOTTING
LOUDENS
LOURING
LOUSING
LOUTING
LOVEINS
LOWHAND
LOWLAND
LOWRENT
MOANING
MOBBING
MOCKING
MODERNE
MODERNS
MOILING
MOLDING
MOLSONS
MOLTING
MONTANA
MONTAND
MONTANO
MONTUNO
MOONING
MOORING
MOOTING
MOPPING
MORAINE
MORDANT
MORDENT
MOREENS
MORGANA
MORGANS
MORMONS
MORNING
MORTONS
MOSCONI
MOSHING
MOSSING
MOTIONS
MOTRINS
MOUSING
NOCKING
NOCOUNT
NODDING
NOGGINS
NOISING
NONBANK
NONFANS
NONSANE
NOONING
NOOSING
NORMAND
NORMANS
NORTONS
NOSHING
NOTAONE
NOTDONE
NOTHING
NOTHINS
NOTIONS
NOTMANY
NOTMINE
NOTTING
NOTURNS
NOVOTNY
POBLANO
POISING
POISONS
POLLENS
POLLING
POMPANO
POMPONS
PONDING
PONTANO
PONYING
POOLING
POOPING
POPGUNS
POPLINS
POPPING
POPPINS
POPSONG
POPTUNE
POPWINE
PORCINE
PORKING
PORSENA
PORTEND
PORTENT
PORTING
POSTING
POTEENS
POTIONS
POTTING
POULENC
POURING
POUTING
ROAMING
ROARING
ROBBING
ROBBINS
ROCKING
RODDING
ROGAINE
ROGUING
ROILING
ROLFING
ROLLAND
ROLLING
ROLLINS
ROLLONS
ROMAINE
ROMAINS
ROMPING
RONSONS
RONZONI
ROOFING
ROOKING
ROOMING
ROOTING
ROSANNA
ROSANNE
ROSSANO
ROSSINI
ROSTAND
ROTTING
ROUGING
ROUSING
ROUTINE
ROUTING
ROWLAND
ROWLING
ROXANNE
SOAKING
SOAPING
SOARING
SOBBING
SOCKING
SODDING
SOFTENS
SOILING
SOLOING
SOLVENT
SOLVING
SOMEONE
SOPPING
SOPRANI
SOPRANO
SORDINI
SORDINO
SORIANO
SORTING
SORVINO
SOURING
SOUSING
SOXFANS
SOYLENT
TOCSINS
TOGGING
TOILING
TOLLING
TOLUENE
TONGANS
TONGING
TONTINE
TOOLING
TOOLONG
TOOMANY
TOOTING
TOPGUNS
TOPLINE
TOPPING
TOPRANK
TOPTENS
TORMENT
TORRENT
TORTONI
TOSSING
TOTTING
TOUCANS
TOURING
TOUTING
TOWLINE
TOYGUNS
TOYLAND
VOGUING
VOICING
VOIDING
VOLCANO
VOLPONE
VOTEDNO
VOTESNO
WOLFING
WONTING
WONTONS
WOODING
WOOFING
WOOLENS
WORDING
WORDONE
WORKING
WORMING
WORSENS
WOULDNT
YOKOONO
YOUMANS
YOURANG
YOWLING
YOYOING
ZONIANS
ZONKING
ZOOMING

•O••••N

BOATMAN
BOATMEN
BOBGOEN
BOGDOWN
BOGYMAN
BOGYMEN
BONDMAN
BONDMEN
BOOKMAN
BOOKMEN
BOOLEAN
BOORMAN
BORNEAN
BORODIN
BOSNIAN
BOSSMAN
BOSSMEN
BOURBON
BOWDOIN
BOWDOWN
BOXEDIN
BOXESIN
BOZEMAN
COALBIN
COARSEN
COCHRAN
COGBURN
COGHLAN
COLEMAN
COLLEEN
COMBIEN
COMESIN
COMESON
COMORAN
COMPLIN
COMPTON
CONCERN
CONDEMN
CONDIGN
CONJOIN
CONKLIN
CONSIGN
CONTAIN
CONTEMN
COONCAN
COPYMAN
COPYMEN
CORAZON
CORNBIN
COSTAIN
COUNTIN
COUNTON
COWSKIN
COWTOWN
DOAGAIN
DODGSON
DOESKIN
DOINGIN
DOLPHIN
DONEGAN
DONJUAN
DONOVAN
DOONEIN
DOORMAN
DOORMEN
DORFMAN
DOTEDON
DOTESON
DOUBLEN
FOCUSON
FOGHORN
FOISTON
FOLDSIN
FONTEYN
FOOTMAN
FOOTMEN
FORCEIN
FORCEON
FOREIGN
FOREMAN
FOREMEN
FORERAN
FORERUN
FORLORN
FORTRAN
FOURMAN
FOURPIN
GOBELIN
GOINGIN
GOINGON
GOLDARN
GOLDMAN
GOLDWYN
GOODMAN
GOODMEN
GOODSON
GOODWIN
GORDIAN
GOTDOWN
GOTEVEN
GOTINON
GOTITON
GOTUPON
HOARSEN
HOBOKEN
HOEDOWN
HOFFMAN
HOFMANN
HOLBEIN
HOLDSIN
HOLDSON
HOLYMAN
HOLYMEN
HOLZMAN
HOMEDIN
HOMERUN
HOMESIN
HONEDIN
HONESIN
HOOKSON
HOOPMAN
HOOPMEN
HORIZON
HORNSIN
HOUSMAN
HOUSTON
HOWTHEN
JOAQUIN
JOCELYN
JOHNSON
JOINSIN
JOTDOWN
JOURDAN
JOYCEAN
KOSYGIN
KOWLOON
LOADSIN
LOAFPAN
LOCKEAN
LOCKLIN
LOCKSIN
LOCKSON
LODGEIN
LONGDEN
LONGRUN
LONGTON
LONIGAN
LOOKSIN
LOOKSON
LORGNON
LOTHIAN
LOWBORN
LOWCHEN
LOWDOWN
MOHEGAN
MOHICAN
MOISSAN
MOISTEN
MOMMSEN
MONACAN
MONCTON
MONSOON
MOORHEN
MORPHIN
MOVEDIN
MOVEDON
MOVESIN
MOVESON
MOWDOWN
NONAGON
NONIRON
NOSEDIN
NOSESIN
NOSTAIN
NOTBEEN
NOTEVEN
NOTOPEN
NOUTURN
NOWTHEN
POISSON
POKEFUN
POKEMON
POLEMAN
POLEMEN
POLYGON
PONTIAN
PONTOON
POOLMAN
POOLMEN
POORMAN
POORMEN
POPCORN
PORTION
PORTMAN
POSTERN
POSTMAN
POSTMEN
POURSIN
POUSSIN
ROBBNEN
ROBESON
ROCKOON
ROLLSIN
ROLLSON
ROMULAN
RONTGEN
ROPEDIN
ROPESIN
ROSALYN
ROUGHEN
ROUNDON
ROYBEAN
ROYCOHN
SOAKSIN
SOCKSIN
SODACAN
SOJOURN
SOLOMON
SONORAN
SOTHERN
SOULMAN
SOUPCAN
SOUPCON
SOUPSON
SOURSON
SOYBEAN
TOATURN
TOHELEN
TOLEDAN
TOLKIEN
TOLLMAN
TOLLMEN
TOOKTEN
TOOSOON
TOPDOWN
TOPEKAN
TOPSPIN
TORSION
TOUCHON
TOUGHEN
TOWEDIN
VOSGIAN
VOTEDIN
VOTEDON
VOTESIN
VOTESON
WOBEGON
WOLFMAN
WOLFMEN
WOODBIN
WOODSON
WOOLLEN
WORKMAN
WORKMEN
WORKSIN
WORKSON
YORKTON
YOUNGUN
YOUREON
YOUTHEN
ZOOMSIN

••ON•••

ACONITE
ADONAIS
AGONIES
AGONISE
AGONISM
AGONIST
AGONIZE
AMONGST
ANONYMS
ARONNAX
ASONANT
ATONERS
ATONICS
ATONIES
ATONING
AVONLEA
BIONICS
BLONDER
BLONDES
BLONDIE
BOONIES
BRONCHI
BRONCHO
BRONCOS
BRONSON
BRONTES
BRONWEN
BRONZED
BRONZER
BRONZES
CLONERS
CLONING
CLONKED
COONCAN
COONCAT
COONDOG
CRONIES
DOONEIN
DRONEON
DRONERS

DRONING
DRONISH
EBONICS
EBONIES
EBONITE
EBONIZE
ECONOMY
EPONINE
EPONYMS
EPONYMY
ETONIAN
ETONICS
EUONYMS
EXONYMS
FRONTAL
FRONTED
FRONTON
GOONEYS
GOONIER
GOONIES
GOONILY
ICONIFY
IRONAGE
IRONBAR
IRONERS
IRONIES
IRONING
IRONIST
IRONMAN
IRONMEN
IRONONS
IRONORE
IRONOUT
IRONSON
ISONOMY
IWONDER
KOONING
LEONARD
LEONATO
LEONDAY
LEONIDS
LEONINE
LEONORA
LEONORE
LIONCUB
LIONELL
LIONELS
LIONESS
LIONETS
LIONISE
LIONIZE
LOONIER
LOONIES
LOONILY
LYONELL
MOONBOW
MOONDOG
MOONERS
MOONEYE
MOONGOD
MOONIER
MOONIES
MOONILY
MOONING
MOONISH
MOONLET
MOONLIT
MOONPIE
MOONSET
NEONATE
NEONGAS
NOONDAY
NOONERS
NOONING
OCONNOR
ODONTIA
OXONIAN
OZONISE
OZONIZE
OZONOUS
PEONAGE
PEONIES
PHONEIN
PHONEME
PHONENO
PHONERS
PHONEYS
PHONICS
PHONIER
PHONIES
PHONILY
PHONING
PHONYUP
PIONEER
PLONKED
PRONATE
PRONAVY
PRONELY
PRONETO
PRONGED
PRONOUN
QUONDAM
QUONSET
SCONCES
SHONUFF
SOONERS
SOONEST
SPONDEE
SPONGED
SPONGER
SPONGES
SPONSOR
STONEAX
STONERS
STONIER
STONILY
STONING
TOONIES
TSONGAS
VRONSKY
WRONGED
WRONGER
WRONGLY
ZIONISM
ZIONIST

••O•N••

ABOUNDS
ACORNED
ADORNED
ADORNER
AMOUNTS
ANOINTS
ARONNAX
ASOFNOW
AWOONOR
BLOWNIN
BLOWNUP
BROSNAN
BROWNED
BROWNER
BROWNIE
CLOONEY
CLOWNED
COOWNED
CROONED
CROONER
CROWNED
CROWNER
DROPNET
DROWNED
ENOUNCE
FLOUNCE
FLOUNCY
FLOWNAT
FLOWNBY
FLOWNIN
FLOWNON
FLOWNTO
FLOWNUP
FROWNAT
FROWNED
FROWNER
FROWNON
GOODNIK
GROANED
GROANER
GROINED
GROUNDS
GROWNON
GROWNUP
OCONNOR
PHOENIX
QUOINED
REOWNED
SCORNED
SCORNER
SHOPNBC
SHOWNIN
SHOWNUP
SPOONED
SPOONER
SWOONED
SWOONER
THORNED
TROUNCE
TWOONIE
TWOUNIT
UNOWNED
WHOKNEW
WOOSNAM
YAOUNDE

••O••N•

ADORING
AJOWANS
ANODYNE
ASONANT
ATONING
AVOWING
BLOWING
BOOKEND
BOOKING
BOOMING
BOOTING
BOOZING
BROGANS
BROMINE
BUOYANT
BUOYING
CHOKING
CHOLINE
CHOPINE
CHORINE
CHOWING
CLONING
CLOSING
CLOYING
COOKING
COOLANT
COOLING
COOPING
CROTONS
CROWING
DIOXINS
DOOMING
DRONING
DROPINS
DUODENA
DUOTONE
ELOPING
EMOTING
EPONINE
ERODENT
ERODING
EVOKING
FIORINA
FLORENZ
FLORINS
FLOWING
FOOLING
FOOTING
FRODING
FROZONE
GAOLING
GLOBING
GLOBINS
GLOVING
GLOWING
GNOMONS
GOODING
GOODONE
GOOFING
GOOSING
GROPING
GROWING
HOODING
HOOFING
HOOKING
HOOPING
HOOTING
IFORONE
ILOCANO
IMOGENE
IRONING
IRONONS
ISOGONS
ISOLINE
ISOTONE
IVORINE
KNOWING
KOONING
LEOGENN
LEONINE
LOOKING
LOOKINS
LOOMING
LOOPING
LOOSENS
LOOSING
LOOTING
MEOWING
MIOCENE
MOONING
MOORING
MOOTING
NEOCENE
NEOCONS
NEOGENE
NOONING
NOOSING
ODORANT
OROGENY
OROTUND
PHONENO
PHONING
PHOTONS
PLOWING
POOLING
POOPING
PROBING
PROBONO
PROFANE
PROGENY
PROLONG
PROPANE
PROPONE
PROSING
PROTONS
PROVINE
PROVING
QUOTING
REOPENS
RIOMUNI
RIOTING
ROOFING
ROOKING
ROOMING
ROOTING
RYOKANS
SCOPING
SCORING
SHOEING
SHOGUNS
SHOOING
SHOOINS
SHORING
SHOVING
SHOWING
SIOUANS
SLOGANS
SLOPING
SLOVENE
SLOVENS
SLOWING
SMOKING
SNOCONE
SNORING
SNOWING
SPOKANE
SPOKING
STOKING
STOLONS
STONING
STORING
STOTINS
STOWING
TOOLING
TOOLONG
TOOMANY
TOOTING
TROJANS
TROWING
TWOLANE
TWOTONE
TWOTONS
UGOLINO
UNOWING
USOPENS
VIOLENT
VIOLINS
VIOLONE
WOODING
WOOFING
WOOLENS
WYOMING
WYOTANA
YAOMING
YEOMANS
ZOOMING

••O•••N

AEOLIAN
APOGEAN
AZOREAN
AZORIAN
BLOUSON
BLOWGUN
BLOWNIN
BLOWSIN
BLOWSON
BOOKMAN
BOOKMEN
BOOLEAN
BOORMAN
BROADEN
BROKEIN
BRONSON
BRONWEN
BROSNAN
CHOKEON
CHOMPON
CLOCKIN
CLOSEIN
COONCAN
CROUTON
CROWDIN
DOONEIN
DOORMAN
DOORMEN
DRONEON
DROPSIN
DROVEIN
ECOTRIN
EMOTION
EROSION
ETONIAN
FLORIAN
FLOWNIN
FLOWNON
FLOWSIN
FOOTMAN
FOOTMEN
FROGMAN
FROGMEN
FRONTON
FROWNON
GGORDON
GLOAMIN
GOODMAN
GOODMEN
GOODSON
GOODWIN
GROOVIN
GROWNON
GROWSON
HOOKSON
HOOPMAN
HOOPMEN
IRONMAN
IRONMEN
IRONSON
IVORIAN
KEOGHAN
KNOCKON
KTOSLIN
LAOCOON
LAOTIAN
LEOGENN
LOOKSIN
LOOKSON
MOORHEN
OXONIAN
PEORIAN
PHONEIN
PLOSION
PLOWMAN
PLOWMEN
PLOWSON
POOLMAN
POOLMEN
POORMAN
POORMEN
PROCYON
PRODSON
PRONOUN
PROPMAN
PROPMEN
PROSCAN
PROTEAN
PROTEIN
RHODIAN
RIORDAN
RIOTGUN
SCOTIAN
SHODDEN
SHOOSIN
SHORTEN
SHOTGUN
SHOVEIN
SHOWMAN
SHOWMEN
SHOWNIN
SHOWSIN
SIOBHAN
SLOEGIN
SLOPSON
SNOWDON
SNOWMAN
SNOWMEN
SNOWSIN
SPORRAN
SPORTIN
STOLEIN
STOLLEN
STOMPIN
STOMPON
STOODIN
STOODON
STOPSIN
STORMIN
STOUTEN
SWOLLEN
SWOOPIN
SWOREIN
THOMSON
THORSON
TIOMKIN
TOOKTEN
TOOSOON
TRODDEN
TROMPIN
TROOPIN
TWOIRON
UNOFTEN
UTOPIAN
WOODBIN
WOODSON
WOOLLEN
WROTEIN
WROTEON
ZOOMSIN

•••ON••

ACRONYM
ADDONTO
AKRONOH
ALFONSE
ALFONSO
ALLONGE
ALLONYM
ALMONDS
ALMONDY
ALMONER
ALMONRY
AMMONIA
AMMONIC
ANIONIC
ANSONIA
ANTONIA
ANTONIN
ANTONIO
ANTONYM
ANYONES
APHONIA
APHONIC
APRONED
ARGONNE
AUTONYM
AVIONIC
AWOONOR
BALONEY
BARONET
BAYONET
BAYONNE
BEGONIA
BELONGS
BEYONCE
BIGONES
BITONAL
BORONIC
BOSONIC
BUJONES
BYGONES
BYRONIC
CACONYM
CANONIC
CANONRY
CHRONIC
CLOONEY
COCONUT
COLONEL
COLONES
COLONNA
COLONUS
CORONAE
CORONAL
CORONAS
CORONER
CORONET
CROONED
CROONER
DEBONED
DEBONES
DEMONIC
DEMONYM
DEPONED
DEPONER
DEPONES
DERONDA
DUGONGS
EDMONDS
ELMONTE
ESTONIA
FACONNE
FATONES
FELONRY
FORONCE
GARONNE
GETONIT
GETONTO
GIRONDE
GOTONIT
GOTONTO
HEDONIC
HERONRY
HOMONYM
HOTONES
HYPONYM
INTONED
INTONER
INTONES
IONONES
ITSONME
JACONET
JTMONEY
KCJONES
KETONES
KETONIC
KIMONOS
LACONIA
LACONIC
LAZONGA
LECONTE
LEMONDE
LOGONTO
MACONGA
MADONNA
MAHONEY
MASONED
MASONIC
MASONRY
MESONIC
MOMONEY
MORONIC
MRBONES
MRJONES
MYKONOS
NOTONCE
OBLONGS
ONEONTA
OOLONGS
ORDONEZ
OSMONDS
PARONYM
PINONES
POCONOS
POLONIA
RAMONES
RANONIN
REDONDO
REHONED
REHONES
REHONOR
RETONED
RETONES
REZONED
REZONES
ROLONDA
RUNONIN
SALONGA
SARONGS
SECONDI
SECONDO
SECONDR
SECONDS
SEDONAS
SIMONIZ
SITONIT
SPOONED
SPOONER
SWOONED
SWOONER
SYNONYM
TACONIC
TALONED
TENONED
TENONER
THRONES
THRONGS
TOPONYM
TORONTO
TWOONIE
UNBONED
UNHONED
UNTONED
UNZONED
UNZONES
UPTONOW
VERONIA
WAGONED
WAGONER
WASONTO
WEEONES
WETONES
WYNONNA
ZEDONKS

•••O•N•

ACCOUNT
ADJOINS
ADNOUNS
AGROUND
ALTOONA
ANTOINE
APPOINT
ARGONNE
ASTOUND
AUTOING
AUTOMNE
BABOONS
BAYONNE
BEMOANS
BEROWNE
BICORNE
BICORNS
BOLOGNA
COCOONS
COFOUND
COLOGNE
COLONNA
CYYOUNG
DADOING
DEHORNS
DEMOING
DEMOUNT
DEYOUNG
DISOWNS
ECHOING
ENJOINS
ENWOUND
EXPOUND
FACONNE
GARONNE
GOROUND
HALOING
HEROINE
HOBOING
HYPOING
IMGOING
IMPOUND
INBOUND
INGOING
INPOINT
KAYOING
KELOWNA
LAGOONS
LEMOYNE
LIVORNO
MACOUNS
MADONNA
MAROONS
MINOANS
MINOTND
NOCOUNT
NOVOTNY
OHIOANS
ONGOING
ONPOINT
OSBORNE
REBOANT
REBOUND
RECOINS
RECOUNT
REDOING
REDOUND
REFOUND
REJOINS
RELOANS
REMOUNT
RENOWNS
REPOINT
RESOUND
REWOUND
SALOONS
SAMOANS
SHOOING
SHOOINS
SILOING
SOLOING
STJOHNS
SUBORNS
THEOMNI
TYCOONS
UNBORNE
UNBOUND
UNDOING
UNFOUND
UNJOINS
UNJOINT
UNROUND
UNSOUND
UNWOUND
UNYOUNG
UPBORNE
UPBOUND
UPGOING
UPTOWNS
VETOING
WYNONNA
XAMOUNT
YESORNO
YOKOONO
YOYOING
ZEROING

•••O••N

ABDOMEN
ADJOURN
ADWOMAN
ADWOMEN
AGNOMEN
ALLOWIN
ALROSEN
ALSORAN
ANGOLAN
ANTONIN
AUTOPEN
BADOMEN
BEDOUIN
BETOKEN
BORODIN
CAROLYN
CAROTIN
COMORAN
CRYOGEN
CUTOPEN
DAKOTAN
DONOVAN
EIDOLON
EUROVAN
FLYOPEN
GASOVEN
GROOVIN
HALOGEN
HOBOKEN
INWOVEN
ISTOMIN
ITSOPEN
JACOBIN
KENOLIN
KILOTON
LANOLIN
LAYOPEN
MAJORIN
MANOLIN
MCCOWEN
MINORIN
MTLOGAN
NOTOPEN
ORTOLAN
OTTOMAN
PELOTON
PIROGEN
PREOPEN
PRYOPEN
RANONIN
REPOMAN
REWOKEN
REWOVEN
RIPOPEN
RUNONIN
SALOMON
SAROYAN
SHOOSIN
SOJOURN
SOLOMON
SONORAN
STOODIN
STOODON
SWOOPIN
THEOMEN
THROWIN
THROWON
TICOTIN
TROOPIN
UNWOVEN
VANOWEN
ZEROSIN

••••ON•

ABALONE
ABSCOND
ACETONE
ACTIONS
AFFRONT
AGELONG
AIRFONE
AKEBONO
ALCYONE
ALIMONY
ALLDONE
ALLGONE
ALTOONA

AMARONE
AMAZONS
AMNIONS
ANEMONE
ANTHONY
ARCHONS
ARIZONA
ARMBONE
ARTSONG
AVALONS
BABOONS
BALCONY
BALLONE
BANKONE
BARNONE
BARRONS
BARYONS
BCLIONS
BEACONS
BECKONS
BELMONT
BELZONI
BESTONE
BICHONS
BLAZONS
BONBONS
BORDONI
BOSTONS
BOSTONU
BOUSONO
BRETONS
BRITONS
BUITONI
BUNIONS
BUTTONS
BUTTONY
BYPHONE
CALZONE
CAMIONS
CANNONS
CANTONS
CANYONS
CANZONA
CANZONE
CANZONI
CARBONS
CARTONS
CATIONS
CHALONS
CHEVONS
CHITONS
CHYRONS
CICCONE
CITRONS
CLIPONS
COCOONS
COLDONE
COMEONS
COMMONS
CONDONE
CORDONS
COTTONS
COTTONY
COUPONS
COWPONY
CRAYONS
CREMONA
CROTONS
CUIBONO
CYCLONE
DACRONS
DAEMONS
DALTONS
DAMSONS
DAYLONG
DAYTONA
DEACONS
DEARONE
DEFCONS
DELMONT
DELTONA
DENTONS
DESMOND
DESPOND
DIAMOND
DINMONT
DOGBONE
DOGGONE
DONJONS
DOWRONG
DRAGONS
DUOTONE
EARBONE
EASYONE
ELEVONS
ENDLONG
ENDZONE
EPIGONE
ERELONG
ETYMONS
EUPHONY
EVELONG
EVILONE
FALCONS
FANIONS
FARGOND
FARGONE
FASTONE
FIVEONE
FLACONS
FLAGONS
FORDONE
FORGONE
FREMONT
FROZONE
FURLONG
FUSIONS
GALLONS
GAMMONS
GARCONS
GASCONS
GASCONY
GASTONE
GETDONE
GIBBONS
GIBSONS
GIDEONS
GNOMONS
GOALONG
GODSONS
GOLDONI
GOODONE
GORGONS
GOTDONE
GOWRONG
HADDONE
HADRONS
HAMBONE
HAMMOND
HARMONY
HASDONE
HAVEONE
HELMOND
HILTONS
HIPBONE
HITSONG
HOBSONS
HOLYONE
HORMONE
HOTZONE
HOWLONG
IFORONE
IFSTONE
ILLDONE
INFRONT
INIRONS
INSTONE
IRONONS
ISECOND
ISOGONS
ISOTONE
ITEMONE
ITSDONE
ITSGONE
JARGONS
JARGONY
JAWBONE
JETSONS
JIMSONS
JUSTONE
KAMFONG
KINMONT
KLAXONS
KMESONS
LADRONE
LAGOONS
LANEONE
LARDONS
LASTONE
LECUONA
LEGBONE
LEGIONS
LENNONS
LEPTONS
LESIONS
LESSONS
LINEONE
LIVEONE
LOTIONS
LYNDONB
MACHONE
MACRONS
MADEONE
MAISONS
MAKEONE
MARCONI
MAROONS
MARRONS
MATRONS
MICRONS
MIGNONS
MINIONS
MISDONE
MISZONE
MOLSONS
MORMONS
MORTONS
MOSCONI
MOTIONS
MRWRONG
MUTTONS
NAMEONE
NATIONS
NEGRONI
NELSONS
NEOCONS
NETTONS
NEURONE
NEURONS
NEWMONT
NEWTONS
NIALONG
NICEONE
NORTONS
NOTAONE
NOTDONE
NOTIONS
OLDSONG
OPTIONS
OPUSONE
ORISONS
OURSONG
OUTDONE
PADRONE
PAGEONE
PANTONE
PARDONS
PARSONS
PARTONE
PATRONS
PCCLONE
PENNONS
PEPTONE
PERSONA
PERSONS
PETPONY
PHOTONS
PIGEONS
PINIONS
PISTONS
PLUSONE
PLUTONS
POISONS
POMPONS
POPSONG
POTIONS
PRESONG
PRISONS
PROBONO
PROLONG
PROPONE
PROTONS
PULLONS
PULMONI
PULMONO
PYTHONS
RAISONS
RAMSONS
RAPSONG
RATIONS
RAYMOND
REASONS
RECKONS
REDBONE
REDMOND
REDPONY
REDZONE
REFRONT
REGIONS
REPHONE
RESPOND
REYMONT
RIBBONS
RIBBONY
RIPSONE
ROLLONS
RONSONS
RONZONI
RULEONE
SADSONG
SAISONS
SALMONP
SALMONS
SALOONS
SAMSONS
SAUCONY
SEASONS
SERMONS
SEXTONS
SHARONA
SIDDONS
SIDEONE
SIMMONS
SIPHONS
SIZEONE
SLIPONS
SNAPONS
SNOCONE
SOMEONE
SPUMONE
SPUMONI
STEPONE
STOLONS
SUBLONG
SUBTONE
SUBZONE
SUMMONS
TAKEONE
TALLONE
TARPONS
TEFLONS
TENDONS
TENTONS
TEUTONS
THATONE
THEFONZ
THEPOND
THISONE
TIGLONS
TOOLONG
TORTONI
TRIGONS
TRITONE
TRITONS
TUCSONS
TURNONS
TWOTONE
TWOTONS
TYCOONS
UNALONE
UNISONS
UNSTONY
UPFRONT
VALLONE
VERMONT
VIOLONE
VISIONS
VOLPONE
WALKONS
WALTONS
WANTONS
WARBOND
WARZONE
WEAKONS
WEAPONS
WILDONE
WILSONS
WISEONE
WONTONS
WORDONE
YEARONE
YOKOONO
ZAMBONI
ZIRCONS

••••O•N

AIRHORN
ALTHORN
ANDSOON
ANYTOWN
ARAGORN
BALLOON
BASSOON
BEDDOWN
BIGHORN
BIGJOHN
BIGTOWN
BOBGOEN
BOGDOWN
BOWDOIN
BOWDOWN
BUFFOON
BUYDOWN
CALHOUN
CARHORN
CARLOAN
CARTOON
CHITOWN
CITROEN
CONJOIN
COWTOWN
CRYDOWN
CUTDOWN
DIEDOWN
DISJOIN
DRAGOON
DRBROWN
DRSLOAN
EMBROWN
FESTOON
FHALOAN
FOGHORN
FORLORN
GETDOWN
GOTDOWN
HARPOON
HITTOWN
HOEDOWN
ICEDOWN
IDAHOAN
IIIJOHN
INBROWN
INGROWN
INKHORN
JOTDOWN
KOWLOON
LAMPOON
LAOCOON
LAYDOWN
LEGHORN
LETDOWN
LIEDOWN
LINCOLN
LOWBORN
LOWDOWN
MAXBORN
MIDMORN
MIDNOON
MIDTOWN
MISCOIN
MISJOIN
MONSOON
MOWDOWN
MRBROWN
MULDOON
NEWBORN
NEWMOON
NEWMOWN
NEWTOWN
OLDMOON
OLDTOWN
ONEDOWN
ONMYOWN
OURTOWN
OUTTORN
OUTWORN
PATDOWN
PATROON
PINDOWN
PLATOON
PONTOON
POPCORN
PREBORN
PRELOAN
PRENOON
PREWORN
PRONOUN
PURLOIN
PUTDOWN
RACCOON
RADIOIN
RAMDOWN
RANDOWN
RANGOON
READORN
REBLOWN
RECROWN
REFLOWN
REGROWN
RESHOWN
RESWORN
RIPTORN
ROCKOON
ROYCOHN
RUBDOWN
RUNDOWN
SANBORN
SASSOON
SATDOWN
SAXHORN
SETDOWN
SIRLOIN
SITDOWN
SUBJOIN
SUNDOWN
TEAGOWN
THEMOON
TIEDOWN
TINHORN
TIPDOWN
TOOSOON
TOPDOWN
TRICORN
TYPHOON
UNBLOWN
UNCROWN
UNFLOWN
UNGROWN
UNICORN
UNKNOWN
UNSHORN
UNSHOWN
UNSWORN
UPGROWN
VIRGOAN
WALLOON
WARTORN
WARWORN
WAYWORN
WETDOWN

•••••ON

ABANDON
ABUTSON
ACHERON
ACHESON
ACTAEON
ACTEDON
ACTINON
ACTUPON
ADAMSON
ADDEDON
ADDISON
AGREEON
AILERON
AJSIMON
ALARCON
ALENCON
ALLISON
ALLSTON
ALLYSON
AMPHION
ANDIRON
ANDSOON
ANISTON
ANTLION
APERSON
AUCTION
AUDUBON
AVEYRON
AVIGNON
BABYLON
BAILSON
BALATON
BALLOON
BANGSON
BANKSON
BASEDON
BASSOON
BASTION
BDALTON
BEALION
BEARSON
BEATSON
BELLSON
BENISON
BERGSON
BILLION
BITESON
BLAMEON
BLANTON
BLOUSON
BLOWSON
BLUSHON
BOURBON
BRANDON
BRANSON
BRAXTON
BRENDON
BRETTON
BRINGON
BRITTON
BRONSON
BUFFOON
BUILDON
BUILTON
BUISSON
BULLION
BURGEON
CAISSON
CALDRON
CALLSON
CAMERON
CAMPION
CAPTION
CARLSON
CARLTON
CARRYON
CARTOON
CASTSON
CATCHON
CAUTION
CELADON
CESSION
CHANSON
CHEATON
CHECKON
CHEERON
CHEVRON
CHEWSON
CHIFFON
CHIGNON
CHOKEON
CHOMPON
CLACTON
CLAMPON
CLANTON
CLAPTON
CLARION
CLASSON
CLAYTON
CLEAVON
CLEMSON
CLICKON
CLIFTON
CLIMBON
CLINTON
CLIPSON
COMESON
COMPTON
CORAZON
COUNTON
CRAMPON
CRATION
CRESTON
CRIMSON
CROUTON
CUSHION
CUTINON
DAVISON
DAWNSON
DECAGON
DENDRON
DENISON
DICKSON
DICTION
DINEDON
DINESON
DODGSON
DOTEDON
DOTESON
DRAGOON
DRAGSON
DRAWNON
DRAWSON
DRAYTON
DREAMON
DREGION
DRIPSON
DRONEON
DUDGEON
DUMPSON
DUNGEON
DWELLON
DWELTON
EARLYON
EASEDON
EASESON
ECHELON
EDITION
EGGEDON
EIDOLON
ELATION
ELCAJON
ELEISON
ELISION
ELLISON
ELUTION
EMERSON
EMOTION
ENDEDON
ENTERON
ENVIRON
EPSILON
EREWHON
ERICSON
ERIKSON
EROSION
ESIASON
EUDEMON
EVASION
FACEDON
FACESON
FACTION
FALLSON
FASHION
FAWNSON
FEASTON
FEEDSON
FENELON
FERMION
FESTOON
FICTION
FINKSON
FIREDON
FIRESON
FISSION
FIXEDON
FIXESON
FIXUPON
FLASHON
FLEURON
FLEXION
FLIESON
FLOWNON
FLUXION
FOCUSON
FOISTON
FORCEON
FRISSON
FRONTON
FROWNON
GAINSON
GALLEON
GAZEDON
GAZESON
GERSHON
GETINON
GETITON
GETUPON
GGORDON
GIGATON
GIVENON
GIVESON
GLEASON
GLUEDON
GLUESON
GLUTTON
GNAWSON
GOINGON
GOODSON
GOTINON
GOTITON
GOTUPON
GRAFTON
GRATEON
GRAYSON
GRIFFON
GROWNON
GROWSON
GRUNION
GRYPHON
GUDGEON
GUERDON
HALCYON
HALFWON
HALSTON
HAMPTON
HANDSON
HANGSON
HARDWON
HARPOON
HARPSON
HEAPSON
HEDISON
HELICON
HELLION
HELPSON
HERNDON
HEXAGON
HINGEON
HIREDON
HIRESON
HITCHON
HITUPON
HOLDSON
HOOKSON
HORIZON
HOUSTON
HURSTON
HYPERON
IRECKON
IRONSON
IVERSON
IZATION
JACKSON
JAMESON
JAMISON
JANSSON
JEMISON
JEWISON
JILLION
JOHNSON
JUMPSON
KARLSON
KEEPSON
KEMPTON
KEYEDON
KEYINON
KILOTON
KINISON
KLINGON
KNOCKON
KOWLOON
KRATION
KRYPTON
LACESON
LAMPOON
LANGDON
LANGTON
LAOCOON
LASTDON
LATCHON
LATERON
LAYITON
LAYUPON
LEADSON
LEANSON
LEAPSON
LEAPTON
LEAVEON
LEBANON
LEBARON
LEGIRON
LETINON
LETUPON
LEXICON
LIAISON
LIGHTON
LIMACON
LIVEDON
LIVESON
LLEYTON
LOCKSON
LONGTON
LOOKSON
LORGNON
LYINGON
LYRICON
MACEDON
MACHAON
MADELON
MADISON
MANSION
MARCHON
MARMION
MARSTON
MCMAHON
MEGALON
MEGATON
MENTION
MGMLION
MIDIRON
MIDNOON
MILLION
MISSION
MONCTON
MONSOON
MOVEDON
MOVESON
MULDOON
MUMESON
MUNCHON
MUSEDON
MUSESON
MYERSON
NEUTRON
NEWMOON
NILSSON
NIPIGON
NONAGON
NONIRON
NUCLEON
OCTAGON
ODINGON
OHANLON
OLDMOON
OMICRON
ONANDON
ONEIRON
OPINION
ORARION
ORATION
ORBISON
OVATION
OWINGON
PACKSON
PALEMON
PARAGON
PARTYON
PASSION
PATROON
PEARSON
PELOTON

PENSION
PERSSON
PETLION
PHAETON
PICKSON
PIDGEON
PIGIRON
PILEDON
PILESON
PILLION
PIMESON
PLANSON
PLATOON
PLAYSON
PLOSION
PLOWSON
PNEUMON
POISSON
POKEMON
POLYGON
PONTOON
PORTION
PRENOON
PRESSON
PRESTON
PREYSON
PROCYON
PRODSON
PULLSON
PUTUPON
PYNCHON
QUINION
QUINTON
RACCOON
RAILSON
RAINSON
RALSTON
RANGOON
READSON
REARDON
RESTSON
REUNION
RIGHTON
ROBESON
ROCKOON
ROLLSON
ROUNDON
RUBICON
RUBUPON
RUCTION
RULEDON
RULESON
SAFFRON
SAILSON
SALOMON
SAMPSON
SASSOON
SATINON
SATUPON
SAVEDON
SAVESON
SEALION
SECTION
SEIZEON
SENDSON
SESSION
SETUPON
SEWEDON

SHANNON
SHEDSON
SHELDON
SHINEON
SIGNSON
SILICON
SIMENON
SIMPSON
SITINON
SITUPON
SIXIRON
SKELTON
SKIMPON
SLAMSON
SLAPSON
SLAYTON
SLEEPON
SLEPTON
SLIPSON
SLOPSON
SMEARON
SMILEON
SNACKON
SNAPSON
SNOWDON
SOLOMON
SOUPCON
SOUPSON
SOURSON
SPENDON
SPENTON
SPIEDON
SPIESON
SPITSON
SPRAYON
SPURSON
SPYUPON
STANDON
STANTON
STARION
STARTON
STATION
STAYSON
STEPSON
STETSON
STICKON
STILTON
STIMSON
STOMPON
STOODON
STRAPON
STSIMON
STUCKON
SUASION
SUCTION
SUELYON
SURGEON
SWANSON
SWEETON
SWENSON
SWINTON
TACHYON
TACKSON
TAKENON
TAKESON
TALKSON
TAPEDON
TAPESON

TAUNTON
TELLSON
TENSION
TEXTRON
THEMOON
THEREON
THOMSON
THORSON
THREWON
THROWON
TIBURON
TOOSOON
TORSION
TOUCHON
TRADEON
TREADON
TREASON
TRENTON
TRIEDON
TRIESON
TRIPSON
TRYITON
TUITION
TURNSON
TWISTON
TWOIRON
TYINGON
TYPHOON
UNCTION
UPSILON
URGEDON
URGESON
VALADON
VENISON
VERGEON
VERIZON
VERSION
VESTRON
VIDICON
VISTEON
VOTEDON
VOTESON
VUITTON
WAITRON
WAITSON
WALKSON
WALLOON
WALSTON
WEARSON
WEIGHON
WEIRTON
WELLWON
WHARTON
WHEATON
WHEREON
WIDGEON
WILLSON
WINSTON
WOBEGON
WOODSON
WORKSON
WRITEON
WROTEON
YANKSON
YANKTON
YORKTON
YOUREON
ZABUTON

ZEBULON
ZILLION

OO•••••

OOBLECK
OOCYTES
OOHLALA
OOLITES
OOLITIC
OOLONGS
OOMPAHS
OOZEOUT
OOZIEST

O•O••••

OBOISTS
OCONNOR
ODONTIA
ODORANT
ODORFUL
ODORIZE
ODOROUS
OLOGIES
OLOROSO
ONORATI
ONORDER
OPOSSUM
OROGENY
OROLOGY
OROTUND
OROURKE
OTOLOGY
OVOIDAL
OXONIAN
OZONISE
OZONIZE
OZONOUS

O••O•••

OBLONGS
OBLOQUY
OCTOBER
OCTOBRE
OCTOPOD
OCTOPUS
OFNOUSE
OFSORTS
OGDOADS
OHIOANS
OHIOART
OKHOTSK
OKTOBER
OLEOOIL
ONBOARD
ONEOCAT
ONEOFFS
ONEOFUS
ONEONTA
ONEOVER
ONGOING
ONLOADS
ONPOINT
ONTOAST
ONTOPIC
ONTOPOF
OOLONGS
OPPOSED
OPPOSER
OPPOSES
ORDONEZ
ORIOLES
ORMOLUS
ORTOLAN
OSBORNE
OSMONDS
OSMOSED
OSMOSES
OSMOSIS
OSMOTIC
OSTOSIS
OTTOIII
OTTOMAN
OUTOFIT
OXFORDS

O•••O••

OAKMOSS
OAKWOOD
OARLOCK
OBVIOUS
OCELOTS
OCHROID
OCHROUS
OCTROIS
ODDJOBS
ODDLOTS
ODDSOCK
ODOROUS
OFASORT
OFFHOUR
OFFLOAD
OFFROAD
OKSHOOT
OLDBOYS
OLDDOGS
OLDFOGY
OLDGOLD
OLDJOKE
OLDMOON
OLDROSE
OLDSONG
OLDTOWN
OLEOOIL
OLICOOK
OLOROSO
OMIGOSH
OMINOUS
ONAROLL
ONATOOT
ONEDOWN
ONEFOLD
ONEFOOT
ONEHOUR
ONEIOTA
ONELOOK
ONELOVE
ONEMORE
ONENOTE
ONEROOM
ONEROUS
ONESOCK
ONETOGO
ONEVOTE
ONEWOOD
ONMYOWN
ONSHORE
OOZEOUT
OPENOUT
OPEROSE
OPTIONS
OPTSOUT
OPUSONE
ORATORS
ORATORY
OREBODY
ORINOCO
ORISONS
OROLOGY
OSCEOLA
OSHKOSH
OSSEOUS
OSTEOID
OTOLOGY
OURSONG
OURTOWN
OUTBOWL
OUTBOWS
OUTCOLD
OUTCOME
OUTCOOK
OUTDOER
OUTDOES
OUTDONE
OUTDOOR
OUTFOOL
OUTFOOT
OUTGOES
OUTHOWL
OUTLOOK
OUTLOUD
OUTLOVE
OUTMODE
OUTMOST
OUTMOVE
OUTPOLL
OUTPOPS
OUTPORT
OUTPOST
OUTPOUR
OUTROAR
OUTROCK
OUTRODE
OUTROLL
OUTROOT
OUTROVE
OUTROWS
OUTSOAR
OUTSOLD
OUTSOLE
OUTTOLD
OUTTOLL
OUTTORE
OUTTORN
OUTVOTE
OUTWORD
OUTWORE
OUTWORK
OUTWORN
OVIFORM
OWNGOAL
OXBLOOD
OXYMORA
OZONOUS

O••••O•

OAKWOOD
OBENTOS
OBLIGOR
OCONNOR
OCTAGON
OCTAVOS
OCTOPOD
ODDSHOE
ODINGON
OFFEROR
OHANLON
OHCAROL
OILSPOT
OKSHOOT
OLDMOON
OLDPROS
OLDSHOE
OLICOOK
OMICRON
ONANDON
ONATOOT
ONEFOOT
ONEIRON
ONELOOK
ONEROOM
ONESHOE
ONESHOT
ONESPOT
ONESTOP
ONETWOS
ONEWOOD
ONLYTOO
ONLYYOU
ONTOPOF
OPENTOE
OPENTOP
OPINION
OPTSFOR
ORARION
ORATION
ORBISON
OUTBLOT
OUTBLOW
OUTCOOK
OUTCROP
OUTCROW
OUTDOOR
OUTDROP
OUTFLOW
OUTFOOL
OUTFOOT
OUTGLOW
OUTGROW
OUTLOOK
OUTPLOD
OUTPLOT
OUTROOT
OUTSHOT
OUTSHOW
OUTTROT
OVATION
OVERCOY
OVERDOG
OVERHOT
OVERJOY
OVERTOP
OWINGON
OXBLOOD

O•••••O

OCCURTO
OCTAVIO
OFFICIO
OFFWEGO
OLOROSO
OMPHALO
ONEKILO
ONETOGO
ONLYTOO
ONTARIO
ONTHEGO
ONVIDEO
OPTEDTO
OPUSTWO
OREGANO
ORINOCO
ORLANDO
ORNITHO
ORVIETO
OTHELLO
OTRANTO
OTTAVIO
OUGHTTO
OUTECHO
OWINGTO
OWNUPTO

•OO••••

BOOBIES
BOOBIRD
BOOBOOS
BOOCOOS
BOODLES
BOOEDAT
BOOGIED
BOOGIES
BOOHBAH
BOOHISS
BOOHOOS
BOOKBAG
BOOKEND
BOOKERS
BOOKERT
BOOKIES
BOOKIII
BOOKING
BOOKISH
BOOKLET
BOOKMAN
BOOKMEN
BOOKVII
BOOLEAN
BOOMBOX
BOOMCAR
BOOMERS
BOOMIER
BOOMING
BOOMLET
BOONIES
BOOPSIE
BOORISH
BOORMAN
BOOSLER
BOOSTED
BOOSTER
BOOSTUP
BOOTCUT
BOOTEES
BOOTERS
BOOTERY
BOOTHIA
BOOTIES
BOOTING
BOOTLEG
BOOTOUT
BOOTSIT
BOOTSUP
BOOTTOP
BOOZERS
BOOZIER
BOOZILY
BOOZING
COOKERS
COOKERY
COOKIES
COOKING
COOKOFF
COOKOUT
COOKPOT
COOKSUP
COOKTOP
COOLAIR
COOLANT
COOLCAT
COOLERS
COOLEST
COOLIES
COOLING
COOLISH
COOLMAX
COOLOUT
COOLPIX
COOLSIT
COONCAN
COONCAT
COONDOG
COOPERS
COOPERY
COOPING
COOPSUP
COOPTED
COOTERS
COOTIES
COOWNED
DOODADS
DOODLED
DOODLER
DOODLES
DOOLIES
DOOMFUL
DOOMIER
DOOMING
DOOMSTO
DOONEIN
DOORDIE
DOORMAN
DOORMAT
DOORMEN
DOORWAY
DOOUTOF
DOOVERS
DOOWOPS
DOOZERS
DOOZIES
FOODIES
FOODWEB
FOOLERS
FOOLERY
FOOLING
FOOLISH
FOOTAGE
FOOTBAG
FOOTERS
FOOTING
FOOTLED
FOOTLER
FOOTLES
FOOTLET
FOOTMAN
FOOTMEN
FOOTPAD
FOOTRUB
FOOTSIE
FOOTSIT
FOOTSUP
FOOTWAY
FOOZLED
FOOZLER
FOOZLES
GOOBERS
GOODAIM
GOODALL
GOODBAR
GOODBUY
GOODBYE
GOODBYS
GOODDAY
GOODDOG
GOODEGG
GOODERS
GOODFOR
GOODGUY
GOODIES
GOODING
GOODISH
GOODJOB
GOODJOE
GOODKID
GOODMAN
GOODMEN
GOODNIK
GOODONE
GOODPAY
GOODSON
GOODTRY
GOODUSE
GOODWIN
GOOFIER
GOOFILY
GOOFING
GOOFOFF
GOOFSUP
GOOFUPS
GOOGLED
GOOGLER
GOOGLES
GOOGOLS
GOOIEST
GOOMBAH
GOOMBAY
GOONEYS
GOONIER
GOONIES
GOONILY
GOOPIER
GOOSIER
GOOSING
HOOCHES
HOODIES
HOODING
HOODLUM
HOODOOS
HOOFERS
HOOFING
HOOFSIT
HOOHAHS
HOOKAHS
HOOKING
HOOKSON
HOOKSUP
HOOKUPS
HOOPERS
HOOPING
HOOPLAS
HOOPMAN
HOOPMEN
HOOPOES
HOOPTOY
HOORAHS
HOORAYS
HOOSIER
HOOTERS
HOOTING
HOOTOWL
HOOTSAT
HOOVERS
KOOKIER
KOOLAID
KOONING
KOOSHES
LOOBIES
LOOFAHS
LOOKERS
LOOKFOR
LOOKING
LOOKINS
LOOKISM
LOOKIST
LOOKOUT
LOOKSAD
LOOKSAT
LOOKSEE
LOOKSIN
LOOKSON
LOOKSTO
LOOKSUP
LOOKUPS
LOOKYOU
LOOMING
LOOMPAS
LOONIER
LOONIES
LOONILY
LOOPERS
LOOPIER
LOOPING
LOOSELY
LOOSENS
LOOSEST
LOOSING
LOOTERS
LOOTING
MOOCHED
MOOCHER
MOOCHES
MOOCOWS
MOODIER
MOODILY
MOONBOW
MOONDOG
MOONERS
MOONEYE
MOONGOD
MOONIER
MOONIES
MOONILY
MOONING
MOONISH
MOONLET
MOONLIT
MOONPIE
MOONSET
MOORAGE
MOORHEN
MOORIER
MOORING
MOORISH
MOOTERS
MOOTING
NOODGED
NOODGES
NOODLED
NOODLES
NOOGIES
NOONDAY
NOONERS
NOONING
NOOSERS
NOOSING
NOOTHER
NOOTKAS
POOCHES
POOCHIE
POODLES
POOHBAH
POOLCUE
POOLERS
POOLING
POOLMAN
POOLMEN
POOPING
POOPOUT
POOPSIE
POORBOX
POORBOY
POOREST
POORISH
POORLAW
POORMAN
POORMEN
POORTAX
ROOFAGE
ROOFERS
ROOFING
ROOFRAT
ROOFTOP
ROOKERY
ROOKIER
ROOKIES
ROOKING
ROOKISH
ROOMBAS
ROOMERS
ROOMFUL
ROOMIER
ROOMIES
ROOMILY
ROOMING
ROOSTED
ROOSTER
ROOTAGE
ROOTCAP
ROOTERS
ROOTFOR
ROOTIER
ROOTING
ROOTLED
ROOTLES
ROOTLET
ROOTOUT
ROOTROT
ROOTSUP
SOONERS
SOONEST
SOOTHED
SOOTHER
SOOTHES
SOOTIER
SOOTILY
TOODLES
TOOEASY
TOOHARD
TOOHIGH
TOOKAIM
TOOKFOR
TOOKILL
TOOKOFF
TOOKOUT
TOOKTEN
TOOLATE
TOOLBAR
TOOLBOX
TOOLERS
TOOLING
TOOLKIT
TOOLONG
TOOLSET
TOOLSUP
TOOMANY
TOOMUCH
TOONIES
TOORDER
TOOSLOW
TOOSOON
TOOTALL
TOOTERS
TOOTHED
TOOTING
TOOTLED
TOOTLER
TOOTLES
TOOTSAT
TOOTSIE
VOODOOS
WOODARD

WOODBIN
WOODBOX
WOODCUT
WOODIER
WOODIES
WOODING
WOODLEY
WOODLOT
WOODROW
WOODSAW
WOODSON
WOODTAR
WOOFERS
WOOFING
WOOKIEE
WOOLENS
WOOLERY
WOOLFAT
WOOLHAT
WOOLIER
WOOLIES
WOOLITE
WOOLLEN
WOOLLEY
WOOLSEY
WOOSHED
WOOSHES
WOOSNAM
WOOSTER
WOOZIER
WOOZILY
YOOHOOS
ZOOIDAL
ZOOIEST
ZOOLOGY
ZOOMING
ZOOMOUT
ZOOMSIN
COPOUTS
COROLLA
CORONAE
CORONAL
CORONAS
CORONER
CORONET
COYOTES
DOLORES
DOLOURS
DONOHOE
DONOTGO
DONOVAN
DOROTHY
FORONCE
FOTOMAT
GOFORIT
GOFORTH
GOROUND
GOSOUTH
GOTOBED
GOTOGAL
GOTOGUY
GOTONIT
GOTONTO
GOTOPOT
GOTOSEA
GOTOSEE
GOTOVER
GOTOWAR
HOBOING
HOBOISM
HOBOKEN
HOMONYM
HONORED
HONOREE
HONORER
HONOURS
HOPOVER
HOTONES
HOTOVER
IOMOTHS
IONONES
JOJOBAS
KOBOLDS
KOSOVAR
LOGOFFS
LOGONTO
LOGOUTS
LOYOLAU
MOLOKAI
MOLOTOV
MOMONEY
MONOCLE
MONODIC
MONOLOG
MONOMER
MONOPOD
MONOSKI
MOROCCO
MORONIC
MOTORED
NOBODYS
NOCOUNT
NODOUBT
NOGOODS
NOKOMIS
NOLOADS
NONOILY
NONOISE
NONORAL
NOTONCE
NOTOPEN
NOTOVER
NOVOTES
NOVOTNY
NOWORSE
OOLONGS
POBOXES
POCONOS
POLOIST
POLONIA
POPOFFS
POPOUTS
POPOVER
POSOLES
POTOMAC
POZOLES
ROBOCOP
ROBOTIC
ROBOTRY
ROCOCOS
RODOLFO
ROLODEX
ROLONDA
SOJOURN
SOLOACT
SOLOING
SOLOIST
SOLOMON
SONORAN
SORORAL
SOSORRY
TOHOMER
TOHORSE
TOPONYM
TOROIDS
TORONTO
TOTOTOO
TOYOTAS
VOCODER
VONOPEL
WONOVER
YOKOONO
YOYOING

•O•O•••

BOLOGNA
BOLOTIE
BORODIN
BOROMIR
BORONIC
BOROUGH
BOSOMED
BOSONIC
BOWOARS
COCONUT
COCOONS
COFOUND
COHORTS
COHOSTS
COLOGNE
COLOMBO
COLONEL
COLONES
COLONNA
COLONUS
COLORED
COLORER
COLORTV
COLOSSI
COLOURS
COMORAN
COMOROS
CONOIDS

•O••O••

BOBDOLE
BOBGOEN
BOBHOPE
BOFFOLA
BOGDOWN
BOGHOLE
BOILOFF
BOILOUT
BONBONS
BONGOES
BONJOUR
BONJOVI
BONMOTS
BONSOIR
BOOBOOS
BOOCOOS
BOOHOOS
BOOTOUT
BORDONI
BOREOUT
BORROWS
BORZOIS
BOSTONS
BOSTONU
BOTTOMS
BOUDOIR
BOUSONO
BOWDOIN
BOWDOWN
BOWSOUT
BOWWOWS
BOXBOYS
BOXCOAT
BOXTOPS
BOYCOTT
BOYHOOD
BOYTOYS
COALOIL
COBCOAL
COCCOID
COCOONS
COINOPS
COLDONE
COLLODI
COLLOID
COLLOPS
COMEOFF
COMEONS
COMEOUT
COMFORT
COMMODE
COMMONS
COMMOVE
COMPORT
COMPOSE
COMPOST
COMPOTE
CONCOCT
CONCORD
CONDOLE
CONDONE
CONDORS
CONFORM
CONGOUS
CONJOBS
CONJOIN
CONKOFF
CONKOUT
CONMOTO
CONNORS
CONNOTE
CONSOLE
CONSORT
CONTORT
CONTOUR
CONVOKE
CONVOYS
COOKOFF
COOKOUT
COOLOUT
COPIOUS
COPPOLA
COPSOUT
CORDOBA
CORDONS
CORKOAK
CORNOIL
CORPORA
CORRODE
COTTONS
COTTONY
COULOMB
COUPONS
COWBOYS
COWPOKE
COWPONY
COWROTE
COWTOWN
COXCOMB
COYDOGS
DOCTORS
DOGBONE
DOGBOOT
DOGBOWL
DOGCOAT
DOGCOMB
DOGDOOR
DOGFOOD
DOGGONE
DOGROSE
DOGTOYS
DOGWOOD
DOLEOUT
DOLLOPS
DONJONS
DONJOSE
DOOWOPS
DOPEOUT
DOSHOTS
DOTBOMB
DOTCOMS
DOWRONG
DOZEOFF
FOBSOFF
FOGBOWS
FOGDOGS
FOGHORN
FOLDOUT
FOLIOED
FOLIOSE
FOLLOWS
FORBORE
FORDOES
FORDONE
FORGOER
FORGOES
FORGONE
FORGOOD
FORKOUT
FORLORN
FORLOVE
FORMOSA
FORSOOK
FORTORD
FOSCOLO
FOULOUT
FOXBORO
FOXHOLE
GOABOUT
GOALONG
GOBROKE
GODHOOD
GODSONS
GOESOFF
GOESOUT
GOLDONI
GONDOLA
GONEOFF
GONEOUT
GONGORA
GOODONE
GOOFOFF
GOOGOLS
GORGONS
GOSFORD
GOTCOLD
GOTDONE
GOTDOWN
GOTGOOD
GOTLOST
GOTSOFT
GOTSORE
GOTTOIT
GOTWORD
GOWRONG
HOBNOBS
HOBSONS
HOEDOWN
HOGNOSE
HOLDOFF
HOLDOUT
HOLEOUT
HOLLOWS
HOLMOAK
HOLYOIL
HOLYOKE
HOLYONE
HOODOOS
HOOPOES
HOOTOWL
HOPSOFF
HOPSOUT
HOPTOIT
HORMONE
HORRORS
HOTCOAL
HOTCOMB
HOTDOGS
HOTFOOT
HOTPOTS
HOTRODS
HOTROLL
HOTSOUP
HOTZONE
HOWCOME
HOWLONG
JOBHOPS
JOBLOCK
JOBLOTS
JOECOOL
JOEROTH
JOPPOLO
JOSBOYS
JOTDOWN
KOWLOON
KOWTOWS
LOANOUT
LOCKOUT
LOGBOOK
LOGROLL
LOGSOFF
LOGSOUT
LONBORG
LOOKOUT
LOPSOFF
LOSEOUT
LOSTOUT
LOTIONS
LOWBORN
LOWBOYS
LOWCOST
LOWDOWN
LOWPOST
LOWROAD
LOWTOPS
MOLDOVA
MOLSONS
MONGOLS
MONROES
MONSOON
MONTOYA
MOOCOWS
MOPTOPS
MORLOCK
MORMONS
MORROWS
MORTONS
MOSCONI
MOTIONS
MOTTOES
MOVEOFF
MOVEOUT
MOWDOWN
NOCUOUS
NODSOFF
NOGOODS
NOISOME
NOKNOCK
NONBODY
NONBOOK
NONCOLA
NONCOMS
NONCORE
NONFOOD
NONFORM
NONGOGO
NONGOLD
NONHOME
NONPOET
NONPOOR
NONVOID
NONWOOL
NONWORD
NONWORK
NORDOFF
NORDOWE
NORFOLK
NORTONS
NORWOOD
NOSCORE
NOSEOUT
NOSHOWS
NOTAONE
NOTDONE
NOTGOOD
NOTHOME
NOTIONS
NOTTOBE
NOWLOOK
NOXIOUS
OOZEOUT
POISONS
POKEOUT
POLLOCK
POMPOMS
POMPONS
POMPOUS
PONTOON
POOPOUT
POPCORN
POPROCK
POPSOFF
POPSONG
POPSOUT
POPTOPS
POSTOPS
POTBOIL
POTHOLE
POTHOOK
POTIONS
POUROUT
POWWOWS
ROANOKE
ROBLOWE
ROBROYS
ROCKOIL
ROCKOON
RODEOFF
RODEOUT
ROLLOFF
ROLLONS
ROLLOUT
ROMCOMS
RONSONS
RONWOOD
RONZONI
ROOTOUT
ROPEOFF
ROSCOES
ROSEOIL
ROSEOLA
ROSTOCK
ROUTOUT
ROWBOAT
ROYCOHN
SOLDOFF
SOLDOUT
SOMEONE
SORROWS
SORTOUT
TOEHOLD
TOELOOP
TOGSOUT
TOLDOFF
TOMBOYS
TOMFOOL
TOMGOLA
TOMJOAD
TOMTOMS
TOOKOFF
TOOKOUT
TOOLONG
TOOSOON
TOPBOOT
TOPCOAT
TOPDOGS
TOPDOWN
TOPFORM
TOPHOLE
TOPMOST
TOPROWS
TOPSOFF
TOPSOIL
TOPSOUT
TOREOFF
TOREOUT
TORNOFF
TORNOUT
TORTOLA
TORTONI
TOSSOFF
TOSSOUT
TOWBOAT
TOWROPE
TOYBOAT
TOYBOOK
TOYDOGS
TOYDOLL
TOYHOOP
TOYTOPS
VOIDOUT
VOLPONE
VOLTORE
VOODOOS
VOTEOUT
WONTONS
WORDONE
WOREOFF
WOREOUT
WORKOFF
WORKOUT
WORNOFF
WORNOUT
YOKOONO
YOMTOVS
YOOHOOS
YOULOSE
ZONEOUT
ZONKOUT
ZOOLOGY
ZOOMOUT

•O•••O•

BOASTOF
BOKCHOY
BOLEROS
BOLSHOI
BONITOS
BOOBOOS
BOOCOOS
BOOHOOS
BOOMBOX
BOOTTOP
BOREDOM
BOURBON
BOUTROS
BOWKNOT
BOWSHOT
BOYHOOD
COINBOX
COJUROR
COMENOW
COMESON
COMOROS
COMPTON
CONCHOS
CONTROL
COOKPOT
COOKTOP
COONDOG
COPILOT
COPSHOP
COPYBOY
CORAZON
CORNCOB
CORNDOG
CORNROW
COTEDOR
COUNTON
DODGSON
DOESFOR
DOESNOT
DOESTOO
DOGBOOT
DOGCHOW
DOGDOOR
DOGFOOD
DOGSHOW
DOGTROT
DOGWOOD
DOINGOK
DOITNOW
DOMINOS
DONATOR
DONEFOR
DONOHOE
DOOUTOF
DORITOS
DOSADOS
DOSIDOS
DOTEDON
DOTESON
DOVECOT
DOWNBOW
FOCUSON
FOISTON
FORCEON
FORETOP
FORGOOD
FORSHOW
FORSOOK
FOXTROT
GOBELOW
GODHOOD
GODUNOV
GOESFOR
GOINFOR
GOINGON
GONEFOR
GOODDOG
GOODFOR
GOODJOB
GOODJOE
GOODSON
GOTAJOB
GOTGOOD
GOTINON
GOTITON
GOTOPOT
GOTUPON
HOLDSON
HOLYCOW
HOLYJOE
HOMEBOY
HONCHOS
HOODOOS
HOOKSON
HOOPTOY
HOPEFOR
HOPENOT
HORIZON
HOTFOOT
HOTSHOT
HOTSPOT
HOUSTON
IOWEYOU
JOBSHOP
JOEBLOW
JOECOOL
JOGTROT
JOHNBOY
JOHNDOE
JOHNSON
JOHNWOO
JOURNOS
KOWLOON
LOADSOF
LOCATOR
LOCKBOX
LOCKSON
LOGBOOK
LONGBOW
LONGFOR
LONGTOM
LONGTON
LOOKFOR
LOOKSON
LOOKYOU
LORGNON
LOSTDOG
LOTHROP
LOVEJOY
LOVEYOU
LOWBLOW
LOWBROW
MOGADOR
MOJITOS
MOLITOR
MOLOTOV
MONCTON
MONITOR
MONOLOG
MONOPOD
MONSOON
MOONBOW
MOONDOG
MOONGOD
MORELOS
MORISOT
MOVADOS
MOVEDON
MOVESON
NOENDOF
NONAGON
NONBOOK
NONCROP
NONFOOD
NONIRON
NONPOOR
NONPROS
NONSTOP
NONWOOL
NORTHOF
NORWOOD
NOSEJOB
NOTALOT
NOTGOOD
NOWLOOK
POCONOS
POISSON
POKEMON
POLYGON
POLYPOD
POMELOS
PONCHOS
PONTOON
POORBOX
POORBOY
POPEDOM
PORTHOS
PORTION
PORTNOY
POSTBOX
POSTDOC
POSTHOC
POTHOOK
POTSHOT
ROADEOS
ROADHOG
ROBESON
ROBOCOP
ROCKCOD
ROCKOON
ROCOCOS
ROLLMOP
ROLLSON
ROLLTOP
ROMANOS
ROMANOV
RONWOOD
ROOFTOP
ROOTFOR
ROOTROT
ROPETOW
ROTATOR
ROUNDON
ROZANOV
SOAPBOX
SOCKHOP
SODAPOP
SOFTTOP
SOLDFOR
SOLOMON
SOMEHOW
SOUPCON
SOUPSON
SOURSON
SOUTHOF
TOELOOP
TOESHOE
TOLEDOS
TOLSTOI
TOLSTOY
TOMFOOL
TONELOC
TONEROW
TONYDOW
TOOKFOR
TOOLBOX
TOOSLOW
TOOSOON
TOPBOOT
TOPKNOT
TOPSPOT
TOREROS
TORINOS
TORSION
TOSSPOT
TOTINOS
TOTOTOO
TOUCHON
TOYBOOK
TOYHOOP
TOYSHOP
VOODOOS
VOSKHOD
VOTEDON
VOTEFOR
VOTESON
WOBEGON
WOLFDOG
WOODBOX
WOODLOT
WOODROW
WOODSON
WORKBOX
WORKFOR
WORKSON
YOOHOOS
YORKTON
YOUKNOW
YOUREON
ZOCALOS

•O••••O

BOIARDO
BOITANO
BONARIO
BONIATO
BOUNDTO
BOUSONO
BOWECHO
BOWEDTO
COLOMBO
COLUMBO
COMESTO
CONBRIO
CONMOTO
CORDERO
CORTICO
DOASIDO
DOESTOO
DOINGSO
DOINGTO
DOMINGO
DONOTGO
DOOMSTO
DOUBLEO
FOLENGO
FOSCOLO
FOXBORO
GOESPRO
GOINGTO
GOLFPRO
GONEPRO
GOTINTO
GOTONTO
GOTTAGO
GOTUPTO

HOLDSTO
HOPEDSO
HOPEDTO
HOPESSO
HOPESTO
HOPINTO
HORATIO
HOWDEDO
HOWDYDO
IONESCO
JOHNWOO
JOPPOLO
KOWADLO
LOATHTO
LOCARNO
LOGONTO
LONGAGO
LOOKSTO
LORENZO
LOSESTO
LOVEDTO
LOVESTO
LOYALTO
MODESTO
MOGAMBO
MONSTRO
MONTANO
MONTEGO
MONTERO
MONTUNO
MORELLO
MOROCCO
MOSCATO
MOVEDTO
MOVESTO
NOCANDO
NOENDTO
NONGOGO
NONHERO
NONZERO
NORELCO
NOTUPTO
NOVARRO
NOVELLO
POBLANO
POINTTO
POMPANO
PONTANO
POPELEO
PORTICO
ROBERTO
ROBUSTO
RODOLFO
RODRIGO
ROSARIO
ROSSANO
ROUGHGO
SOANDSO
SOPRANO
SORDINO
SORENTO
SORIANO
SORVINO
TOBACCO
TORNADO
TORONTO
TORPEDO
TOSHIRO
TOTOTOO
VOLCANO
VOTEDNO
VOTESNO
YOKOONO
YOTEAMO

••OO•••

ALOOFLY
AWOONOR
BLOODED
BLOOMED
BLOOMER
BLOOPED
BLOOPER
BROODED
BROODER
BROOKED
BROOMED
CHOOSER
CHOOSES
CHOOSEY
CLOONEY
CROOKED
CROOKES
CROONED
CROONER
DROOLED
DROOLER
DROOPED
FLOODED
FLOORED
FLOORER
FLOORIT
FROOGLE
GLOOMED
GROOMED
GROOMER
GROOVED
GROOVES
GROOVIN
IDOODIT
IGOOFED
KYOODLE
PROOFED
PROOFER
SCOOBAS
SCOOPED
SCOOPER
SCOOTCH
SCOOTED
SCOOTER
SHOOFLY
SHOOING
SHOOINS
SHOOKUP
SHOOOFF
SHOOSIN
SHOOTAT
SHOOTBY
SHOOTER
SHOOTUP
SMOOTHS
SMOOTHY
SNOOKER
SNOOPED
SNOOPER
SNOOTED
SNOOZED
SNOOZER
SNOOZES
SPOOFED
SPOOFER
SPOOKED
SPOOLED
SPOOLER
SPOONED
SPOONER
STOODBY
STOODIN
STOODON
STOODTO
STOODUP
STOOGED
STOOGES
STOOKEY
STOOLED
STOOLIE
STOOPED
STOOPER
SWOONED
SWOONER
SWOOPED
SWOOPER
SWOOPIN
SWOOSIE
TROOPED
TROOPER
TROOPIN
TWOONIE
VROOMED
WHOOPED
WHOOPEE
WHOOPER
WHOOPIE
WHOOSIS

••O•O••

AMOROSO
AMOROUS
APODOUS
APOLOGY
AXOLOTL
BIOLOGY
BLOTOUT
BLOWOFF
BLOWOUT
BOOBOOS
BOOCOOS
BOOHOOS
BOOTOUT
CHOPOFF
COOKOFF
COOKOUT
COOLOUT
CROTONS
DOOWOPS
DROPOFF
DROPOUT
DUOPOLY
DUOTONE
ECOLOGY
ECONOMY
ENOLOGY
FEODORI
FLOWOUT
FROZONE
GEOCODE
GEOLOGY
GIOCOSO
GLOBOID
GLOBOSE
GLOBOUS
GNOMONS
GOODONE
GOOFOFF
GOOGOLS
GROWOLD
HOODOOS
HOOPOES
HOOTOWL
IFORONE
IGOROTS
IRONONS
IRONORE
IRONOUT
ISOGONS
ISONOMY
ISOPODS
ISOTONE
ISOTOPE
ISOTOPY
LAOCOON
LEONORA
LEONORE
LEOPOLD
LOOKOUT
MOOCOWS
MYOLOGY
NEOCONS
NEOLOGY
ODOROUS
OLOROSO
OROLOGY
OTOLOGY
OZONOUS
PHOTOGS
PHOTOID
PHOTONS
PHOTOOP
POOPOUT
PROBONO
PROBOWL
PROLOGS
PROLONG
PROMOED
PROMOTE
PRONOUN
PROPONE
PROPOSE
PROSODY
PROTONS
PROVOKE
PROVOST
RIOLOBO
RIOTOUS
ROOTOUT
SAOTOME
SHOOOFF
SHOTOUT
SHOWOFF
SHOWOUT
SNOCONE
STOLONS
STOPOFF
TOOKOFF
TOOKOUT
TOOLONG
TOOSOON
TROTOFF
TROTOUT
TWODOOR
TWOFOLD
TWOFOOT
TWOHOUR
TWOMORE
TWOROOM
TWOSOME
TWOTOED
TWOTONE
TWOTONS
UFOLOGY
UPOROUT
UROLOGY
USOTOUR
VIOLONE
VOODOOS
WHOSOUT
YOOHOOS
ZOOLOGY
ZOOMOUT

••O••O•

AFOULOF
AHOSTOF
ALOADOF
ALOHAOE
APOLLOS
ASOFNOW
AWOONOR
BLOSSOM
BLOUSON
BLOWPOP
BLOWSON
BOOBOOS
BOOCOOS
BOOHOOS
BOOMBOX
BOOTTOP
BRONCOS
BRONSON
CHOKEON
CHOMPON
COOKPOT
COOKTOP
COONDOG
CROPTOP
CROUTON
DOOUTOF
DRONEON
DROPBOX
DROPTOP
EMOTION
EROSION
FLOWNON
FRONTON
FROWNON
GGORDON
GIORGOS
GOODDOG
GOODFOR
GOODJOB
GOODJOE
GOODSON
GROTTOS
GROWNON
GROWSON
HOODOOS
HOOKSON
HOOPTOY
IFORGOT
IGOTYOU
IRONSON
KNOCKON
KNOSSOS
KNOWHOW
KNOWSOF
LAOCOON
LOOKFOR
LOOKSON
LOOKYOU
MOONBOW
MOONDOG
MOONGOD
OCONNOR
PHOTOOP
PLOSION
PLOWBOY
PLOWSON
POORBOX
POORBOY
PROCTOR
PROCYON
PRODSON
PROSHOP
PROUDOF
ROOFTOP
ROOTFOR
ROOTROT
SHOEBOX
SHOPFOR
SHOPKOS
SHORTOF
SHOTFOR
SHOWDOG
SHOWHOW
SLOPSON
SNOWDON
SNOWJOB
SPOKEOF
SPONSOR
STOMPON
STOODON
STOPFOR
THOMSON
THORSON
TOOKFOR
TOOLBOX
TOOSLOW
TOOSOON
TROLLOP
TWODOOR
TWOFOOT
TWOIRON
TWOROOM
TWOSHOT
TWOSPOT
USOSHOW
VOODOOS
WOODBOX
WOODLOT
WOODROW
WOODSON
WROTEON
YOOHOOS

••O•••O

ABOUTTO
AMOROSO
AVOCADO
BRONCHO
CHORIZO
CLOSETO
DEODATO
DOOMSTO
DROVETO
ESOBESO
FLOCKTO
FLOWNTO
GIOCOSO
GIORGIO
GROMYKO
GROUCHO
IHOPESO
ILOCANO
ISOLATO
LEONATO
LOOKSTO
OLOROSO
PHONENO
PROBONO
PRONETO
PROVISO
PROXIMO
RIOLOBO
SCORPIO
SPOKETO
STOODTO
SWORETO
UGOLINO
WHOSWHO
WROTETO

•••OO••

ALTOONA
BABOONS
BAZOOKA
BEFOOLS
BEHOOVE
CABOOSE
CAHOOTS
COCOONS
ENROOTS
GALOOTS
INDOORS
LAGOONS
LALOOSH
LLCOOLJ
MAROONS
METOOER
MRMOOSE
NOGOODS
OLEOOIL
PALOOKA
PAPOOSE
REBOOKS
REBOOTS
RECOOKS
RECOOLS
REHOOKS
RELOOKS
REROOFS
REROOTS
RETOOLS
SALOONS
SCHOOLS
SCROOGE
SHNOOKS
SHOOOFF
TABOOED
TVROOMS
TYCOONS
UNCOOPS
UNHOODS
UNHOOKS
UNLOOPS
UNLOOSE
UNMOODY
UNMOORS
UNROOFS
UNROOMY
UNROOTS
UNSOOTY
UNWOOED
UPROOTS
VAMOOSE
YOKOONO
ZEROOUT

•••O•O•

AEROSOL
AFROPOP
AKRONOH
ALCOHOL
ALCOPOP
APROPOS
ARIOSOS
ARROYOS
ATROPOS
AWOONOR
BAROLOS
BICOLOR
COMOROS
CREOSOL
DECOLOR
DESOTOS
DONOHOE
EIDOLON
EMBOSOM
ESPOSOS
EUROPOP
FEDOROV
GASOHOL
GIGOLOS
GOTOPOT
INCOLOR
KILOTON
KIMONOS
LENOVOS
MALODOR
MOLOTOV
MONOLOG
MONOPOD
MYKONOS
NABOKOV
OCTOPOD
ONTOPOF
PELOTON
POCONOS
REBOZOS
RECOLOR
REHONOR
ROBOCOP
ROCOCOS
SALOMON
SOLOMON
STOODON
THEODOR
THROWON
TOTOTOO
UNBOSOM
UPTONOW

•••O••O

ADDONTO
ALFONSO
ANTONIO
ARIOSTO
AUTOBIO
COLOMBO
DONOTGO
GETONTO
GOTONTO
IFYOUGO
LESOTHO
LIVORNO
LOGONTO
MOROCCO
PRIORTO
REDONDO
RIDOTTO
RISOTTO
RODOLFO
SECONDO
SIROCCO
STOODTO
TORONTO
TOTOTOO
WASONTO
YESORNO
YOKOONO

••••OO•

AHCHOOS
AIRCOOL
ALLGOOD
ANDSOON
ARTBOOK
BADMOOD
BALLOON
BAMBOOS
BARROOM
BASSOON
BEDROOM
BIGFOOT
BOOBOOS
BOOCOOS
BOOHOOS
BOYHOOD
BSCHOOL
BUFFOON
BURGOOS
BUTGOOD
CARDOOR
CARPOOL
CARTOON
CATDOOR
CATFOOD
CATFOOT
CHEROOT
CHINOOK
CUCKOOS
DAEWOOS
DAGWOOD
DASBOOT
DAYBOOK
DAYROOM
DIDGOOD
DOGBOOT
DOGDOOR
DOGFOOD
DOGWOOD
DRAGOON
DYEWOOD
ELMWOOD
EYEHOOK
FESTOON
FORGOOD
FORSOOK
FRYCOOK
GETGOOD
GODHOOD
GOTGOOD
GUMBOOT
GUMWOOD
GUNROOM
HADROOM
HALLOOS
HARPOON
HASROOM
HENCOOP
HEYLOOK
HEYWOOD
HIPBOOT
HIPROOF
HOODOOS
HOTFOOT
INAMOOD
INBLOOM
JIBBOOM
JOECOOL
KOWLOON
LADHOOD
LAMPOON
LAOCOON
LAWBOOK
LEAWOOD
LEGROOM
LETGOOF
LOGBOOK
MANHOOD
MIDNOON
MISTOOK
MONSOON
MUDROOM
MULDOON
NEWLOOK
NEWMOON
NONBOOK
NONFOOD
NONPOOR
NONWOOL
NORWOOD
NOTGOOD
NOWLOOK
NUNHOOD
NUTWOOD
OAKWOOD
OKSHOOT
OLDMOON
OLICOOK
ONATOOT
ONEFOOT
ONELOOK
ONEROOM
ONEWOOD
OUTCOOK
OUTDOOR
OUTFOOL
OUTFOOT
OUTLOOK
OUTROOT
OXBLOOD
PARTOOK
PATROON
PETDOOR
PHOTOOP
PLATOON
PLYWOOD
PONTOON
POTHOOK
PREBOOK
PREBOOM
PRECOOK
PRECOOL
PREDOOM
PRENOON
QSCHOOL
RACCOON
RANGOON
RAWFOOD
REBLOOM
RECROOM
REDBOOK
REDROOP
REDROOT
REDWOOD
REFLOOD
REGROOM
REPROOF
RESHOOT
RESPOOL
ROCKOON
RONWOOD
SASSOON
SAWWOOD
SCHNOOK
SEAFOOD
SIXFOOT
SKIBOOT
SKIDOOS
SKYHOOK
SLYLOOK
SUBCOOL
SUBROOT
SUNROOF
SUNROOM
TANDOOR
TAPROOM
TAPROOT
TATTOOS
TEAROOM
TENFOOT
THEFOOL
THEHOOD
THELOOK
THELOOP
THEMOON
THEPOOH
THEROOM
TINROOF
TOELOOP
TOMFOOL
TOOSOON
TOPBOOT
TOYBOOK
TOYHOOP
TWODOOR
TWOFOOT
TWOROOM
TYPHOON
UNFLOOR
UNSPOOL
UPSHOOT
UPSTOOD
VANPOOL
VOODOOS
WALLOON
WARROOM
WAYCOOL
WEBFOOT
WETLOOK
WINWOOD
YOOHOOS

••••O•O

AKEBONO
AMOROSO
BARTOLO
BLTTOGO
BOUSONO
CARDOZO
CONMOTO
CUIBONO
DELTORO
DIABOLO
DIAVOLO
FESTOSO
FLYSOLO
FOSCOLO
FOXBORO
FURIOSO
GIACOMO
GIOCOSO
HANSOLO
HERMOSO
IVANOVO
JOPPOLO
LIMPOPO
MAFIOSO
MINDORO
NICCOLO
NONGOGO
OLOROSO
ONETOGO
ORINOCO
PICCOLO
PIETOSO
PISCOPO
PROBONO
PULMONO
RIOLOBO
SAPPORO
SAYNOTO
THEBOBO
TIEPOLO
TREMOLO
TRIBORO
WAYTOGO
YOKOONO

•••••OO

BUGABOO
BUGALOO
CARABOO
CARIBOO
DOESTOO
ICKYPOO
IDIDTOO
ITISTOO
JACKSOO
JOHNWOO
MINIZOO
MRMAGOO
ONLYTOO
PEKEPOO
SAIDBOO
SAYSBOO
SHAMPOO
SKIDDOO
TOTOTOO

OP•••••

OPACITY
OPALINE
OPALISH
OPAQUES
OPENAIR
OPENBAR
OPENEND
OPENERS
OPENING
OPENNET
OPENOUT
OPENPIT
OPENSEA
OPENSUP
OPENTAP
OPENTOE
OPENTOP
OPERAND
OPERANT
OPERATE
OPEROSE
OPHELIA
OPIATES
OPINERS
OPINING
OPINION
OPOSSUM
OPPOSED
OPPOSER
OPPOSES
OPPRESS
OPPUGNS
OPQRSTU

OPTEDIN
OPTEDTO
OPTICAL
OPTICKS
OPTIMAL
OPTIMAS
OPTIMUM
OPTIONS
OPTSFOR
OPTSOUT
OPULENT
OPUNTIA
OPUSONE
OPUSTWO

O•P••••

OMPHALO
ONPAPER
ONPOINT
OPPOSED
OPPOSER
OPPOSES
OPPRESS
OPPUGNS
ORPHANS
ORPHANT
ORPHEAN
ORPHEUM
ORPHEUS
OSPREYS

O••P•••

OAKPARK
OFFPEAK
OILPALM
OILPANS
OLDPALS
OLDPROS
ONEPAGE
ONEPAIR
ONEPART
ONEPINT
OOMPAHS
OUTPACE
OUTPAID
OUTPASS
OUTPATH
OUTPAYS
OUTPEEP
OUTPICK
OUTPIPE
OUTPITY
OUTPLAN
OUTPLAY
OUTPLOD
OUTPLOT
OUTPOLL
OUTPOPS
OUTPORT
OUTPOST
OUTPOUR
OUTPRAY
OUTPULL
OUTPURL
OUTPUSH
OUTPUTS
OVIPARA

O•••P••

OCCIPUT
OCTOPOD
OCTOPUS
OCTUPLE
OCTUPLY
OEDIPAL
OEDIPUS
OILSPOT
OLYMPIA
OLYMPIC
OLYMPUS
ONEMPTY
ONESPOT
ONPAPER
ONTOPIC
ONTOPOF
OPENPIT
OSHAPED
OSSIPEE
OUTSPED
OUTSPIN
OUTSPIT
OVERPAR
OVERPAY
OVERPLY
OWNUPTO

O••••P•

OILCUPS
ONRAMPS
OUTKEPT
OUTLIPS
OUTPIPE
OUTPOPS
OUTRAPS
OUTWEPT

O•••••P

OFFERUP
OFFRAMP
OILLAMP
OLDCHAP
ONATRIP
ONECHIP
ONELUMP
ONESTEP
ONESTOP
OPENSUP
OPENTAP
OPENTOP
ORDERUP
OUTCROP
OUTDROP
OUTJUMP
OUTKEEP
OUTLEAP
OUTPEEP
OUTSKIP
OUTSTEP
OUTWEEP
OUTYELP
OVERLAP
OVERSUP
OVERTIP
OVERTOP
OWNEDUP

•OP••••

BOPPERS
BOPPING
COPCARS
COPIERS
COPILOT
COPIOUS
COPLAND
COPOUTS
COPPERS
COPPERY
COPPICE
COPPING
COPPOLA
COPSHOP
COPSOUT
COPTERS
COPULAE
COPULAR
COPULAS
COPYBOY
COPYCAT
COPYING
COPYIST
COPYMAN
COPYMEN
DOPEOUT
DOPIEST
DOPPLER
FOPPERY
FOPPISH
GOPHERS
HOPACAB
HOPEDSO
HOPEDTO
HOPEFOR
HOPEFUL
HOPENOT
HOPESSO
HOPESTO
HOPINTO
HOPKINS
HOPLITE
HOPOVER
HOPPERS
HOPPIER
HOPPING
HOPSING
HOPSOFF
HOPSOUT
HOPTOIT
JOPPOLO
KOPECKS
KOPIYKA
LOPPERS
LOPPIER
LOPPING
LOPSOFF
MOPHEAD
MOPIEST
MOPPERS
MOPPETS
MOPPING
MOPTOPS
NOPALES
NOPLACE
NOPQRST
POPCORN
POPDIVA
POPEAFB
POPEDOM
POPELEO
POPEYED
POPEYES
POPGUNS
POPLARS
POPLINS
POPOFFS
POPOUTS
POPOVER
POPPERS
POPPIES
POPPING
POPPINS
POPPLED
POPPLES
POPQUIZ
POPROCK
POPSOFF
POPSONG
POPSOUT
POPSTAR
POPTART
POPTOPS
POPTUNE
POPULAR
POPUPAD
POPWINE
ROPEDIN
ROPEDUP
ROPEOFF
ROPESIN
ROPESUP
ROPETOW
ROPIEST
SOPHIES
SOPHISM
SOPHIST
SOPPIER
SOPPING
SOPRANI
SOPRANO
SOPWITH
TOPAZES
TOPBIDS
TOPBOOT
TOPCOAT
TOPDOGS
TOPDOWN
TOPDRAW
TOPEKAN
TOPFIVE
TOPFORM
TOPGUNS
TOPHATS
TOPHOLE
TOPIARY
TOPICAL
TOPKAPI
TOPKICK
TOPKNOT
TOPLESS
TOPLINE
TOPMAST
TOPMOST
TOPNAME
TOPONYM
TOPPERS
TOPPING
TOPPLED
TOPPLES
TOPRANK
TOPRATE
TOPROWS
TOPSAIL
TOPSEED
TOPSIDE
TOPSOFF
TOPSOIL
TOPSOUT
TOPSPIN
TOPSPOT
TOPTENS
TOPTHIS
YOPLAIT

•O•P•••

BOOPSIE
BOPPERS
BOPPING
COAPTED
COEPTIS
COMPACT
COMPANY
COMPAQS
COMPARE
COMPART
COMPASS
COMPEER
COMPELS
COMPEND
COMPERE
COMPETE
COMPILE
COMPING
COMPLEX
COMPLIN
COMPORT
COMPOSE
COMPOST
COMPOTE
COMPTON
COMPUTE
COOPERS
COOPERY
COOPING
COOPSUP
COOPTED
COPPERS
COPPERY
COPPICE
COPPING
COPPOLA
CORPORA
CORPSES
COUPING
COUPLED
COUPLER
COUPLES
COUPLET
COUPONS
COWPEAS
COWPOKE
COWPONY
DOGPILE
DOLPHIN
DOPPLER
FOPPERY
FOPPISH
GODPAPA
GOMPERS
GOOPIER
GOSPELS
GOTPAST
HOOPERS
HOOPING
HOOPLAS
HOOPMAN
HOOPMEN
HOOPOES
HOOPTOY
HOPPERS
HOPPIER
HOPPING
HOSPICE
HOTPACK
HOTPINK
HOTPOTS
JOPPOLO
JOYPADS
LOOPERS
LOOPIER
LOOPING
LOPPERS
LOPPIER
LOPPING
LOWPAID
LOWPAIR
LOWPOST
MOPPERS
MOPPETS
MOPPING
MORPHED
MORPHIC
MORPHIN
NONPAID
NONPARS
NONPAST
NONPEAK
NONPLAY
NONPLUS
NONPOET
NONPOOR
NONPROS
OOMPAHS
POMPANO
POMPEIA
POMPEII
POMPOMS
POMPONS
POMPOUS
POOPING
POOPOUT
POOPSIE
POPPERS
POPPIES
POPPING
POPPINS
POPPLED
POPPLES
POTPIES
ROMPERS
ROMPING
ROMPISH
SOAPBOX
SOAPERS
SOAPIER
SOAPILY
SOAPING
SOAPNET
SOAPPAD
SOAPSUP
SOPPIER
SOPPING
SOSPADS
SOUPCAN
SOUPCON
SOUPERS
SOUPIER
SOUPMIX
SOUPSON
SOUPSUP
TOEPICK
TOPPERS
TOPPING
TOPPLED
TOPPLES
TORPEDO
TOSPARE
TOUPEES
TOWPATH
TOYPAIL
VOLPONE

•O••P••

COALPIT
COCKPIT
COOKPOT
COOLPIX
DOGAPES
DOWNPAT
FOOTPAD
FOREPAW
FOURPIN
GOESPRO
GOKAPUT
GOLFPRO
GONEPRO
GOODPAY
GOTOPOT
GOTUPON
GOTUPTO
HOTSPOT
HOTSPUR
JODHPUR
JOSEPHA
JOSEPHI
LOAFPAN
LOOMPAS
LOSTPET
MONOPOD
MOONPIE
MOREPAY
MOSHPIT
NONEPIC
NONUPLE
NOTEPAD
NOTOPEN
NOTUPTO
POLYPED
POLYPOD
POPUPAD
PORKPIE
SOAPPAD
SODAPOP
TOPSPIN
TOPSPOT
TOSSPOT
VONOPEL

•O•••P•

BOBHOPE
BOXTOPS
COINOPS
COLLOPS
CONCEPT
CORRUPT
DOGNAPS
DOLLOPS
DOOWOPS
FOLDUPS
FORCEPS
FOULUPS
GODPAPA
GOESAPE
GONEAPE
GOOFUPS
GOSSIPS
GOSSIPY
HOLDUPS
HOOKUPS
HOTCAPS
HOTCUPS
HOTLIPS
HOTTIPS
JOBHOPS
LOCKUPS
LOOKUPS
LOWTOPS
MOCKUPS
MOPTOPS
POPTOPS
POSTOPS
ROLLUPS
TOECAPS
TOETAPS
TOPKAPI
TOSSUPS
TOWROPE
TOYTOPS
WORKUPS

•O••••P

BOARDUP
BOILSUP
BOLTSUP
BONEDUP
BONESUP
BOOSTUP
BOOTSUP
BOOTTOP
BORNEUP
BOTCHUP
BOUNDUP
BOXEDUP
BOXESUP
BOXSTEP
COILSUP
COLDCUP
COMESUP
COOKSUP
COOKTOP
COOPSUP
COPSHOP
CORKSUP
COUGHUP
COUNTUP
COVERUP
COWSLIP
DOINGUP
DOLLSUP
DOUBLEP
FOGLAMP
FOLDSUP
FOOTSUP
FORCEUP
FORETOP
FORKSUP
FOULSUP
FOULTIP
GOINGUP
GOLDTIP
GOOFSUP
GOTATIP
GOTHELP
HOISTUP
HOLDSUP
HOLEDUP
HOLESUP
HOOKSUP
HOTSOUP
JOBSHOP
JOECAMP
JOINSUP
LOADSUP
LOCKSUP
LOOKSUP
LOTHROP
LOUSEUP
LOVETAP
MOCKSUP
MOUNTUP
MOVEDUP
MOVESUP
NONCROP
NONDEEP
NONDRIP
NONSLIP
NONSTOP
NOSEDUP
NOSESUP
NOTRUMP
POINTUP
POWERUP
ROADMAP
ROBOCOP
ROLLMOP
ROLLSUP
ROLLTOP
ROOFTOP
ROOTCAP
ROOTSUP
ROPEDUP
ROPESUP
ROSEHIP
ROUGHUP
ROUNDUP
SOAKSUP
SOAPSUP
SOCKHOP
SODAPOP
SOFTTOP
SONSHIP
SOUPSUP
TOELOOP
TONEDUP
TONESUP
TOOLSUP
TOTALUP
TOTESUP
TOUCHUP
TOYHOOP
TOYSHOP
WOKENUP
WORKSUP
WORSHIP
WOUNDUP

••OP•••

ADOPTED
ADOPTEE
ADOPTER
BIOPICS
BOOPSIE
CHOPINE
CHOPOFF
CHOPPED
CHOPPER
CHOPSUP
CLOPPED
COOPERS
COOPERY
COOPING
COOPSUP
COOPTED
CROPPED
CROPPER
CROPSUP
CROPTOP
DIOPTER
DROPBOX
DROPCAP
DROPINS
DROPLET
DROPNET
DROPOFF
DROPOUT
DROPPED
DROPPER
DROPSBY
DROPSIN
DROPSIT
DROPTOP
DUOPOLY
ELOPERS
ELOPING
EPOPEES
FLOPPED
FLOPPER
GOOPIER
GROPERS
GROPING
GROPIUS
HOOPERS
HOOPING
HOOPLAS
HOOPMAN
HOOPMEN
HOOPOES
HOOPTOY
IHOPESO
ISOPODS
LEOPARD
LEOPOLD
LOOPERS
LOOPIER
LOOPING
MNOPQRS
MYOPIAS
PEOPLED
PEOPLES
PLOPPED
POOPING
POOPOUT
POOPSIE
PROPANE
PROPELS
PROPHET
PROPJET
PROPMAN
PROPMEN
PROPONE
PROPOSE
PROPPED
PROPSUP
REOPENS
SCOPING
SHOPFOR
SHOPFUL
SHOPKOS
SHOPNBC
SHOPPED
SHOPPER
SHOPPES
SHOPSAT
SLOPERS
SLOPING
SLOPPED
SLOPSON
STOPFOR
STOPGAP
STOPOFF
STOPPED
STOPPER
STOPPLE
STOPSAT
STOPSBY
STOPSIN
STOPSIT
STOPSUP
TROPICS
TROPISM
TWOPAIR
TWOPART
UNOPTED
USOPENS
UTOPIAN
UTOPIAS
UTOPISM
UTOPIST
WHOPPED
WHOPPER

••O•P••

ACOUPLE
ADOLPHE
BLOOPED
BLOOPER
BLOWPOP
CHOMPED
CHOMPON
CHOPPED
CHOPPER
CLOMPED
CLOPPED
COOKPOT
COOLPIX
CROPPED
CROPPER
DROOPED
DROPPED
DROPPER
FLOPPED
FLOPPER
FOOTPAD
GOODPAY
GROUPED
GROUPER
GROUPIE
LOOMPAS
MOONPIE
PLOPPED
PROMPTS
PROPPED
PROSPER
SCOOPED
SCOOPER
SCORPIO
SCOUPES
SHOEPAC
SHOPPED
SHOPPER
SHOPPES
SHOTPAR
SHOTPUT
SLOPPED
SNOOPED
SNOOPER
SNOWPEA
STOMPED
STOMPIN
STOMPON
STOOPED
STOOPER
STOPPED
STOPPER
STOPPLE
SWOOPED
SWOOPER
SWOOPIN
TROMPED
TROMPIN
TROOPED
TROOPER
TROOPIN
TROUPED
TROUPER
TROUPES
TWOSPOT
WHOMPED
WHOOPED
WHOOPEE
WHOOPER
WHOOPIE
WHOPPED
WHOPPER

••O••P•

BIOTYPE
BLOWUPS
DOOWOPS
ECOTYPE
GOOFUPS
HOOKUPS
ISOTOPE
ISOTOPY
LOOKUPS
SLOWUPS
SNOCAPS

••O•••P

BIOCHIP
BLOCKUP
BLOTSUP
BLOWNUP
BLOWPOP
BLOWSUP
BOOSTUP
BOOTSUP
BOOTTOP
BROKEUP
BUOYSUP
CHOKEUP
CHOPSUP
CHOSEUP
CLOGSUP
CLOSEUP
CLOTSUP
CLOUDUP
COOKSUP
COOKTOP
COOPSUP
CROPSUP
CROPTOP
CROSSUP
DROPCAP
DROPTOP
DROVEUP
EGOTRIP
EXOCARP
FLOATUP
FLOWNUP
FOOTSUP
FROTHUP
FROZEUP
GOOFSUP
GROWNUP
GROWSUP
HOOKSUP
KNOTSUP
LOOKSUP
PHONYUP
PHOTOOP
PLOWSUP
PROPSUP
PROSHOP
ROOFTOP
ROOTCAP
ROOTSUP

SCOUTUP
SHOOKUP
SHOOTUP
SHOREUP
SHOWNUP
SHOWSUP
SLOWSUP
SMOKEUP
SNOWCAP
SPOKEUP
STOCKUP
STOKEUP
STOODUP
STOPGAP
STOPSUP
STOREUP
TOOLSUP
TROLLOP
TROTSUP
TWODEEP
TWOSTEP
WROTEUP

•••OP••
AFROPOP
ALCOPOP
ALLOPEZ
APROPOS
ATROPHY
ATROPOS
AUTOPEN
AUTOPIA
AUTOPSY
BLOOPED
BLOOPER
CANOPUS
CUTOPEN
DROOPED
EUROPOP
FLYOPEN
GALOPED
GOTOPOT
ITSOPEN
LAYOPEN
LMNOPQR
MEMOPAD
MONOPOD
NOTOPEN
OCTOPOD
OCTOPUS
ONTOPIC
ONTOPOF
PANOPLY
PREOPEN
PRYOPEN
RIPOPEN
SCOOPED
SCOOPER
SNOOPED
SNOOPER
STOOPED
STOOPER
STROPHE
SWOOPED
SWOOPER
SWOOPIN
TROOPED
TROOPER
TROOPIN
UNHOPED
UNROPED
UNROPES
UPTOPAR
VONOPEL
WHOOPED
WHOOPEE
WHOOPER
WHOOPIE
ZATOPEK

•••O•P•
RECOUPS
RESOAPS
RUDOLPH
UNCOOPS
UNLOOPS

•••O••P
AFROPOP
ALCOPOP
EUROPOP
IMHOTEP
ROBOCOP
SHOOKUP
SHOOTUP
STOODUP
THROWUP

••••OP•
AIRPOPS
ANYHOPE
BARHOPS
BIGTOPS
BISHOPS
BOBHOPE
BOXTOPS
CARHOPS
CARTOPS
COINOPS
COLLOPS
CYCLOPS
DAYHOPS
DOLLOPS
DOOWOPS
DRYMOPS
DUNLOPS
ENTROPY
GALLOPS
GUYROPE
HYSSOPS
ICEPOPS
ISOTOPE
ISOTOPY
JOBHOPS
KLMNOPQ
LAPTOPS
LEGROPE
LIMPOPO
LOWTOPS
MANROPE
MISCOPY
MOPTOPS
NEWHOPE
OUTPOPS
PEGTOPS
PISCOPO
POPTOPS
POSTOPS
RAGMOPS
RAGTOPS
READOPT
REDTOPS
SYNCOPE
THEHOPE
THEPOPE
THEROPE
TIEROPE
TIPTOPS
TOWROPE
TOYTOPS
UNCOOPS
UNLOOPS
UNSTOPS
UPPROPS
UPSLOPE
WALLOPS
WETMOPS
ZIPTOPS

••••O•P
BARSOAP
HENCOOP
HOTSOUP
INGROUP
LYESOAP
PEASOUP
PHOTOOP
PRECOUP
REDROOP
REGROUP
SALMONP
THELOOP
TOELOOP
TOYHOOP

•••••OP
AFROPOP
AGALLOP
AIRDROP
ALCOPOP
ARTSHOP
BABYBOP
BEATCOP
BELLHOP
BLOWPOP
BOOTTOP
BRITPOP
BUSSTOP
COOKTOP
COPSHOP
CROPTOP
DAMPMOP
DESKTOP
DEVELOP
DEWDROP
DROPTOP
DUSTMOP
EARDROP
EGGDROP
ENVELOP
ESCALOP
EUROPOP
EYEDROP
FLATTOP
FLIPTOP
FORETOP
GUMDROP
HARDTOP
HENCOOP
HIGHTOP
HILLTOP
IGGYPOP
JKLMNOP
JOBSHOP
KERFLOP
KERPLOP
LETDROP
LIEATOP
LOTHROP
MAINTOP
MILKSOP
NONCROP
NONSTOP
ONESTOP
OPENTOP
OUTCROP
OUTDROP
OVERTOP
PALMTOP
PETSHOP
PHOTOOP
PINETOP
PITSTOP
PROSHOP
RAGSHOP
REDROOP
RIPSTOP
ROBOCOP
ROLLMOP
ROLLTOP
ROOFTOP
RUMSHOP
SATATOP
SCALLOP
SITATOP
SKISHOP
SOCKHOP
SODAPOP
SOFTTOP
TANKTOP
TEASHOP
THEFLOP
THELOOP
TILTTOP
TIMECOP
TOELOOP
TOYHOOP
TOYSHOP
TREETOP
TROLLOP
TUBETOP

O•Q••••
OPQRSTU

O••Q•••
OPAQUES

O•••Q••
OBLIQUE
OBLOQUY

O••••Q•
ONTHEQT

•OQ••••
COQUINA
LOQUATS

•O•Q•••
BOUQUET
COEQUAL
CONQUER
JOAQUIN
JONQUIL
MOSQUES
NOPQRST
POPQUIZ
RORQUAL
TORQUED
TORQUES

•O••Q••
COMIQUE

•O•••Q•
COMPAQS
POSSLQS

•O••••Q
DOUBLEQ

••OQ•••
CROQUET
CROQUIS
EPOQUES

••O•Q••
MNOPQRS

•••OQ••
BAROQUE
OBLOQUY

•••O•Q•
LMNOPQR

••••O•Q
KLMNOPQ

OR•••••
ORACIES
ORACLES
ORALIST
ORANGES
ORANGEY
ORANTES
ORARION
ORARIUM
ORATING
ORATION
ORATORS
ORATORY
ORATRIX
ORBISON
ORBITAL
ORBITED
ORBITER
ORBLESS
ORBLIKE
ORCHARD
ORCHIDS
ORDAINS
ORDEALS
ORDERED
ORDERER
ORDERIN
ORDERLY
ORDERUP
ORDINAL
ORDINES
ORDONEZ
OREBODY
ORECTIC
OREGANO
OREILLY
ORELESS
ORESTES
ORGANDY
ORGANIC
ORGANZA
ORGEATS
ORGIAST
ORIENTE
ORIENTS
ORIFICE
ORIGAMI
ORIGINE
ORIGINS
ORINOCO
ORIOLES
ORISONS
ORKNEYS
ORLANDO
ORLEANS
ORMANDY
ORMOLUS
ORNETTE
ORNITHO
OROGENY
OROLOGY
OROTUND
OROURKE
ORPHANS
ORPHANT
ORPHEAN
ORPHEUM
ORPHEUS
ORRISES
ORTEGAL
ORTOLAN
ORVIETO
ORVILLE

O•R••••
OARLESS
OARLIKE
OARLOCK
OARSMAN
OARSMEN
OERSTED
OGREISH
ONRAMPS
ORRISES
OTRANTO
OURGANG
OURSELF
OURSONG
OURTOWN

O••R•••
OBERLIN
OBTRUDE
OCARINA
OCHROID
OCHROUS
OCTROIS
ODORANT
ODORFUL
ODORIZE
ODOROUS
OFFRAMP
OFFROAD
OILRICH
OILRIGS
OILRING
OILRUBS
OLDROSE
OLOROSO
ONAROLL
ONBREAK
ONEREEL
ONEROOM
ONEROUS
ONORATI
ONORDER
ONTRACK
ONTRIAL
OPERAND
OPERANT
OPERATE
OPEROSE
OPPRESS
OPQRSTU
ORARION
ORARIUM
OSIRIAN
OSPREYS
OSTRAVA
OSTRICH
OTARIES
OUTRACE
OUTRAGE
OUTRAIL
OUTRANG
OUTRANK
OUTRANT
OUTRAPS
OUTRATE
OUTRAVE
OUTREAD
OUTRIBS
OUTRIDE
OUTRIGS
OUTRING
OUTROAR
OUTROCK
OUTRODE
OUTROLL
OUTROOT
OUTROVE
OUTROWS
OUTRUNS
OUTRUSH
OVARIES
OVERACT
OVERAGE
OVERALL
OVERARM
OVERATE
OVERAWE
OVERBED
OVERBET
OVERBID
OVERBIG
OVERBUY
OVERCOY
OVERCUT
OVERDID
OVERDOG
OVERDRY
OVERDUB
OVERDUE
OVERDYE
OVEREAT
OVERFAR
OVERFAT
OVERFED
OVERFEE
OVERFEW
OVERFIT
OVERFIX
OVERFLY
OVERHOT
OVERICE
OVERJOY
OVERLAP
OVERLAX
OVERLAY
OVERLET
OVERLIE
OVERLIT
OVERMAN
OVERMIX
OVERNEW
OVERPAR
OVERPAY
OVERPLY
OVERRAN
OVERRUN
OVERSAD
OVERSAW
OVERSEA
OVERSEE
OVERSET
OVERSEW
OVERSUP
OVERTAX
OVERTIP
OVERTLY
OVERTOP
OVERUSE
OVERWET

O•••R••
OAKTREE
OATBRAN
OBSERVE
OBVERSE
OBVERTS
OCCURTO
OEUVRES
OFFERED
OFFEREE
OFFERER
OFFEROR
OFFERUP
OFSORTS
OHCAROL
OILDRUM
OLDPROS
OMICRON
ONATRIP
ONEARTH
ONEGRAM
ONEIRIC
ONEIRON
ONFIRST
ONSERVE
ONTARIO
ONTHREE
ONWARDS
ORATRIX
ORDERED
ORDERER
ORDERIN
ORDERLY
ORDERUP
OROURKE
OSBORNE
OSETRAS
OSIERED
OUTBRAG
OUTBRAY
OUTBRED
OUTCROP
OUTCROW
OUTDRAG
OUTDRAW
OUTDREW
OUTDROP
OUTGREW
OUTGRIN
OUTGROW
OUTPRAY
OUTTRAY
OUTTROT
OVERRAN
OVERRUN
OXCARTS
OXFORDS

O••••R•
OAKFERN
OAKPARK
OBEYERS
OBSCURA
OBSCURE
OCTOBRE
OCTUBRE
OCULARS
ODDSARE
OFASORT
OHIOART
OILBIRD
OINKERS
OLDCARS
OLDGIRL
OLESTRA
ONADARE
ONAGERS
ONAJURY
ONALARK
ONALERT
ONBOARD
ONEACRE
ONELIRA
ONEMORE
ONEPART
ONETERM
ONEYARD
ONGUARD
ONSHORE
OPENERS
OPINERS
ORATORS
ORATORY
ORCHARD
OSSETRA
OSSUARY
OSTIARY
OSTLERS
OSTMARK
OUSTERS
OUTBARK
OUTBURN
OUTCURE
OUTDARE
OUTEARN
OUTFIRE
OUTHERE
OUTHIRE
OUTHURL
OUTPORT
OUTPURL
OUTSERT
OUTTIRE
OUTTORE
OUTTORN
OUTTURN
OUTWARD
OUTWARS
OUTWORD
OUTWORE
OUTWORK
OUTWORN
OVERARM
OVERDRY
OVIFORM
OVIPARA
OXHEART
OXYMORA
OYSTERS

O•••••R
OBLIGER
OBLIGOR
OBTUSER
OCELLAR
OCONNOR
OCTOBER
OFFERER
OFFEROR
OFFHOUR
OFFICER
OFFYEAR
OFTENER
OKTOBER
OLDSTER
OLIVIER
OMITTER
ONATEAR
ONEHOUR
ONEOVER
ONEPAIR
ONESTAR
ONEYEAR
ONORDER
ONPAPER
ONSAGER
ONWATER
OPENAIR
OPENBAR
OPPOSER
OPTSFOR
ORBITER
ORDERER
OSCULAR
OUTDOER
OUTDOOR
OUTHEAR
OUTLIER
OUTPOUR
OUTROAR
OUTSOAR
OUTTEAR
OUTWEAR
OVERFAR
OVERPAR

•OR••••
BORATES
BORDERS
BORDONI
BOREDOM
BOREOUT
BORGIAS
BORGLUM
BORIDES
BORINGS
BORKING
BORLAUG
BORNEAN
BORNEUP
BORODIN
BOROMIR
BORONIC
BOROUGH
BORROWS
BORSCHT
BORSTAL
BORZAGE
BORZOIS
CORACLE
CORAZON
CORBELS
CORBETT
CORDAGE
CORDATE
CORDELL
CORDERO
CORDERS
CORDIAL
CORDIAS
CORDING
CORDITE
CORDOBA
CORDONS
CORELLI
CORETTA
CORFAMS
CORINNE
CORINTH
CORKAGE
CORKERS
CORKIER
CORKING
CORKOAK
CORKSUP
CORMACK
CORNBIN
CORNCOB
CORNDOG
CORNEAL
CORNEAS
CORNELL
CORNERS
CORNETS
CORNFED
CORNICE
CORNIER
CORNILY
CORNING
CORNISH
CORNOIL
CORNROW
CORNUTE
COROLLA
CORONAE
CORONAL
CORONAS
CORONER
CORONET
CORPORA
CORPSES
CORRADE
CORRALS
CORRECT
CORRIDA
CORRODE
CORRUPT
CORSAGE
CORSAIR
CORSETS
CORSICA
CORTEGE
CORTICO
CORTINA
CORVAIR
CORVEES
CORVIDS
CORVIÑA
CORVINE
CORYELL
CORYZAS
CORZINE
DORFMAN
DORIGHT
DORITOS
DORKIER
DORMANT
DORMERS
DORMICE
DOROTHY
DORSALS
DORSETT
DORSEYS
FORABIT
FORADAY
FORAGED
FORAGER
FORAGES
FORASEC
FORAYED
FORBADE
FORBEAR
FORBIDS
FORBORE
FORBUSH
FORCEIN
FORCEON
FORCEPS
FORCERS
FORCEUP
FORCING
FORDGTS
FORDHAM
FORDING
FORDLTD
FORDOES
FORDONE
FOREACH
FOREARM
FOREBAY
FOREIGN
FORELEG
FOREMAN
FOREMEN
FORENZA
FOREPAW
FORERAN
FORERUN
FORESAW
FORESEE
FORESTS
FORETOP
FOREVER
FORFEIT
FORFEND
FORFREE
FORGAVE
FORGERS
FORGERY
FORGETS
FORGING
FORGIVE
FORGOER
FORGOES
FORGONE
FORGOOD
FORHIRE
FORINTS
FORKERS
FORKFUL
FORKIER
FORKING
FORKOUT
FORKSUP
FORLANI
FORLIFE
FORLORN
FORLOVE
FORMALS
FORMATS

FORMERS
FORMFUL
FORMICA
FORMING
FORMOSA
FORMULA
FORONCE
FORREAL
FORRENT
FORREST
FORSAKE
FORSALE
FORSHOW
FORSIZE
FORSOOK
FORSTER
FORSURE
FORSYTE
FORSYTH
FORTDIX
FORTIES
FORTIFY
FORTIUS
FORTLEE
FORTORD
FORTRAN
FORTUNA
FORTUNE
FORTYAD
FORTYBC
FORWARD
FORWENT
GORDIAN
GORDITA
GORDIUS
GORETEX
GORGERS
GORGING
GORGONS
GORIEST
GORILLA
GORMING
GOROUND
GORSIER
GORTNER
HORATIO
HORDING
HORIZON
HORMONE
HORNETS
HORNIER
HORNING
HORNISH
HORNIST
HORNSBY
HORNSIN
HORNUNG
HORRIFY
HORRORS
HORSIER
HORSILY
HORSING
HORSLEY
HORVITZ
JORDANA
KORANIC
KORDELL
KOREANS

KORUNAS
LORANGE
LORDING
LORDJIM
LORDSIT
LORELAI
LORELEI
LORENTZ
LORENZO
LORETTA
LORGNON
LORIENT
LORISES
LORRIES
LORUSES
MORAINE
MORALES
MORALLY
MORANIS
MORANTE
MORAVIA
MORCERF
MORDANT
MORDENT
MORDRED
MOREENS
MORELLA
MORELLO
MORELOS
MOREPAY
MORESBY
MORETTI
MORGANA
MORGANS
MORGUES
MORISOT
MORLOCK
MORMONS
MORNING
MOROCCO
MORONIC
MORPHED
MORPHIC
MORPHIN
MORROWS
MORSELS
MORTALS
MORTARS
MORTICE
MORTIFY
MORTISE
MORTONS
NORBERT
NORDICA
NORDICS
NORDOFF
NORDOWE
NORELCO
NORFOLK
NORIEGA
NORITES
NORMALS
NORMAND
NORMANS
NORRISH
NORTHER
NORTHOF
NORTONS

NORWALK
NORWICH
NORWOOD
PORCHES
PORCINE
PORGIES
PORIVER
PORKERS
PORKIER
PORKING
PORKISH
PORKPIE
PORSCHE
PORSENA
PORTAGE
PORTALS
PORTEND
PORTENT
PORTERS
PORTHOS
PORTICO
PORTING
PORTION
PORTMAN
PORTNOY
PORTRAY
RORAIMA
RORQUAL
SORBATE
SORBETS
SORCERY
SORDINI
SORDINO
SORENTO
SORGHUM
SORIANO
SORORAL
SORRELL
SORRELS
SORRIER
SORRILY
SORROWS
SORTERS
SORTIED
SORTIES
SORTING
SORTOUT
SORVINO
TORCHED
TORCHER
TORCHES
TOREOFF
TOREOUT
TOREROS
TORINOS
TORMENT
TORNADO
TORNOFF
TORNOUT
TOROIDS
TORONTO
TORPEDO
TORQUED
TORQUES
TORREFY
TORRENT
TORSION
TORTLAW

TORTOLA
TORTONI
TORTUGA
TORTURE
TORVALD
TORVILL
TORYISH
TORYISM
VORLAGE
VORSTER
WORDAGE
WORDIER
WORDILY
WORDING
WORDONE
WOREOFF
WOREOUT
WORKBOX
WORKDAY
WORKERS
WORKFOR
WORKING
WORKMAN
WORKMEN
WORKOFF
WORKOUT
WORKSAT
WORKSHY
WORKSIN
WORKSON
WORKSUP
WORKUPS
WORLDLY
WORMERS
WORMIER
WORMING
WORMISH
WORNOFF
WORNOUT
WORRELL
WORRIED
WORRIER
WORRIES
WORSENS
WORSHIP
WORSLEY
WORSTED
WORTHIT
YORKERS
YORKIES
YORKIST
YORKTON

•O•R•••

BOARDED
BOARDER
BOARDUP
BOARISH
BOERWAR
BOHRIUM
BOORISH
BOORMAN
BORROWS
BOTREES
BOURBON
BOURGET
BOURSES
COARSEN

COARSER
COBRAND
COERCED
COERCER
COERCES
COMRADE
CONRACK
CONRIED
CORRADE
CORRALS
CORRECT
CORRIDA
CORRODE
CORRUPT
COURAGE
COURANT
COURBET
COURIER
COURSED
COURSER
COURSES
COURTED
COURTLY
COURTTV
COWRIES
COWRITE
COWROTE
DOGRACE
DOGREAT
DOGROSE
DOGRUNS
DONRUSS
DOORDIE
DOORMAN
DOORMAT
DOORMEN
DOORWAY
DOTRICE
DOUREST
DOWRIES
DOWRONG
FORREAL
FORRENT
FORREST
FOURAAA
FOURDAY
FOUREEE
FOURIER
FOURMAN
FOURPIN
FOURTHS
FOURWAY
GOBROKE
GOCRAZY
GOIRISH
GOTREAL
GOURAMI
GOURDES
GOURMET
GOWRONG
HOARDED
HOARDER
HOARIER
HOARILY
HOARSEN
HOARSER
HOORAHS
HOORAYS

HORRIFY
HORRORS
HOTRODS
HOTROLL
JODRELL
JOEROTH
JOURDAN
JOURNAL
JOURNEE
JOURNEY
JOURNOS
JOYRIDE
LOGROLL
LORRIES
LOURDES
LOUREED
LOURING
LOWRENT
LOWRISE
LOWRISK
LOWROAD
MOBRULE
MONROES
MOORAGE
MOORHEN
MOORIER
MOORING
MOORISH
MORROWS
MOTRINS
MOURNED
MOURNER
NORRISH
NOTRADE
NOTRARE
NOTREAL
NOTRUMP
NOURISH
PODRIDA
POORBOX
POORBOY
POOREST
POORISH
POORLAW
POORMAN
POORMEN
POORTAX
POPROCK
POURERS
POURING
POUROUT
POURSIN
ROARERS
ROARING
ROARSAT
ROBROYS
RODRIGO
SOARERS
SOAREWE
SOARING
SOIREES
SOPRANI
SOPRANO
SORRELL
SORRELS
SORRIER
SORRILY
SORROWS

SOURALE
SOURCED
SOURCES
SOUREST
SOURING
SOURISH
SOURSON
TOORDER
TOPRANK
TOPRATE
TOPROWS
TORREFY
TORRENT
TOURBUS
TOURERS
TOURING
TOURISM
TOURIST
TOURNEY
TOWROPE
WORRELL
WORRIED
WORRIER
WORRIES
YOURANG
YOUREIT
YOUREON

•O••R••

BODEREK
BODYRUB
BOGARDE
BOGARTS
BOIARDO
BOLEROS
BONARIO
BOUTROS
BOWERED
COCHRAN
CODERED
COHERED
COHERER
COHERES
COHORTS
COJUROR
COLORED
COLORER
COLORTV
COMORAN
COMOROS
COMTREX
CONBRIO
CONFREY
CONTRAS
CONTROL
CONURES
CORNROW
COTERIE
COVERED
COVERER
COVERME
COVERTS
COVERUP
COWARDS
COWERAT
COWERED
DOGTROT
DOHERTY

DOLORES
DOTARDS
DOVERDE
DOWERED
FOGERTY
FOOTRUB
FORERAN
FORERUN
FORFREE
FORTRAN
FOUDRES
FOXTROT
GOCARTS
GODFREY
GOFIRST
GOFORIT
GOFORTH
GOGIRLS
GOKARTS
GONERIL
GOTFREE
GOVERNS
HOFBRAU
HOGARTH
HOMBRES
HOMERED
HOMERIC
HOMERUN
HONORED
HONOREE
HONORER
HOVERED
HOVERER
HOWARDK
HOWARDS
HOWARDU
JOFFREY
JOGBRAS
JOGTROT
JOMARCH
JONERIK
LOCARNO
LONDRES
LONGRUN
LOTHROP
LOUVRED
LOUVRES
LOVERLY
LOWBRED
LOWBROW
LOWERED
MOCHRIE
MODERNE
MODERNS
MOLERAT
MONARCH
MONGREL
MORDRED
MOTORED
MOWBRAY
NOCARBS
NOMBRES
NOMERCY
NOMERGE
NONARAB
NONARTS
NONCROP
NONDRIP

NONDRUG
NONIRON
NONORAL
NONPROS
NOPQRST
NOSIREE
NOSTRIL
NOSTRUM
NOTTRUE
NOTURNS
NOVARRO
NOWORSE
POIVRES
POLARAS
POLARIS
PORTRAY
POUDRES
POVERTY
POWERED
POWERUP
ROBARDS
ROBERTA
ROBERTE
ROBERTF
ROBERTH
ROBERTI
ROBERTO
ROBERTS
ROGERED
ROOFRAT
ROOTROT
ROSARIO
ROSERED
ROSTRAL
ROSTRUM
SOBERED
SOBERER
SOBERLY
SOFARAS
SOLARAS
SOLARIA
SONORAN
SORORAL
SOSORRY
TOHORSE
TONEROW
TOPDRAW
TOREROS
TOUAREG
TOWARDS
TOWERED
TOYSRUS
VOUVRAY
WOLFRAM
WOODROW
YOGURTS

•O•••R•

BOATERS
BOBBERS
BODYART
BOILERS
BOKHARA
BOLTERS
BOMBARD
BOMBERS
BONAIRE
BONDERS

BONEDRY
BONFIRE
BONKERS
BONNARD
BOOBIRD
BOOKERS
BOOKERT
BOOMERS
BOOTERS
BOOTERY
BOOZERS
BOPPERS
BORDERS
BOTHERS
BOWLERS
BOWOARS
BOWYERS
BOXCARS
COALERS
COATERS
COAXERS
COCKERS
CODGERS
COFFERS
COGBURN
COHEIRS
COILERS
COINERS
COLBERT
COLLARD
COLLARS
COLOURS
COMBERS
COMFORT
COMPARE
COMPART
COMPERE
COMPORT
CONAGRA
CONAKRY
CONCERN
CONCERT
CONCORD
CONCURS
CONDORS
CONFERS
CONFIRM
CONFORM
CONGERS
CONJURE
CONJURY
CONKERS
CONNERY
CONNORS
CONSORT
CONTORT
CONVERT
COOKERS
COOKERY
COOLERS
COOPERS
COOPERY
COOTERS
COPCARS
COPIERS
COPPERS
COPPERY
COPTERS

CORDERO
CORDERS
CORKERS
CORNERS
CORPORA
COSHERS
COSTARD
COSTARS
COTTERS
COUGARS
COUNTRY
COUTERS
COUTURE
COWBIRD
COWGIRL
COWHERD
DOCKERS
DOCTORS
DODDERS
DODDERY
DODGERS
DOEUVRE
DOFFERS
DOGBERT
DOGCART
DOGEARS
DOIDARE
DOLLARS
DOLOURS
DONTCRY
DOOVERS
DOOZERS
DORMERS
DOTTERS
DOUSERS
DOWNERS
DOWSERS
FOAMERS
FODDERS
FOGGERS
FOGHORN
FOKKERS
FOLDERS
FOLGERS
FOLKART
FOOLERS
FOOLERY
FOOTERS
FOPPERY
FORBORE
FORCERS
FOREARM
FORGERS
FORGERY
FORHIRE
FORKERS
FORLORN
FORMERS
FORSURE
FORTORD
FORWARD
FOSTERS
FOULARD
FOUNDRY
FOWLERS
FOXBORO
FOXFIRE
GODDARD

GOESPRO
GOITERS
GOLDARN
GOLFERS
GOLFPRO
GOMPERS
GONEPRO
GONGORA
GOOBERS
GOODERS
GOODTRY
GOPHERS
GORGERS
GOSFORD
GOTHURT
GOTSORE
GOTWARM
GOTWORD
GOUGERS
HOAXERS
HOCKERS
HOFSTRA
HOGGERY
HOHNERS
HOLBERG
HOLDERS
HOLLERS
HOLYARK
HOMBURG
HONIARA
HONKERS
HONOURS
HOOFERS
HOOPERS
HOOTERS
HOOVERS
HOPPERS
HORRORS
HOSIERS
HOSIERY
HOTCARS
HOTWARS
HOTWIRE
HOWLERS
JOBBERS
JOBBERY
JOBJARS
JOGGERS
JOINERS
JOINERY
JOLTERS
JOSHERS
JOTTERS
KOSHERS
LOADERS
LOAFERS
LOANERS
LOBBERS
LOCKERS
LODGERS
LOFTERS
LOGGERS
LOITERS
LOLLARD
LOLLERS
LOMBARD
LONBORG
LONGARM

LOOKERS
LOOPERS
LOOTERS
LOPPERS
LOSTART
LOTTERS
LOTTERY
LOUVERS
LOWBORN
LOWCARB
LOWCARD
MOANERS
MOBBERS
MOCKERS
MOCKERY
MOEBERG
MOHAIRS
MOILERS
MOLDERS
MOLIERE
MOLTERS
MONGERS
MONSTRO
MONTERO
MOONERS
MOOTERS
MOPPERS
MORCERF
MORTARS
MOSHERS
MOTHERS
MOTHERY
MOUSERS
NODDERS
NOENTRY
NONCORE
NONDARK
NONFARM
NONFORM
NONHERO
NONJURY
NONPARS
NONWARS
NONWORD
NONWORK
NONZERO
NOONERS
NOOSERS
NORBERT
NOSCORE
NOSEBRA
NOSHERS
NOSTARS
NOTHERE
NOTRARE
NOTSURE
NOUTURN
NOVARRO
NOWHERE
POISERS
POLLARD
POLLERA
POLLERS
POMMARD
PONDERS
PONIARD
POOLERS
POPCORN

POPLARS
POPPERS
POPTART
PORKERS
PORTERS
POSEURS
POSTERN
POSTERS
POSTURE
POTHERB
POTHERS
POTTERS
POTTERY
POULTRY
POURERS
POUTERS
POWDERS
POWDERY
ROADERS
ROAMERS
ROARERS
ROBBERS
ROBBERY
ROBOTRY
ROBSART
ROCKERS
ROCKERY
RODGERS
ROGUERY
ROLFERS
ROLLERS
ROMBERG
ROMPERS
RONDURE
RONSARD
ROOFERS
ROOKERY
ROOMERS
ROOTERS
ROSTERS
ROTHIRA
ROTTERS
ROUSERS
ROUTERS
ROXBURY
SOAKERS
SOAPERS
SOARERS
SOBBERS
SOJOURN
SOLDERS
SOLVERS
SOONERS
SORCERY
SORTERS
SOSORRY
SOTHERE
SOTHERN
SOUPERS
TOATURN
TOGGERY
TOHEART
TOILERS
TOLLERS
TONEARM
TONSURE
TOOHARD
TOOLERS
TOOTERS
TOPFORM
TOPIARY
TOPPERS
TORTURE
TOSHIRO
TOSPARE
TOSSERS
TOSTART
TOTTERS
TOTTERY
TOURERS
TOUTERS
TOWBARS
TOWCARS
TOWNERS
TOYCARS
TOYCART
VOGUERS
VOICERS
VOIDERS
VOITURE
VOLTORE
WONDERS
WOODARD
WOOFERS
WOOLERY
WORKERS
WORMERS
YOGHURT
YONKERS
YORKERS
YOTHERS
YOWLERS

•O••••R

BOARDER
BOASTER
BOBBLER
BOBWEIR
BOCHNER
BODYBAR
BOERWAR
BOGGIER
BOGGLER
BOLIVAR
BOLSTER
BONEYER
BONHEUR
BONJOUR
BONNIER
BONSOIR
BOOMCAR
BOOMIER
BOOSLER
BOOSTER
BOOZIER
BOROMIR
BOSSIER
BOTCHER
BOTTLER
BOUCHER
BOUDOIR
BOULDER
BOUNCER
BOUNDER
BOUVIER
BOWDLER
BOXSTER
COALCAR
COALTAR
COARSER
COASTER
COBBLER
COBUYER
COCHAIR
COCKIER
CODDLER
COERCER
COHERER
COJUROR
COLDWAR
COLLIER
COLLYER
COLORER
COMAKER
COMFIER
COMPEER
CONIFER
CONQUER
CONTOUR
COOLAIR
COPULAR
CORKIER
CORNIER
CORONER
CORSAIR
CORVAIR
COSTNER
COTEDOR
COULTER
COUNTER
COUPLER
COURIER
COURSER
COVERER
COVETER
COZENER
DODGIER
DOESFOR
DOGDOOR
DOGGIER
DOGHAIR
DOGSEAR
DOGSTAR
DOMECAR
DONATOR
DONEFOR
DOODLER
DOOMIER
DOPPLER
DORKIER
DOSSIER
DOTTIER
DOUBLER
DOUBTER
DOUCEUR
DOVEBAR
DOWAGER
DOWDIER
DOWNIER
FOAMIER
FOCUSER
FOGGIER
FOLKIER
FONDLER
FOOTLER
FOOZLER
FORAGER
FORBEAR
FOREVER
FORGOER
FORKIER
FORSTER
FOUNDER
FOURIER
GOAFTER
GOBBLER
GOBYAIR
GOBYCAR
GODLIER
GOESFAR
GOESFOR
GOGGLER
GOINFOR
GOLFCAR
GONEFAR
GONEFOR
GOODBAR
GOODFOR
GOOFIER
GOOGLER
GOONIER
GOOPIER
GOOSIER
GORSIER
GORTNER
GOTOVER
GOTOWAR
GOUNDER
GOUTIER
HOARDER
HOARIER
HOARSER
HOBBLER
HOISTER
HOLSTER
HOLYWAR
HOMAGER
HOMEIER
HONORER
HOOSIER
HOPEFOR
HOPOVER
HOPPIER
HORNIER
HORSIER
HOSTLER
HOTOVER
HOTSPUR
HOUNDER
HOVERER
HOWEVER
IODIZER
IONISER
IONIZER
JOBFAIR
JOCULAR
JODHPUR
JOGGLER
JOINDER
JOINTER
JOLLIER
JOLTIER
JOSTLER
JOUSTER
JOWLIER
KOEHLER
KOOKIER
KOSOVAR
LOAMIER
LOATHER
LOBBYER
LOBSTER
LOCATER
LOCATOR
LOESSER
LOFTIER
LONGFOR
LOOKFOR
LOONIER
LOOPIER
LOPPIER
LOTHAIR
LOUNGER
LOUSIER
LOWGEAR
LOWLIER
LOWPAIR
LOYALER
MOBSTER
MODELER
MODULAR
MOGADOR
MOISTER
MOLDIER
MOLITOR
MONIKER
MONITOR
MONOMER
MONSTER
MOOCHER
MOODIER
MOONIER
MOORIER
MOSSIER
MOTHIER
MOULDER
MOUNTER
MOURNER
MOUSIER
MOUTHER
NOBBIER
NODULAR
NOISIER
NONEVER
NONPOOR
NONUSER
NOOTHER
NORTHER
NOSUGAR
NOTCHER
NOTEVER
NOTFAIR
NOTICER
NOTNEAR
NOTOVER
NOWISER
POACHER
POINTER
POITIER
POLANER
POLECAR
POLICER
POLITER
POLYMER
POPOVER
POPSTAR
POPULAR
PORIVER
PORKIER
POSTWAR
POTTIER
POUNCER
POUNDER
POUTIER
ROADTAR
ROASTER
ROCKIER
ROEDEER
ROILIER
ROISTER
ROLLBAR
ROOKIER
ROOMIER
ROOSTER
ROOTFOR
ROOTIER
ROSSNER
ROTATOR
ROTIFER
ROUGHER
ROUNDER
ROUSTER
ROWDIER
SOAPIER
SOBERER
SODDIER
SOGGIER
SOLACER
SOLDFOR
SOLDIER
SOLIDER
SOOTHER
SOOTIER
SOPPIER
SORRIER
SOUNDER
SOUPIER
SOWSEAR
TOAHAIR
TOASTER
TODDLER
TOFFLER
TOGGLER
TOHOMER
TOLLBAR
TOOKFOR
TOOLBAR
TOORDER
TOOTLER
TORCHER
TOTALER
TOUCHER
TOUGHER
TOWNCAR
TOYFAIR
VOCODER
VOLCKER
VONBAER
VORSTER
VOTEFOR
VOUCHER
VOYAGER
WOBBLER
WONOVER
WOODIER
WOODTAR
WOOLIER
WOOSTER
WOOZIER
WORDIER
WORKFOR
WORMIER
WORRIER
YODELER
YOUNGER
ZOELLER
ZONULAR

••OR•••

ABORTED
ACORNED
ADORERS
ADORING
ADORNED
ADORNER
AMORIST
AMOROSO
AMOROUS
ANORAKS
AZOREAN
AZORIAN
BOORISH
BOORMAN
CHORALE
CHORALS
CHORDAL
CHORDED
CHORINE
CHORIST
CHORIZO
CHORTLE
CLORETS
DEORBIT
DIORAMA
DIORITE
DOORDIE
DOORMAN
DOORMAT
DOORMEN
DOORWAY
EXORDIA
FIORINA
FJORDIC
FLOREAL
FLORENZ
FLORETS
FLORIAN
FLORIDA
FLORINS
FLORIST
GEORGEC
GEORGEI
GEORGEM
GEORGES
GEORGEV
GEORGEW
GEORGIA
GEORGIC
GEORGIE
GFORCES
GGORDON
GIORGIO
GIORGOS
GLORIAS
GLORIED
GLORIES
GLORIFY
GLORYBE
HOORAHS
HOORAYS
IFORGET
IFORGOT
IFORONE
IGOROTS
INORBIT
INORDER
IVORIAN
IVORIES
IVORINE
MOORAGE
MOORHEN
MOORIER
MOORING
MOORISH
ODORANT
ODORFUL
ODORIZE
ODOROUS
OLOROSO
ONORATI
ONORDER
PEORIAN
POORBOX
POORBOY
POOREST
POORISH
POORLAW
POORMAN
POORMEN
POORTAX
PRORATA
PRORATE
QUORUMS
REORDER
RIORDAN
RIORITA
SCORERS
SCORIAS
SCORING
SCORNED
SCORNER
SCORPIO
SHOREUP
SHORING
SHORTED
SHORTEN
SHORTER
SHORTIE
SHORTLY
SHORTOF
SNORERS
SNORING
SNORKEL
SNORTAT
SNORTED
SNORTER
SPORRAN
SPORTED
SPORTIN
STORAGE
STORERS
STOREUP
STORIED
STORIES
STORING
STORMED
STORMIN
SWOREAT
SWOREBY
SWOREIN
SWORETO
THOREAU
THORIUM
THORNED
THORSON
TOORDER
TWOROOM
UNORBED
UPOROUT
UXORIAL
WHORLED

••O•R••

BEOGRAD
CHOIRED
ECOTRIN
EGOTRIP
FLOORED
FLOORER
FLOORIT
FLOURED
FOOTRUB
ISOGRAM
OROURKE
PROARAB
PROGRAM
ROOFRAT
ROOTROT
SCOURED
SCOURER
SCOURGE
SPORRAN
TSOURIS
TWOIRON
WOODROW

••O••R•

ADORERS
ATONERS
AVOWERS
BLOWDRY
BLOWERS
BOOBIRD
BOOKERS
BOOKERT
BOOMERS
BOOTERS
BOOTERY
BOOZERS
BROKERS
BROWARD
CHOKERS
CHOLERA
CHOLERS
CLONERS
CLOSERS
CLOSURE
CLOTURE
CLOVERS
CLOVERY
COOKERS
COOKERY
COOLERS
COOPERS
COOPERY
COOTERS
CROWERS
DEODARS
DOOVERS
DOOZERS
DRONERS
DROVERS
EDOUARD
EGOSURF
ELOPERS
EMOTERS
ERODERS
ESOTERY
EVOKERS
EXOCARP
FEODORI
FLOWERS
FLOWERY
FOOLERS
FOOLERY
FOOTERS
FROWARD
GAOLERS
GLOWERS
GOOBERS
GOODERS
GOODTRY
GROCERS
GROCERY
GROPERS
GROVERS
GROWERS
HOOFERS
HOOPERS
HOOTERS
HOOVERS
IRONERS
IRONORE
ISOBARS
ISOMERS
JROBERT
KNOWERS
LEONARD
LEONORA
LEONORE
LEOPARD
LEOTARD
LOOKERS
LOOPERS
LOOTERS
MEOWERS
MNOPQRS
MOONERS
MOOTERS
NOONERS
NOOSERS
PHONERS
PLOVERS
PLOWERS
POOLERS
PROBERS
PROCURE
PROFARM
PROSERS
PROVERB
PROVERS
QUOTERS
RIOTERS
ROOFERS
ROOKERY
ROOMERS
ROOTERS
SCOLARI
SCORERS
SCOTERS
SHOFARS
SHOVERS
SHOWERS
SHOWERY
SLOPERS
SMOKERS
SNORERS
SOONERS
STOKERS
STONERS
STORERS
STOWERS
TOOHARD
TOOLERS
TOOTERS
TWOACRE
TWOFERS
TWOMORE
TWOPART
TWOTERM
UNOVERT
WOODARD
WOOFERS
WOOLERY

••O•••R

ADOLLAR
ADOPTER
ADORNER
ANOTHER
AROUSER
AVOIDER
AWOONOR
BLOCKER
BLOGGER
BLONDER
BLOOMER
BLOOPER
BLOTTER
BLOWIER
BOOMCAR
BOOMIER
BOOSLER
BOOSTER
BOOZIER
BROADER
BROIDER
BROILER
BRONZER
BROODER
BROTHER
BROWNER
BROWSER
CHOICER
CHOKIER
CHOOSER
CHOPPER
CHOWDER
CLOBBER
CLOCKER
CLOUTER
CLOWDER
COOLAIR
CROAKER
CROCKER
CROFTER
CROONER
CROPPER
CROSIER
CROSSER
CROWBAR
CROWDER
CROWNER
CROZIER
DIOPTER
DOODLER
DOOMIER
DROLLER
DROOLER
DROPPER
ECOTEUR
EVOLVER
EXOILER
FLOATER
FLOGGER
FLOORER
FLOPPER
FLOSSER
FLOUTER
FOOTLER
FOOZLER
FROGGER
FROMMER
FROSTER
FROTHER
FROWNER
GLOATER
GLOSSER
GOODBAR
GOODFOR
GOOFIER
GOOGLER
GOONIER
GOOPIER
GOOSIER
GROANER
GRODIER
GROLIER
GROOMER
GROSSER
GROUPER
GROUSER
GROUTER
GROWLER
HOOSIER
IDOTTER
INORDER
IRONBAR
IWONDER
KNOCKER
KNOTTER
KOOKIER
KROEMER
LOOKFOR
LOONIER
LOOPIER
MOOCHER
MOODIER
MOONIER
MOORIER
NOOTHER
OCONNOR
ONORDER
PHONIER
PIONEER
PLODDER
PLOTTER
PROCTER
PROCTOR
PRODDER
PROFFER
PROOFER
PROSIER
PROSPER
PROUDER
PROWLER
REOCCUR
REOFFER
REORDER
ROOKIER
ROOMIER
ROOSTER
ROOTFOR
ROOTIER
SCOFFER
SCOLDER
SCOOPER
SCOOTER
SCORNER
SCOURER
SCOUTER
SCOWLER
SHOCKER
SHOOTER
SHOPFOR
SHOPPER
SHORTER
SHOTFOR
SHOTPAR
SHOUTER
SHOWIER
SLOBBER
SLOGGER
SLOTCAR
SLOTTER
SMOKIER
SMOLDER
SMOTHER
SNOOKER
SNOOPER
SNOOZER
SNORTER
SNOWIER
SOOTHER

SOOTIER
SPOILER
SPONGER
SPONSOR
SPOOFER
SPOOLER
SPOONER
SPOTTER
SPOUTER
STOCKER
STONIER
STOOPER
STOPFOR
STOPPER
STOUTER
SWOONER
SWOOPER
TOOKFOR
TOOLBAR
TOORDER
TOOTLER
TROLLER
TROOPER
TROTTER
TROUPER
TROUSER
TWODOOR
TWOHOUR
TWOPAIR
TWOSTAR
TWOYEAR
USOTOUR
WHOEVER
WHOOPER
WHOPPER
WOODIER
WOODTAR
WOOLIER
WOOSTER
WOOZIER
WRONGER

•••OR••

ABSORBS
ACCORDS
ACTORLY
ADSORBS
AFFORDS
ALBORAK
ALDORAY
ALFORJA
ALSORAN
ALWORTH
ANDORRA
ANGORAS
ARBORED
ARMORED
ARMORER
ASSORTS
ASTORIA
ATWORST
AURORAE
AURORAL
AURORAS
BEGORRA
BICORNE
BICORNS
BYFORCE
BYFORMS
BYWORDS
CALORIC
CALORIE
CATORCE
CAVORTS
CHLORIC
COHORTS
COLORED
COLORER
COLORTV
COMORAN
COMOROS
CYBORGS
DEBORAH
DECORUM
DEFORMS
DEHORNS
DELORIS
DELORME
DEPORTS
DEVORES
DEWORMS
DIVORCE
DOLORES
EFFORTS
ELNORTE
EMPORIA
ENCORED
ENCORES
ENDORSE
ENFORCE
ENGORGE
ESCORTS
ESTORIL
EXHORTS
EXPORTS
EXTORTS
EXWORKS
FAVORED
FAVORER
FEDORAS
FEDOROV
FEMORAL
FEMORIS
FLOORED
FLOORER
FLOORIT
FTWORTH
FURORES
GOFORIT
GOFORTH
HAWORTH
HONORED
HONOREE
HONORER
HUMORAL
HUMORED
HUMORME
IGNORED
IGNORER
IGNORES
IMBORED
IMFORIT
IMMORAL
IMPORTS
IMSORRY
INDORSE
INFORCE
INFORIT
INFORMS
LABORAT
LABORED
LABORER
LAPORTE
LASORDA
LAVORIS
LIVORNO
MAJORCA
MAJORED
MAJORIN
MAYORAL
MEMOREX
MENORAH
MENORCA
MILORDS
MINORCA
MINORED
MINORIN
MOTORED
MRHORSE
MRNORTH
MRWORDS
MYWORLD
NONORAL
NOWORSE
OFSORTS
OSBORNE
OXFORDS
PCWORLD
PERORAL
PREORAL
PRIORTO
RAZORED
REBORED
REBORES
RECORDS
RECORKS
REFORGE
REFORMS
REMORAS
REMORSE
REPORTS
RESORBS
RESORTS
RETORTS
REWORDS
REWORKS
RUMORED
SATORIS
SAVORED
SAVORER
SCIORRA
SENORAS
SENORES
SONORAN
SORORAL
SOSORRY
SUBORNS
TABORET
THEOREM
TINORES
TOHORSE
TUTORED
UNBORED
UNBORNE
UNCORED
UNCORES
UNCORKS
UNFORKS
UNGORED
UNHORSE
UNSORRY
UNSORTS
UNWORMY
UPBORNE
UPFORIT
UPNORTH
VALOREM
VAPORED
VAPORER
VAPORUB
VISORED
VITORIA
VIZORED
WHWORDS
YESORNO

•••O•R•

ADJOURN
ALMONRY
ANDORRA
ARBOURS
ARDOURS
ARMOIRE
ARMOURS
ARMOURY
BEGORRA
BIGOTRY
BOWOARS
CANOERS
CANONRY
COLOURS
DETOURS
DEVOIRS
DEVOURS
DOLOURS
ECHOERS
FAVOURS
FELONRY
HELOTRY
HERONRY
HONOURS
HUMOURS
IMSORRY
IMYOURS
INBOARD
INCOURT
INDOORS
INPOURS
LABOURS
MASONRY
MCCOURT
MEMOIRE
MEMOIRS
OCTOBRE
OHIOART
ONBOARD
REBOARD
RENOIRS
REPOURS
RETOURS
RIGOURS
ROBOTRY
RUMOURS
SAVOURS
SAVOURY
SCIORRA
SOJOURN
SOSORRY
UNDOERS
UNMOORS
UNSORRY
UPCOURT
UPHOARD
UPROARS
UPSOARS
VALOURS
VAPOURS
VAPOURY
VELOURS
VETOERS
VIGOURS

•••O••R

ALLOVER
ALMONER
ALROKER
ANDOVER
ANNOYER
AREOLAR
ARMORER
ASKOVER
ATEOVER
AWOONOR
BICOLOR
BIPOLAR
BLOOMER
BLOOPER
BOROMIR
BROODER
CAJOLER
CAROLER
CDTOWER
CHOOSER
CNTOWER
COLORER
CORONER
CROONER
CRYOVER
CUTOVER
DECODER
DECOLOR
DECOYER
DEPONER
DEPOSER
DEPOWER
DIDOVER
DIPOLAR
DROOLER
EATOVER
ELBOWER
EMBOWER
EMPOWER
ENCODER
ENDOWER
ENJOYER
EXPOSER
FAVORER
FLOORER
FLYOVER
GETOVER
GOTOVER
GOTOWAR
GROOMER
GYROCAR
HADOVER
HANOVER
HASOVER
HONORER
HOPOVER
HOTOVER
ICEOVER
IGNORER
IMPOSER
INCOLOR
INCOMER
INPOWER
INSOFAR
INTONER
INVOKER
ITSOVER
JAROMIR
JDPOWER
KILOBAR
KOSOVAR
LABORER
LAYOVER
LIEOVER
LMNOPQR
MALODOR
MANOWAR
METOOER
MONOMER
NICOBAR
NOTOVER
OCTOBER
OKTOBER
ONEOVER
OPPOSER
PALOMAR
PIVOTER
POPOVER
PROOFER
PUTOVER
RANOVER
RECOLOR
RECOVER
REHONOR
REMOTER
REMOVER
REPOSER
REPOWER
RESOLER
REVOKER
RUNOVER
SAMOVAR
SAVORER
SAYOVER
SCHOLAR
SCOOPER
SCOOTER
SECONDR
SHOOTER
SNOOKER
SNOOPER
SNOOZER
SPOOFER
SPOOLER
SPOONER
STOOPER
STROKER
SWOONER
SWOOPER
TENONER
THEODOR
THROWER
TIPOVER
TOHOMER
TROOPER
UNCOVER
UNCOYER
UNSOBER
UPTOPAR
VANOCUR
VAPORER
VOCODER
WAGONER
WHOOPER
WIDOWER
WINOVER
WONOVER

••••OR•

ABATORS
AIRHORN
AIRPORT
ALIFORM
ALTDORF
ALTHORN
AMATORY
AMPHORA
ANCHORS
ANDMORE
ANYMORE
APRIORI
ARAGORN
ARDMORE
ARTFORM
ARTWORK
ASHFORD
ATEMORE
AUTHORS
BADFORM
BADWORD
BAILORS
BAYLORU
BBQPORK
BEDFORD
BEDNORZ
BELFORT
BETTORS
BIGHORN
BUDWORM
CANTORS
CAPTORS
CARHORN
CARPORT
CDSTORE
CENSORS
CHICORY
CLAMORS
COMFORT
COMPORT
CONCORD
CONDORS
CONFORM
CONNORS
CONSORT
CONTORT
CORPORA
CREMORA
CURSORS
CURSORY
CUTWORK
CUTWORM
DEBTORS
DELMORE
DELTORO
DEPLORE
DICKORY
DIGGORY
DISCORD
DISPORT
DISTORT
DOCTORS
EATMORE
EDITORS
EELWORM
ELUSORY
ENAMORS
EXPLORE
EYESORE
FACTORS
FACTORY
FARMORE
FAXLORE
FEODORI
FERVORS
FLAVORS
FLAVORY
FLEXORS
FOGHORN
FORBORE
FORLORN
FORTORD
FOXBORO
GAYLORD
GETSORE
GETWORD
GIFFORD
GILFORD
GILMORE
GLAMORS
GONGORA
GOSFORD
GOTSORE
GOTWORD
GREGORY
GUVNORS
HARBORS
HAYFORK
HECTORS
HICKORY
HISTORY
HORRORS
IMPLORE
INAWORD
INDOORS
INKHORN
INSHORE
INSHORT
INSTORE
IRONORE
IRSFORM
ISADORA
ISADORE
ISIDORE
JAILORS
JETPORT
JUNIORS
KENMORE
KEYWORD
LANFORD
LASTORY
LAWFORD
LEADORE
LECTORS
LEEFORD
LEGHORN
LEGWORK
LEONORA
LEONORE
LESSORS
LIENORS
LINDORF
LIQUORS
LONBORG
LOWBORN
LUGWORM
MAHZORS
MAXBORN
MCGRORY
MEDFORD
MENTORS
METEORS
MIDMORN
MINDORO
MIRRORS
MISFORM
MISSORT
MISWORD
MITFORD
MUMFORD
NESTORS
NETWORK
NEWBORN
NEWPORT
NEWWORD
NEWYORK
NONCORE
NONFORM
NONWORD
NONWORK
NOSCORE
OFASORT
ONEMORE
ONSHORE
ORATORS
ORATORY
OUTPORT
OUTTORE
OUTTORN
OUTWORD
OUTWORE
OUTWORK
OUTWORN
OVIFORM
OXYMORA
PALLORS
PANDORA
PARLORS
PASTORS
PAVIORS
PAYMORE
PERFORM
PILLORY
PLEXORS
POPCORN
PREBORN
PREFORM
PRESORT
PRETORS
PREWORK
PREWORN
PURPORT
RADFORD
RANCORS
RAPPORT
RAPTORS
RASBORA
READORN
RECTORS
RECTORY
REDFORD
REDWORM
RESCORE
RESTORE
RESWORE
RESWORN
RHETORS
RIPCORD
RIPTORN
RUMFORD
SAILORS
SALVORS
SAMBORA
SANBORN
SANFORD
SAPPORO
SARTORS
SAVIORS
SAXHORN
SAYMORE
SEABORG
SEAPORT
SECTORS
SEIZORS
SENHORA
SENIORS
SENSORS
SENSORY
SIGNORA
SIGNORE
SIGNORS
STATORS
STUPORS
SUBFORM
SUBSORT
SUCCORS
SUITORS
SUPPORT
TAILORS
TAYLORS
TEMPORE
TENSORS
TERRORS
TINHORN
TINWORK
TOPFORM
TREMORS
TRIBORO
TRICORN
TRIFORM
TWOMORE
UNICORN
UNIFORM
UNMOORS
UNSHORN
UNSHORT
UNSWORE
UNSWORN
VECTORS
VENDORS
VICTORS
VICTORY
VOLTORE
WALDORF
WARLORD
WARTORN
WARWORN
WATFORD
WAXWORK
WAYWORN
WEXFORD
WILFORD

••••O•R

ACTFOUR
AGEFOUR
BALFOUR
BELVOIR
BELVOUR
BIGFOUR
BONJOUR
BONSOIR
BOUDOIR
BUSTOUR
CANDOUR
CARDOOR
CATDOOR
CLAMOUR
CONTOUR
DOGDOOR
ENAMOUR
FABFOUR
FERVOUR
FLAVOUR
FORGOER
GLAMOUR
HARBOUR
LASSOER
MANHOUR
METOOER
MISDOER
NONPOOR
OFFHOUR
ONEHOUR
OUTDOER
OUTDOOR
OUTPOUR
OUTROAR
OUTSOAR
PARFOUR
PARLOUR
PAVIOUR
PETDOOR
PGATOUR
RADIOER
RANCOUR
REDFOUR
SAVIOUR
SEYMOUR
SIXFOUR
SUCCOUR
TANDOOR
TANGOER
TENFOUR
TERROIR
THETOUR
TWODOOR
TWOHOUR
UNFLOOR
USOTOUR
WEEHOUR

•••••OR

ABETTOR
ACHEFOR
ACTSFOR
ADAPTOR
ADJUROR
ADVISOR
AERATOR
AIMSFOR
ALIENOR
ASKSFOR
ASSUROR
AUDITOR
AVIATOR
AWOONOR
BATSFOR
BEGSFOR
BELABOR
BICOLOR
BIDSFOR
BUCKFOR
BURNFOR
CALLFOR
CAMPHOR
CARDOOR
CAREFOR
CATDOOR
CLANGOR
CLAPFOR
COJUROR
COTEDOR
CREATOR
CURATOR
DECOLOR
DEVISOR
DIEDFOR
DIESFOR
DIGSFOR
DILATOR
DILUTOR
DIVISOR
DOESFOR
DOGDOOR
DONATOR
DONEFOR
ECUADOR
EDUCTOR
EJECTOR
ELEANOR
ELECTOR
EMPEROR
ENACTOR
ENARBOR
EQUATOR
ERECTOR
EVERTOR
EVICTOR
EXACTOR
EXCITOR
EXMAYOR
FALLFOR
FEARFOR
FEELFOR
FELLFOR
FELTFOR
FISHFOR
GENITOR
GOESFOR
GOINFOR
GONEFOR
GOODFOR
GRANTOR
GUNSFOR
GYRATOR
HEADFOR
HERITOR
HITSFOR
HOPEFOR
HUMIDOR
HUNTFOR
HURTFOR
IGNITOR
INCISOR
INCOLOR
INERROR
INFAVOR
INLABOR
ITCHFOR
JANITOR
KEILLOR
LAIDFOR
LANGUOR
LAYSFOR
LEAPFOR
LEFTFOR
LEGATOR
LEVATOR
LIEDFOR
LIESFOR
LIVEFOR
LOCATOR
LONGFOR
LOOKFOR
MADEFOR
MAKEFOR
MALODOR
MATADOR
MIRADOR
MOGADOR
MOLITOR
MONITOR
NATATOR
NEGATOR
NONPOOR
OBLIGOR
OCONNOR
OFFEROR
OPTSFOR
OUTDOOR
PAIDFOR

PARADOR
PASSFOR
PAYSFOR
PETDOOR
PICADOR
PINEFOR
PLANFOR
PRAETOR
PRAYFOR
PROCTOR
PULLFOR
PUSHFOR
RANGFOR
REACTOR
READFOR
REALTOR
RECOLOR
REHONOR
RELATOR
REPSFOR
REVISOR
RINGFOR
ROOTFOR
ROTATOR
RUNGFOR
RUNSFOR
SALEMOR
SAVEFOR
SCISSOR
SELLFOR
SENATOR
SENDFOR
SENTFOR
SETTLOR
SHOPFOR
SHOTFOR
SIGHFOR
SIGNFOR
SISENOR
SITSFOR
SOLDFOR
SPECTOR
SPONSOR
SQUALOR
STAYFOR
STENTOR
STERTOR
STOPFOR
SUEDFOR
SUESFOR
TAKEFOR
TANDOOR
TEMBLOR
TESTFOR
THEODOR
TOOKFOR
TRACTOR
TRAITOR
TRAYNOR
TWODOOR
UNFLOOR
USEDFOR
USESFOR
VENTNOR
VIEDFOR
VIESFOR
VISITOR
VOTEFOR
WAITFOR
WARRIOR
WEEPFOR
WENTFOR
WHATFOR
WINDSOR
WISHFOR
WORKFOR
XFACTOR
YELLFOR
YENSFOR

OS•••••

OSAKANS
OSBORNE
OSCEOLA
OSCINES
OSCULAR
OSCULES
OSETRAS
OSHAPED
OSHKOSH
OSIERED
OSIRIAN
OSMATIC
OSMONDS
OSMOSED
OSMOSES
OSMOSIS
OSMOTIC
OSMUNDS
OSPREYS
OSSEOUS
OSSETRA
OSSICLE
OSSIFIC
OSSIPEE
OSSUARY
OSTEOID
OSTIARY
OSTLERS
OSTMARK
OSTOSIS
OSTRAVA
OSTRICH
OSTWALD

O•S••••

OBSCENE
OBSCURA
OBSCURE
OBSERVE
OFSORTS
OISEAUX
OKSHOOT
ONSAGER
ONSERVE
ONSHORE
ONSIDES
ONSIGHT
ONSTAFF
ONSTAGE
OSSEOUS
OSSETRA
OSSICLE
OSSIFIC
OSSIPEE
OSSUARY
OUSTERS
OUSTING
OYSTERS

O••S•••

OARSMAN
OARSMEN
OBESELY
OBESITY
ODDSARE
ODDSHOE
ODDSOCK
ODESSAN
ODYSSEY
OERSTED
OFASORT
OFFSETS
OFFSIDE
OFFSITE
OHMSLAW
OILSAND
OILSEED
OILSKIN
OILSPOT
OLDSALT
OLDSAWS
OLDSHOE
OLDSONG
OLDSTER
OLESTRA
OLMSTED
ONASSIS
ONESELF
ONESHOE
ONESHOT
ONESIZE
ONESOCK
ONESPOT
ONESTAR
ONESTEP
ONESTOP
OPOSSUM
OPTSFOR
OPTSOUT
OPUSONE
OPUSTWO
ORESTES
ORISONS
OURSELF
OURSONG
OUTSAID
OUTSAIL
OUTSANG
OUTSAYS
OUTSEEK
OUTSEEN
OUTSEES
OUTSELL
OUTSERT
OUTSETS
OUTSHOT
OUTSHOW
OUTSIDE
OUTSIFT
OUTSIGH
OUTSING
OUTSINS
OUTSITS
OUTSIZE
OUTSKIP
OUTSOAR
OUTSOLD
OUTSOLE
OUTSPED
OUTSPIN
OUTSPIT
OUTSTAY
OUTSTEP
OUTSULK
OUTSUMS
OUTSUNG
OUTSWAM
OUTSWIM
OUTSWUM
OVISACS

O•••S••

OBLASTS
OBOISTS
OBTESTS
OBTUSER
ODESSAN
ODYSSEY
ONASSIS
OPENSEA
OPENSUP
OPOSSUM
OPPOSED
OPPOSER
OPPOSES
OPQRSTU
ORBISON
ORRISES
OSMOSED
OSMOSES
OSMOSIS
OSTOSIS
OUTASKS
OVERSAD
OVERSAW
OVERSEA
OVERSEE
OVERSET
OVERSEW
OVERSUP

O••••S•

OAKCASK
OAKDESK
OAKIEST
OAKMOSS
OARLESS
OBELISE
OBELISK
OBVERSE
OCULIST
ODDNESS
OFFBASE
OFFCAST
OFFENSE
OFNOUSE
OGREISH
OILBASE
OILIEST
OILLESS
OKHOTSK
OLDNESS
OLDROSE
OLDWEST
OLEMISS
OLOROSO
OMIGOSH
ONEBASE
ONENESS
ONFIRST
ONLEASE
ONLEASH
ONLIEST
ONTOAST
OOZIEST
OPALISH
OPEROSE
OPPRESS
ORALIST
ORBLESS
ORELESS
ORGIAST
OSHKOSH
OUTCAST
OUTFAST
OUTFISH
OUTGUSH
OUTHISS
OUTJEST
OUTKAST
OUTKISS
OUTLASH
OUTLAST
OUTMOST
OUTPASS
OUTPOST
OUTPUSH
OUTRUSH
OUTWASH
OUTWEST
OUTWISH
OVERUSE
OWLIEST
OXIDASE
OXIDISE
OZONISE
OZZFEST

O•••••S

OAHUANS
OAKMOSS
OAKTAGS
OARLESS
OBENTOS
OBEYERS
OBJECTS
OBLASTS
OBLATES
OBLIGES
OBLONGS
OBOISTS
OBTAINS
OBTESTS
OBTUNDS
OBVERTS
OBVIOUS
OCCULTS
OCEANUS
OCELLUS
OCELOTS
OCHROUS
OCICATS
OCTANES
OCTANTS
OCTAVES
OCTAVOS
OCTOPUS
OCTROIS
OCULARS
ODDJOBS
ODDLOTS
ODDNESS
ODELETS
ODOROUS
OEDIPUS
OEUVRES
OFFDAYS
OFFENDS
OFFICES
OFFINGS
OFFSETS
OFSORTS
OGDOADS
OGLALAS
OHIOANS
OHMAGES
OILCANS
OILCUPS
OILLESS
OILPANS
OILRIGS
OILRUBS
OINKERS
OJIBWAS
OLDBATS
OLDBOYS
OLDCARS
OLDDAYS
OLDDOGS
OLDGAGS
OLDNESS
OLDNEWS
OLDPALS
OLDPROS
OLDSAWS
OLDWAYS
OLEATES
OLEFINS
OLEMISS
OLEVELS
OLOGIES
OLYMPUS
OMAHANS
OMELETS
OMINOUS
OMNIBUS
ONABIAS
ONAGERS
ONASSIS
ONEACTS
ONEIDAS
ONENESS
ONEOFFS
ONEOFUS
ONEROUS
ONETWOS
ONLOADS
ONRAMPS
ONSIDES
ONWARDS
OOCYTES
OOLITES
OOLONGS
OOMPAHS
OPAQUES
OPENERS
OPIATES
OPINERS
OPPOSES
OPPRESS
OPPUGNS
OPTICKS
OPTIMAS
OPTIONS
ORACIES
ORACLES
ORANGES
ORANTES
ORATORS
ORBLESS
ORCHIDS
ORDAINS
ORDEALS
ORDINES
ORELESS
ORESTES
ORGEATS
ORIENTS
ORIGINS
ORIOLES
ORISONS
ORKNEYS
ORLEANS
ORMOLUS
ORPHANS
ORPHEUS
ORRISES
OSAKANS
OSCINES
OSCULES
OSETRAS
OSMONDS
OSMOSES
OSMOSIS
OSMUNDS
OSPREYS
OSSEOUS
OSTLERS
OSTOSIS
OTARIES
OTTAWAS
OUSTERS
OUTACTS
OUTADDS
OUTAGES
OUTASKS
OUTAWES
OUTBANS
OUTBATS
OUTBEGS
OUTBIDS
OUTBOWS
OUTBUDS
OUTBUYS
OUTCUTS
OUTDOES
OUTEATS
OUTFITS
OUTGOES
OUTGUNS
OUTHISS
OUTHITS
OUTINGS
OUTJETS
OUTJUTS
OUTKISS
OUTLAWS
OUTLAYS
OUTLETS
OUTLIES
OUTLIPS
OUTMANS
OUTPASS
OUTPAYS
OUTPOPS
OUTPUTS
OUTRAPS
OUTRIBS
OUTRIGS
OUTROWS
OUTRUNS
OUTSAYS
OUTSEES
OUTSETS
OUTSINS
OUTSITS
OUTSUMS
OUTVIES
OUTWARS
OUTWITS
OVARIES
OVISACS
OWLEGGS
OXCARTS
OXFORDS
OXHIDES
OXTAILS
OYSTERS
OZONOUS

•OS••••

BOSCAGE
BOSNIAN
BOSOMED
BOSONIC
BOSSIER
BOSSILY
BOSSING
BOSSISM
BOSSMAN
BOSSMEN
BOSTONS
BOSTONU
BOSWELL
COSETTE
COSHERS
COSHING
COSIEST
COSIGNS
COSINES
COSSACK
COSSETS
COSTAIN
COSTARD
COSTARS
COSTATE
COSTING
COSTIVE
COSTNER
COSTUME
COSYING
DOSADOS
DOSAGES
DOSHOTS
DOSIDOS
DOSSALS
DOSSIER
DOSSING
EOSINES
FOSCOLO
FOSDICK
FOSSILS
FOSTERS
GOSFORD
GOSHAWK
GOSLING
GOSOUTH
GOSPELS
GOSSAGE
GOSSETT
GOSSIPS
GOSSIPY
GOSTALE
HOSANNA
HOSCALE
HOSIERS
HOSIERY
HOSKINS
HOSPICE
HOSTAGE
HOSTELS
HOSTESS
HOSTILE
HOSTING
HOSTLER
JOSBOYS
JOSEPHA
JOSEPHI
JOSHERS
JOSHING
JOSTLED
JOSTLER
JOSTLES
KOSCINA
KOSHERS
KOSHIBA
KOSOVAR
KOSSUTH
KOSYGIN
LOSABLE
LOSEBIG
LOSEOUT
LOSESIT
LOSESTO
LOSINGS
LOSTART
LOSTBIG
LOSTCAT
LOSTDOG
LOSTOUT
LOSTPET
MOSAICS
MOSCATO
MOSCONI
MOSELLE
MOSEYED
MOSHERS
MOSHING
MOSHPIT
MOSLEMS
MOSQUES
MOSSIER
MOSSING
NOSCORE
NOSEATS
NOSEBAG
NOSEBRA
NOSEDIN
NOSEDUP
NOSEEUM
NOSEGAY
NOSEJOB
NOSEOUT
NOSESIN
NOSESUP
NOSHERS
NOSHING
NOSHOWS
NOSIEST
NOSIREE
NOSTAIN
NOSTARS
NOSTRIL
NOSTRUM
NOSUGAR
NOSWEAT
POSABLE
POSADAS
POSEDAS
POSESAS
POSEURS
POSEUSE
POSHEST
POSITED
POSOLES
POSSESS
POSSLQS
POSSUMS
POSTAGE
POSTBAG
POSTBOX
POSTDOC
POSTERN
POSTERS
POSTFIX
POSTHOC
POSTIES
POSTING
POSTITS
POSTMAN
POSTMEN
POSTOPS
POSTURE
POSTWAR
ROSABUD
ROSALIA
ROSALIE
ROSALYN
ROSANNA
ROSANNE
ROSARIO
ROSCOES
ROSEATE
ROSEBAY
ROSEBUD
ROSEHIP
ROSELLA
ROSELLE
ROSEOIL
ROSEOLA
ROSERED
ROSETEA
ROSETTA
ROSETTE
ROSIEST
ROSINED
ROSSANO
ROSSINI
ROSSNER
ROSSSEA
ROSTAND
ROSTERS
ROSTOCK
ROSTRAL
ROSTRUM
ROSWELL
SOSORRY
SOSPADS
SOSUEME
TOSCALE
TOSHIBA
TOSHIRO
TOSPARE
TOSSERS
TOSSING
TOSSOFF
TOSSOUT
TOSSPOT
TOSSUPS
TOSTADA
TOSTART
VOSGIAN
VOSKHOD
ZOSIMUS
ZOSSIMA

•O•S•••

BOASTED
BOASTER
BOASTOF
BOBSLED
BOISEID
BOLSHOI
BOLSTER
BONSOIR
BOOSLER
BOOSTED
BOOSTER
BOOSTUP
BORSCHT
BORSTAL
BOSSIER
BOSSILY
BOSSING
BOSSISM
BOSSMAN
BOSSMEN
BOUSONO
BOWSAWS
BOWSHOT
BOWSOUT
BOXSEAT
BOXSETS
BOXSTEP
BOXSTER
COASTAL
COASTED
COASTER
COMSATS
CONSENT
CONSIGN
CONSIST
CONSOLE
CONSORT
CONSULS
CONSULT
CONSUME
COPSHOP
COPSOUT
CORSAGE
CORSAIR
CORSETS
CORSICA
COSSACK
COSSETS
COUSINE
COUSINS
COWSHED
COWSKIN
COWSLIP
DOASIDO
DOESBAD
DOESFOR
DOESKIN
DOESNOT
DOESTOO
DOGSAGE
DOGSEAR
DOGSHOW
DOGSITS
DOGSLED
DOGSTAR
DORSALS
DORSETT
DORSEYS
DOSSALS
DOSSIER
DOSSING
DOUSERS
DOUSING
DOWSERS
DOWSING
FOBSOFF
FOCSLES
FOISTED
FOISTON
FORSAKE
FORSALE
FORSHOW
FORSIZE
FORSOOK
FORSTER
FORSURE
FORSYTE
FORSYTH
FOSSILS
GODSEND
GODSENT
GODSONS
GOESAFT
GOESAPE
GOESBAD
GOESFAR
GOESFOR
GOESMAD
GOESOFF
GOESOUT
GOESPRO
GOOSIER
GOOSING
GORSIER
GOSSAGE
GOSSETT
GOSSIPS
GOSSIPY
GOTSOFT
GOTSORE
HOBSONS
HOFSTRA
HOISTED
HOISTER
HOISTUP
HOLSTER
HOOSIER
HOPSING
HOPSOFF
HOPSOUT
HORSIER
HORSILY
HORSING
HORSLEY
HOTSEAT
HOTSHOT
HOTSOUP
HOTSPOT
HOTSPUR
HOUSING
HOUSMAN
HOUSSAY
HOUSTON
JOBSHOP
JOISTED
JOUSTED
JOUSTER
KOOSHES
KOSSUTH
LOBSTER
LOESSER
LOESSES
LOGSOFF
LOGSOUT
LOOSELY
LOOSENS
LOOSEST
LOOSING
LOPSOFF
LOUSEUP
LOUSIER
LOUSILY
LOUSING
LOWSIDE
MOBSTER
MOISSAN

MOISTEN
MOISTER
MOISTLY
MOLSONS
MONSOON
MONSTER
MONSTRO
MORSELS
MOSSIER
MOSSING
MOUSERS
MOUSIER
MOUSILY
MOUSING
MOUSSED
MOUSSES
NODSOFF
NOISIER
NOISILY
NOISING
NOISOME
NONSALE
NONSANE
NONSELF
NONSKED
NONSKID
NONSLIP
NONSTOP
NONSUCH
NOOSERS
NOOSING
NOTSAFE
NOTSURE
POESIES
POISERS
POISING
POISONS
POISSON
POPSOFF
POPSONG
POPSOUT
POPSTAR
PORSCHE
PORSENA
POSSESS
POSSLQS
POSSUMS
POTSDAM
POTSHOT
POUSSIN
ROASTED
ROASTER
ROBSART
ROISTER
RONSARD
RONSONS
ROOSTED
ROOSTER
ROSSANO
ROSSINI
ROSSNER
ROSSSEA
ROUSERS
ROUSING
ROUSTED
ROUSTER
SONSHIP
SOUSING

SOWSEAR
TOASTED
TOASTEE
TOASTER
TOCSINS
TOESHOE
TOGSOUT
TOLSTOI
TOLSTOY
TONSILS
TONSURE
TOOSLOW
TOOSOON
TOPSAIL
TOPSEED
TOPSIDE
TOPSOFF
TOPSOIL
TOPSOUT
TOPSPIN
TOPSPOT
TORSION
TOSSERS
TOSSING
TOSSOFF
TOSSOUT
TOSSPOT
TOSSUPS
TOUSLED
TOUSLES
TOYSHOP
TOYSLED
TOYSRUS
VORSTER
WOOSHED
WOOSHES
WOOSNAM
WOOSTER
WORSENS
WORSHIP
WORSLEY
WORSTED
ZOSSIMA
ZOYSIAS

•O••S••

BOBBSEY
BOGUSLY
BOILSUP
BOLTSUP
BOLUSES
BONESET
BONESUP
BONUSES
BOOPSIE
BOOTSIT
BOOTSUP
BOURSES
BOXESIN
BOXESUP
COARSEN
COARSER
COHOSTS
COILSUP
COLOSSI
COMESAS
COMESAT
COMESBY

COMESIN
COMESON
COMESTO
COMESUP
COOKSUP
COOLSIT
COOPSUP
CORKSUP
CORPSES
COUNSEL
COURSED
COURSER
COURSES
DODGSON
DOLLSUP
DOOMSTO
DOTESON
FOCUSED
FOCUSER
FOCUSES
FOCUSON
FOLDSIN
FOLDSUP
FOOTSIE
FOOTSIT
FOOTSUP
FORASEC
FORESAW
FORESEE
FORESTS
FORKSUP
FOULSUP
GOBYSEA
GOODSON
GOOFSUP
GOTOSEA
GOTOSEE
HOARSEN
HOARSER
HOCUSED
HOLDSIN
HOLDSIT
HOLDSON
HOLDSTO
HOLDSUP
HOLESUP
HOLISTS
HOLYSEE
HOMESIN
HONESIN
HONESTY
HONKSAT
HOOFSIT
HOOKSON
HOOKSUP
HOOTSAT
HOPESSO
HOPESTO
HORNSBY
HORNSIN
HOUSSAY
HOWLSAT
IODISED
IODISES
IONESCO
IONISED
IONISER
IONISES

JOCASTA
JOHNSON
JOINSIN
JOINSUP
JONESED
JONESES
LOADSIN
LOADSOF
LOADSUP
LOCKSET
LOCKSIN
LOCKSON
LOCKSUP
LOCUSTS
LOESSER
LOESSES
LOOKSAD
LOOKSAT
LOOKSEE
LOOKSIN
LOOKSON
LOOKSTO
LOOKSUP
LORDSIT
LORISES
LORUSES
LOSESIT
LOSESTO
LOTUSES
LOUISII
LOUISIV
LOUISIX
LOUISVI
LOUISXI
LOUISXV
LOVESET
LOVESIT
LOVESTO
MOCKSUP
MODESTO
MODESTY
MODISTE
MOISSAN
MOLESTS
MOMMSEN
MOMUSES
MONOSKI
MOONSET
MORESBY
MORISOT
MOUSSED
MOUSSES
MOVESIN
MOVESIT
MOVESON
MOVESTO
MOVESUP
NONUSER
NOSESIN
NOSESUP
NOTASTE
NOTUSED
NOVISAD
NOWISEE
NOWISER
POISSON
POKESAT
POLESAT

POLESIT
POLISCI
POLYSCI
POOPSIE
POSESAS
POURSIN
POUSSIN
ROARSAT
ROBESON
ROBUSTA
ROBUSTO
ROLLSBY
ROLLSIN
ROLLSON
ROLLSUP
ROOTSUP
ROPESIN
ROPESUP
ROSSSEA
SOAKSIN
SOAKSUP
SOAPSUP
SOCKSIN
SOMESAY
SOUPSON
SOUPSUP
SOURSON
TOILSAT
TONESUP
TONUSES
TOOLSET
TOOLSUP
TOOTSAT
TOOTSIE
TOTASTE
TOTESUP
VOTESIN
VOTESNO
VOTESON
WOEISME
WOODSAW
WOODSON
WOOLSEY
WORKSAT
WORKSHY
WORKSIN
WORKSON
WORKSUP
ZOOMSIN

•O•••S•

BOARISH
BOGGISH
BOGGUSS
BOLDEST
BOMBAST
BONEASH
BONIEST
BOOHISS
BOOKISH
BOORISH
BOSSISM
BOWLESS
BOXIEST
COCHISE
COCKISH
CODFISH
COEXIST

COKIEST
COLDEST
COLDISH
COLOSSI
COLTISH
COMBUST
COMCAST
COMMISH
COMPASS
COMPOSE
COMPOST
COMTISM
COMTIST
CONCISE
CONCUSS
CONFESS
CONFUSE
CONGEST
CONSIST
CONTEST
CONTUSE
COOLEST
COOLISH
COPYIST
CORNISH
COSIEST
COWFISH
COWIEST
COXLESS
COYNESS
COZIEST
DOGFISH
DOGGISH
DOGLESS
DOGROSE
DOGVEST
DOINGSO
DOLLISH
DOLTISH
DONETSK
DONJOSE
DONNISH
DONRUSS
DONTASK
DOPIEST
DOTDASH
DOUREST
DOZIEST
FOELESS
FOGLESS
FOGYISH
FOGYISM
FOLIOSE
FOLKISH
FONDEST
FOOLISH
FOPPISH
FORBUSH
FORMOSA
FORREST
FOULEST
FOXIEST
GOAMISS
GOATISH
GODDESS
GODLESS
GOFIRST
GOIRISH

GOODISH
GOODUSE
GOOIEST
GORIEST
GOTBUSY
GOTCASH
GOTLOST
GOTPAST
GOTWISE
GOULASH
GOUTISH
HOBOISM
HOGGISH
HOGNOSE
HOGWASH
HOKIEST
HOLIEST
HOMIEST
HOPEDSO
HOPESSO
HORNISH
HORNIST
HOSTESS
HOTNESS
HOTTEST
HOWELSE
JOBLESS
JOKIEST
JOYLESS
KOMATSU
LOGGISH
LOGIEST
LONGEST
LONGISH
LOOKISM
LOOKIST
LOOSEST
LOUDEST
LOUDISH
LOUTISH
LOWCOST
LOWMASS
LOWNESS
LOWPOST
LOWRISE
LOWRISK
MOBBISH
MOBBISM
MOBBIST
MOLLUSC
MOLLUSK
MOMBASA
MONDESI
MONKISH
MOONISH
MOORISH
MOPIEST
MORTISE
NOBLEST
NOCLASS
NONBASE
NONBUSY
NONCASH
NONOISE
NONPAST
NOPQRST
NORRISH
NOSIEST

NOTEASY
NOURISH
NOWNESS
NOWORSE
OOZIEST
PODCAST
POETESS
POETISE
POKIEST
POLOIST
POOREST
POORISH
PORKISH
POSEUSE
POSHEST
POSSESS
RODLESS
ROGUISH
ROMANSH
ROMPISH
ROOKISH
ROPIEST
ROSIEST
SOANDSO
SODLESS
SOFTEST
SOFTISH
SOLNESS
SOLOIST
SONLESS
SOONEST
SOPHISM
SOPHIST
SOTTISH
SOUBISE
SOUREST
SOURISH
TOADISH
TOELESS
TOHORSE
TOLEASE
TONIEST
TOOEASY
TOPLESS
TOPMAST
TOPMOST
TORYISH
TORYISM
TOURISM
TOURIST
TOWNISH
TOYLESS
VOGUISH
VOWLESS
WOLFISH
WORMISH
WOULDST
YOBBISH
YOGIISM
YORKIST
YOULOSE
YOUWISH
ZOOIEST

•O••••S

AOUDADS
BOATELS
BOATERS

BOBBERS
BOBBIES
BOBBINS
BOBBLES
BOBCATS
BOCCIES
BODEGAS
BODICES
BODINGS
BODKINS
BOEINGS
BOFFINS
BOGARTS
BOGGLES
BOGGUSS
BOILERS
BOKKENS
BOLEROS
BOLIDES
BOLTERS
BOLUSES
BOMBERS
BONACIS
BONBONS
BONDERS
BONGOES
BONITOS
BONKERS
BONMOTS
BONNETS
BONUSES
BOOBIES
BOOBOOS
BOOCOOS
BOODLES
BOOGIES
BOOHISS
BOOHOOS
BOOKERS
BOOKIES
BOOMERS
BOONIES
BOOTEES
BOOTERS
BOOTIES
BOOZERS
BOPPERS
BORATES
BORDERS
BORGIAS
BORIDES
BORINGS
BORROWS
BORZOIS
BOSTONS
BOTCHES
BOTHERS
BOTREES
BOTTLES
BOTTOMS
BOUCHES
BOUDINS
BOUFFES
BOUNCES
BOURSES
BOUTROS
BOVINES
BOWFINS

BOWLERS
BOWLESS
BOWOARS
BOWSAWS
BOWTIES
BOWWOWS
BOWYERS
BOXBEDS
BOXBOYS
BOXCARS
BOXFULS
BOXSETS
BOXTOPS
BOYTOYS
COACHES
COALERS
COALGAS
COATEES
COATERS
COAXERS
COBALTS
COBBLES
COBNUTS
COBWEBS
COCKERS
COCKLES
COCOONS
CODDLES
CODGERS
CODICES
COEDITS
COEPTIS
COERCES
COEVALS
COFFEES
COFFERS
COFFINS
COGGLES
COGNACS
COHEIRS
COHERES
COHORTS
COHOSTS
COIGNES
COILERS
COINERS
COINOPS
COLADAS
COLCHIS
COLLARS
COLLETS
COLLIES
COLLINS
COLLOPS
COLONES
COLONUS
COLOURS
COLUMNS
COMBATS
COMBERS
COMEONS
COMESAS
COMFITS
COMICES
COMINGS
COMMITS
COMMONS
COMOROS

COMPAQS
COMPASS
COMPELS
COMSATS
CONCHES
CONCHOS
CONCURS
CONCUSS
CONDORS
CONFABS
CONFERS
CONFESS
CONFITS
CONGERS
CONGOUS
CONJOBS
CONKERS
CONNORS
CONOIDS
CONSULS
CONTACS
CONTRAS
CONURES
CONVEYS
CONVOYS
COOKERS
COOKIES
COOLERS
COOLIES
COOPERS
COOTERS
COOTIES
COPCARS
COPIERS
COPIOUS
COPOUTS
COPPERS
COPTERS
COPULAS
CORBELS
CORDERS
CORDIAS
CORDONS
CORFAMS
CORKERS
CORNEAS
CORNERS
CORNETS
CORONAS
CORPSES
CORRALS
CORSETS
CORVEES
CORVIDS
CORYZAS
COSHERS
COSIGNS
COSINES
COSSETS
COSTARS
COTTERS
COTTONS
COUCHES
COUGARS
COULEES
COUPLES
COUPONS
COURSES

COUSINS
COUTERS
COVERTS
COWARDS
COWBOYS
COWPEAS
COWRIES
COXLESS
COYDOGS
COYNESS
COYOTES
COZZENS
DOBBINS
DOCENTS
DOCKERS
DOCKETS
DOCTORS
DODDERS
DODGEMS
DODGERS
DOFFERS
DOGAPES
DOGBEDS
DOGDAYS
DOGEARS
DOGGIES
DOGLEGS
DOGLESS
DOGNAPS
DOGRUNS
DOGSITS
DOGTAGS
DOGTOYS
DOILIES
DOLLARS
DOLLIES
DOLLOPS
DOLMANS
DOLORES
DOLOURS
DOMAINS
DOMINOS
DOMINUS
DONATES
DONATUS
DONGLES
DONIMUS
DONJONS
DONKEYS
DONRUSS
DOODADS
DOODLES
DOOLIES
DOOVERS
DOOWOPS
DOOZERS
DOOZIES
DORITOS
DORMERS
DORSALS
DORSEYS
DOSADOS
DOSAGES
DOSHOTS
DOSIDOS
DOSSALS
DOTAGES
DOTARDS

DOTCOMS
DOTTERS
DOTTLES
DOUANES
DOUBLES
DOUGLAS
DOUSERS
DOWDIES
DOWNERS
DOWRIES
DOWSERS
EOLITHS
EOSINES
FOAMERS
FOCSLES
FOCUSES
FODDERS
FOELESS
FOGBOWS
FOGDOGS
FOGGERS
FOGLESS
FOIBLES
FOKKERS
FOLATES
FOLDERS
FOLDUPS
FOLGERS
FOLKIES
FOLLIES
FOLLOWS
FOMENTS
FONDLES
FONDUES
FOODIES
FOOLERS
FOOTERS
FOOTLES
FOOZLES
FORAGES
FORBIDS
FORCEPS
FORCERS
FORDGTS
FORDOES
FORESTS
FORGERS
FORGETS
FORGOES
FORINTS
FORKERS
FORMALS
FORMATS
FORMERS
FORTIES
FORTIUS
FOSSILS
FOSTERS
FOUDRES
FOULUPS
FOURTHS
FOWLERS
FOXNEWS
GOALIES
GOAMISS
GOATEES
GOBBLES
GOBLETS

GOBLINS	HOOVERS	KOREANS	MOBILES	NODDERS	POETESS	POURERS	SOFFITS	TOREROS	ZOCALOS	ILOSTIT	BROWSES	LOOKSIN
GOBYBUS	HOPKINS	KORUNAS	MOCKERS	NODDIES	POETICS	POUTERS	SOFTENS	TORINOS	ZODIACS	KNOSSOS	BUOYSUP	LOOKSON
GOCARTS	HOPPERS	KOSHERS	MOCKUPS	NODULES	POINTES	POWDERS	SOFTIES	TOROIDS	ZOMBIES	KOOSHES	CHOMSKY	LOOKSTO
GODDESS	HORNETS	KOWTOWS	MODELAS	NOETICS	POISERS	POWWOWS	SOIREES	TORQUES	ZONIANS	KTOSLIN	CHOOSER	LOOKSUP
GODLESS	HORRORS	LOADERS	MODELBS	NOGALES	POISONS	POZOLES	SOLACES	TOSSERS	ZONULES	LOOSELY	CHOOSES	MAOISTS
GODSONS	HOSIERS	LOAFERS	MODELTS	NOGGINS	POIVRES	ROACHES	SOLARAS	TOSSUPS	ZOSIMUS	LOOSENS	CHOOSEY	MOONSET
GODWITS	HOSKINS	LOANERS	MODERNS	NOGIFTS	POLARAS	ROADEOS	SOLDERS	TOTINOS	ZOYSIAS	LOOSEST	CHOPSUP	OBOISTS
GOGGLES	HOSTELS	LOATHES	MODULES	NOGOODS	POLARIS	ROADERS	SOLNESS	TOTTERS		LOOSING	CLOGSUP	OPOSSUM
GOGIRLS	HOSTESS	LOBBERS	MODULUS	NOHANDS	POLICES	ROADIES	SOLUTES	TOUCANS	••OS•••	MAOSUIT	CLOTSUP	PIOUSLY
GOITERS	HOTBEDS	LOBBIES	MOHAIRS	NOKOMIS	POLLEES	ROAMERS	SOLVERS	TOUCHES	AHOSTOF	NOOSERS	CNOSSUS	PLOESTI
GOKARTS	HOTCAPS	LOBULES	MOHAVES	NOLOADS	POLLENS	ROARERS	SOMALIS	TOUPEES	ANOSMIA	NOOSING	COOKSUP	PLOWSON
GOLFERS	HOTCARS	LOCALES	MOHAWKS	NOMBRES	POLLERS	ROBARDS	SONATAS	TOURBUS	ANOSMIC	OPOSSUM	COOLSIT	PLOWSUP
GOMPERS	HOTCUPS	LOCATES	MOILERS	NONAGES	POMADES	ROBBERS	SONLESS	TOURERS	APOSTLE	PIOSITY	COOPSUP	POOPSIE
GOOBERS	HOTDAYS	LOCKERS	MOJAVES	NONAMES	POMELOS	ROBBINS	SONNETS	TOUSLES	BLOSSOM	PLOSION	CROESUS	PRODSON
GOODBYS	HOTDOGS	LOCKETS	MOJITOS	NONARTS	POMMELS	ROBERTS	SOONERS	TOUTERS	BOOSLER	PLOSIVE	CROPSUP	PROPSUP
GOODERS	HOTKEYS	LOCKINS	MOLDERS	NONCOMS	POMPOMS	ROBROYS	SOOTHES	TOWAGES	BOOSTED	PROSAIC	CROSSAT	QUONSET
GOODIES	HOTLIPS	LOCKUPS	MOLESTS	NONFANS	POMPONS	ROCHETS	SOPHIES	TOWARDS	BOOSTER	PROSCAN	CROSSED	ROOTSUP
GOOFUPS	HOTNESS	LOCULUS	MOLLIES	NONHITS	POMPOUS	ROCKERS	SORBETS	TOWBARS	BOOSTUP	PROSERS	CROSSER	SHOOSIN
GOOGLES	HOTONES	LOCUSTS	MOLSONS	NONJEWS	PONCHOS	ROCKETS	SORRELS	TOWCARS	BROSNAN	PROSHOP	CROSSES	SHOPSAT
GOOGOLS	HOTPOTS	LODGERS	MOLTERS	NONNEWS	PONDERS	ROCKIES	SORROWS	TOWHEES	BROSSES	PROSIER	CROSSLY	SHOWSIN
GOONEYS	HOTRODS	LOESSES	MOMENTS	NONPARS	PONGEES	ROCOCOS	SORTERS	TOWINGS	CHOSEUP	PROSILY	CROSSUP	SHOWSUP
GOONIES	HOTTEAS	LOFTERS	MOMMIES	NONPLUS	PONGIDS	RODENTS	SORTIES	TOWNERS	CLOSEBY	PROSING	DOOMSTO	SLOPSON
GOPHERS	HOTTIES	LOGGERS	MOMUSES	NONPROS	PONTIUS	RODGERS	SOSPADS	TOWNIES	CLOSEIN	PROSODY	DROPSBY	SLOWSUP
GORDIUS	HOTTIPS	LOGGIAS	MONDAYS	NONUKES	POOCHES	RODLESS	SOUPERS	TOYCARS	CLOSELY	PROSPER	DROPSIN	SNOWSIN
GORGERS	HOTTUBS	LOGGINS	MONGERS	NONWARS	POODLES	ROLAIDS	SOURCES	TOYDOGS	CLOSERS	ROOSTED	DROPSIT	SNOWSKI
GORGONS	HOTWARS	LOGJAMS	MONGOLS	NOODGES	POOLERS	ROLEXES	SOVIETS	TOYGUNS	CLOSEST	ROOSTER	DROSSES	SPONSOR
GOSPELS	HOWARDS	LOGOFFS	MONKEES	NOODLES	POPEYES	ROLFERS	SOXFANS	TOYHATS	CLOSETO	SKOSHES	DROWSED	SPOUSAL
GOSSIPS	HOWDAHS	LOGOUTS	MONKEYS	NOOGIES	POPGUNS	ROLLEIS	SOYINKS	TOYLESS	CLOSETS	SLOSHED	DROWSES	SPOUSES
GOTCHAS	HOWELLS	LOITERS	MONROES	NOONERS	POPLARS	ROLLERS	TOADIES	TOYOTAS	CLOSEUP	SLOSHES	EGOISTE	STOPSAT
GOTHICS	HOWLERS	LOLLERS	MOOCHES	NOOSERS	POPLINS	ROLLINS	TOCSINS	TOYSRUS	CLOSING	TOOSLOW	EGOISTS	STOPSBY
GOUGERS	HOYDENS	LOLLIES	MOOCOWS	NOOTKAS	POPOFFS	ROLLONS	TODDIES	TOYTOPS	CLOSURE	TOOSOON	FLOSSED	STOPSIN
GOURDES	IODATES	LONDRES	MOONERS	NOPALES	POPOUTS	ROLLUPS	TODDLES	VOGUERS	CNOSSUS	TWOSHOT	FLOSSER	STOPSIT
GOVERNS	IODIDES	LONGIES	MOONIES	NORDICS	POPPERS	ROMAINS	TOECAPS	VOICERS	CROSIER	TWOSOME	FLOSSES	STOPSUP
HOAGIES	IODISES	LONGUES	MOOTERS	NORITES	POPPIES	ROMAJIS	TOELESS	VOIDERS	CROSSAT	TWOSPOT	FLOSSIE	STOWSIT
HOAXERS	IODIZES	LOOBIES	MOPPERS	NORMALS	POPPINS	ROMANIS	TOETAPS	VOLLEYS	CROSSED	TWOSTAR	FLOTSAM	SWOOSIE
HOBBIES	IOMOTHS	LOOFAHS	MOPPETS	NORMANS	POPPLES	ROMANOS	TOFFEES	VOLUMES	CROSSER	TWOSTEP	FLOWSIN	TAOISTS
HOBBITS	IONIANS	LOOKERS	MOPTOPS	NORTONS	POPTOPS	ROMANUS	TOGGLES	VOLUTES	CROSSES	USOSHOW	FOOTSIE	THOMSON
HOBBLES	IONISES	LOOKINS	MORALES	NOSEATS	PORCHES	ROMCOMS	TOILERS	VOODOOS	CROSSLY	WHOSAID	FOOTSIT	THORSON
HOBNOBS	IONIUMS	LOOKUPS	MORANIS	NOSHERS	PORGIES	ROMNEYS	TOILETS	VOTECHS	CROSSUP	WHOSOUT	FOOTSUP	TOOLSET
HOBSONS	IONIZES	LOOMPAS	MOREENS	NOSHOWS	PORKERS	ROMPERS	TOLEDOS	VOTEYES	CROSTIC	WHOSWHO	GLOSSAE	TOOLSUP
HOCKERS	IONONES	LOONIES	MORELOS	NOSTARS	PORTALS	ROMULUS	TOLLERS	VOTIVES	DROSSES	WOOSHED	GLOSSAL	TOOTSAT
HOGNUTS	JOBBERS	LOOPERS	MORGANS	NOTATES	PORTERS	RONDELS	TOLTECS	VOUCHES	EGOSURF	WOOSHES	GLOSSAS	TOOTSIE
HOGTIES	JOBCUTS	LOOSENS	MORGUES	NOTCHES	PORTHOS	RONSONS	TOMBOYS	VOWLESS	EROSELY	WOOSNAM	GLOSSED	TROTSKY
HOHNERS	JOBHOPS	LOOTERS	MORMONS	NOTHINS	POSADAS	ROOFERS	TOMCATS	VOYAGES	EROSION	WOOSTER	GLOSSER	TROTSUP
HOLDERS	JOBJARS	LOPPERS	MORROWS	NOTICES	POSEDAS	ROOKIES	TOMTITS	WOBBLES	EROSIVE		GLOSSES	TROUSER
HOLDUPS	JOBLESS	LOQUATS	MORSELS	NOTIONS	POSESAS	ROOMBAS	TOMTOMS	WOMBATS	FLOSSED	••O•S••	GNOSSUS	VRONSKY
HOLISTS	JOBLOTS	LORISES	MORTALS	NOTURNS	POSEURS	ROOMERS	TONEMES	WONDERS	FLOSSER	AROUSAL	GOODSON	WHOISIT
HOLLERS	JOCKEYS	LORRIES	MORTARS	NOUGATS	POSOLES	ROOMIES	TONGANS	WONTONS	FLOSSES	AROUSED	GOOFSUP	WHOOSIS
HOLLIES	JOGBRAS	LORUSES	MORTONS	NOUGHTS	POSSESS	ROOTERS	TONGUES	WOODIES	FLOSSIE	AROUSER	GROSSED	WOODSAW
HOLLOWS	JOGGERS	LOSINGS	MOSAICS	NOVALIS	POSSLQS	ROOTLES	TONSILS	WOOFERS	FROSTED	AROUSES	GROSSER	WOODSON
HOMAGES	JOGGLES	LOTIONS	MOSHERS	NOVELAS	POSSUMS	ROSCOES	TONUSES	WOOLENS	FROSTER	BLOSSOM	GROSSES	WOOLSEY
HOMBRES	JOINERS	LOTTERS	MOSLEMS	NOVENAS	POSTERS	ROSTERS	TOODLES	WOOLIES	GHOSTED	BLOTSUP	GROSSLY	ZOOMSIN
HONCHOS	JOJOBAS	LOTUSES	MOSQUES	NOVICES	POSTIES	ROTATES	TOOLERS	WOOSHES	GHOSTLY	BLOUSED	GROUSED	
HONKERS	JOLLIES	LOUDENS	MOTHERS	NOVOTES	POSTITS	ROTGUTS	TOONIES	WORKERS	GLOSSAE	BLOUSES	GROUSER	••O••S•
HONOURS	JOLTERS	LOUNGES	MOTIONS	NOWNESS	POSTOPS	ROTTERS	TOOTERS	WORKUPS	GLOSSAL	BLOUSON	GROUSES	ABOLISH
HOOCHES	JONESES	LOURDES	MOTIVES	NOWTHIS	POTAGES	ROUSERS	TOOTLES	WORMERS	GLOSSAS	BLOWSIN	GROWSON	AGONISE
HOODIES	JOSBOYS	LOUVERS	MOTLEYS	NOXIOUS	POTAMUS	ROUTERS	TOPAZES	WORRIES	GLOSSED	BLOWSIT	GROWSUP	AGONISM
HOODOOS	JOSHERS	LOUVRES	MOTRINS	NOZZLES	POTEENS	ROVINGS	TOPBIDS	WORSENS	GLOSSER	BLOWSON	HOOFSIT	AGONIST
HOOFERS	JOSTLES	LOVAGES	MOTTLES	OOCYTES	POTFULS	ROWDIES	TOPDOGS	YOGINIS	GLOSSES	BLOWSUP	HOOKSON	AMONGST
HOOHAHS	JOTTERS	LOVEINS	MOTTOES	OOLITES	POTHERS	ROYALES	TOPGUNS	YOGURTS	GNOSSUS	BOOPSIE	HOOKSUP	AMORIST
HOOKAHS	JOUNCES	LOWBIDS	MOUSERS	OOLONGS	POTIONS	SOAKERS	TOPHATS	YOMTOVS	GNOSTIC	BOOTSIT	HOOTSAT	AMOROSO
HOOKUPS	JOURNOS	LOWBOYS	MOUSSES	OOMPAHS	POTLIDS	SOAPERS	TOPLESS	YONKERS	GOOSIER	BOOTSUP	IRONSON	ANODISE
HOOPERS	JOYLESS	LOWMASS	MOVADOS	POACHES	POTPIES	SOARERS	TOPPERS	YOOHOOS	GOOSING	BROASTS	KNOSSOS	ATOMISE
HOOPLAS	JOYPADS	LOWNESS	MOWINGS	POBOXES	POTTERS	SOBBERS	TOPPLES	YORKERS	GROSSED	BRODSKY	KNOTSUP	ATOMISM
HOOPOES	KOBOLDS	LOWTOPS	NOBODYS	POCKETS	POTTIES	SOCIALS	TOPROWS	YORKIES	GROSSER	BRONSON	KNOWSOF	ATOMIST
HOORAHS	KODIAKS	LOYALES	NOCARBS	POCONOS	POUCHES	SOCKETS	TOPTENS	YOTHERS	GROSSES	BROSSES	LOOKSAD	BIOMASS
HOORAYS	KOOSHES	MOANERS	NOCLASS	PODIUMS	POUDRES	SODLESS	TOPTHIS	YOUMANS	GROSSLY	BROWSED	LOOKSAT	BOOHISS
HOOTERS	KOPECKS	MOBBERS	NOCUOUS	POESIES	POUNCES	SOFARAS	TORCHES	YOWLERS	HOOSIER	BROWSER	LOOKSEE	BOOKISH

BOORISH
CHORIST
CLOSEST
COOLEST
COOLISH
DIOCESE
DRONISH
EGOTISM
EGOTIST
ESOBESO
EXOTISM
FLORIST
FOOLISH
GEODESY
GIOCOSO
GLOBOSE
GNOMISH
GNOMIST
GOODISH
GOODUSE
GOOIEST
IDOLISE
IDOLIST
IHOPESO
IRONIST
LIONESS
LIONISE
LOOKISM
LOOKIST
LOOSEST
MOONISH
MOORISH
OLOROSO
OZONISE
POOREST
POORISH
PROCESS
PROEAST
PROFESS
PROFUSE
PROMISE
PROPOSE
PROTEST
PROTIST
PROVISO
PROVOST
PROWESS
PROWEST
ROOKISH
SLOWEST
SLOWISH
SOONEST
TOOEASY
TROPISM
TWOBASE
UNOBESE
UTOPISM
UTOPIST
VIOLIST
ZIONISM
ZIONIST
ZOOIEST

••O•••S

ABOUNDS
ADONAIS
ADORERS
AGONIES
AGOUTIS
AJOWANS
AMOEBAS
AMOROUS
AMOUNTS
ANOINTS
ANOMIES
ANONYMS
ANORAKS
APODOUS
APOGEES
APOLLOS
AROUSES
ATOMICS
ATOMIES
ATONERS
ATONICS
ATONIES
AVOCETS
AVOWALS
AVOWERS
AZODYES
BAOBABS
BIOLABS
BIOMASS
BIONICS
BIOPICS
BLONDES
BLOUSES
BLOWERS
BLOWUPS
BMOVIES
BOOBIES
BOOBOOS
BOOCOOS
BOODLES
BOOGIES
BOOHISS
BOOHOOS
BOOKERS
BOOKIES
BOOMERS
BOONIES
BOOTEES
BOOTERS
BOOTIES
BOOZERS
BROADAS
BROASTS
BRODIES
BROGANS
BROGUES
BROKERS
BRONCOS
BRONTES
BRONZES
BROSSES
BROWSES
CHOICES
CHOKERS
CHOLERS
CHOLLAS
CHOOSES
CHORALS
CHOUGHS
CLOCHES
CLONERS
CLORETS
CLOSERS
CLOSETS
CLOTHES
CLOVERS
CNOSSUS
COOKERS
COOKIES
COOLERS
COOLIES
COOPERS
COOTERS
COOTIES
CROESUS
CRONIES
CROOKES
CROQUIS
CROSSES
CROTONS
CROUTES
CROWERS
DEODARS
DIOXINS
DOODADS
DOODLES
DOOLIES
DOOVERS
DOOWOPS
DOOZERS
DOOZIES
DROGUES
DRONERS
DROPINS
DROSSES
DROVERS
DROWSES
DROXIES
EBONICS
EBONIES
EGOISTS
ELOPERS
EMOTERS
EPONYMS
EPOPEES
EPOQUES
EPOXIES
ERODERS
EROTICS
ETOILES
ETONICS
EUONYMS
EVOKERS
EVOLVES
EXOCETS
EXONYMS
EXOTICS
FLORETS
FLORINS
FLOSSES
FLOWERS
FOODIES
FOOLERS
FOOTERS
FOOTLES
FOOZLES
FROLICS
GAOLERS
GEORGES
GFORCES
GIORGOS
GLOBINS
GLOBOUS
GLORIAS
GLORIES
GLOSSAS
GLOSSES
GLOTTIS
GLOWERS
GNOMONS
GNOSSUS
GOOBERS
GOODBYS
GOODERS
GOODIES
GOOFUPS
GOOGLES
GOOGOLS
GOONEYS
GOONIES
GROCERS
GROOVES
GROPERS
GROPIUS
GROSSES
GROTIUS
GROTTOS
GROUNDS
GROUSES
GROVELS
GROVERS
GROWERS
GROWTHS
HOOCHES
HOODIES
HOODOOS
HOOFERS
HOOHAHS
HOOKAHS
HOOKUPS
HOOPERS
HOOPLAS
HOOPOES
HOORAHS
HOORAYS
HOOTERS
HOOVERS
IGOROTS
IRONERS
IRONIES
IRONONS
ISOBARS
ISOGONS
ISOHELS
ISOMERS
ISOPODS
IVORIES
KNOSSOS
KNOWERS
KNOWLES
KOOSHES
LEONIDS
LIONELS
LIONESS
LIONETS
LOOBIES
LOOFAHS
LOOKERS
LOOKINS
LOOKUPS
LOOMPAS
LOONIES
LOOPERS
LOOSENS
LOOTERS
MAOISTS
MEOWERS
MNOPQRS
MOOCHES
MOOCOWS
MOONERS
MOONIES
MOOTERS
MYOPIAS
NEOCONS
NEONGAS
NOODGES
NOODLES
NOOGIES
NOONERS
NOOSERS
NOOTKAS
OBOISTS
ODOROUS
OLOGIES
OZONOUS
PEONIES
PEOPLES
PHOBIAS
PHOBICS
PHOEBES
PHOEBUS
PHONERS
PHONEYS
PHONICS
PHONIES
PHOTICS
PHOTOGS
PHOTONS
PIOLETS
PLOTZES
PLOUGHS
PLOVERS
PLOWERS
POOCHES
POODLES
POOLERS
PROBERS
PROBIES
PROCESS
PROCLUS
PROFESS
PROFITS
PROJETS
PROKEDS
PROLOGS
PROMPTS
PROPELS
PROSERS
PROTEUS
PROTONS
PROVERS
PROWESS
PROXIES
QUORUMS
QUOTEES
QUOTERS
REOPENS
RHOECUS
RHOMBUS
RIOTERS
RIOTOUS
ROOFERS
ROOKIES
ROOMBAS
ROOMERS
ROOMIES
ROOTERS
ROOTLES
RYOKANS
SCONCES
SCOOBAS
SCORERS
SCORIAS
SCOTERS
SCOUPES
SHOFARS
SHOGUNS
SHOOINS
SHOPKOS
SHOPPES
SHOVELS
SHOVERS
SHOWERS
SIOUANS
SKOSHES
SLOGANS
SLOPERS
SLOSHES
SLOUGHS
SLOVAKS
SLOVENS
SLOWUPS
SMOKERS
SMOKEYS
SMOKIES
SMOOTHS
SNOCAPS
SNOCATS
SNOOZES
SNORERS
SOONERS
SOOTHES
SPONGES
SPOUSES
STODGES
STOGIES
STOKERS
STOLONS
STONERS
STOOGES
STORERS
STORIES
STOTINS
STOWERS
TAOISTS
TOODLES
TOOLERS
TOONIES
TOOTERS
TOOTLES
TROCHES
TROIKAS
TROILUS
TROJANS
TROPICS
TROUGHS
TROUPES
TROWELS
TSONGAS
TSOURIS
TWOACTS
TWOBITS
TWODAYS
TWOEGGS
TWOFERS
TWOTONS
USOPENS
UTOPIAS
VIOLETS
VIOLINS
VOODOOS
WHOOSIS
WOODIES
WOOFERS
WOOLENS
WOOLIES
WOOSHES
YEOMANS
YOOHOOS

•••OS••

ACCOSTS
AEROSOL
ALROSEN
ALTOSAX
ALYOSHA
APPOSED
APPOSES
ARIOSOS
ARIOSTO
CHOOSER
CHOOSES
CHOOSEY
COHOSTS
COLOSSI
CREOSOL
DACOSTA
DAMOSEL
DEPOSAL
DEPOSED
DEPOSER
DEPOSES
DEPOSIT
EMBOSOM
ESPOSAS
ESPOSOS
EXPOSED
EXPOSER
EXPOSES
EXPOSIT
GOTOSEA
GOTOSEE
HEXOSES
IMPOSED
IMPOSER
IMPOSES
IMPOSTS
KENOSHA
LACOSTE
LATOSCA
LEGOSET
MEIOSES
MEIOSIS
MIMOSAS
MITOSES
MITOSIS
MONOSKI
NICOSIA
OPPOSED
OPPOSER
OPPOSES
OSMOSED
OSMOSES
OSMOSIS
OSTOSIS
RECOSTS
REDOSED
REDOSES
RELOSES
REPOSED
REPOSER
REPOSES
REPOSIT
REPOSTS
RIPOSTE
RIPOSTS
SAMOSAS
SAMOSET
SHOOSIN
SWOOSIE
UNBOSOM
UNMOSSY
UNNOSED
UNPOSED
UTMOSTS
WHOOSIS
XEROSES
XEROSIS
XYLOSES
ZEROSIN
ZEROSUM

•••O•S•

ALFONSE
ALFONSO
ALTOIST
ATWORST
AUTOPSY
CABOOSE
CAROUSE
COLOSSI
DELOUSE
ECHOISM
ENDORSE
ESPOUSE
FAROESE
FATOUSH
GENOESE
GENOISE
HELOISE
HEROISM
HOBOISM
INDORSE
INHOUSE
JUDOIST
LALOOSH
LITOVSK
MRHORSE
MRMOOSE
NICOISE
NONOISE
NOWORSE
OFNOUSE
OKHOTSK
ONTOAST
PAPOOSE
POLOIST
REHOUSE
REMORSE
RETOAST
SOLOIST
STROUSE
SUMOIST
TITOISM
TITOIST
TOHORSE
UNHORSE
UNHOUSE
UNLOOSE
UNMOIST
UNMOSSY
UNNOISY
UPCOAST
UPROUSE
VAMOOSE
VBLOUSE

•••O••S

ABSORBS
ACCORDS
ACCOSTS
ADJOINS
ADNOUNS
ADSORBS
AEROBES
AFFORDS
ALCOVES
ALLOFUS
ALMONDS
ALTOIDS
ANGORAS
ANYONES
APPOSES
APROPOS
ARBOLES
ARBOURS
ARDOURS
AREOLAS
AREOLES
ARIOSOS
ARMOURS
ARNOLDS
ARROYOS
ASSORTS
ATHOMES
ATROPOS
AURORAS
AUTOBUS
BABOONS
BAROLOS
BECOMES
BEFOOLS
BEFOULS
BEHOLDS
BELONGS
BEMOANS
BENOTES
BICORNS
BIGONES
BOWOARS
BUGOUTS
BUJONES
BULOVAS
BUROAKS
BUYOFFS
BUYOUTS
BYFORMS
BYGONES
BYROADS
BYWORDS
CAHOOTS
CAJOLES
CANOERS
CANOLAS
CANOPUS
CAPOTES
CAVORTS
CHOOSES
CHROMES
COCOONS
COHORTS
COHOSTS
COLONES
COLONUS
COLOURS
COMOROS
CONOIDS
COPOUTS
CORONAS
COYOTES
CREOLES
CROOKES
CUBOIDS
CUPOLAS
CUTOFFS
CUTOUTS
CYBORGS
DAKOTAS
DEBONES
DECOCTS
DECODES
DEFOAMS
DEFOCUS
DEFORMS
DEHORNS
DELORIS
DEMOTES
DEMOTHS
DENOTES
DEPONES
DEPORTS
DEPOSES
DESOTOS
DETOURS
DETOXES
DEVOIRS
DEVORES
DEVOTES
DEVOURS
DEWORMS
DIEOFFS
DIMOUTS
DIPOLES
DISOWNS
DOLORES
DOLOURS
DUGONGS
DUGOUTS
DYNODES
ECHOERS
EDMONDS
EFFORTS
ELFOWLS
ENCODES
ENCORES
ENFOLDS
ENJOINS
ENROBES
ENROLLS
ENROOTS
ENSOULS
ENTOMBS
ESCORTS
ESPOSAS
ESPOSOS
EXHORTS
EXPORTS
EXPOSES
EXTOLLS
EXTORTS
EXWORKS
FANOUTS
FATONES
FAVOURS
FEDORAS
FEMORIS
FURORES
GALOOTS
GENOMES
GIGOLOS
GROOVES
HALOIDS
HEROICS
HEXOSES
HONOURS
HOTONES
HUMOURS
ICEOUTS
IGNORES
IMPORTS
IMPOSES
IMPOSTS
IMYOURS
INBOXES
INCOMES
INDOORS
INFOCUS
INFOLDS
INFORMS
INGOALS
INJOKES
INPOURS
INROADS
INSOLES
INTONES
INVOKES
IOMOTHS
IONONES
JCPOWYS
JOJOBAS
JUDOKAS
KCJONES
KETONES
KIMONOS
KOBOLDS
LABOURS
LAGOONS
LAKOTAS
LAVORIS
LAYODDS
LAYOFFS
LAYOUTS
LEGOLAS
LENOVOS
LIMOGES
LITOTES
LOGOFFS
LOGOUTS
MACOUNS
MAHOUTS
MAROONS
MEGOHMS
MEIOSES
MEIOSIS
MEMOIRS
MIDOFFS
MILORDS
MIMOSAS
MINOANS
MITOSES
MITOSIS
MRBONES
MRHOBBS
MRJONES
MRWORDS
MYKONOS
NICOLAS
NOBODYS
NOGOODS
NOKOMIS
NOLOADS
NOVOTES
NUTOILS
OBLONGS
OCTOPUS
OFSORTS
OGDOADS
OHIOANS
ONEOFFS
ONEOFUS
ONLOADS
OOLONGS
OPPOSES
ORIOLES
ORMOLUS
OSMONDS
OSMOSES
OSMOSIS
OSTOSIS
OXFORDS
PAGODAS
PALOMAS
PAROLES
PAYOFFS
PAYOLAS
PAYOUTS
PELOTAS
PEYOTES
PHLOEMS
PHLOXES
PIGOUTS
PINOAKS
PINONES
POBOXES
POCONOS
POPOFFS
POPOUTS
POSOLES
POZOLES
PTBOATS
PUTOFFS
PUTOUTS
RADOMES
RAGOUTS
RAMONES
RCCOLAS
REBOILS
REBOLTS
REBOOKS
REBOOTS
REBORES
REBOTES
REBOXES
REBOZOS
RECOALS
RECOATS
RECOCKS
RECODES
RECOILS
RECOINS
RECOMBS
RECOOKS
RECOOLS
RECORDS
RECORKS
RECOSTS
RECOUPS
REDOAKS
REDOCKS
REDOSES
REDOUTS
REDOXES
REFOCUS
REFOLDS
REFORMS
REHONES
REHOOKS
REJOINS
RELOADS
RELOANS
RELOCKS
RELOOKS
RELOSES
REMOLDS
REMORAS
REMOTES
REMOVES
RENOIRS
RENOTES
RENOWNS
REPOLLS
REPORTS
REPOSES
REPOSTS
REPOURS
REROLLS
REROOFS
REROOTS
RESOAKS

RESOAPS
RESOILS
RESOLES
RESORBS
RESORTS
RETONES
RETOOLS
RETORTS
RETOURS
REVOKES
REVOLTS
REVOTES
REWORDS
REWORKS
REYOKES
REZONES
RIGOURS
RIPOFFS
RIPOSTS
ROCOCOS
RUMOURS
RUNOFFS
RUNOUTS
SALOONS
SAMOANS
SAMOSAS
SARONGS
SATORIS
SAVOURS
SCHOLES
SCHOOLS
SCOOBAS
SCROLLS
SECONDS
SEDONAS
SENORAS
SENORES
SETOFFS
SETOUTS
SHNOOKS
SHOOINS
SHROUDS
SMOOTHS
SNOOZES
SPROUTS
STJOHNS
STLOUIS
STOOGES
STROBES
STROKES
STROLLS
SUBORNS
SUDOKUS
TACOMAS
TAGOUTS
TANOAKS
TAROILS
TEEOFFS
TFPOWYS
THROATS
THRONES
THRONGS
TINORES
TIPOFFS
TOROIDS
TOYOTAS
TRIODES
TRYOUTS
TVROOMS
TYCOONS
UNBOLTS
UNBOXES
UNCOILS
UNCOOPS
UNCORES
UNCORKS
UNDOCKS
UNDOERS
UNFOLDS
UNFORKS
UNHOODS
UNHOOKS
UNJOINS
UNLOADS
UNLOCKS
UNLOOPS
UNMOLDS
UNMOORS
UNROBES
UNROLLS
UNROOFS
UNROOTS
UNROPES
UNSOLES
UNSORTS
UNYOKES
UNZONES
UPCOILS
UPFOLDS
UPHOLDS
UPLOADS
UPROARS
UPROOTS
UPSOARS
UPTOWNS
UTMOSTS
VALOURS
VAPOURS
VELOURS
VELOXES
VETOERS
VIGOURS
WEEONES
WETONES
WHOOSIS
WHWORDS
XEROSES
XEROSIS
XEROXES
XYLOSES
YUKOLIS
ZEDONKS
ZYGOTES

••••OS•

ACEROSE
ADIPOSE
AFTMOST
AIRHOSE
ALAMOSA
AMBROSE
AMOROSO
ARENOSE
ATACOST
ATALOSS
ATCROSS
AXLROSE
BEDPOST
BIGBOSS
BIGNOSE
BYANOSE
CABOOSE
COMPOSE
COMPOST
CURIOSA
DEFROST
DEGHOST
DISPOSE
DOGROSE
DONJOSE
EGGTOSS
ENCLOSE
ENDMOST
ENGROSS
FESTOSO
FOLIOSE
FORMOSA
FURIOSO
GETLOST
GIOCOSO
GJETOST
GLOBOSE
GLUCOSE
GOTLOST
HERMOSA
HERMOSO
HOGNOSE
INCLOSE
LACTOSE
LALOOSH
LOWCOST
LOWPOST
MAFIOSI
MAFIOSO
MALTOSE
MELROSE
MIDMOST
MRMOOSE
NETCOST
NETLOSS
OAKMOSS
OLDROSE
OLOROSO
OMIGOSH
OPEROSE
OSHKOSH
OUTMOST
OUTPOST
PAPOOSE
PENROSE
PIETOSO
PITBOSS
PLUMOSE
PRELOSS
PREVOST
PROPOSE
PROVOST
PUGNOSE
PURPOSE
REAROSE
RECHOSE
RECROSS
REDNOSE
REDROSE
REGLOSS
REYNOSA
SANJOSE
SEAMOSS
SUBPOST
SUBROSA
SUCROSE
SUPPOSE
TEAROSE
THEBOSS
THEMOST
THEPOST
THEROSE
TOPMOST
UNCLOSE
UNCROSS
UNFROST
UNGROSS
UNLOOSE
UPCLOSE
VAMOOSE
VERBOSE
VFWPOST
VINROSE
YOULOSE

••••O•S

ABATORS
ACTIONS
AHCHOOS
AIRLOGS
AIRPOPS
AIRPOTS
AMATOLS
AMAZONS
AMIDOLS
AMNIONS
AMOROUS
ANALOGS
ANCHORS
ANDROUS
ANTCOWS
ANXIOUS
APODOUS
AQUEOUS
ARCHONS
ARDUOUS
ATALOSS
ATCROSS
AUTHORS
AVALONS
BABOONS
BADBOYS
BADDOGS
BADLOTS
BAGBOYS
BAGJOBS
BAILORS
BALBOAS
BALLOTS
BAMBOOS
BANJOES
BARHOPS
BARRONS
BARROWS
BARYONS
BATBOYS
BBSHOTS
BCLIONS
BEACONS
BECKONS
BEDLOES
BEFOOLS
BELLOWS
BESTOWS
BETTORS
BICHONS
BIGBOSS
BIGBOYS
BIGDOGS
BIGLOTS
BIGTOES
BIGTOPS
BILIOUS
BILLOWS
BIMBOES
BINGOES
BISHOPS
BLAZONS
BONBONS
BONGOES
BONMOTS
BOOBOOS
BOOCOOS
BOOHOOS
BORROWS
BORZOIS
BOSTONS
BOTTOMS
BOWWOWS
BOXBOYS
BOXTOPS
BOYTOYS
BRAVOES
BRETONS
BRITONS
BRUMOUS
BUCKOES
BUGBOYS
BULBOUS
BUNIONS
BURBOTS
BURGOOS
BURROWS
BUSBOYS
BUTTONS
CAHOOTS
CALLOUS
CAMBOYS
CAMIONS
CANNONS
CANTONS
CANTORS
CANYONS
CAPTORS
CARBONS
CARBOYS
CARGOES
CARHOPS
CARIOUS
CARLOTS
CARPOUS
CARROTS
CARTONS
CARTOPS
CASEOUS
CATIONS
CATTOYS
CENSORS
CHALONS
CHAMOIS
CHEVONS
CHIGOES
CHINOIS
CHITONS
CHYRONS
CISCOES
CITRONS
CITROUS
CLAMORS
CLIPONS
COCOONS
COINOPS
COLLOPS
COMEONS
COMMONS
CONDORS
CONGOUS
CONJOBS
CONNORS
CONVOYS
COPIOUS
CORDONS
COTTONS
COUPONS
COWBOYS
COYDOGS
CRAYONS
CROTONS
CUCKOOS
CUPROUS
CURIOUS
CURSORS
CUSTOMS
CYCLOPS
DACRONS
DAEMONS
DAEWOOS
DALTONS
DAMSONS
DAYHOPS
DAYJOBS
DEACONS
DEBTORS
DECLOTS
DEFCONS
DELSOLS
DENMOMS
DENTONS
DEPLOYS
DESMOGS
DESPOTS
DEVIOUS
DIALOGS
DIATOMS
DIGLOTS
DINGOES
DOCTORS
DOGTOYS
DOLLOPS
DONJONS
DOOWOPS
DOSHOTS
DOTCOMS
DRAGONS
DRYFOGS
DRYMOPS
DRYROTS
DUBIOUS
DUNLOPS
DUTEOUS
DYEJOBS
DYELOTS
EDITORS
EELPOTS
EGGNOGS
EGGTOSS
ELEVONS
EMPLOYS
EMULOUS
ENAMORS
ENGROSS
ENROOTS
ENVIOUS
EPILOGS
ESCROWS
ETYMONS
FACTORS
FAEROES
FALCONS
FALLOWS
FANDOMS
FANIONS
FANTODS
FARROWS
FATHOMS
FATUOUS
FELLOWS
FEMBOTS
FERROUS
FERVORS
FIBROUS
FLACONS
FLAGONS
FLAVORS
FLEXORS
FLYBOYS
FLYRODS
FOGBOWS
FOGDOGS
FOLLOWS
FORDOES
FORGOES
FRIVOLS
FUNGOES
FURIOUS
FURROWS
FUSIONS
GALLONS
GALLOPS
GALLOWS
GALOOTS
GAMBOLS
GAMMONS
GARCONS
GASCONS
GASEOUS
GASHOGS
GASLOGS
GECKOES
GESSOES
GIBBONS
GIBBOUS
GIBSONS
GIDEONS
GLAMORS
GLOBOUS
GLYCOLS
GNOMONS
GODSONS
GOOGOLS
GORGONS
GUNDOGS
GUSTOES
GUVNORS
HADRONS
HALLOOS
HALLOWS
HANSOMS
HARBORS
HARLOTS
HARRODS
HARROWS
HAYMOWS
HECTORS
HEINOUS
HELLOES
HIDEOUS
HILTONS
HOBNOBS
HOBSONS
HOLLOWS
HOODOOS
HOOPOES
HORRORS
HOTDOGS
HOTPOTS
HOTRODS
HYDROUS
HYSSOPS
ICEFOGS
ICEPOPS
IGNEOUS
IGOROTS
IMAGOES
IMPIOUS
INDOORS
INFLOWS
INIRONS
INKNOTS
INKPOTS
INSPOTS
IRONONS
ISOGONS
ISOPODS
JAILORS
JARGONS
JEALOUS
JERBOAS
JETSONS
JIMSONS
JINGOES
JOBHOPS
JOBLOTS
JOSBOYS
JUNCOES
JUNIORS
KIDCOMS
KLAXONS
KMESONS
KOWTOWS
LAGOONS
LAPDOGS
LAPTOPS
LARDONS
LASSOES
LAZBOYS
LECTORS
LEGIONS
LENNONS
LEPTONS
LESIONS
LESSONS
LESSORS
LIENORS
LINGOES
LIQUORS
LOTIONS
LOWBOYS
LOWTOPS
MACRONS
MADDOGS
MAGGOTS
MAHZORS
MAISONS
MALLOWS
MANGOES
MARMOTS
MAROONS
MARRONS
MARROWS
MASCOTS
MATRONS
MATZOHS
MAUROIS
MEADOWS
MELLOWS
MENTORS
MERLOTS
METEORS
METHODS
MICRONS
MIGNONS
MILHOUS
MINIONS
MINNOWS
MIRRORS
MISDOES
MOLSONS
MONGOLS
MONROES
MOOCOWS
MOPTOPS
MORMONS
MORROWS
MORTONS
MOTIONS
MOTTOES
MUTTONS
NARROWS
NATIONS
NELSONS
NEOCONS
NERVOUS
NESTORS
NETLOSS
NETTONS
NEURONS
NEWJOBS
NEWTONS
NEWTOYS
NICHOLS
NIMRODS
NITROUS
NIVEOUS
NOCUOUS
NOGOODS
NONCOMS
NORTONS
NOSHOWS
NOTIONS
NOXIOUS
OAKMOSS
OBVIOUS
OCELOTS
OCHROUS
OCTROIS
ODDJOBS
ODDLOTS
ODOROUS
OLDBOYS
OLDDOGS
OMINOUS
ONEROUS
OPTIONS
ORATORS
ORISONS
OSSEOUS
OUTBOWS
OUTDOES
OUTGOES
OUTPOPS
OUTROWS
OZONOUS
PALLORS
PARDONS
PARLORS
PARLOUS
PARROTS
PARSONS
PASTORS
PATROLS
PATRONS
PAVIORS
PEAPODS
PEGTOPS
PENNONS
PEPBOYS
PEQUOTS
PERIODS
PERSONS
PETBOAS
PETCOWS
PETDOGS
PETROLS
PETROUS
PETTOYS
PHENOLS
PHENOMS
PHILOUS
PHOTOGS
PHOTONS
PICEOUS
PIGEONS
PILEOUS
PILLOWS
PINBOYS
PINIONS
PINKOES
PISTOLS
PISTONS
PISTOUS
PITBOSS
PITEOUS
PITROWS
PLEXORS
PLUTONS
POISONS
POMPOMS
POMPONS
POMPOUS
POPTOPS
POSTOPS
POTIONS
POWWOWS
PRELOSS
PRETORS
PRISONS
PROLOGS
PROTONS
PTEROUS
PULLONS
PYEDOGS
PYTHONS
QUAHOGS
RAGMOPS
RAGTOPS
RAISONS
RAMRODS
RAMSONS
RANCORS
RANSOMS
RAPTORS
RATIONS
RAUCOUS
REASONS
REAVOWS
REBOOKS
REBOOTS
RECKONS
RECOOKS
RECOOLS
RECROSS
RECTORS
REDCODS
REDDOGS
REDDOTS
REDHOTS
REDTOPS
REEBOKS
REFLOWS
REGIONS
REGLOSS
REGLOWS
REGROWS
REHOOKS
REKNOTS
RELOOKS
RENVOIS
REPLOTS
REPLOWS
REROOFS
REROOTS
RESHOES
RESHOWS
RESPOTS
RESTOWS
RETOOLS
RHEBOKS
RHETORS
RIBBONS
RIOTOUS
ROBROYS
ROLLONS
ROMCOMS
RONSONS
ROSCOES
RUBIOUS
RUINOUS
SAILORS
SAISONS
SALMONS
SALOONS
SALVOES
SALVORS
SAMSONS
SARTORS
SATCOMS
SAVIORS
SAWLOGS
SCHMOES
SCHOOLS
SEACOWS
SEADOGS
SEAGODS
SEAMOSS
SEASONS
SECTORS
SEIZORS
SENIORS
SENSORS
SERIOUS
SERMONS
SEXPOTS
SEXTONS
SHADOWS
SHAKOES
SHALOMS
SHNOOKS
SIDDONS
SIDIOUS
SIGNORS
SIMMONS
SINUOUS
SIPHONS
SITCOMS
SKIBOBS
SKIDOOS
SKITOWS
SLALOMS
SLIPONS
SNAPONS
SORROWS
SPIGOTS
SPYBOTS
STATORS
STEROLS
STOLONS
STUPORS
SUBGODS
SUBLOTS
SUCCORS
SUITORS
SUMMONS
SUNBOWS
SUNDOGS
SUNGODS
SYMBOLS
TAILORS
TALLOWS
TARPONS
TATTOOS
TAYLORS
TEAPOTS
TEAPOYS
TEDIOUS
TEFLONS
TENDONS
TENSORS
TENTONS
TENUOUS
TERRORS
TEUTONS
THEBOSS
THEBOYS
THEHOGS
TIERODS
TIGLONS
TINGODS
TIPTOES
TIPTOPS
TISSOTS
TOMBOYS
TOMTOMS
TOPDOGS
TOPROWS
TOYDOGS
TOYTOPS
TREMORS
TRICOTS
TRIGONS
TRIPODS
TRITONS
TUCSONS
TURBOTS
TURNONS
TVIDOLS
TVROOMS
TVSHOWS
TVSPOTS
TWOTONS
TYCOONS
UNCLOGS
UNCOOPS
UNCROSS
UNGROSS
UNHOODS
UNHOOKS
UNIPODS
UNISOMS
UNISONS
UNKNOTS
UNLOOPS
UNMOORS
UNPIOUS
UNROOFS
UNROOTS
UNSHOES
UNSTOPS
UNSTOWS

UPFLOWS
UPGROWS
UPPROPS
UPROOTS
UPSHOTS
VACUOUS
VARIOUS
VAUDOIS
VECTORS
VENDORS
VICIOUS
VICTORS
VIDIOTS
VISCOUS
VISIONS
VOODOOS
WALKONS
WALLOPS
WALLOWS
WALTONS
WANTONS
WARGODS
WEAKONS
WEAPONS
WEBLOGS
WETMOPS
WILLOWS
WILSONS
WINDOMS
WINDOWS
WINNOWS
WISDOMS
WONTONS
YARROWS
YELLOWS
YOMTOVS
YOOHOOS
ZEALOTS
ZEALOUS
ZINCOUS
ZIPLOCS
ZIPTOPS
ZIRCONS
ZITCOMS

•••••OS

ACCTNOS
ADAGIOS
AHCHOOS
AIKIDOS
ALBEDOS
ALBINOS
ALNICOS
APOLLOS
APROPOS
ARIOSOS
ARISTOS
ARROYOS
ASIAGOS
ATROPOS
BAGNIOS
BAMBOOS
BAROLOS
BARRIOS
BENTHOS
BISTROS
BOLEROS
BONITOS
BOOBOOS
BOOCOOS
BOOHOOS
BOUTROS
BRILLOS
BRONCOS
BURGOOS
CABRIOS
CALICOS
CAMAROS
CAMINOS
CASINOS
CATALOS
CHARROS
CHEETOS
CHURROS
COMOROS
CONCHOS
CREEPOS
CRYPTOS
CUATROS
CUCKOOS
DACAPOS
DAEWOOS
DESOTOS
DIABLOS
DIARIOS
DISTROS
DOMINOS
DORITOS
DOSADOS
DOSIDOS
DRCHAOS
DUETTOS
DYNAMOS
ELNINOS
EMBRYOS
ENDUROS
ENVIROS
ERYNGOS
ESCUDOS
ESKIMOS
ESPOSOS
ESTADOS
FIASCOS
FRESCOS
FUGATOS
GABBROS
GALANOS
GAUCHOS
GAZEBOS
GELATOS
GHETTOS
GIGOLOS
GINGKOS
GINKGOS
GIORGOS
GITANOS
GRINGOS
GROTTOS
HAIRDOS
HALLOOS
HONCHOS
HOODOOS
INDIGOS
JAZZBOS
JOURNOS
KAKAPOS
KAKUROS
KIARIOS
KIMONOS
KLEPTOS
KNOSSOS
LADINOS
LAREDOS
LATIGOS
LATINOS
LAVABOS
LEANTOS
LEGATOS
LENOVOS
LIBIDOS
LINDROS
LLADROS
MACACOS
MADUROS
MAKEDOS
MARIDOS
MEDICOS
MENUDOS
MERINOS
MIKADOS
MOJITOS
MORELOS
MOVADOS
MTATHOS
MURANOS
MUSTDOS
MYKONOS
NAVAHOS
NAVAJOS
NONPROS
NUMEROS
NUNCIOS
OBENTOS
OCTAVOS
OLDPROS
ONETWOS
PAPAGOS
PGAPROS
PHILCOS
PHYLLOS
PICAROS
PIETROS
POCONOS
POMELOS
PONCHOS
PORTHOS
PRESTOS
PSYCHOS
PUEBLOS
QRATIOS
QUARTOS
QUEIROS
QUIZNOS
RACINOS
RANCHOS
REBOZOS
REREDOS
REZEROS
RIALTOS
ROADEOS
ROCOCOS
ROMANOS
RUBATOS
SABADOS
SHOPKOS
SKIDOOS
SPEEDOS
STEREOS
STERNOS
STUCCOS
STUDIOS
TATTOOS
TEATROS
TECHNOS
TEJANOS
THERMOS
TIEMPOS
TOLEDOS
TOREROS
TORINOS
TOTINOS
TUPELOS
TUXEDOS
VELCROS
VIRAGOS
VOODOOS
WEIRDOS
WENDKOS
XSANDOS
YOOHOOS
ZOCALOS
ZYDECOS

OT•••••

OTALGIA
OTALGIC
OTARIES
OTHELLO
OTOLOGY
OTRANTO
OTTAVIO
OTTAWAN
OTTAWAS
OTTOIII
OTTOMAN
OTTUMWA

O•T••••

OATBRAN
OATCAKE
OATLIKE
OATMEAL
OBTAINS
OBTESTS
OBTRUDE
OBTUNDS
OBTUSER
OCTADIC
OCTAGON
OCTANES
OCTANTS
OCTAVAL
OCTAVES
OCTAVIA
OCTAVIO
OCTAVOS
OCTETTE
OCTOBER
OCTOBRE
OCTOPOD
OCTOPUS
OCTROIS
OCTUBRE
OCTUPLE
OCTUPLY
OFTENER
OKTOBER
ONTARIO
ONTHEDL
ONTHEGO
ONTHEQT
ONTHREE
ONTKEAN
ONTOAST
ONTOPIC
ONTOPOF
ONTRACK
ONTRIAL
OPTEDIN
OPTEDTO
OPTICAL
OPTICKS
OPTIMAL
OPTIMAS
OPTIMUM
OPTIONS
OPTSFOR
OPTSOUT
ORTEGAL
ORTOLAN
OSTEOID
OSTIARY
OSTLERS
OSTMARK
OSTOSIS
OSTRAVA
OSTRICH
OSTWALD
OTTAVIO
OTTAWAN
OTTAWAS
OTTOIII
OTTOMAN
OTTUMWA
OUTACTS
OUTADDS
OUTAGES
OUTASKS
OUTAWED
OUTAWES
OUTBACK
OUTBAKE
OUTBANS
OUTBARK
OUTBATS
OUTBAWL
OUTBEAM
OUTBEGS
OUTBEND
OUTBIDS
OUTBLOT
OUTBLOW
OUTBOWL
OUTBOWS
OUTBRAG
OUTBRAY
OUTBRED
OUTBUDS
OUTBULK
OUTBURN
OUTBUYS
OUTBUZZ
OUTCALL
OUTCANT
OUTCAST
OUTCITY
OUTCOLD
OUTCOME
OUTCOOK
OUTCROP
OUTCROW
OUTCULL
OUTCURE
OUTCUTS
OUTDARE
OUTDATE
OUTDOER
OUTDOES
OUTDONE
OUTDOOR
OUTDRAG
OUTDRAW
OUTDREW
OUTDROP
OUTDUEL
OUTEARN
OUTEATS
OUTECHO
OUTEDGE
OUTFACE
OUTFAST
OUTFAWN
OUTFEED
OUTFEEL
OUTFIND
OUTFIRE
OUTFISH
OUTFITS
OUTFLEE
OUTFLOW
OUTFLUX
OUTFOOL
OUTFOOT
OUTGAIN
OUTGAME
OUTGAVE
OUTGAZE
OUTGIVE
OUTGLOW
OUTGNAW
OUTGOES
OUTGREW
OUTGRIN
OUTGROW
OUTGUNS
OUTGUSH
OUTHAUL
OUTHEAR
OUTHERE
OUTHIRE
OUTHISS
OUTHITS
OUTHOWL
OUTHUNT
OUTHURL
OUTINGS
OUTJEST
OUTJETS
OUTJINX
OUTJUMP
OUTJUTS
OUTKAST
OUTKEEP
OUTKEPT
OUTKICK
OUTKILL
OUTKING
OUTKISS
OUTLAID
OUTLAIN
OUTLAND
OUTLASH
OUTLAST
OUTLAWS
OUTLAYS
OUTLEAD
OUTLEAP
OUTLETS
OUTLIER
OUTLIES
OUTLIMN
OUTLINE
OUTLIPS
OUTLIVE
OUTLOOK
OUTLOUD
OUTLOVE
OUTMANS
OUTMATE
OUTMODE
OUTMOST
OUTMOVE
OUTOFIT
OUTPACE
OUTPAID
OUTPASS
OUTPATH
OUTPAYS
OUTPEEP
OUTPICK
OUTPIPE
OUTPITY
OUTPLAN
OUTPLAY
OUTPLOD
OUTPLOT
OUTPOLL
OUTPOPS
OUTPORT
OUTPOST
OUTPOUR
OUTPRAY
OUTPULL
OUTPURL
OUTPUSH
OUTPUTS
OUTRACE
OUTRAGE
OUTRAIL
OUTRANG
OUTRANK
OUTRANT
OUTRAPS
OUTRATE
OUTRAVE
OUTREAD
OUTRIBS
OUTRIDE
OUTRIGS
OUTRING
OUTROAR
OUTROCK
OUTRODE
OUTROLL
OUTROOT
OUTROVE
OUTROWS
OUTRUNS
OUTRUSH
OUTSAID
OUTSAIL
OUTSANG
OUTSAYS
OUTSEEK
OUTSEEN
OUTSEES
OUTSELL
OUTSERT
OUTSETS
OUTSHOT
OUTSHOW
OUTSIDE
OUTSIFT
OUTSIGH
OUTSING
OUTSINS
OUTSITS
OUTSIZE
OUTSKIP
OUTSOAR
OUTSOLD
OUTSOLE
OUTSPED
OUTSPIN
OUTSPIT
OUTSTAY
OUTSTEP
OUTSULK
OUTSUMS
OUTSUNG
OUTSWAM
OUTSWIM
OUTSWUM
OUTTAKE
OUTTALK
OUTTEAR
OUTTELL
OUTTIRE
OUTTOLD
OUTTOLL
OUTTORE
OUTTORN
OUTTRAY
OUTTROT
OUTTURN
OUTVIED
OUTVIES
OUTVOTE
OUTWAIT
OUTWALK
OUTWARD
OUTWARS
OUTWASH
OUTWAVE
OUTWEAR
OUTWEED
OUTWEEP
OUTWELL
OUTWENT
OUTWEPT
OUTWEST
OUTWILE
OUTWILL
OUTWIND
OUTWING
OUTWISH
OUTWITH
OUTWITS
OUTWORD
OUTWORE
OUTWORK
OUTWORN
OUTYELL
OUTYELP
OXTAILS

O••T•••

OAKTAGS
OAKTREE
OILTANK
OLDTIME
OLDTOWN
OMITTED
OMITTER
ONATEAR
ONATOOT
ONATRIP
ONETERM
ONETIME
ONETOGO
ONETWOS
ONSTAFF
ONSTAGE
ORATING
ORATION
ORATORS
ORATORY
ORATRIX
OROTUND
OSETRAS
OURTOWN
OUSTERS
OUSTING
OUTTAKE
OUTTALK
OUTTEAR
OUTTELL
OUTTIRE
OUTTOLD
OUTTOLL
OUTTORE
OUTTORN
OUTTRAY
OUTTROT
OUTTURN
OVATION
OYSTERS

O•••T••

OBENTOS
OBLATES
OCTETTE
ODONTIA
OERSTED
OKHOTSK
OLDSTER
OLEATES
OLESTRA
OLMSTED
OMITTED
OMITTER
ONESTAR
ONESTEP
ONESTOP
ONLYTOO
ONWATER
OOCYTES
OOLITES
OOLITIC
OPENTAP
OPENTOE
OPENTOP
OPIATES
OPUNTIA
OPUSTWO
ORANTES
ORBITAL
ORBITED
ORBITER
ORECTIC
ORESTES
ORNETTE
ORNITHO
OSMATIC
OSMOTIC
OSSETRA
OUGHTNT
OUGHTTO
OUTSTAY
OUTSTEP
OVERTAX
OVERTIP
OVERTLY
OVERTOP

O••••T•

OBESITY
OBJECTS
OBLASTS
OBOISTS
OBTESTS
OBVERTS
OBVIATE
OCCULTS
OCCURTO
OCELOTS
OCHENTA
OCICATS
OCTANTS
OCTETTE
ODDLOTS
ODELETS
OFFDUTY
OFFSETS
OFFSITE
OFSORTS
OLDBATS
OLDCITY
OMELETS
ONADATE
ONEACTS
ONEARTH
ONEBYTE
ONEIOTA
ONEMPTY
ONENOTE
ONEONTA
ONEVOTE
ONORATI
OPACITY
OPERATE
OPQRSTU
OPTEDTO
ORGEATS
ORIENTE
ORIENTS
ORNETTE
ORVIETO
OTRANTO
OUGHTTO
OUTACTS
OUTBATS
OUTCITY
OUTCUTS
OUTDATE
OUTEATS
OUTFITS
OUTHITS
OUTJETS
OUTJUTS
OUTLETS
OUTMATE
OUTPATH
OUTPITY
OUTPUTS
OUTRATE
OUTSETS
OUTSITS
OUTVOTE
OUTWITH
OUTWITS
OVERATE
OWINGTO
OWNUPTO
OXALATE
OXCARTS
OXIDATE

O•••••T

OAKIEST
OCCIPUT
OCULIST
ODDMENT
ODORANT
OFASORT
OFFBEAT
OFFCAST
OGDENUT
OHIOART
OILHEAT
OILIEST
OILSPOT
OKSHOOT
OLDSALT
OLDWEST
ONADIET
ONALERT
ONATOOT
ONEACAT
ONECENT
ONEFOOT
ONEOCAT
ONEPART
ONEPINT
ONESHOT
ONESPOT
ONEUNIT
ONEWHIT
ONFIRST
ONLIEST
ONPOINT
ONSIGHT
ONTHEQT
ONTOAST
OOZEOUT
OOZIEST
OPENNET
OPENOUT
OPENPIT
OPERANT
OPTSOUT
OPULENT
ORALIST
ORGIAST
ORPHANT
OUGHTNT
OUTBLOT
OUTCANT
OUTCAST
OUTFAST
OUTFOOT
OUTHUNT
OUTJEST
OUTKAST
OUTKEPT
OUTLAST
OUTMOST
OUTOFIT
OUTPLOT
OUTPORT
OUTPOST
OUTRANT
OUTROOT
OUTSERT
OUTSHOT
OUTSIFT
OUTSPIT
OUTTROT
OUTWAIT
OUTWENT
OUTWEPT
OUTWEST
OVERACT
OVERBET
OVERCUT
OVEREAT
OVERFAT
OVERFIT
OVERHOT
OVERLET
OVERLIT
OVERSET
OVERWET
OVIDUCT
OWLIEST
OXHEART
OXIDANT
OZZFEST

•OT••••

BOTANIC
BOTCHED
BOTCHER
BOTCHES
BOTCHUP
BOTHERS
BOTHNIA
BOTREES
BOTTEGA
BOTTLED
BOTTLER
BOTTLES
BOTTOMS
COTEACH
COTEDOR
COTERIE
COTTAGE
COTTERS
COTTONS
COTTONY
DOTAGES
DOTARDS
DOTBOMB
DOTCOMS
DOTDASH
DOTEDON
DOTESON
DOTLIKE
DOTRICE
DOTTERS
DOTTIER
DOTTILY
DOTTING
DOTTLES
FOTOMAT
GOTAHIT
GOTAJOB
GOTATIP
GOTAWAY
GOTBACK
GOTBEAT
GOTBUSY
GOTCASH
GOTCHAS
GOTCOLD
GOTCUTE
GOTDONE
GOTDOWN
GOTEVEN
GOTFREE
GOTGOOD
GOTHELP
GOTHICS
GOTHIKA
GOTHURT
GOTINON
GOTINTO
GOTITON
GOTLOST
GOTMILK
GOTOBED
GOTOGAL
GOTOGUY
GOTONIT

GOTONTO
GOTOPOT
GOTOSEA
GOTOSEE
GOTOVER
GOTOWAR
GOTPAST
GOTREAL
GOTSOFT
GOTSORE
GOTTAGO
GOTTOIT
GOTUPON
GOTUPTO
GOTWARM
GOTWELL
GOTWISE
GOTWORD
HOTBATH
HOTBEDS
HOTCAKE
HOTCAPS
HOTCARS
HOTCOAL
HOTCOMB
HOTCUPS
HOTDATE
HOTDAYS
HOTDOGS
HOTFOOT
HOTGLUE
HOTHAND
HOTHEAD
HOTITEM
HOTKEYS
HOTLEAD
HOTLICK
HOTLINE
HOTLINK
HOTLIPS
HOTMAIL
HOTMEAL
HOTMILK
HOTNESS
HOTONES
HOTOVER
HOTPACK
HOTPINK
HOTPOTS
HOTRODS
HOTROLL
HOTSEAT
HOTSHOT
HOTSOUP
HOTSPOT
HOTSPUR
HOTTEAS
HOTTEST
HOTTIES
HOTTIME
HOTTIPS
HOTTUBS
HOTTUNA
HOTWARS
HOTWIRE
HOTZONE
JOTDOWN
JOTTERS

JOTTING
LOTHAIR
LOTHIAN
LOTHROP
LOTIONS
LOTTERS
LOTTERY
LOTTING
LOTUSES
MOTHERS
MOTHERY
MOTHIER
MOTIONS
MOTIVED
MOTIVES
MOTLEYS
MOTORED
MOTRINS
MOTTLED
MOTTLES
MOTTOES
NOTABIT
NOTABLE
NOTABLY
NOTALIE
NOTALOT
NOTAONE
NOTASTE
NOTATED
NOTATES
NOTBEEN
NOTCHED
NOTCHER
NOTCHES
NOTDONE
NOTEASY
NOTEDLY
NOTEPAD
NOTEVEN
NOTEVER
NOTFAIR
NOTGOOD
NOTHERE
NOTHING
NOTHINS
NOTHOME
NOTICED
NOTICER
NOTICES
NOTIONS
NOTLIKE
NOTLIVE
NOTMANY
NOTMINE
NOTMUCH
NOTNEAR
NOTNICE
NOTONCE
NOTOPEN
NOTOVER
NOTRADE
NOTRARE
NOTREAL
NOTRUMP
NOTSAFE
NOTSURE
NOTTING
NOTTOBE

NOTTRUE
NOTUPTO
NOTURNS
NOTUSED
NOTWELL
NOTWITH
POTABLE
POTAGES
POTAMUS
POTBOIL
POTEENS
POTENCE
POTENCY
POTFULS
POTHERB
POTHERS
POTHOLE
POTHOOK
POTIONS
POTLIDS
POTLUCK
POTOMAC
POTPIES
POTSDAM
POTSHOT
POTTAGE
POTTERS
POTTERY
POTTIER
POTTIES
POTTING
ROTATED
ROTATES
ROTATOR
ROTAWAY
ROTBLAT
ROTELLE
ROTGUTS
ROTHIRA
ROTIFER
ROTTERS
ROTTING
ROTUNDA
SOTHEBY
SOTHERE
SOTHERN
SOTTISH
SOTWEED
TOTABLE
TOTALED
TOTALER
TOTALLY
TOTALUP
TOTASTE
TOTEBAG
TOTEMIC
TOTESUP
TOTINOS
TOTOTOO
TOTTERS
TOTTERY
TOTTING
VOTABLE
VOTEAYE
VOTECHS
VOTEDIN
VOTEDNO
VOTEDON

VOTEFOR
VOTENAY
VOTEOUT
VOTESIN
VOTESNO
VOTESON
VOTEYEA
VOTEYES
VOTIVES
YOTEAMO
YOTHERS

•O•T•••

BOATELS
BOATERS
BOATFUL
BOATING
BOATMAN
BOATMEN
BOBTAIL
BOBTWAY
BOITANO
BOLTERS
BOLTING
BOLTSUP
BOOTCUT
BOOTEES
BOOTERS
BOOTERY
BOOTHIA
BOOTIES
BOOTING
BOOTLEG
BOOTOUT
BOOTSIT
BOOTSUP
BOOTTOP
BOSTONS
BOSTONU
BOTTEGA
BOTTLED
BOTTLER
BOTTLES
BOTTOMS
BOUTROS
BOWTIES
BOXTOPS
BOYTOYS
COATEES
COATERS
COATING
COCTEAU
COETZEE
COLTISH
COMTISM
COMTIST
COMTREX
CONTACS
CONTACT
CONTAIN
CONTEMN
CONTEND
CONTENT
CONTEST
CONTEXT
CONTORT
CONTOUR
CONTRAS

CONTROL
CONTUSE
COOTERS
COOTIES
COPTERS
CORTEGE
CORTICO
CORTINA
COSTAIN
COSTARD
COSTARS
COSTATE
COSTING
COSTIVE
COSTNER
COSTUME
COTTAGE
COTTERS
COTTONS
COTTONY
COUTERS
COUTURE
COWTOWN
DOCTORS
DOGTAGS
DOGTAIL
DOGTICK
DOGTOYS
DOGTROT
DOITNOW
DOLTISH
DONTASK
DONTBEE
DONTCRY
DONTLIE
DOTTERS
DOTTIER
DOTTILY
DOTTING
DOTTLES
FONTANA
FONTANE
FONTEYN
FONTINA
FOOTAGE
FOOTBAG
FOOTERS
FOOTING
FOOTLED
FOOTLER
FOOTLES
FOOTLET
FOOTMAN
FOOTMEN
FOOTPAD
FOOTRUB
FOOTSIE
FOOTSIT
FOOTSUP
FOOTWAY
FORTDIX
FORTIES
FORTIFY
FORTIUS
FORTLEE
FORTORD
FORTRAN
FORTUNA

FORTUNE
FORTYAD
FORTYBC
FOSTERS
FOXTAIL
FOXTROT
GOATEED
GOATEES
GOATISH
GODTHAB
GOITERS
GORTNER
GOSTALE
GOTTAGO
GOTTOIT
GOUTIER
GOUTILY
GOUTISH
HOGTIED
HOGTIES
HOOTERS
HOOTING
HOOTOWL
HOOTSAT
HOPTOIT
HOSTAGE
HOSTELS
HOSTESS
HOSTILE
HOSTING
HOSTLER
HOTTEAS
HOTTEST
HOTTIES
HOTTIME
HOTTIPS
HOTTUBS
HOTTUNA
HOWTHEN
JOGTROT
JOLTERS
JOLTIER
JOLTING
JOSTLED
JOSTLER
JOSTLES
JOTTERS
JOTTING
KONTIKI
KOWTOWS
LOATHED
LOATHER
LOATHES
LOATHLY
LOATHTO
LOFTBED
LOFTERS
LOFTIER
LOFTILY
LOFTING
LOITERS
LOOTERS
LOOTING
LOSTART
LOSTBIG
LOSTCAT
LOSTDOG
LOSTOUT

LOSTPET
LOTTERS
LOTTERY
LOTTING
LOUTING
LOUTISH
LOWTECH
LOWTIDE
LOWTOPS
MOLTERS
MOLTING
MONTAGE
MONTAGU
MONTALE
MONTANA
MONTAND
MONTANO
MONTAUK
MONTEGO
MONTERO
MONTEUX
MONTHLY
MONTOYA
MONTUNO
MOOTERS
MOOTING
MOPTOPS
MORTALS
MORTARS
MORTICE
MORTIFY
MORTISE
MORTONS
MOTTLED
MOTTLES
MOTTOES
MOUTHED
MOUTHER
NOETICS
NOOTHER
NOOTKAS
NORTHER
NORTHOF
NORTONS
NOSTAIN
NOSTARS
NOSTRIL
NOSTRUM
NOTTING
NOTTOBE
NOTTRUE
NOUTURN
NOWTHEN
NOWTHIS
POETESS
POETICA
POETICS
POETISE
POETIZE
POITIER
POLTAVA
PONTANO
PONTIAC
PONTIAN
PONTIFF
PONTIUS
PONTOON
POPTART

POPTOPS
POPTUNE
PORTAGE
PORTALS
PORTEND
PORTENT
PORTERS
PORTHOS
PORTICO
PORTING
PORTION
PORTMAN
PORTNOY
PORTRAY
POSTAGE
POSTBAG
POSTBOX
POSTDOC
POSTERN
POSTERS
POSTFIX
POSTHOC
POSTIES
POSTING
POSTITS
POSTMAN
POSTMEN
POSTOPS
POSTURE
POSTWAR
POTTAGE
POTTERS
POTTERY
POTTIER
POTTIES
POTTING
POUTERS
POUTFUL
POUTIER
POUTING
ROETHKE
RONTGEN
ROOTAGE
ROOTCAP
ROOTERS
ROOTFOR
ROOTIER
ROOTING
ROOTLED
ROOTLES
ROOTLET
ROOTOUT
ROOTROT
ROOTSUP
ROSTAND
ROSTERS
ROSTOCK
ROSTRAL
ROSTRUM
ROTTERS
ROTTING
ROUTERS
ROUTINE
ROUTING
ROUTOUT
SOFTENS
SOFTEST
SOFTGEL

SOFTIES
SOFTISH
SOFTTOP
SOOTHED
SOOTHER
SOOTHES
SOOTIER
SOOTILY
SORTERS
SORTIED
SORTIES
SORTING
SORTOUT
SOTTISH
SOUTHEY
SOUTHOF
TOATURN
TOETAPS
TOLTECS
TOMTITS
TOMTOMS
TONTINE
TOOTALL
TOOTERS
TOOTHED
TOOTING
TOOTLED
TOOTLER
TOOTLES
TOOTSAT
TOOTSIE
TOPTENS
TOPTHIS
TORTLAW
TORTOLA
TORTONI
TORTUGA
TORTURE
TOSTADA
TOSTART
TOTTERS
TOTTERY
TOTTING
TOUTERS
TOUTING
TOYTOPS
VOITURE
VOLTAGE
VOLTAIC
VOLTORE
WOJTYLA
WONTING
WONTONS
WORTHIT
YOMTOVS
YOUTHEN

•O••T••

BOASTED
BOASTER
BOASTOF
BOBATEA
BOLATIE
BOLOTIE
BOLSTER
BONITOS
BOOSTED
BOOSTER

BOOSTUP
BOOTTOP
BORATES
BORSTAL
BOXSTEP
BOXSTER
COACTED
COALTAR
COAPTED
COASTAL
COASTED
COASTER
COEPTIS
COLETTE
COMPTON
COOKTOP
COOPTED
CORETTA
COSETTE
COULTER
COUNTED
COUNTEE
COUNTEM
COUNTER
COUNTIN
COUNTON
COUNTRY
COUNTUP
COURTED
COURTLY
COURTTV
COVETED
COVETER
COYOTES
DOESTOO
DOGSTAR
DONATED
DONATEE
DONATES
DONATOR
DONATUS
DONETSK
DONOTGO
DOOUTOF
DORITOS
DOROTHY
DOUBTED
DOUBTER
DOUBTIT
EOLITHS
FOISTED
FOISTON
FOLATES
FORETOP
FORSTER
FOUETTE
FOULTIP
FOURTHS
GOAFTER
GODUTCH
GOGETEM
GOLDTIP
GOLFTEE
GOODTRY
GORETEX
GOTATIP
GOTITON
HOFSTRA

HOISTED
HOISTER
HOISTUP
HOLSTER
HOOPTOY
HORATIO
HOTITEM
HOUSTON
IODATED
IODATES
IOMOTHS
JOINTED
JOINTER
JOINTLY
JOISTED
JOUSTED
JOUSTER
KOMATSU
LOBATED
LOBSTER
LOCATED
LOCATER
LOCATES
LOCATOR
LONETTE
LONGTOM
LONGTON
LORETTA
LOVETAP
MOBSTER
MOISTEN
MOISTER
MOISTLY
MOJITOS
MOLITOR
MOLOTOV
MONCTON
MONITOR
MONSTER
MONSTRO
MORETTI
MOULTED
MOUNTED
MOUNTER
MOUNTIE
MOUNTUP
MOZETTA
NOCATCH
NOENTRY
NONETTE
NONSTOP
NORITES
NOTATED
NOTATES
NOVOTES
NOVOTNY
OOCYTES
OOLITES
OOLITIC
POINTAT
POINTED
POINTER
POINTES
POINTTO
POINTUP
POLITER
POLITIC
POLLTAX

POORTAX
POPSTAR
POSITED
POULTRY
ROADTAR
ROADTAX
ROASTED
ROASTER
ROBOTIC
ROBOTRY
ROISTER
ROLLTOP
RONETTE
ROOFTOP
ROOSTED
ROOSTER
ROPETOW
ROSETEA
ROSETTA
ROSETTE
ROTATED
ROTATES
ROTATOR
ROUSTED
ROUSTER
ROVETTA
SOFTTOP
SOLUTES
SOMATIC
SONATAS
TOASTED
TOASTEE
TOASTER
TOFUTTI
TOLSTOI
TOLSTOY
TONETTE
TOOKTEN
TOTOTOO
TOYOTAS
VOLUTED
VOLUTES
VORSTER
WOODTAR
WOOSTER
WORSTED
YORKTON

•O•••T•

BOBCATS
BOGARTS
BONIATO
BONMOTS
BONNETS
BOUNDTO
BOWEDTO
BOXKITE
BOXSETS
BOYCOTT
COBALTS
COBNUTS
COEDITS
COGNATE
COHORTS
COHOSTS
COLETTE
COLGATE
COLLATE

COLLETS
COLORTV
COMBATS
COMESTO
COMFITS
COMMITS
COMMUTE
COMPETE
COMPOTE
COMPUTE
COMSATS
CONFITS
CONFUTE
CONMOTO
CONNATE
CONNOTE
COPOUTS
CORBETT
CORDATE
CORDITE
CORETTA
CORINTH
CORNETS
CORNUTE
CORSETS
COSETTE
COSSETS
COSTATE
COURTTV
COVERTS
COWRITE
COWROTE
DOCENTS
DOCKETS
DOGBITE
DOGGATE
DOGGETT
DOGMATA
DOGSITS
DOHERTY
DOINGTO
DOOMSTO
DORSETT
DOSHOTS
DOUGHTY
DOZENTH
FOGCITY
FOGERTY
FOLIATE
FOLLETT
FOMENTS
FORDGTS
FORDLTD
FORESTS
FORGETS
FORINTS
FORMATS
FORSYTE
FORSYTH
FOUETTE
GOBLETS
GOCARTS
GODWITS
GOFORTH
GOINGTO
GOKARTS
GOLIATH
GORDITA

GOSOUTH
GOSSETT
GOTCUTE
GOTINTO
GOTONTO
GOTUPTO
HOBBITS
HOGARTH
HOGNUTS
HOLDSTO
HOLISTS
HONESTY
HOPEDTO
HOPESTO
HOPINTO
HOPLITE
HORNETS
HORVITZ
HOTBATH
HOTDATE
HOTPOTS
JOBCUTS
JOBLOTS
JOCASTA
JOEROTH
JOLLITY
KOLKATA
KOSSUTH
LOATHTO
LOCKETS
LOCUSTS
LOGONTO
LOGOUTS
LONETTE
LOOKSTO
LOQUATS
LORENTZ
LORETTA
LOSESTO
LOVEDTO
LOVESTO
LOYALTO
LOYALTY
MOABITE
MODELTS
MODESTO
MODESTY
MODISTE
MOLESTS
MOMENTA
MOMENTS
MOPPETS
MORANTE
MORETTI
MOSCATO
MOVEDTO
MOVESTO
MOZETTA
NOENDTO
NOGIFTS
NONARTS
NONETTE
NONHITS
NOSEATS
NOTASTE
NOTUPTO
NOTWITH
NOUGATS

NOUGHTS
NOVELTY
POCKETS
POINTTO
POLENTA
POLLUTE
POPOUTS
POSTITS
POVERTY
ROBERTA
ROBERTE
ROBERTF
ROBERTH
ROBERTI
ROBERTO
ROBERTS
ROBUSTA
ROBUSTO
ROCHETS
ROCKETS
RODENTS
RONETTE
ROSEATE
ROSETTA
ROSETTE
ROTGUTS
ROVETTA
ROYALTY
SOCIETY
SOCKETS
SOFFITS
SOLLATI
SONNETS
SOPWITH
SORBATE
SORBETS
SORENTO
SOVIETS
TOCCATA
TOFUTTI
TOILETS
TOMCATS
TOMKITE
TOMTITS
TONETTE
TOOLATE
TOPHATS
TOPRATE
TORONTO
TOTASTE
TOWPATH
TOYHATS
TOYKITE
TOYWITH
VOLANTE
VOLENTE
WOMBATS
WOOLITE
YOGURTS

•O••••T

BODYART
BODYFAT
BODYKIT
BOILOUT
BOLDEST
BOMBAST
BOMBLET

BONELET
BONESET
BONIEST
BOOEDAT
BOOKERT
BOOKLET
BOOMLET
BOOTCUT
BOOTOUT
BOOTSIT
BOREOUT
BORSCHT
BOUQUET
BOURGET
BOWKNOT
BOWSHOT
BOWSOUT
BOXCOAT
BOXIEST
BOXSEAT
BOYCOTT
COAGENT
COALPIT
COCKPIT
COCONUT
COEXIST
COHABIT
COKIEST
COLBERT
COLDCUT
COLDEST
COLLECT
COMBUST
COMCAST
COMEOUT
COMESAT
COMFORT
COMMENT
COMPACT
COMPART
COMPORT
COMPOST
COMTIST
CONCEIT
CONCEPT
CONCERT
CONCOCT
CONDUCT
CONDUIT
CONELET
CONFECT
CONGEST
CONKOUT
CONNECT
CONSENT
CONSIST
CONSORT
CONSULT
CONTACT
CONTENT
CONTEST
CONTEXT
CONTORT
CONVECT
CONVENT
CONVERT
CONVICT
COOKOUT

COOKPOT
COOLANT
COOLCAT
COOLEST
COOLOUT
COOLSIT
COONCAT
COPILOT
COPSOUT
COPYCAT
COPYIST
CORBETT
CORONET
CORRECT
CORRUPT
COSIEST
COULDNT
COUPLET
COURANT
COURBET
COWERAT
COWIEST
COZIEST
DOESNOT
DOGBERT
DOGBOOT
DOGCART
DOGCOAT
DOGGETT
DOGREAT
DOGTROT
DOGVEST
DOLEOUT
DOORMAT
DOPEOUT
DOPIEST
DORIGHT
DORMANT
DORSETT
DOUBLET
DOUBTIT
DOUREST
DOVECOT
DOVELET
DOWNPAT
DOZIEST
FOLDOUT
FOLKART
FOLLETT
FONDANT
FONDEST
FOOTLET
FOOTSIT
FORABIT
FORFEIT
FORKOUT
FORRENT
FORREST
FORWENT
FOTOMAT
FOULEST
FOULOUT
FOXHUNT
FOXIEST
FOXTROT
GOABOUT
GODSENT
GOESAFT

GOESOUT
GOFIRST
GOFORIT
GOINGAT
GOKAPUT
GONEAFT
GONEOUT
GOOIEST
GORIEST
GOSSETT
GOTAHIT
GOTBEAT
GOTHURT
GOTLOST
GOTONIT
GOTOPOT
GOTPAST
GOTSOFT
GOTTOIT
GOURMET
HOKIEST
HOLDOUT
HOLDSIT
HOLEOUT
HOLIEST
HOMIEST
HONKSAT
HOOFSIT
HOOTSAT
HOPENOT
HOPSOUT
HOPTOIT
HORNIST
HOTFOOT
HOTSEAT
HOTSHOT
HOTSPOT
HOTTEST
HOWBEIT
HOWLSAT
IOBJECT
JOBHUNT
JOGTROT
JOKIEST
JOLLIET
KOLANUT
LOANOUT
LOCKLET
LOCKNUT
LOCKOUT
LOCKSET
LOGANUT
LOGIEST
LOGSOUT
LONGEST
LOOKIST
LOOKOUT
LOOKSAT
LOOSEST
LORDSIT
LORIENT
LOSEOUT
LOSESIT
LOSTART
LOSTCAT
LOSTOUT
LOSTPET
LOUDEST

LOVEDIT
LOVESET
LOVESIT
LOWCOST
LOWPOST
LOWRENT
MOBBIST
MOLERAT
MONGKUT
MOONLET
MOONLIT
MOONSET
MOPIEST
MORDANT
MORDENT
MORISOT
MOSHPIT
MOVEDIT
MOVEOUT
MOVESIT
NOBLEST
NOCOUNT
NODOUBT
NOFAULT
NOLIMIT
NONDIET
NONFACT
NONMEAT
NONPAST
NONPOET
NOPQRST
NORBERT
NOSEOUT
NOSIEST
NOSWEAT
NOTABIT
NOTALOT
NOWWHAT
OOZEOUT
OOZIEST
PODCAST
POINTAT
POKEDAT
POKEOUT
POKESAT
POKIEST
POLECAT
POLESAT
POLESIT
POLOIST
POOPOUT
POOREST
POPSOUT
POPTART
PORTENT
POSHEST
POTSHOT
POUROUT
ROARSAT
ROBSART
RODEOUT
ROLLOUT
ROOFRAT
ROOTLET
ROOTOUT
ROOTROT
ROPIEST
ROSIEST

ROTBLAT
ROUAULT
ROUGHIT
ROUTOUT
ROWBOAT
SOAPNET
SOFTEST
SOLDOUT
SOLICIT
SOLOACT
SOLOIST
SOLVEIT
SOLVENT
SOONEST
SOPHIST
SORTOUT
SOUREST
SOYLENT
TOGSOUT
TOHEART
TOILSAT
TONIEST
TONIGHT
TOOKOUT
TOOLKIT
TOOLSET
TOOTSAT
TOPBOOT
TOPCOAT
TOPKNOT
TOPMAST
TOPMOST
TOPSOUT
TOPSPOT
TOREOUT
TORMENT
TORNOUT
TORRENT
TOSSOUT
TOSSPOT
TOSTART
TOURIST
TOWBOAT
TOWNLET
TOYBOAT
TOYCART
VOIDOUT
VOTEOUT
WOODCUT
WOODLOT
WOOLFAT
WOOLHAT
WOREOUT
WORKOUT
WORKSAT
WORNOUT
WORTHIT
WOULDNT
WOULDST
YOGAMAT
YOGHURT
YOPLAIT
YORKIST
YOUREIT
ZONEOUT
ZONKOUT
ZOOIEST
ZOOMOUT

••OT•••

ANOTHER
APOTHEM
BIOTECH
BIOTITE
BIOTYPE
BLOTCHY
BLOTOUT
BLOTSUP
BLOTTED
BLOTTER
BOOTCUT
BOOTEES
BOOTERS
BOOTERY
BOOTHIA
BOOTIES
BOOTING
BOOTLEG
BOOTOUT
BOOTSIT
BOOTSUP
BOOTTOP
BROTHER
CLOTHED
CLOTHES
CLOTSUP
CLOTTED
CLOTURE
COOTERS
COOTIES
CROTONS
DIOTIMA
DUOTONE
ECOTAGE
ECOTEUR
ECOTRIN
ECOTYPE
EGOTISM
EGOTIST
EGOTRIP
EMOTERS
EMOTING
EMOTION
EMOTIVE
EROTICA
EROTICS
ESOTERY
EXOTICA
EXOTICS
EXOTISM
FLOTAGE
FLOTSAM
FOOTAGE
FOOTBAG
FOOTERS
FOOTING
FOOTLED
FOOTLER
FOOTLES
FOOTLET
FOOTMAN
FOOTMEN
FOOTPAD
FOOTRUB
FOOTSIE
FOOTSIT
FOOTSUP

FOOTWAY
FROTHED
FROTHER
FROTHUP
GLOTTAL
GLOTTIS
GROTIUS
GROTTOS
HOOTERS
HOOTING
HOOTOWL
HOOTSAT
IDOTTER
IGOTCHA
IGOTYOU
ISOTONE
ISOTOPE
ISOTOPY
KNOTSUP
KNOTTED
KNOTTER
LAOTIAN
LEOTARD
LOOTERS
LOOTING
MOOTERS
MOOTING
NOOTHER
NOOTKAS
OROTUND
PHOTICS
PHOTOGS
PHOTOID
PHOTONS
PHOTOOP
PLOTFUL
PLOTTED
PLOTTER
PLOTZED
PLOTZES
PROTEAM
PROTEAN
PROTECT
PROTEGE
PROTEIN
PROTEST
PROTEUS
PROTIST
PROTONS
QUOTEES
QUOTERS
QUOTING
RIOTACT
RIOTERS
RIOTGUN
RIOTING
RIOTOUS
ROOTAGE
ROOTCAP
ROOTERS
ROOTFOR
ROOTIER
ROOTING
ROOTLED
ROOTLES
ROOTLET
ROOTOUT
ROOTROT

ROOTSUP
SAOTOME
SCOTERS
SCOTIAN
SCOTTIE
SHOTFOR
SHOTGUN
SHOTOUT
SHOTPAR
SHOTPUT
SLOTCAR
SLOTTED
SLOTTER
SMOTHER
SOOTHED
SOOTHER
SOOTHES
SOOTIER
SOOTILY
SPOTLIT
SPOTTED
SPOTTER
STOTINS
TOOTALL
TOOTERS
TOOTHED
TOOTING
TOOTLED
TOOTLER
TOOTLES
TOOTSAT
TOOTSIE
TROTHED
TROTOFF
TROTOUT
TROTSKY
TROTSUP
TROTTED
TROTTER
TWOTERM
TWOTIME
TWOTOED
TWOTONE
TWOTONS
USOTOUR
WROTEIN
WROTEON
WROTETO
WROTEUP
WYOTANA

••O•T••

ABORTED
ABOUTIT
ABOUTTO
ADOPTED
ADOPTEE
ADOPTER
AGOUTIS
AHOSTOF
APOSTLE
BLOATED
BLOTTED
BLOTTER
BOOSTED
BOOSTER
BOOSTUP
BOOTTOP

BRONTES
CHOCTAW
CHORTLE
CLOTTED
CLOUTED
CLOUTER
COOKTOP
COOPTED
CROATIA
CROFTER
CROPTOP
CROSTIC
CROUTES
CROUTON
DIOPTER
DOOUTOF
DROPTOP
FLOATBY
FLOATED
FLOATER
FLOATUP
FLOUTED
FLOUTER
FRONTAL
FRONTED
FRONTON
FROSTED
FROSTER
GHOSTED
GHOSTLY
GLOATED
GLOATER
GLOTTAL
GLOTTIS
GNOSTIC
GOODTRY
GROTTOS
GROUTED
GROUTER
GROWTHS
HOOPTOY
IDOTTER
ILOSTIT
KNOTTED
KNOTTER
KNOUTED
ODONTIA
PLOTTED
PLOTTER
POORTAX
PROCTER
PROCTOR
QUOITED
ROOFTOP
ROOSTED
ROOSTER
SCOOTCH
SCOOTED
SCOOTER
SCOTTIE
SCOUTED
SCOUTER
SCOUTUP
SHOOTAT
SHOOTBY
SHOOTER
SHOOTUP
SHORTED

SHORTEN
SHORTER
SHORTIE
SHORTLY
SHORTOF
SHOUTAT
SHOUTED
SHOUTER
SLOTTED
SLOTTER
SMOOTHS
SMOOTHY
SNOOTED
SNORTAT
SNORTED
SNORTER
SNOUTED
SPORTED
SPORTIN
SPOTTED
SPOTTER
SPOUTED
SPOUTER
STOUTEN
STOUTER
STOUTLY
TOOKTEN
TROTTED
TROTTER
TWOSTAR
TWOSTEP
UNOFTEN
UNOPTED
WOODTAR
WOOSTER

••O••T•

ABOUTTO
ACOLYTE
ACONITE
AMOUNTS
ANOINTS
AVOCETS
AXOLOTL
BIODATA
BIOLITE
BIOTITE
BROASTS
BROMATE
CLORETS
CLOSETO
CLOSETS
DEODATO
DIORITE
DOOMSTO
DROVETO
EBONITE
EDOMITE
EGOISTE
EGOISTS
ELOCUTE
EVOLUTE
EXOCETS
FLOCKTO
FLORETS
FLOWNTO
GLOBATE
IGOROTS

ISOLATE
ISOLATO
KNOWETH
LEONATO
LIONETS
LOOKSTO
MAOISTS
NEOLITH
NEOLYTE
NEONATE
NIOBITE
OBOISTS
ONORATI
PIOLETS
PIOSITY
PLOESTI
PROBATE
PROBITY
PROCITY
PROFITS
PROJETS
PROLATE
PROMOTE
PROMPTS
PRONATE
PRONETO
PRORATA
PRORATE
RIORITA
SNOCATS
SPOKETO
STOMATA
STOODTO
SWORETO
TAOISTS
TOOLATE
TWOACTS
TWOBITS
VIOLATE
VIOLETS
WOOLITE
WROTETO

••O•••T

ABOUTIT
AGONIST
AMONGST
AMORIST
ASONANT
ATOMIST
BLOTOUT
BLOWOUT
BLOWSIT
BOOEDAT
BOOKERT
BOOKLET
BOOMLET
BOOTCUT
BOOTOUT
BOOTSIT
BROUGHT
BUOYANT
CHORIST
CLOSEST
COOKOUT
COOKPOT
COOLANT
COOLCAT

COOLEST
COOLOUT
COOLSIT
COONCAT
CROCHET
CROCKET
CROQUET
CROSSAT
DEORBIT
DOORMAT
DROPLET
DROPNET
DROPOUT
DROPSIT
DROUGHT
DROVEAT
EGOTIST
ERODENT
FLOORIT
FLORIST
FLOWNAT
FLOWOUT
FOOTLET
FOOTSIT
FROGLET
FROWNAT
GNOMIST
GOOIEST
GROMMET
GROWFAT
HOOFSIT
HOOTSAT
IDOLIST
IDOODIT
IFORGET
IFORGOT
ILOSTIT
ILOVEIT
INORBIT
IRONIST
IRONOUT
JROBERT
LOOKIST
LOOKOUT
LOOKSAT
LOOSEST
MAOSUIT
MOONLET
MOONLIT
MOONSET
ODORANT
POOPOUT
POOREST
PRODUCT
PROEAST
PROJECT
PROPHET
PROPJET
PROTECT
PROTEST
PROTIST
PROVEIT
PROVOST
PROWEST
QUONSET
RIOTACT
ROOFRAT
ROOTLET
ROOTOUT
ROOTROT
SCOFFAT
SHOOTAT
SHOPSAT
SHOTOUT
SHOTPUT
SHOUTAT
SHOWCAT
SHOWOUT
SLOWEST
SNORTAT
SNOWCAT
SNOWHAT
SOONEST
SPOTLIT
STOPSAT
STOPSIT
STOWSIT
SWOREAT
THOUGHT
TOOKOUT
TOOLKIT
TOOLSET
TOOTSAT
TROTOUT
TWOFEET
TWOFOOT
TWOPART
TWOSHOT
TWOSPOT
TWOUNIT
UNOVERT
UPOROUT
UTOPIST
VIOLENT
VIOLIST
WHOISIT
WHOSOUT
WOODCUT
WOODLOT
WOOLFAT
WOOLHAT
WROUGHT
ZIONIST
ZOOIEST
ZOOMOUT

•••OT••

ABBOTCY
ABIOTIC
BENOTED
BENOTES
BIGOTED
BIGOTRY
BOLOTIE
CALOTTE
CAPOTES
CAROTID
CAROTIN
CELOTEX
CHAOTIC
COYOTES
CULOTTE
DAKOTAN
DAKOTAS
DEMOTED
DEMOTES
DEMOTHS
DEMOTIC
DENOTED
DENOTES
DESOTOS
DEVOTED
DEVOTEE
DEVOTES
DONOTGO
DOROTHY
ERGOTIC
FAGOTED
GAROTTE
GAVOTTE
HELOTRY
IDIOTIC
IMHOTEP
INTOTAL
IOMOTHS
KILOTON
LAKOTAS
LAMOTTA
LAMOTTE
LANOTTE
LESOTHO
LITOTES
MEIOTIC
MENOTTI
MINOTND
MITOTIC
MOLOTOV
NEPOTIC
NOVOTES
NOVOTNY
OKHOTSK
OSMOTIC
PAROTID
PELOTAS
PELOTON
PEYOTES
PICOTED
PILOTED
PINOTTA
PIVOTAL
PIVOTED
PIVOTER
PWBOTHA
REBOTES
REMOTER
REMOTES
RENOTED
RENOTES
RETOTAL
REVOTED
REVOTES
RICOTTA
RIDOTTO
RISOTTO
ROBOTIC
ROBOTRY
SCOOTCH
SCOOTED
SCOOTER
SHOOTAT
SHOOTBY
SHOOTER
SHOOTUP
SMOOTHS
SMOOTHY
SNOOTED
SPLOTCH
TICOTIN
TIMOTHY
TOTOTOO
TOYOTAS
UNNOTED
UNVOTED
VALOTTE
XEROTIC
ZAPOTEC
ZYGOTES

•••O•T•

ACCOSTS
ADDONTO
ALWORTH
ARIOSTO
ASSORTS
BUGOUTS
BUYOUTS
BYMOUTH
CAHOOTS
CALOTTE
CAVORTS
COHORTS
COHOSTS
COLORTV
COPOUTS
CULOTTE
CUTOUTS
DACOSTA
DEBOITE
DECOCTS
DEPORTS
DIMOUTS
DUGOUTS
EFFORTS
ELMONTE
ELNORTE
EMBOITE
ENROOTS
ENROUTE
ESCORTS
EXHORTS
EXPORTS
EXTORTS
FANOUTS
FTWORTH
GALOOTS
GAROTTE
GAVOTTE
GETONTO
GOFORTH
GOSOUTH
GOTONTO
HAWORTH
ICEOUTS
IMPORTS
IMPOSTS
LACOSTE
LAMOTTA
LAMOTTE
LANOTTE
LAPORTE
LAYOUTS
LECONTE
LOGONTO
LOGOUTS
MAHOUTS
MENOTTI
MINOLTA
MRNORTH
OFSORTS
ONEONTA
PAYOUTS
PIGOUTS
PINOTTA
POPOUTS
PRIORTO
PTBOATS
PUTOUTS
RAGOUTS
REBOLTS
REBOOTS
RECOATS
RECOSTS
REDOUTS
REPORTS
REPOSTS
REROOTS
REROUTE
RESORTS
RETORTS
REVOLTS
RICOTTA
RIDOTTO
RIPOSTE
RIPOSTS
RISOTTO
RUNOUTS
SETOUTS
SPROUTS
STOODTO
TAGOUTS
THEOATH
THROATS
THROATY
TORONTO
TRYOUTS
UNBOLTS
UNCOUTH
UNLOATH
UNLOFTY
UNROOTS
UNSOOTY
UNSORTS
UPNORTH
UPROOTS
UTMOSTS
VALOTTE
VELOUTE
VICOMTE
WASONTO

•••O••T

ABSOLUT
ACCOUNT
ACROBAT
AEROBAT
ALLOFIT
ALTOIST
APPOINT
ASTOLAT
ATWORST
AUTOMAT
BARONET
BAYONET
CHROMAT
COCONUT
CORONET
DEMOUNT
DEPOSIT
EXPOSIT
FLOORIT
FOTOMAT
GETONIT
GOFORIT
GOTONIT
GOTOPOT
IDOODIT
IKNOWIT
IMFORIT
INCOURT
INDOUBT
INFORIT
INPOINT
JACONET
JUDOIST
KILOBIT
LABORAT
LEGOSET
MCCOURT
NICOLET
NOCOUNT
NODOUBT
OHIOART
ONEOCAT
ONPOINT
ONTOAST
OUTOFIT
POLOIST
PREOMIT
REBOANT
RECOUNT
REDOUBT
REMOUNT
REPOINT
REPOSIT
RESOJET
RETOAST
SAMOSET
SHOOTAT
SITONIT
SOLOACT
SOLOIST
SUMOIST
TABORET
THROWAT
TITOIST
TRIOLET
UNJOINT
UNMOIST
UPCOAST
UPCOURT
UPFORIT
XAMOUNT
ZEROOUT

••••OT•

AIRPOTS
ALIGOTE
AXOLOTL
BADLOTS
BALLOTS
BBSHOTS
BETROTH
BIGLOTS
BONMOTS
BOYCOTT
BURBOTS
CAHOOTS
CARLOTA
CARLOTS
CARROTS
CARROTY
CHAYOTE
COMPOTE
CONMOTO
CONNOTE
COWROTE
DECLOTS
DESPOTS
DIGLOTS
DOSHOTS
DRAGOTI
DRYROTS
DYELOTS
EELPOTS
ELLIOTT
ENDNOTE
ENROOTS
EPIDOTE
FEMBOTS
GALOOTS
GARROTE
HARLOTS
HOTPOTS
IGOROTS
INKNOTS
INKPOTS
INSPOTS
JARROTT
JOBLOTS
JOEROTH
KEYNOTE
MAGGOTS
MAMMOTH
MARMOTS
MASCOTS
MATZOTH
MERLOTS
MRSCOTT
NDAKOTA
OCELOTS
ODDLOTS
ONEIOTA
ONENOTE
ONEVOTE
OUTVOTE
PARROTS
PEQUOTS
PROMOTE
QUIXOTE
REBOOTS
REDDOTS
REDHOTS
REKNOTS
REPLOTS
REQUOTE
REROOTS
RESPOTS
REWROTE
REXROTH
SAYNOTO
SDAKOTA
SEXPOTS
SPIGOTS
SPYBOTS
SUBLOTS
SUCCOTH
SUKKOTH
TEAPOTS
TIMROTH
TISSOTS
TRICOTS
TURBOTS
TVSPOTS
UNKNOTS
UNQUOTE
UNROOTS
UNSOOTY
UPROOTS
UPSHOTS
VIDIOTS
WALCOTT
WESCOTT
YESVOTE
ZEALOTS

••••O•T

ACEDOUT
ACESOUT
ACTSOUT
AFFRONT
AFTMOST
AGEDOUT
AGESOUT
AIRBOAT
AIRPORT
AIRSOUT
ASKSOUT
ATACOST
BACKOUT
BAILOUT
BANGOUT
BAWLOUT
BEAROUT
BEATOUT
BEDPOST
BELFORT
BELMONT
BELTOUT
BERTOLT
BIGFOOT
BLEWOUT
BLOTOUT
BLOWOUT
BOILOUT
BOOTOUT
BOREOUT
BOWSOUT
BOXCOAT
BOYCOTT
BUGSOUT
BUMSOUT
BURNOUT
BUSTOUT
BUTTOUT
BUYSOUT
CALLOUT
CAMEOUT
CAMPOUT
CARCOAT
CARPORT
CASEOUT
CASHOUT
CASTOUT
CATBOAT
CATFOOT
CHEROOT
CHEWOUT
CLIPOUT
COMEOUT
COMFORT
COMPORT
COMPOST
CONCOCT
CONKOUT
CONSORT
CONTORT
COOKOUT
COOLOUT
COPSOUT
CRAPOUT
CUTSOUT
DASBOOT
DEALOUT
DECKOUT
DEFROST
DEGHOST
DELMONT
DETROIT
DIALOUT
DIDTOAT
DIEDOUT
DIESOUT
DIGSOUT
DIMSOUT
DINEOUT
DINMONT
DISHOUT
DISPORT
DISTORT
DOGBOOT
DOGCOAT
DOLEOUT
DOPEOUT
DRAGOUT
DRAWOUT
DREWOUT
DROPOUT
DRUMOUT
DUCKOUT
DUMPOUT
EASEOUT
EATSOUT
EDGEOUT
EDITOUT
EELPOUT
EKEDOUT
EKESOUT
ELLIOTT
ENDMOST
EVENOUT
EXPLOIT
EYEBOLT
FADEOUT
FAKEOUT
FALLOUT
FANSOUT
FARMOUT
FEELOUT
FELLOUT
FELTOUT
FILEOUT
FILLOUT
FINDOUT
FISHOUT
FLATOUT
FLIPOUT
FLOWOUT
FOLDOUT
FORKOUT
FOULOUT
FREMONT
FULLOUT
FURCOAT
GAVEOUT
GETLOST
GETSOFT
GETSOUT
GETTOIT
GIVEOUT
GJETOST
GOABOUT
GOESOUT
GONEOUT
GOTLOST
GOTSOFT
GOTTOIT
GUMBOOT
GUNBOAT
GUSHOUT
HANDOUT
HANGOUT
HASHOUT
HAVEOUT
HAYLOFT
HEADOUT
HEAROUT
HELDOUT
HELPOUT
HIDEOUT
HIKEOUT
HIPBOOT
HIREOUT
HITSOUT
HOLDOUT
HOLEOUT
HOPSOUT
HOPTOIT
HOTFOOT
HUNGOUT
ICEBOAT
ICEDOUT
ICESOUT
ILLDOIT
INFRONT
INSHORT
INTROIT
IRISOUT
IRONOUT
JARROTT
JERKOUT
JETBOAT
JETPORT
JUSTOUT
KEEPOUT
KEPTOUT
KICKOUT
KINMONT
LABCOAT
LAIDOUT
LASHOUT
LAYSOUT
LEADOUT
LEAFOUT
LEFTOUT
LENDOUT
LETSOUT
LINEOUT
LIPSOUT
LIVEOUT
LOANOUT
LOCKOUT
LOGSOUT
LOOKOUT
LOSEOUT
LOSTOUT
LOWCOST
LOWPOST
LUCKOUT
LUGSOUT
MADEOUT
MAILOUT
MAKEOUT
MAPSOUT
MARKOUT
METEOUT
MIDMOST
MISSORT
MISSOUT
MOVEOUT
MRSCOTT
MYCROFT
NETCOST
NEWBOLT
NEWMONT
NEWPORT
NONPOET
NOSEOUT
OFASORT
OKSHOOT
ONATOOT
ONEFOOT
OOZEOUT
OPENOUT
OPTSOUT
OUTFOOT
OUTMOST
OUTPORT
OUTPOST
OUTROOT
PAIDOUT
PANSOUT
PASSOUT
PAYSOUT
PEACOAT
PEEKOUT
PEELOUT
PEEPOUT
PEEROUT
PETGOAT
PICKOUT
PIGSOUT
PLANOUT
PLAYOUT
POKEOUT
POOPOUT
POPSOUT
POUROUT
PRESORT
PREVOST
PROVOST
PUFFOUT
PULLOUT
PUMPOUT
PURPORT
PUSHOUT
PUTSOUT
PUTTOUT
RACKOUT
RAINOUT
RANGOUT
RANKOUT
RAPPORT
RATSOUT
READOPT
READOUT
REAMOUT
REDCOAT
REDROOT
REELOUT
REFLOAT
REFRONT
RENTOUT
RESHOOT
REYMONT
RIDEOUT
RIGSOUT
RINGOUT
RIPSOUT
RODEOUT
ROLLOUT
ROOTOUT
ROUTOUT
ROWBOAT
RUBSOUT
RULEOUT
RUNGOUT
RUNSOUT
RUSHOUT
SACKOUT
SANGOUT
SAWTOIT
SEABOAT
SEAPORT
SEEKOUT
SEENOUT
SEEPOUT
SEESOUT
SEETOIT
SELLOUT
SENDOUT
SENTOUT
SETSOUT
SHEGOAT
SHIPOUT
SHOTOUT
SHOWOUT
SHUTOUT
SICKOUT
SIGNOUT
SINGOUT
SITSOUT
SIXFOOT
SKIBOOT
SKIPOUT
SLIDOUT
SLIPOUT
SOLDOUT
SORTOUT
SPATOUT
SPECOUT
SPEWOUT
SPINOUT
SPITOUT
SPUNOUT
STAYOUT
STEPOUT
SUBPOST
SUBROOT
SUBSORT
SUPPORT
SUSSOUT
TAGSOUT
TAKEOUT
TALKOUT
TAPROOT
TAPSOUT
TEAROUT
TENFOOT
TESTOUT
THAWOUT
THEMOST
THEPOST
THINOUT
TIMEOUT
TIMHOLT
TIREOUT
TOGSOUT
TOOKOUT
TOPBOOT
TOPCOAT
TOPMOST
TOPSOUT
TOREOUT
TORNOUT
TOSSOUT
TOWBOAT
TOYBOAT
TROTOUT
TUGBOAT
TUNEOUT
TURNOUT
TWOFOOT
UNFROST
UNSHORT
UNSTOUT
UPFRONT
UPOROUT
UPSHOOT
VANVOGT
VERMONT
VFWPOST
VOIDOUT
VOTEOUT
WAITOUT

WALCOTT
WALKOUT
WANTOUT
WASHOUT
WEAROUT
WEBFOOT
WEEDOUT
WENTOUT
WESCOTT
WHOSOUT
WIGSOUT
WIMPOUT
WINKOUT
WINSOUT
WIPEOUT
WITEOUT
WITHOUT
WOREOUT
WORKOUT
WORNOUT
XINGOUT
YANKOUT
YELLOUT
ZEROOUT
ZONEOUT
ZONKOUT
ZOOMOUT

•••••OT

AFATLOT
APRICOT
ATEALOT
BACKLOT
BADSHOT
BAGEHOT
BIBELOT
BIENTOT
BIGFOOT
BIGSHOT
BLERIOT
BOWKNOT
BOWSHOT
CAMELOT
CASELOT
CATFOOT
CHARCOT
CHARIOT
CHEROOT
CHEVIOT
COOKPOT
COPILOT
CRABPOT
CYPRIOT
DARENOT
DASBOOT
DASHDOT
DASHPOT
DIDEROT
DOESNOT
DOGBOOT
DOGTROT
DOVECOT
EARSHOT
EATALOT
EYESHOT
EYESPOT
FEARNOT
FEEDLOT
FLUSHOT
FOXTROT
FULLLOT
FUSSPOT
GETSHOT
GOTOPOT
GUMBOOT
GUNSHOT
HARICOT
HAVENOT
HERRIOT
HIPBOOT
HOPENOT
HOTFOOT
HOTSHOT
HOTSPOT
ICANNOT
IFORGOT
INAKNOT
INASPOT
INKBLOT
INKSPOT
ITSALOT
JACKPOT
JEANNOT
JOGTROT
LETSNOT
MAGINOT
MAILLOT
MORISOT
MRHULOT
MUGSHOT
NEEDNOT
NOTALOT
OILSPOT
OKSHOOT
ONATOOT
ONEFOOT
ONESHOT
ONESPOT
OUTBLOT
OUTFOOT
OUTPLOT
OUTROOT
OUTSHOT
OUTTROT
OVERHOT
PATRIOT
PEATPOT
PERIDOT
PEUGEOT
PIERROT
PINCHOT
PLUMCOT
POTSHOT
PREPLOT
PRERIOT
RANRIOT
REALLOT
REDROOT
REDSPOT
RESHOOT
RIMSHOT
ROOTROT
RUNRIOT
SANDLOT
SETSHOT
SHALLOT
SHAVUOT
SIXFOOT
SKIBOOT
SPAMBOT
STEWPOT
SUBPLOT
SUBROOT
SUNSPOT
TAPROOT
TEESHOT
TENFOOT
TENSPOT
TINYTOT
TOPBOOT
TOPKNOT
TOPSPOT
TOSSPOT
TRIVIOT
TSELIOT
TWOFOOT
TWOSHOT
TWOSPOT
UPSHOOT
VERYHOT
WAPSHOT
WEBFOOT
WHATNOT
WOODLOT

OU•••••

OUGHTNT
OUGHTTO
OUGUIYA
OURGANG
OURSELF
OURSONG
OURTOWN
OUSTERS
OUSTING
OUTACTS
OUTADDS
OUTAGES
OUTASKS
OUTAWED
OUTAWES
OUTBACK
OUTBAKE
OUTBANS
OUTBARK
OUTBATS
OUTBAWL
OUTBEAM
OUTBEGS
OUTBEND
OUTBIDS
OUTBLOT
OUTBLOW
OUTBOWL
OUTBOWS
OUTBRAG
OUTBRAY
OUTBRED
OUTBUDS
OUTBULK
OUTBURN
OUTBUYS
OUTBUZZ
OUTCALL
OUTCANT
OUTCAST
OUTCITY
OUTCOLD
OUTCOME
OUTCOOK
OUTCROP
OUTCROW
OUTCULL
OUTCURE
OUTCUTS
OUTDARE
OUTDATE
OUTDOER
OUTDOES
OUTDONE
OUTDOOR
OUTDRAG
OUTDRAW
OUTDREW
OUTDROP
OUTDUEL
OUTEARN
OUTEATS
OUTECHO
OUTEDGE
OUTFACE
OUTFAST
OUTFAWN
OUTFEED
OUTFEEL
OUTFIND
OUTFIRE
OUTFISH
OUTFITS
OUTFLEE
OUTFLOW
OUTFLUX
OUTFOOL
OUTFOOT
OUTGAIN
OUTGAME
OUTGAVE
OUTGAZE
OUTGIVE
OUTGLOW
OUTGNAW
OUTGOES
OUTGREW
OUTGRIN
OUTGROW
OUTGUNS
OUTGUSH
OUTHAUL
OUTHEAR
OUTHERE
OUTHIRE
OUTHISS
OUTHITS
OUTHOWL
OUTHUNT
OUTHURL
OUTINGS
OUTJEST
OUTJETS
OUTJINX
OUTJUMP
OUTJUTS
OUTKAST
OUTKEEP
OUTKEPT
OUTKICK
OUTKILL
OUTKING
OUTKISS
OUTLAID
OUTLAIN
OUTLAND
OUTLASH
OUTLAST
OUTLAWS
OUTLAYS
OUTLEAD
OUTLEAP
OUTLETS
OUTLIER
OUTLIES
OUTLIMN
OUTLINE
OUTLIPS
OUTLIVE
OUTLOOK
OUTLOUD
OUTLOVE
OUTMANS
OUTMATE
OUTMODE
OUTMOST
OUTMOVE
OUTOFIT
OUTPACE
OUTPAID
OUTPASS
OUTPATH
OUTPAYS
OUTPEEP
OUTPICK
OUTPIPE
OUTPITY
OUTPLAN
OUTPLAY
OUTPLOD
OUTPLOT
OUTPOLL
OUTPOPS
OUTPORT
OUTPOST
OUTPOUR
OUTPRAY
OUTPULL
OUTPURL
OUTPUSH
OUTPUTS
OUTRACE
OUTRAGE
OUTRAIL
OUTRANG
OUTRANK
OUTRANT
OUTRAPS
OUTRATE
OUTRAVE
OUTREAD
OUTRIBS
OUTRIDE
OUTRIGS
OUTRING
OUTROAR
OUTROCK
OUTRODE
OUTROLL
OUTROOT
OUTROVE
OUTROWS
OUTRUNS
OUTRUSH
OUTSAID
OUTSAIL
OUTSANG
OUTSAYS
OUTSEEK
OUTSEEN
OUTSEES
OUTSELL
OUTSERT
OUTSETS
OUTSHOT
OUTSHOW
OUTSIDE
OUTSIFT
OUTSIGH
OUTSING
OUTSINS
OUTSITS
OUTSIZE
OUTSKIP
OUTSOAR
OUTSOLD
OUTSOLE
OUTSPED
OUTSPIN
OUTSPIT
OUTSTAY
OUTSTEP
OUTSULK
OUTSUMS
OUTSUNG
OUTSWAM
OUTSWIM
OUTSWUM
OUTTAKE
OUTTALK
OUTTEAR
OUTTELL
OUTTIRE
OUTTOLD
OUTTOLL
OUTTORE
OUTTORN
OUTTRAY
OUTTROT
OUTTURN
OUTVIED
OUTVIES
OUTVOTE
OUTWAIT
OUTWALK
OUTWARD
OUTWARS
OUTWASH
OUTWAVE
OUTWEAR
OUTWEED
OUTWEEP
OUTWELL
OUTWENT
OUTWEPT
OUTWEST
OUTWILE
OUTWILL
OUTWIND
OUTWING
OUTWISH
OUTWITH
OUTWITS
OUTWORD
OUTWORE
OUTWORK
OUTWORN
OUTYELL
OUTYELP

O•U••••

OCULARS
OCULIST
OEUVRES
OPULENT
OPUNTIA
OPUSONE
OPUSTWO

O••U•••

OAHUANS
OBTUNDS
OBTUSER
OCCULTS
OCCURTO
OCTUBRE
OCTUPLE
OCTUPLY
OHFUDGE
OLDUVAI
ONEUNIT
ONGUARD
OPPUGNS
OROURKE
OSCULAR
OSCULES
OSMUNDS
OSSUARY
OTTUMWA
OUGUIYA
OWNUPTO

O•••U••

OBSCURA
OBSCURE
OBTRUDE
OCCLUDE
ODDDUCK
OFFDUTY
OFNOUSE
OILCUPS
OILRUBS
OLEBULL
ONAJURY
ONELUMP
OPAQUES
OROTUND
OUTBUDS
OUTBULK
OUTBURN
OUTBUYS
OUTBUZZ
OUTCULL
OUTCURE
OUTCUTS
OUTDUEL
OUTGUNS
OUTGUSH
OUTHUNT
OUTHURL
OUTJUMP
OUTJUTS
OUTPULL
OUTPURL
OUTPUSH
OUTPUTS
OUTRUNS
OUTRUSH
OUTSULK
OUTSUMS
OUTSUNG
OUTTURN
OVERUSE
OVIDUCT

O••••U•

OBLIQUE
OBLOQUY
OBVIOUS
OCCIPUT
OCEANUS
OCELLUS
OCHROUS
OCTOPUS
ODORFUL
ODOROUS
OEDIPUS
OFFERUP
OFFHOUR
OFVALUE
OGDENUT
OILDRUM
OISEAUX
OKAYGUY
OLDBLUE
OLYMPUS
OMINOUS
OMNIBUS
ONECLUB
ONEHOUR
ONEOFUS
ONEROUS
OOZEOUT
OPENOUT
OPENSUP
OPOSSUM
OPTIMUM
OPTSOUT
ORARIUM
ORDERUP
ORMOLUS
ORPHEUM
ORPHEUS
OSSEOUS
OUTFLUX
OUTHAUL
OUTLOUD
OUTPOUR
OUTSWUM
OVERBUY
OVERCUT
OVERDUB
OVERDUE
OVERRUN
OVERSUP
OWNEDUP
OZONOUS

O•••••U

ONLYYOU
OPQRSTU

•OU••••

AOUDADS
BOUCHER
BOUCHES
BOUDINS
BOUDOIR
BOUFFES
BOUGHED
BOULDER
BOUNCED
BOUNCER
BOUNCES
BOUNDED
BOUNDER
BOUNDTO
BOUNDUP
BOUQUET
BOURBON
BOURGET
BOURSES
BOUSONO
BOUTROS
BOUVIER
COUCHED
COUCHES
COUGARS
COUGHED
COUGHUP
COULDBE
COULDNT
COULEES
COULOMB
COULTER
COUNCIL
COUNSEL
COUNTED
COUNTEE
COUNTEM
COUNTER
COUNTIN
COUNTON
COUNTRY
COUNTUP
COUPING
COUPLED
COUPLER
COUPLES
COUPLET
COUPONS
COURAGE
COURANT
COURBET
COURIER
COURSED
COURSER
COURSES
COURTED
COURTLY
COURTTV
COUSINE
COUSINS
COUTERS
COUTURE
DOUANES
DOUBLEA
DOUBLEB
DOUBLEC
DOUBLED
DOUBLEE
DOUBLEF
DOUBLEG
DOUBLEH
DOUBLEI
DOUBLEJ
DOUBLEK
DOUBLEL
DOUBLEM
DOUBLEN
DOUBLEO
DOUBLEP
DOUBLEQ
DOUBLER
DOUBLES
DOUBLET
DOUBLEU
DOUBLEV
DOUBLEW
DOUBLEX
DOUBLEY
DOUBLEZ
DOUBTED
DOUBTER
DOUBTIT
DOUCEUR
DOUGHTY
DOUGLAS
DOUREST
DOUSERS
DOUSING
FOUDRES
FOUETTE
FOULARD
FOULEST
FOULING
FOULOUT
FOULSUP
FOULTIP
FOULUPS
FOUNDED
FOUNDER
FOUNDRY
FOURAAA
FOURDAY
FOUREEE
FOURIER
FOURMAN
FOURPIN
FOURTHS
FOURWAY
GOUACHE
GOUGERS
GOUGING
GOULASH
GOUNDER
GOURAMI
GOURDES
GOURMET
GOUTIER
GOUTILY
GOUTISH
HOUDINI
HOUNDED
HOUNDER
HOUSING
HOUSMAN
HOUSSAY
HOUSTON
JOUHAUX
JOUNCED
JOUNCES
JOURDAN
JOURNAL
JOURNEE
JOURNEY
JOURNOS
JOUSTED
JOUSTER
LOUDENS
LOUDEST
LOUDISH
LOUELLA
LOUISII
LOUISIV
LOUISIX
LOUISVI
LOUISXI
LOUISXV
LOUNGED
LOUNGER
LOUNGES
LOURDES
LOUREED
LOURING
LOUSEUP
LOUSIER
LOUSILY
LOUSING
LOUTING
LOUTISH
LOUVERS
LOUVRED
LOUVRES
MOULAGE
MOULDED
MOULDER
MOULTED
MOUNDED
MOUNTED
MOUNTER
MOUNTIE
MOUNTUP
MOURNED
MOURNER
MOUSERS
MOUSIER
MOUSILY
MOUSING
MOUSSED
MOUSSES
MOUTHED
MOUTHER
NOUGATS
NOUGHTS
NOURISH
NOUTURN
NOUVEAU
POUCHED
POUCHES
POUDRES
POULENC
POULTRY
POUNCED
POUNCER
POUNCES
POUNDED
POUNDER
POURERS
POURING
POUROUT
POURSIN
POUSSIN
POUTERS
POUTFUL
POUTIER
POUTING
ROUAULT
ROUBAIX
ROUGHED
ROUGHEN
ROUGHER
ROUGHGO
ROUGHIT
ROUGHLY
ROUGHUP
ROUGING
ROULADE
ROULEAU
ROUNDED
ROUNDEL
ROUNDER
ROUNDLY
ROUNDON
ROUNDUP
ROUSERS
ROUSING
ROUSTED
ROUSTER
ROUTERS
ROUTINE
ROUTING
ROUTOUT
SOUBISE
SOUFFLE
SOULFUL
SOULMAN
SOUNDED
SOUNDER
SOUNDLY
SOUPCAN
SOUPCON
SOUPERS
SOUPIER
SOUPMIX
SOUPSON
SOUPSUP
SOURALE
SOURCED
SOURCES
SOUREST
SOURING
SOURISH
SOURSON
SOUSING
SOUTHEY
SOUTHOF
TOUAREG
TOUCANS
TOUCHED
TOUCHER
TOUCHES
TOUCHON
TOUCHUP
TOUGHEN
TOUGHER
TOUGHIE
TOUGHLY
TOUPEES
TOURBUS
TOURERS
TOURING
TOURISM
TOURIST
TOURNEY
TOUSLED
TOUSLES
TOUTERS
TOUTING
VOUCHED
VOUCHER
VOUCHES
VOUVRAY
WOULDBE
WOULDNT
WOULDST
WOUNDED
WOUNDUP
YOUANDI
YOUKNOW
YOULOSE
YOUMANS
YOUNGER
YOUNGMC
YOUNGUN
YOURANG
YOUREIT
YOUREON
YOUTHEN
YOUWISH

•O•U•••

BOGUSLY
BOLUSES
BONUSES
COBUYER
COJUROR
COLUMBA
COLUMBO
COLUMNS
CONURES
COPULAE
COPULAR
COPULAS
COQUINA
COZUMEL
DOEUVRE
DOLUNCH

DOOUTOF
FOCUSED
FOCUSER
FOCUSES
FOCUSON
GODUNOV
GODUTCH
GOTUPON
GOTUPTO
HOCUSED
JOCULAR
KORUNAS
LOBULES
LOCULUS
LOCUSTS
LOQUATS
LORUSES
LOTUSES
MODULAR
MODULES
MODULUS
MOLUCCA
MOMUSES
NOCUOUS
NODULAR
NODULED
NODULES
NOGUCHI
NONUKES
NONUPLE
NONUSER
NOSUGAR
NOTUPTO
NOTURNS
NOTUSED
POPULAR
POPUPAD
ROBUSTA
ROBUSTO
ROGUERY
ROGUING
ROGUISH
ROMULAN
ROMULUS
ROTUNDA
SOLUBLE
SOLUTES
SOSUEME
TOFUTTI
TOLUENE
TONUSES
VOGUERS
VOGUING
VOGUISH
VOLUBLE
VOLUBLY
VOLUMED
VOLUMES
VOLUTED
VOLUTES
YOGURTS
ZONULAR
ZONULES

•O••U••

BOGGUSS
BOROUGH
BOUQUET
BOXFULS
COBNUTS
COEQUAL
COFOUND
COGBURN
COLLUDE
COLOURS
COMBUST
COMMUNE
COMMUTE
COMPUTE
CONCURS
CONCUSS
CONDUCE
CONDUCT
CONDUIT
CONFUSE
CONFUTE
CONJURE
CONJURY
CONQUER
CONSULS
CONSULT
CONSUME
CONTUSE
COPOUTS
CORNUTE
CORRUPT
COSTUME
COUTURE
DOGRUNS
DOLOURS
DONJUAN
DONRUSS
FOLDUPS
FONDUED
FONDUES
FORBUSH
FORMULA
FORSURE
FORTUNA
FORTUNE
FOULUPS
FOXHUNT
GOODUSE
GOOFUPS
GOROUND
GOSOUTH
GOTBUSY
GOTCUTE
GOTHURT
HOGNUTS
HOLDUPS
HOMBURG
HONOURS
HOOKUPS
HORNUNG
HOTCUPS
HOTTUBS
HOTTUNA
HOWDULL
HOWMUCH
IONIUMS
JOAQUIN
JOBCUTS
JOBHUNT
JOEBUCK
JONQUIL
KOSSUTH
LOCKUPS
LOGOUTS
LONGUES
LOOKUPS
MOBRULE
MOCKUPS
MOLLUSC
MOLLUSK
MONTUNO
MORGUES
MOSQUES
NOCOUNT
NODOUBT
NOFAULT
NONBUSY
NONFUEL
NONJURY
NONSUCH
NOTMUCH
NOTRUMP
NOTSURE
NOUTURN
PODIUMS
POLLUTE
POPGUNS
POPOUTS
POPQUIZ
POPTUNE
POSEURS
POSEUSE
POSSUMS
POSTURE
POTFULS
POTLUCK
ROEBUCK
ROLLUPS
RONDURE
RORQUAL
ROTGUTS
ROUAULT
ROXBURY
SOJOURN
TOATURN
TONGUES
TONSURE
TOOMUCH
TOPGUNS
TORQUED
TORQUES
TORTUGA
TORTURE
TOSSUPS
TOYGUNS
VOITURE
WORKUPS
YOGHURT

•O•••U•

BOARDUP
BOATFUL
BODEFUL
BODYRUB
BOHRIUM
BOILOUT
BOILSUP
BOLTSUP
BONEDUP
BONESUP
BONHEUR
BONJOUR
BOOSTUP
BOOTCUT
BOOTOUT
BOOTSUP
BOREOUT
BORGLUM
BORLAUG
BORNEUP
BOTCHUP
BOUNDUP
BOWLFUL
BOWSOUT
BOXEDUP
BOXESUP
COCONUT
COILSUP
COLDCUP
COLDCUT
COLONUS
COMEDUE
COMEOUT
COMESUP
COMIQUE
CONGOUS
CONKOUT
CONTOUR
COOKOUT
COOKSUP
COOLOUT
COOPSUP
COPIOUS
COPSOUT
CORKSUP
COUGHUP
COUNTUP
COVERUP
DOINGUP
DOLEFUL
DOLEOUT
DOLLSUP
DOMINUS
DONAHUE
DONATUS
DONIMUS
DOOMFUL
DOPEOUT
DOUCEUR
FOLDOUT
FOLDSUP
FOOTRUB
FOOTSUP
FORCEUP
FORERUN
FORKFUL
FORKOUT
FORKSUP
FORMFUL
FORTIUS
FOULOUT
FOULSUP
GOABOUT
GOBYBUS
GOESOUT
GOINGUP
GOKAPUT
GOLDBUG
GONEOUT
GOODBUY
GOODGUY
GOOFSUP
GORDIUS
GOTOGUY
HOISTUP
HOLDOUT
HOLDSUP
HOLEDUP
HOLEOUT
HOLESUP
HOLMIUM
HOMERUN
HOODLUM
HOOKSUP
HOPEFUL
HOPSOUT
HOTGLUE
HOTSOUP
HOTSPUR
JODHPUR
JOINSUP
JOUHAUX
KOLANUT
LOADSUP
LOANOUT
LOCKNUT
LOCKOUT
LOCKSUP
LOCULUS
LOGANUT
LOGSOUT
LONGRUN
LOOKOUT
LOOKSUP
LOSEOUT
LOSTOUT
LOUSEUP
LOVEBUG
MOANFUL
MOCKSUP
MODICUM
MODULUS
MONGKUT
MONTAUK
MONTEUX
MOUNTUP
MOVEDUP
MOVEOUT
MOVESUP
NOCUOUS
NONDRUG
NONFLUX
NONPLUS
NOSEDUP
NOSEEUM
NOSEOUT
NOSESUP
NOSTRUM
NOTTRUE
NOXIOUS
OOZEOUT
POINTUP
POKEFUN
POKEOUT
POMPOUS
PONTIUS
POOLCUE
POOPOUT
POPSOUT
POTAMUS
POUROUT
POUTFUL
POWERUP
RODEOUT
ROLLOUT
ROLLSUP
ROMANUS
ROMULUS
ROOMFUL
ROOTOUT
ROOTSUP
ROPEDUP
ROPESUP
ROSABUD
ROSEBUD
ROSTRUM
ROUGHUP
ROUNDUP
ROUTOUT
SOAKSUP
SOAPSUP
SOLDOUT
SONGFUL
SORGHUM
SORTOUT
SOULFUL
SOUPSUP
TOGSOUT
TOILFUL
TONEDUP
TONESUP
TOOKOUT
TOOLSUP
TOPSOUT
TOREOUT
TORNOUT
TOSSOUT
TOTALUP
TOTESUP
TOUCHUP
TOURBUS
TOYSRUS
VOIDOUT
VONLAUE
VOTEOUT
WOKENUP
WOLFCUB
WOODCUT
WOREOUT
WORKOUT
WORKSUP
WORNOUT
WOUNDUP
YOUNGUN
ZONEOUT
ZONKOUT
ZOOMOUT
ZOSIMUS

•O••••U

BOSTONU
COCTEAU
DOUBLEU
HOFBRAU
HOWARDU
IOWEYOU
KOMATSU
LOOKYOU
LOVEYOU
LOYOLAU
MONDIEU
MONTAGU
NOUVEAU
RONDEAU
ROULEAU
TONNEAU

••OU•••

ABOUNDS
ABOUTIT
ABOUTTO
ACOUPLE
AFOULOF
AGOUTIS
AMOUNTS
ANOUILH
AROUSAL
AROUSED
AROUSER
AROUSES
BLOUSED
BLOUSES
BLOUSON
BROUGHT
CHOUGHS
CLOUDED
CLOUDUP
CLOUTED
CLOUTER
CROUTES
CROUTON
DOOUTOF
DROUGHT
EDOUARD
ENOUNCE
FLOUNCE
FLOUNCY
FLOURED
FLOUTED
FLOUTER
GROUCHO
GROUCHY
GROUNDS
GROUPED
GROUPER
GROUPIE
GROUSED
GROUSER
GROUSES
GROUTED
GROUTER
KNOUTED
OROURKE
PIOUSLY
PLOUGHS
PROUDER
PROUDLY
PROUDOF
SCOUPES
SCOURED
SCOURER
SCOURGE
SCOUTED
SCOUTER
SCOUTUP
SHOULDA
SHOULDI
SHOUTAT
SHOUTED
SHOUTER
SIOUANS
SLOUCHY
SLOUGHS
SNOUTED
SPOUSAL
SPOUSES
SPOUTED
SPOUTER
STOUTEN
STOUTER
STOUTLY
THOUGHT
TROUBLE
TROUGHS
TROUNCE
TROUPED
TROUPER
TROUPES
TROUSER
TSOURIS
TWOUNIT
WROUGHT
YAOUNDE

••O•U••

BEOWULF
BIOFUEL
BLOWUPS
BROGUES
CLOSURE
CLOTURE
CROQUET
CROQUIS
DROGUES
EGOSURF
ELOCUTE
EPOQUES
EVOLUTE
GEODUCK
GLOBULE
GOODUSE
GOOFUPS
HOOKUPS
INOCULA
LOOKUPS
MAOSUIT
OROTUND
PROCURE
PRODUCE
PRODUCT
PROFUSE
QUORUMS
RIOMUNI
SHOGUNS
SHONUFF
SLOWUPS
TOOMUCH

••O••U•

AMOROUS
APODOUS
BLOCKUP
BLOTOUT
BLOTSUP
BLOWGUN
BLOWNUP
BLOWOUT
BLOWSUP
BOOSTUP
BOOTCUT
BOOTOUT
BOOTSUP
BROKEUP
BUOYSUP
CHOKEUP
CHOPSUP
CHOSEUP
CLOGSUP
CLOSEUP
CLOTSUP
CLOUDUP
CNOSSUS
COOKOUT
COOKSUP
COOLOUT
COOPSUP
CROESUS
CROPSUP
CROSSUP
DOOMFUL
DROPOUT
DROVEUP
ECOTEUR
FLOATUP
FLOWNUP
FLOWOUT
FOOTRUB
FOOTSUP
FROTHUP
FROZEUP
GLOBOUS
GNOSSUS
GOODBUY
GOODGUY
GOOFSUP
GROPIUS
GROTIUS
GROWNUP
GROWSUP
HOODLUM
HOOKSUP
IRONOUT
KNOTSUP
LIONCUB
LOOKOUT
LOOKSUP
NIOBIUM
ODORFUL
ODOROUS
OPOSSUM
OZONOUS
PHOEBUS
PHONYUP
PLOTFUL
PLOWSUP
POOLCUE
POOPOUT
PROCLUS
PRONOUN
PROPSUP
PROTEUS
REOCCUR
RHODIUM
RHOECUS
RHOMBUS
RIOTGUN
RIOTOUS
ROOMFUL
ROOTOUT
ROOTSUP
SCOUTUP
SHOOKUP
SHOOTUP
SHOPFUL
SHOREUP
SHOTGUN
SHOTOUT
SHOTPUT
SHOWNUP
SHOWOUT
SHOWSUP
SLOWSUP
SMOKEUP
SPOKEUP
STOCKUP
STOKEUP
STOODUP
STOPSUP
STOREUP
THORIUM
TOOKOUT
TOOLSUP
TROILUS
TROTOUT
TROTSUP
TWOHOUR
UPOROUT
USOTOUR
WHOSOUT
WOODCUT
WROTEUP
ZOOMOUT

••O•••U

IGOTYOU
LOOKYOU
THOREAU

•••OU••

ACCOUNT
ADJOURN
ADNOUNS
AGROUND
AMPOULE
ARBOURS
ARDOURS
ARMOURS
ARMOURY
ASTOUND
BEDOUIN
BEFOULS
BIVOUAC
BOROUGH
BUGOUTS
BUYOUTS
BYMOUTH
CAROUSE
COFOUND
COLOURS
COPOUTS
CUTOUTS
CYYOUNG
DEBOULE
DELOUSE
DEMOUNT
DETOURS
DEVOURS
DEYOUNG
DIMOUTS
DOLOURS
DUGOUTS
ENROUTE
ENSOULS
ENWOUND
ESPOUSE
EXPOUND
FANOUTS
FAROUKI
FATOUSH
FAVOURS
GOROUND
GOSOUTH
HONOURS
HUMOURS
ICEOUTS
IFYOUGO
IMPOUND
IMYOURS
INBOUND
INCOURT
INDOUBT
INHOUSE
INPOURS
INTOUCH
KEROUAC
LABOURS
LADOUCE
LAYOUTS
LELOUCH
LOGOUTS
MACOUNS
MAHOUTS
MCCOURT
MIAOUED
NOCOUNT
NODOUBT
OFNOUSE
PAYOUTS
PIGOUTS
POPOUTS
PUTOUTS
RAGOUTS
REBOUND
RECOUNT
RECOUPS
REDOUBT
REDOUND
REDOUTS
REFOUND
REHOUSE
REMOUNT
REPOURS
REROUTE
RESOUND
RETOUCH
RETOURS
REWOUND
RIGOURS
RUMOURS
RUNOUTS
SAVOURS
SAVOURY
SETOUTS
SHROUDS
SOJOURN
SPROUTS
STLOUIS
STROUSE
TABOULI
TAGOUTS
THROUGH
TRYOUTS
UNBOUND
UNCOUTH
UNFOUND
UNHOUSE
UNMOULD
UNROUND
UNSOUND
UNTOUGH
UNWOUND
UNYOUNG
UPBOUND
UPCOURT
UPROUSE
VALOURS
VAPOURS
VAPOURY
VBLOUSE
VELOURS
VELOUTE
VIGOURS
XAMOUNT

•••O•U•

ABSOLUT
ALLOFUS
AUTOBUS
BAROQUE
CANOPUS
COCONUT
COLONUS
DECORUM
DEFOCUS
ECLOGUE
ENVOGUE
GOTOGUY
INFOCUS
INVOGUE
MINOGUE
OBLOQUY
OCTOPUS
ONEOFUS
ORMOLUS
PIROGUE
REFOCUS
SHOOKUP
SHOOTUP
STOODUP
SUDOKUS
THROWUP
VANOCUR
VAPORUB
ZEROOUT
ZEROSUM

•••O••U

LOYOLAU

••••OU•

ACEDOUT
ACESOUT
ACTFOUR
ACTSOUT
AGEDOUT
AGEFOUR
AGESOUT
AIRSOUT
AMOROUS
ANDROUS
ANXIOUS
APODOUS
AQUEOUS
ARDUOUS
ASKSOUT
BACKOUT
BAILOUT
BALFOUR
BANGOUT
BAWLOUT
BEAROUT
BEATOUT
BECLOUD
BELTOUT
BELVOUR
BIGFOUR
BILIOUS
BLEWOUT
BLOTOUT
BLOWOUT
BOILOUT
BONJOUR
BOOTOUT
BOREOUT
BOWSOUT
BRUMOUS
BUGSOUT
BULBOUS
BUMSOUT
BURNOUT
BUSTOUR
BUSTOUT
BUTTOUT
BUYSOUT
CALHOUN
CALLOUS
CALLOUT
CAMEOUT
CAMPOUT
CANDOUR
CARIOUS
CARPOUS
CASEOUS
CASEOUT
CASHOUT
CASTOUT
CHEWOUT
CITROUS

CLAMOUR
CLIPOUT
COMEOUT
CONGOUS
CONKOUT
CONTOUR
COOKOUT
COOLOUT
COPIOUS
COPSOUT
CRAPOUT
CUPROUS
CURIOUS
CUTSOUT
DEALOUT
DECKOUT
DEVIOUS
DIALOUT
DIEDOUT
DIESOUT
DIGSOUT
DIMSOUT
DINEOUT
DISHOUT
DOLEOUT
DOPEOUT
DRAGOUT
DRAWOUT
DREWOUT
DROPOUT
DRUMOUT
DUBIOUS
DUCKOUT
DUMPOUT
DUTEOUS
EASEOUT
EATSOUT
EDGEOUT
EDITOUT
EELPOUT
EKEDOUT
EKESOUT
EMULOUS
ENAMOUR
ENVIOUS
EVENOUT
FABFOUR
FADEOUT
FAKEOUT
FALLOUT
FANSOUT
FARMOUT
FATUOUS
FEELOUT
FELLOUT
FELTOUT
FERROUS
FERVOUR
FIBROUS
FILEOUT
FILLOUT
FINDOUT
FISHOUT
FLATOUT
FLAVOUR
FLIPOUT
FLOWOUT
FOLDOUT
FORKOUT
FOULOUT
FULLOUT
FURIOUS
GASEOUS
GAVEOUT
GETSOUT
GIBBOUS
GIVEOUT
GLAMOUR
GLOBOUS
GOABOUT
GOESOUT
GONEOUT
GUSHOUT
HANDOUT
HANGOUT
HARBOUR
HASHOUT
HAVEOUT
HEADOUT
HEAROUT
HEINOUS
HELDOUT
HELPOUT
HIDEOUS
HIDEOUT
HIKEOUT
HIREOUT
HITSOUT
HOLDOUT
HOLEOUT
HOPSOUT
HOTSOUP
HUNGOUT
HYDROUS
ICEDOUT
ICESOUT
IGNEOUS
IMPIOUS
INGROUP
IRISOUT
IRONOUT
JEALOUS
JERKOUT
JUSTOUT
KEEPOUT
KEPTOUT
KICKOUT
LAIDOUT
LASHOUT
LAYSOUT
LEADOUT
LEAFOUT
LEFTOUT
LENDOUT
LETSOUT
LINEOUT
LIPSOUT
LIVEOUT
LOANOUT
LOCKOUT
LOGSOUT
LOOKOUT
LOSEOUT
LOSTOUT
LUCKOUT
LUGSOUT
MADEOUT
MAHFOUZ
MAILOUT
MAISOUI
MAKEOUT
MANHOUR
MAPSOUT
MARKOUT
MCCLOUD
METEOUT
MILHOUS
MISSOUT
MOVEOUT
NERVOUS
NITROUS
NIVEOUS
NOCUOUS
NOSEOUT
NOXIOUS
OBVIOUS
OCHROUS
ODOROUS
OFFHOUR
OMINOUS
ONEHOUR
ONEROUS
OOZEOUT
OPENOUT
OPTSOUT
OSSEOUS
OUTLOUD
OUTPOUR
OZONOUS
PAIDOUT
PANSOUT
PARFOUR
PARLOUR
PARLOUS
PASSOUT
PAVIOUR
PAYSOUT
PEASOUP
PEEKOUT
PEELOUT
PEEPOUT
PEEROUT
PETROUS
PGATOUR
PHILOUS
PICEOUS
PICKOUT
PIGSOUT
PILEOUS
PISTOUS
PITEOUS
PLANOUT
PLAYOUT
POKEOUT
POMPOUS
POOPOUT
POPSOUT
POUROUT
PRECOUP
PRONOUN
PTEROUS
PUFFOUT
PULLOUT
PUMPOUT
PUSHOUT
PUTSOUT
PUTTOUT
RACKOUT
RAINOUT
RANCOUR
RANGOUT
RANKOUT
RATSOUT
RAUCOUS
READOUT
REAMOUT
REDFOUR
REELOUT
REGROUP
RENTOUT
RIDEOUT
RIGSOUT
RINGOUT
RIOTOUS
RIPSOUT
RODEOUT
ROLLOUT
ROOTOUT
ROUTOUT
RUBIOUS
RUBSOUT
RUINOUS
RULEOUT
RUNGOUT
RUNSOUT
RUSHOUT
SACKOUT
SANGOUT
SAVIOUR
SEEKOUT
SEENOUT
SEEPOUT
SEESOUT
SELLOUT
SENDOUT
SENTOUT
SERIOUS
SETSOUT
SEYMOUR
SHIPOUT
SHOTOUT
SHOWOUT
SHUTOUT
SICKOUT
SIDIOUS
SIGNOUT
SINGOUT
SINUOUS
SITSOUT
SIXFOUR
SKIPOUT
SLIDOUT
SLIPOUT
SOLDOUT
SORTOUT
SPATOUT
SPECOUT
SPEWOUT
SPINOUT
SPITOUT
SPUNOUT
STAYOUT
STCLOUD
STEPOUT
SUCCOUR
SUSSOUT
TAGSOUT
TAKEOUT
TALKOUT
TAPSOUT
TEAROUT
TEDIOUS
TENFOUR
TENUOUS
TESTOUT
THAWOUT
THEROUX
THETOUR
THINOUT
TIMEOUT
TIREOUT
TOGSOUT
TOOKOUT
TOPSOUT
TOREOUT
TORNOUT
TOSSOUT
TROTOUT
TUNEOUT
TURNOUT
TWOHOUR
UNCLOUD
UNPIOUS
UNPROUD
UNSTOUT
UPOROUT
USOTOUR
VACUOUS
VARIOUS
VERDOUX
VICIOUS
VISCOUS
VOIDOUT
VOTEOUT
WAITOUT
WALKOUT
WANTOUT
WASHOUT
WEAROUT
WEEDOUT
WEEHOUR
WENTOUT
WHOSOUT
WIGSOUT
WIMPOUT
WINKOUT
WINSOUT
WIPEOUT
WITEOUT
WITHOUT
WOREOUT
WORKOUT
WORNOUT
XINGOUT
YANKOUT
YELLOUT
ZEALOUS
ZEROOUT
ZINCOUS
ZONEOUT
ZONKOUT
ZOOMOUT

••••O•U

BAYLORU
BOSTONU
CHANOYU
SHIKOKU

•••••OU

ANGELOU
CAILLOU
CARIBOU
EMMYLOU
IBEGYOU
IGOTYOU
IOWEYOU
ISEEYOU
LOOKYOU
LOVEYOU
MARYLOU
MISSYOU
NEARYOU
ONLYYOU
PAXINOU
SAYSYOU
TINAMOU
WILLYOU
YEAHYOU

OV•••••

OVARIES
OVATION
OVERACT
OVERAGE
OVERALL
OVERARM
OVERATE
OVERAWE
OVERBED
OVERBET
OVERBID
OVERBIG
OVERBUY
OVERCOY
OVERCUT
OVERDID
OVERDOG
OVERDRY
OVERDUB
OVERDUE
OVERDYE
OVEREAT
OVERFAR
OVERFAT
OVERFED
OVERFEE
OVERFEW
OVERFIT
OVERFIX
OVERFLY
OVERHOT
OVERICE
OVERJOY
OVERLAP
OVERLAX
OVERLAY
OVERLET
OVERLIE
OVERLIT
OVERMAN
OVERMIX
OVERNEW
OVERPAR
OVERPAY
OVERPLY
OVERRAN
OVERRUN
OVERSAD
OVERSAW
OVERSEA
OVERSEE
OVERSET
OVERSEW
OVERSUP
OVERTAX
OVERTIP
OVERTLY
OVERTOP
OVERUSE
OVERWET
OVIDIAN
OVIDUCT
OVIFORM
OVIPARA
OVISACS
OVOIDAL

O•V••••

OBVERSE
OBVERTS
OBVIATE
OBVIOUS
OFVALUE
ONVIDEO
ORVIETO
ORVILLE

O••V•••

OEUVRES
OLAVIII
OLEVELS
OLIVIER
OLIVINE
ONEVOTE
OUTVIED
OUTVIES
OUTVOTE

O•••V••

OCTAVAL
OCTAVES
OCTAVIA
OCTAVIO
OCTAVOS
OLDUVAI
ONEOVER
OTTAVIO

O••••V•

OBSERVE
OLDNAVY
ONELOVE
ONLEAVE
ONSERVE
OSTRAVA
OUTGAVE
OUTGIVE
OUTLIVE
OUTLOVE
OUTMOVE
OUTRAVE
OUTROVE
OUTWAVE

•OV••••

BOVINES
COVERED
COVERER
COVERME
COVERTS
COVERUP
COVETED
COVETER
DOVEBAR
DOVECOT
DOVELET
DOVERDE
GOVERNS
HOVERED
HOVERER
HOVLANE
LOVABLE
LOVABLY
LOVAGES
LOVEBUG
LOVEDIT
LOVEDTO
LOVEINS
LOVEJOY
LOVERLY
LOVESET
LOVESIT
LOVESTO
LOVETAP
LOVEYOU
MOVABLE
MOVABLY
MOVADOS
MOVEDIN
MOVEDIT
MOVEDON
MOVEDTO
MOVEDUP
MOVEOFF
MOVEOUT
MOVESIN
MOVESIT
MOVESON
MOVESTO
MOVESUP
NOVALIS
NOVARRO
NOVELAS
NOVELLA
NOVELLE
NOVELLO
NOVELTY
NOVENAS
NOVICES
NOVISAD
NOVOTES
NOVOTNY
POVERTY
ROVETTA
ROVINGS
SOVIETS

•O•V•••

BOBVILA
BOUVIER
COEVALS
CONVECT
CONVENE
CONVENT
CONVERT
CONVEYS
CONVICT
CONVOKE
CONVOYS
CORVAIR
CORVEES
CORVIDS
CORVINA
CORVINE
DOGVEST
DOOVERS
HOOVERS
HORVITZ
LOUVERS
LOUVRED
LOUVRES
NONVOID
NOUVEAU
POIVRES
ROLVAAG
SOLVEIT
SOLVENT
SOLVERS
SOLVING
SORVINO
TORVALD
TORVILL
VOUVRAY

•O••V••

BOLIVAR
BOLIVIA
BOOKVII
DOEUVRE
DONOVAN
FOREVER
GODEVIL
GOTEVEN
GOTOVER
HOPOVER
HOTOVER
HOWEVER
JOHNVII
KOSOVAR
MOHAVES
MOJAVES
MORAVIA
MOTIVED
MOTIVES
NONEVER
NONEVIL
NOTEVEN
NOTEVER
NOTOVER
POPOVER
PORIVER
SOHAVEI
VOTIVES
WONOVER

•O•••V•

BONJOVI
COMMOVE
CONCAVE
CONNIVE
COSTIVE
DONLEVY
FORGAVE
FORGIVE
FORLOVE
JOHNXVI
LOUISVI
LOWDIVE
MOLDOVA
MONDAVI
NONLIVE
NOTLIVE
POLTAVA
POPDIVA
TOPFIVE
YOMTOVS

•O••••V

COLORTV
COURTTV
DOUBLEV
GODUNOV
JOHNXIV
LOUISIV
LOUISXV
MOLOTOV
ROCKYIV
ROMANOV
ROYGBIV
ROZANOV

••OV•••

BMOVIES
CLOVERS
CLOVERY
DOOVERS
DROVEAT
DROVEBY
DROVEIN
DROVERS
DROVETO
DROVEUP
GLOVING
GROVELS
GROVERS
HOOVERS
ILOVEIT
ILOVELA
LEOVIII
PLOVDIV
PLOVERS
PROVEIT
PROVERB
PROVERS
PROVIDE
PROVINE
PROVING
PROVISO
PROVOKE
PROVOST
SHOVEIN
SHOVELS
SHOVERS
SHOVING
SLOVAKS
SLOVENE
SLOVENS
UNOVERT

••O•V••

BOOKVII
EVOLVED
EVOLVER
EVOLVES
GROOVED
GROOVES
GROOVIN
WHOEVER

••O••V•

EMOTIVE
EROSIVE
PLOSIVE
PRONAVY

••O•••V

GEORGEV
PLOVDIV

•••OV••

ALCOVES
ALLOVER
ANDOVER
ASKOVER
ATEOVER
BELOVED
BULOVAS
CRYOVER
CUTOVER
DIDOVER
DONOVAN
EATOVER
EUROVAN
FLYOVER
GASOVEN
GETOVER
GOTOVER
GROOVED
GROOVES
GROOVIN
HADOVER
HANOVER
HASOVER
HOPOVER
HOTOVER
ICEOVER
INWOVEN
ITSOVER
KOSOVAR
LAYOVER
LENOVOS
LIEOVER
LITOVSK
MCCOVEY
MRNOVAK
NOTOVER
ONEOVER
POPOVER
PUTOVER
RANOVER
RAYOVAC
RECOVER
REMOVAL
REMOVED
REMOVER
REMOVES
REWOVEN
RUNOVER
SAMOVAR
SAYOVER
SEGOVIA
TIPOVER
TVMOVIE
UNCOVER
UNLOVED
UNMOVED
UNNOVEL
UNWOVEN
WINOVER
WONOVER

•••O•V•

ABSOLVE
BEHOOVE
DEVOLVE
INVOLVE
RESOLVE
REVOLVE

•••O••V

COLORTV
FEDOROV
MOLOTOV
NABOKOV
TUPOLEV

••••OV•

ANCHOVY
APPROVE
BADLOVE
BADMOVE
BEHOOVE
BENBOVA
BIGLOVE
BONJOVI
COMMOVE
FORLOVE
IAMLOVE
IMPROVE
ITSLOVE
IVANOVO
KARLOVY
KEDROVA
MARKOVA
MISMOVE
MOLDOVA
NEWLOVE
ONELOVE
OUTLOVE
OUTMOVE
OUTROVE
PAVLOVA
PETDOVE
REPROVE
ULANOVA
UNGLOVE
UPABOVE
YOMTOVS

•••••OV

AKSAKOV
ALFEROV
BADENOV
BRYUSOV
CHEKHOV
FEDOROV
GODUNOV
GRINKOV
KEMIDOV
KHARKOV
KUTUZOV
MOLOTOV
NABOKOV
NEMEROV
ROMANOV
ROZANOV
SMIRNOV
ULYANOV
USTINOV

OW•••••

OWINGON
OWINGTO
OWLEGGS
OWLEYED
OWLIEST
OWLLIKE
OWNEDUP
OWNGOAL
OWNUPTO

O•W••••

ONWARDS
ONWATER

O••W•••

OAKWOOD
OFFWEGO
OILWELL
OLDWAYS
OLDWEST
ONAWHIM
ONEWEEK
ONEWHIT
ONEWOOD
OSTWALD
OUTWAIT
OUTWALK
OUTWARD
OUTWARS
OUTWASH
OUTWAVE
OUTWEAR
OUTWEED
OUTWEEP
OUTWELL
OUTWENT
OUTWEPT
OUTWEST
OUTWILE
OUTWILL
OUTWIND
OUTWING

OUTWISH
OUTWITH
OUTWITS
OUTWORD
OUTWORE
OUTWORK
OUTWORN

O•••W••
OJIBWAS
OJIBWAY
ONETWOS
OTTAWAN
OTTAWAS
OUTAWED
OUTAWES
OUTSWAM
OUTSWIM
OUTSWUM
OVERWET

O••••W•
OAKLAWN
OKINAWA
OLDNEWS
OLDSAWS
OLDTOWN
ONEDOWN
ONMYOWN
OPUSTWO
OTTUMWA
OURTOWN
OUTBAWL
OUTBOWL
OUTBOWS
OUTFAWN
OUTHOWL
OUTLAWS
OUTROWS
OVERAWE

O•••••W
OHMSLAW
OUTBLOW
OUTCROW
OUTDRAW
OUTDREW
OUTFLOW
OUTGLOW
OUTGNAW
OUTGREW
OUTGROW
OUTSHOW
OVERFEW
OVERNEW
OVERSAW
OVERSEW

•OW••••
BOWDLER
BOWDOIN
BOWDOWN
BOWECHO
BOWEDTO
BOWERED
BOWFINS
BOWHEAD
BOWKNOT
BOWLERS
BOWLESS
BOWLFUL
BOWLIKE
BOWLINE
BOWLING
BOWOARS
BOWSAWS
BOWSHOT
BOWSOUT
BOWTIES
BOWWOWS
BOWYERS
COWARDS
COWBANE
COWBELL
COWBIRD
COWBOYS
COWERAT
COWERED
COWFISH
COWGIRL
COWHAND
COWHERD
COWHIDE
COWIEST
COWLICK
COWLIKE
COWLING
COWPEAS
COWPOKE
COWPONY
COWRIES
COWRITE
COWROTE
COWSHED
COWSKIN
COWSLIP
COWTOWN
DOWAGER
DOWDIER
DOWDIES
DOWDILY
DOWERED
DOWLING
DOWNBOW
DOWNERS
DOWNIER
DOWNING
DOWNPAT
DOWRIES
DOWRONG
DOWSERS
DOWSING
FOWLERS
FOWLING
GOWNING
GOWRONG
HOWARDK
HOWARDS
HOWARDU
HOWBEIT
HOWCOME
HOWDAHS
HOWDEDO
HOWDULL
HOWDYDO
HOWELLS
HOWELSE
HOWEVER
HOWHIGH
HOWLAME
HOWLERS
HOWLING
HOWLONG
HOWLSAT
HOWMANY
HOWMUCH
HOWNICE
HOWTHEN
IOWEYOU
JOWLIER
KOWADLO
KOWLOON
KOWTOWS
LOWBALL
LOWBEAM
LOWBIDS
LOWBLOW
LOWBORN
LOWBOYS
LOWBRED
LOWBROW
LOWCARB
LOWCARD
LOWCHEN
LOWCOST
LOWDIVE
LOWDOWN
LOWEEZY
LOWERED
LOWGEAR
LOWHAND
LOWHEEL
LOWLAND
LOWLIER
LOWLIFE
LOWLILY
LOWMASS
LOWNECK
LOWNESS
LOWPAID
LOWPAIR
LOWPOST
LOWRENT
LOWRISE
LOWRISK
LOWROAD
LOWSIDE
LOWTECH
LOWTIDE
LOWTOPS
MOWBRAY
MOWDOWN
MOWINGS
NOWHERE
NOWISEE
NOWISER
NOWLOOK
NOWNESS
NOWORSE
NOWTHEN
NOWTHIS
NOWWHAT
POWDERS
POWDERY
POWERED
POWERUP
POWWOWS
ROWBOAT
ROWDIER
ROWDIES
ROWDILY
ROWELED
ROWLAND
ROWLING
SOWLIKE
SOWSEAR
TOWABLE
TOWAGES
TOWARDS
TOWAWAY
TOWBARS
TOWBOAT
TOWCARS
TOWEDIN
TOWELED
TOWERED
TOWHEAD
TOWHEES
TOWINGS
TOWLINE
TOWNCAR
TOWNERS
TOWNIES
TOWNISH
TOWNLET
TOWPATH
TOWROPE
VOWELLY
VOWLESS
WOWEDEM
YOWLERS
YOWLING

•O•W•••
BOBWEIR
BOSWELL
BOWWOWS
COBWEBS
COOWNED
DOGWOOD
DOOWOPS
FORWARD
FORWENT
GODWITS
GOTWARM
GOTWELL
GOTWISE
GOTWORD
HOGWASH
HOGWEED
HOGWILD
HOTWARS
HOTWIRE
NONWAGE
NONWARS
NONWOOL
NONWORD
NONWORK
NORWALK
NORWICH
NORWOOD
NOSWEAT
NOTWELL
NOTWITH
NOWWHAT
POPWINE
POWWOWS
RONWOOD
ROSWELL
SOPWITH
SOTWEED
TOYWITH
YOUWISH

•O••W••
BOBTWAY
BOERWAR
COLDWAR
DOORWAY
FOLKWAY
FOODWEB
FOOTWAY
FOURWAY
GOLDWYN
GOODWIN
GOTAWAY
GOTOWAR
HOLYWAR
JOHNWOO
LONGWAY
MOHAWKS
POSTWAR
ROADWAY
ROLLWAY
ROTAWAY
SOMEWAY
TOLLWAY
TOWAWAY

•O•••W•
BOGDOWN
BORROWS
BOWDOWN
BOWSAWS
BOWWOWS
COWTOWN
DOGBOWL
FOGBOWS
FOLLOWS
FOXNEWS
GOSHAWK
GOTDOWN
HOEDOWN
HOLLOWS
HOOTOWL
JOTDOWN
KOWTOWS
LOWDOWN
MOOCOWS
MORROWS
MOWDOWN
NONJEWS
NONNEWS
NORDOWE
NOSHOWS
POWWOWS
ROBLOWE
ROYALWE
SOAREWE
SODIDWE
SORROWS
TOPDOWN
TOPROWS

•O••••W
COMENOW
CORNROW
DOGCHEW
DOGCHOW
DOGSHOW
DOITNOW
DOUBLEW
DOWNBOW
FOREPAW
FORESAW
FORSHOW
GOBELOW
HOLYCOW
JOEBLOW
JOHNLAW
LOCKJAW
LONGBOW
LOWBLOW
LOWBROW
MOONBOW
POORLAW
ROPETOW
SOMEHOW
TONEROW
TONYDOW
TOOSLOW
TOPDRAW
TORTLAW
WOODROW
WOODSAW
YOUKNOW

••OW•••
AJOWANS
AVOWALS
AVOWERS
AVOWING
BEOWULF
BLOWDRY
BLOWERS
BLOWFLY
BLOWGUN
BLOWIER
BLOWING
BLOWNIN
BLOWNUP
BLOWOFF
BLOWOUT
BLOWPOP
BLOWSIN
BLOWSIT
BLOWSON
BLOWSUP
BLOWUPS
BLOWZED
BROWARD
BROWNED
BROWNER
BROWNIE
BROWSED
BROWSER
BROWSES
BROWWAX
CHOWDER
CHOWING
CLOWDER
CLOWNED
COOWNED
CROWBAR
CROWDED
CROWDER
CROWDIN
CROWELL
CROWERS
CROWING
CROWLEY
CROWNED
CROWNER
DOOWOPS
DROWNED
DROWSED
DROWSES
FLOWAGE
FLOWERS
FLOWERY
FLOWING
FLOWNAT
FLOWNBY
FLOWNIN
FLOWNON
FLOWNTO
FLOWNUP
FLOWOUT
FLOWSIN
FROWARD
FROWNAT
FROWNED
FROWNER
FROWNON
GLOWERS
GLOWING
GROWBIG
GROWDIM
GROWERS
GROWFAT
GROWING
GROWLED
GROWLER
GROWNON
GROWNUP
GROWOLD
GROWSON
GROWSUP
GROWTHS
KNOWALL
KNOWERS
KNOWETH
KNOWHOW
KNOWING
KNOWLES
KNOWSOF
MEOWERS
MEOWING
MEOWMIX
PLOWBOY
PLOWERS
PLOWING
PLOWMAN
PLOWMEN
PLOWSON
PLOWSUP
PROWESS
PROWEST
PROWLED
PROWLER
REOWNED
SCOWLED
SCOWLER
SHOWBIZ
SHOWCAT
SHOWDOG
SHOWERS
SHOWERY
SHOWHOW
SHOWIER
SHOWILY
SHOWING
SHOWMAN
SHOWMEN
SHOWNIN
SHOWNUP
SHOWOFF
SHOWOUT
SHOWSIN
SHOWSUP
SLOWDAY
SLOWEST
SLOWING
SLOWISH
SLOWSUP
SLOWUPS
SNOWCAP
SNOWCAT
SNOWDAY
SNOWDON
SNOWHAT
SNOWIER
SNOWILY
SNOWING
SNOWJOB
SNOWMAN
SNOWMEN
SNOWPEA
SNOWSIN
SNOWSKI
STOWAGE
STOWERS
STOWING
STOWSIT
TROWELS
TROWING
TWOWEEK
UNOWING
UNOWNED

••O•W••
BRONWEN
BROWWAX
DOORWAY
FOODWEB
FOOTWAY
GOODWIN
WHOSWHO

••O••W•
HOOTOWL
MOOCOWS
PROBOWL

••O•••W
ASOFNOW
CHOCTAW
GEORGEW
KNOWHOW
MOONBOW
POORLAW
SHOWHOW
TOOSLOW
USOSHOW
WHOKNEW
WOODROW
WOODSAW
WROCLAW

•••OW••
ALLOWAY
ALLOWED
ALLOWIN
ALLOWME
BEROWNE
CDTOWER
CNTOWER
DEPOWER
DISOWNS
ELBOWED
ELBOWER
ELFOWLS
EMBOWER
EMPOWER
ENDOWED
ENDOWER
GOTOWAR
IKNOWIT
INNOWAY
INPOWER
JCPOWYS
JDPOWER
KELOWNA
MANOWAR
MCCOWEN
MIAOWED
REMOWED
RENOWNS
REPOWER
RESOWED
RETOWED
TFPOWYS
THROWAT
THROWER
THROWIN
THROWON
THROWUP
UNBOWED
UNCOWED
UNLOWLY
UNMOWED
UNROWDY
UNSOWED
UNVOWED
UPTOWNS
VANOWEN
WIDOWED
WIDOWER
WIMOWEH

•••O••W
UPTONOW

••••OW•
ANTCOWS
ANYTOWN
BARNOWL
BARROWS
BEDDOWN
BELLOWS
BESTOWS
BIGTOWN
BILLOWS
BILLOWY
BOGDOWN
BORROWS
BOWDOWN
BOWWOWS
BURROWS
BUYDOWN
CATBOWL
CHITOWN
COWTOWN
CRYDOWN
CUTDOWN
DIEDOWN
DOGBOWL
DRBROWN
EMBROWN
ESCROWS
FALLOWS
FARROWS
FELLOWS
FOGBOWS
FOLLOWS
FURROWS
GALLOWS
GETDOWN
GOTDOWN
HALLOWS
HARROWS
HAYMOWS
HITTOWN
HOEDOWN
HOLLOWS
HOOTOWL
ICEDOWN
INBROWN
INCROWD
INFLOWS
INGROWN
JOTDOWN
KOWTOWS
LAYDOWN
LETDOWN
LIEDOWN
LOWDOWN
MALLOWS
MARLOWE
MARROWS
MEADOWS
MEADOWY
MELLOWS
MIDTOWN
MINNOWS
MOOCOWS
MORROWS
MOWDOWN
MRBROWN
NARROWS
NEWMOWN
NEWTOWN
NORDOWE
NOSHOWS
OLDTOWN
ONEDOWN
ONMYOWN
OURTOWN
OUTBOWL
OUTBOWS
OUTHOWL
OUTROWS
PATDOWN
PEAFOWL
PETCOWS
PILLOWS
PILLOWY
PINDOWN
PITROWS
POWWOWS
PROBOWL
PUTDOWN
RAMDOWN
RANDOWN
REAVOWS
REBLOWN
RECROWN
REFLOWN
REFLOWS
REGLOWS
REGROWN
REGROWS
REPLOWS
RESHOWN
RESHOWS
RESTOWS
ROBLOWE
RUBDOWN
RUNDOWN
SATDOWN
SEACOWS
SEAFOWL
SETDOWN
SHADOWS
SHADOWY
SITDOWN
SKITOWS
SORROWS
SUNBOWL
SUNBOWS
SUNDOWN
TALLOWS
TALLOWY
TEAGOWN
TIEDOWN
TIPDOWN
TOPDOWN
TOPROWS
TVSHOWS
UNBLOWN
UNCROWN
UNFLOWN
UNGROWN
UNKNOWN
UNSHOWN
UNSHOWY
UNSTOWS
UPFLOWS
UPGROWN
UPGROWS
WALLOWS
WETDOWN
WILLOWS
WILLOWY
WINDOWS
WINDOWY
WINNOWS
YARROWS
YELLOWS
YELLOWY

•••••OW
AIRFLOW
AIRGLOW
AIRSHOW
ARTSHOW
ASOFNOW
ATECROW
BACKROW
BARSTOW
BIGELOW
BIGSHOW
CALLNOW
CARSHOW
CASHCOW
CATCHOW
CATSHOW
COMENOW
CORNROW
DISAVOW
DOGCHOW
DOGSHOW
DOITNOW
DOWNBOW
EATCROW
EVENNOW
EXITNOW
EYEBROW
FORSHOW
GLASGOW
GLASHOW
GOBELOW
HADACOW
HADAROW
HASACOW
HASAROW
HERENOW
HIGHLOW
HITSHOW
HOLYCOW
ICESHOW
IGNATOW
ILLKNOW
ISEENOW
JANKLOW
JOEBLOW
JUSTNOW
KNEWHOW
KNOWHOW
LAIDLOW
LASTROW
LAYSLOW
LETKNOW
LIESLOW
LIKEWOW
LITHGOW
LONGBOW
LOWBLOW
LOWBROW
LUCKNOW
MANILOW
MILKCOW
MISKNOW
MISTBOW
MOONBOW
MUDFLOW
OUTBLOW
OUTCROW
OUTFLOW
OUTGLOW
OUTGROW
OUTSHOW
PALTROW
PAYSNOW
PETCROW
PILCROW
PRESHOW
RAINBOW
REENDOW
ROPETOW
RUNSLOW
SALCHOW
SHALLOW
SHOWHOW
SKIDROW
SOMEHOW
SPARROW
SUNGLOW
SWALLOW
THECROW
THESHOW
TILLNOW
TONEROW
TONYDOW
TOOSLOW
UPTHROW
UPTONOW
USOSHOW
VERYLOW
WHATNOW
WICKLOW
WINSLOW
WOODROW
YOUKNOW

OX•••••
OXALATE
OXBLOOD
OXCARTS
OXFORDS
OXHEART
OXHIDES
OXIDANT
OXIDASE
OXIDATE
OXIDISE
OXIDIZE
OXONIAN
OXTAILS
OXYMORA

O•X••••
OAXACAN

O•••••X
OISEAUX
OMNIMAX
ORATRIX
OUTFLUX
OUTJINX
OVERFIX
OVERLAX
OVERMIX
OVERTAX

•OX••••
BOXBALL
BOXBEDS
BOXBOYS
BOXCARS
BOXCOAT
BOXEDIN
BOXEDUP
BOXESIN
BOXESUP
BOXFULS
BOXIEST
BOXKITE
BOXLIKE
BOXSEAT
BOXSETS
BOXSTEP
BOXSTER
BOXTOPS
COXCOMB
COXLESS
FOXBORO
FOXFIRE
FOXHOLE
FOXHUNT
FOXIEST
FOXLIKE
FOXNEWS
FOXTAIL
FOXTROT
NOXIOUS
NOXZEMA
ROXANNE
ROXBURY
SOXFANS

•O•X•••
COAXERS
COAXIAL
COAXING
COEXIST
HOAXERS
HOAXING

•O••X••
JOHNXII
JOHNXIV
JOHNXIX
JOHNXVI
JOHNXXI
POBOXES
ROLEXES

•O•••X•
CONTEXT
JOHNXXI
LOUISXI
LOUISXV
POLEAXE

•O••••X
BOOMBOX
COINBOX
COMPLEX
COMTREX
COOLMAX
COOLPIX
DOUBLEX
FORTDIX
GORETEX
JOHNXIX
JOUHAUX
LOCKBOX
LOUISIX
MONTEUX
NONFLUX
POLLTAX
POORBOX
POORTAX
POSTBOX
POSTFIX
ROADTAX
ROLODEX
ROUBAIX
SOAPBOX
SOMINEX
SOUPMIX
TOOLBOX
WOODBOX
WORKBOX

••OX•••
DIOXIDE
DIOXINS
DROXIES
EPOXIED
EPOXIES
LEOXIII
PROXIES
PROXIMA
PROXIMO

••O•••X
ARONNAX
BOOMBOX
BROADAX
BROWWAX
COOLMAX
COOLPIX
DROPBOX
MEOWMIX
PHOENIX
POORBOX
POORTAX
SHOEBOX
STONEAX
TOOLBOX
WOODBOX

•••OX••
DETOXED
DETOXES
INBOXES
PHLOXES
POBOXES
REBOXED
REBOXES
REDOXES
UNBOXED
UNBOXES
UNFOXED
UNTOXIC
VELOXES
XEROXED
XEROXES

•••O••X
ALTOSAX
CELOTEX
FILOFAX
MEMOREX
ROLODEX

••••OX•
BYPROXY

••••O•X
BERVOIX
STCROIX
THEROUX
VERDOUX

•••••OX
BANDBOX
BEATBOX
BLUEFOX
BOOMBOX
BRERFOX
CALLBOX
CASHBOX
COINBOX
DEEDBOX
DROPBOX
EQUINOX
FAREBOX
FIREBOX
FIREFOX
FLUMMOX
FUSEBOX
GEARBOX
GIFTBOX
JUKEBOX
JURYBOX
KICKBOX
LOCKBOX
MAILBOX
PARADOX
PILLBOX
POORBOX
POSTBOX
SALTBOX
SANDBOX
SHOEBOX
SOAPBOX
TOOLBOX
WOODBOX
WORKBOX

OY•••••
OYSTERS

O•Y••••
ODYSSEY
OLYMPIA
OLYMPIC
OLYMPUS
OXYMORA

O••Y•••
OBEYERS
OBEYING
OFFYEAR
OKAYGUY
OKAYING
ONEYARD
ONEYEAR
ONLYTOO
ONLYYOU
ONMYOWN
OOCYTES
OUTYELL
OUTYELP

O•••Y••
OLDLYME
ONEBYTE
ONEEYED
ONLYYOU
OWLEYED

O••••Y•
OFFDAYS
OLDBOYS
OLDDAYS
OLDWAYS
ORKNEYS
OSPREYS
OUGUIYA
OUTBUYS
OUTLAYS
OUTPAYS
OUTSAYS
OVERDYE

O•••••Y
OBESELY
OBESITY
OBLOQUY
OCTUPLY
ODYSSEY
OFFDUTY
OJIBWAY
OKAYGUY
OKELLEY
OLDCITY
OLDFOGY
OLDLADY
OLDNAVY
OLEANNY
OMALLEY
ONAJURY
ONEADAY
ONEMPTY
OPACITY
ORANGEY
ORATORY
ORDERLY
OREBODY
OREILLY
ORGANDY
ORMANDY
OROGENY
OROLOGY
OSSUARY
OSTIARY
OTOLOGY
OUTBRAY
OUTCITY
OUTPITY
OUTPLAY
OUTPRAY
OUTSTAY
OUTTRAY
OVERBUY
OVERCOY
OVERDRY
OVERFLY
OVERJOY
OVERLAY
OVERPAY
OVERPLY
OVERTLY

•OY••••
BOYBAND
BOYCOTT
BOYHOOD
BOYLIKE
BOYTOYS
COYDOGS
COYNESS
COYOTES
DOYENNE
HOYDENS
JOYCEAN
JOYLESS
JOYPADS
JOYRIDE
LOYALER
LOYALES
LOYALLY
LOYALTO
LOYALTY
LOYOLAU
ROYALES
ROYALLY
ROYALTY
ROYALWE
ROYBEAN
ROYCOHN
ROYGBIV
SOYBEAN
SOYINKA
SOYINKS
SOYLENT
SOYMEAL
SOYMILK
TOYBALL
TOYBIKE
TOYBOAT
TOYBOOK
TOYCARS
TOYCART
TOYDOGS
TOYDOLL
TOYFAIR
TOYGUNS
TOYHATS
TOYHOOP
TOYKITE
TOYLAND
TOYLESS
TOYLIKE
TOYNBEE
TOYOTAS
TOYPAIL
TOYSHOP
TOYSLED
TOYSRUS
TOYTOPS
TOYWITH
VOYAGED
VOYAGER
VOYAGES
YOYOING
ZOYSIAS

•O•Y•••
BODYART
BODYBAR
BODYFAT
BODYKIT
BODYRUB
BOGYMAN
BOGYMEN
BOWYERS
COPYBOY
COPYCAT
COPYING
COPYIST
COPYMAN
COPYMEN
CORYELL
CORYZAS
COSYING
COZYING
FOGYISH
FOGYISM
GOBYAIR
GOBYBUS
GOBYCAB
GOBYCAR
GOBYSEA
HOLYARK
HOLYCOW
HOLYDAY
HOLYJOE
HOLYMAN
HOLYMEN
HOLYOIL
HOLYOKE
HOLYONE
HOLYSEE
HOLYWAR
JOEYDEE
KOSYGIN
OOCYTES
POLYGON
POLYMER
POLYPED
POLYPOD
POLYSCI
PONYING
PONYKEG
TONYDOW
TORYISH
TORYISM

•O••Y••
BOGEYED
BONEYER
COBUYER
COLLYER
DOEEYED
FORAYED
FORSYTE
FORSYTH
FORTYAD
FORTYBC
HONEYED
HOWDYDO
IOWEYOU
KOPIYKA
LOBBYER
LOOKYOU
LOVEYOU
MONEYED
MOSEYED
POPEYED
POPEYES
ROCKYII
ROCKYIV
VOTEYEA
VOTEYES
WOJTYLA

•O•••Y•
BOXBOYS
BOYTOYS
CONVEYS
CONVOYS
COWBOYS
DOGDAYS
DOGTOYS
DONKEYS
DORSEYS
FONTEYN
GOLDWYN
GOODBYE
GOODBYS
GOONEYS
HOMONYM
HOORAYS
HOTDAYS
HOTKEYS
JOCELYN
JOCKEYS
JOHNNYB
JOSBOYS
LOWBOYS
MONDAYS
MONKEYS
MONTOYA
MOONEYE
MOTLEYS
NOBODYS
POLANYI
ROBROYS
ROMNEYS
ROSALYN
SOCKEYE
TOMBOYS
TOPONYM
VOLLEYS
VOTEAYE

•O••••Y
BOBBSEY
BOBTWAY
BOGUSLY
BOKCHOY
BONEDRY
BONNILY
BOOTERY
BOOZILY
BOSSILY
COCKILY
COCKNEY
COGENCY
COLDDAY
COLICKY
COMESBY
COMPANY
CONAKRY
CONFREY
CONJURY
CONNERY
COOKERY
COOPERY
COPPERY
COPYBOY
CORNILY
COTTONY
COUNTRY
COURTLY
COWPONY
DODDERY
DOHERTY
DONLEVY
DONTCRY
DOORWAY
DOROTHY
DOTTILY
DOUBLEY
DOUGHTY
DOWDILY
FOAMILY
FOGCITY
FOGERTY
FOGGILY
FOLKWAY
FOOLERY
FOOTWAY
FOPPERY
FORADAY
FOREBAY
FORGERY
FORTIFY
FOUNDRY
FOURDAY
FOURWAY
GOCRAZY
GODFREY
GOINGBY
GOODBUY
GOODDAY
GOODGUY
GOODPAY
GOODTRY
GOOFILY
GOOMBAY
GOONILY
GOSSIPY
GOTAWAY
GOTBUSY
GOTOGUY
GOUTILY
HOARILY
HODADDY
HOGGERY
HOLIDAY
HOLYDAY
HOMEBOY
HONESTY
HOOPTOY
HORNSBY
HORRIFY
HORSILY
HORSLEY
HOSIERY
HOUSSAY
HOWMANY
JOBBERY
JOFFREY
JOHNBOY
JOHNGAY
JOHNJAY
JOINERY
JOINTLY
JOLLIFY
JOLLILY
JOLLITY
JOURNEY
LOATHLY
LOCALLY
LOFTILY
LONGDAY
LONGWAY
LOONILY
LOOSELY
LOTTERY
LOUSILY
LOVABLY
LOVEJOY
LOVERLY
LOWEEZY
LOWLILY
LOYALLY
LOYALTY
MOCKERY
MODESTY
MOISTLY
MOLLIFY
MOMONEY
MONTHLY
MOODILY
MOONILY
MORALLY
MOREPAY
MORESBY
MORTIFY
MOTHERY
MOUSILY
MOVABLY
MOWBRAY
NOENTRY
NOISILY
NOMERCY
NONBODY
NONBUSY
NONJURY
NONOILY
NONPLAY
NOONDAY
NOSEGAY
NOTABLY
NOTEASY
NOTEDLY
NOTMANY
NOVELTY
NOVOTNY
POORBOY
PORTNOY
PORTRAY
POTENCY
POTTERY
POULTRY
POVERTY
POWDERY
ROADWAY
ROBBERY
ROBOTRY
ROCKABY
ROCKERY
ROCKILY
ROGUERY
ROLLSBY
ROLLWAY
ROOKERY
ROOMILY
ROSEBAY
ROTAWAY
ROUGHLY
ROUNDLY
ROWDILY
ROXBURY
ROYALLY
ROYALTY
SOAPILY
SOBERLY
SOCIETY
SOGGILY
SOLIDLY
SOMEDAY
SOMESAY
SOMEWAY
SOOTILY
SORCERY
SORRILY
SOSORRY
SOTHEBY
SOUNDLY
SOUTHEY
TOGGERY
TOLLWAY
TOLSTOY
TONALLY
TOOEASY
TOOMANY
TOPIARY
TORREFY
TOTALLY
TOTTERY
TOUGHLY
TOURNEY
TOWAWAY
VOCABLY
VOCALLY
VOLUBLY
VOTENAY
VOUVRAY
VOWELLY
WOMANLY
WOODLEY
WOOLERY
WOOLLEY
WOOLSEY
WOOZILY
WORDILY
WORKDAY
WORKSHY
WORLDLY
WORSLEY
ZOMBIFY
ZONALLY
ZOOLOGY

••OY•••
BUOYANT
BUOYING
BUOYSUP
CLOYING
TWOYEAR

••O•Y••
ACOLYTE
ANODYNE
ANONYMS
AZODYES
BIOTYPE
ECOTYPE
EPONYMS
EPONYMY
EUONYMS
EXONYMS
GLORYBE
GROMYKO
IGOTYOU
LOOKYOU
NEOLYTE
PHONYUP
PROCYON

••O••Y•
GOODBYE
GOODBYS
GOONEYS
HOORAYS
MOONEYE
PHONEYS
SMOKEYS
TWODAYS

••O•••Y
ALOOFLY
ANOMALY
APOLOGY
BIOLOGY
BLOTCHY
BLOWDRY
BLOWFLY
BOOTERY
BOOZILY
BROADLY
BRODKEY
BRODSKY
CHOMSKY
CHOOSEY
CLOONEY
CLOSEBY
CLOSELY
CLOVERY
COOKERY
COOPERY
CROSSLY
CROWLEY
DOORWAY
DROPSBY
DROVEBY
DUOPOLY
ECOLOGY
ECONOMY
ENOLOGY
EPONYMY
EROSELY
ESOTERY
EXOGAMY
FLOATBY
FLOUNCY
FLOWERY
FLOWNBY
FOOLERY
FOOTWAY
GEODESY
GEOLOGY
GHOSTLY
GLORIFY
GOODBUY
GOODDAY
GOODGUY
GOODPAY
GOODTRY
GOOFILY
GOOMBAY
GOONILY
GROCERY
GROSSLY
GROUCHY
HOOPTOY
ICONIFY
ISONOMY
ISOTOPY
LEONDAY
LOONILY
LOOSELY
MOODILY
MOONILY
MYOLOGY
NEOLOGY
NOONDAY
OROGENY
OROLOGY
OTOLOGY
PHONILY
PIOSITY
PIOUSLY
PLOWBOY
POORBOY
PROBITY
PROCITY
PRODIGY
PROGENY
PRONAVY
PRONELY
PROSILY
PROSODY
PROUDLY
PTOLEMY
ROOKERY
ROOMILY
SHOOFLY
SHOOTBY
SHORTLY
SHOWERY
SHOWILY
SLOUCHY
SLOWDAY
SMOKILY
SMOOTHY
SNOWDAY
SNOWILY
SOOTILY
STOKELY
STONILY
STOODBY
STOOKEY
STOPSBY
STOUTLY
SWOREBY
TOOEASY
TOOMANY
TROLLEY
TROTSKY
UFOLOGY
UROLOGY
VRONSKY
WOODLEY
WOOLERY
WOOLLEY
WOOLSEY
WOOZILY
WRONGLY
ZOOLOGY

•••OY••
ALLOYED
ANNOYED
ANNOYER
ARROYOS
DECOYED
DECOYER
ENJOYED
ENJOYER
LEMOYNE
SAMOYED
SAROYAN
UNCOYER
UNCOYLY
UNJOYED
UNLOYAL

•••O•Y•
ACRONYM
ALLONYM
ANTONYM
AUTONYM
CACONYM
CAROLYN
DEMONYM
HOMONYM
HYPONYM
JCPOWYS
KAROLYI
NOBODYS

PARONYM
SYNONYM
TFPOWYS
TOPONYM

•••O••Y
ABBOTCY
ACTORLY
ALDORAY
ALLOWAY
ALMONDY
ALMONRY
ALOOFLY
ARMOURY
ATROPHY
AUTOPSY
BALONEY
BIGOTRY
BUXOMLY
BYGOLLY
CANONRY
CHOOSEY
CLOONEY
DAHOMEY
DEMOLAY
DISOBEY
DOROTHY
FELONRY
GOTOGUY
HELOTRY
HERONRY
IGNOBLY
IMSORRY
INNOWAY
ITSOKAY
JTMONEY
MAHONEY
MASONRY
MCCOVEY
MOMONEY
MRBODDY
NIKOLAY
NONOILY
NOVOTNY
OBLOQUY
PANOPLY
ROBOTRY
SAVOURY
SHLOCKY
SHOOFLY
SHOOTBY
SMOOTHY
SOSORRY
STOODBY
STOOKEY
THROATY
TIMOTHY
UNBOGGY
UNCOYLY
UNFOGGY
UNGODLY
UNJOLLY
UNLOFTY
UNLOWLY
UNMOLDY
UNMOODY
UNMOSSY
UNNOISY
UNROCKY
UNROOMY
UNROWDY
UNSOGGY
UNSOOTY
UNSORRY
UNWORMY
VAPOURY

••••OY•
AYKROYD
BADBOYS
BAGBOYS
BATBOYS
BIGBOYS
BOXBOYS
BOYTOYS
BUGBOYS
BUSBOYS
CAMBOYS
CARBOYS
CATTOYS
CHANOYU
CONVOYS
COWBOYS
DEPLOYS
DOGTOYS
EMPLOYS
FLYBOYS
JOSBOYS
LAZBOYS
LOWBOYS
MONTOYA
NEWTOYS
OLDBOYS
PEPBOYS
PETTOYS
PINBOYS
ROBROYS
SAMLOYD
SEQUOYA
TEAPOYS
THEBOYS
TOMBOYS

••••O•Y
ALIMONY
AMATORY
ANALOGY
ANATOLY
ANATOMY
ANCHOVY
ANTHONY
ANYBODY
APOLOGY
ASABODY
BALCONY
BILLOWY
BIOLOGY
BUTTONY
BYPROXY
CALPOLY
CARROTY
CHICORY
COTTONY
COWPONY
CURSORY
CUSTODY
DICKORY
DIGGORY
DUOPOLY
ECOLOGY
ECONOMY
ELUSORY
ENOLOGY
ENTROPY
EUPHONY
FACTORY
FLAVORY
GASCONY
GEOLOGY
GREGORY
HARMONY
HICKORY
HISTORY
HYMNODY
ISONOMY
ISOTOPY
JARGONY
KARLOVY
LASTORY
LETGOBY
MCGRORY
MEADOWY
MISCOPY
MYOLOGY
NEOLOGY
NONBODY
OLDFOGY
ORATORY
OREBODY
OROLOGY
OTOLOGY
PALJOEY
PEABODY
PETPONY
PILLORY
PILLOWY
PROSODY
RECTORY
REDPONY
RIBBONY
SAUCONY
SENSORY
SHADOWY
TALLOWY
TEACOZY
THEBODY
TRILOGY
UFOLOGY
UNIBODY
UNMOODY
UNROOMY
UNSHOWY
UNSMOKY
UNSOOTY
UNSTONY
UROLOGY
VICTORY
WILLOWY
WINDOWY
YELLOWY
ZOOLOGY

•••••OY
ATTABOY
BALLBOY
BELLBOY
BESTBOY
BLUEBOY
BOKCHOY
CALLBOY
CHEWTOY
CITYBOY
COPYBOY
DESTROY
DRMCCOY
FARMBOY
FITZROY
FREETOY
GAMEBOY
HAUTBOY
HELLBOY
HIGHBOY
HOMEBOY
HOOPTOY
ITSABOY
JOHNBOY
KILLJOY
LOVEJOY
NEWSBOY
NICEBOY
OVERCOY
OVERJOY
PAGEBOY
PLAYBOY
PLOWBOY
POORBOY
PORTNOY
PULLTOY
REENJOY
TOLSTOY
VICEROY

OZ•••••
OZONISE
OZONIZE
OZONOUS
OZZFEST

O•Z••••
OOZEOUT
OOZIEST
OZZFEST

O••••Z•
OBELIZE
ODORIZE
ONESIZE
ORGANZA
OUTBUZZ
OUTGAZE
OUTSIZE
OXIDIZE
OZONIZE

O•••••Z
ORDONEZ
OUTBUZZ

•OZ••••
BOZEMAN
COZENED
COZENER
COZIEST
COZUMEL
COZYING
COZZENS
DOZENTH
DOZEOFF
DOZIEST
LOZENGE
MOZETTA
MOZILLA
NOZZLES
OOZEOUT
OOZIEST
POZOLES
ROZANOV
ROZELLE
WOZNIAK
WOZZECK

•O•Z•••
BOOZERS
BOOZIER
BOOZILY
BOOZING
BORZAGE
BORZOIS
CORZINE
COZZENS
DOOZERS
DOOZIES
FOOZLED
FOOZLER
FOOZLES
GONZAGA
HOLZMAN
HOTZONE
NONZERO
NOXZEMA
NOZZLES
RONZONI
VONZELL
WOOZIER
WOOZILY
WOZZECK

•O••Z••
COETZEE
CORAZON
CORYZAS
HORIZON
IODIZED
IODIZER
IODIZES
IONIZED
IONIZER
IONIZES
TOPAZES

•O•••Z•
BONANZA
COGNIZE
FORENZA
FORSIZE
GOCRAZY
LORENZO
LOWEEZY
POETIZE

•O••••Z
COBLENZ
DOUBLEZ
HORVITZ
KOBLENZ
LORENTZ
POPQUIZ

••OZ•••
BOOZERS
BOOZIER
BOOZILY
BOOZING
CROZIER
DOOZERS
DOOZIES
FOOZLED
FOOZLER
FOOZLES
FROZEUP
FROZONE
WOOZIER
WOOZILY

••O•Z••
BLOWZED
BRONZED
BRONZER
BRONZES
PLOTZED
PLOTZES
SNOOZED
SNOOZER
SNOOZES

••O••Z•
AGONIZE
ANODIZE
ATOMIZE
CHORIZO
EBONIZE
IDOLIZE
LIONIZE
ODORIZE
OZONIZE

••O•••Z
FLORENZ
SHOWBIZ

•••OZ••
REBOZOS
SNOOZED
SNOOZER
SNOOZES

•••O••Z
ALLOPEZ
ORDONEZ
SIMONIZ

••••OZ•
CARDOZO
SCHNOZZ
SPINOZA
TEACOZY
UNFROZE

••••O•Z
BEDNORZ
MAHFOUZ
SCHNOZZ
THEFONZ

•••••OZ
BERLIOZ
DAVEKOZ
FRANKOZ

PA•••••
PAANGAS
PABLUMS
PABULUM
PACBELL
PACECAR
PACELAP
PACEOFF
PACHISI
PACIEST
PACIFIC
PACKAGE
PACKARD
PACKERS
PACKETS
PACKICE
PACKING
PACKOFF
PACKRAT
PACKSIN
PACKSON
PACKSUP
PACQUIN
PADDERS
PADDIES
PADDING
PADDLED
PADDLER
PADDLES
PADDOCK
PADGETT
PADLOCK
PADRAIC
PADRONE
PADSITE
PADUANS
PADUCAH
PAELLAS
PAGEANT
PAGEBOY
PAGEONE
PAGESIX
PAGETWO
PAGINGS
PAGODAS
PAHLAVI
PAIDADS
PAIDFOR
PAIDOFF
PAIDOUT
PAILFUL
PAINFUL
PAINING
PAINTED
PAINTER
PAIRERS
PAIRING
PAIROFF
PAIRSUP
PAISANO
PAISANS
PAISLEY
PAIUTES
PAJAMAS
PALABRA
PALACES
PALADIN
PALAMAS
PALANCE
PALATAL
PALATES
PALAVER
PALAZZI
PALAZZO
PALEALE
PALEDRY
PALEMON
PALERMO
PALETTE
PALFREY
PALINGS
PALJOEY
PALLETS
PALLIER
PALLING
PALLORS
PALMARY
PALMATE
PALMERS
PALMFUL
PALMIER
PALMING
PALMIST
PALMOFF
PALMOIL
PALMTOP
PALMYRA
PALOMAR
PALOMAS
PALOOKA
PALPATE
PALTERS
PALTROW
PALUDAL
PAMLICO
PAMPERS
PANACEA
PANACHE
PANADAS
PANAMAS
PANARAB
PANCAKE
PANCHAX
PANDERS
PANDITS
PANDORA
PANELED
PANETTA
PANFISH
PANFULS
PANGAEA
PANGRAM
PANICKY
PANICLE
PANIERS
PANINIS
PANNERS
PANNIER
PANNING
PANOPLY
PANPIPE
PANSIES
PANSOUT
PANTENE
PANTERA
PANTERS
PANTHER
PANTIES
PANTILE
PANTING
PANTLEG
PANTONE
PANURGE
PANZERS
PAPADOC
PAPAGOS
PAPAYAS
PAPEETE
PAPELES
PAPERED
PAPERER
PAPIERS
PAPILLA
PAPISTS
PAPOOSE
PAPPIES
PAPRIKA
PAPUANS
PAPYRUS
PARABLE
PARADED
PARADER
PARADES
PARADOR
PARADOX
PARAGON
PARAIBA
PARAMUS
PARAPET
PARAPHS
PARASKI
PARASOL
PARATUS
PARBAKE
PARBOIL
PARCELS
PARCHED
PARCHES
PARDNER
PARDONS
PARENTS
PARFAIT
PARFIVE
PARFOUR
PARFUMS
PARGERS
PARGING
PARIAHS
PARIBUS
PARINGS
PARKADE
PARKAVE
PARKERS
PARKING
PARKINS
PARKMAN
PARKSIT
PARKWAY
PARLAYS
PARLEYS
PARLORS
PARLOUR
PARLOUS
PARODIC
PAROLED
PAROLEE
PAROLES
PARONYM
PAROTID
PARQUET
PARRIED
PARRIER
PARRIES
PARRING
PARRISH
PARROTS
PARSECS
PARSEES
PARSERS
PARSING
PARSLEY
PARSNIP
PARSONS
PARTAKE
PARTIAL
PARTIED
PARTIER
PARTIES
PARTIII
PARTING
PARTITA
PARTITE
PARTNER
PARTONE
PARTOOK
PARTTWO
PARTWAY
PARTYER
PARTYON
PARURES
PARVENU
PASALLE
PASCHAL
PASCOLI
PASSADE
PASSADO
PASSAGE
PASSAIC
PASSANT
PASSATS
PASSELS
PASSERS
PASSEUL
PASSFOR
PASSING
PASSION
PASSIVE
PASSKEY
PASSOFF
PASSOUT
PASTDUE
PASTEIN
PASTELS
PASTERN
PASTERS
PASTEUP
PASTEUR
PASTIER
PASTIES
PASTIME
PASTINA
PASTING
PASTORS
PASTURE
PATACAS
PATCASH
PATCHED
PATCHEN
PATCHER
PATCHES
PATCHUP
PATDOWN
PATELLA
PATENCY
PATENTS
PATERNO
PATHAND
PATHANS
PATHWAY
PATIENT
PATINAS
PATNESS
PATRICE
PATRICK
PATRIES
PATRIOT
PATROLS
PATRONS
PATROON
PATSDRY
PATSIES
PATTERN
PATTERS
PATTIES
PATTING
PATZERS
PAUCITY
PAULIII
PAULINA
PAULINE
PAULING
PAULIST
PAULPRY
PAULSEN
PAUNCHY
PAUPERS
PAUSERS
PAUSING
PAVANES
PAVIDLY
PAVINGS
PAVIORS
PAVIOUR
PAVLOVA
PAWEDAT
PAWNEES
PAWNERS
PAWNING
PAWNOFF
PAWPAWS
PAXINOU
PAYABLE
PAYBACK
PAYCASH
PAYCUTS
PAYDAYS
PAYDIRT
PAYHEED
PAYINTO
PAYLESS
PAYLOAD
PAYMENT
PAYMORE
PAYOFFS
PAYOLAS
PAYOUTS
PAYRATE
PAYROLL
PAYSFOR
PAYSLIP
PAYSNOW
PAYSOFF
PAYSOUT
PAYSTUB
PAYWELL

P•A••••
PAANGAS
PBANDJS
PEABEAN
PEABODY
PEACHED
PEACHES
PEACOAT
PEACOCK
PEAFOWL
PEAHENS
PEAKIER
PEAKING
PEAKISH
PEALIKE
PEALING
PEANUTS
PEAPODS
PEARLED
PEARLER
PEARSON
PEASANT
PEASOUP
PEATBOG
PEATIER
PEATPOT
PGAPROS
PGATOUR
PHAEDRA
PHAETON
PHALANX
PHANTOM
PHARAOH
PHARLAP
PHARYNX
PHASEIN
PHASERS
PHASING
PHATTER
PIAFFED
PIAFFES
PIANISM
PIANIST
PIANOLA
PIASTER
PIASTRE
PIAZZAS
PLACARD
PLACATE
PLACEBO
PLACERS
PLACIDO
PLACING
PLACKET
PLAGUED
PLAGUES
PLAICES
PLAINER
PLAINES
PLAINLY
PLAINTS
PLAISIR
PLAITED
PLAITER
PLAKATS
PLANATE
PLANERS
PLANETS
PLANFOR
PLANING
PLANISH
PLANKED
PLANNED
PLANNER
PLANOUT
PLANSON
PLANSTO
PLANTAR
PLANTED
PLANTER
PLAQUES
PLASHED
PLASHES
PLASMAS
PLASMIC
PLASTER
PLASTIC
PLATEAU
PLATENS
PLATERS
PLATIER
PLATIES
PLATING
PLATOON
PLATTED
PLATTER
PLATYPI
PLAUDIT
PLAUTUS
PLAYACT
PLAYBOY
PLAYDOH
PLAYERS
PLAYFUL
PLAYING
PLAYLET
PLAYOFF
PLAYOUT
PLAYPEN

PLAYSAT
PLAYSBY
PLAYSON
PLAYSTO
PLAYSUP
PLAYTEX
POACHED
POACHER
POACHES
PRACTIC
PRADESH
PRAETOR
PRAIRIE
PRAISED
PRAISER
PRAISES
PRALINE
PRANCED
PRANCER
PRANCES
PRATERS
PRATING
PRATTLE
PRAWNED
PRAYERS
PRAYFOR
PRAYING
PRAYSTO
PSALMIC
PSALTER
PSANDQS

P••A•••

PAJAMAS
PALABRA
PALACES
PALADIN
PALAMAS
PALANCE
PALATAL
PALATES
PALAVER
PALAZZI
PALAZZO
PANACEA
PANACHE
PANADAS
PANAMAS
PANARAB
PAPADOC
PAPAGOS
PAPAYAS
PARABLE
PARADED
PARADER
PARADES
PARADOR
PARADOX
PARAGON
PARAIBA
PARAMUS
PARAPET
PARAPHS
PARASKI
PARASOL
PARATUS
PASALLE
PATACAS
PAVANES
PAYABLE
PDJAMES
PEDALED
PEDALER
PEDANTS
PEGASUS
PEGAWAY
PELAGES
PELAGIC
PENALTY
PENANCE
PENATES
PERAHIA
PERATIO
PESADES
PESANTE
PETALED
PETALES
PETARDS
PGRATED
PHRASAL
PHRASED
PHRASES
PICADOR
PICANTE
PICARAS
PICARDO
PICARDY
PICAROS
PICASSO
PILATES
PILATUS
PINATAS
PIPAGES
PIRAEUS
PIRANHA
PIRATED
PIRATES
PIRATIC
PISANIO
PISARRO
PITAPAT
PITAYAS
PIZARRO
PLEADED
PLEADER
PLEADTO
PLEASED
PLEASER
PLEASES
PLEATED
PLIABLE
PLIABLY
PLIANCY
POLANER
POLANYI
POLARAS
POLARIS
POMADED
POMADES
POSABLE
POSADAS
POTABLE
POTAGES
POTAMUS
PREACHY
PREACID
PREACTS
PREAGED
PREAGES
PREALLY
PREAMPS
PREARMS
PREAVER
PROARAB
PSHAWED
PULASKI
PUPATED
PUPATES
PUTAWAY
PYRAMID
PYRAMUS

P•••A••

PACKAGE
PACKARD
PADRAIC
PADUANS
PAGEANT
PAHLAVI
PAIDADS
PAISANO
PAISANS
PALEALE
PALMARY
PALMATE
PALPATE
PANCAKE
PANGAEA
PAPUANS
PARBAKE
PARFAIT
PARIAHS
PARKADE
PARKAVE
PARLAYS
PARTAKE
PASSADE
PASSADO
PASSAGE
PASSAIC
PASSANT
PASSATS
PATCASH
PATHAND
PATHANS
PAWPAWS
PAYBACK
PAYCASH
PAYDAYS
PAYRATE
PDQBACH
PEASANT
PECCANT
PECCARY
PECCAVI
PEDWAYS
PEERAGE
PELTATE
PENCASE
PENDANT
PENNAME
PENNANT
PENNATE
PENPALS
PENTADS
PENTANE
PEONAGE
PEPBAND
PEPPARD
PEPTALK
PERCALE
PERHAPS
PERIAPT
PERTAIN
PERVADE
PETCAGE
PETCALF
PETCATS
PETGATE
PETHAIR
PETHARE
PETLAMB
PETNAME
PETNAPS
PETRATS
PHALANX
PHARAOH
PICCARD
PICCATA
PICKAXE
PIEBALD
PIEPANS
PIESAFE
PIESALE
PIGTAIL
PILEATE
PILLAGE
PILLARS
PINBALL
PINNACE
PINNATE
PINOAKS
PINTAIL
PINWALE
PIPCARD
PIQUANT
PITFALL
PITSAWS
PIZZAZZ
PLACARD
PLACATE
PLAKATS
PLANATE
PLAYACT
PLENARY
PLICATE
PLUMAGE
PLURALS
POBLANO
PODCAST
POLEAXE
POLKAED
POLLACK
POLLARD
POLTAVA
POMMARD
POMPANO
PONIARD
PONTANO
POPEAFB
POPLARS
POPTART
PORTAGE
PORTALS
POSTAGE
POTTAGE
PREBADE
PREBAKE
PRECAST
PREDARK
PREDATA
PREDATE
PREDAWN
PREFABS
PREFACE
PREFADE
PREGAIN
PREGAME
PRELACY
PRELATE
PREMADE
PREMAKE
PREMATE
PRENAME
PREPACK
PREPAID
PREPARE
PREPAVE
PREPAYS
PRERACE
PRESAGE
PRESALE
PRESALT
PRETAPE
PREVAIL
PREWARM
PREWARN
PREWASH
PRIMACY
PRIMARY
PRIMATE
PRIVACY
PRIVATE
PROBALL
PROBATE
PROEAST
PROFANE
PROFARM
PROLATE
PRONATE
PRONAVY
PROPANE
PRORATA
PRORATE
PROSAIC
PSYWARS
PTBOATS
PUBGAME
PULSARS
PULSATE
PUNJABI
PUTBACK

P••••A•

PAANGAS
PACECAR
PACELAP
PACKRAT
PADUCAH
PAELLAS
PAGODAS
PAJAMAS
PALAMAS
PALATAL
PALOMAR
PALOMAS
PALUDAL
PANADAS
PANAMAS
PANARAB
PANCHAX
PANGRAM
PAPAYAS
PARKMAN
PARKWAY
PARTIAL
PARTWAY
PASCHAL
PATACAS
PATHWAY
PATINAS
PAWEDAT
PAYLOAD
PAYOLAS
PEABEAN
PEACOAT
PECKSAT
PEDICAB
PEEKSAT
PEEPSAT
PEERSAT
PEGAWAY
PELICAN
PELLEAS
PELOTAS
PENZIAS
PEORIAN
PEPITAS
PERLMAN
PERMIAN
PERORAL
PERREAU
PERSIAN
PERUSAL
PERYEAR
PESETAS
PESEWAS
PETBEAR
PETBOAS
PETEMAN
PETGOAT
PETSCAN
PHARLAP
PHIDIAS
PHILEAS
PHINEAS
PHOBIAS
PHRASAL
PIAZZAS
PICARAS
PICKSAT
PIERIAN
PIGMEAT
PINATAS
PINCHAS
PINESAP
PINETAR
PINHEAD
PINKHAM
PINSEAL
PISCEAN
PITAPAT
PITAYAS
PITHEAD
PITTMAN
PIVOTAL
PLANTAR
PLASMAS
PLATEAU
PLAYSAT
PLEBIAN
PLEURAE
PLEURAL
PLOWMAN
PLUSTAX
PLUVIAL
PNEUMAS
PNEUMAT
POINTAT
POKEDAT
POKESAT
POLARAS
POLECAR
POLECAT
POLEMAN
POLESAT
POLLTAX
PONTIAC
PONTIAN
POOHBAH
POOLMAN
POORLAW
POORMAN
POORTAX
POPSTAR
POPULAR
POPUPAD
PORTMAN
PORTRAY
POSADAS
POSEDAS
POSESAS
POSTBAG
POSTMAN
POSTWAR
POTOMAC
POTSDAM
PREHEAL
PREHEAT
PRELOAD
PRELOAN
PREORAL
PREPLAN
PRESEAL
PRESEAT
PRESOAK
PREVIAS
PREWRAP
PRINTAD
PROARAB
PROGRAM
PROPMAN
PROSCAN
PROTEAM
PROTEAN
PULLMAN
PULLTAB
PURITAN
PUTAWAY
PYTHIAN
PYTHIAS

P•••••A

PALABRA
PALMYRA
PALOOKA
PANACEA
PANDORA
PANETTA
PANGAEA
PANTERA
PAPILLA
PAPRIKA
PARAIBA
PARTITA
PASTINA
PATELLA
PAULINA
PAVLOVA
PERAHIA
PERDITA
PERGOLA
PERISSA
PERSONA
PERUGIA
PETULIA
PETUNIA
PHAEDRA
PHRYGIA
PIANOLA
PICCATA
PINOTTA
PIRANHA
PLECTRA
PLUGOLA
PODRIDA
POETICA
POLENTA
POLLERA
POLONIA
POLTAVA
POMPEIA
POPDIVA
PORSENA
PREDATA
PREIDEA
PREPUPA
PRIMERA
PRORATA
PROXIMA
PRUSSIA
PWBOTHA
PYREXIA

•PA••••

APACHES
APAIROF
APATITE
CPAEXAM
EPARCHS
EPARCHY
EPAULET
IPANEMA
OPACITY
OPALINE
OPALISH
OPAQUES
SPACELY
SPACERS
SPACIAL
SPACIER
SPACING
SPACKLE
SPADERS
SPADING
SPAMBOT
SPAMMED
SPAMMER
SPANAIR
SPANDEX
SPANGLE
SPANGLY
SPANIEL
SPANISH
SPANKED
SPANKER
SPANNED
SPANNER
SPARELY
SPAREME
SPARERS
SPAREST
SPARING
SPARKED
SPARKLE
SPARKLY
SPARRED
SPARRER
SPARROW
SPARSER
SPARTAN
SPASSKY
SPATHES
SPATIAL
SPATOUT
SPATTED
SPATTER
SPATULA
SPAWNED
SPAWNER
SPAYERS
SPAYING
UPABOVE
UPAHEAD
UPANDIN
UPATREE

•P•A•••

APHAGIA
APHAGIC
APHASIA
APHASIC
APPALLS
APPARAT
APPAREL
OPIATES
SPEAKER
SPEAKOF
SPEAKTO
SPEAKUP
SPEARED
SPEARER
SPLASHY
SPLAYED
SPRAINS
SPRAWLS
SPRAWLY
SPRAYED
SPRAYER
SPRAYON
UPCARDS
UPCASTS
UPDARTS
UPDATED
UPDATER
UPDATES
UPEARLY
UPGAZED
UPGAZES
UPLANDS
UPRAISE
UPRATED
UPRATES
UPTAKES
UPTALKS
UPVALUE
UPWAFTS
UPWARDS

•P••A••

APPEALS
APPEARS
APPEASE
APPLAUD
CPEBACH
EPHRAIM
EPICARP
EPILADY
EPILATE
EPITAPH
OPENAIR
OPERAND
OPERANT
OPERATE
SPANAIR
SPINACH
SPIRALS
SPOKANE
SPREADS
SPYCAMS
SPYWARE
UPBEARS
UPBEATS
UPBRAID
UPCOAST
UPDRAFT
UPGRADE
UPHEAPS
UPHEAVE
UPHOARD
UPLEAPS
UPLEAPT
UPLOADS
UPPHASE
UPPSALA
UPQUARK
UPREACH
UPREARS
UPROARS
UPSCALE
UPSOARS
UPSTAGE
UPSTAIR
UPSTAND
UPSTARE
UPSTART
UPSTATE
UPTEARS
UPTRADE

•P•••A•

APOGEAL
APOGEAN
APPARAT
APTERAL
APULIAN
CPAEXAM
EPERNAY
EPIGRAM
EPOCHAL
OPENBAR
OPENTAP
OPTICAL
OPTIMAL
OPTIMAS
SPACIAL
SPARTAN
SPATIAL
SPECIAL
SPHERAL
SPIREAS
SPORRAN
SPOUSAL
UPAHEAD
UPTOPAR

•P••••A

APHAGIA
APHASIA
APHELIA
APHONIA
EPHEDRA
IPANEMA
OPENSEA
OPHELIA
OPUNTIA
SPATULA
SPECTRA
SPINOZA
SPLENDA
UPPSALA

••PA•••

ALPACAS
APPALLS
APPARAT
APPAREL
AUPAIRS
BYPATHS
CAPABLE
CAPABLY
CAPADES
CAPAPIE
DEPALMA
DEPARTS
DEPAULU
EMPALED
EMPALES
EMPANEL
EMPATHS
EMPATHY
ESPANOL
ESPARTO
EXPANDS
EXPANSE
EXPARTE
HEPARIN
HEPATIC
HOPACAB
HYPATIA
IMPACTS
IMPAIRS
IMPALAS
IMPALED
IMPALER
IMPALES
IMPANEL
IMPARTS
IMPASSE
IMPASTO
IMPAVID
LAPALMA
LEPANTO
LIPARIS
LIPASES
MCPAPER
MRPADRE
NAPALMS
NEPALIS
NOPALES
ONPAPER
PAPADOC
PAPAGOS
PAPAYAS
PIPAGES
PUPATED
PUPATES
RAPALLO
RAPANUI
REPACKS
REPAGED
REPAGES
REPAINT
REPAIRS
REPANEL
REPAPER
REPARKS
REPASTE
REPASTS
REPATCH
REPAVED
REPAVES
RVPARKS
SEPALED
STPAULS
TOPAZES
UNPACED
UNPACKS
UNPAGAN
UNPAGED
UNPALED
UNPARED
UNPASTE
UNPAVED
UNPAWED
UNPAWNS
ZAPATAS
ZAPATEO

••P•A••

ALPHARD
APPEALS
APPEARS
APPEASE
APPLAUD
ASPHALT
ASPRAWL
ATPEACE
BIPLANE
BYPLAYS
CAPEANN
CAPTAIN
CAPUANA
CEPHALO
CEPHALY
COPCARS
COPLAND
CUPCAKE
DEPLANE
DEPRAVE
ELPRADO
EMPLACE
EMPLANE
ENPLANE
ESPIALS
EXPIATE
EXPLAIN
HEPCATS
HEPTADS
HIPBATH
HUPPAHS
IMPEACH
IMPLANT
INPEACE
INPHASE
INPLACE
LAPCATS
LAPLACA
LAPLACE
LAPLAND
LAPLATA
LAPSANG
LAPWARE
LEPPARD
LIPBALM
LIPMANN
NOPLACE
OMPHALO
ORPHANS
ORPHANT
PAPUANS
PEPBAND
PEPPARD
PEPTALK
PIPCARD
POPEAFB
POPLARS
POPTART
RAPHAEL
REPEALS
REPEATS
REPHASE
REPLACE
REPLANE

REPLANS
REPLANT
REPLATE
REPLAYS
RIPRAPS
RIPSAWN
RIPSAWS
RUPIAHS
SAPSAGO
SOPRANI
SOPRANO
TAPPANS
TIPCART
TIPJARS
TOPHATS
TOPIARY
TOPKAPI
TOPMAST
TOPNAME
TOPRANK
TOPRATE
TOPSAIL
TYPEABS
UNPLAIT
UNPLANS
UPPHASE
UPPSALA
YOPLAIT

••P••A•
ALPACAS
APPARAT
BIPEDAL
BIPOLAR
CAPEMAY
CAPITAL
CAPITAN
CAPSHAW
CAPSTAN
COPULAE
COPULAR
COPULAS
COPYCAT
COPYMAN
CUPOLAS
CUPULAR
CYPRIAN
DEPOSAL
DIPOLAR
ESPOSAS
GAPEDAT
GAPESAT
HOPACAB
IMPALAS
IMPLEAD
KAPITAL
LAPUTAN
LIPREAD
MOPHEAD
NUPTIAL
ORPHEAN
PAPAYAS
PEPITAS
POPSTAR
POPULAR
POPUPAD
RAPIDAN
RAPSTAR
REPLEAD
REPOMAN
SAPHEAD
SEPHIAS
SEPIRAS
TAPEMAN
TOPCOAT
TOPDRAW
TOPEKAN
TOPICAL
TYPICAL
UNPAGAN
ZAPATAS

••P•••A
AMPHORA
CAPELLA
CAPTIVA
CAPUANA
COPPOLA
DAPHNIA
DEPALMA
DIPLOMA
EMPORIA
HYPATIA
IMPREZA
JEPHTHA
KAPITSA
KOPIYKA
LAPALMA
LAPLACA
LAPLATA
NAPHTHA
PAPILLA
PAPRIKA
POPDIVA
REPLICA
TAPIOCA
UPPSALA

•••PA••
ADSPACE
AIRPACK
AIRPARK
ANSPACH
ARAPAHO
ASHPANS
BADPAST
BITPART
BUSPASS
CAMPARI
CARPALS
CARPARK
CASPARY
CHAPALA
CHAPATI
CLIPART
COMPACT
COMPANY
COMPAQS
COMPARE
COMPART
COMPASS
CUSPATE
DAYPACK
DESPAIR
DISPART
FANPALM
FLYPAST
FRYPANS
GALPALS
GASPARD
GETPAST
GODPAPA
GOTPAST
HISPANO
HOTPACK
HUPPAHS
ICEPACK
ILLPASS
INKPADS
INSPACE
INSPANS
JAMPACK
JETPACK
JOYPADS
KAMPALA
KEYPADS
KEYPALS
LEOPARD
LEPPARD
LESPAUL
LETPASS
LOWPAID
LOWPAIR
MALPASO
MISPAGE
MRSPAUL
MUDPACK
MYSPACE
NAIPAUL
NONPAID
NONPARS
NONPAST
OAKPARK
OILPALM
OILPANS
OLDPALS
ONEPAGE
ONEPAIR
ONEPART
OOMPAHS
OUTPACE
OUTPAID
OUTPASS
OUTPATH
OUTPAYS
OVIPARA
PALPATE
PAWPAWS
PENPALS
PEPPARD
PIEPANS
POMPANO
PREPACK
PREPAID
PREPARE
PREPAVE
PREPAYS
PROPANE
QUAPAWS
QUEPASA
RAMPAGE
RAMPANT
RAMPART
RANPAST
RATPACK
RESPACE
RESPADE
RESPANS
RESPARK
RIBPADS
RUNPAST
SAMPANS
SAWPAST
SEEPAGE
SEEPAST
SHEPARD
SIXPACK
SOSPADS
SURPASS
TAMPAFL
TAPPANS
TAXPAID
TENPAST
TIMPANI
TOSPARE
TOWPATH
TOYPAIL
TREPANS
TWOPAIR
TWOPART
TYMPANA
TYMPANI
UNSPANS
WARPAGE
WARPATH
WEBPAGE

•••P•A•
ADEPTAT
AIRPLAY
BEEPSAT
BESPEAK
CARPSAT
CASPIAN
CHAPEAU
CHAPMAN
CHUPPAH
CHUPPAS
COWPEAS
DEEPFAT
DEEPTAN
DIAPHAN
DISPLAY
DRIPPAN
DROPCAP
ENDPLAY
GRAPPAS
GUNPLAY
HITPLAY
HOOPLAS
HOOPMAN
IREPEAT
JUMPSAT
KEEPSAT
LEAPDAY
LEAPSAT
LEAPTAT
LINPIAO
MAUPRAT
MISPLAN
MISPLAY
MYOPIAS
NONPEAK
NONPLAY
NYMPHAL
OFFPEAK
OUTPLAN
OUTPLAY
OUTPRAY
PEEPSAT
PREPLAN
PROPMAN
RESPEAK
RESPRAY
SAMPRAS
SETPLAY
SHIPMAN
SHIPWAY
SHOPSAT
SNAPSAT
SNIPEAT
SOAPPAD
SOUPCAN
STEPDAD
STOPGAP
STOPSAT
TEMPEAZ
TEMPLAR
UNSPEAK
UTOPIAN
UTOPIAS
WHIPSAW

•••P••A
AMAPOLA
CHAPALA
COPPOLA
CORPORA
CRAPOLA
DEEPSEA
DESPINA
GODPAPA
KAMPALA
LEMPIRA
OVIPARA
POMPEIA
PREPUPA
QUEPASA
SCAPULA
SNAPPEA
TEMPERA
TEMPURA
TRIPLEA
TYMPANA
VAMPIRA

••••PA•
BACKPAY
BAKEPAN
BASEPAY
BEARPAW
CAKEPAN
CATSPAW
CHARPAK
CHIAPAS
CHUPPAH
CHUPPAS
DAYSPAS
DEADPAN
DISHPAN
DOWNPAT
DRIPPAN
DUSTPAN
ECTYPAL
ENDUPAT
EVENPAR
FAUXPAS
FOOTPAD
FOREPAW
GOODPAY
GRAMPAS
GRANPAS
GRAPPAS
GRASPAT
HARDPAN
HEELPAD
HELIPAD
HIGHPAY
HINDPAW
KEYSPAN
KNEEPAD
LILYPAD
LOAFPAN
LOOMPAS
MADEPAR
MAKEPAR
MEMOPAD
MOREPAY
NEARPAR
NOTEPAD
OEDIPAL
OVERPAR
OVERPAY
PITAPAT
POPUPAD
SERIPAK
SHERPAS
SHINPAD
SHOEPAC
SHOTPAR
SICKPAY
SITSPAT
SOAPPAD
STEWPAN
TRAMPAS
TUBEPAN
UPTOPAR

••••P•A
AGRIPPA
AUTOPIA
EXEMPLA
JOSEPHA
MAZEPPA
OLYMPIA
SNAPPEA
SNOWPEA
SWEEPEA

•••••PA
AGRIPPA
CATALPA
CHALUPA
CHUTZPA
GODPAPA
GRANDPA
MAANDPA
MAZEPPA
PREPUPA
YUCAIPA

PB•••••
PBANDJS

P•B••••
PABLUMS
PABULUM
PEBBLED
PEBBLES
POBLANO
POBOXES
PTBOATS
PUBERTY
PUBGAME
PUBLICS
PUBLISH
PUBLIUS
PWBOTHA

P••B•••
PACBELL
PARBAKE
PARBOIL
PAYBACK
PDQBACH
PEABEAN
PEABODY
PEBBLED
PEBBLES
PEEBLES
PEPBAND
PEPBOYS
PETBEAR
PETBIRD
PETBOAS
PHOBIAS
PHOBICS
PIEBALD
PINBALL
PINBOYS
PITBOSS
PITBULL
PLEBIAN
POTBOIL
PREBADE
PREBAKE
PREBIDS
PREBILL
PREBIND
PREBOIL
PREBOOK
PREBOOM
PREBORN
PREBURN
PREBUYS
PROBALL
PROBATE
PROBERS
PROBIES
PROBING
PROBITY
PROBLEM
PROBONO
PROBOWL
PUEBLOS
PUTBACK

P•••B••
PAGEBOY
PALABRA
PARABLE
PARIBUS
PAYABLE
PEATBOG
PHILBIN
PHOEBES
PHOEBUS
PILLBOX
PILLBUG
PLAYBOY
PLIABLE
PLIABLY
PLOWBOY
PLUMBED
PLUMBER
PLUMBIC
PLUMBUM
POOHBAH
POORBOX
POORBOY
POSABLE
POSTBAG
POSTBOX
POTABLE
PROMBID

P••••B•
PARAIBA
PLACEBO
PLAYSBY
PREFABS
PUNJABI

P•••••B
PANARAB
PAYSTUB
PEDICAB
PERTURB
PETCOMB
PETLAMB
POPEAFB
POTHERB
PREVERB
PROARAB
PROVERB
PULLTAB

•PB••••
UPBEARS
UPBEATS
UPBORNE
UPBOUND
UPBRAID
UPBUILD
UPBURST

•P•B•••
CPEBACH
SPYBOTS
UPABOVE

•P••B••
EPHEBUS
OPENBAR
SPAMBOT

•P••••B
UPCLIMB

••PB•••
HEPBURN
HIPBATH
HIPBONE
HIPBOOT
LAPBELT
LIPBALM
PEPBAND
PEPBOYS
TOPBIDS
TOPBOOT

••P•B••
CAPABLE
CAPABLY
COPYBOY

••P••B•
LAPROBE
REPROBE
TYPEABS

••P•••B
HOPACAB
POPEAFB
REPLUMB
UNPLUMB
VAPORUB

•••PB••
CAMPBED
DROPBOX
JUMPBID
SOAPBOX

•••P•B•
DROPSBY
SHOPNBC
SKIPSBY
SLIPSBY
STOPSBY

•••P••B
TEMPJOB

••••PB•
CREEPBY

••••P•B
BREWPUB

PC•••••
PCCLONE
PCUSERS
PCWORLD

P•C••••
PACBELL
PACECAR
PACELAP
PACEOFF
PACHISI
PACIEST
PACIFIC
PACKAGE
PACKARD
PACKERS
PACKETS
PACKICE
PACKING
PACKOFF
PACKRAT
PACKSIN
PACKSON
PACKSUP
PACQUIN
PCCLONE
PECCANT
PECCARY
PECCAVI
PECKING
PECKISH
PECKSAT
PECTINS
PICADOR
PICANTE
PICARAS
PICARDO
PICARDY
PICAROS
PICASSO
PICCARD
PICCATA
PICCOLO
PICEOUS
PICKAXE
PICKENS
PICKERS
PICKETS
PICKETT
PICKIER
PICKING
PICKLED
PICKLES
PICKOFF
PICKOUT
PICKSAT
PICKSON
PICKSUP
PICKUPS
PICNICS
PICOTED
PICTISH
PICTURE
POCKETS
POCONOS
PUCCINI
PUCKERS
PUCKERY
PUCKETT
PUCKISH
PVCPIPE

P••C•••
PANCAKE
PANCHAX
PARCELS
PARCHED
PARCHES
PASCHAL
PASCOLI
PATCASH
PATCHED
PATCHEN
PATCHER
PATCHES
PATCHUP
PAUCITY
PAYCASH
PAYCUTS
PEACHED
PEACHES
PEACOAT
PEACOCK
PECCANT
PECCARY
PECCAVI
PENCASE
PENCILS
PEPCIDS
PERCALE
PERCENT
PERCEPT
PERCHED
PERCHER
PERCHES
PERCHIK
PERCUSS
PETCAGE
PETCALF
PETCATS
PETCHEW
PETCOCK
PETCOMB
PETCOWS
PETCROW
PICCARD
PICCATA
PICCOLO
PIECERS
PIECING
PILCROW
PINCERS
PINCHAS
PINCHED
PINCHER
PINCHES
PINCHME
PINCHOT
PINCURL
PIPCARD
PISCEAN
PISCINE
PISCOPO
PITCHED
PITCHER
PITCHES
PITCHIN
PITCHTO
PITCREW
PLACARD
PLACATE
PLACEBO
PLACERS
PLACIDO
PLACING
PLACKET
PLECTRA
PLICATE
PLUCKED
POACHED
POACHER
POACHES
PODCAST
PONCHOS
POOCHES
POOCHIE
POPCORN
PORCHES
PORCINE
POUCHED
POUCHES
PRACTIC
PRECAST
PRECEDE
PRECEPT
PRECISE
PRECITE
PRECODE
PRECOIL
PRECOOK
PRECOOL
PRECOUP
PRECURE
PRECUTS
PRICERS
PRICIER
PRICILY
PRICING
PRICKED
PRICKLE
PRICKLY
PRICKUP
PROCEED
PROCESS
PROCITY
PROCLUS
PROCTER
PROCTOR
PROCURE
PROCYON
PSYCHED
PSYCHES
PSYCHIC
PSYCHOS
PSYCHUP
PUCCINI
PUNCHED
PUNCHER
PUNCHES
PUNCHIN
PUNCHUP
PURCELL
PYNCHON

P•••C••
PACECAR
PADUCAH
PALACES
PANACEA
PANACHE
PANICKY
PANICLE
PATACAS
PAUNCHY
PEDICAB
PELICAN
PENUCHE
PETSCAN
PHILCOS
PIERCED
PIERCER
PIERCES
PLAICES
PLUMCOT
POLECAR
POLECAT
POLICED
POLICER
POLICES
POOLCUE
PORSCHE
POUNCED
POUNCER
POUNCES
PRANCED
PRANCER
PRANCES
PREACHY
PREACID
PREACTS
PRINCES
PROSCAN
PUMICED
PUMICES

P••••C•
PACKICE
PADDOCK
PADLOCK
PALANCE
PAMLICO
PARSECS
PATENCY
PATRICE
PATRICK
PAYBACK
PDQBACH
PEACOCK
PENANCE
PENNOCK
PEPSICO
PEPTICS
PERFECT
PETCOCK
PETDUCK
PETMICE
PETROCK
PHOBICS
PHONICS
PHOTICS
PHYSICS
PICNICS
PIMLICO
PINNACE
PLAYACT
PLIANCY
POETICA
POETICS
POLISCI
POLLACK
POLLOCK
POLYSCI
POPROCK
PORTICO
POTENCE
POTENCY

POTLUCK
PREDICT
PREFACE
PREFECT
PRELACY
PREPACK
PRERACE
PREROCK
PRIMACY
PRIVACY
PRODUCE
PRODUCT
PROJECT
PROTECT
PUBLICS
PUDENCY
PUTBACK

P•••••C
PACIFIC
PADRAIC
PAPADOC
PARODIC
PASSAIC
PELAGIC
PHRENIC
PIRATIC
PLASMIC
PLASTIC
PLUMBIC
POLEMIC
POLITIC
PONTIAC
POSTDOC
POSTHOC
POTOMAC
POULENC
PRACTIC
PROSAIC
PSALMIC
PSYCHIC
PYRETIC
PYRITIC
PYRRHIC

•PC••••
IPCRESS
UPCARDS
UPCASTS
UPCCODE
UPCLIMB
UPCLOSE
UPCOAST
UPCOILS
UPCOURT
UPCURLS
UPCURVE

•P•C•••
APACHES
APECKOF
EPICARP
EPICENE
EPICURE
EPOCHAL
OPACITY
SPACELY
SPACERS
SPACIAL
SPACIER
SPACING
SPACKLE
SPECIAL
SPECIES
SPECIFY
SPECING
SPECKED
SPECKLE
SPECOUT
SPECTER
SPECTOR
SPECTRA
SPECTRE
SPICERS
SPICERY
SPICEUP
SPICIER
SPICILY
SPICING
SPYCAMS
UPCCODE
UPSCALE

•P••C••
APERCUS
APRICOT
EPARCHS
EPARCHY
OPTICAL
OPTICKS
SPENCER
SPLICED
SPLICER
SPLICES
SPRUCED
SPRUCER
SPRUCES
UPTICKS

•P•••C•
CPEBACH
IPSWICH
SPINACH
SPLOTCH
UPREACH

•P••••C
APHAGIC
APHASIC
APHONIC
SPHERIC

••PC•••
COPCARS
CUPCAKE
HEPCATS
LAPCATS
PEPCIDS
PIPCARD
POPCORN
RIPCORD
TIPCART
TOPCOAT
ZIPCODE
ZIPCUFF

••P•C••
ALPACAS
ASPECTS
CAPECOD
CAPUCHE
COPYCAT
DEPECHE
DEPICTS
EXPECTS
HOPACAB
IMPACTS
KOPECKS
REPACKS
REPICKS
TOPICAL
TYPICAL
UNPACED
UNPACKS
UNPICKS

••P••C•
ASPENCO
ATPEACE
CAPRICE
COPPICE
DIPTYCH
EMPLACE
HAPTICS
IMPEACH
INPEACE
INPLACE
LAPLACA
LAPLACE
NIPMUCK
NOPLACE
PEPSICO
PEPTICS
POPROCK
REPATCH
REPLACE
REPLICA
REPRICE
TAPIOCA
TOPKICK
ZIPLOCK
ZIPLOCS

••P•••C
EMPIRIC
HEPATIC
LIPIDIC
LIPSYNC
NEPHRIC
NEPOTIC
PAPADOC
ZAPOTEC

•••PC••
DROPCAP
JUMPCUT
SOUPCAN
SOUPCON

•••P•C•
ADSPACE
AIRPACK
ANSPACH
AUSPICE
BIOPICS
COMPACT
COPPICE
DAYPACK
DRSPOCK
HENPECK
HOSPICE
HOTPACK
ICEPACK
ICEPICK
INSPACE
INSPECT
JAMPACK
JETPACK
MRSPOCK
MUDPACK
MYSPACE
NITPICK
OUTPACE
OUTPICK
PREPACK
RATPACK
RESPACE
RESPECT
RESPICE
SERPICO
SIXPACK
SUSPECT
TAMPICO
TOEPICK
TROPICS
UNSPICY

•••P••C
ASEPTIC
CRYPTIC
DELPHIC
GLYPHIC
GLYPTIC
GRAPHIC
MORPHIC
NYMPHIC
SCEPTIC
SHOPNBC
SKEPTIC
STYPTIC
SYLPHIC

••••P•C
NONEPIC
OLYMPIC
ONTOPIC
SHOEPAC
TELEPIC
WAREPIC

PD•••••
PDJAMES
PDQBACH

P•D••••
PADDERS
PADDIES
PADDING
PADDLED
PADDLER
PADDLES
PADDOCK
PADGETT
PADLOCK
PADRAIC
PADRONE
PADSITE
PADUANS
PADUCAH
PEDALED
PEDALER
PEDANTS
PEDDLED
PEDDLER
PEDDLES
PEDICAB
PEDWAYS
PIDDLED
PIDDLES
PIDGEON
PIDGINS
PODCAST
PODIUMS
PODLIKE
PODRIDA
PUDDING
PUDDLED
PUDDLES
PUDENCY
PUDGIER
PUDGILY

P••D•••
PADDERS
PADDIES
PADDING
PADDLED
PADDLER
PADDLES
PADDOCK
PAIDADS
PAIDFOR
PAIDOFF
PAIDOUT
PANDERS
PANDITS
PANDORA
PARDNER
PARDONS
PATDOWN
PAYDAYS
PAYDIRT
PEDDLED
PEDDLER
PEDDLES
PENDANT
PENDENT
PENDING
PERDIDO
PERDIEM
PERDITA
PERDURE
PETDEER
PETDOGS
PETDOOR
PETDOVE
PETDUCK
PHIDIAS
PIDDLED
PIDDLES
PINDOWN
PLEDGED
PLEDGEE
PLEDGER
PLEDGES
PLODDED
PLODDER
PONDERS
PONDING
POODLES
POPDIVA
POUDRES
POWDERS
POWDERY
PRADESH
PREDARK
PREDATA
PREDATE
PREDAWN
PREDEFY
PREDENY
PREDICT
PREDIET
PREDIVE
PREDOOM
PREDUSK
PRIDING
PRODDED
PRODDER
PRODIGY
PRODSON
PRODUCE
PRODUCT
PRUDENT
PRUDERY
PRUDHOE
PRUDISH
PUDDING
PUDDLED
PUDDLES
PUNDITS
PURDUEU
PUTDOWN
PYEDOGS

P•••D••
PAGODAS
PALADIN
PALEDRY
PALUDAL
PANADAS
PAPADOC
PARADED
PARADER
PARADES
PARADOR
PARADOX
PARODIC
PASTDUE
PATSDRY
PAVIDLY
PAWEDAT
PBANDJS
PERIDOT
PESADES
PHAEDRA
PICADOR
PILEDIN
PILEDON
PILEDUP
PIPEDIN
PIPEDUP
PLAUDIT
PLAYDOH
PLEADED
PLEADER
PLEADTO
PLODDED
PLODDER
PLOVDIV
PLUNDER
POKEDAT
POMADED
POMADES
POPEDOM
POSADAS
POSEDAS
POSTDOC
POTSDAM
POUNDED
POUNDER
PREEDIT
PREIDEA
PRODDED
PRODDER
PROUDER
PROUDLY
PROUDOF
PSANDQS

P••••D•
PAIDADS
PARKADE
PASSADE
PASSADO
PEABODY
PEAPODS
PENTADS
PEPCIDS
PEPTIDE
PERDIDO
PERFIDY
PERIODS
PERVADE
PETARDS
PICARDO
PICARDY
PLACIDO
PODRIDA
PONGIDS
POTLIDS
PREBADE
PREBIDS
PRECEDE
PRECODE
PREFADE
PRELUDE
PREMADE
PREMEDS
PRESIDE
PROKEDS
PROSODY
PROVIDE

P•••••D
PACKARD
PADDLED
PAINTED
PANELED
PAPERED
PARADED
PARCHED
PAROLED
PAROTID
PARRIED
PARTIED
PATCHED
PATHAND
PAYHEED
PAYLOAD
PCWORLD
PEACHED
PEARLED
PEBBLED
PEDALED
PEDDLED
PEOPLED
PEPBAND
PEPPARD
PERCHED
PERILED
PERSEID
PERUSED
PESTLED
PETALED
PETBIRD
PETERED
PGRATED
PHISHED
PHOTOID
PHRASED
PIAFFED
PICCARD
PICKLED
PICOTED
PIDDLED
PIEBALD
PIEEYED
PIERCED
PIFFLED
PIGEYED
PIGWEED
PILOTED
PIMPLED
PINCHED
PINFOLD
PINGUID
PINHEAD
PIPCARD
PIRATED
PITCHED
PITHEAD
PIVOTED
PLACARD
PLAGUED
PLAITED
PLANKED
PLANNED
PLANTED
PLASHED
PLATTED
PLEADED
PLEASED
PLEATED
PLEDGED
PLINKED
PLODDED
PLONKED
PLOPPED
PLOTTED
PLOTZED
PLUCKED
PLUGGED
PLUMBED
PLUMPED
PLUNGED
PLUNKED
PLYWOOD
POACHED
POINTED
POLICED
POLKAED
POLLARD
POLYPED
POLYPOD
POMADED
POMMARD
PONIARD
POPEYED
POPPLED
POPUPAD
PORTEND
POSITED
POUCHED
POUNCED
POUNDED
POWERED
PRAISED
PRANCED
PRAWNED
PREACID
PREAGED
PREBIND
PREENED
PREFUND
PRELOAD
PREPAID
PREPPED
PRESOLD
PRESSED
PRETEND
PRETOLD
PREVOID
PREVUED
PRICKED
PRIMMED
PRIMPED
PRINKED
PRINTAD
PRINTED
PROCEED
PRODDED
PROMBID
PROMOED
PRONGED
PROOFED
PROPPED
PROWLED
PSHAWED
PSYCHED
PUDDLED
PUMICED
PUNCHED
PUPATED
PURFLED
PURPLED
PURSUED
PUSHROD
PUTTIED
PUZZLED
PYRAMID

•PD••••
UPDARTS
UPDATED
UPDATER
UPDATES
UPDIVED
UPDIVES
UPDRAFT
UPDRIED
UPDRIES
UPDRIFT

•P•D•••
APEDIET
APODOUS
EPIDERM
EPIDOTE
SPADERS
SPADING
SPEDOFF
SPIDERS
SPIDERY
SPYDERS

•P••D••
APHIDES
APSIDES
EPHEDRA
IPLEDGE
OPTEDIN
OPTEDTO
SPANDEX
SPEEDED
SPEEDER
SPEEDOS
SPEEDUP
SPENDER
SPENDON
SPIEDON
SPINDLE
SPINDLY
SPINDRY
SPONDEE
UPANDIN
UPENDED
UPSIDES

•P•••D•
APPENDS
EPILADY
EPISODE
SPLENDA
SPREADS
SPYKIDS
UPCARDS
UPCCODE
UPFOLDS
UPGIRDS
UPGRADE
UPHOLDS
UPLANDS
UPLOADS
UPSENDS
UPTRADE
UPWARDS
UPWINDS

•P••••D
APPLAUD
APPLIED
APPOSED
APRONED
EPOXIED
OPENEND
OPERAND
OPPOSED
SPAMMED
SPANKED
SPANNED
SPARKED
SPARRED
SPATTED
SPAWNED
SPEARED
SPECKED
SPEEDED
SPELLED
SPHERED
SPIELED
SPIFFED
SPILLED
SPLAYED
SPLICED
SPOILED
SPONGED
SPOOFED
SPOOKED
SPOOLED
SPOONED
SPORTED
SPOTTED
SPOUTED
SPRAYED
SPRUCED
SPURNED
SPURRED
SPURTED
UPAHEAD
UPBOUND
UPBRAID
UPBUILD
UPDATED
UPDIVED
UPDRIED
UPENDED
UPFIELD
UPGAZED
UPHOARD
UPPILED
UPRATED
UPSIZED
UPSTAND
UPSTOOD
UPTREND

••PD•••
LAPDOGS
POPDIVA
TIPDOWN
TOPDOGS
TOPDOWN
TOPDRAW
ZIPDISK

••P•D••
AMPEDUP
BIPEDAL
CAPADES
GAPEDAT
HOPEDSO
HOPEDTO
HYPEDUP
IMPEDED
IMPEDER
IMPEDES
LEPIDUS
LIPIDIC
MRPADRE
PAPADOC
PIPEDIN
PIPEDUP
POPEDOM
RAPIDAN
RAPIDER
RAPIDLY
ROPEDIN
ROPEDUP
TAPEDON
TAPEDUP
TEPIDLY
TYPEDIN
TYPEDUP
VAPIDLY
WIPEDUP

••P••D•
APPENDS
DEPENDS
ELPRADO
EXPANDS
EXPENDS
EXPLODE
GAPKIDS
HAPKIDO
HEPTADS
IMPENDS
IMPLODE
PEPCIDS
PEPTIDE
RIPTIDE
TOPBIDS
TOPSIDE
ZIPCODE

••P•••D
ALPHARD
APPLAUD
APPLIED
APPOSED
ASPIRED
CAPECOD
CAPERED
COPLAND
CUPELED
DAPPLED
DEPONED
DEPOSED
DEPUTED
DIPLOID
EMPALED
EMPTIED
EXPIRED
EXPOSED
EXPOUND
HAPLOID
HYPNOID
IMPALED
IMPAVID
IMPEDED
IMPLEAD
IMPLIED
IMPOSED
IMPOUND
IMPUTED
LAPELED
LAPLAND
LEPPARD
LIPREAD
MOPHEAD
OPPOSED
PAPERED
PEPBAND
PEPPARD
PIPCARD
POPEYED
POPPLED
POPUPAD
PUPATED
REPAGED
REPAVED
REPINED
REPLEAD
REPLIED
REPOSED
REPUTED
RIPCORD
RIPENED
RIPPLED
SAPHEAD
SEPALED
SUPPLED
TAPERED
TIPPLED
TIPTOED
TOPPLED
TOPSEED
TYPHOID
UMPIRED
UNPACED
UNPAGED
UNPALED
UNPARED
UNPAVED
UNPAWED
UNPILED
UNPIPED
UNPLIED
UNPOLED
UNPOSED
UNPROUD
UPPILED

VAPORED
XIPHOID

•••PD••
DAMPDRY
DRIPDRY
LEAPDAY
STEPDAD

•••P•D•
CUSPIDS
ELAPIDS
INKPADS
ISOPODS
JOYPADS
KEYPADS
PEAPODS
RESPADE
RIBPADS
SOSPADS
STUPIDS
TORPEDO
TRIPODS
UNIPODS
VESPIDS

•••P••D
ADAPTED
ADOPTED
BLIPPED
CAMPBED
CHAPPED
CHIPPED
CHOPPED
CLAPPED
CLIPPED
CLOPPED
COAPTED
COMPEND
COOPTED
COUPLED
CROPPED
DAPPLED
DEEPEND
DEEPRED
DESPOND
DIMPLED
DRIPPED
DROPPED
ELAPSED
ERUPTED
FLAPPED
FLIPPED
FLOPPED
GASPARD
GRAPHED
GRIPPED
HISPEED
HUMPHED
JUMPBID
LEOPARD
LEOPOLD
LEPPARD
LOWPAID
MORPHED
NONPAID
OUTPAID
OUTPLOD
PEOPLED
PEPPARD
PIMPLED
PLOPPED
POPPLED
PREPAID
PREPPED
PROPPED
PURPLED
QUIPPED
RESPOND
REUPPED
RIMPLED
RIPPLED
RUMPEND
RUMPLED
SAMPLED
SHEPARD
SHIPPED
SHOPPED
SKIPPED
SLAPPED
SLIPPED
SLOPPED
SNAPPED
SNIPPED
SOAPPAD
STAPLED
STEPDAD
STEPPED
STIPEND
STOPPED
SUPPLED
SUSPEND
SWAPPED
TAXPAID
TEMPLED
TEMPTED
THEPOND
TIPPLED
TOPPLED
TRAPPED
TRIPLED
TRIPPED
UNOPTED
UNSPIED
WHAPPED
WHIPPED
WHOPPED
WHUPPED
WIMPLED
WRAPPED

••••P•D
BLEEPED
BLIPPED
BLOOPED
CHAMPED
CHAPPED
CHEEPED
CHIPPED
CHIRPED
CHOMPED
CHOPPED
CHUMPED
CLAMPED
CLAPPED
CLASPED
CLIPPED
CLOMPED
CLOPPED
CLUMPED
CRAMPED
CREEPED
CRIMPED
CRISPED
CROPPED
CRUMPED
DECAPOD
DRIPPED
DROOPED
DROPPED
ESCAPED
FLAPPED
FLIPPED
FLOPPED
FOOTPAD
GALOPED
GRASPED
GRIPPED
GROUPED
GRUMPED
HEELPAD
HELIPAD
HEXAPOD
INSIPID
KNEEPAD
LILYPAD
LSHAPED
MEMOPAD
MONOPOD
NOTEPAD
OCTOPOD
OSHAPED
OUTSPED
PLOPPED
PLUMPED
POLYPED
POLYPOD
POPUPAD
PREPPED
PRIMPED
PROPPED
QUIPPED
RETAPED
RETYPED
REUPPED
REWIPED
SCALPED
SCAMPED
SCARPED
SCOOPED
SCRAPED
SCULPED
SEEDPOD
SHARPED
SHINPAD
SHIPPED
SHOPPED
SKIMPED
SKIPPED
SLAPPED
SLIPPED
SLOPPED
SLUMPED
SLURPED
SNAPPED
SNIPPED
SNOOPED
SOAPPAD
SSHAPED
STAMPED
STEEPED
STEPPED
STOMPED
STOOPED
STOPPED
STRIPED
STUMPED
SWAMPED
SWAPPED
SWOOPED
THUMPED
TRAMPED
TRAPPED
TRIPPED
TROMPED
TROOPED
TROUPED
TRUMPED
TSHAPED
UNCAPED
UNDUPED
UNHOPED
UNPIPED
UNROPED
UNTAPED
UNTYPED
UNWIPED
USHAPED
USURPED
VSHAPED
WHAPPED
WHELPED
WHIPPED
WHOMPED
WHOOPED
WHOPPED
WHUPPED
WRAPPED
YSHAPED

PE•••••
PEABEAN
PEABODY
PEACHED
PEACHES
PEACOAT
PEACOCK
PEAFOWL
PEAHENS
PEAKIER
PEAKING
PEAKISH
PEALIKE
PEALING
PEANUTS
PEAPODS
PEARLED
PEARLER
PEARSON
PEASANT
PEASOUP
PEATBOG
PEATIER
PEATPOT
PEBBLED
PEBBLES
PECCANT
PECCARY
PECCAVI
PECKING
PECKISH
PECKSAT
PECTINS
PEDALED
PEDALER
PEDANTS
PEDDLED
PEDDLER
PEDDLES
PEDICAB
PEDWAYS
PEEBLES
PEEKERS
PEEKING
PEEKOUT
PEEKSAT
PEEKSIN
PEELERS
PEELING
PEELOFF
PEELOUT
PEENING
PEEPERS
PEEPING
PEEPLES
PEEPOUT
PEEPSAT
PEERAGE
PEERESS
PEERING
PEEROUT
PEERSAT
PEERSIN
PEEVING
PEEVISH
PEEWEES
PEGASUS
PEGAWAY
PEGGING
PEGLEGS
PEGLESS
PEGLIKE
PEGTOPS
PEIPING
PEKEPOO
PELAGES
PELAGIC
PELICAN
PELISSE
PELLEAS
PELLETS
PELOTAS
PELOTON
PELTATE
PELTERS
PELTING
PELTISH
PENALTY
PENANCE
PENATES
PENCASE
PENCILS
PENDANT
PENDENT
PENDING
PENGUIN
PENLIKE
PENLITE
PENNAME
PENNANT
PENNATE
PENNERS
PENNEYS
PENNIES
PENNINE
PENNING
PENNOCK
PENNONS
PENPALS
PENROSE
PENSEES
PENSION
PENSIVE
PENTADS
PENTANE
PENTELS
PENTIUM
PENUCHE
PENULTS
PENZIAS
PEONAGE
PEONIES
PEOPLED
PEOPLES
PEORIAN
PEPBAND
PEPBOYS
PEPCIDS
PEPITAS
PEPLUMS
PEPPARD
PEPPERS
PEPPERY
PEPPIER
PEPPILL
PEPPILY
PEPPING
PEPPINO
PEPSICO
PEPSINS
PEPTALK
PEPTICS
PEPTIDE
PEPTONE
PEQUOTS
PERAHIA
PERATIO
PERCALE
PERCENT
PERCEPT
PERCHED
PERCHER
PERCHES
PERCHIK
PERCUSS
PERDIDO
PERDIEM
PERDITA
PERDURE
PERETTI
PERFECT
PERFIDY
PERFORM
PERFUME
PERFUMY
PERFUSE
PERGOLA
PERHAPS
PERIAPT
PERIDOT
PERIGEE
PERILED
PERIODS
PERISSA
PERITUS
PERIWIG
PERJURE
PERJURY
PERKIER
PERKILY
PERKING
PERKINS
PERKISH
PERKSUP
PERLITE
PERLMAN
PERMIAN
PERMING
PERMITS
PERMUTE
PERORAL
PERPLEX
PERREAU
PERRIER
PERRINE
PERRINS
PERSEID
PERSEUS
PERSIAN
PERSIST
PERSIUS
PERSOFF
PERSONA
PERSONS
PERSSON
PERTAIN
PERTEST
PERTURB
PERUGIA
PERUKES
PERUSAL
PERUSED
PERUSER
PERUSES
PERVADE
PERWEEK
PERYEAR
PESADES
PESANTE
PESETAS
PESEWAS
PESKIER
PESKILY
PESTERS
PESTLED
PESTLES
PETALED
PETALES
PETARDS
PETBEAR
PETBIRD
PETBOAS
PETCAGE
PETCALF
PETCATS
PETCHEW
PETCOCK
PETCOMB
PETCOWS
PETCROW
PETDEER
PETDOGS
PETDOOR
PETDOVE
PETDUCK
PETEMAN
PETEMEN
PETERED
PETERII
PETFISH
PETFROG
PETGATE
PETGOAT
PETHAIR
PETHARE
PETIOLE
PETITES
PETLAMB
PETLION
PETMICE
PETMULE
PETNAME
PETNAPS
PETPIGS
PETPONY
PETPUPS
PETRATS
PETRELS
PETRIFY
PETROCK
PETROLS
PETROUS
PETSCAN
PETSHOP
PETSITS
PETTERS
PETTIER
PETTILY
PETTING
PETTISH
PETTOYS
PETULIA
PETUNIA
PEUGEOT
PEWTERS
PEYOTES

P•E••••
PAELLAS
PEEBLES
PEEKERS
PEEKING
PEEKOUT
PEEKSAT
PEEKSIN
PEELERS
PEELING
PEELOFF
PEELOUT
PEENING
PEEPERS
PEEPING
PEEPLES
PEEPOUT
PEEPSAT
PEERAGE
PEERESS
PEERING
PEEROUT
PEERSAT
PEERSIN
PEEVING
PEEVISH
PEEWEES
PFENNIG
PHEMIUS
PHENOLS
PHENOMS
PIEBALD
PIECERS
PIECING
PIEEYED
PIEHOLE
PIELIKE
PIEPANS
PIERCED
PIERCER
PIERCES
PIERIAN
PIERROT
PIESAFE
PIESALE
PIETIES
PIETINS
PIETOSO
PIETROS
PLEADED
PLEADER
PLEADTO
PLEASED
PLEASER
PLEASES
PLEATED
PLEBIAN
PLECTRA
PLEDGED
PLEDGEE
PLEDGER
PLEDGES
PLENARY
PLENISH
PLENUMS
PLEURAE
PLEURAL
PLEXORS
PNEUMAS
PNEUMAT
PNEUMON
POESIES
POETESS
POETICA
POETICS
POETISE
POETIZE
PREACHY
PREACID
PREACTS
PREAGED
PREAGES
PREALLY
PREAMPS
PREARMS
PREAVER
PREBADE
PREBAKE
PREBIDS
PREBILL
PREBIND
PREBOIL
PREBOOK
PREBOOM
PREBORN
PREBURN
PREBUYS
PRECAST
PRECEDE
PRECEPT
PRECISE
PRECITE
PRECODE
PRECOIL
PRECOOK
PRECOOL
PRECOUP
PRECURE
PRECUTS
PREDARK
PREDATA
PREDATE
PREDAWN
PREDEFY
PREDENY
PREDICT
PREDIET
PREDIVE
PREDOOM
PREDUSK
PREEDIT
PREEMIE
PREEMPT
PREENED
PREENER
PREFABS
PREFACE
PREFADE
PREFECT
PREFERS
PREFILE
PREFORM
PREFUND
PREGAIN
PREGAME
PREHEAL
PREHEAT
PREIDEA
PRELACY
PRELATE
PRELIFE
PRELIMS
PRELOAD
PRELOAN
PRELOSS
PRELUDE
PREMADE
PREMAKE
PREMATE
PREMEDS
PREMEET
PREMIER
PREMIES
PREMISE
PREMISS
PREMIUM
PRENAME
PRENOON
PRENUPS
PREOMIT
PREOPEN
PREORAL
PREPACK
PREPAID
PREPARE
PREPAVE
PREPAYS
PREPLAN
PREPLOT
PREPPED
PREPPIE
PREPUPA
PREQUEL
PRERACE
PRERENT
PRERIOT
PREROCK
PRESAGE
PRESALE
PRESALT
PRESEAL
PRESEAT
PRESELL
PRESENT
PRESETS
PRESHIP
PRESHOW
PRESIDE
PRESIFT
PRESLEY
PRESOAK
PRESOLD
PRESONG
PRESORT
PRESPUR
PRESQUE
PRESSED
PRESSEL
PRESSER
PRESSES
PRESSON
PRESSUP
PRESTON
PRESTOS
PRESUME
PRETAPE
PRETEEN
PRETELL
PRETEND
PRETERM
PRETEST
PRETEXT
PRETIRE
PRETOLD
PRETORS
PRETRIM
PRETYPE
PRETZEL
PREVAIL
PREVENT
PREVERB
PREVERT
PREVETO
PREVIAS
PREVIEW
PREVOID
PREVOST
PREVUED
PREVUES
PREWARM
PREWARN
PREWASH
PREWHIP
PREWIRE
PREWITT
PREWORK
PREWORN
PREWRAP
PREXIES
PREYERS
PREYING
PREYSON
PTEROUS
PUEBLOS
PUERILE
PYEDOGS

P••E•••
PACECAR
PACELAP
PACEOFF
PAGEANT
PAGEBOY
PAGEONE
PAGESIX
PAGETWO
PALEALE
PALEDRY
PALEMON
PALERMO
PALETTE
PANELED
PANETTA
PAPEETE
PAPELES
PAPERED
PAPERER
PARENTS
PATELLA
PATENCY
PATENTS
PATERNO
PAWEDAT
PEKEPOO
PERETTI
PESETAS
PESEWAS
PETEMAN
PETEMEN
PETERED
PETERII
PHAEDRA
PHAETON
PHLEGMY
PHOEBES
PHOEBUS
PHOENIX
PHRENIC
PICEOUS
PIEEYED
PIGEONS
PIGEYED
PILEATE
PILEDIN
PILEDON
PILEDUP
PILEGGI
PILEOUS
PILESIN
PILESOF
PILESON
PILESUP
PILEUPS
PIMENTO
PIMESON
PINEFOR
PINENUT
PINEOIL
PINESAP
PINESOL
PINETAR
PINETOP
PINETUM
PIPEDIN
PIPEDUP
PIPEFUL
PIPESIN
PIPESUP
PIPETTE
PIRELLI
PITEOUS
PLOESTI
POKEDAT
POKEFUN
POKEMON
POKEOUT
POKESAT
POLEAXE
POLECAR
POLECAT
POLEMAN
POLEMEN
POLEMIC
POLENTA
POLESAT
POLESIT
POMELOS
POPEAFB
POPEDOM
POPELEO
POPEYED
POPEYES
POSEDAS
POSESAS
POSEURS
POSEUSE
POTEENS

POTENCE
POTENCY
POVERTY
POWERED
POWERUP
PRAETOR
PREEDIT
PREEMIE
PREEMPT
PREENED
PREENER
PRIESTS
PROEAST
PUBERTY
PUDENCY
PUTEMUP
PYRETIC
PYREXIA

P•••E••

PACBELL
PACIEST
PACKERS
PACKETS
PADDERS
PADGETT
PAIRERS
PALLETS
PALMERS
PALTERS
PAMPERS
PANDERS
PANIERS
PANNERS
PANTENE
PANTERA
PANTERS
PANZERS
PAPEETE
PAPIERS
PARCELS
PARGERS
PARKERS
PARLEYS
PARSECS
PARSEES
PARSERS
PARVENU
PASSELS
PASSERS
PASSEUL
PASTEIN
PASTELS
PASTERN
PASTERS
PASTEUP
PASTEUR
PATIENT
PATNESS
PATTERN
PATTERS
PATZERS
PAUPERS
PAUSERS
PAWNEES
PAWNERS
PAYHEED
PAYLESS
PAYMENT
PAYWELL
PCUSERS
PEABEAN
PEAHENS
PEEKERS
PEELERS
PEEPERS
PEERESS
PEEWEES
PEGLEGS
PEGLESS
PELLEAS
PELLETS
PELTERS
PENDENT
PENNERS
PENNEYS
PENSEES
PENTELS
PEPPERS
PEPPERY
PERCENT
PERCEPT
PERFECT
PERREAU
PERSEID
PERSEUS
PERTEST
PERWEEK
PERYEAR
PESTERS
PETBEAR
PETDEER
PETRELS
PETTERS
PEUGEOT
PEWTERS
PHASEIN
PHASERS
PHILEAS
PHINEAS
PHLOEMS
PHONEIN
PHONEME
PHONENO
PHONERS
PHONEYS
PICKENS
PICKERS
PICKETS
PICKETT
PIDGEON
PIECERS
PIGGERY
PIGLETS
PIGMEAT
PIGMENT
PIGPENS
PIGWEED
PILFERS
PINCERS
PINGERS
PINHEAD
PINIEST
PINKENS
PINKEST
PINKETT
PINLESS
PINNERS
PINSEAL
PIOLETS
PIONEER
PIPIEST
PIPLESS
PIRAEUS
PISCEAN
PITHEAD
PITIERS
PLACEBO
PLACERS
PLANERS
PLANETS
PLATEAU
PLATENS
PLATERS
PLAYERS
PLOVERS
PLOWERS
POCKETS
POETESS
POISERS
POKIEST
POLLEES
POLLENS
POLLERA
POLLERS
POMMELS
POMPEIA
POMPEII
PONDERS
PONGEES
POOLERS
POOREST
POPPERS
PORKERS
PORSENA
PORTEND
PORTENT
PORTERS
POSHEST
POSSESS
POSTERN
POSTERS
POTEENS
POTHERB
POTHERS
POTTERS
POTTERY
POULENC
POURERS
POUTERS
POWDERS
POWDERY
PRADESH
PRATERS
PRAYERS
PRECEDE
PRECEPT
PREDEFY
PREDENY
PREFECT
PREFERS
PREHEAL
PREHEAT
PREMEDS
PREMEET
PRERENT
PRESEAL
PRESEAT
PRESELL
PRESENT
PRESETS
PRETEEN
PRETELL
PRETEND
PRETERM
PRETEST
PRETEXT
PREVENT
PREVERB
PREVERT
PREVETO
PREYERS
PRICERS
PRIMELY
PRIMERA
PRIMERO
PRIMERS
PRIVETS
PROBERS
PROCEED
PROCESS
PROFESS
PROGENY
PROJECT
PROJETS
PROKEDS
PRONELY
PRONETO
PROPELS
PROSERS
PROTEAM
PROTEAN
PROTECT
PROTEGE
PROTEIN
PROTEST
PROTEUS
PROVEIT
PROVERB
PROVERS
PROWESS
PROWEST
PRUDENT
PRUDERY
PRUNERS
PTOLEMY
PUCKERS
PUCKERY
PUCKETT
PUFFERS
PUFFERY
PULLERS
PULLETS
PULLEYS
PULPERS
PUMMELS
PUMPERS
PUNGENT
PUNIEST
PUNKERS
PUNLESS
PUNNERS
PUNTERS
PUPPETS
PUPTENT
PURCELL
PURRERS
PURSERS
PURVEYS
PUSHERS
PUTREFY
PUTTEES
PUTTERS

P••••E•

PADDIES
PADDLED
PADDLER
PADDLES
PAINTED
PAINTER
PAISLEY
PAIUTES
PALACES
PALATES
PALAVER
PALFREY
PALJOEY
PALLIER
PALMIER
PANACEA
PANELED
PANGAEA
PANNIER
PANSIES
PANTHER
PANTIES
PANTLEG
PAPELES
PAPERED
PAPERER
PAPPIES
PARADED
PARADER
PARADES
PARAPET
PARCHED
PARCHES
PARDNER
PAROLED
PAROLEE
PAROLES
PARQUET
PARRIED
PARRIER
PARRIES
PARSEES
PARSLEY
PARTIED
PARTIER
PARTIES
PARTNER
PARTYER
PARURES
PASSKEY
PASTIER
PASTIES
PATCHED
PATCHEN
PATCHER
PATCHES
PATRIES
PATSIES
PATTIES
PAULSEN
PAVANES
PAWNEES
PAYHEED
PDJAMES
PEACHED
PEACHES
PEAKIER
PEARLED
PEARLER
PEATIER
PEBBLED
PEBBLES
PEDALED
PEDALER
PEDDLED
PEDDLER
PEDDLES
PEEBLES
PEEPLES
PEEWEES
PELAGES
PENATES
PENNIES
PENSEES
PEONIES
PEOPLED
PEOPLES
PEPPIER
PERCHED
PERCHER
PERCHES
PERDIEM
PERIGEE
PERILED
PERKIER
PERPLEX
PERRIER
PERUKES
PERUSED
PERUSER
PERUSES
PERWEEK
PESADES
PESKIER
PESTLED
PESTLES
PETALED
PETALES
PETCHEW
PETDEER
PETEMEN
PETERED
PETITES
PETTIER
PEYOTES
PGRATED
PHATTER
PHILTER
PHISHED
PHISHER
PHISHES
PHLOXES
PHOEBES
PHONIER
PHONIES
PHRASED
PHRASES
PIAFFED
PIAFFES
PIASTER
PICKIER
PICKLED
PICKLES
PICOTED
PIDDLED
PIDDLES
PIEEYED
PIERCED
PIERCER
PIERCES
PIETIES
PIFFLED
PIFFLES
PIGEYED
PIGGIER
PIGGIES
PIGWEED
PILATES
PILOTED
PILSNER
PIMPLED
PIMPLES
PINCHED
PINCHER
PINCHES
PINKIES
PINKOES
PINONES
PIONEER
PIPAGES
PIRATED
PIRATES
PIROGEN
PITCHED
PITCHER
PITCHES
PITCREW
PITHIER
PIVOTED
PIVOTER
PLACKET
PLAGUED
PLAGUES
PLAICES
PLAINER
PLAINES
PLAITED
PLAITER
PLANKED
PLANNED
PLANNER
PLANTED
PLANTER
PLAQUES
PLASHED
PLASHES
PLASTER
PLATIER
PLATIES
PLATTED
PLATTER
PLAYLET
PLAYPEN
PLAYTEX
PLEADED
PLEADER
PLEASED
PLEASER
PLEASES
PLEATED
PLEDGED
PLEDGEE
PLEDGER
PLEDGES
PLINKED
PLISSES
PLODDED
PLODDER
PLONKED
PLOPPED
PLOTTED
PLOTTER
PLOTZED
PLOTZES
PLOWMEN
PLUCKED
PLUGGED
PLUGGER
PLUMBED
PLUMBER
PLUMIER
PLUMMER
PLUMMET
PLUMPED
PLUMPER
PLUNDER
PLUNGED
PLUNGER
PLUNGES
PLUNKED
PLUNKER
PLUSHER
PLUSHES
PLUSSES
POACHED
POACHER
POACHES
POBOXES
POESIES
POINTED
POINTER
POINTES
POITIER
POIVRES
POLANER
POLEMEN
POLICED
POLICER
POLICES
POLITER
POLKAED
POLLEES
POLYMER
POLYPED
POMADED
POMADES
PONGEES
PONYKEG
POOCHES
POODLES
POOLMEN
POORMEN
POPELEO
POPEYED
POPEYES
POPOVER
POPPIES
POPPLED
POPPLES
PORCHES
PORGIES
PORIVER
PORKIER
POSITED
POSOLES
POSTIES
POSTMEN
POTAGES
POTPIES
POTTIER
POTTIES
POUCHED
POUCHES
POUDRES
POUNCED
POUNCER
POUNCES
POUNDED
POUNDER
POUTIER
POWERED
POZOLES
PRAISED
PRAISER
PRAISES
PRANCED
PRANCER
PRANCES
PRAWNED
PREAGED
PREAGES
PREAVER
PREDIET
PREENED
PREENER
PREIDEA
PREMEET
PREMIER
PREMIES
PREOPEN
PREPPED
PREQUEL
PRESLEY
PRESSED
PRESSEL
PRESSER
PRESSES
PRETEEN
PRETZEL
PREVIEW
PREVUED
PREVUES
PREXIES
PRICIER
PRICKED
PRIMMED
PRIMMER
PRIMPED
PRINCES
PRINKED
PRINKER
PRINTED
PRINTER
PRISSES
PRITHEE
PRIUSES
PRIVIER
PRIVIES
PROBIES
PROBLEM
PROCEED
PROCTER
PRODDED
PRODDER
PROFFER
PROMOED
PRONGED
PROOFED
PROOFER
PROPHET
PROPJET
PROPMEN
PROPPED
PROSIER
PROSPER
PROUDER
PROWLED
PROWLER
PROXIES
PRYOPEN
PSALTER
PSHAWED
PSYCHED
PSYCHES
PUDDLED
PUDDLES
PUDGIER
PUFFIER
PUGGLES
PUGSLEY
PULPIER
PUMICED
PUMICES
PUNCHED
PUNCHER
PUNCHES
PUNKIER
PUNKIES
PUNNIER
PUNSTER
PUPATED
PUPATES
PUPPIES
PURDUEU
PURFLED
PURFLER
PURFLES
PURLIEU
PURPLED
PURPLES
PURSIER
PURSUED
PURSUER
PURSUES
PURTIER
PURVIEW
PUSHIER
PUSSIES
PUTOVER
PUTTEES
PUTTIED
PUTTIES
PUZZLED
PUZZLER
PUZZLES
PYGMIES
PYRITES

P•••••E

PACKAGE
PACKICE
PADRONE
PADSITE
PAGEONE
PALANCE
PALEALE
PALETTE
PALMATE
PALPATE
PANACHE
PANCAKE
PANICLE
PANPIPE
PANTENE
PANTILE
PANTONE
PANURGE
PAPEETE
PAPOOSE
PARABLE
PARBAKE
PARFIVE
PARKADE
PARKAVE
PAROLEE
PARTAKE
PARTITE
PARTONE
PASALLE
PASSADE
PASSAGE
PASSIVE
PASTDUE
PASTIME
PASTURE
PATRICE
PAULINE
PAYABLE
PAYMORE
PAYRATE
PCCLONE
PEALIKE
PEERAGE
PEGLIKE
PELISSE
PELTATE
PENANCE
PENCASE
PENLIKE
PENLITE
PENNAME
PENNATE
PENNINE
PENROSE
PENSIVE
PENTANE
PENUCHE
PEONAGE
PEPTIDE
PEPTONE
PERCALE
PERDURE
PERFUME
PERFUSE
PERIGEE
PERJURE
PERLITE
PERMUTE
PERRINE
PERVADE
PESANTE
PETCAGE
PETDOVE
PETGATE
PETHARE
PETIOLE
PETMICE
PETMULE
PETNAME
PHILLIE
PHILTRE
PHONEME
PIASTRE
PICANTE
PICKAXE
PICTURE
PIEHOLE
PIELIKE
PIESAFE
PIESALE
PIGLIKE
PILEATE
PILLAGE
PINCHME
PINHOLE
PINNACE
PINNATE
PINWALE
PIPETTE
PIROGUE
PISCINE
PISMIRE
PISTOLE
PLACATE
PLANATE
PLEDGEE
PLEURAE
PLIABLE
PLICATE
PLOSIVE
PLUMAGE
PLUMOSE
PLUMPIE
PLUMULE
PLUSONE
PODLIKE
POETISE
POETIZE
POLEAXE
POLLUTE
POOCHIE
POOLCUE
POOPSIE
POPTUNE
POPWINE
PORCINE
PORKPIE
PORSCHE
PORTAGE
POSABLE
POSEUSE
POSTAGE
POSTURE
POTABLE
POTENCE
POTHOLE
POTTAGE
PRAIRIE
PRALINE
PRATTLE
PREBADE
PREBAKE
PRECEDE
PRECISE
PRECITE
PRECODE
PRECURE
PREDATE
PREDIVE
PREEMIE
PREFACE
PREFADE
PREFILE
PREGAME
PRELATE
PRELIFE
PRELUDE
PREMADE
PREMAKE
PREMATE
PREMISE
PRENAME
PREPARE
PREPAVE
PREPPIE
PRERACE
PRESAGE
PRESALE
PRESIDE
PRESQUE
PRESUME
PRETAPE
PRETIRE
PRETYPE
PREWIRE
PRICKLE
PRIMATE
PRINGLE
PRITHEE
PRIVATE
PROBATE
PROCURE
PRODUCE
PROFANE
PROFILE
PROFUSE
PROLATE
PROLIFE
PROMISE

PROMOTE
PRONATE
PROPANE
PROPONE
PROPOSE
PRORATE
PROTEGE
PROVIDE
PROVINE
PROVOKE
PRUDHOE
PUBGAME
PUERILE
PUGNOSE
PULSATE
PURPOSE
PVCPIPE

•PE••••

APECKOF
APEDIET
APELETS
APELIKE
APERCUS
APERIES
APERSON
APESUIT
CPEBACH
EPEEIST
EPERGNE
EPERNAY
OPENAIR
OPENBAR
OPENEND
OPENERS
OPENING
OPENNET
OPENOUT
OPENPIT
OPENSEA
OPENSUP
OPENTAP
OPENTOE
OPENTOP
OPERAND
OPERANT
OPERATE
OPEROSE
SPEAKER
SPEAKOF
SPEAKTO
SPEAKUP
SPEARED
SPEARER
SPECIAL
SPECIES
SPECIFY
SPECING
SPECKED
SPECKLE
SPECOUT
SPECTER
SPECTOR
SPECTRA
SPECTRE
SPEDOFF
SPEEDED
SPEEDER
SPEEDOS
SPEEDUP
SPELLED
SPELLER
SPELUNK
SPENCER
SPENDER
SPENDON
SPENSER
SPENTON
SPEWERS
SPEWING
SPEWOUT
UPEARLY
UPENDED

•P•E•••

APHELIA
APLENTY
APPEALS
APPEARS
APPEASE
APPENDS
APPETIT
APTERAL
APTERYX
CPAEXAM
EPEEIST
EPHEBUS
EPHEDRA
EPHESUS
EPPERLY
IPLEDGE
OPHELIA
OPTEDIN
OPTEDTO
SPEEDED
SPEEDER
SPEEDOS
SPEEDUP
SPHERAL
SPHERED
SPHERES
SPHERIC
SPIEDON
SPIEGEL
SPIELED
SPIELER
SPIESON
SPLEENS
SPLEENY
SPLENDA
SPREADS
UPBEARS
UPBEATS
UPHEAPS
UPHEAVE
UPKEEPS
UPLEAPS
UPLEAPT
UPREACH
UPREARS
UPSENDS
UPTEARS
UPTEMPO
UPWELLS

•P••E••

APELETS
APILEOF
APOGEAL
APOGEAN
APOGEES
APPLETS
APTNESS
EPICENE
EPIDERM
EPOPEES
EPSTEIN
IPANEMA
IPCRESS
OPENEND
OPENERS
OPINERS
OPPRESS
OPULENT
SPACELY
SPACERS
SPADERS
SPARELY
SPAREME
SPARERS
SPAREST
SPAYERS
SPEWERS
SPICERS
SPICERY
SPICEUP
SPIDERS
SPIDERY
SPIKERS
SPIKETV
SPIKEUP
SPINELS
SPINETS
SPIREAS
SPLEENS
SPLEENY
SPOKEOF
SPOKETO
SPOKEUP
SPRIEST
SPRYEST
SPYDERS
UPAHEAD
UPFIELD
UPKEEPS
UPSTEPS
UPSWEEP
UPSWELL
UPSWEPT
UPTHERE
UPTREND

•P•••E•

APACHES
APEDIET
APERIES
APHIDES
APLITES
APLUSES
APOGEES
APOTHEM
APPAREL
APPLIED
APPLIER
APPLIES
APPOSED
APPOSES
APRONED
APSIDES
BPLUSES
CPLUSES
DPLUSES
EPAULET
EPITHET
EPOPEES
EPOQUES
EPOXIED
EPOXIES
MPTHREE
OPAQUES
OPENNET
OPENSEA
OPIATES
OPPOSED
OPPOSER
OPPOSES
SPACIER
SPAMMED
SPAMMER
SPANDEX
SPANIEL
SPANKED
SPANKER
SPANNED
SPANNER
SPARKED
SPARRED
SPARRER
SPARSER
SPATHES
SPATTED
SPATTER
SPAWNED
SPAWNER
SPEAKER
SPEARED
SPEARER
SPECIES
SPECKED
SPECTER
SPEEDED
SPEEDER
SPELLED
SPELLER
SPENCER
SPENDER
SPENSER
SPHERED
SPHERES
SPICIER
SPIEGEL
SPIELED
SPIELER
SPIFFED
SPIKIER
SPILLED
SPILLER
SPINIER
SPINNER
SPINNEY
SPIRIER
SPITTER
SPITZES
SPLAYED
SPLICED
SPLICER
SPLICES
SPLINES
SPOILED
SPOILER
SPONDEE
SPONGED
SPONGER
SPONGES
SPOOFED
SPOOFER
SPOOKED
SPOOLED
SPOOLER
SPOONED
SPOONER
SPORTED
SPOTTED
SPOTTER
SPOUSES
SPOUTED
SPOUTER
SPRAYED
SPRAYER
SPRITES
SPRUCED
SPRUCER
SPRUCES
SPUMIER
SPURNED
SPURNER
SPURRED
SPURTED
SPUTTER
UPATREE
UPDATED
UPDATER
UPDATES
UPDIVED
UPDIVES
UPDRIED
UPDRIES
UPENDED
UPGAZED
UPGAZES
UPPILED
UPPILES
UPRATED
UPRATES
UPRISEN
UPRISER
UPRISES
UPRIVER
UPSIDES
UPSIZED
UPSIZES
UPSWEEP
UPTAKES
UPTIMES

•P••••E

APATITE
APELIKE
APOSTLE
APPEASE
APPRISE
APPROVE
EPERGNE
EPICENE
EPICURE
EPIDOTE
EPIGONE
EPILATE
EPISODE
EPISTLE
EPITOME
EPONINE
IPLEDGE
MPTHREE
OPALINE
OPENTOE
OPERATE
OPEROSE
OPUSONE
SPACKLE
SPANGLE
SPAREME
SPARKLE
SPECKLE
SPECTRE
SPINDLE
SPITTLE
SPLURGE
SPOKANE
SPONDEE
SPUMONE
SPYHOLE
SPYWARE
UPABOVE
UPATREE
UPBORNE
UPCCODE
UPCLOSE
UPCURVE
UPGRADE
UPHEAVE
UPPHASE
UPRAISE
UPROUSE
UPSCALE
UPSLOPE
UPSTAGE
UPSTARE
UPSTATE
UPSURGE
UPTHERE
UPTRADE
UPVALUE

••PE•••

AMPEDUP
AMPERES
APPEALS
APPEARS
APPEASE
APPENDS
APPETIT
ASPECTS
ASPENCO
ASPERSE
ATPEACE
BIPEDAL
CAPEANN
CAPECOD
CAPEESH
CAPELET
CAPELLA
CAPEMAY
CAPERED
CUPELED
CUPELER
DEPECHE
DEPENDS
DEPESTS
DOPEOUT
EMPEROR
EPPERLY
EXPECTS
EXPENDS
EXPENSE
EXPERTS
GAPEDAT
GAPESAT
HAPENNY
HOPEDSO
HOPEDTO
HOPEFOR
HOPEFUL
HOPENOT
HOPESSO
HOPESTO
HYPEDUP
HYPERON
HYPESUP
IAPETUS
IIPETER
IMPEACH
IMPEDED
IMPEDER
IMPEDES
IMPENDS
IMPERIL
IMPETUS
INPEACE
INPERIL
KOPECKS
LAPELED
LAPERMS
MTPELEE
PAPEETE
PAPELES
PAPERED
PAPERER
PIPEDIN
PIPEDUP
PIPEFUL
PIPESIN
PIPESUP
PIPETTE
POPEAFB
POPEDOM
POPELEO
POPEYED
POPEYES
REPEALS
REPEATS
REPENTS
REPERKS
RIPENED
RIPENER
ROPEDIN
ROPEDUP
ROPEOFF
ROPESIN
ROPESUP
ROPETOW
STPETER
SUPERGS
TAPEDON
TAPEDUP
TAPEMAN
TAPEMEN
TAPERED
TAPESON
TAPESUP
TOPEKAN
TUPELOS
TYPEABS
TYPEDIN
TYPEDUP
TYPESET
TYPESIN
TYPESUP
UNPEELS
WIPEDUP
WIPEOFF
WIPEOUT
WIPESUP

••P•E••

AMPLEST
APPLETS
BOPPERS
CAPEESH
CAPLESS
CAPLETS
CAPPERS
CEPHEUS
CIPHERS
COPIERS
COPPERS
COPPERY
COPTERS
CYPHERS
CYPRESS
DEPLETE
DEPRESS
DIPNETS
DIPPERS
DOPIEST
EMPRESS
ESPNEWS
EXPRESS
FOPPERY
GAPLESS
GOPHERS
GYPPERS
HAPLESS
HAPPENS
HEPPEST
HIPLESS
HIPNESS
HIPPEST
HOPPERS
HUPPERT
HYPHENS
IMPIETY
IMPLEAD
IMPRESS
IMPREST
IMPREZA
JAPHETH
KIPPERS
LAPBELT
LAPPERS
LAPPETS
LAPSERS
LIPLESS
LIPPERS
LIPREAD
LOPPERS
MAPPERS
MOPHEAD
MOPIEST
MOPPERS
MOPPETS
MUPPETS
NAPIERS
NAPLESS
NAPPERS
NEPHEWS
NIPPERS
OPPRESS
ORPHEAN
ORPHEUM
ORPHEUS
OSPREYS
PAPEETE
PAPIERS
PEPPERS
PEPPERY
PIPIEST
PIPLESS
POPPERS
PUPPETS
PUPTENT
RAPIERS
RAPPELS
RAPPERS
REPLEAD
REPLETE
REPRESS
RIPIENI
RIPIENO
RIPPERS
ROPIEST
SAPHEAD
SAPIENS
SAPIENT
SAPLESS
SAPPERS
SEPTETS
SIPPERS
SUPPERS
SUPREME
TAPPERS
TAPPETS
TIPLESS
TIPPEES
TIPPERS
TIPPETS
TOPLESS
TOPPERS
TOPSEED
TOPTENS
UMPTEEN
UNPEELS
UNPIETY
YAPPERS
ZAPPERS
ZIPPERS

••P••E•

ALPINER
ALPINES
AMPERES
AMPULES
APPAREL
APPLIED
APPLIER
APPLIES
APPOSED
APPOSES
ASPIRED
ASPIRER
ASPIRES
CAPADES
CAPELET
CAPERED
CAPOTES
CAPULET
COPYMEN
CUPELED
CUPELER
CUPPIER
CUPULES
DAPHNES
DAPPLED
DAPPLES
DEPONED
DEPONER
DEPONES
DEPOSED
DEPOSER
DEPOSES
DEPOWER
DEPUTED
DEPUTES
DIPOLES
DIPPIER
DOPPLER
EMPALED
EMPALES
EMPANEL
EMPIRES
EMPOWER
EMPTIED
EMPTIER
EMPTIES
EXPIRED
EXPIRES
EXPOSED
EXPOSER
EXPOSES
FIPPLES
GIPSIES
GUPPIES
GYPSIES
HAPPIER
HIPPIER
HIPPIES
HIPSTER
HOPOVER
HOPPIER
IIPETER
IMPALED
IMPALER
IMPALES
IMPANEL
IMPEDED
IMPEDER
IMPEDES
IMPLIED
IMPLIES
IMPOSED
IMPOSER
IMPOSES
IMPURER
IMPUTED
IMPUTER
IMPUTES
INPOWER
JDPOWER
JUPITER
LAPELED
LIPASES
LIPPIER
LOPPIER
LUPINES
MCPAPER
MTPELEE
NAPPIER
NAPPIES
NAPSTER
NIPPIER
NIPPLES
NOPALES
ONPAPER
OPPOSED
OPPOSER
OPPOSES
PAPELES
PAPERED
PAPERER
PAPPIES
PEPPIER
PIPAGES
POPELEO
POPEYED
POPEYES
POPOVER
POPPIES
POPPLED
POPPLES
PUPATED
PUPATES
PUPPIES
RAPHAEL
RAPIDER
RAPINES
REPAGED
REPAGES
REPANEL
REPAPER
REPAVED
REPAVES
REPINED
REPINER
REPINES
REPLIED
REPLIER
REPLIES
REPOSED
REPOSER
REPOSES
REPOWER
REPUTED
REPUTES
RIPENED
RIPENER
RIPOPEN
RIPPLED
RIPPLES
RIPPLET
SAPPIER
SEPALED
SOPHIES
SOPPIER
STPETER
SUPPLED
SUPPLER
SUPPLES
TAPEMEN
TAPERED
TAPSTER
TIPOVER
TIPPEES
TIPPIER
TIPPLED
TIPPLER
TIPPLES
TIPSIER
TIPSTER
TIPTOED
TIPTOES
TOPAZES
TOPPLED
TOPPLES
TOPSEED
TUPOLEV
TYPESET
UMPIRED
UMPIRES
UMPTEEN
UNPACED
UNPAGED
UNPALED
UNPARED
UNPAVED
UNPAWED
UNPILED
UNPILES
UNPIPED
UNPLIED
UNPOLED
UNPOSED
UPPILED
UPPILES
VAPORED
VAPORER
YIPPIES
YUPPIES
ZAPATEO
ZAPOTEC
ZAPPIER
ZIPPIER

••P•••E

AMPOULE
APPEASE
APPRISE
APPROVE
ASPERSE
ATPEACE
BAPTISE
BAPTIZE
BIPLANE
BYPHONE
CAPABLE
CAPAPIE
CAPRICE
CAPRINE
CAPSIZE
CAPSULE
CAPTIVE
CAPTURE
CAPUCHE
COPPICE
COPULAE
CUPCAKE
CUPLIKE
CUPRITE
DEPECHE
DEPLANE
DEPLETE
DEPLORE
DEPRAVE
DEPRIVE
EMPLACE
EMPLANE
EMPRISE
ENPLANE
ENPRISE
ESPOUSE
EXPANSE
EXPARTE
EXPENSE
EXPIATE
EXPLODE
EXPLORE
EXPUNGE
HIPBONE
HIPLIKE
HOPLITE
IMPASSE
IMPINGE
IMPLODE
IMPLORE
IMPROVE
IMPULSE
INPEACE
INPHASE
INPLACE
KAPTURE
LAPLACE
LAPORTE
LAPROBE
LAPWARE
LIPLIKE
MRPADRE
MTPELEE
NAPTIME
NEPTUNE
NOPLACE
PAPEETE
PAPOOSE
PEPTIDE
PEPTONE

PIPETTE
POPTUNE
POPWINE
RAPTUNE
RAPTURE
REPASTE
REPHASE
REPHONE
REPLACE
REPLANE
REPLATE
REPLETE
REPLUME
REPRICE
REPRIME
REPRISE
REPROBE
REPROVE
REPRUNE
REPTILE
REPULSE
RIPOSTE
RIPSONE
RIPTIDE
RUPTURE
SUPPOSE
SUPREME
TAPSHOE
TIPLINE
TOPFIVE
TOPHOLE
TOPLINE
TOPNAME
TOPRATE
TOPSIDE
UNPASTE
UPPHASE
ZEPPOLE
ZIPCODE

•••PE••

ANAPEST
BEEPERS
BESPEAK
BOPPERS
BUMPERS
CAMPERS
CAPPERS
CARPELS
CARPERS
CARPETS
CHAPEAU
CHAPELS
COMPEER
COMPELS
COMPEND
COMPERE
COMPETE
COOPERS
COOPERY
COPPERS
COPPERY
COWPEAS
DAMPENS
DAMPERS
DAMPEST
DEEPEND
DEEPENS
DEEPEST
DIAPERS
DIPPERS
DISPELS
DRAPERS
DRAPERY
DRYPERS
DUMPERS
ELOPERS
EPOPEES
EXUPERY
FOPPERY
GASPERS
GAWPERS
GELPENS
GOMPERS
GOSPELS
GRAPERY
GRIPERS
GROPERS
GULPERS
GYPPERS
HAMPERS
HAPPENS
HARPERS
HEAPERS
HELPERS
HENPECK
HEPPEST
HERPETO
HIPPEST
HISPEED
HOOPERS
HOPPERS
HUPPERT
IHOPESO
INSPECT
IREPEAT
JASPERS
JASPERY
JEEPERS
JUMPERS
KEEPERS
KIPPERS
LAMPERT
LAPPERS
LAPPETS
LEAPERS
LIMPEST
LIMPETS
LIPPERS
LISPERS
LOOPERS
LOPPERS
LUMPERS
MAPPERS
MOPPERS
MOPPETS
MRSPEEL
MUPPETS
NAPPERS
NIPPERS
NONPEAK
OFFPEAK
OUTPEEP
PAMPERS
PAUPERS
PEEPERS
PEPPERS
PEPPERY
PIGPENS
POMPEIA
POMPEII
POPPERS
PROPELS
PULPERS
PUMPERS
PUPPETS
RAPPELS
RAPPERS
RASPERS
REAPERS
REOPENS
RESPEAK
RESPECT
RESPELL
RESPELT
RIPPERS
ROMPERS
RUMPEND
SAPPERS
SERPENS
SERPENT
SHAPELY
SHAPERS
SHAPEUP
SIMPERS
SIPPERS
SLOPERS
SNIPEAT
SNIPERS
SOAPERS
SOUPERS
STIPEND
STUPEFY
SUPPERS
SUSPECT
SUSPEND
SWIPERS
TAMPERS
TAPPERS
TAPPETS
TEEPEES
TEMPEAZ
TEMPEHS
TEMPERA
TEMPERS
TEMPEST
TIPPEES
TIPPERS
TIPPETS
TOPPERS
TORPEDO
TOUPEES
TRAPEZE
UNSPEAK
UNSPELT
UNSPENT
USOPENS
VAMPERS
VANPELT
VESPERS
WARPERS
WEEPERS
YAPPERS
YAWPERS
YELPERS
ZAPPERS
ZIPPERS

•••P•E•

ADAPTED
ADAPTER
ADEPTER
ADOPTED
ADOPTEE
ADOPTER
BLIPPED
BUMPIER
CAMPBED
CAMPIER
CHAPLET
CHAPMEN
CHAPPED
CHAPTER
CHIPPED
CHIPPER
CHOPPED
CHOPPER
CLAPPED
CLAPPER
CLIPPED
CLIPPER
CLOPPED
COAPTED
COMPEER
COMPLEX
COOPTED
CORPSES
COUPLED
COUPLER
COUPLES
COUPLET
CROPPED
CROPPER
CRUPPER
CUPPIER
DAPPLED
DAPPLES
DEEPRED
DEEPSEA
DEEPSET
DEMPSEY
DIMPLED
DIMPLES
DIOPTER
DIPPIER
DOPPLER
DRIPPED
DRIPPER
DROPLET
DROPNET
DROPPED
DROPPER
DUMPIER
ELAPSED
ELAPSES
EPOPEES
ERUPTED
ERUPTER
FIPPLES
FLAPPED
FLAPPER
FLIPPED
FLIPPEN
FLIPPER
FLOPPED
FLOPPER
FRAPPES
FUNPLEX
GOOPIER
GRAPHED
GRAPIER
GRAPNEL
GRIPPED
GRIPPER
GRIPPES
GULPIER
GUPPIES
HAPPIER
HARPIES
HEMPIER
HIPPIER
HIPPIES
HISPEED
HOOPMEN
HOOPOES
HOPPIER
HUMPHED
HUMPIER
INAPOEM
INAPTER
JUMPIER
KELPIES
KEWPIES
LAMPREY
LIPPIER
LOOPIER
LOPPIER
LUMPIER
MAGPIES
MORPHED
MRSPEEL
MUDPIES
NAPPIER
NAPPIES
NIPPIER
NIPPLES
NONPOET
NTUPLES
OUTPEEP
PAPPIES
PEEPLES
PEOPLED
PEOPLES
PEPPIER
PERPLEX
PIMPLED
PIMPLES
PLOPPED
POPPIES
POPPLED
POPPLES
POTPIES
PREPPED
PROPHET
PROPJET
PROPMEN
PROPPED
PULPIER
PUPPIES
PURPLED
PURPLES
QUIPPED
QUIPPER
RASPIER
REUPPED
RIMPLED
RIMPLES
RIPPLED
RIPPLES
RIPPLET
RUMPLED
RUMPLES
SAMPLED
SAMPLER
SAMPLES
SAPPIER
SCEPTER
SCUPPER
SEEPIER
SHIPMEN
SHIPPED
SHIPPER
SHOPPED
SHOPPER
SHOPPES
SIMPLER
SIMPLES
SIMPLEX
SKIPPED
SKIPPER
SLAPPED
SLAPPER
SLIPPED
SLIPPER
SLOPPED
SNAPPEA
SNAPPED
SNAPPER
SNIPPED
SNIPPER
SNIPPET
SOAPIER
SOAPNET
SOPPIER
SOUPIER
STAPLED
STAPLER
STAPLES
STEPHEN
STEPPED
STEPPER
STEPPES
STOPPED
STOPPER
SUPPLED
SUPPLER
SUPPLES
SWAPPED
SWAPPER
TEEPEES
TEMPLED
TEMPLES
TEMPTED
TEMPTER
TIPPEES
TIPPIER
TIPPLED
TIPPLER
TIPPLES
TOPPLED
TOPPLES
TOUPEES
TRAPPED
TRAPPER
TRIPLEA
TRIPLED
TRIPLES
TRIPLET
TRIPLEX
TRIPPED
TRIPPER
TRIPPET
UNIPLEX
UNOPTED
UNSPIED
VAMPIER
WASPIER
WEEPIER
WHAPPED
WHIPPED
WHIPPER
WHIPPET
WHOPPED
WHOPPER
WHUPPED
WIMPIER
WIMPLED
WIMPLES
WISPIER
WRAPPED
WRAPPER
YIPPIES
YUPPIES
ZAPPIER
ZIPPIER

•••P••E

ADIPOSE
ADOPTEE
ADSPACE
ATIPTOE
AUSPICE
BAGPIPE
BESPOKE
BOOPSIE
CHAPPIE
CHOPINE
COMPARE
COMPERE
COMPETE
COMPILE
COMPOSE
COMPOTE
COMPUTE
COPPICE
COWPOKE
CRAPPIE
CRIPPLE
CUSPATE
DESPISE
DESPITE
DISPOSE
DISPUTE
DOGPILE
GARPIKE
GASPIPE
GRAPPLE
HOSPICE
INAPILE
INAPOKE
INSPACE
INSPIRE
INSPITE
MAYPOLE
MISPAGE
MYSPACE
NUTPINE
ONEPAGE
OUTPACE
OUTPIPE
PALPATE
PANPIPE
POOPSIE
PREPARE
PREPAVE
PREPPIE
PROPANE
PROPONE
PROPOSE
PURPOSE
PVCPIPE
RALPHIE
RAMPAGE
REDPINE
RESPACE
RESPADE
RESPICE
RESPIRE
RESPITE
RESPOKE
RUMPOLE
SCEPTRE
SEEPAGE
SKIPOLE
SNAPPLE
STEPONE
STIPPLE
STOPPLE
SUPPOSE
SUSPIRE
TADPOLE
TEMPORE
THEPOPE
TOSPARE
TRAPEZE
UNSPOKE
VAMPIRE
VOLPONE
VULPINE
WALPOLE
WARPAGE
WEBPAGE
WHIPPLE
WIMPOLE
ZEPPOLE

••••PE•

ALLOPEZ
ARUSPEX
AUTOPEN
BIGAPES
BLEEPED
BLEEPER
BLIPPED
BLOOPED
BLOOPER
BULLPEN
CAGEPET
CALIPER
CANAPES
CHAMPED
CHAMPER
CHAPPED
CHEAPEN
CHEAPER
CHEEPED
CHEEPER
CHIAPET
CHIPPED
CHIPPER
CHIRPED
CHIRPER
CHOMPED
CHOPPED
CHOPPER
CHUMPED
CLAMPED
CLAMPER
CLAPPED
CLAPPER
CLASPED
CLASPER
CLIPPED
CLIPPER
CLOMPED
CLOPPED
CLUMPED
CRAMPED
CREEPED
CREEPER
CRIMPED
CRIMPER
CRISPED
CRISPEN
CRISPER
CROPPED
CROPPER
CRUMPED
CRUMPET
CRUPPER
CUTOPEN
DIGIPET
DNIEPER
DOGAPES
DRIPPED
DRIPPER
DROOPED
DROPPED
DROPPER
ECTYPES
ESCAPED
ESCAPEE
ESCAPER
ESCAPES
FELTPEN
FLAPPED
FLAPPER
FLIPPED
FLIPPEN
FLIPPER
FLOPPED
FLOPPER
FLYOPEN
FRAPPES
GALOPED
GRASPED
GRASPER
GRIPPED
GRIPPER
GRIPPES
GROUPED
GROUPER
GRUMPED
HANAPER
ITSOPEN
JUNIPER
LAYOPEN
LOSTPET
LSHAPED
MCPAPER
NEWSPEG
NOTOPEN
ONPAPER
OSHAPED
OSSIPEE
OUTSPED
PARAPET
PLAYPEN
PLOPPED
PLUMPED
PLUMPER
POLYPED
PREOPEN
PREPPED
PRIMPED
PROPPED
PROSPER
PRYOPEN
QUIPPED
QUIPPER
RECIPES
REEXPEL
REPAPER
RETAPED
RETAPES
RETYPED
RETYPES
REUPPED
REWIPED
REWIPES
RIPOPEN
SCALPED
SCALPEL
SCALPER
SCAMPED
SCAMPER
SCARPED
SCOOPED
SCOOPER
SCOUPES
SCRAPED
SCRAPER
SCRAPES
SCULPED
SCUPPER
SERAPES
SHARPED
SHARPEI
SHARPEN
SHARPER
SHIPPED
SHIPPER
SHOPPED
SHOPPER
SHOPPES
SKIMPED
SKIPPED
SKIPPER
SLAPPED
SLAPPER
SLEEPER
SLIPPED
SLIPPER
SLOPPED
SLUMPED
SLURPED
SLURPEE
SLURPER
SNAPPEA
SNAPPED
SNAPPER
SNIPPED
SNIPPER
SNIPPET
SNOOPED
SNOOPER
SNOWPEA
SSHAPED
STAMPED
STAMPER
STEEPED
STEEPEN
STEEPER
STEMPEL
STEPPED
STEPPER
STEPPES
STOMPED
STOOPED
STOOPER
STOPPED
STOPPER
STRIPED
STRIPER
STRIPES
STUMPED
STUMPER
SWAMPED
SWAPPED
SWAPPER
SWEEPEA
SWEEPER
SWOOPED
SWOOPER
TENTPEG
THIGPEN
THUMPED
THUMPER
TRAMPED
TRAMPER
TRAPPED
TRAPPER
TRIPPED
TRIPPER
TRIPPET
TROMPED
TROOPED
TROOPER
TROUPED
TROUPER
TROUPES
TRUMPED
TRUMPET
TSHAPED
TSHAPES
TVTAPES
UNCAPED
UNDUPED
UNHOPED
UNPIPED
UNRIPER
UNROPED
UNROPES
UNTAPED
UNTAPES
UNTYPED
UNWIPED
USHAPED
USHAPES
USURPED
USURPER
VONOPEL
VSHAPED
VSHAPES
WHAPPED
WHELPED
WHIMPER
WHIPPED
WHIPPER
WHIPPET
WHISPER
WHOMPED
WHOOPED
WHOOPEE
WHOOPER
WHOPPED
WHOPPER
WHUPPED
WRAPPED
WRAPPER
YSHAPED
YSHAPES
ZATOPEK

••••P•E

ACOUPLE
ADOLPHE
BLIMPIE
CAPAPIE
CHAPPIE
CHEAPIE
CRAPPIE
CRIPPLE
CRUMPLE
DECUPLE
ECHAPPE
ECLIPSE
ELLIPSE
ESCAPEE
EXAMPLE
GLIMPSE
GRAPPLE
GROUPIE
LIMEPIE
MANIPLE
MEATPIE
MOONPIE
NONUPLE
OCTUPLE
OSSIPEE
PLUMPIE
PORKPIE
PREPPIE
RELAPSE
SCRUPLE
SHARPIE
SLURPEE
SNAPPLE
STEEPLE
STIPPLE
STOPPLE
STROPHE
SYNAPSE
TRAIPSE
TRAMPLE
WHIPPLE
WHOOPEE
WHOOPIE

•••••PE

ANYHOPE
BAGPIPE
BEDRAPE
BIOTYPE
BOBHOPE
ECHAPPE
ECOTYPE
EUTERPE
GASPIPE
GOESAPE
GONEAPE
GUYROPE
INSHAPE
ISOTOPE
LEGROPE
MANROPE
MISTYPE
NEWHOPE
OUTPIPE
PANPIPE
PRETAPE
PRETYPE
PVCPIPE
REDTAPE
RESHAPE
SETTYPE
SUBTYPE
SYNCOPE
THECAPE
THEHOPE
THEPOPE
THEROPE
TIEROPE
TINTYPE
TOWROPE
UNDRAPE
UPSLOPE
VCRTAPE
WENTAPE

PF•••••

PFENNIG

P•F••••
PIFFLED
PIFFLES
PRFIRMS
PUFFERS
PUFFERY
PUFFIER
PUFFILY
PUFFING
PUFFINS
PUFFOUT
PUFFSUP

P••F•••
PALFREY
PANFISH
PANFULS
PARFAIT
PARFIVE
PARFOUR
PARFUMS
PEAFOWL
PERFECT
PERFIDY
PERFORM
PERFUME
PERFUMY
PERFUSE
PETFISH
PETFROG
PIAFFED
PIAFFES
PIFFLED
PIFFLES
PIGFISH
PILFERS
PINFOLD
PITFALL
POTFULS
PREFABS
PREFACE
PREFADE
PREFECT
PREFERS
PREFILE
PREFORM
PREFUND
PROFANE
PROFARM
PROFESS
PROFFER
PROFILE
PROFITS
PROFUSE
PUFFERS
PUFFERY
PUFFIER
PUFFILY
PUFFING
PUFFINS
PUFFOUT
PUFFSUP
PURFLED
PURFLER
PURFLES

P•••F••
PACIFIC
PAIDFOR
PAILFUL
PAINFUL
PALMFUL
PASSFOR
PAYOFFS
PAYSFOR
PIAFFED
PIAFFES
PINEFOR
PIPEFUL
PITIFUL
PLANFOR
PLAYFUL
PLOTFUL
POKEFUN
POPOFFS
POSTFIX
POUTFUL
PRAYFOR
PROFFER
PROOFED
PROOFER
PULLFOR
PUSHFOR
PUSHFUL
PUTOFFS

P••••F•
PACEOFF
PACKOFF
PAIDOFF
PAIROFF
PALMOFF
PASSOFF
PAWNOFF
PAYOFFS
PAYSOFF
PEELOFF
PERSOFF
PETRIFY
PICKOFF
PIESAFE
PLAYOFF
PONTIFF
POPEAFB
POPOFFS
POPSOFF
PREDEFY
PRELIFE
PRESIFT
PROLIFE
PULLOFF
PULPIFY
PUSHOFF
PUTOFFS
PUTREFY
PUTSOFF

P•••••F
PACEOFF
PACKOFF
PAIDOFF
PAIROFF
PALMOFF
PASSOFF
PAWNOFF
PAYSOFF
PEELOFF
PERSOFF
PETCALF
PICKOFF
PILESOF
PLAYOFF
PONTIFF
POPSOFF
PROUDOF
PULLOFF
PUSHOFF
PUTSOFF

•PF••••
UPFIELD
UPFIRST
UPFLING
UPFLOWS
UPFOLDS
UPFORIT
UPFRONT

•P•F•••
SPIFFED
SPIFFUP

•P••F••
OPTSFOR
SPIFFED
SPIFFUP
SPOOFED
SPOOFER
UPLIFTS
UPWAFTS

•P•••F•
SPECIFY
SPEDOFF
SPINOFF
SPUNOFF
UPDRAFT
UPDRIFT
UPSHIFT

•P••••F
APAIROF
APECKOF
APILEOF
SPEAKOF
SPEDOFF
SPINOFF
SPOKEOF
SPUNOFF

••PF•••
CAPFULS
CUPFULS
LAPFULS
TOPFIVE
TOPFORM

••P•F••
HOPEFOR
HOPEFUL
KEPTFIT
PIPEFUL
POPOFFS
REPSFOR
RIPOFFS
TIPOFFS

••P••F•
AMPLIFY
HAPPIFY
HOPSOFF
KEPTOFF
LIPSOFF
LOPSOFF
POPEAFB
POPOFFS
POPSOFF
RIPOFFS
RIPSOFF
ROPEOFF
TAPSOFF
TIPOFFS
TIPSOFF
TOPSOFF
WIPEOFF
YUPPIFY
ZIPCUFF
ZIPSOFF

••P•••F
HIPROOF
HOPSOFF
KEPTOFF
LIPSOFF
LOPSOFF
POPSOFF
REPROOF
RIPSOFF
ROPEOFF
TAPSOFF
TIPSOFF
TOPSOFF
WIPEOFF
ZIPCUFF
ZIPSOFF

•••PF••
CLAPFOR
DEEPFAT
DEEPFRY
HELPFUL
KEEPFIT
LEAPFOR
SHIPFUL
SHOPFOR
SHOPFUL
STOPFOR
WEEPFOR

•••P•F•
CHOPOFF
CLIPOFF
DAMPOFF
DROPOFF
HAPPIFY
JUMPOFF
KEEPOFF
PULPIFY
SLIPOFF
SNIPOFF
STEPOFF
STOPOFF
STUPEFY
TAMPAFL
YUPPIFY

•••P••F
CHOPOFF
CLIPOFF
DAMPOFF
DROPOFF
HEAPSOF
JUMPOFF
KEEPOFF
SLIPOFF
SNIPOFF
STEPOFF
STOPOFF

••••P•F
ONTOPOF
STRIPOF

PG•••••
PGAPROS
PGATOUR
PGRATED

P•G••••
PAGEANT
PAGEBOY
PAGEONE
PAGESIX
PAGETWO
PAGINGS
PAGODAS
PEGASUS
PEGAWAY
PEGGING
PEGLEGS
PEGLESS
PEGLIKE
PEGTOPS
PIGEONS
PIGEYED
PIGFISH
PIGGERY
PIGGIER
PIGGIES
PIGGING
PIGGISH
PIGIRON
PIGLETS
PIGLIKE
PIGMEAT
PIGMENT
PIGNUTS
PIGOUTS
PIGPENS
PIGSKIN
PIGSOUT
PIGTAIL
PIGWEED
PUGGISH
PUGGLES
PUGNOSE
PUGSLEY
PYGMIES

P••G•••
PADGETT
PANGAEA
PANGRAM
PARGERS
PARGING
PEGGING
PENGUIN
PERGOLA
PETGATE
PETGOAT
PEUGEOT
PIDGEON
PIDGINS
PIGGERY
PIGGIER
PIGGIES
PIGGING
PIGGISH
PILGRIM
PINGERS
PINGING
PINGUID
PLAGUED
PLAGUES
PLIGHTS
PLUGGED
PLUGGER
PLUGINS
PLUGOLA
PLUGSIN
PLUGSUP
PONGEES
PONGIDS
POPGUNS
PORGIES
PREGAIN
PREGAME
PROGENY
PROGRAM
PUBGAME
PUDGIER
PUDGILY
PUGGISH
PUGGLES
PUNGENT
PURGING

P•••G••
PAANGAS
PAPAGOS
PARAGON
PELAGES
PELAGIC
PERIGEE
PERUGIA
PHLEGMY
PHRYGIA
PILEGGI
PIPAGES
PIROGEN
PIROGUE
PLEDGED
PLEDGEE
PLEDGER
PLEDGES
PLOUGHS
PLUGGED
PLUGGER
PLUNGED
PLUNGER
PLUNGES
POLYGON
POTAGES
PREAGED
PREAGES
PRINGLE
PRONGED

P••••G•
PACKAGE
PAGINGS
PALINGS
PANURGE
PARINGS
PASSAGE
PAVINGS
PEERAGE
PEGLEGS
PEONAGE
PETCAGE
PETDOGS
PETPIGS
PHOTOGS
PILEGGI
PILINGS
PILLAGE
PIPINGS
PLUMAGE
PORTAGE
POSTAGE
POTTAGE
PRESAGE
PRODIGY
PROLOGS
PROTEGE
PYEDOGS

P•••••G
PACKING
PADDING
PAINING
PAIRING
PALLING
PALMING
PANNING
PANTING
PANTLEG
PARGING
PARKING
PARRING
PARSING
PARTING
PASSING
PASTING
PATTING
PAULING
PAUSING
PAWNING
PEAKING
PEALING
PEATBOG
PECKING
PEEKING
PEELING
PEENING
PEEPING
PEERING
PEEVING
PEGGING
PEIPING
PELTING
PENDING
PENNING
PEPPING
PERIWIG
PERKING
PERMING
PETFROG
PETTING
PFENNIG
PHASING
PHONING
PICKING
PIECING
PIGGING
PILLBUG
PILLING
PINGING
PINKING
PINNING
PIQUING
PISHING
PITHING
PITTING
PITYING
PLACING
PLANING
PLATING
PLAYING
PLOWING
PLUMING
POISING
POLLING
PONDING
PONYING
PONYKEG
POOLING
POOPING
POPPING
POPSONG
PORKING
PORTING
POSTBAG
POSTING
POTTING
POURING
POUTING
PRATING
PRAYING
PRESONG
PREYING
PRICING
PRIDING
PRIMING
PRIZING
PROBING
PROLONG
PROSING
PROVING
PRUNING
PUDDING
PUFFING
PULLING
PULPING
PULSING
PUMPING
PUNNING
PUNTING
PURGING
PURLING
PURRING
PURSING
PUSHING
PUTTING

•PG••••
UPGAZED
UPGAZES
UPGIRDS
UPGOING
UPGRADE
UPGROWN
UPGROWS

•P•G•••
APOGEAL
APOGEAN
APOGEES
EPIGONE
EPIGRAM
SPIGOTS

•P••G••
APHAGIA
APHAGIC
EPERGNE
OPPUGNS
SPANGLE
SPANGLY
SPIEGEL
SPONGED
SPONGER
SPONGES
UPLIGHT
UPRIGHT
UPTIGHT

•P•••G•
APOLOGY
EPILOGS
IPLEDGE
SPLURGE
SPRINGS
SPRINGY
SPYINGS
UPSTAGE
UPSURGE

•P••••G
APPLING
OPENING
OPINING
SPACING
SPADING
SPARING
SPAYING
SPECING
SPEWING
SPICING
SPIKING
SPITING
SPOKING
SPUMING
SPYRING
UPFLING
UPGOING
UPSWING

••PG•••
CAPGUNS
POPGUNS
TOPGUNS
ZIPGUNS

••P•G••
IMPUGNS
NIPIGON
OPPUGNS
PAPAGOS
PIPAGES
REPAGED
REPAGES
REPUGNS
UNPAGAN
UNPAGED

••P••G•
EXPUNGE
IMPINGE
LAPDOGS
PIPINGS
SAPSAGO
SUPERGS
TAPINGS
TOPDOGS
UNPLUGS

••P•••G
APPLING
BOPPING
CAPPING
COPPING
COPYING
CUPPING
DAPPING
DIPPING
ESPYING
GAPPING
GYPPING
HOPPING
HOPSING
HYPOING
KIPLING
KIPPING
LAPPING
LAPSANG
LAPSING
LAPWING
LIPPING
LOPPING
MAPPING
MOPPING
NAPPING
NIPPING
PEPPING
POPPING
POPSONG
RAPPING
RAPSONG
REPPING
RIPPING
SAPLING
SAPPING
SIPPING
SOPPING
SUPPING
TAPPING
TIPPING
TOPPING
YAPPING
YIPPING
ZAPPING
ZIPPING

•••PG••
BURPGUN
STOPGAP
TRAPGUN

•••P•G•
MISPAGE
ONEPAGE
PETPIGS
RAMPAGE
SEEPAGE
WARPAGE
WEBPAGE

•••P••G
BEEPING
BOPPING
BUMPING
BURPING
CAMPING
CAPPING
CARPING
COMPING
COOPING
COPPING
COUPING
CRAPING
CREPING
CUPPING
DAMPING
DAPPING
DIPPING
DRAPING
DUMPING
EARPLUG
ELOPING
GAPPING
GASPING
GAWPING
GIMPING
GRIPING
GROPING
GULPING
GYPPING
HARPING
HASPING
HEAPING
HELPING
HOOPING
HOPPING
JUMPING
KEEPING
KIPPING
LAPPING
LEAPING
LEIPZIG
LIMPING
LIPPING
LISPING
LOOPING
LOPPING
LUMPING
MAPPING
MOPPING
NAPPING
NIPPING
PEEPING
PEIPING
PEPPING
POOPING
POPPING
PULPING
PUMPING
RAMPING
RAPPING
RASPING
REAPING
REPPING
RIPPING
ROMPING
RSVPING
SAPPING
SCOPING
SEEPING
SHAPING
SIPPING
SLOPING
SNIPING
SOAPING
SOPPING
SUPPING
SWIPING
TAMPING
TAPPING
TEMPING
TIPPING
TOPPING
VAMPING
WARPING
WEEPING
WIMPING
WISPING
YAPPING
YAWPING
YELPING
YIPPING
ZAPPING
ZIPPING

••••P•G
BUSHPIG
MALEPIG
NEWSPEG
TENTPEG
WILDPIG

•••••PG
RATEDPG

PH•••••
PHAEDRA
PHAETON
PHALANX
PHANTOM
PHARAOH
PHARLAP
PHARYNX
PHASEIN
PHASERS
PHASING
PHATTER
PHEMIUS
PHENOLS
PHENOMS
PHIDIAS
PHILBIN
PHILCOS
PHILEAS
PHILIPK
PHILIPS
PHILIPV
PHILLIE
PHILLIP
PHILOUS
PHILTER
PHILTRE
PHINEAS
PHISHED
PHISHER
PHISHES
PHLEGMY
PHLOEMS
PHLOXES
PHOBIAS
PHOBICS
PHOEBES
PHOEBUS
PHOENIX
PHONEIN
PHONEME
PHONENO
PHONERS
PHONEYS
PHONICS
PHONIER
PHONIES
PHONILY
PHONING
PHONYUP
PHOTICS
PHOTOGS
PHOTOID
PHOTONS
PHOTOOP
PHRASAL
PHRASED
PHRASES
PHRENIC
PHRYGIA
PHYLLIS
PHYLLOS
PHYSICS

P•H••••
PAHLAVI
PSHAWED

P••H•••
PACHISI

PATHAND
PATHANS
PATHWAY
PAYHEED
PEAHENS
PERHAPS
PETHAIR
PETHARE
PIEHOLE
PINHEAD
PINHOLE
PISHING
PITHEAD
PITHIER
PITHILY
PITHING
POOHBAH
POSHEST
POTHERB
POTHERS
POTHOLE
POTHOOK
PREHEAL
PREHEAT
PUSHERS
PUSHFOR
PUSHFUL
PUSHIER
PUSHILY
PUSHING
PUSHKIN
PUSHOFF
PUSHOUT
PUSHPIN
PUSHROD
PUSHUPS
PYTHIAN
PYTHIAS
PYTHONS

P•••H••
PANCHAX
PANTHER
PARCHED
PARCHES
PASCHAL
PATCHED
PATCHEN
PATCHER
PATCHES
PATCHUP
PEACHED
PEACHES
PERAHIA
PERCHED
PERCHER
PERCHES
PERCHIK
PETCHEW
PETSHOP
PHISHED
PHISHER
PHISHES
PINCHAS
PINCHED
PINCHER
PINCHES
PINCHME
PINCHOT
PINKHAM
PITCHED
PITCHER
PITCHES
PITCHIN
PITCHTO
PLASHED
PLASHES
PLIGHTS
PLUSHER
PLUSHES
PLUSHLY
POACHED
POACHER
POACHES
PONCHOS
POOCHES
POOCHIE
PORCHES
PORTHOS
POSTHOC
POTSHOT
POUCHED
POUCHES
PRESHIP
PRESHOW
PREWHIP
PRITHEE
PROPHET
PROSHOP
PRUDHOE
PSYCHED
PSYCHES
PSYCHIC
PSYCHOS
PSYCHUP
PUNCHED
PUNCHER
PUNCHES
PUNCHIN
PUNCHUP
PYNCHON
PYRRHIC
PYRRHUS

P••••H•
PANACHE
PARAPHS
PARIAHS
PAUNCHY
PENUCHE
PIRANHA
PLINTHS
PLOUGHS
PORSCHE
PREACHY
PWBOTHA

P•••••H
PADUCAH
PANFISH
PARRISH
PATCASH
PAYCASH
PDQBACH
PEAKISH
PECKISH
PEEVISH
PELTISH
PERKISH
PETFISH
PETTISH
PHARAOH
PICTISH
PIGFISH
PIGGISH
PINKISH
PIXYISH
PLANISH
PLAYDOH
PLENISH
POOHBAH
POORISH
PORKISH
PRADESH
PREWASH
PRUDISH
PUBLISH
PUCKISH
PUGGISH

•PH••••
APHAGIA
APHAGIC
APHASIA
APHASIC
APHELIA
APHIDES
APHILIP
APHONIA
APHONIC
EPHEBUS
EPHEDRA
EPHESUS
EPHRAIM
OPHELIA
SPHERAL
SPHERED
SPHERES
SPHERIC
UPHEAPS
UPHEAVE
UPHILLS
UPHOARD
UPHOLDS

•P•H•••
MPTHREE
SPYHOLE
UPAHEAD
UPPHASE
UPSHIFT
UPSHOOT
UPSHOTS
UPTHERE
UPTHROW
UPWHIRL

•P••H••
APACHES
APISHLY
APOTHEM
EPITHET
EPOCHAL
SPATHES

•P•••H•
EPARCHS
EPARCHY
SPLASHY
UPLIGHT
UPRIGHT
UPTIGHT

•P••••H
CPEBACH
EPITAPH
IPSWICH
OPALISH
SPANISH
SPINACH
SPLOTCH
UPNORTH
UPREACH

••PH•••
ALPHARD
AMPHION
AMPHORA
ASPHALT
BYPHONE
CEPHALO
CEPHALY
CEPHEUS
CIPHERS
CYPHERS
DAPHNES
DAPHNIA
DAPHNIS
EUPHONY
GOPHERS
HYPHENS
INPHASE
JAPHETH
JEPHTHA
MOPHEAD
NAPHTHA
NEPHEWS
NEPHRIC
OMPHALO
ORPHANS
ORPHANT
ORPHEAN
ORPHEUM
ORPHEUS
RAPHAEL
REPHASE
REPHONE
SAPHEAD
SEPHIAS
SIPHONS
SOPHIES
SOPHISM
SOPHIST
TOPHATS
TOPHOLE
TYPHOID
TYPHOON
UPPHASE
XIPHOID
ZEPHYRS

••P•H••
CAPSHAW
COPSHOP
TAPSHOE
TOPTHIS
WAPSHOT

••P••H•
BYPATHS
CAPUCHE
DEPECHE
EMPATHS
EMPATHY
HUPPAHS
JEPHTHA
NAPHTHA
RUPIAHS

••P•••H
CAPEESH
DIPTYCH
FOPPISH
HIPBATH
HIPPISH
IMPEACH
JAPHETH
LAPPISH
REPATCH
SOPWITH

•••PH••
CAMPHOR
DAUPHIN
DELPHIC
DIAPHAN
DOLPHIN
GLYPHIC
GRAPHED
GRAPHIC
GRYPHON
HUMPHED
HUMPHRY
MEMPHIS
MORPHED
MORPHIC
MORPHIN
MURPHYS
NYMPHAL
NYMPHIC
PROPHET
RALPHIE
STEPHEN
SULPHUR
SYLPHIC

•••P•H•
ARAPAHO
HUPPAHS
OOMPAHS
TEMPEHS

•••P••H
ANSPACH
CHUPPAH
DAMPISH
DEEPISH
DUMPISH
FOPPISH
HIPPISH
LAPPISH
LUMPISH
OUTPATH
OUTPUSH
RASPISH
ROMPISH
THEPOOH
TOWPATH
VAMPISH
WARPATH
WASPISH
WIMPISH

••••PH•
ADELPHI
ADOLPHE
ATROPHY
CALIPHS
JOSEPHA
JOSEPHI
PARAPHS
SERAPHS
STROPHE
THIMPHU

••••P•H
CHUPPAH
INDEPTH

•••••PH
DIGRAPH
EPITAPH
GALUMPH
REGRAPH
RUDOLPH
TRIUMPH

PI•••••
PIAFFED
PIAFFES
PIANISM
PIANIST
PIANOLA
PIASTER
PIASTRE
PIAZZAS
PICADOR
PICANTE
PICARAS
PICARDO
PICARDY
PICAROS
PICASSO
PICCARD
PICCATA
PICCOLO
PICEOUS
PICKAXE
PICKENS
PICKERS
PICKETS
PICKETT
PICKIER
PICKING
PICKLED
PICKLES
PICKOFF
PICKOUT
PICKSAT
PICKSON
PICKSUP
PICKUPS
PICNICS
PICOTED
PICTISH
PICTURE
PIDDLED
PIDDLES
PIDGEON
PIDGINS
PIEBALD
PIECERS
PIECING
PIEEYED
PIEHOLE
PIELIKE
PIEPANS
PIERCED
PIERCER
PIERCES
PIERIAN
PIERROT
PIESAFE
PIESALE
PIETIES
PIETINS
PIETOSO
PIETROS
PIFFLED
PIFFLES
PIGEONS
PIGEYED
PIGFISH
PIGGERY
PIGGIER
PIGGIES
PIGGING
PIGGISH
PIGIRON
PIGLETS
PIGLIKE
PIGMEAT
PIGMENT
PIGNUTS
PIGOUTS
PIGPENS
PIGSKIN
PIGSOUT
PIGTAIL
PIGWEED
PILATES
PILATUS
PILCROW
PILEATE
PILEDIN
PILEDON
PILEDUP
PILEGGI
PILEOUS
PILESIN
PILESOF
PILESON
PILESUP
PILEUPS
PILFERS
PILGRIM
PILINGS
PILLAGE
PILLARS
PILLBOX
PILLBUG
PILLING
PILLION
PILLORY
PILLOWS
PILLOWY
PILOTED
PILSNER
PIMENTO
PIMESON
PIMLICO
PIMPLED
PIMPLES
PINATAS
PINBALL
PINBOYS
PINCERS
PINCHAS
PINCHED
PINCHER
PINCHES
PINCHME
PINCHOT
PINCURL
PINDOWN
PINEFOR
PINENUT
PINEOIL
PINESAP
PINESOL
PINETAR
PINETOP
PINETUM
PINFOLD
PINGERS
PINGING
PINGUID
PINHEAD
PINHOLE
PINIEST
PINIONS
PINKENS
PINKEST
PINKETT
PINKHAM
PINKIES
PINKING
PINKISH
PINKOES
PINLESS
PINNACE
PINNATE
PINNERS
PINNING
PINOAKS
PINONES
PINOTTA
PINSEAL
PINTAIL
PINWALE
PIOLETS
PIONEER
PIOSITY
PIOUSLY
PIPAGES
PIPCARD
PIPEDIN
PIPEDUP
PIPEFUL
PIPESIN
PIPESUP
PIPETTE
PIPIEST
PIPINGS
PIPLESS
PIPPINS
PIQUANT
PIQUING
PIRAEUS
PIRANHA
PIRATED
PIRATES
PIRATIC
PIRELLI
PIROGEN
PIROGUE
PISANIO
PISARRO
PISCEAN
PISCINE
PISCOPO
PISHING
PISMIRE
PISTILS
PISTOLE
PISTOLS
PISTONS
PISTOUS
PITAPAT
PITAYAS
PITBOSS
PITBULL
PITCHED
PITCHER
PITCHES
PITCHIN
PITCHTO
PITCREW
PITEOUS
PITFALL
PITHEAD
PITHIER
PITHILY
PITHING
PITIERS
PITIFUL
PITILLO
PITROWS
PITSAWS
PITSTOP
PITTING
PITTMAN
PITYING
PIUSIII
PIUSVII
PIUSXII
PIVOTAL
PIVOTED
PIVOTER
PIXYISH
PIZARRO
PIZZAZZ

P•I••••
PAIDADS
PAIDFOR
PAIDOFF
PAIDOUT
PAILFUL
PAINFUL
PAINING
PAINTED
PAINTER
PAIRERS
PAIRING
PAIROFF
PAIRSUP
PAISANO
PAISANS
PAISLEY
PAIUTES
PEIPING
PHIDIAS
PHILBIN
PHILCOS
PHILEAS
PHILIPK
PHILIPS
PHILIPV
PHILLIE
PHILLIP
PHILOUS
PHILTER
PHILTRE
PHINEAS
PHISHED
PHISHER
PHISHES
PLIABLE
PLIABLY
PLIANCY
PLICATE
PLIGHTS
PLINKED
PLINTHS
PLISSES
POINTAT
POINTED
POINTER
POINTES
POINTTO
POINTUP
POISERS
POISING
POISONS
POISSON
POITIER
POIVRES
PRICERS
PRICIER
PRICILY
PRICING
PRICKED
PRICKLE
PRICKLY
PRICKUP
PRIDING
PRIESTS
PRIMACY
PRIMARY
PRIMATE
PRIMELY
PRIMERA
PRIMERO
PRIMERS
PRIMING
PRIMMED
PRIMMER
PRIMPED
PRINCES
PRINGLE
PRINKED
PRINKER
PRINTAD
PRINTED
PRINTER
PRINTUP
PRIORTO
PRISONS
PRISSES
PRITHEE
PRIUSES
PRIVACY
PRIVATE
PRIVETS
PRIVIER
PRIVIES
PRIVILY
PRIVITY
PRIVYTO
PRIZING
PRIZZIS

P••I•••
PACIEST
PACIFIC
PAGINGS
PALINGS
PANICKY
PANICLE
PANIERS
PANINIS
PAPIERS
PAPILLA
PAPISTS
PARIAHS
PARIBUS
PARINGS
PATIENT
PATINAS
PAVIDLY
PAVINGS
PAVIORS
PAVIOUR
PAXINOU
PAYINTO
PEDICAB
PELICAN
PELISSE
PEPITAS
PERIAPT
PERIDOT
PERIGEE
PERILED
PERIODS
PERISSA
PERITUS
PERIWIG
PETIOLE
PETITES
PIGIRON
PILINGS
PINIEST
PINIONS
PIPIEST
PIPINGS
PITIERS
PITIFUL
PITILLO
PLAICES
PLAINER
PLAINES
PLAINLY
PLAINTS
PLAISIR
PLAITED
PLAITER
PODIUMS
POKIEST
POLICED
POLICER
POLICES
POLISCI
POLITER
POLITIC
PONIARD
PORIVER
POSITED
POTIONS
PRAIRIE
PRAISED
PRAISER
PRAISES
PREIDEA
PRFIRMS
PRYINTO
PUMICED
PUMICES
PUNIEST
PURISTS
PURITAN
PUTITTO
PYRITES
PYRITIC

P•••I••
PACHISI
PACKICE
PACKING
PADDIES
PADDING
PADSITE
PAINING
PAIRING
PALLIER
PALLING
PALMIER
PALMING
PALMIST
PAMLICO
PANDITS
PANFISH
PANNIER
PANNING
PANPIPE
PANSIES
PANTIES
PANTILE
PANTING
PAPPIES
PAPRIKA
PARAIBA
PARFIVE
PARGING
PARKING
PARKINS
PARRIED
PARRIER
PARRIES
PARRING
PARRISH
PARSING
PARTIAL
PARTIED
PARTIER
PARTIES
PARTIII
PARTING
PARTITA
PARTITE
PASSING
PASSION
PASSIVE
PASTIER
PASTIES
PASTIME
PASTINA
PASTING
PATRICE
PATRICK
PATRIES
PATRIOT
PATSIES
PATTIES
PATTING
PAUCITY
PAULIII
PAULINA
PAULINE
PAULING
PAULIST
PAUSING
PAWNING
PAYDIRT
PEAKIER
PEAKING
PEAKISH
PEALIKE
PEALING
PEATIER
PECKING
PECKISH
PECTINS
PEEKING
PEELING
PEENING
PEEPING
PEERING
PEEVING
PEEVISH
PEGGING
PEGLIKE
PEIPING
PELTING
PELTISH

PENCILS PENDING PENLIKE PENLITE PENNIES PENNINE PENNING PENSION PENSIVE PENTIUM PENZIAS PEONIES PEORIAN PEPCIDS PEPPIER PEPPILL PEPPILY PEPPING PEPPINO PEPSICO PEPSINS PEPTICS PEPTIDE PERDIDO PERDIEM PERDITA PERFIDY PERKIER PERKILY PERKING PERKINS PERKISH PERLITE PERMIAN PERMING PERMITS PERRIER PERRINE PERRINS PERSIAN PERSIST PERSIUS PESKIER PESKILY PETBIRD PETFISH PETLION PETMICE PETPIGS PETRIFY PETSITS PETTIER PETTILY PETTING PETTISH PHASING PHEMIUS PHIDIAS PHILIPK PHILIPS PHILIPV PHOBIAS PHOBICS PHONICS PHONIER PHONIES PHONILY PHONING

PHOTICS PHYSICS PIANISM PIANIST PICKIER PICKING PICNICS PICTISH PIDGINS PIECING PIELIKE PIERIAN PIETIES PIETINS PIGFISH PIGGIER PIGGIES PIGGING PIGGISH PIGLIKE PILLING PILLION PIMLICO PINGING PINKIES PINKING PINKISH PINNING PIOSITY PIPPINS PIQUING PISCINE PISHING PISMIRE PISTILS PITHIER PITHILY PITHING PITTING PITYING PIUSIII PIXYISH PLACIDO PLACING PLANING PLANISH PLATIER PLATIES PLATING PLAYING PLEBIAN PLENISH PLOSION PLOSIVE PLOWING PLUGINS PLUMIER PLUMING PLUVIAL PODLIKE PODRIDA POESIES POETICA POETICS POETISE POETIZE POISING POITIER

POLLING POLOIST PONDING PONGIDS PONTIAC PONTIAN PONTIFF PONTIUS PONYING POOLING POOPING POORISH POPDIVA POPLINS POPPIES POPPING POPPINS POPWINE PORCINE PORGIES PORKIER PORKING PORKISH PORTICO PORTING PORTION POSTIES POSTING POSTITS POTLIDS POTPIES POTTIER POTTIES POTTING POURING POUTIER POUTING PRALINE PRATING PRAYING PREBIDS PREBILL PREBIND PRECISE PRECITE PREDICT PREDIET PREDIVE PREFILE PRELIFE PRELIMS PREMIER PREMIES PREMISE PREMISS PREMIUM PRERIOT PRESIDE PRESIFT PRETIRE PREVIAS PREVIEW PREWIRE PREWITT PREXIES PREYING PRICIER PRICILY

PRICING PRIDING PRIMING PRIVIER PRIVIES PRIVILY PRIVITY PRIZING PROBIES PROBING PROBITY PROCITY PRODIGY PROFILE PROFITS PROLIFE PROMISE PROSIER PROSILY PROSING PROTIST PROVIDE PROVINE PROVING PROVISO PROXIES PROXIMA PROXIMO PRUDISH PRUNING PUBLICS PUBLISH PUBLIUS PUCCINI PUCKISH PUDDING PUDGIER PUDGILY PUERILE PUFFIER PUFFILY PUFFING PUFFINS PUGGISH PULLING PULLINS PULPIER PULPIFY PULPING PULPITS PULSING PUMPING PUNDITS PUNKIER PUNKIES PUNNIER PUNNILY PUNNING PUNTING PUPPIES PURGING PURLIEU PURLING PURRING PURSIER PURSING PURTIER PURVIEW

PUSHIER PUSHILY PUSHING PUSSIES PUTTIED PUTTIES PUTTING PVCPIPE PYGMIES PYTHIAN PYTHIAS

P••••I•

PACIFIC PACKSIN PACQUIN PADRAIC PAGESIX PALADIN PALMOIL PANINIS PARBOIL PARFAIT PARKSIT PARODIC PAROTID PARSNIP PARTIII PASSAIC PASTEIN PAULIII PAYSLIP PEEKSIN PEERSIN PELAGIC PENGUIN PERAHIA PERATIO PERCHIK PERIWIG PERSEID PERTAIN PERUGIA PETERII PETHAIR PETULIA PETUNIA PFENNIG PHASEIN PHILBIN PHILLIE PHILLIP PHOENIX PHONEIN PHOTOID PHRENIC PHRYGIA PHYLLIS PIGSKIN PIGTAIL PILEDIN PILESIN PILGRIM PINEOIL PINGUID PINTAIL PIPEDIN PIPESIN

PIRATIC PISANIO PITCHIN PIUSIII PIUSVII PIUSXII PLAISIR PLASMIC PLASTIC PLAUDIT PLOVDIV PLUGSIN PLUMBIC PLUMPIE POLARIS POLEMIC POLESIT POLITIC POLONIA POMPEIA POMPEII POOCHIE POOPSIE POPQUIZ PORKPIE POSTFIX POTBOIL POURSIN POUSSIN PRACTIC PRAIRIE PREACID PREBOIL PRECOIL PREEDIT PREEMIE PREGAIN PREOMIT PREPAID PREPPIE PRESHIP PRETRIM PREVAIL PREVOID PREWHIP PRIZZIS PROMBID PROSAIC PROTEIN PROVEIT PRUSSIA PSALMIC PSYCHIC PULLPIN PULLSIN PUMPKIN PUNCHIN PURLOIN PURSUIT PUSHKIN PUSHPIN PYRAMID PYRETIC PYREXIA PYRITIC PYRRHIC

P•••••I

PACHISI PAHLAVI PALAZZI PARASKI PARTIII PASCOLI PAULIII PECCAVI PERETTI PETERII PILEGGI PIRELLI PIUSIII PIUSVII PIUSXII PLATYPI PLOESTI POLANYI POLISCI POLYSCI POMPEII PUCCINI PULASKI PULMONI PUNJABI

•PI••••

APILEOF APISHLY EPICARP EPICENE EPICURE EPIDERM EPIDOTE EPIGONE EPIGRAM EPILADY EPILATE EPILOGS EPISODE EPISTLE EPITAPH EPITHET EPITOME OPIATES OPINERS OPINING OPINION SPICERS SPICERY SPICEUP SPICIER SPICILY SPICING SPIDERS SPIDERY SPIEDON SPIEGEL SPIELED SPIELER SPIESON SPIFFED SPIFFUP SPIGOTS SPIKERS SPIKETV SPIKEUP

SPIKIER SPIKILY SPIKING SPILLED SPILLER SPINACH SPINDLE SPINDLY SPINDRY SPINELS SPINETS SPINIER SPINNER SPINNEY SPINOFF SPINOUT SPINOZA SPIRALS SPIREAS SPIRIER SPIRITS SPITING SPITOUT SPITSON SPITTER SPITTLE SPITZES

•P•I•••

APAIROF APHIDES APHILIP APLITES APRICOT APRIORI APSIDES EPSILON OPTICAL OPTICKS OPTIMAL OPTIMAS OPTIMUM OPTIONS SPLICED SPLICER SPLICES SPLINES SPLINTS SPLITUP SPOILED SPOILER SPRIEST SPRINGS SPRINGY SPRINTS SPRITES SPYINGS UPDIVED UPDIVES UPFIELD UPFIRST UPGIRDS UPHILLS UPLIFTS UPLIGHT UPLINKS UPPILED UPPILES

UPRIGHT UPRISEN UPRISER UPRISES UPRIVER UPSIDES UPSILON UPSIZED UPSIZES UPTICKS UPTIGHT UPTILTS UPTIMES UPWINDS

•P••I••

APATITE APEDIET APELIKE APERIES APPLIED APPLIER APPLIES APPLING APPOINT APPRISE APULIAN EPEEIST EPONINE EPOXIED EPOXIES IPSWICH OPACITY OPALINE OPALISH OPENING OPINING OPINION SPACIAL SPACIER SPACING SPADING SPANIEL SPANISH SPARING SPATIAL SPAYING SPECIAL SPECIES SPECIFY SPECING SPEWING SPICIER SPICILY SPICING SPIKIER SPIKILY SPIKING SPINIER SPIRIER SPIRITS SPITING SPOKING SPRAINS SPUMIER SPUMING SPYKIDS SPYRING

UPBUILD UPCLIMB UPCOILS UPDRIED UPDRIES UPDRIFT UPFLING UPGOING UPRAISE UPSHIFT UPSPINS UPSTIRS UPSWING UPWHIRL

•P•••I•

APESUIT APHAGIA APHAGIC APHASIA APHASIC APHELIA APHILIP APHONIA APHONIC APPETIT EPHRAIM EPSTEIN OPENAIR OPENPIT OPHELIA OPTEDIN OPUNTIA SPANAIR SPHERIC SPORTIN SPOTLIT SPUTNIK UPANDIN UPBRAID UPFORIT UPSTAIR

•P••••I

APRIORI SPUMONI

••PI•••

ALPINER ALPINES ASPIRED ASPIRER ASPIRES ASPIRIN CAPITAL CAPITAN CAPITOL COPIERS COPILOT COPIOUS DEPICTS DIPINTO DOPIEST EMPIRES EMPIRIC EMPIRIN ESPIALS EXPIATE

EXPIRED EXPIRES HOPINTO IMPIETY IMPINGE IMPIOUS JUPITER KAPITAL KAPITSA KOPIYKA LEPIDUS LIPIDIC LUPINES MOPIEST NAPIERS NIPIGON PAPIERS PAPILLA PAPISTS PEPITAS PIPIEST PIPINGS RAPIDAN RAPIDER RAPIDLY RAPIERS RAPINES RAPINIS REPICKS REPINED REPINER REPINES RIPIENI RIPIENO RIPINTO ROPIEST RUPIAHS SAPIENS SAPIENT SEPIRAS STPIUSI STPIUSV STPIUSX TAPINGS TAPINTO TAPIOCA TEPIDLY TOPIARY TOPICAL TYPICAL TYPISTS UMPIRED UMPIRES UNPICKS UNPIETY UNPILED UNPILES UNPIOUS UNPIPED UPPILED UPPILES VAPIDLY WAPITIS

••P•I••

AMPHION AMPLIFY APPLIED

APPLIER APPLIES APPLING APPOINT APPRISE AUPAIRS BAPTISE BAPTISM BAPTIST BAPTIZE BOPPING CAPPING CAPRICE CAPRINE CAPSIZE CAPTION CAPTIVA CAPTIVE COPPICE COPPING COPYING COPYIST CUPLIKE CUPPIER CUPPING CUPRITE CYPRIAN CYPRIOT DAPPING DEPRIVE DIPPIER DIPPING EMPRISE EMPTIED EMPTIER EMPTIES EMPTILY ENPRISE ESPRITS ESPYING FOPPISH GAPKIDS GAPPING GIPSIES GUPPIES GYPPING GYPSIES HAPKIDO HAPPIER HAPPIFY HAPPILY HAPTICS HIPLIKE HIPPIER HIPPIES HIPPISH HIPPITY HOPKINS HOPLITE HOPPIER HOPPING HOPSING HYPOING IMPAIRS IMPLIED IMPLIES IMPRINT INPOINT

INPRINT KIPLING KIPPING LAPPING LAPPISH LAPSING LAPWING LIPLIKE LIPPIER LIPPING LOPPIER LOPPING MAPPING MOPPING NAPKINS NAPPIER NAPPIES NAPPING NAPTIME NIPPIER NIPPILY NIPPING NUPTIAL ONPOINT PAPPIES PAPRIKA PEPCIDS PEPPIER PEPPILL PEPPILY PEPPING PEPPINO PEPSICO PEPSINS PEPTICS PEPTIDE PIPPINS POPDIVA POPLINS POPPIES POPPING POPPINS POPWINE PUPPIES RAPPING REPAINT REPAIRS REPLICA REPLIED REPLIER REPLIES REPOINT REPPING REPRICE REPRIME REPRINT REPRISE REPTILE RIPPING RIPTIDE SAPLING SAPPIER SAPPILY SAPPING SEPHIAS SIPPING SOPHIES SOPHISM

SOPHIST
SOPPIER
SOPPING
SOPWITH
SUPPING
TAPPING
TIPLINE
TIPPIER
TIPPING
TIPSIER
TIPSILY
TOPBIDS
TOPFIVE
TOPKICK
TOPLINE
TOPPING
TOPSIDE
UNPLIED
YAPPING
YIPPIES
YIPPING
YUPPIES
YUPPIFY
ZAPPIER
ZAPPING
ZIPDISK
ZIPPIER
ZIPPING

••P••I•

APPETIT
ASPIRIN
CAPAPIE
CAPTAIN
DAPHNIA
DAPHNIS
DEPOSIT
DIPLOID
EMPIRIC
EMPIRIN
EMPORIA
EXPLAIN
EXPLOIT
EXPOSIT
HAPLOID
HEPARIN
HEPATIC
HOPTOIT
HYPATIA
HYPNOID
IMPAVID
IMPERIL
INPERIL
KEPTFIT
LIPARIS
LIPIDIC
NEPALIS
NEPHRIC
NEPOTIC
PIPEDIN
PIPESIN
POPQUIZ
RAPINIS
REPOSIT
ROPEDIN
ROPESIN
TOPSAIL
TOPSOIL
TOPSPIN
TOPTHIS
TYPEDIN
TYPESIN
TYPHOID
UNPLAIT
WAPITIS
XIPHOID
YOPLAIT

••P•••I

RAPANUI
RIPIENI
SOPRANI
STPIUSI
TOPKAPI
ZEPPOLI

•••PI••

ARMPITS
ASHPITS
AUSPICE
BAGPIPE
BBQPITS
BEEPING
BIOPICS
BOPPING
BUMPIER
BUMPILY
BUMPING
BURPING
CAMPIER
CAMPILY
CAMPING
CAMPION
CAPPING
CARPING
CASPIAN
CHOPINE
COMPILE
COMPING
COOPING
COPPICE
COPPING
COUPING
CRAPING
CREPING
CUPPIER
CUPPING
CUSPIDS
DAMPING
DAMPISH
DAPPING
DEEPISH
DESPINA
DESPISE
DESPITE
DIPPIER
DIPPING
DOGPILE
DRAPING
DROPINS
DUMPIER
DUMPILY
DUMPING
DUMPISH
ELAPIDS
ELOPING
ENDPINS
EYEPITS
FOPPISH
GAPPING
GARPIKE
GASPING
GASPIPE
GAWPING
GIMPING
GOOPIER
GRAPIER
GRIPING
GROPING
GROPIUS
GULPIER
GULPING
GUPPIES
GYPPING
HAPPIER
HAPPIFY
HAPPILY
HARPIES
HARPING
HARPIST
HASPING
HATPINS
HEAPING
HELPING
HEMPIER
HIPPIER
HIPPIES
HIPPISH
HIPPITY
HOOPING
HOPPIER
HOPPING
HOSPICE
HOTPINK
HUMPIER
ICEPICK
INAPILE
INSPIRE
INSPITE
JUMPIER
JUMPILY
JUMPING
KEEPING
KELPIES
KEWPIES
KIPPING
LAPPING
LAPPISH
LEAPING
LEMPIRA
LIMPING
LINPIAO
LIPPIER
LIPPING
LISPING
LOOPIER
LOOPING
LOPPIER
LOPPING
LUMPIER
LUMPILY
LUMPING
LUMPISH
MAGPIES
MAPPING
MOPPING
MUDPIES
MYOPIAS
NAPPIER
NAPPIES
NAPPING
NIPPIER
NIPPILY
NIPPING
NITPICK
NUTPINE
ONEPINT
OUTPICK
OUTPIPE
OUTPITY
PANPIPE
PAPPIES
PEEPING
PEIPING
PEPPIER
PEPPILL
PEPPILY
PEPPING
PEPPINO
PETPIGS
PIPPINS
POOPING
POPPIES
POPPING
POPPINS
POTPIES
PULPIER
PULPIFY
PULPING
PULPITS
PUMPING
PUPPIES
PVCPIPE
RAMPING
RAPPING
RASPIER
RASPING
RASPISH
REAPING
REDPINE
REPPING
RESPICE
RESPINS
RESPIRE
RESPITE
RIPPING
ROMPING
ROMPISH
RSVPING
SAPPIER
SAPPILY
SAPPING
SAWPITS
SCOPING
SEEPIER
SEEPING
SERPICO
SHAPING
SHAPIRO
SIPPING
SLOPING
SNIPING
SOAPIER
SOAPILY
SOAPING
SOPPIER
SOPPING
SOUPIER
STEPINS
STUPIDS
SUPPING
SUSPIRE
SWIPING
TAMPICO
TAMPING
TAPPING
TARPITS
TEMPING
TENPINS
THEPIPS
THEPITS
TIEPINS
TIPPIER
TIPPING
TIRPITZ
TOEPICK
TOPPING
TROPICS
TROPISM
UNSPICY
UNSPIED
UNSPILT
UPSPINS
UTOPIAN
UTOPIAS
UTOPISM
UTOPIST
VAMPIER
VAMPING
VAMPIRA
VAMPIRE
VAMPISH
VESPIDS
VULPINE
WARPING
WASPIER
WASPILY
WASPISH
WEEPIER
WEEPING
WIMPIER
WIMPING
WIMPISH
WISPIER
WISPILY
WISPING
YAPPING
YAWPING
YELPING
YIPPIES
YIPPING
YUPPIES
YUPPIFY
ZAPPIER
ZAPPING
ZIPPIER
ZIPPING

•••P•I•

ASEPSIS
ASEPTIC
BOOPSIE
BUMPKIN
CHAPLIN
CHAPPIE
CHIPSIN
COEPTIS
COMPLIN
CRAPPIE
CREPTIN
CRYPTIC
CULPRIT
DAUPHIN
DEEPSIX
DELPHIC
DESPAIR
DESPOIL
DOLPHIN
DROPSIN
DROPSIT
GLYPHIC
GLYPTIC
GRAPHIC
HELPSIN
INAPRIL
JUMPBID
JUMPSIN
KEEPFIT
KEEPSIN
LAMPLIT
LAMPOIL
LEAPSIN
LEAPTIN
LEIPZIG
LOWPAID
LOWPAIR
LUMPSIN
LUMPSIT
MEMPHIS
MORPHIC
MORPHIN
NONPAID
NYMPHIC
ONEPAIR
OUTPAID
POMPEIA
POMPEII
POOPSIE
PREPAID
PREPPIE
PUMPKIN
RALPHIE
RESPLIT
SCEPTIC
SEEPSIN
SKEPTIC
SLEPTIN
SLIPSIN
SOUPMIX
STEPSIN
STOPSIN
STOPSIT
STYPSIS
STYPTIC
SYLPHIC
TAXPAID
TOYPAIL
TWOPAIR
UNSPLIT
WHIPSIN

•••P••I

CAMPARI
CHAPATI
POMPEII
TIMPANI
TRIPOLI
TYMPANI
ZEPPOLI

••••PI•

AUTOPIA
BEARPIT
BLIMPIE
BUSHPIG
CAPAPIE
CESSPIT
CHAPPIE
CHEAPIE
CLAYPIT
COALPIT
COCKPIT
COOLPIX
CRAPPIE
CREEPIN
CRESPIN
CRISPIN
CRISPIX
DUCKPIN
FIREPIT
FIVEPIN
FLEAPIT
FOURPIN
GROUPIE
HAIRPIN
HEADPIN
INASPIN
INSIPID
KINGPIN
LIMEPIE
MALEPIG
MEATPIE
MINEPIT
MOONPIE
MOSHPIT
NINEPIN
NONEPIC
OLYMPIA
OLYMPIC
ONTOPIC
OPENPIT
OUTSPIN
OUTSPIT
PLUMPIE
PORKPIE
PREPPIE
PULLPIN
PUSHPIN
SALTPIT
SANDPIT
SCORPIO
SERAPIS
SHARPIE
SLEEPIN
STEEPIN
STOMPIN
STRAPIN
SWOOPIN
TAILPIN
TELEPIC
TELEPIX
THESPIS
TOPSPIN
TROMPIN
TROOPIN
WAREPIC
WHOOPIE
WILDPIG

••••P•I

ADELPHI
JOSEPHI
SHARPEI

•••••PI

PLATYPI
TOPKAPI

P•J••••

PAJAMAS
PDJAMES

P••J•••

PALJOEY
PERJURE
PERJURY
PROJECT
PROJETS
PUNJABI

P•••J••

PROPJET

P••••J•

PBANDJS

••PJ•••

TIPJARS

•••PJ••

PROPJET
TEMPJOB

P•K••••

PEKEPOO
POKEDAT
POKEFUN
POKEMON
POKEOUT
POKESAT
POKIEST

P••K•••

PACKAGE
PACKARD
PACKERS
PACKETS
PACKICE
PACKING
PACKOFF
PACKRAT
PACKSIN
PACKSON
PACKSUP
PARKADE
PARKAVE
PARKERS
PARKING
PARKINS
PARKMAN
PARKSIT
PARKWAY
PEAKIER
PEAKING
PEAKISH
PECKING
PECKISH
PECKSAT
PEEKERS
PEEKING
PEEKOUT
PEEKSAT
PEEKSIN
PERKIER
PERKILY
PERKING
PERKINS
PERKISH
PERKSUP
PESKIER
PESKILY
PICKAXE
PICKENS
PICKERS
PICKETS
PICKETT
PICKIER
PICKING
PICKLED
PICKLES
PICKOFF
PICKOUT
PICKSAT
PICKSON
PICKSUP
PICKUPS
PINKENS
PINKEST
PINKETT
PINKHAM
PINKIES
PINKING
PINKISH
PINKOES
PLAKATS
POCKETS
POLKAED
PORKERS
PORKIER
PORKING
PORKISH
PORKPIE
PROKEDS
PUCKERS
PUCKERY
PUCKETT
PUCKISH
PUNKERS
PUNKIER
PUNKIES

P•••K••

PASSKEY
PERUKES
PIGSKIN
PLACKET
PLANKED
PLINKED
PLONKED
PLUCKED
PLUNKED
PLUNKER
PONYKEG
PRICKED
PRICKLE
PRICKLY
PRICKUP
PRINKED
PRINKER
PUMPKIN
PUSHKIN

P••••K•

PALOOKA
PANCAKE
PANICKY
PAPRIKA
PARASKI
PARBAKE
PARTAKE
PEALIKE
PEGLIKE
PENLIKE
PIELIKE
PIGLIKE
PINOAKS
PODLIKE
PREBAKE
PREMAKE
PROVOKE
PULASKI

P•••••K

PADDOCK
PADLOCK
PARTOOK
PATRICK
PAYBACK
PEACOCK
PENNOCK
PEPTALK
PERCHIK
PERWEEK
PETCOCK
PETDUCK
PETROCK
PHILIPK
POLLACK
POLLOCK
POPROCK
POTHOOK
POTLUCK
PREBOOK
PRECOOK
PREDARK
PREDUSK
PREPACK
PREROCK
PRESOAK
PREWORK
PUTBACK

•PK••••

UPKEEPS

•P•K•••

SPIKERS
SPIKETV
SPIKEUP
SPIKIER
SPIKILY
SPIKING
SPOKANE
SPOKEOF
SPOKETO
SPOKEUP
SPOKING
SPYKIDS

•P••K••

APECKOF
SPACKLE
SPANKED
SPANKER
SPARKED
SPARKLE
SPARKLY
SPEAKER
SPEAKOF
SPEAKTO
SPEAKUP
SPECKED
SPECKLE
SPOOKED
UPTAKES

•P•••K•

APELIKE
OPTICKS
SPASSKY
UPLINKS
UPTALKS
UPTICKS

•P••••K

SPELUNK
SPUTNIK
UPQUARK

••PK•••

GAPKIDS
HAPKIDO
HOPKINS
NAPKINS
TOPKAPI
TOPKICK
TOPKNOT

••P•K••

TOPEKAN

••P••K•

CUPCAKE
CUPLIKE
HIPLIKE
KOPECKS
KOPIYKA
LIPLIKE
PAPRIKA
REPACKS
REPARKS
REPERKS
REPICKS
RVPARKS
UNPACKS
UNPICKS

••P•••K

NIPMUCK
PEPTALK
POPROCK
TOPKICK
TOPRANK
ZIPDISK
ZIPLOCK

•••PK••

BUMPKIN
PUMPKIN
SHOPKOS

•••P•K•

BESPOKE
COWPOKE
DEEPSKY
GARPIKE
INAPOKE
RESPOKE
UNSPOKE

•••P••K

AIRPACK
AIRPARK
BBQPORK
BESPEAK
CARPARK
DAYPACK
DRSPOCK
HENPECK
HOTPACK
HOTPINK
ICEPACK
ICEPICK
JAMPACK
JETPACK
MRSPOCK
MUDPACK
NITPICK
NONPEAK
OAKPARK
OFFPEAK
OUTPICK
PREPACK
RATPACK
RESPARK
RESPEAK
SIXPACK
TOEPICK
UNSPEAK

••••P•K

BTFSPLK
CHARPAK
SERIPAK
ZATOPEK

•••••PK

PHILIPK

PL•••••

PLACARD
PLACATE
PLACEBO
PLACERS
PLACIDO
PLACING
PLACKET
PLAGUED
PLAGUES
PLAICES
PLAINER
PLAINES
PLAINLY
PLAINTS
PLAISIR
PLAITED
PLAITER
PLAKATS
PLANATE
PLANERS
PLANETS
PLANFOR
PLANING
PLANISH
PLANKED
PLANNED
PLANNER
PLANOUT
PLANSON
PLANSTO
PLANTAR
PLANTED
PLANTER
PLAQUES
PLASHED
PLASHES
PLASMAS
PLASMIC
PLASTER
PLASTIC
PLATEAU
PLATENS
PLATERS
PLATIER
PLATIES
PLATING
PLATOON
PLATTED
PLATTER
PLATYPI
PLAUDIT
PLAUTUS
PLAYACT
PLAYBOY
PLAYDOH
PLAYERS
PLAYFUL
PLAYING
PLAYLET
PLAYOFF
PLAYOUT
PLAYPEN
PLAYSAT
PLAYSBY

PLAYSON
PLAYSTO
PLAYSUP
PLAYTEX
PLEADED
PLEADER
PLEADTO
PLEASED
PLEASER
PLEASES
PLEATED
PLEBIAN
PLECTRA
PLEDGED
PLEDGEE
PLEDGER
PLEDGES
PLENARY
PLENISH
PLENUMS
PLEURAE
PLEURAL
PLEXORS
PLIABLE
PLIABLY
PLIANCY
PLICATE
PLIGHTS
PLINKED
PLINTHS
PLISSES
PLODDED
PLODDER
PLOESTI
PLONKED
PLOPPED
PLOSION
PLOSIVE
PLOTFUL
PLOTTED
PLOTTER
PLOTZED
PLOTZES
PLOUGHS
PLOVDIV
PLOVERS
PLOWBOY
PLOWERS
PLOWING
PLOWMAN
PLOWMEN
PLOWSON
PLOWSUP
PLUCKED
PLUGGED
PLUGGER
PLUGINS
PLUGOLA
PLUGSIN
PLUGSUP
PLUMAGE
PLUMBED
PLUMBER
PLUMBIC
PLUMBUM
PLUMCOT
PLUMIER
PLUMING
PLUMMER
PLUMMET
PLUMOSE
PLUMPED
PLUMPER
PLUMPIE
PLUMPLY
PLUMULE
PLUNDER
PLUNGED
PLUNGER
PLUNGES
PLUNKED
PLUNKER
PLURALS
PLUSHER
PLUSHES
PLUSHLY
PLUSONE
PLUSSES
PLUSTAX
PLUSTWO
PLUTONS
PLUVIAL
PLYWOOD

P•L••••

PALABRA
PALACES
PALADIN
PALAMAS
PALANCE
PALATAL
PALATES
PALAVER
PALAZZI
PALAZZO
PALEALE
PALEDRY
PALEMON
PALERMO
PALETTE
PALFREY
PALINGS
PALJOEY
PALLETS
PALLIER
PALLING
PALLORS
PALMARY
PALMATE
PALMERS
PALMFUL
PALMIER
PALMING
PALMIST
PALMOFF
PALMOIL
PALMTOP
PALMYRA
PALOMAR
PALOMAS
PALOOKA
PALPATE
PALTERS
PALTROW
PALUDAL
PELAGES
PELAGIC
PELICAN
PELISSE
PELLEAS
PELLETS
PELOTAS
PELOTON
PELTATE
PELTERS
PELTING
PELTISH
PHLEGMY
PHLOEMS
PHLOXES
PILATES
PILATUS
PILCROW
PILEATE
PILEDIN
PILEDON
PILEDUP
PILEGGI
PILEOUS
PILESIN
PILESOF
PILESON
PILESUP
PILEUPS
PILFERS
PILGRIM
PILINGS
PILLAGE
PILLARS
PILLBOX
PILLBUG
PILLING
PILLION
PILLORY
PILLOWS
PILLOWY
PILOTED
PILSNER
POLANER
POLANYI
POLARAS
POLARIS
POLEAXE
POLECAR
POLECAT
POLEMAN
POLEMEN
POLEMIC
POLENTA
POLESAT
POLESIT
POLICED
POLICER
POLICES
POLISCI
POLITER
POLITIC
POLKAED
POLLACK
POLLARD
POLLEES
POLLENS
POLLERA
POLLERS
POLLING
POLLOCK
POLLTAX
POLLUTE
POLOIST
POLONIA
POLTAVA
POLYGON
POLYMER
POLYPED
POLYPOD
POLYSCI
PULASKI
PULLERS
PULLETS
PULLEYS
PULLFOR
PULLING
PULLINS
PULLMAN
PULLOFF
PULLONS
PULLOUT
PULLPIN
PULLSIN
PULLSON
PULLSUP
PULLTAB
PULLTOY
PULLUPS
PULMONI
PULMONO
PULPERS
PULPIER
PULPIFY
PULPING
PULPITS
PULSARS
PULSATE
PULSING

P••L•••

PABLUMS
PADLOCK
PAELLAS
PAHLAVI
PAILFUL
PALLETS
PALLIER
PALLING
PALLORS
PAMLICO
PARLAYS
PARLEYS
PARLORS
PARLOUR
PARLOUS
PAULIII
PAULINA
PAULINE
PAULING
PAULIST
PAULPRY
PAULSEN
PAVLOVA
PAYLESS
PAYLOAD
PCCLONE
PEALIKE
PEALING
PEELERS
PEELING
PEELOFF
PEELOUT
PEGLEGS
PEGLESS
PEGLIKE
PELLEAS
PELLETS
PENLIKE
PENLITE
PEPLUMS
PERLITE
PERLMAN
PETLAMB
PETLION
PHALANX
PHILBIN
PHILCOS
PHILEAS
PHILIPK
PHILIPS
PHILIPV
PHILLIE
PHILLIP
PHILOUS
PHILTER
PHILTRE
PHYLLIS
PHYLLOS
PIELIKE
PIGLETS
PIGLIKE
PILLAGE
PILLARS
PILLBOX
PILLBUG
PILLING
PILLION
PILLORY
PILLOWS
PILLOWY
PIMLICO
PINLESS
PIOLETS
PIPLESS
POBLANO
PODLIKE
POLLACK
POLLARD
POLLEES
POLLENS
POLLERA
POLLERS
POLLING
POLLOCK
POLLTAX
POLLUTE
POOLCUE
POOLERS
POOLING
POOLMAN
POOLMEN
POPLARS
POPLINS
POTLIDS
POTLUCK
POULENC
POULTRY
PRALINE
PRELACY
PRELATE
PRELIFE
PRELIMS
PRELOAD
PRELOAN
PRELOSS
PRELUDE
PROLATE
PROLIFE
PROLOGS
PROLONG
PSALMIC
PSALTER
PTOLEMY
PUBLICS
PUBLISH
PUBLIUS
PULLERS
PULLETS
PULLEYS
PULLFOR
PULLING
PULLINS
PULLMAN
PULLOFF
PULLONS
PULLOUT
PULLPIN
PULLSIN
PULLSON
PULLSUP
PULLTAB
PULLTOY
PULLUPS
PUNLESS
PURLIEU
PURLING
PURLOIN

P•••L••

PABULUM
PACELAP
PADDLED
PADDLER
PADDLES
PAELLAS
PAISLEY
PANELED
PANTLEG
PAPELES
PAPILLA
PAROLED
PAROLEE
PAROLES
PARSLEY
PASALLE
PATELLA
PAYOLAS
PAYSLIP
PEARLED
PEARLER
PEBBLED
PEBBLES
PEDALED
PEDALER
PEDDLED
PEDDLER
PEDDLES
PEEBLES
PEEPLES
PENALTY
PENULTS
PEOPLED
PEOPLES
PERILED
PERPLEX
PESTLED
PESTLES
PETALED
PETALES
PETULIA
PHARLAP
PHILLIE
PHILLIP
PHYLLIS
PHYLLOS
PICKLED
PICKLES
PIDDLED
PIDDLES
PIFFLED
PIFFLES
PIMPLED
PIMPLES
PIRELLI
PITILLO
PLAYLET
POMELOS
POODLES
POORLAW
POPELEO
POPPLED
POPPLES
POPULAR
POSOLES
POSSLQS
POZOLES
PREALLY
PREPLAN
PREPLOT
PRESLEY
PROBLEM
PROCLUS
PROWLED
PROWLER
PUDDLED
PUDDLES
PUEBLOS
PUGGLES
PUGSLEY
PURFLED
PURFLER
PURFLES
PURPLED
PURPLES
PUZZLED
PUZZLER
PUZZLES

P••••L•

PACBELL
PALEALE
PANFULS
PANICLE
PANOPLY
PANTILE
PAPILLA
PARABLE
PARCELS
PASALLE
PASCOLI
PASSELS
PASTELS
PATELLA
PATROLS
PAVIDLY
PAYABLE
PAYROLL
PAYWELL
PCWORLD
PENCILS
PENPALS
PENTELS
PEPPILL
PEPPILY
PEPTALK
PERCALE
PERGOLA
PERKILY
PESKILY
PETCALF
PETIOLE
PETMULE
PETRELS
PETROLS
PETTILY
PHENOLS
PHONILY
PIANOLA
PICCOLO
PIEBALD
PIEHOLE
PIESALE
PINBALL
PINFOLD
PINHOLE
PINWALE
PIOUSLY
PIRELLI
PISTILS
PISTOLE
PISTOLS
PITBULL
PITFALL
PITHILY
PITILLO
PLAINLY
PLIABLE
PLIABLY
PLUGOLA
PLUMPLY
PLUMULE
PLURALS
PLUSHLY
POMMELS
PORTALS
POSABLE
POTABLE
POTFULS
POTHOLE
PRATTLE
PREALLY
PREBILL
PREFILE
PRESALE
PRESALT
PRESELL
PRESOLD
PRETELL
PRETOLD
PRICILY
PRICKLE
PRICKLY
PRIMELY
PRINGLE
PRIVILY
PROBALL
PROFILE
PRONELY
PROPELS
PROSILY
PROUDLY
PUDGILY
PUERILE
PUFFILY
PUMMELS
PUNNILY
PURCELL
PUSHILY

P•••••L

PACBELL
PAILFUL
PAINFUL
PALATAL
PALMFUL
PALMOIL
PALUDAL
PARASOL
PARBOIL
PARTIAL
PASCHAL
PASSEUL
PAYROLL
PAYWELL
PEAFOWL
PEPPILL
PERORAL
PERUSAL
PHRASAL
PIGTAIL
PINBALL
PINCURL
PINEOIL
PINESOL
PINSEAL
PINTAIL
PIPEFUL
PITBULL
PITFALL
PITIFUL
PIVOTAL
PLAYFUL
PLEURAL
PLOTFUL
PLUVIAL
POTBOIL
POUTFUL
PREBILL
PREBOIL
PRECOIL
PRECOOL
PREHEAL
PREORAL
PREQUEL
PRESEAL
PRESELL
PRESSEL
PRETELL
PRETZEL
PREVAIL
PROBALL
PROBOWL
PURCELL
PUSHFUL

•PL••••

APLENTY
APLITES
APLUSES
BPLUSES
CPLUSES
DPLUSES
IPLEDGE
SPLASHY
SPLAYED
SPLEENS
SPLEENY
SPLENDA
SPLICED
SPLICER
SPLICES
SPLINES
SPLINTS
SPLITUP
SPLOTCH
SPLURGE
UPLANDS
UPLEAPS
UPLEAPT
UPLIFTS
UPLIGHT
UPLINKS
UPLOADS

•P•L•••

APELETS
APELIKE
APILEOF
APOLLOS
APOLOGY
APPLAUD
APPLETS
APPLIED
APPLIER
APPLIES
APPLING
APPLYTO
APULIAN
EPILADY
EPILATE
EPILOGS
OPALINE
OPALISH
OPULENT
SPELLED
SPELLER
SPELUNK
SPILLED
SPILLER
UPCLIMB
UPCLOSE
UPFLING
UPFLOWS
UPSLOPE

•P••L••

APHELIA
APHILIP
APOLLOS
APPALLS
EPAULET
EPSILON
OPHELIA
SPELLED
SPELLER
SPIELED
SPIELER
SPILLED
SPILLER
SPOILED
SPOILER
SPOOLED
SPOOLER
SPOTLIT
UPFOLDS
UPHILLS
UPHOLDS
UPPILED
UPPILES
UPSILON
UPTALKS
UPTILTS
UPVALUE
UPWELLS

•P•••L•

APISHLY
APOSTLE
APPALLS
APPEALS
EPISTLE
EPPERLY
SPACELY
SPACKLE
SPANGLE
SPANGLY
SPARELY
SPARKLE
SPARKLY
SPATULA
SPECKLE
SPICILY
SPIKILY
SPINDLE
SPINDLY
SPINELS
SPIRALS
SPITTLE
SPRAWLS
SPRAWLY
SPYHOLE
UPBUILD
UPCOILS
UPCURLS
UPEARLY
UPFIELD
UPHILLS
UPPSALA
UPSCALE
UPSWELL
UPWELLS

•P••••L

APOGEAL
APPAREL
APTERAL
EPOCHAL
OPTICAL
OPTIMAL
SPACIAL
SPANIEL
SPATIAL
SPECIAL
SPHERAL
SPIEGEL
SPOUSAL
UPSWELL
UPWHIRL

••PL•••

AMPLEST
AMPLIFY
APPLAUD
APPLETS
APPLIED
APPLIER
APPLIES
APPLING
APPLYTO
BIPLANE
BYPLAYS
CAPLESS
CAPLETS
COPLAND
CUPLIKE
DEPLANE
DEPLETE
DEPLORE
DEPLOYS
DIPLOID
DIPLOMA
EMPLACE
EMPLANE
EMPLOYS
ENPLANE
EXPLAIN
EXPLODE
EXPLOIT
EXPLORE
GAPLESS
HAPLESS
HAPLOID
HIPLESS
HIPLIKE
HOPLITE
IMPLANT
IMPLEAD
IMPLIED
IMPLIES
IMPLODE
IMPLORE
INPLACE
KIPLING
LAPLACA
LAPLACE
LAPLAND
LAPLATA
LIPLESS
LIPLIKE
NAPLESS
NOPLACE
PEPLUMS
PIPLESS
POPLARS
POPLINS
REPLACE
REPLANE
REPLANS
REPLANT
REPLATE
REPLAYS
REPLEAD
REPLETE
REPLICA
REPLIED
REPLIER
REPLIES
REPLOTS
REPLOWS
REPLUMB
REPLUME
REPLYTO
SAPLESS
SAPLING
TIPLESS
TIPLINE
TOPLESS
TOPLINE
UNPLAIT
UNPLANS
UNPLIED
UNPLUGS
UNPLUMB
YOPLAIT
ZIPLOCK
ZIPLOCS

••P•L••

AMPULES
APPALLS
BIPOLAR
CAPELET
CAPELLA
CAPULET
COPILOT
COPULAE
COPULAR
COPULAS
CUPELED
CUPELER
CUPOLAS
CUPULAR
CUPULES
DAPPLED
DAPPLES
DEPALMA
DEPULPS
DIPOLAR

DIPOLES
DOPPLER
EMPALED
EMPALES
FIPPLES
IMPALAS
IMPALED
IMPALER
IMPALES
IMPULSE
LAPALMA
LAPELED
MTPELEE
NAPALMS
NEPALIS
NIPPLES
NOPALES
PAPELES
PAPILLA
POPELEO
POPPLED
POPPLES
POPULAR
RAPALLO
REPOLLS
REPULSE
RIPPLED
RIPPLES
RIPPLET
SEPALED
SUPPLED
SUPPLER
SUPPLES
TIPPLED
TIPPLER
TIPPLES
TOPPLED
TOPPLES
TUPELOS
TUPOLEV
UNPALED
UNPILED
UNPILES
UNPOLED
UPPILED
UPPILES

••P••L•

AMPOULE
APPALLS
APPEALS
ASPHALT
CAPABLE
CAPABLY
CAPELLA
CAPFULS
CAPSULE
CEPHALO
CEPHALY
COPPOLA
CUPFULS
DEPAULU
EMPTILY
EPPERLY
ESPIALS
HAPPILY
JOPPOLO
LAPBELT
LAPFULS
LIPBALM
NIPPILY
OMPHALO
PAPILLA
PEPPILL
PEPPILY
PEPTALK
RAPALLO
RAPIDLY
RAPPELS
REPEALS
REPOLLS
REPTILE
SAPPILY
STPAULS
TEPIDLY
TIPSILY
TOPHOLE
UNPEELS
UPPSALA
VAPIDLY
ZEPPOLE
ZEPPOLI

••P•••L

APPAREL
ASPRAWL
BIPEDAL
CAPITAL
CAPITOL
DEPOSAL
EMPANEL
ESPANOL
HOPEFUL
IMPANEL
IMPERIL
INPERIL
KAPITAL
NUPTIAL
PEPPILL
PIPEFUL
RAPHAEL
REPANEL
TOPICAL
TOPSAIL
TOPSOIL
TYPICAL

•••PL••

AIRPLAY
CHAPLET
CHAPLIN
COMPLEX
COMPLIN
COUPLED
COUPLER
COUPLES
COUPLET
DAPPLED
DAPPLES
DIMPLED
DIMPLES
DISPLAY
DOPPLER
DROPLET
EARPLUG
ENDPLAY
FIPPLES
FUNPLEX
GUNPLAY
HITPLAY
HOOPLAS
KERPLOP
LAMPLIT
MISPLAN
MISPLAY
NIPPLES
NONPLAY
NONPLUS
NTUPLES
OUTPLAN
OUTPLAY
OUTPLOD
OUTPLOT
PEEPLES
PEOPLED
PEOPLES
PERPLEX
PIMPLED
PIMPLES
POPPLED
POPPLES
PREPLAN
PREPLOT
PURPLED
PURPLES
RESPLIT
RIMPLED
RIMPLES
RIPPLED
RIPPLES
RIPPLET
RUMPLED
RUMPLES
SAMPLED
SAMPLER
SAMPLES
SETPLAY
SIMPLER
SIMPLES
SIMPLEX
STAPLED
STAPLER
STAPLES
SUBPLOT
SUPPLED
SUPPLER
SUPPLES
SURPLUS
TEMPLAR
TEMPLED
TEMPLES
TIPPLED
TIPPLER
TIPPLES
TOPPLED
TOPPLES
TRIPLEA
TRIPLED
TRIPLES
TRIPLET
TRIPLEX
UNIPLEX
UNSPLIT
WIMPLED
WIMPLES

•••P•L•

ADEPTLY
AMAPOLA
BUMPILY
CALPOLY
CAMPILY
CARPALS
CARPELS
CHAPALA
CHAPELS
COMPELS
COMPILE
COPPOLA
CRAPOLA
CRIPPLE
DISPELS
DOGPILE
DUMPILY
DUOPOLY
FANPALM
GALPALS
GOSPELS
GRAPPLE
HADPULL
HAPPILY
HASPULL
INAPILE
INAPTLY
INEPTLY
JOPPOLO
JUMPILY
KAMPALA
KEYPALS
LEGPULL
LEOPOLD
LUMPILY
MAYPOLE
NIPPILY
OILPALM
OLDPALS
OUTPOLL
OUTPULL
PENPALS
PEPPILL
PEPPILY
PROPELS
RAPPELS
REAPPLY
REDPOLL
RESPELL
RESPELT
RUMPOLE
SAPPILY
SCAPULA
SHAPELY
SKIPOLE
SNAPPLE
SOAPILY
STIPPLE
STOPPLE
TADPOLE
TIEPOLO
TRIPOLI
UNAPTLY
UNSPELT
UNSPILT
VANPELT
WALPOLE
WASPILY
WHIPPLE
WIMPOLE
WISPILY
ZEPPOLE
ZEPPOLI

•••P••L

CARPOOL
DESPOIL
GRAPNEL
HADPULL
HASPULL
HELPFUL
INAPRIL
LAMPOIL
LEGPULL
LESPAUL
MRSPAUL
MRSPEEL
NAIPAUL
NYMPHAL
OUTPOLL
OUTPULL
OUTPURL
PEPPILL
REDPOLL
RESPELL
RESPOOL
SHIPFUL
SHOPFUL
TAMPAFL
TOYPAIL
UNSPOOL
VANPOOL

••••PL•

ACOUPLE
BIASPLY
BTFSPLK
CHEAPLY
CRIPPLE
CRISPLY
CRUMPLE
CRUMPLY
DECUPLE
EJEMPLO
EXAMPLE
EXEMPLA
GRAPPLE
MANIPLE
NONUPLE
OCTUPLE
OCTUPLY
OVERPLY
PANOPLY
PLUMPLY
REAPPLY
REIMPLY
SCRUPLE
SHARPLY
SNAPPLE
STEEPLE
STEEPLY
STIPPLE
STOPPLE
TRAMPLE
WHIPPLE

••••P•L

ECTYPAL
OEDIPAL
REEXPEL
SCALPEL
STEMPEL
VONOPEL

P•M••••

PAMLICO
PAMPERS
PIMENTO
PIMESON
PIMLICO
PIMPLED
PIMPLES
POMADED
POMADES
POMELOS
POMMARD
POMMELS
POMPANO
POMPEIA
POMPEII
POMPOMS
POMPONS
POMPOUS
PUMICED
PUMICES
PUMMELS
PUMPERS
PUMPING
PUMPKIN
PUMPOUT
PUMPSUP

P••M•••

PALMARY
PALMATE
PALMERS
PALMFUL
PALMIER
PALMING
PALMIST
PALMOFF
PALMOIL
PALMTOP
PALMYRA
PAYMENT
PAYMORE
PERMIAN
PERMING
PERMITS
PERMUTE
PETMICE
PETMULE
PHEMIUS
PIGMEAT
PIGMENT
PISMIRE
PLUMAGE
PLUMBED
PLUMBER
PLUMBIC
PLUMBUM
PLUMCOT
PLUMIER
PLUMING
PLUMMER
PLUMMET
PLUMOSE
PLUMPED
PLUMPER
PLUMPIE
PLUMPLY
PLUMULE
POMMARD
POMMELS
PREMADE
PREMAKE
PREMATE
PREMEDS
PREMEET
PREMIER
PREMIES
PREMISE
PREMISS
PREMIUM
PRIMACY
PRIMARY
PRIMATE
PRIMELY
PRIMERA
PRIMERO
PRIMERS
PRIMING
PRIMMED
PRIMMER
PRIMPED
PROMBID
PROMISE
PROMOED
PROMOTE
PROMPTS
PULMONI
PULMONO
PUMMELS
PYGMIES

P•••M••

PAJAMAS
PALAMAS
PALEMON
PALOMAR
PALOMAS
PANAMAS
PARAMUS
PARKMAN
PDJAMES
PERLMAN
PETEMAN
PETEMEN
PITTMAN
PLASMAS
PLASMIC
PLOWMAN
PLOWMEN
PLUMMER
PLUMMET
PNEUMAS
PNEUMAT
PNEUMON
POKEMON
POLEMAN
POLEMEN
POLEMIC
POLYMER
POOLMAN
POOLMEN
POORMAN
POORMEN
PORTMAN
POSTMAN
POSTMEN
POTAMUS
POTOMAC
PREAMPS
PREEMIE
PREEMPT
PREOMIT
PRIMMED
PRIMMER
PROPMAN
PROPMEN
PSALMIC
PULLMAN
PUTEMUP
PYRAMID
PYRAMUS

P••••M•

PABLUMS
PALERMO
PARFUMS
PASTIME
PENNAME
PEPLUMS
PERFUME
PERFUMY
PETCOMB
PETLAMB
PETNAME
PHENOMS
PHLEGMY
PHLOEMS
PHONEME
PINCHME
PLENUMS
PODIUMS
POMPOMS
POSSUMS
PREARMS
PREGAME
PRELIMS
PRENAME
PRESUME
PRFIRMS
PROXIMA
PROXIMO
PTOLEMY
PUBGAME

P•••••M

PABULUM
PANGRAM
PARONYM
PENTIUM
PERDIEM
PERFORM
PHANTOM
PIANISM
PILGRIM
PINETUM
PINKHAM
PLUMBUM
POPEDOM
POTSDAM
PREBOOM
PREDOOM
PREFORM
PREMIUM
PRETERM
PRETRIM
PREWARM
PROBLEM
PROFARM
PROGRAM
PROTEAM

•P•M•••

SPAMBOT
SPAMMED
SPAMMER
SPUMIER
SPUMING
SPUMONE
SPUMONI

•P••M••

OPTIMAL
OPTIMAS
OPTIMUM
SPAMMED
SPAMMER
UPTEMPO
UPTIMES

•P•••M•

EPITOME
EPONYMS
EPONYMY
IPANEMA
SPAREME
SPYCAMS
UPCLIMB

•P••••M

APOTHEM
CPAEXAM
EPHRAIM
EPIDERM
EPIGRAM
OPOSSUM
OPTIMUM

••PM•••

LIPMANN
NIPMUCK
TOPMAST
TOPMOST

••P•M••

CAPEMAY
COPYMAN
COPYMEN
KEPTMUM
REPOMAN
REPUMPS
TAPEMAN
TAPEMEN

••P••M•

DEPALMA
DIPLOMA
GYPSUMS
LAPALMA
LAPERMS
NAPALMS
NAPTIME
PEPLUMS
REPLUMB
REPLUME
REPRIME
SUPREME
TOPNAME
UNPLUMB

••P•••M

BAPTISM
HYPONYM
KEPTMUM
LIPBALM
ORPHEUM
POPEDOM
SOPHISM
TAPROOM
TOPFORM
TOPONYM

•••PM••

CHAPMAN
CHAPMEN
DAMPMOP
HOOPMAN
HOOPMEN
KEEPMUM
PROPMAN
PROPMEN
SHIPMAN
SHIPMEN
SOUPMIX
STEPMOM

•••P•M•

AIRPUMP
GASPUMP
POMPOMS
THEPUMP
WAMPUMS

•••P••M

FANPALM
INAPOEM
KEEPMUM
LUMPSUM
OILPALM
STEPMOM
SYMPTOM
TROPISM
UTOPISM

•••••PM

EIGHTPM
SEVENPM
THREEPM

PN•••••

PNEUMAS
PNEUMAT
PNEUMON

P•N••••

PANACEA
PANACHE
PANADAS
PANAMAS
PANARAB
PANCAKE
PANCHAX
PANDERS
PANDITS
PANDORA
PANELED
PANETTA
PANFISH
PANFULS
PANGAEA
PANGRAM
PANICKY
PANICLE
PANIERS
PANINIS
PANNERS
PANNIER
PANNING
PANOPLY
PANPIPE
PANSIES
PANSOUT
PANTENE
PANTERA
PANTERS
PANTHER
PANTIES
PANTILE
PANTING
PANTLEG
PANTONE
PANURGE
PANZERS
PENALTY
PENANCE
PENATES
PENCASE
PENCILS
PENDANT
PENDENT
PENDING
PENGUIN
PENLIKE
PENLITE
PENNAME
PENNANT
PENNATE
PENNERS
PENNEYS
PENNIES
PENNINE
PENNING
PENNOCK
PENNONS
PENPALS
PENROSE
PENSEES
PENSION
PENSIVE
PENTADS
PENTANE
PENTELS
PENTIUM
PENUCHE
PENULTS
PENZIAS
PINATAS
PINBALL
PINBOYS
PINCERS
PINCHAS
PINCHED
PINCHER
PINCHES
PINCHME
PINCHOT
PINCURL
PINDOWN
PINEFOR
PINENUT
PINEOIL
PINESAP
PINESOL
PINETAR
PINETOP
PINETUM
PINFOLD
PINGERS
PINGING
PINGUID
PINHEAD
PINHOLE
PINIEST
PINIONS
PINKENS
PINKEST
PINKETT
PINKHAM
PINKIES
PINKING
PINKISH
PINKOES
PINLESS
PINNACE
PINNATE
PINNERS
PINNING
PINOAKS
PINONES
PINOTTA
PINSEAL
PINTAIL
PINWALE
PONCHOS
PONDERS
PONDING
PONGEES
PONGIDS
PONIARD
PONTANO
PONTIAC
PONTIAN
PONTIFF
PONTIUS
PONTOON
PONYING
PONYKEG
PUNCHED
PUNCHER
PUNCHES
PUNCHIN
PUNCHUP
PUNDITS
PUNGENT
PUNIEST
PUNJABI
PUNKERS
PUNKIER
PUNKIES
PUNLESS
PUNNERS
PUNNIER
PUNNILY
PUNNING
PUNSTER
PUNTERS
PUNTING
PYNCHON

P••N•••

PAANGAS
PAINFUL
PAINING
PAINTED
PAINTER
PANNERS
PANNIER
PANNING
PATNESS
PAUNCHY
PAWNEES
PAWNERS
PAWNING
PAWNOFF
PBANDJS
PEANUTS
PEENING
PENNAME
PENNANT
PENNATE
PENNERS
PENNEYS
PENNIES
PENNINE
PENNING
PENNOCK
PENNONS
PEONAGE
PEONIES
PETNAME
PETNAPS
PFENNIG
PHANTOM
PHENOLS
PHENOMS
PHINEAS
PHONEIN
PHONEME
PHONENO
PHONERS
PHONEYS
PHONICS
PHONIER

PHONIES	PRONELY	**P••••N•**	PENTANE	POOPING	PURLING	PLEBIAN	**•P•N•••**	SPANNED	UPTOWNS	RAPINIS	NAPPING	ASPIRIN
PHONILY	PRONETO	PACKING	PEPBAND	POPGUNS	PURRING	PLOSION	APTNESS	SPANNER	UPTREND	REPANEL	NEPTUNE	CAPEANN
PHONING	PRONGED	PADDING	PEPPING	POPLINS	PURSING	PLOWMAN	EPONINE	SPAWNED	UPTURNS	REPENTS	NIPPING	CAPITAN
PHONYUP	PRONOUN	PADRONE	PEPPINO	POPPING	PUSHING	PLOWMEN	EPONYMS	SPAWNER		REPINED	ONPOINT	CAPSTAN
PIANISM	PRUNERS	PADUANS	PEPSINS	POPPINS	PUTTING	PLOWSON	EPONYMY	SPINNER	**•P••••N**	REPINER	OPPUGNS	CAPTAIN
PIANIST	PRUNING	PAGEANT	PEPTONE	POPSONG	PYTHONS	PLUGSIN	IPANEMA	SPINNEY	APERSON	REPINES	ORPHANS	CAPTION
PIANOLA	PSANDQS	PAGEONE	PERCENT	POPTUNE		PNEUMON	OPENAIR	SPLENDA	APOGEAN	RIPENED	ORPHANT	COPYMAN
PICNICS	PUGNOSE	PAINING	PERKING	POPWINE	**P•••••N**	POISSON	OPENBAR	SPLINES	APULIAN	RIPENER	PAPUANS	COPYMEN
PIGNUTS	PUNNERS	PAIRING	PERKINS	PORCINE	PACKSIN	POKEFUN	OPENEND	SPLINTS	EPSILON	RIPINTO	PEPBAND	CYPRIAN
PINNACE	PUNNIER	PAISANO	PERMING	PORKING	PACKSON	POKEMON	OPENERS	SPOONED	EPSTEIN	TAPINGS	PEPPING	EMPIRIN
PINNATE	PUNNILY	PAISANS	PERRINE	PORSENA	PACQUIN	POLEMAN	OPENING	SPOONER	OPINION	TAPINTO	PEPPINO	EXPLAIN
PINNERS	PUNNING	PALLING	PERRINS	PORTEND	PALADIN	POLEMEN	OPENNET	SPRINGS	OPTEDIN	TOPKNOT	PEPSINS	HEPARIN
PINNING		PALMING	PERSONA	PORTENT	PALEMON	POLYGON	OPENOUT	SPRINGY	SPARTAN	TOPONYM	PEPTONE	HEPBURN
PIONEER	**P•••N••**	PANNING	PERSONS	PORTING	PARAGON	PONTIAN	OPENPIT	SPRINTS	SPENDON		PIPPINS	HYPERON
PLANATE	PAGINGS	PANTENE	PETPONY	POSTING	PARKMAN	PONTOON	OPENSEA	SPURNED	SPENTON	**••P••N•**	POPGUNS	LAPUTAN
PLANERS	PALANCE	PANTING	PETTING	POTEENS	PARTYON	POOLMAN	OPENSUP	SPURNER	SPIEDON	APPLING	POPLINS	LIPMANN
PLANETS	PALINGS	PANTONE	PHALANX	POTIONS	PASSION	POOLMEN	OPENTAP	SPUTNIK	SPIESON	APPOINT	POPPING	NIPIGON
PLANFOR	PANINIS	PAPUANS	PHARYNX	POTTING	PASTEIN	POORMAN	OPENTOE	SPYINGS	SPITSON	BIPLANE	POPPINS	ORPHEAN
PLANING	PARDNER	PARDONS	PHASING	POULENC	PASTERN	POORMEN	OPENTOP	UPLANDS	SPORRAN	BOPPING	POPSONG	PIPEDIN
PLANISH	PARENTS	PARGING	PHONENO	POURING	PATCHEN	POPCORN	OPINERS	UPLINKS	SPORTIN	BYPHONE	POPTUNE	PIPESIN
PLANKED	PARINGS	PARKING	PHONING	POUTING	PATDOWN	PORTION	OPINING	UPSENDS	SPRAYON	CAPEANN	POPWINE	POPCORN
PLANNED	PARONYM	PARKINS	PHOTONS	PRALINE	PATROON	PORTMAN	OPINION	UPTONOW	SPURSON	CAPGUNS	PUPTENT	RAPIDAN
PLANNER	PARSNIP	PARRING	PICKENS	PRATING	PATTERN	POSTERN	OPUNTIA	UPWINDS	SPYUPON	CAPPING	RAPPING	REPOMAN
PLANOUT	PARTNER	PARSING	PICKING	PRAYING	PAULSEN	POSTMAN	SPANAIR		UPANDIN	CAPRINE	RAPSONG	RIPOPEN
PLANSON	PATENCY	PARSONS	PIDGINS	PREBIND	PEABEAN	POSTMEN	SPANDEX	**•P•••N•**	UPGROWN	CAPUANA	RAPTUNE	RIPSAWN
PLANSTO	PATENTS	PARTING	PIECING	PREDENY	PEARSON	POURSIN	SPANGLE	APPLING	UPRISEN	COPLAND	REPAINT	RIPTORN
PLANTAR	PATINAS	PARTONE	PIEPANS	PREFUND	PEEKSIN	POUSSIN	SPANGLY	APPOINT	UPSILON	COPPING	REPHONE	ROPEDIN
PLANTED	PAVANES	PARVENU	PIETINS	PRERENT	PEERSIN	PREBORN	SPANIEL	EPERGNE		COPYING	REPLANE	ROPESIN
PLANTER	PAVINGS	PASSANT	PIGEONS	PRESENT	PELICAN	PREBURN	SPANISH	EPICENE	**••PN•••**	CUPPING	REPLANS	TAPEDON
PLENARY	PAXINOU	PASSING	PIGGING	PRESONG	PELOTON	PREDAWN	SPANKED	EPIGONE	CAPNUTS	DAPPING	REPLANT	TAPEMAN
PLENISH	PAYINTO	PASTINA	PIGMENT	PRETEND	PENGUIN	PREGAIN	SPANKER	EPONINE	DIPNETS	DEPLANE	REPOINT	TAPEMEN
PLENUMS	PAYSNOW	PASTING	PIGPENS	PREVENT	PENSION	PRELOAN	SPANNED	OPALINE	ESPNEWS	DIPPING	REPPING	TAPESON
PLINKED	PEDANTS	PATERNO	PILLING	PREYING	PEORIAN	PRENOON	SPANNER	OPENEND	HIPNESS	EMPLANE	REPRINT	TIPDOWN
PLINTHS	PENANCE	PATHAND	PINGING	PRICING	PERLMAN	PREOPEN	SPENCER	OPENING	HYPNOID	ENPLANE	REPRUNE	TOPDOWN
PLONKED	PESANTE	PATHANS	PINIONS	PRIDING	PERMIAN	PREPLAN	SPENDER	OPERAND	TOPNAME	ESPYING	REPUGNS	TOPEKAN
PLUNDER	PETUNIA	PATIENT	PINKENS	PRIMING	PERSIAN	PRESSON	SPENDON	OPERANT		EUPHONY	RIPIENI	TOPSPIN
PLUNGED	PFENNIG	PATRONS	PINKING	PRISONS	PERSSON	PRESTON	SPENSER	OPINING	**••P•N••**	EXPOUND	RIPIENO	TYPEDIN
PLUNGER	PHOENIX	PATTING	PINNING	PRIZING	PERTAIN	PRETEEN	SPENTON	OPPUGNS	ALPINER	GAPPING	RIPPING	TYPESIN
PLUNGES	PHRENIC	PAULINA	PIPPINS	PROBING	PETEMAN	PREWARN	SPINACH	OPTIONS	ALPINES	GYPPING	RIPSONE	TYPHOON
PLUNKED	PICANTE	PAULINE	PIQUANT	PROBONO	PETEMEN	PREWORN	SPINDLE	OPULENT	APPENDS	HAPENNY	SAPIENS	UMPTEEN
PLUNKER	PILINGS	PAULING	PIQUING	PROFANE	PETLION	PREYSON	SPINDLY	OPUSONE	ASPENCO	HAPPENS	SAPIENT	UNPAGAN
POINTAT	PILSNER	PAUSING	PISCINE	PROGENY	PETSCAN	PROCYON	SPINDRY	SPACING	DAPHNES	HIPBONE	SAPLING	
POINTED	PIMENTO	PAWNING	PISHING	PROLONG	PHAETON	PRODSON	SPINELS	SPADING	DAPHNIA	HOPKINS	SAPPING	**•••PN••**
POINTER	PINENUT	PAYMENT	PISTONS	PROPANE	PHASEIN	PRONOUN	SPINETS	SPARING	DAPHNIS	HOPPING	SIPHONS	DROPNET
POINTES	PINONES	PCCLONE	PITHING	PROPONE	PHILBIN	PROPMAN	SPINIER	SPAYING	DEPENDS	HOPSING	SIPPING	GRAPNEL
POINTTO	PIPINGS	PEAHENS	PITTING	PROSING	PHONEIN	PROPMEN	SPINNER	SPECING	DEPONED	HYPHENS	SOPPING	SHOPNBC
POINTUP	PIRANHA	PEAKING	PITYING	PROTONS	PICKSON	PROSCAN	SPINNEY	SPELUNK	DEPONER	HYPOING	SOPRANI	SOAPNET
POUNCED	PISANIO	PEALING	PLACING	PROVINE	PIDGEON	PROTEAN	SPINOFF	SPEWING	DEPONES	IMPLANT	SOPRANO	
POUNCER	PLAINER	PEASANT	PLANING	PROVING	PIERIAN	PROTEIN	SPINOUT	SPICING	DIPINTO	IMPOUND	SUPPING	**•••P•N•**
POUNCES	PLAINES	PECCANT	PLATENS	PRUDENT	PIGIRON	PRYOPEN	SPINOZA	SPIKING	EMPANEL	IMPRINT	TAPPANS	ASHPANS
POUNDED	PLAINLY	PECKING	PLATING	PRUNING	PIGSKIN	PULLMAN	SPONDEE	SPITING	ESPANOL	IMPUGNS	TAPPING	BEEPING
POUNDER	PLAINTS	PECTINS	PLAYING	PUCCINI	PILEDIN	PULLPIN	SPONGED	SPLEENS	EXPANDS	INPOINT	TIPLINE	BOPPING
PRANCED	PLANNED	PEEKING	PLOWING	PUDDING	PILEDON	PULLSIN	SPONGER	SPLEENY	EXPANSE	INPRINT	TIPPING	BUMPING
PRANCER	PLANNER	PEELING	PLUGINS	PUFFING	PILESIN	PULLSON	SPONGES	SPOKANE	EXPENDS	KIPLING	TOPGUNS	BURPING
PRANCES	PLIANCY	PEENING	PLUMING	PUFFINS	PILESON	PUMPKIN	SPONSOR	SPOKING	EXPENSE	KIPPING	TOPLINE	CAMPING
PRENAME	POCONOS	PEEPING	PLUSONE	PULLING	PILLION	PUNCHIN	SPUNOFF	SPRAINS	EXPUNGE	LAPLAND	TOPPING	CAPPING
PRENOON	POLANER	PEERING	PLUTONS	PULLINS	PIMESON	PURITAN	SPUNOUT	SPUMING	HAPENNY	LAPPING	TOPRANK	CARPING
PRENUPS	POLANYI	PEEVING	POBLANO	PULLONS	PINDOWN	PURLOIN	UPANDIN	SPUMONE	HOPENOT	LAPSANG	TOPTENS	CHOPINE
PRINCES	POLENTA	PEGGING	POISING	PULMONI	PIPEDIN	PUSHKIN	UPENDED	SPUMONI	HOPINTO	LAPSING	UNPAWNS	CLIPONS
PRINGLE	POLONIA	PEIPING	POISONS	PULMONO	PIPESIN	PUSHPIN		SPYRING	HYPONYM	LAPWING	UNPLANS	COMPANY
PRINKED	PORTNOY	PELTING	POLLENS	PULPING	PIROGEN	PUTDOWN	**•P••N••**	UPBORNE	IMPANEL	LEPTONS	YAPPING	COMPEND
PRINKER	POTENCE	PENDANT	POLLING	PULSING	PISCEAN	PUTUPON	APHONIA	UPBOUND	IMPENDS	LIPMANN	YIPPING	COMPING
PRINTAD	POTENCY	PENDENT	POMPANO	PUMPING	PITCHIN	PYNCHON	APHONIC	UPFLING	IMPINGE	LIPPING	ZAPPING	COOPING
PRINTED	PRAWNED	PENDING	POMPONS	PUNGENT	PITTMAN	PYTHIAN	APLENTY	UPFRONT	LEPANTO	LIPSYNC	ZIPGUNS	COPPING
PRINTER	PREENED	PENNANT	PONDING	PUNNING	PLANSON		APPENDS	UPGOING	LUPINES	LOPPING	ZIPPING	COUPING
PRINTUP	PREENER	PENNINE	PONTANO	PUNTING	PLATOON	**•PN••••**	APRONED	UPSPINS	PIPINGS	MAPPING		COUPONS
PRONATE	PRYINTO	PENNING	PONYING	PUPTENT	PLAYPEN	UPNORTH	EPERNAY	UPSTAND	RAPANUI	MOPPING	**••P•••N**	COWPONY
PRONAVY	PUDENCY	PENNONS	POOLING	PURGING	PLAYSON		OPENNET	UPSWING	RAPINES	NAPKINS	AMPHION	CRAPING

CREPING
CUPPING
DAMPENS
DAMPING
DAPPING
DEEPEND
DEEPENS
DESPINA
DESPOND
DIPPING
DRAPING
DROPINS
DUMPING
ELOPING
ENDPINS
FRYPANS
GAPPING
GASPING
GAWPING
GELPENS
GIMPING
GRIPING
GROPING
GULPING
GYPPING
HAPPENS
HARPING
HASPING
HATPINS
HEAPING
HELPING
HISPANO
HOOPING
HOPPING
HOTPINK
INSPANS
JUMPING
KEEPING
KIPPING
LAPPING
LEAPING
LIMPING
LIPPING
LISPING
LOOPING
LOPPING
LUMPING
MAPPING
MOPPING
NAPPING
NIPPING
NUTPINE
OILPANS
ONEPINT
PEEPING
PEIPING
PEPPING
PEPPINO
PETPONY
PIEPANS
PIGPENS
PIPPINS
POMPANO
POMPONS
POOPING
POPPING
POPPINS
PROPANE
PROPONE
PULPING
PUMPING
RAMPANT
RAMPING
RAPPING
RASPING
REAPING
REDPINE
REDPONY
REOPENS
REPPING
RESPANS
RESPINS
RESPOND
RIPPING
ROMPING
RSVPING
RUMPEND
SAMPANS
SAPPING
SCOPING
SEEPING
SERPENS
SERPENT
SHAPING
SIPPING
SLIPONS
SLOPING
SNAPONS
SNIPING
SOAPING
SOPPING
STEPINS
STEPONE
STIPEND
SUPPING
SUSPEND
SWIPING
TAMPING
TAPPANS
TAPPING
TARPONS
TEMPING
TENPINS
THEPOND
TIEPINS
TIMPANI
TIPPING
TOPPING
TREPANS
TYMPANA
TYMPANI
UNSPANS
UNSPENT
UPSPINS
USOPENS
VAMPING
VOLPONE
VULPINE
WARPING
WEAPONS
WEEPING
WIMPING
WISPING
YAPPING
YAWPING
YELPING
YIPPING
ZAPPING
ZIPPING

•••P••N

BUMPKIN
BURPGUN
CAMPION
CASPIAN
CHAPLIN
CHAPMAN
CHAPMEN
CHIPSIN
CLAPTON
CLIPSON
COMPLIN
COMPTON
CREPTIN
DAUPHIN
DEEPTAN
DIAPHAN
DOLPHIN
DRIPPAN
DRIPSON
DROPSIN
DUMPSON
FLIPPEN
GRYPHON
HAMPTON
HARPOON
HARPSON
HEAPSON
HELPSIN
HELPSON
HOOPMAN
HOOPMEN
JUMPSIN
JUMPSON
KEEPSIN
KEEPSON
KEMPTON
KRYPTON
LAMPOON
LEAPSIN
LEAPSON
LEAPTIN
LEAPTON
LUMPSIN
MISPLAN
MORPHIN
OUTPLAN
PREPLAN
PROPMAN
PROPMEN
PUMPKIN
SAMPSON
SEEPSIN
SHIPMAN
SHIPMEN
SIMPSON
SLAPSON
SLEPTIN
SLEPTON
SLIPSIN
SLIPSON
SLOPSON
SNAPSON
SOUPCAN
SOUPCON
SOUPSON
STEPHEN
STEPSIN
STEPSON
STOPSIN
TRAPGUN
TRIPSON
UTOPIAN
WHIPSIN

••••P•N

ACTUPON
AUTOPEN
BAKEPAN
BULLPEN
CAKEPAN
CHEAPEN
CHOMPON
CLAMPON
CRAMPON
CREEPIN
CRESPIN
CRISPEN
CRISPIN
CUTOPEN
DEADPAN
DISHPAN
DRIPPAN
DUCKPIN
DUSTPAN
FELTPEN
FIVEPIN
FIXUPON
FLIPPEN
FLYOPEN
FOURPIN
GETUPON
GOTUPON
HAIRPIN
HARDPAN
HEADPIN
HITUPON
INASPIN
ITSOPEN
KEYSPAN
KINGPIN
LAYOPEN
LAYUPON
LETUPON
LOAFPAN
NINEPIN
NOTOPEN
OUTSPIN
PLAYPEN
PREOPEN
PRYOPEN
PULLPIN
PUSHPIN
PUTUPON
RIPOPEN
RUBUPON
SATUPON
SETUPON
SHARPEN
SITUPON
SKIMPON
SLEEPIN
SLEEPON
SPYUPON
STEEPEN
STEEPIN
STEWPAN
STOMPIN
STOMPON
STRAPIN
STRAPON
SWOOPIN
TAILPIN
THIGPEN
TOPSPIN
TROMPIN
TROOPIN
TUBEPAN

PO•••••

POACHED
POACHER
POACHES
POBLANO
POBOXES
POCKETS
POCONOS
PODCAST
PODIUMS
PODLIKE
PODRIDA
POESIES
POETESS
POETICA
POETICS
POETISE
POETIZE
POINTAT
POINTED
POINTER
POINTES
POINTTO
POINTUP
POISERS
POISING
POISONS
POISSON
POITIER
POIVRES
POKEDAT
POKEFUN
POKEMON
POKEOUT
POKESAT
POKIEST
POLANER
POLANYI
POLARAS
POLARIS
POLEAXE
POLECAR
POLECAT
POLEMAN
POLEMEN
POLEMIC
POLENTA
POLESAT
POLESIT
POLICED
POLICER
POLICES
POLISCI
POLITER
POLITIC
POLKAED
POLLACK
POLLARD
POLLEES
POLLENS
POLLERA
POLLERS
POLLING
POLLOCK
POLLTAX
POLLUTE
POLOIST
POLONIA
POLTAVA
POLYGON
POLYMER
POLYPED
POLYPOD
POLYSCI
POMADED
POMADES
POMELOS
POMMARD
POMMELS
POMPANO
POMPEIA
POMPEII
POMPOMS
POMPONS
POMPOUS
PONCHOS
PONDERS
PONDING
PONGEES
PONGIDS
PONIARD
PONTANO
PONTIAC
PONTIAN
PONTIFF
PONTIUS
PONTOON
PONYING
PONYKEG
POOCHES
POOCHIE
POODLES
POOHBAH
POOLCUE
POOLERS
POOLING
POOLMAN
POOLMEN
POOPING
POOPOUT
POOPSIE
POORBOX
POORBOY
POOREST
POORISH
POORLAW
POORMAN
POORMEN
POORTAX
POPCORN
POPDIVA
POPEAFB
POPEDOM
POPELEO
POPEYED
POPEYES
POPGUNS
POPLARS
POPLINS
POPOFFS
POPOUTS
POPOVER
POPPERS
POPPIES
POPPING
POPPINS
POPPLED
POPPLES
POPQUIZ
POPROCK
POPSOFF
POPSONG
POPSOUT
POPSTAR
POPTART
POPTOPS
POPTUNE
POPULAR
POPUPAD
POPWINE
PORCHES
PORCINE
PORGIES
PORIVER
PORKERS
PORKIER
PORKING
PORKISH
PORKPIE
PORSCHE
PORSENA
PORTAGE
PORTALS
PORTEND
PORTENT
PORTERS
PORTHOS
PORTICO
PORTING
PORTION
PORTMAN
PORTNOY
PORTRAY
POSABLE
POSADAS
POSEDAS
POSESAS
POSEURS
POSEUSE
POSHEST
POSITED
POSOLES
POSSESS
POSSLQS
POSSUMS
POSTAGE
POSTBAG
POSTBOX
POSTDOC
POSTERN
POSTERS
POSTFIX
POSTHOC
POSTIES
POSTING
POSTITS
POSTMAN
POSTMEN
POSTOPS
POSTURE
POSTWAR
POTABLE
POTAGES
POTAMUS
POTBOIL
POTEENS
POTENCE
POTENCY
POTFULS
POTHERB
POTHERS
POTHOLE
POTHOOK
POTIONS
POTLIDS
POTLUCK
POTOMAC
POTPIES
POTSDAM
POTSHOT
POTTAGE
POTTERS
POTTERY
POTTIER
POTTIES
POTTING
POUCHED
POUCHES
POUDRES
POULENC
POULTRY
POUNCED
POUNCER
POUNCES
POUNDED
POUNDER
POURERS
POURING
POUROUT
POURSIN
POUSSIN
POUTERS
POUTFUL
POUTIER
POUTING
POVERTY
POWDERS
POWDERY
POWERED
POWERUP
POWWOWS
POZOLES

P•O••••

PEONAGE
PEONIES
PEOPLED
PEOPLES
PEORIAN
PHOBIAS
PHOBICS
PHOEBES
PHOEBUS
PHOENIX
PHONEIN
PHONEME
PHONENO
PHONERS
PHONEYS
PHONICS
PHONIER
PHONIES
PHONILY
PHONING
PHONYUP
PHOTICS
PHOTOGS
PHOTOID
PHOTONS
PHOTOOP
PIOLETS
PIONEER
PIOSITY
PIOUSLY
PLODDED
PLODDER
PLOESTI
PLONKED
PLOPPED
PLOSION
PLOSIVE
PLOTFUL
PLOTTED
PLOTTER
PLOTZED
PLOTZES
PLOUGHS
PLOVDIV
PLOVERS
PLOWBOY
PLOWERS
PLOWING
PLOWMAN
PLOWMEN
PLOWSON
PLOWSUP
POOCHES
POOCHIE
POODLES
POOHBAH
POOLCUE
POOLERS
POOLING
POOLMAN
POOLMEN
POOPING
POOPOUT
POOPSIE
POORBOX
POORBOY
POOREST
POORISH
POORLAW
POORMAN
POORMEN
POORTAX
PROARAB
PROBALL
PROBATE
PROBERS
PROBIES
PROBING
PROBITY
PROBLEM
PROBONO
PROBOWL
PROCEED
PROCESS
PROCITY
PROCLUS
PROCTER
PROCTOR
PROCURE
PROCYON
PRODDED
PRODDER
PRODIGY
PRODSON
PRODUCE
PRODUCT
PROEAST
PROFANE
PROFARM
PROFESS
PROFFER
PROFILE
PROFITS
PROFUSE
PROGENY
PROGRAM
PROJECT
PROJETS
PROKEDS
PROLATE
PROLIFE
PROLOGS
PROLONG
PROMBID
PROMISE
PROMOED
PROMOTE
PROMPTS
PRONATE
PRONAVY
PRONELY
PRONETO
PRONGED
PRONOUN
PROOFED
PROOFER
PROPANE
PROPELS
PROPHET
PROPJET
PROPMAN
PROPMEN
PROPONE
PROPOSE
PROPPED
PROPSUP
PRORATA
PRORATE
PROSAIC
PROSCAN
PROSERS
PROSHOP
PROSIER
PROSILY
PROSING
PROSODY
PROSPER
PROTEAM
PROTEAN
PROTECT
PROTEGE
PROTEIN
PROTEST
PROTEUS
PROTIST
PROTONS
PROUDER
PROUDLY
PROUDOF
PROVEIT
PROVERB
PROVERS
PROVIDE
PROVINE
PROVING
PROVISO
PROVOKE
PROVOST
PROWESS
PROWEST
PROWLED
PROWLER
PROXIES
PROXIMA
PROXIMO
PTOLEMY

P••O•••

PAGODAS
PALOMAR
PALOMAS
PALOOKA
PANOPLY
PAPOOSE
PARODIC
PAROLED
PAROLEE
PAROLES
PARONYM
PAROTID
PAYOFFS
PAYOLAS
PAYOUTS
PCWORLD
PELOTAS
PELOTON
PERORAL
PEYOTES
PHLOEMS
PHLOXES
PICOTED
PIGOUTS
PILOTED
PINOAKS
PINONES
PINOTTA
PIROGEN
PIROGUE
PIVOTAL
PIVOTED
PIVOTER
POBOXES
POCONOS
POLOIST
POLONIA
POPOFFS
POPOUTS
POPOVER
POSOLES
POTOMAC
POZOLES
PREOMIT
PREOPEN
PREORAL
PRIORTO
PROOFED
PROOFER
PRYOPEN
PTBOATS
PUTOFFS
PUTOUTS
PUTOVER
PWBOTHA

P•••O••

PACEOFF
PACKOFF
PADDOCK
PADLOCK
PADRONE
PAGEONE
PAIDOFF
PAIDOUT
PAIROFF
PALJOEY
PALLORS
PALMOFF
PALMOIL
PALOOKA
PANDORA
PANSOUT
PANTONE
PAPOOSE
PARBOIL
PARDONS
PARFOUR
PARLORS
PARLOUR
PARLOUS
PARROTS
PARSONS
PARTONE
PARTOOK
PASCOLI
PASSOFF
PASSOUT
PASTORS
PATDOWN
PATROLS
PATRONS
PATROON
PAVIORS
PAVIOUR
PAVLOVA
PAWNOFF
PAYLOAD
PAYMORE
PAYROLL
PAYSOFF
PAYSOUT
PCCLONE
PEABODY
PEACOAT
PEACOCK
PEAFOWL
PEAPODS
PEASOUP
PEEKOUT
PEELOFF
PEELOUT
PEEPOUT
PEEROUT
PEGTOPS
PENNOCK
PENNONS
PENROSE
PEPBOYS
PEPTONE
PEQUOTS
PERFORM
PERGOLA
PERIODS
PERSOFF
PERSONA
PERSONS
PETBOAS
PETCOCK
PETCOMB
PETCOWS
PETDOGS
PETDOOR
PETDOVE
PETGOAT
PETIOLE
PETPONY
PETROCK
PETROLS
PETROUS
PETTOYS
PGATOUR
PHENOLS
PHENOMS
PHILOUS
PHOTOGS
PHOTOID
PHOTONS
PHOTOOP
PIANOLA
PICCOLO
PICEOUS
PICKOFF
PICKOUT
PIEHOLE
PIETOSO
PIGEONS
PIGSOUT
PILEOUS
PILLORY
PILLOWS
PILLOWY
PINBOYS

PINDOWN
PINEOIL
PINFOLD
PINHOLE
PINIONS
PINKOES
PISCOPO
PISTOLE
PISTOLS
PISTONS
PISTOUS
PITBOSS
PITEOUS
PITROWS
PLANOUT
PLATOON
PLAYOFF
PLAYOUT
PLEXORS
PLUGOLA
PLUMOSE
PLUSONE
PLUTONS
PLYWOOD
POISONS
POKEOUT
POLLOCK
POMPOMS
POMPONS
POMPOUS
PONTOON
POOPOUT
POPCORN
POPROCK
POPSOFF
POPSONG
POPSOUT
POPTOPS
POSTOPS
POTBOIL
POTHOLE
POTHOOK
POTIONS
POUROUT
POWWOWS
PREBOIL
PREBOOK
PREBOOM
PREBORN
PRECODE
PRECOIL
PRECOOK
PRECOOL
PRECOUP
PREDOOM
PREFORM
PRELOAD
PRELOAN
PRELOSS
PRENOON
PREROCK
PRESOAK
PRESOLD
PRESONG
PRESORT
PRETOLD
PRETORS
PREVOID
PREVOST
PREWORK
PREWORN
PRISONS
PROBONO
PROBOWL
PROLOGS
PROLONG
PROMOED
PROMOTE
PRONOUN
PROPONE
PROPOSE
PROSODY
PROTONS
PROVOKE
PROVOST
PTEROUS
PUFFOUT
PUGNOSE
PULLOFF
PULLONS
PULLOUT
PULMONI
PULMONO
PUMPOUT
PURLOIN
PURPORT
PURPOSE
PUSHOFF
PUSHOUT
PUTDOWN
PUTSOFF
PUTSOUT
PUTTOUT
PYEDOGS
PYTHONS

P••••O•

PACKSON
PAGEBOY
PAIDFOR
PALEMON
PALMTOP
PALTROW
PAPADOC
PAPAGOS
PARADOR
PARADOX
PARAGON
PARASOL
PARTOOK
PARTYON
PASSFOR
PASSION
PATRIOT
PATROON
PAXINOU
PAYSFOR
PAYSNOW
PEARSON
PEATBOG
PEATPOT
PEKEPOO
PELOTON
PENSION
PERIDOT
PERSSON
PETCROW
PETDOOR
PETFROG
PETLION
PETSHOP
PEUGEOT
PGAPROS
PHAETON
PHANTOM
PHARAOH
PHILCOS
PHOTOOP
PHYLLOS
PICADOR
PICAROS
PICKSON
PIDGEON
PIERROT
PIETROS
PIGIRON
PILCROW
PILEDON
PILESOF
PILESON
PILLBOX
PILLION
PIMESON
PINCHOT
PINEFOR
PINESOL
PINETOP
PITSTOP
PLANFOR
PLANSON
PLATOON
PLAYBOY
PLAYDOH
PLAYSON
PLOSION
PLOWBOY
PLOWSON
PLUMCOT
PLYWOOD
PNEUMON
POCONOS
POISSON
POKEMON
POLYGON
POLYPOD
POMELOS
PONCHOS
PONTOON
POORBOX
POORBOY
POPEDOM
PORTHOS
PORTION
PORTNOY
POSTBOX
POSTDOC
POSTHOC
POTHOOK
POTSHOT
PRAETOR
PRAYFOR
PREBOOK
PREBOOM
PRECOOK
PRECOOL
PREDOOM
PRENOON
PREPLOT
PRERIOT
PRESHOW
PRESSON
PRESTON
PRESTOS
PREYSON
PROCTOR
PROCYON
PRODSON
PROSHOP
PROUDOF
PRUDHOE
PSYCHOS
PUEBLOS
PULLFOR
PULLSON
PULLTOY
PUSHFOR
PUSHROD
PUTUPON
PYNCHON

P•••••O

PAGETWO
PAISANO
PALAZZO
PALERMO
PAMLICO
PARTTWO
PASSADO
PATERNO
PAYINTO
PEKEPOO
PEPPINO
PEPSICO
PERATIO
PERDIDO
PHONENO
PICARDO
PICASSO
PICCOLO
PIETOSO
PIMENTO
PIMLICO
PISANIO
PISARRO
PISCOPO
PITCHTO
PITILLO
PIZARRO
PLACEBO
PLACIDO
PLANSTO
PLAYSTO
PLEADTO
PLUSTWO
POBLANO
POINTTO
POMPANO
PONTANO
POPELEO
PORTICO
PRAYSTO
PREVETO
PRIMERO
PRIORTO
PRIVYTO
PROBONO
PRONETO
PROVISO
PROXIMO
PRYINTO
PULMONO
PUTITTO
PUTUPTO

•PO••••

APODOUS
APOGEAL
APOGEAN
APOGEES
APOLLOS
APOLOGY
APOSTLE
APOTHEM
EPOCHAL
EPONINE
EPONYMS
EPONYMY
EPOPEES
EPOQUES
EPOXIED
EPOXIES
OPOSSUM
SPOILED
SPOILER
SPOKANE
SPOKEOF
SPOKETO
SPOKEUP
SPOKING
SPONDEE
SPONGED
SPONGER
SPONGES
SPONSOR
SPOOFED
SPOOFER
SPOOKED
SPOOLED
SPOOLER
SPOONED
SPOONER
SPORRAN
SPORTED
SPORTIN
SPOTLIT
SPOTTED
SPOTTER
SPOUSAL
SPOUSES
SPOUTED
SPOUTER
UPOROUT

•P•O•••

APHONIA
APHONIC
APPOINT
APPOSED
APPOSES
APRONED
APROPOS
OPPOSED
OPPOSER
OPPOSES
SPLOTCH
SPOOFED
SPOOFER
SPOOKED
SPOOLED
SPOOLER
SPOONED
SPOONER
SPROUTS
UPBORNE
UPBOUND
UPCOAST
UPCOILS
UPCOURT
UPFOLDS
UPFORIT
UPGOING
UPHOARD
UPHOLDS
UPLOADS
UPNORTH
UPROARS
UPROOTS
UPROUSE
UPSOARS
UPTONOW
UPTOPAR
UPTOWNS

•P••O••

APODOUS
APOLOGY
APPROVE
APRIORI
EPIDOTE
EPIGONE
EPILOGS
EPISODE
EPITOME
OPENOUT
OPEROSE
OPTIONS
OPTSOUT
OPUSONE
SPATOUT
SPECOUT
SPEDOFF
SPEWOUT
SPIGOTS
SPINOFF
SPINOUT
SPINOZA
SPITOUT
SPUMONE
SPUMONI
SPUNOFF
SPUNOUT
SPYBOTS
SPYHOLE
UPABOVE
UPCCODE
UPCLOSE
UPFLOWS
UPFRONT
UPGROWN
UPGROWS
UPOROUT
UPPROPS
UPROOTS
UPSHOOT
UPSHOTS
UPSLOPE
UPSTOOD

•P•••O•

APAIROF
APECKOF
APERSON
APILEOF
APOLLOS
APRICOT
APROPOS
EPSILON
OPENTOE
OPENTOP
OPINION
OPTSFOR
SPAMBOT
SPARROW
SPEAKOF
SPECTOR
SPEEDOS
SPENDON
SPENTON
SPIEDON
SPIESON
SPITSON
SPOKEOF
SPONSOR
SPRAYON
SPURSON
SPYUPON
UPSHOOT
UPSILON
UPSTOOD
UPTHROW
UPTONOW

•P••••O

APPLYTO
OPTEDTO
OPUSTWO
SPEAKTO
SPOKETO
UPTEMPO

••PO•••

AMPOULE
APPOINT
APPOSED
APPOSES
BIPOLAR
CAPOTES
COPOUTS
CUPOLAS
DEPONED
DEPONER
DEPONES
DEPORTS
DEPOSAL
DEPOSED
DEPOSER
DEPOSES
DEPOSIT
DEPOWER
DIPOLAR
DIPOLES
EMPORIA
EMPOWER
ESPOSAS
ESPOSOS
ESPOUSE
EXPORTS
EXPOSED
EXPOSER
EXPOSES
EXPOSIT
EXPOUND
HOPOVER
HYPOING
HYPONYM
IMPORTS
IMPOSED
IMPOSER
IMPOSES
IMPOSTS
IMPOUND
INPOINT
INPOURS
INPOWER
JCPOWYS
JDPOWER
LAPORTE
NEPOTIC
ONPOINT
OPPOSED
OPPOSER
OPPOSES
PAPOOSE
POPOFFS
POPOUTS
POPOVER
REPOINT
REPOLLS
REPOMAN
REPORTS
REPOSED
REPOSER
REPOSES
REPOSIT
REPOSTS
REPOURS
REPOWER
RIPOFFS
RIPOPEN
RIPOSTE
RIPOSTS
TFPOWYS
TIPOFFS
TIPOVER
TOPONYM
TUPOLEV
UNPOLED
UNPOSED
VAPORED
VAPORER
VAPORUB
VAPOURS
VAPOURY
ZAPOTEC

••P•O••

AMPHORA
APPROVE
BYPHONE
BYPROXY
CAPTORS
COPIOUS
COPPOLA
COPSOUT
CUPROUS
DEPLORE
DEPLOYS
DIPLOID
DIPLOMA
DOPEOUT
EMPLOYS
EUPHONY
EXPLODE
EXPLOIT
EXPLORE
HAPLOID
HIPBONE
HIPBOOT
HIPROOF
HOPSOFF
HOPSOUT
HOPTOIT
HYPNOID
IMPIOUS
IMPLODE
IMPLORE
IMPROVE
JOPPOLO
KEPTOFF
KEPTOUT
LAPDOGS
LAPROBE
LAPTOPS
LEPTONS
LIPSOFF
LIPSOUT
LOPSOFF
MAPSOUT
MOPTOPS
PAPOOSE
PEPBOYS
PEPTONE
POPCORN
POPROCK
POPSOFF
POPSONG
POPSOUT
POPTOPS
RAPPORT
RAPSONG
RAPTORS
REPHONE
REPLOTS
REPLOWS
REPROBE
REPROOF
REPROVE
RIPCORD
RIPSOFF
RIPSONE
RIPSOUT
RIPTORN
ROPEOFF
SAPPORO
SIPHONS
SUPPORT
SUPPOSE
TAPIOCA
TAPROOM
TAPROOT
TAPSOFF
TAPSOUT
TIPDOWN
TIPSOFF
TIPTOED
TIPTOES
TIPTOPS
TOPBOOT
TOPCOAT
TOPDOGS
TOPDOWN
TOPFORM
TOPHOLE
TOPMOST
TOPROWS
TOPSOFF
TOPSOIL
TOPSOUT
TYPHOID
TYPHOON
UNPIOUS
UNPROUD
UPPROPS
WIPEOFF
WIPEOUT
XIPHOID
ZEPPOLE
ZEPPOLI
ZIPCODE
ZIPLOCK
ZIPLOCS
ZIPSOFF
ZIPTOPS

••P••O•

AMPHION
CAPECOD
CAPITOL
CAPTION
COPILOT
COPSHOP
COPYBOY
CYPRIOT
EMPEROR
ESPANOL
ESPOSOS
HIPBOOT
HIPROOF
HOPEFOR
HOPENOT
HYPERON
NIPIGON
PAPADOC
PAPAGOS
POPEDOM
REPROOF
REPSFOR
RIPSTOP
ROPETOW
TAPEDON
TAPESON
TAPROOM
TAPROOT
TAPSHOE
TOPBOOT
TOPKNOT
TOPSPOT
TUPELOS
TYPHOON
WAPSHOT

••P•••O

APPLYTO
ASPENCO
CEPHALO
DIPINTO
ELPRADO
ESPARTO
HAPKIDO
HAPPYTO
HOPEDSO
HOPEDTO
HOPESSO
HOPESTO
HOPINTO
IMPASTO
JOPPOLO
LEPANTO
OMPHALO
PEPPINO
PEPSICO
POPELEO
RAPALLO
REPLYTO
RIPIENO
RIPINTO
SAPPORO
SAPSAGO
SOPRANO
TAPINTO
ZAPATEO

•••PO••

ADIPOSE
AIRPOPS
AIRPORT
AIRPOTS
AMAPOLA
BBQPORK
BEDPOST
BESPOKE
CALPOLY
CAMPOUT
CARPOOL
CARPORT
CARPOUS
CHOPOFF
CLIPOFF
CLIPONS
CLIPOUT
COMPORT
COMPOSE
COMPOST
COMPOTE
COPPOLA
CORPORA
COUPONS
COWPOKE
COWPONY
CRAPOLA
CRAPOUT
DAMPOFF
DESPOIL
DESPOND
DESPOTS
DISPORT
DISPOSE
DROPOFF
DROPOUT
DRSPOCK
DUMPOUT
DUOPOLY
EELPOTS
EELPOUT
FLIPOUT
HARPOON
HELPOUT
HOOPOES
HOTPOTS
ICEPOPS
INAPOEM
INAPOKE
INKPOTS
INSPOTS
ISOPODS
JETPORT
JOPPOLO
JUMPOFF
KEEPOFF
KEEPOUT
LAMPOIL
LAMPOON
LEOPOLD
LIMPOPO
LOWPOST
MAYPOLE
MRSPOCK
NEWPORT
NONPOET
NONPOOR
OUTPOLL
OUTPOPS
OUTPORT
OUTPOST
OUTPOUR
PEAPODS
PEEPOUT
PETPONY
POMPOMS
POMPONS
POMPOUS
POOPOUT
PROPONE
PROPOSE
PUMPOUT
PURPORT
PURPOSE
RAPPORT
REDPOLL
REDPONY
RESPOKE
RESPOND
RESPOOL
RESPOTS
RUMPOLE
SAPPORO
SEAPORT
SEEPOUT
SEXPOTS
SHIPOUT
SKIPOLE
SKIPOUT
SLIPOFF
SLIPONS
SLIPOUT
SNAPONS
SNIPOFF
STEPOFF
STEPONE
STEPOUT
STOPOFF
STUPORS
SUBPOST
SUPPORT
SUPPOSE
TADPOLE
TARPONS
TEAPOTS
TEAPOYS
TEMPORE
THEPOND
THEPOOH
THEPOPE
THEPOST
TIEPOLO
TRIPODS
TRIPOLI
TVSPOTS
UNIPODS
UNSPOKE
UNSPOOL
VANPOOL
VFWPOST
VOLPONE
WALPOLE
WEAPONS
WIMPOLE
WIMPOUT
ZEPPOLE
ZEPPOLI

•••P•O•

ADAPTOR
ATIPTOE
CAMPHOR
CAMPION
CARPOOL
CLAPFOR
CLAPTON
CLIPSON
COMPTON
CROPTOP
CRYPTOS
DAMPMOP
DRIPSON
DROPBOX
DROPTOP
DUMPSON
FLIPTOP
GRYPHON
HAMPTON
HARPOON
HARPSON
HEAPSOF
HEAPSON

HELPSON
HOOPTOY
JUMPSON
KEEPSON
KEMPTON
KERPLOP
KLEPTOS
KRYPTON
LAMPOON
LEAPFOR
LEAPSON
LEAPTON
NONPOOR
NONPROS
OLDPROS
OUTPLOD
OUTPLOT
PGAPROS
PREPLOT
RESPOOL
SAMPSON
SHOPFOR
SHOPKOS
SIMPSON
SLAPSON
SLEPTON
SLIPSON
SLOPSON
SNAPSON
SOAPBOX
SOUPCON
SOUPSON
STEPMOM
STEPSON
STOPFOR
SUBPLOT
SYMPTOM
TEMPJOB
THEPOOH
TRIPSON
UNSPOOL
VANPOOL
WEEPFOR

•••P••O

ADAPTTO
ARAPAHO
HAPPYTO
HERPETO
HISPANO
IHOPESO
JOPPOLO
KEEPSTO
LIMPOPO
LINPIAO
MALPASO
PEPPINO
POMPANO
SAPPORO
SERPICO
SHAPIRO
SNAPSTO
STEPTWO
TAMPICO
TIEPOLO
TORPEDO

••••PO•

ACTUPON
AFROPOP
ALCOPOP
APROPOS
ATROPOS
BLOWPOP
BRITPOP
CHOMPON
CLAMPON
COOKPOT
CRABPOT
CRAMPON
CREEPOS
DACAPOS
DASHPOT
DECAPOD
EUROPOP
EYESPOT
FIXUPON
FUSSPOT
GETUPON
GOTOPOT
GOTUPON
HEXAPOD
HITUPON
HOTSPOT
ICKYPOO
IGGYPOP
INASPOT
INKSPOT
JACKPOT
KAKAPOS
LAYUPON
LETUPON
MONOPOD
OCTOPOD
OILSPOT
ONESPOT
ONTOPOF
PEATPOT
PEKEPOO
POLYPOD
PUTUPON
REDSPOT
RUBUPON
SATUPON
SEEDPOD
SETUPON
SHAMPOO
SITUPON
SKIMPON
SLEEPON
SODAPOP
SPYUPON
STEWPOT
STOMPON
STRAPON
STRIPOF
SUNSPOT
TENSPOT
TIEMPOS
TOPSPOT
TOSSPOT
TWOSPOT

••••P•O

ADDUPTO
CALYPSO
EJEMPLO
FILIPPO
GOESPRO
GOLFPRO
GONEPRO
GOTUPTO
ICKYPOO
LEDUPTO
NOTUPTO
OWNUPTO
PEKEPOO
PUTUPTO
RANUPTO
RUNUPTO
SCORPIO
SEMIPRO
SHAMPOO
SUMUPTO
TURNPRO
WENTPRO

•••••PO

ELCAMPO
FILIPPO
GESTAPO
LIMPOPO
PISCOPO
RIVERPO
UPTEMPO

P•P••••

PAPADOC
PAPAGOS
PAPAYAS
PAPEETE
PAPELES
PAPERED
PAPERER
PAPIERS
PAPILLA
PAPISTS
PAPOOSE
PAPPIES
PAPRIKA
PAPUANS
PAPYRUS
PEPBAND
PEPBOYS
PEPCIDS
PEPITAS
PEPLUMS
PEPPARD
PEPPERS
PEPPERY
PEPPIER
PEPPILL
PEPPILY
PEPPING
PEPPINO
PEPSICO
PEPSINS
PEPTALK
PEPTICS
PEPTIDE
PEPTONE
PIPAGES
PIPCARD
PIPEDIN
PIPEDUP
PIPEFUL
PIPESIN
PIPESUP
PIPETTE
PIPIEST
PIPINGS
PIPLESS
PIPPINS
POPCORN
POPDIVA
POPEAFB
POPEDOM
POPELEO
POPEYED
POPEYES
POPGUNS
POPLARS
POPLINS
POPOFFS
POPOUTS
POPOVER
POPPERS
POPPIES
POPPING
POPPINS
POPPLED
POPPLES
POPQUIZ
POPROCK
POPSOFF
POPSONG
POPSOUT
POPSTAR
POPTART
POPTOPS
POPTUNE
POPULAR
POPUPAD
POPWINE
PUPATED
PUPATES
PUPPETS
PUPPIES
PUPTENT

P••P•••

PALPATE
PAMPERS
PANPIPE
PAPPIES
PAUPERS
PAWPAWS
PEAPODS
PEEPERS
PEEPING
PEEPLES
PEEPOUT
PEEPSAT
PEIPING
PENPALS
PEOPLED
PEOPLES
PEPPARD
PEPPERS
PEPPERY
PEPPIER
PEPPILL
PEPPILY
PEPPING
PEPPINO
PERPLEX
PETPIGS
PETPONY
PETPUPS
PGAPROS
PIEPANS
PIGPENS
PIMPLED
PIMPLES
PIPPINS
PLOPPED
POMPANO
POMPEIA
POMPEII
POMPOMS
POMPONS
POMPOUS
POOPING
POOPOUT
POOPSIE
POPPERS
POPPIES
POPPING
POPPINS
POPPLED
POPPLES
POTPIES
PREPACK
PREPAID
PREPARE
PREPAVE
PREPAYS
PREPLAN
PREPLOT
PREPPED
PREPPIE
PREPUPA
PROPANE
PROPELS
PROPHET
PROPJET
PROPMAN
PROPMEN
PROPONE
PROPOSE
PROPPED
PROPSUP
PULPERS
PULPIER
PULPIFY
PULPING
PULPITS
PUMPERS
PUMPING
PUMPKIN
PUMPOUT
PUMPSUP
PUPPETS
PUPPIES
PURPLED
PURPLES
PURPORT
PURPOSE
PUTPUTS
PVCPIPE

P•••P••

PANOPLY
PARAPET
PARAPHS
PAULPRY
PEATPOT
PEKEPOO
PITAPAT
PLAYPEN
PLOPPED
PLUMPED
PLUMPER
PLUMPIE
PLUMPLY
POLYPED
POLYPOD
POPUPAD
PORKPIE
PREOPEN
PREPPED
PREPPIE
PRESPUR
PRIMPED
PROMPTS
PROPPED
PROSPER
PRYOPEN
PULLPIN
PUSHPIN
PUTUPON
PUTUPTO

P••••P•

PANPIPE
PEGTOPS
PERCEPT
PERHAPS
PERIAPT
PETNAPS
PETPUPS
PHILIPK
PHILIPS
PHILIPV
PICKUPS
PILEUPS
PISCOPO
PLATYPI
POPTOPS
POSTOPS
PREAMPS
PRECEPT
PREEMPT
PRENUPS
PREPUPA
PRETAPE
PRETYPE
PULLUPS
PUSHUPS
PVCPIPE

P•••••P

PACELAP
PACKSUP
PAIRSUP
PALMTOP
PARSNIP
PASTEUP
PATCHUP
PAYSLIP
PEASOUP
PERKSUP
PETSHOP
PHARLAP
PHILLIP
PHONYUP
PHOTOOP
PICKSUP
PILEDUP
PILESUP
PINESAP
PINETOP
PIPEDUP
PIPESUP
PITSTOP
PLAYSUP
PLOWSUP
PLUGSUP
POINTUP
POWERUP
PRECOUP
PRESHIP
PRESSUP
PREWHIP
PREWRAP
PRICKUP
PRINTUP
PROPSUP
PROSHOP
PSYCHUP
PUFFSUP
PULLSUP
PUMPSUP
PUNCHUP
PUTEMUP

•PP••••

APPALLS
APPARAT
APPAREL
APPEALS
APPEARS
APPEASE
APPENDS
APPETIT
APPLAUD
APPLETS
APPLIED
APPLIER
APPLIES
APPLING
APPLYTO
APPOINT
APPOSED
APPOSES
APPRISE
APPROVE
EPPERLY
OPPOSED
OPPOSER
OPPOSES
OPPRESS
OPPUGNS
UPPHASE
UPPILED
UPPILES
UPPROPS
UPPSALA

•P•P•••

EPOPEES
UPSPINS

•P••P••

APROPOS
OPENPIT
SPYUPON
UPTOPAR

•P•••P•

EPITAPH
UPHEAPS
UPKEEPS
UPLEAPS
UPLEAPT
UPPROPS
UPSLOPE
UPSTEPS
UPSWEPT
UPTEMPO

•P••••P

APHILIP
EPICARP
OPENSUP
OPENTAP
OPENTOP
SPEAKUP
SPEEDUP
SPICEUP
SPIFFUP
SPIKEUP
SPLITUP
SPOKEUP
UPSWEEP

••PP•••

BOPPERS
BOPPING
CAPPERS
CAPPING
COPPERS
COPPERY
COPPICE
COPPING
COPPOLA
CUPPIER
CUPPING
DAPPING
DAPPLED
DAPPLES
DIPPERS
DIPPIER
DIPPING
DOPPLER
FIPPLES
FOPPERY
FOPPISH
GAPPING
GUPPIES
GYPPERS
GYPPING
HAPPENS
HAPPIER
HAPPIFY
HAPPILY
HAPPYTO
HEPPEST
HIPPEST
HIPPIER
HIPPIES
HIPPISH
HIPPITY
HOPPERS
HOPPIER
HOPPING
HUPPAHS
HUPPERT
JOPPOLO
KIPPERS
KIPPING
LAPPERS
LAPPETS
LAPPING
LAPPISH
LEPPARD
LIPPERS
LIPPIER
LIPPING
LOPPERS
LOPPIER
LOPPING
MAPPERS
MAPPING
MOPPERS
MOPPETS
MOPPING
MUPPETS
NAPPERS
NAPPIER
NAPPIES
NAPPING
NIPPERS
NIPPIER
NIPPILY
NIPPING
NIPPLES
PAPPIES
PEPPARD
PEPPERS
PEPPERY
PEPPIER
PEPPILL
PEPPILY
PEPPING
PEPPINO
PIPPINS
POPPERS
POPPIES
POPPING
POPPINS
POPPLED
POPPLES
PUPPETS
PUPPIES
RAPPELS
RAPPERS
RAPPING
RAPPORT
REPPING
RIPPERS
RIPPING
RIPPLED
RIPPLES
RIPPLET
SAPPERS
SAPPIER
SAPPILY
SAPPING
SAPPORO
SIPPERS
SIPPING
SOPPIER
SOPPING
SUPPERS
SUPPING
SUPPLED
SUPPLER
SUPPLES
SUPPORT
SUPPOSE
TAPPANS
TAPPERS
TAPPETS
TAPPING
TIPPEES
TIPPERS
TIPPETS
TIPPIER
TIPPING
TIPPLED
TIPPLER
TIPPLES
TOPPERS
TOPPING
TOPPLED
TOPPLES
YAPPERS
YAPPING
YIPPIES
YIPPING
YUPPIES
YUPPIFY
ZAPPERS
ZAPPIER
ZAPPING
ZEPPOLE
ZEPPOLI
ZIPPERS
ZIPPIER
ZIPPING

••P•P••

CAPAPIE
MCPAPER
ONPAPER
POPUPAD
REPAPER
RIPOPEN
TOPSPIN
TOPSPOT
UNPIPED

••P••P•

DEPULPS
LAPTOPS
MOPTOPS
POPTOPS
REPUMPS
RIPRAPS
TIPTOPS
TOPKAPI
UPPROPS
ZIPTOPS

••P•••P

AMPEDUP
COPSHOP
HYPEDUP
HYPESUP
PIPEDUP
PIPESUP
RIPSTOP
ROPEDUP
ROPESUP
TAPEDUP
TAPESUP
TYPEDUP
TYPESUP
WIPEDUP
WIPESUP

•••PP••

BLIPPED
CHAPPED
CHAPPIE
CHIPPED
CHIPPER
CHOPPED
CHOPPER
CHUPPAH
CHUPPAS
CLAPPED
CLAPPER
CLIPPED
CLIPPER
CLOPPED
CRAPPIE
CRIPPLE
CROPPED
CROPPER
CRUPPER
DRIPPAN
DRIPPED
DRIPPER
DROPPED
DROPPER
FLAPPED
FLAPPER
FLIPPED
FLIPPEN
FLIPPER
FLOPPED
FLOPPER
FRAPPES
GRAPPAS
GRAPPLE
GRIPPED
GRIPPER
GRIPPES
PLOPPED
PREPPED
PREPPIE
PROPPED
QUIPPED
QUIPPER
REAPPLY
REUPPED
SCUPPER
SHIPPED
SHIPPER
SHOPPED
SHOPPER
SHOPPES
SKIPPED
SKIPPER
SLAPPED
SLAPPER
SLIPPED
SLIPPER
SLOPPED
SNAPPEA
SNAPPED
SNAPPER
SNAPPLE
SNIPPED
SNIPPER
SNIPPET
SOAPPAD
STEPPED
STEPPER
STEPPES
STIPPLE
STOPPED
STOPPER
STOPPLE
SWAPPED
SWAPPER
TRAPPED
TRAPPER
TRIPPED
TRIPPER
TRIPPET
WHAPPED
WHIPPED
WHIPPER
WHIPPET
WHIPPLE
WHOPPED
WHOPPER
WHUPPED
WRAPPED
WRAPPER

•••P•P•

AIRPOPS
BAGPIPE
FLIPUPS
GASPIPE
GODPAPA
ICEPOPS
LIMPOPO
OUTPIPE
OUTPOPS
PANPIPE
PETPUPS
PREPUPA
PVCPIPE
SLIPUPS
STEPUPS
THEPIPS
THEPOPE
WRAPUPS

•••P••P

AIRPUMP
BUMPSUP
CAMPSUP
CHIPSUP
CHOPSUP
COOPSUP
CREPTUP
CROPSUP
CROPTOP
DAMPMOP
DROPCAP
DROPTOP
FLIPTOP
GASPUMP
HEAPSUP
HELPSUP
JUMPSUP
KEEPSUP
KERPLOP
LEAPSUP
LEAPTUP
OUTPEEP
PROPSUP
PUMPSUP
RAMPSUP
SHAPEUP
SLIPSUP
SNAPSUP
SOAPSUP
SOUPSUP
STEPSUP
STOPGAP
STOPSUP
SWEPTUP
THEPUMP
TRIPSUP
WHIPSUP
WRAPSUP

••••PP•

AGRIPPA
BEHAPPY
ECHAPPE
FILIPPO
IMHAPPY
MAZEPPA
SCRAPPY
SCRIPPS
UNHAPPY

••••P•P

AFROPOP
ALCOPOP
BLOWPOP
BRITPOP
CREEPUP
EUROPOP
IGGYPOP
SODAPOP
SWEEPUP
TRUMPUP

•••••PP

SCHLEPP

PQ•••••

PQRSTUV

P•Q••••	PREAGES	PREMEDS	PRETZEL	PRIZING	PROSAIC	PARDONS	PERCHER	PHRASED	PYRITIC	POURERS	PROARAB	PHILTRE
PDQBACH	PREALLY	PREMEET	PREVAIL	PRIZZIS	PROSCAN	PARENTS	PERCHES	PHRASES	PYRRHIC	POURING	PROGRAM	PHONERS
PEQUOTS	PREAMPS	PREMIER	PREVENT	PROARAB	PROSERS	PARFAIT	PERCHIK	PHRENIC	PYRRHUS	POUROUT	PUBERTY	PIASTRE
PIQUANT	PREARMS	PREMIES	PREVERB	PROBALL	PROSHOP	PARFIVE	PERCUSS	PHRYGIA		POURSIN	PUSHROD	PICCARD
PIQUING	PREAVER	PREMISE	PREVERT	PROBATE	PROSIER	PARFOUR	PERDIDO	PIRAEUS	**P••R•••**	PRERACE		PICKERS
	PREBADE	PREMISS	PREVETO	PROBERS	PROSILY	PARFUMS	PERDIEM	PIRANHA	PADRAIC	PRERENT	**P••••R•**	PICTURE
P••Q•••	PREBAKE	PREMIUM	PREVIAS	PROBIES	PROSING	PARGERS	PERDITA	PIRATED	PADRONE	PRERIOT	PACKARD	PIECERS
PACQUIN	PREBIDS	PRENAME	PREVIEW	PROBING	PROSODY	PARGING	PERDURE	PIRATES	PAIRERS	PREROCK	PACKERS	PIGGERY
PARQUET	PREBILL	PRENOON	PREVOID	PROBITY	PROSPER	PARIAHS	PERETTI	PIRATIC	PAIRING	PRORATA	PADDERS	PILFERS
PLAQUES	PREBIND	PRENUPS	PREVOST	PROBLEM	PROTEAM	PARIBUS	PERFECT	PIRELLI	PAIROFF	PRORATE	PAIRERS	PILLARS
POPQUIZ	PREBOIL	PREOMIT	PREVUED	PROBONO	PROTEAN	PARINGS	PERFIDY	PIROGEN	PAIRSUP	PTEROUS	PALABRA	PILLORY
PREQUEL	PREBOOK	PREOPEN	PREVUES	PROBOWL	PROTECT	PARKADE	PERFORM	PIROGUE	PAPRIKA	PUERILE	PALEDRY	PINCERS
	PREBOOM	PREORAL	PREWARM	PROCEED	PROTEGE	PARKAVE	PERFUME	PORCHES	PARRIED	PURRERS	PALLORS	PINCURL
P•••Q••	PREBORN	PREPACK	PREWARN	PROCESS	PROTEIN	PARKERS	PERFUMY	PORCINE	PARRIER	PURRING	PALMARY	PINGERS
PRESQUE	PREBURN	PREPAID	PREWASH	PROCITY	PROTEST	PARKING	PERFUSE	PORGIES	PARRIES	PUTREFY	PALMERS	PINNERS
	PREBUYS	PREPARE	PREWHIP	PROCLUS	PROTEUS	PARKINS	PERGOLA	PORIVER	PARRING	PYRRHIC	PALMYRA	PIPCARD
P••••Q•	PRECAST	PREPAVE	PREWIRE	PROCTER	PROTIST	PARKMAN	PERHAPS	PORKERS	PARRISH	PYRRHUS	PALTERS	PISARRO
POSSLQS	PRECEDE	PREPAYS	PREWITT	PROCTOR	PROTONS	PARKSIT	PERIAPT	PORKIER	PARROTS		PAMPERS	PISMIRE
PSANDQS	PRECEPT	PREPLAN	PREWORK	PROCURE	PROUDER	PARKWAY	PERIDOT	PORKING	PATRICE	**P•••R••**	PANDERS	PITIERS
	PRECISE	PREPLOT	PREWORN	PROCYON	PROUDLY	PARLAYS	PERIGEE	PORKISH	PATRICK	PACKRAT	PANDORA	PIZARRO
•PQ••••	PRECITE	PREPPED	PREWRAP	PRODDED	PROUDOF	PARLEYS	PERILED	PORKPIE	PATRIES	PALERMO	PANIERS	PLACARD
OPQRSTU	PRECODE	PREPPIE	PREXIES	PRODDER	PROVEIT	PARLORS	PERIODS	PORSCHE	PATRIOT	PALFREY	PANNERS	PLACERS
UPQUARK	PRECOIL	PREPUPA	PREYERS	PRODIGY	PROVERB	PARLOUR	PERISSA	PORSENA	PATROLS	PALTROW	PANTERA	PLANERS
	PRECOOK	PREQUEL	PREYING	PRODSON	PROVERS	PARLOUS	PERITUS	PORTAGE	PATRONS	PANARAB	PANTERS	PLATERS
•P•Q•••	PRECOOL	PRERACE	PREYSON	PRODUCE	PROVIDE	PARODIC	PERIWIG	PORTALS	PATROON	PANGRAM	PANZERS	PLAYERS
EPOQUES	PRECOUP	PRERENT	PRFIRMS	PRODUCT	PROVINE	PAROLED	PERJURE	PORTEND	PAYRATE	PANURGE	PAPIERS	PLECTRA
OPAQUES	PRECURE	PRERIOT	PRICERS	PROEAST	PROVING	PAROLEE	PERJURY	PORTENT	PAYROLL	PAPERED	PARGERS	PLENARY
	PRECUTS	PREROCK	PRICIER	PROFANE	PROVISO	PAROLES	PERKIER	PORTERS	PEARLED	PAPERER	PARKERS	PLEXORS
••PQ•••	PREDARK	PRESAGE	PRICILY	PROFARM	PROVOKE	PARONYM	PERKILY	PORTHOS	PEARLER	PAPYRUS	PARLORS	PLOVERS
NOPQRST	PREDATA	PRESALE	PRICING	PROFESS	PROVOST	PAROTID	PERKING	PORTICO	PEARSON	PARURES	PARSERS	PLOWERS
POPQUIZ	PREDATE	PRESALT	PRICKED	PROFFER	PROWESS	PARQUET	PERKINS	PORTING	PEERAGE	PATERNO	PASSERS	POISERS
	PREDAWN	PRESEAL	PRICKLE	PROFILE	PROWEST	PARRIED	PERKISH	PORTION	PEERESS	PCWORLD	PASTERN	POLLARD
•••PQ••	PREDEFY	PRESEAT	PRICKLY	PROFITS	PROWLED	PARRIER	PERKSUP	PORTMAN	PEERING	PERORAL	PASTERS	POLLERA
MNOPQRS	PREDENY	PRESELL	PRICKUP	PROFUSE	PROWLER	PARRIES	PERLITE	PORTNOY	PEEROUT	PETARDS	PASTORS	POLLERS
	PREDICT	PRESENT	PRIDING	PROGENY	PROXIES	PARRING	PERLMAN	PORTRAY	PEERSAT	PETCROW	PASTURE	POMMARD
•••P•Q•	PREDIET	PRESETS	PRIESTS	PROGRAM	PROXIMA	PARRISH	PERMIAN	PORSTUV	PEERSIN	PETERED	PATSDRY	PONDERS
COMPAQS	PREDIVE	PRESHIP	PRIMACY	PROJECT	PROXIMO	PARROTS	PERMING	PURCELL	PENROSE	PETERII	PATTERN	PONIARD
	PREDOOM	PRESHOW	PRIMARY	PROJETS	PRUDENT	PARSECS	PERMITS	PURDUEU	PEORIAN	PETFROG	PATTERS	POOLERS
••••PQ•	PREDUSK	PRESIDE	PRIMATE	PROKEDS	PRUDERY	PARSEES	PERMUTE	PURFLED	PERREAU	PGAPROS	PATZERS	POPCORN
LMNOPQR	PREEDIT	PRESIFT	PRIMELY	PROLATE	PRUDHOE	PARSERS	PERORAL	PURFLER	PERRIER	PICARAS	PAULPRY	POPLARS
	PREEMIE	PRESLEY	PRIMERA	PROLIFE	PRUDISH	PARSING	PERPLEX	PURFLES	PERRINE	PICARDO	PAUPERS	POPPERS
•••••PQ	PREEMPT	PRESOAK	PRIMERO	PROLOGS	PRUNERS	PARSLEY	PERREAU	PURGING	PERRINS	PICARDY	PAUSERS	POPTART
KLMNOPQ	PREENED	PRESOLD	PRIMERS	PROLONG	PRUNING	PARSNIP	PERRIER	PURISTS	PETRATS	PICAROS	PAVIORS	PORKERS
	PREENER	PRESONG	PRIMING	PROMBID	PRUSSIA	PARSONS	PERRINE	PURITAN	PETRELS	PIERROT	PAWNERS	PORTERS
PR•••••	PREFABS	PRESORT	PRIMMED	PROMISE	PRYINTO	PARTAKE	PERRINS	PURLIEU	PETRIFY	PIETROS	PAYDIRT	POSEURS
PRACTIC	PREFACE	PRESPUR	PRIMMER	PROMOED	PRYOPEN	PARTIAL	PERSEID	PURLING	PETROCK	PIGIRON	PAYMORE	POSTERN
PRADESH	PREFADE	PRESQUE	PRIMPED	PROMOTE		PARTIED	PERSEUS	PURLOIN	PETROLS	PILCROW	PCUSERS	POSTERS
PRAETOR	PREFECT	PRESSED	PRINCES	PROMPTS	**P•R••••**	PARTIER	PERSIAN	PURPLED	PETROUS	PILGRIM	PECCARY	POSTURE
PRAIRIE	PREFERS	PRESSEL	PRINGLE	PRONATE	PARABLE	PARTIES	PERSIST	PURPLES	PHARAOH	PISARRO	PEEKERS	POTHERB
PRAISED	PREFILE	PRESSER	PRINKED	PRONAVY	PARADED	PARTIII	PERSIUS	PURPORT	PHARLAP	PITCREW	PEELERS	POTHERS
PRAISER	PREFORM	PRESSES	PRINKER	PRONELY	PARADER	PARTING	PERSOFF	PURPOSE	PHARYNX	PIZARRO	PEEPERS	POTTERS
PRAISES	PREFUND	PRESSON	PRINTAD	PRONETO	PARADES	PARTITA	PERSONA	PURRERS	PIERCED	PLEURAE	PELTERS	POTTERY
PRALINE	PREGAIN	PRESSUP	PRINTED	PRONGED	PARADOR	PARTITE	PERSONS	PURRING	PIERCER	PLEURAL	PENNERS	POULTRY
PRANCED	PREGAME	PRESTON	PRINTER	PRONOUN	PARADOX	PARTNER	PERSSON	PURSERS	PIERCES	POIVRES	PEPPARD	POURERS
PRANCER	PREHEAL	PRESTOS	PRINTUP	PROOFED	PARAGON	PARTONE	PERTAIN	PURSIER	PIERIAN	POLARAS	PEPPERS	POUTERS
PRANCES	PREHEAT	PRESUME	PRIORTO	PROOFER	PARAIBA	PARTOOK	PERTEST	PURSING	PIERROT	POLARIS	PEPPERY	POWDERS
PRATERS	PREIDEA	PRETAPE	PRISONS	PROPANE	PARAMUS	PARTTWO	PERTURB	PURSUED	PITROWS	PORTRAY	PERDURE	POWDERY
PRATING	PRELACY	PRETEEN	PRISSES	PROPELS	PARAPET	PARTWAY	PERUGIA	PURSUER	PLURALS	POUDRES	PERFORM	PRATERS
PRATTLE	PRELATE	PRETELL	PRITHEE	PROPHET	PARAPHS	PARTYER	PERUKES	PURSUES	PODRIDA	POVERTY	PERJURE	PRAYERS
PRAWNED	PRELIFE	PRETEND	PRIUSES	PROPJET	PARASKI	PARTYON	PERUSAL	PURSUIT	POORBOX	POWERED	PERJURY	PREBORN
PRAYERS	PRELIMS	PRETERM	PRIVACY	PROPMAN	PARASOL	PARURES	PERUSED	PURTIER	POORBOY	POWERUP	PERTURB	PREBURN
PRAYFOR	PRELOAD	PRETEST	PRIVATE	PROPMEN	PARATUS	PARVENU	PERUSER	PURVEYS	POOREST	PRAIRIE	PESTERS	PRECURE
PRAYING	PRELOAN	PRETEXT	PRIVETS	PROPONE	PARBAKE	PERAHIA	PERUSES	PURVIEW	POORISH	PREARMS	PETBIRD	PREDARK
PRAYSTO	PRELOSS	PRETIRE	PRIVIER	PROPOSE	PARBOIL	PERATIO	PERVADE	PYRAMID	POORLAW	PREORAL	PETHARE	PREFERS
PREACHY	PRELUDE	PRETOLD	PRIVIES	PROPPED	PARCELS	PERCALE	PERWEEK	PYRAMUS	POORMAN	PRETRIM	PETTERS	PREFORM
PREACID	PREMADE	PRETORS	PRIVILY	PROPSUP	PARCHED	PERCENT	PERYEAR	PYRETIC	POORMEN	PREWRAP	PEWTERS	PREPARE
PREACTS	PREMAKE	PRETRIM	PRIVITY	PRORATA	PARCHES	PERCEPT	PGRATED	PYREXIA	POORTAX	PRFIRMS	PHAEDRA	PRESORT
PREAGED	PREMATE	PRETYPE	PRIVYTO	PRORATE	PARDNER	PERCHED	PHRASAL	PYRITES	POPROCK	PRIORTO	PHASERS	PRETERM

PRETIRE
PRETORS
PREVERB
PREVERT
PREWARM
PREWARN
PREWIRE
PREWORK
PREWORN
PREYERS
PRICERS
PRIMARY
PRIMERA
PRIMERO
PRIMERS
PROBERS
PROCURE
PROFARM
PROSERS
PROVERB
PROVERS
PRUDERY
PRUNERS
PSYWARS
PUCKERS
PUCKERY
PUFFERS
PUFFERY
PULLERS
PULPERS
PULSARS
PUMPERS
PUNKERS
PUNNERS
PUNTERS
PURPORT
PURRERS
PURSERS
PUSHERS
PUTTERS

P•••••R

PACECAR
PADDLER
PAIDFOR
PAINTER
PALAVER
PALLIER
PALMIER
PALOMAR
PANNIER
PANTHER
PAPERER
PARADER
PARADOR
PARDNER
PARFOUR
PARLOUR
PARRIER
PARTIER
PARTNER
PARTYER
PASSFOR
PASTEUR
PASTIER
PATCHER
PAVIOUR
PAYSFOR
PEAKIER
PEARLER
PEATIER
PEDALER
PEDDLER
PEPPIER
PERCHER
PERKIER
PERRIER
PERUSER
PERYEAR
PESKIER
PETBEAR
PETDEER
PETDOOR
PETHAIR
PETTIER
PGATOUR
PHATTER
PHILTER
PHISHER
PHONIER
PIASTER
PICADOR
PICKIER
PIERCER
PIGGIER
PILSNER
PINCHER
PINEFOR
PINETAR
PIONEER
PITCHER
PITHIER
PIVOTER
PLAINER
PLAISIR
PLAITER
PLANFOR
PLANNER
PLANTAR
PLANTER
PLASTER
PLATIER
PLATTER
PLEADER
PLEASER
PLEDGER
PLODDER
PLOTTER
PLUGGER
PLUMBER
PLUMIER
PLUMMER
PLUMPER
PLUNDER
PLUNGER
PLUNKER
PLUSHER
POACHER
POINTER
POITIER
POLANER
POLECAR
POLICER
POLITER
POLYMER
POPOVER
POPSTAR
POPULAR
PORIVER
PORKIER
POSTWAR
POTTIER
POUNCER
POUNDER
POUTIER
PRAETOR
PRAISER
PRANCER
PRAYFOR
PREAVER
PREENER
PREMIER
PRESPUR
PRESSER
PRICIER
PRIMMER
PRINKER
PRINTER
PRIVIER
PROCTER
PROCTOR
PRODDER
PROFFER
PROOFER
PROSIER
PROSPER
PROUDER
PROWLER
PSALTER
PUDGIER
PUFFIER
PULLFOR
PULPIER
PUNCHER
PUNKIER
PUNNIER
PUNSTER
PURFLER
PURSIER
PURSUER
PURTIER
PUSHFOR
PUSHIER
PUTOVER
PUZZLER

•PR••••

APRICOT
APRIORI
APRONED
APROPOS
SPRAINS
SPRAWLS
SPRAWLY
SPRAYED
SPRAYER
SPRAYON
SPREADS
SPRIEST
SPRINGS
SPRINGY
SPRINTS
SPRITES
SPROUTS
SPRUCED
SPRUCER
SPRUCES
SPRYEST
UPRAISE
UPRATED
UPRATES
UPREACH
UPREARS
UPRIGHT
UPRISEN
UPRISER
UPRISES
UPRIVER
UPROARS
UPROOTS
UPROUSE

•P•R•••

APERCUS
APERIES
APERSON
APPRISE
APPROVE
EPARCHS
EPARCHY
EPERGNE
EPERNAY
EPHRAIM
IPCRESS
OPERAND
OPERANT
OPERATE
OPEROSE
OPPRESS
OPQRSTU
SPARELY
SPAREME
SPARERS
SPAREST
SPARING
SPARKED
SPARKLE
SPARKLY
SPARRED
SPARRER
SPARROW
SPARSER
SPARTAN
SPIRALS
SPIREAS
SPIRIER
SPIRITS
SPORRAN
SPORTED
SPORTIN
SPURNED
SPURNER
SPURRED
SPURSON
SPURTED
SPYRING
UPBRAID
UPDRAFT
UPDRIED
UPDRIES
UPDRIFT
UPFRONT
UPGRADE
UPGROWN
UPGROWS
UPOROUT
UPPROPS
UPTRADE
UPTREND

•P••R••

APAIROF
APPARAT
APPAREL
APTERAL
APTERYX
EPIGRAM
EPPERLY
MPTHREE
SPARRED
SPARRER
SPARROW
SPEARED
SPEARER
SPHERAL
SPHERED
SPHERES
SPHERIC
SPLURGE
SPORRAN
SPURRED
UPATREE
UPBORNE
UPBURST
UPCARDS
UPCURLS
UPCURVE
UPDARTS
UPEARLY
UPFIRST
UPFORIT
UPGIRDS
UPNORTH
UPSURGE
UPTHROW
UPTURNS
UPWARDS

•P•••R•

APPEARS
APRIORI
EPHEDRA
EPICARP
EPICURE
EPIDERM
OPENERS
OPINERS
SPACERS
SPADERS
SPARERS
SPAYERS
SPECTRA
SPECTRE
SPEWERS
SPICERS
SPICERY
SPIDERS
SPIDERY
SPIKERS
SPINDRY
SPYDERS
SPYWARE
UPBEARS
UPCOURT
UPHOARD
UPQUARK
UPREARS
UPROARS
UPSOARS
UPSTARE
UPSTART
UPSTIRS
UPTEARS
UPTHERE
UPWHIRL

•P••••R

APPLIER
OPENAIR
OPENBAR
OPPOSER
OPTSFOR
SPACIER
SPAMMER
SPANAIR
SPANKER
SPANNER
SPARRER
SPARSER
SPATTER
SPAWNER
SPEAKER
SPEARER
SPECTER
SPECTOR
SPEEDER
SPELLER
SPENCER
SPENDER
SPENSER
SPICIER
SPIELER
SPIKIER
SPILLER
SPINIER
SPINNER
SPIRIER
SPITTER
SPLICER
SPOILER
SPONGER
SPONSOR
SPOOFER
SPOOLER
SPOONER
SPOTTER
SPOUTER
SPRAYER
SPRUCER
SPUMIER
SPURNER
SPUTTER
UPDATER
UPRISER
UPRIVER
UPSTAIR
UPTOPAR

••PR•••

APPRISE
APPROVE
ASPRAWL
BYPROXY
CAPRICE
CAPRINE
CUPRITE
CUPROUS
CYPRESS
CYPRIAN
CYPRIOT
DEPRAVE
DEPRESS
DEPRIVE
ELPRADO
EMPRESS
EMPRISE
ENPRISE
ESPRITS
EXPRESS
HIPROOF
IMPRESS
IMPREST
IMPREZA
IMPRINT
IMPROVE
INPRINT
LAPROBE
LIPREAD
OPPRESS
OSPREYS
PAPRIKA
POPROCK
REPRESS
REPRICE
REPRIME
REPRINT
REPRISE
REPROBE
REPROOF
REPROVE
REPRUNE
RIPRAPS
SOPRANI
SOPRANO
SUPREME
TAPROOM
TAPROOT
TOPRANK
TOPRATE
TOPROWS
UNPROUD
UPPROPS

••P•R••

AMPERES
APPARAT
APPAREL
ASPERSE
ASPIRED
ASPIRER
ASPIRES
ASPIRIN
CAPERED
DEPARTS
DEPORTS
EMPEROR
EMPIRES
EMPIRIC
EMPIRIN
EMPORIA
EPPERLY
ESPARTO
EXPARTE
EXPERTS
EXPIRED
EXPIRES
EXPORTS
HEPARIN
HYPERON
IMPARTS
IMPERIL
IMPORTS
IMPURER
INPERIL
LAPERMS
LAPORTE
LIPARIS
NEPHRIC
NOPQRST
PAPERED
PAPERER
PAPYRUS
REPARKS
REPERKS
REPORTS
RVPARKS
SEPIRAS
SUPERGS
TAPERED
TOPDRAW
UMPIRED
UMPIRES
UNPARED
VAPORED
VAPORER
VAPORUB

••P••R•

ALPHARD
AMPHORA
APPEARS
AUPAIRS
BOPPERS
CAPPERS
CAPTORS
CAPTURE
CIPHERS
COPCARS
COPIERS
COPPERS
COPPERY
COPTERS
CYPHERS
DEPLORE
DIPPERS
EXPLORE
FOPPERY
GOPHERS
GYPPERS
HEPBURN
HOPPERS
HUPPERT
IMPAIRS
IMPLORE
INPOURS
KAPTURE
KIPPERS
LAPPERS
LAPSERS
LAPWARE
LEPPARD
LIPPERS
LOPPERS
MAPPERS
MOPPERS
MRPADRE
NAPIERS
NAPPERS
NIPPERS
PAPIERS
PEPPARD
PEPPERS
PEPPERY
PIPCARD
POPCORN
POPLARS
POPPERS
POPTART
RAPIERS
RAPPERS
RAPPORT
RAPTORS
RAPTURE
REPAIRS
REPOURS
RIPCORD
RIPPERS
RIPTORN
RUPTURE
SAPPERS
SAPPORO
SIPPERS
SUPPERS
SUPPORT
TAPPERS
TIPCART
TIPJARS
TIPPERS
TOPFORM
TOPIARY
TOPPERS
VAPOURS
VAPOURY
YAPPERS
ZAPPERS
ZEPHYRS
ZIPPERS

••P•••R

ALPINER
APPLIER
ASPIRER
BIPOLAR
COPULAR
CUPELER
CUPPIER
CUPULAR
DEPONER
DEPOSER
DEPOWER
DIPOLAR
DIPPIER
DOPPLER
EMPEROR
EMPOWER
EMPTIER
EXPOSER
HAPPIER
HIPPIER
HIPSTER
HOPEFOR
HOPOVER
HOPPIER
IIPETER
IMPALER
IMPEDER
IMPOSER
IMPURER
IMPUTER
INPOWER
JDPOWER
JUPITER
LIPPIER
LOPPIER
MCPAPER
NAPPIER
NAPSTER
NIPPIER
ONPAPER
OPPOSER
PAPERER
PEPPIER
POPOVER
POPSTAR
POPULAR
RAPIDER
RAPSTAR
REPAPER
REPINER
REPLIER
REPOSER
REPOWER
REPSFOR
RIPENER
SAPPIER
SOPPIER
STPETER
SUPPLER
TAPSTER
TIPOVER
TIPPIER
TIPPLER
TIPSIER
TIPSTER
VAPORER
ZAPPIER
ZIPPIER

•••PR••

CULPRIT
DEEPRED
INAPRIL
LAMPREY
MAUPRAT
NONPROS
OLDPROS
OUTPRAY
PGAPROS
RESPRAY
SAMPRAS

•••P•R•

AIRPARK
AIRPORT
BBQPORK
BEEPERS
BITPART
BOPPERS
BUMPERS
CAMPARI
CAMPERS
CAPPERS
CARPARK
CARPERS
CARPORT
CASPARY
CLIPART
COMPARE
COMPART
COMPERE
COMPORT
COOPERS
COOPERY
COPPERS
COPPERY
CORPORA
DAMPDRY
DAMPERS
DEEPFRY
DIAPERS
DIPPERS
DISPART
DISPORT
DRAPERS
DRAPERY
DRIPDRY
DRYPERS
DUMPERS
ELOPERS
EXUPERY
FOPPERY
GASPARD
GASPERS
GAWPERS
GOMPERS
GRAPERY
GRIPERS
GROPERS
GULPERS
GYPPERS
HAMPERS
HARPERS
HEAPERS
HELPERS
HOOPERS
HOPPERS
HUMPHRY
HUPPERT
INSPIRE
JASPERS
JASPERY
JEEPERS
JETPORT
JUMPERS
KEEPERS
KIPPERS
LAMPERT
LAPPERS
LEAPERS
LEMPIRA
LEOPARD
LEPPARD
LIPPERS
LISPERS
LOOPERS
LOPPERS
LUMPERS
MAPPERS
MNOPQRS
MOPPERS
NAPPERS
NEWPORT
NIPPERS
NONPARS
OAKPARK
ONEPART
OUTPORT
OUTPURL
OVIPARA
PAMPERS
PAUPERS
PEEPERS
PEPPARD
PEPPERS
PEPPERY
POPPERS
PREPARE
PULPERS
PUMPERS
PURPORT
RAMPART
RAPPERS
RAPPORT
RASPERS
REAPERS
RESPARK
RESPIRE
RIPPERS
ROMPERS
SAPPERS
SAPPORO
SCEPTRE
SEAPORT
SHAPERS
SHAPIRO
SHEPARD
SIMPERS
SIPPERS
SLOPERS
SNIPERS
SOAPERS
SOUPERS
STUPORS
SUPPERS
SUPPORT
SUSPIRE
SWIPERS
TAMPERS
TAPPERS
TEMPERA
TEMPERS
TEMPORE
TEMPURA
TIPPERS
TOPPERS
TOSPARE
TWOPART
VAMPERS
VAMPIRA
VAMPIRE
VESPERS
WARPERS
WEEPERS
YAPPERS
YAWPERS
YELPERS
ZAPPERS
ZIPPERS

•••P••R

ADAPTER
ADAPTOR
ADEPTER
ADOPTER
BUMPIER
CAMPHOR
CAMPIER
CHAPTER
CHIPPER
CHOPPER
CLAPFOR
CLAPPER
CLIPPER
COMPEER
COUPLER
CROPPER
CRUPPER
CUPPIER
DESPAIR
DIOPTER
DIPPIER
DOPPLER
DRIPPER
DROPPER
DUMPIER
ERUPTER
FLAPPER
FLIPPER
FLOPPER
GOOPIER
GRAPIER
GRIPPER
GULPIER
HAPPIER
HEMPIER
HIPPIER
HOPPIER
HUMPIER
INAPTER
JUMPIER
LEAPFOR
LIPPIER
LOOPIER
LOPPIER
LOWPAIR
LUMPIER
NAPPIER
NIPPIER
NONPOOR
ONEPAIR
OUTPOUR
PEPPIER
PULPIER
QUIPPER
RASPIER

SAMPLER
SAPPIER
SCEPTER
SCUPPER
SEEPIER
SHIPPER
SHOPFOR
SHOPPER
SIMPLER
SKIPPER
SLAPPER
SLIPPER
SNAPPER
SNIPPER
SOAPIER
SOPPIER
SOUPIER
STAPLER
STEPPER
STOPFOR
STOPPER
SULPHUR
SUPPLER
SWAPPER
TEMPLAR
TEMPTER
TIPPIER
TIPPLER
TRAPPER
TRIPPER
TWOPAIR
VAMPIER
WASPIER
WEEPFOR
WEEPIER
WHIPPER
WHOPPER
WIMPIER
WISPIER
WRAPPER
ZAPPIER
ZIPPIER

••••PR•

GOESPRO
GOLFPRO
GONEPRO
PAULPRY
SEMIPRO
TURNPRO
WENTPRO

••••P•R

BLEEPER
BLOOPER
CALIPER
CHAMPER
CHEAPER
CHEEPER
CHIPPER
CHIRPER
CHOPPER
CLAMPER
CLAPPER
CLASPER
CLIPPER
CREEPER
CRIMPER
CRISPER
CROPPER
CRUPPER
DNIEPER
DRIPPER
DROPPER
ESCAPER
EVENPAR
FLAPPER
FLIPPER
FLOPPER
GRASPER
GRIPPER
GROUPER
HANAPER
HOTSPUR
JODHPUR
JUNIPER
LMNOPQR
MADEPAR
MAKEPAR
MANIPUR
MCPAPER
NEARPAR
ONPAPER
OVERPAR
PLUMPER
PRESPUR
PROSPER
QUIPPER
REPAPER
SCALPER
SCAMPER
SCOOPER
SCRAPER
SCUPPER
SHARPER
SHIPPER
SHOPPER
SHOTPAR
SKIPPER
SLAPPER
SLEEPER
SLIPPER
SLURPER
SNAPPER
SNIPPER
SNOOPER
STAMPER
STEEPER
STEPPER
STOOPER
STOPPER
STRIPER
STUMPER
SWAPPER
SWEEPER
SWOOPER
THUMPER
TRAMPER
TRAPPER
TRIPPER
TROOPER
TROUPER
UNRIPER
UPTOPAR
USURPER
WHIMPER
WHIPPER
WHISPER
WHOOPER
WHOPPER
WRAPPER

PS•••••

PSALMIC
PSALTER
PSANDQS
PSHAWED
PSYCHED
PSYCHES
PSYCHIC
PSYCHOS
PSYCHUP
PSYWARS

P•S••••

PASALLE
PASCHAL
PASCOLI
PASSADE
PASSADO
PASSAGE
PASSAIC
PASSANT
PASSATS
PASSELS
PASSERS
PASSEUL
PASSFOR
PASSING
PASSION
PASSIVE
PASSKEY
PASSOFF
PASSOUT
PASTDUE
PASTEIN
PASTELS
PASTERN
PASTERS
PASTEUP
PASTEUR
PASTIER
PASTIES
PASTIME
PASTINA
PASTING
PASTORS
PASTURE
PESADES
PESANTE
PESETAS
PESEWAS
PESKIER
PESKILY
PESTERS
PESTLED
PESTLES
PISANIO
PISARRO
PISCEAN
PISCINE
PISCOPO
PISHING
PISMIRE
PISTILS
PISTOLE
PISTOLS
PISTONS
PISTOUS
POSABLE
POSADAS
POSEDAS
POSESAS
POSEURS
POSEUSE
POSHEST
POSITED
POSOLES
POSSESS
POSSLQS
POSSUMS
POSTAGE
POSTBAG
POSTBOX
POSTDOC
POSTERN
POSTERS
POSTFIX
POSTHOC
POSTIES
POSTING
POSTITS
POSTMAN
POSTMEN
POSTOPS
POSTURE
POSTWAR
PUSHERS
PUSHFOR
PUSHFUL
PUSHIER
PUSHILY
PUSHING
PUSHKIN
PUSHOFF
PUSHOUT
PUSHPIN
PUSHROD
PUSHUPS
PUSSIES

P••S•••

PADSITE
PAISANO
PAISANS
PAISLEY
PANSIES
PANSOUT
PARSECS
PARSEES
PARSERS
PARSING
PARSLEY
PARSNIP
PARSONS
PASSADE
PASSADO
PASSAGE
PASSAIC
PASSANT
PASSATS
PASSELS
PASSERS
PASSEUL
PASSFOR
PASSING
PASSION
PASSIVE
PASSKEY
PASSOFF
PASSOUT
PATSDRY
PATSIES
PAUSERS
PAUSING
PAYSFOR
PAYSLIP
PAYSNOW
PAYSOFF
PAYSOUT
PAYSTUB
PCUSERS
PEASANT
PEASOUP
PENSEES
PENSION
PENSIVE
PEPSICO
PEPSINS
PERSEID
PERSEUS
PERSIAN
PERSIST
PERSIUS
PERSOFF
PERSONA
PERSONS
PERSSON
PETSCAN
PETSHOP
PETSITS
PHASEIN
PHASERS
PHASING
PHISHED
PHISHER
PHISHES
PHYSICS
PIASTER
PIASTRE
PIESAFE
PIESALE
PIGSKIN
PIGSOUT
PILSNER
PINSEAL
PIOSITY
PITSAWS
PITSTOP
PIUSIII
PIUSVII
PIUSXII
PLASHED
PLASHES
PLASMAS
PLASMIC
PLASTER
PLASTIC
PLISSES
PLOSION
PLOSIVE
PLUSHER
PLUSHES
PLUSHLY
PLUSONE
PLUSSES
PLUSTAX
PLUSTWO
POESIES
POISERS
POISING
POISONS
POISSON
POPSOFF
POPSONG
POPSOUT
POPSTAR
PORSCHE
PORSENA
POSSESS
POSSLQS
POSSUMS
POTSDAM
POTSHOT
POUSSIN
PQRSTUV
PRESAGE
PRESALE
PRESALT
PRESEAL
PRESEAT
PRESELL
PRESENT
PRESETS
PRESHIP
PRESHOW
PRESIDE
PRESIFT
PRESLEY
PRESOAK
PRESOLD
PRESONG
PRESORT
PRESPUR
PRESQUE
PRESSED
PRESSEL
PRESSER
PRESSES
PRESSON
PRESSUP
PRESTON
PRESTOS
PRESUME
PRISONS
PRISSES
PROSAIC
PROSCAN
PROSERS
PROSHOP
PROSIER
PROSILY
PROSING
PROSODY
PROSPER
PRUSSIA
PUGSLEY
PULSARS
PULSATE
PULSING
PUNSTER
PURSERS
PURSIER
PURSING
PURSUED
PURSUER
PURSUES
PURSUIT
PUSSIES
PUTSOFF
PUTSOUT

P•••S••

PACKSIN
PACKSON
PACKSUP
PAGESIX
PAIRSUP
PAPISTS
PARASKI
PARASOL
PARKSIT
PAULSEN
PEARSON
PECKSAT
PEEKSAT
PEEKSIN
PEEPSAT
PEERSAT
PEERSIN
PEGASUS
PELISSE
PERISSA
PERKSUP
PERSSON
PERUSAL
PERUSED
PERUSER
PERUSES
PHRASAL
PHRASED
PHRASES
PICASSO
PICKSAT
PICKSON
PICKSUP
PILESIN
PILESOF
PILESON
PILESUP
PIMESON
PINESAP
PINESOL
PIOUSLY
PIPESIN
PIPESUP
PLAISIR
PLANSON
PLANSTO
PLAYSAT
PLAYSBY
PLAYSON
PLAYSTO
PLAYSUP
PLEASED
PLEASER
PLEASES
PLISSES
PLOESTI
PLOWSON
PLOWSUP
PLUGSIN
PLUGSUP
PLUSSES
POISSON
POKESAT
POLESAT
POLESIT
POLISCI
POLYSCI
POOPSIE
POSESAS
POURSIN
POUSSIN
PRAISED
PRAISER
PRAISES
PRAYSTO
PRESSED
PRESSEL
PRESSER
PRESSES
PRESSON
PRESSUP
PREYSON
PRIESTS
PRISSES
PRIUSES
PRODSON
PROPSUP
PRUSSIA
PUFFSUP
PULASKI
PULLSIN
PULLSON
PULLSUP
PUMPSUP
PURISTS

P••••S•

PACHISI
PACIEST
PALMIST
PANFISH
PAPOOSE
PARRISH
PATCASH
PATNESS
PAULIST
PAYCASH
PAYLESS
PEAKISH
PECKISH
PEERESS
PEEVISH
PEGLESS
PELISSE
PELTISH
PENCASE
PENROSE
PERCUSS
PERFUSE
PERISSA
PERKISH
PERSIST
PERTEST
PETFISH
PETTISH
PIANISM
PIANIST
PICASSO
PICTISH
PIETOSO
PIGFISH
PIGGISH
PINIEST
PINKEST
PINKISH
PINLESS
PIPIEST
PIPLESS
PITBOSS
PIXYISH
PLANISH
PLENISH
PLUMOSE
PODCAST
POETESS
POETISE
POKIEST
POLOIST
POOREST
POORISH
PORKISH
POSEUSE
POSHEST
POSSESS
PRADESH
PRECAST
PRECISE
PREDUSK
PRELOSS
PREMISE
PREMISS
PRETEST
PREVOST
PREWASH
PROCESS
PROEAST
PROFESS
PROFUSE
PROMISE
PROPOSE
PROTEST
PROTIST
PROVISO
PROVOST
PROWESS
PROWEST
PRUDISH
PUBLISH
PUCKISH
PUGGISH
PUGNOSE
PUNIEST
PUNLESS
PURPOSE

P•••••S

PAANGAS
PABLUMS
PACKERS
PACKETS
PADDERS
PADDIES
PADDLES
PADUANS
PAELLAS
PAGINGS
PAGODAS
PAIDADS
PAIRERS
PAISANS
PAIUTES
PAJAMAS
PALACES
PALAMAS
PALATES
PALINGS
PALLETS
PALLORS
PALMERS
PALOMAS
PALTERS
PAMPERS
PANADAS
PANAMAS
PANDERS
PANDITS
PANFULS
PANIERS
PANINIS
PANNERS
PANSIES
PANTERS
PANTIES
PANZERS
PAPAGOS
PAPAYAS
PAPELES
PAPIERS
PAPISTS
PAPPIES
PAPUANS
PAPYRUS
PARADES
PARAMUS
PARAPHS
PARATUS
PARCELS
PARCHES
PARDONS
PARENTS
PARFUMS
PARGERS
PARIAHS
PARIBUS
PARINGS
PARKERS
PARKINS
PARLAYS
PARLEYS
PARLORS
PARLOUS
PAROLES
PARRIES
PARROTS
PARSECS
PARSEES
PARSERS
PARSONS
PARTIES
PARURES
PASSATS
PASSELS
PASSERS
PASTELS
PASTERS
PASTIES
PASTORS
PATACAS
PATCHES
PATENTS
PATHANS
PATINAS
PATNESS
PATRIES
PATROLS
PATRONS
PATSIES
PATTERS
PATTIES
PATZERS
PAUPERS
PAUSERS
PAVANES
PAVINGS
PAVIORS
PAWNEES
PAWNERS
PAWPAWS
PAYCUTS
PAYDAYS
PAYLESS
PAYOFFS
PAYOLAS
PAYOUTS
PBANDJS
PCUSERS
PDJAMES
PEACHES
PEAHENS
PEANUTS
PEAPODS
PEBBLES
PECTINS
PEDANTS
PEDDLES
PEDWAYS
PEEBLES
PEEKERS
PEELERS
PEEPERS
PEEPLES
PEERESS
PEEWEES
PEGASUS
PEGLEGS
PEGLESS
PEGTOPS
PELAGES
PELLEAS
PELLETS
PELOTAS
PELTERS
PENATES
PENCILS
PENNERS
PENNEYS
PENNIES
PENNONS
PENPALS
PENSEES
PENTADS
PENTELS
PENULTS
PENZIAS
PEONIES
PEOPLES
PEPBOYS
PEPCIDS
PEPITAS
PEPLUMS
PEPPERS
PEPSINS
PEPTICS
PEQUOTS
PERCHES
PERCUSS
PERHAPS
PERIODS
PERITUS
PERKINS
PERMITS
PERRINS
PERSEUS
PERSIUS
PERSONS
PERUKES
PERUSES
PESADES
PESETAS
PESEWAS
PESTERS
PESTLES
PETALES
PETARDS
PETBOAS
PETCATS
PETCOWS
PETDOGS
PETITES
PETNAPS
PETPIGS
PETPUPS
PETRATS
PETRELS
PETROLS
PETROUS
PETSITS
PETTERS
PETTOYS
PEWTERS
PEYOTES
PGAPROS
PHASERS
PHEMIUS
PHENOLS
PHENOMS
PHIDIAS
PHILCOS
PHILEAS
PHILIPS
PHILOUS
PHINEAS
PHISHES
PHLOEMS
PHLOXES
PHOBIAS
PHOBICS
PHOEBES
PHOEBUS
PHONERS
PHONEYS
PHONICS
PHONIES
PHOTICS
PHOTOGS
PHOTONS
PHRASES
PHYLLIS
PHYLLOS
PHYSICS
PIAFFES
PIAZZAS
PICARAS
PICAROS
PICEOUS
PICKENS
PICKERS
PICKETS
PICKLES
PICKUPS
PICNICS
PIDDLES
PIDGINS
PIECERS
PIEPANS
PIERCES
PIETIES
PIETINS
PIETROS
PIFFLES
PIGEONS
PIGGIES
PIGLETS
PIGNUTS
PIGOUTS
PIGPENS
PILATES
PILATUS
PILEOUS
PILEUPS
PILFERS
PILINGS
PILLARS
PILLOWS
PIMPLES
PINATAS
PINBOYS
PINCERS
PINCHAS
PINCHES
PINGERS
PINIONS
PINKENS
PINKIES
PINKOES
PINLESS
PINNERS
PINOAKS
PINONES
PIOLETS
PIPAGES

PIPINGS
PIPLESS
PIPPINS
PIRAEUS
PIRATES
PISTILS
PISTOLS
PISTONS
PISTOUS
PITAYAS
PITBOSS
PITCHES
PITEOUS
PITIERS
PITROWS
PITSAWS
PLACERS
PLAGUES
PLAICES
PLAINES
PLAINTS
PLAKATS
PLANERS
PLANETS
PLAQUES
PLASHES
PLASMAS
PLATENS
PLATERS
PLATIES
PLAUTUS
PLAYERS
PLEASES
PLEDGES
PLENUMS
PLEXORS
PLIGHTS
PLINTHS
PLISSES
PLOTZES
PLOUGHS
PLOVERS
PLOWERS
PLUGINS
PLUNGES
PLURALS
PLUSHES
PLUSSES
PLUTONS
PNEUMAS
POACHES
POBOXES
POCKETS
POCONOS
PODIUMS
POESIES
POETESS
POETICS
POINTES
POISERS
POISONS
POIVRES
POLARAS
POLARIS
POLICES
POLLEES
POLLENS
POLLERS
POMADES
POMELOS
POMMELS
POMPOMS
POMPONS
POMPOUS
PONCHOS
PONDERS
PONGEES
PONGIDS
PONTIUS
POOCHES
POODLES
POOLERS
POPEYES
POPGUNS
POPLARS
POPLINS
POPOFFS
POPOUTS
POPPERS
POPPIES
POPPINS
POPPLES
POPTOPS
PORCHES
PORGIES
PORKERS
PORTALS
PORTERS
PORTHOS
POSADAS
POSEDAS
POSESAS
POSEURS
POSOLES
POSSESS
POSSLQS
POSSUMS
POSTERS
POSTIES
POSTITS
POSTOPS
POTAGES
POTAMUS
POTEENS
POTFULS
POTHERS
POTIONS
POTLIDS
POTPIES
POTTERS
POTTIES
POUCHES
POUDRES
POUNCES
POURERS
POUTERS
POWDERS
POWWOWS
POZOLES
PRAISES
PRANCES
PRATERS
PRAYERS
PREACTS
PREAGES
PREAMPS
PREARMS
PREBIDS
PREBUYS
PRECUTS
PREFABS
PREFERS
PRELIMS
PRELOSS
PREMEDS
PREMIES
PREMISS
PRENUPS
PREPAYS
PRESETS
PRESSES
PRESTOS
PRETORS
PREVIAS
PREVUES
PREXIES
PREYERS
PRFIRMS
PRICERS
PRIESTS
PRIMERS
PRINCES
PRISONS
PRISSES
PRIUSES
PRIVETS
PRIVIES
PRIZZIS
PROBERS
PROBIES
PROCESS
PROCLUS
PROFESS
PROFITS
PROJETS
PROKEDS
PROLOGS
PROMPTS
PROPELS
PROSERS
PROTEUS
PROTONS
PROVERS
PROWESS
PROXIES
PRUNERS
PSANDQS
PSYCHES
PSYCHOS
PSYWARS
PTBOATS
PTEROUS
PUBLICS
PUBLIUS
PUCKERS
PUDDLES
PUEBLOS
PUFFERS
PUFFINS
PUGGLES
PULLERS
PULLETS
PULLEYS
PULLINS
PULLONS
PULLUPS
PULPERS
PULPITS
PULSARS
PUMICES
PUMMELS
PUMPERS
PUNCHES
PUNDITS
PUNKERS
PUNKIES
PUNLESS
PUNNERS
PUNTERS
PUPATES
PUPPETS
PUPPIES
PURFLES
PURISTS
PURPLES
PURRERS
PURSERS
PURSUES
PURVEYS
PUSHERS
PUSHUPS
PUSSIES
PUTOFFS
PUTOUTS
PUTPUTS
PUTTEES
PUTTERS
PUTTIES
PUZZLES
PYEDOGS
PYGMIES
PYRAMUS
PYRITES
PYRRHUS
PYTHIAS
PYTHONS

•PS••••

APSIDES
EPSILON
EPSTEIN
IPSWICH
UPSCALE
UPSENDS
UPSHIFT
UPSHOOT
UPSHOTS
UPSIDES
UPSILON
UPSIZED
UPSIZES
UPSLOPE
UPSOARS
UPSPINS
UPSTAGE
UPSTAIR
UPSTAND
UPSTARE
UPSTART
UPSTATE
UPSTEPS
UPSTIRS
UPSTOOD
UPSURGE
UPSWEEP
UPSWELL
UPSWEPT
UPSWING

•P•S•••

APESUIT
APISHLY
APOSTLE
EPISODE
EPISTLE
OPOSSUM
OPTSFOR
OPTSOUT
OPUSONE
OPUSTWO
SPASSKY
UPPSALA

•P••S••

APERSON
APHASIA
APHASIC
APLUSES
APPOSED
APPOSES
BPLUSES
CPLUSES
DPLUSES
EPHESUS
OPENSEA
OPENSUP
OPOSSUM
OPPOSED
OPPOSER
OPPOSES
OPQRSTU
SPARSER
SPASSKY
SPENSER
SPIESON
SPITSON
SPLASHY
SPONSOR
SPOUSAL
SPOUSES
SPURSON
UPCASTS
UPRISEN
UPRISER
UPRISES

•P•••S•

APPEASE
APPRISE
APTNESS
EPEEIST
IPCRESS
OPALISH
OPEROSE
OPPRESS
SPANISH
SPAREST
SPRIEST
SPRYEST
UPBURST
UPCLOSE
UPCOAST
UPFIRST
UPPHASE
UPRAISE
UPROUSE

•P••••S

APACHES
APELETS
APERCUS
APERIES
APHIDES
APLITES
APLUSES
APODOUS
APOGEES
APOLLOS
APPALLS
APPEALS
APPEARS
APPENDS
APPLETS
APPLIES
APPOSES
APROPOS
APSIDES
APTNESS
BPLUSES
CPLUSES
DPLUSES
EPARCHS
EPHEBUS
EPHESUS
EPILOGS
EPONYMS
EPOPEES
EPOQUES
EPOXIES
IPCRESS
OPAQUES
OPENERS
OPIATES
OPINERS
OPPOSES
OPPRESS
OPPUGNS
OPTICKS
OPTIMAS
OPTIONS
SPACERS
SPADERS
SPARERS
SPATHES
SPAYERS
SPECIES
SPEEDOS
SPEWERS
SPHERES
SPICERS
SPIDERS
SPIGOTS
SPIKERS
SPINELS
SPINETS
SPIRALS
SPIREAS
SPIRITS
SPITZES
SPLEENS
SPLICES
SPLINES
SPLINTS
SPONGES
SPOUSES
SPRAINS
SPRAWLS
SPREADS
SPRINGS
SPRINTS
SPRITES
SPROUTS
SPRUCES
SPYBOTS
SPYCAMS
SPYDERS
SPYINGS
SPYKIDS
UPBEARS
UPBEATS
UPCARDS
UPCASTS
UPCOILS
UPCURLS
UPDARTS
UPDATES
UPDIVES
UPDRIES
UPFLOWS
UPFOLDS
UPGAZES
UPGIRDS
UPGROWS
UPHEAPS
UPHILLS
UPHOLDS
UPKEEPS
UPLANDS
UPLEAPS
UPLIFTS
UPLINKS
UPLOADS
UPPILES
UPPROPS
UPRATES
UPREARS
UPRISES
UPROARS
UPROOTS
UPSENDS
UPSHOTS
UPSIDES
UPSIZES
UPSOARS
UPSPINS
UPSTEPS
UPSTIRS
UPTAKES
UPTALKS
UPTEARS
UPTICKS
UPTILTS
UPTIMES
UPTOWNS
UPTURNS
UPWAFTS
UPWARDS
UPWELLS
UPWINDS

••PS•••

CAPSHAW
CAPSIZE
CAPSTAN
CAPSULE
COPSHOP
COPSOUT
GIPSIES
GYPSIES
GYPSUMS
HIPSTER
HOPSING
HOPSOFF
HOPSOUT
LAPSANG
LAPSERS
LAPSING
LIPSOFF
LIPSOUT
LIPSYNC
LOPSOFF
MAPSOUT
NAPSTER
PEPSICO
PEPSINS
POPSOFF
POPSONG
POPSOUT
POPSTAR
RAPSONG
RAPSTAR
REPSFOR
RIPSAWN
RIPSAWS
RIPSOFF
RIPSONE
RIPSOUT
RIPSTOP
SAPSAGO
TAPSHOE
TAPSOFF
TAPSOUT
TAPSTER
TIPSIER
TIPSILY
TIPSOFF
TIPSTER
TOPSAIL
TOPSEED
TOPSIDE
TOPSOFF
TOPSOIL
TOPSOUT
TOPSPIN
TOPSPOT
UPPSALA
WAPSHOT
ZIPSOFF

••P•S••

APPOSED
APPOSES
DEPESTS
DEPOSAL
DEPOSED
DEPOSER
DEPOSES
DEPOSIT
ESPOSAS
ESPOSOS
EXPOSED
EXPOSER
EXPOSES
EXPOSIT
GAPESAT
HOPESSO
HOPESTO
HYPESUP
IMPASSE
IMPASTO
IMPOSED
IMPOSER
IMPOSES
IMPOSTS
LIPASES
OPPOSED
OPPOSER
OPPOSES
PAPISTS
PIPESIN
PIPESUP
REPASTE
REPASTS
REPOSED
REPOSER
REPOSES
REPOSIT
REPOSTS
RIPOSTE
RIPOSTS
ROPESIN
ROPESUP
TAPESON
TAPESUP
TYPESET
TYPESIN
TYPESUP
TYPISTS
UNPASTE
UNPOSED
WIPESUP

••P••S•

AMPLEST
APPEASE
APPRISE
ASPERSE
BAPTISE
BAPTISM
BAPTIST
CAPEESH
CAPLESS
COPYIST
CYPRESS
DEPRESS
DOPIEST
EMPRESS
EMPRISE
ENPRISE
ESPOUSE
EXPANSE
EXPENSE
EXPRESS
FOPPISH
GAPLESS
HAPLESS
HEPPEST
HIPLESS
HIPNESS
HIPPEST
HIPPISH
HOPEDSO
HOPESSO
IMPASSE
IMPRESS
IMPREST
IMPULSE
INPHASE
KAPITSA
LAPPISH
LIPLESS
MOPIEST
NAPLESS
NOPQRST
OPPRESS
PAPOOSE
PIPIEST
PIPLESS
REPHASE
REPRESS
REPRISE
REPULSE
ROPIEST
SAPLESS
SOPHISM
SOPHIST
STPIUSI
STPIUSV
STPIUSX
SUPPOSE
TIPLESS
TOPLESS
TOPMAST
TOPMOST
UPPHASE
ZIPDISK

••P•••S

ALPACAS
ALPINES
AMPERES
AMPULES
APPALLS
APPEALS
APPEARS
APPENDS
APPLETS
APPLIES
APPOSES
ASPECTS
ASPIRES
AUPAIRS
BOPPERS
BYPATHS
BYPLAYS
CAPADES
CAPFULS
CAPGUNS
CAPLESS
CAPLETS
CAPNUTS
CAPOTES
CAPPERS
CAPTORS
CEPHEUS
CIPHERS
COPCARS
COPIERS
COPIOUS
COPOUTS
COPPERS
COPTERS
COPULAS
CUPFULS
CUPOLAS
CUPROUS
CUPULES
CYPHERS
CYPRESS
DAPHNES
DAPHNIS
DAPPLES
DEPARTS
DEPENDS
DEPESTS
DEPICTS
DEPLOYS
DEPONES
DEPORTS
DEPOSES
DEPRESS
DEPULPS
DEPUTES
DIPNETS
DIPOLES
DIPPERS
EMPALES
EMPATHS
EMPIRES
EMPLOYS
EMPRESS
EMPTIES
ESPIALS
ESPNEWS
ESPOSAS
ESPOSOS
ESPRITS
EXPANDS
EXPECTS
EXPENDS
EXPERTS
EXPIRES
EXPORTS
EXPOSES
EXPRESS
FIPPLES
GAPKIDS
GAPLESS
GIPSIES
GOPHERS
GUPPIES
GYPPERS
GYPSIES
GYPSUMS
HAPLESS
HAPPENS
HAPTICS
HEPCATS
HEPTADS
HIPLESS
HIPNESS
HIPPIES
HOPKINS
HOPPERS
HUPPAHS
HYPHENS
IAPETUS
IMPACTS
IMPAIRS
IMPALAS
IMPALES
IMPARTS
IMPEDES
IMPENDS
IMPETUS
IMPIOUS
IMPLIES
IMPORTS
IMPOSES
IMPOSTS
IMPRESS
IMPUGNS
IMPUTES
INPOURS
JCPOWYS
KIPPERS
KOPECKS
LAPCATS
LAPDOGS
LAPERMS
LAPFULS
LAPPERS
LAPPETS
LAPSERS
LAPTOPS
LEPIDUS
LEPTONS
LIPARIS
LIPASES
LIPLESS
LIPPERS
LOPPERS
LUPINES
MAPPERS
MOPPERS
MOPPETS
MOPTOPS
MUPPETS
NAPALMS
NAPIERS
NAPKINS
NAPLESS
NAPPERS
NAPPIES
NEPALIS
NEPHEWS
NIPPERS
NIPPLES
NOPALES
OPPOSES
OPPRESS
OPPUGNS
ORPHANS
ORPHEUS
OSPREYS
PAPAGOS
PAPAYAS
PAPELES
PAPIERS
PAPISTS
PAPPIES
PAPUANS
PAPYRUS
PEPBOYS
PEPCIDS
PEPITAS
PEPLUMS
PEPPERS
PEPSINS
PEPTICS
PIPAGES
PIPINGS
PIPLESS
PIPPINS
POPEYES
POPGUNS
POPLARS
POPLINS
POPOFFS
POPOUTS
POPPERS
POPPIES
POPPINS
POPPLES
POPTOPS
PUPATES
PUPPETS
PUPPIES
RAPIERS
RAPINES
RAPINIS
RAPPELS
RAPPERS
RAPTORS
REPACKS
REPAGES
REPAIRS
REPARKS
REPASTS
REPAVES
REPEALS
REPEATS
REPENTS
REPERKS
REPICKS
REPINES
REPLANS
REPLAYS
REPLIES
REPLOTS
REPLOWS
REPOLLS
REPORTS
REPOSES
REPOSTS
REPOURS
REPRESS
REPUGNS
REPUMPS
REPUTES
RIPOFFS
RIPOSTS
RIPPERS
RIPPLES

RIPRAPS
RIPSAWS
RUPIAHS
RVPARKS
SAPIENS
SAPLESS
SAPPERS
SEPHIAS
SEPIRAS
SEPTETS
SIPHONS
SIPPERS
SOPHIES
STPAULS
SUPERGS
SUPPERS
SUPPLES
TAPINGS
TAPPANS
TAPPERS
TAPPETS
TFPOWYS
TIPJARS
TIPLESS
TIPOFFS
TIPPEES
TIPPERS
TIPPETS
TIPPLES
TIPTOES
TIPTOPS
TOPAZES
TOPBIDS
TOPDOGS
TOPGUNS
TOPHATS
TOPLESS
TOPPERS
TOPPLES
TOPROWS
TOPTENS
TOPTHIS
TUPELOS
TYPEABS
TYPISTS
UMPIRES
UNPACKS
UNPAWNS
UNPEELS
UNPICKS
UNPILES
UNPIOUS
UNPLANS
UNPLUGS
UPPILES
UPPROPS
VAPOURS
WAPITIS
YAPPERS
YIPPIES
YUPPIES
ZAPATAS
ZAPPERS
ZEPHYRS
ZIPGUNS
ZIPLOCS
ZIPPERS
ZIPTOPS

•••PS••

ASEPSIS
BEEPSAT
BOOPSIE
BUMPSUP
CAMPSUP
CARPSAT
CHIPSIN
CHIPSUP
CHOPSUP
CLIPSON
COOPSUP
CORPSES
CROPSUP
DEEPSEA
DEEPSET
DEEPSIX
DEEPSKY
DEMPSEY
DRIPSON
DROPSBY
DROPSIN
DROPSIT
DUMPSON
ELAPSED
ELAPSES
HARPSON
HEAPSOF
HEAPSON
HEAPSUP
HELPSIN
HELPSON
HELPSUP
JUMPSAT
JUMPSIN
JUMPSON
JUMPSUP
KEEPSAT
KEEPSIN
KEEPSON
KEEPSTO
KEEPSUP
LEAPSAT
LEAPSIN
LEAPSON
LEAPSUP
LUMPSIN
LUMPSIT
LUMPSUM
PEEPSAT
POOPSIE
PROPSUP
PUMPSUP
RAMPSUP
SAMPSON
SEEPSIN
SHOPSAT
SIMPSON
SKIPSBY
SLAPSON
SLIPSBY
SLIPSIN
SLIPSON
SLIPSUP
SLOPSON
SNAPSAT
SNAPSON
SNAPSTO
SNAPSUP
SOAPSUP
SOUPSON
SOUPSUP
STEPSIN
STEPSON
STEPSUP
STOPSAT
STOPSBY
STOPSIN
STOPSIT
STOPSUP
STYPSIS
TRIPSON
TRIPSUP
WHIPSAW
WHIPSIN
WHIPSUP
WRAPSUP

•••P•S•

ADIPOSE
ANAPEST
BADPAST
BEDPOST
BUSPASS
COMPASS
COMPOSE
COMPOST
DAMPEST
DAMPISH
DEEPEST
DEEPISH
DESPISE
DISPOSE
DUMPISH
FLYPAST
FOPPISH
GETPAST
GOTPAST
HARPIST
HEPPEST
HIPPEST
HIPPISH
IHOPESO
ILLPASS
LAPPISH
LETPASS
LIMPEST
LOWPOST
LUMPISH
MALPASO
NONPAST
OUTPASS
OUTPOST
OUTPUSH
PROPOSE
PURPOSE
QUEPASA
RANPAST
RASPISH
ROMPISH
RUNPAST
SAWPAST
SEEPAST
SUBPOST
SUPPOSE
SURPASS
TEMPEST
TENPAST
THEPOST
TROPISM
UTOPISM
UTOPIST
VAMPISH
VFWPOST
WASPISH
WIMPISH

•••P••S

AIRPOPS
AIRPOTS
ARMPITS
ASEPSIS
ASHPANS
ASHPITS
BBQPITS
BEEPERS
BIOPICS
BOPPERS
BUMPERS
BUSPASS
CAMPERS
CAPPERS
CARPALS
CARPELS
CARPERS
CARPETS
CARPOUS
CHAPELS
CHUPPAS
CLIPONS
COEPTIS
COMPAQS
COMPASS
COMPELS
COOPERS
COPPERS
CORPSES
COUPLES
COUPONS
COWPEAS
CRYPTOS
CUSPIDS
DAMPENS
DAMPERS
DAPPLES
DEEPENS
DESPOTS
DIAPERS
DIMPLES
DIPPERS
DISPELS
DRAPERS
DROPINS
DRYPERS
DUMPERS
EELPOTS
ELAPIDS
ELAPSES
ELOPERS
ENDPINS
EPOPEES
EYEPITS
FIPPLES
FLIPUPS
FRAPPES
FRYPANS
GALPALS
GASPERS
GAWPERS
GELPENS
GOMPERS
GOSPELS
GRAPPAS
GRIPERS
GRIPPES
GROPERS
GROPIUS
GULPERS
GUPPIES
GYPPERS
HAMPERS
HAPPENS
HARPERS
HARPIES
HATPINS
HEAPERS
HELPERS
HIPPIES
HOOPERS
HOOPLAS
HOOPOES
HOPPERS
HOTPOTS
HUPPAHS
ICEPOPS
ILLPASS
INKPADS
INKPOTS
INSPANS
INSPOTS
ISOPODS
JASPERS
JEEPERS
JOYPADS
JUMPERS
KEEPERS
KELPIES
KEWPIES
KEYPADS
KEYPALS
KIPPERS
KLEPTOS
LAPPERS
LAPPETS
LEAPERS
LETPASS
LIMPETS
LIPPERS
LISPERS
LOOPERS
LOPPERS
LUMPERS
MAGPIES
MAPPERS
MEMPHIS
MNOPQRS
MOPPERS
MOPPETS
MUDPIES
MUPPETS
MURPHYS
MYOPIAS
NAPPERS
NAPPIES
NIPPERS
NIPPLES
NONPARS
NONPLUS
NONPROS
NTUPLES
OILPANS
OLDPALS
OLDPROS
OOMPAHS
OUTPASS
OUTPAYS
OUTPOPS
OUTPUTS
PAMPERS
PAPPIES
PAUPERS
PAWPAWS
PEAPODS
PEEPERS
PEEPLES
PENPALS
PEOPLES
PEPPERS
PETPIGS
PETPUPS
PGAPROS
PIEPANS
PIGPENS
PIMPLES
PIPPINS
POMPOMS
POMPONS
POMPOUS
POPPERS
POPPIES
POPPINS
POPPLES
POTPIES
PREPAYS
PROPELS
PULPERS
PULPITS
PUMPERS
PUPPETS
PUPPIES
PURPLES
PUTPUTS
QUAPAWS
RAPPELS
RAPPERS
RASPERS
REAPERS
REOPENS
RESPANS
RESPINS
RESPOTS
RIBPADS
RIMPLES
RIPPERS
RIPPLES
ROMPERS
RUMPLES
SAMPANS
SAMPLES
SAMPRAS
SAPPERS
SAWPITS
SERPENS
SEXPOTS
SHAPERS
SHOPKOS
SHOPPES
SIMPERS
SIMPLES
SIPPERS
SLIPONS
SLIPUPS
SLOPERS
SNAPONS
SNIPERS
SOAPERS
SOSPADS
SOUPERS
STAPLES
STEPINS
STEPPES
STEPUPS
STUPIDS
STUPORS
STYPSIS
SUPPERS
SUPPLES
SURPASS
SURPLUS
SWIPERS
TAMPERS
TAPPANS
TAPPERS
TAPPETS
TARPITS
TARPONS
TEAPOTS
TEAPOYS
TEEPEES
TEMPEHS
TEMPERS
TEMPLES
TENPINS
THEPIPS
THEPITS
TIEPINS
TIPPEES
TIPPERS
TIPPETS
TIPPLES
TOPPERS
TOPPLES
TOUPEES
TREPANS
TRIPLES
TRIPODS
TROPICS
TVSPOTS
UNIPODS
UNSPANS
UPSPINS
USOPENS
UTOPIAS
VAMPERS
VESPERS
VESPIDS
WAMPUMS
WARPERS
WEAPONS
WEEPERS
WIMPLES
WRAPUPS
YAPPERS
YAWPERS
YELPERS
YIPPIES
YUPPIES
ZAPPERS
ZIPPERS

••••PS•

AUTOPSY
CALYPSO
ECLIPSE
ELLIPSE
GLIMPSE
RELAPSE
SYNAPSE
TRAIPSE

••••P•S

ACCEPTS
APROPOS
ATROPOS
BIGAPES
CALIPHS
CANAPES
CANOPUS
CHIAPAS
CHUPPAS
CREEPOS
CRISPUS
DACAPOS
DAYSPAS
DOGAPES
ECTYPES
ESCAPES
EXCEPTS
EXEMPTS
FAUXPAS
FRAPPES
GRAMPAS
GRAMPUS
GRANPAS
GRAPPAS
GRIPPES
INCEPTS
IRRUPTS
KAKAPOS
LOOMPAS
OCTOPUS
OEDIPUS
OLYMPUS
PARAPHS
PROMPTS
RECIPES
RETAPES
RETYPES
REWIPES
SCOUPES
SCRAPES
SCRIPPS
SCRIPTS
SCULPTS
SERAPES
SERAPHS
SERAPIS
SHERPAS
SHOPPES
STEPPES
STRIPES
THESPIS
TIEMPOS
TRAMPAS
TROUPES
TSHAPES
TVTAPES
UNROPES
UNTAPES
USHAPES
VSHAPES
YSHAPES

•••••PS

AAAMAPS
AIRPOPS
ALETAPS
ALLCAPS
BACKUPS
BADRAPS
BARHOPS
BIGTOPS
BISHOPS
BITMAPS
BLOWUPS
BOXTOPS
BUMRAPS
BURLAPS
BUSTUPS
CALLUPS
CARHOPS
CARTOPS
CATNAPS
CATNIPS
CATSUPS
CCLAMPS
CHINUPS
COINOPS
COLLOPS
CUETIPS
CYCLOPS
DAYHOPS
DECAMPS
DEPULPS
DEWLAPS
DIALUPS
DIDLAPS
DOGNAPS
DOLLOPS
DOOWOPS
DRYMOPS
DUNLOPS
DUSTUPS
EARLAPS
EGGCUPS
ENCAMPS
ENTRAPS
ENWRAPS
ESCARPS
EYECUPS
FATLIPS
FILLIPS
FILLUPS
FLIPUPS
FOLDUPS
FORCEPS
FOULUPS
GALLOPS
GASCAPS
GELCAPS
GIVEUPS
GOOFUPS
GOSSIPS
GUNLAPS
HANGUPS
HICCUPS
HOLDUPS
HOOKUPS
HOTCAPS
HOTCUPS
HOTLIPS
HOTTIPS
HUBCAPS
HYSSOPS
ICECAPS
ICEPOPS
INSTEPS
JOBHOPS
KICKUPS
KIDNAPS
LACEUPS
LAPTOPS
LARRUPS
LASHUPS
LEADUPS
LESSEPS
LINEUPS
LINKUPS
LOCKUPS
LOOKUPS
LOWTOPS
MADCAPS
MAKEUPS
MARKUPS
MESSUPS
MIDCAPS
MISHAPS
MOCKUPS
MOPTOPS
MRCHIPS
OILCUPS
ONRAMPS
OUTLIPS
OUTPOPS
OUTRAPS
PEGTOPS
PERHAPS
PETNAPS
PETPUPS
PHILIPS
PICKUPS
PILEUPS
POPTOPS
POSTOPS
PREAMPS
PRENUPS
PULLUPS
PUSHUPS
RAGMOPS
RAGTOPS
RANLAPS
RAVEUPS
RECOUPS
REDCAPS
REDTOPS
REFLIPS
REGRIPS
RELEAPS
REPUMPS
RESHIPS
RESNAPS
RESOAPS
RETRAPS
REVAMPS
REWRAPS
RIPRAPS
ROLLUPS
RUNLAPS
SATRAPS
SCHLEPS
SCHNAPS
SCRIMPS
SCRIPPS
SEAMAPS
SENDUPS
SHRIMPS
SIGNUPS
SKICAPS
SKYCAPS
SKYMAPS
SLIPUPS
SLOWUPS
SNOCAPS
STEPUPS
TEACUPS
THEALPS
THEPIPS
THEVIPS
THEYIPS
TIPTOPS
TOECAPS
TOETAPS
TOSSUPS
TOYTOPS
TRICEPS
TSTRAPS
TUNEUPS
TURNIPS
TURNUPS
UNCLIPS
UNCOOPS
UNGRIPS
UNHASPS
UNLOOPS
UNSHIPS
UNSNAPS
UNSTEPS
UNSTOPS
UNTRAPS
UNWRAPS
UPHEAPS
UPKEEPS
UPLEAPS
UPPROPS
UPSTEPS
WAKEUPS
WALKUPS
WALLOPS
WARMUPS
WASHUPS
WETMOPS
WETNAPS
WINDUPS
WORKUPS
WRAPUPS
ZIPTOPS

PT•••••

PTBOATS
PTEROUS
PTOLEMY

P•T••••

PATACAS
PATCASH
PATCHED
PATCHEN
PATCHER
PATCHES
PATCHUP
PATDOWN
PATELLA
PATENCY
PATENTS
PATERNO
PATHAND
PATHANS
PATHWAY
PATIENT
PATINAS
PATNESS
PATRICE
PATRICK
PATRIES
PATRIOT
PATROLS
PATRONS
PATROON
PATSDRY
PATSIES
PATTERN
PATTERS
PATTIES
PATTING
PATZERS
PETALED
PETALES
PETARDS
PETBEAR
PETBIRD
PETBOAS
PETCAGE
PETCALF
PETCATS
PETCHEW
PETCOCK
PETCOMB
PETCOWS
PETCROW
PETDEER
PETDOGS
PETDOOR
PETDOVE
PETDUCK
PETEMAN
PETEMEN
PETERED
PETERII
PETFISH
PETFROG
PETGATE
PETGOAT
PETHAIR
PETHARE
PETIOLE
PETITES
PETLAMB
PETLION
PETMICE
PETMULE
PETNAME
PETNAPS
PETPIGS
PETPONY
PETPUPS
PETRATS
PETRELS
PETRIFY
PETROCK
PETROLS
PETROUS
PETSCAN
PETSHOP
PETSITS
PETTERS
PETTIER
PETTILY
PETTING
PETTISH
PETTOYS
PETULIA
PETUNIA
PITAPAT
PITAYAS
PITBOSS
PITBULL
PITCHED
PITCHER
PITCHES
PITCHIN
PITCHTO
PITCREW
PITEOUS
PITFALL
PITHEAD
PITHIER
PITHILY
PITHING
PITIERS
PITIFUL
PITILLO
PITROWS
PITSAWS
PITSTOP
PITTING
PITTMAN
PITYING
POTABLE
POTAGES
POTAMUS
POTBOIL
POTEENS
POTENCE
POTENCY
POTFULS
POTHERB

POTHERS
POTHOLE
POTHOOK
POTIONS
POTLIDS
POTLUCK
POTOMAC
POTPIES
POTSDAM
POTSHOT
POTTAGE
POTTERS
POTTERY
POTTIER
POTTIES
POTTING
PUTAWAY
PUTBACK
PUTDOWN
PUTEMUP
PUTITTO
PUTOFFS
PUTOUTS
PUTOVER
PUTPUTS
PUTREFY
PUTSOFF
PUTSOUT
PUTTEES
PUTTERS
PUTTIED
PUTTIES
PUTTING
PUTTOUT
PUTUPON
PUTUPTO
PYTHIAN
PYTHIAS
PYTHONS

P••T•••

PALTERS
PALTROW
PANTENE
PANTERA
PANTERS
PANTHER
PANTIES
PANTILE
PANTING
PANTLEG
PANTONE
PARTAKE
PARTIAL
PARTIED
PARTIER
PARTIES
PARTIII
PARTING
PARTITA
PARTITE
PARTNER
PARTONE
PARTOOK
PARTTWO
PARTWAY
PARTYER
PARTYON
PASTDUE
PASTEIN
PASTELS
PASTERN
PASTERS
PASTEUP
PASTEUR
PASTIER
PASTIES
PASTIME
PASTINA
PASTING
PASTORS
PASTURE
PATTERN
PATTERS
PATTIES
PATTING
PEATBOG
PEATIER
PEATPOT
PECTINS
PEGTOPS
PELTATE
PELTERS
PELTING
PELTISH
PENTADS
PENTANE
PENTELS
PENTIUM
PEPTALK
PEPTICS
PEPTIDE
PEPTONE
PERTAIN
PERTEST
PERTURB
PESTERS
PESTLED
PESTLES
PETTERS
PETTIER
PETTILY
PETTING
PETTISH
PETTOYS
PEWTERS
PGATOUR
PHATTER
PHOTICS
PHOTOGS
PHOTOID
PHOTONS
PHOTOOP
PICTISH
PICTURE
PIETIES
PIETINS
PIETOSO
PIETROS
PIGTAIL
PINTAIL
PISTILS
PISTOLE
PISTOLS
PISTONS
PISTOUS
PITTING
PITTMAN
PLATEAU
PLATENS
PLATERS
PLATIER
PLATIES
PLATING
PLATOON
PLATTED
PLATTER
PLATYPI
PLOTFUL
PLOTTED
PLOTTER
PLOTZED
PLOTZES
PLUTONS
POETESS
POETICA
POETICS
POETISE
POETIZE
POITIER
POLTAVA
PONTANO
PONTIAC
PONTIAN
PONTIFF
PONTIUS
PONTOON
POPTART
POPTOPS
POPTUNE
PORTAGE
PORTALS
PORTEND
PORTENT
PORTERS
PORTHOS
PORTICO
PORTING
PORTION
PORTMAN
PORTNOY
PORTRAY
POSTAGE
POSTBAG
POSTBOX
POSTDOC
POSTERN
POSTERS
POSTFIX
POSTHOC
POSTIES
POSTING
POSTITS
POSTMAN
POSTMEN
POSTOPS
POSTURE
POSTWAR
POTTAGE
POTTERS
POTTERY
POTTIER
POTTIES
POTTING
POUTERS
POUTFUL
POUTIER
POUTING
PRATERS
PRATING
PRATTLE
PRETAPE
PRETEEN
PRETELL
PRETEND
PRETERM
PRETEST
PRETEXT
PRETIRE
PRETOLD
PRETORS
PRETRIM
PRETYPE
PRETZEL
PRITHEE
PROTEAM
PROTEAN
PROTECT
PROTEGE
PROTEIN
PROTEST
PROTEUS
PROTIST
PROTONS
PUNTERS
PUNTING
PUPTENT
PURTIER
PUTTEES
PUTTERS
PUTTIED
PUTTIES
PUTTING
PUTTOUT

P•••T••

PAGETWO
PAINTED
PAINTER
PAIUTES
PALATAL
PALATES
PALETTE
PALMTOP
PANETTA
PARATUS
PAROTID
PARTTWO
PAYSTUB
PELOTAS
PELOTON
PENATES
PEPITAS
PERATIO
PERETTI
PERITUS
PESETAS
PETITES
PEYOTES
PGRATED
PHAETON
PHANTOM
PHATTER
PHILTER
PHILTRE
PIASTER
PIASTRE
PICOTED
PILATES
PILATUS
PILOTED
PINATAS
PINETAR
PINETOP
PINETUM
PINOTTA
PIPETTE
PIRATED
PIRATES
PIRATIC
PITSTOP
PIVOTAL
PIVOTED
PIVOTER
PLAITED
PLAITER
PLANTAR
PLANTED
PLANTER
PLASTER
PLASTIC
PLATTED
PLATTER
PLAUTUS
PLAYTEX
PLEATED
PLECTRA
PLINTHS
PLOTTED
PLOTTER
PLUSTAX
PLUSTWO
POINTAT
POINTED
POINTER
POINTES
POINTTO
POINTUP
POLITER
POLITIC
POLLTAX
POORTAX
POPSTAR
POSITED
POULTRY
PQRSTUV
PRACTIC
PRAETOR
PRATTLE
PRESTON
PRESTOS
PRINTAD
PRINTED
PRINTER
PRINTUP
PROCTER
PROCTOR
PSALTER
PULLTAB
PULLTOY
PUNSTER
PUPATED
PUPATES
PURITAN
PUTITTO
PWBOTHA
PYRETIC
PYRITES
PYRITIC

P••••T•

PACKETS
PADGETT
PADSITE
PALETTE
PALLETS
PALMATE
PALPATE
PANDITS
PANETTA
PAPEETE
PAPISTS
PARENTS
PARROTS
PARTITA
PARTITE
PASSATS
PATENTS
PAUCITY
PAYCUTS
PAYINTO
PAYOUTS
PAYRATE
PEANUTS
PEDANTS
PELLETS
PELTATE
PENALTY
PENLITE
PENNATE
PENULTS
PEQUOTS
PERDITA
PERETTI
PERLITE
PERMITS
PERMUTE
PESANTE
PETCATS
PETGATE
PETRATS
PETSITS
PICANTE
PICCATA
PICKETS
PICKETT
PIGLETS
PIGNUTS
PIGOUTS
PILEATE
PIMENTO
PINKETT
PINNATE
PINOTTA
PIOLETS
PIOSITY
PIPETTE
PITCHTO
PLACATE
PLAINTS
PLAKATS
PLANATE
PLANETS
PLANSTO
PLAYSTO
PLEADTO
PLICATE
PLIGHTS
PLOESTI
POCKETS
POINTTO
POLENTA
POLLUTE
POPOUTS
POSTITS
POVERTY
PRAYSTO
PREACTS
PRECITE
PRECUTS
PREDATA
PREDATE
PRELATE
PREMATE
PRESETS
PREVETO
PREWITT
PRIESTS
PRIMATE
PRIORTO
PRIVATE
PRIVETS
PRIVITY
PRIVYTO
PROBATE
PROBITY
PROCITY
PROFITS
PROJETS
PROLATE
PROMOTE
PROMPTS
PRONATE
PRONETO
PRORATA
PRORATE
PRYINTO
PTBOATS
PUBERTY
PUCKETT
PULLETS
PULPITS
PULSATE
PUNDITS
PUPPETS
PURISTS
PUTITTO
PUTOUTS
PUTPUTS
PUTUPTO

P•••••T

PACIEST
PACKRAT
PADGETT
PAGEANT
PAIDOUT
PALMIST
PANSOUT
PARAPET
PARFAIT
PARKSIT
PARQUET
PASSANT
PASSOUT
PATIENT
PATRIOT
PAULIST
PAWEDAT
PAYDIRT
PAYMENT
PAYSOUT
PEACOAT
PEASANT
PEATPOT
PECCANT
PECKSAT
PEEKOUT
PEEKSAT
PEELOUT
PEEPOUT
PEEPSAT
PEEROUT
PEERSAT
PENDANT
PENDENT
PENNANT
PERCENT
PERCEPT
PERFECT
PERIAPT
PERIDOT
PERSIST
PERTEST
PETGOAT
PEUGEOT
PIANIST
PICKETT
PICKOUT
PICKSAT
PIERROT
PIGMEAT
PIGMENT
PIGSOUT
PINCHOT
PINENUT
PINIEST
PINKEST
PINKETT
PIPIEST
PIQUANT
PITAPAT
PLACKET
PLANOUT
PLAUDIT
PLAYACT
PLAYLET
PLAYOUT
PLAYSAT
PLUMCOT
PLUMMET
PNEUMAT
PODCAST
POINTAT
POKEDAT
POKEOUT
POKESAT
POKIEST
POLECAT
POLESAT
POLESIT
POLOIST
POOPOUT
POOREST
POPSOUT
POPTART
PORTENT
POSHEST
POTSHOT
POUROUT
PRECAST
PRECEPT
PREDICT
PREDIET
PREEDIT
PREEMPT
PREFECT
PREHEAT
PREMEET
PREOMIT
PREPLOT
PRERENT
PRERIOT
PRESALT
PRESEAT
PRESENT
PRESIFT
PRESORT
PRETEST
PRETEXT
PREVENT
PREVERT
PREVOST
PREWITT
PRODUCT
PROEAST
PROJECT
PROPHET
PROPJET
PROTECT
PROTEST
PROTIST
PROVEIT
PROVOST
PROWEST
PRUDENT
PUCKETT
PUFFOUT
PULLOUT
PUMPOUT
PUNGENT
PUNIEST
PUPTENT
PURPORT
PURSUIT
PUSHOUT
PUTSOUT
PUTTOUT

•PT••••

APTERAL
APTERYX
APTNESS
MPTHREE
OPTEDIN
OPTEDTO
OPTICAL
OPTICKS
OPTIMAL
OPTIMAS
OPTIMUM
OPTIONS
OPTSFOR
OPTSOUT
UPTAKES
UPTALKS
UPTEARS
UPTEMPO
UPTHERE
UPTHROW
UPTICKS
UPTIGHT
UPTILTS
UPTIMES
UPTONOW
UPTOPAR
UPTOWNS
UPTRADE
UPTREND
UPTURNS

•P•T•••

APATITE
APOTHEM
EPITAPH
EPITHET
EPITOME
EPSTEIN
SPATHES
SPATIAL
SPATOUT
SPATTED
SPATTER
SPATULA
SPITING
SPITOUT
SPITSON
SPITTER
SPITTLE
SPITZES
SPOTLIT
SPOTTED
SPOTTER
SPUTNIK
SPUTTER
UPATREE
UPSTAGE
UPSTAIR
UPSTAND
UPSTARE
UPSTART
UPSTATE
UPSTEPS
UPSTIRS
UPSTOOD

•P••T••

APLITES
APOSTLE
APPETIT
EPISTLE
OPENTAP
OPENTOE
OPENTOP
OPIATES
OPUNTIA
OPUSTWO
SPARTAN
SPATTED
SPATTER
SPECTER
SPECTOR
SPECTRA
SPECTRE
SPENTON
SPITTER
SPITTLE
SPLITUP
SPLOTCH
SPORTED
SPORTIN
SPOTTED
SPOTTER
SPOUTED
SPOUTER
SPRITES
SPURTED
SPUTTER
UPDATED
UPDATER
UPDATES
UPRATED
UPRATES

•P•••T•

APATITE
APELETS
APLENTY
APPLETS
APPLYTO
EPIDOTE
EPILATE
OPACITY
OPERATE
OPQRSTU
OPTEDTO
SPEAKTO
SPIGOTS
SPIKETV
SPINETS
SPIRITS
SPLINTS
SPOKETO
SPRINTS
SPROUTS
SPYBOTS
UPBEATS
UPCASTS
UPDARTS
UPLIFTS
UPNORTH
UPROOTS
UPSHOTS
UPSTATE
UPTILTS
UPWAFTS

•P••••T

APEDIET
APESUIT
APPARAT
APPETIT
APPOINT
APRICOT
EPAULET
EPEEIST
EPITHET
OPENNET
OPENOUT
OPENPIT
OPERANT
OPTSOUT
OPULENT
SPAMBOT
SPAREST
SPATOUT
SPECOUT
SPEWOUT
SPINOUT
SPITOUT
SPOTLIT
SPRIEST
SPRYEST
SPUNOUT
UPBURST
UPCOAST
UPCOURT
UPDRAFT
UPDRIFT
UPFIRST
UPFORIT
UPFRONT
UPLEAPT
UPLIGHT
UPOROUT
UPRIGHT
UPSHIFT
UPSHOOT
UPSTART
UPSWEPT
UPTIGHT

••PT•••

BAPTISE
BAPTISM
BAPTIST
BAPTIZE
CAPTAIN
CAPTION
CAPTIVA
CAPTIVE
CAPTORS
CAPTURE
COPTERS
DIPTYCH
EMPTIED
EMPTIER
EMPTIES
EMPTILY
HAPTICS
HEPTADS
HOPTOIT
KAPTURE
KEPTFIT
KEPTMUM
KEPTOFF
KEPTOUT
LAPTOPS
LEPTONS
MOPTOPS
NAPTIME
NEPTUNE
NUPTIAL
PEPTALK
PEPTICS
PEPTIDE
PEPTONE
POPTART
POPTOPS
POPTUNE
PUPTENT
RAPTORS
RAPTUNE
RAPTURE
REPTILE
RIPTIDE
RIPTORN
RUPTURE
SEPTETS
TIPTOED
TIPTOES
TIPTOPS
TOPTENS
TOPTHIS
UMPTEEN
ZIPTOPS

••P•T••

APPETIT
BYPATHS
CAPITAL
CAPITAN
CAPITOL
CAPOTES
CAPSTAN
DEPUTED
DEPUTES
EMPATHS
EMPATHY
HEPATIC
HIPSTER
HYPATIA
IAPETUS
IIPETER
IMPETUS
IMPUTED
IMPUTER
IMPUTES
JEPHTHA
JUPITER
KAPITAL
KAPITSA
LAPUTAN
NAPHTHA
NAPSTER
NEPOTIC
PEPITAS
PIPETTE
POPSTAR
PUPATED
PUPATES
RAPSTAR
REPATCH

REPUTED
REPUTES
RIPSTOP
ROPETOW
STPETER
TAPSTER
TIPSTER
WAPITIS
ZAPATAS
ZAPATEO
ZAPOTEC

••P••T•

APPLETS
APPLYTO
ASPECTS
CAPLETS
CAPNUTS
COPOUTS
CUPRITE
DEPARTS
DEPESTS
DEPICTS
DEPLETE
DEPORTS
DIPINTO
DIPNETS
ESPARTO
ESPRITS
EXPARTE
EXPECTS
EXPERTS
EXPIATE
EXPORTS
HAPPYTO
HEPCATS
HIPBATH
HIPPITY
HOPEDTO
HOPESTO
HOPINTO
HOPLITE
IMPACTS
IMPARTS
IMPASTO
IMPIETY
IMPORTS
IMPOSTS
JAPHETH
LAPCATS
LAPLATA
LAPORTE
LAPPETS
LEPANTO
MOPPETS
MUPPETS
PAPEETE
PAPISTS
PIPETTE
POPOUTS
PUPPETS
REPASTE
REPASTS
REPEATS
REPENTS
REPLATE
REPLETE
REPLOTS
REPLYTO
REPORTS
REPOSTS
RIPINTO
RIPOSTE
RIPOSTS
SEPTETS
SOPWITH
TAPINTO
TAPPETS
TIPPETS
TOPHATS
TOPRATE
TYPISTS
UNPASTE
UNPIETY

••P•••T

AMPLEST
APPARAT
APPETIT
APPOINT
ASPHALT
BAPTIST
CAPELET
CAPULET
COPILOT
COPSOUT
COPYCAT
COPYIST
CYPRIOT
DEPOSIT
DOPEOUT
DOPIEST
EXPLOIT
EXPOSIT
GAPEDAT
GAPESAT
HEPPEST
HIPBOOT
HIPPEST
HOPENOT
HOPSOUT
HOPTOIT
HUPPERT
IMPLANT
IMPREST
IMPRINT
INPOINT
INPRINT
KEPTFIT
KEPTOUT
LAPBELT
LIPSOUT
MAPSOUT
MOPIEST
NOPQRST
ONPOINT
ORPHANT
PIPIEST
POPSOUT
POPTART
PUPTENT
RAPPORT
REPAINT
REPLANT
REPOINT
REPOSIT
REPRINT
RIPPLET
RIPSOUT
ROPIEST
SAPIENT
SOPHIST
SUPPORT
TAPROOT
TAPSOUT
TIPCART
TOPBOOT
TOPCOAT
TOPKNOT
TOPMAST
TOPMOST
TOPSOUT
TOPSPOT
TYPESET
UNPLAIT
WAPSHOT
WIPEOUT
YOPLAIT

•••PT••

ADAPTED
ADAPTER
ADAPTOR
ADAPTTO
ADEPTAT
ADEPTER
ADEPTLY
ADOPTED
ADOPTEE
ADOPTER
ASEPTIC
ATIPTOE
CHAPTER
CLAPTON
COAPTED
COEPTIS
COMPTON
COOPTED
CREPTIN
CREPTUP
CROPTOP
CRYPTIC
CRYPTOS
DEEPTAN
DIOPTER
DROPTOP
ERUPTED
ERUPTER
FLIPTOP
GLYPTIC
HAMPTON
HOOPTOY
INAPTER
INAPTLY
INEPTLY
KEMPTON
KLEPTOS
KRYPTON
LEAPTAT
LEAPTIN
LEAPTON
LEAPTUP
SCEPTER
SCEPTIC
SCEPTRE
SKEPTIC
SLEPTIN
SLEPTON
STEPTWO
STYPTIC
SWEPTUP
SYMPTOM
TEMPTED
TEMPTER
UNAPTLY
UNOPTED

•••P•T•

ADAPTTO
AIRPOTS
ARMPITS
ASHPITS
BBQPITS
CARPETS
CHAPATI
COMPETE
COMPOTE
COMPUTE
CUSPATE
DESPITE
DESPOTS
DISPUTE
EELPOTS
EYEPITS
HAPPYTO
HERPETO
HIPPITY
HOTPOTS
INKPOTS
INSPITE
INSPOTS
KEEPSTO
LAPPETS
LIMPETS
MOPPETS
MUPPETS
OUTPATH
OUTPITY
OUTPUTS
PALPATE
PULPITS
PUPPETS
PUTPUTS
RESPITE
RESPOTS
SAWPITS
SEXPOTS
SNAPSTO
TAPPETS
TARPITS
TEAPOTS
THEPITS
TIPPETS
TIRPITZ
TOWPATH
TVSPOTS
WARPATH

•••P••T

ADEPTAT
AIRPORT
ANAPEST
BADPAST
BEDPOST
BEEPSAT
BITPART
CAMPOUT
CARPORT
CARPSAT
CHAPLET
CLIPART
CLIPOUT
COMPACT
COMPART
COMPORT
COMPOST
COUPLET
CRAPOUT
CULPRIT
DAMPEST
DEEPEST
DEEPFAT
DEEPSET
DISPART
DISPORT
DROPLET
DROPNET
DROPOUT
DROPSIT
DUMPOUT
EELPOUT
FLIPOUT
FLYPAST
GETPAST
GOTPAST
HARPIST
HELPOUT
HEPPEST
HIPPEST
HUPPERT
INSPECT
IREPEAT
JETPORT
JUMPCUT
JUMPSAT
KEEPFIT
KEEPOUT
KEEPSAT
LAMPERT
LAMPLIT
LEAPSAT
LEAPTAT
LIMPEST
LOWPOST
LUMPSIT
MAUPRAT
NEWPORT
NONPAST
NONPOET
ONEPART
ONEPINT
OUTPLOT
OUTPORT
OUTPOST
PEEPOUT
PEEPSAT
POOPOUT
PREPLOT
PROPHET
PROPJET
PUMPOUT
PURPORT
RAMPANT
RAMPART
RANPAST
RAPPORT
RESPECT
RESPELT
RESPLIT
RIPPLET
RUNPAST
SAWPAST
SEAPORT
SEEPAST
SEEPOUT
SERPENT
SHIPOUT
SHOPSAT
SKIPOUT
SLIPOUT
SNAPSAT
SNIPEAT
SNIPPET
SOAPNET
STEPOUT
STOPSAT
STOPSIT
SUBPLOT
SUBPOST
SUPPORT
SUSPECT
TEMPEST
TENPAST
THEPOST
TRIPLET
TRIPPET
TWOPART
UNSPELT
UNSPENT
UNSPILT
UNSPLIT
UTOPIST
VANPELT
VFWPOST
WHIPPET
WIMPOUT

••••PT•

ACCEPTS
ADDUPTO
EXCEPTS
EXEMPTS
GOTUPTO
INCEPTS
INDEPTH
IRRUPTS
LEDUPTO
NOTUPTO
ONEMPTY
OWNUPTO
PROMPTS
PUTUPTO
RANUPTO
RUNUPTO
SCRIPTS
SCULPTS
SUMUPTO
UNEMPTY

••••P•T

BEARPIT
CAGEPET
CESSPIT
CHIAPET
CLAYPIT
COALPIT
COCKPIT
COOKPOT
CRABPOT
CRUMPET
DASHPOT
DIGIPET
DOWNPAT
ENDUPAT
EYESPOT
FIREPIT
FLEAPIT
FUSSPOT
GOKAPUT
GOTOPOT
GRASPAT
HARDPUT
HOTSPOT
INASPOT
INKSPOT
JACKPOT
LOSTPET
MINEPIT
MOSHPIT
OCCIPUT
OILSPOT
ONESPOT
OPENPIT
OUTSPIT
PARAPET
PEATPOT
PITAPAT
REDSPOT
SALTPIT
SANDPIT
SHOTPUT
SITSPAT
SNIPPET
STAYPUT
STEWPOT
SUNSPOT
TENSPOT
THRUPUT
TOPSPOT
TOSSPOT
TRIPPET
TRUMPET
TWOSPOT
WELLPUT
WHIPPET

•••••PT

ATTEMPT
CONCEPT
CORRUPT
DECRYPT
DISRUPT
ENCRYPT
EXCERPT
INSWEPT
OUTKEPT
OUTWEPT
PERCEPT
PERIAPT
PRECEPT
PREEMPT
READAPT
READOPT
RECEIPT
REERUPT
UNADEPT
UNCLIPT
UNKEMPT
UNSWEPT
UNWHIPT
UPLEAPT
UPSWEPT

PU•••••

PUBERTY
PUBGAME
PUBLICS
PUBLISH
PUBLIUS
PUCCINI
PUCKERS
PUCKERY
PUCKETT
PUCKISH
PUDDING
PUDDLED
PUDDLES
PUDENCY
PUDGIER
PUDGILY
PUEBLOS
PUERILE
PUFFERS
PUFFERY
PUFFIER
PUFFILY
PUFFING
PUFFINS
PUFFOUT
PUFFSUP
PUGGISH
PUGGLES
PUGNOSE
PUGSLEY
PULASKI
PULLERS
PULLETS
PULLEYS
PULLFOR
PULLING
PULLINS
PULLMAN
PULLOFF
PULLONS
PULLOUT
PULLPIN
PULLSIN
PULLSON
PULLSUP
PULLTAB
PULLTOY
PULLUPS
PULMONI
PULMONO
PULPERS
PULPIER
PULPIFY
PULPING
PULPITS
PULSARS
PULSATE
PULSING
PUMICED
PUMICES
PUMMELS
PUMPERS
PUMPING
PUMPKIN
PUMPOUT
PUMPSUP
PUNCHED
PUNCHER
PUNCHES
PUNCHIN
PUNCHUP
PUNDITS
PUNGENT
PUNIEST
PUNJABI
PUNKERS
PUNKIER
PUNKIES
PUNLESS
PUNNERS
PUNNIER
PUNNILY
PUNNING
PUNSTER
PUNTERS
PUNTING
PUPATED
PUPATES
PUPPETS
PUPPIES
PUPTENT
PURCELL
PURDUEU
PURFLED
PURFLER
PURFLES
PURGING
PURISTS
PURITAN
PURLIEU
PURLING
PURLOIN
PURPLED
PURPLES
PURPORT
PURPOSE
PURRERS
PURRING
PURSERS
PURSIER
PURSING
PURSUED
PURSUER
PURSUES
PURSUIT
PURTIER
PURVEYS
PURVIEW
PUSHERS
PUSHFOR
PUSHFUL
PUSHIER
PUSHILY
PUSHING
PUSHKIN
PUSHOFF
PUSHOUT
PUSHPIN
PUSHROD
PUSHUPS
PUSSIES
PUTAWAY
PUTBACK
PUTDOWN
PUTEMUP
PUTITTO
PUTOFFS
PUTOUTS
PUTOVER
PUTPUTS
PUTREFY
PUTSOFF
PUTSOUT
PUTTEES
PUTTERS
PUTTIED
PUTTIES
PUTTING
PUTTOUT
PUTUPON
PUTUPTO
PUZZLED
PUZZLER
PUZZLES

P•U••••

PAUCITY
PAULIII
PAULINA
PAULINE
PAULING
PAULIST
PAULPRY
PAULSEN
PAUNCHY
PAUPERS
PAUSERS
PAUSING
PCUSERS
PEUGEOT
PIUSIII
PIUSVII
PIUSXII
PLUCKED
PLUGGED
PLUGGER
PLUGINS
PLUGOLA
PLUGSIN
PLUGSUP
PLUMAGE
PLUMBED
PLUMBER
PLUMBIC
PLUMBUM
PLUMCOT
PLUMIER
PLUMING
PLUMMER
PLUMMET
PLUMOSE
PLUMPED
PLUMPER
PLUMPIE
PLUMPLY
PLUMULE
PLUNDER
PLUNGED
PLUNGER
PLUNGES
PLUNKED
PLUNKER
PLURALS
PLUSHER
PLUSHES
PLUSHLY
PLUSONE
PLUSSES
PLUSTAX
PLUSTWO
PLUTONS
PLUVIAL
POUCHED
POUCHES
POUDRES
POULENC
POULTRY
POUNCED
POUNCER
POUNCES
POUNDED
POUNDER
POURERS
POURING
POUROUT
POURSIN
POUSSIN
POUTERS
POUTFUL
POUTIER
POUTING
PRUDENT
PRUDERY
PRUDHOE
PRUDISH
PRUNERS
PRUNING
PRUSSIA

P••U•••

PABULUM
PADUANS
PADUCAH
PAIUTES
PALUDAL
PANURGE
PAPUANS
PARURES
PENUCHE
PENULTS
PEQUOTS
PERUGIA
PERUKES
PERUSAL
PERUSED
PERUSER
PERUSES
PETULIA
PETUNIA
PIOUSLY
PIQUANT
PIQUING
PLAUDIT
PLAUTUS
PLEURAE
PLEURAL
PLOUGHS
PNEUMAS
PNEUMAT
PNEUMON
POPULAR
POPUPAD
PRIUSES
PROUDER
PROUDLY
PROUDOF
PUTUPON
PUTUPTO

P•••U••

PABLUMS
PACQUIN
PANFULS
PARFUMS
PARQUET
PASTURE
PAYCUTS
PAYOUTS
PEANUTS
PENGUIN
PEPLUMS
PERCUSS
PERDURE
PERFUME
PERFUMY
PERFUSE
PERJURE
PERJURY
PERMUTE
PERTURB
PETDUCK
PETMULE
PETPUPS
PICKUPS
PICTURE
PIGNUTS
PIGOUTS
PILEUPS
PINCURL
PINGUID
PITBULL
PLAGUED
PLAGUES
PLAQUES
PLENUMS
PLUMULE
PODIUMS
POLLUTE
POPGUNS
POPOUTS
POPQUIZ
POPTUNE
POSEURS
POSEUSE
POSSUMS
POSTURE
POTFULS
POTLUCK
PREBURN
PREBUYS
PRECURE
PRECUTS
PREDUSK
PREFUND
PRELUDE
PRENUPS
PREPUPA
PREQUEL
PRESUME
PREVUED
PREVUES
PROCURE
PRODUCE
PRODUCT
PROFUSE
PULLUPS
PURDUEU
PURSUED
PURSUER
PURSUES
PURSUIT
PUSHUPS
PUTOUTS
PUTPUTS

P••••U•

PABULUM
PACKSUP
PAIDOUT
PAILFUL
PAINFUL
PAIRSUP
PALMFUL
PANSOUT
PAPYRUS
PARAMUS
PARATUS
PARFOUR
PARIBUS
PARLOUR
PARLOUS
PASSEUL
PASSOUT
PASTDUE
PASTEUP
PASTEUR
PATCHUP
PAVIOUR
PAYSOUT
PAYSTUB
PEASOUP
PEEKOUT
PEELOUT
PEEPOUT
PEEROUT
PEGASUS
PENTIUM
PERITUS
PERKSUP
PERSEUS
PERSIUS

PETROUS
PGATOUR
PHEMIUS
PHILOUS
PHOEBUS
PHONYUP
PICEOUS
PICKOUT
PICKSUP
PIGSOUT
PILATUS
PILEDUP
PILEOUS
PILESUP
PILLBUG
PINENUT
PINETUM
PIPEDUP
PIPEFUL
PIPESUP
PIRAEUS
PIROGUE
PISTOUS
PITEOUS
PITIFUL
PLANOUT
PLAUTUS
PLAYFUL
PLAYOUT
PLAYSUP
PLOTFUL
PLOWSUP
PLUGSUP
PLUMBUM
POINTUP
POKEFUN
POKEOUT
POMPOUS
PONTIUS
POOLCUE
POOPOUT
POPSOUT
POTAMUS
POUROUT
POUTFUL
POWERUP
PQRSTUV
PRECOUP
PREMIUM
PRESPUR
PRESQUE
PRESSUP
PRICKUP
PRINTUP
PROCLUS
PRONOUN
PROPSUP
PROTEUS
PSYCHUP
PTEROUS
PUBLIUS
PUFFOUT
PUFFSUP
PULLOUT
PULLSUP
PUMPOUT
PUMPSUP
PUNCHUP
PUSHFUL
PUSHOUT
PUTEMUP
PUTSOUT
PUTTOUT
PYRAMUS
PYRRHUS

P•••••U
PARVENU
PAXINOU
PERREAU
PLATEAU
PURDUEU
PURLIEU

•PU••••
APULIAN
OPULENT
OPUNTIA
OPUSONE
OPUSTWO
SPUMIER
SPUMING
SPUMONE
SPUMONI
SPUNOFF
SPUNOUT
SPURNED
SPURNER
SPURRED
SPURSON
SPURTED
SPUTNIK
SPUTTER

•P•U•••
APLUSES
BPLUSES
CPLUSES
DPLUSES
EPAULET
OPPUGNS
SPLURGE
SPOUSAL
SPOUSES
SPOUTED
SPOUTER
SPRUCED
SPRUCER
SPRUCES
SPYUPON
UPBUILD
UPBURST
UPCURLS
UPCURVE
UPQUARK
UPSURGE
UPTURNS

•P••U••
APESUIT
EPICURE
EPOQUES
OPAQUES
SPATULA
SPELUNK
SPROUTS
UPBOUND
UPCOURT
UPROUSE

•P•••U•
APERCUS
APODOUS
APPLAUD
EPHEBUS
EPHESUS
OPENOUT
OPENSUP
OPOSSUM
OPTIMUM
OPTSOUT
SPATOUT
SPEAKUP
SPECOUT
SPEEDUP
SPEWOUT
SPICEUP
SPIFFUP
SPIKEUP
SPINOUT
SPITOUT
SPLITUP
SPOKEUP
SPUNOUT
UPOROUT
UPVALUE

•P••••U
OPQRSTU

••PU•••
AMPULES
CAPUANA
CAPUCHE
CAPULET
COPULAE
COPULAR
COPULAS
CUPULAR
CUPULES
DEPULPS
DEPUTED
DEPUTES
EXPUNGE
IMPUGNS
IMPULSE
IMPURER
IMPUTED
IMPUTER
IMPUTES
LAPUTAN
OPPUGNS
PAPUANS
POPULAR
POPUPAD
REPUGNS
REPULSE
REPUMPS
REPUTED
REPUTES

••P•U••
AMPOULE
CAPFULS
CAPGUNS
CAPNUTS
CAPSULE
CAPTURE
COPOUTS
CUPFULS
DEPAULU
ESPOUSE
EXPOUND
GYPSUMS
HEPBURN
IMPOUND
INPOURS
KAPTURE
LAPFULS
NEPTUNE
NIPMUCK
PEPLUMS
POPGUNS
POPOUTS
POPQUIZ
POPTUNE
RAPTUNE
RAPTURE
REPLUMB
REPLUME
REPOURS
REPRUNE
RUPTURE
STPAULS
STPIUSI
STPIUSV
STPIUSX
TOPGUNS
UNPLUGS
UNPLUMB
VAPOURS
VAPOURY
ZIPCUFF
ZIPGUNS

••P••U•
AMPEDUP
APPLAUD
CEPHEUS
COPIOUS
COPSOUT
CUPROUS
DOPEOUT
HOPEFUL
HOPSOUT
HYPEDUP
HYPESUP
IAPETUS
IMPETUS
IMPIOUS
KEPTMUM
KEPTOUT
LEPIDUS
LIPSOUT
MAPSOUT
ORPHEUM
ORPHEUS
PAPYRUS
PIPEDUP
PIPEFUL
PIPESUP
POPSOUT
RAPANUI
RIPSOUT
ROPEDUP
ROPESUP
TAPEDUP
TAPESUP
TAPSOUT
TOPSOUT
TYPEDUP
TYPESUP
UNPIOUS
UNPROUD
VAPORUB
WIPEDUP
WIPEOUT
WIPESUP

••P•••U
DEPAULU

•••PU••
AIRPUMP
COMPUTE
DISPUTE
FLIPUPS
GASPUMP
HADPULL
HASPULL
LEGPULL
OUTPULL
OUTPURL
OUTPUSH
OUTPUTS
PETPUPS
PREPUPA
PUTPUTS
SCAPULA
SLIPUPS
STEPUPS
TEMPURA
THEPUMP
WAMPUMS
WRAPUPS

•••P•U•
BUMPSUP
BURPGUN
CAMPOUT
CAMPSUP
CARPOUS
CHIPSUP
CHOPSUP
CLIPOUT
COOPSUP
CRAPOUT
CREPTUP
CROPSUP
DROPOUT
DUMPOUT
EARPLUG
EELPOUT
FLIPOUT
GROPIUS
HEAPSUP
HELPFUL
HELPOUT
HELPSUP
JUMPCUT
JUMPSUP
KEEPMUM
KEEPOUT
KEEPSUP
LEAPSUP
LEAPTUP
LESPAUL
LUMPSUM
MRSPAUL
NAIPAUL
NONPLUS
OUTPOUR
PEEPOUT
POMPOUS
POOPOUT
PROPSUP
PUMPOUT
PUMPSUP
RAMPSUP
SEEPOUT
SHAPEUP
SHIPFUL
SHIPOUT
SHOPFUL
SKIPOUT
SLIPOUT
SLIPSUP
SNAPSUP
SOAPSUP
SOUPSUP
STEPOUT
STEPSUP
STOPSUP
SULPHUR
SURPLUS
SWEPTUP
TRAPGUN
TRIPSUP
WHIPSUP
WIMPOUT
WRAPSUP

•••P••U
CHAPEAU

••••PU•
BREWPUB
CANOPUS
CREEPUP
CRISPUS
GOKAPUT
GRAMPUS
HARDPUT
HOTSPUR
JODHPUR
MANIPUR
OCCIPUT
OCTOPUS
OEDIPUS
OLYMPUS
PRESPUR
SHOTPUT
STAYPUT
SWEEPUP
THRUPUT
TRUMPUP
WELLPUT

••••P•U
THIMPHU

PV•••••
PVCPIPE

P•V••••
PAVANES
PAVIDLY
PAVINGS
PAVIORS
PAVIOUR
PAVLOVA
PIVOTAL
PIVOTED
PIVOTER
POVERTY

P••V•••
PARVENU
PEEVING
PEEVISH
PERVADE
PLOVDIV
PLOVERS
PLUVIAL
POIVRES
PREVAIL
PREVENT
PREVERB
PREVERT
PREVETO
PREVIAS
PREVIEW
PREVOID
PREVOST
PREVUED
PREVUES
PRIVACY
PRIVATE
PRIVETS
PRIVIER
PRIVIES
PRIVILY
PRIVITY
PRIVYTO
PROVEIT
PROVERB
PROVERS
PROVIDE
PROVINE
PROVING
PROVISO
PROVOKE
PROVOST
PURVEYS
PURVIEW

P•••V••
PALAVER
PIUSVII
POPOVER
PORIVER
PREAVER
PUTOVER

P••••V•
PAHLAVI
PARFIVE
PARKAVE
PASSIVE
PAVLOVA
PECCAVI
PENSIVE
PETDOVE
PLOSIVE
POLTAVA
POPDIVA
PREDIVE
PREPAVE
PRONAVY

P•••••V
PHILIPV
PLOVDIV
PQRSTUV

•PV••••
UPVALUE

•P••V••
UPDIVED
UPDIVES
UPRIVER

•P•••V•
APPROVE
UPABOVE
UPCURVE
UPHEAVE

•P••••V
SPIKETV

••P•V••
HOPOVER
IMPAVID
POPOVER
REPAVED
REPAVES
TIPOVER
UNPAVED

••P••V•
APPROVE
CAPTIVA
CAPTIVE
DEPRAVE
DEPRIVE
IMPROVE
POPDIVA
REPROVE
TOPFIVE

••P•••V
STPIUSV
TUPOLEV

•••P•V•
PREPAVE

•••••PV
PHILIPV

PW•••••
PWBOTHA

P•W••••
PAWEDAT
PAWNEES
PAWNERS
PAWNING
PAWNOFF
PAWPAWS
PCWORLD
PEWTERS
POWDERS
POWDERY
POWERED
POWERUP
POWWOWS

P••W•••
PAYWELL
PEDWAYS
PEEWEES
PERWEEK
PIGWEED
PINWALE
PLOWBOY
PLOWERS
PLOWING
PLOWMAN
PLOWMEN
PLOWSON
PLOWSUP
PLYWOOD
POPWINE
POWWOWS
PRAWNED
PREWARM
PREWARN
PREWASH
PREWHIP
PREWIRE
PREWITT
PREWORK
PREWORN
PREWRAP
PROWESS
PROWEST
PROWLED
PROWLER
PSYWARS

P•••W••
PARKWAY
PARTWAY
PATHWAY
PEGAWAY
PERIWIG
PESEWAS
POSTWAR
PSHAWED
PUTAWAY

P••••W•
PAGETWO
PARTTWO
PATDOWN
PAWPAWS
PEAFOWL
PETCOWS
PILLOWS
PILLOWY
PINDOWN
PITROWS
PITSAWS
PLUSTWO
POWWOWS
PREDAWN
PROBOWL
PUTDOWN

P•••••W
PALTROW
PAYSNOW
PETCHEW
PETCROW
PILCROW
PITCREW
POORLAW
PRESHOW
PREVIEW
PURVIEW

•PW••••
UPWAFTS
UPWARDS
UPWELLS
UPWHIRL
UPWINDS

•P•W•••
IPSWICH
SPAWNED
SPAWNER
SPEWERS
SPEWING
SPEWOUT
SPYWARE
UPSWEEP
UPSWELL
UPSWEPT
UPSWING

•P••W••
SPRAWLS
SPRAWLY
UPTOWNS

•P•••W•
OPUSTWO
UPFLOWS
UPGROWN
UPGROWS

•P••••W
SPARROW
UPTHROW
UPTONOW

••PW•••
LAPWARE
LAPWING
POPWINE
SOPWITH

••P•W••
DEPOWER
EMPOWER
INPOWER
JCPOWYS
JDPOWER
REPOWER
TFPOWYS
UNPAWED
UNPAWNS

••P••W•
ASPRAWL
ESPNEWS
NEPHEWS
REPLOWS
RIPSAWN
RIPSAWS
TIPDOWN
TOPDOWN
TOPROWS

••P•••W
CAPSHAW
ROPETOW
TOPDRAW

•••PW••
SHIPWAY

•••P•W•
PAWPAWS
QUAPAWS
STEPTWO

•••P••W
WHIPSAW

••••P•W
BEARPAW
CATSPAW
FOREPAW
HINDPAW

P•X••••
PAXINOU
PIXYISH

P••X•••
PLEXORS
PREXIES
PROXIES
PROXIMA
PROXIMO

P•••X••
PHLOXES
PIUSXII
POBOXES
PYREXIA

P••••X•
PICKAXE
POLEAXE
PRETEXT

P•••••X
PAGESIX
PANCHAX
PARADOX
PERPLEX
PHALANX
PHARYNX
PHOENIX
PILLBOX
PLAYTEX
PLUSTAX
POLLTAX
POORBOX
POORTAX
POSTBOX
POSTFIX

•P•X•••
EPOXIED
EPOXIES

•P••X••
CPAEXAM

•P••••X
APTERYX
SPANDEX

••P••X•
BYPROXY

••P•••X
STPIUSX

•••P••X
COMPLEX
DEEPSIX
DROPBOX
FUNPLEX
PERPLEX
SIMPLEX
SOAPBOX
SOUPMIX
TRIPLEX
UNIPLEX

••••P•X
ARUSPEX
COOLPIX
CRISPIX
TELEPIX

PY•••••
PYEDOGS
PYGMIES
PYNCHON
PYRAMID
PYRAMUS
PYRETIC
PYREXIA
PYRITES
PYRITIC
PYRRHIC
PYRRHUS
PYTHIAN
PYTHIAS
PYTHONS

P•Y••••
PAYABLE
PAYBACK
PAYCASH
PAYCUTS
PAYDAYS
PAYDIRT
PAYHEED
PAYINTO
PAYLESS
PAYLOAD
PAYMENT
PAYMORE
PAYOFFS
PAYOLAS
PAYOUTS
PAYRATE
PAYROLL
PAYSFOR
PAYSLIP
PAYSNOW
PAYSOFF
PAYSOUT
PAYSTUB
PAYWELL
PEYOTES
PHYLLIS
PHYLLOS
PHYSICS
PLYWOOD
PRYINTO
PRYOPEN
PSYCHED
PSYCHES
PSYCHIC
PSYCHOS
PSYCHUP
PSYWARS

P••Y•••
PAPYRUS
PERYEAR
PHRYGIA
PITYING
PIXYISH
PLAYACT
PLAYBOY
PLAYDOH
PLAYERS
PLAYFUL
PLAYING
PLAYLET
PLAYOFF
PLAYOUT
PLAYPEN
PLAYSAT
PLAYSBY
PLAYSON
PLAYSTO
PLAYSUP
PLAYTEX
POLYGON
POLYMER
POLYPED
POLYPOD
POLYSCI
PONYING
PONYKEG
PRAYERS
PRAYFOR
PRAYING
PRAYSTO
PREYERS
PREYING
PREYSON

P•••Y••
PALMYRA
PAPAYAS
PARTYER
PARTYON
PHARYNX
PHONYUP
PIEEYED
PIGEYED
PITAYAS
PLATYPI
POPEYED
POPEYES
PRETYPE
PRIVYTO
PROCYON

P••••Y•
PARLAYS
PARLEYS
PARONYM
PAYDAYS
PEDWAYS
PENNEYS
PEPBOYS
PETTOYS
PHONEYS
PINBOYS
POLANYI
PREBUYS
PREPAYS
PULLEYS
PURVEYS

P•••••Y
PAGEBOY
PAISLEY
PALEDRY
PALFREY
PALJOEY
PALMARY
PANICKY
PANOPLY
PARKWAY
PARSLEY
PARTWAY
PASSKEY
PATENCY
PATHWAY
PATSDRY
PAUCITY
PAULPRY
PAUNCHY
PAVIDLY
PEABODY
PECCARY
PEGAWAY
PENALTY
PEPPERY
PEPPILY
PERFIDY
PERFUMY
PERJURY
PERKILY
PESKILY
PETPONY
PETRIFY
PETTILY
PHLEGMY
PHONILY
PICARDY
PIGGERY
PILLORY
PILLOWY
PIOSITY
PIOUSLY
PITHILY
PLAINLY
PLAYBOY
PLAYSBY
PLENARY
PLIABLY
PLIANCY
PLOWBOY
PLUMPLY
PLUSHLY
POORBOY
PORTNOY
PORTRAY
POTENCY
POTTERY
POULTRY
POVERTY
POWDERY
PREACHY
PREALLY
PREDEFY
PREDENY
PRELACY
PRESLEY
PRICILY
PRICKLY
PRIMACY
PRIMARY
PRIMELY
PRIVACY
PRIVILY
PRIVITY
PROBITY
PROCITY
PRODIGY
PROGENY
PRONAVY
PRONELY
PROSILY
PROSODY
PROUDLY
PRUDERY
PTOLEMY
PUBERTY
PUCKERY
PUDENCY
PUDGILY
PUFFERY
PUFFILY
PUGSLEY
PULLTOY
PULPIFY
PUNNILY
PUSHILY
PUTAWAY
PUTREFY

•PY••••
SPYBOTS
SPYCAMS
SPYDERS
SPYHOLE
SPYINGS
SPYKIDS
SPYRING
SPYUPON
SPYWARE

•P•Y•••
SPAYERS
SPAYING
SPRYEST

•P••Y••
APPLYTO
EPONYMS
EPONYMY
SPLAYED
SPRAYED
SPRAYER
SPRAYON

•P•••Y•
APTERYX

•P••••Y
APISHLY
APLENTY
APOLOGY
EPARCHY
EPERNAY
EPILADY
EPONYMY
EPPERLY
OPACITY
SPACELY
SPANGLY
SPARELY
SPARKLY
SPASSKY
SPECIFY
SPICERY
SPICILY
SPIDERY
SPIKILY
SPINDLY
SPINDRY
SPINNEY
SPLASHY
SPLEENY
SPRAWLY
SPRINGY
UPEARLY

••PY•••
COPYBOY
COPYCAT
COPYING
COPYIST
COPYMAN
COPYMEN
ESPYING
PAPYRUS

••P•Y••
APPLYTO
DIPTYCH
HAPPYTO
KOPIYKA
LIPSYNC
PAPAYAS
POPEYED
POPEYES
REPLYTO
ZEPHYRS

••P••Y•
BYPLAYS
DEPLOYS
EMPLOYS
HYPONYM
JCPOWYS
OSPREYS
PEPBOYS
REPLAYS
TFPOWYS
TOPONYM

••P•••Y
AMPLIFY
BYPROXY
CAPABLY
CAPEMAY
CEPHALY
COPPERY
COPYBOY
EMPATHY
EMPTILY
EPPERLY
EUPHONY
FOPPERY
HAPENNY
HAPPIFY
HAPPILY
HIPPITY
IMPIETY
NIPPILY
PEPPERY
PEPPILY
RAPIDLY
SAPPILY
TEPIDLY
TIPSILY
TOPIARY
UNPIETY
VAPIDLY
VAPOURY
YUPPIFY

•••PY••
HAPPYTO

•••P•Y•
MURPHYS
OUTPAYS
PREPAYS
TEAPOYS

•••P••Y
ADEPTLY
AIRPLAY
BUMPILY
CALPOLY
CAMPILY
CASPARY
COMPANY
COOPERY
COPPERY
COWPONY
DAMPDRY
DEEPFRY
DEEPSKY
DEMPSEY
DISPLAY
DRAPERY
DRIPDRY
DROPSBY
DUMPILY
DUOPOLY
ENDPLAY
EXUPERY
FOPPERY
GRAPERY
GUNPLAY
HAPPIFY
HAPPILY
HIPPITY
HITPLAY
HOOPTOY
HUMPHRY
INAPTLY
INEPTLY
JASPERY
JUMPILY
LAMPREY
LEAPDAY
LUMPILY
MISPLAY
NIPPILY
NONPLAY
OUTPITY
OUTPLAY
OUTPRAY
PEPPERY
PEPPILY
PETPONY
PULPIFY
REAPPLY
REDPONY
RESPRAY
SAPPILY
SETPLAY
SHAPELY
SHIPWAY
SKIPSBY
SLIPSBY
SOAPILY
STOPSBY
STUPEFY
UNAPTLY
UNSPICY
WASPILY
WISPILY
YUPPIFY

••••P•Y
ATROPHY
AUTOPSY
BACKPAY
BASEPAY
BEHAPPY
BIASPLY
CHEAPLY
CREEPBY
CRISPLY
CRUMPLY
GOODPAY
HIGHPAY
IMHAPPY
MOREPAY
OCTUPLY
ONEMPTY
OVERPAY
OVERPLY
PANOPLY
PAULPRY
PLUMPLY
REAPPLY
REIMPLY
SCRAPPY
SHARPLY
SICKPAY
STEEPLY
UNEMPTY
UNHAPPY

•••••PY
BEHAPPY
ENTROPY
GOSSIPY
IMHAPPY
ISOTOPY
MISCOPY
SATRAPY
SCRAPPY
SCRIMPY
SHRIMPY
THERAPY
UNHAPPY
UNLUMPY
UNRASPY

P•Z••••
PIZARRO
PIZZAZZ
POZOLES
PUZZLED
PUZZLER
PUZZLES

P••Z•••
PANZERS
PATZERS
PENZIAS
PIAZZAS
PIZZAZZ
PRIZING
PRIZZIS
PUZZLED
PUZZLER
PUZZLES

P•••Z••
PALAZZI
PALAZZO
PIAZZAS
PLOTZED
PLOTZES
PRETZEL
PRIZZIS

P••••Z•
PALAZZI
PALAZZO
PIZZAZZ
POETIZE

P•••••Z
PIZZAZZ
POPQUIZ

•P••Z••
SPITZES
UPGAZED
UPGAZES
UPSIZED
UPSIZES

•P•••Z•
SPINOZA

••P•Z••
TOPAZES

••P••Z•
BAPTIZE
CAPSIZE
IMPREZA

••P•••Z
POPQUIZ

•••PZ••
LEIPZIG

•••P•Z•
TRAPEZE

•••P••Z
TEMPEAZ
TIRPITZ

••••P•Z
ALLOPEZ

QA•••••
QABALAH
QABALAS
QADDAFI
QATARIS

Q•A••••
QRATIOS
QUACKED
QUACKER
QUADRIC
QUAFFED
QUAFFER
QUAGGAS
QUAHOGS
QUAILED
QUAKERS
QUAKIER
QUAKIES
QUAKILY
QUAKING
QUALIFY
QUALITY
QUANTUM
QUAPAWS
QUARLES
QUARREL
QUARTAN
QUARTER
QUARTES
QUARTET
QUARTIC
QUARTOS
QUARTZY
QUASARS
QUASHED
QUASHES
QUATRES
QUATTRO
QUAVERS
QUAVERY
QUAYAGE

Q••A•••
QABALAH
QABALAS
QATARIS

Q•••A••
QADDAFI
QINTARS
QUAPAWS
QUASARS
QUAYAGE
QUEPASA
QUINARY
QUINATE

Q••••A•
QABALAH
QABALAS
QBSNEAK
QUAGGAS
QUARTAN
QUENEAU
QUESNAY
QUETZAL
QUINLAN
QUINTAL
QUINTAS
QUONDAM

Q•••••A
QUECHUA
QUEPASA
QUERIDA
QUESERA
QUINELA

•Q•A•••
AQUAMAN
AQUARIA
AQUATIC
AQUAVIT
EQUABLE
EQUABLY
EQUALED
EQUALLY
EQUALTO
EQUATED
EQUATES
EQUATOR
SQUALID
SQUALLS
SQUALLY
SQUALOR
SQUANTO
SQUARED
SQUARER
SQUARES
SQUASHY
SQUATLY
SQUATTY
SQUAWKS
SQUAWKY
UQUARKS

•Q••A••
EQUIANO
SQUEAKS
SQUEAKY
SQUEALS

•Q•••A•
AQUAMAN
AQUINAS
EQUIFAX

•Q••••A
AQUARIA

••Q•A••
EMQUADS
ENQUADS
LIQUATE
LOQUATS
PDQBACH
PIQUANT
TSQUARE
UPQUARK

••Q••A•
BUQSHAS

••Q•••A
COQUINA
SEQUOIA
SEQUOYA
TEQUILA

•••Q•A•
COEQUAL
KUMQUAT
RORQUAL
UNEQUAL

QB•••••
QBSNEAK

Q•B••••
QABALAH
QABALAS

Q••B•••
QUIBBLE

Q•••B••
QUIBBLE

•Q••B••
EQUABLE
EQUABLY

••QB•••
BBQBEEF
PDQBACH

••Q••B•
BBQRIBS

Q•C••••
QSCHOOL

Q••C•••
QUACKED
QUACKER
QUECHUA
QUICHES
QUICKEN
QUICKER
QUICKIE
QUICKLY

Q•••C••
QUINCES
QUINCEY

Q•••••C
QUADRIC
QUARTIC
QUINTIC

•Q•••C•
SQUELCH
SQUINCH

•Q••••C
AQUATIC

••Q••C•
BEQUICK
PDQBACH
UNQUICK

Q•D••••
QADDAFI

Q••D•••
QADDAFI
QUADRIC

Q•••D••
QUONDAM

Q••••D•
QUERIDA
QUERIDO

Q•••••D
QUACKED
QUAFFED
QUAILED
QUASHED
QUEENED
QUEERED
QUELLED
QUERIED
QUESTED
QUIETED
QUILLED
QUILTED
QUIPPED
QUIRTED
QUITTED
QUIZZED
QUOINED
QUOITED

•Q••D••
GQMODEL

•Q••••D
EQUALED
EQUATED
SQUALID
SQUARED
SQUIRED

••Q••D•
EMQUADS
ENQUADS
LIQUIDS

•••Q••D
CASQUED
CLIQUED
TORQUED

Q•E••••
QUECHUA
QUEENED
QUEENIE
QUEENIT
QUEENLY
QUEERED
QUEERER
QUEERLY
QUEIROS
QUELLED
QUELLER
QUELQUE
QUENEAU
QUENTIN
QUEPASA
QUERIDA
QUERIDO
QUERIED
QUERIER
QUERIES
QUERIST
QUESERA
QUESNAY
QUESTED
QUESTER
QUETZAL
QUEUERS
QUEUEUP
QUEUING

Q••E•••
QUEENED
QUEENIE
QUEENIT
QUEENLY
QUEERED
QUEERER
QUEERLY
QUIETED
QUIETEN
QUIETER
QUIETLY
QUIETUS

Q•••E••
QBSNEAK
QUAKERS
QUAVERS
QUAVERY
QUENEAU
QUESERA
QUEUERS
QUEUEUP
QUINELA
QUITESO
QUIVERS
QUIVERY
QUOTEES
QUOTERS

Q••••E•
QUACKED
QUACKER
QUAFFED
QUAFFER
QUAILED
QUAKIER
QUAKIES
QUARLES
QUARREL
QUARTER
QUARTES
QUARTET
QUASHED
QUASHES
QUATRES
QUEENED
QUEERED
QUEERER
QUELLED
QUELLER
QUERIED
QUERIER
QUERIES
QUESTED
QUESTER
QUICHES
QUICKEN
QUICKER
QUIETED
QUIETEN
QUIETER
QUIGLEY
QUILLED
QUILLER
QUILTED
QUILTER
QUINCES
QUINCEY
QUINTES
QUINTET
QUINZES
QUIPPED
QUIPPER
QUIRTED
QUITTED
QUITTER
QUIZZED
QUIZZER
QUIZZES
QUOINED
QUOITED
QUONSET
QUOTEES

Q•••••E
QUAYAGE
QUEENIE
QUELQUE
QUIBBLE
QUICKIE
QUINATE
QUININE
QUINQUE
QUIVIVE
QUIXOTE

•Q•E•••
AQUEOUS
EQUERRY
IQTESTS
SQUEAKS
SQUEAKY
SQUEALS
SQUEERS
SQUEEZE
SQUELCH

•Q••E••
SQUEERS
SQUEEZE

•Q•••E•
AQUIFER
AQUIVER
EQUALED
EQUATED
EQUATES
EQUINES
GQMODEL
SQUARED
SQUARER
SQUARES
SQUIRED
SQUIRES

•Q••••E
EQUABLE
SQUEEZE

••Q•E••
BBQBEEF
BEQUEST
DEQUEUE
ENQUEUE
INQUEST
LIQUEFY
LIQUEUR
MCQUEEN
REQUEST
SEQUELS
VAQUERO

••Q••E•
ASQUIET
BBQBEEF
BEQUIET
MCQUEEN
REQUIEM
UNQUIET

••Q•••E
ACQUIRE
DEQUEUE
ENQUEUE
ENQUIRE
ESQUIRE
INQUIRE
LIQUATE
REQUIRE
REQUITE
REQUOTE
TSQUARE
UNQUOTE

•••Q•E•
BANQUES
BANQUET
BARQUES
BASQUES
BISQUES
BOUQUET
BRIQUET
CASQUED
CASQUES
CHEQUER
CHEQUES
CINQUES
CIRQUES
CLAQUES
CLIQUED
CLIQUES
CLIQUEY
CONQUER
CROQUET
EPOQUES
JACQUES
LACQUER
MARQUEE
MARQUES
MARQUEZ
MASQUER
MASQUES
MOSQUES
OPAQUES
PARQUET
PLAQUES
PREQUEL
RACQUET
SACQUES
TORQUED
TORQUES
UNIQUES
VASQUEZ

•••Q••E
MARQUEE

••••Q•E
ANTIQUE
BAROQUE
BEZIQUE
BRUSQUE
CACIQUE
COMIQUE
DUBUQUE
ENRIQUE
GIAUQUE
LALIQUE
MACAQUE
OBLIQUE
PRESQUE
QUELQUE
QUINQUE

Q••F•••
QUAFFED
QUAFFER

Q•••F••
QUAFFED
QUAFFER

Q••••F•
QADDAFI
QUALIFY

•Q••F••
AQUIFER
EQUIFAX

••Q••F•
LIQUEFY

••Q•••F
BBQBEEF

Q••G•••
QUAGGAS
QUIGLEY

Q•••G••
QUAGGAS

Q••••G•
QUAHOGS
QUAYAGE

Q•••••G
QUAKING
QUEUING
QUOTING

••Q•••G
PIQUING

Q••H•••
QSCHOOL
QUAHOGS

Q•••H••
QUASHED
QUASHES
QUECHUA
QUICHES

Q•••••H
QABALAH

•Q•••H•
SQUASHY
SQUISHY

•Q••••H
SQUELCH
SQUINCH

••Q•H••
BUQSHAS

••Q•••H
ASQUITH
PDQBACH

QI•••••
QINTARS

Q•I••••
QUIBBLE
QUICHES
QUICKEN
QUICKER
QUICKIE
QUICKLY
QUIETED
QUIETEN
QUIETER
QUIETLY
QUIETUS
QUIGLEY
QUILLED
QUILLER
QUILTED
QUILTER
QUINARY
QUINATE
QUINCES
QUINCEY
QUINELA
QUININE
QUINION
QUINLAN
QUINQUE
QUINTAL
QUINTAS
QUINTES
QUINTET
QUINTIC
QUINTON
QUINTUS
QUINZES
QUIPPED
QUIPPER
QUIRTED
QUITESO
QUITSIT
QUITTED
QUITTER
QUIVERS
QUIVERY
QUIVIVE
QUIXOTE
QUIZNOS
QUIZZED
QUIZZER
QUIZZES

Q••I•••
QUAILED
QUEIROS
QUOINED
QUOITED

Q•••I••
QRATIOS
QUAKIER
QUAKIES
QUAKILY
QUAKING
QUALIFY
QUALITY
QUERIDA
QUERIDO
QUERIED
QUERIER
QUERIES
QUERIST
QUEUING
QUININE
QUINION
QUIVIVE
QUOTING

Q••••I•
QATARIS
QUADRIC
QUARTIC
QUEENIE
QUEENIT
QUENTIN
QUICKIE
QUINTIC
QUITSIT

Q•••••I
QADDAFI

•Q•I•••
AQUIFER
AQUINAS
AQUIVER
EQUIANO
EQUIFAX
EQUINES
EQUINOX
SQUINCH
SQUINTS
SQUINTY
SQUIRED
SQUIRES
SQUIRMS
SQUIRMY
SQUIRTS
SQUISHY

•Q•••I•
AQUARIA
AQUATIC
AQUAVIT
SQUALID

••Q•I••
ACQUIRE
ACQUITS
ALQUIST
ASQUIET
ASQUINT
ASQUITH
BBQPITS
BBQRIBS
BEQUICK
BEQUIET
COQUINA
DRQUINN
ENQUIRE
ENQUIRY
ESQUIRE
INQUIRE
INQUIRY
LIQUIDS
MRQUILP
PIQUING
REQUIEM
REQUIRE
REQUITE
SEQUINS
TEQUILA
UNQUICK
UNQUIET

••Q••I•
SEQUOIA

•••Q•I•
CROQUIS
DAYQUIL
JOAQUIN
JONQUIL
MARQUIS
NESQUIK
PACQUIN
POPQUIZ
REEQUIP
YANQUIS

Q••K•••
QUAKERS
QUAKIER
QUAKIES
QUAKILY
QUAKING

Q•••K••
QUACKED
QUACKER
QUICKEN
QUICKER
QUICKIE
QUICKLY

Q•••••K
QBSNEAK

•Q•••K•
SQUAWKS
SQUAWKY
SQUEAKS
SQUEAKY
UQUARKS

••Q•••K
BBQPORK
BEQUICK
UNQUICK
UPQUARK

•••Q••K
NESQUIK

Q••L•••
QUALIFY
QUALITY
QUELLED
QUELLER
QUELQUE
QUILLED
QUILLER
QUILTED
QUILTER

Q•••L••
QABALAH
QABALAS
QUAILED
QUARLES
QUELLED
QUELLER
QUIGLEY
QUILLED
QUILLER
QUINLAN

Q••••L•
QUAKILY
QUEENLY
QUEERLY
QUIBBLE
QUICKLY
QUIETLY
QUINELA

Q•••••L
QSCHOOL
QUARREL
QUETZAL
QUINTAL

•Q••L••
EQUALED
EQUALLY
EQUALTO
SQUALID
SQUALLS
SQUALLY
SQUALOR
SQUELCH

•Q•••L•
EQUABLE
EQUABLY
EQUALLY
SQUALLS
SQUALLY
SQUATLY
SQUEALS

•Q••••L
GQMODEL

••Q••L•
MRQUILP
SEQUELS
TEQUILA

•••Q••L
COEQUAL
DAYQUIL
JONQUIL
PREQUEL
RORQUAL
UNEQUAL

Q••••M•
QUORUMS

Q•••••M
QUANTUM
QUONDAM

•QM••••
GQMODEL

•Q••M••
AQUAMAN

•Q•••M•
SQUIRMS
SQUIRMY

••Q•••M
REQUIEM

Q•N••••
QINTARS

Q••N•••
QBSNEAK
QUANTUM
QUENEAU
QUENTIN
QUINARY
QUINATE
QUINCES
QUINCEY
QUINELA
QUININE
QUINION
QUINLAN
QUINQUE
QUINTAL
QUINTAS
QUINTES
QUINTET
QUINTIC
QUINTON
QUINTUS
QUINZES
QUONDAM
QUONSET

Q•••N••
QUEENED
QUEENIE
QUEENIT
QUEENLY
QUESNAY
QUIZNOS
QUOINED

Q••••N•
QUAKING
QUEUING
QUININE
QUOTING

Q•••••N
QUARTAN
QUENTIN
QUICKEN
QUIETEN
QUINION
QUINLAN
QUINTON

•Q••N••
AQUINAS
EQUINES
EQUINOX
SQUANTO
SQUINCH
SQUINTS
SQUINTY

•Q•••N•
EQUIANO

•Q••••N
AQUAMAN

••Q••N•
ASQUINT
COQUINA
DRQUINN
PIQUANT
PIQUING
SEQUINS

••Q•••N
DRQUINN
MCQUEEN

•••Q••N
JOAQUIN
PACQUIN

Q•O••••
QUOINED
QUOITED
QUONDAM
QUONSET
QUORUMS
QUOTEES
QUOTERS
QUOTING

Q•••O••
QSCHOOL
QUAHOGS
QUIXOTE

Q••••O•
QRATIOS
QSCHOOL
QUARTOS
QUEIROS
QUINION
QUINTON
QUIZNOS

Q•••••O
QUATTRO
QUERIDO
QUITESO

•Q•O•••
GQMODEL

•Q••O••
AQUEOUS

•Q•••O•
EQUATOR
EQUINOX
SQUALOR

•Q••••O
EQUALTO
EQUIANO
SQUANTO

••Q•O••
BBQPORK
LIQUORS
PEQUOTS
REQUOTE
SEQUOIA
SEQUOYA
UNQUOTE

••Q•••O
VAQUERO

Q••P•••
QUAPAWS
QUEPASA
QUIPPED
QUIPPER

Q•••P••
QUIPPED
QUIPPER

Q•••••P
QUEUEUP

••QP•••
BBQPITS
BBQPORK

••Q•••P
MRQUILP

•••Q••P
REEQUIP

Q•••Q••
QUELQUE
QUINQUE

QR•••••
QRATIOS
QRSTUVW

Q••R•••
QUARLES
QUARREL
QUARTAN
QUARTER
QUARTES
QUARTET
QUARTIC
QUARTOS
QUARTZY
QUERIDA
QUERIDO
QUERIED
QUERIER
QUERIES
QUERIST
QUIRTED
QUORUMS

Q•••R••
QATARIS
QUADRIC
QUARREL
QUATRES
QUEERED
QUEERER
QUEERLY
QUEIROS

Q••••R•
QINTARS
QUAKERS
QUASARS
QUATTRO
QUAVERS
QUAVERY
QUESERA
QUEUERS
QUINARY
QUIVERS
QUIVERY
QUOTERS

Q•••••R
QUACKER
QUAFFER
QUAKIER
QUARTER
QUEERER
QUELLER
QUERIER
QUESTER
QUICKER
QUIETER
QUILLER
QUILTER
QUIPPER
QUITTER
QUIZZER

•QR••••
PQRSTUV

•Q•R•••
AQUARIA
EQUERRY
SQUARED
SQUARER
SQUARES
SQUIRED
SQUIRES
SQUIRMS
SQUIRMY
SQUIRTS
UQUARKS

•Q•••R•
EQUERRY
SQUEERS

•Q••••R
AQUIFER
AQUIVER
EQUATOR
SQUALOR
SQUARER

••QR•••
BBQRIBS
OPQRSTU

••Q•R••
ACQUIRE
BBQPORK
ENQUIRE
ENQUIRY
ESQUIRE
INQUIRE
INQUIRY
LIQUORS
REQUIRE
TSQUARE
UPQUARK
VAQUERO

••Q•••R
LIQUEUR

•••QR••
NOPQRST

•••Q••R
CHEQUER
CONQUER
LACQUER
MASQUER

••••QR•
MNOPQRS

•••••QR
LMNOPQR

QS•••••
QSCHOOL

Q•S••••
QBSNEAK
QRSTUVW

Q••S•••
QUASARS
QUASHED
QUASHES
QUESERA
QUESNAY
QUESTED
QUESTER

Q•••S••
QUITSIT
QUONSET

Q••••S•
QUEPASA
QUERIST
QUITESO

Q•••••S
QABALAS
QATARIS
QINTARS
QRATIOS
QUAGGAS
QUAHOGS
QUAKERS
QUAKIES
QUAPAWS
QUARLES
QUARTES
QUARTOS
QUASARS
QUASHES
QUATRES
QUAVERS
QUEIROS
QUERIES
QUEUERS
QUICHES
QUIETUS
QUINCES
QUINTAS
QUINTES
QUINTUS
QUINZES
QUIVERS
QUIZNOS
QUIZZES
QUORUMS
QUOTEES
QUOTERS

•QS••••
PQRSTUV

•Q••S••
IQTESTS
SQUASHY
SQUISHY

•Q••••S
AQUEOUS
AQUINAS
EQUATES
EQUINES
IQTESTS
SQUALLS
SQUARES
SQUAWKS
SQUEAKS
SQUEALS
SQUEERS
SQUINTS
SQUIRES
SQUIRMS
SQUIRTS
UQUARKS

••QS•••
BUQSHAS

••Q•S••
OPQRSTU

••Q••S•
ALQUIST
BEQUEST
INQUEST
REQUEST

••Q•••S
ACQUITS
BBQPITS
BBQRIBS
BUQSHAS
EMQUADS
ENQUADS
LIQUIDS
LIQUORS
LOQUATS
PEQUOTS
SEQUELS
SEQUINS

•••Q•S•
NOPQRST

•••Q••S
BANQUES
BARQUES
BASQUES
BISQUES
CASQUES
CHEQUES
CINQUES
CIRQUES
CLAQUES
CLIQUES
CROQUIS
EPOQUES
JACQUES
MARQUES
MARQUIS
MASQUES
MOSQUES
OPAQUES
PLAQUES
SACQUES
TORQUES
UNIQUES
YANQUIS

••••Q•S
MNOPQRS

•••••QS
COMPAQS
HIGHIQS
POSSLQS
PSANDQS

Q•T••••
QATARIS

Q••T•••
QINTARS

QRATIOS
QRSTUVW
QUATRES
QUATTRO
QUETZAL
QUITESO
QUITSIT
QUITTED
QUITTER
QUOTEES
QUOTERS
QUOTING

Q•••T••
QUANTUM
QUARTAN
QUARTER
QUARTES
QUARTET
QUARTIC
QUARTOS
QUARTZY
QUATTRO
QUENTIN
QUESTED
QUESTER
QUIETED
QUIETEN
QUIETER
QUIETLY
QUIETUS
QUILTED
QUILTER
QUINTAL
QUINTAS
QUINTES
QUINTET
QUINTIC
QUINTON
QUINTUS
QUIRTED
QUITTED
QUITTER
QUOITED

Q••••T•
QUALITY
QUINATE
QUIXOTE

Q•••••T
QUARTET
QUEENIT
QUERIST
QUINTET
QUITSIT
QUONSET

•QT••••
IQTESTS

•Q••T••
AQUATIC
EQUATED
EQUATES
EQUATOR
PQRSTUV
SQUATLY
SQUATTY

•Q•••T•
EQUALTO
IQTESTS
SQUANTO
SQUATTY
SQUINTS
SQUINTY
SQUIRTS

•Q••••T
AQUAVIT

••Q••T•
ACQUITS
ASQUITH
BBQPITS
LIQUATE
LOQUATS
OPQRSTU
PEQUOTS
REQUITE
REQUOTE
UNQUOTE

••Q•••T
ALQUIST
ASQUIET
ASQUINT
BEQUEST
BEQUIET
INQUEST
PIQUANT
REQUEST
UNQUIET

•••Q••T
BANQUET
BOUQUET
BRIQUET
CROQUET
KUMQUAT
NOPQRST
PARQUET
RACQUET

•••••QT
ONTHEQT

QU•••••
QUACKED
QUACKER
QUADRIC
QUAFFED
QUAFFER
QUAGGAS
QUAHOGS
QUAILED
QUAKERS
QUAKIER
QUAKIES
QUAKILY
QUAKING
QUALIFY
QUALITY
QUANTUM
QUAPAWS
QUARLES
QUARREL
QUARTAN
QUARTER
QUARTES
QUARTET
QUARTIC
QUARTOS
QUARTZY
QUASARS
QUASHED
QUASHES
QUATRES
QUATTRO
QUAVERS
QUAVERY
QUAYAGE
QUECHUA
QUEENED
QUEENIE
QUEENIT
QUEENLY
QUEERED
QUEERER
QUEERLY
QUEIROS
QUELLED
QUELLER
QUELQUE
QUENEAU
QUENTIN
QUEPASA
QUERIDA
QUERIDO
QUERIED
QUERIER
QUERIES
QUERIST
QUESERA
QUESNAY
QUESTED
QUESTER
QUETZAL
QUEUERS
QUEUEUP
QUEUING
QUIBBLE
QUICHES
QUICKEN
QUICKER
QUICKIE
QUICKLY
QUIETED
QUIETEN
QUIETER
QUIETLY
QUIETUS
QUIGLEY
QUILLED
QUILLER
QUILTED
QUILTER
QUINARY
QUINATE
QUINCES
QUINCEY
QUINELA
QUININE
QUINION
QUINLAN
QUINQUE
QUINTAL
QUINTAS
QUINTES
QUINTET
QUINTIC
QUINTON
QUINTUS
QUINZES
QUIPPED
QUIPPER
QUIRTED
QUITESO
QUITSIT
QUITTED
QUITTER
QUIVERS
QUIVERY
QUIVIVE
QUIXOTE
QUIZNOS
QUIZZED
QUIZZER
QUIZZES
QUOINED
QUOITED
QUONDAM
QUONSET
QUORUMS
QUOTEES
QUOTERS
QUOTING

Q••U•••
QUEUERS
QUEUEUP
QUEUING

Q•••U••
QRSTUVW
QUORUMS

Q••••U•
QUANTUM
QUECHUA
QUELQUE
QUEUEUP
QUIETUS
QUINQUE
QUINTUS

Q•••••U
QUENEAU

•QU••••
AQUAMAN
AQUARIA
AQUATIC
AQUAVIT
AQUEOUS
AQUIFER
AQUINAS
AQUIVER
EQUABLE
EQUABLY
EQUALED
EQUALLY
EQUALTO
EQUATED
EQUATES
EQUATOR
EQUERRY
EQUIANO
EQUIFAX
EQUINES
EQUINOX
SQUALID
SQUALLS
SQUALLY
SQUALOR
SQUANTO
SQUARED
SQUARER
SQUARES
SQUASHY
SQUATLY
SQUATTY
SQUAWKS
SQUAWKY
SQUEAKS
SQUEAKY
SQUEALS
SQUEERS
SQUEEZE
SQUELCH
SQUINCH
SQUINTS
SQUINTY
SQUIRED
SQUIRES
SQUIRMS
SQUIRMY
SQUIRTS
SQUISHY
UQUARKS

•Q•••U•
AQUEOUS
PQRSTUV

••QU•••
ACQUIRE
ACQUITS
ALQUIST
ASQUIET
ASQUINT
ASQUITH
BEQUEST
BEQUICK
BEQUIET
COQUINA
DEQUEUE
DRQUINN
EMQUADS
ENQUADS
ENQUEUE
ENQUIRE
ENQUIRY
ESQUIRE
INQUEST
INQUIRE
INQUIRY
LIQUATE
LIQUEFY
LIQUEUR
LIQUIDS
LIQUORS
LOQUATS
MCQUEEN
MRQUILP
PEQUOTS
PIQUANT
PIQUING
REQUEST
REQUIEM
REQUIRE
REQUITE
REQUOTE
SEQUELS
SEQUINS
SEQUOIA
SEQUOYA
TEQUILA
TSQUARE
UNQUICK
UNQUIET
UNQUOTE
UPQUARK
VAQUERO

••Q••U•
DEQUEUE
ENQUEUE
LIQUEUR

••Q•••U
OPQRSTU

•••QU••
BANQUES
BANQUET
BARQUES
BASQUES
BISQUES
BOUQUET
BRIQUET
CASQUED
CASQUES
CHEQUER
CHEQUES
CINQUES
CIRQUES
CLAQUES
CLIQUED
CLIQUES
CLIQUEY
COEQUAL
CONQUER
CROQUET
CROQUIS
DAYQUIL
EPOQUES
JACQUES
JOAQUIN
JONQUIL
KUMQUAT
LACQUER
MARQUEE
MARQUES
MARQUEZ
MARQUIS
MASQUER
MASQUES
MOSQUES
NESQUIK
OPAQUES
PACQUIN
PARQUET
PLAQUES
POPQUIZ
PREQUEL
RACQUET
REEQUIP
RORQUAL
SACQUES
TORQUED
TORQUES
UNEQUAL
UNIQUES
VASQUEZ
YANQUIS

••••QU•
ANTIQUE
BAROQUE
BEZIQUE
BRUSQUE
CACIQUE
COMIQUE
DUBUQUE
ENRIQUE
GIAUQUE
LALIQUE
MACAQUE
OBLIQUE
OBLOQUY
PRESQUE
QUELQUE
QUINQUE

Q••V•••
QUAVERS
QUAVERY
QUIVERS
QUIVERY
QUIVIVE

Q••••V•
QRSTUVW
QUIVIVE

•Q••V••
AQUAVIT
AQUIVER

•Q••••V
PQRSTUV

Q••••W•
QUAPAWS

Q•••••W
QRSTUVW

•Q••W••
SQUAWKS
SQUAWKY

Q••X•••
QUIXOTE

•Q••••X
EQUIFAX
EQUINOX

Q••Y•••
QUAYAGE

Q•••••Y
QUAKILY
QUALIFY
QUALITY
QUARTZY
QUAVERY
QUEENLY
QUEERLY
QUESNAY
QUICKLY
QUIETLY
QUIGLEY
QUINARY
QUINCEY
QUIVERY

•Q••••Y
EQUABLY
EQUALLY
EQUERRY
SQUALLY
SQUASHY
SQUATLY
SQUATTY
SQUAWKY
SQUEAKY
SQUINTY
SQUIRMY
SQUISHY

••Q••Y•
SEQUOYA

••Q•••Y
ENQUIRY
INQUIRY
LIQUEFY

•••Q••Y
CLIQUEY

••••Q•Y
OBLOQUY

Q••Z•••
QUIZNOS
QUIZZED
QUIZZER
QUIZZES

Q•••Z••
QUETZAL
QUINZES
QUIZZED
QUIZZER
QUIZZES

Q••••Z•
QUARTZY

•Q•••Z•
SQUEEZE

•••Q••Z
MARQUEZ
POPQUIZ
VASQUEZ

RA•••••
RABBETS
RABBITS
RABBITT
RABBITY
RABBLED
RABBLES
RABIDLY
RACCOON
RACECAR
RACEDBY
RACEDIN
RACEDTO
RACEDUP
RACEMES
RACESBY
RACESTO
RACESUP
RACEWAY
RACHAEL
RACIEST
RACINOS
RACISTS
RACKERS
RACKETS
RACKETY
RACKING
RACKOUT
RACKSUP
RACQUET
RADAMES
RADFORD
RADIALS
RADIANS
RADIANT
RADIATE
RADICAL
RADICES
RADICLE
RADIOAD
RADIODJ
RADIOED
RADIOER
RADIOIN
RADIXES
RADOMES
RAEBURN
RAEDAWN
RAFFIAS
RAFFISH
RAFFLED
RAFFLER
RAFFLES
RAFTERS
RAFTING
RAGBAGS
RAGDOLL
RAGEFUL
RAGGEDY
RAGGIER
RAGGIES
RAGGING
RAGINGS
RAGLANS
RAGMANS
RAGMOPS
RAGOUTS
RAGRUGS
RAGSHOP
RAGTIME
RAGTOPS
RAGWEED
RAIDERS
RAIDING
RAILAGE
RAILBUS
RAILCAR
RAILERS
RAILING
RAILMAN
RAILMEN
RAILSAT
RAILSON
RAILWAY
RAIMENT
RAINBOW
RAINGOD
RAINHAT
RAINIER
RAINILY
RAINING
RAINMAN
RAINOUT
RAINSIN
RAINSON
RAISERS
RAISEUP
RAISING
RAISINS
RAISINY
RAISONS
RAJARAO
RAKABLE
RAKEDIN
RAKEDUP
RAKEOFF
RAKESIN
RAKESUP
RALEIGH
RALLIED
RALLIER
RALLIES
RALLYES
RALLYTO
RALPHIE
RALSTON
RAMADAN
RAMADAS
RAMBLED
RAMBLER
RAMBLES
RAMBLIN
RAMDOWN
RAMEKIN
RAMESES
RAMFANS
RAMHOME
RAMINTO
RAMIREZ
RAMJETS
RAMLIKE
RAMMERS
RAMMING
RAMMISH
RAMONES
RAMPAGE
RAMPANT
RAMPART
RAMPING
RAMPSUP
RAMRODS
RAMSESI
RAMSFAN
RAMSONS
RANAMOK
RANATAB
RANAWAY
RANBACK
RANCHED
RANCHER
RANCHES
RANCHOS
RANCORS
RANCOUR
RANDALL
RANDEEP
RANDIER
RANDOWN
RANFREE
RANGERS
RANGFOR
RANGIER
RANGING
RANGOFF
RANGOON
RANGOUT
RANHOME
RANINTO
RANITUP
RANKERS
RANKEST
RANKINE
RANKING
RANKISH
RANKLED
RANKLES
RANKOUT
RANLAPS
RANLATE
RANONIN
RANOVER
RANPAST
RANRIOT
RANSACK
RANSOMS
RANTERS
RANTING
RANTSAT
RANUPTO
RANWILD
RANWITH
RAPALLO
RAPANUI
RAPHAEL
RAPIDAN
RAPIDER
RAPIDLY
RAPIERS
RAPINES
RAPINIS
RAPPELS
RAPPERS
RAPPING
RAPPORT
RAPSONG
RAPSTAR
RAPTORS
RAPTUNE
RAPTURE
RAREBIT
RAREGAS
RARITAN
RASBORA
RASCALS
RASHERS
RASHEST
RASHIDA
RASPERS
RASPIER
RASPING
RASPISH
RASSLED
RASSLER
RASSLES
RASTERS
RASURES
RATABLE
RATAFIA
RATATAT
RATBERT
RATCHET
RATECAP
RATEDPG
RATFINK
RATHOLE
RATINES
RATINGS
RATIONS
RATITES
RATLIKE
RATLINE
RATLINS
RATPACK
RATRACE
RATSOUT
RATTAIL
RATTANS
RATTERS
RATTIER
RATTING
RATTISH
RATTLED
RATTLER
RATTLES
RATTRAP
RAUCOUS
RAUNCHY
RAVAGED
RAVAGER
RAVAGES
RAVELED
RAVELLY
RAVELOE
RAVENAL
RAVENED
RAVENNA
RAVEUPS
RAVINED
RAVINES
RAVINGS
RAVIOLI
RAWBARS
RAWDATA
RAWDEAL
RAWEGGS
RAWFISH
RAWFOOD
RAWHIDE
RAWISTS
RAWLINS
RAWMEAT
RAWNESS
RAWSILK
RAYBANS
RAYBURN
RAYGUNS
RAYKROC
RAYLESS
RAYLIKE
RAYMOND
RAYNELL
RAYOVAC
RAZORED
RAZZIES
RAZZING

R•A••••
RCADOME
REACHED
REACHER
REACHES
REACHIN
REACHUP
REACTED
REACTOR
REACTTO
READAPT
READDED
READERS
READFOR
READIED
READIER
READIES
READILY
READING
READMIT
READOFF
READOPT
READORN
READOUT
READSIN
READSON
READSTO
READSUP
REAFFIX
REAGANS
REAGENT
REAIMED
REAIRED
REALEST
REALIGN
REALINE

REALISE
REALISM
REALIST
REALITY
REALIZE
REALLOT
REALMAN
REALMEN
REALTER
REALTOR
REAMASS
REAMEND
REAMERS
REAMING
REAMOUT
REANNEX
REAPERS
REAPING
REAPPLY
REARDON
REAREND
REARERS
REARGUE
REARING
REARISE
REARLIT
REARMED
REAROSE
REARSUP
REASKED
REASONS
REASSAY
REATTAS
REAUDIT
REAUMUR
REAVAIL
REAVERS
REAVING
REAVOWS
REAWAKE
REAWOKE
RIALTOS
RIANTLY
ROACHES
ROADBED
ROADEOS
ROADERS
ROADHOG
ROADIES
ROADMAP
ROADTAR
ROADTAX
ROADWAY
ROAMERS
ROAMING
ROANOKE
ROARERS
ROARING
ROARSAT
ROASTED
ROASTER
RRATING
RUANDAS
RVALUES
RWANDAN

R••A•••

RADAMES
RAJARAO
RAKABLE
RAMADAN
RAMADAS
RANAMOK
RANATAB
RANAWAY
RAPALLO
RAPANUI
RATABLE
RATAFIA
RATATAT
RAVAGED
RAVAGER
RAVAGES
RDLAING
REBAITS
REBAKED
REBAKES
REBALED
REBALES
REBANKS
REBASTE
REBATED
REBATER
REBATES
REBATHE
RECABLE
RECAGED
RECAGES
RECALLS
RECANED
RECANES
RECANTS
RECARRY
RECARVE
RECASED
RECASES
RECASTS
REDACTS
REDALGA
REDANTS
REDARED
REDARES
REDARMY
REDARNS
REDATED
REDATES
REEARNS
REFACED
REFACES
REFALLS
REFAXED
REFAXES
REGAINS
REGALED
REGALER
REGALES
REGALIA
REGALLY
REGARDS
REGATTA
REGAUGE
REHANGS
REHAULS
REJAILS
RELABEL
RELACED
RELACES
RELANCE
RELANDS
RELANES
RELAPSE
RELATCH
RELATED
RELATER
RELATES
RELATOR
RELAXED
RELAXER
RELAXES
RELAYED
RELAYER
REMAILS
REMAINS
REMAKES
REMANDS
REMARKS
REMARRY
REMATCH
REMATED
REMATES
RENAILS
RENALDO
RENALLY
RENAMED
RENAMES
RENAULT
REPACKS
REPAGED
REPAGES
REPAINT
REPAIRS
REPANEL
REPAPER
REPARKS
REPASTE
REPASTS
REPATCH
REPAVED
REPAVES
RERACKS
RERAISE
RERAKED
RERAKES
RERANKS
RERATED
RERATES
RESALES
RESALTS
RESANDS
RESAVED
RESAVES
RESAWED
RETABLE
RETACKS
RETAILS
RETAINS
RETAKEN
RETAKER
RETAKES
RETALLY
RETAMED
RETAMES
RETAPED
RETAPES
RETARDS
RETASTE
RETAXED
RETAXES
REVALUE
REVAMPS
REWAGER
REWAKED
REWAKEN
REWAKES
REWARDS
REWARMS
REWARNS
REWATER
REWAXED
REWAXES
RIBALDS
RIBANDS
RICARDO
RIDABLE
RINALDO
RITAGAM
RITALIN
RITAMAE
RITARDS
RIVALED
RIVALRY
ROBARDS
ROGAINE
ROLAIDS
ROMAINE
ROMAINS
ROMAJIS
ROMANCE
ROMANIA
ROMANIC
ROMANIS
ROMANOS
ROMANOV
ROMANSH
ROMANUS
RORAIMA
ROSABUD
ROSALIA
ROSALIE
ROSALYN
ROSANNA
ROSANNE
ROSARIO
ROTATED
ROTATES
ROTATOR
ROTAWAY
ROUAULT
ROXANNE
ROYALES
ROYALLY
ROYALTY
ROYALWE
ROZANOV
RUBADUB
RUBATOS
RUMAKIS
RUMANIA
RUNAMOK
RUNATAB
RUNAWAY
RURALLY
RUTALEE
RVPARKS

R•••A••

RACHAEL
RADIALS
RADIANS
RADIANT
RADIATE
RAEDAWN
RAGBAGS
RAGLANS
RAGMANS
RAILAGE
RAMFANS
RAMPAGE
RAMPANT
RAMPART
RANBACK
RANDALL
RANLAPS
RANLATE
RANPAST
RANSACK
RAPHAEL
RASCALS
RATPACK
RATRACE
RATTAIL
RATTANS
RAWBARS
RAWDATA
RAYBANS
READAPT
REAGANS
REAMASS
REAVAIL
REAWAKE
REBOANT
REBOARD
REBRACE
REBRAND
RECHALK
RECHALL
RECHART
RECLADS
RECLAIM
RECLAME
RECLASP
RECLASS
RECOALS
RECOATS
RECRANK
RECRATE
REDBATS
REDBAYS
REDCAPS
REDCARD
REDDAWN
REDEALS
REDEALT
REDFACE
REDHAIR
REDHATS
REDHAWK
REDIALS
REDJACK
REDOAKS
REDRAFT
REDRAGS
REDRAWN
REDRAWS
REDTABS
REDTAGS
REDTAIL
REDTAPE
REENACT
REFLAGS
REFLATE
REFRACT
REFRAIN
REFRAME
REGEARS
REGLAZE
REGNANT
REGNARD
REGRABS
REGRADE
REGRAFT
REGRANT
REGRAPH
REGRASP
REHEALS
REHEARD
REHEARS
REHEATS
REIMAGE
RELEADS
RELEAPS
RELEARN
RELEASE
RELIANT
RELOADS
RELOANS
REMNANT
RENTALS
REPEALS
REPEATS
REPHASE
REPLACE
REPLANE
REPLANS
REPLANT
REPLATE
REPLAYS
REREADS
RESCALE
RESCANS
RESEALS
RESEAMS
RESEATS
RESEAUS
RESEAUX
RESHAPE
RESHARE
RESHAVE
RESLATE
RESNAIS
RESNAPS
RESOAKS
RESOAPS
RESPACE
RESPADE
RESPANS
RESPARK
RESTABS
RESTACK
RESTAFF
RESTAGE
RESTAIN
RESTAMP
RESTART
RESTATE
RETEACH
RETEARS
RETHANK
RETHAWS
RETIARY
RETOAST
RETRACE
RETRACK
RETRACT
RETRADE
RETRAIN
RETRAPS
REVEALS
REWEARS
REWEAVE
REWRAPS
REXCATS
REYNARD
REYNAUD
RHUBARB
RIBCAGE
RIBPADS
RICHARD
RICRACS
RIEMANN
RIMBAUD
RIOTACT
RIPRAPS
RIPSAWN
RIPSAWS
RITEAID
RITUALS
ROBSART
ROCKABY
ROLLAND
ROLVAAG
RONSARD
ROOFAGE
ROOTAGE
ROSEATE
ROSSANO
ROSTAND
ROUBAIX
ROULADE
ROWLAND
RUDYARD
RUFFALO
RUGRATS
RUINATE
RUMBAED
RUMCAKE
RUMMAGE
RUNBACK
RUNLAPS
RUNLATE
RUNPAST
RUNWAYS
RUPIAHS
RUTHANN
RUTLAND
RYOKANS

R••••A•

RACECAR
RACEWAY
RADICAL
RADIOAD
RAFFIAS
RAILCAR
RAILMAN
RAILSAT
RAILWAY
RAINHAT
RAINMAN
RAJARAO
RAMADAN
RAMADAS
RAMSFAN
RANATAB
RANAWAY
RANTSAT
RAPIDAN
RAPSTAR
RAREGAS
RARITAN
RATATAT
RATECAP
RATTRAP
RAVENAL
RAWDEAL
RAWMEAT
RAYOVAC
RCCOLAS
REALMAN
REASSAY
REATTAS
REBEGAN
REBEKAH
REBREAK
RECITAL
RECLEAN
RECUSAL
REDCLAY
REDCOAT
REDECAY
REDFLAG
REDHEAD
REDHEAT
REDMEAT
REDREAM
REDSFAN
REDSTAR
REEDMAN
REFLOAT
REFUSAL
REFUTAL
REGINAL
REGINAS
REGULAR
REITMAN
REKNEAD
REMORAS
REMOVAL
RENEWAL
REPLEAD
REPOMAN
RESPEAK
RESPRAY
RESTRAP
RESWEAR
RETINAE
RETINAL
RETINAS
RETOTAL
RETREAD
RETREAT
RETRIAL
REVISAL
REVIVAL
RHODIAN
RHUMBAS
RIBMEAT
RICHMAN
RICKMAN
RIDGWAY
RIESMAN
RIKSDAG
RINKRAT
RIORDAN
RITAGAM
RITAMAE
ROADMAP
ROADTAR
ROADTAX
ROADWAY
ROARSAT
ROLLBAR
ROLLWAY
ROLVAAG
ROMULAN
RONDEAU
ROOFRAT
ROOMBAS
ROOTCAP
RORQUAL
ROSEBAY
ROSTRAL
ROTAWAY
ROTBLAT
ROULEAU
ROWBOAT
ROYBEAN
RUANDAS
RUBSRAW
RUFFIAN
RUFIYAA
RUNATAB
RUNAWAY
RUSSIAN
RUSSLAN
RUYBLAS
RWANDAN
RYELOAF

R•••••A

RASBORA
RASHIDA
RATAFIA
RAVENNA
RAWDATA
REBECCA
REDALGA
REGALIA
REGATTA
REPLICA
RESIDUA
RETSINA
REVERSA
REYNOSA
RICKSHA
RICOTTA
RIGVEDA
RIORITA
RIVIERA
ROBERTA
ROBUSTA
ROLONDA
ROMANIA
RORAIMA
ROSALIA
ROSANNA
ROSELLA
ROSEOLA
ROSETEA
ROSETTA
ROSSSEA
ROTHIRA
ROTUNDA
ROVETTA
RUBELLA
RUBEOLA
RUFIYAA
RUMANIA
RUZICKA

•RA••••

ARABIAN
ARABICA
ARABICS
ARABIST
ARABLES
ARACARI
ARACHNE
ARACHNO
ARAFTOF
ARAFURA
ARAGORN
ARALSEA
ARAMAIC
ARAMARK
ARAMEAN
ARAMIDS
ARANEID
ARANTXA
ARAPAHO
BRACERO
BRACERS
BRACEUP
BRACING
BRACKEN
BRACKET
BRADLEE
BRADLEY
BRAEDEN
BRAGGED
BRAGGER
BRAHMAN
BRAHMAS
BRAHMIN
BRAIDED
BRAIDER
BRAILLE
BRAINED
BRAINER
BRAISED
BRAISES
BRAKING
BRALESS
BRAMBLE
BRAMBLY
BRAMLEY
BRANAGH
BRANCHY
BRANDED
BRANDER
BRANDON
BRANIFF
BRANSON
BRASHER
BRASHES
BRASHLY
BRASIER
BRASIZE
BRASSES
BRASSIE
BRATTLE
BRAVADA
BRAVADO
BRAVELY
BRAVERY
BRAVEST
BRAVING
BRAVOED
BRAVOES
BRAVURA
BRAWLED
BRAWLER
BRAWLEY
BRAXTON
BRAYERS
BRAYING
BRAZENS
BRAZIER
BRAZING
CRABBED
CRABBER
CRABPOT
CRACKED
CRACKER
CRACKLE
CRACKLY
CRACKUP
CRADLED
CRADLER
CRADLES
CRAFTED
CRAFTER
CRAFTSY
CRAGGED
CRAIGIE
CRAISIN
CRAMMED
CRAMMER
CRAMPED
CRAMPON
CRAMSIN
CRANIAL
CRANING
CRANIUM
CRANKED
CRANKUP
CRANMER
CRAPING
CRAPOLA
CRAPOUT
CRAPPIE
CRASHAW
CRASHED
CRASHER
CRASHES
CRASSER
CRASSLY
CRASSUS
CRATERS
CRATEUP
CRATING
CRATION
CRAVATS
CRAVENS
CRAVERS
CRAVING
CRAWDAD
CRAWLED
CRAWLER
CRAWLEY
CRAYOLA
CRAYONS
CRAZIER
CRAZIES
CRAZILY
CRAZING
DRABBER
DRABBLE
DRACHMA
DRACULA
DRAFTED
DRAFTEE
DRAFTER
DRAGEES
DRAGGED
DRAGGER
DRAGGLE
DRAGNET
DRAGOFF
DRAGONS
DRAGOON
DRAGOTI
DRAGOUT
DRAGSIN
DRAGSON
DRAGSUP
DRAINED
DRAINER
DRAMADY
DRAMEDY
DRANKIN
DRANKTO
DRANKUP
DRAPERS
DRAPERY
DRAPING
DRASTIC
DRATTED
DRAUGHT
DRAWBAR
DRAWEES
DRAWERS
DRAWING
DRAWLED
DRAWLER
DRAWMAN
DRAWMEN
DRAWNIN
DRAWNON
DRAWNTO
DRAWNUP
DRAWOFF
DRAWOUT
DRAWSIN
DRAWSON
DRAWSTO
DRAWSUP
DRAYAGE
DRAYING
DRAYMAN
DRAYMEN
DRAYTON
ERASERS
ERASING
ERASMUS
ERASTUS
ERASURE
FRACTAL
FRAGGED
FRAGGLE
FRAGILE
FRAICHE
FRAILER
FRAILLY
FRAILTY
FRAISES
FRAMERS
FRAMEUP
FRAMING
FRANCES
FRANCHI
FRANCIS
FRANKED
FRANKEN
FRANKER
FRANKIE
FRANKLY
FRANKOZ
FRANTIC
FRAPPES
FRASIER
FRATERS
FRAUGHT
FRAWLEY
FRAYING
FRAZIER
FRAZZLE
GRABBAG
GRABBAR
GRABBED
GRABBER
GRABSAT
GRACIAS
GRACILE
GRACING
GRACKLE
GRADATE
GRADEAA
GRADERS
GRADING
GRADUAL
GRAFTED
GRAFTER
GRAFTON
GRAHAME

GRAHAMS
GRAINED
GRAINER
GRAMMAR
GRAMMER
GRAMMES
GRAMMYS
GRAMPAS
GRAMPUS
GRANADA
GRANARY
GRANDAM
GRANDEE
GRANDER
GRANDLY
GRANDMA
GRANDPA
GRANGER
GRANGES
GRANITA
GRANITE
GRANNIE
GRANOLA
GRANPAS
GRANTED
GRANTEE
GRANTER
GRANTOR
GRANULE
GRAPERY
GRAPHED
GRAPHIC
GRAPIER
GRAPNEL
GRAPPAS
GRAPPLE
GRASPAT
GRASPED
GRASPER
GRASSED
GRASSES
GRASSLE
GRATEON
GRATERS
GRATEUP
GRATIAS
GRATIFY
GRATING
GRAUMAN
GRAVELS
GRAVELY
GRAVERS
GRAVEST
GRAVIES
GRAVING
GRAVITY
GRAVLAX
GRAVURE
GRAYEST
GRAYING
GRAYISH
GRAYJAY
GRAYLAG
GRAYSON
GRAZERS
GRAZIER
GRAZING
IRANIAN
IRATELY
IRATEST
KRACKEL
KRAKENS
KRAMDEN
KRAMNIK
KRASNER
KRATION
ORACIES
ORACLES
ORALIST
ORANGES
ORANGEY
ORANTES
ORARION
ORARIUM
ORATING
ORATION
ORATORS
ORATORY
ORATRIX
PRACTIC
PRADESH
PRAETOR
PRAIRIE
PRAISED
PRAISER
PRAISES
PRALINE
PRANCED
PRANCER
PRANCES
PRATERS
PRATING
PRATTLE
PRAWNED
PRAYERS
PRAYFOR
PRAYING
PRAYSTO
QRATIOS
RRATING
TRABERT
TRACERS
TRACERY
TRACHEA
TRACING
TRACKED
TRACKER
TRACTOR
TRADEIN
TRADEON
TRADERS
TRADEUP
TRADING
TRADUCE
TRAFFIC
TRAGEDY
TRAILED
TRAILER
TRAINED
TRAINEE
TRAINER
TRAININ
TRAIPSE
TRAITOR
TRALALA
TRAMCAR
TRAMMED
TRAMMEL
TRAMPAS
TRAMPED
TRAMPER
TRAMPLE
TRAMWAY
TRANCED
TRANCES
TRANSAM
TRANSIT
TRANSOM
TRAPEZE
TRAPGUN
TRAPPED
TRAPPER
TRASHED
TRASHER
TRASHES
TRASHTV
TRAUBEL
TRAUMAS
TRAVAIL
TRAVELS
TRAVERS
TRAWLED
TRAWLER
TRAYFUL
TRAYNOR
URACILS
URANITE
URANIUM
WRACKED
WRACKUP
WRAITHS
WRANGEL
WRANGLE
WRAPPED
WRAPPER
WRAPSUP
WRAPUPS
WRASSES
XRATING
XRAYING
XRAYLAB

•R•A•••

ARBACES
ARCADED
ARCADES
ARCADIA
ARCANUM
AREAMAP
AREARUG
AREAWAY
ARGALIS
ARGANTE
ARIADNE
ARIANES
ARMADAS
ARRABAL
ARRACKS
ARRAIGN
ARRANGE
ARRASES
ARRAYAL
ARRAYED
ARRAYER
BREADED
BREADER
BREADTH
BREAKER
BREAKIN
BREAKUP
BREASTS
BREATHE
BREATHS
BREATHY
BRIARDS
BROADAS
BROADAX
BROADEN
BROADER
BROADLY
BROASTS
CREAKED
CREAMED
CREAMER
CREASED
CREASER
CREASES
CREATED
CREATES
CREATOR
CROAKED
CROAKER
CROATIA
DREADED
DREAMED
DREAMER
DREAMIN
DREAMOF
DREAMON
DREAMUP
DRLAURA
DRMARIO
DRYABLE
DRYADES
DRYADIC
ERLANGS
ERRABLE
ERRANCY
ERRANDS
ERRATIC
ERRATUM
FREAKED
FRIABLE
FRIARLY
FRYABLE
GREASED
GREASER
GREASES
GREATEN
GREATER
GREATLY
GREAVES
GROANED
GROANER
MRDARCY
MRHANEY
MRMACHO
MRMAGOO
MRMARCH
MRNANNY
MRPADRE
ORDAINS
ORGANDY
ORGANIC
ORGANZA
ORLANDO
ORMANDY
PREACHY
PREACID
PREACTS
PREAGED
PREAGES
PREALLY
PREAMPS
PREARMS
PREAVER
PROARAB
TREACLE
TREACLY
TREADED
TREADER
TREADLE
TREADON
TREASON
TREATED
TREATER
TRIABLE
TRIADIC
TRIAGES
TRUANCY
TRUANTS
URBANER
URBANII
URBANIV
URBANVI
WREAKED
WREAKER
WREATHE
WREATHS
WREATHY

•R••A••

ARACARI
ARAMAIC
ARAMARK
ARAPAHO
ARCHAIC
ARCLAMP
ARCUATE
ARIGATO
ARIKARA
ARMBAND
ARMYANT
ARREARS
ARTCARS
ARTFAIR
ARTSALE
ARTWALL
ARTWARE
ARUBANS
BRANAGH
BRAVADA
BRAVADO
BREWAGE
BRIDALS
BRIGADE
BRIGAND
BRITAIN
BROCADE
BROGANS
BROMATE
BROWARD
CRAVATS
CREMATE
CRENATE
CRETANS
CRUSADE
CRUZADO
CRUZANS
CRYBABY
DRAMADY
DRAYAGE
DRCHAOS
DRYWALL
DRYWASH
FREEAIR
FRIDAYS
FRIGATE
FROMAGE
FROWARD
FRYPANS
GRADATE
GRAHAME
GRAHAMS
GRANADA
GRANARY
GRENADA
GRENADE
GRIMACE
IRELAND
IRONAGE
MRSBASS
MRSLATE
MRSPAUL
ORCHARD
ORDEALS
OREGANO
ORGEATS
ORGIAST
ORIGAMI
ORLEANS
ORPHANS
ORPHANT
PREBADE
PREBAKE
PRECAST
PREDARK
PREDATA
PREDATE
PREDAWN
PREFABS
PREFACE
PREFADE
PREGAIN
PREGAME
PRELACY
PRELATE
PREMADE
PREMAKE
PREMATE
PRENAME
PREPACK
PREPAID
PREPARE
PREPAVE
PREPAYS
PRERACE
PRESAGE
PRESALE
PRESALT
PRETAPE
PREVAIL
PREWARM
PREWARN
PREWASH
PRIMACY
PRIMARY
PRIMATE
PRIVACY
PRIVATE
PROBALL
PROBATE
PROEAST
PROFANE
PROFARM
PROLATE
PRONATE
PRONAVY
PROPANE
PRORATA
PRORATE
PROSAIC
TRALALA
TRAVAIL
TRENARY
TREPANS
TRINARY
TROJANS
TRUMANS
TRYHARD
TRYSAIL

•R•••A•

ARABIAN
ARAMEAN
ARCHWAY
AREAMAP
AREAWAY
AREOLAE
AREOLAR
AREOLAS
ARISTAE
ARISTAS
ARMADAS
ARMLOAD
ARNICAS
ARONNAX
AROUSAL
ARRABAL
ARRAYAL
ARRIVAL
ARSENAL
ARTISAN
BRAHMAN
BRAHMAS
BRENDAN
BRENNAN
BRIGHAM
BROADAS
BROADAX
BROSNAN
BROWWAX
CRANIAL
CRASHAW
CRAWDAD
CREEDAL
CREWMAN
CRIMEAN
CRITIAS
CROSSAT
CROWBAR
CRUCIAL
CRUSTAL
CRYSTAL
DRAWBAR
DRAWMAN
DRAYMAN
DRESSAS
DRIPPAN
DRISTAN
DRIVEAT
DROPCAP
DROVEAT
DRSLOAN
DRUZEAN
DRUZIAN
DRVEGAS
DRYHEAT
FRACTAL
FREEMAN
FREEWAY
FREITAG
FRENEAU
FRESCAS
FRETSAT
FRETSAW
FREYTAG
FRIEDAN
FRISIAN
FROGMAN
FRONTAL
FROWNAT
GRABBAG
GRABBAR
GRABSAT
GRACIAS
GRADEAA
GRADUAL
GRAMMAR
GRAMPAS
GRANDAM
GRANPAS
GRAPPAS
GRASPAT
GRATIAS
GRAUMAN
GRAVLAX
GRAYJAY
GRAYLAG
GRECIAN
GRESHAM
GREWFAT
GREYLAG
GRIDMAP
GRINSAT
GRISHAM
GROWFAT
GRUMMAN
IRANIAN
IREPEAT
IRONBAR
IRONMAN
MRCLEAN
MRISCAN
MRNOVAK
ORBITAL
ORDINAL
ORPHEAN
ORTEGAL
ORTOLAN
PREHEAL
PREHEAT
PRELOAD
PRELOAN
PREORAL
PREPLAN
PRESEAL
PRESEAT
PRESOAK
PREVIAS
PREWRAP
PRINTAD
PROARAB
PROGRAM
PROPMAN
PROSCAN
PROTEAM
PROTEAN
TRAMCAR
TRAMPAS
TRAMWAY
TRANSAM
TRAUMAS
TREDIAS
TREERAT
TREESAP
TRIGRAM
TRIMTAB
TRISTAN
TRISTAR
TRIVIAL
TROIKAS
TRUDEAU
URSULAK
URUGUAY
WROCLAW
XRAYLAB

•R••••A

ARABICA
ARAFURA
ARALSEA
ARANTXA
ARCADIA
ARIETTA
ARIKARA
ARIZONA
ARMENIA
ARUGULA
BRAVADA
BRAVURA
BRESCIA
CRAPOLA
CRAYOLA
CREMONA
CREMORA
CROATIA
CRUELLA
DRACHMA
DRACULA
DRLAURA
DRYIDEA
ERIGENA
ERITREA
ERMINIA
ERNESTA
EROTICA
FREESIA
GRADEAA
GRANADA
GRANDMA
GRANDPA
GRANITA
GRANOLA
GRENADA
HRYVNIA
KRISHNA
ORGANZA
PREDATA
PREIDEA
PREPUPA
PRIMERA
PRORATA
PROXIMA
PRUSSIA
TRACHEA
TRALALA
TREINTA
TRIBECA
TRIPLEA

••RA•••

AARATED
ABRADED
ABRADER
ABRADES
ABRAHAM
ABRAXAS
ADRATES
AERATED
AERATES
AERATOR
AFRAMES
AIRACES
AMRADIO
ARRABAL
ARRACKS
ARRAIGN
ARRANGE
ARRASES
ARRAYAL
ARRAYED
ARRAYER
AURALEE
AURALLY
BARACUS
BARANOF
BERATED
BERATER
BERATES
BORATES
CARABOO
CARACAS
CARAFES
CARAMBA
CARAMEL
CARAMIA
CARAVAN
CARAVEL
CARAWAY
CBRADIO
CDRACKS
CDRATES
CERAMIC
CERATED
CERATES
CORACLE
CORAZON
CURABLE
CURABLY
CURACAO
CURARES
CURATED
CURATES
CURATOR
DERAILS
DERALTE
DERANGE
DERATED
DERATES
DURABLE
DURABLY
DURANCE
DURANGO
DURANTE
EARACHE
ENRAGED
ENRAGES
ENRANKS
ERRABLE
ERRANCY
ERRANDS
ERRATIC
ERRATUM
EURASIA
FARADAY
FARAWAY
FMRADIO
FORABIT
FORADAY
FORAGED
FORAGER
FORAGES
FORASEC
FORAYED
GARAGED
GARAGES
GERAINT
GERALDO
GIRAFFE
GIRASOL
GYRALLY
GYRATED
GYRATES
GYRATOR
HERALDS
HIRABLE
HORATIO
HYRACES
HYRAXES
IGRAINE
INRANGE
ISRAELI
ISRAFEL
JIRASEK
KARACHI
KARAJAN
KARAKUM
KARAOKE
KARASEA
KARATES
KERATIN
KORANIC
LARAINE
LARAMIE
LORANGE
MARACAS
MARANTZ
MARAUDS
MCRANEY
MIRABEL
MIRACLE
MIRADAS
MIRADOR
MIRAGES
MIRAMAR
MIRAMAX
MIRANDA
MORAINE
MORALES
MORALLY
MORANIS
MORANTE
MORAVIA
MURALED
MURANOS
NARAYAN
ONRAMPS
OTRANTO
PARABLE
PARADED
PARADER
PARADES
PARADOR
PARADOX
PARAGON
PARAIBA
PARAMUS
PARAPET
PARAPHS
PARASKI
PARASOL
PARATUS
PERAHIA
PERATIO
PGRATED
PHRASAL
PHRASED
PHRASES
PIRAEUS
PIRANHA
PIRATED
PIRATES
PIRATIC
PYRAMID
PYRAMUS
RERACKS
RERAISE
RERAKED
RERAKES
RERANKS
RERATED
RERATES
RORAIMA
RURALLY
SARACEN
SARALEE
SARANAC
SARAWAK
SARAZEN
SCRAGGY
SCRAPED
SCRAPER
SCRAPES
SCRAPPY
SCRATCH
SCRAWLS
SCRAWLY
SCRAWNY
SERAPES
SERAPHS
SERAPIS
SPRAINS
SPRAWLS
SPRAWLY
SPRAYED
SPRAYER
SPRAYON
STRAFED
STRAFER
STRAFES
STRAINS
STRAITS
STRANDS
STRANGE
STRAPIN
STRAPON
STRASSE
STRATAS
STRATUM
STRATUS
STRAUSS
STRAYED
STRAYER
TARANTO
TERAOHM
THRALLS
TIRADES
TYRANNY
TYRANTS
UKRAINE
UNRACKS
UNRAINY
UNRAKED
UNRASPY
UNRATED
UNRAVEL
UNRAYED
UNRAZED
UPRAISE
UPRATED
UPRATES
VERANDA
VIRAGOS
WIRABLE
XMRADIO

••R•A••

ABREAST
ABROACH
ACREAGE
ADRIANA
AERIALS
AIRBAGS

AIRBALL
AIRBASE
AIRDAMS
AIRDATE
AIRFARE
AIRLANE
AIRMADA
AIRMAIL
AIRMASS
AIRPACK
AIRPARK
AIRRACE
AIRRAGE
AIRRAID
AIRSACS
AIRTANK
AIRTAXI
AIRWARS
AIRWAVE
AIRWAYS
ALREADY
ARREARS
AUREATE
BARBARA
BARBARY
BARBATE
BARCARS
BARGAIN
BARMAID
BARNABY
BARNARD
BARRACK
BARRAGE
BARTABS
BARWARE
BEREAVE
BERGAMO
BERNARD
BERNAYS
BIRIANI
BIRMANS
BIRYANI
BORLAUG
BORZAGE
BURBAGE
BURBANK
BUREAUS
BUREAUX
BURIALS
BURLAPS
BURMANS
BURNABY
BUROAKS
BURSARS
BYROADS
CARBARN
CARCARE
CARCASS
CARFARE
CARJACK
CARNABY
CARNAGE
CARPALS
CARPARK
CARRARA
CARSALE
CARTAGE
CARTALK
CARWASH
CEREALS
CERTAIN
CIRRATE
CORDAGE
CORDATE
CORFAMS
CORKAGE
CORMACK
CORRADE
CORRALS
CORSAGE
CORSAIR
CORVAIR
CUREALL
CURRANT
CURTAIL
CURTAIN
CURTATE
DARKAGE
DERMATO
DIRHAMS
DORMANT
DORSALS
DURWARD
EARHART
EARLAPS
EARMARK
EARTABS
EARTAGS
FAREAST
FARMAID
FARRAGO
FERMATA
FERMATE
FERMATS
FERNAND
FERRARA
FERRARE
FERRARI
FERRARO
FERRATE
FIRBANK
FIREANT
FIREARM
FORBADE
FOREACH
FOREARM
FORGAVE
FORLANI
FORMALS
FORMATS
FORSAKE
FORSALE
FORWARD
FURBALL
FURCATE
FURFARM
FURNACE
FURTADO
GARBAGE
GARBAGY
GARLAND
GERMAIN
GERMANE
GERMANS
GERMANY
GERVAIS
HARBACH
HARHARS
HARLAND
HARRAHS
HARTACK
HARVARD
HERBAGE
HERBALS
HERBART
HERBAUT
HERMANA
HERMANN
HERMANO
HERMANS
HERNANI
HURRAHS
HURRAYS
IMREADY
INREACH
INROADS
JORDANA
KIRMANS
KOREANS
LARIATS
MARCATO
MARGATE
MARGAUX
MARHAUS
MARIANA
MARIANO
MARMARA
MARSALA
MARYANN
MERCADO
MERMAID
MORDANT
MORGANA
MORGANS
MORTALS
MORTARS
MYRIADS
NARRATE
NARVAEZ
NIRVANA
NORMALS
NORMAND
NORMANS
NORWALK
OURGANG
PARBAKE
PARFAIT
PARIAHS
PARKADE
PARKAVE
PARLAYS
PARTAKE
PERCALE
PERHAPS
PERIAPT
PERTAIN
PERVADE
PORTAGE
PORTALS
REREADS
SARCASM
SCREAKS
SCREAMS
SERFAGE
SERIALS
SERIATE
SERRATE
SERVANT
SORBATE
SORIANO
SPREADS
STREAKS
STREAKY
STREAMS
STRIATE
SURFACE
SURNAME
SURPASS
SYRIANA
SYRIANS
TARBABY
TARMACS
TARSALS
TARTANS
TARTARE
TARTARS
TARZANA
TARZANS
TERNARY
TERNATE
TERRACE
TERRAIN
TERRANS
THREADS
THREADY
THREATS
THROATS
THROATY
TORNADO
TORVALD
TURBANS
UNREADY
UPREACH
UPREARS
UPROARS
VARIANT
VARIATE
VARLAAM
VCRTAPE
VERBALS
VERDANT
VERSACE
VERSANT
VIRGATE
VORLAGE
WARBABY
WARFARE
WARGAME
WARHAWK
WARPAGE
WARPATH
WARRANT
WORDAGE
YARDAGE
YARDARM
ZERMATT

••R••A•

ABRAHAM
ABRAXAS
ACROBAT
ADRENAL
AEROBAT
AFRICAN
AIRBOAT
AIRHEAD
AIRPLAY
AIRTRAP
AMRITAS
ARRABAL
ARRAYAL
ARRIVAL
AURORAE
AURORAL
AURORAS
BARBEAU
BARCLAY
BAREXAM
BARFBAG
BARKSAT
BARSOAP
BARTRAY
BERGMAN
BERIGAN
BERTHAS
BERTRAM
BIRDMAN
BORGIAS
BORNEAN
BORSTAL
BURGLAR
CARACAS
CARAVAN
CARAWAY
CARBRAS
CARCOAT
CARDIAC
CARDIAL
CARINAE
CARINAS
CARLOAD
CARLOAN
CARPSAT
CARSEAT
CHROMAT
CORDIAL
CORDIAS
CORKOAK
CORNEAL
CORNEAS
CORONAE
CORONAL
CORONAS
CORYZAS
CURACAO
CURSEAT
DARESAY
DARKMAN
DARKTAN
DIRTBAG
DORFMAN
EARFLAP
EUREKAS
EUROVAN
FARADAY
FARAWAY
FAREWAR
FARINAS
FARMGAL
FERNBAR
FIREDAT
FIREHAT
FIREMAN
FIRESAT
FORADAY
FORBEAR
FORDHAM
FOREBAY
FOREMAN
FOREPAW
FORERAN
FORESAW
FORREAL
FORTRAN
FORTYAD
FURCOAT
FURSEAL
FURWRAP
GARNEAU
GORDIAN
GURKHAS
GYROCAR
HARDDAY
HARDHAT
HARDPAN
HARDWAY
HARTMAN
HEREIAM
HERNIAE
HERNIAS
JERBOAS
JURYMAN
KARAJAN
KEROUAC
KERSHAW
KORUNAS
LORELAI
LYRICAL
MARACAS
MARCEAU
MARDIAN
MARIDAS
MARINAS
MARITAL
MARKHAM
MARKKAA
MARRYAT
MARSBAR
MARSHAL
MARTIAL
MARTIAN
MARXIAN
MARYKAY
MERCIAN
MERRIAM
MIRADAS
MIRAMAR
MIRAMAX
MOREPAY
NARAYAN
NARWHAL
NKRUMAH
OARSMAN
PARKMAN
PARKWAY
PARTIAL
PARTWAY
PERLMAN
PERMIAN
PERORAL
PERREAU
PERSIAN
PERUSAL
PERYEAR
PHRASAL
PORTMAN
PORTRAY
PURITAN
RAREGAS
RARITAN
RORQUAL
SARANAC
SARAWAK
SAROYAN
SARUMAN
SERBIAN
SERIPAK
SERVEAS
SORORAL
STRATAS
SURECAN
SUREIAM
SURFMAN
SURINAM
SURREAL
THREEAD
THREEAM
THREWAT
THROWAT
THRUWAY
TIREMAN
TORTLAW
TURFMAN
TURFWAR
TURNBAD
UNREGAL
UNRURAL
VARLAAM
VERITAS
VERYBAD
VERYMAD
VERYSAD
VIRGOAN
VIRTUAL
WARHEAD
WIREMAN
WIRETAP
WORKDAY
WORKMAN
WORKSAT
YARDMAN
YEREVAN

••R•••A

ADRIANA
AGRIPPA
AIRMADA
AMREETA
AUREOLA
BARBARA
BARBERA
BARBUDA
BARETTA
BARISTA
BERETTA
BERMUDA
BERNINA
BIRETTA
BURKINA
CARAMBA
CARAMIA
CARIOCA
CARLOTA
CARMELA
CARMINA
CARNERA
CARRARA
CARRERA
CEREBRA
CERVEZA
CHRISTA
CORDOBA
CORETTA
COROLLA
CORPORA
CORRIDA
CORSICA
CORTINA
CORVINA
CURIOSA
DERONDA
DERRIDA
ETRURIA
EURASIA
FERMATA
FERRARA
FIRENZA
FORENZA
FORMICA
FORMOSA
FORMULA
FORTUNA
GARDENA
GORDITA
GORILLA
HERBTEA
HEREDIA
HERMANA
HERMOSA
JERITZA
JORDANA
KARASEA
LARUSSA
LORETTA
MARIANA
MARILLA
MARIMBA
MARKKAA
MARKOVA
MARMARA
MARSALA
MARTINA
MARUSJA
MIRANDA
MORAVIA
MORELLA
MORGANA
NERISSA
NIRVANA
NORDICA
NORIEGA
PARAIBA
PARTITA
PERAHIA
PERDITA
PERGOLA
PERISSA
PERSONA
PERUGIA
PHRYGIA
PIRANHA
PORSENA
PYREXIA
RORAIMA
SYRIANA
TARZANA
THRILLA
TORTOLA
TORTUGA
TURISTA
VERANDA
VERBENA
VERONIA
VERRUCA

•••RA••

ACERATE
AFFRAYS
AIRRACE
AIRRAGE
AIRRAID
AMERADA
AMTRACK
AMTRACS
ANDRADE
ANORAKS
ASHRAMS
ASPRAWL
ATARAXY
ATGRADE
ATTRACT
AVERAGE
AYNRAND
BADRAPS
BAHRAIN
BARRACK
BARRAGE
BEBRAVE
BEDRAIL
BEDRAPE
BETRAYS
BUMRAPS
BUNRAKU
BYTRAIN
CARRARA
CHARADE
CHORALE
CHORALS
CIRRATE
CITRATE
COBRAND
COMRADE
CONRACK
CORRADE
CORRALS
COURAGE
COURANT
CUIRASS
CURRANT
CUTRATE
DEFRAGS
DEFRAME
DEFRAUD
DEFRAYS
DEGRADE
DELRAYS
DEPRAVE
DETRACT
DETRAIN
DIGRAMS
DIGRAPH
DIORAMA
DISRATE
DOGRACE
ELPRADO
ELTRAIN
EMBRACE
EMERALD
EMIRATE
ENFRAME
ENGRAFT
ENGRAIN
ENGRAMS
ENGRAVE
ENTRADA
ENTRAIN
ENTRANT
ENTRAPS
ENWRAPS
EPHRAIM
ESTRADA
ESTRAYS
EXTRACT
FARRAGO
FERRARA
FERRARE
FERRARI
FERRARO
FERRATE
FOURAAA
FTBRAGG
GOCRAZY
GOURAMI
GUARANI
GYMRATS
HARRAHS
HATRACK
HAYRACK
HEBRAIC
HOORAHS
HOORAYS
HURRAHS
HURRAYS
HYDRANT
HYDRATE
INARAGE
INDRAFT
INDRAWN
INFRACT
INGRAFT
INGRAIN
INGRATE
INTRADE
INTRAYS
ITERANT
ITERATE
LABRATS
LEGRAND
LIBRANS
LIBRARY
MACRAME
MALRAUX
MCCRARY
MIGRANT
MIGRATE
MISRATE
MIZRAHI
MOORAGE
NARRATE
NEXRADS
NITRATE
NOTRADE
NOTRARE
ODORANT
OFFRAMP
ONORATI
ONTRACK
OPERAND
OPERANT
OPERATE
OSTRAVA
OUTRACE
OUTRAGE
OUTRAIL
OUTRANG
OUTRANK
OUTRANT
OUTRAPS
OUTRATE
OUTRAVE
OVERACT
OVERAGE
OVERALL
OVERARM
OVERATE
OVERAWE
PADRAIC
PAYRATE
PEERAGE
PETRATS
PHARAOH
PLURALS
PRERACE
PRORATA
PRORATE
RATRACE
REBRACE
REBRAND
RECRANK
RECRATE
REDRAFT
REDRAGS
REDRAWN
REDRAWS
REFRACT
REFRAIN
REFRAME
REGRABS
REGRADE
REGRAFT
REGRANT
REGRAPH
REGRASP
RETRACE
RETRACK
RETRACT
RETRADE
RETRAIN
RETRAPS
REWRAPS
RICRACS
RIPRAPS
RUGRATS
SATRAPS
SATRAPY
SCARABS
SEARACE
SERRATE
SETRATE
SKIRACE
SKIRACK
SOPRANI
SOPRANO
SOURALE
SPIRALS
STORAGE
SUBRACE
SUCRASE
SUNRAYS
TAXRATE
TERRACE
TERRAIN
TERRANS
TETRADS
THERAMS
THERAPY
TIARAED
TIERACK
TITRATE
TOPRANK
TOPRATE
TSTRAPS
UMBRAGE
UNBRACE
UNBRAID
UNBRAKE
UNBRAVE
UNCRAMP
UNCRATE
UNCRAZY
UNDRAPE
UNDRAWN
UNDRAWS
UNFRAIL
UNFRANK
UNGRAND
UNTRACK
UNTRAPS
UNWRAPS
UPBRAID
UPDRAFT
UPGRADE
UPTRADE
USGRANT
VAGRANT
VIBRANT
VIBRATE
VIBRATO
WARRANT
WETRAGS
YOURANG
ZEBRAIC
ZEBRASS

•••R•A•

ACCRUAL
ANDREAS
ANGRYAT
ANYROAD
ASTREAM
AVERNAL
AZOREAN
AZORIAN
BEARCAT
BEARPAW
BEERCAN
BEERTAP
BEHRMAN
BOERWAR
BOORMAN
CHARMAN
CHARPAK
CHORDAL
CSARDAS
CYPRIAN
CZARDAS
DHARMAS
DIURNAL
DOGREAT
DOORMAN
DOORMAT
DOORWAY
EGERIAS
ENTREAT
EPERNAY
ETERNAL
EXURBAN
FAIRFAX
FAIRWAY
FLOREAL
FLORIAN
FMURRAY
FORREAL
FOURAAA
FOURDAY
FOURMAN
FOURWAY
GETREAL
GLAREAT
GLORIAS
GOTREAL
HADRIAN
HEARSAY
IBERIAN
IMGREAT
ISTRIAN
ISUREAM
IVORIAN
JEERSAT
JOURDAN
JOURNAL
LEERSAT
LEFREAK
LIPREAD
LOWROAD
MARRYAT
MAURIAC
MAURIAT
MEERKAT
MEGRYAN
MERRIAM
MISREAD
MYTREAT
NEARPAR

NOTREAL
NUTRIAS
OFFROAD
ONBREAK
ONTRIAL
OSIRIAN
OUTREAD
OUTROAR
OVEREAT
OVERFAR
OVERFAT
OVERLAP
OVERLAX
OVERLAY
OVERMAN
OVERPAR
OVERPAY
OVERRAN
OVERSAD
OVERSAW
OVERTAX
PEERSAT
PEORIAN
PERREAU
PHARLAP
PIERIAN
POORLAW
POORMAN
POORTAX
QUARTAN
REBREAK
REDREAM
RETREAD
RETREAT
RETRIAL
RIORDAN
ROARSAT
SAURIAN
SCORIAS
SHERMAN
SHERPAS
SIERRAS
SNARLAT
SNORTAT
SPARTAN
SPIREAS
SPORRAN
STAREAT
STARMAN
STARMAP
STERNAL
SURREAL
SWOREAT
TAUREAN
TEARGAS
TEARSAT
THEREAT
THERIAC
THERMAL
THOREAU
THURGAU
THURMAN
UMBRIAN
UNTREAD
UNURBAN
UXORIAL
WEIRDAL
WHEREAS

WHEREAT
XTERRAS
YTTRIAS
YZERMAN
ZAIRIAN

•••R••A

ACEROLA
ALFREDA
AMERADA
AMERICA
AMERIKA
CARRARA
CARRERA
CORRIDA
CZARINA
DERRIDA
DIORAMA
EMERITA
ENTRADA
ESTRADA
EXORDIA
EXURBIA
FERRARA
FIORINA
FLORIDA
FOURAAA
GEORGIA
IMPREZA
INERTIA
KATRINA
KEDROVA
OCARINA
OSTRAVA
OVERSEA
PAPRIKA
PODRIDA
PRORATA
QUERIDA
RIORITA
SABRINA
SHARONA
SUBROSA
THERESA
TSARINA
TZARINA
VERRUCA

••••RA•

ADMIRAL
AIRTRAP
ALBORAK
ALDORAY
ALLBRAN
ALSORAN
AMSCRAY
ANAGRAM
ANGORAS
ANITRAS
ANKARAN
ANTHRAX
APPARAT
APTERAL
ASAGRAY
ASFARAS
ASHTRAY
ASMARAN
AUGURAL

AURORAE
AURORAL
AURORAS
AUSTRAL
BARTRAY
BELTRAN
BEOGRAD
BERTRAM
BETARAY
BIAFRAN
BUCKRAM
BUTTRAM
CAMERAE
CAMERAL
CAMERAS
CARBRAS
CATERAS
CENTRAL
CHAKRAS
COCHRAN
COMORAN
CONTRAS
COWERAT
DEBORAH
DEXTRAL
DIAGRAM
DISHRAG
DUSTRAG
ENTHRAL
EPIGRAM
EXEDRAE
FAYWRAY
FEDERAL
FEDORAS
FEMORAL
FIGURAL
FLYTRAP
FMURRAY
FORERAN
FORTRAN
FURWRAP
FUTURAS
GENERAL
GUJARAT
HALFRAW
HEATRAY
HEGIRAS
HOFBRAU
HUMERAL
HUMORAL
ICETRAY
IMMORAL
INATRAP
ISOGRAM
JOGBRAS
KAMERAD
KINGRAT
LABORAT
LATERAL
LATERAN
LAVERAN
LEGTRAP
LIBERAL
LITERAL
LUSTRAL
MACGRAW
MALLRAT
MANTRAP

MANTRAS
MAUPRAT
MAYORAL
MENORAH
MINERAL
MISDRAW
MISTRAL
MITHRAS
MOLERAT
MOWBRAY
MUBARAK
MUSKRAT
NATURAL
NEUTRAL
NONARAB
NONORAL
NUBIRAS
NUMERAL
OATBRAN
ONEGRAM
OSETRAS
OUTBRAG
OUTBRAY
OUTDRAG
OUTDRAW
OUTPRAY
OUTTRAY
OVERRAN
PACKRAT
PANARAB
PANGRAM
PERORAL
PICARAS
PLEURAE
PLEURAL
POLARAS
PORTRAY
PREORAL
PREWRAP
PROARAB
PROGRAM
RAJARAO
RATTRAP
REMORAS
RESPRAY
RESTRAP
RINKRAT
ROOFRAT
ROSTRAL
RUBSRAW
SAHARAN
SAMARAS
SAMPRAS
SAMURAI
SCLERAE
SCLERAL
SCLERAS
SEAGRAM
SEMIRAW
SENORAS
SENTRAS
SEPIRAS
SEVERAL
SHECRAB
SIERRAS
SNEERAT
SOFARAS
SOLARAS

SONORAN
SORORAL
SPHERAL
SPORRAN
SWEARAT
TAMARAC
TANGRAM
TEATRAY
TEHERAN
TELERAN
THEBRAT
THECRAB
TOPDRAW
TREERAT
TRIGRAM
TUNDRAS
UNRURAL
UNSTRAP
VECTRAS
VENTRAD
VENTRAL
VESTRAL
VETERAN
VIHARAS
VITARAS
VOUVRAY
WASHRAG
WOLFRAM
XTERRAS

••••R•A

ALBERTA
ALEGRIA
ALFORJA
ALGERIA
ALMERIA
ANDORRA
AQUARIA
ASSYRIA
ASTORIA
AUSTRIA
BACTRIA
BADAREA
BAVARIA
BAYAREA
BEGORRA
CAMBRIA
CASERTA
CUMBRIA
DELIRIA
ELBERTA
EMPORIA
ENCARTA
ERITREA
ETRURIA
IHEARYA
ILLYRIA
JAKARTA
LACERTA
LASORDA
LIBERIA
LIGURIA
MAJORCA
MALARIA
MAZURKA
MENORCA
MINERVA
MINORCA

NIGERIA
REVERSA
ROBERTA
SAMARIA
SANGRIA
SCHIRRA
SCIORRA
SIBERIA
SKIAREA
SOLARIA
SUBAREA
TALARIA
TAVERNA
VITORIA
VIVARIA
ZIMARRA

•••••RA

ABINTRA
ALGEBRA
ALLEGRA
AMPHORA
ANDORRA
ARAFURA
ARIKARA
BANDERA
BARBARA
BARBERA
BEGORRA
BOKHARA
BRAVURA
BUKHARA
CAESURA
CALDERA
CARNERA
CARRARA
CARRERA
CEREBRA
CHIMERA
CHOLERA
CONAGRA
CORPORA
CREMORA
DRLAURA
DYKSTRA
ELANTRA
ELECTRA
ELEKTRA
EPHEDRA
EXHEDRA
FERRARA
GAZZARA
GONGORA
GUEVARA
HOFSTRA
HONIARA
INTEGRA
ISADORA
KITHARA
KUNDERA
LEMPIRA
LEONORA
LETTERA
LINEARA
MADEIRA
MARMARA
MASCARA
MEGAERA

MIASARA
NIAGARA
NOSEBRA
NUESTRA
OBSCURA
OLESTRA
ONELIRA
OSSETRA
OVIPARA
OXYMORA
PALABRA
PALMYRA
PANDORA
PANTERA
PHAEDRA
PLECTRA
POLLERA
PRIMERA
QUESERA
RASBORA
RIVIERA
ROTHIRA
SAMBORA
SCHIRRA
SCIORRA
SENHORA
SHAKIRA
SIGNORA
SINATRA
SPECTRA
SUMATRA
TANTARA
TEMPERA
TEMPURA
TESSERA
VAMPIRA
VANDURA
VENTURA
VISCERA
ZIMARRA

R•B••••

RABBETS
RABBITS
RABBITT
RABBITY
RABBLED
RABBLES
RABIDLY
REBAITS
REBAKED
REBAKES
REBALED
REBALES
REBANKS
REBASTE
REBATED
REBATER
REBATES
REBATHE
REBECCA
REBEGAN
REBEGIN
REBEGUN
REBEKAH
REBENDS
REBILLS
REBINDS

REBIRTH
REBLOCK
REBLOOM
REBLOWN
REBOANT
REBOARD
REBOILS
REBOLTS
REBOOKS
REBOOTS
REBORED
REBORES
REBOTES
REBOUND
REBOXED
REBOXES
REBOZOS
REBRACE
REBRAND
REBREAK
REBREED
REBREWS
REBROKE
REBRUSH
REBUFFS
REBUILD
REBUILT
REBUKED
REBUKER
REBUKES
REBUSES
RIBALDS
RIBANDS
RIBBERS
RIBBIER
RIBBIES
RIBBING
RIBBONS
RIBBONY
RIBCAGE
RIBCUTS
RIBEYES
RIBLESS
RIBLETS
RIBLIKE
RIBMEAT
RIBPADS
ROBARDS
ROBBERS
ROBBERY
ROBBING
ROBBINS
ROBBNEN
ROBERTA
ROBERTE
ROBERTF
ROBERTH
ROBERTI
ROBERTO
ROBERTS
ROBESON
ROBLOWE
ROBOCOP
ROBOTIC
ROBOTRY
ROBROYS
ROBSART
ROBUSTA

ROBUSTO
RUBADUB
RUBATOS
RUBBERS
RUBBERY
RUBBING
RUBBISH
RUBBLES
RUBDOWN
RUBELLA
RUBEOLA
RUBICON
RUBIOUS
RUBITIN
RUBRICS
RUBSOFF
RUBSOUT
RUBSRAW
RUBUPON
RUBYDEE
RUBYRED

R••B•••

RABBETS
RABBITS
RABBITT
RABBITY
RABBLED
RABBLES
RAEBURN
RAGBAGS
RAMBLED
RAMBLER
RAMBLES
RAMBLIN
RANBACK
RASBORA
RATBERT
RAWBARS
RAYBANS
RAYBURN
REDBATS
REDBAYS
REDBIRD
REDBONE
REDBOOK
REDBUDS
REEBOKS
REUBENS
RHEBOKS
RHUBARB
RIBBERS
RIBBIER
RIBBIES
RIBBING
RIBBONS
RIBBONY
RIMBAUD
ROBBERS
ROBBERY
ROBBING
ROBBINS
ROBBNEN
ROEBUCK
ROMBERG
ROTBLAT
ROUBAIX
ROWBOAT

ROXBURY
ROYBEAN
RUBBERS
RUBBERY
RUBBING
RUBBISH
RUBBLES
RUMBAED
RUMBLED
RUMBLER
RUMBLES
RUNBACK
RUYBLAS
RYEBEER

R•••B••

RAILBUS
RAINBOW
RAKABLE
RAREBIT
RATABLE
RECABLE
REDEBIT
RELABEL
RETABLE
RHOMBIC
RHOMBUS
RHUMBAS
RIDABLE
RIDEBYS
RISIBLE
RISIBLY
ROADBED
ROLLBAR
ROOMBAS
ROSABUD
ROSEBAY
ROSEBUD
ROYGBIV

R••••B•

RACEDBY
RACESBY
RECOMBS
REDOUBT
REDROBE
REDTABS
REGRABS
REPROBE
RESORBS
RESTABS
REVERBS
RIDESBY
RIOLOBO
ROCKABY
ROLLSBY
RULEDBY

R•••••B

RANATAB
RECLIMB
REPLUMB
RESCRUB
RHUBARB
RUBADUB
RUNATAB

•RB••••

ARBACES
ARBITER
ARBOLES
ARBORED
ARBOURS
ARBUTUS
DRBROWN
MRBLISS
MRBODDY
MRBONES
MRBROWN
MRBURNS
MRBUTTS
ORBISON
ORBITAL
ORBITED
ORBITER
ORBLESS
ORBLIKE
URBANER
URBANII
URBANIV
URBANVI

•R•B•••

ARABIAN
ARABICA
ARABICS
ARABIST
ARABLES
ARLBERG
ARMBAND
ARMBONE
ARTBOOK
ARUBANS
BRIBEES
BRIBERS
BRIBERY
BRIBING
BRUBECK
CRABBED
CRABBER
CRABPOT
CRIBBED
CRIBBER
CRYBABY
DRABBER
DRABBLE
DRIBBLE
DRIBLET
DRUBBED
DRUBBER
DRYBULB
FREBERG
FRIBBLE
GRABBAG
GRABBAR
GRABBED
GRABBER
GRABSAT
GRUBBED
GRUBBER
JROBERT
MRSBASS
OREBODY
PREBADE
PREBAKE

PREBIDS
PREBILL
PREBIND
PREBOIL
PREBOOK
PREBOOM
PREBORN
PREBURN
PREBUYS
PROBALL
PROBATE
PROBERS
PROBIES
PROBING
PROBITY
PROBLEM
PROBONO
PROBOWL
TRABERT
TREBLED
TREBLES
TRIBBLE
TRIBECA
TRIBORO
TRIBUNE
TRIBUTE

•R••B••

ARRABAL
BRAMBLE
BRAMBLY
CRABBED
CRABBER
CRIBBED
CRIBBER
CROWBAR
CRUMBED
CRUMBLE
CRUMBLY
CRUMBUM
DRABBER
DRABBLE
DRAWBAR
DRIBBLE
DROPBOX
DRUBBED
DRUBBER
DRYABLE
ERRABLE
FREEBEE
FREEBIE
FRIABLE
FRIBBLE
FRISBEE
FROEBEL
FRYABLE
GRABBAG
GRABBAR
GRABBED
GRABBER
GREWBIG
GROWBIG
GRUBBED
GRUBBER
GRUMBLE
GRUMBLY
IRONBAR
MRHOBBS

MRTIBBS
PROMBID
TRAUBEL
TREMBLE
TREMBLY
TRIABLE
TRIBBLE
TROUBLE

•R•••B•

ARECIBO
CREEPBY
CRYBABY
DRIVEBY
DROPSBY
DROVEBY
DRWELBY
FREDEBB
GRIMSBY
MRHOBBS
MRTIBBS
PREFABS

•R••••B

BREWPUB
DRYBULB
FREDEBB
PREVERB
PROARAB
PROVERB
TRIMTAB
TRUERIB
XRAYLAB

••RB•••

AIRBAGS
AIRBALL
AIRBASE
AIRBILL
AIRBOAT
BARBARA
BARBARY
BARBATE
BARBEAU
BARBELL
BARBERA
BARBERS
BARBETS
BARBIES
BARBILL
BARBING
BARBUDA
BARBULE
BERBERS
BERBICK
BURBAGE
BURBANK
BURBLED
BURBLER
BURBLES
BURBOTS
CARBARN
CARBIDE
CARBINE
CARBONS
CARBOYS
CARBRAS
CORBELS

CORBETT
CURBCUT
CURBING
DERBIES
EARBONE
EARBUDS
FIRBANK
FORBADE
FORBEAR
FORBIDS
FORBORE
FORBUSH
FURBALL
FURBISH
GARBAGE
GARBAGY
GARBING
GARBLED
GARBLER
GARBLES
GERBILS
HARBACH
HARBORS
HARBOUR
HARBURG
HERBAGE
HERBALS
HERBART
HERBAUT
HERBERT
HERBIER
HERBTEA
JERBOAS
MARBLED
MARBLER
MARBLES
NORBERT
PARBAKE
PARBOIL
SERBIAN
SORBATE
SORBETS
TARBABY
TARBELL
TERBIUM
TURBANS
TURBINE
TURBOTS
VERBALS
VERBENA
VERBIDS
VERBIFY
VERBOSE
WARBABY
WARBLED
WARBLER
WARBLES
WARBOND
WARBURG

••R•B••

ACROBAT
AEROBAT
AEROBES
AEROBIC
AGRIBIZ
ARRABAL
BARFBAG
CARABOO
CARIBES
CARIBOO
CARIBOU
CEREBRA
CEREBRO
CORNBIN
CURABLE
CURABLY
DIRTBAG
DURABLE
DURABLY
ENROBED
ENROBES
ERRABLE
FAREBOX
FARMBOY
FERNBAR
FIREBOX
FIREBUG
FORABIT
FOREBAY
HIRABLE
JURYBOX
MARSBAR
MIRABEL
PARABLE
PARIBUS
RAREBIT
SCRIBED
SCRIBER
SCRIBES
SCRUBBY
SCRUBUP
SHRUBBY
STROBES
SUREBET
TURNBAD
UNROBED
UNROBES
VERYBAD
VERYBIG
WIRABLE
WORKBOX

••R••B•

AIRTUBE
BARNABY
BARTABS
BURNABY
CARAMBA
CARNABY
CORDOBA
EARLOBE
EARTABS
FORTYBC
HERNIBS
HORNSBY
MARIMBA
MORESBY
PARAIBA
SCRUBBY
SHRUBBY
TARBABY
THREEBC
WARBABY

••R•••B

CARCLUB
CORNCOB
PERTURB
UNCURBS
WARCLUB

•••RB••

ACERBIC
ALARBUS
BLURBER
BOURBON
COURBET
DEORBIT
ENARBOR
EXURBAN
EXURBIA
GEARBOX
INORBIT
OVERBED
OVERBET
OVERBID
OVERBIG
OVERBUY
POORBOX
POORBOY
SHERBET
THURBER
TOURBUS
UNORBED
UNURBAN

•••R•B•

ASCRIBE
BBQRIBS
CHERUBS
DISROBE
GLORYBE
HEYRUBE
LAPROBE
LATROBE
MICROBE
MIDRIBS
NAIROBI
OILRUBS
OUTRIBS
REDROBE
REGRABS
REPROBE
SCARABS
SWOREBY
THEREBY
THEROBE
WHEREBY

•••R••B

BEARCUB
DECRUMB
MCCRUMB
OVERDUB

••••RB•

ABSORBS
ADSORBS
ADVERBS
BICARBS
ENDERBY
NOCARBS
RESORBS
REVERBS
SUBURBS
SWEARBY
UNCURBS

••••R•B

BACKRUB
BODYRUB
FOOTRUB
NONARAB
PANARAB
PROARAB
RESCRUB
SHECRAB
THECRAB
THETRIB
TRUERIB
VAPORUB

•••••RB

DISTURB
LETTERB
LINEARB
LOWCARB
PERTURB
POTHERB
PREVERB
PROVERB
RHUBARB

RC•••••

RCADOME
RCCOLAS

R•C••••

RACCOON
RACECAR
RACEDBY
RACEDIN
RACEDTO
RACEDUP
RACEMES
RACESBY
RACESTO
RACESUP
RACEWAY
RACHAEL
RACIEST
RACINOS
RACISTS
RACKERS
RACKETS
RACKETY
RACKING
RACKOUT
RACKSUP
RACQUET
RCCOLAS
RECABLE
RECAGED
RECAGES
RECALLS
RECANED
RECANES
RECANTS
RECARRY
RECARVE
RECASED
RECASES
RECASTS
RECEDED
RECEDES
RECEIPT
RECEIVE
RECENCY
RECHALK
RECHALL
RECHART
RECHECK
RECHEWS
RECHOSE
RECIPES
RECITAL
RECITED
RECITER
RECITES
RECKONS
RECLADS
RECLAIM
RECLAME
RECLASP
RECLASS
RECLEAN
RECLIMB
RECLINE
RECLUSE
RECOALS
RECOATS
RECOCKS
RECODED
RECODES
RECOILS
RECOINS
RECOLOR
RECOMBS
RECOOKS
RECOOLS
RECORDS
RECORKS
RECOSTS
RECOUNT
RECOUPS
RECOVER
RECRANK
RECRATE
RECROOM
RECROSS
RECROWN
RECRUIT
RECTIFY
RECTORS
RECTORY
RECURED
RECURES
RECURLS
RECURVE
RECUSAL
RECUSED
RECUSES
RECYCLE
RICARDO
RICHARD
RICHENS
RICHEST
RICHLER
RICHMAN
RICHMEN
RICHTER
RICKETY
RICKEYS
RICKLES
RICKMAN
RICKSHA
RICOTTA
RICRACS
ROCHETS
ROCKABY
ROCKCOD
ROCKERS
ROCKERY
ROCKETS
ROCKIER
ROCKIES
ROCKILY
ROCKING
ROCKOIL
ROCKOON
ROCKYII
ROCKYIV
ROCOCOS
RUCHING
RUCKERT
RUCKING
RUCKSUP
RUCTION

R••C•••

RACCOON
RANCHED
RANCHER
RANCHES
RANCHOS
RANCORS
RANCOUR
RASCALS
RATCHET
RAUCOUS
REACHED
REACHER
REACHES
REACHIN
REACHUP
REACTED
REACTOR
REACTTO
REDCAPS
REDCARD
REDCELL
REDCENT
REDCHIP
REDCLAY
REDCOAT
REDCODS
REICING
REOCCUR
RESCALE
RESCANS
RESCIND
RESCORE
RESCRUB
RESCUED
RESCUER
RESCUES
REXCATS
RIBCAGE
RIBCUTS
RIPCORD
RITCHIE
ROACHES
ROMCOMS
ROSCOES
ROYCOHN
RUMCAKE

R•••C••

RACECAR
RADICAL
RADICES
RADICLE
RAILCAR
RATECAP
RAUNCHY
REBECCA
RECOCKS
RECYCLE
REDACTS
REDECAY
REDOCKS
REDUCED
REDUCER
REDUCES
REFACED
REFACES
REFOCUS
REJECTS
REKICKS
RELACED
RELACES
RELICTS
RELOCKS
RELUCTS
REOCCUR
REPACKS
REPICKS
RERACKS
RESECTS
RETACKS
RETICLE
RHOECUS
ROBOCOP
ROCKCOD
ROCOCOS
ROOTCAP
RUBICON
RUZICKA

R••••C•

RANBACK
RANSACK
RATPACK
RATRACE
REBECCA
REBLOCK
REBRACE
RECENCY
RECHECK
REDFACE
REDJACK
REDNECK
REEJECT
REELECT
REENACT
REERECT
REEVICT
REFENCE
REFLECT
REFRACT
REGENCY
REHITCH
REJOICE
REKNOCK
RELANCE
RELATCH
REMATCH
RENWICK
REPATCH
REPLACE
REPLICA
REPRICE
RESPACE
RESPECT
RESPICE
RESTACK
RESTICK
RESTOCK
RETEACH
RETOUCH
RETRACE
RETRACK
RETRACT
REVOICE
RICRACS
RIDDICK
RIMROCK
RIOTACT
RODDICK
ROEBUCK
ROLLICK
ROMANCE
ROSTOCK
RUBRICS
RUNBACK
RUSTICS

R•••••C

RAYKROC
RAYOVAC
RHEUMIC
RHOMBIC
ROBOTIC
ROMANIC

•RC••••

ARCADED
ARCADES
ARCADIA
ARCANUM
ARCHAIC
ARCHERS
ARCHERY
ARCHEST
ARCHFOE
ARCHIES
ARCHING
ARCHIVE
ARCHONS
ARCHSEE
ARCHWAY
ARCINGS
ARCLAMP
ARCSINE
ARCUATE
ARCWELD
DRCHAOS
MRCHIPS
MRCLEAN
ORCHARD
ORCHIDS
URCHINS

•R•C•••

ARACARI
ARACHNE
ARACHNO
ARECIBO
ARTCARS
BRACERO
BRACERS
BRACEUP
BRACING
BRACKEN
BRACKET
BRICKED
BRICKLE
BRICKUP
BROCADE
CRACKED
CRACKER
CRACKLE
CRACKLY
CRACKUP
CRECHES
CRICKED
CRICKET
CROCHET
CROCKED
CROCKER
CROCKET
CRUCIAL
DRACHMA
DRACULA
DRMCCOY
DRUCKER
DRYCELL
ERECTED
ERECTER
ERECTLY
ERECTOR
ERECTUS
ERICSON
ERUCTED
FRACTAL
FRECKLE
FRECKLY
FRICKER
FROCKED
FRYCOOK
GRACIAS
GRACILE
GRACING
GRACKLE
GRECIAN
GRECISM
GRECIZE
GROCERS
GROCERY
IRECKON
KRACKEL
MRSCOTT
ORACIES
ORACLES
ORECTIC
PRACTIC
PRECAST
PRECEDE
PRECEPT
PRECISE
PRECITE
PRECODE
PRECOIL
PRECOOK
PRECOOL
PRECOUP
PRECURE
PRECUTS
PRICERS
PRICIER
PRICILY
PRICING
PRICKED
PRICKLE
PRICKLY
PRICKUP
PROCEED
PROCESS
PROCITY
PROCLUS
PROCTER
PROCTOR
PROCURE
PROCYON
TRACERS
TRACERY
TRACHEA
TRACING
TRACKED
TRACKER
TRACTOR
TRICEPS
TRICKED
TRICKER
TRICKLE
TRICORN
TRICOTS
TROCHEE
TROCHES
TRUCKED
TRUCKEE
TRUCKER
TRUCKLE
URACILS
WRACKED
WRACKUP
WRECKED
WRECKER
WROCLAW

•R••C••

ARBACES
ARDECHE
ARNICAS
ARRACKS
ARTICLE
BRANCHY
BRESCIA
BRIOCHE
BRITCOM
BRONCHI
BRONCHO
BRONCOS
CREWCUT
CRUNCHY
DRMCCOY
DROPCAP
FRAICHE
FRANCES
FRANCHI
FRANCIS
FRENCHI
FRENCHS
FRESCAS
FRESCOS
GREYCUP
GROUCHO
GROUCHY
MRISCAN
MRLUCKY
MRMACHO
PRANCED
PRANCER
PRANCES
PREACHY
PREACID
PREACTS
PRINCES
PROSCAN
TRAMCAR
TRANCED
TRANCES
TREACLE
TREACLY

•R•••C•

ARABICA
ARABICS
ARDENCY
ARMLOCK
ARTDECO
ARTROCK
BRUBECK
CREVICE
CRITICS
DRIESCH
DRSPOCK
DRYDOCK
ERDRICH
EROTICA
EROTICS
ERRANCY
FROLICS
GRIMACE
IRENICS
MRDARCY
MRMARCH
MRSPOCK
ORIFICE
ORINOCO
PREDICT
PREFACE
PREFECT
PRELACY
PREPACK
PRERACE
PREROCK
PRIMACY
PRIVACY
PRODUCE
PRODUCT
PROJECT
PROTECT
TRADUCE
TRIBECA
TRISECT
TROPICS
TROUNCE
TRUANCY
URGENCY

•R••••C

ARAMAIC
ARCHAIC
ARSENIC
ARTHURC
CROSTIC
CRYPTIC
DRASTIC
DRUIDIC
DRYADIC
ERGOTIC
ERISTIC
ERRATIC
FRANTIC
FREDRIC
GRAPHIC
MRMUSIC
ORECTIC
ORGANIC
PRACTIC
PROSAIC
TRAFFIC
TRIADIC

••RC•••

AIRCOOL
AIRCREW
BARCARS
BARCLAY
BARCODE
BIRCHED
BIRCHEN
BIRCHES
CARCARE
CARCASS
CARCLUB
CARCOAT
CIRCLED
CIRCLER
CIRCLES
CIRCLET
CIRCUIT
CIRCUSY
EARCLIP
FARCEUR
FARCING
FORCEIN
FORCEON
FORCEPS
FORCERS
FORCEUP
FORCING
FURCATE
FURCOAT
GARCONS
HERCULE
HIRCINE
LARCENY
LARCHEN
LARCHES
LURCHED
LURCHER
LURCHES
MARCATO
MARCEAU
MARCELS
MARCHED
MARCHER
MARCHES
MARCHON
MARCONI
MARCUSE
MERCADO
MERCERS
MERCERY
MERCHES
MERCIAN
MERCIES
MERCURE
MERCURY
MORCERF
PARCELS
PARCHED
PARCHES
PERCALE
PERCENT
PERCEPT
PERCHED
PERCHER
PERCHES
PERCHIK
PERCUSS
PORCHES
PORCINE
PURCELL
SARCASM
SORCERY
TERCELS
TORCHED
TORCHER
TORCHES
WARCLUB
ZIRCONS

••R•C••

AFRICAN
AIRACES
APRICOT
ARRACKS
AURICLE
BARACUS
BORSCHT
CARACAS
CDRACKS
CORACLE
CORNCOB
CURACAO
CURBCUT
DERECHO
DIRECTS
DIRECTV
EARACHE

GYROCAR
HARICOT
HYRACES
JERICHO
KARACHI
LAROCHE
LYRICAL
LYRICON
MARACAS
MIRACLE
MOROCCO
PORSCHE
RERACKS
SARACEN
SIROCCO
SPRUCED
SPRUCER
SPRUCES
SURECAN
UNRACKS
UNROCKY
UTRECHT

••R••C•

ABROACH
AIRDUCT
AIRLOCK
AIRPACK
AIRRACE
AIRSACS
AIRSICK
AIRSOCK
AIRWICK
BARLICK
BARRACK
BERBICK
BERWICK
BURDICK
CARIOCA
CARJACK
CORMACK
CORNICE
CORRECT
CORSICA
CORTICO
DERRICK
DERRICO
DORMICE
DURANCE
EARLOCK
EHRLICH
ERRANCY
FIREICE
FOREACH
FORMICA
FORONCE
FURNACE
GARLICS
GARRICK
HARBACH
HARNICK
HARTACK
HEROICS
HERRICK
INREACH
MERRICK
MIRISCH
MORLOCK
MOROCCO
MORTICE
MURDOCH
NORDICA
NORDICS
NORELCO
NORWICH
OARLOCK
PARSECS
PERFECT
PORTICO
SCRATCH
SCREECH
SCRUNCH
SERPICO
SERVICE
SIROCCO
STRETCH
STRITCH
SURFACE
TARMACS
TERENCE
TERRACE
UPREACH
VARRICK
VERDICT
VERRUCA
VERSACE
WARLOCK
WARWICK

••R•••C

ACRYLIC
AEROBIC
BORONIC
BYRONIC
CARDIAC
CERAMIC
CHROMIC
CHRONIC
ERRATIC
FORASEC
FORTYBC
HERETIC
JURIDIC
KEROUAC
KORANIC
MORONIC
MORPHIC
MYRRHIC
PARODIC
PHRENIC
PIRATIC
PYRETIC
PYRITIC
PYRRHIC
SARANAC
THREEBC
VERIDIC
WAREPIC
XEROTIC

•••RC••

AFARCRY
ALARCON
AMERCED
AMERCER
AMERCES
ANARCHS
ANARCHY
APERCUS
BEARCAT
BEARCUB
BEERCAN
CHARCOT
CHURCHY
COERCED
COERCER
COERCES
EPARCHS
EPARCHY
EXARCHS
FIERCER
GFORCES
HAIRCUT
OVERCOY
OVERCUT
PIERCED
PIERCER
PIERCES
SCARCER
SOURCED
SOURCES
STARCHY
TIERCES

•••R•C•

AGARICS
AIRRACE
ALDRICH
AMERICA
AMTRACK
AMTRACS
ARTROCK
ATTRACT
AVARICE
BARRACK
BEDROCK
CAPRICE
CHIRICO
CLARICE
CLERICS
CONRACK
CORRECT
CYMRICS
DEFROCK
DERRICK
DERRICO
DETRACT
DOGRACE
DOTRICE
ELDRICH
ELDRICK
ELGRECO
EMBRACE
ERDRICH
EXTRACT
FABRICS
GARRICK
GEDRICK
HATRACK
HAYRACK
HAYRICK
HENRICH
HERRICK
IATRICS
INFRACT
JIMRICE
KIDROCK
KUBRICK
LEBROCK
MANRICO
MAURICE
MERRICK
METRICS
NEWRICH
OILRICH
ONTRACK
OSTRICH
OUTRACE
OUTROCK
OVERACT
OVERICE
PATRICE
PATRICK
PETROCK
POPROCK
PRERACE
PREROCK
RATRACE
REBRACE
REERECT
REFRACT
REPRICE
RETRACE
RETRACK
RETRACT
RICRACS
RIMROCK
RUBRICS
SEARACE
SECRECY
SKIRACE
SKIRACK
SUBRACE
TERRACE
THEROCK
TIERACK
TIMRICE
UNBRACE
UNERECT
UNFROCK
UNTRACK
VARRICK
VERRUCA
VITRICS

•••R••C

ACERBIC
DHARMIC
FJORDIC
GEORGEC
GEORGIC
HEBRAIC
MAURIAC
MYRRHIC
PADRAIC
PYRRHIC
QUARTIC
THERIAC
THERMIC
ZEBRAIC

••••RC•

AUTARCH
BYFORCE
CATORCE
DEMARCO
DIVORCE
ENFORCE
INFORCE
INMARCH
JOMARCH
LAMARCK
MAJORCA
MENORCA
MINORCA
MONARCH
MRDARCY
MRMARCH
MTMARCY
NOMERCY

••••R•C

AELFRIC
AMHARIC
BALDRIC
CALORIC
CAMBRIC
CENTRIC
CHLORIC
DINARIC
EMPIRIC
ENTERIC
ETHERIC
FREDRIC
GASTRIC
GENERIC
HOMERIC
LAUTREC
LECTRIC
MANTRIC
NEPHRIC
NUMERIC
ONEIRIC
QUADRIC
RAYKROC
SATIRIC
SATYRIC
SPHERIC
STEARIC
TAMARAC
UNLYRIC

•••••RC

ARTHURC
LETTERC

RD•••••

RDLAING

R•D••••

RADAMES
RADFORD
RADIALS
RADIANS
RADIANT
RADIATE
RADICAL
RADICES
RADICLE
RADIOAD
RADIODJ
RADIOED
RADIOER
RADIOIN
RADIXES
RADOMES
REDACTS
REDALGA
REDANTS
REDARED
REDARES
REDARMY
REDARNS
REDATED
REDATES
REDBATS
REDBAYS
REDBIRD
REDBONE
REDBOOK
REDBUDS
REDCAPS
REDCARD
REDCELL
REDCENT
REDCHIP
REDCLAY
REDCOAT
REDCODS
REDDAWN
REDDEER
REDDENS
REDDEST
REDDING
REDDISH
REDDOGS
REDDOTS
REDDUST
REDDYES
REDEALS
REDEALT
REDEBIT
REDECAY
REDEEDS
REDEEMS
REDEYED
REDEYES
REDFACE
REDFERN
REDFINS
REDFIRS
REDFISH
REDFIVE
REDFLAG
REDFORD
REDFOUR
REDHAIR
REDHATS
REDHAWK
REDHEAD
REDHEAT
REDHENS
REDHOTS
REDIALS
REDJACK
REDKING
REDLEGS
REDLINE
REDMEAT
REDMOND
REDNECK
REDNESS
REDNINE
REDNOSE
REDOAKS
REDOCKS
REDOING
REDONDO
REDOSED
REDOSES
REDOUBT
REDOUND
REDOUTS
REDOXES
REDPINE
REDPOLL
REDPONY
REDRAFT
REDRAGS
REDRAWN
REDRAWS
REDREAM
REDRESS
REDRIED
REDRIES
REDRILL
REDRIVE
REDROBE
REDROOP
REDROOT
REDROSE
REDSFAN
REDSKIN
REDSPOT
REDSTAR
REDSUIT
REDSUNS
REDTABS
REDTAGS
REDTAIL
REDTAPE
REDTIDE
REDTIES
REDTOPS
REDUCED
REDUCER
REDUCES
REDUSTS
REDWINE
REDWING
REDWOLF
REDWOOD
REDWORM
REDYING
REDZONE
RIDABLE
RIDDERS
RIDDICK
RIDDING
RIDDLED
RIDDLER
RIDDLES
RIDEBYS
RIDEOFF
RIDEOUT
RIDESBY
RIDESIN
RIDESTO
RIDESUP
RIDGIER
RIDGING
RIDGWAY
RIDINGS
RIDOTTO
RODDICK
RODDING
RODENTS
RODEOFF
RODEOUT
RODGERS
RODLESS
RODLIKE
RODOLFO
RODRIGO
RUDDERS
RUDDIED
RUDDIER
RUDDILY
RUDOLFI
RUDOLPH
RUDYARD

R••D•••

RAEDAWN
RAGDOLL
RAIDERS
RAIDING
RAMDOWN
RANDALL
RANDEEP
RANDIER
RANDOWN
RAWDATA
RAWDEAL
RCADOME
READAPT
READDED
READERS
READFOR
READIED
READIER
READIES
READILY
READING
READMIT
READOFF
READOPT
READORN
READOUT
READSIN
READSON
READSTO
READSUP
REDDAWN
REDDEER
REDDENS
REDDEST
REDDING
REDDISH
REDDOGS
REDDOTS
REDDUST
REDDYES
REEDIER
REEDING
REEDITS
REEDMAN
REEDMEN
RENDELL
RENDERS
RENDING
RHODIAN
RHODIUM
RIDDERS
RIDDICK
RIDDING
RIDDLED
RIDDLER
RIDDLES
RINDIER
RITDYES
ROADBED
ROADEOS
ROADERS
ROADHOG
ROADIES
ROADMAP
ROADTAR
ROADTAX
ROADWAY
RODDICK
RODDING
ROEDEER
RONDEAU
RONDELS
RONDURE
ROWDIER
ROWDIES
ROWDILY
RUBDOWN
RUDDERS
RUDDIED
RUDDIER
RUDDILY
RUNDEEP
RUNDLES
RUNDOWN

R•••D••

RABIDLY
RACEDBY
RACEDIN
RACEDTO
RACEDUP
RAKEDIN
RAKEDUP
RAMADAN
RAMADAS
RAPIDAN
RAPIDER
RAPIDLY
RATEDPG
READDED
REARDON
REAUDIT
RECEDED
RECEDES
RECODED
RECODES
REENDOW
REHIDES
REINDEX
REJUDGE
REMODEL
REORDER
REREDOS
RERIDES
RESIDED
RESIDER
RESIDES
RESIDUA
RESIDUE
REWIDEN
RIGIDLY
RIKSDAG
RILEDUP
RIORDAN
ROLODEX
ROPEDIN
ROPEDUP
ROUNDED
ROUNDEL
ROUNDER
ROUNDLY
ROUNDON
ROUNDUP
RUANDAS
RUBADUB
RUBYDEE
RULEDBY
RULEDON
RUNSDRY
RUSHDIE
RWANDAN

R••••D•

RADIODJ
RAGGEDY
RAMRODS
RASHIDA
RAWHIDE
REBENDS
REBINDS
RECLADS
RECORDS
REDBUDS
REDCODS
REDEEDS
REDONDO
REDTIDE
REFEEDS
REFINDS
REFOLDS
REFUNDS
REGARDS
REGILDS
REGIRDS
REGRADE
REGUIDE
RELANDS
RELEADS
RELENDS
RELOADS
REMANDS
REMENDS
REMINDS
REMOLDS
RENALDO
REREADS
RESANDS
RESEEDS
RESENDS
RESPADE
RESTUDY
RETARDS
RETRADE
REVENDS
REVERDY
REWARDS
REWELDS
REWINDS
REWORDS
RIBALDS
RIBANDS
RIBPADS
RICARDO
RIGVEDA
RINALDO
RIPTIDE
RITARDS
ROBARDS
ROLAIDS
ROLONDA
ROTUNDA
ROULADE

R•••••D

RABBLED
RADFORD
RADIOAD
RADIOED
RAFFLED
RAGWEED
RAINGOD
RALLIED
RAMBLED
RANCHED
RANKLED
RANWILD
RASSLED
RATTLED
RAVAGED
RAVELED
RAVENED
RAVINED
RAWFOOD
RAYMOND
RAZORED
REACHED
REACTED
READDED
READIED
REAIMED
REAIRED
REAMEND
REAREND
REARMED
REASKED
REBAKED
REBALED
REBATED
REBOARD
REBORED
REBOUND
REBOXED
REBRAND
REBREED
REBUILD
REBUKED
RECAGED
RECANED
RECASED
RECEDED
RECITED
RECODED
RECURED
RECUSED
REDARED
REDATED
REDBIRD
REDCARD
REDEYED
REDFORD
REDHEAD
REDMOND
REDOSED
REDOUND
REDRIED
REDUCED
REDWOOD
REFACED
REFAXED
REFILED
REFINED
REFIRED
REFIXED
REFLOOD
REFOUND
REFRIED
REFUGED
REFUSED
REFUTED
REGALED
REGLUED
REGNARD
REGRIND
REHEARD
REHIRED
REHONED
REIFIED
REIGNED
REINKED
REKEYED
REKNEAD
RELACED
RELATED
RELAXED
RELAYED
RELINED
RELIVED
RELUMED
REMATED
REMINED
REMISED
REMIXED
REMOVED
REMOWED
RENAMED
RENEGED
RENEWED
RENOTED
REOILED
REOWNED
REPAGED
REPAVED
REPINED
REPLEAD
REPLIED
REPOSED
REPUTED
RERAKED
RERATED
RESAVED
RESAWED
RESCIND
RESCUED
RESEWED
RESIDED
RESILED
RESINED
RESITED
RESIZED
RESOLED
RESOUND
RESOWED
RESPOND
RESUMED
RETAMED
RETAPED
RETAXED
RETILED
RETIMED
RETIRED
RETONED
RETOWED
RETREAD
RETRIED
RETUNED
RETYPED
REUPPED
REURGED
REVELED
REVERED
REVILED
REVISED
REVIVED
REVOKED
REVOTED
REWAKED
REWAXED
REWIPED
REWIRED
REWOUND
REXREED
REYNARD
REYNAUD
REYOKED
REZONED
RICHARD
RIDDLED
RIFFLED
RIGHTED
RIMBAUD
RIMPLED
RIPCORD
RIPENED
RIPPLED
RITEAID
RIVALED
RIVETED
ROADBED
ROASTED
ROCKCOD

ROGERED
ROLLAND
RONSARD
RONWOOD
ROOSTED
ROOTLED
ROSABUD
ROSEBUD
ROSERED
ROSINED
ROSTAND
ROTATED
ROUGHED
ROUNDED
ROUSTED
ROWELED
ROWLAND
RUBYRED
RUDDIED
RUDYARD
RUFFLED
RUMBAED
RUMBLED
RUMFORD
RUMORED
RUMPEND
RUMPLED
RUNWILD
RUSTLED
RUTLAND

•RD••••

ARDECHE
ARDENCY
ARDMORE
ARDOURS
ARDUOUS
ERDRICH
MRDARCY
MRDEEDS
ORDAINS
ORDEALS
ORDERED
ORDERER
ORDERIN
ORDERLY
ORDERUP
ORDINAL
ORDINES
ORDONEZ

•R•D•••

ARIDEST
ARIDITY
ARTDECO
BRADLEE
BRADLEY
BRIDALS
BRIDGED
BRIDGER
BRIDGES
BRIDGET
BRIDLED
BRIDLER
BRIDLES
BRODIES
BRODKEY
BRODSKY
CRADLED
CRADLER
CRADLES
CREDITS
CRUDELY
CRUDEST
CRUDITY
CRUDSUP
CRYDOWN
DREDGED
DREDGER
DREDGES
DRUDGED
DRUDGER
DRUDGES
DRYDOCK
ERODENT
ERODERS
ERODING
ERUDITE
FREDDIE
FREDEBB
FREDRIC
FRIDAYS
FRIDGES
FRIDLEY
FRODING
GRADATE
GRADEAA
GRADERS
GRADING
GRADUAL
GRIDDED
GRIDDER
GRIDDLE
GRIDMAP
GRODIER
GRUDGED
GRUDGER
GRUDGES
IRIDIUM
PRADESH
PREDARK
PREDATA
PREDATE
PREDAWN
PREDEFY
PREDENY
PREDICT
PREDIET
PREDIVE
PREDOOM
PREDUSK
PRIDING
PRODDED
PRODDER
PRODIGY
PRODSON
PRODUCE
PRODUCT
PRUDENT
PRUDERY
PRUDHOE
PRUDISH
TRADEIN
TRADEON
TRADERS
TRADEUP
TRADING
TRADUCE
TREDIAS
TRIDENT
TRODDEN
TRUDEAU
TRUDGED
TRUDGEN
TRUDGER
TRUDGES

•R••D••

ARCADED
ARCADES
ARCADIA
ARIADNE
ARLEDGE
ARMADAS
ARUNDEL
BRAEDEN
BRAIDED
BRAIDER
BRANDED
BRANDER
BRANDON
BREADED
BREADER
BREADTH
BREEDER
BRENDAN
BRENDEL
BRENDON
BRINDLE
BROADAS
BROADAX
BROADEN
BROADER
BROADLY
BROIDER
BROODED
BROODER
CRAWDAD
CREEDAL
CRIEDUP
CROWDED
CROWDER
CROWDIN
DREADED
DREIDEL
DRESDEN
DRIEDUP
DRIPDRY
DRUIDIC
DRYADES
DRYADIC
DRYIDEA
FREDDIE
FREEDOF
FREEDOM
FREEDUP
FRIEDAN
FRIEDUP
GRANDAM
GRANDEE
GRANDER
GRANDLY
GRANDMA
GRANDPA
GRENDEL
GREWDIM
GRIDDED
GRIDDER
GRIDDLE
GRINDER
GROWDIM
KRAMDEN
MRBODDY
MRPADRE
PREEDIT
PREIDEA
PRODDED
PRODDER
PROUDER
PROUDLY
PROUDOF
TREADED
TREADER
TREADLE
TREADON
TRENDED
TRIADIC
TRIEDIT
TRIEDON
TRIEDTO
TRIODES
TRODDEN
TRUEDUP
TRUNDLE
URGEDON

•R•••D•

ARAMIDS
ARNOLDS
BRAVADA
BRAVADO
BRIARDS
BRIGADE
BROCADE
BROMIDE
CRUSADE
CRUZADO
DRAMADY
DRAMEDY
ERRANDS
FRIENDS
GRANADA
GRENADA
GRENADE
GROUNDS
MRBODDY
MRDEEDS
MRWORDS
ORCHIDS
OREBODY
ORGANDY
ORLANDO
ORMANDY
PREBADE
PREBIDS
PRECEDE
PRECODE
PREFADE
PRELUDE
PREMADE
PREMEDS
PRESIDE
PROKEDS
PROSODY
PROVIDE
TRAGEDY
TRIPODS

•R••••D

ARANEID
ARBORED
ARCADED
ARCWELD
ARMBAND
ARMLOAD
ARMORED
AROUSED
ARRAYED
ARRIVED
BRAGGED
BRAIDED
BRAINED
BRAISED
BRANDED
BRAVOED
BRAWLED
BREADED
BREEZED
BRICKED
BRIDGED
BRIDLED
BRIEFED
BRIGAND
BRIMMED
BRISKED
BROILED
BRONZED
BROODED
BROOKED
BROOMED
BROWARD
BROWNED
BROWSED
BRUISED
BRUITED
BRUSHED
CRABBED
CRACKED
CRADLED
CRAFTED
CRAGGED
CRAMMED
CRAMPED
CRANKED
CRASHED
CRAWDAD
CRAWLED
CREAKED
CREAMED
CREASED
CREATED
CREEPED
CRESTED
CRIBBED
CRICKED
CRIMPED
CRINGED
CRISPED
CROAKED
CROCKED
CROOKED
CROONED
CROPPED
CROSSED
CROWDED
CROWNED
CRUISED
CRUMBED
CRUMPED
CRUSHED
CRUSTED
DRAFTED
DRAGGED
DRAINED
DRATTED
DRAWLED
DREADED
DREAMED
DREDGED
DRESSED
DRFREUD
DRIFTED
DRILLED
DRIPPED
DROOLED
DROOPED
DROPPED
DROWNED
DROWSED
DRUBBED
DRUDGED
DRUGGED
DRUMMED
DRYEYED
ERECTED
ERMINED
ERUCTED
ERUPTED
FRAGGED
FRANKED
FREAKED
FRESHED
FRESSED
FRETTED
FRILLED
FRINGED
FRISKED
FRITTED
FRIZZED
FROCKED
FRONTED
FROSTED
FROTHED
FROWARD
FROWNED
FRUITED
GRABBED
GRAFTED
GRAINED
GRANTED
GRAPHED
GRASPED
GRASSED
GREASED
GREENED
GREETED
GREWOLD
GRIDDED
GRIEVED
GRIFTED
GRILLED
GRINNED
GRIPPED
GRITTED
GROANED
GROINED
GROKKED
GROOMED
GROOVED
GROSSED
GROUPED
GROUSED
GROUTED
GROWLED
GROWOLD
GRUBBED
GRUDGED
GRUMPED
GRUNTED
IRELAND
ORBITED
ORCHARD
ORDERED
OROTUND
PRAISED
PRANCED
PRAWNED
PREACID
PREAGED
PREBIND
PREENED
PREFUND
PRELOAD
PREPAID
PREPPED
PRESOLD
PRESSED
PRETEND
PRETOLD
PREVOID
PREVUED
PRICKED
PRIMMED
PRIMPED
PRINKED
PRINTAD
PRINTED
PROCEED
PRODDED
PROMBID
PROMOED
PRONGED
PROOFED
PROPPED
PROWLED
TRACKED
TRAILED
TRAINED
TRAMMED
TRAMPED
TRANCED
TRAPPED
TRASHED
TRAWLED
TREADED
TREATED
TREBLED
TREKKED
TRENDED
TRESSED
TRICKED
TRIFFID
TRIFLED
TRIFOLD
TRILLED
TRIMMED
TRIPLED
TRIPPED
TROLLED
TROMPED
TROOPED
TROTHED
TROTTED
TROUPED
TRUCKED
TRUDGED
TRUMPED
TRUSSED
TRUSTED
TRYHARD
TRYSTED
VROOMED
WRACKED
WRAPPED
WREAKED
WRECKED
WRESTED
WRITHED
WRONGED

••RD•••

AIRDAMS
AIRDATE
AIRDRIE
AIRDROP
AIRDUCT
BARDEEN
BIRDDOG
BIRDERS
BIRDFLU
BIRDIED
BIRDIES
BIRDING
BIRDMAN
BIRDMEN
BORDERS
BORDONI
BURDENS
BURDICK
CARDERS
CARDIAC
CARDIAL
CARDIFF
CARDING
CARDIUM
CARDKEY
CARDOOR
CARDOZO
CORDAGE
CORDATE
CORDELL
CORDERO
CORDERS
CORDIAL
CORDIAS
CORDING
CORDITE
CORDOBA
CORDONS
CURDIER
CURDING
CURDLED
CURDLER
CURDLES
EARDROP
EARDRUM
FORDGTS
FORDHAM
FORDING
FORDLTD
FORDOES
FORDONE
GARDENA
GARDENS
GARDNER
GIRDERS
GIRDING
GIRDLED
GIRDLER
GIRDLES
GORDIAN
GORDITA
GORDIUS
HARDDAY
HARDEES
HARDENS
HARDEST
HARDHAT
HARDHIT
HARDIER
HARDILY
HARDING
HARDISH
HARDPAN
HARDPUT
HARDSET
HARDSIX
HARDTEN
HARDTOP
HARDWAY
HARDWON
HERDERS
HERDING
HORDING
HURDLED
HURDLER
HURDLES
JARDINE
JARDINS
JORDANA
KORDELL
KURDISH
LARDERS
LARDIER
LARDING
LARDNER
LARDONS
LORDING
LORDJIM
LORDSIT
MARDIAN
MORDANT
MORDENT
MORDRED
MURDERS
MURDOCH
NERDIER
NERDISH
NORDICA
NORDICS
NORDOFF
NORDOWE
PARDNER
PARDONS
PERDIDO
PERDIEM
PERDITA
PERDURE
PURDUEU
SARDINE
SIRDUKE
SORDINI
SORDINO
TARDIER
TARDILY
VERDANT
VERDELL
VERDICT
VERDINS
VERDOUX
VERDUGO
VERDURE
WARDENS
WARDERS
WARDING
WARDOFF
WORDAGE
WORDIER
WORDILY
WORDING
WORDONE
YARDAGE
YARDARM
YARDERS
YARDING
YARDMAN
YARDMEN

••R•D••

ABRADED
ABRADER
ABRADES
ABRIDGE
ACRIDLY
AIREDUP
AMRADIO
BIRDDOG
BOREDOM
BORIDES
BORODIN
CAREDTO
CBRADIO
CCRIDER
CORNDOG
DERIDED
DERIDER
DERIDES
DIRNDLS
EARLDOM
FARADAY
FIREDAT
FIREDOG
FIREDON
FIREDUP
FMRADIO
FORADAY
FORTDIX
HARDDAY
HEREDIA
HERNDON
HIREDON
JURIDIC
LAREDOS
LUREDIN
LURIDLY
MARIDAS
MARIDOS
MARSDEN
MERIDEN
MIRADAS
MIRADOR
PARADED
PARADER
PARADES
PARADOR
PARADOX
PARODIC
PERIDOT
REREDOS
RERIDES
SERFDOM
STRIDER
STRIDES
STRUDEL
TIRADES
TIREDER
TIREDLY
TIREDOF
VERIDIC
VERYDRY
WIREDIN
WIREDUP
WORKDAY
WORLDLY
XMRADIO

••R••D•

AIRMADA
ALREADY
BARBUDA
BARCODE
BERENDT
BERMUDA
BURUNDI
BYROADS
CARBIDE
CERVIDS
CORRADE
CORRIDA
CORRODE
CORVIDS
DERONDA
DERRIDA
EARBUDS
ERRANDS
FARSIDE
FORBADE
FORBIDS
FURTADO
GERALDO
GERUNDS
GIRONDE
HAROLDI
HARRODS
HERALDS
IMREADY
INROADS
MARAUDS
MERCADO
MIRANDA
MYRIADS
NEREIDS
PARKADE
PERDIDO
PERFIDY
PERIODS
PERVADE
REREADS
SCREEDS
SHROUDS
SPREADS
STRANDS
SUREIDO
THREADS
THREADY
TORNADO
TOROIDS
TORPEDO
UNREADY
UNROWDY
VERANDA
VERBIDS
VERYODD
WARGODS

••R•••D

AARATED
ABRADED
AERATED
AGROUND
AIRHEAD
AIRRAID
APRONED
ARRAYED
ARRIVED
BARMAID
BARNARD
BARNRED
BARTEND
BERATED
BERNARD
BERRIED
BERTHED
BIRCHED
BIRDIED
BIRTHED
BURBLED
BURGLED
CARLOAD
CAROLED
CAROMED
CAROTID
CARRIED
CERATED
CHROMED
CIRCLED
CORNFED
CURATED
CURDLED
CURRIED
DARKLED
DARKRED
DARTLED
DERATED
DERIDED
DERIVED
DIRTIED
DURWARD
EARTHED
ENRAGED
ENROBED
FARGOND
FARMAID
FERNAND
FERRIED
FORAGED
FORAYED
FORDLTD
FORFEND
FORGOOD
FORTORD
FORTYAD
FORWARD
GARAGED
GARBLED
GARGLED
GARLAND
GIRDLED
GIRTHED
GOROUND
GURGLED
GYRATED
HARLAND
HARRIED
HARROLD
HARVARD
HURDLED
HURRIED
HURTLED
LURCHED
MARBLED
MARCHED
MARRIED
MARSRED
MERITED
MERMAID
MORDRED
MORPHED
MURALED
MYRRHED
NORMAND
NORWOOD
OERSTED
PARADED
PARCHED
PAROLED
PAROTID
PARRIED
PARTIED
PERCHED
PERILED
PERSEID
PERUSED
PGRATED

PHRASED
PIRATED
PORTEND
PURFLED
PURPLED
PURSUED
PYRAMID
RERAKED
RERATED
SCRAPED
SCREWED
SCRIBED
SHRINED
SIRENED
SORTIED
SPRAYED
SPRUCED
STRAFED
STRAYED
STREWED
STRIPED
STRIVED
STROKED
TARRIED
THREEAD
THRIVED
TORCHED
TORQUED
TORVALD
TURNBAD
TURNRED
TURTLED
UNRAKED
UNRATED
UNRAYED
UNRAZED
UNRIGID
UNRILED
UNRIMED
UNRIVED
UNROBED
UNROPED
UNROUND
UNRULED
UPRATED
VERYBAD
VERYMAD
VERYODD
VERYOLD
VERYRED
VERYSAD
WARBLED
WARBOND
WARHEAD
WARLORD
WORRIED
WORSTED
XEROXED

•••RD••

AWARDED
AWARDEE
AWARDER
BEARDED
BOARDED
BOARDER
BOARDUP
CHORDAL
CHORDED
CSARDAS
CZARDAS
CZARDOM
DEARDEN
DEIRDRE
DOORDIE
EVERDUR
EXORDIA
FJORDIC
FOURDAY
GGORDON
GOURDES
GUARDED
GUARDEE
GUARDER
GUERDON
HAIRDOS
HAIRDYE
HEARDOF
HEIRDOM
HOARDED
HOARDER
INORDER
JOURDAN
LOURDES
MCARDLE
ONORDER
OVERDID
OVERDOG
OVERDRY
OVERDUB
OVERDUE
OVERDYE
REARDON
REORDER
RIORDAN
STARDOM
THIRDLY
TOORDER
TSARDOM
WEIRDAL
WEIRDED
WEIRDER
WEIRDLY
WEIRDOS

•••R•D•

ACARIDS
ALFREDA
ALFREDE
ALFREDO
ALFREDU
AMERADA
ANDRADE
ASTRIDE
ATGRADE
BUSRIDE
CABRIDE
CHARADE
COMRADE
CORRADE
CORRIDA
CORRODE
DEGRADE
DERRIDA
DETRUDE
ELPRADO
ENTRADA
ESTRADA
EXTRUDE
FLORIDA
FLYRODS
HARRODS
HATREDS
HAYRIDE
HOTRODS
HYBRIDS
HYDRIDE
IDAREDS
INTRADE
INTRUDE
ISUREDO
JOYRIDE
LETRIDE
MCBRIDE
NEXRADS
NIMRODS
NITRIDE
NOTRADE
OBTRUDE
OUTRIDE
OUTRODE
PODRIDA
QUERIDA
QUERIDO
RAMRODS
REGRADE
RETRADE
SCAREDY
TETRADS
TETRODE
THEREDS
TIERODS
UNCRUDE
UPGRADE
UPTRADE
USERIDS

•••R••D

ABORTED
ACCRUED
ACORNED
ADORNED
AIRRAID
ALARMED
ALERTED
AMERCED
AMERIND
ANDROID
ANEROID
ANYROAD
AVERRED
AVERTED
AWARDED
AYKROYD
AYNRAND
BEARDED
BERRIED
BLURRED
BLURTED
BOARDED
CAIRNED
CARRIED
CHARGED
CHARMED
CHARRED
CHARTED
CHIRPED
CHIRRED
CHORDED
CHURNED
CLERKED
COBRAND
COERCED
CONRIED
COURSED
COURTED
CURRIED
DEARGOD
DECREED
DECRIED
DEFRAUD
DEGREED
DRFREUD
DWARFED
EMBRUED
EMERALD
EMERGED
EMERSED
ENARMED
EVERTED
EXERTED
FERRIED
FIBROID
FLIRTED
GLORIED
GNARLED
GNARRED
GUARDED
HARRIED
HARROLD
HEARTED
HENREID
HOARDED
HURRIED
IMBRUED
INBREED
INCROWD
KNARRED
KNURLED
LEARNED
LEGRAND
LIPREAD
LOUREED
LOWROAD
MARRIED
MISREAD
MOURNED
MYRRHED
OCHROID
OFFROAD
OPERAND
OUTREAD
OVERBED
OVERBID
OVERDID
OVERFED
OVERSAD
PARRIED
PEARLED
PIERCED
QUERIED
QUIRTED
REAREND
REARMED
REBRAND
REBREED
REDRIED
REFRIED
REGRIND
RETREAD
RETRIED
REURGED
REXREED
SCARFED
SCARPED
SCARRED
SCARWID
SCORNED
SHARPED
SHIRKED
SHIRRED
SHORTED
SKIRLED
SKIRTED
SLURPED
SLURRED
SMARTED
SMIRKED
SNARFED
SNARLED
SNORTED
SOURCED
SPARKED
SPARRED
SPORTED
SPURNED
SPURRED
SPURTED
STARRED
STARTED
STARVED
STEROID
STIRRED
STORIED
STORMED
SWARMED
SWERVED
SWIRLED
TARRIED
THORNED
THYROID
TIARAED
TIMREID
TWIRLED
UNARMED
UNBRAID
UNCRIED
UNDRIED
UNFREED
UNFRIED
UNGRAND
UNORBED
UNPROUD
UNTREAD
UNTREED
UNTRIED
UNURGED
UPBRAID
UPDRIED
UPTREND
USURPED
WEARIED
WEIRDED
WHARFED
WHIRLED
WHIRRED
WHORLED
WORRIED
YEAREND
YEARNED
ZEBROID

••••RD•

ACCORDS
AFFORDS
ALEARDI
BACARDI
BEGIRDS
BOGARDE
BOIARDO
BRIARDS
BYWORDS
CANARDS
COWARDS
DOTARDS
DOVERDE
EDGARDO
EDUARDO
EDWARDG
EDWARDI
EDWARDR
EDWARDS
EDWARDV
ENGARDE
ENGIRDS
HAZARDS
HEYMRDJ
HOWARDK
HOWARDS
HOWARDU
IDCARDS
INNARDS
INWARDS
LASORDA
LIZARDS
MCMURDO
MILORDS
MRWORDS
ONWARDS
OXFORDS
PETARDS
PICARDO
PICARDY
RECORDS
REGARDS
REGIRDS
RETARDS
REVERDY
REWARDS
REWORDS
RICARDO
RITARDS
ROBARDS
SEWARDS
TABARDS
TOWARDS
UNDERDO
UNGIRDS
UNHARDY
UPCARDS
UPGIRDS
UPWARDS
WHWORDS
WIZARDS

••••R•D

ABJURED
ADHERED
ADJURED
ADMIRED
AFEARED
ALLURED
ALTERED
ANGERED
ARBORED
ARMORED
ASCARED
ASPIRED
ASSURED
ATTIRED
AUGURED
AVERRED
AXELROD
BARNRED
BEETRED
BEMIRED
BEOGRAD
BEWARED
BLEARED
BLUERED
BLURRED
BOWERED
CAPERED
CATERED
CEDARED
CENTRED
CHAIRED
CHARRED
CHEERED
CHIRRED
CHOIRED
CLEARED
CODERED
COHERED
COLORED
COVERED
COWERED
DARKRED
DEAIRED
DEEPRED
DEHIRED
DESIRED
DEWIRED
DOWERED
ENCORED
ENDURED
ENSURED
ENTERED
EUCHRED
EXPIRED
FAVORED
FEVERED
FIBERED
FIGURED
FLEERED
FLOORED
FLOURED
FUELROD
GETSRID
GNARRED
HALFROD
HOMERED
HONORED
HOVERED
HUMORED
HUNDRED
IGNORED
ILLBRED
IMBORED
IMMURED
IMTIRED
INHERED
INJURED
INSURED
KAMERAD
KINDRED
KNARRED
LABORED
LAYERED
LEVERED
LIVERED
LOUVRED
LOWBRED
LOWERED
LUSTRED
MAITRED
MAJORED
MANFRED
MANURED
MARSRED
MATURED
METERED
MILDRED
MINORED
MITERED
MORDRED
MOTORED
MYWORLD
NATURED
OFFERED
ORDERED
OSIERED
OUTBRED
PAPERED
PCWORLD
PETERED
POWERED
PUSHROD
QUEERED
RAZORED
REAIRED
REBORED
RECURED
REDARED
REFIRED
REHIRED
RETIRED
REVERED
REWIRED
ROGERED
ROSERED
RUBYRED
RUMORED
SABERED
SAVORED
SCARRED
SCOURED
SECURED
SEESRED
SEVERED
SHEARED
SHEERED
SHIRRED
SLURRED
SMEARED
SNEERED
SOBERED
SPARRED
SPEARED
SPHERED
SPURRED
SQUARED
SQUIRED
STAIRED
STARRED
STEERED
STIRRED
SUBARID
SUGARED
SUTURED
TAPERED
TASERED
TENURED
TOWERED
TURNRED
TUTORED
UMBERED
UMPIRED
UNAIRED
UNBARED
UNBORED
UNCORED
UNCURED
UNDARED
UNFIRED
UNGORED
UNHIRED
UNLURED
UNMIRED
UNPARED
UNTIRED
UNWIRED
USHERED
UTTERED
VAPORED
VENTRAD
VERYRED
VISORED
VIZORED
WAFERED
WAGERED
WATERED
WAVERED
WHIRRED
WILFRED
WINERED

•••••RD

ABELARD
ALEYARD
ALPHARD
ANTBIRD
ASHFORD
ATMCARD
ATTHIRD
AWKWARD
BADWORD
BALLARD
BARNARD
BEDFORD
BEEYARD
BEHEARD
BERNARD
BIGBIRD
BOMBARD
BONNARD
BOOBIRD
BROWARD
BUSTARD
BUZZARD
CATBIRD
COLLARD
CONCORD
COSTARD
COWBIRD
COWHERD
CUECARD
CUSTARD
DASTARD
DEBEARD
DIEHARD
DILLARD
DISCARD
DISCORD
DULLARD
DURWARD
EDOUARD
FORTORD
FORWARD
FOULARD
FROWARD
GASPARD
GAYLORD
GETWORD
GIFFORD
GILFORD
GISCARD
GIZZARD
GODDARD
GOSFORD
GOTWORD
HAGGARD
HALYARD
HARVARD
HAYWARD
HEYWARD
HUBBARD
HUMBARD
INAWORD
INBOARD
INTHIRD
JAYBIRD
JAYWARD
KEYCARD
KEYWORD
LAGGARD
LANFORD
LANYARD
LAWFORD
LEEFORD
LEEWARD
LEONARD
LEOPARD
LEOTARD
LEPPARD
LETTERD
LOLLARD
LOMBARD
LOWCARD
MALLARD
MANSARD
MAYNARD
MEDFORD
MILLARD
MISWORD
MITFORD
MUMFORD
MUSTARD
NEWWORD
NONWORD
OILBIRD
ONBOARD
ONEYARD
ONGUARD
ORCHARD
OUTWARD
OUTWORD
PACKARD
PEPPARD
PETBIRD
PICCARD
PIPCARD
PLACARD
POLLARD
POMMARD
PONIARD
RADFORD
REBOARD
REDBIRD
REDCARD
REDFORD
REGNARD
REHEARD
REYNARD
RICHARD
RIPCORD
RONSARD
RUDYARD
RUMFORD
SAGCARD
SANFORD
SEABIRD
SEAWARD
SHEPARD
SKYNYRD
SKYWARD
STEWARD
SUNBIRD
SUNWARD
SZILARD
TANKARD
THEBARD
TOOHARD
TRYHARD
UNBEARD
UNGUARD
UNHEARD
UNITARD
UPHOARD
VANWARD
VILLARD
WARLORD
WATFORD
WAYWARD
WEXFORD
WILFORD
WILLARD
WOODARD

RE•••••

REACHED
REACHER
REACHES
REACHIN
REACHUP
REACTED
REACTOR
REACTTO
READAPT
READDED
READERS
READFOR
READIED
READIER
READIES
READILY
READING
READMIT
READOFF
READOPT
READORN
READOUT
READSIN
READSON
READSTO
READSUP
REAFFIX
REAGANS
REAGENT
REAIMED
REAIRED
REALEST
REALIGN
REALINE
REALISE
REALISM
REALIST
REALITY
REALIZE
REALLOT
REALMAN
REALMEN
REALTER
REALTOR
REAMASS
REAMEND
REAMERS
REAMING
REAMOUT
REANNEX
REAPERS
REAPING
REAPPLY
REARDON
REAREND
REARERS
REARGUE
REARING
REARISE
REARLIT
REARMED
REAROSE
REARSUP
REASKED
REASONS
REASSAY
REATTAS
REAUDIT
REAUMUR
REAVAIL
REAVERS
REAVING
REAVOWS
REAWAKE
REAWOKE
REBAITS
REBAKED
REBAKES
REBALED
REBALES
REBANKS
REBASTE
REBATED
REBATER
REBATES
REBATHE
REBECCA
REBEGAN
REBEGIN
REBEGUN
REBEKAH
REBENDS
REBILLS
REBINDS
REBIRTH
REBLOCK
REBLOOM
REBLOWN
REBOANT
REBOARD
REBOILS
REBOLTS
REBOOKS
REBOOTS
REBORED
REBORES
REBOTES
REBOUND
REBOXED
REBOXES
REBOZOS
REBRACE
REBRAND
REBREAK
REBREED
REBREWS
REBROKE
REBRUSH
REBUFFS
REBUILD
REBUILT
REBUKED
REBUKER
REBUKES

REBUSES	RECURVE	REDMOND	REEKIER	REFUGED	REHIDES	RELINKS	RENOIRS	REPOSTS	RESENDS	RESTACK	RETINAS	REVERIE
RECABLE	RECUSAL	REDNECK	REEKING	REFUGEE	REHINGE	RELISTS	RENOTED	REPOURS	RESENTS	RESTAFF	RETINGE	REVERSA
RECAGED	RECUSED	REDNESS	REEKSOF	REFUGES	REHIRED	RELIVED	RENOTES	REPOWER	RESERVE	RESTAGE	RETINOL	REVERSE
RECAGES	RECUSES	REDNINE	REELECT	REFUNDS	REHIRES	RELIVES	RENOWNS	REPPING	RESEWED	RESTAIN	RETINTS	REVERTS
RECALLS	RECYCLE	REDNOSE	REELERS	REFUSAL	REHITCH	RELLENO	RENTALS	REPRESS	RESHAPE	RESTAMP	RETINUE	REVESTS
RECANED	REDACTS	REDOAKS	REELING	REFUSED	REHONED	RELOADS	RENTEES	REPRICE	RESHARE	RESTART	RETIRED	REVIEWS
RECANES	REDALGA	REDOCKS	REELOFF	REFUSER	REHONES	RELOANS	RENTERS	REPRIME	RESHAVE	RESTATE	RETIREE	REVILED
RECANTS	REDANTS	REDOING	REELOUT	REFUSES	REHONOR	RELOCKS	RENTIER	REPRINT	RESHIFT	RESTERS	RETIRES	REVILER
RECARRY	REDARED	REDONDO	REELSIN	REFUTAL	REHOOKS	RELOOKS	RENTING	REPRISE	RESHINE	RESTFUL	RETITLE	REVILES
RECARVE	REDARES	REDOSED	REELSUP	REFUTED	REHOUSE	RELOSES	RENTOUT	REPROBE	RESHIPS	RESTICK	RETOAST	REVISAL
RECASED	REDARMY	REDOSES	REEMITS	REFUTER	REICING	RELUCTS	RENTSTO	REPROOF	RESHOES	RESTING	RETONED	REVISED
RECASES	REDARNS	REDOUBT	REENACT	REFUTES	REIFIED	RELUMED	RENUZIT	REPROVE	RESHOOT	RESTIRS	RETONES	REVISER
RECASTS	REDATED	REDOUND	REENDOW	REFYING	REIFIES	RELUMES	RENVOIS	REPRUNE	RESHOWN	RESTIVE	RETOOLS	REVISES
RECEDED	REDATES	REDOUTS	REENJOY	REGAINS	REIGNED	RELYING	RENWICK	REPSFOR	RESHOWS	RESTOCK	RETORTS	REVISIT
RECEDES	REDBATS	REDOXES	REENTER	REGALED	REIMAGE	REMAILS	REOCCUR	REPTILE	RESHUTS	RESTOKE	RETOTAL	REVISOR
RECEIPT	REDBAYS	REDPINE	REENTRY	REGALER	REIMPLY	REMAINS	REOFFER	REPUGNS	RESIDED	RESTORE	RETOUCH	REVITUP
RECEIVE	REDBIRD	REDPOLL	REEQUIP	REGALES	REINDEX	REMAKES	REOILED	REPULSE	RESIDER	RESTOWS	RETOURS	REVIVAL
RECENCY	REDBONE	REDPONY	REERECT	REGALIA	REINING	REMANDS	REOPENS	REPUMPS	RESIDES	RESTRAP	RETOWED	REVIVED
RECHALK	REDBOOK	REDRAFT	REERUPT	REGALLY	REINKED	REMARKS	REORDER	REPUTED	RESIDUA	RESTREW	RETRACE	REVIVER
RECHALL	REDBUDS	REDRAGS	REEVICT	REGARDS	REINSIN	REMARRY	REOWNED	REPUTES	RESIDUE	RESTRIP	RETRACK	REVIVES
RECHART	REDCAPS	REDRAWN	REEVING	REGATTA	REISSUE	REMATCH	REPACKS	REQUEST	RESIFTS	RESTSIN	RETRACT	REVOICE
RECHECK	REDCARD	REDRAWS	REEVOKE	REGAUGE	REITMAN	REMATED	REPAGED	REQUIEM	RESIGHT	RESTSON	RETRADE	REVOKED
RECHEWS	REDCELL	REDREAM	REEXPEL	REGEARS	REJAILS	REMATES	REPAGES	REQUIRE	RESIGNS	RESTSUP	RETRAIN	REVOKER
RECHOSE	REDCENT	REDRESS	REFACED	REGENCY	REJECTS	REMEETS	REPAINT	REQUITE	RESILED	RESTUDY	RETRAPS	REVOKES
RECIPES	REDCHIP	REDRIED	REFACES	REGENTS	REJOICE	REMELTS	REPAIRS	REQUOTE	RESILES	RESTUFF	RETREAD	REVOLTS
RECITAL	REDCLAY	REDRIES	REFALLS	REGIFTS	REJOINS	REMENDS	REPANEL	RERACKS	RESINED	RESTYLE	RETREAT	REVOLVE
RECITED	REDCOAT	REDRILL	REFAXED	REGILDS	REJUDGE	REMERGE	REPAPER	RERAISE	RESINGS	RESUITS	RETRIAL	REVOTED
RECITER	REDCODS	REDRIVE	REFAXES	REGIMEN	REKEYED	REMILLS	REPARKS	RERAKED	RESINKS	RESULTS	RETRIED	REVOTES
RECITES	REDDAWN	REDROBE	REFEEDS	REGIMES	REKICKS	REMINDS	REPASTE	RERAKES	RESISTS	RESUMED	RETRIES	REVVING
RECKONS	REDDEER	REDROOP	REFENCE	REGINAL	REKNEAD	REMINED	REPASTS	RERANKS	RESITED	RESUMES	RETRIMS	REWAGER
RECLADS	REDDENS	REDROOT	REFEREE	REGINAS	REKNITS	REMINES	REPATCH	RERATED	RESIZED	RESURGE	RETSINA	REWAKED
RECLAIM	REDDEST	REDROSE	REFERTO	REGIONS	REKNOCK	REMINTS	REPAVED	RERATES	RESIZER	RESWEAR	RETTING	REWAKEN
RECLAME	REDDING	REDSFAN	REFFING	REGIRDS	REKNOTS	REMISED	REPAVES	REREADS	RESIZES	RESWEEP	RETUNED	REWAKES
RECLASP	REDDISH	REDSKIN	REFIGHT	REGIVEN	RELABEL	REMISES	REPEALS	REREDOS	RESLATE	RESWIMS	RETUNES	REWARDS
RECLASS	REDDOGS	REDSPOT	REFILED	REGIVES	RELACED	REMIXED	REPEATS	REREELS	RESMELT	RESWORE	RETURFS	REWARMS
RECLEAN	REDDOTS	REDSTAR	REFILES	REGLAZE	RELACES	REMIXES	REPENTS	RERENTS	RESNAIS	RESWORN	RETURNS	REWARNS
RECLIMB	REDDUST	REDSUIT	REFILLS	REGLOSS	RELANCE	REMNANT	REPERKS	RERIDES	RESNAPS	RETABLE	RETWINE	REWATER
RECLINE	REDDYES	REDSUNS	REFILMS	REGLOWS	RELANDS	REMODEL	REPHASE	RERINSE	RESOAKS	RETACKS	RETWIST	REWAXED
RECLUSE	REDEALS	REDTABS	REFINDS	REGLUED	RELANES	REMOLDS	REPHONE	RERISEN	RESOAPS	RETAILS	RETYPED	REWAXES
RECOALS	REDEALT	REDTAGS	REFINED	REGLUES	RELAPSE	REMORAS	REPICKS	RERISES	RESOILS	RETAINS	RETYPES	REWEARS
RECOATS	REDEBIT	REDTAIL	REFINER	REGNANT	RELATCH	REMORSE	REPINED	REROLLS	RESOJET	RETAKEN	REUBENS	REWEAVE
RECOCKS	REDECAY	REDTAPE	REFINES	REGNARD	RELATED	REMOTER	REPINER	REROOFS	RESOLED	RETAKER	REUNERS	REWEIGH
RECODED	REDEEDS	REDTIDE	REFIRED	REGNIER	RELATER	REMOTES	REPINES	REROOTS	RESOLER	RETAKES	REUNIFY	REWELDS
RECODES	REDEEMS	REDTIES	REFIRES	REGRABS	RELATES	REMOUNT	REPLACE	REROUTE	RESOLES	RETALLY	REUNION	REWIDEN
RECOILS	REDEYED	REDTOPS	REFIXED	REGRADE	RELATOR	REMOVAL	REPLANE	RESALES	RESOLVE	RETAMED	REUNITE	REWINDS
RECOINS	REDEYES	REDUCED	REFIXES	REGRAFT	RELAXED	REMOVED	REPLANS	RESALTS	RESORBS	RETAMES	REUPPED	REWIPED
RECOLOR	REDFACE	REDUCER	REFLAGS	REGRANT	RELAXER	REMOVER	REPLANT	RESANDS	RESORTS	RETAPED	REURGED	REWIPES
RECOMBS	REDFERN	REDUCES	REFLATE	REGRAPH	RELAXES	REMOVES	REPLATE	RESAVED	RESOUND	RETAPES	REURGES	REWIRED
RECOOKS	REDFINS	REDUSTS	REFLECT	REGRASP	RELAYED	REMOWED	REPLAYS	RESAVES	RESOWED	RETARDS	REUSERS	REWIRES
RECOOLS	REDFIRS	REDWINE	REFLIES	REGREET	RELAYER	RENAILS	REPLEAD	RESAWED	RESPACE	RETASTE	REUSING	REWOKEN
RECORDS	REDFISH	REDWING	REFLIPS	REGRESS	RELEADS	RENALDO	REPLETE	RESCALE	RESPADE	RETAXED	REUTERS	REWORDS
RECORKS	REDFIVE	REDWOLF	REFLOAT	REGRETS	RELEAPS	RENALLY	REPLICA	RESCANS	RESPANS	RETAXES	REUTHER	REWORKS
RECOSTS	REDFLAG	REDWOOD	REFLOOD	REGRIND	RELEARN	RENAMED	REPLIED	RESCIND	RESPARK	RETEACH	REUTTER	REWOUND
RECOUNT	REDFORD	REDWORM	REFLOWN	REGRIPS	RELEASE	RENAMES	REPLIER	RESCORE	RESPEAK	RETEARS	REVALUE	REWOVEN
RECOUPS	REDFOUR	REDYING	REFLOWS	REGROOM	RELENDS	RENAULT	REPLIES	RESCRUB	RESPECT	RETELLS	REVAMPS	REWRAPS
RECOVER	REDHAIR	REDZONE	REFOCUS	REGROUP	RELENTS	RENDELL	REPLOTS	RESCUED	RESPELL	RETESTS	REVEALS	REWRITE
RECRANK	REDHATS	REEARNS	REFOLDS	REGROWN	RELEVEL	RENDERS	REPLOWS	RESCUER	RESPELT	RETHANK	REVELED	REWROTE
RECRATE	REDHAWK	REEBOKS	REFORGE	REGROWS	RELEVER	RENDING	REPLUMB	RESCUES	RESPICE	RETHAWS	REVELER	REXCATS
RECROOM	REDHEAD	REEDIER	REFORMS	REGUIDE	RELEVES	RENEGED	REPLUME	RESEALS	RESPINS	RETHINK	REVELIN	REXREED
RECROSS	REDHEAT	REEDING	REFOUND	REGULAR	RELIANT	RENEGER	REPLYTO	RESEAMS	RESPIRE	RETIARY	REVELRY	REXROTH
RECROWN	REDHENS	REEDITS	REFRACT	REGULUS	RELICTS	RENEGES	REPOINT	RESEATS	RESPITE	RETICLE	REVENDS	REYMONT
RECRUIT	REDHOTS	REEDMAN	REFRAIN	REHANGS	RELIEFS	RENESTS	REPOLLS	RESEAUS	RESPLIT	RETILED	REVENGE	REYNARD
RECTIFY	REDIALS	REEDMEN	REFRAME	REHAULS	RELIERS	RENEWAL	REPOMAN	RESEAUX	RESPOKE	RETILES	REVENUE	REYNAUD
RECTORS	REDJACK	REEFERS	REFRESH	REHEALS	RELIEVE	RENEWED	REPORTS	RESECTS	RESPOND	RETILLS	REVERBS	REYNOSA
RECTORY	REDKING	REEFIER	REFRIED	REHEARD	RELIGHT	RENEWER	REPOSED	RESEEDS	RESPOOL	RETIMED	REVERDY	REYOKED
RECURED	REDLEGS	REEFING	REFRIES	REHEARS	RELIMIT	RENFREW	REPOSER	RESEEKS	RESPOTS	RETIMES	REVERED	REYOKES
RECURES	REDLINE	REEJECT	REFRONT	REHEATS	RELINED	RENNETS	REPOSES	RESEIZE	RESPRAY	RETINAE	REVERER	REZEROS
RECURLS	REDMEAT	REEKERS	REFUELS	REHEELS	RELINES	RENNINS	REPOSIT	RESELLS	RESTABS	RETINAL	REVERES	REZONED

REZONES

R•E••••

RAEBURN
RAEDAWN
REEARNS
REEBOKS
REEDIER
REEDING
REEDITS
REEDMAN
REEDMEN
REEFERS
REEFIER
REEFING
REEJECT
REEKERS
REEKIER
REEKING
REEKSOF
REELECT
REELERS
REELING
REELOFF
REELOUT
REELSIN
REELSUP
REEMITS
REENACT
REENDOW
REENJOY
REENTER
REENTRY
REEQUIP
REERECT
REERUPT
REEVICT
REEVING
REEVOKE
REEXPEL
RHEBOKS
RHENISH
RHENIUM
RHETORS
RHEUMIC
RIEGERT
RIEMANN
RIESENS
RIESMAN
RIESSEN
ROEBUCK
ROEDEER
ROETHKE
RYEBEER
RYELOAF

R••E•••

RACECAR
RACEDBY
RACEDIN
RACEDTO
RACEDUP
RACEMES
RACESBY
RACESTO
RACESUP
RACEWAY
RAGEFUL
RAKEDIN
RAKEDUP
RAKEOFF
RAKESIN
RAKESUP
RALEIGH
RAMEKIN
RAMESES
RAREBIT
RAREGAS
RATECAP
RATEDPG
RAVELED
RAVELLY
RAVELOE
RAVENAL
RAVENED
RAVENNA
RAVEUPS
RAWEGGS
REBECCA
REBEGAN
REBEGIN
REBEGUN
REBEKAH
REBENDS
RECEDED
RECEDES
RECEIPT
RECEIVE
RECENCY
REDEALS
REDEALT
REDEBIT
REDECAY
REDEEDS
REDEEMS
REDEYED
REDEYES
REFEEDS
REFENCE
REFEREE
REFERTO
REGEARS
REGENCY
REGENTS
REHEALS
REHEARD
REHEARS
REHEATS
REHEELS
REJECTS
REKEYED
RELEADS
RELEAPS
RELEARN
RELEASE
RELENDS
RELENTS
RELEVEL
RELEVER
RELEVES
REMEETS
REMELTS
REMENDS
REMERGE
RENEGED
RENEGER
RENEGES
RENESTS
RENEWAL
RENEWED
RENEWER
REPEALS
REPEATS
REPENTS
REPERKS
REREADS
REREDOS
REREELS
RERENTS
RESEALS
RESEAMS
RESEATS
RESEAUS
RESEAUX
RESECTS
RESEEDS
RESEEKS
RESEIZE
RESELLS
RESENDS
RESENTS
RESERVE
RESEWED
RETEACH
RETEARS
RETELLS
RETESTS
REVEALS
REVELED
REVELER
REVELIN
REVELRY
REVENDS
REVENGE
REVENUE
REVERBS
REVERDY
REVERED
REVERER
REVERES
REVERIE
REVERSA
REVERSE
REVERTS
REVESTS
REWEARS
REWEAVE
REWEIGH
REWELDS
REZEROS
RHOECUS
RIBEYES
RIDEBYS
RIDEOFF
RIDEOUT
RIDESBY
RIDESIN
RIDESTO
RIDESUP
RILEDUP
RILESUP
RIPENED
RIPENER
RISENTO
RISESTO
RISESUP
RITEAID
RIVERPO
RIVETED
RIVETER
ROBERTA
ROBERTE
ROBERTF
ROBERTH
ROBERTI
ROBERTO
ROBERTS
ROBESON
RODENTS
RODEOFF
RODEOUT
ROGERED
ROLEXES
RONETTE
ROPEDIN
ROPEDUP
ROPEOFF
ROPESIN
ROPESUP
ROPETOW
ROSEATE
ROSEBAY
ROSEBUD
ROSEHIP
ROSELLA
ROSELLE
ROSEOIL
ROSEOLA
ROSERED
ROSETEA
ROSETTA
ROSETTE
ROTELLE
ROVETTA
ROWELED
ROZELLE
RUBELLA
RUBEOLA
RULEDBY
RULEDON
RULEONE
RULEOUT
RULESON

R•••E••

RABBETS
RACIEST
RACKERS
RACKETS
RACKETY
RAFTERS
RAGGEDY
RAGWEED
RAIDERS
RAILERS
RAIMENT
RAISERS
RAISEUP
RAMJETS
RAMMERS
RAMSESI
RANDEEP
RANGERS
RANKERS
RANKEST
RANTERS
RAPIERS
RAPPELS
RAPPERS
RASHERS
RASHEST
RASPERS
RASTERS
RATBERT
RATTERS
RAWDEAL
RAWMEAT
RAWNESS
RAYLESS
RAYNELL
READERS
REAGENT
REALEST
REAMEND
REAMERS
REAPERS
REAREND
REARERS
REAVERS
REBREAK
REBREED
REBREWS
RECHECK
RECHEWS
RECLEAN
REDCELL
REDCENT
REDDEER
REDDENS
REDDEST
REDEEDS
REDEEMS
REDFERN
REDHEAD
REDHEAT
REDHENS
REDLEGS
REDMEAT
REDNECK
REDNESS
REDREAM
REDRESS
REEFERS
REEJECT
REEKERS
REELECT
REELERS
REERECT
REFEEDS
REFLECT
REFRESH
REFUELS
REGREET
REGRESS
REGRETS
REHEELS
REKNEAD
RELIEFS
RELIERS
RELIEVE
RELLENO
REMEETS
RENDELL
RENDERS
RENNETS
RENTEES
RENTERS
REOPENS
REPLEAD
REPLETE
REPRESS
REQUEST
REREELS
RESEEDS
RESEEKS
RESMELT
RESPEAK
RESPECT
RESPELL
RESPELT
RESTERS
RESWEAR
RESWEEP
RETREAD
RETREAT
REUBENS
REUNERS
REUSERS
REUTERS
REVIEWS
REXREED
RHYMERS
RIBBERS
RIBLESS
RIBLETS
RIBMEAT
RICHENS
RICHEST
RICKETY
RICKEYS
RIDDERS
RIEGERT
RIESENS
RIFLERS
RIFLERY
RIGGERS
RIGUEUR
RIGVEDA
RILIEVO
RILLETS
RIMIEST
RIMLESS
RINGERS
RINSERS
RIOTERS
RIPIENI
RIPIENO
RIPPERS
RISKERS
RIVIERA
RIVIERE
ROADEOS
ROADERS
ROAMERS
ROARERS
ROBBERS
ROBBERY
ROCHETS
ROCKERS
ROCKERY
ROCKETS
RODGERS
RODLESS
ROEDEER
ROGUERY
ROLFERS
ROLLEIS
ROLLERS
ROMBERG
ROMNEYS
ROMPERS
RONDEAU
RONDELS
ROOFERS
ROOKERY
ROOMERS
ROOTERS
ROPIEST
ROSIEST
ROSTERS
ROSWELL
ROTTERS
ROULEAU
ROUSERS
ROUTERS
ROYBEAN
RUBBERS
RUBBERY
RUCKERT
RUDDERS
RUINERS
RULIEST
RUMLESS
RUMMERS
RUMPEND
RUNDEEP
RUNLESS
RUNLETS
RUNNELS
RUNNERS
RUNNETH
RUSHEES
RUSHERS
RUSSELL
RUSSERT
RUSSETS
RUSSETY
RUTGERS
RUTTERS
RYEBEER

R••••E•

RABBLED
RABBLES
RACEMES
RACHAEL
RACQUET
RADAMES
RADICES
RADIOED
RADIOER
RADIXES
RADOMES
RAFFLED
RAFFLER
RAFFLES
RAGGIER
RAGGIES
RAGWEED
RAILMEN
RAINIER
RALLIED
RALLIER
RALLIES
RALLYES
RAMBLED
RAMBLER
RAMBLES
RAMESES
RAMIREZ
RAMONES
RANCHED
RANCHER
RANCHES
RANDEEP
RANDIER
RANFREE
RANGIER
RANKLED
RANKLES
RANOVER
RAPHAEL
RAPIDER
RAPINES
RASPIER
RASSLED
RASSLER
RASSLES
RASURES
RATCHET
RATINES
RATITES
RATTIER
RATTLED
RATTLER
RATTLES
RAVAGED
RAVAGER
RAVAGES
RAVELED
RAVENED
RAVINED
RAVINES
RAZORED
RAZZIES
REACHED
REACHER
REACHES
REACTED
READDED
READIED
READIER
READIES
REAIMED
REAIRED
REALMEN
REALTER
REANNEX
REARMED
REASKED
REBAKED
REBAKES
REBALED
REBALES
REBATED
REBATER
REBATES
REBORED
REBORES
REBOTES
REBOXED
REBOXES
REBREED
REBUKED
REBUKER
REBUKES
REBUSES
RECAGED
RECAGES
RECANED
RECANES
RECASED
RECASES
RECEDED
RECEDES
RECIPES
RECITED
RECITER
RECITES
RECODED
RECODES
RECOVER
RECURED
RECURES
RECUSED
RECUSES
REDARED
REDARES
REDATED
REDATES
REDDEER
REDDYES
REDEYED
REDEYES
REDOSED
REDOSES
REDOXES
REDRIED
REDRIES
REDTIES
REDUCED
REDUCER
REDUCES
REEDIER
REEDMEN
REEFIER
REEKIER
REENTER
REEXPEL
REFACED
REFACES
REFAXED
REFAXES
REFEREE
REFILED
REFILES
REFINED
REFINER
REFINES
REFIRED
REFIRES
REFIXED
REFIXES
REFLIES
REFRIED
REFRIES
REFUGED
REFUGEE
REFUGES
REFUSED
REFUSER
REFUSES
REFUTED
REFUTER
REFUTES
REGALED
REGALER
REGALES
REGIMEN
REGIMES
REGIVEN
REGIVES
REGLUED
REGLUES
REGNIER
REGREET
REHIDES
REHIRED
REHIRES
REHONED
REHONES
REIFIED
REIFIES
REIGNED
REINDEX
REINKED
REKEYED
RELABEL
RELACED
RELACES
RELANES
RELATED
RELATER
RELATES
RELAXED
RELAXER
RELAXES
RELAYED
RELAYER
RELEVEL
RELEVER
RELEVES
RELINED
RELINES
RELIVED
RELIVES
RELOSES
RELUMED
RELUMES
REMAKES
REMATED
REMATES
REMINED
REMINES
REMISED
REMISES
REMIXED
REMIXES
REMODEL
REMOTER
REMOTES
REMOVED
REMOVER
REMOVES
REMOWED
RENAMED
RENAMES
RENEGED
RENEGER
RENEGES
RENEWED
RENEWER
RENFREW
RENOTED
RENOTES
RENTEES
RENTIER
REOFFER
REOILED
REORDER
REOWNED
REPAGED
REPAGES
REPANEL
REPAPER
REPAVED
REPAVES
REPINED
REPINER
REPINES
REPLIED
REPLIER
REPLIES
REPOSED
REPOSER
REPOSES
REPOWER
REPUTED
REPUTES
REQUIEM
RERAKED
RERAKES
RERATED
RERATES
RERIDES
RERISEN
RERISES
RESALES
RESAVED
RESAVES
RESAWED
RESCUED
RESCUER
RESCUES
RESEWED
RESHOES
RESIDED
RESIDER
RESIDES
RESILED
RESILES
RESINED
RESITED
RESIZED
RESIZER
RESIZES
RESOJET
RESOLED
RESOLER
RESOLES
RESOWED
RESTREW
RESUMED
RESUMES
RESWEEP
RETAKEN
RETAKER
RETAKES
RETAMED
RETAMES
RETAPED
RETAPES
RETAXED
RETAXES
RETILED
RETILES
RETIMED
RETIMES
RETIRED
RETIREE
RETIRES
RETONED
RETONES
RETOWED
RETRIED
RETRIES
RETUNED
RETUNES
RETYPED
RETYPES
REUPPED
REURGED
REURGES
REUTHER
REUTTER
REVELED
REVELER
REVERED
REVERER
REVERES
REVILED
REVILER
REVILES
REVISED
REVISER
REVISES
REVIVED
REVIVER
REVIVES
REVOKED
REVOKER
REVOKES
REVOTED
REVOTES
REWAGER
REWAKED
REWAKEN
REWAKES
REWATER
REWAXED
REWAXES
REWIDEN
REWIPED
REWIPES
REWIRED
REWIRES
REWOKEN
REWOVEN
REXREED
REYOKED
REYOKES
REZONED
REZONES
RIBBIER
RIBBIES
RIBEYES
RICHLER
RICHMEN
RICHTER
RICKLES
RIDDLED
RIDDLER
RIDDLES
RIDGIER
RIESSEN
RIFFLED
RIFFLER
RIFFLES
RIGHTED
RIGHTER
RIMPLED
RIMPLES
RINDIER
RINGLET
RIPENED
RIPENER
RIPOPEN
RIPPLED
RIPPLES
RIPPLET
RISKIER
RITDYES
RITZIER
RIVALED
RIVETED
RIVETER
RIVULET
ROACHES
ROADBED
ROADIES
ROASTED
ROASTER
ROBBNEN
ROCKIER
ROCKIES
ROEDEER
ROGERED
ROILIER
ROISTER
ROLEXES
ROLODEX
RONTGEN
ROOKIER
ROOKIES
ROOMIER
ROOMIES
ROOSTED
ROOSTER
ROOTIER
ROOTLED
ROOTLES
ROOTLET
ROSCOES
ROSERED

ROSETEA
ROSINED
ROSSNER
ROSSSEA
ROTATED
ROTATES
ROTIFER
ROUGHED
ROUGHEN
ROUGHER
ROUNDED
ROUNDEL
ROUNDER
ROUSTED
ROUSTER
ROWDIER
ROWDIES
ROWELED
ROYALES
RUBBLES
RUBYDEE
RUBYRED
RUDDIED
RUDDIER
RUFFLED
RUFFLER
RUFFLES
RUGGLES
RUMBAED
RUMBLED
RUMBLER
RUMBLES
RUMMIES
RUMORED
RUMPLED
RUMPLES
RUNDEEP
RUNDLES
RUNFREE
RUNNIER
RUNOVER
RUNTIER
RUSHEES
RUSHIER
RUSTIER
RUSTLED
RUSTLER
RUSTLES
RUTALEE
RUTILES
RUTTIER
RVALUES
RYEBEER

R•••••E

RADIATE
RADICLE
RAGTIME
RAILAGE
RAKABLE
RALPHIE
RAMHOME
RAMLIKE
RAMPAGE
RANFREE
RANHOME
RANKINE
RANLATE
RAPTUNE
RAPTURE
RATABLE
RATHOLE
RATLIKE
RATLINE
RATRACE
RAVELOE
RAWHIDE
RAYLIKE
RCADOME
REALINE
REALISE
REALIZE
REARGUE
REARISE
REAROSE
REAWAKE
REAWOKE
REBASTE
REBATHE
REBRACE
REBROKE
RECABLE
RECARVE
RECEIVE
RECHOSE
RECLAME
RECLINE
RECLUSE
RECRATE
RECURVE
RECYCLE
REDBONE
REDFACE
REDFIVE
REDLINE
REDNINE
REDNOSE
REDPINE
REDRIVE
REDROBE
REDROSE
REDTAPE
REDTIDE
REDWINE
REDZONE
REEVOKE
REFENCE
REFEREE
REFLATE
REFORGE
REFRAME
REFUGEE
REGAUGE
REGLAZE
REGRADE
REGUIDE
REHINGE
REHOUSE
REIMAGE
REISSUE
REJOICE
REJUDGE
RELANCE
RELAPSE
RELEASE
RELIEVE
REMERGE
REMORSE
REPASTE
REPHASE
REPHONE
REPLACE
REPLANE
REPLATE
REPLETE
REPLUME
REPRICE
REPRIME
REPRISE
REPROBE
REPROVE
REPRUNE
REPTILE
REPULSE
REQUIRE
REQUITE
REQUOTE
RERAISE
RERINSE
REROUTE
RESCALE
RESCORE
RESEIZE
RESERVE
RESHAPE
RESHARE
RESHAVE
RESHINE
RESIDUE
RESLATE
RESOLVE
RESPACE
RESPADE
RESPICE
RESPIRE
RESPITE
RESPOKE
RESTAGE
RESTATE
RESTIVE
RESTOKE
RESTORE
RESTYLE
RESURGE
RESWORE
RETABLE
RETASTE
RETICLE
RETINAE
RETINGE
RETINUE
RETIREE
RETITLE
RETRACE
RETRADE
RETWINE
REUNITE
REVALUE
REVENGE
REVENUE
REVERIE
REVERSE
REVOICE
REVOLVE
REWEAVE
REWRITE
REWROTE
RHIZOME
RIBCAGE
RIBLIKE
RIDABLE
RIPOSTE
RIPSONE
RIPTIDE
RISIBLE
RISSOLE
RITAMAE
RITCHIE
RIVIERE
RLSTINE
ROANOKE
ROBERTE
ROBLOWE
RODLIKE
ROETHKE
ROGAINE
ROMAINE
ROMANCE
RONDURE
RONETTE
ROOFAGE
ROOTAGE
ROSALIE
ROSANNE
ROSEATE
ROSELLE
ROSETTE
ROTELLE
ROULADE
ROUTINE
ROXANNE
ROYALWE
ROZELLE
RUBYDEE
RUGLIKE
RUINATE
RULEONE
RUMCAKE
RUMMAGE
RUMPOLE
RUNFREE
RUNHOME
RUNLATE
RUNTIME
RUPTURE
RUSHDIE
RUTALEE

•RE••••

AREAMAP
AREARUG
AREAWAY
ARECIBO
ARENOSE
ARENSKY
AREOLAE
AREOLAR
AREOLAS
AREOLES
ARETINO
BREADED
BREADER
BREADTH
BREAKER
BREAKIN
BREAKUP
BREASTS
BREATHE
BREATHS
BREATHY
BREEDER
BREEZED
BREEZES
BRENDAN
BRENDEL
BRENDON
BRENGUN
BRENNAN
BRENNER
BRERFOX
BRESCIA
BRESLIN
BRETONS
BRETTON
BREVETS
BREVITY
BREWAGE
BREWERS
BREWERY
BREWING
BREWPUB
BREWSKI
BREWSUP
BREYERS
CREAKED
CREAMED
CREAMER
CREASED
CREASER
CREASES
CREATED
CREATES
CREATOR
CRECHES
CREDITS
CREEDAL
CREELEY
CREEPBY
CREEPED
CREEPER
CREEPIN
CREEPOS
CREEPUP
CREMATE
CREMINI
CREMONA
CREMORA
CRENATE
CRENELS
CREOLES
CREOSOL
CREPING
CREPTIN
CREPTUP
CRESPIN
CRESSES
CRESSET
CRESTED
CRESTON
CRETANS
CRETINS
CREVICE
CREWCUT
CREWELS
CREWING
CREWMAN
CREWMEN
DREADED
DREAMED
DREAMER
DREAMIN
DREAMOF
DREAMON
DREAMUP
DREDGED
DREDGER
DREDGES
DREGION
DREIDEL
DREISER
DRESDEN
DRESSAS
DRESSED
DRESSER
DRESSES
DRESSIN
DRESSUP
DREWOFF
DREWOUT
DREXELU
DREXLER
DREYFUS
ERECTED
ERECTER
ERECTLY
ERECTOR
ERECTUS
ERELONG
EREMITE
EREWHON
FREAKED
FREBERG
FRECKLE
FRECKLY
FREDDIE
FREDEBB
FREDRIC
FREEAIR
FREEBEE
FREEBLE
FREEDOF
FREEDOM
FREEDUP
FREEING
FREEMAN
FREEMEN
FREESIA
FREESOF
FREESUP
FREETOY
FREEWAY
FREEZER
FREEZES
FREIGHT
FREITAG
FRELENG
FREMONT
FRENCHI
FRENCHS
FRENEAU
FRENEMY
FRENESI
FRESCAS
FRESCOS
FRESHED
FRESHEN
FRESHER
FRESHES
FRESHET
FRESHLY
FRESNEL
FRESSED
FRESSES
FRETFUL
FRETSAT
FRETSAW
FRETTED
FRETTER
FREYTAG
GREASED
GREASER
GREASES
GREATEN
GREATER
GREATLY
GREAVES
GRECIAN
GRECISM
GRECIZE
GREELEY
GREENED
GREENER
GREENLY
GREETED
GREETER
GREGORY
GREMLIN
GRENADA
GRENADE
GRENDEL
GRESHAM
GRETZKY
GREWBIG
GREWDIM
GREWFAT
GREWOLD
GREYCUP
GREYEST
GREYHEN
GREYING
GREYISH
GREYLAG
HRETHEL
IRECKON
IREFUSE
IRELAND
IRELESS
IRENICS
IREPEAT
IRESIGN
JREWING
KREMLIN
KRESKIN
OREBODY
ORECTIC
OREGANO
OREILLY
ORELESS
ORESTES
PREACHY
PREACID
PREACTS
PREAGED
PREAGES
PREALLY
PREAMPS
PREARMS
PREAVER
PREBADE
PREBAKE
PREBIDS
PREBILL
PREBIND
PREBOIL
PREBOOK
PREBOOM
PREBORN
PREBURN
PREBUYS
PRECAST
PRECEDE
PRECEPT
PRECISE
PRECITE
PRECODE
PRECOIL
PRECOOK
PRECOOL
PRECOUP
PRECURE
PRECUTS
PREDARK
PREDATA
PREDATE
PREDAWN
PREDEFY
PREDENY
PREDICT
PREDIET
PREDIVE
PREDOOM
PREDUSK
PREEDIT
PREEMIE
PREEMPT
PREENED
PREENER
PREFABS
PREFACE
PREFADE
PREFECT
PREFERS
PREFILE
PREFORM
PREFUND
PREGAIN
PREGAME
PREHEAL
PREHEAT
PREIDEA
PRELACY
PRELATE
PRELIFE
PRELIMS
PRELOAD
PRELOAN
PRELOSS
PRELUDE
PREMADE
PREMAKE
PREMATE
PREMEDS
PREMEET
PREMIER
PREMIES
PREMISE
PREMISS
PREMIUM
PRENAME
PRENOON
PRENUPS
PREOMIT
PREOPEN
PREORAL
PREPACK
PREPAID
PREPARE
PREPAVE
PREPAYS
PREPLAN
PREPLOT
PREPPED
PREPPIE
PREPUPA
PREQUEL
PRERACE
PRERENT
PRERIOT
PREROCK
PRESAGE
PRESALE
PRESALT
PRESEAL
PRESEAT
PRESELL
PRESENT
PRESETS
PRESHIP
PRESHOW
PRESIDE
PRESIFT
PRESLEY
PRESOAK
PRESOLD
PRESONG
PRESORT
PRESPUR
PRESQUE
PRESSED
PRESSEL
PRESSER
PRESSES
PRESSON
PRESSUP
PRESTON
PRESTOS
PRESUME
PRETAPE
PRETEEN
PRETELL
PRETEND
PRETERM
PRETEST
PRETEXT
PRETIRE
PRETOLD
PRETORS
PRETRIM
PRETYPE
PRETZEL
PREVAIL
PREVENT
PREVERB
PREVERT
PREVETO
PREVIAS
PREVIEW
PREVOID
PREVOST
PREVUED
PREVUES
PREWARM
PREWARN
PREWASH
PREWHIP
PREWIRE
PREWITT
PREWORK
PREWORN
PREWRAP
PREXIES
PREYERS
PREYING
PREYSON
TREACLE
TREACLY
TREADED
TREADER
TREADLE
TREADON
TREASON
TREATED
TREATER
TREBLED
TREBLES
TREDIAS
TREEING
TREELET
TREERAT
TREESAP
TREETOP
TREFOIL
TREINTA
TREIZES
TREKKED
TREKKER
TREKKIE
TRELLIS
TREMBLE
TREMBLY
TREMOLO
TREMORS
TRENARY
TRENDED
TRENTON
TREPANS
TRESSED
TRESSES
TRESTLE
TREVINO
WREAKED
WREAKER
WREATHE
WREATHS
WREATHY
WRECKED
WRECKER
WRESTED
WRESTER
WRESTLE

•R•E•••

ARDECHE
ARDENCY
ARGENTI
ARGENTO
ARGENTS
ARIETTA
ARIETTE
ARLEDGE
ARMENIA
ARREARS
ARRESTS
ARSENAL
ARSENIC
ARSENIO
ARTEMIS
ARTEMUS
ARTERIO
BRAEDEN
BREEDER
BREEZED
BREEZES
BRIEFED
BRIEFER
BRIEFLY
BRUEGEL
CREEDAL
CREELEY
CREEPBY
CREEPED
CREEPER
CREEPIN
CREEPOS
CREEPUP
CRIEDUP
CRIESUP
CROESUS
CRUELER
CRUELLA
CRUELLY
CRUELTY
DRIEDUP
DRIESCH
DRIESUP
DRMELFI
DRSEUSS
DRTEETH
DRVEGAS
DRWELBY
DRYEYED
DRYEYES
ERNESTA
ERNESTO
ERTEGUN
FREEAIR
FREEBEE
FREEBIE
FREEDOF
FREEDOM
FREEDUP
FREEING
FREEMAN
FREEMEN
FREESIA
FREESOF
FREESUP
FREETOY
FREEWAY
FREEZER
FREEZES
FRIEDAN
FRIEDUP
FRIENDS
FRIESUP
FRIEZES
FROEBEL
GREELEY
GREENED
GREENER
GREENLY
GREETED
GREETER
GRIEVED
GRIEVER
GRIEVES
KROEMER
KRUEGER
MRDEEDS
ORDEALS
ORDERED
ORDERER
ORDERIN
ORDERLY
ORDERUP
ORGEATS
ORIENTE
ORIENTS
ORLEANS
ORNETTE
ORTEGAL
PRAETOR
PREEDIT
PREEMIE
PREEMPT
PREENED
PREENER
PRIESTS
PROEAST
TREEING
TREELET
TREERAT
TREESAP
TREETOP
TRIEDIT
TRIEDON
TRIEDTO
TRIESIT
TRIESON
TRIESTE
TRIESTO
TRUEDUP
TRUEING
TRUERIB
TRUERTO
TRUESUP
URGEDON
URGENCY
URGESON
URTEXTS

•R••E••

ARAMEAN
ARANEID
ARCHERS
ARCHERY
ARCHEST
ARCWELD
ARGUERS
ARIDEST
ARLBERG
ARMLESS
ARMLETS
ARMREST
ARRIERE
ARTDECO
ARTFERN
ARTIEST
ARTLESS
BRACERO
BRACERS
BRACEUP
BRALESS
BRAVELY
BRAVERY
BRAVEST
BRAYERS
BRAZENS
BREVETS
BREWERS
BREWERY
BREYERS
BRIBEES
BRIBERS
BRIBERY
BRINERS
BROKEIN
BROKERS
BROKEUP
BRUBECK
BRUNETS
BRUTELY
CRATERS
CRATEUP
CRAVENS
CRAVERS
CRENELS
CREWELS
CRIMEAN
CROWELL
CROWERS
CRUDELY
CRUDEST
DRAGEES
DRAMEDY
DRAPERS
DRAPERY
DRAWEES
DRAWERS
DREXELU
DRFREUD
DRIVEAT
DRIVEBY
DRIVEIN

DRIVELS
DRIVERS
DRIVETO
DRIVEUP
DRONEON
DRONERS
DROVEAT
DROVEBY
DROVEIN
DROVERS
DROVETO
DROVEUP
DRTEETH
DRUZEAN
DRYCELL
DRYHEAT
DRYNESS
DRYPERS
DRYWELL
ERASERS
ERIGENA
ERODENT
ERODERS
EROSELY
FRAMERS
FRAMEUP
FRATERS
FREBERG
FREDEBB
FRELENG
FRENEAU
FRENEMY
FRENESI
FRISEUR
FROZEUP
GRADEAA
GRADERS
GRAPERY
GRATEON
GRATERS
GRATEUP
GRAVELS
GRAVELY
GRAVERS
GRAVEST
GRAYEST
GRAZERS
GREYEST
GRIPERS
GROCERS
GROCERY
GROPERS
GROVELS
GROVERS
GROWERS
GRUYERE
IRATELY
IRATEST
IRELESS
IREPEAT
IRONERS
JROBERT
KRAKENS
MRCLEAN
MRDEEDS
MRGREEN
MRSPEEL
ORBLESS
ORELESS
ORKNEYS
OROGENY
ORPHEAN
ORPHEUM
ORPHEUS
ORVIETO
PRADESH
PRATERS
PRAYERS
PRECEDE
PRECEPT
PREDEFY
PREDENY
PREFECT
PREFERS
PREHEAL
PREHEAT
PREMEDS
PREMEET
PRERENT
PRESEAL
PRESEAT
PRESELL
PRESENT
PRESETS
PRETEEN
PRETELL
PRETEND
PRETERM
PRETEST
PRETEXT
PREVENT
PREVERB
PREVERT
PREVETO
PREYERS
PRICERS
PRIMELY
PRIMERA
PRIMERO
PRIMERS
PRIVETS
PROBERS
PROCEED
PROCESS
PROFESS
PROGENY
PROJECT
PROJETS
PROKEDS
PRONELY
PRONETO
PROPELS
PROSERS
PROTEAM
PROTEAN
PROTECT
PROTEGE
PROTEIN
PROTEST
PROTEUS
PROVEIT
PROVERB
PROVERS
PROWESS
PROWEST
PRUDENT
PRUDERY
PRUNERS
TRABERT
TRACERS
TRACERY
TRADEIN
TRADEON
TRADERS
TRADEUP
TRAGEDY
TRAPEZE
TRAVELS
TRAVERS
TRIBECA
TRICEPS
TRIDENT
TRIJETS
TRIREME
TRISECT
TRITELY
TRITEST
TRIVETS
TROWELS
TRUDEAU
WRITEIN
WRITEME
WRITEON
WRITERS
WRITETO
WRITEUP
WROTEIN
WROTEON
WROTETO
WROTEUP
WRYNESS

•R•••E

ARABLES
ARALSEA
ARBACES
ARBITER
ARBOLES
ARBORED
ARCADED
ARCADES
ARCHIES
ARCHSEE
AREOLES
ARGUSES
ARGYLES
ARIANES
ARMORED
ARMORER
AROUSED
AROUSER
AROUSES
ARRASES
ARRAYED
ARRAYER
ARRISES
ARRIVED
ARRIVER
ARRIVES
ARTSIER
ARUNDEL
ARUSPEX
BRACKEN
BRACKET
BRADLEE
BRADLEY
BRAEDEN
BRAGGED
BRAGGER
BRAIDED
BRAIDER
BRAINED
BRAINER
BRAISED
BRAISES
BRAMLEY
BRANDED
BRANDER
BRASHER
BRASHES
BRASIER
BRASSES
BRAVOED
BRAVOES
BRAWLED
BRAWLER
BRAWLEY
BRAZIER
BREADED
BREADER
BREAKER
BREEDER
BREEZED
BREEZES
BRENDEL
BRENNER
BRIBEES
BRICKED
BRIDGED
BRIDGER
BRIDGES
BRIDGET
BRIDLED
BRIDLER
BRIDLES
BRIEFED
BRIEFER
BRIMLEY
BRIMMED
BRIMMER
BRINGER
BRINIER
BRINKER
BRIQUET
BRISKED
BRISKER
BRISKET
BRITNEY
BRITTEN
BROADEN
BROADER
BRODIES
BRODKEY
BROGUES
BROIDER
BROILED
BROILER
BRONTES
BRONWEN
BRONZED
BRONZER
BRONZES
BROODED
BROODER
BROOKED
BROOMED
BROSSES
BROTHER
BROWNED
BROWNER
BROWSED
BROWSER
BROWSES
BRUEGEL
BRUISED
BRUISER
BRUISES
BRUITED
BRUMMEL
BRUSHED
BRUSHER
BRUSHES
BRYNNER
CRABBED
CRABBER
CRACKED
CRACKER
CRADLED
CRADLER
CRADLES
CRAFTED
CRAFTER
CRAGGED
CRAMMED
CRAMMER
CRAMPED
CRANKED
CRANMER
CRASHED
CRASHER
CRASHES
CRASSER
CRAWLED
CRAWLER
CRAWLEY
CRAZIER
CRAZIES
CREAKED
CREAMED
CREAMER
CREASED
CREASER
CREASES
CREATED
CREATES
CRECHES
CREELEY
CREEPED
CREEPER
CREOLES
CRESSES
CRESSET
CRESTED
CREWMEN
CRIBBED
CRIBBER
CRICKED
CRICKET
CRIMPED
CRIMPER
CRINGED
CRINGES
CRISPED
CRISPEN
CRISPER
CRITTER
CROAKED
CROAKER
CROCHET
CROCKED
CROCKER
CROCKET
CROFTER
CRONIES
CROOKED
CROOKES
CROONED
CROONER
CROPPED
CROPPER
CROQUET
CROSIER
CROSSED
CROSSER
CROSSES
CROUTES
CROWDED
CROWDER
CROWLEY
CROWNED
CROWNER
CROZIER
CRUELER
CRUGUET
CRUISED
CRUISER
CRUISES
CRULLER
CRUMBED
CRUMPED
CRUMPET
CRUPPER
CRUSHED
CRUSHER
CRUSHES
CRUSTED
CRUTZEN
CRYOGEN
CRYOVER
DRABBER
DRAFTED
DRAFTEE
DRAFTER
DRAGEES
DRAGGED
DRAGGER
DRAGNET
DRAINED
DRAINER
DRATTED
DRAWEES
DRAWLED
DRAWLER
DRAWMEN
DRAYMEN
DREADED
DREAMED
DREAMER
DREDGED
DREDGER
DREDGES
DREIDEL
DREISER
DRESDEN
DRESSED
DRESSER
DRESSES
DREXLER
DRIBLET
DRIFTED
DRIFTER
DRILLED
DRILLER
DRINKER
DRIPPED
DRIPPER
DROGUES
DROLLER
DROOLED
DROOLER
DROOPED
DROPLET
DROPNET
DROPPED
DROPPER
DROSSES
DROWNED
DROWSED
DROWSES
DROXIES
DRUBBED
DRUBBER
DRUCKER
DRUDGED
DRUDGER
DRUDGES
DRUGGED
DRUMMED
DRUMMER
DRUMSET
DRUNKEN
DRUNKER
DRYADES
DRYEYED
DRYEYES
DRYIDEA
ERECTED
ERECTER
ERINYES
ERITREA
ERMINED
ERMINES
ERUCTED
ERUPTED
ERUPTER
FRAGGED
FRAILER
FRAISES
FRANCES
FRANKED
FRANKEN
FRANKER
FRAPPES
FRASIER
FRAWLEY
FRAZIER
FREAKED
FREEBEE
FREEMEN
FREEZER
FREEZES
FRESHED
FRESHEN
FRESHER
FRESHES
FRESHET
FRESNEL
FRESSED
FRESSES
FRETTED
FRETTER
FRICKER
FRIDGES
FRIDLEY
FRIEZES
FRILLED
FRINGED
FRINGES
FRISBEE
FRISKED
FRISKER
FRITTED
FRITTER
FRIZZED
FRIZZER
FRIZZES
FROCKED
FROEBEL
FROGGER
FROGLEG
FROGLET
FROGMEN
FROMMER
FRONTED
FROSTED
FROSTER
FROTHED
FROTHER
FROWNED
FROWNER
FRUITED
GRABBED
GRABBER
GRAFTED
GRAFTER
GRAINED
GRAINER
GRAMMER
GRAMMES
GRANDEE
GRANDER
GRANGER
GRANGES
GRANTED
GRANTEE
GRANTER
GRAPHED
GRAPIER
GRAPNEL
GRASPED
GRASPER
GRASSED
GRASSES
GRAVIES
GRAZIER
GREASED
GREASER
GREASES
GREATEN
GREATER
GREAVES
GREELEY
GREENED
GREENER
GREETED
GREETER
GRENDEL
GREYHEN
GRIDDED
GRIDDER
GRIEVED
GRIEVER
GRIEVES
GRIFFEY
GRIFTED
GRIFTER
GRILLED
GRILLER
GRILLES
GRIMIER
GRIMMER
GRINDER
GRINNED
GRINNER
GRIPPED
GRIPPER
GRIPPES
GRISLET
GRISNEZ
GRISTER
GRITTED
GRITTER
GROANED
GROANER
GRODIER
GROINED
GROKKED
GROLIER
GROMMET
GROOMED
GROOMER
GROOVED
GROOVES
GROSSED
GROSSER
GROSSES
GROUPED
GROUPER
GROUSED
GROUSER
GROUSES
GROUTED
GROUTER
GROWLED
GROWLER
GRUBBED
GRUBBER
GRUDGED
GRUDGER
GRUDGES
GRUFFER
GRUMPED
GRUNGER
GRUNGES
GRUNTED
GRUNTER
HRETHEL
IRISHER
IRONIES
IRONMEN
KRACKEL
KRAMDEN
KRASNER
KROEMER
KRUEGER
MRBONES
MRGREEN
MRHANEY
MRJONES
MRSPEEL
MRTIGER
ORACIES
ORACLES
ORANGES
ORANGEY
ORANTES
ORBITED
ORBITER
ORDERED
ORDERER
ORDINES
ORDONEZ
ORESTES
ORIOLES
ORRISES
PRAISED
PRAISER
PRAISES
PRANCED
PRANCER
PRANCES
PRAWNED
PREAGED
PREAGES
PREAVER
PREDIET
PREENED
PREENER
PREIDEA
PREMEET
PREMIER
PREMIES
PREOPEN
PREPPED
PREQUEL
PRESLEY
PRESSED
PRESSEL
PRESSER
PRESSES
PRETEEN
PRETZEL
PREVIEW
PREVUED
PREVUES
PREXIES
PRICIER
PRICKED
PRIMMED
PRIMMER
PRIMPED
PRINCES
PRINKED
PRINKER
PRINTED
PRINTER
PRISSES
PRITHEE
PRIUSES
PRIVIER
PRIVIES
PROBIES
PROBLEM
PROCEED
PROCTER
PRODDED
PRODDER
PROFFER
PROMOED
PRONGED
PROOFED
PROOFER
PROPHET
PROPJET
PROPMEN
PROPPED
PROSIER
PROSPER
PROUDER
PROWLED
PROWLER
PROXIES
PRYOPEN
TRACHEA
TRACKED
TRACKER
TRAILED
TRAILER
TRAINED
TRAINEE
TRAINER
TRAMMED
TRAMMEL
TRAMPED
TRAMPER
TRANCED
TRANCES
TRAPPED
TRAPPER
TRASHED
TRASHER
TRASHES
TRAUBEL
TRAWLED
TRAWLER
TREADED
TREADER
TREATED
TREATER
TREBLED
TREBLES
TREELET
TREIZES
TREKKED
TREKKER
TRENDED
TRESSED
TRESSES
TRIAGES
TRICKED
TRICKER
TRIFLED
TRIFLER
TRIFLES
TRIGGER
TRILLED
TRILLER
TRIMMED
TRIMMER
TRINKET
TRIODES
TRIOLET
TRIPLEA
TRIPLED
TRIPLES
TRIPLET
TRIPLEX
TRIPPED
TRIPPER
TRIPPET
TROCHEE
TROCHES
TRODDEN
TROLLED
TROLLER
TROLLEY
TROMPED
TROOPED
TROOPER
TROTHED
TROTTED
TROTTER
TROUPED
TROUPER
TROUPES
TROUSER
TRUCKED
TRUCKEE
TRUCKER
TRUDGED
TRUDGEN
TRUDGER
TRUDGES
TRUMPED
TRUMPET
TRUSSED
TRUSSES
TRUSTED
TRUSTEE
TRUSTER
TRYSTED
TRYSTER
URBANER
VROOMED
WRACKED
WRANGEL
WRAPPED
WRAPPER
WRASSES
WREAKED
WREAKER
WRECKED
WRECKER
WRESTED
WRESTER
WRIGLEY
WRINGER
WRITHED
WRITHER
WRITHES
WRITTEN
WRONGED
WRONGER

•R••••E

ARACHNE
ARCHFOE
ARCHIVE
ARCHSEE
ARCSINE
ARCUATE
ARDECHE
ARDMORE
ARENOSE
AREOLAE
ARGANTE
ARGONNE
ARIADNE
ARIETTE
ARISTAE
ARLEDGE
ARMBONE
ARMHOLE
ARMLIKE
ARMOIRE
ARRANGE
ARRIERE
ARSHILE
ARTICLE
ARTISTE
ARTSALE
ARTWARE
BRADLEE
BRAILLE
BRAMBLE
BRASIZE
BRASSIE
BRATTLE
BREATHE
BREWAGE
BRICKLE
BRIGADE
BRINDLE
BRIOCHE
BRISTLE
BRITTLE
BROCADE
BROMATE
BROMIDE
BROMINE
BROWNIE
BRUSQUE
CRACKLE
CRAIGIE
CRAPPIE
CREMATE
CRENATE
CREVICE
CRINKLE
CRIPPLE
CRUMBLE
CRUMPLE
CRUSADE
DRABBLE

DRAFTEE
DRAGGLE
DRAYAGE
DRIBBLE
DRINKME
DRIZZLE
DRYABLE
DRYHOLE
ERASURE
EREMITE
EROSIVE
ERRABLE
ERSKINE
ERUDITE
FRAGGLE
FRAGILE
FRAICHE
FRANKIE
FRAZZLE
FRECKLE
FREDDIE
FREEBEE
FREEBIE
FRIABLE
FRIBBLE
FRIGATE
FRIJOLE
FRISBEE
FRIZZLE
FROMAGE
FROOGLE
FROZONE
FRYABLE
GRACILE
GRACKLE
GRADATE
GRAHAME
GRANDEE
GRANITE
GRANNIE
GRANTEE
GRANULE
GRAPPLE
GRASSLE
GRAVURE
GRECIZE
GRENADE
GRIDDLE
GRIMACE
GRISTLE
GRIZZLE
GROUPIE
GRUMBLE
GRUYERE
IREFUSE
IRKSOME
IRONAGE
IRONORE
KRINGLE
KRYSTLE
MRHORSE
MRMOOSE
MRPADRE
MRSLATE
ORBLIKE
ORIENTE
ORIFICE
ORIGINE
ORNETTE
OROURKE
ORVILLE
PRAIRIE
PRALINE
PRATTLE
PREBADE
PREBAKE
PRECEDE
PRECISE
PRECITE
PRECODE
PRECURE
PREDATE
PREDIVE
PREEMIE
PREFACE
PREFADE
PREFILE
PREGAME
PRELATE
PRELIFE
PRELUDE
PREMADE
PREMAKE
PREMATE
PREMISE
PRENAME
PREPARE
PREPAVE
PREPPIE
PRERACE
PRESAGE
PRESALE
PRESIDE
PRESQUE
PRESUME
PRETAPE
PRETIRE
PRETYPE
PREWIRE
PRICKLE
PRIMATE
PRINGLE
PRITHEE
PRIVATE
PROBATE
PROCURE
PRODUCE
PROFANE
PROFILE
PROFUSE
PROLATE
PROLIFE
PROMISE
PROMOTE
PRONATE
PROPANE
PROPONE
PROPOSE
PRORATE
PROTEGE
PROVIDE
PROVINE
PROVOKE
PRUDHOE
TRADUCE
TRAINEE
TRAIPSE
TRAMPLE
TRAPEZE
TREACLE
TREADLE
TREKKIE
TREMBLE
TRESTLE
TRIABLE
TRIBBLE
TRIBUNE
TRIBUTE
TRICKLE
TRIESTE
TRIREME
TRITONE
TROCHEE
TROUBLE
TROUNCE
TRUCKEE
TRUCKLE
TRUFFLE
TRUNDLE
TRUSTEE
TRUSTME
URANITE
URNLIKE
WRANGLE
WREATHE
WRESTLE
WRIGGLE
WRINKLE
WRITEME

••RE•••

ABREAST
ACREAGE
ADRENAL
AGREEON
AGREERS
AGREETO
AIREDUP
ALREADY
AMREETA
ARREARS
ARRESTS
AUREATE
AUREOLA
AUREOLE
BAREGES
BARENTS
BARETTA
BAREXAM
BEREAVE
BERENDT
BERETTA
BIREMES
BIRETTA
BOREDOM
BOREOUT
BUREAUS
BUREAUX
BURETTE
CAREDTO
CAREENS
CAREERS
CAREFOR
CAREFUL
CARESTO
CEREALS
CEREBRA
CEREBRO
CORELLI
CORETTA
CUREALL
CURETTE
DAREFUL
DARENOT
DARESAY
DARESTO
DAREZZO
DERECHO
DIRECTS
DIRECTV
DIREFUL
EUREKAS
FAREAST
FAREBOX
FAREWAR
FIREANT
FIREARM
FIREBOX
FIREBUG
FIREDAT
FIREDOG
FIREDON
FIREDUP
FIREFLY
FIREFOX
FIREHAT
FIREICE
FIRELIT
FIREMAN
FIREMEN
FIRENZA
FIRENZE
FIREOFF
FIREPIT
FIRESAT
FIRESON
FIRESUP
FOREACH
FOREARM
FOREBAY
FOREIGN
FORELEG
FOREMAN
FOREMEN
FORENZA
FOREPAW
FORERAN
FORERUN
FORESAW
FORESEE
FORESTS
FORETOP
FOREVER
GERENTS
GORETEX
GYRENES
HEREDIA
HEREIAM
HERENOW
HERESTO
HERETIC
HIREDON
HIREOUT
HIRESON
IMREADY
INREACH
KOREANS
LAREDOS
LORELAI
LORELEI
LORENTZ
LORENZO
LORETTA
LUREDIN
LURESIN
LUREXES
MARENGO
MOREENS
MORELLA
MORELLO
MORELOS
MOREPAY
MORESBY
MORETTI
NEREIDS
NORELCO
NUREYEV
OGREISH
PARENTS
PERETTI
PHRENIC
PIRELLI
PYRETIC
PYREXIA
RAREBIT
RAREGAS
REREADS
REREDOS
REREELS
RERENTS
SCREAKS
SCREAMS
SCREECH
SCREEDS
SCREENS
SCREWED
SCREWUP
SERENER
SIRENED
SORENTO
SPREADS
STREAKS
STREAKY
STREAMS
STREETS
STREGIS
STRETCH
STRETTI
STRETTO
STREWED
STREWER
SUREBET
SURECAN
SUREIAM
SUREIDO
SUREROF
TERENCE
THREADS
THREADY
THREATS
THREEAD
THREEAM
THREEBC
THREEEE
THREENO
THREEPM
THREERS
THREEUP
THREWAT
THREWIN
THREWON
THREWUP
TIREDER
TIREDLY
TIREDOF
TIREMAN
TIREMEN
TIREOUT
TIRESOF
TOREOFF
TOREOUT
TOREROS
TUREENS
UNREADY
UNREELS
UNREGAL
UNRESTS
UPREACH
UPREARS
UTRECHT
VEREINE
WAREPIC
WIREDIN
WIREDUP
WIREMAN
WIREMEN
WIRESIN
WIRESUP
WIRETAP
WOREOFF
WOREOUT
YEREVAN

••R•E••

AERIEST
AGREEON
AGREERS
AGREETO
AIRHEAD
AIRIEST
AIRLESS
AIRNESS
AIRVENT
AMREETA
ARRIERE
BARBEAU
BARBELL
BARBERA
BARBERS
BARBETS
BARDEEN
BARGEIN
BARGERS
BARKEEP
BARKERS
BARLESS
BARLEYS
BARNEYS
BARRELS
BARRENS
BARRETS
BARRETT
BARTEND
BARTERS
BERBERS
BERGERE
BERNESE
BERSERK
BIRDERS
BIRLERS
BORDERS
BORNEAN
BORNEUP
BURDENS
BURGEES
BURGEON
BURGERS
BURGESS
BURIERS
BURLERS
BURMESE
BURNERS
BURNETT
CARDERS
CAREENS
CAREERS
CARKEYS
CARLENE
CARLESS
CARMELA
CARNERA
CARNETS
CARPELS
CARPERS
CARPETS
CARRELS
CARRERA
CARRERE
CARSEAT
CARTELS
CARTERS
CARVELS
CARVERS
CERVEZA
CORBELS
CORBETT
CORDELL
CORDERO
CORDERS
CORKERS
CORNEAL
CORNEAS
CORNELL
CORNERS
CORNETS
CORRECT
CORSETS
CORTEGE
CORVEES
CORYELL
CURFEWS
CURLERS
CURLEWS
CURRENT
CURSEAT
CURSERS
CURTEST
CURVETS
DARKENS
DARKEST
DARLEEN
DARLENE
DARNELL
DARNERS
DARTERS
DARWELL
DERWENT
DORMERS
DORSETT
DORSEYS
DURRELL
DURWENT
EARLESS
EARLETS
EARNERS
EARNEST
EERIEST
FARCEUR
FARFELS
FARLEFT
FARMERS
FARMERY
FARNESS
FAROESE
FARRELL
FARSEER
FARWEST
FERMENT
FERNERY
FERRETS
FERRETY
FERVENT
FIRMEST
FORBEAR
FORCEIN
FORCEON
FORCEPS
FORCERS
FORCEUP
FORFEIT
FORFEND
FORGERS
FORGERY
FORGETS
FORKERS
FORMERS
FORREAL
FORRENT
FORREST
FORWENT
FURLERS
FURLESS
FURNESS
FURSEAL
GARDENA
GARDENS
GARMENT
GARNEAU
GARNERS
GARNETS
GARNETT
GARRETS
GARRETT
GARTERS
GIRDERS
GORGERS
GORIEST
GURNEYS
HARDEES
HARDENS
HARDEST
HARKENS
HARLEYS
HARMERS
HARNESS
HARPERS
HARVEST
HARWELL
HERBERT
HERDERS
HERPETO
HERSELF
HORNETS
HURLERS
HURTERS
ISRAELI
JARLESS
JARRELL
JARRETT
JERGENS
JERKERS
JERSEYS
JURGENS
KERNELS
KERTESZ
KORDELL
KURRENT
LARCENY
LARDERS
LARGELY
LARGENT
LARGEOJ
LARGESS
LARGEST
LARKERS
LORIENT
LURKERS
LURLEEN
MARCEAU
MARCELS
MARGERY
MARKERS
MARKETS
MARLENE
MARRERS
MARTENS
MARVELL
MARVELS
MERCERS
MERCERY
MERGEES
MERGERS
MIRIEST
MORCERF
MORDENT
MOREENS
MORSELS
MURDERS
MURIELS
NORBERT
NORIEGA
NURSERS
NURSERY
OARLESS
OURSELF
PARCELS
PARGERS
PARKERS
PARLEYS
PARSECS
PARSEES
PARSERS
PARVENU
PERCENT
PERCEPT
PERFECT
PERREAU
PERSEID
PERSEUS
PERTEST
PERWEEK
PERYEAR
PIRAEUS
PORKERS
PORSENA
PORTEND
PORTENT
PORTERS
PURCELL
PURRERS
PURSERS
PURVEYS
REREELS
SARGENT
SCREECH
SCREEDS
SCREENS
SERIESE
SERIESF
SERIESG
SERIESH
SERIESI
SERIESJ
SERIESK
SERPENS
SERPENT
SERVEAS
SERVERS
SERVEUP
SHRIEKS
SORBETS
SORCERY
SORRELL
SORRELS
SORTERS
SPRIEST
SPRYEST
STREETS
SURFEIT
SURFERS
SURGEON
SURGERY
SURREAL
SURREYS
SURVEIL
SURVEYS
TARBELL
TARGETS
TARHEEL
TARTEST
TERCELS
TERRELL
TERRENE
TERRETS
TERSELY
TERSEST
THREEAD
THREEAM
THREEBC
THREEEE
THREENO
THREEPM
THREERS
THREEUP
TORMENT
TORPEDO
TORREFY
TORRENT
TUREENS
TURKEYS
TURNERS
TURNERY
TURRETS
UNREELS
VARIERS
VARIETY
VARLETS
VERBENA
VERDELL
VERGEON
VERGERS
VERIEST
VERMEER
VERMEIL
VERSETS
WARDENS
WARDERS
WARHEAD
WARHERO
WARIEST
WARLESS
WARMERS
WARMEST
WARPERS
WARRENG
WARRENS
WARVETS
WIRIEST
WORKERS
WORMERS
WORRELL
WORSENS
XERXESI
YARDERS
YARNELL
YORKERS

••R••E•

AARATED
ABRADED
ABRADER
ABRADES
ABRILES
ADRATES
AERATED
AERATES
AEROBES
AFRAMES
AIRACES
AIRCREW
ALROKER
ALROSEN
APRONED
ARRASES
ARRAYED
ARRAYER
ARRISES
ARRIVED
ARRIVER
ARRIVES
AURALEE
BARBIES
BARDEEN
BAREGES
BARITES
BARKEEP
BARKIER
BARKLEY
BARMIER
BARNRED
BARONET
BARQUES
BARRIER
BARTLES
BARTLET
BERATED
BERATER
BERATES
BERKLEY
BERKNER
BERNSEN
BERRIED
BERRIES
BERTHED
BIRCHED
BIRCHEN
BIRCHES
BIRDIED
BIRDIES
BIRDMEN
BIREMES
BIRTHED
BORATES
BORIDES
BURBLED
BURBLER
BURBLES
BURGEES
BURGHER
BURGLED
BURGLES
BURLIER
BURNLEY
BURRIER
BURSTER
CARAFES
CARAMEL
CARAVEL
CARDKEY
CARFREE
CARGOES
CARIBES
CARNIES
CAROLED
CAROLER
CAROMED
CARRIED
CARRIER
CARRIES
CARTIER
CCRIDER
CDRATES
CERATED
CERATES
CERISES
CERUMEN
CHROMED
CHROMES
CIRCLED
CIRCLER
CIRCLES
CIRCLET
CIRQUES
CORKIER
CORNFED
CORNIER
CORONER
CORONET
CORPSES
CORVEES
CURARES
CURATED
CURATES
CURDIER
CURDLED
CURDLER
CURDLES
CURLIER
CURRIED
CURRIER
CURRIES
CURTSEY
CURVIER
DARKLED
DARKLES
DARKRED
DARLEEN
DARTLED
DARTLES
DERATED
DERATES
DERBIES
DERIDED
DERIDER
DERIDES
DERIVED
DERIVER
DERIVES
DERNIER
DIRKSEN
DIRTIED
DIRTIER
DIRTIES
DORKIER
EARLIER
EARLIES
EARTHED
EARTHEN
ENRAGED
ENRAGES
ENROBED
ENROBES
FARRIER
FARSEER

FARTHER
FARTLEK
FERNIER
FERRIED
FERRIES
FERULES
FIREMEN
FIRRIER
FIRTREE
FORAGED
FORAGER
FORAGES
FORASEC
FORAYED
FORDOES
FORELEG
FOREMEN
FORESEE
FOREVER
FORFREE
FORGOER
FORGOES
FORKIER
FORSTER
FORTIES
FORTLEE
FTRILEY
FURORES
FURRIER
FURTHER
GARAGED
GARAGES
GARBLED
GARBLER
GARBLES
GARDNER
GARGLED
GARGLER
GARGLES
GERMIER
GIRDLED
GIRDLER
GIRDLES
GIRLIER
GIRLIES
GIRTHED
GORETEX
GORSIER
GORTNER
GURGLED
GURGLES
GYRATED
GYRATES
GYRENES
HARDEES
HARDIER
HARDSET
HARDTEN
HARPIES
HARRIED
HARRIER
HARRIES
HARRIET
HARSHEN
HARSHER
HARTLEY
HERBIER
HERBTEA

HERSHEY
HORNIER
HORSIER
HORSLEY
HURDLED
HURDLER
HURDLES
HURRIED
HURRIER
HURRIES
HURTLED
HURTLES
HYRACES
HYRAXES
ISRAFEL
JERKIER
JERKIES
JIRASEK
JURYMEN
KARASEA
KARATES
KIRSTEN
KURILES
LARCHEN
LARCHES
LARDIER
LARDNER
LARKIER
LORELEI
LORISES
LORRIES
LORUSES
LURCHED
LURCHER
LURCHES
LUREXES
LURLEEN
MARBLED
MARBLER
MARBLES
MARCHED
MARCHER
MARCHES
MARGRET
MARINER
MARINES
MARLIER
MARNIER
MARQUEE
MARQUES
MARQUEZ
MARRIED
MARRIES
MARSDEN
MARSHES
MARSRED
MARVIER
MCRANEY
MERCHES
MERCIES
MERGEES
MERIDEN
MERIMEE
MERITED
MERRIER
MIRABEL
MIRAGES
MORALES

MORDRED
MORGUES
MORPHED
MURALED
MURKIER
MYRRHED
MYRTLES
NARTHEX
NARVAEZ
NERDIER
NERVIER
NORITES
NORTHER
NUREYEV
OARSMEN
OERSTED
ORRISES
PARADED
PARADER
PARADES
PARAPET
PARCHED
PARCHES
PARDNER
PAROLED
PAROLEE
PAROLES
PARQUET
PARRIED
PARRIER
PARRIES
PARSEES
PARSLEY
PARTIED
PARTIER
PARTIES
PARTNER
PARTYER
PARURES
PERCHED
PERCHER
PERCHES
PERDIEM
PERIGEE
PERILED
PERKIER
PERPLEX
PERRIER
PERUKES
PERUSED
PERUSER
PERUSES
PERWEEK
PGRATED
PHRASED
PHRASES
PIRATED
PIRATES
PIROGEN
PORCHES
PORGIES
PORIVER
PORKIER
PURDUEU
PURFLED
PURFLER
PURFLES
PURLIEU

PURPLED
PURPLES
PURSIER
PURSUED
PURSUER
PURSUES
PURTIER
PURVIEW
PYRITES
RERAKED
RERAKES
RERATED
RERATES
RERIDES
RERISEN
RERISES
SARACEN
SARALEE
SARAZEN
SCRAPED
SCRAPER
SCRAPES
SCREWED
SCRIBED
SCRIBER
SCRIBES
SERAPES
SERENER
SHRIKES
SHRINED
SHRINER
SHRINES
SHRIVEL
SHRIVER
SHRIVES
SIRENED
SORRIER
SORTIED
SORTIES
SPRAYED
SPRAYER
SPRITES
SPRUCED
SPRUCER
SPRUCES
STRAFED
STRAFER
STRAFES
STRAYED
STRAYER
STREWED
STREWER
STRIDER
STRIDES
STRIFES
STRIKER
STRIKES
STRIPED
STRIPER
STRIPES
STRIVED
STRIVEN
STRIVER
STRIVES
STROBES
STROKED
STROKER
STROKES

STRUDEL
SUREBET
SURFIER
SURFMEN
SURLIER
TARDIER
TARHEEL
TARRIED
TARRIER
TARRIES
TARTIER
TARTLET
TERRIER
TERRIES
THREEEE
THRIVED
THRIVEN
THRIVER
THRIVES
THRONES
THROWER
TIRADES
TIREDER
TIREMEN
TORCHED
TORCHER
TORCHES
TORQUED
TORQUES
TURFIER
TURFMEN
TURNKEY
TURNRED
TURTLED
TURTLES
UNRAKED
UNRATED
UNRAVEL
UNRAYED
UNRAZED
UNRILED
UNRIMED
UNRIPER
UNRISEN
UNRIVED
UNRIVEN
UNROBED
UNROBES
UNROPED
UNROPES
UNRULED
UPRATED
UPRATES
UPRISEN
UPRISER
UPRISES
UPRIVER
VARITEK
VERMEER
VERNIER
VERYFEW
VERYNEW
VERYRED
VERYWET
VIRTUES
VIRUSES
VORSTER
WARBLED

WARBLER
WARBLES
WARTIER
WERNHER
WERTHER
WIREMEN
WORDIER
WORKMEN
WORMIER
WORRIED
WORRIER
WORRIES
WORSLEY
WORSTED
XEROSES
XEROXED
XEROXES
YARDMEN
YORKIES

••R•••E

ABRIDGE
ACREAGE
AIRBASE
AIRDATE
AIRDRIE
AIRFARE
AIRFONE
AIRHOLE
AIRHOSE
AIRLANE
AIRLIKE
AIRLINE
AIRMILE
AIRRACE
AIRRAGE
AIRTIME
AIRTUBE
AIRWAVE
ARRANGE
ARRIERE
AURALEE
AUREATE
AUREOLE
AURICLE
AURORAE
BARBATE
BARBULE
BARCODE
BARNONE
BAROQUE
BARRAGE
BARWARE
BEREAVE
BERGERE
BERNESE
BEROWNE
BORZAGE
BURBAGE
BURETTE
BURMESE
CARBIDE
CARBINE
CARCARE
CARFARE
CARFREE
CARINAE
CARIOLE

CARLENE
CARLYLE
CARMINE
CARNAGE
CAROUSE
CARRERE
CARSALE
CARTAGE
CARTIRE
CERVINE
CIRRATE
CORACLE
CORDAGE
CORDATE
CORDITE
CORINNE
CORKAGE
CORNICE
CORNUTE
CORONAE
CORRADE
CORRODE
CORSAGE
CORTEGE
CORVINE
CORZINE
CURABLE
CURETTE
CURLIKE
CURSIVE
CURTATE
DARKAGE
DARLENE
DERALTE
DERANGE
DORMICE
DURABLE
DURANCE
DURANTE
EARACHE
EARBONE
EARHOLE
EARLIKE
EARLOBE
ENRIQUE
ENROUTE
ERRABLE
FARGONE
FARMORE
FAROESE
FARSIDE
FERMATE
FERRARE
FERRATE
FERRITE
FERRULE
FERTILE
FIREICE
FIRENZE
FIRTREE
FORBADE
FORBORE
FORDONE
FORESEE
FORFREE
FORGAVE
FORGIVE
FORGONE

FORHIRE
FORLIFE
FORLOVE
FORONCE
FORSAKE
FORSALE
FORSIZE
FORSURE
FORSYTE
FORTLEE
FORTUNE
FURCATE
FURNACE
FURTIVE
GARBAGE
GARONNE
GAROTTE
GARPIKE
GARROTE
GERMANE
GIRAFFE
GIROLLE
GIRONDE
HARLINE
HERBAGE
HERCULE
HERNIAE
HEROINE
HIRABLE
HIRCINE
HIRSUTE
HORMONE
IGRAINE
INRANGE
JARDINE
KARAOKE
KIRSTIE
LARAINE
LARAMIE
LAROCHE
LORANGE
MARCUSE
MARGATE
MARLENE
MARLOWE
MARQUEE
MARRYME
MARYURE
MERCURE
MERIMEE
MIRACLE
MORAINE
MORANTE
MORTICE
MORTISE
NARRATE
NERVINE
NERVULE
NORDOWE
NURTURE
OARLIKE
PARABLE
PARBAKE
PARFIVE
PARKADE
PARKAVE
PAROLEE
PARTAKE

PARTITE
PARTONE
PERCALE
PERDURE
PERFUME
PERFUSE
PERIGEE
PERJURE
PERLITE
PERMUTE
PERRINE
PERVADE
PIROGUE
PORCINE
PORKPIE
PORSCHE
PORTAGE
PURPOSE
RERAISE
RERINSE
REROUTE
SARALEE
SARDINE
SCROOGE
SCRUPLE
SERFAGE
SERIATE
SERIESE
SERRATE
SERVICE
SERVILE
SIRDUKE
SORBATE
STRANGE
STRASSE
STRIATE
STROPHE
STROUSE
SURFACE
SURMISE
SURNAME
SURVIVE
SYRINGE
TARTARE
TERENCE
TERHUNE
TERMITE
TERNATE
TERRACE
TERRENE
TERRINE
THREEEE
TORTURE
TURBINE
TURFTOE
UKRAINE
UNRHYME
UPRAISE
UPROUSE
VARIATE
VCRTAPE
VERBOSE
VERDURE
VEREINE
VERSACE
VIRGATE
VIRGULE
VORLAGE

WARFARE
WARGAME
WARLIKE
WARPAGE
WARTIME
WARZONE
WIRABLE
WORDAGE
WORDONE
YARDAGE
ZERNIKE

•••RE••

ACCRETE
ACTRESS
ADDRESS
ADORERS
AGGRESS
AIGRETS
ALFREDA
ALFREDE
ALFREDO
ALFREDU
ALGREEN
ANDREAS
ANDRESS
ANDREWS
ARMREST
ASTREAM
AVERELL
AWAREOF
AWAREST
AZOREAN
BAHREIN
BARRELS
BARRENS
BARRETS
BARRETT
BEARERS
BEDREST
BEHRENS
BOTREES
CAIRENE
CARRELS
CARRERA
CARRERE
CLARETS
CLORETS
CORRECT
CURRENT
CYPRESS
DEAREST
DEBRETT
DECREED
DECREER
DECREES
DEGREED
DEGREES
DEPRESS
DIGRESS
DOGREAT
DOUREST
DRFREUD
DURRELL
ELGRECO
EMPRESS
ENTREAT
ENTREES

EVEREST
EVERETT
EXCRETE
EXPRESS
EXTREME
FAIREST
FARRELL
FEARERS
FEBRERO
FERRETS
FERRETY
FLAREUP
FLOREAL
FLORENZ
FLORETS
FORREAL
FORRENT
FORREST
FOUREEE
GAGREEL
GARRETS
GARRETT
GETREAL
GLAREAT
GOTREAL
HATREDS
HEARERS
HEBREWS
HEIRESS
HENREID
IDAREDS
IMARETS
IMGREAT
IMPRESS
IMPREST
IMPREZA
INBREED
INGREEN
INGRESS
IPCRESS
ISUREAM
ISUREDO
JARRELL
JARRETT
JEERERS
JODRELL
KURRENT
LATRELL
LAURELS
LAURENT
LEERERS
LEFREAK
LEGREST
LIPREAD
LOUREED
LOWRENT
MARRERS
MAUREEN
MISREAD
MISRELY
MRGREEN
MYTREAT
NEAREST
NOTREAL
ONBREAK
ONEREEL
OPPRESS
OSPREYS

OUTREAD
OVEREAT
PAIRERS
PEERESS
PERREAU
PETRELS
POOREST
POURERS
PRERENT
PURRERS
PUTREFY
REAREND
REARERS
REBREAK
REBREED
REBREWS
REDREAM
REDRESS
REERECT
REFRESH
REGREET
REGRESS
REGRETS
REPRESS
RETREAD
RETREAT
REXREED
ROARERS
SANREMO
SCAREDY
SCARERS
SCAREUP
SCORERS
SEARERS
SECRECY
SECRETE
SECRETS
SEERESS
SHAREIN
SHARERS
SHOREUP
SNARERS
SNORERS
SOARERS
SOAREWE
SOIREES
SORRELL
SORRELS
SOUREST
SPARELY
SPAREME
SPARERS
SPAREST
SPIREAS
STAREAT
STARERS
STEREOS
STORERS
STOREUP
STYRENE
SUPREME
SURREAL
SURREYS
SWOREAT
SWOREBY
SWOREIN
SWORETO
TAUREAN

TEARERS
TERRELL
TERRENE
TERRETS
THEREAT
THEREBY
THEREDS
THEREIN
THERENT
THEREOF
THEREON
THERESA
THERETO
THOREAU
TIGRESS
TIMREID
TORREFY
TORRENT
TOURERS
TRIREME
TURRETS
TVCREWS
TWERENT
UNDRESS
UNERECT
UNFREED
UNFREES
UNGREEN
UNTREAD
UNTREED
UPTREND
USURERS
WARRENG
WARRENS
WEARERS
WHEREAS
WHEREAT
WHEREBY
WHEREIN
WHERELL
WHEREOF
WHEREON
WHERERE
WHERETO
WHEREVE
WORRELL
YEAREND
YOUREIT
YOUREON

•••R•E•

ABORTED
ACCRUED
ACCRUES
ACORNED
ADORNED
ADORNER
ALARMED
ALARMER
ALERTED
ALERTER
ALGREEN
AMBRIES
AMERCED
AMERCER
AMERCES
ANGRIER
APERIES

AVERRED
AVERTED
AVERTER
AWARDED
AWARDEE
AWARDER
BARRIER
BEARDED
BEERIER
BEERKEG
BERRIED
BERRIES
BEURRES
BLARNEY
BLURBER
BLURRED
BLURTED
BLURTER
BOARDED
BOARDER
BOTREES
BOURGET
BOURSES
BURRIER
CAIRNED
CARRIED
CARRIER
CARRIES
CHARGED
CHARGER
CHARGES
CHARIER
CHARLES
CHARLEY
CHARMED
CHARMEN
CHARMER
CHARRED
CHARRER
CHARTED
CHARTER
CHARVET
CHIRPED
CHIRPER
CHIRRED
CHORDED
CHURNED
CHURNER
CITROEN
CLERKED
COARSEN
COARSER
COERCED
COERCER
COERCES
CONRIED
COURBET
COURIER
COURSED
COURSER
COURSES
COURTED
COWRIES
CURRIED
CURRIER
CURRIES
DAIRIES
DAIRYER
DEARDEN
DEARIES
DEBRIEF
DECREED
DECREER
DECREES
DECRIED
DECRIER
DECRIES
DEGREED
DEGREES
DEVRIES
DIARIES
DOORMEN
DOWRIES
DWARFED
DWARVES
ECARTES
EMBRUED
EMBRUES
EMERGED
EMERGES
EMERIES
EMERSED
ENARMED
ENTREES
ENTRIES
EVERTED
EWERIES
EXERTED
EXERTER
FAERIES
FAEROES
FAIRIES
FAIRSEX
FARRIER
FERRIED
FERRIES
FEVRIER
FIERCER
FIERIER
FIRRIER
FLIRTED
FLIRTER
FOUREEE
FOURIER
FURRIER
GABRIEL
GAGREEL
GEORGEC
GEORGEI
GEORGEM
GEORGES
GEORGEV
GEORGEW
GFORCES
GLORIED
GLORIES
GLURGES
GNARLED
GNARRED
GOURDES
GOURMET
GUARDED
GUARDEE
GUARDER
HAARLEM
HAIRGEL
HAIRIER
HAIRNET
HARRIED
HARRIER
HARRIES
HARRIET
HEARKEN
HEARSES
HEARTED
HEARTEN
HENRIES
HOARDED
HOARDER
HOARIER
HOARSEN
HOARSER
HURRIED
HURRIER
HURRIES
IFORGET
IMBRUED
IMBRUES
INBREED
INBRIEF
INGREEN
INORDER
IVORIES
JOURNEE
JOURNEY
KEARNEY
KNARRED
KNURLED
LAERTES
LEARJET
LEARNED
LEARNER
LEERIER
LORRIES
LOURDES
LOUREED
MAARTEN
MARRIED
MARRIES
MAUREEN
MERRIER
MONROES
MOORHEN
MOORIER
MOURNED
MOURNER
MRGREEN
MYRRHED
ONEREEL
ONORDER
OTARIES
OVARIES
OVERBED
OVERBET
OVERFED
OVERFEE
OVERFEW
OVERLET
OVERNEW
OVERSEA
OVERSEE
OVERSET
OVERSEW
OVERWET
PARRIED
PARRIER
PARRIES
PATRIES
PEARLED
PEARLER
PERRIER
PIERCED
PIERCER
PIERCES
POORMEN
QUARLES
QUARREL
QUARTER
QUARTES
QUARTET
QUERIED
QUERIER
QUERIES
QUIRTED
REARMED
REBREED
REDRIED
REDRIES
REFRIED
REFRIES
REGREET
REORDER
RETRIED
RETRIES
REURGED
REURGES
REXREED
SCARCER
SCARFED
SCARFER
SCARIER
SCARLET
SCARPED
SCARRED
SCARVES
SCORNED
SCORNER
SCURVES
SHARKEY
SHARPED
SHARPEI
SHARPEN
SHARPER
SHERBET
SHIRKED
SHIRKER
SHIRLEY
SHIRRED
SHORTED
SHORTEN
SHORTER
SKIRLED
SKIRTED
SKIRTER
SLURPED
SLURPEE
SLURPER
SLURRED
SMARTED
SMARTEN
SMARTER
SMIRKED
SMIRKER
SNARFED
SNARLED
SNARLER
SNORKEL
SNORTED
SNORTER
SOIREES
SORRIER
SOURCED
SOURCES
SPARKED
SPARRED
SPARRER
SPARSER
SPIRIER
SPORTED
SPURNED
SPURNER
SPURRED
SPURTED
STARKER
STARKEY
STARLET
STARRED
STARTED
STARTER
STARVED
STARVES
STERNER
STIRRED
STIRRER
STORIED
STORIES
STORMED
STURGES
SWARMED
SWARMER
SWERVED
SWERVES
SWIRLED
TARRIED
TARRIER
TARRIES
TEARIER
TERRIER
TERRIES
THORNED
THURBER
TIARAED
TIERCES
TIERNEY
TOORDER
TOURNEY
TWIRLED
TWIRLER
UMBRIEL
UNARMED
UNBRIEF
UNCRIED
UNCRUEL
UNDRIED
UNFREED
UNFREES
UNFRIED
UNGREEN
UNORBED
UNTREED
UNTRIED
UNTRUER
UNURGED
UPDRIED
UPDRIES
USERFEE
USURIES
USURPED
USURPER
VEERIES
VIERNES
WEARIED
WEARIER
WEARIES
WEIRDED
WEIRDER
WHARFED
WHARVES
WHIRLED
WHIRLER
WHIRRED
WHORLED
WORRIED
WORRIER
WORRIES
YEARNED
YEARNER

••R••E

ACCRETE
ACERATE
ACEROSE
AIRRACE
AIRRAGE
ALFREDE
ALLRISE
AMARONE
AMBROSE
ANDRADE
APPRISE
APPROVE
ASARULE
ASCRIBE
ASTRIDE
ATGRADE
ATTRITE
AVARICE
AVERAGE
AWARDEE
AXLROSE
AZURITE
BARRAGE
BEBRAVE
BEDRAPE
BEGRIME
BITROLE
BUSRIDE
CABRIDE
CAIRENE
CAMRYLE
CAPRICE
CAPRINE
CARRERE
CHARADE
CHARLIE
CHORALE
CHORINE
CHORTLE
CIRRATE
CITRATE
CITRINE
CLARICE
COMRADE
CORRADE
CORRODE
COURAGE
COWRITE
COWROTE
CUPRITE
CUTRATE
DEARONE
DEFRAME
DEGRADE
DEIRDRE
DEPRAVE
DEPRIVE
DETRUDE
DHURRIE
DIORITE
DISRATE
DISROBE
DOGRACE
DOGROSE
DOORDIE
DOTRICE
EMBRACE
EMIRATE
EMPRISE
ENFRAME
ENGRAVE
ENPRISE
EPERGNE
EXCRETE
EXTREME
EXTRUDE
FAIRUSE
FEBRILE
FERRARE
FERRATE
FERRITE
FERRULE
FOUREEE
GAGRULE
GARROTE
GEORGIE
GLORYBE
GOBROKE
GUARDEE
GUYROPE
HAIRDYE
HAYRIDE
HEURIGE
HEYRUBE
HYDRATE
HYDRIDE
IFORONE
IMBROKE
IMPROVE
INARAGE
INGRATE
INTRADE
INTRUDE
ITERATE
IVORINE
JIMRICE
JOURNEE
JOYRIDE
JSTROKE
KATRINE
LADRONE
LAPROBE
LATRINE
LATROBE
LEGROPE
LETRIDE
LOWRISE
MACRAME
MANROPE
MARRYME
MAURICE
MCARDLE
MCBRIDE
MELROSE
MICROBE
MIDRISE
MIGRATE
MISRATE
MISRULE
MOBRULE
MOORAGE
NARRATE
NEURONE
NITRATE
NITRIDE
NITRITE
NOTRADE
NOTRARE
OBTRUDE
ODORIZE
OLDROSE
OPERATE
OPEROSE
OUTRACE
OUTRAGE
OUTRATE
OUTRAVE
OUTRIDE
OUTRODE
OUTROVE
OVERAGE
OVERATE
OVERAWE
OVERDUE
OVERDYE
OVERFEE
OVERICE
OVERLIE
OVERSEE
OVERUSE
PADRONE
PATRICE
PAYRATE
PEERAGE
PENROSE
PERRINE
PRERACE
PRORATE
PUERILE
RATRACE
REARGUE
REARISE
REAROSE
REBRACE
REBROKE
RECRATE
REDRIVE
REDROBE
REDROSE
REFRAME
REGRADE
REPRICE
REPRIME
REPRISE
REPROBE
REPROVE
REPRUNE
RETRACE
RETRADE
REWRITE
REWROTE
SEARACE
SECRETE
SERRATE
SETRATE
SHARPIE
SHORTIE
SKIRACE
SLURPEE
SOAREWE
SOURALE
SPAREME
SPARKLE
STARTLE
STERILE
STORAGE
STYRENE
SUBRACE
SUCRASE
SUCROSE
SUNRISE
SUPREME
SVERIGE
TAURINE
TAXRATE
TEAROSE
TERRACE
TERRENE
TERRINE
TETRODE
THEROBE
THEROPE
THEROSE
THERULE
TIEROPE
TIMRICE
TITRATE
TOPRATE
TOWROPE
TRIREME
UMBRAGE
UNBRACE
UNBRAKE
UNBRAVE
UNBROKE
UNCRATE
UNCRUDE
UNDRAPE
UNFROZE
UNTRITE
UPGRADE
UPTRADE
USERFEE
VIBRATE
VINROSE
VITRINE
WHERERE
WHEREVE
YEARONE
ZEBRINE

••••RE•

ABJURED
ABJURER
ABJURES
ADHERED
ADHERER
ADHERES
ADJURED
ADJURER
ADJURES
ADMIRED
ADMIRER
ADMIRES
AFEARED
AIRCREW
ALBIREO
ALLURED
ALLURER
ALLURES
ALTERED
ALTERER
ALVAREZ
AMPERES
ANGERED
ANTARES
APPAREL
ARBORED
ARMORED
ARMORER
ASCARED
ASHTREE
ASPIRED
ASPIRER
ASPIRES
ASSURED
ASSURER
ASSURES
ATTHREE
ATTIRED
ATTIRER
ATTIRES
AUGURED
AUGURER
AVERRED
BADAREA
BARNRED
BAYAREA
BAYTREE
BEETRED
BEETREE
BEMIRED
BEMIRES
BENARES
BESTREW
BEURRES
BEWARED
BEWARES
BLEARED
BLUERED
BLURRED
BODEREK
BOWERED
BUGFREE
CABARET
CAPERED
CARFREE
CATERED
CATERER
CEDARED
CENTRED
CENTRES
CHAIRED
CHARRED
CHARRER
CHEERED
CHEERER
CHEVRES
CHEVRET
CHIRRED
CHOIRED
CLEARED
CLEARER
CODERED
COHERED
COHERER
COHERES
COLORED
COLORER
COMTREX
CONFREY
CONURES
COVERED
COVERER
COWERED
CURARES
DALTREY
DARKRED
DEAIRED
DEEPRED
DEHIRED
DEHIRES
DEMARET
DEMURER
DESERET
DESIRED
DESIREE
DESIRER
DESIRES
DEVORES
DEWIRED
DEWIRES
DOLORES
DOWERED
EAGERER
ELMTREE
EMIGREE
EMIGRES
EMPIRES
ENCORED
ENCORES
ENDURED
ENDURER
ENDURES
ENSURED
ENSURER
ENSURES
ENTERED
ENTERER
ENTIRES
ERITREA
EUCHRED
EUCHRES
EXPIRED
EXPIRES
FABARES
FATFREE
FAVORED
FAVORER
FEEFREE
FEVERED
FIACRES
FIBERED
FIGTREE
FIGURED
FIGURER
FIGURES
FIRTREE
FLEERED
FLOORED
FLOORER
FLOURED
FORFREE
FOUDRES
FURORES
FUTURES
GETFREE
GNARRED
GODFREY
GOTFREE
GUMTREE
HIGHRES
HOMBRES
HOMERED
HONORED
HONOREE
HONORER
HOVERED
HOVERER
HUMORED
HUNDRED
ICEFREE
IGNORED
IGNORER
IGNORES
ILLBRED
IMBORED
IMMURED
IMMURES
IMPURER
IMTIRED
INHERED
INHERES
INJURED
INJURER
INJURES
INSURED
INSURER
INSURES
INTHREE
JEFFREY
JOFFREY
KENDREW
KESTREL
KINDRED
KNARRED
LABORED
LABORER
LACUREE
LAMPREY
LAUTREC
LAYERED
LEDERER
LETTRES
LEVERED
LEVERET
LIVERED
LONDRES
LOUVRED
LOUVRES
LOWBRED
LOWERED
LUSTRED
LUSTRES
MACHREE
MAIGRET
MAITRED
MAITRES
MAJORED
MANDREL
MANFRED
MANURED
MANURES
MARGRET
MARSRED
MATURED
MATURER
MATURES
MCCAREY
MEMOREX
METERED
MILDRED
MINARET
MINORED
MISBREW
MISDREW
MITERED
MONGREL
MORDRED
MOTORED
MPTHREE
MUJERES
MULGREW
NATURED
NATUREL
NATURES
NOMBRES
NOSIREE
NUTTREE
OAKTREE
OEUVRES
OFFERED
OFFEREE
OFFERER
ONTHREE
ORDERED
ORDERER
OSIERED
OUTBRED
OUTDREW
OUTGREW
PALFREY
PAPERED
PAPERER
PARURES

PETERED
PITCREW
POIVRES
POUDRES
POWERED
QUARREL
QUATRES
QUEERED
QUEERER
RAMIREZ
RANFREE
RASURES
RAZORED
REAIRED
REBORED
REBORES
RECURED
RECURES
REDARED
REDARES
REFEREE
REFIRED
REFIRES
REHIRED
REHIRES
RENFREW
RESTREW
RETIRED
RETIREE
RETIRES
REVERED
REVERER
REVERES
REWIRED
REWIRES
ROGERED
ROSERED
RUBYRED
RUMORED
RUNFREE
SABERED
SATIRES
SAVORED
SAVORER
SCARRED
SCOURED
SCOURER
SEAGREN
SECURED
SECURER
SECURES
SEESRED
SENORES
SETFREE
SEVERED
SEVERER
SHEARED
SHEARER
SHEERED
SHEERER
SHIRRED
SKIAREA
SLURRED
SMEARED
SMEARER
SNEERED
SNEERER
SOBERED
SOBERER
SPARRED
SPARRER
SPEARED
SPEARER
SPHERED
SPHERES
SPURRED
SQUARED
SQUARER
SQUARES
SQUIRED
SQUIRES
STAIRED
STARRED
STEERED
STEERER
STIRRED
STIRRER
SUBAREA
SUGARED
SUTURED
SUTURES
SWEARER
TABARET
TABORET
TAPERED
TASERED
TAXFREE
TEATREE
TENURED
TENURES
THEOREM
THETREE
TIMBRES
TINORES
TOUAREG
TOWERED
TUMBREL
TURNRED
TUTORED
UMBERED
UMPIRED
UMPIRES
UNAIRED
UNBARED
UNBARES
UNBORED
UNCORED
UNCORES
UNCURED
UNDARED
UNFIRED
UNGORED
UNHIRED
UNHIRES
UNLURED
UNMIRED
UNPARED
UNSCREW
UNTIRED
UNWIRED
UPATREE
USHERED
UTTERED
UTTERER
VALOREM
VAPORED
VAPORER
VELURES
VERYRED
VICKREY
VISORED
VIZORED
WAFERED
WAGERED
WAGERER
WASTREL
WATERED
WATERER
WAVERED
WAVERER
WHIRRED
WILFRED
WINERED
WINFREY
YEWTREE

••••R•E

AALARGE
ADVERSE
AIRDRIE
ALGARVE
ASHTREE
ASPERSE
ASTARTE
ATLARGE
ATTHREE
AUBERGE
AURORAE
BAYTREE
BEETREE
BICORNE
BIZARRE
BOGARDE
BUGFREE
BYFORCE
CALORIE
CAMERAE
CARFREE
CASERNE
CATORCE
COTERIE
COVERME
DEBARGE
DEFARGE
DELARUE
DELORME
DEMERGE
DESERVE
DESIREE
DETERGE
DHURRIE
DIVERGE
DIVERSE
DIVORCE
DOVERDE
ELMTREE
ELNORTE
EMIGREE
ENCARRE
ENDORSE
ENFORCE
ENGARDE
ENGORGE
ENLARGE
EUTERPE
EXCURSE
EXEDRAE
EXPARTE
EXTERNE
FABERGE
FATFREE
FEEFREE
FIGTREE
FIRTREE
FORFREE
GETFREE
GOTFREE
GUMTREE
GUTHRIE
HONOREE
HUMORME
ICEFREE
IMMERGE
IMMERSE
INCURVE
INDORSE
INFORCE
INLARGE
INNERVE
INTERNE
INTERSE
INTHREE
INVERSE
ITSTRUE
LACUREE
LAFARGE
LAPORTE
LAVERNE
LECARRE
LIBERTE
LUCARNE
LUCERNE
MACHREE
MCENROE
MOCHRIE
MODERNE
MPTHREE
MRHORSE
NAVARRE
NOMERGE
NOSIREE
NOTTRUE
NOWORSE
NUTTREE
OAKTREE
OBSERVE
OBVERSE
OFFEREE
ONSERVE
ONTHREE
OROURKE
OSBORNE
PANURGE
PLEURAE
PRAIRIE
RANFREE
RECARVE
RECURVE
REFEREE
REFORGE
REMERGE
REMORSE
RESERVE
RESURGE
RETIREE
REVERIE
REVERSE
ROBERTE
RUNFREE
SCLERAE
SCOURGE
SETFREE
SHADROE
SPLURGE
TAXFREE
TEATREE
THETREE
TOHORSE
UNBORNE
UNHORSE
UNLARGE
UNMERGE
UNNERVE
UNTERSE
UPATREE
UPBORNE
UPCURVE
UPSURGE
VALERIE
YEWTREE

•••••RE

ACQUIRE
ADAWARE
AFFAIRE
AIRFARE
ALBSURE
ALLHERE
ANDMORE
ANYMORE
ARDMORE
ARMOIRE
ARRIERE
ARTWARE
ASTAIRE
ATEMORE
AUSTERE
BARWARE
BERGERE
BETHERE
BIZARRE
BONAIRE
BONFIRE
BUSFARE
CABFARE
CALIBRE
CAPTURE
CARCARE
CARFARE
CARRERE
CARTIRE
CAVIARE
CDSTORE
CELEBRE
CENSURE
CENTARE
CESAIRE
CHAMBRE
CLOSURE
CLOTURE
COMPARE
COMPERE
CONJURE
COUTURE
CULTURE
DAYCARE
DAYMARE
DECIARE
DECLARE
DEIRDRE
DELMORE
DENTURE
DEPLORE
DOEUVRE
DOIDARE
EATHERE
EATMORE
ENCARRE
ENQUIRE
ENSNARE
EPICURE
ERASURE
ESQUIRE
ETAGERE
EXPLORE
EYECARE
EYESORE
FAILURE
FANFARE
FARMORE
FAXLORE
FEATURE
FENETRE
FERRARE
FISSURE
FIXTURE
FLEXURE
FORBORE
FORHIRE
FORSURE
FOXFIRE
GESTURE
GETSORE
GILMORE
GOTSORE
GRAVURE
GRUYERE
GUNFIRE
HAYWIRE
HECTARE
HILAIRE
HITHERE
HOTWIRE
IMPLORE
IMTHERE
INQUIRE
INSHORE
INSPIRE
INSTORE
INTHERE
IRONORE
ISADORE
ISIDORE
ITSHERE
JETFIRE
KAPTURE
KENMORE
KILDARE
LAPWARE
LAYBARE
LEADORE
LECARRE
LECTURE
LEHAVRE
LEISURE
LEONORE
LESABRE
LETTERE
LUMIERE
MACABRE
MAGUIRE
MAJEURE
MALWARE
MARYURE
MCCLURE
MCGUIRE
MCGWIRE
MEASURE
MEMOIRE
MERCURE
MISFIRE
MISWIRE
MIXTURE
MOLIERE
MRPADRE
MULHARE
NAVARRE
NETWARE
NEWHIRE
NONCORE
NOSCORE
NOTHERE
NOTRARE
NOTSURE
NOWHERE
NURTURE
OBSCURE
OCTOBRE
OCTUBRE
ODDSARE
ONADARE
ONEACRE
ONEMORE
ONSHORE
OUTCURE
OUTDARE
OUTFIRE
OUTHERE
OUTHIRE
OUTTIRE
OUTTORE
OUTWORE
PASTURE
PAYMORE
PERDURE
PERJURE
PETHARE
PHILTRE
PIASTRE
PICTURE
PISMIRE
POSTURE
PRECURE
PREPARE
PRETIRE
PREWIRE
PROCURE
RAPTURE
REQUIRE
RESCORE
RESHARE
RESPIRE
RESTORE
RESWORE
RIVIERE
RONDURE
RUPTURE
SAYMORE
SCEPTRE
SEAFARE
SEEHERE
SEIZURE
SIGNORE
SINCERE
SOTHERE
SPECTRE
SPYWARE
STATURE
SUNFIRE
SUSPIRE
TARTARE
TEMPORE
TENACRE
TEXTURE
THEATRE
TINWARE
TONSURE
TORTURE
TOSPARE
TSQUARE
TWOACRE
TWOMORE
UNAWARE
UNMITRE
UNSWORE
UPSTARE
UPTHERE
VAMPIRE
VENTURE
VERDURE
VESTURE
VOITURE
VOLTORE
VULTURE
WALKURE
WARFARE
WASSURE
WELFARE
WETWARE
WHERERE
YESSIRE

R•F••••

RAFFIAS
RAFFISH
RAFFLED
RAFFLER
RAFFLES
RAFTERS
RAFTING
REFACED
REFACES
REFALLS
REFAXED
REFAXES
REFEEDS
REFENCE
REFEREE
REFERTO
REFFING
REFIGHT
REFILED
REFILES
REFILLS
REFILMS
REFINDS
REFINED
REFINER
REFINES
REFIRED
REFIRES
REFIXED
REFIXES
REFLAGS
REFLATE
REFLECT
REFLIES
REFLIPS
REFLOAT
REFLOOD
REFLOWN
REFLOWS
REFOCUS
REFOLDS
REFORGE
REFORMS
REFOUND
REFRACT
REFRAIN
REFRAME
REFRESH
REFRIED
REFRIES
REFRONT
REFUELS
REFUGED
REFUGEE
REFUGES
REFUNDS
REFUSAL
REFUSED
REFUSER
REFUSES
REFUTAL
REFUTED
REFUTER
REFUTES
REFYING
RIFFING
RIFFLED
RIFFLER
RIFFLES
RIFLERS
RIFLERY
RIFLING
RIFTING
RUFFALO
RUFFIAN
RUFFING
RUFFLED
RUFFLER
RUFFLES
RUFIYAA

R••F•••

RADFORD
RAFFIAS
RAFFISH
RAFFLED
RAFFLER
RAFFLES
RAMFANS
RANFREE
RATFINK
RAWFISH
RAWFOOD
REAFFIX
REDFACE
REDFERN
REDFINS
REDFIRS
REDFISH
REDFIVE
REDFLAG
REDFORD
REDFOUR
REEFERS
REEFIER
REEFING
REFFING
REIFIED
REIFIES
RENFREW
REOFFER
RIFFING
RIFFLED
RIFFLER
RIFFLES
ROLFERS
ROLFING
ROOFAGE
ROOFERS
ROOFING
ROOFRAT
ROOFTOP
RUFFALO
RUFFIAN
RUFFING
RUFFLED
RUFFLER
RUFFLES
RUMFORD
RUNFREE

R•••F••

RAGEFUL
RAMSFAN
RANGFOR
RATAFIA
READFOR
REAFFIX
REBUFFS
REDSFAN
REGIFTS
REOFFER
REPSFOR
RESIFTS
RESTFUL
RINGFOR
RIPOFFS
ROOMFUL
ROOTFOR
ROTIFER
RUNGFOR
RUNOFFS
RUNSFOR
RUTHFUL

R••••F•

RAKEOFF
RANGOFF
READOFF
REBUFFS
RECTIFY
REDRAFT
REELOFF
REGRAFT
RELIEFS
REROOFS
RESHIFT
RESTAFF
RESTUFF
RETURFS
REUNIFY
RIDEOFF
RINGOFF
RIPOFFS
RIPSOFF
RODEOFF
RODOLFO
ROLLOFF
ROPEOFF
RUBSOFF
RUDOLFI
RUNGOFF
RUNOFFS
RUNSOFF
RUSHOFF

R•••••F

RAKEOFF
RANGOFF
READOFF
REDWOLF
REEKSOF
REELOFF
REPROOF
RESTAFF
RESTUFF
RIDEOFF
RINGOFF
RIPSOFF
ROBERTF
RODEOFF
ROLLOFF
ROPEOFF
RUBSOFF
RUNGOFF
RUNSOFF
RUSHOFF
RYELOAF

•RF••••

DRFREUD
DRFRIST
MRFIXIT
PRFIRMS

•R•F•••

ARAFTOF
ARAFURA
ARMFULS
ARTFAIR
ARTFERN
ARTFILM
ARTFORM
CRAFTED
CRAFTER
CRAFTSY
CROFTER
DRAFTED
DRAFTEE
DRAFTER
DRIFTED
DRIFTER
DRIFTIN
DRIFTUP
DRYFOGS
GRAFTED
GRAFTER
GRAFTON
GRIFFEY
GRIFFIN
GRIFFON
GRIFTED
GRIFTER
GRUFFER
GRUFFLY
IREFUSE
IRSFORM
ORIFICE
PREFABS
PREFACE
PREFADE
PREFECT
PREFERS
PREFILE
PREFORM
PREFUND
PROFANE
PROFARM
PROFESS
PROFFER
PROFILE
PROFITS
PROFUSE
TRAFFIC
TREFOIL
TRIFFID
TRIFLED
TRIFLER
TRIFLES
TRIFOLD
TRIFORM
TRUFFLE
URNFULS

•R••F••

ARCHFOE
BRERFOX
BRIEFED
BRIEFER
BRIEFLY
BRIMFUL
DREYFUS
FRETFUL
GREWFAT
GRIFFEY
GRIFFIN
GRIFFON
GROWFAT
GRUFFER
GRUFFLY
PRAYFOR
PROFFER
PROOFED
PROOFER
TRAFFIC
TRAYFUL
TRIFFID
TRUFFLE

•R•••F•

BRANIFF
DRAGOFF
DRAWOFF
DREWOFF
DRMELFI
DROPOFF
GRATIFY
PREDEFY
PRELIFE
PRESIFT
PROLIFE
TRIMOFF
TROTOFF

•R••••F

ARAFTOF
BRANIFF
CRYWOLF
DRAGOFF
DRAWOFF
DREAMOF
DREWOFF
DROPOFF
FREEDOF
FREESOF
PROUDOF
TRIMOFF
TROTOFF

••RF•••

AIRFARE
AIRFLOW
AIRFOIL
AIRFONE
BARFBAG
CARFARE
CARFREE
CARFULS
CORFAMS
CURFEWS
DORFMAN
EARFLAP
EARFULS
FARFELS
FORFEIT
FORFEND
FORFREE
FURFARM
JARFULS
KERFLOP
NORFOLK

PARFAIT
PARFIVE
PARFOUR
PARFUMS
PERFECT
PERFIDY
PERFORM
PERFUME
PERFUMY
PERFUSE
PURFLED
PURFLER
PURFLES
SERFAGE
SERFDOM
SURFACE
SURFEIT
SURFERS
SURFIER
SURFING
SURFMAN
SURFMEN
SURFSUP
TURFIER
TURFING
TURFMAN
TURFMEN
TURFSKI
TURFTOE
TURFWAR
WARFARE

••R•F••

BIRDFLU
BURNFOR
CARAFES
CAREFOR
CAREFUL
CORNFED
DAREFUL
DIREFUL
FIREFLY
FIREFOX
FORKFUL
FORMFUL
GIRAFFE
HARMFUL
HURTFOR
HURTFUL
ISRAFEL
SCRUFFS
SCRUFFY
STRAFED
STRAFER
STRAFES
STRIFES
TARIFFS
THRIFTS
THRIFTY
VERYFEW
VERYFIT
WORKFOR

••R••F•

AIRLIFT
BURNOFF
CARDIFF
CARTOFF
CERTIFY
DARTOFF
EARMUFF
FARLEFT
FIREOFF
FORLIFE
FORTIFY
GIRAFFE
HORRIFY
KARLOFF
MARKOFF
MORTIFY
NORDOFF
PERSOFF
REROOFS
SARNOFF
SCRUFFS
SCRUFFY
TARIFFS
TERRIFY
TOREOFF
TORNOFF
TORREFY
TURNOFF
UNROOFS
VERBIFY
VERSIFY
WARDOFF
WARNOFF
WOREOFF
WORKOFF
WORNOFF

••R•••F

AIRWOLF
BARANOF
BURNOFF
CARDIFF
CARTOFF
DARRYLF
DARTOFF
EARMUFF
FIREOFF
HERSELF
KARLOFF
MARKOFF
MORCERF
NORDOFF
NORTHOF
OURSELF
PERSOFF
SARNOFF
SERIESF
STRIPOF
SUREROF
TIREDOF
TIRESOF
TOREOFF
TORNOFF
TURNOFF
WARDOFF
WARNOFF
WARNSOF
WOREOFF
WORKOFF
WORNOFF

•••RF••

BRERFOX
DEERFLY
DWARFED
FAIRFAX
FEARFOR
FEARFUL
ODORFUL
OVERFAR
OVERFAT
OVERFED
OVERFEE
OVERFEW
OVERFIT
OVERFIX
OVERFLY
SCARFED
SCARFER
SCARFUP
SNARFED
STIRFRY
TEARFUL
USERFEE
WHARFED

•••R•F•

BEAROFF
CLARIFY
ENGRAFT
FAIROFF
GLORIFY
HORRIFY
INDRAFT
INGRAFT
MCGRIFF
MCGRUFF
MIDRIFF
MYCROFT
NITRIFY
PAIROFF
PETRIFY
PUTREFY
REDRAFT
REGRAFT
SCARIFY
SHERIFF
SHERIFS
TEAROFF
TERRIFY
TORREFY
UNGRUFF
UPDRAFT
UPDRIFT
VEEROFF
VITRIFY
WEAROFF

•••R••F

AKERLOF
AWAREOF
BEAROFF
DARRYLF
DEBRIEF
FAIROFF
HEARDOF
HEARSOF
HIPROOF
INBRIEF
LEARNOF
MCGRIFF
MCGRUFF
MIDRIFF
PAIROFF
REPROOF
SHERIFF
SHORTOF
SUNROOF
TEAROFF
THEREOF
TINROOF
UNBRIEF
UNGRUFF
VEEROFF
WEAROFF
WHEREOF

••••RF•

RETURFS

••••R•F

APAIROF
CLEAROF
ROBERTF
SUREROF

•••••RF

ALTDORF
EGOSURF
LETTERF
LINDORF
MORCERF
NETSURF
SKYSURF
WALDORF

R•G••••

RAGBAGS
RAGDOLL
RAGEFUL
RAGGEDY
RAGGIER
RAGGIES
RAGGING
RAGINGS
RAGLANS
RAGMANS
RAGMOPS
RAGOUTS
RAGRUGS
RAGSHOP
RAGTIME
RAGTOPS
RAGWEED
REGAINS
REGALED
REGALER
REGALES
REGALIA
REGALLY
REGARDS
REGATTA
REGAUGE
REGEARS
REGENCY
REGENTS
REGIFTS
REGILDS
REGIMEN
REGIMES
REGINAL
REGINAS
REGIONS
REGIRDS
REGIVEN
REGIVES
REGLAZE
REGLOSS
REGLOWS
REGLUED
REGLUES
REGNANT
REGNARD
REGNIER
REGRABS
REGRADE
REGRAFT
REGRANT
REGRAPH
REGRASP
REGREET
REGRESS
REGRETS
REGRIND
REGRIPS
REGROOM
REGROUP
REGROWN
REGROWS
REGUIDE
REGULAR
REGULUS
RIGGERS
RIGGING
RIGHTED
RIGHTER
RIGHTLY
RIGHTON
RIGIDLY
RIGOURS
RIGSOUT
RIGUEUR
RIGVEDA
ROGAINE
ROGERED
ROGUERY
ROGUING
ROGUISH
RUGGLES
RUGLIKE
RUGRATS

R••G•••

RAGGEDY
RAGGIER
RAGGIES
RAGGING
RANGERS
RANGFOR
RANGIER
RANGING
RANGOFF
RANGOON
RANGOUT
RAYGUNS
REAGANS
REAGENT
REIGNED
RIDGIER
RIDGING
RIDGWAY
RIEGERT
RIGGERS
RIGGING
RINGERS
RINGFOR
RINGING
RINGLET
RINGOFF
RINGOUT
RINGSIN
RINGSUP
RODGERS
ROTGUTS
ROUGHED
ROUGHEN
ROUGHER
ROUGHGO
ROUGHIT
ROUGHLY
ROUGHUP
ROUGING
ROYGBIV
RUGGLES
RUNGFOR
RUNGOFF
RUNGOUT
RUTGERS

R•••G••

RAINGOD
RAREGAS
RAVAGED
RAVAGER
RAVAGES
RAWEGGS
REARGUE
REBEGAN
REBEGIN
REBEGUN
RECAGED
RECAGES
REFIGHT
REFUGED
REFUGEE
REFUGES
RELIGHT
RENEGED
RENEGER
RENEGES
REPAGED
REPAGES
REPUGNS
RESIGHT
RESIGNS
REURGED
REURGES
REWAGER
RIOTGUN
RITAGAM
RONTGEN

R••••G•

RAGBAGS
RAGINGS
RAGRUGS
RAILAGE
RALEIGH
RAMPAGE
RATINGS
RAVINGS
RAWEGGS
REALIGN
REDALGA
REDDOGS
REDLEGS
REDRAGS
REDTAGS
REFLAGS
REFORGE
REGAUGE
REHANGS
REHINGE
REIMAGE
REJUDGE
REMERGE
RESINGS
RESTAGE
RESURGE
RETINGE
REVENGE
REWEIGH
RIBCAGE
RIDINGS
RISINGS
RODRIGO
ROOFAGE
ROOTAGE
ROUGHGO
ROVINGS
RULINGS
RUMMAGE

R•••••G

RACKING
RAFTING
RAGGING
RAIDING
RAILING
RAINING
RAISING
RAMMING
RAMPING
RANGING
RANKING
RANTING
RAPPING
RAPSONG
RASPING
RATEDPG
RATTING
RAZZING
RDLAING
READING
REAMING
REAPING
REARING
REAVING
REDDING
REDFLAG
REDKING
REDOING
REDWING
REDYING
REEDING
REEFING
REEKING
REELING
REEVING
REFFING
REFYING
REICING
REINING
RELYING
RENDING
RENTING
REPPING
RESTING
RETTING
REUSING
REVVING
RHYMING
RIBBING
RIDDING
RIDGING
RIFFING
RIFLING
RIFTING
RIGGING
RIKSDAG
RIMMING
RINGING
RINSING
RIOTING
RIPPING
RISKING
ROADHOG
ROAMING
ROARING
ROBBING
ROCKING
RODDING
ROGUING
ROILING
ROLFING
ROLLING
ROLVAAG
ROMBERG
ROMPING
ROOFING
ROOKING
ROOMING
ROOTING
ROTTING
ROUGING
ROUSING
ROUTING
ROWLING
RRATING
RSVPING
RUBBING
RUCHING
RUCKING
RUFFING
RUINING
RUNNING
RUSHING
RUSTING
RUTTING

•RG••••

ARGALIS
ARGANTE
ARGENTI
ARGENTO
ARGENTS
ARGONNE
ARGUERS
ARGUING
ARGUSES
ARGYLES
ERGOTIC
MRGREEN
ORGANDY
ORGANIC
ORGANZA
ORGEATS
ORGIAST
URGEDON
URGENCY
URGESON
URGINGS

•R•G•••

ARAGORN
ARIGATO
ARUGULA
BRAGGED
BRAGGER
BRIGADE
BRIGAND
BRIGHAM
BRIGHTS
BROGANS
BROGUES
CRAGGED
CRUGUET
DRAGEES
DRAGGED
DRAGGER
DRAGGLE
DRAGNET
DRAGOFF
DRAGONS
DRAGOON
DRAGOTI
DRAGOUT
DRAGSIN
DRAGSON
DRAGSUP
DREGION
DROGUES
DRUGGED
ERIGENA
FRAGGED
FRAGGLE
FRAGILE
FRIGATE
FRIGHTS
FROGGER
FROGLEG
FROGLET
FROGMAN
FROGMEN
GREGORY
GRIGRIS
OREGANO
ORIGAMI
ORIGINE
ORIGINS
OROGENY
PREGAIN
PREGAME
PROGENY
PROGRAM
TRAGEDY
TRIGGER
TRIGONS
TRIGRAM
URUGUAY
WRIGGLE
WRIGGLY
WRIGHTS
WRIGLEY

•R••G••

BRAGGED
BRAGGER
BRENGUN
BRIDGED
BRIDGER
BRIDGES
BRIDGET
BRINGER
BRINGIN
BRINGIT
BRINGON
BRINGTO
BRINGUP
BROUGHT
BRUEGEL
CRAGGED
CRAIGIE
CRINGED
CRINGES
CRYOGEN
DRAGGED
DRAGGER
DRAGGLE
DRAUGHT
DREDGED
DREDGER
DREDGES
DROUGHT
DRUDGED
DRUDGER
DRUDGES
DRUGGED
DRVEGAS
ERTEGUN
ERYNGOS
FRAGGED
FRAGGLE
FRAUGHT
FREIGHT
FRIDGES
FRINGED
FRINGES
FROGGER
FROOGLE
GRANGER
GRANGES
GRINGOS
GRUDGED
GRUDGER
GRUDGES
GRUNGER
GRUNGES
KRINGLE
KRUEGER
MRMAGOO
MRRIGHT
MRTIGER
ORANGES
ORANGEY
ORTEGAL
PREAGED
PREAGES
PRINGLE
PRONGED
TRAPGUN
TRIAGES
TRIGGER
TROUGHS
TRUDGED
TRUDGEN
TRUDGER
TRUDGES
WRANGEL
WRANGLE
WRIGGLE
WRIGGLY
WRINGER
WRONGED
WRONGER
WRONGLY
WROUGHT

•R•••G•

ARCINGS
ARLEDGE
ARRAIGN
ARRANGE
BRANAGH
BREWAGE
DRAYAGE
DRYFOGS
ERLANGS
FROMAGE
IRESIGN
IRONAGE
OROLOGY
PRESAGE
PRODIGY
PROLOGS
PROTEGE
TRILOGY
URGINGS
UROLOGY

•R••••G

ARCHING
AREARUG
ARGUING
ARISING
ARLBERG
ARTSONG
BRACING
BRAKING
BRAVING
BRAYING
BRAZING
BREWING
BRIBING
BRILLIG
BRINING
BRUXING
CRANING
CRAPING
CRATING
CRAVING
CRAZING
CREPING
CREWING
CROWING
DRAPING
DRAWING
DRAYING
DRIVING
DRONING
ERASING
ERELONG
ERODING
FRAMING
FRAYING
FREBERG
FREEING
FREITAG
FRELENG
FREYTAG
FRODING
FROGLEG
GRABBAG
GRACING
GRADING
GRATING
GRAVING
GRAYING
GRAYLAG
GRAZING
GREWBIG
GREYING
GREYLAG
GRIMING
GRIPING
GROPING
GROWBIG
GROWING
IRISING
IRONING
JREWING
MRWRONG
ORATING
PRATING
PRAYING
PRESONG
PREYING
PRICING
PRIDING
PRIMING
PRIZING
PROBING
PROLONG
PROSING
PROVING
PRUNING
RRATING
TRACING
TRADING
TREEING
TROWING
TRUEING
WRITING
XRATING
XRAYING

••RG•••

AIRGLOW
AIRGUNS
BARGAIN
BARGEIN
BARGERS
BARGING
BERGAMO
BERGERE
BERGIUS
BERGMAN
BERGSON
BORGIAS
BORGLUM
BURGEES
BURGEON
BURGERS
BURGESS
BURGHER
BURGLAR
BURGLED
BURGLES
BURGOOS
CARGOES
FARGOND
FARGONE
FORGAVE
FORGERS
FORGERY
FORGETS
FORGING
FORGIVE
FORGOER
FORGOES
FORGONE
FORGOOD
GARGLED
GARGLER
GARGLES
GORGERS
GORGING
GORGONS
GURGLED
GURGLES
JARGONS
JARGONY
JERGENS
JURGENS
LARGELY
LARGENT
LARGEOJ
LARGESS
LARGEST
LARGISH
LORGNON
MARGATE
MARGAUX
MARGERY
MARGINS
MARGRET
MERGEES
MERGERS

MERGING
MORGANA
MORGANS
MORGUES
OURGANG
PARGERS
PARGING
PERGOLA
PORGIES
PURGING
SARGENT
SORGHUM
SURGEON
SURGERY
SURGING
TARGETS
VERGEON
VERGERS
VERGING
VIRGATE
VIRGINS
VIRGOAN
VIRGULE
WARGAME
WARGODS

••R•G••

ALRIGHT
BAREGES
BERIGAN
BURPGUN
BYRIGHT
DARTGUN
DORIGHT
ENRAGED
ENRAGES
ENRIGHT
FARMGAL
FORAGED
FORAGER
FORAGES
FORDGTS
GARAGED
GARAGES
MIRAGES
MRRIGHT
PARAGON
PERIGEE
PERUGIA
PHRYGIA
PIROGEN
PIROGUE
RAREGAS
SCRAGGY
SCRUGGS
STREGIS
UNREGAL
UNRIGID
UPRIGHT
VIRAGOS

••R••G•

ABRIDGE
ACREAGE
AIRBAGS
AIRINGS
AIRLOGS
AIRRAGE
AIRSIGN
ARRAIGN
ARRANGE
BARRAGE
BORINGS
BOROUGH
BORZAGE
BURBAGE
CARNAGE
CARTAGE
CORDAGE
CORKAGE
CORSAGE
CORTEGE
DARKAGE
DERANGE
DURANGO
EARTAGS
EARWIGS
FARRAGO
FIRINGS
FOREIGN
GARBAGE
GARBAGY
HERBAGE
INRANGE
LORANGE
MARENGO
NORIEGA
PARINGS
PORTAGE
SARONGS
SCRAGGY
SCROOGE
SCRUGGS
SERFAGE
SPRINGS
SPRINGY
STRANGE
STRINGS
STRINGY
SYRINGE
THRONGS
THROUGH
TORTUGA
VERDUGO
VERTIGO
VORLAGE
WARPAGE
WIRINGS
WORDAGE
YARDAGE

••R•••G

BARBING
BARFBAG
BARGING
BARKING
BARNING
BARRING
BERMING
BIRDDOG
BIRDING
BIRLING
BIRRING
BORKING
BORLAUG
BURLING
BURNING
BURPING
BURRING
BURYING
CARDING
CARKING
CARLING
CARPING
CARTING
CARVING
CORDING
CORKING
CORNDOG
CORNING
CURBING
CURDING
CURLING
CURRING
CURSING
CURVING
DARLING
DARNING
DARTING
DERRING
DIRKING
DIRTBAG
DURNING
EARNING
EARPLUG
EARRING
FARCING
FARMING
FIREBUG
FIREDOG
FIRMING
FORCING
FORDING
FORELEG
FORGING
FORKING
FORMING
FURLING
FURLONG
FURRING
GARBING
GIRDING
GIRTING
GORGING
GORMING
HARBURG
HARDING
HARKING
HARMING
HARPING
HERDING
HERRING
HORDING
HORNING
HORNUNG
HORSING
HURLING
HURTING
JARRING
JERKING
JURYING
JURYRIG
LARDING
LARKING
LORDING
LURKING
MARKING
MARRING
MERGING
MORNING
NERVING
NURSING
OURGANG
OURSONG
PARGING
PARKING
PARRING
PARSING
PARTING
PERIWIG
PERKING
PERMING
PORKING
PORTING
PURGING
PURLING
PURRING
PURSING
SERIESG
SERLING
SERVING
SORTING
SURFING
SURGING
TARRING
TARTING
TERMING
TURFING
TURNING
VARYING
VERGING
VERSING
VERYBIG
WARBURG
WARDING
WARMING
WARNING
WARPING
WARRENG
WARRING
WARTHOG
WORDING
WORKING
WORMING
YARDING
YARNING
ZEROING

•••RG••

BOURGET
CHARGED
CHARGER
CHARGES
DEARGOD
EMERGED
EMERGES
EPERGNE
GEORGEC
GEORGEI
GEORGEM
GEORGES
GEORGEV
GEORGEW
GEORGIA
GEORGIC
GEORGIE
GIORGIO
GIORGOS
GLURGES
GUARGUM
HAIRGEL
IFORGET
IFORGOT
REARGUE
REURGED
REURGES
STURGES
TEARGAS
THURGAU
UNURGED

•••R•G•

AIRRAGE
AMERIGO
AVERAGE
BARRAGE
BIGRIGS
CATRIGS
COURAGE
DEFRAGS
FARRAGO
FTBRAGG
HEURIGE
INARAGE
MOORAGE
OILRIGS
OUTRAGE
OUTRIGS
OVERAGE
PEERAGE
RAGRUGS
REDRAGS
RODRIGO
STORAGE
SVERIGE
UMBRAGE
WETRAGS

•••R••G

ADORING
BARRING
BEARHUG
BEARING
BEERKEG
BEERMUG
BEHRING
BIRRING
BLARING
BURRING
CHARING
CURRING
DERRING
DOWRONG
EARRING
ENURING
ESTRING
FAIRING
FEARING
FLARING
FTBRAGG
FURRING
GEARING
GLARING
GOWRONG
GSTRING
HEARING
HERRING
INURING
JARRING
JEERING
KEYRING
LAIRING
LEERING
LOURING
MARRING
MITRING
MOORING
MRWRONG
NEARING
OILRING
OUTRANG
OUTRING
OVERBIG
OVERDOG
PAIRING
PARRING
PEERING
POURING
PURRING
REARING
ROARING
SCARING
SCORING
SEARING
SEBRING
SHARING
SHORING
SNARING
SNORING
SOARING
SOURING
SPARING
SPYRING
STARING
STARLOG
STORING
TARRING
TEARING
THERING
TIERING
TITRING
TOURING
UNWRUNG
VEERING
VIERZIG
WARRENG
WARRING
WEARING
YOURANG
ZIERING

••••RG•

AALARGE
ALLERGY
ATLARGE
AUBERGE
CINERGY
CYBORGS
DEBARGE
DEBURGH
DEFARGE
DEMERGE
DETERGE
DIVERGE
EMBARGO
ENGORGE
ENLARGE
FABERGE
IMMERGE
INLARGE
LAFARGE
LITURGY
NOMERGE
PANURGE
REFORGE
REMERGE
RESURGE
SCOURGE
SPLURGE
SUPERGS
SYNERGY
UNDERGO
UNLARGE
UNMERGE
UPSURGE
ZYMURGY

••••R•G

AREARUG
CUTARUG
DISHRAG
DUSTRAG
EDWARDG
JURYRIG
NONDRUG
OUTBRAG
OUTDRAG
PETFROG
SHAGRUG
THEFRUG
TOUAREG
WASHRAG

•••••RG

ARLBERG
FREBERG
HAMBURG
HARBURG
HOLBERG
HOMBURG
ICEBERG
LETTERG
LIMBURG
LONBORG
MCCLURG
MEGAERG
MOEBERG
NEWBURG
ROMBERG
SEABORG
WARBURG

RH•••••

RHEBOKS
RHENISH
RHENIUM
RHETORS
RHEUMIC
RHIZOME
RHODIAN
RHODIUM
RHOECUS
RHOMBIC
RHOMBUS
RHUBARB
RHUMBAS
RHYMERS
RHYMING
RHYMIST
RHYTHMS

R•H••••

REHANGS
REHAULS
REHEALS
REHEARD
REHEARS
REHEATS
REHEELS
REHIDES
REHINGE
REHIRED
REHIRES
REHITCH
REHONED
REHONES
REHONOR
REHOOKS
REHOUSE

R••H•••

RACHAEL
RAMHOME
RANHOME
RAPHAEL
RASHERS
RASHEST
RASHIDA
RATHOLE
RAWHIDE
RECHALK
RECHALL
RECHART
RECHECK
RECHEWS
RECHOSE
REDHAIR
REDHATS
REDHAWK
REDHEAD
REDHEAT
REDHENS
REDHOTS
REPHASE
REPHONE
RESHAPE
RESHARE
RESHAVE
RESHIFT
RESHINE
RESHIPS
RESHOES
RESHOOT
RESHOWN
RESHOWS
RESHUTS
RETHANK
RETHAWS
RETHINK
RICHARD
RICHENS
RICHEST
RICHLER
RICHMAN
RICHMEN
RICHTER
RIGHTED
RIGHTER
RIGHTLY
RIGHTON
ROCHETS
ROTHIRA
RUCHING
RUNHOME
RUSHDIE
RUSHEES
RUSHERS
RUSHIER
RUSHING
RUSHOFF
RUSHOUT
RUTHANN
RUTHFUL

R•••H••

RAGSHOP
RAINHAT
RALPHIE
RANCHED
RANCHER
RANCHES
RANCHOS
RATCHET
REACHED
REACHER
REACHES
REACHIN
REACHUP
REDCHIP
REUTHER
RHYTHMS
RIMSHOT
RITCHIE
ROACHES
ROADHOG
ROETHKE
ROSEHIP
ROUGHED
ROUGHEN
ROUGHER
ROUGHGO
ROUGHIT
ROUGHLY
ROUGHUP
RUMSHOP

R••••H•

RAUNCHY
REBATHE
REFIGHT
RELIGHT
RESIGHT
RICKSHA
ROYCOHN
RUPIAHS

R•••••H

RAFFISH
RALEIGH
RAMMISH
RANKISH
RANWITH
RASPISH
RATTISH
RAWFISH
REBEKAH
REBIRTH
REBRUSH
REDDISH
REDFISH
REFRESH
REGRAPH
REHITCH
RELATCH
REMATCH
REPATCH
RETEACH
RETOUCH
REWEIGH
REXROTH
RHENISH
ROBERTH
ROGUISH
ROMANSH
ROMPISH
ROOKISH
RUBBISH
RUDOLPH
RUNNETH
RUNTISH
RUNWITH
RUTTISH

•RH••••

MRHANEY
MRHOBBS
MRHORSE
MRHULOT

•R•H•••

ARCHAIC
ARCHERS
ARCHERY
ARCHEST
ARCHFOE
ARCHIES
ARCHING
ARCHIVE
ARCHONS
ARCHSEE
ARCHWAY
ARMHOLE
ARSHILE
ARTHURC
ARTHURM
ARTHURS
BRAHMAN
BRAHMAS
BRAHMIN
DRCHAOS
DRYHEAT
DRYHOLE
GRAHAME
GRAHAMS
MRCHIPS
ORCHARD
ORCHIDS
ORPHANS
ORPHANT
ORPHEAN
ORPHEUM
ORPHEUS
PREHEAL
PREHEAT
TRYHARD
URCHINS

•R••H••

ARACHNE
ARACHNO
ARTSHOP
ARTSHOW
BRASHER
BRASHES
BRASHLY
BRIGHAM
BRIGHTS
BROTHER
BRUSHED
BRUSHER
BRUSHES
BRUSHUP
CRASHAW
CRASHED
CRASHER
CRASHES
CRECHES
CROCHET
CRUSHED
CRUSHER
CRUSHES
DRACHMA
EREWHON
ERYTHRO
FRESHED
FRESHEN
FRESHER
FRESHES
FRESHET
FRESHLY
FRIGHTS
FROTHED
FROTHER
FROTHUP
GRAPHED
GRAPHIC
GRESHAM
GREYHEN
GRISHAM
GRYPHON
HRETHEL
IRISHER
KRISHNA
PRESHIP
PRESHOW
PREWHIP
PRITHEE
PROPHET
PROSHOP
PRUDHOE
TRACHEA
TRASHED
TRASHER
TRASHES
TRASHTV
TROCHEE
TROCHES
TROTHED
WRIGHTS
WRITHED
WRITHER
WRITHES

•R•••H•

ARAPAHO
ARDECHE
BRANCHY
BREATHE
BREATHS
BREATHY
BRIOCHE
BRONCHI
BRONCHO
BROUGHT
CRUNCHY
DRAUGHT
DROUGHT
FRAICHE
FRANCHI
FRAUGHT
FREIGHT
FRENCHI
FRENCHS
GROUCHO
GROUCHY
GROWTHS
MRMACHO
MRRIGHT
ORNITHO
PREACHY
TROUGHS
WRAITHS
WREATHE
WREATHS
WREATHY
WROUGHT

•R••••H

BRANAGH
BREADTH
BRINISH
BRITISH
BRUTISH
DRIESCH
DRONISH
DRTEETH
DRYWASH
ERDRICH
GRAYISH
GREYISH
MRMARCH
MRNORTH
MRSMITH
PRADESH
PREWASH
PRUDISH
TRIUMPH

••RH•••

AIRHEAD
AIRHOLE
AIRHORN
AIRHOSE
BARHOPS
CARHOPS
CARHORN
DIRHAMS
EARHART
EARHOLE
FORHIRE
HARHARS
MARHAUS
PERHAPS
TARHEEL
TERHUNE
UNRHYME
WARHAWK
WARHEAD
WARHERO

••R•H••

ABRAHAM
AIRSHIP
AIRSHOW
BERTHAS
BERTHED
BIRCHED
BIRCHEN
BIRCHES
BIRTHED
BURGHER
CARSHOW
EARSHOT
EARTHED
EARTHEN
EARTHLY
FARTHER
FIREHAT
FORDHAM
FORSHOW
FURTHER
GERSHON
GIRTHED
GURKHAS
HARDHAT
HARDHIT
HARSHEN
HARSHER
HARSHLY
HERSHEY
KERSHAW
LARCHEN
LARCHES
LURCHED
LURCHER
LURCHES
MARCHED
MARCHER
MARCHES
MARCHON
MARKHAM
MARSHAL
MARSHES
MERCHES

MORPHED
MORPHIC
MORPHIN
MURPHYS
MYRRHED
MYRRHIC
NARTHEX
NARWHAL
NORTHER
NORTHOF
PARCHED
PARCHES
PERAHIA
PERCHED
PERCHER
PERCHES
PERCHIK
PORCHES
PORTHOS
PYRRHIC
PYRRHUS
SORGHUM
TORCHED
TORCHER
TORCHES
VERYHIP
VERYHOT
WARSHIP
WARTHOG
WERNHER
WERTHER
WORSHIP
WORTHIT

••R••H•

ALRIGHT
ATROPHY
BORSCHT
BYRIGHT
DERECHO
DORIGHT
DOROTHY
EARACHE
ENRIGHT
GIRLSHY
HARRAHS
HURRAHS
JERICHO
KARACHI
LAROCHE
MRRIGHT
PARAPHS
PARIAHS
PIRANHA
PORSCHE
SERAPHS
STROPHE
TERAOHM
UPRIGHT
UTRECHT
VERYSHY
WORKSHY

••R•••H

ABROACH
AKRONOH
BOROUGH
BURNISH
CARWASH
CORINTH
CORNISH
CURRISH
DARKISH
DERVISH
EHRLICH
FORBUSH
FOREACH
FORSYTH
FURBISH
FURNISH
GARNISH
GIRLISH
HARBACH
HARDISH
HORNISH
INREACH
KURDISH
LARGISH
LARKISH
MIRISCH
MURDOCH
MURKISH
NERDISH
NKRUMAH
NORRISH
NORWICH
OGREISH
PARRISH
PERKISH
PORKISH
SCRATCH
SCREECH
SCRUNCH
SERIESH
STRETCH
STRITCH
TARNISH
TARTISH
THROUGH
TORYISH
TURKISH
UPREACH
VARNISH
WARMISH
WARPATH
WORMISH
YERKISH

•••RH••

BASRHIN
BEARHUG
MOORHEN
MYRRHED
MYRRHIC
OVERHOT
PYRRHIC
PYRRHUS

•••R•H•

ANARCHS
ANARCHY
CHURCHY
DEARTHS
EPARCHS
EPARCHY
EXARCHS
FOURTHS
HARRAHS
HEARTHS
HOORAHS
HURRAHS
MIZRAHI
STARCHY
SWARTHY

•••R••H

ALDRICH
BEARISH
BETROTH
BOARISH
BOORISH
BULRUSH
BUMRUSH
CHERISH
CURRISH
DELRUTH
DIGRAPH
ELDRICH
ERDRICH
FAIRISH
GOIRISH
HENRICH
INARUSH
INTRUTH
JOEROTH
MADRUSH
MOORISH
NEWRICH
NORRISH
NOURISH
OILRICH
OSTRICH
OUTRUSH
PARRISH
PHARAOH
POORISH
REBRUSH
REFRESH
REGRAPH
REXROTH
SOURISH
TIMROTH
UNTRUTH

••••R•H

ALWORTH
AUTARCH
BYBIRTH
DEBORAH
DEBURGH
FTWORTH
GOFORTH
HAWORTH
HOGARTH
INMARCH
JOMARCH
MENORAH
MONARCH
MRMARCH
MRNORTH
ONEARTH
REBIRTH
ROBERTH
UNBERTH
UNEARTH
UNFERTH
UNHARSH
UPNORTH

•••••RH

LETTERH

RI•••••

RIALTOS
RIANTLY
RIBALDS
RIBANDS
RIBBERS
RIBBIER
RIBBIES
RIBBING
RIBBONS
RIBBONY
RIBCAGE
RIBCUTS
RIBEYES
RIBLESS
RIBLETS
RIBLIKE
RIBMEAT
RIBPADS
RICARDO
RICHARD
RICHENS
RICHEST
RICHLER
RICHMAN
RICHMEN
RICHTER
RICKETY
RICKEYS
RICKLES
RICKMAN
RICKSHA
RICOTTA
RICRACS
RIDABLE
RIDDERS
RIDDICK
RIDDING
RIDDLED
RIDDLER
RIDDLES
RIDEBYS
RIDEOFF
RIDEOUT
RIDESBY
RIDESIN
RIDESTO
RIDESUP
RIDGIER
RIDGING
RIDGWAY
RIDINGS
RIDOTTO
RIEGERT
RIEMANN
RIESENS
RIESMAN
RIESSEN
RIFFING
RIFFLED
RIFFLER
RIFFLES
RIFLERS
RIFLERY
RIFLING
RIFTING
RIGGERS
RIGGING
RIGHTED
RIGHTER
RIGHTLY
RIGHTON
RIGIDLY
RIGOURS
RIGSOUT
RIGUEUR
RIGVEDA
RIKSDAG
RILEDUP
RILESUP
RILIEVO
RILLETS
RIMBAUD
RIMIEST
RIMLESS
RIMMING
RIMPLED
RIMPLES
RIMROCK
RIMSHOT
RINALDO
RINDIER
RINGERS
RINGFOR
RINGING
RINGLET
RINGOFF
RINGOUT
RINGSIN
RINGSUP
RINKRAT
RINSERS
RINSING
RIOLOBO
RIOMUNI
RIORDAN
RIORITA
RIOTACT
RIOTERS
RIOTGUN
RIOTING
RIOTOUS
RIPCORD
RIPENED
RIPENER
RIPIENI
RIPIENO
RIPINTO
RIPOFFS
RIPOPEN
RIPOSTE
RIPOSTS
RIPPERS
RIPPING
RIPPLED
RIPPLES
RIPPLET
RIPRAPS
RIPSAWN
RIPSAWS
RIPSOFF
RIPSONE
RIPSOUT
RIPSTOP
RIPTIDE
RIPTORN
RISENTO
RISESTO
RISESUP
RISIBLE
RISIBLY
RISINGS
RISKERS
RISKIER
RISKILY
RISKING
RISKSIT
RISOTTO
RISSOLE
RITAGAM
RITALIN
RITAMAE
RITARDS
RITCHIE
RITDYES
RITEAID
RITUALS
RITZIER
RITZILY
RIVALED
RIVALRY
RIVERPO
RIVETED
RIVETER
RIVIERA
RIVIERE
RIVULET
RIZZUTO

R•I••••

RAIDERS
RAIDING
RAILAGE
RAILBUS
RAILCAR
RAILERS
RAILING
RAILMAN
RAILMEN
RAILSAT
RAILSON
RAILWAY
RAIMENT
RAINBOW
RAINGOD
RAINHAT
RAINIER
RAINILY
RAINING
RAINMAN
RAINOUT
RAINSIN
RAINSON
RAISERS
RAISEUP
RAISING
RAISINS
RAISINY
RAISONS
REICING
REIFIED
REIFIES
REIGNED
REIMAGE
REIMPLY
REINDEX
REINING
REINKED
REINSIN
REISSUE
REITMAN
RHIZOME
ROILIER
ROILING
ROISTER
RUINATE
RUINERS
RUINING
RUINOUS

R••I•••

RABIDLY
RACIEST
RACINOS
RACISTS
RADIALS
RADIANS
RADIANT
RADIATE
RADICAL
RADICES
RADICLE
RADIOAD
RADIODJ
RADIOED
RADIOER
RADIOIN
RADIXES
RAGINGS
RAMINTO
RAMIREZ
RANINTO
RANITUP
RAPIDAN
RAPIDER
RAPIDLY
RAPIERS
RAPINES
RAPINIS
RARITAN
RATINES
RATINGS
RATIONS
RATITES
RAVINED
RAVINES
RAVINGS
RAVIOLI
RAWISTS
REAIMED
REAIRED
REBILLS
REBINDS
REBIRTH
RECIPES
RECITAL
RECITED
RECITER
RECITES
REDIALS
REFIGHT
REFILED
REFILES
REFILLS
REFILMS
REFINDS
REFINED
REFINER
REFINES
REFIRED
REFIRES
REFIXED
REFIXES
REGIFTS
REGILDS
REGIMEN
REGIMES
REGINAL
REGINAS
REGIONS
REGIRDS
REGIVEN
REGIVES
REHIDES
REHINGE
REHIRED
REHIRES
REHITCH
REKICKS
RELIANT
RELICTS
RELIEFS
RELIERS
RELIEVE
RELIGHT
RELIMIT
RELINED
RELINES
RELINKS
RELISTS
RELIVED
RELIVES
REMILLS
REMINDS
REMINED
REMINES
REMINTS
REMISED
REMISES
REMIXED
REMIXES
REOILED
REPICKS
REPINED
REPINER
REPINES
RERIDES
RERINSE
RERISEN
RERISES
RESIDED
RESIDER
RESIDES
RESIDUA
RESIDUE
RESIFTS
RESIGHT
RESIGNS
RESILED
RESILES
RESINED
RESINGS
RESINKS
RESISTS
RESITED
RESIZED
RESIZER
RESIZES
RETIARY
RETICLE
RETILED
RETILES
RETILLS
RETIMED
RETIMES
RETINAE
RETINAL
RETINAS
RETINGE
RETINOL
RETINTS
RETINUE
RETIRED
RETIREE
RETIRES
RETITLE
REVIEWS
REVILED
REVILER
REVILES
REVISAL
REVISED
REVISER
REVISES
REVISIT
REVISOR
REVITUP
REVIVAL
REVIVED
REVIVER
REVIVES
REWIDEN
REWINDS
REWIPED
REWIPES
REWIRED
REWIRES
RIDINGS
RIGIDLY
RILIEVO
RIMIEST
RIPIENI
RIPIENO
RIPINTO
RISIBLE
RISIBLY
RISINGS
RIVIERA
RIVIERE
ROPIEST
ROSIEST
ROSINED
ROTIFER
ROVINGS
RUBICON
RUBIOUS
RUBITIN
RUFIYAA
RULIEST
RULINGS
RUNINTO
RUNITUP
RUPIAHS
RUTILES
RUZICKA

R•••I••

RABBITS
RABBITT
RABBITY
RACKING
RAFFIAS
RAFFISH
RAFTING
RAGGIER
RAGGIES
RAGGING
RAGTIME
RAIDING
RAILING
RAINIER
RAINILY
RAINING
RAISING
RAISINS
RAISINY
RALEIGH
RALLIED
RALLIER
RALLIES
RAMLIKE
RAMMING
RAMMISH
RAMPING
RANDIER
RANGIER
RANGING
RANKINE
RANKING
RANKISH
RANRIOT
RANTING
RANWILD
RANWITH
RAPPING
RASHIDA
RASPIER
RASPING
RASPISH
RATFINK
RATLIKE
RATLINE
RATLINS
RATTIER
RATTING
RATTISH
RAWFISH
RAWHIDE
RAWLINS
RAWSILK
RAYLIKE
RAZZIES
RAZZING
RDLAING
READIED
READIER
READIES
READILY
READING
REALIGN
REALINE
REALISE
REALISM
REALIST
REALITY
REALIZE
REAMING
REAPING
REARING
REARISE
REAVING
REBAITS
REBOILS
REBUILD
REBUILT
RECEIPT
RECEIVE
RECLIMB
RECLINE
RECOILS
RECOINS
RECTIFY
REDBIRD
REDDING
REDDISH
REDFINS
REDFIRS
REDFISH
REDFIVE
REDKING
REDLINE
REDNINE
REDOING
REDPINE
REDRIED
REDRIES
REDRILL
REDRIVE
REDTIDE
REDTIES
REDWINE
REDWING
REDYING
REEDIER
REEDING
REEDITS
REEFIER
REEFING
REEKIER
REEKING
REELING
REEMITS
REEVICT
REEVING
REFFING
REFLIES
REFLIPS
REFRIED
REFRIES
REFYING
REGAINS
REGNIER
REGRIND
REGRIPS
REGUIDE
REICING
REIFIED
REIFIES
REINING
REJAILS
REJOICE
REJOINS
REKNITS
RELYING
REMAILS
REMAINS
RENAILS
RENDING
RENNINS
RENOIRS
RENTIER
RENTING
RENWICK
REPAINT
REPAIRS
REPLICA
REPLIED
REPLIER
REPLIES
REPOINT
REPPING
REPRICE
REPRIME
REPRINT
REPRISE
REPTILE
REQUIEM
REQUIRE
REQUITE
RERAISE
RESCIND
RESEIZE
RESHIFT
RESHINE
RESHIPS
RESOILS
RESPICE
RESPINS
RESPIRE
RESPITE
RESTICK
RESTING
RESTIRS
RESTIVE
RESUITS
RESWIMS
RETAILS
RETAINS
RETHINK
RETRIAL
RETRIED
RETRIES
RETRIMS
RETSINA
RETTING
RETWINE
RETWIST
REUNIFY
REUNION
REUNITE
REUSING
REVOICE
REVVING
REWEIGH
REWRITE
RHENISH
RHENIUM
RHODIAN
RHODIUM
RHYMING
RHYMIST
RIBBIER
RIBBIES
RIBBING
RIBLIKE
RIDDICK
RIDDING
RIDGIER
RIDGING
RIFFING
RIFLING
RIFTING
RIGGING
RIMMING
RINDIER
RINGING
RINSING
RIORITA
RIOTING
RIPPING
RIPTIDE
RISKIER
RISKILY
RISKING
RITZIER
RITZILY
RLSTINE
ROADIES
ROAMING
ROARING
ROBBING
ROBBINS
ROCKIER
ROCKIES
ROCKILY
ROCKING
RODDICK
RODDING
RODLIKE
RODRIGO
ROGAINE
ROGUING
ROGUISH
ROILIER
ROILING
ROLAIDS
ROLFING
ROLLICK
ROLLING
ROLLINS
ROMAINE
ROMAINS

ROMPING
ROMPISH
ROOFING
ROOKIER
ROOKIES
ROOKING
ROOKISH
ROOMIER
ROOMIES
ROOMILY
ROOMING
ROOTIER
ROOTING
RORAIMA
ROSSINI
ROTHIRA
ROTTING
ROUGING
ROUSING
ROUTINE
ROUTING
ROWDIER
ROWDIES
ROWDILY
ROWLING
RRATING
RSVPING
RUBBING
RUBBISH
RUBRICS
RUCHING
RUCKING
RUCTION
RUDDIED
RUDDIER
RUDDILY
RUFFIAN
RUFFING
RUGLIKE
RUINING
RUMMIES
RUNNIER
RUNNING
RUNRIOT
RUNTIER
RUNTIME
RUNTISH
RUNWILD
RUNWITH
RUSHIER
RUSHING
RUSSIAN
RUSTICS
RUSTIER
RUSTILY
RUSTING
RUTTIER
RUTTING
RUTTISH

R••••I•

RACEDIN
RADIOIN
RAINSIN
RAKEDIN
RAKESIN
RALPHIE
RAMBLIN
RAMEKIN
RANONIN
RAPINIS
RAREBIT
RATAFIA
RATTAIL
REACHIN
READMIT
READSIN
REAFFIX
REARLIT
REAUDIT
REAVAIL
REBEGIN
RECLAIM
RECRUIT
REDCHIP
REDEBIT
REDHAIR
REDSKIN
REDSUIT
REDTAIL
REELSIN
REEQUIP
REFRAIN
REGALIA
REINSIN
RELIMIT
RENUZIT
RENVOIS
REPOSIT
RESNAIS
RESPLIT
RESTAIN
RESTRIP
RESTSIN
RETRAIN
REVELIN
REVERIE
REVISIT
RHEUMIC
RHOMBIC
RIDESIN
RINGSIN
RISKSIT
RITALIN
RITCHIE
RITEAID
ROBOTIC
ROCKOIL
ROCKYII
ROCKYIV
ROLLEIS
ROLLSIN
ROMAJIS
ROMANIA
ROMANIC
ROMANIS
ROPEDIN
ROPESIN
ROSALIA
ROSALIE
ROSARIO
ROSEHIP
ROSEOIL
ROUBAIX
ROUGHIT
ROYGBIV
RUBITIN
RUMAKIS
RUMANIA
RUNONIN
RUSHDIE

R•••••I

RAMSESI
RAPANUI
RAVIOLI
RIOMUNI
RIPIENI
ROBERTI
ROCKYII
RONZONI
ROSSINI
RUDOLFI

•RI••••

ARIADNE
ARIANES
ARIDEST
ARIDITY
ARIETTA
ARIETTE
ARIGATO
ARIKARA
ARIOSOS
ARIOSTO
ARISING
ARISTAE
ARISTAS
ARISTOS
ARIZONA
BRIARDS
BRIBEES
BRIBERS
BRIBERY
BRIBING
BRICKED
BRICKLE
BRICKUP
BRIDALS
BRIDGED
BRIDGER
BRIDGES
BRIDGET
BRIDLED
BRIDLER
BRIDLES
BRIEFED
BRIEFER
BRIEFLY
BRIGADE
BRIGAND
BRIGHAM
BRIGHTS
BRILLIG
BRILLOS
BRIMFUL
BRIMLEY
BRIMMED
BRIMMER
BRINDLE
BRINERS
BRINGER
BRINGIN
BRINGIT
BRINGON
BRINGTO
BRINGUP
BRINIER
BRINING
BRINISH
BRINKER
BRIOCHE
BRIQUET
BRISKED
BRISKER
BRISKET
BRISKLY
BRISTLE
BRISTLY
BRISTOL
BRITAIN
BRITCOM
BRITISH
BRITNEY
BRITONS
BRITPOP
BRITTEN
BRITTLE
BRITTON
CRIBBED
CRIBBER
CRICKED
CRICKET
CRIEDUP
CRIESUP
CRIMEAN
CRIMINY
CRIMPED
CRIMPER
CRIMSON
CRINGED
CRINGES
CRINKLE
CRINKLY
CRIPPLE
CRISPED
CRISPEN
CRISPER
CRISPIN
CRISPIX
CRISPLY
CRISPUS
CRITIAS
CRITICS
CRITTER
CRITTUR
DRIBBLE
DRIBLET
DRIEDUP
DRIESCH
DRIESUP
DRIFTED
DRIFTER
DRIFTIN
DRIFTUP
DRILLED
DRILLER
DRINKER
DRINKIN
DRINKME
DRINKTO
DRINKUP
DRIPDRY
DRIPPAN
DRIPPED
DRIPPER
DRIPSON
DRISTAN
DRIVEAT
DRIVEBY
DRIVEIN
DRIVELS
DRIVERS
DRIVETO
DRIVEUP
DRIVING
DRIZZLE
DRIZZLY
ERICSON
ERIGENA
ERIKSON
ERINYES
ERISTIC
ERITREA
FRIABLE
FRIARLY
FRIBBLE
FRICKER
FRIDAYS
FRIDGES
FRIDLEY
FRIEDAN
FRIEDUP
FRIENDS
FRIESUP
FRIEZES
FRIGATE
FRIGHTS
FRIJOLE
FRILLED
FRINGED
FRINGES
FRISBEE
FRISEUR
FRISIAN
FRISKED
FRISKER
FRISSON
FRITTED
FRITTER
FRIVOLS
FRIZZED
FRIZZER
FRIZZES
FRIZZLE
FRIZZLY
GRIDDED
GRIDDER
GRIDDLE
GRIDMAP
GRIEVED
GRIEVER
GRIEVES
GRIFFEY
GRIFFIN
GRIFFON
GRIFTED
GRIFTER
GRIGRIS
GRILLED
GRILLER
GRILLES
GRIMACE
GRIMIER
GRIMILY
GRIMING
GRIMMER
GRIMSBY
GRINDER
GRINGOS
GRINKOV
GRINNED
GRINNER
GRINSAT
GRIPERS
GRIPING
GRIPPED
GRIPPER
GRIPPES
GRISHAM
GRISLET
GRISNEZ
GRISSOM
GRISTER
GRISTLE
GRISTLY
GRITTED
GRITTER
GRIZZLE
GRIZZLY
IRIDIUM
IRISHER
IRISING
IRISOUT
KRINGLE
KRISHNA
KRISTIN
MRISCAN
ORIENTE
ORIENTS
ORIFICE
ORIGAMI
ORIGINE
ORIGINS
ORINOCO
ORIOLES
ORISONS
PRICERS
PRICIER
PRICILY
PRICING
PRICKED
PRICKLE
PRICKLY
PRICKUP
PRIDING
PRIESTS
PRIMACY
PRIMARY
PRIMATE
PRIMELY
PRIMERA
PRIMERO
PRIMERS
PRIMING
PRIMMED
PRIMMER
PRIMPED
PRINCES
PRINGLE
PRINKED
PRINKER
PRINTAD
PRINTED
PRINTER
PRINTUP
PRIORTO
PRISONS
PRISSES
PRITHEE
PRIUSES
PRIVACY
PRIVATE
PRIVETS
PRIVIER
PRIVIES
PRIVILY
PRIVITY
PRIVYTO
PRIZING
PRIZZIS
TRIABLE
TRIADIC
TRIAGES
TRIBBLE
TRIBECA
TRIBORO
TRIBUNE
TRIBUTE
TRICEPS
TRICKED
TRICKER
TRICKLE
TRICORN
TRICOTS
TRIDENT
TRIEDIT
TRIEDON
TRIEDTO
TRIESIT
TRIESON
TRIESTE
TRIESTO
TRIFFID
TRIFLED
TRIFLER
TRIFLES
TRIFOLD
TRIFORM
TRIGGER
TRIGONS
TRIGRAM
TRIJETS
TRILLED
TRILLER
TRILLIN
TRILOGY
TRIMMED
TRIMMER
TRIMOFF
TRIMTAB
TRINARY
TRINITY
TRINKET
TRIODES
TRIOLET
TRIPLEA
TRIPLED
TRIPLES
TRIPLET
TRIPLEX
TRIPODS
TRIPOLI
TRIPPED
TRIPPER
TRIPPET
TRIPSON
TRIPSUP
TRIREME
TRISECT
TRISTAN
TRISTAR
TRITELY
TRITEST
TRITIUM
TRITONE
TRITONS
TRIUMPH
TRIVETS
TRIVIAL
TRIVIOT
TRIVIUM
WRIGGLE
WRIGGLY
WRIGHTS
WRIGLEY
WRINGER
WRINKLE
WRINKLY
WRITEIN
WRITEME
WRITEON
WRITERS
WRITETO
WRITEUP
WRITHED
WRITHER
WRITHES
WRITING
WRITTEN

•R•I•••

ARBITER
ARCINGS
ARNICAS
ARRIERE
ARRISES
ARRIVAL
ARRIVED
ARRIVER
ARRIVES
ARTICLE
ARTIEST
ARTISAN
ARTISTE
ARTISTS
BRAIDED
BRAIDER
BRAILLE
BRAINED
BRAINER
BRAISED
BRAISES
BROIDER
BROILED
BROILER
BRUISED
BRUISER
BRUISES
BRUITED
CRAIGIE
CRAISIN
CRUISED
CRUISER
CRUISES
DRAINED
DRAINER
DREIDEL
DREISER
DRUIDIC
DRYIDEA
ERMINED
ERMINES
ERMINIA
FRAICHE
FRAILER
FRAILLY
FRAILTY
FRAISES
FREIGHT
FREITAG
FRUITED
GRAINED
GRAINER
GROINED
MRFIXIT
MRRIGHT
MRTIBBS
MRTIGER
ORBISON
ORBITAL
ORBITED
ORBITER
ORDINAL
ORDINES
OREILLY
ORGIAST
ORNITHO
ORRISES
ORVIETO
ORVILLE
PRAIRIE
PRAISED
PRAISER
PRAISES
PREIDEA
PRFIRMS
PRYINTO
TRAILED
TRAILER
TRAINED
TRAINEE
TRAINER
TRAININ
TRAIPSE
TRAITOR
TREINTA
TREIZES
TROIKAS
TROILUS
TRUISMS
TRYITON
URGINGS
URSINUS
WRAITHS

•R••I••

ARABIAN
ARABICA
ARABICS
ARABIST
ARAMIDS
ARCHIES
ARCHING
ARCHIVE
ARCSINE
ARECIBO
ARETINO
ARGUING
ARIDITY
ARISING
ARMLIKE
ARMOIRE
ARMPITS
ARRAIGN
ARSHILE
ARTFILM
ARTSIER
BRACING
BRAKING
BRANIFF
BRASIER
BRASIZE
BRAVING
BRAYING
BRAZIER
BRAZING
BREVITY
BREWING
BRIBING
BRINIER
BRINING
BRINISH
BRITISH
BRODIES
BROMIDE
BROMINE
BRUTISH
BRUXING
BRUXISM
CRANIAL
CRANING
CRANIUM
CRAPING
CRATING
CRATION
CRAVING
CRAZIER
CRAZIES
CRAZILY
CRAZING
CREDITS
CREMINI
CREPING
CRETINS
CREVICE
CREWING
CRIMINY
CRITIAS
CRITICS
CRONIES
CROSIER
CROWING
CROZIER
CRUCIAL
CRUDITY
DRAPING
DRAWING
DRAYING
DREGION
DRFRIST
DRIVING
DRONING
DRONISH
DROPINS
DROXIES
DRQUINN
DRUZIAN
ERASING
ERDRICH
EREMITE
ERODING
EROSION
EROSIVE
EROTICA
EROTICS
ERSKINE
ERUDITE
FRAGILE
FRAMING
FRASIER
FRAYING
FRAZIER
FREEING
FRISIAN
FRODING
FROLICS
GRACIAS
GRACILE
GRACING
GRADING
GRANITA
GRANITE
GRAPIER
GRATIAS
GRATIFY
GRATING
GRAVIES
GRAVING
GRAVITY
GRAYING
GRAYISH
GRAZIER
GRAZING
GRECIAN
GRECISM
GRECIZE
GREYING
GREYISH
GRIMIER
GRIMILY
GRIMING
GRIPING
GRODIER
GROLIER
GROPING
GROPIUS
GROTIUS
GROWING
GRUNION
IRANIAN
IRENICS
IRESIGN
IRIDIUM
IRISING
IRONIES
IRONING
IRONIST
JREWING
KRATION
MRBLISS
MRCHIPS
MRQUILP
MRSMITH
ORACIES
ORALIST
ORARION
ORARIUM
ORATING
ORATION
ORBLIKE
ORCHIDS
ORDAINS
ORIFICE
ORIGINE
ORIGINS
PRALINE
PRATING
PRAYING
PREBIDS
PREBILL
PREBIND
PRECISE
PRECITE
PREDICT
PREDIET
PREDIVE
PREFILE
PRELIFE
PRELIMS
PREMIER
PREMIES
PREMISE
PREMISS
PREMIUM
PRERIOT
PRESIDE
PRESIFT
PRETIRE
PREVIAS
PREVIEW
PREWIRE
PREWITT
PREXIES
PREYING
PRICIER
PRICILY
PRICING
PRIDING
PRIMING
PRIVIER
PRIVIES
PRIVILY
PRIVITY
PRIZING
PROBIES
PROBING
PROBITY
PROCITY
PRODIGY
PROFILE
PROFITS
PROLIFE
PROMISE
PROSIER
PROSILY
PROSING
PROTIST
PROVIDE
PROVINE
PROVING
PROVISO
PROXIES
PROXIMA
PROXIMO
PRUDISH
PRUNING
QRATIOS
RRATING
TRACING
TRADING
TREDIAS
TREEING
TREVINO
TRINITY
TRITIUM
TRIVIAL
TRIVIOT
TRIVIUM
TROPICS
TROPISM
TROWING
TRUEING
URACILS
URANITE
URANIUM
URCHINS
URNLIKE
WRITING
XRATING
XRAYING

•R•••I•

ARAMAIC
ARANEID
ARCADIA
ARCHAIC
ARGALIS
ARMENIA
ARSENIC
ARSENIO
ARTEMIS
ARTERIO
ARTFAIR
BRAHMIN
BRASSIE
BREAKIN
BRESCIA
BRESLIN
BRILLIG
BRINGIN
BRINGIT
BRITAIN
BROKEIN

BROWNIE
CRAIGIE
CRAISIN
CRAMSIN
CRAPPIE
CREEPIN
CREPTIN
CRESPIN
CRISPIN
CRISPIX
CROATIA
CROQUIS
CROSTIC
CROWDIN
CRYPTIC
DRAGSIN
DRANKIN
DRASTIC
DRAWNIN
DRAWSIN
DREAMIN
DRESSIN
DRIFTIN
DRINKIN
DRIVEIN
DRMARIO
DROPSIN
DROPSIT
DROVEIN
DRUIDIC
DRUMLIN
DRYADIC
DRYSUIT
ERGOTIC
ERISTIC
ERMINIA
ERRATIC
FRANCIS
FRANKIE
FRANTIC
FREDDIE
FREDRIC
FREEAIR
FREEBIE
FREESIA
GRANNIE
GRAPHIC
GREMLIN
GREWBIG
GREWDIM
GRIFFIN
GRIGRIS
GROOVIN
GROUPIE
GROWBIG
GROWDIM
HRYVNIA
KRAMNIK
KREMLIN
KRESKIN
KRISTIN
MRFIXIT
MRMUSIC
MRSMUIR
ORATRIX
ORDERIN
ORECTIC
ORGANIC
PRACTIC
PRAIRIE
PREACID
PREBOIL
PRECOIL
PREEDIT
PREEMIE
PREGAIN
PREOMIT
PREPAID
PREPPIE
PRESHIP
PRETRIM
PREVAIL
PREVOID
PREWHIP
PRIZZIS
PROMBID
PROSAIC
PROTEIN
PROVEIT
PRUSSIA
TRADEIN
TRAFFIC
TRAININ
TRANSIT
TRAVAIL
TREFOIL
TREKKIE
TRELLIS
TRIADIC
TRIEDIT
TRIESIT
TRIFFID
TRILLIN
TROMPIN
TROOPIN
TRUERIB
TRUSTIN
TRYSAIL
URBANII
URBANIV
WRITEIN
WROTEIN

•R••••I

ARACARI
ARGENTI
BREWSKI
BRONCHI
CREMINI
DRAGOTI
DRMELFI
FRANCHI
FRENCHI
FRENESI
ORIGAMI
TRIPOLI
URBANII
URBANVI

••RI•••

ABRIDGE
ABRILES
ACRIDLY
ADRIANA
AERIALS
AERIEST
AFRICAN
AGRIBIZ
AGRIPPA
AIRIEST
AIRINGS
ALRIGHT
AMRITAS
APRICOT
APRIORI
ARRIERE
ARRISES
ARRIVAL
ARRIVED
ARRIVER
ARRIVES
ATRIUMS
AURICLE
AURISTS
BARISTA
BARITES
BERIGAN
BIRIANI
BORIDES
BORINGS
BURIALS
BURIERS
BYRIGHT
CARIBES
CARIBOO
CARIBOU
CARINAE
CARINAS
CARIOCA
CARIOLE
CARIOUS
CCRIDER
CERISES
CHRISMS
CHRISOM
CHRISTA
CHRISTI
CHRISTO
CHRISTY
CORINNE
CORINTH
CURIOSA
CURIOUS
DARIUSI
DERIDED
DERIDER
DERIDES
DERIVED
DERIVER
DERIVES
DORIGHT
DORITOS
EERIEST
ENRIGHT
ENRIQUE
FARINAS
FIRINGS
FORINTS
FTRILEY
FURILLO
FURIOSO
FURIOUS
GERITOL
GORIEST
GORILLA
HARICOT
HERITOR
HORIZON
JERICHO
JERILYN
JERITZA
JURIDIC
JURISTS
KURILES
LARIATS
LORIENT
LORISES
LURIDLY
LYRICAL
LYRICON
LYRISTS
MARIANA
MARIANO
MARIDAS
MARIDOS
MARILLA
MARILYN
MARIMBA
MARINAS
MARINER
MARINES
MARITAL
MERIDEN
MERIMEE
MERINOS
MERITED
MIRIEST
MIRISCH
MORISOT
MRRIGHT
MURIELS
MURILLO
MYRIADS
NERISSA
NORIEGA
NORITES
ORRISES
PARIAHS
PARIBUS
PARINGS
PERIAPT
PERIDOT
PERIGEE
PERILED
PERIODS
PERISSA
PERITUS
PERIWIG
PORIVER
PURISTS
PURITAN
PYRITES
PYRITIC
RARITAN
RERIDES
RERINSE
RERISEN
RERISES
SCRIBED
SCRIBER
SCRIBES
SCRIMPS
SCRIMPY
SCRIPPS
SCRIPTS
SERIALS
SERIATE
SERIESE
SERIESF
SERIESG
SERIESH
SERIESI
SERIESJ
SERIESK
SERIOUS
SERIPAK
SHRIEKS
SHRIKES
SHRILLS
SHRILLY
SHRIMPS
SHRIMPY
SHRINED
SHRINER
SHRINES
SHRINKS
SHRIVEL
SHRIVER
SHRIVES
SORIANO
SPRIEST
SPRINGS
SPRINGY
SPRINTS
SPRITES
STRIATE
STRIDER
STRIDES
STRIFES
STRIKER
STRIKES
STRINGS
STRINGY
STRIPED
STRIPER
STRIPES
STRIPOF
STRITCH
STRIVED
STRIVEN
STRIVER
STRIVES
SURIMIS
SURINAM
SYRIANA
SYRIANS
SYRINGE
TARIFFS
THRIFTS
THRIFTY
THRILLA
THRILLS
THRIVED
THRIVEN
THRIVER
THRIVES
TORINOS
TURISMO
TURISTA
UNRIGID
UNRILED
UNRIMED
UNRIPER
UNRISEN
UNRISKY
UNRIVED
UNRIVEN
UPRIGHT
UPRISEN
UPRISER
UPRISES
UPRIVER
UTRILLO
VARIANT
VARIATE
VARIERS
VARIETY
VARIOUS
VARITEK
VERIDIC
VERIEST
VERISMO
VERISTS
VERITAS
VERIZON
WARIEST
WIRIEST
WIRINGS

••R•I••

AIRBILL
AIRKISS
AIRLIFT
AIRLIKE
AIRLINE
AIRMILE
AIRSICK
AIRSIGN
AIRTIME
AIRWICK
ARRAIGN
BARBIES
BARBILL
BARBING
BARGING
BARKIER
BARKING
BARLICK
BARMIER
BARNING
BARRIER
BARRING
BARRIOS
BERBICK
BERGIUS
BERLIOZ
BERLITZ
BERMING
BERNINA
BERNINI
BERRIED
BERRIES
BERWICK
BIRDIED
BIRDIES
BIRDING
BIRLING
BIRRING
BORGIAS
BORKING
BURDICK
BURKINA
BURLIER
BURLING
BURNING
BURNISH
BURPING
BURRIER
BURRING
BURRITO
BURYING
CARBIDE
CARBINE
CARDIAC
CARDIAL
CARDIFF
CARDING
CARDIUM
CARKING
CARLING
CARMINA
CARMINE
CARNIES
CARPING
CARRIED
CARRIER
CARRIES
CARTIER
CARTING
CARTIRE
CARVING
CERTIFY
CERVIDS
CERVINE
CORDIAL
CORDIAS
CORDING
CORDITE
CORKIER
CORKING
CORNICE
CORNIER
CORNILY
CORNING
CORNISH
CORRIDA
CORSICA
CORTICO
CORTINA
CORVIDS
CORVINA
CORVINE
CORZINE
CURBING
CURDIER
CURDING
CURLIER
CURLIKE
CURLING
CURRIED
CURRIER
CURRIES
CURRING
CURRISH
CURSING
CURSIVE
CURTISS
CURVIER
CURVING
DARKISH
DARLING
DARNING
DARTING
DERAILS
DERBIES
DERNIER
DERRICK
DERRICO
DERRIDA
DERRING
DERVISH
DIRKING
DIRTIED
DIRTIER
DIRTIES
DIRTILY
DORKIER
DORMICE
DURNING
EARLIER
EARLIES
EARLIKE
EARNING
EARRING
EARWIGS
EHRLICH
FARCING
FARMING
FARRIER
FARSIDE
FERMION
FERMIUM
FERNIER
FERRIED
FERRIES
FERRITE
FERTILE
FIREICE
FIRKINS
FIRMING
FIRRIER
FORBIDS
FORCING
FORDING
FOREIGN
FORGING
FORGIVE
FORHIRE
FORKIER
FORKING
FORLIFE
FORMICA
FORMING
FORSIZE
FORTIES
FORTIFY
FORTIUS
FURBISH
FURLING
FURNISH
FURRIER
FURRING
FURTIVE
GARBING
GARLICS
GARLITS
GARNISH
GARPIKE
GARRICK
GERAINT
GERBILS
GERMIER
GIRDING
GIRLIER
GIRLIES
GIRLISH
GIRTING
GORDIAN
GORDITA
GORDIUS
GORGING
GORMING
GORSIER
HARDIER
HARDILY
HARDING
HARDISH
HARKING
HARLINE
HARMING
HARNICK
HARPIES
HARPING
HARPIST
HARRIED
HARRIER
HARRIES
HARRIET
HERBIER
HERDING
HEREIAM
HERMITS
HERNIAE
HERNIAS
HERNIBS
HEROICS
HEROINE
HEROISM
HERRICK
HERRING
HERRIOT
HIRCINE
HORDING
HORNIER
HORNING
HORNISH
HORNIST
HORRIFY
HORSIER
HORSILY
HORSING
HORVITZ
HURLING
HURRIED
HURRIER
HURRIES
HURTING
IGRAINE
INRUINS
JARDINE
JARDINS
JARRING
JERKIER
JERKIES
JERKILY
JERKING
JERKINS
JURYING
KURDISH
LARAINE
LARDIER
LARDING
LARGISH
LARKIER
LARKING
LARKINS
LARKISH
LORDING
LORRIES
LURKING
MARDIAN
MARGINS
MARKIII
MARKING
MARLIER
MARLINS
MARMION
MARNIER
MARRIED
MARRIES
MARRING
MARTIAL
MARTIAN
MARTINA
MARTINI
MARTINO
MARTINS
MARTINU
MARTINV
MARTIUS
MARVIER
MARXIAN
MARXISM
MARXIST
MERCIAN
MERCIES
MERGING
MERLINS
MERRIAM
MERRICK
MERRIER
MERRILL
MERRILY
MORAINE
MORNING
MORTICE
MORTIFY
MORTISE
MURKIER
MURKILY
MURKISH
NERDIER
NERDISH
NEREIDS
NERVIER
NERVILY
NERVINE
NERVING
NORDICA
NORDICS
NORRISH
NORWICH
NURSING
OARLIKE
OGREISH
PARAIBA
PARFIVE
PARGING
PARKING
PARKINS
PARRIED
PARRIER
PARRIES
PARRING
PARRISH
PARSING
PARTIAL
PARTIED
PARTIER
PARTIES
PARTIII
PARTING
PARTITA
PARTITE
PERDIDO
PERDIEM
PERDITA
PERFIDY
PERKIER
PERKILY
PERKING
PERKINS
PERKISH
PERLITE
PERMIAN
PERMING
PERMITS
PERRIER
PERRINE
PERRINS
PERSIAN
PERSIST
PERSIUS
PORCINE
PORGIES
PORKIER
PORKING
PORKISH
PORTICO
PORTING
PORTION
PURGING
PURLIEU
PURLING
PURRING
PURSIER
PURSING
PURTIER
PURVIEW
RERAISE
RORAIMA
SARDINE
SERBIAN
SERLING
SERPICO
SERVICE
SERVILE
SERVING
SORDINI
SORDINO
SORRIER
SORRILY
SORTIED
SORTIES
SORTING
SORVINO
SPRAINS
STRAINS
STRAITS
SUREIAM
SUREIDO
SURFIER
SURFING
SURGING
SURLIER
SURLILY
SURMISE
SURVIVE
TARDIER
TARDILY
TARNISH
TAROILS
TARPITS
TARRIED
TARRIER
TARRIES
TARRING
TARTIER
TARTILY
TARTING
TARTISH
TERBIUM
TERMING
TERMINI
TERMITE
TERRIER
TERRIES
TERRIFY
TERRINE
TIRPITZ
TOROIDS
TORSION
TORVILL
TORYISH
TORYISM
TURBINE
TURFIER
TURFING
TURKISH
TURNING
TURNIPS
UKRAINE
UNRAINY
UPRAISE
VARMINT
VARNISH
VARRICK
VARSITY
VARYING
VERBIDS
VERBIFY
VERDICT
VERDINS
VEREINE
VERGING
VERMINY
VERNIER
VERSIFY
VERSING
VERSION
VERTIGO
VERYILL
VIRGINS
WARDING
WARLIKE
WARMING
WARMISH
WARNING
WARPING
WARRING
WARRIOR
WARTIER
WARTIME
WARWICK
WORDIER
WORDILY
WORDING
WORKING
WORMIER
WORMING
WORMISH
WORRIED
WORRIER
WORRIES
YARDING
YARNING
YERKISH
YORKIES
YORKIST
ZERNIKE
ZEROING

••R••I•

ACRYLIC
AEROBIC
AGRIBIZ
AIRDRIE
AIRFOIL
AIRMAIL
AIRRAID
AIRSHIP
AMRADIO
BARGAIN
BARGEIN
BARMAID
BERVOIX
BORODIN
BOROMIR
BORONIC
BORZOIS
BURNSIN
BURNTIN
BURSTIN
BYRONIC
CARAMIA
CAROLII
CAROTID
CAROTIN
CARRYIN
CARTRIP
CARTSIN
CBRADIO
CERAMIC
CERTAIN

CHROMIC
CHRONIC
CIRCUIT
CORNBIN
CORNOIL
CORSAIR
CORVAIR
CURLSIN
CURTAIL
CURTAIN
CYRUSII
EARCLIP
EARNSIT
ERRATIC
ETRURIA
EURASIA
FARMAID
FIRELIT
FIREPIT
FMRADIO
FORABIT
FORCEIN
FORFEIT
FORTDIX
GERMAIN
GERVAIS
HARDHIT
HARDSIX
HEREDIA
HERETIC
HORATIO
HORNSIN
JAROMIR
JURIDIC
JURYRIG
KERATIN
KIRSTIE
KORANIC
LARAMIE
LORDJIM
LORDSIT
LUREDIN
LURESIN
MARKIII
MARKVII
MARQUIS
MARRYIN
MERMAID
MORANIS
MORAVIA
MORONIC
MORPHIC
MORPHIN
MYRRHIC
PARBOIL
PARFAIT
PARKSIT
PARODIC
PAROTID
PARSNIP
PARTIII
PERAHIA
PERATIO
PERCHIK
PERIWIG
PERSEID
PERTAIN
PERUGIA
PHRENIC
PHRYGIA
PIRATIC
PORKPIE
PURLOIN
PURSUIT
PYRAMID
PYRETIC
PYREXIA
PYRITIC
PYRRHIC
RAREBIT
SERAPIS
SIRLOIN
STRAPIN
STREGIS
SURFEIT
SURIMIS
SURVEIL
TERRAIN
TERROIR
THREWIN
THROWIN
TURMOIL
TURNSIN
UNRIGID
VERIDIC
VERMEIL
VERONIA
VERYBIG
VERYFIT
VERYHIP
WAREPIC
WARSHIP
WIREDIN
WIRESIN
WORKSIN
WORSHIP
WORTHIT
XEROSIS
XEROTIC
XMRADIO
ZEROSIN

••R•••I

ABRUZZI
AIRTAXI
APRIORI
BERNINI
BIRIANI
BIRYANI
BORDONI
BURUNDI
CAROLII
CHRISTI
CORELLI
CYRUSII
DARIUSI
FAROUKI
FERRARI
FORLANI
HAROLDI
HERNANI
ISRAELI
KARACHI
KAROLYI
LORELAI
LORELEI
MARCONI
MARKIII
MARKVII
MARTINI
MORETTI
PARASKI
PARTIII
PERETTI
PIRELLI
SERIESI
SORDINI
STRETTI
TERMINI
TORTONI
TURFSKI
XERXESI

•••RI••

ACARIDS
ADORING
AGARICS
ALDRICH
ALLRISE
AMBRIES
AMERICA
AMERIGO
AMERIKA
AMERIND
AMORIST
ANGRIER
ANGRILY
APERIES
APPRISE
ASCRIBE
ASTRIDE
ATHRILL
ATTRITE
ATTRITS
AVARICE
AVERILL
AZORIAN
AZURITE
BARRIER
BARRING
BARRIOS
BBQRIBS
BEARING
BEARISH
BEERIER
BEGRIME
BEHRING
BERRIED
BERRIES
BIGRIGS
BIRRING
BLARING
BLERIOT
BOARISH
BOHRIUM
BOORISH
BURRIER
BURRING
BURRITO
BUSRIDE
CABRIDE
CABRINI
CABRIOS
CAPRICE
CAPRINE
CARRIED
CARRIER
CARRIES
CATRIGS
CHARIER
CHARILY
CHARING
CHARIOT
CHARITY
CHERISH
CHIRICO
CHORINE
CHORIST
CHORIZO
CITRINE
CLARICE
CLARIFY
CLARION
CLARITY
CLERICS
CLERISY
CONRIED
CORRIDA
COURIER
COWRIES
COWRITE
CUPRITE
CURRIED
CURRIER
CURRIES
CURRING
CURRISH
CYMRICS
CYPRIAN
CYPRIOT
CZARINA
CZARISM
CZARIST
DAIRIES
DATRILS
DEARIES
DEBRIEF
DECRIED
DECRIER
DECRIES
DEPRIVE
DERRICK
DERRICO
DERRIDA
DERRING
DEVRIES
DIARIES
DIARIOS
DIARIST
DIORITE
DOTRICE
DOWRIES
DRFRIST
EARRING
EGERIAS
ELDRICH
ELDRICK
EMERIES
EMERITA
EMERITI
EMPRISE
ENPRISE
ENTRIES
ENURING
ERDRICH
ESPRITS
ESTRING
EWERIES
FABRICS
FABRIZI
FAERIES
FAIRIES
FAIRING
FAIRISH
FARRIER
FEARING
FEBRILE
FERRIED
FERRIES
FERRITE
FEVRIER
FIBRINS
FIERIER
FIERILY
FIORINA
FIRRIER
FLARING
FLORIAN
FLORIDA
FLORINS
FLORIST
FOURIER
FURRIER
FURRING
GABRIEL
GARRICK
GEARING
GEDRICK
GLARING
GLORIAS
GLORIED
GLORIES
GLORIFY
GOIRISH
GSTRING
HADRIAN
HAIRIER
HARRIED
HARRIER
HARRIES
HARRIET
HAYRICK
HAYRIDE
HEARING
HENRICH
HENRIES
HERRICK
HERRING
HERRIOT
HEURIGE
HOARIER
HOARILY
HORRIFY
HURRIED
HURRIER
HURRIES
HYBRIDS
HYDRIDE
IATRICS
IBERIAN
ICERINK
IMPRINT
INBRIEF
INPRINT
INURING
ISTRIAN
IVORIAN
IVORIES
IVORINE
JARRING
JEERING
JIMRICE
JOYRIDE
KATRINA
KATRINE
KEYRING
KIARIOS
KUBRICK
LACRIMO
LAIRING
LATRINE
LAURITZ
LEERIER
LEERILY
LEERING
LETRIDE
LORRIES
LOURING
LOWRISE
LOWRISK
MANRICO
MARRIED
MARRIES
MARRING
MAURIAC
MAURIAT
MAURICE
MCBRIDE
MCGRIFF
MEGRIMS
MERRIAM
MERRICK
MERRIER
MERRILL
MERRILY
METRICS
METRIST
MIDRIBS
MIDRIFF
MIDRISE
MITRING
MOORIER
MOORING
MOORISH
MOTRINS
NATRIUM
NEARING
NEWRICH
NITRIDE
NITRIFY
NITRITE
NORRISH
NOURISH
NUTRIAS
OCARINA
ODORIZE
OILRICH
OILRIGS
OILRING
ONTRIAL
ORARION
ORARIUM
OSIRIAN
OSTRICH
OTARIES
OUTRIBS
OUTRIDE
OUTRIGS
OUTRING
OVARIES
OVERICE
PAIRING
PAPRIKA
PARRIED
PARRIER
PARRIES
PARRING
PARRISH
PATRICE
PATRICK
PATRIES
PATRIOT
PEERING
PEORIAN
PERRIER
PERRINE
PERRINS
PETRIFY
PIERIAN
PODRIDA
POORISH
POURING
PRERIOT
PUERILE
PURRING
QUERIDA
QUERIDO
QUERIED
QUERIER
QUERIES
QUERIST
RANRIOT
REARING
REARISE
REDRIED
REDRIES
REDRILL
REDRIVE
REFRIED
REFRIES
REGRIND
REGRIPS
REPRICE
REPRIME
REPRINT
REPRISE
RETRIAL
RETRIED
RETRIES
RETRIMS
REWRITE
RIORITA
ROARING
RODRIGO
RUBRICS
RUNRIOT
SABRINA
SAURIAN
SCARIER
SCARIFY
SCARILY
SCARING
SCORIAS
SCORING
SEARING
SEBRING
SHARING
SHERIFF
SHERIFS
SHORING
SNARING
SNORING
SOARING
SORRIER
SORRILY
SOURING
SOURISH
SPARING
SPIRIER
SPIRITS
SPYRING
STARING
STARION
STERILE
STORIED
STORIES
STORING
SUNRISE
SVERIGE
TARRIED
TARRIER
TARRIES
TARRING
TAURINE
TEARIER
TEARILY
TEARING
TERRIER
TERRIES
TERRIFY
TERRINE
THERIAC
THERING
THERINK
THERITZ
THORIUM
TIERING
TIMRICE
TITRING
TOURING
TOURISM
TOURIST
TSARINA
TSARISM
TSARIST
TUGRIKS
TZARINA
UMBRIAN
UMBRIEL
UNBRIEF
UNCRIED
UNDRIED
UNFRIED
UNFRILL
UNGRIPS
UNTRIED
UNTRITE
UPDRIED
UPDRIES
UPDRIFT
USERIDS
USURIES
UXORIAL
VANRIJN
VARRICK
VEERIES
VEERING
VITRICS
VITRIFY
VITRINE
VITRIOL
WARRING
WARRIOR
WEARIED
WEARIER
WEARIES
WEARILY
WEARING
WORRIED
WORRIER
WORRIES
YTTRIAS
YTTRIUM
ZAIRIAN
ZEBRINE
ZIERING

•••R•I•

ACERBIC
AIRRAID
ANDROID
ANEROID
BAHRAIN
BAHREIN
BASRHIN
BEARPIT
BEDRAIL
BYTRAIN
CARRYIN
CHARLIE
CHARMIN
CHARNIN
CHERVIL
DEARSIR
DEORBIT
DETRAIN
DETROIT
DHARMIC
DHURRIE
DOORDIE
ELTRAIN
EMBROIL
ENGRAIN
ENTRAIN
EPHRAIM
EXORDIA
EXURBIA
FIBROID
FJORDIC
FOURPIN
GEORGIA
GEORGIC
GEORGIE
GHERKIN
GIORGIO
HAIRPIN
HEBRAIC
HENREID
HENRYII
HENRYIV
INERTIA
INGRAIN
INORBIT
INTROIT
MARRYIN
MAUROIS
MYRRHIC
OBERLIN
OCHROID
OCTROIS
OUTRAIL
OVERBID
OVERBIG
OVERDID
OVERFIT
OVERFIX
OVERLIE
OVERLIT
OVERMIX
OVERTIP
PADRAIC
PEERSIN
POURSIN
PYRRHIC
QUARTIC
REARLIT
RECRUIT
REFRAIN
RETRAIN
SCARWID
SCORPIO
SHAREIN
SHARPIE
SHERWIN
SHORTIE
SPORTIN
STARLIT
STARSIN
STARTIN
STCROIX
STEROID
STIRSIN
STORMIN
SWOREIN
TEARSIT
TERRAIN
TERROIR
THEREIN
THERMIC
THYROID
TIMREID
UNBRAID
UNFRAIL
UPBRAID
VIERZIG
WHEREIN
YOUREIT
ZEBRAIC
ZEBROID

•••R••I

CABRINI
EMERITI
FABRIZI
FERRARI
GEORGEI
GOURAMI
GUARANI
HENRYII
HENRYVI
MIZRAHI
NAIROBI
NEGRONI
ONORATI
SHARPEI
SOPRANI

••••RI•

AELFRIC
AIRDRIE
ALEGRIA
ALGERIA
ALMERIA
AMHARIC
AMNERIS
AQUARIA
ARTERIO
ASPIRIN
ASSYRIA
ASTERIX
ASTORIA
AUSTRIA
BACTRIA
BADTRIP
BALDRIC
BAVARIA
BEATRIX
BONARIO
BUSTRIP
CALORIC
CALORIE
CAMBRIA
CAMBRIC
CANTRIP
CARTRIP
CENTRIC
CETERIS
CHAGRIN
CHEERIO
CHLORIC
CONBRIO
COTERIE
CULPRIT
CUMBRIA
DAYTRIP
DELIRIA
DELORIS
DEMERIT
DENARII
DEXTRIN
DHURRIE
DINARIC
DRMARIO
ECOTRIN
EDITRIX
EGOTRIP
EMPIRIC
EMPIRIN
EMPORIA
ENTERIC
ENTERIN
ESTORIL
ETHERIC
ETRURIA
EUCERIN
FEMORIS
FLOORIT
FREDRIC
GAGARIN
GASTRIC
GENERIC
GENERIS
GETSRID
GOFORIT
GONERIL
GRIGRIS
GUTHRIE
HATBRIM
HENDRIX
HEPARIN
HOMERIC
ILLYRIA
IMFORIT
IMPERIL
INAPRIL
INFORIT
INHERIT
INPERIL
INTERIM
JONERIK
JURYRIG
KEYGRIP
LAVORIS
LECTRIC
LEITRIM
LETSRIP
LIBERIA
LIGURIA
LIPARIS
LITCRIT
MAHARIS
MAJORIN
MALARIA
MANTRIC
MAZARIN
MINORIN
MOCHRIE
NAYARIT
NEPHRIC
NIGERIA
NONDRIP
NOSTRIL
NUMERIC
ONATRIP
ONEIRIC
ONTARIO
ORATRIX
ORDERIN
OUTGRIN
PETERII
PILGRIM
POLARIS
PRAIRIE
PRETRIM
QATARIS
QUADRIC
RESTRIP
REVERIE
ROSARIO
SAFARIS
SAMARIA
SANGRIA
SATIRIC
SATORIS
SATYRIC
SAVARIN
SEATRIP
SEFERIS
SIBERIA
SKITRIP
SOLARIA
SPHERIC
STEARIC
STEARIN
SUBARID
SWEARIN
TALARIA
TENDRIL
THETRIB
TIDERIP
TRUERIB
TSOURIS
UNLYRIC
UPFORIT
USHERIN
VALERIE
VENTRIS
VICTRIX
VITORIA
VIVARIA

••••R•I

ALBERTI
ALEARDI
BACARDI
DENARII
EDWARDI
HAVARTI
PETERII
ROBERTI
SAMURAI
SCHERZI
STUARTI

•••••RI

ALFIERI
APRIORI
ARACARI
BULGARI
CAMPARI
DAKTARI
DIMITRI
FEODORI
FERRARI
LAZZERI
LETTERI
SALIERI
SCOLARI
SHANGRI
SHASTRI
VENTURI
VILLARI

R•J••••
RAJARAO
REJAILS
REJECTS
REJOICE
REJOINS
REJUDGE

R••J•••
RAMJETS
REDJACK
REEJECT

R•••J••
REENJOY
RESOJET
ROMAJIS

R•••••J
RADIODJ

•RJ••••
MRJONES

•R•J•••
FRIJOLE
PROJECT
PROJETS
TRIJETS
TROJANS

•R••J••
GRAYJAY
PROPJET

••RJ•••
CARJACK
PERJURE
PERJURY

••R•J••
KARAJAN
LORDJIM

••R••J•
MARUSJA

••R•••J
LARGEOJ
SERIESJ

•••RJ••
LEARJET
OVERJOY

•••R•J•
VANRIJN

••••RJ•
ALFORJA

••••R•J
HEYMRDJ

•••••RJ
LETTERJ

R•K••••
RAKABLE
RAKEDIN
RAKEDUP
RAKEOFF
RAKESIN
RAKESUP
REKEYED
REKICKS
REKNEAD
REKNITS
REKNOCK
REKNOTS
RIKSDAG

R••K•••
RACKERS
RACKETS
RACKETY
RACKING
RACKOUT
RACKSUP
RANKERS
RANKEST
RANKINE
RANKING
RANKISH
RANKLED
RANKLES
RANKOUT
RAYKROC
RECKONS
REDKING
REEKERS
REEKIER
REEKING
REEKSOF
RICKETY
RICKEYS
RICKLES
RICKMAN
RICKSHA
RINKRAT
RISKERS
RISKIER
RISKILY
RISKING
RISKSIT
ROCKABY
ROCKCOD
ROCKERS
ROCKERY
ROCKETS
ROCKIER
ROCKIES
ROCKILY
ROCKING
ROCKOIL
ROCKOON
ROCKYII
ROCKYIV
ROOKERY
ROOKIER
ROOKIES
ROOKING
ROOKISH
RUCKERT
RUCKING
RUCKSUP
RYOKANS
RYUKYUS

R•••K••
RAMEKIN
REASKED
REBAKED
REBAKES
REBEKAH
REBUKED
REBUKER
REBUKES
REDSKIN
REINKED
REMAKES
RERAKED
RERAKES
RETAKEN
RETAKER
RETAKES
REVOKED
REVOKER
REVOKES
REWAKED
REWAKEN
REWAKES
REWOKEN
REYOKED
REYOKES
RUMAKIS

R••••K•
RAMLIKE
RATLIKE
RAYLIKE
REAWAKE
REAWOKE
REBANKS
REBOOKS
REBROKE
RECOCKS
RECOOKS
RECORKS
REDOAKS
REDOCKS
REEBOKS
REEVOKE
REHOOKS
REKICKS
RELINKS
RELOCKS
RELOOKS
REMARKS
REPACKS
REPARKS
REPERKS
REPICKS
RERACKS
RERANKS
RESEEKS
RESINKS
RESOAKS
RESPOKE
RESTOKE
RETACKS
REWORKS
RHEBOKS
RIBLIKE
ROANOKE
RODLIKE
ROETHKE
RUGLIKE
RUMCAKE
RUZICKA
RVPARKS

R•••••K
RANAMOK
RANBACK
RANSACK
RATFINK
RATPACK
RAWSILK
REBLOCK
REBREAK
RECHALK
RECHECK
RECRANK
REDBOOK
REDHAWK
REDJACK
REDNECK
REKNOCK
RENWICK
RESPARK
RESPEAK
RESTACK
RESTICK
RESTOCK
RETHANK
RETHINK
RETRACK
RIDDICK
RIMROCK
RODDICK
ROEBUCK
ROLLICK
ROSTOCK
RUNAMOK
RUNBACK

•RK••••
IRKSOME
IRKUTSK
ORKNEYS

•R•K•••
ARIKARA
BRAKING
BROKEIN
BROKERS
BROKEUP
ERIKSON
ERSKINE
GROKKED
KRAKENS
PROKEDS
TREKKED
TREKKER
TREKKIE

•R••K••
BRACKEN
BRACKET
BREAKER
BREAKIN
BREAKUP
BRICKED
BRICKLE
BRICKUP
BRINKER
BRISKED
BRISKER
BRISKET
BRISKLY
BRODKEY
BROOKED
CRACKED
CRACKER
CRACKLE
CRACKLY
CRACKUP
CRANKED
CRANKUP
CREAKED
CRICKED
CRICKET
CRINKLE
CRINKLY
CROAKED
CROAKER
CROCKED
CROCKER
CROCKET
CROOKED
CROOKES
DRANKIN
DRANKTO
DRANKUP
DRINKER
DRINKIN
DRINKME
DRINKTO
DRINKUP
DRUCKER
DRUNKEN
DRUNKER
FRANKED
FRANKEN
FRANKER
FRANKIE
FRANKLY
FRANKOZ
FREAKED
FRECKLE
FRECKLY
FRICKER
FRISKED
FRISKER
FROCKED
GRACKLE
GRINKOV
GROKKED
IRECKON
KRACKEL
KRESKIN
PRICKED
PRICKLE
PRICKLY
PRICKUP
PRINKED
PRINKER
TRACKED
TRACKER
TREKKED
TREKKER
TREKKIE
TRICKED
TRICKER
TRICKLE
TRINKET
TROIKAS
TRUCKED
TRUCKEE
TRUCKER
TRUCKLE
WRACKED
WRACKUP
WREAKED
WREAKER
WRECKED
WRECKER
WRINKLE
WRINKLY

•R•••K•
ARENSKY
ARMLIKE
ARRACKS
BREWSKI
BRODSKY
GRETZKY
GROMYKO
MRLUCKY
ORBLIKE
OROURKE
PREBAKE
PREMAKE
PROVOKE
TROTSKY
URNLIKE
VRONSKY

•R••••K
ARAMARK
ARMLOCK
ARTBOOK
ARTROCK
ARTWORK
BRUBECK
DRSPOCK
DRYDOCK
FRYCOOK
IRKUTSK
KRAMNIK
MRNOVAK
MRSPOCK
PREBOOK
PRECOOK
PREDARK
PREDUSK
PREPACK
PREROCK
PRESOAK
PREWORK
URSULAK

••RK•••
AIRKISS
BARKEEP
BARKERS
BARKIER
BARKING
BARKLEY
BARKSAT
BERKLEY
BERKNER
BORKING
BURKINA
CARKEYS
CARKING
CORKAGE
CORKERS
CORKIER
CORKING
CORKOAK
CORKSUP
DARKAGE
DARKENS
DARKEST
DARKISH
DARKLED
DARKLES
DARKMAN
DARKRED
DARKTAN
DIRKING
DIRKSEN
DORKIER
FIRKINS
FORKERS
FORKFUL
FORKIER
FORKING
FORKOUT
FORKSUP
GURKHAS
HARKENS
HARKING
JERKERS
JERKIER
JERKIES
JERKILY
JERKING
JERKINS
JERKOUT
JERKSUP
LARKERS
LARKIER
LARKING
LARKINS
LARKISH
LURKERS
LURKING
MARKERS
MARKETS
MARKHAM
MARKIII
MARKING
MARKKAA
MARKOFF
MARKOUT
MARKOVA
MARKSUP
MARKUPS
MARKVII
MURKIER
MURKILY
MURKISH
PARKADE
PARKAVE
PARKERS
PARKING
PARKINS
PARKMAN
PARKSIT
PARKWAY
PERKIER
PERKILY
PERKING
PERKINS
PERKISH
PERKSUP
PORKERS
PORKIER
PORKING
PORKISH
PORKPIE
TURKEYS
TURKISH
WORKBOX
WORKDAY
WORKERS
WORKFOR
WORKING
WORKMAN
WORKMEN
WORKOFF
WORKOUT
WORKSAT
WORKSHY
WORKSIN
WORKSON
WORKSUP
WORKUPS
YERKISH
YORKERS
YORKIES
YORKIST
YORKTON

••R•K••
ALROKER
CARDKEY
EUREKAS
KARAKUM
MARKKAA
MARYKAY
PERUKES
RERAKED
RERAKES
SHRIKES
STRIKER
STRIKES
STROKED
STROKER
STROKES
TURNKEY
UNRAKED

••R••K•
AIRLIKE
ARRACKS
BUROAKS
CDRACKS
CURLIKE
EARLIKE
ENRANKS
FAROUKI
FORSAKE
GARPIKE
KARAOKE
OARLIKE
PARASKI
PARBAKE
PARTAKE
RERACKS
RERANKS
SCREAKS
SHRIEKS
SHRINKS
SIRDUKE
STREAKS
STREAKY
TURFSKI
UNRACKS
UNRISKY
UNROCKY
WARLIKE
ZERNIKE

••R•••K
AIRLOCK
AIRPACK
AIRPARK
AIRSICK
AIRSOCK
AIRTANK
AIRWICK
BARLICK
BARRACK
BERBICK
BERSERK
BERWICK
BURBANK
BURDICK
CARJACK
CARPARK
CARTALK
CORKOAK
CORMACK
DERRICK
EARLOCK
EARMARK
FARTLEK
FIRBANK
FORSOOK
GARRICK
GARRICK
HARNICK
HARTACK
HERRICK
JIRASEK
MERRICK
MORLOCK
NORFOLK
NORWALK
OARLOCK
PARTOOK
PERCHIK
PERWEEK
SARAWAK
SERIESK
SERIPAK
VARITEK
VARRICK
WARHAWK
WARLOCK
WARWICK

•••RK••
BEERKEG
CLERKED
CLERKLY
GHERKIN
HEARKEN
KHARKOV
MEERKAT
SHARKEY
SHIRKED
SHIRKER
SMIRKED
SMIRKER
SNORKEL
SPARKED
SPARKLE
SPARKLY
STARKER
STARKEY
STARKLY

•••R•K•
AMERIKA
ANORAKS
BUNRAKU
GOBROKE
IMBROKE
JSTROKE
PAPRIKA
REBROKE
STARSKY
TUGRIKS
UNBRAKE
UNBROKE

•••R••K
AMTRACK
ARTROCK
BARRACK
BEDROCK
CHARPAK
CONRACK
DEFROCK
DERRICK
ELDRICK
GARRICK
GEDRICK
HATRACK
HAYRACK
HAYRICK
HERRICK
ICERINK
KIDROCK
KUBRICK
LEBROCK
LEFREAK
LOWRISK
MERRICK
ONBREAK
ONTRACK
OUTRANK
OUTROCK
PATRICK
PETROCK
POPROCK
PREROCK
REBREAK
RECRANK
RETRACK
RIMROCK
SKIRACK
THERINK
THEROCK
TIERACK
TOPRANK
UNDRUNK
UNFRANK
UNFROCK
UNTRACK
VARRICK

••••RK•
AUTARKY
DEBARKS
DEMARKS
EMBARKS
EXWORKS
FEDERKO
MALARKY
MAZURKA
OROURKE
RECORKS
REMARKS
REPARKS
REPERKS
REWORKS
RVPARKS
STMARKS
UNCORKS
UNFORKS
UQUARKS

••••R•K
ALBORAK
BODEREK
DMYTRYK
HOWARDK
JONERIK
LAMARCK
MASARYK
MUBARAK

•••••RK
AIRPARK
ARAMARK
ARTWORK
ASALARK
ATATURK
BBQPORK
BERSERK
BIGJERK
BULWARK
CARPARK
CUTWORK
DEKLERK
DENMARK
DUNKIRK
EARMARK
FALKIRK
FUTHARK
HAYFORK
HOLYARK
INKMARK
LEGWORK
LETTERK
LEXMARK
MISMARK
MUDLARK
NETWORK
NEWYORK
NONDARK
NONWORK
OAKPARK
ONALARK
OSTMARK
OUTBARK
OUTWORK
PREDARK
PREWORK
RESPARK
SELKIRK
SKYLARK
TANBARK
THEJERK
THELARK
TINWORK
TITLARK
UPQUARK
WAXWORK
WIDMARK

RL•••••
RLSTINE

R•L••••
RALEIGH
RALLIED
RALLIER
RALLIES
RALLYES
RALLYTO
RALPHIE
RALSTON
RDLAING
RELABEL
RELACED
RELACES
RELANCE
RELANDS
RELANES
RELAPSE
RELATCH
RELATED
RELATER
RELATES
RELATOR
RELAXED
RELAXER
RELAXES
RELAYED
RELAYER
RELEADS
RELEAPS
RELEARN
RELEASE
RELENDS
RELENTS
RELEVEL
RELEVER
RELEVES
RELIANT
RELICTS
RELIEFS
RELIERS
RELIEVE
RELIGHT
RELIMIT
RELINED
RELINES
RELINKS
RELISTS
RELIVED
RELIVES
RELLENO
RELOADS
RELOANS
RELOCKS
RELOOKS
RELOSES
RELUCTS
RELUMED
RELUMES
RELYING
RILEDUP
RILESUP
RILIEVO
RILLETS
ROLAIDS
ROLEXES
ROLFERS
ROLFING
ROLLAND
ROLLBAR
ROLLEIS
ROLLERS
ROLLICK
ROLLING
ROLLINS
ROLLMOP
ROLLOFF
ROLLONS
ROLLOUT
ROLLSBY
ROLLSIN
ROLLSON
ROLLSUP
ROLLTOP
ROLLUPS
ROLLWAY
ROLODEX
ROLONDA
ROLVAAG
RULEDBY
RULEDON
RULEONE
RULEOUT
RULESON
RULIEST
RULINGS

R••L•••
RAGLANS
RAILAGE
RAILBUS
RAILCAR
RAILERS
RAILING
RAILMAN

RAILMEN
RAILSAT
RAILSON
RAILWAY
RALLIED
RALLIER
RALLIES
RALLYES
RALLYTO
RAMLIKE
RANLAPS
RANLATE
RATLIKE
RATLINE
RATLINS
RAWLINS
RAYLESS
RAYLIKE
REALEST
REALIGN
REALINE
REALISE
REALISM
REALIST
REALITY
REALIZE
REALLOT
REALMAN
REALMEN
REALTER
REALTOR
REBLOCK
REBLOOM
REBLOWN
RECLADS
RECLAIM
RECLAME
RECLASP
RECLASS
RECLEAN
RECLIMB
RECLINE
RECLUSE
REDLEGS
REDLINE
REELECT
REELERS
REELING
REELOFF
REELOUT
REELSIN
REELSUP
REFLAGS
REFLATE
REFLECT
REFLIES
REFLIPS
REFLOAT
REFLOOD
REFLOWN
REFLOWS
REGLAZE
REGLOSS
REGLOWS
REGLUED
REGLUES
RELLENO
REPLACE

REPLANE
REPLANS
REPLANT
REPLATE
REPLAYS
REPLEAD
REPLETE
REPLICA
REPLIED
REPLIER
REPLIES
REPLOTS
REPLOWS
REPLUMB
REPLUME
REPLYTO
RESLATE
RIALTOS
RIBLESS
RIBLETS
RIBLIKE
RIFLERS
RIFLERY
RIFLING
RILLETS
RIMLESS
RIOLOBO
ROBLOWE
RODLESS
RODLIKE
ROILIER
ROILING
ROLLAND
ROLLBAR
ROLLEIS
ROLLERS
ROLLICK
ROLLING
ROLLINS
ROLLMOP
ROLLOFF
ROLLONS
ROLLOUT
ROLLSBY
ROLLSIN
ROLLSON
ROLLSUP
ROLLTOP
ROLLUPS
ROLLWAY
ROULADE
ROULEAU
ROWLAND
ROWLING
RUGLIKE
RUMLESS
RUNLAPS
RUNLATE
RUNLESS
RUNLETS
RUTLAND
RVALUES
RYELOAF

R•••L••

RABBLED
RABBLES
RAFFLED

RAFFLER
RAFFLES
RAMBLED
RAMBLER
RAMBLES
RAMBLIN
RANKLED
RANKLES
RAPALLO
RASSLED
RASSLER
RASSLES
RATTLED
RATTLER
RATTLES
RAVELED
RAVELLY
RAVELOE
RCCOLAS
REALLOT
REARLIT
REBALED
REBALES
REBILLS
REBOLTS
RECALLS
RECOLOR
REDALGA
REDCLAY
REDFLAG
REFALLS
REFILED
REFILES
REFILLS
REFILMS
REFOLDS
REGALED
REGALER
REGALES
REGALIA
REGALLY
REGILDS
REGULAR
REGULUS
REMELTS
REMILLS
REMOLDS
RENALDO
RENALLY
REOILED
REPOLLS
REPULSE
REROLLS
RESALES
RESALTS
RESELLS
RESILED
RESILES
RESOLED
RESOLER
RESOLES
RESOLVE
RESPLIT
RESULTS
RETALLY
RETELLS
RETILED
RETILES

RETILLS
REVALUE
REVELED
REVELER
REVELIN
REVELRY
REVILED
REVILER
REVILES
REVOLTS
REVOLVE
REWELDS
RIBALDS
RICHLER
RICKLES
RIDDLED
RIDDLER
RIDDLES
RIFFLED
RIFFLER
RIFFLES
RIMPLED
RIMPLES
RINALDO
RINGLET
RIPPLED
RIPPLES
RIPPLET
RITALIN
RIVALED
RIVALRY
RIVULET
RODOLFO
ROMULAN
ROMULUS
ROOTLED
ROOTLES
ROOTLET
ROSALIA
ROSALIE
ROSALYN
ROSELLA
ROSELLE
ROTBLAT
ROTELLE
ROWELED
ROYALES
ROYALLY
ROYALTY
ROYALWE
ROZELLE
RUBBLES
RUBELLA
RUDOLFI
RUDOLPH
RUFFLED
RUFFLER
RUFFLES
RUGGLES
RUMBLED
RUMBLER
RUMBLES
RUMPLED
RUMPLES
RUNDLES
RUNSLOW
RURALLY
RUSSLAN

RUSTLED
RUSTLER
RUSTLES
RUTALEE
RUTILES
RUYBLAS

R••••L•

RABIDLY
RADIALS
RADICLE
RAGDOLL
RAINILY
RAKABLE
RANDALL
RANWILD
RAPALLO
RAPIDLY
RAPPELS
RASCALS
RATABLE
RATHOLE
RAVELLY
RAVIOLI
RAWSILK
RAYNELL
READILY
REAPPLY
REBILLS
REBOILS
REBUILD
REBUILT
RECABLE
RECALLS
RECHALK
RECHALL
RECOALS
RECOILS
RECOOLS
RECURLS
RECYCLE
REDCELL
REDEALS
REDEALT
REDIALS
REDPOLL
REDRILL
REDWOLF
REFALLS
REFILLS
REFUELS
REGALLY
REHAULS
REHEALS
REHEELS
REIMPLY
REJAILS
REMAILS
REMILLS
RENAILS
RENALLY
RENAULT
RENDELL
RENTALS
REPEALS
REPOLLS
REPTILE
REREELS

REROLLS
RESCALE
RESEALS
RESELLS
RESMELT
RESOILS
RESPELL
RESPELT
RESTYLE
RETABLE
RETAILS
RETALLY
RETELLS
RETICLE
RETILLS
RETITLE
RETOOLS
REVEALS
RIANTLY
RIDABLE
RIGHTLY
RIGIDLY
RISIBLE
RISIBLY
RISKILY
RISSOLE
RITUALS
RITZILY
ROCKILY
RONDELS
ROOMILY
ROSELLA
ROSELLE
ROSEOLA
ROSWELL
ROTELLE
ROUAULT
ROUGHLY
ROUNDLY
ROWDILY
ROYALLY
ROZELLE
RUBELLA
RUBEOLA
RUDDILY
RUFFALO
RUMPOLE
RUNNELS
RUNWILD
RURALLY
RUSSELL
RUSTILY

R•••••L

RACHAEL
RADICAL
RAGDOLL
RAGEFUL
RANDALL
RAPHAEL
RATTAIL
RAVENAL
RAWDEAL
RAYNELL
REAVAIL
RECHALL
RECITAL
RECUSAL

REDCELL
REDPOLL
REDRILL
REDTAIL
REEXPEL
REFUSAL
REFUTAL
REGINAL
RELABEL
RELEVEL
REMODEL
REMOVAL
RENDELL
RENEWAL
REPANEL
RESPELL
RESPOOL
RESTFUL
RETINAL
RETINOL
RETOTAL
RETRIAL
REVISAL
REVIVAL
ROCKOIL
ROOMFUL
RORQUAL
ROSEOIL
ROSTRAL
ROSWELL
ROUNDEL
RUSSELL
RUTHFUL

•RL••••

ARLBERG
ARLEDGE
DRLAURA
ERLANGS
MRLUCKY
ORLANDO
ORLEANS

•R•L•••

ARALSEA
ARCLAMP
ARMLESS
ARMLETS
ARMLIKE
ARMLOAD
ARMLOCK
ARTLESS
BRALESS
BRILLIG
BRILLOS
CRULLER
DRILLED
DRILLER
DROLLER
DRSLOAN
ERELONG
FRELENG
FRILLED
FROLICS
GRILLED
GRILLER
GRILLES
GROLIER

IRELAND
IRELESS
MRBLISS
MRCLEAN
MRSLATE
ORALIST
ORBLESS
ORBLIKE
ORELESS
OROLOGY
PRALINE
PRELACY
PRELATE
PRELIFE
PRELIMS
PRELOAD
PRELOAN
PRELOSS
PRELUDE
PROLATE
PROLIFE
PROLOGS
PROLONG
TRALALA
TRELLIS
TRILLED
TRILLER
TRILLIN
TRILOGY
TROLLED
TROLLER
TROLLEY
TROLLOP
URNLIKE
UROLOGY

•R••L••

ARABLES
ARBOLES
AREOLAE
AREOLAR
AREOLAS
AREOLES
ARGALIS
ARGYLES
ARNOLDS
BRADLEE
BRADLEY
BRAILLE
BRAMLEY
BRAWLED
BRAWLER
BRAWLEY
BRESLIN
BRIDLED
BRIDLER
BRIDLES
BRILLIG
BRILLOS
BRIMLEY
BROILED
BROILER
CRADLED
CRADLER
CRADLES
CRAWLED
CRAWLER
CRAWLEY

CREELEY
CREOLES
CROWLEY
CRUELER
CRUELLA
CRUELLY
CRUELTY
CRULLER
DRAWLED
DRAWLER
DREXLER
DRIBLET
DRILLED
DRILLER
DRMELFI
DROLLER
DROOLED
DROOLER
DROPLET
DRUMLIN
DRWELBY
FRAILER
FRAILLY
FRAILTY
FRAWLEY
FRIDLEY
FRILLED
FROGLEG
FROGLET
GRAVLAX
GRAYLAG
GREELEY
GREMLIN
GREYLAG
GRILLED
GRILLER
GRILLES
GRISLET
GROWLED
GROWLER
KREMLIN
MRHULOT
ORACLES
OREILLY
ORIOLES
ORMOLUS
ORTOLAN
ORVILLE
PREALLY
PREPLAN
PREPLOT
PRESLEY
PROBLEM
PROCLUS
PROWLED
PROWLER
TRAILED
TRAILER
TRAWLED
TRAWLER
TREBLED
TREBLES
TREELET
TRELLIS
TRIFLED
TRIFLER
TRIFLES
TRILLED

TRILLER
TRILLIN
TRIOLET
TRIPLEA
TRIPLED
TRIPLES
TRIPLET
TRIPLEX
TROILUS
TROLLED
TROLLER
TROLLEY
TROLLOP
URSULAK
WRIGLEY
WROCLAW
XRAYLAB

•R•••L•

ARCWELD
ARMFULS
ARMHOLE
ARSHILE
ARTFILM
ARTICLE
ARTSALE
ARTWALL
ARUGULA
BRAILLE
BRAMBLE
BRAMBLY
BRASHLY
BRATTLE
BRAVELY
BRICKLE
BRIDALS
BRIEFLY
BRINDLE
BRISKLY
BRISTLE
BRISTLY
BRITTLE
BROADLY
BRUTELY
CRACKLE
CRACKLY
CRAPOLA
CRASSLY
CRAYOLA
CRAZILY
CRENELS
CREWELS
CRINKLE
CRINKLY
CRIPPLE
CRISPLY
CROSSLY
CROWELL
CRUDELY
CRUELLA
CRUELLY
CRUMBLE
CRUMBLY
CRUMPLE
CRUMPLY
CRYWOLF
DRABBLE
DRACULA

DRAGGLE
DREXELU
DRIBBLE
DRIVELS
DRIZZLE
DRIZZLY
DRYABLE
DRYBULB
DRYCELL
DRYHOLE
DRYWALL
DRYWELL
ERECTLY
EROSELY
ERRABLE
FRAGGLE
FRAGILE
FRAILLY
FRANKLY
FRAZZLE
FRECKLE
FRECKLY
FRESHLY
FRIABLE
FRIARLY
FRIBBLE
FRIJOLE
FRIVOLS
FRIZZLE
FRIZZLY
FROOGLE
FRYABLE
GRACILE
GRACKLE
GRANDLY
GRANOLA
GRANULE
GRAPPLE
GRASSLE
GRAVELS
GRAVELY
GREATLY
GREENLY
GREWOLD
GRIDDLE
GRIMILY
GRISTLE
GRISTLY
GRIZZLE
GRIZZLY
GROSSLY
GROVELS
GROWOLD
GRUFFLY
GRUMBLE
GRUMBLY
IRATELY
KRINGLE
KRYSTLE
MRQUILP
ORDEALS
ORDERLY
OREILLY
ORVILLE
PRATTLE
PREALLY
PREBILL
PREFILE

PRESALE
PRESALT
PRESELL
PRESOLD
PRETELL
PRETOLD
PRICILY
PRICKLE
PRICKLY
PRIMELY
PRINGLE
PRIVILY
PROBALL
PROFILE
PRONELY
PROPELS
PROSILY
PROUDLY
TRALALA
TRAMPLE
TRAVELS
TREACLE
TREACLY
TREADLE
TREMBLE
TREMBLY
TREMOLO
TRESTLE
TRIABLE
TRIBBLE
TRICKLE
TRIFOLD
TRIPOLI
TRITELY
TROUBLE
TROWELS
TRUCKLE
TRUFFLE
TRUNDLE
URACILS
URNFULS
WRANGLE
WRESTLE
WRIGGLE
WRIGGLY
WRINKLE
WRINKLY
WRONGLY

•R••••L

AROUSAL
ARRABAL
ARRAYAL
ARRIVAL
ARSENAL
ARTWALL
ARUNDEL
BRENDEL
BRIMFUL
BRISTOL
BRUEGEL
BRUMMEL
CRANIAL
CREEDAL
CREOSOL
CROWELL
CRUCIAL
CRUSTAL

CRYSTAL
DREIDEL
DRYCELL
DRYWALL
DRYWELL
FRACTAL
FRESNEL
FRETFUL
FROEBEL
FRONTAL
GRADUAL
GRAPNEL
GRENDEL
HRETHEL
KRACKEL
MRSPAUL
MRSPEEL
ORBITAL
ORDINAL
ORTEGAL
PREBILL
PREBOIL
PRECOIL
PRECOOL
PREHEAL
PREORAL
PREQUEL
PRESEAL
PRESELL
PRESSEL
PRETELL
PRETZEL
PREVAIL
PROBALL
PROBOWL
TRAMMEL
TRAUBEL
TRAVAIL
TRAYFUL
TREFOIL
TRIVIAL
TRYSAIL
WRANGEL

••RL•••

AIRLANE
AIRLESS
AIRLIFT
AIRLIKE
AIRLINE
AIRLOCK
AIRLOGS
BARLESS
BARLEYS
BARLICK
BERLIOZ
BERLITZ
BIRLERS
BIRLING
BORLAUG
BURLAPS
BURLERS
BURLIER
BURLING
CARLENE
CARLESS
CARLING
CARLOAD

CARLOAN
CARLOTA
CARLOTS
CARLSON
CARLTON
CARLYLE
CURLERS
CURLEWS
CURLIER
CURLIKE
CURLING
CURLSIN
CURLSUP
DARLEEN
DARLENE
DARLING
EARLAPS
EARLDOM
EARLESS
EARLETS
EARLIER
EARLIES
EARLIKE
EARLOBE
EARLOCK
EARLYON
EHRLICH
FARLEFT
FORLANI
FORLIFE
FORLORN
FORLOVE
FURLERS
FURLESS
FURLING
FURLONG
GARLAND
GARLICS
GARLITS
GIRLIER
GIRLIES
GIRLISH
GIRLSHY
HARLAND
HARLEYS
HARLINE
HARLOTS
HURLERS
HURLING
JARLESS
KARLOFF
KARLOVY
KARLSON
LURLEEN
MARLENE
MARLIER
MARLINS
MARLOWE
MERLINS
MERLOTS
MORLOCK
OARLESS
OARLIKE
OARLOCK
PARLAYS
PARLEYS
PARLORS
PARLOUR
PARLOUS
PERLITE
PERLMAN
PURLIEU
PURLING
PURLOIN
SERLING
SIRLOIN
SURLIER
SURLILY
VARLAAM
VARLETS
VORLAGE
WARLESS
WARLIKE
WARLOCK
WARLORD
WORLDLY

••R•L••

ABRILES
ACRYLIC
AIRFLOW
AIRGLOW
AIRPLAY
AURALEE
AURALLY
BARCLAY
BARKLEY
BAROLOS
BARTLES
BARTLET
BERKLEY
BORGLUM
BURBLED
BURBLER
BURBLES
BURGLAR
BURGLED
BURGLES
BURNLEY
CARCLUB
CAROLED
CAROLER
CAROLII
CAROLYN
CIRCLED
CIRCLER
CIRCLES
CIRCLET
CORELLI
COROLLA
CURDLED
CURDLER
CURDLES
DARKLED
DARKLES
DARTLED
DARTLES
DERALTE
EARCLIP
EARFLAP
EARPLUG
ENROLLS
FARTLEK
FERULES
FIRELIT
FORDLTD
FORELEG
FORTLEE
FTRILEY
FURILLO
GARBLED
GARBLER
GARBLES
GARGLED
GARGLER
GARGLES
GERALDO
GIRDLED
GIRDLER
GIRDLES
GIROLLE
GORILLA
GURGLED
GURGLES
GYRALLY
HAROLDI
HARTLEY
HERALDS
HORSLEY
HURDLED
HURDLER
HURDLES
HURTLED
HURTLES
JERILYN
KAROLYI
KERFLOP
KERPLOP
KURILES
LORELAI
LORELEI
MARBLED
MARBLER
MARBLES
MARILLA
MARILYN
MARULLO
MARYLOU
MORALES
MORALLY
MORELLA
MORELLO
MORELOS
MURALED
MURILLO
MYRTLES
NORELCO
PAROLED
PAROLEE
PAROLES
PARSLEY
PERILED
PERPLEX
PIRELLI
PURFLED
PURFLER
PURFLES
PURPLED
PURPLES
REROLLS
RURALLY
SARALEE
SCROLLS
SHRILLS
SHRILLY
STROLLS
SURPLUS
TARTLET
THRALLS
THRILLA
THRILLS
TORTLAW
TURTLED
TURTLES
UNRILED
UNROLLS
UNRULED
UTRILLO
VERYLOW
WARBLED
WARBLER
WARBLES
WARCLUB
WORSLEY

••R••L•

ACRIDLY
AERIALS
AIRBALL
AIRBILL
AIRHOLE
AIRMILE
AIRWOLF
AURALLY
AUREOLA
AUREOLE
AURICLE
BARBELL
BARBILL
BARBULE
BARRELS
BARTOLO
BERTOLT
BIRDFLU
BURIALS
CARFULS
CARIOLE
CARLYLE
CARMELA
CARPALS
CARPELS
CARRELS
CARROLL
CARSALE
CARTALK
CARTELS
CARVELS
CEREALS
CORACLE
CORBELS
CORDELL
CORELLI
CORNELL
CORNILY
COROLLA
CORRALS
CORYELL
CURABLE
CURABLY
CUREALL
DARNELL
DARRYLF
DARWELL
DERAILS
DIRNDLS
DIRTILY
DORSALS
DURABLE
DURABLY
DURRELL
EARFULS
EARHOLE
EARTHLY
ENROLLS
ERRABLE
FARFELS
FARRELL
FERRULE
FERTILE
FIREFLY
FIRSTLY
FORMALS
FORMULA
FORSALE
FURBALL
FURILLO
GERBILS
GIROLLE
GORILLA
GYRALLY
HARDILY
HARROLD
HARSHLY
HARWELL
HERBALS
HERCULE
HERSELF
HIRABLE
HORSILY
ISRAELI
JARFULS
JARRELL
JERKILY
KERNELS
KORDELL
LARGELY
LURIDLY
MARCELS
MARILLA
MARSALA
MARULLO
MARVELL
MARVELS
MERRILL
MERRILY
MIRACLE
MORALLY
MORELLA
MORELLO
MORSELS
MORTALS
MURIELS
MURILLO
MURKILY
NERVILY
NERVULE
NORFOLK
NORMALS
NORWALK
OURSELF
PARABLE
PARCELS
PERCALE
PERGOLA
PERKILY
PIRELLI
PORTALS
PURCELL
REREELS
REROLLS
RURALLY
SCRAWLS
SCRAWLY
SCROLLS
SCRUPLE
SERIALS
SERVILE
SHRILLS
SHRILLY
SORRELL
SORRELS
SORRILY
SPRAWLS
SPRAWLY
STROLLS
SURLILY
TARBELL
TARDILY
TAROILS
TARSALS
TARTILY
TERCELS
TERRELL
TERSELY
THRALLS
THRILLA
THRILLS
TIREDLY
TORTOLA
TORVALD
TORVILL
UNREELS
UNROLLS
UTRILLO
VERBALS
VERDELL
VERYILL
VERYOLD
VIRGULE
WIRABLE
WORDILY
WORLDLY
WORRELL
YARNELL

••R•••L

ADRENAL
AEROSOL
AIRBALL
AIRBILL
AIRCOOL
AIRFOIL
AIRMAIL
ARRABAL
ARRAYAL
ARRIVAL
AURORAL
BARBELL
BARBILL
BARNOWL
BORSTAL
CARAMEL
CARAVEL
CARDIAL
CAREFUL
CARPOOL
CARROLL
CORDELL
CORDIAL
CORNEAL
CORNELL
CORNOIL
CORONAL
CORYELL
CUREALL
CURTAIL
DAREFUL
DARNELL
DARWELL
DIREFUL
DURRELL
FARMGAL
FARRELL
FORKFUL
FORMFUL
FORREAL
FURBALL
FURSEAL
GERITOL
GIRASOL
HARMFUL
HARWELL
HURTFUL
ISRAFEL
JARRELL
KORDELL
LYRICAL
MARITAL
MARSHAL
MARTIAL
MARVELL
MERRILL
MIRABEL
NARWHAL
PARASOL
PARBOIL
PARTIAL
PERORAL
PERUSAL
PHRASAL
PURCELL
RORQUAL
SHRIVEL
SORORAL
SORRELL
STRUDEL
SURREAL
SURVEIL
TARBELL
TARHEEL
TERRELL
TORVILL
TURMOIL
UNRAVEL
UNREGAL
UNRURAL
VERDELL
VERMEIL
VERYILL
VIRTUAL
WORRELL
YARNELL

•••RL••

AKERLOF
CHARLES
CHARLEY
CHARLIE
EVERLYS
GNARLED
HAARLEM
KNURLED
OBERLIN
OVERLAP
OVERLAX
OVERLAY
OVERLET
OVERLIE
OVERLIT
PEARLED
PEARLER
PHARLAP
POORLAW
QUARLES
REARLIT
SCARLET
SHIRLEY
SKIRLED
SNARLAT
SNARLED
SNARLER
SNARLUP
STARLET
STARLIT
STARLOG
SWIRLED
TWIRLED
TWIRLER
WHIRLED
WHIRLER
WHORLED

•••R•L•

ACEROLA
ALERTLY
ANGRILY
ASARULE
ATHRILL
AVERELL
AVERILL
BARRELS
BEDROLL
BITROLE
CAMRYLE
CARRELS
CARROLL
CHARILY
CHORALE
CHORALS
CHORTLE
CLERKLY
CORRALS
COURTLY
DARRYLF
DATRILS
DEERFLY
DURRELL
EGGROLL
EMERALD
EYEROLL
FARRELL
FEBRILE
FERRULE
FIERILY
GAGRULE
HARROLD
HOARILY
HOTROLL
INERTLY
JARRELL
JODRELL
LATRELL
LAURELS
LEERILY
LETROLL
LOGROLL
MCARDLE
MERRILL
MERRILY
MISRELY
MISRULE
MOBRULE
ONAROLL
OUTROLL
OVERALL
OVERFLY
OVERPLY
OVERTLY
PATROLS
PAYROLL
PETRELS
PETROLS
PLURALS
PUERILE
REDRILL
SCARILY
SHARPLY
SHORTLY
SMARTLY
SORRELL
SORRELS
SORRILY
SOURALE
SPARELY
SPARKLE
SPARKLY
SPIRALS
STARKLY
STARTLE
STERILE
STERNLY
STEROLS
TEARILY
TERRELL
THERULE
THIRDLY
UNFRILL
UNTRULY
WEARILY
WEIRDLY
WHERELL
WORRELL

•••R••L

ACCRUAL
ASPRAWL
ATHRILL
AVERELL
AVERILL
AVERNAL
BEDRAIL
BEDROLL
CARROLL
CHERVIL
CHORDAL
DIURNAL
DURRELL
EGGROLL
EMBROIL
ETERNAL
EYEROLL
FARRELL
FEARFUL
FLOREAL
FORREAL
GABRIEL
GAGREEL
GETREAL
GOTREAL
HAIRGEL
HOTROLL
JARRELL
JCARROL
JODRELL
JOURNAL
LATRELL
LETROLL
LOGROLL
MERRILL
NOTREAL
ODORFUL
ONAROLL
ONEREEL
ONTRIAL
OUTRAIL
OUTROLL
OVERALL
PAYROLL
QUARREL
REDRILL
RETRIAL
SNORKEL
SORRELL
STERNAL
SURREAL
TEARFUL
TERRELL
THERMAL
UMBRIEL
UNCRUEL
UNFRAIL
UNFRILL
UXORIAL
VITRIOL
WEIRDAL
WHERELL
WORRELL

••••RL•

ACTORLY
BEVERLY
CLEARLY
DECARLO
EAGERLY
ELDERLY
EPPERLY
FRIARLY
GOGIRLS
INNERLY
ITGIRLS
LOVERLY
MISERLY
MYWORLD
ORDERLY
PCWORLD
QUEERLY
RECURLS
SHEERLY
SOBERLY
UNBURLY
UNCURLS
UNFURLS
UNSURLY
UPCURLS
UPEARLY
UTTERLY

••••R•L

ADMIRAL
APPAREL
APTERAL
AUGURAL
AURORAL
AUSTRAL
CAMERAL
CASTROL
CENTRAL
CLAIROL
CONTROL
DEMEROL
DEXTRAL
ENTHRAL
ESTORIL
FEDERAL
FEMORAL
FIGURAL
GENERAL
GONERIL
HUMERAL
HUMORAL
IMMORAL
IMPERIL
INAPRIL
INPERIL
JCARROL
KESTREL
LATERAL
LIBERAL
LITERAL
LUSTRAL
MANDREL
MAYORAL
MINERAL
MISTRAL
MONGREL
NATURAL
NATUREL
NEUTRAL
NONORAL
NOSTRIL
NUMERAL
OHCAROL
PERORAL
PLEURAL
PREORAL
QUARREL
ROSTRAL
SCLERAL
SEVERAL
SORORAL
SPHERAL
TENDRIL
TUMBREL
UNRURAL
VENTRAL
VESTRAL
WASTREL

•••••RL

BADGIRL
BAGGIRL
BATGIRL
BIGGIRL
BUSGIRL
CAMGIRL
COWGIRL
ENSNARL
FLYGIRL
HUSSERL
LETTERL
OLDGIRL
OUTHURL
OUTPURL
PINCURL
UNSNARL
UPWHIRL

R•M••••

RAMADAN
RAMADAS
RAMBLED
RAMBLER
RAMBLES
RAMBLIN
RAMDOWN
RAMEKIN
RAMESES
RAMFANS
RAMHOME
RAMINTO
RAMIREZ
RAMJETS
RAMLIKE
RAMMERS
RAMMING
RAMMISH
RAMONES
RAMPAGE
RAMPANT
RAMPART
RAMPING
RAMPSUP
RAMRODS
RAMSESI
RAMSFAN
RAMSONS
REMAILS
REMAINS
REMAKES
REMANDS
REMARKS
REMARRY
REMATCH
REMATED
REMATES
REMEETS
REMELTS
REMENDS
REMERGE
REMILLS
REMINDS
REMINED
REMINES
REMINTS
REMISED
REMISES
REMIXED
REMIXES
REMNANT
REMODEL
REMOLDS
REMORAS
REMORSE
REMOTER
REMOTES
REMOUNT
REMOVAL
REMOVED
REMOVER
REMOVES
REMOWED
RIMBAUD
RIMIEST
RIMLESS
RIMMING
RIMPLED
RIMPLES
RIMROCK
RIMSHOT
ROMAINE
ROMAINS
ROMAJIS
ROMANCE
ROMANIA
ROMANIC
ROMANIS
ROMANOS
ROMANOV
ROMANSH
ROMANUS
ROMBERG
ROMCOMS
ROMNEYS
ROMPERS
ROMPING
ROMPISH
ROMULAN
ROMULUS
RUMAKIS
RUMANIA
RUMBAED
RUMBLED
RUMBLER
RUMBLES
RUMCAKE

RUMFORD
RUMLESS
RUMMAGE
RUMMERS
RUMMIES
RUMORED
RUMOURS
RUMPEND
RUMPLED
RUMPLES
RUMPOLE
RUMSHOP

R••M•••

RAGMANS
RAGMOPS
RAIMENT
RAMMERS
RAMMING
RAMMISH
RAWMEAT
RAYMOND
REAMASS
REAMEND
REAMERS
REAMING
REAMOUT
REDMEAT
REDMOND
REEMITS
REIMAGE
REIMPLY
RESMELT
REYMONT
RHOMBIC
RHOMBUS
RHUMBAS
RHYMERS
RHYMING
RHYMIST
RIBMEAT
RIEMANN
RIMMING
RIOMUNI
ROAMERS
ROAMING
ROOMBAS
ROOMERS
ROOMFUL
ROOMIER
ROOMIES
ROOMILY
ROOMING
RUMMAGE
RUMMERS
RUMMIES

R•••M••

RACEMES
RADAMES
RADOMES
RAILMAN
RAILMEN
RAINMAN
RANAMOK
READMIT
REAIMED
REALMAN
REALMEN
REARMED
REAUMUR
RECOMBS
REEDMAN
REEDMEN
REGIMEN
REGIMES
REITMAN
RELIMIT
RELUMED
RELUMES
RENAMED
RENAMES
REPOMAN
REPUMPS
RESUMED
RESUMES
RETAMED
RETAMES
RETIMED
RETIMES
REVAMPS
RHEUMIC
RICHMAN
RICHMEN
RICKMAN
RIESMAN
RITAMAE
ROADMAP
ROLLMOP
RUNAMOK

R••••M•

RAGTIME
RAMHOME
RANHOME
RANSOMS
RCADOME
RECLAME
RECLIMB
REDARMY
REDEEMS
REFILMS
REFORMS
REFRAME
REPLUMB
REPLUME
REPRIME
RESEAMS
RESTAMP
RESWIMS
RETRIMS
REWARMS
RHIZOME
RHYTHMS
ROMCOMS
RORAIMA
RUNHOME
RUNTIME

R•••••M

REALISM
REBLOOM
RECLAIM
RECROOM
REDREAM
REDWORM
REGROOM
REQUIEM
RHENIUM
RHODIUM
RITAGAM
ROSTRUM

•RM••••

ARMADAS
ARMBAND
ARMBONE
ARMENIA
ARMFULS
ARMHOLE
ARMLESS
ARMLETS
ARMLIKE
ARMLOAD
ARMLOCK
ARMOIRE
ARMORED
ARMORER
ARMOURS
ARMOURY
ARMPITS
ARMREST
ARMYANT
DRMARIO
DRMCCOY
DRMELFI
ERMINED
ERMINES
ERMINIA
MRMACHO
MRMAGOO
MRMARCH
MRMOOSE
MRMUSIC
ORMANDY
ORMOLUS

•R•M•••

ARAMAIC
ARAMARK
ARAMEAN
ARAMIDS
ARDMORE
BRAMBLE
BRAMBLY
BRAMLEY
BRIMFUL
BRIMLEY
BRIMMED
BRIMMER
BROMATE
BROMIDE
BROMINE
BRUMMEL
BRUMOUS
CRAMMED
CRAMMER
CRAMPED
CRAMPON
CRAMSIN
CREMATE
CREMINI
CREMONA
CREMORA
CRIMEAN
CRIMINY
CRIMPED
CRIMPER
CRIMSON
CRUMBED
CRUMBLE
CRUMBLY
CRUMBUM
CRUMPED
CRUMPET
CRUMPLE
CRUMPLY
DRAMADY
DRAMEDY
DRUMLIN
DRUMMED
DRUMMER
DRUMOUT
DRUMSET
DRUMSUP
DRYMOPS
EREMITE
FRAMERS
FRAMEUP
FRAMING
FREMONT
FROMAGE
FROMMER
GRAMMAR
GRAMMER
GRAMMES
GRAMMYS
GRAMPAS
GRAMPUS
GREMLIN
GRIMACE
GRIMIER
GRIMILY
GRIMING
GRIMMER
GRIMSBY
GROMMET
GROMYKO
GRUMBLE
GRUMBLY
GRUMMAN
GRUMPED
KRAMDEN
KRAMNIK
KREMLIN
MRSMITH
MRSMUIR
PREMADE
PREMAKE
PREMATE
PREMEDS
PREMEET
PREMIER
PREMIES
PREMISE
PREMISS
PREMIUM
PRIMACY
PRIMARY
PRIMATE
PRIMELY
PRIMERA
PRIMERO
PRIMERS
PRIMING
PRIMMED
PRIMMER
PRIMPED
PROMBID
PROMISE
PROMOED
PROMOTE
PROMPTS
TRAMCAR
TRAMMED
TRAMMEL
TRAMPAS
TRAMPED
TRAMPER
TRAMPLE
TRAMWAY
TREMBLE
TREMBLY
TREMOLO
TREMORS
TRIMMED
TRIMMER
TRIMOFF
TRIMTAB
TROMPED
TROMPIN
TRUMANS
TRUMPED
TRUMPET
TRUMPUP

•R••M••

AREAMAP
ARTEMIS
ARTEMUS
BRAHMAN
BRAHMAS
BRAHMIN
BRIMMED
BRIMMER
BROOMED
BRUMMEL
CRAMMED
CRAMMER
CRANMER
CREAMED
CREAMER
CREWMAN
CREWMEN
DRAWMAN
DRAWMEN
DRAYMAN
DRAYMEN
DREAMED
DREAMER
DREAMIN
DREAMOF
DREAMON
DREAMUP
DRUMMED
DRUMMER
ERASMUS
FREEMAN
FREEMEN
FROGMAN
FROGMEN
FROMMER
GRAMMAR
GRAMMER
GRAMMES
GRAMMYS
GRAUMAN
GRIDMAP
GRIMMER
GROMMET
GROOMED
GROOMER
GRUMMAN
IRONMAN
IRONMEN
KROEMER
PREAMPS
PREEMIE
PREEMPT
PREOMIT
PRIMMED
PRIMMER
PROPMAN
PROPMEN
TRAMMED
TRAMMEL
TRAUMAS
TRIMMED
TRIMMER
TRIUMPH
VROOMED

•R•••M•

ARCLAMP
DRACHMA
DRINKME
FRENEMY
GRAHAME
GRAHAMS
GRANDMA
IRKSOME
ORIGAMI
PREARMS
PREGAME
PRELIMS
PRENAME
PRESUME
PRFIRMS
PROXIMA
PROXIMO
TRIREME
TRUISMS
TRUSTME
WRITEME

•R••••M

ARCANUM
ARTFILM
ARTFORM
ARTHURM
BRIGHAM
BRITCOM
BRUXISM
CRANIUM
CRUMBUM
ERRATUM
FREEDOM
FRUSTUM
GRANDAM
GRECISM
GRESHAM
GREWDIM
GRISHAM
GRISSOM
GROWDIM
IRIDIUM
IRSFORM
ORARIUM
ORPHEUM
PREBOOM
PREDOOM
PREFORM
PREMIUM
PRETERM
PRETRIM
PREWARM
PROBLEM
PROFARM
PROGRAM
PROTEAM
TRANSAM
TRANSOM
TRIFORM
TRIGRAM
TRITIUM
TRIVIUM
TROPISM
URANIUM

••RM•••

AIRMADA
AIRMAIL
AIRMASS
AIRMILE
BARMAID
BARMIER
BERMING
BERMUDA
BIRMANS
BURMANS
BURMESE
CARMELA
CARMINA
CARMINE
CORMACK
DERMATO
DORMANT
DORMERS
DORMICE
EARMARK
EARMUFF
FARMAID
FARMBOY
FARMERS
FARMERY
FARMGAL
FARMING
FARMORE
FARMOUT
FERMATA
FERMATE
FERMATS
FERMENT
FERMION
FERMIUM
FIRMEST
FIRMING
FIRMSUP
FORMALS
FORMATS
FORMERS
FORMFUL
FORMICA
FORMING
FORMOSA
FORMULA
GARMENT
GERMAIN
GERMANE
GERMANS
GERMANY
GERMIER
GORMING
HARMERS
HARMFUL
HARMING
HARMONY
HERMANA
HERMANN
HERMANO
HERMANS
HERMITS
HERMOSA
HERMOSO
HORMONE
KIRMANS
MARMARA
MARMION
MARMOTS
MERMAID
MORMONS
MURMURS
NORMALS
NORMAND
NORMANS
PERMIAN
PERMING
PERMITS
PERMUTE
SERMONS
SURMISE
TARMACS
TERMING
TERMINI
TERMITE
TORMENT
TURMOIL
VARMINT
VERMEER
VERMEIL
VERMINY
VERMONT
WARMERS
WARMEST
WARMING
WARMISH
WARMSTO
WARMSUP
WARMUPS
WORMERS
WORMIER
WORMING
WORMISH
ZERMATT

••R•M••

AFRAMES
BERGMAN
BIRDMAN
BIRDMEN
BIREMES
BOROMIR
CARAMBA
CARAMEL
CARAMIA
CAROMED
CERAMIC
CERUMEN
CHROMAT
CHROMED
CHROMES
CHROMIC
DARKMAN
DORFMAN
FIREMAN
FIREMEN
FOREMAN
FOREMEN
HARTMAN
HARTMUT
JAROMIR
JURYMAN
JURYMEN
LARAMIE
MARIMBA
MERIMEE
MIRAMAR
MIRAMAX
NKRUMAH
OARSMAN
OARSMEN
ONRAMPS
PARAMUS
PARKMAN
PERLMAN
PORTMAN
PYRAMID
PYRAMUS
SARUMAN
SCRIMPS
SCRIMPY
SHRIMPS
SHRIMPY
SURFMAN
SURFMEN
SURIMIS
TIREMAN
TIREMEN
TURFMAN
TURFMEN
UNRIMED
VERYMAD
WIREMAN
WIREMEN
WORKMAN
WORKMEN
YARDMAN
YARDMEN

••R••M•

AIRDAMS
AIRPUMP
AIRTIME
ATRIUMS
BARNUMS
BERGAMO
CHRISMS
CORFAMS
DIRHAMS
MARRYME
PARFUMS
PERFUME
PERFUMY
RORAIMA
SCREAMS
STREAMS
SURNAME
TURISMO
TVROOMS
UNRHYME
UNROOMY
VERISMO
WARGAME
WARTIME

••R•••M

ABRAHAM
ACRONYM
BAREXAM
BARROOM
BERTRAM
BOREDOM
BORGLUM
CARDIUM
CHRISOM
EARDRUM
EARLDOM
ERRATUM
FERMIUM
FIREARM
FORDHAM
FOREARM
FURFARM
HEREIAM
HEROISM
KARAKUM
LORDJIM
MARKHAM
MARXISM
MERRIAM
PARONYM
PERDIEM
PERFORM
SARCASM
SERFDOM
SORGHUM
STRATUM
SUREIAM
SURINAM
TERAOHM
TERBIUM
THREEAM
THREEPM
TORYISM
VARLAAM
WARROOM
YARDARM
ZEROSUM

•••RM••

ALARMED
ALARMER
BEERMUG
BEHRMAN
BOORMAN
CHARMAN
CHARMED
CHARMEN
CHARMER
CHARMIN
DHARMAS
DHARMIC
DOORMAN
DOORMAT
DOORMEN
ENARMED
FOURMAN
GOURMET
OVERMAN
OVERMIX
POORMAN
POORMEN
REARMED
SHERMAN
STARMAN
STARMAP
STORMED
STORMIN
SWARMED
SWARMER
THERMAL
THERMIC
THERMOS
THURMAN
UNARMED
YZERMAN

•••R•M•

ALARUMS
ASHRAMS
BAYRUMS
BEGRIME
DECRUMB
DEFRAME
DIGRAMS
DIORAMA
ENFRAME
ENGRAMS
EXTREME
GOURAMI
LACRIMO
MACRAME
MARRYME
MCCRUMB
MEGRIMS
NOTRUMP
OFFRAMP
QUORUMS
REFRAME
REPRIME
RETRIMS
SANREMO
SPAREME
SUPREME
THERAMS
TRIREME
UNCRAMP

•••R••M

ASTREAM
BARROOM
BEDROOM
BOHRIUM
CZARDOM
CZARISM
DAYROOM
EPHRAIM
GEORGEM
GUARGUM
GUNROOM
HAARLEM
HADROOM
HASROOM
HEIRDOM
ISUREAM
LEGROOM
MERRIAM
MUDROOM
NATRIUM
ONEROOM
ORARIUM
OVERARM
RECROOM
REDREAM
REGROOM
STARDOM
STERNUM
SUNROOM
TAPROOM
TEAROOM
THEROOM
THORIUM
TOURISM
TSARDOM
TSARISM
TWOROOM
WARROOM
YTTRIUM

••••RM•

AFFIRMS
BYFORMS
COVERME
DEFORMS
DEGERMS
DELORME
DEWORMS
DISARMS
HUMORME
INFORMS
LAPERMS
PALERMO
PREARMS
PRFIRMS
REDARMY
REFORMS
REWARMS
SEAARMS
SQUIRMS
SQUIRMY
THEARMY
UNWORMY

••••R•M

ANAGRAM
BERTRAM
BUCKRAM
BUTTRAM
CENTRUM
CHETRUM
DECORUM
DIAGRAM
EARDRUM
EATFROM
EPIGRAM
FULCRUM
GETFROM
HATBRIM
HUMDRUM
INTERIM
ISOGRAM
LEITRIM
LUSTRUM
NOSTRUM
OILDRUM
ONEGRAM
PANGRAM
PILGRIM
PRETRIM
PROGRAM
ROSTRUM
SEAGRAM
SHYFROM
TANGRAM
TANTRUM
THEOREM
TRIGRAM
VALOREM
WOLFRAM

•••••RM

ALIFORM
ANTFARM
ARTFORM
ARTHURM
BADFORM
BECHARM
BUDWORM
CONFIRM
CONFORM
CUTWORM
EELWORM
EPIDERM
FATFARM
FIREARM
FOREARM
FURFARM
GETWARM
GOTWARM
IRSFORM
LEFTARM
LETTERM
LONGARM
LUGWORM
MIDTERM
MISFORM
MISTERM
NONFARM
NONFORM
ONETERM
OVERARM
OVIFORM
PERFORM
PREFORM

PRETERM
PREWARM
PROFARM
REDWORM
SIDEARM
SUBFORM
THEFIRM
TONEARM
TOPFORM
TRIFORM
TWOTERM
UNIFORM
YARDARM

R•N••••

RANAMOK
RANATAB
RANAWAY
RANBACK
RANCHED
RANCHER
RANCHES
RANCHOS
RANCORS
RANCOUR
RANDALL
RANDEEP
RANDIER
RANDOWN
RANFREE
RANGERS
RANGFOR
RANGIER
RANGING
RANGOFF
RANGOON
RANGOUT
RANHOME
RANINTO
RANITUP
RANKERS
RANKEST
RANKINE
RANKING
RANKISH
RANKLED
RANKLES
RANKOUT
RANLAPS
RANLATE
RANONIN
RANOVER
RANPAST
RANRIOT
RANSACK
RANSOMS
RANTERS
RANTING
RANTSAT
RANUPTO
RANWILD
RANWITH
RENAILS
RENALDO
RENALLY
RENAMED
RENAMES
RENAULT
RENDELL
RENDERS
RENDING
RENEGED
RENEGER
RENEGES
RENESTS
RENEWAL
RENEWED
RENEWER
RENFREW
RENNETS
RENNINS
RENOIRS
RENOTED
RENOTES
RENOWNS
RENTALS
RENTEES
RENTERS
RENTIER
RENTING
RENTOUT
RENTSTO
RENUZIT
RENVOIS
RENWICK
RINALDO
RINDIER
RINGERS
RINGFOR
RINGING
RINGLET
RINGOFF
RINGOUT
RINGSIN
RINGSUP
RINKRAT
RINSERS
RINSING
RONDEAU
RONDELS
RONDURE
RONETTE
RONSARD
RONSONS
RONTGEN
RONWOOD
RONZONI
RUNAMOK
RUNATAB
RUNAWAY
RUNBACK
RUNDEEP
RUNDLES
RUNDOWN
RUNFREE
RUNGFOR
RUNGOFF
RUNGOUT
RUNHOME
RUNINTO
RUNITUP
RUNLAPS
RUNLATE
RUNLESS
RUNLETS
RUNNELS
RUNNERS
RUNNETH
RUNNIER
RUNNING
RUNOFFS
RUNONIN
RUNOUTS
RUNOVER
RUNPAST
RUNRIOT
RUNSDRY
RUNSFOR
RUNSLOW
RUNSOFF
RUNSOUT
RUNTIER
RUNTIME
RUNTISH
RUNUPTO
RUNWAYS
RUNWILD
RUNWITH

R••N•••

RAINBOW
RAINGOD
RAINHAT
RAINIER
RAINILY
RAINING
RAINMAN
RAINOUT
RAINSIN
RAINSON
RAUNCHY
RAWNESS
RAYNELL
REANNEX
REDNECK
REDNESS
REDNINE
REDNOSE
REENACT
REENDOW
REENJOY
REENTER
REENTRY
REGNANT
REGNARD
REGNIER
REINDEX
REINING
REINKED
REINSIN
REKNEAD
REKNITS
REKNOCK
REKNOTS
REMNANT
RENNETS
RENNINS
RESNAIS
RESNAPS
REUNERS
REUNIFY
REUNION
REUNITE
REYNARD
REYNAUD
REYNOSA
RHENISH
RHENIUM
RIANTLY
ROANOKE
ROMNEYS
ROUNDED
ROUNDEL
ROUNDER
ROUNDLY
ROUNDON
ROUNDUP
RUANDAS
RUINATE
RUINERS
RUINING
RUINOUS
RUNNELS
RUNNERS
RUNNETH
RUNNIER
RUNNING
RWANDAN

R•••N••

RACINOS
RAGINGS
RAMINTO
RAMONES
RANINTO
RANONIN
RAPANUI
RAPINES
RAPINIS
RATINES
RATINGS
RAVENAL
RAVENED
RAVENNA
RAVINED
RAVINES
RAVINGS
REANNEX
REBANKS
REBENDS
REBINDS
RECANED
RECANES
RECANTS
RECENCY
REDANTS
REDONDO
REFENCE
REFINDS
REFINED
REFINER
REFINES
REFUNDS
REGENCY
REGENTS
REGINAL
REGINAS
REHANGS
REHINGE
REHONED
REHONES
REHONOR
REIGNED
RELANCE
RELANDS
RELANES
RELENDS
RELENTS
RELINED
RELINES
RELINKS
REMANDS
REMENDS
REMINDS
REMINED
REMINES
REMINTS
REOWNED
REPANEL
REPENTS
REPINED
REPINER
REPINES
RERANKS
RERENTS
RERINSE
RESANDS
RESENDS
RESENTS
RESINED
RESINGS
RESINKS
RETINAE
RETINAL
RETINAS
RETINGE
RETINOL
RETINTS
RETINUE
RETONED
RETONES
RETUNED
RETUNES
REVENDS
REVENGE
REVENUE
REWINDS
REZONED
REZONES
RIBANDS
RIDINGS
RIPENED
RIPENER
RIPINTO
RISENTO
RISINGS
ROBBNEN
RODENTS
ROLONDA
ROMANCE
ROMANIA
ROMANIC
ROMANIS
ROMANOS
ROMANOV
ROMANSH
ROMANUS
ROSANNA
ROSANNE
ROSINED
ROSSNER
ROTUNDA
ROVINGS
ROXANNE
ROZANOV
RULINGS
RUMANIA
RUNINTO
RUNONIN

R••••N•

RACKING
RADIANS
RADIANT
RAFTING
RAGGING
RAGLANS
RAGMANS
RAIDING
RAILING
RAIMENT
RAINING
RAISING
RAISINS
RAISINY
RAISONS
RAMFANS
RAMMING
RAMPANT
RAMPING
RAMSONS
RANGING
RANKINE
RANKING
RANTING
RAPPING
RAPSONG
RAPTUNE
RASPING
RATFINK
RATIONS
RATLINE
RATLINS
RATTANS
RATTING
RAVENNA
RAWLINS
RAYBANS
RAYGUNS
RAYMOND
RAZZING
RDLAING
READING
REAGANS
REAGENT
REALINE
REAMEND
REAMING
REAPING
REAREND
REARING
REASONS
REAVING
REBOANT
REBOUND
REBRAND
RECKONS
RECLINE
RECOINS
RECOUNT
RECRANK
REDARNS
REDBONE
REDCENT
REDDENS
REDDING
REDFINS
REDHENS
REDKING
REDLINE
REDMOND
REDNINE
REDOING
REDOUND
REDPINE
REDPONY
REDSUNS
REDWINE
REDWING
REDYING
REDZONE
REEARNS
REEDING
REEFING
REEKING
REELING
REEVING
REFFING
REFOUND
REFRONT
REFYING
REGAINS
REGIONS
REGNANT
REGRANT
REGRIND
REICING
REINING
REJOINS
RELIANT
RELLENO
RELOANS
RELYING
REMAINS
REMNANT
REMOUNT
RENDING
RENNINS
RENOWNS
RENTING
REOPENS
REPAINT
REPHONE
REPLANE
REPLANS
REPLANT
REPOINT
REPPING
REPRINT
REPRUNE
REPUGNS
RESCANS
RESCIND
RESHINE
RESIGNS
RESOUND
RESPANS
RESPINS
RESPOND
RESTING
RETAINS
RETHANK
RETHINK
RETSINA
RETTING
RETURNS
RETWINE
REUBENS
REUSING
REVVING
REWARNS
REWOUND
REYMONT
RHYMING
RIBBING
RIBBONS
RIBBONY
RICHENS
RIDDING
RIDGING
RIEMANN
RIESENS
RIFFING
RIFLING
RIFTING
RIGGING
RIMMING
RINGING
RINSING
RIOMUNI
RIOTING
RIPIENI
RIPIENO
RIPPING
RIPSONE
RISKING
RLSTINE
ROAMING
ROARING
ROBBING
ROBBINS
ROCKING
RODDING
ROGAINE
ROGUING
ROILING
ROLFING
ROLLAND
ROLLING
ROLLINS
ROLLONS
ROMAINE
ROMAINS
ROMPING
RONSONS
RONZONI
ROOFING
ROOKING
ROOMING
ROOTING
ROSANNA
ROSANNE
ROSSANO
ROSSINI
ROSTAND
ROTTING
ROUGING
ROUSING
ROUTINE
ROUTING
ROWLAND
ROWLING
ROXANNE
RRATING
RSVPING
RUBBING
RUCHING
RUCKING
RUFFING
RUINING
RULEONE
RUMPEND
RUNNING
RUSHING
RUSTING
RUTHANN
RUTLAND
RUTTING
RYOKANS

R•••••N

RACCOON
RACEDIN
RADIOIN
RAEBURN
RAEDAWN
RAILMAN
RAILMEN
RAILSON
RAINMAN
RAINSIN
RAINSON
RAKEDIN
RAKESIN
RALSTON
RAMADAN
RAMBLIN
RAMDOWN
RAMEKIN
RAMSFAN
RANDOWN
RANGOON
RANONIN
RAPIDAN
RARITAN
RAYBURN
REACHIN
READORN
READSIN
READSON
REALIGN
REALMAN
REALMEN
REARDON
REBEGAN
REBEGIN
REBEGUN
REBLOWN
RECLEAN
RECROWN
REDDAWN
REDFERN
REDRAWN
REDSFAN
REDSKIN
REEDMAN
REEDMEN
REELSIN
REFLOWN
REFRAIN
REGIMEN
REGIVEN
REGROWN
REINSIN
REITMAN
RELEARN
REPOMAN
RERISEN
RESHOWN
RESTAIN
RESTSIN
RESTSON
RESWORN
RETAKEN
RETRAIN
REUNION
REVELIN
REWAKEN
REWIDEN
REWOKEN
REWOVEN
RHODIAN
RICHMAN
RICHMEN
RICKMAN
RIDESIN
RIEMANN
RIESMAN
RIESSEN
RIGHTON
RINGSIN
RIORDAN
RIOTGUN
RIPOPEN
RIPSAWN
RIPTORN
RITALIN
ROBBNEN
ROBESON
ROCKOON
ROLLSIN
ROLLSON
ROMULAN
RONTGEN
ROPEDIN
ROPESIN
ROSALYN
ROUGHEN
ROUNDON
ROYBEAN
ROYCOHN
RUBDOWN
RUBICON
RUBITIN
RUBUPON
RUCTION
RUFFIAN
RULEDON
RULESON
RUNDOWN
RUNONIN
RUSSIAN
RUSSLAN
RUTHANN
RWANDAN

•RN••••

ARNICAS
ARNOLDS
ERNESTA
ERNESTO
MRNANNY
MRNORTH
MRNOVAK
ORNETTE
ORNITHO
URNFULS
URNLIKE

•R•N•••

ARANEID
ARANTXA
ARENOSE
ARENSKY
ARONNAX
ARUNDEL
BRANAGH
BRANCHY
BRANDED
BRANDER
BRANDON
BRANIFF
BRANSON
BRENDAN
BRENDEL
BRENDON
BRENGUN
BRENNAN
BRENNER
BRINDLE
BRINERS
BRINGER
BRINGIN
BRINGIT
BRINGON
BRINGTO
BRINGUP
BRINIER
BRINING
BRINISH
BRINKER
BRONCHI
BRONCHO
BRONCOS
BRONSON
BRONTES
BRONWEN
BRONZED
BRONZER
BRONZES
BRUNETS
BRYNNER
CRANIAL
CRANING
CRANIUM
CRANKED
CRANKUP
CRANMER
CRENATE
CRENELS
CRINGED
CRINGES
CRINKLE
CRINKLY
CRONIES
CRUNCHY
DRANKIN
DRANKTO
DRANKUP
DRINKER
DRINKIN
DRINKME
DRINKTO
DRINKUP
DRONEON
DRONERS
DRONING
DRONISH
DRUNKEN
DRUNKER
DRYNESS
ERINYES
ERYNGOS
FRANCES
FRANCHI
FRANCIS
FRANKED
FRANKEN
FRANKER
FRANKIE
FRANKLY
FRANKOZ
FRANTIC
FRENCHI
FRENCHS
FRENEAU
FRENEMY
FRENESI
FRINGED
FRINGES
FRONTAL
FRONTED
FRONTON
GRANADA
GRANARY
GRANDAM
GRANDEE
GRANDER
GRANDLY
GRANDMA
GRANDPA
GRANGER
GRANGES
GRANITA
GRANITE
GRANNIE
GRANOLA
GRANPAS
GRANTED
GRANTEE
GRANTER
GRANTOR
GRANULE
GRENADA
GRENADE
GRENDEL
GRINDER
GRINGOS
GRINKOV
GRINNED
GRINNER
GRINSAT
GRUNGER
GRUNGES
GRUNION
GRUNTED
GRUNTER
IRANIAN
IRENICS
IRONAGE
IRONBAR
IRONERS
IRONIES
IRONING
IRONIST
IRONMAN
IRONMEN
IRONONS
IRONORE
IRONOUT
IRONSON
KRINGLE
ORANGES
ORANGEY
ORANTES
ORINOCO
ORKNEYS
PRANCED
PRANCER
PRANCES
PRENAME
PRENOON
PRENUPS
PRINCES
PRINGLE
PRINKED
PRINKER
PRINTAD
PRINTED
PRINTER
PRINTUP
PRONATE
PRONAVY
PRONELY
PRONETO
PRONGED
PRONOUN
PRUNERS
PRUNING
TRANCED
TRANCES
TRANSAM
TRANSIT
TRANSOM
TRENARY
TRENDED
TRENTON
TRINARY
TRINITY
TRINKET
TRUNDLE
URANITE
URANIUM
VRONSKY

WRANGEL
WRANGLE
WRINGER
WRINKLE
WRINKLY
WRONGED
WRONGER
WRONGLY
WRYNESS

•R••N••

ARCANUM
ARCINGS
ARDENCY
ARGANTE
ARGENTI
ARGENTO
ARGENTS
ARGONNE
ARIANES
ARMENIA
ARONNAX
ARRANGE
ARSENAL
ARSENIC
ARSENIO
BRAINED
BRAINER
BRENNAN
BRENNER
BRITNEY
BROSNAN
BROWNED
BROWNER
BROWNIE
BRYNNER
CROONED
CROONER
CROWNED
CROWNER
DRAGNET
DRAINED
DRAINER
DRAWNIN
DRAWNON
DRAWNTO
DRAWNUP
DROPNET
DROWNED
ERLANGS
ERMINED
ERMINES
ERMINIA
ERRANCY
ERRANDS
FRESNEL
FRIENDS
FROWNAT
FROWNED
FROWNER
FROWNON
GRAINED
GRAINER
GRANNIE
GRAPNEL
GREENED
GREENER
GREENLY
GRINNED
GRINNER
GRISNEZ
GROANED
GROANER
GROINED
GROUNDS
GROWNON
GROWNUP
HRYVNIA
KRAMNIK
KRASNER
MRBONES
MRHANEY
MRJONES
MRNANNY
ORDINAL
ORDINES
ORDONEZ
ORGANDY
ORGANIC
ORGANZA
ORIENTE
ORIENTS
ORLANDO
ORMANDY
PRAWNED
PREENED
PREENER
PRYINTO
TRAINED
TRAINEE
TRAINER
TRAININ
TRAYNOR
TREINTA
TROUNCE
TRUANCY
TRUANTS
URBANER
URBANII
URBANIV
URBANVI
URGENCY
URGINGS
URSINUS

•R•••N•

ARACHNE
ARACHNO
ARCHING
ARCHONS
ARCSINE
ARETINO
ARGONNE
ARGUING
ARIADNE
ARISING
ARIZONA
ARMBAND
ARMBONE
ARMYANT
ARTSONG
ARUBANS
BRACING
BRAKING
BRAVING
BRAYING
BRAZENS
BRAZING
BRETONS
BREWING
BRIBING
BRIGAND
BRINING
BRITONS
BROGANS
BROMINE
BRUXING
CRANING
CRAPING
CRATING
CRAVENS
CRAVING
CRAYONS
CRAZING
CREMINI
CREMONA
CREPING
CRETANS
CRETINS
CREWING
CRIMINY
CROTONS
CROWING
CRUZANS
DRAGONS
DRAPING
DRAWING
DRAYING
DRIVING
DRONING
DROPINS
DRQUINN
DRYRUNS
ERASING
ERELONG
ERIGENA
ERODENT
ERODING
ERSKINE
FRAMING
FRAYING
FREEING
FRELENG
FREMONT
FRODING
FROZONE
FRYPANS
GRACING
GRADING
GRATING
GRAVING
GRAYING
GRAZING
GREYING
GRIMING
GRIPING
GROPING
GROWING
IRELAND
IRISING
IRONING
IRONONS
JREWING
KRAKENS
KRISHNA
MRBURNS
MRNANNY
MRWRONG
ORATING
ORDAINS
OREGANO
ORIGINE
ORIGINS
ORISONS
ORLEANS
OROGENY
OROTUND
ORPHANS
ORPHANT
PRALINE
PRATING
PRAYING
PREBIND
PREDENY
PREFUND
PRERENT
PRESENT
PRESONG
PRETEND
PREVENT
PREYING
PRICING
PRIDING
PRIMING
PRISONS
PRIZING
PROBING
PROBONO
PROFANE
PROGENY
PROLONG
PROPANE
PROPONE
PROSING
PROTONS
PROVINE
PROVING
PRUDENT
PRUNING
RRATING
TRACING
TRADING
TREEING
TREPANS
TREVINO
TRIBUNE
TRIDENT
TRIGONS
TRITONE
TRITONS
TROJANS
TROWING
TRUEING
TRUMANS
URCHINS
WRITING
XRATING
XRAYING

•R••••N

ARABIAN
ARAGORN
ARAMEAN
ARRAIGN
ARTFERN
ARTISAN
BRACKEN
BRAEDEN
BRAHMAN
BRAHMIN
BRANDON
BRANSON
BRAXTON
BREAKIN
BRENDAN
BRENDON
BRENGUN
BRENNAN
BRESLIN
BRETTON
BRINGIN
BRINGON
BRITAIN
BRITTEN
BRITTON
BROADEN
BROKEIN
BRONSON
BRONWEN
BROSNAN
CRAISIN
CRAMPON
CRAMSIN
CRATION
CREEPIN
CREPTIN
CRESPIN
CRESTON
CREWMAN
CREWMEN
CRIMEAN
CRIMSON
CRISPEN
CRISPIN
CROUTON
CROWDIN
CRUTZEN
CRYDOWN
CRYOGEN
DRAGOON
DRAGSIN
DRAGSON
DRANKIN
DRAWMAN
DRAWMEN
DRAWNIN
DRAWNON
DRAWSIN
DRAWSON
DRAYMAN
DRAYMEN
DRAYTON
DRBROWN
DREAMIN
DREAMON
DREGION
DRESDEN
DRESSIN
DRIFTIN
DRINKIN
DRIPPAN
DRIPSON
DRISTAN
DRIVEIN
DRONEON
DROPSIN
DROVEIN
DRQUINN
DRSLOAN
DRUMLIN
DRUNKEN
DRUZEAN
DRUZIAN
EREWHON
ERICSON
ERIKSON
EROSION
ERTEGUN
FRANKEN
FREEMAN
FREEMEN
FRESHEN
FRIEDAN
FRISIAN
FRISSON
FROGMAN
FROGMEN
FRONTON
FROWNON
GRAFTON
GRATEON
GRAUMAN
GRAYSON
GREATEN
GRECIAN
GREMLIN
GREYHEN
GRIFFIN
GRIFFON
GROOVIN
GROWNON
GROWSON
GRUMMAN
GRUNION
GRYPHON
IRANIAN
IRECKON
IRESIGN
IRONMAN
IRONMEN
IRONSON
KRAMDEN
KRATION
KREMLIN
KRESKIN
KRISTIN
KRYPTON
MRBROWN
MRCLEAN
MRGREEN
MRISCAN
ORARION
ORATION
ORBISON
ORDERIN
ORPHEAN
ORTOLAN
PREBORN
PREBURN
PREDAWN
PREGAIN
PRELOAN
PRENOON
PREOPEN
PREPLAN
PRESSON
PRESTON
PRETEEN
PREWARN
PREWORN
PREYSON
PROCYON
PRODSON
PRONOUN
PROPMAN
PROPMEN
PROSCAN
PROTEAN
PROTEIN
PRYOPEN
TRADEIN
TRADEON
TRAININ
TRAPGUN
TREADON
TREASON
TRENTON
TRICORN
TRIEDON
TRIESON
TRILLIN
TRIPSON
TRISTAN
TRODDEN
TROMPIN
TROOPIN
TRUDGEN
TRUSTIN
TRYITON
URGEDON
URGESON
WRITEIN
WRITEON
WRITTEN
WROTEIN
WROTEON

••RN•••

AIRNESS
BARNABY
BARNARD
BARNEYS
BARNING
BARNONE
BARNOWL
BARNRED
BARNUMS
BERNARD
BERNAYS
BERNESE
BERNINA
BERNINI
BERNSEN
BORNEAN
BORNEUP
BURNABY
BURNERS
BURNETT
BURNFOR
BURNING
BURNISH
BURNLEY
BURNOFF
BURNOUT
BURNSIN
BURNSUP
BURNTIN
BURNTUP
CARNABY
CARNAGE
CARNERA
CARNETS
CARNIES
CORNBIN
CORNCOB
CORNDOG
CORNEAL
CORNEAS
CORNELL
CORNERS
CORNETS
CORNFED
CORNICE
CORNIER
CORNILY
CORNING
CORNISH
CORNOIL
CORNROW
CORNUTE
DARNELL
DARNERS
DARNING
DERNIER
DIRNDLS
DURNING
EARNERS
EARNEST
EARNING
EARNSIT
FARNESS
FERNAND
FERNBAR
FERNERY
FERNIER
FURNACE
FURNESS
FURNISH
GARNEAU
GARNERS
GARNETS
GARNETT
GARNISH
GURNEYS
HARNESS
HARNICK
HERNANI
HERNDON
HERNIAE
HERNIAS
HERNIBS
HORNETS
HORNIER
HORNING
HORNISH
HORNIST
HORNSBY
HORNSIN
HORNUNG
KERNELS
MARNIER
MORNING
SARNOFF
SURNAME
TARNISH
TERNARY
TERNATE
TORNADO
TORNOFF
TORNOUT
TURNBAD
TURNERS
TURNERY
TURNING
TURNIPS
TURNKEY
TURNOFF
TURNONS
TURNOUT
TURNPRO
TURNRED
TURNSIN
TURNSON
TURNSTO
TURNSUP
TURNUPS
VARNISH
VERNIER
WARNING
WARNOFF
WARNSOF
WERNHER
WORNOFF
WORNOUT
YARNELL
YARNING
ZERNIKE

••R•N••

ACRONYM
ADRENAL
AIRINGS
AKRONOH
APRONED
ARRANGE
BARANOF
BARENTS
BARONET
BERENDT
BERKNER
BORINGS
BORONIC
BURUNDI
BYRONIC
CARINAE
CARINAS
CHRONIC
CORINNE
CORINTH
CORONAE
CORONAL
CORONAS
CORONER
CORONET
DARENOT
DERANGE
DERONDA
DURANCE
DURANGO
DURANTE
ENRANKS
ERRANCY
ERRANDS
FARINAS
FIRENZA
FIRENZE
FIRINGS
FORENZA
FORINTS
FORONCE
GARDNER
GARONNE
GERENTS
GERUNDS
GIRONDE
GORTNER
GYRENES
HERENOW
HERONRY
INRANGE
KORANIC
KORUNAS
LARDNER
LORANGE
LORENTZ
LORENZO
LORGNON
MARANTZ
MARENGO
MARINAS
MARINER
MARINES
MCRANEY
MERINOS
MIRANDA
MORANIS
MORANTE
MORONIC
MURANOS
OTRANTO
PARDNER
PARENTS
PARINGS
PARONYM
PARSNIP
PARTNER
PHRENIC
PIRANHA
PORTNOY
RERANKS
RERENTS
RERINSE
SARANAC
SARONGS
SCRUNCH
SERENER
SHRINED
SHRINER
SHRINES
SHRINKS
SIRENED
SORENTO
SPRINGS
SPRINGY
SPRINTS
STRANDS
STRANGE
STRINGS
STRINGY
SURINAM
SYRINGE
TARANTO
TERENCE
THRONES
THRONGS
TORINOS
TORONTO
TYRANNY
TYRANTS
VERANDA
VERONIA
VERYNEW
WIRINGS

••R••N•

ADRIANA
AGROUND
AIRFONE
AIRGUNS
AIRLANE
AIRLINE
AIRTANK
AIRVENT
BARBING
BARGING
BARKING
BARNING
BARNONE
BARRENS
BARRING
BARRONS
BARTEND
BARYONS
BERMING
BERNINA
BERNINI
BEROWNE
BERSUNT
BIRDING
BIRIANI
BIRLING
BIRMANS
BIRRING
BIRYANI
BORDONI
BORKING
BURBANK
BURDENS
BURKINA
BURLING
BURMANS
BURNING
BURPING
BURRING
BURYING
CARBINE
CARBONS
CARDING
CAREENS
CARKING
CARLENE
CARLING
CARMINA
CARMINE
CARPING
CARTING
CARTONS
CARVING
CERVINE
CORDING
CORDONS
CORINNE
CORKING
CORNING
CORTINA
CORVINA
CORVINE
CORZINE
CURBING
CURDING
CURLING
CURRANT
CURRENT
CURRING
CURSING
CURVING
DARKENS
DARLENE
DARLING
DARNING
DARTING
DERRING
DERWENT
DIRKING
DORMANT
DURNING
DURWENT
EARBONE
EARNING
EARRING
FARCING
FARGOND
FARGONE
FARMING
FERMENT
FERNAND
FERVENT
FIRBANK
FIREANT
FIRKINS
FIRMING
FORCING
FORDING
FORDONE
FORFEND
FORGING
FORGONE
FORKING
FORLANI
FORMING
FORRENT
FORTUNA
FORTUNE
FORWENT
FURLING
FURLONG
FURRING
GARBING
GARCONS
GARDENA
GARDENS
GARLAND
GARMENT
GARONNE
GERAINT
GERMANE
GERMANS
GERMANY
GIRDING
GIRTING
GORGING
GORGONS
GORMING
GOROUND
HARDENS
HARDING
HARKENS
HARKING
HARLAND
HARLINE
HARMING
HARMONY
HARPING
HERDING
HERMANA
HERMANN
HERMANO
HERMANS
HERNANI
HEROINE
HERRING
HIRCINE
HORDING
HORMONE
HORNING
HORNUNG
HORSING
HURLING
HURTING
IGRAINE
INRUINS
JARDINE
JARDINS
JARGONS
JARGONY
JARRING
JERGENS
JERKING
JERKINS
JORDANA
JURGENS
JURYING
KIRMANS
KOREANS
KURRENT
LARAINE
LARCENY
LARDING
LARDONS
LARGENT
LARKING
LARKINS
LORDING
LORIENT

LURKING
MARCONI
MARGINS
MARIANA
MARIANO
MARKING
MARLENE
MARLINS
MAROONS
MARRING
MARRONS
MARTENS
MARTINA
MARTINI
MARTINO
MARTINS
MARTINU
MARTINV
MARYANN
MERGING
MERLINS
MORAINE
MORDANT
MORDENT
MOREENS
MORGANA
MORGANS
MORMONS
MORNING
MORTONS
NERVINE
NERVING
NIRVANA
NORMAND
NORMANS
NORTONS
NURSING
OURGANG
OURSONG
PARDONS
PARGING
PARKING
PARKINS
PARRING
PARSING
PARSONS
PARTING
PARTONE
PARVENU
PERCENT
PERKING
PERKINS
PERMING
PERRINE
PERRINS
PERSONA
PERSONS
PORCINE
PORKING
PORSENA
PORTEND
PORTENT
PORTING
PURGING
PURLING
PURRING
PURSING
SARDINE
SARGENT
SCRAWNY
SCREENS
SERLING
SERMONS
SERPENS
SERPENT
SERVANT
SERVING
SORDINI
SORDINO
SORIANO
SORTING
SORVINO
SPRAINS
STRAINS
SURFING
SURGING
SYRIANA
SYRIANS
TARPONS
TARRING
TARTANS
TARTING
TARZANA
TARZANS
TERHUNE
TERMING
TERMINI
TERRANS
TERRENE
TERRINE
THREENO
TORMENT
TORRENT
TORTONI
TURBANS
TURBINE
TUREENS
TURFING
TURNING
TURNONS
TYRANNY
UKRAINE
UNRAINY
UNROUND
VARIANT
VARMINT
VARYING
VERBENA
VERDANT
VERDINS
VEREINE
VERGING
VERMINY
VERMONT
VERSANT
VERSING
VIRGINS
WARBOND
WARDENS
WARDING
WARMING
WARNING
WARPING
WARRANT
WARRENG
WARRENS
WARRING
WARZONE
WORDING
WORDONE
WORKING
WORMING
WORSENS
YARDING
YARNING
ZEROING
ZIRCONS

••R•••N

AFRICAN
AGREEON
AIRHORN
AIRSIGN
ALROSEN
ARRAIGN
BARDEEN
BARGAIN
BARGEIN
BERGMAN
BERGSON
BERIGAN
BERNSEN
BIRCHEN
BIRDMAN
BIRDMEN
BORNEAN
BORODIN
BURGEON
BURNSIN
BURNTIN
BURPGUN
BURSTIN
BURSTYN
CARAVAN
CARBARN
CARHORN
CARLOAN
CARLSON
CARLTON
CAROLYN
CAROTIN
CARRYIN
CARRYON
CARTOON
CARTSIN
CERTAIN
CERUMEN
CORAZON
CORNBIN
CURLSIN
CURTAIN
DARKMAN
DARKTAN
DARLEEN
DARTGUN
DIRKSEN
DORFMAN
EARLYON
EARTHEN
EUROVAN
FERMION
FIREDON
FIREMAN
FIREMEN
FIRESON
FORCEIN
FORCEON
FOREIGN
FOREMAN
FOREMEN
FORERAN
FORERUN
FORLORN
FORTRAN
GERMAIN
GERSHON
GORDIAN
HARDPAN
HARDTEN
HARDWON
HARPOON
HARPSON
HARSHEN
HARTMAN
HERMANN
HERNDON
HIREDON
HIRESON
HORIZON
HORNSIN
HURSTON
JERILYN
JURYMAN
JURYMEN
KARAJAN
KARLSON
KERATIN
KIRSTEN
LARCHEN
LORGNON
LUREDIN
LURESIN
LURLEEN
LYRICON
MARCHON
MARDIAN
MARILYN
MARMION
MARRYIN
MARSDEN
MARSTON
MARTIAN
MARXIAN
MARYANN
MERCIAN
MERIDEN
MORPHIN
NARAYAN
OARSMAN
OARSMEN
OURTOWN
PARAGON
PARKMAN
PARTYON
PERLMAN
PERMIAN
PERSIAN
PERSSON
PERTAIN
PIROGEN
PORTION
PORTMAN
PURITAN
PURLOIN
RARITAN
RERISEN
SARACEN
SARAZEN
SAROYAN
SARUMAN
SERBIAN
SIRLOIN
SPRAYON
STRAPIN
STRAPON
STRIVEN
SURECAN
SURFMAN
SURFMEN
SURGEON
TERRAIN
THREWIN
THREWON
THRIVEN
THROWIN
THROWON
TIREMAN
TIREMEN
TORSION
TURFMAN
TURFMEN
TURNSIN
TURNSON
UNRISEN
UNRIVEN
UPRISEN
VERGEON
VERIZON
VERSION
VIRGOAN
WARTORN
WARWORN
WIREDIN
WIREMAN
WIREMEN
WIRESIN
WORKMAN
WORKMEN
WORKSIN
WORKSON
YARDMAN
YARDMEN
YEREVAN
YORKTON
ZEROSIN

•••RN••

ACORNED
ADORNED
ADORNER
AVERNAL
AVERNUS
BLARNEY
CAIRNED
CHARNIN
CHURNED
CHURNER
CHURNUP
DIURNAL
EPERNAY
ETERNAL
FEARNOT
HAIRNET
JOURNAL
JOURNEE
JOURNEY
JOURNOS
KEARNEY
LEARNED
LEARNER
LEARNOF
LEARNTO
MOURNED
MOURNER
OVERNEW
SCORNED
SCORNER
SMIRNOV
SPURNED
SPURNER
STERNAL
STERNER
STERNLY
STERNOS
STERNUM
THORNED
TIERNEY
TOURNEY
VIERNES
YEARNED
YEARNER
YEARNTO

•••R•N•

ADORING
AFFRONT
AMARONE
AMERIND
AYNRAND
BARRENS
BARRING
BARRONS
BEARING
BEHRENS
BEHRING
BIRRING
BLARING
BURRING
CABRINI
CAIRENE
CAPRINE
CHARING
CHORINE
CHYRONS
CITRINE
CITRONS
COBRAND
COURANT
CURRANT
CURRENT
CURRING
CZARINA
DACRONS
DEARONE
DERRING
DOGRUNS
DOWRONG
DRYRUNS
EARRING
ENDRUNS
ENTRANT
ENURING
EPERGNE
ESTRING
FAIRING
FEARING
FIBRINS
FIORINA
FLARING
FLORENZ
FLORINS
FORRENT
FUNRUNS
FURRING
GEARING
GLARING
GOWRONG
GSTRING
GUARANI
HADRONS
HEARING
HERRING
HYDRANT
ICERINK
ICERUNS
IFORONE
IMPRINT
INFRONT
INIRONS
INPRINT
INURING
ITERANT
IVORINE
JARRING
JEERING
KATRINA
KATRINE
KEYRING
KURRENT
LADRONE
LAIRING
LATRINE
LAURENT
LEERING
LEGRAND
LIBRANS
LOURING
LOWRENT
MACRONS
MARRING
MARRONS
MATRONS
MICRONS
MIGRANT
MITRING
MOORING
MOTRINS
MRWRONG
NEARING
NEGRONI
NEURONE
NEURONS
OCARINA
ODORANT
OILRING
OPERAND
OPERANT
OUTRANG
OUTRANK
OUTRANT
OUTRING
OUTRUNS
PADRONE
PAIRING
PARRING
PATRONS
PEERING
PERRINE
PERRINS
PHARYNX
POURING
PRERENT
PURRING
REAREND
REARING
REBRAND
RECRANK
REFRONT
REGRANT
REGRIND
REPRINT
REPRUNE
ROARING
SABRINA
SCARING
SCORING
SEARING
SEBRING
SHARING
SHARONA
SHORING
SKIRUNS
SNARING
SNORING
SOARING
SOPRANI
SOPRANO
SOURING
SPARING
SPYRING
STARING
STORING
STYRENE
TARRING
TAURINE
TEARING
TERRANS
TERRENE
TERRINE
THERENT
THERING
THERINK
TIERING
TITRING
TOPRANK
TORRENT
TOURING
TSARINA
TWERENT
TZARINA
UNDRUNK
UNFRANK
UNGRAND
UNWRUNG
UPFRONT
UPTREND
USGRANT
VAGRANT
VEERING
VIBRANT
VITRINE
WARRANT
WARRENG
WARRENS
WARRING
WEARING
YEAREND
YEARONE
YOURANG
ZEBRINE
ZIERING

•••R••N

ALARCON
ALGREEN
APERSON
AZOREAN
AZORIAN
BAHRAIN
BAHREIN
BASRHIN
BEARSON
BEERCAN
BEHRMAN
BOORMAN
BOURBON
BYTRAIN
CARRYIN
CARRYON
CHARMAN
CHARMEN
CHARMIN
CHARNIN
CITROEN
CLARION
COARSEN
CYPRIAN
DEARDEN
DETRAIN
DOORMAN
DOORMEN
DRBROWN
ELTRAIN
EMBROWN
EMERSON
ENGRAIN
ENTRAIN
EXURBAN
FLORIAN
FOURMAN
FOURPIN
GGORDON
GHERKIN
GUERDON
HADRIAN
HAIRPIN
HEARKEN
HEARTEN
HOARSEN
IBERIAN
INBROWN
INDRAWN
INGRAIN
INGREEN
INGROWN
ISTRIAN
IVERSON
IVORIAN
JIMRYUN
JOURDAN
MAARTEN
MARRYIN
MAUREEN
MEGRYAN
MOORHEN
MRBROWN
MRGREEN
MYERSON
OBERLIN
ORARION
OSIRIAN
OVERMAN
OVERRAN
OVERRUN
PATROON
PEARSON
PEERSIN
PEORIAN
PIERIAN
POORMAN
POORMEN
POURSIN
QUARTAN
REARDON
RECROWN
REDRAWN
REFRAIN
REGROWN
RETRAIN
RIORDAN
SAURIAN
SHAREIN
SHARPEN
SHERMAN
SHERWIN
SHORTEN
SMARTEN
SOURSON
SPARTAN
SPORRAN
SPORTIN
SPURSON
STARION
STARMAN
STARSIN
STARTIN
STARTON
STIRSIN
STORMIN
SWOREIN
TAUREAN
TERRAIN
THEREIN
THEREON
THORSON
THURMAN
UMBRIAN
UNCROWN
UNDRAWN
UNGREEN
UNGROWN
UNURBAN
UPGROWN
VANRIJN
WEARSON
WEIRTON
WHARTON
WHEREIN
WHEREON
YOUREON
YZERMAN
ZAIRIAN

••••RN•

AUBURNS
AUBURNU
BICORNE
BICORNS
BYTURNS
CASERNE
CASERNS
CAVERNS
DEHORNS
EXTERNE
EXTERNS
GOVERNS
HIBERNO
INFERNO
INTERNE
INTERNS
INTURNS
LAVERNE
LIVORNO
LOCARNO
LUCARNE
LUCERNE
MODERNE
MODERNS
MRBURNS
NOTURNS
OSBORNE
PATERNO
REDARNS
REEARNS
RETURNS
REWARNS
SALERNO
SATURNS
STEARNS
SUBORNS
SUKARNO
TAVERNA
TAVERNS
TEAURNS
UNBORNE
UNBURNT
UPBORNE
UPTURNS
WYVERNS
YESORNO

••••R•N

ACHERON
AILERON
ALLBRAN
ALSORAN
ANDIRON
ANKARAN
ASMARAN
ASPIRIN
AVEYRON
BELTRAN
BIAFRAN
BULLRUN
CALDRON
CAMERON
CHAGRIN
CHEERON
CHEVRON
COCHRAN
COMORAN
DENDRON
DEXTRIN
ECOTRIN
EMPIRIN
ENTERIN
ENTERON
ENVIRON
EUCERIN
FLEURON
FORERAN
FORERUN
FORTRAN
GAGARIN
HEPARIN
HOMERUN
HYPERON
KATHRYN
LATERAN
LATERON
LAVERAN
LEBARON
LEGIRON
LONGRUN
MADERUN
MAJORIN
MAKERUN
MAZARIN
MIDIRON
MILERUN
MILKRUN
MILLRUN
MINORIN
NEUTRON
NONIRON
OATBRAN
OMICRON
ONEIRON
ORDERIN
OUTGRIN
OVERRAN
OVERRUN
PIGIRON
SAFFRON
SAHARAN
SAVARIN
SEAGREN
SIXIRON
SMEARON
SONORAN
SPORRAN
STEARIN
SWEARIN
TEHERAN
TELERAN
TENKRUN
TESTRUN
TEXTRON
TIBURON
TWOIRON
USHERIN
VESTRON
VETERAN
WAITRON
WELLRUN

•••••RN

ADJOURN
AIRHORN
ALTHORN
ARAGORN
ARTFERN
ASHBURN
BIGHORN
BITTERN
CARBARN
CARHORN
CISTERN
CLIBURN
COGBURN
CONCERN
DISCERN
EASTERN
FOGHORN
FORLORN
GOLDARN
HEPBURN
INKHORN
LANTERN
LECTERN
LEGHORN
LETTERN
LOWBORN
MAXBORN
MIDMORN
NEWBERN
NEWBORN
NOUTURN
OAKFERN
OUTBURN
OUTEARN
OUTTORN
OUTTURN
OUTWORN
PASTERN
PATTERN
POPCORN
POSTERN
PREBORN
PREBURN
PREWARN
PREWORN
RAEBURN
RAYBURN
READORN
REDFERN
RELEARN
RESWORN
RIPTORN
SANBORN
SAXHORN
SEAFERN
SOJOURN
SOTHERN

SUNBURN
THETURN
TINHORN
TINTERN
TOATURN
TRICORN
UNCHURN
UNICORN
UNLEARN
UNSHORN
UNSTERN
UNSWORN
WARTORN
WARWORN
WAYWORN
WESTERN

RO•••••

ROACHES
ROADBED
ROADEOS
ROADERS
ROADHOG
ROADIES
ROADMAP
ROADTAR
ROADTAX
ROADWAY
ROAMERS
ROAMING
ROANOKE
ROARERS
ROARING
ROARSAT
ROASTED
ROASTER
ROBARDS
ROBBERS
ROBBERY
ROBBING
ROBBINS
ROBBNEN
ROBERTA
ROBERTE
ROBERTF
ROBERTH
ROBERTI
ROBERTO
ROBERTS
ROBESON
ROBLOWE
ROBOCOP
ROBOTIC
ROBOTRY
ROBROYS
ROBSART
ROBUSTA
ROBUSTO
ROCHETS
ROCKABY
ROCKCOD
ROCKERS
ROCKERY
ROCKETS
ROCKIER
ROCKIES
ROCKILY
ROCKING
ROCKOIL
ROCKOON
ROCKYII
ROCKYIV
ROCOCOS
RODDICK
RODDING
RODENTS
RODEOFF
RODEOUT
RODGERS
RODLESS
RODLIKE
RODOLFO
RODRIGO
ROEBUCK
ROEDEER
ROETHKE
ROGAINE
ROGERED
ROGUERY
ROGUING
ROGUISH
ROILIER
ROILING
ROISTER
ROLAIDS
ROLEXES
ROLFERS
ROLFING
ROLLAND
ROLLBAR
ROLLEIS
ROLLERS
ROLLICK
ROLLING
ROLLINS
ROLLMOP
ROLLOFF
ROLLONS
ROLLOUT
ROLLSBY
ROLLSIN
ROLLSON
ROLLSUP
ROLLTOP
ROLLUPS
ROLLWAY
ROLODEX
ROLONDA
ROLVAAG
ROMAINE
ROMAINS
ROMAJIS
ROMANCE
ROMANIA
ROMANIC
ROMANIS
ROMANOS
ROMANOV
ROMANSH
ROMANUS
ROMBERG
ROMCOMS
ROMNEYS
ROMPERS
ROMPING
ROMPISH
ROMULAN
ROMULUS
RONDEAU
RONDELS
RONDURE
RONETTE
RONSARD
RONSONS
RONTGEN
RONWOOD
RONZONI
ROOFAGE
ROOFERS
ROOFING
ROOFRAT
ROOFTOP
ROOKERY
ROOKIER
ROOKIES
ROOKING
ROOKISH
ROOMBAS
ROOMERS
ROOMFUL
ROOMIER
ROOMIES
ROOMILY
ROOMING
ROOSTED
ROOSTER
ROOTAGE
ROOTCAP
ROOTERS
ROOTFOR
ROOTIER
ROOTING
ROOTLED
ROOTLES
ROOTLET
ROOTOUT
ROOTROT
ROOTSUP
ROPEDIN
ROPEDUP
ROPEOFF
ROPESIN
ROPESUP
ROPETOW
ROPIEST
RORAIMA
RORQUAL
ROSABUD
ROSALIA
ROSALIE
ROSALYN
ROSANNA
ROSANNE
ROSARIO
ROSCOES
ROSEATE
ROSEBAY
ROSEBUD
ROSEHIP
ROSELLA
ROSELLE
ROSEOIL
ROSEOLA
ROSERED
ROSETEA
ROSETTA
ROSETTE
ROSIEST
ROSINED
ROSSANO
ROSSINI
ROSSNER
ROSSSEA
ROSTAND
ROSTERS
ROSTOCK
ROSTRAL
ROSTRUM
ROSWELL
ROTATED
ROTATES
ROTATOR
ROTAWAY
ROTBLAT
ROTELLE
ROTGUTS
ROTHIRA
ROTIFER
ROTTERS
ROTTING
ROTUNDA
ROUAULT
ROUBAIX
ROUGHED
ROUGHEN
ROUGHER
ROUGHGO
ROUGHIT
ROUGHLY
ROUGHUP
ROUGING
ROULADE
ROULEAU
ROUNDED
ROUNDEL
ROUNDER
ROUNDLY
ROUNDON
ROUNDUP
ROUSERS
ROUSING
ROUSTED
ROUSTER
ROUTERS
ROUTINE
ROUTING
ROUTOUT
ROVETTA
ROVINGS
ROWBOAT
ROWDIER
ROWDIES
ROWDILY
ROWELED
ROWLAND
ROWLING
ROXANNE
ROXBURY
ROYALES
ROYALLY
ROYALTY
ROYALWE
ROYBEAN
ROYCOHN
ROYGBIV
ROZANOV
ROZELLE

R•O••••

REOCCUR
REOFFER
REOILED
REOPENS
REORDER
REOWNED
RHODIAN
RHODIUM
RHOECUS
RHOMBIC
RHOMBUS
RIOLOBO
RIOMUNI
RIORDAN
RIORITA
RIOTACT
RIOTERS
RIOTGUN
RIOTING
RIOTOUS
ROOFAGE
ROOFERS
ROOFING
ROOFRAT
ROOFTOP
ROOKERY
ROOKIER
ROOKIES
ROOKING
ROOKISH
ROOMBAS
ROOMERS
ROOMFUL
ROOMIER
ROOMIES
ROOMILY
ROOMING
ROOSTED
ROOSTER
ROOTAGE
ROOTCAP
ROOTERS
ROOTFOR
ROOTIER
ROOTING
ROOTLED
ROOTLES
ROOTLET
ROOTOUT
ROOTROT
ROOTSUP
RYOKANS

R••O•••

RADOMES
RAGOUTS
RAMONES
RANONIN
RANOVER
RAYOVAC
RAZORED
RCCOLAS
REBOANT
REBOARD
REBOILS
REBOLTS
REBOOKS
REBOOTS
REBORED
REBORES
REBOTES
REBOUND
REBOXED
REBOXES
REBOZOS
RECOALS
RECOATS
RECOCKS
RECODED
RECODES
RECOILS
RECOINS
RECOLOR
RECOMBS
RECOOKS
RECOOLS
RECORDS
RECORKS
RECOSTS
RECOUNT
RECOUPS
RECOVER
REDOAKS
REDOCKS
REDOING
REDONDO
REDOSED
REDOSES
REDOUBT
REDOUND
REDOUTS
REDOXES
REFOCUS
REFOLDS
REFORGE
REFORMS
REFOUND
REHONED
REHONES
REHONOR
REHOOKS
REHOUSE
REJOICE
REJOINS
RELOADS
RELOANS
RELOCKS
RELOOKS
RELOSES
REMODEL
REMOLDS
REMORAS
REMORSE
REMOTER
REMOTES
REMOUNT
REMOVAL
REMOVED
REMOVER
REMOVES
REMOWED
RENOIRS
RENOTED
RENOTES
RENOWNS
REPOINT
REPOLLS
REPOMAN
REPORTS
REPOSED
REPOSER
REPOSES
REPOSIT
REPOSTS
REPOURS
REPOWER
REROLLS
REROOFS
REROOTS
REROUTE
RESOAKS
RESOAPS
RESOILS
RESOJET
RESOLED
RESOLER
RESOLES
RESOLVE
RESORBS
RESORTS
RESOUND
RESOWED
RETOAST
RETONED
RETONES
RETOOLS
RETORTS
RETOTAL
RETOUCH
RETOURS
RETOWED
REVOICE
REVOKED
REVOKER
REVOKES
REVOLTS
REVOLVE
REVOTED
REVOTES
REWOKEN
REWORDS
REWORKS
REWOUND
REWOVEN
REYOKED
REYOKES
REZONED
REZONES
RICOTTA
RIDOTTO
RIGOURS
RIPOFFS
RIPOPEN
RIPOSTE
RIPOSTS
RISOTTO
ROBOCOP
ROBOTIC
ROBOTRY
ROCOCOS
RODOLFO
ROLODEX
ROLONDA
RUDOLFI
RUDOLPH
RUMORED
RUMOURS
RUNOFFS
RUNONIN
RUNOUTS
RUNOVER

R•••O••

RACCOON
RACKOUT
RADFORD
RADIOAD
RADIODJ
RADIOED
RADIOER
RADIOIN
RAGDOLL
RAGMOPS
RAGTOPS
RAINOUT
RAISONS
RAKEOFF
RAMDOWN
RAMHOME
RAMRODS
RAMSONS
RANCORS
RANCOUR
RANDOWN
RANGOFF
RANGOON
RANGOUT
RANHOME
RANKOUT
RANSOMS
RAPPORT
RAPSONG
RAPTORS
RASBORA
RATHOLE
RATIONS
RATSOUT
RAUCOUS
RAVIOLI
RAWFOOD
RAYMOND
RCADOME
READOFF
READOPT
READORN
READOUT
REAMOUT
REAROSE
REASONS
REAVOWS
REAWOKE
REBLOCK
REBLOOM
REBLOWN
REBOOKS
REBOOTS
REBROKE
RECHOSE
RECKONS
RECOOKS
RECOOLS
RECROOM
RECROSS
RECROWN
RECTORS
RECTORY
REDBONE
REDBOOK
REDCOAT
REDCODS
REDDOGS
REDDOTS
REDFORD
REDFOUR
REDHOTS
REDMOND
REDNOSE
REDPOLL
REDPONY
REDROBE
REDROOP
REDROOT
REDROSE
REDTOPS
REDWOLF
REDWOOD
REDWORM
REDZONE
REEBOKS
REELOFF
REELOUT
REEVOKE
REFLOAT
REFLOOD
REFLOWN
REFLOWS
REFRONT
REGIONS
REGLOSS
REGLOWS
REGROOM
REGROUP
REGROWN
REGROWS
REHOOKS
REKNOCK
REKNOTS
RELOOKS
RENTOUT
RENVOIS
REPHONE
REPLOTS
REPLOWS
REPROBE
REPROOF
REPROVE
REQUOTE
REROOFS
REROOTS
RESCORE
RESHOES
RESHOOT
RESHOWN
RESHOWS
RESPOKE
RESPOND
RESPOOL
RESPOTS
RESTOCK
RESTOKE
RESTORE
RESTOWS
RESWORE
RESWORN
RETOOLS
REWROTE
REXROTH
REYMONT
REYNOSA
RHEBOKS
RHETORS
RHIZOME
RIBBONS
RIBBONY
RIDEOFF
RIDEOUT
RIGSOUT
RIMROCK
RINGOFF
RINGOUT
RIOLOBO
RIOTOUS
RIPCORD
RIPSOFF
RIPSONE
RIPSOUT
RIPTORN
RISSOLE
ROANOKE
ROBLOWE
ROBROYS
ROCKOIL
ROCKOON
RODEOFF
RODEOUT
ROLLOFF
ROLLONS
ROLLOUT
ROMCOMS
RONSONS
RONWOOD
RONZONI
ROOTOUT
ROPEOFF
ROSCOES
ROSEOIL
ROSEOLA
ROSTOCK
ROUTOUT
ROWBOAT
ROYCOHN
RUBDOWN
RUBEOLA
RUBIOUS
RUBSOFF
RUBSOUT
RUINOUS
RULEONE
RULEOUT
RUMFORD
RUMPOLE
RUNDOWN
RUNGOFF
RUNGOUT
RUNHOME
RUNSOFF
RUNSOUT
RUSHOFF
RUSHOUT
RYELOAF

R••••O•

RACCOON
RACINOS
RAGSHOP
RAILSON
RAINBOW
RAINGOD
RAINSON
RALSTON
RANAMOK
RANCHOS
RANGFOR
RANGOON
RANRIOT
RAVELOE
RAWFOOD
RAYKROC
REACTOR
READFOR
READSON
REALLOT
REALTOR
REARDON
REBLOOM
REBOZOS
RECOLOR
RECROOM
REDBOOK
REDROOP
REDROOT
REDSPOT
REDWOOD
REEKSOF
REENDOW
REENJOY
REFLOOD
REGROOM
REHONOR
RELATOR
REPROOF
REPSFOR
REREDOS
RESHOOT
RESPOOL
RESTSON
RETINOL
REUNION
REVISOR
REZEROS
RIALTOS
RIGHTON
RIMSHOT
RINGFOR
RIPSTOP
ROADEOS
ROADHOG
ROBESON
ROBOCOP
ROCKCOD
ROCKOON
ROCOCOS
ROLLMOP
ROLLSON
ROLLTOP
ROMANOS
ROMANOV
RONWOOD
ROOFTOP
ROOTFOR
ROOTROT
ROPETOW
ROTATOR
ROUNDON
ROZANOV
RUBATOS
RUBICON
RUBUPON
RUCTION
RULEDON
RULESON
RUMSHOP
RUNAMOK
RUNGFOR
RUNRIOT
RUNSFOR
RUNSLOW

R•••••O

RACEDTO
RACESTO
RAJARAO
RALLYTO
RAMINTO
RANINTO
RANUPTO
RAPALLO
REACTTO
READSTO
REDONDO
REFERTO
RELLENO
RENALDO
RENTSTO
REPLYTO
RICARDO
RIDESTO
RIDOTTO
RILIEVO
RINALDO
RIOLOBO
RIPIENO
RIPINTO
RISENTO
RISESTO
RISOTTO
RIVERPO
RIZZUTO
ROBERTO
ROBUSTO
RODOLFO
RODRIGO
ROSARIO
ROSSANO
ROUGHGO
RUFFALO
RUNINTO
RUNUPTO

•RO••••

ARONNAX
AROUSAL
AROUSED
AROUSER
AROUSES
BROADAS
BROADAX
BROADEN
BROADER
BROADLY
BROASTS
BROCADE
BRODIES
BRODKEY
BRODSKY
BROGANS
BROGUES
BROIDER
BROILED
BROILER
BROKEIN
BROKERS
BROKEUP
BROMATE
BROMIDE
BROMINE
BRONCHI
BRONCHO
BRONCOS
BRONSON
BRONTES
BRONWEN
BRONZED
BRONZER
BRONZES
BROODED
BROODER
BROOKED
BROOMED
BROSNAN
BROSSES
BROTHER
BROUGHT
BROWARD
BROWNED
BROWNER
BROWNIE
BROWSED
BROWSER
BROWSES
BROWWAX
CROAKED
CROAKER
CROATIA
CROCHET
CROCKED
CROCKER
CROCKET
CROESUS
CROFTER
CRONIES
CROOKED
CROOKES
CROONED
CROONER

CROPPED CROPPER CROPSUP CROPTOP CROQUET CROQUIS CROSIER CROSSAT CROSSED CROSSER CROSSES CROSSLY CROSSUP CROSTIC CROTONS CROUTES CROUTON CROWBAR CROWDED CROWDER CROWDIN CROWELL CROWERS CROWING CROWLEY CROWNED CROWNER CROZIER DROGUES DROLLER DRONEON DRONERS DRONING DRONISH DROOLED DROOLER DROOPED DROPBOX DROPCAP DROPINS DROPLET DROPNET DROPOFF DROPOUT DROPPED DROPPER DROPSBY DROPSIN DROPSIT DROPTOP DROSSES DROUGHT DROVEAT DROVEBY DROVEIN DROVERS DROVETO DROVEUP DROWNED DROWSED DROWSES DROXIES ERODENT ERODERS ERODING EROSELY EROSION EROSIVE

EROTICA EROTICS FROCKED FRODING FROEBEL FROGGER FROGLEG FROGLET FROGMAN FROGMEN FROLICS FROMAGE FROMMER FRONTAL FRONTED FRONTON FROOGLE FROSTED FROSTER FROTHED FROTHER FROTHUP FROWARD FROWNAT FROWNED FROWNER FROWNON FROZEUP FROZONE GROANED GROANER GROCERS GROCERY GRODIER GROINED GROKKED GROLIER GROMMET GROMYKO GROOMED GROOMER GROOVED GROOVES GROOVIN GROPERS GROPING GROPIUS GROSSED GROSSER GROSSES GROSSLY GROTIUS GROTTOS GROUCHO GROUCHY GROUNDS GROUPED GROUPER GROUPIE GROUSED GROUSER GROUSES GROUTED GROUTER GROVELS GROVERS GROWBIG GROWDIM

GROWERS GROWFAT GROWING GROWLED GROWLER GROWNON GROWNUP GROWOLD GROWSON GROWSUP GROWTHS IRONAGE IRONBAR IRONERS IRONIES IRONING IRONIST IRONMAN IRONMEN IRONONS IRONORE IRONOUT IRONSON JROBERT KROEMER OROGENY OROLOGY OROTUND OROURKE PROARAB PROBALL PROBATE PROBERS PROBIES PROBING PROBITY PROBLEM PROBONO PROBOWL PROCEED PROCESS PROCITY PROCLUS PROCTER PROCTOR PROCURE PROCYON PRODDED PRODDER PRODIGY PRODSON PRODUCE PRODUCT PROEAST PROFANE PROFARM PROFESS PROFFER PROFILE PROFITS PROFUSE PROGENY PROGRAM PROJECT PROJETS PROKEDS PROLATE PROLIFE

PROLOGS PROLONG PROMBID PROMISE PROMOED PROMOTE PROMPTS PRONATE PRONAVY PRONELY PRONETO PRONGED PRONOUN PROOFED PROOFER PROPANE PROPELS PROPHET PROPJET PROPMAN PROPMEN PROPONE PROPOSE PROPPED PROPSUP PRORATA PRORATE PROSAIC PROSCAN PROSERS PROSHOP PROSIER PROSILY PROSING PROSODY PROSPER PROTEAM PROTEAN PROTECT PROTEGE PROTEIN PROTEST PROTEUS PROTIST PROTONS PROUDER PROUDLY PROUDOF PROVEIT PROVERB PROVERS PROVIDE PROVINE PROVING PROVISO PROVOKE PROVOST PROWESS PROWEST PROWLED PROWLER PROXIES PROXIMA PROXIMO TROCHEE TROCHES TRODDEN TROIKAS

TROILUS TROJANS TROLLED TROLLER TROLLEY TROLLOP TROMPED TROMPIN TROOPED TROOPER TROOPIN TROPICS TROPISM TROTHED TROTOFF TROTOUT TROTSKY TROTSUP TROTTED TROTTER TROUBLE TROUGHS TROUNCE TROUPED TROUPER TROUPES TROUSER TROWELS TROWING UROLOGY VRONSKY VROOMED WROCLAW WRONGED WRONGER WRONGLY WROTEIN WROTEON WROTETO WROTEUP WROUGHT

•R•O•••

ARBOLES ARBORED ARBOURS ARDOURS AREOLAE AREOLAR AREOLAS AREOLES ARGONNE ARIOSOS ARIOSTO ARMOIRE ARMORED ARMORER ARMOURS ARMOURY ARNOLDS ARROYOS BRIOCHE BROODED BROODER BROOKED BROOMED CREOLES CREOSOL

CROOKED CROOKES CROONED CROONER CRYOGEN CRYOVER DROOLED DROOLER DROOPED ERGOTIC FROOGLE GROOMED GROOMER GROOVED GROOVES GROOVIN MRBODDY MRBONES MRHOBBS MRHORSE MRJONES MRMOOSE MRNORTH MRNOVAK MRWORDS ORDONEZ ORIOLES ORMOLUS ORTOLAN PREOMIT PREOPEN PREORAL PRIORTO PROOFED PROOFER PRYOPEN TRIODES TRIOLET TROOPED TROOPER TROOPIN TRYOUTS VROOMED

•R••O••

ARAGORN ARCHONS ARDMORE ARDUOUS ARENOSE ARIZONA ARMBONE ARMHOLE ARMLOAD ARMLOCK ARTBOOK ARTFORM ARTROCK ARTSONG ARTWORK BRAVOED BRAVOES BRETONS BRITONS BRUMOUS CRAPOLA CRAPOUT CRAYOLA

CRAYONS CREMONA CREMORA CROTONS CRYDOWN CRYWOLF DRAGOFF DRAGONS DRAGOON DRAGOTI DRAGOUT DRAWOFF DRAWOUT DRBROWN DREWOFF DREWOUT DROPOFF DROPOUT DRSLOAN DRSPOCK DRUMOUT DRYDOCK DRYFOGS DRYHOLE DRYMOPS DRYROTS ERELONG FREMONT FRIJOLE FRIVOLS FROZONE FRYCOOK GRANOLA GREGORY GREWOLD GROWOLD IRISOUT IRKSOME IRONONS IRONORE IRONOUT IRSFORM MRBROWN MRMOOSE MRSCOTT MRSPOCK MRWRONG ORATORS ORATORY OREBODY ORINOCO ORISONS OROLOGY PREBOIL PREBOOK PREBOOM PREBORN PRECODE PRECOIL PRECOOK PRECOOL PRECOUP PREDOOM PREFORM PRELOAD PRELOAN PRELOSS PRENOON

PREROCK PRESOAK PRESOLD PRESONG PRESORT PRETOLD PRETORS PREVOID PREVOST PREWORK PREWORN PRISONS PROBONO PROBOWL PROLOGS PROLONG PROMOED PROMOTE PRONOUN PROPONE PROPOSE PROSODY PROTONS PROVOKE PROVOST TREFOIL TREMOLO TREMORS TRIBORO TRICORN TRICOTS TRIFOLD TRIFORM TRIGONS TRILOGY TRIMOFF TRIPODS TRIPOLI TRITONE TRITONS TROTOFF TROTOUT UROLOGY

•R•••O•

ARAFTOF ARCHFOE ARIOSOS ARISTOS ARROYOS ARTBOOK ARTSHOP ARTSHOW BRANDON BRANSON BRAXTON BRENDON BRERFOX BRETTON BRILLOS BRINGON BRISTOL BRITCOM BRITPOP BRITTON BRONCOS BRONSON BRYUSOV

CRABPOT CRAMPON CRATION CREATOR CREEPOS CREOSOL CRESTON CRIMSON CROPTOP CROUTON CRYPTOS DRAGOON DRAGSON DRAWNON DRAWSON DRAYTON DRCHAOS DREAMOF DREAMON DREGION DRIPSON DRMCCOY DRONEON DROPBOX DROPTOP ERECTOR EREWHON ERICSON ERIKSON EROSION ERYNGOS FRANKOZ FREEDOF FREEDOM FREESOF FREETOY FRESCOS FRISSON FRONTON FROWNON FRYCOOK GRAFTON GRANTOR GRATEON GRAYSON GRIFFON GRINGOS GRINKOV GRISSOM GROTTOS GROWNON GROWSON GRUNION GRYPHON IRECKON IRONSON KRATION KRYPTON MRHULOT MRMAGOO ORARION ORATION ORBISON PRAETOR PRAYFOR PREBOOK PREBOOM PRECOOK

PRECOOL PREDOOM PRENOON PREPLOT PRERIOT PRESHOW PRESSON PRESTON PRESTOS PREYSON PROCTOR PROCYON PRODSON PROSHOP PROUDOF PRUDHOE QRATIOS TRACTOR TRADEON TRAITOR TRANSOM TRAYNOR TREADON TREASON TREETOP TRENTON TRIEDON TRIESON TRIPSON TRIVIOT TROLLOP TRYITON URGEDON URGESON WRITEON WROTEON

•R••••O

ARACHNO ARAPAHO ARECIBO ARETINO ARGENTO ARIGATO ARIOSTO ARSENIO ARTDECO ARTERIO BRACERO BRAVADO BRINGTO BRONCHO CRUZADO DRANKTO DRAWNTO DRAWSTO DRINKTO DRIVETO DRMARIO DROVETO ERNESTO ERYTHRO FRUSTRO GROMYKO GROUCHO MRMACHO MRMAGOO OREGANO

ORINOCO ORLANDO ORNITHO ORVIETO PRAYSTO PREVETO PRIMERO PRIORTO PRIVYTO PROBONO PRONETO PROVISO PROXIMO PRYINTO TREMOLO TREVINO TRIBORO TRIEDTO TRIESTO TRUERTO WRITETO WROTETO

••RO•••

ABROACH ACROBAT ACRONYM AEROBAT AEROBES AEROBIC AEROSOL AFROPOP AGROUND AKRONOH ALROKER ALROSEN APRONED APROPOS ARROYOS ATROPHY ATROPOS AURORAE AURORAL AURORAS BAROLOS BARONET BAROQUE BEROWNE BORODIN BOROMIR BORONIC BOROUGH BUROAKS BYROADS BYRONIC CAROLED CAROLER CAROLII CAROLYN CAROMED CAROTID CAROTIN CAROUSE CHROMAT CHROMED CHROMES CHROMIC CHRONIC

COROLLA CORONAE CORONAL CORONAS CORONER CORONET DERONDA DOROTHY ENROBED ENROBES ENROLLS ENROOTS ENROUTE EUROPOP EUROVAN FAROESE FAROUKI FORONCE FURORES GARONNE GAROTTE GIROLLE GIRONDE GOROUND GYROCAR HAROLDI HEROICS HEROINE HEROISM HERONRY INROADS JAROMIR KAROLYI KEROUAC LAROCHE MAROONS MOROCCO MORONIC PARODIC PAROLED PAROLEE PAROLES PARONYM PAROTID PERORAL PIROGEN PIROGUE REROLLS REROOFS REROOTS REROUTE SARONGS SAROYAN SCROLLS SCROOGE SHROUDS SIROCCO SORORAL SPROUTS STROBES STROKED STROKER STROKES STROLLS STROPHE STROUSE TAROILS THROATS

THROATY THRONES THRONGS THROUGH THROWAT THROWER THROWIN THROWON THROWUP TOROIDS TORONTO TVROOMS UNROBED UNROBES UNROCKY UNROLLS UNROOFS UNROOMY UNROOTS UNROPED UNROPES UNROUND UNROWDY UPROARS UPROOTS UPROUSE VERONIA XEROSES XEROSIS XEROTIC XEROXED XEROXES ZEROING ZEROOUT ZEROSIN ZEROSUM

••R•O••

AIRBOAT AIRCOOL AIRFOIL AIRFONE AIRHOLE AIRHORN AIRHOSE AIRLOCK AIRLOGS AIRPOPS AIRPORT AIRPOTS AIRSOCK AIRSOUT AIRWOLF APRIORI AUREOLA AUREOLE BARCODE BARHOPS BARNONE BARNOWL BARRONS BARROOM BARROWS BARSOAP BARTOLO BARYONS BERTOLT BERVOIX

BORDONI
BOREOUT
BORROWS
BORZOIS
BURBOTS
BURGOOS
BURNOFF
BURNOUT
BURROWS
CARBONS
CARBOYS
CARCOAT
CARDOOR
CARDOZO
CARGOES
CARHOPS
CARHORN
CARIOCA
CARIOLE
CARIOUS
CARLOAD
CARLOAN
CARLOTA
CARLOTS
CARPOOL
CARPORT
CARPOUS
CARROLL
CARROTS
CARROTY
CARTOFF
CARTONS
CARTOON
CARTOPS
CORDOBA
CORDONS
CORKOAK
CORNOIL
CORPORA
CORRODE
CURIOSA
CURIOUS
CURSORS
CURSORY
DARTOFF
EARBONE
EARHOLE
EARLOBE
EARLOCK
ENROOTS
FARGOND
FARGONE
FARMORE
FARMOUT
FARROWS
FERROUS
FERVORS
FERVOUR
FIREOFF
FORBORE
FORDOES
FORDONE
FORGOER
FORGOES
FORGONE
FORGOOD
FORKOUT
FORLORN

FORLOVE
FORMOSA
FORSOOK
FORTORD
FURCOAT
FURIOSO
FURIOUS
FURLONG
FURROWS
GARCONS
GARROTE
GORGONS
HARBORS
HARBOUR
HARLOTS
HARMONY
HARPOON
HARRODS
HARROLD
HARROWS
HERMOSA
HERMOSO
HIREOUT
HORMONE
HORRORS
JARGONS
JARGONY
JARROTT
JERBOAS
JERKOUT
KARAOKE
KARLOFF
KARLOVY
LARDONS
MARCONI
MARKOFF
MARKOUT
MARKOVA
MARLOWE
MARMOTS
MAROONS
MARRONS
MARROWS
MERLOTS
MIRRORS
MORLOCK
MORMONS
MORROWS
MORTONS
MURDOCH
NARROWS
NERVOUS
NORDOFF
NORDOWE
NORFOLK
NORTONS
NORWOOD
OARLOCK
OURSONG
OURTOWN
PARBOIL
PARDONS
PARFOUR
PARLORS
PARLOUR
PARLOUS
PARROTS
PARSONS

PARTONE
PARTOOK
PERFORM
PERGOLA
PERIODS
PERSOFF
PERSONA
PERSONS
PURLOIN
PURPORT
PURPOSE
REROOFS
REROOTS
SARNOFF
SARTORS
SCROOGE
SERIOUS
SERMONS
SIRLOIN
SORROWS
SORTOUT
TARPONS
TERAOHM
TERROIR
TERRORS
TIREOUT
TOREOFF
TOREOUT
TORNOFF
TORNOUT
TORTOLA
TORTONI
TURBOTS
TURMOIL
TURNOFF
TURNONS
TURNOUT
TVROOMS
UNROOFS
UNROOMY
UNROOTS
UPROOTS
VARIOUS
VERBOSE
VERDOUX
VERMONT
VERYODD
VERYOLD
VIRGOAN
WARBOND
WARDOFF
WARGODS
WARLOCK
WARLORD
WARNOFF
WARROOM
WARTORN
WARWORN
WARZONE
WORDONE
WOREOFF
WOREOUT
WORKOFF
WORKOUT
WORNOFF
WORNOUT
YARROWS
ZEROOUT

ZIRCONS

••R••O•

AERATOR
AEROSOL
AFROPOP
AGREEON
AIRCOOL
AIRDROP
AIRFLOW
AIRGLOW
AIRSHOW
AKRONOH
APRICOT
APROPOS
ARROYOS
ATROPOS
BARANOF
BAROLOS
BARRIOS
BARROOM
BARSTOW
BERGSON
BERLIOZ
BIRDDOG
BOREDOM
BURGEON
BURGOOS
BURNFOR
CARABOO
CARDOOR
CAREFOR
CARIBOO
CARIBOU
CARLSON
CARLTON
CARPOOL
CARRYON
CARSHOW
CARTOON
CHRISOM
CORAZON
CORNCOB
CORNDOG
CORNROW
CURATOR
DARENOT
DORITOS
EARDROP
EARLDOM
EARLYON
EARSHOT
EUROPOP
FAREBOX
FARMBOY
FERMION
FIREBOX
FIREDOG
FIREDON
FIREFOX
FIRESON
FORCEON
FORETOP
FORGOOD
FORSHOW
FORSOOK
GERITOL
GERSHON

GIRASOL
GYRATOR
HARDTOP
HARDWON
HARICOT
HARPOON
HARPSON
HERENOW
HERITOR
HERNDON
HERRIOT
HIREDON
HIRESON
HORIZON
HURSTON
HURTFOR
JURYBOX
KARLSON
KERFLOP
KERPLOP
LAREDOS
LARGEOJ
LORGNON
LYRICON
MARCHON
MARIDOS
MARMION
MARSTON
MARYLOU
MERINOS
MIRADOR
MORELOS
MORISOT
MURANOS
NORTHOF
NORWOOD
PARADOR
PARADOX
PARAGON
PARASOL
PARTOOK
PARTYON
PERIDOT
PERSSON
PORTHOS
PORTION
PORTNOY
REREDOS
SERFDOM
SPRAYON
STRAPON
STRIPOF
SUREROF
SURGEON
THREWON
THROWON
TIREDOF
TIRESOF
TOREROS
TORINOS
TORSION
TURFTOE
TURNSON
VERGEON
VERIZON
VERSION
VERYHOT
VERYLOW

VIRAGOS
WARNSOF
WARRIOR
WARROOM
WARTHOG
WORKBOX
WORKFOR
WORKSON
YORKTON

••R•••O

AGREETO
AMRADIO
BARTOLO
BERGAMO
BURRITO
CARABOO
CARDOZO
CAREDTO
CARESTO
CARIBOO
CBRADIO
CEREBRO
CHRISTO
CORDERO
CORTICO
CURACAO
DARESTO
DAREZZO
DERECHO
DERMATO
DERRICO
DURANGO
FARRAGO
FERRARO
FMRADIO
FURILLO
FURIOSO
FURTADO
GERALDO
HERESTO
HERMANO
HERMOSO
HERPETO
HORATIO
JERICHO
LORENZO
MARCATO
MARENGO
MARIANO
MARTINO
MARULLO
MERCADO
MORELLO
MOROCCO
MURILLO
NORELCO
OTRANTO
PARTTWO
PERATIO
PERDIDO
PORTICO
SERPICO
SIROCCO
SORDINO
SORENTO
SORIANO
SORVINO

STRETTO
SUREIDO
TARANTO
THREENO
TORNADO
TORONTO
TORPEDO
TURISMO
TURNPRO
TURNSTO
UTRILLO
VERDUGO
VERISMO
VERTIGO
WARHERO
WARMSTO
XMRADIO

•••RO••

ACEROLA
ACEROSE
AFFRONT
AMARONE
AMBROSE
AMOROSO
AMOROUS
ANDROID
ANDROUS
ANEROID
ANYROAD
APPROVE
ARTROCK
ATCROSS
AXLROSE
AYKROYD
BARRONS
BARROOM
BARROWS
BEAROFF
BEAROUT
BEDROCK
BEDROLL
BEDROOM
BETROTH
BITROLE
BORROWS
BURROWS
BYPROXY
CARROLL
CARROTS
CARROTY
CHEROOT
CHYRONS
CITROEN
CITRONS
CITROUS
CORRODE
COWROTE
CUPROUS
DACRONS
DAYROOM
DEARONE
DEFROCK
DEFROST
DETROIT
DISROBE
DOGROSE
DOWRONG

DRBROWN
DRYROTS
EGGROLL
EMBROIL
EMBROWN
ENGROSS
ENTROPY
ESCROWS
EYEROLL
FAEROES
FAIROFF
FARROWS
FERROUS
FIBROID
FIBROUS
FLYRODS
FURROWS
GARROTE
GOBROKE
GOWRONG
GUNROOM
GUYROPE
HADRONS
HADROOM
HARRODS
HARROLD
HARROWS
HASROOM
HEAROUT
HIPROOF
HORRORS
HOTRODS
HOTROLL
HYDROUS
IFORONE
IGOROTS
IMBROKE
IMPROVE
INBROWN
INCROWD
INFRONT
INGROUP
INGROWN
INIRONS
INTROIT
JARROTT
JOEROTH
JSTROKE
KEDROVA
KIDROCK
LADRONE
LAPROBE
LATROBE
LEBROCK
LEGROOM
LEGROPE
LETROLL
LOGROLL
LOWROAD
MACRONS
MANROPE
MARRONS
MARROWS
MATRONS
MAUROIS
MCGRORY
MELROSE
MICROBE

MICRONS
MIRRORS
MONROES
MORROWS
MRBROWN
MRWRONG
MUDROOM
MYCROFT
NAIROBI
NARROWS
NEGRONI
NEURONE
NEURONS
NIMRODS
NITROUS
OCHROID
OCHROUS
OCTROIS
ODOROUS
OFFROAD
OLDROSE
OLOROSO
ONAROLL
ONEROOM
ONEROUS
OPEROSE
OUTROAR
OUTROCK
OUTRODE
OUTROLL
OUTROOT
OUTROVE
OUTROWS
PADRONE
PAIROFF
PARROTS
PATROLS
PATRONS
PATROON
PAYROLL
PEEROUT
PENROSE
PETROCK
PETROLS
PETROUS
PITROWS
POPROCK
POUROUT
PREROCK
PTEROUS
RAMRODS
REAROSE
REBROKE
RECROOM
RECROSS
RECROWN
REDROBE
REDROOP
REDROOT
REDROSE
REFRONT
REGROOM
REGROUP
REGROWN
REGROWS
REPROBE
REPROOF
REPROVE

REWROTE
REXROTH
RIMROCK
ROBROYS
SHARONA
SORROWS
STCROIX
STEROID
STEROLS
SUBROOT
SUBROSA
SUCROSE
SUNROOF
SUNROOM
TAPROOM
TAPROOT
TEAROFF
TEAROOM
TEAROSE
TEAROUT
TERROIR
TERRORS
TETRODE
THEROBE
THEROCK
THEROOM
THEROPE
THEROSE
THEROUX
THYROID
TIERODS
TIEROPE
TIMROTH
TINROOF
TOPROWS
TOWROPE
TWOROOM
UNBROKE
UNCROSS
UNCROWN
UNFROCK
UNFROST
UNFROZE
UNGROSS
UNGROWN
UNPROUD
UPFRONT
UPGROWN
UPGROWS
UPOROUT
UPPROPS
VEEROFF
VINROSE
WARROOM
WEAROFF
WEAROUT
YARROWS
YEARONE
ZEBROID

•••R•O•

AKERLOF
ALARCON
APERSON
AWAREOF
BARRIOS
BARROOM
BEARSON

BEDROOM
BLERIOT
BOURBON
BRERFOX
CABRIOS
CARRYON
CHARCOT
CHARIOT
CHARROS
CHEROOT
CHURROS
CLARION
CYPRIOT
CZARDOM
DAYROOM
DEARGOD
DIARIOS
EMBRYOS
EMERSON
ENARBOR
EVERTOR
FEARFOR
FEARNOT
GEARBOX
GGORDON
GIORGOS
GUERDON
GUNROOM
HADROOM
HAIRDOS
HASROOM
HEARDOF
HEARSOF
HEIRDOM
HERRIOT
HIPROOF
IFORGOT
INERROR
IVERSON
JCARROL
JOURNOS
KHARKOV
KIARIOS
LEARNOF
LEGROOM
MUDROOM
MYERSON
NEARYOU
ONEROOM
ORARION
OUTROOT
OVERCOY
OVERDOG
OVERHOT
OVERJOY
OVERTOP
PATRIOT
PATROON
PEARSON
PHARAOH
PIERROT
POORBOX
POORBOY
PRERIOT
QUARTOS
RANRIOT
REARDON
RECROOM

REDROOP
REDROOT
REGROOM
REPROOF
RUNRIOT
SHORTOF
SMIRNOV
SOURSON
SPARROW
SPURSON
STARDOM
STARION
STARLOG
STARTON
STEREOS
STERNOS
STERTOR
SUBROOT
SUNROOF
SUNROOM
TAPROOM
TAPROOT
TEAROOM
THEREOF
THEREON
THERMOS
THEROOM
THORSON
TINROOF
TSARDOM
TWOROOM
VITRIOL
WARRIOR
WARROOM
WEARSON
WEIRDOS
WEIRTON
WHARTON
WHEREOF
WHEREON
YOUREON

•••R••O

ALERTTO
ALFREDO
AMERIGO
AMOROSO
BURRITO
CHIRICO
CHORIZO
DERRICO
ELGRECO
ELPRADO
FARRAGO
FEBRERO
FERRARO
GEARSTO
GIORGIO
ISUREDO
LACRIMO
LEARNTO
MANRICO
OLOROSO
QUERIDO
RODRIGO
SANREMO
SCORPIO
SOPRANO

STARTTO
SWORETO
THERETO
VIBRATO
WHERETO
YEARNTO

••••RO•

ACHERON
ADJUROR
AILERON
AIRDROP
ALFEROV
ANDIRON
APAIROF
ASSUROR
ATECROW
AVEYRON
AXELROD
BACKROW
BISTROS
BOLEROS
BOUTROS
CALDRON
CAMAROS
CAMERON
CASTROL
CHARROS
CHEERON
CHEVRON
CHURROS
CLAIROL
CLEAROF
COJUROR
COMOROS
CONTROL
CORNROW
CUATROS
DEMEROL
DENDRON
DESTROY
DEWDROP
DIDEROT
DISTROS
DOGTROT
EARDROP
EATCROW
EATFROM
EGGDROP
EMPEROR
ENDUROS
ENTERON
ENVIRON
ENVIROS
EYEBROW
EYEDROP
FEDOROV
FITZROY
FLEURON
FOXTROT
FUELROD
GABBROS
GETFROM
GUMDROP
HADAROW
HALFROD
HASAROW
HYPERON

7
RO

INERROR
JCARROL
JOGTROT
KAKUROS
LASTROW
LATERON
LEBARON
LEGIRON
LETDROP
LINDROS
LLADROS
LOTHROP
LOWBROW
MADUROS
MCENROE
MIDIRON
NEMEROV
NEUTRON
NONCROP
NONIRON
NONPROS
NUMEROS
OFFEROR
OHCAROL
OLDPROS
OMICRON
ONEIRON
OUTCROP
OUTCROW
OUTDROP
OUTGROW
OUTTROT
PALTROW
PETCROW
PETFROG
PGAPROS
PICAROS
PIERROT
PIETROS
PIGIRON
PILCROW
PUSHROD
QUEIROS
RAYKROC
REZEROS
ROOTROT
SAFFRON
SHADROE
SHYFROM
SIXIRON
SKIDROW
SMEARON
SPARROW
SUREROF
TEATROS
TEXTRON
THECROW
TIBURON
TONEROW
TOREROS
TWOIRON
UPTHROW
VELCROS
VESTRON
VICEROY
WAITRON
WOODROW

••••R•O

ALBERTO
ALBIREO
ARTERIO
BIZARRO
BOIARDO
BONARIO
CATERTO
CHEERIO
CONBRIO
DECARLO
DEFERTO
DEMARCO
DRMARIO
EDGARDO
EDUARDO
EMBARGO
ESPARTO
FEDERKO
HIBERNO
IGNARRO
INFERNO
LIVORNO
LOCARNO
MCMURDO
NOVARRO
OCCURTO
ONTARIO
PALERMO
PATERNO
PICARDO
PISARRO
PIZARRO
PRIORTO
RAJARAO
REFERTO
RICARDO
RIVERPO
ROBERTO
ROSARIO
SALERNO
SCHERZO
SUHARTO
SUKARNO
SWEARTO
TRUERTO
UMBERTO
UNDERDO
UNDERGO
YESORNO

•••••RO

ALLEGRO
BEAHERO
BIZARRO
BRACERO
CALABRO
CEREBRO
CORDERO
DELTORO
DEUTERO
ELECTRO
ERYTHRO
FEBRERO
FERRARO
FOXBORO
FRUSTRO
GASTERO
GENNARO
GOESPRO
GOLFPRO
GONEPRO
HHMUNRO
IGNARRO
INUTERO
INVITRO
JANEIRO
LETTERO
LLANERO
MAESTRO
MILAGRO
MINDORO
MONSTRO
MONTERO
NETZERO
NONHERO
NONZERO
NOVARRO
NUESTRO
PISARRO
PIZARRO
PRIMERO
QUATTRO
SAGUARO
SAPPORO
SEAHERO
SEMIPRO
SHAPIRO
SUBZERO
THEHERO
TOSHIRO
TRIBORO
TURNPRO
VACCARO
VAQUERO
WARHERO
WENTPRO

R•P••••

RAPALLO
RAPANUI
RAPHAEL
RAPIDAN
RAPIDER
RAPIDLY
RAPIERS
RAPINES
RAPINIS
RAPPELS
RAPPERS
RAPPING
RAPPORT
RAPSONG
RAPSTAR
RAPTORS
RAPTUNE
RAPTURE
REPACKS
REPAGED
REPAGES
REPAINT
REPAIRS
REPANEL
REPAPER
REPARKS
REPASTE
REPASTS
REPATCH
REPAVED
REPAVES
REPEALS
REPEATS
REPENTS
REPERKS
REPHASE
REPHONE
REPICKS
REPINED
REPINER
REPINES
REPLACE
REPLANE
REPLANS
REPLANT
REPLATE
REPLAYS
REPLEAD
REPLETE
REPLICA
REPLIED
REPLIER
REPLIES
REPLOTS
REPLOWS
REPLUMB
REPLUME
REPLYTO
REPOINT
REPOLLS
REPOMAN
REPORTS
REPOSED
REPOSER
REPOSES
REPOSIT
REPOSTS
REPOURS
REPOWER
REPPING
REPRESS
REPRICE
REPRIME
REPRINT
REPRISE
REPROBE
REPROOF
REPROVE
REPRUNE
REPSFOR
REPTILE
REPUGNS
REPULSE
REPUMPS
REPUTED
REPUTES
RIPCORD
RIPENED
RIPENER
RIPIENI
RIPIENO
RIPINTO
RIPOFFS
RIPOPEN
RIPOSTE
RIPOSTS
RIPPERS
RIPPING
RIPPLED
RIPPLES
RIPPLET
RIPRAPS
RIPSAWN
RIPSAWS
RIPSOFF
RIPSONE
RIPSOUT
RIPSTOP
RIPTIDE
RIPTORN
ROPEDIN
ROPEDUP
ROPEOFF
ROPESIN
ROPESUP
ROPETOW
ROPIEST
RUPIAHS
RUPTURE
RVPARKS

R••P•••

RALPHIE
RAMPAGE
RAMPANT
RAMPART
RAMPING
RAMPSUP
RANPAST
RAPPELS
RAPPERS
RAPPING
RAPPORT
RASPERS
RASPIER
RASPING
RASPISH
RATPACK
REAPERS
REAPING
REAPPLY
REDPINE
REDPOLL
REDPONY
REOPENS
REPPING
RESPACE
RESPADE
RESPANS
RESPARK
RESPEAK
RESPECT
RESPELL
RESPELT
RESPICE
RESPINS
RESPIRE
RESPITE
RESPLIT
RESPOKE
RESPOND
RESPOOL
RESPOTS
RESPRAY
REUPPED
RIBPADS
RIMPLED
RIMPLES
RIPPERS
RIPPING
RIPPLED
RIPPLES
RIPPLET
ROMPERS
ROMPING
ROMPISH
RSVPING
RUMPEND
RUMPLED
RUMPLES
RUMPOLE
RUNPAST

R•••P••

RANUPTO
REAPPLY
RECIPES
REDSPOT
REEXPEL
REIMPLY
RELAPSE
REPAPER
RETAPED
RETAPES
RETYPED
RETYPES
REUPPED
REWIPED
REWIPES
RIPOPEN
RUBUPON
RUNUPTO

R••••P•

RAGMOPS
RAGTOPS
RANLAPS
RATEDPG
RAVEUPS
READAPT
READOPT
RECEIPT
RECOUPS
REDCAPS
REDTAPE
REDTOPS
REERUPT
REFLIPS
REGRAPH
REGRIPS
RELEAPS
REPUMPS
RESHAPE
RESHIPS
RESNAPS
RESOAPS
RETRAPS
REVAMPS
REWRAPS
RIPRAPS
RIVERPO
ROLLUPS
RUDOLPH
RUNLAPS

R•••••P

RACEDUP
RACESUP
RACKSUP
RAGSHOP
RAISEUP
RAKEDUP
RAKESUP
RAMPSUP
RANDEEP
RANITUP
RATECAP
RATTRAP
REACHUP
READSUP
REARSUP
RECLASP
REDCHIP
REDROOP
REELSUP
REEQUIP
REGRASP
REGROUP
RESTAMP
RESTRAP
RESTRIP
RESTSUP
RESWEEP
REVITUP
RIDESUP
RILEDUP
RILESUP
RINGSUP
RIPSTOP
RISESUP
ROADMAP
ROBOCOP
ROLLMOP
ROLLSUP
ROLLTOP
ROOFTOP
ROOTCAP
ROOTSUP
ROPEDUP
ROPESUP
ROSEHIP
ROUGHUP
ROUNDUP
RUCKSUP
RUMSHOP
RUNDEEP
RUNITUP

•RP••••

MRPADRE
ORPHANS
ORPHANT
ORPHEAN
ORPHEUM
ORPHEUS

•R•P•••

ARAPAHO
ARMPITS
CRAPING
CRAPOLA
CRAPOUT
CRAPPIE
CREPING
CREPTIN
CREPTUP
CRIPPLE
CROPPED
CROPPER
CROPSUP
CROPTOP
CRUPPER
CRYPTIC
CRYPTOS
DRAPERS
DRAPERY
DRAPING
DRIPDRY
DRIPPAN
DRIPPED
DRIPPER
DRIPSON
DROPBOX
DROPCAP
DROPINS
DROPLET
DROPNET
DROPOFF
DROPOUT
DROPPED
DROPPER
DROPSBY
DROPSIN
DROPSIT
DROPTOP
DRSPOCK
DRYPERS
ERUPTED
ERUPTER
FRAPPES
FRYPANS
GRAPERY
GRAPHED
GRAPHIC
GRAPIER
GRAPNEL
GRAPPAS
GRAPPLE
GRIPERS
GRIPING
GRIPPED
GRIPPER
GRIPPES
GROPERS
GROPING
GROPIUS
GRYPHON
IREPEAT
KRYPTON
MRSPAUL
MRSPEEL
MRSPOCK
PREPACK
PREPAID
PREPARE
PREPAVE
PREPAYS
PREPLAN
PREPLOT
PREPPED
PREPPIE
PREPUPA
PROPANE
PROPELS
PROPHET
PROPJET
PROPMAN
PROPMEN
PROPONE
PROPOSE
PROPPED
PROPSUP
TRAPEZE
TRAPGUN
TRAPPED
TRAPPER
TREPANS
TRIPLEA
TRIPLED
TRIPLES
TRIPLET
TRIPLEX
TRIPODS
TRIPOLI
TRIPPED
TRIPPER
TRIPPET
TRIPSON
TRIPSUP
TROPICS
TROPISM
WRAPPED
WRAPPER
WRAPSUP
WRAPUPS

•R••P••

ARUSPEX
BREWPUB
BRITPOP
CRABPOT
CRAMPED
CRAMPON
CRAPPIE
CREEPBY
CREEPED
CREEPER
CREEPIN
CREEPOS
CREEPUP
CRESPIN
CRIMPED
CRIMPER
CRIPPLE
CRISPED
CRISPEN
CRISPER
CRISPIN
CRISPIX
CRISPLY
CRISPUS
CROPPED
CROPPER
CRUMPED
CRUMPET
CRUMPLE
CRUMPLY
CRUPPER
DRIPPAN
DRIPPED
DRIPPER
DROOPED
DROPPED
DROPPER
FRAPPES
GRAMPAS
GRAMPUS
GRANPAS
GRAPPAS
GRAPPLE
GRASPAT
GRASPED
GRASPER
GRIPPED
GRIPPER
GRIPPES
GROUPED
GROUPER
GROUPIE
GRUMPED
IRRUPTS
PREOPEN
PREPPED
PREPPIE
PRESPUR
PRIMPED
PROMPTS
PROPPED
PROSPER
PRYOPEN
TRAIPSE
TRAMPAS
TRAMPED
TRAMPER
TRAMPLE
TRAPPED
TRAPPER
TRIPPED
TRIPPER
TRIPPET
TROMPED
TROMPIN
TROOPED
TROOPER
TROOPIN
TROUPED
TROUPER
TROUPES
TRUMPED
TRUMPET
TRUMPUP
WRAPPED
WRAPPER

•R•••P•

DRYMOPS
GRANDPA
MRCHIPS
PREAMPS
PRECEPT
PREEMPT
PRENUPS
PREPUPA
PRETAPE
PRETYPE
TRICEPS
TRIUMPH
WRAPUPS

•R••••P

ARCLAMP
AREAMAP
ARTSHOP
BRACEUP
BREAKUP
BREWSUP
BRICKUP
BRINGUP
BRITPOP
BROKEUP
BRUSHUP
CRACKUP
CRANKUP
CRATEUP
CREEPUP
CREPTUP
CRIEDUP
CRIESUP
CROPSUP
CROPTOP
CROSSUP
CRUDSUP
DRAGSUP
DRANKUP
DRAWNUP
DRAWSUP
DREAMUP
DRESSUP
DRIEDUP
DRIESUP
DRIFTUP
DRINKUP
DRIVEUP
DROPCAP
DROPTOP
DROVEUP
DRUMSUP
FRAMEUP
FREEDUP
FREESUP
FRIEDUP
FRIESUP
FROTHUP
FROZEUP
GRATEUP
GREYCUP
GRIDMAP
GROWNUP
GROWSUP
MRQUILP
ORDERUP
PRECOUP
PRESHIP
PRESSUP
PREWHIP
PREWRAP
PRICKUP
PRINTUP
PROPSUP
PROSHOP
TRADEUP
TREESAP
TREETOP
TRIPSUP
TROLLOP
TROTSUP
TRUEDUP
TRUESUP
TRUMPUP
TRUSSUP
WRACKUP
WRAPSUP
WRITEUP
WROTEUP

••RP•••

AIRPACK
AIRPARK
AIRPLAY
AIRPOPS
AIRPORT
AIRPOTS
AIRPUMP
BURPGUN
BURPING
CARPALS
CARPARK
CARPELS
CARPERS
CARPETS
CARPING
CARPOOL
CARPORT
CARPOUS
CARPSAT
CORPORA
CORPSES
EARPLUG
GARPIKE
HARPERS
HARPIES
HARPING
HARPIST
HARPOON
HARPSON
HERPETO
KERPLOP
MORPHED
MORPHIC
MORPHIN
MURPHYS
PERPLEX
PURPLED
PURPLES
PURPORT
PURPOSE
SERPENS
SERPENT
SERPICO
SURPASS
SURPLUS
TARPITS
TARPONS
TIRPITZ
TORPEDO
WARPAGE
WARPATH
WARPERS
WARPING

••R•P••

AFROPOP
AGRIPPA
APROPOS
ATROPHY
ATROPOS
EUROPOP
FIREPIT
FOREPAW
HARDPAN
HARDPUT
IRRUPTS
MOREPAY
PARAPET
PARAPHS
PORKPIE
SCRAPED
SCRAPER
SCRAPES
SCRAPPY
SCRIPPS
SCRIPTS
SCRUPLE
SERAPES
SERAPHS
SERAPIS
SERIPAK
STRAPIN
STRAPON
STRIPED
STRIPER
STRIPES
STRIPOF
STROPHE
THRUPUT
TURNPRO
UNRIPER
UNROPED
UNROPES
WAREPIC

••R••P•

AGRIPPA
AIRPOPS
BARHOPS
BURLAPS
CARHOPS
CARTOPS
CORRUPT
EARLAPS
FORCEPS
LARRUPS
MARKUPS
ONRAMPS
PERCEPT
PERHAPS
PERIAPT
SCRAPPY
SCRIMPS
SCRIMPY
SCRIPPS
SHRIMPS
SHRIMPY
THREEPM
TURNIPS
TURNUPS
UNRASPY
VCRTAPE

WARMUPS
WORKUPS

••R•••P

AFROPOP
AIRDROP
AIREDUP
AIRPUMP
AIRSHIP
AIRTRAP
BARKEEP
BARSOAP
BORNEUP
BURNSUP
BURNTUP
CARTRIP
CORKSUP
CURLSUP
EARCLIP
EARDROP
EARFLAP
EUROPOP
FIREDUP
FIRESUP
FIRMSUP
FIRSTUP
FORCEUP
FORETOP
FORKSUP
FURWRAP
HARDTOP
HURRYUP
JERKSUP
KERFLOP
KERPLOP
MARKSUP
PARSNIP
PERKSUP
SCREWUP
SCRUBUP
SERVEUP
SURFSUP
TARTSUP
THREEUP
THREWUP
THROWUP
TURNSUP
VERYHIP
WARMSUP
WARSHIP
WIREDUP
WIRESUP
WIRETAP
WORKSUP
WORSHIP

•••RP••

BEARPAW
BEARPIT
CHARPAK
CHIRPED
CHIRPER
FOURPIN
HAIRPIN
NEARPAR
OVERPAR
OVERPAY
OVERPLY
SCARPED
SCORPIO
SHARPED
SHARPEI
SHARPEN
SHARPER
SHARPIE
SHARPLY
SHERPAS
SLURPED
SLURPEE
SLURPER
USURPED
USURPER

•••R•P•

BADRAPS
BEDRAPE
BUMRAPS
CORRUPT
DECRYPT
DIGRAPH
DISRUPT
ENCRYPT
ENTRAPS
ENTROPY
ENWRAPS
GUYROPE
LARRUPS
LEGROPE
MANROPE
OUTRAPS
REERUPT
REGRAPH
REGRIPS
RETRAPS
REWRAPS
RIPRAPS
SATRAPS
SATRAPY
THERAPY
THEROPE
TIEROPE
TOWROPE
TSTRAPS
UNDRAPE
UNGRIPS
UNTRAPS
UNWRAPS
UPPROPS

•••R••P

BEARSUP
BEERTAP
BOARDUP
CHIRRUP
CHURNUP
FAIRSUP
FLAREUP
GEARSUP
HURRYUP
INGROUP
NOTRUMP
OFFRAMP
OVERLAP
OVERSUP
OVERTIP
OVERTOP
PAIRSUP
PHARLAP
REARSUP
REDROOP
REGRASP
REGROUP
SCAREUP
SCARFUP
SHOREUP
SNARLUP
STARMAP
STARTUP
STIRRUP
STIRSUP
STOREUP
TEARSUP
UNCRAMP

••••RP•

ESCARPS
EUTERPE
EXCERPT
RIVERPO

••••R•P

AIRDROP
AIRTRAP
BADTRIP
BUSTRIP
CANTRIP
CARTRIP
CHEERUP
CHIRRUP
CLEARUP
COVERUP
DAYTRIP
DEWDROP
EARDROP
EGGDROP
EGOTRIP
EYEDROP
FLYTRAP
FURWRAP
GUMDROP
INATRAP
KEYGRIP
LEGTRAP
LETDROP
LETSRIP
LOTHROP
MANTRAP
NONCROP
NONDRIP
OFFERUP
ONATRIP
ORDERUP
OUTCROP
OUTDROP
POWERUP
PREWRAP
RATTRAP
RESTRAP
RESTRIP
SEATRIP
SKITRIP
STIRRUP
TIDERIP
UNSTRAP

•••••RP

ANTWERP
ASSHARP
EPICARP
EXOCARP
HANSARP
JEANARP
LETTERP
MASTERP
UNSHARP

R•Q••••

REQUEST
REQUIEM
REQUIRE
REQUITE
REQUOTE

R••Q•••

RACQUET
REEQUIP
RORQUAL

•RQ••••

DRQUINN
MRQUILP

•R•Q•••

BRIQUET
CROQUET
CROQUIS
PREQUEL

•R••Q••

BRUSQUE
PRESQUE

••RQ•••

BARQUES
CIRQUES
MARQUEE
MARQUES
MARQUEZ
MARQUIS
PARQUET
RORQUAL
TORQUED
TORQUES

••R•Q••

BAROQUE
ENRIQUE

•••••RQ

LETTERQ

RR•••••

RRATING

R•R••••

RAREBIT
RAREGAS
RARITAN
RERACKS
RERAISE
RERAKED
RERAKES
RERANKS
RERATED
RERATES
REREADS
REREDOS
REREELS
RERENTS
RERIDES
RERINSE
RERISEN
RERISES
REROLLS
REROOFS
REROOTS
REROUTE
RORAIMA
RORQUAL
RURALLY

R••R•••

RAGRUGS
RAMRODS
RANRIOT
RATRACE
REARDON
REAREND
REARERS
REARGUE
REARING
REARISE
REARLIT
REARMED
REAROSE
REARSUP
REBRACE
REBRAND
REBREAK
REBREED
REBREWS
REBROKE
REBRUSH
RECRANK
RECRATE
RECROOM
RECROSS
RECROWN
RECRUIT
REDRAFT
REDRAGS
REDRAWN
REDRAWS
REDREAM
REDRESS
REDRIED
REDRIES
REDRILL
REDRIVE
REDROBE
REDROOP
REDROOT
REDROSE
REERECT
REERUPT
REFRACT
REFRAIN
REFRAME
REFRESH
REFRIED
REFRIES
REFRONT
REGRABS
REGRADE
REGRAFT
REGRANT
REGRAPH
REGRASP
REGREET
REGRESS
REGRETS
REGRIND
REGRIPS
REGROOM
REGROUP
REGROWN
REGROWS
REORDER
REPRESS
REPRICE
REPRIME
REPRINT
REPRISE
REPROBE
REPROOF
REPROVE
REPRUNE
RETRACE
RETRACK
RETRACT
RETRADE
RETRAIN
RETRAPS
RETREAD
RETREAT
RETRIAL
RETRIED
RETRIES
RETRIMS
REURGED
REURGES
REWRAPS
REWRITE
REWROTE
REXREED
REXROTH
RICRACS
RIMROCK
RIORDAN
RIORITA
RIPRAPS
ROARERS
ROARING
ROARSAT
ROBROYS
RODRIGO
RUBRICS
RUGRATS
RUNRIOT

R•••R••

RAJARAO
RAMIREZ
RANFREE
RASURES
RATTRAP
RAYKROC
RAZORED
REAIRED
REBIRTH
REBORED
REBORES
RECARRY
RECARVE
RECORDS
RECORKS
RECURED
RECURES
RECURLS
RECURVE
REDARED
REDARES
REDARMY
REDARNS
REEARNS
REFEREE
REFERTO
REFIRED
REFIRES
REFORGE
REFORMS
REGARDS
REGIRDS
REHIRED
REHIRES
REMARKS
REMARRY
REMERGE
REMORAS
REMORSE
RENFREW
REPARKS
REPERKS
REPORTS
RESCRUB
RESERVE
RESORBS
RESORTS
RESPRAY
RESTRAP
RESTREW
RESTRIP
RESURGE
RETARDS
RETIRED
RETIREE
RETIRES
RETORTS
RETURFS
RETURNS
REVERBS
REVERDY
REVERED
REVERER
REVERES
REVERIE
REVERSA
REVERSE
REVERTS
REWARDS
REWARMS
REWARNS
REWIRED
REWIRES
REWORDS
REWORKS
REZEROS
RICARDO
RINKRAT
RITARDS
RIVERPO
ROBARDS
ROBERTA
ROBERTE
ROBERTF
ROBERTH
ROBERTI
ROBERTO
ROBERTS
ROGERED
ROOFRAT
ROOTROT
ROSARIO
ROSERED
ROSTRAL
ROSTRUM
RUBSRAW
RUBYRED
RUMORED
RUNFREE
RVPARKS

R••••R•

RACKERS
RADFORD
RAEBURN
RAFTERS
RAIDERS
RAILERS
RAISERS
RAMMERS
RAMPART
RANCORS
RANGERS
RANKERS
RANTERS
RAPIERS
RAPPERS
RAPPORT
RAPTORS
RAPTURE
RASBORA
RASHERS
RASPERS
RASTERS
RATBERT
RATTERS
RAWBARS
RAYBURN
READERS
READORN
REAMERS
REAPERS
REARERS
REAVERS
REBOARD
RECARRY
RECHART
RECTORS
RECTORY
REDBIRD
REDCARD
REDFERN
REDFIRS
REDFORD
REDWORM
REEFERS
REEKERS
REELERS
REENTRY
REGEARS
REGNARD
REHEARD
REHEARS
RELEARN
RELIERS
REMARRY
RENDERS
RENOIRS
RENTERS
REPAIRS
REPOURS
REQUIRE
RESCORE
RESHARE
RESPARK
RESPIRE
RESTART
RESTERS
RESTIRS
RESTORE
RESWORE
RESWORN
RETEARS
RETIARY
RETOURS
REUNERS
REUSERS
REUTERS
REVELRY
REWEARS
REYNARD
RHETORS
RHUBARB
RHYMERS
RIBBERS
RICHARD
RIDDERS
RIEGERT
RIFLERS
RIFLERY
RIGGERS
RIGOURS
RINGERS
RINSERS
RIOTERS
RIPCORD
RIPPERS
RIPTORN
RISKERS
RIVALRY
RIVIERA
RIVIERE
ROADERS
ROAMERS
ROARERS
ROBBERS
ROBBERY
ROBOTRY
ROBSART
ROCKERS
ROCKERY
RODGERS
ROGUERY
ROLFERS
ROLLERS
ROMBERG
ROMPERS
RONDURE
RONSARD
ROOFERS
ROOKERY
ROOMERS
ROOTERS
ROSTERS
ROTHIRA
ROTTERS
ROUSERS
ROUTERS
ROXBURY
RUBBERS
RUBBERY
RUCKERT
RUDDERS
RUDYARD
RUINERS
RUMFORD
RUMMERS
RUMOURS
RUNNERS
RUNSDRY
RUPTURE
RUSHERS
RUSSERT
RUTGERS
RUTTERS

R•••••R

RACECAR
RADIOER
RAFFLER
RAGGIER
RAILCAR
RAINIER
RALLIER
RAMBLER
RANCHER
RANCOUR
RANDIER
RANGFOR
RANGIER
RANOVER
RAPIDER
RAPSTAR
RASPIER
RASSLER
RATTIER
RATTLER
RAVAGER
REACHER
REACTOR
READFOR
READIER
REALTER
REALTOR
REAUMUR
REBATER
REBUKER
RECITER
RECOLOR
RECOVER
REDDEER
REDFOUR
REDHAIR
REDSTAR
REDUCER
REEDIER
REEFIER
REEKIER
REENTER
REFINER
REFUSER
REFUTER
REGALER
REGNIER
REGULAR
REHONOR
RELATER
RELATOR
RELAXER
RELAYER
RELEVER
REMOTER
REMOVER
RENEGER
RENEWER
RENTIER
REOCCUR
REOFFER
REORDER
REPAPER
REPINER
REPLIER
REPOSER
REPOWER
REPSFOR
RESCUER
RESIDER
RESIZER
RESOLER
RESWEAR
RETAKER
REUTHER
REUTTER
REVELER
REVERER
REVILER
REVISER
REVISOR
REVIVER
REVOKER
REWAGER
REWATER
RIBBIER
RICHLER
RICHTER
RIDDLER
RIDGIER
RIFFLER
RIGHTER
RIGUEUR
RINDIER
RINGFOR
RIPENER
RISKIER
RITZIER
RIVETER
ROADTAR
ROASTER
ROCKIER
ROEDEER
ROILIER
ROISTER
ROLLBAR
ROOKIER
ROOMIER
ROOSTER
ROOTFOR
ROOTIER
ROSSNER
ROTATOR
ROTIFER
ROUGHER
ROUNDER
ROUSTER
ROWDIER
RUDDIER
RUFFLER
RUMBLER
RUNGFOR
RUNNIER
RUNOVER
RUNSFOR
RUNTIER
RUSHIER
RUSTIER
RUSTLER
RUTTIER
RYEBEER

•RR••••

ARRABAL
ARRACKS
ARRAIGN
ARRANGE
ARRASES
ARRAYAL
ARRAYED
ARRAYER
ARREARS
ARRESTS
ARRIERE
ARRISES
ARRIVAL
ARRIVED
ARRIVER
ARRIVES
ARROYOS
ERRABLE
ERRANCY
ERRANDS
ERRATIC
ERRATUM
IRRUPTS
MRRIGHT
ORRISES

•R•R•••

ARMREST
ARTROCK
BRERFOX
DRBROWN
DRFREUD
DRFRIST
DRYROTS
DRYRUNS
ERDRICH
MRBROWN
MRGREEN
MRWRONG
ORARION
ORARIUM
PRERACE
PRERENT
PRERIOT
PREROCK
PRORATA
PRORATE
TRIREME

•R••R••

ARBORED
AREARUG
ARMORED
ARMORER
ARTERIO
BRIARDS
DRMARIO
ERITREA
FREDRIC
FRIARLY
GRIGRIS
MRBURNS
MRDARCY
MRHORSE
MRMARCH
MRNORTH
MRWORDS
ORATRIX
ORDERED
ORDERER
ORDERIN
ORDERLY
ORDERUP
OROURKE
PRAIRIE
PREARMS
PREORAL
PRETRIM
PREWRAP
PRFIRMS
PRIORTO
PROARAB
PROGRAM
TREERAT
TRIGRAM
TRUERIB
TRUERTO

•R•••R•

ARACARI
ARAFURA
ARAGORN
ARAMARK
ARBOURS
ARCHERS
ARCHERY
ARDMORE
ARDOURS
ARGUERS
ARIKARA
ARLBERG
ARMOIRE
ARMOURS
ARMOURY

ARREARS
ARRIERE
ARTCARS
ARTFERN
ARTFORM
ARTHURC
ARTHURM
ARTHURS
ARTWARE
ARTWORK
BRACERO
BRACERS
BRAVERY
BRAVURA
BRAYERS
BREWERS
BREWERY
BREYERS
BRIBERS
BRIBERY
BRINERS
BROKERS
BROWARD
CRATERS
CRAVERS
CREMORA
CROWERS
DRAPERS
DRAPERY
DRAWERS
DRIPDRY
DRIVERS
DRLAURA
DRONERS
DROVERS
DRYPERS
ERASERS
ERASURE
ERODERS
ERYTHRO
FRAMERS
FRATERS
FREBERG
FROWARD
FRUSTRO
GRADERS
GRANARY
GRAPERY
GRATERS
GRAVERS
GRAVURE
GRAZERS
GREGORY
GRIPERS
GROCERS
GROCERY
GROPERS
GROVERS
GROWERS
GRUYERE
IRONERS
IRONORE
IRSFORM
JROBERT
MRPADRE
ORATORS
ORATORY
ORCHARD

PRATERS
PRAYERS
PREBORN
PREBURN
PRECURE
PREDARK
PREFERS
PREFORM
PREPARE
PRESORT
PRETERM
PRETIRE
PRETORS
PREVERB
PREVERT
PREWARM
PREWARN
PREWIRE
PREWORK
PREWORN
PREYERS
PRICERS
PRIMARY
PRIMERA
PRIMERO
PRIMERS
PROBERS
PROCURE
PROFARM
PROSERS
PROVERB
PROVERS
PRUDERY
PRUNERS
TRABERT
TRACERS
TRACERY
TRADERS
TRAVERS
TREMORS
TRENARY
TRIBORO
TRICORN
TRIFORM
TRINARY
TRYHARD
WRITERS

•R••••R

ARBITER
AREOLAR
ARMORER
AROUSER
ARRAYER
ARRIVER
ARTFAIR
ARTSIER
BRAGGER
BRAIDER
BRAINER
BRANDER
BRASHER
BRASIER
BRAWLER
BRAZIER
BREADER
BREAKER
BREEDER
BRENNER
BRIDGER
BRIDLER
BRIEFER
BRIMMER
BRINGER
BRINIER
BRINKER
BRISKER
BROADER
BROIDER
BROILER
BRONZER
BROODER
BROTHER
BROWNER
BROWSER
BRUISER
BRUSHER
BRYNNER
CRABBER
CRACKER
CRADLER
CRAFTER
CRAMMER
CRANMER
CRASHER
CRASSER
CRAWLER
CRAZIER
CREAMER
CREASER
CREATOR
CREEPER
CRIBBER
CRIMPER
CRISPER
CRITTER
CRITTUR
CROAKER
CROCKER
CROFTER
CROONER
CROPPER
CROSIER
CROSSER
CROWBAR
CROWDER
CROWNER
CROZIER
CRUELER
CRUISER
CRULLER
CRUPPER
CRUSHER
CRYOVER
DRABBER
DRAFTER
DRAGGER
DRAINER
DRAWBAR
DRAWLER
DREAMER
DREDGER
DREISER
DRESSER
DREXLER
DRIFTER
DRILLER
DRINKER
DRIPPER
DROLLER
DROOLER
DROPPER
DRUBBER
DRUCKER
DRUDGER
DRUMMER
DRUNKER
ERECTER
ERECTOR
ERUPTER
FRAILER
FRANKER
FRASIER
FRAZIER
FREEAIR
FREEZER
FRESHER
FRETTER
FRICKER
FRISEUR
FRISKER
FRITTER
FRIZZER
FROGGER
FROMMER
FROSTER
FROTHER
FROWNER
GRABBAR
GRABBER
GRAFTER
GRAINER
GRAMMAR
GRAMMER
GRANDER
GRANGER
GRANTER
GRANTOR
GRAPIER
GRASPER
GRAZIER
GREASER
GREATER
GREENER
GREETER
GRIDDER
GRIEVER
GRIFTER
GRILLER
GRIMIER
GRIMMER
GRINDER
GRINNER
GRIPPER
GRISTER
GRITTER
GROANER
GRODIER
GROLIER
GROOMER
GROSSER
GROUPER
GROUSER
GROUTER
GROWLER
GRUBBER
GRUDGER
GRUFFER
GRUNGER
GRUNTER
IRISHER
IRONBAR
KRASNER
KROEMER
KRUEGER
MRSMUIR
MRTIGER
ORBITER
ORDERER
PRAETOR
PRAISER
PRANCER
PRAYFOR
PREAVER
PREENER
PREMIER
PRESPUR
PRESSER
PRICIER
PRIMMER
PRINKER
PRINTER
PRIVIER
PROCTER
PROCTOR
PRODDER
PROFFER
PROOFER
PROSIER
PROSPER
PROUDER
PROWLER
TRACKER
TRACTOR
TRAILER
TRAINER
TRAITOR
TRAMCAR
TRAMPER
TRAPPER
TRASHER
TRAWLER
TRAYNOR
TREADER
TREATER
TREKKER
TRICKER
TRIFLER
TRIGGER
TRILLER
TRIMMER
TRIPPER
TRISTAR
TROLLER
TROOPER
TROTTER
TROUPER
TROUSER
TRUCKER
TRUDGER
TRUSTER
TRYSTER
URBANER
WRAPPER
WREAKER
WRECKER
WRESTER
WRINGER
WRITHER
WRONGER

••RR•••

AIRRACE
AIRRAGE
AIRRAID
BARRACK
BARRAGE
BARRELS
BARRENS
BARRETS
BARRETT
BARRIER
BARRING
BARRIOS
BARRONS
BARROOM
BARROWS
BERRIED
BERRIES
BIRRING
BORROWS
BURRIER
BURRING
BURRITO
BURROWS
CARRARA
CARRELS
CARRERA
CARRERE
CARRIED
CARRIER
CARRIES
CARROLL
CARROTS
CARROTY
CARRYIN
CARRYON
CIRRATE
CORRADE
CORRALS
CORRECT
CORRIDA
CORRODE
CORRUPT
CURRANT
CURRENT
CURRIED
CURRIER
CURRIES
CURRING
CURRISH
DARRYLF
DERRICK
DERRICO
DERRIDA
DERRING
DURRELL
EARRING
FARRAGO
FARRELL
FARRIER
FARROWS
FERRARA
FERRARE
FERRARI
FERRARO
FERRATE
FERRETS
FERRETY
FERRIED
FERRIES
FERRITE
FERROUS
FERRULE
FIRRIER
FORREAL
FORRENT
FORREST
FURRIER
FURRING
FURROWS
GARRETS
GARRETT
GARRICK
GARROTE
HARRAHS
HARRIED
HARRIER
HARRIES
HARRIET
HARRODS
HARROLD
HARROWS
HERRICK
HERRING
HERRIOT
HORRIFY
HORRORS
HURRAHS
HURRAYS
HURRIED
HURRIER
HURRIES
HURRYUP
JARRELL
JARRETT
JARRING
JARROTT
KURRENT
LARRUPS
LORRIES
MARRERS
MARRIED
MARRIES
MARRING
MARRONS
MARROWS
MARRYAT
MARRYIN
MARRYME
MERRIAM
MERRICK
MERRIER
MERRILL
MERRILY
MIRRORS
MORROWS
MYRRHED
MYRRHIC
NARRATE
NARROWS
NORRISH
PARRIED
PARRIER
PARRIES
PARRING
PARRISH
PARROTS
PERREAU
PERRIER
PERRINE
PERRINS
PURRERS
PURRING
PYRRHIC
PYRRHUS
SERRATE
SORRELL
SORRELS
SORRIER
SORRILY
SORROWS
SURREAL
SURREYS
TARRIED
TARRIER
TARRIES
TARRING
TERRACE
TERRAIN
TERRANS
TERRELL
TERRENE
TERRETS
TERRIER
TERRIES
TERRIFY
TERRINE
TERROIR
TERRORS
TORREFY
TORRENT
TURRETS
VARRICK
VERRUCA
WARRANT
WARRENG
WARRENS
WARRING
WARRIOR
WARROOM
WORRELL
WORRIED
WORRIER
WORRIES
YARROWS

••R•R••

AIRCREW
AIRDRIE
AIRDROP
AIRTRAP
AURORAE
AURORAL
AURORAS
BARNRED
BARTRAY
BERTRAM
CARBRAS
CARFREE
CARTRIP
CORNROW
CURARES
DARKRED
EARDROP
EARDRUM
ETRURIA
FIRTREE
FORERAN
FORERUN
FORFREE
FORTRAN
FURORES
FURWRAP
JURYRIG
MARGRET
MARSRED
MORDRED
PARURES
PERORAL
PORTRAY
SORORAL
SUREROF
TOREROS
TURNRED
UNRURAL
VERYRED

••R••R•

AGREERS
AIRFARE
AIRHORN
AIRPARK
AIRPORT
AIRWARS
APRIORI
ARREARS
ARRIERE
BARBARA
BARBARY
BARBERA
BARBERS
BARCARS
BARGERS
BARKERS
BARNARD
BARTERS
BARWARE
BERBERS
BERGERE
BERNARD
BERSERK
BIRDERS
BIRLERS
BORDERS
BURGERS
BURIERS
BURLERS
BURNERS
BURSARS
CARBARN
CARCARE
CARDERS
CAREERS
CARFARE
CARHORN
CARNERA
CARPARK
CARPERS
CARPORT
CARRARA
CARRERA
CARRERE
CARTERS
CARTIRE
CARVERS
CEREBRA
CEREBRO
CORDERO
CORDERS
CORKERS
CORNERS
CORPORA
CURLERS
CURSERS
CURSORS
CURSORY
DARNERS
DARTERS
DORMERS
DURWARD
EARHART
EARMARK
EARNERS
FARMERS
FARMERY
FARMORE
FERNERY
FERRARA
FERRARE
FERRARI
FERRARO
FERVORS
FIREARM
FORBORE
FORCERS
FOREARM
FORGERS
FORGERY
FORHIRE
FORKERS
FORLORN
FORMERS
FORSURE
FORTORD
FORWARD
FURFARM
FURLERS
GARNERS
GARTERS
GIRDERS
GORGERS
HARBORS
HARBURG
HARHARS
HARMERS
HARPERS
HARVARD
HERBART
HERBERT
HERDERS
HERONRY
HORRORS
HURLERS
HURTERS
JERKERS
LARDERS
LARKERS
LURKERS
MARGERY
MARKERS
MARMARA
MARRERS
MARTYRS
MARYURE
MERCERS
MERCERY
MERCURE
MERCURY
MERGERS
MIRRORS
MORCERF
MORTARS
MURDERS
MURMURS
NORBERT
NURSERS
NURSERY
NURTURE
PARGERS
PARKERS
PARLORS
PARSERS
PERDURE
PERFORM
PERJURE
PERJURY
PERTURB
PORKERS
PORTERS
PURPORT
PURRERS
PURSERS
SARTORS
SERVERS
SORCERY
SORTERS
SURFERS
SURGERY
TARTARE
TARTARS
TERNARY
TERRORS
THREERS
TORTURE
TURNERS
TURNERY
TURNPRO
UPREARS
UPROARS
VARIERS
VERDURE
VERGERS
VERYDRY
WARBURG
WARDERS
WARFARE
WARHERO
WARLORD
WARMERS
WARPERS
WARTORN
WARWORN
WORKERS
WORMERS
YARDARM
YARDERS
YORKERS

••R•••R

ABRADER
AERATOR
ALROKER
ARRAYER
ARRIVER
BARKIER
BARMIER
BARRIER
BERATER
BERKNER
BOROMIR
BURBLER
BURGHER
BURGLAR
BURLIER
BURNFOR
BURRIER
BURSTER
CARDOOR
CAREFOR
CAROLER
CARRIER
CARTIER
CCRIDER
CIRCLER
CORKIER
CORNIER
CORONER
CORSAIR
CORVAIR
CURATOR
CURDIER
CURDLER
CURLIER
CURRIER
CURVIER
DERIDER
DERIVER
DERNIER
DIRTIER
DORKIER
EARLIER
FARCEUR
FAREWAR
FARRIER
FARSEER
FARTHER
FERNBAR
FERNIER
FERVOUR
FIRRIER
FORAGER
FORBEAR
FOREVER
FORGOER
FORKIER
FORSTER
FURRIER
FURTHER
GARBLER
GARDNER
GARGLER
GERMIER
GIRDLER
GIRLIER
GORSIER
GORTNER
GYRATOR
GYROCAR
HARBOUR
HARDIER
HARRIER
HARSHER
HERBIER
HERITOR
HORNIER
HORSIER
HURDLER
HURRIER
HURTFOR
JAROMIR
JERKIER
LARDIER
LARDNER
LARKIER
LURCHER
MARBLER
MARCHER
MARINER
MARLIER
MARNIER
MARSBAR
MARVIER
MERRIER
MIRADOR
MIRAMAR
MURKIER
NERDIER
NERVIER
NORTHER
PARADER
PARADOR
PARDNER
PARFOUR
PARLOUR
PARRIER
PARTIER
PARTNER
PARTYER
PERCHER
PERKIER
PERRIER
PERUSER
PERYEAR
PORIVER
PORKIER
PURFLER
PURSIER
PURSUER
PURTIER
SCRAPER
SCRIBER
SERENER
SHRINER
SHRIVER
SORRIER

SPRAYER
SPRUCER
STRAFER
STRAYER
STREWER
STRIDER
STRIKER
STRIPER
STRIVER
STROKER
SURFIER
SURLIER
TARDIER
TARRIER
TARTIER
TERRIER
TERROIR
THRIVER
THROWER
TIREDER
TORCHER
TURFIER
TURFWAR
UNRIPER
UPRISER
UPRIVER
VERMEER
VERNIER
VORSTER
WARBLER
WARRIOR
WARTIER
WERNHER
WERTHER
WORDIER
WORKFOR
WORMIER
WORRIER

•••RR••

AVERRED
BEURRES
BLURRED
CHARRED
CHARRER
CHARROS
CHIRRED
CHIRRUP
CHURROS
DHURRIE
FMURRAY
GNARRED
INERROR
JCARROL
KNARRED
OVERRAN
OVERRUN
PIERROT
QUARREL
SCARRED
SHIRRED
SIERRAS
SLURRED
SPARRED
SPARRER
SPARROW
SPORRAN
SPURRED
STARRED
STIRRED
STIRRER
STIRRUP
WHIRRED
XTERRAS

•••R•R•

ADORERS
AFARCRY
BEARERS
CARRARA
CARRERA
CARRERE
DEIRDRE
FEARERS
FEBRERO
FERRARA
FERRARE
FERRARI
FERRARO
HEARERS
HORRORS
JEERERS
LEERERS
LIBRARY
MARRERS
MCCRARY
MCGRORY
MIRRORS
NOTRARE
OVERARM
OVERDRY
PAIRERS
POURERS
PURRERS
REARERS
ROARERS
SCARERS
SCORERS
SEARERS
SHARERS
SNARERS
SNORERS
SOARERS
SPARERS
STARERS
STIRFRY
STORERS
TEARERS
TERRORS
TOURERS
USURERS
WEARERS
WHERERE

•••R••R

ADORNER
ALARMER
ALERTER
AMERCER
ANGRIER
AVERTER
AWARDER
BARRIER
BEERIER
BLURBER
BLURTER
BOARDER
BOERWAR
BURRIER
CARRIER
CHARGER
CHARIER
CHARMER
CHARRER
CHARTER
CHIRPER
CHURNER
COARSER
COERCER
COURIER
COURSER
CURRIER
DAIRYER
DEARSIR
DECREER
DECRIER
ENARBOR
EVERDUR
EVERTOR
EXERTER
FARRIER
FEARFOR
FEVRIER
FIERCER
FIERIER
FIRRIER
FLIRTER
FOURIER
FURRIER
GUARDER
HAIRIER
HARRIER
HOARDER
HOARIER
HOARSER
HURRIER
INERROR
INORDER
LEARNER
LEERIER
MERRIER
MOORIER
MOURNER
NEARPAR
ONORDER
OUTROAR
OVERFAR
OVERPAR
PARRIER
PEARLER
PERRIER
PIERCER
QUARTER
QUERIER
REORDER
SCARCER
SCARFER
SCARIER
SCORNER
SHARPER
SHIRKER
SHORTER
SKIRTER
SLURPER
SMARTER
SMIRKER
SNARLER
SNORTER
SORRIER
SPARRER
SPARSER
SPIRIER
SPURNER
STARKER
STARTER
STERNER
STERTOR
STIRRER
SWARMER
TARRIER
TEARIER
TERRIER
TERROIR
THURBER
TOORDER
TWIRLER
UNTRUER
USURPER
WARRIOR
WEARIER
WEIRDER
WHIRLER
WORRIER
YEARNER

••••RR•

ANDORRA
BEGORRA
BIZARRE
BIZARRO
DEBURRS
DUBARRY
ENCARRE
EQUERRY
IGNARRO
IMSORRY
LECARRE
NAVARRE
NOVARRO
PISARRO
PIZARRO
RECARRY
REMARRY
SCHIRRA
SCIORRA
SOSORRY
THIERRY
UNMERRY
UNSORRY
ZIMARRA

••••R•R

ABJURER
ADHERER
ADJURER
ADJUROR
ADMIRER
ALLURER
ALTERER
ARMORER
ASPIRER
ASSURER
ASSUROR
ATTIRER
AUGURER
CATERER
CHARRER
CHEERER
CLEARER
COHERER
COJUROR
COLORER
COVERER
DEMURER
DESIRER
EAGERER
EDWARDR
EMPEROR
ENDURER
ENSURER
ENTERER
FAVORER
FIGURER
FLOORER
HONORER
HOVERER
IGNORER
IMPURER
INERROR
INJURER
INSURER
LABORER
LEDERER
MATURER
OFFERER
OFFEROR
ORDERER
PAPERER
QUEERER
REVERER
SAVORER
SCOURER
SECURER
SEVERER
SHEARER
SHEERER
SMEARER
SNEERER
SOBERER
SPARRER
SPEARER
SQUARER
STEERER
STIRRER
SWEARER
UTTERER
VAPORER
WAGERER
WATERER
WAVERER

•••••RR

LETTERR

RS•••••

RSTUVWX
RSVPING

R•S••••

RASBORA
RASCALS
RASHERS
RASHEST
RASHIDA
RASPERS
RASPIER
RASPING
RASPISH
RASSLED
RASSLER
RASSLES
RASTERS
RASURES
RESALES
RESALTS
RESANDS
RESAVED
RESAVES
RESAWED
RESCALE
RESCANS
RESCIND
RESCORE
RESCRUB
RESCUED
RESCUER
RESCUES
RESEALS
RESEAMS
RESEATS
RESEAUS
RESEAUX
RESECTS
RESEEDS
RESEEKS
RESEIZE
RESELLS
RESENDS
RESENTS
RESERVE
RESEWED
RESHAPE
RESHARE
RESHAVE
RESHIFT
RESHINE
RESHIPS
RESHOES
RESHOOT
RESHOWN
RESHOWS
RESHUTS
RESIDED
RESIDER
RESIDES
RESIDUA
RESIDUE
RESIFTS
RESIGHT
RESIGNS
RESILED
RESILES
RESINED
RESINGS
RESINKS
RESISTS
RESITED
RESIZED
RESIZER
RESIZES
RESLATE
RESMELT
RESNAIS
RESNAPS
RESOAKS
RESOAPS
RESOILS
RESOJET
RESOLED
RESOLER
RESOLES
RESOLVE
RESORBS
RESORTS
RESOUND
RESOWED
RESPACE
RESPADE
RESPANS
RESPARK
RESPEAK
RESPECT
RESPELL
RESPELT
RESPICE
RESPINS
RESPIRE
RESPITE
RESPLIT
RESPOKE
RESPOND
RESPOOL
RESPOTS
RESPRAY
RESTABS
RESTACK
RESTAFF
RESTAGE
RESTAIN
RESTAMP
RESTART
RESTATE
RESTERS
RESTFUL
RESTICK
RESTING
RESTIRS
RESTIVE
RESTOCK
RESTOKE
RESTORE
RESTOWS
RESTRAP
RESTREW
RESTRIP
RESTSIN
RESTSON
RESTSUP
RESTUDY
RESTUFF
RESTYLE
RESUITS
RESULTS
RESUMED
RESUMES
RESURGE
RESWEAR
RESWEEP
RESWIMS
RESWORE
RESWORN
RISENTO
RISESTO
RISESUP
RISIBLE
RISIBLY
RISINGS
RISKERS
RISKIER
RISKILY
RISKING
RISKSIT
RISOTTO
RISSOLE
RLSTINE
ROSABUD
ROSALIA
ROSALIE
ROSALYN
ROSANNA
ROSANNE
ROSARIO
ROSCOES
ROSEATE
ROSEBAY
ROSEBUD
ROSEHIP
ROSELLA
ROSELLE
ROSEOIL
ROSEOLA
ROSERED
ROSETEA
ROSETTA
ROSETTE
ROSIEST
ROSINED
ROSSANO
ROSSINI
ROSSNER
ROSSSEA
ROSTAND
ROSTERS
ROSTOCK
ROSTRAL
ROSTRUM
ROSWELL
RUSHDIE
RUSHEES
RUSHERS
RUSHIER
RUSHING
RUSHOFF
RUSHOUT
RUSSELL
RUSSERT
RUSSETS
RUSSETY
RUSSIAN
RUSSLAN
RUSTICS
RUSTIER
RUSTILY
RUSTING
RUSTLED
RUSTLER
RUSTLES

R••S•••

RAGSHOP
RAISERS
RAISEUP
RAISING
RAISINS
RAISINY
RAISONS
RALSTON
RAMSESI
RAMSFAN
RAMSONS
RANSACK
RANSOMS
RAPSONG
RAPSTAR
RASSLED
RASSLER
RASSLES
RATSOUT
RAWSILK
REASKED
REASONS
REASSAY
REDSFAN
REDSKIN
REDSPOT
REDSTAR
REDSUIT
REDSUNS
REISSUE
REPSFOR
RETSINA
REUSERS
REUSING
RIESENS
RIESMAN
RIESSEN
RIGSOUT
RIKSDAG
RIMSHOT
RINSERS
RINSING
RIPSAWN
RIPSAWS
RIPSOFF
RIPSONE
RIPSOUT
RIPSTOP
RISSOLE
ROASTED
ROASTER
ROBSART
ROISTER
RONSARD
RONSONS
ROOSTED
ROOSTER
ROSSANO
ROSSINI
ROSSNER
ROSSSEA
ROUSERS
ROUSING
ROUSTED
ROUSTER
RUBSOFF
RUBSOUT
RUBSRAW
RUMSHOP
RUNSDRY
RUNSFOR
RUNSLOW
RUNSOFF
RUNSOUT
RUSSELL
RUSSERT
RUSSETS
RUSSETY
RUSSIAN
RUSSLAN

R•••S••

RACESBY
RACESTO
RACESUP
RACISTS
RACKSUP
RAILSAT
RAILSON
RAINSIN
RAINSON
RAKESIN
RAKESUP
RAMESES
RAMPSUP
RANTSAT
RAWISTS
READSIN
READSON
READSTO
READSUP
REARSUP
REASSAY
REBASTE
REBUSES
RECASED
RECASES
RECASTS
RECOSTS
RECUSAL
RECUSED
RECUSES
REDOSED
REDOSES
REDUSTS
REEKSOF
REELSIN
REELSUP
REFUSAL
REFUSED
REFUSER
REFUSES
REINSIN
REISSUE
RELISTS
RELOSES
REMISED
REMISES
RENESTS
RENTSTO
REPASTE
REPASTS
REPOSED
REPOSER
REPOSES
REPOSIT
REPOSTS
RERISEN
RERISES
RESISTS
RESTSIN
RESTSON
RESTSUP
RETASTE
RETESTS
REVESTS
REVISAL
REVISED
REVISER
REVISES
REVISIT
REVISOR
RICKSHA
RIDESBY
RIDESIN
RIDESTO
RIDESUP
RIESSEN
RILESUP
RINGSIN
RINGSUP
RIPOSTE
RIPOSTS
RISESTO
RISESUP
RISKSIT
ROARSAT
ROBESON
ROBUSTA
ROBUSTO
ROLLSBY
ROLLSIN
ROLLSON
ROLLSUP
ROOTSUP
ROPESIN
ROPESUP
ROSSSEA
RUCKSUP
RULESON

R••••S•

RACIEST
RAFFISH
RAMMISH
RAMSESI
RANKEST
RANKISH
RANPAST
RASHEST
RASPISH
RATTISH
RAWFISH
RAWNESS
RAYLESS
REALEST
REALISE
REALISM
REALIST
REAMASS
REARISE
REAROSE
REBRUSH
RECHOSE
RECLASP
RECLASS
RECLUSE
RECROSS
REDDEST
REDDISH
REDDUST
REDFISH
REDNESS
REDNOSE
REDRESS
REDROSE
REFRESH
REGLOSS
REGRASP
REGRESS
REHOUSE
RELAPSE
RELEASE
REMORSE
REPHASE
REPRESS
REPRISE
REPULSE
REQUEST
RERAISE
RERINSE
RETOAST
RETWIST
REVERSA
REVERSE
REYNOSA
RHENISH
RHYMIST
RIBLESS
RICHEST
RIMIEST
RIMLESS
RODLESS
ROGUISH
ROMANSH
ROMPISH
ROOKISH
ROPIEST
ROSIEST
RUBBISH
RULIEST
RUMLESS
RUNLESS
RUNPAST
RUNTISH
RUTTISH

R•••••S

RABBETS
RABBITS
RABBLES
RACEMES
RACINOS
RACISTS
RACKERS
RACKETS
RADAMES
RADIALS
RADIANS
RADICES
RADIXES
RADOMES
RAFFIAS
RAFFLES
RAFTERS
RAGBAGS
RAGGIES
RAGINGS
RAGLANS
RAGMANS
RAGMOPS
RAGOUTS
RAGRUGS
RAGTOPS
RAIDERS
RAILBUS
RAILERS
RAISERS
RAISINS
RAISONS
RALLIES
RALLYES
RAMADAS
RAMBLES
RAMESES
RAMFANS
RAMJETS
RAMMERS
RAMONES
RAMRODS
RAMSONS
RANCHES
RANCHOS
RANCORS
RANGERS
RANKERS
RANKLES
RANLAPS
RANSOMS
RANTERS
RAPIERS
RAPINES
RAPINIS
RAPPELS
RAPPERS
RAPTORS
RAREGAS
RASCALS
RASHERS
RASPERS
RASSLES
RASTERS
RASURES
RATINES
RATINGS
RATIONS
RATITES
RATLINS
RATTANS
RATTERS
RATTLES
RAUCOUS
RAVAGES
RAVEUPS
RAVINES

RAVINGS RAWBARS RAWEGGS RAWISTS RAWLINS RAWNESS RAYBANS RAYGUNS RAYLESS RAZZIES RCCOLAS REACHES READERS READIES REAGANS REAMASS REAMERS REAPERS REARERS REASONS REATTAS REAVERS REAVOWS REBAITS REBAKES REBALES REBANKS REBATES REBENDS REBILLS REBINDS REBOILS REBOLTS REBOOKS REBOOTS REBORES REBOTES REBOXES REBOZOS REBREWS REBUFFS REBUKES REBUSES RECAGES RECALLS RECANES RECANTS RECASES RECASTS RECEDES RECHEWS RECIPES RECITES RECKONS RECLADS RECLASS RECOALS RECOATS RECOCKS RECODES RECOILS RECOINS RECOMBS RECOOKS RECOOLS RECORDS RECORKS RECOSTS

RECOUPS RECROSS RECTORS RECURES RECURLS RECUSES REDACTS REDANTS REDARES REDARNS REDATES REDBATS REDBAYS REDBUDS REDCAPS REDCODS REDDENS REDDOGS REDDOTS REDDYES REDEALS REDEEDS REDEEMS REDEYES REDFINS REDFIRS REDHATS REDHENS REDHOTS REDIALS REDLEGS REDNESS REDOAKS REDOCKS REDOSES REDOUTS REDOXES REDRAGS REDRAWS REDRESS REDRIES REDSUNS REDTABS REDTAGS REDTIES REDTOPS REDUCES REDUSTS REEARNS REEBOKS REEDITS REEFERS REEKERS REELERS REEMITS REFACES REFALLS REFAXES REFEEDS REFILES REFILLS REFILMS REFINDS REFINES REFIRES REFIXES REFLAGS REFLIES

REFLIPS REFLOWS REFOCUS REFOLDS REFORMS REFRIES REFUELS REFUGES REFUNDS REFUSES REFUTES REGAINS REGALES REGARDS REGEARS REGENTS REGIFTS REGILDS REGIMES REGINAS REGIONS REGIRDS REGIVES REGLOSS REGLOWS REGLUES REGRABS REGRESS REGRETS REGRIPS REGROWS REGULUS REHANGS REHAULS REHEALS REHEARS REHEATS REHEELS REHIDES REHIRES REHONES REHOOKS REIFIES REJAILS REJECTS REJOINS REKICKS REKNITS REKNOTS RELACES RELANDS RELANES RELATES RELAXES RELEADS RELEAPS RELENDS RELENTS RELEVES RELICTS RELIEFS RELIERS RELINES RELINKS RELISTS RELIVES RELOADS RELOANS

RELOCKS RELOOKS RELOSES RELUCTS RELUMES REMAILS REMAINS REMAKES REMANDS REMARKS REMATES REMEETS REMELTS REMENDS REMILLS REMINDS REMINES REMINTS REMISES REMIXES REMOLDS REMORAS REMOTES REMOVES RENAILS RENAMES RENDERS RENEGES RENESTS RENNETS RENNINS RENOIRS RENOTES RENOWNS RENTALS RENTEES RENTERS RENVOIS REOPENS REPACKS REPAGES REPAIRS REPARKS REPASTS REPAVES REPEALS REPEATS REPENTS REPERKS REPICKS REPINES REPLANS REPLAYS REPLIES REPLOTS REPLOWS REPOLLS REPORTS REPOSES REPOSTS REPOURS REPRESS REPUGNS REPUMPS REPUTES RERACKS RERAKES RERANKS

RERATES REREADS REREDOS REREELS RERENTS RERIDES RERISES REROLLS REROOFS REROOTS RESALES RESALTS RESANDS RESAVES RESCANS RESCUES RESEALS RESEAMS RESEATS RESEAUS RESECTS RESEEDS RESEEKS RESELLS RESENDS RESENTS RESHIPS RESHOES RESHOWS RESHUTS RESIDES RESIFTS RESIGNS RESILES RESINGS RESINKS RESISTS RESIZES RESNAIS RESNAPS RESOAKS RESOAPS RESOILS RESOLES RESORBS RESORTS RESPANS RESPINS RESPOTS RESTABS RESTERS RESTIRS RESTOWS RESUITS RESULTS RESUMES RESWIMS RETACKS RETAILS RETAINS RETAKES RETAMES RETAPES RETARDS RETAXES RETEARS RETELLS RETESTS

RETHAWS RETILES RETILLS RETIMES RETINAS RETINTS RETIRES RETONES RETOOLS RETORTS RETOURS RETRAPS RETRIES RETRIMS RETUNES RETURFS RETURNS RETYPES REUBENS REUNERS REURGES REUSERS REUTERS REVAMPS REVEALS REVENDS REVERBS REVERES REVERTS REVESTS REVIEWS REVILES REVISES REVIVES REVOKES REVOLTS REVOTES REWAKES REWARDS REWARMS REWARNS REWAXES REWEARS REWELDS REWINDS REWIPES REWIRES REWORDS REWORKS REWRAPS REXCATS REYOKES REZEROS REZONES RHEBOKS RHETORS RHOECUS RHOMBUS RHUMBAS RHYMERS RHYTHMS RIALTOS RIBALDS RIBANDS RIBBERS RIBBIES RIBBONS RIBCUTS

RIBEYES RIBLESS RIBLETS RIBPADS RICHENS RICKEYS RICKLES RICRACS RIDDERS RIDDLES RIDEBYS RIDINGS RIESENS RIFFLES RIFLERS RIGGERS RIGOURS RILLETS RIMLESS RIMPLES RINGERS RINSERS RIOTERS RIOTOUS RIPOFFS RIPOSTS RIPPERS RIPPLES RIPRAPS RIPSAWS RISINGS RISKERS RITARDS RITDYES RITUALS ROACHES ROADEOS ROADERS ROADIES ROAMERS ROARERS ROBARDS ROBBERS ROBBINS ROBERTS ROBROYS ROCHETS ROCKERS ROCKETS ROCKIES ROCOCOS RODENTS RODGERS RODLESS ROLAIDS ROLEXES ROLFERS ROLLEIS ROLLERS ROLLINS ROLLONS ROLLUPS ROMAINS ROMAJIS ROMANIS ROMANOS ROMANUS ROMCOMS

ROMNEYS ROMPERS ROMULUS RONDELS RONSONS ROOFERS ROOKIES ROOMBAS ROOMERS ROOMIES ROOTERS ROOTLES ROSCOES ROSTERS ROTATES ROTGUTS ROTTERS ROUSERS ROUTERS ROVINGS ROWDIES ROYALES RUANDAS RUBATOS RUBBERS RUBBLES RUBIOUS RUBRICS RUDDERS RUFFLES RUGGLES RUGRATS RUINERS RUINOUS RULINGS RUMAKIS RUMBLES RUMLESS RUMMERS RUMMIES RUMOURS RUMPLES RUNDLES RUNLAPS RUNLESS RUNLETS RUNNELS RUNNERS RUNOFFS RUNOUTS RUNWAYS RUPIAHS RUSHEES RUSHERS RUSSETS RUSTICS RUSTLES RUTGERS RUTILES RUTTERS RUYBLAS RVALUES RVPARKS RYOKANS RYUKYUS

•RS••••

ARSENAL ARSENIC ARSENIO ARSHILE DRSEUSS DRSLOAN DRSPOCK ERSKINE IRSFORM MRSBASS MRSCOTT MRSLATE MRSMITH MRSMUIR MRSPAUL MRSPEEL MRSPOCK QRSTUVW URSINUS URSULAK

•R•S•••

ARCSINE ARISING ARISTAE ARISTAS ARISTOS ARTSALE ARTSHOP ARTSHOW ARTSIER ARTSONG ARUSPEX BRASHER BRASHES BRASHLY BRASIER BRASIZE BRASSES BRASSIE BRESCIA BRESLIN BRISKED BRISKER BRISKET BRISKLY BRISTLE BRISTLY BRISTOL BROSNAN BROSSES BRUSHED BRUSHER BRUSHES BRUSHUP BRUSQUE CRASHAW CRASHED CRASHER CRASHES CRASSER CRASSLY CRASSUS CRESPIN CRESSES CRESSET CRESTED CRESTON CRISPED

CRISPEN CRISPER CRISPIN CRISPIX CRISPLY CRISPUS CROSIER CROSSAT CROSSED CROSSER CROSSES CROSSLY CROSSUP CROSTIC CRUSADE CRUSHED CRUSHER CRUSHES CRUSTAL CRUSTED CRYSTAL DRASTIC DRESDEN DRESSAS DRESSED DRESSER DRESSES DRESSIN DRESSUP DRISTAN DROSSES DRYSUIT ERASERS ERASING ERASMUS ERASTUS ERASURE ERISTIC EROSELY EROSION EROSIVE FRASIER FRESCAS FRESCOS FRESHED FRESHEN FRESHER FRESHES FRESHET FRESHLY FRESNEL FRESSED FRESSES FRISBEE FRISEUR FRISIAN FRISKED FRISKER FRISSON FROSTED FROSTER FRUSTRO FRUSTUM GRASPAT GRASPED GRASPER GRASSED GRASSES

GRASSLE GRESHAM GRISHAM GRISLET GRISNEZ GRISSOM GRISTER GRISTLE GRISTLY GROSSED GROSSER GROSSES GROSSLY IRESIGN IRISHER IRISING IRISOUT IRKSOME KRASNER KRESKIN KRISHNA KRISTIN KRYSTLE MRISCAN ORESTES ORISONS PRESAGE PRESALE PRESALT PRESEAL PRESEAT PRESELL PRESENT PRESETS PRESHIP PRESHOW PRESIDE PRESIFT PRESLEY PRESOAK PRESOLD PRESONG PRESORT PRESPUR PRESQUE PRESSED PRESSEL PRESSER PRESSES PRESSON PRESSUP PRESTON PRESTOS PRESUME PRISONS PRISSES PROSAIC PROSCAN PROSERS PROSHOP PROSIER PROSILY PROSING PROSODY PROSPER PRUSSIA TRASHED TRASHER

TRASHES TRASHTV TRESSED TRESSES TRESTLE TRISECT TRISTAN TRISTAR TRUSSED TRUSSES TRUSSUP TRUSTED TRUSTEE TRUSTER TRUSTIN TRUSTME TRYSAIL TRYSTED TRYSTER WRASSES WRESTED WRESTER WRESTLE

•R••S••

ARALSEA ARCHSEE ARENSKY ARGUSES ARIOSOS ARIOSTO AROUSAL AROUSED AROUSER AROUSES ARRASES ARRESTS ARRISES ARTISAN ARTISTE ARTISTS BRAISED BRAISES BRANSON BRASSES BRASSIE BREASTS BREWSKI BREWSUP BROASTS BRODSKY BRONSON BROSSES BROWSED BROWSER BROWSES BRUISED BRUISER BRUISES BRYUSOV CRAISIN CRAMSIN CRASSER CRASSLY CRASSUS CREASED CREASER CREASES

CREOSOL CRESSES CRESSET CRIESUP CRIMSON CROESUS CROPSUP CROSSAT CROSSED CROSSER CROSSES CROSSLY CROSSUP CRUDSUP CRUISED CRUISER CRUISES DRAGSIN DRAGSON DRAGSUP DRAWSIN DRAWSON DRAWSTO DRAWSUP DREISER DRESSAS DRESSED DRESSER DRESSES DRESSIN DRESSUP DRIESCH DRIESUP DRIPSON DROPSBY DROPSIN DROPSIT DROSSES DROWSED DROWSES DRUMSET DRUMSUP ERICSON ERIKSON ERNESTA ERNESTO FRAISES FREESIA FREESOF FREESUP FRESSED FRESSES FRETSAT FRETSAW FRIESUP FRISSON GRABSAT GRASSED GRASSES GRASSLE GRAYSON GREASED GREASER GREASES GRIMSBY GRINSAT GRISSOM GROSSED

GROSSER
GROSSES
GROSSLY
GROUSED
GROUSER
GROUSES
GROWSON
GROWSUP
IRONSON
MRMUSIC
ORBISON
ORRISES
PRAISED
PRAISER
PRAISES
PRAYSTO
PRESSED
PRESSEL
PRESSER
PRESSES
PRESSON
PRESSUP
PREYSON
PRIESTS
PRISSES
PRIUSES
PRODSON
PROPSUP
PRUSSIA
TRANSAM
TRANSIT
TRANSOM
TREASON
TREESAP
TRESSED
TRESSES
TRIESIT
TRIESON
TRIESTE
TRIESTO
TRIPSON
TRIPSUP
TROTSKY
TROTSUP
TROUSER
TRUESUP
TRUISMS
TRUSSED
TRUSSES
TRUSSUP
URGESON
VRONSKY
WRAPSUP
WRASSES

•R•••S•

ARABIST
ARCHEST
ARENOSE
ARIDEST
ARMLESS
ARMREST
ARTIEST
ARTLESS
BRALESS
BRAVEST
BRINISH
BRITISH
BRUTISH
BRUXISM
CRAFTSY
CRUDEST
DRFRIST
DRONISH
DRSEUSS
DRYNESS
DRYWASH
FRENESI
GRAVEST
GRAYEST
GRAYISH
GRECISM
GREYEST
GREYISH
IRATEST
IREFUSE
IRELESS
IRKUTSK
IRONIST
MRBLISS
MRHORSE
MRMOOSE
MRSBASS
ORALIST
ORBLESS
ORELESS
ORGIAST
PRADESH
PRECAST
PRECISE
PREDUSK
PRELOSS
PREMISE
PREMISS
PRETEST
PREVOST
PREWASH
PROCESS
PROEAST
PROFESS
PROFUSE
PROMISE
PROPOSE
PROTEST
PROTIST
PROVISO
PROVOST
PROWESS
PROWEST
PRUDISH
TRAIPSE
TRITEST
TROPISM
WRYNESS

•R••••S

ARABICS
ARABLES
ARAMIDS
ARBACES
ARBOLES
ARBOURS
ARBUTUS
ARCADES
ARCHERS
ARCHIES
ARCHONS
ARCINGS
ARDOURS
ARDUOUS
AREOLAS
AREOLES
ARGALIS
ARGENTS
ARGUERS
ARGUSES
ARGYLES
ARIANES
ARIOSOS
ARISTAS
ARISTOS
ARMADAS
ARMFULS
ARMLESS
ARMLETS
ARMOURS
ARMPITS
ARNICAS
ARNOLDS
AROUSES
ARRACKS
ARRASES
ARREARS
ARRESTS
ARRISES
ARRIVES
ARROYOS
ARTCARS
ARTEMIS
ARTEMUS
ARTHURS
ARTISTS
ARTLESS
ARUBANS
BRACERS
BRAHMAS
BRAISES
BRALESS
BRASHES
BRASSES
BRAVOES
BRAYERS
BRAZENS
BREASTS
BREATHS
BREEZES
BRETONS
BREVETS
BREWERS
BREYERS
BRIARDS
BRIBEES
BRIBERS
BRIDALS
BRIDGES
BRIDLES
BRIGHTS
BRILLOS
BRINERS
BRITONS
BROADAS
BROASTS
BRODIES
BROGANS
BROGUES
BROKERS
BRONCOS
BRONTES
BRONZES
BROSSES
BROWSES
BRUISES
BRUMOUS
BRUNETS
BRUSHES
CRADLES
CRASHES
CRASSUS
CRATERS
CRAVATS
CRAVENS
CRAVERS
CRAYONS
CRAZIES
CREASES
CREATES
CRECHES
CREDITS
CREEPOS
CRENELS
CREOLES
CRESSES
CRETANS
CRETINS
CREWELS
CRINGES
CRISPUS
CRITIAS
CRITICS
CROESUS
CRONIES
CROOKES
CROQUIS
CROSSES
CROTONS
CROUTES
CROWERS
CRUISES
CRUSHES
CRUZANS
CRYPTOS
DRAGEES
DRAGONS
DRAPERS
DRAWEES
DRAWERS
DRCHAOS
DREDGES
DRESSAS
DRESSES
DREYFUS
DRIVELS
DRIVERS
DROGUES
DRONERS
DROPINS
DROSSES
DROVERS
DROWSES
DROXIES
DRSEUSS
DRUDGES
DRVEGAS
DRYADES
DRYEYES
DRYFOGS
DRYMOPS
DRYNESS
DRYPERS
DRYROTS
DRYRUNS
ERASERS
ERASMUS
ERASTUS
ERECTUS
ERINYES
ERLANGS
ERMINES
ERODERS
EROTICS
ERRANDS
ERYNGOS
FRAISES
FRAMERS
FRANCES
FRANCIS
FRAPPES
FRATERS
FREEZES
FRENCHS
FRESCAS
FRESCOS
FRESHES
FRESSES
FRIDAYS
FRIDGES
FRIENDS
FRIEZES
FRIGHTS
FRINGES
FRIVOLS
FRIZZES
FROLICS
FRYPANS
GRACIAS
GRADERS
GRAHAMS
GRAMMES
GRAMMYS
GRAMPAS
GRAMPUS
GRANGES
GRANPAS
GRAPPAS
GRASSES
GRATERS
GRATIAS
GRAVELS
GRAVERS
GRAVIES
GRAZERS
GREASES
GREAVES
GRIEVES
GRIGRIS
GRILLES
GRINGOS
GRIPERS
GRIPPES
GROCERS
GROOVES
GROPERS
GROPIUS
GROSSES
GROTIUS
GROTTOS
GROUNDS
GROUSES
GROVELS
GROVERS
GROWERS
GROWTHS
GRUDGES
GRUNGES
IRELESS
IRENICS
IRONERS
IRONIES
IRONONS
IRRUPTS
KRAKENS
MRBLISS
MRBONES
MRBURNS
MRBUTTS
MRCHIPS
MRDEEDS
MRHOBBS
MRJONES
MRSBASS
MRTIBBS
MRWORDS
ORACIES
ORACLES
ORANGES
ORANTES
ORATORS
ORBLESS
ORCHIDS
ORDAINS
ORDEALS
ORDINES
ORELESS
ORESTES
ORGEATS
ORIENTS
ORIGINS
ORIOLES
ORISONS
ORKNEYS
ORLEANS
ORMOLUS
ORPHANS
ORPHEUS
ORRISES
PRAISES
PRANCES
PRATERS
PRAYERS
PREACTS
PREAGES
PREAMPS
PREARMS
PREBIDS
PREBUYS
PRECUTS
PREFABS
PREFERS
PRELIMS
PRELOSS
PREMEDS
PREMIES
PREMISS
PRENUPS
PREPAYS
PRESETS
PRESSES
PRESTOS
PRETORS
PREVIAS
PREVUES
PREXIES
PREYERS
PRFIRMS
PRICERS
PRIESTS
PRIMERS
PRINCES
PRISONS
PRISSES
PRIUSES
PRIVETS
PRIVIES
PRIZZIS
PROBERS
PROBIES
PROCESS
PROCLUS
PROFESS
PROFITS
PROJETS
PROKEDS
PROLOGS
PROMPTS
PROPELS
PROSERS
PROTEUS
PROTONS
PROVERS
PROWESS
PROXIES
PRUNERS
ORATIOS
TRACERS
TRADERS
TRAMPAS
TRANCES
TRASHES
TRAUMAS
TRAVELS
TRAVERS
TREBLES
TREDIAS
TREIZES
TRELLIS
TREMORS
TREPANS
TRESSES
TRIAGES
TRICEPS
TRICOTS
TRIFLES
TRIGONS
TRIJETS
TRIODES
TRIPLES
TRIPODS
TRITONS
TRIVETS
TROCHES
TROIKAS
TROILUS
TROJANS
TROPICS
TROUGHS
TROUPES
TROWELS
TRUANTS
TRUDGES
TRUISMS
TRUMANS
TRUSSES
TRYOUTS
URACILS
URCHINS
URGINGS
URNFULS
URSINUS
URTEXTS
WRAITHS
WRAPUPS
WRASSES
WREATHS
WRIGHTS
WRITERS
WRITHES
WRYNESS

••RS•••

AIRSACS
AIRSHIP
AIRSHOW
AIRSICK
AIRSIGN
AIRSOCK
AIRSOUT
BARSOAP
BARSTOW
BERSERK
BERSUNT
BORSCHT
BORSTAL
BURSARS
BURSTER
BURSTIN
BURSTYN
CARSALE
CARSEAT
CARSHOW
CORSAGE
CORSAIR
CORSETS
CORSICA
CURSEAT
CURSERS
CURSING
CURSIVE
CURSORS
CURSORY
DORSALS
DORSETT
DORSEYS
EARSHOT
FARSEER
FARSIDE
FIRSTLY
FIRSTUP
FORSAKE
FORSALE
FORSHOW
FORSIZE
FORSOOK
FORSTER
FORSURE
FORSYTE
FORSYTH
FURSEAL
GERSHON
GORSIER
HARSHEN
HARSHER
HARSHLY
HERSELF
HERSHEY
HIRSUTE
HORSIER
HORSILY
HORSING
HORSLEY
HURSTON
JERSEYS
KERSHAW
KIRSTEN
KIRSTIE
MARSALA
MARSBAR
MARSDEN
MARSHAL
MARSHES
MARSRED
MARSTON
MORSELS
NURSERS
NURSERY
NURSING
OARSMAN
OARSMEN
OERSTED
OURSELF
OURSONG
PARSECS
PARSEES
PARSERS
PARSING
PARSLEY
PARSNIP
PARSONS
PERSEID
PERSEUS
PERSIAN
PERSIST
PERSIUS
PERSOFF
PERSONA
PERSONS
PERSSON
PORSCHE
PORSENA
PQRSTUV
PURSERS
PURSIER
PURSING
PURSUED
PURSUER
PURSUES
PURSUIT
TARSALS
TERSELY
TERSEST
TORSION
VARSITY
VERSACE
VERSANT
VERSETS
VERSIFY
VERSING
VERSION
VORSTER
WARSHIP
WORSENS
WORSHIP
WORSLEY
WORSTED

••R•S••

AEROSOL
ALROSEN
ARRASES
ARRESTS
ARRISES
AURISTS
BARISTA
BARKSAT
BERGSON
BERNSEN
BURNSIN
BURNSUP
CARESTO
CARLSON
CARPSAT
CARTSIN
CERISES
CHRISMS
CHRISOM
CHRISTA
CHRISTI
CHRISTO
CHRISTY
CORKSUP
CORPSES
CURLSIN
CURLSUP
CURTSEY
CYRUSII
DARESAY
DARESTO
DERUSTS
DIRKSEN
EARNSIT
EURASIA
FIRESAT
FIRESON
FIRESUP
FIRMSUP
FORASEC
FORESAW
FORESEE
FORESTS
FORKSUP
GIRASOL
GIRLSHY
HARDSET
HARDSIX
HARPSON
HERESTO
HIRESON
HORNSBY
HORNSIN
JERKSUP
JIRASEK
JURISTS
KARASEA
KARLSON
LARUSSA
LORDSIT
LORISES
LORUSES
LURESIN
LYRISTS
MARKSUP
MARUSJA
MIRISCH
MORESBY
MORISOT
NERISSA
ORRISES
PARASKI
PARASOL
PARKSIT
PERISSA
PERKSUP
PERSSON
PERUSAL
PERUSED
PERUSER
PERUSES
PHRASAL
PHRASED
PHRASES
PURISTS
RERISEN
RERISES
STRASSE
SURFSUP
TARTSUP
THRUSTS
TIRESOF
TURFSKI
TURISMO
TURISTA
TURNSIN
TURNSON
TURNSTO
TURNSUP
UNRASPY
UNRESTS
UNRISEN
UNRISKY
UPRISEN
UPRISER
UPRISES
VERISMO
VERISTS
VERYSAD
VERYSHY
VIRUSES
WARMSTO
WARMSUP
WARNSOF
WIRESIN
WIRESUP
WORKSAT
WORKSHY
WORKSIN
WORKSON
WORKSUP
XEROSES
XEROSIS
ZEROSIN
ZEROSUM

••R••S•

ABREAST
AERIEST
AIRBASE
AIRHOSE
AIRIEST
AIRKISS
AIRLESS
AIRMASS
AIRNESS
BARLESS
BERNESE
BURGESS
BURMESE
BURNISH
CARCASS
CARLESS
CAROUSE
CARWASH
CIRCUSY
CORNISH
CURIOSA
CURRISH
CURTEST
CURTISS
DARIUSI
DARKEST
DARKISH
DERVISH
EARLESS
EARNEST
EERIEST
FAREAST
FARNESS
FAROESE
FARWEST
FIRMEST
FORBUSH
FORMOSA
FORREST
FURBISH
FURIOSO
FURLESS
FURNESS
FURNISH
GARNISH
GIRLISH
GORIEST
HARDEST
HARDISH
HARNESS
HARPIST
HARVEST
HERMOSA
HERMOSO
HEROISM
HORNISH
HORNIST
JARLESS
KERTESZ
KURDISH
LARGESS
LARGEST
LARGISH
LARKISH
LARUSSA
MARCUSE
MARXISM
MARXIST
MIRIEST
MORTISE
MURKISH
NERDISH
NERISSA
NORRISH
OARLESS
OGREISH
PARRISH
PERCUSS
PERFUSE
PERISSA
PERKISH
PERSIST
PERTEST
PORKISH
PURPOSE
RERAISE
RERINSE
SARCASM
SERIESE
SERIESF
SERIESG
SERIESH
SERIESI
SERIESJ
SERIESK
SPRIEST
SPRYEST
STRASSE
STRAUSS
STROUSE
SURMISE
SURPASS
TARNISH
TARTEST
TARTISH
TERSEST
TORYISH
TORYISM
TURKISH
UPRAISE
UPROUSE
VARNISH
VERBOSE
VERIEST
WARIEST
WARLESS
WARMEST
WARMISH
WIRIEST
WORMISH
XERXESI
YERKISH

YORKIST

••R•••S

ABRADES
ABRAXAS
ABRILES
ADRATES
AERATES
AERIALS
AEROBES
AFRAMES
AGREERS
AIRACES
AIRBAGS
AIRDAMS
AIRGUNS
AIRINGS
AIRKISS
AIRLESS
AIRLOGS
AIRMASS
AIRNESS
AIRPOPS
AIRPOTS
AIRSACS
AIRWARS
AIRWAYS
AMRITAS
APROPOS
ARRACKS
ARRASES
ARREARS
ARRESTS
ARRISES
ARRIVES
ARROYOS
ATRIUMS
ATROPOS
AURISTS
AURORAS
BARACUS
BARBERS
BARBETS
BARBIES
BARCARS
BAREGES
BARENTS
BARGERS
BARHOPS
BARITES
BARKERS
BARLESS
BARLEYS
BARNEYS
BARNUMS
BAROLOS
BARQUES
BARRELS
BARRENS
BARRETS
BARRIOS
BARRONS
BARROWS
BARTABS
BARTERS
BARTLES
BARYONS
BERATES
BERBERS
BERGIUS
BERNAYS
BERRIES
BERTHAS
BIRCHES
BIRDERS
BIRDIES
BIREMES
BIRLERS
BIRMANS
BORATES
BORDERS
BORGIAS
BORIDES
BORINGS
BORROWS
BORZOIS
BURBLES
BURBOTS
BURDENS
BUREAUS
BURGEES
BURGERS
BURGESS
BURGLES
BURGOOS
BURIALS
BURIERS
BURLAPS
BURLERS
BURMANS
BURNERS
BUROAKS
BURROWS
BURSARS
BYROADS
CARACAS
CARAFES
CARBONS
CARBOYS
CARBRAS
CARCASS
CARDERS
CAREENS
CAREERS
CARFULS
CARGOES
CARHOPS
CARIBES
CARINAS
CARIOUS
CARKEYS
CARLESS
CARLOTS
CARNETS
CARNIES
CARPALS
CARPELS
CARPERS
CARPETS
CARPOUS
CARRELS
CARRIES
CARROTS
CARTELS
CARTERS
CARTONS
CARTOPS
CARVELS
CARVERS
CDRACKS
CDRATES
CERATES
CEREALS
CERISES
CERVIDS
CHRISMS
CHROMES
CIRCLES
CIRQUES
CORBELS
CORDERS
CORDIAS
CORDONS
CORFAMS
CORKERS
CORNEAS
CORNERS
CORNETS
CORONAS
CORPSES
CORRALS
CORSETS
CORVEES
CORVIDS
CORYZAS
CURARES
CURATES
CURDLES
CURFEWS
CURIOUS
CURLERS
CURLEWS
CURRIES
CURSERS
CURSORS
CURTISS
CURVETS
DARKENS
DARKLES
DARNERS
DARTERS
DARTLES
DERAILS
DERATES
DERBIES
DERIDES
DERIVES
DERUSTS
DIRECTS
DIRHAMS
DIRNDLS
DIRTIES
DORITOS
DORMERS
DORSALS
DORSEYS
EARBUDS
EARFULS
EARLAPS
EARLESS
EARLETS
EARLIES
EARNERS
EARTABS
EARTAGS
EARWIGS
ENRAGES
ENRANKS
ENROBES
ENROLLS
ENROOTS
ERRANDS
EUREKAS
FARFELS
FARINAS
FARMERS
FARNESS
FARROWS
FERMATS
FERRETS
FERRIES
FERROUS
FERULES
FERVORS
FIRINGS
FIRKINS
FORAGES
FORBIDS
FORCEPS
FORCERS
FORDGTS
FORDOES
FORESTS
FORGERS
FORGETS
FORGOES
FORINTS
FORKERS
FORMALS
FORMATS
FORMERS
FORTIES
FORTIUS
FURIOUS
FURLERS
FURLESS
FURNESS
FURORES
FURROWS
GARAGES
GARBLES
GARCONS
GARDENS
GARGLES
GARLICS
GARLITS
GARNERS
GARNETS
GARRETS
GARTERS
GERBILS
GERENTS
GERMANS
GERUNDS
GERVAIS
GIRDERS
GIRDLES
GIRLIES
GORDIUS
GORGERS
GORGONS
GURGLES
GURKHAS
GURNEYS
GYRATES
GYRENES
HARBORS
HARDEES
HARDENS
HARHARS
HARKENS
HARLEYS
HARLOTS
HARMERS
HARNESS
HARPERS
HARPIES
HARRAHS
HARRIES
HARRODS
HARROWS
HERALDS
HERBALS
HERDERS
HERMANS
HERMITS
HERNIAS
HERNIBS
HEROICS
HORNETS
HORRORS
HURDLES
HURLERS
HURRAHS
HURRAYS
HURRIES
HURTERS
HURTLES
HYRACES
HYRAXES
INROADS
INRUINS
IRRUPTS
JARDINS
JARFULS
JARGONS
JARLESS
JERBOAS
JERGENS
JERKERS
JERKIES
JERKINS
JERSEYS
JURGENS
JURISTS
KARATES
KERNELS
KIRMANS
KOREANS
KORUNAS
KURILES
LARCHES
LARDERS
LARDONS
LAREDOS
LARGESS
LARIATS
LARKERS
LARKINS
LARRUPS
LORISES
LORRIES
LORUSES
LURCHES
LUREXES
LURKERS
LYRISTS
MARACAS
MARAUDS
MARBLES
MARCELS
MARCHES
MARGINS
MARHAUS
MARIDAS
MARIDOS
MARINAS
MARINES
MARKERS
MARKETS
MARKUPS
MARLINS
MARMOTS
MAROONS
MARQUES
MARQUIS
MARRERS
MARRIES
MARRONS
MARROWS
MARSHES
MARTENS
MARTINS
MARTIUS
MARTYRS
MARVELS
MERCERS
MERCHES
MERCIES
MERGEES
MERGERS
MERINOS
MERLINS
MERLOTS
MIRADAS
MIRAGES
MIRRORS
MORALES
MORANIS
MOREENS
MORELOS
MORGANS
MORGUES
MORMONS
MORROWS
MORSELS
MORTALS
MORTARS
MORTONS
MURANOS
MURDERS
MURIELS
MURMURS
MURPHYS
MYRIADS
MYRTLES
NARROWS
NEREIDS
NERVOUS
NORDICS
NORITES
NORMALS
NORMANS
NORTONS
NURSERS
OARLESS
ONRAMPS
ORRISES
PARADES
PARAMUS
PARAPHS
PARATUS
PARCELS
PARCHES
PARDONS
PARENTS
PARFUMS
PARGERS
PARIAHS
PARIBUS
PARINGS
PARKERS
PARKINS
PARLAYS
PARLEYS
PARLORS
PARLOUS
PAROLES
PARRIES
PARROTS
PARSECS
PARSEES
PARSERS
PARSONS
PARTIES
PARURES
PERCHES
PERCUSS
PERHAPS
PERIODS
PERITUS
PERKINS
PERMITS
PERRINS
PERSEUS
PERSIUS
PERSONS
PERUKES
PERUSES
PHRASES
PIRAEUS
PIRATES
PORCHES
PORGIES
PORKERS
PORTALS
PORTERS
PORTHOS
PURFLES
PURISTS
PURPLES
PURRERS
PURSERS
PURSUES
PURVEYS
PYRAMUS
PYRITES
PYRRHUS
RAREGAS
RERACKS
RERAKES
RERANKS
RERATES
REREADS
REREDOS
REREELS
RERENTS
RERIDES
RERISES
REROLLS
REROOFS
REROOTS
SARONGS
SARTORS
SCRAPES
SCRAWLS
SCREAKS
SCREAMS
SCREEDS
SCREENS
SCRIBES
SCRIMPS
SCRIPPS
SCRIPTS
SCROLLS
SCRUFFS
SCRUGGS
SERAPES
SERAPHS
SERAPIS
SERIALS
SERIOUS
SERMONS
SERPENS
SERVEAS
SERVERS
SHRIEKS
SHRIKES
SHRILLS
SHRIMPS
SHRINES
SHRINKS
SHRIVES
SHROUDS
SORBETS
SORRELS
SORROWS
SORTERS
SORTIES
SPRAINS
SPRAWLS
SPREADS
SPRINGS
SPRINTS
SPRITES
SPROUTS
SPRUCES
STRAFES
STRAINS
STRAITS
STRANDS
STRATAS
STRATUS
STRAUSS
STREAKS
STREAMS
STREETS
STREGIS
STRIDES
STRIFES
STRIKES
STRINGS
STRIPES
STRIVES
STROBES
STROKES
STROLLS
SURFERS
SURIMIS
SURPASS
SURPLUS
SURREYS
SURVEYS
SYRIANS
TARGETS
TARIFFS
TARMACS
TAROILS
TARPITS
TARPONS
TARRIES
TARSALS
TARTANS
TARTARS
TARZANS
TERCELS
TERRANS
TERRETS
TERRIES
TERRORS
THRALLS
THREADS
THREATS
THREERS
THRIFTS
THRILLS
THRIVES
THROATS
THRONES
THRONGS
THRUSTS
TIRADES
TORCHES
TOREROS
TORINOS
TOROIDS
TORQUES
TURBANS
TURBOTS
TUREENS
TURKEYS
TURNERS
TURNIPS
TURNONS
TURNUPS
TURRETS
TURTLES
TVROOMS
TYRANTS
UNRACKS
UNREELS
UNRESTS
UNROBES
UNROLLS
UNROOFS
UNROOTS
UNROPES
UPRATES
UPREARS
UPRISES
UPROARS
UPROOTS
VARIERS
VARIOUS
VARLETS
VERBALS
VERBIDS
VERDINS
VERGERS
VERISTS
VERITAS
VERSETS
VIRAGOS
VIRGINS
VIRTUES
VIRUSES
WARBLES
WARDENS
WARDERS
WARGODS
WARLESS
WARMERS
WARMUPS
WARPERS
WARRENS
WARVETS
WIRINGS
WORKERS
WORKUPS
WORMERS
WORRIES
WORSENS
XEROSES
XEROSIS
XEROXES
YARDERS
YARROWS
YORKERS
YORKIES
ZIRCONS

•••RS••

APERSON
BEARSON
BEARSUP
BOURSES
COARSEN
COARSER
COURSED
COURSER
COURSES
DEARSIR
EMERSED
EMERSON
FAIRSEX
FAIRSUP
GEARSTO
GEARSUP
HEARSAY
HEARSES
HEARSOF
HOARSEN
HOARSER
IVERSON
JEERSAT
LEERSAT
MYERSON
OPQRSTU
OVERSAD
OVERSAW
OVERSEA
OVERSEE
OVERSET
OVERSEW
OVERSUP
PAIRSUP
PEARSON
PEERSAT
PEERSIN
POURSIN
REARSUP
ROARSAT
SOURSON
SPARSER
SPURSON
STARSIN
STARSKY
STIRSIN
STIRSUP
TEARSAT
TEARSIT
TEARSUP
THIRSTS
THIRSTY
THORSON
WEARSON

•••R•S•

ACEROSE
ACTRESS
ADDRESS
AGGRESS
ALLRISE
AMBROSE
AMORIST
AMOROSO
ANDRESS
APPRISE
ARMREST
ATCROSS
AWAREST
AXLROSE
BEARISH
BEDREST
BOARISH
BOORISH
BULRUSH
BUMRUSH
CHERISH
CHORIST
CLERISY
CUIRASS
CURRISH
CYPRESS
CZARISM
CZARIST
DEAREST
DEFROST
DEPRESS
DIARIST
DIGRESS
DOGROSE
DONRUSS
DOUREST
DRFRIST
EMPRESS
EMPRISE
ENCRUST
ENGROSS
ENPRISE
ENTRUST
EVEREST
EXPRESS
FAIREST
FAIRISH
FAIRUSE
FLORIST
FORREST
GOIRISH
HEIRESS
IMPRESS
IMPREST
INARUSH
INCRUST
INGRESS
INTRUST
IPCRESS
LEGREST
LOWRISE
LOWRISK
MADRUSH
MELROSE
METRIST
MIDRISE
MOORISH
NEAREST
NORRISH
NOURISH
OLDROSE
OLOROSO
OPEROSE
OPPRESS
OUTRUSH
OVERUSE
PARRISH
PEERESS
PENROSE
POOREST
POORISH
QUERIST
REARISE
REAROSE
REBRUSH
RECROSS
REDRESS
REDROSE
REFRESH
REGRASP
REGRESS
REPRESS
REPRISE
SEERESS
SOUREST
SOURISH
SPAREST
SUBROSA
SUCRASE
SUCROSE
SUNRISE
TEAROSE
THERESA
THEROSE
TIGRESS
TOURISM
TOURIST
TSARISM
TSARIST
UNCROSS
UNDRESS
UNFROST
UNGROSS
UNTRUSS
VINROSE
ZEBRASS

•••R••S

ACARIDS
ACCRUES
ACTRESS
ADDRESS
ADORERS
AFFRAYS
AGARICS
AGGRESS
AIGRETS
ALARBUS
ALARUMS
AMBRIES
AMERCES
AMOROUS
AMTRACS
ANARCHS
ANDREAS
ANDRESS
ANDREWS
ANDROUS
ANORAKS
APERCUS
APERIES
ASHRAMS
ATCROSS
ATTRITS
AVERNUS
BADRAPS
BARRELS
BARRENS
BARRETS
BARRIOS
BARRONS
BARROWS
BAYRUMS
BBQRIBS
BEARERS
BEHRENS
BERRIES
BETRAYS
BEURRES
BIGRIGS
BORROWS
BOTREES
BOURSES
BUMRAPS
BURROWS
CABRIOS

CARRELS	ESTRAYS	LABRATS	RAGRUGS	TERRETS	MRHORSE	CETERIS	GENERIS	OSETRAS	SEFERIS	•••••RS	BEATERS	BURGERS
CARRIES	EVERLYS	LAERTES	RAMRODS	TERRIES	NOPQRST	CHAKRAS	GOCARTS	OXCARTS	SENORAS	ABASERS	BEAVERS	BURIERS
CARROTS	EWERIES	LARRUPS	REARERS	TERRORS	NOWORSE	CHARROS	GOGIRLS	OXFORDS	SENORES	ABATERS	BEEMERS	BURLERS
CATRIGS	EXARCHS	LAURELS	REBREWS	TETRADS	OBVERSE	CHEVRES	GOKARTS	PAPYRUS	SENTRAS	ABATORS	BEEPERS	BURNERS
CHARGES	EXPRESS	LEERERS	RECROSS	THERAMS	ONFIRST	CHURROS	GOVERNS	PARURES	SEPIRAS	ABIDERS	BEEZERS	BURSARS
CHARLES	FABRICS	LIBRANS	REDRAGS	THEREDS	REMORSE	COHERES	GRIGRIS	PETARDS	SEVERUS	ABUSERS	BEGGARS	BUSHERS
CHARROS	FAERIES	LORRIES	REDRAWS	THERMOS	REVERSA	COHORTS	HAZARDS	PGAPROS	SEWARDS	ADORERS	BELAIRS	BUSKERS
CHERUBS	FAEROES	LOURDES	REDRESS	THIRSTS	REVERSE	COMOROS	HEGIRAS	PICARAS	SIERRAS	AFFAIRS	BELIERS	BUSSERS
CHORALS	FAIRIES	MACRONS	REDRIES	TIERCES	TOHORSE	CONTRAS	HIGHRES	PICAROS	SOFARAS	AGREERS	BELTERS	BUSTERS
CHURROS	FARROWS	MARRERS	REFRIES	TIERODS	UNBURST	CONURES	HOMBRES	PIETROS	SOLARAS	AIRWARS	BENDERS	BUTLERS
CHYRONS	FEARERS	MARRIES	REGRABS	TIGRESS	UNHARSH	COVERTS	HOWARDS	POIVRES	SPHERES	ALEGARS	BERBERS	BUTTERS
CITRONS	FERRETS	MARRONS	REGRESS	TOPROWS	UNHORSE	COWARDS	HUMERUS	POLARAS	SQUARES	ALGIERS	BESTIRS	BUZZERS
CITROUS	FERRIES	MARROWS	REGRETS	TOURBUS	UNTERSE	CUATROS	ICTERUS	POLARIS	SQUIRES	ALINERS	BETTERS	CABLERS
CLARETS	FERROUS	MATRONS	REGRIPS	TOURERS	UPBURST	CURARES	IDCARDS	POUDRES	SQUIRMS	ALLEARS	BETTORS	CADGERS
CLERICS	FIBRINS	MAUROIS	REGROWS	TSTRAPS	UPFIRST	CYBORGS	IGNORES	PREARMS	SQUIRTS	AMBLERS	BEZIERS	CAESARS
CLORETS	FIBROUS	MEGRIMS	REPRESS	TUGRIKS		DEBARKS	IMMURES	PRFIRMS	STBARTS	AMUSERS	BIBBERS	CAHIERS
COERCES	FLORETS	METRICS	RETRAPS	TURRETS	••••R•S	DEBURRS	IMPARTS	QATARIS	STEARNS	ANCHORS	BICKERS	CALDERS
CORRALS	FLORINS	MICRONS	RETRIES	TVCREWS	ABJURES	DEFORMS	IMPORTS	QUATRES	STMARKS	ANGLERS	BIDDERS	CALKERS
COURSES	FLYRODS	MIDRIBS	RETRIMS	UNCROSS	ABSORBS	DEGERMS	INFORMS	QUEIROS	STMARYS	ANKLERS	BIGCARS	CALLERS
COWRIES	FOURTHS	MIRRORS	REURGES	UNDRAWS	ACCORDS	DEHIRES	INHERES	RASURES	SUBARUS	ANSWERS	BIGEARS	CAMBERS
CSARDAS	FUNRUNS	MONROES	REWRAPS	UNDRESS	ADHERES	DEHORNS	INJURES	REBORES	SUBORNS	ANTHERS	BIGGERS	CAMPERS
CUIRASS	FURROWS	MORROWS	RICRACS	UNFREES	ADJURES	DELORIS	INNARDS	RECORDS	SUBURBS	ANTLERS	BILKERS	CANCERS
CUPROUS	GARRETS	MOTRINS	RIPRAPS	UNGRIPS	ADMIRES	DEMARKS	INSERTS	RECORKS	SUPERGS	APPEARS	BILLERS	CANKERS
CURRIES	GEORGES	NARROWS	ROARERS	UNGROSS	ADSORBS	DEPARTS	INSURES	RECURES	SUTURES	ARBOURS	BINDERS	CANNERS
CYMRICS	GFORCES	NEURONS	ROBROYS	UNTRAPS	ADVERBS	DEPORTS	INTERNS	RECURLS	TABARDS	ARCHERS	BINGERS	CANOERS
CYPRESS	GIORGOS	NEXRADS	RUBRICS	UNTRUSS	ADVERTS	DESERTS	INTURNS	REDARES	TAVERNS	ARDOURS	BIRDERS	CANTERS
CZARDAS	GLORIAS	NIMRODS	RUGRATS	UNWRAPS	AFFIRMS	DESIRES	INVERTS	REDARNS	TEATROS	ARGUERS	BIRLERS	CANTORS
DACRONS	GLORIES	NITROUS	SATRAPS	UPDRIES	AFFORDS	DEVORES	INWARDS	REEARNS	TEAURNS	ARMOURS	BITTERS	CAPPERS
DAIRIES	GLURGES	NUTRIAS	SCARABS	UPGROWS	ALLURES	DEWIRES	ITGIRLS	REFIRES	TENURES	ARREARS	BLADERS	CAPTORS
DATRILS	GOURDES	OCHROUS	SCARERS	UPPROPS	AMNERIS	DEWORMS	JOGBRAS	REFORMS	THEARTS	ARTCARS	BLAMERS	CARDERS
DEARIES	GYMRATS	OCTROIS	SCARVES	USERIDS	AMPERES	DISARMS	KAKUROS	REGARDS	THWARTS	ARTHURS	BLAZERS	CAREERS
DEARTHS	HADRONS	ODOROUS	SCORERS	USURERS	ANGORAS	DISTROS	KIDSRUS	REGIRDS	TIMBRES	ASHLARS	BLOWERS	CARPERS
DECREES	HAIRDOS	OILRIGS	SCORIAS	USURIES	ANITRAS	DIVERTS	LAPERMS	REHIRES	TINORES	ATONERS	BOATERS	CARTERS
DECRIES	HARRAHS	OILRUBS	SCURVES	VEERIES	ANTARES	DOLORES	LAVORIS	REMARKS	TOREROS	AUPAIRS	BOBBERS	CARVERS
DEFRAGS	HARRIES	ONEROUS	SEARERS	VIERNES	ANTERUS	DOTARDS	LAZARUS	REMORAS	TOWARDS	AUSTERS	BOILERS	CASTERS
DEFRAYS	HARRODS	OPPRESS	SECRETS	VITRICS	ASFARAS	EDWARDS	LETTRES	REPARKS	TOYSRUS	AUTEURS	BOLTERS	CAUSERS
DEGREES	HARROWS	OSPREYS	SEERESS	WARRENS	ASPIRES	EFFORTS	LINDROS	REPERKS	TSHIRTS	AUTHORS	BOMBERS	CAVIARS
DELRAYS	HATREDS	OTARIES	SHARERS	WEARERS	ASSERTS	EMBARKS	LIPARIS	REPORTS	TSOURIS	AVATARS	BONDERS	CELLARS
DEPRESS	HEARERS	OUTRAPS	SHERIFS	WEARIES	ASSORTS	EMIGRES	LIZARDS	RESORBS	TUNDRAS	AVOWERS	BONKERS	CENSERS
DEVRIES	HEARSES	OUTRIBS	SHERPAS	WEIRDOS	ASSURES	EMPIRES	LLADROS	RESORTS	UMPIRES	AWAKERS	BOOKERS	CENSORS
DHARMAS	HEARTHS	OUTRIGS	SIERRAS	WETRAGS	ATTIRES	ENCORES	LONDRES	RETARDS	UNBARES	BACKERS	BOOMERS	CENTERS
DIARIES	HEBREWS	OUTROWS	SKIRUNS	WHARVES	AUBURNS	ENDURES	LOUVRES	RETIRES	UNCORES	BADGERS	BOOTERS	CHAFERS
DIARIOS	HEIRESS	OUTRUNS	SNARERS	WHEREAS	AURORAS	ENDUROS	LUSTRES	RETORTS	UNCORKS	BAFFERS	BOOZERS	CHASERS
DIGRAMS	HENRIES	OVARIES	SNORERS	WORRIES	BEGIRDS	ENGIRDS	MADUROS	RETURFS	UNCURBS	BAGGERS	BOPPERS	CHEDERS
DIGRESS	HOORAHS	PAIRERS	SOARERS	XTERRAS	BELARUS	ENSURES	MAHARIS	RETURNS	UNCURLS	BAILERS	BORDERS	CHEWERS
DOGRUNS	HOORAYS	PARRIES	SOIREES	YARROWS	BEMIRES	ENTIRES	MAITRES	REVERBS	UNFORKS	BAILORS	BOTHERS	CHIDERS
DONRUSS	HORRORS	PARROTS	SORRELS	YTTRIAS	BENARES	ENVIROS	MANTRAS	REVERES	UNFURLS	BAITERS	BOWLERS	CHIMERS
DOWRIES	HOTRODS	PATRIES	SORROWS	ZEBRASS	BEURRES	ESCARPS	MANURES	REVERTS	UNGIRDS	BALKERS	BOWOARS	CHOKERS
DRYROTS	HURRAHS	PATROLS	SOURCES		BEWARES	ESCORTS	MATURES	REWARDS	UNHIRES	BANDERS	BOWYERS	CHOLERS
DRYRUNS	HURRAYS	PATRONS	SPARERS	••••RS•	BICARBS	EUCHRES	MILORDS	REWARMS	UNSORTS	BANGERS	BOXCARS	CINDERS
DWARVES	HURRIES	PEERESS	SPIRALS	ACCURST	BICORNS	EXHORTS	MITHRAS	REWARNS	UPCARDS	BANKERS	BRACERS	CIPHERS
ECARTES	HYBRIDS	PERRINS	SPIREAS	ADVERSE	BISTROS	EXPERTS	MODERNS	REWIRES	UPCURLS	BANNERS	BRAYERS	CLAMORS
EGERIAS	HYDROUS	PETRATS	SPIRITS	AMHERST	BOGARTS	EXPIRES	MRBURNS	REWORDS	UPDARTS	BANTERS	BREWERS	CLAWERS
EMBRUES	IATRICS	PETRELS	STARERS	ASPERSE	BOLEROS	EXPORTS	MRWORDS	REWORKS	UPGIRDS	BARBERS	BREYERS	CLONERS
EMBRYOS	ICERUNS	PETROLS	STARVES	ATFIRST	BOUTROS	EXSERTS	MUJERES	REZEROS	UPTURNS	BARCARS	BRIBERS	CLOSERS
EMERGES	IDAREDS	PETROUS	STEREOS	ATHIRST	BRIARDS	EXTERNS	NATURES	RITARDS	UPWARDS	BARGERS	BRINERS	CLOVERS
EMERIES	IGOROTS	PIERCES	STERNOS	ATWORST	BYFORMS	EXTORTS	NOCARBS	ROBARDS	UQUARKS	BARKERS	BROKERS	COALERS
EMPRESS	IMARETS	PITROWS	STEROLS	BAKERST	BYTURNS	EXWORKS	NOMBRES	ROBERTS	VECTRAS	BARTERS	BUCKERS	COATERS
ENDRUNS	IMBRUES	PLURALS	STORERS	DIVERSE	BYWORDS	FABARES	NONARTS	RVPARKS	VELCROS	BASHERS	BUDDERS	COAXERS
ENGRAMS	IMPRESS	POURERS	STORIES	ENDORSE	CAMAROS	FEDORAS	NONPROS	SAFARIS	VELURES	BASTERS	BUDGERS	COCKERS
ENGROSS	INGRESS	PTEROUS	STURGES	EXCURSE	CAMERAS	FEMORIS	NOTURNS	SAMARAS	VENTRIS	BATHERS	BUFFERS	CODGERS
ENTRAPS	INIRONS	PURRERS	SUNRAYS	GOFIRST	CANARDS	FIACRES	NUBIRAS	SAMPRAS	VIHARAS	BATTERS	BUGLERS	COFFERS
ENTREES	INTRAYS	PYRRHUS	SURREYS	IMMERSE	CARBRAS	FIGURES	NUMEROS	SATIRES	VITARAS	BAWLERS	BULGARS	COHEIRS
ENTRIES	IPCRESS	QUARLES	SWERVES	INDORSE	CASERNS	FOUDRES	OBVERTS	SATORIS	WHWORDS	BAZAARS	BULGURS	COILERS
ENWRAPS	IVORIES	QUARTES	TARRIES	INFIRST	CATERAS	FURORES	OEUVRES	SATURNS	WIZARDS	BEADERS	BUMMERS	COINERS
EPARCHS	JEERERS	QUARTOS	TEARERS	INTERSE	CAVERNS	FUTURAS	OFSORTS	SCLERAS	WYVERNS	BEAKERS	BUMPERS	COLLARS
ESCROWS	JOURNOS	QUERIES	TEARGAS	INVERSE	CAVORTS	FUTURES	OLDPROS	SEAARMS	XTERRAS	BEAMERS	BUNKERS	COLOURS
ESPRITS	KIARIOS	QUORUMS	TERRANS	MEFIRST	CENTRES	GABBROS	ONWARDS	SECURES	YOGURTS	BEARERS	BUNTERS	COMBERS

CONCURS	DIFFERS	FATHERS	GATHERS	HEDGERS	JITTERS	LITTERS	MOBBERS	PAIRERS	PREFERS	RETEARS	SEEKERS	SPYDERS
CONDORS	DIGGERS	FAVOURS	GAUGERS	HEEDERS	JOBBERS	LOADERS	MOCKERS	PALLORS	PRETORS	RETOURS	SEINERS	SQUEERS
CONFERS	DIMMERS	FAWNERS	GAWKERS	HEELERS	JOBJARS	LOAFERS	MOHAIRS	PALMERS	PREYERS	REUNERS	SEIZERS	STAGERS
CONGERS	DINGERS	FEARERS	GAWPERS	HEFTERS	JOGGERS	LOANERS	MOILERS	PALTERS	PRICERS	REUSERS	SEIZORS	STARERS
CONKERS	DINNERS	FEDDERS	GEEZERS	HEIFERS	JOINERS	LOBBERS	MOLDERS	PAMPERS	PRIMERS	REUTERS	SELLERS	STATERS
CONNORS	DIPPERS	FEEDERS	GENDERS	HELPERS	JOLTERS	LOCKERS	MOLTERS	PANDERS	PROBERS	REWEARS	SENDERS	STATORS
COOKERS	DISBARS	FEELERS	GENXERS	HEMMERS	JOSHERS	LODGERS	MONGERS	PANIERS	PROSERS	RHETORS	SENIORS	STAYERS
COOLERS	DISEURS	FELLERS	GETTERS	HERDERS	JOTTERS	LOFTERS	MOONERS	PANNERS	PROVERS	RHYMERS	SENSORS	STEWERS
COOPERS	DITHERS	FENCERS	GEYSERS	HINDERS	JUDGERS	LOGGERS	MOOTERS	PANTERS	PRUNERS	RIBBERS	SERVERS	STOKERS
COOTERS	DOCKERS	FENDERS	GIBBERS	HINTERS	JUICERS	LOITERS	MOPPERS	PANZERS	PSYWARS	RIDDERS	SETTERS	STONERS
COPCARS	DOCTORS	FERVORS	GILDERS	HISSERS	JUMPERS	LOLLERS	MORTARS	PAPIERS	PUCKERS	RIFLERS	SHADERS	STORERS
COPIERS	DODDERS	FESTERS	GINGERS	HITTERS	JUNIORS	LOOKERS	MOSHERS	PARGERS	PUFFERS	RIGGERS	SHAKERS	STOWERS
COPPERS	DODGERS	FETTERS	GIRDERS	HOAXERS	JUNKERS	LOOPERS	MOTHERS	PARKERS	PULLERS	RIGOURS	SHAPERS	STUPORS
COPTERS	DOFFERS	FIBBERS	GLAMORS	HOCKERS	KAISERS	LOOTERS	MOUSERS	PARLORS	PULPERS	RINGERS	SHARERS	STYLERS
CORDERS	DOGEARS	FIGBARS	GLAZERS	HOHNERS	KEDGERS	LOPPERS	MSIEURS	PARSERS	PULSARS	RINSERS	SHAVERS	SUBWARS
CORKERS	DOLLARS	FILLERS	GLIDERS	HOLDERS	KEENERS	LOTTERS	MUCKERS	PASSERS	PUMPERS	RIOTERS	SHINERS	SUCCORS
CORNERS	DOLOURS	FILTERS	GLOWERS	HOLLERS	KEEPERS	LOUVERS	MUDDERS	PASTERS	PUNKERS	RIPPERS	SHIVERS	SUCKERS
COSHERS	DOOVERS	FINDERS	GNAWERS	HONKERS	KEGGERS	LUBBERS	MUGGERS	PASTORS	PUNNERS	RISKERS	SHOFARS	SUDSERS
COSTARS	DOOZERS	FINGERS	GOITERS	HONOURS	KEGLERS	LUGGERS	MULLERS	PATTERS	PUNTERS	ROADERS	SHOVERS	SUFFERS
COTTERS	DORMERS	FISHERS	GOLFERS	HOOFERS	KICKERS	LULLERS	MUMMERS	PATZERS	PURRERS	ROAMERS	SHOWERS	SUITORS
COUGARS	DOTTERS	FITTERS	GOMPERS	HOOPERS	KIDDERS	LUMBARS	MURDERS	PAUPERS	PURSERS	ROARERS	SIDDURS	SULKERS
COUTERS	DOUSERS	FIZZERS	GOOBERS	HOOTERS	KILLERS	LUMBERS	MURMURS	PAUSERS	PUSHERS	ROBBERS	SIFTERS	SUMMERS
CRATERS	DOWNERS	FLAKERS	GOODERS	HOOVERS	KIPPERS	LUMPERS	MUSHERS	PAVIORS	PUTTERS	ROCKERS	SIGHERS	SUNDERS
CRAVERS	DOWSERS	FLAMERS	GOPHERS	HOPPERS	KISSERS	LUNGERS	MUSTERS	PAWNERS	QINTARS	RODGERS	SIGNERS	SUPPERS
CROWERS	DRAPERS	FLAVORS	GORGERS	HORRORS	KNIFERS	LUNKERS	MUTTERS	PCUSERS	QUAKERS	ROLFERS	SIGNORS	SURFERS
CULLERS	DRAWERS	FLAYERS	GOUGERS	HOSIERS	KNOWERS	LURKERS	MYSTARS	PEEKERS	QUASARS	ROLLERS	SILVERS	SWAYERS
CUMBERS	DRIVERS	FLEXORS	GRADERS	HOTCARS	KOSHERS	LUSTERS	NABBERS	PEELERS	QUAVERS	ROMPERS	SIMMERS	SWIPERS
CURLERS	DRONERS	FLOWERS	GRATERS	HOTWARS	LABOURS	MADDERS	NAGGERS	PEEPERS	QUEUERS	ROOFERS	SIMPERS	TACKERS
CURSERS	DROVERS	FLUTERS	GRAVERS	HOWLERS	LADDERS	MAGYARS	NAILERS	PELTERS	QUIVERS	ROOMERS	SINGERS	TAGGERS
CURSORS	DRYPERS	FOAMERS	GRAZERS	HUGGERS	LADLERS	MAHZORS	NAPIERS	PENNERS	QUOTERS	ROOTERS	SINKERS	TAILERS
CUSSERS	DUBBERS	FODDERS	GRIPERS	HULLERS	LAGGERS	MAILERS	NAPPERS	PEPPERS	RACKERS	ROSTERS	SINNERS	TAILORS
CUSTERS	DUCKERS	FOGGERS	GROCERS	HUMMERS	LANCERS	MAIMERS	NATTERS	PESTERS	RAFTERS	ROTTERS	SIPPERS	TALKERS
CUTLERS	DUELERS	FOKKERS	GROPERS	HUMOURS	LANDERS	MAINERS	NECKERS	PETTERS	RAIDERS	ROUSERS	SISTERS	TAMPERS
CUTTERS	DUFFERS	FOLDERS	GROVERS	HUNGERS	LAPPERS	MANGERS	NECTARS	PEWTERS	RAILERS	ROUTERS	SITTERS	TANKERS
CYCLERS	DUMPERS	FOLGERS	GROWERS	HUNKERS	LAPSERS	MANNERS	NEEDERS	PHASERS	RAISERS	RUBBERS	SKATERS	TANNERS
CYPHERS	DUNKERS	FOOLERS	GUIDERS	HUNTERS	LARDERS	MAPPERS	NESTERS	PHONERS	RAMMERS	RUDDERS	SKEWERS	TAPPERS
DABBERS	DUNNERS	FOOTERS	GUITARS	HURLERS	LARKERS	MARKERS	NESTORS	PICKERS	RANCORS	RUINERS	SLAKERS	TARTARS
DAGGERS	DUSTERS	FORCERS	GULPERS	HURTERS	LASCARS	MARRERS	NETTERS	PIECERS	RANGERS	RUMMERS	SLATERS	TASTERS
DAMMERS	EARNERS	FORGERS	GUNNERS	HUSKERS	LASHERS	MARTYRS	NEUTERS	PILFERS	RANKERS	RUMOURS	SLAVERS	TATTERS
DAMNERS	EASTERS	FORKERS	GUSHERS	HUSSARS	LATHERS	MASHERS	NEWCARS	PILLARS	RANTERS	RUNNERS	SLAYERS	TAYLORS
DAMPERS	EBAYERS	FORMERS	GUTTERS	IMAGERS	LAUDERS	MASKERS	NICKERS	PINCERS	RAPIERS	RUSHERS	SLICERS	TEARERS
DANCERS	ECHOERS	FOSTERS	GUVNORS	IMPAIRS	LAWYERS	MASTERS	NIPPERS	PINGERS	RAPPERS	RUTGERS	SLIDERS	TEASERS
DANDERS	ECLAIRS	FOWLERS	GYPPERS	IMYOURS	LEADERS	MATHERS	NODDERS	PINNERS	RAPTORS	RUTTERS	SLIVERS	TEENERS
DANGERS	EDITORS	FRAMERS	HACKERS	INCHERS	LEAKERS	MATTERS	NONPARS	PITIERS	RASHERS	SACKERS	SLOPERS	TEETERS
DANVERS	EGGLERS	FRATERS	HAILERS	INDOORS	LEANERS	MAULERS	NONWARS	PLACERS	RASPERS	SAILERS	SMILERS	TELLERS
DARNERS	ELATERS	FTMYERS	HALTERS	INPOURS	LEAPERS	MAUSERS	NOONERS	PLANERS	RASTERS	SAILORS	SMITERS	TEMPERS
DARTERS	ELIDERS	FUDGERS	HALVERS	INTEARS	LEASERS	MEETERS	NOOSERS	PLATERS	RATTERS	SALTERS	SMOKERS	TENDERS
DASHERS	ELIXIRS	FUELERS	HAMMERS	INYEARS	LECHERS	MELDERS	NOSHERS	PLAYERS	RAWBARS	SALVERS	SNAKERS	TENNERS
DAUBERS	ELOPERS	FULMARS	HAMPERS	IRONERS	LECTORS	MELTERS	NOSTARS	PLEXORS	READERS	SALVORS	SNARERS	TENSORS
DEALERS	ELUDERS	FUNDERS	HANDERS	ISOBARS	LEDGERS	MEMBERS	NUBBERS	PLOVERS	REAMERS	SANDERS	SNIPERS	TENTERS
DEBEERS	EMOTERS	FUNFURS	HANGARS	ISOMERS	LEERERS	MEMOIRS	NUDGERS	PLOWERS	REAPERS	SAPPERS	SNORERS	TERRORS
DEBLURS	ENAMORS	FURLERS	HANGERS	ISSUERS	LENDERS	MENDERS	NUMBERS	POISERS	REARERS	SARTORS	SOAKERS	TESTERS
DEBTORS	ENDEARS	FUSSERS	HANKERS	JABBERS	LESSORS	MENTORS	NURSERS	POLLERS	REAVERS	SASSERS	SOAPERS	TETHERS
DEBURRS	ENVIERS	GABBERS	HARBORS	JAEGERS	LETTERS	MEOWERS	NUTTERS	PONDERS	RECTORS	SAUCERS	SOARERS	THALERS
DECKERS	ERASERS	GADDERS	HARHARS	JAGUARS	LEVIERS	MERCERS	OBEYERS	POOLERS	REDFIRS	SAVIORS	SOBBERS	THAWERS
DEFIERS	ERODERS	GAFFERS	HARMERS	JAILERS	LIBBERS	MERGERS	OCULARS	POPLARS	REEFERS	SAVOURS	SOLDERS	THECARS
DEHAIRS	ESCHERS	GAGGERS	HARPERS	JAILORS	LICKERS	METEORS	OINKERS	POPPERS	REEKERS	SAWYERS	SOLVERS	THREERS
DEICERS	ETCHERS	GAINERS	HATTERS	JAMMERS	LIENORS	METIERS	OLDCARS	PORKERS	REELERS	SCALARS	SOONERS	TICKERS
DELVERS	EVADERS	GAITERS	HAULERS	JASPERS	LIFTERS	MEWLERS	ONAGERS	PORTERS	REGEARS	SCALERS	SORTERS	TIEBARS
DENIERS	EVENERS	GAMMERS	HAWKERS	JAZZERS	LIMBERS	MILKERS	OPENERS	POSEURS	REHEARS	SCARERS	SOUPERS	TILLERS
DEODARS	EVOKERS	GANDERS	HAWSERS	JEEPERS	LIMNERS	MILLERS	OPINERS	POSTERS	RELIERS	SCORERS	SPACERS	TILTERS
DETOURS	EXILERS	GANGERS	HEADERS	JEERERS	LINGERS	MINCERS	ORATORS	POTHERS	RENDERS	SCOTERS	SPADERS	TIMBERS
DEVOIRS	FABLERS	GAOLERS	HEALERS	JEFFERS	LINKERS	MINDERS	OSTLERS	POTTERS	RENOIRS	SEALERS	SPARERS	TINDERS
DEVOURS	FACTORS	GARNERS	HEAPERS	JERKERS	LINTERS	MINTERS	OUSTERS	POURERS	RENTERS	SEAMERS	SPAYERS	TINEARS
DIALERS	FALLERS	GARTERS	HEARERS	JESTERS	LIPPERS	MIRRORS	OUTWARS	POUTERS	REPAIRS	SEARERS	SPEWERS	TINKERS
DIAPERS	FALTERS	GASPERS	HEATERS	JIGGERS	LIQUORS	MISTERS	OYSTERS	POWDERS	REPOURS	SEATERS	SPICERS	TINNERS
DICKERS	FANNERS	GASSERS	HEAVERS	JILTERS	LISPERS	MNOPQRS	PACKERS	PRATERS	RESTERS	SECTORS	SPIDERS	TINTERS
DIETERS	FARMERS	GASWARS	HECTORS	JINXERS	LISTERS	MOANERS	PADDERS	PRAYERS	RESTIRS	SEEDERS	SPIKERS	TIPJARS

TIPPERS
TITHERS
TITTERS
TOILERS
TOLLERS
TOOLERS
TOOTERS
TOPPERS
TOSSERS
TOTTERS
TOURERS
TOUTERS
TOWBARS
TOWCARS
TOWNERS
TOYCARS
TRACERS
TRADERS
TRAVERS
TREMORS
TUCKERS
TUGGERS
TURNERS
TUSKERS
TVSTARS
TWINERS
TWOFERS
ULSTERS
UNDOERS
UNHAIRS
UNITERS
UNMOORS
UNTIERS
UPBEARS
UPREARS
UPROARS
UPSOARS
UPSTIRS
UPTEARS
USURERS
VALOURS
VALUERS
VAMPERS
VAPOURS
VARIERS
VEADARS
VECTORS
VEILERS
VELOURS
VENDERS
VENDORS
VENEERS
VENTERS
VERGERS
VESPERS
VETOERS
VETTERS
VICKERS
VICTORS
VIEWERS
VIGOURS
VIZIERS
VOGUERS
VOICERS
VOIDERS
WADDERS
WAFTERS
WAGGERS

WAILERS
WAITERS
WAIVERS
WALKERS
WALTERS
WANDERS
WANTERS
WARDERS
WARMERS
WARPERS
WASHERS
WASTERS
WEANERS
WEARERS
WEAVERS
WEDDERS
WEEDERS
WEEPERS
WELDERS
WELTERS
WENDERS
WESTERS
WETBARS
WHALERS
WHINERS
WICKERS
WIENERS
WILLERS
WINCERS
WINDERS
WINGERS
WINKERS
WINNERS
WINTERS
WISHERS
WITHERS
WONDERS
WOOFERS
WORKERS
WORMERS
WRITERS
XYSTERS
YAKKERS
YAMMERS
YANKERS
YAPPERS
YARDERS
YATTERS
YAWNERS
YAWPERS
YELLERS
YELPERS
YONKERS
YORKERS
YOTHERS
YOWLERS
ZAPPERS
ZEPHYRS
ZESTERS
ZINGERS
ZIPPERS
ZITHERS

R•T••••

RATABLE
RATAFIA
RATATAT
RATBERT

RATCHET
RATECAP
RATEDPG
RATFINK
RATHOLE
RATINES
RATINGS
RATIONS
RATITES
RATLIKE
RATLINE
RATLINS
RATPACK
RATRACE
RATSOUT
RATTAIL
RATTANS
RATTERS
RATTIER
RATTING
RATTISH
RATTLED
RATTLER
RATTLES
RATTRAP
RETABLE
RETACKS
RETAILS
RETAINS
RETAKEN
RETAKER
RETAKES
RETALLY
RETAMED
RETAMES
RETAPED
RETAPES
RETARDS
RETASTE
RETAXED
RETAXES
RETEACH
RETEARS
RETELLS
RETESTS
RETHANK
RETHAWS
RETHINK
RETIARY
RETICLE
RETILED
RETILES
RETILLS
RETIMED
RETIMES
RETINAE
RETINAL
RETINAS
RETINGE
RETINOL
RETINTS
RETINUE
RETIRED
RETIREE
RETIRES
RETITLE
RETOAST
RETONED

RETONES
RETOOLS
RETORTS
RETOTAL
RETOUCH
RETOURS
RETOWED
RETRACE
RETRACK
RETRACT
RETRADE
RETRAIN
RETRAPS
RETREAD
RETREAT
RETRIAL
RETRIED
RETRIES
RETRIMS
RETSINA
RETTING
RETUNED
RETUNES
RETURFS
RETURNS
RETWINE
RETWIST
RETYPED
RETYPES
RITAGAM
RITALIN
RITAMAE
RITARDS
RITCHIE
RITDYES
RITEAID
RITUALS
RITZIER
RITZILY
ROTATED
ROTATES
ROTATOR
ROTAWAY
ROTBLAT
ROTELLE
ROTGUTS
ROTHIRA
ROTIFER
ROTTERS
ROTTING
ROTUNDA
RSTUVWX
RUTALEE
RUTGERS
RUTHANN
RUTHFUL
RUTILES
RUTLAND
RUTTERS
RUTTIER
RUTTING
RUTTISH

R••T•••

RAFTERS
RAFTING
RAGTIME
RAGTOPS

RANTERS
RANTING
RANTSAT
RAPTORS
RAPTUNE
RAPTURE
RASTERS
RATTAIL
RATTANS
RATTERS
RATTIER
RATTING
RATTISH
RATTLED
RATTLER
RATTLES
RATTRAP
REATTAS
RECTIFY
RECTORS
RECTORY
REDTABS
REDTAGS
REDTAIL
REDTAPE
REDTIDE
REDTIES
REDTOPS
REITMAN
RENTALS
RENTEES
RENTERS
RENTIER
RENTING
RENTOUT
RENTSTO
REPTILE
RESTABS
RESTACK
RESTAFF
RESTAGE
RESTAIN
RESTAMP
RESTART
RESTATE
RESTERS
RESTFUL
RESTICK
RESTING
RESTIRS
RESTIVE
RESTOCK
RESTOKE
RESTORE
RESTOWS
RESTRAP
RESTREW
RESTRIP
RESTSIN
RESTSON
RESTSUP
RESTUDY
RESTUFF
RESTYLE
RETTING
REUTERS
REUTHER
REUTTER

RHETORS
RHYTHMS
RIFTING
RIOTACT
RIOTERS
RIOTGUN
RIOTING
RIOTOUS
RIPTIDE
RIPTORN
RLSTINE
ROETHKE
RONTGEN
ROOTAGE
ROOTCAP
ROOTERS
ROOTFOR
ROOTIER
ROOTING
ROOTLED
ROOTLES
ROOTLET
ROOTOUT
ROOTROT
ROOTSUP
ROSTAND
ROSTERS
ROSTOCK
ROSTRAL
ROSTRUM
ROTTERS
ROTTING
ROUTERS
ROUTINE
ROUTING
ROUTOUT
RRATING
RUCTION
RUNTIER
RUNTIME
RUNTISH
RUPTURE
RUSTICS
RUSTIER
RUSTILY
RUSTING
RUSTLED
RUSTLER
RUSTLES
RUTTERS
RUTTIER
RUTTING
RUTTISH

R•••T••

RALSTON
RANATAB
RANITUP
RAPSTAR
RARITAN
RATATAT
RATITES
REACTED
REACTOR
REACTTO
REALTER
REALTOR
REATTAS

REBATED
REBATER
REBATES
REBATHE
REBOTES
RECITAL
RECITED
RECITER
RECITES
REDATED
REDATES
REDSTAR
REENTER
REENTRY
REFUTAL
REFUTED
REFUTER
REFUTES
REGATTA
REHITCH
RELATCH
RELATED
RELATER
RELATES
RELATOR
REMATCH
REMATED
REMATES
REMOTER
REMOTES
RENOTED
RENOTES
REPATCH
REPUTED
REPUTES
RERATED
RERATES
RESITED
RETITLE
RETOTAL
REUTTER
REVITUP
REVOTED
REVOTES
REWATER
RIALTOS
RIANTLY
RICHTER
RICOTTA
RIDOTTO
RIGHTED
RIGHTER
RIGHTLY
RIGHTON
RIPSTOP
RISOTTO
RIVETED
RIVETER
ROADTAR
ROADTAX
ROASTED
ROASTER
ROBOTIC
ROBOTRY
ROISTER
ROLLTOP
RONETTE
ROOFTOP

ROOSTED
ROOSTER
ROPETOW
ROSETEA
ROSETTA
ROSETTE
ROTATED
ROTATES
ROTATOR
ROUSTED
ROUSTER
ROVETTA
RUBATOS
RUBITIN
RUNATAB
RUNITUP

R••••T•

RABBETS
RABBITS
RABBITT
RABBITY
RACEDTO
RACESTO
RACISTS
RACKETS
RACKETY
RADIATE
RAGOUTS
RALLYTO
RAMINTO
RAMJETS
RANINTO
RANLATE
RANUPTO
RANWITH
RAWDATA
RAWISTS
REACTTO
READSTO
REALITY
REBAITS
REBASTE
REBIRTH
REBOLTS
REBOOTS
RECANTS
RECASTS
RECOATS
RECOSTS
RECRATE
REDACTS
REDANTS
REDBATS
REDDOTS
REDHATS
REDHOTS
REDOUTS
REDUSTS
REEDITS
REEMITS
REFERTO
REFLATE
REGATTA
REGENTS
REGIFTS
REGRETS
REHEATS

REJECTS
REKNITS
REKNOTS
RELENTS
RELICTS
RELISTS
RELUCTS
REMEETS
REMELTS
REMINTS
RENESTS
RENNETS
RENTSTO
REPASTE
REPASTS
REPEATS
REPENTS
REPLATE
REPLETE
REPLOTS
REPLYTO
REPORTS
REPOSTS
REQUITE
REQUOTE
RERENTS
REROOTS
REROUTE
RESALTS
RESEATS
RESECTS
RESENTS
RESHUTS
RESIFTS
RESISTS
RESLATE
RESORTS
RESPITE
RESPOTS
RESTATE
RESUITS
RESULTS
RETASTE
RETESTS
RETINTS
RETORTS
REUNITE
REVERTS
REVESTS
REVOLTS
REWRITE
REWROTE
REXCATS
REXROTH
RIBCUTS
RIBLETS
RICKETY
RICOTTA
RIDESTO
RIDOTTO
RILLETS
RIORITA
RIPINTO
RIPOSTE
RIPOSTS
RISENTO
RISESTO
RISOTTO

RIZZUTO
ROBERTA
ROBERTE
ROBERTF
ROBERTH
ROBERTI
ROBERTO
ROBERTS
ROBUSTA
ROBUSTO
ROCHETS
ROCKETS
RODENTS
RONETTE
ROSEATE
ROSETTA
ROSETTE
ROTGUTS
ROVETTA
ROYALTY
RUGRATS
RUINATE
RUNINTO
RUNLATE
RUNLETS
RUNNETH
RUNOUTS
RUNUPTO
RUNWITH
RUSSETS
RUSSETY

R•••••T

RABBITT
RACIEST
RACKOUT
RACQUET
RADIANT
RAILSAT
RAIMENT
RAINHAT
RAINOUT
RAMPANT
RAMPART
RANGOUT
RANKEST
RANKOUT
RANPAST
RANRIOT
RANTSAT
RAPPORT
RAREBIT
RASHEST
RATATAT
RATBERT
RATCHET
RATSOUT
RAWMEAT
READAPT
READMIT
READOPT
READOUT
REAGENT
REALEST
REALIST
REALLOT
REAMOUT
REARLIT

REAUDIT
REBOANT
REBUILT
RECEIPT
RECHART
RECOUNT
RECRUIT
REDCENT
REDCOAT
REDDEST
REDDUST
REDEALT
REDEBIT
REDHEAT
REDMEAT
REDOUBT
REDRAFT
REDROOT
REDSPOT
REDSUIT
REEJECT
REELECT
REELOUT
REENACT
REERECT
REERUPT
REEVICT
REFIGHT
REFLECT
REFLOAT
REFRACT
REFRONT
REGNANT
REGRAFT
REGRANT
REGREET
RELIANT
RELIGHT
RELIMIT
REMNANT
REMOUNT
RENAULT
RENTOUT
RENUZIT
REPAINT
REPLANT
REPOINT
REPOSIT
REPRINT
REQUEST
RESHIFT
RESHOOT
RESIGHT
RESMELT
RESOJET
RESPECT
RESPELT
RESPLIT
RESTART
RETOAST
RETRACT
RETREAT
RETWIST
REVISIT
REYMONT
RHYMIST
RIBMEAT
RICHEST

RIDEOUT
RIEGERT
RIGSOUT
RIMIEST
RIMSHOT
RINGLET
RINGOUT
RINKRAT
RIOTACT
RIPPLET
RIPSOUT
RISKSIT
RIVULET
ROARSAT
ROBSART
RODEOUT
ROLLOUT
ROOFRAT
ROOTLET
ROOTOUT
ROOTROT
ROPIEST
ROSIEST
ROTBLAT
ROUAULT
ROUGHIT
ROUTOUT
ROWBOAT
RUBSOUT
RUCKERT
RULEOUT
RULIEST
RUNGOUT
RUNPAST
RUNRIOT
RUNSOUT
RUSHOUT
RUSSERT

•RT••••

ARTBOOK
ARTCARS
ARTDECO
ARTEMIS
ARTEMUS
ARTERIO
ARTFAIR
ARTFERN
ARTFILM
ARTFORM
ARTHURC
ARTHURM
ARTHURS
ARTICLE
ARTIEST
ARTISAN
ARTISTE
ARTISTS
ARTLESS
ARTROCK
ARTSALE
ARTSHOP
ARTSHOW
ARTSIER
ARTSONG
ARTWALL
ARTWARE
ARTWORK

DRTEETH
ERTEGUN
MRTIBBS
MRTIGER
ORTEGAL
ORTOLAN
URTEXTS

•R•T•••

ARETINO
BRATTLE
BRETONS
BRETTON
BRITAIN
BRITCOM
BRITISH
BRITNEY
BRITONS
BRITPOP
BRITTEN
BRITTLE
BRITTON
BROTHER
BRUTELY
BRUTISH
CRATERS
CRATEUP
CRATING
CRATION
CRETANS
CRETINS
CRITIAS
CRITICS
CRITTER
CRITTUR
CROTONS
CRUTZEN
DRATTED
ERITREA
EROTICA
EROTICS
ERYTHRO
FRATERS
FRETFUL
FRETSAT
FRETSAW
FRETTED
FRETTER
FRITTED
FRITTER
FROTHED
FROTHER
FROTHUP
GRATEON
GRATERS
GRATEUP
GRATIAS
GRATIFY
GRATING
GRETZKY
GRITTED
GRITTER
GROTIUS
GROTTOS
HRETHEL
IRATELY
IRATEST
KRATION

ORATING
ORATION
ORATORS
ORATORY
ORATRIX
OROTUND
PRATERS
PRATING
PRATTLE
PRETAPE
PRETEEN
PRETELL
PRETEND
PRETERM
PRETEST
PRETEXT
PRETIRE
PRETOLD
PRETORS
PRETRIM
PRETYPE
PRETZEL
PRITHEE
PROTEAM
PROTEAN
PROTECT
PROTEGE
PROTEIN
PROTEST
PROTEUS
PROTIST
PROTONS
QRATIOS
QRSTUVW
RRATING
TRITELY
TRITEST
TRITIUM
TRITONE
TRITONS
TROTHED
TROTOFF
TROTOUT
TROTSKY
TROTSUP
TROTTED
TROTTER
WRITEIN
WRITEME
WRITEON
WRITERS
WRITETO
WRITEUP
WRITHED
WRITHER
WRITHES
WRITING
WRITTEN
WROTEIN
WROTEON
WROTETO
WROTEUP
XRATING

•R••T••

ARAFTOF
ARANTXA
ARBITER
ARBUTUS
ARIETTA
ARIETTE
ARISTAE
ARISTAS
ARISTOS
BRATTLE
BRAXTON
BREATHE
BREATHS
BREATHY
BRETTON
BRISTLE
BRISTLY
BRISTOL
BRITTEN
BRITTLE
BRITTON
BRONTES
BRUITED
CRAFTED
CRAFTER
CRAFTSY
CREATED
CREATES
CREATOR
CREPTIN
CREPTUP
CRESTED
CRESTON
CRITTER
CRITTUR
CROATIA
CROFTER
CROPTOP
CROSTIC
CROUTES
CROUTON
CRUSTAL
CRUSTED
CRYPTIC
CRYPTOS
CRYSTAL
DRAFTED
DRAFTEE
DRAFTER
DRASTIC
DRATTED
DRAYTON
DRIFTED
DRIFTER
DRIFTIN
DRIFTUP
DRISTAN
DROPTOP
ERASTUS
ERECTED
ERECTER
ERECTLY
ERECTOR
ERECTUS
ERGOTIC
ERISTIC
ERRATIC
ERRATUM
ERUCTED
ERUPTED
ERUPTER
FRACTAL
FRANTIC
FREETOY
FREITAG
FRETTED
FRETTER
FREYTAG
FRITTED
FRITTER
FRONTAL
FRONTED
FRONTON
FROSTED
FROSTER
FRUITED
FRUSTRO
FRUSTUM
GRAFTED
GRAFTER
GRAFTON
GRANTED
GRANTEE
GRANTER
GRANTOR
GREATEN
GREATER
GREATLY
GREETED
GREETER
GRIFTED
GRIFTER
GRISTER
GRISTLE
GRISTLY
GRITTED
GRITTER
GROTTOS
GROUTED
GROUTER
GROWTHS
GRUNTED
GRUNTER
IRKUTSK
KRISTIN
KRYPTON
KRYSTLE
MRBUTTS
ORANTES
ORBITAL
ORBITED
ORBITER
ORECTIC
ORESTES
ORNETTE
ORNITHO
PRACTIC
PRAETOR
PRATTLE
PRESTON
PRESTOS
PRINTAD
PRINTED
PRINTER
PRINTUP
PROCTER
PROCTOR
TRACTOR
TRAITOR
TREATED
TREATER
TREETOP
TRENTON
TRESTLE
TRIMTAB
TRISTAN
TRISTAR
TROTTED
TROTTER
TRUSTED
TRUSTEE
TRUSTER
TRUSTIN
TRUSTME
TRYITON
TRYSTED
TRYSTER
WRAITHS
WREATHE
WREATHS
WREATHY
WRESTED
WRESTER
WRESTLE
WRITTEN

•R•••T•

ARCUATE
ARGANTE
ARGENTI
ARGENTO
ARGENTS
ARIDITY
ARIETTA
ARIETTE
ARIGATO
ARIOSTO
ARMLETS
ARMPITS
ARRESTS
ARTISTE
ARTISTS
BREADTH
BREASTS
BREVETS
BREVITY
BRIGHTS
BRINGTO
BROASTS
BROMATE
BRUNETS
CRAVATS
CREDITS
CREMATE
CRENATE
CRUDITY
CRUELTY
DRAGOTI
DRANKTO
DRAWNTO
DRAWSTO
DRINKTO
DRIVETO
DROVETO
DRTEETH
DRYROTS
EREMITE
ERNESTA
ERNESTO
ERUDITE
FRAILTY
FRIGATE
FRIGHTS
GRADATE
GRANITA
GRANITE
GRAVITY
IRRUPTS
MRBUTTS
MRNORTH
MRSCOTT
MRSLATE
MRSMITH
ORGEATS
ORIENTE
ORIENTS
ORNETTE
ORVIETO
PRAYSTO
PREACTS
PRECITE
PRECUTS
PREDATA
PREDATE
PRELATE
PREMATE
PRESETS
PREVETO
PREWITT
PRIESTS
PRIMATE
PRIORTO
PRIVATE
PRIVETS
PRIVITY
PRIVYTO
PROBATE
PROBITY
PROCITY
PROFITS
PROJETS
PROLATE
PROMOTE
PROMPTS
PRONATE
PRONETO
PRORATA
PRORATE
PRYINTO
TRASHTV
TREINTA
TRIBUTE
TRICOTS
TRIEDTO
TRIESTE
TRIESTO
TRIJETS
TRINITY
TRIVETS
TRUANTS
TRUERTO
TRYOUTS
URANITE
URTEXTS
WRIGHTS
WRITETO
WROTETO

•R••••T

ARABIST
ARCHEST
ARIDEST
ARMREST
ARMYANT
ARTIEST
BRACKET
BRAVEST
BRIDGET
BRINGIT
BRIQUET
BRISKET
BROUGHT
CRABPOT
CRAPOUT
CRESSET
CREWCUT
CRICKET
CROCHET
CROCKET
CROQUET
CROSSAT
CRUDEST
CRUGUET
CRUMPET
DRAGNET
DRAGOUT
DRAUGHT
DRAWOUT
DREWOUT
DRFRIST
DRIBLET
DRIVEAT
DROPLET
DROPNET
DROPOUT
DROPSIT
DROUGHT
DROVEAT
DRUMOUT
DRUMSET
DRYHEAT
DRYSUIT
ERODENT
FRAUGHT
FREIGHT
FREMONT
FRESHET
FRETSAT
FROGLET
FROWNAT
GRABSAT
GRASPAT
GRAVEST
GRAYEST
GREWFAT
GREYEST
GRINSAT
GRISLET
GROMMET
GROWFAT
IRATEST
IREPEAT
IRISOUT
IRONIST
IRONOUT
JROBERT
MRFIXIT
MRHULOT
MRRIGHT
MRSCOTT
ORALIST
ORGIAST
ORPHANT
PRECAST
PRECEPT
PREDICT
PREDIET
PREEDIT
PREEMPT
PREFECT
PREHEAT
PREMEET
PREOMIT
PREPLOT
PRERENT
PRERIOT
PRESALT
PRESEAT
PRESENT
PRESIFT
PRESORT
PRETEST
PRETEXT
PREVENT
PREVERT
PREVOST
PREWITT
PRODUCT
PROEAST
PROJECT
PROPHET
PROPJET
PROTECT
PROTEST
PROTIST
PROVEIT
PROVOST
PROWEST
PRUDENT
TRABERT
TRANSIT
TREELET
TREERAT
TRIDENT
TRIEDIT
TRIESIT
TRINKET
TRIOLET
TRIPLET
TRIPPET
TRISECT
TRITEST
TRIVIOT
TROTOUT
TRUMPET
WROUGHT

••RT•••

AIRTANK
AIRTAXI
AIRTIME
AIRTRAP
AIRTUBE
BARTABS
BARTEND
BARTERS
BARTLES
BARTLET
BARTOLO
BARTRAY
BERTHAS
BERTHED
BERTOLT
BERTRAM
BIRTHED
CARTAGE
CARTALK
CARTELS
CARTERS
CARTIER
CARTING
CARTIRE
CARTOFF
CARTONS
CARTOON
CARTOPS
CARTRIP
CARTSIN
CERTAIN
CERTIFY
CORTEGE
CORTICO
CORTINA
CURTAIL
CURTAIN
CURTATE
CURTEST
CURTISS
CURTSEY
DARTERS
DARTGUN
DARTING
DARTLED
DARTLES
DARTOFF
DIRTBAG
DIRTIED
DIRTIER
DIRTIES
DIRTILY
EARTABS
EARTAGS
EARTHED
EARTHEN
EARTHLY
FARTHER
FARTLEK
FERTILE
FIRTREE
FORTDIX
FORTIES
FORTIFY
FORTIUS
FORTLEE
FORTORD
FORTRAN
FORTUNA
FORTUNE
FORTYAD
FORTYBC
FURTADO
FURTHER
FURTIVE
GARTERS
GIRTHED
GIRTING
GORTNER
HARTACK
HARTLEY
HARTMAN
HARTMUT
HURTERS
HURTFOR
HURTFUL
HURTING
HURTLED
HURTLES
KERTESZ
MARTENS
MARTIAL
MARTIAN
MARTINA
MARTINI
MARTINO
MARTINS
MARTINU
MARTINV
MARTIUS
MARTYRS
MORTALS
MORTARS
MORTICE
MORTIFY
MORTISE
MORTONS
MYRTLES
NARTHEX
NORTHER
NORTHOF
NORTONS
NURTURE
OURTOWN
PARTAKE
PARTIAL
PARTIED
PARTIER
PARTIES
PARTIII
PARTING
PARTITA
PARTITE
PARTNER
PARTONE
PARTOOK
PARTTWO
PARTWAY
PARTYER
PARTYON
PERTAIN
PERTEST
PERTURB
PORTAGE
PORTALS
PORTEND
PORTENT
PORTERS
PORTHOS
PORTICO
PORTING
PORTION
PORTMAN
PORTNOY
PORTRAY
PURTIER
SARTORS
SORTERS
SORTIED
SORTIES
SORTING
SORTOUT
TARTANS
TARTARE
TARTARS
TARTEST
TARTIER
TARTILY
TARTING
TARTISH
TARTLET
TARTSUP
TORTLAW
TORTOLA
TORTONI
TORTUGA
TORTURE
TURTLED
TURTLES
VCRTAPE
VERTIGO
VIRTUAL
VIRTUES
WARTHOG
WARTIER
WARTIME
WARTORN
WERTHER
WORTHIT

••R•T••

AARATED
ADRATES
AERATED
AERATES
AERATOR
AMRITAS
BARETTA
BARITES
BARSTOW
BERATED
BERATER
BERATES
BERETTA
BIRETTA
BORATES
BORSTAL
BURETTE
BURNTIN
BURNTUP
BURSTER
BURSTIN
BURSTYN
CARLTON
CAROTID
CAROTIN
CDRATES
CERATED
CERATES
CORETTA
CURATED
CURATES
CURATOR
CURETTE
DARKTAN
DERATED
DERATES
DORITOS
DOROTHY
ERRATIC
ERRATUM
FIRSTLY
FIRSTUP
FORETOP
FORSTER
GAROTTE
GERITOL
GORETEX
GYRATED
GYRATES
GYRATOR
HARDTEN
HARDTOP
HERBTEA
HERETIC
HERITOR
HORATIO
HURSTON
JERITZA
KARATES
KERATIN
KIRSTEN
KIRSTIE
LORETTA
MARITAL
MARSTON
MERITED
MORETTI
NORITES
OERSTED
PARATUS
PAROTID
PARTTWO
PERATIO
PERETTI
PERITUS
PGRATED
PIRATED
PIRATES
PIRATIC
PQRSTUV
PURITAN
PYRETIC
PYRITES
PYRITIC
RARITAN
RERATED
RERATES
SCRATCH
SPRITES
STRATAS
STRATUM
STRATUS
STRETCH
STRETTI
STRETTO
STRITCH
TURFTOE
UNRATED
UPRATED
UPRATES
VARITEK
VERITAS
VORSTER
WIRETAP
WORSTED
XEROTIC
YORKTON

••R••T•

AGREETO
AIRDATE
AIRPOTS
AMREETA
ARRESTS
AUREATE
AURISTS
BARBATE
BARBETS
BARENTS
BARETTA
BARISTA
BARRETS
BARRETT
BERETTA
BERLITZ
BIRETTA
BURBOTS
BURETTE
BURNETT
BURRITO
CAREDTO
CARESTO
CARLOTA
CARLOTS
CARNETS
CARPETS
CARROTS
CARROTY
CHRISTA
CHRISTI
CHRISTO
CHRISTY
CIRRATE
CORBETT
CORDATE
CORDITE
CORETTA
CORINTH
CORNETS
CORNUTE
CORSETS
CURETTE
CURTATE
CURVETS
DARESTO
DERALTE
DERMATO
DERUSTS
DIRECTS
DIRECTV
DORSETT
DURANTE
EARLETS
ENROOTS
ENROUTE
FERMATA
FERMATE
FERMATS
FERRATE
FERRETS
FERRETY
FERRITE
FORDGTS
FORDLTD
FORESTS
FORGETS
FORINTS
FORMATS
FORSYTE
FORSYTH
FURCATE
GARLITS
GARNETS
GARNETT
GAROTTE
GARRETS
GARRETT
GARROTE
GERENTS
GORDITA
HARLOTS
HERESTO
HERMITS
HERPETO
HIRSUTE
HORNETS
HORVITZ
IRRUPTS
JARRETT
JARROTT
JURISTS
LARIATS
LORENTZ
LORETTA
LYRISTS
MARANTZ
MARCATO
MARGATE
MARKETS
MARMOTS
MERLOTS
MORANTE
MORETTI
NARRATE
OTRANTO
PARENTS
PARROTS
PARTITA
PARTITE
PERDITA
PERETTI
PERLITE
PERMITS
PERMUTE
PURISTS
RERENTS
REROOTS
REROUTE
SCRIPTS
SERIATE

SERRATE
SORBATE
SORBETS
SORENTO
SPRINTS
SPROUTS
STRAITS
STREETS
STRETTI
STRETTO
STRIATE
TARANTO
TARGETS
TARPITS
TERMITE
TERNATE
TERRETS
THREATS
THRIFTS
THRIFTY
THROATS
THROATY
THRUSTS
TIRPITZ
TORONTO
TURBOTS
TURISTA
TURNSTO
TURRETS
TYRANTS
UNRESTS
UNROOTS
UPROOTS
VARIATE
VARIETY
VARLETS
VARSITY
VERISTS
VERSETS
VIRGATE
WARMSTO
WARPATH
WARVETS
ZERMATT

••R•••T

ABREAST
ACROBAT
AERIEST
AEROBAT
AIRBOAT
AIRDUCT
AIRIEST
AIRLIFT
AIRPORT
AIRSOUT
AIRVENT
ALRIGHT
APRICOT
BARKSAT
BARONET
BARRETT
BARTLET
BERENDT
BERSUNT
BERTOLT
BOREOUT
BORSCHT
BURNETT
BURNOUT
BYRIGHT
CARCOAT
CARPORT
CARPSAT
CARSEAT
CHROMAT
CIRCLET
CIRCUIT
CORBETT
CORONET
CORRECT
CORRUPT
CURBCUT
CURRANT
CURRENT
CURSEAT
CURTEST
DARENOT
DARKEST
DERWENT
DORIGHT
DORMANT
DORSETT
DURWENT
EARHART
EARNEST
EARNSIT
EARSHOT
EERIEST
ENRIGHT
FAREAST
FARLEFT
FARMOUT
FARWEST
FERMENT
FERVENT
FIREANT
FIREDAT
FIREHAT
FIRELIT
FIREPIT
FIRESAT
FIRMEST
FORABIT
FORFEIT
FORKOUT
FORRENT
FORREST
FORWENT
FURCOAT
GARMENT
GARNETT
GARRETT
GERAINT
GORIEST
HARDEST
HARDHAT
HARDHIT
HARDPUT
HARDSET
HARICOT
HARPIST
HARRIET
HARTMUT
HARVEST
HERBART
HERBAUT
HERBERT
HERRIOT
HIREOUT
HORNIST
JARRETT
JARROTT
JERKOUT
KURRENT
LARGENT
LARGEST
LORDSIT
LORIENT
MARGRET
MARKOUT
MARRYAT
MARXIST
MIRIEST
MORDANT
MORDENT
MORISOT
MRRIGHT
NORBERT
PARAPET
PARFAIT
PARKSIT
PARQUET
PERCENT
PERCEPT
PERFECT
PERIAPT
PERIDOT
PERSIST
PERTEST
PORTENT
PURPORT
PURSUIT
RAREBIT
SARGENT
SERPENT
SERVANT
SORTOUT
SPRIEST
SPRYEST
SUREBET
SURFEIT
TARTEST
TARTLET
TERSEST
THREWAT
THROWAT
THRUPUT
TIREOUT
TOREOUT
TORMENT
TORNOUT
TORRENT
TURNOUT
UPRIGHT
UTRECHT
VARIANT
VARMINT
VERDANT
VERDICT
VERIEST
VERMONT
VERSANT
VERYFIT
VERYHOT
VERYWET
WARIEST
WARMEST
WARRANT
WIRIEST
WOREOUT
WORKOUT
WORKSAT
WORNOUT
WORTHIT
YORKIST
ZERMATT
ZEROOUT

•••RT••

ABORTED
ALERTED
ALERTER
ALERTLY
ALERTTO
AVERTED
AVERTER
BEERTAP
BLURTED
BLURTER
CHARTED
CHARTER
CHORTLE
COURTED
COURTLY
COURTTV
DEARTHS
ECARTES
EVERTED
EVERTOR
EXERTED
EXERTER
FLIRTED
FLIRTER
FOURTHS
HEARTED
HEARTEN
HEARTHS
INERTIA
INERTLY
LAERTES
MAARTEN
OVERTAX
OVERTIP
OVERTLY
OVERTOP
POORTAX
QUARTAN
QUARTER
QUARTES
QUARTET
QUARTIC
QUARTOS
QUARTZY
QUIRTED
SHORTED
SHORTEN
SHORTER
SHORTIE
SHORTLY
SHORTOF
SKIRTED
SKIRTER
SMARTED
SMARTEN
SMARTER
SMARTLY
SNORTAT
SNORTED
SNORTER
SPARTAN
SPORTED
SPORTIN
SPURTED
STARTED
STARTER
STARTIN
STARTLE
STARTON
STARTTO
STARTUP
STERTOR
SWARTHY
WEIRTON
WHARTON

•••R•T•

ACCRETE
ACERATE
AIGRETS
ALERTTO
ATTRITE
ATTRITS
AZURITE
BARRETS
BARRETT
BETROTH
BURRITO
CARROTS
CARROTY
CHARITY
CIRRATE
CITRATE
CLARETS
CLARITY
CLORETS
COURTTV
COWRITE
COWROTE
CUPRITE
CUTRATE
DEBRETT
DELRUTH
DIORITE
DISRATE
DRYROTS
EMERITA
EMERITI
EMIRATE
ESPRITS
EVERETT
EXCRETE
FERRATE
FERRETS
FERRETY
FERRITE
FLORETS
GARRETS
GARRETT
GARROTE
GEARSTO
GYMRATS
HYDRATE
IGOROTS
IMARETS
INGRATE
INTRUTH
ITERATE
JARRETT
JARROTT
JOEROTH
LABRATS
LAURITZ
LEARNTO
MIGRATE
MISRATE
NARRATE
NITRATE
NITRITE
ONORATI
OPERATE
OPQRSTU
OUTRATE
OVERATE
PARROTS
PAYRATE
PETRATS
PRORATA
PRORATE
RECRATE
REGRETS
REWRITE
REWROTE
REXROTH
RIORITA
RUGRATS
SECRETE
SECRETS
SERRATE
SETRATE
SPIRITS
STARTTO
SWORETO
TAXRATE
TERRETS
THERETO
THERITZ
THIRSTS
THIRSTY
TIMROTH
TITRATE
TOPRATE
TURRETS
UNCRATE
UNTRITE
UNTRUTH
VIBRATE
VIBRATO
WHERETO
YEARNTO

•••R••T

AFFRONT
AMORIST
ANGRYAT
ARMREST
ATTRACT
AWAREST
BARRETT
BEARCAT
BEAROUT
BEARPIT
BEDREST
BLERIOT
BOURGET
CHARCOT
CHARIOT
CHARVET
CHEROOT
CHORIST
CORRECT
CORRUPT
COURANT
COURBET
CURRANT
CURRENT
CYPRIOT
CZARIST
DEAREST
DEBRETT
DECRYPT
DEFROST
DEORBIT
DETRACT
DETROIT
DIARIST
DISRUPT
DOGREAT
DOORMAT
DOUREST
DRFRIST
ENCRUST
ENCRYPT
ENGRAFT
ENTRANT
ENTREAT
ENTRUST
EVEREST
EVERETT
EXTRACT
FAIREST
FEARNOT
FLORIST
FORRENT
FORREST
GARRETT
GLAREAT
GOURMET
HAIRCUT
HAIRNET
HARRIET
HEAROUT
HERRIOT
HYDRANT
IFORGET
IFORGOT
IMGREAT
IMPREST
IMPRINT
INCRUST
INDRAFT
INFRACT
INFRONT
INGRAFT
INORBIT
INPRINT
INTROIT
INTRUST
ITERANT
JARRETT
JARROTT
JEERSAT
KURRENT
LAURENT
LEARJET
LEERSAT
LEGREST
LOWRENT
MARRYAT
MAURIAT
MEERKAT
METRIST
MIGRANT
MYCROFT
MYTREAT
NEAREST
ODORANT
OPERANT
OUTRANT
OUTROOT
OVERACT
OVERBET
OVERCUT
OVEREAT
OVERFAT
OVERFIT
OVERHOT
OVERLET
OVERLIT
OVERSET
OVERWET
PATRIOT
PEEROUT
PEERSAT
PIERROT
POOREST
POUROUT
PRERENT
PRERIOT
QUARTET
QUERIST
RANRIOT
REARLIT
RECRUIT
REDRAFT
REDROOT
REERECT
REERUPT
REFRACT
REFRONT
REGRAFT
REGRANT
REGREET
REPRINT
RETRACT
RETREAT
ROARSAT
RUNRIOT
SCARLET
SHERBET
SNARLAT
SNORTAT
SOUREST
SPAREST
STAREAT
STARLET
STARLIT
SUBROOT
SWOREAT
TAPROOT
TEAROUT
TEARSAT
TEARSIT
THEREAT
THERENT
TORRENT
TOURIST
TSARIST
TWERENT
UNERECT
UNFROST
UPDRAFT
UPDRIFT
UPFRONT
UPOROUT
USGRANT
VAGRANT
VIBRANT
WARRANT
WEAROUT
WHEREAT
YOUREIT

••••RT•

ADVERTS
ALBERTA
ALBERTI
ALBERTO
ALWORTH
ASSERTS
ASSORTS
ASTARTE
BOGARTS
BYBIRTH
CASERTA
CATERTO
CAVORTS
COHORTS
COLORTV
COVERTS
DEFERTO
DEPARTS
DEPORTS
DESERTS
DIVERTS
DOHERTY
EFFORTS
ELBERTA
ELNORTE
ENCARTA
ESCORTS
ESPARTO
EXHORTS
EXPARTE
EXPERTS
EXPORTS
EXSERTS
EXTORTS
FOGERTY
FTWORTH
GOCARTS
GOFORTH
GOKARTS
HAGERTY
HAVARTI
HAWORTH
HOGARTH
IMPARTS
IMPORTS
INSERTS
INVERTS
ITHIRTY
JAKARTA
LACERTA
LAPORTE
LIBERTE
LIBERTY
MRNORTH
NONARTS
OBVERTS
OCCURTO
OFSORTS
ONEARTH
OXCARTS
POVERTY
PRIORTO
PUBERTY
REBIRTH
REFERTO
REPORTS
RESORTS
RETORTS
REVERTS
ROBERTA
ROBERTE
ROBERTF
ROBERTH
ROBERTI
ROBERTO
ROBERTS
SQUIRTS
STBARTS
STUARTI
SUHARTO
SWEARTO
THEARTS
THWARTS
TRUERTO
TSHIRTS
UMBERTO
UNBERTH
UNEARTH
UNFERTH
UNSORTS
UPDARTS
UPNORTH
YOGURTS

••••R•T

ACCURST
AMHERST
APPARAT
ATFIRST
ATHIRST
ATWORST
BAKERST
CABARET
CHEVRET
COWERAT
CULPRIT
DEMARET
DEMERIT
DESERET
DIDEROT
DOGTROT
EXCERPT
FLOORIT
FOXTROT
GOFIRST
GOFORIT
GUJARAT
IMFORIT
INFIRST
INFORIT
INHERIT
JOGTROT
KINGRAT
LABORAT
LEVERET
LITCRIT
MAIGRET
MALLRAT
MARGRET
MAUPRAT
MEFIRST
MINARET
MOLERAT
MUSKRAT
NAYARIT
NOPQRST
ONFIRST
OUTTROT
PACKRAT
PIERROT
RINKRAT
ROOFRAT
ROOTROT
SNEERAT
SWEARAT
TABARET
TABORET
THEBRAT
TREERAT
UNBURNT
UNBURST
UPBURST
UPFIRST
UPFORIT

•••••RT

AIRPORT
ANTIART
ATEDIRT
ATHEART
ATHWART
BELFORT
BITPART
BODYART
BOOKERT
BYHEART
CALVERT
CARPORT
CATBERT
CAVEART
CLIPART
COLBERT
COMFORT
COMPART
COMPORT
CONCERT
CONSORT
CONTORT
CONVERT
CULVERT
DADAART
DELBERT
DESSERT
DEWAART
DILBERT
DISPART
DISPORT
DISSERT
DISTORT
DOGBERT
DOGCART
EARHART
EATDIRT
ECKHART
ELKHART
FILBERT
FINEART
FOLKART
GETHURT
GILBERT
GOTHURT
HASTERT
HECKART
HERBART
HERBERT
HIGHART
HILBERT
HUMBERT
HUPPERT
INCOURT
INSHORT
JETPORT
JROBERT
JUNKART
LAMBERT
LAMPERT
LETTERT
LOSTART
MCCOURT
MISSORT
NEWHART
NEWPORT
NORBERT
OFASORT
OHIOART
ONALERT
ONEPART
OUTPORT
OUTSERT
OXHEART
PAYDIRT
POPTART
PRESORT
PREVERT
PURPORT
RAMPART
RAPPORT
RATBERT
RECHART
RESTART
RIEGERT
ROBSART
RUCKERT
RUSSERT
SEAGIRT
SEAPORT
SHUBERT
STEWART
SUBSORT
SUBVERT
SUPPORT
SWIGERT
TEACART
TIPCART
TOHEART
TOSTART
TOYCART
TRABERT
TWOPART
UNALERT
UNINERT
UNOVERT
UNSHORT
UNSMART
UPCOURT
UPSTART
WALMART
WILBERT
YOGHURT

RU•••••

RUANDAS
RUBADUB
RUBATOS
RUBBERS
RUBBERY
RUBBING
RUBBISH
RUBBLES
RUBDOWN
RUBELLA
RUBEOLA
RUBICON
RUBIOUS
RUBITIN
RUBRICS
RUBSOFF
RUBSOUT
RUBSRAW
RUBUPON
RUBYDEE
RUBYRED
RUCHING
RUCKERT
RUCKING
RUCKSUP
RUCTION
RUDDERS
RUDDIED
RUDDIER
RUDDILY
RUDOLFI
RUDOLPH
RUDYARD
RUFFALO
RUFFIAN
RUFFING
RUFFLED
RUFFLER
RUFFLES

RUFIYAA
RUGGLES
RUGLIKE
RUGRATS
RUINATE
RUINERS
RUINING
RUINOUS
RULEDBY
RULEDON
RULEONE
RULEOUT
RULESON
RULIEST
RULINGS
RUMAKIS
RUMANIA
RUMBAED
RUMBLED
RUMBLER
RUMBLES
RUMCAKE
RUMFORD
RUMLESS
RUMMAGE
RUMMERS
RUMMIES
RUMORED
RUMOURS
RUMPEND
RUMPLED
RUMPLES
RUMPOLE
RUMSHOP
RUNAMOK
RUNATAB
RUNAWAY
RUNBACK
RUNDEEP
RUNDLES
RUNDOWN
RUNFREE
RUNGFOR
RUNGOFF
RUNGOUT
RUNHOME
RUNINTO
RUNITUP
RUNLAPS
RUNLATE
RUNLESS
RUNLETS
RUNNELS
RUNNERS
RUNNETH
RUNNIER
RUNNING
RUNOFFS
RUNONIN
RUNOUTS
RUNOVER
RUNPAST
RUNRIOT
RUNSDRY
RUNSFOR
RUNSLOW
RUNSOFF
RUNSOUT
RUNTIER
RUNTIME
RUNTISH
RUNUPTO
RUNWAYS
RUNWILD
RUNWITH
RUPIAHS
RUPTURE
RURALLY
RUSHDIE
RUSHEES
RUSHERS
RUSHIER
RUSHING
RUSHOFF
RUSHOUT
RUSSELL
RUSSERT
RUSSETS
RUSSETY
RUSSIAN
RUSSLAN
RUSTICS
RUSTIER
RUSTILY
RUSTING
RUSTLED
RUSTLER
RUSTLES
RUTALEE
RUTGERS
RUTHANN
RUTHFUL
RUTILES
RUTLAND
RUTTERS
RUTTIER
RUTTING
RUTTISH
RUYBLAS
RUZICKA

R•U••••

RAUCOUS
RAUNCHY
REUBENS
REUNERS
REUNIFY
REUNION
REUNITE
REUPPED
REURGED
REURGES
REUSERS
REUSING
REUTERS
REUTHER
REUTTER
RHUBARB
RHUMBAS
ROUAULT
ROUBAIX
ROUGHED
ROUGHEN
ROUGHER
ROUGHGO
ROUGHIT
ROUGHLY
ROUGHUP
ROUGING
ROULADE
ROULEAU
ROUNDED
ROUNDEL
ROUNDER
ROUNDLY
ROUNDON
ROUNDUP
ROUSERS
ROUSING
ROUSTED
ROUSTER
ROUTERS
ROUTINE
ROUTING
ROUTOUT
RYUKYUS

R••U•••

RANUPTO
RASURES
REAUDIT
REAUMUR
REBUFFS
REBUILD
REBUILT
REBUKED
REBUKER
REBUKES
REBUSES
RECURED
RECURES
RECURLS
RECURVE
RECUSAL
RECUSED
RECUSES
REDUCED
REDUCER
REDUCES
REDUSTS
REFUELS
REFUGED
REFUGEE
REFUGES
REFUNDS
REFUSAL
REFUSED
REFUSER
REFUSES
REFUTAL
REFUTED
REFUTER
REFUTES
REGUIDE
REGULAR
REGULUS
REJUDGE
RELUCTS
RELUMED
RELUMES
RENUZIT
REPUGNS
REPULSE
REPUMPS
REPUTED
REPUTES
REQUEST
REQUIEM
REQUIRE
REQUITE
REQUOTE
RESUITS
RESULTS
RESUMED
RESUMES
RESURGE
RETUNED
RETUNES
RETURFS
RETURNS
RHEUMIC
RIGUEUR
RITUALS
RIVULET
ROBUSTA
ROBUSTO
ROGUERY
ROGUING
ROGUISH
ROMULAN
ROMULUS
ROTUNDA
RSTUVWX
RUBUPON
RUNUPTO

R•••U••

RACQUET
RAEBURN
RAGOUTS
RAGRUGS
RAPTUNE
RAPTURE
RAVEUPS
RAYBURN
RAYGUNS
REBOUND
REBRUSH
RECLUSE
RECOUNT
RECOUPS
RECRUIT
REDBUDS
REDDUST
REDOUBT
REDOUND
REDOUTS
REDSUIT
REDSUNS
REEQUIP
REERUPT
REFOUND
REGAUGE
REGLUED
REGLUES
REHAULS
REHOUSE
REMOUNT
RENAULT
REPLUMB
REPLUME
REPOURS
REPRUNE
REROUTE
RESCUED
RESCUER
RESCUES
RESHUTS
RESOUND
RESTUDY
RESTUFF
RETOUCH
RETOURS
REWOUND
RIBCUTS
RIGOURS
RIOMUNI
RIZZUTO
ROEBUCK
ROLLUPS
RONDURE
RORQUAL
ROTGUTS
ROUAULT
ROXBURY
RUMOURS
RUNOUTS
RUPTURE
RVALUES

R••••U•

RACEDUP
RACESUP
RACKOUT
RACKSUP
RAGEFUL
RAILBUS
RAINOUT
RAISEUP
RAKEDUP
RAKESUP
RAMPSUP
RANCOUR
RANGOUT
RANITUP
RANKOUT
RAPANUI
RATSOUT
RAUCOUS
REACHUP
READOUT
READSUP
REAMOUT
REARGUE
REARSUP
REAUMUR
REBEGUN
REDFOUR
REELOUT
REELSUP
REFOCUS
REGROUP
REGULUS
REISSUE
RENTOUT
REOCCUR
RESCRUB
RESEAUS
RESEAUX
RESIDUA
RESIDUE
RESTFUL
RESTSUP
RETINUE
REVALUE
REVENUE
REVITUP
REYNAUD
RHENIUM
RHODIUM
RHOECUS
RHOMBUS
RIDEOUT
RIDESUP
RIGSOUT
RIGUEUR
RILEDUP
RILESUP
RIMBAUD
RINGOUT
RINGSUP
RIOTGUN
RIOTOUS
RIPSOUT
RISESUP
RODEOUT
ROLLOUT
ROLLSUP
ROMANUS
ROMULUS
ROOMFUL
ROOTOUT
ROOTSUP
ROPEDUP
ROPESUP
ROSABUD
ROSEBUD
ROSTRUM
ROUGHUP
ROUNDUP
ROUTOUT
RUBADUB
RUBIOUS
RUBSOUT
RUCKSUP
RUINOUS
RULEOUT
RUNGOUT
RUNITUP
RUNSOUT
RUSHOUT
RUTHFUL
RYUKYUS

R•••••U

RONDEAU
ROULEAU

•RU••••

ARUBANS
ARUGULA
ARUNDEL
ARUSPEX
BRUBECK
BRUEGEL
BRUISED
BRUISER
BRUISES
BRUITED
BRUMMEL
BRUMOUS
BRUNETS
BRUSHED
BRUSHER
BRUSHES
BRUSHUP
BRUSQUE
BRUTELY
BRUTISH
BRUXING
BRUXISM
CRUCIAL
CRUDELY
CRUDEST
CRUDITY
CRUDSUP
CRUELER
CRUELLA
CRUELLY
CRUELTY
CRUGUET
CRUISED
CRUISER
CRUISES
CRULLER
CRUMBED
CRUMBLE
CRUMBLY
CRUMBUM
CRUMPED
CRUMPET
CRUMPLE
CRUMPLY
CRUNCHY
CRUPPER
CRUSADE
CRUSHED
CRUSHER
CRUSHES
CRUSTAL
CRUSTED
CRUTZEN
CRUZADO
CRUZANS
DRUBBED
DRUBBER
DRUCKER
DRUDGED
DRUDGER
DRUDGES
DRUGGED
DRUIDIC
DRUMLIN
DRUMMED
DRUMMER
DRUMOUT
DRUMSET
DRUMSUP
DRUNKEN
DRUNKER
DRUZEAN
DRUZIAN
ERUCTED
ERUDITE
ERUPTED
ERUPTER
FRUITED
FRUSTRO
FRUSTUM
GRUBBED
GRUBBER
GRUDGED
GRUDGER
GRUDGES
GRUFFER
GRUFFLY
GRUMBLE
GRUMBLY
GRUMMAN
GRUMPED
GRUNGER
GRUNGES
GRUNION
GRUNTED
GRUNTER
GRUYERE
KRUEGER
PRUDENT
PRUDERY
PRUDHOE
PRUDISH
PRUNERS
PRUNING
PRUSSIA
TRUANCY
TRUANTS
TRUCKED
TRUCKEE
TRUCKER
TRUCKLE
TRUDEAU
TRUDGED
TRUDGEN
TRUDGER
TRUDGES
TRUEDUP
TRUEING
TRUERIB
TRUERTO
TRUESUP
TRUFFLE
TRUISMS
TRUMANS
TRUMPED
TRUMPET
TRUMPUP
TRUNDLE
TRUSSED
TRUSSES
TRUSSUP
TRUSTED
TRUSTEE
TRUSTER
TRUSTIN
TRUSTME
URUGUAY

•R•U•••

ARBUTUS
ARCUATE
ARDUOUS
ARGUERS
ARGUING
ARGUSES
AROUSAL
AROUSED
AROUSER
AROUSES
BROUGHT
BRYUSOV
CROUTES
CROUTON
DRAUGHT
DROUGHT
DRQUINN
FRAUGHT
GRAUMAN
GROUCHO
GROUCHY
GROUNDS
GROUPED
GROUPER
GROUPIE
GROUSED
GROUSER
GROUSES
GROUTED
GROUTER
IRKUTSK
IRRUPTS
MRBURNS
MRBUTTS
MRHULOT
MRLUCKY
MRMUSIC
MRQUILP
OROURKE
PRIUSES
PROUDER
PROUDLY
PROUDOF
TRAUBEL
TRAUMAS
TRIUMPH
TROUBLE
TROUGHS
TROUNCE
TROUPED
TROUPER
TROUPES
TROUSER
URSULAK
WROUGHT

•R••U••

ARAFURA
ARBOURS
ARDOURS
ARMFULS
ARMOURS
ARMOURY
ARTHURC
ARTHURM
ARTHURS
ARUGULA
BRAVURA
BRIQUET
BROGUES
CROQUET
CROQUIS
CRUGUET
DRACULA
DRLAURA
DROGUES
DRSEUSS
DRYBULB
DRYRUNS
DRYSUIT
ERASURE
GRADUAL
GRANULE
GRAVURE
IREFUSE
MRSMUIR
OROTUND
PREBURN
PREBUYS
PRECURE
PRECUTS
PREDUSK
PREFUND
PRELUDE
PRENUPS
PREPUPA
PREQUEL
PRESUME
PREVUED
PREVUES
PROCURE
PRODUCE
PRODUCT
PROFUSE
QRSTUVW
TRADUCE
TRIBUNE
TRIBUTE
TRYOUTS
URNFULS
URUGUAY
WRAPUPS

•R•••U•

ARBUTUS
ARCANUM
ARDUOUS
AREARUG
ARTEMUS
BRACEUP
BREAKUP
BRENGUN
BREWPUB
BREWSUP
BRICKUP
BRIMFUL
BRINGUP
BROKEUP
BRUMOUS
BRUSHUP
BRUSQUE
CRACKUP
CRANIUM
CRANKUP
CRAPOUT
CRASSUS
CRATEUP
CREEPUP
CREPTUP
CREWCUT
CRIEDUP
CRIESUP
CRISPUS
CRITTUR
CROESUS
CROPSUP
CROSSUP
CRUDSUP
CRUMBUM
DRAGOUT
DRAGSUP
DRANKUP
DRAWNUP
DRAWOUT
DRAWSUP
DREAMUP
DRESSUP
DREWOUT
DREYFUS
DRFREUD
DRIEDUP
DRIESUP
DRIFTUP
DRINKUP
DRIVEUP
DROPOUT
DROVEUP
DRUMOUT
DRUMSUP
ERASMUS
ERASTUS
ERECTUS
ERRATUM
ERTEGUN
FRAMEUP
FREEDUP
FREESUP
FRETFUL
FRIEDUP
FRIESUP
FRISEUR
FROTHUP
FROZEUP
FRUSTUM
GRAMPUS
GRATEUP
GREYCUP
GROPIUS
GROTIUS
GROWNUP
GROWSUP
IRIDIUM
IRISOUT
IRONOUT
MRSPAUL
ORARIUM
ORDERUP
ORMOLUS
ORPHEUM
ORPHEUS
PRECOUP
PREMIUM
PRESPUR
PRESQUE
PRESSUP
PRICKUP
PRINTUP
PROCLUS
PRONOUN
PROPSUP
PROTEUS
TRADEUP
TRAPGUN
TRAYFUL
TRIPSUP
TRITIUM
TRIVIUM
TROILUS
TROTOUT
TROTSUP
TRUEDUP
TRUESUP
TRUMPUP
TRUSSUP
URANIUM
URSINUS
WRACKUP
WRAPSUP
WRITEUP
WROTEUP

•R••••U

DREXELU
FRENEAU
TRUDEAU

••RU•••

ABRUZZI
BURUNDI
CERUMEN
CYRUSII
DERUSTS
ETRURIA
FERULES
GERUNDS
INRUINS
IRRUPTS
KORUNAS
LARUSSA
LORUSES
MARULLO
MARUSJA
NKRUMAH
PARURES
PERUGIA
PERUKES
PERUSAL
PERUSED
PERUSER
PERUSES
SARUMAN
SCRUBBY
SCRUBUP
SCRUFFS
SCRUFFY
SCRUGGS
SCRUNCH
SCRUPLE
SHRUBBY
SPRUCED
SPRUCER
SPRUCES
STRUDEL
THRUPUT
THRUSTS
THRUWAY
UNRULED
UNRURAL
VIRUSES

••R•U••

AGROUND
AIRDUCT
AIRGUNS
AIRPUMP
AIRTUBE
ATRIUMS
BARBUDA
BARBULE
BARNUMS
BARQUES
BERMUDA
BERSUNT
BOROUGH
CARFULS
CAROUSE
CIRCUIT
CIRCUSY
CIRQUES
CORNUTE
CORRUPT
DARIUSI
EARBUDS
EARFULS
EARMUFF
ENROUTE
FAROUKI
FERRULE
FORBUSH
FORMULA
FORSURE
FORTUNA
FORTUNE
GOROUND
HARBURG
HERCULE
HIRSUTE
HORNUNG
JARFULS
KEROUAC
LARRUPS
MARAUDS
MARCUSE
MARKUPS
MARQUEE
MARQUES
MARQUEZ
MARQUIS
MARYURE
MERCURE
MERCURY
MORGUES
MURMURS
NERVULE
NURTURE
PARFUMS
PARQUET
PERCUSS
PERDURE
PERFUME
PERFUMY
PERFUSE
PERJURE
PERJURY
PERMUTE
PERTURB

PURDUEU
PURSUED
PURSUER
PURSUES
PURSUIT
REROUTE
RORQUAL
SHROUDS
SIRDUKE
SPROUTS
STRAUSS
STROUSE
TERHUNE
THROUGH
TORQUED
TORQUES
TORTUGA
TORTURE
TURNUPS
UNROUND
UPROUSE
VERDUGO
VERDURE
VERRUCA
VIRGULE
VIRTUAL
VIRTUES
WARBURG
WARMUPS
WORKUPS

••R••U•

AIREDUP
AIRSOUT
BARACUS
BAROQUE
BERGIUS
BOREOUT
BORGLUM
BORLAUG
BORNEUP
BUREAUS
BUREAUX
BURNOUT
BURNSUP
BURNTUP
BURPGUN
CARCLUB
CARDIUM
CAREFUL
CARIOUS
CARPOUS
CORKSUP
CURBCUT
CURIOUS
CURLSUP
DAREFUL
DARTGUN
DIREFUL
EARDRUM
EARPLUG
ENRIQUE
ERRATUM
FARCEUR
FARMOUT
FERMIUM
FERROUS
FERVOUR
FIREBUG
FIREDUP
FIRESUP
FIRMSUP
FIRSTUP
FORCEUP
FORERUN
FORKFUL
FORKOUT
FORKSUP
FORMFUL
FORTIUS
FURIOUS
GORDIUS
HARBOUR
HARDPUT
HARMFUL
HARTMUT
HERBAUT
HIREOUT
HURRYUP
HURTFUL
JERKOUT
JERKSUP
KARAKUM
MARGAUX
MARHAUS
MARKOUT
MARKSUP
MARTIUS
NERVOUS
PARAMUS
PARATUS
PARFOUR
PARIBUS
PARLOUR
PARLOUS
PERITUS
PERKSUP
PERSEUS
PERSIUS
PIRAEUS
PIROGUE
PQRSTUV
PYRAMUS
PYRRHUS
SCREWUP
SCRUBUP
SERIOUS
SERVEUP
SORGHUM
SORTOUT
STRATUM
STRATUS
SURFSUP
SURPLUS
TARTSUP
TERBIUM
THREEUP
THREWUP
THROWUP
THRUPUT
TIREOUT
TOREOUT
TORNOUT
TURNOUT
TURNSUP
VARIOUS
VERDOUX
WARCLUB
WARMSUP
WIREDUP
WIRESUP
WOREOUT
WORKOUT
WORKSUP
WORNOUT
ZEROOUT
ZEROSUM

••R•••U

BARBEAU
BIRDFLU
CARIBOU
GARNEAU
MARCEAU
MARTINU
MARYLOU
PARVENU
PERREAU
PURDUEU
PURLIEU

•••RU••

ACCRUAL
ACCRUED
ACCRUES
ALARUMS
ASARULE
BAYRUMS
BULRUSH
BUMRUSH
CHERUBS
CORRUPT
DECRUMB
DELRUTH
DETRUDE
DISRUPT
DOGRUNS
DONRUSS
DRYRUNS
EMBRUED
EMBRUES
ENCRUST
ENDRUNS
ENTRUST
EXTRUDE
FAIRUSE
FERRULE
FUNRUNS
GAGRULE
HEYRUBE
ICERUNS
IMBRUED
IMBRUES
INARUSH
INCRUST
INTRUDE
INTRUST
INTRUTH
LARRUPS
MADRUSH
MCCRUMB
MCGRUFF
MISRULE
MOBRULE
NOTRUMP
OBTRUDE
OILRUBS
OUTRUNS
OUTRUSH
OVERUSE
QUORUMS
RAGRUGS
REBRUSH
RECRUIT
REERUPT
REPRUNE
SKIRUNS
THERULE
UNCRUDE
UNCRUEL
UNDRUNK
UNGRUFF
UNTRUER
UNTRULY
UNTRUSS
UNTRUTH
UNWRUNG
VERRUCA

•••R•U•

ALARBUS
AMOROUS
ANDROUS
APERCUS
AVERNUS
BEARCUB
BEARHUG
BEAROUT
BEARSUP
BEERMUG
BOARDUP
BOHRIUM
CHIRRUP
CHURNUP
CITROUS
CUPROUS
DEFRAUD
DRFREUD
EVERDUR
FAIRSUP
FEARFUL
FERROUS
FIBROUS
FLAREUP
GEARSUP
GUARGUM
HAIRCUT
HEAROUT
HURRYUP
HYDROUS
INGROUP
JIMRYUN
MALRAUX
NATRIUM
NITROUS
OCHROUS
ODORFUL
ODOROUS
ONEROUS
ORARIUM
OVERBUY
OVERCUT
OVERDUB
OVERDUE
OVERRUN
OVERSUP
PAIRSUP
PEEROUT
PETROUS
POUROUT
PTEROUS
PYRRHUS
REARGUE
REARSUP
REGROUP
SCAREUP
SCARFUP
SHOREUP
SNARLUP
STARTUP
STERNUM
STIRRUP
STIRSUP
STOREUP
TEARFUL
TEAROUT
TEARSUP
THEROUX
THORIUM
TOURBUS
UNPROUD
UPOROUT
WEAROUT
YTTRIUM

•••R••U

ALFREDU
BUNRAKU
NEARYOU
OPQRSTU
PERREAU
THOREAU
THURGAU

••••RU•

ANTERUS
AREARUG
BACKRUB
BELARUS
BODYRUB
BULLRUN
CENTRUM
CHEERUP
CHETRUM
CHIRRUP
CLEARUP
COVERUP
CUTARUG
DECORUM
DELARUE
EARDRUM
FOOTRUB
FORERUN
FULCRUM
HOMERUN
HUMDRUM
HUMERUS
ICTERUS
ITSTRUE
KIDSRUS
LAZARUS
LONGRUN
LUSTRUM
MADERUN
MAKERUN
MILERUN
MILKRUN
MILLRUN
NONDRUG
NOSTRUM
NOTTRUE
OFFERUP
OILDRUM
ORDERUP
OVERRUN
PAPYRUS
POWERUP
RESCRUB
ROSTRUM
SEVERUS
SHAGRUG
STIRRUP
SUBARUS
TANTRUM
TENKRUN
TESTRUN
THEFRUG
TOYSRUS
VAPORUB
WELLRUN

••••R•U

AUBURNU
HOFBRAU
HOWARDU

•••••RU

BAYLORU
LETTERU
SEETHRU
XAVIERU

RV•••••

RVALUES
RVPARKS

R•V••••

RAVAGED
RAVAGER
RAVAGES
RAVELED
RAVELLY
RAVELOE
RAVENAL
RAVENED
RAVENNA
RAVEUPS
RAVINED
RAVINES
RAVINGS
RAVIOLI
REVALUE
REVAMPS
REVEALS
REVELED
REVELER
REVELIN
REVELRY
REVENDS
REVENGE
REVENUE
REVERBS
REVERDY
REVERED
REVERER
REVERES
REVERIE
REVERSA
REVERSE
REVERTS
REVESTS
REVIEWS
REVILED
REVILER
REVILES
REVISAL
REVISED
REVISER
REVISES
REVISIT
REVISOR
REVITUP
REVIVAL
REVIVED
REVIVER
REVIVES
REVOICE
REVOKED
REVOKER
REVOKES
REVOLTS
REVOLVE
REVOTED
REVOTES
REVVING
RIVALED
RIVALRY
RIVERPO
RIVETED
RIVETER
RIVIERA
RIVIERE
RIVULET
ROVETTA
ROVINGS
RSVPING

R••V•••

REAVAIL
REAVERS
REAVING
REAVOWS
REEVICT
REEVING
REEVOKE
RENVOIS
REVVING
RIGVEDA
ROLVAAG

R•••V••

RANOVER
RAYOVAC
RECOVER
REGIVEN
REGIVES
RELEVEL
RELEVER
RELEVES
RELIVED
RELIVES
REMOVAL
REMOVED
REMOVER
REMOVES
REPAVED
REPAVES
RESAVED
RESAVES
REVIVAL
REVIVED
REVIVER
REVIVES
REWOVEN
RSTUVWX
RUNOVER

R••••V•

RECARVE
RECEIVE
RECURVE
REDFIVE
REDRIVE
RELIEVE
REPROVE
RESERVE
RESHAVE
RESOLVE
RESTIVE
REVOLVE
REWEAVE
RILIEVO

R•••••V

ROCKYIV
ROMANOV
ROYGBIV
ROZANOV

•RV••••

DRVEGAS
ORVIETO
ORVILLE

•R•V•••

BRAVADA
BRAVADO
BRAVELY
BRAVERY
BRAVEST
BRAVING
BRAVOED
BRAVOES
BRAVURA
BREVETS
BREVITY
CRAVATS
CRAVENS
CRAVERS
CRAVING
CREVICE
DRIVEAT
DRIVEBY
DRIVEIN
DRIVELS
DRIVERS
DRIVETO
DRIVEUP
DRIVING
DROVEAT
DROVEBY
DROVEIN
DROVERS
DROVETO
DROVEUP
FRIVOLS
GRAVELS
GRAVELY
GRAVERS
GRAVEST
GRAVIES
GRAVING
GRAVITY
GRAVLAX
GRAVURE
GROVELS
GROVERS
HRYVNIA
PREVAIL
PREVENT
PREVERB
PREVERT
PREVETO
PREVIAS
PREVIEW
PREVOID
PREVOST
PREVUED
PREVUES
PRIVACY
PRIVATE
PRIVETS
PRIVIER
PRIVIES
PRIVILY
PRIVITY
PRIVYTO
PROVEIT
PROVERB
PROVERS
PROVIDE
PROVINE
PROVING
PROVISO
PROVOKE
PROVOST
TRAVAIL
TRAVELS
TRAVERS
TREVINO
TRIVETS
TRIVIAL
TRIVIOT
TRIVIUM

•R••V••

ARRIVAL
ARRIVED
ARRIVER
ARRIVES
CRYOVER
GREAVES
GRIEVED
GRIEVER
GRIEVES
GROOVED
GROOVES
GROOVIN
MRNOVAK
PREAVER

•R•••V•

ARCHIVE
EROSIVE
PREDIVE
PREPAVE
PRONAVY
QRSTUVW
URBANVI

•R••••V

BRYUSOV
GRINKOV
TRASHTV
URBANIV

••RV•••

AIRVENT
BERVOIX
CARVELS
CARVERS
CARVING
CERVEZA
CERVIDS
CERVINE
CORVAIR
CORVEES
CORVIDS
CORVINA
CORVINE
CURVETS
CURVIER
CURVING
DERVISH
FERVENT
FERVORS
FERVOUR
GERVAIS
HARVARD
HARVEST
HORVITZ
MARVELL
MARVELS
MARVIER
NARVAEZ
NERVIER
NERVILY
NERVINE
NERVING
NERVOUS
NERVULE
NIRVANA
PARVENU
PERVADE
PURVEYS
PURVIEW
SERVANT
SERVEAS
SERVERS
SERVEUP
SERVICE
SERVILE
SERVING
SORVINO
SURVEIL
SURVEYS
SURVIVE
TORVALD
TORVILL
WARVETS

••R•V••

ARRIVAL
ARRIVED
ARRIVER
ARRIVES
CARAVAN
CARAVEL
DERIVED
DERIVER
DERIVES
EUROVAN
FOREVER
MARKVII
MORAVIA
PORIVER
SHRIVEL
SHRIVER
SHRIVES
STRIVED
STRIVEN
STRIVER
STRIVES
THRIVED
THRIVEN
THRIVER
THRIVES
UNRAVEL
UNRIVED
UNRIVEN
UPRIVER
YEREVAN

••R••V•

AIRWAVE
BEREAVE
CURSIVE
FORGAVE
FORGIVE
FORLOVE
FURTIVE
KARLOVY
MARKOVA
PARFIVE
PARKAVE
SURVIVE

••R•••V

DIRECTV
MARTINV
NUREYEV
PQRSTUV

•••RV••

CHARVET
CHERVIL
DWARVES
SCARVES
SCURVES
STARVED
STARVES
SWERVED
SWERVES
WHARVES

•••R•V•

APPROVE
BEBRAVE
DEPRAVE
DEPRIVE
ENGRAVE
HENRYVI
IMPROVE
KEDROVA
OSTRAVA
OUTRAVE
OUTROVE
REDRIVE
REPROVE
UNBRAVE
WHEREVE

•••R••V

COURTTV
GEORGEV
HENRYIV
KHARKOV
SMIRNOV

••••RV•

ALGARVE
DESERVE
INCURVE
INNERVE
MINERVA
OBSERVE
ONSERVE
RECARVE
RECURVE
RESERVE
UNNERVE
UPCURVE

••••R•V

ALFEROV
COLORTV
EDWARDV
FEDOROV
NEMEROV

•••••RV

LETTERV

RW•••••

RWANDAN

R•W••••

RAWBARS
RAWDATA
RAWDEAL
RAWEGGS
RAWFISH
RAWFOOD
RAWHIDE
RAWISTS
RAWLINS
RAWMEAT
RAWNESS
RAWSILK
REWAGER
REWAKED
REWAKEN
REWAKES
REWARDS
REWARMS
REWARNS
REWATER
REWAXED
REWAXES
REWEARS
REWEAVE
REWEIGH
REWELDS
REWIDEN
REWINDS
REWIPED
REWIPES
REWIRED
REWIRES
REWOKEN
REWORDS
REWORKS
REWOUND
REWOVEN
REWRAPS
REWRITE
REWROTE
ROWBOAT
ROWDIER
ROWDIES
ROWDILY
ROWELED
ROWLAND
ROWLING

R••W•••

RAGWEED
RANWILD
RANWITH
REAWAKE
REAWOKE
REDWINE
REDWING
REDWOLF
REDWOOD
REDWORM
RENWICK
REOWNED
RESWEAR
RESWEEP
RESWIMS
RESWORE
RESWORN
RETWINE
RETWIST
RONWOOD
ROSWELL
RUNWAYS
RUNWILD
RUNWITH

R•••W••

RACEWAY
RAILWAY

RANAWAY
REMOWED
RENEWAL
RENEWED
RENEWER
RENOWNS
REPOWER
RESAWED
RESEWED
RESOWED
RETOWED
RIDGWAY
ROADWAY
ROLLWAY
ROTAWAY
RUNAWAY

R••••W•
RAEDAWN
RAMDOWN
RANDOWN
REAVOWS
REBLOWN
REBREWS
RECHEWS
RECROWN
REDDAWN
REDHAWK
REDRAWN
REDRAWS
REFLOWN
REFLOWS
REGLOWS
REGROWN
REGROWS
REPLOWS
RESHOWN
RESHOWS
RESTOWS
RETHAWS
REVIEWS
RIPSAWN
RIPSAWS
ROBLOWE
ROYALWE
RSTUVWX
RUBDOWN
RUNDOWN

R•••••W
RAINBOW
REENDOW
RENFREW
RESTREW
ROPETOW
RUBSRAW
RUNSLOW

•RW••••
DRWELBY
MRWORDS
MRWRONG

•R•W•••
ARCWELD
ARTWALL
ARTWARE
ARTWORK
BRAWLED
BRAWLER
BRAWLEY
BREWAGE
BREWERS
BREWERY
BREWING
BREWPUB
BREWSKI
BREWSUP
BROWARD
BROWNED
BROWNER
BROWNIE
BROWSED
BROWSER
BROWSES
BROWWAX
CRAWDAD
CRAWLED
CRAWLER
CRAWLEY
CREWCUT
CREWELS
CREWING
CREWMAN
CREWMEN
CROWBAR
CROWDED
CROWDER
CROWDIN
CROWELL
CROWERS
CROWING
CROWLEY
CROWNED
CROWNER
CRYWOLF
DRAWBAR
DRAWEES
DRAWERS
DRAWING
DRAWLED
DRAWLER
DRAWMAN
DRAWMEN
DRAWNIN
DRAWNON
DRAWNTO
DRAWNUP
DRAWOFF
DRAWOUT
DRAWSIN
DRAWSON
DRAWSTO
DRAWSUP
DREWOFF
DREWOUT
DROWNED
DROWSED
DROWSES
DRYWALL
DRYWASH
DRYWELL
EREWHON
FRAWLEY
FROWARD
FROWNAT
FROWNED
FROWNER
FROWNON
GREWBIG
GREWDIM
GREWFAT
GREWOLD
GROWBIG
GROWDIM
GROWERS
GROWFAT
GROWING
GROWLED
GROWLER
GROWNON
GROWNUP
GROWOLD
GROWSON
GROWSUP
GROWTHS
JREWING
PRAWNED
PREWARM
PREWARN
PREWASH
PREWHIP
PREWIRE
PREWITT
PREWORK
PREWORN
PREWRAP
PROWESS
PROWEST
PROWLED
PROWLER
TRAWLED
TRAWLER
TROWELS
TROWING

•R••W••
ARCHWAY
AREAWAY
BRONWEN
BROWWAX
FREEWAY
TRAMWAY

•R•••W•
CRYDOWN
DRBROWN
MRBROWN
PREDAWN
PROBOWL

•R••••W
ARTSHOW
CRASHAW
FRETSAW
PRESHOW
PREVIEW
QRSTUVW
WROCLAW

••RW•••
AIRWARS
AIRWAVE
AIRWAYS
AIRWICK
AIRWOLF
BARWARE
BERWICK
CARWASH
DARWELL
DERWENT
DURWARD
DURWENT
EARWIGS
FARWEST
FORWARD
FORWENT
FURWRAP
HARWELL
NARWHAL
NORWALK
NORWICH
NORWOOD
PERWEEK
WARWICK
WARWORN

••R•W••
BEROWNE
CARAWAY
FARAWAY
FAREWAR
HARDWAY
HARDWON
PARKWAY
PARTWAY
PERIWIG
SARAWAK
SCRAWLS
SCRAWLY
SCRAWNY
SCREWED
SCREWUP
SPRAWLS
SPRAWLY
STREWED
STREWER
THREWAT
THREWIN
THREWON
THREWUP
THROWAT
THROWER
THROWIN
THROWON
THROWUP
THRUWAY
TURFWAR
UNROWDY
VERYWET

••R••W•
BARNOWL
BARROWS
BORROWS
BURROWS
CURFEWS
CURLEWS
FARROWS
FURROWS
HARROWS
MARLOWE
MARROWS
MORROWS
NARROWS
NORDOWE
OURTOWN
PARTTWO
SORROWS
WARHAWK
YARROWS

••R•••W
AIRCREW
AIRFLOW
AIRGLOW
AIRSHOW
BARSTOW
CARSHOW
CORNROW
FOREPAW
FORESAW
FORSHOW
HERENOW
KERSHAW
PURVIEW
TORTLAW
VERYFEW
VERYLOW
VERYNEW

•••RW••
BOERWAR
DOORWAY
FAIRWAY
FOURWAY
OVERWET
SCARWID
SHERWIN

•••R•W•
ANDREWS
ASPRAWL
BARROWS
BORROWS
BURROWS
DRBROWN
EMBROWN
ESCROWS
FARROWS
FURROWS
HARROWS
HEBREWS
INBROWN
INCROWD
INDRAWN
INGROWN
MARROWS
MORROWS
MRBROWN
NARROWS
OUTROWS
OVERAWE
PITROWS
REBREWS
RECROWN
REDRAWN
REDRAWS
REGROWN
REGROWS
SOAREWE
SORROWS
TOPROWS
TVCREWS
UNCROWN
UNDRAWN
UNDRAWS
UNGROWN
UPGROWN
UPGROWS
YARROWS

•••R••W
BEARPAW
GEORGEW
OVERFEW
OVERNEW
OVERSAW
OVERSEW
POORLAW
SPARROW

••••R•W
AIRCREW
ATECROW
BACKROW
BESTREW
CORNROW
EATCROW
EYEBROW
HADAROW
HALFRAW
HASAROW
KENDREW
LASTROW
LOWBROW
MACGRAW
MISBREW
MISDRAW
MISDREW
MULGREW
OUTCROW
OUTDRAW
OUTDREW
OUTGREW
OUTGROW
PALTROW
PETCROW
PILCROW
PITCREW
RENFREW
RESTREW
RUBSRAW
SEMIRAW
SKIDROW
SPARROW
THECROW
TONEROW
TOPDRAW
UNSCREW
UPTHROW
WOODROW

•••••RW
LETTERW

R•X••••
REXCATS
REXREED
REXROTH
ROXANNE
ROXBURY

R••X•••
REEXPEL

R•••X••
RADIXES
REBOXED
REBOXES
REDOXES
REFAXED
REFAXES
REFIXED
REFIXES
RELAXED
RELAXER
RELAXES
REMIXED
REMIXES
RETAXED
RETAXES
REWAXED
REWAXES
ROLEXES

R•••••X
REAFFIX
REANNEX
REINDEX
RESEAUX
ROADTAX
ROLODEX
ROUBAIX
RSTUVWX

•R•X•••
BRAXTON
BRUXING
BRUXISM
DREXELU
DREXLER
DROXIES
PREXIES
PROXIES
PROXIMA
PROXIMO

•R••X••
MRFIXIT
URTEXTS

•R•••X•
ARANTXA
PRETEXT

•R••••X
ARONNAX
ARUSPEX
BRERFOX
BROADAX
BROWWAX
CRISPIX
DROPBOX
GRAVLAX
ORATRIX
TRIPLEX

••RX•••
MARXIAN
MARXISM
MARXIST
XERXESI

••R•X••
ABRAXAS
BAREXAM
HYRAXES
LUREXES
PYREXIA
XEROXED
XEROXES

••R••X•
AIRTAXI

••R•••X
BERVOIX
BUREAUX
FAREBOX
FIREBOX
FIREFOX
FORTDIX
GORETEX
HARDSIX
JURYBOX
MARGAUX
MIRAMAX
NARTHEX
PARADOX
PERPLEX
VERDOUX
WORKBOX

•••R•X•
ATARAXY
BYPROXY

•••R••X
BRERFOX
FAIRFAX
FAIRSEX
GEARBOX
MALRAUX
OVERFIX
OVERLAX
OVERMIX
OVERTAX
PHARYNX
POORBOX
POORTAX
STCROIX
THEROUX

••••R•X
ANTHRAX
APTERYX
ASTERIX
BEATRIX
COMTREX
EDITRIX
HENDRIX
HENDRYX
MEMOREX
ORATRIX
VICTRIX

•••••RX
LETTERX
LEXUSRX
MISTERX

RY•••••
RYEBEER
RYELOAF
RYOKANS
RYUKYUS

R•Y••••
RAYBANS
RAYBURN
RAYGUNS
RAYKROC
RAYLESS
RAYLIKE
RAYMOND
RAYNELL
RAYOVAC
REYMONT
REYNARD
REYNAUD
REYNOSA
REYOKED
REYOKES
RHYMERS
RHYMING
RHYMIST
RHYTHMS
ROYALES
ROYALLY
ROYALTY
ROYALWE
ROYBEAN
ROYCOHN
ROYGBIV
RUYBLAS

R••Y•••
RECYCLE
REDYING
REFYING
RELYING
RETYPED
RETYPES
RUBYDEE
RUBYRED
RUDYARD

R•••Y••
RALLYES
RALLYTO
REDDYES
REDEYED
REDEYES
REKEYED
RELAYED
RELAYER
REPLYTO
RESTYLE
RIBEYES
RITDYES
ROCKYII
ROCKYIV
RUFIYAA
RYUKYUS

R••••Y•
REDBAYS
REPLAYS
RICKEYS
RIDEBYS
ROBROYS
ROMNEYS
ROSALYN
RUNWAYS

R•••••Y
RABBITY
RABIDLY
RACEDBY
RACESBY
RACEWAY
RACKETY
RAGGEDY
RAILWAY
RAINILY
RAISINY
RANAWAY
RAPIDLY
RAUNCHY
RAVELLY
READILY
REALITY
REAPPLY
REASSAY
RECARRY
RECENCY
RECTIFY
RECTORY
REDARMY
REDCLAY
REDECAY
REDPONY
REENJOY
REENTRY
REGALLY
REGENCY
REIMPLY
REMARRY
RENALLY
RESPRAY
RESTUDY
RETALLY
RETIARY
REUNIFY
REVELRY
REVERDY
RIANTLY
RIBBONY
RICKETY
RIDESBY
RIDGWAY
RIFLERY
RIGHTLY
RIGIDLY
RISIBLY
RISKILY
RITZILY
RIVALRY
ROADWAY
ROBBERY
ROBOTRY
ROCKABY
ROCKERY
ROCKILY
ROGUERY
ROLLSBY
ROLLWAY
ROOKERY
ROOMILY
ROSEBAY
ROTAWAY
ROUGHLY
ROUNDLY
ROWDILY
ROXBURY
ROYALLY
ROYALTY
RUBBERY
RUDDILY
RULEDBY
RUNAWAY
RUNSDRY
RURALLY
RUSSETY
RUSTILY

•RY••••
BRYNNER
BRYUSOV
CRYBABY
CRYDOWN
CRYOGEN
CRYOVER
CRYPTIC
CRYPTOS
CRYSTAL
CRYWOLF
DRYABLE
DRYADES
DRYADIC
DRYBULB
DRYCELL
DRYDOCK
DRYEYED
DRYEYES
DRYFOGS
DRYHEAT
DRYHOLE
DRYIDEA
DRYMOPS
DRYNESS
DRYPERS
DRYROTS
DRYRUNS
DRYSUIT
DRYWALL
DRYWASH
DRYWELL
ERYNGOS
ERYTHRO
FRYABLE
FRYCOOK
FRYPANS
GRYPHON
HRYVNIA
KRYPTON
KRYSTLE
PRYINTO
PRYOPEN
TRYHARD
TRYITON
TRYOUTS
TRYSAIL
TRYSTED
TRYSTER
WRYNESS

•R•Y•••
ARGYLES
ARMYANT
BRAYERS
BRAYING
BREYERS
CRAYOLA
CRAYONS
DRAYAGE
DRAYING
DRAYMAN
DRAYMEN
DRAYTON
DREYFUS
FRAYING
FREYTAG
GRAYEST
GRAYING
GRAYISH
GRAYJAY
GRAYLAG
GRAYSON
GREYCUP
GREYEST
GREYHEN
GREYING
GREYISH
GREYLAG
GRUYERE
PRAYERS
PRAYFOR
PRAYING
PRAYSTO
PREYERS
PREYING
PREYSON
TRAYFUL
TRAYNOR
XRAYING
XRAYLAB

•R••Y••
ARRAYAL
ARRAYED
ARRAYER
ARROYOS
DRYEYED
DRYEYES
ERINYES
GROMYKO
PRETYPE
PRIVYTO
PROCYON

•R•••Y•
FRIDAYS
GRAMMYS
ORKNEYS
PREBUYS
PREPAYS

•R••••Y
ARCHERY
ARCHWAY
ARDENCY
AREAWAY
ARENSKY
ARIDITY
ARMOURY
BRADLEY
BRAMBLY
BRAMLEY
BRANCHY
BRASHLY
BRAVELY
BRAVERY
BRAWLEY
BREATHY
BREVITY
BREWERY
BRIBERY
BRIEFLY
BRIMLEY
BRISKLY
BRISTLY
BRITNEY
BROADLY
BRODKEY
BRODSKY
BRUTELY
CRACKLY
CRAFTSY
CRASSLY
CRAWLEY
CRAZILY
CREELEY
CREEPBY
CRIMINY
CRINKLY
CRISPLY
CROSSLY
CROWLEY
CRUDELY
CRUDITY
CRUELLY
CRUELTY
CRUMBLY
CRUMPLY
CRUNCHY
CRYBABY
DRAMADY
DRAMEDY
DRAPERY
DRIPDRY
DRIVEBY
DRIZZLY
DRMCCOY
DROPSBY
DROVEBY
DRWELBY
ERECTLY
EROSELY
ERRANCY
FRAILLY
FRAILTY
FRANKLY

7 RW

FRAWLEY
FRECKLY
FREETOY
FREEWAY
FRENEMY
FRESHLY
FRIARLY
FRIDLEY
FRIZZLY
GRANARY
GRANDLY
GRAPERY
GRATIFY
GRAVELY
GRAVITY
GRAYJAY
GREATLY
GREELEY
GREENLY
GREGORY
GRETZKY
GRIFFEY
GRIMILY
GRIMSBY
GRISTLY
GRIZZLY
GROCERY
GROSSLY
GROUCHY
GRUFFLY
GRUMBLY
IRATELY
MRBODDY
MRDARCY
MRHANEY
MRLUCKY
MRNANNY
ORANGEY
ORATORY
ORDERLY
OREBODY
OREILLY
ORGANDY
ORMANDY
OROGENY
OROLOGY
PREACHY
PREALLY
PREDEFY
PREDENY
PRELACY
PRESLEY
PRICILY
PRICKLY
PRIMACY
PRIMARY
PRIMELY
PRIVACY
PRIVILY
PRIVITY
PROBITY
PROCITY
PRODIGY
PROGENY
PRONAVY
PRONELY
PROSILY
PROSODY
PROUDLY
PRUDERY
TRACERY
TRAGEDY
TRAMWAY
TREACLY
TREMBLY
TRENARY
TRILOGY
TRINARY
TRINITY
TRITELY
TROLLEY
TROTSKY
TRUANCY
URGENCY
UROLOGY
URUGUAY
VRONSKY
WREATHY
WRIGGLY
WRIGLEY
WRINKLY
WRONGLY

••RY•••

ACRYLIC
BARYONS
BIRYANI
BURYING
CORYELL
CORYZAS
JURYBOX
JURYING
JURYMAN
JURYMEN
JURYRIG
MARYANN
MARYKAY
MARYLOU
MARYURE
PERYEAR
PHRYGIA
SPRYEST
TORYISH
TORYISM
VARYING
VERYBAD
VERYBIG
VERYDRY
VERYFEW
VERYFIT
VERYHIP
VERYHOT
VERYILL
VERYLOW
VERYMAD
VERYNEW
VERYODD
VERYOLD
VERYRED
VERYSAD
VERYSHY
VERYWET

••R•Y••

ARRAYAL
ARRAYED
ARRAYER
ARROYOS
CARLYLE
CARRYIN
CARRYON
DARRYLF
EARLYON
FORAYED
FORSYTE
FORSYTH
FORTYAD
FORTYBC
HURRYUP
MARRYAT
MARRYIN
MARRYME
MARTYRS
NARAYAN
NUREYEV
PARTYER
PARTYON
SAROYAN
SPRAYED
SPRAYER
SPRAYON
STRAYED
STRAYER
UNRAYED
UNRHYME

••R••Y•

ACRONYM
AIRWAYS
BARLEYS
BARNEYS
BERNAYS
BURSTYN
CARBOYS
CARKEYS
CAROLYN
DORSEYS
GURNEYS
HARLEYS
HURRAYS
JERILYN
JERSEYS
KAROLYI
MARILYN
MURPHYS
PARLAYS
PARLEYS
PARONYM
PURVEYS
SURREYS
SURVEYS
TURKEYS

••R•••Y

ACRIDLY
AIRPLAY
ALREADY
ATROPHY
AURALLY
BARBARY
BARCLAY
BARKLEY
BARNABY
BARTRAY
BERKLEY
BURNABY
BURNLEY
CARAWAY
CARDKEY
CARNABY
CARROTY
CERTIFY
CHRISTY
CIRCUSY
CORNILY
CURABLY
CURSORY
CURTSEY
DARESAY
DIRTILY
DOROTHY
DURABLY
EARTHLY
ERRANCY
FARADAY
FARAWAY
FARMBOY
FARMERY
FERNERY
FERRETY
FIREFLY
FIRSTLY
FORADAY
FOREBAY
FORGERY
FORTIFY
FTRILEY
GARBAGY
GERMANY
GIRLSHY
GYRALLY
HARDDAY
HARDILY
HARDWAY
HARMONY
HARSHLY
HARTLEY
HERONRY
HERSHEY
HORNSBY
HORRIFY
HORSILY
HORSLEY
IMREADY
JARGONY
JERKILY
KARLOVY
LARCENY
LARGELY
LURIDLY
MARGERY
MARYKAY
MCRANEY
MERCERY
MERCURY
MERRILY
MORALLY
MOREPAY
MORESBY
MORTIFY
MURKILY
NERVILY
NURSERY
PARKWAY
PARSLEY
PARTWAY
PERFIDY
PERFUMY
PERJURY
PERKILY
PORTNOY
PORTRAY
RURALLY
SCRAGGY
SCRAPPY
SCRAWLY
SCRAWNY
SCRIMPY
SCRUBBY
SCRUFFY
SHRILLY
SHRIMPY
SHRUBBY
SORCERY
SORRILY
SPRAWLY
SPRINGY
STREAKY
STRINGY
SURGERY
SURLILY
TARBABY
TARDILY
TARTILY
TERNARY
TERRIFY
TERSELY
THREADY
THRIFTY
THROATY
THRUWAY
TIREDLY
TORREFY
TURNERY
TURNKEY
TYRANNY
UNRAINY
UNRASPY
UNREADY
UNRISKY
UNROCKY
UNROOMY
UNROWDY
VARIETY
VARSITY
VERBIFY
VERMINY
VERSIFY
VERYDRY
VERYSHY
WARBABY
WORDILY
WORKDAY
WORKSHY
WORLDLY
WORSLEY

•••RY••

ANGRYAT
CAMRYLE
CARRYIN
CARRYON
DAIRYER
DARRYLF
DECRYPT
EMBRYOS
ENCRYPT
GLORYBE
HENRYII
HENRYIV
HENRYVI
HURRYUP
JIMRYUN
MARRYAT
MARRYIN
MARRYME
MEGRYAN
NEARYOU
PHARYNX

•••R•Y•

AFFRAYS
AYKROYD
BETRAYS
DEFRAYS
DELRAYS
ESTRAYS
EVERLYS
HAIRDYE
HOORAYS
HURRAYS
INTRAYS
OSPREYS
OVERDYE
ROBROYS
SUNRAYS
SURREYS

•••R••Y

AFARCRY
ALERTLY
ANARCHY
ANGRILY
ATARAXY
BLARNEY
BYPROXY
CARROTY
CHARILY
CHARITY
CHARLEY
CHURCHY
CLARIFY
CLARITY
CLERISY
CLERKLY
COURTLY
DEERFLY
DOORWAY
ENTROPY
EPARCHY
EPERNAY
FAIRWAY
FERRETY
FIERILY
FMURRAY
FOURDAY
FOURWAY
GLORIFY
GOCRAZY
HEARSAY
HOARILY
HORRIFY
INERTLY
JOURNEY
KEARNEY
LEERILY
LIBRARY
MCCRARY
MCGRORY
MERRILY
MISRELY
NITRIFY
OVERBUY
OVERCOY
OVERDRY
OVERFLY
OVERJOY
OVERLAY
OVERPAY
OVERPLY
OVERTLY
PETRIFY
POORBOY
PUTREFY
QUARTZY
SATRAPY
SCAREDY
SCARIFY
SCARILY
SECRECY
SHARKEY
SHARPLY
SHIRLEY
SHORTLY
SMARTLY
SORRILY
SPARELY
SPARKLY
STARCHY
STARKEY
STARKLY
STARSKY
STERNLY
STIRFRY
SWARTHY
SWOREBY
TEARILY
TERRIFY
THERAPY
THEREBY
THIRDLY
THIRSTY
TIERNEY
TORREFY
TOURNEY
UNCRAZY
UNTRULY
VITRIFY
WEARILY
WEIRDLY
WHEREBY

••••RY•

APTERYX
DMYTRYK
HENDRYX
IHEARYA
KATHRYN
MASARYK
STMARYS

••••R•Y

ACTORLY
ALDORAY
ALLERGY
AMSCRAY
ASAGRAY
ASHTRAY
AUTARKY
BARTRAY
BETARAY
BEVERLY
CINERGY
CLEARLY
CONFREY
DALTREY
DESTROY
DOHERTY
DUBARRY
EAGERLY
ELDERLY
ENDERBY
EPPERLY
EQUERRY
FAYWRAY
FITZROY
FMURRAY
FOGERTY
FRIARLY
GODFREY
HAGERTY
HEATRAY
ICETRAY
IMSORRY
INNERLY
ITHIRTY
JEFFREY
JOFFREY
LAMPREY
LIBERTY
LITURGY
LOVERLY
MALARKY
MCCAREY
MISERLY
MOWBRAY
MRDARCY
MTMARCY
NOMERCY
ORDERLY
OUTBRAY
OUTPRAY
OUTTRAY
PALFREY
PICARDY
PORTRAY
POVERTY
PUBERTY
QUEERLY
RECARRY
REDARMY
REMARRY
RESPRAY
REVERDY
SHEERLY
SOBERLY
SOSORRY
SQUIRMY
SWEARBY
SYNERGY
TEATRAY
THEARMY
THIERRY
UNBURLY
UNHARDY
UNMERRY
UNSORRY
UNSURLY
UNWORMY
UPEARLY
UTTERLY
VICEROY
VICKREY
VOUVRAY
WINFREY
ZYMURGY

•••••RY

ACTUARY
AFARCRY
AGENTRY
ALMONRY
AMATORY
ARCHERY
ARMOURY
ASHBERY
ASHBURY
BANBURY
BARBARY
BATTERY
BEANERY
BEGGARY
BIGOTRY
BINDERY
BLOWDRY
BONEDRY
BOOTERY
BRAVERY
BREWERY
BRIBERY
BUTTERY
CADBURY
CALGARY
CALVARY
CANNERY
CANONRY
CASPARY
CAVALRY
CENTURY
CHANTRY
CHICORY
CILIARY
CINDERY
CLOVERY
CONAKRY
CONJURY
CONNERY
COOKERY
COOPERY
COPPERY
COUNTRY
CURSORY
CUTLERY
DAMPDRY
DANBURY
DEANERY
DEEPFRY
DEVILRY
DICKORY
DIETARY
DIGGORY
DITHERY
DODDERY
DONTCRY
DRAPERY
DRIPDRY
DUBARRY
ELUSORY
ENQUIRY
EQUERRY
ESOTERY
ESTUARY
EXUPERY
FACTORY
FARMERY
FELONRY
FERNERY
FISHERY
FISHFRY
FLAVORY
FLOWERY
FOOLERY
FOPPERY
FORGERY
FOUNDRY
FTHENRY
GALLERY
GAUDERY
GINGERY
GOODTRY
GRANARY
GRAPERY
GREGORY
GROCERY
GUNNERY
HELOTRY
HENNERY
HERONRY
HICKORY
HILLARY
HISTORY
HOGGERY
HOSIERY
HUMPHRY
HUNGARY
HYMNARY
IMAGERY
IMSORRY
INAFURY
INQUIRY
JANUARY
JASPERY
JEWELRY
JIGGERY
JITTERY
JOBBERY
JOINERY
KILNDRY
KITTERY
KNAVERY
LANGTRY
LASTORY
LATHERY
LAUNDRY
LETTERY
LIBRARY
LINEDRY
LITTERY
LOTTERY
MARGERY
MASONRY
MASTERY
MCCRARY
MCGRORY
MCHENRY
MERCERY
MERCURY
MIMICRY
MOCKERY
MOTHERY
MUMMERY
MYSTERY
NECTARY
NEWBERY
NICETRY
NOENTRY
NONJURY
NUNNERY
NURSERY
ONAJURY
ORATORY
OSSUARY
OSTIARY
OVERDRY
PALEDRY
PALMARY
PATSDRY
PAULPRY
PECCARY
PEPPERY
PERJURY
PIGGERY
PILLORY
PLENARY
POTTERY
POULTRY
POWDERY
PRIMARY
PRUDERY
PUCKERY
PUFFERY
QUAVERY
QUINARY
QUIVERY
RECARRY
RECTORY
REENTRY
REMARRY
RETIARY
REVELRY
RIFLERY
RIVALRY
ROBBERY
ROBOTRY
ROCKERY
ROGUERY
ROOKERY
ROXBURY
RUBBERY
RUNSDRY
SAVOURY
SCENERY
SEALERY
SEMIDRY
SENSORY
SHIVERY
SHOWERY
SILVERY
SLAVERY
SORCERY
SOSORRY
SPICERY
SPIDERY
SPINDRY
STAYDRY
STIRFRY
SUCKDRY
SUDBURY
SUMMARY
SUMMERY
SURGERY
SWELTRY
SWINERY
TANNERY
TATTERY
TERNARY
THIERRY
TIMBERY
TINDERY
TOGGERY
TOPIARY
TOTTERY
TRACERY
TRENARY
TRINARY
TURNERY
TUSHERY
UNANGRY
UNCHARY
UNFIERY
UNHAIRY
UNITARY
UNMERRY
UNSORRY
UNWEARY
VAPOURY
VERYDRY
VICTORY
WAGGERY
WIGGERY
WINTERY
WOOLERY
ZACHARY

R•Z••••

RAZORED
RAZZIES
RAZZING
REZEROS
REZONED
REZONES
RIZZUTO
ROZANOV
ROZELLE
RUZICKA

R••Z•••

RAZZIES
RAZZING
REDZONE
RHIZOME
RITZIER
RITZILY
RIZZUTO
RONZONI

R•••Z••

REBOZOS
RENUZIT
RESIZED
RESIZER
RESIZES

R••••Z•

REALIZE
REGLAZE
RESEIZE

R•••••Z

RAMIREZ

•R•Z•••

ARIZONA
BRAZENS
BRAZIER
BRAZING
CRAZIER
CRAZIES
CRAZILY
CRAZING
CROZIER
CRUZADO
CRUZANS
DRIZZLE
DRIZZLY
DRUZEAN
DRUZIAN
FRAZIER
FRAZZLE
FRIZZED
FRIZZER
FRIZZES
FRIZZLE
FRIZZLY
FROZEUP
FROZONE
GRAZERS
GRAZIER
GRAZING
GRIZZLE
GRIZZLY
PRIZING
PRIZZIS

•R••Z••

BREEZED
BREEZES
BRONZED
BRONZER
BRONZES
CRUTZEN
DRIZZLE
DRIZZLY
FRAZZLE

FREEZER
FREEZES
FRIEZES
FRIZZED
FRIZZER
FRIZZES
FRIZZLE
FRIZZLY
GRETZKY
GRIZZLE
GRIZZLY
PRETZEL
PRIZZIS
TREIZES

•R•••Z•

BRASIZE
GRECIZE
ORGANZA
TRAPEZE

•R••••Z

FRANKOZ
GRISNEZ
ORDONEZ

••RZ•••

BORZAGE
BORZOIS
CORZINE
TARZANA
TARZANS
WARZONE

••R•Z••

ABRUZZI
CORAZON
CORYZAS
DAREZZO
HORIZON
SARAZEN
UNRAZED
VERIZON

••R••Z•

ABRUZZI
CARDOZO
CERVEZA
DAREZZO
FIRENZA
FIRENZE
FORENZA
FORSIZE
JERITZA
LORENZO

••R•••Z

AGRIBIZ
BERLIOZ
BERLITZ
HORVITZ
KERTESZ
LORENTZ
MARANTZ
MARQUEZ
NARVAEZ
TIRPITZ

•••RZ••

VIERZIG

•••R•Z•

CHORIZO
FABRIZI
GOCRAZY
IMPREZA
ODORIZE
QUARTZY
UNCRAZY
UNFROZE

•••R••Z

FLORENZ
LAURITZ
THERITZ

••••RZ•

SCHERZI
SCHERZO

••••R•Z

ALVAREZ
RAMIREZ

•••••RZ

BEDNORZ
LETTERZ

SA•••••

SAATCHI
SABADOS
SABBATH
SABERED
SABINES
SABRINA
SACCADE
SACHEMS
SACHETS
SACKERS
SACKFUL
SACKING
SACKOUT
SACKSUP
SACLIKE
SACQUES
SADCAFE
SADDENS
SADDEST
SADDLED
SADDLER
SADDLES
SADEYED
SADEYES
SADFATE
SADISTS
SADNESS
SADSACK
SADSONG
SAFARIS
SAFEBET
SAFEWAY
SAFFRON
SAGCARD
SAGEHEN
SAGETEA
SAGGIER
SAGGING
SAGIEST
SAGINAW
SAGUARO
SAHARAN
SAIDAAH
SAIDAYE
SAIDBOO
SAIDIDO
SAIDNAY
SAILERS
SAILING
SAILORS
SAILSON
SAILSTO
SAINTED
SAINTES
SAINTLO
SAINTLY
SAISONS
SALAAMS
SALABLE
SALADES
SALADIN
SALAMIS
SALAZAR
SALCHOW
SALEMOR
SALERNO
SALIENT
SALIERI
SALINAS
SALINES
SALIVAS
SALLIED
SALLIER
SALLIES
SALMONP
SALMONS
SALOMON
SALONGA
SALOONS
SALSODA
SALTANT
SALTBOX
SALTERS
SALTIER
SALTILY
SALTINE
SALTING
SALTISH
SALTPIT
SALTSEA
SALUKIS
SALUTED
SALUTER
SALUTES
SALVAGE
SALVERS
SALVING
SALVOES
SALVORS
SAMARAS
SAMARIA
SAMBAED
SAMBASS
SAMBORA
SAMBUCA
SAMEDAY
SAMEDIS
SAMEKHS
SAMEOLD
SAMHILL
SAMHUFF
SAMISEN
SAMLETS
SAMLOYD
SAMMYJO
SAMNUNN
SAMOANS
SAMOSAS
SAMOSET
SAMOVAR
SAMOYED
SAMPANS
SAMPLED
SAMPLER
SAMPLES
SAMPRAS
SAMPSON
SAMSONS
SAMSUNG
SAMUELL
SAMURAI
SAMWISE
SANBLAS
SANBORN
SANCTUM
SANCTUS
SANDALS
SANDBAG
SANDBAR
SANDBOX
SANDBUR
SANDDAB
SANDERS
SANDFLY
SANDHOG
SANDIER
SANDING
SANDLER
SANDLOT
SANDMAN
SANDMEN
SANDPIT
SANFORD
SANGOUT
SANGRIA
SANIBEL
SANJOSE
SANJUAN
SANREMO
SANSEIS
SANTAFE
SANTANA
SANTINI
SAOTOME
SAPHEAD
SAPIENS
SAPIENT
SAPLESS
SAPLING
SAPPERS
SAPPIER
SAPPILY
SAPPING
SAPPORO
SAPSAGO
SARACEN
SARALEE
SARANAC
SARAWAK
SARAZEN
SARCASM
SARDINE
SARGENT
SARNOFF
SARONGS
SAROYAN
SARTORS
SARUMAN
SASHAYS
SASHIMI
SASHING
SASSERS
SASSIER
SASSILY
SASSING
SASSOON
SATANIC
SATATOP
SATBACK
SATCHEL
SATCHMO
SATCOMS
SATDOWN
SATEENS
SATHOME
SATIATE
SATIETY
SATINET
SATINON
SATIRES
SATIRIC
SATISFY
SATORIS
SATRAPS
SATRAPY
SATSUMA
SATUPON
SATURNS
SATWELL
SATWITH
SATYRIC
SAUCERS
SAUCIER
SAUCILY
SAUCING
SAUCONY
SAUNAED
SAUNTER
SAURIAN
SAUSAGE
SAUTEED
SAVABLE
SAVAGED
SAVAGER
SAVAGES
SAVALAS
SAVANAS
SAVANNA
SAVANTS
SAVARIN
SAVEDON
SAVEDUP
SAVEFOR
SAVESON
SAVESUP
SAVINGS
SAVIORS
SAVIOUR
SAVORED
SAVORER
SAVOURS
SAVOURY
SAVVIED
SAVVIER
SAVVIES
SAVVILY
SAWATCH
SAWBUCK
SAWCHUK
SAWDUST
SAWFISH
SAWINTO
SAWLIKE
SAWLOGS
SAWMILL
SAWNOFF
SAWPAST
SAWPITS
SAWSOFF
SAWTOIT
SAWWOOD
SAWYERS
SAXHORN
SAXTUBA
SAYABLE
SAYAMEN
SAYHITO
SAYINGS
SAYMASS
SAYMORE
SAYNOTO
SAYOVER
SAYSAAH
SAYSAYE
SAYSBOO
SAYSIDO
SAYSNAY
SAYSWHO
SAYSYES
SAYSYOU
SAYWAIT
SAYWHAT
SAYWHEN

S•A••••

SAATCHI
SCACCHI
SCADSOF
SCALAGE
SCALARS
SCALDED
SCALDER
SCALENE
SCALERS
SCALEUP
SCALIER
SCALING
SCALLOP
SCALPED
SCALPEL
SCALPER
SCAMMED
SCAMMER
SCAMPED
SCAMPER
SCANDAL
SCANNED
SCANNER
SCANTED
SCANTER
SCANTLY
SCAPULA
SCARABS
SCARCER
SCAREDY
SCARERS
SCAREUP
SCARFED
SCARFER
SCARFUP
SCARIER
SCARIFY
SCARILY
SCARING
SCARLET
SCARPED
SCARRED
SCARVES
SCARWID
SCATHED
SCATHES
SCATMAN
SCATTED
SCATTER
SDAKOTA
SEAARMS
SEABAGS
SEABASS
SEABEDS
SEABEES
SEABIRD
SEABLUE
SEABOAT
SEABORG
SEACALM
SEACATS
SEACOWS
SEADOGS
SEADUCK
SEADUTY
SEAEELS
SEAFARE
SEAFERN
SEAFOAM
SEAFOOD
SEAFOWL
SEAGATE
SEAGIRT
SEAGODS
SEAGRAM
SEAGREN
SEAGULL
SEAHAWK
SEAHERO
SEAHUNT
SEALABS
SEALANE
SEALANT
SEALEGS
SEALERS
SEALERY
SEALIFE
SEALIFT
SEALIKE
SEALILY
SEALING
SEALION
SEALOFF
SEALSIN
SEALSUP
SEAMAPS
SEAMERS
SEAMIER
SEAMILE
SEAMING
SEAMIST
SEAMOSS
SEANCES
SEAPORT
SEARACE
SEARERS
SEARING
SEASALT
SEASICK
SEASIDE
SEASLUG
SEASONS
SEASTAR
SEATERS
SEATING
SEATRIP
SEATTLE
SEAWALL
SEAWARD
SEAWAYS
SEAWEED
SEAWOLF
SHABBAT
SHACKED
SHACKLE
SHADERS
SHADIER
SHADILY
SHADING
SHADOWS
SHADOWY
SHADROE
SHAFFER
SHAFTED
SHAGGED
SHAGRUG
SHAHDOM
SHAKERS
SHAKEUP
SHAKIER
SHAKILY
SHAKING
SHAKIRA
SHAKOES
SHALALA
SHALIER
SHALLOT
SHALLOW
SHALLWE
SHALOMS
SHAMANS
SHAMBLE
SHAMING
SHAMMED
SHAMPOO
SHANANA
SHANGRI
SHANKAR
SHANKED
SHANNEN
SHANNON
SHANTER
SHAPELY
SHAPERS
SHAPEUP
SHAPING
SHAPIRO
SHAREIN
SHARERS
SHARING
SHARKEY
SHARONA
SHARPED
SHARPEI
SHARPEN
SHARPER
SHARPIE
SHARPLY
SHASTRI
SHATNER
SHATTER
SHAVERS
SHAVIAN
SHAVING
SHAVUOT
SHAWLED
SHAWNEE
SIAMESE
SKAGWAY
SKATERS
SKATING
SLABBED
SLACKED
SLACKEN
SLACKER
SLACKLY
SLACKUP
SLAKERS
SLAKING
SLALOMS
SLAMMED
SLAMMER
SLAMSON
SLANDER
SLANTED
SLANTLY
SLANTUP
SLAPPED
SLAPPER
SLAPSON
SLASHED
SLASHER
SLASHES
SLATERS
SLATHER
SLATIER
SLATING
SLATKIN
SLATTED
SLAVERS
SLAVERY
SLAVING
SLAVISH
SLAYERS
SLAYING
SLAYTON
SMACKED
SMACKER
SMACKOF
SMACKUP
SMALLAD
SMALLER
SMALLOJ
SMARTED
SMARTEN
SMARTER
SMARTLY
SMASHED
SMASHER
SMASHES
SMASHUP
SMATTER
SNACKED
SNACKER
SNACKON
SNAFUED
SNAGGED
SNAGGER
SNAGSUP
SNAKERS
SNAKIER
SNAKILY
SNAKING
SNAPONS
SNAPPEA
SNAPPED
SNAPPER
SNAPPLE
SNAPSAT
SNAPSON
SNAPSTO
SNAPSUP
SNARERS
SNARFED
SNARING
SNARLAT
SNARLED
SNARLER
SNARLUP
SNAZZUP
SOAKERS
SOAKING
SOAKSIN
SOAKSUP
SOANDSO
SOAPBOX
SOAPERS
SOAPIER
SOAPILY
SOAPING
SOAPNET
SOAPPAD
SOAPSUP
SOARERS
SOAREWE
SOARING
SPACELY
SPACERS
SPACIAL
SPACIER
SPACING
SPACKLE
SPADERS
SPADING
SPAMBOT
SPAMMED
SPAMMER
SPANAIR
SPANDEX
SPANGLE
SPANGLY
SPANIEL
SPANISH
SPANKED
SPANKER
SPANNED
SPANNER
SPARELY
SPAREME
SPARERS
SPAREST
SPARING
SPARKED
SPARKLE
SPARKLY
SPARRED
SPARRER
SPARROW
SPARSER
SPARTAN
SPASSKY
SPATHES
SPATIAL
SPATOUT
SPATTED
SPATTER
SPATULA
SPAWNED
SPAWNER
SPAYERS
SPAYING
STABBED
STABBER
STABILE
STABLED
STABLER
STABLES
STACKED
STACKER
STACKUP
STADIUM
STADLER
STAFFED
STAFFER
STAGERS
STAGGED
STAGGER
STAGIER
STAGILY
STAGING
STAGNES
STAIDER
STAIDLY
STAINED
STAINER
STAIRED
STAKING
STALAGS
STALELY
STALEST
STALKED
STALKER
STALLED
STALLER
STAMENS
STAMINA
STAMMER
STAMPED
STAMPER
STANCES
STANDBY
STANDEE
STANDER
STANDIN
STANDON
STANDTO
STANDUP
STANINE
STANKUP
STANLEE
STANLEY
STANNIC
STANNUM
STANTON
STANZAS
STAPLED
STAPLER
STAPLES
STARCHY
STARDOM
STAREAT
STARERS
STARING
STARION
STARKER
STARKEY
STARKLY
STARLET
STARLIT
STARLOG
STARMAN
STARMAP
STARRED
STARSIN
STARSKY
STARTED
STARTER
STARTIN
STARTLE
STARTON
STARTTO
STARTUP
STARVED
STARVES
STASHED
STASHES
STASSEN
STATELY
STATERS
STATICE
STATICS
STATING
STATINS
STATION
STATISM
STATIST
STATLER
STATORS
STATUES
STATURE
STATUTE
STAUNCH
STAVING
STAYDRY
STAYERS
STAYFOR
STAYING
STAYOFF
STAYOUT
STAYPUT
STAYSAT
STAYSIN
STAYSON
STAYSUP
SUASION
SUASIVE
SUAVELY
SUAVEST
SUAVITY
SWABBED
SWABBER
SWADDLE
SWAGGER
SWAGMAN
SWAGMEN
SWAHILI
SWALLOW
SWAMPED
SWANKED
SWANKER
SWANKUP
SWANSEA
SWANSON
SWAPPED
SWAPPER
SWARMED
SWARMER
SWARTHY
SWASHED
SWASHES
SWATHED
SWATHES
SWATSAT
SWATTED
SWATTER
SWAYBAR
SWAYERS
SWAYING

S••A•••

SABADOS
SAFARIS
SAHARAN
SALAAMS
SALABLE
SALADES
SALADIN
SALAMIS
SALAZAR
SAMARAS

SAMARIA
SARACEN
SARALEE
SARANAC
SARAWAK
SARAZEN
SATANIC
SATATOP
SAVABLE
SAVAGED
SAVAGER
SAVAGES
SAVALAS
SAVANAS
SAVANNA
SAVANTS
SAVARIN
SAWATCH
SAYABLE
SAYAMEN
SCHAYES
SCIATIC
SCLAFFS
SCRAGGY
SCRAPED
SCRAPER
SCRAPES
SCRAPPY
SCRATCH
SCRAWLS
SCRAWLY
SCRAWNY
SEAARMS
SECANTS
SEDALIA
SEDATED
SEDATER
SEDATES
SEEABLE
SEEALSO
SEMANAS
SENATES
SENATOR
SEPALED
SERAPES
SERAPHS
SERAPIS
SESAMES
SEWARDS
SHEAFED
SHEARED
SHEARER
SHEATHE
SHEATHS
SHEAVED
SHEAVES
SHIATSU
SHOALED
SHYAWAY
SINATRA
SITATOP
SIZABLE
SIZABLY
SKIABLE
SKIAREA
SLEAZES
SMEAGOL
SMEARED
SMEARER
SMEARON
SNEAKBY
SNEAKED
SNEAKER
SNEAKIN
SNEAKUP
SODACAN
SODAPOP
SOFABED
SOFARAS
SOHAVEI
SOLACED
SOLACER
SOLACES
SOLARAS
SOLARIA
SOMALIA
SOMALIS
SOMATIC
SONANCE
SONATAS
SPEAKER
SPEAKOF
SPEAKTO
SPEAKUP
SPEARED
SPEARER
SPLASHY
SPLAYED
SPRAINS
SPRAWLS
SPRAWLY
SPRAYED
SPRAYER
SPRAYON
SQUALID
SQUALLS
SQUALLY
SQUALOR
SQUANTO
SQUARED
SQUARER
SQUARES
SQUASHY
SQUATLY
SQUATTY
SQUAWKS
SQUAWKY
SSHAPED
STBARTS
STBASIL
STEADED
STEALER
STEALIN
STEALTH
STEAMED
STEAMER
STEAMUP
STEANNE
STEARIC
STEARIN
STEARNS
STJAMES
STMARKS
STMARYS
STPAULS
STRAFED
STRAFER
STRAFES
STRAINS
STRAITS
STRANDS
STRANGE
STRAPIN
STRAPON
STRASSE
STRATAS
STRATUM
STRATUS
STRAUSS
STRAYED
STRAYER
STUARTI
SUBAREA
SUBARID
SUBARUS
SUDAFED
SUGARED
SUHARTO
SUKARNO
SUMATRA
SUSANNA
SUSANNE
SUZANNE
SWEARAT
SWEARBY
SWEARER
SWEARIN
SWEARTO
SWEATED
SWEATER
SWEATIT
SYNAPSE

S•••A••

SABBATH
SACCADE
SADCAFE
SADFATE
SADSACK
SAGCARD
SAGUARO
SAIDAAH
SAIDAYE
SALAAMS
SALTANT
SALVAGE
SAMBAED
SAMBASS
SAMOANS
SAMPANS
SANDALS
SANTAFE
SANTANA
SAPSAGO
SARCASM
SASHAYS
SATBACK
SATIATE
SATRAPS
SATRAPY
SAUNAED
SAUSAGE
SAWPAST
SAYMASS
SAYSAAH
SAYSAYE
SAYWAIT
SCALAGE
SCALARS
SCARABS
SCHNAPS
SCHWANN
SCOLARI
SCREAKS
SCREAMS
SCUBAED
SEABAGS
SEABASS
SEACALM
SEACATS
SEAFARE
SEAGATE
SEAHAWK
SEALABS
SEALANE
SEALANT
SEAMAPS
SEARACE
SEASALT
SEAWALL
SEAWARD
SEAWAYS
SEENALL
SEEPAGE
SEEPAST
SEESALL
SEESAWS
SEGWAYS
SELMAAL
SELVAGE
SENSATE
SERFAGE
SERIALS
SERIATE
SERRATE
SERVANT
SETBACK
SETBAIL
SETRATE
SETSAIL
SEXTANS
SEXTANT
SHALALA
SHAMANS
SHANANA
SHEBANG
SHEPARD
SHEVATS
SHOFARS
SIDEARM
SIGNAGE
SIGNALS
SIMIANS
SINKAGE
SINUATE
SIOUANS
SITBACK
SITUATE
SIXBALL
SIXLANE
SIXPACK
SKICAPS
SKIHATS
SKIMASK
SKIRACE
SKIRACK
SKYCAMS
SKYCAPS
SKYJACK
SKYLARK
SKYMAPS
SKYWALK
SKYWARD
SKYWAYS
SLOGANS
SLOVAKS
SMETANA
SNOBALL
SNOCAPS
SNOCATS
SOCIALS
SOILAGE
SOLLATI
SOLOACT
SOPRANI
SOPRANO
SORBATE
SORIANO
SOSPADS
SOURALE
SOXFANS
SPANAIR
SPINACH
SPIRALS
SPOKANE
SPREADS
SPYCAMS
SPYWARE
SQUEAKS
SQUEAKY
SQUEALS
STALAGS
STEFANI
STEWARD
STEWART
STOMACH
STOMATA
STORAGE
STOWAGE
STREAKS
STREAKY
STREAMS
STRIATE
SUBBAND
SUBBANK
SUBBASE
SUBBASS
SUBCASE
SUBCASH
SUBCAST
SUBDATE
SUBHALL
SUBRACE
SUBTASK
SUBWARS
SUBWAYS
SUCRASE
SULFATE
SULTANA
SULTANS
SUMMAND
SUMMARY
SUMMATE
SUNBATH
SUNDAES
SUNDAYS
SUNFANS
SUNFAST
SUNHATS
SUNLAMP
SUNMAID
SUNRAYS
SUNTANS
SUNWARD
SURFACE
SURNAME
SURPASS
SUSTAIN
SYLLABI
SYRIANA
SYRIANS
SZILARD

S••••A•

SAFEWAY
SAGINAW
SAHARAN
SAIDAAH
SAIDNAY
SALAZAR
SALINAS
SALIVAS
SAMARAS
SAMEDAY
SAMOSAS
SAMOVAR
SAMPRAS
SAMURAI
SANBLAS
SANDBAG
SANDBAR
SANDDAB
SANDMAN
SANJUAN
SAPHEAD
SARANAC
SARAWAK
SAROYAN
SARUMAN
SAURIAN
SAVALAS
SAVANAS
SAYSAAH
SAYSNAY
SAYWHAT
SCANDAL
SCATMAN
SCHEMAS
SCHMEAR
SCHOLAR
SCLERAE
SCLERAL
SCLERAS
SCOFFAT
SCOOBAS
SCORIAS
SCOTIAN
SEABOAT
SEAFOAM
SEAGRAM
SEASTAR
SECULAR
SEDONAS
SEISMAL
SELMAAL
SEMANAS
SEMINAL
SEMINAR
SEMIRAW
SENECAN
SENECAS
SENEGAL
SENORAS
SENSUAL
SENTRAS
SEPHIAS
SEPIRAS
SERBIAN
SERIPAK
SERVEAS
SETPLAY
SEVENAD
SEVENAM
SEVERAL
SHABBAT
SHANKAR
SHAVIAN
SHEBEAR
SHECRAB
SHEEHAN
SHEGOAT
SHEILAE
SHEILAS
SHELLAC
SHERMAN
SHERPAS
SHINPAD
SHIPMAN
SHIPWAY
SHOEPAC
SHOOTAT
SHOPSAT
SHOTPAR
SHOUTAT
SHOWCAT
SHOWMAN
SHULMAN
SHYAWAY
SICKBAY
SICKDAY
SICKPAY
SIDEBAR
SIDECAR
SIDEMAN
SIDEWAY
SIENNAS
SIERRAS
SIESTAS
SIGHSAT
SILICAS
SILKHAT
SIMILAC
SIMILAR
SINDBAD
SINUTAB
SIOBHAN
SITEMAP
SITSPAT
SIXTYAD
SIXYEAR
SKAGWAY
SKIWEAR
SLOTCAR
SLOWDAY
SMALLAD
SMILEAT
SMILLAS
SNAPSAT
SNARLAT
SNEERAT
SNIFFAT
SNIPEAT
SNORTAT
SNOWCAP
SNOWCAT
SNOWDAY
SNOWHAT
SNOWMAN
SOAPPAD
SODACAN
SOFARAS
SOLARAS
SOLEDAD
SOMEDAY
SOMESAY
SOMEWAY
SONATAS
SONORAN
SORORAL
SOULMAN
SOUPCAN
SOWSEAR
SOYBEAN
SOYMEAL
SPACIAL
SPARTAN
SPATIAL
SPECIAL
SPHERAL
SPIREAS
SPORRAN
SPOUSAL
STANZAS
STAREAT
STARMAN
STARMAP
STAYSAT
STELIAS
STELLAR
STEPDAD
STERNAL
STEWPAN
STIGMAS
STOICAL
STONEAX
STOPGAP
STOPSAT
STRATAS
STYGIAN
SUBBIAS
SUBCLAN
SUBDUAL
SUBGOAL
SUBHEAD
SUNBEAM
SUNDIAL
SUNSFAN
SURECAN
SUREIAM
SURFMAN
SURINAM
SURREAL
SWAGMAN
SWATSAT
SWAYBAR
SWEARAT
SWINGAT
SWOREAT
SWUNGAT
SYNGMAN
SYNODAL
SZYSLAK

S•••••A

SABRINA
SAGETEA
SALONGA
SALSODA
SALTSEA
SAMARIA
SAMBORA
SAMBUCA
SANGRIA
SANTANA
SATSUMA
SAVANNA
SAXTUBA
SCAPULA
SCHIRRA
SCIORRA
SDAKOTA
SEDALIA
SEGOVIA
SENHORA
SEQUOIA
SEQUOYA
SESTINA
SETENTA
SEVILLA
SHAKIRA
SHALALA
SHANANA
SHARONA
SHINOLA
SHOULDA
SIBERIA
SICILIA
SIGNORA
SILENTA
SILESIA
SINATRA
SKIAREA
SMETANA
SNAPPEA
SNOWPEA
SOLARIA
SOMALIA
SOYINKA
SPATULA
SPECTRA
SPINOZA
SPLENDA
STAMINA
STLUCIA
STOMATA
SUBAREA
SUBIDEA
SUBROSA
SULTANA
SULUSEA
SUMATRA
SUSANNA
SWANSEA
SWEEPEA
SYRIANA

•SA••••

ASABODY
ASAGIFT
ASAGRAY
ASAJOKE
ASALARK
ASANTES
ASARULE
ASATEAM
CSARDAS
ISABEAU
ISADORA
ISADORE
ISAHEAD
ISAIDNO
OSAKANS
PSALMIC
PSALTER
PSANDOS
TSARDOM
TSARINA
TSARISM
TSARIST
USABLES
USANCES
XSANDOS

•S•A•••

ASCARED
ASFARAS
ASHAMED
ASHANTI
ASIAGOS
ASIATIC
ASKANCE
ASKAWAY
ASMARAN
ASSAILS
ASSANTE
ASSAULT
ASSAYED
ASSAYER
ASTAIRE
ASTARTE
ESCALOP
ESCALUS
ESCAPED
ESCAPEE
ESCAPER
ESCAPES
ESCARPS
ESIASON
ESPANOL
ESPARTO
ESSAYED
ESSAYER
ESTADOS
ESTAMIN
ESTATED
ESTATES
ISFAHAN
ISLAMIC
ISLANDS
ISRAELI
ISRAFEL
LSHAPED
OSHAPED
OSMATIC
PSHAWED
SSHAPED
TSHAPED
TSHAPES
USHAPED
USHAPES
USUALLY
VSHAPED
VSHAPES
YSHAPED
YSHAPES

•S••A••

ASALARK
ASBYATT
ASHCAKE
ASHCANS
ASHLAND
ASHLARS
ASHPANS
ASHRAMS
ASISAID
ASONANT
ASPHALT
ASPRAWL
ASSHARP
ASSUAGE
ESPIALS
ESTRADA
ESTRAYS
ESTUARY
ISHMAEL
ISITAGO
ISOBARS
ISOLATE
ISOLATO
ISSUANT
OSAKANS
OSSUARY
OSTIARY
OSTMARK
OSTRAVA
OSTWALD
PSYWARS
TSQUARE
TSTRAPS
TSUNAMI
USFLAGS
USGRANT
USSTATE

•S•••A•

ASAGRAY
ASATEAM
ASEXUAL
ASFARAS
ASHHEAP
ASHTRAY
ASKAWAY
ASMARAN
ASOCIAL
ASSTDAS
ASTHMAS
ASTOLAT
ASTREAM
ASUSUAL
CSARDAS
ESCHEAT
ESPOSAS
ESTEBAN
ESTEFAN
ESTIVAL
ISABEAU
ISAHEAD
ISCHIAL
ISFAHAN
ISOGRAM
ISSUEAD
ISTRIAN
ISUREAM
OSCULAR
OSETRAS
OSIRIAN
TSONGAS
USEDCAR

•S••••A

ASSUNTA
ASSYRIA
ASTORIA
ESCUELA
ESTELLA
ESTONIA
ESTRADA
ISADORA
OSCEOLA
OSSETRA
OSTRAVA
TSARINA

••SA•••

ABSALOM
AKSAKOV
ALSATIA
ASSAILS
ASSANTE
ASSAULT
ASSAYED
ASSAYER
AUSABLE
BASALLY
BASALTS
CASABAS
CASAVAS
CESAIRE
DESALTS
DISABLE
DISARMS
DISAVOW
DOSADOS
DOSAGES
ESSAYED
ESSAYER
HASACOW
HASAFIT
HASAGAS
HASANIP
HASAROW
HASASAY
HASASET
HASATIT
HOSANNA
IDSAYSO
INSALES
INSANER
ITSABOY
ITSAHIT
ITSALIE
ITSALOT
ITSASIN
ITSATIE
LASAGNA
LASAGNE
LASALLE
LESABRE
LISAGAY
LOSABLE
MASARYK
MESAMIS
MISACTS
MISADDS
MISAIMS
MISALLY
MISAVER
MOSAICS
MUSANTE
NASALLY
ONSAGER
PASALLE
PESADES
PESANTE
PISANIO
PISARRO
POSABLE
POSADAS
RESALES
RESALTS
RESANDS
RESAVED
RESAVES
RESAWED
ROSABUD
ROSALIA
ROSALIE
ROSALYN
ROSANNA
ROSANNE
ROSARIO
SESAMES
SUSANNA
SUSANNE
TISANES
UNSADLY
UNSAFER
UNSALTY
UNSATED
UNSAVED
UNSAVVY
UNSAWED
VISAGED

VISAGES
VISAING
VISALIA
VISAVIS
VISAYAN
WASABIS
WASATCH

••S•A••

ABSTAIN
ADSPACE
ALSHAIN
ANSPACH
ASSHARP
ASSUAGE
ATSTAKE
BASMATI
BASSALE
BASSANI
BASSANO
BISTATE
BOSCAGE
BUSFARE
BUSLANE
BUSMANS
BUSPASS
BUSTARD
CASCADE
CASEATE
CASPARY
CASSABA
CASSATT
CASSAVA
CASUALS
CISEAUX
COSSACK
COSTAIN
COSTARD
COSTARS
COSTATE
CTSCANS
CUSHAWS
CUSPATE
CUSTARD
DASTARD
DESCANT
DESPAIR
DESTAEL
DESTAIN
DISBAND
DISBARS
DISCARD
DISDAIN
DISEASE
DISMALS
DISMAST
DISMAYS
DISPART
DISRATE
DISTAFF
DISTANT
DOSSALS
ECSTASY
ENSEALS
ENSEATS
ENSLAVE
ENSNARE
ENSNARL
EUSTACE
GASBAGS
GASCANS
GASCAPS
GASLAMP
GASMAIN
GASMASK
GASPARD
GASTANK
GASWARS
GESTALT
GESTAPO
GESTATE
GISCARD
GOSHAWK
GOSSAGE
GOSTALE
GUSTAVE
HESSAFE
HISPANO
HOSCALE
HOSTAGE
HUSBAND
HUSHABY
HUSSARS
INSCALE
INSEAMS
INSHAPE
INSPACE
INSPANS
INSTALL
INSTALS
INSTANT
INSTATE
ISSUANT
ITSEASY
ITSLATE
LASCALA
LASCARS
LASCAUX
LASTACT
LESCAUT
LESPAUL
LOSTART
MASCARA
MASSAGE
MCSHANE
MESCALS
MESHACH
MESSAGE
MESSALA
MISCALL
MISCAST
MISDATE
MISGAVE
MISHAPS
MISLAID
MISLAYS
MISMARK
MISMATE
MISNAME
MISPAGE
MISRATE
MISSAID
MISSALS
MISSAYS
MISTAKE
MOSCATO
MRSBASS
MRSLATE
MRSPAUL
MUSCATS
MUSTAFA
MUSTANG
MUSTARD
MYSPACE
MYSTARS
NASTASE
NESCAFE
NISSANS
NISSANZ
NOSEATS
NOSTAIN
NOSTARS
OISEAUX
ONSTAFF
ONSTAGE
OSSUARY
PASSADE
PASSADO
PASSAGE
PASSAIC
PASSANT
PASSATS
POSTAGE
RASCALS
RESCALE
RESCANS
RESEALS
RESEAMS
RESEATS
RESEAUS
RESEAUX
RESHAPE
RESHARE
RESHAVE
RESLATE
RESNAIS
RESNAPS
RESOAKS
RESOAPS
RESPACE
RESPADE
RESPANS
RESPARK
RESTABS
RESTACK
RESTAFF
RESTAGE
RESTAIN
RESTAMP
RESTART
RESTATE
ROSEATE
ROSSANO
ROSTAND
SASHAYS
SOSPADS
SUSTAIN
TESTACY
TESTATE
TOSCALE
TOSPARE
TOSTADA
TOSTART
TUSCANS
TUSCANY
TUSSAUD
TVSTARS
UNSCALY
UNSEALS
UNSEAMS
UNSEATS
UNSHADE
UNSHADY
UNSHARP
UNSLACK
UNSLAIN
UNSMART
UNSNAGS
UNSNAKY
UNSNAPS
UNSNARL
UNSPANS
UNSTACK
UNSTAGY
UNSTAID
UNSTATE
UPSCALE
UPSOARS
UPSTAGE
UPSTAIR
UPSTAND
UPSTARE
UPSTART
UPSTATE
USSTATE
VASSALS
VESTALS
VISTAED
VISUALS
WASFAIR
WASLATE
WASSAIL
WASTAGE
YESMAAM

••S••A•

ALSORAN
AMSCRAY
ARSENAL
ASSTDAS
AUSTRAL
BASEMAN
BASEPAY
BASINAL
BASSSAX
BESMEAR
BESPEAK
BESTIAL
BESTMAN
BOSNIAN
BOSSMAN
BUSHMAN
BUSHWAH
BUSLOAD
CASABAS
CASAVAS
CASELAW
CASHBAR
CASITAS
CASPIAN
CASSIAS
CESSNAS
DISCMAN
DISHPAN
DISHRAG
DISPLAY
DRSLOAN
DUSTMAN
DUSTPAN
DUSTRAG
EASTHAM
EASTMAN
FASCIAE
FASCIAL
FASCIAS
FASTCAR
FUSTIAN
FUSUMAS
GASHEAT
GASLEAK
GASSMAN
HASAGAS
HASASAY
HESHVAN
HESSIAN
INSOFAR
INSTEAD
INSULAR
ISSUEAD
ITSOKAY
KOSOVAR
LASTGAS
LASTLAP
LASTMAY
LESSFAT
LESSTAR
LISAGAY
LOSTCAT
LUSTRAL
MESSIAH
MISDEAL
MISDIAL
MISDRAW
MISHEAR
MISHNAH
MISLEAD
MISPLAN
MISPLAY
MISREAD
MISSEAT
MISTRAL
MTSINAI
MUSICAL
MUSKRAT
NESSMAN
NOSEBAG
NOSEGAY
NOSUGAR
NOSWEAT
PASCHAL
PESETAS
PESEWAS
PISCEAN
POSADAS
POSEDAS
POSESAS
POSTBAG
POSTMAN
POSTWAR
QBSNEAK
RESPEAK
RESPRAY
RESTRAP
RESWEAR
ROSEBAY
ROSTRAL
RUSSIAN
RUSSLAN
TASKBAR
TESTBAN
TESTLAB
UNSPEAK
UNSTRAP
UNSWEAR
URSULAK
VESTRAL
VISAYAN
VOSGIAN
WASHDAY
WASHRAG
WISEMAN
YASHMAK
YESDEAR
YESICAN
YESMAAM

••S•••A

ALSATIA
ANSONIA
ASSUNTA
ASSYRIA
AUSTRIA
CASELLA
CASERTA
CASSABA
CASSAVA
CASSOLA
DASILVA
DESPINA
DESYLVA
FESTINA
FESTIVA
HOSANNA
INSECTA
JESSICA
JOSEPHA
KOSCINA
KOSHIBA
LASAGNA
LASCALA
LASORDA
MASCARA
MESHUGA
MESSALA
MESSINA
MISHIMA
MISSUSA
MUSCIDA
MUSETTA
MUSTAFA
NOSEBRA
OBSCURA
OSSETRA
PASTINA
RASBORA
RASHIDA
RESIDUA
ROSALIA
ROSANNA
ROSELLA
ROSEOLA
ROSETEA
ROSETTA
ROSSSEA
SESTINA
SUSANNA
TESSERA
TOSHIBA
TOSTADA
VISALIA
VISCERA
VISTULA
YASHICA
YESHIVA
ZOSSIMA

•••SA••

ADDSALT
AGESAGO
AIRSACS
ANASAZI
ARTSALE
ASISAID
AZUSACA
BALSAMS
BALSAMY
BASSALE
BASSANI
BASSANO
BIGSALE
BOWSAWS
BURSARS
CAESARS
CARSALE
CASSABA
CASSATT
CASSAVA
COMSATS
CORSAGE
CORSAIR
COSSACK
CRUSADE
DAYSAIL
DOGSAGE
DORSALS
DOSSALS
EGGSACS
FAISALI
FORSAKE
FORSALE
GETSANA
GETSANF
GOESAFT
GOESAPE
GOSSAGE
HANSARP
HESSAFE
HUSSARS
IBNSAUD
INKSACS
JIGSAWS
KANSANS
LAPSANG
LHASANS
LUGSAIL
MANSARD
MARSALA
MASSAGE
MENSANS
MESSAGE
MESSALA
MIASARA
MISSAID
MISSALS
MISSAYS
NAYSAID
NAYSAYS
NISSANS
NISSANZ
NONSALE
NONSANE
NOTSAFE
ODDSARE
OILSAND
OLDSALT
OLDSAWS
OUTSAID
OUTSAIL
OUTSANG
OUTSAYS
OVISACS
PAISANO
PAISANS
PASSADE
PASSADO
PASSAGE
PASSAIC
PASSANT
PASSATS
PEASANT
PIESAFE
PIESALE
PITSAWS
PRESAGE
PRESALE
PRESALT
PROSAIC
PULSARS
PULSATE
QUASARS
RANSACK
RIPSAWN
RIPSAWS
ROBSART
RONSARD
ROSSANO
SADSACK
SAPSAGO
SAUSAGE
SAYSAAH
SAYSAYE
SEASALT
SEESALL
SEESAWS
SENSATE
SETSAIL
TAGSALE
TARSALS
TAXSALE
THESACK
THESAME
TOPSAIL
TRYSAIL
TULSANS
TULSAOK
TUSSAUD
UPPSALA
VANSANT
VASSALS
VERSACE
VERSANT
WASSAIL
WHOSAID

•••S•A•

ABYSMAL
ABYSSAL
ALASKAN
ALASKAS
ALASSAD
ALLSTAR
ALMSMAN
AMESLAN
AMISTAD
ARISTAE
ARISTAS
ASUSUAL
AVESTAN
AVESTAS
BARSOAP
BASSSAX
BATSMAN
BEESWAX
BIGSTAR
BORSTAL
BOSSMAN
BOXSEAT
BROSNAN
BUQSHAS
CAPSHAW
CAPSTAN
CARSEAT
CASSIAS
CATSCAN
CATSPAW
CESSNAS
CHASMAL
COASTAL
CRASHAW
CROSSAT
CRUSTAL
CRYSTAL
CUBSFAN
CUESTAS
CUMSHAW
CURSEAT
DAYSPAS
DAYSTAR
DOESBAD
DOGSEAR
DOGSTAR
DRESSAS
DRISTAN
DUNSTAN
ELYSIAN
ETESIAN
FIESTAS
FRESCAS
FRISIAN
FURSEAL
GASSMAN
GEISHAS
GETSFAR
GETSMAD
GLOSSAE
GLOSSAL
GLOSSAS
GOESBAD
GOESFAR
GOESMAD
GRASPAT
GRESHAM
GRISHAM
GUESSAT
HEISMAN
HESSIAN
HOTSEAT
HOUSMAN
HOUSSAY
INASNAP
JETSFAN
JETSTAR
KEESHAN
KEESLAR
KERSHAW
KEYSPAN
KIDSEAT
KINSMAN
LENSCAP
LENSMAN
LESSFAT
LESSTAR
LETSEAT
LYESOAP
MANSMAN
MARSBAR
MARSHAL
MESSIAH
METSFAN
MIASMAL
MIASMAS
MISSEAT
MOISSAN
MRISCAN
NAUSEAM
NESSMAN
NEWSDAY
NEWSMAN
OARSMAN
ODESSAN
OHMSLAW
ONESTAR
OUTSOAR
OUTSTAY
OUTSWAM
PERSIAN
PETSCAN
PINSEAL
PLASMAS
PLUSTAX
POPSTAR
POTSDAM
PRESEAL
PRESEAT
PRESOAK
PROSCAN
QUESNAY
RAMSFAN
RAPSTAR
REASSAY
REDSFAN
REDSTAR
RIESMAN
RIKSDAG
RUBSRAW
RUSSIAN
RUSSLAN
SAYSAAH
SAYSNAY
SEASTAR
SEISMAL
SENSUAL
SIESTAS
SITSPAT
SOWSEAR
SUNSFAN
SZYSLAK
TELSTAR
THESTAR
THESWAN
THISDAY
THISWAY
THUSFAR
TINSTAR
TRISTAN
TRISTAR
TUESDAY
TWOSTAR
UNUSUAL
VIZSLAS
WAKSMAN
WHISKAS
WOOSNAM
ZOYSIAS

•••S••A

ANOSMIA
AZUSACA
BRESCIA
CAESURA
CASSABA
CASSAVA
CASSOLA
CORSICA
DYKSTRA
GETSANA
HOFSTRA
JESSICA
KRISHNA
MARSALA
MESSALA
MESSINA
MIASARA
MISSUSA
NUESTRA
OLESTRA
PERSONA
PORSENA
PRUSSIA
QUESERA
RETSINA
ROSSSEA
SALSODA
SATSUMA
TESSERA
UPPSALA
ZOSSIMA

••••SA•

ABYSSAL
ACCUSAL
ALASSAD
ALTOSAX
AROUSAL
ARTISAN
BABYSAT
BACKSAW
BALKSAT
BANDSAW
BARKSAT
BASSSAX
BEATSAT
BEEPSAT
BELTSAW
BUCKSAW
BUZZSAW
CANTSAY
CARPSAT
CLAUSAL
CLAWSAT
COMESAS
COMESAT
CROSSAT
DARESAY
DEPOSAL
DINESAT
DRESSAS
ESPOSAS
EXCUSAL
EXCUSAS
FIRESAT
FLIESAT
FLOTSAM
FORESAW
FRETSAT
FRETSAW
FUJISAN
FUMESAT
GAINSAY
GANGSAW
GAPESAT
GAWKSAT
GAZESAT
GIBESAT
GLOSSAE
GLOSSAL
GLOSSAS
GNAWSAT
GRABSAT
GRINSAT
GUESSAT
HACKSAW
HADASAY
HANDSAW
HASASAY
HEADSAW
HEARSAY
HINTSAT
HONKSAT
HOOTSAT
HOUSSAY
HOWLSAT
JEERSAT
JIBESAT
JUMPSAT
KEEPSAT
LANDSAT
LEAPSAT
LEERSAT
LINDSAY
LIVESAT
LOOKSAD
LOOKSAT
MEDUSAE
MEDUSAN
MEDUSAS
MIKASAS
MIMOSAS
MOISSAN
NOVISAD
ODESSAN
OVERSAD
OVERSAW
PECKSAT
PEEKSAT
PEEPSAT
PEERSAT
PERUSAL
PHRASAL
PICKSAT
PINESAP
PLAYSAT
POKESAT
POLESAT
POSESAS
RAILSAT
RANTSAT
REASSAY
RECUSAL
REFUSAL
REVISAL
ROARSAT
SAMOSAS
SHOPSAT
SIGHSAT
SNAPSAT
SOMESAY
SPOUSAL
STAYSAT
STOPSAT
SWATSAT
TALKSAT
TEARSAT
THEYSAY
TILTSAT
TOILSAT
TOOTSAT
TRANSAM
TREESAP
UNNASAL
VERYSAD
WAVESAT
WHATSAY
WHIPSAW
WINESAP
WINKSAT
WOODSAW
WORKSAT
YANKSAT
YELLSAT

••••S•A

ALYOSHA
AMNESIA

APHASIA
ARALSEA
AUGUSTA
BARISTA
BATISTA
CALISTA
CALMSEA
CANASTA
CELESTA
CHELSEA
CHRISTA
CINESIA
DACOSTA
DEADSEA
DEEPSEA
EMMUSKA
ERNESTA
EURASIA
FREESIA
FUCHSIA
GANGSTA
GOBYSEA
GOTOSEA
HIGHSEA
INGESTA
JOCASTA
KARASEA
KATISHA
KENOSHA
LARUSSA
LATOSCA
LUNESTA
MARUSJA
MELISMA
MELISSA
NATASHA
NERISSA
NICOSIA
OPENSEA
OVERSEA
PERISSA
PRUSSIA
RICKSHA
ROBUSTA
ROSSSEA
SALTSEA
SILESIA
SULUSEA
SWANSEA
TUNISIA
TURISTA
VANESSA
WABASHA
ZAKUSKA

•••••SA
ALAMOSA
CURIOSA
FORMOSA
HERMOSA
KAPITSA
LARUSSA
MELISSA
MISSUSA
MOMBASA
NERISSA
PERISSA
QUEPASA
REVERSA
REYNOSA
SUBROSA
TEAMUSA
THERESA
VANESSA

S•B••••
SABADOS
SABBATH
SABERED
SABINES
SABRINA
SEBRING
SIBERIA
SIBLING
SIBYLIC
SOBBERS
SOBBING
SOBERED
SOBERER
SOBERLY
STBARTS
STBASIL
SUBAREA
SUBARID
SUBARUS
SUBBAND
SUBBANK
SUBBASE
SUBBASS
SUBBIAS
SUBBING
SUBCASE
SUBCASH
SUBCAST
SUBCELL
SUBCLAN
SUBCODE
SUBCOOL
SUBDATE
SUBDEBS
SUBDUAL
SUBDUCT
SUBDUED
SUBDUER
SUBDUES
SUBECHO
SUBFILE
SUBFORM
SUBGOAL
SUBGODS
SUBHALL
SUBHEAD
SUBIDEA
SUBITEM
SUBJECT
SUBJOIN
SUBKING
SUBLETS
SUBLIDS
SUBLIME
SUBLONG
SUBLOTS
SUBMITS
SUBNETS
SUBORNS
SUBPLOT
SUBPOST
SUBRACE
SUBROOT
SUBROSA
SUBSECT
SUBSETS
SUBSIDE
SUBSIDY
SUBSIST
SUBSOIL
SUBSORT
SUBSUME
SUBTASK
SUBTEEN
SUBTEND
SUBTEXT
SUBTLER
SUBTONE
SUBTYPE
SUBUNIT
SUBURBS
SUBVENE
SUBVERT
SUBWARS
SUBWAYS
SUBZERO
SUBZONE

S••B•••
SABBATH
SAMBAED
SAMBASS
SAMBORA
SAMBUCA
SANBLAS
SANBORN
SATBACK
SAWBUCK
SCUBAED
SEABAGS
SEABASS
SEABEDS
SEABEES
SEABIRD
SEABLUE
SEABOAT
SEABORG
SERBIAN
SETBACK
SETBAIL
SHABBAT
SHEBANG
SHEBEAR
SHUBERT
SIEBZIG
SIOBHAN
SITBACK
SIXBALL
SKIBIBS
SKIBOBS
SKIBOOT
SKIBUMS
SKYBLUE
SLABBED
SLOBBER
SNOBALL
SNUBBED
SNUBBER
SOBBERS
SOBBING
SORBATE
SORBETS
SOUBISE
SOYBEAN
SPYBOTS
STABBED
STABBER
STABILE
STABLED
STABLER
STABLES
STUBBED
STUBBLE
STUBBLY
STUBING
SUBBAND
SUBBANK
SUBBASE
SUBBASS
SUBBIAS
SUBBING
SUDBURY
SUNBATH
SUNBEAM
SUNBELT
SUNBIRD
SUNBOWL
SUNBOWS
SUNBURN
SWABBED
SWABBER
SYMBOLS

S•••B••
SAFEBET
SAIDBOO
SALABLE
SALTBOX
SANDBAG
SANDBAR
SANDBOX
SANDBUR
SANIBEL
SAVABLE
SAYABLE
SAYSBOO
SCOOBAS
SCRIBED
SCRIBER
SCRIBES
SCRUBBY
SCRUBUP
SEEABLE
SEEDBED
SHABBAT
SHAMBLE
SHERBET
SHOEBOX
SHOWBIZ
SHRUBBY
SICKBAY
SICKBED
SIDEBAR
SIDEBET
SINDBAD
SIZABLE
SIZABLY
SKIABLE
SLABBED
SLOBBER
SLUMBER
SNUBBED
SNUBBER
SOAPBOX
SOFABED
SOLUBLE
SPAMBOT
STABBED
STABBER
STEUBEN
STROBES
STUBBED
STUBBLE
STUBBLY
STUMBLE
SUREBET
SWABBED
SWABBER
SWAYBAR

S••••B•
SAXTUBA
SCARABS
SCHLUBS
SCRUBBY
SEALABS
SENDSBY
SEVENBC
SHOOTBY
SHOPNBC
SHRUBBY
SIXTYBC
SKIBIBS
SKIBOBS
SKIPSBY
SLIDEBY
SLIPSBY
SNEAKBY
SOTHEBY
STANDBY
STICKBY
STOODBY
STOPSBY
STUCKBY
SUBDEBS
SUBURBS
SWEARBY
SWINGBY
SWOREBY
SWUNGBY
SYLLABI

S•••••B
SANDDAB
SHECRAB
SILENTB
SINUTAB
SNOWJOB
SUCCUMB

•SB••••
ASBYATT
OSBORNE

•S•B•••
ASABODY
ASHBERY
ASHBINS
ASHBURN
ASHBURY
ESOBESO
ISABEAU
ISOBARS
USABLES

•S••B••
ESTEBAN

•S•••B•
ASCRIBE

••SB•••
BUSBIES
BUSBOYS
DASBOOT
DISBAND
DISBARS
DISBUDS
GASBAGS
HASBEEN
HUSBAND
ITSBEST
JOSBOYS
LISBETH
MISBILL
MISBIND
MISBREW
MRSBASS
NESBITT
RASBORA
YASBECK

••S•B••
AUSABLE
BESTBET
BESTBOY
BESTBUD
BESTBUY
BUSYBEE
CASABAS
CASHBAR
CASHBOX
DISABLE
DISOBEY
DUSTBIN
FUSEBOX
FUSIBLE
ITSABOY
LESABRE
LOSABLE
LOSEBIG
LOSTBIG
MISTBOW
NOSEBAG
NOSEBRA
POSABLE
POSTBAG
POSTBOX
RISIBLE
RISIBLY
ROSABUD
ROSEBAY
ROSEBUD
TASKBAR
TESTBAN
TESTBED
UNSOBER
VISIBLE
VISIBLY
WASABIS

••S••B•
ABSORBS
ADSORBS
CASSABA
DISROBE
EASEDBY
EASESBY
HASTOBE
HISNIBS
HUSHABY
KOSHIBA
RESORBS
RESTABS
TOSHIBA

••S•••B
DISTURB
EASYJOB
NOSEJOB
RESCRUB
TESTLAB
WASHTUB

•••SB••
DOESBAD
FRISBEE
GEMSBOK
GOESBAD
MARSBAR
NEWSBOY
SAYSBOO
WINSBIG

•••S•B•
CASSABA
CLOSEBY

•••S••B
PAYSTUB

••••SB•
COMESBY
DROPSBY
EASESBY
FILESBY
FLIESBY
FLITSBY
GRIMSBY
HANGSBY
HORNSBY
MORESBY
PLAYSBY
RACESBY
RIDESBY
ROLLSBY
SENDSBY
SKIPSBY
SLIPSBY
STOPSBY
TICKSBY
WALKSBY

••••S•B
MINISUB
TUNASUB

SC•••••
SCACCHI
SCADSOF
SCALAGE
SCALARS
SCALDED
SCALDER
SCALENE
SCALERS
SCALEUP
SCALIER
SCALING
SCALLOP
SCALPED
SCALPEL
SCALPER
SCAMMED
SCAMMER
SCAMPED
SCAMPER
SCANDAL
SCANNED
SCANNER
SCANTED
SCANTER
SCANTLY
SCAPULA
SCARABS
SCARCER
SCAREDY
SCARERS
SCAREUP
SCARFED
SCARFER
SCARFUP
SCARIER
SCARIFY
SCARILY
SCARING
SCARLET
SCARPED
SCARRED
SCARVES
SCARWID
SCATHED
SCATHES
SCATMAN
SCATTED
SCATTER
SCENEII
SCENEIV
SCENERY
SCENEVI
SCENICS
SCENTED
SCENTER
SCEPTER
SCEPTIC
SCEPTRE
SCHAYES
SCHELDT
SCHEMAS
SCHEMED
SCHEMER
SCHEMES
SCHERZI
SCHERZO
SCHICKS
SCHIRRA
SCHISMS
SCHISTS
SCHLEPP
SCHLEPS
SCHLITZ
SCHLOCK
SCHLUBS
SCHLUMP
SCHMEAR
SCHMEER
SCHMIDT
SCHMITT
SCHMOES
SCHNAPS
SCHNOOK
SCHNOZZ
SCHOLAR
SCHOLES
SCHOOLS
SCHTICK
SCHULTZ
SCHUMER
SCHWANN
SCHWINN
SCIATIC
SCIENCE
SCIORRA
SCISSOR
SCITECH
SCLAFFS
SCLERAE
SCLERAL
SCLERAS
SCOFFAT
SCOFFED
SCOFFER
SCOLARI
SCOLDED
SCOLDER
SCONCES
SCOOBAS
SCOOPED
SCOOPER
SCOOTCH
SCOOTED
SCOOTER
SCOPING
SCORERS
SCORIAS
SCORING
SCORNED
SCORNER
SCORPIO
SCOTERS
SCOTIAN
SCOTTIE
SCOUPES
SCOURED
SCOURER
SCOURGE
SCOUTED
SCOUTER
SCOUTUP
SCOWLED
SCOWLER
SCRAGGY
SCRAPED
SCRAPER
SCRAPES
SCRAPPY
SCRATCH
SCRAWLS
SCRAWLY
SCRAWNY
SCREAKS
SCREAMS
SCREECH
SCREEDS
SCREENS
SCREWED
SCREWUP
SCRIBED
SCRIBER
SCRIBES
SCRIMPS
SCRIMPY
SCRIPPS
SCRIPTS
SCROLLS
SCROOGE
SCRUBBY
SCRUBUP
SCRUFFS
SCRUFFY
SCRUGGS
SCRUNCH
SCRUPLE
SCUBAED
SCUDDED
SCUDDER
SCUFFED
SCUFFER
SCUFFLE
SCULLED
SCULLER
SCULPED
SCULPTS
SCUPPER
SCURVES
SCUSEME
SCUTTLE
SCUZZES
SCYTHED
SCYTHES

S•C••••
SACCADE
SACHEMS
SACHETS
SACKERS
SACKFUL
SACKING
SACKOUT
SACKSUP
SACLIKE
SACQUES
SECANTS
SECEDED
SECEDER
SECEDES
SECHZIG
SECKELS
SECLUDE
SECONDI
SECONDO
SECONDR
SECONDS
SECRECY
SECRETE
SECRETS
SECTION
SECTORS
SECULAR
SECURED
SECURER
SECURES
SICCING
SICILIA
SICKBAY
SICKBED
SICKDAY
SICKENS
SICKEST
SICKISH
SICKLES
SICKOUT
SICKPAY
SOCIALS
SOCIETY
SOCKETS
SOCKEYE
SOCKHOP
SOCKING
SOCKSIN
STCLOUD
STCROIX
SUCCEED
SUCCESS
SUCCORS
SUCCOTH
SUCCOUR
SUCCUMB
SUCKDRY
SUCKERS
SUCKIER
SUCKING
SUCKSIN
SUCKSUP
SUCRASE
SUCROSE
SUCTION

S••C•••
SACCADE
SADCAFE
SAGCARD
SALCHOW
SANCTUM
SANCTUS
SARCASM
SATCHEL
SATCHMO
SATCOMS
SAUCERS
SAUCIER
SAUCILY
SAUCING
SAUCONY
SAWCHUK
SCACCHI
SEACALM
SEACATS
SEACOWS
SHACKED
SHACKLE
SHECRAB
SHOCKED
SHOCKER
SHUCKED
SHUCKER
SICCING
SIMCITY
SINCERE
SINCITY
SITCOMS
SKICAPS
SKYCAMS
SKYCAPS
SLACKED
SLACKEN
SLACKER
SLACKLY
SLACKUP
SLICERS
SLICEUP
SLICING
SLICKED
SLICKER
SLICKLY
SMACKED
SMACKER
SMACKOF
SMACKUP
SMUCKER
SNACKED
SNACKER
SNACKON
SNICKER
SNICKET
SNOCAPS
SNOCATS
SNOCONE
SNUCKUP
SORCERY
SPACELY
SPACERS
SPACIAL
SPACIER
SPACING
SPACKLE
SPECIAL
SPECIES
SPECIFY
SPECING
SPECKED
SPECKLE
SPECOUT
SPECTER
SPECTOR
SPECTRA
SPECTRE
SPICERS
SPICERY
SPICEUP
SPICIER
SPICILY
SPICING
SPYCAMS
STACKED
STACKER
STACKUP
STICKBY
STICKER
STICKIN
STICKON
STICKTO
STICKUM
STICKUP
STOCKED
STOCKER
STOCKUP
STUCCOS
STUCKBY
STUCKIN
STUCKON
STUCKTO
STUCKUP
SUBCASE
SUBCASH
SUBCAST
SUBCELL
SUBCLAN
SUBCODE
SUBCOOL
SUCCEED
SUCCESS
SUCCORS
SUCCOTH
SUCCOUR
SUCCUMB
SUNCITY
SYNCHED
SYNCING
SYNCOPE

S•••C••
SAATCHI
SARACEN
SCACCHI
SCARCER
SCHICKS
SCONCES
SEANCES
SEDUCED
SEDUCER
SEDUCES
SELECTS
SENECAN
SENECAS
SHLOCKY
SHOWCAT
SHTICKS
SHTICKY
SIDECAR
SILICAS
SILICON
SIROCCO
SKETCHY
SLOTCAR
SLOUCHY
SLUICED
SLUICES

SNOWCAP
SNOWCAT
SODACAN
SOLACED
SOLACER
SOLACES
SOLICIT
SOUPCAN
SOUPCON
SOURCED
SOURCES
SPENCER
SPLICED
SPLICER
SPLICES
SPRUCED
SPRUCER
SPRUCES
STANCES
STARCHY
STENCIL
STLUCIA
STOICAL
STUCCOS
SUBECHO
SURECAN

S••••C•

SADSACK
SAMBUCA
SATBACK
SAWATCH
SAWBUCK
SCENICS
SCHLOCK
SCHTICK
SCIENCE
SCITECH
SCOOTCH
SCRATCH
SCREECH
SCRUNCH
SEADUCK
SEARACE
SEASICK
SECRECY
SELLECK
SENESCE
SERPICO
SERVICE
SETBACK
SHYLOCK
SILENCE
SIROCCO
SITBACK
SIXPACK
SKIRACE
SKIRACK
SKYJACK
SNEETCH
SOLOACT
SONANCE
SPINACH
SPLOTCH
SQUELCH
SQUINCH
STATICE
STATICS
STAUNCH
STOMACH
STRETCH
STRITCH
SUBDUCT
SUBJECT
SUBRACE
SUBSECT
SUFFICE
SUNDECK
SURFACE
SUSPECT
SYNDICS

S•••••C

SARANAC
SATANIC
SATIRIC
SATYRIC
SCEPTIC
SCIATIC
SEISMIC
SELENIC
SEMITIC
SEVENBC
SHELLAC
SHOEPAC
SHOPNBC
SIBYLIC
SILENTC
SIMILAC
SIXTYBC
SKEPTIC
SOMATIC
SPHERIC
STANNIC
STEARIC
STYPTIC
SYLPHIC
SYNODIC

•SC••••

ASCARED
ASCENDS
ASCENTS
ASCETIC
ASCRIBE
BSCHOOL
ESCALOP
ESCALUS
ESCAPED
ESCAPEE
ESCAPER
ESCAPES
ESCARPS
ESCENCE
ESCHEAT
ESCHERS
ESCHEWS
ESCORTS
ESCROWS
ESCUDOS
ESCUELA
ISCHIAL
ISCHIUM
OSCEOLA
OSCINES
OSCULAR
OSCULES
OSCHOOL

•S•C•••

ASHCAKE
ASHCANS
ASOCIAL
ISECOND
PSYCHED
PSYCHES
PSYCHIC
PSYCHOS
PSYCHUP

•S••C••

ASPECTS
OSSICLE
USANCES
USEDCAR
USEDCDS

•S•••C•

ASKANCE
ASPENCO
ESCENCE
ESSENCE
OSTRICH

•S••••C

ASCETIC
ASEPTIC
ASIATIC
ISLAMIC
OSMATIC
OSMOTIC
OSSIFIC
PSALMIC
PSYCHIC

••SC•••

ABSCISE
ABSCOND
AMSCRAY
BISCUIT
BOSCAGE
BUSCEMI
CASCADE
CISCOES
CTSCANS
DASCHLE
DESCANT
DESCEND
DESCENT
DISCARD
DISCERN
DISCING
DISCMAN
DISCOED
DISCOID
DISCORD
DISCUSS
EXSCIND
FASCIAE
FASCIAL
FASCIAS
FASCISM
FASCIST
FESCUES
FISCHER
FOSCOLO
GASCANS
GASCAPS
GASCONS
GASCONY
GISCARD
HOSCALE
INSCALE
ITSCOLD
KOSCINA
LASCALA
LASCARS
LASCAUX
LESCAUT
MASCARA
MASCOTS
MESCALS
MISCALL
MISCAST
MISCITE
MISCODE
MISCOIN
MISCOPY
MISCUED
MISCUES
MISCUTS
MOSCATO
MOSCONI
MRSCOTT
MUSCATS
MUSCIDA
MUSCLED
MUSCLES
NASCENT
NESCAFE
NOSCORE
OBSCENE
OBSCURA
OBSCURE
PASCHAL
PASCOLI
PISCEAN
PISCINE
PISCOPO
RASCALS
RESCALE
RESCANS
RESCIND
RESCORE
RESCRUB
RESCUED
RESCUER
RESCUES
ROSCOES
TOSCALE
TUSCANS
TUSCANY
UNSCALY
UNSCREW
UPSCALE
VISCERA
VISCOUS
VISCUSO
WESCOTT

••S•C••

BESTCUT
BISECTS
CASHCOW
EXSECTS
FASTCAR
HASACOW
INSECTA
INSECTS
LOSTCAT
MISACTS
MUSICAL
MUSICKS
OSSICLE
RESECTS
VESICLE
YESICAN

••S••C•

ABSENCE
ADSPACE
ANSPACH
AUSPICE
BESEECH
CASSOCK
COSSACK
DESTOCK
DISSECT
DISTICH
DRSPOCK
ESSENCE
EUSTACE
FOSDICK
HASSOCK
HOSPICE
INSHOCK
INSPACE
INSPECT
INSTOCK
INSYNCH
IPSWICH
JESSICA
JUSTICE
LASTACT
MASTICS
MESHACH
MESSICK
MOSAICS
MRSPOCK
MYSPACE
MYSTICS
RESPACE
RESPECT
RESPICE
RESTACK
RESTICK
RESTOCK
ROSTOCK
RUSTICS
SUSPECT
TESTACY
TUSSOCK
UNSLACK
UNSLICK
UNSPICY
UNSTACK
UNSTICK
UNSTUCK
WASATCH
YASBECK
YASHICA

••S•••C

ARSENIC
BASILIC
BOSONIC
GASTRIC
HASIDIC
MASONIC
MESONIC
MISKOLC
OSSIFIC
PASSAIC
POSTDOC
POSTHOC
UNSTOIC

•••SC••

BORSCHT
BRESCIA
CATSCAN
FIASCOS
FRESCAS
FRESCOS
KITSCHY
LENSCAP
MENSCHY
MRISCAN
PETSCAN
PORSCHE
PROSCAN

•••S•C•

AIRSACS
AIRSICK
AIRSOCK
ANDSUCH
AZUSACA
CANSECO
CASSOCK
CORSICA
COSSACK
DISSECT
EGGSACS
GYMSOCK
HASSOCK
INKSACS
JESSICA
MESSICK
NONSUCH
ODDSOCK
ONESOCK
OVISACS
PARSECS
PEPSICO
PHYSICS
RANSACK
SADSACK
SEASICK
SUBSECT
THESACK
TRISECT
TUSSOCK
VERSACE

•••S••C

ANOSMIC
CAUSTIC
CHASMIC
CLASSIC
CROSTIC
DEISTIC
DRASTIC
EKISTIC
ELASTIC
ERISTIC
GNOSTIC
LIPSYNC
MIASMIC
PASSAIC
PLASMIC
PLASTIC
PROSAIC
SEISMIC

••••SC•

BELASCO
DEHISCE
DEUTSCH
DRIESCH
ILIESCU
IONESCO
JALISCO
KLATSCH
KLENSCH
LATOSCA
MENISCI
MIRISCH
NABISCO
POLISCI
POLYSCI
SENESCE
TABASCO
TUMESCE

••••S•C

AMNESIC
APHASIC
CLASSIC
FORASEC
KINESIC
LEXUSSC
MRMUSIC

•••••SC

LEXUSSC
MOLLUSC

SD•••••

SDAKOTA

S•D••••

SADCAFE
SADDENS
SADDEST
SADDLED
SADDLER
SADDLES
SADEYED
SADEYES
SADFATE
SADISTS
SADNESS
SADSACK
SADSONG
SEDALIA
SEDATED
SEDATER
SEDATES
SEDGIER
SEDONAS
SEDUCED
SEDUCER
SEDUCES
SIDDONS
SIDDURS
SIDEARM
SIDEBAR
SIDEBET
SIDECAR
SIDEMAN
SIDEMEN
SIDEONE
SIDETWO
SIDEWAY
SIDINGS
SIDIOUS
SIDLING
SODACAN
SODAPOP
SODDIER
SODDING
SODIDWE
SODLESS
STDENIS
SUDAFED
SUDBURY
SUDOKUS
SUDSERS
SUDSIER
SUDSING
SYDHOFF

S••D•••

SADDENS
SADDEST
SADDLED
SADDLER
SADDLES
SAIDAAH
SAIDAYE
SAIDBOO
SAIDIDO
SAIDNAY
SANDALS
SANDBAG
SANDBAR
SANDBOX
SANDBUR
SANDDAB
SANDERS
SANDFLY
SANDHOG
SANDIER
SANDING
SANDLER
SANDLOT
SANDMAN
SANDMEN
SANDPIT
SARDINE
SATDOWN
SAWDUST
SCADSOF
SCUDDED
SCUDDER
SEADOGS
SEADUCK
SEADUTY
SEEDBED
SEEDERS
SEEDIER
SEEDILY
SEEDING
SEEDLET
SEEDPOD
SENDEES
SENDERS
SENDFOR
SENDING
SENDOFF
SENDOUT
SENDSBY
SENDSIN
SENDSON
SENDSTO
SENDSUP
SENDUPS
SETDOWN
SHADERS
SHADIER
SHADILY
SHADING
SHADOWS
SHADOWY
SHADROE
SHEDDER
SHEDSON
SHODDEN
SHUDDER
SIDDONS
SIDDURS
SINDBAD
SIRDUKE
SITDOWN
SKIDDED
SKIDDER
SKIDDOO
SKIDLID
SKIDOOS
SKIDROW
SKYDIVE
SKYDOME
SLEDDED
SLEDDER
SLEDDOG
SLEDFUL
SLEDGED
SLEDGES
SLIDEBY
SLIDEIN
SLIDERS
SLIDING
SLIDOFF
SLIDOUT
SLUDGES
SMIDGEN
SMIDGES
SMUDGED
SMUDGES
SNIDELY
SNIDEST
SODDIER
SODDING
SOLDERS
SOLDFOR
SOLDIER
SOLDOFF
SOLDOUT
SORDINI
SORDINO
SPADERS
SPADING
SPEDOFF
SPIDERS
SPIDERY
SPYDERS
STADIUM
STADLER
STODGED
STODGES
STUDDED
STUDENT
STUDIED
STUDIER
STUDIES
STUDIOS
SUBDATE
SUBDEBS
SUBDUAL
SUBDUCT
SUBDUED
SUBDUER
SUBDUES
SUEDFOR
SUNDAES
SUNDAYS
SUNDECK
SUNDERS
SUNDIAL
SUNDOGS
SUNDOWN
SWADDLE
SWEDISH
SYNDICS

S•••D••

SABADOS
SALADES
SALADIN
SAMEDAY
SAMEDIS
SANDDAB
SAVEDON
SAVEDUP
SCALDED
SCALDER
SCANDAL
SCOLDED
SCOLDER
SCUDDED
SCUDDER
SECEDED
SECEDER
SECEDES
SEMIDRY
SERFDOM
SEWEDON
SEWEDUP
SHAHDOM
SHEDDER
SHELDON
SHINDIG
SHODDEN
SHOWDOG
SHUDDER
SICKDAY
SINEDIE
SIZEDUP
SKIDDED
SKIDDER
SKIDDOO
SLANDER
SLEDDED
SLEDDER
SLEDDOG
SLENDER
SLOWDAY
SMOLDER
SNOWDAY
SNOWDON
SOANDSO
SODIDWE
SOLEDAD
SOLIDER
SOLIDLY
SOMEDAY
SOUNDED
SOUNDER
SOUNDLY
SPANDEX
SPEEDED
SPEEDER
SPEEDOS
SPEEDUP
SPENDER
SPENDON
SPIEDON
SPINDLE
SPINDLY
SPINDRY
SPONDEE
STAIDER
STAIDLY
STANDBY
STANDEE
STANDER
STANDIN
STANDON
STANDTO
STANDUP
STARDOM
STAYDRY
STEADED
STEPDAD
STOODBY
STOODIN
STOODON
STOODTO
STOODUP
STRIDER
STRIDES
STRUDEL
STUDDED
SUBIDEA
SUCKDRY
SWADDLE
SWINDLE
SYNODAL
SYNODIC

S••••D•

SACCADE
SAIDIDO
SALSODA
SAYSIDO
SCAREDY
SCHELDT
SCHMIDT
SCREEDS
SEABEDS
SEAGODS
SEASIDE
SECLUDE
SECONDI
SECONDO
SECONDR
SECONDS
SEWARDS
SHIELDS
SHOULDA
SHOULDI
SHROUDS
SOSPADS
SPLENDA
SPREADS
SPYKIDS
STRANDS
STUPIDS
SUBCODE
SUBGODS
SUBLIDS
SUBSIDE
SUBSIDY
SULFIDE
SUNGODS
SUREIDO

S•••••D

SABERED
SADDLED
SADEYED
SAGCARD
SAINTED
SALLIED
SALUTED
SAMBAED
SAMEOLD
SAMLOYD
SAMOYED
SAMPLED
SANFORD
SAPHEAD
SAUNAED
SAUTEED
SAVAGED
SAVORED
SAVVIED
SAWWOOD
SCALDED
SCALPED
SCAMMED
SCAMPED
SCANNED
SCANTED
SCARFED
SCARPED
SCARRED
SCARWID
SCATHED
SCATTED
SCENTED
SCHEMED
SCOFFED
SCOLDED
SCOOPED
SCOOTED
SCORNED
SCOURED
SCOUTED
SCOWLED
SCRAPED
SCREWED
SCRIBED
SCUBAED
SCUDDED
SCUFFED
SCULLED
SCULPED
SCYTHED
SEABIRD
SEAFOOD
SEAWARD
SEAWEED
SECEDED
SECURED
SEDATED
SEDUCED
SEEDBED
SEEDPOD
SEESRED
SEETHED
SEPALED
SETTLED
SEVENAD
SEVERED
SHACKED
SHAFTED
SHAGGED
SHAMMED
SHANKED
SHARPED
SHAWLED
SHEAFED
SHEARED
SHEAVED
SHEERED
SHEETED
SHELLED
SHELVED
SHEPARD
SHIFTED
SHILLED
SHINNED
SHINPAD
SHIPPED
SHIRKED
SHIRRED
SHOALED
SHOCKED
SHOPPED
SHORTED
SHOUTED
SHRINED

SHUCKED
SHUNNED
SHUNTED
SHUSHED
SICKBED
SIGHTED
SIGMOID
SIGMUND
SILENTD
SINDBAD
SINEWED
SINGLED
SIRENED
SIXFOLD
SIXTYAD
SIZZLED
SKIDDED
SKIDLID
SKIFFED
SKILLED
SKIMMED
SKIMPED
SKINNED
SKIPPED
SKIRLED
SKIRTED
SKULKED
SKULLED
SKUNKED
SKYNYRD
SKYWARD
SLABBED
SLACKED
SLAMMED
SLANTED
SLAPPED
SLASHED
SLATTED
SLEDDED
SLEDGED
SLEEKED
SLEETED
SLEEVED
SLICKED
SLIMMED
SLINKED
SLIPPED
SLITTED
SLOGGED
SLOPPED
SLOSHED
SLOTTED
SLUGGED
SLUICED
SLUMMED
SLUMPED
SLURPED
SLURRED
SLUSHED
SMACKED
SMALLAD
SMARTED
SMASHED
SMEARED
SMELLED
SMELTED
SMIRKED
SMITHED

SMUDGED
SMUSHED
SNACKED
SNAFUED
SNAGGED
SNAPPED
SNARFED
SNARLED
SNEAKED
SNEERED
SNEEZED
SNIFFED
SNIPPED
SNOOPED
SNOOTED
SNOOZED
SNORTED
SNOUTED
SNUBBED
SNUFFED
SNUGGED
SOAPPAD
SOBERED
SOFABED
SOLACED
SOLEDAD
SOOTHED
SORTIED
SOTWEED
SOUNDED
SOURCED
SPAMMED
SPANKED
SPANNED
SPARKED
SPARRED
SPATTED
SPAWNED
SPEARED
SPECKED
SPEEDED
SPELLED
SPHERED
SPIELED
SPIFFED
SPILLED
SPLAYED
SPLICED
SPOILED
SPONGED
SPOOFED
SPOOKED
SPOOLED
SPOONED
SPORTED
SPOTTED
SPOUTED
SPRAYED
SPRUCED
SPURNED
SPURRED
SPURTED
SQUALID
SQUARED
SQUIRED
SSHAPED
STABBED
STABLED

STACKED
STAFFED
STAGGED
STAINED
STAIRED
STALKED
STALLED
STAMPED
STAPLED
STARRED
STARTED
STARVED
STASHED
STCLOUD
STEADED
STEAMED
STEELED
STEEPED
STEERED
STEEVED
STEMMED
STEPDAD
STEPPED
STEROID
STETTED
STEWARD
STIFFED
STIFLED
STILLED
STILTED
STINTED
STIPEND
STIRRED
STOCKED
STODGED
STOMPED
STOOGED
STOOLED
STOOPED
STOPPED
STORIED
STORMED
STRAFED
STRAYED
STREWED
STRIPED
STRIVED
STROKED
STUBBED
STUDDED
STUDIED
STUFFED
STUMPED
STUNNED
STUNTED
STYMIED
SUBARID
SUBBAND
SUBDUED
SUBHEAD
SUBTEND
SUCCEED
SUDAFED
SUGARED
SULLIED
SUMMAND
SUNBIRD
SUNMAID

SUNWARD
SUPPLED
SUSPEND
SUTURED
SWABBED
SWAMPED
SWANKED
SWAPPED
SWARMED
SWASHED
SWATHED
SWATTED
SWEATED
SWELLED
SWERVED
SWIGGED
SWILLED
SWIRLED
SWISHED
SWOONED
SWOOPED
SYNCHED
SZILARD

•S•D•••

ISADORA
ISADORE
ISIDORE
USEDCAR
USEDCDS
USEDFOR

•S••D••

ASKEDIN
ASKEDOF
ASKEDUP
ASSTDAS
ASUNDER
CSARDAS
ESCUDOS
ESTADOS
ISAIDNO
PSANDQS
TSARDOM
USTEDES
XSANDOS

•S•••D•

ASABODY
ASCENDS
ASTRIDE
ESTRADA
ISLANDS
ISOPODS
ISUREDO
OSMONDS
OSMUNDS
USEDCDS
USERIDS

•S••••D

ASCARED
ASHAMED
ASHFORD
ASHLAND
ASISAID
ASPIRED
ASSAYED

ASSUMED
ASSURED
ASTOUND
ESCAPED
ESSAYED
ESTATED
ISAHEAD
ISECOND
ISLETED
ISSUEAD
LSHAPED
OSHAPED
OSIERED
OSMOSED
OSTEOID
OSTWALD
PSHAWED
PSYCHED
SSHAPED
TSHAPED
USHAPED
USHERED
USURPED
VSHAPED
YSHAPED

••SD•••

DISDAIN
FOSDICK
HASDONE
ITSDONE
MISDATE
MISDEAL
MISDEED
MISDEEM
MISDIAL
MISDOER
MISDOES
MISDONE
MISDRAW
MISDREW
WISDOMS
YESDEAR

••S•D••

APSIDES
ASSTDAS
BASEDON
BESIDES
DASHDOT
DOSADOS
DOSIDOS
EASEDBY
EASEDIN
EASEDON
EASEDUP
GASEDUP
HASIDIC
HASIDIM
INSIDER
INSIDES
LASTDON
LOSTDOG
MISADDS
MISEDIT
MUSEDON
MUSTDOS
NOSEDIN

NOSEDUP
ONSIDES
PASTDUE
PESADES
POSADAS
POSEDAS
POSTDOC
RESIDED
RESIDER
RESIDES
RESIDUA
RESIDUE
RUSHDIE
UNSADLY
UNSIDED
UPSIDES
WASHDAY
WISEDUP
YESIDID

••S••D•

AXSEEDS
BUSHIDO
BUSRIDE
CASCADE
CASSIDY
CUSPIDS
CUSTODY
DESEEDS
DISBUDS
LASORDA
MISADDS
MISCODE
MUSCIDA
PASSADE
PASSADO
RASHIDA
RESANDS
RESEEDS
RESENDS
RESPADE
RESTUDY
SOSPADS
TOSTADA
UNSHADE
UNSHADY
UPSENDS
VESPIDS

••S•••D

ABSCOND
ASSAYED
ASSUMED
ASSURED
BESTBUD
BOSOMED
BUSLOAD
BUSTARD
BUSTLED
CASQUED
CASTLED
COSTARD
CUSTARD
DASTARD
DESCEND
DESEXED
DESIRED
DESMOND

DESPOND
DISBAND
DISCARD
DISCOED
DISCOID
DISCORD
DISTEND
DISUSED
EASELED
EASTEND
ENSILED
ENSKIED
ENSURED
ESSAYED
EXSCIND
GASPARD
GESSOED
GISCARD
GOSFORD
GUSSIED
HASSLED
HISPEED
HUSBAND
HUSTLED
INSIPID
INSTEAD
INSURED
ISSUEAD
ITSCOLD
JOSTLED
LASSOED
LUSTRED
MASONED
MASTOID
MISBIND
MISCUED
MISDEED
MISFEED
MISLAID
MISLEAD
MISREAD
MISSAID
MISSEND
MISTOLD
MISUSED
MISWORD
MOSEYED
MUSCLED
MUSTARD
NESTLED
PESTLED
POSITED
PUSHROD
RASSLED
RESAVED
RESAWED
RESCIND
RESCUED
RESEWED
RESIDED
RESILED
RESINED
RESITED
RESIZED
RESOLED
RESOUND
RESOWED
RESPOND

RESUMED
ROSABUD
ROSEBUD
ROSERED
ROSINED
ROSTAND
RUSTLED
SUSPEND
TASERED
TESTBED
TUSSAUD
TUSSLED
UNSATED
UNSAVED
UNSAWED
UNSEWED
UNSHOED
UNSIDED
UNSIZED
UNSOLED
UNSOLID
UNSOUND
UNSOWED
UNSPIED
UNSTAID
UPSIZED
UPSTAND
UPSTOOD
VISAGED
VISITED
VISORED
VISTAED
VOSKHOD
WESTEND
YESIDID

•••SD••

DRESDEN
GADSDEN
MARSDEN
NEWSDAY
PATSDRY
POTSDAM
RIKSDAG
RUNSDRY
THISDAY
TUESDAY

•••S•D•

BEDSIDE
CASSIDY
CRUSADE
DAYSIDE
DOASIDO
EPISODE
FARSIDE
LOWSIDE
OFFSIDE
OUTSIDE
PASSADE
PASSADO
PRESIDE
PROSODY
SALSODA
SAYSIDO
SEASIDE
SUBSIDE
SUBSIDY

TOPSIDE
WAYSIDE

•••S••D

ABASHED
ALASSAD
AMASSED
AMISTAD
ANISEED
ASISAID
BIASSED
BLASTED
BLESSED
BLISSED
BLUSHED
BOASTED
BOBSLED
BOISEID
BOOSTED
BRISKED
BRUSHED
CHASSED
CHESTED
CLASHED
CLASPED
CLASSED
COASTED
COWSHED
CRASHED
CRESTED
CRISPED
CROSSED
CRUSHED
CRUSTED
DAYSEND
DOESBAD
DOGSLED
DRESSED
EGESTED
ENISLED
EXISTED
FEASTED
FLASHED
FLESHED
FLOSSED
FLUSHED
FOISTED
FRESHED
FRESSED
FRISKED
FROSTED
GESSOED
GETSMAD
GETSOLD
GETSRID
GHOSTED
GLASSED
GLOSSED
GNASHED
GODSEND
GOESBAD
GOESMAD
GRASPED
GRASSED
GROSSED
GUESSED
GUESTED
GUSSIED

HASSLED
HAYSEED
HEISTED
HOISTED
IBNSAUD
JOISTED
JOUSTED
LASSOED
LEASHED
LINSEED
MANSARD
MARSRED
MISSAID
MISSEND
MOUSSED
NAYSAID
NONSKED
NONSKID
OERSTED
OILSAND
OILSEED
OLMSTED
OUTSAID
OUTSOLD
OUTSPED
PERSEID
PHISHED
PLASHED
PRESOLD
PRESSED
PURSUED
QUASHED
QUESTED
RASSLED
REASKED
ROASTED
RONSARD
ROOSTED
ROUSTED
SEESRED
SHUSHED
SLASHED
SLOSHED
SLUSHED
SMASHED
SMUSHED
STASHED
SWASHED
SWISHED
TOASTED
TOPSEED
TOUSLED
TOYSLED
TRASHED
TRESSED
TRUSSED
TRUSTED
TRYSTED
TUSSAUD
TUSSLED
TWISTED
UNASKED
WAISTED
WHISHED
WHISKED
WHOSAID
WITSEND
WOOSHED

WORSTED
WRESTED
YEASTED

••••SD•

MAKESDO

••••S•D

ACCUSED
ADVISED
ALASSAD
AMASSED
APPOSED
AROUSED
AULDSOD
AVULSED
BEMUSED
BIASSED
BLESSED
BLISSED
BLOUSED
BRAISED
BROWSED
BRUISED
CHASSED
CHEESED
CLASSED
COURSED
CREASED
CROSSED
CRUISED
DEBASED
DEFUSED
DEMISED
DEPOSED
DEVISED
DISUSED
DRESSED
DROWSED
EFFUSED
ELAPSED
EMERSED
ENCASED
EVULSED
EXCISED
EXCUSED
EXPOSED
FINISHD
FLENSED
FLOSSED
FOCUSED
FRESSED
GLASSED
GLOSSED
GRASSED
GREASED
GROSSED
GROUSED
GUESSED
HOCUSED
ILLUSED
IMPOSED
INCASED
INCISED
INCUSED
INFUSED
IODISED
IONISED

JONESED
LIAISED
LOOKSAD
MISUSED
MOUSSED
NOTUSED
NOVISAD
OPPOSED
OSMOSED
OVERSAD
PERUSED
PHRASED
PLEASED
PRAISED
PRESSED
RECASED
RECUSED
REDOSED
REFUSED
REMISED
REPOSED
REVISED
TRESSED
TRUSSED
UNBASED
UNCASED
UNFUSED
UNNOSED
UNPOSED
VERYSAD

SE•••••

SEAARMS
SEABAGS
SEABASS
SEABEDS
SEABEES
SEABIRD
SEABLUE
SEABOAT
SEABORG
SEACALM
SEACATS
SEACOWS
SEADOGS
SEADUCK
SEADUTY
SEAEELS
SEAFARE
SEAFERN
SEAFOAM
SEAFOOD
SEAFOWL
SEAGATE
SEAGIRT
SEAGODS
SEAGRAM
SEAGREN
SEAGULL
SEAHAWK
SEAHERO
SEAHUNT
SEALABS
SEALANE
SEALANT
SEALEGS
SEALERS
SEALERY

SEALIFE
SEALIFT
SEALIKE
SEALILY
SEALING
SEALION
SEALOFF
SEALSIN
SEALSUP
SEAMAPS
SEAMERS
SEAMIER
SEAMILE
SEAMING
SEAMIST
SEAMOSS
SEANCES
SEAPORT
SEARACE
SEARERS
SEARING
SEASALT
SEASICK
SEASIDE
SEASLUG
SEASONS
SEASTAR
SEATERS
SEATING
SEATRIP
SEATTLE
SEAWALL
SEAWARD
SEAWAYS
SEAWEED
SEAWOLF
SEBRING
SECANTS
SECEDED
SECEDER
SECEDES
SECHZIG
SECKELS
SECLUDE
SECONDI
SECONDO
SECONDR
SECONDS
SECRECY
SECRETE
SECRETS
SECTION
SECTORS
SECULAR
SECURED
SECURER
SECURES
SEDALIA
SEDATED
SEDATER
SEDATES
SEDGIER
SEDONAS
SEDUCED
SEDUCER
SEDUCES
SEEABLE
SEEALSO

SEEDBED
SEEDERS
SEEDIER
SEEDILY
SEEDING
SEEDLET
SEEDPOD
SEEHERE
SEEINTO
SEEKERS
SEEKING
SEEKOUT
SEEMING
SEEMSTO
SEENALL
SEENFIT
SEENOFF
SEENOUT
SEEPAGE
SEEPAST
SEEPIER
SEEPING
SEEPOUT
SEEPSIN
SEERESS
SEESALL
SEESAWS
SEESFIT
SEESOFF
SEESOUT
SEESRED
SEETHED
SEETHES
SEETHRU
SEETOIT
SEFERIS
SEGMENT
SEGOVIA
SEGWAYS
SEINERS
SEINING
SEISMAL
SEISMIC
SEIZEON
SEIZERS
SEIZING
SEIZORS
SEIZURE
SELECTS
SELENIC
SELFISH
SELKIRK
SELLECK
SELLERS
SELLFOR
SELLING
SELLOFF
SELLOUT
SELLSIT
SELLSTO
SELMAAL
SELTZER
SELVAGE
SEMANAS
SEMIDRY
SEMILOG
SEMINAL
SEMINAR
SEMIPRO
SEMIRAW
SEMITES
SEMITIC
SENATES
SENATOR
SENDEES
SENDERS
SENDFOR
SENDING
SENDOFF
SENDOUT
SENDSBY
SENDSIN
SENDSON
SENDSTO
SENDSUP
SENDUPS
SENECAN
SENECAS
SENEGAL
SENESCE
SENHORA
SENIORS
SENNETT
SENORAS
SENORES
SENSATE
SENSEIS
SENSENS
SENSING
SENSORS
SENSORY
SENSUAL
SENTFOR
SENTOFF
SENTOUT
SENTRAS
SEPALED
SEPHIAS
SEPIRAS
SEPTETS
SEQUELS
SEQUINS
SEQUOIA
SEQUOYA
SERAPES
SERAPHS
SERAPIS
SERBIAN
SERENER
SERFAGE
SERFDOM
SERIALS
SERIATE
SERIESE
SERIESF
SERIESG
SERIESH
SERIESI
SERIESJ
SERIESK
SERIOUS
SERIPAK
SERLING
SERMONS
SERPENS
SERPENT
SERPICO
SERRATE
SERVANT
SERVEAS
SERVERS
SERVEUP
SERVICE
SERVILE
SERVING
SESAMES
SESSILE
SESSION
SESTETS
SESTINA
SETBACK
SETBAIL
SETDOWN
SETENTA
SETFEES
SETFREE
SETINTO
SETOFFS
SETOUTS
SETPLAY
SETRATE
SETSAIL
SETSHOT
SETSOFF
SETSOUT
SETTEES
SETTERS
SETTING
SETTLED
SETTLER
SETTLES
SETTLOR
SETTYPE
SETUPON
SEVENAD
SEVENAM
SEVENBC
SEVENEE
SEVENNO
SEVENPM
SEVENTH
SEVENTY
SEVENUP
SEVERAL
SEVERED
SEVERER
SEVERUS
SEVIGNY
SEVILLA
SEVILLE
SEWARDS
SEWEDON
SEWEDUP
SEWISTS
SEXIEST
SEXISTS
SEXLESS
SEXPOTS
SEXTANS
SEXTANT
SEXTETS
SEXTONS
SEYMOUR

S•E••••

SCENEII
SCENEIV
SCENERY
SCENEVI
SCENICS
SCENTED
SCENTER
SCEPTER
SCEPTIC
SCEPTRE
SEEABLE
SEEALSO
SEEDBED
SEEDERS
SEEDIER
SEEDILY
SEEDING
SEEDLET
SEEDPOD
SEEHERE
SEEINTO
SEEKERS
SEEKING
SEEKOUT
SEEMING
SEEMSTO
SEENALL
SEENFIT
SEENOFF
SEENOUT
SEEPAGE
SEEPAST
SEEPIER
SEEPING
SEEPOUT
SEEPSIN
SEERESS
SEESALL
SEESAWS
SEESFIT
SEESOFF
SEESOUT
SEESRED
SEETHED
SEETHES
SEETHRU
SEETOIT
SHEAFED
SHEARED
SHEARER
SHEATHE
SHEATHS
SHEAVED
SHEAVES
SHEBANG
SHEBEAR
SHECRAB
SHEDDER
SHEDSON
SHEEHAN
SHEERED
SHEERER
SHEERLY
SHEETED
SHEFFER
SHEGOAT
SHEIKHS
SHEILAE
SHEILAS
SHEKELS
SHELDON
SHELLAC
SHELLED
SHELLER
SHELLEY
SHELTER
SHELTIE
SHELVED
SHELVER
SHELVES
SHEPARD
SHERBET
SHERIFF
SHERIFS
SHERMAN
SHERPAS
SHERWIN
SHEVATS
SHEWOLF
SIEBZIG
SIEGING
SIEMENS
SIENESE
SIENNAS
SIERRAS
SIESTAS
SIEVING
SKEETER
SKEEZIX
SKELTER
SKELTON
SKEPTIC
SKETCHY
SKEWERS
SKEWING
SLEAZES
SLEDDED
SLEDDER
SLEDDOG
SLEDFUL
SLEDGED
SLEDGES
SLEEKED
SLEEKEN
SLEEKER
SLEEKLY
SLEEPER
SLEEPIN
SLEEPON
SLEETED
SLEEVED
SLEEVES
SLEIGHS
SLEIGHT
SLENDER
SLEPTIN
SLEPTON
SLEUTHS
SLEWING
SMEAGOL
SMEARED
SMEARER
SMEARON
SMELLED
SMELLER
SMELTED
SMELTER
SMETANA
SNEAKBY
SNEAKED
SNEAKER
SNEAKIN
SNEAKUP
SNEERAT
SNEERED
SNEERER
SNEETCH
SNEEZED
SNEEZER
SNEEZES
SNELLEN
SPEAKER
SPEAKOF
SPEAKTO
SPEAKUP
SPEARED
SPEARER
SPECIAL
SPECIES
SPECIFY
SPECING
SPECKED
SPECKLE
SPECOUT
SPECTER
SPECTOR
SPECTRA
SPECTRE
SPEDOFF
SPEEDED
SPEEDER
SPEEDOS
SPEEDUP
SPELLED
SPELLER
SPELUNK
SPENCER
SPENDER
SPENDON
SPENSER
SPENTON
SPEWERS
SPEWING
SPEWOUT
STEADED
STEALER
STEALIN
STEALTH
STEAMED
STEAMER
STEAMUP
STEANNE
STEARIC
STEARIN
STEARNS
STEELED
STEELER
STEELIE
STEEPED
STEEPEN
STEEPER
STEEPIN
STEEPLE
STEEPLY
STEERED
STEERER
STEEVED
STEEVES
STEFANI
STEIGER
STEINEM
STEINER
STELIAS
STELLAR
STEMMED
STEMPEL
STENCIL
STENGEL
STENGUN
STENNIS
STENTOR
STEPDAD
STEPHEN
STEPINS
STEPMOM
STEPOFF
STEPONE
STEPOUT
STEPPED
STEPPER
STEPPES
STEPSIN
STEPSON
STEPSUP
STEPTWO
STEPUPS
STEREOS
STERILE
STERNAL
STERNER
STERNLY
STERNOS
STERNUM
STEROID
STEROLS
STERTOR
STETSON
STETTED
STEUBEN
STEVENS
STEWARD
STEWART
STEWERS
STEWIER
STEWING
STEWPAN
STEWPOT
SUEDFOR
SUELLEN
SUELYON
SUESFOR
SVELTER
SVERIGE
SWEARAT
SWEARBY
SWEARER
SWEARIN
SWEARTO
SWEATED
SWEATER
SWEATIT
SWEDISH
SWEENEY
SWEEPEA
SWEEPER
SWEEPUP
SWEETEN
SWEETER
SWEETIE
SWEETLY
SWEETON
SWELLED
SWELLER
SWELLUP
SWELTER
SWELTRY
SWENSON
SWEPTUP
SWERVED
SWERVES

S••E•••

SABERED
SADEYED
SADEYES
SAFEBET
SAFEWAY
SAGEHEN
SAGETEA
SALEMOR
SALERNO
SAMEDAY
SAMEDIS
SAMEKHS
SAMEOLD
SATEENS
SAVEDON
SAVEDUP
SAVEFOR
SAVESON
SAVESUP
SCHELDT
SCHEMAS
SCHEMED
SCHEMER
SCHEMES
SCHERZI
SCHERZO
SCIENCE
SCLERAE
SCLERAL
SCLERAS
SCREAKS
SCREAMS
SCREECH
SCREEDS
SCREENS
SCREWED
SCREWUP
SEAEELS
SECEDED
SECEDER
SECEDES
SEFERIS
SELECTS
SELENIC
SENECAN
SENECAS
SENEGAL
SENESCE
SERENER
SETENTA
SEVENAD
SEVENAM
SEVENBC
SEVENEE
SEVENNO
SEVENPM
SEVENTH
SEVENTY
SEVENUP
SEVERAL
SEVERED
SEVERER
SEVERUS
SEWEDON
SEWEDUP
SHEEHAN
SHEERED
SHEERER
SHEERLY
SHEETED
SHIELDS
SHOEBOX
SHOEING
SHOEPAC
SHTETLS
SIBERIA
SIDEARM
SIDEBAR
SIDEBET
SIDECAR
SIDEMAN
SIDEMEN
SIDEONE
SIDETWO
SIDEWAY
SILENCE
SILENTA
SILENTB
SILENTC
SILENTD
SILENTE
SILENTF
SILENTG
SILENTH
SILENTI
SILENTJ
SILENTK
SILENTL
SILENTM
SILENTN
SILENTO
SILENTP
SILENTQ
SILENTR
SILENTS
SILENTT
SILENTU
SILENTV
SILENTW
SILENTX
SILENTY
SILENTZ
SILESIA
SIMENON
SINEDIE
SINEWED
SIRENED
SISENOR
SITEMAP
SIXEEEE
SIZEDUP
SIZEONE
SIZESIX
SIZESUP
SIZETEN
SIZETWO
SKEETER
SKEEZIX
SLEEKED
SLEEKEN
SLEEKER
SLEEKLY
SLEEPER
SLEEPIN
SLEEPON
SLEETED
SLEEVED
SLEEVES
SLOEGIN
SNEERAT
SNEERED
SNEERER
SNEETCH
SNEEZED
SNEEZER
SNEEZES
SOBERED
SOBERER
SOBERLY
SOLEDAD
SOMEDAY
SOMEHOW
SOMEONE
SOMESAY
SOMEWAY
SORENTO
SPEEDED
SPEEDER
SPEEDOS
SPEEDUP
SPHERAL
SPHERED
SPHERES
SPHERIC
SPIEDON
SPIEGEL
SPIELED
SPIELER
SPIESON
SPLEENS
SPLEENY
SPLENDA
SPREADS
SQUEAKS
SQUEAKY
SQUEALS
SQUEERS
SQUEEZE
SQUELCH
STDENIS
STEELED
STEELER
STEELIE
STEEPED
STEEPEN
STEEPER
STEEPIN
STEEPLE
STEEPLY
STEERED
STEERER
STEEVED
STEEVES
STPETER
STREAKS
STREAKY
STREAMS
STREETS
STREGIS
STRETCH
STRETTI
STRETTO
STREWED
STREWER
SUBECHO
SUPERGS
SUREBET
SURECAN
SUREIAM
SUREIDO
SUREROF
SUZETTE
SWEENEY
SWEEPEA
SWEEPER
SWEEPUP
SWEETEN
SWEETER
SWEETIE
SWEETLY
SWEETON
SYNERGY

S•••E••

SACHEMS
SACHETS
SACKERS
SADDENS
SADDEST
SADNESS
SAGIEST
SAILERS
SALIENT
SALIERI
SALTERS
SALVERS
SAMLETS
SAMUELL
SANDERS
SANREMO
SANSEIS
SAPHEAD
SAPIENS
SAPIENT
SAPLESS
SAPPERS
SARGENT
SASSERS
SATEENS
SATIETY
SATWELL
SAUCERS
SAUTEED
SAWYERS
SCALENE
SCALERS
SCALEUP
SCAREDY
SCARERS
SCAREUP
SCENEII
SCENEIV
SCENERY
SCENEVI
SCHLEPP
SCHLEPS
SCHMEAR
SCHMEER
SCITECH
SCORERS
SCOTERS
SCREECH
SCREEDS
SCREENS
SCUSEME
SEABEDS
SEABEES
SEAEELS
SEAFERN
SEAHERO
SEALEGS
SEALERS
SEALERY
SEAMERS
SEARERS
SEATERS
SEAWEED
SECKELS
SECRECY
SECRETE
SECRETS
SEEDERS
SEEHERE
SEEKERS
SEERESS
SEGMENT
SEINERS
SEIZEON
SEIZERS
SELLECK
SELLERS
SENDEES
SENDERS
SENNETT
SENSEIS
SENSENS
SEPTETS
SEQUELS
SERIESE
SERIESF
SERIESG
SERIESH
SERIESI
SERIESJ
SERIESK
SERPENS
SERPENT
SERVEAS
SERVERS
SERVEUP
SESTETS
SETFEES
SETTEES
SETTERS
SEXIEST
SEXLESS
SEXTETS
SHADERS
SHAKERS
SHAKEUP
SHAPELY
SHAPERS
SHAPEUP
SHAREIN
SHARERS
SHAVERS
SHEBEAR
SHEKELS
SHINEON
SHINERS
SHINEUP
SHIVERS
SHIVERY
SHOREUP
SHOVEIN
SHOVELS
SHOVERS
SHOWERS
SHOWERY
SHRIEKS
SHUBERT
SHUTEYE
SHYNESS
SIAMESE
SICKENS
SICKEST
SIEMENS
SIENESE
SIFTERS
SIGHERS
SIGNEES
SIGNERS
SIGNETS
SILVERS
SILVERY
SIMMERS
SIMPERS
SINCERE
SINGERS
SINKERS
SINLESS
SINNERS
SIPPERS
SISTERS
SITTERS
SITWELL
SIXEEEE
SIXFEET
SIXTEEN
SIXWEEK
SIXYEAR
SKATERS
SKEWERS
SKIVEST
SKIWEAR
SKYLESS
SLAKERS

SLATERS
SLAVERS
SLAVERY
SLAYERS
SLICERS
SLICEUP
SLIDEBY
SLIDEIN
SLIDERS
SLIVERS
SLOPERS
SLOVENE
SLOVENS
SLOWEST
SLYNESS
SMILEAT
SMILEON
SMILERS
SMILEYS
SMITERS
SMOKERS
SMOKEUP
SMOKEYS
SNAKERS
SNARERS
SNIDELY
SNIDEST
SNIPEAT
SNIPERS
SNIVELS
SNORERS
SOAKERS
SOAPERS
SOARERS
SOAREWE
SOBBERS
SOCIETY
SOCKETS
SOCKEYE
SODLESS
SOFTENS
SOFTEST
SOIREES
SOLDERS
SOLFEGE
SOLNESS
SOLVEIT
SOLVENT
SOLVERS
SONLESS
SONNETS
SOONERS
SOONEST
SORBETS
SORCERY
SORRELL
SORRELS
SORTERS
SOSUEME
SOTHEBY
SOTHERE
SOTHERN
SOTWEED
SOUPERS
SOUREST
SOVIETS
SOWSEAR
SOYBEAN
SOYLENT
SOYMEAL
SPACELY
SPACERS
SPADERS
SPARELY
SPAREME
SPARERS
SPAREST
SPAYERS
SPEWERS
SPICERS
SPICERY
SPICEUP
SPIDERS
SPIDERY
SPIKERS
SPIKETV
SPIKEUP
SPINELS
SPINETS
SPIREAS
SPLEENS
SPLEENY
SPOKEOF
SPOKETO
SPOKEUP
SPRIEST
SPRYEST
SPYDERS
SQUEERS
SQUEEZE
STAGERS
STALELY
STALEST
STAMENS
STAREAT
STARERS
STATELY
STATERS
STAYERS
STEREOS
STEVENS
STEWERS
STIPEND
STOKELY
STOKERS
STOKEUP
STOLEIN
STONEAX
STONERS
STORERS
STOREUP
STOWERS
STREETS
STUDENT
STUPEFY
STYLERS
STYLETS
STYRENE
SUAVELY
SUAVEST
SUBCELL
SUBDEBS
SUBHEAD
SUBJECT
SUBLETS
SUBNETS
SUBSECT
SUBSETS
SUBTEEN
SUBTEND
SUBTEXT
SUBVENE
SUBVERT
SUBZERO
SUCCEED
SUCCESS
SUCKERS
SUDSERS
SUFFERS
SUGGEST
SULKERS
SUMLESS
SUMMERS
SUMMERY
SUNBEAM
SUNBELT
SUNDECK
SUNDERS
SUNLESS
SUNSETS
SUPPERS
SUPREME
SURFEIT
SURFERS
SURGEON
SURGERY
SURREAL
SURREYS
SURVEIL
SURVEYS
SUSPECT
SUSPEND
SWAYERS
SWIGERT
SWINERY
SWIPERS
SWIVELS
SWIVETS
SWOREAT
SWOREBY
SWOREIN
SWORETO
SYSTEMS

S••••E•

SABERED
SABINES
SACQUES
SADDLED
SADDLER
SADDLES
SADEYED
SADEYES
SAFEBET
SAGEHEN
SAGETEA
SAGGIER
SAINTED
SAINTES
SALADES
SALINES
SALLIED
SALLIER
SALLIES
SALTIER
SALTSEA
SALUTED
SALUTER
SALUTES
SALVOES
SAMBAED
SAMISEN
SAMOSET
SAMOYED
SAMPLED
SAMPLER
SAMPLES
SANDIER
SANDLER
SANDMEN
SANIBEL
SAPPIER
SARACEN
SARALEE
SARAZEN
SASSIER
SATCHEL
SATINET
SATIRES
SAUCIER
SAUNAED
SAUNTER
SAUTEED
SAVAGED
SAVAGER
SAVAGES
SAVORED
SAVORER
SAVVIED
SAVVIER
SAVVIES
SAYAMEN
SAYOVER
SAYSYES
SAYWHEN
SCALDED
SCALDER
SCALIER
SCALPED
SCALPEL
SCALPER
SCAMMED
SCAMMER
SCAMPED
SCAMPER
SCANNED
SCANNER
SCANTED
SCANTER
SCARCER
SCARFED
SCARFER
SCARIER
SCARLET
SCARPED
SCARRED
SCARVES
SCATHED
SCATHES
SCATTED
SCATTER
SCENTED
SCENTER
SCEPTER
SCHAYES
SCHEMED
SCHEMER
SCHEMES
SCHMEER
SCHMOES
SCHOLES
SCHUMER
SCOFFED
SCOFFER
SCOLDED
SCOLDER
SCONCES
SCOOPED
SCOOPER
SCOOTED
SCOOTER
SCORNED
SCORNER
SCOUPES
SCOURED
SCOURER
SCOUTED
SCOUTER
SCOWLED
SCOWLER
SCRAPED
SCRAPER
SCRAPES
SCREWED
SCRIBED
SCRIBER
SCRIBES
SCUBAED
SCUDDED
SCUDDER
SCUFFED
SCUFFER
SCULLED
SCULLER
SCULPED
SCUPPER
SCURVES
SCUZZES
SCYTHED
SCYTHES
SEABEES
SEAGREN
SEAMIER
SEANCES
SEAWEED
SECEDED
SECEDER
SECEDES
SECURED
SECURER
SECURES
SEDATED
SEDATER
SEDATES
SEDGIER
SEDUCED
SEDUCER
SEDUCES
SEEDBED
SEEDIER
SEEDLET
SEEPIER
SEESRED
SEETHED
SEETHES
SELTZER
SEMITES
SENATES
SENDEES
SENORES
SEPALED
SERAPES
SERENER
SESAMES
SETFEES
SETFREE
SETTEES
SETTLED
SETTLER
SETTLES
SEVENEE
SEVERED
SEVERER
SHACKED
SHADIER
SHAFFER
SHAFTED
SHAGGED
SHAKIER
SHAKOES
SHALIER
SHAMMED
SHANKED
SHANNEN
SHANTER
SHARKEY
SHARPED
SHARPEI
SHARPEN
SHARPER
SHATNER
SHATTER
SHAWLED
SHAWNEE
SHEAFED
SHEARED
SHEARER
SHEAVED
SHEAVES
SHEDDER
SHEERED
SHEERER
SHEETED
SHEFFER
SHELLED
SHELLER
SHELLEY
SHELTER
SHELVED
SHELVER
SHELVES
SHERBET
SHIFTED
SHIFTER
SHIITES
SHILLED
SHIMMER
SHINIER
SHINNED
SHIPMEN
SHIPPED
SHIPPER
SHIRKED
SHIRKER
SHIRLEY
SHIRRED
SHOALED
SHOCKED
SHOCKER
SHODDEN
SHOOTER
SHOPPED
SHOPPER
SHOPPES
SHORTED
SHORTEN
SHORTER
SHOUTED
SHOUTER
SHOWIER
SHOWMEN
SHRIKES
SHRINED
SHRINER
SHRINES
SHRIVEL
SHRIVER
SHRIVES
SHUCKED
SHUCKER
SHUDDER
SHUNNED
SHUNTED
SHUNTER
SHUSHED
SHUSHES
SHUSTER
SHUTTER
SHYSTER
SICKBED
SICKLES
SIDEBET
SIDEMEN
SIGHTED
SIGHTER
SIGNEES
SILKIER
SILLIER
SILLIES
SILTIER
SIMILES
SIMPLER
SIMPLES
SIMPLEX
SINEWED
SINGLED
SINGLES
SINGLET
SINUSES
SIRENED
SISSIER
SISSIES
SIXEEEE
SIXFEET
SIXTEEN
SIXTIES
SIXWEEK
SIZETEN
SIZZLED
SIZZLER
SIZZLES
SKEETER
SKELTER
SKIAREA
SKIDDED
SKIDDER
SKIFFED
SKILLED
SKILLET
SKIMMED
SKIMMER
SKIMPED
SKINNED
SKINNER
SKIPPED
SKIPPER
SKIRLED
SKIRTED
SKIRTER
SKITTER
SKOSHES
SKULKED
SKULKER
SKULLED
SKUNKED
SLABBED
SLACKED
SLACKEN
SLACKER
SLAMMED
SLAMMER
SLANDER
SLANTED
SLAPPED
SLAPPER
SLASHED
SLASHER
SLASHES
SLATHER
SLATIER
SLATTED
SLEAZES
SLEDDED
SLEDDER
SLEDGED
SLEDGES
SLEEKED
SLEEKEN
SLEEKER
SLEEPER
SLEETED
SLEEVED
SLEEVES
SLENDER
SLICKED
SLICKER
SLIMIER
SLIMMED
SLIMMER
SLINGER
SLINKED
SLINKER
SLIPPED
SLIPPER
SLITHER
SLITTED
SLITTER
SLOBBER
SLOGGED
SLOGGER
SLOPPED
SLOSHED
SLOSHES
SLOTTED
SLOTTER
SLUDGES
SLUGGED
SLUGGER
SLUICED
SLUICES
SLUMBER
SLUMMED
SLUMMER
SLUMPED
SLURPED
SLURPEE
SLURPER
SLURRED
SLUSHED
SLUSHES
SMACKED
SMACKER
SMALLER
SMARTED
SMARTEN
SMARTER
SMASHED
SMASHER
SMASHES
SMATTER
SMEARED
SMEARER
SMELLED
SMELLER
SMELTED
SMELTER
SMIDGEN
SMIDGES
SMIRKED
SMIRKER
SMITHED
SMITTEN
SMOKIER
SMOKIES
SMOLDER
SMOTHER
SMUCKER
SMUDGED
SMUDGES
SMUGGER
SMUSHED
SMUSHES
SNACKED
SNACKER
SNAFUED
SNAGGED
SNAGGER
SNAKIER
SNAPPEA
SNAPPED
SNAPPER
SNARFED
SNARLED
SNARLER
SNEAKED
SNEAKER
SNEERED
SNEERER
SNEEZED
SNEEZER
SNEEZES
SNELLEN
SNICKER
SNICKET
SNIFFED
SNIFFER
SNIFTER
SNIGLET
SNIPPED
SNIPPER
SNIPPET
SNOOKER
SNOOPED
SNOOPER
SNOOTED
SNOOZED
SNOOZER
SNOOZES
SNORKEL
SNORTED
SNORTER
SNOUTED
SNOWIER
SNOWMEN
SNOWPEA
SNUBBED
SNUBBER
SNUFFED
SNUFFER
SNUGGED
SNUGGER
SOAPIER
SOAPNET
SOBERED
SOBERER
SODDIER
SOFABED
SOFTGEL
SOFTIES
SOGGIER
SOHAVEI
SOIGNEE
SOIREES
SOLACED
SOLACER
SOLACES
SOLDIER
SOLIDER
SOLUTES
SOMINEX
SOOTHED
SOOTHER
SOOTHES
SOOTIER
SOPHIES
SOPPIER
SORRIER
SORTIED
SORTIES
SOTWEED
SOUNDED
SOUNDER
SOUPIER
SOURCED
SOURCES
SOUTHEY
SPACIER
SPAMMED
SPAMMER
SPANDEX
SPANIEL
SPANKED
SPANKER
SPANNED
SPANNER
SPARKED
SPARRED
SPARRER
SPARSER
SPATHES
SPATTED
SPATTER
SPAWNED
SPAWNER
SPEAKER
SPEARED
SPEARER
SPECIES
SPECKED
SPECTER
SPEEDED
SPEEDER
SPELLED
SPELLER
SPENCER
SPENDER
SPENSER
SPHERED
SPHERES
SPICIER
SPIEGEL
SPIELED
SPIELER
SPIFFED
SPIKIER
SPILLED
SPILLER
SPINIER
SPINNER
SPINNEY
SPIRIER
SPITTER
SPITZES
SPLAYED
SPLICED
SPLICER
SPLICES
SPLINES
SPOILED
SPOILER
SPONDEE
SPONGED
SPONGER
SPONGES
SPOOFED
SPOOFER
SPOOKED
SPOOLED
SPOOLER
SPOONED
SPOONER
SPORTED
SPOTTED
SPOTTER
SPOUSES
SPOUTED
SPOUTER
SPRAYED
SPRAYER
SPRITES
SPRUCED
SPRUCER
SPRUCES
SPUMIER
SPURNED
SPURNER
SPURRED
SPURTED
SPUTTER
SQUARED
SQUARER
SQUARES
SQUIRED
SQUIRES
SSHAPED
STABBED
STABBER
STABLED
STABLER
STABLES
STACKED
STACKER
STADLER
STAFFED
STAFFER
STAGGED
STAGGER
STAGIER
STAGNES
STAIDER
STAINED
STAINER
STAIRED
STALKED
STALKER
STALLED
STALLER
STAMMER
STAMPED
STAMPER
STANCES
STANDEE
STANDER
STANLEE
STANLEY
STAPLED
STAPLER
STAPLES
STARKER
STARKEY
STARLET
STARRED
STARTED
STARTER
STARVED
STARVES
STASHED
STASHES
STASSEN
STATLER
STATUES
STEADED
STEALER
STEAMED
STEAMER
STEELED
STEELER
STEEPED
STEEPEN
STEEPER
STEERED
STEERER
STEEVED
STEEVES
STEIGER
STEINEM
STEINER
STEMMED
STEMPEL
STENGEL
STEPHEN
STEPPED
STEPPER
STEPPES
STERNER
STETTED
STEUBEN
STEWIER
STICKER
STIFFED
STIFFEL
STIFFEN
STIFFER
STIFLED
STIFLES
STILLED
STILLER
STILTED
STINGER
STINKER
STINTED
STINTER
STIRRED
STIRRER
STJAMES
STLUKES
STOCKED
STOCKER
STODGED
STODGES
STOGIES
STOLLEN
STOMPED
STONIER
STOOGED
STOOGES
STOOKEY
STOOLED
STOOPED
STOOPER
STOPPED
STOPPER
STORIED
STORIES

STORMED
STOUTEN
STOUTER
STPETER
STRAFED
STRAFER
STRAFES
STRAYED
STRAYER
STREWED
STREWER
STRIDER
STRIDES
STRIFES
STRIKER
STRIKES
STRIPED
STRIPER
STRIPES
STRIVED
STRIVEN
STRIVER
STRIVES
STROBES
STROKED
STROKER
STROKES
STRUDEL
STUBBED
STUDDED
STUDIED
STUDIER
STUDIES
STUFFED
STUFFER
STUMPED
STUMPER
STUNNED
STUNNER
STUNTED
STURGES
STUTTER
STUTZES
STYMIED
STYMIES
SUBAREA
SUBDUED
SUBDUER
SUBDUES
SUBIDEA
SUBITEM
SUBTEEN
SUBTLER
SUCCEED
SUCKIER
SUDAFED
SUDSIER
SUELLEN
SUGARED
SULKIER
SULKIES
SULLIED
SULLIES
SULUSEA
SUNDAES
SUNNIER
SUPPLED
SUPPLER

SUPPLES
SUREBET
SURFIER
SURFMEN
SURLIER
SUTURED
SUTURES
SVELTER
SWABBED
SWABBER
SWAGGER
SWAGMEN
SWAMPED
SWANKED
SWANKER
SWANSEA
SWAPPED
SWAPPER
SWARMED
SWARMER
SWASHED
SWASHES
SWATHED
SWATHES
SWATTED
SWATTER
SWEARER
SWEATED
SWEATER
SWEENEY
SWEEPEA
SWEEPER
SWEETEN
SWEETER
SWELLED
SWELLER
SWELTER
SWERVED
SWERVES
SWIFTER
SWIGGED
SWILLED
SWILLER
SWIMMER
SWINGER
SWIRLED
SWISHED
SWISHES
SWITZER
SWOLLEN
SWOONED
SWOONER
SWOOPED
SWOOPER
SYNCHED
SYNFUEL

S•••••E

SACCADE
SACLIKE
SADCAFE
SADFATE
SAIDAYE
SALABLE
SALTINE
SALVAGE
SAMWISE
SANJOSE

SANTAFE
SAOTOME
SARALEE
SARDINE
SATHOME
SATIATE
SAUSAGE
SAVABLE
SAWLIKE
SAYABLE
SAYMORE
SAYSAYE
SCALAGE
SCALENE
SCEPTRE
SCIENCE
SCLERAE
SCOTTIE
SCOURGE
SCROOGE
SCRUPLE
SCUFFLE
SCUSEME
SCUTTLE
SEABLUE
SEAFARE
SEAGATE
SEALANE
SEALIFE
SEALIKE
SEAMILE
SEARACE
SEASIDE
SEATTLE
SECLUDE
SECRETE
SEEABLE
SEEHERE
SEEPAGE
SEIZURE
SELVAGE
SENESCE
SENSATE
SERFAGE
SERIATE
SERIESE
SERRATE
SERVICE
SERVILE
SESSILE
SETFREE
SETRATE
SETTYPE
SEVENEE
SEVILLE
SHACKLE
SHADROE
SHALLWE
SHAMBLE
SHARPIE
SHAWNEE
SHEATHE
SHEILAE
SHELTIE
SHINGLE
SHORTIE
SHUFFLE
SHUTEYE

SHUTTLE
SIAMESE
SIDEONE
SIENESE
SIGNAGE
SIGNORE
SILENCE
SILENTE
SILKTIE
SILLYME
SINCERE
SINEDIE
SINKAGE
SINLIKE
SINUATE
SIRDUKE
SISTINE
SITHOME
SITUATE
SIXEEEE
SIXFIVE
SIXLANE
SIXNINE
SIZABLE
SIZEONE
SKIABLE
SKIFFLE
SKIPOLE
SKIRACE
SKITTLE
SKYBLUE
SKYDIVE
SKYDOME
SKYLIKE
SKYLINE
SLOVENE
SLURPEE
SMUGGLE
SNAPPLE
SNIFFLE
SNOCONE
SNUFFLE
SNUGGLE
SOAREWE
SOCKEYE
SODIDWE
SOIGNEE
SOILAGE
SOLFEGE
SOLUBLE
SOMEONE
SONANCE
SONLIKE
SORBATE
SOSUEME
SOTHERE
SOUBISE
SOUFFLE
SOURALE
SOWLIKE
SPACKLE
SPANGLE
SPAREME
SPARKLE
SPECKLE
SPECTRE
SPINDLE
SPITTLE

SPLURGE
SPOKANE
SPONDEE
SPUMONE
SPYHOLE
SPYWARE
SQUEEZE
STABILE
STANDEE
STANINE
STANLEE
STARTLE
STATICE
STATURE
STATUTE
STEANNE
STEELIE
STEEPLE
STEPONE
STERILE
STIPPLE
STOOLIE
STOPPLE
STORAGE
STOWAGE
STRANGE
STRASSE
STRIATE
STROPHE
STROUSE
STUBBLE
STUMBLE
STYLISE
STYLIZE
STYRENE
SUASIVE
SUBBASE
SUBCASE
SUBCODE
SUBDATE
SUBFILE
SUBLIME
SUBRACE
SUBSIDE
SUBSUME
SUBTONE
SUBTYPE
SUBVENE
SUBZONE
SUCRASE
SUCROSE
SUFFICE
SUFFUSE
SUITSME
SULFATE
SULFIDE
SULFITE
SUMMATE
SUNFIRE
SUNLIKE
SUNRISE
SUPPOSE
SUPREME
SURFACE
SURMISE
SURNAME
SURVIVE
SUSANNE

SUSPIRE
SUZANNE
SUZETTE
SVERIGE
SWADDLE
SWEETIE
SWINDLE
SWIZZLE
SWOOSIE
SYNAPSE
SYNCOPE
SYRINGE
SYSTOLE

•SE••••

ASEETHE
ASEPSIS
ASEPTIC
ASEXUAL
ISECOND
ISEENOW
ISEEYOU
OSETRAS
TSELIOT
TSETSES
TSETUNG
USEDCAR
USEDCDS
USEDFOR
USELESS
USERFEE
USERIDS
USESFOR

•S•E•••

ASCENDS
ASCENTS
ASCETIC
ASEETHE
ASKEDIN
ASKEDOF
ASKEDUP
ASLEWOF
ASPECTS
ASPENCO
ASPERSE
ASSENTS
ASSERTS
ASTERIX
CSLEWIS
ESCENCE
ESSENCE
ESSENES
ESTEBAN
ESTEEMS
ESTEFAN
ESTELLA
ESTELLE
ESTEVEZ
ISEENOW
ISEEYOU
ISLETED
MSIEURS
OSCEOLA
OSIERED
OSSEOUS
OSSETRA
OSTEOID

USHERED
USHERIN
USTEDES

•S••E••

ASATEAM
ASHBERY
ASHHEAP
ASHIEST
ASHLESS
ASSWEET
ASTREAM
ESCHEAT
ESCHERS
ESCHEWS
ESCUELA
ESOBESO
ESOTERY
ESPNEWS
ESTEEMS
ESTHETE
ISABEAU
ISAHEAD
ISOHELS
ISOMERS
ISRAELI
ISSUEAD
ISSUERS
ISUREAM
ISUREDO
OSPREYS
OSTLERS
USELESS
USOPENS
USSTEEL
USURERS

•S•••E•

ASANTES
ASCARED
ASHAMED
ASHIVER
ASHTREE
ASIMMER
ASKOVER
ASPIRED
ASPIRER
ASPIRES
ASQUIET
ASSAYED
ASSAYER
ASSIZES
ASSUMED
ASSUMER
ASSUMES
ASSURED
ASSURER
ASSURES
ASSWEET
ASTUTER
ASUNDER
ESCAPED
ESCAPEE
ESCAPER
ESCAPES
ESSAYED
ESSAYER
ESSENES

ESTATED
ESTATES
ESTEVEZ
ISHMAEL
ISLETED
ISRAFEL
LSHAPED
OSCINES
OSCULES
OSHAPED
OSIERED
OSMOSED
OSMOSES
OSSIPEE
PSALTER
PSHAWED
PSYCHED
PSYCHES
SSHAPED
TSETSES
TSHAPED
TSHAPES
USABLES
USANCES
USERFEE
USHAPED
USHAPES
USHERED
USSTEEL
USTEDES
USURIES
USURPED
USURPER
VSHAPED
VSHAPES
YSHAPED
YSHAPES

•S••••E

ASAJOKE
ASARULE
ASCRIBE
ASEETHE
ASHCAKE
ASHTREE
ASININE
ASKANCE
ASPERSE
ASSANTE
ASSLIKE
ASSUAGE
ASTAIRE
ASTARTE
ASTRIDE
ESCAPEE
ESCENCE
ESPOUSE
ESQUIRE
ESSENCE
ESTELLE
ESTHETE
ISADORE
ISIDORE
ISOLATE
ISOLINE
ISOTONE
ISOTOPE
JSTROKE

OSBORNE
OSSICLE
OSSIPEE
TSQUARE
USERFEE
USSTATE

••SE•••

ABSENCE
ABSENTS
ANSELMO
ARSENAL
ARSENIC
ARSENIO
ASSENTS
ASSERTS
ATSEVEN
AXSEEDS
BASEDON
BASEHIT
BASEMAN
BASEMEN
BASENJI
BASEPAY
BASESIX
BASETEN
BASETWO
BESEECH
BISECTS
CASEATE
CASEINS
CASELAW
CASELLA
CASELOT
CASEOUS
CASEOUT
CASERNE
CASERNS
CASERTA
CISEAUX
COSETTE
DESEEDS
DESERET
DESERTS
DESERVE
DESEXED
DESEXES
DISEASE
DISEURS
DISEUSE
DRSEUSS
EASEDBY
EASEDIN
EASEDON
EASEDUP
EASEFUL
EASELED
EASEOFF
EASEOUT
EASESBY
EASESIN
EASESON
EASESUP
ENSEALS
ENSEATS
ESSENCE
ESSENES
EXSECTS

EXSERTS
FUSEBOX
GASEDUP
GASEITY
GASEOUS
GASESUP
GISELLE
INSEAMS
INSECTA
INSECTS
INSERTS
ITSEASY
JOSEPHA
JOSEPHI
LISENTE
LOSEBIG
LOSEOUT
LOSESIT
LOSESTO
LYSENKO
MESEEMS
MISEDIT
MISERLY
MOSELLE
MOSEYED
MUSEDON
MUSEFUL
MUSESON
MUSETTA
MUSETTE
MUSEUMS
NOSEATS
NOSEBAG
NOSEBRA
NOSEDIN
NOSEDUP
NOSEEUM
NOSEGAY
NOSEJOB
NOSEOUT
NOSESIN
NOSESUP
OBSERVE
OISEAUX
ONSERVE
OSSEOUS
OSSETRA
PESETAS
PESEWAS
POSEDAS
POSESAS
POSEURS
POSEUSE
RESEALS
RESEAMS
RESEATS
RESEAUS
RESEAUX
RESECTS
RESEEDS
RESEEKS
RESEIZE
RESELLS
RESENDS
RESENTS
RESERVE
RESEWED
RISENTO

RISESTO
RISESUP
ROSEATE
ROSEBAY
ROSEBUD
ROSEHIP
ROSELLA
ROSELLE
ROSEOIL
ROSEOLA
ROSERED
ROSETEA
ROSETTA
ROSETTE
SISENOR
TASERED
UNSEALS
UNSEAMS
UNSEATS
UNSELLS
UNSEWED
UPSENDS
WISEDUP
WISEGUY
WISEMAN
WISEMEN
WISEONE
WISESUP

••S•E••

AMSTELS
ANSWERS
ASSWEET
AUSLESE
AUSTERE
AUSTERS
AXSEEDS
BASHERS
BASKETS
BASKETT
BASSETS
BASSETT
BASTERS
BESEECH
BESIEGE
BESMEAR
BESPEAK
BESSELL
BISSELL
BOSWELL
BUSCEMI
BUSHELS
BUSHERS
BUSIEST
BUSKERS
BUSSERS
BUSTERS
CASHEWS
CASKETS
CASTERS
CBSNEWS
CISTERN
COSHERS
COSIEST
COSSETS
CUSSERS
CUSTERS
DASHERS

DESCEND
DESCENT
DESEEDS
DESHELL
DESSERT
DESTEMS
DISCERN
DISPELS
DISSECT
DISSENT
DISSERT
DISTEND
DUSTERS
EASIEST
EASTEGG
EASTEND
EASTERN
EASTERS
EPSTEIN
FASTENS
FASTEST
FESTERS
FISHERS
FISHERY
FISHEYE
FOSTERS
FUSSERS
GASHEAT
GASJETS
GASKELL
GASKETS
GASLEAK
GASLESS
GASPERS
GASSERS
GASTERO
GOSPELS
GOSSETT
GUSHERS
GUSSETS
HASBEEN
HASKELL
HASTENS
HASTERT
HISPEED
HISSERS
HOSIERS
HOSIERY
HOSTELS
HOSTESS
HUSKERS
HUSSEIN
HUSSERL
IMSWELL
INSPECT
INSTEAD
INSTEPS
INSWEPT
ISSUEAD
ISSUERS
ITSBEST
ITSHERE
JASPERS
JASPERY
JESTERS
JOSHERS
JUSTEST
KISLEVS

KISMETS
KISSELS
KISSERS
KOSHERS
LASHERS
LESSEES
LESSENS
LESSEPS
LISBETH
LISPERS
LISTEES
LISTENS
LISTERS
LUSHEST
LUSTERS
MASHERS
MASKERS
MASSEUR
MASTERP
MASTERS
MASTERY
MESEEMS
MISDEAL
MISDEED
MISDEEM
MISFEED
MISHEAR
MISKEYS
MISLEAD
MISMESH
MISREAD
MISRELY
MISSEAT
MISSEND
MISSENT
MISSETS
MISTELL
MISTERM
MISTERS
MISTERX
MOSHERS
MOSLEMS
MRSPEEL
MUSHERS
MUSKEGO
MUSKETS
MUSSELS
MUSTERS
MYSTERY
NASCENT
NESTEGG
NESTERS
NOSEEUM
NOSHERS
NOSIEST
NOSWEAT
OBSCENE
OUSTERS
OYSTERS
PASSELS
PASSERS
PASSEUL
PASTEIN
PASTELS
PASTERN
PASTERS
PASTEUP
PASTEUR

PESTERS
PISCEAN
POSHEST
POSSESS
POSTERN
POSTERS
PUSHERS
QBSNEAK
RASHERS
RASHEST
RASPERS
RASTERS
RESEEDS
RESEEKS
RESMELT
RESPEAK
RESPECT
RESPELL
RESPELT
RESTERS
RESWEAR
RESWEEP
RISKERS
ROSIEST
ROSTERS
ROSWELL
RUSHEES
RUSHERS
RUSSELL
RUSSERT
RUSSETS
RUSSETY
SASSERS
SESTETS
SISTERS
SOSUEME
SUSPECT
SUSPEND
SYSTEMS
TASSELS
TASTEIT
TASTERS
TESSERA
TESTEES
TESTERS
TOSSERS
TUSHERY
TUSKERS
ULSTERS
UNSHEER
UNSHELL
UNSKEWS
UNSLEEK
UNSPEAK
UNSPELT
UNSPENT
UNSTEEL
UNSTEPS
UNSTERN
UNSWEAR
UNSWEET
UNSWEPT
UPSTEPS
UPSWEEP
UPSWELL
UPSWEPT
USSTEEL
VASTEST
VESPERS
VESSELS
VESTEES
VISCERA
VISTEON
WASHERS
WASTERS
WESTEGG
WESTEND
WESTERN
WESTERS
WISHERS
XYSTERS
YASBECK
YESDEAR
YESLETS
ZESTERS

••S••E•

APSIDES
ASSAYED
ASSAYER
ASSIZES
ASSUMED
ASSUMER
ASSUMES
ASSURED
ASSURER
ASSURES
ASSWEET
ATSEVEN
AUSSIES
BASEMEN
BASETEN
BASQUES
BASSIER
BESIDES
BESTBET
BESTMEN
BESTREW
BISHKEK
BISQUES
BOSOMED
BOSSIER
BOSSMEN
BUSBIES
BUSHIER
BUSHMEN
BUSTIER
BUSTLED
BUSTLER
BUSTLES
BUSYBEE
CASHIER
CASQUED
CASQUES
CASTLED
CASTLES
CISCOES
COSINES
COSTNER
CUSHIER
CUSSLER
DASHIER
DESERET
DESEXED
DESEXES
DESIRED
DESIREE
DESIRER
DESIRES
DESKSET
DESTAEL
DISCOED
DISHIER
DISOBEY
DISUSED
DISUSES
DOSAGES
DOSSIER
DUSKIER
DUSTIER
DUSTMEN
EASELED
ENSILED
ENSILES
ENSKIED
ENSKIES
ENSURED
ENSURER
ENSURES
EOSINES
ESSAYED
ESSAYER
ESSENES
FASTNET
FESCUES
FISCHER
FISHIER
FISHNET
FUSSIER
FUSTIER
GASOVEN
GASSIER
GESSOED
GESSOES
GUSHIER
GUSSIED
GUSSIES
GUSTIER
GUSTOES
HASASET
HASBEEN
HASOVER
HASSLED
HASSLES
HASTIER
HISPEED
HISSIER
HOSTLER
HUSKIER
HUSKIES
HUSSIES
HUSTLED
HUSTLER
HUSTLES
INSALES
INSANER
INSIDER
INSIDES
INSOLES
INSURED
INSURER
INSURES
ITSOPEN
ITSOVER
JOSTLED
JOSTLER
JOSTLES
KASTLER
KESTREL
KISHKES
LASSIES
LASSOED
LASSOER
LASSOES
LASTLEG
LESSEES
LISTEES
LOSTPET
LUSHIER
LUSTIER
LUSTRED
LUSTRES
MASHIES
MASONED
MASQUER
MASQUES
MASSIER
MESHIER
MESSIER
MISAVER
MISBREW
MISCUED
MISCUES
MISDEED
MISDEEM
MISDOER
MISDOES
MISDREW
MISFEED
MISKNEW
MISSIES
MISSTEP
MISTIER
MISUSED
MISUSER
MISUSES
MOSEYED
MOSQUES
MOSSIER
MRSPEEL
MUSCLED
MUSCLES
MUSHIER
MUSKIER
MUSKIES
MUSSIER
MUSTIER
MUSTSEE
NASTIER
NASTIES
NESTLED
NESTLER
NESTLES
NOSIREE
ONSAGER
ONSIDES
OSSIPEE
PASSKEY
PASTIER
PASTIES
PESADES
PESKIER
PESTLED
PESTLES
POSITED
POSOLES
POSTIES
POSTMEN
PUSHIER
PUSSIES
RASPIER
RASSLED
RASSLER
RASSLES
RASURES
RESALES
RESAVED
RESAVES
RESAWED
RESCUED
RESCUER
RESCUES
RESEWED
RESHOES
RESIDED
RESIDER
RESIDES
RESILED
RESILES
RESINED
RESITED
RESIZED
RESIZER
RESIZES
RESOJET
RESOLED
RESOLER
RESOLES
RESOWED
RESTREW
RESUMED
RESUMES
RESWEEP
RISKIER
ROSCOES
ROSERED
ROSETEA
ROSINED
ROSSNER
ROSSSEA
RUSHEES
RUSHIER
RUSTIER
RUSTLED
RUSTLER
RUSTLES
SASSIER
SESAMES
SISSIER
SISSIES
TASERED
TASTIER
TESTBED
TESTEES
TESTIER
TISANES
TISSUES
TISSUEY
TUSHIES
TUSSLED
TUSSLES
UNSAFER
UNSATED
UNSAVED
UNSAWED
UNSCREW
UNSEWED
UNSHEER
UNSHIER
UNSHOED
UNSHOES
UNSHYER
UNSIDED
UNSIZED
UNSLEEK
UNSLIER
UNSLYER
UNSOBER
UNSOLED
UNSOLES
UNSOWED
UNSPIED
UNSTEEL
UNSWEET
UPSIDES
UPSIZED
UPSIZES
UPSWEEP
USSTEEL
VASQUEZ
VASTIER
VESTEES
VISAGED
VISAGES
VISITED
VISORED
VISTAED
WASHIER
WASPIER
WASTREL
WESTIES
WISEMEN
WISPIER
YESISEE
ZESTIER

••S•••E

ABSCISE
ABSENCE
ABSOLVE
ADSPACE
ARSHILE
ASSANTE
ASSLIKE
ASSUAGE
ATSTAKE
AUSABLE
AUSLESE
AUSPICE
AUSTERE
BASSALE
BESIEGE
BESPOKE
BESTONE
BISTATE
BOSCAGE
BUSFARE
BUSLANE
BUSLINE
BUSRIDE
BUSYBEE
CASCADE
CASEATE
CASERNE
CASTILE
CDSTORE
CESAIRE
COSETTE
COSTATE
COSTIVE
COSTUME
CUSPATE
DASCHLE
DESERVE
DESIREE
DESPISE
DESPITE
DESTINE
DISABLE
DISEASE
DISEUSE
DISLIKE
DISPOSE
DISPUTE
DISRATE
DISROBE
EASYONE
ENSLAVE
ENSNARE
ENSUITE
ERSKINE
ESSENCE
EUSTACE
FASCIAE
FASTONE
FESTIVE
FISHEYE
FISSILE
FISSURE
FUSIBLE
GASLINE
GASPIPE
GASTONE
GESTATE
GESTURE
GISELLE
GOSSAGE
GOSTALE
GUSTAVE
HASDONE
HASTIME
HASTOBE
HESSAFE
HOSCALE
HOSPICE
HOSTAGE
HOSTILE
HUSSITE
IFSTONE
INSCALE
INSHAPE
INSHORE
INSIGNE
INSPACE
INSPIRE
INSPITE
INSTATE
INSTONE
INSTORE
INSTYLE
ITSALIE
ITSATIE
ITSDONE
ITSFINE
ITSGONE
ITSHERE
ITSLATE
ITSLOVE
ITSONME
ITSTIME
ITSTRUE
JASMINE
JUSTICE
JUSTINE
JUSTONE
LASAGNE
LASALLE
LASTONE
LESABRE
LISENTE
LISSOME
LOSABLE
MASSAGE
MASSINE
MASSIVE
MCSHANE
MCSWINE
MESSAGE
MISCITE
MISCODE
MISDATE
MISDONE
MISFILE
MISFIRE
MISGAVE
MISGIVE
MISLIKE
MISMATE
MISMOVE
MISNAME
MISPAGE
MISRATE
MISRULE
MISSILE
MISSIVE
MISTAKE
MISTIME
MISTUNE
MISTYPE
MISWIRE
MISZONE
MOSELLE
MRSLATE
MUSANTE
MUSETTE
MUSTSEE
MYSPACE
NASTASE
NESCAFE
NOSCORE
NOSIREE
OBSCENE
OBSCURE
OBSERVE
ONSERVE
ONSHORE
ONSTAGE
OSSICLE
OSSIPEE
PASALLE
PASSADE
PASSAGE
PASSIVE
PASTDUE
PASTIME
PASTURE
PESANTE
PISCINE
PISMIRE
PISTOLE
POSABLE
POSEUSE
POSTAGE
POSTURE
RESCALE
RESCORE
RESEIZE
RESERVE
RESHAPE
RESHARE
RESHAVE
RESHINE
RESIDUE
RESLATE
RESOLVE
RESPACE
RESPADE
RESPICE
RESPIRE
RESPITE
RESPOKE
RESTAGE
RESTATE
RESTIVE
RESTOKE
RESTORE
RESTYLE
RESURGE
RESWORE
RISIBLE
RISSOLE
RLSTINE
ROSALIE
ROSANNE
ROSEATE
ROSELLE
ROSETTE
RUSHDIE
SESSILE
SISTINE
SOSUEME
SUSANNE
SUSPIRE
SYSTOLE
TESTATE
TOSCALE
TOSPARE
TUSSIVE
UNSHADE
UNSPOKE
UNSTATE
UNSWORE
UPSCALE
UPSLOPE
UPSTAGE
UPSTARE
UPSTATE
UPSURGE
USSTATE
VESICLE
VESTIGE
VESTURE
VISIBLE
WASLATE
WASSURE
WASTAGE
WISEONE
YASMINE
YESISEE
YESSIRE
YESVOTE

•••SE••

ABASERS
ABUSERS
AMUSEME
AMUSERS
ANISEED
BASSETS
BASSETT
BERSERK
BESSELL
BISSELL
BOISEID
BOXSEAT
BOXSETS
BUSSERS
CANSECO
CARSEAT
CATSEYE
CAUSERS
CENSERS
CHASERS
CHISELS
CHOSEUP
CLOSEBY
CLOSEIN
CLOSELY
CLOSERS
CLOSEST
CLOSETO
CLOSETS
CLOSEUP
CONSENT
CORSETS
COSSETS
CURSEAT
CURSERS
CUSSERS
DAMSELS
DANSEUR
DAYSEND
DENSELY
DENSEST
DESSERT
DIESELS
DISSECT
DISSENT
DISSERT
DOGSEAR
DORSETT
DORSEYS
DOUSERS
DOWSERS
ELYSEES
ERASERS
EROSELY
FALSELY
FALSEST
FARSEER
FRISEUR
FURSEAL
FUSSERS
GASSERS
GEYSERS
GINSENG
GODSEND
GODSENT
GOSSETT
GUNSELS
GUSSETS
HAWSERS
HAYSEED
HERSELF
HIMSELF
HISSERS
HOTSEAT
HUSSEIN
HUSSERL
JERSEYS
JETSETS
KAISERS
KIDSEAT
KISSELS
KISSERS
LAPSERS
LEASERS
LEASETO
LESSEES
LESSENS
LESSEPS
LETSEAT
LINSEED
LOOSELY
LOOSENS
LOOSEST
LOUSEUP
MASSEUR
MAUSERS
MISSEAT
MISSEND
MISSENT
MISSETS
MORSELS
MOUSERS
MUSSELS
NAUSEAM
NONSELF
NOOSERS
NURSERS
NURSERY
OBESELY
OFFSETS
OILSEED
ONESELF
OURSELF
OUTSEEK
OUTSEEN
OUTSEES
OUTSELL
OUTSERT
OUTSETS
PARSECS
PARSEES
PARSERS
PASSELS
PASSERS
PASSEUL
PAUSERS
PCUSERS
PENSEES
PERSEID
PERSEUS
PHASEIN
PHASERS
PINSEAL
POISERS
PORSENA
POSSESS
PRESEAL
PRESEAT
PRESELL
PRESENT
PRESETS
PROSERS
PURSERS
QUESERA
RAISERS
RAISEUP
RAMSESI
REUSERS
RIESENS
RINSERS
ROUSERS
RUSSELL
RUSSERT
RUSSETS
RUSSETY
SANSEIS
SASSERS
SCUSEME
SENSEIS
SENSENS
SOWSEAR
SUBSECT
SUBSETS
SUDSERS
SUNSETS
TABSETS
TASSELS
TEASELS
TEASERS
TEASETS
TEASEUP
TENSELY
TENSEST
TENSEUP
TERSELY
TERSEST
TESSERA
THESELF
THESEUS
THYSELF
TINSELS
TOPSEED
TOSSERS
TRISECT
VERSETS
VESSELS
WEASELS
WITSEND
WORSENS

•••S•E•

ABASHED
ABASHES
ABYSSES
ALMSMEN
AMASSED
AMASSER
AMASSES
ANISEED
ANTSIER
ARTSIER
ARUSPEX
AUSSIES
BANSHEE
BASSIER
BATSMEN
BEASLEY
BIASSED
BIASSES
BITSIER
BLASTED
BLASTER
BLESSED
BLESSER
BLESSES
BLISSED
BLISSES
BLISTER
BLUSHED
BLUSHER
BLUSHES
BLUSTER
BOASTED
BOASTER
BOBSLED
BOLSTER
BOOSLER
BOOSTED
BOOSTER
BOSSIER
BOSSMEN
BOXSTEP
BOXSTER
BRASHER
BRASHES
BRASIER
BRASSES
BRISKED
BRISKER
BRISKET
BROSSES
BRUSHED
BRUSHER
BRUSHES
BURSTER
CHASSED
CHASSES
CHASTEN
CHASTER
CHESTED
CHESTER

CLASHED
CLASHER
CLASHES
CLASPED
CLASPER
CLASSED
CLASSER
CLASSES
CLUSTER
COASTED
COASTER
COWSHED
CRASHED
CRASHER
CRASHES
CRASSER
CRESSES
CRESSET
CRESTED
CRISPED
CRISPEN
CRISPER
CROSIER
CROSSED
CROSSER
CROSSES
CRUSHED
CRUSHER
CRUSHES
CRUSTED
CUSSLER
DAISIES
DAUSSET
DITSIER
DOGSLED
DOSSIER
DRESDEN
DRESSED
DRESSER
DRESSES
DROSSES
EDASNER
EGESTED
ELYSEES
ENISLED
ENISLES
EXISTED
FANSLER
FARSEER
FEASTED
FEASTER
FIBSTER
FLASHED
FLASHER
FLASHES
FLESHED
FLESHES
FLOSSED
FLOSSER
FLOSSES
FLUSHED
FLUSHER
FLUSHES
FLUSTER
FOCSLES
FOISTED
FORSTER
FRASIER
FRESHED
FRESHEN
FRESHER
FRESHES
FRESHET
FRESNEL
FRESSED
FRESSES
FRISBEE
FRISKED
FRISKER
FROSTED
FROSTER
FUBSIER
FUNSTER
FUSSIER
GADSDEN
GAGSTER
GASSIER
GAUSSES
GESSOED
GESSOES
GETSHEP
GETSSET
GETSWET
GHOSTED
GIPSIES
GLASSED
GLASSES
GLISTEN
GLISTER
GLOSSED
GLOSSER
GLOSSES
GNASHED
GNASHER
GNASHES
GOOSIER
GORSIER
GRASPED
GRASPER
GRASSED
GRASSES
GRISLET
GRISNEZ
GRISTER
GROSSED
GROSSER
GROSSES
GUESSED
GUESSER
GUESSES
GUESTED
GUSSIED
GUSSIES
GUTSIER
GYPSIES
HAMSTER
HARSHEN
HARSHER
HASSLED
HASSLES
HAYSEED
HEISTED
HEMSLEY
HENSLEY
HERSHEY
HIPSTER
HISSIER
HOISTED
HOISTER
HOLSTER
HOOSIER
HORSIER
HORSLEY
HUSSIES
INASTEW
INKSTER
IRISHER
JANSSEN
JOISTED
JOUSTED
JOUSTER
KAISHEK
KEESLER
KEISTER
KINSMEN
KIRSTEN
KLISTER
KNESSET
KNISHES
KOOSHES
KRASNER
KVASSES
LAISSEZ
LASSIES
LASSOED
LASSOER
LASSOES
LEASHED
LEASHES
LEISTER
LENSMEN
LESSEES
LETSSEE
LINSEED
LOBSTER
LOESSER
LOESSES
LOUSIER
MARSDEN
MARSHES
MARSRED
MASSIER
MEASLES
MEISSEN
MEISTER
MESSIER
MINSTER
MISSIES
MISSTEP
MOBSTER
MOISTEN
MOISTER
MONSTER
MOSSIER
MOUSIER
MOUSSED
MOUSSES
MUNSTER
MUSSIER
NAPSTER
NETSTER
NEWSIER
NEWSIES
NEWSMEN
NEWSPEG
NOISIER
NONSKED
NUTSIER
OARSMEN
ODYSSEY
OERSTED
OILSEED
OLDSTER
OLMSTED
ONESTEP
ORESTES
OUTSEEK
OUTSEEN
OUTSEES
OUTSPED
OUTSTEP
PAISLEY
PANSIES
PARSEES
PARSLEY
PASSKEY
PATSIES
PENSEES
PHISHED
PHISHER
PHISHES
PIASTER
PILSNER
PLASHED
PLASHES
PLASTER
PLISSES
PLUSHER
PLUSHES
PLUSSES
POESIES
PRESLEY
PRESSED
PRESSEL
PRESSER
PRESSES
PRISSES
PROSIER
PROSPER
PUGSLEY
PUNSTER
PURSIER
PURSUED
PURSUER
PURSUES
PUSSIES
QUASHED
QUASHES
QUESTED
QUESTER
RASSLED
RASSLER
RASSLES
REASKED
RIESSEN
ROASTED
ROASTER
ROISTER
ROOSTED
ROOSTER
ROSSNER
ROSSSEA
ROUSTED
ROUSTER
SASSIER
SAYSYES
SEESRED
SHUSHED
SHUSHES
SHUSTER
SHYSTER
SISSIER
SISSIES
SKOSHES
SLASHED
SLASHER
SLASHES
SLOSHED
SLOSHES
SLUSHED
SLUSHES
SMASHED
SMASHER
SMASHES
SMUSHED
SMUSHES
STASHED
STASHES
STASSEN
SUDSIER
SWASHED
SWASHES
SWISHED
SWISHES
TANSIES
TAPSTER
TIPSIER
TIPSTER
TISSUES
TISSUEY
TOASTED
TOASTEE
TOASTER
TOPSEED
TOUSLED
TOUSLES
TOYSLED
TRASHED
TRASHER
TRASHES
TRESSED
TRESSES
TRUSSED
TRUSSES
TRUSTED
TRUSTEE
TRUSTER
TRYSTED
TRYSTER
TUSSLED
TUSSLES
TWISTED
TWISTER
TWOSTEP
ULYSSES
UNASKED
VORSTER
WAISTED
WEBSTER
WHISHED
WHISHES
WHISKED
WHISKER
WHISKEY
WHISPER
WINSLET
WOOSHED
WOOSHES
WOOSTER
WORSLEY
WORSTED
WRASSES
WRESTED
WRESTER
YEASTED

•••S••E

ABUSIVE
AHASSLE
ALBSURE
AMUSEME
APOSTLE
ARCSINE
ARISTAE
ARTSALE
ATISSUE
AWESOME
BANSHEE
BASSALE
BEASTIE
BEDSIDE
BIGSALE
BRASIZE
BRASSIE
BRISTLE
BRUSQUE
CAPSIZE
CAPSULE
CARSALE
CATSEYE
CENSURE
CLOSURE
CONSOLE
CONSUME
CORSAGE
COUSINE
CRUSADE
CUISINE
CURSIVE
DAYSIDE
DOGSAGE
ELUSIVE
EPISODE
EPISTLE
ERASURE
EROSIVE
EVASIVE
EYESORE
FARSIDE
FISSILE
FISSURE
FLOSSIE
FORSAKE
FORSALE
FORSIZE
FORSURE
FORSYTE
FRISBEE
FULSOME
GETSORE
GLOSSAE
GOESAPE
GOSSAGE
GOTSORE
GRASSLE
GRISTLE
GUMSHOE
GYMSHOE
HADSOME
HATSIZE
HESSAFE
HIRSUTE
HUSSITE
INASHOE
IRKSOME
KIRSTIE
KRYSTLE
LEISURE
LETSSEE
LETSUSE
LISSOME
LOWSIDE
MANSIZE
MASSAGE
MASSINE
MASSIVE
MEASURE
MESSAGE
MIDSIZE
MIDSOLE
MISSILE
MISSIVE
NATSUME
NETSUKE
NEWSOME
NOISOME
NONSALE
NONSANE
NOTSAFE
NOTSURE
ODDSARE
ODDSHOE
OFFSIDE
OFFSITE
OLDSHOE
ONESHOE
ONESIZE
OPUSONE
OUTSIDE
OUTSIZE
OUTSOLE
PADSITE
PASSADE
PASSAGE
PASSIVE
PENSIVE
PIASTRE
PIESAFE
PIESALE
PLOSIVE
PLUSONE
PORSCHE
PRESAGE
PRESALE
PRESIDE
PRESQUE
PRESUME
PULSATE
REISSUE
RIPSONE
RISSOLE
SAUSAGE
SAYSAYE
SCUSEME
SEASIDE
SENSATE
SESSILE
SUASIVE
SUBSIDE
SUBSUME
TAGSALE
TAPSHOE
TAXSALE
TENSILE
TENSIVE
THESAME
THISONE
THISTLE
TOASTEE
TOESHOE
TONSURE
TOPSIDE
TRESTLE
TRUSTEE
TRUSTME
TUSSIVE
TWOSOME
UNISIZE
VERSACE
WASSURE
WAYSIDE
WEBSITE
WHISTLE
WINSOME
WRESTLE
YESSIRE

••••SE•

ABYSSES
ACCUSED
ACCUSER
ACCUSES
ADAMSES
ADVISED
ADVISEE
ADVISER
ADVISES
AEGISES
ALEKSEI
ALIASES
ALROSEN
ALUNSER
AMASSED
AMASSER
AMASSES
APLUSES
APPOSED
APPOSES
ARALSEA
ARCHSEE
ARGUSES
AROUSED
AROUSER
AROUSES
ARRASES
ARRISES
ATLASES
AVGASES
AVULSED
AVULSES
BALASES
BEMUSED
BEMUSES
BENTSEN
BERNSEN
BIASSED
BIASSES
BLESSED
BLESSER
BLESSES
BLISSED
BLISSES
BLOUSED
BLOUSES
BOBBSEY
BOLUSES
BONESET
BONUSES
BOURSES
BPLUSES
BRAISED
BRAISES
BRASSES
BROSSES
BROWSED
BROWSER
BROWSES
BRUISED
BRUISER
BRUISES
CALMSEA
CAMISES
CAYUSES
CDCASES
CERISES
CHAISES
CHASSED
CHASSES
CHEESED
CHEESES
CHELSEA
CHOOSER
CHOOSES
CHOOSEY
CLASSED
CLASSER
CLASSES
CLAUSES
COARSEN
COARSER
CORPSES
COUNSEL
COURSED
COURSER
COURSES
CPLUSES
CRASSER
CREASED
CREASER
CREASES
CRESSES
CRESSET
CROSSED
CROSSER
CROSSES
CRUISED
CRUISER
CRUISES
CURTSEY
CUTISES
DAMOSEL
DATASET
DAUSSET
DEADSEA
DEADSET
DEBASED
DEBASER
DEBASES
DEBUSES
DEEPSEA
DEEPSET
DEFUSED
DEFUSER
DEFUSES
DEMISED
DEMISES
DEMPSEY
DEPOSED
DEPOSER
DEPOSES
DESKSET
DEVISED
DEVISEE
DEVISER
DEVISES
DIDASET
DINESEN
DIRKSEN
DISUSED
DISUSES
DNAASES
DPLUSES
DREISER
DRESSED
DRESSER
DRESSES
DROSSES
DROWSED
DROWSES
DRUMSET
DUFUSES
ECDYSES
EFFUSED
EFFUSES
EGLISES
ELAPSED
ELAPSES
EMERSED
ENCASED
ENCASES
ENDUSER
ENDUSES
EVULSED
EVULSES
EXCISED
EXCISES
EXCUSED
EXCUSER
EXCUSES
EXCUSEZ
EXPOSED
EXPOSER
EXPOSES
FAIRSEX
FETUSES
FICUSES
FILMSET
FLENSED
FLENSER
FLENSES
FLOSSED
FLOSSER
FLOSSES
FOCUSED
FOCUSER
FOCUSES
FORASEC
FORESEE
FRAISES
FRESSED
FRESSES
GAUSSES
GENESEE
GENESES
GENESET
GENUSES
GETSSET
GIBUSES
GIFTSET
GLASSED
GLASSES
GLOSSED
GLOSSER
GLOSSES
GOBYSEA
GOTOSEA
GOTOSEE
GRASSED
GRASSES
GREASED
GREASER
GREASES
GROSSED
GROSSER
GROSSES
GROUSED
GROUSER
GROUSES
GUESSED
GUESSER
GUESSES
GUNUSER
HADASET
HANDSEL
HANDSET
HARDSET
HASASET
HAYESES
HDTVSET
HEADSET
HEARSES
HEXOSES
HIGHSEA
HOARSEN
HOARSER
HOCUSED
HOLYSEE
HUMUSES
ICTUSES
ILLUSED
ILLUSES
IMPOSED
IMPOSER
IMPOSES
INCASED
INCASES
INCISED
INCISES
INCUSED
INCUSES
INFUSED
INFUSER
INFUSES
IODISED
IODISES
IONISED
IONISER
IONISES
JANSSEN
JIRASEK
JONESED
JONESES
JUDASES
KARASEA
KINESES
KLEISER
KNESSET
KVASSES
LAISSEZ
LEGOSET
LETSSEE
LEXISES
LEXUSES
LIAISED
LIAISES
LINDSEY
LIPASES
LIVESET
LIVESEY
LOCKSET
LOESSER
LOESSES
LOOKSEE
LORISES
LORUSES
LOTUSES
LOVESET
MACUSER
MALMSEY
MAVISES
MEIOSES
MEISSEN
MIDASES
MIMESES
MINDSET
MINUSES
MISUSED
MISUSER
MISUSES
MITOSES
MOMMSEN
MOMUSES
MOONSET
MOUSSED
MOUSSES
MUSTSEE
NAILSET
NEGUSES
NEMESES
NEXUSES
NIELSEN
NONUSER
NOTUSED
NOWISEE
NOWISER
NULLSET
OBTUSER
ODYSSEY
OPENSEA
OPPOSED
OPPOSER
OPPOSES
ORRISES
OSMOSED
OSMOSES
OVERSEA
OVERSEE
OVERSET
OVERSEW
PAULSEN
PERUSED
PERUSER
PERUSES
PHRASED
PHRASES
PLEASED
PLEASER
PLEASES
PLISSES
PLUSSES
PRAISED
PRAISER
PRAISES
PRESSED
PRESSEL
PRESSER
PRESSES
PRISSES
PRIUSES
QUONSET
RAMESES
REBUSES
RECASED
RECASES
RECUSED
RECUSES
REDOSED
REDOSES
REFUSED
REFUSER
REFUSES
RELOSES
REMISED
REMISES
REPOSED
REPOSER
REPOSES
RERISEN
RERISES
REVISED
REVISER
REVISES
RIESSEN
ROSSSEA

SALTSEA
SAMISEN
SAMOSET
SINUSES
SPARSER
SPENSER
SPOUSES
STASSEN
SULUSEA
SWANSEA
TALUSES
TONUSES
TOOLSET
TRESSED
TRESSES
TROUSER
TRUSSED
TRUSSES
TSETSES
TWINSET
TYPESET
ULYSSES
UNBASED
UNBESET
UNCASED
UNCASES
UNEASES
UNFUSED
UNNOSED
UNPOSED
UNRISEN
UNWISER
UPRISEN
UPRISER
UPRISES
VALISES
VENUSES
VIRUSES
WELLSEE
WELLSET
WOOLSEY
WRASSES
XEROSES
XYLOSES
YESISEE

••••S•E

ADVISEE
AHASSLE
ALCESTE
ARCHSEE
ARTISTE
ATISSUE
AUGUSTE
BATISTE
BEATSME
BLEDSOE
BOOPSIE
BRASSIE
CELESTE
DEHISCE
DEMESNE
DEVISEE
EGOISTE
ENMASSE
FINESSE
FLOSSIE
FOOTSIE
FORESEE
GENESEE
GLOSSAE
GOTOSEE
GRASSLE
HOLYSEE
IDLESSE
IMPASSE
INHASTE
INTASTE
LACOSTE
LAGASSE
LETSSEE
LOOKSEE
MAJESTE
MATISSE
MEDUSAE
MODISTE
MUSTSEE
NOTASTE
NOWISEE
OVERSEE
PELISSE
POOPSIE
REBASTE
REISSUE
REPASTE
RETASTE
RIPOSTE
SENESCE
STRASSE
SUITSME
SWOOSIE
TEENSIE
TOOTSIE
TOTASTE
TRIESTE
TUMESCE
UNPASTE
WELLSEE
WOEISME
YESISEE

•••••SE

ABSCISE
ACEROSE
ADIPOSE
ADVERSE
AGONISE
AIRBASE
AIRHOSE
ALFONSE
ALLELSE
ALLRISE
ALLWISE
AMBROSE
AMYLASE
ANALYSE
ANATASE
ANODISE
ANYWISE
APPEASE
APPRISE
ARENOSE
ASPERSE
ATOMISE
AUSLESE
AXLROSE
BADCASE
BAPTISE
BECAUSE
BERNESE
BIGNOSE
BUDVASE
BURMESE
BYANOSE
CABOOSE
CAROUSE
CHEMISE
CHINESE
CLEANSE
COCHISE
COMPOSE
CONCISE
CONFUSE
CONTUSE
DECEASE
DEFENSE
DELOUSE
DELUISE
DESPISE
DIFFUSE
DIOCESE
DISEASE
DISEUSE
DISPOSE
DIVERSE
DIVULSE
DOGROSE
DONJOSE
ECLIPSE
EDMEESE
EGGCASE
ELLIPSE
EMPRISE
ENCHASE
ENCLOSE
ENDORSE
ENDWISE
ENMASSE
ENPRISE
ENTHUSE
ESPOUSE
EXCURSE
EXPANSE
EXPENSE
FAIRUSE
FANBASE
FANWISE
FAROESE
FBICASE
FINESSE
FOLIOSE
GENOESE
GENOISE
GETWISE
GLIMPSE
GLOBOSE
GLUCOSE
GOODUSE
GOTWISE
GUNCASE
HELOISE
HOGNOSE
HOWELSE
IDLESSE
IDOLISE
IMMENSE
IMMERSE
IMPASSE
IMPULSE
INCENSE
INCLOSE
INDORSE
INGLESE
INHOUSE
INPHASE
INTENSE
INTERSE
INULASE
INVERSE
IREFUSE
ITEMISE
JACCUSE
KEYCASE
LACTASE
LACTOSE
LAGASSE
LAVALSE
LAWCASE
LETSUSE
LICENSE
LIONISE
LOWRISE
MALAISE
MALTASE
MALTESE
MALTOSE
MARCUSE
MATISSE
MELROSE
MIDRISE
MORTISE
MRHORSE
MRMOOSE
NASTASE
NICOISE
NONBASE
NONOISE
NOWORSE
OBELISE
OBVERSE
OFFBASE
OFFENSE
OFNOUSE
OILBASE
OLDROSE
ONEBASE
ONLEASE
OPEROSE
OVERUSE
OXIDASE
OXIDISE
OZONISE
PAPOOSE
PELISSE
PENCASE
PENROSE
PERFUSE
PLUMOSE
POETISE
POSEUSE
PRECISE
PREMISE
PROFUSE
PROMISE
PROPOSE
PUGNOSE
PURPOSE
REALISE
REARISE
REAROSE
RECHOSE
RECLUSE
REDNOSE
REDROSE
REHOUSE
RELAPSE
RELEASE
REMORSE
REPHASE
REPRISE
REPULSE
RERAISE
RERINSE
REVERSE
SAMWISE
SANJOSE
SERIESE
SIAMESE
SIENESE
SOUBISE
STRASSE
STROUSE
STYLISE
SUBBASE
SUBCASE
SUCRASE
SUCROSE
SUFFUSE
SUNRISE
SUPPOSE
SURMISE
SYNAPSE
TAXBASE
TEAROSE
THEROSE
TOHORSE
TOLEASE
TRAIPSE
TWOBASE
UNCLOSE
UNHORSE
UNHOUSE
UNITISE
UNLOOSE
UNOBESE
UNTENSE
UNTERSE
UPCLOSE
UPPHASE
UPRAISE
UPROUSE
UTILISE
VAMOOSE
VBLOUSE
VERBOSE
VINROSE
YOULOSE

S•F••••

SAFARIS
SAFEBET
SAFEWAY
SAFFRON
SEFERIS
SIFTERS
SIFTING
SOFABED
SOFARAS
SOFFITS
SOFTENS
SOFTEST
SOFTGEL
SOFTIES
SOFTISH
SOFTTOP
SUFFERS
SUFFICE
SUFFOLK
SUFFUSE

S••F•••

SADFATE
SAFFRON
SANFORD
SAWFISH
SCOFFAT
SCOFFED
SCOFFER
SCUFFED
SCUFFER
SCUFFLE
SEAFARE
SEAFERN
SEAFOAM
SEAFOOD
SEAFOWL
SELFISH
SERFAGE
SERFDOM
SETFEES
SETFREE
SHAFFER
SHAFTED
SHEFFER
SHIFTED
SHIFTER
SHOFARS
SHUFFLE
SHYFROM
SIXFEET
SIXFIVE
SIXFOLD
SIXFOOT
SIXFOUR
SKIFFED
SKIFFLE
SNAFUED
SNIFFAT
SNIFFED
SNIFFER
SNIFFLE
SNIFFLY
SNIFFUP
SNIFTER
SNUFFED
SNUFFER
SNUFFLE
SOFFITS
SOLFEGE
SOUFFLE
SOXFANS
SPIFFED
SPIFFUP
STAFFED
STAFFER
STEFANI
STIFFED
STIFFEL
STIFFEN
STIFFER
STIFFLY
STIFLED
STIFLES
STUFFED
STUFFER
STUFFIN
SUBFILE
SUBFORM
SUFFERS
SUFFICE
SUFFOLK
SUFFUSE
SULFATE
SULFIDE
SULFITE
SUNFANS
SUNFAST
SUNFIRE
SUNFISH
SURFACE
SURFEIT
SURFERS
SURFIER
SURFING
SURFMAN
SURFMEN
SURFSUP
SWIFTER
SWIFTLY
SYNFUEL

S•••F••

SACKFUL
SANDFLY
SAVEFOR
SCARFED
SCARFER
SCARFUP
SCLAFFS
SCOFFAT
SCOFFED
SCOFFER
SCRUFFS
SCRUFFY
SCUFFED
SCUFFER
SCUFFLE
SEENFIT
SEESFIT
SELLFOR
SENDFOR
SENTFOR
SETOFFS
SHAFFER
SHEAFED
SHEFFER
SHIPFUL
SHOOFLY
SHOPFOR
SHOPFUL
SHOTFOR
SHUFFLE
SIGHFOR
SIGHFUL
SIGNFOR
SITSFOR
SKIFFED
SKIFFLE
SKILFUL
SLEDFUL
SNARFED
SNIFFAT
SNIFFED
SNIFFER
SNIFFLE
SNIFFLY
SNIFFUP
SNUFFED
SNUFFER
SNUFFLE
SNUGFIT
SOLDFOR
SONGFUL
SOUFFLE
SOULFUL
SPIFFED
SPIFFUP
SPOOFED
SPOOFER
STAFFED
STAFFER
STAYFOR
STIFFED
STIFFEL
STIFFEN
STIFFER
STIFFLY
STIRFRY
STOPFOR
STRAFED
STRAFER
STRAFES
STRIFES
STUFFED
STUFFER
STUFFIN
SUDAFED
SUEDFOR
SUESFOR
SUNSFAN

S••••F•

SADCAFE
SAMHUFF
SANTAFE
SARNOFF
SATISFY
SAWNOFF
SAWSOFF
SCARIFY
SCLAFFS
SCRUFFS
SCRUFFY
SEALIFE
SEALIFT
SEALOFF
SEENOFF
SEESOFF
SELLOFF
SENDOFF
SENTOFF
SETOFFS
SETSOFF
SHERIFF
SHERIFS
SHONUFF
SHOOOFF
SHOWOFF
SHUTOFF
SIGNIFY
SIGNOFF
SKILIFT
SLIDOFF
SLIPOFF
SNIPOFF
SOLDOFF
SPECIFY
SPEDOFF
SPINOFF
SPUNOFF
STAYOFF
STEPOFF
STOPOFF
STUPEFY
SYDHOFF

S•••••F

SAMHUFF
SARNOFF
SAWNOFF
SAWSOFF
SCADSOF
SEALOFF
SEAWOLF
SEENOFF
SEESOFF
SELLOFF
SENDOFF
SENTOFF
SERIESF
SETSOFF
SHERIFF
SHEWOLF
SHONUFF
SHOOOFF
SHORTOF
SHOWOFF
SHUTOFF
SIGNOFF
SILENTF
SKYSURF
SLIDOFF
SLIPOFF
SMACKOF
SNIPOFF
SOLDOFF
SOUTHOF
SPEAKOF
SPEDOFF
SPINOFF
SPOKEOF
SPUNOFF
STAYOFF
STEPOFF
STOPOFF
STRIPOF
SUNROOF
SUREROF
SYDHOFF

•SF••••

ASFARAS
ISFAHAN
USFLAGS

•S•F•••

ASHFORD
ASOFNOW

•S••F••

ASKSFOR
ESTEFAN
ISRAFEL
OSSIFIC
USEDFOR
USERFEE
USESFOR

•S•••F•

ASAGIFT
ASSTIFF

•S••••F

ASKEDOF
ASLEWOF
ASSTIFF

••SF•••

BUSFARE
GOSFORD
HASFITS
IRSFORM
ITSFINE
MISFEED
MISFILE
MISFIRE
MISFITS
MISFORM
WASFAIR

••S•F••

BASHFUL
DESKFUL
DISHFUL
EASEFUL
FISHFOR
FISHFRY
FISTFUL
HASAFIT
HUSHFUL
INSOFAR
LESSFAT
LUSTFUL
MUSEFUL
NESTFUL
OSSIFIC
PASSFOR
POSTFIX
PUSHFOR
PUSHFUL
RESIFTS
RESTFUL
TESTFLY
TESTFOR
UNSAFER
WISHFOR
WISHFUL
WISTFUL
ZESTFUL

••S••F•

ASSTIFF
BESTOFF
CASTOFF
DASHOFF
DISTAFF
DUSTOFF
EASEOFF
EASYOFF
HESSAFE
JUSTIFY
KISSOFF
MASSIFS
MASTIFF
MUSTAFA
MYSTIFY
NESCAFE
ONSTAFF
PASSOFF
PUSHOFF
RESHIFT
RESTAFF
RESTUFF
RUSHOFF
TESTIFY
TOSSOFF
UNSHIFT
UNSTIFF
UPSHIFT
WASHOFF

••S•••F

ASSTIFF
BESTOFF
CASTOFF
DASHOFF
DISTAFF
DUSTOFF
EASEOFF
EASYOFF
KISSOFF
MASTIFF
ONSTAFF
PASSOFF
PUSHOFF
RESTAFF
RESTUFF
RUSHOFF
TOSSOFF
UNSTIFF
WASHOFF

•••SF••

ACTSFOR
AIMSFOR
ASKSFOR
BATSFOR
BEGSFOR
BIDSFOR
CUBSFAN
DIESFOR
DIGSFOR
DOESFOR
GETSFAR
GETSFIT
GOESFAR
GOESFOR
GUNSFOR
HITSFOR
JETSFAN
LAYSFOR
LESSFAT
LETSFLY
LIESFOR
METSFAN
OPTSFOR
PASSFOR
PAYSFOR
RAMSFAN
REDSFAN
REPSFOR
RUNSFOR
SEESFIT
SITSFOR
SUESFOR
SUNSFAN
THUSFAR
USESFOR
VIESFOR
YENSFOR

•••S•F•

BEGSOFF
BUGSOFF
BUYSOFF
CUTSOFF
DAYSOFF
DENSIFY
DIESOFF
FALSIFY
FOBSOFF
GETSOFF
GETSOFT
GOESAFT
GOESOFF
GOTSOFT
HATSOFF
HESSAFE
HITSOFF
HOPSOFF
KISSOFF
LAYSOFF
LETSOFF
LIPSOFF
LOGSOFF
LOPSOFF
MASSIFS
NODSOFF
NOTSAFE
OUTSIFT
PASSOFF
PAYSOFF
PERSOFF
PIESAFE
POPSOFF
PRESIFT
PUTSOFF
RIPSOFF
RUBSOFF
RUNSOFF
SAWSOFF
SEESOFF
SETSOFF
TAPSOFF
TEESOFF
TIESOFF
TIPSOFF
TOPSOFF
TOSSOFF
VERSIFY
ZIPSOFF

•••S••F

AHOSTOF
BEGSOFF
BOASTOF
BUGSOFF
BUYSOFF
CUTSOFF
DAYSOFF
DIESOFF
EGOSURF
FOBSOFF
GETSANF
GETSOFF
GOESOFF
HATSOFF
HERSELF
HIMSELF
HITSOFF
HOPSOFF
KISSOFF
LAYSOFF
LETSOFF
LIPSOFF
LOGSOFF
LOPSOFF
NETSURF
NODSOFF
NONSELF
ONESELF
OURSELF
PASSOFF
PAYSOFF
PERSOFF
POPSOFF
PUTSOFF
RIPSOFF
RUBSOFF
RUNSOFF
SAWSOFF
SEESOFF
SETSOFF
SKYSURF
TAPSOFF
TEESOFF
THESELF
THYSELF
TIESOFF
TIPSOFF
TOPSOFF
TOSSOFF
ZIPSOFF

••••SF•
SATISFY

••••S•F
FREESOF
GIVESOF
HEAPSOF
HEARSOF
KNOWSOF
LOADSOF
PILESOF
REEKSOF
SCADSOF
TALKSOF
TELLSOF
TIRESOF
WARNSOF

•••••SF
SERIESF

S•G••••
SAGCARD
SAGEHEN
SAGETEA
SAGGIER
SAGGING
SAGIEST
SAGINAW
SAGUARO
SEGMENT
SEGOVIA
SEGWAYS
SIGHERS
SIGHFOR
SIGHFUL
SIGHING
SIGHSAT
SIGHTED
SIGHTER
SIGHTLY
SIGMOID
SIGMUND
SIGNAGE
SIGNALS
SIGNEES
SIGNERS
SIGNETS
SIGNFOR
SIGNIFY
SIGNING
SIGNOFF
SIGNORA
SIGNORE
SIGNORS
SIGNOUT
SIGNSIN
SIGNSON
SIGNSUP
SIGNUPS
SOGGIER
SOGGILY
SUGARED
SUGGEST

S••G•••
SAGGIER
SAGGING
SANGOUT
SANGRIA
SARGENT
SEAGATE
SEAGIRT
SEAGODS
SEAGRAM
SEAGREN
SEAGULL
SEDGIER
SHAGGED
SHAGRUG
SHEGOAT
SHOGUNS
SIEGING
SINGERS
SINGING
SINGLED
SINGLES
SINGLET
SINGOUT
SINGSTO
SIXGUNS
SKAGWAY
SLIGHTS
SLOGANS
SLOGGED
SLOGGER
SLUGGED
SLUGGER
SMUGGER
SMUGGLE
SNAGGED
SNAGGER
SNAGSUP
SNIGLET
SNUGFIT
SNUGGED
SNUGGER
SNUGGLE
SNUGGLY
SNUGLIS
SOGGIER
SOGGILY
SOIGNEE
SONGFUL
SORGHUM
SPIGOTS
STAGERS
STAGGED
STAGGER
STAGIER
STAGILY
STAGING
STAGNES
STIGMAS
STOGIES
STYGIAN
SUBGOAL
SUBGODS
SUGGEST
SUNGLOW
SUNGODS
SURGEON
SURGERY
SURGING
SWAGGER
SWAGMAN
SWAGMEN
SWIGERT
SWIGGED
SYNGMAN

S•••G••
SAVAGED
SAVAGER
SAVAGES
SCRAGGY
SCRUGGS
SENEGAL
SEVIGNY
SHAGGED
SHANGRI
SHINGLE
SHINGLY
SHOTGUN
SLEDGED
SLEDGES
SLEIGHS
SLEIGHT
SLINGER
SLOEGIN
SLOGGED
SLOGGER
SLOUGHS
SLUDGES
SLUGGED
SLUGGER
SMEAGOL
SMIDGEN
SMIDGES
SMUDGED
SMUDGES
SMUGGER
SMUGGLE
SNAGGED
SNAGGER
SNUGGED
SNUGGER
SNUGGLE
SNUGGLY
SOFTGEL
SPANGLE
SPANGLY
SPIEGEL
SPONGED
SPONGER
SPONGES
STAGGED
STAGGER
STEIGER
STENGEL
STENGUN
STINGER
STODGED
STODGES
STOOGED
STOOGES
STOPGAP
STREGIS
STUNGUN
STURGES
SWAGGER
SWIGGED
SWINGAT
SWINGBY
SWINGER
SWINGIT
SWUNGAT
SWUNGBY
SWUNGIT

S••••G•
SALONGA
SALVAGE
SAPSAGO
SARONGS
SAUSAGE
SAVINGS
SAWLOGS
SAYINGS
SCALAGE
SCOURGE
SCRAGGY
SCROOGE
SCRUGGS
SEABAGS
SEADOGS
SEALEGS
SEEPAGE
SELVAGE
SERFAGE
SIDINGS
SIGNAGE
SINKAGE
SKYHIGH
SOILAGE
SOLFEGE
SPLURGE
SPRINGS
SPRINGY
SPYINGS
STALAGS
STORAGE
STOWAGE
STRANGE
STRINGS
STRINGY
SUNDOGS
SUPERGS
SVERIGE
SYNERGY
SYRINGE

S•••••G
SACKING
SADSONG
SAGGING
SAILING
SALTING
SALVING
SAMSUNG
SANDBAG
SANDHOG
SANDING
SAPLING
SAPPING
SASHING
SASSING
SAUCING
SCALING
SCARING
SCOPING
SCORING
SEABORG
SEALING
SEAMING
SEARING
SEASLUG
SEATING
SEBRING
SECHZIG
SEEDING
SEEKING
SEEMING
SEEPING
SEINING
SEIZING
SELLING
SEMILOG
SENDING
SENSING
SERIESG
SERLING
SERVING
SETTING
SHADING
SHAGRUG
SHAKING
SHAMING
SHAPING
SHARING
SHAVING
SHEBANG
SHINDIG
SHINING
SHOEING
SHOOING
SHORING
SHOVING
SHOWDOG
SHOWING
SIBLING
SICCING
SIDLING
SIEBZIG
SIEGING
SIEVING
SIFTING
SIGHING
SIGNING
SILENTG
SILOING
SILTING
SINGING
SINKING
SINNING
SIPPING
SITTING
SKATING
SKEWING
SLAKING
SLATING
SLAVING
SLAYING
SLEDDOG
SLEWING
SLICING
SLIDING
SLIMING
SLOPING
SLOWING
SMILING
SMITING
SMOKING
SNAKING
SNARING
SNIPING
SNORING
SNOWING
SOAKING
SOAPING
SOARING
SOBBING
SOCKING
SODDING
SOILING
SOLOING
SOLVING
SOPPING
SORTING
SOURING
SOUSING
SPACING
SPADING
SPARING
SPAYING
SPECING
SPEWING
SPICING
SPIKING
SPITING
SPOKING
SPUMING
SPYRING
STAGING
STAKING
STARING
STARLOG
STATING
STAVING
STAYING
STEWING
STOKING
STONING
STORING
STOWING
STUBING
STYLING
SUBBING
SUBKING
SUBLONG
SUCKING
SUDSING
SUITING
SULKING
SUMMING
SUNNING
SUPPING
SURFING
SURGING
SUSSING
SWAYING
SWIPING
SYNCING

•SG••••
USGRANT

•S•G•••
ASAGIFT
ASAGRAY
ISOGONS
ISOGRAM

•S••G••
ASIAGOS
ASSIGNS
TSONGAS
USINGIN
USINGUP

•S•••G•
ASSUAGE
ISITAGO
USFLAGS

•S••••G
ESPYING
ESTRING
GSTRING
ISSUING
RSVPING
TSETUNG

••SG•••
BUSGIRL
DISGUST
ITSGONE
MISGAVE
MISGIVE
VOSGIAN

••S•G••
ASSIGNS
ATSIGHT
ATSIGNS
COSIGNS
DESIGNS
DOSAGES
DUSTGUN
ENSIGNS
HASAGAS
INSIGHT
INSIGNE
KOSYGIN
LASAGNA
LASAGNE
LASTGAS
LISAGAY
MUSIGNY
NOSEGAY
NOSUGAR
ONSAGER
ONSIGHT
RESIGHT
RESIGNS
UNSIGHT
UNSOGGY
VISAGED
VISAGES
WISEGUY

••S••G•
ASSUAGE
BESIEGE
BOSCAGE
CASINGS
DESMOGS
EASTEGG
GASBAGS
GASHOGS
GASLOGS
GOSSAGE
HOSTAGE
LOSINGS
MASSAGE
MESHUGA
MESSAGE
MISPAGE
MUSINGS
MUSKEGO
NESTEGG
ONSTAGE
PASSAGE
POSTAGE
RESINGS
RESTAGE
RESURGE
RISINGS
UNSNAGS
UNSOGGY
UNSTAGY
UPSTAGE
UPSURGE
VESTIGE
WASTAGE
WESTEGG

••S•••G
BASHING
BASKING
BASTING
BESTING
BOSSING
BUSHHOG
BUSHING
BUSHPIG
BUSKING
BUSSING
BUSTING
BUSYING
CASHING
CASKING
CASTING
CESSING
COSHING
COSTING
COSYING
CUSHING
CUSSING
DASHING
DISCING
DISHING
DISHRAG
DISKING
DISSING
DOSSING
DUSKING
DUSTING
DUSTRAG
EASTEGG
EASTING
ENSUING
FASTING
FESSING
FISHING
FUSSING
GASHING
GASPING
GASSING
GISSING
GOSLING
GUSHING
GUSTING
HASHING
HASPING
HASTING
HISSING
HOSTING
HUSHING
HUSKING
ISSUING
JESTING
JOSHING
KISSING
LASHING
LASTING
LASTLEG
LESSING
LISPING
LISTING
LOSEBIG
LOSTBIG
LOSTDOG
LUSTING
MASHING
MASKING
MASSING
MASTING
MESHING
MESSING
MISSING
MISTING
MOSHING
MOSSING
MUSHING
MUSSING
MUSTANG
NESTEGG
NESTING
NOSEBAG
NOSHING
OUSTING
PASSING
PASTING
PISHING
POSTBAG
POSTING
PUSHING
RASPING
RESTING
RISKING
RUSHING
RUSTING
SASHING
SASSING
SUSSING
TASKING
TASTING
TESTING
TOSSING
TUSKING
UNSLING
UNSLUNG
UNSTUNG
UNSWUNG
UPSWING
VESTING
VISAING
WASHING
WASHRAG
WASTING
WESTEGG
WISHING
WISPING
WYSIWYG
YESSING
ZESTING

•••SG••
GLASGOW

•••S•G•
AGESAGO
AIRSIGN
BADSIGN
CONSIGN
CORSAGE
DOGSAGE
GOSSAGE
HEXSIGN
IMUSTGO
IRESIGN
MASSAGE
MESSAGE
OUTSIGH
PASSAGE
PRESAGE
SAPSAGO
SAUSAGE

•••S••G
ABASING
ABUSING
AMUSING
ARISING
ARTSONG
BIASING
BOSSING
BUSSING
CAUSING
CEASING
CENSING
CESSING
CHASING
CLOSING
CURSING
CUSSING
DISSING
DOSSING
DOUSING
DOWSING
ERASING
FESSING
FUSSING
GASSING
GINSENG
GISSING
GOOSING
HELSING
HISSING
HITSONG
HOPSING
HORSING
HOUSING
IRISING
KISSING
LANSING
LAPSANG
LAPSING
LEASING
LESSING
LOOSING
LOUSING
MASSING
MESSING
MISSING
MOSSING
MOUSING
MUSSING
NEWSPEG
NOISING
NOOSING
NURSING
OLDSONG
OURSONG
OUTSANG
OUTSING
OUTSUNG
PARSING
PASSING
PAUSING
PHASING
POISING
POPSONG
PRESONG
PROSING
PULSING
PURSING
RAISING
RAPSONG
REUSING
RIKSDAG
RINSING
ROUSING
SADSONG
SAMSUNG
SASSING
SEASLUG
SENSING
SOUSING
SUDSING
SUSSING
TEASING
TENSING
TOSSING
VERSING
WINSBIG
YESSING

••••SG•
LEXUSGS
LEXUSGX
MAKESGO

•••••SG
SERIESG

SH•••••
SHABBAT
SHACKED
SHACKLE
SHADERS
SHADIER
SHADILY
SHADING
SHADOWS
SHADOWY
SHADROE
SHAFFER
SHAFTED
SHAGGED
SHAGRUG
SHAHDOM
SHAKERS
SHAKEUP
SHAKIER
SHAKILY
SHAKING
SHAKIRA
SHAKOES
SHALALA
SHALIER
SHALLOT
SHALLOW
SHALLWE
SHALOMS
SHAMANS
SHAMBLE
SHAMING
SHAMMED
SHAMPOO
SHANANA
SHANGRI
SHANKAR
SHANKED
SHANNEN
SHANNON
SHANTER
SHAPELY
SHAPERS
SHAPEUP
SHAPING
SHAPIRO
SHAREIN
SHARERS
SHARING
SHARKEY
SHARONA
SHARPED
SHARPEI
SHARPEN
SHARPER
SHARPIE
SHARPLY
SHASTRI
SHATNER
SHATTER
SHAVERS
SHAVIAN
SHAVING
SHAVUOT
SHAWLED
SHAWNEE
SHEAFED
SHEARED
SHEARER
SHEATHE
SHEATHS
SHEAVED
SHEAVES
SHEBANG
SHEBEAR
SHECRAB
SHEDDER
SHEDSON
SHEEHAN
SHEERED
SHEERER
SHEERLY
SHEETED
SHEFFER
SHEGOAT
SHEIKHS
SHEILAE
SHEILAS
SHEKELS
SHELDON
SHELLAC
SHELLED
SHELLER
SHELLEY
SHELTER
SHELTIE
SHELVED
SHELVER
SHELVES
SHEPARD
SHERBET
SHERIFF
SHERIFS
SHERMAN
SHERPAS
SHERWIN
SHEVATS
SHEWOLF
SHHHHHH
SHIATSU
SHIELDS
SHIFTED
SHIFTER
SHIHTZU
SHIITES
SHIKOKU
SHILLED
SHIMMER
SHINDIG
SHINEON
SHINERS
SHINEUP
SHINGLE
SHINGLY
SHINIER
SHINILY
SHINING
SHINNED
SHINOLA
SHINPAD
SHIPFUL
SHIPMAN
SHIPMEN
SHIPOUT
SHIPPED
SHIPPER

SHIPWAY
SHIRKED
SHIRKER
SHIRLEY
SHIRRED
SHIVERS
SHIVERY
SHLOCKY
SHNOOKS
SHOALED
SHOCKED
SHOCKER
SHODDEN
SHOEBOX
SHOEING
SHOEPAC
SHOFARS
SHOGUNS
SHONUFF
SHOOFLY
SHOOING
SHOOINS
SHOOKUP
SHOOOFF
SHOOSIN
SHOOTAT
SHOOTBY
SHOOTER
SHOOTUP
SHOPFOR
SHOPFUL
SHOPKOS
SHOPNBC
SHOPPED
SHOPPER
SHOPPES
SHOPSAT
SHOREUP
SHORING
SHORTED
SHORTEN
SHORTER
SHORTIE
SHORTLY
SHORTOF
SHOTFOR
SHOTGUN
SHOTOUT
SHOTPAR
SHOTPUT
SHOULDA
SHOULDI
SHOUTAT
SHOUTED
SHOUTER
SHOVEIN
SHOVELS
SHOVERS
SHOVING
SHOWBIZ
SHOWCAT
SHOWDOG
SHOWERS
SHOWERY
SHOWHOW
SHOWIER
SHOWILY
SHOWING
SHOWMAN
SHOWMEN
SHOWNIN
SHOWNUP
SHOWOFF
SHOWOUT
SHOWSIN
SHOWSUP
SHRIEKS
SHRIKES
SHRILLS
SHRILLY
SHRIMPS
SHRIMPY
SHRINED
SHRINER
SHRINES
SHRINKS
SHRIVEL
SHRIVER
SHRIVES
SHROUDS
SHRUBBY
SHTETLS
SHTICKS
SHTICKY
SHUBERT
SHUCKED
SHUCKER
SHUDDER
SHUFFLE
SHULMAN
SHUNNED
SHUNTED
SHUNTER
SHUSHED
SHUSHES
SHUSTER
SHUTEYE
SHUTINS
SHUTOFF
SHUTOUT
SHUTSIN
SHUTSUP
SHUTTER
SHUTTLE
SHYAWAY
SHYFROM
SHYLOCK
SHYNESS
SHYSTER

S•H••••

SAHARAN
SCHAYES
SCHELDT
SCHEMAS
SCHEMED
SCHEMER
SCHEMES
SCHERZI
SCHERZO
SCHICKS
SCHIRRA
SCHISMS
SCHISTS
SCHLEPP
SCHLEPS
SCHLITZ
SCHLOCK
SCHLUBS
SCHLUMP
SCHMEAR
SCHMEER
SCHMIDT
SCHMITT
SCHMOES
SCHNAPS
SCHNOOK
SCHNOZZ
SCHOLAR
SCHOLES
SCHOOLS
SCHTICK
SCHULTZ
SCHUMER
SCHWANN
SCHWINN
SHHHHHH
SOHAVEI
SPHERAL
SPHERED
SPHERES
SPHERIC
SSHAPED
SUHARTO

S••H•••

SACHEMS
SACHETS
SAMHILL
SAMHUFF
SAPHEAD
SASHAYS
SASHIMI
SASHING
SATHOME
SAXHORN
SAYHITO
SEAHAWK
SEAHERO
SEAHUNT
SECHZIG
SEEHERE
SENHORA
SEPHIAS
SHAHDOM
SHHHHHH
SHIHTZU
SIGHERS
SIGHFOR
SIGHFUL
SIGHING
SIGHSAT
SIGHTED
SIGHTER
SIGHTLY
SIKHISM
SIPHONS
SITHOME
SKIHATS
SKYHIGH
SKYHOOK
SOPHIES
SOPHISM
SOPHIST
SOTHEBY
SOTHERE
SOTHERN
SPYHOLE
SUBHALL
SUBHEAD
SUNHATS
SWAHILI
SYDHOFF

S•••H••

SAGEHEN
SALCHOW
SANDHOG
SATCHEL
SATCHMO
SAWCHUK
SAYWHAT
SAYWHEN
SCATHED
SCATHES
SCYTHED
SCYTHES
SEETHED
SEETHES
SEETHRU
SETSHOT
SHEEHAN
SHHHHHH
SHOWHOW
SHUSHED
SHUSHES
SILKHAT
SIOBHAN
SIXTHLY
SKISHOP
SKOSHES
SLASHED
SLASHER
SLASHES
SLATHER
SLIGHTS
SLITHER
SLOSHED
SLOSHES
SLUSHED
SLUSHES
SMASHED
SMASHER
SMASHES
SMASHUP
SMITHED
SMOTHER
SMUSHED
SMUSHES
SNOWHAT
SOCKHOP
SOMEHOW
SONSHIP
SOOTHED
SOOTHER
SOOTHES
SORGHUM
SOUTHEY
SOUTHOF
SPATHES
STASHED
STASHES
STEPHEN
STJOHNS
SULPHUR
SWASHED
SWASHES
SWATHED
SWATHES
SWISHED
SWISHES
SYLPHIC
SYNCHED

S••••H•

SAATCHI
SAMEKHS
SAYSWHO
SCACCHI
SERAPHS
SHEATHE
SHEATHS
SHEIKHS
SHHHHHH
SKETCHY
SLEIGHS
SLEIGHT
SLEUTHS
SLOUCHY
SLOUGHS
SMOOTHS
SMOOTHY
SPLASHY
SQUASHY
SQUISHY
STARCHY
STROPHE
SUBECHO
SWARTHY

S•••••H

SABBATH
SAIDAAH
SALTISH
SATWITH
SAWATCH
SAWFISH
SAYSAAH
SCITECH
SCOOTCH
SCRATCH
SCREECH
SCRUNCH
SELFISH
SERIESH
SEVENTH
SHHHHHH
SICKISH
SILENTH
SITWITH
SKYHIGH
SLAVISH
SLOWISH
SNEETCH
SOFTISH
SOPWITH
SOTTISH
SOURISH
SPANISH
SPINACH
SPLOTCH
SQUELCH
SQUINCH
STAUNCH
STEALTH
STOMACH
STRETCH
STRITCH
STYLISH
SUBCASH
SUCCOTH
SUKKOTH
SUNBATH
SUNFISH
SWEDISH
SWINISH

•SH••••

ASHAMED
ASHANTI
ASHBERY
ASHBINS
ASHBURN
ASHBURY
ASHCAKE
ASHCANS
ASHFORD
ASHHEAP
ASHIEST
ASHIVER
ASHLAND
ASHLARS
ASHLESS
ASHPANS
ASHPITS
ASHRAMS
ASHTRAY
ASHTREE
ISHMAEL
LSHAPED
OSHAPED
OSHKOSH
PSHAWED
SSHAPED
TSHAPED
TSHAPES
TSHIRTS
USHAPED
USHAPES
USHERED
USHERIN
VSHAPED
VSHAPES
YSHAPED
YSHAPES

•S•H•••

ASHHEAP
ASPHALT
ASSHARP
ASTHMAS
BSCHOOL
ESCHEAT
ESCHERS
ESCHEWS
ESTHETE
ISAHEAD
ISCHIAL
ISCHIUM
ISOHELS
ISTHMUS
QSCHOOL

•S••H••

ISFAHAN
PSYCHED
PSYCHES
PSYCHIC
PSYCHOS
PSYCHUP
USOSHOW

•S•••H•

ASEETHE

•S••••H

ASQUITH
OSHKOSH
OSTRICH

••SH•••

ALSHAIN
ARSHILE
ASSHARP
BASHERS
BASHFUL
BASHING
BBSHOTS
BISHKEK
BISHOPS
BUSHELS
BUSHERS
BUSHHOG
BUSHIDO
BUSHIER
BUSHILY
BUSHING
BUSHMAN
BUSHMEN
BUSHPIG
BUSHWAH
CASHBAR
CASHBOX
CASHCOW
CASHEWS
CASHIER
CASHING
CASHINS
CASHOUT
COSHERS
COSHING
CUSHAWS
CUSHIER
CUSHILY
CUSHING
CUSHION
DASHDOT
DASHERS
DASHIER
DASHIKI
DASHING
DASHOFF
DASHPOT
DESHELL
DISHFUL
DISHIER
DISHING
DISHOUT
DISHPAN
DISHRAG
DOSHOTS
FASHION
FISHERS
FISHERY
FISHEYE
FISHFOR
FISHFRY
FISHIER
FISHILY
FISHING
FISHNET
FISHOIL
FISHOUT
GASHEAT
GASHING
GASHOGS
GOSHAWK
GUSHERS
GUSHIER
GUSHILY
GUSHING
GUSHOUT
HASHING
HASHISH
HASHOUT
HESHVAN
HUSHABY
HUSHFUL
HUSHING
INSHAPE
INSHOCK
INSHORE
INSHORT
ITSHERE
JOSHERS
JOSHING
KASHMIR
KISHKES
KOSHERS
KOSHIBA
LASHERS
LASHING
LASHOUT
LASHUPS
LUSHEST
LUSHIER
MASHERS
MASHIES
MASHING
MCSHANE
MESHACH
MESHIER
MESHING
MESHUGA
MISHAPS
MISHEAR
MISHIMA
MISHITS
MISHNAH
MOSHERS
MOSHING
MOSHPIT
MUSHERS
MUSHIER
MUSHILY
MUSHING
NOSHERS
NOSHING
NOSHOWS
OKSHOOT
ONSHORE
PISHING
POSHEST
PUSHERS
PUSHFOR
PUSHFUL
PUSHIER
PUSHILY
PUSHING
PUSHKIN
PUSHOFF
PUSHOUT
PUSHPIN
PUSHROD
PUSHUPS
RASHERS
RASHEST
RASHIDA
RESHAPE
RESHARE
RESHAVE
RESHIFT
RESHINE
RESHIPS
RESHOES
RESHOOT
RESHOWN
RESHOWS
RESHUTS
RUSHDIE
RUSHEES
RUSHERS
RUSHIER
RUSHING
RUSHOFF
RUSHOUT
SASHAYS
SASHIMI
SASHING
TASHLIN
TOSHIBA
TOSHIRO
TUSHERY
TUSHIES
TVSHOWS
UNSHADE
UNSHADY
UNSHARP
UNSHEER
UNSHELL
UNSHIER
UNSHIFT
UNSHINY
UNSHIPS
UNSHOED
UNSHOES
UNSHORN
UNSHORT
UNSHOWN
UNSHOWY
UNSHYER
UNSHYLY
UPSHIFT
UPSHOOT
UPSHOTS
WASHDAY
WASHERS
WASHIER
WASHING
WASHOFF
WASHOUT
WASHRAG
WASHTUB
WASHUPS
WISHERS
WISHFOR
WISHFUL
WISHING
YASHICA
YASHMAK
YESHIVA

••S•H••

BASEHIT
BASRHIN
BUSHHOG
DASCHLE
EASTHAM
FISCHER
GASOHOL
ITSAHIT
MISSHIP
PASCHAL
POSTHOC
ROSEHIP
VOSKHOD

••S••H•

ATSIGHT
INSIGHT
JOSEPHA
JOSEPHI
LESOTHO
ONSIGHT
RESIGHT
UNSIGHT

••S•••H

ABSINTH
ALSMITH
ANSPACH
BESEECH
BISMUTH
BUSHWAH
DISTICH
DUSKISH
GOSOUTH
HASHISH
INSYNCH
IPSWICH
KOSSUTH
LISBETH
MESHACH
MESSIAH
MISHNAH
MISMESH
MISSISH
MRSMITH
NESMITH
RASPISH
WASATCH
WASPISH

•••SH••

ABASHED
ABASHES
AIRSHIP
AIRSHOW
APISHLY
ARTSHOP
ARTSHOW
AWASHIN
BADSHOT
BANSHEE
BIGSHOT
BIGSHOW
BLUSHED
BLUSHER
BLUSHES
BLUSHON
BOLSHOI
BOWSHOT
BRASHER
BRASHES
BRASHLY
BRUSHED
BRUSHER
BRUSHES
BRUSHUP
BUQSHAS
CAPSHAW
CARSHOW
CATSHOW
CLASHED
CLASHER
CLASHES
COPSHOP
COWSHED
CRASHAW
CRASHED
CRASHER
CRASHES
CRUSHED
CRUSHER
CRUSHES
CUMSHAW
DOGSHOW
EARSHOT
EYESHOT
FLASHED
FLASHER
FLASHES
FLASHON
FLESHED
FLESHES
FLESHLY
FLUSHED
FLUSHER
FLUSHES
FLUSHOT
FORSHOW
FRESHED
FRESHEN
FRESHER
FRESHES
FRESHET
FRESHLY
GEISHAS
GERSHON
GETSHEP
GETSHIP
GETSHOT
GLASHOW
GNASHED
GNASHER
GNASHES
GRESHAM
GRISHAM
GUMSHOE
GUNSHIP
GUNSHOT
GYMSHOE
HARSHEN
HARSHER
HARSHLY
HERSHEY
HITSHOW
HOTSHOT
ICESHOW
INASHOE
IRISHER
JOBSHOP
KAISHEK
KEESHAN
KERSHAW
KINSHIP
KNISHES
KOOSHES
KRISHNA
LAKSHMI
LEASHED
LEASHES
MARSHAL
MARSHES
MIDSHIP
MISSHIP
MUGSHOT
NUNSHIP
ODDSHOE
OLDSHOE
ONESHOE
ONESHOT
OUTSHOT
OUTSHOW
PETSHOP
PHISHED
PHISHER
PHISHES
PLASHED
PLASHES
PLUSHER
PLUSHES
PLUSHLY
POTSHOT
PRESHIP
PRESHOW
PROSHOP
QUASHED
QUASHES
RAGSHOP
RIMSHOT
RUMSHOP
SETSHOT
SHUSHED
SHUSHES
SKISHOP
SKOSHES
SLASHED
SLASHER
SLASHES
SLOSHED
SLOSHES
SLUSHED
SLUSHES
SMASHED
SMASHER
SMASHES
SMASHUP
SMUSHED
SMUSHES
SONSHIP
STASHED
STASHES
SWASHED
SWASHES
SWISHED
SWISHES
TAPSHOE
TEASHOP
TEESHOT
THESHOW
TOESHOE
TOYSHOP
TRASHED
TRASHER
TRASHES
TRASHTV
TWOSHOT
USOSHOW
WAPSHOT
WARSHIP
WHISHED
WHISHES
WOOSHED
WOOSHES.
WORSHIP

•••S•H•

BORSCHT
KITSCHY
MENSCHY
PORSCHE
SAYSWHO
WHOSWHO.

•••S••H

ANDSUCH
FORSYTH
KOSSUTH
MESSIAH
MISSISH
NONSUCH
OUTSIGH
SAYSAAH

••••SH•

ALYOSHA
BELUSHI
FINISHD
GIRLSHY
HALFSHY
KATISHA
KENOSHA
NATASHA

RICKSHA
SPLASHY
SQUASHY
SQUISHY
VERYSHY
WABASHA
WORKSHY

••••S•H
DEUTSCH
DRIESCH
KLATSCH
KLENSCH
MIRISCH
NILESOH

•••••SH
ABOLISH
ALLCASH
ANGUISH
BAALISH
BABYISH
BADDISH
BALDISH
BEAMISH
BEARISH
BEAUISH
BIGFISH
BIGGISH
BLEMISH
BLUEISH
BOARISH
BOGGISH
BONEASH
BOOKISH
BOORISH
BRINISH
BRITISH
BRUTISH
BULLISH
BULRUSH
BUMRUSH
BURNISH
CADDISH
CAPEESH
CARWASH
CATFISH
CATTISH
CHERISH
CHUMASH
CLAYISH
COCKISH
CODFISH
COLDISH
COLTISH
COMMISH
COOLISH
CORNISH
COWFISH
CUBBISH
CULTISH
CURRISH
DAMPISH
DARKISH
DEEPISH
DERVISH
DOGFISH
DOGGISH
DOLLISH
DOLTISH
DONNISH
DOTDASH
DRONISH
DRYWASH
DULLISH
DUMPISH
DUNCISH
DUSKISH
ENGLISH
EVANISH
EYELASH
EYEWASH
FADDISH
FAIRISH
FATOUSH
FATTISH
FINNISH
FLEMISH
FLYFISH
FOGYISH
FOLKISH
FOOLISH
FOPPISH
FORBUSH
FURBISH
FURNISH
GARNISH
GAULISH
GAWKISH
GETCASH
GIRLISH
GNOMISH
GOATISH
GOIRISH
GOODISH
GOTCASH
GOULASH
GOUTISH
GRAYISH
GREYISH
HAGGISH
HAIMISH
HARDISH
HASHISH
HAWKISH
HELLISH
HENNISH
HIGHISH
HIPPISH
HOGGISH
HOGWASH
HORNISH
HUFFISH
HUNNISH
INARUSH
JAZZISH
JEBBUSH
JETWASH
JIGGISH
KADDISH
KENTISH
KIDDISH
KNAVISH
KURDISH
LADDISH
LADYISH
LALOOSH
LAPPISH
LARGISH
LARKISH
LAZYISH
LEFTISH
LETTISH
LOGGISH
LONGISH
LOUDISH
LOUTISH
LUMPISH
MADDASH
MADDISH
MADRUSH
MAIDISH
MANNISH
MAWKISH
MINXISH
MISMESH
MISSISH
MOBBISH
MONKISH
MOONISH
MOORISH
MUDFISH
MUGGISH
MURKISH
NAGGISH
NEBBISH
NERDISH
NONCASH
NORRISH
NOURISH
NUNNISH
OGREISH
OMIGOSH
ONLEASH
OPALISH
OSHKOSH
OUTFISH
OUTGUSH
OUTLASH
OUTPUSH
OUTRUSH
OUTWASH
OUTWISH
PANFISH
PARRISH
PATCASH
PAYCASH
PEAKISH
PECKISH
PEEVISH
PELTISH
PERKISH
PETFISH
PETTISH
PICTISH
PIGFISH
PIGGISH
PINKISH
PIXYISH
PLANISH
PLENISH
POORISH
PORKISH
PRADESH
PREWASH
PRUDISH
PUBLISH
PUCKISH
PUGGISH
RAFFISH
RAMMISH
RANKISH
RASPISH
RATTISH
RAWFISH
REBRUSH
REDDISH
REDFISH
REFRESH
RHENISH
ROGUISH
ROMANSH
ROMPISH
ROOKISH
RUBBISH
RUNTISH
RUTTISH
SALTISH
SAWFISH
SELFISH
SERIESH
SICKISH
SLAVISH
SLOWISH
SOFTISH
SOTTISH
SOURISH
SPANISH
STYLISH
SUBCASH
SUNFISH
SWEDISH
SWINISH
TALLISH
TANNISH
TARNISH
TARTISH
THEBUSH
TINFISH
TOADISH
TORYISH
TOWNISH
TURKISH
UNHARSH
UNLEASH
VAMPISH
VARNISH
VOGUISH
WAGGISH
WAIFISH
WANNISH
WARMISH
WASPISH
WEAKISH
WETTISH
WETWASH
WHEYISH
WHITISH
WILDISH
WIMPISH
WOLFISH
WORMISH
YERKISH
YIDDISH
YOBBISH
YOUWISH
ZANYISH

SI•••••
SIAMESE
SIBERIA
SIBLING
SIBYLIC
SICCING
SICILIA
SICKBAY
SICKBED
SICKDAY
SICKENS
SICKEST
SICKISH
SICKLES
SICKOUT
SICKPAY
SIDDONS
SIDDURS
SIDEARM
SIDEBAR
SIDEBET
SIDECAR
SIDEMAN
SIDEMEN
SIDEONE
SIDETWO
SIDEWAY
SIDINGS
SIDIOUS
SIDLING
SIEBZIG
SIEGING
SIEMENS
SIENESE
SIENNAS
SIERRAS
SIESTAS
SIEVING
SIFTERS
SIFTING
SIGHERS
SIGHFOR
SIGHFUL
SIGHING
SIGHSAT
SIGHTED
SIGHTER
SIGHTLY
SIGMOID
SIGMUND
SIGNAGE
SIGNALS
SIGNEES
SIGNERS
SIGNETS
SIGNFOR
SIGNIFY
SIGNING
SIGNOFF
SIGNORA
SIGNORE
SIGNORS
SIGNOUT
SIGNSIN
SIGNSON
SIGNSUP
SIGNUPS
SIKHISM
SILENCE
SILENTA
SILENTB
SILENTC
SILENTD
SILENTE
SILENTF
SILENTG
SILENTH
SILENTI
SILENTJ
SILENTK
SILENTL
SILENTM
SILENTN
SILENTO
SILENTP
SILENTQ
SILENTR
SILENTS
SILENTT
SILENTU
SILENTV
SILENTW
SILENTX
SILENTY
SILENTZ
SILESIA
SILICAS
SILICON
SILKHAT
SILKIER
SILKILY
SILKTIE
SILLIER
SILLIES
SILLYME
SILOING
SILTIER
SILTING
SILVERS
SILVERY
SIMCITY
SIMENON
SIMIANS
SIMILAC
SIMILAR
SIMILES
SIMMERS
SIMMONS
SIMONIZ
SIMPERS
SIMPLER
SIMPLES
SIMPLEX
SIMPSON
SINATRA
SINCERE
SINCITY
SINDBAD
SINEDIE
SINEWED
SINGERS
SINGING
SINGLED
SINGLES
SINGLET
SINGOUT
SINGSTO
SINKAGE
SINKERS
SINKING
SINKSIN
SINLESS
SINLIKE
SINNERS
SINNING
SINUATE
SINUOUS
SINUSES
SINUTAB
SIOBHAN
SIOUANS
SIPHONS
SIPPERS
SIPPING
SIRDUKE
SIRENED
SIRLOIN
SIROCCO
SISENOR
SISSIER
SISSIES
SISTERS
SISTINE
SITATOP
SITBACK
SITCOMS
SITDOWN
SITEMAP
SITHOME
SITINON
SITONIT
SITSFOR
SITSOUT
SITSPAT
SITTERS
SITTING
SITUATE
SITUPON
SITWELL
SITWITH
SIXBALL
SIXEEEE
SIXFEET
SIXFIVE
SIXFOLD
SIXFOOT
SIXFOUR
SIXGUNS
SIXIRON
SIXLANE
SIXNINE
SIXPACK
SIXTEEN
SIXTHLY
SIXTIES
SIXTYAD
SIXTYBC
SIXWEEK
SIXYEAR
SIZABLE
SIZABLY
SIZEDUP
SIZEONE
SIZESIX
SIZESUP
SIZETEN
SIZETWO
SIZZLED
SIZZLER
SIZZLES

S•I••••
SAIDAAH
SAIDAYE
SAIDBOO
SAIDIDO
SAIDNAY
SAILERS
SAILING
SAILORS
SAILSON
SAILSTO
SAINTED
SAINTES
SAINTLO
SAINTLY
SAISONS
SCIATIC
SCIENCE
SCIORRA
SCISSOR
SCITECH
SEINERS
SEINING
SEISMAL
SEISMIC
SEIZEON
SEIZERS
SEIZING
SEIZORS
SEIZURE
SHIATSU
SHIELDS
SHIFTED
SHIFTER
SHIHTZU
SHIITES
SHIKOKU
SHILLED
SHIMMER
SHINDIG
SHINEON
SHINERS
SHINEUP
SHINGLE
SHINGLY
SHINIER
SHINILY
SHINING
SHINNED
SHINOLA
SHINPAD
SHIPFUL
SHIPMAN
SHIPMEN
SHIPOUT
SHIPPED
SHIPPER
SHIPWAY
SHIRKED
SHIRKER
SHIRLEY
SHIRRED
SHIVERS
SHIVERY
SKIABLE
SKIAREA
SKIBIBS
SKIBOBS
SKIBOOT
SKIBUMS
SKICAPS
SKIDDED
SKIDDER
SKIDDOO
SKIDLID
SKIDOOS
SKIDROW
SKIFFED
SKIFFLE
SKIHATS
SKIJUMP
SKILFUL
SKILIFT
SKILLED
SKILLET
SKIMASK
SKIMMED
SKIMMER
SKIMPED
SKIMPON
SKINNED
SKINNER
SKIPOLE
SKIPOUT
SKIPPED
SKIPPER
SKIPSBY
SKIRACE
SKIRACK
SKIRLED
SKIRTED
SKIRTER
SKIRUNS
SKISHOP
SKISUIT
SKITOWS
SKITRIP
SKITTER
SKITTLE
SKIVEST
SKIWEAR
SLICERS
SLICEUP
SLICING
SLICKED
SLICKER
SLICKLY
SLIDEBY
SLIDEIN
SLIDERS
SLIDING
SLIDOFF
SLIDOUT
SLIGHTS
SLIMIER
SLIMILY
SLIMING
SLIMJIM
SLIMMED
SLIMMER
SLINGER
SLINKED
SLINKER
SLINKIN
SLINKUP
SLIPOFF
SLIPONS
SLIPOUT
SLIPPED
SLIPPER
SLIPSBY
SLIPSIN
SLIPSON
SLIPSUP
SLIPUPS
SLITHER
SLITTED
SLITTER
SLIVERS
SMIDGEN
SMIDGES
SMILEAT
SMILEON
SMILERS
SMILEYS
SMILING
SMILLAS
SMIRKED
SMIRKER
SMIRNOV
SMITERS
SMITHED
SMITING
SMITTEN
SNICKER
SNICKET
SNIDELY
SNIDEST
SNIFFAT
SNIFFED
SNIFFER
SNIFFLE
SNIFFLY
SNIFFUP
SNIFTER
SNIGLET
SNIPEAT
SNIPERS
SNIPING
SNIPOFF
SNIPPED
SNIPPER
SNIPPET
SNIVELS
SOIGNEE
SOILAGE
SOILING
SOIREES
SPICERS
SPICERY
SPICEUP
SPICIER
SPICILY
SPICING
SPIDERS
SPIDERY
SPIEDON
SPIEGEL
SPIELED
SPIELER
SPIESON
SPIFFED
SPIFFUP
SPIGOTS
SPIKERS
SPIKETV
SPIKEUP
SPIKIER
SPIKILY
SPIKING
SPILLED
SPILLER
SPINACH
SPINDLE
SPINDLY
SPINDRY
SPINELS
SPINETS
SPINIER
SPINNER
SPINNEY
SPINOFF
SPINOUT
SPINOZA
SPIRALS
SPIREAS
SPIRIER
SPIRITS
SPITING
SPITOUT
SPITSON
SPITTER
SPITTLE
SPITZES
STICKBY
STICKER
STICKIN
STICKON
STICKTO
STICKUM
STICKUP
STIFFED
STIFFEL
STIFFEN
STIFFER
STIFFLY
STIFLED
STIFLES
STIGMAS
STILLED
STILLER
STILLUP
STILTED
STILTON
STIMSON
STIMULI
STINGER
STINKER
STINKUP
STINTED
STINTER
STIPEND
STIPPLE
STIRFRY
STIRRED
STIRRER
STIRRUP
STIRSIN
STIRSUP
SUITING
SUITORS
SUITSME
SUITSUP
SWIFTER
SWIFTLY
SWIGERT
SWIGGED
SWILLED
SWILLER
SWIMMER
SWIMSUP
SWINDLE
SWINERY
SWINGAT
SWINGBY
SWINGER
SWINGIT
SWINISH
SWINTON
SWIPERS
SWIPING
SWIRLED
SWISHED
SWISHES
SWITZER
SWIVELS
SWIVETS
SWIZZLE
SZILARD

S••I•••
SABINES
SADISTS
SAGIEST
SAGINAW
SALIENT
SALIERI
SALINAS
SALINES
SALIVAS
SAMISEN
SANIBEL
SAPIENS
SAPIENT
SATIATE
SATIETY
SATINET
SATINON
SATIRES
SATIRIC
SATISFY
SAVINGS
SAVIORS
SAVIOUR
SAWINTO
SAYINGS
SCHICKS
SCHIRRA
SCHISMS
SCHISTS
SCRIBED
SCRIBER
SCRIBES
SCRIMPS
SCRIMPY
SCRIPPS
SCRIPTS
SEEINTO
SEMIDRY
SEMILOG
SEMINAL
SEMINAR
SEMIPRO
SEMIRAW
SEMITES
SEMITIC
SENIORS
SEPIRAS
SERIALS
SERIATE
SERIESE
SERIESF
SERIESG
SERIESH
SERIESI
SERIESJ
SERIESK
SERIOUS
SERIPAK
SETINTO
SEVIGNY
SEVILLA
SEVILLE
SEWISTS
SEXIEST
SEXISTS
SHEIKHS
SHEILAE
SHEILAS
SHIITES
SHRIEKS
SHRIKES
SHRILLS
SHRILLY
SHRIMPS
SHRIMPY
SHRINED
SHRINER
SHRINES
SHRINKS
SHRIVEL
SHRIVER
SHRIVES
SHTICKS
SHTICKY
SICILIA
SIDINGS
SIDIOUS
SILICAS
SILICON
SIMIANS
SIMILAC
SIMILAR
SIMILES
SITINON

SIXIRON
SLEIGHS
SLEIGHT
SLUICED
SLUICES
SOCIALS
SOCIETY
SODIDWE
SOLICIT
SOLIDER
SOLIDLY
SOMINEX
SORIANO
SOVIETS
SOYINKA
SOYINKS
SPLICED
SPLICER
SPLICES
SPLINES
SPLINTS
SPLITUP
SPOILED
SPOILER
SPRIEST
SPRINGS
SPRINGY
SPRINTS
SPRITES
SPYINGS
SQUINCH
SQUINTS
SQUINTY
SQUIRED
SQUIRES
SQUIRMS
SQUIRMY
SQUIRTS
SQUISHY
STAIDER
STAIDLY
STAINED
STAINER
STAIRED
STEIGER
STEINEM
STEINER
STKITTS
STOICAL
STPIUSI
STPIUSV
STPIUSX
STRIATE
STRIDER
STRIDES
STRIFES
STRIKER
STRIKES
STRINGS
STRINGY
STRIPED
STRIPER
STRIPES
STRIPOF
STRITCH
STRIVED
STRIVEN
STRIVER
STRIVES
STSIMON
SUBIDEA
SUBITEM
SUMITUP
SURIMIS
SURINAM
SYRIANA
SYRIANS
SYRINGE

S•••I••

SABRINA
SACKING
SACLIKE
SAGGIER
SAGGING
SAIDIDO
SAILING
SALLIED
SALLIER
SALLIES
SALTIER
SALTILY
SALTINE
SALTING
SALTISH
SALVING
SAMHILL
SAMWISE
SANDIER
SANDING
SANTINI
SAPLING
SAPPIER
SAPPILY
SAPPING
SARDINE
SASHIMI
SASHING
SASSIER
SASSILY
SASSING
SATWITH
SAUCIER
SAUCILY
SAUCING
SAURIAN
SAVVIED
SAVVIER
SAVVIES
SAVVILY
SAWFISH
SAWLIKE
SAWMILL
SAWPITS
SAYHITO
SAYSIDO
SCALIER
SCALING
SCARIER
SCARIFY
SCARILY
SCARING
SCENICS
SCHLITZ
SCHMIDT
SCHMITT
SCHTICK
SCHWINN
SCOPING
SCORIAS
SCORING
SCOTIAN
SEABIRD
SEAGIRT
SEALIFE
SEALIFT
SEALIKE
SEALILY
SEALING
SEALION
SEAMIER
SEAMILE
SEAMING
SEAMIST
SEARING
SEASICK
SEASIDE
SEATING
SEBRING
SECTION
SEDGIER
SEEDIER
SEEDILY
SEEDING
SEEKING
SEEMING
SEEPIER
SEEPING
SEINING
SEIZING
SELFISH
SELKIRK
SELLING
SENDING
SENSING
SEPHIAS
SEQUINS
SERBIAN
SERLING
SERPICO
SERVICE
SERVILE
SERVING
SESSILE
SESSION
SESTINA
SETTING
SHADIER
SHADILY
SHADING
SHAKIER
SHAKILY
SHAKING
SHAKIRA
SHALIER
SHAMING
SHAPING
SHAPIRO
SHARING
SHAVIAN
SHAVING
SHERIFF
SHERIFS
SHINIER
SHINILY
SHINING
SHOEING
SHOOING
SHOOINS
SHORING
SHOVING
SHOWIER
SHOWILY
SHOWING
SHUTINS
SIBLING
SICCING
SICKISH
SIDLING
SIEGING
SIEVING
SIFTING
SIGHING
SIGNIFY
SIGNING
SIKHISM
SILKIER
SILKILY
SILLIER
SILLIES
SILOING
SILTIER
SILTING
SIMCITY
SINCITY
SINGING
SINKING
SINLIKE
SINNING
SIPPING
SISSIER
SISSIES
SISTINE
SITTING
SITWITH
SIXFIVE
SIXNINE
SIXTIES
SKATING
SKEWING
SKIBIBS
SKILIFT
SKYDIVE
SKYHIGH
SKYLIKE
SKYLINE
SLAKING
SLATIER
SLATING
SLAVING
SLAVISH
SLAYING
SLEWING
SLICING
SLIDING
SLIMIER
SLIMILY
SLIMING
SLOPING
SLOWING
SLOWISH
SMILING
SMITING
SMOKIER
SMOKIES
SMOKILY
SMOKING
SNAKIER
SNAKILY
SNAKING
SNARING
SNIPING
SNORING
SNOWIER
SNOWILY
SNOWING
SOAKING
SOAPIER
SOAPILY
SOAPING
SOARING
SOBBING
SOCKING
SODDIER
SODDING
SOFFITS
SOFTIES
SOFTISH
SOGGIER
SOGGILY
SOILING
SOLDIER
SOLOING
SOLOIST
SOLVING
SONLIKE
SOOTIER
SOOTILY
SOPHIES
SOPHISM
SOPHIST
SOPPIER
SOPPING
SOPWITH
SORDINI
SORDINO
SORRIER
SORRILY
SORTIED
SORTIES
SORTING
SORVINO
SOTTISH
SOUBISE
SOUPIER
SOURING
SOURISH
SOUSING
SOWLIKE
SOYMILK
SPACIAL
SPACIER
SPACING
SPADING
SPANIEL
SPANISH
SPARING
SPATIAL
SPAYING
SPECIAL
SPECIES
SPECIFY
SPECING
SPEWING
SPICIER
SPICILY
SPICING
SPIKIER
SPIKILY
SPIKING
SPINIER
SPIRIER
SPIRITS
SPITING
SPOKING
SPRAINS
SPUMIER
SPUMING
SPYKIDS
SPYRING
STABILE
STADIUM
STAGIER
STAGILY
STAGING
STAKING
STAMINA
STANINE
STARING
STARION
STATICE
STATICS
STATING
STATINS
STATION
STATISM
STATIST
STAVING
STAYING
STELIAS
STEPINS
STERILE
STEWIER
STEWING
STOGIES
STOKING
STONIER
STONILY
STONING
STORIED
STORIES
STORING
STOTINS
STOWING
STRAINS
STRAITS
STUBING
STUDIED
STUDIER
STUDIES
STUDIOS
STUPIDS
STYGIAN
STYLING
STYLISE
STYLISH
STYLIST
STYLIZE
STYMIED
STYMIES
SUASION
SUASIVE
SUAVITY
SUBBIAS
SUBBING
SUBFILE
SUBKING
SUBLIDS
SUBLIME
SUBMITS
SUBSIDE
SUBSIDY
SUBSIST
SUCKIER
SUCKING
SUCTION
SUDSIER
SUDSING
SUFFICE
SUITING
SULFIDE
SULFITE
SULKIER
SULKIES
SULKILY
SULKING
SULLIED
SULLIES
SUMMING
SUMMITS
SUMOIST
SUNBIRD
SUNCITY
SUNDIAL
SUNFIRE
SUNFISH
SUNKIST
SUNLIKE
SUNNIER
SUNNILY
SUNNING
SUNRISE
SUPPING
SUREIAM
SUREIDO
SURFIER
SURFING
SURGING
SURLIER
SURLILY
SURMISE
SURVIVE
SUSPIRE
SUSSING
SVERIGE
SWAHILI
SWAYING
SWEDISH
SWINISH
SWIPING
SYNCING
SYNDICS

S••••I•

SAFARIS
SALADIN
SALAMIS
SALTPIT
SALUKIS
SAMARIA
SAMEDIS
SANDPIT
SANGRIA
SANSEIS
SATANIC
SATIRIC
SATORIS
SATYRIC
SAVARIN
SAWTOIT
SAYWAIT
SCARWID
SCENEII
SCENEIV
SCEPTIC
SCIATIC
SCORPIO
SCOTTIE
SEALSIN
SEATRIP
SECHZIG
SEDALIA
SEENFIT
SEEPSIN
SEESFIT
SEETOIT
SEFERIS
SEGOVIA
SEISMIC
SELENIC
SELLSIT
SEMITIC
SENDSIN
SENSEIS
SEQUOIA
SERAPIS
SETBAIL
SETSAIL
SHAREIN
SHARPIE
SHELTIE
SHERWIN
SHINDIG
SHOOSIN
SHORTIE
SHOVEIN
SHOWBIZ
SHOWNIN
SHOWSIN
SHUTSIN
SIBERIA
SIBYLIC
SICILIA
SIEBZIG
SIGMOID
SIGNSIN
SILESIA
SILKTIE
SIMONIZ
SINEDIE
SINKSIN
SIRLOIN
SITONIT
SIZESIX
SKEEZIX
SKEPTIC
SKIDLID
SKISUIT
SKITRIP
SLATKIN
SLEEPIN
SLEPTIN
SLIDEIN
SLIMJIM
SLINKIN
SLIPSIN
SLOEGIN
SLUNKIN
SNEAKIN
SNOWSIN
SNUGFIT
SNUGLIS
SOAKSIN
SOCKSIN
SOLARIA
SOLICIT
SOLVEIT
SOMALIA
SOMALIS
SOMATIC
SONSHIP
SOUPMIX
SPANAIR
SPHERIC
SPORTIN
SPOTLIT
SPUTNIK
SQUALID
STANDIN
STANNIC
STARLIT
STARSIN
STARTIN
STAYSIN
STBASIL
STCROIX
STDENIS
STEALIN
STEARIC
STEARIN
STEELIE
STEEPIN
STENCIL
STENNIS
STEPSIN
STEROID
STICKIN
STIRSIN
STLOUIS
STLUCIA
STOLEIN
STOMPIN
STOODIN
STOOLIE
STOPSIN
STOPSIT
STORMIN
STOWSIT
STRAPIN
STREGIS
STUCKIN
STUFFIN
STYPSIS
STYPTIC
SUBARID
SUBJOIN
SUBSOIL
SUBUNIT
SUCKSIN
SUNMAID
SUNSUIT
SURFEIT
SURIMIS
SURVEIL
SUSTAIN
SUZUKIS
SWEARIN
SWEATIT
SWEETIE
SWINGIT
SWOOPIN
SWOOSIE
SWOREIN
SWUNGIT
SYLPHIC
SYNODIC

S•••••I

SAATCHI
SALIERI
SAMURAI
SANTINI
SASHIMI
SCACCHI
SCENEII
SCENEVI
SCHERZI
SCOLARI
SECONDI
SERIESI
SHANGRI
SHARPEI
SHASTRI
SHOULDI
SILENTI
SNOWSKI
SOHAVEI
SOLLATI
SOPRANI
SORDINI
SPUMONI
STEFANI
STIMULI
STPIUSI
STRETTI
STUARTI
SWAHILI
SYLLABI

•SI••••

ASIAGOS
ASIATIC
ASIMMER
ASININE
ASISAID
ESIASON
ISIDORE
ISITAGO
MSIEURS
OSIERED
OSIRIAN
USINGIN
USINGUP

•S•I•••

ASHIEST
ASHIVER
ASPIRED
ASPIRER
ASPIRES
ASPIRIN
ASSIGNS
ASSISTS
ASSIZES
ESKIMOS
ESPIALS
ESTIVAL
ISAIDNO
OSCINES
OSSICLE
OSSIFIC
OSSIPEE
OSTIARY
TSHIRTS
USTINOV

•S••I••

ASAGIFT
ASCRIBE
ASHBINS
ASHPITS
ASININE
ASOCIAL
ASQUIET
ASQUINT
ASQUITH
ASSAILS
ASSLIKE
ASSTIFF
ASTAIRE
ASTRIDE
ESPRITS
ESPYING
ESQUIRE
ESTRING
GSTRING
ISCHIAL
ISCHIUM
ISOLINE
ISSUING
ISTRIAN
OSIRIAN
OSTRICH
RSVPING
TSARINA
TSARISM
TSARIST
TSELIOT
USERIDS
USURIES

•S•••I•

ASCETIC
ASEPSIS
ASEPTIC
ASIATIC
ASISAID
ASKEDIN
ASPIRIN
ASSYRIA
ASTERIX
ASTORIA
CSLEWIS
ESTAMIN
ESTONIA
ESTORIL
ISLAMIC
ISTOMIN
OSMATIC
OSMOSIS
OSMOTIC
OSSIFIC
OSTEOID
OSTOSIS
PSALMIC
PSYCHIC
TSOURIS
USHERIN
USINGIN

•S••••I

ASHANTI
ISRAELI
TSUNAMI

••SI•••

ABSINTH
AJSIMON
APSIDES
ASSIGNS
ASSISTS
ASSIZES
ATSIGHT
ATSIGNS
BASILIC
BASILIO
BASINAL
BESIDES
BESIEGE
BUSIEST
CASIMIR
CASINGS
CASINOS
CASITAS
COSIEST
COSIGNS
COSINES
DASILVA
DESIGNS
DESILTS
DESIRED
DESIREE
DESIRER
DESIRES
DESISTS
DOSIDOS
EASIEST
ENSIGNS
ENSILED
ENSILES
EOSINES
EPSILON
FUSIBLE
FUSILLI
FUSIONS
HASIDIC
HASIDIM
HOSIERS
HOSIERY
INSIDER
INSIDES
INSIGHT
INSIGNE
INSIPID
INSISTS
LESIONS
LOSINGS
MTSINAI
MUSICAL
MUSICKS
MUSIGNY
MUSINGS
NOSIEST
NOSIREE
ONSIDES
ONSIGHT
OSSICLE
OSSIFIC
OSSIPEE
POSITED
RESIDED
RESIDER
RESIDES
RESIDUA
RESIDUE
RESIFTS
RESIGHT
RESIGNS
RESILED
RESILES
RESINED
RESINGS
RESINKS
RESISTS
RESITED
RESIZED
RESIZER
RESIZES
RISIBLE
RISIBLY
RISINGS
ROSIEST
ROSINED
STSIMON
UNSIDED
UNSIGHT
UNSILLY
UNSIZED
UPSIDES
UPSILON
UPSIZED
UPSIZES
URSINUS
VESICLE
VISIBLE
VISIBLY
VISIONS
VISITED
VISITOR
WYSIWYG
YESICAN
YESIDID
YESISEE
YESITIS

ZOSIMUS

••S•I••

ABSCISE
ALSMITH
ARSHILE
ASSAILS
ASSLIKE
ASSTIFF
AUSPICE
AUSSIES
AUSTINS
BASHING
BASKING
BASSIER
BASSIST
BASTING
BASTION
BESTIAL
BESTILL
BESTING
BESTIRS
BOSNIAN
BOSSIER
BOSSILY
BOSSING
BOSSISM
BUSBIES
BUSGIRL
BUSHIDO
BUSHIER
BUSHILY
BUSHING
BUSKING
BUSLINE
BUSRIDE
BUSSING
BUSTIER
BUSTING
BUSYING
CASEINS
CASHIER
CASHING
CASHINS
CASKING
CASPIAN
CASSIAS
CASSIDY
CASSINI
CASSINO
CASSIUS
CASTILE
CASTING
CASUIST
CESAIRE
CESSING
CESSION
COSHING
COSTING
COSTIVE
COSYING
CUSHIER
CUSHILY
CUSHING
CUSHION
CUSPIDS
CUSSING
DASHIER
DASHIKI
DASHING
DESPINA
DESPISE
DESPITE
DESTINE
DESTINO
DESTINY
DISCING
DISHIER
DISHING
DISKING
DISLIKE
DISMISS
DISSING
DISTICH
DISTILL
DISTILS
DOSSIER
DOSSING
DUSKIER
DUSKILY
DUSKING
DUSKISH
DUSTIER
DUSTILY
DUSTING
EASTING
ENSKIED
ENSKIES
ENSUING
ENSUITE
ERSKINE
EXSCIND
FASCIAE
FASCIAL
FASCIAS
FASCISM
FASCIST
FASHION
FASTING
FESSING
FESTINA
FESTIVA
FESTIVE
FISHIER
FISHILY
FISHING
FISSILE
FISSION
FOSDICK
FOSSILS
FUSSIER
FUSSILY
FUSSING
FUSTIAN
FUSTIER
FUSTILY
GASEITY
GASHING
GASLINE
GASPING
GASPIPE
GASSIER
GASSING
GISSING
GOSLING
GOSSIPS
GOSSIPY
GUSHIER
GUSHILY
GUSHING
GUSSIED
GUSSIES
GUSTIER
GUSTILY
GUSTING
HASFITS
HASHING
HASHISH
HASPING
HASSIUM
HASTIER
HASTILY
HASTIME
HASTING
HESSIAN
HISNIBS
HISSIER
HISSING
HOSKINS
HOSPICE
HOSTILE
HOSTING
HUSHING
HUSKIER
HUSKIES
HUSKILY
HUSKING
HUSSIES
HUSSITE
INSPIRE
INSPITE
INSTILL
INSTILS
IPSWICH
ISSUING
ITSFINE
ITSTIME
JASMINE
JESSICA
JESTING
JESUITS
JOSHING
JUSTICE
JUSTIFY
JUSTINE
KISSING
KOSCINA
KOSHIBA
LASHING
LASSIES
LASTING
LESSING
LISPING
LISTING
LUSHIER
LUSTIER
LUSTILY
LUSTING
MASHIES
MASHING
MASKING
MASSIER
MASSIFS
MASSINE
MASSING
MASSIVE
MASTICS
MASTIFF
MASTING
MCSWINE
MESHIER
MESHING
MESSIAH
MESSICK
MESSIER
MESSILY
MESSINA
MESSING
MISAIMS
MISBILL
MISBIND
MISCITE
MISDIAL
MISFILE
MISFIRE
MISFITS
MISGIVE
MISHIMA
MISHITS
MISLIKE
MISSIES
MISSILE
MISSING
MISSION
MISSISH
MISSIVE
MISTIER
MISTILY
MISTIME
MISTING
MISWIRE
MOSAICS
MOSHING
MOSSIER
MOSSING
MRSMITH
MUSCIDA
MUSHIER
MUSHILY
MUSHING
MUSKIER
MUSKIES
MUSLIMS
MUSLINS
MUSSIER
MUSSILY
MUSSING
MUSTIER
MUSTILY
MYSTICS
MYSTIFY
NASTIER
NASTIES
NASTILY
NESBITT
NESMITH
NESTING
NOSHING
OUSTING
PASSING
PASSION
PASSIVE
PASTIER
PASTIES
PASTIME
PASTINA
PASTING
PESKIER
PESKILY
PISCINE
PISHING
PISMIRE
PISTILS
POSTIES
POSTING
POSTITS
PUSHIER
PUSHILY
PUSHING
PUSSIES
RASHIDA
RASPIER
RASPING
RASPISH
RESCIND
RESEIZE
RESHIFT
RESHINE
RESHIPS
RESOILS
RESPICE
RESPINS
RESPIRE
RESPITE
RESTICK
RESTING
RESTIRS
RESTIVE
RESUITS
RESWIMS
RISKIER
RISKILY
RISKING
RLSTINE
ROSSINI
RUSHIER
RUSHING
RUSSIAN
RUSTICS
RUSTIER
RUSTILY
RUSTING
SASHIMI
SASHING
SASSIER
SASSILY
SASSING
SESSILE
SESSION
SESTINA
SISSIER
SISSIES
SISTINE
SUSPIRE
SUSSING
TASKING
TASTIER
TASTILY
TASTING
TESTIER
TESTIFY
TESTILY
TESTING
TOSHIBA
TOSHIRO
TOSSING
TUSHIES
TUSKING
TUSSIVE
UNSHIER
UNSHIFT
UNSHINY
UNSHIPS
UNSLICK
UNSLIER
UNSLING
UNSPICY
UNSPIED
UNSPILT
UNSTICK
UNSTIFF
UPSHIFT
UPSPINS
UPSTIRS
UPSWING
VASTIER
VASTITY
VESPIDS
VESTIGE
VESTING
VISAING
VOSGIAN
WASHIER
WASHING
WASPIER
WASPILY
WASPISH
WASSILY
WASTING
WESKITS
WESTIES
WESTINS
WISHING
WISPIER
WISPILY
WISPING
YASHICA
YASMINE
YESHIVA
YESSING
YESSIRE
ZESTIER
ZESTILY
ZESTING
ZOSSIMA

••S••I•

ABSTAIN
ALSATIA
ALSHAIN
ANSONIA
ARSENIC
ARSENIO
ASSYRIA
AUSTRIA
BASEHIT
BASESIX
BASILIC
BASILIO
BASRHIN
BISCUIT
BOSONIC
BUSHPIG
BUSTRIP
BUSTSIN
CASIMIR
CESSPIT
COSTAIN
DESPAIR
DESPOIL
DESTAIN
DISCOID
DISDAIN
DISJOIN
DUSTBIN
EASEDIN
EASESIN
EPSTEIN
FISHOIL
GASMAIN
GASTRIC
HASAFIT
HASANIP
HASATIT
HASIDIC
HASIDIM
HUSSEIN
INSIPID
INSULIN
ITSAHIT
ITSALIE
ITSASIN
ITSATIE
KASHMIR
KOSYGIN
LESTOIL
LOSEBIG
LOSESIT
LOSTBIG
MASONIC
MASTOID
MESAMIS
MESONIC
MESSKIT
MISCOIN
MISEDIT
MISJOIN
MISLAID
MISSAID
MISSHIP
MOSHPIT
MRSMUIR
NESQUIK
NESTSIN
NOSEDIN
NOSESIN
NOSTAIN
NOSTRIL
OSSIFIC
PASSAIC
PASTEIN
PISANIO
POSTFIX
PUSHKIN
PUSHPIN
RESNAIS
RESPLIT
RESTAIN
RESTRIP
RESTSIN
RISKSIT
ROSALIA
ROSALIE
ROSARIO
ROSEHIP
ROSEOIL
RUSHDIE
SUSTAIN
TASHLIN
TASTEIT
TESTKIT
UNSLAIN
UNSOLID
UNSPLIT
UNSTAID
UNSTOIC
UPSTAIR
VISALIA
VISAVIS
WASABIS
WASFAIR
WASSAIL
YESIDID
YESITIS

••S•••I

BASENJI
BASMATI
BASSANI
BUSCEMI
CASSINI
CESTMOI
DASHIKI
FUSILLI
JOSEPHI
MOSCONI
MTSINAI
PASCOLI
ROSSINI
SASHIMI
XYSTUSI

•••SI••

ABASING
ABUSING
ABUSIVE
AIRSICK
AIRSIGN
AMUSING
ANTSIER
ARCSINE
ARISING
ARTSIER
AUSSIES
BADSIGN
BASSIER
BASSIST
BEDSIDE
BEDSITS
BIASING
BITSIER
BOSSIER
BOSSILY
BOSSING
BOSSISM
BRASIER
BRASIZE
BUSSING
CAPSIZE
CASSIAS
CASSIDY
CASSINI
CASSINO
CASSIUS
CATSITS
CAUSING
CEASING
CELSIUS
CENSING
CESSING
CESSION
CHASING
CLOSING
CONSIGN
CONSIST
CORSICA
COUSINE
COUSINS
CROSIER
CUISINE
CURSING
CURSIVE
CUSSING
DAISIES
DAYSIDE
DAYSINN
DENSIFY
DENSITY
DISSING
DITSIER
DOASIDO
DOGSITS
DOSSIER
DOSSING
DOUSING
DOWSING
ELISION
ELUSIVE
ELYSIAN
ELYSIUM
ERASING
EROSION
EROSIVE
ETESIAN
EVASION
EVASIVE
FALSIFY
FALSITY
FARSIDE
FESSING
FISSILE
FISSION
FORSIZE
FOSSILS
FRASIER
FRISIAN
FUBSIER
FUSSIER
FUSSILY
FUSSING
GASSIER
GASSING
GIPSIES
GISSING
GOOSIER
GOOSING
GORSIER
GOSSIPS
GOSSIPY
GUSSIED
GUSSIES
GUTSIER
GUTSILY
GYPSIES
HASSIUM
HATSIZE
HELSING
HESSIAN
HEXSIGN
HISSIER
HISSING
HOOSIER
HOPSING
HORSIER
HORSILY
HORSING
HOUSING
HUSSIES
HUSSITE
IINSIST
IRESIGN
IRISING
JESSICA
KISSING
LANSING
LAPSING
LASSIES
LEASING
LESSING
LOOSING
LOUSIER
LOUSILY
LOUSING
LOWSIDE
MANSION
MANSIZE
MASSIER
MASSIFS
MASSINE
MASSING
MASSIVE
MESSIAH
MESSICK
MESSIER
MESSILY
MESSINA
MESSING
MIDSIZE
MISSIES
MISSILE
MISSING
MISSION
MISSISH
MISSIVE
MOSSIER
MOSSING
MOUSIER
MOUSILY
MOUSING
MUSSIER
MUSSILY
MUSSING
NEWSIER
NEWSIES
NOISIER
NOISILY
NOISING
NOOSING
NURSING
NUTSIER
OBESITY
OFFSIDE
OFFSITE
ONESIZE
OUTSIDE
OUTSIFT
OUTSIGH
OUTSING
OUTSINS
OUTSITS
OUTSIZE
PADSITE
PANSIES
PARSING
PASSING
PASSION
PASSIVE
PATSIES
PAUSING
PENSION
PENSIVE
PEPSICO
PEPSINS
PERSIAN
PERSIST
PERSIUS
PETSITS
PHASING
PHYSICS
PIOSITY
PIUSIII
PLOSION
PLOSIVE
POESIES
POISING
PRESIDE
PRESIFT
PROSIER
PROSILY
PROSING
PULSING
PURSIER
PURSING
PUSSIES
RAISING
RAISINS
RAISINY
RAWSILK
RETSINA
REUSING
RINSING
ROSSINI
ROUSING
RUSSIAN
SASSIER
SASSILY
SASSING
SAYSIDO
SEASICK
SEASIDE
SENSING
SESSILE
SESSION
SISSIER
SISSIES
SOUSING
SUASION
SUASIVE
SUBSIDE
SUBSIDY
SUBSIST
SUDSIER
SUDSING
SUSSING
TANSIES
TEASING
TENSILE
TENSING
TENSION
TENSITY
TENSIVE
THESIMS
TILSITS
TIPSIER
TIPSILY
TOCSINS
TONSILS
TOPSIDE
TORSION
TOSSING
TUSSIVE
UNISIZE
VARSITY
VERSIFY
VERSING
VERSION
WASSILY
WAYSIDE
WEBSITE
YESSING
YESSIRE
ZOSSIMA
ZOYSIAS

•••S•I•

AGASSIZ
AIRSHIP
ANOSMIA
ANOSMIC
APESUIT
ASISAID
AWASHIN
BATSUIT
BEASTIE
BOISEID
BONSOIR
BRASSIE
BRESCIA
BRESLIN
BURSTIN
CATSUIT
CAUSTIC
CESSPIT
CHASMIC
CHASSIS
CLASSIC
CLOSEIN
CORSAIR
COWSKIN
COWSLIP
CRESPIN
CRISPIN
CRISPIX
CROSTIC
DAYSAIL
DEISTIC
DOESKIN
DRASTIC
DRESSIN
DRYSUIT
EELSKIN
EKISTIC
ELASTIC
ELASTIN
ERISTIC
FLOSSIE
GETSFIT
GETSHIP
GETSRID
GNOSTIC
GUNSHIP
GYMSUIT
HUSSEIN
ILOSTIT
INASNIT
INASPIN
INASTIR
INASUIT
JETSKIS
KIDSKIN
KINSHIP
KIRSTIE
KRESKIN
KRISTIN
KTOSLIN
LAWSUIT
LETSLIP
LETSRIP
LUGSAIL
MAOSUIT
MESSKIT
MIASMIC
MIDSHIP
MISSAID
MISSHIP
MUESLIS
MUESLIX
NAYSAID
NONSKID
NONSLIP
NUNSHIP
OILSKIN
ONASSIS
OUTSAID
OUTSAIL
OUTSKIP
OUTSPIN
OUTSPIT
OUTSWIM
PARSNIP
PASSAIC
PAYSLIP
PERSEID
PHASEIN

PIGSKIN
PIUSIII
PIUSVII
PIUSXII
PLASMIC
PLASTIC
POUSSIN
PRESHIP
PROSAIC
PRUSSIA
PURSUIT
REDSKIN
REDSUIT
SANSEIS
SEESFIT
SEISMIC
SENSEIS
SETSAIL
SKISUIT
SONSHIP
SUBSOIL
SUNSUIT
THESPIS
TOPSAIL
TOPSOIL
TOPSPIN
TRUSTIN
TRYSAIL
WARSHIP
WASSAIL
WETSUIT
WHOSAID
WINSBIG
WORSHIP

•••S••I

ANASAZI
BASSANI
BOLSHOI
CASSINI
FAISALI
LAKSHMI
MAISOUI
PIUSIII
PIUSVII
PIUSXII
RAMSESI
ROSSINI
SHASTRI
TOLSTOI

••••SI•

AGASSIZ
AMNESIA
AMNESIC
APHASIA
APHASIC
ASEPSIS
BABYSIT
BACKSIN
BASESIX
BEATSIT
BITESIN
BLOWSIN
BLOWSIT
BOOPSIE
BOOTSIT
BOXESIN
BRASSIE
BURNSIN
BUSTSIN
BUTTSIN
CALLSIN
CALLSIT
CARTSIN
CAVESIN
CHASSIS
CHIPSIN
CINESIA
CLASSIC
CLUESIN
COMESIN
COOLSIT
CRAISIN
CRAMSIN
CURLSIN
CYRUSII
DALASIS
DEALSIN
DEARSIR
DEEPSIX
DEPOSIT
DIALSIN
DINESIN
DIVESIN
DRAGSIN
DRAWSIN
DRESSIN
DROPSIN
DROPSIT
EARNSIT
EASESIN
ECDYSIS
EDGESIN
EURASIA
EXPOSIT
FACESIT
FADESIN
FAKESIT
FALLSIN
FEEDSIN
FILESIN
FILLSIN
FIVESIX
FLIESIN
FLITSIN
FLOSSIE
FLOWSIN
FOLDSIN
FOOTSIE
FOOTSIT
FREESIA
FUCHSIA
GELUSIL
GENESIS
GIVESIN
HACKSIT
HANDSIN
HANGSIN
HARDSIX
HATESIT
HAULSIN
HEADSIN
HELPSIN
HOLDSIN
HOLDSIT
HOMESIN
HONESIN
HOOFSIT
HORNSIN
ITSASIN
JAMESII
JAMESIV
JOINSIN
JUMPSIN
KEEPSIN
KICKSIN
KINESIC
KINESIS
LEADSIN
LEAKSIN
LEANSIN
LEAPSIN
LEXUSIS
LIVESIN
LOADSIN
LOCKSIN
LOOKSIN
LORDSIT
LOSESIT
LOUISII
LOUISIV
LOUISIX
LOVESIT
LUMPSIN
LUMPSIT
LURESIN
MACHSIX
MAILSIN
MAKESIT
MEANSIT
MEIOSIS
MIMESIS
MITOSIS
MIXESIN
MOVESIN
MOVESIT
MRMUSIC
NAILSIN
NAILSIT
NEMESIS
NESTSIN
NICOSIA
NOSESIN
ONASSIS
OSMOSIS
OSTOSIS
PACKSIN
PAGESIX
PARKSIT
PEEKSIN
PEERSIN
PILESIN
PIPESIN
PLAISIR
PLUGSIN
POLESIT
POOPSIE
POURSIN
POUSSIN
PRUSSIA
PULLSIN
QUITSIT
RAINSIN
RAKESIN
READSIN
REELSIN
REINSIN
REPOSIT
RESTSIN
REVISIT
RIDESIN
RINGSIN
RISKSIT
ROLLSIN
ROPESIN
SEALSIN
SEEPSIN
SELLSIT
SENDSIN
SHOOSIN
SHOWSIN
SHUTSIN
SIGNSIN
SILESIA
SINKSIN
SIZESIX
SLIPSIN
SNOWSIN
SOAKSIN
SOCKSIN
STARSIN
STAYSIN
STBASIL
STEPSIN
STIRSIN
STOPSIN
STOPSIT
STOWSIT
STYPSIS
SUCKSIN
SWOOSIE
TAKESIN
TAKESIT
TEARSIT
TEENSIE
TELLSIT
THATSIT
TOOTSIE
TRANSIT
TRIESIT
TUCKSIN
TUNESIN
TUNISIA
TURNSIN
TYPESIN
UTENSIL
VOTESIN
WADESIN
WALLSIN
WANTSIN
WATUSIS
WAVESIN
WHATSIS
WHATSIT
WHIPSIN
WHOISIT
WHOOSIS
WHYISIT
WINGSIT
WIRESIN
WORKSIN
XEROSIS
YELTSIN
ZEROSIN
ZOOMSIN

••••S•I

ALEKSEI
BELUSHI
BREWSKI
CHRISTI
COLOSSI
CYRUSII
ELMISTI
JAMESII
JAMESVI
LOUISII
LOUISVI
LOUISXI
MENISCI
MINISKI
MONOSKI
PARASKI
PLOESTI
POLISCI
POLYSCI
PULASKI
SNOWSKI
TURFSKI

•••••SI

COLOSSI
DARIUSI
ECCLESI
EKWENSI
FRENESI
LUCIUSI
MAFIOSI
MONDESI
PACHISI
RAMSESI
SERIESI
STPIUSI
TBILISI
XERXESI
XYSTUSI

S•J••••

SOJOURN
STJAMES
STJOHNS

S••J•••

SANJOSE
SANJUAN
SKIJUMP
SKYJACK
SUBJECT
SUBJOIN

S•••J••

SLIMJIM
SNOWJOB

S••••J•

SAMMYJO

S•••••J

SERIESJ
SILENTJ
SMALLOJ

•S•J•••

ASAJOKE

••SJ•••

DISJOIN
GASJETS
MISJOIN

••S•J••

EASYJOB
NOSEJOB
RESOJET

••S••J•

BASENJI

••••SJ•

MARUSJA

•••••SJ

SERIESJ

SK•••••

SKAGWAY
SKATERS
SKATING
SKEETER
SKEEZIX
SKELTER
SKELTON
SKEPTIC
SKETCHY
SKEWERS
SKEWING
SKIABLE
SKIAREA
SKIBIBS
SKIBOBS
SKIBOOT
SKIBUMS
SKICAPS
SKIDDED
SKIDDER
SKIDDOO
SKIDLID
SKIDOOS
SKIDROW
SKIFFED
SKIFFLE
SKIHATS
SKIJUMP
SKILFUL
SKILIFT
SKILLED
SKILLET
SKIMASK
SKIMMED
SKIMMER
SKIMPED
SKIMPON
SKINNED
SKINNER
SKIPOLE
SKIPOUT
SKIPPED
SKIPPER
SKIPSBY
SKIRACE
SKIRACK
SKIRLED
SKIRTED
SKIRTER
SKIRUNS
SKISHOP
SKISUIT
SKITOWS
SKITRIP
SKITTER
SKITTLE
SKIVEST
SKIWEAR
SKOSHES
SKULKED
SKULKER
SKULLED
SKUNKED
SKYBLUE
SKYCAMS
SKYCAPS
SKYDIVE
SKYDOME
SKYHIGH
SKYHOOK
SKYJACK
SKYLARK
SKYLESS
SKYLIKE
SKYLINE
SKYMAPS
SKYNYRD
SKYSURF
SKYWALK
SKYWARD
SKYWAYS

S•K••••

SIKHISM
STKITTS
SUKARNO
SUKKOTH

S••K•••

SACKERS
SACKFUL
SACKING
SACKOUT
SACKSUP
SDAKOTA
SECKELS
SEEKERS
SEEKING
SEEKOUT
SELKIRK
SHAKERS
SHAKEUP
SHAKIER
SHAKILY
SHAKING
SHAKIRA
SHAKOES
SHEKELS
SHIKOKU
SICKBAY
SICKBED
SICKDAY
SICKENS
SICKEST
SICKISH
SICKLES
SICKOUT
SICKPAY
SILKHAT
SILKIER
SILKILY
SILKTIE
SINKAGE
SINKERS
SINKING
SINKSIN
SLAKERS
SLAKING
SMOKERS
SMOKEUP
SMOKEYS
SMOKIER
SMOKIES
SMOKILY
SMOKING
SNAKERS
SNAKIER
SNAKILY
SNAKING
SOAKERS
SOAKING
SOAKSIN
SOAKSUP
SOCKETS
SOCKEYE
SOCKHOP
SOCKING
SOCKSIN
SPIKERS
SPIKETV
SPIKEUP
SPIKIER
SPIKILY
SPIKING
SPOKANE
SPOKEOF
SPOKETO
SPOKEUP
SPOKING
SPYKIDS
STAKING
STOKELY
STOKERS
STOKEUP
STOKING
SUBKING
SUCKDRY
SUCKERS
SUCKIER
SUCKING
SUCKSIN
SUCKSUP
SUKKOTH
SULKERS
SULKIER
SULKIES
SULKILY
SULKING
SUNKIST

S•••K••

SALUKIS
SAMEKHS
SHACKED
SHACKLE
SHANKAR
SHANKED
SHARKEY
SHEIKHS
SHIRKED
SHIRKER
SHOCKED
SHOCKER
SHOOKUP
SHOPKOS
SHRIKES
SHUCKED
SHUCKER
SKULKED
SKULKER
SKUNKED
SLACKED
SLACKEN
SLACKER
SLACKLY
SLACKUP
SLATKIN
SLEEKED
SLEEKEN
SLEEKER
SLEEKLY
SLICKED
SLICKER
SLICKLY
SLINKED
SLINKER
SLINKIN
SLINKUP
SLUNKIN
SLUNKUP
SMACKED
SMACKER
SMACKOF
SMACKUP
SMIRKED
SMIRKER
SMUCKER
SNACKED
SNACKER
SNACKON
SNEAKBY
SNEAKED
SNEAKER
SNEAKIN
SNEAKUP
SNICKER
SNICKET
SNOOKER
SNORKEL
SNUCKUP
SPACKLE
SPANKED
SPANKER
SPARKED
SPARKLE
SPARKLY
SPEAKER
SPEAKOF
SPEAKTO
SPEAKUP
SPECKED
SPECKLE
SPOOKED
STACKED
STACKER
STACKUP
STALKED
STALKER
STANKUP
STARKER
STARKEY
STARKLY
STICKBY
STICKER
STICKIN
STICKON
STICKTO
STICKUM
STICKUP
STINKER
STINKUP
STLUKES
STOCKED
STOCKER
STOCKUP
STOOKEY
STRIKER
STRIKES
STROKED
STROKER
STROKES
STUCKBY
STUCKIN
STUCKON
STUCKTO
STUCKUP
SUDOKUS
SUZUKIS
SWANKED
SWANKER
SWANKUP

S••••K•

SACLIKE
SAWLIKE
SCHICKS
SCREAKS
SEALIKE
SHIKOKU
SHLOCKY
SHNOOKS
SHRIEKS
SHRINKS
SHTICKS
SHTICKY
SINLIKE
SIRDUKE
SKYLIKE
SLOVAKS
SNOWSKI
SONLIKE
SOWLIKE
SOYINKA
SOYINKS
SPASSKY
SQUAWKS
SQUAWKY
SQUEAKS
SQUEAKY
STARSKY
STMARKS
STREAKS
STREAKY
SUNLIKE

S•••••K

SADSACK
SARAWAK
SATBACK
SAWBUCK
SAWCHUK
SCHLOCK
SCHNOOK
SCHTICK
SEADUCK
SEAHAWK
SEASICK
SELKIRK
SELLECK
SERIESK
SERIPAK
SETBACK
SHYLOCK
SILENTK
SITBACK
SIXPACK
SIXWEEK
SKIMASK
SKIRACK
SKYHOOK
SKYJACK
SKYLARK
SKYWALK
SLYLOOK
SOYMILK
SPELUNK
SPUTNIK
SUBBANK
SUBTASK
SUFFOLK
SUNDECK
SZYSLAK

•SK••••

ASKANCE
ASKAWAY
ASKEDIN
ASKEDOF
ASKEDUP
ASKOVER
ASKSFOR
ASKSOUT
ESKIMOS
TSKTSKS

•S•K•••

OSAKANS
OSHKOSH

•S•••K•

ASAJOKE
ASHCAKE
ASSLIKE
JSTROKE
TSKTSKS

•S••••K

ASALARK
OSTMARK

••SK•••

BASKETS
BASKETT
BASKING
BUSKERS
BUSKING
CASKETS
CASKING
DESKFUL
DESKSET
DESKTOP
DISKING
DUSKIER
DUSKILY
DUSKING
DUSKISH
ENSKIED
ENSKIES
ERSKINE
GASKELL
GASKETS
HASKELL
HOSKINS
HUSKERS
HUSKIER
HUSKIES
HUSKILY
HUSKING
MASKERS
MASKING
MISKEYS
MISKNEW
MISKNOW
MISKOLC
MUSKEGO
MUSKETS
MUSKIER
MUSKIES
MUSKRAT
PESKIER
PESKILY
RISKERS
RISKIER
RISKILY
RISKING
RISKSIT
TASKBAR
TASKING
TUSKERS
TUSKING
UNSKEWS
VOSKHOD
WESKITS

••S•K••

AKSAKOV
BISHKEK
ITSOKAY
KISHKES
MESSKIT
PASSKEY
PUSHKIN
TESTKIT

••S••K•

ASSLIKE
ATSTAKE
BESPOKE
DASHIKI
DISLIKE
LYSENKO
MISLIKE
MISTAKE
MUSICKS
RESEEKS
RESINKS
RESOAKS
RESPOKE
RESTOKE
UNSMOKY
UNSNAKY
UNSPOKE
UNSULKY

••S•••K

BESPEAK
BISHKEK
CASSOCK
COSSACK
DESTOCK
DRSPOCK
FOSDICK
GASLEAK
GASMASK
GASTANK
GOSHAWK
HASSOCK
INSHOCK
INSTOCK
MASARYK
MESSICK
MISMARK
MISTOOK
MRSPOCK
NESQUIK
QBSNEAK
RESPARK
RESPEAK
RESTACK
RESTICK
RESTOCK
ROSTOCK
TUSSOCK
UNSLACK
UNSLEEK
UNSLICK
UNSPEAK
UNSTACK
UNSTICK
UNSTUCK
URSULAK
YASBECK
YASHMAK

•••SK••

ALASKAN
ALASKAS
BRISKED

BRISKER
BRISKET
BRISKLY
COWSKIN
DOESKIN
EELSKIN
FRISKED
FRISKER
JETSKIS
KIDSKIN
KRESKIN
MESSKIT
MINSKYS
NONSKED
NONSKID
OILSKIN
OUTSKIP
PASSKEY
PIGSKIN
REASKED
REDSKIN
UNASKED
WHISKAS
WHISKED
WHISKER
WHISKEY

•••S•K•

FORSAKE
NETSUKE
SPASSKY

•••S••K

AIRSICK
AIRSOCK
BERSERK
BTFSPLK
CASSOCK
COSSACK
FORSOOK
GEMSBOK
GYMSOCK
HASSOCK
KAISHEK
MESSICK
ODDSOCK
ONESOCK
OUTSEEK
OUTSULK
PRESOAK
RANSACK
RAWSILK
SADSACK
SEASICK
SZYSLAK
THESACK
TULSAOK
TUSSOCK

••••SK•

ARENSKY
BLUESKY
BREWSKI
BRODSKY
CHOMSKY
DAMASKS
DEEPSKY
EMMUSKA
MINISKI
MONOSKI
OUTASKS
PARASKI
PULASKI
SNOWSKI
SPASSKY
STARSKY
TROTSKY
TSKTSKS
TURFSKI
UNCASKS
UNHUSKS
UNMASKS
UNRISKY
VRONSKY
ZAKUSKA

••••S•K

FEELSOK
JIRASEK
THATSOK

•••••SK

DONETSK
DONTASK
EYEMASK
GASMASK
IRKUTSK
LITOVSK
LOWRISK
MOLLUSK
OAKCASK
OAKDESK
OBELISK
OKHOTSK
PREDUSK
SERIESK
SKIMASK
SUBTASK
THEMASK
VITEBSK
YAKUTSK
ZIPDISK

SL•••••

SLABBED
SLACKED
SLACKEN
SLACKER
SLACKLY
SLACKUP
SLAKERS
SLAKING
SLALOMS
SLAMMED
SLAMMER
SLAMSON
SLANDER
SLANTED
SLANTLY
SLANTUP
SLAPPED
SLAPPER
SLAPSON
SLASHED
SLASHER
SLASHES
SLATERS
SLATHER
SLATIER
SLATING
SLATKIN
SLATTED
SLAVERS
SLAVERY
SLAVING
SLAVISH
SLAYERS
SLAYING
SLAYTON
SLEAZES
SLEDDED
SLEDDER
SLEDDOG
SLEDFUL
SLEDGED
SLEDGES
SLEEKED
SLEEKEN
SLEEKER
SLEEKLY
SLEEPER
SLEEPIN
SLEEPON
SLEETED
SLEEVED
SLEEVES
SLEIGHS
SLEIGHT
SLENDER
SLEPTIN
SLEPTON
SLEUTHS
SLEWING
SLICERS
SLICEUP
SLICING
SLICKED
SLICKER
SLICKLY
SLIDEBY
SLIDEIN
SLIDERS
SLIDING
SLIDOFF
SLIDOUT
SLIGHTS
SLIMIER
SLIMILY
SLIMING
SLIMJIM
SLIMMED
SLIMMER
SLINGER
SLINKED
SLINKER
SLINKIN
SLINKUP
SLIPOFF
SLIPONS
SLIPOUT
SLIPPED
SLIPPER
SLIPSBY
SLIPSIN
SLIPSON
SLIPSUP
SLIPUPS
SLITHER
SLITTED
SLITTER
SLIVERS
SLOBBER
SLOEGIN
SLOGANS
SLOGGED
SLOGGER
SLOPERS
SLOPING
SLOPPED
SLOPSON
SLOSHED
SLOSHES
SLOTCAR
SLOTTED
SLOTTER
SLOUCHY
SLOUGHS
SLOVAKS
SLOVENE
SLOVENS
SLOWDAY
SLOWEST
SLOWING
SLOWISH
SLOWSUP
SLOWUPS
SLUDGES
SLUGGED
SLUGGER
SLUICED
SLUICES
SLUMBER
SLUMMED
SLUMMER
SLUMPED
SLUNKIN
SLUNKUP
SLURPED
SLURPEE
SLURPER
SLURRED
SLUSHED
SLUSHES
SLYLOOK
SLYNESS

S•L••••

SALAAMS
SALABLE
SALADES
SALADIN
SALAMIS
SALAZAR
SALCHOW
SALEMOR
SALERNO
SALIENT
SALIERI
SALINAS
SALINES
SALIVAS
SALLIED
SALLIER
SALLIES
SALMONP
SALMONS
SALOMON
SALONGA
SALOONS
SALSODA
SALTANT
SALTBOX
SALTERS
SALTIER
SALTILY
SALTINE
SALTING
SALTISH
SALTPIT
SALTSEA
SALUKIS
SALUTED
SALUTER
SALUTES
SALVAGE
SALVERS
SALVING
SALVOES
SALVORS
SCLAFFS
SCLERAE
SCLERAL
SCLERAS
SELECTS
SELENIC
SELFISH
SELKIRK
SELLECK
SELLERS
SELLFOR
SELLING
SELLOFF
SELLOUT
SELLSIT
SELLSTO
SELMAAL
SELTZER
SELVAGE
SHLOCKY
SILENCE
SILENTA
SILENTB
SILENTC
SILENTD
SILENTE
SILENTF
SILENTG
SILENTH
SILENTI
SILENTJ
SILENTK
SILENTL
SILENTM
SILENTN
SILENTO
SILENTP
SILENTQ
SILENTR
SILENTS
SILENTT
SILENTU
SILENTV
SILENTW
SILENTX
SILENTY
SILENTZ
SILESIA
SILICAS
SILICON
SILKHAT
SILKIER
SILKILY
SILKTIE
SILLIER
SILLIES
SILLYME
SILOING
SILTIER
SILTING
SILVERS
SILVERY
SOLACED
SOLACER
SOLACES
SOLARAS
SOLARIA
SOLDERS
SOLDFOR
SOLDIER
SOLDOFF
SOLDOUT
SOLEDAD
SOLFEGE
SOLICIT
SOLIDER
SOLIDLY
SOLLATI
SOLNESS
SOLOACT
SOLOING
SOLOIST
SOLOMON
SOLUBLE
SOLUTES
SOLVEIT
SOLVENT
SOLVERS
SOLVING
SPLASHY
SPLAYED
SPLEENS
SPLEENY
SPLENDA
SPLICED
SPLICER
SPLICES
SPLINES
SPLINTS
SPLITUP
SPLOTCH
SPLURGE
STLOUIS
STLUCIA
STLUKES
SULFATE
SULFIDE
SULFITE
SULKERS
SULKIER
SULKIES
SULKILY
SULKING
SULLIED
SULLIES
SULPHUR
SULTANA
SULTANS
SULUSEA
SYLLABI
SYLPHIC

S••L•••

SACLIKE
SAILERS
SAILING
SAILORS
SAILSON
SAILSTO
SALLIED
SALLIER
SALLIES
SAMLETS
SAMLOYD
SAPLESS
SAPLING
SAWLIKE
SAWLOGS
SCALAGE
SCALARS
SCALDED
SCALDER
SCALENE
SCALERS
SCALEUP
SCALIER
SCALING
SCALLOP
SCALPED
SCALPEL
SCALPER
SCHLEPP
SCHLEPS
SCHLITZ
SCHLOCK
SCHLUBS
SCHLUMP
SCOLARI
SCOLDED
SCOLDER
SCULLED
SCULLER
SCULPED
SCULPTS
SEALABS
SEALANE
SEALANT
SEALEGS
SEALERS
SEALERY
SEALIFE
SEALIFT
SEALIKE
SEALILY
SEALING
SEALION
SEALOFF
SEALSIN
SEALSUP
SECLUDE
SELLECK
SELLERS
SELLFOR
SELLING
SELLOFF
SELLOUT
SELLSIT
SELLSTO
SERLING
SEXLESS
SHALALA
SHALIER
SHALLOT
SHALLOW
SHALLWE
SHALOMS
SHELDON
SHELLAC
SHELLED
SHELLER
SHELLEY
SHELTER
SHELTIE
SHELVED
SHELVER
SHELVES
SHILLED
SHULMAN
SHYLOCK
SIBLING
SIDLING
SILLIER
SILLIES
SILLYME
SINLESS
SINLIKE
SIRLOIN
SIXLANE
SKELTER
SKELTON
SKILFUL
SKILIFT
SKILLED
SKILLET
SKULKED
SKULKER
SKULLED
SKYLARK
SKYLESS
SKYLIKE
SKYLINE
SLALOMS
SLYLOOK
SMALLAD
SMALLER
SMALLOJ
SMELLED
SMELLER
SMELTED
SMELTER
SMILEAT
SMILEON
SMILERS
SMILEYS
SMILING
SMILLAS
SMOLDER
SNELLEN
SODLESS
SOILAGE
SOILING
SOLLATI
SONLESS
SONLIKE
SOULFUL
SOULMAN
SOWLIKE
SOYLENT
SPELLED
SPELLER
SPELUNK
SPILLED
SPILLER
STALAGS
STALELY
STALEST
STALKED
STALKER
STALLED
STALLER
STCLOUD
STELIAS
STELLAR
STILLED
STILLER
STILLUP
STILTED
STILTON
STOLEIN
STOLLEN
STOLONS
STYLERS
STYLETS
STYLING
STYLISE
STYLISH
STYLIST
STYLIZE
SUBLETS
SUBLIDS
SUBLIME
SUBLONG
SUBLOTS
SUELLEN
SUELYON
SULLIED
SULLIES
SUMLESS
SUNLAMP
SUNLESS
SUNLIKE
SURLIER
SURLILY
SVELTER
SWALLOW
SWELLED
SWELLER
SWELLUP
SWELTER
SWELTRY
SWILLED
SWILLER
SWOLLEN
SYLLABI
SZILARD

S•••L••

SADDLED
SADDLER
SADDLES
SAMPLED
SAMPLER
SAMPLES
SANBLAS
SANDLER
SANDLOT
SARALEE
SAVALAS
SCALLOP
SCARLET
SCHELDT
SCHOLAR
SCHOLES
SCHULTZ
SCOWLED
SCOWLER
SCROLLS
SCULLED
SCULLER
SEABLUE
SEASLUG
SECULAR
SEDALIA
SEEALSO
SEEDLET
SEMILOG
SEPALED
SETPLAY
SETTLED
SETTLER
SETTLES
SETTLOR
SEVILLA
SEVILLE
SHALLOT
SHALLOW
SHALLWE
SHAWLED
SHEILAE
SHEILAS
SHELLAC
SHELLED
SHELLER
SHELLEY
SHIELDS
SHILLED
SHIRLEY
SHOALED
SHOULDA
SHOULDI
SHRILLS
SHRILLY
SIBYLIC
SICILIA
SICKLES
SIMILAC
SIMILAR
SIMILES
SIMPLER
SIMPLES
SIMPLEX
SINGLED
SINGLES
SINGLET
SIZZLED
SIZZLER
SIZZLES
SKIDLID
SKILLED
SKILLET
SKIRLED
SKULLED
SKYBLUE
SMALLAD
SMALLER
SMALLOJ
SMELLED
SMELLER
SMILLAS
SNARLAT
SNARLED
SNARLER
SNARLUP
SNELLEN
SNIGLET
SNUGLIS
SOMALIA
SOMALIS
SPELLED
SPELLER
SPIELED
SPIELER
SPILLED
SPILLER
SPOILED
SPOILER
SPOOLED
SPOOLER
SPOTLIT
SQUALID
SQUALLS
SQUALLY
SQUALOR
SQUELCH
STABLED
STABLER
STABLES
STADLER
STALLED
STALLER
STANLEE
STANLEY
STAPLED
STAPLER
STAPLES
STARLET
STARLIT
STARLOG
STATLER
STEALER
STEALIN
STEALTH
STEELED
STEELER
STEELIE
STELLAR
STIFLED
STIFLES
STILLED
STILLER
STILLUP
STOLLEN
STOOLED
STOOLIE
STROLLS
SUBCLAN
SUBPLOT
SUBTLER
SUELLEN
SUNGLOW
SUPPLED
SUPPLER
SUPPLES
SURPLUS
SWALLOW
SWELLED
SWELLER
SWELLUP
SWILLED
SWILLER
SWIRLED
SWOLLEN
SZYSLAK

S••••L•

SAINTLO
SAINTLY
SALABLE
SALTILY
SAMEOLD
SAMHILL
SAMUELL
SANDALS
SANDFLY
SAPPILY
SASSILY
SATWELL
SAUCILY
SAVABLE
SAVVILY
SAWMILL
SAYABLE
SCANTLY
SCAPULA
SCARILY
SCHOOLS
SCRAWLS
SCRAWLY
SCROLLS
SCRUPLE
SCUFFLE
SCUTTLE
SEACALM
SEAEELS
SEAGULL
SEALILY
SEAMILE
SEASALT
SEATTLE
SEAWALL
SEAWOLF
SECKELS
SEEABLE
SEEDILY
SEENALL
SEESALL
SEQUELS
SERIALS
SERVILE
SESSILE
SEVILLA
SEVILLE
SHACKLE
SHADILY
SHAKILY
SHALALA
SHAMBLE
SHAPELY
SHARPLY
SHEERLY
SHEKELS
SHEWOLF
SHINGLE
SHINGLY
SHINILY
SHINOLA
SHOOFLY
SHORTLY
SHOVELS
SHOWILY
SHRILLS
SHRILLY
SHTETLS
SHUFFLE
SHUTTLE
SIGHTLY
SIGNALS
SILKILY
SITWELL
SIXBALL
SIXFOLD
SIXTHLY
SIZABLE
SIZABLY
SKIABLE
SKIFFLE
SKIPOLE
SKITTLE
SKYWALK
SLACKLY
SLANTLY
SLEEKLY
SLICKLY
SLIMILY
SMARTLY
SMOKILY
SMUGGLE
SNAKILY
SNAPPLE
SNIDELY
SNIFFLE
SNIFFLY
SNIVELS
SNOBALL
SNOWILY
SNUFFLE
SNUGGLE
SNUGGLY
SOAPILY
SOBERLY
SOCIALS
SOGGILY
SOLIDLY
SOLUBLE
SOOTILY

SORRELL
SORRELS
SORRILY
SOUFFLE
SOUNDLY
SOURALE
SOYMILK
SPACELY
SPACKLE
SPANGLE
SPANGLY
SPARELY
SPARKLE
SPARKLY
SPATULA
SPECKLE
SPICILY
SPIKILY
SPINDLE
SPINDLY
SPINELS
SPIRALS
SPITTLE
SPRAWLS
SPRAWLY
SPYHOLE
SQUALLS
SQUALLY
SQUATLY
SQUEALS
STABILE
STAGILY
STAIDLY
STALELY
STARKLY
STARTLE
STATELY
STEEPLE
STEEPLY
STERILE
STERNLY
STEROLS
STIFFLY
STIMULI
STIPPLE
STOKELY
STONILY
STOPPLE
STOUTLY
STPAULS
STROLLS
STUBBLE
STUBBLY
STUMBLE
SUAVELY
SUBCELL
SUBFILE
SUBHALL
SUFFOLK
SULKILY
SUNBELT
SUNNILY
SURLILY
SWADDLE
SWAHILI
SWEETLY
SWIFTLY
SWINDLE
SWIVELS
SWIZZLE
SYMBOLS
SYSTOLE

S•••••L

SACKFUL
SAMHILL
SAMUELL
SANIBEL
SATCHEL
SATWELL
SAWMILL
SCALPEL
SCANDAL
SCLERAL
SEAFOWL
SEAGULL
SEAWALL
SEENALL
SEESALL
SEISMAL
SELMAAL
SEMINAL
SENEGAL
SENSUAL
SETBAIL
SETSAIL
SEVERAL
SHIPFUL
SHOPFUL
SHRIVEL
SIGHFUL
SILENTL
SITWELL
SIXBALL
SKILFUL
SLEDFUL
SMEAGOL
SNOBALL
SNORKEL
SOFTGEL
SONGFUL
SORORAL
SORRELL
SOULFUL
SOYMEAL
SPACIAL
SPANIEL
SPATIAL
SPECIAL
SPHERAL
SPIEGEL
SPOUSAL
STBASIL
STEMPEL
STENCIL
STENGEL
STERNAL
STIFFEL
STOICAL
STRUDEL
SUBCELL
SUBCOOL
SUBDUAL
SUBGOAL
SUBHALL
SUBSOIL
SUNBOWL
SUNDIAL
SURREAL
SURVEIL
SYNFUEL
SYNODAL

•SL••••

ASLEWOF
CSLEWIS
ISLAMIC
ISLANDS
ISLETED

•S•L•••

ASALARK
ASHLAND
ASHLARS
ASHLESS
ASSLIKE
ASYLUMS
ISOLATE
ISOLATO
ISOLINE
OSTLERS
PSALMIC
PSALTER
TSELIOT
USELESS
USFLAGS

•S••L••

ASTOLAT
ESCALOP
ESCALUS
ESTELLA
ESTELLE
OSCULAR
OSCULES
USABLES
USUALLY

•S•••L•

ASARULE
ASPHALT
ASSAILS
ASSAULT
ESCUELA
ESPIALS
ESTELLA
ESTELLE
ISOHELS
ISRAELI
OSCEOLA
OSSICLE
OSTWALD
USUALLY

•S••••L

ASEXUAL
ASOCIAL
ASPRAWL
ASUSUAL
BSCHOOL
ESPANOL
ESTIVAL
ESTORIL
ISCHIAL
ISHMAEL
ISRAFEL
QSCHOOL
USSTEEL

••SL•••

ASSLIKE
AUSLESE
BUSLANE
BUSLINE
BUSLOAD
DESLUMS
DISLIKE
DRSLOAN
ENSLAVE
GASLAMP
GASLEAK
GASLESS
GASLINE
GASLOGS
GOSLING
ITSLATE
ITSLOVE
KISLEVS
MISLAID
MISLAYS
MISLEAD
MISLIKE
MOSLEMS
MRSLATE
MUSLIMS
MUSLINS
RESLATE
UNSLACK
UNSLAIN
UNSLEEK
UNSLICK
UNSLIER
UNSLING
UNSLUNG
UNSLYER
UNSLYLY
UPSLOPE
WASLATE
YESLETS

••S•L••

ABSALOM
ABSOLUT
ABSOLVE
ANSELMO
BASALLY
BASALTS
BASILIC
BASILIO
BUSTLED
BUSTLER
BUSTLES
CASELAW
CASELLA
CASELOT
CASTLED
CASTLES
CUSSLER
DASILVA
DESALTS
DESILTS
DESYLVA
DISPLAY
EASELED
ENSILED
ENSILES
EPSILON
FUSILLI
GISELLE
HASSLED
HASSLES
HOSTLER
HUSTLED
HUSTLER
HUSTLES
INSALES
INSOLES
INSULAR
INSULIN
INSULTS
ITSALIE
ITSALOT
JOSTLED
JOSTLER
JOSTLES
KASTLER
LASALLE
LASTLAP
LASTLEG
MISALLY
MISPLAN
MISPLAY
MOSELLE
MUSCLED
MUSCLES
NASALLY
NESTLED
NESTLER
NESTLES
PASALLE
PESTLED
PESTLES
POSOLES
POSSLQS
RASSLED
RASSLER
RASSLES
RESALES
RESALTS
RESELLS
RESILED
RESILES
RESOLED
RESOLER
RESOLES
RESOLVE
RESPLIT
RESULTS
ROSALIA
ROSALIE
ROSALYN
ROSELLA
ROSELLE
RUSSLAN
RUSTLED
RUSTLER
RUSTLES
TASHLIN
TESTLAB
TUSSLED
TUSSLES
UNSALTY
UNSELLS
UNSILLY
UNSOLED
UNSOLES
UNSOLID
UNSPLIT
UNSULKY
UPSILON
URSULAK
VISALIA

••S••L•

AMSTELS
ARSHILE
ASSAILS
ASSAULT
AUSABLE
BASALLY
BASSALE
BESSELL
BESTILL
BISSELL
BOSSILY
BOSWELL
BUSHELS
BUSHILY
CASELLA
CASSOLA
CASTILE
CASUALS
CUSHILY
DASCHLE
DESHELL
DISABLE
DISMALS
DISPELS
DISTILL
DISTILS
DOSSALS
DUSKILY
DUSTILY
ENSEALS
ENSOULS
FISHILY
FISSILE
FOSCOLO
FOSSILS
FUSIBLE
FUSILLI
FUSSILY
FUSTILY
GASKELL
GESTALT
GISELLE
GOSPELS
GOSTALE
GUSHILY
GUSTILY
HASKELL
HASPULL
HASTILY
HOSCALE
HOSTELS
HOSTILE
HUSKILY
IMSWELL
INSCALE
INSTALL
INSTALS
INSTILL
INSTILS
INSTYLE
ITSCOLD
KISSELS
LASALLE
LASCALA
LOSABLE
LUSTILY
MESCALS
MESSALA
MESSILY
MISALLY
MISBILL
MISCALL
MISERLY
MISFILE
MISKOLC
MISRELY
MISRULE
MISSALS
MISSILE
MISTELL
MISTILY
MISTOLD
MOSELLE
MUSHILY
MUSSELS
MUSSILY
MUSTILY
NASALLY
NASTILY
OSSICLE
PASALLE
PASCOLI
PASSELS
PASTELS
PESKILY
PISTILS
PISTOLE
PISTOLS
POSABLE
PUSHILY
RASCALS
RESCALE
RESEALS
RESELLS
RESMELT
RESOILS
RESPELL
RESPELT
RESTYLE
RISIBLE
RISIBLY
RISKILY
RISSOLE
ROSELLA
ROSELLE
ROSEOLA
ROSWELL
RUSSELL
RUSTILY
SASSILY
SESSILE
SYSTOLE
TASSELS
TASTILY
TESTFLY
TESTILY
TOSCALE
UNSADLY
UNSCALY
UNSEALS
UNSELLS
UNSHELL
UNSHYLY
UNSILLY
UNSLYLY
UNSPELT
UNSPILT
UNSURLY
UPSCALE
UPSWELL
VASSALS
VESICLE
VESSELS
VESTALS
VISIBLE
VISIBLY
VISTULA
VISUALS
WASPILY
WASSILY
WISPILY
ZESTILY

••S•••L

ARSENAL
AUSTRAL
BASHFUL
BASINAL
BESSELL
BESTIAL
BESTILL
BISSELL
BOSWELL
BUSGIRL
CASTROL
DESHELL
DESKFUL
DESPOIL
DESTAEL
DISHFUL
DISTILL
EASEFUL
ENSNARL
FASCIAL
FISHOIL
FISTFUL
GASKELL
GASOHOL
HASKELL
HASPULL
HUSHFUL
HUSSERL
IMSWELL
INSTALL
INSTILL
KESTREL
LESPAUL
LESTOIL
LUSTFUL
LUSTRAL
MISBILL
MISCALL
MISDEAL
MISDIAL
MISTELL
MISTRAL
MRSPAUL
MRSPEEL
MUSEFUL
MUSICAL
NESTFUL
NOSTRIL
PASCHAL
PASSEUL
PUSHFUL
RESPELL
RESPOOL
RESTFUL
ROSEOIL
ROSTRAL
ROSWELL
RUSSELL
UNSHELL
UNSNARL
UNSPOOL
UNSTEEL
UPSWELL
USSTEEL
VESTRAL
WASSAIL
WASTREL
WISHFUL
WISTFUL
ZESTFUL

•••SL••

AMESLAN
BEASLEY
BOBSLED
BOOSLER
BRESLIN
COWSLIP
CUSSLER
DOGSLED
ENISLED
ENISLES
FANSLER
FOCSLES
GRISLET
HASSLED
HASSLES
HEMSLEY
HENSLEY
HORSLEY
KEESLAR
KEESLER
KTOSLIN
LAYSLOW
LETSLIP
LIESLOW
MEASLES
MUESLIS
MUESLIX
NONSLIP
OHMSLAW
PAISLEY
PARSLEY
PAYSLIP
POSSLQS
PRESLEY
PUGSLEY
RASSLED
RASSLER
RASSLES
RUNSLOW
RUSSLAN
SEASLUG
SZYSLAK
TOOSLOW
TOUSLED
TOUSLES
TOYSLED
TUSSLED
TUSSLES
VIZSLAS
WINSLET
WINSLOW
WORSLEY

•••S•L•

ADDSALT
AHASSLE
APISHLY
APOSTLE
ARTSALE
BASSALE
BEASTLY
BESSELL
BIASPLY
BIGSALE
BISSELL
BOSSILY
BRASHLY
BRISKLY
BRISTLE
BRISTLY
BTFSPLK
CAPSULE
CARSALE
CASSOLA
CHISELS
CLOSELY
CONSOLE
CONSULS
CONSULT
CRASSLY
CRISPLY
CROSSLY
DAMSELS
DELSOLS
DENSELY
DIESELS
DORSALS
DOSSALS
EPISTLE
EROSELY
FAISALI
FALSELY
FIRSTLY
FISSILE
FLESHLY
FLYSOLO
FORSALE
FOSSILS
FRESHLY
FUSSILY
GETSOLD
GHASTLY
GHOSTLY
GRASSLE
GRISTLE
GRISTLY
GROSSLY
GUNSELS
GUTSILY
HANSOLO
HARSHLY
HERSELF
HIMSELF
HORSILY
KISSELS
KRYSTLE
LETSFLY
LOOSELY
LOUSILY
MARSALA
MESSALA
MESSILY
MIDSOLE
MISSALS
MISSILE
MOISTLY
MORSELS
MOUSILY
MUSSELS
MUSSILY
NOISILY
NONSALE
NONSELF
OBESELY
OLDSALT
ONESELF
OURSELF
OUTSELL
OUTSOLD
OUTSOLE
OUTSULK
PASSELS
PIESALE
PLUSHLY
PRESALE
PRESALT
PRESELL
PRESOLD
PROSILY
RAWSILK
RISSOLE
RUSSELL
SASSILY
SEASALT
SEESALL
SESSILE
TAGSALE
TARSALS
TASSELS
TAXSALE
TEASELS
TENSELY
TENSILE
TERSELY
THESELF
THISTLE
THISTLY
THYSELF
TINSELS
TIPSILY
TONSILS
TRESTLE
UPPSALA
VASSALS
VESSELS
WASSILY
WEASELS
WHISTLE
WRESTLE

•••S••L

ABYSMAL
ABYSSAL
ASUSUAL
BESSELL
BISSELL
BORSTAL
BRISTOL
CHASMAL
COASTAL
CRUSTAL
CRYSTAL
DAYSAIL
FRESNEL
FURSEAL
GLOSSAL
HUSSERL
LUGSAIL
MARSHAL
MIASMAL
OUTSAIL
OUTSELL
PASSEUL
PINSEAL
PRESEAL
PRESELL
PRESSEL
RUSSELL
SEESALL
SEISMAL
SENSUAL
SETSAIL
SUBSOIL
TOPSAIL
TOPSOIL
TRYSAIL
UNUSUAL
WASSAIL

••••SL•

AHASSLE
BOGUSLY
CRASSLY
CROSSLY
GRASSLE
GROSSLY
LEXUSLS
LEXUSLX
PIOUSLY

••••S•L

ABYSSAL
ACCUSAL
AEROSOL
ANBESOL
AROUSAL
CLAUSAL
COUNSEL
CREOSOL
DAMOSEL
DEPOSAL
EXCUSAL
GELUSIL
GIRASOL
GLOSSAL
HANDSEL
PARASOL
PERUSAL
PHRASAL
PINESOL
PRESSEL
RECUSAL
REFUSAL
REVISAL
SPOUSAL
STBASIL
UNNASAL
UTENSIL

SM•••••

SMACKED
SMACKER
SMACKOF
SMACKUP
SMALLAD
SMALLER
SMALLOJ
SMARTED
SMARTEN
SMARTER
SMARTLY
SMASHED
SMASHER
SMASHES
SMASHUP
SMATTER
SMEAGOL
SMEARED
SMEARER
SMEARON
SMELLED
SMELLER
SMELTED
SMELTER
SMETANA
SMIDGEN
SMIDGES
SMILEAT
SMILEON
SMILERS
SMILEYS
SMILING
SMILLAS
SMIRKED
SMIRKER
SMIRNOV
SMITERS
SMITHED
SMITING
SMITTEN
SMOKERS
SMOKEUP
SMOKEYS
SMOKIER

SMOKIES
SMOKILY
SMOKING
SMOLDER
SMOOTHS
SMOOTHY
SMOTHER
SMUCKER
SMUDGED
SMUDGES
SMUGGER
SMUGGLE
SMUSHED
SMUSHES

S•M••••

SAMARAS
SAMARIA
SAMBAED
SAMBASS
SAMBORA
SAMBUCA
SAMEDAY
SAMEDIS
SAMEKHS
SAMEOLD
SAMHILL
SAMHUFF
SAMISEN
SAMLETS
SAMLOYD
SAMMYJO
SAMNUNN
SAMOANS
SAMOSAS
SAMOSET
SAMOVAR
SAMOYED
SAMPANS
SAMPLED
SAMPLER
SAMPLES
SAMPRAS
SAMPSON
SAMSONS
SAMSUNG
SAMUELL
SAMURAI
SAMWISE
SEMANAS
SEMIDRY
SEMILOG
SEMINAL
SEMINAR
SEMIPRO
SEMIRAW
SEMITES
SEMITIC
SIMCITY
SIMENON
SIMIANS
SIMILAC
SIMILAR
SIMILES
SIMMERS
SIMMONS
SIMONIZ
SIMPERS
SIMPLER
SIMPLES
SIMPLEX
SIMPSON
SOMALIA
SOMALIS
SOMATIC
SOMEDAY
SOMEHOW
SOMEONE
SOMESAY
SOMEWAY
SOMINEX
STMARKS
STMARYS
SUMATRA
SUMITUP
SUMLESS
SUMMAND
SUMMARY
SUMMATE
SUMMERS
SUMMERY
SUMMING
SUMMITS
SUMMONS
SUMOIST
SUMUPTO
SYMBOLS
SYMPTOM

S••M•••

SALMONP
SALMONS
SAMMYJO
SAWMILL
SAYMASS
SAYMORE
SCAMMED
SCAMMER
SCAMPED
SCAMPER
SCHMEAR
SCHMEER
SCHMIDT
SCHMITT
SCHMOES
SEAMAPS
SEAMERS
SEAMIER
SEAMILE
SEAMING
SEAMIST
SEAMOSS
SEEMING
SEEMSTO
SEGMENT
SELMAAL
SERMONS
SEYMOUR
SHAMANS
SHAMBLE
SHAMING
SHAMMED
SHAMPOO
SHIMMER
SIAMESE
SIEMENS
SIGMOID
SIGMUND
SIMMERS
SIMMONS
SKIMASK
SKIMMED
SKIMMER
SKIMPED
SKIMPON
SKYMAPS
SLAMMED
SLAMMER
SLAMSON
SLIMIER
SLIMILY
SLIMING
SLIMJIM
SLIMMED
SLIMMER
SLUMBER
SLUMMED
SLUMMER
SLUMPED
SOYMEAL
SOYMILK
SPAMBOT
SPAMMED
SPAMMER
SPUMIER
SPUMING
SPUMONE
SPUMONI
STAMENS
STAMINA
STAMMER
STAMPED
STAMPER
STEMMED
STEMPEL
STIMSON
STIMULI
STOMACH
STOMATA
STOMPED
STOMPIN
STOMPON
STUMBLE
STUMPED
STUMPER
STYMIED
STYMIES
SUBMITS
SUMMAND
SUMMARY
SUMMATE
SUMMERS
SUMMERY
SUMMING
SUMMITS
SUMMONS
SUNMAID
SURMISE
SWAMPED
SWIMMER
SWIMSUP

S•••M••

SALAMIS
SALEMOR
SALOMON
SANDMAN
SANDMEN
SARUMAN
SAYAMEN
SCAMMED
SCAMMER
SCATMAN
SCHEMAS
SCHEMED
SCHEMER
SCHEMES
SCHUMER
SCRIMPS
SCRIMPY
SEISMAL
SEISMIC
SESAMES
SHAMMED
SHERMAN
SHIMMER
SHIPMAN
SHIPMEN
SHOWMAN
SHOWMEN
SHRIMPS
SHRIMPY
SHULMAN
SIDEMAN
SIDEMEN
SITEMAP
SKIMMED
SKIMMER
SLAMMED
SLAMMER
SLIMMED
SLIMMER
SLUMMED
SLUMMER
SNOWMAN
SNOWMEN
SOLOMON
SOULMAN
SOUPMIX
SPAMMED
SPAMMER
STAMMER
STARMAN
STARMAP
STEAMED
STEAMER
STEAMUP
STEMMED
STEPMOM
STIGMAS
STJAMES
STORMED
STORMIN
STSIMON
SURFMAN
SURFMEN
SURIMIS
SWAGMAN
SWAGMEN
SWARMED
SWARMER
SWIMMER
SYNGMAN

S••••M•

SACHEMS
SALAAMS
SANREMO
SAOTOME
SASHIMI
SATCHMO
SATCOMS
SATHOME
SATSUMA
SCHISMS
SCHLUMP
SCREAMS
SCUSEME
SEAARMS
SHALOMS
SILLYME
SITCOMS
SITHOME
SKIBUMS
SKIJUMP
SKYCAMS
SKYDOME
SLALOMS
SOSUEME
SPAREME
SPYCAMS
SQUIRMS
SQUIRMY
STREAMS
SUBLIME
SUBSUME
SUCCUMB
SUITSME
SUNLAMP
SUPREME
SURNAME
SYSTEMS

S•••••M

SANCTUM
SARCASM
SEACALM
SEAFOAM
SEAGRAM
SERFDOM
SEVENAM
SEVENPM
SHAHDOM
SHYFROM
SIDEARM
SIKHISM
SILENTM
SLIMJIM
SOPHISM
SORGHUM
STADIUM
STANNUM
STARDOM
STATISM
STEINEM
STEPMOM
STERNUM
STICKUM
STRATUM
SUBFORM
SUBITEM
SUNBEAM
SUNROOM
SUREIAM
SURINAM
SYMPTOM
SYNONYM

•SM••••

ASMARAN
OSMATIC
OSMONDS
OSMOSED
OSMOSES
OSMOSIS
OSMOTIC
OSMUNDS

•S•M•••

ASIMMER
ISHMAEL
ISOMERS
OSTMARK

•S••M••

ASHAMED
ASIMMER
ASSUMED
ASSUMER
ASSUMES
ASTHMAS
ESKIMOS
ESTAMIN
ISLAMIC
ISTHMUS
ISTOMIN
PSALMIC

•S•••M•

ASHRAMS
ASYLUMS
ESTEEMS
ISONOMY
TSUNAMI

•S••••M

ASATEAM
ASTREAM
ISCHIUM
ISOGRAM
ISUREAM
TSARDOM
TSARISM

••SM•••

ALSMITH
BASMATI
BESMEAR
BISMUTH
BUSMANS
DESMOGS
DESMOND
DISMALS
DISMAST
DISMAYS
DISMISS
GASMAIN
GASMASK
JASMINE
KISMETS
MISMARK
MISMATE
MISMESH
MISMOVE
MRSMITH
MRSMUIR
NESMITH
PISMIRE
RESMELT
UNSMART
UNSMOKY
YASMINE
YESMAAM

••S•M••

AJSIMON
ASSUMED
ASSUMER
ASSUMES
BASEMAN
BASEMEN
BESTMAN
BESTMEN
BOSOMED
BOSSMAN
BOSSMEN
BUSHMAN
BUSHMEN
CASIMIR
CESTMOI
DISCMAN
DUSTMAN
DUSTMEN
DUSTMOP
EASTMAN
FUSUMAS
GASSMAN
KASHMIR
LASTMAY
MESAMIS
NESSMAN
POSTMAN
POSTMEN
RESUMED
RESUMES
SESAMES
STSIMON
WISEMAN
WISEMEN
YASHMAK
ZOSIMUS

••S••M•

ANSELMO
BUSCEMI
COSTUME
CUSTOMS
DESLUMS
DESTEMS
DISARMS
GASLAMP
GASPUMP
HASTIME
INSEAMS
ITSONME
ITSTIME
LISSOME
MESEEMS
MISAIMS
MISHIMA
MISNAME
MISTIME
MOSLEMS
MUSEUMS
MUSLIMS
PASTIME
POSSUMS
RESEAMS
RESTAMP
RESWIMS
SASHIMI
SOSUEME
SYSTEMS
UNSEAMS
WISDOMS
ZOSSIMA

••S•••M

ABSALOM
BOSSISM
EASTHAM
FASCISM
HASIDIM
HASROOM
HASSIUM
IRSFORM
LUSTRUM
MISDEEM
MISFORM
MISTERM
NOSEEUM
NOSTRUM
ROSTRUM
YESMAAM

•••SM••

ABYSMAL
ALMSMAN
ALMSMEN
ANOSMIA
ANOSMIC
BATSMAN
BATSMEN
BOSSMAN
BOSSMEN
CHASMAL
CHASMIC
ERASMUS
GASSMAN
GETSMAD
GOESMAD
HEISMAN
HOUSMAN
KINSMAN
KINSMEN
LENSMAN
LENSMEN
MANSMAN
MIASMAL
MIASMAS
MIASMIC
NESSMAN
NEWSMAN
NEWSMEN
OARSMAN
OARSMEN
PLASMAS
PLASMIC
RIESMAN
SEISMAL
SEISMIC
WAKSMAN

•••S•M•

AMUSEME
AWESOME
BALSAMS
BALSAMY
CONSUME
DIDSUMS
FULSOME
GYPSUMS
HADSOME
HANSOMS
IRKSOME
LAKSHMI
LISSOME
NATSUME
NEWSOME
NOISOME
OUTSUMS
POSSUMS
PRESUME
RANSOMS
SATSUMA
SCUSEME
SUBSUME
THESAME
THESIMS
TRUSTME
TWOSOME
UNISOMS
WINSOME
ZOSSIMA

•••S••M

ALYSSUM
BLOSSOM
BOSSISM
ELYSIUM
FRUSTUM
GRESHAM
GRISHAM
GRISSOM
HASSIUM
NAUSEAM
OPOSSUM
OUTSWAM
OUTSWIM
OUTSWUM
POTSDAM
WOOSNAM

••••SM•

BEATSME
CHRISMS
MELISMA
SCHISMS
SUITSME
THEISMS
TRUISMS
TURISMO
VERISMO
WOEISME

••••S•M

ALYSSUM
BLOSSOM
CHRISOM
EMBOSOM
FLOTSAM
GRISSOM
LUMPSUM
OPOSSUM
TIDYSUM
TRANSAM
TRANSOM
UNBOSOM
ZEROSUM

•••••SM

AGONISM
ANIMISM
ATAVISM
ATHEISM
ATOMISM
BAALISM
BAHAISM
BAPTISM
BOSSISM
BRUXISM
COMTISM
CULTISM
CZARISM
DADAISM
DUALISM
ECHOISM
EGOTISM
ELITISM
EXOTISM
FADDISM
FANTASM
FASCISM
FAUVISM
FOGYISM
GRECISM
HEROISM
HOBOISM
IMAGISM
JAINISM
JUDAISM
LAMAISM
LEFTISM
LOOKISM
LUDDISM
MAHDISM
MARXISM
MOBBISM
PIANISM
REALISM
SARCASM
SIKHISM
SOPHISM
STATISM
TITOISM
TORYISM
TOURISM
TROPISM
TSARISM
UTOPISM
YOGIISM
ZANYISM
ZIONISM

SN•••••

SNACKED
SNACKER
SNACKON
SNAFUED
SNAGGED
SNAGGER
SNAGSUP
SNAKERS
SNAKIER
SNAKILY
SNAKING
SNAPONS
SNAPPEA
SNAPPED
SNAPPER
SNAPPLE
SNAPSAT
SNAPSON
SNAPSTO
SNAPSUP
SNARERS
SNARFED
SNARING
SNARLAT
SNARLED
SNARLER
SNARLUP
SNAZZUP
SNEAKBY
SNEAKED
SNEAKER
SNEAKIN
SNEAKUP
SNEERAT
SNEERED
SNEERER
SNEETCH
SNEEZED
SNEEZER
SNEEZES
SNELLEN
SNICKER
SNICKET
SNIDELY
SNIDEST
SNIFFAT
SNIFFED
SNIFFER
SNIFFLE
SNIFFLY
SNIFFUP
SNIFTER
SNIGLET
SNIPEAT
SNIPERS
SNIPING
SNIPOFF
SNIPPED
SNIPPER
SNIPPET
SNIVELS
SNOBALL
SNOCAPS
SNOCATS
SNOCONE
SNOOKER
SNOOPED
SNOOPER
SNOOTED
SNOOZED
SNOOZER
SNOOZES
SNORERS
SNORING
SNORKEL
SNORTAT
SNORTED
SNORTER
SNOUTED
SNOWCAP
SNOWCAT
SNOWDAY
SNOWDON
SNOWHAT
SNOWIER
SNOWILY
SNOWING
SNOWJOB
SNOWMAN
SNOWMEN
SNOWPEA
SNOWSIN
SNOWSKI
SNUBBED
SNUBBER
SNUCKUP
SNUFFED
SNUFFER
SNUFFLE
SNUGFIT
SNUGGED
SNUGGER
SNUGGLE
SNUGGLY
SNUGLIS

S•N••••

SANBLAS
SANBORN
SANCTUM
SANCTUS
SANDALS
SANDBAG
SANDBAR
SANDBOX
SANDBUR
SANDDAB
SANDERS
SANDFLY
SANDHOG
SANDIER
SANDING
SANDLER
SANDLOT
SANDMAN
SANDMEN
SANDPIT
SANFORD
SANGOUT
SANGRIA
SANIBEL
SANJOSE
SANJUAN
SANREMO
SANSEIS
SANTAFE
SANTANA
SANTINI
SENATES
SENATOR
SENDEES
SENDERS
SENDFOR
SENDING
SENDOFF
SENDOUT
SENDSBY
SENDSIN
SENDSON
SENDSTO
SENDSUP
SENDUPS
SENECAN
SENECAS
SENEGAL
SENESCE
SENHORA
SENIORS
SENNETT
SENORAS
SENORES
SENSATE
SENSEIS
SENSENS
SENSING
SENSORS
SENSORY
SENSUAL
SENTFOR
SENTOFF
SENTOUT
SENTRAS
SHNOOKS
SINATRA
SINCERE
SINCITY
SINDBAD
SINEDIE
SINEWED
SINGERS
SINGING
SINGLED
SINGLES
SINGLET
SINGOUT
SINGSTO
SINKAGE
SINKERS
SINKING
SINKSIN
SINLESS
SINLIKE
SINNERS
SINNING
SINUATE
SINUOUS
SINUSES
SINUTAB
SONANCE

SONATAS
SONGFUL
SONLESS
SONLIKE
SONNETS
SONORAN
SONSHIP
SUNBATH
SUNBEAM
SUNBELT
SUNBIRD
SUNBOWL
SUNBOWS
SUNBURN
SUNCITY
SUNDAES
SUNDAYS
SUNDECK
SUNDERS
SUNDIAL
SUNDOGS
SUNDOWN
SUNFANS
SUNFAST
SUNFIRE
SUNFISH
SUNGLOW
SUNGODS
SUNHATS
SUNKIST
SUNLAMP
SUNLESS
SUNLIKE
SUNMAID
SUNNIER
SUNNILY
SUNNING
SUNRAYS
SUNRISE
SUNROOF
SUNROOM
SUNSETS
SUNSFAN
SUNSPOT
SUNSUIT
SUNTANS
SUNWARD
SYNAPSE
SYNCHED
SYNCING
SYNCOPE
SYNDICS
SYNERGY
SYNFUEL
SYNGMAN
SYNODAL
SYNODIC
SYNONYM

S••N•••

SADNESS
SAINTED
SAINTES
SAINTLO
SAINTLY
SAMNUNN
SARNOFF
SAUNAED
SAUNTER
SAWNOFF
SAYNOTO
SCANDAL
SCANNED
SCANNER
SCANTED
SCANTER
SCANTLY
SCENEII
SCENEIV
SCENERY
SCENEVI
SCENICS
SCENTED
SCENTER
SCHNAPS
SCHNOOK
SCHNOZZ
SCONCES
SEANCES
SEENALL
SEENFIT
SEENOFF
SEENOUT
SEINERS
SEINING
SENNETT
SHANANA
SHANGRI
SHANKAR
SHANKED
SHANNEN
SHANNON
SHANTER
SHINDIG
SHINEON
SHINERS
SHINEUP
SHINGLE
SHINGLY
SHINIER
SHINILY
SHINING
SHINNED
SHINOLA
SHINPAD
SHONUFF
SHUNNED
SHUNTED
SHUNTER
SHYNESS
SIENESE
SIENNAS
SIGNAGE
SIGNALS
SIGNEES
SIGNERS
SIGNETS
SIGNFOR
SIGNIFY
SIGNING
SIGNOFF
SIGNORA
SIGNORE
SIGNORS
SIGNOUT
SIGNSIN
SIGNSON
SIGNSUP
SIGNUPS
SINNERS
SINNING
SIXNINE
SKINNED
SKINNER
SKUNKED
SKYNYRD
SLANDER
SLANTED
SLANTLY
SLANTUP
SLENDER
SLINGER
SLINKED
SLINKER
SLINKIN
SLINKUP
SLUNKIN
SLUNKUP
SLYNESS
SOANDSO
SOLNESS
SONNETS
SOONERS
SOONEST
SOUNDED
SOUNDER
SOUNDLY
SPANAIR
SPANDEX
SPANGLE
SPANGLY
SPANIEL
SPANISH
SPANKED
SPANKER
SPANNED
SPANNER
SPENCER
SPENDER
SPENDON
SPENSER
SPENTON
SPINACH
SPINDLE
SPINDLY
SPINDRY
SPINELS
SPINETS
SPINIER
SPINNER
SPINNEY
SPINOFF
SPINOUT
SPINOZA
SPONDEE
SPONGED
SPONGER
SPONGES
SPONSOR
SPUNOFF
SPUNOUT
STANCES
STANDBY
STANDEE
STANDER
STANDIN
STANDON
STANDTO
STANDUP
STANINE
STANKUP
STANLEE
STANLEY
STANNIC
STANNUM
STANTON
STANZAS
STENCIL
STENGEL
STENGUN
STENNIS
STENTOR
STINGER
STINKER
STINKUP
STINTED
STINTER
STONEAX
STONERS
STONIER
STONILY
STONING
STUNGUN
STUNNED
STUNNER
STUNTED
SUBNETS
SUNNIER
SUNNILY
SUNNING
SURNAME
SWANKED
SWANKER
SWANKUP
SWANSEA
SWANSON
SWENSON
SWINDLE
SWINERY
SWINGAT
SWINGBY
SWINGER
SWINGIT
SWINISH
SWINTON
SWUNGAT
SWUNGBY
SWUNGIT

S•••N••

SABINES
SAGINAW
SAIDNAY
SALINAS
SALINES
SALONGA
SARANAC
SARONGS
SATANIC
SATINET
SATINON
SAVANAS
SAVANNA
SAVANTS
SAVINGS
SAWINTO
SAYINGS
SAYSNAY
SCANNED
SCANNER
SCIENCE
SCORNED
SCORNER
SCRUNCH
SECANTS
SECONDI
SECONDO
SECONDR
SECONDS
SEDONAS
SEEINTO
SELENIC
SEMANAS
SEMINAL
SEMINAR
SERENER
SETENTA
SETINTO
SEVENAD
SEVENAM
SEVENBC
SEVENEE
SEVENNO
SEVENPM
SEVENTH
SEVENTY
SEVENUP
SHANNEN
SHANNON
SHATNER
SHAWNEE
SHINNED
SHOPNBC
SHOWNIN
SHOWNUP
SHRINED
SHRINER
SHRINES
SHRINKS
SHUNNED
SIDINGS
SIENNAS
SILENCE
SILENTA
SILENTB
SILENTC
SILENTD
SILENTE
SILENTF
SILENTG
SILENTH
SILENTI
SILENTJ
SILENTK
SILENTL
SILENTM
SILENTN
SILENTO
SILENTP
SILENTQ
SILENTR
SILENTS
SILENTT
SILENTU
SILENTV
SILENTW
SILENTX
SILENTY
SILENTZ
SIMENON
SIMONIZ
SIRENED
SISENOR
SITINON
SITONIT
SKINNED
SKINNER
SMIRNOV
SOAPNET
SOIGNEE
SOMINEX
SONANCE
SORENTO
SOYINKA
SOYINKS
SPANNED
SPANNER
SPAWNED
SPAWNER
SPINNER
SPINNEY
SPLENDA
SPLINES
SPLINTS
SPOONED
SPOONER
SPRINGS
SPRINGY
SPRINTS
SPURNED
SPURNER
SPUTNIK
SPYINGS
SQUANTO
SQUINCH
SQUINTS
SQUINTY
STAGNES
STAINED
STAINER
STANNIC
STANNUM
STAUNCH
STDENIS
STEANNE
STEINEM
STEINER
STENNIS
STERNAL
STERNER
STERNLY
STERNOS
STERNUM
STRANDS
STRANGE
STRINGS
STRINGY
STUNNED
STUNNER
SUBUNIT
SURINAM
SUSANNA
SUSANNE
SUZANNE
SWEENEY
SWOONED
SWOONER
SYNONYM
SYRINGE

S••••N•

SABRINA
SACKING
SADDENS
SADSONG
SAGGING
SAILING
SAISONS
SALERNO
SALIENT
SALMONP
SALMONS
SALOONS
SALTANT
SALTINE
SALTING
SALVING
SAMNUNN
SAMOANS
SAMPANS
SAMSONS
SAMSUNG
SANDING
SANTANA
SANTINI
SAPIENS
SAPIENT
SAPLING
SAPPING
SARDINE
SARGENT
SASHING
SASSING
SATEENS
SATURNS
SAUCING
SAUCONY
SAVANNA
SCALENE
SCALING
SCARING
SCHWANN
SCHWINN
SCOPING
SCORING
SCRAWNY
SCREENS
SEAHUNT
SEALANE
SEALANT
SEALING
SEAMING
SEARING
SEASONS
SEATING
SEBRING
SEEDING
SEEKING
SEEMING
SEEPING
SEGMENT
SEINING
SEIZING
SELLING
SENDING
SENSENS
SENSING
SEQUINS
SERLING
SERMONS
SERPENS
SERPENT
SERVANT
SERVING
SESTINA
SETTING
SEVENNO
SEVIGNY
SEXTANS
SEXTANT
SEXTONS
SHADING
SHAKING
SHAMANS
SHAMING
SHANANA
SHAPING
SHARING
SHARONA
SHAVING
SHEBANG
SHINING
SHOEING
SHOGUNS
SHOOING
SHOOINS
SHORING
SHOVING
SHOWING
SHUTINS
SIBLING
SICCING
SICKENS
SIDDONS
SIDEONE
SIDLING
SIEGING
SIEMENS
SIEVING
SIFTING
SIGHING
SIGMUND
SIGNING
SILOING
SILTING
SIMIANS
SIMMONS
SINGING
SINKING
SINNING
SIOUANS
SIPHONS
SIPPING
SISTINE
SITTING
SIXGUNS
SIXLANE
SIXNINE
SIZEONE
SKATING
SKEWING
SKIRUNS
SKYLINE
SLAKING
SLATING
SLAVING
SLAYING
SLEWING
SLICING
SLIDING
SLIMING
SLIPONS
SLOGANS
SLOPING
SLOVENE
SLOVENS
SLOWING
SMETANA
SMILING
SMITING
SMOKING
SNAKING
SNAPONS
SNARING
SNIPING
SNOCONE
SNORING
SNOWING
SOAKING
SOAPING
SOARING
SOBBING
SOCKING
SODDING
SOFTENS
SOILING
SOLOING
SOLVENT
SOLVING
SOMEONE
SOPPING
SOPRANI
SOPRANO
SORDINI
SORDINO
SORIANO
SORTING
SORVINO
SOURING
SOUSING
SOXFANS
SOYLENT
SPACING
SPADING
SPARING
SPAYING
SPECING
SPELUNK
SPEWING
SPICING
SPIKING
SPITING
SPLEENS
SPLEENY
SPOKANE
SPOKING
SPRAINS
SPUMING
SPUMONE
SPUMONI
SPYRING
STAGING
STAKING
STAMENS
STAMINA
STANINE
STARING
STATING
STATINS
STAVING
STAYING
STEANNE
STEARNS
STEFANI
STEPINS
STEPONE
STEVENS
STEWING
STIPEND
STJOHNS
STOKING
STOLONS
STONING
STORING
STOTINS
STOWING
STRAINS
STUBING
STUDENT
STYLING
STYRENE
SUBBAND
SUBBANK
SUBBING
SUBKING
SUBLONG
SUBORNS
SUBTEND
SUBTONE
SUBVENE
SUBZONE
SUCKING
SUDSING
SUITING
SUKARNO
SULKING
SULTANA
SULTANS
SUMMAND
SUMMING
SUMMONS
SUNFANS
SUNNING
SUNTANS
SUPPING
SURFING
SURGING
SUSANNA
SUSANNE
SUSPEND
SUSSING
SUZANNE
SWAYING
SWIPING
SYNCING
SYRIANA
SYRIANS

S•••••N

SAFFRON
SAGEHEN
SAHARAN
SAILSON
SALADIN
SALOMON
SAMISEN
SAMNUNN
SAMPSON
SANBORN
SANDMAN
SANDMEN
SANJUAN
SARACEN
SARAZEN
SAROYAN
SARUMAN
SASSOON
SATDOWN
SATINON
SATUPON
SAURIAN
SAVARIN
SAVEDON
SAVESON
SAXHORN
SAYAMEN
SAYWHEN
SCATMAN
SCHWANN
SCHWINN
SCOTIAN
SEAFERN
SEAGREN
SEALION
SEALSIN
SECTION
SEEPSIN
SEIZEON
SENDSIN
SENDSON
SENECAN
SERBIAN
SESSION
SETDOWN
SETUPON
SEWEDON
SHANNEN
SHANNON
SHAREIN
SHARPEN
SHAVIAN
SHEDSON
SHEEHAN
SHELDON
SHERMAN
SHERWIN
SHINEON
SHIPMAN
SHIPMEN
SHODDEN
SHOOSIN
SHORTEN
SHOTGUN
SHOVEIN
SHOWMAN
SHOWMEN
SHOWNIN
SHOWSIN
SHULMAN
SHUTSIN
SIDEMAN
SIDEMEN
SIGNSIN
SIGNSON
SILENTN
SILICON
SIMENON
SIMPSON
SINKSIN
SIOBHAN
SIRLOIN
SITDOWN
SITINON
SITUPON
SIXIRON
SIXTEEN
SIZETEN
SKELTON
SKIMPON
SLACKEN
SLAMSON
SLAPSON
SLATKIN
SLAYTON
SLEEKEN
SLEEPIN
SLEEPON
SLEPTIN
SLEPTON
SLIDEIN
SLINKIN
SLIPSIN
SLIPSON
SLOEGIN
SLOPSON
SLUNKIN
SMARTEN
SMEARON
SMIDGEN
SMILEON
SMITTEN
SNACKON
SNAPSON
SNEAKIN
SNELLEN
SNOWDON
SNOWMAN
SNOWMEN
SNOWSIN
SOAKSIN
SOCKSIN
SODACAN
SOJOURN
SOLOMON
SONORAN
SOTHERN
SOULMAN
SOUPCAN
SOUPCON
SOUPSON
SOURSON
SOYBEAN
SPARTAN
SPENDON
SPENTON
SPIEDON
SPIESON
SPITSON
SPORRAN
SPORTIN
SPRAYON
SPURSON
SPYUPON
STANDIN
STANDON
STANTON
STARION
STARMAN
STARSIN
STARTIN
STARTON
STASSEN
STATION
STAYSIN
STAYSON
STEALIN
STEARIN
STEEPEN
STEEPIN
STENGUN
STEPHEN
STEPSIN
STEPSON
STETSON
STEUBEN
STEWPAN
STICKIN
STICKON
STIFFEN
STILTON
STIMSON
STIRSIN
STOLEIN
STOLLEN
STOMPIN
STOMPON
STOODIN
STOODON
STOPSIN
STORMIN
STOUTEN
STRAPIN
STRAPON
STRIVEN
STSIMON
STUCKIN
STUCKON
STUFFIN
STUNGUN
STYGIAN
SUASION
SUBCLAN
SUBJOIN
SUBTEEN

SUCKSIN
SUCTION
SUELLEN
SUELYON
SUNBURN
SUNDOWN
SUNSFAN
SURECAN
SURFMAN
SURFMEN
SURGEON
SUSTAIN
SWAGMAN
SWAGMEN
SWANSON
SWEARIN
SWEETEN
SWEETON
SWENSON
SWINTON
SWOLLEN
SWOOPIN
SWOREIN
SYNGMAN

•S•N•••

ASANTES
ASININE
ASONANT
ASUNDER
ESPNEWS
ISONOMY
PSANDQS
TSONGAS
TSUNAMI
USANCES
USINGIN
USINGUP
XSANDOS

•S••N••

ASCENDS
ASCENTS
ASHANTI
ASKANCE
ASOFNOW
ASPENCO
ASSANTE
ASSENTS
ASSUNTA
ESCENCE
ESPANOL
ESSENCE
ESSENES
ESTONIA
ISEENOW
ISLANDS
OSCINES
OSMONDS
OSMUNDS
USTINOV

•S•••N•

ASHBINS
ASHCANS
ASHLAND
ASHPANS
ASININE
ASONANT
ASQUINT
ASSIGNS
ASTOUND
ESPYING
ESTRING
GSTRING
ISAIDNO
ISECOND
ISOGONS
ISOLINE
ISOTONE
ISSUANT
ISSUING
OSAKANS
OSBORNE
RSVPING
TSARINA
TSETUNG
USGRANT
USOPENS

•S••••N

ASHBURN
ASKEDIN
ASMARAN
ASPIRIN
ESIASON
ESTAMIN
ESTEBAN
ESTEFAN
ISFAHAN
ISTOMIN
ISTRIAN
OSIRIAN
USHERIN
USINGIN

••SN•••

BOSNIAN
CBSNEWS
ENSNARE
ENSNARL
HISNIBS
MISNAME
OBSNEAK
RESNAIS
RESNAPS
UNSNAGS
UNSNAKY
UNSNAPS
UNSNARL

••S•N••

ABSENCE
ABSENTS
ABSINTH
ANSONIA
ARSENAL
ARSENIC
ARSENIO
ASSANTE
ASSENTS
ASSUNTA
BASENJI
BASINAL
BOSONIC
CASINGS
CASINOS
CESSNAS
COSINES
COSTNER
EOSINES
ESSENCE
ESSENES
FASTNET
FISHNET
HASANIP
HOSANNA
INSANER
INSYNCH
ITSONME
JUSTNOW
LISENTE
LOSINGS
LYSENKO
MASONED
MASONIC
MASONRY
MESONIC
MISHNAH
MISKNEW
MISKNOW
MTSINAI
MUSANTE
MUSINGS
PESANTE
PISANIO
RESANDS
RESENDS
RESENTS
RESINED
RESINGS
RESINKS
RISENTO
RISINGS
ROSANNA
ROSANNE
ROSINED
ROSSNER
SISENOR
SUSANNA
SUSANNE
TISANES
UNSUNNY
UPSENDS
URSINUS
WASONTO

••S••N•

ABSCOND
ASSIGNS
ATSIGNS
AUSTINS
BASHING
BASKING
BASSANI
BASSANO
BASTING
BESTING
BESTONE
BOSSING
BOSTONS
BOSTONU
BUSHING
BUSKING
BUSLANE
BUSLINE
BUSMANS
BUSSING
BUSTING
BUSYING
CASEINS
CASERNE
CASERNS
CASHING
CASHINS
CASKING
CASSINI
CASSINO
CASTING
CESSING
COSHING
COSIGNS
COSTING
COSYING
CTSCANS
CUSHING
CUSSING
DASHING
DESCANT
DESCEND
DESCENT
DESIGNS
DESMOND
DESPINA
DESPOND
DESTINE
DESTINO
DESTINY
DISBAND
DISCING
DISHING
DISKING
DISOWNS
DISSENT
DISSING
DISTANT
DISTEND
DOSSING
DUSKING
DUSTING
EASTEND
EASTING
EASYONE
ENSIGNS
ENSUING
ERSKINE
EXSCIND
FASTENS
FASTING
FASTONE
FESSING
FESTINA
FISHING
FUSIONS
FUSSING
GASCANS
GASCONS
GASCONY
GASHING
GASLINE
GASPING
GASSING
GASTANK
GASTONE
GISSING
GOSLING
GUSHING
GUSTING
HASDONE
HASHING
HASPING
HASTENS
HASTING
HISPANO
HISSING
HOSANNA
HOSKINS
HOSTING
HUSBAND
HUSHING
HUSKING
IFSTONE
INSIGNE
INSPANS
INSTANT
INSTONE
ISSUANT
ISSUING
ITSDONE
ITSFINE
ITSGONE
JASMINE
JESTING
JOSHING
JUSTINE
JUSTONE
KISSING
KOSCINA
LASAGNA
LASAGNE
LASHING
LASTING
LASTONE
LESIONS
LESSENS
LESSING
LESSONS
LISPING
LISTENS
LISTING
LUSTING
MASHING
MASKING
MASSINE
MASSING
MASTING
MCSHANE
MCSWINE
MESHING
MESSINA
MESSING
MISBIND
MISDONE
MISSEND
MISSENT
MISSING
MISTING
MISTUNE
MISZONE
MOSCONI
MOSHING
MOSSING
MUSHING
MUSIGNY
MUSLINS
MUSSING
MUSTANG
NASCENT
NESTING
NISSANS
NISSANZ
NOSHING
OBSCENE
OUSTING
PASSANT
PASSING
PASTINA
PASTING
PISCINE
PISHING
PISTONS
POSTING
PUSHING
RASPING
RESCANS
RESCIND
RESHINE
RESIGNS
RESOUND
RESPANS
RESPINS
RESPOND
RESTING
RISKING
RLSTINE
ROSANNA
ROSANNE
ROSSANO
ROSSINI
ROSTAND
RUSHING
RUSTING
SASHING
SASSING
SESTINA
SISTINE
SUSANNA
SUSANNE
SUSPEND
SUSSING
TASKING
TASTING
TESTING
TOSSING
TUSCANS
TUSCANY
TUSKING
UNSHINY
UNSLING
UNSLUNG
UNSOUND
UNSPANS
UNSPENT
UNSTONY
UNSTUNG
UNSUNNY
UNSWUNG
UPSPINS
UPSTAND
UPSWING
VESTING
VISAING
VISIONS
WASHING
WASTING
WESTEND
WESTINS
WISEONE
WISHING
WISPING
YASMINE
YESORNO
YESSING
ZESTING

••S•••N

ABSTAIN
AJSIMON
ALSHAIN
ALSORAN
ATSEVEN
BASEDON
BASEMAN
BASEMEN
BASETEN
BASRHIN
BASSOON
BASTION
BESTMAN
BESTMEN
BOSNIAN
BOSSMAN
BOSSMEN
BUSHMAN
BUSHMEN
BUSTSIN
CASPIAN
CASTSON
CESSION
CISTERN
COSTAIN
CUSHION
DESTAIN
DISCERN
DISCMAN
DISDAIN
DISHPAN
DISJOIN
DRSLOAN
DUSTBIN
DUSTGUN
DUSTMAN
DUSTMEN
DUSTPAN
EASEDIN
EASEDON
EASESIN
EASESON
EASTERN
EASTMAN
EPSILON
EPSTEIN
FASHION
FESTOON
FISSION
FUSTIAN
GASMAIN
GASOVEN
GASSMAN
HASBEEN
HESHVAN
HESSIAN
HUSSEIN
INSULIN
ITSASIN
ITSOPEN
KOSYGIN
LASTDON
MISCOIN
MISJOIN
MISPLAN
MISSION
MUSEDON
MUSESON
NESSMAN
NESTSIN
NOSEDIN
NOSESIN
NOSTAIN
PASSION
PASTEIN
PASTERN
PISCEAN
POSTERN
POSTMAN
POSTMEN
PUSHKIN
PUSHPIN
RESHOWN
RESTAIN
RESTSIN
RESTSON
RESWORN
ROSALYN
RUSSIAN
RUSSLAN
SASSOON
SESSION
STSIMON
SUSTAIN
TASHLIN
TESTBAN
TESTRUN
UNSHORN
UNSHOWN
UNSLAIN
UNSTERN
UNSWORN
UPSILON
VESTRON
VISAYAN
VISTEON
VOSGIAN
WESTERN
WISEMAN
WISEMEN
YESICAN

•••SN••

BROSNAN
CESSNAS
DOESNOT
EDASNER
FRESNEL
GRISNEZ
INASNAP
INASNIT
KRASNER
LETSNOT
PARSNIP
PAYSNOW
PILSNER
QUESNAY
ROSSNER
SAYSNAY
WOOSNAM

•••S•N•

ABASING
ABUSING
AMUSING
ARCSINE
ARISING
ARTSONG
BASSANI
BASSANO
BERSUNT
BIASING
BOSSING
BOUSONO
BUSSING
CASSINI
CASSINO
CAUSING
CEASING
CENSING
CESSING
CHASING
CLOSING
CONSENT
COUSINE
COUSINS
CUISINE
CURSING
CUSSING
DAMSONS
DATSUNS
DAYSEND
DAYSINN
DISSENT
DISSING
DOSSING
DOUSING
DOWSING
ERASING
FESSING
FUSSING
GASSING
GETSANA
GETSANF
GIBSONS
GINSENG
GISSING
GODSEND
GODSENT
GODSONS
GOOSING
HELSING
HISSING
HITSONG
HOBSONS
HOPSING
HORSING
HOUSING
IRISING
JETSONS
JIMSONS
KANSANS
KISSING
KMESONS
KRISHNA
LANSING
LAPSANG
LAPSING
LEASING
LESSENS
LESSING
LESSONS
LHASANS
LIPSYNC
LOOSENS
LOOSING
LOUSING
MAISONS
MASSINE
MASSING
MENSANS
MESSINA
MESSING
MISSEND
MISSENT
MISSING
MOLSONS
MOSSING
MOUSING
MUSSING
NELSONS
NISSANS
NISSANZ
NOISING
NONSANE
NOOSING
NURSING
OILSAND
OLDSONG
OPUSONE
ORISONS
OURSONG
OUTSANG
OUTSING
OUTSINS
OUTSUNG
PAISANO
PAISANS
PARSING
PARSONS
PASSANT
PASSING
PAUSING
PEASANT
PEPSINS
PERSONA
PERSONS
PHASING
PLUSONE
POISING
POISONS
POPSONG
PORSENA
PRESENT
PRESONG
PRISONS
PROSING
PULSING
PURSING
RAISING
RAISINS
RAISINY
RAISONS
RAMSONS
RAPSONG
REASONS
REDSUNS
RETSINA
REUSING
RIESENS
RINSING
RIPSONE
RONSONS
ROSSANO
ROSSINI
ROUSING
SADSONG
SAISONS
SAMSONS
SAMSUNG
SASSING
SEASONS
SENSENS
SENSING
SOUSING
SUDSING
SUSSING
TEASING
TENSING
THESUNS
THISONE
TOCSINS
TOSSING
TUCSONS
TULSANS
UNISONS
VANSANT
VERSANT
VERSING
WILSONS
WITSEND
WORSENS
YESSING

•••S••N

AIRSIGN
ALASKAN
ALLSTON
ALMSMAN
ALMSMEN
AMESLAN
ANDSOON
ANISTON
AVESTAN
AWASHIN
BADSIGN
BASSOON
BATSMAN
BATSMEN
BLUSHON
BOSSMAN
BOSSMEN
BRESLIN
BROSNAN
BUISSON
BURSTIN
BURSTYN
CAISSON
CAPSTAN
CATSCAN
CESSION
CHASTEN
CLASSON
CLOSEIN
CONSIGN
COWSKIN
CRESPIN
CRESTON
CRISPEN
CRISPIN
CUBSFAN
DAYSINN
DOESKIN
DRESDEN
DRESSIN
DRISTAN
DUNSTAN
EELSKIN
ELASTIN
ELISION
ELYSIAN
EROSION
ETESIAN
EVASION
FEASTON
FISSION
FLASHON
FOISTON
FRESHEN
FRISIAN
FRISSON
GADSDEN
GASSMAN
GERSHON
GLISTEN
HALSTON
HARSHEN
HEISMAN
HESSIAN
HEXSIGN
HOUSMAN
HOUSTON
HURSTON
HUSSEIN
INASPIN
IRESIGN
JANSSEN
JANSSON
JETSFAN
KEESHAN
KEYSPAN
KIDSKIN
KINSMAN
KINSMEN
KIRSTEN
KRESKIN
KRISTIN
KTOSLIN
LENSMAN
LENSMEN
MANSION
MANSMAN
MARSDEN
MARSTON
MEISSEN
METSFAN
MISSION
MOISSAN
MOISTEN
MONSOON
MRISCAN
NESSMAN
NEWSMAN
NEWSMEN
NILSSON
OARSMAN
OARSMEN
ODESSAN
OILSKIN
OUTSEEN
OUTSPIN
PASSION
PENSION
PERSIAN
PERSSON
PETSCAN
PHASEIN
PIGSKIN
PLOSION
POISSON
POUSSIN
PRESSON
PRESTON
PROSCAN
RALSTON
RAMSFAN
REDSFAN
REDSKIN
RIESMAN
RIESSEN
RIPSAWN
RUSSIAN
RUSSLAN
SASSOON
SESSION
STASSEN
SUASION
SUNSFAN
TENSION
THESWAN
TOOSOON
TOPSPIN
TORSION
TRISTAN
TRUSTIN
TWISTON
VERSION
WAKSMAN
WALSTON
WINSTON

••••SN•

DEMESNE
VOTESNO

••••S•N

ABUTSON
ACHESON

ADAMSON
ADDISON
ALLISON
ALLYSON
ALROSEN
APERSON
ARTISAN
BACKSIN
BAILSON
BANGSON
BANKSON
BEARSON
BEATSON
BELLSON
BENISON
BENTSEN
BERGSON
BERNSEN
BITESIN
BITESON
BLOUSON
BLOWSIN
BLOWSON
BLUESUN
BOXESIN
BRANSON
BRONSON
BUISSON
BURNSIN
BUSTSIN
BUTTSIN
CAISSON
CALLSIN
CALLSON
CARLSON
CARTSIN
CASTSON
CAVESIN
CHANSON
CHEWSON
CHIPSIN
CLASSON
CLEMSON
CLIPSON
CLUESIN
COARSEN
COMESIN
COMESON
CRAISIN
CRAMSIN
CRIMSON
CURLSIN
DAVISON
DAWNSON
DEALSIN
DENISON
DIALSIN
DICKSON
DINESEN
DINESIN
DINESON
DIRKSEN
DIVESIN
DODGSON
DOTESON
DRAGSIN
DRAGSON
DRAWSIN
DRAWSON
DRESSIN
DRIPSON
DROPSIN
DUMPSON
EASESIN
EASESON
EDGESIN
ELEISON
ELLISON
EMERSON
ERICSON
ERIKSON
ESIASON
FACESON
FADESIN
FALLSIN
FALLSON
FAWNSON
FEEDSIN
FEEDSON
FILESIN
FILLSIN
FINKSON
FIRESON
FIXESON
FLIESIN
FLIESON
FLITSIN
FLOWSIN
FOCUSON
FOLDSIN
FRISSON
FUJISAN
GAINSON
GAZESON
GIVESIN
GIVESON
GLEASON
GLUESON
GNAWSON
GOODSON
GRAYSON
GROWSON
HANDSIN
HANDSON
HANGSIN
HANGSON
HARPSON
HAULSIN
HEADSIN
HEAPSON
HEDISON
HELPSIN
HELPSON
HIRESON
HOARSEN
HOLDSIN
HOLDSON
HOMESIN
HONESIN
HOOKSON
HORNSIN
IRONSON
ITSASIN
IVERSON
JACKSON
JAMESON
JAMISON
JANSSEN
JANSSON
JEMISON
JEWISON
JOHNSON
JOINSIN
JUMPSIN
JUMPSON
KARLSON
KEEPSIN
KEEPSON
KICKSIN
KINISON
LACESON
LEADSIN
LEADSON
LEAKSIN
LEANSIN
LEANSON
LEAPSIN
LEAPSON
LIAISON
LIVESIN
LIVESON
LOADSIN
LOCKSIN
LOCKSON
LOOKSIN
LOOKSON
LUMPSIN
LURESIN
MADISON
MAILSIN
MEDUSAN
MEISSEN
MIXESIN
MOISSAN
MOMMSEN
MOVESIN
MOVESON
MUMESON
MUSESON
MYERSON
NAILSIN
NESTSIN
NIELSEN
NILSSON
NOSESIN
ODESSAN
ORBISON
PACKSIN
PACKSON
PAULSEN
PEARSON
PEEKSIN
PEERSIN
PERSSON
PICKSON
PILESIN
PILESON
PIMESON
PIPESIN
PLANSON
PLAYSON
PLOWSON
PLUGSIN
POISSON
POURSIN
POUSSIN
PRESSON
PREYSON
PRODSON
PULLSIN
PULLSON
RAILSON
RAINSIN
RAINSON
RAKESIN
READSIN
READSON
REELSIN
REINSIN
RERISEN
RESTSIN
RESTSON
RIDESIN
RIESSEN
RINGSIN
ROBESON
ROLLSIN
ROLLSON
ROPESIN
RULESON
SAILSON
SAMISEN
SAMPSON
SAVESON
SEALSIN
SEEPSIN
SENDSIN
SENDSON
SHEDSON
SHOOSIN
SHOWSIN
SHUTSIN
SIGNSIN
SIGNSON
SIMPSON
SINKSIN
SLAMSON
SLAPSON
SLIPSIN
SLIPSON
SLOPSON
SNAPSON
SNOWSIN
SOAKSIN
SOCKSIN
SOUPSON
SOURSON
SPIESON
SPITSON
SPURSON
STARSIN
STASSEN
STAYSIN
STAYSON
STEPSIN
STEPSON
STETSON
STIMSON
STIRSIN
STOPSIN
SUCKSIN
SWANSON
SWENSON
TACKSON
TAKESIN
TAKESON
TALKSON
TAPESON
TELLSON
THOMSON
THORSON
TREASON
TRIESON
TRIPSON
TUCKSIN
TUNESIN
TURNSIN
TURNSON
TYPESIN
UNRISEN
UPRISEN
URGESON
VENISON
VOTESIN
VOTESON
WADESIN
WAITSON
WALKSON
WALLSIN
WANTSIN
WAVESIN
WEARSON
WHIPSIN
WHITSUN
WILLSON
WIRESIN
WOODSON
WORKSIN
WORKSON
YANKSON
YELTSIN
ZEROSIN
ZOOMSIN

SO•••••

SOAKERS
SOAKING
SOAKSIN
SOAKSUP
SOANDSO
SOAPBOX
SOAPERS
SOAPIER
SOAPILY
SOAPING
SOAPNET
SOAPPAD
SOAPSUP
SOARERS
SOAREWE
SOARING
SOBBERS
SOBBING
SOBERED
SOBERER
SOBERLY
SOCIALS
SOCIETY
SOCKETS
SOCKEYE
SOCKHOP
SOCKING
SOCKSIN
SODACAN
SODAPOP
SODDIER
SODDING
SODIDWE
SODLESS
SOFABED
SOFARAS
SOFFITS
SOFTENS
SOFTEST
SOFTGEL
SOFTIES
SOFTISH
SOFTTOP
SOGGIER
SOGGILY
SOHAVEI
SOIGNEE
SOILAGE
SOILING
SOIREES
SOJOURN
SOLACED
SOLACER
SOLACES
SOLARAS
SOLARIA
SOLDERS
SOLDFOR
SOLDIER
SOLDOFF
SOLDOUT
SOLEDAD
SOLFEGE
SOLICIT
SOLIDER
SOLIDLY
SOLLATI
SOLNESS
SOLOACT
SOLOING
SOLOIST
SOLOMON
SOLUBLE
SOLUTES
SOLVEIT
SOLVENT
SOLVERS
SOLVING
SOMALIA
SOMALIS
SOMATIC
SOMEDAY
SOMEHOW
SOMEONE
SOMESAY
SOMEWAY
SOMINEX
SONANCE
SONATAS
SONGFUL
SONLESS
SONLIKE
SONNETS
SONORAN
SONSHIP
SOONERS
SOONEST
SOOTHED
SOOTHER
SOOTHES
SOOTIER
SOOTILY
SOPHIES
SOPHISM
SOPHIST
SOPPIER
SOPPING
SOPRANI
SOPRANO
SOPWITH
SORBATE
SORBETS
SORCERY
SORDINI
SORDINO
SORENTO
SORGHUM
SORIANO
SORORAL
SORRELL
SORRELS
SORRIER
SORRILY
SORROWS
SORTERS
SORTIED
SORTIES
SORTING
SORTOUT
SORVINO
SOSORRY
SOSPADS
SOSUEME
SOTHEBY
SOTHERE
SOTHERN
SOTTISH
SOTWEED
SOUBISE
SOUFFLE
SOULFUL
SOULMAN
SOUNDED
SOUNDER
SOUNDLY
SOUPCAN
SOUPCON
SOUPERS
SOUPIER
SOUPMIX
SOUPSON
SOUPSUP
SOURALE
SOURCED
SOURCES
SOUREST
SOURING
SOURISH
SOURSON
SOUSING
SOUTHEY
SOUTHOF
SOVIETS
SOWLIKE
SOWSEAR
SOXFANS
SOYBEAN
SOYINKA
SOYINKS
SOYLENT
SOYMEAL
SOYMILK

S•O••••

SAOTOME
SCOFFAT
SCOFFED
SCOFFER
SCOLARI
SCOLDED
SCOLDER
SCONCES
SCOOBAS
SCOOPED
SCOOPER
SCOOTCH
SCOOTED
SCOOTER
SCOPING
SCORERS
SCORIAS
SCORING
SCORNED
SCORNER
SCORPIO
SCOTERS
SCOTIAN
SCOTTIE
SCOUPES
SCOURED
SCOURER
SCOURGE
SCOUTED
SCOUTER
SCOUTUP
SCOWLED
SCOWLER
SHOALED
SHOCKED
SHOCKER
SHODDEN
SHOEBOX
SHOEING
SHOEPAC
SHOFARS
SHOGUNS
SHONUFF
SHOOFLY
SHOOING
SHOOINS
SHOOKUP
SHOOOFF
SHOOSIN
SHOOTAT
SHOOTBY
SHOOTER
SHOOTUP
SHOPFOR
SHOPFUL
SHOPKOS
SHOPNBC
SHOPPED
SHOPPER
SHOPPES
SHOPSAT
SHOREUP
SHORING
SHORTED
SHORTEN
SHORTER
SHORTIE
SHORTLY
SHORTOF
SHOTFOR
SHOTGUN
SHOTOUT
SHOTPAR
SHOTPUT
SHOULDA
SHOULDI
SHOUTAT
SHOUTED
SHOUTER
SHOVEIN
SHOVELS
SHOVERS
SHOVING
SHOWBIZ
SHOWCAT
SHOWDOG
SHOWERS
SHOWERY
SHOWHOW
SHOWIER
SHOWILY
SHOWING
SHOWMAN
SHOWMEN
SHOWNIN
SHOWNUP
SHOWOFF
SHOWOUT
SHOWSIN
SHOWSUP
SIOBHAN
SIOUANS
SKOSHES
SLOBBER
SLOEGIN
SLOGANS
SLOGGED
SLOGGER
SLOPERS
SLOPING
SLOPPED
SLOPSON
SLOSHED
SLOSHES
SLOTCAR
SLOTTED
SLOTTER
SLOUCHY
SLOUGHS
SLOVAKS
SLOVENE
SLOVENS
SLOWDAY
SLOWEST
SLOWING
SLOWISH
SLOWSUP
SLOWUPS
SMOKERS
SMOKEUP
SMOKEYS
SMOKIER
SMOKIES
SMOKILY
SMOKING
SMOLDER
SMOOTHS
SMOOTHY
SMOTHER
SNOBALL
SNOCAPS
SNOCATS
SNOCONE
SNOOKER
SNOOPED
SNOOPER
SNOOTED
SNOOZED
SNOOZER
SNOOZES
SNORERS
SNORING
SNORKEL
SNORTAT
SNORTED
SNORTER
SNOUTED
SNOWCAP
SNOWCAT
SNOWDAY
SNOWDON
SNOWHAT
SNOWIER
SNOWILY
SNOWING
SNOWJOB
SNOWMAN
SNOWMEN
SNOWPEA
SNOWSIN
SNOWSKI
SOONERS
SOONEST
SOOTHED
SOOTHER
SOOTHES
SOOTIER
SOOTILY
SPOILED
SPOILER
SPOKANE
SPOKEOF
SPOKETO
SPOKEUP
SPOKING
SPONDEE
SPONGED
SPONGER
SPONGES
SPONSOR
SPOOFED
SPOOFER
SPOOKED
SPOOLED
SPOOLER
SPOONED
SPOONER
SPORRAN
SPORTED
SPORTIN
SPOTLIT
SPOTTED
SPOTTER
SPOUSAL
SPOUSES
SPOUTED
SPOUTER
STOCKED
STOCKER
STOCKUP
STODGED
STODGES
STOGIES
STOICAL
STOKELY
STOKERS
STOKEUP
STOKING
STOLEIN
STOLLEN
STOLONS
STOMACH
STOMATA
STOMPED
STOMPIN
STOMPON
STONEAX
STONERS
STONIER
STONILY
STONING
STOODBY
STOODIN
STOODON
STOODTO
STOODUP
STOOGED
STOOGES
STOOKEY
STOOLED
STOOLIE
STOOPED
STOOPER
STOPFOR
STOPGAP
STOPOFF
STOPPED
STOPPER
STOPPLE
STOPSAT
STOPSBY
STOPSIN
STOPSIT
STOPSUP
STORAGE
STORERS
STOREUP
STORIED
STORIES
STORING
STORMED
STORMIN
STOTINS
STOUTEN
STOUTER
STOUTLY
STOWAGE
STOWERS
STOWING
STOWSIT
SWOLLEN
SWOONED
SWOONER
SWOOPED
SWOOPER
SWOOPIN
SWOOSIE
SWOREAT
SWOREBY
SWOREIN
SWORETO

S••O•••

SALOMON
SALONGA
SALOONS
SAMOANS
SAMOSAS
SAMOSET
SAMOVAR
SAMOYED
SARONGS
SAROYAN
SATORIS
SAVORED
SAVORER
SAVOURS
SAVOURY
SAYOVER
SCHOLAR
SCHOLES
SCHOOLS
SCIORRA
SCOOBAS
SCOOPED
SCOOPER
SCOOTCH
SCOOTED
SCOOTER
SCROLLS
SCROOGE
SECONDI
SECONDO
SECONDR
SECONDS
SEDONAS
SEGOVIA
SENORAS
SENORES
SETOFFS
SETOUTS
SHLOCKY
SHNOOKS
SHOOFLY
SHOOING
SHOOINS
SHOOKUP
SHOOOFF
SHOOSIN
SHOOTAT
SHOOTBY
SHOOTER
SHOOTUP
SHROUDS
SILOING
SIMONIZ
SIROCCO
SITONIT
SMOOTHS
SMOOTHY
SNOOKER
SNOOPED
SNOOPER
SNOOTED
SNOOZED
SNOOZER
SNOOZES
SOJOURN
SOLOACT
SOLOING
SOLOIST
SOLOMON
SONORAN
SORORAL
SOSORRY
SPLOTCH
SPOOFED
SPOOFER
SPOOKED
SPOOLED
SPOOLER
SPOONED
SPOONER
SPROUTS
STJOHNS
STLOUIS
STOODBY
STOODIN
STOODON
STOODTO
STOODUP
STOOGED
STOOGES
STOOKEY
STOOLED
STOOLIE
STOOPED
STOOPER
STROBES
STROKED
STROKER
STROKES
STROLLS
STROPHE
STROUSE
SUBORNS
SUDOKUS
SUMOIST
SWOONED
SWOONER
SWOOPED
SWOOPER
SWOOPIN
SWOOSIE
SYNODAL

SYNODIC
SYNONYM

S•••O••

SACKOUT
SADSONG
SAILORS
SAISONS
SALMONP
SALMONS
SALOONS
SALSODA
SALVOES
SALVORS
SAMBORA
SAMEOLD
SAMLOYD
SAMSONS
SANBORN
SANFORD
SANGOUT
SANJOSE
SAOTOME
SAPPORO
SARNOFF
SARTORS
SASSOON
SATCOMS
SATDOWN
SATHOME
SAUCONY
SAVIORS
SAVIOUR
SAWLOGS
SAWNOFF
SAWSOFF
SAWTOIT
SAWWOOD
SAXHORN
SAYMORE
SAYNOTO
SCHLOCK
SCHMOES
SCHNOOK
SCHNOZZ
SCHOOLS
SCROOGE
SDAKOTA
SEABOAT
SEABORG
SEACOWS
SEADOGS
SEAFOAM
SEAFOOD
SEAFOWL
SEAGODS
SEALOFF
SEAMOSS
SEAPORT
SEASONS
SEAWOLF
SECTORS
SEEKOUT
SEENOFF
SEENOUT
SEEPOUT
SEESOFF
SEESOUT
SEETOIT
SEIZORS
SELLOFF
SELLOUT
SENDOFF
SENDOUT
SENHORA
SENIORS
SENSORS
SENSORY
SENTOFF
SENTOUT
SEQUOIA
SEQUOYA
SERIOUS
SERMONS
SETDOWN
SETSOFF
SETSOUT
SEXPOTS
SEXTONS
SEYMOUR
SHADOWS
SHADOWY
SHAKOES
SHALOMS
SHARONA
SHEGOAT
SHEWOLF
SHIKOKU
SHINOLA
SHIPOUT
SHNOOKS
SHOOOFF
SHOTOUT
SHOWOFF
SHOWOUT
SHUTOFF
SHUTOUT
SHYLOCK
SICKOUT
SIDDONS
SIDEONE
SIDIOUS
SIGMOID
SIGNOFF
SIGNORA
SIGNORE
SIGNORS
SIGNOUT
SIMMONS
SINGOUT
SINUOUS
SIPHONS
SIRLOIN
SITCOMS
SITDOWN
SITHOME
SITSOUT
SIXFOLD
SIXFOOT
SIXFOUR
SIZEONE
SKIBOBS
SKIBOOT
SKIDOOS
SKIPOLE
SKIPOUT
SKITOWS
SKYDOME
SKYHOOK
SLALOMS
SLIDOFF
SLIDOUT
SLIPOFF
SLIPONS
SLIPOUT
SLYLOOK
SNAPONS
SNIPOFF
SNOCONE
SOLDOFF
SOLDOUT
SOMEONE
SORROWS
SORTOUT
SPATOUT
SPECOUT
SPEDOFF
SPEWOUT
SPIGOTS
SPINOFF
SPINOUT
SPINOZA
SPITOUT
SPUMONE
SPUMONI
SPUNOFF
SPUNOUT
SPYBOTS
SPYHOLE
STATORS
STAYOFF
STAYOUT
STCLOUD
STCROIX
STEPOFF
STEPONE
STEPOUT
STEROID
STEROLS
STOLONS
STOPOFF
STUPORS
SUBCODE
SUBCOOL
SUBFORM
SUBGOAL
SUBGODS
SUBJOIN
SUBLONG
SUBLOTS
SUBPOST
SUBROOT
SUBROSA
SUBSOIL
SUBSORT
SUBTONE
SUBZONE
SUCCORS
SUCCOTH
SUCCOUR
SUCROSE
SUFFOLK
SUITORS
SUKKOTH
SUMMONS
SUNBOWL
SUNBOWS
SUNDOGS
SUNDOWN
SUNGODS
SUNROOF
SUNROOM
SUPPORT
SUPPOSE
SUSSOUT
SYDHOFF
SYMBOLS
SYNCOPE
SYSTOLE

S••••O•

SABADOS
SAFFRON
SAIDBOO
SAILSON
SALCHOW
SALEMOR
SALOMON
SALTBOX
SAMPSON
SANDBOX
SANDHOG
SANDLOT
SASSOON
SATATOP
SATINON
SATUPON
SAVEDON
SAVEFOR
SAVESON
SAWWOOD
SAYSBOO
SAYSYOU
SCADSOF
SCALLOP
SCHNOOK
SCISSOR
SEAFOOD
SEALION
SECTION
SEEDPOD
SEIZEON
SELLFOR
SEMILOG
SENATOR
SENDFOR
SENDSON
SENTFOR
SERFDOM
SESSION
SETSHOT
SETTLOR
SETUPON
SEWEDON
SHADROE
SHAHDOM
SHALLOT
SHALLOW
SHAMPOO
SHANNON
SHAVUOT
SHEDSON
SHELDON
SHINEON
SHOEBOX
SHOPFOR
SHOPKOS
SHORTOF
SHOTFOR
SHOWDOG
SHOWHOW
SHYFROM
SIGHFOR
SIGNFOR
SIGNSON
SILICON
SIMENON
SIMPSON
SISENOR
SITATOP
SITINON
SITSFOR
SITUPON
SIXFOOT
SIXIRON
SKELTON
SKIBOOT
SKIDDOO
SKIDOOS
SKIDROW
SKIMPON
SKISHOP
SKYHOOK
SLAMSON
SLAPSON
SLAYTON
SLEDDOG
SLEEPON
SLEPTON
SLIPSON
SLOPSON
SLYLOOK
SMACKOF
SMALLOJ
SMEAGOL
SMEARON
SMILEON
SMIRNOV
SNACKON
SNAPSON
SNOWDON
SNOWJOB
SOAPBOX
SOCKHOP
SODAPOP
SOFTTOP
SOLDFOR
SOLOMON
SOMEHOW
SOUPCON
SOUPSON
SOURSON
SOUTHOF
SPAMBOT
SPARROW
SPEAKOF
SPECTOR
SPEEDOS
SPENDON
SPENTON
SPIEDON
SPIESON
SPITSON
SPOKEOF
SPONSOR
SPRAYON
SPURSON
SPYUPON
SQUALOR
STANDON
STANTON
STARDOM
STARION
STARLOG
STARTON
STATION
STAYFOR
STAYSON
STENTOR
STEPMOM
STEPSON
STEREOS
STERNOS
STERTOR
STETSON
STEWPOT
STICKON
STILTON
STIMSON
STOMPON
STOODON
STOPFOR
STRAPON
STRIPOF
STSIMON
STUCCOS
STUCKON
STUDIOS
SUASION
SUBCOOL
SUBPLOT
SUBROOT
SUCTION
SUEDFOR
SUELYON
SUESFOR
SUNGLOW
SUNROOF
SUNROOM
SUNSPOT
SUREROF
SURGEON
SWALLOW
SWANSON
SWEETON
SWENSON
SWINTON
SYMPTOM

S•••••O

SAGUARO
SAIDBOO
SAIDIDO
SAILSTO
SAINTLO
SALERNO
SAMMYJO
SANREMO
SAPPORO
SAPSAGO
SATCHMO
SAWINTO
SAYHITO
SAYNOTO
SAYSBOO
SAYSIDO
SAYSWHO
SCHERZO
SCORPIO
SEAHERO
SECONDO
SEEALSO
SEEINTO
SEEMSTO
SELLSTO
SEMIPRO
SENDSTO
SERPICO
SETINTO
SEVENNO
SHAMPOO
SHAPIRO
SIDETWO
SILENTO
SINGSTO
SIROCCO
SIZETWO
SKIDDOO
SNAPSTO
SOANDSO
SOPRANO
SORDINO
SORENTO
SORIANO
SORVINO
SPEAKTO
SPOKETO
SQUANTO
STANDTO
STARTTO
STEPTWO
STICKTO
STOODTO
STRETTO
STUCKTO
SUBECHO
SUBZERO
SUHARTO
SUKARNO
SUMUPTO
SUREIDO
SWEARTO
SWORETO

•SO••••

ASOCIAL
ASOFNOW
ASONANT
ESOBESO
ESOTERY
ISOBARS
ISOGONS
ISOGRAM
ISOHELS
ISOLATE
ISOLATO
ISOLINE
ISOMERS
ISONOMY
ISOPODS
ISOTONE
ISOTOPE
ISOTOPY
TSONGAS
TSOURIS
USOPENS
USOSHOW
USOTOUR

•S•O•••

ASKOVER
ASSORTS
ASTOLAT
ASTORIA
ASTOUND
ESCORTS
ESPOSAS
ESPOSOS
ESPOUSE
ESTONIA
ESTORIL
ISTOMIN
OSBORNE
OSMONDS
OSMOSED
OSMOSES
OSMOSIS
OSMOTIC
OSTOSIS

•S••O••

ASABODY
ASAJOKE
ASHFORD
ASKSOUT
BSCHOOL
ESCROWS
ISADORA
ISADORE
ISECOND
ISIDORE
ISOGONS
ISONOMY
ISOPODS
ISOTONE
ISOTOPE
ISOTOPY
JSTROKE
OSCEOLA
OSHKOSH
OSSEOUS
OSTEOID
QSCHOOL
USOTOUR

•S•••O•

ASIAGOS
ASKEDOF
ASKSFOR
ASLEWOF
ASOFNOW
ASSUROR
BSCHOOL
ESCALOP
ESCUDOS
ESIASON
ESKIMOS
ESPANOL
ESPOSOS
ESTADOS
ISEENOW
ISEEYOU
PSYCHOS
QSCHOOL
TSARDOM
TSELIOT
USEDFOR
USESFOR
USOSHOW
USTINOV
XSANDOS

•S••••O

ASPENCO
ESOBESO
ESPARTO
ISAIDNO
ISITAGO
ISOLATO
ISUREDO

••SO•••

ABSOLUT
ABSOLVE
ABSORBS
ADSORBS
ALSORAN
ANSONIA
ASSORTS
BOSOMED
BOSONIC
DESOTOS
DISOBEY
DISOWNS
ENSOULS
GASOHOL
GASOVEN
GOSOUTH
HASOVER
IMSORRY
INSOFAR
INSOLES
ITSOKAY
ITSONME
ITSOPEN
ITSOVER
KOSOVAR
LASORDA
LESOTHO
MASONED
MASONIC
MASONRY
MESONIC
OFSORTS
POSOLES
RESOAKS
RESOAPS
RESOILS
RESOJET
RESOLED
RESOLER
RESOLES
RESOLVE
RESORBS
RESORTS
RESOUND
RESOWED
RISOTTO
SOSORRY
UNSOBER
UNSOGGY
UNSOLED
UNSOLES
UNSOLID
UNSOOTY
UNSORRY
UNSORTS
UNSOUND
UNSOWED
UPSOARS
VISORED
WASONTO
YESORNO

••S•O••

ABSCOND
BASSOON
BBSHOTS
BESPOKE
BESTOFF
BESTONE
BESTOWS
BISHOPS
BOSTONS
BOSTONU
BUSBOYS
BUSLOAD
BUSTOUR
BUSTOUT
CASEOUS
CASEOUT
CASHOUT
CASSOCK
CASSOLA
CASTOFF
CASTOUT
CDSTORE
CISCOES
CUSTODY
CUSTOMS
DASBOOT
DASHOFF
DESMOGS
DESMOND
DESPOIL
DESPOND
DESPOTS
DESTOCK
DISCOED
DISCOID
DISCORD
DISHOUT
DISJOIN
DISPORT
DISPOSE
DISROBE
DISTORT
DOSHOTS
DRSLOAN
DRSPOCK
DUSTOFF
EASEOFF
EASEOUT
EASYOFF
EASYONE
FASTONE
FESTOON
FESTOSO
FISHOIL
FISHOUT
FOSCOLO
FUSIONS
GASCONS
GASCONY
GASEOUS
GASHOGS
GASLOGS
GASTONE
GESSOED
GESSOES
GOSFORD
GUSHOUT
GUSTOES
HASDONE
HASHOUT
HASROOM
HASSOCK
HASTOBE
HISTORY
HYSSOPS
IFSTONE
INSHOCK
INSHORE
INSHORT
INSPOTS
INSTOCK
INSTONE
INSTORE
IRSFORM
ITSCOLD
ITSDONE
ITSGONE
ITSLOVE
JOSBOYS
JUSTONE
JUSTOUT
KISSOFF
LASHOUT
LASSOED
LASSOER
LASSOES
LASTONE
LASTORY
LESIONS
LESSONS
LESSORS
LESTOIL
LISSOME
LOSEOUT
LOSTOUT
MASCOTS
MASTOID
MISCODE
MISCOIN
MISCOPY
MISDOER
MISDOES
MISDONE
MISFORM
MISJOIN
MISKOLC
MISMOVE
MISSORT
MISSOUT
MISTOLD
MISTOOK
MISWORD
MISZONE
MOSCONI
MRSCOTT
MRSPOCK
NESTORS
NOSCORE
NOSEOUT
NOSHOWS
OKSHOOT
ONSHORE
OSSEOUS
PASCOLI
PASSOFF
PASSOUT
PASTORS
PISCOPO
PISTOLE
PISTOLS
PISTONS
PISTOUS
POSTOPS
PUSHOFF
PUSHOUT
RASBORA
RESCORE
RESHOES
RESHOOT
RESHOWN
RESHOWS
RESPOKE
RESPOND
RESPOOL
RESPOTS
RESTOCK
RESTOKE
RESTORE
RESTOWS
RESWORE
RESWORN
RISSOLE
ROSCOES
ROSEOIL
ROSEOLA
ROSTOCK
RUSHOFF
RUSHOUT
SASSOON
SUSSOUT
SYSTOLE
TESTOUT
TISSOTS
TOSSOFF
TOSSOUT
TUSSOCK
TVSHOWS
TVSPOTS
UNSHOED
UNSHOES
UNSHORN
UNSHORT
UNSHOWN
UNSHOWY
UNSMOKY
UNSOOTY
UNSPOKE
UNSPOOL
UNSTOIC
UNSTONY
UNSTOPS
UNSTOUT
UNSTOWS
UNSWORE
UNSWORN
UPSHOOT
UPSHOTS
UPSLOPE
UPSTOOD
VISCOUS
VISIONS
WASHOFF
WASHOUT
WESCOTT
WISDOMS
WISEONE
YESVOTE

••S••O•

ABSALOM
AJSIMON
AKSAKOV
ASSUROR
BASEDON
BASSOON
BASTION
BESTBOY
BISTROS
BUSHHOG
BUSSTOP
CASELOT
CASHBOX
CASHCOW
CASINOS
CASTROL
CASTSON
CESSION
CESTMOI
CUSHION
DASBOOT
DASHDOT
DASHPOT
DESKTOP
DESOTOS
DESTROY
DISAVOW
DISTROS
DOSADOS
DOSIDOS
DUSTMOP
EASEDON
EASESON
EASYJOB
EPSILON
FASHION
FESTOON
FISHFOR
FISSION
FUSEBOX

FUSSPOT
GASOHOL
HASACOW
HASAROW
HASROOM
ITSABOY
ITSALOT
JUSTNOW
LASTDON
LASTROW
LOSTDOG
MISKNOW
MISSION
MISSYOU
MISTBOW
MISTOOK
MUSEDON
MUSESON
MUSTDOS
NOSEJOB
OKSHOOT
PASSFOR
PASSION
POSTBOX
POSTDOC
POSTHOC
PUSHFOR
PUSHROD
RESHOOT
RESPOOL
RESTSON
SASSOON
SESSION
SISENOR
STSIMON
TESTFOR
TOSSPOT
UNSPOOL
UPSHOOT
UPSILON
UPSTOOD
VESTRON
VISITOR
VISTEON
VOSKHOD
WISHFOR

••S•••O

ANSELMO
ARSENIO
BASETWO
BASILIO
BASSANO
BUSHIDO
CASSINO
DESTINO
FESTOSO
FOSCOLO
GASTERO
GESTAPO
HISPANO
IDSAYSO
LESOTHO
LOSESTO
LYSENKO
MOSCATO
MUSKEGO
PASSADO
P!SANIO
PISARRO
PISCOPO
RISENTO
RISESTO
RISOTTO
ROSARIO
ROSSANO
TOSHIRO
VISCUSO
WASONTO
YESORNO

•••SO••

ACESOUT
ACTSOUT
AGESOUT
AIRSOCK
AIRSOUT
ANDSOON
ARTSONG
ASKSOUT
AWESOME
BARSOAP
BASSOON
BEGSOFF
BONSOIR
BOUSONO
BOWSOUT
BUGSOFF
BUGSOUT
BUMSOUT
BUYSOFF
BUYSOUT
CASSOCK
CASSOLA
CENSORS
CONSOLE
CONSORT
COPSOUT
CURSORS
CURSORY
CUTSOFF
CUTSOUT
DAMSONS
DAYSOFF
DELSOLS
DIESOFF
DIESOUT
DIGSOUT
DIMSOUT
EATSOUT
EKESOUT
ELUSORY
EPISODE
EYESORE
FANSOUT
FLYSOLO
FOBSOFF
FORSOOK
FULSOME
GESSOED
GESSOES
GETSOFF
GETSOFT
GETSOLD
GETSORE
GETSOUT
GIBSONS
GODSONS
GOESOFF
GOESOUT
GOTSOFT
GOTSORE
GYMSOCK
HADSOME
HANSOLO
HANSOMS
HASSOCK
HATSOFF
HITSOFF
HITSONG
HITSOUT
HOBSONS
HOPSOFF
HOPSOUT
HOTSOUP
HYSSOPS
ICESOUT
IRISOUT
IRKSOME
JETSONS
JIMSONS
KISSOFF
KMESONS
LASSOED
LASSOER
LASSOES
LAYSOFF
LAYSOUT
LESSONS
LESSORS
LETSOFF
LETSOUT
LIPSOFF
LIPSOUT
LISSOME
LOGSOFF
LOGSOUT
LOPSOFF
LUGSOUT
LYESOAP
MAISONS
MAISOUI
MAPSOUT
MIDSOLE
MISSORT
MISSOUT
MOLSONS
MONSOON
NELSONS
NEWSOME
NODSOFF
NOISOME
ODDSOCK
OFASORT
OLDSONG
ONESOCK
OPTSOUT
OPUSONE
ORISONS
OURSONG
OUTSOAR
OUTSOLD
OUTSOLE
PANSOUT
PARSONS
PASSOFF
PASSOUT
PAYSOFF
PAYSOUT
PEASOUP
PERSOFF
PERSONA
PERSONS
PIGSOUT
PLUSONE
POISONS
POPSOFF
POPSONG
POPSOUT
PRESOAK
PRESOLD
PRESONG
PRESORT
PRISONS
PROSODY
PUTSOFF
PUTSOUT
RAISONS
RAMSONS
RANSOMS
RAPSONG
RATSOUT
REASONS
RIGSOUT
RIPSOFF
RIPSONE
RIPSOUT
RISSOLE
RONSONS
RUBSOFF
RUBSOUT
RUNSOFF
RUNSOUT
SADSONG
SAISONS
SALSODA
SAMSONS
SASSOON
SAWSOFF
SEASONS
SEESOFF
SEESOUT
SENSORS
SENSORY
SETSOFF
SETSOUT
SITSOUT
SUBSOIL
SUBSORT
SUSSOUT
TAGSOUT
TAPSOFF
TAPSOUT
TEESOFF
TENSORS
THISONE
TIESOFF
TIPSOFF
TISSOTS
TOGSOUT
TOOSOON
TOPSOFF
TOPSOIL
TOPSOUT
TOSSOFF
TOSSOUT
TUCSONS
TUSSOCK
TWOSOME
UNISOMS
UNISONS
WHOSOUT
WIGSOUT
WILSONS
WINSOME
WINSOUT
ZIPSOFF

•••S•O•

ACTSFOR
AHOSTOF
AIMSFOR
AIRSHOW
ALLSTON
ANDSOON
ANISTON
ARISTOS
ARTSHOP
ARTSHOW
ASKSFOR
BADSHOT
BARSTOW
BASSOON
BATSFOR
BEGSFOR
BIDSFOR
BIGSHOT
BIGSHOW
BLOSSOM
BLUSHON
BOASTOF
BOLSHOI
BOWSHOT
BRISTOL
BUISSON
BUSSTOP
CAISSON
CARSHOW
CATSHOW
CESSION
CLASSON
COPSHOP
CRESTON
DIESFOR
DIGSFOR
DOESFOR
DOESNOT
DOESTOO
DOGSHOW
EARSHOT
ELISION
EROSION
EVASION
EYESHOT
EYESPOT
FEASTON
FIASCOS
FISSION
FLASHON
FLUSHOT
FOISTON
FORSHOW
FORSOOK
FRESCOS
FRISSON
FUSSPOT
GEMSBOK
GERSHON
GETSHOT
GLASGOW
GLASHOW
GOESFOR
GRISSOM
GUMSHOE
GUNSFOR
GUNSHOT
GYMSHOE
HALSTON
HITSFOR
HITSHOW
HOTSHOT
HOTSPOT
HOUSTON
HURSTON
ICESHOW
INASHOE
INASPOT
INKSPOT
ITISTOO
JANSSON
JOBSHOP
KNOSSOS
LAYSFOR
LAYSLOW
LETSNOT
LIESFOR
LIESLOW
MANSION
MARSTON
MISSION
MISSYOU
MONSOON
MUGSHOT
NEWSBOY
NILSSON
NONSTOP
ODDSHOE
OILSPOT
OLDSHOE
ONESHOE
ONESHOT
ONESPOT
ONESTOP
OPTSFOR
OUTSHOT
OUTSHOW
PASSFOR
PASSION
PAYSFOR
PAYSNOW
PENSION
PERSSON
PETSHOP
PITSTOP
PLOSION
POISSON
POTSHOT
PRESHOW
PRESSON
PRESTON
PRESTOS
PROSHOP
RAGSHOP
RALSTON
REDSPOT
REPSFOR
RIMSHOT
RIPSTOP
RUMSHOP
RUNSFOR
RUNSLOW
SASSOON
SAYSBOO
SAYSYOU
SCISSOR
SESSION
SETSHOT
SITSFOR
SKISHOP
SUASION
SUESFOR
SUNSPOT
TAPSHOE
TEASHOP
TEESHOT
TENSION
TENSPOT
THESHOW
TOESHOE
TOLSTOI
TOLSTOY
TOOSLOW
TOOSOON
TOPSPOT
TORSION
TOSSPOT
TOYSHOP
TULSAOK
TWISTON
TWOSHOT
TWOSPOT
USESFOR
USOSHOW
VERSION
VIESFOR
WALSTON
WAPSHOT
WINSLOW
WINSTON
YENSFOR

•••S••O

AGESAGO
BASSANO
BOUSONO
CANSECO
CASSINO
CLOSETO
DOASIDO
DOESTOO
FLYSOLO
FRUSTRO
GOESPRO
GUESSSO
HANSOLO
IMUSTGO
ITISTOO
LEASETO
MAESTRO
MONSTRO
NUESTRO
OPUSTWO
PAISANO
PASSADO
PEPSICO
PLUSTWO
ROSSANO
SAPSAGO
SAYSBOO
SAYSIDO
SAYSWHO
WHOSWHO
ZEMSTVO

••••SO•

ABUTSON
ACHESON
ADAMSON
ADDISON
ADVISOR
AEROSOL
ALLISON
ALLYSON
ANBESOL
APERSON
ARIOSOS
AULDSOD
BAILSON
BANGSON
BANKSON
BEARSON
BEATSON
BELLSON
BENISON
BERGSON
BITESON
BLEDSOE
BLOSSOM
BLOUSON
BLOWSON
BRANSON
BRONSON
BRYUSOV
BUISSON
CAISSON
CALLSON
CARLSON
CASTSON
CHANSON
CHEWSON
CHRISOM
CLASSON
CLEMSON
CLIPSON
COMESON
CREOSOL
CRIMSON
DAVISON
DAWNSON
DENISON
DEVISOR
DICKSON
DINESON
DIVISOR
DODGSON
DOTESON
DRAGSON
DRAWSON
DRIPSON
DUMPSON
EASESON
ELEISON
ELLISON
EMBOSOM
EMERSON
ERICSON
ERIKSON
ESIASON
ESPOSOS
FACESON
FALLSON
FAWNSON
FEEDSON
FEELSOK
FINKSON
FIRESON
FIXESON
FLIESON
FOCUSON
FREESOF
FRISSON
GAINSON
GAZESON
GIRASOL
GIVESOF
GIVESON
GLEASON
GLUESON
GNAWSON
GOODSON
GRAYSON
GRISSOM
GROWSON
HANDSON
HANGSON
HARPSON
HEAPSOF
HEAPSON
HEARSOF
HEDISON
HELPSON
HIRESON
HOLDSON
HOOKSON
INCISOR
IRONSON
IVERSON
JACKSON
JACKSOO
JAMESON
JAMISON
JANSSON
JEMISON
JEWISON
JOHNSON
JUMPSON
KARLSON
KEEPSON
KINISON
KNOSSOS
KNOWSOF
LACESON
LEADSON
LEANSON
LEAPSON
LIAISON
LIVESON
LOADSOF
LOCKSON
LOOKSON
MADISON
MILKSOP
MORISOT
MOVESON
MUMESON
MUSESON
MYERSON
NILESOH
NILSSON
ORBISON
PACKSON
PARASOL
PEARSON
PERSSON
PICKSON
PILESOF
PILESON
PIMESON
PINESOL
PLANSON
PLAYSON
PLOWSON
POISSON
PRESSON
PREYSON
PRODSON
PULLSON
RAILSON
RAINSON
READSON
REEKSOF
RESTSON
REVISOR
ROBESON
ROLLSON
RULESON
SAILSON
SAMPSON
SAVESON
SCADSOF
SCISSOR
SENDSON
SHEDSON
SIGNSON
SIMPSON
SLAMSON
SLAPSON
SLIPSON
SLOPSON
SNAPSON
SOUPSON
SOURSON
SPIESON
SPITSON
SPONSOR
SPURSON
STAYSON
STEPSON
STETSON
STIMSON
SWANSON
SWENSON
TACKSON
TAKESON
TALKSOF
TALKSON
TAPESON
TELLSOF
TELLSON
THATSOK
THOMSON
THORSON
TIRESOF
TRANSOM
TREASON
TRIESON
TRIPSON
TURNSON
UNBOSOM
URGESON
VENISON
VOTESON
WAITSON
WALKSON
WARNSOF
WEARSON
WILLSON
WINDSOR
WOODSON
WORKSON
YANKSON

••••S•O

ARIOSTO
AUGUSTO
BELASCO
BINDSTO
CALLSTO
CARESTO
CHRISTO
COMESTO
DARESTO
DEALSTO
DOOMSTO
DRAWSTO
ERNESTO
FAILSTO
FALLSTO
FEEDSTO
FLIESTO
GEARSTO
GIVESTO
GLUESTO
GUESSSO
HEADSTO
HERESTO
HOLDSTO
HOPESSO
HOPESTO
IMPASTO
IONESCO
JACKSOO
JALISCO
KEEPSTO
LEADSTO
LEANSTO
LOOKSTO
LOSESTO
LOVESTO
MAKESDO
MAKESGO
MEANSTO
MODESTO
MOVESTO
NABISCO
NEEDSTO
PICASSO
PLANSTO
PLAYSTO
PRAYSTO
RACESTO
READSTO
RENTSTO
RIDESTO
RISESTO
ROBUSTO
SAILSTO
SEEMSTO
SELLSTO
SENDSTO
SINGSTO
SNAPSTO
TABASCO
TAKESTO
TALKSTO
TELESTO
TENDSTO
TRIESTO
TUNESTO
TURISMO
TURNSTO
VERISMO
VOTESNO
WALKSTO
WANTSTO
WARMSTO
WAVESTO

•••••SO

ALFONSO
AMOROSO
CALYPSO
DOINGSO
ESOBESO
EXTENSO
FESTOSO
FURIOSO
GIOCOSO
GUESSSO
HERMOSO
HOPEDSO
HOPESSO
IDSAYSO
IHOPESO
IZZATSO
MAFIOSO
MALPASO
MANCUSO
MAYBESO
OLOROSO
PICASSO
PIETOSO
PROVISO
QUITESO
SEEALSO
SOANDSO
THINKSO
VISCUSO

SP•••••

SPACELY
SPACERS
SPACIAL
SPACIER
SPACING
SPACKLE
SPADERS
SPADING
SPAMBOT
SPAMMED
SPAMMER
SPANAIR
SPANDEX
SPANGLE
SPANGLY
SPANIEL
SPANISH
SPANKED
SPANKER
SPANNED
SPANNER
SPARELY
SPAREME
SPARERS
SPAREST
SPARING
SPARKED
SPARKLE
SPARKLY
SPARRED
SPARRER
SPARROW
SPARSER
SPARTAN
SPASSKY
SPATHES
SPATIAL
SPATOUT
SPATTED
SPATTER
SPATULA
SPAWNED
SPAWNER
SPAYERS
SPAYING
SPEAKER
SPEAKOF
SPEAKTO
SPEAKUP
SPEARED
SPEARER
SPECIAL
SPECIES
SPECIFY
SPECING
SPECKED
SPECKLE
SPECOUT
SPECTER
SPECTOR
SPECTRA
SPECTRE
SPEDOFF
SPEEDED

SPEEDER
SPEEDOS
SPEEDUP
SPELLED
SPELLER
SPELUNK
SPENCER
SPENDER
SPENDON
SPENSER
SPENTON
SPEWERS
SPEWING
SPEWOUT
SPHERAL
SPHERED
SPHERES
SPHERIC
SPICERS
SPICERY
SPICEUP
SPICIER
SPICILY
SPICING
SPIDERS
SPIDERY
SPIEDON
SPIEGEL
SPIELED
SPIELER
SPIESON
SPIFFED
SPIFFUP
SPIGOTS
SPIKERS
SPIKETV
SPIKEUP
SPIKIER
SPIKILY
SPIKING
SPILLED
SPILLER
SPINACH
SPINDLE
SPINDLY
SPINDRY
SPINELS
SPINETS
SPINIER
SPINNER
SPINNEY
SPINOFF
SPINOUT
SPINOZA
SPIRALS
SPIREAS
SPIRIER
SPIRITS
SPITING
SPITOUT
SPITSON
SPITTER
SPITTLE
SPITZES
SPLASHY
SPLAYED
SPLEENS
SPLEENY
SPLENDA
SPLICED
SPLICER
SPLICES
SPLINES
SPLINTS
SPLITUP
SPLOTCH
SPLURGE
SPOILED
SPOILER
SPOKANE
SPOKEOF
SPOKETO
SPOKEUP
SPOKING
SPONDEE
SPONGED
SPONGER
SPONGES
SPONSOR
SPOOFED
SPOOFER
SPOOKED
SPOOLED
SPOOLER
SPOONED
SPOONER
SPORRAN
SPORTED
SPORTIN
SPOTLIT
SPOTTED
SPOTTER
SPOUSAL
SPOUSES
SPOUTED
SPOUTER
SPRAINS
SPRAWLS
SPRAWLY
SPRAYED
SPRAYER
SPRAYON
SPREADS
SPRIEST
SPRINGS
SPRINGY
SPRINTS
SPRITES
SPROUTS
SPRUCED
SPRUCER
SPRUCES
SPRYEST
SPUMIER
SPUMING
SPUMONE
SPUMONI
SPUNOFF
SPUNOUT
SPURNED
SPURNER
SPURRED
SPURSON
SPURTED
SPUTNIK
SPUTTER
SPYBOTS
SPYCAMS
SPYDERS
SPYHOLE
SPYINGS
SPYKIDS
SPYRING
SPYUPON
SPYWARE

S•P••••

SAPHEAD
SAPIENS
SAPIENT
SAPLESS
SAPLING
SAPPERS
SAPPIER
SAPPILY
SAPPING
SAPPORO
SAPSAGO
SEPALED
SEPHIAS
SEPIRAS
SEPTETS
SIPHONS
SIPPERS
SIPPING
SOPHIES
SOPHISM
SOPHIST
SOPPIER
SOPPING
SOPRANI
SOPRANO
SOPWITH
STPAULS
STPETER
STPIUSI
STPIUSV
STPIUSX
SUPERGS
SUPPERS
SUPPING
SUPPLED
SUPPLER
SUPPLES
SUPPORT
SUPPOSE
SUPREME

S••P•••

SAMPANS
SAMPLED
SAMPLER
SAMPLES
SAMPRAS
SAMPSON
SAPPERS
SAPPIER
SAPPILY
SAPPING
SAPPORO
SAWPAST
SAWPITS
SCAPULA
SCEPTER
SCEPTIC
SCEPTRE
SCOPING
SCUPPER
SEAPORT
SEEPAGE
SEEPAST
SEEPIER
SEEPING
SEEPOUT
SEEPSIN
SERPENS
SERPENT
SERPICO
SETPLAY
SEXPOTS
SHAPELY
SHAPERS
SHAPEUP
SHAPING
SHAPIRO
SHEPARD
SHIPFUL
SHIPMAN
SHIPMEN
SHIPOUT
SHIPPED
SHIPPER
SHIPWAY
SHOPFOR
SHOPFUL
SHOPKOS
SHOPNBC
SHOPPED
SHOPPER
SHOPPES
SHOPSAT
SIMPERS
SIMPLER
SIMPLES
SIMPLEX
SIMPSON
SIPPERS
SIPPING
SIXPACK
SKEPTIC
SKIPOLE
SKIPOUT
SKIPPED
SKIPPER
SKIPSBY
SLAPPED
SLAPPER
SLAPSON
SLEPTIN
SLEPTON
SLIPOFF
SLIPONS
SLIPOUT
SLIPPED
SLIPPER
SLIPSBY
SLIPSIN
SLIPSON
SLIPSUP
SLIPUPS
SLOPERS
SLOPING
SLOPPED
SLOPSON
SNAPONS
SNAPPEA
SNAPPED
SNAPPER
SNAPPLE
SNAPSAT
SNAPSON
SNAPSTO
SNAPSUP
SNIPEAT
SNIPERS
SNIPING
SNIPOFF
SNIPPED
SNIPPER
SNIPPET
SOAPBOX
SOAPERS
SOAPIER
SOAPILY
SOAPING
SOAPNET
SOAPPAD
SOAPSUP
SOPPIER
SOPPING
SOSPADS
SOUPCAN
SOUPCON
SOUPERS
SOUPIER
SOUPMIX
SOUPSON
SOUPSUP
STAPLED
STAPLER
STAPLES
STEPDAD
STEPHEN
STEPINS
STEPMOM
STEPOFF
STEPONE
STEPOUT
STEPPED
STEPPER
STEPPES
STEPSIN
STEPSON
STEPSUP
STEPTWO
STEPUPS
STIPEND
STIPPLE
STOPFOR
STOPGAP
STOPOFF
STOPPED
STOPPER
STOPPLE
STOPSAT
STOPSBY
STOPSIN
STOPSIT
STOPSUP
STUPEFY
STUPIDS
STUPORS
STYPSIS
STYPTIC
SUBPLOT
SUBPOST
SULPHUR
SUPPERS
SUPPING
SUPPLED
SUPPLER
SUPPLES
SUPPORT
SUPPOSE
SURPASS
SURPLUS
SUSPECT
SUSPEND
SUSPIRE
SWAPPED
SWAPPER
SWEPTUP
SWIPERS
SWIPING
SYLPHIC
SYMPTOM

S•••P••

SALTPIT
SANDPIT
SATUPON
SCALPED
SCALPEL
SCALPER
SCAMPED
SCAMPER
SCARPED
SCOOPED
SCOOPER
SCORPIO
SCOUPES
SCRAPED
SCRAPER
SCRAPES
SCRAPPY
SCRIPPS
SCRIPTS
SCRUPLE
SCULPED
SCULPTS
SCUPPER
SEEDPOD
SEMIPRO
SERAPES
SERAPHS
SERAPIS
SERIPAK
SETUPON
SHAMPOO
SHARPED
SHARPEI
SHARPEN
SHARPER
SHARPIE
SHARPLY
SHERPAS
SHINPAD
SHIPPED
SHIPPER
SHOEPAC
SHOPPED
SHOPPER
SHOPPES
SHOTPAR
SHOTPUT
SICKPAY
SITSPAT
SITUPON
SKIMPED
SKIMPON
SKIPPED
SKIPPER
SLAPPED
SLAPPER
SLEEPER
SLEEPIN
SLEEPON
SLIPPED
SLIPPER
SLOPPED
SLUMPED
SLURPED
SLURPEE
SLURPER
SNAPPEA
SNAPPED
SNAPPER
SNAPPLE
SNIPPED
SNIPPER
SNIPPET
SNOOPED
SNOOPER
SNOWPEA
SOAPPAD
SODAPOP
SPYUPON
SSHAPED
STAMPED
STAMPER
STAYPUT
STEEPED
STEEPEN
STEEPER
STEEPIN
STEEPLE
STEEPLY
STEMPEL
STEPPED
STEPPER
STEPPES
STEWPAN
STEWPOT
STIPPLE
STOMPED
STOMPIN
STOMPON
STOOPED
STOOPER
STOPPED
STOPPER
STOPPLE
STRAPIN
STRAPON
STRIPED
STRIPER
STRIPES
STRIPOF
STROPHE
STUMPED
STUMPER
SUMUPTO
SUNSPOT
SWAMPED
SWAPPED
SWAPPER
SWEEPEA
SWEEPER
SWEEPUP
SWOOPED
SWOOPER
SWOOPIN
SYNAPSE

S••••P•

SATRAPS
SATRAPY
SCHLEPP
SCHLEPS
SCHNAPS
SCRAPPY
SCRIMPS
SCRIMPY
SCRIPPS
SEAMAPS
SENDUPS
SETTYPE
SEVENPM
SHRIMPS
SHRIMPY
SIGNUPS
SKICAPS
SKYCAPS
SKYMAPS
SLIPUPS
SLOWUPS
SNOCAPS
STEPUPS
SUBTYPE
SYNCOPE

S•••••P

SACKSUP
SALMONP
SATATOP
SAVEDUP
SAVESUP
SCALEUP
SCALLOP
SCAREUP
SCARFUP
SCHLEPP
SCHLUMP
SCOUTUP
SCREWUP
SCRUBUP
SEALSUP
SEATRIP
SENDSUP
SERVEUP
SEVENUP
SEWEDUP
SHAKEUP
SHAPEUP
SHINEUP
SHOOKUP
SHOOTUP
SHOREUP
SHOWNUP
SHOWSUP
SHUTSUP
SIGNSUP
SILENTP
SITATOP
SITEMAP
SIZEDUP
SIZESUP
SKIJUMP
SKISHOP
SKITRIP
SLACKUP
SLANTUP
SLICEUP
SLINKUP
SLIPSUP
SLOWSUP
SLUNKUP
SMACKUP
SMASHUP
SMOKEUP
SNAGSUP
SNAPSUP
SNARLUP
SNAZZUP
SNEAKUP
SNIFFUP
SNOWCAP
SNUCKUP
SOAKSUP
SOAPSUP
SOCKHOP
SODAPOP
SOFTTOP
SONSHIP
SOUPSUP
SPEAKUP
SPEEDUP
SPICEUP
SPIFFUP
SPIKEUP
SPLITUP
SPOKEUP
STACKUP
STANDUP
STANKUP
STARMAP
STARTUP
STAYSUP
STEAMUP
STEPSUP
STICKUP
STILLUP
STINKUP
STIRRUP
STIRSUP
STOCKUP
STOKEUP
STOODUP
STOPGAP
STOPSUP
STOREUP
STUCKUP
SUCKSUP
SUITSUP
SUMITUP
SUNLAMP
SURFSUP
SWANKUP
SWEEPUP
SWELLUP
SWEPTUP
SWIMSUP

•SP••••

ASPECTS
ASPENCO
ASPERSE
ASPHALT
ASPIRED
ASPIRER
ASPIRES
ASPIRIN
ASPRAWL
ESPANOL
ESPARTO
ESPIALS
ESPNEWS
ESPOSAS
ESPOSOS
ESPOUSE
ESPRITS
ESPYING
OSPREYS

•S•P•••

ASEPSIS
ASEPTIC
ASHPANS
ASHPITS
ISOPODS
RSVPING
USOPENS

•S••P••

ESCAPED
ESCAPEE
ESCAPER
ESCAPES
LSHAPED
OSHAPED
OSSIPEE
SSHAPED
TSHAPED
TSHAPES
USHAPED
USHAPES
USURPED
USURPER
VSHAPED
VSHAPES
YSHAPED
YSHAPES

•S•••P•

ESCARPS
ISOTOPE
ISOTOPY
TSTRAPS

•S••••P

ASHHEAP
ASKEDUP
ASSHARP
ESCALOP
PSYCHUP
USINGUP

••SP•••

ADSPACE
ANSPACH
AUSPICE
BESPEAK
BESPOKE
BUSPASS
CASPARY
CASPIAN
CUSPATE
CUSPIDS
DESPAIR
DESPINA
DESPISE
DESPITE
DESPOIL
DESPOND
DESPOTS
DISPART
DISPELS
DISPLAY
DISPORT
DISPOSE
DISPUTE
DRSPOCK
GASPARD
GASPERS
GASPING
GASPIPE
GASPUMP
GOSPELS
HASPING
HASPULL
HISPANO
HISPEED
HOSPICE
INSPACE
INSPANS
INSPECT
INSPIRE
INSPITE
INSPOTS
JASPERS
JASPERY
LESPAUL
LISPERS
LISPING
MISPAGE
MISPLAN
MISPLAY
MRSPAUL
MRSPEEL
MRSPOCK
MYSPACE
RASPERS
RASPIER
RASPING
RASPISH
RESPACE
RESPADE
RESPANS
RESPARK
RESPEAK
RESPECT
RESPELL
RESPELT
RESPICE
RESPINS
RESPIRE
RESPITE
RESPLIT
RESPOKE
RESPOND
RESPOOL
RESPOTS
RESPRAY
SOSPADS
SUSPECT
SUSPEND
SUSPIRE
TOSPARE
TVSPOTS
UNSPANS
UNSPEAK
UNSPELT
UNSPENT
UNSPICY
UNSPIED
UNSPILT
UNSPLIT
UNSPOKE
UNSPOOL
UPSPINS
VESPERS
VESPIDS
WASPIER
WASPILY
WASPISH
WISPIER
WISPILY
WISPING

••S•P••

BASEPAY
BUSHPIG
CESSPIT
DASHPOT
DISHPAN
DUSTPAN
FUSSPOT
INSIPID
ITSOPEN
JOSEPHA
JOSEPHI
LOSTPET
MOSHPIT
OSSIPEE
PUSHPIN
TOSSPOT

••S••P•

BISHOPS
BUSTUPS
DISRUPT
DUSTUPS
GASCAPS
GASPIPE
GESTAPO
GOSSIPS
GOSSIPY
HYSSOPS
INSHAPE
INSTEPS
INSWEPT
LASHUPS
LESSEPS
MESSUPS
MISCOPY
MISHAPS
MISTYPE
PISCOPO
POSTOPS
PUSHUPS
RESHAPE
RESHIPS
RESNAPS
RESOAPS
TOSSUPS
UNSHIPS
UNSNAPS
UNSTEPS
UNSTOPS
UNSWEPT
UPSLOPE
UPSTEPS
UPSWEPT
WASHUPS

••S•••P

ASSHARP
BUSSTOP
BUSTRIP
BUSTSUP
CASTSUP
DESKTOP
DUSTMOP
EASEDUP
EASESUP
GASEDUP
GASESUP
GASLAMP
GASPUMP
GUSSYUP
HASANIP
LASTLAP
MASTERP
MISSHIP
MISSTEP
MISTSUP
NOSEDUP
NOSESUP
PASTEUP
RESTAMP
RESTRAP
RESTRIP
RESTSUP
RESWEEP
RISESUP
ROSEHIP
UNSHARP
UNSTRAP
UPSWEEP
WISEDUP
WISESUP

•••SP••
ARUSPEX
BIASPLY
BTFSPLK
CATSPAW
CESSPIT
CLASPED
CLASPER
CRESPIN
CRISPED
CRISPEN
CRISPER
CRISPIN
CRISPIX
CRISPLY
CRISPUS
DAYSPAS
EYESPOT
FUSSPOT
GOESPRO
GRASPAT
GRASPED
GRASPER
HOTSPOT
HOTSPUR
INASPIN
INASPOT
INKSPOT
KEYSPAN
NEWSPEG
OILSPOT
ONESPOT
OUTSPED
OUTSPIN
OUTSPIT
PRESPUR
PROSPER
REDSPOT
SITSPAT
SUNSPOT
TENSPOT
THESPIS
TOPSPIN
TOPSPOT
TOSSPOT
TWOSPOT
WHISPER

•••S•P•
CATSUPS
GOESAPE
GOSSIPS
GOSSIPY
HYSSOPS
LESSEPS
MESSUPS
TOSSUPS

•••S••P
AIRSHIP
ARTSHOP
BARSOAP
BOOSTUP
BOXSTEP
BRUSHUP
BUSSTOP
CHOSEUP
CLOSEUP
COPSHOP
COWSLIP
CROSSUP
DRESSUP
FIRSTUP
GETSHEP
GETSHIP
GUNSHIP
GUSSYUP
HANSARP
HOISTUP
HOTSOUP
INASNAP
JOBSHOP
KINSHIP
LENSCAP
LETSLIP
LETSRIP
LOUSEUP
LYESOAP
MIDSHIP
MISSHIP
MISSTEP
NONSLIP
NONSTOP
NUNSHIP
ONESTEP
ONESTOP
OUTSKIP
OUTSTEP
PARSNIP
PAYSLIP
PEASOUP
PETSHOP
PITSTOP
PRESHIP
PRESSUP
PROSHOP
RAGSHOP
RAISEUP
RIPSTOP
RUMSHOP
SKISHOP
SMASHUP
SONSHIP
TEASEUP
TEASHOP
TENSEUP
TOYSHOP
TRUSSUP
TWISTUP
TWOSTEP
WARSHIP
WORSHIP

••••SP•
UNHASPS
UNRASPY

••••S•P
ANTESUP
BACKSUP
BALLSUP
BANGSUP
BANKSUP
BEADSUP
BEAMSUP
BEARSUP
BEATSUP
BEEFSUP
BELTSUP
BINDSUP
BITESUP
BLOTSUP
BLOWSUP
BOILSUP
BOLTSUP
BONESUP
BOOTSUP
BOXESUP
BREWSUP
BUCKSUP
BUFFSUP
BULKSUP
BUMPSUP
BUOYSUP
BURNSUP
BUSTSUP
CAGESUP
CAKESUP
CALLSUP
CAMPSUP
CASTSUP
CHATSUP
CHEWSUP
CHIPSUP
CHOPSUP
CLAMSUP
CLOGSUP
CLOTSUP
CLUBSUP
COILSUP
COMESUP
COOKSUP
COOPSUP
CORKSUP
CRIESUP
CROPSUP
CROSSUP
CRUDSUP
CURLSUP
DEALSUP
DIALSUP
DOLLSUP
DRAGSUP
DRAWSUP
DRESSUP
DRIESUP
DRUMSUP
DUDESUP
EASESUP
EVENSUP
FAIRSUP
FILLSUP
FIRESUP
FIRMSUP
FIXESUP
FLIESUP
FOLDSUP
FOOTSUP
FORKSUP
FOULSUP
FREESUP
FRIESUP
FUELSUP
GANGSUP
GASESUP
GEARSUP
GIVESUP
GLAMSUP
GOOFSUP
GROWSUP
HACKSUP
HANDSUP
HANGSUP
HAULSUP
HEADSUP
HEALSUP
HEAPSUP
HEATSUP
HELPSUP
HIKESUP
HOLDSUP
HOLESUP
HOOKSUP
HUNTSUP
HYPESUP
JACKSUP
JERKSUP
JOINSUP
JUMPSUP
KEEPSUP
KICKSUP
KNEESUP
KNOTSUP
LACESUP
LANDSUP
LEADSUP
LEAPSUP
LICKSUP
LIFTSUP
LINESUP
LINKSUP
LOADSUP
LOCKSUP
LOOKSUP
MAKESUP
MARKSUP
MEETSUP
MILKSOP
MISTSUP
MIXESUP
MOCKSUP
MOVESUP
MUCKSUP
NAILSUP
NOSESUP
OPENSUP
OVERSUP
PACKSUP
PAIRSUP
PERKSUP
PICKSUP
PILESUP
PINESAP
PIPESUP
PLAYSUP
PLOWSUP
PLUGSUP
PRESSUP
PROPSUP
PUFFSUP
PULLSUP
PUMPSUP
RACESUP
RACKSUP
RAKESUP
RAMPSUP
READSUP
REARSUP
REELSUP
RESTSUP
RIDESUP
RILESUP
RINGSUP
RISESUP
ROLLSUP
ROOTSUP
ROPESUP
RUCKSUP
SACKSUP
SAVESUP
SEALSUP
SENDSUP
SHOWSUP
SHUTSUP
SIGNSUP
SIZESUP
SLIPSUP
SLOWSUP
SNAGSUP
SNAPSUP
SOAKSUP
SOAPSUP
SOUPSUP
STAYSUP
STEPSUP
STIRSUP
STOPSUP
SUCKSUP
SUITSUP
SURFSUP
SWIMSUP
TACKSUP
TAKESUP
TALKSUP
TANKSUP
TAPESUP
TARTSUP
TEAMSUP
TEARSUP
TILTSUP
TIMESUP
TONESUP
TOOLSUP
TOTESUP
TREESAP
TRIPSUP
TROTSUP
TRUESUP
TRUSSUP
TUNESUP
TURNSUP
TYPESUP
WAITSUP
WAKESUP
WALLSUP
WARMSUP
WAXESUP
WELLSUP
WHATSUP
WHIPSUP
WINDSUP
WINESAP
WIPESUP
WIRESUP
WISESUP
WORKSUP
WRAPSUP

•••••SP
ENCLASP
MUDWASP
RECLASP
REGRASP
UNCLASP

SQ•••••
SQUALID
SQUALLS
SQUALLY
SQUALOR
SQUANTO
SQUARED
SQUARER
SQUARES
SQUASHY
SQUATLY
SQUATTY
SQUAWKS
SQUAWKY
SQUEAKS
SQUEAKY
SQUEALS
SQUEERS
SQUEEZE
SQUELCH
SQUINCH
SQUINTS
SQUINTY
SQUIRED
SQUIRES
SQUIRMS
SQUIRMY
SQUIRTS
SQUISHY

S•Q••••
SEQUELS
SEQUINS
SEQUOIA
SEQUOYA

S••Q•••
SACQUES

S•••••Q
SILENTQ

•SQ••••
ASQUIET
ASQUINT
ASQUITH
ESQUIRE
TSQUARE

•S•••Q•
PSANDQS

••SQ•••
BASQUES
BISQUES
CASQUED
CASQUES
MASQUER
MASQUES
MOSQUES
NESQUIK
VASQUEZ

••S••Q•
POSSLQS

•••SQ••
BRUSQUE
PRESQUE

•••S•Q•
POSSLQS

S•R••••
SARACEN
SARALEE
SARANAC
SARAWAK
SARAZEN
SARCASM
SARDINE
SARGENT
SARNOFF
SARONGS
SAROYAN
SARTORS
SARUMAN
SCRAGGY
SCRAPED
SCRAPER
SCRAPES
SCRAPPY
SCRATCH
SCRAWLS
SCRAWLY
SCRAWNY
SCREAKS
SCREAMS
SCREECH
SCREEDS
SCREENS
SCREWED
SCREWUP
SCRIBED
SCRIBER
SCRIBES
SCRIMPS
SCRIMPY
SCRIPPS
SCRIPTS
SCROLLS
SCROOGE
SCRUBBY
SCRUBUP
SCRUFFS
SCRUFFY
SCRUGGS
SCRUNCH
SCRUPLE
SERAPES
SERAPHS
SERAPIS
SERBIAN
SERENER
SERFAGE
SERFDOM
SERIALS
SERIATE
SERIESE
SERIESF
SERIESG
SERIESH
SERIESI
SERIESJ
SERIESK
SERIOUS
SERIPAK
SERLING
SERMONS
SERPENS
SERPENT
SERPICO
SERRATE
SERVANT
SERVEAS
SERVERS
SERVEUP
SERVICE
SERVILE
SERVING
SHRIEKS
SHRIKES
SHRILLS
SHRILLY
SHRIMPS
SHRIMPY
SHRINED
SHRINER
SHRINES
SHRINKS
SHRIVEL
SHRIVER
SHRIVES
SHROUDS
SHRUBBY
SIRDUKE
SIRENED
SIRLOIN
SIROCCO
SORBATE
SORBETS
SORCERY
SORDINI
SORDINO
SORENTO
SORGHUM
SORIANO
SORORAL
SORRELL
SORRELS
SORRIER
SORRILY
SORROWS
SORTERS
SORTIED
SORTIES
SORTING
SORTOUT
SORVINO
SPRAINS
SPRAWLS
SPRAWLY
SPRAYED
SPRAYER
SPRAYON
SPREADS
SPRIEST
SPRINGS
SPRINGY
SPRINTS
SPRITES
SPROUTS
SPRUCED
SPRUCER
SPRUCES
SPRYEST
STRAFED
STRAFER
STRAFES
STRAINS
STRAITS
STRANDS
STRANGE
STRAPIN
STRAPON
STRASSE
STRATAS
STRATUM
STRATUS
STRAUSS
STRAYED
STRAYER
STREAKS
STREAKY
STREAMS
STREETS
STREGIS
STRETCH
STRETTI
STRETTO
STREWED
STREWER
STRIATE
STRIDER
STRIDES
STRIFES
STRIKER
STRIKES
STRINGS
STRINGY
STRIPED
STRIPER
STRIPES
STRIPOF
STRITCH
STRIVED
STRIVEN
STRIVER
STRIVES
STROBES
STROKED
STROKER
STROKES
STROLLS
STROPHE
STROUSE
STRUDEL
SUREBET
SURECAN
SUREIAM
SUREIDO
SUREROF
SURFACE
SURFEIT
SURFERS
SURFIER
SURFING
SURFMAN
SURFMEN
SURFSUP
SURGEON
SURGERY
SURGING
SURIMIS
SURINAM
SURLIER
SURLILY
SURMISE
SURNAME
SURPASS
SURPLUS
SURREAL
SURREYS
SURVEIL
SURVEYS
SURVIVE
SYRIANA
SYRIANS
SYRINGE

S••R•••
SABRINA
SANREMO
SATRAPS
SATRAPY
SAURIAN
SCARABS
SCARCER
SCAREDY
SCARERS
SCAREUP
SCARFED
SCARFER
SCARFUP
SCARIER
SCARIFY
SCARILY
SCARING
SCARLET
SCARPED
SCARRED
SCARVES
SCARWID
SCORERS
SCORIAS
SCORING
SCORNED
SCORNER
SCORPIO
SCURVES
SEARACE
SEARERS
SEARING
SEBRING
SECRECY
SECRETE
SECRETS
SEERESS
SERRATE
SETRATE
SHAREIN
SHARERS
SHARING
SHARKEY
SHARONA
SHARPED
SHARPEI
SHARPEN
SHARPER
SHARPIE
SHARPLY
SHERBET
SHERIFF
SHERIFS
SHERMAN
SHERPAS
SHERWIN
SHIRKED
SHIRKER
SHIRLEY
SHIRRED
SHOREUP
SHORING
SHORTED
SHORTEN
SHORTER
SHORTIE
SHORTLY
SHORTOF
SIERRAS
SKIRACE
SKIRACK
SKIRLED
SKIRTED
SKIRTER
SKIRUNS
SLURPED
SLURPEE
SLURPER
SLURRED
SMARTED
SMARTEN
SMARTER
SMARTLY
SMIRKED
SMIRKER
SMIRNOV
SNARERS
SNARFED
SNARING
SNARLAT
SNARLED
SNARLER
SNARLUP
SNORERS
SNORING
SNORKEL
SNORTAT
SNORTED
SNORTER
SOARERS
SOAREWE
SOARING
SOIREES
SOPRANI
SOPRANO
SORRELL
SORRELS
SORRIER
SORRILY
SORROWS
SOURALE
SOURCED
SOURCES
SOUREST
SOURING
SOURISH
SOURSON
SPARELY
SPAREME
SPARERS
SPAREST
SPARING
SPARKED
SPARKLE
SPARKLY
SPARRED
SPARRER
SPARROW
SPARSER
SPARTAN
SPIRALS
SPIREAS
SPIRIER
SPIRITS
SPORRAN
SPORTED
SPORTIN
SPURNED
SPURNER
SPURRED
SPURSON
SPURTED
SPYRING
STARCHY
STARDOM
STAREAT
STARERS
STARING
STARION
STARKER
STARKEY
STARKLY
STARLET
STARLIT
STARLOG
STARMAN
STARMAP
STARRED
STARSIN
STARSKY
STARTED
STARTER
STARTIN
STARTLE
STARTON
STARTTO
STARTUP
STARVED
STARVES
STCROIX
STEREOS
STERILE
STERNAL
STERNER
STERNLY
STERNOS
STERNUM
STEROID
STEROLS
STERTOR
STIRFRY
STIRRED
STIRRER
STIRRUP
STIRSIN
STIRSUP
STORAGE
STORERS
STOREUP
STORIED
STORIES
STORING
STORMED
STORMIN
STURGES
STYRENE
SUBRACE
SUBROOT
SUBROSA
SUCRASE
SUCROSE
SUNRAYS
SUNRISE
SUNROOF
SUNROOM
SUPREME
SURREAL
SURREYS
SVERIGE
SWARMED
SWARMER
SWARTHY
SWERVED
SWERVES
SWIRLED
SWOREAT
SWOREBY
SWOREIN
SWORETO

S•••R••
SABERED
SAFARIS
SAFFRON
SAHARAN
SALERNO
SAMARAS
SAMARIA
SAMPRAS
SAMURAI
SANGRIA
SATIRES
SATIRIC
SATORIS
SATURNS
SATYRIC
SAVARIN

SAVORED
SAVORER
SCARRED
SCHERZI
SCHERZO
SCHIRRA
SCIORRA
SCLERAE
SCLERAL
SCLERAS
SCOURED
SCOURER
SCOURGE
SEAARMS
SEAGRAM
SEAGREN
SEATRIP
SECURED
SECURER
SECURES
SEESRED
SEFERIS
SEMIRAW
SENORAS
SENORES
SENTRAS
SEPIRAS
SETFREE
SEVERAL
SEVERED
SEVERER
SEVERUS
SEWARDS
SHADROE
SHAGRUG
SHEARED
SHEARER
SHECRAB
SHEERED
SHEERER
SHEERLY
SHIRRED
SHYFROM
SIBERIA
SIERRAS
SIXIRON
SKIAREA
SKIDROW
SKITRIP
SLURRED
SMEARED
SMEARER
SMEARON
SNEERAT
SNEERED
SNEERER
SOBERED
SOBERER
SOBERLY
SOFARAS
SOLARAS
SOLARIA
SONORAN
SORORAL
SOSORRY
SPARRED
SPARRER
SPARROW
SPEARED
SPEARER
SPHERAL
SPHERED
SPHERES
SPHERIC
SPLURGE
SPORRAN
SPURRED
SQUARED
SQUARER
SQUARES
SQUIRED
SQUIRES
SQUIRMS
SQUIRMY
SQUIRTS
STAIRED
STARRED
STBARTS
STEARIC
STEARIN
STEARNS
STEERED
STEERER
STIRRED
STIRRER
STIRRUP
STMARKS
STMARYS
STUARTI
SUBAREA
SUBARID
SUBARUS
SUBORNS
SUBURBS
SUGARED
SUHARTO
SUKARNO
SUPERGS
SUREROF
SUTURED
SUTURES
SWEARAT
SWEARBY
SWEARER
SWEARIN
SWEARTO
SYNERGY

S••••R•

SACKERS
SAGCARD
SAGUARO
SAILERS
SAILORS
SALIERI
SALTERS
SALVERS
SALVORS
SAMBORA
SANBORN
SANDERS
SANFORD
SAPPERS
SAPPORO
SARTORS
SASSERS
SAUCERS
SAVIORS
SAVOURS
SAVOURY
SAWYERS
SAXHORN
SAYMORE
SCALARS
SCALERS
SCARERS
SCENERY
SCEPTRE
SCHIRRA
SCIORRA
SCOLARI
SCORERS
SCOTERS
SEABIRD
SEABORG
SEAFARE
SEAFERN
SEAGIRT
SEAHERO
SEALERS
SEALERY
SEAMERS
SEAPORT
SEARERS
SEATERS
SEAWARD
SECTORS
SEEDERS
SEEHERE
SEEKERS
SEETHRU
SEINERS
SEIZERS
SEIZORS
SEIZURE
SELKIRK
SELLERS
SEMIDRY
SEMIPRO
SENDERS
SENHORA
SENIORS
SENSORS
SENSORY
SERVERS
SETTERS
SHADERS
SHAKERS
SHAKIRA
SHANGRI
SHAPERS
SHAPIRO
SHARERS
SHASTRI
SHAVERS
SHEPARD
SHINERS
SHIVERS
SHIVERY
SHOFARS
SHOVERS
SHOWERS
SHOWERY
SHUBERT
SIDDURS
SIDEARM
SIFTERS
SIGHERS
SIGNERS
SIGNORA
SIGNORE
SIGNORS
SILVERS
SILVERY
SIMMERS
SIMPERS
SINATRA
SINCERE
SINGERS
SINKERS
SINNERS
SIPPERS
SISTERS
SITTERS
SKATERS
SKEWERS
SKYLARK
SKYNYRD
SKYSURF
SKYWARD
SLAKERS
SLATERS
SLAVERS
SLAVERY
SLAYERS
SLICERS
SLIDERS
SLIVERS
SLOPERS
SMILERS
SMITERS
SMOKERS
SNAKERS
SNARERS
SNIPERS
SNORERS
SOAKERS
SOAPERS
SOARERS
SOBBERS
SOJOURN
SOLDERS
SOLVERS
SOONERS
SORCERY
SORTERS
SOSORRY
SOTHERE
SOTHERN
SOUPERS
SPACERS
SPADERS
SPARERS
SPAYERS
SPECTRA
SPECTRE
SPEWERS
SPICERS
SPICERY
SPIDERS
SPIDERY
SPIKERS
SPINDRY
SPYDERS
SPYWARE
SQUEERS
STAGERS
STARERS
STATERS
STATORS
STATURE
STAYDRY
STAYERS
STEWARD
STEWART
STEWERS
STIRFRY
STOKERS
STONERS
STORERS
STOWERS
STUPORS
STYLERS
SUBFORM
SUBSORT
SUBVERT
SUBWARS
SUBZERO
SUCCORS
SUCKDRY
SUCKERS
SUDBURY
SUDSERS
SUFFERS
SUITORS
SULKERS
SUMATRA
SUMMARY
SUMMERS
SUMMERY
SUNBIRD
SUNBURN
SUNDERS
SUNFIRE
SUNWARD
SUPPERS
SUPPORT
SURFERS
SURGERY
SUSPIRE
SWAYERS
SWELTRY
SWIGERT
SWINERY
SWIPERS
SZILARD

S•••••R

SADDLER
SAGGIER
SALAZAR
SALEMOR
SALLIER
SALTIER
SALUTER
SAMOVAR
SAMPLER
SANDBAR
SANDBUR
SANDIER
SANDLER
SAPPIER
SASSIER
SAUCIER
SAUNTER
SAVAGER
SAVEFOR
SAVIOUR
SAVORER
SAVVIER
SAYOVER
SCALDER
SCALIER
SCALPER
SCAMMER
SCAMPER
SCANNER
SCANTER
SCARCER
SCARFER
SCARIER
SCATTER
SCENTER
SCEPTER
SCHEMER
SCHMEAR
SCHMEER
SCHOLAR
SCHUMER
SCISSOR
SCOFFER
SCOLDER
SCOOPER
SCOOTER
SCORNER
SCOURER
SCOUTER
SCOWLER
SCRAPER
SCRIBER
SCUDDER
SCUFFER
SCULLER
SCUPPER
SEAMIER
SEASTAR
SECEDER
SECONDR
SECULAR
SECURER
SEDATER
SEDGIER
SEDUCER
SEEDIER
SEEPIER
SELLFOR
SELTZER
SEMINAR
SENATOR
SENDFOR
SENTFOR
SERENER
SETTLER
SETTLOR
SEVERER
SEYMOUR
SHADIER
SHAFFER
SHAKIER
SHALIER
SHANKAR
SHANTER
SHARPER
SHATNER
SHATTER
SHEARER
SHEBEAR
SHEDDER
SHEERER
SHEFFER
SHELLER
SHELTER
SHELVER
SHIFTER
SHIMMER
SHINIER
SHIPPER
SHIRKER
SHOCKER
SHOOTER
SHOPFOR
SHOPPER
SHORTER
SHOTFOR
SHOTPAR
SHOUTER
SHOWIER
SHRINER
SHRIVER
SHUCKER
SHUDDER
SHUNTER
SHUSTER
SHUTTER
SHYSTER
SIDEBAR
SIDECAR
SIGHFOR
SIGHTER
SIGNFOR
SILENTR
SILKIER
SILLIER
SILTIER
SIMILAR
SIMPLER
SISENOR
SISSIER
SITSFOR
SIXFOUR
SIXYEAR
SIZZLER
SKEETER
SKELTER
SKIDDER
SKIMMER
SKINNER
SKIPPER
SKIRTER
SKITTER
SKIWEAR
SKULKER
SLACKER
SLAMMER
SLANDER
SLAPPER
SLASHER
SLATHER
SLATIER
SLEDDER
SLEEKER
SLEEPER
SLENDER
SLICKER
SLIMIER
SLIMMER
SLINGER
SLINKER
SLIPPER
SLITHER
SLITTER
SLOBBER
SLOGGER
SLOTCAR
SLOTTER
SLUGGER
SLUMBER
SLUMMER
SLURPER
SMACKER
SMALLER
SMARTER
SMASHER
SMATTER
SMEARER
SMELLER
SMELTER
SMIRKER
SMOKIER
SMOLDER
SMOTHER
SMUCKER
SMUGGER
SNACKER
SNAGGER
SNAKIER
SNAPPER
SNARLER
SNEAKER
SNEERER
SNEEZER
SNICKER
SNIFFER
SNIFTER
SNIPPER
SNOOKER
SNOOPER
SNOOZER
SNORTER
SNOWIER
SNUBBER
SNUFFER
SNUGGER
SOAPIER
SOBERER
SODDIER
SOGGIER
SOLACER
SOLDFOR
SOLDIER
SOLIDER
SOOTHER
SOOTIER
SOPPIER
SORRIER
SOUNDER
SOUPIER
SOWSEAR
SPACIER
SPAMMER
SPANAIR
SPANKER
SPANNER
SPARRER
SPARSER
SPATTER
SPAWNER
SPEAKER
SPEARER
SPECTER
SPECTOR
SPEEDER
SPELLER
SPENCER
SPENDER
SPENSER
SPICIER
SPIELER
SPIKIER
SPILLER
SPINIER
SPINNER
SPIRIER
SPITTER
SPLICER
SPOILER
SPONGER
SPONSOR
SPOOFER
SPOOLER
SPOONER
SPOTTER
SPOUTER
SPRAYER
SPRUCER
SPUMIER
SPURNER
SPUTTER
SQUALOR
SQUARER
STABBER
STABLER
STACKER
STADLER
STAFFER
STAGGER
STAGIER
STAIDER
STAINER
STALKER
STALLER
STAMMER
STAMPER
STANDER
STAPLER
STARKER
STARTER
STATLER
STAYFOR
STEALER
STEAMER
STEELER
STEEPER
STEERER
STEIGER
STEINER
STELLAR
STENTOR
STEPPER
STERNER
STERTOR
STEWIER
STICKER
STIFFER
STILLER
STINGER
STINKER
STINTER
STIRRER
STOCKER
STONIER
STOOPER
STOPFOR
STOPPER
STOUTER
STPETER
STRAFER
STRAYER
STREWER
STRIDER
STRIKER
STRIPER
STRIVER
STROKER
STUDIER
STUFFER
STUMPER
STUNNER
STUTTER
SUBDUER
SUBTLER
SUCCOUR
SUCKIER
SUDSIER
SUEDFOR
SUESFOR
SULKIER
SULPHUR
SUNNIER
SUPPLER
SURFIER
SURLIER
SVELTER
SWABBER
SWAGGER
SWANKER
SWAPPER
SWARMER
SWATTER
SWAYBAR
SWEARER
SWEATER
SWEEPER
SWEETER
SWELLER
SWELTER
SWIFTER
SWILLER
SWIMMER
SWINGER
SWITZER
SWOONER
SWOOPER

•SR••••

ISRAELI
ISRAFEL

•S•R•••

ASARULE
ASCRIBE
ASHRAMS
ASPRAWL
ASTREAM
ASTRIDE
CSARDAS
ESCROWS
ESPRITS
ESTRADA
ESTRAYS
ESTRING
GSTRING
ISTRIAN
ISUREAM
ISUREDO
JSTROKE
OSIRIAN
OSPREYS
OSTRAVA
OSTRICH
TSARDOM
TSARINA
TSARISM
TSARIST
TSTRAPS
USERFEE
USERIDS
USGRANT
USURERS
USURIES
USURPED
USURPER

•S••R••

ASAGRAY
ASCARED
ASFARAS
ASHTRAY
ASHTREE
ASMARAN
ASPERSE
ASPIRED
ASPIRER
ASPIRES
ASPIRIN
ASSERTS
ASSORTS
ASSURED
ASSURER
ASSURES
ASSUROR
ASSYRIA
ASTARTE
ASTERIX
ASTORIA
ESCARPS
ESCORTS
ESPARTO
ESTORIL
ISOGRAM
OSBORNE
OSETRAS
OSIERED
TSHIRTS
TSOURIS
USHERED
USHERIN

•S•••R•

ASALARK
ASHBERY
ASHBURN
ASHBURY
ASHFORD
ASHLARS
ASSHARP
ASTAIRE
ESCHERS
ESOTERY
ESQUIRE
ESTUARY
ISADORA
ISADORE
ISIDORE
ISOBARS
ISOMERS
ISSUERS
MSIEURS
OSSETRA
OSSUARY
OSTIARY
OSTLERS
OSTMARK
PSYWARS
TSQUARE
USURERS

•S••••R

ASHIVER
ASIMMER
ASKOVER
ASKSFOR
ASPIRER
ASSAYER
ASSUMER
ASSURER
ASSUROR
ASTUTER
ASUNDER
ESCAPER
ESSAYER
OSCULAR
PSALTER
USEDCAR
USEDFOR
USESFOR
USOTOUR
USURPER

••SR•••

BASRHIN
BUSRIDE
DISRATE
DISROBE
DISRUPT
HASROOM
MISRATE
MISREAD
MISRELY
MISRULE

••S•R••

ABSORBS
ADSORBS
ALSORAN
AMSCRAY
ASSERTS
ASSORTS
ASSURED
ASSURER
ASSURES
ASSUROR
ASSYRIA
AUSTRAL
AUSTRIA
BESTREW
BISTROS
BUSTRIP
CASERNE
CASERNS
CASERTA
CASTROL
DESERET
DESERTS
DESERVE
DESIRED
DESIREE
DESIRER
DESIRES
DESTROY
DISARMS
DISHRAG
DISTROS
DUSTRAG
ENSURED
ENSURER
ENSURES
EXSERTS
GASTRIC
HASAROW
IMSORRY
INSERTS
INSURED
INSURER
INSURES
ITSTRUE
KESTREL
LASORDA
LASTROW
LUSTRAL
LUSTRED
LUSTRES
LUSTRUM
MASARYK
MISBREW
MISDRAW
MISDREW
MISERLY
MISTRAL
MUSKRAT
NOSIREE
NOSTRIL
NOSTRUM
OBSERVE

OFSORTS
ONSERVE
PISARRO
PUSHROD
RASURES
RESCRUB
RESERVE
RESORBS
RESORTS
RESPRAY
RESTRAP
RESTREW
RESTRIP
RESURGE
ROSARIO
ROSERED
ROSTRAL
ROSTRUM
SOSORRY
TASERED
TESTRUN
UNSCREW
UNSORRY
UNSORTS
UNSTRAP
UNSURLY
UPSURGE
VESTRAL
VESTRON
VISORED
WASHRAG
WASTREL
YESORNO

••S••R•

ANSWERS
ASSHARP
AUSTERE
AUSTERS
BASHERS
BASTERS
BESTIRS
BUSFARE
BUSGIRL
BUSHERS
BUSKERS
BUSSERS
BUSTARD
BUSTERS
CASPARY
CASTERS
CDSTORE
CESAIRE
CISTERN
COSHERS
COSTARD
COSTARS
CUSSERS
CUSTARD
CUSTERS
DASHERS
DASTARD
DESSERT
DISBARS
DISCARD
DISCERN
DISCORD
DISEURS
DISPART
DISPORT
DISSERT
DISTORT
DISTURB
DUSTERS
EASTERN
EASTERS
ENSNARE
ENSNARL
FESTERS
FISHERS
FISHERY
FISHFRY
FISSURE
FOSTERS
FUSSERS
GASPARD
GASPERS
GASSERS
GASTERO
GASWARS
GESTURE
GISCARD
GOSFORD
GUSHERS
HASTERT
HISSERS
HISTORY
HOSIERS
HOSIERY
HUSKERS
HUSSARS
HUSSERL
IMSORRY
INSHORE
INSHORT
INSPIRE
INSTORE
IRSFORM
ISSUERS
ITSHERE
JASPERS
JASPERY
JESTERS
JOSHERS
KISSERS
KOSHERS
LASCARS
LASHERS
LASTORY
LESABRE
LESSORS
LISPERS
LISTERS
LOSTART
LUSTERS
MASCARA
MASHERS
MASKERS
MASONRY
MASTERP
MASTERS
MASTERY
MISFIRE
MISFORM
MISMARK
MISSORT
MISTERM
MISTERS
MISTERX
MISWIRE
MISWORD
MOSHERS
MUSHERS
MUSTARD
MUSTERS
MYSTARS
MYSTERY
NESTERS
NESTORS
NOSCORE
NOSEBRA
NOSHERS
NOSTARS
OBSCURA
OBSCURE
ONSHORE
OSSETRA
OSSUARY
OUSTERS
OYSTERS
PASSERS
PASTERN
PASTERS
PASTORS
PASTURE
PESTERS
PISARRO
PISMIRE
POSEURS
POSTERN
POSTERS
POSTURE
PUSHERS
RASBORA
RASHERS
RASPERS
RASTERS
RESCORE
RESHARE
RESPARK
RESPIRE
RESTART
RESTERS
RESTIRS
RESTORE
RESWORE
RESWORN
RISKERS
ROSTERS
RUSHERS
RUSSERT
SASSERS
SISTERS
SOSORRY
SUSPIRE
TASTERS
TESSERA
TESTERS
TOSHIRO
TOSPARE
TOSSERS
TOSTART
TUSHERY
TUSKERS
TVSTARS
ULSTERS
UNSHARP
UNSHORN
UNSHORT
UNSMART
UNSNARL
UNSORRY
UNSTERN
UNSWORE
UNSWORN
UPSOARS
UPSTARE
UPSTART
UPSTIRS
VESPERS
VESTURE
VISCERA
WASHERS
WASSURE
WASTERS
WESTERN
WESTERS
WISHERS
XYSTERS
YESSIRE
ZESTERS

••S•••R

ASSAYER
ASSUMER
ASSURER
ASSUROR
BASSIER
BESMEAR
BOSSIER
BUSHIER
BUSTIER
BUSTLER
BUSTOUR
CASHBAR
CASHIER
CASIMIR
COSTNER
CUSHIER
CUSSLER
DASHIER
DESIRER
DESPAIR
DISHIER
DOSSIER
DUSKIER
DUSTIER
ENSURER
ESSAYER
FASTCAR
FISCHER
FISHFOR
FISHIER
FUSSIER
FUSTIER
GASSIER
GUSHIER
GUSTIER
HASOVER
HASTIER
HISSIER
HOSTLER
HUSKIER
HUSTLER
INSANER
INSIDER
INSOFAR
INSULAR
INSURER
ITSOVER
JOSTLER
KASHMIR
KASTLER
KOSOVAR
LASSOER
LESSTAR
LUSHIER
LUSTIER
MASQUER
MASSEUR
MASSIER
MESHIER
MESSIER
MISAVER
MISDOER
MISHEAR
MISTIER
MISUSER
MOSSIER
MRSMUIR
MUSHIER
MUSKIER
MUSSIER
MUSTIER
NASTIER
NESTLER
NOSUGAR
ONSAGER
PASSFOR
PASTEUR
PASTIER
PESKIER
POSTWAR
PUSHFOR
PUSHIER
RASPIER
RASSLER
RESCUER
RESIDER
RESIZER
RESOLER
RESWEAR
RISKIER
ROSSNER
RUSHIER
RUSTIER
RUSTLER
SASSIER
SISENOR
SISSIER
TASKBAR
TASTIER
TESTFOR
TESTIER
UNSAFER
UNSHEER
UNSHIER
UNSHYER
UNSLIER
UNSLYER
UNSOBER
UNSWEAR
UPSTAIR
VASTIER
VISITOR
WASFAIR
WASHIER
WASPIER
WISHFOR
WISPIER
YESDEAR
ZESTIER

•••SR••

GETSRID
KIDSRUS
LETSRIP
MARSRED
RUBSRAW
SEESRED
TOYSRUS

•••S•R•

ABASERS
ABUSERS
ALBSURE
AMUSERS
BERSERK
BURSARS
BUSSERS
CAESARS
CAESURA
CAUSERS
CENSERS
CENSORS
CENSURE
CHASERS
CLOSERS
CLOSURE
CONSORT
CURSERS
CURSORS
CURSORY
CUSSERS
DESSERT
DISSERT
DOUSERS
DOWSERS
DYKSTRA
EGOSURF
ELUSORY
ERASERS
ERASURE
EYESORE
FISSURE
FORSURE
FRUSTRO
FUSSERS
GASSERS
GETSORE
GEYSERS
GOESPRO
GOTSORE
HANSARP
HAWSERS
HISSERS
HOFSTRA
HUSSARS
HUSSERL
KAISERS
KISSERS
LAPSERS
LEASERS
LEISURE
LESSORS
MAESTRO
MANSARD
MAUSERS
MEASURE
MIASARA
MISSORT
MONSTRO
MOUSERS
NETSURF
NOOSERS
NOTSURE
NUESTRA
NUESTRO
NURSERS
NURSERY
ODDSARE
OFASORT
OLESTRA
OUTSERT
PARSERS
PASSERS
PATSDRY
PAUSERS
PCUSERS
PHASERS
PIASTRE
POISERS
PRESORT
PROSERS
PULSARS
PURSERS
QUASARS
QUESERA
RAISERS
REUSERS
RINSERS
ROBSART
RONSARD
ROUSERS
RUNSDRY
RUSSERT
SASSERS
SENSORS
SENSORY
SHASTRI
SKYSURF
SUBSORT
SUDSERS
TEASERS
TENSORS
TESSERA
TONSURE
TOSSERS
WASSURE
YESSIRE

•••S••R

ACTSFOR
AIMSFOR
ALLSTAR
AMASSER
ANTSIER
ARTSIER
ASKSFOR
BASSIER
BATSFOR
BEGSFOR
BIDSFOR
BIGSTAR
BITSIER
BLASTER
BLESSER
BLISTER
BLUSHER
BLUSTER
BOASTER
BOLSTER
BONSOIR
BOOSLER
BOOSTER
BOSSIER
BOXSTER
BRASHER
BRASIER
BRISKER
BRUSHER
BURSTER
CHASTER
CHESTER
CLASHER
CLASPER
CLASSER
CLUSTER
COASTER
CORSAIR
CRASHER
CRASSER
CRISPER
CROSIER
CROSSER
CRUSHER
CUSSLER
DANSEUR
DAYSTAR
DIESFOR
DIGSFOR
DITSIER
DOESFOR
DOGSEAR
DOGSTAR
DOSSIER
DRESSER
EDASNER
FANSLER
FARSEER
FEASTER
FIBSTER
FLASHER
FLOSSER
FLUSHER
FLUSTER
FORSTER
FRASIER
FRESHER
FRISEUR
FRISKER
FROSTER
FUBSIER
FUNSTER
FUSSIER
GAGSTER
GASSIER
GETSFAR
GLISTER
GLOSSER
GNASHER
GOESFAR
GOESFOR
GOOSIER
GORSIER
GRASPER
GRISTER
GROSSER
GUESSER
GUNSFOR
GUTSIER
HAMSTER
HARSHER
HIPSTER
HISSIER
HITSFOR
HOISTER
HOLSTER
HOOSIER
HORSIER
HOTSPUR
INASTIR
INKSTER
IRISHER
JETSTAR
JOUSTER
KEESLAR
KEESLER
KEISTER
KLISTER
KRASNER
LASSOER
LAYSFOR
LEISTER
LESSTAR
LIESFOR
LOBSTER
LOESSER
LOUSIER
MARSBAR
MASSEUR
MASSIER
MEISTER
MESSIER
MINSTER
MOBSTER
MOISTER
MONSTER
MOSSIER
MOUSIER
MUNSTER
MUSSIER
NAPSTER
NETSTER
NEWSIER
NOISIER
NUTSIER
OLDSTER
ONESTAR
OPTSFOR
OUTSOAR
PASSFOR
PAYSFOR
PHISHER
PIASTER
PILSNER
PLASTER
PLUSHER
POPSTAR
PRESPUR
PRESSER
PROSIER
PROSPER
PUNSTER
PURSIER
PURSUER
QUESTER
RAPSTAR
RASSLER
REDSTAR
REPSFOR
ROASTER
ROISTER
ROOSTER
ROSSNER
ROUSTER
RUNSFOR
SASSIER
SCISSOR
SEASTAR
SHUSTER
SHYSTER
SISSIER
SITSFOR
SLASHER
SMASHER
SOWSEAR
SUDSIER
SUESFOR
TAPSTER
TELSTAR
THESTAR
THUSFAR
TINSTAR
TIPSIER
TIPSTER
TOASTER
TRASHER
TRISTAR
TRUSTER
TRYSTER
TWISTER
TWOSTAR
USESFOR
VIESFOR
VORSTER
WEBSTER
WHISKER
WHISPER
WOOSTER
WRESTER
YENSFOR

••••SR•

LEXUSRX

••••S•R

ACCUSER
ADVISER
ADVISOR
ALUNSER
AMASSER
AROUSER
BLESSER
BROWSER
BRUISER
CHOOSER
CLASSER
COARSER
COURSER
CRASSER
CREASER
CROSSER
CRUISER
DEARSIR
DEBASER
DEFUSER
DEPOSER
DEVISER
DEVISOR
DIVISOR
DREISER
DRESSER
ENDUSER
EXCUSER
EXPOSER
FLENSER
FLOSSER
FOCUSER
GLOSSER
GREASER
GROSSER
GROUSER
GUESSER
GUNUSER
HOARSER
IMPOSER
INCISOR
INFUSER
IONISER
KLEISER
LOESSER
MACUSER
MISUSER
NONUSER
NOWISER
OBTUSER
OPPOSER
PERUSER
PLAISIR
PLEASER
PRAISER
PRESSER
REFUSER
REPOSER
REVISER
REVISOR
SCISSOR
SPARSER
SPENSER
SPONSOR
THEUSSR
TROUSER
UNWISER
UPRISER
WINDSOR

•••••SR

THEUSSR

SS•••••

SSHAPED
SSSSSSS

S•S••••

SASHAYS
SASHIMI
SASHING
SASSERS
SASSIER
SASSILY
SASSING
SASSOON
SESAMES
SESSILE
SESSION
SESTETS
SESTINA
SISENOR
SISSIER
SISSIES
SISTERS
SISTINE
SOSORRY
SOSPADS
SOSUEME
SSSSSSS
STSIMON
SUSANNA
SUSANNE
SUSPECT
SUSPEND
SUSPIRE
SUSSING
SUSSOUT
SUSTAIN
SYSTEMS
SYSTOLE

S••S•••

SADSACK
SADSONG
SAISONS
SALSODA
SAMSONS
SAMSUNG
SANSEIS
SAPSAGO
SASSERS
SASSIER
SASSILY
SASSING
SASSOON
SATSUMA
SAUSAGE
SAWSOFF
SAYSAAH
SAYSAYE
SAYSBOO
SAYSIDO
SAYSNAY
SAYSWHO
SAYSYES
SAYSYOU
SCISSOR
SCUSEME
SEASALT
SEASICK
SEASIDE
SEASLUG
SEASONS
SEASTAR
SEESALL
SEESAWS
SEESFIT
SEESOFF
SEESOUT
SEESRED
SEISMAL
SEISMIC
SENSATE
SENSEIS
SENSENS
SENSING
SENSORS
SENSORY
SENSUAL
SESSILE
SESSION
SETSAIL
SETSHOT
SETSOFF
SETSOUT
SHASTRI
SHUSHED
SHUSHES
SHUSTER
SHYSTER
SIESTAS
SISSIER
SISSIES
SITSFOR
SITSOUT
SITSPAT
SKISHOP
SKISUIT
SKOSHES
SKYSURF
SLASHED
SLASHER
SLASHES
SLOSHED
SLOSHES
SLUSHED
SLUSHES
SMASHED
SMASHER
SMASHES
SMASHUP
SMUSHED
SMUSHES
SONSHIP
SOUSING
SOWSEAR
SPASSKY
SSSSSSS
STASHED
STASHES
STASSEN
SUASION
SUASIVE
SUBSECT
SUBSETS

SUBSIDE
SUBSIDY
SUBSIST
SUBSOIL
SUBSORT
SUBSUME
SUDSERS
SUDSIER
SUDSING
SUESFOR
SUNSETS
SUNSFAN
SUNSPOT
SUNSUIT
SUSSING
SUSSOUT
SWASHED
SWASHES
SWISHED
SWISHES
SZYSLAK

S•••S••

SACKSUP
SADISTS
SAILSON
SAILSTO
SALTSEA
SAMISEN
SAMOSAS
SAMOSET
SAMPSON
SATISFY
SAVESON
SAVESUP
SCADSOF
SCHISMS
SCHISTS
SCISSOR
SEALSIN
SEALSUP
SEEMSTO
SEEPSIN
SELLSIT
SELLSTO
SENDSBY
SENDSIN
SENDSON
SENDSTO
SENDSUP
SENESCE
SEWISTS
SEXISTS
SHEDSON
SHOOSIN
SHOPSAT
SHOWSIN
SHOWSUP
SHUTSIN
SHUTSUP
SIGHSAT
SIGNSIN
SIGNSON
SIGNSUP
SILESIA
SIMPSON
SINGSTO
SINKSIN
SINUSES
SIZESIX
SIZESUP
SKIPSBY
SLAMSON
SLAPSON
SLIPSBY
SLIPSIN
SLIPSON
SLIPSUP
SLOPSON
SLOWSUP
SNAGSUP
SNAPSAT
SNAPSON
SNAPSTO
SNAPSUP
SNOWSIN
SNOWSKI
SOAKSIN
SOAKSUP
SOAPSUP
SOCKSIN
SOMESAY
SOUPSON
SOUPSUP
SOURSON
SPARSER
SPASSKY
SPENSER
SPIESON
SPITSON
SPLASHY
SPONSOR
SPOUSAL
SPOUSES
SPURSON
SQUASHY
SQUISHY
SSSSSSS
STARSIN
STARSKY
STASSEN
STAYSAT
STAYSIN
STAYSON
STAYSUP
STBASIL
STEPSIN
STEPSON
STEPSUP
STETSON
STIMSON
STIRSIN
STIRSUP
STOPSAT
STOPSBY
STOPSIN
STOPSIT
STOPSUP
STOWSIT
STRASSE
STYPSIS
SUCKSIN
SUCKSUP
SUITSME
SUITSUP
SULUSEA
SURFSUP
SWANSEA
SWANSON
SWATSAT
SWENSON
SWIMSUP
SWOOSIE

S••••S•

SADDEST
SADNESS
SAGIEST
SALTISH
SAMBASS
SAMWISE
SANJOSE
SAPLESS
SARCASM
SAWDUST
SAWFISH
SAWPAST
SAYMASS
SEABASS
SEAMIST
SEAMOSS
SEEALSO
SEEPAST
SEERESS
SELFISH
SERIESE
SERIESF
SERIESG
SERIESH
SERIESI
SERIESJ
SERIESK
SEXIEST
SEXLESS
SHIATSU
SHYNESS
SIAMESE
SICKEST
SICKISH
SIENESE
SIKHISM
SINLESS
SKIMASK
SKIVEST
SKYLESS
SLAVISH
SLOWEST
SLOWISH
SLYNESS
SNIDEST
SOANDSO
SODLESS
SOFTEST
SOFTISH
SOLNESS
SOLOIST
SONLESS
SOONEST
SOPHISM
SOPHIST
SOTTISH
SOUBISE
SOUREST
SOURISH
SPANISH
SPAREST
SPRIEST
SPRYEST
SSSSSSS
STALEST
STATISM
STATIST
STPIUSI
STPIUSV
STPIUSX
STRASSE
STRAUSS
STROUSE
STYLISE
STYLISH
STYLIST
SUAVEST
SUBBASE
SUBBASS
SUBCASE
SUBCASH
SUBCAST
SUBPOST
SUBROSA
SUBSIST
SUBTASK
SUCCESS
SUCRASE
SUCROSE
SUFFUSE
SUGGEST
SUMLESS
SUMOIST
SUNFAST
SUNFISH
SUNKIST
SUNLESS
SUNRISE
SUPPOSE
SURMISE
SURPASS
SWEDISH
SWINISH
SYNAPSE

S•••••S

SABADOS
SABINES
SACHEMS
SACHETS
SACKERS
SACQUES
SADDENS
SADDLES
SADEYES
SADISTS
SADNESS
SAFARIS
SAILERS
SAILORS
SAINTES
SAISONS
SALAAMS
SALADES
SALAMIS
SALINAS
SALINES
SALIVAS
SALLIES
SALMONS
SALOONS
SALTERS
SALUKIS
SALUTES
SALVERS
SALVOES
SALVORS
SAMARAS
SAMBASS
SAMEDIS
SAMEKHS
SAMLETS
SAMOANS
SAMOSAS
SAMPANS
SAMPLES
SAMPRAS
SAMSONS
SANBLAS
SANCTUS
SANDALS
SANDERS
SANSEIS
SAPIENS
SAPLESS
SAPPERS
SARONGS
SARTORS
SASHAYS
SASSERS
SATCOMS
SATEENS
SATIRES
SATORIS
SATRAPS
SATURNS
SAUCERS
SAVAGES
SAVALAS
SAVANAS
SAVANTS
SAVINGS
SAVIORS
SAVOURS
SAVVIES
SAWLOGS
SAWPITS
SAWYERS
SAYINGS
SAYMASS
SAYSYES
SCALARS
SCALERS
SCARABS
SCARERS
SCARVES
SCATHES
SCENICS
SCHAYES
SCHEMAS
SCHEMES
SCHICKS
SCHISMS
SCHISTS
SCHLEPS
SCHLUBS
SCHMOES
SCHNAPS
SCHOLES
SCHOOLS
SCLAFFS
SCLERAS
SCONCES
SCOOBAS
SCORERS
SCORIAS
SCOTERS
SCOUPES
SCRAPES
SCRAWLS
SCREAKS
SCREAMS
SCREEDS
SCREENS
SCRIBES
SCRIMPS
SCRIPPS
SCRIPTS
SCROLLS
SCRUFFS
SCRUGGS
SCULPTS
SCURVES
SCUZZES
SCYTHES
SEAARMS
SEABAGS
SEABASS
SEABEDS
SEABEES
SEACATS
SEACOWS
SEADOGS
SEAEELS
SEAGODS
SEALABS
SEALEGS
SEALERS
SEAMAPS
SEAMERS
SEAMOSS
SEANCES
SEARERS
SEASONS
SEATERS
SEAWAYS
SECANTS
SECEDES
SECKELS
SECONDS
SECRETS
SECTORS
SECURES
SEDATES
SEDONAS
SEDUCES
SEEDERS
SEEKERS
SEERESS
SEESAWS
SEETHES
SEFERIS
SEGWAYS
SEINERS
SEIZERS
SEIZORS
SELECTS
SELLERS
SEMANAS
SEMITES
SENATES
SENDEES
SENDERS
SENDUPS
SENECAS
SENIORS
SENORAS
SENORES
SENSEIS
SENSENS
SENSORS
SENTRAS
SEPHIAS
SEPIRAS
SEPTETS
SEQUELS
SEQUINS
SERAPES
SERAPHS
SERAPIS
SERIALS
SERIOUS
SERMONS
SERPENS
SERVEAS
SERVERS
SESAMES
SESTETS
SETFEES
SETOFFS
SETOUTS
SETTEES
SETTERS
SETTLES
SEVERUS
SEWARDS
SEWISTS
SEXISTS
SEXLESS
SEXPOTS
SEXTANS
SEXTETS
SEXTONS
SHADERS
SHADOWS
SHAKERS
SHAKOES
SHALOMS
SHAMANS
SHAPERS
SHARERS
SHAVERS
SHEATHS
SHEAVES
SHEIKHS
SHEILAS
SHEKELS
SHELVES
SHERIFS
SHERPAS
SHEVATS
SHIELDS
SHIITES
SHINERS
SHIVERS
SHNOOKS
SHOFARS
SHOGUNS
SHOOINS
SHOPKOS
SHOPPES
SHOVELS
SHOVERS
SHOWERS
SHRIEKS
SHRIKES
SHRILLS
SHRIMPS
SHRINES
SHRINKS
SHRIVES
SHROUDS
SHTETLS
SHTICKS
SHUSHES
SHUTINS
SHYNESS
SICKENS
SICKLES
SIDDONS
SIDDURS
SIDINGS
SIDIOUS
SIEMENS
SIENNAS
SIERRAS
SIESTAS
SIFTERS
SIGHERS
SIGNALS
SIGNEES
SIGNERS
SIGNETS
SIGNORS
SIGNUPS
SILENTS
SILICAS
SILLIES
SILVERS
SIMIANS
SIMILES
SIMMERS
SIMMONS
SIMPERS
SIMPLES
SINGERS
SINGLES
SINKERS
SINLESS
SINNERS
SINUOUS
SINUSES
SIOUANS
SIPHONS
SIPPERS
SISSIES
SISTERS
SITCOMS
SITTERS
SIXGUNS
SIXTIES
SIZZLES
SKATERS
SKEWERS
SKIBIBS
SKIBOBS
SKIBUMS
SKICAPS
SKIDOOS
SKIHATS
SKIRUNS
SKITOWS
SKOSHES
SKYCAMS
SKYCAPS
SKYLESS
SKYMAPS
SKYWAYS
SLAKERS
SLALOMS
SLASHES
SLATERS
SLAVERS
SLAYERS
SLEAZES
SLEDGES
SLEEVES
SLEIGHS
SLEUTHS
SLICERS
SLIDERS
SLIGHTS
SLIPONS
SLIPUPS
SLIVERS
SLOGANS
SLOPERS
SLOSHES
SLOUGHS
SLOVAKS
SLOVENS
SLOWUPS
SLUDGES
SLUICES
SLUSHES
SLYNESS
SMASHES
SMIDGES
SMILERS
SMILEYS
SMILLAS
SMITERS
SMOKERS
SMOKEYS
SMOKIES
SMOOTHS
SMUDGES
SMUSHES
SNAKERS
SNAPONS
SNARERS
SNEEZES
SNIPERS
SNIVELS
SNOCAPS
SNOCATS
SNOOZES
SNORERS
SNUGLIS
SOAKERS
SOAPERS
SOARERS
SOBBERS
SOCIALS
SOCKETS
SODLESS
SOFARAS
SOFFITS
SOFTENS
SOFTIES
SOIREES
SOLACES
SOLARAS
SOLDERS
SOLNESS
SOLUTES
SOLVERS
SOMALIS
SONATAS
SONLESS
SONNETS
SOONERS
SOOTHES
SOPHIES
SORBETS
SORRELS
SORROWS
SORTERS
SORTIES
SOSPADS
SOUPERS
SOURCES
SOVIETS
SOXFANS
SOYINKS
SPACERS
SPADERS
SPARERS
SPATHES
SPAYERS
SPECIES
SPEEDOS
SPEWERS
SPHERES
SPICERS
SPIDERS
SPIGOTS
SPIKERS
SPINELS
SPINETS
SPIRALS
SPIREAS
SPIRITS
SPITZES
SPLEENS
SPLICES
SPLINES
SPLINTS
SPONGES
SPOUSES
SPRAINS
SPRAWLS
SPREADS
SPRINGS
SPRINTS
SPRITES
SPROUTS
SPRUCES
SPYBOTS
SPYCAMS
SPYDERS
SPYINGS
SPYKIDS
SQUALLS
SQUARES
SQUAWKS
SQUEAKS
SQUEALS
SQUEERS
SQUINTS
SQUIRES
SQUIRMS
SQUIRTS
SSSSSSS
STABLES
STAGERS
STAGNES
STALAGS
STAMENS
STANCES
STANZAS
STAPLES
STARERS
STARVES
STASHES
STATERS
STATICS
STATINS
STATORS
STATUES
STAYERS
STBARTS
STDENIS
STEARNS
STEEVES
STELIAS
STENNIS
STEPINS
STEPPES
STEPUPS
STEREOS
STERNOS
STEROLS
STEVENS
STEWERS
STIFLES
STIGMAS
STJAMES
STJOHNS
STKITTS
STLOUIS
STLUKES
STMARKS
STMARYS
STODGES
STOGIES
STOKERS
STOLONS
STONERS
STOOGES
STORERS
STORIES
STOTINS
STOWERS
STPAULS
STRAFES
STRAINS
STRAITS
STRANDS
STRATAS
STRATUS
STRAUSS
STREAKS
STREAMS
STREETS
STREGIS
STRIDES
STRIFES
STRIKES
STRINGS
STRIPES
STRIVES
STROBES
STROKES
STROLLS
STUCCOS
STUDIES
STUDIOS
STUPIDS
STUPORS
STURGES
STUTZES
STYLERS
STYLETS
STYMIES
STYPSIS
SUBARUS
SUBBASS
SUBBIAS
SUBDEBS
SUBDUES
SUBGODS
SUBLETS
SUBLIDS
SUBLOTS
SUBMITS
SUBNETS
SUBORNS
SUBSETS
SUBURBS
SUBWARS
SUBWAYS
SUCCESS
SUCCORS
SUCKERS
SUDOKUS
SUDSERS
SUFFERS
SUITORS
SULKERS
SULKIES
SULLIES
SULTANS
SUMLESS
SUMMERS
SUMMITS
SUMMONS
SUNBOWS
SUNDAES
SUNDAYS
SUNDERS
SUNDOGS
SUNFANS
SUNGODS
SUNHATS
SUNLESS
SUNRAYS
SUNSETS
SUNTANS
SUPERGS
SUPPERS
SUPPLES
SURFERS
SURIMIS
SURPASS
SURPLUS
SURREYS
SURVEYS
SUTURES
SUZUKIS
SWASHES
SWATHES
SWAYERS
SWERVES
SWIPERS
SWISHES
SWIVELS
SWIVETS
SYMBOLS
SYNDICS
SYRIANS
SYSTEMS

•SS••••

ASSAILS
ASSANTE
ASSAULT
ASSAYED
ASSAYER
ASSENTS
ASSERTS
ASSHARP
ASSIGNS
ASSISTS
ASSIZES
ASSLIKE
ASSORTS
ASSTDAS
ASSTIFF
ASSUAGE
ASSUMED
ASSUMER
ASSUMES
ASSUNTA
ASSURED
ASSURER
ASSURES
ASSUROR
ASSWEET
ASSYRIA
ESSAYED
ESSAYER
ESSENCE
ESSENES
ISSUANT
ISSUEAD
ISSUERS
ISSUING
OSSEOUS

OSSETRA
OSSICLE
OSSIFIC
OSSIPEE
OSSUARY
SSSSSSS
USSTATE
USSTEEL

•S•S•••
ASISAID
ASKSFOR
ASKSOUT
ASUSUAL
SSSSSSS
USESFOR
USOSHOW

•S••S••
ASEPSIS
ASSISTS
ESIASON
ESPOSAS
ESPOSOS
OSMOSED
OSMOSES
OSMOSIS
OSTOSIS
SSSSSSS
TSETSES
TSKTSKS

•S•••S•
ASHIEST
ASHLESS
ASPERSE
ESOBESO
ESPOUSE
OSHKOSH
SSSSSSS
TSARISM
TSARIST
USELESS

•S••••S
ASANTES
ASCENDS
ASCENTS
ASEPSIS
ASFARAS
ASHBINS
ASHCANS
ASHLARS
ASHLESS
ASHPANS
ASHPITS
ASHRAMS
ASIAGOS
ASPECTS
ASPIRES
ASSAILS
ASSENTS
ASSERTS
ASSIGNS
ASSISTS
ASSIZES
ASSORTS
ASSTDAS
ASSUMES
ASSURES
ASTHMAS
ASYLUMS
CSARDAS
CSLEWIS
ESCALUS
ESCAPES
ESCARPS
ESCHERS
ESCHEWS
ESCORTS
ESCROWS
ESCUDOS
ESKIMOS
ESPIALS
ESPNEWS
ESPOSAS
ESPOSOS
ESPRITS
ESSENES
ESTADOS
ESTATES
ESTEEMS
ESTRAYS
ISLANDS
ISOBARS
ISOGONS
ISOHELS
ISOMERS
ISOPODS
ISSUERS
ISTHMUS
MSIEURS
OSAKANS
OSCINES
OSCULES
OSETRAS
OSMONDS
OSMOSES
OSMOSIS
OSMUNDS
OSPREYS
OSSEOUS
OSTLERS
OSTOSIS
PSANDQS
PSYCHES
PSYCHOS
PSYWARS
SSSSSSS
TSETSES
TSHAPES
TSHIRTS
TSKTSKS
TSONGAS
TSOURIS
TSTRAPS
USABLES
USANCES
USEDCDS
USELESS
USERIDS
USFLAGS
USHAPES
USOPENS
USTEDES
USURERS
USURIES
VSHAPES
XSANDOS
YSHAPES

••SS•••
AUSSIES
BASSALE
BASSANI
BASSANO
BASSETS
BASSETT
BASSIER
BASSIST
BASSOON
BASSSAX
BESSELL
BISSELL
BOSSIER
BOSSILY
BOSSING
BOSSISM
BOSSMAN
BOSSMEN
BUSSERS
BUSSING
BUSSTOP
CASSABA
CASSATT
CASSAVA
CASSIAS
CASSIDY
CASSINI
CASSINO
CASSIUS
CASSOCK
CASSOLA
CESSING
CESSION
CESSNAS
CESSPIT
COSSACK
COSSETS
CUSSERS
CUSSING
CUSSLER
DESSERT
DISSECT
DISSENT
DISSERT
DISSING
DOSSALS
DOSSIER
DOSSING
FESSING
FISSILE
FISSION
FISSURE
FOSSILS
FUSSERS
FUSSIER
FUSSILY
FUSSING
FUSSPOT
GASSERS
GASSIER
GASSING
GASSMAN
GESSOED
GESSOES
GISSING
GOSSAGE
GOSSETT
GOSSIPS
GOSSIPY
GUSSETS
GUSSIED
GUSSIES
GUSSYUP
HASSIUM
HASSLED
HASSLES
HASSOCK
HESSAFE
HESSIAN
HISSERS
HISSIER
HISSING
HUSSARS
HUSSEIN
HUSSERL
HUSSIES
HUSSITE
HYSSOPS
JESSICA
KISSELS
KISSERS
KISSING
KISSOFF
KOSSUTH
LASSIES
LASSOED
LASSOER
LASSOES
LESSEES
LESSENS
LESSEPS
LESSFAT
LESSING
LESSONS
LESSORS
LESSTAR
LISSOME
MASSAGE
MASSEUR
MASSIER
MASSIFS
MASSINE
MASSING
MASSIVE
MESSAGE
MESSALA
MESSIAH
MESSICK
MESSIER
MESSILY
MESSINA
MESSING
MESSKIT
MESSUPS
MISSAID
MISSALS
MISSAYS
MISSEAT
MISSEND
MISSENT
MISSETS
MISSHIP
MISSIES
MISSILE
MISSING
MISSION
MISSISH
MISSIVE
MISSORT
MISSOUT
MISSTEP
MISSUSA
MISSYOU
MOSSIER
MOSSING
MUSSELS
MUSSIER
MUSSILY
MUSSING
NESSMAN
NISSANS
NISSANZ
PASSADE
PASSADO
PASSAGE
PASSAIC
PASSANT
PASSATS
PASSELS
PASSERS
PASSEUL
PASSFOR
PASSING
PASSION
PASSIVE
PASSKEY
PASSOFF
PASSOUT
POSSESS
POSSLQS
POSSUMS
PUSSIES
RASSLED
RASSLER
RASSLES
RISSOLE
ROSSANO
ROSSINI
ROSSNER
ROSSSEA
RUSSELL
RUSSERT
RUSSETS
RUSSETY
RUSSIAN
RUSSLAN
SASSERS
SASSIER
SASSILY
SASSING
SASSOON
SESSILE
SESSION
SISSIER
SISSIES
SSSSSSS
SUSSING
SUSSOUT
TASSELS
TESSERA
TISSOTS
TISSUES
TISSUEY
TOSSERS
TOSSING
TOSSOFF
TOSSOUT
TOSSPOT
TOSSUPS
TUSSAUD
TUSSIVE
TUSSLED
TUSSLES
TUSSOCK
VASSALS
VESSELS
WASSAIL
WASSILY
WASSURE
YESSING
YESSIRE
ZOSSIMA

••S•S••
ASSISTS
BASESIX
BASSSAX
BUSTSIN
BUSTSUP
CASTSON
CASTSUP
DESISTS
DESKSET
DISUSED
DISUSES
EASESBY
EASESIN
EASESON
EASESUP
GASESUP
HASASAY
HASASET
INSISTS
ITSASIN
LOSESIT
LOSESTO
MISTSUP
MISUSED
MISUSER
MISUSES
MUSESON
MUSTSEE
NESTSIN
NOSESIN
NOSESUP
POSESAS
RESISTS
RESTSIN
RESTSON
RESTSUP
RISESTO
RISESUP
RISKSIT
ROSSSEA
SSSSSSS
WISESUP
YESISEE

••S••S•
ABSCISE
AUSLESE
BASSIST
BOSSISM
BUSIEST
BUSPASS
CASUIST
COSIEST
DESPISE
DISCUSS
DISEASE
DISEUSE
DISGUST
DISMAST
DISMISS
DISPOSE
DRSEUSS
DUSKISH
EASIEST
ECSTASY
FASCISM
FASCIST
FASTEST
FESTOSO
GASLESS
GASMASK
HASHISH
HOSTESS
IDSAYSO
ITSBEST
ITSEASY
JUSTEST
LUSHEST
MISCAST
MISMESH
MISSISH
MISSUSA
MRSBASS
NASTASE
NOSIEST
POSEUSE
POSHEST
POSSESS
RASHEST
RASPISH
ROSIEST
SSSSSSS
VASTEST
VISCUSO
WASPISH
XYSTUSI

••S•••S
ABSENTS
ABSORBS
ADSORBS
AMSTELS
ANSWERS
APSIDES
ASSAILS
ASSENTS
ASSERTS
ASSIGNS
ASSISTS
ASSIZES
ASSORTS
ASSTDAS
ASSUMES
ASSURES
ATSIGNS
AUSSIES
AUSTERS
AUSTINS
AXSEEDS
BASALTS
BASHERS
BASKETS
BASQUES
BASSETS
BASTERS
BBSHOTS
BESIDES
BESTIRS
BESTOWS
BISECTS
BISHOPS
BISQUES
BISTROS
BOSTONS
BUSBIES
BUSBOYS
BUSHELS
BUSHERS
BUSKERS
BUSMANS
BUSPASS
BUSSERS
BUSTERS
BUSTLES
BUSTUPS
CASABAS
CASAVAS
CASEINS
CASEOUS
CASERNS
CASHEWS
CASHINS
CASINGS
CASINOS
CASITAS
CASKETS
CASQUES
CASSIAS
CASSIUS
CASTERS
CASTLES
CASUALS
CBSNEWS
CESSNAS
CISCOES
COSHERS
COSIGNS
COSINES
COSSETS
COSTARS
CTSCANS
CUSHAWS
CUSPIDS
CUSSERS
CUSTERS
CUSTOMS
DASHERS
DESALTS
DESEEDS
DESERTS
DESEXES
DESIGNS
DESILTS
DESIRES
DESISTS
DESLUMS
DESMOGS
DESOTOS
DESPOTS
DESTEMS
DISARMS
DISBARS
DISBUDS
DISCUSS
DISEURS
DISMALS
DISMAYS
DISMISS
DISOWNS
DISPELS
DISTILS
DISTROS
DISUSES
DOSADOS
DOSAGES
DOSHOTS
DOSIDOS
DOSSALS
DRSEUSS
DUSTERS
DUSTUPS
EASTERS
ENSEALS
ENSEATS
ENSIGNS
ENSILES
ENSKIES
ENSOULS
ENSURES
EOSINES
ESSENES
EXSECTS
EXSERTS
FASCIAS
FASTENS
FESCUES
FESTERS
FISHERS
FOSSILS
FOSTERS
FUSIONS
FUSSERS
FUSUMAS
GASBAGS
GASCANS
GASCAPS
GASCONS
GASEOUS
GASHOGS
GASJETS
GASKETS
GASLESS
GASLOGS
GASPERS
GASSERS
GASWARS
GESSOES
GOSPELS
GOSSIPS
GUSHERS
GUSSETS
GUSSIES
GUSTOES
HASAGAS
HASFITS
HASSLES
HASTENS
HISNIBS
HISSERS
HOSIERS
HOSKINS
HOSTELS
HOSTESS
HUSKERS
HUSKIES
HUSSARS
HUSSIES
HUSTLES
HYSSOPS
INSALES
INSEAMS
INSECTS
INSERTS
INSIDES
INSISTS
INSOLES
INSPANS
INSPOTS
INSTALS
INSTEPS
INSTILS
INSULTS
INSURES
ISSUERS
JASPERS
JESTERS
JESUITS
JOSBOYS
JOSHERS
JOSTLES
KISHKES
KISLEVS
KISMETS
KISSELS
KISSERS
KOSHERS
LASCARS
LASHERS
LASHUPS
LASSIES
LASSOES
LASTGAS
LESIONS
LESSEES
LESSENS
LESSEPS
LESSONS
LESSORS
LISPERS
LISTEES
LISTENS
LISTERS
LOSINGS
LUSTERS
LUSTRES
MASCOTS
MASHERS
MASHIES
MASKERS
MASQUES
MASSIFS
MASTERS
MASTICS
MESAMIS
MESCALS
MESEEMS
MESSUPS
MISACTS
MISADDS
MISAIMS
MISCUES
MISCUTS
MISDOES
MISFITS
MISHAPS
MISHITS
MISKEYS
MISLAYS
MISSALS
MISSAYS
MISSETS
MISSIES
MISTERS
MISUSES
MOSAICS
MOSHERS
MOSLEMS
MOSQUES
MRSBASS
MUSCATS
MUSCLES
MUSEUMS
MUSHERS
MUSICKS
MUSINGS
MUSKETS
MUSKIES
MUSLIMS
MUSLINS
MUSSELS
MUSTDOS
MUSTERS
MYSTARS
MYSTICS
NASTIES
NESTERS
NESTLES
NESTORS
NISSANS
NOSEATS
NOSHERS
NOSHOWS
NOSTARS
OFSORTS
ONSIDES
OSSEOUS
OUSTERS
OYSTERS
PASSATS
PASSELS
PASSERS
PASTELS
PASTERS
PASTIES
PASTORS
PESADES
PESETAS
PESEWAS
PESTERS
PESTLES
PISTILS
PISTOLS
PISTONS
PISTOUS
POSADAS
POSEDAS
POSESAS
POSEURS
POSOLES
POSSESS
POSSLQS
POSSUMS
POSTERS
POSTIES
POSTITS
POSTOPS
PUSHERS
PUSHUPS
PUSSIES
RASCALS
RASHERS
RASPERS
RASSLES
RASTERS
RASURES
RESALES
RESALTS
RESANDS
RESAVES
RESCANS
RESCUES
RESEALS
RESEAMS
RESEATS
RESEAUS
RESECTS
RESEEDS
RESEEKS
RESELLS
RESENDS
RESENTS
RESHIPS
RESHOES
RESHOWS
RESHUTS
RESIDES
RESIFTS
RESIGNS
RESILES
RESINGS
RESINKS
RESISTS
RESIZES
RESNAIS
RESNAPS
RESOAKS
RESOAPS
RESOILS
RESOLES
RESORBS
RESORTS
RESPANS
RESPINS
RESPOTS
RESTABS
RESTERS
RESTIRS
RESTOWS
RESUITS
RESULTS
RESUMES
RESWIMS
RISINGS
RISKERS
ROSCOES
ROSTERS
RUSHEES
RUSHERS
RUSSETS
RUSTICS
RUSTLES
SASHAYS
SASSERS
SESAMES
SESTETS
SISSIES
SISTERS
SOSPADS
SSSSSSS
SYSTEMS
TASSELS
TASTERS
TESTEES
TESTERS
TISANES
TISSOTS
TISSUES
TOSSERS
TOSSUPS
TUSCANS
TUSHIES
TUSKERS
TUSSLES
TVSHOWS
TVSPOTS
TVSTARS
ULSTERS
UNSEALS
UNSEAMS
UNSEATS
UNSELLS
UNSHIPS
UNSHOES
UNSKEWS
UNSNAGS
UNSNAPS
UNSOLES
UNSORTS
UNSPANS
UNSTEPS
UNSTOPS
UNSTOWS
UPSENDS
UPSHOTS
UPSIDES
UPSIZES
UPSOARS
UPSPINS

UPSTEPS
UPSTIRS
URSINUS
VASSALS
VESPERS
VESPIDS
VESSELS
VESTALS
VESTEES
VISAGES
VISAVIS
VISCOUS
VISIONS
VISUALS
WASABIS
WASHERS
WASHUPS
WASTERS
WESKITS
WESTERS
WESTIES
WESTINS
WISDOMS
WISHERS
XYSTERS
YESITIS
YESLETS
ZESTERS
ZOSIMUS

•••SS••

ABYSSAL
ABYSSES
AGASSIZ
AHASSLE
ALASSAD
ALYSSUM
AMASSED
AMASSER
AMASSES
ATISSUE
BASSSAX
BIASSED
BIASSES
BLESSED
BLESSER
BLESSES
BLISSED
BLISSES
BLOSSOM
BRASSES
BRASSIE
BROSSES
BUISSON
CAISSON
CHASSED
CHASSES
CHASSIS
CLASSED
CLASSER
CLASSES
CLASSIC
CLASSON
CNOSSUS
CRASSER
CRASSLY
CRASSUS
CRESSES
CRESSET
CROSSAT
CROSSED
CROSSER
CROSSES
CROSSLY
CROSSUP
DAUSSET
DRESSAS
DRESSED
DRESSER
DRESSES
DRESSIN
DRESSUP
DROSSES
FLOSSED
FLOSSER
FLOSSES
FLOSSIE
FRESSED
FRESSES
FRISSON
GAUSSES
GETSSET
GLASSED
GLASSES
GLOSSAE
GLOSSAL
GLOSSAS
GLOSSED
GLOSSER
GLOSSES
GNOSSUS
GRASSED
GRASSES
GRASSLE
GRISSOM
GROSSED
GROSSER
GROSSES
GROSSLY
GUESSAT
GUESSED
GUESSER
GUESSES
GUESSSO
HOUSSAY
JANSSEN
JANSSON
KNESSET
KNOSSOS
KVASSES
LAISSEZ
LETSSEE
LOESSER
LOESSES
MEISSEN
MOISSAN
MOUSSED
MOUSSES
NILSSON
ODESSAN
ODYSSEY
ONASSIS
OPOSSUM
PERSSON
PLISSES
PLUSSES
POISSON
POUSSIN
PRESSED
PRESSEL
PRESSER
PRESSES
PRESSON
PRESSUP
PRISSES
PRUSSIA
REASSAY
REISSUE
RIESSEN
ROSSSEA
SCISSOR
SPASSKY
SSSSSSS
STASSEN
TRESSED
TRESSES
TRUSSED
TRUSSES
TRUSSUP
ULYSSES
WRASSES

•••S•S•

BASSIST
BOSSISM
CLOSEST
CONSIST
DENSEST
FALSEST
GUESSSO
IINSIST
LETSUSE
LOOSEST
MISSISH
MISSUSA
PERSIST
POSSESS
RAMSESI
SSSSSSS
SUBSIST
TENSEST
TERSEST

•••S••S

ABASERS
ABASHES
ABUSERS
ABYSSES
AIRSACS
ALASKAS
AMASSES
AMUSERS
ARISTAS
ARISTOS
AUSSIES
AVESTAS
BALSAMS
BASSETS
BEDSITS
BIASSES
BLESSES
BLISSES
BLUSHES
BOWSAWS
BOXSETS
BRASHES
BRASSES
BROSSES
BRUSHES
BUQSHAS
BURSARS
BUSSERS
CAESARS
CASSIAS
CASSIUS
CATSITS
CATSUPS
CAUSERS
CELSIUS
CENSERS
CENSORS
CESSNAS
CHASERS
CHASSES
CHASSIS
CHISELS
CLASHES
CLASSES
CLOSERS
CLOSETS
CNOSSUS
COMSATS
CONSULS
CORSETS
COSSETS
COUSINS
CRASHES
CRASSUS
CRESSES
CRISPUS
CROSSES
CRUSHES
CUESTAS
CURSERS
CURSORS
CUSSERS
DAISIES
DAMSELS
DAMSONS
DATSUNS
DAYSPAS
DELSOLS
DIDSUMS
DIESELS
DOGSITS
DORSALS
DORSEYS
DOSSALS
DOUSERS
DOWSERS
DRESSAS
DRESSES
DROSSES
EGGSACS
ELYSEES
ENISLES
ERASERS
ERASMUS
ERASTUS
FAUSTUS
FIASCOS
FIESTAS
FLASHES
FLESHES
FLOSSES
FLUSHES
FOCSLES
FOSSILS
FRESCAS
FRESCOS
FRESHES
FRESSES
FUSSERS
GASSERS
GAUSSES
GEISHAS
GESSOES
GEYSERS
GIBSONS
GIPSIES
GLASSES
GLOSSAS
GLOSSES
GNASHES
GNOSSUS
GODSONS
GOSSIPS
GRASSES
GROSSES
GUESSES
GUNSELS
GUSSETS
GUSSIES
GYPSIES
GYPSUMS
HANSOMS
HASSLES
HAWSERS
HISSERS
HOBSONS
HUSSARS
HUSSIES
HYSSOPS
INKSACS
JERSEYS
JETSETS
JETSKIS
JETSONS
JIGSAWS
JIMSONS
KAISERS
KANSANS
KIDSRUS
KISSELS
KISSERS
KMESONS
KNISHES
KNOSSOS
KOOSHES
KVASSES
LAPSERS
LASSIES
LASSOES
LEASERS
LEASHES
LESSEES
LESSENS
LESSEPS
LESSONS
LESSORS
LHASANS
LOESSES
LOOSENS
MAISONS
MARSHES
MASSIFS
MAUSERS
MEASLES
MENSANS
MESSUPS
MIASMAS
MINSKYS
MISSALS
MISSAYS
MISSETS
MISSIES
MOLSONS
MORSELS
MOUSERS
MOUSSES
MUESLIS
MUSSELS
NAYSAYS
NELSONS
NEWSIES
NISSANS
NOOSERS
NURSERS
OFFSETS
OLDSAWS
ONASSIS
ORESTES
ORISONS
OUTSAYS
OUTSEES
OUTSETS
OUTSINS
OUTSITS
OUTSUMS
OVISACS
PAISANS
PANSIES
PARSECS
PARSEES
PARSERS
PARSONS
PASSATS
PASSELS
PASSERS
PATSIES
PAUSERS
PCUSERS
PENSEES
PEPSINS
PERSEUS
PERSIUS
PERSONS
PETSITS
PHASERS
PHISHES
PHYSICS
PITSAWS
PLASHES
PLASMAS
PLISSES
PLUSHES
PLUSSES
POESIES
POISERS
POISONS
POSSESS
POSSLQS
POSSUMS
PRESETS
PRESSES
PRESTOS
PRISONS
PRISSES
PROSERS
PULSARS
PURSERS
PURSUES
PUSSIES
QUASARS
QUASHES
RAISERS
RAISINS
RAISONS
RAMSONS
RANSOMS
RASSLES
REASONS
REDSUNS
REUSERS
RIESENS
RINSERS
RIPSAWS
RONSONS
ROUSERS
RUSSETS
SAISONS
SAMSONS
SANSEIS
SASSERS
SAYSYES
SEASONS
SEESAWS
SENSEIS
SENSENS
SENSORS
SHUSHES
SIESTAS
SISSIES
SKOSHES
SLASHES
SLOSHES
SLUSHES
SMASHES
SMUSHES
SSSSSSS
STASHES
SUBSETS
SUDSERS
SUNSETS
SWASHES
SWISHES
TABSETS
TANSIES
TARSALS
TASSELS
TEASELS
TEASERS
TEASETS
TENSORS
THESEUS
THESIMS
THESPIS
THESUNS
TILSITS
TINSELS
TISSOTS
TISSUES
TOCSINS
TONSILS
TOSSERS
TOSSUPS
TOUSLES
TOYSRUS
TRASHES
TRESSES
TRUSSES
TUCSONS
TULSANS
TUSSLES
ULYSSES
UNISOMS
UNISONS
VASSALS
VERSETS
VESSELS
VIZSLAS
WEASELS
WHISHES
WHISKAS
WILSONS
WOOSHES
WORSENS
WRASSES
ZOYSIAS

••••SS•

COLOSSI
DEBUSSY
EMBASSY
ENMASSE
FINESSE
GUESSSO
HOPESSO
IDLESSE
IGUASSU
IMPASSE
LAGASSE
LARUSSA
LEXUSSC
MATISSE
MELISSA
NERISSA
PELISSE
PERISSA
PICASSO
SSSSSSS
STRASSE
THEUSSR
UNFUSSY
UNMOSSY
VANESSA

••••S•S

ABYSSES
ACCOSTS
ACCUSES
ADAMSES
ADJUSTS
ADVISES
AEGISES
AGEISTS
ALIASES
AMASSES
APLUSES
APPOSES
ARGUSES
ARIOSOS
AROUSES
ARRASES
ARRESTS
ARRISES
ARTISTS
ASEPSIS
ASSISTS
ATLASES
ATTESTS
AUGUSTS
AURISTS
AUTISTS
AVGASES
AVULSES
BALASES
BEHESTS
BEMUSES
BIASSES
BLESSES
BLISSES
BLOUSES
BOLUSES
BONUSES
BOURSES
BPLUSES
BRAISES
BRASSES
BREASTS
BROASTS
BROSSES
BROWSES
BRUISES
CAMISES
CAYUSES
CDCASES
CERISES
CHAISES
CHASSES
CHASSIS
CHEESES
CHOOSES
CHRISMS
CLASSES
CLAUSES
CNOSSUS
COHOSTS
COMESAS
CORPSES
COURSES
CPLUSES
CRASSUS
CREASES
CRESSES
CROESUS
CROSSES
CRUISES
CUBISTS
CUTISES
DALASIS
DAMASKS
DAMASUS
DEBASES
DEBUSES
DEFUSES
DEGUSTS
DELISTS
DEMASTS
DEMISES
DEMISTS
DEPESTS
DEPOSES
DERUSTS
DESISTS
DETESTS
DEVESTS
DEVISES
DIGESTS
DISUSES
DIVESTS
DNAASES
DPLUSES
DRESSAS
DRESSES
DROSSES
DROWSES
DUFUSES
DYNASTS
ECDYSES
ECDYSIS
EFFUSES
EGLISES
EGOISTS
ELAPSES
ENCASES
ENDUSES
ENLISTS
EPHESUS
ESPOSAS
ESPOSOS
EVULSES
EXCISES
EXCUSAS
EXCUSES
EXPOSES
FETUSES
FICUSES
FLENSES
FLOSSES
FOCUSES
FORESTS
FRAISES
FRESSES
GAUSSES
GENESES
GENESIS
GENUSES
GIBUSES
GLASSES
GLOSSAS
GLOSSES
GNOSSUS
GRASSES
GREASES
GROSSES
GROUSES
GUESSES
HAYESES
HEARSES
HEXOSES
HOLISTS
HUMUSES
ICTUSES
ILLUSES
IMPOSES
IMPOSTS
INCASES
INCISES
INCUSES
INFESTS
INFUSES
INGESTS
INSISTS
INVESTS
IODISES
IONISES
IQTESTS
JONESES
JUDASES
JURISTS
KINESES
KINESIS
KNOSSOS
KVASSES
LAKISTS
LEGISTS
LEXISES
LEXUSES
LEXUSGS
LEXUSIS
LEXUSLS
LIAISES
LIPASES
LOCUSTS
LOESSES
LORISES
LORUSES
LOTUSES
LUTISTS
LYRISTS
MAOISTS
MAVISES
MEDUSAS
MEIOSES
MEIOSIS
MIDASES
MIKASAS
MIMESES
MIMESIS
MIMOSAS
MINUSES
MISUSES
MITOSES
MITOSIS
MOLESTS
MOMUSES
MOUSSES
NEGUSES
NEMESES
NEMESIS
NEXUSES
NUDISTS
OBLASTS
OBOISTS
OBTESTS
ONASSIS
OPPOSES
ORRISES
OSMOSES
OSMOSIS
OSTOSIS
OUTASKS
PAPISTS
PEGASUS
PERUSES
PHRASES
PLEASES
PLISSES
PLUSSES
POSESAS
PRAISES
PRESSES
PRIESTS
PRISSES
PRIUSES
PURISTS
RACISTS
RAMESES
RAWISTS
REBUSES
RECASES
RECASTS
RECOSTS
RECUSES
REDOSES
REDUSTS
REFUSES
RELISTS
RELOSES
REMISES
RENESTS
REPASTS
REPOSES
REPOSTS
RERISES
RESISTS
RETESTS
REVESTS
REVISES
RIPOSTS
SADISTS
SAMOSAS
SCHISMS
SCHISTS
SEWISTS
SEXISTS
SINUSES
SPOUSES
SSSSSSS
STYPSIS
TALUSES
TAOISTS
THEISMS
THEISTS
THIRSTS
THRUSTS
TONUSES
TRESSES
TRUISMS
TRUSSES
TSETSES
TSKTSKS
TUBISTS
TYPISTS
ULYSSES
UNCASES
UNCASKS
UNEASES
UNHASPS
UNHUSKS
UNMASKS
UNMASTS
UNRESTS
UPCASTS
UPRISES
UTMOSTS
VALISES
VEDISTS
VENUSES
VERISTS
VIBISTS
VIRUSES
WATUSIS
WHATSIS
WHOOSIS
WRASSES
XEROSES
XEROSIS
XYLOSES
ZENISTS

•••••SS

ACTRESS
ADDRESS
AGELESS
AGGRESS
AIDLESS
AIMLESS
AIRKISS
AIRLESS
AIRMASS
AIRNESS
ALLNESS
ANDRESS
APTNESS
ARMLESS
ARTLESS
ASHLESS
ATALOSS
ATCROSS
ATELESS
AWELESS
AWNLESS
BADNESS
BARLESS
BEDLESS
BIBLESS
BIGBOSS
BIGMESS
BIGNESS
BIOMASS
BITLESS
BOGGUSS
BOOHISS
BOWLESS
BRALESS
BUDLESS
BURGESS
BUSPASS
CANVASS
CAPLESS
CARCASS
CARLESS

COMPASS
CONCUSS
CONFESS
COXLESS
COYNESS
CUIRASS
CURTISS
CUTLASS
CYPRESS
DECLASS
DEGAUSS
DEPRESS
DEWLESS
DIGRESS
DIMNESS
DISCUSS
DISMISS
DOGLESS
DONRUSS
DRSEUSS
DRYNESS
DUCHESS
EARLESS
EATLESS
EGGLESS
EGGTOSS
EMPRESS
ENDLESS
ENGROSS
EXPRESS
EYELESS
FARNESS
FATLESS
FATNESS
FEELESS
FEWNESS
FEYNESS
FINLESS
FITNESS
FLYLESS
FOELESS
FOGLESS
FTBLISS
FULNESS
FURLESS
FURNESS
GAPLESS
GASLESS
GAYNESS
GEMLESS
GOAMISS
GODDESS
GODLESS
GUMLESS
GUNLESS
GUTLESS
HAPLESS
HARNESS
HATLESS
HEIRESS
HIPLESS
HIPNESS
HITLESS
HOSTESS
HOTNESS
HUELESS
ICELESS
ICINESS

ILLNESS
ILLPASS
IMAMESS
IMPRESS
INAMESS
INCLASS
INGRESS
INKLESS
INNLESS
IPCRESS
IRELESS
JACKASS
JAGLESS
JARLESS
JAWLESS
JOBLESS
JOYLESS
KEYLESS
KINLESS
LARGESS
LAWLESS
LAXNESS
LEGLESS
LETPASS
LIDLESS
LIONESS
LIPLESS
LOWMASS
LOWNESS
MADNESS
MANLESS
MATLESS
MRBLISS
MRSBASS
NAPLESS
NETLESS
NETLOSS
NEWNESS
NOCLASS
NOWNESS
OAKMOSS
OARLESS
ODDNESS
OILLESS
OLDNESS
OLEMISS
ONENESS
OPPRESS
ORBLESS
ORELESS
OUTHISS
OUTKISS
OUTPASS
PATNESS
PAYLESS
PEERESS
PEGLESS
PERCUSS
PINLESS
PIPLESS
PITBOSS
POETESS
POSSESS
PRELOSS
PREMISS
PROCESS
PROFESS
PROWESS

PUNLESS
RAWNESS
RAYLESS
REAMASS
RECLASS
RECROSS
REDNESS
REDRESS
REGLOSS
REGRESS
REPRESS
RIBLESS
RIMLESS
RODLESS
RUMLESS
RUNLESS
SADNESS
SAMBASS
SAPLESS
SAYMASS
SEABASS
SEAMOSS
SEERESS
SEXLESS
SHYNESS
SINLESS
SKYLESS
SLYNESS
SODLESS
SOLNESS
SONLESS
SSSSSSS
STRAUSS
SUBBASS
SUCCESS
SUMLESS
SUNLESS
SURPASS
TAXLESS
TEALESS
THEBOSS
THEKISS
TIELESS
TIGRESS
TIPLESS
TOELESS
TOPLESS
TOYLESS
TUGLESS
UNCROSS
UNDRESS
UNGROSS
UNTRUSS
USELESS
VOWLESS
WANNESS
WARLESS
WAYLESS
WEBLESS
WEENESS
WETKISS
WETNESS
WIGLESS
WINLESS
WITLESS
WITNESS
WRYNESS
ZEBRASS

ST•••••

STABBED
STABBER
STABILE
STABLED
STABLER
STABLES
STACKED
STACKER
STACKUP
STADIUM
STADLER
STAFFED
STAFFER
STAGERS
STAGGED
STAGGER
STAGIER
STAGILY
STAGING
STAGNES
STAIDER
STAIDLY
STAINED
STAINER
STAIRED
STAKING
STALAGS
STALELY
STALEST
STALKED
STALKER
STALLED
STALLER
STAMENS
STAMINA
STAMMER
STAMPED
STAMPER
STANCES
STANDBY
STANDEE
STANDER
STANDIN
STANDON
STANDTO
STANDUP
STANINE
STANKUP
STANLEE
STANLEY
STANNIC
STANNUM
STANTON
STANZAS
STAPLED
STAPLER
STAPLES
STARCHY
STARDOM
STAREAT
STARERS
STARING
STARION
STARKER
STARKEY
STARKLY
STARLET

STARLIT
STARLOG
STARMAN
STARMAP
STARRED
STARSIN
STARSKY
STARTED
STARTER
STARTIN
STARTLE
STARTON
STARTTO
STARTUP
STARVED
STARVES
STASHED
STASHES
STASSEN
STATELY
STATERS
STATICE
STATICS
STATING
STATINS
STATION
STATISM
STATIST
STATLER
STATORS
STATUES
STATURE
STATUTE
STAUNCH
STAVING
STAYDRY
STAYERS
STAYFOR
STAYING
STAYOFF
STAYOUT
STAYPUT
STAYSAT
STAYSIN
STAYSON
STAYSUP
STBARTS
STBASIL
STCLOUD
STCROIX
STDENIS
STEADED
STEALER
STEALIN
STEALTH
STEAMED
STEAMER
STEAMUP
STEANNE
STEARIC
STEARIN
STEARNS
STEELED
STEELER
STEELIE
STEEPED
STEEPEN
STEEPER

STEEPIN
STEEPLE
STEEPLY
STEERED
STEERER
STEEVED
STEEVES
STEFANI
STEIGER
STEINEM
STEINER
STELIAS
STELLAR
STEMMED
STEMPEL
STENCIL
STENGEL
STENGUN
STENNIS
STENTOR
STEPDAD
STEPHEN
STEPINS
STEPMOM
STEPOFF
STEPONE
STEPOUT
STEPPED
STEPPER
STEPPES
STEPSIN
STEPSON
STEPSUP
STEPTWO
STEPUPS
STEREOS
STERILE
STERNAL
STERNER
STERNLY
STERNOS
STERNUM
STEROID
STEROLS
STERTOR
STETSON
STETTED
STEUBEN
STEVENS
STEWARD
STEWART
STEWERS
STEWIER
STEWING
STEWPAN
STEWPOT
STICKBY
STICKER
STICKIN
STICKON
STICKTO
STICKUM
STICKUP
STIFFED
STIFFEL
STIFFEN
STIFFER
STIFFLY

STIFLED
STIFLES
STIGMAS
STILLED
STILLER
STILLUP
STILTED
STILTON
STIMSON
STIMULI
STINGER
STINKER
STINKUP
STINTED
STINTER
STIPEND
STIPPLE
STIRFRY
STIRRED
STIRRER
STIRRUP
STIRSIN
STIRSUP
STJAMES
STJOHNS
STKITTS
STLOUIS
STLUCIA
STLUKES
STMARKS
STMARYS
STOCKED
STOCKER
STOCKUP
STODGED
STODGES
STOGIES
STOICAL
STOKELY
STOKERS
STOKEUP
STOKING
STOLEIN
STOLLEN
STOLONS
STOMACH
STOMATA
STOMPED
STOMPIN
STOMPON
STONEAX
STONERS
STONIER
STONILY
STONING
STOODBY
STOODIN
STOODON
STOODTO
STOODUP
STOOGED
STOOGES
STOOKEY
STOOLED
STOOLIE
STOOPED
STOOPER
STOPFOR

STOPGAP
STOPOFF
STOPPED
STOPPER
STOPPLE
STOPSAT
STOPSBY
STOPSIN
STOPSIT
STOPSUP
STORAGE
STORERS
STOREUP
STORIED
STORIES
STORING
STORMED
STORMIN
STOTINS
STOUTEN
STOUTER
STOUTLY
STOWAGE
STOWERS
STOWING
STOWSIT
STPAULS
STPETER
STPIUSI
STPIUSV
STPIUSX
STRAFED
STRAFER
STRAFES
STRAINS
STRAITS
STRANDS
STRANGE
STRAPIN
STRAPON
STRASSE
STRATAS
STRATUM
STRATUS
STRAUSS
STRAYED
STRAYER
STREAKS
STREAKY
STREAMS
STREETS
STREGIS
STRETCH
STRETTI
STRETTO
STREWED
STREWER
STRIATE
STRIDER
STRIDES
STRIFES
STRIKER
STRIKES
STRINGS
STRINGY
STRIPED
STRIPER
STRIPES

STRIPOF
STRITCH
STRIVED
STRIVEN
STRIVER
STRIVES
STROBES
STROKED
STROKER
STROKES
STROLLS
STROPHE
STROUSE
STRUDEL
STSIMON
STUARTI
STUBBED
STUBBLE
STUBBLY
STUBING
STUCCOS
STUCKBY
STUCKIN
STUCKON
STUCKTO
STUCKUP
STUDDED
STUDENT
STUDIED
STUDIER
STUDIES
STUDIOS
STUFFED
STUFFER
STUFFIN
STUMBLE
STUMPED
STUMPER
STUNGUN
STUNNED
STUNNER
STUNTED
STUPEFY
STUPIDS
STUPORS
STURGES
STUTTER
STUTZES
STUVWXY
STYGIAN
STYLERS
STYLETS
STYLING
STYLISE
STYLISH
STYLIST
STYLIZE
STYMIED
STYMIES
STYPSIS
STYPTIC
STYRENE

S•T••••

SATANIC
SATATOP
SATBACK
SATCHEL
SATCHMO
SATCOMS
SATDOWN
SATEENS
SATHOME
SATIATE
SATIETY
SATINET
SATINON
SATIRES
SATIRIC
SATISFY
SATORIS
SATRAPS
SATRAPY
SATSUMA
SATUPON
SATURNS
SATWELL
SATWITH
SATYRIC
SETBACK
SETBAIL
SETDOWN
SETENTA
SETFEES
SETFREE
SETINTO
SETOFFS
SETOUTS
SETPLAY
SETRATE
SETSAIL
SETSHOT
SETSOFF
SETSOUT
SETTEES
SETTERS
SETTING
SETTLED
SETTLER
SETTLES
SETTLOR
SETTYPE
SETUPON
SHTETLS
SHTICKS
SHTICKY
SITATOP
SITBACK
SITCOMS
SITDOWN
SITEMAP
SITHOME
SITINON
SITONIT
SITSFOR
SITSOUT
SITSPAT
SITTERS
SITTING
SITUATE
SITUPON
SITWELL
SITWITH
SOTHEBY
SOTHERE
SOTHERN
SOTTISH
SOTWEED
SUTURED
SUTURES

S••T•••

SAATCHI
SALTANT
SALTBOX
SALTERS
SALTIER
SALTILY
SALTINE
SALTING
SALTISH
SALTPIT
SALTSEA
SANTAFE
SANTANA
SANTINI
SAOTOME
SARTORS
SAUTEED
SAWTOIT
SAXTUBA
SCATHED
SCATHES
SCATMAN
SCATTED
SCATTER
SCHTICK
SCITECH
SCOTERS
SCOTIAN
SCOTTIE
SCUTTLE
SCYTHED
SCYTHES
SEATERS
SEATING
SEATRIP
SEATTLE
SECTION
SECTORS
SEETHED
SEETHES
SEETHRU
SEETOIT
SELTZER
SENTFOR
SENTOFF
SENTOUT
SENTRAS
SEPTETS
SESTETS
SESTINA
SETTEES
SETTERS
SETTING
SETTLED
SETTLER
SETTLES
SETTLOR
SETTYPE
SEXTANS
SEXTANT
SEXTETS
SEXTONS
SHATNER
SHATTER
SHOTFOR
SHOTGUN
SHOTOUT
SHOTPAR
SHOTPUT
SHUTEYE
SHUTINS
SHUTOFF
SHUTOUT
SHUTSIN
SHUTSUP
SHUTTER
SHUTTLE
SIFTERS
SIFTING
SILTIER
SILTING
SISTERS
SISTINE
SITTERS
SITTING
SIXTEEN
SIXTHLY
SIXTIES
SIXTYAD
SIXTYBC
SKATERS
SKATING
SKETCHY
SKITOWS
SKITRIP
SKITTER
SKITTLE
SLATERS
SLATHER
SLATIER
SLATING
SLATKIN
SLATTED
SLITHER
SLITTED
SLITTER
SLOTCAR
SLOTTED
SLOTTER
SMATTER
SMETANA
SMITERS
SMITHED
SMITING
SMITTEN
SMOTHER
SOFTENS
SOFTEST
SOFTGEL
SOFTIES
SOFTISH
SOFTTOP
SOOTHED
SOOTHER
SOOTHES
SOOTIER
SOOTILY
SORTERS
SORTIED
SORTIES
SORTING
SORTOUT
SOTTISH
SOUTHEY
SOUTHOF
SPATHES
SPATIAL
SPATOUT
SPATTED
SPATTER
SPATULA
SPITING
SPITOUT
SPITSON
SPITTER
SPITTLE
SPITZES
SPOTLIT
SPOTTED
SPOTTER
SPUTNIK
SPUTTER
STATELY
STATERS
STATICE
STATICS
STATING
STATINS
STATION
STATISM
STATIST
STATLER
STATORS
STATUES
STATURE
STATUTE
STETSON
STETTED
STOTINS
STUTTER
STUTZES
SUBTASK
SUBTEEN
SUBTEND
SUBTEXT
SUBTLER
SUBTONE
SUBTYPE
SUCTION
SUITING
SUITORS
SUITSME
SUITSUP
SULTANA
SULTANS
SUNTANS
SUSTAIN
SWATHED
SWATHES
SWATSAT
SWATTED
SWATTER
SWITZER
SYSTEMS
SYSTOLE

S•••T••

SAGETEA

SAINTED
SAINTES
SAINTLO
SAINTLY
SALUTED
SALUTER
SALUTES
SANCTUM
SANCTUS
SATATOP
SAUNTER
SAWATCH
SCANTED
SCANTER
SCANTLY
SCATTED
SCATTER
SCENTED
SCENTER
SCEPTER
SCEPTIC
SCEPTRE
SCIATIC
SCOOTCH
SCOOTED
SCOOTER
SCOTTIE
SCOUTED
SCOUTER
SCOUTUP
SCRATCH
SCUTTLE
SEASTAR
SEATTLE
SEDATED
SEDATER
SEDATES
SEMITES
SEMITIC
SENATES
SENATOR
SHAFTED
SHANTER
SHASTRI
SHATTER
SHEATHE
SHEATHS
SHEETED
SHELTER
SHELTIE
SHIATSU
SHIFTED
SHIFTER
SHIHTZU
SHIITES
SHOOTAT
SHOOTBY
SHOOTER
SHOOTUP
SHORTED
SHORTEN
SHORTER
SHORTIE
SHORTLY
SHORTOF
SHOUTAT
SHOUTED
SHOUTER
SHTETLS
SHUNTED
SHUNTER
SHUSTER
SHUTTER
SHUTTLE
SHYSTER
SIDETWO
SIESTAS
SIGHTED
SIGHTER
SIGHTLY
SILKTIE
SINATRA
SINUTAB
SITATOP
SIZETEN
SIZETWO
SKEETER
SKELTER
SKELTON
SKEPTIC
SKIRTED
SKIRTER
SKITTER
SKITTLE
SLANTED
SLANTLY
SLANTUP
SLATTED
SLAYTON
SLEETED
SLEPTIN
SLEPTON
SLEUTHS
SLITTED
SLITTER
SLOTTED
SLOTTER
SMARTED
SMARTEN
SMARTER
SMARTLY
SMATTER
SMELTED
SMELTER
SMITTEN
SMOOTHS
SMOOTHY
SNEETCH
SNIFTER
SNOOTED
SNORTAT
SNORTED
SNORTER
SNOUTED
SOFTTOP
SOLUTES
SOMATIC
SONATAS
SPARTAN
SPATTED
SPATTER
SPECTER
SPECTOR
SPECTRA
SPECTRE
SPENTON
SPITTER
SPITTLE
SPLITUP
SPLOTCH
SPORTED
SPORTIN
SPOTTED
SPOTTER
SPOUTED
SPOUTER
SPRITES
SPURTED
SPUTTER
SQUATLY
SQUATTY
STANTON
STARTED
STARTER
STARTIN
STARTLE
STARTON
STARTTO
STARTUP
STENTOR
STEPTWO
STERTOR
STETTED
STILTED
STILTON
STINTED
STINTER
STKITTS
STOUTEN
STOUTER
STOUTLY
STPETER
STRATAS
STRATUM
STRATUS
STRETCH
STRETTI
STRETTO
STRITCH
STUNTED
STUTTER
STYPTIC
SUBITEM
SUMATRA
SUMITUP
SUZETTE
SVELTER
SWARTHY
SWATTED
SWATTER
SWEATED
SWEATER
SWEATIT
SWEETEN
SWEETER
SWEETIE
SWEETLY
SWEETON
SWELTER
SWELTRY
SWEPTUP
SWIFTER
SWIFTLY
SWINTON
SYMPTOM

S••••T•

SABBATH
SACHETS
SADFATE
SADISTS
SAILSTO
SAMLETS
SATIATE
SATIETY
SATWITH
SAVANTS
SAWINTO
SAWPITS
SAYHITO
SAYNOTO
SCHISTS
SCHLITZ
SCHMITT
SCHULTZ
SCRIPTS
SCULPTS
SDAKOTA
SEACATS
SEADUTY
SEAGATE
SECANTS
SECRETE
SECRETS
SEEINTO
SEEMSTO
SELECTS
SELLSTO
SENDSTO
SENNETT
SENSATE
SEPTETS
SERIATE
SERRATE
SESTETS
SETENTA
SETINTO
SETOUTS
SETRATE
SEVENTH
SEVENTY
SEWISTS
SEXISTS
SEXPOTS
SEXTETS
SHEVATS
SIGNETS
SILENTA
SILENTB
SILENTC
SILENTD
SILENTE
SILENTF
SILENTG
SILENTH
SILENTI
SILENTJ
SILENTK
SILENTL
SILENTM
SILENTN
SILENTO
SILENTP
SILENTQ
SILENTR
SILENTS
SILENTT
SILENTU
SILENTV
SILENTW
SILENTX
SILENTY
SILENTZ
SIMCITY
SINCITY
SINGSTO
SINUATE
SITUATE
SITWITH
SKIHATS
SLIGHTS
SNAPSTO
SNOCATS
SOCIETY
SOCKETS
SOFFITS
SOLLATI
SONNETS
SOPWITH
SORBATE
SORBETS
SORENTO
SOVIETS
SPEAKTO
SPIGOTS
SPIKETV
SPINETS
SPIRITS
SPLINTS
SPOKETO
SPRINTS
SPROUTS
SPYBOTS
SQUANTO
SQUATTY
SQUINTS
SQUINTY
SQUIRTS
STANDTO
STARTTO
STATUTE
STBARTS
STEALTH
STICKTO
STKITTS
STOMATA
STOODTO
STRAITS
STREETS
STRETTI
STRETTO
STRIATE
STUARTI
STUCKTO
STYLETS
SUAVITY
SUBDATE
SUBLETS
SUBLOTS
SUBMITS
SUBNETS
SUBSETS
SUCCOTH
SUHARTO
SUKKOTH
SULFATE
SULFITE
SUMMATE
SUMMITS
SUMUPTO
SUNBATH
SUNCITY
SUNHATS
SUNSETS
SUZETTE
SWEARTO
SWIVETS
SWORETO

S•••••T

SACKOUT
SADDEST
SAFEBET
SAGIEST
SALIENT
SALTANT
SALTPIT
SAMOSET
SANDLOT
SANDPIT
SANGOUT
SAPIENT
SARGENT
SATINET
SAWDUST
SAWPAST
SAWTOIT
SAYWAIT
SAYWHAT
SCARLET
SCHELDT
SCHMIDT
SCHMITT
SCOFFAT
SEABOAT
SEAGIRT
SEAHUNT
SEALANT
SEALIFT
SEAMIST
SEAPORT
SEASALT
SEEDLET
SEEKOUT
SEENFIT
SEENOUT
SEEPAST
SEEPOUT
SEESFIT
SEESOUT
SEETOIT
SEGMENT
SELLOUT
SELLSIT
SENDOUT
SENNETT
SENTOUT
SERPENT
SERVANT
SETSHOT
SETSOUT
SEXIEST
SEXTANT
SHABBAT
SHALLOT
SHAVUOT
SHEGOAT
SHERBET
SHIPOUT
SHOOTAT
SHOPSAT
SHOTOUT
SHOTPUT
SHOUTAT
SHOWCAT
SHOWOUT
SHUBERT
SHUTOUT
SICKEST
SICKOUT
SIDEBET
SIGHSAT
SIGNOUT
SILENTT
SILKHAT
SINGLET
SINGOUT
SITONIT
SITSOUT
SITSPAT
SIXFEET
SIXFOOT
SKIBOOT
SKILIFT
SKILLET
SKIPOUT
SKISUIT
SKIVEST
SLEIGHT
SLIDOUT
SLIPOUT
SLOWEST
SMILEAT
SNAPSAT
SNARLAT
SNEERAT
SNICKET
SNIDEST
SNIFFAT
SNIGLET
SNIPEAT
SNIPPET
SNORTAT
SNOWCAT
SNOWHAT
SNUGFIT
SOAPNET
SOFTEST
SOLDOUT
SOLICIT
SOLOACT
SOLOIST
SOLVEIT
SOLVENT
SOONEST
SOPHIST
SORTOUT
SOUREST
SOYLENT
SPAMBOT
SPAREST
SPATOUT
SPECOUT
SPEWOUT
SPINOUT
SPITOUT
SPOTLIT
SPRIEST
SPRYEST
SPUNOUT
STALEST
STAREAT
STARLET
STARLIT
STATIST
STAYOUT
STAYPUT
STAYSAT
STEPOUT
STEWART
STEWPOT
STOPSAT
STOPSIT
STOWSIT
STUDENT
STYLIST
SUAVEST
SUBCAST
SUBDUCT
SUBJECT
SUBPLOT
SUBPOST
SUBROOT
SUBSECT
SUBSIST
SUBSORT
SUBTEXT
SUBUNIT
SUBVERT
SUGGEST
SUMOIST
SUNBELT
SUNFAST
SUNKIST
SUNSPOT
SUNSUIT
SUPPORT
SUREBET
SURFEIT
SUSPECT
SUSSOUT
SWATSAT
SWEARAT
SWEATIT
SWIGERT
SWINGAT
SWINGIT
SWOREAT
SWUNGAT
SWUNGIT

•ST••••

ASTAIRE
ASTARTE
ASTERIX
ASTHMAS
ASTOLAT
ASTORIA
ASTOUND
ASTREAM
ASTRIDE
ASTUTER
ESTADOS
ESTAMIN
ESTATED
ESTATES
ESTEBAN
ESTEEMS
ESTEFAN
ESTELLA
ESTELLE
ESTEVEZ
ESTHETE
ESTIVAL
ESTONIA
ESTORIL
ESTRADA
ESTRAYS
ESTRING
ESTUARY
GSTRING
ISTHMUS
ISTOMIN
ISTRIAN
JSTROKE
OSTEOID
OSTIARY
OSTLERS
OSTMARK
OSTOSIS
OSTRAVA
OSTRICH
OSTWALD
RSTUVWX
TSTRAPS
USTEDES
USTINOV

•S•T•••

ASATEAM
ASHTRAY
ASHTREE
ASSTDAS
ASSTIFF
ESOTERY
ISITAGO
ISOTONE
ISOTOPE
ISOTOPY
OSETRAS
TSETSES
TSETUNG
TSKTSKS
USOTOUR
USSTATE
USSTEEL

•S••T••

ASANTES
ASCETIC
ASEETHE
ASEPTIC
ASIATIC
ASTUTER
ESTATED
ESTATES
ISLETED
OSMATIC
OSMOTIC
OSSETRA
PSALTER

•S•••T•

ASBYATT
ASCENTS
ASHANTI
ASHPITS
ASPECTS
ASQUITH
ASSANTE
ASSENTS
ASSERTS
ASSISTS
ASSORTS
ASSUNTA
ASTARTE
ESCORTS
ESPARTO
ESPRITS
ESTHETE
ISOLATE
ISOLATO
TSHIRTS
USSTATE

•S••••T

ASAGIFT
ASBYATT
ASHIEST
ASKSOUT
ASONANT
ASPHALT
ASQUIET
ASQUINT
ASSAULT
ASSWEET
ASTOLAT
ESCHEAT
ISSUANT
TSARIST
TSELIOT
USGRANT

••ST•••

ABSTAIN
AMSTELS
ASSTDAS
ASSTIFF
ATSTAKE
AUSTERE
AUSTERS
AUSTINS
AUSTRAL
AUSTRIA
BASTERS
BASTING
BASTION
BESTBET
BESTBOY
BESTBUD
BESTBUY
BESTCUT
BESTIAL
BESTILL
BESTING
BESTIRS
BESTMAN
BESTMEN
BESTOFF
BESTONE
BESTOWS
BESTREW
BISTATE
BISTROS
BOSTONS
BOSTONU
BUSTARD
BUSTERS
BUSTIER
BUSTING
BUSTLED
BUSTLER
BUSTLES
BUSTOUR
BUSTOUT
BUSTRIP
BUSTSIN
BUSTSUP
BUSTUPS
CASTERS
CASTILE
CASTING
CASTLED
CASTLES
CASTOFF
CASTOUT
CASTROL
CASTSON
CASTSUP
CDSTORE
CESTMOI
CISTERN
COSTAIN
COSTARD
COSTARS
COSTATE
COSTING
COSTIVE
COSTNER
COSTUME
CUSTARD
CUSTERS
CUSTODY
CUSTOMS
DASTARD
DESTAEL
DESTAIN
DESTEMS
DESTINE
DESTINO
DESTINY
DESTOCK
DESTROY
DISTAFF
DISTANT
DISTEND
DISTICH
DISTILL
DISTILS
DISTORT
DISTROS
DISTURB
DUSTBIN
DUSTERS
DUSTGUN
DUSTIER
DUSTILY
DUSTING
DUSTMAN
DUSTMEN
DUSTMOP
DUSTOFF
DUSTPAN
DUSTRAG
DUSTUPS
EASTEGG
EASTEND
EASTERN
EASTERS
EASTHAM
EASTING
EASTMAN
ECSTASY
EPSTEIN
EUSTACE
FASTCAR
FASTENS
FASTEST
FASTING
FASTNET
FASTONE
FESTERS
FESTINA
FESTIVA
FESTIVE
FESTOON
FESTOSO
FISTFUL
FOSTERS
FUSTIAN
FUSTIER
FUSTILY
GASTANK
GASTERO
GASTONE
GASTRIC
GESTALT
GESTAPO
GESTATE
GESTURE
GOSTALE
GUSTAVE
GUSTIER
GUSTILY
GUSTING
GUSTOES
HASTENS
HASTERT
HASTIER
HASTILY
HASTIME
HASTING
HASTOBE
HISTORY
HOSTAGE
HOSTELS
HOSTESS
HOSTILE
HOSTING
HOSTLER
HUSTLED
HUSTLER
HUSTLES
IFSTONE
INSTALL
INSTALS
INSTANT
INSTATE
INSTEAD
INSTEPS
INSTILL
INSTILS
INSTOCK
INSTONE
INSTORE
INSTYLE
ITSTIME
ITSTRUE
JESTERS
JESTING
JOSTLED
JOSTLER
JOSTLES
JUSTEST
JUSTICE
JUSTIFY
JUSTINE
JUSTNOW
JUSTONE
JUSTOUT
KASTLER
KESTREL
LASTACT
LASTDON
LASTGAS
LASTING
LASTLAP
LASTLEG
LASTMAY
LASTONE
LASTORY
LASTROW
LESTOIL
LISTEES
LISTENS
LISTERS
LISTING
LOSTART
LOSTBIG
LOSTCAT
LOSTDOG
LOSTOUT
LOSTPET
LUSTERS
LUSTFUL
LUSTIER
LUSTILY
LUSTING
LUSTRAL
LUSTRED
LUSTRES
LUSTRUM
MASTERP
MASTERS

MASTERY
MASTICS
MASTIFF
MASTING
MASTOID
MISTAKE
MISTBOW
MISTELL
MISTERM
MISTERS
MISTERX
MISTIER
MISTILY
MISTIME
MISTING
MISTOLD
MISTOOK
MISTRAL
MISTSUP
MISTUNE
MISTYPE
MUSTAFA
MUSTANG
MUSTARD
MUSTDOS
MUSTERS
MUSTIER
MUSTILY
MUSTSEE
MYSTARS
MYSTERY
MYSTICS
MYSTIFY
NASTASE
NASTIER
NASTIES
NASTILY
NESTEGG
NESTERS
NESTFUL
NESTING
NESTLED
NESTLER
NESTLES
NESTORS
NESTSIN
NOSTAIN
NOSTARS
NOSTRIL
NOSTRUM
ONSTAFF
ONSTAGE
OUSTERS
OUSTING
OYSTERS
PASTDUE
PASTEIN
PASTELS
PASTERN
PASTERS
PASTEUP
PASTEUR
PASTIER
PASTIES
PASTIME
PASTINA
PASTING
PASTORS
PASTURE
PESTERS
PESTLED
PESTLES
PISTILS
PISTOLE
PISTOLS
PISTONS
PISTOUS
POSTAGE
POSTBAG
POSTBOX
POSTDOC
POSTERN
POSTERS
POSTFIX
POSTHOC
POSTIES
POSTING
POSTITS
POSTMAN
POSTMEN
POSTOPS
POSTURE
POSTWAR
QRSTUVW
RASTERS
RESTABS
RESTACK
RESTAFF
RESTAGE
RESTAIN
RESTAMP
RESTART
RESTATE
RESTERS
RESTFUL
RESTICK
RESTING
RESTIRS
RESTIVE
RESTOCK
RESTOKE
RESTORE
RESTOWS
RESTRAP
RESTREW
RESTRIP
RESTSIN
RESTSON
RESTSUP
RESTUDY
RESTUFF
RESTYLE
RLSTINE
ROSTAND
ROSTERS
ROSTOCK
ROSTRAL
ROSTRUM
RUSTICS
RUSTIER
RUSTILY
RUSTING
RUSTLED
RUSTLER
RUSTLES
SESTETS
SESTINA
SISTERS
SISTINE
SUSTAIN
SYSTEMS
SYSTOLE
TASTEIT
TASTERS
TASTIER
TASTILY
TASTING
TESTACY
TESTATE
TESTBAN
TESTBED
TESTEES
TESTERS
TESTFLY
TESTFOR
TESTIER
TESTIFY
TESTILY
TESTING
TESTKIT
TESTLAB
TESTOUT
TESTRUN
TOSTADA
TOSTART
TVSTARS
ULSTERS
UNSTACK
UNSTAGY
UNSTAID
UNSTATE
UNSTEEL
UNSTEPS
UNSTERN
UNSTICK
UNSTIFF
UNSTOIC
UNSTONY
UNSTOPS
UNSTOUT
UNSTOWS
UNSTRAP
UNSTUCK
UNSTUNG
UPSTAGE
UPSTAIR
UPSTAND
UPSTARE
UPSTART
UPSTATE
UPSTEPS
UPSTIRS
UPSTOOD
USSTATE
USSTEEL
VASTEST
VASTIER
VASTITY
VESTALS
VESTEES
VESTIGE
VESTING
VESTRAL
VESTRON
VESTURE
VISTAED
VISTEON
VISTULA
WASTAGE
WASTERS
WASTING
WASTREL
WESTEGG
WESTEND
WESTERN
WESTERS
WESTIES
WESTINS
WISTFUL
XYSTERS
XYSTUSI
ZESTERS
ZESTFUL
ZESTIER
ZESTILY
ZESTING

••S•T••

ALSATIA
BASETEN
BASETWO
BUSSTOP
CASITAS
COSETTE
DESKTOP
DESOTOS
HASATIT
ITSATIE
LESOTHO
LESSTAR
MISSTEP
MUSETTA
MUSETTE
OSSETRA
PESETAS
POSITED
RESITED
RISOTTO
ROSETEA
ROSETTA
ROSETTE
UNSATED
VISITED
VISITOR
WASATCH
WASHTUB
YESITIS

••S••T•

ABSENTS
ABSINTH
ALSMITH
ASSANTE
ASSENTS
ASSERTS
ASSISTS
ASSORTS
ASSUNTA
BASALTS
BASKETS
BASKETT
BASMATI
BASSETS
BASSETT
BBSHOTS
BISECTS
BISMUTH
BISTATE
CASEATE
CASERTA
CASKETS
CASSATT
COSETTE
COSSETS
COSTATE
CUSPATE
DESALTS
DESERTS
DESILTS
DESISTS
DESPITE
DESPOTS
DISPUTE
DISRATE
DOSHOTS
ENSEATS
ENSUITE
EXSECTS
EXSERTS
GASEITY
GASJETS
GASKETS
GESTATE
GOSOUTH
GOSSETT
GUSSETS
HASFITS
HUSSITE
INSECTA
INSECTS
INSERTS
INSISTS
INSPITE
INSPOTS
INSTATE
INSULTS
ITSLATE
JESUITS
KISMETS
KOSSUTH
LISBETH
LISENTE
LOSESTO
MASCOTS
MISACTS
MISCITE
MISCUTS
MISDATE
MISFITS
MISHITS
MISMATE
MISRATE
MISSETS
MOSCATO
MRSCOTT
MRSLATE
MRSMITH
MUSANTE
MUSCATS
MUSETTA
MUSETTE
MUSKETS
NESBITT
NESMITH
NOSEATS
OFSORTS
PASSATS
PESANTE
POSTITS
RESALTS
RESEATS
RESECTS
RESENTS
RESHUTS
RESIFTS
RESISTS
RESLATE
RESORTS
RESPITE
RESPOTS
RESTATE
RESUITS
RESULTS
RISENTO
RISESTO
RISOTTO
ROSEATE
ROSETTA
ROSETTE
RUSSETS
RUSSETY
SESTETS
TESTATE
TISSOTS
TVSPOTS
UNSALTY
UNSEATS
UNSOOTY
UNSORTS
UNSTATE
UPSHOTS
UPSTATE
USSTATE
VASTITY
WASLATE
WASONTO
WESCOTT
WESKITS
YESLETS
YESVOTE

••S•••T

ABSOLUT
ASSAULT
ASSWEET
ATSIGHT
BASEHIT
BASKETT
BASSETT
BASSIST
BESTBET
BESTCUT
BISCUIT
BUSIEST
BUSTOUT
CASELOT
CASEOUT
CASHOUT
CASSATT
CASTOUT
CASUIST
CESSPIT
COSIEST
DASBOOT
DASHDOT
DASHPOT
DESCANT
DESCENT
DESERET
DESKSET
DESSERT
DISGUST
DISHOUT
DISMAST
DISPART
DISPORT
DISRUPT
DISSECT
DISSENT
DISSERT
DISTANT
DISTORT
EASEOUT
EASIEST
FASCIST
FASTEST
FASTNET
FISHNET
FISHOUT
FUSSPOT
GASHEAT
GESTALT
GOSSETT
GUSHOUT
HASAFIT
HASASET
HASATIT
HASHOUT
HASTERT
INSHORT
INSIGHT
INSPECT
INSTANT
INSWEPT
ISSUANT
ITSAHIT
ITSALOT
ITSBEST
JUSTEST
JUSTOUT
LASHOUT
LASTACT
LESCAUT
LESSFAT
LOSEOUT
LOSESIT
LOSTART
LOSTCAT
LOSTOUT
LOSTPET
LUSHEST
MESSKIT
MISCAST
MISEDIT
MISSEAT
MISSENT
MISSORT
MISSOUT
MOSHPIT
MRSCOTT
MUSKRAT
NASCENT
NESBITT
NOSEOUT
NOSIEST
NOSWEAT
OKSHOOT
ONSIGHT
PASSANT
PASSOUT
POSHEST
PUSHOUT
RASHEST
RESHIFT
RESHOOT
RESIGHT
RESMELT
RESOJET
RESPECT
RESPELT
RESPLIT
RESTART
RISKSIT
ROSIEST
RUSHOUT
RUSSERT
SUSPECT
SUSSOUT
TASTEIT
TESTKIT
TESTOUT
TOSSOUT
TOSSPOT
TOSTART
UNSHIFT
UNSHORT
UNSIGHT
UNSMART
UNSPELT
UNSPENT
UNSPILT
UNSPLIT
UNSTOUT
UNSWEET
UNSWEPT
UPSHIFT
UPSHOOT
UPSTART
UPSWEPT
VASTEST
WASHOUT
WESCOTT

•••ST••

AHOSTOF
ALLSTAR
ALLSTON
AMISTAD
ANISTON
APOSTLE
ARISTAE
ARISTAS
ARISTOS
AVESTAN
AVESTAS
BARSTOW
BEASTIE
BEASTLY
BIGSTAR
BLASTED
BLASTER
BLISTER
BLUSTER
BOASTED
BOASTER
BOASTOF
BOLSTER
BOOSTED
BOOSTER
BOOSTUP
BORSTAL
BOXSTEP
BOXSTER
BRISTLE
BRISTLY
BRISTOL
BURSTER
BURSTIN
BURSTYN
BUSSTOP
CAPSTAN
CAUSTIC
CHASTEN
CHASTER
CHESTED
CHESTER
CLUSTER
COASTAL
COASTED
COASTER
CRESTED
CRESTON
CROSTIC
CRUSTAL
CRUSTED
CRYSTAL
CUESTAS
DAYSTAR
DEISTIC
DOESTOO
DOGSTAR
DRASTIC
DRISTAN
DUNSTAN
DYKSTRA
EGESTED
EKISTIC
ELASTIC
ELASTIN
EPISTLE
ERASTUS
ERISTIC
EXISTED
FAUSTUS
FEASTED
FEASTER
FEASTON
FIBSTER
FIESTAS
FIRSTLY
FIRSTUP
FLUSTER
FOISTED
FOISTON
FORSTER
FROSTED
FROSTER
FRUSTRO
FRUSTUM
FUNSTER
GAGSTER
GHASTLY
GHOSTED
GHOSTLY
GLISTEN
GLISTER
GNOSTIC
GRISTER
GRISTLE
GRISTLY
GUESTED
HALSTON
HAMSTER
HEISTED
HIPSTER
HOFSTRA
HOISTED
HOISTER
HOISTUP
HOLSTER
HOUSTON
HURSTON
ILOSTIT
IMUSTGO
INASTEW
INASTIR
INKSTER
ITISTOO
JETSTAR
JOISTED
JOUSTED
JOUSTER
KEISTER
KIRSTEN
KIRSTIE
KLISTER
KRISTIN
KRYSTLE
LEISTER
LESSTAR
LOBSTER
MAESTRO
MARSTON
MEISTER
MINSTER
MISSTEP
MOBSTER
MOISTEN
MOISTER
MOISTLY
MONSTER
MONSTRO
MUNSTER
NAPSTER
NETSTER
NONSTOP
NUESTRA
NUESTRO
OERSTED
OLDSTER
OLESTRA
OLMSTED
ONESTAR
ONESTEP
ONESTOP
OPUSTWO
ORESTES
OUTSTAY
OUTSTEP
PAYSTUB
PIASTER
PIASTRE
PITSTOP
PLASTER
PLASTIC
PLUSTAX
PLUSTWO
POPSTAR
PQRSTUV
PRESTON
PRESTOS
PUNSTER
QUESTED
QUESTER
RALSTON
RAPSTAR
REDSTAR
RIPSTOP
ROASTED
ROASTER
ROISTER
ROOSTED
ROOSTER
ROUSTED
ROUSTER
SEASTAR
SHASTRI
SHUSTER
SHYSTER
SIESTAS
TAPSTER
TELSTAR
THESTAR
THISTLE
THISTLY
TINSTAR
TIPSTER
TOASTED
TOASTEE
TOASTER
TOLSTOI
TOLSTOY
TRESTLE
TRISTAN
TRISTAR
TRUSTED
TRUSTEE
TRUSTER
TRUSTIN
TRUSTME
TRYSTED
TRYSTER
TWISTED
TWISTER
TWISTON
TWISTUP
TWOSTAR
TWOSTEP
VORSTER
WAISTED
WALSTON
WEBSTER
WHISTLE
WINSTON
WOOSTER
WORSTED
WRESTED
WRESTER
WRESTLE
YEASTED
ZEMSTVO

•••S•T•

BASSETS
BASSETT
BEDSITS
BOXSETS
CASSATT
CATSITS
CLOSETO
CLOSETS
COMSATS
CORSETS
COSSETS
DENSITY
DOGSITS
DORSETT
FALSITY
FORSYTE
FORSYTH
GOSSETT
GUSSETS
HIRSUTE
HUSSITE
JETSETS
KOSSUTH
LEASETO
MISSETS
OBESITY
OFFSETS
OFFSITE
OUTSETS
OUTSITS
PADSITE
PASSATS
PETSITS
PIOSITY
PRESETS
PULSATE
RUSSETS
RUSSETY
SENSATE
SUBSETS
SUNSETS
TABSETS
TEASETS
TENSITY
TILSITS
TISSOTS
TRASHTV
VARSITY
VERSETS
WEBSITE

•••S••T

ACESOUT
ACTSOUT
ADDSALT
AGESOUT
AIRSOUT
APESUIT
ASKSOUT
BADSHOT
BASSETT
BASSIST
BATSUIT
BERSUNT
BIGSHOT
BORSCHT
BOWSHOT
BOWSOUT
BOXSEAT
BRISKET
BUGSOUT
BUMSOUT
BUYSOUT
CARSEAT
CASSATT
CATSUIT
CESSPIT
CLOSEST
CONSENT
CONSIST
CONSORT
CONSULT
COPSOUT
CRESSET
CROSSAT
CURSEAT
CUTSOUT
DAUSSET
DENSEST
DESSERT
DIESOUT
DIGSOUT
DIMSOUT
DISSECT
DISSENT
DISSERT
DOESNOT
DORSETT
DRYSUIT
EARSHOT
EATSOUT
EKESOUT
EYESHOT
EYESPOT
FALSEST
FANSOUT
FLUSHOT
FRESHET
FUSSPOT
GETSFIT
GETSHOT
GETSOFT
GETSOUT
GETSSET
GETSWET
GODSENT
GOESAFT
GOESOUT
GOSSETT
GOTSOFT
GRASPAT

GRISLET
GUESSAT
GUNSHOT
GYMSUIT
HITSOUT
HOPSOUT
HOTSEAT
HOTSHOT
HOTSPOT
ICESOUT
IINSIST
ILOSTIT
INASNIT
INASPOT
INASUIT
INKSPOT
IRISOUT
KIDSEAT
KNESSET
LAWSUIT
LAYSOUT
LESSFAT
LETSEAT
LETSNOT
LETSOUT
LIPSOUT
LOGSOUT
LOOSEST
LUGSOUT
MAOSUIT
MAPSOUT
MESSKIT
MISSEAT
MISSENT
MISSORT
MISSOUT
MUGSHOT
OFASORT
OILSPOT
OLDSALT
ONESHOT
ONESPOT
OPTSOUT
OUTSERT
OUTSHOT
OUTSIFT
OUTSPIT
PANSOUT
PASSANT
PASSOUT
PAYSOUT
PEASANT
PERSIST
PIGSOUT
POPSOUT
POTSHOT
PRESALT
PRESEAT
PRESENT
PRESIFT
PRESORT
PURSUIT
PUTSOUT
RATSOUT
REDSPOT
REDSUIT
RIGSOUT
RIMSHOT
RIPSOUT
ROBSART
RUBSOUT
RUNSOUT
RUSSERT
SEASALT
SEESFIT
SEESOUT
SETSHOT
SETSOUT
SITSOUT
SITSPAT
SKISUIT
SUBSECT
SUBSIST
SUBSORT
SUNSPOT
SUNSUIT
SUSSOUT
TAGSOUT
TAPSOUT
TEESHOT
TENSEST
TENSPOT
TERSEST
TOGSOUT
TOPSOUT
TOPSPOT
TOSSOUT
TOSSPOT
TRISECT
TWOSHOT
TWOSPOT
VANSANT
VERSANT
WAPSHOT
WETSUIT
WHOSOUT
WIGSOUT
WINSLET
WINSOUT

••••ST•

ACCOSTS
ADJUSTS
AGEISTS
ALCESTE
AMNESTY
ARIOSTO
ARRESTS
ARTISTE
ARTISTS
ASSISTS
ATTESTS
AUGUSTA
AUGUSTE
AUGUSTO
AUGUSTS
AURISTS
AUTISTS
BARISTA
BATISTA
BATISTE
BEHESTS
BINDSTO
BREASTS
BROASTS
CALISTA
CALLSTO
CANASTA
CARESTO
CELESTA
CELESTE
CHRISTA
CHRISTI
CHRISTO
CHRISTY
COHOSTS
COMESTO
CUBISTS
DACOSTA
DARESTO
DEALSTO
DEGUSTS
DELISTS
DEMASTS
DEMISTS
DEPESTS
DERUSTS
DESISTS
DETESTS
DEVESTS
DIGESTS
DIVESTS
DOOMSTO
DRAWSTO
DYNASTS
DYNASTY
EGOISTE
EGOISTS
ELMISTI
ENLISTS
ERNESTA
ERNESTO
FAILSTO
FALLSTO
FEEDSTO
FLIESTO
FORESTS
GANGSTA
GEARSTO
GIVESTO
GLUESTO
HEADSTO
HERESTO
HOLDSTO
HOLISTS
HONESTY
HOPESTO
IMPASTO
IMPOSTS
INFESTS
INGESTA
INGESTS
INHASTE
INSISTS
INTASTE
INVESTS
IQTESTS
JOCASTA
JURISTS
KEEPSTO
LACOSTE
LAKISTS
LEADSTO
LEANSTO
LEGISTS
LOCUSTS
LOOKSTO
LOSESTO
LOVESTO
LUNESTA
LUTISTS
LYRISTS
MAJESTE
MAJESTY
MAOISTS
MEANSTO
MODESTO
MODESTY
MODISTE
MOLESTS
MOVESTO
NEEDSTO
NOTASTE
NUDISTS
OBLASTS
OBOISTS
OBTESTS
OPQRSTU
PAPISTS
PLANSTO
PLAYSTO
PLOESTI
PRAYSTO
PRIESTS
PURISTS
RACESTO
RACISTS
RAWISTS
READSTO
REBASTE
RECASTS
RECOSTS
REDUSTS
RELISTS
RENESTS
RENTSTO
REPASTE
REPASTS
REPOSTS
RESISTS
RETASTE
RETESTS
REVESTS
RIDESTO
RIPOSTE
RIPOSTS
RISESTO
ROBUSTA
ROBUSTO
SADISTS
SAILSTO
SCHISTS
SEEMSTO
SELLSTO
SENDSTO
SEWISTS
SEXISTS
SINGSTO
SNAPSTO
TAKESTO
TALKSTO
TAOISTS
TELESTO
TENDSTO
THEISTS
THIRSTS
THIRSTY
THRUSTS
TOTASTE
TRIESTE
TRIESTO
TUBISTS
TUNESTO
TURISTA
TURNSTO
TYPISTS
UNDUSTY
UNHASTY
UNLUSTY
UNMASTS
UNPASTE
UNRESTS
UNTASTY
UPCASTS
UTMOSTS
VEDISTS
VERISTS
VIBISTS
WALKSTO
WANTSTO
WARMSTO
WAVESTO
ZENISTS

••••S•T

BABYSAT
BABYSIT
BALKSAT
BARKSAT
BEATSAT
BEATSIT
BEEPSAT
BLOWSIT
BONESET
BOOTSIT
CALLSIT
CARPSAT
CLAWSAT
COMESAT
COOLSIT
CRESSET
CROSSAT
DATASET
DAUSSET
DEADSET
DEEPSET
DEPOSIT
DESKSET
DIDASET
DINESAT
DROPSIT
DRUMSET
EARNSIT
EXPOSIT
FACESIT
FAKESIT
FILMSET
FIRESAT
FLIESAT
FOOTSIT
FRETSAT
FUMESAT
GAPESAT
GAWKSAT
GAZESAT
GENESET
GETSSET
GIBESAT
GIFTSET
GNAWSAT
GRABSAT
GRINSAT
GUESSAT
HACKSIT
HADASET
HANDSET
HARDSET
HASASET
HATESIT
HDTVSET
HEADSET
HINTSAT
HOLDSIT
HONKSAT
HOOFSIT
HOOTSAT
HOWLSAT
JEERSAT
JIBESAT
JUMPSAT
KEEPSAT
KNESSET
LANDSAT
LEAPSAT
LEERSAT
LEGOSET
LIVESAT
LIVESET
LOCKSET
LOOKSAT
LORDSIT
LOSESIT
LOVESET
LOVESIT
LUMPSIT
MAKESIT
MEANSIT
MINDSET
MOONSET
MORISOT
MOVESIT
NAILSET
NAILSIT
NULLSET
OVERSET
PARKSIT
PECKSAT
PEEKSAT
PEEPSAT
PEERSAT
PICKSAT
PLAYSAT
POKESAT
POLESAT
POLESIT
QUITSIT
QUONSET
RAILSAT
RANTSAT
REPOSIT
REVISIT
RISKSIT
ROARSAT
SAMOSET
SELLSIT
SHOPSAT
SIGHSAT
SNAPSAT
STAYSAT
STOPSAT
STOPSIT
STOWSIT
SWATSAT
TAKESIT
TALKSAT
TEARSAT
TEARSIT
TELLSIT
THATSIT
TILTSAT
TOILSAT
TOOLSET
TOOTSAT
TRANSIT
TRIESIT
TWINSET
TYPESET
UNBESET
WAVESAT
WELLSET
WHATSIT
WHOISIT
WHYISIT
WINGSIT
WINKSAT
WORKSAT
YANKSAT
YELLSAT

•••••ST

ABREAST
ACCURST
ACHIEST
ACUTEST
AERIEST
AFTMOST
AGAINST
AGILEST
AGONIST
AIRIEST
ALQUIST
ALTOIST
AMHERST
AMONGST
AMORIST
AMPLEST
ANALYST
ANAPEST
ANIMIST
ARABIST
ARCHEST
ARIDEST
ARMREST
ARTIEST
ASHIEST
ATACOST
ATAVIST
ATFIRST
ATHEIST
ATHIRST
ATLEAST
ATOMIST
ATWORST
AVIDEST
AWAREST
BAALIST
BABIEST
BADDEST
BADPAST
BAHAIST
BAKERST
BALDEST
BALLAST
BAPTIST
BASSIST
BEDPOST
BEDREST
BELFAST
BEQUEST
BIGEAST
BIGGEST
BOLDEST
BOMBAST
BONIEST
BOXIEST
BRAVEST
BUFFEST
BUSIEST
CAGIEST
CAKIEST
CALMEST
CANIEST
CASUIST
CELLIST
CHEMIST
CHICEST
CHORIST
CHUTIST
CLOSEST
COEXIST
COKIEST
COLDEST
COMBUST
COMCAST
COMPOST
COMTIST
CONGEST
CONSIST
CONTEST
COOLEST
COPYIST
COSIEST
COWIEST
COZIEST
CRUDEST
CULTIST
CURTEST
CYCLIST
CZARIST
DADAIST
DAFTEST
DAMPEST
DANKEST
DARKEST
DEADEST
DEAFEST
DEAREST
DEEPEST
DEFFEST
DEFROST
DEFTEST
DEGHOST
DENSEST
DENTIST
DEWIEST
DIARIST
DICIEST
DIECAST
DIMMEST
DISGUST
DISMAST
DNATEST
DOGVEST
DOPIEST
DOUREST
DOZIEST
DRFRIST
DUALIST
DUEEAST
DUELIST
DUEWEST
DULLEST
DUMBEST
EARNEST
EASIEST
EDGIEST
EELIEST
EERIEST
EGGIEST
EGOTIST
ELEGIST
ELITEST
ELITIST
ELMIEST
ENCRUST
ENDMOST
ENTRUST
ENTWIST
EPEEIST
EVENEST
EVEREST
EVILEST
EXHAUST
EYETEST
FABBEST
FADDIST
FAINEST
FAIREST
FALSEST
FANFEST
FANTAST
FAREAST
FARWEST
FASCIST
FASTEST
FATTEST
FAUVIST
FEUDIST
FIRMEST
FITTEST
FLORIST
FLUTIST
FLYCAST
FLYPAST
FONDEST
FORREST
FOULEST
FOXIEST
FULLEST
FUMIEST
FUNFEST
GABFEST
GAMIEST
GETLOST
GETPAST
GJETOST
GLUIEST
GNOMIST
GOFIRST
GOOIEST
GORIEST
GOTLOST
GOTPAST
GRAVEST
GRAYEST
GREYEST
GYMNAST
HADBEST
HARDEST
HARPIST
HARVEST
HAZIEST
HEPPEST
HIGHEST
HIPPEST
HITLIST
HOKIEST
HOLIEST
HOMIEST
HORNIST
HOTTEST
IAMBIST
ICKIEST
IDOLIST
IDYLIST
IFFIEST
IINSIST
IMAGIST
IMPREST
INACAST
INANEST
INCRUST
INFIRST
INKIEST
INQUEST
INTRUST
IRATEST
IRONIST
ITSBEST
JAINIST
JIVIEST
JOKIEST
JUDOIST
JUSTEST
KEENEST
KEYWEST
KINDEST
LABTEST
LACIEST
LAKIEST
LAMAIST
LANKEST
LARGEST
LAZIEST
LEANEST
LEFTEST
LEFTIST
LEGREST
LEWDEST
LIEFEST
LIETEST
LIMIEST
LIMPEST
LINIEST
LITHEST
LOGIEST
LONGEST
LOOKIST
LOOSEST
LOUDEST
LOWCOST
LOWPOST
LUSHEST
MADDEST
MAEWEST
MAHDIST
MARXIST
MAZIEST
MEANEST
MEEKEST
MEFIRST
METRIST
MIDEAST
MIDLIST
MIDMOST
MIDWEST
MILDEST
MIRIEST
MISCAST
MOBBIST
MOPIEST
NAIVEST
NEAREST
NEATEST
NETCOST
NIGHEST
NOBLEST
NONPAST
NOPQRST
NOSIEST
NUMBEST
OAKIEST
OCULIST
OFFCAST
OILIEST
OLDWEST
ONFIRST
ONLIEST
ONTOAST
OOZIEST
ORALIST
ORGIAST
OUTCAST
OUTFAST
OUTJEST
OUTKAST
OUTLAST
OUTMOST
OUTPOST
OUTWEST
OWLIEST
OZZFEST
PACIEST
PALMIST
PAULIST
PERSIST
PERTEST
PIANIST
PINIEST
PINKEST
PIPIEST
PODCAST
POKIEST
POLOIST
POOREST
POSHEST
PRECAST
PRETEST
PREVOST
PROEAST
PROTEST
PROTIST
PROVOST
PROWEST
PUNIEST
QUERIST
RACIEST
RANKEST
RANPAST
RASHEST
REALEST
REALIST
REDDEST
REDDUST
REQUEST
RETOAST
RETWIST
RHYMIST
RICHEST
RIMIEST
ROPIEST
ROSIEST
RULIEST
RUNPAST
SADDEST
SAGIEST
SAWDUST
SAWPAST
SEAMIST
SEEPAST
SEXIEST
SICKEST
SKIVEST
SLOWEST
SNIDEST
SOFTEST
SOLOIST
SOONEST
SOPHIST
SOUREST
SPAREST
SPRIEST
SPRYEST
STALEST
STATIST
STYLIST
SUAVEST
SUBCAST
SUBPOST
SUBSIST
SUGGEST
SUMOIST
SUNFAST
SUNKIST
TALLEST
TANNEST
TARTEST
TAUTEST
TEMPEST
TENPAST
TENSEST
TERSEST
THEBEST
THEEAST
THEMOST
THEPOST
TIDIEST
TINIEST
TITLIST
TITOIST
TONIEST
TOPMAST
TOPMOST
TOURIST
TRITEST
TSARIST
TUBAIST
UGLIEST
UNBLEST
UNBURST
UNFROST
UNMOIST
UNTWIST
UPBURST
UPCOAST
UPFIRST
UTOPIST
VAGUEST
VAINEST
VASTEST
VERIEST
VFWPOST
VINIEST
VIOLIST
WACKEST
WANIEST
WANNEST
WARIEST
WARMEST
WAVIEST
WAXIEST
WEAKEST
WEBCAST
WETTEST
WHITEST
WILDEST
WILIEST
WINIEST
WIRIEST
WOULDST
YORKIST
ZANIEST
ZIONIST
ZOOIEST

SU•••••
SUASION
SUASIVE
SUAVELY
SUAVEST
SUAVITY
SUBAREA
SUBARID
SUBARUS
SUBBAND
SUBBANK
SUBBASE
SUBBASS
SUBBIAS
SUBBING
SUBCASE
SUBCASH
SUBCAST
SUBCELL
SUBCLAN
SUBCODE
SUBCOOL
SUBDATE
SUBDEBS
SUBDUAL
SUBDUCT
SUBDUED
SUBDUER
SUBDUES
SUBECHO
SUBFILE
SUBFORM
SUBGOAL
SUBGODS
SUBHALL
SUBHEAD
SUBIDEA
SUBITEM
SUBJECT
SUBJOIN
SUBKING
SUBLETS
SUBLIDS
SUBLIME
SUBLONG
SUBLOTS
SUBMITS
SUBNETS
SUBORNS
SUBPLOT
SUBPOST
SUBRACE
SUBROOT
SUBROSA
SUBSECT
SUBSETS
SUBSIDE
SUBSIDY
SUBSIST
SUBSOIL
SUBSORT
SUBSUME
SUBTASK
SUBTEEN
SUBTEND
SUBTEXT
SUBTLER
SUBTONE
SUBTYPE
SUBUNIT
SUBURBS
SUBVENE
SUBVERT
SUBWARS
SUBWAYS
SUBZERO
SUBZONE
SUCCEED
SUCCESS
SUCCORS
SUCCOTH
SUCCOUR
SUCCUMB
SUCKDRY
SUCKERS
SUCKIER
SUCKING
SUCKSIN
SUCKSUP
SUCRASE
SUCROSE
SUCTION
SUDAFED
SUDBURY
SUDOKUS
SUDSERS
SUDSIER
SUDSING
SUEDFOR
SUELLEN
SUELYON
SUESFOR
SUFFERS
SUFFICE
SUFFOLK
SUFFUSE
SUGARED
SUGGEST
SUHARTO
SUITING
SUITORS
SUITSME
SUITSUP
SUKARNO
SUKKOTH
SULFATE
SULFIDE
SULFITE
SULKERS
SULKIER
SULKIES
SULKILY
SULKING
SULLIED
SULLIES
SULPHUR
SULTANA
SULTANS
SULUSEA
SUMATRA
SUMITUP
SUMLESS
SUMMAND
SUMMARY
SUMMATE
SUMMERS
SUMMERY
SUMMING
SUMMITS
SUMMONS
SUMOIST
SUMUPTO
SUNBATH
SUNBEAM
SUNBELT
SUNBIRD
SUNBOWL
SUNBOWS
SUNBURN
SUNCITY
SUNDAES
SUNDAYS
SUNDECK
SUNDERS
SUNDIAL
SUNDOGS
SUNDOWN
SUNFANS
SUNFAST
SUNFIRE
SUNFISH
SUNGLOW
SUNGODS
SUNHATS
SUNKIST
SUNLAMP
SUNLESS
SUNLIKE
SUNMAID
SUNNIER
SUNNILY
SUNNING
SUNRAYS
SUNRISE
SUNROOF
SUNROOM
SUNSETS
SUNSFAN
SUNSPOT
SUNSUIT
SUNTANS
SUNWARD
SUPERGS
SUPPERS
SUPPING
SUPPLED
SUPPLER
SUPPLES
SUPPORT
SUPPOSE
SUPREME
SUREBET
SURECAN
SUREIAM
SUREIDO
SUREROF
SURFACE
SURFEIT
SURFERS
SURFIER
SURFING
SURFMAN
SURFMEN
SURFSUP
SURGEON
SURGERY
SURGING
SURIMIS
SURINAM
SURLIER
SURLILY
SURMISE
SURNAME
SURPASS
SURPLUS
SURREAL
SURREYS
SURVEIL
SURVEYS
SURVIVE
SUSANNA
SUSANNE
SUSPECT
SUSPEND
SUSPIRE
SUSSING
SUSSOUT
SUSTAIN
SUTURED
SUTURES
SUZANNE
SUZETTE
SUZUKIS

S•U••••
SAUCERS
SAUCIER
SAUCILY
SAUCING
SAUCONY
SAUNAED
SAUNTER
SAURIAN
SAUSAGE
SAUTEED
SCUBAED
SCUDDED
SCUDDER
SCUFFED
SCUFFER
SCUFFLE
SCULLED
SCULLER
SCULPED
SCULPTS
SCUPPER
SCURVES
SCUSEME
SCUTTLE
SCUZZES
SHUBERT
SHUCKED
SHUCKER
SHUDDER
SHUFFLE
SHULMAN
SHUNNED
SHUNTED
SHUNTER
SHUSHED
SHUSHES
SHUSTER
SHUTEYE
SHUTINS
SHUTOFF
SHUTOUT
SHUTSIN
SHUTSUP
SHUTTER
SHUTTLE
SKULKED
SKULKER
SKULLED
SKUNKED
SLUDGES
SLUGGED
SLUGGER
SLUICED
SLUICES
SLUMBER
SLUMMED
SLUMMER
SLUMPED
SLUNKIN
SLUNKUP
SLURPED
SLURPEE
SLURPER
SLURRED
SLUSHED
SLUSHES
SMUCKER
SMUDGED
SMUDGES
SMUGGER
SMUGGLE
SMUSHED
SMUSHES
SNUBBED
SNUBBER
SNUCKUP
SNUFFED
SNUFFER
SNUFFLE
SNUGFIT
SNUGGED
SNUGGER
SNUGGLE
SNUGGLY
SNUGLIS
SOUBISE
SOUFFLE
SOULFUL
SOULMAN
SOUNDED
SOUNDER
SOUNDLY
SOUPCAN
SOUPCON
SOUPERS
SOUPIER
SOUPMIX
SOUPSON
SOUPSUP
SOURALE
SOURCED
SOURCES
SOUREST
SOURING
SOURISH
SOURSON
SOUSING
SOUTHEY
SOUTHOF
SPUMIER
SPUMING
SPUMONE
SPUMONI
SPUNOFF
SPUNOUT
SPURNED
SPURNER
SPURRED
SPURSON
SPURTED
SPUTNIK
SPUTTER
SQUALID
SQUALLS
SQUALLY
SQUALOR
SQUANTO
SQUARED
SQUARER
SQUARES
SQUASHY
SQUATLY
SQUATTY
SQUAWKS
SQUAWKY
SQUEAKS
SQUEAKY
SQUEALS
SQUEERS
SQUEEZE
SQUELCH
SQUINCH
SQUINTS
SQUINTY
SQUIRED
SQUIRES
SQUIRMS
SQUIRMY
SQUIRTS
SQUISHY
STUARTI
STUBBED
STUBBLE
STUBBLY
STUBING
STUCCOS
STUCKBY
STUCKIN
STUCKON
STUCKTO
STUCKUP
STUDDED
STUDENT
STUDIED
STUDIER
STUDIES
STUDIOS
STUFFED
STUFFER
STUFFIN
STUMBLE
STUMPED
STUMPER
STUNGUN
STUNNED
STUNNER
STUNTED
STUPEFY
STUPIDS
STUPORS
STURGES
STUTTER
STUTZES
STUVWXY
SWUNGAT
SWUNGBY
SWUNGIT

S••U•••
SAGUARO
SALUKIS
SALUTED
SALUTER
SALUTES
SAMUELL
SAMURAI
SARUMAN
SATUPON
SATURNS
SCHULTZ
SCHUMER
SCOUPES
SCOURED
SCOURER
SCOURGE
SCOUTED
SCOUTER
SCOUTUP
SCRUBBY
SCRUBUP
SCRUFFS
SCRUFFY
SCRUGGS
SCRUNCH
SCRUPLE
SECULAR
SECURED
SECURER
SECURES
SEDUCED
SEDUCER
SEDUCES
SEQUELS
SEQUINS
SEQUOIA
SEQUOYA
SETUPON
SHOULDA
SHOULDI
SHOUTAT
SHOUTED
SHOUTER
SHRUBBY
SINUATE
SINUOUS
SINUSES
SINUTAB
SIOUANS
SITUATE
SITUPON
SLEUTHS
SLOUCHY
SLOUGHS
SNOUTED
SOLUBLE
SOLUTES
SOSUEME
SPLURGE
SPOUSAL
SPOUSES
SPOUTED
SPOUTER
SPRUCED
SPRUCER
SPRUCES
SPYUPON
STAUNCH
STEUBEN
STLUCIA
STLUKES
STOUTEN
STOUTER
STOUTLY
STRUDEL
SUBUNIT
SUBURBS
SULUSEA
SUMUPTO
SUTURED
SUTURES
SUZUKIS

S•••U••
SACQUES
SAMBUCA
SAMHUFF
SAMNUNN
SAMSUNG
SANJUAN
SATSUMA
SAVOURS
SAVOURY
SAWBUCK
SAWDUST
SAXTUBA
SCAPULA
SCHLUBS
SCHLUMP
SEADUCK
SEADUTY
SEAGULL
SEAHUNT
SECLUDE
SEIZURE
SENDUPS
SENSUAL
SETOUTS
SHAVUOT
SHOGUNS
SHONUFF
SHROUDS
SIDDURS
SIGMUND
SIGNUPS
SIRDUKE
SIXGUNS
SKIBUMS
SKIJUMP
SKIRUNS
SKISUIT
SKYSURF
SLIPUPS
SLOWUPS
SNAFUED
SOJOURN
SPATULA
SPELUNK
SPROUTS
STATUES
STATURE
STATUTE
STEPUPS
STIMULI
STLOUIS
STPAULS
STPIUSI
STPIUSV
STPIUSX
STRAUSS
STROUSE
SUBDUAL
SUBDUCT
SUBDUED
SUBDUER
SUBDUES
SUBSUME
SUCCUMB
SUDBURY
SUFFUSE
SUNBURN
SUNSUIT
SYNFUEL

S••••U•
SACKFUL
SACKOUT
SACKSUP
SANCTUM
SANCTUS
SANDBUR
SANGOUT
SAVEDUP
SAVESUP
SAVIOUR
SAWCHUK
SCALEUP
SCAREUP
SCARFUP
SCOUTUP
SCREWUP
SCRUBUP
SEABLUE
SEALSUP
SEASLUG
SEEKOUT
SEENOUT
SEEPOUT
SEESOUT
SELLOUT
SENDOUT
SENDSUP
SENTOUT
SERIOUS
SERVEUP
SETSOUT
SEVENUP
SEVERUS
SEWEDUP
SEYMOUR
SHAGRUG
SHAKEUP
SHAPEUP
SHINEUP
SHIPFUL
SHIPOUT
SHOOKUP
SHOOTUP
SHOPFUL
SHOREUP
SHOTGUN
SHOTOUT
SHOTPUT
SHOWNUP
SHOWOUT
SHOWSUP
SHUTOUT
SHUTSUP
SICKOUT
SIDIOUS
SIGHFUL
SIGNOUT
SIGNSUP
SINGOUT
SINUOUS
SITSOUT
SIXFOUR
SIZEDUP
SIZESUP
SKILFUL
SKIPOUT
SKYBLUE
SLACKUP
SLANTUP
SLEDFUL
SLICEUP
SLIDOUT
SLINKUP
SLIPOUT
SLIPSUP
SLOWSUP
SLUNKUP
SMACKUP
SMASHUP
SMOKEUP
SNAGSUP
SNAPSUP
SNARLUP
SNAZZUP
SNEAKUP
SNIFFUP
SNUCKUP
SOAKSUP
SOAPSUP
SOLDOUT
SONGFUL
SORGHUM
SORTOUT
SOULFUL
SOUPSUP
SPATOUT
SPEAKUP
SPECOUT
SPEEDUP
SPEWOUT
SPICEUP
SPIFFUP
SPIKEUP
SPINOUT
SPITOUT
SPLITUP
SPOKEUP
SPUNOUT
STACKUP
STADIUM
STANDUP
STANKUP
STANNUM
STARTUP
STAYOUT
STAYPUT
STAYSUP
STCLOUD
STEAMUP
STENGUN
STEPOUT
STEPSUP
STERNUM
STICKUM
STICKUP
STILLUP
STINKUP
STIRRUP
STIRSUP
STOCKUP
STOKEUP
STOODUP
STOPSUP
STOREUP
STRATUM
STRATUS
STUCKUP
STUNGUN
SUBARUS
SUCCOUR
SUCKSUP
SUDOKUS
SUITSUP
SULPHUR
SUMITUP
SURFSUP
SURPLUS
SUSSOUT
SWANKUP
SWEEPUP
SWELLUP
SWEPTUP
SWIMSUP

S•••••U
SAYSYOU
SEETHRU
SHIATSU
SHIHTZU
SHIKOKU
SILENTU

•SU••••
ASUNDER
ASUSUAL
ISUREAM
ISUREDO
TSUNAMI
USUALLY
USURERS
USURIES
USURPED
USURPER

•S•U•••
ASQUIET
ASQUINT
ASQUITH
ASSUAGE
ASSUMED
ASSUMER
ASSUMES
ASSUNTA
ASSURED
ASSURER
ASSURES
ASSUROR
ASTUTER
ESCUDOS
ESCUELA
ESQUIRE
ESTUARY
ISSUANT
ISSUEAD
ISSUERS
ISSUING
OSCULAR
OSCULES
OSMUNDS
OSSUARY
RSTUVWX
TSOURIS
TSQUARE

•S••U••
ASARULE
ASEXUAL
ASHBURN
ASHBURY
ASSAULT
ASTOUND
ASUSUAL
ASYLUMS
ESPOUSE
MSIEURS
TSETUNG

•S•••U•
ASKEDUP
ASKSOUT
ESCALUS
ISCHIUM
ISTHMUS
OSSEOUS
PSYCHUP
USINGUP
USOTOUR

•S••••U
ISABEAU
ISEEYOU

••SU•••
ASSUAGE
ASSUMED
ASSUMER
ASSUMES
ASSUNTA
ASSURED
ASSURER
ASSURES
ASSUROR
CASUALS
CASUIST
DISUSED
DISUSES
ENSUING
ENSUITE
ENSURED
ENSURER
ENSURES
FUSUMAS
INSULAR
INSULIN
INSULTS
INSURED
INSURER
INSURES
ISSUANT
ISSUEAD
ISSUERS
ISSUING
JESUITS
MISUSED
MISUSER
MISUSES
NOSUGAR
OSSUARY
RASURES
RESUITS
RESULTS
RESUMED
RESUMES
RESURGE
SOSUEME
UNSULKY
UNSUNNY
UNSURLY
UPSURGE
URSULAK
VISUALS

••S•U••
ASSAULT
BASQUES
BISCUIT
BISMUTH
BISQUES
BUSTUPS
CASQUED
CASQUES
COSTUME
DESLUMS
DISBUDS
DISCUSS
DISEURS
DISEUSE
DISGUST
DISPUTE
DISRUPT
DISTURB
DRSEUSS
DUSTUPS
ENSOULS
FESCUES

FISSURE
GASPUMP
GESTURE
GOSOUTH
HASPULL
KOSSUTH
LASHUPS
MASQUER
MASQUES
MESHUGA
MESSUPS
MISCUED
MISCUES
MISCUTS
MISRULE
MISSUSA
MISTUNE
MOSQUES
MRSMUIR
MUSEUMS
NESQUIK
OBSCURA
OBSCURE
PASTURE
POSEURS
POSEUSE
POSSUMS
POSTURE
PUSHUPS
QRSTUVW
RESCUED
RESCUER
RESCUES
RESHUTS
RESOUND
RESTUDY
RESTUFF
TISSUES
TISSUEY
TOSSUPS
UNSLUNG
UNSOUND
UNSTUCK
UNSTUNG
UNSWUNG
VASQUEZ
VESTURE
VISCUSO
VISTULA
WASHUPS
WASSURE
XYSTUSI

••S••U•
ABSOLUT
BASHFUL
BESTBUD
BESTBUY
BESTCUT
BUSTOUR
BUSTOUT
BUSTSUP
CASEOUS
CASEOUT
CASHOUT
CASSIUS
CASTOUT
CASTSUP
CISEAUX
DESKFUL
DISHFUL
DISHOUT
DUSTGUN
EASEDUP
EASEFUL
EASEOUT
EASESUP
FISHOUT
FISTFUL
GASEDUP
GASEOUS
GASESUP
GUSHOUT
GUSSYUP
HASHOUT
HASSIUM
HUSHFUL
ITSTRUE
JUSTOUT
LASCAUX
LASHOUT
LESCAUT
LESPAUL
LOSEOUT
LOSTOUT
LUSTFUL
LUSTRUM
MASSEUR
MISSOUT
MISTSUP
MRSPAUL
MUSEFUL
NESTFUL
NOSEDUP
NOSEEUM
NOSEOUT
NOSESUP
NOSTRUM
OISEAUX
OSSEOUS
PASSEUL
PASSOUT
PASTDUE
PASTEUP
PASTEUR
PISTOUS
PUSHFUL
PUSHOUT
RESCRUB
RESEAUS
RESEAUX
RESIDUA
RESIDUE
RESTFUL
RESTSUP
RISESUP
ROSABUD
ROSEBUD
ROSTRUM
RUSHOUT
SUSSOUT
TESTOUT
TESTRUN
TOSSOUT
TUSSAUD
UNSTOUT
URSINUS
VISCOUS
WASHOUT
WASHTUB
WISEDUP
WISEGUY
WISESUP
WISHFUL
WISTFUL
ZESTFUL
ZOSIMUS

••S•••U
BOSTONU
MISSYOU

•••SU••
ALBSURE
ANDSUCH
APESUIT
ASUSUAL
BATSUIT
BERSUNT
CAESURA
CAPSULE
CATSUIT
CATSUPS
CENSURE
CLOSURE
CONSULS
CONSULT
CONSUME
DATSUNS
DIDSUMS
DRYSUIT
EGOSURF
ERASURE
FISSURE
FORSURE
GYMSUIT
GYPSUMS
HIRSUTE
INASUIT
KOSSUTH
LAWSUIT
LEISURE
LETSUSE
MAOSUIT
MEASURE
MESSUPS
MISSUSA
NATSUME
NETSUKE
NETSURF
NONSUCH
NOTSURE
OUTSULK
OUTSUMS
OUTSUNG
POSSUMS
PRESUME
PURSUED
PURSUER
PURSUES
PURSUIT
REDSUIT
REDSUNS
SAMSUNG
SATSUMA
SENSUAL
SKISUIT
SKYSURF
SUBSUME
SUNSUIT
THESUNS
TISSUES
TISSUEY
TONSURE
TOSSUPS
UNUSUAL
WASSURE
WETSUIT

•••S•U•
ACESOUT
ACTSOUT
AGESOUT
AIRSOUT
ALYSSUM
ASKSOUT
ATISSUE
BOOSTUP
BOWSOUT
BRUSHUP
BRUSQUE
BUGSOUT
BUMSOUT
BUYSOUT
CASSIUS
CELSIUS
CHOSEUP
CLOSEUP
CNOSSUS
COPSOUT
CRASSUS
CRISPUS
CROSSUP
CUTSOUT
DANSEUR
DIESOUT
DIGSOUT
DIMSOUT
DRESSUP
EATSOUT
EKESOUT
ELYSIUM
ERASMUS
ERASTUS
FANSOUT
FAUSTUS
FIRSTUP
FRISEUR
FRUSTUM
GETSOUT
GNOSSUS
GOESOUT
GUSSYUP
HASSIUM
HITSOUT
HOISTUP
HOPSOUT
HOTSOUP
HOTSPUR
IBNSAUD
ICESOUT
IRISOUT
KIDSRUS
LAYSOUT
LETSOUT
LIPSOUT
LOGSOUT
LOUSEUP
LUGSOUT
MAISOUI
MAPSOUT
MASSEUR
MISSOUT
OPOSSUM
OPTSOUT
OUTSWUM
PANSOUT
PASSEUL
PASSOUT
PAYSOUT
PAYSTUB
PEASOUP
PERSEUS
PERSIUS
PIGSOUT
POPSOUT
PQRSTUV
PRESPUR
PRESQUE
PRESSUP
PUTSOUT
RAISEUP
RATSOUT
REISSUE
RIGSOUT
RIPSOUT
RUBSOUT
RUNSOUT
SEASLUG
SEESOUT
SETSOUT
SITSOUT
SMASHUP
SUSSOUT
TAGSOUT
TAPSOUT
TEASEUP
TENSEUP
THESEUS
TOGSOUT
TOPSOUT
TOSSOUT
TOYSRUS
TRUSSUP
TUSSAUD
TWISTUP
WHOSOUT
WIGSOUT
WINSOUT

•••S••U
MISSYOU
SAYSYOU

••••SU•
ALYSSUM
ANTESUP
ATISSUE
BACKSUP
BALLSUP
BANGSUP
BANKSUP
BEADSUP
BEAMSUP
BEARSUP
BEATSUP
BEEFSUP
BELTSUP
BINDSUP
BITESUP
BLOTSUP
BLOWSUP
BLUESUN
BOILSUP
BOLTSUP
BONESUP
BOOTSUP
BOXESUP
BREWSUP
BUCKSUP
BUFFSUP
BULKSUP
BUMPSUP
BUOYSUP
BURNSUP
BUSTSUP
CAGESUP
CAKESUP
CALLSUP
CAMPSUP
CASTSUP
CHATSUP
CHEWSUP
CHIPSUP
CHOPSUP
CLAMSUP
CLOGSUP
CLOTSUP
CLUBSUP
CNOSSUS
COILSUP
COMESUP
COOKSUP
COOPSUP
CORKSUP
CRASSUS
CRIESUP
CROESUS
CROPSUP
CROSSUP
CRUDSUP
CURLSUP
DAMASUS
DEALSUP
DIALSUP
DOLLSUP
DRAGSUP
DRAWSUP
DRESSUP
DRIESUP
DRUMSUP
DUDESUP
EASESUP
EPHESUS
EVENSUP
FAIRSUP
FILLSUP
FIRESUP
FIRMSUP
FIXESUP
FLIESUP
FOLDSUP
FOOTSUP
FORKSUP
FOULSUP
FREESUP
FRIESUP
FUELSUP
GANGSUP
GASESUP
GEARSUP
GIVESUP
GLAMSUP
GNOSSUS
GOOFSUP
GROWSUP
HACKSUP
HANDSUP
HANGSUP
HAULSUP
HEADSUP
HEALSUP
HEAPSUP
HEATSUP
HELPSUP
HIKESUP
HOLDSUP
HOLESUP
HOOKSUP
HUNTSUP
HYPESUP
JACKSUP
JERKSUP
JOINSUP
JUMPSUP
KEEPSUP
KICKSUP
KNEESUP
KNOTSUP
LACESUP
LANDSUP
LEADSUP
LEAPSUP
LICKSUP
LIFTSUP
LINESUP
LINKSUP
LOADSUP
LOCKSUP
LOOKSUP
LUMPSUM
MAKESUP
MARKSUP
MEETSUP
MINISUB
MISTSUP
MIXESUP
MOCKSUP
MOVESUP
MUCKSUP
NAILSUP
NOSESUP
OPENSUP
OPOSSUM
OVERSUP
PACKSUP
PAIRSUP
PEGASUS
PERKSUP
PICKSUP
PILESUP
PIPESUP
PLAYSUP
PLOWSUP
PLUGSUP
PRESSUP
PROPSUP
PUFFSUP
PULLSUP
PUMPSUP
RACESUP
RACKSUP
RAKESUP
RAMPSUP
READSUP
REARSUP
REELSUP
REISSUE
RESTSUP
RIDESUP
RILESUP
RINGSUP
RISESUP
ROLLSUP
ROOTSUP
ROPESUP
RUCKSUP
SACKSUP
SAVESUP
SEALSUP
SENDSUP
SHOWSUP
SHUTSUP
SIGNSUP
SIZESUP
SLIPSUP
SLOWSUP
SNAGSUP
SNAPSUP
SOAKSUP
SOAPSUP
SOUPSUP
STAYSUP
STEPSUP
STIRSUP
STOPSUP
SUCKSUP
SUITSUP
SURFSUP
SWIMSUP
TACKSUP
TAKESUP
TALKSUP
TANKSUP
TAPESUP
TARTSUP
TEAMSUP
TEARSUP
TIDYSUM
TILTSUP
TIMESUP
TONESUP
TOOLSUP
TOTESUP
TRIPSUP
TROTSUP
TRUESUP
TRUSSUP
TUNASUB
TUNESUP
TURNSUP
TYPESUP
WAITSUP
WAKESUP
WALLSUP
WARMSUP
WAXESUP
WELLSUP
WHATSUP
WHIPSUP
WHITSUN
WINDSUP
WIPESUP
WIRESUP
WISESUP
WORKSUP
WRAPSUP
ZEROSUM

••••S•U
IGUASSU
ILIESCU
OPQRSTU

•••••SU
FUJITSU
IGUASSU
JUJITSU
KOMATSU
SHIATSU

SV•••••
SVELTER
SVERIGE

S•V••••
SAVABLE
SAVAGED
SAVAGER
SAVAGES
SAVALAS
SAVANAS
SAVANNA
SAVANTS
SAVARIN
SAVEDON
SAVEDUP
SAVEFOR
SAVESON
SAVESUP
SAVINGS
SAVIORS
SAVIOUR
SAVORED
SAVORER
SAVOURS
SAVOURY
SAVVIED
SAVVIER
SAVVIES
SAVVILY
SEVENAD
SEVENAM
SEVENBC
SEVENEE
SEVENNO
SEVENPM
SEVENTH
SEVENTY
SEVENUP
SEVERAL
SEVERED
SEVERER
SEVERUS
SEVIGNY
SEVILLA
SEVILLE
SOVIETS

S••V•••
SALVAGE
SALVERS
SALVING
SALVOES
SALVORS
SAVVIED
SAVVIER
SAVVIES
SAVVILY
SELVAGE
SERVANT
SERVEAS
SERVERS
SERVEUP
SERVICE
SERVILE
SERVING
SHAVERS
SHAVIAN
SHAVING
SHAVUOT
SHEVATS
SHIVERS
SHIVERY
SHOVEIN
SHOVELS
SHOVERS
SHOVING
SIEVING
SILVERS
SILVERY
SKIVEST
SLAVERS
SLAVERY
SLAVING
SLAVISH
SLIVERS
SLOVAKS
SLOVENE
SLOVENS
SNIVELS
SOLVEIT
SOLVENT
SOLVERS
SOLVING
SORVINO
STAVING
STEVENS
STUVWXY
SUAVELY
SUAVEST
SUAVITY
SUBVENE
SUBVERT
SURVEIL
SURVEYS
SURVIVE
SWIVELS
SWIVETS

S•••V••
SALIVAS
SAMOVAR
SAYOVER
SCARVES
SCURVES
SEGOVIA
SHEAVED
SHEAVES
SHELVED
SHELVER
SHELVES
SHRIVEL
SHRIVER
SHRIVES
SLEEVED
SLEEVES
SOHAVEI
STARVED
STARVES
STEEVED
STEEVES
STRIVED
STRIVEN
STRIVER
STRIVES
SWERVED
SWERVES

S••••V•
SCENEVI
SIXFIVE
SKYDIVE
SUASIVE
SURVIVE

S•••••V
SCENEIV
SILENTV
SMIRNOV
SPIKETV
STPIUSV

•SV••••
RSVPING

•S••V••
ASHIVER
ASKOVER
ESTEVEZ
ESTIVAL
RSTUVWX

•S•••V•
OSTRAVA

•S••••V
USTINOV

••SV•••
YESVOTE

••S•V••
ATSEVEN
CASAVAS
DISAVOW
GASOVEN
HASOVER
HESHVAN
ITSOVER
KOSOVAR
MISAVER
RESAVED
RESAVES
UNSAVED
UNSAVVY
VISAVIS

••S••V•
ABSOLVE
CASSAVA
COSTIVE
DASILVA
DESERVE
DESYLVA
ENSLAVE
FESTIVA
FESTIVE
GUSTAVE
ITSLOVE
KISLEVS
MASSIVE
MISGAVE
MISGIVE
MISMOVE
MISSIVE
OBSERVE
ONSERVE
PASSIVE
QRSTUVW
RESERVE
RESHAVE
RESOLVE
RESTIVE
TUSSIVE
UNSAVVY
YESHIVA

••S•••V
AKSAKOV

•••SV••
PIUSVII

•••S•V•
ABUSIVE
CASSAVA
CURSIVE
ELUSIVE
EROSIVE
EVASIVE
MASSIVE
MISSIVE
PASSIVE
PENSIVE
PLOSIVE
SUASIVE
TENSIVE
TUSSIVE
ZEMSTVO

•••S••V
PQRSTUV
TRASHTV

••••SV•
JAMESVI
LOUISVI

••••S•V
BRYUSOV
JAMESIV
LOUISIV
LOUISXV

•••••SV
STPIUSV

SW•••••
SWABBED
SWABBER
SWADDLE
SWAGGER
SWAGMAN
SWAGMEN
SWAHILI
SWALLOW
SWAMPED
SWANKED
SWANKER
SWANKUP
SWANSEA
SWANSON
SWAPPED
SWAPPER
SWARMED
SWARMER
SWARTHY
SWASHED
SWASHES
SWATHED
SWATHES
SWATSAT
SWATTED
SWATTER
SWAYBAR
SWAYERS
SWAYING
SWEARAT
SWEARBY
SWEARER
SWEARIN
SWEARTO
SWEATED
SWEATER
SWEATIT
SWEDISH
SWEENEY
SWEEPEA
SWEEPER
SWEEPUP
SWEETEN
SWEETER
SWEETIE
SWEETLY

SWEETON
SWELLED
SWELLER
SWELLUP
SWELTER
SWELTRY
SWENSON
SWEPTUP
SWERVED
SWERVES
SWIFTER
SWIFTLY
SWIGERT
SWIGGED
SWILLED
SWILLER
SWIMMER
SWIMSUP
SWINDLE
SWINERY
SWINGAT
SWINGBY
SWINGER
SWINGIT
SWINISH
SWINTON
SWIPERS
SWIPING
SWIRLED
SWISHED
SWISHES
SWITZER
SWIVELS
SWIVETS
SWIZZLE
SWOLLEN
SWOONED
SWOONER
SWOOPED
SWOOPER
SWOOPIN
SWOOSIE
SWOREAT
SWOREBY
SWOREIN
SWORETO
SWUNGAT
SWUNGBY
SWUNGIT

S•W••••
SAWATCH
SAWBUCK
SAWCHUK
SAWDUST
SAWFISH
SAWINTO
SAWLIKE
SAWLOGS
SAWMILL
SAWNOFF
SAWPAST
SAWPITS
SAWSOFF
SAWTOIT
SAWWOOD
SAWYERS
SEWARDS
SEWEDON
SEWEDUP
SEWISTS
SOWLIKE
SOWSEAR

S••W•••
SAMWISE
SATWELL
SATWITH
SAWWOOD
SAYWAIT
SAYWHAT
SAYWHEN
SCHWANN
SCHWINN
SCOWLED
SCOWLER
SEAWALL
SEAWARD
SEAWAYS
SEAWEED
SEAWOLF
SEGWAYS
SHAWLED
SHAWNEE
SHEWOLF
SHOWBIZ
SHOWCAT
SHOWDOG
SHOWERS
SHOWERY
SHOWHOW
SHOWIER
SHOWILY
SHOWING
SHOWMAN
SHOWMEN
SHOWNIN
SHOWNUP
SHOWOFF
SHOWOUT
SHOWSIN
SHOWSUP
SITWELL
SITWITH
SIXWEEK
SKEWERS
SKEWING
SKIWEAR
SKYWALK
SKYWARD
SKYWAYS
SLEWING
SLOWDAY
SLOWEST
SLOWING
SLOWISH
SLOWSUP
SLOWUPS
SNOWCAP
SNOWCAT
SNOWDAY
SNOWDON
SNOWHAT
SNOWIER
SNOWILY
SNOWING
SNOWJOB
SNOWMAN
SNOWMEN
SNOWPEA
SNOWSIN
SNOWSKI
SOPWITH
SOTWEED
SPAWNED
SPAWNER
SPEWERS
SPEWING
SPEWOUT
SPYWARE
STEWARD
STEWART
STEWERS
STEWIER
STEWING
STEWPAN
STEWPOT
STOWAGE
STOWERS
STOWING
STOWSIT
SUBWARS
SUBWAYS
SUNWARD

S•••W••
SAFEWAY
SARAWAK
SAYSWHO
SCARWID
SCRAWLS
SCRAWLY
SCRAWNY
SCREWED
SCREWUP
SHERWIN
SHIPWAY
SHYAWAY
SIDEWAY
SINEWED
SKAGWAY
SOMEWAY
SPRAWLS
SPRAWLY
SQUAWKS
SQUAWKY
STREWED
STREWER
STUVWXY

S••••W•
SATDOWN
SEACOWS
SEAFOWL
SEAHAWK
SEESAWS
SETDOWN
SHADOWS
SHADOWY
SHALLWE
SIDETWO
SITDOWN
SIZETWO
SKITOWS
SOAREWE
SODIDWE
SORROWS
STEPTWO
SUNBOWL
SUNBOWS
SUNDOWN

S•••••W
SAGINAW
SALCHOW
SEMIRAW
SHALLOW
SHOWHOW
SILENTW
SKIDROW
SOMEHOW
SPARROW
SUNGLOW
SWALLOW

•S•W•••
ASSWEET
OSTWALD
PSYWARS

•S••W••
ASKAWAY
ASLEWOF
CSLEWIS
PSHAWED

•S•••W•
ASPRAWL
ESCHEWS
ESCROWS
ESPNEWS
RSTUVWX

•S••••W
ASOFNOW
ISEENOW
USOSHOW

••SW•••
ANSWERS
ASSWEET
BOSWELL
GASWARS
IMSWELL
INSWEPT
IPSWICH
MCSWINE
MISWIRE
MISWORD
NOSWEAT
RESWEAR
RESWEEP
RESWIMS
RESWORE
RESWORN
ROSWELL
UNSWEAR
UNSWEET
UNSWEPT
UNSWORE
UNSWORN
UNSWUNG
UPSWEEP
UPSWELL
UPSWEPT
UPSWING

••S•W••
BUSHWAH
DISOWNS
PESEWAS
POSTWAR
RESAWED
RESEWED
RESOWED
UNSAWED
UNSEWED
UNSOWED
WYSIWYG

••S••W•
BASETWO
BESTOWS
CASHEWS
CBSNEWS
CUSHAWS
GOSHAWK
NOSHOWS
RESHOWN
RESHOWS
RESTOWS
TVSHOWS
UNSHOWN
UNSHOWY
UNSKEWS
UNSTOWS

••S•••W
BESTREW
CASELAW
CASHCOW
DISAVOW
HASACOW
HASAROW
JUSTNOW
LASTROW
MISBREW
MISDRAW
MISDREW
MISKNEW
MISKNOW
MISTBOW
QRSTUVW
RESTREW
UNSCREW

•••SW••
BEESWAX
GETSWET
OUTSWAM
OUTSWIM
OUTSWUM
SAYSWHO
THESWAN
THISWAY
WHOSWHO

•••S•W•
BOWSAWS
JIGSAWS
OLDSAWS
OPUSTWO
PITSAWS
PLUSTWO
RIPSAWN
RIPSAWS
SEESAWS

•••S••W
AIRSHOW
ARTSHOW
BARSTOW
BIGSHOW
CAPSHAW
CARSHOW
CATSHOW
CATSPAW
CRASHAW
CUMSHAW
DOGSHOW
FORSHOW
GLASGOW
GLASHOW
HITSHOW
ICESHOW
INASTEW
KERSHAW
LAYSLOW
LIESLOW
OHMSLAW
OUTSHOW
PAYSNOW
PRESHOW
RUBSRAW
RUNSLOW
THESHOW
TOOSLOW
USOSHOW
WINSLOW

••••S•W
BACKSAW
BANDSAW
BELTSAW
BUCKSAW
BUZZSAW
FORESAW
FRETSAW
GANGSAW
HACKSAW
HANDSAW
HEADSAW
OVERSAW
OVERSEW
WHIPSAW
WOODSAW

S•X••••
SAXHORN
SAXTUBA
SEXIEST
SEXISTS
SEXLESS
SEXPOTS
SEXTANS
SEXTANT
SEXTETS
SEXTONS
SIXBALL
SIXEEEE
SIXFEET
SIXFIVE
SIXFOLD
SIXFOOT
SIXFOUR
SIXGUNS
SIXIRON
SIXLANE
SIXNINE
SIXPACK
SIXTEEN
SIXTHLY
SIXTIES
SIXTYAD
SIXTYBC
SIXWEEK
SIXYEAR
SOXFANS

S••••X•
STUVWXY
SUBTEXT

S•••••X
SALTBOX
SANDBOX
SHOEBOX
SILENTX
SIMPLEX
SIZESIX
SKEEZIX
SOAPBOX
SOMINEX
SOUPMIX
SPANDEX
STCROIX
STONEAX
STPIUSX

•S•X•••
ASEXUAL

•S••••X
ASTERIX
RSTUVWX

••S•X••
DESEXED
DESEXES

••S•••X
BASESIX
BASSSAX
CASHBOX
CISEAUX
FUSEBOX
LASCAUX
MISTERX
OISEAUX
POSTBOX
POSTFIX
RESEAUX

•••SX••
PIUSXII

•••S••X
ARUSPEX
BASSSAX
BEESWAX
CRISPIX
MUESLIX
PLUSTAX

••••SX•
LOUISXI
LOUISXV

••••S•X
ALTOSAX
BASESIX
BASSSAX
DEEPSIX
FAIRSEX
FIVESIX
HARDSIX
LEXUSGX
LEXUSLX
LEXUSRX
LOUISIX
MACHSIX
PAGESIX
SIZESIX

•••••SX
STPIUSX

SY•••••
SYDHOFF
SYLLABI
SYLPHIC
SYMBOLS
SYMPTOM
SYNAPSE
SYNCHED
SYNCING
SYNCOPE
SYNDICS
SYNERGY
SYNFUEL
SYNGMAN
SYNODAL
SYNODIC
SYNONYM
SYRIANA
SYRIANS
SYRINGE
SYSTEMS
SYSTOLE

S•Y••••
SAYABLE
SAYAMEN
SAYHITO
SAYINGS
SAYMASS
SAYMORE
SAYNOTO
SAYOVER
SAYSAAH
SAYSAYE
SAYSBOO
SAYSIDO
SAYSNAY
SAYSWHO
SAYSYES
SAYSYOU
SAYWAIT
SAYWHAT
SAYWHEN
SCYTHED
SCYTHES
SEYMOUR
SHYAWAY
SHYFROM
SHYLOCK
SHYNESS
SHYSTER
SKYBLUE
SKYCAMS
SKYCAPS
SKYDIVE
SKYDOME
SKYHIGH
SKYHOOK
SKYJACK
SKYLARK
SKYLESS
SKYLIKE
SKYLINE
SKYMAPS
SKYNYRD
SKYSURF
SKYWALK
SKYWARD
SKYWAYS
SLYLOOK
SLYNESS
SOYBEAN
SOYINKA
SOYINKS
SOYLENT
SOYMEAL
SOYMILK
SPYBOTS
SPYCAMS
SPYDERS
SPYHOLE
SPYINGS
SPYKIDS
SPYRING
SPYUPON
SPYWARE
STYGIAN
STYLERS
STYLETS
STYLING
STYLISE
STYLISH
STYLIST
STYLIZE
STYMIED
STYMIES
STYPSIS
STYPTIC
STYRENE
SZYSLAK

S••Y•••
SATYRIC
SAWYERS
SIBYLIC
SIXYEAR
SLAYERS
SLAYING
SLAYTON
SPAYERS
SPAYING
SPRYEST
STAYDRY
STAYERS
STAYFOR
STAYING
STAYOFF
STAYOUT
STAYPUT
STAYSAT
STAYSIN
STAYSON
STAYSUP
SWAYBAR
SWAYERS
SWAYING

S•••Y••
SADEYED
SADEYES
SAMMYJO
SAMOYED
SAROYAN
SAYSYES
SAYSYOU
SCHAYES
SETTYPE
SILLYME
SIXTYAD
SIXTYBC
SKYNYRD
SPLAYED
SPRAYED
SPRAYER
SPRAYON
STRAYED
STRAYER
SUBTYPE
SUELYON

S••••Y•
SAIDAYE
SAMLOYD
SASHAYS
SAYSAYE
SEAWAYS
SEGWAYS
SEQUOYA
SHUTEYE
SKYWAYS
SMILEYS
SMOKEYS
SOCKEYE
STMARYS
SUBWAYS
SUNDAYS
SUNRAYS
SURREYS
SURVEYS
SYNONYM

S•••••Y
SAFEWAY
SAIDNAY
SAINTLY
SALTILY
SAMEDAY
SANDFLY
SAPPILY
SASSILY
SATIETY
SATISFY
SATRAPY
SAUCILY
SAUCONY
SAVOURY
SAVVILY
SAYSNAY
SCANTLY
SCAREDY
SCARIFY
SCARILY
SCENERY
SCRAGGY
SCRAPPY
SCRAWLY
SCRAWNY
SCRIMPY
SCRUBBY
SCRUFFY
SEADUTY
SEALERY
SEALILY
SECRECY
SEEDILY
SEMIDRY
SENDSBY
SENSORY
SETPLAY
SEVENTY
SEVIGNY
SHADILY
SHADOWY
SHAKILY
SHAPELY
SHARKEY
SHARPLY
SHEERLY
SHELLEY
SHINGLY
SHINILY
SHIPWAY
SHIRLEY
SHIVERY
SHLOCKY
SHOOFLY
SHOOTBY
SHORTLY
SHOWERY
SHOWILY
SHRILLY
SHRIMPY
SHRUBBY
SHTICKY
SHYAWAY
SICKBAY
SICKDAY
SICKPAY
SIDEWAY
SIGHTLY
SIGNIFY
SILENTY
SILKILY
SILVERY
SIMCITY
SINCITY
SIXTHLY
SIZABLY
SKAGWAY
SKETCHY
SKIPSBY
SLACKLY
SLANTLY
SLAVERY
SLEEKLY
SLICKLY
SLIDEBY
SLIMILY
SLIPSBY
SLOUCHY
SLOWDAY
SMARTLY
SMOKILY
SMOOTHY
SNAKILY
SNEAKBY
SNIDELY
SNIFFLY
SNOWDAY
SNOWILY
SNUGGLY
SOAPILY
SOBERLY
SOCIETY
SOGGILY
SOLIDLY
SOMEDAY
SOMESAY
SOMEWAY
SOOTILY
SORCERY
SORRILY
SOSORRY
SOTHEBY
SOUNDLY
SOUTHEY
SPACELY
SPANGLY
SPARELY
SPARKLY
SPASSKY
SPECIFY
SPICERY
SPICILY
SPIDERY
SPIKILY
SPINDLY
SPINDRY
SPINNEY
SPLASHY
SPLEENY
SPRAWLY
SPRINGY
SQUALLY
SQUASHY
SQUATLY
SQUATTY
SQUAWKY
SQUEAKY
SQUINTY
SQUIRMY
SQUISHY
STAGILY
STAIDLY
STALELY
STANDBY
STANLEY
STARCHY
STARKEY
STARKLY
STARSKY
STATELY
STAYDRY
STEEPLY
STERNLY
STICKBY
STIFFLY
STIRFRY
STOKELY
STONILY
STOODBY
STOOKEY
STOPSBY
STOUTLY
STREAKY
STRINGY
STUBBLY
STUCKBY
STUPEFY
STUVWXY
SUAVELY
SUAVITY
SUBSIDY
SUCKDRY
SUDBURY
SULKILY
SUMMARY
SUMMERY
SUNCITY
SUNNILY
SURGERY
SURLILY
SWARTHY
SWEARBY
SWEENEY
SWEETLY
SWELTRY
SWIFTLY
SWINERY
SWINGBY
SWOREBY
SWUNGBY
SYNERGY

•SY••••
ASYLUMS
PSYCHED
PSYCHES
PSYCHIC
PSYCHOS
PSYCHUP
PSYWARS

•S•Y•••
ASBYATT
ASSYRIA
ESPYING

•S••Y••
ASSAYED
ASSAYER
ESSAYED
ESSAYER
ISEEYOU

•S•••Y•
ESTRAYS
OSPREYS

•S••••Y
ASABODY
ASAGRAY
ASHBERY
ASHBURY
ASHTRAY
ASKAWAY
ESOTERY
ESTUARY
ISONOMY
ISOTOPY
OSSUARY
OSTIARY
USUALLY

••SY•••
ASSYRIA
BUSYBEE
BUSYING
COSYING
DESYLVA
EASYJOB
EASYOFF
EASYONE
INSYNCH
KOSYGIN

••S•Y••
ASSAYED
ASSAYER
ESSAYED
ESSAYER
GUSSYUP
IDSAYSO
INSTYLE
MISSYOU
MISTYPE
MOSEYED
RESTYLE
UNSHYER
UNSHYLY
UNSLYER
UNSLYLY
VISAYAN

••S••Y•
BUSBOYS
DISMAYS
FISHEYE
JOSBOYS
MASARYK
MISKEYS
MISLAYS
MISSAYS
ROSALYN
SASHAYS
WYSIWYG

••S•••Y
AMSCRAY
BASALLY
BASEPAY
BESTBOY
BESTBUY
BOSSILY
BUSHILY
CASPARY
CASSIDY
CUSHILY
CUSTODY
DESTINY
DESTROY
DISOBEY
DISPLAY
DUSKILY
DUSTILY
EASEDBY
EASESBY
ECSTASY
FISHERY
FISHFRY
FISHILY
FUSSILY
FUSTILY
GASCONY
GASEITY
GOSSIPY
GUSHILY
GUSTILY
HASASAY
HASTILY
HISTORY
HOSIERY
HUSHABY
HUSKILY
IMSORRY
ITSABOY
ITSEASY
ITSOKAY
JASPERY
JUSTIFY
LASTMAY
LASTORY
LISAGAY
LUSTILY
MASONRY
MASTERY
MESSILY
MISALLY
MISCOPY
MISERLY
MISPLAY
MISRELY
MISTILY
MUSHILY
MUSIGNY
MUSSILY
MUSTILY
MYSTERY
MYSTIFY
NASALLY
NASTILY
NOSEGAY
OSSUARY
PASSKEY
PESKILY
PUSHILY
RESPRAY
RESTUDY
RISIBLY
RISKILY
ROSEBAY
RUSSETY
RUSTILY
SASSILY
SOSORRY
TASTILY
TESTACY
TESTFLY
TESTIFY
TESTILY
TISSUEY
TUSCANY
TUSHERY
UNSADLY
UNSALTY
UNSAVVY
UNSCALY
UNSHADY
UNSHINY
UNSHOWY
UNSHYLY
UNSILLY
UNSLYLY
UNSMOKY
UNSNAKY
UNSOGGY
UNSOOTY
UNSORRY
UNSPICY
UNSTAGY
UNSTONY
UNSULKY
UNSUNNY
UNSURLY
VASTITY
VISIBLY
WASHDAY
WASPILY
WASSILY
WISEGUY
WISPILY
ZESTILY

•••SY••
FORSYTE
FORSYTH
GUSSYUP
LIPSYNC
MISSYOU
SAYSYES
SAYSYOU

•••S•Y•
BURSTYN
CATSEYE
DORSEYS
JERSEYS
MINSKYS
MISSAYS
NAYSAYS
OUTSAYS
SAYSAYE

•••S••Y
APISHLY
BALSAMY
BEASLEY
BEASTLY
BIASPLY
BOSSILY
BRASHLY
BRISKLY
BRISTLY
CASSIDY
CLOSEBY
CLOSELY
CRASSLY
CRISPLY
CROSSLY
CURSORY
DENSELY
DENSIFY
DENSITY
ELUSORY
EROSELY
FALSELY
FALSIFY
FALSITY
FIRSTLY
FLESHLY
FRESHLY
FUSSILY
GHASTLY
GHOSTLY
GOSSIPY
GRISTLY
GROSSLY
GUTSILY
HARSHLY
HEMSLEY
HENSLEY
HERSHEY
HORSILY
HORSLEY
HOUSSAY
KITSCHY
LETSFLY
LOOSELY
LOUSILY
MENSCHY
MESSILY
MOISTLY
MOUSILY
MUSSILY
NEWSBOY
NEWSDAY
NOISILY
NURSERY
OBESELY
OBESITY
ODYSSEY
OUTSTAY
PAISLEY
PARSLEY
PASSKEY
PATSDRY
PIOSITY
PLUSHLY
PRESLEY
PROSILY
PROSODY
PUGSLEY
QUESNAY
RAISINY
REASSAY
RUNSDRY
RUSSETY
SASSILY
SAYSNAY
SENSORY
SPASSKY
SUBSIDY
TENSELY
TENSITY
TERSELY
THISDAY
THISTLY
THISWAY
TIPSILY
TISSUEY
TOLSTOY
TUESDAY
VARSITY
VERSIFY
WASSILY
WHISKEY
WORSLEY

••••S•Y
AMNESTY
ARENSKY
BLUESKY
BOBBSEY
BOGUSLY
BRODSKY
CANTSAY
CHOMSKY
CHOOSEY
CHRISTY
COMESBY
CRASSLY
CROSSLY
CURTSEY
DARESAY
DEBUSSY
DEEPSKY
DEMPSEY
DROPSBY
DYNASTY
EASESBY
EMBASSY
FILESBY
FLIESBY
FLITSBY
GAINSAY
GIRLSHY
GRIMSBY
GROSSLY
HADASAY
HALFSHY
HANGSBY
HASASAY
HEARSAY
HONESTY
HORNSBY
HOUSSAY
LINDSAY
LINDSEY
LIVESEY
MAJESTY
MALMSEY
MODESTY
MORESBY
ODYSSEY
PIOUSLY
PLAYSBY
RACESBY
REASSAY
RIDESBY
ROLLSBY
SATISFY
SENDSBY
SKIPSBY
SLIPSBY
SOMESAY
SPASSKY
SPLASHY
SQUASHY
SQUISHY
STARSKY
STOPSBY
THEYSAY
THIRSTY
TICKSBY
TROTSKY
UNDUSTY
UNFUSSY
UNHASTY
UNLUSTY
UNMOSSY
UNRASPY
UNRISKY
UNTASTY
VERYSHY
VRONSKY
WALKSBY
WHATSAY
WOOLSEY
WORKSHY

•••••SY
AUTOPSY
BIGEASY
CIRCUSY
CLERISY
CRAFTSY
DEBUSSY
ECSTASY
EMBASSY
FANTASY
GEODESY
GETBUSY
GOTBUSY
ITSEASY
NONBUSY
NOTEASY
TOOEASY
UNFUSSY
UNMOSSY
UNNOISY

SZ•••••
SZILARD
SZYSLAK

S•Z••••
SIZABLE
SIZABLY
SIZEDUP
SIZEONE
SIZESIX
SIZESUP
SIZETEN
SIZETWO
SIZZLED
SIZZLER
SIZZLES
SUZANNE
SUZETTE
SUZUKIS

S••Z•••
SCUZZES
SEIZEON
SEIZERS
SEIZING
SEIZORS
SEIZURE
SIZZLED
SIZZLER
SIZZLES
SNAZZUP
SUBZERO
SUBZONE
SWIZZLE

S•••Z••
SALAZAR
SARAZEN
SCUZZES
SECHZIG
SELTZER
SIEBZIG
SKEEZIX
SLEAZES
SNAZZUP
SNEEZED
SNEEZER
SNEEZES
SNOOZED
SNOOZER
SNOOZES
SPITZES
STANZAS
STUTZES
SWITZER
SWIZZLE

S••••Z•
SCHERZI
SCHERZO
SCHNOZZ
SHIHTZU
SPINOZA
SQUEEZE
STYLIZE

S•••••Z
SCHLITZ
SCHNOZZ
SCHULTZ
SHOWBIZ
SILENTZ
SIMONIZ

•S••Z••
ASSIZES

•S••••Z
ESTEVEZ

••SZ•••
MISZONE

••S•Z••
ASSIZES
RESIZED
RESIZER
RESIZES
UNSIZED
UPSIZED
UPSIZES

••S••Z•
RESEIZE

••S•••Z
NISSANZ
VASQUEZ

•••S•Z•
ANASAZI
BRASIZE
CAPSIZE
FORSIZE
HATSIZE
MANSIZE
MIDSIZE
ONESIZE
OUTSIZE
UNISIZE

•••S••Z
AGASSIZ
GRISNEZ
LAISSEZ
NISSANZ

••••S•Z
AGASSIZ
EXCUSEZ
LAISSEZ

•••••SZ
KERTESZ

TA•••••
TABARDS
TABARET
TABASCO
TABBIES
TABBING
TABITHA
TABKEYS
TABLEAU
TABLETS
TABLING
TABLOID
TABOOED
TABORET
TABOULI
TABSETS
TABUING
TABULAR
TACHYON
TACITLY
TACITUS
TACKERS
TACKIER
TACKILY
TACKING
TACKLED
TACKLER
TACKLES
TACKSON
TACKSUP
TACOMAS
TACONIC
TACTFUL
TACTICS
TACTILE
TACTUAL
TADPOLE
TAFFETA
TAFFIES
TAGALOG
TAGAMET
TAGDAYS
TAGENDS
TAGGANT
TAGGERS
TAGGING
TAGLIKE
TAGLINE
TAGOUTS
TAGSALE
TAGSOUT
TAGTEAM
TAHINIS
TAILEND
TAILERS
TAILFIN
TAILING
TAILOFF
TAILORS
TAILPIN
TAILWAG
TAINTED
TAKABLE
TAKEAIM
TAKEFOR
TAKEILL
TAKEINS
TAKENBY
TAKENIN
TAKENON
TAKENTO
TAKENUP
TAKEOFF
TAKEONE
TAKEOUT
TAKESIN
TAKESIT
TAKESON
TAKESTO
TAKESUP
TAKETEA
TAKETEN
TAKINGS
TALARIA
TALCKED
TALCUMS
TALENTS
TALIBAN
TALKBIG
TALKERS
TALKIER
TALKIES
TALKING
TALKOUT
TALKSAT
TALKSOF
TALKSON
TALKSTO
TALKSUP
TALLEST
TALLIED
TALLIER
TALLIES
TALLINN
TALLISH
TALLITH
TALLONE
TALLOWS
TALLOWY
TALLYHO
TALLYUP
TALONED
TALUSES
TAMABLE
TAMALES
TAMARAC
TAMBALA
TAMBLYN
TAMGLEN
TAMIAMI
TAMMANY
TAMPAFL
TAMPERS
TAMPICO
TAMPING
TAMTAMS
TANAGER
TANBARK
TANDEMS
TANDOOR
TANGELO
TANGENT
TANGIER
TANGING
TANGLED
TANGLER
TANGLES
TANGOED
TANGOER
TANGRAM
TANKAGE
TANKARD
TANKCAR
TANKERS
TANKFUL
TANKING
TANKINI
TANKSUP
TANKTOP
TANLINE
TANNERS
TANNERY
TANNEST
TANNING
TANNINS
TANNISH
TANOAKS
TANSIES
TANTARA
TANTIVY
TANTRUM
TAOISTS
TAPEDON
TAPEDUP
TAPEMAN
TAPEMEN
TAPERED
TAPESON
TAPESUP
TAPINGS
TAPINTO
TAPIOCA
TAPPANS
TAPPERS
TAPPETS
TAPPING
TAPROOM
TAPROOT
TAPSHOE
TAPSOFF
TAPSOUT
TAPSTER
TARANTO
TARBABY
TARBELL
TARDIER
TARDILY
TARGETS
TARHEEL
TARIFFS
TARMACS
TARNISH
TAROILS
TARPITS
TARPONS
TARRIED
TARRIER
TARRIES
TARRING
TARSALS
TARTANS
TARTARE
TARTARS
TARTEST
TARTIER
TARTILY
TARTING
TARTISH
TARTLET
TARTSUP
TARZANA
TARZANS
TASERED
TASHLIN
TASKBAR
TASKING
TASSELS
TASTEIT
TASTERS
TASTIER
TASTILY
TASTING
TATAMIS
TATIANA
TATTERS
TATTERY
TATTIER
TATTILY
TATTING
TATTLED
TATTLER
TATTLES
TATTOOS
TAUNTED
TAUNTER
TAUNTON
TAUREAN
TAURINE
TAUTENS
TAUTEST
TAVERNA
TAVERNS
TAWNIER
TAWNILY
TAXABLE
TAXBASE
TAXCODE
TAXCUTS
TAXFREE
TAXHIKE
TAXICAB
TAXIING
TAXIMAN
TAXIMEN
TAXIWAY
TAXLAWS
TAXLESS
TAXLEVY
TAXPAID
TAXRATE
TAXSALE
TAXYEAR
TAYBACK
TAYLORS

T•A••••
TEABAGS
TEABALL
TEACAKE
TEACART
TEACHER
TEACHES
TEACHIN
TEACOZY
TEACUPS
TEAGOWN
TEALEAF
TEALESS
TEAMING
TEAMSUP
TEAMUSA
TEANECK
TEAPOTS
TEAPOYS
TEARERS
TEARFUL
TEARGAS
TEARIER
TEARILY
TEARING
TEAROFF
TEAROOM
TEAROSE
TEAROUT
TEARSAT
TEARSIT
TEARSUP
TEASELS
TEASERS
TEASETS
TEASEUP
TEASHOP
TEASING
TEATIME
TEATRAY
TEATREE
TEATROS
TEAURNS
THALERS
THANDIE
THANKED
THANKER
THATCHY
THATONE
THATSIT
THATSOK
THATWAY
THAWERS
THAWING
THAWOUT
TIARAED
TOADIED
TOADIES
TOADISH
TOAHAIR
TOASTED
TOASTEE
TOASTER
TOATURN
TRABERT
TRACERS
TRACERY
TRACHEA
TRACING
TRACKED
TRACKER
TRACTOR
TRADEIN
TRADEON
TRADERS
TRADEUP
TRADING
TRADUCE
TRAFFIC
TRAGEDY
TRAILED
TRAILER
TRAINED
TRAINEE
TRAINER
TRAININ
TRAIPSE
TRAITOR
TRALALA
TRAMCAR
TRAMMED
TRAMMEL

TRAMPAS
TRAMPED
TRAMPER
TRAMPLE
TRAMWAY
TRANCED
TRANCES
TRANSAM
TRANSIT
TRANSOM
TRAPEZE
TRAPGUN
TRAPPED
TRAPPER
TRASHED
TRASHER
TRASHES
TRASHTV
TRAUBEL
TRAUMAS
TRAVAIL
TRAVELS
TRAVERS
TRAWLED
TRAWLER
TRAYFUL
TRAYNOR
TSARDOM
TSARINA
TSARISM
TSARIST
TWADDLE
TWANGED
TWANGER
TZARINA

T••A•••

TABARDS
TABARET
TABASCO
TAGALOG
TAGAMET
TAKABLE
TALARIA
TAMABLE
TAMALES
TAMARAC
TANAGER
TARANTO
TATAMIS
TAXABLE
TEBALDI
TEJANAS
TEJANOS
TELAVIV
TENABLE
TENABLY
TENACES
TENACRE
TENANCY
TENANTS
TERAOHM
TETANUS
THEABCS
THEAGES
THEALPS
THEARMY
THEARTS
THEATER
THEATRE
THEAXIS
THIAMIN
THRALLS
THWACKS
THWARTS
TIDALLY
TINAFEY
TINAMOU
TIRADES
TISANES
TITANAE
TITANIA
TITANIC
TOBACCO
TONALLY
TOPAZES
TOTABLE
TOTALED
TOTALER
TOTALLY
TOTALUP
TOTASTE
TOUAREG
TOWABLE
TOWAGES
TOWARDS
TOWAWAY
TREACLE
TREACLY
TREADED
TREADER
TREADLE
TREADON
TREASON
TREATED
TREATER
TRIABLE
TRIADIC
TRIAGES
TRUANCY
TRUANTS
TSHAPED
TSHAPES
TUBAIST
TULANEU
TUNABLE
TUNAOIL
TUNASUB
TVGAMES
TVTABLE
TVTAPES
TWEAKED
TWOACRE
TWOACTS
TYRANNY
TYRANTS

T•••A••

TAGDAYS
TAGGANT
TAGSALE
TAKEAIM
TAMBALA
TAMIAMI
TAMMANY
TAMPAFL
TAMTAMS
TANBARK
TANKAGE
TANKARD
TANOAKS
TANTARA
TAPPANS
TARBABY
TARMACS
TARSALS
TARTANS
TARTARE
TARTARS
TARZANA
TARZANS
TATIANA
TAXBASE
TAXLAWS
TAXPAID
TAXRATE
TAXSALE
TAYBACK
TEABAGS
TEABALL
TEACAKE
TEACART
TEDMACK
TEENAGE
TELLALL
TENBALL
TENDAYS
TENNANT
TENPAST
TERNARY
TERNATE
TERRACE
TERRAIN
TERRANS
TESTACY
TESTATE
TETRADS
THEBABE
THEBABY
THEBAND
THEBANS
THEBARD
THECAPE
THECARS
THECAVS
THEEAST
THEFALL
THEGAME
THEGANG
THELAMB
THELARK
THEMAGI
THEMALL
THEMASK
THEMAVS
THEMAYO
THEOATH
THERAMS
THERAPY
THESACK
THESAME
THEWALL
THEWAVE
THINAIR
THREADS
THREADY
THREATS
THROATS
THROATY
TIARAED
TICTACS
TIEBACK
TIEBARS
TIEGAME
TIERACK
TIETACK
TIETACS
TIFFANY
TIJUANA
TILLAGE
TIMBALE
TIMBALS
TIMPANI
TINCANS
TINEARS
TINHATS
TINWARE
TIPCART
TIPJARS
TITIANS
TITLARK
TITRATE
TOAHAIR
TOBLAME
TOCCATA
TOECAPS
TOENAIL
TOETAPS
TOHEART
TOLDALL
TOLEASE
TOLLAGE
TOMCATS
TONEARM
TONGANS
TONNAGE
TOOEASY
TOOHARD
TOOKAIM
TOOLATE
TOOMANY
TOOTALL
TOPHATS
TOPIARY
TOPKAPI
TOPMAST
TOPNAME
TOPRANK
TOPRATE
TOPSAIL
TORNADO
TORVALD
TOSCALE
TOSPARE
TOSTADA
TOSTART
TOUCANS
TOWBARS
TOWCARS
TOWPATH
TOYBALL
TOYCARS
TOYCART
TOYFAIR
TOYHATS
TOYLAND
TOYPAIL
TRALALA
TRAVAIL
TRENARY
TREPANS
TRINARY
TROJANS
TRUMANS
TRYHARD
TRYSAIL
TSQUARE
TSTRAPS
TSUNAMI
TULSANS
TULSAOK
TURBANS
TUSCANS
TUSCANY
TUSSAUD
TVSTARS
TWOBALL
TWOBASE
TWODAYS
TWOFACE
TWOLANE
TWOPAIR
TWOPART
TYMPANA
TYMPANI
TYNDALL
TYPEABS

T••••A•

TABLEAU
TABULAR
TACOMAS
TACTUAL
TAGTEAM
TAILWAG
TALIBAN
TALKSAT
TAMARAC
TANGRAM
TANKCAR
TAPEMAN
TASKBAR
TAUREAN
TAXICAB
TAXIMAN
TAXIWAY
TAXYEAR
TEALEAF
TEARGAS
TEARSAT
TEATRAY
TEHERAN
TEJANAS
TELEFAX
TELERAN
TELSTAR
TEMPEAZ
TEMPLAR
TENYEAR
TESTBAN
TESTLAB
TEXTUAL
THATWAY
THEBEAR
THEBRAT
THECRAB
THEHEAT
THEREAT
THERIAC
THERMAL
THESTAR
THESWAN
THEYSAY
THINMAN
THISDAY
THISWAY
THOREAU
THREEAD
THREEAM
THREWAT
THROWAT
THRUWAY
THURGAU
THURMAN
THUSFAR
TIBETAN
TIEBEAM
TIENDAS
TILTSAT
TIMELAG
TIMEWAS
TINSTAR
TIREMAN
TITANAE
TITULAR
TOBEHAD
TOILSAT
TOLEDAN
TOLLBAR
TOLLMAN
TOLLWAY
TOMJOAD
TONNEAU
TOOLBAR
TOOTSAT
TOPCOAT
TOPDRAW
TOPEKAN
TOPICAL
TORTLAW
TOTEBAG
TOWAWAY
TOWBOAT
TOWHEAD
TOWNCAR
TOYBOAT
TOYOTAS
TRAMCAR
TRAMPAS
TRAMWAY
TRANSAM
TRAUMAS
TREDIAS
TREERAT
TREESAP
TRIGRAM
TRIMTAB
TRISTAN
TRISTAR
TRIVIAL
TROIKAS
TRUDEAU
TSONGAS
TUBEPAN
TUBULAR
TUCHMAN
TUESDAY
TUGBOAT
TUNDRAS
TURFMAN
TURFWAR
TURNBAD
TUTELAR
TWOSTAR
TWOYEAR
TYPICAL

T•••••A

TABITHA
TAFFETA
TAKETEA
TALARIA
TAMBALA
TANTARA
TAPIOCA
TARZANA
TATIANA
TAVERNA
TEAMUSA
TEMPERA
TEMPURA
TEQUILA
TESSERA
THEBIGA
THEFLEA
THEIDEA
THERESA
THRILLA
TIJUANA
TITANIA
TOCCATA
TOCELIA
TOMGOLA
TORTOLA
TORTUGA
TOSHIBA
TOSTADA
TRACHEA
TRALALA
TREINTA
TRIBECA
TRIPLEA
TSARINA
TUNISIA
TURISTA
TUTUILA
TWELVEA
TYMPANA
TZARINA

•TA••••

ATABOIL
ATACAMA
ATACLIP
ATACOST
ATALOSS
ATAMANS
ATANEND
ATARAXY
ATATILT
ATATIME
ATATURK
ATAVISM
ATAVIST
ETAGERE
ETAILED
ETAILER
ETALIBI
ETAMINE
ITALIAN
ITALICS
MTADAMS
MTATHOS
OTALGIA
OTALGIC
OTARIES
STABBED
STABBER
STABILE
STABLED
STABLER
STABLES
STACKED
STACKER
STACKUP
STADIUM
STADLER
STAFFED
STAFFER
STAGERS
STAGGED
STAGGER
STAGIER
STAGILY
STAGING
STAGNES
STAIDER
STAIDLY
STAINED
STAINER
STAIRED
STAKING
STALAGS
STALELY
STALEST
STALKED
STALKER
STALLED
STALLER
STAMENS
STAMINA
STAMMER
STAMPED
STAMPER
STANCES
STANDBY
STANDEE
STANDER
STANDIN
STANDON
STANDTO
STANDUP
STANINE
STANKUP
STANLEE
STANLEY
STANNIC
STANNUM
STANTON
STANZAS
STAPLED
STAPLER
STAPLES
STARCHY
STARDOM
STAREAT
STARERS
STARING
STARION
STARKER
STARKEY
STARKLY
STARLET
STARLIT
STARLOG
STARMAN
STARMAP
STARRED
STARSIN
STARSKY
STARTED
STARTER
STARTIN
STARTLE
STARTON
STARTTO
STARTUP
STARVED
STARVES
STASHED
STASHES
STASSEN
STATELY
STATERS
STATICE
STATICS
STATING
STATINS
STATION
STATISM
STATIST
STATLER
STATORS
STATUES
STATURE
STATUTE
STAUNCH
STAVING
STAYDRY
STAYERS
STAYFOR
STAYING
STAYOFF
STAYOUT
STAYPUT
STAYSAT
STAYSIN
STAYSON
STAYSUP
UTAHANS

•T•A•••

ATEABIT
ATEALOT
ATEAWAY
ATFAULT
ATLANTA
ATLARGE
ATLASES
ATTABOY
ATTACHE
ATTACKS
ATTAINS
ATTAINT
ATWATER
ETHANES
ETHANOL
FTWAYNE
ITHACAN
ITMAYBE
ITSABOY
ITSAHIT
ITSALIE
ITSALOT
ITSASIN
ITSATIE
MTBALDY
MTMARCY
OTRANTO
OTTAVIO
OTTAWAN
OTTAWAS
STBARTS
STBASIL
STEADED
STEALER
STEALIN
STEALTH
STEAMED
STEAMER
STEAMUP
STEANNE
STEARIC
STEARIN
STEARNS
STJAMES
STMARKS
STMARYS
STPAULS
STRAFED
STRAFER
STRAFES
STRAINS
STRAITS
STRANDS
STRANGE
STRAPIN
STRAPON
STRASSE
STRATAS
STRATUM
STRATUS
STRAUSS
STRAYED
STRAYER
STUARTI

•T••A••

ATACAMA
ATAMANS
ATARAXY
ATELATE
ATGRADE
ATHEART
ATHWART
ATLEAST
ATMCARD
ATPEACE
ATSTAKE
ATTRACT
CTSCANS
ETCHANT
FTBRAGG
FTMEADE
ITERANT
ITERATE
ITSEASY
ITSLATE
MTADAMS
MTBLANC
MTEVANS
PTBOATS
STALAGS
STEFANI
STEWARD
STEWART
STOMACH
STOMATA
STORAGE
STOWAGE
STREAKS
STREAKY
STREAMS
STRIATE
UTAHANS
UTICANS
UTICANY

•T•••A•

ATEAWAY
ETERNAL
ETESIAN
ETHICAL
ETONIAN
ITALIAN
ITHACAN
ITSOKAY
LTKOJAK
MTLOGAN
MTSINAI
OTTAWAN
OTTAWAS
OTTOMAN
STANZAS
STAREAT
STARMAN
STARMAP
STAYSAT
STELIAS
STELLAR
STEPDAD
STERNAL
STEWPAN
STIGMAS
STOICAL
STONEAX
STOPGAP
STOPSAT
STRATAS
STYGIAN
UTOPIAN
UTOPIAS
XTERRAS
YTTRIAS

•T••••A

ATACAMA
ATLANTA
ETRURIA
ETVOILA
MTKENYA
OTALGIA
OTTUMWA
STAMINA
STLUCIA
STOMATA

••TA•••

ACTABLE
ACTAEON
ANTACID
ANTARES
ASTAIRE
ASTARTE
ATTABOY
ATTACHE
ATTACKS
ATTAINS
ATTAINT
AUTARCH
AUTARKY
BATAVIA
BETAKEN
BETAKES
BETAMAX
BETARAY
BOTANIC
BUTANES
BYTALKS
CATALAN
CATALOG
CATALOS
CATALPA
CATANIA
CATAWBA
CETANES
CITABLE
CITADEL
CUTARUG
CUTAWAY
DATABLE
DATABUS
DATASET
DETAILS
DETAINS
DOTAGES
DOTARDS
EATABIT
EATABLE
EATALOT
EATAWAY
ENTAILS
ESTADOS
ESTAMIN
ESTATED
ESTATES
FATALES
FATALLY
GETABLE
GETAHIT
GETAJOB
GETATIP
GETAWAY
GITANOS
GOTAHIT
GOTAJOB
GOTATIP
GOTAWAY
HATABLE
HITACHI
INTAILS
INTAKES
INTASTE
KATAYEV
MATADOR
MATALIN
METALED
METATES
MUTABLE
MUTABLY
MUTAGEN
MUTANTS
MUTATED
MUTATES
NATALIA
NATALIE
NATASHA
NATATOR
NOTABIT
NOTABLE
NOTABLY
NOTALIE
NOTALOT
NOTAONE
NOTASTE
NOTATED
NOTATES
NUTATED
NUTATES
OBTAINS
OCTADIC
OCTAGON
OCTANES
OCTANTS
OCTAVAL
OCTAVES
OCTAVIA
OCTAVIO
OCTAVOS
ONTARIO
OTTAVIO
OTTAWAN
OTTAWAS
OUTACTS
OUTADDS
OUTAGES
OUTASKS
OUTAWED
OUTAWES
OXTAILS
PATACAS
PETALED
PETALES

PETARDS
PITAPAT
PITAYAS
POTABLE
POTAGES
POTAMUS
PUTAWAY
QATARIS
RATABLE
RATAFIA
RATATAT
RETABLE
RETACKS
RETAILS
RETAINS
RETAKEN
RETAKER
RETAKES
RETALLY
RETAMED
RETAMES
RETAPED
RETAPES
RETARDS
RETASTE
RETAXED
RETAXES
RITAGAM
RITALIN
RITAMAE
RITARDS
ROTATED
ROTATES
ROTATOR
ROTAWAY
RUTALEE
SATANIC
SATATOP
SITATOP
TATAMIS
TETANUS
TITANAE
TITANIA
TITANIC
TOTABLE
TOTALED
TOTALER
TOTALLY
TOTALUP
TOTASTE
TVTABLE
TVTAPES
UNTACKS
UNTAKEN
UNTAMED
UNTAMES
UNTAPED
UNTAPES
UNTASTY
UNTAXED
UNTAXES
UPTAKES
UPTALKS
VITALIS
VITALLY
VITAMIN
VITARAS
VOTABLE

••T•A••

ACTUARY
ACTUATE
ALTTABS
AMTRACK
AMTRACS
ANTFARM
ANTIART
ARTCARS
ARTFAIR
ARTSALE
ARTWALL
ARTWARE
ATTRACT
BATDAYS
BATEAUX
BETHANY
BETRAYS
BETTANY
BITMAPS
BITPART
BYTRAIN
CATCALL
CATHAIR
CATNAPS
CATTAIL
CATTALO
CATWALK
CITRATE
COTEACH
COTTAGE
CUTBACK
CUTLASS
CUTRATE
DETRACT
DETRAIN
DOTDASH
EATCAKE
EATLATE
ELTRAIN
ENTRADA
ENTRAIN
ENTRANT
ENTRAPS
ESTRADA
ESTRAYS
ESTUARY
EXTRACT
FATBACK
FATCATS
FATFARM
FUTHARK
GATEAUX
GATTACA
GETBACK
GETCASH
GETPAST
GETSANA
GETSANF
GETWARM
GOTBACK
GOTCASH
GOTPAST
GOTTAGO
GOTWARM
HATBAND
HATRACK
HITBACK
HOTBATH
HOTCAKE
HOTCAPS
HOTCARS
HOTDATE
HOTDAYS
HOTHAND
HOTMAIL
HOTPACK
HOTWARS
INTEARS
INTRADE
INTRAYS
JETFANS
JETLAGS
JETPACK
JETWASH
JETWAYS
JUTLAND
KITBAGS
KITHARA
KITKATS
LETFALL
LETHAVE
LETPASS
LOTHAIR
METCALF
METFANS
METHANE
MUTUALS
NATHANS
NETBALL
NETCAFE
NETGAIN
NETGAME
NETWARE
NITRATE
NITTANY
NOTEASY
NOTFAIR
NOTMANY
NOTRADE
NOTRARE
NOTSAFE
OATCAKE
ONTOAST
ONTRACK
OSTIARY
OSTMARK
OSTRAVA
OSTWALD
OUTBACK
OUTBAKE
OUTBANS
OUTBARK
OUTBATS
OUTBAWL
OUTCALL
OUTCANT
OUTCAST
OUTDARE
OUTDATE
OUTEARN
OUTEATS
OUTFACE
OUTFAST
OUTFAWN
OUTGAIN
OUTGAME
OUTGAVE
OUTGAZE
OUTHAUL
OUTKAST
OUTLAID
OUTLAIN
OUTLAND
OUTLASH
OUTLAST
OUTLAWS
OUTLAYS
OUTMANS
OUTMATE
OUTPACE
OUTPAID
OUTPASS
OUTPATH
OUTPAYS
OUTRACE
OUTRAGE
OUTRAIL
OUTRANG
OUTRANK
OUTRANT
OUTRAPS
OUTRATE
OUTRAVE
OUTSAID
OUTSAIL
OUTSANG
OUTSAYS
OUTTAKE
OUTTALK
OUTWAIT
OUTWALK
OUTWARD
OUTWARS
OUTWASH
OUTWAVE
PATCASH
PATHAND
PATHANS
PETCAGE
PETCALF
PETCATS
PETGATE
PETHAIR
PETHARE
PETLAMB
PETNAME
PETNAPS
PETRATS
PITFALL
PITSAWS
POTTAGE
PUTBACK
RATPACK
RATRACE
RATTAIL
RATTANS
RETEACH
RETEARS
RETHANK
RETHAWS
RETIARY
RETOAST
RETRACE
RETRACK
RETRACT
RETRADE
RETRAIN
RETRAPS
RITEAID
RITUALS
RUTHANN
RUTLAND
SATBACK
SATIATE
SATRAPS
SATRAPY
SETBACK
SETBAIL
SETRATE
SETSAIL
SITBACK
SITUATE
TATIANA
TETRADS
TITIANS
TITLARK
TITRATE
TSTRAPS
UNTEACH
UNTHAWS
UNTRACK
UNTRAPS
UPTEARS
UPTRADE
VITIATE
VOTEAYE
WATTAGE
WETBARS
WETLAND
WETNAPS
WETRAGS
WETWARE
WETWASH
YOTEAMO

••T••A•

ACTEDAS
ACTIVAS
ALTIMAS
ALTOSAX
ANTBEAR
ANTHRAX
ANTITAX
ANTIWAR
APTERAL
ARTISAN
ASTHMAS
ASTOLAT
ASTREAM
AUTOMAT
AZTECAN
BATEMAN
BATHMAT
BATSMAN
BETAMAX
BETARAY
BITONAL
BUTTRAM
CATALAN
CATBOAT
CATENAE
CATENAS
CATERAS
CATFLAP
CATHEAD
CATSCAN
CATSPAW
CITYGAL
CUTAWAY
EATAWAY
EATENAT
ECTYPAL
ENTHRAL
ENTREAT
ESTEBAN
ESTEFAN
ESTIVAL
FATHEAD
FOTOMAT
FUTURAS
GATEMAN
GATEWAY
GETAWAY
GETBEAT
GETREAL
GETSFAR
GETSMAD
GOTAWAY
GOTBEAT
GOTCHAS
GOTOGAL
GOTOWAR
GOTREAL
HITPLAY
HOTCOAL
HOTHEAD
HOTLEAD
HOTMEAL
HOTSEAT
HOTTEAS
INTOTAL
ISTRIAN
JETBOAT
JETSFAN
JETSTAR
KETCHAM
LATERAL
LATERAN
LATETAG
LATIFAH
LATINAS
LATVIAN
LETHEAN
LETSEAT
LITERAL
LOTHIAN
MATEWAN
MATHIAS
MATINAL
MATTHAU
METSFAN
MITHRAS
MITZVAH
MYTREAT
NATURAL
NOTEPAD
NOTNEAR
NOTREAL
NUTMEAT
NUTRIAS
OATBRAN
OATMEAL
OCTAVAL
ONTKEAN
ONTRIAL
OPTICAL
OPTIMAL
OPTIMAS
ORTEGAL
ORTOLAN
OTTAWAN
OTTAWAS
OTTOMAN
OUTBEAM
OUTBRAG
OUTBRAY
OUTDRAG
OUTDRAW
OUTGNAW
OUTHEAR
OUTLEAD
OUTLEAP
OUTPLAN
OUTPLAY
OUTPRAY
OUTREAD
OUTROAR
OUTSOAR
OUTSTAY
OUTSWAM
OUTTEAR
OUTTRAY
OUTWEAR
PATACAS
PATHWAY
PATINAS
PETBEAR
PETBOAS
PETEMAN
PETGOAT
PETSCAN
PITAPAT
PITAYAS
PITHEAD
PITTMAN
POTOMAC
POTSDAM
PUTAWAY
PYTHIAN
PYTHIAS
RATATAT
RATECAP
RATTRAP
RETINAE
RETINAL
RETINAS
RETOTAL
RETREAD
RETREAT
RETRIAL
RITAGAM
RITAMAE
ROTAWAY
ROTBLAT
SETPLAY
SITEMAP
SITSPAT
TITANAE
TITULAR
TOTEBAG
TUTELAR
ULTIMAS
UNTREAD
UPTOPAR
VATICAL
VATICAN
VETERAN
VITARAS
VOTENAY
WATTEAU
YITZHAK
YTTRIAS

••T•••A

ALTOONA
ANTENNA
ANTIGUA
ANTONIA
ASTORIA
AUTOPIA
BATAVIA
BATISTA
BOTHNIA
BOTTEGA
CATALPA
CATANIA
CATAWBA
CATFLEA
ENTRADA
ESTELLA
ESTONIA
ESTRADA
GATTACA
GETSANA
GOTHIKA
GOTOSEA
HOTTUNA
INTEGRA
KATISHA
KATRINA
KITHARA
LATOSCA
LETITIA
LETTERA
LUTETIA
MATILDA
NATALIA
NATASHA
OCTAVIA
OSTRAVA
OTTUMWA
PATELLA
PETULIA
PETUNIA
RATAFIA
RETSINA
ROTHIRA
ROTUNDA
SATSUMA
SETENTA
TATIANA
TITANIA
TUTUILA
VITORIA
VOTEYEA

•••TA••

ABSTAIN
ACETALS
ACETATE
AGITATE
AGITATO
AIRTANK
AIRTAXI
ALETAPS
ALTTABS
ANATASE
ATSTAKE
AVATARS
BANTAMS
BARTABS
BEATALL
BELTANE
BETTANY
BHUTANI
BIGTALK
BISTATE
BLATANT
BOBTAIL
BOITANO
BRITAIN
BUSTARD
CAFTANS
CANTABS
CANTALS
CANTATA
CAPTAIN
CARTAGE
CARTALK
CATTAIL
CATTALO
CENTALS
CENTARE
CENTAUR
CENTAVO
CERTAIN
CONTACS
CONTACT
CONTAIN
COSTAIN
COSTARD
COSTARS
COSTATE
COTTAGE
CRETANS
CURTAIL
CURTAIN
CURTATE
CUSTARD
DAKTARI
DASTARD
DELTAIC
DENTALS
DENTATE
DESTAEL
DESTAIN
DICTATE
DIETARY
DIKTATS
DISTAFF
DISTANT
DOGTAGS
DOGTAIL
DONTASK
EARTABS
EARTAGS
ECOTAGE
ECSTASY
EPITAPH
EUSTACE
FANTAIL
FANTANS
FANTASM
FANTAST
FANTASY
FLOTAGE
FONTANA
FONTANE
FOOTAGE
FOXTAIL
FURTADO
GAETANO
GASTANK
GATTACA
GAUTAMA
GESTALT
GESTAPO
GESTATE
GOSTALE
GOTTAGO
GUITARS
GUSTAVE
HARTACK
HECTARE
HEPTADS
HOSTAGE
IMITATE
INSTALL
INSTALS
INSTANT
INSTATE
ISITAGO
KHATAMI
LACTAID
LACTASE
LACTATE
LANTANA
LASTACT
LEFTARM
LEOTARD
LOSTART
MAITAIS
MALTASE
MAYTAGS
MEATAXE
MELTAGE
MINTAGE
MISTAKE
MONTAGE
MONTAGU
MONTALE
MONTANA
MONTAND
MONTANO
MONTAUK
MORTALS
MORTARS
MUSTAFA
MUSTANG
MUSTARD
MYSTARS
NASTASE
NECTARS
NECTARY
NICTATE
NITTANY
NOSTAIN
NOSTARS
OAKTAGS
OILTANK
ONSTAFF
ONSTAGE
OUTTAKE
OUTTALK
PARTAKE
PELTATE
PENTADS
PENTANE
PEPTALK
PERTAIN
PIGTAIL
PINTAIL
POLTAVA
PONTANO
POPTART
PORTAGE
PORTALS
POSTAGE
POTTAGE
PRETAPE
QINTARS
RATTAIL
RATTANS
REDTABS
REDTAGS
REDTAIL
REDTAPE
RENTALS
RESTABS
RESTACK
RESTAFF
RESTAGE
RESTAIN
RESTAMP
RESTART
RESTATE
RIOTACT
ROOTAGE
ROSTAND
SALTANT
SANTAFE
SANTANA
SEXTANS
SEXTANT
SMETANA
SUBTASK
SULTANA
SULTANS
SUNTANS
SUSTAIN
TAMTAMS
TANTARA
TARTANS
TARTARE
TARTARS
TESTACY
TESTATE
TICTACS
TIETACK
TIETACS
TOETAPS
TOOTALL
TOSTADA
TOSTART
TVSTARS
UNITARD
UNITARY
UNSTACK
UNSTAGY
UNSTAID
UNSTATE
UPSTAGE
UPSTAIR
UPSTAND
UPSTARE
UPSTART
UPSTATE
USSTATE
VANTAGE
VCRTAPE
VENTAGE
VESTALS
VINTAGE
VISTAED
VOLTAGE
VOLTAIC
WANTADS
WANTAGH
WASTAGE
WATTAGE
WENTAFT
WENTAPE
WHATAMI
WYOTANA

•••T•A•

ABETTAL
ABUTTAL
AFCTEAM
AINTHAY
AIRTRAP
ALLTHAT
ANITRAS
ASATEAM
ASHTRAY
ASSTDAS
AUSTRAL
BAITCAR
BARTRAY
BEATSAT
BELTBAG
BELTRAN
BELTSAW
BELTWAY
BENTHAM
BERTHAS
BERTRAM
BESTIAL
BESTMAN
BOATMAN
BOBTWAY
BUTTRAM
CANTSAY
CENTRAL
CHATEAU
CHATHAM
COCTEAU
CONTRAS
CRITIAS
CULTJAM
DANTEAN
DEXTRAL
DIDTOAT
DIRTBAG
DUSTMAN
DUSTPAN
DUSTRAG
EASTHAM
EASTMAN
FACTUAL
FASTCAR
FELTBAD
FELTHAT
FIFTYAD
FLATCAR
FLATHAT
FLATTAX
FLOTSAM
FLYTRAP
FOOTBAG
FOOTMAN
FOOTPAD
FOOTWAY
FORTRAN
FORTYAD
FRETSAT
FRETSAW
FUSTIAN
GENTIAN
GIFTTAX
GLOTTAL
GLUTEAL
GODTHAB
GRATIAS
HAITIAN
HARTMAN
HEATFAN
HEATRAY
HINTSAT
HOOTSAT
HOTTEAS
ICETEAS
ICETRAY
INATRAP
INITIAL
INSTEAD
KANTIAN
LACTEAL
LAOTIAN
LASTGAS
LASTLAP
LASTMAY
LEFTEAR
LEFTJAB
LEGTRAP
LOSTCAT
LUSTRAL
MANTRAP
MANTRAS
MANTUAN
MARTIAL
MARTIAN
MATTHAU
MEATMAN
MISTRAL
NBATEAM

NEUTRAL	YEATEAM	ARISTAE	OVERTAX	BERETTA	BERETTA	TAFFETA	THEBIGA	TOLLBAR	STUBBLY	OUTBOWS	HOTTUBS	RESTABS
NEXTDAY		ARISTAS	PALATAL	BIRETTA	BIODATA	TOCCATA	THEBLOB	TOOLBAR	STUBING	OUTBRAG	LATROBE	SAXTUBA
NFCTEAM	**•••T••A**	AVESTAN	PELOTAS	BOBATEA	BIRETTA	TREINTA	THEBOBO	TOOLBOX		OUTBRAY	LETGOBY	SIXTYBC
NFLTEAM	AUSTRIA	AVESTAS	PEPITAS	CORETTA	CALISTA	TURISTA	THEBODY	TOTABLE	**•T••B••**	OUTBRED	LETITBE	THETUBE
NHLTEAM	BACTRIA	BALATAS	PESETAS	CROATIA	CANASTA	WICHITA	THEBOMB	TOTEBAG	ATEABIT	OUTBUDS	LETMEBE	
NOOTKAS	BOOTHIA	BEERTAP	PINATAS	DYKSTRA	CANTATA		THEBOSS	TOURBUS	ATTABOY	OUTBULK	MRTIBBS	**•••T••B**
NUPTIAL	BOTTEGA	BENATAR	PINETAR	ELANTRA	CARLOTA	**TB•••••**	THEBOYS	TOWABLE	ITSABOY	OUTBURN	NOTTOBE	DISTURB
ONATEAR	CANTATA	BIGSTAR	PIVOTAL	ELECTRA	CASERTA	TBILISI	THEBRAT	TOYNBEE	STABBED	OUTBUYS	OUTRIBS	FOOTRUB
OSETRAS	CANTINA	BIMETAL	PLANTAR	ELEKTRA	CELESTA		THEBUSH	TRAUBEL	STABBER	OUTBUZZ	SOTHEBY	GODTHAB
OUTTEAR	CAPTIVA	BORSTAL	PLUSTAX	GALATEA	CHRISTA	**T•B••••**	TIBBETT	TREMBLE	STEUBEN	PETBEAR		LEFTJAB
OUTTRAY	CHUTZPA	CAPITAL	POINTAT	GALATIA	CORETTA	TABARDS	TIDBITS	TREMBLY	STROBES	PETBIRD	**••T•••B**	LETTERB
PARTIAL	CORTINA	CAPITAN	POLLTAX	HERBTEA	DACOSTA	TABARET	TIEBACK	TRIABLE	STUBBED	PETBOAS	BATHTUB	PERTURB
PARTWAY	CYNTHIA	CAPSTAN	POORTAX	HIGHTEA	DOGMATA	TABASCO	TIEBARS	TRIBBLE	STUBBLE	PITBOSS	CATCOMB	TESTLAB
PITTMAN	DAYTONA	CASITAS	POPSTAR	HOFSTRA	EDEMATA	TABBIES	TIEBEAM	TROUBLE	STUBBLY	PITBULL	DOTBOMB	THETRIB
PLATEAU	DELTONA	CHEETAH	PRINTAD	HYPATIA	ELBERTA	TABBING	TIMBALE	TUNABLE	STUMBLE	POTBOIL	GETAJOB	
PONTIAC	DIOTIMA	CHEETAS	PULLTAB	ICEDTEA	EMERITA	TABITHA	TIMBALS	TURNBAD		PUTBACK	GOTAJOB	**••••TB•**
PONTIAN	ERITREA	CHOCTAW	PURITAN	INERTIA	ENCARTA	TABKEYS	TIMBERS	TVTABLE	**•T•••B•**	RATBERT	HOTCOMB	CANITBE
PORTMAN	EROTICA	COALTAR	QUARTAN	JEPHTHA	ERNESTA	TABLEAU	TIMBERY	TWINBED	ETALIBI	ROTBLAT	LETTERB	EIGHTBC
PORTRAY	EXOTICA	COASTAL	QUINTAL	JERITZA	FERMATA	TABLETS	TIMBRES		ITMAYBE	SATBACK	PETCOMB	FLOATBY
POSTBAG	FESTINA	CRUSTAL	QUINTAS	KAPITSA	GANGSTA	TABLING	TMOBILE	**T••••B•**	STANDBY	SETBACK	PETLAMB	LETITBE
POSTMAN	FESTIVA	CRYSTAL	RANATAB	LAMOTTA	GORDITA	TABLOID	TOMBOYS	TAKENBY	STICKBY	SETBAIL	POTHERB	SHOOTBY
POSTWAR	FONTANA	CUBITAL	RAPSTAR	LETITIA	GRANITA	TABOOED	TOPBIDS	TARBABY	STOODBY	SITBACK	WETBULB	
PROTEAM	FONTINA	CUESTAS	RARITAN	LORETTA	INEDITA	TABORET	TOPBOOT	THEBABE	STOPSBY	WETBARS		**••••T•B**
PROTEAN	FORTUNA	DAKOTAN	RATATAT	LUCETTA	INFANTA	TABOULI	TOWBARS	THEBABY	STUCKBY	WETBULB	**•••TB••**	BATHTUB
QUETZAL	GATTACA	DAKOTAS	REATTAS	LUTETIA	INGESTA	TABSETS	TOWBOAT	THEBOBO			AUNTBEE	PAYSTUB
RANTSAT	GAUTAMA	DARKTAN	RECITAL	MAHATMA	INSECTA	TABUING	TOYBALL	THECUBS	**••TB•••**	**••T•B••**	BEATBOX	PULLTAB
RATTRAP	HOTTUNA	DAYSTAR	REDSTAR	MELITTA	INVICTA	TABULAR	TOYBIKE	THEREBY	ANTBEAR	ACTABLE	BELTBAG	RANATAB
REATTAS	IGOTCHA	DEEPTAN	REFUTAL	MILITIA	JAKARTA	TEBALDI	TOYBOAT	THEROBE	ANTBIRD	ANTIBES	BESTBET	RUNATAB
REITMAN	LANTANA	DIGITAL	RETOTAL	MINTTEA	JOCASTA	TIBBETT	TOYBOOK	THETUBE	ARTBOOK	ATTABOY	BESTBOY	SINUTAB
RESTRAP	LETTERA	DOGSTAR	ROADTAR	MINUTIA	KOLKATA	TIBETAN	TRABERT	THREEBC	BATBOYS	AUTOBIO	BESTBUD	TRIMTAB
ROOTCAP	MANTECA	DRISTAN	ROADTAX	MOZETTA	LACERTA	TIBURON	TREBLED	TICKSBY	CATBEDS	AUTOBUS	BESTBUY	WASHTUB
ROSTRAL	MARTINA	DUNSTAN	RUNATAB	MUSETTA	LAMOTTA	TOBACCO	TREBLES	TOSHIBA	CATBERT	CITABLE	DIRTBAG	
SCATMAN	MINTTEA	EDICTAL	SEASTAR	NAPHTHA	LAPLATA	TOBEHAD	TRIBBLE	TYPEABS	CATBIRD	CITYBOY	DONTBEE	**•••••TB**
SCOTIAN	MONTANA	EIGHTAD	SHOOTAT	NUESTRA	LEMMATA	TOBLAME	TRIBECA		CATBOAT	DATABLE	DUSTBIN	SILENTB
SENTRAS	MONTOYA	EIGHTAM	SHOUTAT	ODONTIA	LORETTA	TUBAIST	TRIBORO	**T•••••B**	CATBOWL	DATABUS	FELTBAD	
SHOTPAR	MUSTAFA	EXACTAS	SIESTAS	OLESTRA	LUCETTA	TUBBIER	TRIBUNE	TAXICAB	CUTBACK	EATABIT	FLATBED	**T•C••••**
SIXTYAD	NAUTICA	FAJITAS	SINUTAB	OPUNTIA	LUNESTA	TUBBING	TRIBUTE	TEMPJOB	DOTBOMB	EATABLE	FOOTBAG	TACHYON
SLOTCAR	PANTERA	FIESTAS	SNORTAT	OSSETRA	MAGENTA	TUBEPAN	TUBBIER	TESTLAB	FATBACK	ENTEBBE	GIFTBOX	TACITLY
SPATIAL	PARTITA	FLATTAX	SONATAS	PANETTA	MELITTA	TUBETOP	TUBBING	THEBLOB	GETBACK	ESTEBAN	HAUTBOY	TACITUS
SWATSAT	PASTINA	FLAUTAS	SPARTAN	PINOTTA	MINOLTA	TUBFULS	TUGBOAT	THEBOMB	GETBEAT	GETABLE	LOFTBED	TACKERS
TACTUAL	POETICA	FRACTAL	STRATAS	PLECTRA	MOMENTA	TUBISTS	TUMBLED	THECRAB	GETBENT	GOTOBED	LOSTBIG	TACKIER
TAGTEAM	POLTAVA	FREITAG	TELSTAR	PWBOTHA	MOZETTA	TUBLIKE	TUMBLER	THELAMB	GETBUSY	HATABLE	MALTBIE	TACKILY
TEATRAY	SALTSEA	FREYTAG	THESTAR	REGATTA	MUSETTA	TUBULAR	TUMBLES	THETRIB	GOTBACK	IVTUBES	MISTBOW	TACKING
TESTBAN	SANTANA	FRONTAL	TIBETAN	RICOTTA	MYLANTA	TUBULES	TUMBREL	TRIMTAB	GOTBEAT	MRTIBBS	PEATBOG	TACKLED
TESTLAB	SAXTUBA	GAMETAL	TINSTAR	ROSETEA	NDAKOTA		TURBANS	TRUERIB	GOTBUSY	MUTABLE	POSTBAG	TACKLER
TEXTUAL	SESTINA	GIFTTAX	TOYOTAS	ROSETTA	OCHENTA	**T••B•••**	TURBINE	TUNASUB	HATBAND	MUTABLY	POSTBOX	TACKLES
THATWAY	SMETANA	GLOTTAL	TRIMTAB	ROVETTA	ONEIOTA	TABBIES	TURBOTS	TWELVEB	HATBRIM	NOTABIT	SALTBOX	TACKSON
TILTSAT	SPATULA	HABITAT	TRISTAN	SAGETEA	ONEONTA	TABBING	TWOBALL		HITBACK	NOTABLE	TENTBED	TACKSUP
TOOTSAT	SULTANA	HEELTAP	TRISTAR	SINATRA	PANETTA	TAMBALA	TWOBASE	**•TB••••**	HOTBATH	NOTABLY	TESTBAN	TACOMAS
TORTLAW	TANTARA	INTOTAL	TWOSTAR	SPECTRA	PARTITA	TAMBLYN	TWOBITS	FTBLISS	HOTBEDS	OCTOBER	TESTBED	TACONIC
UNSTRAP	TORTOLA	JACKTAR	UNVITAL	SUMATRA	PERDITA	TANBARK		FTBRAGG	JETBOAT	OCTOBRE	WENTBAD	TACTFUL
VECTRAS	TORTUGA	JETSTAR	VEGETAL	TABITHA	PICCATA	TARBABY	**T•••B••**	MTBALDY	KITBAGS	OCTUBRE		TACTICS
VELTMAN	TOSTADA	KAPITAL	VERITAS	TAKETEA	PINOTTA	TARBELL	TAKABLE	MTBLANC	NETBALL	OKTOBER	**•••T•B•**	TACTILE
VENTRAD	VENTURA	LAKOTAS	VIVITAR		POLENTA	TAXBASE	TALIBAN	PTBOATS	NOTBEEN	POTABLE	ABITIBI	TACTUAL
VENTRAL	VIATICA	LANDTAG	WIRETAP	**•••••TA**	PREDATA	TAYBACK	TALKBIG	STBARTS	OATBRAN	RATABLE	AIRTUBE	TECHIES
VESTRAL	VISTULA	LANDTAX	WOODTAR	ALBERTA	PRORATA	TEABAGS	TAMABLE	STBASIL	OUTBACK	RETABLE	ALTTABS	TECHNOS
VICTUAL	WOJTYLA	LAPUTAN	YUCATAN	ALMAATA	RAWDATA	TEABALL	TASKBAR		OUTBAKE	TOTABLE	BARTABS	TICCING
VIETNAM	WYOTANA	LATETAG	YUKATAS	AMANITA	REGATTA	TEMBLOR	TAXABLE	**•T•B•••**	OUTBANS	TOTEBAG	CANTABS	TICKERS
VIRTUAL		LEAPTAT	ZAPATAS	AMREETA	RICOTTA	TENBALL	TENABLE	ATABOIL	OUTBARK	TVTABLE	EARTABS	TICKETS
WALTHAM	**••••TA•**	LESSTAR		ARIETTA	RIORITA	TERBIUM	TENABLY	ITSBEST	OUTBATS	VITEBSK	FIFTYBC	TICKING
WATTEAU	ABETTAL	LOVETAP	**••••T•A**	ASSUNTA	ROBERTA	THEBABE	TENTBED	STABBED	OUTBAWL	VOTABLE	FLITSBY	TICKLED
WENTBAD	ABUTTAL	MARITAL	ABINTRA	ATLANTA	ROBUSTA	THEBABY	TESTBAN	STABBER	OUTBEAM		FORTYBC	TICKLER
WENTFAR	ADEPTAT	MULETAS	ALSATIA	AUGUSTA	ROSETTA	THEBAND	TESTBED	STABILE	OUTBEGS	**••T••B•**	HADTOBE	TICKLES
WENTMAD	ALLSTAR	NAMETAG	ARANTXA	AULETTA	ROVETTA	THEBANS	THEABCS	STABLED	OUTBEND	ALTTABS	HASTOBE	TICKOFF
WHATSAY	ALNITAK	ONESTAR	ARIETTA	BACHATA	SDAKOTA	THEBARD	THIMBLE	STABLER	OUTBIDS	BYTHEBY	HOTTUBS	TICKSBY
WHITMAN	AMISTAD	OPENTAP	AULETTA	BARETTA	SETENTA	THEBEAR	THUMBED	STABLES	OUTBLOT	CATAWBA	LABTUBE	TICOTIN
XANTHAN	AMRITAS	ORBITAL	BARETTA	BARISTA	SILENTA	THEBELL	THURBER	STUBBED	OUTBLOW	ENTEBBE	NOTTOBE	TICTACS
YAYTEAM	ANTITAX	OUTSTAY	BEEFTEA	BATISTA	STOMATA	THEBEST	TINYBIT	STUBBLE	OUTBOWL	ENTOMBS	REDTABS	TOCCATA

TOCELIA
TOCSINS
TUCHMAN
TUCKERS
TUCKING
TUCKSIN
TUCSONS
TVCREWS
TYCOONS

T••C•••

TALCKED
TALCUMS
TAXCODE
TAXCUTS
TEACAKE
TEACART
TEACHER
TEACHES
TEACHIN
TEACOZY
TEACUPS
TEICHER
TENCENT
TENCHES
TENCODE
TERCELS
THECAPE
THECARS
THECAVS
THECITY
THECRAB
THECROW
THECUBS
THICKEN
THICKER
THICKET
THICKLY
TICCING
TIECLIP
TINCANS
TINCTED
TIPCART
TOCCATA
TOECAPS
TOMCATS
TOPCOAT
TORCHED
TORCHER
TORCHES
TOSCALE
TOUCANS
TOUCHED
TOUCHER
TOUCHES
TOUCHON
TOUCHUP
TOWCARS
TOYCARS
TOYCART
TRACERS
TRACERY
TRACHEA
TRACING
TRACKED
TRACKER
TRACTOR
TRICEPS
TRICKED
TRICKER
TRICKLE
TRICORN
TRICOTS
TROCHEE
TROCHES
TRUCKED
TRUCKEE
TRUCKER
TRUCKLE
TUSCANS
TUSCANY

T•••C••

TANKCAR
TAXICAB
TELECOM
TENACES
TENACRE
THATCHY
THWACKS
TIERCES
TIMECOP
TOBACCO
TOPICAL
TOWNCAR
TRAMCAR
TRANCED
TRANCES
TREACLE
TREACLY
TUNICLE
TWITCHY
TWOACRE
TWOACTS
TYPICAL

T••••C•

TABASCO
TACTICS
TAMPICO
TAPIOCA
TARMACS
TAYBACK
TEANECK
TEDMACK
TENANCY
TENNECO
TERENCE
TERRACE
TESTACY
THEABCS
THEMICK
THEROCK
THESACK
THINICE
TICTACS
TIEBACK
TIERACK
TIETACK
TIETACS
TIMRICE
TITMICE
TOBACCO
TOEPICK
TOLTECS
TOOMUCH
TOPKICK
TRADUCE
TRIBECA
TRISECT
TROPICS
TROUNCE
TRUANCY
TUMESCE
TUSSOCK
TWOFACE

T•••••C

TACONIC
TAMARAC
TELEPIC
THERIAC
THERMIC
THREEBC
TITANIC
TONELOC
TOTEMIC
TRAFFIC
TRIADIC
TWELVEC

•TC••••

ATCROSS
ETCHANT
ETCHERS
ETCHING
ITCHFOR
ITCHIER
ITCHING
STCLOUD
STCROIX

•T•C•••

ATACAMA
ATACLIP
ATACOST
ATECROW
ATMCARD
CTSCANS
ETICKET
ITSCOLD
STACKED
STACKER
STACKUP
STICKBY
STICKER
STICKIN
STICKON
STICKTO
STICKUM
STICKUP
STOCKED
STOCKER
STOCKUP
STUCCOS
STUCKBY
STUCKIN
STUCKON
STUCKTO
STUCKUP
UTICANS
UTICANY

•T••C••

ATTACHE
ATTACKS
ATTICUS
ATTUCKS
ETHICAL
ITHACAN
STANCES
STARCHY
STENCIL
STLUCIA
STOICAL
STUCCOS
UTRECHT

•T•••C•

ATDEUCE
ATLUNCH
ATOMICS
ATONICS
ATPEACE
ATTRACT
ETHNICS
ETONICS
ITALICS
MTMARCY
STATICE
STATICS
STAUNCH
STOMACH
STRETCH
STRITCH

•T••••C

ETHERIC
MTBLANC
OTALGIC
STANNIC
STEARIC
STYPTIC

••TC•••

AITCHES
ANTCOWS
ARTCARS
BATCHED
BATCHES
BOTCHED
BOTCHER
BOTCHES
BOTCHUP
BUTCHER
BUTCHES
CATCALL
CATCHER
CATCHES
CATCHON
CATCHOW
CATCHUP
CATCOMB
DITCHED
DITCHER
DITCHES
DOTCOMS
EATCAKE
EATCROW
FATCATS
FATCELL
FATCITY
FETCHED
FETCHER
FETCHES
GETCASH
GETCOLD
GETCUTE
GOTCASH
GOTCHAS
GOTCOLD
GOTCUTE
HATCHED
HATCHER
HATCHES
HATCHET
HITCHED
HITCHER
HITCHES
HITCHON
HITCHUP
HOTCAKE
HOTCAPS
HOTCARS
HOTCOAL
HOTCOMB
HOTCUPS
HUTCHES
KETCHAM
KETCHES
KETCHUM
KETCHUP
KITCHEN
KUTCHER
LATCHED
LATCHES
LATCHON
LITCHIS
LITCRIT
MATCHED
MATCHER
MATCHES
MATCHUP
METCALF
MITCHUM
NATCHEZ
NETCAFE
NETCOST
NOTCHED
NOTCHER
NOTCHES
OATCAKE
OUTCALL
OUTCANT
OUTCAST
OUTCITY
OUTCOLD
OUTCOME
OUTCOOK
OUTCROP
OUTCROW
OUTCULL
OUTCURE
OUTCUTS
PATCASH
PATCHED
PATCHEN
PATCHER
PATCHES
PATCHUP
PETCAGE
PETCALF
PETCATS
PETCHEW
PETCOCK
PETCOMB
PETCOWS
PETCROW
PITCHED
PITCHER
PITCHES
PITCHIN
PITCHTO
PITCREW
RATCHET
RITCHIE
SATCHEL
SATCHMO
SATCOMS
SITCOMS
VETCHES
WATCHED
WATCHER
WATCHES
WATCHIT
WATCHTV
WETCELL
WITCHED
WITCHES
ZITCOMS

••T•C••

ANTACID
ARTICLE
ATTACHE
ATTACKS
ATTICUS
ATTUCKS
AZTECAN
CATSCAN
CUTICLE
DETECTO
DETECTS
ENTICED
ENTICER
ENTICES
HITACHI
KITSCHY
LATICES
NOTICED
NOTICER
NOTICES
OPTICAL
OPTICKS
OUTACTS
OUTECHO
PATACAS
PETSCAN
RATECAP
RETACKS
RETICLE
SHTICKS
SHTICKY
UNTACKS
UNTUCKS
UPTICKS
VATICAL
VATICAN
VOTECHS

••T••C•

AMTRACK
AMTRACS
ANTIOCH
ARTDECO
ARTROCK
ATTRACT
AUTARCH
CATORCE
COTEACH
CUTBACK
DETRACT
DOTRICE
EXTINCT
EXTRACT
FATBACK
FETLOCK
GATTACA
GATWICK
GETBACK
GOTBACK
GOTHICS
HATRACK
HITBACK
HOTLICK
HOTPACK
IATRICS
INTOUCH
JETPACK
LATENCY
LATOSCA
LATTICE
LETTUCE
MATLOCK
MATTOCK
METRICS
NATWICK
NITPICK
NOTMUCH
NOTNICE
NOTONCE
ONTRACK
OSTRICH
OUTBACK
OUTFACE
OUTKICK
OUTPACE
OUTPICK
OUTRACE
OUTROCK
PATENCY
PATRICE
PATRICK
PETCOCK
PETDUCK
PETMICE
PETROCK
POTENCE
POTENCY
POTLUCK
PUTBACK
RATPACK
RATRACE
RETEACH
RETOUCH
RETRACE
RETRACK
RETRACT
SATBACK
SETBACK
SITBACK
TITMICE
UNTEACH
UNTHICK
UNTRACK
VITRICS

••T•••C

ARTHURC
BOTANIC
ENTERIC
FATIDIC
KETONIC
LETTERC
MITOTIC
OCTADIC
ONTOPIC
POTOMAC
SATANIC
SATIRIC
SATYRIC
TITANIC
TOTEMIC
UNTOXIC

•••TC••

BAITCAR
BEATCOP
BESTCUT
BLOTCHY
BOOTCUT
BRITCOM
CLUTCHY
DONTCRY
FASTCAR
FLATCAR
GLITCHY
IGOTCHA
KVETCHY
LOSTCAT
ROOTCAP
SAATCHI
SKETCHY
SLOTCAR
THATCHY
TWITCHY

•••T•C•

BIOTECH
CALTECH
CELTICS
CONTACS
CONTACT
CORTICO
CRITICS
DESTOCK
DEUTSCH
DIPTYCH
DISTICH
DOGTICK
EMETICS
EROTICA
EROTICS
EUSTACE
EXOTICA
EXOTICS
EYETUCK
GATTACA
HAPTICS
HARTACK
INSTOCK
JUSTICE
KLATSCH
LABTECH
LASTACT
LATTICE
LETTUCE
LOWTECH
MANTECA
MASTICS
MATTOCK
MIXTECS
MORTICE
MYSTICS
NAUTICA
NOETICS
PEPTICS
PHOTICS
POETICA
POETICS
PORTICO
PROTECT
RESTACK
RESTICK
RESTOCK
RIOTACT
ROSTOCK
RUSTICS
SCHTICK
SCITECH
STATICE
STATICS
TACTICS
TESTACY
TICTACS
TIETACK
TIETACS
TOLTECS
UNSTACK
UNSTICK
UNSTUCK
VIATICA

•••T••C

CENTRIC
DELTAIC
FIFTYBC
FORTYBC
GASTRIC
LAUTREC
LECTRIC
LETTERC
MANTRIC
PONTIAC
POSTDOC
POSTHOC
SIXTYBC
UNSTOIC
VOLTAIC
XANTHIC

••••TC•

ABBOTCY
BADITCH
BEWITCH
BYCATCH
GODUTCH
INDUTCH
NIDETCH
NOCATCH
REHITCH
RELATCH
REMATCH
REPATCH
SAWATCH
SCOOTCH
SCRATCH
SNEETCH
SPLOTCH
STRETCH
STRITCH
UNHITCH
UNLATCH
WASATCH

••••T•C

ABIOTIC
AGNATIC
AQUATIC
ASCETIC
ASEPTIC
ASIATIC
AVIATIC
CAUSTIC
CHAOTIC
CROSTIC
CRYPTIC
DEISTIC
DEMOTIC
DRASTIC
EIDETIC
EIGHTBC
EKISTIC
ELASTIC
ERGOTIC
ERISTIC
ERRATIC
FANATIC
FRANTIC
GENETIC
GLYPTIC
GNOSTIC
HAMITIC
HEMATIC
HEPATIC
HERETIC
IDENTIC
IDIOTIC
KINETIC
LEVITIC
LUNATIC
MEIOTIC
MIMETIC
MITOTIC
NEPOTIC
NIANTIC
OOLITIC
ORECTIC
OSMATIC
OSMOTIC
PIRATIC
PLASTIC
POLITIC
PRACTIC
PYRETIC
PYRITIC
QUARTIC
QUINTIC
ROBOTIC
SCEPTIC
SCIATIC
SEMITIC
SKEPTIC
SOMATIC
STYPTIC
VENATIC
XEROTIC
YUCATEC
ZAPOTEC

•••••TC

SILENTC

T•D••••

TADPOLE
TEDDIES
TEDEUMS
TEDIOUS
TEDIUMS
TEDMACK
TIDALLY
TIDBITS
TIDERIP
TIDIEST
TIDINGS
TIDYING
TIDYSUM
TODDIES
TODDLED
TODDLER
TODDLES

T••D•••

TAGDAYS
TANDEMS
TANDOOR
TARDIER
TARDILY
TEDDIES
TEEDOFF
TENDAYS
TENDERS
TENDING
TENDONS
TENDRIL
TENDSTO
THEDEEP
THEDELL
THEDIET
THEDOLE
THEDUKE
THUDDED
TIEDOFF
TIEDOWN
TIEDYED
TIEDYES
TINDERS
TINDERY
TIPDOWN
TOADIED
TOADIES
TOADISH
TODDIES
TODDLED
TODDLER
TODDLES
TOLDALL
TOLDOFF
TOODLES
TOPDOGS
TOPDOWN
TOPDRAW
TOYDOGS
TOYDOLL
TRADEIN
TRADEON
TRADERS
TRADEUP
TRADING
TRADUCE
TREDIAS
TRIDENT
TRODDEN
TRUDEAU
TRUDGED
TRUDGEN
TRUDGER
TRUDGES
TUNDRAS
TVIDOLS
TWADDLE
TWIDDLE
TWODAYS
TWODEEP
TWODOOR
TYNDALL

T•••D••

TAPEDON
TAPEDUP
TEPIDLY
THANDIE
THEEDGE
THEIDEA
THEODOR
THIRDLY
THISDAY
THUDDED
THUNDER
TIENDAS
TIMIDER
TIMIDLY
TIRADES
TIREDER
TIREDLY
TIREDOF
TOLEDAN
TOLEDOS
TONEDUP
TONYDOW
TOORDER
TOWEDIN
TREADED
TREADER
TREADLE
TREADON
TRENDED
TRIADIC
TRIEDIT
TRIEDON
TRIEDTO
TRIODES
TRODDEN
TRUEDUP
TRUNDLE
TSARDOM
TUESDAY
TUNEDIN
TUNEDTO
TUNEDUP
TUXEDOS
TWADDLE
TWEEDLE
TWIDDLE
TYPEDIN
TYPEDUP

T••••D•

TABARDS
TAGENDS
TAXCODE
TEBALDI
TENCODE
TETRADS
TETRODE
THEBODY
THEFEDS
THEREDS
THREADS
THREADY
TIERODS
TINGODS
TOPBIDS
TOPSIDE
TORNADO
TOROIDS
TORPEDO
TOSTADA
TOWARDS
TRAGEDY
TRIPODS
TVGUIDE

T•••••D

TABLOID
TABOOED
TACKLED
TAILEND
TAINTED
TALCKED
TALLIED
TALONED
TANGLED
TANGOED
TANKARD
TAPERED
TARRIED
TASERED
TATTLED
TAUNTED
TAXPAID
TEEHEED
TEETHED

TELEXED
TEMPLED
TEMPTED
TENFOLD
TENONED
TENTBED
TENURED
TESTBED
THANKED
THEBAND
THEBARD
THEGOLD
THEHOOD
THEPOND
THEWIND
THIEVED
THINNED
THORNED
THREEAD
THRIVED
THUDDED
THUMBED
THUMPED
THUNKED
THYROID
TIARAED
TICKLED
TIEDYED
TIMREID
TINCTED
TINGLED
TINKLED
TIPPLED
TIPTOED
TOADIED
TOASTED
TOBEHAD
TODDLED
TOEHOLD
TOGGLED
TOKENED
TOMJOAD
TOOHARD
TOOTHED
TOOTLED
TOPPLED
TOPSEED
TORCHED
TORQUED
TORVALD
TOTALED
TOUCHED
TOUSLED
TOWELED
TOWERED
TOWHEAD
TOYLAND
TOYSLED
TRACKED
TRAILED
TRAINED
TRAMMED
TRAMPED
TRANCED
TRAPPED
TRASHED
TRAWLED
TREADED
TREATED
TREBLED
TREKKED
TRENDED
TRESSED
TRICKED
TRIFFID
TRIFLED
TRIFOLD
TRILLED
TRIMMED
TRIPLED
TRIPPED
TROLLED
TROMPED
TROOPED
TROTHED
TROTTED
TROUPED
TRUCKED
TRUDGED
TRUMPED
TRUSSED
TRUSTED
TRYHARD
TRYSTED
TSHAPED
TUMBLED
TURNBAD
TURNRED
TURTLED
TUSSAUD
TUSSLED
TUTORED
TWANGED
TWEAKED
TWEETED
TWEEZED
TWELVED
TWILLED
TWINBED
TWINGED
TWINNED
TWIRLED
TWISTED
TWITTED
TWOFOLD
TWOTOED
TYPHOID

•TD••••

ATDEUCE
FTDIXNJ
FTDODGE
STDENIS

•T•D•••

ATEDIRT
ITSDONE
MTADAMS
STADIUM
STADLER
STODGED
STODGES
STUDDED
STUDENT
STUDIED
STUDIER
STUDIES
STUDIOS

•T••D••

FTDODGE
STAIDER
STAIDLY
STANDBY
STANDEE
STANDER
STANDIN
STANDON
STANDTO
STANDUP
STARDOM
STAYDRY
STEADED
STEPDAD
STOODBY
STOODIN
STOODON
STOODTO
STOODUP
STRIDER
STRIDES
STRUDEL
STUDDED

•T•••D•

ATGRADE
ATTENDS
FTMEADE
MTBALDY
STRANDS
STUPIDS

•T••••D

ATANEND
ATMCARD
ATTHIRD
ATTIRED
ATTUNED
CTENOID
ETAILED
ETHMOID
ITSCOLD
STABBED
STABLED
STACKED
STAFFED
STAGGED
STAINED
STAIRED
STALKED
STALLED
STAMPED
STAPLED
STARRED
STARTED
STARVED
STASHED
STCLOUD
STEADED
STEAMED
STEELED
STEEPED
STEERED
STEEVED
STEMMED
STEPDAD
STEPPED
STEROID
STETTED
STEWARD
STIFFED
STIFLED
STILLED
STILTED
STINTED
STIPEND
STIRRED
STOCKED
STODGED
STOMPED
STOOGED
STOOLED
STOOPED
STOPPED
STORIED
STORMED
STRAFED
STRAYED
STREWED
STRIPED
STRIVED
STROKED
STUBBED
STUDDED
STUDIED
STUFFED
STUMPED
STUNNED
STUNTED
STYMIED
UTTERED

••TD•••

ALTDORF
ARTDECO
BATDAYS
CATDOOR
CUTDOWN
DOTDASH
EATDIRT
GETDONE
GETDOWN
GOTDONE
GOTDOWN
HOTDATE
HOTDAYS
HOTDOGS
JOTDOWN
LETDOWN
LETDROP
NOTDONE
OUTDARE
OUTDATE
OUTDOER
OUTDOES
OUTDONE
OUTDOOR
OUTDRAG
OUTDRAW
OUTDREW
OUTDROP
OUTDUEL
PATDOWN
PETDEER
PETDOGS
PETDOOR
PETDOVE
PETDUCK
PUTDOWN
RITDYES
SATDOWN
SETDOWN
SITDOWN
VATDYED
VATDYES
WETDOWN

••T•D••

ACTEDAS
ACTEDIN
ACTEDON
ACTEDUP
ANTEDUP
BETIDED
BETIDES
CITADEL
COTEDOR
DATEDLY
DOTEDON
ESTADOS
FATIDIC
FETIDLY
HATEDIT
KATYDID
MATADOR
MUTEDLY
NOTEDLY
OCTADIC
OPTEDIN
OPTEDTO
OUTADDS
OUTEDGE
PATSDRY
POTSDAM
RATEDPG
USTEDES
VOTEDIN
VOTEDNO
VOTEDON

••T••D•

ALTOIDS
ASTRIDE
ATTENDS
CATBEDS
CATHODE
DETRUDE
DOTARDS
ENTRADA
ESTRADA
EXTENDS
EXTRUDE
HATREDS
HOTBEDS
HOTRODS
INTENDS
INTRADE
INTRUDE
LETRIDE
MATILDA
METHODS
NITRIDE
NOTRADE
OBTRUDE
OBTUNDS
ONTHEDL
OUTADDS
OUTBIDS
OUTBUDS
OUTMODE
OUTRIDE
OUTRODE
OUTSIDE
PETARDS
POTLIDS
RETARDS
RETRADE
RITARDS
ROTUNDA
TETRADS
TETRODE
UPTRADE

••T•••D

ACTIFED
ALTERED
ANTACID
ANTBIRD
ASTOUND
ATTHIRD
ATTIRED
ATTUNED
BATCHED
BATIKED
BATTLED
BETIDED
BOTCHED
BOTTLED
BUTGOOD
CATBIRD
CATERED
CATEYED
CATFOOD
CATHEAD
DETOXED
DETUNED
DITCHED
DITTOED
ENTERED
ENTICED
ESTATED
FATHEAD
FETCHED
GETCOLD
GETGOOD
GETSMAD
GETSOLD
GETSRID
GETWORD
GOTCOLD
GOTGOOD
GOTOBED
GOTWORD
HATBAND
HATCHED
HITCHED
HOTHAND
HOTHEAD
HOTLEAD
IMTIRED
INTHIRD
INTONED
JETTIED
JUTLAND
KATYDID
LATCHED
LATENED
LETTERD
LITHOID
MATCHED
MATURED
METALED
METERED
MITERED
MITFORD
MOTIVED
MOTORED
MOTTLED
MUTATED
NATURED
NETTLED
NOTATED
NOTCHED
NOTEPAD
NOTGOOD
NOTICED
NOTUSED
NUTATED
NUTWOOD
OCTOPOD
OSTEOID
OSTWALD
OUTAWED
OUTBEND
OUTBRED
OUTCOLD
OUTFEED
OUTFIND
OUTLAID
OUTLAND
OUTLEAD
OUTLOUD
OUTPAID
OUTPLOD
OUTREAD
OUTSAID
OUTSOLD
OUTSPED
OUTTOLD
OUTVIED
OUTWARD
OUTWEED
OUTWIND
OUTWORD
PATCHED
PATHAND
PETALED
PETBIRD
PETERED
PITCHED
PITHEAD
PUTTIED
RATTLED
RETAMED
RETAPED
RETAXED
RETILED
RETIMED
RETIRED
RETONED
RETOWED
RETREAD
RETRIED
RETUNED
RETYPED
RITEAID
ROTATED
RUTLAND
SETTLED
SOTWEED
SUTURED
TATTLED
TOTALED
TUTORED
UNTAMED
UNTAPED
UNTAXED
UNTILED
UNTIMED
UNTIMID
UNTIRED
UNTONED
UNTREAD
UNTREED
UNTRIED
UNTUNED
UNTYPED
UPTREND
UTTERED
VATDYED
WATCHED
WATERED
WATFORD
WATTLED
WETEYED
WETLAND
WITCHED
WITSEND

•••TD••

ASSTDAS
FORTDIX
IFITDIE
LASTDON
LOSTDOG
MUSTDOS
NEXTDAY
PASTDUE
POSTDOC

•••T•D•

CUSTODY
EBBTIDE
FANTODS
FURTADO
HEPTADS
LEETIDE
LOWTIDE
MALTEDS
PENTADS
PEPTIDE
REDTIDE
RESTUDY
RIPTIDE
TOSTADA
WANTADS

•••T••D

ABETTED
ABUTTED
ALLTIED
ALLTOLD
BARTEND
BATTLED
BEETRED
BERTHED
BESTBUD
BIRTHED
BLATTED
BLITZED
BLOTTED
BOTTLED
BUSTARD
BUSTLED
CASTLED
CENTRED
CHATTED
CLOTHED
CLOTTED
CONTEND
COSTARD
CUSTARD
DARTLED
DASTARD
DELTOID
DENTOID
DIRTIED
DISTEND
DITTOED
DRATTED
DUETTED
EARTHED
EASTEND
EMITTED
EMPTIED
FACTOID
FELTBAD
FIFTYAD
FLATBED
FLATTED
FLITTED
FOOTLED
FOOTPAD
FORTORD
FORTYAD
FRETTED
FRITTED
FROTHED
GENTLED
GIRTHED
GLITZED
GLUTTED
GOATEED
GRITTED
HOGTIED
HURTLED
HUSTLED
INSTEAD
JETTIED
JOSTLED
KNITTED
KNOTTED
LACTAID
LEFTEND
LEOTARD
LETTERD
LOATHED
LOFTBED
LUSTRED
MAITRED
MANTLED
MASTOID
MISTOLD
MONTAND
MOTTLED
MOUTHED
MUSTARD
NESTLED
NETTLED
OMITTED
OROTUND
OUTTOLD
PARTIED
PESTLED
PHOTOID
PLATTED
PLOTTED
PLOTZED
PORTEND
PRETEND
PRETOLD
PUTTIED
QUITTED
RATTLED
ROOTLED
ROSTAND
RUSTLED
SAUTEED
SCATHED
SCATTED
SCYTHED
SEETHED
SETTLED
SIXTYAD
SLATTED
SLITTED
SLOTTED
SMITHED
SOOTHED
SORTIED
SPATTED
SPOTTED
STETTED
SUBTEND
SWATHED
SWATTED
TATTLED
TEETHED
TENTBED
TESTBED
TIPTOED
TOOTHED
TOOTLED
TROTHED
TROTTED
TURTLED
TWITTED
TWOTOED
UNITARD
UNSTAID
UPSTAND
UPSTOOD
VENTRAD
VISTAED
WALTZED
WATTLED
WEBTOED
WENTBAD
WENTMAD
WESTEND
WHETTED
WRITHED

••••T•D

AARATED
ABETTED
ABLATED
ABORTED
ABUTTED
ADAPTED
ADOPTED
AERATED
AGENTED
ALERTED
AMISTAD
AUDITED
AVERTED
AVIATED
AWAITED
BELATED
BENOTED
BERATED
BIGOTED
BLASTED
BLATTED
BLEATED
BLOATED
BLOTTED
BLUNTED
BLURTED
BOASTED
BOOSTED
BRUITED
CAROTID
CERATED
CHANTED
CHARTED
CHATTED
CHEATED
CHESTED
CLEATED
CLOTTED
CLOUTED
COACTED
COAPTED
COASTED
COOPTED
COUNTED
COURTED
COVETED
CRAFTED
CREATED
CRESTED
CRUSTED
CURATED
DAUNTED
DEBATED
DEBITED
DEBUTED
DELETED
DEMOTED
DENOTED
DEPUTED
DERATED
DEVOTED
DILATED
DILUTED
DONATED
DOUBTED
DRAFTED
DRATTED
DRIFTED
DUETTED
EDUCTED
EGESTED
EIGHTAD
EJECTED
ELECTED
EMITTED
ENACTED
EQUATED
ERECTED
ERUCTED
ERUPTED
ESTATED
EVERTED
EVICTED
EXACTED
EXALTED
EXCITED
EXERTED
EXISTED
EXULTED
FACETED
FAGOTED
FAINTED
FAULTED
FEASTED
FEINTED
FIXATED
FLATTED
FLEETED
FLIRTED
FLITTED
FLOATED
FLOUTED
FOISTED
FRETTED
FRITTED
FRONTED
FROSTED
FRUITED
GELATED
GHOSTED
GLINTED
GLOATED
GLUTTED
GRAFTED
GRANTED
GREETED
GRIFTED
GRITTED
GROUTED
GRUNTED
GUESTED
GYRATED
HABITED
HAUNTED
HEARTED
HEISTED
HOISTED
IDEATED
IGNITED
IMPUTED
INCITED
INDITED
INVITED
IODATED
ISLETED
JAUNTED
JOINTED
JOISTED
JOUSTED
KNITTED
KNOTTED
KNOUTED
LIGATED
LIGHTED
LIMITED
LOBATED
LOCATED
LUNATED
LUXATED
MERITED
MINOTND
MINUTED
MOULTED
MOUNTED
MULCTED
MUTATED
NEGATED
NOTATED
NUTATED
OERSTED
OLMSTED
OMITTED
ORBITED
PAINTED
PAROTID
PGRATED
PICOTED
PILOTED
PIRATED
PIVOTED
PLAITED
PLANTED
PLATTED
PLEATED
PLOTTED
POINTED
POSITED
PRINTAD
PRINTED
PUPATED
QUESTED
QUIETED
QUILTED
QUIRTED
QUITTED
QUOITED
REACTED
REBATED
RECITED
REDATED

REFUTED
RELATED
REMATED
RENOTED
REPUTED
RERATED
RESITED
REVOTED
RIGHTED
RIVETED
ROASTED
ROOSTED
ROTATED
ROUSTED
SAINTED
SALUTED
SCANTED
SCATTED
SCENTED
SCOOTED
SCOUTED
SEDATED
SHAFTED
SHEETED
SHIFTED
SHORTED
SHOUTED
SHUNTED
SIGHTED
SKIRTED
SLANTED
SLATTED
SLEETED
SLITTED
SLOTTED
SMARTED
SMELTED
SNOOTED
SNORTED
SNOUTED
SPATTED
SPORTED
SPOTTED
SPOUTED
SPURTED
STARTED
STETTED
STILTED
STINTED
STUNTED
SWATTED
SWEATED
TAINTED
TAUNTED
TEMPTED
TINCTED
TOASTED
TREATED
TROTTED
TRUSTED
TRYSTED
TWEETED
TWISTED
TWITTED
UNACTED
UNBATED
UNCITED
UNDATED
UNFATED
UNFETED
UNGATED
UNHATED
UNMATED
UNMUTED
UNNOTED
UNOPTED
UNRATED
UNSATED
UNVOTED
UPDATED
UPRATED
VACATED
VALETED
VAULTED
VAUNTED
VISITED
VOLUTED
WAISTED
WHETTED
WORSTED
WRESTED
YACHTED
YEASTED

•••••TD

DWIGHTD
FORDLTD
SILENTD

TE•••••

TEABAGS
TEABALL
TEACAKE
TEACART
TEACHER
TEACHES
TEACHIN
TEACOZY
TEACUPS
TEAGOWN
TEALEAF
TEALESS
TEAMING
TEAMSUP
TEAMUSA
TEANECK
TEAPOTS
TEAPOYS
TEARERS
TEARFUL
TEARGAS
TEARIER
TEARILY
TEARING
TEAROFF
TEAROOM
TEAROSE
TEAROUT
TEARSAT
TEARSIT
TEARSUP
TEASELS
TEASERS
TEASETS
TEASEUP
TEASHOP
TEASING
TEATIME
TEATRAY
TEATREE
TEATROS
TEAURNS
TEBALDI
TECHIES
TECHNOS
TEDDIES
TEDEUMS
TEDIOUS
TEDIUMS
TEDMACK
TEEDOFF
TEEHEED
TEEHEES
TEEITUP
TEEMING
TEENAGE
TEENERS
TEENIER
TEENSIE
TEEOFFS
TEEPEES
TEESHOT
TEESOFF
TEETERS
TEETHED
TEETHER
TEETHES
TEETIME
TEEVEES
TEFLONS
TEHERAN
TEICHER
TEJANAS
TEJANOS
TEKKIES
TELAVIV
TELECOM
TELEFAX
TELEPIC
TELEPIX
TELERAN
TELESTO
TELEXED
TELEXES
TELLALL
TELLERS
TELLIES
TELLING
TELLOFF
TELLSIT
TELLSOF
TELLSON
TELSTAR
TEMBLOR
TEMPEAZ
TEMPEHS
TEMPERA
TEMPERS
TEMPEST
TEMPING
TEMPJOB
TEMPLAR
TEMPLED
TEMPLES
TEMPORE
TEMPTED
TEMPTER
TEMPURA
TENABLE
TENABLY
TENACES
TENACRE
TENANCY
TENANTS
TENBALL
TENCENT
TENCHES
TENCODE
TENDAYS
TENDERS
TENDING
TENDONS
TENDRIL
TENDSTO
TENEEEE
TENFEET
TENFOLD
TENFOOT
TENFOUR
TENKRUN
TENMILE
TENNANT
TENNECO
TENNERS
TENNIEL
TENNIES
TENONED
TENONER
TENPAST
TENPINS
TENSELY
TENSEST
TENSEUP
TENSILE
TENSING
TENSION
TENSITY
TENSIVE
TENSORS
TENSPOT
TENTBED
TENTERS
TENTFUL
TENTHLY
TENTING
TENTONS
TENTPEG
TENUITY
TENUOUS
TENURED
TENURES
TENWEEK
TENYEAR
TENZING
TEPIDLY
TEQUILA
TERAOHM
TERBIUM
TERCELS
TERENCE
TERHUNE
TERMING
TERMINI
TERMITE
TERNARY
TERNATE
TERRACE
TERRAIN
TERRANS
TERRELL
TERRENE
TERRETS
TERRIER
TERRIES
TERRIFY
TERRINE
TERROIR
TERRORS
TERSELY
TERSEST
TESSERA
TESTACY
TESTATE
TESTBAN
TESTBED
TESTEES
TESTERS
TESTFLY
TESTFOR
TESTIER
TESTIFY
TESTILY
TESTING
TESTKIT
TESTLAB
TESTOUT
TESTRUN
TETANUS
TETHERS
TETRADS
TETRODE
TEUTONS
TEXTILE
TEXTING
TEXTRON
TEXTUAL
TEXTURE

T•E••••

TEEDOFF
TEEHEED
TEEHEES
TEEITUP
TEEMING
TEENAGE
TEENERS
TEENIER
TEENSIE
TEEOFFS
TEEPEES
TEESHOT
TEESOFF
TEETERS
TEETHED
TEETHER
TEETHES
TEETIME
TEEVEES
THEABCS
THEAGES
THEALPS
THEARMY
THEARTS
THEATER
THEATRE
THEAXIS
THEBABE
THEBABY
THEBAND
THEBANS
THEBARD
THEBEAR
THEBELL
THEBEST
THEBIGA
THEBLOB
THEBOBO
THEBODY
THEBOMB
THEBOSS
THEBOYS
THEBRAT
THEBUSH
THECAPE
THECARS
THECAVS
THECITY
THECRAB
THECROW
THECUBS
THEDEEP
THEDELL
THEDIET
THEDOLE
THEDUKE
THEEAST
THEEDGE
THEFALL
THEFEDS
THEFIRM
THEFIVE
THEFLEA
THEFLOP
THEFONZ
THEFOOL
THEFRUG
THEGAME
THEGANG
THEGIFT
THEGOLD
THEHEAT
THEHELP
THEHERO
THEHILL
THEHOGS
THEHOOD
THEHOPE
THEHULK
THEIDEA
THEISMS
THEISTS
THEJERK
THEJETS
THEKING
THEKISS
THELAMB
THELARK
THELEFT
THELIKE
THELOOK
THELOOP
THEMAGI
THEMALL
THEMASK
THEMAVS
THEMAYO
THEMETS
THEMICK
THEMOON
THEMOST
THENETS
THENEWS
THENILE
THEOATH
THEODOR
THEOMEN
THEOMNI
THEOREM
THEPIPS
THEPITS
THEPOND
THEPOOH
THEPOPE
THEPOST
THEPUMP
THERAMS
THERAPY
THEREAT
THEREBY
THEREDS
THEREIN
THERENT
THEREOF
THEREON
THERESA
THERETO
THERIAC
THERING
THERINK
THERITZ
THERMAL
THERMIC
THERMOS
THEROBE
THEROCK
THEROOM
THEROPE
THEROSE
THEROUX
THERULE
THESACK
THESAME
THESELF
THESEUS
THESHOW
THESIMS
THESPIS
THESTAR
THESUNS
THESWAN
THETOUR
THETREE
THETRIB
THETUBE
THETURN
THEUSSR
THEVIEW
THEVIPS
THEWALL
THEWAVE
THEWIND
THEYIPS
THEYSAY
TIEBACK
TIEBARS
TIEBEAM
TIECLIP
TIEDOFF
TIEDOWN
TIEDYED
TIEDYES
TIEGAME
TIEINTO
TIELESS
TIELINE
TIEMPOS
TIENDAS
TIEPINS
TIEPOLO
TIERACK
TIERCES
TIERING
TIERNEY
TIERODS
TIEROPE
TIESOFF
TIETACK
TIETACS
TOECAPS
TOEHOLD
TOELESS
TOELIKE
TOELOOP
TOENAIL
TOEPICK
TOESHOE
TOETAPS
TREACLE
TREACLY
TREADED
TREADER
TREADLE
TREADON
TREASON
TREATED
TREATER
TREBLED
TREBLES
TREDIAS
TREEING
TREELET
TREERAT
TREESAP
TREETOP
TREFOIL
TREINTA
TREIZES
TREKKED
TREKKER
TREKKIE
TRELLIS
TREMBLE
TREMBLY
TREMOLO
TREMORS
TRENARY
TRENDED
TRENTON
TREPANS
TRESSED
TRESSES
TRESTLE
TREVINO
TSELIOT
TSETSES
TSETUNG
TUESDAY
TWEAKED
TWEEDLE
TWEENER
TWEETED
TWEETER
TWEEZED
TWEEZER
TWEEZES
TWELFTH
TWELVEA
TWELVEB
TWELVEC
TWELVED
TWELVEE
TWELVES
TWERENT

T••E•••

TAGENDS
TAKEAIM
TAKEFOR
TAKEILL
TAKEINS
TAKENBY
TAKENIN
TAKENON
TAKENTO
TAKENUP
TAKEOFF
TAKEONE
TAKEOUT
TAKESIN
TAKESIT
TAKESON
TAKESTO
TAKESUP
TAKETEA
TAKETEN
TALENTS
TAPEDON
TAPEDUP
TAPEMAN
TAPEMEN
TAPERED
TAPESON
TAPESUP
TASERED
TAVERNA
TAVERNS
TEDEUMS
TEHERAN
TELECOM
TELEFAX
TELEPIC
TELEPIX
TELERAN
TELESTO
TELEXED
TELEXES
TENEEEE
TERENCE
THEEAST
THEEDGE
THIERRY
THIEVED
THIEVES
THREADS
THREADY
THREATS
THREEAD
THREEAM
THREEBC
THREEEE
THREENO
THREEPM
THREERS
THREEUP
THREWAT
THREWIN
THREWON
THREWUP
TIBETAN
TIDERIP
TIMECOP
TIMELAG
TIMEOFF
TIMEOUT
TIMESUP
TIMEWAS
TIMEXES
TINEARS
TIREDER
TIREDLY
TIREDOF
TIREMAN
TIREMEN
TIREOUT
TIRESOF
TOBEHAD
TOCELIA
TOHEART
TOHELEN
TOKENED
TOLEASE
TOLEDAN
TOLEDOS
TONEARM
TONEDUP
TONELOC
TONEMES
TONEROW
TONESUP
TONETTE
TOOEASY
TOPEKAN
TOREOFF
TOREOUT
TOREROS
TOTEBAG
TOTEMIC
TOTESUP
TOWEDIN
TOWELED
TOWERED
TREEING
TREELET
TREERAT
TREESAP
TREETOP
TRIEDIT
TRIEDON
TRIEDTO
TRIESIT
TRIESON
TRIESTE
TRIESTO
TRUEDUP
TRUEING
TRUERIB
TRUERTO
TRUESUP
TUBEPAN
TUBETOP
TUMESCE
TUNEDIN
TUNEDTO
TUNEDUP
TUNEFUL
TUNEOUT
TUNESIN
TUNESTO
TUNESUP
TUNEUPS
TUPELOS
TUREENS
TUTELAR
TUXEDOS
TWEEDLE
TWEENER
TWEETED
TWEETER
TWEEZED
TWEEZER
TWEEZES
TWOEEEE
TWOEGGS
TYLENOL
TYPEABS
TYPEDIN
TYPEDUP
TYPESET
TYPESIN
TYPESUP

T•••E••

TABKEYS
TABLEAU
TABLETS
TABSETS
TACKERS
TAFFETA
TAGGERS
TAGTEAM
TAILEND
TAILERS
TALKERS
TALLEST
TAMPERS
TANDEMS
TANGELO
TANGENT
TANKERS
TANNERS
TANNERY
TANNEST
TAPPERS
TAPPETS
TARBELL
TARGETS
TARHEEL
TARTEST
TASSELS
TASTEIT
TASTERS
TATTERS
TATTERY
TAUREAN
TAUTENS
TAUTEST
TAXLESS
TAXLEVY
TAXYEAR
TEALEAF
TEALESS
TEANECK
TEARERS
TEASELS
TEASERS
TEASETS
TEASEUP
TEEHEED
TEEHEES
TEENERS
TEEPEES
TEETERS
TEEVEES
TELLERS
TEMPEAZ
TEMPEHS
TEMPERA
TEMPERS
TEMPEST
TENCENT
TENDERS
TENEEEE
TENFEET
TENNECO
TENNERS
TENSELY
TENSEST
TENSEUP
TENTERS
TENWEEK
TENYEAR
TERCELS
TERRELL
TERRENE
TERRETS
TERSELY
TERSEST
TESSERA
TESTEES
TESTERS
TETHERS
THALERS
THAWERS
THEBEAR
THEBELL
THEBEST
THEDEEP
THEDELL
THEFEDS
THEHEAT
THEHELP
THEHERO
THEJERK
THEJETS
THELEFT
THEMETS
THENETS
THENEWS
THEREAT
THEREBY
THEREDS
THEREIN
THERENT
THEREOF
THEREON
THERESA
THERETO
THESELF
THESEUS
THOREAU
THREEAD
THREEAM
THREEBC
THREEEE
THREENO
THREEPM
THREERS
THREEUP
THYSELF
TIBBETT
TICKERS
TICKETS
TIDIEST
TIEBEAM
TIELESS
TIGRESS
TILLERS
TILLETS
TILTERS
TIMBERS
TIMBERY
TIMREID
TINDERS
TINDERY
TINIEST
TINKERS
TINNERS
TINSELS
TINTERN
TINTERS
TIPLESS
TIPPEES
TIPPERS
TIPPETS
TITHERS
TITTERS
TOELESS
TOFFEES
TOGGERY
TOILERS
TOILETS
TOLLERS
TOLTECS
TOLUENE

TONIEST
TONNEAU
TOOLERS
TOOTERS
TOPLESS
TOPPERS
TOPSEED
TOPTENS
TORMENT
TORPEDO
TORREFY
TORRENT
TOSSERS
TOTTERS
TOTTERY
TOUPEES
TOURERS
TOUTERS
TOWHEAD
TOWHEES
TOWNERS
TOYLESS
TRABERT
TRACERS
TRACERY
TRADEIN
TRADEON
TRADERS
TRADEUP
TRAGEDY
TRAPEZE
TRAVELS
TRAVERS
TRIBECA
TRICEPS
TRIDENT
TRIJETS
TRIREME
TRISECT
TRITELY
TRITEST
TRIVETS
TROWELS
TRUDEAU
TUCKERS
TUFFETS
TUGGERS
TUGLESS
TUNNELS
TUREENS
TURKEYS
TURNERS
TURNERY
TURRETS
TUSHERY
TUSKERS
TVCREWS
TWERENT
TWINERS
TWODEEP
TWOEEEE
TWOFEET
TWOFERS
TWOTERM
TWOWEEK
TWOYEAR

T••••E•

TABARET
TABBIES
TABOOED
TABORET
TACKIER
TACKLED
TACKLER
TACKLES
TAFFIES
TAGAMET
TAINTED
TAKETEA
TAKETEN
TALCKED
TALKIER
TALKIES
TALLIED
TALLIER
TALLIES
TALONED
TALUSES
TAMALES
TAMGLEN
TANAGER
TANGIER
TANGLED
TANGLER
TANGLES
TANGOED
TANGOER
TANSIES
TAPEMEN
TAPERED
TAPSTER
TARDIER
TARHEEL
TARRIED
TARRIER
TARRIES
TARTIER
TARTLET
TASERED
TASTIER
TATTIER
TATTLED
TATTLER
TATTLES
TAUNTED
TAUNTER
TAWNIER
TAXFREE
TAXIMEN
TEACHER
TEACHES
TEARIER
TEATREE
TECHIES
TEDDIES
TEEHEED
TEEHEES
TEENIER
TEEPEES
TEETHED
TEETHER
TEETHES
TEEVEES
TEICHER
TEKKIES
TELEXED
TELEXES
TELLIES
TEMPLED
TEMPLES
TEMPTED
TEMPTER
TENACES
TENCHES
TENEEEE
TENFEET
TENNIEL
TENNIES
TENONED
TENONER
TENTBED
TENTPEG
TENURED
TENURES
TENWEEK
TERRIER
TERRIES
TESTBED
TESTEES
TESTIER
THANKED
THANKER
THEAGES
THEATER
THEDEEP
THEDIET
THEFLEA
THEIDEA
THEOMEN
THEOREM
THETREE
THEVIEW
THICKEN
THICKER
THICKET
THIEVED
THIEVES
THIGPEN
THINKER
THINNED
THINNER
THITHER
THORNED
THREEEE
THRIVED
THRIVEN
THRIVER
THRIVES
THRONES
THROWER
THUDDED
THUMBED
THUMPED
THUMPER
THUNDER
THUNKED
THURBER
TIARAED
TICKLED
TICKLER
TICKLES
TIEDYED
TIEDYES
TIERCES
TIERNEY
TIGHTEN
TIGHTER
TIMBRES
TIMEXES
TIMIDER
TINAFEY
TINCTED
TINGLED
TINGLER
TINGLES
TINKLED
TINKLER
TINKLES
TINNIER
TINORES
TIPOVER
TIPPEES
TIPPIER
TIPPLED
TIPPLER
TIPPLES
TIPSIER
TIPSTER
TIPTOED
TIPTOES
TIRADES
TIREDER
TIREMEN
TISANES
TISSUES
TISSUEY
TITTLES
TIZZIES
TOADIED
TOADIES
TOASTED
TOASTEE
TOASTER
TODDIES
TODDLED
TODDLER
TODDLES
TOFFEES
TOFFLER
TOGGLED
TOGGLER
TOGGLES
TOHELEN
TOHOMER
TOKENED
TOLKIEN
TOLLMEN
TONEMES
TONGUES
TONUSES
TOODLES
TOOKTEN
TOOLSET
TOONIES
TOORDER
TOOTHED
TOOTLED
TOOTLER
TOOTLES
TOPAZES
TOPPLED
TOPPLES
TOPSEED
TORCHED
TORCHER
TORCHES
TORQUED
TORQUES
TOTALED
TOTALER
TOUAREG
TOUCHED
TOUCHER
TOUCHES
TOUGHEN
TOUGHER
TOUPEES
TOURNEY
TOUSLED
TOUSLES
TOWAGES
TOWELED
TOWERED
TOWHEES
TOWNIES
TOWNLET
TOYNBEE
TOYSLED
TRACHEA
TRACKED
TRACKER
TRAILED
TRAILER
TRAINED
TRAINEE
TRAINER
TRAMMED
TRAMMEL
TRAMPED
TRAMPER
TRANCED
TRANCES
TRAPPED
TRAPPER
TRASHED
TRASHER
TRASHES
TRAUBEL
TRAWLED
TRAWLER
TREADED
TREADER
TREATED
TREATER
TREBLED
TREBLES
TREELET
TREIZES
TREKKED
TREKKER
TRENDED
TRESSED
TRESSES
TRIAGES
TRICKED
TRICKER
TRIFLED
TRIFLER
TRIFLES
TRIGGER
TRILLED
TRILLER
TRIMMED
TRIMMER
TRINKET
TRIODES
TRIOLET
TRIPLEA
TRIPLED
TRIPLES
TRIPLET
TRIPLEX
TRIPPED
TRIPPER
TRIPPET
TROCHEE
TROCHES
TRODDEN
TROLLED
TROLLER
TROLLEY
TROMPED
TROOPED
TROOPER
TROTHED
TROTTED
TROTTER
TROUPED
TROUPER
TROUPES
TROUSER
TRUCKED
TRUCKEE
TRUCKER
TRUDGED
TRUDGEN
TRUDGER
TRUDGES
TRUMPED
TRUMPET
TRUSSED
TRUSSES
TRUSTED
TRUSTEE
TRUSTER
TRYSTED
TRYSTER
TSETSES
TSHAPED
TSHAPES
TUBBIER
TUBULES
TUFTIER
TUILLES
TULANEU
TUMBLED
TUMBLER
TUMBLES
TUMBREL
TUMMIES
TUMMLER
TUPOLEV
TURFIER
TURFMEN
TURNKEY
TURNRED
TURTLED
TURTLES
TUSHIES
TUSSLED
TUSSLES
TUTORED
TVGAMES
TVTAPES
TWANGED
TWANGER
TWEAKED
TWEENER
TWEETED
TWEETER
TWEEZED
TWEEZER
TWEEZES
TWELVEA
TWELVEB
TWELVEC
TWELVED
TWELVEE
TWELVES
TWILLED
TWINBED
TWINGED
TWINGES
TWINIER
TWINJET
TWINNED
TWINSET
TWIRLED
TWIRLER
TWISTED
TWISTER
TWITTED
TWITTER
TWODEEP
TWOEEEE
TWOFEET
TWOSTEP
TWOTOED
TWOWEEK
TYPESET
TZIMMES

T•••••E

TACTILE
TADPOLE
TAGLIKE
TAGLINE
TAGSALE
TAKABLE
TAKEONE
TALLONE
TAMABLE
TANKAGE
TANLINE
TAPSHOE
TARTARE
TAURINE
TAXABLE
TAXBASE
TAXCODE
TAXFREE
TAXHIKE
TAXRATE
TAXSALE
TEACAKE
TEAROSE
TEATIME
TEATREE
TEENAGE
TEENSIE
TEETIME
TEMPORE
TENABLE
TENACRE
TENCODE
TENEEEE
TENMILE
TENSILE
TENSIVE
TERENCE
TERHUNE
TERMITE
TERNATE
TERRACE
TERRENE
TERRINE
TESTATE
TETRODE
TEXTILE
TEXTURE
THANDIE
THATONE
THEATRE
THEBABE
THECAPE
THEDOLE
THEDUKE
THEEDGE
THEFIVE
THEGAME
THEHOPE
THELIKE
THENILE
THEPOPE
THEROBE
THEROPE
THEROSE
THERULE
THESAME
THETREE
THETUBE
THEWAVE
THIMBLE
THINICE
THISONE
THISTLE
THREEEE
THWHITE
THYMINE
TIEGAME
TIELINE
TIEROPE
TILLAGE
TIMBALE
TIMRICE
TINLIKE
TINMINE
TINTYPE
TINWARE
TIPLINE
TITANAE
TITMICE
TITRATE
TMOBILE
TOASTEE
TOBLAME
TOELIKE
TOESHOE
TOHORSE
TOLEASE
TOLLAGE
TOLUENE
TOMKITE
TONETTE
TONNAGE
TONSURE
TONTINE
TOOLATE
TOOTSIE
TOPFIVE
TOPHOLE
TOPLINE
TOPNAME
TOPRATE
TOPSIDE
TORTURE
TOSCALE
TOSPARE
TOTABLE
TOTASTE
TOUGHIE
TOWABLE
TOWLINE
TOWROPE
TOYBIKE
TOYKITE
TOYLIKE
TOYNBEE
TRADUCE
TRAINEE
TRAIPSE
TRAMPLE
TRAPEZE
TREACLE
TREADLE
TREKKIE
TREMBLE
TRESTLE
TRIABLE
TRIBBLE
TRIBUNE
TRIBUTE
TRICKLE
TRIESTE
TRIREME
TRITONE
TROCHEE
TROUBLE
TROUNCE
TRUCKEE
TRUCKLE
TRUFFLE
TRUNDLE
TRUSTEE
TRUSTME
TSQUARE
TUBLIKE
TUMESCE
TUNABLE
TUNICLE
TURBINE
TURFTOE
TUSSIVE
TVGUIDE
TVMOVIE
TVTABLE
TWADDLE
TWEEDLE
TWELVEE
TWIDDLE
TWINKIE
TWINKLE
TWOACRE
TWOBASE
TWOEEEE
TWOFACE
TWOLANE
TWOMORE
TWOONIE
TWOSOME
TWOTIME
TWOTONE

•TE••••

ATEABIT
ATEALOT
ATEAWAY
ATECROW
ATEDIRT
ATEIGHT
ATEINTO
ATEITUP
ATELATE
ATELESS
ATELIER
ATEMORE
ATEOVER
CTENOID
ETERNAL
ETESIAN
ITEMING
ITEMISE
ITEMIZE
ITEMONE
ITERANT
ITERATE
MTEVANS
PTEROUS
STEADED
STEALER
STEALIN
STEALTH
STEAMED
STEAMER
STEAMUP
STEANNE
STEARIC
STEARIN
STEARNS
STEELED
STEELER
STEELIE
STEEPED
STEEPEN
STEEPER
STEEPIN
STEEPLE
STEEPLY
STEERED
STEERER
STEEVED
STEEVES
STEFANI
STEIGER
STEINEM
STEINER
STELIAS
STELLAR
STEMMED
STEMPEL
STENCIL
STENGEL
STENGUN
STENNIS
STENTOR
STEPDAD
STEPHEN
STEPINS
STEPMOM
STEPOFF
STEPONE
STEPOUT
STEPPED
STEPPER
STEPPES
STEPSIN
STEPSON
STEPSUP
STEPTWO
STEPUPS
STEREOS
STERILE
STERNAL
STERNER
STERNLY
STERNOS
STERNUM
STEROID
STEROLS
STERTOR
STETSON
STETTED
STEUBEN
STEVENS
STEWARD
STEWART
STEWERS
STEWIER
STEWING
STEWPAN
STEWPOT
UTENSIL
XTERRAS

•T•E•••

ATDEUCE
ATHEART
ATHEISM
ATHEIST
ATLEAST
ATPEACE
ATSEVEN
ATTEMPT
ATTENDS
ATTESTS
BTWELVE
ETHENES
ETHERIC
ETIENNE
FTHENRY
FTMEADE
ITSEASY
ITWELVE
ITWENTY
MTKENYA
MTPELEE
OTHELLO
STDENIS
STEELED
STEELER
STEELIE
STEEPED
STEEPEN
STEEPER
STEEPIN
STEEPLE
STEEPLY
STEERED
STEERER
STEEVED
STEEVES
STPETER
STREAKS
STREAKY
STREAMS
STREETS
STREGIS
STRETCH
STRETTI
STRETTO
STREWED
STREWER
UTRECHT
UTTERED
UTTERER
UTTERLY

•T••E••

ATANEND
ATELESS
ATHLETE
ATMFEES
ATONERS
ETAGERE
ETCHERS
FTMYERS
ITSBEST
ITSHERE
PTOLEMY
STAGERS
STALELY
STALEST
STAMENS
STAREAT
STARERS
STATELY
STATERS
STAYERS
STEREOS
STEVENS
STEWERS
STIPEND
STOKELY
STOKERS
STOKEUP
STOLEIN
STONEAX
STONERS
STORERS
STOREUP
STOWERS
STREETS
STUDENT
STUPEFY
STYLERS
STYLETS
STYRENE

•T•••E•

ATELIER
ATEOVER
ATHOMES
ATLASES
ATMFEES
ATOMIES
ATONIES
ATSEVEN
ATTHREE
ATTIMES
ATTIRED
ATTIRER
ATTIRES
ATTUNED
ATTUNES
ATTYGEN
ATWATER
ETAILED
ETAILER
ETHANES
ETHENES
ETICKET
ETOILES
FTRILEY
ITCHIER
ITSOPEN
ITSOVER
JTMONEY
MTPELEE
NTUPLES
OTARIES
STABBED
STABBER
STABLED
STABLER
STABLES
STACKED
STACKER
STADLER
STAFFED
STAFFER
STAGGED
STAGGER
STAGIER
STAGNES
STAIDER
STAINED
STAINER
STAIRED
STALKED
STALKER
STALLED
STALLER

STAMMER
STAMPED
STAMPER
STANCES
STANDEE
STANDER
STANLEE
STANLEY
STAPLED
STAPLER
STAPLES
STARKER
STARKEY
STARLET
STARRED
STARTED
STARTER
STARVED
STARVES
STASHED
STASHES
STASSEN
STATLER
STATUES
STEADED
STEALER
STEAMED
STEAMER
STEELED
STEELER
STEEPED
STEEPEN
STEEPER
STEERED
STEERER
STEEVED
STEEVES
STEIGER
STEINEM
STEINER
STEMMED
STEMPEL
STENGEL
STEPHEN
STEPPED
STEPPER
STEPPES
STERNER
STETTED
STEUBEN
STEWIER
STICKER
STIFFED
STIFFEL
STIFFEN
STIFFER
STIFLED
STIFLES
STILLED
STILLER
STILTED
STINGER
STINKER
STINTED
STINTER
STIRRED
STIRRER
STJAMES
STLUKES
STOCKED
STOCKER
STODGED
STODGES
STOGIES
STOLLEN
STOMPED
STONIER
STOOGED
STOOGES
STOOKEY
STOOLED
STOOPED
STOOPER
STOPPED
STOPPER
STORIED
STORIES
STORMED
STOUTEN
STOUTER
STPETER
STRAFED
STRAFER
STRAFES
STRAYED
STRAYER
STREWED
STREWER
STRIDER
STRIDES
STRIFES
STRIKER
STRIKES
STRIPED
STRIPER
STRIPES
STRIVED
STRIVEN
STRIVER
STRIVES
STROBES
STROKED
STROKER
STROKES
STRUDEL
STUBBED
STUDDED
STUDIED
STUDIER
STUDIES
STUFFED
STUFFER
STUMPED
STUMPER
STUNNED
STUNNER
STUNTED
STURGES
STUTTER
STUTZES
STYMIED
STYMIES
UTTERED
UTTERER

•T••••E

ATATIME
ATDEUCE
ATELATE
ATEMORE
ATGRADE
ATHLETE
ATINGLE
ATIPTOE
ATISSUE
ATLARGE
ATOMISE
ATOMIZE
ATPEACE
ATSTAKE
ATTACHE
ATTHREE
ATTRITE
BTWELVE
ETAGERE
ETAMINE
ETIENNE
FTDODGE
FTMEADE
FTWAYNE
ITEMISE
ITEMIZE
ITEMONE
ITERATE
ITMAYBE
ITSALIE
ITSATIE
ITSDONE
ITSFINE
ITSGONE
ITSHERE
ITSLATE
ITSLOVE
ITSONME
ITSTIME
ITSTRUE
ITWELVE
MTPELEE
STABILE
STANDEE
STANINE
STANLEE
STARTLE
STATICE
STATURE
STATUTE
STEANNE
STEELIE
STEEPLE
STEPONE
STERILE
STIPPLE
STOOLIE
STOPPLE
STORAGE
STOWAGE
STRANGE
STRASSE
STRIATE
STROPHE
STROUSE
STUBBLE
STUMBLE
STYLISE
STYLIZE
STYRENE
UTILISE
UTILIZE

••TE•••

ACTEDAS
ACTEDIN
ACTEDON
ACTEDUP
ALTERED
ALTERER
ANTEDUP
ANTEING
ANTENNA
ANTERUS
ANTESUP
APTERAL
APTERYX
ARTEMIS
ARTEMUS
ARTERIO
ASTERIX
ATTEMPT
ATTENDS
ATTESTS
AUTEURS
AZTECAN
BATEAUX
BATEMAN
BITEOFF
BITESIN
BITESON
BITESUP
BUTENES
CATENAE
CATENAS
CATERAS
CATERED
CATERER
CATERTO
CATEYED
CETERIS
COTEACH
COTEDOR
COTERIE
DATEDLY
DETECTO
DETECTS
DETENTE
DETENTS
DETERGE
DETESTS
DOTEDON
DOTESON
DRTEETH
DUTEOUS
EATENAT
EATENUP
ENTEBBE
ENTENTE
ENTERED
ENTERER
ENTERIC
ENTERIN
ENTERON
ERTEGUN
ESTEBAN
ESTEEMS
ESTEFAN
ESTELLA
ESTELLE
ESTEVEZ
EUTERPE
EXTENDS
EXTENSO
EXTENTS
EXTERNE
EXTERNS
FATEFUL
GATEAUX
GATELEG
GATEMAN
GATEMEN
GATEWAY
GETEVEN
GOTEVEN
HATEDIT
HATEFUL
HATESIT
ICTERUS
INTEARS
INTEGER
INTEGRA
INTENDS
INTENSE
INTENTS
INTERIM
INTERNE
INTERNS
INTERSE
IQTESTS
LATEENS
LATEFEE
LATENCY
LATENED
LATENTS
LATERAL
LATERAN
LATERON
LATETAG
LATEXES
LETEMIN
LITERAL
LUTETIA
MATEWAN
METEORS
METEOUT
METERED
MITERED
MUTEDLY
NOTEASY
NOTEDLY
NOTEPAD
NOTEVEN
NOTEVER
OBTESTS
OCTETTE
OFTENER
OPTEDIN
OPTEDTO
ORTEGAL
OSTEOID
OUTEARN
OUTEATS
OUTECHO
OUTEDGE
PATELLA
PATENCY
PATENTS
PATERNO
PETEMAN
PETEMEN
PETERED
PETERII
PITEOUS
POTEENS
POTENCE
POTENCY
PUTEMUP
RATECAP
RATEDPG
RETEACH
RETEARS
RETELLS
RETESTS
RITEAID
ROTELLE
SATEENS
SETENTA
SHTETLS
SITEMAP
TOTEBAG
TOTEMIC
TOTESUP
TUTELAR
UNTEACH
UNTENSE
UNTERSE
UPTEARS
UPTEMPO
URTEXTS
USTEDES
UTTERED
UTTERER
UTTERLY
VETERAN
VITEBSK
VOTEAYE
VOTECHS
VOTEDIN
VOTEDNO
VOTEDON
VOTEFOR
VOTENAY
VOTEOUT
VOTESIN
VOTESNO
VOTESON
VOTEYEA
VOTEYES
WATERED
WATERER
WETEYED
WITEOUT
YOTEAMO

••T•E••

ACTAEON
ACTRESS
ALTKEYS
ANTBEAR
ANTHEIL
ANTHEMS
ANTHERS
ANTLERS
ANTWERP
APTNESS
ARTDECO
ARTFERN
ARTIEST
ARTLESS
ASTREAM
BATHERS
BATNEXT
BATTENS
BATTERS
BATTERY
BETHELS
BETHERE
BETTERS
BETWEEN
BITLESS
BITTERN
BITTERS
BOTHERS
BOTREES
BOTTEGA
BUTLERS
BUTTEMT
BUTTERS
BUTTERY
BYTHEBY
CATBEDS
CATBERT
CATFEET
CATHEAD
CATSEYE
COTTERS
CUTLERS
CUTLERY
CUTLETS
CUTTERS
DITHERS
DITHERY
DOTTERS
DRTEETH
EATHERE
EATLESS
ENTREAT
ENTREES
ESTEEMS
ESTHETE
EXTREME
FATCELL
FATHEAD
FATHERS
FATLESS
FATNESS
FATTENS
FATTEST
FETTERS
FITNESS
FITTERS
FITTEST
FITWELL
GATHERS
GETBEAT
GETBENT
GETHELP
GETREAL
GETTERS
GETWELL
GOTBEAT
GOTHELP
GOTREAL
GOTWELL
GUTLESS
GUTTERS
HATLESS
HATREDS
HATTERS
HITHERE
HITLESS
HITTERS
HOTBEDS
HOTHEAD
HOTKEYS
HOTLEAD
HOTMEAL
HOTNESS
HOTSEAT
HOTTEAS
HOTTEST
IDTHEFT
IMTHERE
INTHERE
JETSETS
JITNEYS
JITTERS
JITTERY
JOTTERS
KITTENS
KITTERY
LATEENS
LATHERS
LATHERY
LATRELL
LETHEAN
LETMEBE
LETMEGO
LETMEIN
LETSEAT
LETTERA
LETTERB
LETTERC
LETTERD
LETTERE
LETTERF
LETTERG
LETTERH
LETTERI
LETTERJ
LETTERK
LETTERL
LETTERM
LETTERN
LETTERO
LETTERP
LETTERQ
LETTERR
LETTERS
LETTERT
LETTERU
LETTERV
LETTERW
LETTERX
LETTERY
LETTERZ
LITHELY
LITHEST
LITTERS
LITTERY
LOTTERS
LOTTERY
MATHERS
MATHEWS
MATLESS
MATTERS
METIERS
MITTENS
MOTHERS
MOTHERY
MOTLEYS
MUTTERS
MYTREAT
NATTERS
NETLESS
NETTERS
NETZERO
NOTBEEN
NOTHERE
NOTNEAR
NOTREAL
NOTWELL
NUTLETS
NUTMEAT
NUTMEGS
NUTTERS
OATMEAL
ONTHEDL
ONTHEGO
ONTHEQT
ONTKEAN
OSTLERS
OUTBEAM
OUTBEGS
OUTBEND
OUTFEED
OUTFEEL
OUTHEAR
OUTHERE
OUTJEST
OUTJETS
OUTKEEP
OUTKEPT
OUTLEAD
OUTLEAP
OUTLETS
OUTPEEP
OUTREAD
OUTSEEK
OUTSEEN
OUTSEES
OUTSELL
OUTSERT
OUTSETS
OUTTEAR
OUTTELL
OUTWEAR
OUTWEED
OUTWEEP
OUTWELL
OUTWENT
OUTWEPT
OUTWEST
OUTYELL
OUTYELP
PATIENT
PATNESS
PATTERN
PATTERS
PATZERS
PETBEAR
PETDEER
PETRELS
PETTERS
PITHEAD
PITIERS
POTEENS
POTHERB
POTHERS
POTTERS
POTTERY
PUTREFY
PUTTEES
PUTTERS
RATBERT
RATTERS
RETREAD
RETREAT
ROTTERS
RUTGERS
RUTTERS
SATEENS
SATIETY
SATWELL
SETFEES
SETTEES
SETTERS
SITTERS
SITWELL
SOTHEBY
SOTHERE
SOTHERN
SOTWEED
TATTERS
TATTERY
TETHERS
TITHERS
TITTERS
TOTTERS
TOTTERY
UNTIERS
UNTREAD
UNTREED
UPTHERE
UPTREND
VETOERS
VETTERS
WATTEAU
WETCELL
WETNESS
WETTEST
WITHERS
WITLESS
WITNESS
WITSEND
YATTERS
YOTHERS
ZITHERS

••T••E•

ACTIFED
ACTIVES
AITCHES
ALTERED
ALTERER
ANTARES
ANTIBES
ANTIGEN
ANTSIER
ARTSIER
ASTUTER
ATTHREE
ATTIMES
ATTIRED
ATTIRER
ATTIRES
ATTUNED
ATTUNES
ATTYGEN
AUTOPEN
BATCHED
BATCHES
BATIKED
BATSMEN
BATTIER
BATTLED
BATTLER
BATTLES
BETAKEN
BETAKES
BETIDED
BETIDES
BETIMES
BETOKEN
BETTGER
BETWEEN
BITSIER
BITTIER
BOTCHED
BOTCHER
BOTCHES
BOTREES
BOTTLED
BOTTLER
BOTTLES
BUTANES
BUTCHER
BUTCHES
BUTENES
CATCHER
CATCHES
CATERED
CATERER
CATEYED
CATFEET
CATFLEA
CATTIER
CDTOWER
CETANES
CITADEL
CITIZEN
CITROEN
CNTOWER
CUTISES
CUTOPEN
CUTOVER
DATASET
DATIVES
DETOXED
DETOXES
DETUNED
DETUNES
DITCHED
DITCHER
DITCHES
DITSIER
DITTIES
DITTOED
DITZIER
DOTAGES
DOTTIER
DOTTLES
EATOVER
ECTYPES
ENTERED
ENTERER
ENTICED
ENTICER
ENTICES
ENTIRES
ENTREES
ENTRIES
ESTATED
ESTATES
ESTEVEZ
FATALES
FATFREE
FATONES
FATTIER
FETCHED
FETCHER
FETCHES
FETTLES
FETUSES
FUTURES
GATELEG
GATEMEN
GETEVEN
GETFREE
GETOVER
GETSHEP
GETSSET
GETSWET
GOTEVEN
GOTFREE
GOTOBED
GOTOSEA
GOTOSEE
GOTOVER
GUTSIER
GUTTIER
HATCHED
HATCHER
HATCHES
HATCHET
HDTVSET
HITCHED
HITCHER
HITCHES
HOTITEM
HOTONES
HOTOVER
HOTTIES
HUTCHES
ICTUSES
IMTIRED
INTAKES
INTEGER
INTHREE
INTONED
INTONER
INTONES
IVTUBES
JETTIED
JETTIES
KATAYEV
KETCHES
KETONES
KETTLES
KITCHEN
KITTIES
KUTCHER
LATCHED
LATCHES
LATEFEE
LATENED
LATEXES
LATICES
LATIMES
LETSSEE
LETTRES
LITOTES
LITTLER
LITTLES
LOTUSES
LUTHIER
MATCHED
MATCHER
MATCHES
MATHIEU
MATINEE
MATTHEW
MATURED
MATURER
MATURES
METALED
METATES
METERED
METOOER
METTLER
METTLES
MITERED
MITOSES
MOTHIER
MOTIVED
MOTIVES
MOTORED
MOTTLED
MOTTLES
MOTTOES
MPTHREE
MRTIGER
MUTAGEN
MUTATED
MUTATES
NATCHEZ
NATIVES
NATTIER
NATURED
NATUREL
NATURES
NETIZEN
NETSTER
NETTLED
NETTLES
NITTIER

NOTATED
NOTATES
NOTBEEN
NOTCHED
NOTCHER
NOTCHES
NOTEVEN
NOTEVER
NOTICED
NOTICER
NOTICES
NOTOPEN
NOTOVER
NOTUSED
NUTATED
NUTATES
NUTSIER
NUTTIER
NUTTREE
NYTIMES
OBTUSER
OCTANES
OCTAVES
OCTOBER
OFTENER
OKTOBER
ONTHREE
OUTAGES
OUTAWED
OUTAWES
OUTBRED
OUTDOER
OUTDOES
OUTDREW
OUTDUEL
OUTFEED
OUTFEEL
OUTFLEE
OUTGOES
OUTGREW
OUTKEEP
OUTLIER
OUTLIES
OUTPEEP
OUTSEEK
OUTSEEN
OUTSEES
OUTSPED
OUTSTEP
OUTVIED
OUTVIES
OUTWEED
OUTWEEP
PATCHED
PATCHEN
PATCHER
PATCHES
PATRIES
PATSIES
PATTIES
PETALED
PETALES
PETCHEW
PETDEER
PETEMEN
PETERED
PETITES
PETTIER

PITCHED
PITCHER
PITCHES
PITCREW
PITHIER
POTAGES
POTPIES
POTTIER
POTTIES
PUTOVER
PUTTEES
PUTTIED
PUTTIES
RATCHET
RATINES
RATITES
RATTIER
RATTLED
RATTLER
RATTLES
RETAKEN
RETAKER
RETAKES
RETAMED
RETAMES
RETAPED
RETAPES
RETAXED
RETAXES
RETILED
RETILES
RETIMED
RETIMES
RETIRED
RETIREE
RETIRES
RETONED
RETONES
RETOWED
RETRIED
RETRIES
RETUNED
RETUNES
RETYPED
RETYPES
RITDYES
RITZIER
ROTATED
ROTATES
ROTIFER
RUTALEE
RUTILES
RUTTIER
SATCHEL
SATINET
SATIRES
SETFEES
SETFREE
SETTEES
SETTLED
SETTLER
SETTLES
SOTWEED
SUTURED
SUTURES
TATTIER
TATTLED
TATTLER

TATTLES
TITTLES
TOTALED
TOTALER
TUTORED
TVTAPES
UNTAKEN
UNTAMED
UNTAMES
UNTAPED
UNTAPES
UNTAXED
UNTAXES
UNTILED
UNTIMED
UNTIRED
UNTONED
UNTREED
UNTRIED
UNTRUER
UNTUNED
UNTUNES
UNTYPED
UPTAKES
UPTIMES
USTEDES
UTTERED
UTTERER
VATDYED
VATDYES
VETCHES
VITTLES
VOTEYEA
VOTEYES
VOTIVES
WATCHED
WATCHER
WATCHES
WATERED
WATERER
WATTLED
WATTLES
WETEYED
WETONES
WITCHED
WITCHES
WITHIES
WITTIER
YETTIES
ZATOPEK

••T•••E

ACTABLE
ACTFIVE
ACTLIKE
ACTUATE
ANTIQUE
ANTLIKE
ANTOINE
ARTICLE
ARTISTE
ARTSALE
ARTWARE
ASTAIRE
ASTARTE
ASTRIDE
ATTACHE
ATTHREE

ATTRITE
AUTOMNE
BATISTE
BATLIKE
BETHERE
BETHUNE
BITROLE
CATENAE
CATHODE
CATLIKE
CATORCE
CATSEYE
CITABLE
CITRATE
CITRINE
COTERIE
COTTAGE
CUTICLE
CUTRATE
CUTTIME
DATABLE
DETENTE
DETERGE
DETRUDE
DOTLIKE
DOTRICE
EATABLE
EATCAKE
EATHERE
EATLATE
EATMORE
ENTEBBE
ENTENTE
ENTHUSE
ENTITLE
ENTWINE
ESTELLE
ESTHETE
EUTERPE
EXTERNE
EXTREME
EXTRUDE
FATFREE
FATIGUE
FATLIKE
GETABLE
GETCUTE
GETDONE
GETFREE
GETSORE
GETWISE
GOTCUTE
GOTDONE
GOTFREE
GOTOSEE
GOTSORE
GOTWISE
GUTHRIE
HATABLE
HATLIKE
HATSIZE
HITHERE
HITHOME
HITTITE
HITTUNE
HOTCAKE
HOTDATE
HOTGLUE

HOTLINE
HOTTIME
HOTWIRE
HOTZONE
HUTLIKE
IMTHERE
INTASTE
INTENSE
INTERNE
INTERSE
INTHERE
INTHREE
INTRADE
INTRUDE
JETFIRE
JSTROKE
KATRINE
LATEFEE
LATRINE
LATROBE
LATTICE
LETHAVE
LETITBE
LETLIVE
LETMEBE
LETRIDE
LETSSEE
LETSUSE
LETTERE
LETTUCE
MATINEE
MATISSE
METHANE
METLIFE
MPTHREE
MUTABLE
NATALIE
NATSUME
NETCAFE
NETGAME
NETLIKE
NETSUKE
NETWARE
NITRATE
NITRIDE
NITRITE
NOTABLE
NOTALIE
NOTAONE
NOTASTE
NOTDONE
NOTHERE
NOTHOME
NOTLIKE
NOTLIVE
NOTMINE
NOTNICE
NOTONCE
NOTRADE
NOTRARE
NOTSAFE
NOTSURE
NOTTOBE
NOTTRUE
NUTLIKE
NUTPINE
NUTTREE
OATCAKE

OATLIKE
OBTRUDE
OCTETTE
OCTOBRE
OCTUBRE
OCTUPLE
ONTHREE
OUTBAKE
OUTCOME
OUTCURE
OUTDARE
OUTDATE
OUTDONE
OUTEDGE
OUTFACE
OUTFIRE
OUTFLEE
OUTGAME
OUTGAVE
OUTGAZE
OUTGIVE
OUTHERE
OUTHIRE
OUTLINE
OUTLIVE
OUTLOVE
OUTMATE
OUTMODE
OUTMOVE
OUTPACE
OUTPIPE
OUTRACE
OUTRAGE
OUTRATE
OUTRAVE
OUTRIDE
OUTRODE
OUTROVE
OUTSIDE
OUTSIZE
OUTSOLE
OUTTAKE
OUTTIRE
OUTTORE
OUTVOTE
OUTWAVE
OUTWILE
OUTWORE
PATRICE
PETCAGE
PETDOVE
PETGATE
PETHARE
PETIOLE
PETMICE
PETMULE
PETNAME
POTABLE
POTENCE
POTHOLE
POTTAGE
RATABLE
RATHOLE
RATLIKE
RATLINE
RATRACE
RETABLE
RETASTE

RETICLE
RETINAE
RETINGE
RETINUE
RETIREE
RETITLE
RETRACE
RETRADE
RETWINE
RITAMAE
RITCHIE
ROTELLE
RUTALEE
SATHOME
SATIATE
SETFREE
SETRATE
SETTYPE
SITHOME
SITUATE
SOTHERE
TETRODE
TITANAE
TITMICE
TITRATE
TOTABLE
TOTASTE
TVTABLE
UNTENSE
UNTERSE
UNTRITE
UNTWINE
UPTHERE
UPTRADE
VITIATE
VITRINE
VOTABLE
VOTEAYE
WATTAGE
WETWARE

•••TE••

ABATERS
ACUTELY
ACUTEST
AFCTEAM
ALATEEN
AMATEUR
AMSTELS
ASATEAM
AUSTERE
AUSTERS
BAITERS
BANTERS
BARTEND
BARTERS
BASTERS
BATTENS
BATTERS
BATTERY
BEATERS
BELTERS
BETTERS
BIGTENT
BIOTECH
BITTERN
BITTERS
BOATELS

BOATERS
BOLTERS
BOOTEES
BOOTERS
BOOTERY
BOTTEGA
BRUTELY
BUNTERS
BUSTERS
BUTTEMT
BUTTERS
BUTTERY
CALTECH
CANTEEN
CANTERS
CARTELS
CARTERS
CASTERS
CENTERS
CHATEAU
CISTERN
COATEES
COATERS
COCTEAU
CONTEMN
CONTEND
CONTENT
CONTEST
CONTEXT
COOTERS
COPTERS
CORTEGE
COTTERS
COUTERS
CRATERS
CRATEUP
CURTEST
CUSTERS
CUTTERS
DAFTEST
DANTEAN
DANTEII
DARTERS
DEBTEES
DEFTEST
DESTEMS
DEUTERO
DIETERS
DISTEND
DNATEST
DOTTERS
DUSTERS
EASTEGG
EASTEND
EASTERN
EASTERS
ECOTEUR
ELATERS
ELITEST
EMOTERS
EPSTEIN
ESOTERY
EYETEST
FALTERS
FASTENS
FASTEST
FATTENS
FATTEST

FESTERS
FETTERS
FIFTEEN
FILTERS
FITTERS
FITTEST
FLUTERS
FONTEYN
FOOTERS
FOSTERS
FRATERS
GAITERS
GARTERS
GASTERO
GENTEEL
GETTERS
GIFTEES
GLUTEAL
GLUTENS
GLUTEUS
GOATEED
GOATEES
GOITERS
GRATEON
GRATERS
GRATEUP
GUTTERS
HALTERS
HASTENS
HASTERT
HATTERS
HAUTEUR
HEATERS
HEFTERS
HINTERS
HITTERS
HOOTERS
HOSTELS
HOSTESS
HOTTEAS
HOTTEST
HUNTERS
HURTERS
ICETEAS
IHATEIT
ILLTELL
INSTEAD
INSTEPS
INUTERO
IRATELY
IRATEST
JESTERS
JILTERS
JITTERS
JITTERY
JOLTERS
JOTTERS
JUSTEST
KERTESZ
KITTENS
KITTERY
LABTECH
LABTEST
LACTEAL
LANTERN
LECTERN
LEFTEAR
LEFTEND

LEFTEST
LEFTEYE
LETTERA
LETTERB
LETTERC
LETTERD
LETTERE
LETTERF
LETTERG
LETTERH
LETTERI
LETTERJ
LETTERK
LETTERL
LETTERM
LETTERN
LETTERO
LETTERP
LETTERQ
LETTERR
LETTERS
LETTERT
LETTERU
LETTERV
LETTERW
LETTERX
LETTERY
LETTERZ
LIETEST
LIFTERS
LINTELS
LINTERS
LISTEES
LISTENS
LISTERS
LITTERS
LITTERY
LOFTERS
LOITERS
LOOTERS
LOTTERS
LOTTERY
LOWTECH
LUSTERS
MALTEDS
MALTESE
MANTECA
MANTELS
MARTENS
MASTERP
MASTERS
MASTERY
MATTERS
MEETERS
MELTERS
MENTEES
MIDTEEN
MIDTERM
MINTERS
MISTELL
MISTERM
MISTERS
MISTERX
MITTENS
MIXTECS
MOLTERS
MONTEGO
MONTERO

MONTEUX
MOOTERS
MUSTERS
MUTTERS
MYSTERY
NATTERS
NBATEAM
NEATENS
NEATEST
NESTEGG
NESTERS
NETTERS
NEUTERS
NFCTEAM
NFLTEAM
NHLTEAM
NUTTERS
ONATEAR
ONETERM
OUSTERS
OUTTEAR
OUTTELL
OYSTERS
PALTERS
PANTENE
PANTERA
PANTERS
PASTEIN
PASTELS
PASTERN
PASTERS
PASTEUP
PASTEUR
PATTERN
PATTERS
PELTERS
PENTELS
PERTEST
PESTERS
PETTERS
PEWTERS
PLATEAU
PLATENS
PLATERS
POETESS
PORTEND
PORTENT
PORTERS
POSTERN
POSTERS
POTTERS
POTTERY
POUTERS
PRATERS
PRETEEN
PRETELL
PRETEND
PRETERM
PRETEST
PRETEXT
PROTEAM
PROTEAN
PROTECT
PROTEGE
PROTEIN
PROTEST
PROTEUS
PUNTERS

PUPTENT
PUTTEES
PUTTERS
QUITESO
QUOTEES
QUOTERS
RAFTERS
RANTERS
RASTERS
RATTERS
RENTEES
RENTERS
RESTERS
REUTERS
RIOTERS
ROOTERS
ROSTERS
ROTTERS
ROUTERS
RUTTERS
SALTERS
SAUTEED
SCITECH
SCOTERS
SEATERS
SEPTETS
SESTETS
SETTEES
SETTERS
SEXTETS
SHUTEYE
SIFTERS
SISTERS
SITTERS
SIXTEEN
SKATERS
SLATERS
SMITERS
SOFTENS
SOFTEST
SORTERS
STATELY
STATERS
SUBTEEN
SUBTEND
SUBTEXT
SYSTEMS
TAGTEAM
TARTEST
TASTEIT
TASTERS
TATTERS
TATTERY
TAUTENS
TAUTEST
TEETERS
TENTERS
TESTEES
TESTERS
TILTERS
TINTERN
TINTERS
TITTERS
TOLTECS
TOOTERS
TOPTENS
TOTTERS
TOTTERY

TOUTERS
TRITELY
TRITEST
TWOTERM
ULSTERS
UMPTEEN
UNITERS
UNSTEEL
UNSTEPS
UNSTERN
UPSTEPS
USSTEEL
VASTEST
VENTERS
VESTEES
VETTERS
VISTEON
WAFTERS
WAITERS
WALTERS
WANTERS
WASTERS
WATTEAU
WELTERS
WESTEGG
WESTEND
WESTERN
WESTERS
WETTEST
WHITELY
WHITENS
WHITEST
WINTERS
WINTERY
WRITEIN
WRITEME
WRITEON
WRITERS
WRITETO
WRITEUP
WROTEIN
WROTEON
WROTETO
WROTEUP
XYSTERS
YATTERS
YAYTEAM
YEATEAM
ZESTERS

•••T•E•

ABETTED
ABETTER
ABUTTED
ABUTTER
AGUTTER
ALATEEN
ALETTES
ALLTIED
AMITIES
ANDTHEN
ANOTHER
APOTHEM
ASHTREE
AUNTBEE
AUNTIES
BARTLES
BARTLET

BATTIER	CRITTER	FUSTIER	LISTEES	PATTIES	SETTLES	TIPTOES	APATITE	FESTIVE	MINTAGE	ROETHKE	WRITEME	BOASTED
BATTLED	CRUTZEN	GANTLET	LITTLER	PEATIER	SHATNER	TITTLES	ASHTREE	FICTILE	MISTAKE	ROOTAGE	YAHTZEE	BOASTER
BATTLER	CURTSEY	GAUTIER	LITTLES	PESTLED	SHATTER	TOOTHED	ATATIME	FICTIVE	MISTIME	ROUTINE	YEWTREE	BOBATEA
BATTLES	DALTREY	GENTEEL	LOATHED	PESTLES	SHUTTER	TOOTLED	ATSTAKE	FIGTREE	MISTUNE	RUNTIME		BOLSTER
BAYTREE	DARTLED	GENTLED	LOATHER	PETTIER	SILTIER	TOOTLER	AUNTBEE	FIRTREE	MISTYPE	RUPTURE	**••••TE•**	BOOSTED
BEATLES	DARTLES	GENTLER	LOATHES	PHATTER	SIXTEEN	TOOTLES	AUSTERE	FIXTURE	MIXTURE	SALTINE	AARATED	BOOSTER
BEETIER	DEBTEES	GENTLES	LOFTBED	PIETIES	SIXTIES	TROTHED	BADTIME	FLOTAGE	MONTAGE	SANTAFE	ABETTED	BORATES
BEETLES	DEITIES	GIFTEES	LOFTIER	PLATIER	SKITTER	TROTTED	BAPTISE	FONTANE	MONTALE	SAOTOME	ABETTER	BOXSTEP
BEETRED	DESTAEL	GIFTSET	LOSTPET	PLATIES	SLATHER	TROTTER	BAPTIZE	FOOTAGE	MORTICE	SCOTTIE	ABLATED	BOXSTER
BEETREE	DIRTIED	GIRTHED	LUSTIER	PLATTED	SLATIER	TSETSES	BAYTREE	FOOTSIE	MORTISE	SCUTTLE	ABLATES	BRITTEN
BENTLEY	DIRTIER	GLITTER	LUSTRED	PLATTER	SLATTED	TUFTIER	BEATSME	FORTLEE	MUSTSEE	SEATTLE	ABORTED	BRONTES
BENTSEN	DIRTIES	GLITZED	LUSTRES	PLOTTED	SLITHER	TURTLED	BEATTIE	FORTUNE	NAPTIME	SETTYPE	ABUTTED	BRUITED
BERTHED	DITTIES	GLITZES	MAITRED	PLOTTER	SLITTED	TURTLES	BEDTIME	FUNTIME	NASTASE	SHUTEYE	ABUTTER	BURSTER
BESTBET	DITTOED	GLUTTED	MAITRES	PLOTZED	SLITTER	TWITTED	BEETREE	FURTIVE	NEPTUNE	SHUTTLE	ADAPTED	CAPOTES
BESTMEN	DONTBEE	GOATEED	MALTIER	PLOTZES	SLOTTED	TWITTER	BELTANE	GASTONE	NICTATE	SISTINE	ADAPTER	CDRATES
BESTREW	DOTTIER	GOATEES	MANTLED	POITIER	SLOTTER	TWOTOED	BESTONE	GENTILE	NOTTOBE	SKITTLE	ADEPTER	CELOTEX
BETTGER	DOTTLES	GORTNER	MANTLES	POSTIES	SMATTER	UMPTEEN	BIGTIME	GESTATE	NOTTRUE	SPITTLE	ADOPTED	CERATED
BIGTOES	DRATTED	GOUTIER	MANTLET	POSTMEN	SMITHED	UNITIES	BIOTITE	GESTURE	NURTURE	STATICE	ADOPTEE	CERATES
BIRTHED	DUETTED	GRITTED	MATTHEW	POTTIER	SMITTEN	UNSTEEL	BIOTYPE	GOSTALE	NUTTREE	STATURE	ADOPTER	CHANTED
BITTIER	DUSTIER	GRITTER	MEATIER	POTTIES	SMOTHER	UPATREE	BISTATE	GUMTREE	OAKTREE	STATUTE	ADRATES	CHANTER
BLATHER	DUSTMEN	GUMTREE	MEATMEN	POUTIER	SOFTGEL	USSTEEL	BRATTLE	GUSTAVE	OLDTIME	SUBTONE	AERATED	CHANTEY
BLATTED	EARTHED	GUNTHER	MEITNER	PRETEEN	SOFTIES	VASTIER	BRITTLE	HADTIME	ONETIME	SUBTYPE	AERATES	CHAPTER
BLITHER	EARTHEN	GUSTIER	MENTEES	PRETZEL	SOOTHED	VESTEES	BUDTIME	HADTOBE	ONSTAGE	SUITSME	AGENTED	CHARTED
BLITZED	ELMTREE	GUSTOES	METTLER	PRITHEE	SOOTHER	VINTNER	BUYTIME	HASTIME	OUTTAKE	SYSTOLE	AGNATES	CHARTER
BLITZEN	EMITTED	GUTTIER	METTLES	PURTIER	SOOTHES	VIRTUES	CAPTIVE	HASTOBE	OUTTIRE	TACTILE	AGUTTER	CHASTEN
BLITZER	EMITTER	HARTLEY	MIDTEEN	PUTTEES	SOOTIER	VISTAED	CAPTURE	HECTARE	OUTTORE	TARTARE	ALERTED	CHASTER
BLITZES	EMPTIED	HASTIER	MINTIER	PUTTIED	SORTIED	VITTLES	CARTAGE	HITTITE	PANTENE	TEATIME	ALERTER	CHATTED
BLOTTED	EMPTIER	HEATHEN	MINTTEA	PUTTIES	SORTIES	WALTHER	CARTIRE	HITTUNE	PANTILE	TEATREE	ALETTES	CHATTEL
BLOTTER	EMPTIES	HEATHER	MISTIER	QUATRES	SOUTHEY	WALTZED	CASTILE	HOSTAGE	PANTONE	TEETIME	AMMETER	CHATTER
BOATMEN	EPITHET	HEATTER	MOTTLED	QUITTED	SPATHES	WALTZER	CDSTORE	HOSTILE	PARTAKE	TESTATE	APLITES	CHEATED
BOOTEES	ERITREA	HEFTIER	MOTTLES	QUITTER	SPATTED	WALTZES	CENTARE	HOTTIME	PARTITE	TEXTILE	ARBITER	CHEATER
BOOTIES	EXITFEE	HOGTIED	MOTTOES	QUOTEES	SPATTER	WARTIER	CENTIME	IFITDIE	PARTONE	TEXTURE	ASANTES	CHESTED
BOOTLEG	FARTHER	HOGTIES	MOUTHED	RATTIER	SPITTER	WASTREL	CLOTURE	IFSTONE	PASTDUE	THATONE	ASTUTER	CHESTER
BOTTLED	FARTLEK	HOSTLER	MOUTHER	RATTLED	SPITZES	WATTLED	COETZEE	IMITATE	PASTIME	THETREE	ATWATER	CHITTER
BOTTLER	FASTNET	HOTTIES	MUSTIER	RATTLER	SPOTTED	WATTLES	CONTUSE	INSTATE	PASTURE	THETUBE	AUDITED	CLATTER
BOTTLES	FATTIER	HOWTHEN	MUSTSEE	RATTLES	SPOTTER	WEATHER	CORTEGE	INSTONE	PELTATE	TINTYPE	AUDITEE	CLEATED
BOWTIES	FEATHER	HRETHEL	MYRTLES	REDTIES	SPUTTER	WEBTOED	COSTATE	INSTORE	PENTANE	TONTINE	AUGITES	CLOTTED
BRITNEY	FELTPEN	HUNTLEY	NARTHEX	RENTEES	STATLER	WERTHER	COSTIVE	INSTYLE	PEPTIDE	TOOTSIE	AVERTED	CLOUTED
BRITTEN	FETTLES	HURTLED	NASTIER	RENTIER	STATUES	WESTIES	COSTUME	INUTILE	PEPTONE	TORTURE	AVERTER	CLOUTER
BROTHER	FIFTEEN	HURTLES	NASTIES	RESTREW	STETTED	WHETHER	COTTAGE	ISOTONE	PICTURE	TRITONE	AVIATED	CLUSTER
BUSTIER	FIFTIES	HUSTLED	NATTIER	REUTHER	STUTTER	WHETTED	COUTURE	ISOTOPE	PISTOLE	TWOTIME	AVIATES	CLUTTER
BUSTLED	FIGTREE	HUSTLER	NEITHER	REUTTER	STUTZES	WHETTER	CULTURE	ITSTIME	POETISE	TWOTONE	AWAITED	COACTED
BUSTLER	FIRTREE	HUSTLES	NESTLED	RONTGEN	SUBTEEN	WHITHER	CURTATE	ITSTRUE	POETIZE	UNITISE	AWAITER	COAPTED
BUSTLES	FLATBED	IDOTTER	NESTLER	ROOTIER	SUBTLER	WHITNEY	CUTTIME	JIGTIME	POPTUNE	UNITIVE	BAINTER	COASTED
CANTEEN	FLATLET	JETTIED	NESTLES	ROOTLED	SWATHED	WITTIER	DAYTIME	JUSTICE	PORTAGE	UNITIZE	BARITES	COASTER
CANTLES	FLATTED	JETTIES	NETTLED	ROOTLES	SWATHES	WRITHED	DENTATE	JUSTINE	POSTAGE	UNSTATE	BASETEN	COOPTED
CARTIER	FLATTEN	JOLTIER	NETTLES	ROOTLET	SWATTED	WRITHER	DENTINE	JUSTONE	POSTURE	UPATREE	BEEFTEA	COULTER
CASTLED	FLATTER	JOSTLED	NIFTIER	RUNTIER	SWATTER	WRITHES	DENTURE	KAPTURE	POTTAGE	UPSTAGE	BELATED	COUNTED
CASTLES	FLITTED	JOSTLER	NIFTIES	RUSTIER	SWITZER	WRITTEN	DENTYNE	LABTUBE	PRATTLE	UPSTARE	BENOTED	COUNTEE
CATTIER	FLITTER	JOSTLES	NITTIER	RUSTLED	TARTIER	YAHTZEE	DESTINE	LACTASE	PRETAPE	UPSTATE	BENOTES	COUNTEM
CAUTHEN	FLUTIER	KASTLER	NOOTHER	RUSTLER	TARTLET	YETTIES	DICTATE	LACTATE	PRETIRE	USSTATE	BERATED	COUNTER
CENTRED	FLUTIES	KESTREL	NORTHER	RUSTLES	TASTIER	YEWTREE	DIDTIME	LACTOSE	PRETYPE	VANTAGE	BERATER	COURTED
CENTRES	FLUTTER	KETTLES	NOWTHEN	RUTTIER	TATTIER	YOUTHEN	DONTBEE	LASTONE	PRITHEE	VCRTAPE	BERATES	COVETED
CHATTED	FLYTIER	KILTIES	NUTTIER	SALTIER	TATTLED	ZESTIER	DONTLIE	LATTICE	PROTEGE	VENTAGE	BIGOTED	COVETER
CHATTEL	FOOTLED	KITTIES	NUTTREE	SALTSEA	TATTLER		DUCTILE	LECTURE	RAGTIME	VENTURE	BLASTED	COYOTES
CHATTER	FOOTLER	KLUTZES	OAKTREE	SAUTEED	TATTLES	**•••T••E**	DUOTONE	LEETIDE	RAPTUNE	VESTIGE	BLASTER	CRAFTED
CHITTER	FOOTLES	KNITTED	OMITTED	SCATHED	TEATREE	ACETATE	EBBTIDE	LEFTEYE	RAPTURE	VESTURE	BLATTED	CRAFTER
CHUTNEY	FOOTLET	KNITTER	OMITTER	SCATHES	TEETHED	ACETONE	ECOTAGE	LETTERE	REDTAPE	VINTAGE	BLEATED	CREATED
CLATTER	FOOTMEN	KNOTTED	PANTHER	SCATTED	TEETHER	AGATINE	ECOTYPE	LETTUCE	REDTIDE	VOITURE	BLEATER	CREATES
CLOTHED	FORTIES	KNOTTER	PANTIES	SCATTER	TEETHES	AGITATE	ELMTREE	LOWTIDE	REPTILE	VOLTAGE	BLISTER	CRESTED
CLOTHES	FORTLEE	LAITIES	PANTLEG	SCYTHED	TENTBED	AIRTIME	EMOTIVE	MALTASE	RESTAGE	VOLTORE	BLOATED	CRITTER
CLOTTED	FRETTED	LASTLEG	PARTIED	SCYTHES	TENTPEG	AIRTUBE	EPITOME	MALTBIE	RESTATE	VULTURE	BLOTTED	CROFTER
CLUTTER	FRETTER	LAUTREC	PARTIER	SEETHED	TESTBED	ALITTLE	EUSTACE	MALTESE	RESTIVE	WARTIME	BLOTTER	CROUTES
COATEES	FRITTED	LEATHER	PARTIES	SEETHES	TESTEES	ALLTIME	EXITFEE	MALTOSE	RESTOKE	WASTAGE	BLUNTED	CRUSTED
COETZEE	FRITTER	LEFTIES	PARTNER	SELTZER	TESTIER	AMATIVE	FANTINE	MAYTIME	RESTORE	WATTAGE	BLUNTER	CURATED
COMTREX	FROTHED	LEFTLEG	PARTYER	SETTEES	THETREE	ANATASE	FASTONE	MEATAXE	RESTYLE	WENTAPE	BLURTED	CURATES
COOTIES	FROTHER	LETTRES	PASTIER	SETTLED	THITHER	ANATOLE	FEATURE	MEATPIE	RIPTIDE	WHATTHE	BLURTER	DANITES
COSTNER	FURTHER	LINTIER	PASTIES	SETTLER	TIPTOED	ANYTIME	FERTILE	MELTAGE	RLSTINE	WHITTLE	BLUSTER	DAUNTED

DAUNTER
DEBATED
DEBATER
DEBATES
DEBITED
DEBUTED
DELETED
DELETES
DEMETER
DEMOTED
DEMOTES
DENOTED
DENOTES
DEPUTED
DEPUTES
DERATED
DERATES
DEVOTED
DEVOTEE
DEVOTES
DEWATER
DICHTER
DILATED
DILATES
DILUTED
DILUTER
DILUTES
DIMETER
DIOPTER
DONATED
DONATEE
DONATES
DOUBTED
DOUBTER
DRAFTED
DRAFTEE
DRAFTER
DRATTED
DRIFTED
DRIFTER
DUETTED
ECARTES
EDUCTED
EGESTED
EIGHTEE
EJECTED
ELECTED
ELECTEE
ELUATES
EMITTED
EMITTER
ENACTED
EQUATED
EQUATES
ERECTED
ERECTER
ERUCTED
ERUPTED
ERUPTER
ESTATED
ESTATES
EVERTED
EVICTED
EVICTEE
EXACTED
EXACTER
EXALTED
EXALTER

EXCITED
EXCITER
EXCITES
EXERTED
EXERTER
EXISTED
EXMATES
EXULTED
FACETED
FAGOTED
FAINTED
FAINTER
FAULTED
FEASTED
FEASTER
FEINTED
FIBSTER
FIGHTER
FINITES
FIVETEN
FIXATED
FIXATES
FLATTED
FLATTEN
FLATTER
FLEETED
FLEETER
FLIRTED
FLIRTER
FLITTED
FLITTER
FLOATED
FLOATER
FLOUTED
FLOUTER
FLUSTER
FLUTTER
FOISTED
FOLATES
FORSTER
FRETTED
FRETTER
FRITTED
FRITTER
FRONTED
FROSTED
FROSTER
FRUITED
FUENTES
FUNSTER
GAGSTER
GALATEA
GAMETES
GAUNTER
GELATED
GELATES
GHOSTED
GLINTED
GLISTEN
GLISTER
GLITTER
GLOATED
GLOATER
GLUTTED
GOAFTER
GOGETEM
GOLFTEE
GORETEX

GRAFTED
GRAFTER
GRANTED
GRANTEE
GRANTER
GREATEN
GREATER
GREETED
GREETER
GRIFTED
GRIFTER
GRISTER
GRITTED
GRITTER
GROUTED
GROUTER
GRUNTED
GRUNTER
GUESTED
GUNITES
GYRATED
GYRATES
HABITED
HALITES
HAMITES
HAMSTER
HANGTEN
HARDTEN
HAUNTED
HAUNTER
HEARTED
HEARTEN
HEATTER
HEISTED
HERBTEA
HIGHTEA
HIPSTER
HOISTED
HOISTER
HOLSTER
HOTITEM
HUNGTEN
ICEDTEA
IDEATED
IDEATES
IDOTTER
IGNITED
IGNITER
IGNITES
IIPETER
IMHOTEP
IMPUTED
IMPUTER
IMPUTES
INAPTER
INASTEW
INCITED
INCITER
INCITES
INDITED
INDITER
INDITES
INGATES
INKSTER
INMATES
INVITED
INVITEE
INVITER

INVITES
IODATED
IODATES
ISLETED
JAUNTED
JOINTED
JOINTER
JOISTED
JOUSTED
JOUSTER
JUPITER
KARATES
KEISTER
KIRSTEN
KLISTER
KNITTED
KNITTER
KNOTTED
KNOTTER
KNOUTED
LAERTES
LEGATEE
LEGATES
LEISTER
LEVITES
LIGATED
LIGATES
LIGHTED
LIGHTEN
LIGHTER
LILETEE
LIMITED
LIMITER
LITOTES
LOBATED
LOBSTER
LOCATED
LOCATER
LOCATES
LUCITES
LUNATED
LUNATES
LUXATED
LUXATES
MAARTEN
MANATEE
MEISTER
MERITED
METATES
MINSTER
MINTTEA
MINUTED
MINUTER
MINUTES
MISSTEP
MOBSTER
MOISTEN
MOISTER
MONSTER
MOULTED
MOUNTED
MOUNTER
MULCTED
MUNSTER
MUTATED
MUTATES
NAPSTER
NEGATED

NEGATER
NEGATES
NETSTER
NIGHTER
NORITES
NOTATED
NOTATES
NOVOTES
NUTATED
NUTATES
OBLATES
OERSTED
OLDSTER
OLEATES
OLMSTED
OMITTED
OMITTER
ONESTEP
ONWATER
OOCYTES
OOLITES
OPIATES
ORANTES
ORBITED
ORBITER
ORESTES
OUTSTEP
PAINTED
PAINTER
PAIUTES
PALATES
PENATES
PETITES
PEYOTES
PGRATED
PHATTER
PHILTER
PIASTER
PICOTED
PILATES
PILOTED
PIRATED
PIRATES
PIVOTED
PIVOTER
PLAITED
PLAITER
PLANTED
PLANTER
PLASTER
PLATTED
PLATTER
PLAYTEX
PLEATED
PLOTTED
PLOTTER
POINTED
POINTER
POINTES
POLITER
POSITED
PRINTED
PRINTER
PROCTER
PSALTER
PUNSTER
PUPATED
PUPATES

PYRITES
QUARTER
QUARTES
QUARTET
QUESTED
QUESTER
QUIETED
QUIETEN
QUIETER
QUILTED
QUILTER
QUINTES
QUINTET
QUIRTED
QUITTED
QUITTER
QUOITED
RATITES
REACTED
REALTER
REBATED
REBATER
REBATES
REBOTES
RECITED
RECITER
RECITES
REDATED
REDATES
REENTER
REFUTED
REFUTER
REFUTES
RELATED
RELATER
RELATES
REMATED
REMATES
REMOTER
REMOTES
RENOTED
RENOTES
REPUTED
REPUTES
RERATED
RERATES
RESITED
REUTTER
REVOTED
REVOTES
REWATER
RICHTER
RIGHTED
RIGHTER
RIVETED
RIVETER
ROASTED
ROASTER
ROISTER
ROOSTED
ROOSTER
ROSETEA
ROTATED
ROTATES
ROUSTED
ROUSTER
SAGETEA
SAINTED

SAINTES
SALUTED
SALUTER
SALUTES
SAUNTER
SCANTED
SCANTER
SCATTED
SCATTER
SCENTED
SCENTER
SCEPTER
SCOOTED
SCOOTER
SCOUTED
SCOUTER
SEDATED
SEDATER
SEDATES
SEMITES
SENATES
SHAFTED
SHANTER
SHATTER
SHEETED
SHELTER
SHIFTED
SHIFTER
SHIITES
SHOOTER
SHORTED
SHORTEN
SHORTER
SHOUTED
SHOUTER
SHUNTED
SHUNTER
SHUSTER
SHUTTER
SHYSTER
SIGHTED
SIGHTER
SIZETEN
SKEETER
SKELTER
SKIRTED
SKIRTER
SKITTER
SLANTED
SLATTED
SLEETED
SLITTED
SLITTER
SLOTTED
SLOTTER
SMARTED
SMARTEN
SMARTER
SMATTER
SMELTED
SMELTER
SMITTEN
SNIFTER
SNOOTED
SNORTED
SNORTER
SNOUTED
SOLUTES

SPATTED
SPATTER
SPECTER
SPITTER
SPORTED
SPOTTED
SPOTTER
SPOUTED
SPOUTER
SPRITES
SPURTED
SPUTTER
STARTED
STARTER
STETTED
STILTED
STINTED
STINTER
STOUTEN
STOUTER
STPETER
STUNTED
STUTTER
SUBITEM
SVELTER
SWATTED
SWATTER
SWEATED
SWEATER
SWEETEN
SWEETER
SWELTER
SWIFTER
TAINTED
TAKETEA
TAKETEN
TAPSTER
TAUNTED
TAUNTER
TEMPTED
TEMPTER
THEATER
TIGHTEN
TIGHTER
TINCTED
TIPSTER
TOASTED
TOASTEE
TOASTER
TOOKTEN
TREATED
TREATER
TROTTED
TROTTER
TRUSTED
TRUSTEE
TRUSTER
TRYSTED
TRYSTER
TWEETED
TWEETER
TWISTED
TWISTER
TWITTED
TWITTER
TWOSTEP
UNACTED
UNBATED

UNCITED
UNDATED
UNEATEN
UNFATED
UNFETED
UNGATED
UNHATED
UNIATES
UNMATED
UNMATES
UNMITER
UNMUTED
UNNOTED
UNOFTEN
UNOPTED
UNRATED
UNSATED
UNVOTED
UPDATED
UPDATER
UPDATES
UPRATED
UPRATES
VACATED
VACATES
VALETED
VARITEK
VAULTED
VAULTER
VAUNTED
VAUNTER
VECHTEN
VEINTES
VISITED
VOLUTED
VOLUTES
VORSTER
VUMETER
WAISTED
WEBSTER
WHEATEN
WHETTED
WHETTER
WINDTEE
WOOSTER
WORSTED
WRESTED
WRESTER
WRITTEN
YACHTED
YACHTER
YEASTED
YUCATEC
ZAPATEO
ZAPOTEC
ZYGOTES

••••T•E

ADOPTEE
ALITTLE
ANNETTE
APOSTLE
ARIETTE
ARISTAE
ASEETHE
ATIPTOE
AUDITEE
BABETTE
BEASTIE
BEATTIE
BLINTZE
BOLATIE
BOLOTIE
BRATTLE
BREATHE
BRISTLE
BRITTLE
BURETTE
CADETTE
CALOTTE
CANITBE
CHORTLE
COLETTE
COSETTE
COUNTEE
CULOTTE
CURETTE
CUVETTE
DEVOTEE
DINETTE
DONATEE
DRAFTEE
EIGHTEE
ELECTEE
ELECTME
ENTITLE
EPISTLE
EVICTEE
FAYETTE
FENETRE
FOUETTE
GALETTE
GAROTTE
GAVOTTE
GAZETTE
GOLFTEE
GRANTEE
GRISTLE
HABITUE
INVITEE
ITSATIE
KIRSTIE
KRYSTLE
LAFITTE
LAMOTTE
LANOTTE
LAYETTE
LEGATEE
LETITBE
LILETEE
LIZETTE
LONETTE
LUNETTE
LYNETTE
MANATEE
MANETTE
MOUNTIE
MUSETTE
NANETTE
NECKTIE
NIGHTIE
NONETTE
OCTETTE
OPENTOE
ORNETTE
PALETTE
PHILTRE
PIASTRE
PIPETTE
PRATTLE
REBATHE
RETITLE
RONETTE
ROSETTE
SCEPTRE
SCOTTIE
SCUTTLE
SEATTLE
SHEATHE
SHELTIE
SHORTIE
SHUTTLE
SILKTIE
SKITTLE
SPECTRE
SPITTLE
STARTLE
SUZETTE
SWEETIE
THEATRE
THISTLE
TOASTEE
TONETTE
TRESTLE
TRUSTEE
TRUSTME
TURFTOE
UNMITRE
VALOTTE
VEDETTE
VIDETTE
WHATTHE
WHISTLE
WHITTLE
WINDTEE
WREATHE
WRESTLE
WYNETTE
YACHTIE
YANGTZE

•••••TE

ACCRETE
ACERATE
ACETATE
ACOLYTE
ACONITE
ACTUATE
ADAMITE
ADULATE
AGEMATE
AGITATE
AIRDATE
ALCESTE
ALDENTE
ALIGOTE
ALLANTE
AMILATE
AMINUTE
ANALYTE
ANDANTE
ANIMATE
ANNETTE
APATITE
ARCUATE
ARGANTE
ARIETTE
ARTISTE
ASSANTE
ASTARTE
ATELATE
ATHLETE
ATTRITE
AUGUSTE
AUREATE
AZURITE
BAALITE
BABETTE
BARBATE
BATISTE
BAUXITE
BEDMATE
BIOLITE
BIOTITE
BISTATE
BOXKITE
BROMATE
BURETTE
CADETTE
CALCITE
CALOTTE
CASEATE
CAUDATE
CELESTE
CHAYOTE
CHELATE
CILIATE
CIRRATE
CITRATE
CLAVATE
CLEANTE
CLIMATE
COGNATE
COLETTE
COLGATE
COLLATE
COMMUTE
COMPETE
COMPOTE
COMPUTE
CONFUTE
CONNATE
CONNOTE
CORDATE
CORDITE
CORNUTE
COSETTE
COSTATE
COWRITE
COWROTE
CREMATE
CRENATE
CULOTTE
CUNEATE
CUPRITE
CURETTE
CURTATE
CUSPATE
CUTRATE
CUVETTE
DEBOITE
DEFLATE
DENTATE
DEPLETE
DERALTE
DESPITE
DETENTE
DEVIATE
DICTATE
DINETTE
DIORITE
DISPUTE
DISRATE
DOGBITE
DOGGATE
DUEDATE
DURANTE
EATLATE
EBONITE
EBWHITE
EDOMITE
EDUCATE
EGALITE
EGOISTE
ELAMITE
ELEVATE
ELMONTE
ELNORTE
ELOCUTE
EMANATE
EMBOITE
EMIRATE
EMULATE
ENDLATE
ENDNOTE
ENROUTE
ENSUITE
ENTENTE
EPIDOTE
EPILATE
EREMITE
ERUDITE
ESTHETE
EVOLUTE
EXABYTE
EXCRETE
EXECUTE
EXEGETE
EXPARTE
EXPIATE
EXUDATE
FALCATE
FAYETTE
FEEBATE
FERMATE
FERRATE
FERRITE
FOLIATE
FORSYTE
FOUETTE
FRIGATE
FURCATE
GALEATE
GALETTE
GAROTTE
GARROTE
GAVOTTE
GAZETTE
GEFILTE
GEMMATE

GESTATE
GETCUTE
GLOBATE
GOTCUTE
GRADATE
GRANITE
HIRSUTE
HITTITE
HOPLITE
HOTDATE
HUSSITE
HYALITE
HYDRATE
ILLBITE
IMAMATE
IMITATE
INFANTE
INFLATE
INGRATE
INHASTE
INSPITE
INSTATE
INTASTE
INWHITE
ISOLATE
ITERATE
ITSLATE
JADEITE
KEYNOTE
KHANATE
LABIATE
LACOSTE
LACTATE
LAFITTE
LAMOTTE
LANOTTE
LAPORTE
LAYETTE
LECONTE
LIBERTE
LIGNITE
LIMNITE
LINEATE
LIQUATE
LISENTE
LIZETTE
LONETTE
LUDDITE
LUNETTE
LYDDITE
LYNETTE
MACHETE
MAGNATE
MAJESTE
MANDATE
MANETTE
MARGATE
MEDIATE
MIGRATE
MISCITE
MISDATE
MISMATE
MISRATE
MOABITE
MODISTE
MORANTE
MRSLATE
MUSANTE
MUSETTE
NAIVETE
NANETTE
NARRATE
NEOLYTE
NEONATE
NEWGATE
NICTATE
NIOBITE
NITRATE
NITRITE
NONETTE
NOTASTE
OBVIATE
OCTETTE
OFFSITE
ONADATE
ONEBYTE
ONENOTE
ONEVOTE
OPERATE
ORIENTE
ORNETTE
OUTDATE
OUTMATE
OUTRATE
OUTVOTE
OVERATE
OXALATE
OXIDATE
PADSITE
PALETTE
PALMATE
PALPATE
PAPEETE
PARTITE
PAYRATE
PELTATE
PENLITE
PENNATE
PERLITE
PERMUTE
PESANTE
PETGATE
PICANTE
PILEATE
PINNATE
PIPETTE
PLACATE
PLANATE
PLICATE
POLLUTE
PRECITE
PREDATE
PRELATE
PREMATE
PRIMATE
PRIVATE
PROBATE
PROLATE
PROMOTE
PRONATE
PRORATE
PULSATE
QUINATE
QUIXOTE
RADIATE
RANLATE
REBASTE
RECRATE
REFLATE
REPASTE
REPLATE
REPLETE
REQUITE
REQUOTE
REROUTE
RESLATE
RESPITE
RESTATE
RETASTE
REUNITE
REWRITE
REWROTE
RIPOSTE
ROBERTE
RONETTE
ROSEATE
ROSETTE
RUINATE
RUNLATE
SADFATE
SATIATE
SEAGATE
SECRETE
SENSATE
SERIATE
SERRATE
SETRATE
SILENTE
SINUATE
SITUATE
SORBATE
STATUTE
STRIATE
SUBDATE
SULFATE
SULFITE
SUMMATE
SUZETTE
TAXRATE
TERMITE
TERNATE
TESTATE
THWHITE
TITRATE
TOMKITE
TONETTE
TOOLATE
TOPRATE
TOTASTE
TOYKITE
TRIBUTE
TRIESTE
ULULATE
UNCRATE
UNPASTE
UNQUOTE
UNSTATE
UNTRITE
UNWHITE
UPSTATE
URANITE
USSTATE
VALENTE
VALOTTE
VALUATE
VALVATE
VARIATE
VEDETTE
VELOUTE
VIBRATE
VICENTE
VICOMTE
VIDETTE
VIOLATE
VIRGATE
VITIATE
VOLANTE
VOLENTE
VULGATE
WASLATE
WEBSITE
WOOLITE
WYNETTE
YESVOTE
ZINCITE

TF•••••

TFPOWYS

T•F••••

TAFFETA
TAFFIES
TEFLONS
TIFFANY
TIFFING
TIFFINS
TOFFEES
TOFFLER
TOFUTTI
TUFFETS
TUFTIER
TUFTING

T••F•••

TAFFETA
TAFFIES
TAXFREE
TENFEET
TENFOLD
TENFOOT
TENFOUR
THEFALL
THEFEDS
THEFIRM
THEFIVE
THEFLEA
THEFLOP
THEFONZ
THEFOOL
THEFRUG
TIFFANY
TIFFING
TIFFINS
TINFISH
TINFOIL
TOFFEES
TOFFLER
TOMFOOL
TOPFIVE
TOPFORM
TOYFAIR
TRAFFIC
TREFOIL
TRIFFID
TRIFLED
TRIFLER
TRIFLES
TRIFOLD
TRIFORM
TRUFFLE
TUBFULS
TUFFETS
TURFIER
TURFING
TURFMAN
TURFMEN
TURFSKI
TURFTOE
TURFWAR
TWOFACE
TWOFEET
TWOFERS
TWOFOLD
TWOFOOT

T•••F••

TACTFUL
TAILFIN
TAKEFOR
TANKFUL
TARIFFS
TEARFUL
TEEOFFS
TELEFAX
TENTFUL
TESTFLY
TESTFOR
THRIFTS
THRIFTY
THUSFAR
TINAFEY
TIPOFFS
TOILFUL
TOOKFOR
TRAFFIC
TRAYFUL
TRIFFID
TRUFFLE
TUNEFUL
TWELFTH

T••••F•

TAILOFF
TAKEOFF
TAMPAFL
TAPSOFF
TARIFFS
TEAROFF
TEEDOFF
TEEOFFS
TEESOFF
TELLOFF
TERRIFY
TESTIFY
THEGIFT
THELEFT
TICKOFF
TIEDOFF
TIESOFF
TIMEOFF
TIPOFFS
TIPSOFF
TOLDOFF
TOOKOFF
TOPSOFF
TOREOFF
TORNOFF
TORREFY
TOSSOFF
TRIMOFF
TROTOFF
TURNOFF

T•••••F

TAILOFF
TAKEOFF
TALKSOF
TAPSOFF
TEALEAF
TEAROFF
TEEDOFF
TEESOFF
TELLOFF
TELLSOF
THEREOF
THESELF
THINKOF
THYSELF
TICKOFF
TIEDOFF
TIESOFF
TIMEOFF
TINROOF
TIPSOFF
TIREDOF
TIRESOF
TOLDOFF
TOOKOFF
TOPSOFF
TOREOFF
TORNOFF
TOSSOFF
TRIMOFF
TROTOFF
TURNOFF

•TF••••

ATFAULT
ATFIRST
BTFSPLK

•T•F•••

ATMFEES
ITSFINE
STAFFED
STAFFER
STEFANI
STIFFED
STIFFEL
STIFFEN
STIFFER
STIFFLY
STIFLED
STIFLES
STUFFED
STUFFER
STUFFIN

•T••F••

ITCHFOR
STAFFED
STAFFER
STAYFOR
STIFFED
STIFFEL
STIFFEN
STIFFER
STIFFLY
STIRFRY
STOPFOR
STRAFED
STRAFER
STRAFES
STRIFES
STUFFED
STUFFER
STUFFIN

•T•••F•

STAYOFF
STEPOFF
STOPOFF
STUPEFY

•T••••F

STAYOFF
STEPOFF
STOPOFF
STRIPOF

••TF•••

ACTFIVE
ACTFOUR
ANTFARM
ARTFAIR
ARTFERN
ARTFILM
ARTFORM
CATFEET
CATFISH
CATFITS
CATFLAP
CATFLEA
CATFOOD
CATFOOT
EATFROM
FATFARM
FATFREE
GETFREE
GETFROM
GOTFREE
HATFULS
HITFILM
HOTFOOT
JETFANS
JETFIRE
JETFOIL
LETFALL
METFANS
MITFORD
NETFLIX
NETFULS
NOTFAIR
OUTFACE
OUTFAST
OUTFAWN
OUTFEED
OUTFEEL
OUTFIND
OUTFIRE
OUTFISH
OUTFITS
OUTFLEE
OUTFLOW
OUTFLUX
OUTFOOL
OUTFOOT
PETFISH
PETFROG
PITFALL
POTFULS
RATFINK
SETFEES
SETFREE
VATFULS
WATFORD

••T•F••

ACTIFED
ACTSFOR
ANTIFOG
BATSFOR
CUTOFFS
DUTIFUL
ESTEFAN
FATEFUL
GETSFAR
GETSFIT
HATEFUL
HITSFOR
JETSFAN
LATEFEE
LATIFAH
LETSFLY
METSFAN
OPTSFOR
OUTOFIT
PITIFUL
PUTOFFS
RATAFIA
ROTIFER
RUTHFUL
SETOFFS
SITSFOR
VOTEFOR

••T••F•

BITEOFF
CUTOFFS
CUTSOFF
GETSOFF
GETSOFT
GOTSOFT
HATSOFF
HITSOFF
IDTHEFT
LETSOFF
METLIFE
MYTHIFY
NETCAFE
NITRIFY
NOTSAFE
OUTSIFT
PETRIFY
PUTOFFS
PUTREFY
PUTSOFF
RETURFS
SATISFY
SETOFFS
SETSOFF
VITRIFY

••T•••F

ALTDORF
BITEOFF
CUTSOFF
GETSANF
GETSOFF
HATSOFF
HITSOFF
LETGOOF
LETSOFF
LETTERF
METCALF
NETSURF
ONTOPOF
PETCALF
PUTSOFF
SETSOFF

•••TF••

BOATFUL
EXITFEE
FACTFUL
FELTFOR
FISTFUL
FRETFUL
HEATFAN
HEATFUL
HUNTFOR
HURTFOR
HURTFUL
KEPTFIT
LEFTFOR
LUSTFUL
NESTFUL
PLOTFUL
POSTFIX
POUTFUL
RESTFUL
ROOTFOR
SENTFOR
SHOTFOR
TACTFUL
TENTFUL
TESTFLY
TESTFOR
WAITFOR
WENTFAR
WENTFOR
WHATFOR
WISTFUL
ZESTFUL

•••T•F•

ACETIFY
ASSTIFF
BEATIFY
BEATOFF
BESTOFF
CARTOFF
CASTOFF
CERTIFY
DARTOFF
DISTAFF
DUSTOFF
FELTOFF
FORTIFY
GRATIFY
HENTOFF
JUSTIFY
KEPTOFF
LEFTOFF
LIFTOFF
MASTIFF
MORTIFY
MUSTAFA
MYSTIFY
ONSTAFF
PONTIFF
RECTIFY
RESTAFF
RESTUFF
SANTAFE
SENTOFF
SHUTOFF
TESTIFY
TROTOFF
UNSTIFF
WENTAFT
WENTOFF
WHATIFS

•••T••F

ASSTIFF
BEATOFF
BESTOFF
CARTOFF
CASTOFF
DARTOFF
DISTAFF
DUSTOFF
FELTOFF
HENTOFF
KEPTOFF
LEFTOFF
LETTERF
LIFTOFF
MASTIFF
NORTHOF
ONSTAFF
PONTIFF
RESTAFF
RESTUFF
SENTOFF
SHUTOFF
SOUTHOF
TROTOFF
UNSTIFF
WENTOFF

••••T•F

AHOSTOF
ARAFTOF
BOASTOF
DOOUTOF
SHORTOF

•••••TF

ROBERTF
SILENTF

T•G••••

TAGALOG
TAGAMET
TAGDAYS
TAGENDS
TAGGANT
TAGGERS
TAGGING
TAGLIKE
TAGLINE
TAGOUTS
TAGSALE
TAGSOUT
TAGTEAM
TIGHTEN
TIGHTER
TIGHTLY
TIGLONS
TIGRESS
TOGGERY
TOGGING
TOGGLED
TOGGLER
TOGGLES
TOGSOUT
TUGBOAT
TUGGERS
TUGGING
TUGLESS
TUGRIKS
TVGAMES
TVGUIDE

T••G•••

TAGGANT
TAGGERS
TAGGING
TAMGLEN
TANGELO
TANGENT
TANGIER
TANGING
TANGLED
TANGLER
TANGLES
TANGOED
TANGOER
TANGRAM
TARGETS
TEAGOWN
THEGAME
THEGANG
THEGIFT
THEGOLD
THIGPEN
TIEGAME
TINGING
TINGLED
TINGLER
TINGLES
TINGODS
TOGGERY
TOGGING
TOGGLED
TOGGLER
TOGGLES
TOMGOLA
TONGANS
TONGING
TONGUES
TOPGUNS
TOUGHEN
TOUGHER
TOUGHIE
TOUGHLY
TOYGUNS
TRAGEDY
TRIGGER
TRIGONS
TRIGRAM
TUGGERS
TUGGING
TUNGOIL

T•••G••

TANAGER
TEARGAS
THEAGES
THOUGHT
THURGAU
TLINGIT
TONIGHT
TOWAGES
TRAPGUN
TRIAGES
TRIGGER
TROUGHS
TRUDGED
TRUDGEN
TRUDGER
TRUDGES
TSONGAS
TWANGED
TWANGER
TWINGED
TWINGES
TWOEGGS
TYINGIN
TYINGON
TYINGTO
TYINGUP

T••••G•

TAKINGS
TANKAGE
TAPINGS
TEABAGS
TEENAGE
THEBIGA
THEEDGE
THEHOGS
THEMAGI
THRONGS
THROUGH
TIDINGS
TILINGS
TILLAGE
TIMINGS
TOLLAGE
TONNAGE
TOOHIGH
TOPDOGS
TORTUGA
TOWINGS
TOYDOGS
TRILOGY
TWOEGGS

T•••••G

TABBING
TABLING
TABUING
TACKING
TAGALOG
TAGGING
TAILING
TAILWAG
TALKBIG
TALKING
TAMPING
TANGING
TANKING
TANNING
TAPPING
TARRING
TARTING
TASKING
TASTING
TATTING
TAXIING
TEAMING
TEARING
TEASING
TEEMING
TELLING
TEMPING
TENDING
TENSING
TENTING
TENTPEG
TENZING
TERMING
TESTING
TEXTING
THAWING
THEFRUG
THEGANG
THEKING
THERING
TICCING
TICKING
TIDYING
TIERING
TIFFING
TILLING
TILTING
TIMELAG
TINGING
TINNING
TINTING
TIPPING
TITHING
TITLING
TITRING
TOGGING
TOILING
TOLLING
TONGING
TOOLING
TOOLONG

TOOTING
TOPPING
TOSSING
TOTEBAG
TOTTING
TOUAREG
TOURING
TOUTING
TRACING
TRADING
TREEING
TROWING
TRUEING
TSETUNG
TUBBING
TUCKING
TUFTING
TUGGING
TURFING
TURNING
TUSKING
TUTTING
TWINING

•TG••••

ATGRADE
ITGIRLS

•T•G•••

ETAGERE
ITSGONE
STAGERS
STAGGED
STAGGER
STAGIER
STAGILY
STAGING
STAGNES
STIGMAS
STOGIES
STYGIAN

•T••G••

ATEIGHT
ATINGLE
ATNIGHT
ATSIGHT
ATSIGNS
ATTYGEN
MTLOGAN
OTALGIA
OTALGIC
STAGGED
STAGGER
STEIGER
STENGEL
STENGUN
STINGER
STODGED
STODGES
STOOGED
STOOGES
STOPGAP
STREGIS
STUNGUN
STURGES

•T•••G•

ATLARGE
FTBRAGG
FTDODGE
OTOLOGY
STALAGS
STORAGE
STOWAGE
STRANGE
STRINGS
STRINGY

•T••••G

ATONING
ETCHING
FTBRAGG
ITCHING
ITEMING
STAGING
STAKING
STARING
STARLOG
STATING
STAVING
STAYING
STEWING
STOKING
STONING
STORING
STOWING
STUBING
STYLING

••TG•••

BATGIRL
BUTGOOD
CATGUTS
GETGOOD
GOTGOOD
HOTGLUE
JETGUNS
LETGOBY
LETGOOF
NETGAIN
NETGAME
NOTGOOD
OUTGAIN
OUTGAME
OUTGAVE
OUTGAZE
OUTGIVE
OUTGLOW
OUTGNAW
OUTGOES
OUTGREW
OUTGRIN
OUTGROW
OUTGUNS
OUTGUSH
PETGATE
PETGOAT
ROTGUTS
RUTGERS

••T•G••

ANTIGEN
ANTIGUA
ANTIGUN
ATTYGEN
BETTGER
CITYGAL
DOTAGES
ERTEGUN
FATIGUE
GOTOGAL
GOTOGUY
INTEGER
INTEGRA
LATIGOS
LITHGOW
MRTIGER
MUTAGEN
OCTAGON
ORTEGAL
OUTAGES
POTAGES
RITAGAM
UPTIGHT

••T••G•

BLTTOGO
BOTTEGA
CATRIGS
COTTAGE
DATINGS
DETERGE
GATINGS
GOTTAGO
HOTDOGS
JETLAGS
KITBAGS
LETITGO
LETMEGO
LITURGY
NUTMEGS
ONTHEGO
OUTBEGS
OUTEDGE
OUTINGS
OUTRAGE
OUTRIGS
OUTSIGH
PETCAGE
PETDOGS
PETPIGS
POTTAGE
RATINGS
RETINGE
UNTOUGH
WATTAGE
WETRAGS

••T•••G

ALTHING
ANTEING
ANTIFOG
ANTILOG
ARTSONG
AUTOING
BATHING
BATTING
BATWING
BETTING
BITTING
BUTTING
CATALOG
CUTARUG
CUTTING
DOTTING
ESTRING
FATLING
FATTING
FITTING
FUTZING
GATELEG
GATLING
GETTING
GITTING
GSTRING
GUTTING
HATTING
HITSONG
HITTING
HUTTING
INTHING
JETTING
JOTTING
JUTTING
KITTING
LATETAG
LATHING
LETTERG
LETTING
LOTTING
MATTING
MITRING
NETTING
NOTHING
NOTTING
NUTTING
OUTBRAG
OUTDRAG
OUTKING
OUTRANG
OUTRING
OUTSANG
OUTSING
OUTSUNG
OUTWING
PATTING
PETFROG
PETTING
PITHING
PITTING
PITYING
POTTING
PUTTING
RATEDPG
RATTING
RETTING
ROTTING
RUTTING
SETTING
SITTING
TATTING
TITHING
TITLING
TITRING
TOTEBAG
TOTTING
TUTTING
UNTYING
VATTING
VETOING
VETTING
WETTING
WITLING
WITTING

•••TG••

BETTGER
DARTGUN
DUSTGUN
LASTGAS
RJOTGUN
RONTGEN
SHOTGUN
SOFTGEL

•••T•G•

BLTTOGO
BOTTEGA
CARTAGE
CORTEGE
COTTAGE
DOGTAGS
EARTAGS
EASTEGG
ECOTAGE
FLOTAGE
FOOTAGE
GOTTAGO
HOSTAGE
ISITAGO
LENTIGO
MAYTAGS
MELTAGE
MINTAGE
MONTAGE
MONTAGU
MONTEGO
NESTEGG
OAKTAGS
ONETOGO
ONSTAGE
PHOTOGS
PORTAGE
POSTAGE
POTTAGE
PROTEGE
REDTAGS
RESTAGE
ROOTAGE
TORTUGA
UNSTAGY
UPSTAGE
VANTAGE
VENTAGE
VERTIGO
VESTIGE
VINTAGE
VOLTAGE
WANTAGH
WASTAGE
WATTAGE
WAYTOGO
WESTEGG

•••T••G

ABATING
ACHTUNG
BAITING
BANTING
BASTING
BATTING
BEATING
BELTBAG
BELTING
BESTING
BETTING
BITTING
BOATING
BOLTING
BOOTING
BOOTLEG
BUNTING
BUSTING
BUTTING
CANTING
CARTING
CASTING
CHUTING
COATING
COSTING
CRATING
CUTTING
DARTING
DENTING
DIETING
DINTING
DIRTBAG
DOTTING
DUCTING
DUETING
DUSTING
DUSTRAG
EASTEGG
EASTING
EDITING
ELATING
ELUTING
EMOTING
EXITING
FASTING
FATTING
FELTING
FITTING
FLUTING
FOOTBAG
FOOTING
GAITING
GETTING
GIFTING
GIRTING
GITTING
GRATING
GUSTING
GUTTING
HAFTING
HALTING
HASTING
HATTING
HEATING
HEFTING
HILTING
HINTING
HITTING
HOOTING
HOSTING
HUNTING
HURTING
HUTTING
JESTING
JETTING
JILTING
JOLTING
JOTTING
JUTTING
KILTING
KITTING
LASTING
LASTLEG
LEFTLEG
LETTERG
LETTING
LIFTING
LILTING
LINTING
LISTING
LOFTING
LOOTING
LOSTBIG
LOSTDOG
LOTTING
LOUTING
LUSTING
MALTING
MASTING
MATTING
MEETING
MELTING
MINTING
MISTING
MOLTING
MOOTING
MUSTANG
NESTEGG
NESTING
NETTING
NOTTING
NUTTING
ORATING
OUSTING
PANTING
PANTLEG
PARTING
PASTING
PATTING
PEATBOG
PELTING
PETTING
PITTING
PLATING
PORTING
POSTBAG
POSTING
POTTING
POUTING
PRATING
PUNTING
PUTTING
QUOTING
RAFTING
RANTING
RATTING
RENTING
RESTING
RETTING
RIFTING
RIOTING
ROOTING
ROTTING
ROUTING
RRATING
RUSTING
RUTTING
SALTING
SEATING
SETTING
SIFTING
SILTING
SITTING
SKATING
SLATING
SMITING
SORTING
SPITING
STATING
SUITING
TARTING
TASTING
TATTING
TENTING
TENTPEG
TESTING
TEXTING
TILTING
TINTING
TOOTING
TOTTING
TOUTING
TSETUNG
TUFTING
TUTTING
UNITING
UNSTUNG
VATTING
VENTING
VESTING
VETTING
WAFTING
WAITING
WANTING
WARTHOG
WASTING
WELTING
WESTEGG
WETTING
WHITING
WILTING
WITTING
WONTING
WRITING
XRATING
ZEITUNG
ZESTING

••••TG•

DONOTGO
IMUSTGO
LETITGO

••••T•G

FREITAG
FREYTAG
LANDTAG
LATETAG
NAMETAG

•••••TG

SILENTG

TH•••••

THALERS
THANDIE
THANKED
THANKER
THATCHY
THATONE
THATSIT
THATSOK
THATWAY
THAWERS
THAWING
THAWOUT
THEABCS
THEAGES
THEALPS
THEARMY
THEARTS
THEATER
THEATRE
THEAXIS
THEBABE
THEBABY
THEBAND
THEBANS
THEBARD
THEBEAR
THEBELL
THEBEST
THEBIGA
THEBLOB
THEBOBO
THEBODY
THEBOMB
THEBOSS
THEBOYS
THEBRAT
THEBUSH
THECAPE
THECARS
THECAVS
THECITY
THECRAB
THECROW
THECUBS
THEDEEP
THEDELL
THEDIET
THEDOLE
THEDUKE
THEEAST
THEEDGE
THEFALL
THEFEDS
THEFIRM
THEFIVE
THEFLEA
THEFLOP
THEFONZ
THEFOOL
THEFRUG
THEGAME
THEGANG
THEGIFT
THEGOLD
THEHEAT
THEHELP
THEHERO
THEHILL
THEHOGS
THEHOOD
THEHOPE
THEHULK
THEIDEA
THEISMS
THEISTS
THEJERK
THEJETS
THEKING
THEKISS
THELAMB
THELARK
THELEFT
THELIKE
THELOOK
THELOOP
THEMAGI
THEMALL
THEMASK
THEMAVS
THEMAYO
THEMETS
THEMICK
THEMOON
THEMOST
THENETS
THENEWS
THENILE
THEOATH
THEODOR
THEOMEN
THEOMNI
THEOREM
THEPIPS
THEPITS
THEPOND
THEPOOH
THEPOPE
THEPOST
THEPUMP
THERAMS
THERAPY
THEREAT
THEREBY
THEREDS
THEREIN
THERENT
THEREOF
THEREON
THERESA
THERETO
THERIAC
THERING
THERINK
THERITZ
THERMAL
THERMIC
THERMOS
THEROBE
THEROCK
THEROOM
THEROPE
THEROSE
THEROUX
THERULE
THESACK
THESAME
THESELF
THESEUS
THESHOW
THESIMS
THESPIS
THESTAR
THESUNS
THESWAN
THETOUR
THETREE
THETRIB
THETUBE
THETURN
THEUSSR
THEVIEW
THEVIPS
THEWALL
THEWAVE
THEWIND
THEYIPS
THEYSAY
THIAMIN
THICKEN
THICKER
THICKET
THICKLY
THIERRY
THIEVED
THIEVES
THIGPEN
THIMBLE
THIMPHU
THINAIR
THINICE
THINKER
THINKOF
THINKSO
THINKUP
THINMAN
THINNED
THINNER
THINOUT
THIRDLY
THIRSTS
THIRSTY
THISDAY
THISONE
THISTLE
THISTLY
THISWAY
THITHER
THOMSON
THOREAU
THORIUM
THORNED
THORSON
THOUGHT
THRALLS
THREADS
THREADY
THREATS
THREEAD
THREEAM
THREEBC
THREEEE
THREENO
THREEPM
THREERS
THREEUP
THREWAT
THREWIN
THREWON
THREWUP
THRIFTS
THRIFTY
THRILLA
THRILLS
THRIVED
THRIVEN
THRIVER
THRIVES
THROATS
THROATY
THRONES
THRONGS
THROUGH
THROWAT
THROWER
THROWIN
THROWON
THROWUP
THRUPUT
THRUSTS
THRUWAY
THUDDED
THULIUM
THUMBED
THUMPED
THUMPER
THUNDER
THUNKED
THURBER
THURGAU
THURMAN
THUSFAR
THWACKS
THWARTS
THWHITE
THYMINE
THYROID
THYSELF

T•H••••

TAHINIS
TEHERAN
TOHEART
TOHELEN
TOHOMER
TOHORSE
TSHAPED
TSHAPES
TSHIRTS

T••H•••

TACHYON
TARHEEL
TASHLIN
TAXHIKE
TECHIES
TECHNOS
TEEHEED
TEEHEES
TERHUNE
TETHERS
THEHEAT
THEHELP
THEHERO
THEHILL
THEHOGS
THEHOOD
THEHOPE
THEHULK
THWHITE
TIGHTEN
TIGHTER
TIGHTLY
TIMHOLT
TINHATS
TINHORN
TITHERS
TITHING
TOAHAIR
TOEHOLD
TOOHARD
TOOHIGH
TOPHATS
TOPHOLE
TOSHIBA
TOSHIRO
TOWHEAD
TOWHEES
TOYHATS
TOYHOOP
TRYHARD
TUCHMAN
TUSHERY
TUSHIES
TVSHOWS
TWOHOUR
TYPHOID
TYPHOON

T•••H••

TAPSHOE
TEACHER
TEACHES
TEACHIN
TEASHOP
TEESHOT
TEETHED
TEETHER
TEETHES
TEICHER
TENCHES
TENTHLY
THESHOW
THITHER
TOBEHAD
TOESHOE
TOOTHED
TOPTHIS
TORCHED
TORCHER
TORCHES
TOUCHED
TOUCHER
TOUCHES

TOUCHON
TOUCHUP
TOUGHEN
TOUGHER
TOUGHIE
TOUGHLY
TOYSHOP
TRACHEA
TRASHED
TRASHER
TRASHES
TRASHTV
TROCHEE
TROCHES
TROTHED
TWOSHOT

T••••H•

TABITHA
TALLYHO
TEMPEHS
TERAOHM
THATCHY
THIMPHU
THOUGHT
TIMOTHY
TONIGHT
TROUGHS
TWITCHY

T•••••H

TALLISH
TALLITH
TANNISH
TARNISH
TARTISH
THEBUSH
THEOATH
THEPOOH
THROUGH
TIMROTH
TINFISH
TOADISH
TOOHIGH
TOOMUCH
TORYISH
TOWNISH
TOWPATH
TOYWITH
TRIUMPH
TURKISH
TWELFTH

•TH••••

ATHEART
ATHEISM
ATHEIST
ATHIRST
ATHLETE
ATHOMES
ATHRILL
ATHWART
ETHANES
ETHANOL
ETHENES
ETHERIC
ETHICAL
ETHMOID
ETHNICS
ETHENRY
ITHACAN
ITHIRTY
OTHELLO

•T•H•••

ATTHIRD
ATTHREE
ETCHANT
ETCHERS
ETCHING
ITCHFOR
ITCHIER
ITCHING
ITSHERE
UTAHANS

•T••H••

ITSAHIT
MTATHOS
STASHED
STASHES
STEPHEN
STJOHNS

•T•••H•

ATEIGHT
ATNIGHT
ATROPHY
ATSIGHT
ATTACHE
STARCHY
STROPHE
UTRECHT

•T••••H

ATLUNCH
FTWORTH
STAUNCH
STEALTH
STOMACH
STRETCH
STRITCH
STYLISH

••TH•••

ALTHING
ALTHORN
ANTHEIL
ANTHEMS
ANTHERS
ANTHILL
ANTHONY
ANTHRAX
ARTHURC
ARTHURM
ARTHURS
ASTHMAS
ATTHIRD
ATTHREE
AUTHORS
BATHERS
BATHING
BATHMAT
BATHOIL
BATHTUB
BETHANY
BETHELS
BETHERE
BETHINK
BETHUNE
BOTHERS
BOTHNIA
BYTHEBY
CATHAIR
CATHEAD
CATHODE
DITHERS
DITHERY
EATHERE
ENTHRAL
ENTHUSE
ESTHETE
FATHEAD
FATHERS
FATHOMS
FUTHARK
GATHERS
GETHELP
GETHURT
GOTHELP
GOTHICS
GOTHIKA
GOTHURT
GUTHRIE
HITHERE
HITHOME
HOTHAND
HOTHEAD
IDTHEFT
IMTHERE
INTHERE
INTHING
INTHIRD
INTHREE
ISTHMUS
KATHRYN
KITHARA
LATHERS
LATHERY
LATHING
LETHAVE
LETHEAN
LITHELY
LITHEST
LITHGOW
LITHIUM
LITHOID
LOTHAIR
LOTHIAN
LOTHROP
LUTHIER
LUTHULI
MATHERS
MATHEWS
MATHIAS
MATHIEU
METHANE
METHODS
MITHRAS
MOTHERS
MOTHERY
MOTHIER
MPTHREE
MYTHIFY
NATHANS
NOTHERE
NOTHING
NOTHINS
NOTHOME
ONTHEDL
ONTHEGO
ONTHEQT
ONTHREE
OUTHAUL
OUTHEAR
OUTHERE
OUTHIRE
OUTHISS
OUTHITS
OUTHOWL
OUTHUNT
OUTHURL
PATHAND
PATHANS
PATHWAY
PETHAIR
PETHARE
PITHEAD
PITHIER
PITHILY
PITHING
POTHERB
POTHERS
POTHOLE
POTHOOK
PYTHIAN
PYTHIAS
PYTHONS
RATHOLE
RETHANK
RETHAWS
RETHINK
ROTHIRA
RUTHANN
RUTHFUL
SATHOME
SITHOME
SOTHEBY
SOTHERE
SOTHERN
TETHERS
TITHERS
TITHING
UNTHAWS
UNTHICK
UNTHINK
UPTHERE
UPTHROW
WITHERS
WITHIES
WITHOUT
YOTHERS
ZITHERS

••T•H••

AITCHES
ARTSHOP
ARTSHOW
BATCHED
BATCHES
BOTCHED
BOTCHER
BOTCHES
BOTCHUP
BUTCHER
BUTCHES
CATCHER
CATCHES
CATCHON
CATCHOW
CATCHUP
CATSHOW
DITCHED
DITCHER
DITCHES
FETCHED
FETCHER
FETCHES
GETAHIT
GETSHEP
GETSHIP
GETSHOT
GETTHIS
GOTAHIT
GOTCHAS
HATCHED
HATCHER
HATCHES
HATCHET
HITCHED
HITCHER
HITCHES
HITCHON
HITCHUP
HITSHOW
HOTSHOT
HUTCHES
KETCHAM
KETCHES
KETCHUM
KETCHUP
KITCHEN
KUTCHER
LATCHED
LATCHES
LATCHON
LITCHIS
MATCHED
MATCHER
MATCHES
MATCHUP
MATTHAU
MATTHEW
MITCHUM
NATCHEZ
NOTCHED
NOTCHER
NOTCHES
OUTSHOT
OUTSHOW
PATCHED
PATCHEN
PATCHER
PATCHES
PATCHUP
PETCHEW
PETSHOP
PITCHED
PITCHER
PITCHES
PITCHIN
PITCHTO
POTSHOT
RATCHET
RITCHIE
SATCHEL
SATCHMO
SETSHOT
VETCHES
WATCHED
WATCHER
WATCHES
WATCHIT
WATCHTV
WITCHED
WITCHES
YITZHAK

••T••H•

ATTACHE
HITACHI
KATISHA
KITSCHY
MATZOHS
NATASHA
OUTECHO
UPTIGHT
VOTECHS

••T•••H

ANTIOCH
AUTARCH
BETROTH
CATFISH
CATTISH
COTEACH
DOTDASH
DRTEETH
FATOUSH
FATTISH
GETCASH
GOTCASH
HOTBATH
INTOUCH
INTRUTH
JETWASH
LATIFAH
LETTERH
LETTISH
MATZOTH
METWITH
MITZVAH
NOTMUCH
NOTWITH
OSTRICH
OUTFISH
OUTGUSH
OUTLASH
OUTPATH
OUTPUSH
OUTRUSH
OUTSIGH
OUTWASH
OUTWISH
OUTWITH
PATCASH
PETFISH
PETTISH
RATTISH
RETEACH
RETOUCH
RUTTISH
SATWITH
SITWITH
SOTTISH
UNTEACH
UNTOUGH
UNTRUTH
WETTISH
WETWASH

•••TH••

AINTHAY
ALLTHAT
ALLTHIS
ANDTHEN
ANOTHER
APOTHEM
BENTHAM
BENTHOS
BERTHAS
BERTHED
BIRTHED
BLATHER
BLITHER
BOOTHIA
BROTHER
CAUTHEN
CHATHAM
CLOTHED
CLOTHES
CYNTHIA
EARTHED
EARTHEN
EARTHLY
EASTHAM
EPITHET
ERYTHRO
FARTHER
FEATHER
FELTHAT
FIFTHLY
FLATHAT
FROTHED
FROTHER
FROTHUP
FURTHER
GETTHIS
GIRTHED
GODTHAB
GUNTHER
HEATHEN
HEATHER
HOWTHEN
HRETHEL
LEATHER
LEFTHIP
LOATHED
LOATHER
LOATHES
LOATHLY
LOATHTO
MALTHUS
MATTHAU
MATTHEW
MENTHOL
MONTHLY
MOUTHED
MOUTHER
MTATHOS
NARTHEX
NEITHER
NINTHLY
NOOTHER
NORTHER
NORTHOF
NOWTHEN
NOWTHIS
PANTHER
PORTHOS
POSTHOC
PRITHEE
REUTHER
RHYTHMS
ROETHKE
SCATHED
SCATHES
SCYTHED
SCYTHES
SEETHED
SEETHES
SEETHRU
SIXTHLY
SLATHER
SLITHER
SMITHED
SMOTHER
SOOTHED
SOOTHER
SOOTHES
SOUTHEY
SOUTHOF
SPATHES
SWATHED
SWATHES
TEETHED
TEETHER
TEETHES
TENTHLY
THITHER
TOOTHED
TOPTHIS
TROTHED
WALTHAM
WALTHER
WARTHOG
WEATHER
WERTHER
WHETHER
WHITHER
WORTHIT
WRITHED
WRITHER
WRITHES
XANTHAN
XANTHIC
YOUTHEN

•••T•H•

BLOTCHY
CLUTCHY
GLITCHY
IGOTCHA
KVETCHY
SAATCHI
SKETCHY
THATCHY
TWITCHY
WHATTHE

•••T••H

BIOTECH
BRITISH
BRUTISH
CALTECH
CATTISH
COLTISH
CULTISH
DEUTSCH
DIPTYCH
DISTICH
DOLTISH
EPITAPH
FATTISH
GOATISH
GOUTISH
KENTISH
KLATSCH
LABTECH
LEFTISH
LETTERH
LETTISH
LOUTISH
LOWTECH
PELTISH
PETTISH
PICTISH
RATTISH
RUNTISH
RUTTISH
SALTISH
SCITECH
SOFTISH
SOTTISH
TARTISH
WANTAGH
WETTISH
WHITISH

••••TH•

ACANTHI
ASEETHE
BREATHE
BREATHS
BREATHY
BYPATHS
DALETHS
DEARTHS
DEMOTHS
DOROTHY
EIGHTHS
EMPATHS
EMPATHY
EOLITHS
FOURTHS
GROWTHS
HEALTHY
HEARTHS
IOMOTHS
JEPHTHA
LENGTHS
LENGTHY
LESOTHO
NAPHTHA
ORNITHO
PLINTHS
PWBOTHA
REBATHE
SHEATHE
SHEATHS
SLEUTHS
SMOOTHS
SMOOTHY
SWARTHY
TABITHA
TIMOTHY
WEALTHS
WEALTHY
WHATTHE
WRAITHS
WREATHE
WREATHS
WREATHY
ZENITHS

••••T•H

BADITCH
BEWITCH
BYCATCH
CHEETAH
GODUTCH
INDUTCH
NIDETCH
NOCATCH
REHITCH
RELATCH
REMATCH
REPATCH
SAWATCH
SCOOTCH
SCRATCH
SNEETCH
SPLOTCH
STRETCH
STRITCH
UNHITCH
UNLATCH
WASATCH

•••••TH

ABSINTH
ALSMITH
ALWORTH
ASQUITH
AZIMUTH
BEDBATH
BENEATH
BETROTH
BISMUTH
BREADTH
BYBIRTH
BYMOUTH
CORINTH
DELRUTH
DOZENTH
DRTEETH
DYEBATH
FORSYTH
FTWORTH
GOFORTH
GOLIATH
GOSOUTH
GWYNETH
HAWORTH
HIPBATH
HOGARTH
HOTBATH
ICEBATH
INDEPTH
INFAITH
INTRUTH
JACINTH
JAPHETH
JOEROTH
KENNETH
KLAMATH
KNOWETH
KOSSUTH
LAMBETH
LEADETH
LISBETH
MACBETH
MAMMOTH
MATZOTH
METWITH
MRNORTH
MRSMITH
MUDBATH
NCWYETH
NEOLITH
NESMITH
NEWMATH
NOTWITH
ONEARTH
OUTPATH
OUTWITH
RANWITH
REBIRTH
REXROTH
ROBERTH
RUNNETH
RUNWITH
SABBATH
SATWITH
SEVENTH
SILENTH
SITWITH
SOPWITH
STEALTH
SUCCOTH
SUKKOTH
SUNBATH
TALLITH
THEOATH
TIMROTH
TOWPATH
TOYWITH
TWELFTH
UNBERTH
UNCOUTH
UNEARTH
UNFAITH
UNFERTH
UNLOATH
UNTRUTH
UPNORTH
VIEWITH
WARPATH

TI•••••

TIARAED
TIBBETT
TIBETAN
TIBURON
TICCING
TICKERS
TICKETS
TICKING
TICKLED
TICKLER
TICKLES
TICKOFF
TICKSBY
TICOTIN
TICTACS
TIDALLY
TIDBITS
TIDERIP
TIDIEST
TIDINGS
TIDYING
TIDYSUM
TIEBACK
TIEBARS
TIEBEAM
TIECLIP
TIEDOFF
TIEDOWN
TIEDYED
TIEDYES
TIEGAME
TIEINTO
TIELESS
TIELINE
TIEMPOS
TIENDAS
TIEPINS
TIEPOLO
TIERACK
TIERCES
TIERING
TIERNEY
TIERODS
TIEROPE
TIESOFF
TIETACK
TIETACS
TIFFANY
TIFFING
TIFFINS
TIGHTEN
TIGHTER
TIGHTLY
TIGLONS
TIGRESS
TIJUANA
TILINGS
TILLAGE
TILLERS
TILLETS
TILLING
TILLNOW
TILSITS
TILTERS
TILTING
TILTSAT
TILTSUP
TILTTOP
TIMBALE
TIMBALS
TIMBERS
TIMBERY
TIMBRES
TIMECOP
TIMELAG
TIMEOFF
TIMEOUT
TIMESUP
TIMEWAS
TIMEXES
TIMHOLT
TIMIDER
TIMIDLY
TIMINGS
TIMMINS
TIMOTHY
TIMPANI
TIMREID
TIMRICE
TIMROTH
TINAFEY
TINAMOU
TINCANS
TINCTED
TINDERS
TINDERY
TINEARS
TINFISH
TINFOIL
TINGING
TINGLED
TINGLER
TINGLES
TINGODS
TINHATS
TINHORN
TINIEST
TINKERS
TINKLED
TINKLER
TINKLES
TINLIKE
TINMINE
TINNERS
TINNIER
TINNILY
TINNING
TINORES
TINROOF
TINSELS
TINSTAR
TINTERN
TINTERS
TINTING
TINTYPE
TINWARE
TINWORK
TINYBIT
TINYTIM
TINYTOT
TIOMKIN
TIPCART
TIPDOWN
TIPJARS
TIPLESS

TIPLINE
TIPOFFS
TIPOVER
TIPPEES
TIPPERS
TIPPETS
TIPPIER
TIPPING
TIPPLED
TIPPLER
TIPPLES
TIPSIER
TIPSILY
TIPSOFF
TIPSTER
TIPTOED
TIPTOES
TIPTOPS
TIRADES
TIREDER
TIREDLY
TIREDOF
TIREMAN
TIREMEN
TIREOUT
TIRESOF
TIRPITZ
TISANES
TISSOTS
TISSUES
TISSUEY
TITANAE
TITANIA
TITANIC
TITHERS
TITHING
TITIANS
TITLARK
TITLING
TITLIST
TITMICE
TITOISM
TITOIST
TITRATE
TITRING
TITTERS
TITTLES
TITULAR
TIZZIES

T•I••••

TAILEND
TAILERS
TAILFIN
TAILING
TAILOFF
TAILORS
TAILPIN
TAILWAG
TAINTED
TBILISI
TEICHER
THIAMIN
THICKEN
THICKER
THICKET
THICKLY
THIERRY
THIEVED
THIEVES
THIGPEN
THIMBLE
THIMPHU
THINAIR
THINICE
THINKER
THINKOF
THINKSO
THINKUP
THINMAN
THINNED
THINNER
THINOUT
THIRDLY
THIRSTS
THIRSTY
THISDAY
THISONE
THISTLE
THISTLY
THISWAY
THITHER
TLINGIT
TOILERS
TOILETS
TOILFUL
TOILING
TOILSAT
TRIABLE
TRIADIC
TRIAGES
TRIBBLE
TRIBECA
TRIBORO
TRIBUNE
TRIBUTE
TRICEPS
TRICKED
TRICKER
TRICKLE
TRICORN
TRICOTS
TRIDENT
TRIEDIT
TRIEDON
TRIEDTO
TRIESIT
TRIESON
TRIESTE
TRIESTO
TRIFFID
TRIFLED
TRIFLER
TRIFLES
TRIFOLD
TRIFORM
TRIGGER
TRIGONS
TRIGRAM
TRIJETS
TRILLED
TRILLER
TRILLIN
TRILOGY
TRIMMED
TRIMMER
TRIMOFF
TRIMTAB
TRINARY
TRINITY
TRINKET
TRIODES
TRIOLET
TRIPLEA
TRIPLED
TRIPLES
TRIPLET
TRIPLEX
TRIPODS
TRIPOLI
TRIPPED
TRIPPER
TRIPPET
TRIPSON
TRIPSUP
TRIREME
TRISECT
TRISTAN
TRISTAR
TRITELY
TRITEST
TRITIUM
TRITONE
TRITONS
TRIUMPH
TRIVETS
TRIVIAL
TRIVIOT
TRIVIUM
TUILLES
TUITION
TVIDOLS
TWIDDLE
TWILLED
TWINBED
TWINERS
TWINGED
TWINGES
TWINIER
TWINING
TWINJET
TWINKIE
TWINKLE
TWINKLY
TWINNED
TWINSET
TWIRLED
TWIRLER
TWISTED
TWISTER
TWISTON
TWISTUP
TWITCHY
TWITTED
TWITTER
TYINGIN
TYINGON
TYINGTO
TYINGUP
TZIMMES

T••I•••

TABITHA
TACITLY
TACITUS
TAHINIS
TAKINGS
TALIBAN
TAMIAMI
TAOISTS
TAPINGS
TAPINTO
TAPIOCA
TARIFFS
TATIANA
TAXICAB
TAXIING
TAXIMAN
TAXIMEN
TAXIWAY
TEDIOUS
TEDIUMS
TEEITUP
TEPIDLY
THEIDEA
THEISMS
THEISTS
THRIFTS
THRIFTY
THRILLA
THRILLS
THRIVED
THRIVEN
THRIVER
THRIVES
TIDIEST
TIDINGS
TIEINTO
TILINGS
TIMIDER
TIMIDLY
TIMINGS
TINIEST
TITIANS
TONIEST
TONIGHT
TOPIARY
TOPICAL
TORINOS
TOTINOS
TOWINGS
TRAILED
TRAILER
TRAINED
TRAINEE
TRAINER
TRAININ
TRAIPSE
TRAITOR
TREINTA
TREIZES
TROIKAS
TROILUS
TRUISMS
TRYITON
TSHIRTS
TUBISTS
TUNICLE
TUNISIA
TURISMO
TURISTA
TWOIRON
TYPICAL
TYPISTS

T•••I••

TABBIES
TABBING
TABLING
TABUING
TACKIER
TACKILY
TACKING
TACTICS
TACTILE
TAFFIES
TAGGING
TAGLIKE
TAGLINE
TAILING
TAKEILL
TAKEINS
TALKIER
TALKIES
TALKING
TALLIED
TALLIER
TALLIES
TALLINN
TALLISH
TALLITH
TAMPICO
TAMPING
TANGIER
TANGING
TANKING
TANKINI
TANLINE
TANNING
TANNINS
TANNISH
TANSIES
TANTIVY
TAPPING
TARDIER
TARDILY
TARNISH
TAROILS
TARPITS
TARRIED
TARRIER
TARRIES
TARRING
TARTIER
TARTILY
TARTING
TARTISH
TASKING
TASTIER
TASTILY
TASTING
TATTIER
TATTILY
TATTING
TAURINE
TAWNIER
TAWNILY
TAXHIKE
TAXIING
TBILISI
TEAMING
TEARIER
TEARILY
TEARING
TEASING
TEATIME
TECHIES
TEDDIES
TEEMING
TEENIER
TEETIME
TEKKIES
TELLIES
TELLING
TEMPING
TENDING
TENMILE
TENNIEL
TENNIES
TENPINS
TENSILE
TENSING
TENSION
TENSITY
TENSIVE
TENTING
TENUITY
TENZING
TEQUILA
TERBIUM
TERMING
TERMINI
TERMITE
TERRIER
TERRIES
TERRIFY
TERRINE
TESTIER
TESTIFY
TESTILY
TESTING
TEXTILE
TEXTING
THAWING
THEBIGA
THECITY
THEDIET
THEFIRM
THEFIVE
THEGIFT
THEHILL
THEKING
THEKISS
THELIKE
THEMICK
THENILE
THEPIPS
THEPITS
THERIAC
THERING
THERINK
THERITZ
THESIMS
THEVIEW
THEVIPS
THEWIND
THEYIPS
THINICE
THORIUM
THULIUM
THWHITE
THYMINE
TICCING
TICKING
TIDBITS
TIDYING
TIELINE
TIEPINS
TIERING
TIFFING
TIFFINS
TILLING
TILSITS
TILTING
TIMMINS
TIMRICE
TINFISH
TINGING
TINLIKE
TINMINE
TINNIER
TINNILY
TINNING
TINTING
TIPLINE
TIPPIER
TIPPING
TIPSIER
TIPSILY
TIRPITZ
TITHING
TITLING
TITLIST
TITMICE
TITOISM
TITOIST
TITRING
TIZZIES
TMOBILE
TOADIED
TOADIES
TOADISH
TOCSINS
TODDIES
TOELIKE
TOEPICK
TOGGING
TOILING
TOLKIEN
TOLLING
TOMKITE
TOMTITS
TONGING
TONSILS
TONTINE
TOOHIGH
TOOKILL
TOOLING
TOONIES
TOOTING
TOPBIDS
TOPFIVE
TOPKICK
TOPLINE
TOPPING
TOPSIDE
TOROIDS
TORSION
TORVILL
TORYISH
TORYISM
TOSHIBA
TOSHIRO
TOSSING
TOTTING
TOURING
TOURISM
TOURIST
TOUTING
TOWLINE
TOWNIES
TOWNISH
TOYBIKE
TOYKITE
TOYLIKE
TOYWITH
TRACING
TRADING
TREDIAS
TREEING
TREVINO
TRINITY
TRITIUM
TRIVIAL
TRIVIOT
TRIVIUM
TROPICS
TROPISM
TROWING
TRUEING
TSARINA
TSARISM
TSARIST
TSELIOT
TUBAIST
TUBBIER
TUBBING
TUBLIKE
TUCKING
TUFTIER
TUFTING
TUGGING
TUGRIKS
TUITION
TUMMIES
TURBINE
TURFIER
TURFING
TURKISH
TURNING
TURNIPS
TUSHIES
TUSKING
TUSSIVE
TUTTING
TUTUILA
TVGUIDE
TWINIER
TWINING
TWOBITS
TWOTIME
TZARINA

T••••I•

TABLOID
TACONIC
TAHINIS
TAILFIN
TAILPIN
TAKEAIM
TAKENIN
TAKESIN
TAKESIT
TALARIA
TALKBIG
TASHLIN
TASTEIT
TATAMIS
TAXPAID
TEACHIN
TEARSIT
TEENSIE
TELAVIV
TELEPIC
TELEPIX
TELLSIT
TENDRIL
TERRAIN
TERROIR
TESTKIT
THANDIE
THATSIT
THEAXIS
THEREIN
THERMIC
THESPIS
THETRIB
THIAMIN
THINAIR
THREWIN
THROWIN
THYROID
TICOTIN
TIDERIP
TIECLIP
TIMREID
TINFOIL
TINYBIT
TINYTIM
TIOMKIN
TITANIA
TITANIC
TLINGIT
TOAHAIR
TOCELIA
TOENAIL
TOOKAIM
TOOLKIT
TOOTSIE
TOPSAIL
TOPSOIL
TOPSPIN
TOPTHIS
TOTEMIC
TOUGHIE
TOWEDIN
TOYFAIR
TOYPAIL
TRADEIN
TRAFFIC
TRAININ
TRANSIT
TRAVAIL
TREFOIL
TREKKIE
TRELLIS
TRIADIC
TRIEDIT
TRIESIT
TRIFFID
TRILLIN
TROMPIN
TROOPIN
TRUERIB
TRUSTIN
TRYSAIL
TSOURIS
TUCKSIN
TUNAOIL
TUNEDIN
TUNESIN
TUNGOIL
TUNISIA
TURMOIL
TURNSIN
TVMOVIE
TWINKIE
TWOONIE
TWOPAIR
TWOUNIT
TYINGIN
TYPEDIN
TYPESIN
TYPHOID

T•••••I

TABOULI
TAMIAMI
TANKINI
TBILISI
TEBALDI
TERMINI
THEMAGI
THEOMNI
TIMPANI
TOFUTTI
TOLSTOI
TOPKAPI
TORTONI
TRIPOLI
TSUNAMI
TURFSKI
TYMPANI

•TI••••

ATINGLE
ATIPTOE
ATISSUE
ETICKET
ETIENNE
ITISTOO
STICKBY
STICKER
STICKIN
STICKON
STICKTO
STICKUM
STICKUP
STIFFED
STIFFEL
STIFFEN
STIFFER
STIFFLY
STIFLED
STIFLES
STIGMAS
STILLED
STILLER
STILLUP
STILTED
STILTON
STIMSON
STIMULI
STINGER
STINKER
STINKUP
STINTED
STINTER
STIPEND
STIPPLE
STIRFRY
STIRRED
STIRRER
STIRRUP
STIRSIN
STIRSUP
UTICANS
UTICANY
UTILISE
UTILITY
UTILIZE

•T•I•••

ATEIGHT
ATEINTO
ATEITUP
ATFIRST
ATHIRST
ATNIGHT
ATRIUMS
ATSIGHT
ATSIGNS
ATTICUS
ATTIMES
ATTIRED
ATTIRER
ATTIRES
ETAILED
ETAILER
ETHICAL
ETOILES
FTDIXNJ
FTRILEY
ITGIRLS
ITHIRTY
MTSINAI
STAIDER
STAIDLY
STAINED
STAINER
STAIRED
STEIGER
STEINEM
STEINER
STKITTS
STOICAL
STPIUSI
STPIUSV
STPIUSX
STRIATE
STRIDER
STRIDES
STRIFES
STRIKER
STRIKES
STRINGS
STRINGY
STRIPED
STRIPER
STRIPES
STRIPOF
STRITCH
STRIVED
STRIVEN
STRIVER
STRIVES
STSIMON
UTRILLO

•T••I••

ATATILT
ATATIME
ATAVISM
ATAVIST
ATEDIRT
ATELIER
ATHEISM
ATHEIST
ATHRILL
ATOMICS
ATOMIES
ATOMISE
ATOMISM
ATOMIST
ATOMIZE
ATONICS
ATONIES
ATONING
ATTAINS
ATTAINT
ATTHIRD
ATTRITE
ATTRITS
ETALIBI
ETAMINE
ETCHING
ETESIAN
ETHNICS
ETONIAN
ETONICS
ETVOILA
FTBLISS
ITALIAN
ITALICS
ITCHIER
ITCHING
ITEMING
ITEMISE
ITEMIZE
ITSFINE
ITSTIME
OTARIES
OTTOIII
STABILE
STADIUM
STAGIER
STAGILY
STAGING
STAKING
STAMINA
STANINE
STARING
STARION
STATICE
STATICS
STATING
STATINS
STATION
STATISM
STATIST
STAVING
STAYING
STELIAS
STEPINS
STERILE
STEWIER
STEWING
STOGIES
STOKING
STONIER
STONILY
STONING
STORIED
STORIES
STORING
STOTINS
STOWING
STRAINS
STRAITS
STUBING
STUDIED
STUDIER
STUDIES
STUDIOS
STUPIDS
STYGIAN
STYLING
STYLISE
STYLISH
STYLIST
STYLIZE
STYMIED
STYMIES
UTILISE
UTILITY
UTILIZE
UTOPIAN
UTOPIAS
UTOPISM
UTOPIST
YTTRIAS
YTTRIUM

•T•••I•

ATABOIL
ATACLIP
ATEABIT
CTENOID
ETHERIC
ETHMOID
ETRURIA
ITSAHIT
ITSALIE

ITSASIN
ITSATIE
KTOSLIN
OTALGIA
OTALGIC
OTTAVIO
OTTOIII
STANDIN
STANNIC
STARLIT
STARSIN
STARTIN
STAYSIN
STBASIL
STCROIX
STDENIS
STEALIN
STEARIC
STEARIN
STEELIE
STEEPIN
STENCIL
STENNIS
STEPSIN
STEROID
STICKIN
STIRSIN
STLOUIS
STLUCIA
STOLEIN
STOMPIN
STOODIN
STOOLIE
STOPSIN
STOPSIT
STORMIN
STOWSIT
STRAPIN
STREGIS
STUCKIN
STUFFIN
STYPSIS
STYPTIC
UTENSIL

•T••••I

ETALIBI
MTSINAI
OTTOIII
STEFANI
STIMULI
STPIUSI
STRETTI
STUARTI

••TI•••

ACTIFED
ACTINON
ACTIONS
ACTIVAS
ACTIVES
ALTIMAS
ANTIART
ANTIBES
ANTIFOG
ANTIGEN
ANTIGUA
ANTIGUN
ANTILOG
ANTIOCH
ANTIQUE
ANTITAX
ANTIWAR
ARTICLE
ARTIEST
ARTISAN
ARTISTE
ARTISTS
ATTICUS
ATTIMES
ATTIRED
ATTIRER
ATTIRES
AUTISTS
BATIKED
BATISTA
BATISTE
BETIDED
BETIDES
BETIMES
CATIONS
CITIZEN
CUTICLE
CUTINON
CUTINTO
CUTISES
DATINGS
DATIVES
DUTIFUL
EATINTO
EATITUP
ENTICED
ENTICER
ENTICES
ENTIRES
ENTITLE
ESTIVAL
EXTINCT
FATIDIC
FATIGUE
FETIDLY
FITINTO
GATINGS
GETINON
GETINTO
GETITON
GOTINON
GOTINTO
GOTITON
HITINTO
HOTITEM
ICTINUS
IMTIRED
KATISHA
LATICES
LATIFAH
LATIGOS
LATIMES
LATINAS
LATINII
LATINOS
LATINUS
LETINON
LETITBE
LETITGO
LETITIA
LITINTO
LOTIONS
LUTISTS
MATILDA
MATINAL
MATINEE
MATISSE
METIERS
MOTIONS
MOTIVED
MOTIVES
MRTIBBS
MRTIGER
NATIONS
NATIVES
NETIZEN
NOTICED
NOTICER
NOTICES
NOTIONS
NYTIMES
OPTICAL
OPTICKS
OPTIMAL
OPTIMAS
OPTIMUM
OPTIONS
OSTIARY
OUTINGS
PATIENT
PATINAS
PETIOLE
PETITES
PITIERS
PITIFUL
PITILLO
POTIONS
PUTITTO
RATINES
RATINGS
RATIONS
RATITES
RETIARY
RETICLE
RETILED
RETILES
RETILLS
RETIMED
RETIMES
RETINAE
RETINAL
RETINAS
RETINGE
RETINOL
RETINTS
RETINUE
RETIRED
RETIREE
RETIRES
RETITLE
ROTIFER
RUTILES
SATIATE
SATIETY
SATINET
SATINON
SATIRES
SATIRIC
SATISFY
SETINTO
SHTICKS
SHTICKY
SITINON
TATIANA
TITIANS
TOTINOS
ULTIMAS
UNTIERS
UNTILED
UNTIMED
UNTIMID
UNTIRED
UPTICKS
UPTIGHT
UPTILTS
UPTIMES
USTINOV
VATICAL
VATICAN
VITIATE
VOTIVES

••T•I••

ACTFIVE
ACTLIKE
ALTHING
ALTOIDS
ALTOIST
ANTBIRD
ANTEING
ANTHILL
ANTLIKE
ANTLION
ANTOINE
ANTSIER
ARTFILM
ARTSIER
ASTAIRE
ASTRIDE
ATTAINS
ATTAINT
ATTHIRD
ATTRITE
ATTRITS
AUTOING
BATGIRL
BATHING
BATLIKE
BATTIER
BATTING
BATWING
BETHINK
BETTING
BETWIXT
BITSIER
BITTIER
BITTING
BUTTING
CATBIRD
CATFISH
CATFITS
CATKINS
CATLIKE
CATMINT
CATNIPS
CATRIGS
CATSITS
CATTIER
CATTILY
CATTISH
CITRINE
CUTTIME
CUTTING
DATRILS
DETAILS
DETAINS
DITSIER
DITTIES
DITZIER
DOTLIKE
DOTRICE
DOTTIER
DOTTILY
DOTTING
EATDIRT
ENTAILS
ENTRIES
ENTWINE
ENTWIST
ESTRING
FATCITY
FATLIKE
FATLING
FATLIPS
FATTIER
FATTILY
FATTING
FATTISH
FATUITY
FITTING
FUTZING
GATLING
GATLINS
GATWICK
GETTING
GETWISE
GITTING
GOTHICS
GOTHIKA
GOTMILK
GOTWISE
GSTRING
GUTSIER
GUTSILY
GUTTIER
GUTTING
HATLIKE
HATPINS
HATSIZE
HATTING
HITFILM
HITLIST
HITTING
HITTITE
HOTLICK
HOTLINE
HOTLINK
HOTLIPS
HOTMILK
HOTPINK
HOTTIES
HOTTIME
HOTTIPS
HOTWIRE
HUTLIKE
HUTTING
IATRICS
INTAILS
INTHING
INTHIRD
INTUITS
ISTRIAN
JETFIRE
JETTIED
JETTIES
JETTING
JOTTING
JUTTING
KATRINA
KATRINE
KITTIES
KITTING
LATHING
LATRINE
LATTICE
LATVIAN
LETLIVE
LETRIDE
LETTING
LETTISH
LITHIUM
LOTHIAN
LOTTING
LUTHIER
MATHIAS
MATHIEU
MATTING
METLIFE
METRICS
METRIST
METWITH
MITRING
MOTHIER
MOTRINS
MYTHIFY
NATRIUM
NATTIER
NATTILY
NATWICK
NETLIKE
NETTING
NITPICK
NITRIDE
NITRIFY
NITRITE
NITTIER
NITWITS
NOTHING
NOTHINS
NOTLIKE
NOTLIVE
NOTMINE
NOTNICE
NOTTING
NOTWITH
NUTLIKE
NUTOILS
NUTPINE
NUTRIAS
NUTSIER
NUTTIER
NUTTILY
NUTTING
OATLIKE
OBTAINS
ONTRIAL
OSTRICH
OTTOIII
OUTBIDS
OUTCITY
OUTFIND
OUTFIRE
OUTFISH
OUTFITS
OUTGIVE
OUTHIRE
OUTHISS
OUTHITS
OUTJINX
OUTKICK
OUTKILL
OUTKING
OUTKISS
OUTLIER
OUTLIES
OUTLIMN
OUTLINE
OUTLIPS
OUTLIVE
OUTPICK
OUTPIPE
OUTPITY
OUTRIBS
OUTRIDE
OUTRIGS
OUTRING
OUTSIDE
OUTSIFT
OUTSIGH
OUTSING
OUTSINS
OUTSITS
OUTSIZE
OUTTIRE
OUTVIED
OUTVIES
OUTWILE
OUTWILL
OUTWIND
OUTWING
OUTWISH
OUTWITH
OUTWITS
OXTAILS
PATRICE
PATRICK
PATRIES
PATRIOT
PATSIES
PATTIES
PATTING
PETBIRD
PETFISH
PETLION
PETMICE
PETPIGS
PETRIFY
PETSITS
PETTIER
PETTILY
PETTING
PETTISH
PITHIER
PITHILY
PITHING
PITTING
PITYING
POTLIDS
POTPIES
POTTIER
POTTIES
POTTING
PUTTIED
PUTTIES
PUTTING
PYTHIAN
PYTHIAS
RATFINK
RATLIKE
RATLINE
RATLINS
RATTIER
RATTING
RATTISH
RETAILS
RETAINS
RETHINK
RETRIAL
RETRIED
RETRIES
RETRIMS
RETSINA
RETTING
RETWINE
RETWIST
RITZIER
RITZILY
ROTHIRA
ROTTING
RUTTIER
RUTTING
RUTTISH
SATWITH
SETTING
SITTING
SITWITH
SOTTISH
TATTIER
TATTILY
TATTING
TITHING
TITLING
TITLIST
TITMICE
TITOISM
TITOIST
TITRING
TOTTING
TUTTING
TUTUILA
UNTHICK
UNTHINK
UNTRIED
UNTRITE
UNTWINE
UNTWIST
UNTYING
VATTING
VETOING
VETTING
VITRICS
VITRIFY
VITRINE
VITRIOL
WATKINS
WETKISS
WETTING
WETTISH
WITHIES
WITLING
WITTIER
WITTILY
WITTING
YETTIES
YTTRIAS
YTTRIUM

••T••I•

ACTEDIN
ANTACID
ANTHEIL
ANTONIA
ANTONIN
ANTONIO
ARTEMIS
ARTERIO
ARTFAIR
ASTERIX
ASTORIA
AUTOBIO
AUTOPIA
BATAVIA
BATHOIL
BATSUIT
BITESIN
BOTANIC
BOTHNIA
BUTTSIN
BYTRAIN
CATANIA
CATHAIR
CATSUIT
CATTAIL
CETERIS
COTERIE
DETRAIN
DETROIT
EATABIT
ELTRAIN
ENTERIC
ENTERIN
ENTRAIN
ESTAMIN
ESTONIA
ESTORIL
FATIDIC
GETAHIT
GETATIP
GETONIT
GETSFIT
GETSHIP
GETSRID
GETTHIS
GETTOIT
GOTAHIT
GOTATIP
GOTONIT
GOTTOIT
GUTHRIE
HATBRIM
HATEDIT
HATESIT
HOTMAIL
INTERIM
INTROIT
ISTOMIN
JETFOIL
JETSKIS
KATYDID
KETONIC
LATINII
LETEMIN
LETITIA
LETMEIN
LETSLIP
LETSRIP
LITCHIS
LITCRIT
LITHOID
LOTHAIR
LUTETIA
MATALIN
MITOSIS
MITOTIC
NATALIA
NATALIE
NETFLIX
NETGAIN
NOTABIT
NOTALIE
NOTFAIR
OCTADIC
OCTAVIA
OCTAVIO
OCTROIS
ONTARIO
ONTOPIC
OPTEDIN
OSTEOID
OSTOSIS
OTTAVIO
OTTOIII
OUTGAIN
OUTGRIN
OUTLAID
OUTLAIN
OUTOFIT
OUTPAID
OUTRAIL
OUTSAID
OUTSAIL
OUTSKIP
OUTSPIN
OUTSPIT
OUTSWIM
OUTWAIT
PETERII
PETHAIR
PETULIA
PETUNIA
PITCHIN
POTBOIL
QATARIS
RATAFIA
RATTAIL
RETRAIN
RITALIN
RITCHIE
RITEAID
SATANIC
SATIRIC
SATORIS
SATYRIC
SETBAIL
SETSAIL
SITONIT
TATAMIS
TITANIA
TITANIC
TOTEMIC
UNTIMID
UNTOXIC
VITALIS
VITAMIN
VITORIA
VOTEDIN
VOTESIN
WATCHIT
WATUSIS
WETSUIT

••T•••I

HITACHI
LATINII
LETTERI
LUTHULI
OTTOIII
PETERII

•••TI••

ABATING
ABITIBI
ACETIFY
AGATINE
AIRTIME
ALLTIED
ALLTIME
AMATIVE
AMITIES
ANYTIME
APATITE
ARETINO
ASSTIFF
ATATILT
ATATIME
AUCTION
AUNTIES
AUSTINS
BADTIME
BAITING
BANTING
BAPTISE
BAPTISM
BAPTIST
BAPTIZE
BASTING
BASTION
BATTIER
BATTING
BEATIFY
BEATING
BEDTIME
BEETIER
BELTING
BESTIAL
BESTILL
BESTING
BESTIRS
BETTING
BIGTIME
BIOTITE
BITTIER
BITTING
BOATING
BOLTING
BOOTIES
BOOTING
BOWTIES
BRITISH
BRUTISH
BUDTIME
BUNTING
BUSTIER
BUSTING
BUTTING
BUYTIME
CANTILY
CANTINA
CANTING
CANTINO
CAPTION
CAPTIVA
CAPTIVE
CARTIER
CARTING
CARTIRE
CASTILE
CASTING
CATTIER
CATTILY
CATTISH
CAUTION
CELTICS
CENTIME
CENTIMO
CERTIFY
CHUTING
CHUTIST
COATING
COLTISH
COMTISM
COMTIST
COOTIES
CORTICO
CORTINA
COSTING
COSTIVE
CRATING
CRATION
CRETINS
CRITIAS
CRITICS
CUETIPS
CULTISH
CULTISM
CULTIST
CURTISS
CUTTIME
CUTTING
DARTING
DAYTIME
DEITIES
DENTINE
DENTING
DENTINS
DENTIST
DESTINE
DESTINO
DESTINY
DICTION
DIDTIME
DIETING
DINTING
DIOTIMA
DIRTIED
DIRTIER
DIRTIES
DIRTILY
DISTICH
DISTILL
DISTILS
DITTIES
DOGTICK
DOLTISH
DOTTIER
DOTTILY
DOTTING
DUCTILE
DUCTING
DUETING
DUSTIER
DUSTILY
DUSTING
EASTING
EBBTIDE
EDITING
EDITION
EGOTISM
EGOTIST
ELATING
ELATION
ELITISM
ELITIST
ELUTING
ELUTION
EMETICS
EMOTING
EMOTION
EMOTIVE
EMPTIED
EMPTIER
EMPTIES
EMPTILY
EROTICA
EROTICS
EXITING
EXOTICA
EXOTICS
EXOTISM
FACTION
FANTINE
FASTING
FATTIER
FATTILY
FATTING
FATTISH
FELTILL
FELTING

FERTILE
FESTINA
FESTIVA
FESTIVE
FICTILE
FICTION
FICTIVE
FIFTIES
FITTING
FLUTIER
FLUTIES
FLUTING
FLUTIST
FLYTIER
FONTINA
FOOTING
FORTIES
FORTIFY
FORTIUS
FUNTIME
FURTIVE
FUSTIAN
FUSTIER
FUSTILY
GAITING
GAUTIER
GENTIAN
GENTILE
GETTING
GIFTING
GIRTING
GITTING
GOATISH
GOUTIER
GOUTILY
GOUTISH
GRATIAS
GRATIFY
GRATING
GROTIUS
GUSTIER
GUSTILY
GUSTING
GUTTIER
GUTTING
HADTIME
HAFTING
HAITIAN
HALTING
HAPTICS
HASTIER
HASTILY
HASTIME
HASTING
HATTING
HEATING
HEFTIER
HEFTILY
HEFTING
HILTING
HINTING
HITTING
HITTITE
HOGTIED
HOGTIES
HOOTING
HOSTILE
HOSTING
HOTTIES
HOTTIME
HOTTIPS
HUNTING
HURTING
HUTTING
INITIAL
INSTILL
INSTILS
INUTILE
ITSTIME
IZATION
JESTING
JETTIED
JETTIES
JETTING
JIGTIME
JILTING
JOLTIER
JOLTING
JOTTING
JUSTICE
JUSTIFY
JUSTINE
JUTTING
KANTIAN
KENTISH
KILTIES
KILTING
KITTIES
KITTING
KONTIKI
KRATION
LAITIES
LAOTIAN
LASTING
LATTICE
LEETIDE
LEFTIES
LEFTISH
LEFTISM
LEFTIST
LENTIGO
LENTILS
LETTING
LETTISH
LIFTING
LILTING
LINTIER
LINTING
LISTING
LOFTIER
LOFTILY
LOFTING
LOOTING
LOTTING
LOUTING
LOUTISH
LOWTIDE
LUSTIER
LUSTILY
LUSTING
MALTIER
MALTING
MARTIAL
MARTIAN
MARTINA
MARTINI
MARTINO
MARTINS
MARTINU
MARTINV
MARTIUS
MASTICS
MASTIFF
MASTING
MATTING
MAYTIME
MEATIER
MEATILY
MEETING
MELTING
MENTION
MINTIER
MINTING
MISTIER
MISTILY
MISTIME
MISTING
MOLTING
MOOTING
MORTICE
MORTIFY
MORTISE
MUSTIER
MUSTILY
MYSTICS
MYSTIFY
NAPTIME
NASTIER
NASTIES
NASTILY
NATTIER
NATTILY
NAUTICA
NAUTILI
NESTING
NETTING
NIFTIER
NIFTIES
NIFTILY
NITTIER
NOETICS
NOTTING
NUPTIAL
NUTTIER
NUTTILY
NUTTING
OLDTIME
ONETIME
ORATING
ORATION
OUSTING
OUTTIRE
OVATION
PANTIES
PANTILE
PANTING
PARTIAL
PARTIED
PARTIER
PARTIES
PARTIII
PARTING
PARTITA
PARTITE
PASTIER
PASTIES
PASTIME
PASTINA
PASTING
PATTIES
PATTING
PEATIER
PECTINS
PELTING
PELTISH
PENTIUM
PEPTICS
PEPTIDE
PETTIER
PETTILY
PETTING
PETTISH
PHOTICS
PICTISH
PIETIES
PIETINS
PISTILS
PITTING
PLATIER
PLATIES
PLATING
POETICA
POETICS
POETISE
POETIZE
POITIER
PONTIAC
PONTIAN
PONTIFF
PONTIUS
PORTICO
PORTING
PORTION
POSTIES
POSTING
POSTITS
POTTIER
POTTIES
POTTING
POUTIER
POUTING
PRATING
PRETIRE
PROTIST
PUNTING
PURTIER
PUTTIED
PUTTIES
PUTTING
QRATIOS
QUOTING
RAFTING
RAGTIME
RANTING
RATTIER
RATTING
RATTISH
RECTIFY
REDTIDE
REDTIES
RENTIER
RENTING
REPTILE
RESTICK
RESTING
RESTIRS
RESTIVE
RETTING
RIFTING
RIOTING
RIPTIDE
RLSTINE
ROOTIER
ROOTING
ROTTING
ROUTINE
ROUTING
RRATING
RUCTION
RUNTIER
RUNTIME
RUNTISH
RUSTICS
RUSTIER
RUSTILY
RUSTING
RUTTIER
RUTTING
RUTTISH
SALTIER
SALTILY
SALTINE
SALTING
SALTISH
SANTINI
SCHTICK
SCOTIAN
SEATING
SECTION
SESTINA
SETTING
SHUTINS
SIFTING
SILTIER
SILTING
SISTINE
SITTING
SIXTIES
SKATING
SLATIER
SLATING
SMITING
SOFTIES
SOFTISH
SOOTIER
SOOTILY
SORTIED
SORTIES
SORTING
SOTTISH
SPATIAL
SPITING
STATICE
STATICS
STATING
STATINS
STATION
STATISM
STATIST
STOTINS
SUCTION
SUITING
TACTICS
TACTILE
TANTIVY
TARTIER
TARTILY
TARTING
TARTISH
TASTIER
TASTILY
TASTING
TATTIER
TATTILY
TATTING
TEATIME
TEETIME
TENTING
TESTIER
TESTIFY
TESTILY
TESTING
TEXTILE
TEXTING
TILTING
TINTING
TOMTITS
TONTINE
TOOTING
TOTTING
TOUTING
TRITIUM
TUFTIER
TUFTING
TUITION
TUTTING
TWOTIME
UNCTION
UNITIES
UNITING
UNITISE
UNITIVE
UNITIZE
UNSTICK
UNSTIFF
UPSTIRS
VASTIER
VASTITY
VATTING
VENTING
VERTIGO
VESTIGE
VESTING
VETTING
VIATICA
VICTIMS
WAFTING
WAITING
WANTING
WARTIER
WARTIME
WASTING
WELTING
WESTIES
WESTINS
WETTING
WETTISH
WHATIFS
WHITING
WHITISH
WILTING
WITTIER
WITTILY
WITTING
WONTING
WRITING
XRATING
YETTIES
ZESTIER
ZESTILY
ZESTING

•••T•I•

ABSTAIN
ALLTHIS
AUSTRIA
BACTRIA
BADTRIP
BEATNIK
BEATRIX
BEATSIT
BEATTIE
BOBTAIL
BOOTHIA
BOOTSIT
BRITAIN
BUSTRIP
BUSTSIN
BUTTSIN
CANTRIP
CAPTAIN
CARTRIP
CARTSIN
CATTAIL
CENTRIC
CERTAIN
CHATWIN
CHITLIN
CONTAIN
COSTAIN
CURTAIL
CURTAIN
CYNTHIA
DANTEII
DAYTRIP
DELTAIC
DELTOID
DENTOID
DESTAIN
DEXTRIN
DOGTAIL
DONTLIE
DUSTBIN
ECOTRIN
EDITRIX
EGOTRIP
EPSTEIN
FACTOID
FANTAIL
FELTTIP
FLITSIN
FOOTSIE
FOOTSIT
FORTDIX
FOXTAIL
GASTRIC
GETTHIS
GETTOIT
GLOTTIS
GOTTOIT
HOPTOIT
IFITDIE
IHATEIT
KEPTFIT
LACTAID
LECTRIC
LEFTHIP
LEITRIM
LESTOIL
LOSTBIG
MAITAIS
MALTBIE
MANTRIC
MASTOID
MEATPIE
NEATNIK
NESTSIN
NOSTAIN
NOSTRIL
NOWTHIS
ONATRIP
ORATRIX
PARTIII
PASTEIN
PERTAIN
PHOTOID
PIGTAIL
PINTAIL
POSTFIX
PRETRIM
PROTEIN
QUITSIT
RATTAIL
REDTAIL
RESTAIN
RESTRIP
RESTSIN
SALTPIT
SAWTOIT
SCOTTIE
SEATRIP
SEETOIT
SHUTSIN
SKITRIP
SLATKIN
SPOTLIT
SPUTNIK
SUSTAIN
TASTEIT
TESTKIT
THATSIT
THETRIB
TOOTSIE
TOPTHIS
UNSTAID
UNSTOIC
UPSTAIR
VENTRIS
VICTRIX
VOLTAIC
WANTSIN
WHATSIS
WHATSIT
WORTHIT
WRITEIN
WROTEIN
XANTHIC
YELTSIN

•••T••I

ABITIBI
AIRTAXI
BHUTANI
BUITONI
CESTMOI
DAKTARI
DANTEII
KHATAMI
KONTIKI
LETTERI
MARTINI
NAUTILI
PARTIII
PLATYPI
SAATCHI
SANTINI
TORTONI
VENTURI
WHATAMI
XYSTUSI

••••TI•

ABIOTIC
ABOUTIT
AGNATIC
AGOUTIS
ALSATIA
AMANTIS
APPETIT
AQUATIC
ASCETIC
ASEPTIC
ASIATIC
AVANTIS
AVIATIC
BEASTIE
BEATTIE
BLENTIN
BLUETIT
BOLATIE
BOLOTIE
BUILTIN
BURNTIN
BURSTIN
CAKETIN
CAROTID
CAROTIN
CAUSTIC
CHAOTIC
CHEATIN
COEPTIS
COUNTIN
CREPTIN
CROATIA
CROSTIC
CRYPTIC
DEALTIN
DEISTIC
DEMOTIC
DOUBTIT
DRASTIC
DRIFTIN
EIDETIC
EKISTIC
ELASTIC
ELASTIN
ERGOTIC
ERISTIC
ERRATIC
FANATIC
FELTTIP
FOULTIP
FRANTIC
GALATIA
GELATIN
GELATIS
GENETIC
GETATIP
GLOTTIS
GLYPTIC
GNOSTIC
GOLDTIP
GOTATIP
HADATIT
HAMITIC
HASATIT
HEMATIC
HEMATIN
HEPATIC
HERETIC
HORATIO
HYPATIA
IDENTIC
IDIOTIC
ILOSTIT
INASTIR
INERTIA
ITSATIE
IWANTIT
KERATIN
KINETIC
KIRSTIE
KRISTIN
LEAPTIN
LETITIA
LEVITIC
LUNATIC
LUTETIA
MEANTIT
MEIOTIC
MILITIA
MIMETIC
MINUTIA
MITOTIC
MOUNTIE
NAILTIP
NECKTIE
NEPOTIC
NIANTIC
NIGHTIE
ODONTIA
OOLITIC
OPUNTIA
ORECTIC
OSMATIC
OSMOTIC
OVERTIP
PAROTID
PERATIO
PIRATIC
PLASTIC
POLITIC
PRACTIC
PYRETIC
PYRITIC
QUARTIC
QUENTIN
QUINTIC
ROBOTIC
RUBITIN
SCEPTIC
SCIATIC
SCOTTIE
SEMITIC
SHELTIE
SHORTIE
SILKTIE
SKEPTIC
SLEPTIN
SOMATIC
SPORTIN
STARTIN
STYPTIC
SWEATIT
SWEETIE
TICOTIN
TINYTIM
TRUSTIN
VENATIC
WAPITIS
WINGTIP
XEROTIC
YACHTIE
YESITIS

••••T•I

ACANTHI
BUGATTI
CANETTI
DIMITRI
FLINTMI
MENOTTI
MORETTI
PERETTI
SHASTRI
STRETTI
TOFUTTI
TOLSTOI

•••••TI

ALBERTI
ARGENTI
ASHANTI
BASMATI
BUGATTI
CANETTI
CHAPATI
CHIANTI
CHRISTI
DELICTI
DRAGOTI
ELMISTI
EMERITI
HAVARTI
HUANGTI
KUWAITI
MAIMITI
MENOTTI
MORETTI
ONORATI
PERETTI
PLOESTI
ROBERTI
SILENTI
SOLLATI
STRETTI
STUARTI
TOFUTTI
VALENTI

T•J••••

TEJANAS
TEJANOS
TIJUANA

T••J•••

THEJERK
THEJETS
TIPJARS
TOMJOAD
TRIJETS
TROJANS

T•••J••

TEMPJOB
TWINJET

•TJ••••

STJAMES
STJOHNS

•T••J••

LTKOJAK

•T••••J

FTDIXNJ

••TJ•••

OUTJEST
OUTJETS
OUTJINX
OUTJUMP
OUTJUTS

••T•J••

GETAJOB
GOTAJOB

••T•••J

LETTERJ

•••TJ••

CULTJAM
LEFTJAB

•••T••J

LETTERJ

•••••TJ

SILENTJ

T•K••••

TAKABLE
TAKEAIM
TAKEFOR
TAKEILL
TAKEINS
TAKENBY
TAKENIN
TAKENON
TAKENTO
TAKENUP
TAKEOFF
TAKEONE
TAKEOUT
TAKESIN
TAKESIT
TAKESON
TAKESTO
TAKESUP
TAKETEA
TAKETEN
TAKINGS
TEKKIES
TOKENED
TSKTSKS

T••K•••

TABKEYS
TACKERS
TACKIER
TACKILY
TACKING
TACKLED
TACKLER
TACKLES
TACKSON
TACKSUP
TALKBIG
TALKERS
TALKIER
TALKIES
TALKING
TALKOUT
TALKSAT
TALKSOF
TALKSON
TALKSTO
TALKSUP
TANKAGE
TANKARD
TANKCAR
TANKERS
TANKFUL
TANKING
TANKINI
TANKSUP
TANKTOP
TASKBAR
TASKING
TEKKIES
TENKRUN
THEKING
THEKISS
TICKERS
TICKETS
TICKING
TICKLED
TICKLER
TICKLES
TICKOFF
TICKSBY
TINKERS
TINKLED

TINKLER
TINKLES
TOLKIEN
TOMKITE
TOOKAIM
TOOKFOR
TOOKILL
TOOKOFF
TOOKOUT
TOOKTEN
TOPKAPI
TOPKICK
TOPKNOT
TOYKITE
TREKKED
TREKKER
TREKKIE
TUCKERS
TUCKING
TUCKSIN
TURKEYS
TURKISH
TUSKERS
TUSKING

T•••K••

TALCKED
TESTKIT
THANKED
THANKER
THICKEN
THICKER
THICKET
THICKLY
THINKER
THINKOF
THINKSO
THINKUP
THUNKED
TIOMKIN
TOOLKIT
TOPEKAN
TRACKED
TRACKER
TREKKED
TREKKER
TREKKIE
TRICKED
TRICKER
TRICKLE
TRINKET
TROIKAS
TRUCKED
TRUCKEE
TRUCKER
TRUCKLE
TURNKEY
TWEAKED
TWINKIE
TWINKLE
TWINKLY

T••••K•

TAGLIKE
TANOAKS
TAXHIKE
TEACAKE
THEDUKE
THELIKE
THWACKS
TINLIKE
TOELIKE
TOYBIKE
TOYLIKE
TROTSKY
TSKTSKS
TUBLIKE
TUGRIKS
TURFSKI

T•••••K

TANBARK
TAYBACK
TEANECK
TEDMACK
TENWEEK
THATSOK
THEHULK
THEJERK
THELARK
THELOOK
THEMASK
THEMICK
THERINK
THEROCK
THESACK
TIEBACK
TIERACK
TIETACK
TINWORK
TITLARK
TOEPICK
TOPKICK
TOPRANK
TOYBOOK
TULSAOK
TUSSOCK
TWOWEEK

•TK••••

LTKOJAK
MTKENYA
STKITTS

•T•K•••

STAKING
STOKELY
STOKERS
STOKEUP
STOKING

•T••K••

ETICKET
ITSOKAY
STACKED
STACKER
STACKUP
STALKED
STALKER
STANKUP
STARKER
STARKEY
STARKLY
STICKBY
STICKER
STICKIN
STICKON
STICKTO
STICKUM
STICKUP
STINKER
STINKUP
STLUKES
STOCKED
STOCKER
STOCKUP
STOOKEY
STRIKER
STRIKES
STROKED
STROKER
STROKES
STUCKBY
STUCKIN
STUCKON
STUCKTO
STUCKUP

•T•••K•

ATSTAKE
ATTACKS
ATTUCKS
STARSKY
STMARKS
STREAKS
STREAKY

•T••••K

ATATURK
BTFSPLK
LTKOJAK

••TK•••

ALTKEYS
CATKINS
HOTKEYS
KITKATS
LETKNOW
ONTKEAN
OUTKAST
OUTKEEP
OUTKEPT
OUTKICK
OUTKILL
OUTKING
OUTKISS
WATKINS
WETKISS

••T•K••

BATIKED
BETAKEN
BETAKES
BETOKEN
INTAKES
JETSKIS
OUTSKIP
RETAKEN
RETAKER
RETAKES
UNTAKEN
UPTAKES

••T••K•

ACTLIKE
ANTLIKE
ATTACKS
ATTUCKS
AUTARKY
BATLIKE
BYTALKS
CATLIKE
DOTLIKE
EATCAKE
FATLIKE
GOTHIKA
HATLIKE
HOTCAKE
HUTLIKE
JSTROKE
NETLIKE
NETSUKE
NOTLIKE
NUTLIKE
OATCAKE
OATLIKE
OPTICKS
OUTASKS
OUTBAKE
OUTTAKE
RATLIKE
RETACKS
SHTICKS
SHTICKY
UNTACKS
UNTUCKS
UPTALKS
UPTICKS

••T•••K

AMTRACK
ARTBOOK
ARTROCK
ARTWORK
BETHINK
CATWALK
CUTBACK
CUTWORK
FATBACK
FETLOCK
FUTHARK
GATWICK
GETBACK
GOTBACK
GOTMILK
HATRACK
HITBACK
HOTLICK
HOTLINK
HOTMILK
HOTPACK
HOTPINK
JETPACK
LETTERK
LITOVSK
MATLOCK
MATTOCK
NATWICK
NETWORK
NITPICK
ONTRACK
OSTMARK
OUTBACK
OUTBARK
OUTBULK
OUTCOOK
OUTKICK
OUTLOOK
OUTPICK
OUTRANK
OUTROCK
OUTSEEK
OUTSULK
OUTTALK
OUTWALK
OUTWORK
PATRICK
PETCOCK
PETDUCK
PETROCK
POTHOOK
POTLUCK
PUTBACK
RATFINK
RATPACK
RETHANK
RETHINK
RETRACK
SATBACK
SETBACK
SITBACK
TITLARK
UNTHICK
UNTHINK
UNTRACK
VITEBSK
WETLOOK
YITZHAK
ZATOPEK

•••TK••

NOOTKAS
SLATKIN
TESTKIT

•••T•K•

ATSTAKE
GRETZKY
KONTIKI
MISTAKE
OUTTAKE
PARTAKE
RESTOKE
ROETHKE
TROTSKY
TSKTSKS

•••T••K

AIRTANK
ATATURK
BEATNIK
BIGTALK
CARTALK
DESTOCK
DMYTRYK
DOGTICK
DONTASK
EYETUCK
FARTLEK
GASTANK
HARTACK
INSTOCK
LETTERK
MATTOCK
MISTOOK
MONTAUK
NEATNIK
OILTANK
OUTTALK
PARTOOK
PEPTALK
RESTACK
RESTICK
RESTOCK
ROSTOCK
SCHTICK
SPUTNIK
SUBTASK
THATSOK
TIETACK
UNSTACK
UNSTICK
UNSTUCK

••••T•K

ALNITAK
DONETSK
GANGTOK
IRKUTSK
OKHOTSK
VARITEK
YAKUTSK

•••••TK

SILENTK

TL•••••

TLINGIT

T•L••••

TALARIA
TALCKED
TALCUMS
TALENTS
TALIBAN
TALKBIG
TALKERS
TALKIER
TALKIES
TALKING
TALKOUT
TALKSAT
TALKSOF
TALKSON
TALKSTO
TALKSUP
TALLEST
TALLIED
TALLIER
TALLIES
TALLINN
TALLISH
TALLITH
TALLONE
TALLOWS
TALLOWY
TALLYHO
TALLYUP
TALONED
TALUSES
TELAVIV
TELECOM
TELEFAX
TELEPIC
TELEPIX
TELERAN
TELESTO
TELEXED
TELEXES
TELLALL
TELLERS
TELLIES
TELLING
TELLOFF
TELLSIT
TELLSOF
TELLSON
TELSTAR
TILINGS
TILLAGE
TILLERS
TILLETS
TILLING
TILLNOW
TILSITS
TILTERS
TILTING
TILTSAT
TILTSUP
TILTTOP
TOLDALL
TOLDOFF
TOLEASE
TOLEDAN
TOLEDOS
TOLKIEN
TOLLAGE
TOLLBAR
TOLLERS
TOLLING
TOLLMAN
TOLLMEN
TOLLWAY
TOLSTOI
TOLSTOY
TOLTECS
TOLUENE
TULANEU
TULSANS
TULSAOK
TYLENOL

T••L•••

TABLEAU
TABLETS
TABLING
TABLOID
TAGLIKE
TAGLINE
TAILEND
TAILERS
TAILFIN
TAILING
TAILOFF
TAILORS
TAILPIN
TAILWAG
TALLEST
TALLIED
TALLIER
TALLIES
TALLINN
TALLISH
TALLITH
TALLONE
TALLOWS
TALLOWY
TALLYHO
TALLYUP
TANLINE
TAXLAWS
TAXLESS
TAXLEVY
TAYLORS
TBILISI
TEALEAF
TEALESS
TEFLONS
TELLALL
TELLERS
TELLIES
TELLING
TELLOFF
TELLSIT
TELLSOF
TELLSON
THALERS
THELAMB
THELARK
THELEFT
THELIKE
THELOOK
THELOOP
THULIUM
TIELESS
TIELINE
TIGLONS
TILLAGE
TILLERS
TILLETS
TILLING
TILLNOW
TINLIKE
TIPLESS
TIPLINE
TITLARK
TITLING
TITLIST
TOBLAME
TOELESS
TOELIKE
TOELOOP
TOILERS
TOILETS
TOILFUL
TOILING
TOILSAT
TOLLAGE
TOLLBAR
TOLLERS
TOLLING
TOLLMAN
TOLLMEN
TOLLWAY
TOOLATE
TOOLBAR
TOOLBOX
TOOLERS
TOOLING
TOOLKIT
TOOLONG
TOOLSET
TOOLSUP
TOPLESS
TOPLINE
TOWLINE
TOYLAND
TOYLESS
TOYLIKE
TRALALA
TRELLIS
TRILLED
TRILLER
TRILLIN
TRILOGY
TROLLED
TROLLER
TROLLEY
TROLLOP
TSELIOT
TUBLIKE
TUGLESS
TUILLES
TWELFTH
TWELVEA
TWELVEB
TWELVEC
TWELVED
TWELVEE
TWELVES
TWILLED
TWOLANE

T•••L••

TABULAR
TACKLED
TACKLER
TACKLES
TAGALOG
TAMALES
TAMBLYN
TAMGLEN
TANGLED
TANGLER
TANGLES
TARTLET
TASHLIN
TATTLED
TATTLER
TATTLES
TEBALDI
TEMBLOR
TEMPLAR
TEMPLED
TEMPLES
TESTLAB
THEALPS
THEBLOB
THEFLEA
THEFLOP
THRALLS
THRILLA
THRILLS
TICKLED
TICKLER
TICKLES
TIDALLY
TIECLIP
TIMELAG
TINGLED
TINGLER
TINGLES
TINKLED
TINKLER
TINKLES
TIPPLED
TIPPLER
TIPPLES
TITTLES
TITULAR
TOCELIA
TODDLED
TODDLER
TODDLES
TOFFLER
TOGGLED
TOGGLER
TOGGLES
TOHELEN
TONALLY
TONELOC
TOODLES
TOOSLOW
TOOTLED
TOOTLER
TOOTLES
TOPPLED
TOPPLES
TORTLAW
TOTALED
TOTALER
TOTALLY
TOTALUP
TOUSLED
TOUSLES
TOWELED
TOWNLET
TOYSLED
TRAILED
TRAILER
TRAWLED
TRAWLER
TREBLED
TREBLES
TREELET
TRELLIS
TRIFLED
TRIFLER
TRIFLES
TRILLED
TRILLER
TRILLIN
TRIOLET
TRIPLEA
TRIPLED
TRIPLES
TRIPLET
TRIPLEX
TROILUS
TROLLED
TROLLER
TROLLEY
TROLLOP
TUBULAR
TUBULES
TUILLES
TUMBLED
TUMBLER
TUMBLES
TUMMLER
TUMULTS
TUPELOS
TUPOLEV
TURTLED
TURTLES
TUSSLED
TUSSLES
TUTELAR
TWILLED
TWIRLED
TWIRLER

T••••L•

TABOULI
TACITLY
TACKILY
TACTILE
TADPOLE
TAGSALE
TAKABLE
TAKEILL
TAMABLE
TAMBALA
TANGELO
TARBELL
TARDILY
TAROILS
TARSALS
TARTILY
TASSELS
TASTILY
TATTILY
TAWNILY
TAXABLE
TAXSALE
TEABALL
TEARILY
TEASELS
TELLALL
TENABLE
TENABLY
TENBALL
TENFOLD
TENMILE
TENSELY
TENSILE
TENTHLY
TEPIDLY
TEQUILA
TERCELS
TERRELL
TERSELY
TESTFLY
TESTILY
TEXTILE
THEBELL
THEDELL
THEDOLE
THEFALL
THEGOLD
THEHELP
THEHILL
THEHULK
THEMALL
THENILE
THERULE
THESELF
THEWALL
THICKLY
THIMBLE
THIRDLY
THISTLE
THISTLY
THRALLS
THRILLA
THRILLS
THYSELF
TIDALLY
TIEPOLO
TIGHTLY
TIMBALE
TIMBALS
TIMHOLT
TIMIDLY
TINNILY
TINSELS
TIPSILY
TIREDLY
TMOBILE
TOEHOLD
TOLDALL
TOMGOLA
TONALLY
TONSILS
TOOKILL
TOOTALL
TOPHOLE
TORTOLA
TORVALD
TORVILL
TOSCALE
TOTABLE
TOTALLY
TOUGHLY
TOWABLE
TOYBALL
TOYDOLL
TRALALA
TRAMPLE
TRAVELS
TREACLE
TREACLY
TREADLE
TREMBLE
TREMBLY
TREMOLO
TRESTLE
TRIABLE
TRIBBLE
TRICKLE
TRIFOLD
TRIPOLI
TRITELY
TROUBLE
TROWELS
TRUCKLE
TRUFFLE
TRUNDLE
TUBFULS
TUNABLE
TUNICLE
TUNNELS
TUTUILA
TVIDOLS
TVTABLE
TWADDLE
TWEEDLE
TWIDDLE
TWINKLE
TWINKLY
TWOBALL
TWOFOLD
TYNDALL

T•••••L

TACTFUL
TACTUAL
TAKEILL
TAMPAFL
TANKFUL
TARBELL
TARHEEL
TEABALL
TEARFUL
TELLALL
TENBALL
TENDRIL
TENNIEL
TENTFUL
TERRELL
TEXTUAL
THEBELL
THEDELL
THEFALL
THEFOOL
THEHILL
THEMALL
THERMAL
THEWALL
TINFOIL
TOENAIL
TOILFUL
TOLDALL
TOMFOOL
TOOKILL
TOOTALL
TOPICAL
TOPSAIL
TOPSOIL
TORVILL
TOYBALL
TOYDOLL
TOYPAIL
TRAMMEL
TRAUBEL
TRAVAIL
TRAYFUL
TREFOIL
TRIVIAL
TRYSAIL
TUMBREL
TUNAOIL
TUNEFUL

TUNGOIL
TURMOIL
TWOBALL
TYLENOL
TYNDALL
TYPICAL

•TL••••

ATLANTA
ATLARGE
ATLASES
ATLEAST
ATLUNCH
MTLOGAN
STLOUIS
STLUCIA
STLUKES

•T•L•••

ATALOSS
ATELATE
ATELESS
ATELIER
ATHLETE
ETALIBI
FTBLISS
ITALIAN
ITALICS
ITSLATE
ITSLOVE
MTBLANC
OTALGIA
OTALGIC
OTOLOGY
PTOLEMY
STALAGS
STALELY
STALEST
STALKED
STALKER
STALLED
STALLER
STCLOUD
STELIAS
STELLAR
STILLED
STILLER
STILLUP
STILTED
STILTON
STOLEIN
STOLLEN
STOLONS
STYLERS
STYLETS
STYLING
STYLISE
STYLISH
STYLIST
STYLIZE
UTILISE
UTILITY
UTILIZE

•T••L••

ATACLIP
ATEALOT
BTWELVE
ETAILED
ETAILER
ETOILES
FTRILEY
ITSALIE
ITSALOT
ITWELVE
KTOSLIN
MTBALDY
MTPELEE
NTUPLES
OTHELLO
STABLED
STABLER
STABLES
STADLER
STALLED
STALLER
STANLEE
STANLEY
STAPLED
STAPLER
STAPLES
STARLET
STARLIT
STARLOG
STATLER
STEALER
STEALIN
STEALTH
STEELED
STEELER
STEELIE
STELLAR
STIFLED
STIFLES
STILLED
STILLER
STILLUP
STOLLEN
STOOLED
STOOLIE
STROLLS
UTRILLO

•T•••L•

ATATILT
ATFAULT
ATHRILL
ATINGLE
BTFSPLK
ETVOILA
ITGIRLS
ITSCOLD
OTHELLO
STABILE
STAGILY
STAIDLY
STALELY
STARKLY
STARTLE
STATELY
STEEPLE
STEEPLY
STERILE
STERNLY
STEROLS
STIFFLY
STIMULI
STIPPLE
STOKELY
STONILY
STOPPLE
STOUTLY
STPAULS
STROLLS
STUBBLE
STUBBLY
STUMBLE
UTRILLO
UTTERLY

•T••••L

ATABOIL
ATHRILL
ETERNAL
ETHANOL
ETHICAL
STBASIL
STEMPEL
STENCIL
STENGEL
STERNAL
STIFFEL
STOICAL
STRUDEL
UTENSIL

••TL•••

ACTLIKE
ANTLERS
ANTLIKE
ANTLION
ARTLESS
BATLIKE
BITLESS
BUTLERS
CATLIKE
CUTLASS
CUTLERS
CUTLERY
CUTLETS
DOTLIKE
EATLATE
EATLESS
FATLESS
FATLIKE
FATLING
FATLIPS
FETLOCK
GATLING
GATLINS
GETLOST
GOTLOST
GUTLESS
HATLESS
HATLIKE
HITLESS
HITLIST
HOTLEAD
HOTLICK
HOTLINE
HOTLINK
HOTLIPS
HUTLIKE
JETLAGS
JUTLAND
LETLIVE
MATLESS
MATLOCK
METLIFE
MOTLEYS
NETLESS
NETLIKE
NETLOSS
NOTLIKE
NOTLIVE
NUTLETS
NUTLIKE
OATLIKE
OSTLERS
OUTLAID
OUTLAIN
OUTLAND
OUTLASH
OUTLAST
OUTLAWS
OUTLAYS
OUTLEAD
OUTLEAP
OUTLETS
OUTLIER
OUTLIES
OUTLIMN
OUTLINE
OUTLIPS
OUTLIVE
OUTLOOK
OUTLOUD
OUTLOVE
PETLAMB
PETLION
POTLIDS
POTLUCK
RATLIKE
RATLINE
RATLINS
RUTLAND
TITLARK
TITLING
TITLIST
WETLAND
WETLOOK
WITLESS
WITLING

••T•L••

ANTILOG
ASTOLAT
BATTLED
BATTLER
BATTLES
BOTTLED
BOTTLER
BOTTLES
BYTALKS
CATALAN
CATALOG
CATALOS
CATALPA
CATFLAP
CATFLEA
DOTTLES
EATALOT
ESTELLA
ESTELLE
EXTOLLS
FATALES
FATALLY
FETTLES
GATELEG
HITPLAY
HOTGLUE
KETTLES
LETSLIP
LITTLER
LITTLES
MATALIN
MATILDA
METALED
METTLER
METTLES
MOTTLED
MOTTLES
NATALIA
NATALIE
NETFLIX
NETTLED
NETTLES
NOTALIE
NOTALOT
ORTOLAN
OUTBLOT
OUTBLOW
OUTFLEE
OUTFLOW
OUTFLUX
OUTGLOW
OUTPLAN
OUTPLAY
OUTPLOD
OUTPLOT
PATELLA
PETALED
PETALES
PETULIA
PITILLO
RATTLED
RATTLER
RATTLES
RETALLY
RETELLS
RETILED
RETILES
RETILLS
RITALIN
ROTBLAT
ROTELLE
RUTALEE
RUTILES
SETPLAY
SETTLED
SETTLER
SETTLES
SETTLOR
TATTLED
TATTLER
TATTLES
TITTLES
TITULAR
TOTALED
TOTALER
TOTALLY
TOTALUP
TUTELAR
UNTILED
UPTALKS
UPTILTS
VITALIS
VITALLY
VITTLES
WATTLED
WATTLES

••T••L•

ACTABLE
ACTORLY
ANTHILL
ARTFILM
ARTICLE
ARTSALE
ARTWALL
BETHELS
BITROLE
CATCALL
CATTALO
CATTILY
CATWALK
CITABLE
CUTICLE
DATABLE
DATEDLY
DATRILS
DETAILS
DOTTILY
EATABLE
ENTAILS
ENTITLE
ESTELLA
ESTELLE
EXTOLLS
FATALLY
FATCELL
FATTILY
FETIDLY
FITWELL
GETABLE
GETCOLD
GETHELP
GETSOLD
GETWELL
GOTCOLD
GOTHELP
GOTMILK
GOTWELL
GUTSILY
HATABLE
HATFULS
HITFILM
HOTMILK
HOTROLL
INTAILS
LATRELL
LETFALL
LETROLL
LETSFLY
LITHELY
LUTHULI
METCALF
MUTABLE
MUTABLY
MUTEDLY
MUTUALS
NATTILY
NETBALL
NETFULS
NOTABLE
NOTABLY
NOTEDLY
NOTWELL
NUTOILS
NUTTILY
OCTUPLE
OCTUPLY
OSTWALD
OUTBULK
OUTCALL
OUTCOLD
OUTCULL
OUTKILL
OUTPOLL
OUTPULL
OUTROLL
OUTSELL
OUTSOLD
OUTSOLE
OUTSULK
OUTTALK
OUTTELL
OUTTOLD
OUTTOLL
OUTWALK
OUTWELL
OUTWILE
OUTWILL
OUTYELL
OUTYELP
OXTAILS
PATELLA
PATROLS
PETCALF
PETIOLE
PETMULE
PETRELS
PETROLS
PETTILY
PITBULL
PITFALL
PITHILY
PITILLO
POTABLE
POTFULS
POTHOLE
RATABLE
RATHOLE
RETABLE
RETAILS
RETALLY
RETELLS
RETICLE
RETILLS
RETITLE
RETOOLS
RITUALS
RITZILY
ROTELLE
SATWELL
SHTETLS
SITWELL
TATTILY
TOTABLE
TOTALLY
TUTUILA
TVTABLE
UNTRULY
UTTERLY
VATFULS
VITALLY
VOTABLE
WETBULB
WETCELL
WITTILY

••T•••L

ANTHEIL
ANTHILL
APTERAL
ARTWALL
BATGIRL
BATHOIL
BITONAL
CATBOWL
CATCALL
CATTAIL
CITADEL
CITYGAL
DUTIFUL
ECTYPAL
ENTHRAL
ESTIVAL
ESTORIL
FATCELL
FATEFUL
FITWELL
GETREAL
GETWELL
GOTOGAL
GOTREAL
GOTWELL
HATEFUL
HOTCOAL
HOTMAIL
HOTMEAL
HOTROLL
INTOTAL
JETFOIL
LATERAL
LATRELL
LETFALL
LETROLL
LETTERL
LITERAL
MATINAL
NATURAL
NATUREL
NETBALL
NOTREAL
NOTWELL
OATMEAL
OCTAVAL
ONTHEDL
ONTRIAL
OPTICAL
OPTIMAL
ORTEGAL
OUTBAWL
OUTBOWL
OUTCALL
OUTCULL
OUTDUEL
OUTFEEL
OUTFOOL
OUTHAUL
OUTHOWL
OUTHURL
OUTKILL
OUTPOLL
OUTPULL
OUTPURL
OUTRAIL
OUTROLL
OUTSAIL
OUTSELL
OUTTELL
OUTTOLL
OUTWELL
OUTWILL
OUTYELL
PITBULL
PITFALL
PITIFUL
POTBOIL
RATTAIL
RETINAL
RETINOL
RETOTAL
RETRIAL
RUTHFUL
SATCHEL
SATWELL
SETBAIL
SETSAIL
SITWELL
VATICAL
VITRIOL
WETCELL

•••TL••

AFATLOT
BARTLES
BARTLET
BATTLED
BATTLER
BATTLES
BEATLES
BEETLES
BENTLEY
BOOTLEG
BOTTLED
BOTTLER
BOTTLES
BUSTLED
BUSTLER
BUSTLES
CANTLES
CASTLED
CASTLES
CHITLIN
DARTLED
DARTLES
DONTLIE
DOTTLES
FARTLEK
FETTLES
FIATLUX
FLATLET
FOOTLED
FOOTLER
FOOTLES
FOOTLET
FORTLEE
GANTLET
GENTLED
GENTLER
GENTLES
HARTLEY
HOSTLER
HUNTLEY
HURTLED
HURTLES
HUSTLED
HUSTLER
HUSTLES
JOSTLED
JOSTLER
JOSTLES
KASTLER
KETTLES
LASTLAP
LASTLEG
LEFTLEG
LITTLER
LITTLES
MANTLED
MANTLES
MANTLET
METTLER
METTLES
MOTTLED
MOTTLES
MYRTLES
NESTLED
NESTLER
NESTLES
NETTLED
NETTLES
PANTLEG
PESTLED
PESTLES
RATTLED
RATTLER
RATTLES
ROOTLED
ROOTLES
ROOTLET
RUSTLED
RUSTLER
RUSTLES
SETTLED
SETTLER
SETTLES
SETTLOR
SPOTLIT
STATLER
SUBTLER
TARTLET
TATTLED
TATTLER
TATTLES
TESTLAB
TITTLES
TOOTLED
TOOTLER
TOOTLES
TORTLAW
TURTLED
TURTLES
VITTLES
WATTLED
WATTLES

•••T•L•

ACETALS
ACUTELY
ALITTLE
ALLTOLD
AMATOLS
AMSTELS
ANATOLE
ANATOLY
ATATILT
BARTOLO
BEATALL
BERTOLT
BESTILL
BIGTALK
BOATELS
BRATTLE
BRITTLE
BRUTELY
CANTALS
CANTILY
CARTALK
CARTELS
CASTILE
CATTALO
CATTILY
CENTALS
DACTYLS
DENTALS
DIRTILY
DISTILL
DISTILS
DOTTILY
DUCTILE
DUSTILY
EARTHLY
EMPTILY
FATTILY
FELTILL
FERTILE
FICTILE
FIFTHLY
FUSTILY
GENTILE
GESTALT
GOSTALE
GOUTILY
GUSTILY
HASTILY
HEFTILY
HOSTELS
HOSTILE
ILLTELL
INSTALL
INSTALS
INSTILL
INSTILS
INSTYLE
INUTILE
IRATELY
LENTILS
LINTELS
LOATHLY
LOFTILY
LUSTILY
MANTELS
MEATILY
MISTELL
MISTILY
MISTOLD
MONTALE
MONTHLY
MORTALS
MUSTILY
NASTILY
NATTILY
NAUTILI
NIFTILY
NINTHLY
NUTTILY
OUTTALK
OUTTELL
OUTTOLD
OUTTOLL
PANTILE
PASTELS
PENTELS
PEPTALK
PETTILY
PISTILS
PISTOLE
PISTOLS
PORTALS
PRATTLE
PRETELL
PRETOLD
RENTALS
REPTILE
RESTYLE
RUSTILY
SALTILY
SCUTTLE
SEATTLE
SHUTTLE
SIXTHLY
SKITTLE
SOOTILY
SPATULA
SPITTLE
STATELY
SYSTOLE
TACTILE
TARTILY
TASTILY
TATTILY
TENTHLY
TESTFLY
TESTILY
TEXTILE
TOOTALL
TORTOLA
TRITELY
VESTALS
VISTULA
WHITELY
WHITTLE
WITTILY
WOJTYLA
ZESTILY

•••T••L

ABETTAL
ABUTTAL
AUSTRAL
BEATALL
BESTIAL
BESTILL
BOATFUL
BOBTAIL
CASTROL
CATTAIL
CENTRAL
CHATTEL
CONTROL
CURTAIL
DESTAEL
DEXTRAL
DISTILL
DOGTAIL
FACTFUL
FACTUAL
FANTAIL
FELTILL
FISTFUL
FOXTAIL
FRETFUL
GENTEEL
GLOTTAL
GLUTEAL
HEATFUL
HOOTOWL
HRETHEL
HURTFUL
ILLTELL
INITIAL
INSTALL
INSTILL
KESTREL
LACTEAL
LESTOIL
LETTERL
LUSTFUL
LUSTRAL
MARTIAL
MENTHOL
MISTELL
MISTRAL
NESTFUL
NEUTRAL
NOSTRIL
NUPTIAL
OUTTELL
OUTTOLL
PARTIAL
PIGTAIL
PINTAIL
PLOTFUL
POUTFUL
PRETELL
PRETZEL
QUETZAL
RATTAIL
REDTAIL
RESTFUL
ROSTRAL

SOFTGEL
SPATIAL
TACTFUL
TACTUAL
TENTFUL
TEXTUAL
TOOTALL
UNSTEEL
USSTEEL
VENTRAL
VESTRAL
VICTUAL
VIRTUAL
WASTREL
WISTFUL
ZESTFUL

••••TL•

ADEPTLY
ADULTLY
ALERTLY
ALITTLE
APOSTLE
BEASTLY
BLUNTLY
BRATTLE
BRISTLE
BRISTLY
BRITTLE
CHORTLE
COURTLY
ENTITLE
EPISTLE
ERECTLY
EXACTLY
FAINTLY
FIRSTLY
FLEETLY
GAUNTLY
GHASTLY
GHOSTLY
GREATLY
GRISTLE
GRISTLY
INAPTLY
INEPTLY
INERTLY
JOINTLY
KRYSTLE
LICITLY
LIGHTLY
MOISTLY
NIGHTLY
OVERTLY
PRATTLE
QUIETLY
RETITLE
RIANTLY
RIGHTLY
SAINTLO
SAINTLY
SCANTLY
SCUTTLE
SEATTLE
SHORTLY
SHTETLS
SHUTTLE
SIGHTLY
SKITTLE
SLANTLY
SMARTLY
SPITTLE
SQUATLY
STARTLE
STOUTLY
SWEETLY
SWIFTLY
TACITLY
THISTLE
THISTLY
TIGHTLY
TRESTLE
UNAPTLY
UNFITLY
WHISTLE
WHITTLE
WRESTLE

••••T•L

ABETTAL
ABUTTAL
BIMETAL
BORSTAL
BRISTOL
CAPITAL
CAPITOL
CHATTEL
COASTAL
CRUSTAL
CRYSTAL
CUBITAL
DIGITAL
EDICTAL
FRACTAL
FRONTAL
GAMETAL
GERITOL
GLOTTAL
INTOTAL
KAPITAL
MARITAL
ORBITAL
PALATAL
PIVOTAL
QUINTAL
RECITAL
REFUTAL
RETOTAL
UNVITAL
VEGETAL

•••••TL

AXOLOTL
NAHUATL
SILENTL

TM•••••

TMOBILE

T•M••••

TAMABLE
TAMALES
TAMARAC
TAMBALA
TAMBLYN
TAMGLEN
TAMIAMI
TAMMANY
TAMPAFL
TAMPERS
TAMPICO
TAMPING
TAMTAMS
TEMBLOR
TEMPEAZ
TEMPEHS
TEMPERA
TEMPERS
TEMPEST
TEMPING
TEMPJOB
TEMPLAR
TEMPLED
TEMPLES
TEMPORE
TEMPTED
TEMPTER
TEMPURA
TIMBALE
TIMBALS
TIMBERS
TIMBERY
TIMBRES
TIMECOP
TIMELAG
TIMEOFF
TIMEOUT
TIMESUP
TIMEWAS
TIMEXES
TIMHOLT
TIMIDER
TIMIDLY
TIMINGS
TIMMINS
TIMOTHY
TIMPANI
TIMREID
TIMRICE
TIMROTH
TOMBOYS
TOMCATS
TOMFOOL
TOMGOLA
TOMJOAD
TOMKITE
TOMTITS
TOMTOMS
TUMBLED
TUMBLER
TUMBLES
TUMBREL
TUMESCE
TUMMIES
TUMMLER
TUMULTS
TVMOVIE
TYMPANA
TYMPANI

T••M•••

TAMMANY
TARMACS
TEAMING
TEAMSUP
TEAMUSA
TEDMACK
TEEMING
TENMILE
TERMING
TERMINI
TERMITE
THEMAGI
THEMALL
THEMASK
THEMAVS
THEMAYO
THEMETS
THEMICK
THEMOON
THEMOST
THIMBLE
THIMPHU
THOMSON
THUMBED
THUMPED
THUMPER
THYMINE
TIEMPOS
TIMMINS
TINMINE
TIOMKIN
TITMICE
TOOMANY
TOOMUCH
TOPMAST
TOPMOST
TORMENT
TRAMCAR
TRAMMED
TRAMMEL
TRAMPAS
TRAMPED
TRAMPER
TRAMPLE
TRAMWAY
TREMBLE
TREMBLY
TREMOLO
TREMORS
TRIMMED
TRIMMER
TRIMOFF
TRIMTAB
TROMPED
TROMPIN
TRUMANS
TRUMPED
TRUMPET
TRUMPUP
TUMMIES
TUMMLER
TURMOIL
TWOMORE
TZIMMES

T•••M••

TACOMAS
TAGAMET
TAPEMAN
TAPEMEN
TATAMIS
TAXIMAN
TAXIMEN
THEOMEN
THEOMNI
THERMAL
THERMIC
THERMOS
THIAMIN
THINMAN
THURMAN
TINAMOU
TIREMAN
TIREMEN
TOHOMER
TOLLMAN
TOLLMEN
TONEMES
TOTEMIC
TRAMMED
TRAMMEL
TRAUMAS
TRIMMED
TRIMMER
TRIUMPH
TUCHMAN
TURFMAN
TURFMEN
TVGAMES
TZIMMES

T••••M•

TALCUMS
TAMIAMI
TAMTAMS
TANDEMS
TEATIME
TEDEUMS
TEDIUMS
TEETIME
THEARMY
THEBOMB
THEGAME
THEISMS
THELAMB
THEPUMP
THERAMS
THESAME
THESIMS
TIEGAME
TOBLAME
TOMTOMS
TOPNAME
TRIREME
TRUISMS
TRUSTME
TSUNAMI
TURISMO
TVROOMS
TWOSOME
TWOTIME

T•••••M

TAGTEAM
TAKEAIM
TANGRAM
TANTRUM
TAPROOM
TEAROOM
TELECOM
TERAOHM
TERBIUM
THEFIRM
THEOREM
THEROOM
THORIUM
THREEAM
THREEPM
THULIUM
TIDYSUM
TIEBEAM
TINYTIM
TITOISM
TONEARM
TOOKAIM
TOPFORM
TOPONYM
TORYISM
TOURISM
TRANSAM
TRANSOM
TRIFORM
TRIGRAM
TRITIUM
TRIVIUM
TROPISM
TSARDOM
TSARISM
TWOROOM
TWOTERM

•TM••••

ATMCARD
ATMFEES
FTMEADE
FTMYERS
ITMAYBE
JTMONEY
MTMARCY
STMARKS
STMARYS
UTMOSTS

•T•M•••

ATAMANS
ATEMORE
ATOMICS
ATOMIES
ATOMISE
ATOMISM
ATOMIST
ATOMIZE
ETAMINE
ETHMOID
ETYMONS
ITEMING
ITEMISE
ITEMIZE
ITEMONE
STAMENS
STAMINA
STAMMER
STAMPED
STAMPER
STEMMED
STEMPEL
STIMSON
STIMULI
STOMACH
STOMATA
STOMPED
STOMPIN
STOMPON
STUMBLE
STUMPED
STUMPER
STYMIED
STYMIES

•T••M••

ATHOMES
ATTEMPT
ATTIMES
OTTOMAN
OTTUMWA
STAMMER
STARMAN
STARMAP
STEAMED
STEAMER
STEAMUP
STEMMED
STEPMOM
STIGMAS
STJAMES
STORMED
STORMIN
STSIMON

•T•••M•

ATACAMA
ATATIME
ATRIUMS
ITSONME
ITSTIME
MTADAMS
PTOLEMY
STREAMS

•T••••M

ATAVISM
ATHEISM
ATOMISM
STADIUM
STANNUM
STARDOM
STATISM
STEINEM
STEPMOM
STERNUM
STICKUM
STRATUM
UTOPISM
YTTRIUM

••TM•••

AFTMOST
BITMAPS
CATMINT
EATMORE
GOTMILK
HOTMAIL
HOTMEAL
HOTMILK
LETMEBE
LETMEGO
LETMEIN
NOTMANY
NOTMINE
NOTMUCH
NUTMEAT
NUTMEGS
OATMEAL
OSTMARK
OUTMANS
OUTMATE
OUTMODE
OUTMOST
OUTMOVE
PETMICE
PETMULE
TITMICE
WETMOPS

••T•M••

ALTIMAS
ARTEMIS
ARTEMUS
ASTHMAS
ATTEMPT
ATTIMES
AUTOMAT
AUTOMNE
AUTUMNS
BATEMAN
BATHMAT
BATSMAN
BATSMEN
BETAMAX
BETIMES
ENTOMBS
ESTAMIN
FOTOMAT
GATEMAN
GATEMEN
GETSMAD
ISTHMUS
ISTOMIN
LATIMES
LETEMIN
NYTIMES
OPTIMAL
OPTIMAS
OPTIMUM
OTTOMAN
OTTUMWA
PETEMAN
PETEMEN
PITTMAN
POTAMUS
POTOMAC
PUTEMUP
RETAMED
RETAMES
RETIMED
RETIMES
RITAMAE
SITEMAP
TATAMIS
TOTEMIC
ULTIMAS
UNTAMED
UNTAMES
UNTIMED
UNTIMID
UPTEMPO
UPTIMES
VITAMIN

••T••M•

ANTHEMS
BOTTOMS
BUTTEMT
CATCOMB
CUTTIME
DOTBOMB
DOTCOMS
ESTEEMS
EXTREME
FATHOMS
HITHOME
HOTCOMB
HOTTIME
NATSUME
NETGAME
NOTHOME
NOTRUMP
OUTCOME
OUTGAME
OUTJUMP
OUTLIMN
OUTSUMS
PETCOMB
PETLAMB
PETNAME
RETRIMS
SATCHMO
SATCOMS
SATHOME
SATSUMA
SITCOMS
SITHOME
YOTEAMO
ZITCOMS

••T•••M

ANTFARM
ANTONYM
ARTFILM
ARTFORM
ARTHURM
ASTREAM
AUTONYM
BUTTRAM
CUTWORM
EATFROM
FATFARM
GETFROM
GETWARM
GOTWARM
HATBRIM
HITFILM
HOTITEM
INTERIM
KETCHAM
KETCHUM
LETTERM
LITHIUM
MITCHUM
NATRIUM
OPTIMUM
OUTBEAM
OUTSWAM
OUTSWIM
OUTSWUM
POTSDAM
RITAGAM
TITOISM
YTTRIUM

•••TM••

BESTMAN
BESTMEN
BOATMAN
BOATMEN
CESTMOI
DUSTMAN
DUSTMEN
DUSTMOP
EASTMAN
FOOTMAN
FOOTMEN
HARTMAN
HARTMUT
KEPTMUM
LASTMAY
MEATMAN
MEATMEN
PITTMAN
PORTMAN
POSTMAN
POSTMEN
REITMAN
SCATMAN
VELTMAN
WENTMAD
WHITMAN

•••T•M•

AIRTIME
ALLTIME
ANATOMY
ANYTIME
ATATIME
BADTIME
BANTAMS
BEATSME
BEDTIME
BIGTIME
BOTTOMS
BUDTIME
BUTTEMT
BUYTIME
CENTIME
CENTIMO
CONTEMN
COSTUME
CUSTOMS
CUTTIME
DAYTIME
DESTEMS
DIATOMS
DICTUMS
DIDTIME
DIOTIMA
EPITOME
FUNTIME
GAUTAMA
HADTIME
HASTIME
HOTTIME
ITSTIME
JIGTIME
KHATAMI
MAYTIME
MISTIME
NAPTIME
OLDTIME
ONETIME
PASTIME
RAGTIME
RESTAMP
RHYTHMS
RUNTIME
SAOTOME
SUITSME
SYSTEMS
TAMTAMS
TEATIME
TEETIME
TOMTOMS
TWOTIME
VICTIMS
WARTIME
WHATAMI
WRITEME

•••T••M

AFCTEAM
APOTHEM
ASATEAM
BAPTISM
BENTHAM
BERTRAM
BRITCOM
BUTTRAM
CENTRUM
CHATHAM
CHETRUM
COMTISM
CULTISM
CULTJAM
EASTHAM
EGOTISM
ELITISM
EXOTISM
FANTASM
FLOTSAM
KEPTMUM
LEFTARM
LEFTISM
LEITRIM
LETTERM
LUSTRUM
MIDTERM
MISTERM
NBATEAM
NFCTEAM
NFLTEAM
NHLTEAM
NOSTRUM
ONETERM
PENTIUM
PRETERM
PRETRIM
PROTEAM
ROSTRUM
STATISM
TAGTEAM
TANTRUM
TRITIUM
TWOTERM
VIETNAM
WALTHAM
YAYTEAM
YEATEAM

••••TM•

ELECTME
FLINTMI
MAHATMA
TRUSTME

••••T•M

COUNTEM
EIGHTAM
EIGHTPM
ERRATUM
FRUSTUM
GOGETEM
HOTITEM
LONGTOM
PHANTOM
PINETUM
QUANTUM
SANCTUM
STRATUM
SUBITEM
SYMPTOM
TINYTIM

•••••TM

SILENTM

T•N••••

TANAGER
TANBARK
TANDEMS
TANDOOR
TANGELO
TANGENT
TANGIER
TANGING
TANGLED
TANGLER
TANGLES
TANGOED
TANGOER
TANGRAM
TANKAGE
TANKARD
TANKCAR
TANKERS
TANKFUL
TANKING
TANKINI
TANKSUP
TANKTOP
TANLINE
TANNERS
TANNERY
TANNEST
TANNING
TANNINS
TANNISH
TANOAKS
TANSIES
TANTARA
TANTIVY
TANTRUM
TENABLE
TENABLY
TENACES
TENACRE
TENANCY
TENANTS
TENBALL
TENCENT
TENCHES
TENCODE
TENDAYS
TENDERS
TENDING
TENDONS
TENDRIL
TENDSTO
TENEEEE
TENFEET
TENFOLD
TENFOOT
TENFOUR
TENKRUN
TENMILE
TENNANT
TENNECO
TENNERS
TENNIEL
TENNIES
TENONED
TENONER
TENPAST
TENPINS
TENSELY
TENSEST
TENSEUP
TENSILE
TENSING
TENSION
TENSITY
TENSIVE
TENSORS
TENSPOT
TENTBED
TENTERS
TENTFUL
TENTHLY
TENTING
TENTONS
TENTPEG
TENUITY
TENUOUS
TENURED
TENURES
TENWEEK
TENYEAR
TENZING
TINAFEY
TINAMOU
TINCANS
TINCTED
TINDERS
TINDERY
TINEARS

TINFISH
TINFOIL
TINGING
TINGLED
TINGLER
TINGLES
TINGODS
TINHATS
TINHORN
TINIEST
TINKERS
TINKLED
TINKLER
TINKLES
TINLIKE
TINMINE
TINNERS
TINNIER
TINNILY
TINNING
TINORES
TINROOF
TINSELS
TINSTAR
TINTERN
TINTERS
TINTING
TINTYPE
TINWARE
TINWORK
TINYBIT
TINYTIM
TINYTOT
TONALLY
TONEARM
TONEDUP
TONELOC
TONEMES
TONEROW
TONESUP
TONETTE
TONGANS
TONGING
TONGUES
TONIEST
TONIGHT
TONNAGE
TONNEAU
TONSILS
TONSURE
TONTINE
TONUSES
TONYDOW
TUNABLE
TUNAOIL
TUNASUB
TUNDRAS
TUNEDIN
TUNEDTO
TUNEDUP
TUNEFUL
TUNEOUT
TUNESIN
TUNESTO
TUNESUP
TUNEUPS
TUNGOIL
TUNICLE
TUNISIA
TUNNELS
TYNDALL

T••N•••

TAINTED
TANNERS
TANNERY
TANNEST
TANNING
TANNINS
TANNISH
TARNISH
TAUNTED
TAUNTER
TAUNTON
TAWNIER
TAWNILY
TEANECK
TEENAGE
TEENERS
TEENIER
TEENSIE
TENNANT
TENNECO
TENNERS
TENNIEL
TENNIES
TERNARY
TERNATE
THANDIE
THANKED
THANKER
THENETS
THENEWS
THENILE
THINAIR
THINICE
THINKER
THINKOF
THINKSO
THINKUP
THINMAN
THINNED
THINNER
THINOUT
THUNDER
THUNKED
TIENDAS
TINNERS
TINNIER
TINNILY
TINNING
TLINGIT
TOENAIL
TONNAGE
TONNEAU
TOONIES
TOPNAME
TORNADO
TORNOFF
TORNOUT
TOWNCAR
TOWNERS
TOWNIES
TOWNISH
TOWNLET
TOYNBEE
TRANCED
TRANCES
TRANSAM
TRANSIT
TRANSOM
TRENARY
TRENDED
TRENTON
TRINARY
TRINITY
TRINKET
TRUNDLE
TSONGAS
TSUNAMI
TUNNELS
TURNBAD
TURNERS
TURNERY
TURNING
TURNIPS
TURNKEY
TURNOFF
TURNONS
TURNOUT
TURNPRO
TURNRED
TURNSIN
TURNSON
TURNSTO
TURNSUP
TURNUPS
TWANGED
TWANGER
TWINBED
TWINERS
TWINGED
TWINGES
TWINIER
TWINING
TWINJET
TWINKIE
TWINKLE
TWINKLY
TWINNED
TWINSET
TYINGIN
TYINGON
TYINGTO
TYINGUP

T•••N••

TACONIC
TAGENDS
TAHINIS
TAKENBY
TAKENIN
TAKENON
TAKENTO
TAKENUP
TAKINGS
TALENTS
TALONED
TAPINGS
TAPINTO
TARANTO
TECHNOS
TEJANAS
TEJANOS
TENANCY
TENANTS
TENONED
TENONER
TERENCE
TETANUS
THINNED
THINNER
THORNED
THRONES
THRONGS
TIDINGS
TIEINTO
TIERNEY
TILINGS
TILLNOW
TIMINGS
TISANES
TITANAE
TITANIA
TITANIC
TOKENED
TOPKNOT
TOPONYM
TORINOS
TORONTO
TOTINOS
TOURNEY
TOWINGS
TRAINED
TRAINEE
TRAINER
TRAININ
TRAYNOR
TREINTA
TROUNCE
TRUANCY
TRUANTS
TULANEU
TWEENER
TWINNED
TWOONIE
TWOUNIT
TYLENOL
TYRANNY
TYRANTS

T••••N•

TABBING
TABLING
TABUING
TACKING
TAGGANT
TAGGING
TAGLINE
TAILEND
TAILING
TAKEINS
TAKEONE
TALKING
TALLINN
TALLONE
TAMMANY
TAMPING
TANGENT
TANGING
TANKING
TANKINI
TANLINE
TANNING
TANNINS
TAPPANS
TAPPING
TARPONS
TARRING
TARTANS
TARTING
TARZANA
TARZANS
TASKING
TASTING
TATIANA
TATTING
TAURINE
TAUTENS
TAVERNA
TAVERNS
TAXIING
TEAMING
TEARING
TEASING
TEAURNS
TEEMING
TEFLONS
TELLING
TEMPING
TENCENT
TENDING
TENDONS
TENNANT
TENPINS
TENSING
TENTING
TENTONS
TENZING
TERHUNE
TERMING
TERMINI
TERRANS
TERRENE
TERRINE
TESTING
TEUTONS
TEXTING
THATONE
THAWING
THEBAND
THEBANS
THEFONZ
THEGANG
THEKING
THEOMNI
THEPOND
THERENT
THERING
THERINK
THESUNS
THEWIND
THISONE
THREENO
THYMINE
TICCING
TICKING
TIDYING
TIELINE
TIEPINS
TIERING
TIFFANY
TIFFING
TIFFINS
TIGLONS
TIJUANA
TILLING
TILTING
TIMMINS
TIMPANI
TINCANS
TINGING
TINMINE
TINNING
TINTING
TIPLINE
TIPPING
TITHING
TITIANS
TITLING
TITRING
TOCSINS
TOGGING
TOILING
TOLLING
TOLUENE
TONGANS
TONGING
TONTINE
TOOLING
TOOLONG
TOOMANY
TOOTING
TOPGUNS
TOPLINE
TOPPING
TOPRANK
TOPTENS
TORMENT
TORRENT
TORTONI
TOSSING
TOTTING
TOUCANS
TOURING
TOUTING
TOWLINE
TOYGUNS
TOYLAND
TRACING
TRADING
TREEING
TREPANS
TREVINO
TRIBUNE
TRIDENT
TRIGONS
TRITONE
TRITONS
TROJANS
TROWING
TRUEING
TRUMANS
TSARINA
TSETUNG
TUBBING
TUCKING
TUCSONS
TUFTING
TUGGING
TULSANS
TURBANS
TURBINE
TUREENS
TURFING
TURNING
TURNONS
TUSCANS
TUSCANY
TUSKING
TUTTING
TWERENT
TWINING
TWOLANE
TWOTONE
TWOTONS
TYCOONS
TYMPANA
TYMPANI
TYRANNY
TZARINA

T•••••N

TACHYON
TACKSON
TAILFIN
TAILPIN
TAKENIN
TAKENON
TAKESIN
TAKESON
TAKETEN
TALIBAN
TALKSON
TALLINN
TAMBLYN
TAMGLEN
TAPEDON
TAPEMAN
TAPEMEN
TAPESON
TASHLIN
TAUNTON
TAUREAN
TAXIMAN
TAXIMEN
TEACHIN
TEAGOWN
TEHERAN
TELERAN
TELLSON
TENKRUN
TENSION
TERRAIN
TESTBAN
TESTRUN
TEXTRON
THEMOON
THEOMEN
THEREIN
THEREON
THESWAN
THETURN
THIAMIN
THICKEN
THIGPEN
THINMAN
THOMSON
THORSON
THREWIN
THREWON
THRIVEN
THROWIN
THROWON
THURMAN
TIBETAN
TIBURON
TICOTIN
TIEDOWN
TIGHTEN
TINHORN
TINTERN
TIOMKIN
TIPDOWN
TIREMAN
TIREMEN
TOATURN
TOHELEN
TOLEDAN
TOLKIEN
TOLLMAN
TOLLMEN
TOOKTEN
TOOSOON
TOPDOWN
TOPEKAN
TOPSPIN
TORSION
TOUCHON
TOUGHEN
TOWEDIN
TRADEIN
TRADEON
TRAININ
TRAPGUN
TREADON
TREASON
TRENTON
TRICORN
TRIEDON
TRIESON
TRILLIN
TRIPSON
TRISTAN
TRODDEN
TROMPIN
TROOPIN
TRUDGEN
TRUSTIN
TRYITON
TUBEPAN
TUCHMAN
TUCKSIN
TUITION
TUNEDIN
TUNESIN
TURFMAN
TURFMEN
TURNSIN
TURNSON
TWISTON
TWOIRON
TYINGIN
TYINGON
TYPEDIN
TYPESIN
TYPHOON

•TN••••

ATNIGHT

•T•N•••

ATANEND
ATINGLE
ATONERS
ATONICS
ATONIES
ATONING
CTENOID
ETHNICS
ETONIAN
ETONICS
STANCES
STANDBY
STANDEE
STANDER
STANDIN
STANDON
STANDTO
STANDUP
STANINE
STANKUP
STANLEE
STANLEY
STANNIC
STANNUM
STANTON
STANZAS
STENCIL
STENGEL
STENGUN
STENNIS
STENTOR
STINGER
STINKER
STINKUP
STINTED
STINTER
STONEAX
STONERS
STONIER
STONILY
STONING
STUNGUN
STUNNED
STUNNER
STUNTED
UTENSIL

•T••N••

ATEINTO
ATLANTA
ATLUNCH
ATTENDS
ATTUNED
ATTUNES
ETERNAL
ETHANES
ETHANOL
ETHENES
ETIENNE
FTHENRY
ITSONME
ITWENTY
JTMONEY
MTKENYA
MTSINAI
OTRANTO
STAGNES
STAINED
STAINER
STANNIC
STANNUM
STAUNCH
STDENIS
STEANNE
STEINEM
STEINER
STENNIS
STERNAL
STERNER
STERNLY
STERNOS
STERNUM
STRANDS
STRANGE
STRINGS
STRINGY
STUNNED
STUNNER

•T•••N•

ATAMANS
ATANEND
ATONING
ATSIGNS
ATTAINS
ATTAINT
CTSCANS
ETAMINE
ETCHANT
ETCHING
ETIENNE
ETYMONS
FTDIXNJ
FTWAYNE
ITCHING
ITEMING
ITEMONE
ITERANT
ITSDONE
ITSFINE
ITSGONE
MTBLANC
MTEVANS
STAGING
STAKING
STAMENS
STAMINA
STANINE
STARING
STATING
STATINS
STAVING
STAYING
STEANNE
STEARNS
STEFANI
STEPINS
STEPONE
STEVENS
STEWING
STIPEND
STJOHNS
STOKING
STOLONS
STONING
STORING
STOTINS
STOWING
STRAINS
STUBING
STUDENT
STYLING
STYRENE
UTAHANS
UTICANS
UTICANY

•T••••N

ATSEVEN
ATTYGEN
ETESIAN
ETONIAN
ITALIAN
ITHACAN
ITSASIN
ITSOPEN
KTOSLIN
MTLOGAN
OTTAWAN
OTTOMAN
STANDIN
STANDON
STANTON
STARION
STARMAN
STARSIN
STARTIN
STARTON
STASSEN
STATION
STAYSIN
STAYSON
STEALIN
STEARIN
STEEPEN
STEEPIN
STENGUN
STEPHEN
STEPSIN
STEPSON
STETSON
STEUBEN
STEWPAN
STICKIN
STICKON
STIFFEN
STILTON
STIMSON
STIRSIN
STOLEIN
STOLLEN
STOMPIN
STOMPON
STOODIN
STOODON
STOPSIN
STORMIN
STOUTEN
STRAPIN
STRAPON
STRIVEN
STSIMON
STUCKIN
STUCKON
STUFFIN
STUNGUN
STYGIAN
UTOPIAN

••TN•••

APTNESS
BATNEXT
CATNAPS
CATNIPS
FATNESS
FITNESS
HOTNESS
JITNEYS
NOTNEAR
NOTNICE
PATNESS
PETNAME
PETNAPS
WETNAPS
WETNESS
WITNESS

••T•N••

ACTINON
ANTENNA
ANTONIA
ANTONIN
ANTONIO
ANTONYM
ATTENDS
ATTUNED
ATTUNES
AUTONYM
BITONAL
BOTANIC
BOTHNIA
BUTANES
BUTENES
CATANIA
CATENAE
CATENAS
CETANES
CUTINON
CUTINTO
DATINGS
DETENTE
DETENTS
DETUNED
DETUNES
EATENAT
EATENUP
EATINTO
ENTENTE
ESTONIA
EXTENDS
EXTENSO
EXTENTS
EXTINCT
FATONES
FITINTO
GATINGS
GETINON
GETINTO
GETONIT
GETONTO
GITANOS
GOTINON
GOTINTO
GOTONIT
GOTONTO
HITINTO
HOTONES
ICTINUS
INTENDS
INTENSE
INTENTS
INTONED
INTONER
INTONES
KETONES
KETONIC
LATENCY
LATENED
LATENTS
LATINAS
LATINII
LATINOS
LATINUS
LETINON
LETKNOW
LETSNOT
LITINTO
MATINAL
MATINEE
MUTANTS
NOTONCE
OBTUNDS
OCTANES
OCTANTS
OFTENER
OUTGNAW
OUTINGS
PATENCY
PATENTS
PATINAS
PETUNIA
POTENCE
POTENCY
RATINES
RATINGS
RETINAE
RETINAL
RETINAS
RETINGE
RETINOL
RETINTS
RETINUE
RETONED
RETONES
RETUNED
RETUNES
ROTUNDA
SATANIC
SATINET
SATINON
SETENTA
SETINTO

SITINON
SITONIT
TETANUS
TITANAE
TITANIA
TITANIC
TOTINOS
UNTENSE
UNTONED
UNTUNED
UNTUNES
UPTONOW
USTINOV
VOTENAY
WETONES

••T••N•

ACTIONS
ALTHING
ALTOONA
ANTEING
ANTENNA
ANTHONY
ANTOINE
ARTSONG
ASTOUND
ATTAINS
ATTAINT
AUTOING
AUTOMNE
AUTUMNS
BATHING
BATTENS
BATTING
BATWING
BETHANY
BETHINK
BETHUNE
BETTANY
BETTING
BITTING
BUTTING
BUTTONS
BUTTONY
BYTURNS
CATIONS
CATKINS
CATMINT
CITRINE
CITRONS
COTTONS
COTTONY
CUTTING
DATSUNS
DETAINS
DOTTING
ENTRANT
ENTWINE
ESTRING
EXTERNE
EXTERNS
FATLING
FATTENS
FATTING
FITTING
FUTZING
GATLING
GATLINS
GETBENT
GETDONE
GETSANA
GETSANF
GETTING
GITTING
GOTDONE
GSTRING
GUTTING
HATBAND
HATPINS
HATTING
HITSONG
HITTING
HITTUNE
HOTHAND
HOTLINE
HOTLINK
HOTPINK
HOTTUNA
HOTZONE
HUTTING
INTERNE
INTERNS
INTHING
INTURNS
JETFANS
JETGUNS
JETSONS
JETTING
JOTTING
JUTLAND
JUTTING
KATRINA
KATRINE
KITTENS
KITTING
LATEENS
LATHING
LATRINE
LETTING
LOTIONS
LOTTING
MATRONS
MATTING
METFANS
METHANE
MITRING
MITTENS
MOTIONS
MOTRINS
MUTTONS
NATHANS
NATIONS
NETTING
NETTONS
NITTANY
NOTAONE
NOTDONE
NOTHING
NOTHINS
NOTIONS
NOTMANY
NOTMINE
NOTTING
NOTURNS
NUTPINE
NUTTING
OBTAINS
OPTIONS
OUTBANS
OUTBEND
OUTCANT
OUTDONE
OUTFIND
OUTGUNS
OUTHUNT
OUTJINX
OUTKING
OUTLAND
OUTLINE
OUTMANS
OUTRANG
OUTRANK
OUTRANT
OUTRING
OUTRUNS
OUTSANG
OUTSING
OUTSINS
OUTSUNG
OUTWENT
OUTWIND
OUTWING
PATERNO
PATHAND
PATHANS
PATIENT
PATRONS
PATTING
PETPONY
PETTING
PITHING
PITTING
PITYING
POTEENS
POTIONS
POTTING
PUTTING
PYTHONS
RATFINK
RATIONS
RATLINE
RATLINS
RATTANS
RATTING
RETAINS
RETHANK
RETHINK
RETSINA
RETTING
RETURNS
RETWINE
ROTTING
RUTHANN
RUTLAND
RUTTING
SATEENS
SATURNS
SETTING
SITTING
TATIANA
TATTING
TITHING
TITIANS
TITLING
TITRING
TOTTING
TUTTING
UNTHINK
UNTWINE
UNTYING
UPTOWNS
UPTREND
UPTURNS
VATTING
VETOING
VETTING
VITRINE
VOTEDNO
VOTESNO
WATKINS
WETLAND
WETTING
WITLING
WITSEND
WITTING

••T•••N

ACTAEON
ACTEDIN
ACTEDON
ACTINON
ACTUPON
ALTHORN
ANTIGEN
ANTIGUN
ANTLION
ANTONIN
ARTFERN
ARTISAN
ATTYGEN
AUTOPEN
AZTECAN
BATEMAN
BATSMAN
BATSMEN
BETAKEN
BETOKEN
BETWEEN
BITESIN
BITESON
BITTERN
BUTTSIN
BYTRAIN
CATALAN
CATCHON
CATSCAN
CITIZEN
CITROEN
CUTDOWN
CUTINON
CUTOPEN
DETRAIN
DOTEDON
DOTESON
ELTRAIN
ENTERIN
ENTERON
ENTRAIN
ERTEGUN
ESTAMIN
ESTEBAN
ESTEFAN
GATEMAN
GATEMEN
GETDOWN
GETEVEN
GETINON
GETITON
GETUPON
GOTDOWN
GOTEVEN
GOTINON
GOTITON
GOTUPON
HITCHON
HITTOWN
HITUPON
ISTOMIN
ISTRIAN
JETSFAN
JOTDOWN
KATHRYN
KITCHEN
LATCHON
LATERAN
LATERON
LATVIAN
LETDOWN
LETEMIN
LETHEAN
LETINON
LETMEIN
LETTERN
LETUPON
LOTHIAN
MATALIN
MATEWAN
METSFAN
MUTAGEN
NETGAIN
NETIZEN
NOTBEEN
NOTEVEN
NOTOPEN
OATBRAN
OCTAGON
ONTKEAN
OPTEDIN
ORTOLAN
OTTAWAN
OTTOMAN
OUTBURN
OUTEARN
OUTFAWN
OUTGAIN
OUTGRIN
OUTLAIN
OUTLIMN
OUTPLAN
OUTSEEN
OUTSPIN
OUTTORN
OUTTURN
OUTWORN
PATCHEN
PATDOWN
PATROON
PATTERN
PETEMAN
PETEMEN
PETLION
PETSCAN
PITCHIN
PITTMAN
PUTDOWN
PUTUPON
PYTHIAN
RETAKEN
RETRAIN
RITALIN
RUTHANN
SATDOWN
SATINON
SATUPON
SETDOWN
SETUPON
SITDOWN
SITINON
SITUPON
SOTHERN
UNTAKEN
VATICAN
VETERAN
VITAMIN
VOTEDIN
VOTEDON
VOTESIN
VOTESON
WETDOWN

•••TN••

ACCTNOS
BEATNIK
BRITNEY
CHUTNEY
COSTNER
DOITNOW
EXITNOW
FASTNET
GORTNER
JUSTNOW
MEITNER
NEATNIK
PARTNER
PORTNOY
SHATNER
SPUTNIK
VENTNOR
VIETNAM
VINTNER
WHATNOT
WHATNOW
WHITNEY

•••T•N•

ABATING
ACETONE
ACHTUNG
AGATINE
AIRTANK
ARETINO
AUSTINS
BAITING
BANTING
BARTEND
BASTING
BATTENS
BATTING
BEATING
BELTANE
BELTING
BESTING
BESTONE
BETTANY
BETTING
BHUTANI
BIGTENT
BITTING
BLATANT
BOATING
BOITANO
BOLTING
BOOTING
BOSTONS
BOSTONU
BRETONS
BRITONS
BUITONI
BUNTING
BUSTING
BUTTING
BUTTONS
BUTTONY
CAFTANS
CANTINA
CANTING
CANTINO
CANTONS
CARTING
CARTONS
CASTING
CHITONS
CHUTING
COATING
CONTEND
CONTENT
CORTINA
COSTING
COTTONS
COTTONY
CRATING
CRETANS
CRETINS
CROTONS
CUTTING
DALTONS
DARTING
DAYTONA
DELTONA
DENTINE
DENTING
DENTINS
DENTONS
DENTYNE
DESTINE
DESTINO
DESTINY
DIETING
DINTING
DISTANT
DISTEND
DOTTING
DUCTING
DUETING
DUOTONE
DUSTING
EASTEND
EASTING
EDITING
ELATING
ELUTING
EMOTING
EXITING
FANTANS
FANTINE
FASTENS
FASTING
FASTONE
FATTENS
FATTING
FELTING
FESTINA
FITTING
FLUTING
FONTANA
FONTANE
FONTINA
FOOTING
FORTUNA
FORTUNE
GAETANO
GAITING
GASTANK
GASTONE
GETTING
GIFTING
GIRTING
GITTING
GLUTENS
GRATING
GUSTING
GUTTING
HAFTING
HALTING
HASTENS
HASTING
HATTING
HEATING
HEFTING
HILTING
HILTONS
HINTING
HITTING
HITTUNE
HOOTING
HOSTING
HOTTUNA
HUNTING
HURTING
HUTTING
IFSTONE
INSTANT
INSTONE
ISOTONE
JESTING
JETTING
JILTING
JOLTING
JOTTING
JUSTINE
JUSTONE
JUTTING
KILTING
KITTENS
KITTING
LANTANA
LASTING
LASTONE
LEFTEND
LEPTONS
LETTING
LIFTING
LILTING
LINTING
LISTENS
LISTING
LOFTING
LOOTING
LOTTING
LOUTING
LUSTING
MALTING
MARTENS
MARTINA
MARTINI
MARTINO
MARTINS
MARTINU
MARTINV
MASTING
MATTING
MEETING
MELTING
MINTING
MISTING
MISTUNE
MITTENS
MOLTING
MONTANA
MONTAND
MONTANO
MONTUNO
MOOTING
MORTONS
MUSTANG
MUTTONS
NEATENS
NEPTUNE
NESTING
NETTING
NETTONS
NEWTONS
NITTANY
NORTONS
NOTTING
NUTTING
OILTANK
ORATING
OROTUND
OUSTING
PANTENE
PANTING
PANTONE
PARTING
PARTONE
PASTINA
PASTING
PATTING
PECTINS
PELTING
PENTANE
PEPTONE
PETTING
PHOTONS
PIETINS
PISTONS
PITTING
PLATENS
PLATING
PLUTONS
PONTANO
POPTUNE
PORTEND
PORTENT
PORTING
POSTING
POTTING
POUTING
PRATING
PRETEND
PROTONS
PUNTING
PUPTENT
PUTTING
QUOTING
RAFTING
RANTING
RAPTUNE
RATTANS
RATTING
RENTING
RESTING
RETTING
RIFTING
RIOTING
RLSTINE
ROOTING
ROSTAND
ROTTING
ROUTINE
ROUTING
RRATING
RUSTING
RUTTING
SALTANT
SALTINE
SALTING
SANTANA
SANTINI
SEATING
SESTINA
SETTING
SEXTANS
SEXTANT
SEXTONS
SHUTINS
SIFTING
SILTING
SISTINE
SITTING
SKATING
SLATING
SMETANA
SMITING
SOFTENS
SORTING
SPITING
STATING
STATINS
STOTINS
SUBTEND
SUBTONE
SUITING
SULTANA
SULTANS
SUNTANS
TARTANS
TARTING
TASTING
TATTING
TAUTENS
TENTING
TENTONS
TESTING
TEUTONS
TEXTING
THATONE
TILTING
TINTING
TONTINE
TOOTING
TOPTENS
TORTONI
TOTTING
TOUTING
TRITONE
TRITONS
TSETUNG
TUFTING
TUTTING
TWOTONE
TWOTONS
UNITING
UNSTONY
UNSTUNG
UPSTAND
VATTING
VENTING
VESTING
VETTING
WAFTING
WAITING
WALTONS
WANTING
WANTONS
WASTING
WELTING
WESTEND
WESTINS
WETTING
WHITENS
WHITING
WILTING
WITTING
WONTING
WONTONS
WRITING
WYOTANA
XRATING
ZEITUNG
ZESTING

•••T••N

ABSTAIN
ABUTSON
ALATEEN
ANDTHEN
ANYTOWN
AUCTION
BASTION
BEATSON
BELTRAN
BENTSEN
BESTMAN
BESTMEN
BIGTOWN
BITTERN
BLITZEN
BOATMAN
BOATMEN
BRETTON
BRITAIN
BRITTEN
BRITTON
BUSTSIN
BUTTSIN
CANTEEN
CAPTAIN
CAPTION
CARTOON
CARTSIN
CASTSON
CAUTHEN
CAUTION
CERTAIN
CHATWIN
CHITLIN
CHITOWN
CISTERN
CONTAIN
CONTEMN
COSTAIN
COWTOWN
CRATION
CRUTZEN
CURTAIN
DANTEAN
DARTGUN
DESTAIN
DEXTRIN
DICTION
DUSTBIN
DUSTGUN
DUSTMAN
DUSTMEN
DUSTPAN
EARTHEN
EASTERN
EASTMAN
ECOTRIN
EDITION
ELATION
ELUTION
EMOTION
EPSTEIN
FACTION
FELTPEN
FESTOON
FICTION
FIFTEEN
FLATTEN
FLITSIN
FONTEYN
FOOTMAN
FOOTMEN
FORTRAN
FUSTIAN
GENTIAN
GLUTTON
GRATEON
HAITIAN
HARTMAN
HEATFAN
HEATHEN
HITTOWN
HOWTHEN
IZATION
KANTIAN
KRATION
LANTERN
LAOTIAN
LASTDON
LECTERN
LETTERN
MANTUAN
MARTIAN
MEATMAN
MEATMEN
MENTION
MIDTEEN
MIDTOWN
NESTSIN
NEUTRON
NEWTOWN
NOSTAIN
NOUTURN
NOWTHEN
OLDTOWN
ORATION
OURTOWN
OUTTORN
OUTTURN
OVATION
PARTYON
PASTEIN
PASTERN
PATTERN
PERTAIN
PITTMAN
PLATOON
PONTIAN
PONTOON
PORTION
PORTMAN
POSTERN
POSTMAN
POSTMEN
PRETEEN
PROTEAN
PROTEIN
REITMAN
RESTAIN
RESTSIN
RESTSON
RIOTGUN
RIPTORN
RONTGEN
RUCTION
SCATMAN
SCOTIAN
SECTION
SHOTGUN
SHUTSIN
SIXTEEN

SLATKIN
SMITTEN
SPITSON
STATION
STETSON
SUBTEEN
SUCTION
SUSTAIN
TESTBAN
TESTRUN
TEXTRON
THETURN
TINTERN
TOATURN
TUITION
UMPTEEN
UNCTION
UNSTERN
VELTMAN
VESTRON
VISTEON
VUITTON
WAITRON
WAITSON
WANTSIN
WARTORN
WESTERN
WHITMAN
WHITSUN
WRITEIN
WRITEON
WRITTEN
WROTEIN
WROTEON
XANTHAN
YELTSIN
YOUTHEN

••••TN•

MIGHTNT
MINOTND
NOVOTNY
OUGHTNT

••••T•N

ALLSTON
ANISTON
AVESTAN
BALATON
BASETEN
BDALTON
BLANTON
BLENTIN
BRAXTON
BRETTON
BRITTEN
BRITTON
BUILTIN
BUILTON
BURNTIN
BURSTIN
BURSTYN
CAKETIN
CAPITAN
CAPSTAN
CARLTON
CAROTIN
CHASTEN
CHEATIN
CHEATON
CLACTON
CLANTON
CLAPTON
CLAYTON
CLIFTON
CLINTON
COMPTON
COUNTIN
COUNTON
CREPTIN
CRESTON
CROUTON
DAKOTAN
DARKTAN
DEALTIN
DEEPTAN
DRAYTON
DRIFTIN
DRISTAN
DUNSTAN
DWELTON
ELASTIN
FEASTON
FIVETEN
FLATTEN
FOISTON
FRONTON
GELATIN
GETITON
GIGATON
GLISTEN
GLUTTON
GOTITON
GRAFTON
GREATEN
HALSTON
HAMPTON
HANGTEN
HARDTEN
HEARTEN
HEMATIN
HOUSTON
HUNGTEN
HURSTON
KEMPTON
KERATIN
KILOTON
KIRSTEN
KRISTIN
KRYPTON
LANGTON
LAPUTAN
LAYITON
LEAPTIN
LEAPTON
LIGHTEN
LIGHTON
LLEYTON
LONGTON
MAARTEN
MARSTON
MEGATON
MOISTEN
MONCTON
PELOTON
PHAETON
PRESTON
PURITAN
QUARTAN
QUENTIN
QUIETEN
QUINTON
RALSTON
RARITAN
RIGHTON
RUBITIN
SHORTEN
SIZETEN
SKELTON
SLAYTON
SLEPTIN
SLEPTON
SMARTEN
SMITTEN
SPARTAN
SPENTON
SPORTIN
STANTON
STARTIN
STARTON
STILTON
STOUTEN
SWEETEN
SWEETON
SWINTON
TAKETEN
TAUNTON
TIBETAN
TICOTIN
TIGHTEN
TOOKTEN
TRENTON
TRISTAN
TRUSTIN
TRYITON
TWISTON
UNEATEN
UNOFTEN
VECHTEN
VUITTON
WALSTON
WEIRTON
WHARTON
WHEATEN
WHEATON
WINSTON
WRITTEN
YANKTON
YORKTON
YUCATAN
ZABUTON

•••••TN

SILENTN

TO•••••

TOADIED
TOADIES
TOADISH
TOAHAIR
TOASTED
TOASTEE
TOASTER
TOATURN
TOBACCO
TOBEHAD
TOBLAME
TOCCATA
TOCELIA
TOCSINS
TODDIES
TODDLED
TODDLER
TODDLES
TOECAPS
TOEHOLD
TOELESS
TOELIKE
TOELOOP
TOENAIL
TOEPICK
TOESHOE
TOETAPS
TOFFEES
TOFFLER
TOFUTTI
TOGGERY
TOGGING
TOGGLED
TOGGLER
TOGGLES
TOGSOUT
TOHEART
TOHELEN
TOHOMER
TOHORSE
TOILERS
TOILETS
TOILFUL
TOILING
TOILSAT
TOKENED
TOLDALL
TOLDOFF
TOLEASE
TOLEDAN
TOLEDOS
TOLKIEN
TOLLAGE
TOLLBAR
TOLLERS
TOLLING
TOLLMAN
TOLLMEN
TOLLWAY
TOLSTOI
TOLSTOY
TOLTECS
TOLUENE
TOMBOYS
TOMCATS
TOMFOOL
TOMGOLA
TOMJOAD
TOMKITE
TOMTITS
TOMTOMS
TONALLY
TONEARM
TONEDUP
TONELOC
TONEMES
TONEROW
TONESUP
TONETTE
TONGANS
TONGING
TONGUES
TONIEST
TONIGHT
TONNAGE
TONNEAU
TONSILS
TONSURE
TONTINE
TONUSES
TONYDOW
TOODLES
TOOEASY
TOOHARD
TOOHIGH
TOOKAIM
TOOKFOR
TOOKILL
TOOKOFF
TOOKOUT
TOOKTEN
TOOLATE
TOOLBAR
TOOLBOX
TOOLERS
TOOLING
TOOLKIT
TOOLONG
TOOLSET
TOOLSUP
TOOMANY
TOOMUCH
TOONIES
TOORDER
TOOSLOW
TOOSOON
TOOTALL
TOOTERS
TOOTHED
TOOTING
TOOTLED
TOOTLER
TOOTLES
TOOTSAT
TOOTSIE
TOPAZES
TOPBIDS
TOPBOOT
TOPCOAT
TOPDOGS
TOPDOWN
TOPDRAW
TOPEKAN
TOPFIVE
TOPFORM
TOPGUNS
TOPHATS
TOPHOLE
TOPIARY
TOPICAL
TOPKAPI
TOPKICK
TOPKNOT
TOPLESS
TOPLINE
TOPMAST
TOPMOST
TOPNAME
TOPONYM
TOPPERS
TOPPING
TOPPLED
TOPPLES
TOPRANK
TOPRATE
TOPROWS
TOPSAIL
TOPSEED
TOPSIDE
TOPSOFF
TOPSOIL
TOPSOUT
TOPSPIN
TOPSPOT
TOPTENS
TOPTHIS
TORCHED
TORCHER
TORCHES
TOREOFF
TOREOUT
TOREROS
TORINOS
TORMENT
TORNADO
TORNOFF
TORNOUT
TOROIDS
TORONTO
TORPEDO
TORQUED
TORQUES
TORREFY
TORRENT
TORSION
TORTLAW
TORTOLA
TORTONI
TORTUGA
TORTURE
TORVALD
TORVILL
TORYISH
TORYISM
TOSCALE
TOSHIBA
TOSHIRO
TOSPARE
TOSSERS
TOSSING
TOSSOFF
TOSSOUT
TOSSPOT
TOSSUPS
TOSTADA
TOSTART
TOTABLE
TOTALED
TOTALER
TOTALLY
TOTALUP
TOTASTE
TOTEBAG
TOTEMIC
TOTESUP
TOTINOS
TOTOTOO
TOTTERS
TOTTERY
TOTTING
TOUAREG
TOUCANS
TOUCHED
TOUCHER
TOUCHES
TOUCHON
TOUCHUP
TOUGHEN
TOUGHER
TOUGHIE
TOUGHLY
TOUPEES
TOURBUS
TOURERS
TOURING
TOURISM
TOURIST
TOURNEY
TOUSLED
TOUSLES
TOUTERS
TOUTING
TOWABLE
TOWAGES
TOWARDS
TOWAWAY
TOWBARS
TOWBOAT
TOWCARS
TOWEDIN
TOWELED
TOWERED
TOWHEAD
TOWHEES
TOWINGS
TOWLINE
TOWNCAR
TOWNERS
TOWNIES
TOWNISH
TOWNLET
TOWPATH
TOWROPE
TOYBALL
TOYBIKE
TOYBOAT
TOYBOOK
TOYCARS
TOYCART
TOYDOGS
TOYDOLL
TOYFAIR
TOYGUNS
TOYHATS
TOYHOOP
TOYKITE
TOYLAND
TOYLESS
TOYLIKE
TOYNBEE
TOYOTAS
TOYPAIL
TOYSHOP
TOYSLED
TOYSRUS
TOYTOPS
TOYWITH

T•O••••

TAOISTS
THOMSON
THOREAU
THORIUM
THORNED
THORSON
THOUGHT
TIOMKIN
TMOBILE
TOODLES
TOOEASY
TOOHARD
TOOHIGH
TOOKAIM
TOOKFOR
TOOKILL
TOOKOFF
TOOKOUT
TOOKTEN
TOOLATE
TOOLBAR
TOOLBOX
TOOLERS
TOOLING
TOOLKIT
TOOLONG
TOOLSET
TOOLSUP
TOOMANY
TOOMUCH
TOONIES
TOORDER
TOOSLOW
TOOSOON
TOOTALL
TOOTERS
TOOTHED
TOOTING
TOOTLED
TOOTLER
TOOTLES
TOOTSAT
TOOTSIE
TROCHEE
TROCHES
TRODDEN
TROIKAS
TROILUS
TROJANS
TROLLED
TROLLER
TROLLEY
TROLLOP
TROMPED
TROMPIN
TROOPED
TROOPER
TROOPIN
TROPICS
TROPISM
TROTHED
TROTOFF
TROTOUT
TROTSKY
TROTSUP
TROTTED
TROTTER
TROUBLE
TROUGHS
TROUNCE
TROUPED
TROUPER
TROUPES
TROUSER
TROWELS
TROWING
TSONGAS
TSOURIS
TWOACRE
TWOACTS
TWOBALL
TWOBASE
TWOBITS
TWODAYS
TWODEEP
TWODOOR
TWOEEEE
TWOEGGS
TWOFACE
TWOFEET
TWOFERS
TWOFOLD
TWOFOOT
TWOHOUR
TWOIRON
TWOLANE
TWOMORE
TWOONIE
TWOPAIR
TWOPART
TWOROOM
TWOSHOT
TWOSOME
TWOSPOT
TWOSTAR
TWOSTEP
TWOTERM
TWOTIME
TWOTOED
TWOTONE
TWOTONS
TWOUNIT
TWOWEEK
TWOYEAR

T••O•••

TABOOED
TABORET
TABOULI
TACOMAS
TACONIC
TAGOUTS
TALONED
TANOAKS
TAROILS
TEEOFFS
TENONED
TENONER
TFPOWYS
THEOATH
THEODOR
THEOMEN
THEOMNI
THEOREM
THROATS
THROATY
THRONES
THRONGS
THROUGH
THROWAT
THROWER
THROWIN
THROWON
THROWUP
TICOTIN
TIMOTHY
TINORES
TIPOFFS
TIPOVER
TITOISM
TITOIST
TOHOMER
TOHORSE
TOPONYM
TOROIDS
TORONTO
TOTOTOO
TOYOTAS
TRIODES
TRIOLET
TROOPED
TROOPER
TROOPIN
TRYOUTS
TUPOLEV
TUTORED
TVMOVIE
TVROOMS
TWOONIE
TYCOONS

T•••O••

TABLOID
TABOOED
TADPOLE
TAGSOUT
TAILOFF
TAILORS
TAKEOFF
TAKEONE
TAKEOUT
TALKOUT
TALLONE
TALLOWS
TALLOWY
TANDOOR
TANGOED
TANGOER
TAPIOCA
TAPROOM
TAPROOT
TAPSOFF
TAPSOUT
TARPONS
TATTOOS
TAXCODE
TAYLORS
TEACOZY
TEAGOWN
TEAPOTS
TEAPOYS
TEAROFF
TEAROOM
TEAROSE
TEAROUT
TEDIOUS
TEEDOFF
TEESOFF
TEFLONS
TELLOFF
TEMPORE
TENCODE
TENDONS
TENFOLD
TENFOOT
TENFOUR
TENSORS
TENTONS
TENUOUS
TERAOHM
TERROIR
TERRORS
TESTOUT
TETRODE
TEUTONS
THATONE
THAWOUT
THEBOBO
THEBODY
THEBOMB
THEBOSS
THEBOYS
THEDOLE
THEFONZ
THEFOOL
THEGOLD
THEHOGS
THEHOOD
THEHOPE
THELOOK
THELOOP
THEMOON
THEMOST
THEPOND
THEPOOH
THEPOPE
THEPOST
THEROBE
THEROCK
THEROOM
THEROPE
THEROSE
THEROUX
THETOUR
THINOUT
THISONE
THYROID
TICKOFF
TIEDOFF
TIEDOWN
TIEPOLO
TIERODS
TIEROPE
TIESOFF
TIGLONS
TIMEOFF
TIMEOUT
TIMHOLT
TIMROTH
TINFOIL
TINGODS
TINHORN
TINROOF
TINWORK
TIPDOWN
TIPSOFF
TIPTOED
TIPTOES
TIPTOPS
TIREOUT
TISSOTS
TOEHOLD
TOELOOP
TOGSOUT
TOLDOFF
TOMBOYS
TOMFOOL
TOMGOLA
TOMJOAD
TOMTOMS
TOOKOFF
TOOKOUT
TOOLONG
TOOSOON
TOPBOOT
TOPCOAT
TOPDOGS
TOPDOWN
TOPFORM
TOPHOLE
TOPMOST
TOPROWS
TOPSOFF
TOPSOIL
TOPSOUT
TOREOFF
TOREOUT
TORNOFF
TORNOUT
TORTOLA
TORTONI
TOSSOFF
TOSSOUT
TOWBOAT
TOWROPE
TOYBOAT
TOYBOOK
TOYDOGS
TOYDOLL
TOYHOOP
TOYTOPS
TREFOIL
TREMOLO
TREMORS
TRIBORO
TRICORN
TRICOTS
TRIFOLD
TRIFORM
TRIGONS
TRILOGY
TRIMOFF
TRIPODS
TRIPOLI
TRITONE
TRITONS
TROTOFF
TROTOUT
TUCSONS
TUGBOAT
TUNAOIL
TUNEOUT
TUNGOIL
TURBOTS
TURMOIL
TURNOFF
TURNONS
TURNOUT
TUSSOCK
TVIDOLS
TVROOMS
TVSHOWS
TVSPOTS
TWODOOR
TWOFOLD
TWOFOOT
TWOHOUR
TWOMORE
TWOROOM
TWOSOME
TWOTOED
TWOTONE
TWOTONS
TYCOONS
TYPHOID
TYPHOON

T••••O•

TACHYON
TACKSON
TAGALOG
TAKEFOR
TAKENON
TAKESON
TALKSOF
TALKSON
TANDOOR
TANKTOP
TAPEDON
TAPESON
TAPROOM
TAPROOT
TAPSHOE
TATTOOS
TAUNTON
TEAROOM
TEASHOP
TEATROS
TECHNOS
TEESHOT
TEJANOS
TELECOM
TELLSOF
TELLSON
TEMBLOR
TEMPJOB
TENFOOT
TENSION
TENSPOT

TESTFOR
TEXTRON
THATSOK
THEBLOB
THECROW
THEFLOP
THEFOOL
THEHOOD
THELOOK
THELOOP
THEMOON
THEODOR
THEPOOH
THEREOF
THEREON
THERMOS
THEROOM
THESHOW
THINKOF
THOMSON
THORSON
THREWON
THROWON
TIBURON
TIEMPOS
TILLNOW
TILTTOP
TIMECOP
TINAMOU
TINROOF
TINYTOT
TIREDOF
TIRESOF
TOELOOP
TOESHOE
TOLEDOS
TOLSTOI
TOLSTOY
TOMFOOL
TONELOC
TONEROW
TONYDOW
TOOKFOR
TOOLBOX
TOOSLOW
TOOSOON
TOPBOOT
TOPKNOT
TOPSPOT
TOREROS
TORINOS
TORSION
TOSSPOT
TOTINOS
TOTOTOO
TOUCHON
TOYBOOK
TOYHOOP
TOYSHOP
TRACTOR
TRADEON
TRAITOR
TRANSOM
TRAYNOR
TREADON
TREASON
TREETOP
TRENTON
TRIEDON
TRIESON
TRIPSON
TRIVIOT
TROLLOP
TRYITON
TSARDOM
TSELIOT
TUBETOP
TUITION
TULSAOK
TUPELOS
TURFTOE
TURNSON
TUXEDOS
TWISTON
TWODOOR
TWOFOOT
TWOIRON
TWOROOM
TWOSHOT
TWOSPOT
TYINGON
TYLENOL
TYPHOON

T•••••O

TABASCO
TAKENTO
TAKESTO
TALKSTO
TALLYHO
TAMPICO
TANGELO
TAPINTO
TARANTO
TELESTO
TENDSTO
TENNECO
THEBOBO
THEHERO
THEMAYO
THERETO
THINKSO
THREENO
TIEINTO
TIEPOLO
TOBACCO
TORNADO
TORONTO
TORPEDO
TOSHIRO
TOTOTOO
TREMOLO
TREVINO
TRIBORO
TRIEDTO
TRIESTO
TRUERTO
TUNEDTO
TUNESTO
TURISMO
TURNPRO
TURNSTO
TYINGTO

•TO••••

ATOMICS
ATOMIES
ATOMISE
ATOMISM
ATOMIST
ATOMIZE
ATONERS
ATONICS
ATONIES
ATONING
ETOILES
ETONIAN
ETONICS
KTOSLIN
OTOLOGY
PTOLEMY
STOCKED
STOCKER
STOCKUP
STODGED
STODGES
STOGIES
STOICAL
STOKELY
STOKERS
STOKEUP
STOKING
STOLEIN
STOLLEN
STOLONS
STOMACH
STOMATA
STOMPED
STOMPIN
STOMPON
STONEAX
STONERS
STONIER
STONILY
STONING
STOODBY
STOODIN
STOODON
STOODTO
STOODUP
STOOGED
STOOGES
STOOKEY
STOOLED
STOOLIE
STOOPED
STOOPER
STOPFOR
STOPGAP
STOPOFF
STOPPED
STOPPER
STOPPLE
STOPSAT
STOPSBY
STOPSIN
STOPSIT
STOPSUP
STORAGE
STORERS
STOREUP
STORIED
STORIES
STORING
STORMED
STORMIN
STOTINS
STOUTEN
STOUTER
STOUTLY
STOWAGE
STOWERS
STOWING
STOWSIT
UTOPIAN
UTOPIAS
UTOPISM
UTOPIST

•T•O•••

ATEOVER
ATHOMES
ATROPHY
ATROPOS
ATWORST
ETVOILA
FTDODGE
FTWORTH
ITSOKAY
ITSONME
ITSOPEN
ITSOVER
JTMONEY
LTKOJAK
MTLOGAN
OTTOIII
OTTOMAN
PTBOATS
STJOHNS
STLOUIS
STOODBY
STOODIN
STOODON
STOODTO
STOODUP
STOOGED
STOOGES
STOOKEY
STOOLED
STOOLIE
STOOPED
STOOPER
STROBES
STROKED
STROKER
STROKES
STROLLS
STROPHE
STROUSE
UTMOSTS

•T••O••

ATABOIL
ATACOST
ATALOSS
ATCROSS
ATEMORE
CTENOID
ETHMOID
ETYMONS
ITEMONE
ITSCOLD
ITSDONE
ITSGONE
ITSLOVE
OTOLOGY
PTEROUS
STATORS
STAYOFF
STAYOUT
STCLOUD
STCROIX
STEPOFF
STEPONE
STEPOUT
STEROID
STEROLS
STOLONS
STOPOFF
STUPORS

•T•••O•

ATEALOT
ATECROW
ATIPTOE
ATROPOS
ATTABOY
ETHANOL
ITCHFOR
ITISTOO
ITSABOY
ITSALOT
MTATHOS
STANDON
STANTON
STARDOM
STARION
STARLOG
STARTON
STATION
STAYFOR
STAYSON
STENTOR
STEPMOM
STEPSON
STEREOS
STERNOS
STERTOR
STETSON
STEWPOT
STICKON
STILTON
STIMSON
STOMPON
STOODON
STOPFOR
STRAPON
STRIPOF
STSIMON
STUCCOS
STUCKON
STUDIOS

•T••••O

ATEINTO
ITISTOO
OTHELLO
OTRANTO
OTTAVIO
STANDTO
STARTTO
STEPTWO
STICKTO
STOODTO
STRETTO
STUCKTO
UTRILLO

••TO•••

ACTORLY
ALTOIDS
ALTOIST
ALTOONA
ALTOSAX
ANTOINE
ANTONIA
ANTONIN
ANTONIO
ANTONYM
ASTOLAT
ASTORIA
ASTOUND
AUTOBIO
AUTOBUS
AUTOING
AUTOMAT
AUTOMNE
AUTONYM
AUTOPEN
AUTOPIA
AUTOPSY
BETOKEN
BITONAL
CATORCE
CDTOWER
CNTOWER
CUTOFFS
CUTOPEN
CUTOUTS
CUTOVER
DETOURS
DETOXED
DETOXES
EATOVER
ENTOMBS
ESTONIA
ESTORIL
EXTOLLS
EXTORTS
FATONES
FATOUSH
FOTOMAT
GETONIT
GETONTO
GETOVER
GOTOBED
GOTOGAL
GOTOGUY
GOTONIT
GOTONTO
GOTOPOT
GOTOSEA
GOTOSEE
GOTOVER
GOTOWAR
HOTONES
HOTOVER
INTONED
INTONER
INTONES
INTOTAL
INTOUCH
ISTOMIN
KETONES
KETONIC
LATOSCA
LITOTES
LITOVSK
METOOER
MITOSES
MITOSIS
MITOTIC
MOTORED
NOTONCE
NOTOPEN
NOTOVER
NUTOILS
OCTOBER
OCTOBRE
OCTOPOD
OCTOPUS
OKTOBER
ONTOAST
ONTOPIC
ONTOPOF
ORTOLAN
OSTOSIS
OTTOIII
OTTOMAN
OUTOFIT
POTOMAC
PUTOFFS
PUTOUTS
PUTOVER
RETOAST
RETONED
RETONES
RETOOLS
RETORTS
RETOTAL
RETOUCH
RETOURS
RETOWED
SATORIS
SETOFFS
SETOUTS
SITONIT
TITOISM
TITOIST
TOTOTOO
TUTORED
UNTONED
UNTOUGH
UNTOXIC
UPTONOW
UPTOPAR
UPTOWNS
VETOERS
VETOING
VITORIA
WETONES
ZATOPEK

••T•O••

ACTFOUR
ACTIONS
ACTSOUT
AFTMOST
ALTDORF
ALTHORN
ALTOONA
ANTCOWS
ANTHONY
ANTIOCH
ARTBOOK
ARTFORM
ARTROCK
ARTSONG
ARTWORK
AUTHORS
BATBOYS
BATHOIL
BETROTH
BETTORS
BITEOFF
BITROLE
BLTTOGO
BOTTOMS
BUTGOOD
BUTTONS
BUTTONY
BUTTOUT
CATBOAT
CATBOWL
CATCOMB
CATDOOR
CATFOOD
CATFOOT
CATHODE
CATIONS
CATTOYS
CITROEN
CITRONS
CITROUS
COTTONS
COTTONY
CUTDOWN
CUTSOFF
CUTSOUT
CUTWORK
CUTWORM
DETROIT
DITTOED
DOTBOMB
DOTCOMS
DUTEOUS
EATMORE
EATSOUT
ENTROPY
FATHOMS
FATUOUS
FETLOCK
GETCOLD
GETDONE
GETDOWN
GETGOOD
GETLOST
GETSOFF
GETSOFT
GETSOLD
GETSORE
GETSOUT
GETTOIT
GETWORD
GOTCOLD
GOTDONE
GOTDOWN
GOTGOOD
GOTLOST
GOTSOFT
GOTSORE
GOTTOIT
GOTWORD
HATSOFF
HITHOME
HITSOFF
HITSONG
HITSOUT
HITTOWN
HOTCOAL
HOTCOMB
HOTDOGS
HOTFOOT
HOTPOTS
HOTRODS
HOTROLL
HOTSOUP
HOTZONE
INTROIT
JETBOAT
JETFOIL
JETPORT
JETSONS
JOTDOWN
JSTROKE
LATROBE
LETDOWN
LETGOBY
LETGOOF
LETROLL
LETSOFF
LETSOUT
LITHOID
LOTIONS
MATLOCK
MATRONS
MATTOCK
MATZOHS
MATZOTH
METEORS
METEOUT
METHODS
METOOER
MITFORD
MOTIONS
MOTTOES
MUTTONS
NATIONS
NETCOST
NETLOSS
NETTONS
NETWORK
NITROUS
NOTAONE
NOTDONE
NOTGOOD
NOTHOME
NOTIONS
NOTTOBE
NUTWOOD
OCTROIS
OPTIONS
OPTSOUT
OSTEOID
OUTBOWL
OUTBOWS
OUTCOLD
OUTCOME
OUTCOOK
OUTDOER
OUTDOES
OUTDONE
OUTDOOR
OUTFOOL
OUTFOOT
OUTGOES
OUTHOWL
OUTLOOK
OUTLOUD
OUTLOVE
OUTMODE
OUTMOST
OUTMOVE
OUTPOLL
OUTPOPS
OUTPORT
OUTPOST
OUTPOUR
OUTROAR
OUTROCK
OUTRODE
OUTROLL
OUTROOT
OUTROVE
OUTROWS
OUTSOAR
OUTSOLD
OUTSOLE
OUTTOLD
OUTTOLL
OUTTORE
OUTTORN
OUTVOTE
OUTWORD
OUTWORE
OUTWORK
OUTWORN
PATDOWN
PATROLS
PATRONS
PATROON
PETBOAS
PETCOCK
PETCOMB
PETCOWS
PETDOGS
PETDOOR
PETDOVE
PETGOAT
PETIOLE
PETPONY
PETROCK
PETROLS
PETROUS
PETTOYS
PITBOSS
PITEOUS
PITROWS
POTBOIL
POTHOLE
POTHOOK
POTIONS
PUTDOWN
PUTSOFF
PUTSOUT
PUTTOUT
PYTHONS
RATHOLE
RATIONS
RATSOUT
RETOOLS
SATCOMS
SATDOWN
SATHOME
SETDOWN
SETSOFF
SETSOUT
SITCOMS
SITDOWN
SITHOME
SITSOUT
TATTOOS
TETRODE
VOTEOUT
WATFORD
WETDOWN
WETLOOK
WETMOPS
WITEOUT
WITHOUT
ZITCOMS

••T••O•

ACTAEON
ACTEDON
ACTINON
ACTSFOR
ACTUPON
ANTIFOG
ANTILOG
ANTLION
ARTBOOK
ARTSHOP
ARTSHOW
ATTABOY
BATSFOR
BITESON
BUTGOOD
CATALOG
CATALOS
CATCHON
CATCHOW
CATDOOR
CATFOOD
CATFOOT
CATSHOW
CITYBOY
COTEDOR
CUTINON
DOTEDON
DOTESON
EATALOT
EATCROW
EATFROM
ENTERON
ESTADOS
FITZROY
GETAJOB
GETFROM
GETGOOD
GETINON
GETITON
GETSHOT
GETUPON
GITANOS
GOTAJOB
GOTGOOD
GOTINON
GOTITON
GOTOPOT
GOTUPON
HITCHON
HITSFOR
HITSHOW
HITUPON
HOTFOOT
HOTSHOT
HOTSPOT
KUTUZOV
LATCHON
LATERON
LATIGOS
LATINOS
LETDROP
LETGOOF
LETINON
LETKNOW
LETSNOT
LETUPON
LITHGOW
LOTHROP
MATADOR
NATATOR
NOTALOT
NOTGOOD
NUTWOOD
OCTAGON
OCTAVOS
OCTOPOD
ONTOPOF
OPTSFOR
OUTBLOT
OUTBLOW
OUTCOOK
OUTCROP
OUTCROW
OUTDOOR
OUTDROP
OUTFLOW
OUTFOOL
OUTFOOT
OUTGLOW
OUTGROW
OUTLOOK
OUTPLOD
OUTPLOT
OUTROOT
OUTSHOT
OUTSHOW
OUTTROT
PATRIOT
PATROON
PETCROW
PETDOOR
PETFROG
PETLION
PETSHOP
PITSTOP
POTHOOK
POTSHOT
PUTUPON
RETINOL
ROTATOR
SATATOP
SATINON
SATUPON
SETSHOT
SETTLOR
SETUPON
SITATOP
SITINON
SITSFOR
SITUPON
TATTOOS
TOTINOS
TOTOTOO
UPTHROW
UPTONOW
USTINOV
VITRIOL
VOTEDON
VOTEFOR
VOTESON
WETLOOK

••T•••O

ANTONIO
ARTDECO
ARTERIO
AUTOBIO
BLTTOGO
CATERTO
CATTALO
CUTINTO
DETECTO
EATINTO
EXTENSO
FITINTO
GETINTO
GETONTO
GOTINTO
GOTONTO
GOTTAGO
GOTUPTO
HITINTO
LETITGO
LETMEGO
LETTERO
LITINTO
NETZERO
NOTUPTO
OCTAVIO
ONTARIO
ONTHEGO
OPTEDTO
OTTAVIO
OUTECHO
PATERNO
PITCHTO
PITILLO
PUTITTO
PUTUPTO
SATCHMO
SETINTO

TOTOTOO
UPTEMPO
VOTEDNO
VOTESNO
YOTEAMO

•••TO••

ABATORS
ACETONE
ALLTOLD
AMATOLS
AMATORY
ANATOLE
ANATOLY
ANATOMY
ANYTOWN
BARTOLO
BEATOFF
BEATOUT
BELTOUT
BERTOLT
BESTOFF
BESTONE
BESTOWS
BETTORS
BIGTOES
BIGTOPS
BIGTOWN
BLOTOUT
BLTTOGO
BOOTOUT
BOSTONS
BOSTONU
BOTTOMS
BOXTOPS
BOYTOYS
BRETONS
BRITONS
BUITONI
BUSTOUR
BUSTOUT
BUTTONS
BUTTONY
BUTTOUT
CANTONS
CANTORS
CAPTORS
CARTOFF
CARTONS
CARTOON
CARTOPS
CASTOFF
CASTOUT
CATTOYS
CDSTORE
CHITONS
CHITOWN
CONTORT
CONTOUR
COTTONS
COTTONY
COWTOWN
CROTONS
CUSTODY
CUSTOMS
DALTONS
DARTOFF
DAYTONA
DEBTORS
DELTOID
DELTONA
DELTORO
DENTOID
DENTONS
DESTOCK
DIATOMS
DIDTOAT
DISTORT
DITTOED
DOCTORS
DOGTOYS
DUOTONE
DUSTOFF
EDITORS
EDITOUT
EGGTOSS
EPITOME
FACTOID
FACTORS
FACTORY
FANTODS
FASTONE
FELTOFF
FELTOUT
FESTOON
FESTOSO
FLATOUT
FORTORD
GASTONE
GETTOIT
GJETOST
GOTTOIT
GUSTOES
HADTOBE
HASTOBE
HECTORS
HENTOFF
HILTONS
HISTORY
HITTOWN
HOOTOWL
HOPTOIT
IFSTONE
INSTOCK
INSTONE
INSTORE
ISOTONE
ISOTOPE
ISOTOPY
JUSTONE
JUSTOUT
KEPTOFF
KEPTOUT
KOWTOWS
LACTOSE
LAPTOPS
LASTONE
LASTORY
LECTORS
LEFTOFF
LEFTOUT
LEPTONS
LESTOIL
LIFTOFF
LOSTOUT
LOWTOPS
MALTOSE
MASTOID
MATTOCK
MENTORS
MIDTOWN
MISTOLD
MISTOOK
MONTOYA
MOPTOPS
MORTONS
MOTTOES
MUTTONS
NESTORS
NETTONS
NEWTONS
NEWTOWN
NEWTOYS
NORTONS
NOTTOBE
OLDTOWN
ONATOOT
ONETOGO
ORATORS
ORATORY
OURTOWN
OUTTOLD
OUTTOLL
OUTTORE
OUTTORN
PANTONE
PARTONE
PARTOOK
PASTORS
PEGTOPS
PEPTONE
PETTOYS
PGATOUR
PHOTOGS
PHOTOID
PHOTONS
PHOTOOP
PIETOSO
PISTOLE
PISTOLS
PISTONS
PISTOUS
PLATOON
PLUTONS
PONTOON
POPTOPS
POSTOPS
PRETOLD
PRETORS
PROTONS
PUTTOUT
RAGTOPS
RAPTORS
RECTORS
RECTORY
REDTOPS
RENTOUT
RESTOCK
RESTOKE
RESTORE
RESTOWS
RHETORS
RIOTOUS
RIPTORN
ROOTOUT
ROSTOCK
ROUTOUT
SAOTOME
SARTORS
SAWTOIT
SECTORS
SEETOIT
SENTOFF
SENTOUT
SEXTONS
SHOTOUT
SHUTOFF
SHUTOUT
SKITOWS
SORTOUT
SPATOUT
SPITOUT
STATORS
SUBTONE
SUITORS
SYSTOLE
TATTOOS
TENTONS
TESTOUT
TEUTONS
THATONE
THETOUR
TIPTOED
TIPTOES
TIPTOPS
TOMTOMS
TORTOLA
TORTONI
TOYTOPS
TRITONE
TRITONS
TROTOFF
TROTOUT
TWOTOED
TWOTONE
TWOTONS
UNSTOIC
UNSTONY
UNSTOPS
UNSTOUT
UNSTOWS
UPSTOOD
USOTOUR
VECTORS
VICTORS
VICTORY
VOLTORE
WAITOUT
WALTONS
WANTONS
WANTOUT
WARTORN
WAYTOGO
WEBTOED
WENTOFF
WENTOUT
WONTONS
YOMTOVS
ZIPTOPS

•••T•O•

ABETTOR
ABUTSON
ACCTNOS
AFATLOT
AUCTION
BASTION
BEATBOX
BEATCOP
BEATSON
BENTHOS
BESTBOY
BISTROS
BOOTTOP
BOUTROS
BRETTON
BRITCOM
BRITPOP
BRITTON
CAPTION
CARTOON
CASTROL
CASTSON
CAUTION
CESTMOI
CONTROL
CRATION
CUATROS
DESTROY
DICTION
DISTROS
DOGTROT
DOITNOW
DUETTOS
DUSTMOP
EDITION
ELATION
ELUTION
EMOTION
EXITNOW
FACTION
FELTFOR
FESTOON
FICTION
FLATTOP
FOXTROT
GHETTOS
GIFTBOX
GLUTTON
GRATEON
GROTTOS
HAUTBOY
HUNTFOR
HURTFOR
IGOTYOU
IZATION
JOGTROT
JUSTNOW
KRATION
LASTDON
LASTROW
LEFTFOR
LOSTDOG
MENTHOL
MENTION
MISTBOW
MISTOOK
MTATHOS
MUSTDOS
NEUTRON
NORTHOF
ONATOOT
ONETWOS
ORATION
OUTTROT
OVATION
PALTROW
PARTOOK
PARTYON
PEATBOG
PEATPOT
PHOTOOP
PIETROS
PLATOON
PONTOON
PORTHOS
PORTION
PORTNOY
POSTBOX
POSTDOC
POSTHOC
QRATIOS
RESTSON
ROOTFOR
ROOTROT
RUCTION
SALTBOX
SECTION
SENTFOR
SETTLOR
SHOTFOR
SOFTTOP
SOUTHOF
SPITSON
STATION
STETSON
SUCTION
TATTOOS
TEATROS
TESTFOR
TEXTRON
THATSOK
TILTTOP
TUITION
UNCTION
UPSTOOD
VENTNOR
VESTRON
VISTEON
VUITTON
WAITFOR
WAITRON
WAITSON
WARTHOG
WENTFOR
WHATFOR
WHATNOT
WHATNOW
WRITEON
WROTEON

•••T••O

AGITATO
ARETINO
BARTOLO
BLTTOGO
BOITANO
CANTINO
CATTALO
CENTAVO
CENTIMO
CORTICO
DELTORO
DESTINO
DEUTERO
ERYTHRO
FESTOSO
FURTADO
GAETANO
GASTERO
GESTAPO
GOTTAGO
INUTERO
ISITAGO
LENTIGO
LETTERO
LOATHTO
MARTINO
MONTANO
MONTEGO
MONTERO
MONTUNO
ONETOGO
PARTTWO
PIETOSO
PONTANO
PORTICO
QUATTRO
QUITESO
RENTSTO
VERTIGO
WANTSTO
WAYTOGO
WENTPRO
WRITETO
WROTETO

••••TO•

ABETTOR
ADAPTOR
AERATOR
AHOSTOF
ALLSTON
ANISTON
ARAFTOF
ARISTOS
ATIPTOE
AUDITOR
AVIATOR
BALATON
BARSTOW
BDALTON
BIENTOT
BLANTON
BOASTOF
BONITOS
BOOTTOP
BRAXTON
BRETTON
BRISTOL
BRITTON
BUILTON
BUSSTOP
CAPITOL
CARLTON
CHEATON
CHEETOS
CHEWTOY
CLACTON
CLANTON
CLAPTON
CLAYTON
CLIFTON
CLINTON
COMPTON
COOKTOP
COUNTON
CREATOR
CRESTON
CROPTOP
CROUTON
CRYPTOS
CURATOR
DESKTOP
DESOTOS
DILATOR
DILUTOR
DOESTOO
DONATOR
DOOUTOF
DORITOS
DRAYTON
DROPTOP
DUETTOS
DWELTON
EDUCTOR
EJECTOR
ELECTOR
ENACTOR
EQUATOR
ERECTOR
EVERTOR
EVICTOR
EXACTOR
EXCITOR
FEASTON
FLATTOP
FLIPTOP
FOISTON
FORETOP
FREETOY
FRONTON
FUGATOS
GANGTOK
GELATOS
GENITOR
GERITOL
GETITON
GHETTOS
GIGATON
GLUTTON
GOTITON
GRAFTON
GRANTOR
GROTTOS
GYRATOR
HALSTON
HAMPTON
HARDTOP
HERITOR
HIGHTOP
HILLTOP
HOOPTOY
HOUSTON
HURSTON
IDIDTOO
IGNATOW
IGNITOR
ITISTOO
JANITOR
KEMPTON
KILOTON
KLEPTOS
KRYPTON
LANGTON
LAYITON
LEANTOS
LEAPTON
LEGATOR
LEGATOS
LEVATOR
LIEATOP
LIGHTON
LLEYTON
LOCATOR
LONGTOM
LONGTON
MAINTOP
MARSTON
MEGATON
MOJITOS
MOLITOR
MOLOTOV
MONCTON
MONITOR
NATATOR
NEGATOR
NONSTOP
OBENTOS
ONESTOP
ONLYTOO
OPENTOE
OPENTOP
OVERTOP
PALMTOP
PELOTON
PHAETON
PHANTOM
PINETOP
PITSTOP
PRAETOR
PRESTON
PRESTOS
PROCTOR
PULLTOY
QUARTOS
QUINTON
RALSTON
REACTOR
REALTOR
RELATOR
RIALTOS
RIGHTON
RIPSTOP
ROLLTOP
ROOFTOP
ROPETOW
ROTATOR
RUBATOS
SATATOP
SENATOR
SHORTOF
SITATOP
SKELTON
SLAYTON
SLEPTON
SOFTTOP
SPECTOR
SPENTON
STANTON
STARTON
STENTOR
STERTOR
STILTON
SWEETON
SWINTON
SYMPTOM
TANKTOP
TAUNTON
TILTTOP
TINYTOT
TOLSTOI
TOLSTOY
TOTOTOO
TRACTOR
TRAITOR
TREETOP
TRENTON
TRYITON
TUBETOP
TURFTOE
TWISTON
VISITOR
VUITTON
WALSTON
WEIRTON
WHARTON
WHEATON
WINSTON
XFACTOR
YANKTON
YORKTON
ZABUTON

••••T•O

ABOUTTO
ADAPTTO
ADMITTO
ALERTTO
ANNATTO
BALLTWO
BASETWO
DEALTTO
DOESTOO
DONOTGO
ELECTRO
FIVETWO
FRUSTRO
HORATIO
IDIDTOO
IMUSTGO
INVITRO
ITISTOO
IWANTTO
IZZATSO
LANETWO
LESOTHO
LETITGO
LINETWO
MACHTWO
MAESTRO
MEANTTO
MONSTRO
MULATTO
NUESTRO
ONLYTOO
OPUSTWO
ORNITHO
OUGHTTO
PAGETWO
PARTTWO
PERATIO
PLUSTWO
POINTTO
PUTITTO
QUATTRO
REACTTO
RIDOTTO
RISOTTO
SAINTLO
SIDETWO
SIZETWO
STARTTO
STEPTWO
STRETTO
TOTOTOO
ZANETTO
ZAPATEO
ZEMSTVO

•••••TO

ABOUTTO
ADAPTTO
ADDEDTO
ADDONTO
ADDUPTO
ADMITTO
AGITATO
AGREETO
AKIHITO
ALBERTO
ALERTTO
ALIENTO
ALIVETO
ANIMATO
ANNATTO
APPLYTO
ARGENTO
ARIGATO
ARIOSTO
ATEINTO
AUGUSTO
BANDITO
BEGANTO
BINDSTO
BLINDTO
BONIATO
BOUNDTO
BOWEDTO
BRINGTO
BURRITO
BUYINTO
CALLSTO
CAREDTO
CARESTO
CATERTO
CHRISTO
CILENTO
CLAMATO
CLIMBTO
CLINGTO
CLOSETO
CLUNGTO
COMESTO
CONMOTO
CUTINTO
DARESTO
DEALSTO
DEALTTO
DEFACTO
DEFERTO
DEIGNTO
DELICTO
DEMENTO
DEODATO
DERMATO
DETECTO
DIGINTO
DIPINTO
DOINGTO
DOOMSTO
DRANKTO
DRAWNTO
DRAWSTO
DRINKTO
DRIVETO
DROVETO
DUGINTO
EATINTO
EQUALTO
ERNESTO
ESPARTO
EXFACTO
FAILSTO
FALLSTO
FEDINTO
FEEDSTO
FITINTO
FLIEDTO
FLIESTO
FLOCKTO
FLOWNTO
FLYINTO
GALENTO
GEARSTO
GETINTO
GETONTO
GIVENTO
GIVESTO
GLUEDTO
GLUESTO
GOINGTO
GOTINTO
GOTONTO
GOTUPTO
HANDYTO
HAPPYTO
HEADSTO
HEAVETO
HERESTO
HERPETO
HEWEDTO
HITINTO
HOLDSTO
HOPEDTO
HOPESTO
HOPINTO
IMPASTO
ISOLATO
IWANTTO
JACINTO
KEEPSTO
LAMINTO
LAYINTO
LEADSTO
LEANSTO
LEARNTO
LEASETO
LEDINTO
LEDUPTO
LEONATO
LEPANTO
LIKENTO
LITINTO
LOATHTO
LOGONTO
LOOKSTO
LOSESTO
LOVEDTO
LOVESTO
LOYALTO
LYINGTO
MAGNETO
MANKATO
MARCATO
MEANSTO
MEANTTO
MEMENTO
MODESTO
MOSCATO
MOVEDTO
MOVESTO
MULATTO
NEEDSTO
NOENDTO
NOTUPTO
OCCURTO
OPTEDTO
ORVIETO
OTRANTO
OUGHTTO
OWINGTO
OWNUPTO
PAYINTO
PIMENTO
PITCHTO
PLANSTO
PLAYSTO
PLEADTO
POINTTO
PRAYSTO
PREVETO
PRIORTO
PRIVYTO
PRONETO
PRYINTO
PUTITTO
PUTUPTO
RACEDTO
RACESTO
RALLYTO
RAMINTO
RANINTO
RANUPTO

REACTTO
READSTO
REFERTO
RENTSTO
REPLYTO
RIDESTO
RIDOTTO
RIPINTO
RISENTO
RISESTO
RISOTTO
RIZZUTO
ROBERTO
ROBUSTO
RUNINTO
RUNUPTO
SAILSTO
SAWINTO
SAYHITO
SAYNOTO
SEEINTO
SEEMSTO
SELLSTO
SENDSTO
SETINTO
SILENTO
SINGSTO
SNAPSTO
SORENTO
SPEAKTO
SPOKETO
SQUANTO
STANDTO
STARTTO
STICKTO
STOODTO
STRETTO
STUCKTO
SUHARTO
SUMUPTO
SWEARTO
SWORETO
TAKENTO
TAKESTO
TALKSTO
TAPINTO
TARANTO
TELESTO
TENDSTO
THERETO
TIEINTO
TORONTO
TRIEDTO
TRIESTO
TRUERTO
TUNEDTO
TUNESTO
TURNSTO
TYINGTO
UMBERTO
VIBRATO
WAIKATO
WALKSTO
WANTSTO
WARMSTO
WASONTO
WAVEDTO
WAVESTO
WHERETO
WRITETO
WROTETO
YEARNTO
YIELDTO
ZANETTO

T•P••••

TAPEDON
TAPEDUP
TAPEMAN
TAPEMEN
TAPERED
TAPESON
TAPESUP
TAPINGS
TAPINTO
TAPIOCA
TAPPANS
TAPPERS
TAPPETS
TAPPING
TAPROOM
TAPROOT
TAPSHOE
TAPSOFF
TAPSOUT
TAPSTER
TEPIDLY
TFPOWYS
TIPCART
TIPDOWN
TIPJARS
TIPLESS
TIPLINE
TIPOFFS
TIPOVER
TIPPEES
TIPPERS
TIPPETS
TIPPIER
TIPPING
TIPPLED
TIPPLER
TIPPLES
TIPSIER
TIPSILY
TIPSOFF
TIPSTER
TIPTOED
TIPTOES
TIPTOPS
TOPAZES
TOPBIDS
TOPBOOT
TOPCOAT
TOPDOGS
TOPDOWN
TOPDRAW
TOPEKAN
TOPFIVE
TOPFORM
TOPGUNS
TOPHATS
TOPHOLE
TOPIARY
TOPICAL
TOPKAPI
TOPKICK
TOPKNOT
TOPLESS
TOPLINE
TOPMAST
TOPMOST
TOPNAME
TOPONYM
TOPPERS
TOPPING
TOPPLED
TOPPLES
TOPRANK
TOPRATE
TOPROWS
TOPSAIL
TOPSEED
TOPSIDE
TOPSOFF
TOPSOIL
TOPSOUT
TOPSPIN
TOPSPOT
TOPTENS
TOPTHIS
TUPELOS
TUPOLEV
TYPEABS
TYPEDIN
TYPEDUP
TYPESET
TYPESIN
TYPESUP
TYPHOID
TYPHOON
TYPICAL
TYPISTS

T••P•••

TADPOLE
TAMPAFL
TAMPERS
TAMPICO
TAMPING
TAPPANS
TAPPERS
TAPPETS
TAPPING
TARPITS
TARPONS
TAXPAID
TEAPOTS
TEAPOYS
TEEPEES
TEMPEAZ
TEMPEHS
TEMPERA
TEMPERS
TEMPEST
TEMPING
TEMPJOB
TEMPLAR
TEMPLED
TEMPLES
TEMPORE
TEMPTED
TEMPTER
TEMPURA
TENPAST
TENPINS
THEPIPS
THEPITS
THEPOND
THEPOOH
THEPOPE
THEPOST
THEPUMP
TIEPINS
TIEPOLO
TIMPANI
TIPPEES
TIPPERS
TIPPETS
TIPPIER
TIPPING
TIPPLED
TIPPLER
TIPPLES
TIRPITZ
TOEPICK
TOPPERS
TOPPING
TOPPLED
TOPPLES
TORPEDO
TOSPARE
TOUPEES
TOWPATH
TOYPAIL
TRAPEZE
TRAPGUN
TRAPPED
TRAPPER
TREPANS
TRIPLEA
TRIPLED
TRIPLES
TRIPLET
TRIPLEX
TRIPODS
TRIPOLI
TRIPPED
TRIPPER
TRIPPET
TRIPSON
TRIPSUP
TROPICS
TROPISM
TVSPOTS
TWOPAIR
TWOPART
TYMPANA
TYMPANI

T•••P••

TAILPIN
TELEPIC
TELEPIX
TENSPOT
TENTPEG
THESPIS
THIGPEN
THIMPHU
THRUPUT
THUMPED
THUMPER
TIEMPOS
TOPSPIN
TOPSPOT
TOSSPOT
TRAIPSE
TRAMPAS
TRAMPED
TRAMPER
TRAMPLE
TRAPPED
TRAPPER
TRIPPED
TRIPPER
TRIPPET
TROMPED
TROMPIN
TROOPED
TROOPER
TROOPIN
TROUPED
TROUPER
TROUPES
TRUMPED
TRUMPET
TRUMPUP
TSHAPED
TSHAPES
TUBEPAN
TURNPRO
TVTAPES
TWOSPOT

T••••P•

TEACUPS
THEALPS
THECAPE
THEHOPE
THEPIPS
THEPOPE
THERAPY
THEROPE
THEVIPS
THEYIPS
THREEPM
TIEROPE
TINTYPE
TIPTOPS
TOECAPS
TOETAPS
TOPKAPI
TOSSUPS
TOWROPE
TOYTOPS
TRICEPS
TRIUMPH
TSTRAPS
TUNEUPS
TURNIPS
TURNUPS

T•••••P

TACKSUP
TAKENUP
TAKESUP
TALKSUP
TALLYUP
TANKSUP
TANKTOP
TAPEDUP
TAPESUP
TARTSUP
TEAMSUP
TEARSUP
TEASEUP
TEASHOP
TEEITUP
TENSEUP
THEDEEP
THEFLOP
THEHELP
THELOOP
THEPUMP
THINKUP
THREEUP
THREWUP
THROWUP
TIDERIP
TIECLIP
TILTSUP
TILTTOP
TIMECOP
TIMESUP
TOELOOP
TONEDUP
TONESUP
TOOLSUP
TOTALUP
TOTESUP
TOUCHUP
TOYHOOP
TOYSHOP
TRADEUP
TREESAP
TREETOP
TRIPSUP
TROLLOP
TROTSUP
TRUEDUP
TRUESUP
TRUMPUP
TRUSSUP
TUBETOP
TUNEDUP
TUNESUP
TURNSUP
TWISTUP
TWODEEP
TWOSTEP
TYINGUP
TYPEDUP
TYPESUP

•TP••••

ATPEACE
MTPELEE
STPAULS
STPETER
STPIUSI
STPIUSV
STPIUSX

•T•P•••

ATIPTOE
NTUPLES
STAPLED
STAPLER
STAPLES
STEPDAD
STEPHEN
STEPINS
STEPMOM
STEPOFF
STEPONE
STEPOUT
STEPPED
STEPPER
STEPPES
STEPSIN
STEPSON
STEPSUP
STEPTWO
STEPUPS
STIPEND
STIPPLE
STOPFOR
STOPGAP
STOPOFF
STOPPED
STOPPER
STOPPLE
STOPSAT
STOPSBY
STOPSIN
STOPSIT
STOPSUP
STUPEFY
STUPIDS
STUPORS
STYPSIS
STYPTIC
UTOPIAN
UTOPIAS
UTOPISM
UTOPIST

•T••P••

ATROPHY
ATROPOS
BTFSPLK
ITSOPEN
STAMPED
STAMPER
STAYPUT
STEEPED
STEEPEN
STEEPER
STEEPIN
STEEPLE
STEEPLY
STEMPEL
STEPPED
STEPPER
STEPPES
STEWPAN
STEWPOT
STIPPLE
STOMPED
STOMPIN
STOMPON
STOOPED
STOOPER
STOPPED
STOPPER
STOPPLE
STRAPIN
STRAPON
STRIPED
STRIPER
STRIPES
STRIPOF
STROPHE
STUMPED
STUMPER

•T•••P•

ATTEMPT
STEPUPS

•T••••P

ATACLIP
ATEITUP
STACKUP
STANDUP
STANKUP
STARMAP
STARTUP
STAYSUP
STEAMUP
STEPSUP
STICKUP
STILLUP
STINKUP
STIRRUP
STIRSUP
STOCKUP
STOKEUP
STOODUP
STOPGAP
STOPSUP
STOREUP
STUCKUP

••TP•••

BITPART
GETPAST
GOTPAST
HATPINS
HITPLAY
HOTPACK
HOTPINK
HOTPOTS
JETPACK
JETPORT
LETPASS
NITPICK
NUTPINE
OUTPACE
OUTPAID
OUTPASS
OUTPATH
OUTPAYS
OUTPEEP
OUTPICK
OUTPIPE
OUTPITY
OUTPLAN
OUTPLAY
OUTPLOD
OUTPLOT
OUTPOLL
OUTPOPS
OUTPORT
OUTPOST
OUTPOUR
OUTPRAY
OUTPULL
OUTPURL
OUTPUSH
OUTPUTS
PETPIGS
PETPONY
PETPUPS
POTPIES
PUTPUTS
RATPACK
SETPLAY

••T•P••

ACTUPON
AUTOPEN
AUTOPIA
AUTOPSY
CATSPAW
CUTOPEN
ECTYPAL
ECTYPES
GETUPON
GOTOPOT
GOTUPON
GOTUPTO
HITUPON
HOTSPOT
HOTSPUR
LETUPON
NOTEPAD
NOTOPEN
NOTUPTO
OCTOPOD
OCTOPUS
OCTUPLE
OCTUPLY
ONTOPIC
ONTOPOF
OUTSPED
OUTSPIN
OUTSPIT
PITAPAT
PUTUPON
PUTUPTO
RETAPED
RETAPES
RETYPED
RETYPES
SATUPON
SETUPON
SITSPAT
SITUPON
TVTAPES
UNTAPED
UNTAPES
UNTYPED
UPTOPAR
ZATOPEK

••T••P•

ATTEMPT
BITMAPS
CATALPA
CATNAPS
CATNIPS
CATSUPS
ENTRAPS
ENTROPY
EUTERPE
FATLIPS
HOTCAPS
HOTCUPS
HOTLIPS
HOTTIPS
OUTKEPT
OUTLIPS
OUTPIPE
OUTPOPS
OUTRAPS
OUTWEPT
PETNAPS
PETPUPS
RATEDPG
RETRAPS
SATRAPS
SATRAPY
SETTYPE
TSTRAPS
UNTRAPS
UPTEMPO
WETMOPS
WETNAPS

••T•••P

ACTEDUP
ANTEDUP
ANTESUP
ANTWERP
ARTSHOP
BITESUP
BOTCHUP
CATCHUP
CATFLAP
EATENUP
EATITUP
GETATIP
GETHELP
GETSHEP
GETSHIP
GOTATIP
GOTHELP
HITCHUP
HOTSOUP
KETCHUP
LETDROP
LETSLIP
LETSRIP
LETTERP
LOTHROP
MATCHUP
NOTRUMP
OUTCROP
OUTDROP
OUTJUMP
OUTKEEP
OUTLEAP
OUTPEEP
OUTSKIP
OUTSTEP
OUTWEEP
OUTYELP
PATCHUP
PETSHOP
PITSTOP
PUTEMUP
RATECAP
RATTRAP
SATATOP
SITATOP
SITEMAP
TOTALUP
TOTESUP

•••TP••

BRITPOP
DUSTPAN
FELTPEN
FOOTPAD
LOSTPET
MEATPIE
PEATPOT
SALTPIT
SHOTPAR
SHOTPUT
TENTPEG
WENTPRO

•••T•P•

ALETAPS
BIGTOPS
BIOTYPE
BOXTOPS
BUSTUPS
CARTOPS
CHUTZPA
CUETIPS
DUSTUPS
ECOTYPE
EPITAPH
GESTAPO
HOTTIPS
INSTEPS
ISOTOPE
ISOTOPY
LAPTOPS
LOWTOPS
MISTYPE
MOPTOPS
PEGTOPS
PLATYPI
POPTOPS
POSTOPS
PRETAPE
PRETYPE
RAGTOPS
REDTAPE
REDTOPS
SETTYPE
SUBTYPE
TINTYPE
TIPTOPS
TOETAPS
TOYTOPS
UNSTEPS
UNSTOPS
UPSTEPS
VCRTAPE
WENTAPE
ZIPTOPS

•••T••P

AIRTRAP
BADTRIP
BEATCOP
BEATSUP
BELTSUP
BLOTSUP
BOLTSUP
BOOTSUP
BOOTTOP
BRITPOP
BUSTRIP
BUSTSUP
CANTRIP
CARTRIP
CASTSUP
CHATSUP
CLOTSUP
CRATEUP
DAYTRIP
DUSTMOP
EGOTRIP
FELTTIP
FLATTOP
FLYTRAP
FOOTSUP
FROTHUP
GRATEUP
HEATSUP
HUNTSUP
INATRAP
KNOTSUP
LASTLAP
LEFTHIP
LEGTRAP
LETTERP
LIFTSUP
MANTRAP
MASTERP
MEETSUP
MISTSUP
ONATRIP
PASTEUP
PHOTOOP
RATTRAP
RESTAMP
RESTRAP
RESTRIP
RESTSUP
ROOTCAP
ROOTSUP
SEATRIP
SHUTSUP
SKITRIP
SOFTTOP
SUITSUP
TARTSUP
TILTSUP
TILTTOP
TROTSUP
UNSTRAP
WAITSUP
WHATSUP
WRITEUP
WROTEUP

••••TP•

EIGHTPM

••••T•P

ATEITUP
BEERTAP
BOOSTUP
BOOTTOP
BOXSTEP
BUILTUP
BURNTUP
BUSSTOP
COOKTOP
COUNTUP
CREPTUP
CROPTOP
DEALTUP
DESKTOP
DRIFTUP
DROPTOP
EATITUP
EIGHTUP
FELTTIP
FIRSTUP
FLATTOP
FLIPTOP
FLOATUP
FORETOP
FOULTIP
GETATIP
GOLDTIP
GOTATIP
HAMITUP
HARDTOP
HEELTAP
HIGHTOP
HILLTOP
HOISTUP
IMHOTEP
LEAPTUP
LIEATOP
LIGHTUP
LOVETAP
MAINTOP
MISSTEP
MIXITUP
MOUNTUP
NAILTIP
NONSTOP
ONESTEP
ONESTOP
OPENTAP
OPENTOP
OUTSTEP
OVERTIP
OVERTOP
PALMTOP
PINETOP
PITSTOP
POINTUP
PRINTUP
RANITUP
REVITUP
RIPSTOP
ROLLTOP
ROOFTOP
RUNITUP
SATATOP
SCOUTUP
SHOOTUP
SITATOP

SLANTUP
SOFTTOP
SPLITUP
STARTUP
SUMITUP
SWEPTUP
TANKTOP
TEEITUP
TILTTOP
TREETOP
TUBETOP
TWISTUP
TWOSTEP
WINGTIP
WIRETAP

•••••TP
SILENTP

T•Q••••
TEQUILA
TSQUARE

T••Q•••
TORQUED
TORQUES

••T•Q••
ANTIQUE

••T••Q•
ONTHEQT

••T•••Q
LETTERQ

•••T••Q
LETTERQ

•••••TQ
SILENTQ

TR•••••
TRABERT
TRACERS
TRACERY
TRACHEA
TRACING
TRACKED
TRACKER
TRACTOR
TRADEIN
TRADEON
TRADERS
TRADEUP
TRADING
TRADUCE
TRAFFIC
TRAGEDY
TRAILED
TRAILER
TRAINED
TRAINEE
TRAINER
TRAININ
TRAIPSE
TRAITOR
TRALALA
TRAMCAR
TRAMMED
TRAMMEL
TRAMPAS
TRAMPED
TRAMPER
TRAMPLE
TRAMWAY
TRANCED
TRANCES
TRANSAM
TRANSIT
TRANSOM
TRAPEZE
TRAPGUN
TRAPPED
TRAPPER
TRASHED
TRASHER
TRASHES
TRASHTV
TRAUBEL
TRAUMAS
TRAVAIL
TRAVELS
TRAVERS
TRAWLED
TRAWLER
TRAYFUL
TRAYNOR
TREACLE
TREACLY
TREADED
TREADER
TREADLE
TREADON
TREASON
TREATED
TREATER
TREBLED
TREBLES
TREDIAS
TREEING
TREELET
TREERAT
TREESAP
TREETOP
TREFOIL
TREINTA
TREIZES
TREKKED
TREKKER
TREKKIE
TRELLIS
TREMBLE
TREMBLY
TREMOLO
TREMORS
TRENARY
TRENDED
TRENTON
TREPANS
TRESSED
TRESSES
TRESTLE
TREVINO
TRIABLE
TRIADIC
TRIAGES
TRIBBLE
TRIBECA
TRIBORO
TRIBUNE
TRIBUTE
TRICEPS
TRICKED
TRICKER
TRICKLE
TRICORN
TRICOTS
TRIDENT
TRIEDIT
TRIEDON
TRIEDTO
TRIESIT
TRIESON
TRIESTE
TRIESTO
TRIFFID
TRIFLED
TRIFLER
TRIFLES
TRIFOLD
TRIFORM
TRIGGER
TRIGONS
TRIGRAM
TRIJETS
TRILLED
TRILLER
TRILLIN
TRILOGY
TRIMMED
TRIMMER
TRIMOFF
TRIMTAB
TRINARY
TRINITY
TRINKET
TRIODES
TRIOLET
TRIPLEA
TRIPLED
TRIPLES
TRIPLET
TRIPLEX
TRIPODS
TRIPOLI
TRIPPED
TRIPPER
TRIPPET
TRIPSON
TRIPSUP
TRIREME
TRISECT
TRISTAN
TRISTAR
TRITELY
TRITEST
TRITIUM
TRITONE
TRITONS
TRIUMPH
TRIVETS
TRIVIAL
TRIVIOT
TRIVIUM
TROCHEE
TROCHES
TRODDEN
TROIKAS
TROILUS
TROJANS
TROLLED
TROLLER
TROLLEY
TROLLOP
TROMPED
TROMPIN
TROOPED
TROOPER
TROOPIN
TROPICS
TROPISM
TROTHED
TROTOFF
TROTOUT
TROTSKY
TROTSUP
TROTTED
TROTTER
TROUBLE
TROUGHS
TROUNCE
TROUPED
TROUPER
TROUPES
TROUSER
TROWELS
TROWING
TRUANCY
TRUANTS
TRUCKED
TRUCKEE
TRUCKER
TRUCKLE
TRUDEAU
TRUDGED
TRUDGEN
TRUDGER
TRUDGES
TRUEDUP
TRUEING
TRUERIB
TRUERTO
TRUESUP
TRUFFLE
TRUISMS
TRUMANS
TRUMPED
TRUMPET
TRUMPUP
TRUNDLE
TRUSSED
TRUSSES
TRUSSUP
TRUSTED
TRUSTEE
TRUSTER
TRUSTIN
TRUSTME
TRYHARD
TRYITON
TRYOUTS
TRYSAIL
TRYSTED
TRYSTER

T•R••••
TARANTO
TARBABY
TARBELL
TARDIER
TARDILY
TARGETS
TARHEEL
TARIFFS
TARMACS
TARNISH
TAROILS
TARPITS
TARPONS
TARRIED
TARRIER
TARRIES
TARRING
TARSALS
TARTANS
TARTARE
TARTARS
TARTEST
TARTIER
TARTILY
TARTING
TARTISH
TARTLET
TARTSUP
TARZANA
TARZANS
TERAOHM
TERBIUM
TERCELS
TERENCE
TERHUNE
TERMING
TERMINI
TERMITE
TERNARY
TERNATE
TERRACE
TERRAIN
TERRANS
TERRELL
TERRENE
TERRETS
TERRIER
TERRIES
TERRIFY
TERRINE
TERROIR
TERRORS
TERSELY
TERSEST
THRALLS
THREADS
THREADY
THREATS
THREEAD
THREEAM
THREEBC
THREEEE
THREENO
THREEPM
THREERS
THREEUP
THREWAT
THREWIN
THREWON
THREWUP
THRIFTS
THRIFTY
THRILLA
THRILLS
THRIVED
THRIVEN
THRIVER
THRIVES
THROATS
THROATY
THRONES
THRONGS
THROUGH
THROWAT
THROWER
THROWIN
THROWON
THROWUP
THRUPUT
THRUSTS
THRUWAY
TIRADES
TIREDER
TIREDLY
TIREDOF
TIREMAN
TIREMEN
TIREOUT
TIRESOF
TIRPITZ
TORCHED
TORCHER
TORCHES
TOREOFF
TOREOUT
TOREROS
TORINOS
TORMENT
TORNADO
TORNOFF
TORNOUT
TOROIDS
TORONTO
TORPEDO
TORQUED
TORQUES
TORREFY
TORRENT
TORSION
TORTLAW
TORTOLA
TORTONI
TORTUGA
TORTURE
TORVALD
TORVILL
TORYISH
TORYISM
TURBANS
TURBINE
TURBOTS
TUREENS
TURFIER
TURFING
TURFMAN
TURFMEN
TURFSKI
TURFTOE
TURFWAR
TURISMO
TURISTA
TURKEYS
TURKISH
TURMOIL
TURNBAD
TURNERS
TURNERY
TURNING
TURNIPS
TURNKEY
TURNOFF
TURNONS
TURNOUT
TURNPRO
TURNRED
TURNSIN
TURNSON
TURNSTO
TURNSUP
TURNUPS
TURRETS
TURTLED
TURTLES
TVROOMS
TYRANNY
TYRANTS

T••R•••
TAPROOM
TAPROOT
TARRIED
TARRIER
TARRIES
TARRING
TAUREAN
TAURINE
TAXRATE
TEARERS
TEARFUL
TEARGAS
TEARIER
TEARILY
TEARING
TEAROFF
TEAROOM
TEAROSE
TEAROUT
TEARSAT
TEARSIT
TEARSUP
TERRACE
TERRAIN
TERRANS
TERRELL
TERRENE
TERRETS
TERRIER
TERRIES
TERRIFY
TERRINE
TERROIR
TERRORS
TETRADS
TETRODE
THERAMS
THERAPY
THEREAT
THEREBY
THEREDS
THEREIN
THERENT
THEREOF
THEREON
THERESA
THERETO
THERIAC
THERING
THERINK
THERITZ
THERMAL
THERMIC
THERMOS
THEROBE
THEROCK
THEROOM
THEROPE
THEROSE
THEROUX
THERULE
THIRDLY
THIRSTS
THIRSTY
THOREAU
THORIUM
THORNED
THORSON
THURBER
THURGAU
THURMAN
THYROID
TIARAED
TIERACK
TIERCES
TIERING
TIERNEY
TIERODS
TIEROPE
TIGRESS
TIMREID
TIMRICE
TIMROTH
TINROOF
TITRATE
TITRING
TOORDER
TOPRANK
TOPRATE
TOPROWS
TORREFY
TORRENT
TOURBUS
TOURERS
TOURING
TOURISM
TOURIST
TOURNEY
TOWROPE
TRIREME
TSARDOM
TSARINA
TSARISM
TSARIST
TSTRAPS
TUGRIKS
TURRETS
TVCREWS
TWERENT
TWIRLED
TWIRLER
TWOROOM
TZARINA

T•••R••
TABARDS
TABARET
TABORET
TALARIA
TAMARAC
TANGRAM
TANTRUM
TAPERED
TASERED
TAVERNA
TAVERNS
TAXFREE
TEATRAY
TEATREE
TEATROS
TEAURNS
TEHERAN
TELERAN
TENDRIL
TENKRUN
TENURED
TENURES
TESTRUN
TEXTRON
THEARMY
THEARTS
THEBRAT
THECRAB
THECROW
THEFRUG
THEOREM
THETREE
THETRIB
THIERRY
THWARTS
TIBURON
TIDERIP
TIMBRES
TINORES
TOHORSE
TONEROW
TOPDRAW
TOREROS
TOUAREG
TOWARDS
TOWERED
TOYSRUS
TREERAT
TRIGRAM
TRUERIB
TRUERTO
TSHIRTS
TSOURIS
TUMBREL
TUNDRAS
TURNRED
TUTORED
TWOIRON

T••••R•
TACKERS
TAGGERS
TAILERS
TAILORS
TALKERS
TAMPERS
TANBARK
TANKARD
TANKERS
TANNERS
TANNERY
TANTARA
TAPPERS
TARTARE
TARTARS
TASTERS
TATTERS
TATTERY
TAYLORS
TEACART
TEARERS
TEASERS
TEENERS
TEETERS
TELLERS
TEMPERA
TEMPERS
TEMPORE
TEMPURA
TENACRE
TENDERS
TENNERS
TENSORS
TENTERS
TERNARY
TERRORS
TESSERA
TESTERS
TETHERS
TEXTURE
THALERS
THAWERS
THEATRE
THEBARD
THECARS
THEFIRM
THEHERO
THEJERK
THELARK
THETURN
THIERRY
THREERS
TICKERS
TIEBARS
TILLERS
TILTERS
TIMBERS
TIMBERY
TINDERS
TINDERY
TINEARS
TINHORN
TINKERS
TINNERS
TINTERN
TINTERS
TINWARE
TINWORK
TIPCART
TIPJARS
TIPPERS
TITHERS
TITLARK
TITTERS
TOATURN
TOGGERY
TOHEART
TOILERS
TOLLERS
TONEARM
TONSURE
TOOHARD
TOOLERS
TOOTERS
TOPFORM
TOPIARY
TOPPERS
TORTURE
TOSHIRO
TOSPARE
TOSSERS
TOSTART
TOTTERS
TOTTERY
TOURERS
TOUTERS
TOWBARS
TOWCARS
TOWNERS
TOYCARS
TOYCART
TRABERT
TRACERS
TRACERY
TRADERS
TRAVERS
TREMORS
TRENARY
TRIBORO
TRICORN
TRIFORM
TRINARY
TRYHARD
TSQUARE
TUCKERS
TUGGERS
TURNERS
TURNERY
TURNPRO
TUSHERY
TUSKERS
TVSTARS
TWINERS
TWOACRE
TWOFERS
TWOMORE
TWOPART
TWOTERM

T•••••R
TABULAR
TACKIER
TACKLER
TAKEFOR
TALKIER
TALLIER
TANAGER
TANDOOR
TANGIER
TANGLER
TANGOER
TANKCAR
TAPSTER
TARDIER
TARRIER
TARTIER
TASKBAR
TASTIER
TATTIER
TATTLER
TAUNTER
TAWNIER
TAXYEAR
TEACHER
TEARIER
TEENIER
TEETHER
TEICHER
TELSTAR
TEMBLOR
TEMPLAR
TEMPTER
TENFOUR
TENONER
TENYEAR
TERRIER
TERROIR
TESTFOR
TESTIER
THANKER
THEATER
THEBEAR
THEODOR
THESTAR
THETOUR
THEUSSR
THICKER
THINAIR
THINKER
THINNER
THITHER
THRIVER
THROWER
THUMPER
THUNDER
THURBER
THUSFAR
TICKLER
TIGHTER
TIMIDER
TINGLER
TINKLER
TINNIER
TINSTAR
TIPOVER
TIPPIER
TIPPLER
TIPSIER
TIPSTER
TIREDER
TITULAR
TOAHAIR
TOASTER
TODDLER
TOFFLER
TOGGLER
TOHOMER
TOLLBAR
TOOKFOR
TOOLBAR
TOORDER
TOOTLER
TORCHER
TOTALER
TOUCHER
TOUGHER
TOWNCAR
TOYFAIR
TRACKER
TRACTOR
TRAILER
TRAINER
TRAITOR
TRAMCAR
TRAMPER
TRAPPER
TRASHER
TRAWLER
TRAYNOR
TREADER
TREATER
TREKKER
TRICKER
TRIFLER
TRIGGER
TRILLER
TRIMMER
TRIPPER
TRISTAR
TROLLER
TROOPER
TROTTER
TROUPER
TROUSER
TRUCKER
TRUDGER
TRUSTER
TRYSTER
TUBBIER
TUBULAR
TUFTIER
TUMBLER
TUMMLER
TURFIER
TURFWAR
TUTELAR
TWANGER
TWEENER
TWEETER
TWEEZER
TWINIER
TWIRLER
TWISTER
TWITTER
TWODOOR

TWOHOUR
TWOPAIR
TWOSTAR
TWOYEAR

•TR••••

ATRIUMS
ATROPHY
ATROPOS
ETRURIA
FTRILEY
OTRANTO
STRAFED
STRAFER
STRAFES
STRAINS
STRAITS
STRANDS
STRANGE
STRAPIN
STRAPON
STRASSE
STRATAS
STRATUM
STRATUS
STRAUSS
STRAYED
STRAYER
STREAKS
STREAKY
STREAMS
STREETS
STREGIS
STRETCH
STRETTI
STRETTO
STREWED
STREWER
STRIATE
STRIDER
STRIDES
STRIFES
STRIKER
STRIKES
STRINGS
STRINGY
STRIPED
STRIPER
STRIPES
STRIPOF
STRITCH
STRIVED
STRIVEN
STRIVER
STRIVES
STROBES
STROKED
STROKER
STROKES
STROLLS
STROPHE
STROUSE
STRUDEL
UTRECHT
UTRILLO

•T•R•••

ATARAXY
ATCROSS
ATGRADE
ATHRILL
ATTRACT
ATTRITE
ATTRITS
ETERNAL
FTBRAGG
ITERANT
ITERATE
OTARIES
PTEROUS
STARCHY
STARDOM
STAREAT
STARERS
STARING
STARION
STARKER
STARKEY
STARKLY
STARLET
STARLIT
STARLOG
STARMAN
STARMAP
STARRED
STARSIN
STARSKY
STARTED
STARTER
STARTIN
STARTLE
STARTON
STARTTO
STARTUP
STARVED
STARVES
STCROIX
STEREOS
STERILE
STERNAL
STERNER
STERNLY
STERNOS
STERNUM
STEROID
STEROLS
STERTOR
STIRFRY
STIRRED
STIRRER
STIRRUP
STIRSIN
STIRSUP
STORAGE
STORERS
STOREUP
STORIED
STORIES
STORING
STORMED
STORMIN
STURGES
STYRENE
XTERRAS
YTTRIAS
YTTRIUM

•T••R••

ATECROW
ATFIRST
ATHIRST
ATLARGE
ATTHREE
ATTIRED
ATTIRER
ATTIRES
ATWORST
ETHERIC
ETRURIA
FTWORTH
ITGIRLS
ITHIRTY
ITSTRUE
MTMARCY
STAIRED
STARRED
STBARTS
STEARIC
STEARIN
STEARNS
STEERED
STEERER
STIRRED
STIRRER
STIRRUP
STMARKS
STMARYS
STUARTI
UTTERED
UTTERER
UTTERLY
XTERRAS

•T•••R•

ATATURK
ATEDIRT
ATEMORE
ATHEART
ATHWART
ATMCARD
ATONERS
ATTHIRD
ETAGERE
ETCHERS
FTHENRY
FTMYERS
ITSHERE
STAGERS
STARERS
STATERS
STATORS
STATURE
STAYDRY
STAYERS
STEWARD
STEWART
STEWERS
STIRFRY
STOKERS
STONERS
STORERS
STOWERS
STUPORS
STYLERS

•T••••R

ATELIER
ATEOVER
ATTIRER
ATWATER
ETAILER
ITCHFOR
ITCHIER
ITSOVER
STABBER
STABLER
STACKER
STADLER
STAFFER
STAGGER
STAGIER
STAIDER
STAINER
STALKER
STALLER
STAMMER
STAMPER
STANDER
STAPLER
STARKER
STARTER
STATLER
STAYFOR
STEALER
STEAMER
STEELER
STEEPER
STEERER
STEIGER
STEINER
STELLAR
STENTOR
STEPPER
STERNER
STERTOR
STEWIER
STICKER
STIFFER
STILLER
STINGER
STINKER
STINTER
STIRRER
STOCKER
STONIER
STOOPER
STOPFOR
STOPPER
STOUTER
STPETER
STRAFER
STRAYER
STREWER
STRIDER
STRIKER
STRIPER
STRIVER
STROKER
STUDIER
STUFFER
STUMPER
STUNNER
STUTTER
UTTERER

••TR•••

ACTRESS
AMTRACK
AMTRACS
ARTROCK
ASTREAM
ASTRIDE
ATTRACT
ATTRITE
ATTRITS
BETRAYS
BETROTH
BITROLE
BOTREES
BYTRAIN
CATRIGS
CITRATE
CITRINE
CITROEN
CITRONS
CITROUS
CUTRATE
DATRILS
DETRACT
DETRAIN
DETROIT
DETRUDE
DOTRICE
ELTRAIN
ENTRADA
ENTRAIN
ENTRANT
ENTRAPS
ENTREAT
ENTREES
ENTRIES
ENTROPY
ENTRUST
ESTRADA
ESTRAYS
ESTRING
EXTRACT
EXTREME
EXTRUDE
GETREAL
GOTREAL
GSTRING
HATRACK
HATREDS
HOTRODS
HOTROLL
IATRICS
INTRADE
INTRAYS
INTROIT
INTRUDE
INTRUST
INTRUTH
ISTRIAN
JSTROKE
KATRINA
KATRINE
LATRELL
LATRINE
LATROBE
LETRIDE
LETROLL
MATRONS
METRICS
METRIST
MITRING
MOTRINS
MYTREAT
NATRIUM
NITRATE
NITRIDE
NITRIFY
NITRITE
NITROUS
NOTRADE
NOTRARE
NOTREAL
NOTRUMP
NUTRIAS
OBTRUDE
OCTROIS
ONTRACK
ONTRIAL
OSTRAVA
OSTRICH
OUTRACE
OUTRAGE
OUTRAIL
OUTRANG
OUTRANK
OUTRANT
OUTRAPS
OUTRATE
OUTRAVE
OUTREAD
OUTRIBS
OUTRIDE
OUTRIGS
OUTRING
OUTROAR
OUTROCK
OUTRODE
OUTROLL
OUTROOT
OUTROVE
OUTROWS
OUTRUNS
OUTRUSH
PATRICE
PATRICK
PATRIES
PATRIOT
PATROLS
PATRONS
PATROON
PETRATS
PETRELS
PETRIFY
PETROCK
PETROLS
PETROUS
PITROWS
PUTREFY
RATRACE
RETRACE
RETRACK
RETRACT
RETRADE
RETRAIN
RETRAPS
RETREAD
RETREAT
RETRIAL
RETRIED
RETRIES
RETRIMS
SATRAPS
SATRAPY
SETRATE
TETRADS
TETRODE
TITRATE
TITRING
TSTRAPS
UNTRACK
UNTRAPS
UNTREAD
UNTREED
UNTRIED
UNTRITE
UNTRUER
UNTRULY
UNTRUSS
UNTRUTH
UPTRADE
UPTREND
VITRICS
VITRIFY
VITRINE
VITRIOL
WETRAGS
YTTRIAS
YTTRIUM

••T•R••

ACTORLY
ALTERED
ALTERER
ANTARES
ANTERUS
ANTHRAX
APTERAL
APTERYX
ARTERIO
ASTARTE
ASTERIX
ASTORIA
ATTHREE
ATTIRED
ATTIRER
ATTIRES
AUTARCH
AUTARKY
BETARAY
BUTTRAM
BYTURNS
CATERAS
CATERED
CATERER
CATERTO
CATORCE
CETERIS
COTERIE
CUTARUG
DETERGE
DOTARDS
EATCROW
EATFROM
ENTERED
ENTERER
ENTERIC
ENTERIN
ENTERON
ENTHRAL
ENTIRES
ESTORIL
EUTERPE
EXTERNE
EXTERNS
EXTORTS
FATFREE
FITZROY
FUTURAS
FUTURES
GETFREE
GETFROM
GETSRID
GOTFREE
GUTHRIE
HATBRIM
ICTERUS
IMTIRED
INTERIM
INTERNE
INTERNS
INTERSE
INTHREE
INTURNS
KATHRYN
LATERAL
LATERAN
LATERON
LETDROP
LETSRIP
LETTRES
LITCRIT
LITERAL
LITURGY
LOTHROP
MATURED
MATURER
MATURES
METERED
MITERED
MITHRAS
MOTORED
MPTHREE
NATURAL
NATURED
NATUREL
NATURES
NOTTRUE
NOTURNS
NUTTREE
OATBRAN
ONTARIO
ONTHREE
OUTBRAG
OUTBRAY
OUTBRED
OUTCROP
OUTCROW
OUTDRAG
OUTDRAW
OUTDREW
OUTDROP
OUTGREW
OUTGRIN
OUTGROW
OUTPRAY
OUTTRAY
OUTTROT
PATERNO
PETARDS
PETCROW
PETERED
PETERII
PETFROG
PITCREW
QATARIS
RATTRAP
RETARDS
RETIRED
RETIREE
RETIRES
RETORTS
RETURFS
RETURNS
RITARDS
SATIRES
SATIRIC
SATORIS
SATURNS
SATYRIC
SETFREE
SUTURED
SUTURES
TUTORED
UNTERSE
UNTIRED
UPTHROW
UPTURNS
UTTERED
UTTERER
UTTERLY
VETERAN
VITARAS
VITORIA
WATERED
WATERER

••T••R•

ACTUARY
ALTDORF
ALTHORN
ANTBIRD
ANTFARM
ANTHERS
ANTIART
ANTLERS
ANTWERP
ARTCARS
ARTFERN
ARTFORM
ARTHURC
ARTHURM
ARTHURS
ARTWARE
ARTWORK
ASTAIRE
ATTHIRD
AUTEURS
AUTHORS
BATGIRL
BATHERS
BATTERS
BATTERY
BETHERE
BETTERS
BETTORS
BITPART
BITTERN
BITTERS
BOTHERS
BUTLERS
BUTTERS
BUTTERY
CATBERT
CATBIRD
COTTERS
CUTLERS
CUTLERY
CUTTERS
CUTWORK
CUTWORM
DETOURS
DITHERS
DITHERY
DOTTERS
EATDIRT
EATHERE
EATMORE
ESTUARY
FATFARM
FATHERS
FETTERS
FITTERS
FUTHARK
GATHERS
GETHURT
GETSORE
GETTERS
GETWARM
GETWORD
GOTHURT
GOTSORE
GOTWARM
GOTWORD
GUTTERS
HATTERS
HITHERE
HITTERS
HOTCARS
HOTWARS
HOTWIRE
IMTHERE
INTEARS
INTEGRA
INTHERE
INTHIRD
JETFIRE
JETPORT
JITTERS
JITTERY
JOTTERS
KITHARA
KITTERY
LATHERS
LATHERY
LETTERA
LETTERB
LETTERC
LETTERD
LETTERE
LETTERF
LETTERG
LETTERH
LETTERI
LETTERJ
LETTERK
LETTERL
LETTERM
LETTERN
LETTERO
LETTERP
LETTERQ
LETTERR
LETTERS
LETTERT
LETTERU
LETTERV
LETTERW
LETTERX
LETTERY
LETTERZ
LITTERS
LITTERY
LOTTERS
LOTTERY
MATHERS
MATTERS
METEORS
METIERS
MITFORD
MOTHERS
MOTHERY
MUTTERS
NATTERS
NETSURF
NETTERS
NETWARE
NETWORK
NETZERO
NOTHERE
NOTRARE
NOTSURE
NUTTERS
OCTOBRE
OCTUBRE
OSTIARY
OSTLERS
OSTMARK
OUTBARK
OUTBURN
OUTCURE
OUTDARE
OUTEARN
OUTFIRE
OUTHERE
OUTHIRE
OUTHURL
OUTPORT
OUTPURL
OUTSERT
OUTTIRE
OUTTORE
OUTTORN
OUTTURN
OUTWARD
OUTWARS
OUTWORD
OUTWORE
OUTWORK
OUTWORN
PATSDRY
PATTERN
PATTERS
PATZERS
PETBIRD
PETHARE
PETTERS
PITIERS
POTHERB
POTHERS
POTTERS
POTTERY
PUTTERS
RATBERT
RATTERS
RETEARS
RETIARY
RETOURS
ROTHIRA
ROTTERS
RUTGERS
RUTTERS
SETTERS
SITTERS
SOTHERE
SOTHERN
TATTERS
TATTERY
TETHERS
TITHERS
TITLARK
TITTERS
TOTTERS
TOTTERY
UNTIERS
UPTEARS
UPTHERE
VETOERS
VETTERS
WATFORD
WETBARS
WETWARE
WITHERS
YATTERS
YOTHERS
ZITHERS

••T•••R

ACTFOUR
ACTSFOR
ALTERER
ANTBEAR
ANTIWAR
ANTSIER
ARTFAIR
ARTSIER
ASTUTER
ATTIRER
BATSFOR
BATTIER
BATTLER
BETTGER
BITSIER
BITTIER
BOTCHER
BOTTLER
BUTCHER
CATCHER
CATDOOR
CATERER
CATHAIR
CATTIER
CDTOWER
CNTOWER
COTEDOR
CUTOVER
DITCHER
DITSIER
DITZIER
DOTTIER
EATOVER
ENTERER
ENTICER
FATTIER
FETCHER
GETOVER
GETSFAR
GOTOVER
GOTOWAR
GUTSIER
GUTTIER
HATCHER
HITCHER
HITSFOR
HOTOVER
HOTSPUR
INTEGER
INTONER
JETSTAR
KUTCHER
LETTERR
LITTLER
LOTHAIR
LUTHIER
MATADOR
MATCHER
MATURER
METOOER
METTLER
MOTHIER
MRTIGER
NATATOR
NATTIER
NETSTER
NITTIER
NOTCHER
NOTEVER
NOTFAIR
NOTICER
NOTNEAR
NOTOVER
NUTSIER
NUTTIER
OBTUSER
OCTOBER
OFTENER
OKTOBER
OPTSFOR
OUTDOER
OUTDOOR
OUTHEAR

OUTLIER
OUTPOUR
OUTROAR
OUTSOAR
OUTTEAR
OUTWEAR
PATCHER
PETBEAR
PETDEER
PETDOOR
PETHAIR
PETTIER
PITCHER
PITHIER
POTTIER
PUTOVER
RATTIER
RATTLER
RETAKER
RITZIER
ROTATOR
ROTIFER
RUTTIER
SETTLER
SETTLOR
SITSFOR
TATTIER
TATTLER
TITULAR
TOTALER
TUTELAR
UNTRUER
UPTOPAR
UTTERER
VOTEFOR
WATCHER
WATERER
WITTIER

•••TR••

AIRTRAP
ANITRAS
ASHTRAY
ASHTREE
AUSTRAL
AUSTRIA
BACTRIA
BADTRIP
BARTRAY
BAYTREE
BEATRIX
BEETRED
BEETREE
BELTRAN
BERTRAM
BESTREW
BISTROS
BOUTROS
BUSTRIP
BUTTRAM
CANTRIP
CARTRIP
CASTROL
CENTRAL
CENTRED
CENTRES
CENTRIC
CENTRUM
CHETRUM
COMTREX
CONTRAS
CONTROL
CUATROS
DALTREY
DAYTRIP
DESTROY
DEXTRAL
DEXTRIN
DISTROS
DMYTRYK
DOGTROT
DUSTRAG
ECOTRIN
EDITRIX
EGOTRIP
ELMTREE
ERITREA
FIGTREE
FIRTREE
FLYTRAP
FOOTRUB
FORTRAN
FOXTROT
GASTRIC
GUMTREE
HEATRAY
ICETRAY
INATRAP
ITSTRUE
JOGTROT
KESTREL
LASTROW
LAUTREC
LECTRIC
LEGTRAP
LEITRIM
LETTRES
LUSTRAL
LUSTRED
LUSTRES
LUSTRUM
MAITRED
MAITRES
MANTRAP
MANTRAS
MANTRIC
MISTRAL
NEUTRAL
NEUTRON
NOSTRIL
NOSTRUM
NOTTRUE
NUTTREE
OAKTREE
ONATRIP
ORATRIX
OSETRAS
OUTTRAY
OUTTROT
PALTROW
PIETROS
PORTRAY
PRETRIM
QUATRES
RATTRAP
RESTRAP
RESTREW
RESTRIP
ROOTROT
ROSTRAL
ROSTRUM
SEATRIP
SENTRAS
SKITRIP
TANTRUM
TEATRAY
TEATREE
TEATROS
TESTRUN
TEXTRON
THETREE
THETRIB
UNSTRAP
UPATREE
VECTRAS
VENTRAD
VENTRAL
VENTRIS
VESTRAL
VESTRON
VICTRIX
WAITRON
WASTREL
YEWTREE

•••T•R•

ABATERS
ABATORS
AMATORY
ATATURK
AUSTERE
AUSTERS
AVATARS
BAITERS
BANTERS
BARTERS
BASTERS
BATTERS
BATTERY
BEATERS
BELTERS
BESTIRS
BETTERS
BETTORS
BITTERN
BITTERS
BOATERS
BOLTERS
BOOTERS
BOOTERY
BUNTERS
BUSTARD
BUSTERS
BUTTERS
BUTTERY
CANTERS
CANTORS
CAPTORS
CAPTURE
CARTERS
CARTIRE
CASTERS
CDSTORE
CENTARE
CENTERS
CENTURY
CISTERN
CLOTURE
COATERS
CONTORT
COOTERS
COPTERS
COSTARD
COSTARS
COTTERS
COUTERS
COUTURE
CRATERS
CULTURE
CUSTARD
CUSTERS
CUTTERS
DAKTARI
DARTERS
DASTARD
DEBTORS
DELTORO
DENTURE
DEUTERO
DIETARY
DIETERS
DISTORT
DISTURB
DOCTORS
DONTCRY
DOTTERS
DUSTERS
EASTERN
EASTERS
EDITORS
ELATERS
EMOTERS
ERYTHRO
ESOTERY
FACTORS
FACTORY
FALTERS
FEATURE
FESTERS
FETTERS
FILTERS
FITTERS
FIXTURE
FLUTERS
FOOTERS
FORTORD
FOSTERS
FRATERS
GAITERS
GARTERS
GASTERO
GESTURE
GETTERS
GOITERS
GRATERS
GUITARS
GUTTERS
HALTERS
HASTERT
HATTERS
HEATERS
HECTARE
HECTORS
HEFTERS
HINTERS
HISTORY
HITTERS
HOOTERS
HUNTERS
HURTERS
INSTORE
INUTERO
JESTERS
JILTERS
JITTERS
JITTERY
JOLTERS
JOTTERS
KAPTURE
KITTERY
LANTERN
LASTORY
LECTERN
LECTORS
LECTURE
LEFTARM
LEOTARD
LETTERA
LETTERB
LETTERC
LETTERD
LETTERE
LETTERF
LETTERG
LETTERH
LETTERI
LETTERJ
LETTERK
LETTERL
LETTERM
LETTERN
LETTERO
LETTERP
LETTERQ
LETTERR
LETTERS
LETTERT
LETTERU
LETTERV
LETTERW
LETTERX
LETTERY
LETTERZ
LIFTERS
LINTERS
LISTERS
LITTERS
LITTERY
LOFTERS
LOITERS
LOOTERS
LOSTART
LOTTERS
LOTTERY
LUSTERS
MARTYRS
MASTERP
MASTERS
MASTERY
MATTERS
MEETERS
MELTERS
MENTORS
MIDTERM
MINTERS
MISTERM
MISTERS
MISTERX
MIXTURE
MOLTERS
MONTERO
MOOTERS
MORTARS
MUSTARD
MUSTERS
MUTTERS
MYSTARS
MYSTERY
NATTERS
NECTARS
NECTARY
NESTERS
NESTORS
NETTERS
NEUTERS
NOSTARS
NOUTURN
NURTURE
NUTTERS
ONETERM
ORATORS
ORATORY
OUSTERS
OUTTIRE
OUTTORE
OUTTORN
OUTTURN
OYSTERS
PALTERS
PANTERA
PANTERS
PASTERN
PASTERS
PASTORS
PASTURE
PATTERN
PATTERS
PELTERS
PERTURB
PESTERS
PETTERS
PEWTERS
PICTURE
PLATERS
POPTART
PORTERS
POSTERN
POSTERS
POSTURE
POTTERS
POTTERY
POUTERS
PRATERS
PRETERM
PRETIRE
PRETORS
PUNTERS
PUTTERS
QINTARS
QUATTRO
QUOTERS
RAFTERS
RANTERS
RAPTORS
RAPTURE
RASTERS
RATTERS
RECTORS
RECTORY
RENTERS
RESTART
RESTERS
RESTIRS
RESTORE
REUTERS
RHETORS
RIOTERS
RIPTORN
ROOTERS
ROSTERS
ROTTERS
ROUTERS
RUPTURE
RUTTERS
SALTERS
SARTORS
SCOTERS
SEATERS
SECTORS
SEETHRU
SETTERS
SIFTERS
SISTERS
SITTERS
SKATERS
SLATERS
SMITERS
SORTERS
STATERS
STATORS
STATURE
SUITORS
TANTARA
TARTARE
TARTARS
TASTERS
TATTERS
TATTERY
TEETERS
TENTERS
TESTERS
TEXTURE
THETURN
TILTERS
TINTERN
TINTERS
TITTERS
TOATURN
TOOTERS
TORTURE
TOSTART
TOTTERS
TOTTERY
TOUTERS
TVSTARS
TWOTERM
ULSTERS
UNITARD
UNITARY
UNITERS
UNSTERN
UPSTARE
UPSTART
UPSTIRS
VECTORS
VENTERS
VENTURA
VENTURE
VENTURI
VESTURE
VETTERS
VICTORS
VICTORY
VOITURE
VOLTORE
VULTURE
WAFTERS
WAITERS
WALTERS
WANTERS
WARTORN
WASTERS
WELTERS
WENTPRO
WESTERN
WESTERS
WINTERS
WINTERY
WRITERS
XYSTERS
YATTERS
ZESTERS

•••T••R

ABETTER
ABETTOR
ABUTTER
AGUTTER
AMATEUR
ANOTHER
BAITCAR
BATTIER
BATTLER
BEETIER
BETTGER
BITTIER
BLATHER
BLITHER
BLITZER
BLOTTER
BOTTLER
BROTHER
BUSTIER
BUSTLER
BUSTOUR
CARTIER
CATTIER
CENTAUR
CHATTER
CHITTER
CLATTER
CLUTTER
CONTOUR
COSTNER
CRITTER
CRITTUR
DIRTIER
DOTTIER
DUSTIER
ECOTEUR
EMITTER
EMPTIER
FARTHER
FASTCAR
FATTIER
FEATHER
FELTFOR
FLATCAR
FLATTER
FLITTER
FLUTIER
FLUTTER
FLYTIER
FOOTLER
FRETTER
FRITTER
FROTHER
FURTHER
FUSTIER
GAUTIER
GENTLER
GLITTER
GORTNER
GOUTIER
GRITTER
GUNTHER
GUSTIER
GUTTIER
HASTIER
HAUTEUR
HEATHER
HEATTER
HEFTIER
HOSTLER
HUNTFOR
HURTFOR
HUSTLER
IDOTTER
JOLTIER
JOSTLER
KASTLER
KNITTER
KNOTTER
LEATHER
LEFTEAR
LEFTFOR
LETTERR
LINTIER
LITTLER
LOATHER
LOFTIER
LUSTIER
MALTIER
MEATIER
MEITNER
METTLER
MINTIER
MISTIER
MOUTHER
MUSTIER
NASTIER
NATTIER
NEITHER
NESTLER
NIFTIER
NITTIER
NOOTHER
NORTHER
NUTTIER
OMITTER
ONATEAR
OUTTEAR
PANTHER
PARTIER
PARTNER
PARTYER
PASTEUR
PASTIER
PEATIER
PETTIER
PGATOUR
PHATTER
PLATIER
PLATTER
PLOTTER
POITIER
POSTWAR
POTTIER
POUTIER
PURTIER
QUITTER
RATTIER
RATTLER
RENTIER
REUTHER
REUTTER
ROOTFOR
ROOTIER
RUNTIER
RUSTIER
RUSTLER
RUTTIER
SALTIER
SCATTER
SELTZER
SENTFOR
SETTLER
SETTLOR
SHATNER
SHATTER
SHOTFOR
SHOTPAR
SHUTTER
SILTIER
SKITTER
SLATHER
SLATIER
SLITHER
SLITTER
SLOTCAR
SLOTTER
SMATTER
SMOTHER
SOOTHER
SOOTIER
SPATTER
SPITTER
SPOTTER
SPUTTER
STATLER
STUTTER
SUBTLER
SWATTER
SWITZER
TARTIER
TASTIER
TATTIER
TATTLER
TEETHER
TESTFOR
TESTIER
THETOUR
THITHER
TOOTLER
TROTTER
TUFTIER
TWITTER
UPSTAIR
USOTOUR
VASTIER
VENTNOR
VINTNER
WAITFOR
WALTHER
WALTZER
WARTIER
WEATHER
WENTFAR
WENTFOR
WERTHER
WHATFOR
WHETHER
WHETTER
WHITHER
WITTIER
WRITHER
ZESTIER

••••TR•

ABINTRA
AGENTRY
BIGOTRY
CHANTRY
COUNTRY
DIMITRI
DYKSTRA
ELANTRA
ELECTRA
ELECTRO
ELEKTRA
FENETRE
FRUSTRO
GOODTRY
HELOTRY
HOFSTRA
INVITRO
LANGTRY
MAESTRO
MONSTRO
NICETRY
NOENTRY
NUESTRA
NUESTRO
OLESTRA
OSSETRA
PHILTRE
PIASTRE
PLECTRA
POULTRY
QUATTRO
REENTRY
ROBOTRY
SCEPTRE
SHASTRI
SINATRA
SPECTRA
SPECTRE
SUMATRA
SWELTRY
THEATRE
UNMITRE

••••T•R

ABETTER
ABETTOR
ABUTTER
ADAPTER
ADAPTOR
ADEPTER
ADOPTER
AERATOR
AGUTTER
ALERTER
ALLSTAR
AMMETER
ARBITER
ASTUTER
ATWATER
AUDITOR
AVERTER
AVIATOR
AWAITER
BAINTER
BENATAR
BERATER
BIGSTAR
BLASTER
BLEATER
BLISTER
BLOTTER
BLUNTER
BLURTER
BLUSTER
BOASTER
BOLSTER
BOOSTER
BOXSTER
BURSTER
CHANTER
CHAPTER
CHARTER
CHASTER
CHATTER
CHEATER
CHESTER
CHITTER
CLATTER
CLOUTER
CLUSTER
CLUTTER
COALTAR
COASTER
COULTER
COUNTER
COVETER
CRAFTER
CREATOR
CRITTER
CRITTUR
CROFTER
CURATOR
DAUNTER
DAYSTAR
DEBATER
DECATUR
DEMETER
DEWATER
DICHTER
DILATOR
DILUTER
DILUTOR
DIMETER
DIOPTER
DOGSTAR
DONATOR
DOUBTER
DRAFTER
DRIFTER
EDUCTOR
EJECTOR
ELECTOR
EMITTER
ENACTOR
EQUATOR
ERECTER
ERECTOR
ERUPTER
EVERTOR
EVICTOR
EXACTER
EXACTOR
EXALTER
EXCITER
EXCITOR
EXERTER
FAINTER
FEASTER
FIBSTER
FIGHTER
FLATTER
FLEETER
FLIRTER
FLITTER
FLOATER
FLOUTER
FLUSTER
FLUTTER
FORSTER
FRETTER
FRITTER
FROSTER
FUNSTER
GAGSTER
GAUNTER
GENITOR
GLISTER
GLITTER
GLOATER
GOAFTER
GRAFTER
GRANTER
GRANTOR
GREATER
GREETER

GRIFTER
GRISTER
GRITTER
GROUTER
GRUNTER
GYRATOR
HAMSTER
HAUNTER
HEATTER
HERITOR
HIPSTER
HOISTER
HOLSTER
IDOTTER
IGNITER
IGNITOR
IIPETER
IMPUTER
INAPTER
INASTIR
INCITER
INDITER
INKSTER
INVITER
JACKTAR
JANITOR
JETSTAR
JOINTER
JOUSTER
JUPITER
KEISTER
KLISTER
KNITTER
KNOTTER
LEGATOR
LEISTER
LESSTAR
LEVATOR
LIGHTER
LIMITER
LOBSTER
LOCATER
LOCATOR
MEISTER
MINSTER
MINUTER
MOBSTER
MOISTER
MOLITOR
MONITOR
MONSTER
MOUNTER
MUNSTER
NAPSTER
NATATOR
NEGATER
NEGATOR
NETSTER
NIGHTER
OLDSTER
OMITTER
ONESTAR
ONWATER
ORBITER
PAINTER
PHATTER
PHILTER
PIASTER
PINETAR
PIVOTER
PLAITER
PLANTAR
PLANTER
PLASTER
PLATTER
PLOTTER
POINTER
POLITER
POPSTAR
PRAETOR
PRINTER
PROCTER
PROCTOR
PSALTER
PUNSTER
QUARTER
QUESTER
QUIETER
QUILTER
QUITTER
RAPSTAR
REACTOR
REALTER
REALTOR
REBATER
RECITER
REDSTAR
REENTER
REFUTER
RELATER
RELATOR
REMOTER
REUTTER
REWATER
RICHTER
RIGHTER
RIVETER
ROADTAR
ROASTER
ROISTER
ROOSTER
ROTATOR
ROUSTER
SALUTER
SAUNTER
SCANTER
SCATTER
SCENTER
SCEPTER
SCOOTER
SCOUTER
SEASTAR
SEDATER
SENATOR
SHANTER
SHATTER
SHELTER
SHIFTER
SHOOTER
SHORTER
SHOUTER
SHUNTER
SHUSTER
SHUTTER
SHYSTER
SIGHTER
SKEETER
SKELTER
SKIRTER
SKITTER
SLITTER
SLOTTER
SMARTER
SMATTER
SMELTER
SNIFTER
SNORTER
SPATTER
SPECTER
SPECTOR
SPITTER
SPOTTER
SPOUTER
SPUTTER
STARTER
STENTOR
STERTOR
STINTER
STOUTER
STPETER
STUTTER
SVELTER
SWATTER
SWEATER
SWEETER
SWELTER
SWIFTER
TAPSTER
TAUNTER
TELSTAR
TEMPTER
THEATER
THESTAR
TIGHTER
TINSTAR
TIPSTER
TOASTER
TRACTOR
TRAITOR
TREATER
TRISTAR
TROTTER
TRUSTER
TRYSTER
TWEETER
TWISTER
TWITTER
TWOSTAR
UNMITER
UPDATER
VAULTER
VAUNTER
VISITOR
VIVITAR
VORSTER
VUMETER
WEBSTER
WHETTER
WOODTAR
WOOSTER
WRESTER
XFACTOR
YACHTER

•••••TR

SILENTR

TS•••••

TSARDOM
TSARINA
TSARISM
TSARIST
TSELIOT
TSETSES
TSETUNG
TSHAPED
TSHAPES
TSHIRTS
TSKTSKS
TSONGAS
TSOURIS
TSQUARE
TSTRAPS
TSUNAMI

T•S••••

TASERED
TASHLIN
TASKBAR
TASKING
TASSELS
TASTEIT
TASTERS
TASTIER
TASTILY
TASTING
TESSERA
TESTACY
TESTATE
TESTBAN
TESTBED
TESTEES
TESTERS
TESTFLY
TESTFOR
TESTIER
TESTIFY
TESTILY
TESTING
TESTKIT
TESTLAB
TESTOUT
TESTRUN
TISANES
TISSOTS
TISSUES
TISSUEY
TOSCALE
TOSHIBA
TOSHIRO
TOSPARE
TOSSERS
TOSSING
TOSSOFF
TOSSOUT
TOSSPOT
TOSSUPS
TOSTADA
TOSTART
TUSCANS
TUSCANY
TUSHERY
TUSHIES
TUSKERS
TUSKING
TUSSAUD
TUSSIVE
TUSSLED
TUSSLES
TUSSOCK
TVSHOWS
TVSPOTS
TVSTARS

T••S•••

TABSETS
TAGSALE
TAGSOUT
TANSIES
TAPSHOE
TAPSOFF
TAPSOUT
TAPSTER
TARSALS
TASSELS
TAXSALE
TEASELS
TEASERS
TEASETS
TEASEUP
TEASHOP
TEASING
TEESHOT
TEESOFF
TELSTAR
TENSELY
TENSEST
TENSEUP
TENSILE
TENSING
TENSION
TENSITY
TENSIVE
TENSORS
TENSPOT
TERSELY
TERSEST
TESSERA
THESACK
THESAME
THESELF
THESEUS
THESHOW
THESIMS
THESPIS
THESTAR
THESUNS
THESWAN
THISDAY
THISONE
THISTLE
THISTLY
THISWAY
THUSFAR
THYSELF
TIESOFF
TILSITS
TINSELS
TINSTAR
TIPSIER
TIPSILY
TIPSOFF
TIPSTER
TISSOTS
TISSUES
TISSUEY
TOASTED
TOASTEE
TOASTER
TOCSINS
TOESHOE
TOGSOUT
TOLSTOI
TOLSTOY
TONSILS
TONSURE
TOOSLOW
TOOSOON
TOPSAIL
TOPSEED
TOPSIDE
TOPSOFF
TOPSOIL
TOPSOUT
TOPSPIN
TOPSPOT
TORSION
TOSSERS
TOSSING
TOSSOFF
TOSSOUT
TOSSPOT
TOSSUPS
TOUSLED
TOUSLES
TOYSHOP
TOYSLED
TOYSRUS
TRASHED
TRASHER
TRASHES
TRASHTV
TRESSED
TRESSES
TRESTLE
TRISECT
TRISTAN
TRISTAR
TRUSSED
TRUSSES
TRUSSUP
TRUSTED
TRUSTEE
TRUSTER
TRUSTIN
TRUSTME
TRYSAIL
TRYSTED
TRYSTER
TUCSONS
TUESDAY
TULSANS
TULSAOK
TUSSAUD
TUSSIVE
TUSSLED
TUSSLES
TUSSOCK
TWISTED
TWISTER
TWISTON
TWISTUP
TWOSHOT
TWOSOME
TWOSPOT
TWOSTAR
TWOSTEP

T•••S••

TABASCO
TACKSON
TACKSUP
TAKESIN
TAKESIT
TAKESON
TAKESTO
TAKESUP
TALKSAT
TALKSOF
TALKSON
TALKSTO
TALKSUP
TALUSES
TANKSUP
TAOISTS
TAPESON
TAPESUP
TARTSUP
TEAMSUP
TEARSAT
TEARSIT
TEARSUP
TEENSIE
TELESTO
TELLSIT
TELLSOF
TELLSON
TENDSTO
THATSIT
THATSOK
THEISMS
THEISTS
THEUSSR
THEYSAY
THIRSTS
THIRSTY
THOMSON
THORSON
THRUSTS
TICKSBY
TIDYSUM
TILTSAT
TILTSUP
TIMESUP
TIRESOF
TOILSAT
TONESUP
TONUSES
TOOLSET
TOOLSUP
TOOTSAT
TOOTSIE
TOTASTE
TOTESUP
TRANSAM
TRANSIT
TRANSOM
TREASON
TREESAP
TRESSED
TRESSES
TRIESIT
TRIESON
TRIESTE
TRIESTO
TRIPSON
TRIPSUP
TROTSKY
TROTSUP
TROUSER
TRUESUP
TRUISMS
TRUSSED
TRUSSES
TRUSSUP
TSETSES
TSKTSKS
TUBISTS
TUCKSIN
TUMESCE
TUNASUB
TUNESIN
TUNESTO
TUNESUP
TUNISIA
TURFSKI
TURISMO
TURISTA
TURNSIN
TURNSON
TURNSTO
TURNSUP
TWINSET
TYPESET
TYPESIN
TYPESUP
TYPISTS

T••••S•

TALLEST
TALLISH
TANNEST
TANNISH
TARNISH
TARTEST
TARTISH
TAUTEST
TAXBASE
TAXLESS
TBILISI
TEALESS
TEAMUSA
TEAROSE
TEMPEST
TENPAST
TENSEST
TERSEST
THEBEST
THEBOSS
THEBUSH
THEEAST
THEKISS
THEMASK
THEMOST
THEPOST
THERESA
THEROSE
THEUSSR
THINKSO
TIDIEST
TIELESS
TIGRESS
TINFISH
TINIEST
TIPLESS
TITLIST
TITOISM
TITOIST
TOADISH
TOELESS
TOHORSE
TOLEASE
TONIEST
TOOEASY
TOPLESS
TOPMAST
TOPMOST
TORYISH
TORYISM
TOURISM
TOURIST
TOWNISH
TOYLESS
TRAIPSE
TRITEST
TROPISM
TSARISM
TSARIST
TUBAIST
TUGLESS
TURKISH
TWOBASE

T•••••S

TABARDS
TABBIES
TABKEYS
TABLETS
TABSETS
TACITUS
TACKERS
TACKLES
TACOMAS
TACTICS
TAFFIES
TAGDAYS
TAGENDS
TAGGERS
TAGOUTS
TAHINIS
TAILERS
TAILORS
TAKEINS
TAKINGS
TALCUMS
TALENTS
TALKERS
TALKIES
TALLIES
TALLOWS
TALUSES
TAMALES
TAMPERS
TAMTAMS
TANDEMS
TANGLES
TANKERS
TANNERS
TANNINS
TANOAKS
TANSIES
TAOISTS
TAPINGS
TAPPANS
TAPPERS
TAPPETS
TARGETS
TARIFFS
TARMACS
TAROILS
TARPITS
TARPONS
TARRIES
TARSALS
TARTANS
TARTARS
TARZANS
TASSELS
TASTERS
TATAMIS
TATTERS
TATTLES
TATTOOS
TAUTENS
TAVERNS
TAXCUTS
TAXLAWS
TAXLESS
TAYLORS
TEABAGS
TEACHES
TEACUPS
TEALESS
TEAPOTS
TEAPOYS
TEARERS
TEARGAS
TEASELS
TEASERS
TEASETS
TEATROS
TEAURNS
TECHIES
TECHNOS
TEDDIES
TEDEUMS
TEDIOUS
TEDIUMS
TEEHEES
TEENERS
TEEOFFS
TEEPEES
TEETERS
TEETHES
TEEVEES
TEFLONS
TEJANAS
TEJANOS
TEKKIES
TELEXES
TELLERS
TELLIES
TEMPEHS
TEMPERS
TEMPLES
TENACES
TENANTS
TENCHES
TENDAYS
TENDERS
TENDONS
TENNERS
TENNIES
TENPINS
TENSORS
TENTERS
TENTONS
TENUOUS
TENURES
TERCELS
TERRANS
TERRETS
TERRIES
TERRORS
TESTEES
TESTERS
TETANUS
TETHERS
TETRADS
TEUTONS
TFPOWYS
THALERS
THAWERS
THEABCS
THEAGES
THEALPS
THEARTS
THEAXIS
THEBANS
THEBOSS
THEBOYS
THECARS
THECAVS
THECUBS
THEFEDS
THEHOGS
THEISMS
THEISTS
THEJETS
THEKISS
THEMAVS
THEMETS
THENETS
THENEWS
THEPIPS
THEPITS
THERAMS
THEREDS
THERMOS
THESEUS
THESIMS
THESPIS
THESUNS
THEVIPS
THEYIPS
THIEVES
THIRSTS
THRALLS
THREADS
THREATS
THREERS
THRIFTS
THRILLS
THRIVES
THROATS
THRONES
THRONGS
THRUSTS
THWACKS
THWARTS
TICKERS
TICKETS
TICKLES
TICTACS
TIDBITS
TIDINGS
TIEBARS
TIEDYES
TIELESS
TIEMPOS
TIENDAS
TIEPINS
TIERCES
TIERODS
TIETACS
TIFFINS
TIGLONS
TIGRESS
TILINGS
TILLERS
TILLETS
TILSITS
TILTERS
TIMBALS
TIMBERS
TIMBRES
TIMEWAS
TIMEXES
TIMINGS
TIMMINS
TINCANS
TINDERS
TINEARS
TINGLES
TINGODS
TINHATS
TINKERS
TINKLES
TINNERS
TINORES
TINSELS
TINTERS
TIPJARS
TIPLESS
TIPOFFS
TIPPEES
TIPPERS
TIPPETS
TIPPLES
TIPTOES
TIPTOPS
TIRADES
TISANES
TISSOTS
TISSUES
TITHERS
TITIANS
TITTERS
TITTLES
TIZZIES
TOADIES
TOCSINS
TODDIES
TODDLES
TOECAPS
TOELESS
TOETAPS
TOFFEES
TOGGLES
TOILERS
TOILETS
TOLEDOS
TOLLERS
TOLTECS
TOMBOYS
TOMCATS
TOMTITS
TOMTOMS
TONEMES
TONGANS
TONGUES
TONSILS
TONUSES
TOODLES
TOOLERS
TOONIES
TOOTERS
TOOTLES
TOPAZES
TOPBIDS
TOPDOGS
TOPGUNS
TOPHATS
TOPLESS
TOPPERS
TOPPLES
TOPROWS
TOPTENS
TOPTHIS
TORCHES
TOREROS
TORINOS
TOROIDS
TORQUES
TOSSERS
TOSSUPS
TOTINOS
TOTTERS
TOUCANS
TOUCHES
TOUPEES
TOURBUS
TOURERS
TOUSLES
TOUTERS
TOWAGES
TOWARDS
TOWBARS
TOWCARS
TOWHEES
TOWINGS
TOWNERS
TOWNIES
TOYCARS

TOYDOGS
TOYGUNS
TOYHATS
TOYLESS
TOYOTAS
TOYSRUS
TOYTOPS
TRACERS
TRADERS
TRAMPAS
TRANCES
TRASHES
TRAUMAS
TRAVELS
TRAVERS
TREBLES
TREDIAS
TREIZES
TRELLIS
TREMORS
TREPANS
TRESSES
TRIAGES
TRICEPS
TRICOTS
TRIFLES
TRIGONS
TRIJETS
TRIODES
TRIPLES
TRIPODS
TRITONS
TRIVETS
TROCHES
TROIKAS
TROILUS
TROJANS
TROPICS
TROUGHS
TROUPES
TROWELS
TRUANTS
TRUDGES
TRUISMS
TRUMANS
TRUSSES
TRYOUTS
TSETSES
TSHAPES
TSHIRTS
TSKTSKS
TSONGAS
TSOURIS
TSTRAPS
TUBFULS
TUBISTS
TUBULES
TUCKERS
TUCSONS
TUFFETS
TUGGERS
TUGLESS
TUGRIKS
TUILLES
TULSANS
TUMBLES
TUMMIES
TUMULTS
TUNDRAS
TUNEUPS
TUNNELS
TUPELOS
TURBANS
TURBOTS
TUREENS
TURKEYS
TURNERS
TURNIPS
TURNONS
TURNUPS
TURRETS
TURTLES
TUSCANS
TUSHIES
TUSKERS
TUSSLES
TUTTUTS
TUXEDOS
TVCREWS
TVGAMES
TVIDOLS
TVROOMS
TVSHOWS
TVSPOTS
TVSTARS
TVTAPES
TWEEZES
TWELVES
TWINERS
TWINGES
TWOACTS
TWOBITS
TWODAYS
TWOEGGS
TWOFERS
TWOTONS
TYCOONS
TYPEABS
TYPISTS
TYRANTS
TZIMMES

•TS••••

ATSEVEN
ATSIGHT
ATSIGNS
ATSTAKE
CTSCANS
ITSABOY
ITSAHIT
ITSALIE
ITSALOT
ITSASIN
ITSATIE
ITSBEST
ITSCOLD
ITSDONE
ITSEASY
ITSFINE
ITSGONE
ITSHERE
ITSLATE
ITSLOVE
ITSOKAY
ITSONME
ITSOPEN
ITSOVER
ITSTIME
ITSTRUE
MTSINAI
STSIMON

•T•S•••

ATISSUE
BTFSPLK
ETESIAN
ITISTOO
KTOSLIN
STASHED
STASHES
STASSEN

•T••S••

ATISSUE
ATLASES
ATTESTS
ITSASIN
STARSIN
STARSKY
STASSEN
STAYSAT
STAYSIN
STAYSON
STAYSUP
STBASIL
STEPSIN
STEPSON
STEPSUP
STETSON
STIMSON
STIRSIN
STIRSUP
STOPSAT
STOPSBY
STOPSIN
STOPSIT
STOPSUP
STOWSIT
STRASSE
STYPSIS
UTENSIL
UTMOSTS

•T•••S•

ATACOST
ATALOSS
ATAVISM
ATAVIST
ATCROSS
ATELESS
ATFIRST
ATHEISM
ATHEIST
ATHIRST
ATLEAST
ATOMISE
ATOMISM
ATOMIST
ATWORST
FTBLISS
ITEMISE
ITSBEST
ITSEASY
STALEST
STATISM
STATIST
STPIUSI
STPIUSV
STPIUSX
STRASSE
STRAUSS
STROUSE
STYLISE
STYLISH
STYLIST
UTILISE
UTOPISM
UTOPIST

•T••••S

ATALOSS
ATAMANS
ATCROSS
ATELESS
ATHOMES
ATLASES
ATMFEES
ATOMICS
ATOMIES
ATONERS
ATONICS
ATONIES
ATRIUMS
ATROPOS
ATSIGNS
ATTACKS
ATTAINS
ATTENDS
ATTESTS
ATTICUS
ATTIMES
ATTIRES
ATTRITS
ATTUCKS
ATTUNES
CTSCANS
ETCHERS
ETHANES
ETHENES
ETHNICS
ETOILES
ETONICS
ETYMONS
FTBLISS
FTMYERS
ITALICS
ITGIRLS
MTADAMS
MTATHOS
MTEVANS
NTUPLES
OTARIES
OTTAWAS
PTBOATS
PTEROUS
STABLES
STAGERS
STAGNES
STALAGS
STAMENS
STANCES
STANZAS
STAPLES
STARERS
STARVES
STASHES
STATERS
STATICS
STATINS
STATORS
STATUES
STAYERS
STBARTS
STDENIS
STEARNS
STEEVES
STELIAS
STENNIS
STEPINS
STEPPES
STEPUPS
STEREOS
STERNOS
STEROLS
STEVENS
STEWERS
STIFLES
STIGMAS
STJAMES
STJOHNS
STKITTS
STLOUIS
STLUKES
STMARKS
STMARYS
STODGES
STOGIES
STOKERS
STOLONS
STONERS
STOOGES
STORERS
STORIES
STOTINS
STOWERS
STPAULS
STRAFES
STRAINS
STRAITS
STRANDS
STRATAS
STRATUS
STRAUSS
STREAKS
STREAMS
STREETS
STREGIS
STRIDES
STRIFES
STRIKES
STRINGS
STRIPES
STRIVES
STROBES
STROKES
STROLLS
STUCCOS
STUDIES
STUDIOS
STUPIDS
STUPORS
STURGES
STUTZES
STYLERS
STYLETS
STYMIES
STYPSIS
UTAHANS
UTICANS
UTMOSTS
UTOPIAS
XTERRAS
YTTRIAS

••TS•••

ACTSFOR
ACTSOUT
ANTSIER
ARTSALE
ARTSHOP
ARTSHOW
ARTSIER
ARTSONG
BATSFOR
BATSMAN
BATSMEN
BATSUIT
BITSIER
CATSCAN
CATSEYE
CATSHOW
CATSITS
CATSPAW
CATSUIT
CATSUPS
CUTSOFF
CUTSOUT
DATSUNS
DITSIER
EATSOUT
GETSANA
GETSANF
GETSFAR
GETSFIT
GETSHEP
GETSHIP
GETSHOT
GETSMAD
GETSOFF
GETSOFT
GETSOLD
GETSORE
GETSOUT
GETSRID
GETSSET
GETSWET
GOTSOFT
GOTSORE
GUTSIER
GUTSILY
HATSIZE
HATSOFF
HITSFOR
HITSHOW
HITSOFF
HITSONG
HITSOUT
HOTSEAT
HOTSHOT
HOTSOUP
HOTSPOT
HOTSPUR
JETSETS
JETSFAN
JETSKIS
JETSONS
JETSTAR
KITSCHY
LETSEAT
LETSFLY
LETSLIP
LETSNOT
LETSOFF
LETSOUT
LETSRIP
LETSSEE
LETSUSE
METSFAN
NATSUME
NETSTER
NETSUKE
NETSURF
NOTSAFE
NOTSURE
NUTSIER
OPTSFOR
OPTSOUT
OUTSAID
OUTSAIL
OUTSANG
OUTSAYS
OUTSEEK
OUTSEEN
OUTSEES
OUTSELL
OUTSERT
OUTSETS
OUTSHOT
OUTSHOW
OUTSIDE
OUTSIFT
OUTSIGH
OUTSING
OUTSINS
OUTSITS
OUTSIZE
OUTSKIP
OUTSOAR
OUTSOLD
OUTSOLE
OUTSPED
OUTSPIN
OUTSPIT
OUTSTAY
OUTSTEP
OUTSULK
OUTSUMS
OUTSUNG
OUTSWAM
OUTSWIM
OUTSWUM
PATSDRY
PATSIES
PETSCAN
PETSHOP
PETSITS
PITSAWS
PITSTOP
POTSDAM
POTSHOT
PUTSOFF
PUTSOUT
RATSOUT
RETSINA
SATSUMA
SETSAIL
SETSHOT
SETSOFF
SETSOUT
SITSFOR
SITSOUT
SITSPAT
WETSUIT
WITSEND

••T•S••

ALTOSAX
ANTESUP
ARTISAN
ARTISTE
ARTISTS
ATTESTS
AUTISTS
BATISTA
BATISTE
BITESIN
BITESON
BITESUP
BUTTSIN
CUTISES
DATASET
DETESTS
DOTESON
FETUSES
GETSSET
GOTOSEA
GOTOSEE
HATESIT
HDTVSET
ICTUSES
INTASTE
IQTESTS
KATISHA
LATOSCA
LETSSEE
LOTUSES
LUTISTS
MATISSE
MITOSES
MITOSIS
NATASHA
NOTASTE
NOTUSED
OBTESTS
OBTUSER
OSTOSIS
OUTASKS
RETASTE
RETESTS
SATISFY
TOTASTE
TOTESUP
UNTASTY
VOTESIN
VOTESNO
VOTESON
WATUSIS

••T••S•

ACTRESS
AFTMOST
ALTOIST
APTNESS
ARTIEST
ARTLESS
AUTOPSY
BITLESS
CATFISH
CATTISH
CUTLASS
DOTDASH
EATLESS
ENTHUSE
ENTRUST
ENTWIST
EXTENSO
FATLESS
FATNESS
FATOUSH
FATTEST
FATTISH
FITNESS
FITTEST
GETBUSY
GETCASH
GETLOST
GETPAST
GETWISE
GOTBUSY
GOTCASH
GOTLOST
GOTPAST
GOTWISE
GUTLESS
HATLESS
HITLESS
HITLIST
HOTNESS
HOTTEST
INTENSE
INTERSE
INTRUST
JETWASH
LETPASS
LETSUSE
LETTISH
LITHEST
LITOVSK
MATISSE
MATLESS
METRIST
NETCOST
NETLESS
NETLOSS
NOTEASY
ONTOAST
OUTCAST
OUTFAST
OUTFISH
OUTGUSH
OUTHISS
OUTJEST
OUTKAST
OUTKISS
OUTLASH
OUTLAST
OUTMOST
OUTPASS
OUTPOST
OUTPUSH
OUTRUSH
OUTWASH
OUTWEST
OUTWISH
PATCASH
PATNESS
PETFISH
PETTISH
PITBOSS
RATTISH
RETOAST
RETWIST
RUTTISH
SOTTISH
TITLIST
TITOISM
TITOIST
UNTENSE
UNTERSE
UNTRUSS
UNTWIST
VITEBSK
WETKISS
WETNESS
WETTEST
WETTISH
WETWASH
WITLESS
WITNESS

••T•••S

ACTEDAS
ACTIONS
ACTIVAS
ACTIVES
ACTRESS
AITCHES
ALTIMAS
ALTKEYS
ALTOIDS
ALTTABS
AMTRACS
ANTARES
ANTCOWS
ANTERUS
ANTHEMS
ANTHERS
ANTIBES
ANTLERS
APTNESS
ARTCARS
ARTEMIS
ARTEMUS
ARTHURS
ARTISTS
ARTLESS
ASTHMAS
ATTACKS
ATTAINS
ATTENDS
ATTESTS
ATTICUS
ATTIMES
ATTIRES
ATTRITS
ATTUCKS
ATTUNES
AUTEURS
AUTHORS
AUTISTS
AUTOBUS
AUTUMNS
BATBOYS
BATCHES
BATDAYS
BATHERS
BATTENS
BATTERS
BATTLES
BETAKES
BETHELS
BETIDES
BETIMES
BETRAYS
BETTERS
BETTORS
BITLESS
BITMAPS
BITTERS
BOTCHES
BOTHERS
BOTREES
BOTTLES
BOTTOMS
BUTANES
BUTCHES
BUTENES
BUTLERS
BUTTERS
BUTTONS
BYTALKS
BYTURNS
CATALOS
CATBEDS
CATCHES
CATENAS
CATERAS
CATFITS
CATGUTS
CATIONS
CATKINS
CATNAPS
CATNIPS
CATRIGS
CATSITS
CATSUPS
CATTOYS
CETANES
CETERIS
CITRONS
CITROUS
COTTERS
COTTONS
CUTISES
CUTLASS
CUTLERS
CUTLETS
CUTOFFS
CUTOUTS
CUTTERS
DATABUS
DATINGS
DATIVES
DATRILS
DATSUNS
DETAILS
DETAINS
DETECTS
DETENTS
DETESTS
DETOURS
DETOXES
DETUNES
DITCHES
DITHERS
DITTIES
DOTAGES
DOTARDS
DOTCOMS
DOTTERS
DOTTLES
DUTEOUS
EATLESS
ECTYPES
ENTAILS
ENTICES
ENTIRES
ENTOMBS
ENTRAPS
ENTREES
ENTRIES
ESTADOS
ESTATES
ESTEEMS
ESTRAYS
EXTENDS
EXTENTS
EXTERNS
EXTOLLS
EXTORTS
FATALES
FATCATS
FATHERS
FATHOMS
FATLESS
FATLIPS
FATNESS
FATONES
FATTENS
FATUOUS
FETCHES
FETTERS
FETTLES
FETUSES
FITNESS
FITTERS
FUTURAS
FUTURES
GATHERS
GATINGS
GATLINS
GETTERS
GETTHIS
GITANOS
GOTCHAS
GOTHICS
GUTLESS
GUTTERS
HATCHES
HATFULS
HATLESS
HATPINS
HATREDS
HATTERS
HITCHES
HITLESS
HITTERS
HOTBEDS
HOTCAPS
HOTCARS
HOTCUPS
HOTDAYS
HOTDOGS
HOTKEYS
HOTLIPS
HOTNESS
HOTONES
HOTPOTS
HOTRODS
HOTTEAS
HOTTIES
HOTTIPS
HOTTUBS
HOTWARS
HUTCHES
IATRICS
ICTERUS
ICTINUS
ICTUSES
INTAILS
INTAKES
INTEARS
INTENDS
INTENTS
INTERNS
INTONES
INTRAYS
INTUITS
INTURNS
IQTESTS
ISTHMUS
IVTUBES
JETFANS
JETGUNS
JETLAGS
JETSETS
JETSKIS
JETSONS
JETTIES
JETWAYS
JITNEYS
JITTERS
JOTTERS
KETCHES
KETONES
KETTLES
KITBAGS
KITKATS
KITTENS
KITTIES
LATCHES
LATEENS
LATENTS
LATEXES

LATHERS
LATICES
LATIGOS
LATIMES
LATINAS
LATINOS
LATINUS
LETPASS
LETTERS
LETTRES
LITCHIS
LITOTES
LITTERS
LITTLES
LOTIONS
LOTTERS
LOTUSES
LUTISTS
MATCHES
MATHERS
MATHEWS
MATHIAS
MATLESS
MATRONS
MATTERS
MATURES
MATZOHS
METATES
METEORS
METFANS
METHODS
METIERS
METRICS
METTLES
MITHRAS
MITOSES
MITOSIS
MITTENS
MOTHERS
MOTIONS
MOTIVES
MOTLEYS
MOTRINS
MOTTLES
MOTTOES
MRTIBBS
MUTANTS
MUTATES
MUTTERS
MUTTONS
MUTUALS
NATHANS
NATIONS
NATIVES
NATTERS
NATURES
NETFULS
NETLESS
NETLOSS
NETTERS
NETTLES
NETTONS
NITROUS
NITWITS
NOTATES
NOTCHES
NOTHINS
NOTICES

NOTIONS
NOTURNS
NUTATES
NUTLETS
NUTMEGS
NUTOILS
NUTRIAS
NUTTERS
NYTIMES
OBTAINS
OBTESTS
OBTUNDS
OCTANES
OCTANTS
OCTAVES
OCTAVOS
OCTOPUS
OCTROIS
OPTICKS
OPTIMAS
OPTIONS
OSTLERS
OSTOSIS
OTTAWAS
OUTACTS
OUTADDS
OUTAGES
OUTASKS
OUTAWES
OUTBANS
OUTBATS
OUTBEGS
OUTBIDS
OUTBOWS
OUTBUDS
OUTBUYS
OUTCUTS
OUTDOES
OUTEATS
OUTFITS
OUTGOES
OUTGUNS
OUTHISS
OUTHITS
OUTINGS
OUTJETS
OUTJUTS
OUTKISS
OUTLAWS
OUTLAYS
OUTLETS
OUTLIES
OUTLIPS
OUTMANS
OUTPASS
OUTPAYS
OUTPOPS
OUTPUTS
OUTRAPS
OUTRIBS
OUTRIGS
OUTROWS
OUTRUNS
OUTSAYS
OUTSEES
OUTSETS
OUTSINS
OUTSITS

OUTSUMS
OUTVIES
OUTWARS
OUTWITS
OXTAILS
PATACAS
PATCHES
PATENTS
PATHANS
PATINAS
PATNESS
PATRIES
PATROLS
PATRONS
PATSIES
PATTERS
PATTIES
PATZERS
PETALES
PETARDS
PETBOAS
PETCATS
PETCOWS
PETDOGS
PETITES
PETNAPS
PETPIGS
PETPUPS
PETRATS
PETRELS
PETROLS
PETROUS
PETSITS
PETTERS
PETTOYS
PITAYAS
PITBOSS
PITCHES
PITEOUS
PITIERS
PITROWS
PITSAWS
POTAGES
POTAMUS
POTEENS
POTFULS
POTHERS
POTIONS
POTLIDS
POTPIES
POTTERS
POTTIES
PUTOFFS
PUTOUTS
PUTPUTS
PUTTEES
PUTTERS
PUTTIES
PYTHIAS
PYTHONS
QATARIS
RATINES
RATINGS
RATIONS
RATITES
RATLINS
RATTANS
RATTERS

RATTLES
RETACKS
RETAILS
RETAINS
RETAKES
RETAMES
RETAPES
RETARDS
RETAXES
RETEARS
RETELLS
RETESTS
RETHAWS
RETILES
RETILLS
RETIMES
RETINAS
RETINTS
RETIRES
RETONES
RETOOLS
RETORTS
RETOURS
RETRAPS
RETRIES
RETRIMS
RETUNES
RETURFS
RETURNS
RETYPES
RITARDS
RITDYES
RITUALS
ROTATES
ROTGUTS
ROTTERS
RUTGERS
RUTILES
RUTTERS
SATCOMS
SATEENS
SATIRES
SATORIS
SATRAPS
SATURNS
SETFEES
SETOFFS
SETOUTS
SETTEES
SETTERS
SETTLES
SHTETLS
SHTICKS
SITCOMS
SITTERS
SUTURES
TATAMIS
TATTERS
TATTLES
TATTOOS
TETANUS
TETHERS
TETRADS
TITHERS
TITIANS
TITTERS
TITTLES
TOTINOS

TOTTERS
TSTRAPS
TUTTUTS
TVTAPES
ULTIMAS
UNTACKS
UNTAMES
UNTAPES
UNTAXES
UNTHAWS
UNTIERS
UNTRAPS
UNTRUSS
UNTUCKS
UNTUNES
UPTAKES
UPTALKS
UPTEARS
UPTICKS
UPTILTS
UPTIMES
UPTOWNS
UPTURNS
URTEXTS
USTEDES
VATDYES
VATFULS
VETCHES
VETOERS
VETTERS
VITALIS
VITARAS
VITRICS
VITTLES
VOTECHS
VOTEYES
VOTIVES
WATCHES
WATKINS
WATTLES
WATUSIS
WETBARS
WETKISS
WETMOPS
WETNAPS
WETNESS
WETONES
WETRAGS
WITCHES
WITHERS
WITHIES
WITLESS
WITNESS
YATTERS
YETTIES
YOTHERS
YTTRIAS
ZITCOMS
ZITHERS

•••TS••

ABUTSON
BEATSAT
BEATSIT
BEATSME
BEATSON
BEATSUP
BELTSAW

BELTSUP
BENTSEN
BLOTSUP
BOLTSUP
BOOTSIT
BOOTSUP
BUSTSIN
BUSTSUP
BUTTSIN
CANTSAY
CARTSIN
CASTSON
CASTSUP
CHATSUP
CLOTSUP
CURTSEY
DEUTSCH
FLITSBY
FLITSIN
FLOTSAM
FOOTSIE
FOOTSIT
FOOTSUP
FRETSAT
FRETSAW
GIFTSET
HEATSUP
HINTSAT
HOOTSAT
HUNTSUP
KLATSCH
KNOTSUP
LIFTSUP
MEETSUP
MISTSUP
MUSTSEE
NESTSIN
QUITSIT
RANTSAT
RENTSTO
RESTSIN
RESTSON
RESTSUP
ROOTSUP
SALTSEA
SHUTSIN
SHUTSUP
SPITSON
STETSON
SUITSME
SUITSUP
SWATSAT
TARTSUP
THATSIT
THATSOK
TILTSAT
TILTSUP
TOOTSAT
TOOTSIE
TROTSKY
TROTSUP
TSETSES
TSKTSKS
WAITSON
WAITSUP
WANTSIN
WANTSTO
WHATSAY

WHATSIS
WHATSIT
WHATSUP
WHITSUN
YELTSIN

•••T•S•

ACUTEST
ANATASE
BAPTISE
BAPTISM
BAPTIST
BRITISH
BRUTISH
CATTISH
CHUTIST
COLTISH
COMTISM
COMTIST
CONTEST
CONTUSE
CULTISH
CULTISM
CULTIST
CURTEST
CURTISS
DAFTEST
DEFTEST
DENTIST
DNATEST
DOLTISH
DONTASK
ECSTASY
EGGTOSS
EGOTISM
EGOTIST
ELITEST
ELITISM
ELITIST
EXOTISM
EYETEST
FANTASM
FANTAST
FANTASY
FASTEST
FATTEST
FATTISH
FESTOSO
FITTEST
FLUTIST
GJETOST
GOATISH
GOUTISH
HOSTESS
HOTTEST
IRATEST
JUSTEST
KENTISH
KERTESZ
LABTEST
LACTASE
LACTOSE
LEFTEST
LEFTISH
LEFTISM
LEFTIST
LETTISH
LIETEST

LOUTISH
MALTASE
MALTESE
MALTOSE
MORTISE
NASTASE
NEATEST
PELTISH
PERTEST
PETTISH
PICTISH
PIETOSO
POETESS
POETISE
PRETEST
PROTEST
PROTIST
QUITESO
RATTISH
RUNTISH
RUTTISH
SALTISH
SOFTEST
SOFTISH
SOTTISH
STATISM
STATIST
SUBTASK
TARTEST
TARTISH
TAUTEST
TRITEST
UNITISE
VASTEST
WETTEST
WETTISH
WHITEST
WHITISH
XYSTUSI

•••T••S

ABATERS
ABATORS
ACCTNOS
ACETALS
ALETAPS
ALETTES
ALLTHIS
ALTTABS
AMATOLS
AMITIES
AMSTELS
ANITRAS
ASSTDAS
AUNTIES
AUSTERS
AUSTINS
AVATARS
BAITERS
BANTAMS
BANTERS
BARTABS
BARTERS
BARTLES
BASTERS
BATTENS
BATTERS
BATTLES

BEATERS
BEATLES
BEETLES
BELTERS
BENTHOS
BERTHAS
BESTIRS
BESTOWS
BETTERS
BETTORS
BIGTOES
BIGTOPS
BISTROS
BITTERS
BLITZES
BOATELS
BOATERS
BOLTERS
BOOTEES
BOOTERS
BOOTIES
BOSTONS
BOTTLES
BOTTOMS
BOUTROS
BOWTIES
BOXTOPS
BOYTOYS
BRETONS
BRITONS
BUNTERS
BUSTERS
BUSTLES
BUSTUPS
BUTTERS
BUTTONS
CAFTANS
CANTABS
CANTALS
CANTERS
CANTLES
CANTONS
CANTORS
CAPTORS
CARTELS
CARTERS
CARTONS
CARTOPS
CASTERS
CASTLES
CATTOYS
CELTICS
CENTALS
CENTERS
CENTRES
CHITONS
CLOTHES
COATEES
COATERS
CONTACS
CONTRAS
COOTERS
COOTIES
COPTERS
COSTARS
COTTERS
COTTONS
COUTERS

CRATERS
CRETANS
CRETINS
CRITIAS
CRITICS
CROTONS
CUATROS
CUETIPS
CURTISS
CUSTERS
CUSTOMS
CUTTERS
DACTYLS
DALTONS
DARTERS
DARTLES
DEBTEES
DEBTORS
DEITIES
DENTALS
DENTINS
DENTONS
DESTEMS
DIATOMS
DICTUMS
DIETERS
DIKTATS
DIRTIES
DISTILS
DISTROS
DITTIES
DOCTORS
DOGTAGS
DOGTOYS
DOTTERS
DOTTLES
DUETTOS
DUSTERS
DUSTUPS
EARTABS
EARTAGS
EASTERS
EDITORS
EGGTOSS
ELATERS
EMETICS
EMOTERS
EMPTIES
EROTICS
EXOTICS
FACTORS
FALTERS
FANTANS
FANTODS
FASTENS
FATTENS
FESTERS
FETTERS
FETTLES
FIFTIES
FILTERS
FITTERS
FLATTVS
FLUTERS
FLUTIES
FOOTERS
FOOTLES
FORTIES

FORTIUS
FOSTERS
FRATERS
GAITERS
GARTERS
GENTLES
GETTERS
GETTHIS
GHETTOS
GIFTEES
GLITZES
GLOTTIS
GLUTENS
GLUTEUS
GOATEES
GOITERS
GRATERS
GRATIAS
GROTIUS
GROTTOS
GUITARS
GUSTOES
GUTTERS
HALTERS
HAPTICS
HASTENS
HATTERS
HEATERS
HECTORS
HEFTERS
HEPTADS
HILTONS
HINTERS
HITTERS
HOGTIES
HOOTERS
HOSTELS
HOSTESS
HOTTEAS
HOTTIES
HOTTIPS
HOTTUBS
HUNTERS
HURTERS
HURTLES
HUSTLES
ICETEAS
INSTALS
INSTEPS
INSTILS
JESTERS
JETTIES
JILTERS
JITTERS
JOLTERS
JOSTLES
JOTTERS
KETTLES
KILTIES
KITTENS
KITTIES
KLUTZES
KOWTOWS
LAITIES
LAPTOPS
LASTGAS
LECTORS
LEFTIES

LENTILS
LEPTONS
LETTERS
LETTRES
LIFTERS
LINTELS
LINTERS
LISTEES
LISTENS
LISTERS
LITTERS
LITTLES
LOATHES
LOFTERS
LOITERS
LOOTERS
LOTTERS
LOWTOPS
LUSTERS
LUSTRES
MAITAIS
MAITRES
MALTEDS
MALTHUS
MANTELS
MANTLES
MANTRAS
MARTENS
MARTINS
MARTIUS
MARTYRS
MASTERS
MASTICS
MATTERS
MAYTAGS
MEETERS
MELTERS
MENTEES
MENTORS
METTLES
MINTERS
MISTERS
MITTENS
MIXTECS
MOLTERS
MOOTERS
MOPTOPS
MORTALS
MORTARS
MORTONS
MOTTLES
MOTTOES
MTATHOS
MUSTDOS
MUSTERS
MUTTERS
MUTTONS
MYRTLES
MYSTARS
MYSTICS
NASTIES
NATTERS
NEATENS
NECTARS
NESTERS
NESTLES
NESTORS
NETTERS

NETTLES
NETTONS
NEUTERS
NEWTONS
NEWTOYS
NIFTIES
NOETICS
NOOTKAS
NORTONS
NOSTARS
NOWTHIS
NUTTERS
OAKTAGS
ONETWOS
ORATORS
OSETRAS
OUSTERS
OYSTERS
PALTERS
PANTERS
PANTIES
PARTIES
PASTELS
PASTERS
PASTIES
PASTORS
PATTERS
PATTIES
PECTINS
PEGTOPS
PELTERS
PENTADS
PENTELS
PEPTICS
PESTERS
PESTLES
PETTERS
PETTOYS
PEWTERS
PHOTICS
PHOTOGS
PHOTONS
PIETIES
PIETINS
PIETROS
PISTILS
PISTOLS
PISTONS
PISTOUS
PLATENS
PLATERS
PLATIES
PLOTZES
PLUTONS
POETESS
POETICS
PONTIUS
POPTOPS
PORTALS
PORTERS
PORTHOS
POSTERS
POSTIES
POSTITS
POSTOPS
POTTERS
POTTIES
POUTERS

PRATERS
PRETORS
PROTEUS
PROTONS
PUNTERS
PUTTEES
PUTTERS
PUTTIES
QINTARS
QRATIOS
QUATRES
QUOTEES
QUOTERS
RAFTERS
RAGTOPS
RANTERS
RAPTORS
RASTERS
RATTANS
RATTERS
RATTLES
REATTAS
RECTORS
REDTABS
REDTAGS
REDTIES
REDTOPS
RENTALS
RENTEES
RENTERS
RESTABS
RESTERS
RESTIRS
RESTOWS
REUTERS
RHETORS
RHYTHMS
RIOTERS
RIOTOUS
ROOTERS
ROOTLES
ROSTERS
ROTTERS
ROUTERS
RUSTICS
RUSTLES
RUTTERS
SALTERS
SARTORS
SCATHES
SCOTERS
SCYTHES
SEATERS
SECTORS
SEETHES
SENTRAS
SEPTETS
SESTETS
SETTEES
SETTERS
SETTLES
SEXTANS
SEXTETS
SEXTONS
SHUTINS
SIFTERS
SISTERS
SITTERS
SIXTIES
SKATERS
SKITOWS
SLATERS
SMITERS
SOFTENS
SOFTIES
SOOTHES
SORTERS
SORTIES
SPATHES
SPITZES
STATERS
STATICS
STATINS
STATORS
STATUES
STOTINS
STUTZES
SUITORS
SULTANS
SUNTANS
SWATHES
SYSTEMS
TACTICS
TAMTAMS
TARTANS
TARTARS
TASTERS
TATTERS
TATTLES
TATTOOS
TAUTENS
TEATROS
TEETERS
TEETHES
TENTERS
TENTONS
TESTEES
TESTERS
TEUTONS
TICTACS
TIETACS
TILTERS
TINTERS
TIPTOES
TIPTOPS
TITTERS
TITTLES
TOETAPS
TOLTECS
TOMTITS
TOMTOMS
TOOTERS
TOOTLES
TOPTENS
TOPTHIS
TOTTERS
TOUTERS
TOYTOPS
TRITONS
TSETSES
TSKTSKS
TURTLES
TUTTUTS
TVSTARS
TWOTONS
ULSTERS
UNITERS
UNITIES
UNSTEPS
UNSTOPS
UNSTOWS
UPSTEPS
UPSTIRS
VECTORS
VECTRAS
VENTERS
VENTRIS
VESTALS
VESTEES
VETTERS
VICTIMS
VICTORS
VIRTUES
VITTLES
WAFTERS
WAITERS
WALTERS
WALTONS
WALTZES
WANTADS
WANTERS
WANTONS
WASTERS
WATTLES
WELTERS
WESTERS
WESTIES
WESTINS
WHATIFS
WHATSIS
WHITENS
WINTERS
WONTONS
WRITERS
WRITHES
XYSTERS
YATTERS
YETTIES
YOMTOVS
ZESTERS
ZIPTOPS

••••TS•

CRAFTSY
DONETSK
FUJITSU
IRKUTSK
IZZATSO
JUJITSU
KAPITSA
KOMATSU
OKHOTSK
SHIATSU
YAKUTSK

••••T•S

ABLATES
ADRATES
AERATES
AGNATES
AGOUTIS
ALETTES
AMANTIS
AMRITAS
APLITES
ARBUTUS
ARISTAS
ARISTOS
ASANTES
AUGITES
AVANTIS
AVESTAS
AVIATES
BALATAS
BARITES
BENOTES
BERATES
BONITOS
BORATES
BREATHS
BRONTES
BYPATHS
CAPOTES
CASITAS
CDRATES
CERATES
CHEETAS
CHEETOS
COEPTIS
COYOTES
CREATES
CROUTES
CRYPTOS
CUBITUS
CUESTAS
CURATES
DAKOTAS
DALETHS
DANITES
DEARTHS
DEBATES
DELETES
DEMOTES
DEMOTHS
DENOTES
DEPUTES
DERATES
DESOTOS
DEVOTES
DILATES
DILUTES
DONATES
DONATUS
DORITOS
DUETTOS
ECARTES
EIGHTHS
ELUATES
EMPATHS
EOLITHS
EQUATES
ERASTUS
ERECTUS
ESTATES
EXACTAS
EXCITES
EXMATES
FAJITAS
FAUSTUS
FIESTAS
FINITES
FIXATES
FLATTVS
FLAUTAS
FOLATES
FOURTHS
FUENTES
FUGATOS
GAMETES
GELATES
GELATIS
GELATOS
GHETTOS
GLOTTIS
GROTTOS
GROWTHS
GUNITES
GYRATES
HALITES
HAMITES
HEARTHS
IAPETUS
IDEATES
IGNITES
IMPETUS
IMPUTES
INCITES
INDITES
INGATES
INMATES
INVITES
IODATES
IOMOTHS
KADETTS
KARATES
KLEPTOS
LABATTS
LAERTES
LAKOTAS
LEANTOS
LEGATES
LEGATOS
LENGTHS
LEVITES
LIGATES
LITOTES
LOCATES
LUCITES
LUNATES
LUXATES
METATES
MINITVS
MINUTES
MOJITOS
MRBUTTS
MULETAS
MUTATES
NEGATES
NORITES
NOTATES
NOVOTES
NUTATES
OBENTOS
OBLATES
OLEATES
OOCYTES
OOLITES
OPIATES
ORANTES
ORESTES
PAIUTES
PALATES
PARATUS
PELOTAS
PENATES
PEPITAS
PERITUS
PESETAS
PETITES
PEYOTES
PILATES
PILATUS
PINATAS
PIRATES
PLAUTUS
PLINTHS
POINTES
PRESTOS
PUPATES
PYRITES
QUARTES
QUARTOS
QUIETUS
QUINTAS
QUINTES
QUINTUS
RATITES
REATTAS
REBATES
REBOTES
RECITES
REDATES
REFUTES
RELATES
REMATES
REMOTES
RENOTES
REPUTES
RERATES
REVOTES
RIALTOS
ROTATES
RUBATOS
SAINTES
SALUTES
SANCTUS
SEDATES
SEMITES
SENATES
SHEATHS
SHIITES
SHTETLS
SIESTAS
SLEUTHS
SMOOTHS
SOLUTES
SONATAS
SPRITES
STKITTS
STRATAS
STRATUS
TACITUS
TOYOTAS
UNIATES
UNMATES
UPDATES
UPRATES
VACATES
VEINTES
VERITAS
VOLUTES
WAPITIS
WEALTHS
WRAITHS
WREATHS
YESITIS
YUKATAS
ZAPATAS
ZENITHS
ZYGOTES

•••••TS

ABDUCTS
ABSENTS
ACCENTS
ACCEPTS
ACCOSTS
ACQUITS
ADDICTS
ADDUCTS
ADJUSTS
ADVENTS
ADVERTS
AFFECTS
AGEISTS
AIGLETS
AIGRETS
AIRPOTS
ALIGHTS
AMOUNTS
AMULETS
ANKLETS
ANOINTS
APELETS
APPLETS
ARGENTS
ARMLETS
ARMPITS
ARRESTS
ARTISTS
ASCENTS
ASHPITS
ASPECTS
ASSENTS
ASSERTS
ASSISTS
ASSORTS
ATTESTS
ATTRITS
AUGUSTS
AUKLETS
AURISTS
AUTISTS
AVOCETS
BADFITS
BADHATS
BADLOTS
BALLETS
BALLOTS
BANDITS
BANKITS
BARBETS
BARENTS
BARRETS
BASALTS
BASKETS
BASSETS
BBQPITS
BBSHOTS
BEDSITS
BEHESTS
BIGBETS
BIGCATS
BIGHITS
BIGLOTS
BILLETS
BISECTS
BLIGHTS
BOBCATS
BOGARTS
BONMOTS
BONNETS
BOXSETS
BREASTS
BREVETS
BRIGHTS
BROASTS
BRUNETS
BUCKETS
BUDGETS
BUFFETS
BUGOUTS
BULLETS
BURBOTS
BUYOUTS
CABLETS
CACHETS
CAHOOTS
CAPLETS
CAPNUTS
CARLOTS
CARNETS
CARPETS
CARROTS
CASKETS
CATFITS
CATGUTS
CATSITS
CAVEATS
CAVORTS
CEMENTS
CHALETS
CHEVETS
CLARETS
CLIENTS
CLIMATS
CLORETS
CLOSETS
COBALTS
COBNUTS
COEDITS
COHORTS
COHOSTS
COLLETS
COMBATS
COMFITS
COMMITS
COMSATS
CONFITS
COPOUTS
CORNETS
CORSETS
COSSETS
COVERTS
CRAVATS
CREDITS
CUBISTS
CULLETS
CURVETS
CUTLETS
CUTOUTS
CYGNETS
DECANTS
DECEITS
DECLOTS
DECOCTS
DEDUCTS
DEFEATS
DEFECTS
DEGUSTS
DEJECTS
DELICTS
DELINTS
DELISTS
DEMASTS
DEMISTS
DEPARTS
DEPESTS
DEPICTS
DEPORTS
DERUSTS
DESALTS
DESERTS
DESILTS
DESISTS
DESPOTS
DETECTS
DETENTS
DETESTS
DEVESTS
DIDACTS
DIECUTS
DIGESTS
DIGLOTS
DIKTATS
DIMOUTS
DIMWITS
DIPNETS
DIRECTS
DIVERTS
DIVESTS
DOCENTS
DOCKETS
DOGSITS
DOSHOTS
DRYROTS
DUGOUTS
DYELOTS
DYEVATS
DYNASTS
EAGLETS
EARLETS
EELPOTS
EFFECTS
EFFORTS
EGOISTS
ELANETS
ELEGITS
ELICITS
ELUANTS
ENDCUTS
ENFANTS
ENGLUTS
ENLISTS
ENROOTS
ENSEATS
ESCORTS
ESPRITS
EXCEPTS
EXEMPTS
EXEUNTS
EXHORTS
EXOCETS
EXPECTS
EXPERTS
EXPORTS
EXSECTS
EXSERTS
EXTENTS
EXTORTS
EYELETS
EYEPITS
FANJETS
FANOUTS
FATCATS
FAUCETS
FEMBOTS
FERMATS
FERRETS
FIDGETS
FILLETS
FLAUNTS
FLIGHTS
FLORETS
FLYNETS
FOMENTS
FORDGTS
FORESTS
FORGETS
FORINTS
FORMATS
FRIGHTS
GADGETS
GALANTS
GALOOTS
GAMBITS
GANNETS
GARLITS
GARNETS
GARRETS
GASJETS
GASKETS
GERENTS
GIBLETS
GIMLETS
GOBLETS
GOCARTS
GODWITS
GOKARTS
GULLETS
GUSSETS
GYMRATS
HADFITS
HAMLETS
HARLOTS
HASFITS
HAZMATS
HEIGHTS
HELMETS
HENBITS
HEPCATS
HERMITS
HEXNUTS
HOBBITS
HOGNUTS
HOLISTS
HORNETS
HOTPOTS
ICEOUTS
IGOROTS
IMARETS
IMPACTS
IMPARTS
IMPORTS
IMPOSTS
INCANTS
INCENTS
INCEPTS
INDENTS
INDICTS
INDUCTS
INFANTS
INFECTS
INFESTS
INGESTS
INJECTS
INKJETS
INKNOTS
INKPOTS
INSECTS
INSERTS
INSISTS
INSPOTS
INSULTS
INTENTS
INTUITS
INVENTS
INVERTS
INVESTS
IQTESTS
IRRUPTS
JACKETS
JENNETS
JESUITS
JETSETS
JOBCUTS
JOBLOTS
JUNKETS
JURISTS
KADETTS
KEYDETS
KIDULTS
KISMETS
KITKATS
KNIGHTS
KUZNETS
LABATTS
LABRATS
LAKISTS
LAMENTS
LANCETS
LAPCATS
LAPPETS
LARIATS
LATENTS
LAYOUTS
LEGISTS
LIMPETS
LINNETS
LIONETS
LOCKETS
LOCUSTS
LOGOUTS
LOQUATS
LUGNUTS
LUTISTS
LYRISTS
MAGGOTS
MAGNETS
MAHOUTS
MALLETS
MAOISTS
MARKETS
MARMOTS
MASCOTS
MERLOTS
MIDGETS
MILLETS
MINUETS
MISACTS
MISCUTS
MISFITS
MISHITS
MISSETS
MODELTS
MOLESTS
MOMENTS
MOPPETS
MRBUTTS
MUDCATS
MULLETS
MUPPETS
MUSCATS
MUSKETS
MUTANTS
NAUGHTS
NEWHATS
NIBLETS
NITWITS
NOGIFTS
NONARTS
NONHITS
NOSEATS
NOUGATS
NOUGHTS
NUDISTS
NUGGETS
NUMBATS
NUTLETS
OBJECTS
OBLASTS
OBOISTS
OBTESTS
OBVERTS
OCCULTS
OCELOTS
OCICATS
OCTANTS
ODDLOTS
ODELETS
OFFSETS
OFSORTS
OLDBATS
OMELETS
ONEACTS
ORGEATS
ORIENTS
OUTACTS
OUTBATS
OUTCUTS
OUTEATS
OUTFITS
OUTHITS
OUTJETS
OUTJUTS
OUTLETS
OUTPUTS
OUTSETS
OUTSITS
OUTWITS
OXCARTS
PACKETS
PALLETS
PANDITS
PAPISTS
PARENTS
PARROTS
PASSATS
PATENTS
PAYCUTS
PAYOUTS
PEANUTS
PEDANTS
PELLETS
PENULTS
PEQUOTS
PERMITS
PETCATS
PETRATS
PETSITS
PICKETS
PIGLETS
PIGNUTS
PIGOUTS
PIOLETS
PLAINTS
PLAKATS
PLANETS
PLIGHTS
POCKETS
POPOUTS
POSTITS
PREACTS
PRECUTS
PRESETS
PRIESTS
PRIVETS
PROFITS
PROJETS
PROMPTS
PTBOATS
PULLETS
PULPITS
PUNDITS
PUPPETS
PURISTS
PUTOUTS
PUTPUTS
RABBETS
RABBITS
RACISTS
RACKETS
RAGOUTS
RAMJETS

RAWISTS
REBAITS
REBOLTS
REBOOTS
RECANTS
RECASTS
RECOATS
RECOSTS
REDACTS
REDANTS
REDBATS
REDDOTS
REDHATS
REDHOTS
REDOUTS
REDUSTS
REEDITS
REEMITS
REGENTS
REGIFTS
REGRETS
REHEATS
REJECTS
REKNITS
REKNOTS
RELENTS
RELICTS
RELISTS
RELUCTS
REMEETS
REMELTS
REMINTS
RENESTS
RENNETS
REPASTS
REPEATS
REPENTS
REPLOTS
REPORTS
REPOSTS
RERENTS
REROOTS
RESALTS
RESEATS
RESECTS
RESENTS
RESHUTS
RESIFTS
RESISTS
RESORTS
RESPOTS
RESUITS
RESULTS
RETESTS
RETINTS
RETORTS
REVERTS
REVESTS
REVOLTS
REXCATS
RIBCUTS
RIBLETS
RILLETS
RIPOSTS
ROBERTS
ROCHETS
ROCKETS
RODENTS
ROTGUTS
RUGRATS
RUNLETS
RUNOUTS
RUSSETS
SACHETS
SADISTS
SAMLETS
SAVANTS
SAWPITS
SCHISTS
SCRIPTS
SCULPTS
SEACATS
SECANTS
SECRETS
SELECTS
SEPTETS
SESTETS
SETOUTS
SEWISTS
SEXISTS
SEXPOTS
SEXTETS
SHEVATS
SIGNETS
SILENTS
SKIHATS
SLIGHTS
SNOCATS
SOCKETS
SOFFITS
SONNETS
SORBETS
SOVIETS
SPIGOTS
SPINETS
SPIRITS
SPLINTS
SPRINTS
SPROUTS
SPYBOTS
SQUINTS
SQUIRTS
STBARTS
STKITTS
STRAITS
STREETS
STYLETS
SUBLETS
SUBLOTS
SUBMITS
SUBNETS
SUBSETS
SUMMITS
SUNHATS
SUNSETS
SWIVETS
TABLETS
TABSETS
TAGOUTS
TALENTS
TAOISTS
TAPPETS
TARGETS
TARPITS
TAXCUTS
TEAPOTS
TEASETS
TENANTS
TERRETS
THEARTS
THEISTS
THEJETS
THEMETS
THENETS
THEPITS
THIRSTS
THREATS
THRIFTS
THROATS
THRUSTS
THWARTS
TICKETS
TIDBITS
TILLETS
TILSITS
TINHATS
TIPPETS
TISSOTS
TOILETS
TOMCATS
TOMTITS
TOPHATS
TOYHATS
TRICOTS
TRIJETS
TRIVETS
TRUANTS
TRYOUTS
TSHIRTS
TUBISTS
TUFFETS
TUMULTS
TURBOTS
TURRETS
TUTTUTS
TVSPOTS
TWOACTS
TWOBITS
TYPISTS
TYRANTS
UMLAUTS
UNBAITS
UNBELTS
UNBOLTS
UNFACTS
UNKNITS
UNKNOTS
UNMASTS
UNRESTS
UNROOTS
UNSEATS
UNSORTS
UPBEATS
UPCASTS
UPDARTS
UPLIFTS
UPROOTS
UPSHOTS
UPTILTS
UPWAFTS
URTEXTS
UTMOSTS
VARLETS
VEDISTS
VEIGHTS
VELVETS
VERISTS
VERSETS
VIBISTS
VIDIOTS
VIOLETS
VIVANTS
WABBITS
WALLETS
WALNUTS
WARVETS
WBYEATS
WEEBITS
WEIGHTS
WESKITS
WICKETS
WIDGETS
WIGLETS
WOMBATS
WRIGHTS
YESLETS
YOGURTS
ZAGNUTS
ZEALOTS
ZENISTS

T•T••••

TATAMIS
TATIANA
TATTERS
TATTERY
TATTIER
TATTILY
TATTING
TATTLED
TATTLER
TATTLES
TATTOOS
TETANUS
TETHERS
TETRADS
TETRODE
TITANAE
TITANIA
TITANIC
TITHERS
TITHING
TITIANS
TITLARK
TITLING
TITLIST
TITMICE
TITOISM
TITOIST
TITRATE
TITRING
TITTERS
TITTLES
TITULAR
TOTABLE
TOTALED
TOTALER
TOTALLY
TOTALUP
TOTASTE
TOTEBAG
TOTEMIC
TOTESUP
TOTINOS
TOTOTOO
TOTTERS
TOTTERY
TOTTING
TSTRAPS
TUTELAR
TUTORED
TUTTING
TUTTUTS
TUTUILA
TVTABLE
TVTAPES

T••T•••

TACTFUL
TACTICS
TACTILE
TACTUAL
TAGTEAM
TAMTAMS
TANTARA
TANTIVY
TANTRUM
TARTANS
TARTARE
TARTARS
TARTEST
TARTIER
TARTILY
TARTING
TARTISH
TARTLET
TARTSUP
TASTEIT
TASTERS
TASTIER
TASTILY
TASTING
TATTERS
TATTERY
TATTIER
TATTILY
TATTING
TATTLED
TATTLER
TATTLES
TATTOOS
TAUTENS
TAUTEST
TEATIME
TEATRAY
TEATREE
TEATROS
TEETERS
TEETHED
TEETHER
TEETHES
TEETIME
TENTBED
TENTERS
TENTFUL
TENTHLY
TENTING
TENTONS
TENTPEG
TESTACY
TESTATE
TESTBAN
TESTBED
TESTEES
TESTERS
TESTFLY
TESTFOR
TESTIER
TESTIFY
TESTILY
TESTING
TESTKIT
TESTLAB
TESTOUT
TESTRUN
TEUTONS
TEXTILE
TEXTING
TEXTRON
TEXTUAL
TEXTURE
THATCHY
THATONE
THATSIT
THATSOK
THATWAY
THETOUR
THETREE
THETRIB
THETUBE
THETURN
THITHER
TICTACS
TIETACK
TIETACS
TILTERS
TILTING
TILTSAT
TILTSUP
TILTTOP
TINTERN
TINTERS
TINTING
TINTYPE
TIPTOED
TIPTOES
TIPTOPS
TITTERS
TITTLES
TOATURN
TOETAPS
TOLTECS
TOMTITS
TOMTOMS
TONTINE
TOOTALL
TOOTERS
TOOTHED
TOOTING
TOOTLED
TOOTLER
TOOTLES
TOOTSAT
TOOTSIE
TOPTENS
TOPTHIS
TORTLAW
TORTOLA
TORTONI
TORTUGA
TORTURE
TOSTADA
TOSTART
TOTTERS
TOTTERY
TOTTING
TOUTERS
TOUTING
TOYTOPS
TRITELY
TRITEST
TRITIUM
TRITONE
TRITONS
TROTHED
TROTOFF
TROTOUT
TROTSKY
TROTSUP
TROTTED
TROTTER
TSETSES
TSETUNG
TSKTSKS
TUFTIER
TUFTING
TUITION
TURTLED
TURTLES
TUTTING
TUTTUTS
TVSTARS
TWITCHY
TWITTED
TWITTER
TWOTERM
TWOTIME
TWOTOED
TWOTONE
TWOTONS

T•••T••

TABITHA
TACITLY
TACITUS
TAINTED
TAKETEA
TAKETEN
TANKTOP
TAPSTER
TAUNTED
TAUNTER
TAUNTON
TEEITUP
TELSTAR
TEMPTED
TEMPTER
THEATER
THEATRE
THESTAR
THISTLE
THISTLY
TIBETAN
TICOTIN
TIGHTEN
TIGHTER
TIGHTLY
TILTTOP
TIMOTHY
TINCTED
TINSTAR
TINYTIM
TINYTOT
TIPSTER
TOASTED
TOASTEE
TOASTER
TOFUTTI
TOLSTOI
TOLSTOY
TONETTE
TOOKTEN
TOTOTOO
TOYOTAS
TRACTOR
TRAITOR
TREATED
TREATER
TREETOP
TRENTON
TRESTLE
TRIMTAB
TRISTAN
TRISTAR
TROTTED
TROTTER
TRUSTED
TRUSTEE
TRUSTER
TRUSTIN
TRUSTME
TRYITON
TRYSTED
TRYSTER
TUBETOP
TURFTOE
TWEETED
TWEETER
TWISTED
TWISTER
TWISTON
TWISTUP
TWITTED
TWITTER
TWOSTAR
TWOSTEP

T••••T•

TABLETS
TABSETS
TAFFETA
TAGOUTS
TAKENTO
TAKESTO
TALENTS
TALKSTO
TALLITH
TAOISTS
TAPINTO
TAPPETS
TARANTO
TARGETS
TARPITS
TAXCUTS
TAXRATE
TEAPOTS
TEASETS
TELESTO
TENANTS
TENDSTO
TENSITY
TENUITY
TERMITE
TERNATE
TERRETS
TESTATE
THEARTS
THECITY
THEISTS
THEJETS
THEMETS
THENETS
THEOATH
THEPITS
THERETO
THERITZ
THIRSTS
THIRSTY
THREATS
THRIFTS
THRIFTY
THROATS
THROATY
THRUSTS
THWARTS
THWHITE
TIBBETT
TICKETS
TIDBITS
TIEINTO
TILLETS
TILSITS
TIMROTH
TINHATS
TIPPETS
TIRPITZ
TISSOTS
TITRATE
TOCCATA
TOFUTTI
TOILETS
TOMCATS
TOMKITE
TOMTITS
TONETTE
TOOLATE
TOPHATS
TOPRATE
TORONTO
TOTASTE
TOWPATH
TOYHATS
TOYKITE
TOYWITH
TRASHTV
TREINTA
TRIBUTE
TRICOTS
TRIEDTO
TRIESTE
TRIESTO
TRIJETS
TRINITY
TRIVETS
TRUANTS
TRUERTO
TRYOUTS
TSHIRTS
TUBISTS
TUFFETS
TUMULTS
TUNEDTO
TUNESTO
TURBOTS
TURISTA
TURNSTO
TURRETS
TUTTUTS
TVSPOTS
TWELFTH
TWOACTS
TWOBITS
TYINGTO
TYPISTS
TYRANTS

T•••••T

TABARET
TABORET
TAGAMET
TAGGANT
TAGSOUT
TAKEOUT
TAKESIT
TALKOUT
TALKSAT
TALLEST
TANGENT
TANNEST
TAPROOT
TAPSOUT
TARTEST
TARTLET
TASTEIT
TAUTEST
TEACART
TEAROUT
TEARSAT
TEARSIT
TEESHOT
TELLSIT
TEMPEST
TENCENT
TENFEET
TENFOOT
TENNANT
TENPAST
TENSEST
TENSPOT
TERSEST
TESTKIT
TESTOUT
THATSIT
THAWOUT
THEBEST
THEBRAT
THEDIET
THEEAST
THEGIFT
THEHEAT
THELEFT
THEMOST
THEPOST
THEREAT
THERENT
THICKET
THINOUT
THOUGHT
THREWAT
THROWAT
THRUPUT
TIBBETT
TIDIEST
TILTSAT
TIMEOUT
TIMHOLT
TINIEST
TINYBIT
TINYTOT
TIPCART
TIREOUT
TITLIST
TITOIST
TLINGIT
TOGSOUT
TOHEART
TOILSAT
TONIEST
TONIGHT
TOOKOUT
TOOLKIT
TOOLSET
TOOTSAT
TOPBOOT
TOPCOAT
TOPKNOT
TOPMAST
TOPMOST
TOPSOUT
TOPSPOT
TOREOUT
TORMENT
TORNOUT
TORRENT
TOSSOUT
TOSSPOT
TOSTART
TOURIST
TOWBOAT
TOWNLET
TOYBOAT
TOYCART
TRABERT
TRANSIT
TREELET
TREERAT
TRIDENT
TRIEDIT
TRIESIT
TRINKET
TRIOLET
TRIPLET
TRIPPET
TRISECT
TRITEST
TRIVIOT
TROTOUT
TRUMPET
TSARIST
TSELIOT
TUBAIST
TUGBOAT
TUNEOUT
TURNOUT
TWERENT
TWINJET
TWINSET
TWOFEET
TWOFOOT
TWOPART
TWOSHOT
TWOSPOT
TWOUNIT
TYPESET

•TT••••

ATTABOY
ATTACHE
ATTACKS
ATTAINS
ATTAINT
ATTEMPT
ATTENDS
ATTESTS
ATTHIRD
ATTHREE
ATTICUS
ATTIMES
ATTIRED
ATTIRER
ATTIRES
ATTRACT
ATTRITE
ATTRITS
ATTUCKS
ATTUNED
ATTUNES
ATTYGEN
OTTAVIO
OTTAWAN
OTTAWAS
OTTOIII
OTTOMAN
OTTUMWA
UTTERED
UTTERER
UTTERLY
YTTRIAS
YTTRIUM

•T•T•••

ATATILT
ATATIME
ATATURK
ATSTAKE
ITSTIME
ITSTRUE
MTATHOS
STATELY
STATERS
STATICE
STATICS
STATING
STATINS
STATION
STATISM
STATIST
STATLER
STATORS
STATUES
STATURE
STATUTE
STETSON
STETTED
STOTINS
STUTTER
STUTZES

•T••T••

ATEITUP
ATIPTOE
ATWATER
ITISTOO
ITSATIE
STANTON
STARTED
STARTER
STARTIN
STARTLE
STARTON
STARTTO
STARTUP
STENTOR
STEPTWO
STERTOR
STETTED
STILTED
STILTON
STINTED
STINTER
STKITTS
STOUTEN
STOUTER
STOUTLY
STPETER
STRATAS
STRATUM
STRATUS
STRETCH
STRETTI
STRETTO
STRITCH
STUNTED
STUTTER
STYPTIC

•T•••T•

ATEINTO
ATELATE
ATHLETE
ATLANTA
ATTESTS
ATTRITE
ATTRITS
FTWORTH
ITERATE
ITHIRTY
ITSLATE
ITWENTY
OTRANTO
PTBOATS
STANDTO
STARTTO
STATUTE

STBARTS
STEALTH
STICKTO
STKITTS
STOMATA
STOODTO
STRAITS
STREETS
STRETTI
STRETTO
STRIATE
STUARTI
STUCKTO
STYLETS
UTILITY
UTMOSTS

•T••••T

ATACOST
ATATILT
ATAVIST
ATEABIT
ATEALOT
ATEDIRT
ATEIGHT
ATFAULT
ATFIRST
ATHEART
ATHEIST
ATHIRST
ATHWART
ATLEAST
ATNIGHT
ATOMIST
ATSIGHT
ATTAINT
ATTEMPT
ATTRACT
ATWORST
ETCHANT
ETICKET
ITERANT
ITSAHIT
ITSALOT
ITSBEST
STALEST
STAREAT
STARLET
STARLIT
STATIST
STAYOUT
STAYPUT
STAYSAT
STEPOUT
STEWART
STEWPOT
STOPSAT
STOPSIT
STOWSIT
STUDENT
STYLIST
UTOPIST
UTRECHT

••TT•••

ALTTABS
BATTENS
BATTERS
BATTERY
BATTIER
BATTING
BATTLED
BATTLER
BATTLES
BETTANY
BETTERS
BETTGER
BETTING
BETTORS
BITTERN
BITTERS
BITTIER
BITTING
BLTTOGO
BOTTEGA
BOTTLED
BOTTLER
BOTTLES
BOTTOMS
BUTTEMT
BUTTERS
BUTTERY
BUTTING
BUTTONS
BUTTONY
BUTTOUT
BUTTRAM
BUTTSIN
CATTAIL
CATTALO
CATTIER
CATTILY
CATTISH
CATTOYS
COTTAGE
COTTERS
COTTONS
COTTONY
CUTTERS
CUTTIME
CUTTING
DITTIES
DITTOED
DOTTERS
DOTTIER
DOTTILY
DOTTING
DOTTLES
FATTENS
FATTEST
FATTIER
FATTILY
FATTING
FATTISH
FETTERS
FETTLES
FITTERS
FITTEST
FITTING
GATTACA
GETTERS
GETTHIS
GETTING
GETTOIT
GITTING
GOTTAGO
GOTTOIT
GUTTERS
GUTTIER
GUTTING
HATTERS
HATTING
HITTERS
HITTING
HITTITE
HITTOWN
HITTUNE
HOTTEAS
HOTTEST
HOTTIES
HOTTIME
HOTTIPS
HOTTUBS
HOTTUNA
HUTTING
JETTIED
JETTIES
JETTING
JITTERS
JITTERY
JOTTERS
JOTTING
JUTTING
KETTLES
KITTENS
KITTERY
KITTIES
KITTING
LATTICE
LETTERA
LETTERB
LETTERC
LETTERD
LETTERE
LETTERF
LETTERG
LETTERH
LETTERI
LETTERJ
LETTERK
LETTERL
LETTERM
LETTERN
LETTERO
LETTERP
LETTERQ
LETTERR
LETTERS
LETTERT
LETTERU
LETTERV
LETTERW
LETTERX
LETTERY
LETTERZ
LETTING
LETTISH
LETTRES
LETTUCE
LITTERS
LITTERY
LITTLER
LITTLES
LOTTERS
LOTTERY
LOTTING
MATTERS
MATTHAU
MATTHEW
MATTING
MATTOCK
METTLER
METTLES
MITTENS
MOTTLED
MOTTLES
MOTTOES
MUTTERS
MUTTONS
NATTERS
NATTIER
NATTILY
NETTERS
NETTING
NETTLED
NETTLES
NETTONS
NITTANY
NITTIER
NOTTING
NOTTOBE
NOTTRUE
NUTTERS
NUTTIER
NUTTILY
NUTTING
NUTTREE
OUTTAKE
OUTTALK
OUTTEAR
OUTTELL
OUTTIRE
OUTTOLD
OUTTOLL
OUTTORE
OUTTORN
OUTTRAY
OUTTROT
OUTTURN
PATTERN
PATTERS
PATTIES
PATTING
PETTERS
PETTIER
PETTILY
PETTING
PETTISH
PETTOYS
PITTING
PITTMAN
POTTAGE
POTTERS
POTTERY
POTTIER
POTTIES
POTTING
PUTTEES
PUTTERS
PUTTIED
PUTTIES
PUTTING
PUTTOUT
RATTAIL
RATTANS
RATTERS
RATTIER
RATTING
RATTISH
RATTLED
RATTLER
RATTLES
RATTRAP
RETTING
ROTTERS
ROTTING
RUTTERS
RUTTIER
RUTTING
RUTTISH
SETTEES
SETTERS
SETTING
SETTLED
SETTLER
SETTLES
SETTLOR
SETTYPE
SITTERS
SITTING
SOTTISH
TATTERS
TATTERY
TATTIER
TATTILY
TATTING
TATTLED
TATTLER
TATTLES
TATTOOS
TITTERS
TITTLES
TOTTERS
TOTTERY
TOTTING
TUTTING
TUTTUTS
VATTING
VETTERS
VETTING
VITTLES
WATTAGE
WATTEAU
WATTLED
WATTLES
WETTEST
WETTING
WETTISH
WITTIER
WITTILY
WITTING
YATTERS
YETTIES

••T•T••

ANTITAX
ASTUTER
BATHTUB
EATITUP
ENTITLE
ESTATED
ESTATES
GETATIP
GETITON
GOTATIP
GOTITON
HOTITEM
INTOTAL
JETSTAR
LATETAG
LETITBE
LETITGO
LETITIA
LITOTES
LUTETIA
METATES
MITOTIC
MUTATED
MUTATES
NATATOR
NETSTER
NOTATED
NOTATES
NUTATED
NUTATES
OCTETTE
OUTSTAY
OUTSTEP
PETITES
PITSTOP
PUTITTO
RATATAT
RATITES
RETITLE
RETOTAL
ROTATED
ROTATES
ROTATOR
SATATOP
SHTETLS
SITATOP
TOTOTOO

••T••T•

ACTUATE
ARTISTE
ARTISTS
ASTARTE
ATTESTS
ATTRITE
ATTRITS
AUTISTS
BATISTA
BATISTE
BETROTH
CATERTO
CATFITS
CATGUTS
CATSITS
CITRATE
CUTINTO
CUTLETS
CUTOUTS
CUTRATE
DETECTO
DETECTS
DETENTE
DETENTS
DETESTS
DRTEETH
EATINTO
EATLATE
ENTENTE
ESTHETE
EXTENTS
EXTORTS
FATCATS
FATCITY
FATUITY
FITINTO
GETCUTE
GETINTO
GETONTO
GOTCUTE
GOTINTO
GOTONTO
GOTUPTO
HITINTO
HITTITE
HOTBATH
HOTDATE
HOTPOTS
INTASTE
INTENTS
INTRUTH
INTUITS
IQTESTS
JETSETS
KITKATS
LATENTS
LITINTO
LUTISTS
MATZOTH
METWITH
MUTANTS
NITRATE
NITRITE
NITWITS
NOTASTE
NOTUPTO
NOTWITH
NUTLETS
OBTESTS
OCTANTS
OCTETTE
OPTEDTO
OUTACTS
OUTBATS
OUTCITY
OUTCUTS
OUTDATE
OUTEATS
OUTFITS
OUTHITS
OUTJETS
OUTJUTS
OUTLETS
OUTMATE
OUTPATH
OUTPITY
OUTPUTS
OUTRATE
OUTSETS
OUTSITS
OUTVOTE
OUTWITH
OUTWITS
PATENTS
PETCATS
PETGATE
PETRATS
PETSITS
PITCHTO
PUTITTO
PUTOUTS
PUTPUTS
PUTUPTO
RETASTE
RETESTS
RETINTS
RETORTS
ROTGUTS
SATIATE
SATIETY
SATWITH
SETENTA
SETINTO
SETOUTS
SETRATE
SITUATE
SITWITH
TITRATE
TOTASTE
TUTTUTS
UNTASTY
UNTRITE
UNTRUTH
UPTILTS
URTEXTS
VITIATE
WATCHTV

••T•••T

ACTSOUT
AFTMOST
ALTOIST
ANTIART
ARTIEST
ASTOLAT
ATTAINT
ATTEMPT
ATTRACT
AUTOMAT
BATHMAT
BATNEXT
BATSUIT
BETWIXT
BITPART
BUTTEMT
BUTTOUT
CATBERT
CATBOAT
CATFEET
CATFOOT
CATMINT
CATSUIT
CUTSOUT
DATASET
DETRACT
DETROIT
EATABIT
EATALOT
EATDIRT
EATENAT
EATSOUT
ENTRANT
ENTREAT
ENTRUST
ENTWIST
EXTINCT
EXTRACT
FATTEST
FITTEST
FOTOMAT
GETAHIT
GETBEAT
GETBENT
GETHURT
GETLOST
GETONIT
GETPAST
GETSFIT
GETSHOT
GETSOFT
GETSOUT
GETSSET
GETSWET
GETTOIT
GOTAHIT
GOTBEAT
GOTHURT
GOTLOST
GOTONIT
GOTOPOT
GOTPAST
GOTSOFT
GOTTOIT
HATCHET
HATEDIT
HATESIT
HDTVSET
HITLIST
HITSOUT
HOTFOOT
HOTSEAT
HOTSHOT
HOTSPOT
HOTTEST
IDTHEFT
INTROIT
INTRUST
JETBOAT
JETPORT
LETSEAT
LETSNOT
LETSOUT
LETTERT
LITCRIT
LITHEST
METEOUT
METRIST
MYTREAT
NETCOST
NOTABIT
NOTALOT
NUTMEAT
ONTHEQT
ONTOAST
OPTSOUT
OUTBLOT
OUTCANT
OUTCAST
OUTFAST
OUTFOOT
OUTHUNT
OUTJEST
OUTKAST
OUTKEPT
OUTLAST
OUTMOST
OUTOFIT
OUTPLOT
OUTPORT
OUTPOST
OUTRANT
OUTROOT
OUTSERT
OUTSHOT
OUTSIFT
OUTSPIT
OUTTROT
OUTWAIT
OUTWENT
OUTWEPT
OUTWEST
PATIENT
PATRIOT
PETGOAT
PITAPAT
POTSHOT
PUTSOUT
PUTTOUT
RATATAT
RATBERT
RATCHET
RATSOUT
RETOAST
RETRACT
RETREAT
RETWIST
ROTBLAT
SATINET
SETSHOT
SETSOUT
SITONIT
SITSOUT
SITSPAT
TITLIST
TITOIST
UNTWIST
UPTIGHT
VOTEOUT
WATCHIT
WETSUIT
WETTEST
WITEOUT
WITHOUT

•••TT••

ABETTAL
ABETTED
ABETTER
ABETTOR
ABUTTAL
ABUTTED
ABUTTER
AGUTTER
ALETTES
ALITTLE
BEATTIE
BLATTED
BLOTTED
BLOTTER
BOOTTOP
BRATTLE
BRETTON
BRITTEN
BRITTLE
BRITTON
CHATTED
CHATTEL
CHATTER
CHITTER
CLATTER
CLOTTED
CLUTTER
CRITTER
CRITTUR
DRATTED
DUETTED
DUETTOS
EMITTED
EMITTER
FELTTIP
FLATTAX
FLATTED
FLATTEN
FLATTER
FLATTOP
FLATTVS
FLITTED
FLITTER
FLUTTER
FRETTED
FRETTER
FRITTED
FRITTER
GHETTOS
GIFTTAX
GLITTER
GLOTTAL
GLOTTIS
GLUTTED
GLUTTON
GRITTED
GRITTER
GROTTOS
HEATTER
IDOTTER
KNITTED
KNITTER
KNOTTED
KNOTTER
MINTTEA
OMITTED
OMITTER
PARTTWO
PHATTER
PLATTED
PLATTER
PLOTTED
PLOTTER
PRATTLE
QUATTRO
QUITTED
QUITTER
REATTAS
REUTTER
SCATTED
SCATTER
SCOTTIE
SCUTTLE
SEATTLE
SHATTER
SHUTTER
SHUTTLE
SKITTER
SKITTLE
SLATTED
SLITTED
SLITTER
SLOTTED
SLOTTER
SMATTER
SMITTEN
SOFTTOP
SPATTED
SPATTER
SPITTER
SPITTLE
SPOTTED
SPOTTER
SPUTTER
STETTED
STUTTER
SWATTED
SWATTER
TILTTOP
TROTTED
TROTTER
TWITTED
TWITTER
VUITTON
WHATTHE
WHETTED
WHETTER
WHITTLE
WRITTEN

•••T•T•

ACETATE
AGITATE
AGITATO
APATITE
BIOTITE
BISTATE
CANTATA
COSTATE
CURTATE
DENTATE
DICTATE
DIKTATS
GESTATE
HITTITE
IMITATE
INSTATE
LACTATE
LOATHTO
NICTATE
PARTITA
PARTITE
PELTATE
POSTITS
RENTSTO
RESTATE
SEPTETS
SESTETS
SEXTETS
STATUTE
TESTATE
TOMTITS
TUTTUTS
UNSTATE
UPSTATE
USSTATE
VASTITY
WANTSTO
WRITETO
WROTETO

•••T••T

ACUTEST
AFATLOT
ALLTHAT
ATATILT
BAPTIST
BARTLET
BEATOUT
BEATSAT
BEATSIT
BELTOUT
BERTOLT
BESTBET
BESTCUT
BIGTENT
BLATANT
BLOTOUT
BOOTCUT
BOOTOUT
BOOTSIT
BUSTOUT
BUTTEMT
BUTTOUT
CASTOUT
CHUTIST
COMTIST
CONTACT
CONTENT
CONTEST
CONTEXT
CONTORT
CULTIST
CURTEST
DAFTEST
DEFTEST
DENTIST
DIDTOAT
DISTANT
DISTORT
DNATEST
DOGTROT
EDITOUT
EGOTIST
ELITEST
ELITIST
EPITHET
EYETEST
FANTAST
FASTEST
FASTNET
FATTEST
FELTHAT
FELTOUT
FITTEST

FLATHAT
FLATLET
FLATOUT
FLUTIST
FOOTLET
FOOTSIT
FOXTROT
FRETSAT
GANTLET
GESTALT
GETTOIT
GIFTSET
GJETOST
GOTTOIT
HARTMUT
HASTERT
HINTSAT
HOOTSAT
HOPTOIT
HOTTEST
IHATEIT
INSTANT
IRATEST
JOGTROT
JUSTEST
JUSTOUT
KEPTFIT
KEPTOUT
LABTEST
LASTACT
LEFTEST
LEFTIST
LEFTOUT
LETTERT
LIETEST
LOSTART
LOSTCAT
LOSTOUT
LOSTPET
MANTLET
NEATEST
ONATOOT
OUTTROT
PEATPOT
PERTEST
POPTART
PORTENT
PRETEST
PRETEXT
PROTECT
PROTEST
PROTIST
PUPTENT
PUTTOUT
QUITSIT
RANTSAT
RENTOUT
RESTART
RIOTACT
ROOTLET
ROOTOUT
ROOTROT
ROUTOUT
SALTANT
SALTPIT
SAWTOIT
SEETOIT
SENTOUT
SEXTANT
SHOTOUT
SHOTPUT
SHUTOUT
SOFTEST
SORTOUT
SPATOUT
SPITOUT
SPOTLIT
STATIST
SUBTEXT
SWATSAT
TARTEST
TARTLET
TASTEIT
TAUTEST
TESTKIT
TESTOUT
THATSIT
TILTSAT
TOOTSAT
TOSTART
TRITEST
TROTOUT
UNSTOUT
UPSTART
VASTEST
WAITOUT
WANTOUT
WENTAFT
WENTOUT
WETTEST
WHATNOT
WHATSIT
WHITEST
WORTHIT

••••TT•

ABOUTTO
ADAPTTO
ADMITTO
ALERTTO
ANNATTO
ANNETTE
ARIETTA
ARIETTE
AULETTA
BABETTE
BARETTA
BERETTA
BIRETTA
BUGATTI
BURETTE
CADETTE
CALOTTE
CANETTI
COLETTE
CORETTA
COSETTE
COURTTV
CULOTTE
CURETTE
CUVETTE
DEALTTO
DINETTE
FAYETTE
FOUETTE
GALETTE
GAROTTE
GAVOTTE
GAZETTE
IWANTTO
KADETTS
LABATTS
LAFITTE
LAMOTTA
LAMOTTE
LANOTTE
LAYETTE
LIZETTE
LONETTE
LORETTA
LUCETTA
LUNETTE
LYNETTE
MANETTE
MEANTTO
MELITTA
MENOTTI
MORETTI
MOZETTA
MRBUTTS
MULATTO
MUSETTA
MUSETTE
NANETTE
NONETTE
OCTETTE
ORNETTE
OUGHTTO
PALETTE
PANETTA
PERETTI
PINOTTA
PIPETTE
POINTTO
PUTITTO
REACTTO
REGATTA
RICOTTA
RIDOTTO
RISOTTO
RONETTE
ROSETTA
ROSETTE
ROVETTA
SQUATTY
STARTTO
STKITTS
STRETTI
STRETTO
SUZETTE
TOFUTTI
TONETTE
UNFATTY
UNWITTY
VALOTTE
VEDETTE
VIDETTE
WYNETTE
ZANETTO

••••T•T

ABOUTIT
ADEPTAT
APPETIT
BIENTOT
BLUETIT
DOUBTIT
HABITAT
HADATIT
HASATIT
ILOSTIT
IWANTIT
KINGTUT
LEAPTAT
MEANTIT
MIGHTNT
OUGHTNT
POINTAT
QUARTET
QUINTET
RATATAT
SHOOTAT
SHOUTAT
SNORTAT
SWEATIT
TINYTOT

•••••TT

ASBYATT
BABBITT
BARRETT
BASKETT
BASSETT
BECKETT
BENNETT
BOYCOTT
BUFFETT
BULLITT
BURNETT
CASSATT
CORBETT
DEBRETT
DOGGETT
DORSETT
ELLIOTT
EVERETT
FAWCETT
FOLLETT
GANNETT
GARNETT
GARRETT
GOSSETT
HACKETT
HAMMETT
HAZLITT
HEWLETT
JARRETT
JARROTT
LIGGETT
MILLETT
MRSCOTT
NESBITT
PADGETT
PICKETT
PINKETT
PREWITT
PUCKETT
RABBITT
SCHMITT
SENNETT
SILENTT
TIBBETT
WALCOTT
WESCOTT
ZERMATT

TU•••••

TUBAIST
TUBBIER
TUBBING
TUBEPAN
TUBETOP
TUBFULS
TUBISTS
TUBLIKE
TUBULAR
TUBULES
TUCHMAN
TUCKERS
TUCKING
TUCKSIN
TUCSONS
TUESDAY
TUFFETS
TUFTIER
TUFTING
TUGBOAT
TUGGERS
TUGGING
TUGLESS
TUGRIKS
TUILLES
TUITION
TULANEU
TULSANS
TULSAOK
TUMBLED
TUMBLER
TUMBLES
TUMBREL
TUMESCE
TUMMIES
TUMMLER
TUMULTS
TUNABLE
TUNAOIL
TUNASUB
TUNDRAS
TUNEDIN
TUNEDTO
TUNEDUP
TUNEFUL
TUNEOUT
TUNESIN
TUNESTO
TUNESUP
TUNEUPS
TUNGOIL
TUNICLE
TUNISIA
TUNNELS
TUPELOS
TUPOLEV
TURBANS
TURBINE
TURBOTS
TUREENS
TURFIER
TURFING
TURFMAN
TURFMEN
TURFSKI
TURFTOE
TURFWAR
TURISMO
TURISTA
TURKEYS
TURKISH
TURMOIL
TURNBAD
TURNERS
TURNERY
TURNING
TURNIPS
TURNKEY
TURNOFF
TURNONS
TURNOUT
TURNPRO
TURNRED
TURNSIN
TURNSON
TURNSTO
TURNSUP
TURNUPS
TURRETS
TURTLED
TURTLES
TUSCANS
TUSCANY
TUSHERY
TUSHIES
TUSKERS
TUSKING
TUSSAUD
TUSSIVE
TUSSLED
TUSSLES
TUSSOCK
TUTELAR
TUTORED
TUTTING
TUTTUTS
TUTUILA
TUVWXYZ
TUXEDOS

T•U••••

TAUNTED
TAUNTER
TAUNTON
TAUREAN
TAURINE
TAUTENS
TAUTEST
TEUTONS
THUDDED
THULIUM
THUMBED
THUMPED
THUMPER
THUNDER
THUNKED
THURBER
THURGAU
THURMAN
THUSFAR
TOUAREG
TOUCANS
TOUCHED
TOUCHER
TOUCHES
TOUCHON
TOUCHUP
TOUGHEN
TOUGHER
TOUGHIE
TOUGHLY
TOUPEES
TOURBUS
TOURERS
TOURING
TOURISM
TOURIST
TOURNEY
TOUSLED
TOUSLES
TOUTERS
TOUTING
TRUANCY
TRUANTS
TRUCKED
TRUCKEE
TRUCKER
TRUCKLE
TRUDEAU
TRUDGED
TRUDGEN
TRUDGER
TRUDGES
TRUEDUP
TRUEING
TRUERIB
TRUERTO
TRUESUP
TRUFFLE
TRUISMS
TRUMANS
TRUMPED
TRUMPET
TRUMPUP
TRUNDLE
TRUSSED
TRUSSES
TRUSSUP
TRUSTED
TRUSTEE
TRUSTER
TRUSTIN
TRUSTME
TSUNAMI

T••U•••

TABUING
TABULAR
TALUSES
TEAURNS
TENUITY
TENUOUS
TENURED
TENURES
TEQUILA
THEUSSR
THOUGHT
THRUPUT
THRUSTS
THRUWAY
TIBURON
TIJUANA
TITULAR
TOFUTTI
TOLUENE
TONUSES
TRAUBEL
TRAUMAS
TRIUMPH
TROUBLE
TROUGHS
TROUNCE
TROUPED
TROUPER
TROUPES
TROUSER
TSOURIS
TSQUARE
TUBULAR
TUBULES
TUMULTS
TUTUILA
TVGUIDE
TWOUNIT

T•••U••

TABOULI
TACTUAL
TAGOUTS
TALCUMS
TAXCUTS
TEACUPS
TEAMUSA
TEDEUMS
TEDIUMS
TEMPURA
TERHUNE
TEXTUAL
TEXTURE
THEBUSH
THECUBS
THEDUKE
THEHULK
THEPUMP
THERULE
THESUNS
THETUBE
THETURN
THROUGH
TISSUES
TISSUEY
TOATURN
TONGUES
TONSURE
TOOMUCH
TOPGUNS
TORQUED
TORQUES
TORTUGA
TORTURE
TOSSUPS
TOYGUNS
TRADUCE
TRIBUNE
TRIBUTE
TRYOUTS
TSETUNG
TUBFULS
TUNEUPS
TURNUPS
TUTTUTS

T••••U•

TACITUS
TACKSUP
TACTFUL
TAGSOUT
TAKENUP
TAKEOUT
TAKESUP
TALKOUT
TALKSUP
TALLYUP
TANKFUL
TANKSUP
TANTRUM
TAPEDUP
TAPESUP
TAPSOUT
TARTSUP
TEAMSUP
TEARFUL
TEAROUT
TEARSUP
TEASEUP
~~TEDIOUS~~
TEEITUP
TENFOUR
TENKRUN
TENSEUP
TENTFUL
TENUOUS
TERBIUM
TESTOUT
TESTRUN
TETANUS
THAWOUT
THEFRUG
THEROUX
THESEUS
THETOUR
THINKUP
THINOUT
THORIUM
THREEUP
THREWUP
THROWUP
THRUPUT
THULIUM
TIDYSUM
TILTSUP
TIMEOUT
TIMESUP
TIREOUT
TOGSOUT
TOILFUL
TONEDUP
TONESUP
TOOKOUT
TOOLSUP
TOPSOUT
TOREOUT
TORNOUT
TOSSOUT
TOTALUP
TOTESUP
TOUCHUP
TOURBUS
TOYSRUS
TRADEUP
TRAPGUN
TRAYFUL
TRIPSUP
TRITIUM
TRIVIUM
TROILUS
TROTOUT
TROTSUP
TRUEDUP
TRUESUP
TRUMPUP
TRUSSUP
TUNASUB
TUNEDUP
TUNEFUL
TUNEOUT
TUNESUP
TURNOUT
TURNSUP
TUSSAUD
TWISTUP
TWOHOUR
TYINGUP
TYPEDUP
TYPESUP

T•••••U

TABLEAU
THIMPHU
THOREAU
THURGAU
TINAMOU
TONNEAU
TRUDEAU
TULANEU

•TU••••

NTUPLES
STUARTI
STUBBED
STUBBLE
STUBBLY
STUBING
STUCCOS
STUCKBY
STUCKIN
STUCKON
STUCKTO
STUCKUP
STUDDED
STUDENT
STUDIED
STUDIER
STUDIES
STUDIOS
STUFFED
STUFFER
STUFFIN
STUMBLE
STUMPED
STUMPER
STUNGUN
STUNNED
STUNNER
STUNTED
STUPEFY
STUPIDS
STUPORS
STURGES
STUTTER
STUTZES
STUVWXY

•T•U•••

ATLUNCH
ATTUCKS
ATTUNED
ATTUNES
ETRURIA
OTTUMWA
STAUNCH
STEUBEN
STLUCIA
STLUKES
STOUTEN
STOUTER
STOUTLY
STRUDEL

•T••U••

ATATURK
ATDEUCE
ATFAULT
ATRIUMS
STATUES
STATURE
STATUTE
STEPUPS
STIMULI
STLOUIS
STPAULS
STPIUSI
STPIUSV
STPIUSX
STRAUSS
STROUSE

•T•••U•

ATEITUP
ATISSUE
ATTICUS
ITSTRUE
PTEROUS
STACKUP
STADIUM
STANDUP
STANKUP
STANNUM
STARTUP
STAYOUT
STAYPUT
STAYSUP
STCLOUD
STEAMUP
STENGUN
STEPOUT
STEPSUP
STERNUM
STICKUM
STICKUP
STILLUP
STINKUP
STIRRUP
STIRSUP
STOCKUP
STOKEUP
STOODUP
STOPSUP
STOREUP
STRATUM
STRATUS
STUCKUP
STUNGUN
YTTRIUM

••TU•••

ACTUARY
ACTUATE
ACTUPON
ASTUTER
ATTUCKS
ATTUNED
ATTUNES
AUTUMNS
BYTURNS
DETUNED
DETUNES
ESTUARY
FATUITY
FATUOUS
FETUSES
FUTURAS
FUTURES
GETUPON
GOTUPON
GOTUPTO
HITUPON
ICTUSES
INTUITS
INTURNS
IVTUBES
KUTUZOV
LETUPON
LITURGY
LOTUSES
MATURED
MATURER
MATURES
MUTUALS
NATURAL
NATURED
NATUREL
NATURES
NOTUPTO
NOTURNS
NOTUSED
OBTUNDS
OBTUSER
OCTUBRE
OCTUPLE
OCTUPLY
OTTUMWA
PETULIA
PETUNIA
PUTUPON
PUTUPTO
RETUNED
RETUNES
RETURFS
RETURNS
RITUALS
ROTUNDA
RSTUVWX
SATUPON
SATURNS
SETUPON
SITUATE
SITUPON
SUTURED
SUTURES
TITULAR
TUTUILA
UNTUCKS
UNTUNED
UNTUNES
UPTURNS
WATUSIS

••T•U••

ARTHURC
ARTHURM
ARTHURS
ASTOUND
AUTEURS
BATSUIT
BETHUNE
CATGUTS
CATSUIT
CATSUPS
CUTOUTS
DATSUNS
DETOURS
DETRUDE
ENTHUSE
ENTRUST
EXTRUDE
FATOUSH
GETBUSY
GETCUTE
GETHURT
GOTBUSY
GOTCUTE
GOTHURT
HATFULS
HITTUNE
HOTCUPS
HOTTUBS
HOTTUNA
INTOUCH
INTRUDE
INTRUST
INTRUTH
JETGUNS
LETSUSE
LETTUCE
LUTHULI
NATSUME
NETFULS
NETSUKE
NETSURF
NOTMUCH
NOTRUMP
NOTSURE
OBTRUDE
OUTBUDS
OUTBULK
OUTBURN

OUTBUYS
OUTBUZZ
OUTCULL
OUTCURE
OUTCUTS
OUTDUEL
OUTGUNS
OUTGUSH
OUTHUNT
OUTHURL
OUTJUMP
OUTJUTS
OUTPULL
OUTPURL
OUTPUSH
OUTPUTS
OUTRUNS
OUTRUSH
OUTSULK
OUTSUMS
OUTSUNG
OUTTURN
PETDUCK
PETMULE
PETPUPS
PITBULL
POTFULS
POTLUCK
PUTOUTS
PUTPUTS
RETOUCH
RETOURS
ROTGUTS
SATSUMA
SETOUTS
TUTTUTS
UNTOUGH
UNTRUER
UNTRULY
UNTRUSS
UNTRUTH
VATFULS
WETBULB
WETSUIT

••T••U•
ACTEDUP
ACTFOUR
ACTSOUT
ANTEDUP
ANTERUS
ANTESUP
ANTIGUA
ANTIGUN
ANTIQUE
ARTEMUS
ATTICUS
AUTOBUS
BATEAUX
BATHTUB
BITESUP
BOTCHUP
BUTTOUT
CATCHUP
CITROUS
CUTARUG
CUTSOUT
DATABUS
DUTEOUS
DUTIFUL
EATENUP
EATITUP
EATSOUT
ERTEGUN
FATEFUL
FATIGUE
FATUOUS
GATEAUX
GETSOUT
GOTOGUY
HATEFUL
HITCHUP
HITSOUT
HOTGLUE
HOTSOUP
HOTSPUR
ICTERUS
ICTINUS
ISTHMUS
KETCHUM
KETCHUP
LATINUS
LETSOUT
LITHIUM
MATCHUP
METEOUT
MITCHUM
NATRIUM
NITROUS
NOTTRUE
OCTOPUS
OPTIMUM
OPTSOUT
OUTFLUX
OUTHAUL
OUTLOUD
OUTPOUR
OUTSWUM
PATCHUP
PETROUS
PITEOUS
PITIFUL
POTAMUS
PUTEMUP
PUTSOUT
PUTTOUT
RATSOUT
RETINUE
RUTHFUL
SETSOUT
SITSOUT
TETANUS
TOTALUP
TOTESUP
VOTEOUT
WITEOUT
WITHOUT
YTTRIUM

••T•••U
LETTERU
MATHIEU
MATTHAU
WATTEAU

•••TU••
ACHTUNG
AIRTUBE
ATATURK
BUSTUPS
CAPTURE
CENTURY
CLOTURE
CONTUSE
COSTUME
COUTURE
CULTURE
DENTURE
DICTUMS
DISTURB
DUSTUPS
EYETUCK
FACTUAL
FEATURE
FIXTURE
FORTUNA
FORTUNE
GESTURE
HITTUNE
HOTTUBS
HOTTUNA
KAPTURE
LABTUBE
LECTURE
LETTUCE
MANTUAN
MISTUNE
MIXTURE
MONTUNO
NEPTUNE
NOUTURN
NURTURE
OROTUND
OUTTURN
PASTURE
PERTURB
PICTURE
POPTUNE
POSTURE
QRSTUVW
RAPTUNE
RAPTURE
RESTUDY
RESTUFF
RUPTURE
SAXTUBA
SPATULA
STATUES
STATURE
STATUTE
TACTUAL
TEXTUAL
TEXTURE
THETUBE
THETURN
TOATURN
TORTUGA
TORTURE
TSETUNG
TUTTUTS
UNSTUCK
UNSTUNG
VENTURA
VENTURE
VENTURI
VESTURE
VICTUAL
VIRTUAL
VIRTUES
VISTULA
VOITURE
VULTURE
XYSTUSI
ZEITUNG

•••T•U•
AMATEUR
BEATOUT
BEATSUP
BELTOUT
BELTSUP
BESTBUD
BESTBUY
BESTCUT
BLOTOUT
BLOTSUP
BOATFUL
BOLTSUP
BOOTCUT
BOOTOUT
BOOTSUP
BUSTOUR
BUSTOUT
BUSTSUP
BUTTOUT
CASTOUT
CASTSUP
CENTAUR
CENTRUM
CHATSUP
CHETRUM
CLOTSUP
CONTOUR
CRATEUP
CRITTUR
DARTGUN
DUSTGUN
ECOTEUR
EDITOUT
FACTFUL
FELTOUT
FIATLUX
FISTFUL
FLATOUT
FOOTRUB
FOOTSUP
FORTIUS
FRETFUL
FROTHUP
GLUTEUS
GRATEUP
GROTIUS
HARTMUT
HAUTEUR
HEATFUL
HEATSUP
HUNTSUP
HURTFUL
ITSTRUE
JUSTOUT
KEPTMUM
KEPTOUT
KNOTSUP
LEFTOUT
LIFTSUP
LOSTOUT
LUSTFUL
LUSTRUM
MALTHUS
MARTIUS
MEETSUP
MISTSUP
MONTAUK
MONTEUX
NESTFUL
NOSTRUM
NOTTRUE
PASTDUE
PASTEUP
PASTEUR
PENTIUM
PGATOUR
PISTOUS
PLOTFUL
PONTIUS
POUTFUL
PROTEUS
PUTTOUT
RENTOUT
RESTFUL
RESTSUP
RIOTGUN
RIOTOUS
ROOTOUT
ROOTSUP
ROSTRUM
ROUTOUT
SENTOUT
SHOTGUN
SHOTOUT
SHOTPUT
SHUTOUT
SHUTSUP
SORTOUT
SPATOUT
SPITOUT
SUITSUP
TACTFUL
TANTRUM
TARTSUP
TENTFUL
TESTOUT
TESTRUN
THETOUR
TILTSUP
TRITIUM
TROTOUT
TROTSUP
UNSTOUT
USOTOUR
WAITOUT
WAITSUP
WANTOUT
WENTOUT
WHATSUP
WHITSUN
WISTFUL
WRITEUP
WROTEUP
ZESTFUL

•••T••U
BOSTONU
CHATEAU
COCTEAU
IGOTYOU
LETTERU
MARTINU
MATTHAU
MONTAGU
PLATEAU
SEETHRU
WATTEAU

••••TU•
ARBUTUS
ATEITUP
BATHTUB
BOOSTUP
BUILTUP
BURNTUP
COUNTUP
CREPTUP
CRITTUR
CUBITUS
DEALTUP
DECATUR
DONATUS
DRIFTUP
EATITUP
EIGHTUP
ERASTUS
ERECTUS
ERRATUM
FAUSTUS
FIRSTUP
FLOATUP
FRUSTUM
HABITUE
HAMITUP
HOISTUP
IAPETUS
IMPETUS
KINGTUT
LEAPTUP
LIGHTUP
MIXITUP
MOUNTUP
PARATUS
PAYSTUB
PERITUS
PILATUS
PINETUM
PLAUTUS
POINTUP
PQRSTUV
PRINTUP
QUANTUM
QUIETUS
QUINTUS
RANITUP
REVITUP
RUNITUP
SANCTUM
SANCTUS
SCOUTUP
SHOOTUP
SLANTUP
SPLITUP
STARTUP
STRATUM
STRATUS
SUMITUP
SWEPTUP
TACITUS
TEEITUP
TWISTUP
WASHTUB

••••T•U
FUJITSU
JUJITSU
KOMATSU
SHIATSU
SHIHTZU

•••••TU
OPQRSTU
SILENTU
VANUATU

TV•••••
TVCREWS
TVGAMES
TVGUIDE
TVIDOLS
TVMOVIE
TVROOMS
TVSHOWS
TVSPOTS
TVSTARS
TVTABLE
TVTAPES

T•V••••
TAVERNA
TAVERNS
TUVWXYZ

T••V•••
TEEVEES
THEVIEW
THEVIPS
TORVALD
TORVILL
TRAVAIL
TRAVELS
TRAVERS
TREVINO
TRIVETS
TRIVIAL
TRIVIOT
TRIVIUM

T•••V••
TELAVIV
THIEVED
THIEVES
THRIVED
THRIVEN
THRIVER
THRIVES
TIPOVER
TVMOVIE
TWELVEA
TWELVEB
TWELVEC
TWELVED
TWELVEE
TWELVES

T••••V•
TANTIVY
TAXLEVY
TENSIVE
THECAVS
THEFIVE
THEMAVS
THEWAVE
TOPFIVE
TUSSIVE

T•••••V
TELAVIV
TRASHTV
TUPOLEV

•TV••••
ETVOILA

•T•V•••
ATAVISM
ATAVIST
MTEVANS
STAVING
STEVENS
STUVWXY

•T••V••
ATEOVER
ATSEVEN
ITSOVER
OTTAVIO
STARVED
STARVES
STEEVED
STEEVES
STRIVED
STRIVEN
STRIVER
STRIVES

•T•••V•
BTWELVE
ITSLOVE
ITWELVE

•T••••V
STPIUSV

••TV•••
HDTVSET
LATVIAN
OUTVIED
OUTVIES
OUTVOTE

••T•V••
ACTIVAS
ACTIVES
BATAVIA
CUTOVER
DATIVES
EATOVER
ESTEVEZ
ESTIVAL
GETEVEN
GETOVER
GOTEVEN
GOTOVER
HOTOVER
LITOVSK
MITZVAH
MOTIVED
MOTIVES
NATIVES
NOTEVEN
NOTEVER
NOTOVER
OCTAVAL
OCTAVES
OCTAVIA
OCTAVIO
OCTAVOS
OTTAVIO
PUTOVER
RSTUVWX
VOTIVES

••T••V•
ACTFIVE
LETHAVE
LETLIVE
NOTLIVE
OSTRAVA
OUTGAVE
OUTGIVE
OUTLIVE
OUTLOVE
OUTMOVE
OUTRAVE
OUTROVE
OUTWAVE
PETDOVE

••T•••V
KATAYEV
KUTUZOV
LETTERV
USTINOV
WATCHTV

•••T•V•
AMATIVE
CAPTIVA
CAPTIVE
CENTAVO
COSTIVE
EMOTIVE
FESTIVA
FESTIVE
FICTIVE
FLATTVS
FURTIVE
GUSTAVE
POLTAVA
QRSTUVW
RESTIVE
TANTIVY
UNITIVE
YOMTOVS

•••T••V
LETTERV
MARTINV

••••TV•
FLATTVS
MINITVS
ZEMSTVO

••••T•V
COURTTV
MOLOTOV
PQRSTUV

•••••TV
CABLETV
COLORTV
COURTTV
DIRECTV
SILENTV
SPIKETV
TRASHTV
WATCHTV

TW•••••
TWADDLE
TWANGED
TWANGER
TWEAKED
TWEEDLE
TWEENER
TWEETED
TWEETER
TWEEZED
TWEEZER
TWEEZES
TWELFTH
TWELVEA
TWELVEB
TWELVEC
TWELVED
TWELVEE
TWELVES
TWERENT
TWIDDLE
TWILLED
TWINBED
TWINERS
TWINGED
TWINGES
TWINIER
TWINING
TWINJET
TWINKIE
TWINKLE
TWINKLY
TWINNED
TWINSET
TWIRLED
TWIRLER
TWISTED
TWISTER
TWISTON
TWISTUP
TWITCHY
TWITTED
TWITTER
TWOACRE
TWOACTS
TWOBALL
TWOBASE
TWOBITS
TWODAYS
TWODEEP
TWODOOR
TWOEEEE
TWOEGGS
TWOFACE
TWOFEET
TWOFERS
TWOFOLD
TWOFOOT
TWOHOUR
TWOIRON
TWOLANE
TWOMORE
TWOONIE
TWOPAIR
TWOPART
TWOROOM
TWOSHOT
TWOSOME
TWOSPOT
TWOSTAR
TWOSTEP
TWOTERM
TWOTIME
TWOTOED
TWOTONE
TWOTONS
TWOUNIT
TWOWEEK
TWOYEAR

T•W••••
TAWNIER
TAWNILY
THWACKS
THWARTS
THWHITE
TOWABLE
TOWAGES
TOWARDS
TOWAWAY
TOWBARS
TOWBOAT
TOWCARS
TOWEDIN
TOWELED
TOWERED
TOWHEAD
TOWHEES
TOWINGS
TOWLINE
TOWNCAR
TOWNERS
TOWNIES
TOWNISH
TOWNLET
TOWPATH
TOWROPE

T••W•••
TENWEEK
THAWERS
THAWING
THAWOUT
THEWALL
THEWAVE
THEWIND
TINWARE
TINWORK
TOYWITH
TRAWLED
TRAWLER
TROWELS
TROWING
TUVWXYZ
TWOWEEK

T•••W••
TAILWAG
TAXIWAY
TFPOWYS
THATWAY
THESWAN
THISWAY
THREWAT
THREWIN
THREWON
THREWUP
THROWAT
THROWER
THROWIN
THROWON
THROWUP
THRUWAY
TIMEWAS
TOLLWAY
TOWAWAY
TRAMWAY
TURFWAR

T••••W•
TALLOWS
TALLOWY
TAXLAWS
TEAGOWN
THENEWS
TIEDOWN
TIPDOWN
TOPDOWN
TOPROWS
TVCREWS
TVSHOWS

T•••••W
THECROW
THESHOW
THEVIEW
TILLNOW
TONEROW
TONYDOW
TOOSLOW
TOPDRAW
TORTLAW

•TW••••
ATWATER
ATWORST
BTWELVE
FTWAYNE
FTWORTH
ITWELVE
ITWENTY

•T•W•••
ATHWART
STEWARD
STEWART
STEWERS
STEWIER
STEWING
STEWPAN
STEWPOT
STOWAGE
STOWERS
STOWING
STOWSIT

•T••W••
ATEAWAY
OTTAWAN
OTTAWAS
STREWED
STREWER
STUVWXY

•T•••W•
OTTUMWA
STEPTWO

•T••••W
ATECROW

••TW•••
ANTWERP
ARTWALL
ARTWARE
ARTWORK
BATWING
BETWEEN
BETWIXT
CATWALK
CUTWORK
CUTWORM
ENTWINE
ENTWIST
FITWELL
GATWICK
GETWARM
GETWELL
GETWISE
GETWORD
GOTWARM
GOTWELL
GOTWISE
GOTWORD
HOTWARS
HOTWIRE
JETWASH
JETWAYS
METWITH
NATWICK
NETWARE
NETWORK
NITWITS
NOTWELL
NOTWITH
NUTWOOD
OSTWALD
OUTWAIT

OUTWALK
OUTWARD
OUTWARS
OUTWASH
OUTWAVE
OUTWEAR
OUTWEED
OUTWEEP
OUTWELL
OUTWENT
OUTWEPT
OUTWEST
OUTWILE
OUTWILL
OUTWIND
OUTWING
OUTWISH
OUTWITH
OUTWITS
OUTWORD
OUTWORE
OUTWORK
OUTWORN
RETWINE
RETWIST
SATWELL
SATWITH
SITWELL
SITWITH
SOTWEED
UNTWINE
UNTWIST
WETWARE
WETWASH

••T•W••
ANTIWAR
CATAWBA
CDTOWER
CNTOWER
CUTAWAY
EATAWAY
GATEWAY
GETAWAY
GETSWET
GOTAWAY
GOTOWAR
MATEWAN
OTTAWAN
OTTAWAS
OUTAWED
OUTAWES
OUTSWAM
OUTSWIM
OUTSWUM
PATHWAY
PUTAWAY
RETOWED
ROTAWAY
UPTOWNS

••T••W•
ANTCOWS
CATBOWL
CUTDOWN
GETDOWN
GOTDOWN
HITTOWN
JOTDOWN
LETDOWN
MATHEWS
OTTUMWA
OUTBAWL
OUTBOWL
OUTBOWS
OUTFAWN
OUTHOWL
OUTLAWS
OUTROWS
PATDOWN
PETCOWS
PITROWS
PITSAWS
PUTDOWN
RETHAWS
RSTUVWX
SATDOWN
SETDOWN
SITDOWN
UNTHAWS
WETDOWN

••T•••W
ARTSHOW
CATCHOW
CATSHOW
CATSPAW
EATCROW
HITSHOW
LETKNOW
LETTERW
LITHGOW
MATTHEW
OUTBLOW
OUTCROW
OUTDRAW
OUTDREW
OUTFLOW
OUTGLOW
OUTGNAW
OUTGREW
OUTGROW
OUTSHOW
PETCHEW
PETCROW
PITCREW
UPTHROW
UPTONOW

•••TW••
BELTWAY
BOBTWAY
CHATWIN
FOOTWAY
ONETWOS
PARTWAY
POSTWAR
THATWAY

•••T•W•
ANYTOWN
BESTOWS
BIGTOWN
CHITOWN
COWTOWN
HITTOWN
HOOTOWL
KOWTOWS
MIDTOWN
NEWTOWN
OLDTOWN
OURTOWN
PARTTWO
RESTOWS
SKITOWS
UNSTOWS

•••T••W
BELTSAW
BESTREW
DOITNOW
EXITNOW
FRETSAW
JUSTNOW
LASTROW
LETTERW
MATTHEW
MISTBOW
PALTROW
QRSTUVW
RESTREW
TORTLAW
WHATNOW

••••TW•
BALLTWO
BASETWO
FIVETWO
LANETWO
LINETWO
MACHTWO
OPUSTWO
PAGETWO
PARTTWO
PLUSTWO
SIDETWO
SIZETWO
STEPTWO

••••T•W
BARSTOW
CHOCTAW
IGNATOW
INASTEW
ROPETOW

•••••TW
SILENTW

T•X••••
TAXABLE
TAXBASE
TAXCODE
TAXCUTS
TAXFREE
TAXHIKE
TAXICAB
TAXIING
TAXIMAN
TAXIMEN
TAXIWAY
TAXLAWS
TAXLESS
TAXLEVY
TAXPAID
TAXRATE
TAXSALE
TAXYEAR
TEXTILE
TEXTING
TEXTRON
TEXTUAL
TEXTURE
TUXEDOS

T•••X••
TELEXED
TELEXES
THEAXIS
TIMEXES
TUVWXYZ

T•••••X
TELEFAX
TELEPIX
THEROUX
TOOLBOX
TRIPLEX

•T••X••
FTDIXNJ

•T•••X•
ATARAXY
STUVWXY

•T••••X
STCROIX
STONEAX
STPIUSX

••T•X••
DETOXED
DETOXES
LATEXES
RETAXED
RETAXES
UNTAXED
UNTAXES
UNTOXIC
URTEXTS

••T••X•
BATNEXT
BETWIXT

••T•••X
ALTOSAX
ANTHRAX
ANTITAX
APTERYX
ASTERIX
BATEAUX
BETAMAX
GATEAUX
LETTERX
NETFLIX
OUTFLUX
OUTJINX
RSTUVWX

•••T•X•
AIRTAXI
CONTEXT
MEATAXE
PRETEXT
SUBTEXT

•••T••X
BEATBOX
BEATRIX
COMTREX
EDITRIX
FIATLUX
FLATTAX
FORTDIX
GIFTBOX
GIFTTAX
LETTERX
MISTERX
MONTEUX
NARTHEX
ORATRIX
POSTBOX
POSTFIX
SALTBOX
VICTRIX

••••TX•
ARANTXA

••••T•X
ANTITAX
CELOTEX
FLATTAX
GIFTTAX
GORETEX
LANDTAX
OVERTAX
PLAYTEX
PLUSTAX
POLLTAX
POORTAX
ROADTAX

•••••TX
SILENTX

TY•••••
TYCOONS
TYINGIN
TYINGON
TYINGTO
TYINGUP
TYLENOL
TYMPANA
TYMPANI
TYNDALL
TYPEABS
TYPEDIN
TYPEDUP
TYPESET
TYPESIN
TYPESUP
TYPHOID
TYPHOON
TYPICAL
TYPISTS
TYRANNY
TYRANTS

T•Y••••
TAYBACK
TAYLORS
THYMINE
THYROID
THYSELF
TOYBALL
TOYBIKE
TOYBOAT
TOYBOOK
TOYCARS
TOYCART
TOYDOGS
TOYDOLL
TOYFAIR
TOYGUNS
TOYHATS
TOYHOOP
TOYKITE
TOYLAND
TOYLESS
TOYLIKE
TOYNBEE
TOYOTAS
TOYPAIL
TOYSHOP
TOYSLED
TOYSRUS
TOYTOPS
TOYWITH
TRYHARD
TRYITON
TRYOUTS
TRYSAIL
TRYSTED
TRYSTER

T••Y•••
TAXYEAR
TENYEAR
THEYIPS
THEYSAY
TIDYING
TIDYSUM
TINYBIT
TINYTIM
TINYTOT
TONYDOW
TORYISH
TORYISM
TRAYFUL
TRAYNOR
TWOYEAR

T•••Y••
TACHYON
TALLYHO
TALLYUP
TIEDYED
TIEDYES
TINTYPE

T••••Y•
TABKEYS
TAGDAYS
TAMBLYN
TEAPOYS
TENDAYS
TFPOWYS
THEBOYS
THEMAYO
TOMBOYS
TOPONYM
TURKEYS
TUVWXYZ
TWODAYS

T•••••Y
TACITLY
TACKILY
TAKENBY
TALLOWY
TAMMANY
TANNERY
TANTIVY
TARBABY
TARDILY
TARTILY
TASTILY
TATTERY
TATTILY
TAWNILY
TAXIWAY
TAXLEVY
TEACOZY
TEARILY
TEATRAY
TENABLY
TENANCY
TENSELY
TENSITY
TENTHLY
TENUITY
TEPIDLY
TERNARY
TERRIFY
TERSELY
TESTACY
TESTFLY
TESTIFY
TESTILY
THATCHY
THATWAY
THEARMY
THEBABY
THEBODY
THECITY
THERAPY
THEREBY
THEYSAY
THICKLY
THIERRY
THIRDLY
THIRSTY
THISDAY
THISTLY
THISWAY
THREADY
THRIFTY
THROATY
THRUWAY
TICKSBY
TIDALLY
TIERNEY
TIFFANY
TIGHTLY
TIMBERY
TIMIDLY
TIMOTHY
TINAFEY
TINDERY
TINNILY
TIPSILY
TIREDLY
TISSUEY
TOGGERY
TOLLWAY
TOLSTOY
TONALLY
TOOEASY
TOOMANY
TOPIARY
TORREFY
TOTALLY
TOTTERY
TOUGHLY
TOURNEY
TOWAWAY
TRACERY
TRAGEDY
TRAMWAY
TREACLY
TREMBLY
TRENARY
TRILOGY
TRINARY
TRINITY
TRITELY
TROLLEY
TROTSKY
TRUANCY
TUESDAY
TURNERY
TURNKEY
TUSCANY
TUSHERY
TWINKLY
TWITCHY
TYRANNY

•TY••••
ETYMONS
STYGIAN
STYLERS
STYLETS
STYLING
STYLISE
STYLISH
STYLIST
STYLIZE
STYMIED
STYMIES
STYPSIS
STYPTIC
STYRENE

•T•Y•••
ATTYGEN
FTMYERS
STAYDRY
STAYERS
STAYFOR
STAYING
STAYOFF
STAYOUT
STAYPUT
STAYSAT
STAYSIN
STAYSON
STAYSUP

•T••Y••
FTWAYNE
ITMAYBE
STRAYED
STRAYER

•T•••Y•
MTKENYA
STMARYS

•T••••Y
ATARAXY
ATEAWAY
ATROPHY
ATTABOY
FTHENRY
FTRILEY
ITHIRTY
ITSABOY
ITSEASY
ITSOKAY
ITWENTY
JTMONEY
MTBALDY
MTMARCY
OTOLOGY
PTOLEMY
STAGILY
STAIDLY
STALELY
STANDBY
STANLEY
STARCHY
STARKEY
STARKLY
STARSKY
STATELY
STAYDRY
STEEPLY
STERNLY
STICKBY
STIFFLY
STIRFRY
STOKELY
STONILY
STOODBY
STOOKEY
STOPSBY
STOUTLY
STREAKY
STRINGY
STUBBLY
STUCKBY
STUPEFY
STUVWXY
UTICANY
UTILITY
UTTERLY

••TY•••
ATTYGEN
CITYBOY
CITYGAL
ECTYPAL
ECTYPES
KATYDID
OUTYELL
OUTYELP
PITYING
RETYPED
RETYPES
SATYRIC
UNTYING
UNTYPED

••T•Y••
CATEYED
KATAYEV
PITAYAS
RITDYES
SETTYPE
VATDYED
VATDYES
VOTEYEA
VOTEYES
WETEYED

••T••Y•
ALTKEYS
ANTONYM
APTERYX
AUTONYM
BATBOYS
BATDAYS
BETRAYS
CATSEYE
CATTOYS
ESTRAYS
HOTDAYS
HOTKEYS
INTRAYS
JETWAYS
JITNEYS
KATHRYN
MOTLEYS
OUTBUYS
OUTLAYS
OUTPAYS
OUTSAYS
PETTOYS
VOTEAYE

••T•••Y
ACTORLY
ACTUARY
ANTHONY
ATTABOY
AUTARKY
AUTOPSY
BATTERY
BETARAY
BETHANY
BETTANY
BUTTERY
BUTTONY
BYTHEBY
CATTILY
CITYBOY
COTTONY
CUTAWAY
CUTLERY
DATEDLY
DITHERY
DOTTILY
EATAWAY
ENTROPY
ESTUARY
FATALLY
FATCITY
FATTILY
FATUITY
FETIDLY
FITZROY
GATEWAY
GETAWAY
GETBUSY
GOTAWAY
GOTBUSY
GOTOGUY
GUTSILY
HITPLAY
JITTERY
KITSCHY
KITTERY
LATENCY
LATHERY
LETGOBY
LETSFLY
LETTERY
LITHELY
LITTERY
LITURGY
LOTTERY
MOTHERY
MUTABLY
MUTEDLY
MYTHIFY
NATTILY
NITRIFY
NITTANY
NOTABLY
NOTEASY
NOTEDLY
NOTMANY
NUTTILY
OCTUPLY
OSTIARY
OUTBRAY
OUTCITY
OUTPITY
OUTPLAY
OUTPRAY
OUTSTAY
OUTTRAY
PATENCY
PATHWAY
PATSDRY
PETPONY
PETRIFY
PETTILY
PITHILY
POTENCY
POTTERY
PUTAWAY
PUTREFY
RETALLY
RETIARY
RITZILY
ROTAWAY
SATIETY
SATISFY
SATRAPY
SETPLAY
SHTICKY
SOTHEBY
TATTERY
TATTILY
TOTALLY
TOTTERY
UNTASTY
UNTRULY
UTTERLY
VITALLY
VITRIFY
VOTENAY
WITTILY

•••TY••
BIOTYPE
DACTYLS
DENTYNE
DIPTYCH
ECOTYPE
FIFTYAD
FIFTYBC
FORTYAD
FORTYBC
IGOTYOU
INSTYLE
MARTYRS
MISTYPE
PARTYER
PARTYON
PLATYPI
PRETYPE
RESTYLE
SETTYPE
SIXTYAD
SIXTYBC
SUBTYPE
TINTYPE
WOJTYLA

•••T•Y•
BOYTOYS
CATTOYS
DMYTRYK
DOGTOYS
FONTEYN
LEFTEYE
MONTOYA
NEWTOYS
PETTOYS
SHUTEYE

•••T••Y
ACETIFY
ACUTELY
AINTHAY
AMATORY
ANATOLY
ANATOMY
ASHTRAY
BARTRAY
BATTERY
BEATIFY
BELTWAY
BENTLEY
BESTBOY
BESTBUY
BETTANY
BLOTCHY
BOBTWAY
BOOTERY
BRITNEY
BRUTELY
BUTTERY
BUTTONY
CANTILY
CANTSAY
CATTILY
CENTURY
CERTIFY
CHUTNEY
CLUTCHY
COTTONY
CURTSEY
CUSTODY
DALTREY
DESTINY
DESTROY
DIETARY
DIRTILY
DONTCRY
DOTTILY
DUSTILY
EARTHLY
ECSTASY
EMPTILY
ESOTERY
FACTORY
FANTASY
FATTILY
FIFTHLY
FLITSBY
FOOTWAY
FORTIFY
FUSTILY
GLITCHY
GOUTILY
GRATIFY
GRETZKY
GUSTILY
HARTLEY
HASTILY
HAUTBOY
HEATRAY
HEFTILY
HISTORY
HUNTLEY
ICETRAY
IRATELY
ISOTOPY
JITTERY
JUSTIFY
KITTERY
KVETCHY
LASTMAY
LASTORY
LETTERY
LITTERY

LOATHLY
LOFTILY
LOTTERY
LUSTILY
MASTERY
MEATILY
MISTILY
MONTHLY
MORTIFY
MUSTILY
MYSTERY
MYSTIFY
NASTILY
NATTILY
NECTARY
NEXTDAY
NIFTILY
NINTHLY
NITTANY
NUTTILY
ORATORY
OUTTRAY
PARTWAY
PETTILY
PORTNOY
PORTRAY
POTTERY
RECTIFY
RECTORY
RESTUDY
RUSTILY
SALTILY
SIXTHLY
SKETCHY
SOOTILY
SOUTHEY
STATELY
TANTIVY
TARTILY
TASTILY
TATTERY
TATTILY
TEATRAY
TENTHLY
TESTACY
TESTFLY
TESTIFY
TESTILY
THATCHY
THATWAY
TOTTERY
TRITELY
TROTSKY
TWITCHY
UNITARY
UNSTAGY
UNSTONY
VASTITY
VICTORY
WHATSAY
WHITELY
WHITNEY
WINTERY
WITTILY
ZESTILY

••••TY•
BURSTYN

••••T•Y
ABBOTCY
ADEPTLY
ADULTLY
AGENTRY
ALERTLY
BEASTLY
BIGOTRY
BLUNTLY
BREATHY
BRISTLY
CHANTEY
CHANTRY
CHEWTOY
CHINTZY
COUNTRY
COURTLY
CRAFTSY
DOROTHY
EMPATHY
ERECTLY
EXACTLY
FAINTLY
FIRSTLY
FLEETLY
FLOATBY
FREETOY
GAUNTLY
GHASTLY
GHOSTLY
GOODTRY
GREATLY
GRISTLY
HEALTHY
HELOTRY
HOOPTOY
INAPTLY
INEPTLY
INERTLY
JOINTLY
LANGTRY
LENGTHY
LICITLY
LIGHTLY
MOISTLY
NICETRY
NIGHTLY
NOENTRY
NOVOTNY
OUTSTAY
OVERTLY
POULTRY
PULLTOY
QUARTZY
QUIETLY
REENTRY
RIANTLY
RIGHTLY
ROBOTRY
SAINTLY
SCANTLY
SHOOTBY
SHORTLY
SIGHTLY
SLANTLY
SMARTLY
SMOOTHY
SQUATLY
SQUATTY
STOUTLY
SWARTHY
SWEETLY
SWELTRY
SWIFTLY
TACITLY
THISTLY
TIGHTLY
TIMOTHY
TOLSTOY
UNAPTLY
UNFATTY
UNFITLY
UNWITTY
WEALTHY
WREATHY

•••••TY
ABILITY
ACIDITY
AGILITY
AMENITY
AMNESTY
ANILITY
ANNUITY
ANXIETY
APLENTY
ARIDITY
AVIDITY
BAYCITY
BIGCITY
BIGGITY
BLIGHTY
BREVITY
CARROTY
CHARITY
CHRISTY
CLARITY
CRUDITY
CRUELTY
DELCITY
DENSITY
DIGGITY
DIGNITY
DOHERTY
DOUGHTY
DUALITY
DUBIETY
DYNASTY
EDACITY
ELMCITY
FACULTY
FALSITY
FATCITY
FATUITY
FERRETY
FIDGETY
FLAUNTY
FLIGHTY
FOGCITY
FOGERTY
FRAILTY
GADGETY
GASEITY
GRAVITY
HAGERTY
HAUGHTY
HIPPITY
HONESTY
IBILITY
IEIGHTY
IMPIETY
INANITY
ININETY
ITHIRTY
ITWENTY
JOLLITY
KKKKATY
LIBERTY
LICKETY
LOYALTY
MAJESTY
MODESTY
NAIVETY
NAUGHTY
NIMIETY
NOVELTY
NUGGETY
NULLITY
OBESITY
OFFDUTY
OLDCITY
ONEMPTY
OPACITY
OUTCITY
OUTPITY
PAUCITY
PENALTY
PIOSITY
POVERTY
PRIVITY
PROBITY
PROCITY
PUBERTY
QUALITY
RABBITY
RACKETY
REALITY
RICKETY
ROYALTY
RUSSETY
SATIETY
SEADUTY
SEVENTY
SILENTY
SIMCITY
SINCITY
SOCIETY
SQUATTY
SQUINTY
SUAVITY
SUNCITY
TENSITY
TENUITY
THECITY
THIRSTY
THRIFTY
THROATY
TRINITY
UNDUSTY
UNEMPTY
UNFATTY
UNHASTY
UNLOFTY
UNLUSTY
UNPIETY
UNSALTY
UNSOOTY
UNTASTY
UNWITTY
UTILITY
VACUITY
VARIETY
VARSITY
VASTITY
VELVETY
WEIGHTY

TZ•••••
TZARINA
TZIMMES

T•Z••••
TIZZIES

T••Z•••
TARZANA
TARZANS
TENZING
TIZZIES

T•••Z••
TOPAZES
TREIZES
TWEEZED
TWEEZER
TWEEZES

T••••Z•
TEACOZY
TRAPEZE

T•••••Z
TEMPEAZ
THEFONZ
THERITZ
TIRPITZ
TUVWXYZ

•T••Z••
STANZAS
STUTZES

•T•••Z•
ATOMIZE
ITEMIZE
STYLIZE
UTILIZE

••TZ•••
DITZIER
FITZROY
FUTZING
HOTZONE
MATZOHS
MATZOTH
MITZVAH
NETZERO
PATZERS
RITZIER
RITZILY
YITZHAK

••T•Z••
CITIZEN
KUTUZOV
NETIZEN

••T••Z•
HATSIZE
OUTBUZZ
OUTGAZE
OUTSIZE

••T•••Z
ESTEVEZ
LETTERZ
NATCHEZ
OUTBUZZ

•••TZ••
BLITZED
BLITZEN
BLITZER
BLITZES
CHUTZPA
COETZEE
CRUTZEN
GLITZED
GLITZES
GRETZKY
KLUTZES
PLOTZED
PLOTZES
PRETZEL
QUETZAL
SELTZER
SPITZES
STUTZES
SWITZER
WALTZED
WALTZER
WALTZES
YAHTZEE

•••T•Z•
BAPTIZE
POETIZE
UNITIZE

•••T••Z
KERTESZ
LETTERZ

••••TZ•
BLINTZE
CHINTZY
JERITZA
QUARTZY
SHIHTZU
YANGTZE

•••••TZ
BERLITZ
HEIFETZ
HORVITZ
KIBBUTZ
LAURITZ
LORENTZ
MARANTZ
SCHLITZ
SCHULTZ
SILENTZ
THERITZ
TIRPITZ

U•A••••
UGANDAN
ULALUME
ULANOVA
ULANUDE
UNACTED
UNADDED
UNADEPT
UNADULT
UNAGILE
UNAGING
UNAIDED
UNAIMED
UNAIRED
UNALERT
UNALIKE
UNALONE
UNAMUNO
UNANGRY
UNAPTLY
UNARMED
UNASKED
UNAWAKE
UNAWARE
UNAWFUL
UNAXLED
UPABOVE
UPAHEAD
UPANDIN
UPATREE
URACILS
URANITE
URANIUM
USABLES
USANCES
UTAHANS
UVALUES

U••A•••
UKRAINE
ULLAGES
ULYANOV
ULZANAS
UMLAUTS
UNBAITS
UNBAKED
UNBALED
UNBALES
UNBARED
UNBARES
UNBASED
UNBATED
UNCAGED
UNCAGES
UNCAKED
UNCAKES
UNCANED
UNCANNY
UNCAPED
UNCASED
UNCASES
UNCASKS
UNDARED
UNDATED
UNDAZED
UNEAGER
UNEARTH
UNEASES
UNEATEN
UNEAVED
UNFACED
UNFACTS
UNFADED
UNFAITH
UNFAKED
UNFAMED
UNFANCY
UNFATED
UNFATTY
UNFAZED
UNGATED
UNGAUDY
UNHAIRS
UNHAIRY
UNHANDS
UNHANDY
UNHAPPY
UNHARDY
UNHARSH
UNHASPS
UNHASTY
UNHATED
UNHAYED
UNHAZED
UNIATES
UNJADED
UNLACED
UNLACES
UNLADED
UNLADEN
UNLADES
UNLARGE
UNLATCH
UNLAVED
UNLAXED
UNLAXES
UNMACHO
UNMADLY
UNMAKER
UNMAKES
UNMANED
UNMANLY
UNMASKS
UNMASTS
UNMATED
UNMATES
UNNAILS
UNNAIVE
UNNAMED
UNNASAL
UNPACED
UNPACKS
UNPAGAN
UNPAGED
UNPALED
UNPARED
UNPASTE
UNPAVED
UNPAWED
UNPAWNS
UNRACKS
UNRAINY
UNRAKED
UNRASPY
UNRATED
UNRAVEL
UNRAYED
UNRAZED
UNSADLY
UNSAFER
UNSALTY
UNSATED
UNSAVED
UNSAVVY
UNSAWED
UNTACKS
UNTAKEN
UNTAMED
UNTAMES
UNTAPED
UNTAPES
UNTASTY
UNTAXED
UNTAXES
UNVAGUE
UNWADED
UNWAGED
UNWAKED
UNWALLS
UNWANED
UNWAVED
UNWAXED
UPCARDS
UPCASTS
UPDARTS
UPDATED
UPDATER
UPDATES
UPEARLY
UPGAZED
UPGAZES
UPLANDS
UPRAISE
UPRATED
UPRATES
UPTAKES
UPTALKS
UPVALUE
UPWAFTS
UPWARDS
UQUARKS
URBANER
URBANII
URBANIV
URBANVI
USHAPED
USHAPES
USUALLY

U•••A••
ULLMANN
ULULANT
ULULATE
UMBRAGE
UNAWAKE
UNAWARE
UNBEARD
UNBLADE
UNBRACE
UNBRAID
UNBRAKE
UNBRAVE
UNCHAIN
UNCHAIR
UNCHARY
UNCIALS
UNCLAMP
UNCLASP
UNCRAMP
UNCRATE
UNCRAZY
UNDEALT
UNDRAPE
UNDRAWN
UNDRAWS
UNFLAKY
UNFRAIL
UNFRANK
UNGRAND
UNGUARD
UNHEADY
UNHEARD
UNHEAVY
UNIBALL
UNITARD
UNITARY
UNIVACS
UNLEADS
UNLEAFS
UNLEAKY
UNLEARN
UNLEASH
UNLOADS
UNLOATH
UNMEANT
UNPLAIT
UNPLANS
UNREADY
UNSCALY
UNSEALS
UNSEAMS
UNSEATS
UNSHADE
UNSHADY
UNSHARP
UNSLACK
UNSLAIN
UNSMART
UNSNAGS
UNSNAKY
UNSNAPS
UNSNARL
UNSPANS
UNSTACK
UNSTAGY
UNSTAID
UNSTATE
UNTEACH
UNTHAWS
UNTRACK
UNTRAPS
UNWEARY
UNWEAVE
UNWRAPS
UPBEARS
UPBEATS
UPBRAID
UPCOAST
UPDRAFT
UPGRADE
UPHEAPS
UPHEAVE
UPHOARD
UPLEAPS
UPLEAPT
UPLOADS
UPPHASE
UPPSALA
UPQUARK
UPREACH
UPREARS
UPROARS
UPSCALE
UPSOARS
UPSTAGE
UPSTAIR
UPSTAND
UPSTARE
UPSTART
UPSTATE
UPTEARS
UPTRADE
USFLAGS
USGRANT
USSTATE
UTAHANS
UTICANS
UTICANY

U••••A•
UGANDAN
ULTIMAS
ULZANAS
UMBRIAN
UNCLEAN
UNCLEAR
UNCLOAK
UNDULAR
UNEQUAL
UNGULAE
UNGULAR
UNHUMAN
UNIDEAL
UNLEGAL
UNLOCAL
UNLOYAL
UNNASAL
UNPAGAN
UNREGAL
UNRURAL
UNSPEAK
UNSTRAP
UNSWEAR
UNTREAD
UNURBAN
UNUSUAL
UNVENAL
UNVITAL
UNVOCAL
UPAHEAD
UPTOPAR
URSULAK
URUGUAY
USEDCAR
UTOPIAN
UTOPIAS
UXORIAL

U•••••A
ULANOVA
UPPSALA

•UA••••
CUATROS
DUALISM
DUALIST
DUALITY
DUALIZE
GUANACO
GUANINE
GUARANI
GUARDED
GUARDEE
GUARDER
GUARGUM
HUANGHE
HUANGTI
MUAMMAR
NUANCED
NUANCES
QUACKED
QUACKER
QUADRIC
QUAFFED
QUAFFER
QUAGGAS
QUAHOGS
QUAILED
QUAKERS
QUAKIER
QUAKIES
QUAKILY
QUAKING
QUALIFY
QUALITY
QUANTUM
QUAPAWS
QUARLES
QUARREL
QUARTAN
QUARTER
QUARTES
QUARTET
QUARTIC
QUARTOS
QUARTZY
QUASARS
QUASHED
QUASHES
QUATRES
QUATTRO
QUAVERS
QUAVERY
QUAYAGE
RUANDAS
SUASION
SUASIVE
SUAVELY
SUAVEST
SUAVITY

•U•A•••
AUBADES
AUPAIRS
AURALEE
AURALLY
AUSABLE
AUTARCH
AUTARKY
BUGABOO
BUGALOO
BUGATTI
BUTANES
BUYABLE
CUBAGES
CURABLE
CURABLY
CURACAO
CURARES
CURATED
CURATES
CURATOR
CUTARUG
CUTAWAY
DUBARRY
DUCALLY
DUHAMEL
DUKAKIS
DUNAWAY
DURABLE
DURABLY
DURANCE
DURANGO
DURANTE
EUBANKS
EULABUS
EURASIA
FUGALLY
FUGATOS
GUJARAT
HUMANLY
HUMANUM
JUDAICA
JUDAISM
JUDASES
JUMADAS
JUMANJI
KUWAITI
LUCANIA
LUCARNE
LUNATED
LUNATES
LUNATIC
LUXATED
LUXATES
MUBARAK
MULATTO
MURALED
MURANOS
MUSANTE
MUTABLE
MUTABLY
MUTAGEN
MUTANTS
MUTATED
MUTATES
NUNAVUT
NUTATED
NUTATES
OUTACTS
OUTADDS

OUTAGES
OUTASKS
OUTAWED
OUTAWES
PULASKI
PUPATED
PUPATES
PUTAWAY
RUBADUB
RUBATOS
RUMAKIS
RUMANIA
RUNAMOK
RUNATAB
RUNAWAY
RURALLY
RUTALEE
SUBAREA
SUBARID
SUBARUS
SUDAFED
SUGARED
SUHARTO
SUKARNO
SUMATRA
SUSANNA
SUSANNE
SUZANNE
TUBAIST
TULANEU
TUNABLE
TUNAOIL
TUNASUB
YUCAIPA
YUCATAN
YUCATEC
YUKATAS

•U••A••

AUREATE
BUDVASE
BUFFALO
BUKHARA
BULGARI
BULGARS
BULWARK
BUMRAPS
BUNRAKU
BUOYANT
BURBAGE
BURBANK
BUREAUS
BUREAUX
BURIALS
BURLAPS
BURMANS
BURNABY
BUROAKS
BURSARS
BUSFARE
BUSLANE
BUSMANS
BUSPASS
BUSTARD
BUYBACK
BUZZARD
CUBFANS
CUEBALL
CUECARD
CUIRASS
CUNEATE
CUPCAKE
CUREALL
CURRANT
CURTAIL
CURTAIN
CURTATE
CUSHAWS
CUSPATE
CUSTARD
CUTBACK
CUTLASS
CUTRATE
DUCHAMP
DUEDATE
DUEEAST
DULLARD
DUNDALK
DUNNAGE
DURWARD
EUSTACE
FULMARS
FUNFAIR
FURBALL
FURCATE
FURFARM
FURNACE
FURTADO
FUTHARK
GUANACO
GUARANI
GUEVARA
GUFFAWS
GUITARS
GULLAHS
GUMBALL
GUNCASE
GUNLAPS
GUNLAWS
GUNWALE
GUSTAVE
HUBBARD
HUBCAPS
HUMBARD
HUNGARY
HUPPAHS
HURRAHS
HURRAYS
HUSBAND
HUSHABY
HUSSARS
HUZZAHS
JUDEANS
JUGBAND
JULIANA
JUNKART
JUTLAND
LUCIANA
LUCIANO
LUGGAGE
LUGSAIL
LULLABY
LUMBAGO
LUMBARS
MUDBATH
MUDCATS
MUDLARK
MUDPACK
MUDWASP
MULCAHY
MULDAUR
MULHARE
MULLAHS
MUNDANE
MUSCATS
MUSTAFA
MUSTANG
MUSTARD
MUTUALS
NUBIANS
NUMBATS
OURGANG
OUTBACK
OUTBAKE
OUTBANS
OUTBARK
OUTBATS
OUTBAWL
OUTCALL
OUTCANT
OUTCAST
OUTDARE
OUTDATE
OUTEARN
OUTEATS
OUTFACE
OUTFAST
OUTFAWN
OUTGAIN
OUTGAME
OUTGAVE
OUTGAZE
OUTHAUL
OUTKAST
OUTLAID
OUTLAIN
OUTLAND
OUTLASH
OUTLAST
OUTLAWS
OUTLAYS
OUTMANS
OUTMATE
OUTPACE
OUTPAID
OUTPASS
OUTPATH
OUTPAYS
OUTRACE
OUTRAGE
OUTRAIL
OUTRANG
OUTRANK
OUTRANT
OUTRAPS
OUTRATE
OUTRAVE
OUTSAID
OUTSAIL
OUTSANG
OUTSAYS
OUTTAKE
OUTTALK
OUTWAIT
OUTWALK
OUTWARD
OUTWARS
OUTWASH
OUTWAVE
PUBGAME
PULSARS
PULSATE
PUNJABI
PUTBACK
QUAPAWS
QUASARS
QUAYAGE
QUEPASA
QUINARY
QUINATE
RUDYARD
RUFFALO
RUGRATS
RUINATE
RUMBAED
RUMCAKE
RUMMAGE
RUNBACK
RUNLAPS
RUNLATE
RUNPAST
RUNWAYS
RUPIAHS
RUTHANN
RUTLAND
SUBBAND
SUBBANK
SUBBASE
SUBBASS
SUBCASE
SUBCASH
SUBCAST
SUBDATE
SUBHALL
SUBRACE
SUBTASK
SUBWARS
SUBWAYS
SUCRASE
SULFATE
SULTANA
SULTANS
SUMMAND
SUMMARY
SUMMATE
SUNBATH
SUNDAES
SUNDAYS
SUNFANS
SUNFAST
SUNHATS
SUNLAMP
SUNMAID
SUNRAYS
SUNTANS
SUNWARD
SURFACE
SURNAME
SURPASS
SUSTAIN
TULSANS
TULSAOK
TURBANS
TUSCANS
TUSCANY
TUSSAUD
VULCANS
VULGATE
ZUMWALT
ZUNIANS

•U•••A•

AUGURAL
AURORAE
AURORAL
AURORAS
AUSTRAL
AUTOMAT
BUCHMAN
BUCKRAM
BUCKSAW
BUDDHAS
BUGBEAR
BULOVAS
BUMDEAL
BUQSHAS
BURGLAR
BUSHMAN
BUSHWAH
BUSLOAD
BUTTRAM
BUZZSAW
CUBICAL
CUBITAL
CUBSFAN
CUESTAS
CULTJAM
CUMBIAS
CUMSHAW
CUPOLAS
CUPULAR
CURACAO
CURSEAT
CUTAWAY
DUENNAS
DUNAWAY
DUNSTAN
DUSTMAN
DUSTPAN
DUSTRAG
EUREKAS
EUROVAN
FUJISAN
FULLDAY
FUMEDAT
FUMESAT
FURCOAT
FURSEAL
FURWRAP
FUSTIAN
FUSUMAS
FUTURAS
GUESSAT
GUINEAN
GUINEAS
GUJARAT
GULFWAR
GUNBOAT
GUNPLAY
GURKHAS
HUFFMAN
HUMERAL
HUMORAL
JUDELAW
JUDOKAS
JUGHEAD
JUGULAR
JULYDAY
JUMADAS
JUMPSAT
JUNEDAY
JUNGIAN
JUNKCAR
JUNKFAX
JUNKMAN
JURYMAN
JUVENAL
KUMQUAT
LUCIDAE
LUCKMAN
LUMINAS
LUNGEAT
LUNULAE
LUNULAR
LUSTRAL
MUAMMAR
MUBARAK
MUDFLAP
MUDFLAT
MULETAS
MUSICAL
MUSKRAT
NUBIRAS
NUCLEAR
NUMERAL
NUPTIAL
NUTMEAT
NUTRIAS
OUTBEAM
OUTBRAG
OUTBRAY
OUTDRAG
OUTDRAW
OUTGNAW
OUTHEAR
OUTLEAD
OUTLEAP
OUTPLAN
OUTPLAY
OUTPRAY
OUTREAD
OUTROAR
OUTSOAR
OUTSTAY
OUTSWAM
OUTTEAR
OUTTRAY
OUTWEAR
PULLMAN
PULLTAB
PURITAN
PUTAWAY
QUAGGAS
QUARTAN
QUENEAU
QUESNAY
QUETZAL
QUINLAN
QUINTAL
QUINTAS
QUONDAM
RUANDAS
RUBSRAW
RUFFIAN
RUFIYAA
RUNATAB
RUNAWAY
RUSSIAN
RUSSLAN
RUYBLAS
SUBBIAS
SUBCLAN
SUBDUAL
SUBGOAL
SUBHEAD
SUNBEAM
SUNDIAL
SUNSFAN
SURECAN
SUREIAM
SURFMAN
SURINAM
SURREAL
TUBEPAN
TUBULAR
TUCHMAN
TUESDAY
TUGBOAT
TUNDRAS
TURFMAN
TURFWAR
TURNBAD
TUTELAR
YUCATAN
YUKATAS

•U••••A

AUGUSTA
AULETTA
AUREOLA
AUSTRIA
AUTOPIA
BUKHARA
BURKINA
CUMBRIA
CURIOSA
DUODENA
EUGENIA
EUGLENA
EUNOMIA
EURASIA
FUCHSIA
GUEVARA
JUDAICA
JULIANA
JUNKDNA
KUNDERA
LUCANIA
LUCETTA
LUCIANA
LUCINDA
LUNESTA
LUTETIA
MUSCIDA
MUSETTA
MUSTAFA
NUESTRA
OUGUIYA
QUECHUA
QUEPASA
QUERIDA
QUESERA
QUINELA
RUBELLA
RUBEOLA
RUFIYAA
RUMANIA
RUZICKA
SUBAREA
SUBIDEA
SUBROSA
SULTANA
SULUSEA
SUMATRA
SUSANNA
TUNISIA
TURISTA
TUTUILA
YUCAIPA

••UA•••

AQUAMAN
AQUARIA
AQUATIC
AQUAVIT
DOUANES
ECUADOR
EDUARDO
ELUANTS
ELUATES
EQUABLE
EQUABLY
EQUALED
EQUALLY
EQUALTO
EQUATED
EQUATES
EQUATOR
GOUACHE
IGUANAS
IGUANID
IGUASSU
ROUAULT
SQUALID
SQUALLS
SQUALLY
SQUALOR
SQUANTO
SQUARED
SQUARER
SQUARES
SQUASHY
SQUATLY
SQUATTY
SQUAWKS
SQUAWKY
STUARTI
TOUAREG
TRUANCY
TRUANTS
UQUARKS
USUALLY
YOUANDI

••U•A••

ADULATE
AOUDADS
ARUBANS
AZUSACA
BAUHAUS
BHUTANI
CAUDATE
CHUMASH
COUGARS
COURAGE
COURANT
CRUSADE
CRUZADO
CRUZANS
EDUCATE
EMULATE
EQUIANO
EXUDATE
FOULARD
FOURAAA
GAUTAMA
GOULASH
GOURAMI
HAULAGE
INULASE
JOUHAUX
LAULAUS
MAUMAUS
MAUVAIS
MOULAGE
NEUMANN
NOUGATS
OCULARS
PLUMAGE
PLURALS
RHUBARB
ROUBAIX
ROULADE
SAUNAED
SAUSAGE
SCUBAED
SOURALE
SQUEAKS
SQUEAKY
SQUEALS
TOUCANS
TRUMANS
TSUNAMI
ULULANT
ULULATE
YOUMANS
YOURANG

••U••A•

ABUTTAL
AGULHAS
ALUMNAE
ALUMNAL
APULIAN
AQUAMAN
AQUINAS
ASUSUAL
BLUEJAY
BLUELAW
CHUPPAH
CHUPPAS
CLUBCAR
CRUCIAL
CRUSTAL
DIURNAL
DOUGLAS
DRUZEAN
DRUZIAN
ELUVIAL
EQUIFAX
EXURBAN
FAUXPAS
FLUIDAL
FLUNGAT
FLUVIAL
FMURRAY
FOURAAA
FOURDAY
FOURMAN
FOURWAY
GLUTEAL
GRUMMAN
HOUSMAN
HOUSSAY
HYUNDAI
IGUANAS
ISUREAM
JOURDAN
JOURNAL
KAUFMAN
KLUGMAN
LAUGHAT
MAUGHAM
MAUPRAT
MAURIAC
MAURIAT
NAUSEAM
NEUTRAL
NOUVEAU
PLUSTAX
PLUVIAL
RHUMBAS
ROULEAU
SAURIAN
SHULMAN
SOULMAN
SOUPCAN
SWUNGAT
TAUREAN
THURGAU
THURMAN
THUSFAR
TRUDEAU
UNURBAN
UNUSUAL
URUGUAY
VAUGHAN
VOUVRAY

••U•••A

ALUMINA
AQUARIA
ARUGULA
AZUSACA
CHUTZPA
CRUELLA
DOUBLEA
EXURBIA
FOURAAA
GAUTAMA
LOUELLA
NAUTICA
OPUNTIA
PAULINA
PLUGOLA
PRUSSIA

•••UA••

ACTUARY
ACTUATE
ANNUALS
ARCUATE
ASSUAGE
CAPUANA
CASUALS
EDOUARD
EMQUADS
ENQUADS
ESTUARY
ISSUANT
JAGUARS
JANUARY
LIQUATE
LOQUATS
MANUALS
MUTUALS
NAHUATL
OAHUANS
ONGUARD
OSSUARY
PADUANS
PAPUANS
PIQUANT
RITUALS
SAGUARO
SINUATE
SIOUANS
SITUATE
TIJUANA
TSQUARE
UNGUARD
UPQUARK
VALUATE
VANUATU
VISUALS

•••U•A•

ACAUDAL
ACCUSAL
ANGULAR
ANNULAR
AROUSAL
AUGURAL
BELUGAS
CANULAE
CANULAS
CAYUGAS
CLAUSAL
COPULAE
COPULAR
COPULAS
CUPULAR
ENDUPAT
EXCUSAL
EXCUSAS
FACULAE
FIBULAE
FIBULAR
FIBULAS
FIGURAL
FLAUTAS
FUSUMAS
FUTURAS
GRAUMAN
HANUKAH
INHUMAN
INSULAR
ISSUEAD
JOCULAR
JUGULAR
KAHUNAS
KORUNAS
LACUNAE
LACUNAL
LACUNAR
LACUNAS
LAGUNAS
LAPUTAN
LUNULAE
LUNULAR
MACULAE
MACULAR
MCLUHAN
MEDUSAE
MEDUSAN
MEDUSAS
MENUBAR
MEZUZAH
MEZUZAS
MIZUNAS
MODULAR
NATURAL
NEBULAE
NEBULAR
NEBULAS
NKRUMAH
NODULAR
NOSUGAR
OLDUVAI
OSCULAR
PADUCAH
PALUDAL
PERUSAL
PLEURAE
PLEURAL
PNEUMAS
PNEUMAT
POPULAR
POPUPAD
RECUSAL
REFUSAL
REFUTAL
REGULAR
ROMULAN
SAMURAI
SARUMAN
SECULAR
SHOUTAT
SINUTAB
SPOUSAL
TABULAR
THRUWAY
TITULAR
TRAUMAS
TUBULAR
UNDULAR
UNGULAE
UNGULAR
UNHUMAN
UNRURAL
URSULAK
VICUNAS
ZONULAR

•••U••A

ALLUVIA
ASSUNTA
AUGUSTA
CAPUANA
CLAUDIA
COLUMBA
COQUINA
EMMUSKA
ESCUELA
ETRURIA
LARUSSA
LECUONA
LIGURIA
MARUSJA
MAZURKA
MEDULLA
MINUTIA
MOLUCCA
OTTUMWA
OUGUIYA
PERUGIA
PETULIA
PETUNIA
ROBUSTA
ROTUNDA
SEQUOIA
SEQUOYA
SHOULDA
STLUCIA
SULUSEA
TEQUILA
TIJUANA
TUTUILA
ZAKUSKA

••••UA•

ACCRUAL
ASEXUAL
ASUSUAL
BIVOUAC
COEQUAL
DONJUAN
FACTUAL
GRADUAL
KEROUAC
KUMQUAT
LENGUAS
LINGUAE
LINGUAL
MANTUAN
RORQUAL
SANJUAN
SENSUAL
SUBDUAL
TACTUAL
TEXTUAL
UNEQUAL
UNUSUAL
URUGUAY

VICTUAL
VIRTUAL

••••U•A
ARAFURA
ARUGULA
BARBUDA
BERMUDA
BLACULA
BRAVURA
CAESURA
CANNULA
CHALUPA
DRACULA
DRLAURA
EVALUNA
FORMULA
FORTUNA
HECKUVA
HELLUVA
HOTTUNA
INOCULA
KILAUEA
LINGULA
MESHUGA
MISSUSA
OBSCURA
PREPUPA
SAMBUCA
SATSUMA
SAXTUBA
SCAPULA
SPATULA
TEAMUSA
TEMPURA
TORTUGA
VALVULA
VANDURA
VENTURA
VERRUCA
VINCULA
VISTULA

•••••UA
ANTIGUA
MANAGUA
QUECHUA
RESIDUA

U•B••••
UMBERED
UMBERTO
UMBRAGE
UMBRIAN
UMBRIEL
UNBAITS
UNBAKED
UNBALED
UNBALES
UNBARED
UNBARES
UNBASED
UNBATED
UNBEARD
UNBELDI
UNBELTS
UNBENCH
UNBENDS
UNBERTH
UNBESET
UNBINDS
UNBLADE
UNBLENT
UNBLEST
UNBLOCK
UNBLOWN
UNBLUED
UNBOGGY
UNBOLTS
UNBONED
UNBORED
UNBORNE
UNBOSOM
UNBOUND
UNBOWED
UNBOXED
UNBOXES
UNBRACE
UNBRAID
UNBRAKE
UNBRAVE
UNBRIEF
UNBROKE
UNBUILD
UNBUILT
UNBULKY
UNBURLY
UNBURNT
UNBURST
UPBEARS
UPBEATS
UPBORNE
UPBOUND
UPBRAID
UPBUILD
UPBURST
URBANER
URBANII
URBANIV
URBANVI

U••B•••
UNEBBED
UNIBALL
UNIBODY
UNOBESE
UPABOVE
USABLES

U•••B••
UNCUBIC
UNEBBED
UNLOBED
UNORBED
UNROBED
UNROBES
UNSOBER
UNURBAN

U••••B•
UNCURBS

U•••••B
UNPLUMB
UPCLIMB

•UB••••
AUBADES
AUBERGE
AUBURNS
AUBURNU
BUBBLED
BUBBLES
CUBAGES
CUBBIES
CUBBING
CUBBINS
CUBBISH
CUBFANS
CUBICAL
CUBICLE
CUBICLY
CUBISTS
CUBITAL
CUBITUS
CUBOIDS
CUBSFAN
DUBARRY
DUBBERS
DUBBING
DUBIETY
DUBIOUS
DUBNIUM
DUBUQUE
EUBANKS
FUBSIER
HUBBARD
HUBBELL
HUBBIES
HUBBUBS
HUBCAPS
JUBILEE
KUBELIK
KUBRICK
LUBBERS
LUBBOCK
LUBEJOB
MUBARAK
NUBBERS
NUBBIER
NUBBINS
NUBBLES
NUBIANS
NUBIRAS
PUBERTY
PUBGAME
PUBLICS
PUBLISH
PUBLIUS
RUBADUB
RUBATOS
RUBBERS
RUBBERY
RUBBING
RUBBISH
RUBBLES
RUBDOWN
RUBELLA
RUBEOLA
RUBICON
RUBIOUS
RUBITIN
RUBRICS
RUBSOFF
RUBSOUT
RUBSRAW
RUBUPON
RUBYDEE
RUBYRED
SUBAREA
SUBARID
SUBARUS
SUBBAND
SUBBANK
SUBBASE
SUBBASS
SUBBIAS
SUBBING
SUBCASE
SUBCASH
SUBCAST
SUBCELL
SUBCLAN
SUBCODE
SUBCOOL
SUBDATE
SUBDEBS
SUBDUAL
SUBDUCT
SUBDUED
SUBDUER
SUBDUES
SUBECHO
SUBFILE
SUBFORM
SUBGOAL
SUBGODS
SUBHALL
SUBHEAD
SUBIDEA
SUBITEM
SUBJECT
SUBJOIN
SUBKING
SUBLETS
SUBLIDS
SUBLIME
SUBLONG
SUBLOTS
SUBMITS
SUBNETS
SUBORNS
SUBPLOT
SUBPOST
SUBRACE
SUBROOT
SUBROSA
SUBSECT
SUBSETS
SUBSIDE
SUBSIDY
SUBSIST
SUBSOIL
SUBSORT
SUBSUME
SUBTASK
SUBTEEN
SUBTEND
SUBTEXT
SUBTLER
SUBTONE
SUBTYPE
SUBUNIT
SUBURBS
SUBVENE
SUBVERT
SUBWARS
SUBWAYS
SUBZERO
SUBZONE
TUBAIST
TUBBIER
TUBBING
TUBEPAN
TUBETOP
TUBFULS
TUBISTS
TUBLIKE
TUBULAR
TUBULES

•U•B•••
BUBBLED
BUBBLES
BUGBEAR
BUGBOYS
BULBLET
BULBOUS
BUMBLED
BUMBLER
BUMBLES
BURBAGE
BURBANK
BURBLED
BURBLER
BURBLES
BURBOTS
BUSBIES
BUSBOYS
BUYBACK
CUBBIES
CUBBING
CUBBINS
CUBBISH
CUEBALL
CUEBIDS
CUIBONO
CUMBERS
CUMBIAS
CUMBRIA
CURBCUT
CURBING
CUTBACK
DUBBERS
DUBBING
DUMBEST
DUMBING
FUMBLED
FUMBLER
FUMBLES
FURBALL
FURBISH
GUMBALL
GUMBOOT
GUNBELT
GUNBOAT
HUBBARD
HUBBELL
HUBBIES
HUBBUBS
HUMBARD
HUMBERT
HUMBLED
HUMBLER
HUMBLES
HUMBUGS
HUSBAND
JUGBAND
JUMBLED
JUMBLER
JUMBLES
JUMBUCK
LUBBERS
LUBBOCK
LUMBAGO
LUMBARS
LUMBERS
MUDBATH
MUMBLED
MUMBLER
MUMBLES
MUYBIEN
NUBBERS
NUBBIER
NUBBINS
NUBBLES
NUMBATS
NUMBERS
NUMBEST
NUMBING
OUTBACK
OUTBAKE
OUTBANS
OUTBARK
OUTBATS
OUTBAWL
OUTBEAM
OUTBEGS
OUTBEND
OUTBIDS
OUTBLOT
OUTBLOW
OUTBOWL
OUTBOWS
OUTBRAG
OUTBRAY
OUTBRED
OUTBUDS
OUTBULK
OUTBURN
OUTBUYS
OUTBUZZ
PUEBLOS
PUTBACK
QUIBBLE
RUBBERS
RUBBERY
RUBBING
RUBBISH
RUBBLES
RUMBAED
RUMBLED
RUMBLER
RUMBLES
RUNBACK
RUYBLAS
SUBBAND
SUBBANK
SUBBASE
SUBBASS
SUBBIAS
SUBBING
SUDBURY
SUNBATH
SUNBEAM
SUNBELT
SUNBIRD
SUNBOWL
SUNBOWS
SUNBURN
TUBBIER
TUBBING
TUGBOAT
TUMBLED
TUMBLER
TUMBLES
TUMBREL
TURBANS
TURBINE
TURBOTS

•U••B••
AUDIBLE
AUDIBLY
AUDUBON
AUNTBEE
AUSABLE
AUTOBIO
AUTOBUS
BUGABOO
BUNKBED
BUSYBEE
BUYABLE
CURABLE
CURABLY
DURABLE
DURABLY
DUSTBIN
EULABUS
FUSEBOX
FUSIBLE
JUJUBES
JUKEBOX
JUMPBID
JUNEBUG
JURYBOX
MUTABLE
MUTABLY
QUIBBLE
SUREBET
TUNABLE
TURNBAD

•U•••B•
BURNABY
HUBBUBS
HUNNYBS
HUSHABY
LULLABY
OUTRIBS
PUNJABI
RULEDBY
SUBDEBS
SUBURBS

•U••••B
LUBEJOB
PULLTAB
RUBADUB
RUNATAB
SUCCUMB
TUNASUB

••UB•••
ARUBANS
BAUBLES
BLUBBER
BRUBECK
CLUBBED
CLUBBER
CLUBCAR
CLUBMED
CLUBSUP
DAUBERS
DAUBING
DOUBLEA
DOUBLEB
DOUBLEC
DOUBLED
DOUBLEE
DOUBLEF
DOUBLEG
DOUBLEH
DOUBLEI
DOUBLEJ
DOUBLEK
DOUBLEL
DOUBLEM
DOUBLEN
DOUBLEO
DOUBLEP
DOUBLEQ
DOUBLER
DOUBLES
DOUBLET
DOUBLEU
DOUBLEV
DOUBLEW
DOUBLEX
DOUBLEY
DOUBLEZ
DOUBTED
DOUBTER
DOUBTIT
DRUBBED
DRUBBER
FLUBBED
FLUBBER
FLUBDUB
FLUBUGS
GRUBBED
GRUBBER
REUBENS
RHUBARB
ROUBAIX
SCUBAED
SHUBERT
SNUBBED
SNUBBER
SOUBISE
STUBBED
STUBBLE
STUBBLY
STUBING

••U•B••
BLUBBER
BLUEBOY
BLURBER
BOURBON
CLUBBED
CLUBBER
COURBET
CRUMBED
CRUMBLE
CRUMBLY
CRUMBUM
DRUBBED
DRUBBER
EQUABLE
EQUABLY
EXURBAN
EXURBIA
FLUBBED
FLUBBER
FNUMBER
GRUBBED
GRUBBER
GRUMBLE
GRUMBLY
HAUTBOY
PLUMBED
PLUMBER
PLUMBIC
PLUMBUM
RHUMBAS
SLUMBER
SNUBBED
SNUBBER
STUBBED
STUBBLE
STUBBLY
STUMBLE
THUMBED
THURBER
TOURBUS
UNURBAN

••U••B•
COULDBE
STUCKBY
SWUNGBY
WOULDBE

••U•••B
COULOMB
DOUBLEB
FLUBDUB
RHUBARB
TRUERIB

•••UB••
ALDUBIN
AUDUBON
BLAUBOK
INCUBUS
IVTUBES
JUJUBES
MENUBAR
OCTUBRE
SCRUBBY
SCRUBUP
SHRUBBY
SOLUBLE
STEUBEN
TRAUBEL
TROUBLE
UNCUBIC
VOLUBLE
VOLUBLY

•••U•B•
AAJUMBO
BENUMBS
COLUMBA
COLUMBO
SCRUBBY
SHRUBBY
SUBURBS
UNCURBS

•••U••B
SINUTAB

••••UB•
AIRTUBE
BEDAUBS
CHERUBS
HEYRUBE
HOTTUBS
HUBBUBS
ICECUBE
INDOUBT
LABTUBE
NODOUBT
OILRUBS
REDOUBT
SAXTUBA
SCHLUBS
THECUBS
THETUBE

••••U•B
DECRUMB
DIMBULB
DISTURB
DRYBULB
MCCRUMB
PERTURB
REPLUMB
SUCCUMB
UNPLUMB
WETBULB

•••••UB
BACKRUB
BATHTUB
BEARCUB
BODYRUB
BREWPUB
CARCLUB
FANCLUB
FLUBDUB
FOOTRUB
GYMCLUB
KEYCLUB
LIONCUB
MINISUB
ONECLUB
OVERDUB
PAYSTUB
RESCRUB
RUBADUB
TUNASUB
VAPORUB
WARCLUB
WASHTUB
WOLFCUB

UC•••••
UCCELLO

U•C••••
UCCELLO
UNCAGED
UNCAGES
UNCAKED
UNCAKES
UNCANED
UNCANNY
UNCAPED
UNCASED
UNCASES
UNCASKS
UNCEDED
UNCHAIN
UNCHAIR
UNCHARY
UNCHECK
UNCHOKE
UNCHURN
UNCIALS
UNCINCH
UNCITED
UNCIVIC
UNCIVIL
UNCLAMP
UNCLASP
UNCLEAN
UNCLEAR
UNCLEFT
UNCLIPS
UNCLIPT
UNCLOAK
UNCLOGS
UNCLOSE
UNCLOUD
UNCODED
UNCOILS
UNCOMIC
UNCOOPS
UNCORED
UNCORES
UNCORKS
UNCOUTH
UNCOVER
UNCOWED
UNCOYER
UNCOYLY
UNCRAMP
UNCRATE
UNCRAZY
UNCRIED
UNCROSS
UNCROWN
UNCRUDE
UNCRUEL
UNCTION
UNCUBIC
UNCUFFS
UNCURBS
UNCURED
UNCURLS
UPCARDS
UPCASTS
UPCCODE
UPCLIMB
UPCLOSE
UPCOAST
UPCOILS
UPCOURT
UPCURLS
UPCURVE
URCHINS

U••C•••
UNACTED
UNICODE
UNICORN
UNSCALY
UNSCREW
UPCCODE
UPSCALE
URACILS
UTICANS
UTICANY

U•••C••
UNDOCKS
UNFACED
UNFACTS
UNLACED
UNLACES
UNLOCAL
UNLOCKS
UNLUCID
UNLUCKY
UNMACHO
UNPACED
UNPACKS
UNPICKS
UNRACKS
UNROCKY
UNTACKS
UNTUCKS
UNVOCAL
UPTICKS
USANCES
USEDCAR
USEDCDS
UTRECHT

U••••C•
UNBENCH
UNBLOCK
UNBRACE
UNCHECK
UNCINCH
UNERECT
UNFANCY
UNFENCE
UNFROCK
UNHITCH
UNIVACS
UNJUICY
UNLATCH
UNQUICK
UNSLACK
UNSLICK
UNSPICY
UNSTACK
UNSTICK
UNSTUCK
UNTEACH
UNTHICK
UNTRACK
UNVOICE
UPREACH
URGENCY

U•••••C
UNCIVIC
UNCOMIC
UNCUBIC
UNLYRIC
UNSTOIC
UNTOXIC

•UC••••
AUCTION
BUCHMAN
BUCHNER
BUCKERS
BUCKETS
BUCKEYE
BUCKFOR
BUCKING
BUCKLED
BUCKLES
BUCKLEY
BUCKNER
BUCKOES
BUCKRAM
BUCKSAW
BUCKSUP
BUCOLIC
CUCKOOS
DUCALLY
DUCHAMP
DUCHESS
DUCHIES
DUCKERS
DUCKIER
DUCKIES
DUCKING
DUCKOUT
DUCKPIN
DUCTILE
DUCTING
EUCERIN
EUCHRED
EUCHRES
FUCHSIA
GUCKIER
KUCHENS
LUCANIA
LUCARNE
LUCENCY
LUCERNE
LUCETTA
LUCHINO
LUCIANA
LUCIANO

LUCIDAE
LUCIDLY
LUCIFER
LUCILLE
LUCINDA
LUCITES
LUCIUSI
LUCKIER
LUCKILY
LUCKING
LUCKMAN
LUCKNOW
LUCKOUT
LUCYLIU
MUCKERS
MUCKIER
MUCKING
MUCKSUP
NUCLEAR
NUCLEIC
NUCLEON
NUCLEUS
NUCLIDE
PUCCINI
PUCKERS
PUCKERY
PUCKETT
PUCKISH
RUCHING
RUCKERT
RUCKING
RUCKSUP
RUCTION
SUCCEED
SUCCESS
SUCCORS
SUCCOTH
SUCCOUR
SUCCUMB
SUCKDRY
SUCKERS
SUCKIER
SUCKING
SUCKSIN
SUCKSUP
SUCRASE
SUCROSE
SUCTION
TUCHMAN
TUCKERS
TUCKING
TUCKSIN
TUCSONS
YUCAIPA
YUCATAN
YUCATEC
YUCKIER

•U•C•••

BUNCHED
BUNCHES
BUNCHUP
BUNCOED
BUSCEMI
BUTCHER
BUTCHES
CUECARD
CULCHES
CUPCAKE
DULCIFY
DUNCISH
FULCRUM
FURCATE
FURCOAT
GULCHES
GUNCASE
HUBCAPS
HUNCHED
HUNCHES
HUTCHES
JUICERS
JUICEUP
JUICIER
JUICILY
JUICING
JUNCOES
KUTCHER
LUNCHED
LUNCHER
LUNCHES
LURCHED
LURCHER
LURCHES
MUDCATS
MULCAHY
MULCHED
MULCHES
MULCTED
MUNCHED
MUNCHEN
MUNCHER
MUNCHES
MUNCHIE
MUNCHON
MUSCATS
MUSCIDA
MUSCLED
MUSCLES
NUNCIOS
OUTCALL
OUTCANT
OUTCAST
OUTCITY
OUTCOLD
OUTCOME
OUTCOOK
OUTCROP
OUTCROW
OUTCULL
OUTCURE
OUTCUTS
PUCCINI
PUNCHED
PUNCHER
PUNCHES
PUNCHIN
PUNCHUP
PURCELL
QUACKED
QUACKER
QUECHUA
QUICHES
QUICKEN
QUICKER
QUICKIE
QUICKLY
RUMCAKE
SUBCASE
SUBCASH
SUBCAST
SUBCELL
SUBCLAN
SUBCODE
SUBCOOL
SUCCEED
SUCCESS
SUCCORS
SUCCOTH
SUCCOUR
SUCCUMB
SUNCITY
TUSCANS
TUSCANY
VULCANS

•U••C••

AURICLE
BUZZCUT
CUBICAL
CUBICLE
CUBICLY
CURACAO
CURBCUT
CUTICLE
JUMPCUT
JUNKCAR
MUSICAL
MUSICKS
NUANCED
NUANCES
OUTACTS
OUTECHO
PUMICED
PUMICES
QUINCES
QUINCEY
RUBICON
RUZICKA
SUBECHO
SURECAN
TUNICLE

•U•••C•

AUSPICE
AUTARCH
BULLOCK
BURDICK
BUYBACK
CUTBACK
DURANCE
EUSTACE
FURNACE
GUANACO
GUNLOCK
JUDAICA
JUMBUCK
JUSTICE
KUBRICK
LUBBOCK
LUCENCY
MUDPACK
MURDOCH
NUMLOCK
OUTBACK
OUTFACE
OUTKICK
OUTPACE
OUTPICK
OUTRACE
OUTROCK
PUBLICS
PUDENCY
PUTBACK
RUBRICS
RUNBACK
RUSTICS
SUBDUCT
SUBJECT
SUBRACE
SUBSECT
SUFFICE
SUNDECK
SURFACE
SUSPECT
TUMESCE
TUSSOCK

•U••••C

BUCOLIC
EUGENIC
JURIDIC
LUNATIC
NUCLEIC
NUMERIC
QUADRIC
QUARTIC
QUINTIC
YUCATEC

••UC•••

BOUCHER
BOUCHES
CHUCKED
CHUCKIT
CHUCKLE
CLUCKED
CLUCKER
COUCHED
COUCHES
CRUCIAL
DEUCING
DOUCEUR
DRUCKER
EDUCATE
EDUCING
EDUCTED
EDUCTOR
ERUCTED
FAUCETS
GAUCHER
GAUCHOS
GLUCOSE
KNUCKLE
KNUCKLY
LEUCINE
PAUCITY
PLUCKED
POUCHED
POUCHES
RAUCOUS
SAUCERS
SAUCIER
SAUCILY
SAUCING
SAUCONY
SHUCKED
SHUCKER
SMUCKER
SNUCKUP
STUCCOS
STUCKBY
STUCKIN
STUCKON
STUCKTO
STUCKUP
TOUCANS
TOUCHED
TOUCHER
TOUCHES
TOUCHON
TOUCHUP
TRUCKED
TRUCKEE
TRUCKER
TRUCKLE
VOUCHED
VOUCHER
VOUCHES

••U•C••

BOUNCED
BOUNCER
BOUNCES
CHURCHY
CLUBCAR
CLUTCHY
COUNCIL
CRUNCHY
GOUACHE
JOUNCED
JOUNCES
PAUNCHY
PLUMCOT
POUNCED
POUNCER
POUNCES
RAUNCHY
SLUICED
SLUICES
SOUPCAN
SOUPCON
SOURCED
SOURCES
STUCCOS

••U••C•

AZUSACA
BLUEICE
BRUBECK
DEUTSCH
FLUENCY
MAURICE
NAUTICA
SQUELCH
SQUINCH
TRUANCY

••U•••C

AQUATIC
CAUSTIC
DOUBLEC
DRUIDIC
FLUIDIC
LAUTREC
MAURIAC
PLUMBIC
POULENC
YOUNGMC

•••UC••

ABDUCED
ABDUCES
ABDUCTS
ADDUCED
ADDUCER
ADDUCES
ADDUCTS
ATTUCKS
CADUCEI
CANUCKS
CAPUCHE
CHAUCER
DEDUCED
DEDUCER
DEDUCES
DEDUCTS
GROUCHO
GROUCHY
INDUCED
INDUCER
INDUCES
INDUCTS
MOLUCCA
MRLUCKY
NABUCCO
NOGUCHI
PADUCAH
PENUCHE
REDUCED
REDUCER
REDUCES
RELUCTS
SEDUCED
SEDUCER
SEDUCES
SLOUCHY
SPRUCED
SPRUCER
SPRUCES
STLUCIA
UNLUCID
UNLUCKY
UNTUCKS

•••U•C•

ADJUNCT
ATLUNCH
BEQUICK
DEFUNCT
DOLUNCH
ENOUNCE
FLOUNCE
FLOUNCY
GODUTCH
INDUTCH
MOLUCCA
NABUCCO
SCRUNCH
STAUNCH
TROUNCE
UNJUICY
UNQUICK

•••U••C

LEXUSSC
MRMUSIC
RHEUMIC
UNCUBIC

••••UC•

AIRDUCT
ANDSUCH
ANYLUCK
ATDEUCE
BADLUCK
CONDUCE
CONDUCT
DEBAUCH
EYETUCK
GEODUCK
HOWMUCH
ILLLUCK
INTOUCH
JOEBUCK
JUMBUCK
LADOUCE
LELOUCH
LETTUCE
NIPMUCK
NONSUCH
NOTMUCH
ODDDUCK
OVIDUCT
PETDUCK
POTLUCK
PRODUCE
PRODUCT
RETOUCH
ROEBUCK
SAMBUCA
SAWBUCK
SEADUCK
SUBDUCT
TOOMUCH
TRADUCE
UNSTUCK
VERRUCA
VIADUCT

••••U•C

ARTHURC
BIVOUAC
KEROUAC
MOLLUSC

•••••UC

JEANLUC

U•D••••

UNDARED
UNDATED
UNDAZED
UNDEALT
UNDERDO
UNDERGO
UNDEWED
UNDIKED
UNDINES
UNDOCKS
UNDOERS
UNDOING
UNDOMED
UNDRAPE
UNDRAWN
UNDRAWS
UNDRESS
UNDRIED
UNDRUNK
UNDULAR
UNDUPED
UNDUSTY
UNDYING
UPDARTS
UPDATED
UPDATER
UPDATES
UPDIVED
UPDIVES
UPDRAFT
UPDRIED
UPDRIES
UPDRIFT

U••D•••

UNADDED
UNADEPT
UNADULT
UNEDGED
UNEDGES
UNIDEAL
USEDCAR
USEDCDS
USEDFOR

U•••D••

UGANDAN
UNADDED
UNAIDED
UNCEDED
UNCODED
UNENDED
UNFADED
UNGIDDY
UNGODLY
UNJADED
UNLADED
UNLADEN
UNLADES
UNMADLY
UNMUDDY
UNSADLY
UNSIDED
UNWADED
UNWEDGE
UPANDIN
UPENDED
UPSIDES
URGEDON
USTEDES
UVINDEX

U••••D•

ULANUDE
UNBELDI
UNBENDS
UNBINDS
UNBLADE
UNCRUDE
UNDERDO
UNFOLDS
UNGAUDY
UNGIDDY
UNGIRDS
UNHANDS
UNHANDY
UNHARDY
UNHEADY
UNHEEDS
UNHOODS
UNIBODY
UNICODE
UNIPODS
UNLEADS
UNLOADS
UNMOLDS
UNMOLDY
UNMOODY
UNMUDDY
UNNEEDY
UNREADY
UNROWDY
UNSHADE
UNSHADY
UNWINDS
UNWINDY
UPCARDS
UPCCODE
UPFOLDS
UPGIRDS
UPGRADE
UPHOLDS
UPLANDS
UPLOADS
UPSENDS
UPTRADE
UPWARDS
UPWINDS
USEDCDS
USERIDS

U•••••D

UMBERED
UMPIRED
UNACTED
UNADDED
UNAIDED
UNAIMED
UNAIRED
UNARMED
UNASKED
UNAXLED
UNBAKED
UNBALED
UNBARED
UNBASED
UNBATED
UNBEARD
UNBLUED
UNBONED
UNBORED
UNBOUND
UNBOWED
UNBOXED
UNBRAID
UNBUILD
UNCAGED
UNCAKED
UNCANED
UNCAPED
UNCASED
UNCEDED
UNCITED
UNCLOUD
UNCODED
UNCORED
UNCOWED
UNCRIED
UNCURED
UNDARED
UNDATED
UNDAZED
UNDEWED
UNDIKED
UNDOMED
UNDRIED
UNDUPED
UNEAVED
UNEBBED
UNEDGED
UNENDED
UNFACED
UNFADED
UNFAKED
UNFAMED
UNFATED
UNFAZED
UNFETED
UNFILED
UNFINED
UNFIRED
UNFIXED
UNFLUID
UNFOUND
UNFOXED
UNFREED
UNFRIED
UNFUSED
UNGATED
UNGLUED
UNGORED
UNGRAND
UNGUARD
UNGUYED
UNGYVED
UNHATED
UNHAYED
UNHAZED
UNHEARD
UNHEWED
UNHIRED
UNHONED
UNHOPED
UNHUMID
UNIFIED
UNINKED
UNITARD
UNJADED
UNJOYED
UNKEYED
UNLACED
UNLADED
UNLAVED
UNLAXED
UNLIKED
UNLINED
UNLIVED
UNLOBED
UNLOVED
UNLUCID
UNLURED
UNMANED
UNMATED
UNMEWED
UNMIKED
UNMINED
UNMIRED
UNMIXED
UNMOULD
UNMOVED
UNMOWED
UNMUTED
UNNAMED
UNNOSED
UNNOTED
UNOGLED
UNOILED
UNOPTED
UNORBED
UNOWNED
UNPACED
UNPAGED
UNPALED
UNPARED
UNPAVED
UNPAWED
UNPILED
UNPIPED
UNPLIED
UNPOLED
UNPOSED
UNPROUD
UNRAKED
UNRATED
UNRAYED
UNRAZED
UNRIGID
UNRILED
UNRIMED
UNRIVED
UNROBED
UNROPED
UNROUND
UNRULED
UNSATED
UNSAVED
UNSAWED
UNSEWED
UNSHOED
UNSIDED
UNSIZED
UNSOLED
UNSOLID
UNSOUND
UNSOWED
UNSPIED
UNSTAID
UNTAMED
UNTAPED
UNTAXED
UNTILED
UNTIMED
UNTIMID
UNTIRED
UNTONED
UNTREAD
UNTREED
UNTRIED
UNTUNED
UNTYPED
UNURGED
UNVEXED
UNVIVID
UNVOTED
UNVOWED
UNWADED
UNWAGED
UNWAKED
UNWANED
UNWAVED
UNWAXED
UNWIPED
UNWIRED
UNWOOED
UNWOUND
UNYOKED
UNZONED
UPAHEAD
UPBOUND
UPBRAID
UPBUILD
UPDATED
UPDIVED
UPDRIED
UPENDED
UPFIELD
UPGAZED
UPHOARD
UPPILED
UPRATED
UPSIZED
UPSTAND
UPSTOOD
UPTREND
USHAPED
USHERED
USURPED
UTTERED

•UD••••

AUDIBLE
AUDIBLY
AUDILES
AUDITED
AUDITEE
AUDITOR
AUDUBON
BUDDERS
BUDDHAS
BUDDIED
BUDDIES
BUDDING
BUDDYUP
BUDGERS
BUDGETS
BUDGIES
BUDGING
BUDLESS
BUDLIKE
BUDTIME
BUDVASE
BUDWORM
CUDDIES
CUDDLED
CUDDLES
CUDGELS
DUDEDUP
DUDESUP
DUDGEON
EUDEMON
FUDDIES
FUDDLED
FUDDLES
FUDGERS
FUDGING
GUDGEON
HUDDLED
HUDDLER
HUDDLES
JUDAICA
JUDAISM
JUDASES
JUDEANS
JUDELAW
JUDGERS
JUDGING
JUDOIST
JUDOKAS
LUDDISM
LUDDITE
MUDBATH
MUDCATS
MUDDERS
MUDDIED
MUDDIER
MUDDIES
MUDDILY
MUDDING
MUDDLED
MUDDLER
MUDDLES
MUDEELS
MUDFISH
MUDFLAP
MUDFLAT
MUDFLOW
MUDHENS
MUDHOLE
MUDLARK
MUDPACK
MUDPIES
MUDROOM
MUDWASP
NUDGERS
NUDGING
NUDISTS
NUDNIKS
NUDZHED
NUDZHES
PUDDING
PUDDLED
PUDDLES
PUDENCY
PUDGIER
PUDGILY

RUDDERS
RUDDIED
RUDDIER
RUDDILY
RUDOLFI
RUDOLPH
RUDYARD
SUDAFED
SUDBURY
SUDOKUS
SUDSERS
SUDSIER
SUDSING

•U•D•••

AULDSOD
BUDDERS
BUDDHAS
BUDDIED
BUDDIES
BUDDING
BUDDYUP
BUMDEAL
BUNDLED
BUNDLER
BUNDLES
BURDENS
BURDICK
BUYDOWN
CUDDIES
CUDDLED
CUDDLES
CURDIER
CURDING
CURDLED
CURDLER
CURDLES
CUTDOWN
DUEDATE
DUMDUMS
DUNDALK
DUODENA
FUDDIES
FUDDLED
FUDDLES
FUNDERS
FUNDING
GUIDERS
GUIDING
GULDENS
GUMDROP
GUNDOGS
HUDDLED
HUDDLER
HUDDLES
HUMDRUM
HUNDRED
HURDLED
HURDLER
HURDLES
KUNDERA
KURDISH
LUDDISM
LUDDITE
MUDDERS
MUDDIED
MUDDIER
MUDDIES
MUDDILY
MUDDING
MUDDLED
MUDDLER
MUDDLES
MULDAUR
MULDOON
MUNDANE
MURDERS
MURDOCH
OUTDARE
OUTDATE
OUTDOER
OUTDOES
OUTDONE
OUTDOOR
OUTDRAG
OUTDRAW
OUTDREW
OUTDROP
OUTDUEL
PUDDING
PUDDLED
PUDDLES
PUNDITS
PURDUEU
PUTDOWN
QUADRIC
RUBDOWN
RUDDERS
RUDDIED
RUDDIER
RUDDILY
RUNDEEP
RUNDLES
RUNDOWN
SUBDATE
SUBDEBS
SUBDUAL
SUBDUCT
SUBDUED
SUBDUER
SUBDUES
SUEDFOR
SUNDAES
SUNDAYS
SUNDECK
SUNDERS
SUNDIAL
SUNDOGS
SUNDOWN
TUNDRAS

•U••D••

AUBADES
BUILDER
BUILDIN
BUILDON
BUILDUP
BULLDOG
DUDEDUP
DUKEDOM
DUNEDIN
FULLDAY
FUMEDAT
GUARDED
GUARDEE
GUARDER
GUERDON
GUILDER
HUMIDEX
HUMIDLY
HUMIDOR
JULYDAY
JUMADAS
JUNEDAY
JUNKDNA
JURIDIC
LUCIDAE
LUCIDLY
LUREDIN
LURIDLY
MUSEDON
MUSTDOS
MUTEDLY
OUTADDS
OUTEDGE
QUONDAM
RUANDAS
RUBADUB
RUBYDEE
RULEDBY
RULEDON
RUNSDRY
RUSHDIE
SUBIDEA
SUCKDRY
TUESDAY
TUNEDIN
TUNEDTO
TUNEDUP
TUXEDOS

•U•••D•

AUGENDS
BURUNDI
BUSHIDO
BUSRIDE
CUBOIDS
CUEBIDS
CUSPIDS
CUSTODY
FURTADO
LUCINDA
MUSCIDA
NUCLIDE
OUTADDS
OUTBIDS
OUTBUDS
OUTMODE
OUTRIDE
OUTRODE
OUTSIDE
QUERIDA
QUERIDO
SUBCODE
SUBGODS
SUBLIDS
SUBSIDE
SUBSIDY
SULFIDE
SUNGODS
SUREIDO

•U••••D

AUDITED
AUGURED
AULDSOD
BUBBLED
BUCKLED
BUDDIED
BUGEYED
BULLIED
BUMBLED
BUNCHED
BUNCOED
BUNDLED
BUNGLED
BUNKBED
BUNKOED
BURBLED
BURGLED
BUSLOAD
BUSTARD
BUSTLED
BUTGOOD
BUZZARD
CUDDLED
CUECARD
CULLIED
CUPELED
CURATED
CURDLED
CURRIED
CUSTARD
DUELLED
DUETTED
DULLARD
DUMMIED
DURWARD
EUCHRED
FUDDLED
FUELLED
FUELROD
FUMBLED
GUARDED
GUESSED
GUESTED
GULLIED
GUMWOOD
GURGLED
GUSSIED
GUZZLED
HUBBARD
HUDDLED
HULLOED
HUMBARD
HUMBLED
HUMORED
HUMPHED
HUNCHED
HUNDRED
HURDLED
HURRIED
HURTLED
HUSBAND
HUSTLED
JUGBAND
JUGGLED
JUGHEAD
JUMBLED
JUMPBID
JUTLAND
LUNATED
LUNCHED
LURCHED
LUSTRED
LUXATED
MUDDIED
MUDDLED
MUFFLED
MULCHED
MULCTED
MUMBLED
MUMFORD
MUNCHED
MURALED
MUSCLED
MUSTARD
MUTATED
MUZZLED
NUANCED
NUDZHED
NUNHOOD
NUTATED
NUTWOOD
NUZZLED
OUTAWED
OUTBEND
OUTBRED
OUTCOLD
OUTFEED
OUTFIND
OUTLAID
OUTLAND
OUTLEAD
OUTLOUD
OUTPAID
OUTPLOD
OUTREAD
OUTSAID
OUTSOLD
OUTSPED
OUTTOLD
OUTVIED
OUTWARD
OUTWEED
OUTWIND
OUTWORD
PUDDLED
PUMICED
PUNCHED
PUPATED
PURFLED
PURPLED
PURSUED
PUSHROD
PUTTIED
PUZZLED
QUACKED
QUAFFED
QUAILED
QUASHED
QUEENED
QUEERED
QUELLED
QUERIED
QUESTED
QUIETED
QUILLED
QUILTED
QUIPPED
QUIRTED
QUITTED
QUIZZED
QUOINED
QUOITED
RUBYRED
RUDDIED
RUDYARD
RUFFLED
RUMBAED
RUMBLED
RUMFORD
RUMORED
RUMPEND
RUMPLED
RUNWILD
RUSTLED
RUTLAND
SUBARID
SUBBAND
SUBDUED
SUBHEAD
SUBTEND
SUCCEED
SUDAFED
SUGARED
SULLIED
SUMMAND
SUNBIRD
SUNMAID
SUNWARD
SUPPLED
SUSPEND
SUTURED
TUMBLED
TURNBAD
TURNRED
TURTLED
TUSSAUD
TUSSLED
TUTORED

••UD•••

ALUDELS
AOUDADS
BLUDGED
BLUDGER
BLUDGES
BOUDINS
BOUDOIR
CAUDATE
CRUDELY
CRUDEST
CRUDITY
CRUDSUP
DRUDGED
DRUDGER
DRUDGES
ELUDERS
ELUDING
ERUDITE
EXUDATE
EXUDING
FEUDING
FEUDIST
FOUDRES
GAUDENS
GAUDERY
GAUDIER
GAUDIES
GAUDILY
GRUDGED
GRUDGER
GRUDGES
HOUDINI
KLUDGED
KLUDGES
LAUDERS
LAUDING
LOUDENS
LOUDEST
LOUDISH
MAUDLIN
POUDRES
PRUDENT
PRUDERY
PRUDHOE
PRUDISH
SCUDDED
SCUDDER
SHUDDER
SLUDGES
SMUDGED
SMUDGES
STUDDED
STUDENT
STUDIED
STUDIER
STUDIES
STUDIOS
THUDDED
TRUDEAU
TRUDGED
TRUDGEN
TRUDGER
TRUDGES
VAUDOIS

••U•D••

ARUNDEL
ASUNDER
BLUNDEN
BLUNDER
BOULDER
BOUNDED
BOUNDER
BOUNDTO
BOUNDUP
CLUEDIN
COULDBE
COULDNT
DRUIDIC
ECUADOR
FLUBDUB
FLUIDAL
FLUIDIC
FLUIDLY
FOUNDED
FOUNDER
FOUNDRY
FOURDAY
GLUEDON
GLUEDTO
GOUNDER
GOURDES
HOUNDED
HOUNDER
HYUNDAI
JOURDAN
LAUNDER
LAUNDRY
LOURDES
MAULDIN
MAUNDER
MOULDED
MOULDER
MOUNDED
PLUNDER
POUNDED
POUNDER
ROUNDED
ROUNDEL
ROUNDER
ROUNDLY
ROUNDON
ROUNDUP
SCUDDED
SCUDDER
SHUDDER
SOUNDED
SOUNDER
SOUNDLY
STUDDED
THUDDED
THUNDER
TRUEDUP
TRUNDLE
WOULDBE
WOULDNT
WOULDST
WOUNDED
WOUNDUP

••U••D•

AOUDADS
CRUSADE
CRUZADO
EDUARDO
ISUREDO
ROULADE
STUPIDS
YOUANDI

••U•••D

ABUTTED
AVULSED
BAULKED
BLUDGED
BLUERED
BLUFFED
BLUNTED
BLURRED
BLURTED
BLUSHED
BOUGHED
BOUNCED
BOUNDED
BRUISED
BRUITED
BRUSHED
CAULKED
CHUCKED
CHUFFED
CHUGGED
CHUMMED
CHUMPED
CHUNKED
CHURNED
CLUBBED
CLUBMED
CLUCKED
CLUMPED
CLUNKED
COUCHED
COUGHED
COUNTED
COUPLED
COURSED
COURTED
CRUISED
CRUMBED
CRUMPED
CRUSHED
CRUSTED
DAUNTED
DOUBLED
DOUBTED
DRUBBED
DRUDGED
DRUGGED
DRUMMED
EDUCTED
EQUALED
EQUATED
ERUCTED
ERUPTED
EVULSED
EXULTED
FAULTED
FLUBBED
FLUFFED
FLUNKED
FLUSHED
FOULARD
FOUNDED
FRUITED
GLUGGED
GLUMMED
GLUTTED
GRUBBED
GRUDGED
GRUMPED
GRUNTED
HAUNTED
HOUNDED
IGUANID
JAUNTED
JOUNCED
JOUSTED
KLUDGED
KNURLED
LAUGHED
LOUNGED
LOUREED
LOUVRED
MOULDED
MOULTED
MOUNDED
MOUNTED
MOURNED
MOUSSED
MOUTHED
PLUCKED
PLUGGED
PLUMBED
PLUMPED
PLUNGED
PLUNKED
POUCHED
POUNCED
POUNDED
REUPPED
REURGED
ROUGHED
ROUNDED
ROUSTED
SAUNAED
SAUTEED
SCUBAED
SCUDDED
SCUFFED
SCULLED
SCULPED
SHUCKED
SHUNNED
SHUNTED
SHUSHED
SKULKED
SKULLED
SKUNKED
SLUGGED
SLUICED
SLUMMED
SLUMPED
SLURPED
SLURRED
SLUSHED
SMUDGED
SMUSHED
SNUBBED
SNUFFED
SNUGGED
SOUNDED
SOURCED
SPURNED
SPURRED
SPURTED
SQUALID
SQUARED
SQUIRED
STUBBED
STUDDED
STUDIED
STUFFED
STUMPED
STUNNED
STUNTED
TAUNTED
THUDDED
THUMBED
THUMPED
THUNKED
TOUCHED
TOUSLED
TRUCKED
TRUDGED
TRUMPED
TRUSSED
TRUSTED
UNURGED
USURPED
VAULTED
VAUNTED
VOUCHED
WHUPPED
WOUNDED

•••UD••

ACAUDAL
ADJUDGE
ALLUDED
ALLUDES
CLAUDEL
CLAUDIA
CLAUDIO
CLOUDED
CLOUDUP
DELUDED
DELUDER
DELUDES
DENUDED
DENUDER
DENUDES
ELFUDGE
ESCUDOS
ILLUDED
ILLUDES
INCUDES
MENUDOS
MYBUDDY
OHFUDGE
PALUDAL
PLAUDIT
PROUDER
PROUDLY
PROUDOF
REAUDIT
REJUDGE
STRUDEL
UNMUDDY
WHAUDEN

•••U•D•

ABOUNDS
ALBUNDY
BURUNDI
DEFUNDS
EDMUNDI
EDMUNDS
ELMUNDO
EMQUADS
ENQUADS
GERUNDS
GROUNDS
LIQUIDS
MCMURDO
MYBUDDY
OBTUNDS
OSMUNDS
REFUNDS
REGUIDE
ROTUNDA
SHOULDA
SHOULDI
TVGUIDE
UNMUDDY
YAOUNDE

•••U••D

ABDUCED
ABJURED
ACCUSED
ADDUCED
ADJURED
ALLUDED
ALLURED
AROUSED
ASSUMED
ASSURED
ATTUNED
AUGURED
BEMUSED
BLOUSED
CLOUDED
CLOUTED
DEBUTED
DEDUCED
DEFUSED
DELUDED
DELUGED
DENUDED
DEPUTED
DETUNED
DILUTED
DISUSED
EDOUARD
EFFUSED
ENDURED
ENSURED
EXCUSED
EXHUMED
FIGURED
FLOURED
FLOUTED
FOCUSED
GROUPED
GROUSED
GROUTED
HOCUSED
ILLUDED
ILLUMED
ILLUSED
IMMURED
IMPUTED
INCUSED
INDUCED
INFUSED
INHUMED
INJURED
INSURED
ISSUEAD
KNOUTED
MANURED
MATURED
MINUEND
MINUTED
MISUSED
NATURED
NODULED
NOTUSED
ONGUARD
PERUSED
POPUPAD
REBUILD
REBUKED
RECURED
RECUSED
REDUCED
REFUGED
REFUSED
REFUTED
RELUMED
REPUTED
RESUMED
RETUNED
SALUTED
SCOURED
SCOUTED
SECURED
SEDUCED
SHOUTED
SNOUTED
SPOUTED
SPRUCED
SUTURED
TENURED
TROUPED
UNBUILD
UNCURED
UNDUPED
UNFUSED
UNGUARD
UNGUYED
UNHUMID
UNLUCID
UNLURED
UNMUTED
UNRULED
UNTUNED
UPBUILD
VOLUMED
VOLUTED

••••UD•

BARBUDA
BERMUDA
COLLUDE
DETRUDE
DISBUDS
EARBUDS
EXCLUDE
EXTRUDE
HEYJUDE
INCLUDE
INTRUDE
MARAUDS
OBTRUDE
OCCLUDE
OUTBUDS
PRELUDE
REDBUDS
RESTUDY
SECLUDE
SHROUDS
ULANUDE
UNCRUDE
UNGAUDY

••••U•D

ACCRUED
AGROUND
ASTOUND
CASQUED
CLIQUED

COFOUND
EANMUND
EMBRUED
ENGLUND
ENWOUND
EXPOUND
FONDUED
GOROUND
IMBRUED
IMPOUND
INBOUND
LANGUID
LEAGUED
MIAOUED
MISCUED
OROTUND
PINGUID
PLAGUED
PREFUND
PREVUED
PURSUED
REBOUND
REDOUND
REFOUND
REGLUED
RESCUED
RESOUND
REWOUND
SIGMUND
SNAFUED
SUBDUED
TORQUED
UNBLUED
UNBOUND
UNFLUID
UNFOUND
UNGLUED
UNMOULD
UNROUND
UNSOUND
UNWOUND
UPBOUND

•••••UD

APPLAUD
BECLOUD
BESTBUD
DEFRAUD
DRFREUD
GIELGUD
IBNSAUD
MALAMUD
MCCLOUD
MILHAUD
MILKDUD
OUTLOUD
REYNAUD
RIMBAUD
ROSABUD
ROSEBUD
STCLOUD
TUSSAUD
UNCLOUD
UNPROUD

U•E••••

UKELELE
UNEAGER
UNEARTH
UNEASES
UNEATEN
UNEAVED
UNEBBED
UNEDGED
UNEDGES
UNEMPTY
UNENDED
UNEQUAL
UNERECT
UPEARLY
UPENDED
USEDCAR
USEDCDS
USEDFOR
USELESS
USERFEE
USERIDS
USESFOR
UTENSIL

U••E•••

UCCELLO
UMBERED
UMBERTO
UNBEARD
UNBELDI
UNBELTS
UNBENCH
UNBENDS
UNBERTH
UNBESET
UNCEDED
UNDEALT
UNDERDO
UNDERGO
UNDEWED
UNFENCE
UNFERTH
UNFETED
UNHEADY
UNHEARD
UNHEAVY
UNHEEDS
UNHELMS
UNHEWED
UNKEMPT
UNKEYED
UNLEADS
UNLEAFS
UNLEAKY
UNLEARN
UNLEASH
UNLEGAL
UNLEVEL
UNMEANT
UNMERGE
UNMERRY
UNMEWED
UNNEEDY
UNNERVE
UNPEELS
UNREADY
UNREELS
UNREGAL
UNRESTS
UNSEALS
UNSEAMS
UNSEATS
UNSELLS
UNSEWED
UNTEACH
UNTENSE
UNTERSE
UNVEILS
UNVENAL
UNVEXED
UNWEARY
UNWEAVE
UNWEDGE
UPBEARS
UPBEATS
UPHEAPS
UPHEAVE
UPKEEPS
UPLEAPS
UPLEAPT
UPREACH
UPREARS
UPSENDS
UPTEARS
UPTEMPO
UPWELLS
URGEDON
URGENCY
URGESON
URTEXTS
USHERED
USHERIN
USTEDES
UTRECHT
UTTERED
UTTERER
UTTERLY

U•••E••

UGLIEST
UKELELE
UKULELE
ULSTERS
UMPTEEN
UNADEPT
UNALERT
UNBLENT
UNBLEST
UNCHECK
UNCLEAN
UNCLEAR
UNCLEFT
UNDOERS
UNDRESS
UNERECT
UNFIERY
UNFREED
UNFREES
UNGREEN
UNGUENT
UNHEEDS
UNIDEAL
UNINERT
UNITERS
UNNEEDY
UNOBESE
UNOVERT
UNPEELS
UNPIETY
UNREELS
UNSHEER
UNSHELL
UNSKEWS
UNSLEEK
UNSPEAK
UNSPELT
UNSPENT
UNSTEEL
UNSTEPS
UNSTERN
UNSWEAR
UNSWEET
UNSWEPT
UNTIERS
UNTREAD
UNTREED
UNWHEEL
UPAHEAD
UPFIELD
UPKEEPS
UPSTEPS
UPSWEEP
UPSWELL
UPSWEPT
UPTHERE
UPTREND
USELESS
USOPENS
USSTEEL
USURERS

U••••E•

ULLAGES
ULYSSES
UMBERED
UMBRIEL
UMPIRED
UMPIRES
UMPTEEN
UNACTED
UNADDED
UNAIDED
UNAIMED
UNAIRED
UNARMED
UNASKED
UNAXLED
UNBAKED
UNBALED
UNBALES
UNBARED
UNBARES
UNBASED
UNBATED
UNBESET
UNBLUED
UNBONED
UNBORED
UNBOWED
UNBOXED
UNBOXES
UNBRIEF
UNCAGED
UNCAGES
UNCAKED
UNCAKES
UNCANED
UNCAPED
UNCASED
UNCASES
UNCEDED
UNCITED
UNCODED
UNCORED
UNCORES
UNCOVER
UNCOWED
UNCOYER
UNCRIED
UNCRUEL
UNCURED
UNDARED
UNDATED
UNDAZED
UNDEWED
UNDIKED
UNDINES
UNDOMED
UNDRIED
UNDUPED
UNEAGER
UNEASES
UNEATEN
UNEAVED
UNEBBED
UNEDGED
UNEDGES
UNENDED
UNFACED
UNFADED
UNFAKED
UNFAMED
UNFATED
UNFAZED
UNFETED
UNFILED
UNFILES
UNFINED
UNFINES
UNFIRED
UNFIXED
UNFIXES
UNFOXED
UNFREED
UNFREES
UNFRIED
UNFUSED
UNGATED
UNGIVEN
UNGLUED
UNGLUES
UNGORED
UNGREEN
UNGUYED
UNGYVED
UNHATED
UNHAYED
UNHAZED
UNHEWED
UNHIRED
UNHIRES
UNHONED
UNHOPED
UNIATES
UNIFIED
UNIFIER
UNIFIES
UNINKED
UNIPLEX
UNIQUES
UNITIES
UNJADED
UNJOYED
UNKEYED
UNLACED
UNLACES
UNLADED
UNLADEN
UNLADES
UNLAVED
UNLAXED
UNLAXES
UNLEVEL
UNLIKED
UNLIKES
UNLINED
UNLIVED
UNLIVES
UNLOBED
UNLOVED
UNLURED
UNMAKER
UNMAKES
UNMANED
UNMATED
UNMATES
UNMEWED
UNMIKED
UNMINED
UNMIRED
UNMITER
UNMIXED
UNMIXES
UNMOVED
UNMOWED
UNMUTED
UNNAMED
UNNOSED
UNNOTED
UNNOVEL
UNOFTEN
UNOGLED
UNOILED
UNOPTED
UNORBED
UNOWNED
UNPACED
UNPAGED
UNPALED
UNPARED
UNPAVED
UNPAWED
UNPILED
UNPILES
UNPIPED
UNPLIED
UNPOLED
UNPOSED
UNQUIET
UNRAKED
UNRATED
UNRAVEL
UNRAYED
UNRAZED
UNRILED
UNRIMED
UNRIPER
UNRISEN
UNRIVED
UNRIVEN
UNROBED
UNROBES
UNROPED
UNROPES
UNRULED
UNSAFER
UNSATED
UNSAVED
UNSAWED
UNSCREW
UNSEWED
UNSHEER
UNSHIER
UNSHOED
UNSHOES
UNSHYER
UNSIDED
UNSIZED
UNSLEEK
UNSLIER
UNSLYER
UNSOBER
UNSOLED
UNSOLES
UNSOWED
UNSPIED
UNSTEEL
UNSWEET
UNTAKEN
UNTAMED
UNTAMES
UNTAPED
UNTAPES
UNTAXED
UNTAXES
UNTILED
UNTIMED
UNTIRED
UNTONED
UNTREED
UNTRIED
UNTRUER
UNTUNED
UNTUNES
UNTYPED
UNURGED
UNVEXED
UNVOTED
UNVOWED
UNWADED
UNWAGED
UNWAKED
UNWANED
UNWAVED
UNWAXED
UNWHEEL
UNWIPED
UNWIRED
UNWISER
UNWOOED
UNWOVEN
UNYOKED
UNYOKES
UNZONED
UNZONES
UPATREE
UPDATED
UPDATER
UPDATES
UPDIVED
UPDIVES
UPDRIED
UPDRIES
UPENDED
UPGAZED
UPGAZES
UPPILED
UPPILES
UPRATED
UPRATES
UPRISEN
UPRISER
UPRISES
UPRIVER
UPSIDES
UPSIZED
UPSIZES
UPSWEEP
UPTAKES
UPTIMES
URBANER
USABLES
USANCES
USERFEE
USHAPED
USHAPES
USHERED
USSTEEL
USTEDES
USURIES
USURPED
USURPER
UTTERED
UTTERER
UVALUES
UVINDEX

U•••••E

UKELELE
UKRAINE
UKULELE
ULALUME
ULANUDE
ULULATE
UMBRAGE
UNAGILE
UNALIKE
UNALONE
UNAWAKE
UNAWARE
UNBLADE
UNBORNE
UNBRACE
UNBRAKE
UNBRAVE
UNBROKE
UNCHOKE
UNCLOSE
UNCRATE
UNCRUDE
UNDRAPE
UNFENCE
UNFROZE
UNGLOVE
UNGULAE
UNHINGE
UNHORSE
UNHOUSE
UNICODE
UNISIZE
UNITISE
UNITIVE
UNITIZE
UNLARGE
UNLOOSE
UNMERGE
UNMITRE
UNNAIVE
UNNERVE
UNOBESE
UNPASTE
UNQUOTE
UNRHYME
UNSHADE
UNSPOKE
UNSTATE
UNSWORE
UNTENSE
UNTERSE
UNTRITE
UNTWINE
UNVAGUE
UNVOICE
UNWEAVE
UNWEDGE
UNWHITE
UNWHOLE
UPABOVE
UPATREE
UPBORNE
UPCCODE
UPCLOSE
UPCURVE
UPGRADE
UPHEAVE
UPPHASE
UPRAISE
UPROUSE
UPSCALE
UPSLOPE
UPSTAGE
UPSTARE
UPSTATE
UPSURGE
UPTHERE
UPTRADE
UPVALUE
URANITE
URNLIKE
USERFEE
USSTATE
UTILISE
UTILIZE

•UE••••

BUELLER
CUEBALL
CUEBIDS
CUECARD
CUESTAS
CUETIPS
DUEDATE
DUEEAST
DUELERS
DUELING
DUELIST
DUELLED
DUENNAS
DUETING
DUETTED
DUETTOS
DUEWEST
FUELERS
FUELING
FUELLED
FUELOIL
FUELROD
FUELSUP
FUENTES
GUERDON
GUESSAT
GUESSED
GUESSER
GUESSES
GUESSSO
GUESTED
GUEVARA
HUELESS
MUELLER
MUESLIS
MUESLIX
MUEZZIN
NUESTRA
NUESTRO
PUEBLOS
PUERILE
QUECHUA
QUEENED
QUEENIE
QUEENIT
QUEENLY
QUEERED
QUEERER
QUEERLY
QUEIROS
QUELLED
QUELLER
QUELQUE
QUENEAU
QUENTIN
QUEPASA
QUERIDA
QUERIDO
QUERIED
QUERIER
QUERIES
QUERIST
QUESERA
QUESNAY
QUESTED
QUESTER
QUETZAL
QUEUERS
QUEUEUP
QUEUING
SUEDFOR
SUELLEN
SUELYON
SUESFOR
TUESDAY

•U•E•••

AUBERGE
AUGENDS
AULETTA
AUREATE
AUREOLA
AUREOLE
AUTEURS
BUGEYED
BUREAUS
BUREAUX
BURETTE
BUTENES
CULEXES
CUNEATE
CUPELED
CUPELER
CUREALL
CURETTE
CUVETTE
DUDEDUP
DUDESUP
DUEEAST
DUKEDOM
DUNEDIN
DUTEOUS
EUCERIN
EUDEMON
EUGENIA
EUGENIC
EUGENIE
EUREKAS
EUTERPE
FUMEDAT
FUMESAT
FUSEBOX
HUMERAL
HUMERUS
JUDEANS
JUDELAW
JUKEBOX
JUNEBUG
JUNEDAY
JUVENAL
KUBELIK
LUBEJOB
LUCENCY
LUCERNE
LUCETTA
LUNESTA
LUNETTE
LUREDIN
LURESIN
LUREXES
LUTETIA
MUDEELS
MUJERES
MULETAS
MUMESON
MUSEDON
MUSEFUL
MUSESON
MUSETTA
MUSETTE
MUSEUMS
MUTEDLY
NUMERAL
NUMERIC
NUMEROS
NUREYEV
OUTEARN
OUTEATS
OUTECHO
OUTEDGE
PUBERTY
PUDENCY
PUTEMUP
QUEENED
QUEENIE
QUEENIT
QUEENLY
QUEERED
QUEERER
QUEERLY
QUIETED
QUIETEN
QUIETER
QUIETLY
QUIETUS
RUBELLA
RUBEOLA
RULEDBY
RULEDON
RULEONE
RULEOUT
RULESON
SUBECHO
SUPERGS
SUREBET
SURECAN
SUREIAM
SUREIDO
SUREROF
SUZETTE
TUBEPAN
TUBETOP
TUMESCE
TUNEDIN
TUNEDTO
TUNEDUP
TUNEFUL
TUNEOUT
TUNESIN
TUNESTO
TUNESUP
TUNEUPS
TUPELOS
TUREENS
TUTELAR
TUXEDOS
VUMETER
YULELOG

•U••E••

AUGMENT
AUKLETS
AUSLESE
AUSTERE
AUSTERS
BUCKERS
BUCKETS
BUCKEYE
BUDDERS
BUDGERS
BUDGETS
BUDLESS
BUFFERS
BUFFEST
BUFFETS
BUFFETT
BUGBEAR
BUGLERS
BULLETS
BUMDEAL
BUMLEGS
BUMMERS
BUMPERS
BUNGEES
BUNKERS
BUNTERS
BUNUELO
BURDENS
BURGEES
BURGEON
BURGERS
BURGESS
BURIERS
BURLERS
BURMESE
BURNERS
BURNETT
BUSCEMI
BUSHELS
BUSHERS
BUSIEST
BUSKERS
BUSSERS
BUSTERS
BUTLERS
BUTTEMT
BUTTERS
BUTTERY
BUZZELL
BUZZERS
CUDGELS
CULLERS
CULLETS
CULVERT
CUMBERS
CURFEWS
CURLERS
CURLEWS
CURRENT
CURSEAT
CURSERS
CURTEST
CURVETS
CUSSERS
CUSTERS
CUTLERS
CUTLERY
CUTLETS
CUTTERS
DUBBERS
DUBIETY
DUCHESS
DUCKERS

DUDGEON
DUELERS
DUEWEST
DUFFELS
DUFFERS
DULLEST
DUMBEST
DUMPERS
DUNGEON
DUNKERS
DUNNERS
DUODENA
DURRELL
DURWENT
DUSTERS
EUGLENA
FUDGERS
FUELERS
FULGENT
FULLEST
FULNESS
FUMIEST
FUNDERS
FUNFEST
FUNNELS
FURLERS
FURLESS
FURNESS
FURSEAL
FUSSERS
GUDGEON
GUIDERS
GUINEAN
GUINEAS
GULDENS
GULLETS
GULPERS
GUMLESS
GUNBELT
GUNLESS
GUNNERS
GUNNERY
GUNSELS
GURNEYS
GUSHERS
GUSSETS
GUTLESS
GUTTERS
HUBBELL
HUELESS
HUGGERS
HULLERS
HUMBERT
HUMMELS
HUMMERS
HUMVEES
HUNGERS
HUNKERS
HUNTERS
HUPPERT
HURLERS
HURTERS
HUSKERS
HUSSEIN
HUSSERL
HUYGENS
JUDGERS
JUGHEAD
JUICERS
JUICEUP
JUMPERS
JUNKERS
JUNKETS
JURGENS
JUSTEST
KUCHENS
KUMMELS
KUNDERA
KURRENT
KUZNETS
LUBBERS
LUGGERS
LULLERS
LUMBERS
LUMIERE
LUMPERS
LUNGEAT
LUNGERS
LUNKERS
LURKERS
LURLEEN
LUSHEST
LUSTERS
MUCKERS
MUDDERS
MUDEELS
MUDHENS
MUGGERS
MULLERS
MULLETS
MUMMERS
MUMMERY
MUPPETS
MURDERS
MURIELS
MUSHERS
MUSKEGO
MUSKETS
MUSSELS
MUSTERS
MUTTERS
NUBBERS
NUCLEAR
NUCLEIC
NUCLEON
NUCLEUS
NUDGERS
NUGGETS
NUGGETY
NUMBERS
NUMBEST
NUNNERY
NURSERS
NURSERY
NUTLETS
NUTMEAT
NUTMEGS
NUTTERS
OURSELF
OUSTERS
OUTBEAM
OUTBEGS
OUTBEND
OUTFEED
OUTFEEL
OUTHEAR
OUTHERE
OUTJEST
OUTJETS
OUTKEEP
OUTKEPT
OUTLEAD
OUTLEAP
OUTLETS
OUTPEEP
OUTREAD
OUTSEEK
OUTSEEN
OUTSEES
OUTSELL
OUTSERT
OUTSETS
OUTTEAR
OUTTELL
OUTWEAR
OUTWEED
OUTWEEP
OUTWELL
OUTWENT
OUTWEPT
OUTWEST
OUTYELL
OUTYELP
PUCKERS
PUCKERY
PUCKETT
PUFFERS
PUFFERY
PULLERS
PULLETS
PULLEYS
PULPERS
PUMMELS
PUMPERS
PUNGENT
PUNIEST
PUNKERS
PUNLESS
PUNNERS
PUNTERS
PUPPETS
PUPTENT
PURCELL
PURRERS
PURSERS
PURVEYS
PUSHERS
PUTREFY
PUTTEES
PUTTERS
QUAKERS
QUAVERS
QUAVERY
QUENEAU
QUESERA
QUEUERS
QUEUEUP
QUINELA
QUITESO
QUIVERS
QUIVERY
QUOTEES
QUOTERS
RUBBERS
RUBBERY
RUCKERT
RUDDERS
RUINERS
RULIEST
RUMLESS
RUMMERS
RUMPEND
RUNDEEP
RUNLESS
RUNLETS
RUNNELS
RUNNERS
RUNNETH
RUSHEES
RUSHERS
RUSSELL
RUSSERT
RUSSETS
RUSSETY
RUTGERS
RUTTERS
SUAVELY
SUAVEST
SUBCELL
SUBDEBS
SUBHEAD
SUBJECT
SUBLETS
SUBNETS
SUBSECT
SUBSETS
SUBTEEN
SUBTEND
SUBTEXT
SUBVENE
SUBVERT
SUBZERO
SUCCEED
SUCCESS
SUCKERS
SUDSERS
SUFFERS
SUGGEST
SULKERS
SUMLESS
SUMMERS
SUMMERY
SUNBEAM
SUNBELT
SUNDECK
SUNDERS
SUNLESS
SUNSETS
SUPPERS
SUPREME
SURFEIT
SURFERS
SURGEON
SURGERY
SURREAL
SURREYS
SURVEIL
SURVEYS
SUSPECT
SUSPEND
TUCKERS
TUFFETS
TUGGERS
TUGLESS
TUNNELS
TUREENS
TURKEYS
TURNERS
TURNERY
TURRETS
TUSHERY
TUSKERS

•U•••E•

AUBADES
AUDILES
AUDITED
AUDITEE
AUGITES
AUGURED
AUGURER
AUNTBEE
AUNTIES
AURALEE
AUSSIES
AUTOPEN
BUBBLED
BUBBLES
BUCHNER
BUCKLED
BUCKLES
BUCKLEY
BUCKNER
BUCKOES
BUDDIED
BUDDIES
BUDGIES
BUELLER
BUGEYED
BUGFREE
BUGGIER
BUGGIES
BUGGLES
BUILDER
BUJONES
BULBLET
BULGIER
BULKIER
BULLIED
BULLIES
BULLPEN
BUMBLED
BUMBLER
BUMBLES
BUMPIER
BUNCHED
BUNCHES
BUNCOED
BUNDLED
BUNDLER
BUNDLES
BUNGEES
BUNGLED
BUNGLER
BUNGLES
BUNKBED
BUNKOED
BUNNIES
BURBLED
BURBLER
BURBLES
BURGEES
BURGHER
BURGLED
BURGLES
BURLIER
BURNLEY
BURRIER
BURSTER
BUSBIES
BUSHIER
BUSHMEN
BUSTIER
BUSTLED
BUSTLER
BUSTLES
BUSYBEE
BUTANES
BUTCHER
BUTCHES
BUTENES
BUZZIER
CUBAGES
CUBBIES
CUDDIES
CUDDLED
CUDDLES
CULCHES
CULEXES
CULLIED
CULLIES
CUPELED
CUPELER
CUPPIER
CUPULES
CURARES
CURATED
CURATES
CURDIER
CURDLED
CURDLER
CURDLES
CURLIER
CURRIED
CURRIER
CURRIES
CURTSEY
CURVIER
CUSHIER
CUSSLER
CUTISES
CUTOPEN
CUTOVER
DUCHIES
DUCKIER
DUCKIES
DUELLED
DUETTED
DUFFLES
DUFUSES
DUHAMEL
DUMMIED
DUMMIES
DUMPIER
DUSKIER
DUSTIER
DUSTMEN
EUCHRED
EUCHRES
FUBSIER
FUDDIES
FUDDLED
FUDDLES
FUELLED
FUENTES
FUMBLED
FUMBLER
FUMBLES
FUNGOES
FUNKIER
FUNNIER
FUNNIES
FUNPLEX
FUNSTER
FURORES
FURRIER
FURTHER
FUSSIER
FUSTIER
FUTURES
FUZZIER
GUARDED
GUARDEE
GUARDER
GUCKIER
GUESSED
GUESSER
GUESSES
GUESTED
GUILDER
GULCHES
GULLIED
GULLIES
GULPIER
GUMMIER
GUMTREE
GUNITES
GUNKIER
GUNNIES
GUNTHER
GUNUSER
GUPPIES
GURGLED
GURGLES
GUSHIER
GUSSIED
GUSSIES
GUSTIER
GUSTOES
GUTSIER
GUTTIER
GUZZLED
GUZZLER
GUZZLES
HUBBIES
HUDDLED
HUDDLER
HUDDLES
HUFFIER
HUGGIES
HULKIER
HULLOED
HUMBLED
HUMBLER
HUMBLES
HUMIDEX
HUMORED
HUMPHED
HUMPIER
HUMUSES
HUMVEES
HUNCHED
HUNCHES
HUNDRED
HUNGTEN
HUNKIER
HUNTLEY
HURDLED
HURDLER
HURDLES
HURRIED
HURRIER
HURRIES
HURTLED
HURTLES
HUSKIER
HUSKIES
HUSSIES
HUSTLED
HUSTLER
HUSTLES
HUTCHES
JUBILEE
JUDASES
JUGGLED
JUGGLER
JUGGLES
JUICIER
JUILLET
JUJUBES
JUMBLED
JUMBLER
JUMBLES
JUMPIER
JUNCOES
JUNGLES
JUNIPER
JUNKIER
JUNKIES
JUNKMEN
JUPITER
JURYMEN
KURILES
KUTCHER
LUCIFER
LUCITES
LUCKIER
LUMPIER
LUNATED
LUNATES
LUNCHED
LUNCHER
LUNCHES
LUPINES
LURCHED
LURCHER
LURCHES
LUREXES
LURLEEN
LUSHIER
LUSTIER
LUSTRED
LUSTRES
LUTHIER
LUXATED
LUXATES
MUCKIER
MUDDIED
MUDDIER
MUDDIES
MUDDLED
MUDDLER
MUDDLES
MUDPIES
MUELLER
MUFFLED
MUFFLER
MUFFLES
MUGGIER
MUGGLES
MUJERES
MULCHED
MULCHES
MULCTED
MULGREW
MUMBLED
MUMBLER
MUMBLES
MUMMIES
MUNCHED
MUNCHEN
MUNCHER
MUNCHES
MUNSTER
MURALED
MURKIER
MUSCLED
MUSCLES
MUSHIER
MUSKIER
MUSKIES
MUSSIER
MUSTIER
MUSTSEE
MUTAGEN
MUTATED
MUTATES
MUYBIEN
MUZZIER
MUZZLED
MUZZLER
MUZZLES
NUANCED
NUANCES
NUBBIER
NUBBLES
NUDZHED
NUDZHES
NULLSET
NUNGWEN
NUREYEV
NUTATED
NUTATES
NUTSIER
NUTTIER
NUTTREE
NUZZLED
NUZZLER
NUZZLES
OUTAGES
OUTAWED
OUTAWES
OUTBRED
OUTDOER
OUTDOES
OUTDREW
OUTDUEL
OUTFEED
OUTFEEL
OUTFLEE
OUTGOES
OUTGREW
OUTKEEP
OUTLIER
OUTLIES
OUTPEEP
OUTSEEK
OUTSEEN
OUTSEES
OUTSPED
OUTSTEP
OUTVIED
OUTVIES
OUTWEED
OUTWEEP
PUDDLED
PUDDLES
PUDGIER
PUFFIER
PUGGLES
PUGSLEY
PULPIER
PUMICED
PUMICES
PUNCHED
PUNCHER
PUNCHES
PUNKIER
PUNKIES
PUNNIER
PUNSTER
PUPATED
PUPATES
PUPPIES
PURDUEU
PURFLED
PURFLER
PURFLES
PURLIEU
PURPLED
PURPLES
PURSIER
PURSUED
PURSUER
PURSUES
PURTIER
PURVIEW
PUSHIER
PUSSIES
PUTOVER
PUTTEES
PUTTIED
PUTTIES
PUZZLED
PUZZLER
PUZZLES
QUACKED
QUACKER
QUAFFED
QUAFFER
QUAILED
QUAKIER
QUAKIES
QUARLES
QUARREL
QUARTER
QUARTES
QUARTET
QUASHED
QUASHES
QUATRES
QUEENED
QUEERED
QUEERER
QUELLED
QUELLER
QUERIED
QUERIER
QUERIES
QUESTED
QUESTER
QUICHES
QUICKEN
QUICKER
QUIETED
QUIETEN
QUIETER
QUIGLEY
QUILLED
QUILLER
QUILTED
QUILTER
QUINCES
QUINCEY
QUINTES
QUINTET
QUINZES
QUIPPED
QUIPPER
QUIRTED
QUITTED
QUITTER
QUIZZED
QUIZZER
QUIZZES
QUOINED
QUOITED
QUONSET
QUOTEES
RUBBLES
RUBYDEE
RUBYRED
RUDDIED
RUDDIER
RUFFLED
RUFFLER
RUFFLES
RUGGLES
RUMBAED
RUMBLED
RUMBLER
RUMBLES
RUMMIES
RUMORED
RUMPLED
RUMPLES
RUNDEEP
RUNDLES
RUNFREE
RUNNIER
RUNOVER
RUNTIER
RUSHEES
RUSHIER
RUSTIER
RUSTLED
RUSTLER
RUSTLES
RUTALEE
RUTILES
RUTTIER
SUBAREA
SUBDUED
SUBDUER
SUBDUES
SUBIDEA
SUBITEM
SUBTEEN
SUBTLER
SUCCEED
SUCKIER
SUDAFED
SUDSIER
SUELLEN
SUGARED
SULKIER
SULKIES
SULLIED
SULLIES
SULUSEA
SUNDAES
SUNNIER
SUPPLED
SUPPLER
SUPPLES
SUREBET
SURFIER
SURFMEN
SURLIER
SUTURED
SUTURES
TUBBIER
TUBULES
TUFTIER
TUILLES
TULANEU
TUMBLED
TUMBLER
TUMBLES
TUMBREL
TUMMIES
TUMMLER
TUPOLEV
TURFIER
TURFMEN
TURNKEY
TURNRED
TURTLED
TURTLES
TUSHIES
TUSSLED
TUSSLES
TUTORED
VUMETER
YUCATEC
YUCKIER
YUMMIER
YUPPIES

•U••••E

AUBERGE
AUDIBLE
AUDITEE
AUGUSTE
AUNTBEE
AURALEE
AUREATE
AUREOLE
AURICLE
AURORAE
AUSABLE
AUSLESE
AUSPICE
AUSTERE
AUTOMNE
BUCKEYE
BUDLIKE
BUDTIME
BUDVASE
BUGFREE
BURBAGE
BURETTE
BURMESE
BUSFARE
BUSLANE
BUSLINE
BUSRIDE
BUSYBEE
BUYABLE
BUYTIME
CUBICLE
CUISINE
CULOTTE
CULTURE
CUNEATE
CUPCAKE
CUPLIKE
CUPRITE
CURABLE
CURETTE
CURLIKE
CURSIVE
CURTATE
CUSPATE
CUTICLE
CUTRATE
CUTTIME
CUVETTE
DUALIZE
DUBUQUE
DUCTILE
DUEDATE
DUNNAGE
DUOTONE
DURABLE
DURANCE
DURANTE
EUGENIE
EUSTACE
EUTERPE
FULSOME
FUNTIME
FURCATE
FURNACE

FURTIVE
FUSIBLE
GUANINE
GUARDEE
GUMLIKE
GUMSHOE
GUMTREE
GUNCASE
GUNFIRE
GUNWALE
GUSTAVE
GUTHRIE
GUYROPE
HUANGHE
HUMORME
HUNLIKE
HUSSITE
HUTLIKE
JUBILEE
JUGWINE
JUSTICE
JUSTINE
JUSTONE
LUCARNE
LUCERNE
LUCIDAE
LUCILLE
LUDDITE
LUGGAGE
LUMIERE
LUNETTE
LUNULAE
MUDHOLE
MULHARE
MUNCHIE
MUNDANE
MUSANTE
MUSETTE
MUSTSEE
MUTABLE
NUCLIDE
NUNLIKE
NURTURE
NUTLIKE
NUTPINE
NUTTREE
OUTBAKE
OUTCOME
OUTCURE
OUTDARE
OUTDATE
OUTDONE
OUTEDGE
OUTFACE
OUTFIRE
OUTFLEE
OUTGAME
OUTGAVE
OUTGAZE
OUTGIVE
OUTHERE
OUTHIRE
OUTLINE
OUTLIVE
OUTLOVE
OUTMATE
OUTMODE
OUTMOVE
OUTPACE
OUTPIPE
OUTRACE
OUTRAGE
OUTRATE
OUTRAVE
OUTRIDE
OUTRODE
OUTROVE
OUTSIDE
OUTSIZE
OUTSOLE
OUTTAKE
OUTTIRE
OUTTORE
OUTVOTE
OUTWAVE
OUTWILE
OUTWORE
PUBGAME
PUERILE
PUGNOSE
PULSATE
PURPOSE
QUAYAGE
QUEENIE
QUELQUE
QUIBBLE
QUICKIE
QUINATE
QUININE
QUINQUE
QUIVIVE
QUIXOTE
RUBYDEE
RUGLIKE
RUINATE
RULEONE
RUMCAKE
RUMMAGE
RUMPOLE
RUNFREE
RUNHOME
RUNLATE
RUNTIME
RUPTURE
RUSHDIE
RUTALEE
SUASIVE
SUBBASE
SUBCASE
SUBCODE
SUBDATE
SUBFILE
SUBLIME
SUBRACE
SUBSIDE
SUBSUME
SUBTONE
SUBTYPE
SUBVENE
SUBZONE
SUCRASE
SUCROSE
SUFFICE
SUFFUSE
SUITSME
SULFATE
SULFIDE
SULFITE
SUMMATE
SUNFIRE
SUNLIKE
SUNRISE
SUPPOSE
SUPREME
SURFACE
SURMISE
SURNAME
SURVIVE
SUSANNE
SUSPIRE
SUZANNE
SUZETTE
TUBLIKE
TUMESCE
TUNABLE
TUNICLE
TURBINE
TURFTOE
TUSSIVE
VULGATE
VULPINE
VULTURE

••UE•••

AQUEOUS
BLUEBOY
BLUEFIN
BLUEFLU
BLUEFOX
BLUEHEN
BLUEICE
BLUEING
BLUEISH
BLUEJAY
BLUELAW
BLUERED
BLUESKY
BLUESUN
BLUETIT
BRUEGEL
CLUEDIN
CLUEFUL
CLUEING
CLUESIN
CRUELER
CRUELLA
CRUELLY
CRUELTY
ECUELLE
EKUELES
EQUERRY
FLUENCY
FOUETTE
GLUEDON
GLUEDTO
GLUEGUN
GLUESON
GLUESTO
KRUEGER
LOUELLA
SQUEAKS
SQUEAKY
SQUEALS
SQUEERS
SQUEEZE
SQUELCH
TRUEDUP
TRUEING
TRUERIB
TRUERTO
TRUESUP

••U•E••

ABUSERS
ACUMENS
ACUTELY
ACUTEST
ALUDELS
AMULETS
AMUSEME
AMUSERS
AZULEJO
BRUBECK
BRUNETS
BRUTELY
CAUSERS
COULEES
COUTERS
CRUDELY
CRUDEST
DAUBERS
DEUTERO
DOUCEUR
DOUREST
DOUSERS
DRUZEAN
ELUDERS
EXUPERY
FAUCETS
FLUTERS
FOULEST
FOUREEE
GAUDENS
GAUDERY
GAUGERS
GLUIEST
GLUTEAL
GLUTENS
GLUTEUS
GOUGERS
GRUYERE
HAULERS
HAUTEUR
INUTERO
ISUREAM
ISUREDO
LAUDERS
LAURELS
LAURENT
LOUDENS
LOUDEST
LOUREED
LOUSEUP
LOUVERS
MAULERS
MAUREEN
MAUSERS
MOUSERS
NAUSEAM
NEUTERS
NOUVEAU
OPULENT
PAUPERS
PAUSERS
PCUSERS
PEUGEOT
POULENC
POURERS
POUTERS
PRUDENT
PRUDERY
PRUNERS
REUBENS
REUNERS
REUSERS
REUTERS
ROULEAU
ROUSERS
ROUTERS
SAUCERS
SAUTEED
SCUSEME
SHUBERT
SHUTEYE
SOUPERS
SOUREST
SQUEERS
SQUEEZE
STUDENT
STUPEFY
TAUREAN
TAUTENS
TAUTEST
TOUPEES
TOURERS
TOUTERS
TRUDEAU
UKULELE
USURERS
YOUREIT
YOUREON

••U••E•

ABUTTED
ABUTTER
AGUTTER
ALUNSER
AQUIFER
AQUIVER
ARUNDEL
ARUSPEX
ASUNDER
AVULSED
AVULSES
BAUBLES
BAULKED
BAULKER
BEURRES
BLUBBER
BLUDGED
BLUDGER
BLUDGES
BLUEHEN
BLUERED
BLUFFED
BLUFFER
BLUNDEN
BLUNDER
BLUNTED
BLUNTER
BLURBER
BLURRED
BLURTED
BLURTER
BLUSHED
BLUSHER
BLUSHES
BLUSTER
BOUCHER
BOUCHES
BOUFFES
BOUGHED
BOULDER
BOUNCED
BOUNCER
BOUNCES
BOUNDED
BOUNDER
BOUQUET
BOURGET
BOURSES
BOUVIER
BRUEGEL
BRUISED
BRUISER
BRUISES
BRUITED
BRUMMEL
BRUSHED
BRUSHER
BRUSHES
CAULKED
CAULKER
CAUTHEN
CHUCKED
CHUFFED
CHUGGED
CHUGGER
CHUKKER
CHUMMED
CHUMPED
CHUNKED
CHUNNEL
CHURNED
CHURNER
CHUTNEY
CLUBBED
CLUBBER
CLUBMED
CLUCKED
CLUCKER
CLUMPED
CLUNKED
CLUNKER
CLUSTER
CLUTTER
COUCHED
COUCHES
COUGHED
COULEES
COULTER
COUNSEL
COUNTED
COUNTEE
COUNTEM
COUNTER
COUPLED
COUPLER
COUPLES
COUPLET
COURBET
COURIER
COURSED
COURSER
COURSES
COURTED
CRUELER
CRUGUET
CRUISED
CRUISER
CRUISES
CRULLER
CRUMBED
CRUMPED
CRUMPET
CRUPPER
CRUSHED
CRUSHER
CRUSHES
CRUSTED
CRUTZEN
DAUMIER
DAUNTED
DAUNTER
DAUSSET
DOUANES
DOUBLEA
DOUBLEB
DOUBLEC
DOUBLED
DOUBLEE
DOUBLEF
DOUBLEG
DOUBLEH
DOUBLEI
DOUBLEJ
DOUBLEK
DOUBLEL
DOUBLEM
DOUBLEN
DOUBLEO
DOUBLEP
DOUBLEQ
DOUBLER
DOUBLES
DOUBLET
DOUBLEU
DOUBLEV
DOUBLEW
DOUBLEX
DOUBLEY
DOUBLEZ
DOUBTED
DOUBTER
DRUBBED
DRUBBER
DRUCKER
DRUDGED
DRUDGER
DRUDGES
DRUGGED
DRUMMED
DRUMMER
DRUMSET
DRUNKEN
DRUNKER
EDUCTED
EKUELES
ELUATES
EQUALED
EQUATED
EQUATES
EQUINES
ERUCTED
ERUPTED
ERUPTER
EVULSED
EVULSES
EXULTED
FAULTED
FLUBBED
FLUBBER
FLUFFED
FLUFFER
FLUKIER
FLUNKED
FLUNKER
FLUSHED
FLUSHER
FLUSHES
FLUSTER
FLUTIER
FLUTIES
FLUTTER
FNUMBER
FOUDRES
FOUNDED
FOUNDER
FOUREEE
FOURIER
FRUITED
GAUCHER
GAUDIER
GAUDIES
GAUNTER
GAUSSES
GAUTIER
GAUZIER
GLUGGED
GLUMMED
GLUMMER
GLURGES
GLUTTED
GOUNDER
GOURDES
GOURMET
GOUTIER
GRUBBED
GRUBBER
GRUDGED
GRUDGER
GRUDGES
GRUFFER
GRUMPED
GRUNGER
GRUNGES
GRUNTED
GRUNTER
HAUNTED
HAUNTER
HOUNDED
HOUNDER
JAUNTED
JOUNCED
JOUNCES
JOURNEE
JOURNEY
JOUSTED
JOUSTER
KLUDGED
KLUDGES
KLUTZES
KNURLED
KRUEGER
LAUGHED
LAUGHER
LAUNDER
LAUTREC
LOUNGED
LOUNGER
LOUNGES
LOURDES
LOUREED
LOUSIER
LOUVRED
LOUVRES
MAUNDER
MAUREEN
MOULDED
MOULDER
MOULTED
MOUNDED
MOUNTED
MOUNTER
MOURNED
MOURNER
MOUSIER
MOUSSED
MOUSSES
MOUTHED
MOUTHER
NTUPLES
OEUVRES
PAULSEN
PLUCKED
PLUGGED
PLUGGER
PLUMBED
PLUMBER
PLUMIER
PLUMMER
PLUMMET
PLUMPED
PLUMPER
PLUNDER
PLUNGED
PLUNGER
PLUNGES
PLUNKED
PLUNKER
PLUSHER
PLUSHES
PLUSSES
POUCHED
POUCHES
POUDRES
POUNCED
POUNCER
POUNCES
POUNDED
POUNDER
POUTIER
REUPPED
REURGED
REURGES
REUTHER
REUTTER
ROUGHED
ROUGHEN
ROUGHER
ROUNDED
ROUNDEL
ROUNDER
ROUSTED
ROUSTER
SAUCIER
SAUNAED
SAUNTER
SAUTEED
SCUBAED
SCUDDED
SCUDDER
SCUFFED
SCUFFER
SCULLED
SCULLER
SCULPED
SCUPPER
SCURVES
SCUZZES
SHUCKED
SHUCKER
SHUDDER
SHUNNED
SHUNTED
SHUNTER
SHUSHED
SHUSHES
SHUSTER
SHUTTER
SKULKED
SKULKER
SKULLED
SKUNKED
SLUDGES
SLUGGED
SLUGGER
SLUICED
SLUICES
SLUMBER
SLUMMED
SLUMMER
SLUMPED
SLURPED
SLURPEE
SLURPER
SLURRED
SLUSHED
SLUSHES
SMUCKER
SMUDGED
SMUDGES
SMUGGER
SMUSHED
SMUSHES
SNUBBED
SNUBBER
SNUFFED
SNUFFER
SNUGGED
SNUGGER
SOUNDED
SOUNDER
SOUPIER
SOURCED
SOURCES
SOUTHEY
SPUMIER
SPURNED
SPURNER
SPURRED
SPURTED
SPUTTER
SQUARED
SQUARER
SQUARES
SQUIRED
SQUIRES
STUBBED
STUDDED
STUDIED
STUDIER
STUDIES
STUFFED
STUFFER
STUMPED
STUMPER
STUNNED
STUNNER
STUNTED
STURGES
STUTTER
STUTZES
TAUNTED
TAUNTER
THUDDED
THUMBED
THUMPED
THUMPER
THUNDER
THUNKED
THURBER
TOUAREG
TOUCHED
TOUCHER
TOUCHES
TOUGHEN
TOUGHER
TOUPEES
TOURNEY
TOUSLED
TOUSLES
TRUCKED
TRUCKEE
TRUCKER
TRUDGED
TRUDGEN
TRUDGER
TRUDGES
TRUMPED
TRUMPET
TRUSSED
TRUSSES
TRUSTED
TRUSTEE
TRUSTER
UNURGED
USURIES
USURPED
USURPER
VAULTED
VAULTER
VAUNTED
VAUNTER
VOUCHED
VOUCHER
VOUCHES
WHUPPED
WOUNDED
YOUNGER
YOUTHEN

••U•••E

ABUSIVE
ADULATE
ALUMNAE
AMUSEME
AZURITE
BAUXITE
BLUEICE
BRUSQUE
CAUDATE
CHUCKLE
COULDBE
COUNTEE
COURAGE
COUSINE
COUTURE
CRUMBLE
CRUMPLE
CRUSADE
DHURRIE
DOUBLEE
ECUELLE
EDUCATE
ELUSIVE
EMULATE
EQUABLE
ERUDITE
EXUDATE
FOUETTE
FOUREEE
GLUCOSE
GOUACHE
GRUMBLE
GRUYERE
HAULAGE
HEURIGE
INULASE
INUTILE
JOURNEE
KNUCKLE
LEUCINE
MAURICE
MOULAGE
MOUNTIE
NEURONE
OPUSONE
PAULINE
PLUMAGE
PLUMOSE
PLUMPIE
PLUMULE
PLUSONE
PRUDHOE
REUNITE
ROULADE
ROUTINE
SAUSAGE
SCUFFLE
SCUSEME
SCUTTLE
SHUFFLE
SHUTEYE
SHUTTLE
SLURPEE
SMUGGLE
SNUFFLE
SNUGGLE
SOUBISE
SOUFFLE
SOURALE
SPUMONE
SQUEEZE
STUBBLE
STUMBLE
TAURINE
TOUGHIE
TRUCKEE
TRUCKLE
TRUFFLE
TRUNDLE
TRUSTEE
TRUSTME
UKULELE
ULULATE
WOULDBE
YOULOSE

•••UE••

ARGUERS
BEQUEST
BUNUELO
DEFUELS
DEQUEUE
DILUENT
ENQUEUE
ESCUELA
INQUEST
ISSUEAD
ISSUERS
LIQUEFY
LIQUEUR
MCQUEEN
MINUEND
MINUETS
QUEUERS
QUEUEUP
REFUELS
REQUEST
RIGUEUR
ROGUERY
SAMUELL
SEQUELS
SOSUEME
TOLUENE
UNGUENT
VAGUELY
VAGUEST
VALUERS
VAQUERO
VOGUERS

•••U•E•

ABDUCED
ABDUCES
ABJURED
ABJURER
ABJURES
ACCUSED
ACCUSER
ACCUSES
ADDUCED
ADDUCER
ADDUCES
ADJURED
ADJURER
ADJURES
ALBUMEN
ALLUDED
ALLUDES
ALLURED
ALLURER
ALLURES
AMPULES
ANNULET
APLUSES
ARGUSES
AROUSED
AROUSER
AROUSES
ASQUIET
ASSUMED
ASSUMER
ASSUMES
ASSURED
ASSURER
ASSURES
ASTUTER
ATTUNED
ATTUNES
AUGURED
AUGURER
BEMUSED
BEMUSES
BEQUIET
BLOUSED
BLOUSES
BOLUSES
BONUSES
BPLUSES
CADUCEI
CALUMET
CAPULET
CAYUSES
CERUMEN
CHAUCER
CLAUDEL
CLAUSES
CLOUDED
CLOUTED
CLOUTER
COBUYER
CONURES
COZUMEL
CPLUSES
CROUTES
CUPULES
DEBUSES
DEBUTED
DEDUCED
DEDUCER
DEDUCES
DEFUSED
DEFUSER
DEFUSES
DELUDED
DELUDER
DELUDES
DELUGED
DELUGES
DEMURER
DENUDED
DENUDER
DENUDES
DEPUTED
DEPUTES
DETUNED
DETUNES
DILUTED
DILUTER
DILUTES
DISUSED
DISUSES
DPLUSES
DUFUSES
EFFUSED
EFFUSES
ENDURED
ENDURER
ENDURES
ENDUSER
ENDUSES
ENSURED
ENSURER
ENSURES
EPAULET
EXCUSED
EXCUSER
EXCUSES
EXCUSEZ
EXHUMED
EXHUMER
EXHUMES
FERULES
FETUSES
FICUSES
FIGURED
FIGURER
FIGURES
FLOURED
FLOUTED
FLOUTER
FOCUSED
FOCUSER
FOCUSES
FUTURES
GENUSES
GIBUSES
GROUPED
GROUPER
GROUSED
GROUSER
GROUSES
GROUTED
GROUTER
GUNUSER
HOCUSED
HUMUSES
ICTUSES
ILLUDED
ILLUDES
ILLUMED
ILLUMES
ILLUSED
ILLUSES
IMMUNES
IMMURED
IMMURES
IMPURER
IMPUTED
IMPUTER
IMPUTES
INCUDES
INCUSED
INCUSES
INDUCED
INDUCER
INDUCES
INFUSED
INFUSER
INFUSES
INHUMED
INHUMER
INHUMES
INJURED
INJURER
INJURES
INSURED
INSURER
INSURES
IVTUBES
JUJUBES
KNOUTED
LACUREE
LEGUMES
LEXUSES
LOBULES
LORUSES
LOTUSES
MACUSER
MANURED
MANURES
MATURED
MATURER
MATURES
MCQUEEN
MINUSES
MINUTED
MINUTER
MINUTES
MISUSED
MISUSER
MISUSES
MODULES
MOMUSES
NATURED
NATUREL
NATURES
NEGUSES
NEXUSES
NODULED
NODULES
NONUKES
NONUSER
NOTUSED
OBTUSER
OSCULES
PAIUTES
PARURES
PERUKES
PERUSED
PERUSER
PERUSES
PRIUSES
PROUDER
RASURES
REBUKED
REBUKER
REBUKES
REBUSES
RECURED
RECURES
RECUSED
RECUSES
REDUCED
REDUCER
REDUCES
REFUGED
REFUGEE
REFUGES
REFUSED
REFUSER
REFUSES
REFUTED
REFUTER
REFUTES
RELUMED
RELUMES
REPUTED
REPUTES
REQUIEM
RESUMED
RESUMES
RETUNED
RETUNES
RIVULET
SALUTED
SALUTER
SALUTES
SCHUMER
SCOUPES
SCOURED
SCOURER
SCOUTED
SCOUTER
SECURED
SECURER
SECURES
SEDUCED
SEDUCER
SEDUCES
SHOUTED
SHOUTER
SINUSES
SNOUTED
SOLUTES
SPOUSES
SPOUTED
SPOUTER
SPRUCED
SPRUCER
SPRUCES
STEUBEN
STLUKES
STOUTEN
STOUTER
STRUDEL
SULUSEA
SUTURED
SUTURES
TALUSES
TENURED
TENURES
TONUSES
TRAUBEL
TROUPED
TROUPER
TROUPES
TROUSER
TUBULES
UNCURED
UNDUPED
UNFUSED
UNGUYED
UNLURED
UNMUTED
UNQUIET
UNRULED
UNTUNED
UNTUNES
VELURES
VENULES
VENUSES
VIRUSES
VOLUMED
VOLUMES
VOLUTED
VOLUTES
WHAUDEN
ZONULES

•••U••E

ACOUPLE
ACQUIRE
ACTUATE
ADJUDGE
ARCUATE
ASSUAGE
AUGUSTE
BEGUILE
BEGUINE
CANULAE
CAPUCHE
COPULAE
DECUPLE
DELUISE
DEQUEUE
DIVULGE
DIVULSE
DOEUVRE
DUBUQUE
ELFUDGE
ENOUNCE
ENQUEUE
ENQUIRE
ENSUITE
ESQUIRE
EXCURSE
EXPUNGE
FACULAE
FIBULAE
FLOUNCE
GENUINE
GIAUQUE
GROUPIE
IMPULSE
INCURVE
INDULGE
INQUIRE
LACUNAE
LACUREE
LIQUATE
LUNULAE
MACULAE
MAGUIRE
MCGUIRE
MEDUSAE
NEBULAE
NONUPLE
OCTUBRE
OCTUPLE
OHFUDGE
OROURKE
PANURGE
PENUCHE
PLEURAE
RECURVE
REFUGEE
REGUIDE
REJUDGE
REPULSE
REQUIRE
REQUITE
REQUOTE
RESURGE
SCOURGE
SCRUPLE
SINUATE
SITUATE
SOLUBLE
SOSUEME
SPLURGE
TOLUENE
TROUBLE
TROUNCE
TSQUARE
TVGUIDE
UNGULAE
UNQUOTE
UPCURVE
UPSURGE
VACUOLE
VALUATE
VOLUBLE
YAOUNDE

••••UE•

ACCRUED
ACCRUES
AVENUEQ
AVENUES
BALLUET
BANQUES
BANQUET
BARQUES
BASQUES
BIOFUEL
BISQUES
BOUQUET
BRIQUET
BROGUES
CASQUED
CASQUES
CHEQUER
CHEQUES
CINQUES
CIRQUES
CLAQUES
CLIQUED
CLIQUES
CLIQUEY
CONQUER
CROQUET
CRUGUET
DROGUES
EMANUEL
EMBRUED
EMBRUES
EPOQUES
EVACUEE
FESCUES
FONDUED
FONDUES
GIBLUES
IMBRUED
IMBRUES
JACQUES
KILAUEA
LACQUER
LEAGUED
LEAGUER
LEAGUES
LONGUES
MARQUEE
MARQUES
MARQUEZ
MASQUER
MASQUES
MIAOUED
MISCUED
MISCUES
MORGUES
MOSQUES
NONFUEL
OPAQUES
OUTDUEL
PARQUET
PLAGUED
PLAGUES
PLAQUES
PREQUEL
PREVUED
PREVUES
PURDUEU
PURSUED
PURSUER
PURSUES
RACQUET
REGLUED
REGLUES
RESCUED
RESCUER
RESCUES
RVALUES
SACQUES
SNAFUED
STATUES
SUBDUED
SUBDUER
SUBDUES
SYNFUEL
TISSUES
TISSUEY
TONGUES
TORQUED
TORQUES
UNBLUED
UNCRUEL
UNGLUED
UNGLUES
UNIQUES
UNTRUER
UVALUES
VASQUEZ
VENDUES
VIRTUES

••••U•E

AIRTUBE
ALBSURE
AMINUTE
AMPOULE
ASARULE
ATDEUCE
BARBULE
BECAUSE
BETHUNE
CAPSULE
CAPTURE
CAROUSE
CELLULE
CENSURE
CLOSURE
CLOTURE
COLLUDE
COMMUNE
COMMUTE
COMPUTE
CONDUCE
CONFUSE
CONFUTE
CONJURE
CONSUME
CONTUSE
CORNUTE
COSTUME
COUTURE
CULTURE
DEBOULE
DELOUSE
DENEUVE
DENTURE
DETRUDE
DIFFUSE
DISEUSE
DISPUTE
ELOCUTE
ENROUTE
ENTHUSE
EPICURE
ERASURE
ESPOUSE
EVACUEE
EVOLUTE
EXCLUDE
EXECUTE
EXTRUDE
FAILURE
FAIRUSE
FEATURE
FERRULE
FISSURE
FIXTURE
FLEXURE
FORSURE
FORTUNE
GAGRULE
GESTURE
GETCUTE
GLOBULE
GOODUSE
GOTCUTE
GRANULE
GRAVURE
HERCULE
HEYJUDE
HEYRUBE
HIRSUTE
HITTUNE
ICECUBE
INCLUDE
INHOUSE
INTRUDE
IREFUSE
JACCUSE
KAPTURE
LABTUBE
LADOUCE
LECTURE
LEISURE
LEJEUNE
LETSUSE
LETTUCE
LINGUAE
MAJEURE
MARCUSE
MARQUEE
MARYURE
MCCLURE
MEASURE
MERCURE
MIDJUNE
MISRULE
MISTUNE
MIXTURE
MOBRULE
NATSUME
NEPTUNE
NERVULE
NETSUKE
NOTSURE
NURTURE
OBSCURE
OBTRUDE
OCCLUDE
OFNOUSE
OUTCURE
OVERUSE
PASTURE
PERDURE
PERFUME
PERFUSE
PERJURE
PERMUTE
PETMULE
PICTURE
PLUMULE
POLLUTE
POPTUNE
POSEUSE
POSTURE
PRECURE
PRELUDE
PRESUME
PROCURE
PRODUCE
PROFUSE
RAPTUNE
RAPTURE
RECLUSE
REGAUGE
REHOUSE
REPLUME
REPRUNE
REROUTE
RONDURE
RUPTURE
SECLUDE
SEIZURE
SIRDUKE
STATURE
STATUTE
STROUSE
SUBSUME
SUFFUSE
TERHUNE
TEXTURE
THEDUKE
THERULE
THETUBE
TONSURE
TORTURE
TRADUCE
TRIBUNE
TRIBUTE
ULALUME
ULANUDE
UNCRUDE
UNHOUSE
UPROUSE
VALVULE
VBLOUSE
VEINULE
VELOUTE
VENTURE
VERDURE
VESTURE
VIRGULE
VOITURE
VULTURE
WALKURE
WASSURE

•••••UE

AMIBLUE
ANTIQUE
ATISSUE
BAROQUE
BENBLUE
BEZIQUE
BIGBLUE
BRUSQUE
CACIQUE
CAMEDUE
CIMABUE
COMEDUE
COMIQUE
DELARUE
DEQUEUE
DEVALUE
DONAHUE
DUBUQUE
ECLOGUE
ENQUEUE
ENRIQUE
ENVOGUE
FALLDUE
FATIGUE
FELLDUE
GIAUQUE
HABITUE
HOTGLUE
ICEBLUE
INGENUE
INVOGUE
ITSTRUE
LALIQUE
MACAQUE
MINOGUE
NBCBLUE
NOTTRUE
OBLIQUE
OFVALUE
OLDBLUE
OVERDUE
PASTDUE
PIROGUE
POOLCUE
PRESQUE
QUELQUE
QUINQUE
REARGUE
REISSUE
RESIDUE
RETINUE
REVALUE
REVENUE
SEABLUE
SKYBLUE
UNVAGUE
UPVALUE
VONLAUE

UF•••••

UFOLOGY

U•F••••

UNFACED
UNFACTS
UNFADED
UNFAITH
UNFAKED
UNFAMED
UNFANCY
UNFATED
UNFATTY
UNFAZED
UNFENCE
UNFERTH
UNFETED
UNFIERY
UNFILED
UNFILES
UNFINED
UNFINES
UNFIRED
UNFITLY
UNFIXED
UNFIXES
UNFLAKY
UNFLOOR
UNFLOWN
UNFLUID
UNFOGGY
UNFOLDS
UNFORKS
UNFOUND
UNFOXED
UNFRAIL
UNFRANK
UNFREED
UNFREES
UNFRIED
UNFRILL
UNFROCK
UNFROST
UNFROZE
UNFULLY
UNFUNNY
UNFURLS
UNFUSED
UNFUSSY
UPFIELD
UPFIRST
UPFLING
UPFLOWS
UPFOLDS
UPFORIT
UPFRONT
USFLAGS

U••F•••

UNIFIED
UNIFIER
UNIFIES
UNIFORM
UNOFTEN
URNFULS

U•••F••

UNAWFUL
UNCUFFS
UNLOFTY
UNSAFER
UPLIFTS
UPWAFTS
USEDFOR
USERFEE
USESFOR

U••••F•

UNCLEFT
UNCUFFS
UNGRUFF
UNLEAFS
UNROOFS
UNSHIFT
UNSTIFF
UPDRAFT
UPDRIFT
UPSHIFT

U•••••F

UNBRIEF
UNGRUFF
UNSTIFF

•UF••••

BUFFALO
BUFFERS
BUFFEST
BUFFETS
BUFFETT
BUFFING
BUFFOON
BUFFSUP
CUFFING
DUFFELS
DUFFERS
DUFFLES
DUFUSES
GUFFAWS
HUFFIER
HUFFILY
HUFFING
HUFFISH
HUFFMAN
LUFFING
MUFFING
MUFFINS
MUFFLED
MUFFLER
MUFFLES
PUFFERS
PUFFERY
PUFFIER
PUFFILY
PUFFING
PUFFINS
PUFFOUT
PUFFSUP
RUFFALO
RUFFIAN
RUFFING
RUFFLED
RUFFLER
RUFFLES
RUFIYAA
SUFFERS
SUFFICE
SUFFOLK
SUFFUSE
TUFFETS
TUFTIER
TUFTING

•U•F•••

BUFFALO
BUFFERS
BUFFEST
BUFFETS
BUFFETT
BUFFING
BUFFOON
BUFFSUP
BUGFREE

BUSFARE
CUBFANS
CUFFING
CUPFULS
CURFEWS
DUFFELS
DUFFERS
DUFFLES
FULFILL
FULFILS
FUNFAIR
FUNFEST
FUNFURS
FUNFZIG
FURFARM
GUFFAWS
GULFING
GULFOIL
GULFWAR
GUNFIRE
HUFFIER
HUFFILY
HUFFING
HUFFISH
HUFFMAN
JUGFULS
LUFFING
MUDFISH
MUDFLAP
MUDFLAT
MUDFLOW
MUFFING
MUFFINS
MUFFLED
MUFFLER
MUFFLES
MUGFULS
MUMFORD
OUTFACE
OUTFAST
OUTFAWN
OUTFEED
OUTFEEL
OUTFIND
OUTFIRE
OUTFISH
OUTFITS
OUTFLEE
OUTFLOW
OUTFLUX
OUTFOOL
OUTFOOT
PUFFERS
PUFFERY
PUFFIER
PUFFILY
PUFFING
PUFFINS
PUFFOUT
PUFFSUP
PURFLED
PURFLER
PURFLES
QUAFFED
QUAFFER
RUFFALO
RUFFIAN
RUFFING
RUFFLED
RUFFLER
RUFFLES
RUMFORD
RUNFREE
SUBFILE
SUBFORM
SUFFERS
SUFFICE
SUFFOLK
SUFFUSE
SULFATE
SULFIDE
SULFITE
SUNFANS
SUNFAST
SUNFIRE
SUNFISH
SURFACE
SURFEIT
SURFERS
SURFIER
SURFING
SURFMAN
SURFMEN
SURFSUP
TUBFULS
TUFFETS
TURFIER
TURFING
TURFMAN
TURFMEN
TURFSKI
TURFTOE
TURFWAR

•U••F••

BUCKFOR
BURNFOR
BUYOFFS
CUBSFAN
CUTOFFS
DUTIFUL
GUNSFOR
HUNTFOR
HURTFOR
HURTFUL
HUSHFUL
JUNKFAX
LUCIFER
LUSTFUL
MUSEFUL
OUTOFIT
PULLFOR
PUSHFOR
PUSHFUL
PUTOFFS
QUAFFED
QUAFFER
RUNGFOR
RUNOFFS
RUNSFOR
RUTHFUL
SUDAFED
SUEDFOR
SUESFOR
SUNSFAN
TUNEFUL

•U•••F•

BUGSOFF
BURNOFF
BUYOFFS
BUYSOFF
BUZZOFF
CUTOFFS
CUTSOFF
DULCIFY
DUSTOFF
HUNGOFF
JUMPOFF
JUSTIFY
MUMMIFY
MUSTAFA
NULLIFY
OUTSIFT
PULLOFF
PULPIFY
PUSHOFF
PUTOFFS
PUTREFY
PUTSOFF
QUALIFY
RUBSOFF
RUDOLFI
RUNGOFF
RUNOFFS
RUNSOFF
RUSHOFF
TURNOFF
YUPPIFY

•U••••F

BUGSOFF
BURNOFF
BUYSOFF
BUZZOFF
CUTSOFF
DUSTOFF
HUNGOFF
JUMPOFF
OURSELF
PULLOFF
PUSHOFF
PUTSOFF
RUBSOFF
RUNGOFF
RUNSOFF
RUSHOFF
SUNROOF
SUREROF
TURNOFF

••UF•••

BLUFFED
BLUFFER
BLUFFLY
BOUFFES
CHUFFED
FLUFFED
FLUFFER
FLUFFUP
GRUFFER
GRUFFLY
KAUFMAN
SCUFFED
SCUFFER
SCUFFLE
SHUFFLE
SNUFFED
SNUFFER
SNUFFLE
SOUFFLE
STUFFED
STUFFER
STUFFIN
TRUFFLE

••U•F••

AQUIFER
BLUEFIN
BLUEFLU
BLUEFOX
BLUFFED
BLUFFER
BLUFFLY
BOUFFES
CHUFFED
CLUEFUL
EQUIFAX
FAUXFUR
FLUFFED
FLUFFER
FLUFFUP
GRUFFER
GRUFFLY
POUTFUL
SCUFFED
SCUFFER
SCUFFLE
SHUFFLE
SNUFFED
SNUFFER
SNUFFLE
SNUGFIT
SOUFFLE
SOULFUL
STUFFED
STUFFER
STUFFIN
THUSFAR
TRUFFLE

••U••F•

HAULOFF
REUNIFY
SHUTOFF
SPUNOFF
STUPEFY

••U•••F

DOUBLEF
HAULOFF
SHUTOFF
SOUTHOF
SPUNOFF

•••UF••

REBUFFS
SCRUFFS
SCRUFFY
UNCUFFS

•••U•F•

ENGULFS
INGULFS
LIQUEFY
REBUFFS
RETURFS
SCRUFFS
SCRUFFY
UNCUFFS

•••U••F

AFOULOF
DOOUTOF
PROUDOF

••••UF•

EARMUFF
INAHUFF
MACDUFF
MCGRUFF
RESTUFF
SAMHUFF
SHONUFF
UNGRUFF
ZIPCUFF

••••U•F

BEOWULF
EARMUFF
EGOSURF
INAHUFF
MACDUFF
MCGRUFF
NETSURF
RESTUFF
SAMHUFF
SHONUFF
SKYSURF
UNGRUFF
ZIPCUFF

UG•••••

UGANDAN
UGLIEST
UGOLINO

U•G••••

UNGATED
UNGAUDY
UNGIDDY
UNGIRDS
UNGIVEN
UNGLOVE
UNGLUED
UNGLUES
UNGODLY
UNGORED
UNGRAND
UNGREEN
UNGRIPS
UNGROSS
UNGROWN
UNGRUFF
UNGUARD
UNGUENT
UNGULAE
UNGULAR
UNGUYED
UNGYVED
UPGAZED
UPGAZES
UPGIRDS
UPGOING
UPGRADE
UPGROWN
UPGROWS
URGEDON
URGENCY
URGESON
URGINGS
USGRANT

U••G•••

UNAGILE
UNAGING
UNOGLED
URUGUAY

U•••G••

ULLAGES
UNANGRY
UNBOGGY
UNCAGED
UNCAGES
UNEAGER
UNEDGED
UNEDGES
UNFOGGY
UNLEGAL
UNLIGHT
UNPAGAN
UNPAGED
UNREGAL
UNRIGID
UNSIGHT
UNSOGGY
UNURGED
UNVAGUE
UNWAGED
UPLIGHT
UPRIGHT
UPTIGHT
USINGIN
USINGUP

U••••G•

UFOLOGY
UMBRAGE
UNBOGGY
UNCLOGS
UNDERGO
UNFOGGY
UNHINGE
UNLARGE
UNMERGE
UNPLUGS
UNSNAGS
UNSOGGY
UNSTAGY
UNTOUGH
UNWEDGE
UPSTAGE
UPSURGE
URGINGS
UROLOGY
USFLAGS

U•••••G

UNAGING
UNDOING
UNDYING
UNITING
UNLYING
UNOWING
UNSLING
UNSLUNG
UNSTUNG
UNSWUNG
UNTYING
UNVYING
UNWRUNG
UNYOUNG
UPFLING
UPGOING
UPSWING

•UG••••

AUGENDS
AUGITES
AUGMENT
AUGURAL
AUGURED
AUGURER
AUGUSTA
AUGUSTE
AUGUSTO
AUGUSTS
BUGABOO
BUGALOO
BUGATTI
BUGBEAR
BUGBOYS
BUGEYED
BUGFREE
BUGGIER
BUGGIES
BUGGING
BUGGLES
BUGLERS
BUGLING
BUGOUTS
BUGSOFF
BUGSOUT
DUGINTO
DUGONGS
DUGOUTS
EUGENIA
EUGENIC
EUGENIE
EUGLENA
FUGALLY
FUGATOS
HUGGERS
HUGGIES
HUGGING
HUGGINS
JUGBAND
JUGFULS
JUGGING
JUGGLED
JUGGLER
JUGGLES
JUGHEAD
JUGULAR
JUGWINE
LUGGAGE
LUGGERS
LUGGING
LUGNUTS
LUGSAIL
LUGSOUT
LUGWORM
MUGFULS
MUGGERS
MUGGIER
MUGGING
MUGGISH
MUGGLES
MUGSHOT
MUGWUMP
NUGGETS
NUGGETY
OUGHTNT
OUGHTTO
OUGUIYA
PUGGISH
PUGGLES
PUGNOSE
PUGSLEY
RUGGLES
RUGLIKE
RUGRATS
SUGARED
SUGGEST
TUGBOAT
TUGGERS
TUGGING
TUGLESS
TUGRIKS

•U•G•••

BUDGERS
BUDGETS
BUDGIES
BUDGING
BUGGIER
BUGGIES
BUGGING
BUGGLES
BULGARI
BULGARS
BULGHUR
BULGIER
BULGING
BULGURS
BUNGEES
BUNGING
BUNGLED
BUNGLER
BUNGLES
BURGEES
BURGEON
BURGERS
BURGESS
BURGHER
BURGLAR
BURGLED
BURGLES
BURGOOS
BUSGIRL
BUTGOOD
CUDGELS
DUDGEON
DUNGEON
FUDGERS
FUDGING
FULGENT
FULGHUM
FUNGOES
GUDGEON
GUIGNOL
GURGLED
GURGLES
HUGGERS
HUGGIES
HUGGING
HUGGINS
HUNGARY
HUNGERS
HUNGOFF
HUNGOUT
HUNGTEN
HUYGENS
JUDGERS
JUDGING
JUGGING
JUGGLED
JUGGLER
JUGGLES
JUNGIAN
JUNGLES
JURGENS
LUGGAGE
LUGGERS
LUGGING
LUNGEAT
LUNGERS
LUNGING
MUGGERS
MUGGIER
MUGGING
MUGGISH
MUGGLES
MULGREW
NUDGERS
NUDGING
NUGGETS
NUGGETY
NUNGWEN
OURGANG
OUTGAIN
OUTGAME
OUTGAVE
OUTGAZE
OUTGIVE
OUTGLOW
OUTGNAW
OUTGOES
OUTGREW
OUTGRIN
OUTGROW
OUTGUNS
OUTGUSH
PUBGAME
PUDGIER
PUDGILY
PUGGISH
PUGGLES
PUNGENT
PURGING
QUAGGAS
QUIGLEY
RUGGLES
RUNGFOR
RUNGOFF
RUNGOUT
RUTGERS
SUBGOAL
SUBGODS
SUGGEST
SUNGLOW
SUNGODS
SURGEON
SURGERY
SURGING
TUGGERS
TUGGING
TUNGOIL
VULGATE

•U••G••

BURPGUN
CUBAGES
CUINGIN
DUSTGUN
GUARGUM
HUANGHE
HUANGTI
MUSIGNY
MUTAGEN
OUTAGES
QUAGGAS

•U•••G•

AUBERGE
BUMLEGS
BURBAGE
DUGONGS
DUNNAGE
DURANGO
GUNDOGS
HUMBUGS
LUGGAGE
LUMBAGO
MUSINGS
MUSKEGO
NUTMEGS
OUTBEGS
OUTEDGE
OUTINGS
OUTRAGE
OUTRIGS
OUTSIGH
QUAHOGS
QUAYAGE
RULINGS
RUMMAGE
SUNDOGS
SUPERGS

•U••••G

AUTOING
BUCKING
BUDDING
BUDGING
BUFFING
BUGGING
BUGLING
BULGING
BULKING
BULLDOG
BULLING
BUMMING
BUMPING
BUNGING
BUNKING
BUNNING
BUNTING
BUOYING
BURLING
BURNING
BURPING
BURRING
BURYING
BUSHHOG
BUSHING
BUSHPIG
BUSKING
BUSSING
BUSTING
BUSYING
BUTTING
BUZZING
CUBBING
CUFFING
CULLING
CUNNING
CUPPING
CURBING
CURDING
CURLING
CURRING
CURSING
CURVING
CUSHING
CUSSING
CUTARUG
CUTTING
DUBBING
DUCKING
DUCTING
DUELING
DUETING
DULLING
DUMBING
DUMPING
DUNKING
DUNNING
DURNING
DUSKING
DUSTING
DUSTRAG
FUDGING
FUELING
FUNDING
FUNFZIG
FUNKING
FUNNING
FURLING
FURLONG
FURRING
FUSSING
FUTZING
FUZZING
GUIDING
GUILING
GULFING
GULLING
GULPING
GUMMING
GUNNING
GUSHING
GUSTING
GUTTING
HUFFING
HUGGING
HULKING
HULLING
HUMMING
HUNTING
HURLING
HURTING
HUSHING
HUSKING
HUTTING
JUDGING
JUGGING
JUICING
JUMPING
JUNEBUG
JUNKING
JURYING
JURYRIG
JUTTING
LUCKING
LUFFING
LUGGING
LULLING
LUMPING
LUNGING
LURKING
LUSTING
MUCKING
MUDDING
MUFFING
MUGGING
MULLING
MUMMING
MUSHING
MUSSING
MUSTANG
NUDGING
NULLING
NUMBING
NURSING
NUTTING
OURGANG
OURSONG
OUSTING
OUTBRAG
OUTDRAG
OUTKING
OUTRANG
OUTRING
OUTSANG
OUTSING
OUTSUNG
OUTWING
PUDDING
PUFFING
PULLING
PULPING
PULSING
PUMPING
PUNNING
PUNTING
PURGING
PURLING
PURRING
PURSING
PUSHING
PUTTING
QUAKING
QUEUING
QUOTING
RUBBING
RUCHING
RUCKING
RUFFING
RUINING
RUNNING
RUSHING
RUSTING
RUTTING
SUBBING
SUBKING
SUBLONG
SUCKING
SUDSING
SUITING
SULKING
SUMMING
SUNNING
SUPPING
SURFING
SURGING
SUSSING
TUBBING
TUCKING
TUFTING
TUGGING
TURFING
TURNING
TUSKING
TUTTING
YUKKING
YULELOG

••UG•••

ARUGULA
BOUGHED
CHUGGED
CHUGGER
COUGARS
COUGHED
COUGHUP
CRUGUET
DOUGHTY
DOUGLAS
DRUGGED
GAUGERS
GAUGING
GAUGUIN
GLUGGED
GOUGERS
GOUGING
HAUGHTY
KLUGMAN
LAUGHAT
LAUGHED
LAUGHER
LAUGHIN
MAUGHAM

NAUGHTS
NAUGHTY
NOUGATS
NOUGHTS
PEUGEOT
PLUGGED
PLUGGER
PLUGINS
PLUGOLA
PLUGSIN
PLUGSUP
ROUGHED
ROUGHEN
ROUGHER
ROUGHGO
ROUGHIT
ROUGHLY
ROUGHUP
ROUGING
SLUGGED
SLUGGER
SMUGGER
SMUGGLE
SNUGFIT
SNUGGED
SNUGGER
SNUGGLE
SNUGGLY
SNUGLIS
TOUGHEN
TOUGHER
TOUGHIE
TOUGHLY
URUGUAY
VAUGHAN

••U•G••

BLUDGED
BLUDGER
BLUDGES
BOURGET
BRUEGEL
CHUGGED
CHUGGER
CLUNGTO
DRUDGED
DRUDGER
DRUDGES
DRUGGED
FLUNGAT
GLUEGUN
GLUGGED
GLURGES
GRUDGED
GRUDGER
GRUDGES
GRUNGER
GRUNGES
KLUDGED
KLUDGES
KRUEGER
LOUNGED
LOUNGER
LOUNGES
PLUGGED
PLUGGER
PLUNGED
PLUNGER
PLUNGES
REURGED
REURGES
SLUDGES
SLUGGED
SLUGGER
SMUDGED
SMUDGES
SMUGGER
SMUGGLE
SNUGGED
SNUGGER
SNUGGLE
SNUGGLY
STUNGUN
STURGES
SWUNGAT
SWUNGBY
SWUNGIT
THURGAU
TRUDGED
TRUDGEN
TRUDGER
TRUDGES
UNURGED
YOUNGER
YOUNGMC
YOUNGUN

••U•G•

BLUINGS
COURAGE
FLUBUGS
HAULAGE
HEURIGE
IMUSTGO
MOULAGE
PLUMAGE
ROUGHGO
SAUSAGE

••U•••G

ABUSING
AMUSING
BLUEING
BRUXING
CAUSING
CHUTING
CLUEING
COUPING
DAUBING
DEUCING
DOUBLEG
DOUSING
EDUCING
ELUDING
ELUTING
ENURING
EXUDING
FEUDING
FLUTING
FLUXING
FOULING
GAUGING
GOUGING
HAULING
HOUSING
INURING
LAUDING
LOURING
LOUSING
LOUTING
MAULING
MOUSING
PAULING
PAUSING
PLUMING
POURING
POUTING
PRUNING
REUSING
ROUGING
ROUSING
ROUTING
SAUCING
SOURING
SOUSING
SPUMING
STUBING
TOUAREG
TOURING
TOUTING
TRUEING
YOURANG

•••UG••

BELUGAS
BROUGHT
CAYUGAS
CHOUGHS
DELUGED
DELUGES
DRAUGHT
DROUGHT
FRAUGHT
IMPUGNS
NOSUGAR
OPPUGNS
PERUGIA
PLOUGHS
REFUGED
REFUGEE
REFUGES
REPUGNS
SCRUGGS
SLOUGHS
THOUGHT
TROUGHS
WROUGHT

•••U•G•

ADJUDGE
ASSUAGE
DEBURGH
DIVULGE
ELFUDGE
EXPUNGE
INDULGE
LEXUSGS
LEXUSGX
LITURGY
OHFUDGE
PANURGE
REJUDGE
RESURGE
SCOURGE
SCRUGGS
SPLURGE
UPSURGE
ZYMURGY

•••U•G

ARGUING
ENDUING
ENSUING
IMBUING
ISSUING
PIQUING
QUEUING
ROGUING
TABUING
VALUING
VOGUING

••••UG•

BEDBUGS
BIGHUGS
BOROUGH
FLUBUGS
HUMBUGS
IFYOUGO
MESHUGA
RAGRUGS
REGAUGE
THROUGH
TORTUGA
UNPLUGS
UNTOUGH
VERDUGO

••••U•G

ACHTUNG
CYYOUNG
DEYOUNG
HAMBURG
HARBURG
HOMBURG
HORNUNG
LIMBURG
MCCLURG
NEWBURG
OUTSUNG
SAMSUNG
TSETUNG
UNSLUNG
UNSTUNG
UNSWUNG
UNWRUNG
UNYOUNG
WARBURG
ZEITUNG

•••••UG

AREARUG
BEARHUG
BEERMUG
BORLAUG
CUTARUG
EARPLUG
FIREBUG
GOLDBUG
HALFDUG
JUNEBUG
LADYBUG
LOVEBUG
NONDRUG
PILLBUG
SEASLUG
SHAGRUG
THEFRUG

U•H••••

UNHAIRS
UNHAIRY
UNHANDS
UNHANDY
UNHAPPY
UNHARDY
UNHARSH
UNHASPS
UNHASTY
UNHATED
UNHAYED
UNHAZED
UNHEADY
UNHEARD
UNHEAVY
UNHEEDS
UNHELMS
UNHEWED
UNHILLY
UNHINGE
UNHIRED
UNHIRES
UNHITCH
UNHONED
UNHOODS
UNHOOKS
UNHOPED
UNHORSE
UNHOUSE
UNHULLS
UNHUMAN
UNHUMID
UNHUSKS
UPHEAPS
UPHEAVE
UPHILLS
UPHOARD
UPHOLDS
USHAPED
USHAPES
USHERED
USHERIN

U••H•••

UNCHAIN
UNCHAIR
UNCHARY
UNCHECK
UNCHOKE
UNCHURN
UNRHYME
UNSHADE
UNSHADY
UNSHARP
UNSHEER
UNSHELL
UNSHIER
UNSHIFT
UNSHINY
UNSHIPS
UNSHOED
UNSHOES
UNSHORN
UNSHORT
UNSHOWN
UNSHOWY
UNSHYER
UNSHYLY
UNTHAWS
UNTHICK
UNTHINK
UNWHEEL
UNWHIPT
UNWHITE
UNWHOLE
UPAHEAD
UPPHASE
UPSHIFT
UPSHOOT
UPSHOTS
UPTHERE
UPTHROW
UPWHIRL
URCHINS
UTAHANS

U•••H••

USOSHOW

U••••H•

UNLIGHT
UNMACHO
UNSIGHT
UPLIGHT
UPRIGHT
UPTIGHT
UTRECHT

U•••••H

UNBENCH
UNBERTH
UNCINCH
UNCOUTH
UNEARTH
UNFAITH
UNFERTH
UNHARSH
UNHITCH
UNLATCH
UNLEASH
UNLOATH
UNTEACH
UNTOUGH
UNTRUTH
UPNORTH
UPREACH

•UH••••

DUHAMEL
SUHARTO

•U•H•••

AUTHORS
BUCHMAN
BUCHNER
BUKHARA
BUSHELS
BUSHERS
BUSHHOG
BUSHIDO
BUSHIER
BUSHILY
BUSHING
BUSHMAN
BUSHMEN
BUSHPIG
BUSHWAH
CUSHAWS
CUSHIER
CUSHILY
CUSHING
CUSHION
DUCHAMP
DUCHESS
DUCHIES
EUCHRED
EUCHRES
EUPHONY
FUCHSIA
FUTHARK
GUSHERS
GUSHIER
GUSHILY
GUSHING
GUSHOUT
GUTHRIE
HUSHABY
HUSHFUL
HUSHING
JUGHEAD
KUCHENS
LUCHINO
LUSHEST
LUSHIER
LUTHIER
LUTHULI
MUDHENS
MUDHOLE
MULHARE
MUSHERS
MUSHIER
MUSHILY
MUSHING
NUNHOOD
OUGHTNT
OUGHTTO
OUTHAUL
OUTHEAR
OUTHERE
OUTHIRE
OUTHISS
OUTHITS
OUTHOWL
OUTHUNT
OUTHURL
PUSHERS
PUSHFOR
PUSHFUL
PUSHIER
PUSHILY
PUSHING
PUSHKIN
PUSHOFF
PUSHOUT
PUSHPIN
PUSHROD
PUSHUPS
QUAHOGS
RUCHING
RUNHOME
RUSHDIE
RUSHEES
RUSHERS
RUSHIER
RUSHING
RUSHOFF
RUSHOUT
RUTHANN
RUTHFUL
SUBHALL
SUBHEAD
SUNHATS
TUCHMAN
TUSHERY
TUSHIES

•U••H••

BUDDHAS
BULGHUR
BUNCHED
BUNCHES
BUNCHUP
BUQSHAS
BURGHER
BUSHHOG
BUTCHER
BUTCHES
CULCHES
CUMSHAW
FULGHUM
FURTHER
GULCHES
GUMSHOE
GUNSHIP
GUNSHOT
GUNTHER
GURKHAS
HUMPHED
HUMPHRY
HUNCHED
HUNCHES
HUTCHES
KUTCHER
LUNCHED
LUNCHER
LUNCHES
LURCHED
LURCHER
LURCHES
MUGSHOT
MULCHED
MULCHES
MUNCHED
MUNCHEN
MUNCHER
MUNCHES
MUNCHIE
MUNCHON
MURPHYS
NUDZHED
NUDZHES
NUNSHIP
OUTSHOT
OUTSHOW
PUNCHED
PUNCHER
PUNCHES
PUNCHIN
PUNCHUP
QUASHED
QUASHES
QUECHUA
QUICHES
RUMSHOP
SULPHUR

•U•••H•

GULLAHS
HUANGHE
HUPPAHS
HURRAHS
HUZZAHS
MULCAHY
MULLAHS
OUTECHO
RUPIAHS
SUBECHO

•U••••H

AUTARCH
BULLISH
BULRUSH
BUMRUSH
BURNISH
BUSHWAH
CUBBISH
CULTISH
CURRISH
DULLISH
DUMPISH
DUNCISH
DUSKISH
FURBISH
FURNISH
HUFFISH
HUNNISH
KURDISH
LUMPISH
MUDBATH
MUDFISH
MUGGISH
MURDOCH
MURKISH
NUNNISH
OUTFISH
OUTGUSH
OUTLASH
OUTPATH
OUTPUSH
OUTRUSH
OUTSIGH
OUTWASH
OUTWISH
OUTWITH
PUBLISH
PUCKISH
PUGGISH
RUBBISH
RUDOLPH
RUNNETH
RUNTISH
RUNWITH
RUTTISH
SUBCASH
SUCCOTH
SUKKOTH
SUNBATH
SUNFISH
TURKISH

••UH•••

BAUHAUS
JOUHAUX

••U•H••

AGULHAS
BLUEHEN
BLUSHED
BLUSHER
BLUSHES
BLUSHON
BOUCHER
BOUCHES
BOUGHED
BRUSHED
BRUSHER
BRUSHES
BRUSHUP
CAUTHEN
COUCHED
COUCHES
COUGHED
COUGHUP
CRUSHED
CRUSHER
CRUSHES
DAUPHIN
DOUGHTY
FLUSHED
FLUSHER
FLUSHES
FLUSHOT
GAUCHER
GAUCHOS
HAUGHTY
LAUGHAT
LAUGHED
LAUGHER
LAUGHIN
MAUGHAM
MOUTHED
MOUTHER
NAUGHTS
NAUGHTY
NOUGHTS
PLUSHER
PLUSHES
PLUSHLY
POUCHED
POUCHES
PRUDHOE
REUTHER
ROUGHED
ROUGHEN
ROUGHER
ROUGHGO
ROUGHIT
ROUGHLY
ROUGHUP
SHUSHED
SHUSHES
SLUSHED
SLUSHES
SMUSHED
SMUSHES
SOUTHEY
SOUTHOF
TOUCHED
TOUCHER
TOUCHES
TOUCHON
TOUCHUP
TOUGHEN
TOUGHER
TOUGHIE
TOUGHLY
VAUGHAN
VOUCHED
VOUCHER
VOUCHES
YOUTHEN

••U••H•

CHURCHY
CLUTCHY
CRUNCHY
FOURTHS
GOUACHE
PAUNCHY
RAUNCHY
SQUASHY
SQUISHY

••U•••H

BLUEISH
BRUTISH
CHUMASH
CHUPPAH
DEUTSCH
DOUBLEH
GAULISH
GOULASH
GOUTISH
LOUDISH
LOUTISH
NOURISH
PRUDISH
SOURISH
SQUELCH
SQUINCH
YOUWISH

•••UH••

MCLUHAN
MENUHIN

•••U•H•

BELUSHI
BROUGHT
CAPUCHE
CHOUGHS
DRAUGHT
DROUGHT
FRAUGHT
GROUCHO
GROUCHY
NOGUCHI
PENUCHE
PLOUGHS
SLEUTHS
SLOUCHY
SLOUGHS
THOUGHT
TROUGHS
WROUGHT

•••U••H

ANGUISH
ANOUILH
ASQUITH
ATLUNCH
BEAUISH
DEBURGH
DOLUNCH
GALUMPH
GODUTCH
HANUKAH
INDUTCH
MEZUZAH
NKRUMAH
PADUCAH
ROGUISH
SCRUNCH
STAUNCH
TRIUMPH
VOGUISH

••••UH•

NIEBUHR

••••U•H

ANDSUCH
AZIMUTH
BISMUTH
BOROUGH
BULRUSH
BUMRUSH
BYMOUTH
DEBAUCH
DELRUTH
FATOUSH
FORBUSH
GOSOUTH
HOWMUCH
INARUSH
INTOUCH
INTRUTH
JEBBUSH
KOSSUTH
LELOUCH
MADRUSH
NONSUCH
NOTMUCH
OUTGUSH
OUTPUSH
OUTRUSH
REBRUSH
RETOUCH
THEBUSH
THROUGH
TOOMUCH
UNCOUTH
UNTOUGH
UNTRUTH

U•I••••

UNIATES
UNIBALL
UNIBODY
UNICODE
UNICORN
UNIDEAL
UNIFIED
UNIFIER
UNIFIES
UNIFORM
UNINERT
UNINKED
UNIPLEX
UNIPODS
UNIQUES
UNISIZE
UNISOMS
UNISONS
UNITARD
UNITARY
UNITERS
UNITIES
UNITING
UNITISE
UNITIVE
UNITIZE
UNIVACS
USINGIN
USINGUP
UTICANS
UTICANY
UTILISE
UTILITY
UTILIZE
UVINDEX

U••I•••

UGLIEST
ULTIMAS
UMPIRED
UMPIRES
UNAIDED
UNAIMED
UNAIRED
UNBINDS
UNCIALS
UNCINCH
UNCITED
UNCIVIC
UNCIVIL
UNDIKED
UNDINES
UNFIERY
UNFILED
UNFILES
UNFINED
UNFINES
UNFIRED
UNFITLY
UNFIXED
UNFIXES
UNGIDDY
UNGIRDS
UNGIVEN
UNHILLY
UNHINGE
UNHIRED

UNHIRES
UNHITCH
UNKINKS
UNLIGHT
UNLIKED
UNLIKES
UNLINED
UNLINKS
UNLIVED
UNLIVES
UNMIKED
UNMINED
UNMIRED
UNMITER
UNMITRE
UNMIXED
UNMIXES
UNOILED
UNPICKS
UNPIETY
UNPILED
UNPILES
UNPIOUS
UNPIPED
UNRIGID
UNRILED
UNRIMED
UNRIPER
UNRISEN
UNRISKY
UNRIVED
UNRIVEN
UNSIDED
UNSIGHT
UNSILLY
UNSIZED
UNTIERS
UNTILED
UNTIMED
UNTIMID
UNTIRED
UNVITAL
UNVIVID
UNWINDS
UNWINDY
UNWIPED
UNWIRED
UNWISER
UNWITTY
UPDIVED
UPDIVES
UPFIELD
UPFIRST
UPGIRDS
UPHILLS
UPLIFTS
UPLIGHT
UPLINKS
UPPILED
UPPILES
UPRIGHT
UPRISEN
UPRISER
UPRISES
UPRIVER
UPSIDES
UPSILON
UPSIZED
UPSIZES
UPTICKS
UPTIGHT
UPTILTS
UPTIMES
UPWINDS
URGINGS
URSINUS
USTINOV
UTRILLO

U•••I••

UGOLINO
UKRAINE
UMBRIAN
UMBRIEL
UNAGILE
UNAGING
UNALIKE
UNBAITS
UNBRIEF
UNBUILD
UNBUILT
UNCLIPS
UNCLIPT
UNCOILS
UNCRIED
UNCTION
UNDOING
UNDRIED
UNDYING
UNFAITH
UNFRIED
UNFRILL
UNGRIPS
UNHAIRS
UNHAIRY
UNIFIED
UNIFIER
UNIFIES
UNISIZE
UNITIES
UNITING
UNITISE
UNITIVE
UNITIZE
UNJOINS
UNJOINT
UNJUICY
UNKNITS
UNLYING
UNMOIST
UNNAILS
UNNAIVE
UNNOISY
UNOWING
UNPLIED
UNQUICK
UNQUIET
UNRAINY
UNSHIER
UNSHIFT
UNSHINY
UNSHIPS
UNSLICK
UNSLIER
UNSLING
UNSPICY
UNSPIED
UNSPILT
UNSTICK
UNSTIFF
UNTHICK
UNTHINK
UNTRIED
UNTRITE
UNTWINE
UNTWIST
UNTYING
UNVEILS
UNVOICE
UNVYING
UNWHIPT
UNWHITE
UPBUILD
UPCLIMB
UPCOILS
UPDRIED
UPDRIES
UPDRIFT
UPFLING
UPGOING
UPRAISE
UPSHIFT
UPSPINS
UPSTIRS
UPSWING
UPWHIRL
URACILS
URANITE
URANIUM
URCHINS
URNLIKE
USERIDS
USURIES
UTILISE
UTILITY
UTILIZE
UTOPIAN
UTOPIAS
UTOPISM
UTOPIST
UXORIAL

U••••I•

UNBRAID
UNCHAIN
UNCHAIR
UNCIVIC
UNCIVIL
UNCOMIC
UNCUBIC
UNFLUID
UNFRAIL
UNHUMID
UNLUCID
UNLYRIC
UNPLAIT
UNRIGID
UNSLAIN
UNSOLID
UNSPLIT
UNSTAID
UNSTOIC
UNTIMID
UNTOXIC
UNVIVID
UPANDIN
UPBRAID
UPFORIT
UPSTAIR
URBANII
URBANIV
USHERIN
USINGIN
UTENSIL

U•••••I

UNBELDI
URBANII
URBANVI

•UI••••

BUILDER
BUILDIN
BUILDON
BUILDUP
BUILTIN
BUILTON
BUILTUP
BUISSON
BUITONI
CUIBONO
CUINGIN
CUIRASS
CUISINE
GUIDERS
GUIDING
GUIGNOL
GUILDER
GUILING
GUINEAN
GUINEAS
GUITARS
JUICERS
JUICEUP
JUICIER
JUICILY
JUICING
JUILLET
QUIBBLE
QUICHES
QUICKEN
QUICKER
QUICKIE
QUICKLY
QUIETED
QUIETEN
QUIETER
QUIETLY
QUIETUS
QUIGLEY
QUILLED
QUILLER
QUILTED
QUILTER
QUINARY
QUINATE
QUINCES
QUINCEY
QUINELA
QUININE
QUINION
QUINLAN
QUINQUE
QUINTAL
QUINTAS
QUINTES
QUINTET
QUINTIC
QUINTON
QUINTUS
QUINZES
QUIPPED
QUIPPER
QUIRTED
QUITESO
QUITSIT
QUITTED
QUITTER
QUIVERS
QUIVERY
QUIVIVE
QUIXOTE
QUIZNOS
QUIZZED
QUIZZER
QUIZZES
RUINATE
RUINERS
RUINING
RUINOUS
SUITING
SUITORS
SUITSME
SUITSUP
TUILLES
TUITION
VUITTON

•U•I•••

AUDIBLE
AUDIBLY
AUDILES
AUDITED
AUDITEE
AUDITOR
AUGITES
AURICLE
AURISTS
AUTISTS
BUNIONS
BURIALS
BURIERS
BUSIEST
BUYINTO
CUBICAL
CUBICLE
CUBICLY
CUBISTS
CUBITAL
CUBITUS
CURIOSA
CURIOUS
CUTICLE
CUTINON
CUTINTO
CUTISES
DUBIETY
DUBIOUS
DUGINTO
DUTIFUL
FUJISAN
FUJITSU
FUMIEST
FURILLO
FURIOSO
FURIOUS
FUSIBLE
FUSILLI
FUSIONS
GUNITES
HUMIDEX
HUMIDLY
HUMIDOR
JUBILEE
JUJITSU
JULIANA
JUNIORS
JUNIPER
JUPITER
JURIDIC
JURISTS
KURILES
LUCIANA
LUCIANO
LUCIDAE
LUCIDLY
LUCIFER
LUCILLE
LUCINDA
LUCITES
LUCIUSI
LUMIERE
LUMINAS
LUPINES
LURIDLY
LUTISTS
MURIELS
MURILLO
MUSICAL
MUSICKS
MUSIGNY
MUSINGS
NUBIANS
NUBIRAS
NUDISTS
OUTINGS
PUMICED
PUMICES
PUNIEST
PURISTS
PURITAN
PUTITTO
QUAILED
QUEIROS
QUOINED
QUOITED
RUBICON
RUBIOUS
RUBITIN
RUFIYAA
RULIEST
RULINGS
RUNINTO
RUNITUP
RUPIAHS
RUTILES
RUZICKA
SUBIDEA
SUBITEM
SUMITUP
SURIMIS
SURINAM
TUBISTS
TUNICLE
TUNISIA
TURISMO
TURISTA
ZUNIANS

•U••I••

AUCTION
AUNTIES
AUPAIRS
AUSPICE
AUSSIES
AUSTINS
AUTOING
BUCKING
BUDDIED
BUDDIES
BUDDING
BUDGIES
BUDGING
BUDLIKE
BUDTIME
BUFFING
BUGGIER
BUGGIES
BUGGING
BUGLING
BULGIER
BULGING
BULKIER
BULKING
BULLIED
BULLIES
BULLING
BULLINS
BULLION
BULLISH
BULLITT
BUMMING
BUMPIER
BUMPILY
BUMPING
BUNGING
BUNKING
BUNNIES
BUNNING
BUNTING
BUOYING
BURDICK
BURKINA
BURLIER
BURLING
BURNING
BURNISH
BURPING
BURRIER
BURRING
BURRITO
BURYING
BUSBIES
BUSGIRL
BUSHIDO
BUSHIER
BUSHILY
BUSHING
BUSKING
BUSLINE
BUSRIDE
BUSSING
BUSTIER
BUSTING
BUSYING
BUTTING
BUYTIME
BUZZIER
BUZZING
CUBBIES
CUBBING
CUBBINS
CUBBISH
CUBOIDS
CUDDIES
CUEBIDS
CUETIPS
CUFFING
CUISINE
CULLIED
CULLIES
CULLING
CULTISH
CULTISM
CULTIST
CUMBIAS
CUNNING
CUPLIKE
CUPPIER
CUPPING
CUPRITE
CURBING
CURDIER
CURDING
CURLIER
CURLIKE
CURLING
CURRIED
CURRIER
CURRIES
CURRING
CURRISH
CURSING
CURSIVE
CURTISS
CURVIER
CURVING
CUSHIER
CUSHILY
CUSHING
CUSHION
CUSPIDS
CUSSING
CUTTIME
CUTTING
DUALISM
DUALIST
DUALITY
DUALIZE
DUBBING
DUBNIUM
DUCHIES
DUCKIER
DUCKIES
DUCKING
DUCTILE
DUCTING
DUELING
DUELIST
DUETING
DULCIFY
DULLING
DULLISH
DUMBING
DUMMIED
DUMMIES
DUMPIER
DUMPILY
DUMPING
DUMPISH
DUNCISH
DUNKING
DUNKIRK
DUNLINS
DUNNING
DURNING
DUSKIER
DUSKILY
DUSKING
DUSKISH
DUSTIER
DUSTILY
DUSTING
FUBSIER
FUDDIES
FUDGING
FUELING
FULFILL
FULFILS
FUNDING
FUNKIER
FUNKILY
FUNKING
FUNNIER
FUNNIES
FUNNILY
FUNNING
FUNTIME
FURBISH
FURLING
FURNISH
FURRIER
FURRING
FURTIVE
FUSSIER
FUSSILY
FUSSING
FUSTIAN
FUSTIER
FUSTILY
FUTZING
FUZZIER
FUZZILY
FUZZING
GUANINE
GUCKIER
GUIDING
GUILING
GULFING
GULLIED
GULLIES
GULLING
GULPIER
GULPING
GUMLIKE
GUMMIER
GUMMING
GUNFIRE
GUNKIER
GUNNIES
GUNNING
GUPPIES
GUSHIER
GUSHILY
GUSHING
GUSSIED
GUSSIES
GUSTIER
GUSTILY
GUSTING
GUTSIER
GUTSILY
GUTTIER
GUTTING
HUBBIES
HUFFIER
HUFFILY
HUFFING
HUFFISH
HUGGIES
HUGGING
HUGGINS
HULKIER
HULKING
HULLING
HUMMING
HUMPIER
HUNKIER
HUNLIKE
HUNNISH
HUNTING
HURLING
HURRIED
HURRIER
HURRIES
HURTING
HUSHING
HUSKIER
HUSKIES
HUSKILY
HUSKING
HUSSIES
HUSSITE
HUTLIKE
HUTTING
JUDAICA
JUDAISM
JUDGING
JUDOIST
JUGGING
JUGWINE
JUICIER
JUICILY
JUICING
JUMPIER
JUMPILY
JUMPING
JUNGIAN
JUNKIER
JUNKIES
JUNKING
JURYING
JUSTICE
JUSTIFY
JUSTINE
JUTTING
KUBRICK
KURDISH
KUWAITI
LUCHINO
LUCKIER
LUCKILY
LUCKING
LUDDISM
LUDDITE
LUFFING
LUGGING
LULLING
LUMPIER
LUMPILY
LUMPING
LUMPISH
LUNGING
LURKING
LUSHIER
LUSTIER
LUSTILY
LUSTING
LUTHIER
MUCKIER
MUCKING
MUDDIED
MUDDIER
MUDDIES
MUDDILY
MUDDING
MUDFISH
MUDPIES
MUFFING
MUFFINS
MUGGIER
MUGGING
MUGGISH
MULLING
MULLINS
MUMMIES
MUMMIFY
MUMMING
MURKIER
MURKILY
MURKISH
MUSCIDA
MUSHIER
MUSHILY
MUSHING
MUSKIER
MUSKIES
MUSLIMS
MUSLINS
MUSSIER
MUSSILY
MUSSING
MUSTIER
MUSTILY
MUYBIEN
MUZZIER
MUZZILY
NUBBIER
NUBBINS
NUCLIDE
NUDGING
NUDNIKS
NULLIFY
NULLING
NULLITY
NUMBING
NUNCIOS
NUNLIKE
NUNNISH
NUPTIAL
NURSING
NUTLIKE
NUTOILS
NUTPINE
NUTRIAS
NUTSIER
NUTTIER
NUTTILY
NUTTING
OUGUIYA
OUSTING
OUTBIDS
OUTCITY
OUTFIND
OUTFIRE
OUTFISH
OUTFITS
OUTGIVE
OUTHIRE
OUTHISS
OUTHITS
OUTJINX
OUTKICK
OUTKILL
OUTKING
OUTKISS
OUTLIER
OUTLIES
OUTLIMN
OUTLINE
OUTLIPS
OUTLIVE
OUTPICK
OUTPIPE
OUTPITY
OUTRIBS
OUTRIDE
OUTRIGS
OUTRING
OUTSIDE
OUTSIFT
OUTSIGH
OUTSING
OUTSINS
OUTSITS
OUTSIZE
OUTTIRE
OUTVIED
OUTVIES
OUTWILE
OUTWILL
OUTWIND
OUTWING
OUTWISH
OUTWITH
OUTWITS
PUBLICS
PUBLISH
PUBLIUS
PUCCINI
PUCKISH
PUDDING
PUDGIER
PUDGILY
PUERILE
PUFFIER
PUFFILY
PUFFING
PUFFINS
PUGGISH
PULLING
PULLINS
PULPIER
PULPIFY
PULPING
PULPITS
PULSING
PUMPING
PUNDITS
PUNKIER
PUNKIES
PUNNIER
PUNNILY
PUNNING
PUNTING
PUPPIES
PURGING
PURLIEU
PURLING
PURRING
PURSIER
PURSING
PURTIER
PURVIEW
PUSHIER
PUSHILY
PUSHING
PUSSIES
PUTTIED
PUTTIES
PUTTING
QUAKIER
QUAKIES
QUAKILY
QUAKING
QUALIFY
QUALITY
QUERIDA
QUERIDO
QUERIED
QUERIER
QUERIES
QUERIST
QUEUING
QUININE
QUINION
QUIVIVE
QUOTING
RUBBING
RUBBISH
RUBRICS
RUCHING
RUCKING
RUCTION

RUDDIED
RUDDIER
RUDDILY
RUFFIAN
RUFFING
RUGLIKE
RUINING
RUMMIES
RUNNIER
RUNNING
RUNRIOT
RUNTIER
RUNTIME
RUNTISH
RUNWILD
RUNWITH
RUSHIER
RUSHING
RUSSIAN
RUSTICS
RUSTIER
RUSTILY
RUSTING
RUTTIER
RUTTING
RUTTISH
SUASION
SUASIVE
SUAVITY
SUBBIAS
SUBBING
SUBFILE
SUBKING
SUBLIDS
SUBLIME
SUBMITS
SUBSIDE
SUBSIDY
SUBSIST
SUCKIER
SUCKING
SUCTION
SUDSIER
SUDSING
SUFFICE
SUITING
SULFIDE
SULFITE
SULKIER
SULKIES
SULKILY
SULKING
SULLIED
SULLIES
SUMMING
SUMMITS
SUMOIST
SUNBIRD
SUNCITY
SUNDIAL
SUNFIRE
SUNFISH
SUNKIST
SUNLIKE
SUNNIER
SUNNILY
SUNNING
SUNRISE
SUPPING
SUREIAM
SUREIDO
SURFIER
SURFING
SURGING
SURLIER
SURLILY
SURMISE
SURVIVE
SUSPIRE
SUSSING
TUBAIST
TUBBIER
TUBBING
TUBLIKE
TUCKING
TUFTIER
TUFTING
TUGGING
TUGRIKS
TUITION
TUMMIES
TURBINE
TURFIER
TURFING
TURKISH
TURNING
TURNIPS
TUSHIES
TUSKING
TUSSIVE
TUTTING
TUTUILA
VULPINE
YUCAIPA
YUCKIER
YUKKING
YUMMIER
YUPPIES
YUPPIFY

•U•••I•

AUSTRIA
AUTOBIO
AUTOPIA
BUCOLIC
BUILDIN
BUILTIN
BUMPKIN
BURNSIN
BURNTIN
BURSTIN
BUSHPIG
BUSTRIP
BUSTSIN
BUTTSIN
CUINGIN
CULPRIT
CUMBRIA
CURLSIN
CURTAIL
CURTAIN
DUCKPIN
DUKAKIS
DUNEDIN
DUSTBIN
DUUMVIR
EUCERIN
EUGENIA
EUGENIC
EUGENIE
EUNOMIA
EURASIA
FUCHSIA
FUELOIL
FUNFAIR
FUNFZIG
GULFOIL
GUNSHIP
GUTHRIE
HUSSEIN
JUMPBID
JUMPSIN
JURIDIC
JURYRIG
KUBELIK
LUCANIA
LUCYLIU
LUGSAIL
LUMPSIN
LUMPSIT
LUNATIC
LUREDIN
LURESIN
LUTETIA
MUESLIS
MUESLIX
MUEZZIN
MUNCHIE
NUCLEIC
NUMERIC
NUNSHIP
OUTGAIN
OUTGRIN
OUTLAID
OUTLAIN
OUTOFIT
OUTPAID
OUTRAIL
OUTSAID
OUTSAIL
OUTSKIP
OUTSPIN
OUTSPIT
OUTSWIM
OUTWAIT
PULLPIN
PULLSIN
PUMPKIN
PUNCHIN
PURLOIN
PURSUIT
PUSHKIN
PUSHPIN
QUADRIC
QUARTIC
QUEENIE
QUEENIT
QUENTIN
QUICKIE
QUINTIC
QUITSIT
RUBITIN
RUMAKIS
RUMANIA
RUNONIN
RUSHDIE
SUBARID
SUBJOIN
SUBSOIL
SUBUNIT
SUCKSIN
SUNMAID
SUNSUIT
SURFEIT
SURIMIS
SURVEIL
SUSTAIN
SUZUKIS
TUCKSIN
TUNAOIL
TUNEDIN
TUNESIN
TUNGOIL
TUNISIA
TURMOIL
TURNSIN
YUKOLIS

•U••••I

BUGATTI
BUITONI
BULGARI
BURUNDI
BUSCEMI
FUSILLI
GUARANI
HUANGTI
JUMANJI
KUWAITI
LUCIUSI
LUTHULI
PUCCINI
PULASKI
PULMONI
PUNJABI
RUDOLFI
TURFSKI

••UI•••

AQUIFER
AQUINAS
AQUIVER
BLUINGS
BRUISED
BRUISER
BRUISES
BRUITED
CRUISED
CRUISER
CRUISES
DRUIDIC
EQUIANO
EQUIFAX
EQUINES
EQUINOX
FLUIDAL
FLUIDIC
FLUIDLY
FRUITED
GLUIEST
LOUISII
LOUISIV
LOUISIX
LOUISVI
LOUISXI
LOUISXV
NEUILLY
SLUICED
SLUICES
SQUINCH
SQUINTS
SQUINTY
SQUIRED
SQUIRES
SQUIRMS
SQUIRMY
SQUIRTS
SQUISHY
TRUISMS

••U•I••

ABUSING
ABUSIVE
ALUMINA
AMUSING
APULIAN
AZURITE
BAUXITE
BLUEICE
BLUEING
BLUEISH
BOUDINS
BOUVIER
BRUTISH
BRUXING
BRUXISM
CAUSING
CAUTION
CHUTING
CHUTIST
CLUEING
COUPING
COURIER
COUSINE
COUSINS
CRUCIAL
CRUDITY
DAUBING
DAUMIER
DEUCING
DOUSING
DRUZIAN
EDUCING
ELUDING
ELUSIVE
ELUTING
ELUTION
ELUVIAL
ELUVIUM
ENURING
ERUDITE
EXUDING
FAUVISM
FAUVIST
FEUDING
FEUDIST
FLUKIER
FLUKILY
FLUTIER
FLUTIES
FLUTING
FLUTIST
FLUVIAL
FLUXING
FLUXION
FOULING
FOURIER
GAUDIER
GAUDIES
GAUDILY
GAUGING
GAULISH
GAUTIER
GAUZIER
GAUZILY
GOUGING
GOUTIER
GOUTILY
GOUTISH
GRUNION
HAULING
HEURIGE
HOUDINI
HOUSING
INURING
INUTILE
LAUDING
LAURITZ
LEUCINE
LOUDISH
LOURING
LOUSIER
LOUSILY
LOUSING
LOUTING
LOUTISH
MAULING
MAURIAC
MAURIAT
MAURICE
MOUSIER
MOUSILY
MOUSING
NAUTICA
NAUTILI
NOURISH
OCULIST
PAUCITY
PAULIII
PAULINA
PAULINE
PAULING
PAULIST
PAUSING
PIUSIII
PLUGINS
PLUMIER
PLUMING
PLUVIAL
POURING
POUTIER
POUTING
PRUDISH
PRUNING
REUNIFY
REUNION
REUNITE
REUSING
ROUGING
ROUSING
ROUTINE
ROUTING
SAUCIER
SAUCILY
SAUCING
SAURIAN
SHUTINS
SOUBISE
SOUPIER
SOURING
SOURISH
SOUSING
SPUMIER
SPUMING
STUBING
STUDIED
STUDIER
STUDIES
STUDIOS
STUPIDS
TAURINE
THULIUM
TOURING
TOURISM
TOURIST
TOUTING
TRUEING
USURIES
YOUWISH

••U••I•

AQUARIA
AQUATIC
AQUAVIT
BLUEFIN
BLUETIT
BOUDOIR
CAUSTIC
CHUCKIT
CLUEDIN
CLUESIN
COUNCIL
COUNTIN
DAUPHIN
DHURRIE
DOUBTIT
DRUIDIC
DRUMLIN
DUUMVIR
EXURBIA
FLUIDIC
FOULTIP
FOURPIN
GAUGUIN
HAULSIN
IGUANID
LAUGHIN
LOUISII
LOUISIV
LOUISIX
MAUDLIN
MAULDIN
MAUROIS
MAUVAIS
MOUNTIE
OPUNTIA
PAULIII
PIUSIII
PIUSVII
PIUSXII
PLUGSIN
PLUMBIC
PLUMPIE
POURSIN
POUSSIN
PRUSSIA
ROUBAIX
ROUGHIT
SHUTSIN
SLUNKIN
SNUGFIT
SNUGLIS
SOUPMIX
SPUTNIK
SQUALID
STUCKIN
STUFFIN
SWUNGIT
TOUGHIE
TRUERIB
TRUSTIN
VAUDOIS
YOUREIT

••U•••I

BHUTANI
DOUBLEI
GOURAMI
HOUDINI
HYUNDAI
LOUISII
LOUISVI
LOUISXI
NAUTILI
PAULIII
PIUSIII
PIUSVII
PIUSXII
SPUMONI
STUARTI
TSUNAMI
YOUANDI

•••UI••

ACQUIRE
ACQUITS
ALQUIST
ANGUISH
ANNUITY
ANOUILH
ARGUING
ASQUIET
ASQUINT
ASQUITH
BEAUISH
BEGUILE
BEGUINE
BEQUICK
BEQUIET
CASUIST
COQUINA
DELUISE
DRQUINN
ENDUING
ENQUIRE
ENQUIRY
ENSUING
ENSUITE
ESQUIRE
FATUITY
GENUINE
IMBUING
INBUILT
INQUIRE
INQUIRY
INRUINS
INTUITS
ISSUING
JESUITS
LIQUIDS
MAGUIRE
MCGUIRE
MRQUILP
OUGUIYA
PIQUING
QUEUING
REBUILD
REBUILT
REGUIDE
REQUIEM
REQUIRE
REQUITE
RESUITS
ROGUING
ROGUISH
SEQUINS
TABUING
TENUITY
TEQUILA
TUTUILA
TVGUIDE
UNBUILD
UNBUILT
UNJUICY
UNQUICK
UNQUIET
UPBUILD
VACUITY
VALUING
VOGUING
VOGUISH

•••U•I•

ABOUTIT
ADZUKIS
AGOUTIS
ALBUMIN
ALDUBIN
ALLUVIA
BIGUNIT
CLAUDIA
CLAUDIO
CYRUSII
ETRURIA
GELUSIL
GROUPIE
INSULIN
KABUKIS
LEXUSIS
LIGURIA
MANUMIT
MENUHIN
MINUTIA
MRMUSIC
ONEUNIT
PERUGIA
PETULIA
PETUNIA
PLAUDIT
READUIT
RENUZIT
RHEUMIC
SALUKIS
SEQUOIA
STLUCIA
SUBUNIT
SUZUKIS
TSOURIS
TWOUNIT
UNCUBIC
UNHUMID
UNLUCID
WATUSIS

•••U••I

ABRUZZI
BELUSHI
BURUNDI
CADUCEI
CYRUSII
EDMUNDI
JACUZZI
NOGUCHI
OLDUVAI
SAMURAI
SHOULDI
TOFUTTI

••••UI•

APESUIT
BATSUIT
BEDOUIN
BISCUIT
CATSUIT
CIRCUIT
CONDUIT
CROQUIS
DAYQUIL
DRYSUIT
FANEUIL
GAUGUIN
GYMSUIT
INASUIT
JOAQUIN
JONQUIL
LANGUID
LAWSUIT
MAOSUIT
MARQUIS
MRSMUIR
NESQUIK
PACQUIN
PENGUIN
PINGUID
POPQUIZ
PURSUIT
RECRUIT
REDSUIT
REEQUIP
SKISUIT
STLOUIS
SUNSUIT
UNFLUID
WETSUIT
YANQUIS

••••U•I

CALCULI
DARIUSI
FAROUKI
LUCIUSI
LUTHULI
RIOMUNI
STIMULI
STPIUSI
TABOULI
VENTURI
XYSTUSI

•••••UI

MAISOUI
RAPANUI

U•J••••

UNJADED
UNJOINS
UNJOINT
UNJOLLY
UNJOYED
UNJUICY

•UJ••••

BUJONES
FUJISAN
FUJITSU
GUJARAT
JUJITSU
JUJUBES
MUJERES

•U•J•••

OUTJEST
OUTJETS
OUTJINX
OUTJUMP
OUTJUTS
PUNJABI
SUBJECT
SUBJOIN

•U••J••

CULTJAM
LUBEJOB

•U•••J•

JUMANJI

••U•J••

BLUEJAY

••U••J•

AZULEJO

••U•••J

DOUBLEJ

•••U•J•

MARUSJA

UK•••••

UKELELE
UKRAINE
UKULELE

U•K••••

UNKEMPT
UNKEYED
UNKINKS
UNKNITS
UNKNOTS
UNKNOWN
UPKEEPS

U••K•••

UNSKEWS

U•••K••

UNASKED
UNBAKED
UNCAKED
UNCAKES
UNDIKED
UNFAKED
UNINKED
UNLIKED
UNLIKES
UNMAKER
UNMAKES
UNMIKED
UNRAKED
UNTAKEN
UNWAKED
UNYOKED
UNYOKES
UPTAKES

U••••K•

UNALIKE
UNAWAKE
UNBRAKE
UNBROKE
UNBULKY
UNCASKS
UNCHOKE
UNCORKS
UNDOCKS
UNFLAKY
UNFORKS
UNHOOKS
UNHUSKS
UNKINKS
UNLEAKY
UNLINKS
UNLOCKS
UNLUCKY
UNMASKS
UNPACKS
UNPICKS
UNRACKS
UNRISKY
UNROCKY
UNSMOKY
UNSNAKY
UNSPOKE
UNSULKY
UNTACKS
UNTUCKS
UPLINKS
UPTALKS
UPTICKS
UQUARKS
URNLIKE

U•••••K

UNBLOCK
UNCHECK
UNCLOAK
UNDRUNK
UNFRANK
UNFROCK
UNQUICK
UNSLACK
UNSLEEK
UNSLICK
UNSPEAK
UNSTACK
UNSTICK
UNSTUCK
UNTHICK
UNTHINK
UNTRACK
UPQUARK
URSULAK

•UK••••

AUKLETS
BUKHARA
DUKAKIS
DUKEDOM
JUKEBOX
MUKLUKS
SUKARNO
SUKKOTH
YUKATAS
YUKKING
YUKOLIS

•U•K•••

BUCKERS
BUCKETS
BUCKEYE
BUCKFOR
BUCKING
BUCKLED
BUCKLES
BUCKLEY
BUCKNER
BUCKOES
BUCKRAM
BUCKSAW
BUCKSUP
BULKIER
BULKING
BULKSUP
BUNKBED
BUNKERS
BUNKING
BUNKOED
BUNKUMS
BURKINA
BUSKERS
BUSKING
CUCKOOS
DUCKERS
DUCKIER

DUCKIES
DUCKING
DUCKOUT
DUCKPIN
DUNKERS
DUNKING
DUNKIRK
DUSKIER
DUSKILY
DUSKING
DUSKISH
FUNKIER
FUNKILY
FUNKING
GUCKIER
GUNKIER
GURKHAS
HULKIER
HULKING
HUNKERS
HUNKIER
HUSKERS
HUSKIER
HUSKIES
HUSKILY
HUSKING
JUNKART
JUNKCAR
JUNKDNA
JUNKERS
JUNKETS
JUNKFAX
JUNKIER
JUNKIES
JUNKING
JUNKMAN
JUNKMEN
LUCKIER
LUCKILY
LUCKING
LUCKMAN
LUCKNOW
LUCKOUT
LUNKERS
LURKERS
LURKING
MUCKERS
MUCKIER
MUCKING
MUCKSUP
MURKIER
MURKILY
MURKISH
MUSKEGO
MUSKETS
MUSKIER
MUSKIES
MUSKRAT
OUTKAST
OUTKEEP
OUTKEPT
OUTKICK
OUTKILL
OUTKING
OUTKISS
PUCKERS
PUCKERY
PUCKETT
PUCKISH
PUNKERS
PUNKIER
PUNKIES
QUAKERS
QUAKIER
QUAKIES
QUAKILY
QUAKING
RUCKERT
RUCKING
RUCKSUP
SUBKING
SUCKDRY
SUCKERS
SUCKIER
SUCKING
SUCKSIN
SUCKSUP
SUKKOTH
SULKERS
SULKIER
SULKIES
SULKILY
SULKING
SUNKIST
TUCKERS
TUCKING
TUCKSIN
TURKEYS
TURKISH
TUSKERS
TUSKING
YUCKIER
YUKKING

•U••K••
BUMPKIN
DUKAKIS
EUREKAS
JUDOKAS
OUTSKIP
PUMPKIN
PUSHKIN
QUACKED
QUACKER
QUICKEN
QUICKER
QUICKIE
QUICKLY
RUMAKIS
SUDOKUS
SUZUKIS
TURNKEY

•U•••K•
AUTARKY
BUDLIKE
BUNRAKU
BUROAKS
CUPCAKE
CUPLIKE
CURLIKE
EUBANKS
GUMLIKE
HUNLIKE
HUTLIKE
MUKLUKS
MUSICKS
NUDNIKS
NUNLIKE
NUTLIKE
OUTASKS
OUTBAKE
OUTTAKE
PULASKI
RUGLIKE
RUMCAKE
RUZICKA
SUNLIKE
TUBLIKE
TUGRIKS
TURFSKI

•U••••K
BULLOCK
BULWARK
BURBANK
BURDICK
BUYBACK
CUTBACK
CUTWORK
DUNDALK
DUNKIRK
FUTHARK
GUNLOCK
JUMBUCK
KUBELIK
KUBRICK
LUBBOCK
MUBARAK
MUDLARK
MUDPACK
NUMLOCK
OUTBACK
OUTBARK
OUTBULK
OUTCOOK
OUTKICK
OUTLOOK
OUTPICK
OUTRANK
OUTROCK
OUTSEEK
OUTSULK
OUTTALK
OUTWALK
OUTWORK
PUTBACK
RUNAMOK
RUNBACK
SUBBANK
SUBTASK
SUFFOLK
SUNDECK
TULSAOK
TUSSOCK

••UK•••
CHUKKER
FLUKIER
FLUKILY
RYUKYUS
YOUKNOW

••U•K••
BAULKED
BAULKER
CAULKED
CAULKER
CHUCKED
CHUCKIT
CHUCKLE
CHUKKER
CHUNKED
CLUCKED
CLUCKER
CLUNKED
CLUNKER
DRUCKER
DRUNKEN
DRUNKER
FLUNKED
FLUNKER
KNUCKLE
KNUCKLY
PLUCKED
PLUNKED
PLUNKER
SHUCKED
SHUCKER
SKULKED
SKULKER
SKUNKED
SLUNKIN
SLUNKUP
SMUCKER
SNUCKUP
STUCKBY
STUCKIN
STUCKON
STUCKTO
STUCKUP
THUNKED
TRUCKED
TRUCKEE
TRUCKER
TRUCKLE

••U••K•
BLUESKY
SQUAWKS
SQUAWKY
SQUEAKS
SQUEAKY
UQUARKS

••U•••K
BRUBECK
DOUBLEK
SPUTNIK

•••UK••
ADZUKIS
HANUKAH
KABUKIS
NONUKES
PERUKES
REBUKED
REBUKER
REBUKES
SALUKIS
STLUKES
SUZUKIS

•••U•K•
ATTUCKS
CANUCKS
DEBUNKS
DEJUNKS
EMMUSKA
MAZURKA
MRLUCKY
OROURKE
UNBULKY
UNHUSKS
UNLUCKY
UNSULKY
UNTUCKS
ZAKUSKA

•••U••K
BEQUICK
BLAUBOK
IRKUTSK
UNQUICK
UPQUARK
URSULAK
YAKUTSK

••••UK•
DYBBUKS
FAROUKI
MUKLUKS
NETSUKE
SIRDUKE
THEDUKE

••••U•K
ANYLUCK
ATATURK
BADLUCK
EYETUCK
GEODUCK
ILLLUCK
INAFUNK
JOEBUCK
JUMBUCK
MOLLUSK
NESQUIK
NIPMUCK
ODDDUCK
OUTBULK
OUTSULK
PETDUCK
POTLUCK
PREDUSK
ROEBUCK
SAWBUCK
SEADUCK
SPELUNK
THEHULK
UNDRUNK
UNSTUCK

•••••UK
MONTAUK
SAWCHUK

UL•••••
ULALUME
ULANOVA
ULANUDE
ULLAGES
ULLMANN
ULSTERS
ULTIMAS
ULULANT
ULULATE
ULYANOV
ULYSSES
ULZANAS

U•L••••
UGLIEST
ULLAGES
ULLMANN
UMLAUTS
UNLACED
UNLACES
UNLADED
UNLADEN
UNLADES
UNLARGE
UNLATCH
UNLAVED
UNLAXED
UNLAXES
UNLEADS
UNLEAFS
UNLEAKY
UNLEARN
UNLEASH
UNLEGAL
UNLEVEL
UNLIGHT
UNLIKED
UNLIKES
UNLINED
UNLINKS
UNLIVED
UNLIVES
UNLOADS
UNLOATH
UNLOBED
UNLOCAL
UNLOCKS
UNLOFTY
UNLOOPS
UNLOOSE
UNLOVED
UNLOWLY
UNLOYAL
UNLUCID
UNLUCKY
UNLUMPY
UNLURED
UNLUSTY
UNLYING
UNLYRIC
UPLANDS
UPLEAPS
UPLEAPT
UPLIFTS
UPLIGHT
UPLINKS
UPLOADS

U••L•••
UFOLOGY
UGOLINO
UKELELE
UKULELE
ULALUME
ULULANT
ULULATE
UNALERT
UNALIKE
UNALONE
UNBLADE
UNBLENT
UNBLEST
UNBLOCK
UNBLOWN
UNBLUED
UNCLAMP
UNCLASP
UNCLEAN
UNCLEAR
UNCLEFT
UNCLIPS
UNCLIPT
UNCLOAK
UNCLOGS
UNCLOSE
UNCLOUD
UNFLAKY
UNFLOOR
UNFLOWN
UNFLUID
UNGLOVE
UNGLUED
UNGLUES
UNPLAIT
UNPLANS
UNPLIED
UNPLUGS
UNPLUMB
UNSLACK
UNSLAIN
UNSLEEK
UNSLICK
UNSLIER
UNSLING
UNSLUNG
UNSLYER
UNSLYLY
UPCLIMB
UPCLOSE
UPFLING
UPFLOWS
UPSLOPE
URNLIKE
UROLOGY
USELESS
USFLAGS
UTILISE
UTILITY
UTILIZE
UVALUES

U•••L••
UCCELLO
UNAXLED
UNBALED
UNBALES
UNBELDI
UNBELTS
UNBOLTS
UNBULKY
UNDULAR
UNFILED
UNFILES
UNFOLDS
UNFULLY
UNGULAE
UNGULAR
UNHELMS
UNHILLY
UNHULLS
UNIPLEX
UNJOLLY
UNMOLDS
UNMOLDY
UNOGLED
UNOILED
UNPALED
UNPILED
UNPILES
UNPOLED
UNRILED
UNROLLS
UNRULED
UNSALTY
UNSELLS
UNSILLY
UNSOLED
UNSOLES
UNSOLID
UNSPLIT
UNSULKY
UNTILED
UNWALLS
UPFOLDS
UPHILLS
UPHOLDS
UPPILED
UPPILES
UPSILON
UPTALKS
UPTILTS
UPVALUE
UPWELLS
URSULAK
USABLES
USUALLY
UTRILLO

U••••L•
UCCELLO
UKELELE
UKULELE
UNADULT
UNAGILE
UNAPTLY
UNBUILD
UNBUILT
UNBURLY
UNCIALS
UNCOILS
UNCOYLY
UNCURLS
UNDEALT
UNFITLY
UNFRILL
UNFULLY
UNFURLS
UNGODLY
UNHILLY
UNHULLS
UNIBALL
UNJOLLY
UNLOWLY
UNMADLY
UNMANLY
UNMOULD
UNNAILS
UNPEELS
UNREELS
UNROLLS
UNSADLY
UNSCALY
UNSEALS
UNSELLS
UNSHELL
UNSHYLY
UNSILLY
UNSLYLY
UNSPELT
UNSPILT
UNSURLY
UNTRULY
UNVEILS
UNWALLS
UNWHOLE
UPBUILD
UPCOILS
UPCURLS
UPEARLY
UPFIELD
UPHILLS
UPPSALA
UPSCALE
UPSWELL
UPWELLS
URACILS
URNFULS
USUALLY
UTRILLO
UTTERLY

U•••••L
UMBRIEL
UNAWFUL
UNCIVIL
UNCRUEL
UNEQUAL
UNFRAIL
UNFRILL
UNIBALL
UNIDEAL
UNLEGAL
UNLEVEL
UNLOCAL
UNLOYAL
UNNASAL
UNNOVEL
UNRAVEL
UNREGAL
UNRURAL
UNSHELL
UNSNARL
UNSPOOL
UNSTEEL
UNUSUAL
UNVENAL
UNVITAL
UNVOCAL
UNWHEEL
UPSWELL
UPWHIRL
USSTEEL
UTENSIL
UXORIAL

•UL••••
AULDSOD
AULETTA
BULBLET
BULBOUS
BULGARI
BULGARS
BULGHUR
BULGIER
BULGING
BULGURS
BULKIER
BULKING
BULKSUP
BULLDOG
BULLETS
BULLIED
BULLIES
BULLING
BULLINS
BULLION
BULLISH
BULLITT
BULLOCK
BULLPEN
BULLRUN
BULOVAS
BULRUSH
BULWARK
CULCHES
CULEXES
CULLERS
CULLETS
CULLIED
CULLIES
CULLING
CULOTTE
CULPRIT
CULTISH
CULTISM
CULTIST
CULTJAM
CULTURE
CULVERT
DULCIFY
DULLARD
DULLEST
DULLING
DULLISH
EULABUS
FULCRUM
FULFILL
FULFILS
FULGENT
FULGHUM
FULLDAY
FULLEST
FULLLOT
FULLOUT
FULMARS
FULNESS
FULSOME
GULCHES
GULDENS
GULFING
GULFOIL
GULFWAR
GULLAHS
GULLETS
GULLIED
GULLIES
GULLING
GULPERS
GULPIER
GULPING
HULKIER
HULKING
HULLERS
HULLING
HULLOED
JULIANA
JULYDAY
LULLABY
LULLERS
LULLING
MULATTO
MULCAHY
MULCHED
MULCHES
MULCTED
MULDAUR
MULDOON
MULETAS
MULGREW
MULHARE
MULLAHS
MULLERS
MULLETS
MULLING
MULLINS
NULLIFY
NULLING
NULLITY
NULLSET
PULASKI
PULLERS
PULLETS
PULLEYS
PULLFOR
PULLING
PULLINS
PULLMAN
PULLOFF
PULLONS
PULLOUT
PULLPIN
PULLSIN
PULLSON
PULLSUP
PULLTAB
PULLTOY
PULLUPS
PULMONI
PULMONO
PULPERS
PULPIER
PULPIFY
PULPING
PULPITS
PULSARS
PULSATE
PULSING
RULEDBY
RULEDON
RULEONE
RULEOUT
RULESON
RULIEST
RULINGS
SULFATE
SULFIDE
SULFITE
SULKERS
SULKIER
SULKIES
SULKILY
SULKING
SULLIED
SULLIES
SULPHUR
SULTANA
SULTANS
SULUSEA
TULANEU
TULSANS
TULSAOK
VULCANS
VULGATE
VULPINE
VULTURE
YULELOG

•U•L•••
AUKLETS
AUSLESE
BUDLESS
BUDLIKE
BUELLER
BUGLERS
BUGLING
BUILDER
BUILDIN
BUILDON
BUILDUP
BUILTIN
BUILTON
BUILTUP
BULLDOG
BULLETS
BULLIED
BULLIES
BULLING
BULLINS
BULLION
BULLISH
BULLITT
BULLOCK
BULLPEN
BULLRUN
BUMLEGS
BURLAPS
BURLERS
BURLIER
BURLING
BUSLANE
BUSLINE
BUSLOAD
BUTLERS
CULLERS
CULLETS
CULLIED
CULLIES
CULLING
CUPLIKE
CURLERS
CURLEWS
CURLIER
CURLIKE
CURLING
CURLSIN
CURLSUP
CUTLASS
CUTLERS
CUTLERY
CUTLETS
DUALISM
DUALIST
DUALITY
DUALIZE
DUELERS
DUELING
DUELIST
DUELLED
DULLARD
DULLEST
DULLING
DULLISH
DUNLINS
DUNLOPS
EUGLENA
FUELERS
FUELING
FUELLED
FUELOIL
FUELROD
FUELSUP
FULLDAY
FULLEST
FULLLOT
FULLOUT
FURLERS
FURLESS
FURLING
FURLONG
GUILDER
GUILING
GULLAHS
GULLETS
GULLIED
GULLIES
GULLING
GUMLESS
GUMLIKE
GUNLAPS
GUNLAWS
GUNLESS
GUNLOCK
GUTLESS
HUELESS

HULLERS
HULLING
HULLOED
HUNLIKE
HURLERS
HURLING
HUTLIKE
JUILLET
JUTLAND
LULLABY
LULLERS
LULLING
LURLEEN
MUDLARK
MUELLER
MUKLUKS
MULLAHS
MULLERS
MULLETS
MULLING
MULLINS
MUSLIMS
MUSLINS
NUCLEAR
NUCLEIC
NUCLEON
NUCLEUS
NUCLIDE
NULLIFY
NULLING
NULLITY
NULLSET
NUMLOCK
NUNLIKE
NUTLETS
NUTLIKE
OUTLAID
OUTLAIN
OUTLAND
OUTLASH
OUTLAST
OUTLAWS
OUTLAYS
OUTLEAD
OUTLEAP
OUTLETS
OUTLIER
OUTLIES
OUTLIMN
OUTLINE
OUTLIPS
OUTLIVE
OUTLOOK
OUTLOUD
OUTLOVE
PUBLICS
PUBLISH
PUBLIUS
PULLERS
PULLETS
PULLEYS
PULLFOR
PULLING
PULLINS
PULLMAN
PULLOFF
PULLONS
PULLOUT

PULLPIN
PULLSIN
PULLSON
PULLSUP
PULLTAB
PULLTOY
PULLUPS
PUNLESS
PURLIEU
PURLING
PURLOIN
QUALIFY
QUALITY
QUELLED
QUELLER
QUELQUE
QUILLED
QUILLER
QUILTED
QUILTER
RUGLIKE
RUMLESS
RUNLAPS
RUNLATE
RUNLESS
RUNLETS
RUTLAND
SUBLETS
SUBLIDS
SUBLIME
SUBLONG
SUBLOTS
SUELLEN
SUELYON
SULLIED
SULLIES
SUMLESS
SUNLAMP
SUNLESS
SUNLIKE
SURLIER
SURLILY
TUBLIKE
TUGLESS
TUILLES

•U••L••

AUDILES
AURALEE
AURALLY
BUBBLED
BUBBLES
BUCKLED
BUCKLES
BUCKLEY
BUCOLIC
BUELLER
BUGALOO
BUGGLES
BULBLET
BUMBLED
BUMBLER
BUMBLES
BUNDLED
BUNDLER
BUNDLES
BUNGLED
BUNGLER
BUNGLES
BURBLED
BURBLER
BURBLES
BURGLAR
BURGLED
BURGLES
BURNLEY
BUSTLED
BUSTLER
BUSTLES
CUDDLED
CUDDLES
CUMULUS
CUPELED
CUPELER
CUPOLAS
CUPULAR
CUPULES
CURDLED
CURDLER
CURDLES
CUSSLER
DUCALLY
DUELLED
DUFFLES
FUDDLED
FUDDLES
FUELLED
FUGALLY
FULLLOT
FUMBLED
FUMBLER
FUMBLES
FUNPLEX
FURILLO
FUSILLI
GUNPLAY
GURGLED
GURGLES
GUZZLED
GUZZLER
GUZZLES
HUDDLED
HUDDLER
HUDDLES
HUMBLED
HUMBLER
HUMBLES
HUNTLEY
HURDLED
HURDLER
HURDLES
HURTLED
HURTLES
HUSTLED
HUSTLER
HUSTLES
JUBILEE
JUDELAW
JUGGLED
JUGGLER
JUGGLES
JUGULAR
JUILLET
JUMBLED
JUMBLER
JUMBLES
JUNGLES
KUBELIK
KURILES
LUCILLE
LUCYLIU
LUNULAE
LUNULAR
MUDDLED
MUDDLER
MUDDLES
MUDFLAP
MUDFLAT
MUDFLOW
MUELLER
MUESLIS
MUESLIX
MUFFLED
MUFFLER
MUFFLES
MUGGLES
MUMBLED
MUMBLER
MUMBLES
MURALED
MURILLO
MUSCLED
MUSCLES
MUZZLED
MUZZLER
MUZZLES
NUBBLES
NUZZLED
NUZZLER
NUZZLES
OUTBLOT
OUTBLOW
OUTFLEE
OUTFLOW
OUTFLUX
OUTGLOW
OUTPLAN
OUTPLAY
OUTPLOD
OUTPLOT
PUDDLED
PUDDLES
PUEBLOS
PUGGLES
PUGSLEY
PURFLED
PURFLER
PURFLES
PURPLED
PURPLES
PUZZLED
PUZZLER
PUZZLES
QUAILED
QUARLES
QUELLED
QUELLER
QUIGLEY
QUILLED
QUILLER
QUINLAN
RUBBLES
RUBELLA
RUDOLFI
RUDOLPH
RUFFLED
RUFFLER
RUFFLES
RUGGLES
RUMBLED
RUMBLER
RUMBLES
RUMPLED
RUMPLES
RUNDLES
RUNSLOW
RURALLY
RUSSLAN
RUSTLED
RUSTLER
RUSTLES
RUTALEE
RUTILES
RUYBLAS
SUBCLAN
SUBPLOT
SUBTLER
SUELLEN
SUNGLOW
SUPPLED
SUPPLER
SUPPLES
SURPLUS
TUBULAR
TUBULES
TUILLES
TUMBLED
TUMBLER
TUMBLES
TUMMLER
TUMULTS
TUPELOS
TUPOLEV
TURTLED
TURTLES
TUSSLED
TUSSLES
TUTELAR
YUKOLIS
YULELOG

•U•••L•

AUDIBLE
AUDIBLY
AURALLY
AUREOLA
AUREOLE
AURICLE
AUSABLE
BUFFALO
BUMPILY
BUNUELO
BURIALS
BUSHELS
BUSHILY
BUXOMLY
BUYABLE
BUZZELL
CUBICLE
CUBICLY
CUDGELS
CUEBALL
CUPFULS
CURABLE
CURABLY
CUREALL
CUSHILY
CUTICLE
DUCALLY
DUCTILE
DUFFELS
DUMPILY
DUNDALK
DUOPOLY
DURABLE
DURABLY
DURRELL
DUSKILY
DUSTILY
FUGALLY
FULFILL
FULFILS
FUNKILY
FUNNELS
FUNNILY
FURBALL
FURILLO
FUSIBLE
FUSILLI
FUSSILY
FUSTILY
FUZZILY
GUMBALL
GUNBELT
GUNMOLL
GUNSELS
GUNWALE
GUSHILY
GUSTILY
GUTSILY
HUBBELL
HUFFILY
HUMANLY
HUMIDLY
HUMMELS
HUSKILY
JUGFULS
JUICILY
JUMPILY
KUMMELS
LUCIDLY
LUCILLE
LUCKILY
LUMPILY
LURIDLY
LUSTILY
LUTHULI
MUDDILY
MUDEELS
MUDHOLE
MUGFULS
MURIELS
MURILLO
MURKILY
MUSHILY
MUSSELS
MUSSILY
MUSTILY
MUTABLE
MUTABLY
MUTEDLY
MUTUALS
MUZZILY
NUTOILS
NUTTILY
OURSELF
OUTBULK
OUTCALL
OUTCOLD
OUTCULL
OUTKILL
OUTPOLL
OUTPULL
OUTROLL
OUTSELL
OUTSOLD
OUTSOLE
OUTSULK
OUTTALK
OUTTELL
OUTTOLD
OUTTOLL
OUTWALK
OUTWELL
OUTWILE
OUTWILL
OUTYELL
OUTYELP
PUDGILY
PUERILE
PUFFILY
PUMMELS
PUNNILY
PURCELL
PUSHILY
QUAKILY
QUEENLY
QUEERLY
QUIBBLE
QUICKLY
QUIETLY
QUINELA
RUBELLA
RUBEOLA
RUDDILY
RUFFALO
RUMPOLE
RUNNELS
RUNWILD
RURALLY
RUSSELL
RUSTILY
SUAVELY
SUBCELL
SUBFILE
SUBHALL
SUFFOLK
SULKILY
SUNBELT
SUNNILY
SURLILY
TUBFULS
TUNABLE
TUNICLE
TUNNELS
TUTUILA
ZUMWALT

•U••••L

AUGURAL
AURORAL
AUSTRAL
BUMDEAL
BUSGIRL
BUZZELL
CUBICAL
CUBITAL
CUEBALL
CUREALL
CURTAIL
DUHAMEL
DURRELL
DUTIFUL
FUELOIL
FULFILL
FURBALL
FURSEAL
GUIGNOL
GULFOIL
GUMBALL
GUNMOLL
HUBBELL
HUMERAL
HUMORAL
HURTFUL
HUSHFUL
HUSSERL
JUVENAL
LUGSAIL
LUSTFUL
LUSTRAL
MUSEFUL
MUSICAL
NUMERAL
NUPTIAL
OUTBAWL
OUTBOWL
OUTCALL
OUTCULL
OUTDUEL
OUTFEEL
OUTFOOL
OUTHAUL
OUTHOWL
OUTHURL
OUTKILL
OUTPOLL
OUTPULL
OUTPURL
OUTRAIL
OUTROLL
OUTSAIL
OUTSELL
OUTTELL
OUTTOLL
OUTWELL
OUTWILL
OUTYELL
PURCELL
PUSHFUL
QUARREL
QUETZAL
QUINTAL
RUSSELL
RUTHFUL
SUBCELL
SUBCOOL
SUBDUAL
SUBGOAL
SUBHALL
SUBSOIL
SUNBOWL
SUNDIAL
SURREAL
SURVEIL
TUMBREL
TUNAOIL
TUNEFUL
TUNGOIL
TURMOIL

••UL•••

ADULATE
ADULTLY
AGULHAS
AMULETS
APULIAN
AVULSED
AVULSES
AZULEJO
BAULKED
BAULKER
BOULDER
CAULKED
CAULKER
COULDBE
COULDNT
COULEES
COULOMB
COULTER
CRULLER
EMULATE
EMULOUS
EVULSED
EVULSES
EXULTED
FAULTED
FOULARD
FOULEST
FOULING
FOULOUT
FOULSUP
FOULTIP
FOULUPS
GAULISH
GOULASH
HAULAGE
HAULERS
HAULING
HAULOFF
HAULSIN
HAULSUP
INULASE
LAULAUS
MAULDIN
MAULERS
MAULING
MOULAGE
MOULDED
MOULDER
MOULTED
OCULARS
OCULIST
OPULENT
PAULIII
PAULINA
PAULINE
PAULING
PAULIST
PAULPRY
PAULSEN
POULENC
POULTRY
ROULADE
ROULEAU
SCULLED
SCULLER
SCULPED
SCULPTS
SHULMAN
SKULKED
SKULKER
SKULLED
SOULFUL
SOULMAN
THULIUM
UKULELE
ULULANT
ULULATE
VAULTED
VAULTER
WOULDBE
WOULDNT
WOULDST
YOULOSE

••U•L••

BAUBLES
BLUELAW
COUPLED
COUPLER
COUPLES
COUPLET
CRUELER
CRUELLA
CRUELLY
CRUELTY
CRULLER
DOUBLEA
DOUBLEB
DOUBLEC
DOUBLED
DOUBLEE
DOUBLEF
DOUBLEG
DOUBLEH
DOUBLEI
DOUBLEJ
DOUBLEK
DOUBLEL
DOUBLEM
DOUBLEN
DOUBLEO
DOUBLEP
DOUBLEQ
DOUBLER
DOUBLES
DOUBLET
DOUBLEU
DOUBLEV
DOUBLEW
DOUBLEX
DOUBLEY
DOUBLEZ
DOUGLAS
DRUMLIN
ECUELLE
EKUELES
EQUALED
EQUALLY
EQUALTO
KNURLED
LOUELLA
MAUDLIN
NEUILLY
NTUPLES
SCULLED
SCULLER
SKULLED
SNUGLIS
SQUALID
SQUALLS
SQUALLY
SQUALOR
SQUELCH
TOUSLED
TOUSLES
USUALLY

••U••L•

ACUTELY
ADULTLY
ALUDELS
ARUGULA
BLUEFLU
BLUFFLY
BLUNTLY
BRUTELY
CHUCKLE
COURTLY
CRUDELY
CRUELLA
CRUELLY
CRUMBLE
CRUMBLY
CRUMPLE
CRUMPLY
ECUELLE
EQUABLE
EQUABLY
EQUALLY
FLUIDLY
FLUKILY
GAUDILY
GAUNTLY
GAUZILY
GOUTILY
GRUFFLY
GRUMBLE
GRUMBLY
INUTILE
KNUCKLE
KNUCKLY
LAURELS
LOUELLA
LOUSILY
MOUSILY
NAUTILI
NEUILLY
PLUGOLA
PLUMPLY
PLUMULE
PLURALS
PLUSHLY
ROUAULT
ROUGHLY
ROUNDLY
SAUCILY
SCUFFLE
SCUTTLE
SHUFFLE
SHUTTLE
SMUGGLE
SNUFFLE
SNUGGLE
SNUGGLY
SOUFFLE
SOUNDLY
SOURALE
SQUALLS
SQUALLY
SQUATLY
SQUEALS
STUBBLE
STUBBLY
STUMBLE
TOUGHLY
TRUCKLE
TRUFFLE
TRUNDLE
UKULELE
USUALLY

••U•••L

ABUTTAL
ALUMNAL
ARUNDEL
ASUSUAL
BRUEGEL
BRUMMEL
CHUNNEL
CLUEFUL
COUNCIL
COUNSEL
CRUCIAL
CRUSTAL
DIURNAL
DOUBLEL
ELUVIAL
FLUIDAL
FLUVIAL
GLUTEAL
JOURNAL
NEUTRAL
PLUVIAL
POUTFUL
ROUNDEL
SOULFUL
UNUSUAL

•••UL••

AFOULOF
AMPULES
ANGULAR
ANNULAR
ANNULET
ANNULUS
AWFULLY
CANULAE
CANULAS
CAPULET
COPULAE
COPULAR
COPULAS
CUMULUS
CUPULAR
CUPULES
DEPULPS
DIVULGE
DIVULSE
ENGULFS
EPAULET
FACULAE
FACULTY
FAMULUS
FERULES
FIBULAE
FIBULAR
FIBULAS
HAMULUS
IMPULSE
INDULGE
INGULFS
INSULAR
INSULIN
INSULTS
JOCULAR
JUGULAR
KIDULTS
LOBULES
LOCULUS
LUNULAE
LUNULAR
MACULAE
MACULAR
MARULLO
MEDULLA
MODULAR
MODULES
MODULUS
MRHULOT
NEBULAE
NEBULAR
NEBULAS
NODULAR
NODULED
NODULES
OCCULTS
OSCULAR
OSCULES
PABULUM
PENULTS
PETULIA
POPULAR
REGULAR
REGULUS
REPULSE
RESULTS
RIVULET
ROMULAN
ROMULUS
SCHULTZ
SECULAR
SHOULDA
SHOULDI
TABULAR

TITULAR
TUBULAR
TUBULES
TUMULTS
UNBULKY
UNDULAR
UNFULLY
UNGULAE
UNGULAR
UNHULLS
UNRULED
UNSULKY
URSULAK
VENULES
ZEBULON
ZEBULUN
ZONULAR
ZONULES

•••U•L•
ACOUPLE
ANNUALS
ANOUILH
AWFULLY
BEGUILE
BOGUSLY
BUNUELO
CASUALS
DECUPLE
DEFUELS
ESCUELA
INBUILT
LEXUSLS
LEXUSLX
MANUALS
MARULLO
MEDULLA
MRQUILP
MUTUALS
NONUPLE
OCTUPLE
OCTUPLY
PIOUSLY
PROUDLY
REBUILD
REBUILT
RECURLS
REFUELS
RITUALS
SAMUELL
SCRUPLE
SEQUELS
SOLUBLE
STOUTLY
TEQUILA
TROUBLE
TUTUILA
UNBUILD
UNBUILT
UNBURLY
UNCURLS
UNFULLY
UNFURLS
UNHULLS
UNSURLY
UPBUILD
UPCURLS
VACUOLE

VAGUELY
VISUALS
VOLUBLE
VOLUBLY

•••U••L
ACAUDAL
ACCUSAL
AROUSAL
AUGURAL
CLAUDEL
CLAUSAL
COZUMEL
EXCUSAL
FIGURAL
GELUSIL
LACUNAL
NAHUATL
NATURAL
NATUREL
PALUDAL
PERUSAL
PLEURAL
RECUSAL
REFUSAL
REFUTAL
SAMUELL
SPOUSAL
STRUDEL
TRAUBEL
UNRURAL

••••UL•
AMPOULE
ARMFULS
ARUGULA
ASARULE
ASSAULT
ATFAULT
BAGFULS
BARBULE
BEFOULS
BEOWULF
BIGGULP
BLACULA
BOXFULS
CALCULI
CANFULS
CANNULA
CAPFULS
CAPSULE
CARFULS
CELLULE
CONSULS
CONSULT
CUPFULS
DEBOULE
DEFAULT
DEPAULU
DIMBULB
DRACULA
DRYBULB
EARFULS
ENSOULS
EYEFULS
FERRULE
FORMULA
GAGRULE

GLOBULE
GRANULE
HADPULL
HASPULL
HATFULS
HERCULE
HOWDULL
INOCULA
JARFULS
JUGFULS
LAPFULS
LEGPULL
LINGULA
LUTHULI
MIDJULY
MISRULE
MOBRULE
MUGFULS
MYFAULT
NERVULE
NETFULS
NOFAULT
OLEBULL
OUTBULK
OUTCULL
OUTPULL
OUTSULK
PANFULS
PETMULE
PITBULL
PLUMULE
POTFULS
REHAULS
RENAULT
ROUAULT
SCAPULA
SEAGULL
SPATULA
STIMULI
STPAULS
TABOULI
THEHULK
THERULE
TUBFULS
UNADULT
UNMOULD
UNTRULY
URNFULS
VALVULA
VALVULE
VATFULS
VEINULE
VINCULA
VIRGULE
VISTULA
WETBULB

••••U•L
ACCRUAL
ASEXUAL
ASUSUAL
BIOFUEL
COEQUAL
DAYQUIL
EMANUEL
FACTUAL
FANEUIL
GRADUAL

HADPULL
HASPULL
HOWDULL
JONQUIL
LEGPULL
LINGUAL
NONFUEL
OLEBULL
OUTCULL
OUTDUEL
OUTHURL
OUTPULL
OUTPURL
PINCURL
PITBULL
PREQUEL
RORQUAL
SEAGULL
SENSUAL
SUBDUAL
SYNFUEL
TACTUAL
TEXTUAL
UNCRUEL
UNEQUAL
UNUSUAL
VICTUAL
VIRTUAL

•••••UL
BALEFUL
BANEFUL
BASHFUL
BOATFUL
BODEFUL
BOWLFUL
BRIMFUL
CAREFUL
CLUEFUL
DAREFUL
DESKFUL
DIREFUL
DISHFUL
DOLEFUL
DOOMFUL
DUTIFUL
EASEFUL
FACTFUL
FATEFUL
FEARFUL
FISTFUL
FORKFUL
FORMFUL
FRETFUL
GAINFUL
GLEEFUL
HANDFUL
HARMFUL
HATEFUL
HEADFUL
HEATFUL
HEEDFUL
HELPFUL
HOPEFUL
HURTFUL
HUSHFUL
LESPAUL
LIFEFUL

LUSTFUL
MINDFUL
MOANFUL
MRSPAUL
MUSEFUL
NAIPAUL
NEEDFUL
NESTFUL
ODORFUL
OUTHAUL
PAILFUL
PAINFUL
PALMFUL
PASSEUL
PIPEFUL
PITIFUL
PLAYFUL
PLOTFUL
POUTFUL
PUSHFUL
RAGEFUL
RESTFUL
ROOMFUL
RUTHFUL
SACKFUL
SHIPFUL
SHOPFUL
SIGHFUL
SKILFUL
SLEDFUL
SONGFUL
SOULFUL
TACTFUL
TANKFUL
TEARFUL
TENTFUL
TOILFUL
TRAYFUL
TUNEFUL
UNAWFUL
VIALFUL
WAILFUL
WAKEFUL
WILLFUL
WISHFUL
WISTFUL
YAWNFUL
ZESTFUL

UM•••••
UMBERED
UMBERTO
UMBRAGE
UMBRIAN
UMBRIEL
UMLAUTS
UMPIRED
UMPIRES
UMPTEEN

U•M••••
UNMACHO
UNMADLY
UNMAKER
UNMAKES
UNMANED
UNMANLY
UNMASKS

UNMASTS
UNMATED
UNMATES
UNMEANT
UNMERGE
UNMERRY
UNMEWED
UNMIKED
UNMINED
UNMIRED
UNMITER
UNMITRE
UNMIXED
UNMIXES
UNMOIST
UNMOLDS
UNMOLDY
UNMOODY
UNMOORS
UNMOSSY
UNMOULD
UNMOVED
UNMOWED
UNMUDDY
UNMUTED
UTMOSTS

U••M•••
ULLMANN
UNAMUNO
UNEMPTY
UNSMART
UNSMOKY

U•••M••
ULTIMAS
UNAIMED
UNARMED
UNCOMIC
UNDOMED
UNFAMED
UNHUMAN
UNHUMID
UNKEMPT
UNLUMPY
UNNAMED
UNRIMED
UNTAMED
UNTAMES
UNTIMED
UNTIMID
UPTEMPO
UPTIMES

U••••M•
ULALUME
UNCLAMP
UNCRAMP
UNHELMS
UNISOMS
UNPLUMB
UNRHYME
UNROOMY
UNSEAMS
UNWORMY
UPCLIMB

U•••••M
UNBOSOM
UNIFORM
URANIUM
UTOPISM

•UM••••
BUMBLED
BUMBLER
BUMBLES
BUMDEAL
BUMLEGS
BUMMERS
BUMMING
BUMPERS
BUMPIER
BUMPILY
BUMPING
BUMPKIN
BUMPSUP
BUMRAPS
BUMRUSH
BUMSOUT
CUMBERS
CUMBIAS
CUMBRIA
CUMSHAW
CUMULUS
DUMBEST
DUMBING
DUMDUMS
DUMMIED
DUMMIES
DUMMYUP
DUMPERS
DUMPIER
DUMPILY
DUMPING
DUMPISH
DUMPOUT
DUMPSON
FUMBLED
FUMBLER
FUMBLES
FUMEDAT
FUMESAT
FUMIEST
GUMBALL
GUMBOOT
GUMDROP
GUMLESS
GUMLIKE
GUMMIER
GUMMING
GUMSHOE
GUMTREE
GUMWOOD
HUMANLY
HUMANUM
HUMBARD
HUMBERT
HUMBLED
HUMBLER
HUMBLES
HUMBUGS
HUMDRUM
HUMERAL
HUMERUS

HUMIDEX
HUMIDLY
HUMIDOR
HUMMELS
HUMMERS
HUMMING
HUMORAL
HUMORED
HUMORME
HUMOURS
HUMPHED
HUMPHRY
HUMPIER
HUMUSES
HUMVEES
JUMADAS
JUMANJI
JUMBLED
JUMBLER
JUMBLES
JUMBUCK
JUMPBID
JUMPCUT
JUMPERS
JUMPIER
JUMPILY
JUMPING
JUMPOFF
JUMPSAT
JUMPSIN
JUMPSON
JUMPSUP
KUMMELS
KUMQUAT
LUMBAGO
LUMBARS
LUMBERS
LUMIERE
LUMINAS
LUMPERS
LUMPIER
LUMPILY
LUMPING
LUMPISH
LUMPSIN
LUMPSIT
LUMPSUM
MUMBLED
MUMBLER
MUMBLES
MUMESON
MUMFORD
MUMMERS
MUMMERY
MUMMIES
MUMMIFY
MUMMING
NUMBATS
NUMBERS
NUMBEST
NUMBING
NUMERAL
NUMERIC
NUMEROS
NUMLOCK
PUMICED
PUMICES
PUMMELS

PUMPERS
PUMPING
PUMPKIN
PUMPOUT
PUMPSUP
RUMAKIS
RUMANIA
RUMBAED
RUMBLED
RUMBLER
RUMBLES
RUMCAKE
RUMFORD
RUMLESS
RUMMAGE
RUMMERS
RUMMIES
RUMORED
RUMOURS
RUMPEND
RUMPLED
RUMPLES
RUMPOLE
RUMSHOP
SUMATRA
SUMITUP
SUMLESS
SUMMAND
SUMMARY
SUMMATE
SUMMERS
SUMMERY
SUMMING
SUMMITS
SUMMONS
SUMOIST
SUMUPTO
TUMBLED
TUMBLER
TUMBLES
TUMBREL
TUMESCE
TUMMIES
TUMMLER
TUMULTS
VUMETER
YUMMIER
ZUMWALT

•U•M•••
AUGMENT
BUMMERS
BUMMING
BURMANS
BURMESE
BUSMANS
DUMMIED
DUMMIES
DUMMYUP
DUUMVIR
FULMARS
GUMMIER
GUMMING
GUNMOLL
HUMMELS
HUMMERS
HUMMING
KUMMELS

MUAMMAR
MUMMERS
MUMMERY
MUMMIES
MUMMIFY
MUMMING
MURMURS
MUUMUUS
NUTMEAT
NUTMEGS
OUTMANS
OUTMATE
OUTMODE
OUTMOST
OUTMOVE
PULMONI
PULMONO
PUMMELS
RUMMAGE
RUMMERS
RUMMIES
SUBMITS
SUMMAND
SUMMARY
SUMMATE
SUMMERS
SUMMERY
SUMMING
SUMMITS
SUMMONS
SUNMAID
SURMISE
TUMMIES
TUMMLER
TURMOIL
YUMMIER

•U••M••
AUTOMAT
AUTOMNE
AUTUMNS
BUCHMAN
BUSHMAN
BUSHMEN
BUXOMLY
DUHAMEL
DUSTMAN
DUSTMEN
DUSTMOP
EUDEMON
EUNOMIA
FUSUMAS
HUFFMAN
JUNKMAN
JUNKMEN
JURYMAN
JURYMEN
LUCKMAN
MUAMMAR
PULLMAN
PUTEMUP
RUNAMOK
SURFMAN
SURFMEN
SURIMIS
TUCHMAN
TURFMAN
TURFMEN

•U•••M•
BUDTIME
BUNKUMS
BUSCEMI
BUTTEMT
BUYTIME
CUSTOMS
CUTTIME
DUCHAMP
DUMDUMS
EUONYMS
FULSOME
FUNTIME
HUMORME
MUGWUMP
MUSEUMS
MUSLIMS
OUTCOME
OUTGAME
OUTJUMP
OUTLIMN
OUTSUMS
PUBGAME
QUORUMS
RUNHOME
RUNTIME
SUBLIME
SUBSUME
SUCCUMB
SUITSME
SUNLAMP
SUPREME
SURNAME
TURISMO

•U••••M
AUTONYM
BUCKRAM
BUDWORM
BUTTRAM
CULTISM
CULTJAM
CUTWORM
DUALISM
DUBNIUM
DUKEDOM
FULCRUM
FULGHUM
FURFARM
GUARGUM
GUNROOM
HUMANUM
HUMDRUM
JUDAISM
LUDDISM
LUGWORM
LUMPSUM
LUSTRUM
MUDROOM
OUTBEAM
OUTSWAM
OUTSWIM
OUTSWUM
QUANTUM
QUONDAM
SUBFORM
SUBITEM
SUNBEAM

SUNROOM
SUREIAM
SURINAM

••UM•••
ACUMENS
ALUMINA
ALUMNAE
ALUMNAL
ALUMNUS
BRUMMEL
BRUMOUS
CHUMASH
CHUMMED
CHUMPED
CLUMPED
CRUMBED
CRUMBLE
CRUMBLY
CRUMBUM
CRUMPED
CRUMPET
CRUMPLE
CRUMPLY
DAUMIER
DRUMLIN
DRUMMED
DRUMMER
DRUMOUT
DRUMSET
DRUMSUP
DUUMVIR
FLUMMOX
FNUMBER
GLUMMED
GLUMMER
GRUMBLE
GRUMBLY
GRUMMAN
GRUMPED
MAUMAUS
MUUMUUS
NEUMANN
PLUMAGE
PLUMBED
PLUMBER
PLUMBIC
PLUMBUM
PLUMCOT
PLUMIER
PLUMING
PLUMMER
PLUMMET
PLUMOSE
PLUMPED
PLUMPER
PLUMPIE
PLUMPLY
PLUMULE
RHUMBAS
SLUMBER
SLUMMED
SLUMMER
SLUMPED
SPUMIER
SPUMING
SPUMONE
SPUMONI

STUMBLE
STUMPED
STUMPER
THUMBED
THUMPED
THUMPER
TRUMANS
TRUMPED
TRUMPET
TRUMPUP
YOUMANS

••U•M••
AQUAMAN
BRUMMEL
CHUMMED
CLUBMED
DRUMMED
DRUMMER
FLUMMOX
FOURMAN
GLUMMED
GLUMMER
GOURMET
GRUMMAN
HOUSMAN
KAUFMAN
KLUGMAN
PLUMMER
PLUMMET
SHULMAN
SLUMMED
SLUMMER
SOULMAN
SOUPMIX
THURMAN

••U••M•
AMUSEME
COULOMB
GAUTAMA
GOURAMI
SCUSEME
SQUIRMS
SQUIRMY
TRUISMS
TRUSTME
TSUNAMI
YOUNGMC

••U•••M
BRUXISM
COUNTEM
CRUMBUM
DOUBLEM
ELUVIUM
FAUVISM
FRUSTUM
ISUREAM
MAUGHAM
NAUSEAM
PLUMBUM
THULIUM
TOURISM

•••UM••
AAJUMBO
ALBUMEN

ALBUMIN
ASSUMED
ASSUMER
ASSUMES
AUTUMNS
BENUMBS
CALUMET
CALUMNY
CERUMEN
COLUMBA
COLUMBO
COLUMNS
COZUMEL
EXHUMED
EXHUMER
EXHUMES
FUSUMAS
GALUMPH
GRAUMAN
ILLUMED
ILLUMES
INHUMAN
INHUMED
INHUMER
INHUMES
LEGUMES
MANUMIT
NKRUMAH
OTTUMWA
PNEUMAS
PNEUMAT
PNEUMON
REAUMUR
RELUMED
RELUMES
REPUMPS
RESUMED
RESUMES
RHEUMIC
SARUMAN
SCHUMER
TRAUMAS
TRIUMPH
UNHUMAN
UNHUMID
UNLUMPY
VOLUMED
VOLUMES

•••U•M•

SOSUEME
VACUUMS

•••U••M

JEJUNUM
PABULUM
REQUIEM

••••UM•

AIRPUMP
ALARUMS
ALLIUMS
ASYLUMS
ATRIUMS
BARNUMS
BAYRUMS
BUNKUMS
CONSUME
COSTUME
DECRUMB
DEMBUMS
DESLUMS
DICTUMS
DIDSUMS
DUMDUMS
GASPUMP
GYPSUMS
IONIUMS
LYCEUMS
MAGNUMS
MCCRUMB
MEDIUMS
MUGWUMP
MUSEUMS
NATSUME
NOTRUMP
ONELUMP
OUTJUMP
OUTSUMS
PABLUMS
PARFUMS
PEPLUMS
PERFUME
PERFUMY
PLENUMS
PODIUMS
POSSUMS
PRESUME
QUORUMS
REPLUMB
REPLUME
SATSUMA
SCHLUMP
SKIBUMS
SKIJUMP
SUBSUME
SUCCUMB
TALCUMS
TEDEUMS
TEDIUMS
THEPUMP
ULALUME
UNPLUMB
VACUUMS
VELLUMS
WAMPUMS

••••U•M

ARTHURM

•••••UM

AGENDUM
ALYSSUM
ARCANUM
BELGIUM
BOHRIUM
BORGLUM
CADMIUM
CALCIUM
CARDIUM
CDALBUM
CENTRUM
CHETRUM
CHEWGUM
CHILLUM
CRANIUM
CRUMBUM
DECORUM
DUBNIUM
EARDRUM
ELUVIUM
ELYSIUM
ERRATUM
FEMINUM
FERMIUM
FRUSTUM
FULCRUM
FULGHUM
GALLIUM
GUARGUM
HAFNIUM
HAHNIUM
HASSIUM
HOLMIUM
HOODLUM
HUMANUM
HUMDRUM
IRIDIUM
ISCHIUM
JEJUNUM
KARAKUM
KEEPMUM
KEPTMUM
KETCHUM
LITHIUM
LUMPSUM
LUSTRUM
MAXIMUM
MINIMUM
MITCHUM
MODICUM
NATRIUM
NIOBIUM
NOSEEUM
NOSTRUM
OILDRUM
OPOSSUM
OPTIMUM
ORARIUM
ORPHEUM
OUTSWUM
PABULUM
PENTIUM
PINETUM
PLUMBUM
PREMIUM
QUANTUM
RHENIUM
RHODIUM
ROSTRUM
SANCTUM
SORGHUM
STADIUM
STANNUM
STERNUM
STICKUM
STRATUM
TANTRUM
TERBIUM
THORIUM
THULIUM
TIDYSUM
TRITIUM
TRIVIUM
URANIUM
YTTRIUM
ZEROSUM

UN•••••

UNACTED
UNADDED
UNADEPT
UNADULT
UNAGILE
UNAGING
UNAIDED
UNAIMED
UNAIRED
UNALERT
UNALIKE
UNALONE
UNAMUNO
UNANGRY
UNAPTLY
UNARMED
UNASKED
UNAWAKE
UNAWARE
UNAWFUL
UNAXLED
UNBAITS
UNBAKED
UNBALED
UNBALES
UNBARED
UNBARES
UNBASED
UNBATED
UNBEARD
UNBELDI
UNBELTS
UNBENCH
UNBENDS
UNBERTH
UNBESET
UNBINDS
UNBLADE
UNBLENT
UNBLEST
UNBLOCK
UNBLOWN
UNBLUED
UNBOGGY
UNBOLTS
UNBONED
UNBORED
UNBORNE
UNBOSOM
UNBOUND
UNBOWED
UNBOXED
UNBOXES
UNBRACE
UNBRAID
UNBRAKE
UNBRAVE
UNBRIEF
UNBROKE
UNBUILD
UNBUILT
UNBULKY
UNBURLY
UNBURNT
UNBURST
UNCAGED
UNCAGES
UNCAKED
UNCAKES
UNCANED
UNCANNY
UNCAPED
UNCASED
UNCASES
UNCASKS
UNCEDED
UNCHAIN
UNCHAIR
UNCHARY
UNCHECK
UNCHOKE
UNCHURN
UNCIALS
UNCINCH
UNCITED
UNCIVIC
UNCIVIL
UNCLAMP
UNCLASP
UNCLEAN
UNCLEAR
UNCLEFT
UNCLIPS
UNCLIPT
UNCLOAK
UNCLOGS
UNCLOSE
UNCLOUD
UNCODED
UNCOILS
UNCOMIC
UNCOOPS
UNCORED
UNCORES
UNCORKS
UNCOUTH
UNCOVER
UNCOWED
UNCOYER
UNCOYLY
UNCRAMP
UNCRATE
UNCRAZY
UNCRIED
UNCROSS
UNCROWN
UNCRUDE
UNCRUEL
UNCTION
UNCUBIC
UNCUFFS
UNCURBS
UNCURED
UNCURLS
UNDARED
UNDATED
UNDAZED
UNDEALT
UNDERDO
UNDERGO
UNDEWED
UNDIKED
UNDINES
UNDOCKS
UNDOERS
UNDOING
UNDOMED
UNDRAPE
UNDRAWN
UNDRAWS
UNDRESS
UNDRIED
UNDRUNK
UNDULAR
UNDUPED
UNDUSTY
UNDYING
UNEAGER
UNEARTH
UNEASES
UNEATEN
UNEAVED
UNEBBED
UNEDGED
UNEDGES
UNEMPTY
UNENDED
UNEQUAL
UNERECT
UNFACED
UNFACTS
UNFADED
UNFAITH
UNFAKED
UNFAMED
UNFANCY
UNFATED
UNFATTY
UNFAZED
UNFENCE
UNFERTH
UNFETED
UNFIERY
UNFILED
UNFILES
UNFINED
UNFINES
UNFIRED
UNFITLY
UNFIXED
UNFIXES
UNFLAKY
UNFLOOR
UNFLOWN
UNFLUID
UNFOGGY
UNFOLDS
UNFORKS
UNFOUND
UNFOXED
UNFRAIL
UNFRANK
UNFREED
UNFREES
UNFRIED
UNFRILL
UNFROCK
UNFROST
UNFROZE
UNFULLY
UNFUNNY
UNFURLS
UNFUSED
UNFUSSY
UNGATED
UNGAUDY
UNGIDDY
UNGIRDS
UNGIVEN
UNGLOVE
UNGLUED
UNGLUES
UNGODLY
UNGORED
UNGRAND
UNGREEN
UNGRIPS
UNGROSS
UNGROWN
UNGRUFF
UNGUARD
UNGUENT
UNGULAE
UNGULAR
UNGUYED
UNGYVED
UNHAIRS
UNHAIRY
UNHANDS
UNHANDY
UNHAPPY
UNHARDY
UNHARSH
UNHASPS
UNHASTY
UNHATED
UNHAYED
UNHAZED
UNHEADY
UNHEARD
UNHEAVY
UNHEEDS
UNHELMS
UNHEWED
UNHILLY
UNHINGE
UNHIRED
UNHIRES
UNHITCH
UNHONED
UNHOODS
UNHOOKS
UNHOPED
UNHORSE
UNHOUSE
UNHULLS
UNHUMAN
UNHUMID
UNHUSKS
UNIATES
UNIBALL
UNIBODY
UNICODE
UNICORN
UNIDEAL
UNIFIED
UNIFIER
UNIFIES
UNIFORM
UNINERT
UNINKED
UNIPLEX
UNIPODS
UNIQUES
UNISIZE
UNISOMS
UNISONS
UNITARD
UNITARY
UNITERS
UNITIES
UNITING
UNITISE
UNITIVE
UNITIZE
UNIVACS
UNJADED
UNJOINS
UNJOINT
UNJOLLY
UNJOYED
UNJUICY
UNKEMPT
UNKEYED
UNKINKS
UNKNITS
UNKNOTS
UNKNOWN
UNLACED
UNLACES
UNLADED
UNLADEN
UNLADES
UNLARGE
UNLATCH
UNLAVED
UNLAXED
UNLAXES
UNLEADS
UNLEAFS
UNLEAKY
UNLEARN
UNLEASH
UNLEGAL
UNLEVEL
UNLIGHT
UNLIKED
UNLIKES
UNLINED
UNLINKS
UNLIVED
UNLIVES
UNLOADS
UNLOATH
UNLOBED
UNLOCAL
UNLOCKS
UNLOFTY
UNLOOPS
UNLOOSE
UNLOVED
UNLOWLY
UNLOYAL
UNLUCID
UNLUCKY
UNLUMPY
UNLURED
UNLUSTY
UNLYING
UNLYRIC
UNMACHO
UNMADLY
UNMAKER
UNMAKES
UNMANED
UNMANLY
UNMASKS
UNMASTS
UNMATED
UNMATES
UNMEANT
UNMERGE
UNMERRY
UNMEWED
UNMIKED
UNMINED
UNMIRED
UNMITER
UNMITRE
UNMIXED
UNMIXES
UNMOIST
UNMOLDS
UNMOLDY
UNMOODY
UNMOORS
UNMOSSY
UNMOULD
UNMOVED
UNMOWED
UNMUDDY
UNMUTED
UNNAILS
UNNAIVE
UNNAMED
UNNASAL
UNNEEDY
UNNERVE
UNNOISY
UNNOSED
UNNOTED
UNNOVEL
UNOBESE
UNOFTEN
UNOGLED
UNOILED
UNOPTED
UNORBED
UNOVERT
UNOWING
UNOWNED
UNPACED
UNPACKS
UNPAGAN
UNPAGED
UNPALED
UNPARED
UNPASTE
UNPAVED
UNPAWED
UNPAWNS
UNPEELS
UNPICKS
UNPIETY
UNPILED
UNPILES
UNPIOUS
UNPIPED
UNPLAIT
UNPLANS
UNPLIED
UNPLUGS
UNPLUMB
UNPOLED
UNPOSED
UNPROUD
UNQUICK
UNQUIET
UNQUOTE
UNRACKS
UNRAINY
UNRAKED
UNRASPY
UNRATED
UNRAVEL
UNRAYED
UNRAZED
UNREADY
UNREELS
UNREGAL
UNRESTS
UNRHYME
UNRIGID
UNRILED
UNRIMED
UNRIPER
UNRISEN
UNRISKY
UNRIVED
UNRIVEN
UNROBED
UNROBES
UNROCKY
UNROLLS
UNROOFS
UNROOMY
UNROOTS
UNROPED
UNROPES
UNROUND
UNROWDY
UNRULED
UNRURAL
UNSADLY
UNSAFER
UNSALTY
UNSATED
UNSAVED
UNSAVVY
UNSAWED
UNSCALY
UNSCREW
UNSEALS
UNSEAMS
UNSEATS
UNSELLS
UNSEWED
UNSHADE
UNSHADY
UNSHARP
UNSHEER
UNSHELL
UNSHIER
UNSHIFT
UNSHINY
UNSHIPS
UNSHOED
UNSHOES
UNSHORN
UNSHORT
UNSHOWN
UNSHOWY
UNSHYER
UNSHYLY
UNSIDED
UNSIGHT
UNSILLY
UNSIZED
UNSKEWS
UNSLACK
UNSLAIN
UNSLEEK
UNSLICK
UNSLIER
UNSLING
UNSLUNG
UNSLYER
UNSLYLY
UNSMART
UNSMOKY
UNSNAGS
UNSNAKY
UNSNAPS
UNSNARL
UNSOBER
UNSOGGY
UNSOLED
UNSOLES
UNSOLID
UNSOOTY
UNSORRY
UNSORTS
UNSOUND
UNSOWED
UNSPANS
UNSPEAK
UNSPELT
UNSPENT
UNSPICY
UNSPIED
UNSPILT
UNSPLIT
UNSPOKE
UNSPOOL
UNSTACK
UNSTAGY
UNSTAID
UNSTATE
UNSTEEL
UNSTEPS
UNSTERN
UNSTICK
UNSTIFF
UNSTOIC
UNSTONY
UNSTOPS
UNSTOUT
UNSTOWS
UNSTRAP
UNSTUCK
UNSTUNG
UNSULKY
UNSUNNY
UNSURLY
UNSWEAR
UNSWEET
UNSWEPT
UNSWORE
UNSWORN
UNSWUNG
UNTACKS
UNTAKEN
UNTAMED
UNTAMES
UNTAPED
UNTAPES
UNTASTY
UNTAXED
UNTAXES
UNTEACH
UNTENSE
UNTERSE
UNTHAWS
UNTHICK
UNTHINK
UNTIERS
UNTILED
UNTIMED
UNTIMID
UNTIRED
UNTONED
UNTOUGH
UNTOXIC
UNTRACK
UNTRAPS
UNTREAD
UNTREED
UNTRIED
UNTRITE
UNTRUER
UNTRULY
UNTRUSS
UNTRUTH
UNTUCKS
UNTUNED
UNTUNES
UNTWINE
UNTWIST
UNTYING
UNTYPED
UNURBAN
UNURGED
UNUSUAL
UNVAGUE
UNVEILS
UNVENAL
UNVEXED
UNVITAL
UNVIVID
UNVOCAL
UNVOICE
UNVOTED
UNVOWED
UNVYING
UNWADED
UNWAGED
UNWAKED
UNWALLS
UNWANED
UNWAVED
UNWAXED
UNWEARY
UNWEAVE
UNWEDGE
UNWHEEL
UNWHIPT
UNWHITE
UNWHOLE
UNWINDS
UNWINDY
UNWIPED
UNWIRED
UNWISER
UNWITTY
UNWOOED
UNWORMY
UNWOUND
UNWOVEN
UNWRAPS
UNWRUNG
UNYOKED
UNYOKES
UNYOUNG
UNZONED
UNZONES

U•N••••

UNNAILS
UNNAIVE
UNNAMED
UNNASAL
UNNEEDY
UNNERVE
UNNOISY
UNNOSED
UNNOTED
UNNOVEL
UPNORTH
URNFULS
URNLIKE

U••N•••

UGANDAN
ULANOVA
ULANUDE
UNANGRY
UNENDED
UNINERT
UNINKED
UNKNITS
UNKNOTS
UNKNOWN
UNSNAGS
UNSNAKY
UNSNAPS
UNSNARL
UPANDIN
UPENDED
URANITE
URANIUM
USANCES
USINGIN
USINGUP
UTENSIL
UVINDEX

U•••N••

ULYANOV
ULZANAS
UNBENCH
UNBENDS
UNBINDS
UNBONED
UNCANED
UNCANNY
UNCINCH
UNDINES
UNFANCY
UNFENCE
UNFINED
UNFINES
UNFUNNY
UNHANDS
UNHANDY
UNHINGE
UNHONED
UNKINKS
UNLINED
UNLINKS
UNMANED
UNMANLY
UNMINED
UNOWNED
UNSUNNY
UNTENSE
UNTONED
UNTUNED
UNTUNES
UNVENAL
UNWANED
UNWINDS
UNWINDY
UNZONED
UNZONES
UPLANDS
UPLINKS
UPSENDS
UPTONOW
UPWINDS
URBANER
URBANII
URBANIV
URBANVI
URGENCY
URGINGS
URSINUS
USTINOV
UNFOUND
UNFRANK
UNFUNNY
UNGRAND
UNGUENT
UNISONS
UNITING
UNJOINS
UNJOINT
UNLYING
UNMEANT
UNOWING
UNPAWNS
UNPLANS
UNRAINY
UNROUND
UNSHINY
UNSLING
UNSLUNG
UNSOUND
UNSPANS
UNSPENT
UNSTONY
UNSTUNG
UNSUNNY
UNSWUNG
UNTHINK
UNTWINE
UNTYING
UNVYING
UNWOUND
UNWRUNG
UNYOUNG
UPBORNE
UPBOUND
UPFLING
UPFRONT
UPGOING
UPSPINS
UPSTAND
UPSWING
UPTOWNS
UPTREND
UPTURNS
URCHINS
USGRANT
USOPENS
UTAHANS
UTICANS
UTICANY
UNHUMAN
UNICORN
UNKNOWN
UNLADEN
UNLEARN
UNOFTEN
UNPAGAN
UNRISEN
UNRIVEN
UNSHORN
UNSHOWN
UNSLAIN
UNSTERN
UNSWORN
UNTAKEN
UNURBAN
UNWOVEN
UPANDIN
UPGROWN
UPRISEN
UPSILON
URGEDON
URGESON
USHERIN
USINGIN
UTOPIAN

U•••N•

UGOLINO
UKRAINE
ULLMANN
ULULANT
UNAGING
UNALONE
UNAMUNO
UNBLENT
UNBORNE
UNBOUND
UNBURNT
UNCANNY
UNDOING
UNDRUNK
UNDYING

U•••••N

UGANDAN
ULLMANN
UMBRIAN
UMPTEEN
UNBLOWN
UNCHAIN
UNCHURN
UNCLEAN
UNCROWN
UNCTION
UNDRAWN
UNEATEN
UNFLOWN
UNGIVEN
UNGREEN
UNGROWN

•UN••••

AUNTBEE
AUNTIES
BUNCHED
BUNCHES
BUNCHUP
BUNCOED
BUNDLED
BUNDLER
BUNDLES
BUNGEES
BUNGING
BUNGLED
BUNGLER
BUNGLES
BUNIONS
BUNKBED
BUNKERS
BUNKING
BUNKOED
BUNKUMS
BUNNIES
BUNNING
BUNRAKU
BUNTERS
BUNTING
BUNUELO
CUNEATE
CUNNING
DUNAWAY
DUNCISH
DUNDALK
DUNEDIN
DUNGEON
DUNKERS
DUNKING
DUNKIRK
DUNLINS
DUNLOPS
DUNNAGE
DUNNERS
DUNNING
DUNSTAN
EUNOMIA
FUNDERS
FUNDING
FUNFAIR
FUNFEST
FUNFURS
FUNFZIG
FUNGOES
FUNKIER
FUNKILY
FUNKING
FUNNELS
FUNNIER
FUNNIES
FUNNILY
FUNNING
FUNPLEX
FUNRUNS
FUNSTER
FUNTIME
GUNBELT
GUNBOAT
GUNCASE
GUNDOGS
GUNFIRE
GUNITES
GUNKIER
GUNLAPS
GUNLAWS
GUNLESS
GUNLOCK
GUNMOLL
GUNNERS
GUNNERY
GUNNIES
GUNNING
GUNPLAY
GUNROOM
GUNSELS
GUNSFOR
GUNSHIP
GUNSHOT
GUNTHER
GUNUSER
GUNWALE
HUNCHED
HUNCHES
HUNDRED
HUNGARY
HUNGERS
HUNGOFF
HUNGOUT
HUNGTEN
HUNKERS
HUNKIER
HUNLIKE
HUNNISH
HUNNYBS
HUNTERS
HUNTFOR
HUNTING
HUNTLEY
HUNTSUP
JUNCOES
JUNEBUG
JUNEDAY
JUNGIAN
JUNGLES
JUNIORS
JUNIPER
JUNKART
JUNKCAR
JUNKDNA
JUNKERS
JUNKETS
JUNKFAX
JUNKIER
JUNKIES
JUNKING
JUNKMAN
JUNKMEN
KUNDERA
LUNATED
LUNATES
LUNATIC
LUNCHED
LUNCHER
LUNCHES
LUNESTA
LUNETTE
LUNGEAT
LUNGERS
LUNGING
LUNKERS
LUNULAE
LUNULAR
MUNCHED
MUNCHEN
MUNCHER
MUNCHES
MUNCHIE
MUNCHON
MUNDANE
MUNSTER
NUNAVUT
NUNCIOS
NUNGWEN
NUNHOOD
NUNLIKE
NUNNERY
NUNNISH
NUNSHIP
PUNCHED
PUNCHER
PUNCHES
PUNCHIN
PUNCHUP
PUNDITS
PUNGENT
PUNIEST
PUNJABI
PUNKERS
PUNKIER
PUNKIES
PUNLESS
PUNNERS
PUNNIER
PUNNILY
PUNNING
PUNSTER
PUNTERS
PUNTING
RUNAMOK
RUNATAB
RUNAWAY
RUNBACK
RUNDEEP
RUNDLES
RUNDOWN
RUNFREE
RUNGFOR
RUNGOFF
RUNGOUT
RUNHOME
RUNINTO
RUNITUP
RUNLAPS
RUNLATE
RUNLESS
RUNLETS
RUNNELS
RUNNERS
RUNNETH
RUNNIER
RUNNING
RUNOFFS
RUNONIN
RUNOUTS
RUNOVER
RUNPAST
RUNRIOT
RUNSDRY
RUNSFOR
RUNSLOW
RUNSOFF
RUNSOUT
RUNTIER
RUNTIME
RUNTISH
RUNUPTO
RUNWAYS
RUNWILD
RUNWITH
SUNBATH
SUNBEAM
SUNBELT
SUNBIRD
SUNBOWL
SUNBOWS
SUNBURN
SUNCITY
SUNDAES
SUNDAYS
SUNDECK
SUNDERS
SUNDIAL
SUNDOGS
SUNDOWN
SUNFANS
SUNFAST
SUNFIRE
SUNFISH
SUNGLOW
SUNGODS
SUNHATS
SUNKIST
SUNLAMP
SUNLESS
SUNLIKE
SUNMAID
SUNNIER
SUNNILY
SUNNING
SUNRAYS
SUNRISE
SUNROOF
SUNROOM
SUNSETS
SUNSFAN
SUNSPOT
SUNSUIT
SUNTANS
SUNWARD
TUNABLE
TUNAOIL
TUNASUB
TUNDRAS
TUNEDIN
TUNEDTO
TUNEDUP
TUNEFUL
TUNEOUT
TUNESIN
TUNESTO
TUNESUP
TUNEUPS
TUNGOIL
TUNICLE
TUNISIA
TUNNELS
ZUNIANS

•U•N•••

BUNNIES
BUNNING
BURNABY
BURNERS
BURNETT
BURNFOR
BURNING
BURNISH
BURNLEY
BURNOFF
BURNOUT
BURNSIN
BURNSUP
BURNTIN
BURNTUP
CUINGIN
CUNNING
DUBNIUM
DUENNAS
DUNNAGE
DUNNERS
DUNNING
DURNING
EUONYMS
FUENTES
FULNESS
FUNNELS
FUNNIER
FUNNIES
FUNNILY
FUNNING
FURNACE
FURNESS
FURNISH
GUANACO
GUANINE
GUINEAN
GUINEAS
GUNNERS
GUNNERY
GUNNIES
GUNNING
GURNEYS
GUVNORS
HUANGHE
HUANGTI
HUNNISH
HUNNYBS
KUZNETS
LUGNUTS
NUANCED
NUANCES
NUDNIKS
NUNNERY
NUNNISH
PUGNOSE
PUNNERS
PUNNIER
PUNNILY
PUNNING
QUANTUM
QUENEAU
QUENTIN
QUINARY
QUINATE
QUINCES
QUINCEY
QUINELA
QUININE
QUINION
QUINLAN
QUINQUE
QUINTAL
QUINTAS
QUINTES
QUINTET
QUINTIC
QUINTON
QUINTUS
QUINZES
QUONDAM
QUONSET
RUANDAS
RUINATE
RUINERS
RUINING
RUINOUS
RUNNELS
RUNNERS
RUNNETH
RUNNIER
RUNNING
SUBNETS
SUNNIER
SUNNILY
SUNNING
SURNAME
TUNNELS
TURNBAD
TURNERS
TURNERY
TURNING
TURNIPS
TURNKEY
TURNOFF
TURNONS
TURNOUT
TURNPRO
TURNRED
TURNSIN
TURNSON
TURNSTO
TURNSUP
TURNUPS

•U••N••

AUGENDS
AUTONYM
BUCHNER
BUCKNER
BUJONES
BURUNDI
BUTANES
BUTENES
BUYINTO
CUTINON
CUTINTO
DUENNAS
DUGINTO
DUGONGS
DURANCE
DURANGO
DURANTE
EUBANKS
EUGENIA
EUGENIC
EUGENIE
GUIGNOL
HUMANLY
HUMANUM
JUMANJI
JUSTNOW
JUVENAL
LUCANIA
LUCENCY
LUCINDA
LUCKNOW
LUMINAS
LUPINES
MURANOS
MUSANTE
MUSINGS
MUTANTS
OUTGNAW
OUTINGS
PUDENCY
QUEENED
QUEENIE
QUEENIT
QUEENLY
QUESNAY
QUIZNOS
QUOINED
RULINGS
RUMANIA
RUNINTO
RUNONIN
SUBUNIT
SURINAM
SUSANNA
SUSANNE
SUZANNE
TULANEU

•U•••N•

AUBURNS
AUBURNU
AUGMENT
AUSTINS
AUTOING
AUTOMNE
AUTUMNS
BUCKING
BUDDING
BUDGING
BUFFING
BUGGING
BUGLING
BUITONI
BULGING
BULKING
BULLING
BULLINS
BUMMING
BUMPING
BUNGING
BUNIONS
BUNKING
BUNNING
BUNTING
BUOYANT
BUOYING
BURBANK
BURDENS
BURKINA
BURLING
BURMANS
BURNING
BURPING
BURRING
BURYING
BUSHING
BUSKING
BUSLANE
BUSLINE
BUSMANS
BUSSING
BUSTING
BUSYING
BUTTING
BUTTONS
BUTTONY
BUZZING
CUBBING
CUBBINS
CUBFANS
CUFFING
CUIBONO
CUISINE
CULLING
CUNNING
CUPPING
CURBING
CURDING
CURLING
CURRANT
CURRENT
CURRING
CURSING
CURVING
CUSHING
CUSSING
CUTTING
DUBBING
DUCKING
DUCTING
DUELING
DUETING
DULLING
DUMBING
DUMPING
DUNKING
DUNLINS
DUNNING
DUODENA
DUOTONE
DURNING
DURWENT
DUSKING
DUSTING
EUGLENA
EUPHONY
FUDGING
FUELING
FULGENT
FUNDING
FUNKING
FUNNING
FUNRUNS
FURLING
FURLONG
FURRING
FUSIONS
FUSSING
FUTZING
FUZZING
GUANINE
GUARANI
GUIDING
GUILING
GULDENS
GULFING
GULLING
GULPING
GUMMING
GUNNING
GUSHING
GUSTING
GUTTING
HUFFING
HUGGING
HUGGINS
HULKING
HULLING
HUMMING
HUNTING
HURLING
HURTING
HUSBAND
HUSHING
HUSKING
HUTTING
HUYGENS
JUDEANS
JUDGING
JUGBAND
JUGGING
JUGWINE
JUICING
JULIANA
JUMPING
JUNKDNA
JUNKING
JURGENS
JURYING
JUSTINE
JUSTONE
JUTLAND
JUTTING
KUCHENS
KURRENT
LUCARNE
LUCERNE
LUCHINO
LUCIANA
LUCIANO
LUCKING
LUFFING
LUGGING
LULLING
LUMPING
LUNGING
LURKING
LUSTING
MUCKING
MUDDING
MUDHENS
MUFFING
MUFFINS
MUGGING
MULLING
MULLINS
MUMMING
MUNDANE
MUSHING
MUSIGNY
MUSLINS
MUSSING
MUSTANG
MUTTONS
NUBBINS
NUBIANS
NUDGING
NULLING
NUMBING
NURSING
NUTPINE
NUTTING
OUGHTNT
OURGANG
OURSONG
OUSTING
OUTBANS
OUTBEND
OUTCANT
OUTDONE
OUTFIND
OUTGUNS
OUTHUNT
OUTJINX
OUTKING
OUTLAND
OUTLINE
OUTMANS
OUTRANG
OUTRANK
OUTRANT
OUTRING
OUTRUNS
OUTSANG
OUTSING
OUTSINS
OUTSUNG
OUTWENT
OUTWIND
OUTWING
PUCCINI
PUDDING
PUFFING
PUFFINS
PULLING
PULLINS
PULLONS
PULMONI
PULMONO
PULPING
PULSING
PUMPING
PUNGENT
PUNNING
PUNTING
PUPTENT
PURGING
PURLING
PURRING
PURSING
PUSHING
PUTTING
QUAKING
QUEUING
QUININE
QUOTING
RUBBING
RUCHING
RUCKING
RUFFING
RUINING
RULEONE
RUMPEND
RUNNING
RUSHING
RUSTING
RUTHANN
RUTLAND
RUTTING
SUBBAND
SUBBANK
SUBBING
SUBKING
SUBLONG
SUBORNS
SUBTEND
SUBTONE
SUBVENE
SUBZONE
SUCKING
SUDSING
SUITING
SUKARNO
SULKING
SULTANA
SULTANS
SUMMAND
SUMMING
SUMMONS
SUNFANS

SUNNING
SUNTANS
SUPPING
SURFING
SURGING
SUSANNA
SUSANNE
SUSPEND
SUSSING
SUZANNE
TUBBING
TUCKING
TUCSONS
TUFTING
TUGGING
TULSANS
TURBANS
TURBINE
TUREENS
TURFING
TURNING
TURNONS
TUSCANS
TUSCANY
TUSKING
TUTTING
VULCANS
VULPINE
YUKKING
ZUNIANS

•U••••N

AUCTION
AUDUBON
AUTOPEN
BUCHMAN
BUFFOON
BUILDIN
BUILDON
BUILTIN
BUILTON
BUISSON
BULLION
BULLPEN
BULLRUN
BUMPKIN
BURGEON
BURNSIN
BURNTIN
BURPGUN
BURSTIN
BURSTYN
BUSHMAN
BUSHMEN
BUSTSIN
BUTTSIN
BUYDOWN
CUBSFAN
CUINGIN
CURLSIN
CURTAIN
CUSHION
CUTDOWN
CUTINON
CUTOPEN
DUCKPIN
DUDGEON
DUMPSON
DUNEDIN
DUNGEON
DUNSTAN
DUSTBIN
DUSTGUN
DUSTMAN
DUSTMEN
DUSTPAN
EUCERIN
EUDEMON
EUROVAN
FUJISAN
FUSTIAN
GUDGEON
GUERDON
GUINEAN
HUFFMAN
HUNGTEN
HURSTON
HUSSEIN
JUMPSIN
JUMPSON
JUNGIAN
JUNKMAN
JUNKMEN
JURYMAN
JURYMEN
LUCKMAN
LUMPSIN
LUREDIN
LURESIN
LURLEEN
MUEZZIN
MULDOON
MUMESON
MUNCHEN
MUNCHON
MUSEDON
MUSESON
MUTAGEN
MUYBIEN
NUCLEON
NUNGWEN
OURTOWN
OUTBURN
OUTEARN
OUTFAWN
OUTGAIN
OUTGRIN
OUTLAIN
OUTLIMN
OUTPLAN
OUTSEEN
OUTSPIN
OUTTORN
OUTTURN
OUTWORN
PULLMAN
PULLPIN
PULLSIN
PULLSON
PUMPKIN
PUNCHIN
PURITAN
PURLOIN
PUSHKIN
PUSHPIN
PUTDOWN
PUTUPON
QUARTAN
QUENTIN
QUICKEN
QUIETEN
QUINION
QUINLAN
QUINTON
RUBDOWN
RUBICON
RUBITIN
RUBUPON
RUCTION
RUFFIAN
RULEDON
RULESON
RUNDOWN
RUNONIN
RUSSIAN
RUSSLAN
RUTHANN
SUASION
SUBCLAN
SUBJOIN
SUBTEEN
SUCKSIN
SUCTION
SUELLEN
SUELYON
SUNBURN
SUNDOWN
SUNSFAN
SURECAN
SURFMAN
SURFMEN
SURGEON
SUSTAIN
TUBEPAN
TUCHMAN
TUCKSIN
TUITION
TUNEDIN
TUNESIN
TURFMAN
TURFMEN
TURNSIN
TURNSON
VUITTON
YUCATAN

••UN•••

ALUNSER
ARUNDEL
ASUNDER
BLUNDEN
BLUNDER
BLUNTED
BLUNTER
BLUNTLY
BOUNCED
BOUNCER
BOUNCES
BOUNDED
BOUNDER
BOUNDTO
BOUNDUP
BRUNETS
CHUNKED
CHUNNEL
CLUNGTO
CLUNKED
CLUNKER
COUNCIL
COUNSEL
COUNTED
COUNTEE
COUNTEM
COUNTER
COUNTIN
COUNTON
COUNTRY
COUNTUP
CRUNCHY
DAUNTED
DAUNTER
DRUNKEN
DRUNKER
FLUNGAT
FLUNKED
FLUNKER
FOUNDED
FOUNDER
FOUNDRY
GAUNTER
GAUNTLY
GOUNDER
GRUNGER
GRUNGES
GRUNION
GRUNTED
GRUNTER
HAUNTED
HAUNTER
HOUNDED
HOUNDER
HYUNDAI
JAUNTED
JOUNCED
JOUNCES
LAUNDER
LAUNDRY
LOUNGED
LOUNGER
LOUNGES
MAUNDER
MOUNDED
MOUNTED
MOUNTER
MOUNTIE
MOUNTUP
OPUNTIA
PAUNCHY
PLUNDER
PLUNGED
PLUNGER
PLUNGES
PLUNKED
PLUNKER
POUNCED
POUNCER
POUNCES
POUNDED
POUNDER
PRUNERS
PRUNING
RAUNCHY
REUNERS
REUNIFY
REUNION
REUNITE
ROUNDED
ROUNDEL
ROUNDER
ROUNDLY
ROUNDON
ROUNDUP
SAUNAED
SAUNTER
SHUNNED
SHUNTED
SHUNTER
SKUNKED
SLUNKIN
SLUNKUP
SOUNDED
SOUNDER
SOUNDLY
SPUNOFF
SPUNOUT
STUNGUN
STUNNED
STUNNER
STUNTED
SWUNGAT
SWUNGBY
SWUNGIT
TAUNTED
TAUNTER
TAUNTON
THUNDER
THUNKED
TRUNDLE
TSUNAMI
VAUNTED
VAUNTER
WOUNDED
WOUNDUP
YOUNGER
YOUNGMC
YOUNGUN

••U•N••

ALUMNAE
ALUMNAL
ALUMNUS
AQUINAS
BLUINGS
CHUNNEL
CHURNED
CHURNER
CHURNUP
CHUTNEY
DIURNAL
DOUANES
ELUANTS
EQUINES
EQUINOX
FLUENCY
IGUANAS
IGUANID
JOURNAL
JOURNEE
JOURNEY
JOURNOS
MOURNED
MOURNER
SHUNNED
SPURNED
SPURNER
SPUTNIK
SQUANTO
SQUINCH
SQUINTS
SQUINTY
STUNNED
STUNNER
TOURNEY
TRUANCY
TRUANTS
YOUANDI
YOUKNOW

••U••N•

ABUSING
ACUMENS
ALUMINA
AMUSING
ARUBANS
BHUTANI
BLUEING
BOUDINS
BOUSONO
BRUXING
CAUSING
CHUTING
CLUEING
COULDNT
COUPING
COUPONS
COURANT
COUSINE
COUSINS
CRUZANS
DAUBING
DEUCING
DOUSING
EDUCING
ELUDING
ELUTING
ENURING
EQUIANO
EXUDING
FEUDING
FLUTING
FLUXING
FOULING
GAUDENS
GAUGING
GLUTENS
GOUGING
HAULING
HOUDINI
HOUSING
INURING
LAUDING
LAURENT
LEUCINE
LOUDENS
LOURING
LOUSING
LOUTING
MAULING
MOUSING
NEUMANN
NEURONE
NEURONS
OPULENT
OPUSONE
PAULINA
PAULINE
PAULING
PAUSING
PLUGINS
PLUMING
PLUSONE
PLUTONS
POULENC
POURING
POUTING
PRUDENT
PRUNING
REUBENS
REUSING
ROUGING
ROUSING
ROUTINE
ROUTING
SAUCING
SAUCONY
SHUTINS
SOURING
SOUSING
SPUMING
SPUMONE
SPUMONI
STUBING
STUDENT
TAURINE
TAUTENS
TEUTONS
TOUCANS
TOURING
TOUTING
TRUEING
TRUMANS
ULULANT
WOULDNT
YOUMANS
YOURANG

••U•••N

ABUTSON
APULIAN
AQUAMAN
BLUEFIN
BLUEHEN
BLUESUN
BLUNDEN
BLUSHON
BOURBON
CAUTHEN
CAUTION
CLUEDIN
CLUESIN
COUNTIN
COUNTON
CRUTZEN
DAUPHIN
DOUBLEN
DRUMLIN
DRUNKEN
DRUZEAN
DRUZIAN
ELUTION
EXURBAN
FLUXION
FOURMAN
FOURPIN
GAUGUIN
GLUEDON
GLUEGUN
GLUESON
GLUTTON
GRUMMAN
GRUNION
HAULSIN
HOUSMAN
HOUSTON
JOURDAN
KAUFMAN
KLUGMAN
LAUGHIN
MAUDLIN
MAULDIN
MAUREEN
NEUMANN
NEUTRON
NOUTURN
PAULSEN
PLUGSIN
POURSIN
POUSSIN
REUNION
ROUGHEN
ROUNDON
SAURIAN
SHULMAN
SHUTSIN
SLUNKIN
SOULMAN
SOUPCAN
SOUPCON
SOUPSON
SOURSON
SPURSON
STUCKIN
STUCKON
STUFFIN
STUNGUN
TAUNTON
TAUREAN
THURMAN
TOUCHON
TOUGHEN
TRUDGEN
TRUSTIN
UNURBAN
VAUGHAN
YOUNGUN
YOUREON
YOUTHEN

•••UN••

ABOUNDS
ADJUNCT
ALBUNDY
AMOUNTS
ASSUNTA
ATLUNCH
ATTUNED
ATTUNES
BIGUNIT
BURUNDI
DEBUNKS
DEFUNCT
DEFUNDS
DEJUNKS
DETUNED
DETUNES
DOLUNCH
EDMUNDI
EDMUNDS
ELMUNDO
ENOUNCE
EXEUNTS
EXPUNGE
FLAUNTS
FLAUNTY
FLOUNCE
FLOUNCY
GERUNDS
GODUNOV
GROUNDS
HHMUNRO
IMMUNES
JEJUNUM
KAHUNAS
KORUNAS
LACUNAE
LACUNAL
LACUNAR
LACUNAS
LAGUNAS
MIZUNAS
OBTUNDS
ONEUNIT
OSMUNDS
PETUNIA
REFUNDS
RETUNED
RETUNES
ROTUNDA
SCRUNCH
STAUNCH
SUBUNIT
TROUNCE
TWOUNIT
UNFUNNY
UNSUNNY
UNTUNED
UNTUNES
VICUNAS
YAOUNDE

•••U•N•

ARGUING
ASQUINT
AUBURNS
AUBURNU
AUTUMNS
BEGUINE
BYTURNS
CALUMNY
CAPUANA
COLUMNS
COQUINA
DILUENT
DRQUINN
ENDUING
ENSUING
GENUINE
IMBUING
IMPUGNS
INRUINS
INTURNS
ISSUANT
ISSUING
LECUONA
MINUEND
MRBURNS
NOTURNS
OAHUANS
OPPUGNS
PADUANS
PAPUANS
PIQUANT
PIQUING
QUEUING
REPUGNS
RETURNS
ROGUING
SATURNS
SEQUINS
SIOUANS
TABUING
TEAURNS
TIJUANA
TOLUENE
UNBURNT
UNFUNNY
UNGUENT
UNSUNNY
UPTURNS
VALUING
VOGUING

•••U••N

ACTUPON
ALBUMEN
ALBUMIN
ALDUBIN
AUDUBON
BLOUSON
CERUMEN
CROUTON
DRQUINN
FIXUPON
FLEURON
FOCUSON
GETUPON
GOTUPON
GRAUMAN
HITUPON
INHUMAN
INSULIN
LAPUTAN
LAYUPON
LETUPON
MCLUHAN
MCQUEEN
MEDUSAN
MENUHIN
PNEUMON
PUTUPON
ROMULAN
RUBUPON
SARUMAN
SATUPON
SETUPON
SITUPON
SPYUPON
STEUBEN
STOUTEN
TIBURÓN
UNHUMAN
WHAUDEN
ZABUTON
ZEBULON
ZEBULUN

••••UN•

ACCOUNT
ACHTUNG
ADNOUNS
AGROUND
AIRGUNS
ASTOUND
BENGUNN
BERSUNT
BETHUNE
BIGGUNS
CAPGUNS
COFOUND
COMMUNE
CYYOUNG
DATSUNS
DEMOUNT
DEYOUNG
DOGRUNS
DRYRUNS
EANMUND
EGGHUNT
ENDRUNS
ENGLUND
ENWOUND
EVALUNA
EXPOUND
FORTUNA
FORTUNE
FOXHUNT
FUNRUNS
GOROUND
HITTUNE
HORNUNG
HOTTUNA
ICERUNS
IMPOUND
INAFUNK
INBOUND
JETGUNS
JOBHUNT
LEJEUNE
MACOUNS
MANHUNT
MIDJUNE
MISTUNE
MONTUNO
NEPTUNE
NOCOUNT
OROTUND
OUTGUNS
OUTHUNT
OUTRUNS
OUTSUNG
POPGUNS
POPTUNE
PREFUND
RAPTUNE
RAYGUNS
REBOUND
RECOUNT
REDOUND
REDSUNS
REFOUND
REMOUNT
REPRUNE
RESOUND
REWOUND
RIOMUNI
SAMNUNN
SAMSUNG
SEAHUNT
SHOGUNS
SIGMUND
SIXGUNS
SKIRUNS
SPELUNK
TERHUNE
THESUNS
TOPGUNS
TOYGUNS
TRIBUNE
TSETUNG
UNAMUNO
UNBOUND
UNDRUNK
UNFOUND
UNROUND
UNSLUNG
UNSOUND
UNSTUNG
UNSWUNG
UNWOUND
UNWRUNG
UNYOUNG
UPBOUND
XAMOUNT
ZEITUNG
ZIPGUNS

••••U•N

ADJOURN
ASHBURN
BEDOUIN
BENGUNN
CLIBURN
COGBURN
DONJUAN
GAUGUIN
HEPBURN
JOAQUIN
MANTUAN
NOUTURN
OUTBURN
OUTTURN
PACQUIN
PENGUIN
PREBURN
RAEBURN
RAYBURN
SAMNUNN
SANJUAN
SOJOURN
SUNBURN
THETURN
TOATURN
UNCHURN
VANDUYN

•••••UN

ANTIGUN
BLOWGUN
BLUESUN
BRENGUN
BULLRUN
BURPGUN
CALHOUN
DARTGUN
DUSTGUN
ELAAIUN
ERTEGUN
FORERUN
GLUEGUN
HANDGUN
HAVEFUN
HOMERUN
JIMRYUN
LONGRUN
MADEFUN
MADERUN
MAKEFUN
MAKERUN
MILERUN
MILKRUN
MILLRUN
NAILGUN
OVERRUN
POKEFUN
PRONOUN
REBEGUN
RIOTGUN
SHOTGUN
STENGUN
STUNGUN
TENKRUN
TESTRUN
TRAPGUN
WELLRUN
WHITSUN
YOUNGUN
ZEBULUN

U•O••••

UFOLOGY
UGOLINO
UNOBESE
UNOFTEN
UNOGLED
UNOILED
UNOPTED
UNORBED
UNOVERT
UNOWING
UNOWNED
UPOROUT
UROLOGY
USOPENS
USOSHOW

USOTOUR
UTOPIAN
UTOPIAS
UTOPISM
UTOPIST
UXORIAL

U••O•••

UNBOGGY
UNBOLTS
UNBONED
UNBORED
UNBORNE
UNBOSOM
UNBOUND
UNBOWED
UNBOXED
UNBOXES
UNCODED
UNCOILS
UNCOMIC
UNCOOPS
UNCORED
UNCORES
UNCORKS
UNCOUTH
UNCOVER
UNCOWED
UNCOYER
UNCOYLY
UNDOCKS
UNDOERS
UNDOING
UNDOMED
UNFOGGY
UNFOLDS
UNFORKS
UNFOUND
UNFOXED
UNGODLY
UNGORED
UNHONED
UNHOODS
UNHOOKS
UNHOPED
UNHORSE
UNHOUSE
UNJOINS
UNJOINT
UNJOLLY
UNJOYED
UNLOADS
UNLOATH
UNLOBED
UNLOCAL
UNLOCKS
UNLOFTY
UNLOOPS
UNLOOSE
UNLOVED
UNLOWLY
UNLOYAL
UNMOIST
UNMOLDS
UNMOLDY
UNMOODY
UNMOORS
UNMOSSY
UNMOULD
UNMOVED
UNMOWED
UNNOISY
UNNOSED
UNNOTED
UNNOVEL
UNPOLED
UNPOSED
UNROBED
UNROBES
UNROCKY
UNROLLS
UNROOFS
UNROOMY
UNROOTS
UNROPED
UNROPES
UNROUND
UNROWDY
UNSOBER
UNSOGGY
UNSOLED
UNSOLES
UNSOLID
UNSOOTY
UNSORRY
UNSORTS
UNSOUND
UNSOWED
UNTONED
UNTOUGH
UNTOXIC
UNVOCAL
UNVOICE
UNVOTED
UNVOWED
UNWOOED
UNWORMY
UNWOUND
UNWOVEN
UNYOKED
UNYOKES
UNYOUNG
UNZONED
UNZONES
UPBORNE
UPBOUND
UPCOAST
UPCOILS
UPCOURT
UPFOLDS
UPFORIT
UPGOING
UPHOARD
UPHOLDS
UPLOADS
UPNORTH
UPROARS
UPROOTS
UPROUSE
UPSOARS
UPTONOW
UPTOPAR
UPTOWNS
UTMOSTS

U•••O••

UFOLOGY
ULANOVA
UNALONE
UNBLOCK
UNBLOWN
UNBROKE
UNCHOKE
UNCLOAK
UNCLOGS
UNCLOSE
UNCLOUD
UNCOOPS
UNCROSS
UNCROWN
UNFLOOR
UNFLOWN
UNFROCK
UNFROST
UNFROZE
UNGLOVE
UNGROSS
UNGROWN
UNHOODS
UNHOOKS
UNIBODY
UNICODE
UNICORN
UNIFORM
UNIPODS
UNISOMS
UNISONS
UNKNOTS
UNKNOWN
UNLOOPS
UNLOOSE
UNMOODY
UNMOORS
UNPIOUS
UNPROUD
UNQUOTE
UNROOFS
UNROOMY
UNROOTS
UNSHOED
UNSHOES
UNSHORN
UNSHORT
UNSHOWN
UNSHOWY
UNSMOKY
UNSOOTY
UNSPOKE
UNSPOOL
UNSTOIC
UNSTONY
UNSTOPS
UNSTOUT
UNSTOWS
UNSWORE
UNSWORN
UNWHOLE
UNWOOED
UPABOVE
UPCCODE
UPCLOSE
UPFLOWS
UPFRONT
UPGROWN
UPGROWS
UPOROUT
UPPROPS
UPROOTS
UPSHOOT
UPSHOTS
UPSLOPE
UPSTOOD
UROLOGY
USOTOUR

U••••O•

ULYANOV
UNBOSOM
UNCTION
UNFLOOR
UNSPOOL
UPSHOOT
UPSILON
UPSTOOD
UPTHROW
UPTONOW
URGEDON
URGESON
USEDFOR
USESFOR
USOSHOW
USTINOV

U•••••O

UCCELLO
UGOLINO
UMBERTO
UNAMUNO
UNDERDO
UNDERGO
UNMACHO
UPTEMPO
UTRILLO

•UO••••

BUOYANT
BUOYING
BUOYSUP
DUODENA
DUOPOLY
DUOTONE
EUONYMS
QUOINED
QUOITED
QUONDAM
QUONSET
QUORUMS
QUOTEES
QUOTERS
QUOTING

•U•O•••

AURORAE
AURORAL
AURORAS
AUTOBIO
AUTOBUS
AUTOING
AUTOMAT
AUTOMNE
AUTONYM
AUTOPEN
AUTOPIA
AUTOPSY
BUCOLIC
BUGOUTS
BUJONES
BULOVAS
BUROAKS
BUXOMLY
BUYOFFS
BUYOUTS
CUBOIDS
CULOTTE
CUPOLAS
CUTOFFS
CUTOPEN
CUTOUTS
CUTOVER
DUGONGS
DUGOUTS
EUNOMIA
EUROPOP
EUROVAN
FURORES
HUMORAL
HUMORED
HUMORME
HUMOURS
JUDOIST
JUDOKAS
NUTOILS
OUTOFIT
PUTOFFS
PUTOUTS
PUTOVER
RUDOLFI
RUDOLPH
RUMORED
RUMOURS
RUNOFFS
RUNONIN
RUNOUTS
RUNOVER
SUBORNS
SUDOKUS
SUMOIST
TUPOLEV
TUTORED
YUKOLIS

•U••O••

AUREOLA
AUREOLE
AUTHORS
BUCKOES
BUDWORM
BUFFOON
BUGBOYS
BUGSOFF
BUGSOUT
BUITONI
BULBOUS
BULLOCK
BUMSOUT
BUNCOED
BUNIONS
BUNKOED
BURBOTS
BURGOOS
BURNOFF
BURNOUT
BURROWS
BUSBOYS
BUSLOAD
BUSTOUR
BUSTOUT
BUTGOOD
BUTTONS
BUTTONY
BUTTOUT
BUYDOWN
BUYSOFF
BUYSOUT
BUZZOFF
CUCKOOS
CUIBONO
CUPROUS
CURIOSA
CURIOUS
CURSORS
CURSORY
CUSTODY
CUSTOMS
CUTDOWN
CUTSOFF
CUTSOUT
CUTWORK
CUTWORM
DUBIOUS
DUCKOUT
DUMPOUT
DUNLOPS
DUOPOLY
DUOTONE
DUSTOFF
DUTEOUS
EUPHONY
FUELOIL
FULLOUT
FULSOME
FUNGOES
FURCOAT
FURIOSO
FURIOUS
FURLONG
FURROWS
FUSIONS
GULFOIL
GUMBOOT
GUMWOOD
GUNBOAT
GUNDOGS
GUNLOCK
GUNMOLL
GUNROOM
GUSHOUT
GUSTOES
GUVNORS
GUYROPE
HULLOED
HUNGOFF
HUNGOUT
JUMPOFF
JUNCOES
JUNIORS
JUSTONE
JUSTOUT
LUBBOCK
LUCKOUT
LUGSOUT
LUGWORM
MUDHOLE
MUDROOM
MULDOON
MUMFORD
MURDOCH
MUTTONS
NUMLOCK
NUNHOOD
NUTWOOD
OURSONG
OURTOWN
OUTBOWL
OUTBOWS
OUTCOLD
OUTCOME
OUTCOOK
OUTDOER
OUTDOES
OUTDONE
OUTDOOR
OUTFOOL
OUTFOOT
OUTGOES
OUTHOWL
OUTLOOK
OUTLOUD
OUTLOVE
OUTMODE
OUTMOST
OUTMOVE
OUTPOLL
OUTPOPS
OUTPORT
OUTPOST
OUTPOUR
OUTROAR
OUTROCK
OUTRODE
OUTROLL
OUTROOT
OUTROVE
OUTROWS
OUTSOAR
OUTSOLD
OUTSOLE
OUTTOLD
OUTTOLL
OUTTORE
OUTTORN
OUTVOTE
OUTWORD
OUTWORE
OUTWORK
OUTWORN
PUFFOUT
PUGNOSE
PULLOFF
PULLONS
PULLOUT
PULMONI
PULMONO
PUMPOUT
PURLOIN
PURPORT
PURPOSE
PUSHOFF
PUSHOUT
PUTDOWN
PUTSOFF
PUTSOUT
PUTTOUT
QUAHOGS
QUIXOTE
RUBDOWN
RUBEOLA
RUBIOUS
RUBSOFF
RUBSOUT
RUINOUS
RULEONE
RULEOUT
RUMFORD
RUMPOLE
RUNDOWN
RUNGOFF
RUNGOUT
RUNHOME
RUNSOFF
RUNSOUT
RUSHOFF
RUSHOUT
SUBCODE
SUBCOOL
SUBFORM
SUBGOAL
SUBGODS
SUBJOIN
SUBLONG
SUBLOTS
SUBPOST
SUBROOT
SUBROSA
SUBSOIL
SUBSORT
SUBTONE
SUBZONE
SUCCORS
SUCCOTH
SUCCOUR
SUCROSE
SUFFOLK
SUITORS
SUKKOTH
SUMMONS
SUNBOWL
SUNBOWS
SUNDOGS
SUNDOWN
SUNGODS
SUNROOF
SUNROOM
SUPPORT
SUPPOSE
SUSSOUT
TUCSONS
TUGBOAT
TUNAOIL
TUNEOUT
TUNGOIL
TURBOTS
TURMOIL
TURNOFF
TURNONS
TURNOUT
TUSSOCK

•U•••O•

AUCTION
AUDITOR
AUDUBON
AULDSOD
BUCKFOR
BUFFOON
BUGABOO
BUGALOO
BUILDON
BUILTON
BUISSON
BULLDOG
BULLION
BURGEON
BURGOOS
BURNFOR
BUSHHOG
BUSSTOP
BUTGOOD
CUATROS
CUCKOOS
CURATOR
CUSHION
CUTINON
DUDGEON
DUETTOS
DUKEDOM
DUMPSON
DUNGEON
DUSTMOP
EUDEMON
EUROPOP
FUELROD
FUGATOS
FULLLOT
FUSEBOX
FUSSPOT
GUDGEON
GUERDON
GUIGNOL
GUMBOOT
GUMDROP
GUMSHOE
GUMWOOD
GUNROOM
GUNSFOR
GUNSHOT
HUMIDOR
HUNTFOR
HURSTON
HURTFOR
JUKEBOX
JUMPSON
JURYBOX
JUSTNOW
KUTUZOV
LUBEJOB
LUCKNOW
MUDFLOW
MUDROOM
MUGSHOT
MULDOON
MUMESON
MUNCHON
MURANOS
MUSEDON
MUSESON
MUSTDOS
NUCLEON
NUMEROS
NUNCIOS
NUNHOOD
NUTWOOD
OUTBLOT
OUTBLOW
OUTCOOK
OUTCROP
OUTCROW
OUTDOOR
OUTDROP
OUTFLOW
OUTFOOL
OUTFOOT
OUTGLOW
OUTGROW
OUTLOOK
OUTPLOD
OUTPLOT
OUTROOT
OUTSHOT
OUTSHOW
OUTTROT
PUEBLOS
PULLFOR
PULLSON
PULLTOY
PUSHFOR
PUSHROD
PUTUPON
QUARTOS
QUEIROS
QUINION
QUINTON
QUIZNOS
RUBATOS
RUBICON
RUBUPON
RUCTION
RULEDON
RULESON
RUMSHOP
RUNAMOK
RUNGFOR
RUNRIOT
RUNSFOR
RUNSLOW
SUASION
SUBCOOL
SUBPLOT
SUBROOT
SUCTION
SUEDFOR
SUELYON
SUESFOR
SUNGLOW
SUNROOF
SUNROOM
SUNSPOT
SUREROF
SURGEON
TUBETOP
TUITION
TULSAOK
TUPELOS
TURFTOE
TURNSON
TUXEDOS
VUITTON
YULELOG

•U••••O

AUGUSTO
AUTOBIO
BUFFALO
BUGABOO
BUGALOO
BUNUELO
BURRITO
BUSHIDO
BUYINTO
CUIBONO
CURACAO
CUTINTO
DUGINTO
DURANGO
FURILLO
FURIOSO
FURTADO
GUANACO
GUESSSO
LUCHINO
LUCIANO
LUMBAGO
MULATTO
MURILLO
MUSKEGO
NUESTRO
OUGHTTO
OUTECHO
PULMONO
PUTITTO
PUTUPTO
QUATTRO
QUERIDO
QUITESO
RUFFALO
RUNINTO
RUNUPTO
SUBECHO
SUBZERO
SUHARTO
SUKARNO
SUMUPTO
SUREIDO
TUNEDTO
TUNESTO
TURISMO
TURNPRO
TURNSTO

••U•O••

AQUEOUS
BOUDOIR
BOUSONO
BRUMOUS
COULOMB
COUPONS
DRUMOUT
ELUSORY
EMULOUS
FOULOUT
GLUCOSE
HAULOFF
MAUROIS
NEURONE
NEURONS
OPUSONE
PLUGOLA
PLUMOSE
PLUSONE
PLUTONS
POUROUT
RAUCOUS
ROUTOUT
SAUCONY
SHUTOFF
SHUTOUT
SPUMONE
SPUMONI
SPUNOFF
SPUNOUT
STUPORS
TEUTONS
VAUDOIS
YOULOSE

••U••O•

ABUTSON
BLUEBOY
BLUEFOX
BLUSHON
BOURBON
BOUTROS
CAUTION
CHURROS
COUNTON
ECUADOR
EDUCTOR
ELUTION
EQUATOR
EQUINOX
FLUMMOX
FLUSHOT
FLUXION
GAUCHOS
GLUEDON
GLUESON
GLUTTON
GRUNION
HAUTBOY
HOUSTON
JOURNOS
NEUTRON
PEUGEOT
PLUMCOT
PRUDHOE
REUNION
ROUNDON
SOUPCON
SOUPSON
SOURSON
SOUTHOF
SPURSON
SQUALOR
STUCCOS
STUCKON
STUDIOS
TAUNTON
TOUCHON
YOUKNOW
YOUREON

••U•••O

AZULEJO
BOUNDTO
BOUSONO
CLUNGTO
CRUZADO
DEUTERO
DOUBLEO
EDUARDO
EQUALTO
EQUIANO
FRUSTRO
GLUEDTO
GLUESTO
IMUSTGO
INUTERO
ISUREDO
OPUSTWO
PLUSTWO
ROUGHGO
SQUANTO
STUCKTO
TRUERTO

•••UO••

ARDUOUS
FATUOUS
LECUONA
LIQUORS
NOCUOUS
PEQUOTS
REQUOTE
SEQUOIA
SEQUOYA
SINUOUS
TENUOUS
UNQUOTE
VACUOLE
VACUOUS

•••U•O•

ACTUPON
ADJUROR
AFOULOF
ASSUROR
AUDUBON
BLAUBOK
BLOUSON
BRYUSOV
COJUROR
CROUTON
DILUTOR
DOOUTOF
ENDUROS
ESCUDOS
FIXUPON
FLEURON
FOCUSON
GETUPON
GODUNOV
GOTUPON
HITUPON

KAKUROS
KUTUZOV
LAYUPON
LETUPON
MADUROS
MENUDOS
MRHULOT
PNEUMON
PROUDOF
PUTUPON
RUBUPON
SATUPON
SETUPON
SITUPON
SPYUPON
TIBURON
ZABUTON
ZEBULON

•••U••O

AAJUMBO
ABOUTTO
ADDUPTO
AUGUSTO
BUNUELO
CLAUDIO
COLUMBO
ELMUNDO
GOTUPTO
GROUCHO
HHMUNRO
LEDUPTO
MARULLO
MCMURDO
NABUCCO
NOTUPTO
OCCURTO
OWNUPTO
PUTUPTO
RANUPTO
ROBUSTO
RUNUPTO
SAGUARO
SUMUPTO
VAQUERO

••••UO•

LANGUOR
SHAVUOT

••••U•O

IFYOUGO
MANCUSO
MONTUNO
RIZZUTO
UNAMUNO
VERDUGO
VISCUSO

•••••UO

INVACUO

UP•••••

UPABOVE
UPAHEAD
UPANDIN
UPATREE
UPBEARS
UPBEATS
UPBORNE
UPBOUND
UPBRAID
UPBUILD
UPBURST
UPCARDS
UPCASTS
UPCCODE
UPCLIMB
UPCLOSE
UPCOAST
UPCOILS
UPCOURT
UPCURLS
UPCURVE
UPDARTS
UPDATED
UPDATER
UPDATES
UPDIVED
UPDIVES
UPDRAFT
UPDRIED
UPDRIES
UPDRIFT
UPEARLY
UPENDED
UPFIELD
UPFIRST
UPFLING
UPFLOWS
UPFOLDS
UPFORIT
UPFRONT
UPGAZED
UPGAZES
UPGIRDS
UPGOING
UPGRADE
UPGROWN
UPGROWS
UPHEAPS
UPHEAVE
UPHILLS
UPHOARD
UPHOLDS
UPKEEPS
UPLANDS
UPLEAPS
UPLEAPT
UPLIFTS
UPLIGHT
UPLINKS
UPLOADS
UPNORTH
UPOROUT
UPPHASE
UPPILED
UPPILES
UPPROPS
UPPSALA
UPQUARK
UPRAISE
UPRATED
UPRATES
UPREACH
UPREARS
UPRIGHT
UPRISEN
UPRISER
UPRISES
UPRIVER
UPROARS
UPROOTS
UPROUSE
UPSCALE
UPSENDS
UPSHIFT
UPSHOOT
UPSHOTS
UPSIDES
UPSILON
UPSIZED
UPSIZES
UPSLOPE
UPSOARS
UPSPINS
UPSTAGE
UPSTAIR
UPSTAND
UPSTARE
UPSTART
UPSTATE
UPSTEPS
UPSTIRS
UPSTOOD
UPSURGE
UPSWEEP
UPSWELL
UPSWEPT
UPSWING
UPTAKES
UPTALKS
UPTEARS
UPTEMPO
UPTHERE
UPTHROW
UPTICKS
UPTIGHT
UPTILTS
UPTIMES
UPTONOW
UPTOPAR
UPTOWNS
UPTRADE
UPTREND
UPTURNS
UPVALUE
UPWAFTS
UPWARDS
UPWELLS
UPWHIRL
UPWINDS

U•P••••

UMPIRED
UMPIRES
UMPTEEN
UNPACED
UNPACKS
UNPAGAN
UNPAGED
UNPALED
UNPARED
UNPASTE
UNPAVED
UNPAWED
UNPAWNS
UNPEELS
UNPICKS
UNPIETY
UNPILED
UNPILES
UNPIOUS
UNPIPED
UNPLAIT
UNPLANS
UNPLIED
UNPLUGS
UNPLUMB
UNPOLED
UNPOSED
UNPROUD
UPPHASE
UPPILED
UPPILES
UPPROPS
UPPSALA

U••P•••

UNAPTLY
UNIPLEX
UNIPODS
UNOPTED
UNSPANS
UNSPEAK
UNSPELT
UNSPENT
UNSPICY
UNSPIED
UNSPILT
UNSPLIT
UNSPOKE
UNSPOOL
UPSPINS
USOPENS
UTOPIAN
UTOPIAS
UTOPISM
UTOPIST

U•••P••

UNCAPED
UNDUPED
UNEMPTY
UNHAPPY
UNHOPED
UNPIPED
UNRIPER
UNROPED
UNROPES
UNTAPED
UNTAPES
UNTYPED
UNWIPED
UPTOPAR
USHAPED
USHAPES
USURPED
USURPER

U••••P•

UNADEPT
UNCLIPS
UNCLIPT
UNCOOPS
UNDRAPE
UNGRIPS
UNHAPPY
UNHASPS
UNKEMPT
UNLOOPS
UNLUMPY
UNRASPY
UNSHIPS
UNSNAPS
UNSTEPS
UNSTOPS
UNSWEPT
UNTRAPS
UNWHIPT
UNWRAPS
UPHEAPS
UPKEEPS
UPLEAPS
UPLEAPT
UPPROPS
UPSLOPE
UPSTEPS
UPSWEPT
UPTEMPO

U•••••P

UNCLAMP
UNCLASP
UNCRAMP
UNSHARP
UNSTRAP
UPSWEEP
USINGUP

•UP••••

AUPAIRS
CUPCAKE
CUPELED
CUPELER
CUPFULS
CUPLIKE
CUPOLAS
CUPPIER
CUPPING
CUPRITE
CUPROUS
CUPULAR
CUPULES
EUPHONY
GUPPIES
HUPPAHS
HUPPERT
JUPITER
LUPINES
MUPPETS
NUPTIAL
PUPATED
PUPATES
PUPPETS
PUPPIES
PUPTENT
RUPIAHS
RUPTURE
SUPERGS
SUPPERS
SUPPING
SUPPLED
SUPPLER
SUPPLES
SUPPORT
SUPPOSE
SUPREME
TUPELOS
TUPOLEV
YUPPIES
YUPPIFY

•U•P•••

AUSPICE
BUMPERS
BUMPIER
BUMPILY
BUMPING
BUMPKIN
BUMPSUP
BURPGUN
BURPING
BUSPASS
CULPRIT
CUPPIER
CUPPING
CUSPATE
CUSPIDS
DUMPERS
DUMPIER
DUMPILY
DUMPING
DUMPISH
DUMPOUT
DUMPSON
DUOPOLY
FUNPLEX
GULPERS
GULPIER
GULPING
GUNPLAY
GUPPIES
HUMPHED
HUMPHRY
HUMPIER
HUPPAHS
HUPPERT
JUMPBID
JUMPCUT
JUMPERS
JUMPIER
JUMPILY
JUMPING
JUMPOFF
JUMPSAT
JUMPSIN
JUMPSON
JUMPSUP
LUMPERS
LUMPIER
LUMPILY
LUMPING
LUMPISH
LUMPSIN
LUMPSIT
LUMPSUM
MUDPACK
MUDPIES
MUPPETS
MURPHYS
NUTPINE
OUTPACE
OUTPAID
OUTPASS
OUTPATH
OUTPAYS
OUTPEEP
OUTPICK
OUTPIPE
OUTPITY
OUTPLAN
OUTPLAY
OUTPLOD
OUTPLOT
OUTPOLL
OUTPOPS
OUTPORT
OUTPOST
OUTPOUR
OUTPRAY
OUTPULL
OUTPURL
OUTPUSH
OUTPUTS
PULPERS
PULPIER
PULPIFY
PULPING
PULPITS
PUMPERS
PUMPING
PUMPKIN
PUMPOUT
PUMPSUP
PUPPETS
PUPPIES
PURPLED
PURPLES
PURPORT
PURPOSE
PUTPUTS
QUAPAWS
QUEPASA
QUIPPED
QUIPPER
RUMPEND
RUMPLED
RUMPLES
RUMPOLE
RUNPAST
SUBPLOT
SUBPOST
SULPHUR
SUPPERS
SUPPING
SUPPLED
SUPPLER
SUPPLES
SUPPORT
SUPPOSE
SURPASS
SURPLUS
SUSPECT
SUSPEND
SUSPIRE
VULPINE
YUPPIES
YUPPIFY

•U••P••

AUTOPEN
AUTOPIA
AUTOPSY
BULLPEN
BUSHPIG
CUTOPEN
DUCKPIN
DUSTPAN
EUROPOP
FUSSPOT
JUNIPER
OUTSPED
OUTSPIN
OUTSPIT
PULLPIN
PUSHPIN
PUTUPON
PUTUPTO
QUIPPED
QUIPPER
RUBUPON
RUNUPTO
SUMUPTO
SUNSPOT
TUBEPAN
TURNPRO

•U•••P•

BUMRAPS
BURLAPS
BUSTUPS
CUETIPS
DUNLOPS
DUSTUPS
EUTERPE
GUNLAPS
GUYROPE
HUBCAPS
OUTKEPT
OUTLIPS
OUTPIPE
OUTPOPS
OUTRAPS
OUTWEPT
PULLUPS
PUSHUPS
RUDOLPH
RUNLAPS
SUBTYPE
TUNEUPS
TURNIPS
TURNUPS
YUCAIPA

•U••••P

BUCKSUP
BUDDYUP
BUFFSUP
BUILDUP
BUILTUP
BULKSUP
BUMPSUP
BUNCHUP
BUOYSUP
BURNSUP
BURNTUP
BUSSTOP
BUSTRIP
BUSTSUP
CURLSUP
DUCHAMP
DUDEDUP
DUDESUP
DUMMYUP
DUSTMOP
EUROPOP
FUELSUP
FURWRAP
GUMDROP
GUNSHIP
GUSSYUP
HUNTSUP
HURRYUP
JUICEUP
JUMPSUP
MUCKSUP
MUDFLAP
MUDWASP
MUGWUMP
NUNSHIP
OUTCROP
OUTDROP
OUTJUMP
OUTKEEP
OUTLEAP
OUTPEEP
OUTSKIP
OUTSTEP
OUTWEEP
OUTYELP
PUFFSUP
PULLSUP
PUMPSUP
PUNCHUP
PUTEMUP
QUEUEUP
RUCKSUP
RUMSHOP
RUNDEEP
RUNITUP
SUCKSUP
SUITSUP
SUMITUP
SUNLAMP
SURFSUP
TUBETOP
TUNEDUP
TUNESUP
TURNSUP

••UP•••

CHUPPAH
CHUPPAS
COUPING
COUPLED
COUPLER
COUPLES
COUPLET
COUPONS
CRUPPER
DAUPHIN
ERUPTED
ERUPTER
EXUPERY
MAUPRAT
NTUPLES
PAUPERS
REUPPED
SCUPPER
SOUPCAN
SOUPCON
SOUPERS
SOUPIER
SOUPMIX
SOUPSON
SOUPSUP
STUPEFY
STUPIDS
STUPORS
TOUPEES
WHUPPED

••U•P••

ARUSPEX
CHUMPED
CHUPPAH
CHUPPAS
CLUMPED
CRUMPED
CRUMPET
CRUMPLE
CRUMPLY
CRUPPER
FAUXPAS
FOURPIN
GRUMPED
PAULPRY
PLUMPED
PLUMPER
PLUMPIE
PLUMPLY
REUPPED
SCULPED
SCULPTS
SCUPPER
SLUMPED
SLURPED
SLURPEE
SLURPER
STUMPED
STUMPER
THUMPED
THUMPER
TRUMPED
TRUMPET
TRUMPUP
USURPED
USURPER
WHUPPED

••U••P•

CHUTZPA
FOULUPS

••U•••P

BOUNDUP
BRUSHUP
CHURNUP
CLUBSUP
COUGHUP
COUNTUP
CRUDSUP
DOUBLEP
DRUMSUP
FLUFFUP
FOULSUP
FOULTIP
HAULSUP
LOUSEUP
MOUNTUP
PLUGSUP
ROUGHUP
ROUNDUP
SHUTSUP
SLUNKUP
SNUCKUP
SOUPSUP
STUCKUP
TOUCHUP
TRUEDUP
TRUESUP
TRUMPUP
TRUSSUP
WOUNDUP

•••UP••

ACOUPLE
ACTUPON
ADDUPTO
DECUPLE
ENDUPAT
FIXUPON
GETUPON
GOTUPON
GOTUPTO
GROUPED
GROUPER
GROUPIE
HITUPON
IRRUPTS
LAYUPON
LEDUPTO
LETUPON
NONUPLE
NOTUPTO
OCTUPLE
OCTUPLY
OWNUPTO
POPUPAD
PUTUPON
PUTUPTO
RANUPTO
RUBUPON
RUNUPTO
SATUPON
SCOUPES
SCRUPLE
SETUPON
SITUPON
SPYUPON
SUMUPTO
THRUPUT
TROUPED
TROUPER
TROUPES
UNDUPED

•••U•P•

DEPULPS
GALUMPH
REPUMPS
TRIUMPH
UNLUMPY

•••U••P

CLOUDUP
MRQUILP
QUEUEUP
SCOUTUP
SCRUBUP

••••UP•

BACKUPS
BLOWUPS
BUSTUPS
CALLUPS
CATSUPS
CHALUPA
CHINUPS
CORRUPT
DIALUPS
DISRUPT
DUSTUPS
EGGCUPS
EYECUPS
FILLUPS
FLIPUPS
FOLDUPS
FOULUPS
GIVEUPS
GOOFUPS
HANGUPS
HICCUPS
HOLDUPS
HOOKUPS
HOTCUPS
KICKUPS
LACEUPS
LARRUPS
LASHUPS
LEADUPS
LINEUPS
LINKUPS
LOCKUPS
LOOKUPS
MAKEUPS
MARKUPS
MESSUPS
MOCKUPS
OILCUPS
PETPUPS
PICKUPS
PILEUPS
PRENUPS
PREPUPA
PULLUPS
PUSHUPS
RAVEUPS
RECOUPS
REERUPT
ROLLUPS
SENDUPS
SIGNUPS
SLIPUPS
SLOWUPS
STEPUPS
TEACUPS
TOSSUPS
TUNEUPS
TURNUPS
WAKEUPS
WALKUPS
WARMUPS
WASHUPS
WINDUPS
WORKUPS
WRAPUPS

••••U•P

AIRPUMP
BIGGULP
GASPUMP
MUGWUMP
NOTRUMP
ONELUMP
OUTJUMP
REEQUIP
SCHLUMP
SKIJUMP
THEPUMP

•••••UP

ACTEDUP
ADDEDUP
AIREDUP
AMPEDUP
ANTEDUP
ANTESUP
ASKEDUP
ATEITUP
BACKSUP
BALLSUP
BANGSUP
BANKSUP
BEADSUP
BEAMSUP
BEARSUP
BEATSUP
BEEFSUP
BELLYUP
BELTSUP
BINDSUP
BITESUP
BLAZEUP
BLOCKUP
BLOTSUP
BLOWNUP
BLOWSUP
BOARDUP
BOILSUP
BOLTSUP
BONEDUP
BONESUP
BOOSTUP
BOOTSUP
BORNEUP
BOTCHUP
BOUNDUP
BOXEDUP
BOXESUP
BRACEUP
BREAKUP
BREWSUP

BRICKUP
BRINGUP
BROKEUP
BRUSHUP
BUCKSUP
BUDDYUP
BUFFSUP
BUILDUP
BUILTUP
BULKSUP
BUMPSUP
BUNCHUP
BUOYSUP
BURNSUP
BURNTUP
BUSTSUP
CAGEDUP
CAGESUP
CAKEDUP
CAKESUP
CALLSUP
CAMPSUP
CASTSUP
CATCHUP
CHAINUP
CHALKUP
CHATSUP
CHECKUP
CHEERUP
CHEWSUP
CHIPSUP
CHIRRUP
CHOKEUP
CHOPSUP
CHOSEUP
CHURNUP
CLAMSUP
CLEANUP
CLEARUP
CLIMBUP
CLOGSUP
CLOSEUP
CLOTSUP
CLOUDUP
CLUBSUP
COILSUP
COLDCUP
COMESUP
COOKSUP
COOPSUP
CORKSUP
COUGHUP
COUNTUP
COVERUP
CRACKUP
CRANKUP
CRATEUP
CREEPUP
CREPTUP
CRIEDUP
CRIESUP
CROPSUP
CROSSUP
CRUDSUP
CURLSUP
DEALSUP
DEALTUP
DIALSUP

DICECUP
DIVVYUP
DOINGUP
DOLLSUP
DRAGSUP
DRANKUP
DRAWNUP
DRAWSUP
DREAMUP
DRESSUP
DRIEDUP
DRIESUP
DRIFTUP
DRINKUP
DRIVEUP
DROVEUP
DRUMSUP
DUDEDUP
DUDESUP
DUMMYUP
EASEDUP
EASESUP
EATENUP
EATITUP
EIGHTUP
ENDEDUP
EVENSUP
FAIRSUP
FANCYUP
FENCEUP
FILLSUP
FIREDUP
FIRESUP
FIRMSUP
FIRSTUP
FIXEDUP
FIXESUP
FLAMEUP
FLAREUP
FLIESUP
FLOATUP
FLOWNUP
FLUFFUP
FOLDSUP
FOOTSUP
FORCEUP
FORKSUP
FOULSUP
FRAMEUP
FREEDUP
FREESUP
FRIEDUP
FRIESUP
FROTHUP
FROZEUP
FUELSUP
GANGSUP
GASEDUP
GASESUP
GEARSUP
GIDDYUP
GIVENUP
GIVESUP
GLAMSUP
GOINGUP
GOOFSUP
GRATEUP
GREYCUP

GROWNUP
GROWSUP
GUSSYUP
HACKSUP
HAMITUP
HANDSUP
HANGSUP
HAULSUP
HEADSUP
HEALSUP
HEAPSUP
HEATSUP
HELPSUP
HIKEDUP
HIKESUP
HITCHUP
HOISTUP
HOLDSUP
HOLEDUP
HOLESUP
HOOKSUP
HOTSOUP
HUNTSUP
HURRYUP
HYPEDUP
HYPESUP
ICINGUP
IGIVEUP
INGROUP
JACKSUP
JERKSUP
JOINSUP
JUICEUP
JUMPSUP
KEEPSUP
KETCHUP
KEYEDUP
KICKSUP
KNEESUP
KNOTSUP
LACEDUP
LACESUP
LANDSUP
LEADSUP
LEAPSUP
LEAPTUP
LICKSUP
LIFTSUP
LIGHTUP
LINEDUP
LINESUP
LINKSUP
LIVENUP
LOADSUP
LOCKSUP
LOOKSUP
LOUSEUP
LYINGUP
MAKESUP
MARKSUP
MATCHUP
MEETSUP
MISTSUP
MIXEDUP
MIXESUP
MIXITUP
MOCKSUP
MOUNTUP

MOVEDUP
MOVESUP
MUCKSUP
NAILSUP
NOSEDUP
NOSESUP
OFFERUP
OPENSUP
ORDERUP
OVERSUP
OWNEDUP
PACKSUP
PAIRSUP
PASTEUP
PATCHUP
PEASOUP
PERKSUP
PHONYUP
PICKSUP
PILEDUP
PILESUP
PIPEDUP
PIPESUP
PLAYSUP
PLOWSUP
PLUGSUP
POINTUP
POWERUP
PRECOUP
PRESSUP
PRICKUP
PRINTUP
PROPSUP
PSYCHUP
PUFFSUP
PULLSUP
PUMPSUP
PUNCHUP
PUTEMUP
QUEUEUP
RACEDUP
RACESUP
RACKSUP
RAISEUP
RAKEDUP
RAKESUP
RAMPSUP
RANITUP
REACHUP
READSUP
REARSUP
REELSUP
REGROUP
RESTSUP
REVITUP
RIDESUP
RILEDUP
RILESUP
RINGSUP
RISESUP
ROLLSUP
ROOTSUP
ROPEDUP
ROPESUP
ROUGHUP
ROUNDUP
RUCKSUP
RUNITUP

SACKSUP
SAVEDUP
SAVESUP
SCALEUP
SCAREUP
SCARFUP
SCOUTUP
SCREWUP
SCRUBUP
SEALSUP
SENDSUP
SERVEUP
SEVENUP
SEWEDUP
SHAKEUP
SHAPEUP
SHINEUP
SHOOKUP
SHOOTUP
SHOREUP
SHOWNUP
SHOWSUP
SHUTSUP
SIGNSUP
SIZEDUP
SIZESUP
SLACKUP
SLANTUP
SLICEUP
SLINKUP
SLIPSUP
SLOWSUP
SLUNKUP
SMACKUP
SMASHUP
SMOKEUP
SNAGSUP
SNAPSUP
SNARLUP
SNAZZUP
SNEAKUP
SNIFFUP
SNUCKUP
SOAKSUP
SOAPSUP
SOUPSUP
SPEAKUP
SPEEDUP
SPICEUP
SPIFFUP
SPIKEUP
SPLITUP
SPOKEUP
STACKUP
STANDUP
STANKUP
STARTUP
STAYSUP
STEAMUP
STEPSUP
STICKUP
STILLUP
STINKUP
STIRRUP
STIRSUP
STOCKUP
STOKEUP
STOODUP

STOPSUP
STOREUP
STUCKUP
SUCKSUP
SUITSUP
SUMITUP
SURFSUP
SWANKUP
SWEEPUP
SWELLUP
SWEPTUP
SWIMSUP
TACKSUP
TAKENUP
TAKESUP
TALKSUP
TALLYUP
TANKSUP
TAPEDUP
TAPESUP
TARTSUP
TEAMSUP
TEARSUP
TEASEUP
TEEITUP
TENSEUP
THINKUP
THREEUP
THREWUP
THROWUP
TILTSUP
TIMESUP
TONEDUP
TONESUP
TOOLSUP
TOTALUP
TOTESUP
TOUCHUP
TRADEUP
TRIPSUP
TROTSUP
TRUEDUP
TRUESUP
TRUMPUP
TRUSSUP
TUNEDUP
TUNESUP
TURNSUP
TWISTUP
TYINGUP
TYPEDUP
TYPESUP
USINGUP
WAITSUP
WAKEDUP
WAKESUP
WALLSUP
WARMSUP
WAXEDUP
WAXESUP
WEIGHUP
WELLSUP
WHATSUP
WHIPSUP
WICKIUP
WINDSUP
WIPEDUP
WIPESUP

WIREDUP
WIRESUP
WISEDUP
WISESUP
WOKENUP
WORKSUP
WOUNDUP
WRACKUP
WRAPSUP
WRITEUP
WROTEUP

UQ•••••
UQUARKS

U•Q••••
UNQUICK
UNQUIET
UNQUOTE
UPQUARK

U••Q•••
UNEQUAL
UNIQUES

•UQ••••
BUQSHAS

•U•Q•••
KUMQUAT

•U••Q••
DUBUQUE
QUELQUE
QUINQUE

••UQ•••
BOUQUET

••U•Q••
BRUSQUE

••U•••Q
DOUBLEQ

•••UQ••
DUBUQUE
GIAUQUE

••••U•Q
AVENUEQ

UR•••••
URACILS
URANITE
URANIUM
URBANER
URBANII
URBANIV
URBANVI
URCHINS
URGEDON
URGENCY
URGESON
URGINGS
URNFULS
URNLIKE
UROLOGY
URSINUS
URSULAK
URTEXTS
URUGUAY

U•R••••
UKRAINE
UNRACKS
UNRAINY
UNRAKED
UNRASPY
UNRATED
UNRAVEL
UNRAYED
UNRAZED
UNREADY
UNREELS
UNREGAL
UNRESTS
UNRHYME
UNRIGID
UNRILED
UNRIMED
UNRIPER
UNRISEN
UNRISKY
UNRIVED
UNRIVEN
UNROBED
UNROBES
UNROCKY
UNROLLS
UNROOFS
UNROOMY
UNROOTS
UNROPED
UNROPES
UNROUND
UNROWDY
UNRULED
UNRURAL
UPRAISE
UPRATED
UPRATES
UPREACH
UPREARS
UPRIGHT
UPRISEN
UPRISER
UPRISES
UPRIVER
UPROARS
UPROOTS
UPROUSE
UTRECHT
UTRILLO

U••R•••
UMBRAGE
UMBRIAN
UMBRIEL
UNARMED
UNBRACE
UNBRAID
UNBRAKE
UNBRAVE
UNBRIEF
UNBROKE
UNCRAMP
UNCRATE
UNCRAZY
UNCRIED
UNCROSS
UNCROWN
UNCRUDE
UNCRUEL
UNDRAPE
UNDRAWN
UNDRAWS
UNDRESS
UNDRIED
UNDRUNK
UNERECT
UNFRAIL
UNFRANK
UNFREED
UNFREES
UNFRIED
UNFRILL
UNFROCK
UNFROST
UNFROZE
UNGRAND
UNGREEN
UNGRIPS
UNGROSS
UNGROWN
UNGRUFF
UNORBED
UNPROUD
UNTRACK
UNTRAPS
UNTREAD
UNTREED
UNTRIED
UNTRITE
UNTRUER
UNTRULY
UNTRUSS
UNTRUTH
UNURBAN
UNURGED
UNWRAPS
UNWRUNG
UPBRAID
UPDRAFT
UPDRIED
UPDRIES
UPDRIFT
UPFRONT
UPGRADE
UPGROWN
UPGROWS
UPOROUT
UPPROPS
UPTRADE
UPTREND
USERFEE
USERIDS
USGRANT
USURERS
USURIES
USURPED
USURPER
UXORIAL

U•••R••
UMBERED
UMBERTO
UMPIRED
UMPIRES
UNAIRED
UNBARED
UNBARES
UNBERTH
UNBORED
UNBORNE
UNBURLY
UNBURNT
UNBURST
UNCORED
UNCORES
UNCORKS
UNCURBS
UNCURED
UNCURLS
UNDARED
UNDERDO
UNDERGO
UNEARTH
UNFERTH
UNFIRED
UNFORKS
UNFURLS
UNGIRDS
UNGORED
UNHARDY
UNHARSH
UNHIRED
UNHIRES
UNHORSE
UNLARGE
UNLURED
UNLYRIC
UNMERGE
UNMERRY
UNMIRED
UNNERVE
UNPARED
UNRURAL
UNSCREW
UNSORRY
UNSORTS
UNSTRAP
UNSURLY
UNTERSE
UNTIRED
UNWIRED
UNWORMY
UPATREE
UPBORNE
UPBURST
UPCARDS
UPCURLS
UPCURVE
UPDARTS
UPEARLY
UPFIRST
UPFORIT
UPGIRDS
UPNORTH
UPSURGE
UPTHROW
UPTURNS
UPWARDS
UQUARKS
USHERED
USHERIN
UTTERED
UTTERER
UTTERLY

U••••R•
ULSTERS
UNALERT
UNANGRY
UNAWARE
UNBEARD
UNCHARY
UNCHURN
UNDOERS
UNFIERY
UNGUARD
UNHAIRS
UNHAIRY
UNHEARD
UNICORN
UNIFORM
UNINERT
UNITARD
UNITARY
UNITERS
UNLEARN
UNMERRY
UNMITRE
UNMOORS
UNOVERT
UNSHARP
UNSHORN
UNSHORT
UNSMART
UNSNARL
UNSORRY
UNSTERN
UNSWORE
UNSWORN
UNTIERS
UNWEARY
UPBEARS
UPCOURT
UPHOARD
UPQUARK
UPREARS
UPROARS
UPSOARS
UPSTARE
UPSTART
UPSTIRS
UPTEARS
UPTHERE
UPWHIRL
USURERS

U•••••R
UNCHAIR
UNCLEAR
UNCOVER
UNCOYER
UNDULAR
UNEAGER
UNFLOOR
UNGULAR
UNIFIER
UNMAKER
UNMITER
UNRIPER
UNSAFER
UNSHEER
UNSHIER
UNSHYER
UNSLIER
UNSLYER
UNSOBER
UNSWEAR
UNTRUER
UNWISER
UPDATER
UPRISER
UPRIVER
UPSTAIR
UPTOPAR
URBANER
USEDCAR
USEDFOR
USESFOR
USOTOUR
USURPER
UTTERER

•UR••••
AURALEE
AURALLY
AUREATE
AUREOLA
AUREOLE
AURICLE
AURISTS
AURORAE
AURORAL
AURORAS
BURBAGE
BURBANK
BURBLED
BURBLER
BURBLES
BURBOTS
BURDENS
BURDICK
BUREAUS
BUREAUX
BURETTE
BURGEES
BURGEON
BURGERS
BURGESS
BURGHER
BURGLAR
BURGLED
BURGLES
BURGOOS
BURIALS
BURIERS
BURKINA
BURLAPS
BURLERS
BURLIER
BURLING
BURMANS
BURMESE
BURNABY
BURNERS
BURNETT
BURNFOR
BURNING
BURNISH
BURNLEY
BURNOFF
BURNOUT
BURNSIN
BURNSUP
BURNTIN
BURNTUP
BUROAKS
BURPGUN
BURPING
BURRIER
BURRING
BURRITO
BURROWS
BURSARS
BURSTER
BURSTIN
BURSTYN
BURUNDI
BURYING
CURABLE
CURABLY
CURACAO
CURARES
CURATED
CURATES
CURATOR
CURBCUT
CURBING
CURDIER
CURDING
CURDLED
CURDLER
CURDLES
CUREALL
CURETTE
CURFEWS
CURIOSA
CURIOUS
CURLERS
CURLEWS
CURLIER
CURLIKE
CURLING
CURLSIN
CURLSUP
CURRANT
CURRENT
CURRIED
CURRIER
CURRIES
CURRING
CURRISH
CURSEAT
CURSERS
CURSING
CURSIVE
CURSORS
CURSORY
CURTAIL
CURTAIN
CURTATE
CURTEST

CURTISS
CURTSEY
CURVETS
CURVIER
CURVING
DURABLE
DURABLY
DURANCE
DURANGO
DURANTE
DURNING
DURRELL
DURWARD
DURWENT
EURASIA
EUREKAS
EUROPOP
EUROVAN
FURBALL
FURBISH
FURCATE
FURCOAT
FURFARM
FURILLO
FURIOSO
FURIOUS
FURLERS
FURLESS
FURLING
FURLONG
FURNACE
FURNESS
FURNISH
FURORES
FURRIER
FURRING
FURROWS
FURSEAL
FURTADO
FURTHER
FURTIVE
FURWRAP
GURGLED
GURGLES
GURKHAS
GURNEYS
HURDLED
HURDLER
HURDLES
HURLERS
HURLING
HURRAHS
HURRAYS
HURRIED
HURRIER
HURRIES
HURRYUP
HURSTON
HURTERS
HURTFOR
HURTFUL
HURTING
HURTLED
HURTLES
JURGENS
JURIDIC
JURISTS
JURYBOX
JURYING
JURYMAN
JURYMEN
JURYRIG
KURDISH
KURILES
KURRENT
LURCHED
LURCHER
LURCHES
LUREDIN
LURESIN
LUREXES
LURIDLY
LURKERS
LURKING
LURLEEN
MURALED
MURANOS
MURDERS
MURDOCH
MURIELS
MURILLO
MURKIER
MURKILY
MURKISH
MURMURS
MURPHYS
NUREYEV
NURSERS
NURSERY
NURSING
NURTURE
OURGANG
OURSELF
OURSONG
OURTOWN
PURCELL
PURDUEU
PURFLED
PURFLER
PURFLES
PURGING
PURISTS
PURITAN
PURLIEU
PURLING
PURLOIN
PURPLED
PURPLES
PURPORT
PURPOSE
PURRERS
PURRING
PURSERS
PURSIER
PURSING
PURSUED
PURSUER
PURSUES
PURSUIT
PURTIER
PURVEYS
PURVIEW
RURALLY
SUREBET
SURECAN
SUREIAM
SUREIDO
SUREROF
SURFACE
SURFEIT
SURFERS
SURFIER
SURFING
SURFMAN
SURFMEN
SURFSUP
SURGEON
SURGERY
SURGING
SURIMIS
SURINAM
SURLIER
SURLILY
SURMISE
SURNAME
SURPASS
SURPLUS
SURREAL
SURREYS
SURVEIL
SURVEYS
SURVIVE
TURBANS
TURBINE
TURBOTS
TUREENS
TURFIER
TURFING
TURFMAN
TURFMEN
TURFSKI
TURFTOE
TURFWAR
TURISMO
TURISTA
TURKEYS
TURKISH
TURMOIL
TURNBAD
TURNERS
TURNERY
TURNING
TURNIPS
TURNKEY
TURNOFF
TURNONS
TURNOUT
TURNPRO
TURNRED
TURNSIN
TURNSON
TURNSTO
TURNSUP
TURNUPS
TURRETS
TURTLED
TURTLES

•U•R•••

BULRUSH
BUMRAPS
BUMRUSH
BUNRAKU
BURRIER
BURRING
BURRITO
BURROWS
BUSRIDE
CUIRASS
CUPRITE
CUPROUS
CURRANT
CURRENT
CURRIED
CURRIER
CURRIES
CURRING
CURRISH
CUTRATE
DURRELL
FUNRUNS
FURRIER
FURRING
FURROWS
GUARANI
GUARDED
GUARDEE
GUARDER
GUARGUM
GUERDON
GUNROOM
GUYROPE
HURRAHS
HURRAYS
HURRIED
HURRIER
HURRIES
HURRYUP
KUBRICK
KURRENT
MUDROOM
NUTRIAS
OUTRACE
OUTRAGE
OUTRAIL
OUTRANG
OUTRANK
OUTRANT
OUTRAPS
OUTRATE
OUTRAVE
OUTREAD
OUTRIBS
OUTRIDE
OUTRIGS
OUTRING
OUTROAR
OUTROCK
OUTRODE
OUTROLL
OUTROOT
OUTROVE
OUTROWS
OUTRUNS
OUTRUSH
PUERILE
PURRERS
PURRING
PUTREFY
QUARLES
QUARREL
QUARTAN
QUARTER
QUARTES
QUARTET
QUARTIC
QUARTOS
QUARTZY
QUERIDA
QUERIDO
QUERIED
QUERIER
QUERIES
QUERIST
QUIRTED
QUORUMS
RUBRICS
RUGRATS
RUNRIOT
SUBRACE
SUBROOT
SUBROSA
SUCRASE
SUCROSE
SUNRAYS
SUNRISE
SUNROOF
SUNROOM
SUPREME
SURREAL
SURREYS
TUGRIKS
TURRETS

•U••R••

AUBERGE
AUBURNS
AUBURNU
AUGURAL
AUGURED
AUGURER
AURORAE
AURORAL
AURORAS
AUSTRAL
AUSTRIA
AUTARCH
AUTARKY
BUCKRAM
BUGFREE
BULLRUN
BUSTRIP
BUTTRAM
CUATROS
CULPRIT
CUMBRIA
CURARES
CUTARUG
DUBARRY
DUSTRAG
EUCERIN
EUCHRED
EUCHRES
EUTERPE
FUELROD
FULCRUM
FURORES
FURWRAP
FUTURAS
FUTURES
GUJARAT
GUMDROP
GUMTREE
GUTHRIE
HUMDRUM
HUMERAL
HUMERUS
HUMORAL
HUMORED
HUMORME
HUNDRED
JURYRIG
LUCARNE
LUCERNE
LUSTRAL
LUSTRED
LUSTRES
LUSTRUM
MUBARAK
MUJERES
MULGREW
MUSKRAT
NUBIRAS
NUMERAL
NUMERIC
NUMEROS
NUTTREE
OUTBRAG
OUTBRAY
OUTBRED
OUTCROP
OUTCROW
OUTDRAG
OUTDRAW
OUTDREW
OUTDROP
OUTGREW
OUTGRIN
OUTGROW
OUTPRAY
OUTTRAY
OUTTROT
PUBERTY
PUSHROD
QUADRIC
QUARREL
QUATRES
QUEERED
QUEERER
QUEERLY
QUEIROS
RUBSRAW
RUBYRED
RUMORED
RUNFREE
SUBAREA
SUBARID
SUBARUS
SUBORNS
SUBURBS
SUGARED
SUHARTO
SUKARNO
SUPERGS
SUREROF
SUTURED
SUTURES
TUMBREL
TUNDRAS
TURNRED
TUTORED

•U•••R•

AUPAIRS
AUSTERE
AUSTERS
AUTEURS
AUTHORS
BUCKERS
BUDDERS
BUDGERS
BUDWORM
BUFFERS
BUGLERS
BUKHARA
BULGARI
BULGARS
BULGURS
BULWARK
BUMMERS
BUMPERS
BUNKERS
BUNTERS
BURGERS
BURIERS
BURLERS
BURNERS
BURSARS
BUSFARE
BUSGIRL
BUSHERS
BUSKERS
BUSSERS
BUSTARD
BUSTERS
BUTLERS
BUTTERS
BUTTERY
BUZZARD
BUZZERS
CUECARD
CULLERS
CULTURE
CULVERT
CUMBERS
CURLERS
CURSERS
CURSORS
CURSORY
CUSSERS
CUSTARD
CUSTERS
CUTLERS
CUTLERY
CUTTERS
CUTWORK
CUTWORM
DUBARRY
DUBBERS
DUCKERS
DUELERS
DUFFERS
DULLARD
DUMPERS
DUNKERS
DUNKIRK
DUNNERS
DURWARD
DUSTERS
FUDGERS
FUELERS
FULMARS
FUNDERS
FUNFURS
FURFARM
FURLERS
FUSSERS
FUTHARK
GUEVARA
GUIDERS
GUITARS
GULPERS
GUNFIRE
GUNNERS
GUNNERY
GUSHERS
GUTTERS
GUVNORS
HUBBARD
HUGGERS
HULLERS
HUMBARD
HUMBERT
HUMMERS
HUMOURS
HUMPHRY
HUNGARY
HUNGERS
HUNKERS
HUNTERS
HUPPERT
HURLERS
HURTERS
HUSKERS
HUSSARS
HUSSERL
JUDGERS
JUICERS
JUMPERS
JUNIORS
JUNKART
JUNKERS
KUNDERA
LUBBERS
LUGGERS
LUGWORM
LULLERS
LUMBARS
LUMBERS
LUMIERE
LUMPERS
LUNGERS
LUNKERS
LURKERS
LUSTERS
MUCKERS
MUDDERS
MUDLARK
MUGGERS
MULHARE
MULLERS
MUMFORD
MUMMERS
MUMMERY
MURDERS
MURMURS
MUSHERS
MUSTARD
MUSTERS
MUTTERS
NUBBERS
NUDGERS
NUESTRA
NUESTRO
NUMBERS
NUNNERY
NURSERS
NURSERY
NURTURE
NUTTERS
OUSTERS
OUTBARK
OUTBURN
OUTCURE
OUTDARE
OUTEARN
OUTFIRE
OUTHERE
OUTHIRE
OUTHURL
OUTPORT
OUTPURL
OUTSERT
OUTTIRE
OUTTORE
OUTTORN
OUTTURN
OUTWARD
OUTWARS
OUTWORD
OUTWORE
OUTWORK
OUTWORN
PUCKERS
PUCKERY
PUFFERS
PUFFERY
PULLERS
PULPERS
PULSARS
PUMPERS
PUNKERS
PUNNERS
PUNTERS
PURPORT
PURRERS
PURSERS
PUSHERS
PUTTERS
QUAKERS
QUASARS
QUATTRO
QUAVERS
QUAVERY
QUESERA
QUEUERS
QUINARY
QUIVERS
QUIVERY
QUOTERS
RUBBERS
RUBBERY
RUCKERT
RUDDERS
RUDYARD
RUINERS
RUMFORD
RUMMERS
RUMOURS
RUNNERS
RUNSDRY
RUPTURE
RUSHERS
RUSSERT
RUTGERS
RUTTERS
SUBFORM
SUBSORT
SUBVERT
SUBWARS
SUBZERO
SUCCORS
SUCKDRY
SUCKERS
SUDBURY
SUDSERS
SUFFERS
SUITORS
SULKERS
SUMATRA
SUMMARY
SUMMERS
SUMMERY
SUNBIRD
SUNBURN
SUNDERS
SUNFIRE
SUNWARD
SUPPERS
SUPPORT
SURFERS
SURGERY
SUSPIRE
TUCKERS
TUGGERS
TURNERS
TURNERY
TURNPRO
TUSHERY
TUSKERS
VULTURE

•U••••R

AUDITOR
AUGURER
BUCHNER
BUCKFOR
BUCKNER
BUELLER
BUGBEAR
BUGGIER
BUILDER
BULGHUR
BULGIER
BULKIER
BUMBLER
BUMPIER
BUNDLER
BUNGLER
BURBLER
BURGHER
BURGLAR
BURLIER
BURNFOR
BURRIER
BURSTER
BUSHIER
BUSTIER
BUSTLER
BUSTOUR
BUTCHER
BUZZIER
CUPELER
CUPPIER
CUPULAR
CURATOR
CURDIER
CURDLER
CURLIER
CURRIER
CURVIER
CUSHIER
CUSSLER
CUTOVER
DUCKIER
DUMPIER
DUSKIER
DUSTIER
DUUMVIR
FUBSIER
FUMBLER
FUNFAIR
FUNKIER
FUNNIER
FUNSTER
FURRIER
FURTHER
FUSSIER
FUSTIER
FUZZIER
GUARDER
GUCKIER
GUESSER
GUILDER
GULFWAR
GULPIER
GUMMIER
GUNKIER
GUNSFOR
GUNTHER
GUNUSER
GUSHIER
GUSTIER
GUTSIER
GUTTIER
GUZZLER
HUDDLER
HUFFIER
HULKIER
HUMBLER
HUMIDOR
HUMPIER
HUNKIER
HUNTFOR
HURDLER
HURRIER
HURTFOR
HUSKIER
HUSTLER
JUGGLER
JUGULAR
JUICIER
JUMBLER
JUMPIER
JUNIPER
JUNKCAR
JUNKIER
JUPITER
KUTCHER
LUCIFER
LUCKIER
LUMPIER
LUNCHER
LUNULAR
LURCHER
LUSHIER
LUSTIER
LUTHIER
MUAMMAR
MUCKIER
MUDDIER
MUDDLER
MUELLER
MUFFLER
MUGGIER
MULDAUR
MUMBLER
MUNCHER
MUNSTER
MURKIER
MUSHIER
MUSKIER
MUSSIER
MUSTIER
MUZZIER
MUZZLER
NUBBIER
NUCLEAR
NUTSIER
NUTTIER
NUZZLER
OUTDOER
OUTDOOR
OUTHEAR
OUTLIER
OUTPOUR
OUTROAR
OUTSOAR
OUTTEAR
OUTWEAR
PUDGIER
PUFFIER
PULLFOR
PULPIER
PUNCHER
PUNKIER
PUNNIER
PUNSTER
PURFLER
PURSIER
PURSUER
PURTIER
PUSHFOR
PUSHIER
PUTOVER
PUZZLER
QUACKER
QUAFFER
QUAKIER
QUARTER
QUEERER
QUELLER
QUERIER
QUESTER
QUICKER
QUIETER
QUILLER
QUILTER
QUIPPER
QUITTER
QUIZZER
RUDDIER
RUFFLER
RUMBLER
RUNGFOR
RUNNIER
RUNOVER
RUNSFOR
RUNTIER
RUSHIER
RUSTIER
RUSTLER
RUTTIER
SUBDUER
SUBTLER
SUCCOUR
SUCKIER
SUDSIER
SUEDFOR
SUESFOR
SULKIER
SULPHUR
SUNNIER
SUPPLER
SURFIER
SURLIER
TUBBIER
TUBULAR
TUFTIER
TUMBLER
TUMMLER
TURFIER
TURFWAR
TUTELAR
VUMETER
YUCKIER
YUMMIER

••UR•••

AZURITE
BEURRES
BLURBER
BLURRED
BLURTED
BLURTER
BOURBON
BOURGET
BOURSES
CHURCHY
CHURNED
CHURNER
CHURNUP
CHURROS
COURAGE

COURANT
COURBET
COURIER
COURSED
COURSER
COURSES
COURTED
COURTLY
COURTTV
DHURRIE
DIURNAL
DOUREST
ENURING
EXURBAN
EXURBIA
FMURRAY
FOURAAA
FOURDAY
FOUREEE
FOURIER
FOURMAN
FOURPIN
FOURTHS
FOURWAY
GLURGES
GOURAMI
GOURDES
GOURMET
HEURIGE
INURING
ISUREAM
ISUREDO
JOURDAN
JOURNAL
JOURNEE
JOURNEY
JOURNOS
KNURLED
LAURELS
LAURENT
LAURITZ
LOURDES
LOUREED
LOURING
MAUREEN
MAURIAC
MAURIAT
MAURICE
MAUROIS
MOURNED
MOURNER
NEURONE
NEURONS
NOURISH
PLURALS
POURERS
POURING
POUROUT
POURSIN
REURGED
REURGES
SAURIAN
SCURVES
SLURPED
SLURPEE
SLURPER
SLURRED
SOURALE
SOURCED
SOURCES
SOUREST
SOURING
SOURISH
SOURSON
SPURNED
SPURNER
SPURRED
SPURSON
SPURTED
STURGES
TAUREAN
TAURINE
THURBER
THURGAU
THURMAN
TOURBUS
TOURERS
TOURING
TOURISM
TOURIST
TOURNEY
UNURBAN
UNURGED
USURERS
USURIES
USURPED
USURPER
YOURANG
YOUREIT
YOUREON

••U•R••

AQUARIA
BEURRES
BLUERED
BLURRED
BOUTROS
CHURROS
DHURRIE
EDUARDO
EQUERRY
FMURRAY
FOUDRES
LAUTREC
LOUVRED
LOUVRES
MAUPRAT
NEUTRAL
NEUTRON
OEUVRES
POUDRES
SLURRED
SPURRED
SQUARED
SQUARER
SQUARES
SQUIRED
SQUIRES
SQUIRMS
SQUIRMY
SQUIRTS
STUARTI
TOUAREG
TRUERIB
TRUERTO
UQUARKS
VOUVRAY

••U••R•

ABUSERS
AMUSERS
CAUSERS
COUGARS
COUNTRY
COUTERS
COUTURE
DAUBERS
DEUTERO
DOUSERS
ELUDERS
ELUSORY
EQUERRY
EXUPERY
FLUTERS
FOULARD
FOUNDRY
FRUSTRO
GAUDERY
GAUGERS
GOUGERS
GRUYERE
HAULERS
INUTERO
LAUDERS
LAUNDRY
LOUVERS
MAULERS
MAUSERS
MOUSERS
NEUTERS
NOUTURN
OCULARS
PAULPRY
PAUPERS
PAUSERS
PCUSERS
POULTRY
POURERS
POUTERS
PRUDERY
PRUNERS
REUNERS
REUSERS
REUTERS
RHUBARB
ROUSERS
ROUTERS
SAUCERS
SHUBERT
SOUPERS
SQUEERS
STUPORS
TOURERS
TOUTERS
USURERS

••U•••R

ABUTTER
AGUTTER
ALUNSER
AQUIFER
AQUIVER
ASUNDER
BAULKER
BLUBBER
BLUDGER
BLUFFER
BLUNDER
BLUNTER
BLURBER
BLURTER
BLUSHER
BLUSTER
BOUCHER
BOUDOIR
BOULDER
BOUNCER
BOUNDER
BOUVIER
BRUISER
BRUSHER
CAULKER
CHUGGER
CHUKKER
CHURNER
CLUBBER
CLUBCAR
CLUCKER
CLUNKER
CLUSTER
CLUTTER
COULTER
COUNTER
COUPLER
COURIER
COURSER
CRUELER
CRUISER
CRULLER
CRUPPER
CRUSHER
DAUMIER
DAUNTER
DOUBLER
DOUBTER
DOUCEUR
DRUBBER
DRUCKER
DRUDGER
DRUMMER
DRUNKER
DUUMVIR
ECUADOR
EDUCTOR
EQUATOR
ERUPTER
FAUXFUR
FLUBBER
FLUFFER
FLUKIER
FLUNKER
FLUSHER
FLUSTER
FLUTIER
FLUTTER
FNUMBER
FOUNDER
FOURIER
GAUCHER
GAUDIER
GAUNTER
GAUTIER
GAUZIER
GLUMMER
GOUNDER
GOUTIER
GRUBBER
GRUDGER
GRUFFER
GRUNGER
GRUNTER
HAUNTER
HAUTEUR
HOUNDER
JOUSTER
KRUEGER
LAUGHER
LAUNDER
LOUNGER
LOUSIER
MAUNDER
MOULDER
MOUNTER
MOURNER
MOUSIER
MOUTHER
PLUGGER
PLUMBER
PLUMIER
PLUMMER
PLUMPER
PLUNDER
PLUNGER
PLUNKER
PLUSHER
POUNCER
POUNDER
POUTIER
REUTHER
REUTTER
ROUGHER
ROUNDER
ROUSTER
SAUCIER
SAUNTER
SCUDDER
SCUFFER
SCULLER
SCUPPER
SHUCKER
SHUDDER
SHUNTER
SHUSTER
SHUTTER
SKULKER
SLUGGER
SLUMBER
SLUMMER
SLURPER
SMUCKER
SMUGGER
SNUBBER
SNUFFER
SNUGGER
SOUNDER
SOUPIER
SPUMIER
SPURNER
SPUTTER
SQUALOR
SQUARER
STUDIER
STUFFER
STUMPER
STUNNER
STUTTER
TAUNTER
THUMPER
THUNDER
THURBER
THUSFAR
TOUCHER
TOUGHER
TRUCKER
TRUDGER
TRUSTER
USURPER
VAULTER
VAUNTER
VOUCHER
YOUNGER

•••UR••

ABJURED
ABJURER
ABJURES
ACCURST
ADJURED
ADJURER
ADJURES
ADJUROR
ALLURED
ALLURER
ALLURES
ASSURED
ASSURER
ASSURES
ASSUROR
AUBURNS
AUBURNU
AUGURAL
AUGURED
AUGURER
BYTURNS
COJUROR
CONURES
DEBURGH
DEBURRS
DEMURER
ENDURED
ENDURER
ENDURES
ENDUROS
ENSURED
ENSURER
ENSURES
ETRURIA
EXCURSE
FIGURAL
FIGURED
FIGURER
FIGURES
FLEURON
FLOURED
FUTURAS
FUTURES
IMMURED
IMMURES
IMPURER
INCURVE
INJURED
INJURER
INJURES
INSURED
INSURER
INSURES
INTURNS
KAKUROS
LACUREE
LIGURIA
LITURGY
MADUROS
MANURED
MANURES
MATURED
MATURER
MATURES
MAZURKA
MCMURDO
MRBURNS
NATURAL
NATURED
NATUREL
NATURES
NOTURNS
OCCURTO
OROURKE
PANURGE
PARURES
PLEURAE
PLEURAL
RASURES
RECURED
RECURES
RECURLS
RECURVE
RESURGE
RETURFS
RETURNS
SAMURAI
SATURNS
SCOURED
SCOURER
SCOURGE
SECURED
SECURER
SECURES
SPLURGE
SUBURBS
SUTURED
SUTURES
TEAURNS
TENURED
TENURES
TIBURON
TSOURIS
UNBURLY
UNBURNT
UNBURST
UNCURBS
UNCURED
UNCURLS
UNFURLS
UNLURED
UNRURAL
UNSURLY
UPBURST
UPCURLS
UPCURVE
UPSURGE
UPTURNS
VELURES
YOGURTS
ZYMURGY

•••U•R•

ACQUIRE
ACTUARY
ARGUERS
DEBURRS
DOEUVRE
EDOUARD
ENQUIRE
ENQUIRY
ESQUIRE
ESTUARY
HHMUNRO
INQUIRE
INQUIRY
ISSUERS
JAGUARS
JANUARY
LEXUSRX
LIQUORS
MAGUIRE
MCGUIRE
OCTUBRE
ONGUARD
OSSUARY
QUEUERS
REQUIRE
ROGUERY
SAGUARO
TSQUARE
UNGUARD
UPQUARK
VALUERS
VAQUERO
VOGUERS

•••U••R

ABJURER
ACCUSER
ADDUCER
ADJURER
ADJUROR
ALLURER
ANGULAR
ANNULAR
AROUSER
ASSUMER
ASSURER
ASSUROR
ASTUTER
AUGURER
CHAUCER
CLOUTER
COBUYER
COJUROR
COPULAR
CUPULAR
DEDUCER
DEFUSER
DELUDER
DEMURER
DENUDER
DILUTER
DILUTOR
ENDURER
ENDUSER
ENSURER
EXCUSER
EXHUMER
FIBULAR
FIGURER
FLOUTER
FOCUSER
GROUPER
GROUSER
GROUTER
GUNUSER
IMPURER
IMPUTER
INDUCER
INFUSER
INHUMER
INJURER
INSULAR
INSURER
JOCULAR
JUGULAR
LACUNAR
LIQUEUR
LUNULAR
MACULAR
MACUSER
MATURER
MENUBAR
MINUTER
MISUSER
MODULAR
NEBULAR
NODULAR
NONUSER
NOSUGAR
OBTUSER
OSCULAR
PERUSER
POPULAR
PROUDER
REAUMUR
REBUKER
REDUCER
REFUSER
REFUTER
REGULAR
RIGUEUR
SALUTER
SCHUMER
SCOURER
SCOUTER
SECULAR
SECURER
SEDUCER
SHOUTER
SPOUTER
SPRUCER
STOUTER
TABULAR
THEUSSR
TITULAR
TROUPER
TROUSER
TUBULAR
UNDULAR
UNGULAR
ZONULAR

••••UR•

ADJOURN
ALBSURE
ARAFURA
ARBOURS
ARDOURS
ARMOURS
ARMOURY
ARTHURC
ARTHURM
ARTHURS
ASHBURN
ASHBURY
ATATURK
AUTEURS
BANBURY
BRAVURA
BULGURS
CADBURY
CAESURA
CAPTURE
CENSURE
CENTURY
CLIBURN
CLOSURE
CLOTURE
COGBURN
COLOURS
CONCURS
CONJURE
CONJURY
COUTURE
CULTURE
DANBURY
DEBLURS
DENTURE
DETOURS
DEVOURS
DISEURS
DISTURB
DOLOURS
DRLAURA
EGOSURF
EPICURE
ERASURE
FAILURE
FAVOURS
FEATURE
FISSURE
FIXTURE
FLEXURE
FORSURE
FUNFURS
GESTURE
GETHURT
GOTHURT
GRAVURE
HAMBURG
HARBURG
HEPBURN
HOMBURG
HONOURS
HUMOURS
IMYOURS
INAFURY
INCOURT
INPOURS
KAPTURE
LABOURS
LECTURE
LEISURE
LIMBURG
MAJEURE
MARYURE
MCCLURE
MCCLURG
MCCOURT
MEASURE
MERCURE
MERCURY
MIXTURE
MSIEURS
MURMURS
NETSURF
NEWBURG
NONJURY
NOTSURE
NOUTURN
NURTURE
OBSCURA
OBSCURE
ONAJURY
OUTBURN
OUTCURE
OUTHURL
OUTPURL
OUTTURN
PASTURE
PERDURE
PERJURE
PERJURY
PERTURB
PICTURE
PINCURL
POSEURS
POSTURE
PREBURN
PRECURE
PROCURE
RAEBURN
RAPTURE
RAYBURN
REPOURS
RETOURS
RIGOURS
RONDURE
ROXBURY
RUMOURS
RUPTURE
SAVOURS
SAVOURY
SEIZURE
SIDDURS
SKYSURF
SOJOURN
STATURE
SUDBURY
SUNBURN
TEMPURA
TEXTURE
THETURN
TOATURN
TONSURE
TORTURE
UNCHURN
UPCOURT
VALOURS
VANDURA
VAPOURS
VAPOURY
VELOURS
VENTURA
VENTURE
VENTURI
VERDURE
VESTURE
VIGOURS
VOITURE
VULTURE
WALKURE
WARBURG
WASSURE
YOGHURT

••••U•R

CHEQUER
CONQUER
LACQUER
LANGUOR
LEAGUER
MASQUER
MRSMUIR
NIEBUHR
PURSUER
RESCUER
SUBDUER
UNTRUER

•••••UR

ACTFOUR
AGEFOUR
AMATEUR
BALFOUR
BELVOUR
BIGFOUR
BONHEUR
BONJOUR
BULGHUR
BUSTOUR
CANDOUR
CENTAUR
CLAMOUR
CONTOUR
CRITTUR
DANSEUR
DECATUR
DOUCEUR
ECOTEUR
ENAMOUR
EVERDUR
FABFOUR
FAKEFUR
FARCEUR
FAUXFUR
FERVOUR
FLANEUR
FLAVOUR
FRISEUR
GLAMOUR
HARBOUR
HAUTEUR
HOTSPUR
JODHPUR
LAFLEUR
LIQUEUR
MANHOUR
MANIPUR
MASSEUR
MULDAUR
OFFHOUR
ONEHOUR
OUTPOUR
PARFOUR
PARLOUR
PASTEUR
PAVIOUR
PGATOUR
PRESPUR
RANCOUR
REAUMUR
REDFOUR
REOCCUR
RIGUEUR
SANDBUR
SAVIOUR
SEYMOUR
SIXFOUR
SUCCOUR
SULPHUR
TENFOUR
THETOUR
TWOHOUR
USOTOUR
VANOCUR
WEEHOUR

US•••••

USABLES
USANCES
USEDCAR
USEDCDS
USEDFOR
USELESS
USERFEE
USERIDS
USESFOR
USFLAGS
USGRANT
USHAPED
USHAPES
USHERED
USHERIN
USINGIN
USINGUP
USOPENS
USOSHOW
USOTOUR
USSTATE
USSTEEL
USTEDES
USTINOV
USUALLY
USURERS
USURIES
USURPED
USURPER

7
UR

U•S••••

ULSTERS
UNSADLY
UNSAFER
UNSALTY
UNSATED
UNSAVED
UNSAVVY
UNSAWED
UNSCALY
UNSCREW
UNSEALS
UNSEAMS
UNSEATS
UNSELLS
UNSEWED
UNSHADE
UNSHADY
UNSHARP
UNSHEER
UNSHELL
UNSHIER
UNSHIFT
UNSHINY
UNSHIPS
UNSHOED
UNSHOES
UNSHORN
UNSHORT
UNSHOWN
UNSHOWY
UNSHYER
UNSHYLY
UNSIDED
UNSIGHT
UNSILLY
UNSIZED
UNSKEWS
UNSLACK
UNSLAIN
UNSLEEK
UNSLICK
UNSLIER
UNSLING
UNSLUNG
UNSLYER
UNSLYLY
UNSMART
UNSMOKY
UNSNAGS
UNSNAKY
UNSNAPS
UNSNARL
UNSOBER
UNSOGGY
UNSOLED
UNSOLES
UNSOLID
UNSOOTY
UNSORRY
UNSORTS
UNSOUND
UNSOWED
UNSPANS
UNSPEAK
UNSPELT
UNSPENT
UNSPICY
UNSPIED
UNSPILT
UNSPLIT
UNSPOKE
UNSPOOL
UNSTACK
UNSTAGY
UNSTAID
UNSTATE
UNSTEEL
UNSTEPS
UNSTERN
UNSTICK
UNSTIFF
UNSTOIC
UNSTONY
UNSTOPS
UNSTOUT
UNSTOWS
UNSTRAP
UNSTUCK
UNSTUNG
UNSULKY
UNSUNNY
UNSURLY
UNSWEAR
UNSWEET
UNSWEPT
UNSWORE
UNSWORN
UNSWUNG
UPSCALE
UPSENDS
UPSHIFT
UPSHOOT
UPSHOTS
UPSIDES
UPSILON
UPSIZED
UPSIZES
UPSLOPE
UPSOARS
UPSPINS
UPSTAGE
UPSTAIR
UPSTAND
UPSTARE
UPSTART
UPSTATE
UPSTEPS
UPSTIRS
UPSTOOD
UPSURGE
UPSWEEP
UPSWELL
UPSWEPT
UPSWING
URSINUS
URSULAK
USSTATE
USSTEEL

U••S•••

ULYSSES
UNASKED
UNISIZE
UNISOMS
UNISONS
UNUSUAL
UPPSALA
USESFOR
USOSHOW

U•••S••

ULYSSES
UNBASED
UNBESET
UNBOSOM
UNCASED
UNCASES
UNCASKS
UNDUSTY
UNEASES
UNFUSED
UNFUSSY
UNHASPS
UNHASTY
UNHUSKS
UNLUSTY
UNMASKS
UNMASTS
UNMOSSY
UNNASAL
UNNOSED
UNPASTE
UNPOSED
UNRASPY
UNRESTS
UNRISEN
UNRISKY
UNTASTY
UNWISER
UPCASTS
UPRISEN
UPRISER
UPRISES
URGESON
UTENSIL
UTMOSTS

U••••S•

UGLIEST
UNBLEST
UNBURST
UNCLASP
UNCLOSE
UNCROSS
UNDRESS
UNFROST
UNFUSSY
UNGROSS
UNHARSH
UNHORSE
UNHOUSE
UNITISE
UNLEASH
UNLOOSE
UNMOIST
UNMOSSY
UNNOISY
UNOBESE
UNTENSE
UNTERSE
UNTRUSS
UNTWIST
UPBURST
UPCLOSE
UPCOAST
UPFIRST
UPPHASE
UPRAISE
UPROUSE
USELESS
UTILISE
UTOPISM
UTOPIST

U•••••S

ULLAGES
ULSTERS
ULTIMAS
ULYSSES
ULZANAS
UMLAUTS
UMPIRES
UNBAITS
UNBALES
UNBARES
UNBELTS
UNBENDS
UNBINDS
UNBOLTS
UNBOXES
UNCAGES
UNCAKES
UNCASES
UNCASKS
UNCIALS
UNCLIPS
UNCLOGS
UNCOILS
UNCOOPS
UNCORES
UNCORKS
UNCROSS
UNCUFFS
UNCURBS
UNCURLS
UNDINES
UNDOCKS
UNDOERS
UNDRAWS
UNDRESS
UNEASES
UNEDGES
UNFACTS
UNFILES
UNFINES
UNFIXES
UNFOLDS
UNFORKS
UNFREES
UNFURLS
UNGIRDS
UNGLUES
UNGRIPS
UNGROSS
UNHAIRS
UNHANDS
UNHASPS
UNHEEDS
UNHELMS
UNHIRES
UNHOODS
UNHOOKS
UNHULLS
UNHUSKS
UNIATES
UNIFIES
UNIPODS
UNIQUES
UNISOMS
UNISONS
UNITERS
UNITIES
UNIVACS
UNJOINS
UNKINKS
UNKNITS
UNKNOTS
UNLACES
UNLADES
UNLAXES
UNLEADS
UNLEAFS
UNLIKES
UNLINKS
UNLIVES
UNLOADS
UNLOCKS
UNLOOPS
UNMAKES
UNMASKS
UNMASTS
UNMATES
UNMIXES
UNMOLDS
UNMOORS
UNNAILS
UNPACKS
UNPAWNS
UNPEELS
UNPICKS
UNPILES
UNPIOUS
UNPLANS
UNPLUGS
UNRACKS
UNREELS
UNRESTS
UNROBES
UNROLLS
UNROOFS
UNROOTS
UNROPES
UNSEALS
UNSEAMS
UNSEATS
UNSELLS
UNSHIPS
UNSHOES
UNSKEWS
UNSNAGS
UNSNAPS
UNSOLES
UNSORTS
UNSPANS
UNSTEPS
UNSTOPS
UNSTOWS
UNTACKS
UNTAMES
UNTAPES
UNTAXES
UNTHAWS
UNTIERS
UNTRAPS
UNTRUSS
UNTUCKS
UNTUNES
UNVEILS
UNWALLS
UNWINDS
UNWRAPS
UNYOKES
UNZONES
UPBEARS
UPBEATS
UPCARDS
UPCASTS
UPCOILS
UPCURLS
UPDARTS
UPDATES
UPDIVES
UPDRIES
UPFLOWS
UPFOLDS
UPGAZES
UPGIRDS
UPGROWS
UPHEAPS
UPHILLS
UPHOLDS
UPKEEPS
UPLANDS
UPLEAPS
UPLIFTS
UPLINKS
UPLOADS
UPPILES
UPPROPS
UPRATES
UPREARS
UPRISES
UPROARS
UPROOTS
UPSENDS
UPSHOTS
UPSIDES
UPSIZES
UPSOARS
UPSPINS
UPSTEPS
UPSTIRS
UPTAKES
UPTALKS
UPTEARS
UPTICKS
UPTILTS
UPTIMES
UPTOWNS
UPTURNS
UPWAFTS
UPWARDS
UPWELLS
UPWINDS
UQUARKS
URACILS
URCHINS
URGINGS
URNFULS
URSINUS
URTEXTS
USABLES
USANCES
USEDCDS
USELESS
USERIDS
USFLAGS
USHAPES
USOPENS
USTEDES
USURERS
USURIES
UTAHANS
UTICANS
UTMOSTS
UTOPIAS
UVALUES

•US••••

AUSABLE
AUSLESE
AUSPICE
AUSSIES
AUSTERE
AUSTERS
AUSTINS
AUSTRAL
AUSTRIA
BUSBIES
BUSBOYS
BUSCEMI
BUSFARE
BUSGIRL
BUSHELS
BUSHERS
BUSHHOG
BUSHIDO
BUSHIER
BUSHILY
BUSHING
BUSHMAN
BUSHMEN
BUSHPIG
BUSHWAH
BUSIEST
BUSKERS
BUSKING
BUSLANE
BUSLINE
BUSLOAD
BUSMANS
BUSPASS
BUSRIDE
BUSSERS
BUSSING
BUSSTOP
BUSTARD
BUSTERS
BUSTIER
BUSTING
BUSTLED
BUSTLER
BUSTLES
BUSTOUR
BUSTOUT
BUSTRIP
BUSTSIN
BUSTSUP
BUSTUPS
BUSYBEE
BUSYING
CUSHAWS
CUSHIER
CUSHILY
CUSHING
CUSHION
CUSPATE
CUSPIDS
CUSSERS
CUSSING
CUSSLER
CUSTARD
CUSTERS
CUSTODY
CUSTOMS
DUSKIER
DUSKILY
DUSKING
DUSKISH
DUSTBIN
DUSTERS
DUSTGUN
DUSTIER
DUSTILY
DUSTING
DUSTMAN
DUSTMEN
DUSTMOP
DUSTOFF
DUSTPAN
DUSTRAG
DUSTUPS
EUSTACE
FUSEBOX
FUSIBLE
FUSILLI
FUSIONS
FUSSERS
FUSSIER
FUSSILY
FUSSING
FUSSPOT
FUSTIAN
FUSTIER
FUSTILY
FUSUMAS
GUSHERS
GUSHIER
GUSHILY
GUSHING
GUSHOUT
GUSSETS
GUSSIED
GUSSIES
GUSSYUP
GUSTAVE
GUSTIER
GUSTILY
GUSTING
GUSTOES
HUSBAND
HUSHABY
HUSHFUL
HUSHING
HUSKERS
HUSKIER
HUSKIES
HUSKILY
HUSKING
HUSSARS
HUSSEIN
HUSSERL
HUSSIES
HUSSITE
HUSTLED
HUSTLER
HUSTLES
JUSTEST
JUSTICE
JUSTIFY
JUSTINE
JUSTNOW
JUSTONE
JUSTOUT
LUSHEST
LUSHIER
LUSTERS
LUSTFUL
LUSTIER
LUSTILY
LUSTING
LUSTRAL
LUSTRED
LUSTRES
LUSTRUM
MUSANTE
MUSCATS
MUSCIDA
MUSCLED
MUSCLES
MUSEDON
MUSEFUL
MUSESON
MUSETTA
MUSETTE
MUSEUMS
MUSHERS
MUSHIER
MUSHILY
MUSHING
MUSICAL
MUSICKS
MUSIGNY
MUSINGS
MUSKEGO
MUSKETS
MUSKIER
MUSKIES
MUSKRAT
MUSLIMS
MUSLINS
MUSSELS
MUSSIER
MUSSILY
MUSSING
MUSTAFA
MUSTANG
MUSTARD
MUSTDOS
MUSTERS
MUSTIER
MUSTILY
MUSTSEE
OUSTERS
OUSTING
PUSHERS
PUSHFOR
PUSHFUL
PUSHIER
PUSHILY
PUSHING
PUSHKIN
PUSHOFF
PUSHOUT
PUSHPIN
PUSHROD
PUSHUPS
PUSSIES
RUSHDIE
RUSHEES
RUSHERS
RUSHIER
RUSHING
RUSHOFF
RUSHOUT
RUSSELL
RUSSERT
RUSSETS
RUSSETY
RUSSIAN
RUSSLAN
RUSTICS
RUSTIER
RUSTILY
RUSTING
RUSTLED
RUSTLER
RUSTLES
SUSANNA
SUSANNE
SUSPECT
SUSPEND
SUSPIRE
SUSSING
SUSSOUT
SUSTAIN
TUSCANS
TUSCANY
TUSHERY
TUSHIES
TUSKERS
TUSKING
TUSSAUD
TUSSIVE
TUSSLED
TUSSLES
TUSSOCK

•U•S•••

AUSSIES
BUGSOFF
BUGSOUT
BUISSON
BUMSOUT
BUQSHAS
BURSARS
BURSTER
BURSTIN
BURSTYN
BUSSERS
BUSSING
BUSSTOP
BUYSOFF
BUYSOUT
CUBSFAN
CUESTAS
CUISINE
CUMSHAW
CURSEAT
CURSERS
CURSING
CURSIVE
CURSORS
CURSORY
CUSSERS
CUSSING
CUSSLER
CUTSOFF
CUTSOUT
DUNSTAN
FUBSIER
FULSOME
FUNSTER
FURSEAL
FUSSERS
FUSSIER
FUSSILY
FUSSING
FUSSPOT
GUESSAT
GUESSED
GUESSER
GUESSES
GUESSSO
GUESTED
GUMSHOE
GUNSELS
GUNSFOR
GUNSHIP
GUNSHOT
GUSSETS
GUSSIED
GUSSIES
GUSSYUP
GUTSIER
GUTSILY
HURSTON
HUSSARS
HUSSEIN
HUSSERL
HUSSIES
HUSSITE
LUGSAIL
LUGSOUT
MUESLIS
MUESLIX
MUGSHOT
MUNSTER
MUSSELS
MUSSIER
MUSSILY
MUSSING
NUESTRA
NUESTRO
NUNSHIP
NURSERS
NURSERY
NURSING
NUTSIER
OURSELF
OURSONG
OUTSAID
OUTSAIL
OUTSANG
OUTSAYS
OUTSEEK
OUTSEEN
OUTSEES
OUTSELL
OUTSERT
OUTSETS
OUTSHOT
OUTSHOW
OUTSIDE
OUTSIFT
OUTSIGH
OUTSING
OUTSINS
OUTSITS
OUTSIZE
OUTSKIP
OUTSOAR
OUTSOLD
OUTSOLE
OUTSPED
OUTSPIN
OUTSPIT
OUTSTAY
OUTSTEP
OUTSULK
OUTSUMS
OUTSUNG
OUTSWAM
OUTSWIM
OUTSWUM
PUGSLEY
PULSARS
PULSATE
PULSING
PUNSTER
PURSERS
PURSIER
PURSING
PURSUED
PURSUER
PURSUES
PURSUIT
PUSSIES
PUTSOFF
PUTSOUT
QUASARS
QUASHED
QUASHES
QUESERA
QUESNAY
QUESTED
QUESTER
RUBSOFF
RUBSOUT
RUBSRAW
RUMSHOP
RUNSDRY
RUNSFOR
RUNSLOW
RUNSOFF
RUNSOUT
RUSSELL
RUSSERT
RUSSETS
RUSSETY
RUSSIAN
RUSSLAN
SUASION
SUASIVE
SUBSECT
SUBSETS
SUBSIDE
SUBSIDY
SUBSIST
SUBSOIL
SUBSORT
SUBSUME
SUDSERS
SUDSIER
SUDSING
SUESFOR
SUNSETS
SUNSFAN
SUNSPOT
SUNSUIT
SUSSING
SUSSOUT
TUCSONS
TUESDAY
TULSANS
TULSAOK
TUSSAUD
TUSSIVE
TUSSLED
TUSSLES
TUSSOCK

•U••S••

AUGUSTA
AUGUSTE
AUGUSTO
AUGUSTS
AULDSOD
AURISTS
AUTISTS
BUCKSAW
BUCKSUP
BUFFSUP
BUISSON
BULKSUP
BUMPSUP
BUOYSUP
BURNSIN
BURNSUP
BUSTSIN
BUSTSUP
BUTTSIN
BUZZSAW
CUBISTS
CURLSIN
CURLSUP
CURTSEY
CUTISES
DUDESUP
DUFUSES
DUMPSON
EURASIA
FUCHSIA

FUELSUP
FUJISAN
FUMESAT
GUESSAT
GUESSED
GUESSER
GUESSES
GUESSSO
GUNUSER
HUMUSES
HUNTSUP
JUDASES
JUMPSAT
JUMPSIN
JUMPSON
JUMPSUP
JURISTS
LUMPSIN
LUMPSIT
LUMPSUM
LUNESTA
LURESIN
LUTISTS
MUCKSUP
MUMESON
MUSESON
MUSTSEE
NUDISTS
NULLSET
OUTASKS
PUFFSUP
PULASKI
PULLSIN
PULLSON
PULLSUP
PUMPSUP
PURISTS
QUITSIT
QUONSET
RUCKSUP
RULESON
SUCKSIN
SUCKSUP
SUITSME
SUITSUP
SULUSEA
SURFSUP
TUBISTS
TUCKSIN
TUMESCE
TUNASUB
TUNESIN
TUNESTO
TUNESUP
TUNISIA
TURFSKI
TURISMO
TURISTA
TURNSIN
TURNSON
TURNSTO
TURNSUP

•U•••S•

AUSLESE
AUTOPSY
BUDLESS
BUDVASE
BUFFEST
BULLISH
BULRUSH
BUMRUSH
BURGESS
BURMESE
BURNISH
BUSIEST
BUSPASS
CUBBISH
CUIRASS
CULTISH
CULTISM
CULTIST
CURIOSA
CURRISH
CURTEST
CURTISS
CUTLASS
DUALISM
DUALIST
DUCHESS
DUEEAST
DUELIST
DUEWEST
DULLEST
DULLISH
DUMBEST
DUMPISH
DUNCISH
DUSKISH
FUJITSU
FULLEST
FULNESS
FUMIEST
FUNFEST
FURBISH
FURIOSO
FURLESS
FURNESS
FURNISH
GUESSSO
GUMLESS
GUNCASE
GUNLESS
GUTLESS
HUELESS
HUFFISH
HUNNISH
JUDAISM
JUDOIST
JUJITSU
JUSTEST
KURDISH
LUCIUSI
LUDDISM
LUMPISH
LUSHEST
MUDFISH
MUDWASP
MUGGISH
MURKISH
NUMBEST
NUNNISH
OUTCAST
OUTFAST
OUTFISH
OUTGUSH
OUTHISS
OUTJEST
OUTKAST
OUTKISS
OUTLASH
OUTLAST
OUTMOST
OUTPASS
OUTPOST
OUTPUSH
OUTRUSH
OUTWASH
OUTWEST
OUTWISH
PUBLISH
PUCKISH
PUGGISH
PUGNOSE
PUNIEST
PUNLESS
PURPOSE
QUEPASA
QUERIST
QUITESO
RUBBISH
RULIEST
RUMLESS
RUNLESS
RUNPAST
RUNTISH
RUTTISH
SUAVEST
SUBBASE
SUBBASS
SUBCASE
SUBCASH
SUBCAST
SUBPOST
SUBROSA
SUBSIST
SUBTASK
SUCCESS
SUCRASE
SUCROSE
SUFFUSE
SUGGEST
SUMLESS
SUMOIST
SUNFAST
SUNFISH
SUNKIST
SUNLESS
SUNRISE
SUPPOSE
SURMISE
SURPASS
TUBAIST
TUGLESS
TURKISH

•U••••S

AUBADES
AUBURNS
AUDILES
AUGENDS
AUGITES
AUGUSTS
AUKLETS
AUNTIES
AUPAIRS
AURISTS
AURORAS
AUSSIES
AUSTERS
AUSTINS
AUTEURS
AUTHORS
AUTISTS
AUTOBUS
AUTUMNS
BUBBLES
BUCKERS
BUCKETS
BUCKLES
BUCKOES
BUDDERS
BUDDHAS
BUDDIES
BUDGERS
BUDGETS
BUDGIES
BUDLESS
BUFFERS
BUFFETS
BUGBOYS
BUGGIES
BUGGLES
BUGLERS
BUGOUTS
BUJONES
BULBOUS
BULGARS
BULGURS
BULLETS
BULLIES
BULLINS
BULOVAS
BUMBLES
BUMLEGS
BUMMERS
BUMPERS
BUMRAPS
BUNCHES
BUNDLES
BUNGEES
BUNGLES
BUNIONS
BUNKERS
BUNKUMS
BUNNIES
BUNTERS
BUQSHAS
BURBLES
BURBOTS
BURDENS
BUREAUS
BURGEES
BURGERS
BURGESS
BURGLES
BURGOOS
BURIALS
BURIERS
BURLAPS
BURLERS
BURMANS
BURNERS
BUROAKS
BURROWS
BURSARS
BUSBIES
BUSBOYS
BUSHELS
BUSHERS
BUSKERS
BUSMANS
BUSPASS
BUSSERS
BUSTERS
BUSTLES
BUSTUPS
BUTANES
BUTCHES
BUTENES
BUTLERS
BUTTERS
BUTTONS
BUYOFFS
BUYOUTS
BUZZERS
CUATROS
CUBAGES
CUBBIES
CUBBINS
CUBFANS
CUBISTS
CUBITUS
CUBOIDS
CUCKOOS
CUDDIES
CUDDLES
CUDGELS
CUEBIDS
CUESTAS
CUETIPS
CUIRASS
CULCHES
CULEXES
CULLERS
CULLETS
CULLIES
CUMBERS
CUMBIAS
CUMULUS
CUPFULS
CUPOLAS
CUPROUS
CUPULES
CURARES
CURATES
CURDLES
CURFEWS
CURIOUS
CURLERS
CURLEWS
CURRIES
CURSERS
CURSORS
CURTISS
CURVETS
CUSHAWS
CUSPIDS
CUSSERS
CUSTERS
CUSTOMS
CUTISES
CUTLASS
CUTLERS
CUTLETS
CUTOFFS
CUTOUTS
CUTTERS
DUBBERS
DUBIOUS
DUCHESS
DUCHIES
DUCKERS
DUCKIES
DUELERS
DUENNAS
DUETTOS
DUFFELS
DUFFERS
DUFFLES
DUFUSES
DUGONGS
DUGOUTS
DUKAKIS
DUMDUMS
DUMMIES
DUMPERS
DUNKERS
DUNLINS
DUNLOPS
DUNNERS
DUSTERS
DUSTUPS
DUTEOUS
EUBANKS
EUCHRES
EULABUS
EUONYMS
EUREKAS
FUDDIES
FUDDLES
FUDGERS
FUELERS
FUENTES
FUGATOS
FULFILS
FULMARS
FULNESS
FUMBLES
FUNDERS
FUNFURS
FUNGOES
FUNNELS
FUNNIES
FUNRUNS
FURIOUS
FURLERS
FURLESS
FURNESS
FURORES
FURROWS
FUSIONS
FUSSERS
FUSUMAS
FUTURAS
FUTURES
GUESSES
GUFFAWS
GUIDERS
GUINEAS
GUITARS
GULCHES
GULDENS
GULLAHS
GULLETS
GULLIES
GULPERS
GUMLESS
GUNDOGS
GUNITES
GUNLAPS
GUNLAWS
GUNLESS
GUNNERS
GUNNIES
GUNSELS
GUPPIES
GURGLES
GURKHAS
GURNEYS
GUSHERS
GUSSETS
GUSSIES
GUSTOES
GUTLESS
GUTTERS
GUVNORS
GUZZLES
HUBBIES
HUBBUBS
HUBCAPS
HUDDLES
HUELESS
HUGGERS
HUGGIES
HUGGINS
HULLERS
HUMBLES
HUMBUGS
HUMERUS
HUMMELS
HUMMERS
HUMOURS
HUMUSES
HUMVEES
HUNCHES
HUNGERS
HUNKERS
HUNNYBS
HUNTERS
HUPPAHS
HURDLES
HURLERS
HURRAHS
HURRAYS
HURRIES
HURTERS
HURTLES
HUSKERS
HUSKIES
HUSSARS
HUSSIES
HUSTLES
HUTCHES
HUYGENS
HUZZAHS
JUDASES
JUDEANS
JUDGERS
JUDOKAS
JUGFULS
JUGGLES
JUICERS
JUJUBES
JUMADAS
JUMBLES
JUMPERS
JUNCOES
JUNGLES
JUNIORS
JUNKERS
JUNKETS
JUNKIES
JURGENS
JURISTS
KUCHENS
KUMMELS
KURILES
KUZNETS
LUBBERS
LUCITES
LUGGERS
LUGNUTS
LULLERS
LUMBARS
LUMBERS
LUMINAS
LUMPERS
LUNATES
LUNCHES
LUNGERS
LUNKERS
LUPINES
LURCHES
LUREXES
LURKERS
LUSTERS
LUSTRES
LUTISTS
LUXATES
MUCKERS
MUDCATS
MUDDERS
MUDDIES
MUDDLES
MUDEELS
MUDHENS
MUDPIES
MUESLIS
MUFFINS
MUFFLES
MUGFULS
MUGGERS
MUGGLES
MUJERES
MUKLUKS
MULCHES
MULETAS
MULLAHS
MULLERS
MULLETS
MULLINS
MUMBLES
MUMMERS
MUMMIES
MUNCHES
MUPPETS
MURANOS
MURDERS
MURIELS
MURMURS
MURPHYS
MUSCATS
MUSCLES
MUSEUMS
MUSHERS
MUSICKS
MUSINGS
MUSKETS
MUSKIES
MUSLIMS
MUSLINS
MUSSELS
MUSTDOS
MUSTERS
MUTANTS
MUTATES
MUTTERS
MUTTONS
MUTUALS
MUUMUUS
MUZZLES
NUANCES
NUBBERS
NUBBINS
NUBBLES
NUBIANS
NUBIRAS
NUCLEUS
NUDGERS
NUDISTS
NUDNIKS
NUDZHES
NUGGETS
NUMBATS
NUMBERS
NUMEROS
NUNCIOS
NURSERS
NUTATES
NUTLETS
NUTMEGS
NUTOILS
NUTRIAS
NUTTERS
NUZZLES
OUSTERS
OUTACTS
OUTADDS
OUTAGES
OUTASKS
OUTAWES
OUTBANS
OUTBATS
OUTBEGS
OUTBIDS
OUTBOWS
OUTBUDS
OUTBUYS
OUTCUTS
OUTDOES
OUTEATS
OUTFITS
OUTGOES
OUTGUNS
OUTHISS
OUTHITS
OUTINGS
OUTJETS
OUTJUTS
OUTKISS
OUTLAWS
OUTLAYS
OUTLETS
OUTLIES
OUTLIPS
OUTMANS
OUTPASS
OUTPAYS
OUTPOPS
OUTPUTS
OUTRAPS
OUTRIBS
OUTRIGS
OUTROWS
OUTRUNS
OUTSAYS
OUTSEES
OUTSETS
OUTSINS
OUTSITS
OUTSUMS
OUTVIES
OUTWARS
OUTWITS
PUBLICS
PUBLIUS
PUCKERS
PUDDLES
PUEBLOS
PUFFERS
PUFFINS
PUGGLES
PULLERS
PULLETS
PULLEYS
PULLINS
PULLONS
PULLUPS
PULPERS
PULPITS
PULSARS
PUMICES
PUMMELS
PUMPERS
PUNCHES
PUNDITS
PUNKERS
PUNKIES
PUNLESS
PUNNERS
PUNTERS
PUPATES
PUPPETS
PUPPIES
PURFLES
PURISTS
PURPLES
PURRERS
PURSERS
PURSUES
PURVEYS
PUSHERS
PUSHUPS
PUSSIES
PUTOFFS
PUTOUTS
PUTPUTS
PUTTEES
PUTTERS
PUTTIES
PUZZLES
QUAGGAS
QUAHOGS
QUAKERS
QUAKIES
QUAPAWS
QUARLES
QUARTES
QUARTOS
QUASARS
QUASHES
QUATRES
QUAVERS
QUEIROS
QUERIES
QUEUERS
QUICHES
QUIETUS
QUINCES
QUINTAS
QUINTES
QUINTUS
QUINZES
QUIVERS
QUIZNOS
QUIZZES
QUORUMS
QUOTEES
QUOTERS
RUANDAS
RUBATOS
RUBBERS
RUBBLES
RUBIOUS
RUBRICS
RUDDERS
RUFFLES
RUGGLES
RUGRATS
RUINERS
RUINOUS
RULINGS
RUMAKIS
RUMBLES
RUMLESS
RUMMERS
RUMMIES
RUMOURS
RUMPLES
RUNDLES
RUNLAPS
RUNLESS
RUNLETS
RUNNELS
RUNNERS
RUNOFFS
RUNOUTS
RUNWAYS
RUPIAHS
RUSHEES
RUSHERS
RUSSETS
RUSTICS
RUSTLES
RUTGERS
RUTILES
RUTTERS
RUYBLAS
SUBARUS
SUBBASS
SUBBIAS
SUBDEBS
SUBDUES
SUBGODS
SUBLETS
SUBLIDS
SUBLOTS
SUBMITS
SUBNETS
SUBORNS
SUBSETS
SUBURBS
SUBWARS
SUBWAYS
SUCCESS
SUCCORS
SUCKERS
SUDOKUS
SUDSERS
SUFFERS
SUITORS
SULKERS
SULKIES
SULLIES
SULTANS
SUMLESS
SUMMERS
SUMMITS
SUMMONS
SUNBOWS
SUNDAES
SUNDAYS
SUNDERS
SUNDOGS
SUNFANS
SUNGODS
SUNHATS
SUNLESS
SUNRAYS
SUNSETS
SUNTANS
SUPERGS
SUPPERS
SUPPLES
SURFERS
SURIMIS
SURPASS
SURPLUS
SURREYS
SURVEYS
SUTURES
SUZUKIS
TUBFULS
TUBISTS
TUBULES
TUCKERS
TUCSONS
TUFFETS
TUGGERS
TUGLESS
TUGRIKS
TUILLES
TULSANS
TUMBLES
TUMMIES
TUMULTS
TUNDRAS
TUNEUPS
TUNNELS
TUPELOS
TURBANS
TURBOTS
TUREENS
TURKEYS
TURNERS
TURNIPS
TURNONS
TURNUPS
TURRETS
TURTLES
TUSCANS
TUSHIES
TUSKERS
TUSSLES
TUTTUTS
TUXEDOS
VULCANS
YUKATAS
YUKOLIS
YUPPIES
ZUNIANS

••US•••

ABUSERS
ABUSING
ABUSIVE
AMUSEME
AMUSERS
AMUSING
ARUSPEX
ASUSUAL
AZUSACA
BLUSHED
BLUSHER
BLUSHES
BLUSHON
BLUSTER
BOUSONO
BRUSHED
BRUSHER
BRUSHES
BRUSHUP
BRUSQUE
CAUSERS
CAUSING
CAUSTIC
CLUSTER
COUSINE
COUSINS
CRUSADE
CRUSHED
CRUSHER
CRUSHES

CRUSTAL
CRUSTED
DAUSSET
DOUSERS
DOUSING
ELUSIVE
ELUSORY
FAUSTUS
FLUSHED
FLUSHER
FLUSHES
FLUSHOT
FLUSTER
FRUSTRO
FRUSTUM
GAUSSES
HOUSING
HOUSMAN
HOUSSAY
HOUSTON
IMUSTGO
JOUSTED
JOUSTER
LOUSEUP
LOUSIER
LOUSILY
LOUSING
MAUSERS
MOUSERS
MOUSIER
MOUSILY
MOUSING
MOUSSED
MOUSSES
NAUSEAM
OPUSONE
OPUSTWO
PAUSERS
PAUSING
PCUSERS
PIUSIII
PIUSVII
PIUSXII
PLUSHER
PLUSHES
PLUSHLY
PLUSONE
PLUSSES
PLUSTAX
PLUSTWO
POUSSIN
PRUSSIA
REUSERS
REUSING
ROUSERS
ROUSING
ROUSTED
ROUSTER
SAUSAGE
SCUSEME
SHUSHED
SHUSHES
SHUSTER
SLUSHED
SLUSHES
SMUSHED
SMUSHES
SOUSING

THUSFAR
TOUSLED
TOUSLES
TRUSSED
TRUSSES
TRUSSUP
TRUSTED
TRUSTEE
TRUSTER
TRUSTIN
TRUSTME
UNUSUAL

••U•S••

ABUTSON
ALUNSER
AVULSED
AVULSES
BLUESKY
BLUESUN
BOURSES
BRUISED
BRUISER
BRUISES
CLUBSUP
CLUESIN
COUNSEL
COURSED
COURSER
COURSES
CRUDSUP
CRUISED
CRUISER
CRUISES
DAUSSET
DEUTSCH
DRUMSET
DRUMSUP
EVULSED
EVULSES
FOULSUP
GAUSSES
GLUESON
GLUESTO
HAULSIN
HAULSUP
HOUSSAY
IGUASSU
LOUISII
LOUISIV
LOUISIX
LOUISVI
LOUISXI
LOUISXV
MOUSSED
MOUSSES
PAULSEN
PLUGSIN
PLUGSUP
PLUSSES
POURSIN
POUSSIN
PRUSSIA
SHUTSIN
SHUTSUP
SOUPSON
SOUPSUP
SOURSON

SPURSON
SQUASHY
SQUISHY
TRUESUP
TRUISMS
TRUSSED
TRUSSES
TRUSSUP

••U••S•

ACUTEST
BLUEISH
BRUTISH
BRUXISM
CHUMASH
CHUTIST
CRUDEST
DOUREST
FAUVISM
FAUVIST
FEUDIST
FLUTIST
FOULEST
GAULISH
GLUCOSE
GLUIEST
GOULASH
GOUTISH
IGUASSU
INULASE
LOUDEST
LOUDISH
LOUTISH
NOURISH
OCULIST
PAULIST
PLUMOSE
PRUDISH
SOUBISE
SOUREST
SOURISH
TAUTEST
TOURISM
TOURIST
WOULDST
YOULOSE
YOUWISH

••U•••S

ABUSERS
ACUMENS
AGULHAS
ALUDELS
ALUMNUS
AMULETS
AMUSERS
AOUDADS
AQUEOUS
AQUINAS
ARUBANS
AVULSES
BAUBLES
BAUHAUS
BEURRES
BLUDGES
BLUINGS
BLUSHES
BOUCHES

BOUDINS
BOUFFES
BOUNCES
BOURSES
BOUTROS
BRUISES
BRUMOUS
BRUNETS
BRUSHES
CAUSERS
CHUPPAS
CHURROS
COUCHES
COUGARS
COULEES
COUPLES
COUPONS
COURSES
COUSINS
COUTERS
CRUISES
CRUSHES
CRUZANS
DAUBERS
DOUANES
DOUBLES
DOUGLAS
DOUSERS
DRUDGES
EKUELES
ELUANTS
ELUATES
ELUDERS
EMULOUS
EQUATES
EQUINES
EVULSES
FAUCETS
FAUSTUS
FAUXPAS
FLUBUGS
FLUSHES
FLUTERS
FLUTIES
FOUDRES
FOULUPS
FOURTHS
GAUCHOS
GAUDENS
GAUDIES
GAUGERS
GAUSSES
GLURGES
GLUTENS
GLUTEUS
GOUGERS
GOURDES
GRUDGES
GRUNGES
HAULERS
IGUANAS
JOUNCES
JOURNOS
KLUDGES
KLUTZES
LAUDERS
LAULAUS
LAURELS

LOUDENS
LOUNGES
LOURDES
LOUVERS
LOUVRES
MAULERS
MAUMAUS
MAUROIS
MAUSERS
MAUVAIS
MOUSERS
MOUSSES
MUUMUUS
NAUGHTS
NEURONS
NEUTERS
NOUGATS
NOUGHTS
NTUPLES
OCULARS
OEUVRES
PAUPERS
PAUSERS
PCUSERS
PLUGINS
PLUNGES
PLURALS
PLUSHES
PLUSSES
PLUTONS
POUCHES
POUDRES
POUNCES
POURERS
POUTERS
PRUNERS
RAUCOUS
REUBENS
REUNERS
REURGES
REUSERS
REUTERS
RHUMBAS
ROUSERS
ROUTERS
RYUKYUS
SAUCERS
SCULPTS
SCURVES
SCUZZES
SHUSHES
SHUTINS
SLUDGES
SLUICES
SLUSHES
SMUDGES
SMUSHES
SNUGLIS
SOUPERS
SOURCES
SQUALLS
SQUARES
SQUAWKS
SQUEAKS
SQUEALS
SQUEERS
SQUINTS
SQUIRES

SQUIRMS
SQUIRTS
STUCCOS
STUDIES
STUDIOS
STUPIDS
STUPORS
STURGES
STUTZES
TAUTENS
TEUTONS
TOUCANS
TOUCHES
TOUPEES
TOURBUS
TOURERS
TOUSLES
TOUTERS
TRUANTS
TRUDGES
TRUISMS
TRUMANS
TRUSSES
UQUARKS
USURERS
USURIES
VAUDOIS
VOUCHES
YOUMANS

•••US••

ACCUSAL
ACCUSED
ACCUSER
ACCUSES
ADJUSTS
APLUSES
ARGUSES
AROUSAL
AROUSED
AROUSER
AROUSES
AUGUSTA
AUGUSTE
AUGUSTO
AUGUSTS
BELUSHI
BEMUSED
BEMUSES
BLOUSED
BLOUSES
BLOUSON
BOGUSLY
BOLUSES
BONUSES
BPLUSES
BRYUSOV
CAYUSES
CLAUSAL
CLAUSES
CPLUSES
CYRUSII
DEBUSES
DEBUSSY
DEFUSED
DEFUSER
DEFUSES
DEGUSTS

DERUSTS
DISUSED
DISUSES
DPLUSES
DUFUSES
EFFUSED
EFFUSES
EMMUSKA
ENDUSER
ENDUSES
EXCUSAL
EXCUSAS
EXCUSED
EXCUSER
EXCUSES
EXCUSEZ
FETUSES
FICUSES
FOCUSED
FOCUSER
FOCUSES
FOCUSON
GELUSIL
GENUSES
GIBUSES
GROUSED
GROUSER
GROUSES
GUNUSER
HOCUSED
HUMUSES
ICTUSES
ILLUSED
ILLUSES
INCUSED
INCUSES
INFUSED
INFUSER
INFUSES
LARUSSA
LEXUSES
LEXUSGS
LEXUSGX
LEXUSIS
LEXUSLS
LEXUSLX
LEXUSRX
LEXUSSC
LOCUSTS
LORUSES
LOTUSES
MACUSER
MARUSJA
MEDUSAE
MEDUSAN
MEDUSAS
MINUSES
MISUSED
MISUSER
MISUSES
MOMUSES
MRMUSIC
NEGUSES
NEXUSES
NONUSER
NOTUSED
OBTUSER
PERUSAL

PERUSED
PERUSER
PERUSES
PIOUSLY
PRIUSES
REBUSES
RECUSAL
RECUSED
RECUSES
REDUSTS
REFUSAL
REFUSED
REFUSER
REFUSES
ROBUSTA
ROBUSTO
SINUSES
SPOUSAL
SPOUSES
SULUSEA
TALUSES
THEUSSR
THRUSTS
TONUSES
TROUSER
UNDUSTY
UNFUSED
UNFUSSY
UNHUSKS
UNLUSTY
VENUSES
VIRUSES
WATUSIS
ZAKUSKA

•••U•S•

ACCURST
ALQUIST
ANGUISH
BEAUISH
BEQUEST
CASUIST
DEBUSSY
DELUISE
DIVULSE
EXCURSE
IMPULSE
INQUEST
IRKUTSK
LARUSSA
LEXUSSC
REPULSE
REQUEST
ROGUISH
THEUSSR
UNBURST
UNFUSSY
UPBURST
VAGUEST
VOGUISH
YAKUTSK

•••U••S

ABDUCES
ABDUCTS
ABJURES
ABOUNDS
ACCUSES

ACQUITS
ADDUCES
ADDUCTS
ADJURES
ADJUSTS
ADZUKIS
AGOUTIS
ALLUDES
ALLURES
AMOUNTS
AMPULES
ANNUALS
ANNULUS
APLUSES
ARBUTUS
ARDUOUS
ARGUERS
ARGUSES
AROUSES
ASSUMES
ASSURES
ATTUCKS
ATTUNES
AUBURNS
AUGUSTS
AUTUMNS
BELUGAS
BEMUSES
BENUMBS
BLOUSES
BOLUSES
BONUSES
BPLUSES
BYTURNS
CANUCKS
CANULAS
CASUALS
CAYUGAS
CAYUSES
CHOUGHS
CLAUSES
COLUMNS
CONURES
COPULAS
CPLUSES
CROUTES
CUMULUS
CUPULES
DEBUNKS
DEBURRS
DEBUSES
DEDUCES
DEDUCTS
DEFUELS
DEFUNDS
DEFUSES
DEGUSTS
DEJUNKS
DELUDES
DELUGES
DENUDES
DEPULPS
DEPUTES
DERUSTS
DETUNES
DILUTES
DISUSES
DPLUSES

DUFUSES
EDMUNDS
EFFUSES
EMQUADS
ENDURES
ENDUROS
ENDUSES
ENGULFS
ENQUADS
ENSURES
ESCUDOS
EXCUSAS
EXCUSES
EXEUNTS
EXHUMES
FAMULUS
FATUOUS
FERULES
FETUSES
FIBULAS
FICUSES
FIGURES
FLAUNTS
FLAUTAS
FOCUSES
FUSUMAS
FUTURAS
FUTURES
GENUSES
GERUNDS
GIBUSES
GROUNDS
GROUSES
HAMULUS
HUMUSES
ICTUSES
ILLUDES
ILLUMES
ILLUSES
IMMUNES
IMMURES
IMPUGNS
IMPUTES
INCUBUS
INCUDES
INCUSES
INDUCES
INDUCTS
INFUSES
INGULFS
INHUMES
INJURES
INRUINS
INSULTS
INSURES
INTUITS
INTURNS
IRRUPTS
ISSUERS
IVTUBES
JAGUARS
JESUITS
JUJUBES
KABUKIS
KAHUNAS
KAKUROS
KIDULTS
KIKUYUS

KORUNAS
LACUNAS
LAGUNAS
LEGUMES
LEXUSES
LEXUSGS
LEXUSIS
LEXUSLS
LIQUIDS
LIQUORS
LOBULES
LOCULUS
LOCUSTS
LOQUATS
LORUSES
LOTUSES
MADUROS
MANUALS
MANURES
MATURES
MEDUSAS
MENUDOS
MEZUZAS
MINUETS
MINUSES
MINUTES
MISUSES
MIZUNAS
MODULES
MODULUS
MOMUSES
MRBURNS
MRBUTTS
MUTUALS
NATURES
NEBULAS
NEGUSES
NEXUSES
NOCUOUS
NODULES
NONUKES
NOTURNS
OAHUANS
OBTUNDS
OCCULTS
OPPUGNS
OSCULES
OSMUNDS
PADUANS
PAIUTES
PAPUANS
PARURES
PENULTS
PEQUOTS
PERUKES
PERUSES
PLAUTUS
PLOUGHS
PNEUMAS
PRIUSES
QUEUERS
RASURES
REBUFFS
REBUKES
REBUSES
RECURES
RECURLS
RECUSES

REDUCES
REDUSTS
REFUELS
REFUGES
REFUNDS
REFUSES
REFUTES
REGULUS
RELUCTS
RELUMES
REPUGNS
REPUMPS
REPUTES
RESUITS
RESULTS
RESUMES
RETUNES
RETURFS
RETURNS
RITUALS
ROMULUS
SALUKIS
SALUTES
SATURNS
SCOUPES
SCRUFFS
SCRUGGS
SECURES
SEDUCES
SEQUELS
SEQUINS
SINUOUS
SINUSES
SIOUANS
SLEUTHS
SLOUGHS
SOLUTES
SPOUSES
SPRUCES
STLUKES
SUBURBS
SUTURES
SUZUKIS
TALUSES
TEAURNS
TENUOUS
TENURES
THRUSTS
TONUSES
TRAUMAS
TROUGHS
TROUPES
TSOURIS
TUBULES
TUMULTS
UNCUFFS
UNCURBS
UNCURLS
UNFURLS
UNHULLS
UNHUSKS
UNTUCKS
UNTUNES
UPCURLS
UPTURNS
VACUOUS
VACUUMS
VALUERS

VELURES
VENULES
VENUSES
VICUNAS
VIRUSES
VISUALS
VOGUERS
VOLUMES
VOLUTES
WATUSIS
YOGURTS
ZONULES

••••US•

BECAUSE
BOGGUSS
BULRUSH
BUMRUSH
CAROUSE
CIRCUSY
COMBUST
CONCUSS
CONFUSE
CONTUSE
DARIUSI
DEGAUSS
DELOUSE
DIFFUSE
DISCUSS
DISEUSE
DISGUST
DONRUSS
DRSEUSS
ENCRUST
ENTHUSE
ENTRUST
ESPOUSE
EXHAUST
FAIRUSE
FATOUSH
FORBUSH
GETBUSY
GOODUSE
GOTBUSY
INARUSH
INCRUST
INHOUSE
INTRUST
IREFUSE
JACCUSE
JEBBUSH
LETSUSE
LUCIUSI
MADRUSH
MANCUSO
MARCUSE
MISSUSA
MOLLUSC
MOLLUSK
NONBUSY
OFNOUSE
OUTGUSH
OUTPUSH
OUTRUSH
OVERUSE
PERCUSS
PERFUSE
POSEUSE

PREDUSK
PROFUSE
REBRUSH
RECLUSE
REDDUST
REHOUSE
SAWDUST
STPIUSI
STPIUSV
STPIUSX
STRAUSS
STROUSE
SUFFUSE
TEAMUSA
THEBUSH
UNHOUSE
UNTRUSS
UPROUSE
VBLOUSE
VISCUSO
XYSTUSI

••••U•S

ACCRUES
ADNOUNS
AIRGUNS
ALARUMS
ALLIUMS
ARBOURS
ARDOURS
ARMFULS
ARMOURS
ARTHURS
ASYLUMS
ATRIUMS
AUTEURS
AVENUES
BACKUPS
BADGUYS
BAGFULS
BANQUES
BARNUMS
BARQUES
BASQUES
BAYRUMS
BEDAUBS
BEDBUGS
BEFOULS
BIGGUNS
BIGHUGS
BISQUES
BLOWUPS
BOGGUSS
BOXFULS
BROGUES
BUGOUTS
BULGURS
BUNKUMS
BUSTUPS
BUYOUTS
CALLUPS
CANFULS
CAPFULS
CAPGUNS
CAPNUTS
CARFULS
CASQUES
CATGUTS
CATSUPS
CHEQUES
CHERUBS
CHINUPS
CINQUES
CIRQUES
CLAQUES
CLIQUES
COBNUTS
COLOURS
CONCURS
CONCUSS
CONSULS
COPOUTS
CROQUIS
CUPFULS
CUTOUTS
DATSUNS
DEBLURS
DEGAUSS
DEMBUMS
DESLUMS
DETOURS
DEVOURS
DIALUPS
DICTUMS
DIDSUMS
DIECUTS
DIMOUTS
DISBUDS
DISCUSS
DISEURS
DOGRUNS
DOLOURS
DONRUSS
DROGUES
DRSEUSS
DRYRUNS
DUGOUTS
DUMDUMS
DUSTUPS
DYBBUKS
EARBUDS
EARFULS
EGGCUPS
EMBRUES
ENDCUTS
ENDRUNS
ENGLUTS
ENSOULS
EPOQUES
EYECUPS
EYEFULS
FANOUTS
FAVOURS
FESCUES
FILLUPS
FLIPUPS
FLUBUGS
FOLDUPS
FONDUES
FOULUPS
FUNFURS
FUNRUNS
GIBLUES
GIVEUPS
GOOFUPS
GYPSUMS
HANGUPS
HATFULS
HEXNUTS
HICCUPS
HOGNUTS
HOLDUPS
HONOURS
HOOKUPS
HOTCUPS
HOTTUBS
HUBBUBS
HUMBUGS
HUMOURS
ICEOUTS
ICERUNS
IMBRUES
IMYOURS
INPOURS
IONIUMS
JACQUES
JARFULS
JETGUNS
JOBCUTS
JUGFULS
KICKUPS
LABOURS
LACEUPS
LAPFULS
LARRUPS
LASHUPS
LAYOUTS
LEADUPS
LEAGUES
LENGUAS
LINEUPS
LINKUPS
LOCKUPS
LOGOUTS
LONGUES
LOOKUPS
LUGNUTS
LYCEUMS
MACOUNS
MAGNUMS
MAHOUTS
MAKEUPS
MARAUDS
MARKUPS
MARQUES
MARQUIS
MASQUES
MEDIUMS
MESSUPS
MISCUES
MISCUTS
MOCKUPS
MORGUES
MOSQUES
MSIEURS
MUGFULS
MUKLUKS
MURMURS
MUSEUMS
MUUMUUS
NETFULS
OILCUPS
OILRUBS
OPAQUES
OUTBUDS
OUTBUYS
OUTCUTS
OUTGUNS
OUTJUTS
OUTPUTS
OUTRUNS
OUTSUMS
PABLUMS
PANFULS
PARFUMS
PAYCUTS
PAYOUTS
PEANUTS
PEPLUMS
PERCUSS
PETPUPS
PICKUPS
PIGNUTS
PIGOUTS
PILEUPS
PLAGUES
PLAQUES
PLENUMS
PODIUMS
POPGUNS
POPOUTS
POSEURS
POSSUMS
POTFULS
PREBUYS
PRECUTS
PRENUPS
PREVUES
PULLUPS
PURSUES
PUSHUPS
PUTOUTS
PUTPUTS
QUORUMS
RAGOUTS
RAGRUGS
RAVEUPS
RAYGUNS
RECOUPS
REDBUDS
REDOUTS
REDSUNS
REGLUES
REHAULS
REPOURS
RESCUES
RESHUTS
RETOURS
RIBCUTS
RIGOURS
ROLLUPS
ROTGUTS
RUMOURS
RUNOUTS
RVALUES
SACQUES
SAVOURS
SCHLUBS
SENDUPS
SETOUTS
SHOGUNS
SHROUDS
SIDDURS
SIGNUPS
SIXGUNS
SKIBUMS
SKIRUNS
SLIPUPS
SLOWUPS
SPROUTS
STATUES
STEPUPS
STLOUIS
STPAULS
STRAUSS
SUBDUES
TAGOUTS
TALCUMS
TAXCUTS
TEACUPS
TEDEUMS
TEDIUMS
THECUBS
THESUNS
TISSUES
TONGUES
TOPGUNS
TORQUES
TOSSUPS
TOYGUNS
TRYOUTS
TUBFULS
TUNEUPS
TURNUPS
TUTTUTS
UMLAUTS
UNGLUES
UNIQUES
UNPLUGS
UNTRUSS
URNFULS
UVALUES
VACUUMS
VALOURS
VAPOURS
VATFULS
VELLUMS
VELOURS
VENDUES
VIGOURS
VIRTUES
WAKEUPS
WALKUPS
WALNUTS
WAMPUMS
WARMUPS
WASHUPS
WINDUPS
WORKUPS
WRAPUPS
YANQUIS
ZAGNUTS
ZIPGUNS

•••••US

ALARBUS
ALLOFUS
ALUMNUS
AMADEUS
AMOROUS
ANDROUS
ANGELUS
ANNULUS
ANTERUS
ANXIOUS
APERCUS
APODOUS
AQUEOUS
ARBUTUS
ARDUOUS
ARTEMUS
ATTICUS
AUTOBUS
AVERNUS
BACCHUS
BARACUS
BAUHAUS
BELARUS
BERGIUS
BILIOUS
BRUMOUS
BULBOUS
BUREAUS
CALLOUS
CANOPUS
CARIOUS
CARPOUS
CASEOUS
CASSIUS
CELSIUS
CEPHEUS
CITROUS
CNOSSUS
COLONUS
CONGOUS
COPIOUS
CRASSUS
CRISPUS
CROESUS
CUBITUS
CUMULUS
CUPROUS
CURIOUS
DAMASUS
DATABUS
DEDALUS
DEFOCUS
DEVIOUS
DOMINUS
DONATUS
DONIMUS
DREYFUS
DUBIOUS
DUTEOUS
ELIGIUS
EMULOUS
ENVIOUS
EPHEBUS
EPHESUS
ERASMUS
ERASTUS
ERECTUS
ESCALUS
EULABUS
FAMULUS
FATUOUS
FAUSTUS
FERROUS
FIBROUS
FLAVIUS
FORTIUS
FURIOUS
GASEOUS
GIBBOUS
GLOBOUS
GLUTEUS
GNOSSUS
GOBYBUS
GORDIUS
GRAMPUS
GROPIUS
GROTIUS
HAMULUS
HEINOUS
HIDEOUS
HUMERUS
HYDROUS
HYGINUS
IAPETUS
ICTERUS
ICTINUS
IGNEOUS
IMPETUS
IMPIOUS
INCUBUS
INFOCUS
ISTHMUS
JEALOUS
KIDSRUS
KIKUYUS
LANDAUS
LATINUS
LAULAUS
LAZARUS
LEPIDUS
LOCULUS
MALLEUS
MALTHUS
MARHAUS
MARTIUS
MAUMAUS
MAXIMUS
MENCIUS
MILHOUS
MILIEUS
MINIBUS
MINIMUS
MODULUS
MUUMUUS
NENNIUS
NERVOUS
NITROUS
NIVEOUS
NOCUOUS
NONPLUS
NOXIOUS
NUCLEUS
OBVIOUS
OCEANUS
OCELLUS
OCHROUS
OCTOPUS
ODOROUS
OEDIPUS
OLYMPUS
OMINOUS
OMNIBUS
ONEOFUS
ONEROUS
ORMOLUS
ORPHEUS
OSSEOUS
OZONOUS
PAPYRUS
PARAMUS
PARATUS
PARIBUS
PARLOUS
PEGASUS
PERITUS
PERSEUS
PERSIUS
PETROUS
PHEMIUS
PHILOUS
PHOEBUS
PICEOUS
PILATUS
PILEOUS
PIRAEUS
PISTOUS
PITEOUS
PLAUTUS
POMPOUS
PONTIUS
POTAMUS
PROCLUS
PROTEUS
PTEROUS
PUBLIUS
PYRAMUS
PYRRHUS
QUIETUS
QUINTUS
RAILBUS
RAUCOUS
REFOCUS
REGULUS
RESEAUS
RHOECUS
RHOMBUS
RIOTOUS
ROMANUS
ROMULUS
RUBIOUS
RUINOUS
RYUKYUS
SANCTUS
SERIOUS
SEVERUS
SIDIOUS
SINUOUS
STRATUS
SUBARUS
SUDOKUS
SURPLUS
TACITUS
TEDIOUS
TENUOUS
TETANUS
THESEUS
TOURBUS
TOYSRUS
TROILUS
UNPIOUS
URSINUS
VACUOUS
VARIOUS
VICIOUS
VILNIUS
VISCOUS
WINDAUS
XANADUS
ZEALOUS
ZINCOUS
ZOSIMUS

UT•••••

UTAHANS
UTENSIL
UTICANS
UTICANY
UTILISE
UTILITY
UTILIZE
UTMOSTS
UTOPIAN
UTOPIAS
UTOPISM
UTOPIST
UTRECHT
UTRILLO
UTTERED
UTTERER
UTTERLY

U•T••••

ULTIMAS
UNTACKS
UNTAKEN
UNTAMED
UNTAMES
UNTAPED
UNTAPES
UNTASTY
UNTAXED
UNTAXES
UNTEACH
UNTENSE
UNTERSE
UNTHAWS
UNTHICK
UNTHINK
UNTIERS
UNTILED
UNTIMED
UNTIMID
UNTIRED
UNTONED
UNTOUGH
UNTOXIC
UNTRACK
UNTRAPS
UNTREAD
UNTREED
UNTRIED
UNTRITE
UNTRUER
UNTRULY
UNTRUSS
UNTRUTH
UNTUCKS
UNTUNED
UNTUNES
UNTWINE
UNTWIST
UNTYING
UNTYPED
UPTAKES
UPTALKS
UPTEARS
UPTEMPO
UPTHERE
UPTHROW
UPTICKS
UPTIGHT
UPTILTS
UPTIMES
UPTONOW
UPTOPAR
UPTOWNS
UPTRADE
UPTREND
UPTURNS
URTEXTS
USTEDES
USTINOV
UTTERED
UTTERER
UTTERLY

U••T•••

ULSTERS
UMPTEEN
UNCTION
UNITARD
UNITARY
UNITERS
UNITIES
UNITING
UNITISE
UNITIVE
UNITIZE
UNSTACK
UNSTAGY
UNSTAID
UNSTATE
UNSTEEL
UNSTEPS
UNSTERN
UNSTICK
UNSTIFF
UNSTOIC
UNSTONY
UNSTOPS
UNSTOUT
UNSTOWS
UNSTRAP
UNSTUCK
UNSTUNG
UPATREE
UPSTAGE
UPSTAIR
UPSTAND
UPSTARE
UPSTART
UPSTATE
UPSTEPS
UPSTIRS
UPSTOOD
USOTOUR
USSTATE
USSTEEL

U•••T••

UNACTED
UNAPTLY
UNBATED
UNCITED
UNDATED
UNEATEN
UNFATED
UNFATTY
UNFETED
UNFITLY
UNGATED
UNHATED
UNHITCH
UNIATES
UNLATCH
UNMATED
UNMATES
UNMITER
UNMITRE
UNMUTED
UNNOTED
UNOFTEN
UNOPTED
UNRATED
UNSATED
UNVITAL
UNVOTED
UNWITTY
UPDATED
UPDATER
UPDATES
UPRATED
UPRATES

U••••T•

ULULATE
UMBERTO
UMLAUTS
UNBAITS
UNBELTS
UNBERTH
UNBOLTS
UNCOUTH
UNCRATE
UNDUSTY
UNEARTH
UNEMPTY
UNFACTS
UNFAITH
UNFATTY
UNFERTH
UNHASTY
UNKNITS
UNKNOTS
UNLOATH
UNLOFTY
UNLUSTY
UNMASTS
UNPASTE
UNPIETY
UNQUOTE
UNRESTS
UNROOTS
UNSALTY
UNSEATS
UNSOOTY
UNSORTS
UNSTATE
UNTASTY
UNTRITE
UNTRUTH
UNWHITE
UNWITTY
UPBEATS
UPCASTS
UPDARTS
UPLIFTS
UPNORTH
UPROOTS
UPSHOTS
UPSTATE
UPTILTS
UPWAFTS
URANITE
URTEXTS
USSTATE
UTILITY
UTMOSTS

U•••••T

UGLIEST
ULULANT
UNADEPT
UNADULT
UNALERT
UNBESET
UNBLENT
UNBLEST
UNBUILT
UNBURNT
UNBURST
UNCLEFT
UNCLIPT
UNDEALT
UNERECT
UNFROST
UNGUENT
UNINERT
UNJOINT
UNKEMPT
UNLIGHT
UNMEANT
UNMOIST
UNOVERT
UNPLAIT
UNQUIET
UNSHIFT
UNSHORT
UNSIGHT
UNSMART
UNSPELT
UNSPENT
UNSPILT
UNSPLIT
UNSTOUT
UNSWEET
UNSWEPT
UNTWIST
UNWHIPT
UPBURST
UPCOAST
UPCOURT
UPDRAFT
UPDRIFT
UPFIRST
UPFORIT
UPFRONT
UPLEAPT
UPLIGHT
UPOROUT
UPRIGHT
UPSHIFT
UPSHOOT
UPSTART
UPSWEPT
UPTIGHT
USGRANT
UTOPIST
UTRECHT

•UT••••

AUTARCH
AUTARKY
AUTEURS
AUTHORS
AUTISTS
AUTOBIO
AUTOBUS
AUTOING
AUTOMAT
AUTOMNE
AUTONYM
AUTOPEN
AUTOPIA
AUTOPSY
AUTUMNS
BUTANES
BUTCHER
BUTCHES
BUTENES
BUTGOOD
BUTLERS
BUTTEMT
BUTTERS
BUTTERY
BUTTING
BUTTONS
BUTTONY
BUTTOUT
BUTTRAM
BUTTSIN
CUTARUG
CUTAWAY
CUTBACK
CUTDOWN
CUTICLE
CUTINON
CUTINTO
CUTISES
CUTLASS
CUTLERS
CUTLERY
CUTLETS
CUTOFFS
CUTOPEN
CUTOUTS
CUTOVER
CUTRATE
CUTSOFF

CUTSOUT
CUTTERS
CUTTIME
CUTTING
CUTWORK
CUTWORM
DUTEOUS
DUTIFUL
EUTERPE
FUTHARK
FUTURAS
FUTURES
FUTZING
GUTHRIE
GUTLESS
GUTSIER
GUTSILY
GUTTERS
GUTTIER
GUTTING
HUTCHES
HUTLIKE
HUTTING
JUTLAND
JUTTING
KUTCHER
KUTUZOV
LUTETIA
LUTHIER
LUTHULI
LUTISTS
MUTABLE
MUTABLY
MUTAGEN
MUTANTS
MUTATED
MUTATES
MUTEDLY
MUTTERS
MUTTONS
MUTUALS
NUTATED
NUTATES
NUTLETS
NUTLIKE
NUTMEAT
NUTMEGS
NUTOILS
NUTPINE
NUTRIAS
NUTSIER
NUTTERS
NUTTIER
NUTTILY
NUTTING
NUTTREE
NUTWOOD
OUTACTS
OUTADDS
OUTAGES
OUTASKS
OUTAWED
OUTAWES
OUTBACK
OUTBAKE
OUTBANS
OUTBARK
OUTBATS
OUTBAWL
OUTBEAM
OUTBEGS
OUTBEND
OUTBIDS
OUTBLOT
OUTBLOW
OUTBOWL
OUTBOWS
OUTBRAG
OUTBRAY
OUTBRED
OUTBUDS
OUTBULK
OUTBURN
OUTBUYS
OUTBUZZ
OUTCALL
OUTCANT
OUTCAST
OUTCITY
OUTCOLD
OUTCOME
OUTCOOK
OUTCROP
OUTCROW
OUTCULL
OUTCURE
OUTCUTS
OUTDARE
OUTDATE
OUTDOER
OUTDOES
OUTDONE
OUTDOOR
OUTDRAG
OUTDRAW
OUTDREW
OUTDROP
OUTDUEL
OUTEARN
OUTEATS
OUTECHO
OUTEDGE
OUTFACE
OUTFAST
OUTFAWN
OUTFEED
OUTFEEL
OUTFIND
OUTFIRE
OUTFISH
OUTFITS
OUTFLEE
OUTFLOW
OUTFLUX
OUTFOOL
OUTFOOT
OUTGAIN
OUTGAME
OUTGAVE
OUTGAZE
OUTGIVE
OUTGLOW
OUTGNAW
OUTGOES
OUTGREW
OUTGRIN
OUTGROW
OUTGUNS
OUTGUSH
OUTHAUL
OUTHEAR
OUTHERE
OUTHIRE
OUTHISS
OUTHITS
OUTHOWL
OUTHUNT
OUTHURL
OUTINGS
OUTJEST
OUTJETS
OUTJINX
OUTJUMP
OUTJUTS
OUTKAST
OUTKEEP
OUTKEPT
OUTKICK
OUTKILL
OUTKING
OUTKISS
OUTLAID
OUTLAIN
OUTLAND
OUTLASH
OUTLAST
OUTLAWS
OUTLAYS
OUTLEAD
OUTLEAP
OUTLETS
OUTLIER
OUTLIES
OUTLIMN
OUTLINE
OUTLIPS
OUTLIVE
OUTLOOK
OUTLOUD
OUTLOVE
OUTMANS
OUTMATE
OUTMODE
OUTMOST
OUTMOVE
OUTOFIT
OUTPACE
OUTPAID
OUTPASS
OUTPATH
OUTPAYS
OUTPEEP
OUTPICK
OUTPIPE
OUTPITY
OUTPLAN
OUTPLAY
OUTPLOD
OUTPLOT
OUTPOLL
OUTPOPS
OUTPORT
OUTPOST
OUTPOUR
OUTPRAY
OUTPULL
OUTPURL
OUTPUSH
OUTPUTS
OUTRACE
OUTRAGE
OUTRAIL
OUTRANG
OUTRANK
OUTRANT
OUTRAPS
OUTRATE
OUTRAVE
OUTREAD
OUTRIBS
OUTRIDE
OUTRIGS
OUTRING
OUTROAR
OUTROCK
OUTRODE
OUTROLL
OUTROOT
OUTROVE
OUTROWS
OUTRUNS
OUTRUSH
OUTSAID
OUTSAIL
OUTSANG
OUTSAYS
OUTSEEK
OUTSEEN
OUTSEES
OUTSELL
OUTSERT
OUTSETS
OUTSHOT
OUTSHOW
OUTSIDE
OUTSIFT
OUTSIGH
OUTSING
OUTSINS
OUTSITS
OUTSIZE
OUTSKIP
OUTSOAR
OUTSOLD
OUTSOLE
OUTSPED
OUTSPIN
OUTSPIT
OUTSTAY
OUTSTEP
OUTSULK
OUTSUMS
OUTSUNG
OUTSWAM
OUTSWIM
OUTSWUM
OUTTAKE
OUTTALK
OUTTEAR
OUTTELL
OUTTIRE
OUTTOLD
OUTTOLL
OUTTORE
OUTTORN
OUTTRAY
OUTTROT
OUTTURN
OUTVIED
OUTVIES
OUTVOTE
OUTWAIT
OUTWALK
OUTWARD
OUTWARS
OUTWASH
OUTWAVE
OUTWEAR
OUTWEED
OUTWEEP
OUTWELL
OUTWENT
OUTWEPT
OUTWEST
OUTWILE
OUTWILL
OUTWIND
OUTWING
OUTWISH
OUTWITH
OUTWITS
OUTWORD
OUTWORE
OUTWORK
OUTWORN
OUTYELL
OUTYELP
PUTAWAY
PUTBACK
PUTDOWN
PUTEMUP
PUTITTO
PUTOFFS
PUTOUTS
PUTOVER
PUTPUTS
PUTREFY
PUTSOFF
PUTSOUT
PUTTEES
PUTTERS
PUTTIED
PUTTIES
PUTTING
PUTTOUT
PUTUPON
PUTUPTO
RUTALEE
RUTGERS
RUTHANN
RUTHFUL
RUTILES
RUTLAND
RUTTERS
RUTTIER
RUTTING
RUTTISH
SUTURED
SUTURES
TUTELAR
TUTORED
TUTTING
TUTTUTS
TUTUILA

•U•T•••

AUCTION
AUNTBEE
AUNTIES
AUSTERE
AUSTERS
AUSTINS
AUSTRAL
AUSTRIA
BUDTIME
BUITONI
BUNTERS
BUNTING
BUSTARD
BUSTERS
BUSTIER
BUSTING
BUSTLED
BUSTLER
BUSTLES
BUSTOUR
BUSTOUT
BUSTRIP
BUSTSIN
BUSTSUP
BUSTUPS
BUTTEMT
BUTTERS
BUTTERY
BUTTING
BUTTONS
BUTTONY
BUTTOUT
BUTTRAM
BUTTSIN
BUYTIME
CUATROS
CUETIPS
CULTISH
CULTISM
CULTIST
CULTJAM
CULTURE
CURTAIL
CURTAIN
CURTATE
CURTEST
CURTISS
CURTSEY
CUSTARD
CUSTERS
CUSTODY
CUSTOMS
CUTTERS
CUTTIME
CUTTING
DUCTILE
DUCTING
DUETING
DUETTED
DUETTOS
DUOTONE
DUSTBIN
DUSTERS
DUSTGUN
DUSTIER
DUSTILY
DUSTING
DUSTMAN
DUSTMEN
DUSTMOP
DUSTOFF
DUSTPAN
DUSTRAG
DUSTUPS
EUSTACE
FUNTIME
FURTADO
FURTHER
FURTIVE
FUSTIAN
FUSTIER
FUSTILY
GUITARS
GUMTREE
GUNTHER
GUSTAVE
GUSTIER
GUSTILY
GUSTING
GUSTOES
GUTTERS
GUTTIER
GUTTING
HUNTERS
HUNTFOR
HUNTING
HUNTLEY
HUNTSUP
HURTERS
HURTFOR
HURTFUL
HURTING
HURTLED
HURTLES
HUSTLED
HUSTLER
HUSTLES
HUTTING
JUSTEST
JUSTICE
JUSTIFY
JUSTINE
JUSTNOW
JUSTONE
JUSTOUT
JUTTING
LUSTERS
LUSTFUL
LUSTIER
LUSTILY
LUSTING
LUSTRAL
LUSTRED
LUSTRES
LUSTRUM
MUSTAFA
MUSTANG
MUSTARD
MUSTDOS
MUSTERS
MUSTIER
MUSTILY
MUSTSEE
MUTTERS
MUTTONS
NUPTIAL
NURTURE
NUTTERS
NUTTIER
NUTTILY
NUTTING
NUTTREE
OURTOWN
OUSTERS
OUSTING
OUTTAKE
OUTTALK
OUTTEAR
OUTTELL
OUTTIRE
OUTTOLD
OUTTOLL
OUTTORE
OUTTORN
OUTTRAY
OUTTROT
OUTTURN
PUNTERS
PUNTING
PUPTENT
PURTIER
PUTTEES
PUTTERS
PUTTIED
PUTTIES
PUTTING
PUTTOUT
QUATRES
QUATTRO
QUETZAL
QUITESO
QUITSIT
QUITTED
QUITTER
QUOTEES
QUOTERS
QUOTING
RUCTION
RUNTIER
RUNTIME
RUNTISH
RUPTURE
RUSTICS
RUSTIER
RUSTILY
RUSTING
RUSTLED
RUSTLER
RUSTLES
RUTTERS
RUTTIER
RUTTING
RUTTISH
SUBTASK
SUBTEEN
SUBTEND
SUBTEXT
SUBTLER
SUBTONE
SUBTYPE
SUCTION
SUITING
SUITORS
SUITSME
SUITSUP
SULTANA
SULTANS
SUNTANS
SUSTAIN
TUFTIER
TUFTING
TUITION
TURTLED
TURTLES
TUTTING
TUTTUTS
VUITTON
VULTURE

•U••T••

AUDITED
AUDITEE
AUDITOR
AUGITES
AULETTA
BUGATTI
BUILTIN
BUILTON
BUILTUP
BURETTE
BURNTIN
BURNTUP
BURSTER
BURSTIN
BURSTYN
BUSSTOP
CUBITAL
CUBITUS
CUESTAS
CULOTTE
CURATED
CURATES
CURATOR
CURETTE
CUVETTE
DUETTED
DUETTOS
DUNSTAN
FUENTES
FUGATOS
FUJITSU
FUNSTER
GUESTED
GUNITES
HUNGTEN
HURSTON
JUJITSU
JUPITER
LUCETTA
LUCITES
LUNATED
LUNATES
LUNATIC
LUNETTE
LUTETIA
LUXATED
LUXATES
MULATTO
MULCTED
MULETAS
MUNSTER
MUSETTA
MUSETTE
MUTATED
MUTATES
NUESTRA
NUESTRO
NUTATED
NUTATES
OUGHTNT
OUGHTTO
OUTSTAY
OUTSTEP
PULLTAB
PULLTOY
PUNSTER
PUPATED
PUPATES
PURITAN
PUTITTO
QUANTUM
QUARTAN
QUARTER
QUARTES
QUARTET
QUARTIC
QUARTOS
QUARTZY
QUATTRO
QUENTIN
QUESTED
QUESTER
QUIETED
QUIETEN
QUIETER
QUIETLY
QUIETUS
QUILTED
QUILTER
QUINTAL
QUINTAS
QUINTES
QUINTET
QUINTIC
QUINTON
QUINTUS
QUIRTED
QUITTED
QUITTER
QUOITED
RUBATOS
RUBITIN
RUNATAB
RUNITUP
SUBITEM
SUMATRA
SUMITUP
SUZETTE
TUBETOP
TURFTOE
VUITTON
VUMETER
YUCATAN
YUCATEC
YUKATAS

•U•••T•

AUGUSTA
AUGUSTE
AUGUSTO
AUGUSTS
AUKLETS
AULETTA
AUREATE
AURISTS
AUTISTS
BUCKETS
BUDGETS
BUFFETS
BUFFETT
BUGATTI
BUGOUTS
BULLETS
BULLITT
BURBOTS
BURETTE
BURNETT
BURRITO
BUYINTO
BUYOUTS
CUBISTS
CULLETS
CULOTTE
CUNEATE
CUPRITE
CURETTE
CURTATE
CURVETS
CUSPATE
CUTINTO
CUTLETS
CUTOUTS
CUTRATE
CUVETTE
DUALITY
DUBIETY
DUEDATE
DUGINTO
DUGOUTS
DURANTE
FURCATE
GULLETS
GUSSETS
HUANGTI
HUSSITE
JUNKETS
JURISTS
KUWAITI
KUZNETS
LUCETTA
LUDDITE
LUGNUTS
LUNESTA
LUNETTE
LUTISTS
MUDBATH
MUDCATS
MULATTO
MULLETS
MUPPETS
MUSANTE
MUSCATS
MUSETTA
MUSETTE
MUSKETS
MUTANTS
NUDISTS
NUGGETS
NUGGETY
NULLITY
NUMBATS
NUTLETS
OUGHTTO
OUTACTS
OUTBATS
OUTCITY
OUTCUTS
OUTDATE
OUTEATS
OUTFITS
OUTHITS
OUTJETS
OUTJUTS
OUTLETS
OUTMATE
OUTPATH
OUTPITY
OUTPUTS
OUTRATE
OUTSETS
OUTSITS
OUTVOTE
OUTWITH
OUTWITS
PUBERTY
PUCKETT
PULLETS
PULPITS
PULSATE
PUNDITS
PUPPETS
PURISTS
PUTITTO
PUTOUTS
PUTPUTS
PUTUPTO
QUALITY
QUINATE
QUIXOTE
RUGRATS
RUINATE
RUNINTO
RUNLATE
RUNLETS
RUNNETH
RUNOUTS
RUNUPTO
RUNWITH
RUSSETS
RUSSETY
SUAVITY
SUBDATE
SUBLETS
SUBLOTS
SUBMITS
SUBNETS
SUBSETS
SUCCOTH
SUHARTO
SUKKOTH
SULFATE
SULFITE
SUMMATE
SUMMITS
SUMUPTO
SUNBATH
SUNCITY
SUNHATS
SUNSETS
SUZETTE
TUBISTS
TUFFETS
TUMULTS
TUNEDTO
TUNESTO
TURBOTS
TURISTA
TURNSTO
TURRETS
TUTTUTS
VULGATE

•U••••T

AUGMENT
AUTOMAT
BUFFEST
BUFFETT
BUGSOUT
BULBLET
BULLITT
BUMSOUT
BUOYANT
BURNETT
BURNOUT
BUSIEST
BUSTOUT
BUTTEMT
BUTTOUT
BUYSOUT
BUZZCUT
CULPRIT
CULTIST
CULVERT
CURBCUT
CURRANT
CURRENT
CURSEAT
CURTEST
CUTSOUT
DUALIST
DUCKOUT
DUEEAST
DUELIST
DUEWEST
DULLEST
DUMBEST
DUMPOUT
DURWENT
FULGENT
FULLEST
FULLLOT
FULLOUT
FUMEDAT
FUMESAT
FUMIEST
FUNFEST
FURCOAT
FUSSPOT

GUESSAT
GUJARAT
GUMBOOT
GUNBELT
GUNBOAT
GUNSHOT
GUSHOUT
HUMBERT
HUNGOUT
HUPPERT
JUDOIST
JUILLET
JUMPCUT
JUMPSAT
JUNKART
JUSTEST
JUSTOUT
KUMQUAT
KURRENT
LUCKOUT
LUGSOUT
LUMPSIT
LUNGEAT
LUSHEST
MUDFLAT
MUGSHOT
MUSKRAT
NULLSET
NUMBEST
NUNAVUT
NUTMEAT
OUGHTNT
OUTBLOT
OUTCANT
OUTCAST
OUTFAST
OUTFOOT
OUTHUNT
OUTJEST
OUTKAST
OUTKEPT
OUTLAST
OUTMOST
OUTOFIT
OUTPLOT
OUTPORT
OUTPOST
OUTRANT
OUTROOT
OUTSERT
OUTSHOT
OUTSIFT
OUTSPIT
OUTTROT
OUTWAIT
OUTWENT
OUTWEPT
OUTWEST
PUCKETT
PUFFOUT
PULLOUT
PUMPOUT
PUNGENT
PUNIEST
PUPTENT
PURPORT
PURSUIT
PUSHOUT
PUTSOUT
PUTTOUT
QUARTET
QUEENIT
QUERIST
QUINTET
QUITSIT
QUONSET
RUBSOUT
RUCKERT
RULEOUT
RULIEST
RUNGOUT
RUNPAST
RUNRIOT
RUNSOUT
RUSHOUT
RUSSERT
SUAVEST
SUBCAST
SUBDUCT
SUBJECT
SUBPLOT
SUBPOST
SUBROOT
SUBSECT
SUBSIST
SUBSORT
SUBTEXT
SUBUNIT
SUBVERT
SUGGEST
SUMOIST
SUNBELT
SUNFAST
SUNKIST
SUNSPOT
SUNSUIT
SUPPORT
SUREBET
SURFEIT
SUSPECT
SUSSOUT
TUBAIST
TUGBOAT
TUNEOUT
TURNOUT
ZUMWALT

••UT•••

ABUTSON
ABUTTAL
ABUTTED
ABUTTER
ACUTELY
ACUTEST
AGUTTER
BHUTANI
BOUTROS
BRUTELY
BRUTISH
CAUTHEN
CAUTION
CHUTING
CHUTIST
CHUTNEY
CHUTZPA
CLUTCHY
CLUTTER
COUTERS
COUTURE
CRUTZEN
DEUTERO
DEUTSCH
ELUTING
ELUTION
FLUTERS
FLUTIER
FLUTIES
FLUTING
FLUTIST
FLUTTER
GAUTAMA
GAUTIER
GLUTEAL
GLUTENS
GLUTEUS
GLUTTED
GLUTTON
GOUTIER
GOUTILY
GOUTISH
HAUTBOY
HAUTEUR
INUTERO
INUTILE
KLUTZES
LAUTREC
LOUTING
LOUTISH
MOUTHED
MOUTHER
NAUTICA
NAUTILI
NEUTERS
NEUTRAL
NEUTRON
NOUTURN
PLUTONS
POUTERS
POUTFUL
POUTIER
POUTING
REUTERS
REUTHER
REUTTER
ROUTERS
ROUTINE
ROUTING
ROUTOUT
SAUTEED
SCUTTLE
SHUTEYE
SHUTINS
SHUTOFF
SHUTOUT
SHUTSIN
SHUTSUP
SHUTTER
SHUTTLE
SOUTHEY
SOUTHOF
SPUTNIK
SPUTTER
STUTTER
STUTZES
TAUTENS
TAUTEST
TEUTONS
TOUTERS
TOUTING
YOUTHEN

••U•T••

ABUTTAL
ABUTTED
ABUTTER
ADULTLY
AGUTTER
AQUATIC
BLUETIT
BLUNTED
BLUNTER
BLUNTLY
BLURTED
BLURTER
BLUSTER
BRUITED
CAUSTIC
CLUSTER
CLUTTER
COULTER
COUNTED
COUNTEE
COUNTEM
COUNTER
COUNTIN
COUNTON
COUNTRY
COUNTUP
COURTED
COURTLY
COURTTV
CRUSTAL
CRUSTED
DAUNTED
DAUNTER
DOUBTED
DOUBTER
DOUBTIT
EDUCTED
EDUCTOR
ELUATES
EQUATED
EQUATES
EQUATOR
ERUCTED
ERUPTED
ERUPTER
EXULTED
FAULTED
FAUSTUS
FLUSTER
FLUTTER
FOUETTE
FOULTIP
FOURTHS
FRUITED
FRUSTRO
FRUSTUM
GAUNTER
GAUNTLY
GLUTTED
GLUTTON
GRUNTED
GRUNTER
HAUNTED
HAUNTER
HOUSTON
IMUSTGO
JAUNTED
JOUSTED
JOUSTER
MOULTED
MOUNTED
MOUNTER
MOUNTIE
MOUNTUP
OPUNTIA
OPUSTWO
PLUSTAX
PLUSTWO
POULTRY
REUTTER
ROUSTED
ROUSTER
SAUNTER
SCUTTLE
SHUNTED
SHUNTER
SHUSTER
SHUTTER
SHUTTLE
SPURTED
SPUTTER
SQUATLY
SQUATTY
STUNTED
STUTTER
TAUNTED
TAUNTER
TAUNTON
TRUSTED
TRUSTEE
TRUSTER
TRUSTIN
TRUSTME
VAULTED
VAULTER
VAUNTED
VAUNTER

••U••T•

ADULATE
AMULETS
AZURITE
BAUXITE
BOUNDTO
BRUNETS
CAUDATE
CLUNGTO
COURTTV
CRUDITY
CRUELTY
DOUGHTY
EDUCATE
ELUANTS
EMULATE
EQUALTO
ERUDITE
EXUDATE
FAUCETS
FOUETTE
GLUEDTO
GLUESTO
HAUGHTY
LAURITZ
NAUGHTS
NAUGHTY
NOUGATS
NOUGHTS
PAUCITY
REUNITE
SCULPTS
SQUANTO
SQUATTY
SQUINTS
SQUINTY
SQUIRTS
STUARTI
STUCKTO
TRUANTS
TRUERTO
ULULATE

••U•••T

ACUTEST
AQUAVIT
BLUETIT
BOUQUET
BOURGET
CHUCKIT
CHUTIST
COULDNT
COUPLET
COURANT
COURBET
CRUDEST
CRUGUET
CRUMPET
DAUSSET
DOUBLET
DOUBTIT
DOUREST
DRUMOUT
DRUMSET
FAUVIST
FEUDIST
FLUNGAT
FLUSHOT
FLUTIST
FOULEST
FOULOUT
GLUIEST
GOURMET
LAUGHAT
LAURENT
LOUDEST
MAUPRAT
MAURIAT
OCULIST
OPULENT
PAULIST
PEUGEOT
PLUMCOT
PLUMMET
POUROUT
PRUDENT
ROUAULT
ROUGHIT
ROUTOUT
SHUBERT
SHUTOUT
SNUGFIT
SOUREST
SPUNOUT
STUDENT
SWUNGAT
SWUNGIT
TAUTEST
TOURIST
TRUMPET
ULULANT
WOULDNT
WOULDST
YOUREIT

•••UT••

ABOUTIT
ABOUTTO
AGOUTIS
ARBUTUS
ASTUTER
CLOUTED
CLOUTER
CROUTES
CROUTON
DEBUTED
DEPUTED
DEPUTES
DILUTED
DILUTER
DILUTES
DILUTOR
DOOUTOF
FLAUTAS
FLOUTED
FLOUTER
GODUTCH
GROUTED
GROUTER
IMPUTED
IMPUTER
IMPUTES
INDUTCH
IRKUTSK
KNOUTED
LAPUTAN
MINUTED
MINUTER
MINUTES
MINUTIA
MRBUTTS
PAIUTES
PLAUTUS
REFUTAL
REFUTED
REFUTER
REFUTES
REPUTED
REPUTES
SALUTED
SALUTER
SALUTES
SCOUTED
SCOUTER
SCOUTUP
SHOUTAT
SHOUTED
SHOUTER
SINUTAB
SLEUTHS
SNOUTED
SOLUTES
SPOUTED
SPOUTER
STOUTEN
STOUTER
STOUTLY
TOFUTTI
UNMUTED
VOLUTED
VOLUTES
YAKUTSK
ZABUTON

•••U•T•

ABDUCTS
ABOUTTO
ACQUITS
ACTUATE
ADDUCTS
ADDUPTO
ADJUSTS
AMOUNTS
ANNUITY
ARCUATE
ASQUITH
ASSUNTA
AUGUSTA
AUGUSTE
AUGUSTO
AUGUSTS
DEDUCTS
DEGUSTS
DERUSTS
ENSUITE
EXEUNTS
FACULTY
FATUITY
FLAUNTS
FLAUNTY
GOTUPTO
INDUCTS
INSULTS
INTUITS
IRRUPTS
JESUITS
KIDULTS
LEDUPTO
LIQUATE
LOCUSTS
LOQUATS
MINUETS
MRBUTTS
NAHUATL
NOTUPTO
OCCULTS
OCCURTO
OWNUPTO
PENULTS
PEQUOTS
PUTUPTO
RANUPTO
REDUSTS
RELUCTS
REQUITE
REQUOTE
RESUITS
RESULTS
ROBUSTA
ROBUSTO
RUNUPTO
SCHULTZ
SINUATE
SITUATE
SUMUPTO
TENUITY
THRUSTS
TOFUTTI
TUMULTS
UNDUSTY
UNLUSTY
UNQUOTE
VACUITY
VALUATE
VANUATU
YOGURTS

•••U••T

ABOUTIT
ACCURST
ADJUNCT
ALQUIST
ANNULET
ASQUIET
ASQUINT
BEQUEST
BEQUIET
BIGUNIT
BROUGHT
CALUMET
CAPULET
CASUIST
DEFUNCT
DILUENT
DRAUGHT
DROUGHT
ENDUPAT
EPAULET
FRAUGHT
INBUILT
INQUEST
ISSUANT
MANUMIT
MRHULOT
ONEUNIT
PIQUANT
PLAUDIT
PNEUMAT
REAUDIT
REBUILT
RENUZIT
REQUEST
RIVULET
SHOUTAT
SUBUNIT
THOUGHT
THRUPUT
TWOUNIT
UNBUILT
UNBURNT
UNBURST
UNGUENT
UNQUIET
UPBURST
VAGUEST
WROUGHT

••••UT•

AMINUTE
AZIMUTH
BISMUTH
BUGOUTS
BUYOUTS
BYMOUTH
CAPNUTS
CATGUTS
COBNUTS
COMMUTE
COMPUTE
CONFUTE
COPOUTS
CORNUTE
CUTOUTS
DELRUTH
DIECUTS
DIMOUTS
DISPUTE
DUGOUTS
ELOCUTE
ENDCUTS
ENGLUTS
ENROUTE
EVOLUTE
EXECUTE
FANOUTS
GETCUTE
GOSOUTH
GOTCUTE
HEXNUTS
HIRSUTE
HOGNUTS
ICEOUTS
INTRUTH
JOBCUTS
KIBBUTZ
KOSSUTH
LAYOUTS
LOGOUTS
LUGNUTS
MAHOUTS
MISCUTS
OFFDUTY
OUTCUTS
OUTJUTS
OUTPUTS
PAYCUTS
PAYOUTS
PEANUTS
PERMUTE
PIGNUTS
PIGOUTS
POLLUTE
POPOUTS
PRECUTS
PUTOUTS
PUTPUTS
RAGOUTS
REDOUTS
REROUTE
RESHUTS
RIBCUTS
RIZZUTO
ROTGUTS
RUNOUTS
SEADUTY
SETOUTS
SPROUTS
STATUTE
TAGOUTS
TAXCUTS
TRIBUTE
TRYOUTS
TUTTUTS
UMLAUTS
UNCOUTH
UNTRUTH
VELOUTE
WALNUTS
ZAGNUTS

••••U•T

ACCOUNT
AIRDUCT
APESUIT
ASSAULT
ATFAULT
BALLUET
BANQUET
BATSUIT
BERSUNT
BISCUIT
BOUQUET
BRIQUET
CATSUIT
CIRCUIT
COMBUST
CONDUCT
CONDUIT
CONSULT
CORRUPT
CROQUET
CRUGUET
DEFAULT
DEMOUNT
DISGUST
DISRUPT
DRYSUIT
EGGHUNT
ENCRUST
ENTRUST
EXHAUST
FOXHUNT
GETHURT
GOTHURT
GYMSUIT
INASUIT
INCOURT
INCRUST
INDOUBT
INTRUST
JOBHUNT
KUMQUAT
LAWSUIT
MANHUNT
MAOSUIT
MCCOURT
MYFAULT
NOCOUNT
NODOUBT
NOFAULT
OUTHUNT
OVIDUCT
PARQUET
PRODUCT
PURSUIT
RACQUET
RECOUNT
RECRUIT
REDDUST
REDOUBT
REDSUIT
REERUPT
REMOUNT
RENAULT
ROUAULT
SAWDUST
SEAHUNT
SHAVUOT
SKISUIT
SUBDUCT
SUNSUIT
UNADULT
UPCOURT
VIADUCT
WETSUIT
XAMOUNT
YOGHURT

•••••UT

ABSOLUT
ACEDOUT
ACESOUT
ACTSOUT
AGEDOUT
AGESOUT
AIRSOUT
ASKSOUT
BACKOUT
BAILOUT
BANGOUT
BAWLOUT
BEAROUT
BEATOUT
BELTOUT
BESTCUT
BLEWOUT
BLOTOUT
BLOWOUT
BOILOUT
BOOTCUT
BOOTOUT
BOREOUT
BOWSOUT
BUGSOUT
BUMSOUT
BURNOUT
BUSTOUT
BUTTOUT
BUYSOUT
BUZZCUT
CALLOUT
CAMEOUT
CAMPOUT
CASEOUT
CASHOUT
CASTOUT
CHEWOUT
CLIPOUT
COCONUT
COLDCUT
COMEOUT
CONKOUT
COOKOUT
COOLOUT
COPSOUT
CRAPOUT
CREWCUT
CURBCUT
CUTSOUT
DEALOUT
DECKOUT
DIALOUT
DIEDOUT
DIESOUT
DIGSOUT
DIMSOUT
DINEOUT
DISHOUT
DOLEOUT
DOPEOUT
DRAGOUT
DRAWOUT
DREWOUT
DROPOUT
DRUMOUT
DUCKOUT
DUMPOUT
EASEOUT
EATSOUT
EDGEOUT
EDITOUT
EELPOUT
EKEDOUT
EKESOUT
EVENOUT
FADEOUT
FAKEOUT
FALLOUT
FANSOUT
FARMOUT
FEELOUT
FELLOUT
FELTOUT
FILEOUT
FILLOUT
FINDOUT
FISHOUT
FLATOUT
FLIPOUT
FLOWOUT
FOLDOUT
FORKOUT
FOULOUT
FULLOUT
GAVEOUT
GETSOUT
GIVEOUT
GOABOUT
GOESOUT
GOKAPUT
GONEOUT
GUSHOUT
HAIRCUT
HALFCUT

HALIBUT
HANDOUT
HANGOUT
HARDPUT
HARTMUT
HASHOUT
HAVEOUT
HEADOUT
HEAROUT
HELDOUT
HELPOUT
HERBAUT
HIDEOUT
HIKEOUT
HIREOUT
HITSOUT
HOLDOUT
HOLEOUT
HOPSOUT
HUNGOUT
ICEDOUT
ICESOUT
IRISOUT
IRONOUT
JERKOUT
JUMPCUT
JUSTOUT
KEEPOUT
KEPTOUT
KICKOUT
KINGTUT
KOLANUT
LAIDOUT
LASHOUT
LAYSOUT
LEADOUT
LEAFOUT
LEANCUT
LEFTOUT
LENDOUT
LESCAUT
LETSOUT
LINECUT
LINEOUT
LIPSOUT
LIVEOUT
LOANOUT
LOCKNUT
LOCKOUT
LOGANUT
LOGSOUT
LOOKOUT
LOSEOUT
LOSTOUT
LUCKOUT
LUGSOUT
MADEOUT
MAILOUT
MAKEOUT
MAPSOUT
MARKOUT
METEOUT
MISSOUT
MONGKUT
MOVEOUT
NOSEOUT
NUNAVUT
OCCIPUT

OGDENUT
OOZEOUT
OPENOUT
OPTSOUT
OVERCUT
PAIDOUT
PANSOUT
PASSOUT
PAYSOUT
PEEKOUT
PEELOUT
PEEPOUT
PEEROUT
PICKOUT
PIGSOUT
PINENUT
PLANOUT
PLAYOUT
POKEOUT
POOPOUT
POPSOUT
POUROUT
PUFFOUT
PULLOUT
PUMPOUT
PUSHOUT
PUTSOUT
PUTTOUT
RACKOUT
RAINOUT
RANGOUT
RANKOUT
RATSOUT
READOUT
REAMOUT
REELOUT
RENTOUT
RIDEOUT
RIGSOUT
RINGOUT
RIPSOUT
RODEOUT
ROLLOUT
ROOTOUT
ROUTOUT
RUBSOUT
RULEOUT
RUNGOUT
RUNSOUT
RUSHOUT
SACKOUT
SANGOUT
SEEKOUT
SEENOUT
SEEPOUT
SEESOUT
SELLOUT
SENDOUT
SENTOUT
SETSOUT
SHIPOUT
SHOTOUT
SHOTPUT
SHOWOUT
SHUTOUT
SICKOUT
SIGNOUT
SINGOUT

SITSOUT
SKIPOUT
SLIDOUT
SLIPOUT
SOLDOUT
SORTOUT
SPATOUT
SPECOUT
SPEWOUT
SPINOUT
SPITOUT
SPUNOUT
STAYOUT
STAYPUT
STEPOUT
SUSSOUT
TAGSOUT
TAKEOUT
TALKOUT
TAPSOUT
TEAROUT
TESTOUT
THAWOUT
THINOUT
THRUPUT
TIMEOUT
TIREOUT
TOGSOUT
TOOKOUT
TOPSOUT
TOREOUT
TORNOUT
TOSSOUT
TROTOUT
TUNEOUT
TURNOUT
UNSTOUT
UPOROUT
VOIDOUT
VOTEOUT
WAITOUT
WALKOUT
WANTOUT
WASHOUT
WEAROUT
WEEDOUT
WELLCUT
WELLPUT
WENTOUT
WHOSOUT
WIGSOUT
WIMPOUT
WINGNUT
WINKOUT
WINSOUT
WIPEOUT
WITEOUT
WITHOUT
WOODCUT
WOREOUT
WORKOUT
WORNOUT
XINGOUT
YANKOUT
YEAHBUT
YELLOUT
ZEROOUT
ZONEOUT

ZONKOUT
ZOOMOUT

U•U••••
UKULELE
ULULANT
ULULATE
UNURBAN
UNURGED
UNUSUAL
UQUARKS
URUGUAY
USUALLY
USURERS
USURIES
USURPED
USURPER

U••U•••
UNBUILD
UNBUILT
UNBULKY
UNBURLY
UNBURNT
UNBURST
UNCUBIC
UNCUFFS
UNCURBS
UNCURED
UNCURLS
UNDULAR
UNDUPED
UNDUSTY
UNFULLY
UNFUNNY
UNFURLS
UNFUSED
UNFUSSY
UNGUARD
UNGUENT
UNGULAE
UNGULAR
UNGUYED
UNHULLS
UNHUMAN
UNHUMID
UNHUSKS
UNJUICY
UNLUCID
UNLUCKY
UNLUMPY
UNLURED
UNLUSTY
UNMUDDY
UNMUTED
UNQUICK
UNQUIET
UNQUOTE
UNRULED
UNRURAL
UNSULKY
UNSUNNY
UNSURLY
UNTUCKS
UNTUNED
UNTUNES
UPBUILD
UPBURST

UPCURLS
UPCURVE
UPQUARK
UPSURGE
UPTURNS
URSULAK

U•••U••
ULALUME
ULANUDE
UMLAUTS
UNADULT
UNAMUNO
UNBLUED
UNBOUND
UNCHURN
UNCOUTH
UNCRUDE
UNCRUEL
UNDRUNK
UNEQUAL
UNFLUID
UNFOUND
UNGAUDY
UNGLUED
UNGLUES
UNGRUFF
UNHOUSE
UNIQUES
UNMOULD
UNPLUGS
UNPLUMB
UNROUND
UNSLUNG
UNSOUND
UNSTUCK
UNSTUNG
UNSWUNG
UNTOUGH
UNTRUER
UNTRULY
UNTRUSS
UNTRUTH
UNUSUAL
UNWOUND
UNWRUNG
UNYOUNG
UPBOUND
UPCOURT
UPROUSE
URNFULS
URUGUAY
UVALUES

U••••U•
UNAWFUL
UNCLOUD
UNPIOUS
UNPROUD
UNSTOUT
UNVAGUE
UPOROUT
UPVALUE
URANIUM
URSINUS
USINGUP
USOTOUR

•UU••••
DUUMVIR
MUUMUUS

•U•U•••
AUBURNS
AUBURNU
AUDUBON
AUGURAL
AUGURED
AUGURER
AUGUSTA
AUGUSTE
AUGUSTO
AUGUSTS
AUTUMNS
BUNUELO
BURUNDI
CUMULUS
CUPULAR
CUPULES
DUBUQUE
DUFUSES
FUSUMAS
FUTURAS
FUTURES
GUNUSER
HUMUSES
JUGULAR
JUJUBES
KUTUZOV
LUNULAE
LUNULAR
MUTUALS
OUGUIYA
PUTUPON
PUTUPTO
QUEUERS
QUEUEUP
QUEUING
RUBUPON
RUNUPTO
SUBUNIT
SUBURBS
SULUSEA
SUMUPTO
SUTURED
SUTURES
SUZUKIS
TUBULAR
TUBULES
TUMULTS
TUTUILA

•U••U••
AUTEURS
BUGOUTS
BULGURS
BULRUSH
BUMRUSH
BUNKUMS
BUSTUPS
BUYOUTS
CULTURE
CUPFULS
CUTOUTS
DUGOUTS
DUMDUMS

DUSTUPS
FUNFURS
FUNRUNS
HUBBUBS
HUMBUGS
HUMOURS
JUGFULS
JUMBUCK
KUMQUAT
LUCIUSI
LUGNUTS
LUTHULI
MUGFULS
MUGWUMP
MUKLUKS
MURMURS
MUSEUMS
MUUMUUS
NURTURE
OUTBUDS
OUTBULK
OUTBURN
OUTBUYS
OUTBUZZ
OUTCULL
OUTCURE
OUTCUTS
OUTDUEL
OUTGUNS
OUTGUSH
OUTHUNT
OUTHURL
OUTJUMP
OUTJUTS
OUTPULL
OUTPURL
OUTPUSH
OUTPUTS
OUTRUNS
OUTRUSH
OUTSULK
OUTSUMS
OUTSUNG
OUTTURN
PULLUPS
PURDUEU
PURSUED
PURSUER
PURSUES
PURSUIT
PUSHUPS
PUTOUTS
PUTPUTS
QUORUMS
RUMOURS
RUNOUTS
RUPTURE
SUBDUAL
SUBDUCT
SUBDUED
SUBDUER
SUBDUES
SUBSUME
SUCCUMB
SUDBURY
SUFFUSE
SUNBURN
SUNSUIT

TUBFULS
TUNEUPS
TURNUPS
TUTTUTS
VULTURE

•U•••U•
AUTOBUS
BUCKSUP
BUDDYUP
BUFFSUP
BUGSOUT
BUILDUP
BUILTUP
BULBOUS
BULGHUR
BULKSUP
BULLRUN
BUMPSUP
BUMSOUT
BUNCHUP
BUOYSUP
BUREAUS
BUREAUX
BURNOUT
BURNSUP
BURNTUP
BURPGUN
BUSTOUR
BUSTOUT
BUSTSUP
BUTTOUT
BUYSOUT
BUZZCUT
CUBITUS
CUMULUS
CUPROUS
CURBCUT
CURIOUS
CURLSUP
CUTARUG
CUTSOUT
DUBIOUS
DUBNIUM
DUBUQUE
DUCKOUT
DUDEDUP
DUDESUP
DUMMYUP
DUMPOUT
DUSTGUN
DUTEOUS
DUTIFUL
EULABUS
FUELSUP
FULCRUM
FULGHUM
FULLOUT
FURIOUS
GUARGUM
GUSHOUT
GUSSYUP
HUMANUM
HUMDRUM
HUMERUS
HUNGOUT
HUNTSUP
HURRYUP

HURTFUL
HUSHFUL
JUICEUP
JUMPCUT
JUMPSUP
JUNEBUG
JUSTOUT
LUCKOUT
LUGSOUT
LUMPSUM
LUSTFUL
LUSTRUM
MUCKSUP
MULDAUR
MUSEFUL
MUUMUUS
NUCLEUS
NUNAVUT
OUTFLUX
OUTHAUL
OUTLOUD
OUTPOUR
OUTSWUM
PUBLIUS
PUFFOUT
PUFFSUP
PULLOUT
PULLSUP
PUMPOUT
PUMPSUP
PUNCHUP
PUSHFUL
PUSHOUT
PUTEMUP
PUTSOUT
PUTTOUT
QUANTUM
QUECHUA
QUELQUE
QUEUEUP
QUIETUS
QUINQUE
QUINTUS
RUBADUB
RUBIOUS
RUBSOUT
RUCKSUP
RUINOUS
RULEOUT
RUNGOUT
RUNITUP
RUNSOUT
RUSHOUT
RUTHFUL
SUBARUS
SUCCOUR
SUCKSUP
SUDOKUS
SUITSUP
SULPHUR
SUMITUP
SURFSUP
SURPLUS
SUSSOUT
TUNASUB
TUNEDUP
TUNEFUL
TUNEOUT

TUNESUP
TURNOUT
TURNSUP
TUSSAUD

•U••••U
AUBURNU
BUNRAKU
FUJITSU
JUJITSU
LUCYLIU
PURDUEU
PURLIEU
QUENEAU
TULANEU

••U•U••
ARUGULA
ASUSUAL
BOUQUET
COUTURE
CRUGUET
FLUBUGS
FOULUPS
GAUGUIN
MUUMUUS
NOUTURN
PLUMULE
ROUAULT
UNUSUAL
URUGUAY

••U••U•
ALUMNUS
AQUEOUS
BAUHAUS
BLUESUN
BOUNDUP
BRUMOUS
BRUSHUP
BRUSQUE
CHURNUP
CLUBSUP
CLUEFUL
COUGHUP
COUNTUP
CRUDSUP
CRUMBUM
DOUCEUR
DRUMOUT
DRUMSUP
ELUVIUM
EMULOUS
FAUSTUS
FAUXFUR
FLUBDUB
FLUFFUP
FOULOUT
FOULSUP
FRUSTUM
GLUEGUN
GLUTEUS
HAULSUP
HAUTEUR
JOUHAUX
LAULAUS
LOUSEUP
MAUMAUS

MOUNTUP
MUUMUUS
PLUGSUP
PLUMBUM
POUROUT
POUTFUL
RAUCOUS
ROUGHUP
ROUNDUP
ROUTOUT
RYUKYUS
SHUTOUT
SHUTSUP
SLUNKUP
SNUCKUP
SOULFUL
SOUPSUP
SPUNOUT
STUCKUP
STUNGUN
THULIUM
TOUCHUP
TOURBUS
TRUEDUP
TRUESUP
TRUMPUP
TRUSSUP
WOUNDUP
YOUNGUN

••U•••U
BLUEFLU
DOUBLEU
IGUASSU
NOUVEAU
ROULEAU
THURGAU
TRUDEAU

•••UU••
VACUUMS

•••U•U•
ANNULUS
ARBUTUS
ARDUOUS
CLOUDUP
CUMULUS
DEQUEUE
DUBUQUE
ENQUEUE
FAMULUS
FATUOUS
GIAUQUE
HAMULUS
INCUBUS
JEJUNUM
KIKUYUS
LIQUEUR
LOCULUS
MODULUS
NOCUOUS
PABULUM
PLAUTUS
QUEUEUP
REAUMUR
REGULUS
RIGUEUR

ROMULUS
SCOUTUP
SCRUBUP
SINUOUS
TENUOUS
THRUPUT
VACUOUS
ZEBULUN

•••U••U
AUBURNU
VANUATU

••••UU•
MUUMUUS

••••U•U
DEPAULU
PURDUEU

UV•••••
UVALUES
UVINDEX

U•V••••
UNVAGUE
UNVEILS
UNVENAL
UNVEXED
UNVITAL
UNVIVID
UNVOCAL
UNVOICE
UNVOTED
UNVOWED
UNVYING
UPVALUE

U••V•••
UNIVACS
UNOVERT

U•••V••
UNCIVIC
UNCIVIL
UNCOVER
UNEAVED
UNGIVEN
UNGYVED
UNLAVED
UNLEVEL
UNLIVED
UNLIVES
UNLOVED
UNMOVED
UNNOVEL
UNPAVED
UNRAVEL
UNRIVED
UNRIVEN
UNSAVED
UNSAVVY
UNVIVID
UNWAVED
UNWOVEN
UPDIVED
UPDIVES
UPRIVER

U••••V•
ULANOVA
UNBRAVE
UNGLOVE
UNHEAVY
UNITIVE
UNNAIVE
UNNERVE
UNSAVVY
UNWEAVE
UPABOVE
UPCURVE
UPHEAVE
URBANVI

U•••••V
ULYANOV
URBANIV
USTINOV

•UV••••
CUVETTE
GUVNORS
JUVENAL
TUVWXYZ

•U•V•••
BUDVASE
CULVERT
CURVETS
CURVIER
CURVING
GUEVARA
HUMVEES
OUTVIED
OUTVIES
OUTVOTE
PURVEYS
PURVIEW
QUAVERS
QUAVERY
QUIVERS
QUIVERY
QUIVIVE
SUAVELY
SUAVEST
SUAVITY
SUBVENE
SUBVERT
SURVEIL
SURVEYS
SURVIVE

•U••V••
BULOVAS
CUTOVER
DUUMVIR
EUROVAN
NUNAVUT
PUTOVER
RUNOVER

•U•••V•
CURSIVE
FURTIVE
GUSTAVE
OUTGAVE
OUTGIVE

OUTLIVE
OUTLOVE
OUTMOVE
OUTRAVE
OUTROVE
OUTWAVE
QUIVIVE
SUASIVE
SURVIVE
TUSSIVE

•U••••V
KUTUZOV
NUREYEV
TUPOLEV

••UV•••
BOUVIER
ELUVIAL
ELUVIUM
FAUVISM
FAUVIST
FLUVIAL
LOUVERS
LOUVRED
LOUVRES
MAUVAIS
NOUVEAU
OEUVRES
PLUVIAL
STUVWXY
VOUVRAY

••U•V••
AQUAVIT
AQUIVER
DUUMVIR
PIUSVII
SCURVES

••U••V•
ABUSIVE
ELUSIVE
LOUISVI

••U•••V
COURTTV
DOUBLEV
LOUISIV
LOUISXV

•••UV••
ALLUVIA
DOEUVRE
OLDUVAI
RSTUVWX

•••U•V•
INCURVE
RECURVE
UPCURVE

•••U••V
BRYUSOV
GODUNOV
KUTUZOV

••••UV•
DENEUVE
HECKUVA
HELLUVA
QRSTUVW

••••U•V
STPIUSV

•••••UV
PQRSTUV

U•W••••
UNWADED
UNWAGED
UNWAKED
UNWALLS
UNWANED
UNWAVED
UNWAXED
UNWEARY
UNWEAVE
UNWEDGE
UNWHEEL
UNWHIPT
UNWHITE
UNWHOLE
UNWINDS
UNWINDY
UNWIPED
UNWIRED
UNWISER
UNWITTY
UNWOOED
UNWORMY
UNWOUND
UNWOVEN
UNWRAPS
UNWRUNG
UPWAFTS
UPWARDS
UPWELLS
UPWHIRL
UPWINDS

U••W•••
UNAWAKE
UNAWARE
UNAWFUL
UNOWING
UNOWNED
UNSWEAR
UNSWEET
UNSWEPT
UNSWORE
UNSWORN
UNSWUNG
UNTWINE
UNTWIST
UPSWEEP
UPSWELL
UPSWEPT
UPSWING

U•••W••
UNBOWED
UNCOWED
UNDEWED
UNHEWED
UNLOWLY
UNMEWED
UNMOWED
UNPAWED
UNPAWNS
UNROWDY
UNSAWED
UNSEWED
UNSOWED
UNVOWED
UPTOWNS

U••••W•
UNBLOWN
UNCROWN
UNDRAWN
UNDRAWS
UNFLOWN
UNGROWN
UNKNOWN
UNSHOWN
UNSHOWY
UNSKEWS
UNSTOWS
UNTHAWS
UPFLOWS
UPGROWN
UPGROWS

U•••••W
UNSCREW
UPTHROW
UPTONOW
USOSHOW

•UW••••
KUWAITI

•U•W•••
BUDWORM
BULWARK
CUTWORK
CUTWORM
DUEWEST
DURWARD
DURWENT
FURWRAP
GUMWOOD
GUNWALE
JUGWINE
LUGWORM
MUDWASP
MUGWUMP
NUTWOOD
OUTWAIT
OUTWALK
OUTWARD
OUTWARS
OUTWASH
OUTWAVE
OUTWEAR
OUTWEED
OUTWEEP
OUTWELL
OUTWENT
OUTWEPT
OUTWEST
OUTWILE
OUTWILL
OUTWIND
OUTWING
OUTWISH
OUTWITH
OUTWITS
OUTWORD
OUTWORE
OUTWORK
OUTWORN
RUNWAYS
RUNWILD
RUNWITH
SUBWARS
SUBWAYS
SUNWARD
TUVWXYZ
ZUMWALT

•U••W••
BUSHWAH
CUTAWAY
DUNAWAY
GULFWAR
NUNGWEN
OUTAWED
OUTAWES
OUTSWAM
OUTSWIM
OUTSWUM
PUTAWAY
RUNAWAY
TURFWAR

•U•••W•
BURROWS
BUYDOWN
CURFEWS
CURLEWS
CUSHAWS
CUTDOWN
FURROWS
GUFFAWS
GUNLAWS
OURTOWN
OUTBAWL
OUTBOWL
OUTBOWS
OUTFAWN
OUTHOWL
OUTLAWS
OUTROWS
PUTDOWN
QUAPAWS
RUBDOWN
RUNDOWN
SUNBOWL
SUNBOWS
SUNDOWN

•U••••W
BUCKSAW
BUZZSAW
CUMSHAW
JUDELAW
JUSTNOW
LUCKNOW
MUDFLOW
MULGREW
OUTBLOW
OUTCROW
OUTDRAW
OUTDREW
OUTFLOW
OUTGLOW
OUTGNAW
OUTGREW
OUTGROW
OUTSHOW
PURVIEW
RUBSRAW
RUNSLOW
SUNGLOW

••UW•••
YOUWISH

••U•W••
FOURWAY
SQUAWKS
SQUAWKY
STUVWXY

••U••W•
OPUSTWO
PLUSTWO

••U•••W
BLUELAW
DOUBLEW
YOUKNOW

•••UW••
THRUWAY

•••U•W•
OTTUMWA
RSTUVWX

••••U•W
QRSTUVW

UX•••••
UXORIAL

U••X•••
UNAXLED

U•••X••
UNBOXED
UNBOXES
UNFIXED
UNFIXES
UNFOXED
UNLAXED
UNLAXES
UNMIXED
UNMIXES
UNTAXED
UNTAXES
UNTOXIC
UNVEXED
UNWAXED
URTEXTS

U•••••X
UNIPLEX
UVINDEX

•UX••••
BUXOMLY
LUXATED
LUXATES
TUXEDOS

•U•X•••
QUIXOTE

•U••X••
CULEXES
LUREXES
TUVWXYZ

•U•••X•
SUBTEXT

•U••••X
BUREAUX
FUNPLEX
FUSEBOX
HUMIDEX
JUKEBOX
JUNKFAX
JURYBOX
MUESLIX
OUTFLUX
OUTJINX

••UX•••
BAUXITE
BRUXING
BRUXISM
FAUXFUR
FAUXPAS
FLUXING
FLUXION

••U•X••
PIUSXII

••U••X•
LOUISXI
LOUISXV
STUVWXY

••U•••X
ARUSPEX
BLUEFOX
DOUBLEX
EQUIFAX
EQUINOX
FLUMMOX
JOUHAUX
LOUISIX
PLUSTAX
ROUBAIX
SOUPMIX

•••U••X
LEXUSGX
LEXUSLX
LEXUSRX
RSTUVWX

••••U•X
STPIUSX

•••••UX
BATEAUX
BENELUX
BUREAUX
CADEAUX
CHEVAUX
CISEAUX
FIATLUX
GATEAUX
JOUHAUX
LASCAUX
LEMIEUX
MALRAUX
MARGAUX
MICHAUX
MILIEUX
MIMIEUX
MONTEUX
NONFLUX
OISEAUX
OUTFLUX
RESEAUX
THEROUX
VERDOUX

U•Y••••
ULYANOV
ULYSSES
UNYOKED
UNYOKES
UNYOUNG

U••Y•••
UNDYING
UNGYVED
UNLYING
UNLYRIC
UNTYING
UNTYPED
UNVYING

U•••Y••
UNCOYER
UNCOYLY
UNGUYED
UNHAYED
UNJOYED
UNKEYED
UNLOYAL
UNRAYED
UNRHYME
UNSHYER
UNSHYLY
UNSLYER
UNSLYLY

U•••••Y
UFOLOGY
UNANGRY
UNAPTLY
UNBOGGY
UNBULKY
UNBURLY
UNCANNY
UNCHARY
UNCOYLY
UNCRAZY
UNDUSTY
UNEMPTY
UNFANCY
UNFATTY
UNFIERY
UNFITLY
UNFLAKY
UNFOGGY
UNFULLY
UNFUNNY
UNFUSSY
UNGAUDY
UNGIDDY
UNGODLY
UNHAIRY
UNHANDY
UNHAPPY
UNHARDY
UNHASTY
UNHEADY
UNHEAVY
UNHILLY
UNIBODY
UNITARY
UNJOLLY
UNJUICY
UNLEAKY
UNLOFTY
UNLOWLY
UNLUCKY
UNLUMPY
UNLUSTY
UNMADLY
UNMANLY
UNMERRY
UNMOLDY
UNMOODY
UNMOSSY
UNMUDDY
UNNEEDY
UNNOISY
UNPIETY
UNRAINY
UNRASPY
UNREADY
UNRISKY
UNROCKY
UNROOMY
UNROWDY
UNSADLY
UNSALTY
UNSAVVY
UNSCALY
UNSHADY
UNSHINY
UNSHOWY
UNSHYLY
UNSILLY
UNSLYLY
UNSMOKY
UNSNAKY
UNSOGGY
UNSOOTY
UNSORRY
UNSPICY
UNSTAGY
UNSTONY
UNSULKY
UNSUNNY
UNSURLY
UNTASTY
UNTRULY
UNWEARY
UNWINDY
UNWITTY
UNWORMY
UPEARLY
URGENCY
UROLOGY
URUGUAY
USUALLY
UTICANY
UTILITY
UTTERLY

•UY••••
BUYABLE
BUYBACK
BUYDOWN
BUYINTO
BUYOFFS
BUYOUTS
BUYSOFF
BUYSOUT
BUYTIME
GUYROPE
HUYGENS
MUYBIEN
RUYBLAS

•U•Y•••
BUOYANT
BUOYING
BUOYSUP
BURYING
BUSYBEE
BUSYING
JULYDAY
JURYBOX
JURYING
JURYMAN
JURYMEN
JURYRIG
LUCYLIU
OUTYELL
OUTYELP
QUAYAGE
RUBYDEE
RUBYRED
RUDYARD

•U••Y••
BUDDYUP
BUGEYED
DUMMYUP
EUONYMS
GUSSYUP
HUNNYBS
HURRYUP
NUREYEV
RUFIYAA
SUBTYPE
SUELYON

•U•••Y•
AUTONYM
BUCKEYE
BUGBOYS
BURSTYN
BUSBOYS
GURNEYS
HURRAYS
MURPHYS
OUGUIYA
OUTBUYS
OUTLAYS
OUTPAYS
OUTSAYS
PULLEYS
PURVEYS
RUNWAYS
SUBWAYS
SUNDAYS
SUNRAYS
SURREYS
SURVEYS
TURKEYS
TUVWXYZ

•U••••Y
AUDIBLY
AURALLY
AUTARKY
AUTOPSY
BUCKLEY
BUMPILY
BURNABY
BURNLEY
BUSHILY
BUTTERY
BUTTONY
BUXOMLY
CUBICLY
CURABLY
CURSORY
CURTSEY
CUSHILY
CUSTODY
CUTAWAY
CUTLERY
DUALITY
DUBARRY
DUBIETY
DUCALLY
DULCIFY
DUMPILY
DUNAWAY
DUOPOLY
DURABLY
DUSKILY
DUSTILY
EUPHONY
FUGALLY
FULLDAY
FUNKILY
FUNNILY
FUSSILY
FUSTILY
FUZZILY
GUNNERY
GUNPLAY
GUSHILY
GUSTILY
GUTSILY
HUFFILY
HUMANLY
HUMIDLY
HUMPHRY
HUNGARY
HUNTLEY
HUSHABY
HUSKILY
JUICILY
JULYDAY
JUMPILY
JUNEDAY
JUSTIFY
LUCENCY
LUCIDLY
LUCKILY
LULLABY
LUMPILY
LURIDLY
LUSTILY
MUDDILY
MULCAHY
MUMMERY
MUMMIFY
MURKILY
MUSHILY
MUSIGNY
MUSSILY
MUSTILY
MUTABLY
MUTEDLY
MUZZILY
NUGGETY
NULLIFY
NULLITY
NUNNERY
NURSERY
NUTTILY
OUTBRAY
OUTCITY
OUTPITY
OUTPLAY
OUTPRAY
OUTSTAY
OUTTRAY
PUBERTY
PUCKERY
PUDENCY
PUDGILY
PUFFERY
PUFFILY
PUGSLEY
PULLTOY
PULPIFY
PUNNILY
PUSHILY
PUTAWAY
PUTREFY
QUAKILY
QUALIFY
QUALITY
QUARTZY
QUAVERY
QUEENLY
QUEERLY
QUESNAY
QUICKLY
QUIETLY
QUIGLEY
QUINARY
QUINCEY
QUIVERY
RUBBERY
RUDDILY
RULEDBY
RUNAWAY
RUNSDRY
RURALLY
RUSSETY
RUSTILY
SUAVELY
SUAVITY
SUBSIDY
SUCKDRY
SUDBURY
SULKILY
SUMMARY
SUMMERY
SUNCITY
SUNNILY
SURGERY
SURLILY
TUESDAY
TURNERY
TURNKEY
TUSCANY
TUSHERY
YUPPIFY

••UY•••
GRUYERE

••U•Y••
RYUKYUS

••U••Y•
SHUTEYE

••U•••Y
ACUTELY
ADULTLY
BLUEBOY
BLUEJAY
BLUESKY
BLUFFLY
BLUNTLY
BRUTELY
CHURCHY
CHUTNEY
CLUTCHY
COUNTRY
COURTLY
CRUDELY
CRUDITY
CRUELLY
CRUELTY
CRUMBLY
CRUMPLY
CRUNCHY
DOUBLEY
DOUGHTY
ELUSORY
EQUABLY
EQUALLY
EQUERRY
EXUPERY
FLUENCY
FLUIDLY
FLUKILY
FMURRAY
FOUNDRY
FOURDAY
FOURWAY
GAUDERY
GAUDILY
GAUNTLY
GAUZILY
GOUTILY
GRUFFLY
GRUMBLY
HAUGHTY
HAUTBOY
HOUSSAY
JOURNEY
KNUCKLY
LAUNDRY
LOUSILY
MOUSILY
NAUGHTY
NEUILLY
PAUCITY
PAULPRY
PAUNCHY
PLUMPLY
PLUSHLY
POULTRY
PRUDERY
RAUNCHY
REUNIFY
ROUGHLY
ROUNDLY
SAUCILY
SAUCONY
SNUGGLY
SOUNDLY
SOUTHEY
SQUALLY
SQUASHY
SQUATLY
SQUATTY
SQUAWKY
SQUEAKY
SQUINTY
SQUIRMY
SQUISHY
STUBBLY
STUCKBY
STUPEFY
STUVWXY
SWUNGBY
TOUGHLY
TOURNEY
TRUANCY
URUGUAY
USUALLY
VOUVRAY

•••UY••
COBUYER
KIKUYUS
UNGUYED

•••U•Y•
OUGUIYA
SEQUOYA

•••U••Y
ACTUARY
ALBUNDY
ANNUITY
AWFULLY
BOGUSLY
CALUMNY
DEBUSSY
ENQUIRY
ESTUARY
FACULTY
FATUITY
FLAUNTY
FLOUNCY
GROUCHY
INQUIRY
JANUARY
LIQUEFY
LITURGY
MRLUCKY
MYBUDDY
OCTUPLY
OSSUARY
PIOUSLY
PROUDLY
ROGUERY
SCRUBBY
SCRUFFY
SHRUBBY
SLOUCHY
STOUTLY
TENUITY
THRUWAY
UNBULKY
UNBURLY
UNDUSTY
UNFULLY
UNFUNNY
UNFUSSY
UNJUICY
UNLUCKY
UNLUMPY
UNLUSTY
UNMUDDY
UNSULKY
UNSUNNY
UNSURLY
VACUITY
VAGUELY
VOLUBLY
ZYMURGY

••••UY•
BADGUYS
OUTBUYS
PREBUYS
VANDUYN

••••U•Y
ARMOURY
ASHBURY
BANBURY
CADBURY
CENTURY
CIRCUSY
CLIQUEY
CONJURY
DANBURY
GETBUSY
GOTBUSY
INAFURY
MERCURY
MIDJULY
NONBUSY
NONJURY
OFFDUTY
ONAJURY
PERFUMY
PERJURY
RESTUDY
ROXBURY
SAVOURY
SEADUTY
SUDBURY
TISSUEY
UNGAUDY
UNTRULY
URUGUAY
VAPOURY

•••••UY
BESTBUY
FALLGUY
GOODBUY
GOODGUY
GOTOGUY
NICEGUY
OBLOQUY
OKAYGUY
OVERBUY
WISEGUY

U•Z••••
ULZANAS
UNZONED
UNZONES

U•••Z••
UNDAZED
UNFAZED
UNHAZED
UNRAZED
UNSIZED
UPGAZED
UPGAZES
UPSIZED
UPSIZES

U••••Z•
UNCRAZY
UNFROZE
UNISIZE
UNITIZE
UTILIZE

•UZ••••
BUZZARD
BUZZCUT
BUZZELL
BUZZERS
BUZZIER
BUZZING
BUZZOFF
BUZZSAW
FUZZIER
FUZZILY
FUZZING
GUZZLED
GUZZLER
GUZZLES
HUZZAHS
KUZNETS
MUZZIER
MUZZILY
MUZZLED
MUZZLER
MUZZLES
NUZZLED
NUZZLER
NUZZLES
PUZZLED
PUZZLER
PUZZLES
RUZICKA
SUZANNE
SUZETTE
SUZUKIS

•U•Z•••
BUZZARD
BUZZCUT
BUZZELL
BUZZERS
BUZZIER
BUZZING
BUZZOFF
BUZZSAW
FUTZING
FUZZIER
FUZZILY
FUZZING
GUZZLED
GUZZLER
GUZZLES
HUZZAHS
MUEZZIN
MUZZIER
MUZZILY
MUZZLED
MUZZLER
MUZZLES
NUDZHED
NUDZHES
NUZZLED
NUZZLER
NUZZLES
PUZZLED
PUZZLER
PUZZLES
QUIZNOS
QUIZZED
QUIZZER
QUIZZES
SUBZERO
SUBZONE

•U••Z••
FUNFZIG
KUTUZOV
MUEZZIN
QUETZAL
QUINZES
QUIZZED
QUIZZER
QUIZZES

•U•••Z•
DUALIZE
OUTBUZZ
OUTGAZE
OUTSIZE
QUARTZY

•U••••Z
OUTBUZZ
TUVWXYZ

••UZ•••
CRUZADO
CRUZANS
DRUZEAN
DRUZIAN
GAUZIER
GAUZILY
SCUZZES

••U•Z••
CHUTZPA
CRUTZEN
KLUTZES
SCUZZES
STUTZES

••U••Z•
SQUEEZE

••U•••Z
DOUBLEZ
LAURITZ

•••UZ••
ABRUZZI
JACUZZI
KUTUZOV
MEZUZAH
MEZUZAS
RENUZIT

•••U•Z•
ABRUZZI
JACUZZI

•••U••Z
EXCUSEZ
SCHULTZ

••••UZ•
OUTBUZZ

••••U•Z
KIBBUTZ
MARQUEZ
OUTBUZZ
POPQUIZ
VASQUEZ

•••••UZ
MAHFOUZ

VA•••••
VACANCY
VACATED
VACATES
VACCARO
VACCINE
VACUITY
VACUOLE
VACUOUS
VACUUMS
VAGRANT
VAGUELY
VAGUEST
VAINEST
VALADON
VALANCE
VALENCE
VALENTE
VALENTI
VALERIE
VALETED
VALIANT
VALIDID
VALIDLY
VALINES
VALISES
VALJEAN
VALLEJO
VALLEYS
VALLONE
VALMIKI
VALOREM
VALOTTE
VALOURS
VALUATE
VALUERS
VALUING
VALVATE
VALVULA
VALVULE
VAMOOSE
VAMPERS
VAMPIER
VAMPING
VAMPIRA
VAMPIRE
VAMPISH
VANADIC
VANCAMP
VANDALS
VANDIEN
VANDINE
VANDURA
VANDUYN
VANDYCK
VANDYKE
VANESSA
VANEXEL
VANEYCK
VANGOGH
VANILLA
VANILLI
VANLINE
VANLOAD
VANNING
VANOCUR
VANOWEN
VANPELT
VANPOOL
VANRIJN
VANSANT
VANTAGE
VANUATU
VANVOGT
VANWARD
VANWYCK
VANZANT
VAPIDLY
VAPORED
VAPORER
VAPORUB
VAPOURS
VAPOURY
VAQUERO
VARIANT
VARIATE
VARIERS
VARIETY
VARIOUS
VARITEK
VARLAAM
VARLETS
VARMINT
VARNISH
VARRICK
VARSITY
VARYING
VASQUEZ
VASSALS
VASTEST
VASTIER
VASTITY
VATDYED
VATDYES
VATFULS
VATICAL
VATICAN
VATTING
VAUDOIS
VAUGHAN
VAULTED
VAULTER
VAUNTED
VAUNTER

V•A••••
VEADARS
VEALIER
VIADENT
VIADUCT
VIALFUL
VIALING
VIALLED
VIATICA

V••A•••
VACANCY
VACATED
VACATES
VALADON
VALANCE
VANADIC
VENABLE
VENALLY
VENATIC
VERANDA
VIDALIA
VIHARAS
VIRAGOS
VISAGED
VISAGES
VISAING
VISALIA
VISAVIS
VISAYAN
VITALIS
VITALLY
VITAMIN
VITARAS
VIVALDI
VIVANTS
VIVARIA
VOCABLE
VOCABLY
VOCALIC
VOCALLY
VOLANTE
VOTABLE
VOYAGED
VOYAGER
VOYAGES
VSHAPED
VSHAPES

V•••A••
VACCARO
VAGRANT
VALIANT
VALUATE
VALVATE
VANCAMP
VANDALS
VANSANT
VANTAGE
VANUATU
VANWARD
VANZANT
VARIANT
VARIATE
VARLAAM
VASSALS
VCRTAPE
VEADARS
VEEJAYS
VENTAGE
VERBALS
VERDANT
VERSACE
VERSANT
VESTALS
VFWHALL
VIBRANT
VIBRATE
VIBRATO
VICDANA
VILLAGE
VILLAIN
VILLARD
VILLARI
VINLAND
VINTAGE
VIOLATE
VIRGATE
VISTAED
VISUALS
VITIATE
VOLCANO
VOLTAGE
VOLTAIC
VONBAER
VONLAUE
VORLAGE
VOTEAYE
VULCANS
VULGATE

V••••A•
VALJEAN
VANLOAD
VARLAAM
VATICAL
VATICAN
VAUGHAN
VECTRAS
VEGETAL
VELTMAN
VENEMAN
VENTRAD
VENTRAL
VERITAS
VERYBAD
VERYMAD
VERYSAD
VESTRAL
VETERAN
VICINAL
VICTUAL
VICUNAS
VIETNAM
VIHARAS
VIMINAL
VINEGAR
VIRGOAN
VIRTUAL
VISAYAN
VITARAS
VIVICAA
VIVITAR
VIZSLAS
VOSGIAN
VOTENAY
VOUVRAY

V•••••A
VALVULA
VAMPIRA
VANDURA
VANESSA
VANILLA
VENEZIA
VENTURA
VERANDA
VERBENA
VERONIA
VERRUCA
VIATICA
VICDANA
VICENZA
VIDALIA
VIGNOLA
VINCULA
VISALIA
VISCERA
VISTULA
VITORIA
VIVARIA
VIVICAA
VOTEYEA

•VA••••
AVAILED
AVALONS
AVANTIS
AVARICE
AVATARS
EVACUEE
EVADERS
EVADING
EVALUNA
EVANDER
EVANGEL
EVANISH
EVASION
EVASIVE
IVANHOE
IVANIII
IVANOVO
KVASSES
OVARIES
OVATION
RVALUES
UVALUES

•V•A•••
AVGASES
AVIANCA
AVIATED
AVIATES
AVIATIC
AVIATOR
RVPARKS
TVGAMES
TVTABLE
TVTAPES

•V••A••
AVATARS
AVERAGE
AVOCADO
AVOWALS
OVERACT
OVERAGE
OVERALL
OVERARM
OVERATE
OVERAWE
OVIPARA
OVISACS
TVSTARS

•V•••A•
AVERNAL
AVESTAN
AVESTAS
AVIDFAN
AVIVIAN
EVENPAR
IVORIAN
OVEREAT
OVERFAR
OVERFAT
OVERLAP
OVERLAX
OVERLAY
OVERMAN
OVERPAR
OVERPAY
OVERRAN
OVERSAD
OVERSAW
OVERTAX
OVIDIAN
OVOIDAL

•V••••A
AVENIDA
AVIANCA
AVONLEA
EVALUNA
OVERSEA
OVIPARA

••VA•••
ADVANCE
ALVAREZ
BAVARIA
BIVALVE
CAVALRY
DEVALUE
HAVANAN
HAVANAS
HAVARTI
INVACUO
INVADED
INVADER
INVADES
INVALID
JAVAMAN
LAVABOS
LAVACHE
LAVAGES
LAVAINE
LAVALSE
LEVADES
LEVATOR
LIVABLE
LOVABLE
LOVABLY
LOVAGES
MOVABLE
MOVABLY
MOVADOS
NAVAHOS
NAVAIDS
NAVAJOS
NAVARRE
NEVADAN
NOVALIS
NOVARRO
OFVALUE
PAVANES
RAVAGED
RAVAGER
RAVAGES
REVALUE
REVAMPS
RIVALED
RIVALRY
SAVABLE
SAVAGED
SAVAGER
SAVAGES
SAVALAS
SAVANAS
SAVANNA
SAVANTS
SAVARIN
UNVAGUE
UPVALUE
VIVALDI
VIVANTS
VIVARIA

••V•A••
CAVEART
CAVEATS
CAVIARE
CAVIARS
DEVIANT
DEVIATE
FIVEAAA
GAVIALS
HAVEAGO
HOVLANE
LIVEAID
OBVIATE
REVEALS

••V••A•
BIVOUAC
CAVEMAN
CAVILAT
DOVEBAR
DRVEGAS
FIVEAAA
FIVEDAY
FIVEMAN
FIVEWAY
GAVEEAR
GAVEWAY
GAVILAN
GIVEEAR
GIVEWAY
HAVANAN
HAVANAS
JAVAMAN
JUVENAL
LAVERAN
LIVEOAK
LIVESAT
LOVETAP
NAVIDAD
NAVYMAN
NEVADAN
NOVELAS
NOVENAS
NOVISAD
PIVOTAL
RAVENAL
REVISAL
REVIVAL
SAVALAS
SAVANAS
SEVENAD
SEVENAM
SEVERAL
UNVENAL
UNVITAL
UNVOCAL
VIVICAA
VIVITAR
WAVEDAT
WAVESAT

••V•••A
BAVARIA
ETVOILA
FIVEAAA
INVICTA
LAVINIA
NOVELLA
PAVLOVA
RAVENNA
REVERSA
RIVIERA
ROVETTA
SAVANNA
SEVILLA
TAVERNA
VIVARIA
VIVICAA

•••VA••
BRAVADA
BRAVADO
BUDVASE
CALVARY
CANVASS
CHEVAUX
CLAVATE
COEVALS
CORVAIR
CRAVATS
DYEVATS
ELEVATE
GALVANI
GALVANO
GERVAIS
GUEVARA
HALVAHS
HARVARD
INAVALE
MAUVAIS
MTEVANS
NARVAEZ
NIRVANA
PERVADE
PREVAIL
PRIVACY
PRIVATE
REAVAIL
ROLVAAG
SALVAGE
SELVAGE
SERVANT
SHEVATS
SLOVAKS
TORVALD
TRAVAIL
UNIVACS
VALVATE
ZHIVAGO

•••V•A•
AVIVIAN
DRIVEAT
DROVEAT
ELUVIAL
FLUVIAL
GRAVLAX
LATVIAN
NOUVEAU
PLUVIAL
PREVIAS
ROLVAAG
SERVEAS
SHAVIAN
TRIVIAL
VOUVRAY

•••V••A
BOBVILA
BRAVADA
BRAVURA
CERVEZA
CORVINA
ELEVENA
GUEVARA
HRYVNIA
ILOVELA
MALVINA
NIRVANA
RIGVEDA
VALVULA

••••VA•
ACTIVAS
ARRIVAL
BOLIVAR
BULOVAS
CARAVAN
CASAVAS
DONOVAN
ESTIVAL
EUROVAN
GENEVAN
HALAVAH
HESHVAN
KOSOVAR
MEDEVAC
MEDIVAC
MINIVAC
MINIVAN
MITZVAH
MRNOVAK
OCTAVAL
OLDUVAI
RAYOVAC
REMOVAL
REVIVAL
SALIVAS
SAMOVAR
WINEVAT
YEREVAN

••••V•A
ALLUVIA
BATAVIA
BOLIVIA
MORAVIA
OCTAVIA

SEGOVIA
TWELVEA

•••••VA
ACHIEVA
BAKLAVA
BENBOVA
CAPTIVA
CASSAVA
DASILVA
DESYLVA
FESTIVA
GINGIVA
HECKUVA
HELLUVA
KEDROVA
MARKOVA
MINERVA
MOLDOVA
OSTRAVA
PAVLOVA
POLTAVA
POPDIVA
ULANOVA
YESHIVA

VB•••••
VBLOUSE

V•B••••
VIBISTS
VIBRANT
VIBRATE
VIBRATO

V••B•••
VERBALS
VERBENA
VERBIDS
VERBIFY
VERBOSE
VONBAER

V•••B••
VENABLE
VERYBAD
VERYBIG
VISIBLE
VISIBLY
VITEBSK
VOCABLE
VOCABLY
VOLUBLE
VOLUBLY
VOTABLE

V•••••B
VAPORUB

•V••B••
EVENBET
IVTUBES
OVERBED
OVERBET
OVERBID
OVERBIG
OVERBUY
TVTABLE

•V••••B
OVERDUB

••V•B••
DOVEBAR
LAVABOS
LIVABLE
LOVABLE
LOVABLY
LOVEBUG
MOVABLE
MOVABLY
SAVABLE

••V••B•
ADVERBS
GIVENBY
REVERBS
SEVENBC

•••V•B•
DRIVEBY
DROVEBY
LEAVEBE

•••V••B
ELEVENB
PREVERB
PROVERB

••••V•B
TWELVEB

VC•••••
VCRTAPE

V•C••••
VACANCY
VACATED
VACATES
VACCARO
VACCINE
VACUITY
VACUOLE
VACUOUS
VACUUMS
VECHTEN
VECTORS
VECTRAS
VICDANA
VICENTE
VICENZA
VICEROY
VICINAL
VICIOUS
VICKERS
VICKREY
VICOMTE
VICTIMS
VICTORS
VICTORY
VICTRIX
VICTUAL
VICUNAS
VOCABLE
VOCABLY
VOCALIC
VOCALLY
VOCODER

V••C•••
VACCARO
VACCINE
VANCAMP
VELCROS
VETCHES
VINCENT
VINCULA
VISCERA
VISCOUS
VISCUSO
VNECKED
VOICERS
VOICING
VOLCANO
VOLCKER
VOUCHED
VOUCHER
VOUCHES
VULCANS

V•••C••
VANOCUR
VATICAL
VATICAN
VEHICLE
VESICLE
VIDICON
VIVICAA
VOTECHS

V••••C•
VACANCY
VALANCE
VALENCE
VANDYCK
VANEYCK
VANWYCK
VARRICK
VEENECK
VERDICT
VERRUCA
VERSACE
VIADUCT
VIATICA
VITRICS

V•••••C
VANADIC
VENATIC
VERIDIC
VINYLIC
VOCALIC
VOLTAIC

•VC••••
PVCPIPE
TVCREWS

•V•C•••
AVOCADO
AVOCETS
EVACUEE
EVICTED
EVICTEE
EVICTOR

•V••C••
EVINCED
EVINCES
KVETCHY
OVERCOY
OVERCUT

•V•••C•
AVARICE
AVIANCA
OVERACT
OVERICE
OVIDUCT
OVISACS

•V••••C
AVIATIC
AVIONIC

••V•C••
ADVICES
CEVICHE
DEVICES
DOVECOT
INVACUO
INVICTA
LAVACHE
NOVICES
UNVOCAL
VIVICAA
WAVICLE

••V••C•
ADVANCE
DAVINCI
DIVORCE
INVOICE
REVOICE
UNVOICE

••V•••C
BIVOUAC
LEVITIC
SEVENBC

•••V•C•
CONVECT
CONVICT
CREVICE
PRIVACY
REEVICT
SERVICE
UNIVACS

•••V••C
ELEVENC

••••V•C
MEDEVAC
MEDIVAC
MINIVAC
RAYOVAC
TWELVEC
UNCIVIC

V•D••••
VEDETTE
VEDISTS
VIDALIA
VIDEOED
VIDETTE
VIDICON
VIDIOTS

V••D•••
VANDALS
VANDIEN
VANDINE
VANDURA
VANDUYN
VANDYCK
VANDYKE
VATDYED
VATDYES
VAUDOIS
VEADARS
VENDEES
VENDERS
VENDING
VENDOME
VENDORS
VENDUES
VERDANT
VERDELL
VERDICT
VERDINS
VERDOUX
VERDUGO
VERDURE
VIADENT
VIADUCT
VICDANA
VIEDFOR
VOIDERS
VOIDING
VOIDOUT
VOODOOS

V•••D••
VALADON
VALIDID
VALIDLY
VANADIC
VAPIDLY
VERIDIC
VERYDRY
VEXEDLY
VIVIDER
VIVIDLY
VOCODER
VOTEDIN
VOTEDNO
VOTEDON

V••••D•
VERANDA
VERBIDS
VERYODD
VESPIDS
VIVALDI
VIVENDI

V•••••D
VACATED
VALETED
VALIDID
VANLOAD
VANWARD
VAPORED
VATDYED
VAULTED
VAUNTED
VENTRAD
VERYBAD
VERYMAD
VERYODD
VERYOLD
VERYRED
VERYSAD
VIALLED
VIDEOED
VILLARD
VINLAND
VISAGED
VISITED
VISORED
VISTAED
VIZORED
VNECKED
VOLUMED
VOLUTED
VOSKHOD
VOUCHED
VOYAGED
VROOMED
VSHAPED

•V•D•••
AVIDEST
AVIDFAN
AVIDITY
EVADERS
EVADING
EVIDENT
OVIDIAN
OVIDUCT
TVIDOLS

•V••D••
AVOIDED
AVOIDER
EVANDER
EVERDUR
OVERDID
OVERDOG
OVERDRY
OVERDUB
OVERDUE
OVERDYE
OVOIDAL
UVINDEX

•V•••D•
AVENIDA
AVOCADO
TVGUIDE

•V••••D
AVAILED
AVENGED
AVERRED
AVERTED
AVIATED
AVOIDED
AVULSED
EVERTED
EVICTED
EVINCED
EVOLVED
EVULSED
KVELLED
OVERBED
OVERBID
OVERDID
OVERFED
OVERSAD

••V•D••
CAVEDIN
DIVEDIN
DIVIDED
DIVIDER
DIVIDES
FIVEDAY
INVADED
INVADER
INVADES
LEVADES
LIVEDIN
LIVEDON
LIVIDLY
LOVEDIT
LOVEDTO
MOVADOS
MOVEDIN
MOVEDIT
MOVEDON
MOVEDTO
MOVEDUP
NAVIDAD
NEVADAN
ONVIDEO
PAVIDLY
SAVEDON
SAVEDUP
VIVIDER
VIVIDLY
WAVEDAT
WAVEDIN
WAVEDTO

••V••D•
DOVERDE
NAVAIDS
REVENDS
REVERDY
VIVALDI
VIVENDI

••V•••D
ADVISED
BEVELED
CAVILED
COVERED
COVETED
DEVILED
DEVISED
DEVOTED
DIVIDED
DIVINED
DIVVIED
FAVORED
FEVERED
GAVELED
HOVERED
INVADED
INVALID
INVITED
INVOKED
LEVELED
LEVERED
LIVEAID
LIVENED
LIVERED
NAVIDAD
NOVISAD
PIVOTED
RAVAGED
RAVELED
RAVENED
RAVINED
REVELED
REVERED
REVILED
REVISED
REVIVED
REVOKED
REVOTED
RIVALED
RIVETED
SAVAGED
SAVORED
SAVVIED
SEVENAD
SEVERED
UNVEXED
UNVIVID
UNVOTED
UNVOWED
WAVERED

•••VD••
PLOVDIV

•••V•D•
BRAVADA
BRAVADO
CERVIDS
CORVIDS
KIDVIDS
PERVADE
PROVIDE
RIGVEDA

•••V••D
BRAVOED
CHIVIED
DIVVIED
ELEVEND
HARVARD
LOUVRED
NONVOID
OUTVIED
PREVOID
PREVUED
SAVVIED
TORVALD

••••V•D
ARRIVED
BEHAVED
BELOVED
CLEAVED
DERIVED
EVOLVED
GRIEVED
GROOVED
IMPAVID
MOTIVED
RELIVED
REMOVED
REPAVED
RESAVED
REVIVED
SHEAVED
SHELVED
SLEEVED
STARVED
STEEVED
STRIVED
SWERVED
THIEVED
THRIVED
TWELVED
UNEAVED
UNGYVED
UNLAVED
UNLIVED
UNLOVED
UNMOVED
UNPAVED
UNRIVED
UNSAVED
UNVIVID
UNWAVED
UPDIVED

VE•••••
VEADARS
VEALIER
VECHTEN
VECTORS
VECTRAS
VEDETTE
VEDISTS
VEEJAYS
VEENECK
VEERIES
VEERING
VEEROFF
VEGETAL
VEGGIES
VEGGING
VEHICLE
VEIGHTS
VEILERS
VEILING
VEINIER
VEINING
VEINLET
VEINTES
VEINULE
VELCROS
VELLUMS
VELOURS
VELOUTE
VELOXES
VELTMAN
VELURES
VELVETS
VELVETY
VENABLE
VENALLY
VENATIC
VENDEES
VENDERS
VENDING
VENDOME
VENDORS
VENDUES
VENEERS
VENEMAN
VENEZIA
VENISON
VENTAGE
VENTERS
VENTING
VENTNOR
VENTRAD
VENTRAL
VENTRIS
VENTURA
VENTURE
VENTURI
VENULES
VENUSES
VERANDA
VERBALS
VERBENA
VERBIDS
VERBIFY
VERBOSE
VERDANT
VERDELL
VERDICT
VERDINS
VERDOUX
VERDUGO
VERDURE
VEREINE
VERGEON
VERGERS
VERGING
VERIDIC
VERIEST
VERISMO
VERISTS
VERITAS
VERIZON
VERMEER
VERMEIL
VERMINY
VERMONT
VERNIER
VERONIA
VERRUCA
VERSACE
VERSANT
VERSETS
VERSIFY
VERSING
VERSION
VERTIGO
VERYBAD
VERYBIG
VERYDRY
VERYFEW
VERYFIT
VERYHIP
VERYHOT
VERYILL
VERYLOW
VERYMAD
VERYNEW
VERYODD
VERYOLD
VERYRED
VERYSAD
VERYSHY
VERYWET
VESICLE
VESPERS
VESPIDS
VESSELS
VESTALS
VESTEES
VESTIGE
VESTING
VESTRAL
VESTRON
VESTURE
VETCHES
VETERAN
VETOERS
VETOING
VETTERS
VETTING
VEXEDLY

V•E••••
VEEJAYS
VEENECK
VEERIES
VEERING
VEEROFF
VIEDFOR
VIELLES
VIERNES
VIERZIG
VIESFOR
VIETNAM
VIEWERS
VIEWIER
VIEWING
VIEWITH
VNECKED

V••E•••
VALENCE
VALENTE
VALENTI
VALERIE
VALETED
VANESSA
VANEXEL
VANEYCK
VEDETTE
VEGETAL
VENEERS
VENEMAN
VENEZIA
VEREINE
VETERAN
VEXEDLY
VICENTE
VICENZA
VICEROY
VIDEOED
VIDETTE
VINEGAR
VITEBSK
VIVENDI
VIXENLY
VOLENTE
VOTEAYE
VOTECHS
VOTEDIN
VOTEDNO
VOTEDON
VOTEFOR
VOTENAY
VOTEOUT
VOTESIN
VOTESNO
VOTESON
VOTEYEA
VOTEYES
VOWELLY
VUMETER

V•••E••
VAGUELY
VAGUEST
VAINEST
VALJEAN
VALLEJO
VALLEYS
VALUERS
VAMPERS
VANPELT
VAQUERO
VARIERS
VARIETY
VARLETS
VASTEST
VEENECK
VEILERS
VELVETS
VELVETY
VENDEES
VENDERS
VENEERS
VENTERS
VERBENA
VERDELL
VERGEON
VERGERS
VERIEST
VERMEER
VERMEIL
VERSETS
VESPERS
VESSELS
VESTEES
VETOERS
VETTERS
VIADENT
VICKERS
VIEWERS
VILLEIN
VINCENT
VINIEST
VIOLENT
VIOLETS
VISCERA
VISTEON
VIZIERS
VOGUERS
VOICERS
VOIDERS
VOLLEYS
VONZELL
VOWLESS

V••••E•
VACATED
VACATES
VALETED
VALINES
VALISES
VALOREM
VAMPIER
VANDIEN
VANEXEL
VANOWEN
VAPORED
VAPORER
VARITEK
VASQUEZ
VASTIER
VATDYED
VATDYES
VAULTED
VAULTER
VAUNTED
VAUNTER
VEALIER
VECHTEN
VEERIES
VEGGIES
VEINIER
VEINLET
VEINTES
VELOXES
VELURES
VENDEES
VENDUES
VENULES
VENUSES
VERMEER
VERNIER
VERYFEW
VERYNEW
VERYRED
VERYWET
VESTEES
VETCHES
VIALLED
VICKREY
VIDEOED
VIELLES
VIERNES
VIEWIER
VINTNER
VIRTUES
VIRUSES
VISAGED
VISAGES
VISITED
VISORED

VISTAED
VITTLES
VIVIDER
VIZORED
VNECKED
VOCODER
VOLCKER
VOLUMED
VOLUMES
VOLUTED
VOLUTES
VONBAER
VONOPEL
VORSTER
VOTEYEA
VOTEYES
VOTIVES
VOUCHED
VOUCHER
VOUCHES
VOYAGED
VOYAGER
VOYAGES
VROOMED
VSHAPED
VSHAPES
VUMETER

V•••••E

VACCINE
VACUOLE
VALANCE
VALENCE
VALENTE
VALERIE
VALLONE
VALOTTE
VALUATE
VALVATE
VALVULE
VAMOOSE
VAMPIRE
VANDINE
VANDYKE
VANLINE
VANTAGE
VARIATE
VBLOUSE
VCRTAPE
VEDETTE
VEHICLE
VEINULE
VELOUTE
VENABLE
VENDOME
VENTAGE
VENTURE
VERBOSE
VERDURE
VEREINE
VERSACE
VESICLE
VESTIGE
VESTURE
VIBRATE
VICENTE
VICOMTE
VIDETTE
VILLAGE
VINROSE
VINTAGE
VIOLATE
VIOLONE
VIRGATE
VIRGULE
VISIBLE
VITIATE
VITRINE
VOCABLE
VOITURE
VOLANTE
VOLENTE
VOLPONE
VOLTAGE
VOLTORE
VOLUBLE
VONLAUE
VORLAGE
VOTABLE
VOTEAYE
VULGATE
VULPINE
VULTURE

•VE••••

AVENGED
AVENGER
AVENGES
AVENIDA
AVENUEQ
AVENUES
AVERAGE
AVERELL
AVERILL
AVERNAL
AVERNUS
AVERRED
AVERTED
AVERTER
AVESTAN
AVESTAS
AVEYRON
EVELONG
EVENBET
EVENERS
EVENEST
EVENING
EVENNOW
EVENOFF
EVENOUT
EVENPAR
EVENSUP
EVERDUR
EVEREST
EVERETT
EVERLYS
EVERTED
EVERTOR
IVERSON
KVELLED
KVETCHY
OVERACT
OVERAGE
OVERALL
OVERARM
OVERATE
OVERAWE
OVERBED
OVERBET
OVERBID
OVERBIG
OVERBUY
OVERCOY
OVERCUT
OVERDID
OVERDOG
OVERDRY
OVERDUB
OVERDUE
OVERDYE
OVEREAT
OVERFAR
OVERFAT
OVERFED
OVERFEE
OVERFEW
OVERFIT
OVERFIX
OVERFLY
OVERHOT
OVERICE
OVERJOY
OVERLAP
OVERLAX
OVERLAY
OVERLET
OVERLIE
OVERLIT
OVERMAN
OVERMIX
OVERNEW
OVERPAR
OVERPAY
OVERPLY
OVERRAN
OVERRUN
OVERSAD
OVERSAW
OVERSEA
OVERSEE
OVERSET
OVERSEW
OVERSUP
OVERTAX
OVERTIP
OVERTLY
OVERTOP
OVERUSE
OVERWET
SVELTER
SVERIGE

•V••E••

AVERELL
AVIDEST
AVOCETS
AVOWERS
EVADERS
EVENERS
EVENEST
EVEREST
EVERETT
EVIDENT
EVILEST
EVILEYE
EVOKERS
OVEREAT
TVCREWS

•V•••E•

AVAILED
AVENGED
AVENGER
AVENGES
AVENUEQ
AVENUES
AVERRED
AVERTED
AVERTER
AVGASES
AVIATED
AVIATES
AVOIDED
AVOIDER
AVONLEA
AVULSED
AVULSES
EVACUEE
EVANDER
EVANGEL
EVENBET
EVERTED
EVICTED
EVICTEE
EVILLER
EVINCED
EVINCES
EVOLVED
EVOLVER
EVOLVES
EVULSED
EVULSES
IVORIES
IVTUBES
KVASSES
KVELLED
OVARIES
OVERBED
OVERBET
OVERFED
OVERFEE
OVERFEW
OVERLET
OVERNEW
OVERSEA
OVERSEE
OVERSET
OVERSEW
OVERWET
RVALUES
SVELTER
TVGAMES
TVTAPES
UVALUES
UVINDEX

•V••••E

AVARICE
AVERAGE
EVACUEE
EVASIVE
EVICTEE
EVILEYE
EVILONE
EVOLUTE
IVANHOE
IVORINE
IVYLIKE
OVERAGE
OVERATE
OVERAWE
OVERDUE
OVERDYE
OVERFEE
OVERICE
OVERLIE
OVERSEE
OVERUSE
PVCPIPE
SVERIGE
TVGUIDE
TVMOVIE
TVTABLE

••VE•••

ADVENTS
ADVERBS
ADVERSE
ADVERTS
ALVEOLI
BEVELED
BEVELER
BEVERLY
CAVEART
CAVEATS
CAVEDIN
CAVEINS
CAVEMAN
CAVEMEN
CAVERNS
CAVESIN
COVERED
COVERER
COVERME
COVERTS
COVERUP
COVETED
COVETER
CUVETTE
DAVEKOZ
DEVEINS
DEVELOP
DEVESTS
DIVEDIN
DIVERGE
DIVERSE
DIVERTS
DIVESIN
DIVESTS
DOVEBAR
DOVECOT
DOVELET
DOVERDE
DRVEGAS
ENVEILS
ENVELOP
ENVENOM
FEVERED
FIVEAAA
FIVEDAY
FIVEEEE
FIVEMAN
FIVEONE
FIVEPIN
FIVESIX
FIVETEN
FIVETWO
FIVEWAY
GAVEEAR
GAVELED
GAVEOFF
GAVEOUT
GAVEWAY
GIVEEAR
GIVENBY
GIVENIN
GIVENOF
GIVENON
GIVENTO
GIVENUP
GIVEOFF
GIVEOUT
GIVESIN
GIVESOF
GIVESON
GIVESTO
GIVESUP
GIVEUPS
GIVEWAY
GOVERNS
HAVEAGO
HAVEFUN
HAVENER
HAVENOT
HAVEONE
HAVEOUT
HIVEOFF
HOVERED
HOVERER
INVEIGH
INVENTS
INVERSE
INVERTS
INVESTS
JAVELIN
JUVENAL
LAVELLI
LAVERAN
LAVERNE
LEVELED
LEVELER
LEVELLY
LEVERED
LEVERET
LIVEAID
LIVEDIN
LIVEDON
LIVEFOR
LIVENED
LIVENER
LIVENUP
LIVEOAK
LIVEONE
LIVEOUT
LIVERED
LIVESAT
LIVESET
LIVESEY
LIVESIN
LIVESON
LOVEBUG
LOVEDIT
LOVEDTO
LOVEINS
LOVEJOY
LOVERLY
LOVESET
LOVESIT
LOVESTO
LOVETAP
LOVEYOU
MOVEDIN
MOVEDIT
MOVEDON
MOVEDTO
MOVEDUP
MOVEOFF
MOVEOUT
MOVESIN
MOVESIT
MOVESON
MOVESTO
MOVESUP
NIVEOUS
NOVELAS
NOVELLA
NOVELLE
NOVELLO
NOVELTY
NOVENAS
OBVERSE
OBVERTS
POVERTY
RAVELED
RAVELLY
RAVELOE
RAVENAL
RAVENED
RAVENNA
RAVEUPS
REVEALS
REVELED
REVELER
REVELIN
REVELRY
REVENDS
REVENGE
REVENUE
REVERBS
REVERDY
REVERED
REVERER
REVERES
REVERIE
REVERSA
REVERSE
REVERTS
REVESTS
RIVERPO
RIVETED
RIVETER
ROVETTA
SAVEDON
SAVEDUP
SAVEFOR
SAVESON
SAVESUP
SEVENAD
SEVENAM
SEVENBC
SEVENEE
SEVENNO
SEVENPM
SEVENTH
SEVENTY
SEVENUP
SEVERAL
SEVERED
SEVERER
SEVERUS
TAVERNA
TAVERNS
UNVEILS
UNVENAL
UNVEXED
VIVENDI
WAVEDAT
WAVEDIN
WAVEDTO
WAVELET
WAVEOFF
WAVERED
WAVERER
WAVESAT
WAVESIN
WAVESTO
WYVERNS

••V•E••

ENVIERS
FIVEEEE
GAVEEAR
GIVEEAR
JIVIEST
LEVIERS
ORVIETO
REVIEWS
RIVIERA
RIVIERE
SOVIETS
WAVIEST
XAVIERU
YEVGENY

••V••E•

ADVICES
ADVISED
ADVISEE
ADVISER
ADVISES
ALVAREZ
BEVELED
BEVELER
BOVINES
CAVEMEN
CAVILED
CAVILER
CIVVIES
COVERED
COVERER
COVETED
COVETER
DEVICES
DEVILED
DEVISED
DEVISEE
DEVISER
DEVISES
DEVORES
DEVOTED
DEVOTEE
DEVOTES
DEVRIES
DIVIDED
DIVIDER
DIVIDES
DIVINED
DIVINER
DIVINES
DIVVIED
DIVVIES
DOVELET
FAVORED
FAVORER
FEVERED
FEVRIER
FIVEEEE
FIVETEN
GAVELED
HAVENER
HOVERED
HOVERER
INVADED
INVADER
INVADES
INVITED
INVITEE
INVITER
INVITES
INVOKED
INVOKER
INVOKES
LAVAGES
LEVADES
LEVELED
LEVELER
LEVERED
LEVERET
LEVITES
LIVENED
LIVENER
LIVERED
LIVESET
LIVESEY
LOVAGES
LOVESET
MAVISES
NAVYMEN
NOVICES
NOVOTES
ONVIDEO
PAVANES
PIVOTED
PIVOTER
RAVAGED
RAVAGER
RAVAGES
RAVELED
RAVENED
RAVINED
RAVINES
REVELED
REVELER
REVERED
REVERER
REVERES
REVILED
REVILER
REVILES
REVISED
REVISER
REVISES
REVIVED
REVIVER
REVIVES
REVOKED
REVOKER
REVOKES
REVOTED
REVOTES
RIVALED
RIVETED
RIVETER
RIVULET
SAVAGED
SAVAGER
SAVAGES
SAVORED
SAVORER
SAVVIED
SAVVIER
SAVVIES
SEVENEE
SEVERED
SEVERER
UNVEXED
UNVOTED
UNVOWED
VIVIDER
WAVELET
WAVERED
WAVERER

••V•••E

ADVANCE
ADVERSE
ADVISEE
BIVALVE
CAVIARE
CEVICHE
COVERME
CUVETTE
DEVALUE
DEVIATE
DEVILLE
DEVISEE
DEVOLVE
DEVOTEE
DIVERGE
DIVERSE
DIVORCE
DIVULGE
DIVULSE
DOVERDE
ENVOGUE
FIVEEEE
FIVEONE
GAVOTTE
HAVEONE
HOVLANE
INVERSE
INVITEE
INVOGUE
INVOICE
INVOLVE
LAVACHE
LAVAINE
LAVALSE
LAVERNE
LIVABLE
LIVEONE
LOVABLE
MOVABLE
NAVARRE
NEVILLE
NOVELLE
OBVERSE
OBVIATE
OFVALUE
ORVILLE
RAVELOE
REVALUE
REVENGE
REVENUE
REVERIE
REVERSE
REVOICE
REVOLVE
RIVIERE
SAVABLE
SEVENEE
SEVILLE
UNVAGUE
UNVOICE
UPVALUE
WAVICLE

•••VE••

AIRVENT
ALEVELS
ALIVETO
BEAVERS
BRAVELY
BRAVERY
BRAVEST
BREVETS
CALVERT
CARVELS
CARVERS
CERVEZA
CHEVETS
CLAVELL
CLOVERS
CLOVERY
CONVECT
CONVENE
CONVENT
CONVERT
CONVEYS
CORVEES
CRAVENS
CRAVERS
CULVERT
CURVETS
DANVERS
DELVERS
DOGVEST
DOOVERS
DRIVEAT
DRIVEBY
DRIVEIN
DRIVELS
DRIVERS
DRIVETO
DRIVEUP
DROVEAT
DROVEBY
DROVEIN
DROVERS
DROVETO
DROVEUP
ELEVENA
ELEVENB
ELEVENC
ELEVEND
ELEVENE
ELEVENS
FERVENT
GRAVELS
GRAVELY
GRAVERS
GRAVEST
GROVELS
GROVERS
HALVERS
HARVEST
HEAVEHO
HEAVENS
HEAVERS
HEAVETO
HOOVERS
HUMVEES
IGIVEUP
IHAVEIT
ILOVEIT
ILOVELA
JAYVEES
KNAVERY
LEAVEBE
LEAVEIN
LEAVEIT
LEAVENS
LEAVEON
LOUVERS
MARVELL
MARVELS
NAIVELY
NAIVEST
NAIVETE
NAIVETY
NOUVEAU
OLEVELS
PARVENU
PLOVERS
PREVENT
PREVERB
PREVERT
PREVETO
PRIVETS
PROVEIT
PROVERB
PROVERS
PURVEYS
QUAVERS
QUAVERY
QUIVERS
QUIVERY
REAVERS
RIGVEDA
SALVERS
SERVEAS
SERVERS
SERVEUP
SHAVERS
SHIVERS
SHIVERY
SHOVEIN
SHOVELS
SHOVERS
SILVERS
SILVERY
SKIVEST
SLAVERS
SLAVERY
SLIVERS
SLOVENE
SLOVENS
SNIVELS
SOLVEIT
SOLVENT
SOLVERS
STEVENS
SUAVELY
SUAVEST
SUBVENE
SUBVERT
SURVEIL
SURVEYS
SWIVELS
SWIVETS
TEEVEES
TRAVELS
TRAVERS
TRIVETS
UNOVERT
VELVETS
VELVETY
WAIVERS
WARVETS
WEAVERS

•••V•E•

BMOVIES
BOUVIER
BRAVOED
BRAVOES
CHEVRES
CHEVRET
CHIVIED
CHIVIES
CIVVIES
CLAVIER
CORVEES
CURVIER
DIMVIEW
DIVVIED
DIVVIES
FLIVVER
GRAVIES
HDTVSET
HEAVIER
HEAVIES
HUMVEES
JANVIER

JAYVEES
LOUVRED
LOUVRES
MARVIER
NARVAEZ
NERVIER
OEUVRES
OLIVIER
OUTVIED
OUTVIES
POIVRES
PREVIEW
PREVUED
PREVUES
PRIVIER
PRIVIES
PURVIEW
SALVOES
SAVVIED
SAVVIER
SAVVIES
TEEVEES
THEVIEW

•••V••E
BUDVASE
CERVINE
CLAVATE
CONVENE
CONVOKE
CORVINE
CREVICE
ELEVATE
ELEVENE
GLAVINE
GRAVURE
INAVALE
LEAVEBE
NAIVETE
NERVINE
NERVULE
OLIVINE
ONEVOTE
OUTVOTE
PERVADE
PRIVATE
PROVIDE
PROVINE
PROVOKE
QUIVIVE
REEVOKE
SALVAGE
SELVAGE
SERVICE
SERVILE
SLOVENE
SUBVENE
SURVIVE
VALVATE
VALVULE
YESVOTE

••••VE•
ACTIVES
ALCOVES
ALLOVER
ANDOVER
AQUIVER
ARRIVED
ARRIVER
ARRIVES
ASHIVER
ASKOVER
ATEOVER
ATSEVEN
BEHAVED
BEHAVES
BELEVEN
BELOVED
BILEVEL
BYFIVES
CADAVER
CARAVEL
CHARVET
CHEEVER
CLEAVED
CLEAVER
CLEAVES
CRYOVER
CUTOVER
DATIVES
DEHAVEN
DELIVER
DERIVED
DERIVER
DERIVES
DIDOVER
DWARVES
EATOVER
ENDIVES
ENLIVEN
ESTEVEZ
EVOLVED
EVOLVER
EVOLVES
EXWIVES
FLIVVER
FLYOVER
FOREVER
GASOVEN
GETEVEN
GETOVER
GOTEVEN
GOTOVER
GREAVES
GRIEVED
GRIEVER
GRIEVES
GROOVED
GROOVES
HADOVER
HANOVER
HASOVER
HOPOVER
HOTOVER
HOWEVER
ICEOVER
INFIVES
INWOVEN
ITSOVER
KNIEVEL
LAYOVER
LIEOVER
MCCOVEY
MINIVER
MISAVER
MOHAVES
MOJAVES
MOTIVED
MOTIVES
NATIVES
NINEVEH
NONEVER
NOTEVEN
NOTEVER
NOTOVER
OCTAVES
ONEOVER
PALAVER
POPOVER
PORIVER
PREAVER
PUTOVER
RANOVER
RECOVER
REGIVEN
REGIVES
RELEVEL
RELEVER
RELEVES
RELIVED
RELIVES
REMOVED
REMOVER
REMOVES
REPAVED
REPAVES
RESAVED
RESAVES
REVIVED
REVIVER
REVIVES
REWOVEN
RUNOVER
SAYOVER
SCARVES
SCURVES
SHEAVED
SHEAVES
SHELVED
SHELVER
SHELVES
SHRIVEL
SHRIVER
SHRIVES
SLEEVED
SLEEVES
SOHAVEI
STARVED
STARVES
STEEVED
STEEVES
STRIVED
STRIVEN
STRIVER
STRIVES
SWERVED
SWERVES
THIEVED
THIEVES
THRIVED
THRIVEN
THRIVER
THRIVES
TIPOVER
TWELVEA
TWELVEB
TWELVEC
TWELVED
TWELVEE
TWELVES
UNCOVER
UNEAVED
UNGIVEN
UNGYVED
UNLAVED
UNLEVEL
UNLIVED
UNLIVES
UNLOVED
UNMOVED
UNNOVEL
UNPAVED
UNRAVEL
UNRIVED
UNRIVEN
UNSAVED
UNWAVED
UNWOVEN
UPDIVED
UPDIVES
UPRIVER
VOTIVES
WHARVES
WHOEVER
WHYEVER
WINOVER
WONOVER

••••V•E
DOEUVRE
LEHAVRE
TVMOVIE
TWELVEE

•••••VE
ABSOLVE
ABUSIVE
ACHIEVE
ACTFIVE
AGEFIVE
AIRWAVE
ALGARVE
AMATIVE
APPROVE
ARCHIVE
BADLOVE
BADMOVE
BEBRAVE
BEEHIVE
BEHOOVE
BELIEVE
BEREAVE
BIGFIVE
BIGLOVE
BIVALVE
BTWELVE
CAPTIVE
COMMOVE
CONCAVE
CONNIVE
COSTIVE
CURSIVE
DECEIVE
DENEUVE
DEPRAVE
DEPRIVE
DESERVE
DEVOLVE
ELUSIVE
EMOTIVE
ENCLAVE
ENGRAVE
ENSLAVE
EROSIVE
EVASIVE
EXCLAVE
FESTIVE
FICTIVE
FORGAVE
FORGIVE
FORLOVE
FURTIVE
GUSTAVE
IAMLOVE
ICECAVE
ILLLIVE
IMPROVE
INCURVE
INNERVE
INVOLVE
INWEAVE
ITSLOVE
ITWELVE
KHEDIVE
LETHAVE
LETLIVE
LOWDIVE
MALDIVE
MASSIVE
MISGAVE
MISGIVE
MISMOVE
MISSIVE
NBALIVE
NEWLOVE
NEWWAVE
NONLIVE
NOTLIVE
OBSERVE
ONELOVE
ONLEAVE
ONSERVE
OUTGAVE
OUTGIVE
OUTLIVE
OUTLOVE
OUTMOVE
OUTRAVE
OUTROVE
OUTWAVE
PARFIVE
PARKAVE
PASSIVE
PENSIVE
PETDOVE
PLOSIVE
PREDIVE
PREPAVE
QUIVIVE
RECARVE
RECEIVE
RECURVE
REDFIVE
REDRIVE
RELIEVE
REPROVE
RESERVE
RESHAVE
RESOLVE
RESTIVE
REVOLVE
REWEAVE
SIXFIVE
SKYDIVE
SUASIVE
SURVIVE
TENSIVE
THEFIVE
THEWAVE
TOPFIVE
TUSSIVE
UNBRAVE
UNGLOVE
UNITIVE
UNNAIVE
UNNERVE
UNWEAVE
UPABOVE
UPCURVE
UPHEAVE
WHEREVE

VF•••••
VFWHALL
VFWPOST

V••F•••
VATFULS

V•••F••
VERYFEW
VERYFIT
VIALFUL
VIEDFOR
VIESFOR
VOTEFOR

V••••F•
VEEROFF
VERBIFY
VERSIFY
VITRIFY

V•••••F
VEEROFF

•V•F•••
OVIFORM

•V••F••
AVIDFAN
OVERFAR
OVERFAT
OVERFED
OVERFEE
OVERFEW
OVERFIT
OVERFIX
OVERFLY

•V•••F•
EVENOFF

•V••••F
EVENOFF

••V•F••
HAVEFUN
LIVEFOR
SAVEFOR

••V••F•
GAVEOFF
GIVEOFF
HIVEOFF
MOVEOFF
WAVEOFF

••V•••F
GAVEOFF
GIVENOF
GIVEOFF
GIVESOF
HIVEOFF
MOVEOFF
WAVEOFF

V•G••••
VAGRANT
VAGUELY
VAGUEST
VEGETAL
VEGGIES
VEGGING
VIGNOLA
VIGOURS
VOGUERS
VOGUING
VOGUISH

V••G•••
VANGOGH
VAUGHAN
VEGGIES
VEGGING
VEIGHTS
VERGEON
VERGERS
VERGING
VIRGATE
VIRGINS
VIRGOAN
VIRGULE
VOSGIAN
VULGATE

V•••G••
VINEGAR
VIRAGOS
VISAGED
VISAGES
VOYAGED
VOYAGER
VOYAGES

V••••G•
VANGOGH
VANTAGE
VANVOGT
VENTAGE
VERDUGO
VERTIGO
VESTIGE
VIKINGS
VILLAGE
VINTAGE
VOLTAGE
VORLAGE

V•••••G
VALUING
VAMPING
VANNING
VARYING
VATTING
VEERING
VEGGING
VEILING
VEINING
VENDING
VENTING
VERGING
VERSING
VERYBIG
VESTING
VETOING
VETTING
VIALING
VIERZIG
VIEWING
VISAING
VOGUING
VOICING
VOIDING

•VG••••
AVGASES
TVGAMES
TVGUIDE

•V•G•••
AVIGNON

•V••G••
AVENGED
AVENGER
AVENGES
EVANGEL

•V•••G•
AVERAGE
OVERAGE
SVERIGE

•V••••G
AVOWING
EVADING
EVELONG
EVENING
EVOKING
OVERBIG
OVERDOG

••VG•••
YEVGENY

••V•G••
DRVEGAS
ENVOGUE
INVOGUE
LAVAGES
LOVAGES
RAVAGED
RAVAGER
RAVAGES
SAVAGED
SAVAGER
SAVAGES
SEVIGNY
UNVAGUE

••V••G•
DIVERGE
DIVULGE
HAVEAGO
INVEIGH
LIVINGS
PAVINGS
RAVINGS
REVENGE
ROVINGS
SAVINGS

••V•••G
ENVYING
LEVYING
LOVEBUG
REVVING
RSVPING
UNVYING

•••V•G•
SALVAGE
SELVAGE
VANVOGT
ZHIVAGO

•••V••G
BRAVING
CALVING
CARVING
CRAVING
CURVING
DELVING
DRIVING
GLOVING
GRAVING
HALVING
HEAVING
LEAVING
NERVING
PEEVING
PROVING
REAVING
REEVING
REVVING
ROLVAAG
SALVING
SERVING
SHAVING
SHOVING
SIEVING
SLAVING
SOLVING
STAVING
WAIVING
WEAVING

V•H••••
VEHICLE
VIHARAS
VSHAPED
VSHAPES

V••H•••
VECHTEN
VFWHALL

V•••H••
VAUGHAN
VEIGHTS
VERYHIP
VERYHOT
VETCHES
VOSKHOD
VOUCHED
VOUCHER
VOUCHES

V••••H•
VERYSHY
VOTECHS

V•••••H
VAMPISH
VANGOGH
VARNISH
VIEWITH
VOGUISH

•V•H•••
TVSHOWS

•V••H••
IVANHOE
OVERHOT

•V•••H•
KVETCHY

•V••••H
EVANISH

••V•H••
NAVAHOS

••V••H•
CEVICHE
LAVACHE

••V•••H
INVEIGH
SEVENTH

•••V•H•
HALVAHS
HEAVEHO

•••V••H
DERVISH
KNAVISH
PEEVISH
SLAVISH

••••V•H
HALAVAH
MITZVAH
NINEVEH

VI•••••
VIADENT
VIADUCT
VIALFUL
VIALING
VIALLED
VIATICA
VIBISTS
VIBRANT
VIBRATE
VIBRATO
VICDANA
VICENTE
VICENZA
VICEROY
VICINAL
VICIOUS
VICKERS
VICKREY
VICOMTE
VICTIMS
VICTORS
VICTORY
VICTRIX
VICTUAL
VICUNAS
VIDALIA
VIDEOED
VIDETTE
VIDICON
VIDIOTS
VIEDFOR
VIELLES
VIERNES
VIERZIG
VIESFOR
VIETNAM
VIEWERS
VIEWIER
VIEWING
VIEWITH
VIGNOLA
VIGOURS
VIHARAS
VIKINGS
VILLAGE
VILLAIN
VILLARD
VILLARI
VILLEIN
VILNIUS
VIMINAL
VINCENT
VINCULA
VINEGAR
VINIEST
VINLAND
VINROSE
VINTAGE
VINTNER
VINYLIC
VIOLATE
VIOLENT
VIOLETS
VIOLINS
VIOLIST
VIOLONE
VIRAGOS
VIRGATE
VIRGINS
VIRGOAN
VIRGULE
VIRTUAL
VIRTUES
VIRUSES
VISAGED
VISAGES
VISAING
VISALIA
VISAVIS
VISAYAN
VISCERA
VISCOUS
VISCUSO
VISIBLE
VISIBLY
VISIONS
VISITED
VISITOR
VISORED
VISTAED
VISTEON
VISTULA
VISUALS
VITALIS
VITALLY
VITAMIN
VITARAS
VITEBSK
VITIATE
VITORIA
VITRICS
VITRIFY
VITRINE
VITRIOL
VITTLES
VIVALDI
VIVANTS
VIVARIA
VIVENDI
VIVICAA
VIVIDER
VIVIDLY
VIVITAR
VIXENLY
VIZIERS
VIZORED
VIZSLAS

V•I••••
VAINEST
VEIGHTS
VEILERS
VEILING
VEINIER
VEINING
VEINLET
VEINTES
VEINULE
VOICERS
VOICING
VOIDERS
VOIDING
VOIDOUT
VOITURE
VUITTON

V••I•••
VALIANT
VALIDID
VALIDLY
VALINES
VALISES
VANILLA
VANILLI
VAPIDLY
VARIANT
VARIATE
VARIERS
VARIETY
VARIOUS
VARITEK
VATICAL
VATICAN
VEDISTS
VEHICLE
VENISON
VERIDIC
VERIEST
VERISMO
VERISTS
VERITAS
VERIZON
VESICLE
VIBISTS
VICINAL
VICIOUS
VIDICON
VIDIOTS
VIKINGS
VIMINAL
VINIEST
VISIBLE
VISIBLY
VISIONS
VISITED
VISITOR
VITIATE
VIVICAA
VIVIDER
VIVIDLY
VIVITAR
VIZIERS
VOTIVES

V•••I••
VACCINE
VACUITY
VALMIKI
VALUING
VAMPIER
VAMPING
VAMPIRA

VAMPIRE
VAMPISH
VANDIEN
VANDINE
VANLINE
VANNING
VANRIJN
VARMINT
VARNISH
VARRICK
VARSITY
VARYING
VASTIER
VASTITY
VATTING
VEALIER
VEERIES
VEERING
VEGGIES
VEGGING
VEILING
VEINIER
VEINING
VENDING
VENTING
VERBIDS
VERBIFY
VERDICT
VERDINS
VEREINE
VERGING
VERMINY
VERNIER
VERSIFY
VERSING
VERSION
VERTIGO
VERYILL
VESPIDS
VESTIGE
VESTING
VETOING
VETTING
VIALING
VIATICA
VICTIMS
VIEWIER
VIEWING
VIEWITH
VILNIUS
VIOLINS
VIOLIST
VIRGINS
VISAING
VITRICS
VITRIFY
VITRINE
VITRIOL
VOGUING
VOGUISH
VOICING
VOIDING
VOSGIAN
VULPINE

V••••I•

VALERIE
VALIDID
VANADIC
VAUDOIS
VENATIC
VENEZIA
VENTRIS
VERIDIC
VERMEIL
VERONIA
VERYBIG
VERYFIT
VERYHIP
VICTRIX
VIDALIA
VIERZIG
VILLAIN
VILLEIN
VINYLIC
VISALIA
VISAVIS
VITALIS
VITAMIN
VITORIA
VIVARIA
VOCALIC
VOLTAIC
VOTEDIN
VOTESIN

V•••••I

VALENTI
VALMIKI
VANILLI
VENTURI
VILLARI
VIVALDI
VIVENDI

•VI••••

AVIANCA
AVIATED
AVIATES
AVIATIC
AVIATOR
AVIDEST
AVIDFAN
AVIDITY
AVIGNON
AVIONIC
AVIVIAN
EVICTED
EVICTEE
EVICTOR
EVIDENT
EVILEST
EVILEYE
EVILLER
EVILONE
EVINCED
EVINCES
OVIDIAN
OVIDUCT
OVIFORM
OVIPARA
OVISACS
TVIDOLS
UVINDEX

•V•I•••

AVAILED
AVOIDED
AVOIDER
OVOIDAL

•V••I••

AVARICE
AVENIDA
AVERILL
AVIDITY
AVIVIAN
AVOWING
EVADING
EVANISH
EVASION
EVASIVE
EVENING
EVOKING
IVANIII
IVORIAN
IVORIES
IVORINE
IVYLIKE
OVARIES
OVATION
OVERICE
OVIDIAN
PVCPIPE
SVERIGE
TVGUIDE

•V•••I•

AVANTIS
AVIATIC
AVIONIC
IVANIII
OVERBID
OVERBIG
OVERDID
OVERFIT
OVERFIX
OVERLIE
OVERLIT
OVERMIX
OVERTIP
TVMOVIE

•V••••I

IVANIII

••VI•••

ADVICES
ADVISED
ADVISEE
ADVISER
ADVISES
ADVISOR
BOVINES
CAVIARE
CAVIARS
CAVILAT
CAVILED
CAVILER
CEVICHE
CIVILLY
DAVINCI
DAVISON
DEVIANT
DEVIATE
DEVICES
DEVILED
DEVILLE
DEVILRY
DEVIOUS
DEVISED
DEVISEE
DEVISER
DEVISES
DEVISOR
DIVIDED
DIVIDER
DIVIDES
DIVINED
DIVINER
DIVINES
DIVISOR
ENVIERS
ENVIOUS
ENVIRON
ENVIROS
GAVIALS
GAVILAN
INVICTA
INVITED
INVITEE
INVITER
INVITES
INVITRO
JIVIEST
LAVINIA
LEVIERS
LEVILLI
LEVITES
LEVITIC
LIVIDLY
LIVINGS
MAVISES
NAVIDAD
NEVILLE
NOVICES
NOVISAD
OBVIATE
OBVIOUS
ONVIDEO
ORVIETO
ORVILLE
PAVIDLY
PAVINGS
PAVIORS
PAVIOUR
RAVINED
RAVINES
RAVINGS
RAVIOLI
REVIEWS
REVILED
REVILER
REVILES
REVISAL
REVISED
REVISER
REVISES
REVISIT
REVISOR
REVITUP
REVIVAL
REVIVED
REVIVER
REVIVES
RIVIERA
RIVIERE
ROVINGS
SAVINGS
SAVIORS
SAVIOUR
SEVIGNY
SEVILLA
SEVILLE
SOVIETS
UNVITAL
UNVIVID
VIVICAA
VIVIDER
VIVIDLY
VIVITAR
WAVICLE
WAVIEST
XAVIERU

••V•I••

CAVEINS
CIVVIES
DEVEINS
DEVOIRS
DEVRIES
DIVVIED
DIVVIES
ENVEILS
ENVYING
ETVOILA
FEVRIER
INVEIGH
INVOICE
LAVAINE
LEVYING
LOVEINS
NAVAIDS
REVOICE
REVVING
RSVPING
SAVVIED
SAVVIER
SAVVIES
SAVVILY
UNVEILS
UNVOICE
UNVYING

••V••I•

BAVARIA
CAVEDIN
CAVESIN
DIVEDIN
DIVESIN
FIVEPIN
FIVESIX
GIVENIN
GIVESIN
INVALID
JAVELIN
LAVINIA
LAVORIS
LEVITIC
LIVEAID
LIVEDIN
LIVESIN
LOVEDIT
LOVESIT
MOVEDIN
MOVEDIT
MOVESIN
MOVESIT
NOVALIS
REVELIN
REVERIE
REVISIT
SAVARIN
UNVIVID
VIVARIA
WAVEDIN
WAVESIN

••V•••I

ALVEOLI
DAVINCI
HAVARTI
LAVELLI
LEVILLI
RAVIOLI
VIVALDI
VIVENDI

•••VI••

ATAVISM
ATAVIST
AVIVIAN
BMOVIES
BOBVILA
BOUVIER
BRAVING
BREVITY
CALVING
CALVINO
CARVING
CERVIDS
CERVINE
CHEVIOT
CHIVIED
CHIVIES
CIVVIES
CLAVIER
CONVICT
CORVIDS
CORVINA
CORVINE
CRAVING
CREVICE
CURVIER
CURVING
DELVING
DERVISH
DIMVIEW
DIVVIED
DIVVIES
DRIVING
ELUVIAL
ELUVIUM
FAUVISM
FAUVIST
FLAVIUS
FLUVIAL
GLAVINE
GLOVING
GRAVIES
GRAVING
GRAVITY
HALVING
HEAVIER
HEAVIES
HEAVILY
HEAVING
HORVITZ
JANVIER
KELVINS
KIDVIDS
KNAVISH
LANVINS
LATVIAN
LEAVING
LEOVIII
MALVINA
MARVIER
NERVIER
NERVILY
NERVINE
NERVING
OLAVIII
OLIVIER
OLIVINE
OUTVIED
OUTVIES
PEEVING
PEEVISH
PLUVIAL
PREVIAS
PREVIEW
PRIVIER
PRIVIES
PRIVILY
PRIVITY
PROVIDE
PROVINE
PROVING
PROVISO
PURVIEW
QUIVIVE
REAVING
REEVICT
REEVING
REVVING
SALVING
SAVVIED
SAVVIER
SAVVIES
SAVVILY
SERVICE
SERVILE
SERVING
SHAVIAN
SHAVING
SHOVING
SIEVING
SLAVING
SLAVISH
SOLVING
SORVINO
STAVING
SUAVITY
SURVIVE
THEVIEW
THEVIPS
TORVILL
TREVINO
TRIVIAL
TRIVIOT
TRIVIUM
WAIVING
WEAVING
WEEVILS

•••V•I•

BELVOIR
BERVOIX
CORVAIR
DRIVEIN
DROVEIN
GERVAIS
HRYVNIA
IHAVEIT
ILOVEIT
LEAVEIN
LEAVEIT
LEOVIII
MAUVAIS
NONVOID
OLAVIII
PLOVDIV
PREVAIL
PREVOID
PROVEIT
REAVAIL
RENVOIS
SHOVEIN
SOLVEIT
SURVEIL
TRAVAIL

•••V••I

GALVANI
LEOVIII
OLAVIII

••••VI•

ALDAVIS
ALLUVIA
AQUAVIT
BATAVIA
BEDEVIL
BOLIVIA
BOOKVII
CHERVIL
DUUMVIR
GODEVIL
GROOVIN
IMPAVID
INCIVIL
JOHNVII
MARKVII
MCGAVIN
MORAVIA
NONEVIL
OCTAVIA
OCTAVIO
OTTAVIO
PIUSVII
SEGOVIA
TELAVIV
TVMOVIE
UNCIVIC
UNCIVIL
UNVIVID
VISAVIS

••••V•I

BOOKVII
JOHNVII
MARKVII
OLDUVAI
PIUSVII
SOHAVEI

•••••VI

BONJOVI
HENRYVI
JAMESVI
JOHNXVI
LOUISVI
MONDAVI
PAHLAVI
PECCAVI
SCENEVI
URBANVI

V••J•••

VALJEAN
VEEJAYS

V••••J•

VALLEJO
VANRIJN

•V••J••

OVERJOY

••V•J••

LOVEJOY
NAVAJOS

V•K••••

VIKINGS

V••K•••

VICKERS
VICKREY
VOSKHOD

V•••K••

VNECKED
VOLCKER

V••••K•

VALMIKI
VANDYKE
VRONSKY

V•••••K

VANDYCK
VANEYCK
VANWYCK
VARITEK
VARRICK
VEENECK
VITEBSK

•V•K•••

EVOKERS
EVOKING

•V•••K•

IVYLIKE
RVPARKS

••V•K••

DAVEKOZ
INVOKED
INVOKER
INVOKES
REVOKED
REVOKER
REVOKES

••V•••K

LIVEOAK

•••V•K•

CONVOKE
PROVOKE
REEVOKE
SLOVAKS

••••V•K

LITOVSK
MRNOVAK

V•L••••

VALADON
VALANCE
VALENCE
VALENTE
VALENTI
VALERIE
VALETED
VALIANT
VALIDID
VALIDLY
VALINES
VALISES
VALJEAN
VALLEJO
VALLEYS
VALLONE
VALMIKI
VALOREM
VALOTTE
VALOURS
VALUATE
VALUERS
VALUING
VALVATE
VALVULA
VALVULE
VBLOUSE
VELCROS
VELLUMS
VELOURS
VELOUTE
VELOXES
VELTMAN
VELURES
VELVETS
VELVETY
VILLAGE
VILLAIN
VILLARD
VILLARI
VILLEIN
VILNIUS
VOLANTE
VOLCANO
VOLCKER
VOLENTE
VOLLEYS
VOLPONE
VOLTAGE
VOLTAIC
VOLTORE
VOLUBLE
VOLUBLY
VOLUMED
VOLUMES
VOLUTED
VOLUTES
VULCANS
VULGATE
VULPINE
VULTURE

V••L•••

VALLEJO
VALLEYS
VALLONE
VANLINE
VANLOAD
VARLAAM
VARLETS
VAULTED
VAULTER
VEALIER
VEILERS
VEILING
VELLUMS
VIALFUL
VIALING
VIALLED
VIELLES
VILLAGE
VILLAIN
VILLARD
VILLARI
VILLEIN
VINLAND
VIOLATE
VIOLENT
VIOLETS
VIOLINS
VIOLIST
VIOLONE
VOLLEYS
VONLAUE
VORLAGE
VOWLESS

V•••L••

VANILLA
VANILLI
VEINLET
VENALLY
VENULES
VERYLOW
VIALLED
VIDALIA
VIELLES
VINYLIC
VISALIA
VITALIS
VITALLY
VITTLES
VIVALDI
VIZSLAS
VOCALIC
VOCALLY
VOWELLY

V••••L•

VACUOLE
VAGUELY
VALIDLY
VALVULA
VALVULE
VANDALS
VANILLA
VANILLI
VANPELT
VAPIDLY
VASSALS
VATFULS
VEHICLE
VEINULE
VENABLE
VENALLY
VERBALS
VERDELL
VERYILL
VERYOLD
VESICLE
VESSELS
VESTALS
VEXEDLY
VFWHALL
VIGNOLA
VINCULA
VIRGULE
VISIBLE
VISIBLY
VISTULA
VISUALS
VITALLY
VIVIDLY
VIXENLY
VOCABLE
VOCABLY
VOCALLY
VOLUBLE
VOLUBLY
VONZELL
VOTABLE
VOWELLY

V•••••L

VANEXEL
VANPOOL
VATICAL
VEGETAL
VENTRAL
VERDELL
VERMEIL
VERYILL
VESTRAL
VFWHALL
VIALFUL
VICINAL
VICTUAL
VIMINAL
VIRTUAL
VITRIOL
VONOPEL
VONZELL

•V•L•••

AVALONS
AVULSED
AVULSES
EVALUNA
EVELONG
EVILEST
EVILEYE
EVILLER
EVILONE
EVOLUTE
EVOLVED
EVOLVER
EVOLVES
EVULSED
EVULSES
IVYLIKE
KVELLED
RVALUES
SVELTER
UVALUES

•V••L••

AVAILED
AVONLEA
EVERLYS
EVILLER
KVELLED
OVERLAP
OVERLAX
OVERLAY
OVERLET
OVERLIE
OVERLIT

•V•••L•

AVERELL
AVERILL
AVOWALS
OVERALL
OVERFLY
OVERPLY
OVERTLY
TVIDOLS
TVTABLE

•V••••L

AVERELL
AVERILL
AVERNAL
EVANGEL
OVERALL
OVOIDAL

••VL•••

HOVLANE
PAVLOVA

••V•L••
BEVELED
BEVELER
BIVALVE
CAVALRY
CAVILAT
CAVILED
CAVILER
CIVILLY
DEVALUE
DEVELOP
DEVILED
DEVILLE
DEVILRY
DEVOLVE
DIVULGE
DIVULSE
DOVELET
ENVELOP
GAVELED
GAVILAN
INVALID
INVOLVE
JAVELIN
LAVALSE
LAVELLI
LEVELED
LEVELER
LEVELLY
LEVILLI
NEVILLE
NOVALIS
NOVELAS
NOVELLA
NOVELLE
NOVELLO
NOVELTY
OFVALUE
ORVILLE
RAVELED
RAVELLY
RAVELOE
REVALUE
REVELED
REVELER
REVELIN
REVELRY
REVILED
REVILER
REVILES
REVOLTS
REVOLVE
RIVALED
RIVALRY
RIVULET
SAVALAS
SEVILLA
SEVILLE
UPVALUE
VIVALDI
WAVELET

••V••L•
ALVEOLI
BEVERLY
CIVILLY
DEVILLE
ENVEILS
ETVOILA
GAVIALS
LAVELLI
LEVELLY
LEVILLI
LIVABLE
LIVIDLY
LOVABLE
LOVABLY
LOVERLY
MOVABLE
MOVABLY
NEVILLE
NOVELLA
NOVELLE
NOVELLO
ORVILLE
PAVIDLY
RAVELLY
RAVIOLI
REVEALS
SAVABLE
SAVVILY
SEVILLA
SEVILLE
UNVEILS
VIVIDLY
WAVICLE

••V•••L
JUVENAL
PIVOTAL
RAVENAL
REVISAL
REVIVAL
SEVERAL
UNVENAL
UNVITAL
UNVOCAL

•••VL••
GRAVLAX

•••V•L•
ALEVELS
BOBVILA
BRAVELY
CARVELS
CLAVELL
COEVALS
DIAVOLO
DRIVELS
FRIVOLS
GRAVELS
GRAVELY
GROVELS
HEAVILY
ILOVELA
INAVALE
MARVELL
MARVELS
NAIVELY
NERVILY
NERVULE
OLEVELS
PRIVILY
SAVVILY
SERVILE
SHOVELS
SNIVELS
SUAVELY
SWIVELS
TORVALD
TORVILL
TRAVELS
VALVULA
VALVULE
WEEVILS

•••V••L
CLAVELL
ELUVIAL
FLUVIAL
MARVELL
PLUVIAL
PREVAIL
REAVAIL
SURVEIL
TORVILL
TRAVAIL
TRIVIAL

••••V•L
ARRIVAL
BEDEVIL
BILEVEL
CARAVEL
CHERVIL
ESTIVAL
GODEVIL
INCIVIL
KNIEVEL
NONEVIL
OCTAVAL
RELEVEL
REMOVAL
REVIVAL
SHRIVEL
UNCIVIL
UNLEVEL
UNNOVEL
UNRAVEL

V•M••••
VAMOOSE
VAMPERS
VAMPIER
VAMPING
VAMPIRA
VAMPIRE
VAMPISH
VIMINAL
VUMETER

V••M•••
VALMIKI
VARMINT
VERMEER
VERMEIL
VERMINY
VERMONT

V•••M••
VELTMAN
VENEMAN
VERYMAD
VICOMTE
VITAMIN
VOLUMED
VOLUMES
VROOMED

V••••M•
VACUUMS
VANCAMP
VELLUMS
VENDOME
VERISMO
VICTIMS

V•••••M
VALOREM
VARLAAM
VIETNAM

•VM••••
TVMOVIE

•V••M••
OVERMAN
OVERMIX
TVGAMES

•V•••M•
TVROOMS

•V••••M
OVERARM
OVIFORM

••V•M••
CAVEMAN
CAVEMEN
FIVEMAN
JAVAMAN
NAVYMAN
NAVYMEN
REVAMPS

••V••M•
COVERME

••V•••M
ENVENOM
SEVENAM
SEVENPM

•••V••M
ATAVISM
ELUVIUM
FAUVISM
TRIVIUM

VN•••••
VNECKED

V•N••••
VANADIC
VANCAMP
VANDALS
VANDIEN
VANDINE
VANDURA
VANDUYN
VANDYCK
VANDYKE
VANESSA
VANEXEL
VANEYCK
VANGOGH
VANILLA
VANILLI
VANLINE
VANLOAD
VANNING
VANOCUR
VANOWEN
VANPELT
VANPOOL
VANRIJN
VANSANT
VANTAGE
VANUATU
VANVOGT
VANWARD
VANWYCK
VANZANT
VENABLE
VENALLY
VENATIC
VENDEES
VENDERS
VENDING
VENDOME
VENDORS
VENDUES
VENEERS
VENEMAN
VENEZIA
VENISON
VENTAGE
VENTERS
VENTING
VENTNOR
VENTRAD
VENTRAL
VENTRIS
VENTURA
VENTURE
VENTURI
VENULES
VENUSES
VINCENT
VINCULA
VINEGAR
VINIEST
VINLAND
VINROSE
VINTAGE
VINTNER
VINYLIC
VONBAER
VONLAUE
VONOPEL
VONZELL

V••N•••
VAINEST
VANNING
VARNISH
VAUNTED
VAUNTER
VEENECK
VEINIER
VEINING
VEINLET
VEINTES
VEINULE
VERNIER
VIGNOLA
VILNIUS
VRONSKY

V•••N••
VACANCY
VALANCE
VALENCE
VALENTE
VALENTI
VALINES
VENTNOR
VERANDA
VERONIA
VERYNEW
VICENTE
VICENZA
VICINAL
VICUNAS
VIERNES
VIETNAM
VIKINGS
VIMINAL
VINTNER
VIVANTS
VIVENDI
VIXENLY
VOLANTE
VOLENTE
VOTENAY

V••••N•
VACCINE
VAGRANT
VALIANT
VALLONE
VALUING
VAMPING
VANDINE
VANLINE
VANNING
VANSANT
VANZANT
VARIANT
VARMINT
VARYING
VATTING
VEERING
VEGGING
VEILING
VEINING
VENDING
VENTING
VERBENA
VERDANT
VERDINS
VEREINE
VERGING
VERMINY
VERMONT
VERSANT
VERSING
VESTING
VETOING
VETTING
VIADENT
VIALING
VIBRANT
VICDANA
VIEWING
VINCENT
VINLAND
VIOLENT
VIOLINS
VIOLONE
VIRGINS
VISAING
VISIONS
VITRINE
VOGUING
VOICING
VOIDING
VOLCANO
VOLPONE
VOTEDNO
VOTESNO
VULCANS
VULPINE

V•••••N
VALADON
VALJEAN
VANDIEN
VANDUYN
VANOWEN
VANRIJN
VATICAN
VAUGHAN
VECHTEN
VELTMAN
VENEMAN
VENISON
VERGEON
VERIZON
VERSION
VESTRON
VETERAN
VIDICON
VILLAIN
VILLEIN
VIRGOAN
VISAYAN
VISTEON
VITAMIN
VOSGIAN
VOTEDIN
VOTEDON
VOTESIN
VOTESON
VUITTON

•V•N•••
AVANTIS
AVENGED
AVENGER
AVENGES
AVENIDA
AVENUEQ
AVENUES
AVONLEA
EVANDER
EVANGEL
EVANISH
EVENBET
EVENERS
EVENEST
EVENING
EVENNOW
EVENOFF
EVENOUT
EVENPAR
EVENSUP
EVINCED
EVINCES
IVANHOE
IVANIII
IVANOVO
UVINDEX

•V••N••
AVERNAL
AVERNUS
AVIANCA
AVIGNON
AVIONIC
EVENNOW
OVERNEW

•V•••N•
AVALONS
AVOWING
EVADING
EVALUNA
EVELONG
EVENING
EVIDENT
EVILONE
EVOKING
IVORINE

•V••••N
AVESTAN
AVEYRON
AVIDFAN
AVIGNON
AVIVIAN
EVASION
IVERSON
IVORIAN
OVATION
OVERMAN
OVERRAN
OVERRUN
OVIDIAN

••VN•••
GUVNORS

••V•N••
ADVANCE
ADVENTS
BOVINES
DAVINCI
DIVINED
DIVINER
DIVINES
ENVENOM
GIVENBY
GIVENIN
GIVENOF
GIVENON
GIVENTO
GIVENUP
HAVANAN
HAVANAS
HAVENER
HAVENOT
INVENTS
JUVENAL
LAVINIA
LIVENED
LIVENER
LIVENUP
LIVINGS
NOVENAS
PAVANES
PAVINGS
RAVENAL
RAVENED
RAVENNA
RAVINED
RAVINES
RAVINGS
REVENDS
REVENGE
REVENUE
ROVINGS
SAVANAS
SAVANNA
SAVANTS
SAVINGS
SEVENAD
SEVENAM
SEVENBC
SEVENEE
SEVENNO
SEVENPM
SEVENTH
SEVENTY
SEVENUP
UNVENAL
VIVANTS
VIVENDI

••V••N•
CAVEINS
CAVERNS
DEVEINS
DEVIANT
ENVYING
FIVEONE
GOVERNS
HAVEONE
HOVLANE
LAVAINE
LAVERNE
LEVYING
LIVEONE
LIVORNO
LOVEINS
NOVOTNY
RAVENNA
REVVING
RSVPING
SAVANNA
SEVENNO
SEVIGNY
TAVERNA
TAVERNS
UNVYING
WYVERNS
YEVGENY

••V•••N
CAVEDIN
CAVEMAN
CAVEMEN
CAVESIN
DAVISON
DIVEDIN
DIVESIN
ENVIRON
FIVEMAN
FIVEPIN
FIVETEN
GAVILAN
GIVENIN
GIVENON
GIVESIN
GIVESON
HAVANAN
HAVEFUN
JAVAMAN
JAVELIN
LAVERAN
LIVEDIN
LIVEDON
LIVESIN
LIVESON
MOVEDIN
MOVEDON
MOVESIN
MOVESON
NAVYMAN
NAVYMEN
NEVADAN
REVELIN
SAVARIN
SAVEDON
SAVESON
WAVEDIN
WAVESIN

•••VN••
HRYVNIA

•••V•N•
AIRVENT
BRAVING
CALVING
CALVINO
CARVING
CERVINE
CHEVONS
CONVENE
CONVENT
CORVINA
CORVINE
CRAVENS
CRAVING
CURVING
DELVING
DRIVING
ELEVENA
ELEVENB
ELEVENC
ELEVEND
ELEVENE
ELEVENS
ELEVONS
FERVENT
GALVANI
GALVANO
GLAVINE
GLOVING
GRAVING
HALVING
HEAVENS
HEAVING
KELVINS
LANVINS
LEAVENS
LEAVING
MALVINA
MTEVANS
NERVINE
NERVING
NIRVANA
OLIVINE
PARVENU
PEEVING
PREVENT
PROVINE
PROVING
REAVING
REEVING
REVVING
SALVING
SERVANT
SERVING
SHAVING
SHOVING
SIEVING
SLAVING
SLOVENE
SLOVENS
SOLVENT
SOLVING
SORVINO
STAVING
STEVENS
SUBVENE
TREVINO
WAIVING
WEAVING

•••V••N
AVIVIAN
CHEVRON
DRIVEIN
DROVEIN
LATVIAN
LEAVEIN
LEAVEON
SHAVIAN
SHOVEIN

••••V•N
ATSEVEN
BELEVEN
CARAVAN
CLEAVON
DEHAVEN
DONOVAN
ENLIVEN
EUROVAN
GASOVEN
GENEVAN
GETEVEN
GOTEVEN
GROOVIN
HESHVAN
INWOVEN
MCGAVIN
MINIVAN
NOTEVEN
REGIVEN
REWOVEN
STRIVEN
THRIVEN
UNGIVEN
UNRIVEN
UNWOVEN
YEREVAN

VO•••••
VOCABLE
VOCABLY
VOCALIC
VOCALLY
VOCODER
VOGUERS
VOGUING
VOGUISH
VOICERS
VOICING
VOIDERS
VOIDING
VOIDOUT
VOITURE
VOLANTE
VOLCANO
VOLCKER
VOLENTE
VOLLEYS
VOLPONE
VOLTAGE
VOLTAIC
VOLTORE
VOLUBLE
VOLUBLY
VOLUMED
VOLUMES
VOLUTED
VOLUTES
VONBAER
VONLAUE
VONOPEL
VONZELL
VOODOOS
VORLAGE
VORSTER
VOSGIAN
VOSKHOD
VOTABLE
VOTEAYE
VOTECHS
VOTEDIN
VOTEDNO
VOTEDON
VOTEFOR
VOTENAY
VOTEOUT
VOTESIN
VOTESNO
VOTESON
VOTEYEA
VOTEYES
VOTIVES
VOUCHED
VOUCHER
VOUCHES
VOUVRAY
VOWELLY
VOWLESS
VOYAGED
VOYAGER
VOYAGES

V•O••••
VIOLATE
VIOLENT
VIOLETS
VIOLINS
VIOLIST
VIOLONE
VOODOOS
VRONSKY
VROOMED

V••O•••
VALOREM
VALOTTE
VALOURS
VAMOOSE
VANOCUR
VANOWEN
VAPORED
VAPORER
VAPORUB
VAPOURS
VAPOURY
VBLOUSE
VELOURS
VELOUTE
VELOXES
VERONIA
VETOERS
VETOING
VICOMTE
VIGOURS
VISORED
VITORIA
VIZORED
VOCODER
VONOPEL
VROOMED

V•••O••
VACUOLE
VACUOUS
VALLONE
VAMOOSE
VANGOGH
VANLOAD
VANPOOL
VANVOGT

VARIOUS
VAUDOIS
VECTORS
VEEROFF
VENDOME
VENDORS
VERBOSE
VERDOUX
VERMONT
VERYODD
VERYOLD
VFWPOST
VICIOUS
VICTORS
VICTORY
VIDEOED
VIDIOTS
VIGNOLA
VINROSE
VIOLONE
VIRGOAN
VISCOUS
VISIONS
VOIDOUT
VOLPONE
VOLTORE
VOODOOS
VOTEOUT

V••••O•
VALADON
VANPOOL
VELCROS
VENISON
VENTNOR
VERGEON
VERIZON
VERSION
VERYHOT
VERYLOW
VESTRON
VICEROY
VIDICON
VIEDFOR
VIESFOR
VIRAGOS
VISITOR
VISTEON
VITRIOL
VOODOOS
VOSKHOD
VOTEDON
VOTEFOR
VOTESON
VUITTON

V•••••O
VACCARO
VALLEJO
VAQUERO
VERDUGO
VERISMO
VERTIGO
VIBRATO
VISCUSO
VOLCANO
VOTEDNO
VOTESNO

•VO••••
AVOCADO
AVOCETS
AVOIDED
AVOIDER
AVONLEA
AVOWALS
AVOWERS
AVOWING
EVOKERS
EVOKING
EVOLUTE
EVOLVED
EVOLVER
EVOLVES
IVORIAN
IVORIES
IVORINE
OVOIDAL

•V•O•••
AVIONIC
TVMOVIE
TVROOMS

•V••O••
AVALONS
EVELONG
EVENOFF
EVENOUT
EVILONE
IVANOVO
OVIFORM
TVIDOLS
TVROOMS
TVSHOWS
TVSPOTS

•V•••O•
AVEYRON
AVIATOR
AVIGNON
EVASION
EVENNOW
EVERTOR
EVICTOR
IVANHOE
IVERSON
OVATION
OVERCOY
OVERDOG
OVERHOT
OVERJOY
OVERTOP

•V••••O
AVOCADO
IVANOVO

••VO•••
BIVOUAC
CAVORTS
DEVOIRS
DEVOLVE
DEVORES
DEVOTED
DEVOTEE
DEVOTES
DEVOURS
DIVORCE
ENVOGUE
ETVOILA
FAVORED
FAVORER
FAVOURS
GAVOTTE
INVOGUE
INVOICE
INVOKED
INVOKER
INVOKES
INVOLVE
LAVORIS
LIVORNO
NOVOTES
NOVOTNY
PIVOTAL
PIVOTED
PIVOTER
REVOICE
REVOKED
REVOKER
REVOKES
REVOLTS
REVOLVE
REVOTED
REVOTES
SAVORED
SAVORER
SAVOURS
SAVOURY
UNVOCAL
UNVOICE
UNVOTED
UNVOWED

••V•O••
ALVEOLI
DEVIOUS
ENVIOUS
FIVEONE
GAVEOFF
GAVEOUT
GIVEOFF
GIVEOUT
GUVNORS
HAVEONE
HAVEOUT
HIVEOFF
LIVEOAK
LIVEONE
LIVEOUT
MOVEOFF
MOVEOUT
NIVEOUS
OBVIOUS
PAVIORS
PAVIOUR
PAVLOVA
RAVIOLI
SAVIORS
SAVIOUR
WAVEOFF

••V••O•
ADVISOR
DAVEKOZ
DAVISON
DEVELOP
DEVISOR
DIVISOR
DOVECOT
ENVELOP
ENVENOM
ENVIRON
ENVIROS
GIVENOF
GIVENON
GIVESOF
GIVESON
HAVENOT
LAVABOS
LEVATOR
LIVEDON
LIVEFOR
LIVESON
LOVEJOY
LOVEYOU
MOVADOS
MOVEDON
MOVESON
NAVAHOS
NAVAJOS
RAVELOE
REVISOR
SAVEDON
SAVEFOR
SAVESON

••V•••O
FIVETWO
GIVENTO
GIVESTO
HAVEAGO
INVACUO
INVITRO
LIVORNO
LOVEDTO
LOVESTO
MOVEDTO
MOVESTO
NOVARRO
NOVELLO
ONVIDEO
ORVIETO
RIVERPO
SEVENNO
WAVEDTO
WAVESTO

•••VO••
BELVOIR
BELVOUR
BERVOIX
BRAVOED
BRAVOES
CHEVONS
CONVOKE
CONVOYS
DIAVOLO
ELEVONS
FERVORS
FERVOUR
FLAVORS
FLAVORY
FLAVOUR
FRIVOLS
NERVOUS
NONVOID
ONEVOTE
OUTVOTE
PREVOID
PREVOST
PROVOKE
PROVOST
REAVOWS
REEVOKE
RENVOIS
SALVOES
SALVORS
VANVOGT
YESVOTE

•••V•O•
CHEVIOT
CHEVRON
LEAVEON
SHAVUOT
TRIVIOT

•••V••O
ALIVETO
BRAVADO
CALVINO
DIAVOLO
DRIVETO
DROVETO
GALVANO
HEAVEHO
HEAVETO
PREVETO
PRIVYTO
PROVISO
SORVINO
TREVINO
ZHIVAGO

••••VO•
CLEAVON
DISAVOW
INFAVOR
LENOVOS
OCTAVOS

••••V•O
OCTAVIO
OTTAVIO

•••••VO
CENTAVO
IVANOVO
RILIEVO
ZEMSTVO

VP•••••
VAPIDLY
VAPORED
VAPORER
VAPORUB
VAPOURS
VAPOURY

V••P•••
VAMPERS
VAMPIER
VAMPING
VAMPIRA
VAMPIRE
VAMPISH
VANPELT
VANPOOL
VESPERS
VESPIDS
VFWPOST
VOLPONE
VULPINE

V•••P••
VONOPEL
VSHAPED
VSHAPES

V••••P•
VCRTAPE

V•••••P
VANCAMP
VERYHIP

•VP••••
RVPARKS

•V•P•••
OVIPARA
PVCPIPE
TVSPOTS

•V••P••
EVENPAR
OVERPAR
OVERPAY
OVERPLY
TVTAPES

•V•••P•
PVCPIPE

•V••••P
EVENSUP
OVERLAP
OVERSUP
OVERTIP
OVERTOP

••VP•••
RSVPING

••V•P••
FIVEPIN

••V••P•
GIVEUPS
RAVEUPS
REVAMPS
RIVERPO
SEVENPM

••V•••P
COVERUP
DEVELOP
DIVVYUP
ENVELOP
GIVENUP
GIVESUP
LIVENUP
LOVETAP
MOVEDUP
MOVESUP
REVITUP
SAVEDUP
SAVESUP
SEVENUP

•••V•P•
THEVIPS

•••V••P
DIVVYUP
DRIVEUP
DROVEUP
IGIVEUP
SERVEUP

V•Q••••
VAQUERO

V••Q•••
VASQUEZ

•V••••Q
AVENUEQ

VR•••••
VRONSKY
VROOMED

V•R••••
VARIANT
VARIATE
VARIERS
VARIETY
VARIOUS
VARITEK
VARLAAM
VARLETS
VARMINT
VARNISH
VARRICK
VARSITY
VARYING
VCRTAPE
VERANDA
VERBALS
VERBENA
VERBIDS
VERBIFY
VERBOSE
VERDANT
VERDELL
VERDICT
VERDINS
VERDOUX
VERDUGO
VERDURE
VEREINE
VERGEON
VERGERS
VERGING
VERIDIC
VERIEST
VERISMO
VERISTS
VERITAS
VERIZON
VERMEER
VERMEIL
VERMINY
VERMONT
VERNIER
VERONIA
VERRUCA
VERSACE
VERSANT
VERSETS
VERSIFY
VERSING
VERSION
VERTIGO
VERYBAD
VERYBIG
VERYDRY
VERYFEW
VERYFIT
VERYHIP
VERYHOT
VERYILL
VERYLOW
VERYMAD
VERYNEW
VERYODD
VERYOLD
VERYRED
VERYSAD
VERYSHY
VERYWET
VIRAGOS
VIRGATE
VIRGINS
VIRGOAN
VIRGULE
VIRTUAL
VIRTUES
VIRUSES
VORLAGE
VORSTER

V••R•••
VAGRANT
VANRIJN
VARRICK
VEERIES
VEERING
VEEROFF
VERRUCA
VIBRANT
VIBRATE
VIBRATO
VIERNES
VIERZIG
VINROSE
VITRICS
VITRIFY
VITRINE
VITRIOL

V•••R••
VALERIE
VALOREM
VAPORED
VAPORER
VAPORUB
VECTRAS
VELCROS
VELURES
VENTRAD
VENTRAL
VENTRIS
VERYRED
VESTRAL
VESTRON
VETERAN
VICEROY
VICKREY
VICTRIX
VIHARAS
VISORED
VITARAS
VITORIA
VIVARIA
VIZORED
VOUVRAY

V••••R•
VACCARO
VALOURS
VALUERS
VAMPERS
VAMPIRA
VAMPIRE
VANDURA
VANWARD
VAPOURS
VAPOURY
VAQUERO
VARIERS
VEADARS
VECTORS
VEILERS
VELOURS
VENDERS
VENDORS
VENEERS
VENTERS
VENTURA
VENTURE
VENTURI
VERDURE
VERGERS
VERYDRY
VESPERS
VESTURE
VETOERS
VETTERS
VICKERS
VICTORS
VICTORY
VIEWERS
VIGOURS
VILLARD
VILLARI
VISCERA
VIZIERS
VOGUERS
VOICERS
VOIDERS
VOITURE
VOLTORE
VULTURE

V•••••R
VAMPIER
VANOCUR
VAPORER
VASTIER
VAULTER
VAUNTER
VEALIER
VEINIER
VENTNOR
VERMEER
VERNIER
VIEDFOR
VIESFOR
VIEWIER
VINEGAR
VINTNER
VISITOR
VIVIDER
VIVITAR
VOCODER
VOLCKER
VONBAER
VORSTER
VOTEFOR
VOUCHER
VOYAGER
VUMETER

•VR••••
TVROOMS

•V•R•••
AVARICE
AVERAGE
AVERELL
AVERILL
AVERNAL
AVERNUS
AVERRED
AVERTED
AVERTER
EVERDUR
EVEREST
EVERETT
EVERLYS
EVERTED
EVERTOR
IVERSON
IVORIAN
IVORIES
IVORINE
OVARIES
OVERACT
OVERAGE
OVERALL
OVERARM
OVERATE
OVERAWE
OVERBED
OVERBET
OVERBID
OVERBIG
OVERBUY
OVERCOY
OVERCUT
OVERDID
OVERDOG
OVERDRY
OVERDUB
OVERDUE
OVERDYE
OVEREAT
OVERFAR
OVERFAT
OVERFED
OVERFEE
OVERFEW
OVERFIT
OVERFIX
OVERFLY
OVERHOT
OVERICE
OVERJOY
OVERLAP
OVERLAX
OVERLAY
OVERLET
OVERLIE
OVERLIT
OVERMAN
OVERMIX
OVERNEW
OVERPAR
OVERPAY
OVERPLY
OVERRAN
OVERRUN
OVERSAD
OVERSAW
OVERSEA
OVERSEE
OVERSET
OVERSEW
OVERSUP
OVERTAX
OVERTIP
OVERTLY
OVERTOP
OVERUSE
OVERWET
SVERIGE
TVCREWS

•V••R••
AVERRED
AVEYRON
OVERRAN
OVERRUN
RVPARKS

•V•••R•
AVATARS
AVOWERS
EVADERS
EVENERS
EVOKERS
OVERARM
OVERDRY
OVIFORM
OVIPARA
TVSTARS

•V••••R
AVENGER
AVERTER
AVIATOR
AVOIDER
EVANDER
EVENPAR
EVERDUR
EVERTOR
EVICTOR
EVILLER
EVOLVER
OVERFAR
OVERPAR
SVELTER

••VR•••
DEVRIES
FEVRIER

••V•R••
ADVERBS
ADVERSE
ADVERTS
ALVAREZ
BAVARIA
BEVERLY
CAVERNS
CAVORTS
COVERED
COVERER
COVERME
COVERTS
COVERUP
DEVORES
DIVERGE
DIVERSE
DIVERTS
DIVORCE
DOVERDE
ENVIRON
ENVIROS
FAVORED
FAVORER
FEVERED
GOVERNS
HAVARTI
HOVERED
HOVERER
INVERSE
INVERTS
LAVERAN
LAVERNE
LAVORIS
LEVERED
LEVERET
LIVERED
LIVORNO
LOVERLY
NAVARRE
NOVARRO
OBVERSE
OBVERTS
POVERTY
REVERBS
REVERDY
REVERED
REVERER
REVERES
REVERIE
REVERSA
REVERSE
REVERTS
RIVERPO
SAVARIN
SAVORED
SAVORER
SEVERAL
SEVERED
SEVERER
SEVERUS
TAVERNA
TAVERNS
VIVARIA
WAVERED
WAVERER
WYVERNS

••V••R•
CAVALRY
CAVEART
CAVIARE
CAVIARS
DEVILRY
DEVOIRS
DEVOURS
ENVIERS
FAVOURS
GUVNORS
INVITRO
LEVIERS
NAVARRE
NOVARRO
PAVIORS
REVELRY
RIVALRY
RIVIERA
RIVIERE
SAVIORS
SAVOURS
SAVOURY
XAVIERU

••V•••R
ADVISER
ADVISOR
BEVELER
CAVILER
COVERER
COVETER
DEVISER
DEVISOR
DIVIDER
DIVINER
DIVISOR
DOVEBAR
FAVORER
FEVRIER
GAVEEAR
GIVEEAR
HAVENER
HOVERER
INVADER

INVITER
INVOKER
LEVATOR
LEVELER
LIVEFOR
LIVENER
PAVIOUR
PIVOTER
RAVAGER
REVELER
REVERER
REVILER
REVISER
REVISOR
REVIVER
REVOKER
RIVETER
SAVAGER
SAVEFOR
SAVIOUR
SAVORER
SAVVIER
SEVERER
VIVIDER
VIVITAR
WAVERER

•••VR••
CHEVRES
CHEVRET
CHEVRON
LOUVRED
LOUVRES
OEUVRES
POIVRES
VOUVRAY

•••V•R•
BEAVERS
BRAVERY
BRAVURA
CALVARY
CALVERT
CARVERS
CLOVERS
CLOVERY
CONVERT
CRAVERS
CULVERT
DANVERS
DELVERS
DOOVERS
DRIVERS
DROVERS
FERVORS
FLAVORS
FLAVORY
GRAVERS
GRAVURE
GROVERS
GUEVARA
HALVERS
HARVARD
HEAVERS
HOOVERS
KNAVERY
LOUVERS
PLOVERS
PREVERB
PREVERT
PROVERB
PROVERS
QUAVERS
QUAVERY
QUIVERS
QUIVERY
REAVERS
SALVERS
SALVORS
SERVERS
SHAVERS
SHIVERS
SHIVERY
SHOVERS
SILVERS
SILVERY
SLAVERS
SLAVERY
SLIVERS
SOLVERS
SUBVERT
TRAVERS
UNOVERT
WAIVERS
WEAVERS

•••V••R
BELVOIR
BELVOUR
BOUVIER
CLAVIER
CORVAIR
CURVIER
FERVOUR
FLAVOUR
FLIVVER
HEAVIER
JANVIER
MARVIER
NERVIER
OLIVIER
PRIVIER
SAVVIER

••••VR•
DOEUVRE
LEHAVRE

••••V•R
ALLOVER
ANDOVER
AQUIVER
ARRIVER
ASHIVER
ASKOVER
ATEOVER
BOLIVAR
CADAVER
CHEEVER
CLEAVER
CRYOVER
CUTOVER
DELIVER
DERIVER
DIDOVER
DUUMVIR
EATOVER
EVOLVER
FLIVVER
FLYOVER
FOREVER
GETOVER
GOTOVER
GRIEVER
HADOVER
HANOVER
HASOVER
HOPOVER
HOTOVER
HOWEVER
ICEOVER
INFAVOR
ITSOVER
KOSOVAR
LAYOVER
LIEOVER
MINIVER
MISAVER
NONEVER
NOTEVER
NOTOVER
ONEOVER
PALAVER
POPOVER
PORIVER
PREAVER
PUTOVER
RANOVER
RECOVER
RELEVER
REMOVER
REVIVER
RUNOVER
SAMOVAR
SAYOVER
SHELVER
SHRIVER
STRIVER
THRIVER
TIPOVER
UNCOVER
UPRIVER
WHOEVER
WHYEVER
WINOVER
WONOVER

VS•••••
VSHAPED
VSHAPES

V•S••••
VASQUEZ
VASSALS
VASTEST
VASTIER
VASTITY
VESICLE
VESPERS
VESPIDS
VESSELS
VESTALS
VESTEES
VESTIGE
VESTING
VESTRAL
VESTRON
VESTURE
VISAGED
VISAGES
VISAING
VISALIA
VISAVIS
VISAYAN
VISCERA
VISCOUS
VISCUSO
VISIBLE
VISIBLY
VISIONS
VISITED
VISITOR
VISORED
VISTAED
VISTEON
VISTULA
VISUALS
VOSGIAN
VOSKHOD

V••S•••
VANSANT
VARSITY
VASSALS
VERSACE
VERSANT
VERSETS
VERSIFY
VERSING
VERSION
VESSELS
VIESFOR
VIZSLAS
VORSTER

V•••S••
VALISES
VANESSA
VEDISTS
VENISON
VENUSES
VERISMO
VERISTS
VERYSAD
VERYSHY
VIBISTS
VIRUSES
VOTESIN
VOTESNO
VOTESON
VRONSKY

V••••S•
VAGUEST
VAINEST
VAMOOSE
VAMPISH
VANESSA
VARNISH
VASTEST
VBLOUSE
VERBOSE
VERIEST
VFWPOST
VINIEST
VINROSE
VIOLIST
VISCUSO
VITEBSK
VOGUISH
VOWLESS

V•••••S
VACATES
VACUOUS
VACUUMS
VALINES
VALISES
VALLEYS
VALOURS
VALUERS
VAMPERS
VANDALS
VAPOURS
VARIERS
VARIOUS
VARLETS
VASSALS
VATDYES
VATFULS
VAUDOIS
VEADARS
VECTORS
VECTRAS
VEDISTS
VEEJAYS
VEERIES
VEGGIES
VEIGHTS
VEILERS
VEINTES
VELCROS
VELLUMS
VELOURS
VELOXES
VELURES
VELVETS
VENDEES
VENDERS
VENDORS
VENDUES
VENEERS
VENTERS
VENTRIS
VENULES
VENUSES
VERBALS
VERBIDS
VERDINS
VERGERS
VERISTS
VERITAS
VERSETS
VESPERS
VESPIDS
VESSELS
VESTALS
VESTEES
VETCHES
VETOERS
VETTERS
VIBISTS
VICIOUS
VICKERS
VICTIMS
VICTORS
VICUNAS
VIDIOTS
VIELLES
VIERNES
VIEWERS
VIGOURS
VIHARAS
VIKINGS
VILNIUS
VIOLETS
VIOLINS
VIRAGOS
VIRGINS
VIRTUES
VIRUSES
VISAGES
VISAVIS
VISCOUS
VISIONS
VISUALS
VITALIS
VITARAS
VITRICS
VITTLES
VIVANTS
VIZIERS
VIZSLAS
VOGUERS
VOICERS
VOIDERS
VOLLEYS
VOLUMES
VOLUTES
VOODOOS
VOTECHS
VOTEYES
VOTIVES
VOUCHES
VOWLESS
VOYAGES
VSHAPES
VULCANS

•VS••••
TVSHOWS
TVSPOTS
TVSTARS

•V•S•••
AVESTAN
AVESTAS
EVASION
EVASIVE
KVASSES
OVISACS

•V••S••
AVGASES
AVULSED
AVULSES
EVENSUP
EVULSED
EVULSES
IVERSON
KVASSES
OVERSAD
OVERSAW
OVERSEA
OVERSEE
OVERSET
OVERSEW
OVERSUP

•V•••S•
AVIDEST
EVANISH
EVENEST
EVEREST
EVILEST
OVERUSE

•V••••S
AVALONS
AVANTIS
AVATARS
AVENGES
AVENUES
AVERNUS
AVESTAS
AVGASES
AVIATES
AVOCETS
AVOWALS
AVOWERS
AVULSES
EVADERS
EVENERS
EVERLYS
EVINCES
EVOKERS
EVOLVES
EVULSES
IVORIES
IVTUBES
KVASSES
OVARIES
OVISACS
RVALUES
RVPARKS
TVCREWS
TVGAMES
TVIDOLS
TVROOMS
TVSHOWS
TVSPOTS
TVSTARS
TVTAPES
UVALUES

••V•S••
ADVISED
ADVISEE
ADVISER
ADVISES
ADVISOR
CAVESIN
DAVISON
DEVESTS
DEVISED
DEVISEE
DEVISER
DEVISES
DEVISOR
DIVESIN
DIVESTS
DIVISOR
FIVESIX
GIVESIN
GIVESOF
GIVESON
GIVESTO
GIVESUP
INVESTS
LIVESAT
LIVESET
LIVESEY
LIVESIN
LIVESON
LOVESET
LOVESIT
LOVESTO
MAVISES
MOVESIN
MOVESIT
MOVESON
MOVESTO
MOVESUP
NOVISAD
REVESTS
REVISAL
REVISED
REVISER
REVISES
REVISIT
REVISOR
SAVESON
SAVESUP
WAVESAT
WAVESIN
WAVESTO

••V••S•
ADVERSE
DIVERSE
DIVULSE
INVERSE
JIVIEST
LAVALSE
OBVERSE
REVERSA
REVERSE
WAVIEST

••V•••S
ADVENTS
ADVERBS
ADVERTS
ADVICES
ADVISES
BOVINES
CAVEATS
CAVEINS
CAVERNS
CAVIARS
CAVORTS
CIVVIES
COVERTS
DEVEINS
DEVESTS
DEVICES
DEVIOUS
DEVISES
DEVOIRS
DEVORES
DEVOTES
DEVOURS
DEVRIES
DIVERTS
DIVESTS
DIVIDES
DIVINES
DIVVIES
DRVEGAS
ENVEILS
ENVIERS
ENVIOUS
ENVIROS
FAVOURS
GAVIALS
GIVEUPS
GOVERNS
GUVNORS
HAVANAS
INVADES
INVENTS
INVERTS
INVESTS
INVITES
INVOKES
LAVABOS
LAVAGES
LAVORIS
LEVADES
LEVIERS
LEVITES
LIVINGS
LOVAGES
LOVEINS
MAVISES
MOVADOS
NAVAHOS
NAVAIDS
NAVAJOS
NIVEOUS
NOVALIS
NOVELAS
NOVENAS
NOVICES
NOVOTES
OBVERTS
OBVIOUS
PAVANES
PAVINGS
PAVIORS
RAVAGES
RAVEUPS
RAVINES
RAVINGS
REVAMPS
REVEALS
REVENDS
REVERBS
REVERES
REVERTS
REVESTS
REVIEWS
REVILES
REVISES
REVIVES
REVOKES
REVOLTS
REVOTES
ROVINGS
SAVAGES
SAVALAS
SAVANAS
SAVANTS
SAVINGS
SAVIORS
SAVOURS
SAVVIES
SEVERUS
SOVIETS
TAVERNS
UNVEILS
VIVANTS
WYVERNS

•••VS••
HDTVSET

•••V•S•
ATAVISM
ATAVIST
BRAVEST
BUDVASE
CANVASS
DERVISH
DOGVEST
FAUVISM
FAUVIST
GRAVEST
HARVEST
KNAVISH
NAIVEST
PEEVISH
PREVOST
PROVISO
PROVOST
SKIVEST
SLAVISH
SUAVEST

•••V••S
ALEVELS
BEAVERS
BMOVIES
BRAVOES
BREVETS
CANVASS
CARVELS
CARVERS
CERVIDS
CHEVETS
CHEVONS
CHEVRES
CHIVIES
CIVVIES
CLOVERS
COEVALS
CONVEYS
CONVOYS
CORVEES
CORVIDS
CRAVATS
CRAVENS
CRAVERS
CURVETS
DANVERS
DELVERS
DIVVIES
DOOVERS
DRIVELS
DRIVERS
DROVERS
DYEVATS
ELEVENS
ELEVONS
FERVORS
FLAVIUS
FLAVORS
FRIVOLS
GERVAIS
GRAVELS
GRAVERS
GRAVIES
GROVELS
GROVERS
HALVAHS
HALVERS
HEAVENS
HEAVERS
HEAVIES
HOOVERS
HUMVEES
JAYVEES
KELVINS
KIDVIDS
LANVINS
LEAVENS
LOUVERS
LOUVRES
MARVELS
MAUVAIS
MTEVANS
NERVOUS
OEUVRES
OLEVELS
OUTVIES
PLOVERS
POIVRES
PREVIAS
PREVUES
PRIVETS
PRIVIES
PROVERS
PURVEYS
QUAVERS
QUIVERS
REAVERS
REAVOWS
RENVOIS
SALVERS
SALVOES
SALVORS
SAVVIES
SERVEAS
SERVERS
SHAVERS
SHEVATS
SHIVERS
SHOVELS
SHOVERS
SILVERS
SLAVERS
SLIVERS
SLOVAKS
SLOVENS
SNIVELS
SOLVERS
STEVENS
SURVEYS
SWIVELS
SWIVETS
TEEVEES
THEVIPS
TRAVELS
TRAVERS
TRIVETS
UNIVACS
VELVETS
WAIVERS
WARVETS
WEAVERS
WEEVILS

••••VS•
LITOVSK

••••V•S
ACTIVAS
ACTIVES
ALCOVES
ALDAVIS
ARRIVES
BEHAVES
BULOVAS
BYFIVES
CASAVAS
CLEAVES
DATIVES
DERIVES
DWARVES
ENDIVES
EVOLVES
EXWIVES
GREAVES
GRIEVES
GROOVES
INFIVES
LENOVOS
MOHAVES
MOJAVES
MOTIVES
NATIVES
OCTAVES
OCTAVOS
REGIVES
RELEVES
RELIVES
REMOVES
REPAVES
RESAVES
REVIVES
SALIVAS
SCARVES
SCURVES
SHEAVES
SHELVES
SHRIVES
SLEEVES
STARVES
STEEVES
STRIVES
SWERVES
THIEVES
THRIVES
TWELVES
UNLIVES
UPDIVES
VISAVIS
VOTIVES
WHARVES

•••••VS
FLATTVS
KISLEVS
MAGLEVS
MINITVS
THECAVS
THEMAVS
YOMTOVS

V•T••••
VATDYED
VATDYES
VATFULS
VATICAL
VATICAN
VATTING
VETCHES
VETERAN
VETOERS
VETOING
VETTERS
VETTING
VITALIS
VITALLY
VITAMIN
VITARAS
VITEBSK
VITIATE
VITORIA
VITRICS
VITRIFY
VITRINE
VITRIOL
VITTLES
VOTABLE
VOTEAYE
VOTECHS
VOTEDIN
VOTEDNO
VOTEDON
VOTEFOR
VOTENAY
VOTEOUT
VOTESIN
VOTESNO
VOTESON
VOTEYEA
VOTEYES
VOTIVES

V••T•••
VANTAGE
VASTEST
VASTIER

VASTITY
VATTING
VCRTAPE
VECTORS
VECTRAS
VELTMAN
VENTAGE
VENTERS
VENTING
VENTNOR
VENTRAD
VENTRAL
VENTRIS
VENTURA
VENTURE
VENTURI
VERTIGO
VESTALS
VESTEES
VESTIGE
VESTING
VESTRAL
VESTRON
VESTURE
VETTERS
VETTING
VIATICA
VICTIMS
VICTORS
VICTORY
VICTRIX
VICTUAL
VIETNAM
VINTAGE
VINTNER
VIRTUAL
VIRTUES
VISTAED
VISTEON
VISTULA
VITTLES
VOITURE
VOLTAGE
VOLTAIC
VOLTORE
VUITTON
VULTURE

V•••T••
VACATED
VACATES
VALETED
VALOTTE
VARITEK
VAULTED
VAULTER
VAUNTED
VAUNTER
VECHTEN
VEDETTE
VEGETAL
VEINTES
VENATIC
VERITAS
VIDETTE
VISITED
VISITOR
VIVITAR
VOLUTED
VOLUTES
VORSTER
VUITTON
VUMETER

V••••T•
VACUITY
VALENTE
VALENTI
VALOTTE
VALUATE
VALVATE
VANUATU
VARIATE
VARIETY
VARLETS
VARSITY
VASTITY
VEDETTE
VEDISTS
VEIGHTS
VELOUTE
VELVETS
VELVETY
VERISTS
VERSETS
VIBISTS
VIBRATE
VIBRATO
VICENTE
VICOMTE
VIDETTE
VIDIOTS
VIEWITH
VIOLATE
VIOLETS
VIRGATE
VITIATE
VIVANTS
VOLANTE
VOLENTE
VULGATE

V•••••T
VAGRANT
VAGUEST
VAINEST
VALIANT
VANPELT
VANSANT
VANVOGT
VANZANT
VARIANT
VARMINT
VASTEST
VEINLET
VERDANT
VERDICT
VERIEST
VERMONT
VERSANT
VERYFIT
VERYHOT
VERYWET
VFWPOST
VIADENT
VIADUCT
VIBRANT
VINCENT
VINIEST
VIOLENT
VIOLIST
VOIDOUT
VOTEOUT

•VT••••
IVTUBES
TVTABLE
TVTAPES

•V•T•••
AVATARS
KVETCHY
OVATION
TVSTARS

•V••T••
AVANTIS
AVERTED
AVERTER
AVESTAN
AVESTAS
AVIATED
AVIATES
AVIATIC
AVIATOR
EVERTED
EVERTOR
EVICTED
EVICTEE
EVICTOR
OVERTAX
OVERTIP
OVERTLY
OVERTOP
SVELTER

•V•••T•
AVIDITY
AVOCETS
EVERETT
EVOLUTE
OVERATE
TVSPOTS

•V••••T
AVIDEST
EVENBET
EVENEST
EVENOUT
EVEREST
EVERETT
EVIDENT
EVILEST
OVERACT
OVERBET
OVERCUT
OVEREAT
OVERFAT
OVERFIT
OVERHOT
OVERLET
OVERLIT
OVERSET
OVERWET
OVIDUCT

••V•T••
COVETED
COVETER
CUVETTE
DEVOTED
DEVOTEE
DEVOTES
FIVETEN
FIVETWO
GAVOTTE
INVITED
INVITEE
INVITER
INVITES
INVITRO
LEVATOR
LEVITES
LEVITIC
LOVETAP
NOVOTES
NOVOTNY
PIVOTAL
PIVOTED
PIVOTER
REVITUP
REVOTED
REVOTES
RIVETED
RIVETER
ROVETTA
UNVITAL
UNVOTED
VIVITAR

••V••T•
ADVENTS
ADVERTS
CAVEATS
CAVORTS
COVERTS
CUVETTE
DEVESTS
DEVIATE
DIVERTS
DIVESTS
GAVOTTE
GIVENTO
GIVESTO
HAVARTI
INVENTS
INVERTS
INVESTS
INVICTA
LOVEDTO
LOVESTO
MOVEDTO
MOVESTO
NOVELTY
OBVERTS
OBVIATE
ORVIETO
POVERTY
REVERTS
REVESTS
REVOLTS
ROVETTA
SAVANTS
SEVENTH
SEVENTY
SOVIETS
VIVANTS
WAVEDTO
WAVESTO

••V•••T
CAVEART
CAVILAT
DEVIANT
DOVECOT
DOVELET
GAVEOUT
GIVEOUT
HAVENOT
HAVEOUT
JIVIEST
LEVERET
LIVEOUT
LIVESAT
LIVESET
LOVEDIT
LOVESET
LOVESIT
MOVEDIT
MOVEOUT
MOVESIT
REVISIT
RIVULET
WAVEDAT
WAVELET
WAVESAT
WAVIEST

•••V•T•
ALIVETO
BREVETS
BREVITY
CHEVETS
CLAVATE
CRAVATS
CURVETS
DRIVETO
DROVETO
DYEVATS
ELEVATE
GRAVITY
HEAVETO
HORVITZ
NAIVETE
NAIVETY
ONEVOTE
OUTVOTE
PREVETO
PRIVATE
PRIVETS
PRIVITY
PRIVYTO
SHEVATS
SUAVITY
SWIVETS
TRIVETS
VALVATE
VELVETS
VELVETY
WARVETS
YESVOTE

•••V••T
AIRVENT
ATAVIST
BRAVEST
CALVERT
CHEVIOT
CHEVRET
CONVECT
CONVENT
CONVERT
CONVICT
CULVERT
DOGVEST
DRIVEAT
DROVEAT
FAUVIST
FERVENT
GRAVEST
HARVEST
HDTVSET
IHAVEIT
ILOVEIT
LEAVEIT
NAIVEST
PREVENT
PREVERT
PREVOST
PROVEIT
PROVOST
REEVICT
SERVANT
SHAVUOT
SKIVEST
SOLVEIT
SOLVENT
SUAVEST
SUBVERT
TRIVIOT
UNOVERT
VANVOGT

••••V•T
AQUAVIT
CHARVET
NUNAVUT
WINEVAT

VU•••••
VUITTON
VULCANS
VULGATE
VULPINE
VULTURE
VUMETER

V•U••••
VAUDOIS
VAUGHAN
VAULTED
VAULTER
VAUNTED
VAUNTER
VOUCHED
VOUCHER
VOUCHES
VOUVRAY

V••U•••
VACUITY
VACUOLE
VACUOUS
VACUUMS
VAGUELY
VAGUEST
VALUATE
VALUERS
VALUING
VANUATU
VAQUERO
VELURES
VENULES
VENUSES
VICUNAS
VIRUSES
VISUALS
VOGUERS
VOGUING
VOGUISH
VOLUBLE
VOLUBLY
VOLUMED
VOLUMES
VOLUTED
VOLUTES

V•••U••
VACUUMS
VALOURS
VALVULA
VALVULE
VANDURA
VANDUYN
VAPOURS
VAPOURY
VASQUEZ
VATFULS
VBLOUSE
VEINULE
VELLUMS
VELOURS
VELOUTE
VENDUES
VENTURA
VENTURE
VENTURI
VERDUGO
VERDURE
VERRUCA
VESTURE
VIADUCT
VICTUAL
VIGOURS
VINCULA
VIRGULE
VIRTUAL
VIRTUES
VISCUSO
VISTULA
VOITURE
VULTURE

V••••U•
VACUOUS
VANOCUR
VAPORUB
VARIOUS
VERDOUX
VIALFUL
VICIOUS
VILNIUS
VISCOUS
VOIDOUT
VONLAUE
VOTEOUT

V•••••U
VANUATU

•VU••••
AVULSED
AVULSES
EVULSED
EVULSES

•V•U•••
IVTUBES
TVGUIDE

•V••U••
AVENUEQ
AVENUES
EVACUEE
EVALUNA
EVOLUTE
OVERUSE
OVIDUCT
RVALUES
UVALUES

•V•••U•
AVERNUS
EVENOUT
EVENSUP
EVERDUR
OVERBUY
OVERCUT
OVERDUB
OVERDUE
OVERRUN
OVERSUP

••VU•••
DIVULGE
DIVULSE
RIVULET

••V•U••
BIVOUAC
DEVOURS
FAVOURS
GIVEUPS
RAVEUPS
SAVOURS
SAVOURY

••V••U•
COVERUP
DEVALUE
DEVIOUS
DIVVYUP
ENVIOUS
ENVOGUE
GAVEOUT
GIVENUP
GIVEOUT
GIVESUP
HAVEFUN
HAVEOUT
INVACUO
INVOGUE
LIVENUP
LIVEOUT
LOVEBUG
MOVEDUP
MOVEOUT
MOVESUP
NIVEOUS
OBVIOUS
OFVALUE
PAVIOUR
REVALUE
REVENUE
REVITUP
SAVEDUP
SAVESUP
SAVIOUR
SEVENUP
SEVERUS
UNVAGUE
UPVALUE

••V•••U
LOVEYOU
XAVIERU

•••VU••
BRAVURA
GRAVURE
NERVULE
PREVUED
PREVUES
SHAVUOT
VALVULA
VALVULE

•••V•U•
BELVOUR
CHEVAUX
DIVVYUP
DRIVEUP
DROVEUP
ELUVIUM
FERVOUR
FLAVIUS
FLAVOUR
IGIVEUP
NERVOUS
SERVEUP
TRIVIUM

•••V••U
NOUVEAU
PARVENU

••••VU•
NUNAVUT

V•V••••
VIVALDI
VIVANTS
VIVARIA
VIVENDI
VIVICAA
VIVIDER
VIVIDLY
VIVITAR

V••V•••
VALVATE
VALVULA
VALVULE
VANVOGT
VELVETS
VELVETY
VOUVRAY

V•••V••
VISAVIS
VOTIVES

•V•V•••
AVIVIAN

•V••V••
EVOLVED
EVOLVER
EVOLVES
TVMOVIE

•V•••V•
EVASIVE
IVANOVO

••VV•••
CIVVIES
DIVVIED
DIVVIES
DIVVYUP
REVVING
SAVVIED
SAVVIER
SAVVIES
SAVVILY

••V•V••
REVIVAL
REVIVED
REVIVER
REVIVES
UNVIVID

••V••V•
BIVALVE
DEVOLVE
INVOLVE
PAVLOVA
REVOLVE

•••VV••
FLIVVER

•••V•V•
QUIVIVE
SURVIVE

•••V••V
PLOVDIV

••••VV•
UNSAVVY

••••V•V
TELAVIV

V•W••••
VFWHALL
VFWPOST
VOWELLY
VOWLESS

V••W•••
VANWARD
VANWYCK
VIEWERS
VIEWIER
VIEWING
VIEWITH

V•••W••
VANOWEN
VERYWET

V•••••W
VERYFEW
VERYLOW
VERYNEW

•V•W•••
AVOWALS
AVOWERS
AVOWING

•V••W••
OVERWET

•V•••W•
OVERAWE
TVCREWS
TVSHOWS

•V••••W
EVENNOW
OVERFEW
OVERNEW
OVERSAW
OVERSEW

••VW•••
TUVWXYZ

••V•W••
FIVEWAY
GAVEWAY
GIVEWAY
UNVOWED

••V••W•
FIVETWO
REVIEWS

•••VW••
STUVWXY

•••V•W•
REAVOWS

•••V••W
DIMVIEW
PREVIEW
PURVIEW
THEVIEW

••••VW•
RSTUVWX

••••V•W
DISAVOW

•••••VW
QRSTUVW

V•X••••
VEXEDLY
VIXENLY

V•••X••
VANEXEL
VELOXES

V•••••X
VERDOUX
VICTRIX

•V••••X
OVERFIX
OVERLAX
OVERMIX
OVERTAX
UVINDEX

••V•X••
TUVWXYZ
UNVEXED

••V•••X
FIVESIX

•••V•X•
STUVWXY

•••V••X
BERVOIX
CHEVAUX
GRAVLAX

••••V•X
RSTUVWX

V•Y••••
VOYAGED
VOYAGER
VOYAGES

V••Y•••
VARYING
VERYBAD
VERYBIG
VERYDRY
VERYFEW
VERYFIT
VERYHIP
VERYHOT
VERYILL
VERYLOW
VERYMAD
VERYNEW
VERYODD
VERYOLD
VERYRED
VERYSAD
VERYSHY
VERYWET
VINYLIC

V•••Y••
VANDYCK
VANDYKE
VANEYCK
VANWYCK
VATDYED
VATDYES
VISAYAN
VOTEYEA
VOTEYES

V••••Y•
VALLEYS
VANDUYN
VEEJAYS
VOLLEYS
VOTEAYE

V•••••Y
VACANCY
VACUITY
VAGUELY
VALIDLY
VAPIDLY
VAPOURY
VARIETY
VARSITY
VASTITY
VELVETY
VENALLY
VERBIFY
VERMINY
VERSIFY
VERYDRY
VERYSHY
VEXEDLY
VICEROY
VICKREY
VICTORY
VISIBLY
VITALLY
VITRIFY
VIVIDLY
VIXENLY
VOCABLY
VOCALLY
VOLUBLY
VOTENAY
VOUVRAY
VOWELLY
VRONSKY

•VY••••
IVYLIKE

•V•Y•••
AVEYRON

•V•••Y•
EVERLYS
EVILEYE
OVERDYE

•V••••Y
AVIDITY
KVETCHY
OVERBUY
OVERCOY
OVERDRY
OVERFLY
OVERJOY
OVERLAY
OVERPAY
OVERPLY
OVERTLY

••VY•••
ENVYING
LEVYING
NAVYMAN
NAVYMEN
UNVYING

••V•Y••
DIVVYUP
LOVEYOU

••V••Y•
TUVWXYZ

••V•••Y
BEVERLY
CAVALRY
CIVILLY
DEVILRY
FIVEDAY
FIVEWAY
GAVEWAY
GIVENBY
GIVEWAY
LEVELLY
LIVESEY
LIVIDLY
LOVABLY
LOVEJOY
LOVERLY
MOVABLY
NOVELTY
NOVOTNY
PAVIDLY
POVERTY
RAVELLY
REVELRY
REVERDY
RIVALRY
SAVOURY
SAVVILY
SEVENTY
SEVIGNY
VIVIDLY
YEVGENY

•••VY••
DIVVYUP
PRIVYTO

•••V•Y•
CONVEYS
CONVOYS
PURVEYS
SURVEYS

•••V••Y
BRAVELY
BRAVERY
BREVITY
CALVARY
CLOVERY
DRIVEBY
DROVEBY
FLAVORY
GRAVELY
GRAVITY
HEAVILY
KNAVERY
NAIVELY
NAIVETY
NERVILY
PRIVACY
PRIVILY
PRIVITY
QUAVERY
QUIVERY
SAVVILY
SHIVERY
SILVERY
SLAVERY
STUVWXY
SUAVELY
SUAVITY
VELVETY
VOUVRAY

••••V•Y
MCCOVEY
UNSAVVY

•••••VY
ANCHOVY
DONLEVY
KARLOVY
OLDNAVY
PRONAVY
TANTIVY
TAXLEVY
UNHEAVY
UNSAVVY

V•Z••••
VIZIERS
VIZORED
VIZSLAS

V••Z•••
VANZANT
VONZELL

V•••Z••
VENEZIA
VERIZON
VIERZIG

V••••Z•
VICENZA

V•••••Z
VASQUEZ

••V•••Z
ALVAREZ
DAVEKOZ
TUVWXYZ

•••V•Z•
CERVEZA

•••V••Z
HORVITZ
NARVAEZ

••••V•Z
ESTEVEZ

WA•••••
WABASHA
WABBITS
WACKEST
WACKIER
WACKILY
WADDELL
WADDERS
WADDING
WADDLED
WADDLER
WADDLES
WADEDIN
WADESIN
WADKINS
WAFERED
WAFFLED
WAFFLER
WAFFLES
WAFTERS
WAFTING
WAGERED
WAGERER
WAGEWAR
WAGGERS
WAGGERY
WAGGING
WAGGISH
WAGGLED
WAGGLER
WAGGLES
WAGONED
WAGONER
WAHINES
WAHWAHS
WAIFISH
WAIKATO
WAIKIKI
WAILERS
WAILFUL
WAILING
WAISTED
WAITERS
WAITFOR
WAITING
WAITOUT
WAITRON
WAITSON
WAITSUP
WAIVERS
WAIVING
WAKAMES
WAKEDUP
WAKEFUL
WAKENED
WAKENER
WAKESUP
WAKEUPS
WAKINGS
WAKSMAN
WALCOTT
WALDORF
WALKERS
WALKING
WALKINS
WALKMAN
WALKOFF
WALKONS
WALKOUT
WALKSBY
WALKSON
WALKSTO
WALKUPS
WALKURE
WALKWAY
WALLABY
WALLACE
WALLACH
WALLETS
WALLEYE
WALLING
WALLMAP
WALLOFF
WALLOON
WALLOPS
WALLOWS
WALLSIN
WALLSUP
WALMART
WALNUTS
WALPOLE
WALSTON
WALTERS
WALTHAM
WALTHER
WALTONS
WALTZED
WALTZER
WALTZES
WAMBLED
WAMBLES
WAMPUMS
WANDERS
WANGLED
WANGLER
WANGLES
WANIEST
WANKELS
WANNABE
WANNESS
WANNEST
WANNING
WANNISH
WANTADS
WANTAGH
WANTERS
WANTING
WANTONS
WANTOUT
WANTSIN
WANTSTO
WAPITIS
WAPSHOT
WARBABY
WARBLED
WARBLER
WARBLES
WARBOND
WARBURG
WARCLUB
WARDENS
WARDERS
WARDING
WARDOFF
WAREPIC
WARFARE
WARGAME
WARGODS
WARHAWK
WARHEAD
WARHERO
WARIEST
WARLESS
WARLIKE
WARLOCK
WARLORD
WARMERS
WARMEST
WARMING
WARMISH
WARMSTO
WARMSUP
WARMUPS
WARNING
WARNOFF
WARNSOF
WARPAGE
WARPATH
WARPERS
WARPING
WARRANT
WARRENG
WARRENS
WARRING
WARRIOR
WARROOM
WARSHIP
WARTHOG
WARTIER
WARTIME
WARTORN
WARVETS
WARWICK
WARWORN
WARZONE
WASABIS
WASATCH
WASFAIR
WASHDAY
WASHERS
WASHIER
WASHING
WASHOFF
WASHOUT
WASHRAG
WASHTUB
WASHUPS
WASLATE
WASONTO
WASPIER
WASPILY
WASPISH
WASSAIL
WASSILY
WASSURE
WASTAGE
WASTERS
WASTING
WASTREL
WATCHED
WATCHER
WATCHES
WATCHIT
WATCHTV
WATERED
WATERER
WATFORD
WATKINS
WATTAGE
WATTEAU
WATTLED
WATTLES
WATUSIS
WAVEDAT
WAVEDIN
WAVEDTO
WAVELET
WAVEOFF
WAVERED
WAVERER
WAVESAT
WAVESIN
WAVESTO
WAVICLE
WAVIEST
WAXABLE
WAXBEAN
WAXEDUP
WAXESUP
WAXIEST
WAXINGS
WAXLIKE
WAXWING
WAXWORK
WAYBACK
WAYBILL
WAYCOOL
WAYLAID
WAYLAND
WAYLAYS
WAYLESS
WAYSIDE
WAYTOGO
WAYWARD
WAYWORN

W•A••••
WEAKENS
WEAKEST
WEAKISH
WEAKONS
WEALTHS
WEALTHY
WEANERS
WEANING
WEAPONS
WEARERS
WEARIED
WEARIER
WEARIES
WEARILY
WEARING
WEAROFF
WEAROUT
WEARSON
WEASELS
WEATHER
WEAVERS
WEAVING
WHACKED
WHACKER
WHALERS
WHALING
WHALLEY
WHAMMED
WHANGED
WHAPPED
WHARFED
WHARTON
WHARVES
WHATAMI
WHATFOR
WHATIFS
WHATNOT
WHATNOW
WHATSAY
WHATSIS
WHATSIT
WHATSUP
WHATTHE
WHAUDEN
WRACKED
WRACKUP
WRAITHS
WRANGEL
WRANGLE
WRAPPED
WRAPPER
WRAPSUP
WRAPUPS
WRASSES

W••A•••
WABASHA
WAKAMES
WASABIS
WASATCH
WAXABLE
WCHANDY
WHEATEN
WHEATON
WIRABLE
WIZARDS
WOMANLY
WREAKED
WREAKER
WREATHE
WREATHS
WREATHY

W•••A••
WAHWAHS
WAIKATO
WALLABY
WALLACE
WALLACH
WALMART
WANNABE
WANTADS
WANTAGH
WARBABY
WARFARE
WARGAME
WARHAWK
WARPAGE
WARPATH
WARRANT
WASFAIR
WASLATE
WASSAIL
WASTAGE
WATTAGE
WAYBACK
WAYLAID
WAYLAND
WAYLAYS
WAYWARD
WBYEATS
WEBCAMS
WEBCAST
WEBMAIL
WEBPAGE
WELFARE
WELLAND
WENTAFT
WENTAPE
WETBARS
WETLAND
WETNAPS
WETRAGS
WETWARE
WETWASH
WHATAMI
WHOSAID
WHYWAIT
WICCANS
WIDMARK
WIELAND
WIGWAGS
WIGWAMS
WILLARD
WINBACK
WINDAGE
WINDAUS
WOMBATS
WOODARD
WORDAGE
WYOTANA

W••••A•
WAGEWAR
WAKSMAN
WALKMAN
WALKWAY
WALLMAP
WALTHAM
WARHEAD
WASHDAY
WASHRAG
WATTEAU
WAVEDAT
WAVESAT
WAXBEAN
WEEKDAY
WEIDMAN
WEIRDAL
WELLMAN
WENTBAD
WENTFAR
WENTMAD
WHATSAY
WHEREAS
WHEREAT
WHIPSAW
WHISKAS
WHITMAN
WILDCAT
WILDMAN
WILLIAM
WINDBAG
WINEBAR
WINESAP
WINEVAT
WINGMAN
WINKSAT
WIREMAN
WIRETAP
WISEMAN
WOLFGAL
WOLFMAN
WOLFRAM
WOODSAW
WOODTAR
WOOLFAT
WOOLHAT
WOOSNAM
WORKDAY
WORKMAN
WORKSAT
WOZNIAK
WROCLAW
WYNDHAM

W•••••A
WABASHA
WICHITA
WOJTYLA
WYNONNA
WYOTANA

•WA••••
AWAITED
AWAITER
AWAKENS
AWAKERS
AWAKING
AWARDED
AWARDEE
AWARDER
AWAREOF
AWAREST
AWASHIN
DWARFED
DWARVES
IWANTIT
IWANTTO
KWACHAS
KWANZAA
KWANZAS
RWANDAN
SWABBED
SWABBER
SWADDLE
SWAGGER
SWAGMAN
SWAGMEN
SWAHILI
SWALLOW
SWAMPED
SWANKED
SWANKER
SWANKUP
SWANSEA
SWANSON
SWAPPED
SWAPPER
SWARMED
SWARMER
SWARTHY
SWASHED
SWASHES
SWATHED
SWATHES
SWATSAT
SWATTED
SWATTER
SWAYBAR
SWAYERS
SWAYING
TWADDLE
TWANGED
TWANGER
ZWANZIG

•W•A•••
SWEARAT
SWEARBY
SWEARER
SWEARIN
SWEARTO
SWEATED
SWEATER
SWEATIT
TWEAKED
TWOACRE
TWOACTS

•W••A••
AWKWARD
EWELAMB
TWOBALL
TWOBASE
TWODAYS
TWOFACE
TWOLANE
TWOPAIR
TWOPART

•W•••A•
DWELLAT
KWACHAS
KWANZAA
KWANZAS
OWNGOAL
RWANDAN
SWAGMAN
SWATSAT
SWAYBAR
SWEARAT
SWINGAT
SWOREAT
SWUNGAT
TWOSTAR
TWOYEAR
ZWICKAU

•W••••A
IWOJIMA
KWANZAA
PWBOTHA
SWANSEA
SWEEPEA
TWELVEA

••WA•••
ATWATER
BEWAILS
BEWARED
BEWARES
BYWAYOF
COWARDS
DEWAART
DEWATER
DEWAXED
DEWAXES
DOWAGER
EDWARDG
EDWARDI
EDWARDR
EDWARDS
EDWARDV
FTWAYNE
HOWARDK
HOWARDS
HOWARDU
INWARDS
KIWANIS
KOWADLO
KUWAITI
LAWANDA
NEWAGER
NEWAGEY
ONWARDS
ONWATER
REWAGER
REWAKED
REWAKEN
REWAKES
REWARDS
REWARMS
REWARNS
REWATER
REWAXED
REWAXES
SAWATCH
SEWARDS
THWACKS
THWARTS
TOWABLE
TOWAGES
TOWARDS
TOWAWAY
UNWADED
UNWAGED
UNWAKED
UNWALLS
UNWANED
UNWAVED
UNWAXED
UPWAFTS
UPWARDS

••W•A••
BOWOARS
BOWSAWS
COWBANE
COWHAND
DEWAART
DEWFALL
DEWLAPS
ENWRAPS
GEWGAWS
HAWHAWS
HOWDAHS
HOWLAME
HOWMANY
INWEAVE
LAWCASE
LOWBALL
LOWCARB
LOWCARD
LOWHAND
LOWLAND
LOWMASS
LOWPAID
LOWPAIR
NEWCARS
NEWFACE
NEWGATE
NEWHAND
NEWHART
NEWHATS
NEWLAID
NEWMADE
NEWMANS
NEWMATH
NEWNAME
NEWWAVE
PAWPAWS
RAWBARS
RAWDATA
REWEARS
REWEAVE
REWRAPS
ROWLAND
SAWPAST
TOWBARS
TOWCARS
TOWPATH
UNWEARY
UNWEAVE
UNWRAPS
VFWHALL

••W••A•
ADWOMAN
BOWHEAD
COWERAT
COWPEAS
DEWCLAW
DOWNPAT
GAWKSAT
HAWKMAN
HOWLSAT
IFWEMAY
JAWEDAT
LEWHOAD
LOWBEAM
LOWGEAR
LOWROAD
MOWBRAY
NEWDEAL
NEWLEAF
NEWSDAY
NEWSMAN
NEWYEAR
NOWWHAT
PAWEDAT
RAWDEAL
RAWMEAT
ROWBOAT
SOWSEAR
TOWAWAY
TOWBOAT
TOWHEAD
TOWNCAR

••W•••A
LAWANDA
NEWIDEA
RAWDATA

•••WA••
ADAWARE
AIRWARS
AIRWAVE
AIRWAYS
AJOWANS
ANYWAYS
ARTWALL
ARTWARE
ATHWART
AVOWALS
AWKWARD
BARWARE
BREWAGE
BROWARD
BULWARK
CARWASH
CATWALK
DRYWALL
DRYWASH
DURWARD
ENDWAYS
EYEWALL
EYEWASH
FLOWAGE
FLYWAYS
FORWARD
FROWARD
GASWARS
GETWARM
GOTWARM
GUNWALE
HAYWARD
HEYWARD
HOGWASH
HOTWARS
JAYWALK
JAYWARD

JETWASH
JETWAYS
KENWAHL
KEYWAYS
KNOWALL
LAPWARE
LEEWARD
LEEWAYS
MALWARE
MIDWAYS
MUDWASP
NETWARE
NEWWAVE
NONWAGE
NONWARS
NORWALK
OLDWAYS
OSTWALD
OUTWAIT
OUTWALK
OUTWARD
OUTWARS
OUTWASH
OUTWAVE
PEDWAYS
PINWALE
PREWARM
PREWARN
PREWASH
PSYWARS
REAWAKE
RUNWAYS
SAYWAIT
SCHWANN
SEAWALL
SEAWARD
SEAWAYS
SEGWAYS
SKYWALK
SKYWARD
SKYWAYS
SPYWARE
STEWARD
STEWART
STOWAGE
SUBWARS
SUBWAYS
SUNWARD
THEWALL
THEWAVE
TINWARE
UNAWAKE
UNAWARE
VANWARD
WAHWAHS
WAYWARD
WETWARE
WETWASH
WHYWAIT
WIGWAGS
WIGWAMS
ZUMWALT

•••W•A•
BROWWAX
CLAWSAT
CRAWDAD
CREWMAN
CROWBAR
DAYWEAR
DRAWBAR
DRAWMAN
EYEWEAR
FAYWRAY
FLOWNAT
FROWNAT
FURWRAP
GNAWSAT
GREWFAT
GROWFAT
LEGWEAR
NARWHAL
NOSWEAT
NOWWHAT
OUTWEAR
PLOWMAN
PREWRAP
RESWEAR
SAYWHAT
SHOWCAT
SHOWMAN
SKIWEAR
SLOWDAY
SNOWCAP
SNOWCAT
SNOWDAY
SNOWHAT
SNOWMAN
STEWPAN
UNSWEAR

•••W••A
LIDWINA
SNOWPEA

••••WA•
ALLOWAY
ANTIWAR
ARCHWAY
AREAWAY
ASKAWAY
ATEAWAY
BACKWAY
BEESWAX
BELTWAY
BIKEWAY
BOBTWAY
BOERWAR
BROWWAX
BUSHWAH
CARAWAY
CHINWAG
COLDWAR
CUTAWAY
DIEAWAY
DOORWAY
DUNAWAY
EATAWAY
FAIRWAY
FARAWAY
FAREWAR
FIVEWAY
FLYAWAY
FOLKWAY
FOOTWAY
FOURWAY
FREEWAY
GANGWAY
GATEWAY
GAVEWAY
GETAWAY
GIVEWAY
GOTAWAY
GOTOWAR
GULFWAR
HALFWAY
HALLWAY
HARDWAY
HEADWAY
HIDAWAY
HIGHWAY
HOLYWAR
INNOWAY
JANEWAY
LANGWAY
LAYAWAY
LEDAWAY
LONGWAY
MADEWAR
MADEWAY
MAKEWAR
MAKEWAY
MANOWAR
MATEWAN
MEDAWAR
OJIBWAS
OJIBWAY
OTTAWAN
OTTAWAS
OUTSWAM
PARKWAY
PARTWAY
PATHWAY
PEGAWAY
PESEWAS
POSTWAR
PUTAWAY
RACEWAY
RAILWAY
RANAWAY
RENEWAL
RIDGWAY
ROADWAY
ROLLWAY
ROTAWAY
RUNAWAY
SAFEWAY
SARAWAK
SHIPWAY
SHYAWAY
SIDEWAY
SKAGWAY
SOMEWAY
TAILWAG
TAXIWAY
THATWAY
THESWAN
THISWAY
THREWAT
THROWAT
THRUWAY
TIMEWAS
TOLLWAY
TOWAWAY
TRAMWAY
TURFWAR
WAGEWAR
WALKWAY

••••W•A
CATAWBA
KELOWNA

•••••WA
OKINAWA
OTTUMWA

WB•••••
WBYEATS

W•B••••
WABASHA
WABBITS
WEBBIER
WEBBING
WEBCAMS
WEBCAST
WEBFEET
WEBFOOT
WEBLESS
WEBLIKE
WEBLOGS
WEBMAIL
WEBPAGE
WEBSITE
WEBSTER
WEBTOED
WEBZINE
WOBBLED
WOBBLER
WOBBLES
WOBEGON

W••B•••
WABBITS
WAMBLED
WAMBLES
WARBABY
WARBLED
WARBLER
WARBLES
WARBOND
WARBURG
WAXBEAN
WAYBACK
WAYBILL
WEBBIER
WEBBING
WEEBITS
WEMBLEY
WETBARS
WETBULB
WILBERT
WINBACK
WOBBLED
WOBBLER
WOBBLES
WOMBATS

W•••B••
WASABIS
WAXABLE
WENTBAD
WINDBAG
WINEBAR
WINSBIG
WIRABLE
WOODBIN
WOODBOX
WORKBOX

W••••B•
WALKSBY
WALLABY
WANNABE
WARBABY
WHEREBY
WOULDBE

W•••••B
WARCLUB
WASHTUB
WETBULB
WOLFCUB

•WB••••
PWBOTHA

•W•B•••
SWABBED
SWABBER
TWOBALL
TWOBASE
TWOBITS

•W••B••
AWEEBIT
SWABBED
SWABBER
SWAYBAR
TWINBED

•W•••B•
SWEARBY
SWINGBY
SWOREBY
SWUNGBY

•W••••B
EWELAMB
TWELVEB

••WB•••
COWBANE
COWBELL
COWBIRD
COWBOYS
HOWBEIT
JAWBONE
LAWBOOK
LOWBALL
LOWBEAM
LOWBIDS
LOWBLOW
LOWBORN
LOWBOYS
LOWBRED
LOWBROW
MOWBRAY
NEWBERN
NEWBERY
NEWBIES
NEWBOLT
NEWBORN
NEWBURG
RAWBARS
ROWBOAT
SAWBUCK
TOWBARS
TOWBOAT

••W•B••
DOWNBOW
NEWSBOY
TOWABLE

••W••B•
DRWELBY
NEWJOBS

••W•••B
LOWCARB

•••WB••
CROWBAR
DRAWBAR
GREWBIG
GROWBIG
PLOWBOY
SHOWBIZ

•••W•B•
COBWEBS
FLOWNBY

•••W••B
BREWPUB
SNOWJOB

••••WB•
CATAWBA

••••W•B
FOODWEB

WC•••••
WCHANDY

W•C••••
WACKEST
WACKIER
WACKILY
WICCANS
WICHITA
WICKERS
WICKETS
WICKING
WICKIUP
WICKLOW

W••C•••
WALCOTT
WARCLUB
WATCHED
WATCHER
WATCHES
WATCHIT
WATCHTV
WAYCOOL
WEBCAMS
WEBCAST
WELCOME
WENCHES
WESCOTT
WETCELL
WHACKED
WHACKER
WICCANS
WINCERS
WINCHED
WINCHER
WINCHES
WINCING
WITCHED
WITCHES
WRACKED
WRACKUP
WRECKED
WRECKER
WROCLAW

W•••C••
WAVICLE
WELLCUT
WILDCAT
WOLFCUB
WOODCUT

W••••C•
WALLACE
WALLACH
WARLOCK
WARWICK
WASATCH
WAYBACK
WEDLOCK
WINBACK
WOZZECK

W•••••C
WAREPIC

•W•C•••
KWACHAS
ZWICKAU

•W••C••
TWITCHY
TWOACRE
TWOACTS

•W•••C•
EWENECK
TWOFACE

•W••••C
TWELVEC

••WC•••
DEWCLAW
FAWCETT
HOWCOME
LAWCASE
LOWCARB
LOWCARD
LOWCHEN
LOWCOST
NEWCARS
SAWCHUK
TOWCARS

••W•C••
BOWECHO
THWACKS
TOWNCAR

••W••C•
BEWITCH
COWLICK
HOWMUCH
HOWNICE
LOWNECK
LOWTECH
NEWFACE
NEWRICH
SAWATCH
SAWBUCK

•••WC••
CREWCUT
SHOWCAT
SNOWCAP
SNOWCAT

•••W•C•
AIRWICK
BERWICK
GATWICK
IPSWICH
MEDWICK
NATWICK
NORWICH
RENWICK
VANWYCK
WARWICK

W•D••••
WADDELL
WADDERS
WADDING
WADDLED
WADDLER
WADDLES
WADEDIN
WADESIN
WADKINS
WEDDELL
WEDDERS
WEDDING
WEDELED
WEDELNS
WEDGEIN
WEDGIER
WEDGIES
WEDGING
WEDIDIT
WEDLOCK
WIDENED
WIDENER
WIDGEON
WIDGETS
WIDMARK
WIDOWED
WIDOWER

W••D•••
WADDELL
WADDERS
WADDING
WADDLED
WADDLER
WADDLES
WALDORF
WANDERS
WARDENS
WARDERS
WARDING
WARDOFF
WEDDELL
WEDDERS
WEDDING
WEEDERS
WEEDIER
WEEDILY
WEEDING
WEEDOUT
WEIDMAN
WELDERS
WELDING
WENDELL
WENDERS
WENDING
WENDKOS
WETDOWN
WILDCAT
WILDDOG
WILDEST
WILDING
WILDISH
WILDMAN
WILDMEN
WILDONE
WILDPIG
WINDAGE
WINDAUS
WINDBAG
WINDERS
WINDGOD
WINDIER
WINDIGO
WINDILY
WINDING
WINDOMS
WINDOWS
WINDOWY
WINDSOR
WINDSUP
WINDTEE
WINDUPS
WISDOMS
WONDERS
WOODARD
WOODBIN
WOODBOX
WOODCUT
WOODIER
WOODIES
WOODING
WOODLEY
WOODLOT
WOODROW
WOODSAW
WOODSON
WOODTAR
WORDAGE
WORDIER
WORDILY
WORDING
WORDONE
WYNDHAM

W•••D••
WADEDIN
WAKEDUP
WASHDAY
WAVEDAT
WAVEDIN
WAVEDTO
WAXEDUP
WEDIDIT
WEEKDAY
WEIRDAL
WEIRDED
WEIRDER
WEIRDLY
WEIRDOS
WHAUDEN
WHEEDLE
WIELDED
WIELDER
WILDDOG
WIPEDUP
WIREDIN
WIREDUP
WISEDUP
WOLFDOG
WORKDAY
WORLDLY
WOULDBE
WOULDNT
WOULDST
WOUNDED
WOUNDUP
WOWEDEM

W••••D•
WANTADS
WARGODS
WAYSIDE
WCHANDY
WHWORDS
WIZARDS

W•••••D
WADDLED
WAFERED
WAFFLED
WAGERED
WAGGLED
WAGONED
WAISTED
WAKENED
WALTZED
WAMBLED
WANGLED
WARBLED
WARBOND
WARHEAD
WARLORD
WATCHED
WATERED
WATFORD
WATTLED
WAVERED
WAYLAID
WAYLAND
WAYWARD
WEARIED
WEBTOED
WEDELED
WEEKEND
WEIGHED
WEIRDED
WELLAND
WELLFED
WELLHID
WELLLED
WENTBAD
WENTMAD
WESTEND
WETEYED
WETLAND
WEXFORD
WHACKED
WHAMMED
WHANGED
WHAPPED
WHARFED
WHEELED
WHEEZED
WHELMED
WHELPED
WHETTED
WHIFFED
WHIPPED
WHIRLED
WHIRRED
WHISHED
WHISKED
WHIZKID
WHIZZED
WHOMPED
WHOOPED
WHOPPED
WHORLED
WHOSAID
WHUPPED
WIDENED
WIDOWED
WIELAND
WIELDED
WIGGLED
WILFORD
WILFRED
WILLARD
WIMPLED
WINCHED
WINDGOD
WINERED
WINWOOD
WITCHED
WITSEND
WIZENED
WOBBLED
WOODARD
WOOSHED
WORRIED
WORSTED
WOUNDED
WRACKED
WRAPPED
WREAKED
WRECKED
WRESTED
WRITHED
WRONGED

•W•D•••
SWADDLE
SWEDISH
TWADDLE
TWIDDLE
TWODAYS
TWODEEP
TWODOOR

•W••D••
AWARDED
AWARDEE
AWARDER
DWINDLE
IWONDER
OWNEDUP
RWANDAN
SWADDLE
SWINDLE
TWADDLE
TWEEDLE
TWIDDLE

•W••••D
AWAITED
AWARDED
AWKWARD
DWARFED
DWELLED
DWIGHTD
OWLEYED
SWABBED
SWAMPED
SWANKED
SWAPPED
SWARMED
SWASHED
SWATHED
SWATTED
SWEATED
SWELLED
SWERVED
SWIGGED
SWILLED
SWIRLED
SWISHED
SWOONED
SWOOPED
TWANGED
TWEAKED
TWEETED
TWEEZED
TWELVED
TWILLED
TWINBED
TWINGED
TWINNED
TWIRLED
TWISTED
TWITTED
TWOFOLD
TWOTOED

••WD•••
BAWDIER
BAWDILY
BOWDLER
BOWDOIN
BOWDOWN
DAWDLED
DAWDLER
DAWDLES
DEWDROP
DOWDIER
DOWDIES
DOWDILY
HOWDAHS
HOWDEDO
HOWDULL
HOWDYDO
LEWDEST
LOWDIVE
LOWDOWN
MOWDOWN
NEWDEAL
POWDERS
POWDERY
RAWDATA
RAWDEAL
ROWDIER
ROWDIES
ROWDILY
SAWDUST

••W•D••
BOWEDTO
HEWEDTO
JAWEDAT
KOWADLO
NEWIDEA
NEWSDAY
PAWEDAT
REWIDEN
SEWEDON
SEWEDUP
TOWEDIN
UNWADED
UNWEDGE
WOWEDEM

••W••D•
BYWORDS
COWARDS
COWHIDE
DEWILDE
EDWARDG
EDWARDI
EDWARDR
EDWARDS
EDWARDV
ENWINDS
HOWARDK
HOWARDS
HOWARDU
HOWDEDO
HOWDYDO
INWARDS
LAWANDA

LOWBIDS
LOWSIDE
LOWTIDE
MRWORDS
NEWKIDS
NEWMADE
ONWARDS
RAWHIDE
REWARDS
REWELDS
REWINDS
REWORDS
SEWARDS
TOWARDS
UNWINDS
UNWINDY
UPWARDS
UPWINDS
WHWORDS

••W•••D

BEWARED
BOWERED
BOWHEAD
COWBIRD
COWERED
COWHAND
COWHERD
COWSHED
DAWDLED
DEWAXED
DEWIRED
DOWERED
ENWOUND
JEWELED
LAWFORD
LEWHOAD
LOWBRED
LOWCARD
LOWERED
LOWHAND
LOWLAND
LOWPAID
LOWROAD
MYWORLD
NEWHAND
NEWLAID
NEWWORD
PCWORLD
POWERED
RAWFOOD
REWAKED
REWAXED
REWIPED
REWIRED
REWOUND
ROWELED
ROWLAND
SAWWOOD
TOWELED
TOWERED
TOWHEAD
UNWADED
UNWAGED
UNWAKED
UNWANED
UNWAVED
UNWAXED
UNWIPED
UNWIRED
UNWOOED
UNWOUND

•••WD••

BLOWDRY
CHOWDER
CLOWDER
CRAWDAD
CROWDED
CROWDER
CROWDIN
GREWDIM
GROWDIM
SHOWDOG
SLOWDAY
SNOWDAY
SNOWDON

•••W•D

ARCWELD
AWKWARD
BADWORD
BLOWZED
BRAWLED
BROWARD
BROWNED
BROWSED
CLOWNED
COOWNED
CRAWDAD
CRAWLED
CROWDED
CROWNED
DAGWOOD
DOGWOOD
DRAWLED
DROWNED
DROWSED
DURWARD
DYEWOOD
ELMWOOD
FORWARD
FROWARD
FROWNED
GETWORD
GOTWORD
GREWOLD
GROWLED
GROWOLD
GUMWOOD
HAYWARD
HEYWARD
HEYWOOD
HOGWEED
HOGWILD
ICYWIND
ILLWIND
INAWORD
JAYWARD
KEYWORD
LEAWOOD
LEEWARD
MISWORD
NEWWORD
NONWORD
NORWOOD
NUTWOOD
OAKWOOD
ONEWOOD
OSTWALD
OUTWARD
OUTWEED
OUTWIND
OUTWORD
PIGWEED
PLYWOOD
PRAWNED
PROWLED
RAGWEED
RANWILD
REDWOOD
REOWNED
RONWOOD
RUNWILD
SAWWOOD
SCOWLED
SEAWARD
SEAWEED
SHAWLED
SKYWARD
SOTWEED
SPAWNED
STEWARD
SUNWARD
THEWIND
TRAWLED
UNOWNED
VANWARD
WAYWARD
WINWOOD

••••WD•

UNROWDY

••••W•D

ALLOWED
BEDEWED
ELBOWED
ENDOWED
MIAOWED
OUTAWED
PSHAWED
REMOWED
RENEWED
RESAWED
RESEWED
RESOWED
RETOWED
SCARWID
SCREWED
SINEWED
STREWED
UNBOWED
UNCOWED
UNDEWED
UNHEWED
UNMEWED
UNMOWED
UNPAWED
UNSAWED
UNSEWED
UNSOWED
UNVOWED
WIDOWED

•••••WD

INCROWD

WE•••••

WEAKENS
WEAKEST
WEAKISH
WEAKONS
WEALTHS
WEALTHY
WEANERS
WEANING
WEAPONS
WEARERS
WEARIED
WEARIER
WEARIES
WEARILY
WEARING
WEAROFF
WEAROUT
WEARSON
WEASELS
WEATHER
WEAVERS
WEAVING
WEBBIER
WEBBING
WEBCAMS
WEBCAST
WEBFEET
WEBFOOT
WEBLESS
WEBLIKE
WEBLOGS
WEBMAIL
WEBPAGE
WEBSITE
WEBSTER
WEBTOED
WEBZINE
WEDDELL
WEDDERS
WEDDING
WEDELED
WEDELNS
WEDGEIN
WEDGIER
WEDGIES
WEDGING
WEDIDIT
WEDLOCK
WEEBITS
WEEDERS
WEEDIER
WEEDILY
WEEDING
WEEDOUT
WEEFOLK
WEEHOUR
WEEKDAY
WEEKEND
WEENESS
WEENIES
WEEONES
WEEPERS
WEEPFOR
WEEPIER
WEEPING
WEEVILS
WEGENER
WEIDMAN
WEIGHED
WEIGHER
WEIGHIN
WEIGHON
WEIGHTS
WEIGHTY
WEIGHUP
WEIRDAL
WEIRDED
WEIRDER
WEIRDLY
WEIRDOS
WEIRTON
WELCOME
WELDERS
WELDING
WELFARE
WELLAND
WELLCUT
WELLFED
WELLHID
WELLHIT
WELLING
WELLLED
WELLLIT
WELLMAN
WELLOFF
WELLPUT
WELLRUN
WELLSEE
WELLSET
WELLSUP
WELLWON
WELLYES
WELTERS
WELTING
WEMBLEY
WENCHES
WENDELL
WENDERS
WENDING
WENDKOS
WENTAFT
WENTAPE
WENTBAD
WENTFAR
WENTFOR
WENTMAD
WENTOFF
WENTOUT
WENTPRO
WERNHER
WERTHER
WESCOTT
WESKITS
WESTEGG
WESTEND
WESTERN
WESTERS
WESTIES
WESTINS
WETBARS
WETBULB
WETCELL
WETDOWN
WETEYED
WETKISS
WETLAND
WETLOOK
WETMOPS
WETNAPS
WETNESS
WETONES
WETRAGS
WETSUIT
WETTEST
WETTING
WETTISH
WETWARE
WETWASH
WEXFORD

W•E••••

WEEBITS
WEEDERS
WEEDIER
WEEDILY
WEEDING
WEEDOUT
WEEFOLK
WEEHOUR
WEEKDAY
WEEKEND
WEENESS
WEENIES
WEEONES
WEEPERS
WEEPFOR
WEEPIER
WEEPING
WEEVILS
WHEATEN
WHEATON
WHEEDLE
WHEELED
WHEELER
WHEELIE
WHEELIN
WHEEZED
WHEEZER
WHEEZES
WHELMED
WHELPED
WHEREAS
WHEREAT
WHEREBY
WHEREIN
WHERELL
WHEREOF
WHEREON
WHERERE
WHERETO
WHEREVE
WHETHER
WHETTED
WHETTER
WHEYISH
WIELAND
WIELDED
WIELDER
WIENERS
WIENIES
WOEISME
WREAKED
WREAKER
WREATHE
WREATHS
WREATHY
WRECKED
WRECKER
WRESTED
WRESTER
WRESTLE

W••E•••

WADEDIN
WADESIN
WAFERED
WAGERED
WAGERER
WAGEWAR
WAKEDUP
WAKEFUL
WAKENED
WAKENER
WAKESUP
WAKEUPS
WAREPIC
WATERED
WATERER
WAVEDAT
WAVEDIN
WAVEDTO
WAVELET
WAVEOFF
WAVERED
WAVERER
WAVESAT
WAVESIN
WAVESTO
WAXEDUP
WAXESUP
WBYEATS
WEDELED
WEDELNS
WEGENER
WETEYED
WHEEDLE
WHEELED
WHEELER
WHEELIE
WHEELIN
WHEEZED
WHEEZER
WHEEZES
WHOEVER
WHYEVER
WIDENED
WIDENER
WINEBAR
WINERED
WINESAP
WINEVAT
WIPEDUP
WIPEOFF
WIPEOUT
WIPESUP
WIREDIN
WIREDUP
WIREMAN
WIREMEN
WIRESIN
WIRESUP
WIRETAP
WISEDUP
WISEGUY
WISEMAN
WISEMEN
WISEONE
WISESUP
WITEOUT
WIZENED
WOBEGON
WOKENUP
WOREOFF
WOREOUT
WOWEDEM
WYNETTE
WYVERNS

W•••E••

WACKEST
WADDELL
WADDERS
WAFTERS
WAGGERS
WAGGERY
WAILERS
WAITERS
WAIVERS
WALKERS
WALLETS
WALLEYE
WALTERS
WANDERS
WANIEST
WANKELS
WANNESS
WANNEST
WANTERS
WARDENS
WARDERS
WARHEAD
WARHERO
WARIEST
WARLESS
WARMERS
WARMEST
WARPERS
WARRENG
WARRENS
WARVETS
WASHERS
WASTERS
WATTEAU
WAVIEST
WAXBEAN
WAXIEST
WAYLESS
WEAKENS
WEAKEST
WEANERS
WEARERS
WEASELS
WEAVERS
WEBFEET
WEBLESS
WEDDELL
WEDDERS
WEDGEIN
WEEDERS
WEEKEND
WEENESS
WEEPERS
WELDERS
WELTERS
WENDELL
WENDERS
WESTEGG
WESTEND
WESTERN
WESTERS
WETCELL
WETNESS
WETTEST
WHALERS
WHEREAS
WHEREAT
WHEREBY
WHEREIN
WHERELL
WHEREOF
WHEREON
WHERERE
WHERETO
WHEREVE
WHINERS
WHITELY
WHITENS
WHITEST
WICKERS
WICKETS
WIDGEON
WIDGETS
WIENERS
WIGGERY
WIGLESS
WIGLETS
WILBERT
WILDEST
WILHELM
WILIEST
WILKENS
WILLERS
WINCERS
WINDERS
WINGERS
WINIEST
WINKERS
WINLESS
WINNERS
WINTERS
WINTERY
WIRIEST
WISHERS
WITHERS
WITLESS
WITNESS
WITSEND
WONDERS
WOOFERS
WOOLENS
WOOLERY
WORKERS
WORMERS
WORRELL
WORSENS
WOZZECK
WRITEIN
WRITEME
WRITEON
WRITERS
WRITETO
WRITEUP
WROTEIN
WROTEON
WROTETO
WROTEUP
WRYNESS

W••••E•

WACKIER
WADDLED
WADDLER
WADDLES
WAFERED
WAFFLED
WAFFLER
WAFFLES
WAGERED
WAGERER
WAGGLED
WAGGLER
WAGGLES
WAGONED
WAGONER
WAHINES
WAISTED
WAKAMES
WAKENED
WAKENER
WALTHER
WALTZED
WALTZER
WALTZES
WAMBLED
WAMBLES
WANGLED
WANGLER
WANGLES
WARBLED
WARBLER
WARBLES
WARTIER
WASHIER
WASPIER
WASTREL
WATCHED
WATCHER
WATCHES
WATERED
WATERER
WATTLED
WATTLES
WAVELET
WAVERED
WAVERER
WEARIED
WEARIER
WEARIES
WEATHER
WEBBIER
WEBFEET
WEBSTER
WEBTOED
WEDELED
WEDGIER
WEDGIES
WEEDIER
WEENIES
WEEONES
WEEPIER
WEGENER
WEIGHED
WEIGHER
WEIRDED
WEIRDER
WELLFED
WELLLED
WELLSEE
WELLSET
WELLYES
WEMBLEY
WENCHES
WERNHER
WERTHER
WESTIES
WETEYED
WETONES
WHACKED
WHACKER
WHALLEY
WHAMMED
WHANGED
WHAPPED
WHARFED
WHARVES
WHAUDEN
WHEATEN
WHEELED
WHEELER
WHEEZED
WHEEZER
WHEEZES
WHELMED
WHELPED
WHETHER
WHETTED
WHETTER
WHIFFED
WHIFFER
WHIMPER
WHINIER
WHIPPED
WHIPPER
WHIPPET
WHIRLED
WHIRLER
WHIRRED
WHISHED
WHISHES
WHISKED
WHISKER
WHISKEY
WHISPER
WHITHER
WHITNEY
WHIZZED
WHIZZER
WHIZZES
WHOEVER
WHOKNEW
WHOMPED
WHOOPED
WHOOPEE
WHOOPER
WHOPPED
WHOPPER
WHORLED
WHUPPED
WHYEVER
WIDENED
WIDENER
WIDOWED
WIDOWER
WIELDED
WIELDER
WIENIES
WIGGIER
WIGGLED
WIGGLER
WIGGLES
WILDMEN
WILFRED
WILLIES
WIMOWEH
WIMPIER
WIMPLED
WIMPLES
WINCHED
WINCHER
WINCHES
WINDIER
WINDTEE
WINERED
WINFREY
WINGLET
WINGMEN
WINKLER
WINOVER
WINSLET
WIREMEN
WISEMEN
WISPIER
WITCHED
WITCHES
WITHIES
WITTIER
WIZENED
WOBBLED
WOBBLER
WOBBLES
WOLFMEN
WONOVER
WOODIER
WOODIES
WOODLEY
WOOKIEE
WOOLIER
WOOLIES
WOOLLEN
WOOLLEY
WOOLSEY
WOOSHED
WOOSHES
WOOSTER
WOOZIER
WORDIER
WORKMEN
WORMIER
WORRIED
WORRIER
WORRIES
WORSLEY
WORSTED
WOUNDED
WOWEDEM
WRACKED
WRANGEL
WRAPPED
WRAPPER
WRASSES
WREAKED
WREAKER
WRECKED
WRECKER
WRESTED
WRESTER
WRIGLEY
WRINGER
WRITHED
WRITHER
WRITHES
WRITTEN
WRONGED
WRONGER

W•••••E

WALKURE
WALLACE
WALLEYE
WALPOLE
WANNABE
WARFARE
WARGAME
WARLIKE
WARPAGE
WARTIME
WARZONE
WASLATE
WASSURE
WASTAGE
WATTAGE
WAVICLE
WAXABLE
WAXLIKE
WAYSIDE
WEBLIKE
WEBPAGE
WEBSITE
WEBZINE
WELCOME
WELFARE
WELLSEE
WENTAPE
WETWARE
WHATTHE
WHEEDLE
WHEELIE
WHERERE
WHEREVE
WHIFFLE
WHIPPLE
WHISTLE
WHITTLE
WHOOPEE
WHOOPIE
WIGLIKE

WILDONE
WILLKIE
WIMPOLE
WINDAGE
WINDTEE
WINSOME
WIRABLE
WISEONE
WOEISME
WOOKIEE
WOOLITE
WORDAGE
WORDONE
WOULDBE
WRANGLE
WREATHE
WRESTLE
WRIGGLE
WRINKLE
WRITEME
WYNETTE

•WE••••

AWEEBIT
AWELESS
AWESOME
DWEEZIL
DWELLAT
DWELLED
DWELLER
DWELLIN
DWELLON
DWELTON
EWELAMB
EWENECK
EWERIES
SWEARAT
SWEARBY
SWEARER
SWEARIN
SWEARTO
SWEATED
SWEATER
SWEATIT
SWEDISH
SWEENEY
SWEEPEA
SWEEPER
SWEEPUP
SWEETEN
SWEETER
SWEETIE
SWEETLY
SWEETON
SWELLED
SWELLER
SWELLUP
SWELTER
SWELTRY
SWENSON
SWEPTUP
SWERVED
SWERVES
TWEAKED
TWEEDLE
TWEENER
TWEETED
TWEETER
TWEEZED
TWEEZER
TWEEZES
TWELFTH
TWELVEA
TWELVEB
TWELVEC
TWELVED
TWELVEE
TWELVES
TWERENT

•W•E•••

AWEEBIT
DWEEZIL
OWLEGGS
OWLEYED
OWNEDUP
SWEENEY
SWEEPEA
SWEEPER
SWEEPUP
SWEETEN
SWEETER
SWEETIE
SWEETLY
SWEETON
TWEEDLE
TWEENER
TWEETED
TWEETER
TWEEZED
TWEEZER
TWEEZES
TWOEEEE
TWOEGGS

•W••E••

AWAKENS
AWAKERS
AWAREOF
AWAREST
AWELESS
AWNLESS
EWENECK
GWYNETH
OWLIEST
SWAYERS
SWIGERT
SWINERY
SWIPERS
SWIVELS
SWIVETS
SWOREAT
SWOREBY
SWOREIN
SWORETO
TWERENT
TWINERS
TWODEEP
TWOEEEE
TWOFEET
TWOFERS
TWOTERM
TWOWEEK
TWOYEAR

•W•••E•

AWAITED
AWAITER
AWARDED
AWARDEE
AWARDER
DWARFED
DWARVES
DWELLED
DWELLER
EWERIES
IWONDER
OWLEYED
SWABBED
SWABBER
SWAGGER
SWAGMEN
SWAMPED
SWANKED
SWANKER
SWANSEA
SWAPPED
SWAPPER
SWARMED
SWARMER
SWASHED
SWASHES
SWATHED
SWATHES
SWATTED
SWATTER
SWEARER
SWEATED
SWEATER
SWEENEY
SWEEPEA
SWEEPER
SWEETEN
SWEETER
SWELLED
SWELLER
SWELTER
SWERVED
SWERVES
SWIFTER
SWIGGED
SWILLED
SWILLER
SWIMMER
SWINGER
SWIRLED
SWISHED
SWISHES
SWITZER
SWOLLEN
SWOONED
SWOONER
SWOOPED
SWOOPER
TWANGED
TWANGER
TWEAKED
TWEENER
TWEETED
TWEETER
TWEEZED
TWEEZER
TWEEZES
TWELVEA
TWELVEB
TWELVEC
TWELVED
TWELVEE
TWELVES
TWILLED
TWINBED
TWINGED
TWINGES
TWINIER
TWINJET
TWINNED
TWINSET
TWIRLED
TWIRLER
TWISTED
TWISTER
TWITTED
TWITTER
TWODEEP
TWOEEEE
TWOFEET
TWOSTEP
TWOTOED
TWOWEEK

•W••••E

AWARDEE
AWESOME
DWINDLE
OWLLIKE
SWADDLE
SWEETIE
SWINDLE
SWIZZLE
SWOOSIE
TWADDLE
TWEEDLE
TWELVEE
TWIDDLE
TWINKIE
TWINKLE
TWOACRE
TWOBASE
TWOEEEE
TWOFACE
TWOLANE
TWOMORE
TWOONIE
TWOSOME
TWOTIME
TWOTONE

••WE•••

BOWECHO
BOWEDTO
BOWERED
BTWELVE
COWERAT
COWERED
DOWERED
DRWELBY
EKWENSI
HEWEDTO
HGWELLS
HOWELLS
HOWELSE
HOWEVER
IFWEMAY
INWEAVE
IOWEYOU
ITWELVE
ITWENTY
JAWEDAT
JEWELED
JEWELER
JEWELRY
LOWEEZY
LOWERED
PAWEDAT
POWERED
POWERUP
RAWEGGS
REWEARS
REWEAVE
REWEIGH
REWELDS
ROWELED
SEWEDON
SEWEDUP
TOWEDIN
TOWELED
TOWERED
UNWEARY
UNWEAVE
UNWEDGE
UPWELLS
VOWELLY
WOWEDEM

••W•E••

BAWLERS
BOWHEAD
BOWLERS
BOWLESS
BOWYERS
COWBELL
COWHERD
COWIEST
COWPEAS
DEWIEST
DEWLESS
DOWNERS
DOWSERS
FAWCETT
FAWNERS
FEWNESS
FOWLERS
GAWKERS
GAWPERS
HAWKERS
HAWKEYE
HAWSERS
HEWLETT
HOWBEIT
HOWDEDO
HOWLERS
JAWLESS
LAWLESS
LAWYERS
LEWDEST
LOWBEAM
LOWEEZY
LOWGEAR
LOWHEEL
LOWNECK
LOWNESS
LOWRENT
LOWTECH
MEWLERS
NCWYETH
NEWBERN
NEWBERY
NEWDEAL
NEWLEAF
NEWLEFT
NEWNESS
NEWWEEK
NEWYEAR
NOWHERE
NOWNESS
PAWNEES
PAWNERS
PEWTERS
POWDERS
POWDERY
RAWDEAL
RAWMEAT
RAWNESS
SAWYERS
SOWSEAR
TOWHEAD
TOWHEES
TOWNERS
UNWHEEL
VOWLESS
YAWNERS
YAWPERS
YOWLERS

••W••E•

ADWOMEN
ATWATER
BAWDIER
BEWARED
BEWARES
BOWDLER
BOWERED
BOWTIES
COWERED
COWRIES
COWSHED
DAWDLED
DAWDLER
DAWDLES
DEWATER
DEWAXED
DEWAXES
DEWIRED
DEWIRES
DOWAGER
DOWDIER
DOWDIES
DOWERED
DOWNIER
DOWRIES
EXWIVES
GAWKIER
HOWEVER
HOWTHEN
INWOVEN
JEWELED
JEWELER
JOWLIER
KEWPIES
LOWBRED
LOWCHEN
LOWERED
LOWHEEL
LOWLIER
NEWAGER
NEWAGEY
NEWBIES
NEWIDEA
NEWSIER
NEWSIES
NEWSMEN
NEWSPEG
NEWWEEK
NOWISEE
NOWISER
NOWTHEN
ONWATER
PAWNEES
POWERED
REWAGER
REWAKED
REWAKEN
REWAKES
REWATER
REWAXED
REWAXES
REWIDEN
REWIPED
REWIPES
REWIRED
REWIRES
REWOKEN
REWOVEN
ROWDIER
ROWDIES
ROWELED
TAWNIER
TOWAGES
TOWELED
TOWERED
TOWHEES
TOWNIES
TOWNLET
UNWADED
UNWAGED
UNWAKED
UNWANED
UNWAVED
UNWAXED
UNWHEEL
UNWIPED
UNWIRED
UNWISER
UNWOOED
UNWOVEN
WOWEDEM
YAWNIER
YEWTREE

••W•••E

BOWLIKE
BOWLINE
BTWELVE
COWBANE
COWHIDE
COWLIKE
COWPOKE
COWRITE
COWROTE
DEWILDE
DEWLINE
EBWHITE
FTWAYNE
HAWKEYE
HOWCOME
HOWELSE
HOWLAME
HOWNICE
INWEAVE
INWHITE
ITWELVE
JAWBONE
JAWLIKE
JAWLINE
LAWCASE
LAWLIKE
LOWDIVE
LOWLIFE
LOWRISE
LOWSIDE
LOWTIDE
NEWFACE
NEWGATE
NEWHIRE
NEWHOPE
NEWLIFE
NEWLINE
NEWLOVE
NEWMADE
NEWNAME
NEWSOME
NEWWAVE
NOWHERE
NOWISEE
NOWORSE
RAWHIDE
REWEAVE
REWRITE
REWROTE
SAWLIKE
SOWLIKE
THWHITE
TOWABLE
TOWLINE
TOWROPE
UNWEAVE
UNWEDGE
UNWHITE
UNWHOLE
YEWTREE

•••WE••

ANSWERS
ANTWERP
ARCWELD
ASSWEET
AVOWERS
BAGWELL
BETWEEN
BLOWERS
BOBWEIR
BOSWELL
BREWERS
BREWERY
CHEWERS
CLAWERS
COBWEBS
CREWELS
CROWELL
CROWERS
DARWELL
DAYWEAR
DERWENT
DIDWELL
DRAWEES
DRAWERS
DRYWELL
DUEWEST
DURWENT
EYEWEAR
FALWELL
FARWEST
FITWELL
FLOWERS
FLOWERY
FORWENT
GETWELL
GLOWERS
GNAWERS
GOTWELL
GROWERS
HARWELL
HOGWEED
IMSWELL
INAWEOF
INDWELL
INDWELT
INKWELL
INSWEPT
KEYWEST
KNOWERS
KNOWETH
LEGWEAR
MAEWEST
MAXWELL
MEOWERS
MIDWEEK
MIDWEST
NEWWEEK
NOSWEAT
NOTWELL
OFFWEGO
OILWELL
OLDWEST
ONEWEEK
OUTWEAR
OUTWEED
OUTWEEP
OUTWELL
OUTWENT
OUTWEPT
OUTWEST
PAYWELL
PEEWEES
PERWEEK
PIGWEED
PLOWERS
PROWESS
PROWEST
RAGWEED
RESWEAR
RESWEEP
ROSWELL
SATWELL
SEAWEED
SHOWERS
SHOWERY
SITWELL
SIXWEEK
SKEWERS
SKIWEAR
SLOWEST
SOTWEED
SPEWERS
STEWERS
STOWERS
TENWEEK
THAWERS
TROWELS
TWOWEEK
UNSWEAR
UNSWEET
UNSWEPT
UPSWEEP
UPSWELL
UPSWEPT
VIEWERS

•••W•E•

ASSWEET
BETWEEN
BLOWIER
BLOWZED
BRAWLED
BRAWLER
BRAWLEY
BROWNED
BROWNER
BROWSED
BROWSER
BROWSES
CHEWIER
CHOWDER
CLOWDER
CLOWNED
COOWNED
CRAWLED
CRAWLER
CRAWLEY
CREWMEN
CROWDED
CROWDER
CROWLEY
CROWNED
CROWNER
DRAWEES
DRAWLED
DRAWLER
DRAWMEN
DROWNED
DROWSED
DROWSES
FLAWIER
FRAWLEY
FROWNED
FROWNER
GROWLED
GROWLER
HOGWEED
KNOWLES
MIDWEEK
NEWWEEK
ONEWEEK
OUTWEED
OUTWEEP
PEEWEES
PERWEEK
PIGWEED
PLOWMEN
PRAWNED
PROWLED
PROWLER
RAGWEED
REOWNED
RESWEEP
SAYWHEN
SCOWLED
SCOWLER
SEAWEED
SHAWLED
SHAWNEE
SHOWIER
SHOWMEN
SIXWEEK
SNOWIER
SNOWMEN
SNOWPEA
SOTWEED
SPAWNED
SPAWNER
STEWIER
TENWEEK
TRAWLED
TRAWLER
TWOWEEK
UNOWNED
UNSWEET
UPSWEEP
VIEWIER

•••W••E

ADAWARE
AIRWAVE
ALEWIFE
ALLWISE
ANYWISE
ARTWARE
BARWARE
BREWAGE
BROWNIE
ENDWISE
ENTWINE
FANWISE
FLOWAGE
GETWISE
GOTWISE
GUNWALE
HAYWIRE
HOTWIRE
ICEWINE
JUGWINE
LAPWARE
MALWARE
MAYWINE
MCGWIRE
MCSWINE
MIDWIFE
MISWIRE
NETWARE
NEWWAVE
NONWAGE
OUTWAVE
OUTWILE
OUTWORE
PINWALE
POPWINE
PREWIRE
REAWAKE
REAWOKE
REDWINE
RESWORE
RETWINE
SAMWISE
SHAWNEE
SPYWARE
STOWAGE
THEWAVE
TINWARE
UNAWAKE
UNAWARE
UNSWORE
UNTWINE
WETWARE

••••WE•

ALLOWED
BEDEWED
BEJEWEL
BRONWEN
CDTOWER
CNTOWER
DEPOWER
ELBOWED
ELBOWER
EMBOWER
EMPOWER
ENDOWED
ENDOWER
FOODWEB
GETSWET
INPOWER
JDPOWER
MCCOWEN
MIAOWED
NUNGWEN
OUTAWED
OUTAWES
OVERWET
PSHAWED
REMOWED
RENEWED
RENEWER
REPOWER
RESAWED
RESEWED
RESOWED
RETOWED
SCREWED
SINEWED
STREWED
STREWER
THROWER
UNBOWED
UNCOWED
UNDEWED
UNHEWED
UNMEWED
UNMOWED
UNPAWED
UNSAWED
UNSEWED
UNSOWED
UNVOWED
VANOWEN
VERYWET
WIDOWED
WIDOWER
WIMOWEH

••••W•E

ALLOWME
BEROWNE

•••••WE

MARLOWE
NORDOWE
OVERAWE
ROBLOWE
ROYALWE
SHALLWE
SOAREWE
SODIDWE

W•F••••

WAFERED
WAFFLED
WAFFLER
WAFFLES
WAFTERS
WAFTING
WIFYING

W••F•••

WAFFLED
WAFFLER
WAFFLES
WAIFISH
WARFARE
WASFAIR
WATFORD
WEBFEET
WEBFOOT
WEEFOLK
WELFARE
WEXFORD
WHIFFED
WHIFFER
WHIFFLE
WILFORD
WILFRED
WINFREY
WOLFCUB
WOLFDOG
WOLFGAL
WOLFING
WOLFISH
WOLFMAN
WOLFMEN
WOLFRAM
WOOFERS
WOOFING

W•••F••
WAILFUL
WAITFOR
WAKEFUL
WEEPFOR
WELLFED
WENTFAR
WENTFOR
WHARFED
WHATFOR
WHIFFED
WHIFFER
WHIFFLE
WILLFUL
WISHFOR
WISHFUL
WISTFUL
WOOLFAT
WORKFOR

W••••F•
WALKOFF
WALLOFF
WARDOFF
WARNOFF
WASHOFF
WAVEOFF
WEAROFF
WELLOFF
WENTAFT
WENTOFF
WHATIFS
WIPEOFF
WOREOFF
WORKOFF
WORNOFF

W•••••F
WALDORF
WALKOFF
WALLOFF
WARDOFF
WARNOFF
WARNSOF
WASHOFF
WAVEOFF
WEAROFF
WELLOFF
WENTOFF
WHEREOF
WIPEOFF
WOREOFF
WORKOFF
WORNOFF

•WF••••
AWFULLY

•W•F•••
SWIFTER
SWIFTLY
TWOFACE
TWOFEET
TWOFERS
TWOFOLD
TWOFOOT

•W••F••
DWARFED
TWELFTH

•W••••F
AWAREOF

••WF•••
BOWFINS
COWFISH
DEWFALL
LAWFORD
NEWFACE
RAWFISH
RAWFOOD
SAWFISH

••W•F••
BOWLFUL
UPWAFTS
YAWNFUL

••W••F•
LOWLIFE
NEWLEFT
NEWLIFE
PAWNOFF
SAWNOFF
SAWSOFF

••W•••F
BYWAYOF
NEWLEAF
PAWNOFF
SAWNOFF
SAWSOFF

•••WF••
BLOWFLY
GREWFAT
GROWFAT
UNAWFUL

•••W•F•
ALEWIFE
BLEWOFF
BLOWOFF
DRAWOFF
DREWOFF
MIDWIFE
SHOWOFF

•••W••F
AIRWOLF
BEOWULF
BLEWOFF
BLOWOFF
CRYWOLF
DRAWOFF
DREWOFF
INAWEOF
KNOWSOF
REDWOLF
SEAWOLF
SHEWOLF
SHOWOFF

••••W•F
ASLEWOF

W•G••••
WAGERED
WAGERER
WAGEWAR
WAGGERS
WAGGERY
WAGGING
WAGGISH
WAGGLED
WAGGLER
WAGGLES
WAGONED
WAGONER
WEGENER
WIGGERY
WIGGIER
WIGGING
WIGGLED
WIGGLER
WIGGLES
WIGLESS
WIGLETS
WIGLIKE
WIGSOUT
WIGWAGS
WIGWAMS

W••G•••
WAGGERS
WAGGERY
WAGGING
WAGGISH
WAGGLED
WAGGLER
WAGGLES
WANGLED
WANGLER
WANGLES
WARGAME
WARGODS
WEDGEIN
WEDGIER
WEDGIES
WEDGING
WEIGHED
WEIGHER
WEIGHIN
WEIGHON
WEIGHTS
WEIGHTY
WEIGHUP
WIDGEON
WIDGETS
WIGGERY
WIGGIER
WIGGING
WIGGLED
WIGGLER
WIGGLES
WINGERS
WINGING
WINGLET
WINGMAN
WINGMEN
WINGNUT
WINGSIT
WINGTIP
WRIGGLE
WRIGGLY
WRIGHTS
WRIGLEY

W•••G••
WHANGED
WINDGOD
WISEGUY
WOBEGON
WOLFGAL
WRANGEL
WRANGLE
WRIGGLE
WRIGGLY
WRINGER
WRONGED
WRONGER
WRONGLY
WROUGHT

W••••G•
WAKINGS
WANTAGH
WARPAGE
WASTAGE
WATTAGE
WAXINGS
WAYTOGO
WEBLOGS
WEBPAGE
WESTEGG
WETRAGS
WIGWAGS
WINDAGE
WINDIGO
WIRINGS
WORDAGE

W•••••G
WADDING
WAFTING
WAGGING
WAILING
WAITING
WAIVING
WALKING
WALLING
WANNING
WANTING
WARBURG
WARDING
WARMING
WARNING
WARPING
WARRENG
WARRING
WARTHOG
WASHING
WASHRAG
WASTING
WAXWING
WEANING
WEARING
WEAVING
WEBBING
WEDDING
WEDGING
WEEDING
WEEPING
WELDING
WELLING
WELTING
WENDING
WESTEGG
WETTING
WHALING
WHILING
WHINING
WHITING
WICKING
WIFYING
WIGGING
WILDDOG
WILDING
WILDPIG
WILLING
WILTING
WIMPING
WINCING
WINDBAG
WINDING
WINGING
WINKING
WINNING
WINSBIG
WISHING
WISPING
WITLING
WITTING
WOLFDOG
WOLFING
WONTING
WOODING
WOOFING
WORDING
WORKING
WORMING
WRITING
WYOMING
WYSIWYG

•W•G•••
DWIGHTD
OWNGOAL
SWAGGER
SWAGMAN
SWAGMEN
SWIGERT
SWIGGED

•W••G••
OWINGON
OWINGTO
OWLEGGS
SWAGGER
SWIGGED
SWINGAT
SWINGBY
SWINGER
SWINGIT
SWUNGAT
SWUNGBY
SWUNGIT
TWANGED
TWANGER
TWINGED
TWINGES
TWOEGGS
ZWINGLI

•W•••G•
AWNINGS
OWLEGGS
TWOEGGS

•W••••G
AWAKING
SWAYING
SWIPING
TWINING
ZWANZIG

••WG•••
COWGIRL
GEWGAWS
LOWGEAR
NEWGATE

••W•G••
DOWAGER
NEWAGER
NEWAGEY
RAWEGGS
REWAGER
TOWAGES
UNWAGED

••W••G•
HOWHIGH
MOWINGS
RAWEGGS
REWEIGH
SAWLOGS
TOWINGS
UNWEDGE

••W•••G
BAWLING
BOWLING
COWLING
DAWNING
DOWLING
DOWNING
DOWRONG
DOWSING
EDWARDG
FAWNING
FOWLING
GAWKING
GAWPING
GOWNING
GOWRONG
HAWKING
HOWLING
HOWLONG
MEWLING
MRWRONG
NEWBURG
NEWSPEG
PAWNING
ROWLING
UNWRUNG
YAWNING
YAWPING
YOWLING

•••WG••
BLOWGUN
CHEWGUM

•••W•G•
BAGWIGS
BIGWIGS
BREWAGE
EARWIGS
FLOWAGE
NONWAGE
OFFWEGO
STOWAGE
WIGWAGS

•••W••G
AVOWING
BATWING
BLOWING
BREWING
CHAWING
CHEWING
CHOWING
CLAWING
CLEWING
CREWING
CROWING
DRAWING
FLAWING
FLOWING
GLOWING
GNAWING
GREWBIG
GROWBIG
GROWING
JREWING
KNOWING
LAPWING
MEOWING
OUTWING
PLOWING
REDWING
SHOWDOG
SHOWING
SKEWING
SLEWING
SLOWING
SNOWING
SPEWING
STEWING
STOWING
THAWING
TROWING
UNOWING
UNSWUNG
UPSWING
VIEWING
WAXWING

••••W•G
CHINWAG
PERIWIG
TAILWAG
WYSIWYG

WH•••••
WHACKED
WHACKER
WHALERS
WHALING
WHALLEY
WHAMMED
WHANGED
WHAPPED
WHARFED
WHARTON
WHARVES
WHATAMI
WHATFOR
WHATIFS
WHATNOT
WHATNOW
WHATSAY
WHATSIS
WHATSIT
WHATSUP
WHATTHE
WHAUDEN
WHEATEN
WHEATON
WHEEDLE
WHEELED
WHEELER
WHEELIE
WHEELIN
WHEEZED
WHEEZER
WHEEZES
WHELMED
WHELPED
WHEREAS
WHEREAT
WHEREBY
WHEREIN
WHERELL
WHEREOF
WHEREON
WHERERE
WHERETO
WHEREVE
WHETHER
WHETTED
WHETTER
WHEYISH
WHIFFED
WHIFFER
WHIFFLE
WHILING
WHIMPER
WHINERS
WHINIER
WHINING
WHIPPED
WHIPPER
WHIPPET
WHIPPLE
WHIPSAW
WHIPSIN
WHIPSUP
WHIRLED
WHIRLER
WHIRRED
WHISHED
WHISHES
WHISKAS
WHISKED
WHISKER
WHISKEY
WHISPER
WHISTLE
WHITELY
WHITENS
WHITEST
WHITHER
WHITING
WHITISH
WHITMAN
WHITNEY
WHITSUN
WHITTLE
WHIZKID
WHIZZED
WHIZZER
WHIZZES
WHOEVER
WHOISIT
WHOKNEW
WHOMPED
WHOOPED
WHOOPEE
WHOOPER
WHOOPIE
WHOOSIS
WHOPPED
WHOPPER
WHORLED
WHOSAID
WHOSOUT
WHOSWHO
WHUPPED
WHWORDS
WHYEVER
WHYISIT
WHYWAIT

W•H••••
WAHINES
WAHWAHS
WCHANDY

W••H•••
WARHAWK
WARHEAD
WARHERO
WASHDAY
WASHERS
WASHIER
WASHING
WASHOFF
WASHOUT
WASHRAG
WASHTUB
WASHUPS
WEEHOUR
WICHITA
WILHELM
WISHERS
WISHFOR
WISHFUL
WISHING
WITHERS
WITHIES
WITHOUT

W•••H••
WALTHAM
WALTHER
WAPSHOT
WARSHIP
WARTHOG
WATCHED
WATCHER
WATCHES
WATCHIT
WATCHTV
WEATHER
WEIGHED
WEIGHER
WEIGHIN
WEIGHON
WEIGHTS
WEIGHTY
WEIGHUP
WELLHID
WELLHIT
WENCHES
WERNHER
WERTHER
WHETHER
WHISHED
WHISHES
WHITHER
WINCHED
WINCHER
WINCHES
WITCHED
WITCHES
WOOLHAT
WOOSHED
WOOSHES
WORSHIP
WORTHIT
WRIGHTS
WRITHED
WRITHER
WRITHES
WYNDHAM

W••••H•
WABASHA
WAHWAHS
WEALTHS
WEALTHY
WHATTHE
WHOSWHO
WORKSHY
WRAITHS
WREATHE
WREATHS
WREATHY
WROUGHT

W•••••H
WAGGISH
WAIFISH
WALLACH
WANNISH
WANTAGH
WARMISH
WARPATH
WASATCH
WASPISH
WEAKISH
WETTISH
WETWASH
WHEYISH
WHITISH
WILDISH
WIMOWEH
WIMPISH
WOLFISH
WORMISH

•W•H•••
SWAHILI
TWOHOUR

•W••H••
AWASHIN
DWIGHTD
KWACHAS
SWASHED
SWASHES
SWATHED
SWATHES
SWISHED
SWISHES
TWOSHOT

•W•••H•
PWBOTHA
SWARTHY
TWITCHY

•W••••H
GWYNETH
SWEDISH
SWINISH
TWELFTH

••WH•••
BOWHEAD
COWHAND
COWHERD
COWHIDE
EBWHITE
HAWHAWS
HOWHIGH
INWHITE
LEWHOAD
LOWHAND
LOWHEEL
NEWHAND
NEWHART
NEWHATS
NEWHIRE
NEWHOPE
NOWHERE
RAWHIDE
THWHITE
TOWHEAD
TOWHEES
UNWHEEL
UNWHIPT
UNWHITE
UNWHOLE
UPWHIRL
VFWHALL

••W•H••
BOWSHOT
COWSHED
HOWTHEN
LOWCHEN
NOWTHEN
NOWTHIS
NOWWHAT
SAWCHUK

••W••H•
BOWECHO
HOWDAHS

••W•••H
ALWORTH
BEWITCH
COWFISH
FTWORTH
GAWKISH
HAWKISH
HAWORTH
HOWHIGH
HOWMUCH
LOWTECH
MAWKISH
NCWYETH
NEWMATH
NEWRICH
RAWFISH
REWEIGH
SAWATCH
SAWFISH
TOWNISH
TOWPATH

•••WH••
EREWHON
GEEWHIZ
KNEWHOW
KNOWHOW
NARWHAL
NOWWHAT
ONAWHIM
ONEWHIT
PREWHIP
SAYWHAT
SAYWHEN
SHOWHOW
SNOWHAT

•••W•H•
GROWTHS
KENWAHL
WAHWAHS

•••W••H
CARWASH
DRYWASH
EYEWASH
HOGWASH
IPSWICH
JETWASH
KNOWETH
METWITH
NORWICH
NOTWITH
OUTWASH
OUTWISH
OUTWITH
PREWASH
RANWITH
RUNWITH
SATWITH
SITWITH
SLOWISH
SOPWITH
TOYWITH
VIEWITH
WETWASH
YOUWISH

••••WH•
SAYSWHO
WHOSWHO

••••W•H
BUSHWAH
WIMOWEH

WI•••••
WICCANS
WICHITA
WICKERS
WICKETS
WICKING
WICKIUP
WICKLOW
WIDENED
WIDENER
WIDGEON
WIDGETS
WIDMARK
WIDOWED
WIDOWER
WIELAND
WIELDED
WIELDER
WIENERS
WIENIES
WIFYING
WIGGERY
WIGGIER
WIGGING
WIGGLED
WIGGLER
WIGGLES
WIGLESS
WIGLETS
WIGLIKE
WIGSOUT
WIGWAGS
WIGWAMS
WILBERT
WILDCAT
WILDDOG
WILDEST
WILDING
WILDISH
WILDMAN
WILDMEN
WILDONE

WILDPIG
WILFORD
WILFRED
WILHELM
WILIEST
WILKENS
WILKINS
WILLARD
WILLERS
WILLFUL
WILLIAM
WILLIES
WILLING
WILLKIE
WILLOWS
WILLOWY
WILLSON
WILLYOU
WILSONS
WILTING
WIMOWEH
WIMPIER
WIMPING
WIMPISH
WIMPLED
WIMPLES
WIMPOLE
WIMPOUT
WINBACK
WINCERS
WINCHED
WINCHER
WINCHES
WINCING
WINDAGE
WINDAUS
WINDBAG
WINDERS
WINDGOD
WINDIER
WINDIGO
WINDILY
WINDING
WINDOMS
WINDOWS
WINDOWY
WINDSOR
WINDSUP
WINDTEE
WINDUPS
WINEBAR
WINERED
WINESAP
WINEVAT
WINFREY
WINGERS
WINGING
WINGLET
WINGMAN
WINGMEN
WINGNUT
WINGSIT
WINGTIP
WINIEST
WINKERS
WINKING
WINKLER
WINKOUT

WINKSAT
WINLESS
WINNERS
WINNING
WINNOWS
WINOVER
WINSBIG
WINSLET
WINSLOW
WINSOME
WINSOUT
WINSTON
WINTERS
WINTERY
WINWOOD
WIPEDUP
WIPEOFF
WIPEOUT
WIPESUP
WIRABLE
WIREDIN
WIREDUP
WIREMAN
WIREMEN
WIRESIN
WIRESUP
WIRETAP
WIRIEST
WIRINGS
WISDOMS
WISEDUP
WISEGUY
WISEMAN
WISEMEN
WISEONE
WISESUP
WISHERS
WISHFOR
WISHFUL
WISHING
WISPIER
WISPILY
WISPING
WISTFUL
WITCHED
WITCHES
WITEOUT
WITHERS
WITHIES
WITHOUT
WITLESS
WITLING
WITNESS
WITSEND
WITTIER
WITTILY
WITTING
WIZARDS
WIZENED

W•I••••
WAIFISH
WAIKATO
WAIKIKI
WAILERS
WAILFUL
WAILING
WAISTED
WAITERS
WAITFOR
WAITING
WAITOUT
WAITRON
WAITSON
WAITSUP
WAIVERS
WAIVING
WEIDMAN
WEIGHED
WEIGHER
WEIGHIN
WEIGHON
WEIGHTS
WEIGHTY
WEIGHUP
WEIRDAL
WEIRDED
WEIRDER
WEIRDLY
WEIRDOS
WEIRTON
WHIFFED
WHIFFER
WHIFFLE
WHILING
WHIMPER
WHINERS
WHINIER
WHINING
WHIPPED
WHIPPER
WHIPPET
WHIPPLE
WHIPSAW
WHIPSIN
WHIPSUP
WHIRLED
WHIRLER
WHIRRED
WHISHED
WHISHES
WHISKAS
WHISKED
WHISKER
WHISKEY
WHISPER
WHISTLE
WHITELY
WHITENS
WHITEST
WHITHER
WHITING
WHITISH
WHITMAN
WHITNEY
WHITSUN
WHITTLE
WHIZKID
WHIZZED
WHIZZER
WHIZZES
WRIGGLE
WRIGGLY
WRIGHTS
WRIGLEY
WRINGER
WRINKLE
WRINKLY
WRITEIN
WRITEME
WRITEON
WRITERS
WRITETO
WRITEUP
WRITHED
WRITHER
WRITHES
WRITING
WRITTEN

W••I•••
WAHINES
WAKINGS
WANIEST
WAPITIS
WARIEST
WAVICLE
WAVIEST
WAXIEST
WAXINGS
WEDIDIT
WHOISIT
WHYISIT
WILIEST
WINIEST
WIRIEST
WIRINGS
WOEISME
WRAITHS
WYSIWYG

W•••I••
WABBITS
WACKIER
WACKILY
WADDING
WADKINS
WAFTING
WAGGING
WAGGISH
WAIFISH
WAIKIKI
WAILING
WAITING
WAIVING
WALKING
WALKINS
WALLING
WANNING
WANNISH
WANTING
WARDING
WARLIKE
WARMING
WARMISH
WARNING
WARPING
WARRING
WARRIOR
WARTIER
WARTIME
WARWICK
WASHIER
WASHING
WASPIER
WASPILY
WASPISH
WASSILY
WASTING
WATKINS
WAXLIKE
WAXWING
WAYBILL
WAYSIDE
WEAKISH
WEANING
WEARIED
WEARIER
WEARIES
WEARILY
WEARING
WEAVING
WEBBIER
WEBBING
WEBLIKE
WEBSITE
WEBZINE
WEDDING
WEDGIER
WEDGIES
WEDGING
WEEBITS
WEEDIER
WEEDILY
WEEDING
WEENIES
WEEPIER
WEEPING
WEEVILS
WELDING
WELLING
WELTING
WENDING
WESKITS
WESTIES
WESTINS
WETKISS
WETTING
WETTISH
WHALING
WHATIFS
WHEYISH
WHILING
WHINIER
WHINING
WHITING
WHITISH
WICHITA
WICKING
WICKIUP
WIENIES
WIFYING
WIGGIER
WIGGING
WIGLIKE
WILDING
WILDISH
WILKINS
WILLIAM
WILLIES
WILLING
WILTING
WIMPIER
WIMPING
WIMPISH
WINCING
WINDIER
WINDIGO
WINDILY
WINDING
WINGING
WINKING
WINNING
WISHING
WISPIER
WISPILY
WISPING
WITHIES
WITLING
WITTIER
WITTILY
WITTING
WOLFING
WOLFISH
WONTING
WOODIER
WOODIES
WOODING
WOOFING
WOOKIEE
WOOLIER
WOOLIES
WOOLITE
WOOZIER
WOOZILY
WORDIER
WORDILY
WORDING
WORKING
WORMIER
WORMING
WORMISH
WORRIED
WORRIER
WORRIES
WOZNIAK
WRITING
WYOMING

W••••I•
WADEDIN
WADESIN
WALLSIN
WANTSIN
WAPITIS
WAREPIC
WARSHIP
WASABIS
WASFAIR
WASSAIL
WATCHIT
WATUSIS
WAVEDIN
WAVESIN
WAYLAID
WEBMAIL
WEDGEIN
WEDIDIT
WEIGHIN
WELLHID
WELLHIT
WELLLIT
WETSUIT
WHATSIS
WHATSIT
WHEELIE
WHEELIN
WHEREIN
WHIPSIN
WHIZKID
WHOISIT
WHOOPIE
WHOOSIS
WHOSAID
WHYISIT
WHYWAIT
WILDPIG
WILLKIE
WINGSIT
WINGTIP
WINSBIG
WIREDIN
WIRESIN
WOODBIN
WORKSIN
WORSHIP
WORTHIT
WRITEIN
WROTEIN

W•••••I
WAIKIKI
WHATAMI

•WI••••
DWIGHTD
DWINDLE
OWINGON
OWINGTO
SWIFTER
SWIFTLY
SWIGERT
SWIGGED
SWILLED
SWILLER
SWIMMER
SWIMSUP
SWINDLE
SWINERY
SWINGAT
SWINGBY
SWINGER
SWINGIT
SWINISH
SWINTON
SWIPERS
SWIPING
SWIRLED
SWISHED
SWISHES
SWITZER
SWIVELS
SWIVETS
SWIZZLE
TWIDDLE
TWILLED
TWINBED
TWINERS
TWINGED
TWINGES
TWINIER
TWINING
TWINJET
TWINKIE
TWINKLE
TWINKLY
TWINNED
TWINSET
TWIRLED
TWIRLER
TWISTED
TWISTER
TWISTON
TWISTUP
TWITCHY
TWITTED
TWITTER
ZWICKAU
ZWINGLI

•W•I•••
AWAITED
AWAITER
AWNINGS
OWLIEST
TWOIRON

•W••I••
AWAKING
EWERIES
IWOJIMA
OWLLIKE
SWAHILI
SWAYING
SWEDISH
SWINISH
SWIPING
TWINIER
TWINING
TWOBITS
TWOTIME

•W•••I•
AWASHIN
AWEEBIT
DWEEZIL
DWELLIN
IWANTIT
SWEARIN
SWEATIT
SWEETIE
SWINGIT
SWOOPIN
SWOOSIE
SWOREIN
SWUNGIT
TWINKIE
TWOONIE
TWOPAIR
TWOUNIT
ZWANZIG

•W••••I
SWAHILI
ZWINGLI

••WI•••
BEWITCH
COWIEST
DEWIEST
DEWILDE
DEWIRED
DEWIRES
ENWINDS
EXWIVES
JEWISON
MOWINGS
NEWIDEA
NOWISEE
NOWISER
RAWISTS
REWIDEN
REWINDS
REWIPED
REWIPES
REWIRED
REWIRES
SAWINTO
SEWISTS
TOWINGS
UNWINDS
UNWINDY
UNWIPED
UNWIRED
UNWISER
UNWITTY
UPWINDS

••W•I••
BAWDIER
BAWDILY
BAWLING
BEWAILS
BOWFINS
BOWLIKE
BOWLINE
BOWLING
BOWTIES
COWBIRD
COWFISH
COWGIRL
COWHIDE
COWLICK
COWLIKE
COWLING
COWRIES
COWRITE
DAWKINS
DAWNING
DEWLINE
DOWDIER
DOWDIES
DOWDILY
DOWLING
DOWNIER
DOWNING
DOWRIES
DOWSING
EBWHITE
FAWNING
FOWLING
GAWKIER
GAWKILY
GAWKING
GAWKISH
GAWPING
GOWNING
HAWKING
HAWKINS
HAWKISH
HOWHIGH
HOWLING
HOWNICE
INWHITE
JAWLIKE
JAWLINE
JOWLIER
KEWPIES
KUWAITI
LAWLIKE
LOWBIDS
LOWDIVE
LOWLIER
LOWLIFE
LOWLILY
LOWRISE
LOWRISK
LOWSIDE
LOWTIDE
MAWKISH
MEWLING
NEWBIES
NEWHIRE
NEWKIDS
NEWLIFE
NEWLINE
NEWMINT
NEWRICH
NEWSIER
NEWSIES
PAWNING
RAWFISH
RAWHIDE
RAWLINS
RAWSILK
REWEIGH
REWRITE
ROWDIER
ROWDIES
ROWDILY
ROWLING
SAWFISH
SAWLIKE
SAWMILL
SAWPITS
SOWLIKE
TAWNIER
TAWNILY
THWHITE
TOWLINE
TOWNIES
TOWNISH
UNWHIPT
UNWHITE
UPWHIRL
YAWNIER
YAWNING
YAWPING
YOWLING

••W••I•
BOWDOIN
COWSKIN
COWSLIP
HOWBEIT
KIWANIS
LAWSUIT
LOWPAID
LOWPAIR
NEWLAID
NOWTHIS
SAWTOIT
TOWEDIN

••W•••I
EDWARDI
EKWENSI
KUWAITI

•••WI••
AIRWICK
ALEWIFE
ALLWISE
ANYWISE
AVOWING
BAGWIGS
BATWING
BERWICK
BETWIXT
BIGWIGS
BIGWINS
BLOWIER
BLOWING
BREWING
CHAWING
CHEWIER
CHEWING
CHOWING
CLAWING
CLEWING
CREWING
CROWING
DIMWITS
DRAWING
EARWIGS
ENDWISE
ENTWINE
ENTWIST
EYEWINK
FANWISE
FLAWIER
FLAWING
FLOWING
GATWICK
GETWISE
GLOWING
GNAWING
GODWITS
GOTWISE
GROWING
HAYWIRE
HOGWILD
HOTWIRE
ICEWINE
ICYWIND
ILLWILL
ILLWIND
INAWINK
IPSWICH
JREWING
JUGWINE
KNOWING
LAPWING
LIDWINA
MAYWINE
MCGWIRE
MCSWINE
MEDWICK
MEOWING
METWITH
MIDWIFE
MISWIRE
NATWICK
NITWITS
NORWICH
NOTWITH
OUTWILE
OUTWILL
OUTWIND
OUTWING
OUTWISH
OUTWITH
OUTWITS
PLOWING
POPWINE
PREWIRE
PREWITT
RANWILD
RANWITH
REDWINE
REDWING
RENWICK
RESWIMS
RETWINE
RETWIST
RUNWILD
RUNWITH
SAMWISE
SATWITH
SCHWINN
SHOWIER
SHOWILY
SHOWING
SITWITH
SKEWING
SLEWING
SLOWING
SLOWISH
SNOWIER
SNOWILY
SNOWING
SOPWITH
SPEWING
STEWIER
STEWING
STOWING
THAWING
THEWIND
TOYWITH
TROWING
UNOWING
UNTWINE
UNTWIST
UPSWING
VIEWIER
VIEWING
VIEWITH
WARWICK
WAXWING
YOUWISH

•••W•I•
BLOWNIN
BLOWSIN
BLOWSIT
BOBWEIR
BROWNIE
CROWDIN
DRAWNIN
DRAWSIN
FLOWNIN
FLOWSIN
GEEWHIZ
GREWBIG
GREWDIM
GROWBIG
GROWDIM
MEOWMIX
ONAWHIM
ONEWHIT
OUTWAIT
PREWHIP
SAYWAIT
SHOWBIZ
SHOWNIN
SHOWSIN
SNOWSIN
STOWSIT
WHYWAIT

•••W••I
BREWSKI
SNOWSKI

••••WI•
ALLEWIS
ALLOWIN
BALDWIN
CHATWIN
CSLEWIS
GOODWIN
HALFWIT
IKNEWIT
IKNOWIT
LACKWIT
OUTSWIM
PERIWIG
SCARWID
SHERWIN
THREWIN
THROWIN

W•J••••
WOJTYLA

•W•J•••
IWOJIMA

•W••J••
TWINJET

••WJ•••
NEWJOBS

•••WJ••
SNOWJOB

W•K••••
WAKAMES
WAKEDUP
WAKEFUL
WAKENED
WAKENER
WAKESUP
WAKEUPS
WAKINGS
WAKSMAN
WOKENUP

W••K•••
WACKEST
WACKIER
WACKILY
WADKINS
WAIKATO
WAIKIKI
WALKERS
WALKING
WALKINS
WALKMAN
WALKOFF
WALKONS
WALKOUT
WALKSBY
WALKSON
WALKSTO
WALKUPS
WALKURE
WALKWAY
WANKELS
WATKINS
WEAKENS
WEAKEST
WEAKISH
WEAKONS
WEEKDAY
WEEKEND
WESKITS
WETKISS
WHOKNEW
WICKERS
WICKETS
WICKING
WICKIUP
WICKLOW
WILKENS
WILKINS
WINKERS
WINKING
WINKLER
WINKOUT
WINKSAT
WOOKIEE
WORKBOX
WORKDAY
WORKERS
WORKFOR
WORKING
WORKMAN
WORKMEN
WORKOFF
WORKOUT
WORKSAT
WORKSHY
WORKSIN
WORKSON
WORKSUP
WORKUPS

W•••K••
WENDKOS
WHACKED
WHACKER
WHISKAS
WHISKED
WHISKER
WHISKEY
WHIZKID
WILLKIE
WRACKED
WRACKUP
WREAKED
WREAKER
WRECKED
WRECKER
WRINKLE
WRINKLY

W••••K•
WAIKIKI
WARLIKE
WAXLIKE
WEBLIKE
WIGLIKE

W•••••K
WARHAWK
WARLOCK
WARWICK
WAXWORK
WAYBACK
WEDLOCK
WEEFOLK
WETLOOK
WIDMARK
WINBACK
WOZNIAK
WOZZECK

•WK••••
AWKWARD

•W•K•••
AWAKENS
AWAKERS
AWAKING

•W••K••
SWANKED
SWANKER
SWANKUP
TWEAKED
TWINKIE
TWINKLE
TWINKLY
ZWICKAU

•W•••K•
OWLLIKE

•W••••K
EWENECK
TWOWEEK

••WK•••
BOWKNOT
DAWKINS
GAWKERS
GAWKIER
GAWKILY
GAWKING
GAWKISH
GAWKSAT
HAWKERS
HAWKEYE
HAWKING
HAWKINS
HAWKISH
HAWKMAN
MAWKISH
NEWKIDS

••W•K••
COWSKIN
REWAKED
REWAKEN
REWAKES
REWOKEN
UNWAKED

••W••K•
BOWLIKE
COWLIKE
COWPOKE
EXWORKS
JAWLIKE
LAWLIKE
REWORKS
SAWLIKE
SOWLIKE
THWACKS

••W•••K
COWLICK
HOWARDK
LAWBOOK
LOWNECK
LOWRISK
NEWLOOK
NEWWEEK
NEWYORK
NOWLOOK
RAWSILK
SAWBUCK
SAWCHUK

•••W•K•
BREWSKI
REAWAKE
REAWOKE
SNOWSKI
UNAWAKE

•••W••K
AIRWICK
ARTWORK
BERWICK
BULWARK
CATWALK
CUTWORK
EYEWINK
GATWICK
INAWINK
JAYWALK
LEGWORK
MEDWICK
MIDWEEK
NATWICK
NETWORK
NEWWEEK
NONWORK
NORWALK
ONEWEEK
OUTWALK
OUTWORK
PERWEEK
PREWORK
RENWICK
SIXWEEK
SKYWALK
TENWEEK
TINWORK
TWOWEEK
VANWYCK
WARWICK
WAXWORK

••••WK•
MOHAWKS
SQUAWKS
SQUAWKY

••••W•K
SARAWAK

•••••WK
GOSHAWK
REDHAWK
SEAHAWK
WARHAWK

W•L••••
WALCOTT
WALDORF
WALKERS
WALKING
WALKINS
WALKMAN
WALKOFF
WALKONS
WALKOUT
WALKSBY
WALKSON
WALKSTO
WALKUPS
WALKURE
WALKWAY
WALLABY
WALLACE
WALLACH
WALLETS
WALLEYE
WALLING
WALLMAP
WALLOFF
WALLOON
WALLOPS
WALLOWS
WALLSIN
WALLSUP
WALMART
WALNUTS
WALPOLE
WALSTON
WALTERS
WALTHAM
WALTHER
WALTONS
WALTZED
WALTZER
WALTZES
WELCOME
WELDERS
WELDING
WELFARE
WELLAND
WELLCUT
WELLFED
WELLHID
WELLHIT
WELLING
WELLLED
WELLLIT
WELLMAN
WELLOFF
WELLPUT
WELLRUN
WELLSEE
WELLSET
WELLSUP
WELLWON
WELLYES
WELTERS
WELTING
WILBERT
WILDCAT
WILDDOG
WILDEST
WILDING
WILDISH
WILDMAN
WILDMEN
WILDONE
WILDPIG
WILFORD
WILFRED
WILHELM
WILIEST
WILKENS
WILKINS
WILLARD
WILLERS
WILLFUL
WILLIAM
WILLIES
WILLING
WILLKIE
WILLOWS
WILLOWY
WILLSON
WILLYOU
WILSONS
WILTING
WOLFCUB
WOLFDOG
WOLFGAL
WOLFING
WOLFISH
WOLFMAN
WOLFMEN
WOLFRAM

W••L•••
WAILERS
WAILFUL
WAILING
WALLABY
WALLACE
WALLACH
WALLETS
WALLEYE
WALLING
WALLMAP
WALLOFF
WALLOON
WALLOPS
WALLOWS
WALLSIN
WALLSUP
WARLESS
WARLIKE
WARLOCK
WARLORD
WASLATE
WAXLIKE
WAYLAID
WAYLAND
WAYLAYS
WAYLESS
WEALTHS
WEALTHY
WEBLESS
WEBLIKE
WEBLOGS
WEDLOCK
WELLAND
WELLCUT
WELLFED
WELLHID
WELLHIT
WELLING
WELLLED
WELLLIT
WELLMAN
WELLOFF
WELLPUT
WELLRUN
WELLSEE
WELLSET
WELLSUP
WELLWON
WELLYES
WETLAND
WETLOOK
WHALERS
WHALING
WHALLEY
WHELMED
WHELPED
WHILING
WIELAND
WIELDED
WIELDER
WIGLESS
WIGLETS
WIGLIKE
WILLARD
WILLERS
WILLFUL
WILLIAM
WILLIES
WILLING
WILLKIE
WILLOWS
WILLOWY
WILLSON
WILLYOU
WINLESS
WITLESS
WITLING
WOOLENS
WOOLERY
WOOLFAT
WOOLHAT
WOOLIER
WOOLIES
WOOLITE
WOOLLEN
WOOLLEY
WOOLSEY
WORLDLY
WOULDBE
WOULDNT
WOULDST

W•••L••
WADDLED
WADDLER
WADDLES
WAFFLED
WAFFLER
WAFFLES
WAGGLED
WAGGLER
WAGGLES
WAMBLED
WAMBLES
WANGLED
WANGLER
WANGLES
WARBLED
WARBLER
WARBLES
WARCLUB
WATTLED
WATTLES
WAVELET
WEDELED
WEDELNS
WELLLED
WELLLIT
WEMBLEY
WHALLEY
WHEELED
WHEELER
WHEELIE
WHEELIN
WHIRLED
WHIRLER
WHORLED
WICKLOW
WIGGLED
WIGGLER
WIGGLES
WIMPLED
WIMPLES
WINGLET
WINKLER
WINSLET
WINSLOW
WOBBLED
WOBBLER
WOBBLES
WOODLEY
WOODLOT
WOOLLEN
WOOLLEY
WORSLEY
WRIGLEY
WROCLAW

W••••L•
WACKILY
WADDELL
WALPOLE
WANKELS
WASPILY
WASSILY
WAVICLE
WAXABLE
WAYBILL
WEARILY
WEASELS
WEDDELL
WEEDILY
WEEFOLK
WEEVILS
WEIRDLY
WENDELL
WETBULB
WETCELL
WHEEDLE
WHERELL
WHIFFLE
WHIPPLE
WHISTLE
WHITELY
WHITTLE
WILHELM
WIMPOLE
WINDILY
WIRABLE
WISPILY
WITTILY
WOJTYLA
WOMANLY
WOOZILY
WORDILY
WORLDLY
WORRELL
WRANGLE
WRESTLE
WRIGGLE
WRIGGLY
WRINKLE
WRINKLY
WRONGLY

W•••••L
WADDELL
WAILFUL
WAKEFUL
WASSAIL
WASTREL
WAYBILL
WAYCOOL
WEBMAIL
WEDDELL
WEIRDAL
WENDELL
WETCELL
WHERELL
WILLFUL
WISHFUL
WISTFUL
WOLFGAL
WORRELL
WRANGEL

•WL••••
OWLEGGS
OWLEYED
OWLIEST
OWLLIKE

•W•L•••
AWELESS
AWNLESS
DWELLAT
DWELLED
DWELLER
DWELLIN
DWELLON
DWELTON
EWELAMB
OWLLIKE
SWALLOW
SWELLED
SWELLER
SWELLUP
SWELTER
SWELTRY
SWILLED
SWILLER
SWOLLEN
TWELFTH
TWELVEA
TWELVEB
TWELVEC
TWELVED
TWELVEE
TWELVES
TWILLED
TWOLANE

•W••L••
AWFULLY
DWELLAT
DWELLED
DWELLER
DWELLIN
DWELLON
SWALLOW
SWELLED
SWELLER
SWELLUP
SWILLED
SWILLER
SWIRLED
SWOLLEN
TWILLED
TWIRLED
TWIRLER

•W•••L•
AWFULLY
DWINDLE
SWADDLE
SWAHILI
SWEETLY
SWIFTLY
SWINDLE
SWIVELS
SWIZZLE
TWADDLE
TWEEDLE
TWIDDLE
TWINKLE
TWINKLY
TWOBALL
TWOFOLD
ZWINGLI

•W••••L
DWEEZIL
OWNGOAL
TWOBALL

••WL•••
BAWLERS
BAWLING
BAWLOUT
BOWLERS
BOWLESS
BOWLFUL
BOWLIKE
BOWLINE
BOWLING
COWLICK
COWLIKE
COWLING
DEWLAPS
DEWLESS
DEWLINE
DOWLING
FOWLERS
FOWLING
HEWLETT
HOWLAME
HOWLERS
HOWLING
HOWLONG
HOWLSAT
JAWLESS
JAWLIKE
JAWLINE
JOWLIER
KOWLOON
LAWLESS
LAWLIKE
LOWLAND
LOWLIER
LOWLIFE
LOWLILY
MEWLERS
MEWLING
NEWLAID
NEWLEAF
NEWLEFT
NEWLIFE
NEWLINE
NEWLOOK
NEWLOVE
NOWLOOK
RAWLINS
ROWLAND
ROWLING
SAWLIKE
SAWLOGS
SOWLIKE
TOWLINE
VOWLESS
YOWLERS
YOWLING

••W•L••
BOWDLER
BTWELVE
COWSLIP
DAWDLED
DAWDLER
DAWDLES
DEWCLAW
DEWILDE
DRWELBY
HGWELLS
HOWELLS
HOWELSE
ITWELVE
JEWELED
JEWELER
JEWELRY
LOWBLOW
REWELDS
ROWELED
TOWELED
TOWNLET
UNWALLS
UPWELLS
VOWELLY

••W••L•
BAWDILY
BEWAILS
COWBELL
DEWFALL
DOWDILY
GAWKILY
HGWELLS
HOWDULL
HOWELLS
KOWADLO
LOWBALL
LOWLILY
MYWORLD
NEWBOLT
PCWORLD
RAWSILK
ROWDILY
SAWMILL
TAWNILY
TOWABLE
UNWALLS
UNWHOLE
UPWELLS
VFWHALL
VOWELLY

••W•••L
BOWLFUL
COWBELL
COWGIRL
DEWFALL
HOWDULL
LOWBALL
LOWHEEL
NEWDEAL
RAWDEAL
SAWMILL
UNWHEEL
UPWHIRL
VFWHALL
YAWNFUL

•••WL••
BRAWLED
BRAWLER
BRAWLEY
CRAWLED
CRAWLER
CRAWLEY
CROWLEY
DRAWLED
DRAWLER
FRAWLEY
GROWLED
GROWLER
KNOWLES
PROWLED
PROWLER
SCOWLED
SCOWLER
SHAWLED
TRAWLED
TRAWLER

•••W•L•
AIRWOLF
ARCWELD
ARTWALL
AVOWALS
BAGWELL
BEOWULF
BLOWFLY
BOSWELL
CATWALK
CREWELS
CROWELL
CRYWOLF
DARWELL
DIDWELL
DRYWALL
DRYWELL
EYEWALL
FALWELL
FITWELL
GETWELL
GOTWELL
GREWOLD
GROWOLD
GUNWALE
HARWELL
HOGWILD
ILLWILL
IMSWELL
INDWELL
INDWELT
INKWELL
JAYWALK
KNOWALL
MAXWELL
NORWALK
NOTWELL
OILWELL
OSTWALD
OUTWALK
OUTWELL
OUTWILE
OUTWILL
PAYWELL
PINWALE
RANWILD
REDWOLF
ROSWELL
RUNWILD
SATWELL
SEAWALL
SEAWOLF
SHEWOLF
SHOWILY
SITWELL
SKYWALK
SNOWILY
THEWALL
TROWELS
UPSWELL
ZUMWALT

•••W••L
ARTWALL
BAGWELL
BOSWELL
CROWELL
DARWELL
DIDWELL
DRYWALL
DRYWELL
EYEWALL
FALWELL
FITWELL
GETWELL
GOTWELL
HARWELL
ILLWILL
IMSWELL
INDWELL
INKWELL
KENWAHL
KNOWALL
MAXWELL
NARWHAL
NONWOOL
NOTWELL
OILWELL
OUTWELL
OUTWILL
PAYWELL
ROSWELL
SATWELL
SEAWALL
SITWELL
THEWALL

UNAWFUL
UPSWELL

••••WL•
ELFOWLS
SCRAWLS
SCRAWLY
SPRAWLS
SPRAWLY
UNLOWLY

••••W•L
BEJEWEL
RENEWAL

•••••WL
ASPRAWL
BARNOWL
CATBOWL
DOGBOWL
HOOTOWL
OUTBAWL
OUTBOWL
OUTHOWL
PEAFOWL
PROBOWL
SEAFOWL
SUNBOWL

W•M••••
WAMBLED
WAMBLES
WAMPUMS
WEMBLEY
WIMOWEH
WIMPIER
WIMPING
WIMPISH
WIMPLED
WIMPLES
WIMPOLE
WIMPOUT
WOMANLY
WOMBATS

W••M•••
WALMART
WARMERS
WARMEST
WARMING
WARMISH
WARMSTO
WARMSUP
WARMUPS
WEBMAIL
WETMOPS
WHAMMED
WHIMPER
WHOMPED
WIDMARK
WORMERS
WORMIER
WORMING
WORMISH
WYOMING

W•••M••
WAKAMES
WAKSMAN
WALKMAN
WALLMAP
WEIDMAN
WELLMAN
WENTMAD
WHAMMED
WHELMED
WHITMAN
WILDMAN
WILDMEN
WINGMAN
WINGMEN
WIREMAN
WIREMEN
WISEMAN
WISEMEN
WOLFMAN
WOLFMEN
WORKMAN
WORKMEN

W••••M•
WAMPUMS
WARGAME
WARTIME
WEBCAMS
WELCOME
WHATAMI
WIGWAMS
WINDOMS
WINSOME
WISDOMS
WOEISME
WRITEME

W•••••M
WALTHAM
WARROOM
WILHELM
WILLIAM
WOLFRAM
WOOSNAM
WOWEDEM
WYNDHAM

•W•M•••
SWAMPED
SWIMMER
SWIMSUP
TWOMORE

•W••M••
SWAGMAN
SWAGMEN
SWARMED
SWARMER
SWIMMER

•W•••M•
AWESOME
EWELAMB
IWOJIMA
TWOSOME
TWOTIME

•W••••M
TWOROOM
TWOTERM

••WM•••
HOWMANY
HOWMUCH
LOWMASS
NEWMADE
NEWMANS
NEWMATH
NEWMINT
NEWMONT
NEWMOON
NEWMOWN
RAWMEAT
SAWMILL

••W•M••
ADWOMAN
ADWOMEN
HAWKMAN
IFWEMAY
NEWSMAN
NEWSMEN

••W••M•
DEWORMS
HOWCOME
HOWLAME
NEWNAME
NEWSOME
REWARMS
UNWORMY

••W•••M
LOWBEAM
WOWEDEM

•••WM••
CREWMAN
CREWMEN
DRAWMAN
DRAWMEN
MEOWMIX
PLOWMAN
PLOWMEN
SHOWMAN
SHOWMEN
SNOWMAN
SNOWMEN

•••W•M•
MUGWUMP
RESWIMS
WIGWAMS

•••W••M
BUDWORM
CHEWGUM
CUTWORM
EELWORM
GETWARM
GOTWARM
GREWDIM
GROWDIM
LUGWORM
ONAWHIM
PREWARM
REDWORM

••••WM•
ALLOWME

••••W•M
OUTSWAM
OUTSWIM
OUTSWUM

W•N••••
WANDERS
WANGLED
WANGLER
WANGLES
WANIEST
WANKELS
WANNABE
WANNESS
WANNEST
WANNING
WANNISH
WANTADS
WANTAGH
WANTERS
WANTING
WANTONS
WANTOUT
WANTSIN
WANTSTO
WENCHES
WENDELL
WENDERS
WENDING
WENDKOS
WENTAFT
WENTAPE
WENTBAD
WENTFAR
WENTFOR
WENTMAD
WENTOFF
WENTOUT
WENTPRO
WINBACK
WINCERS
WINCHED
WINCHER
WINCHES
WINCING
WINDAGE
WINDAUS
WINDBAG
WINDERS
WINDGOD
WINDIER
WINDIGO
WINDILY
WINDING
WINDOMS
WINDOWS
WINDOWY
WINDSOR
WINDSUP
WINDTEE
WINDUPS
WINEBAR
WINERED
WINESAP
WINEVAT
WINFREY
WINGERS
WINGING
WINGLET
WINGMAN
WINGMEN
WINGNUT
WINGSIT
WINGTIP
WINIEST
WINKERS
WINKING
WINKLER
WINKOUT
WINKSAT
WINLESS
WINNERS
WINNING
WINNOWS
WINOVER
WINSBIG
WINSLET
WINSLOW
WINSOME
WINSOUT
WINSTON
WINTERS
WINTERY
WINWOOD
WONDERS
WONOVER
WONTING
WONTONS
WYNDHAM
WYNETTE
WYNONNA

W••N•••
WALNUTS
WANNABE
WANNESS
WANNEST
WANNING
WANNISH
WARNING
WARNOFF
WARNSOF
WEANERS
WEANING
WEENESS
WEENIES
WERNHER
WETNAPS
WETNESS
WHANGED
WHINERS
WHINIER
WHINING
WIENERS
WIENIES
WINNERS
WINNING
WINNOWS
WITNESS
WORNOFF
WORNOUT
WOUNDED
WOUNDUP
WOZNIAK
WRANGEL
WRANGLE
WRINGER
WRINKLE
WRINKLY
WRONGED
WRONGER
WRONGLY
WRYNESS

W•••N••
WAGONED
WAGONER
WAHINES
WAKENED
WAKENER
WAKINGS
WASONTO
WAXINGS
WCHANDY
WEEONES
WEGENER
WETONES
WHATNOT
WHATNOW
WHITNEY
WHOKNEW
WIDENED
WIDENER
WINGNUT
WIRINGS
WIZENED
WOKENUP
WOMANLY
WOOSNAM
WYNONNA

W••••N•
WADDING
WADKINS
WAFTING
WAGGING
WAILING
WAITING
WAIVING
WALKING
WALKINS
WALKONS
WALLING
WALTONS
WANNING
WANTING
WANTONS
WARBOND
WARDENS
WARDING
WARMING
WARNING
WARPING
WARRANT
WARRENG
WARRENS
WARRING
WARZONE
WASHING
WASTING
WATKINS
WAXWING
WAYLAND
WEAKENS
WEAKONS
WEANING
WEAPONS
WEARING
WEAVING
WEBBING
WEBZINE
WEDDING
WEDELNS
WEDGING
WEEDING
WEEKEND
WEEPING
WELDING
WELLAND
WELLING
WELTING
WENDING
WESTEND
WESTINS
WETLAND
WETTING
WHALING
WHILING
WHINING
WHITENS
WHITING
WICCANS
WICKING
WIELAND
WIFYING
WIGGING
WILDING
WILDONE
WILKENS
WILKINS
WILLING
WILSONS
WILTING
WIMPING
WINCING
WINDING
WINGING
WINKING
WINNING
WISEONE
WISHING
WISPING
WITLING
WITSEND
WITTING
WOLFING
WONTING
WONTONS
WOODING
WOOFING
WOOLENS
WORDING
WORDONE
WORKING
WORMING
WORSENS
WOULDNT
WRITING
WYNONNA
WYOMING
WYOTANA
WYVERNS

W•••••N
WADEDIN
WADESIN
WAITRON
WAITSON
WAKSMAN
WALKMAN
WALKSON
WALLOON
WALLSIN
WALSTON
WANTSIN
WARTORN
WARWORN
WAVEDIN
WAVESIN
WAXBEAN
WAYWORN
WEARSON
WEDGEIN
WEIDMAN
WEIGHIN
WEIGHON
WEIRTON
WELLMAN
WELLRUN
WELLWON
WESTERN
WETDOWN
WHARTON
WHAUDEN
WHEATEN
WHEATON
WHEELIN
WHEREIN
WHEREON
WHIPSIN
WHITMAN
WHITSUN
WIDGEON
WILDMAN
WILDMEN
WILLSON
WINGMAN
WINGMEN
WINSTON
WIREDIN
WIREMAN
WIREMEN
WIRESIN
WISEMAN
WISEMEN
WOBEGON
WOLFMAN
WOLFMEN
WOODBIN
WOODSON
WOOLLEN
WORKMAN
WORKMEN
WORKSIN
WORKSON
WRITEIN
WRITEON
WRITTEN
WROTEIN
WROTEON

•WN••••
AWNINGS
AWNLESS
OWNEDUP
OWNGOAL
OWNUPTO

•W•N•••
DWINDLE
EWENECK
GWYNETH
IWANTIT
IWANTTO
IWONDER
KWANZAA
KWANZAS
OWINGON
OWINGTO
RWANDAN
SWANKED
SWANKER
SWANKUP
SWANSEA
SWANSON
SWENSON
SWINDLE
SWINERY
SWINGAT
SWINGBY
SWINGER
SWINGIT
SWINISH
SWINTON
SWUNGAT
SWUNGBY
SWUNGIT
TWANGED
TWANGER
TWINBED
TWINERS
TWINGED
TWINGES
TWINIER
TWINING
TWINJET
TWINKIE
TWINKLE
TWINKLY
TWINNED
TWINSET
ZWANZIG
ZWINGLI

•W••N••
AWNINGS
AWOONOR
SWEENEY
SWOONED
SWOONER
TWEENER
TWINNED
TWOONIE
TWOUNIT

•W•••N•
AWAKENS
AWAKING
SWAYING
SWIPING
TWERENT
TWINING
TWOLANE
TWOTONE
TWOTONS

•W••••N
AWASHIN
DWELLIN
DWELLON
DWELTON
OWINGON
RWANDAN
SWAGMAN
SWAGMEN
SWANSON
SWEARIN
SWEETEN
SWEETON
SWENSON
SWINTON
SWOLLEN
SWOOPIN
SWOREIN
TWISTON
TWOIRON

••WN•••
DAWNING
DAWNSON
DOWNBOW
DOWNERS
DOWNIER
DOWNING
DOWNPAT
FAWNERS
FAWNING
FAWNSON
FEWNESS
GOWNING
HOWNICE
LOWNECK
LOWNESS
NEWNAME
NEWNESS
NOWNESS
PAWNEES
PAWNERS
PAWNING
PAWNOFF
RAWNESS
SAWNOFF
TAWNIER
TAWNILY
TOWNCAR
TOWNERS
TOWNIES
TOWNISH
TOWNLET
YAWNERS
YAWNFUL
YAWNIER
YAWNING

••W•N••
BOWKNOT
EKWENSI
ENWINDS
ITWENTY
KIWANIS
LAWANDA
MOWINGS
REWINDS
SAWINTO
TOWINGS
UNWANED
UNWINDS
UNWINDY
UPWINDS

••W••N•
BAWLING
BOWFINS
BOWLINE
BOWLING
COWBANE
COWHAND
COWLING
COWPONY
DAWKINS
DAWNING
DEWLINE
DOWLING
DOWNING
DOWRONG
DOWSING
ENWOUND
FAWNING
FOWLING
FTWAYNE
GAWKING
GAWPING
GOWNING
GOWRONG
HAWKING
HAWKINS
HOWLING
HOWLONG
HOWMANY
JAWBONE
JAWLINE
LOWHAND
LOWLAND
LOWRENT
MEWLING
MRWRONG
NEWHAND
NEWLINE
NEWMANS
NEWMINT
NEWMONT
NEWTONS
PAWNING
RAWLINS
REWARNS
REWOUND
ROWLAND
ROWLING
TOWLINE
UNWOUND
UNWRUNG
YAWNING
YAWPING
YOWLING

••W•••N
ADWOMAN
ADWOMEN
BOWDOIN
BOWDOWN
COWSKIN
COWTOWN
DAWNSON
FAWNSON
HAWKMAN
HOWTHEN
INWOVEN
JEWISON
KOWLOON
LOWBORN
LOWCHEN
LOWDOWN
MOWDOWN
NEWBERN
NEWBORN
NEWMOON
NEWMOWN
NEWSMAN
NEWSMEN
NEWTOWN
NOWTHEN
REWAKEN
REWIDEN
REWOKEN
REWOVEN
SEWEDON
TOWEDIN
UNWOVEN

•••WN••
BLOWNIN
BLOWNUP
BROWNED
BROWNER
BROWNIE
CLOWNED
COOWNED
CROWNED
CROWNER
DRAWNIN
DRAWNON
DRAWNTO
DRAWNUP
DROWNED
FLOWNAT
FLOWNBY
FLOWNIN
FLOWNON
FLOWNTO
FLOWNUP
FROWNAT
FROWNED
FROWNER
FROWNON
GROWNON
GROWNUP
PRAWNED
REOWNED
SHAWNEE
SHOWNIN
SHOWNUP
SPAWNED
SPAWNER
UNOWNED

•••W•N•
AJOWANS
AVOWING
BATWING
BIGWINS
BLOWING
BREWING
CHAWING
CHEWING
CHOWING
CLAWING
CLEWING
CREWING
CROWING
DERWENT
DRAWING
DURWENT
ENTWINE
EYEWINK
FLAWING
FLOWING
FORWENT
GLOWING
GNAWING
GROWING
ICEWINE
ICYWIND
ILLWIND
INAWINK
JREWING
JUGWINE
KNOWING
LAPWING
LIDWINA
MAYWINE
MCSWINE
MEOWING
OUTWENT
OUTWIND
OUTWING
PLOWING
POPWINE
REDWINE
REDWING
RETWINE
SCHWANN
SCHWINN
SHOWING
SKEWING
SLEWING
SLOWING
SNOWING
SPEWING
STEWING
STOWING
THAWING
THEWIND
TROWING
UNOWING
UNSWUNG
UNTWINE
UPSWING
VIEWING

WAXWING

•••W••N
BETWEEN
BLOWGUN
BLOWNIN
BLOWSIN
BLOWSON
CHEWSON
CREWMAN
CREWMEN
CROWDIN
DRAWMAN
DRAWMEN
DRAWNIN
DRAWNON
DRAWSIN
DRAWSON
EREWHON
FLOWNIN
FLOWNON
FLOWSIN
FROWNON
GNAWSON
GROWNON
GROWSON
OUTWORN
PLOWMAN
PLOWMEN
PLOWSON
PREWARN
PREWORN
RESWORN
SAYWHEN
SCHWANN
SCHWINN
SHOWMAN
SHOWMEN
SHOWNIN
SHOWSIN
SNOWDON
SNOWMAN
SNOWMEN
SNOWSIN
STEWPAN
UNSWORN
WARWORN
WAYWORN

••••WN•
BEROWNE
DISOWNS
KELOWNA
RENOWNS
SCRAWNY
UNPAWNS
UPTOWNS

••••W•N
ALLOWIN
BALDWIN
BRONWEN
CHATWIN
GOLDWYN
GOODWIN
HALFWON
HARDWON
MATEWAN
MCCOWEN
NUNGWEN
OTTAWAN
SHERWIN
THESWAN
THREWIN
THREWON
THROWIN
THROWON
VANOWEN
WELLWON

•••••WN
ANYTOWN
BEDDOWN
BIGTOWN
BOGDOWN
BOWDOWN
BUYDOWN
CHITOWN
COWTOWN
CRYDOWN
CUTDOWN
DIEDOWN
DRBROWN
EMBROWN
GETDOWN
GOTDOWN
HITTOWN
HOEDOWN
ICEDOWN
INBROWN
INDRAWN
INGROWN
JOTDOWN
LAYDOWN
LETDOWN
LIEDOWN
LOWDOWN
MIDTOWN
MOWDOWN
MRBROWN
NEWMOWN
NEWTOWN
OAKLAWN
OLDTOWN
ONEDOWN
ONMYOWN
OURTOWN
OUTFAWN
PATDOWN
PINDOWN
PREDAWN
PUTDOWN
RAEDAWN
RAMDOWN
RANDOWN
REBLOWN
RECROWN
REDDAWN
REDRAWN
REFLOWN
REGROWN
RESHOWN
RIPSAWN
RUBDOWN
RUNDOWN
SATDOWN
SETDOWN
SITDOWN
SUNDOWN
TEAGOWN
TIEDOWN
TIPDOWN
TOPDOWN
UNBLOWN
UNCROWN
UNDRAWN
UNFLOWN
UNGROWN
UNKNOWN
UNSHOWN
UPGROWN
WETDOWN

WO•••••
WOBBLED
WOBBLER
WOBBLES
WOBEGON
WOEISME
WOJTYLA
WOKENUP
WOLFCUB
WOLFDOG
WOLFGAL
WOLFING
WOLFISH
WOLFMAN
WOLFMEN
WOLFRAM
WOMANLY
WOMBATS
WONDERS
WONOVER
WONTING
WONTONS
WOODARD
WOODBIN
WOODBOX
WOODCUT
WOODIER
WOODIES
WOODING
WOODLEY
WOODLOT
WOODROW
WOODSAW
WOODSON
WOODTAR
WOOFERS
WOOFING
WOOKIEE
WOOLENS
WOOLERY
WOOLFAT
WOOLHAT
WOOLIER
WOOLIES
WOOLITE
WOOLLEN
WOOLLEY
WOOLSEY
WOOSHED
WOOSHES
WOOSNAM
WOOSTER
WOOZIER
WOOZILY
WORDAGE
WORDIER
WORDILY
WORDING
WORDONE
WOREOFF
WOREOUT
WORKBOX
WORKDAY
WORKERS
WORKFOR
WORKING
WORKMAN
WORKMEN
WORKOFF
WORKOUT
WORKSAT
WORKSHY
WORKSIN
WORKSON
WORKSUP
WORKUPS
WORLDLY
WORMERS
WORMIER
WORMING
WORMISH
WORNOFF
WORNOUT
WORRELL
WORRIED
WORRIER
WORRIES
WORSENS
WORSHIP
WORSLEY
WORSTED
WORTHIT
WOULDBE
WOULDNT
WOULDST
WOUNDED
WOUNDUP
WOWEDEM
WOZNIAK
WOZZECK

W•O••••
WHOEVER
WHOISIT
WHOKNEW
WHOMPED
WHOOPED
WHOOPEE
WHOOPER
WHOOPIE
WHOOSIS
WHOPPED
WHOPPER
WHORLED
WHOSAID
WHOSOUT
WHOSWHO
WOODARD
WOODBIN
WOODBOX
WOODCUT
WOODIER
WOODIES
WOODING
WOODLEY
WOODLOT
WOODROW
WOODSAW
WOODSON
WOODTAR
WOOFERS
WOOFING
WOOKIEE
WOOLENS
WOOLERY
WOOLFAT
WOOLHAT
WOOLIER
WOOLIES
WOOLITE
WOOLLEN
WOOLLEY
WOOLSEY
WOOSHED
WOOSHES
WOOSNAM
WOOSTER
WOOZIER
WOOZILY
WROCLAW
WRONGED
WRONGER
WRONGLY
WROTEIN
WROTEON
WROTETO
WROTEUP
WROUGHT
WYOMING
WYOTANA.

W••O•••
WAGONED
WAGONER
WASONTO
WEEONES
WETONES
WHOOPED
WHOOPEE
WHOOPER
WHOOPIE
WHOOSIS
WHWORDS
WIDOWED
WIDOWER
WIMOWEH
WINOVER
WONOVER
WYNONNA

W•••O••
WAITOUT
WALCOTT
WALDORF
WALKOFF
WALKONS
WALKOUT
WALLOFF
WALLOON
WALLOPS
WALLOWS
WALPOLE
WALTONS
WANTONS
WANTOUT
WARBOND
WARDOFF
WARGODS
WARLOCK
WARLORD
WARNOFF
WARROOM
WARTORN
WARWORN
WARZONE
WASHOFF
WASHOUT
WATFORD
WAVEOFF
WAXWORK
WAYCOOL
WAYTOGO
WAYWORN
WEAKONS
WEAPONS
WEAROFF
WEAROUT
WEBFOOT
WEBLOGS
WEBTOED
WEDLOCK
WEEDOUT
WEEFOLK
WEEHOUR
WELCOME
WELLOFF
WENTOFF
WENTOUT
WESCOTT
WETDOWN
WETLOOK
WETMOPS
WEXFORD
WHOSOUT
WIGSOUT
WILDONE
WILFORD
WILLOWS
WILLOWY
WILSONS
WIMPOLE
WIMPOUT
WINDOMS
WINDOWS
WINDOWY
WINKOUT
WINNOWS
WINSOME
WINSOUT
WINWOOD
WIPEOFF
WIPEOUT
WISDOMS
WISEONE
WITEOUT
WITHOUT
WONTONS
WORDONE
WOREOFF
WOREOUT
WORKOFF
WORKOUT
WORNOFF
WORNOUT

W••••O•
WAITFOR
WAITRON
WAITSON
WALKSON
WALLOON
WALSTON
WAPSHOT
WARNSOF
WARRIOR
WARROOM
WARTHOG
WAYCOOL
WEARSON
WEBFOOT
WEEPFOR
WEIGHON
WEIRDOS
WEIRTON
WELLWON
WENDKOS
WENTFOR
WETLOOK
WHARTON
WHATFOR
WHATNOT
WHATNOW
WHEATON
WHEREOF
WHEREON
WICKLOW
WIDGEON
WILDDOG
WILLSON
WILLYOU
WINDGOD
WINDSOR
WINSLOW
WINSTON
WINWOOD
WISHFOR
WOBEGON
WOLFDOG
WOODBOX
WOODLOT
WOODROW
WOODSON
WORKBOX
WORKFOR
WORKSON
WRITEON
WROTEON

W•••••O
WAIKATO
WALKSTO
WANTSTO
WARHERO
WARMSTO
WASONTO
WAVEDTO
WAVESTO
WAYTOGO
WENTPRO
WHERETO
WHOSWHO
WINDIGO
WRITETO
WROTETO

•WO••••
AWOONOR
IWOJIMA
IWONDER
SWOLLEN
SWOONED
SWOONER
SWOOPED
SWOOPER
SWOOPIN
SWOOSIE
SWOREAT
SWOREBY
SWOREIN
SWORETO
TWOACRE
TWOACTS
TWOBALL
TWOBASE
TWOBITS
TWODAYS
TWODEEP
TWODOOR
TWOEEEE
TWOEGGS
TWOFACE
TWOFEET
TWOFERS
TWOFOLD
TWOFOOT
TWOHOUR
TWOIRON
TWOLANE
TWOMORE
TWOONIE
TWOPAIR
TWOPART
TWOROOM
TWOSHOT
TWOSOME
TWOSPOT
TWOSTAR
TWOSTEP
TWOTERM
TWOTIME
TWOTOED
TWOTONE
TWOTONS
TWOUNIT
TWOWEEK
TWOYEAR

•W•O•••
AWOONOR
PWBOTHA
SWOONED
SWOONER
SWOOPED
SWOOPER
SWOOPIN
SWOOSIE
TWOONIE

•W••O••
AWESOME
OWNGOAL
TWODOOR
TWOFOLD
TWOFOOT
TWOHOUR
TWOMORE
TWOROOM
TWOSOME
TWOTOED
TWOTONE
TWOTONS

•W•••O•
AWAREOF
AWOONOR
DWELLON
DWELTON
OWINGON
SWALLOW
SWANSON
SWEETON
SWENSON
SWINTON
TWISTON
TWODOOR
TWOFOOT
TWOIRON
TWOROOM
TWOSHOT
TWOSPOT

•W••••O
IWANTTO
OWINGTO
OWNUPTO
SWEARTO
SWORETO

••WO•••
ADWOMAN
ADWOMEN
ALWORTH
ATWORST
BOWOARS
BYWORDS
DEWORMS
ENWOUND
EXWORKS
FTWORTH
HAWORTH
INWOVEN
MRWORDS
MYWORLD
NOWORSE
PCWORLD
REWOKEN
REWORDS
REWORKS
REWOUND
REWOVEN
UNWOOED
UNWORMY
UNWOUND
UNWOVEN
WHWORDS

••W•O••
BAWLOUT
BOWDOIN
BOWDOWN
BOWSOUT
BOWWOWS
COWBOYS
COWPOKE
COWPONY
COWROTE
COWTOWN
DOWRONG
GOWRONG
HOWCOME
HOWLONG
JAWBONE
KOWLOON
KOWTOWS
LAWBOOK
LAWFORD
LEWHOAD
LOWBORN
LOWBOYS
LOWCOST
LOWDOWN
LOWPOST
LOWROAD
LOWTOPS
MOWDOWN
MRWRONG
NEWBOLT
NEWBORN
NEWHOPE
NEWJOBS
NEWLOOK
NEWLOVE
NEWMONT
NEWMOON
NEWMOWN
NEWPORT
NEWSOME
NEWTONS
NEWTOWN
NEWTOYS
NEWWORD
NEWYORK
NOWLOOK
PAWNOFF
POWWOWS
RAWFOOD
REWROTE
ROWBOAT
SAWLOGS
SAWNOFF
SAWSOFF
SAWTOIT
SAWWOOD
TOWBOAT
TOWROPE
UNWHOLE
UNWOOED
VFWPOST

••W••O•
BOWKNOT
BOWSHOT
BYWAYOF
DAWNSON
DEWDROP
DOWNBOW
FAWNSON
IOWEYOU
JEWISON
KOWLOON
LAWBOOK
LOWBLOW
LOWBROW
NEWLOOK
NEWMOON
NEWSBOY
NOWLOOK
RAWFOOD
SAWWOOD
SEWEDON

••W•••O
BOWECHO
BOWEDTO
HEWEDTO
HOWDEDO
HOWDYDO
KOWADLO
SAWINTO

•••WO••
AIRWOLF
ARTWORK
BADWORD
BLEWOFF
BLEWOUT
BLOWOFF
BLOWOUT
BOWWOWS
BUDWORM
CHEWOUT
CRYWOLF
CUTWORK
CUTWORM
DAEWOOS
DAGWOOD
DOGWOOD
DOOWOPS
DRAWOFF
DRAWOUT
DREWOFF
DREWOUT
DYEWOOD
EELWORM
ELMWOOD
FLOWOUT
GETWORD
GOTWORD
GREWOLD
GROWOLD
GUMWOOD
HEYWOOD
INAWORD
KEYWORD
LEAWOOD
LEGWORK
LUGWORM
MISWORD
NETWORK
NEWWORD
NONWOOL
NONWORD
NONWORK
NORWOOD
NUTWOOD
OAKWOOD
ONEWOOD
OUTWORD
OUTWORE
OUTWORK
OUTWORN
PLYWOOD
POWWOWS
PREWORK
PREWORN
REAWOKE
REDWOLF
REDWOOD
REDWORM
RESWORE
RESWORN
RONWOOD
SAWWOOD
SEAWOLF
SHEWOLF
SHOWOFF
SHOWOUT
SPEWOUT
THAWOUT
TINWORK
UNSWORE
UNSWORN
WARWORN
WAXWORK
WAYWORN
WINWOOD

•••W•O•
BLOWPOP
BLOWSON
CHEWSON
CHEWTOY
DAEWOOS
DAGWOOD
DOGWOOD
DRAWNON
DRAWSON
DYEWOOD
ELMWOOD
EREWHON
FLOWNON
FROWNON
GNAWSON
GROWNON
GROWSON
GUMWOOD
HEYWOOD
INAWEOF
KNEWHOW
KNOWHOW
KNOWSOF
LEAWOOD
NONWOOL
NORWOOD
NUTWOOD
OAKWOOD
ONEWOOD
PLOWBOY
PLOWSON
PLYWOOD
REDWOOD
RONWOOD
SAWWOOD
SHOWDOG
SHOWHOW
SNOWDON
SNOWJOB
STEWPOT
WINWOOD

•••W••O
DRAWNTO
DRAWSTO
FLOWNTO
OFFWEGO

••••WO•
ASLEWOF
HALFWON
HARDWON
JOHNWOO
LIKEWOW
ONETWOS
THREWON
THROWON
WELLWON

••••W•O
JOHNWOO
SAYSWHO
WHOSWHO

•••••WO
BALLTWO
BASETWO
FIVETWO
LANETWO
LINETWO
MACHTWO
OPUSTWO
PAGETWO
PARTTWO
PLUSTWO
SIDETWO
SIZETWO
STEPTWO

W•P••••
WAPITIS
WAPSHOT
WIPEDUP
WIPEOFF
WIPEOUT
WIPESUP

W••P•••
WALPOLE
WAMPUMS
WARPAGE
WARPATH
WARPERS

WARPING WASPIER WASPILY WASPISH WEAPONS WEBPAGE WEEPERS WEEPFOR WEEPIER WEEPING WHAPPED WHIPPED WHIPPER WHIPPET WHIPPLE WHIPSAW WHIPSIN WHIPSUP WHOPPED WHOPPER WHUPPED WIMPIER WIMPING WIMPISH WIMPLED WIMPLES WIMPOLE WIMPOUT WISPIER WISPILY WISPING WRAPPED WRAPPER WRAPSUP WRAPUPS

W•••P••

WAREPIC WELLPUT WENTPRO WHAPPED WHELPED WHIMPER WHIPPED WHIPPER WHIPPET WHIPPLE WHISPER WHOMPED WHOOPED WHOOPEE WHOOPER WHOOPIE WHOPPED WHOPPER WHUPPED WILDPIG WRAPPED WRAPPER

W••••P•

WAKEUPS WALKUPS WALLOPS WARMUPS WASHUPS WENTAPE WETMOPS WETNAPS WINDUPS WORKUPS WRAPUPS

W•••••P

WAITSUP WAKEDUP WAKESUP WALLMAP WALLSUP WARMSUP WARSHIP WAXEDUP WAXESUP WEIGHUP WELLSUP WHATSUP WHIPSUP WICKIUP WINDSUP WINESAP WINGTIP WIPEDUP WIPESUP WIREDUP WIRESUP WIRETAP WISEDUP WISESUP WOKENUP WORKSUP WORSHIP WOUNDUP WRACKUP WRAPSUP WRITEUP WROTEUP

•W•P•••

SWAPPED SWAPPER SWEPTUP SWIPERS SWIPING TWOPAIR TWOPART

•W••P••

OWNUPTO SWAMPED SWAPPED SWAPPER SWEEPEA SWEEPER SWEEPUP SWOOPED SWOOPER SWOOPIN TWOSPOT

•W••••P

OWNEDUP SWANKUP SWEEPUP SWELLUP SWEPTUP SWIMSUP TWISTUP TWODEEP TWOSTEP

••WP•••

COWPEAS COWPOKE COWPONY GAWPERS GAWPING KEWPIES LOWPAID LOWPAIR LOWPOST NEWPORT PAWPAWS SAWPAST SAWPITS TOWPATH VFWPOST YAWPERS YAWPING

••W•P••

DOWNPAT NEWSPEG REWIPED REWIPES UNWIPED

••W••P•

DEWLAPS ENWRAPS LOWTOPS NEWHOPE REWRAPS TOWROPE UNWHIPT UNWRAPS

••W•••P

COWSLIP DEWDROP POWERUP SEWEDUP

•••WP••

BLOWPOP BREWPUB SNOWPEA STEWPAN STEWPOT

•••W•P•

BLOWUPS DOOWOPS INSWEPT OUTWEPT SLOWUPS UNSWEPT UPSWEPT

•••W••P

ANTWERP BLOWNUP BLOWPOP BLOWSUP BREWSUP CHEWSUP DRAWNUP DRAWSUP FLOWNUP FURWRAP GROWNUP GROWSUP MUDWASP MUGWUMP OUTWEEP PLOWSUP PREWHIP PREWRAP RESWEEP SHOWNUP SHOWSUP SLOWSUP SNOWCAP UPSWEEP

••••W•P

SCREWUP THREWUP THROWUP

WR•••••

WRACKED WRACKUP WRAITHS WRANGEL WRANGLE WRAPPED WRAPPER WRAPSUP WRAPUPS WRASSES WREAKED WREAKER WREATHE WREATHS WREATHY WRECKED WRECKER WRESTED WRESTER WRESTLE WRIGGLE WRIGGLY WRIGHTS WRIGLEY WRINGER WRINKLE WRINKLY WRITEIN WRITEME WRITEON WRITERS WRITETO WRITEUP WRITHED WRITHER WRITHES WRITING WRITTEN WROCLAW WRONGED WRONGER WRONGLY WROTEIN WROTEON WROTETO WROTEUP WROUGHT WRYNESS

W•R••••

WARBABY WARBLED WARBLER WARBLES WARBOND WARBURG WARCLUB WARDENS WARDERS WARDING WARDOFF WAREPIC WARFARE WARGAME WARGODS WARHAWK WARHEAD WARHERO WARIEST WARLESS WARLIKE WARLOCK WARLORD WARMERS WARMEST WARMING WARMISH WARMSTO WARMSUP WARMUPS WARNING WARNOFF WARNSOF WARPAGE WARPATH WARPERS WARPING WARRANT WARRENG WARRENS WARRING WARRIOR WARROOM WARSHIP WARTHOG WARTIER WARTIME WARTORN WARVETS WARWICK WARWORN WARZONE WERNHER WERTHER WIRABLE WIREDIN WIREDUP WIREMAN WIREMEN WIRESIN WIRESUP WIRETAP WIRIEST WIRINGS WORDAGE WORDIER WORDILY WORDING WORDONE WOREOFF WOREOUT WORKBOX WORKDAY WORKERS WORKFOR WORKING WORKMAN WORKMEN WORKOFF WORKOUT WORKSAT WORKSHY WORKSIN WORKSON WORKSUP WORKUPS WORLDLY WORMERS WORMIER WORMING WORMISH WORNOFF WORNOUT WORRELL WORRIED WORRIER WORRIES WORSENS WORSHIP WORSLEY WORSTED WORTHIT

W••R•••

WARRANT WARRENG WARRENS WARRING WARRIOR WARROOM WEARERS WEARIED WEARIER WEARIES WEARILY WEARING WEAROFF WEAROUT WEARSON WEIRDAL WEIRDED WEIRDER WEIRDLY WEIRDOS WEIRTON WETRAGS WHARFED WHARTON WHARVES WHEREAS WHEREAT WHEREBY WHEREIN WHERELL WHEREOF WHEREON WHERERE WHERETO WHEREVE WHIRLED WHIRLER WHIRRED WHORLED WORRELL WORRIED WORRIER WORRIES

W•••R••

WAFERED WAGERED WAGERER WAITRON WASHRAG WASTREL WATERED WATERER WAVERED WAVERER WELLRUN WHIRRED WHWORDS WILFRED WINERED WINFREY WIZARDS WOLFRAM WOODROW WYVERNS

W••••R•

WADDERS WAFTERS WAGGERS WAGGERY WAILERS WAITERS WAIVERS WALDORF WALKERS WALKURE WALMART WALTERS WANDERS WANTERS WARBURG WARDERS WARFARE WARHERO WARLORD WARMERS WARPERS WARTORN WARWORN WASHERS WASSURE WASTERS WATFORD WAXWORK WAYWARD WAYWORN WEANERS WEARERS WEAVERS WEDDERS WEEDERS WEEPERS WELDERS WELFARE WELTERS WENDERS WENTPRO WESTERN WESTERS WETBARS WETWARE WEXFORD WHALERS WHERERE WHINERS WICKERS WIDMARK WIENERS WIGGERY WILBERT WILFORD WILLARD WILLERS WINCERS WINDERS WINGERS WINKERS WINNERS WINTERS WINTERY WISHERS WITHERS WONDERS WOODARD WOOFERS WOOLERY WORKERS WORMERS WRITERS

W•••••R

WACKIER WADDLER WAFFLER WAGERER WAGEWAR WAGGLER WAGONER WAITFOR WAKENER WALTHER WALTZER WANGLER WARBLER WARRIOR WARTIER WASFAIR WASHIER WASPIER WATCHER WATERER WAVERER WEARIER WEATHER WEBBIER WEBSTER WEDGIER WEEDIER WEEHOUR WEEPFOR WEEPIER WEGENER WEIGHER WEIRDER WENTFAR WENTFOR WERNHER WERTHER WHACKER WHATFOR WHEELER WHEEZER WHETHER WHETTER WHIFFER WHIMPER WHINIER WHIPPER WHIRLER WHISKER WHISPER WHITHER WHIZZER WHOEVER WHOOPER WHOPPER WHYEVER WIDENER WIDOWER WIELDER WIGGIER WIGGLER WIMPIER WINCHER WINDIER WINDSOR WINEBAR WINKLER WINOVER WISHFOR WISPIER WITTIER WOBBLER WONOVER WOODIER WOODTAR WOOLIER WOOSTER WOOZIER WORDIER WORKFOR WORMIER WORRIER WRAPPER WREAKER WRECKER WRESTER WRINGER WRITHER WRONGER

•W•R•••

AWARDED AWARDEE AWARDER AWAREOF AWAREST DWARFED DWARVES EWERIES SWARMED SWARMER SWARTHY SWERVED SWERVES SWIRLED SWOREAT SWOREBY SWOREIN SWORETO TWERENT TWIRLED TWIRLER TWOROOM

•W••R••

SWEARAT SWEARBY SWEARER SWEARIN SWEARTO TWOIRON

•W•••R•

AWAKERS AWKWARD SWAYERS SWELTRY SWIGERT SWINERY SWIPERS TWINERS TWOACRE TWOFERS TWOMORE TWOPART TWOTERM

•W••••R

AWAITER AWARDER AWOONOR DWELLER IWONDER SWABBER SWAGGER SWANKER SWAPPER SWARMER SWATTER SWAYBAR SWEARER SWEATER SWEEPER SWEETER SWELLER SWELTER SWIFTER SWILLER SWIMMER SWINGER SWITZER SWOONER SWOOPER TWANGER TWEENER TWEETER TWEEZER TWINIER TWIRLER TWISTER TWITTER TWODOOR TWOHOUR TWOPAIR TWOSTAR TWOYEAR

••WR•••

COWRIES COWRITE COWROTE DOWRIES DOWRONG ENWRAPS GOWRONG LOWRENT LOWRISE LOWRISK LOWROAD MRWRONG NEWRICH REWRAPS REWRITE REWROTE TOWROPE UNWRAPS UNWRUNG

••W•R••

ALWORTH ATWORST BEWARED BEWARES BOWERED BYWORDS COWARDS COWERAT COWERED DEWDROP DEWIRED DEWIRES DEWORMS DOWERED EDWARDG EDWARDI EDWARDR EDWARDS EDWARDV EXWORKS FTWORTH HAWORTH HOWARDK HOWARDS HOWARDU INWARDS LOWBRED LOWBROW LOWERED MOWBRAY MRWORDS MYWORLD NOWORSE ONWARDS PCWORLD POWERED POWERUP REWARDS REWARMS REWARNS REWIRED REWIRES REWORDS REWORKS SEWARDS THWARTS TOWARDS TOWERED UNWIRED UNWORMY UPWARDS WHWORDS YEWTREE

••W••R•

BAWLERS BOWLERS BOWOARS BOWYERS COWBIRD COWGIRL COWHERD DEWAART DOWNERS DOWSERS FAWNERS FOWLERS GAWKERS GAWPERS HAWKERS HAWSERS HOWLERS JEWELRY LAWFORD LAWYERS LOWBORN LOWCARB LOWCARD MEWLERS NEWBERN NEWBERY NEWBORN NEWBURG NEWCARS NEWHART NEWHIRE NEWPORT NEWWORD NEWYORK NOWHERE PAWNERS PEWTERS POWDERS POWDERY RAWBARS REWEARS SAWYERS TOWBARS TOWCARS TOWNERS UNWEARY UPWHIRL YAWNERS YAWPERS YOWLERS

••W•••R

ATWATER BAWDIER BOWDLER DAWDLER DEWATER DOWAGER DOWDIER DOWNIER EDWARDR GAWKIER HOWEVER JEWELER JOWLIER LOWGEAR LOWLIER LOWPAIR NEWAGER NEWSIER NEWYEAR NOWISER ONWATER REWAGER REWATER ROWDIER SOWSEAR TAWNIER TOWNCAR UNWISER YAWNIER

•••WR••

FAYWRAY FURWRAP PREWRAP

•••W•R•

ADAWARE AIRWARS ANSWERS ANTWERP ARTWARE ARTWORK ATHWART AVOWERS AWKWARD BADWORD BARWARE BLOWDRY BLOWERS BREWERS BREWERY BROWARD

BUDWORM
BULWARK
CHEWERS
CLAWERS
CROWERS
CUTWORK
CUTWORM
DRAWERS
DURWARD
EELWORM
FLOWERS
FLOWERY
FORWARD
FROWARD
GASWARS
GETWARM
GETWORD
GLOWERS
GNAWERS
GOTWARM
GOTWORD
GROWERS
HAYWARD
HAYWIRE
HEYWARD
HOTWARS
HOTWIRE
INAWORD
JAYWARD
KEYWORD
KNOWERS
LAPWARE
LEEWARD
LEGWORK
LUGWORM
MALWARE
MCGWIRE
MEOWERS
MISWIRE
MISWORD
NETWARE
NETWORK
NEWWORD
NONWARS
NONWORD
NONWORK
OUTWARD
OUTWARS
OUTWORD
OUTWORE
OUTWORK
OUTWORN
PLOWERS
PREWARM
PREWARN
PREWIRE
PREWORK
PREWORN
PSYWARS
REDWORM
RESWORE
RESWORN
SEAWARD
SHOWERS
SHOWERY
SKEWERS
SKYWARD
SPEWERS
SPYWARE
STEWARD
STEWART
STEWERS
STOWERS
SUBWARS
SUNWARD
THAWERS
TINWARE
TINWORK
UNAWARE
UNSWORE
UNSWORN
VANWARD
VIEWERS
WARWORN
WAXWORK
WAYWARD
WAYWORN
WETWARE

•••W••R

BLOWIER
BOBWEIR
BRAWLER
BROWNER
BROWSER
CHEWIER
CHOWDER
CLOWDER
CRAWLER
CROWBAR
CROWDER
CROWNER
DAYWEAR
DRAWBAR
DRAWLER
EYEWEAR
FLAWIER
FROWNER
GROWLER
LEGWEAR
OUTWEAR
PROWLER
RESWEAR
SCOWLER
SHOWIER
SKIWEAR
SNOWIER
SPAWNER
STEWIER
TRAWLER
UNSWEAR
VIEWIER

••••W•R

ANTIWAR
BOERWAR
CDTOWER
CNTOWER
COLDWAR
DEPOWER
ELBOWER
EMBOWER
EMPOWER
ENDOWER
FAREWAR
GOTOWAR
GULFWAR
HOLYWAR
INPOWER
JDPOWER
MADEWAR
MAKEWAR
MANOWAR
MEDAWAR
POSTWAR
RENEWER
REPOWER
STREWER
THROWER
TURFWAR
WAGEWAR
WIDOWER

W•S••••

WASABIS
WASATCH
WASFAIR
WASHDAY
WASHERS
WASHIER
WASHING
WASHOFF
WASHOUT
WASHRAG
WASHTUB
WASHUPS
WASLATE
WASONTO
WASPIER
WASPILY
WASPISH
WASSAIL
WASSILY
WASSURE
WASTAGE
WASTERS
WASTING
WASTREL
WESCOTT
WESKITS
WESTEGG
WESTEND
WESTERN
WESTERS
WESTIES
WESTINS
WISDOMS
WISEDUP
WISEGUY
WISEMAN
WISEMEN
WISEONE
WISESUP
WISHERS
WISHFOR
WISHFUL
WISHING
WISPIER
WISPILY
WISPING
WISTFUL
WYSIWYG

W••S•••

WAISTED
WAKSMAN
WALSTON
WAPSHOT
WARSHIP
WASSAIL
WASSILY
WASSURE
WAYSIDE
WEASELS
WEBSITE
WEBSTER
WETSUIT
WHISHED
WHISHES
WHISKAS
WHISKED
WHISKER
WHISKEY
WHISPER
WHISTLE
WHOSAID
WHOSOUT
WHOSWHO
WIGSOUT
WILSONS
WINSBIG
WINSLET
WINSLOW
WINSOME
WINSOUT
WINSTON
WITSEND
WOOSHED
WOOSHES
WOOSNAM
WOOSTER
WORSENS
WORSHIP
WORSLEY
WORSTED
WRASSES
WRESTED
WRESTER
WRESTLE

W•••S••

WABASHA
WADESIN
WAITSON
WAITSUP
WAKESUP
WALKSBY
WALKSON
WALKSTO
WALLSIN
WALLSUP
WANTSIN
WANTSTO
WARMSTO
WARMSUP
WARNSOF
WATUSIS
WAVESAT
WAVESIN
WAVESTO
WAXESUP
WEARSON
WELLSEE
WELLSET
WELLSUP
WHATSAY
WHATSIS
WHATSIT
WHATSUP
WHIPSAW
WHIPSIN
WHIPSUP
WHITSUN
WHOISIT
WHOOSIS
WHYISIT
WILLSON
WINDSOR
WINDSUP
WINESAP
WINGSIT
WINKSAT
WIPESUP
WIRESIN
WIRESUP
WISESUP
WOEISME
WOODSAW
WOODSON
WOOLSEY
WORKSAT
WORKSHY
WORKSIN
WORKSON
WORKSUP
WRAPSUP
WRASSES

W••••S•

WACKEST
WAGGISH
WAIFISH
WANIEST
WANNESS
WANNEST
WANNISH
WARIEST
WARLESS
WARMEST
WARMISH
WASPISH
WAVIEST
WAXIEST
WAYLESS
WEAKEST
WEAKISH
WEBCAST
WEBLESS
WEENESS
WETKISS
WETNESS
WETTEST
WETTISH
WETWASH
WHEYISH
WHITEST
WHITISH
WIGLESS
WILDEST
WILDISH
WILIEST
WIMPISH
WINIEST
WINLESS
WIRIEST
WITLESS
WITNESS
WOLFISH
WORMISH
WOULDST
WRYNESS

W•••••S

WABBITS
WADDERS
WADDLES
WADKINS
WAFFLES
WAFTERS
WAGGERS
WAGGLES
WAHINES
WAHWAHS
WAILERS
WAITERS
WAIVERS
WAKAMES
WAKEUPS
WAKINGS
WALKERS
WALKINS
WALKONS
WALKUPS
WALLETS
WALLOPS
WALLOWS
WALNUTS
WALTERS
WALTONS
WALTZES
WAMBLES
WAMPUMS
WANDERS
WANGLES
WANKELS
WANNESS
WANTADS
WANTERS
WANTONS
WAPITIS
WARBLES
WARDENS
WARDERS
WARGODS
WARLESS
WARMERS
WARMUPS
WARPERS
WARRENS
WARVETS
WASABIS
WASHERS
WASHUPS
WASTERS
WATCHES
WATKINS
WATTLES
WATUSIS
WAXINGS
WAYLAYS
WAYLESS
WBYEATS
WEAKENS
WEAKONS
WEALTHS
WEANERS
WEAPONS
WEARERS
WEARIES
WEASELS
WEAVERS
WEBCAMS
WEBLESS
WEBLOGS
WEDDERS
WEDELNS
WEDGIES
WEEBITS
WEEDERS
WEENESS
WEENIES
WEEONES
WEEPERS
WEEVILS
WEIGHTS
WEIRDOS
WELDERS
WELLYES
WELTERS
WENCHES
WENDERS
WENDKOS
WESKITS
WESTERS
WESTIES
WESTINS
WETBARS
WETKISS
WETMOPS
WETNAPS
WETNESS
WETONES
WETRAGS
WHALERS
WHARVES
WHATIFS
WHATSIS
WHEEZES
WHEREAS
WHINERS
WHISHES
WHISKAS
WHITENS
WHIZZES
WHOOSIS
WHWORDS
WICCANS
WICKERS
WICKETS
WIDGETS
WIENERS
WIENIES
WIGGLES
WIGLESS
WIGLETS
WIGWAGS
WIGWAMS
WILKENS
WILKINS
WILLERS
WILLIES
WILLOWS
WILSONS
WIMPLES
WINCERS
WINCHES
WINDAUS
WINDERS
WINDOMS
WINDOWS
WINDUPS
WINGERS
WINKERS
WINLESS
WINNERS
WINNOWS
WINTERS
WIRINGS
WISDOMS
WISHERS
WITCHES
WITHERS
WITHIES
WITLESS
WITNESS
WIZARDS
WOBBLES
WOMBATS
WONDERS
WONTONS
WOODIES
WOOFERS
WOOLENS
WOOLIES
WOOSHES
WORKERS
WORKUPS
WORMERS
WORRIES
WORSENS
WRAITHS
WRAPUPS
WRASSES
WREATHS
WRIGHTS
WRITERS
WRITHES
WRYNESS
WYVERNS

•W•S•••

AWASHIN
AWESOME
SWASHED
SWASHES
SWISHED
SWISHES
TWISTED
TWISTER
TWISTON
TWISTUP
TWOSHOT
TWOSOME
TWOSPOT
TWOSTAR
TWOSTEP

•W••S••

SWANSEA
SWANSON
SWATSAT
SWENSON
SWIMSUP
SWOOSIE
TWINSET

•W•••S•

AWAREST
AWELESS
AWNLESS
OWLIEST
SWEDISH
SWINISH
TWOBASE

•W••••S

AWAKENS
AWAKERS
AWELESS
AWNINGS
AWNLESS
DWARVES
EWERIES
KWACHAS
KWANZAS
OWLEGGS
SWASHES
SWATHES
SWAYERS
SWERVES
SWIPERS
SWISHES
SWIVELS
SWIVETS
TWEEZES
TWELVES
TWINERS
TWINGES
TWOACTS
TWOBITS
TWODAYS
TWOEGGS
TWOFERS
TWOTONS

••WS•••

BOWSAWS
BOWSHOT
BOWSOUT
COWSHED
COWSKIN
COWSLIP
DOWSERS
DOWSING
HAWSERS
LAWSUIT
LOWSIDE
NEWSBOY
NEWSDAY
NEWSIER
NEWSIES
NEWSMAN
NEWSMEN
NEWSOME
NEWSPEG
RAWSILK
SAWSOFF
SOWSEAR

••W•S••

DAWNSON
FAWNSON
GAWKSAT
HOWLSAT
JEWISON
NOWISEE
NOWISER
RAWISTS
SEWISTS
UNWISER

••W••S•

ATWORST
BOWLESS
COWFISH
COWIEST
DEWIEST
DEWLESS
EKWENSI
FEWNESS
GAWKISH
HAWKISH
HOWELSE
JAWLESS
LAWCASE
LAWLESS
LEWDEST
LOWCOST
LOWMASS
LOWNESS
LOWPOST
LOWRISE
LOWRISK
MAWKISH
NEWNESS
NOWNESS
NOWORSE
RAWFISH
RAWNESS
SAWDUST
SAWFISH
SAWPAST
TOWNISH
VFWPOST
VOWLESS

••W•••S

BAWLERS
BEWAILS
BEWARES
BOWFINS
BOWLERS
BOWLESS
BOWOARS
BOWSAWS
BOWTIES
BOWWOWS
BOWYERS
BYWORDS
COWARDS
COWBOYS
COWPEAS
COWRIES
DAWDLES
DAWKINS
DEWAXES
DEWIRES
DEWLAPS
DEWLESS
DEWORMS
DOWDIES
DOWNERS
DOWRIES
DOWSERS
EDWARDS
ENWINDS
ENWRAPS
EXWIVES
EXWORKS
FAWNERS
FEWNESS
FOWLERS
GAWKERS
GAWPERS
GEWGAWS
HAWHAWS
HAWKERS
HAWKINS
HAWSERS
HGWELLS
HOWARDS
HOWDAHS
HOWELLS
HOWLERS
INWARDS
JAWLESS
KEWPIES
KIWANIS
KOWTOWS
LAWLESS
LAWYERS
LOWBIDS
LOWBOYS
LOWMASS
LOWNESS
LOWTOPS
MEWLERS
MOWINGS
MRWORDS
NEWBIES
NEWCARS
NEWHATS
NEWJOBS
NEWKIDS
NEWMANS
NEWNESS
NEWSIES
NEWTONS
NEWTOYS
NOWNESS
NOWTHIS
ONWARDS
PAWNEES
PAWNERS
PAWPAWS
PEWTERS
POWDERS
POWWOWS
RAWBARS
RAWEGGS
RAWISTS
RAWLINS
RAWNESS
REWAKES
REWARDS
REWARMS
REWARNS
REWAXES
REWEARS
REWELDS
REWINDS
REWIPES
REWIRES
REWORDS
REWORKS
REWRAPS
ROWDIES
SAWLOGS
SAWPITS
SAWYERS
SEWARDS
SEWISTS
THWACKS
THWARTS
TOWAGES
TOWARDS
TOWBARS
TOWCARS
TOWHEES
TOWINGS
TOWNERS
TOWNIES
UNWALLS
UNWINDS
UNWRAPS
UPWAFTS
UPWARDS
UPWELLS
UPWINDS
VOWLESS
WHWORDS
YAWNERS
YAWPERS
YOWLERS

•••WS••

BLOWSIN
BLOWSIT
BLOWSON
BLOWSUP
BREWSKI
BREWSUP
BROWSED
BROWSER
BROWSES
CHEWSON
CHEWSUP
CLAWSAT
DRAWSIN
DRAWSON
DRAWSTO
DRAWSUP
DROWSED
DROWSES
FLOWSIN
GNAWSAT
GNAWSON
GROWSON
GROWSUP
KNOWSOF
PLOWSON
PLOWSUP
SHOWSIN
SHOWSUP
SLOWSUP
SNOWSIN
SNOWSKI
STOWSIT

•••W•S•

ALLWISE
ANYWISE
CARWASH
DRYWASH
DUEWEST
ENDWISE
ENTWIST
EYEWASH
FANWISE
FARWEST
GETWISE
GOTWISE
HOGWASH
JETWASH
KEYWEST
MAEWEST
MIDWEST
MUDWASP
OLDWEST
OUTWASH
OUTWEST
OUTWISH
PREWASH
PROWESS
PROWEST
RETWIST
SAMWISE
SLOWEST
SLOWISH
UNTWIST
WETWASH
YOUWISH

•••W••S

AIRWARS
AIRWAYS
AJOWANS
ANSWERS
ANYWAYS
AVOWALS
AVOWERS
BAGWIGS
BIGWIGS
BIGWINS
BLOWERS
BLOWUPS
BOWWOWS
BREWERS
BROWSES
CHEWERS
CLAWERS
COBWEBS
CREWELS

CROWERS
DAEWOOS
DIMWITS
DOOWOPS
DRAWEES
DRAWERS
DROWSES
EARWIGS
ENDWAYS
FLOWERS
FLYWAYS
GASWARS
GLOWERS
GNAWERS
GODWITS
GROWERS
GROWTHS
HOTWARS
JETWAYS
KEYWAYS
KNOWERS
KNOWLES
LEEWAYS
MEOWERS
MIDWAYS
NITWITS
NONWARS
OLDWAYS
OUTWARS
OUTWITS
PEDWAYS
PEEWEES
PLOWERS
POWWOWS
PROWESS
PSYWARS
RESWIMS
RUNWAYS
SEAWAYS
SEGWAYS
SHOWERS
SKEWERS
SKYWAYS
SLOWUPS
SPEWERS
STEWERS
STOWERS
SUBWARS
SUBWAYS
THAWERS
TROWELS
VIEWERS
WAHWAHS
WIGWAGS
WIGWAMS

••••W•S

ALLEWIS
CSLEWIS
DISOWNS
ELFOWLS
JCPOWYS
MOHAWKS
OJIBWAS
ONETWOS
OTTAWAS
OUTAWES
PESEWAS
RENOWNS
SCRAWLS
SPRAWLS
SQUAWKS
TFPOWYS
TIMEWAS
UNPAWNS
UPTOWNS

•••••WS

ABCNEWS
ALLNEWS
ANDREWS
ANTCOWS
ANYNEWS
BADNEWS
BARROWS
BELLOWS
BESTOWS
BIGNEWS
BILLOWS
BORROWS
BOWSAWS
BOWWOWS
BURROWS
CASHEWS
CBSNEWS
CURFEWS
CURLEWS
CUSHAWS
DECLAWS
ESCHEWS
ESCROWS
ESPNEWS
FALLOWS
FARROWS
FELLOWS
FOGBOWS
FOLLOWS
FOXNEWS
FURROWS
GAGLAWS
GALLOWS
GEEGAWS
GEWGAWS
GUFFAWS
GUNLAWS
HALLOWS
HARROWS
HAWHAWS
HAYMOWS
HEBREWS
HEEHAWS
HOLLOWS
INFLOWS
JIGSAWS
KOWTOWS
MALLOWS
MARROWS
MATHEWS
MEADOWS
MELLOWS
MILDEWS
MINNOWS
MOOCOWS
MORROWS
NARROWS
NBCNEWS
NEPHEWS
NONJEWS
NONNEWS
NOSHOWS
OLDNEWS
OLDSAWS
OUTBOWS
OUTLAWS
OUTROWS
PAWPAWS
PETCOWS
PILLOWS
PITROWS
PITSAWS
POWWOWS
QUAPAWS
REAVOWS
REBREWS
RECHEWS
REDRAWS
REFLOWS
REGLOWS
REGROWS
REPLOWS
RESHOWS
RESTOWS
RETHAWS
REVIEWS
RIPSAWS
SEACOWS
SEESAWS
SHADOWS
SKITOWS
SORROWS
SUNBOWS
TALLOWS
TAXLAWS
THENEWS
TOPROWS
TVCREWS
TVSHOWS
UNDRAWS
UNSKEWS
UNSTOWS
UNTHAWS
UPFLOWS
UPGROWS
WALLOWS
WILLOWS
WINDOWS
WINNOWS
YARROWS
YELLOWS

W•T••••

WATCHED
WATCHER
WATCHES
WATCHIT
WATCHTV
WATERED
WATERER
WATFORD
WATKINS
WATTAGE
WATTEAU
WATTLED
WATTLES
WATUSIS
WETBARS
WETBULB
WETCELL
WETDOWN
WETEYED
WETKISS
WETLAND
WETLOOK
WETMOPS
WETNAPS
WETNESS
WETONES
WETRAGS
WETSUIT
WETTEST
WETTING
WETTISH
WETWARE
WETWASH
WITCHED
WITCHES
WITEOUT
WITHERS
WITHIES
WITHOUT
WITLESS
WITLING
WITNESS
WITSEND
WITTIER
WITTILY
WITTING

W••T•••

WAFTERS
WAFTING
WAITERS
WAITFOR
WAITING
WAITOUT
WAITRON
WAITSON
WAITSUP
WALTERS
WALTHAM
WALTHER
WALTONS
WALTZED
WALTZER
WALTZES
WANTADS
WANTAGH
WANTERS
WANTING
WANTONS
WANTOUT
WANTSIN
WANTSTO
WARTHOG
WARTIER
WARTIME
WARTORN
WASTAGE
WASTERS
WASTING
WASTREL
WATTAGE
WATTEAU
WATTLED
WATTLES
WAYTOGO
WEATHER
WEBTOED
WELTERS
WELTING
WENTAFT
WENTAPE
WENTBAD
WENTFAR
WENTFOR
WENTMAD
WENTOFF
WENTOUT
WENTPRO
WERTHER
WESTEGG
WESTEND
WESTERN
WESTERS
WESTIES
WESTINS
WETTEST
WETTING
WETTISH
WHATAMI
WHATFOR
WHATIFS
WHATNOT
WHATNOW
WHATSAY
WHATSIS
WHATSIT
WHATSUP
WHATTHE
WHETHER
WHETTED
WHETTER
WHITELY
WHITENS
WHITEST
WHITHER
WHITING
WHITISH
WHITMAN
WHITNEY
WHITSUN
WHITTLE
WILTING
WINTERS
WINTERY
WISTFUL
WITTIER
WITTILY
WITTING
WOJTYLA
WONTING
WONTONS
WORTHIT
WRITEIN
WRITEME
WRITEON
WRITERS
WRITETO
WRITEUP
WRITHED
WRITHER
WRITHES
WRITING
WRITTEN
WROTEIN
WROTEON
WROTETO
WROTEUP
WYOTANA

W•••T••

WAISTED
WALSTON
WAPITIS
WASATCH
WASHTUB
WEALTHS
WEALTHY
WEBSTER
WEIRTON
WHARTON
WHATTHE
WHEATEN
WHEATON
WHETTED
WHETTER
WHISTLE
WHITTLE
WINDTEE
WINGTIP
WINSTON
WIRETAP
WOODTAR
WOOSTER
WORSTED
WRAITHS
WREATHE
WREATHS
WREATHY
WRESTED
WRESTER
WRESTLE
WRITTEN
WYNETTE

W••••T•

WABBITS
WAIKATO
WALCOTT
WALKSTO
WALLETS
WALNUTS
WANTSTO
WARMSTO
WARPATH
WARVETS
WASLATE
WASONTO
WATCHTV
WAVEDTO
WAVESTO
WBYEATS
WEBSITE
WEEBITS
WEIGHTS
WEIGHTY
WESCOTT
WESKITS
WHERETO
WICHITA
WICKETS
WIDGETS
WIGLETS
WOMBATS
WOOLITE
WRIGHTS
WRITETO
WROTETO
WYNETTE

W•••••T

WACKEST
WAITOUT
WALCOTT
WALKOUT
WALMART
WANIEST
WANNEST
WANTOUT
WAPSHOT
WARIEST
WARMEST
WARRANT
WASHOUT
WATCHIT
WAVEDAT
WAVELET
WAVESAT
WAVIEST
WAXIEST
WEAKEST
WEAROUT
WEBCAST
WEBFEET
WEBFOOT
WEDIDIT
WEEDOUT
WELLCUT
WELLHIT
WELLLIT
WELLPUT
WELLSET
WENTAFT
WENTOUT
WESCOTT
WETSUIT
WETTEST
WHATNOT
WHATSIT
WHEREAT
WHIPPET
WHITEST
WHOISIT
WHOSOUT
WHYISIT
WHYWAIT
WIGSOUT
WILBERT
WILDCAT
WILDEST
WILIEST
WIMPOUT
WINEVAT
WINGLET
WINGNUT
WINGSIT
WINIEST
WINKOUT
WINKSAT
WINSLET
WINSOUT
WIPEOUT
WIRIEST
WITEOUT
WITHOUT
WOODCUT
WOODLOT
WOOLFAT
WOOLHAT
WOREOUT
WORKOUT
WORKSAT
WORNOUT
WORTHIT
WOULDNT
WOULDST
WROUGHT

•W•T•••

SWATHED
SWATHES
SWATSAT
SWATTED
SWATTER
SWITZER
TWITCHY
TWITTED
TWITTER
TWOTERM
TWOTIME
TWOTOED
TWOTONE
TWOTONS

•W••T••

AWAITED
AWAITER
DWELTON
IWANTIT
IWANTTO
PWBOTHA
SWARTHY
SWATTED
SWATTER
SWEATED
SWEATER
SWEATIT
SWEETEN
SWEETER
SWEETIE
SWEETLY
SWEETON
SWELTER
SWELTRY
SWEPTUP
SWIFTER
SWIFTLY
SWINTON
TWEETED
TWEETER
TWISTED
TWISTER
TWISTON
TWISTUP
TWITTED
TWITTER
TWOSTAR
TWOSTEP

•W•••T•

DWIGHTD
GWYNETH
IWANTTO
OWINGTO
OWNUPTO
SWEARTO
SWIVETS
SWORETO
TWELFTH
TWOACTS
TWOBITS

•W••••T

AWAREST
AWEEBIT
DWELLAT
IWANTIT
OWLIEST
SWATSAT
SWEARAT
SWEATIT
SWIGERT
SWINGAT
SWINGIT
SWOREAT
SWUNGAT
SWUNGIT
TWERENT
TWINJET
TWINSET
TWOFEET
TWOFOOT
TWOPART
TWOSHOT
TWOSPOT
TWOUNIT

••WT•••

BOWTIES
COWTOWN
HOWTHEN
KOWTOWS
LOWTECH
LOWTIDE
LOWTOPS
NEWTONS
NEWTOWN
NEWTOYS
NOWTHEN
NOWTHIS
PEWTERS
SAWTOIT
YEWTREE

••W•T••

ATWATER
BEWITCH
DEWATER
ONWATER
REWATER
SAWATCH
UNWITTY

••W••T•

ALWORTH
BOWEDTO
COWRITE
COWROTE
EBWHITE
FAWCETT
FTWORTH
HAWORTH
HEWEDTO
HEWLETT
INWHITE
ITWENTY
KUWAITI
NCWYETH
NEWGATE
NEWHATS
NEWMATH
RAWDATA
RAWISTS
REWRITE
REWROTE
SAWINTO
SAWPITS
SEWISTS
THWARTS
THWHITE
TOWPATH
UNWHITE
UNWITTY
UPWAFTS

••W•••T

ATWORST
BAWLOUT
BOWKNOT
BOWSHOT
BOWSOUT
COWERAT
COWIEST
DEWAART
DEWIEST
DOWNPAT
FAWCETT
GAWKSAT
HEWLETT
HOWBEIT
HOWLSAT
JAWEDAT
LAWSUIT
LEWDEST
LOWCOST
LOWPOST
LOWRENT
NEWBOLT
NEWHART
NEWLEFT
NEWMINT
NEWMONT
NEWPORT
NOWWHAT
PAWEDAT
RAWMEAT
ROWBOAT
SAWDUST
SAWPAST
SAWTOIT
TOWBOAT
TOWNLET
UNWHIPT
VFWPOST

•••WT••

CHEWTOY
GROWTHS

•••W•T•

DIMWITS
DRAWNTO
DRAWSTO
FLOWNTO
GODWITS
KNOWETH
METWITH
NITWITS
NOTWITH
OUTWITH
OUTWITS
PREWITT
RANWITH
RUNWITH
SATWITH
SITWITH
SOPWITH
TOYWITH
VIEWITH

•••W••T

ASSWEET
ATHWART
BETWIXT
BLEWOUT
BLOWOUT
BLOWSIT
CHEWOUT
CLAWSAT
CREWCUT
DERWENT
DRAWOUT
DREWOUT
DUEWEST
DURWENT
ENTWIST
FARWEST
FLOWNAT
FLOWOUT
FORWENT
FROWNAT
GNAWSAT
GREWFAT
GROWFAT
INDWELT
INSWEPT
KEYWEST
MAEWEST
MIDWEST
NOSWEAT
NOWWHAT
OLDWEST
ONEWHIT
OUTWAIT
OUTWENT
OUTWEPT
OUTWEST
PREWITT
PROWEST
RETWIST
SAYWAIT
SAYWHAT
SHOWCAT
SHOWOUT
SLOWEST
SNOWCAT
SNOWHAT
SPEWOUT
STEWART
STEWPOT
STOWSIT
THAWOUT
UNSWEET
UNSWEPT
UNTWIST
UPSWEPT
WHYWAIT
ZUMWALT

••••W•T

GETSWET
HALFWIT
IKNEWIT
IKNOWIT
LACKWIT
OVERWET
THREWAT
THROWAT
VERYWET

W•U••••

WHUPPED
WOULDBE
WOULDNT
WOULDST
WOUNDED
WOUNDUP

W••U•••

WATUSIS
WHAUDEN
WROUGHT

W•••U••

WAKEUPS
WALKUPS
WALKURE
WALNUTS
WAMPUMS
WARBURG
WARMUPS
WASHUPS
WASSURE
WETBULB
WETSUIT
WINDUPS
WORKUPS
WRAPUPS

W••••U•

WAILFUL
WAITOUT
WAITSUP
WAKEDUP
WAKEFUL
WAKESUP
WALKOUT
WALLSUP
WANTOUT
WARCLUB
WARMSUP
WASHOUT
WASHTUB
WAXEDUP
WAXESUP
WEAROUT
WEEDOUT
WEEHOUR
WEIGHUP
WELLCUT
WELLPUT
WELLRUN
WELLSUP
WENTOUT
WHATSUP
WHIPSUP
WHITSUN
WHOSOUT
WICKIUP
WIGSOUT
WILLFUL
WIMPOUT
WINDAUS
WINDSUP
WINGNUT
WINKOUT
WINSOUT
WIPEDUP
WIPEOUT
WIPESUP
WIREDUP
WIRESUP
WISEDUP
WISEGUY
WISESUP
WISHFUL
WISTFUL
WITEOUT
WITHOUT
WOKENUP
WOLFCUB
WOODCUT
WOREOUT
WORKOUT
WORKSUP
WORNOUT
WOUNDUP
WRACKUP
WRAPSUP
WRITEUP
WROTEUP

W•••••U

WATTEAU
WILLYOU

•WU••••

SWUNGAT
SWUNGBY
SWUNGIT

•W•U•••

AWFULLY
OWNUPTO
TWOUNIT

•W•••U•
OWNEDUP
SWANKUP
SWEEPUP
SWELLUP
SWEPTUP
SWIMSUP
TWISTUP
TWOHOUR

•W••••U
ZWICKAU

••W•U••
ENWOUND
HOWDULL
HOWMUCH
LAWSUIT
NEWBURG
REWOUND
SAWBUCK
SAWDUST
UNWOUND
UNWRUNG

••W••U•
BAWLOUT
BOWLFUL
BOWSOUT
POWERUP
SAWCHUK
SEWEDUP
YAWNFUL

••W•••U
HOWARDU
IOWEYOU

•••WU••
BEOWULF
BLOWUPS
MUGWUMP
SLOWUPS
UNSWUNG

•••W•U•
BLEWOUT
BLOWGUN
BLOWNUP
BLOWOUT
BLOWSUP
BREWPUB
BREWSUP
CHEWGUM
CHEWOUT
CHEWSUP
CREWCUT
DRAWNUP
DRAWOUT
DRAWSUP
DREWOUT
FLOWNUP
FLOWOUT
GROWNUP
GROWSUP
PLOWSUP
SHOWNUP
SHOWOUT
SHOWSUP
SLOWSUP
SPEWOUT
THAWOUT
UNAWFUL

••••WU•
OUTSWUM
SCREWUP
THREWUP
THROWUP

W•V••••
WAVEDAT
WAVEDIN
WAVEDTO
WAVELET
WAVEOFF
WAVERED
WAVERER
WAVESAT
WAVESIN
WAVESTO
WAVICLE
WAVIEST
WYVERNS

W••V•••
WAIVERS
WAIVING
WARVETS
WEAVERS
WEAVING
WEEVILS

W•••V••
WHARVES
WHOEVER
WHYEVER
WINEVAT
WINOVER
WONOVER

W••••V•
WHEREVE

W•••••V
WATCHTV

•W•V•••
SWIVELS
SWIVETS

•W••V••
DWARVES
SWERVED
SWERVES
TWELVEA
TWELVEB
TWELVEC
TWELVED
TWELVEE
TWELVES

••W•V••
EXWIVES
HOWEVER
INWOVEN
REWOVEN
UNWAVED
UNWOVEN

••W••V•
BTWELVE
INWEAVE
ITWELVE
LOWDIVE
NEWLOVE
NEWWAVE
REWEAVE
UNWEAVE

••W•••V
EDWARDV

•••W•V•
AIRWAVE
NEWWAVE
OUTWAVE
THEWAVE

W•W••••
WHWORDS
WOWEDEM

W••W•••
WAHWAHS
WARWICK
WARWORN
WAXWING
WAXWORK
WAYWARD
WAYWORN
WETWARE
WETWASH
WHYWAIT
WIGWAGS
WIGWAMS
WINWOOD

W•••W••
WAGEWAR
WALKWAY
WELLWON
WHOSWHO
WIDOWED
WIDOWER
WIMOWEH
WYSIWYG

W••••W•
WALLOWS
WARHAWK
WETDOWN
WILLOWS
WILLOWY
WINDOWS
WINDOWY
WINNOWS

W•••••W
WHATNOW
WHIPSAW
WHOKNEW
WICKLOW
WINSLOW
WOODROW
WOODSAW
WROCLAW

•W•W•••
AWKWARD
TWOWEEK

•W••••W
SWALLOW

••WW•••
BOWWOWS
NEWWAVE
NEWWEEK
NEWWORD
NOWWHAT
POWWOWS
SAWWOOD

••W•W••
TOWAWAY

••W••W•
BOWDOWN
BOWSAWS
BOWWOWS
COWTOWN
GEWGAWS
HAWHAWS
KOWTOWS
LOWDOWN
MOWDOWN
NEWMOWN
NEWTOWN
PAWPAWS
POWWOWS

••W•••W
DEWCLAW
DOWNBOW
LOWBLOW
LOWBROW

•••WW••
BROWWAX

•••W•W•
BOWWOWS
POWWOWS

•••W••W
KNEWHOW
KNOWHOW
SHOWHOW

••••W•W
LIKEWOW

W•X••••
WAXABLE
WAXBEAN
WAXEDUP
WAXESUP
WAXIEST
WAXINGS
WAXLIKE
WAXWING
WAXWORK
WEXFORD

W•••••X
WOODBOX
WORKBOX

••W•X••
DEWAXED
DEWAXES
REWAXED
REWAXES
UNWAXED

•••WX••
TUVWXYZ

•••W•X•
BETWIXT

•••W••X
BROWWAX
MEOWMIX

••••WX•
STUVWXY

••••W•X
BEESWAX
BROWWAX

•••••WX
RSTUVWX

WY•••••
WYNDHAM
WYNETTE
WYNONNA
WYOMING
WYOTANA
WYSIWYG
WYVERNS

W•Y••••
WAYBACK
WAYBILL
WAYCOOL
WAYLAID
WAYLAND
WAYLAYS
WAYLESS
WAYSIDE
WAYTOGO
WAYWARD
WAYWORN
WBYEATS
WHYEVER
WHYISIT
WHYWAIT
WRYNESS

W••Y•••
WHEYISH
WIFYING

W•••Y••
WELLYES
WETEYED
WILLYOU
WOJTYLA

W••••Y•
WALLEYE
WAYLAYS
WYSIWYG

W•••••Y
WACKILY
WAGGERY
WALKSBY
WALKWAY
WALLABY
WARBABY
WASHDAY
WASPILY
WASSILY
WCHANDY
WEALTHY
WEARILY
WEEDILY
WEEKDAY
WEIGHTY
WEIRDLY
WEMBLEY
WHALLEY
WHATSAY
WHEREBY
WHISKEY
WHITELY
WHITNEY
WIGGERY
WILLOWY
WINDILY
WINDOWY
WINFREY
WINTERY
WISEGUY
WISPILY
WITTILY
WOMANLY
WOODLEY
WOOLERY
WOOLLEY
WOOLSEY
WOOZILY
WORDILY
WORKDAY
WORKSHY
WORLDLY
WORSLEY
WREATHY
WRIGGLY
WRIGLEY
WRINKLY
WRONGLY

•WY••••
GWYNETH

•W•Y•••
SWAYBAR
SWAYERS
SWAYING
TWOYEAR

•W••Y••
OWLEYED

•W•••Y•
TWODAYS

•W••••Y
AWFULLY
SWARTHY
SWEARBY
SWEENEY
SWEETLY
SWELTRY
SWIFTLY
SWINERY
SWINGBY
SWOREBY
SWUNGBY
TWINKLY
TWITCHY

••WY•••
BOWYERS
LAWYERS
NCWYETH
NEWYEAR
NEWYORK
SAWYERS

••W•Y••
BYWAYOF
FTWAYNE
HOWDYDO
IOWEYOU

••W••Y•
COWBOYS
HAWKEYE
LOWBOYS
NEWTOYS

••W•••Y
BAWDILY
COWPONY
DOWDILY
DRWELBY
GAWKILY
HOWMANY
IFWEMAY
ITWENTY
JEWELRY
LOWEEZY
LOWLILY
MOWBRAY
NEWAGEY
NEWBERY
NEWSBOY
NEWSDAY
POWDERY
ROWDILY
TAWNILY
TOWAWAY
UNWEARY
UNWINDY
UNWITTY
UNWORMY
VOWELLY

•••WY••
VANWYCK

•••W•Y•
AIRWAYS
ANYWAYS
ENDWAYS
FLYWAYS
JETWAYS
KEYWAYS
LEEWAYS
MIDWAYS
OLDWAYS
PEDWAYS
RUNWAYS
SEAWAYS
SEGWAYS
SKYWAYS
SUBWAYS
TUVWXYZ

•••W••Y
BLOWDRY
BLOWFLY
BRAWLEY
BREWERY
CHEWTOY
CRAWLEY
CROWLEY
FAYWRAY
FLOWERY
FLOWNBY
FRAWLEY
PLOWBOY
SHOWERY
SHOWILY
SLOWDAY
SNOWDAY
SNOWILY

••••WY•
GOLDWYN
JCPOWYS
TFPOWYS
WYSIWYG

••••W•Y
ALLOWAY
ARCHWAY
AREAWAY
ASKAWAY
ATEAWAY
BACKWAY
BELTWAY
BIKEWAY
BOBTWAY
CARAWAY
CUTAWAY
DIEAWAY
DOORWAY
DUNAWAY
EATAWAY
FAIRWAY
FARAWAY
FIVEWAY
FLYAWAY
FOLKWAY
FOOTWAY
FOURWAY
FREEWAY
GANGWAY
GATEWAY
GAVEWAY
GETAWAY
GIVEWAY
GOTAWAY
HALFWAY
HALLWAY
HARDWAY
HEADWAY
HIDAWAY
HIGHWAY
INNOWAY
JANEWAY
LANGWAY
LAYAWAY
LEDAWAY
LONGWAY
MADEWAY
MAKEWAY
OJIBWAY
PARKWAY
PARTWAY
PATHWAY
PEGAWAY
PUTAWAY
RACEWAY
RAILWAY
RANAWAY
RIDGWAY
ROADWAY
ROLLWAY
ROTAWAY
RUNAWAY
SAFEWAY
SCRAWLY
SCRAWNY
SHIPWAY
SHYAWAY
SIDEWAY
SKAGWAY
SOMEWAY
SPRAWLY
SQUAWKY
STUVWXY
TAXIWAY
THATWAY
THISWAY
THRUWAY
TOLLWAY
TOWAWAY
TRAMWAY
UNLOWLY
UNROWDY
WALKWAY

•••••WY
BILLOWY
MEADOWY
MILDEWY
PILLOWY
SHADOWY
TALLOWY
UNSHOWY
WILLOWY
WINDOWY
YELLOWY

W•Z••••
WIZARDS
WIZENED
WOZNIAK
WOZZECK

W••Z•••
WARZONE
WEBZINE
WHIZKID
WHIZZED
WHIZZER
WHIZZES
WOOZIER
WOOZILY
WOZZECK

W•••Z••
WALTZED
WALTZER
WALTZES
WHEEZED
WHEEZER
WHEEZES
WHIZZED
WHIZZER
WHIZZES

•W•Z•••
SWIZZLE

•W••Z••
DWEEZIL
KWANZAA
KWANZAS
SWITZER
SWIZZLE
TWEEZED
TWEEZER
TWEEZES
ZWANZIG

••W••Z•
LOWEEZY

•••WZ••
BLOWZED

•••W••Z
GEEWHIZ
SHOWBIZ
TUVWXYZ

XA•••••
XAMOUNT
XANADUS
XANTHAN
XANTHIC
XAVIERU

X•A••••
XFACTOR
XRATING
XRAYING
XRAYLAB
XSANDOS

X••A•••
XANADUS
XMRADIO

X•••A••
XENIAOH

X••••A•
XANTHAN
XENICAL
XRAYLAB
XTERRAS

•XA••••
EXABYTE
EXACTAS
EXACTED
EXACTER
EXACTLY
EXACTOR
EXALTED
EXALTER
EXAMINE
EXAMPLE
EXANIMO
EXARCHS
OXALATE

•X•A•••
AXIALLY
EXFACTO
EXHALED
EXHALES
EXHAUST
EXMATES
EXMAYOR
EXPANDS
EXPANSE
EXPARTE
EXYANKS
OXCARTS
OXTAILS

•X••A••
AXHEADS
EXCLAIM
EXCLAVE
EXOCARP
EXOGAMY
EXPIATE
EXPLAIN
EXTRACT
EXUDATE
OXALATE
OXHEART
OXIDANT
OXIDASE
OXIDATE

•X•••A•
AXEHEAD
AXILLAE
AXILLAR
AXILLAS
EXACTAS
EXCELAT
EXCUSAL
EXCUSAS
EXEDRAE
EXURBAN
OXONIAN
UXORIAL

•X••••A
EXEMPLA
EXHEDRA
EXORDIA
EXOTICA
EXURBIA
OXYMORA

••XA•••
FIXABLE
FIXATED
FIXATES
HEXADIC
HEXAGON
HEXANES
HEXAPOD
LUXATED
LUXATES
MIXABLE
OAXACAN
ROXANNE
TAXABLE
WAXABLE

••X•A••
BOXBALL
BOXCARS
FOXTAIL
LEXMARK
MAXBAER
NEXRADS
REXCATS
SEXTANS
SEXTANT
SIXBALL
SIXLANE
SIXPACK
SOXFANS
TAXBASE
TAXLAWS
TAXPAID
TAXRATE
TAXSALE

••X••A•
BOXCOAT
BOXSEAT
DEXTRAL
LEXICAL
MAXIMAL
MAXIMAS
MEXICAN
NEXTDAY
OAXACAN
SIXTYAD
SIXYEAR
TAXICAB
TAXIMAN
TAXIWAY
TAXYEAR
TEXTUAL
WAXBEAN

••X•••A
MAXILLA
NOXZEMA
SAXTUBA

•••XA••
INEXACT

•••X•A•
ASEXUAL
BIAXIAL
COAXIAL
FAUXPAS
MANXCAT
MANXMAN
MARXIAN

•••X••A
PROXIMA

••••XA•
ABRAXAS
BAREXAM
CPAEXAM
EYEEXAM

••••X•A
PYREXIA

•••••XA
ARANTXA

X•••••B
XRAYLAB

•XB••••
OXBLOOD

•X•B•••
EXABYTE

•X••B••
EXHIBIT
EXURBAN
EXURBIA

••XB•••
BOXBALL
BOXBEDS
BOXBOYS
FOXBORO
MAXBAER
MAXBORN
ROXBURY
SIXBALL
TAXBASE
WAXBEAN

••X•B••
FIXABLE
MIXABLE
TAXABLE
WAXABLE

••X••B•
SAXTUBA
SIXTYBC

••X•••B
COXCOMB
TAXICAB

X••C•••
XFACTOR

X•••C••
XENICAL

X•••••C
XANTHIC
XEROTIC

•XC••••
EXCEEDS
EXCELAT
EXCELIN
EXCEPTS
EXCERPT
EXCIDED
EXCIDES
EXCISED
EXCISES
EXCITED
EXCITER
EXCITES
EXCITOR
EXCLAIM
EXCLAVE
EXCLUDE
EXCRETE
EXCURSE
EXCUSAL
EXCUSAS
EXCUSED
EXCUSER
EXCUSES
EXCUSEZ
OXCARTS

•X•C•••
EXACTAS
EXACTED
EXACTER
EXACTLY
EXACTOR
EXECUTE
EXOCARP
EXOCETS
EXSCIND

•X••C••
EXARCHS
EXFACTO
EXPECTS
EXSECTS

•X•••C•
EXOTICA
EXOTICS
EXTINCT
EXTRACT

••XC•••
BOXCARS
BOXCOAT
COXCOMB
REXCATS
TAXCODE
TAXCUTS

••X•C••
LEXICAL
LEXICON
MEXICAN
OAXACAN
TAXICAB

••X••C•
MIXTECS
SIXPACK

••X•••C
HEXADIC
LEXUSSC
SIXTYBC

•••XC••
MANXCAT

•••X•C•
INEXACT

••••X•C
UNTOXIC

X•••D••
XANADUS
XMRADIO
XSANDOS

X•••••D
XEROXED
XIPHOID

•X•D•••
EXEDRAE
EXUDATE
EXUDING
OXIDANT
OXIDASE
OXIDATE
OXIDISE
OXIDIZE

•X••D••
EXCIDED
EXCIDES
EXHEDRA
EXORDIA
OXHIDES

•X•••D•
AXHEADS
AXSEEDS
EXCEEDS
EXCLUDE
EXPANDS
EXPENDS
EXPLODE
EXTENDS
EXTRUDE
OXFORDS

•X••••D
AXEHEAD
AXELROD
EXACTED
EXALTED
EXCIDED
EXCISED
EXCITED
EXCUSED
EXERTED
EXHALED
EXHUMED
EXISTED
EXPIRED
EXPOSED
EXPOUND
EXSCIND
EXULTED
OXBLOOD

••X•D••
BOXEDIN
BOXEDUP
FIXEDLY
FIXEDON
FIXEDUP
HEXADIC
MIXEDIN
MIXEDLY
MIXEDUP
NEXTDAY
TUXEDOS
VEXEDLY
WAXEDUP

••X••D•
BOXBEDS
NEXRADS
TAXCODE

••X•••D
FIXATED
HEXAPOD
LUXATED
REXREED
SIXFOLD
SIXTYAD
TAXPAID
WEXFORD

•••X•D•
DIOXIDE

•••X••D
EPOXIED
UNAXLED

••••X•D
ADMIXED
AFFIXED
ANNEXED
DEHEXED
DESEXED
DETOXED
DEWAXED
FEDEXED
IMMIXED
INDEXED
INFIXED
REBOXED
REFAXED
REFIXED
RELAXED
REMIXED
RETAXED
REWAXED
TELEXED
UNBOXED
UNFIXED
UNFOXED
UNLAXED
UNMIXED
UNTAXED
UNVEXED
UNWAXED
XEROXED

XE•••••
XENIAOH
XENICAL
XEROSES
XEROSIS
XEROTIC
XEROXED
XEROXES
XERXESI

X•E••••
XTERRAS

X••E•••
XIMENES

X•••E••
XAVIERU
XERXESI
XYSTERS

X••••E•
XEROSES
XEROXED
XEROXES
XIMENES
XYLOSES

•XE••••
AXEHEAD
AXELIKE
AXELROD
EXECUTE
EXEDRAE
EXEGETE
EXEMPLA
EXEMPTS
EXENEMY
EXERTED
EXERTER
EXEUNTS

•X•E•••
AXHEADS
AXSEEDS
EXCEEDS
EXCELAT
EXCELIN
EXCEPTS
EXCERPT
EXHEDRA
EXPECTS
EXPENDS
EXPENSE
EXPERTS
EXSECTS
EXSERTS
EXTENDS
EXTENSO
EXTENTS
EXTERNE
EXTERNS
OXHEART

•X••E••
AXEHEAD
AXSEEDS
EXCEEDS
EXCRETE
EXEGETE
EXENEMY
EXIGENT
EXILERS
EXOCETS
EXPRESS
EXTREME
EXUPERY

•X•••E•
EXACTED
EXACTER
EXALTED
EXALTER
EXCIDED
EXCIDES
EXCISED
EXCISES
EXCITED
EXCITER
EXCITES
EXCUSED
EXCUSER
EXCUSES
EXCUSEZ
EXERTED
EXERTER
EXHALED
EXHALES
EXHUMED
EXHUMER
EXHUMES
EXISTED
EXITFEE
EXMATES
EXOILER
EXPIRED
EXPIRES
EXPOSED
EXPOSER
EXPOSES
EXULTED
EXWIVES
OXHIDES

•X••••E
AXELIKE
AXILLAE
AXLROSE
EXABYTE
EXAMINE
EXAMPLE
EXCLAVE
EXCLUDE
EXCRETE
EXCURSE
EXECUTE
EXEDRAE
EXEGETE
EXITFEE
EXPANSE
EXPARTE
EXPENSE
EXPIATE
EXPLODE
EXPLORE
EXPUNGE
EXTERNE
EXTREME
EXTRUDE
EXUDATE
OXALATE
OXIDASE
OXIDATE
OXIDISE
OXIDIZE

••XE•••
BOXEDIN
BOXEDUP
BOXESIN
BOXESUP
FIXEDLY
FIXEDON
FIXEDUP
FIXESON
FIXESUP
MIXEDIN
MIXEDLY
MIXEDUP
MIXESIN
MIXESUP
SIXEEEE
TUXEDOS
VEXEDLY
VIXENLY
WAXEDUP
WAXESUP

••X•E••
ANXIETY
BOXBEDS
BOXIEST
BOXSEAT
BOXSETS
COXLESS
FOXIEST
FOXNEWS
LAXNESS
MAXWELL
MIXTECS
NOXZEMA
REXREED
SEXIEST
SEXLESS
SEXTETS
SIXEEEE
SIXFEET
SIXTEEN
SIXWEEK
SIXYEAR
TAXLESS
TAXLEVY
TAXYEAR
WAXBEAN
WAXIEST

••X••E•
BOXSTEP
BOXSTER
FIXATED
FIXATES
HEXANES
HEXOSES
LEXISES
LEXUSES
LUXATED
LUXATES
MAXBAER
MAXIXES
NEXUSES
REXREED
SIXEEEE
SIXFEET
SIXTEEN
SIXTIES
SIXWEEK
TAXFREE
TAXIMEN

••X•••E
BOXKITE
BOXLIKE
FAXLORE
FIXABLE
FIXTURE
FOXFIRE
FOXHOLE
FOXLIKE
MIXABLE
MIXTURE
ROXANNE
SIXEEEE
SIXFIVE
SIXLANE
SIXNINE
TAXABLE
TAXBASE
TAXCODE
TAXFREE
TAXHIKE
TAXRATE
TAXSALE
TEXTILE
TEXTURE
WAXABLE
WAXLIKE

•••XE••
COAXERS
DREXELU
GENXERS
HOAXERS
JINXERS
XERXESI

•••X•E•
DREXLER
DROXIES
EPOXIED
EPOXIES
FLAXIER
FLEXNER
MANXMEN
PREXIES
PROXIES
REEXPEL
UNAXLED

•••X••E
BAUXITE
DIOXIDE
FLEXILE
FLEXURE
INEXILE
QUIXOTE

••••XE•
ADDAXES
ADMIXED
ADMIXES
AFFIXED
AFFIXER
AFFIXES
ANNEXED
ANNEXES
CALYXES
CULEXES
DEHEXED
DEHEXES
DESEXED
DESEXES
DETOXED
DETOXES
DEWAXED
DEWAXES
FEDEXED
FEDEXES
GALAXES
HELIXES
HYRAXES
ICEAXES
IMMIXED
IMMIXES
INBOXES
INDEXED
INDEXER
INDEXES
INFIXED
INFIXES
LATEXES
LUREXES
MAXIXES
PHLOXES
POBOXES
RADIXES
REBOXED
REBOXES
REDOXES
REFAXED
REFAXES
REFIXED
REFIXES
RELAXED
RELAXER
RELAXES
REMIXED
REMIXES
RETAXED
RETAXES
REWAXED
REWAXES
ROLEXES
TELEXED
TELEXES
TIMEXES
UNBOXED
UNBOXES
UNFIXED
UNFIXES
UNFOXED
UNLAXED
UNLAXES
UNMIXED
UNMIXES
UNTAXED
UNTAXES
UNVEXED
UNWAXED
VANEXEL
VELOXES
XEROXED
XEROXES

••••X•E
GALAXIE

•••••XE
HANDAXE
MEATAXE
PICKAXE
POLEAXE

XF•••••
XFACTOR

•XF••••
EXFACTO
OXFORDS

•X••F••
EXITFEE

••XF•••
BOXFULS
FOXFIRE
SIXFEET
SIXFIVE
SIXFOLD
SIXFOOT
SIXFOUR
SOXFANS
TAXFREE
WEXFORD

•••XF••
FAUXFUR

X••G•••
XINGOUT

X•••••G
XRATING
XRAYING

•X•G•••
EXEGETE
EXIGENT
EXOGAMY

•X•••G•
EXPUNGE

•X••••G
EXILING
EXITING
EXUDING

••XG•••
SIXGUNS

••X•G••
HEXAGON

••X••G•
FIXINGS
HEXSIGN
LEXUSGS
LEXUSGX
WAXINGS

••X•••G
TAXIING
TEXTING
WAXWING

•••X••G
BRUXING
COAXING
FLEXING
FLUXING
HOAXING
JINXING

X••H•••
XIPHOID

X•••H••
XANTHAN
XANTHIC

X•••••H
XENIAOH

•XH••••
AXHEADS
EXHALED
EXHALES
EXHAUST
EXHEDRA
EXHIBIT
EXHORTS
EXHUMED
EXHUMER
EXHUMES
OXHEART
OXHIDES

•X•H•••
AXEHEAD

•X•••H•
EXARCHS

••XH•••
FOXHOLE
FOXHUNT
SAXHORN
TAXHIKE

••X•H••
SIXTHLY

••X•••H
PIXYISH
REXROTH

•••X••H
MINXISH

XI•••••
XIMENES
XINGOUT
XIPHOID

X••I•••
XAVIERU
XENIAOH
XENICAL

X•••I••
XRATING
XRAYING

X••••I•
XANTHIC
XEROSIS
XEROTIC
XIPHOID
XMRADIO

X•••••I
XERXESI
XYSTUSI

•XI••••
AXIALLY
AXILLAE
AXILLAR
AXILLAS
EXIGENT
EXILERS
EXILING
EXISTED
EXITFEE
EXITING
EXITNOW
OXIDANT
OXIDASE
OXIDATE
OXIDISE
OXIDIZE

•X•I•••
EXCIDED
EXCIDES
EXCISED
EXCISES
EXCITED
EXCITER
EXCITES
EXCITOR
EXHIBIT
EXOILER
EXPIATE
EXPIRED
EXPIRES
EXTINCT
EXWIVES
OXHIDES

•X••I••
AXELIKE
EXAMINE
EXANIMO
EXILING
EXITING
EXOTICA
EXOTICS
EXOTISM
EXSCIND
EXUDING
OXIDISE
OXIDIZE
OXONIAN
OXTAILS
UXORIAL

•X•••I•
EXCELIN
EXCLAIM
EXHIBIT
EXORDIA
EXPLAIN
EXPLOIT
EXPOSIT
EXURBIA

••XI•••
ANXIETY
ANXIOUS
BOXIEST
FIXINGS
FOXIEST
LEXICAL
LEXICON
LEXISES
MAXILLA
MAXIMAL
MAXIMAS
MAXIMUM
MAXIMUS
MAXIXES
MEXICAN
MIXITUP
NOXIOUS
PAXINOU
SEXIEST
SEXISTS
SIXIRON
TAXICAB
TAXIING
TAXIMAN
TAXIMEN
TAXIWAY
WAXIEST
WAXINGS

••X•I••
BOXKITE
BOXLIKE
FOXFIRE
FOXLIKE
HEXSIGN
PIXYISH
SIXFIVE
SIXNINE
SIXTIES
TAXHIKE
TAXIING
TEXTILE
TEXTING
WAXLIKE
WAXWING

••X••I•
BOXEDIN
BOXESIN
DEXTRIN
FOXTAIL
HEXADIC
LEXUSIS
MIXEDIN
MIXESIN
TAXPAID

•••XI••
BAUXITE
BIAXIAL
BRUXING
BRUXISM
COAXIAL
COAXING
COEXIST
DIOXIDE
DIOXINS
DROXIES
ELIXIRS
EPOXIED
EPOXIES
FLAXIER
FLEXILE
FLEXING
FLEXION
FLUXING
FLUXION
HOAXING
INEXILE
JINXING
LEOXIII
MARXIAN
MARXISM
MARXIST
MINXISH
PREXIES
PROXIES
PROXIMA
PROXIMO

•••X•I•
CHEXMIX
LEOXIII

•••X••I
LEOXIII
XERXESI

••••XI•
GALAXIE
JOHNXII
JOHNXIV
JOHNXIX
MRFIXIT
PIUSXII
PYREXIA
THEAXIS
UNTOXIC

••••X•I
JOHNXII
JOHNXVI
JOHNXXI
PIUSXII

•••••XI
AIRTAXI
JOHNXXI
LOUISXI

••••X•J
FTDIXNJ

•X•••K•
AXELIKE
EXWORKS
EXYANKS

••XK•••
BOXKITE

••X••K•
BOXLIKE
FOXLIKE
TAXHIKE
WAXLIKE

••X•••K
LEXMARK
SIXPACK
SIXWEEK
WAXWORK

X•L••••
XYLOSES

X•••L••
XRAYLAB

X•••••L
XENICAL

•XL••••
AXLROSE

•X•L•••
AXELIKE
AXELROD
AXILLAE
AXILLAR
AXILLAS
AXOLOTL
EXALTED
EXALTER
EXCLAIM
EXCLAVE
EXCLUDE
EXILERS
EXILING
EXPLAIN
EXPLODE
EXPLOIT
EXPLORE
EXULTED
OXALATE
OXBLOOD

•X••L••
AXIALLY
AXILLAE
AXILLAR
AXILLAS
EXCELAT
EXCELIN
EXHALED
EXHALES
EXOILER
EXTOLLS

•X•••L•
AXIALLY
EXACTLY
EXAMPLE
EXEMPLA
EXTOLLS
OXTAILS

•X••••L
AXOLOTL
EXCUSAL
UXORIAL

••XL•••
BOXLIKE
COXLESS
FAXLORE
FOXLIKE
SEXLESS
SIXLANE
TAXLAWS
TAXLESS
TAXLEVY
WAXLIKE

••X•L••
MAXILLA

••X••L•
BOXBALL
BOXFULS
BUXOMLY
FIXABLE
FIXEDLY
FOXHOLE
LEXUSLS
LEXUSLX
MAXILLA
MAXWELL
MIXABLE
MIXEDLY
SIXBALL
SIXFOLD
SIXTHLY
TAXABLE
TAXSALE
TEXTILE
VEXEDLY
VIXENLY
WAXABLE

••X•••L
BOXBALL
DEXTRAL
FOXTAIL
LEXICAL
MAXIMAL
MAXWELL
SIXBALL
TEXTUAL

•••XL••
DREXLER
UNAXLED

•••X•L•
DREXELU
FLEXILE
INEXILE

•••X••L
ASEXUAL
BIAXIAL
COAXIAL
REEXPEL

••••X•L
VANEXEL

XM•••••
XMRADIO

X•M••••
XAMOUNT
XIMENES

•XM••••
EXMATES
EXMAYOR

•X•M•••
EXAMINE
EXAMPLE
EXEMPLA
EXEMPTS
OXYMORA

•X••M••
EXHUMED
EXHUMER
EXHUMES

•X•••M•
EXANIMO
EXENEMY
EXOGAMY
EXONYMS
EXTREME

•X••••M
EXCLAIM
EXOTISM

••XM•••
LEXMARK

••X•M••
BUXOMLY
MAXIMAL
MAXIMAS
MAXIMUM
MAXIMUS
TAXIMAN
TAXIMEN

••X••M•
COXCOMB
NOXZEMA

••X•••M
MAXIMUM

•••XM••
CHEXMIX
MANXMAN
MANXMEN

•••X•M•
PROXIMA
PROXIMO

•••X••M
BRUXISM
MARXISM

••••X•M
BAREXAM
CPAEXAM
EYEEXAM

X•N••••
XANADUS
XANTHAN
XANTHIC
XENIAOH
XENICAL
XINGOUT

X••N•••
XSANDOS

X•••N••
XIMENES

X••••N•
XAMOUNT
XRATING
XRAYING

X•••••N
XANTHAN

•X•N•••
EXANIMO
EXENEMY
EXONYMS
OXONIAN

•X••N••
EXEUNTS
EXITNOW
EXPANDS
EXPANSE
EXPENDS
EXPENSE
EXPUNGE
EXTENDS
EXTENSO
EXTENTS
EXTINCT
EXYANKS

•X•••N•
EXAMINE
EXIGENT
EXILING
EXITING
EXPOUND
EXSCIND
EXTERNE
EXTERNS
EXUDING
OXIDANT

•X••••N
EXCELIN
EXPLAIN
EXURBAN
OXONIAN

••XN•••
FOXNEWS
HEXNUTS
LAXNESS
SIXNINE

••X•N••
FIXINGS
HEXANES
PAXINOU
ROXANNE
VIXENLY
WAXINGS

••X••N•
FOXHUNT
ROXANNE
SEXTANS
SEXTANT
SEXTONS
SIXGUNS
SIXLANE
SIXNINE
SOXFANS
TAXIING
TEXTING
WAXWING

••X•••N
BOXEDIN
BOXESIN
DEXTRIN
FIXEDON
FIXESON
FIXUPON
HEXAGON
HEXSIGN
LEXICON
MAXBORN
MEXICAN
MIXEDIN
MIXESIN
OAXACAN
SAXHORN
SIXIRON
SIXTEEN
TAXIMAN
TAXIMEN
TEXTRON
WAXBEAN

•••XN••
FLEXNER

•••X•N•
BRUXING
COAXING
DIOXINS
FLEXING
FLUXING
HOAXING
JINXING
KLAXONS

•••X••N
BRAXTON
FLEXION
FLUXION
MANXMAN
MANXMEN
MARXIAN

••••XN•
FTDIXNJ

X••O•••
XAMOUNT
XEROSES
XEROSIS
XEROTIC
XEROXED
XEROXES
XYLOSES

X•••O••
XINGOUT
XIPHOID

X••••O•
XENIAOH
XFACTOR
XSANDOS

X•••••O
XMRADIO

•XO••••
AXOLOTL
EXOCARP
EXOCETS
EXOGAMY
EXOILER
EXONYMS
EXORDIA
EXOTICA
EXOTICS
EXOTISM
OXONIAN
UXORIAL

•X•O•••
EXHORTS
EXPORTS
EXPOSED
EXPOSER
EXPOSES
EXPOSIT
EXPOUND
EXTOLLS
EXTORTS
EXWORKS
OXFORDS

•X••O••
AXLROSE
AXOLOTL
EXPLODE
EXPLOIT
EXPLORE
OXBLOOD
OXYMORA

•X•••O•
AXELROD
EXACTOR
EXCITOR
EXITNOW
EXMAYOR
OXBLOOD

•X••••O
EXANIMO
EXFACTO
EXTENSO

••XO•••
BUXOMLY
HEXOSES

••X•O••
ANXIOUS
BOXBOYS
BOXCOAT
BOXTOPS
COXCOMB
FAXLORE
FOXBORO
FOXHOLE
MAXBORN
NOXIOUS
REXROTH
SAXHORN
SEXPOTS
SEXTONS
SIXFOLD
SIXFOOT
SIXFOUR
TAXCODE
WAXWORK
WEXFORD

••X••O•
FIXEDON
FIXESON
FIXUPON
FOXTROT
HEXAGON
HEXAPOD
LEXICON
PAXINOU
SIXFOOT
SIXIRON
TEXTRON
TUXEDOS

••X•••O
FOXBORO

•••XO••
FLEXORS
KLAXONS
PLEXORS
QUIXOTE

•••X•O•
BRAXTON
FLEXION
FLUXION

•••X••O
PROXIMO

X•P••••
XIPHOID

•XP••••
EXPANDS
EXPANSE
EXPARTE
EXPECTS
EXPENDS
EXPENSE
EXPERTS
EXPIATE
EXPIRED
EXPIRES
EXPLAIN
EXPLODE
EXPLOIT
EXPLORE
EXPORTS
EXPOSED
EXPOSER
EXPOSES
EXPOSIT
EXPOUND
EXPRESS
EXPUNGE

•X•P•••
EXUPERY

•X••P••
EXAMPLE
EXCEPTS
EXEMPLA
EXEMPTS

•X•••P•
EXCERPT

•X••••P
EXOCARP

••XP•••
SEXPOTS
SIXPACK
TAXPAID

••X•P••
FIXUPON
HEXAPOD

••X••P•
BOXTOPS

••X•••P
BOXEDUP
BOXESUP
BOXSTEP
FIXEDUP
FIXESUP
MIXEDUP
MIXESUP
MIXITUP
WAXEDUP
WAXESUP

•••XP••
FAUXPAS
REEXPEL

XR•••••
XRATING
XRAYING
XRAYLAB

X•R••••
XEROSES
XEROSIS
XEROTIC
XEROXED
XEROXES
XERXESI
XMRADIO

X••R•••
XTERRAS

X•••R••
XTERRAS

X••••R•
XAVIERU
XYSTERS

X•••••R
XFACTOR

•X•R•••
AXLROSE
EXARCHS
EXCRETE
EXERTED
EXERTER
EXORDIA
EXPRESS
EXTRACT
EXTREME
EXTRUDE
EXURBAN
EXURBIA
UXORIAL

•X••R••
AXELROD
EXCERPT
EXCURSE
EXEDRAE
EXHORTS
EXPARTE
EXPERTS
EXPIRED
EXPIRES
EXPORTS
EXSERTS
EXTERNE
EXTERNS
EXTORTS
EXWORKS
OXCARTS
OXFORDS

•X•••R•
EXHEDRA
EXILERS
EXOCARP
EXPLORE
EXUPERY
OXHEART
OXYMORA

•X••••R
AXILLAR
EXACTER
EXACTOR
EXALTER
EXCITER
EXCITOR
EXCUSER
EXERTER
EXHUMER
EXMAYOR
EXOILER
EXPOSER

••XR•••
NEXRADS
REXREED
REXROTH
TAXRATE

••X•R••
DEXTRAL
DEXTRIN
FOXTROT
SIXIRON
TAXFREE
TEXTRON

••X••R•
BOXCARS
FAXLORE
FIXTURE
FOXBORO
FOXFIRE
LEXMARK
LEXUSRX
MAXBORN
MIXTURE
ROXBURY
SAXHORN
TEXTURE
WAXWORK
WEXFORD

••X•••R
BOXSTER
MAXBAER
SIXFOUR
SIXYEAR
TAXYEAR

•••X•R•
COAXERS
ELIXIRS
FLEXORS
FLEXURE
GENXERS
HOAXERS
JINXERS
PLEXORS

•••X••R
DREXLER
FAUXFUR
FLAXIER
FLEXNER

••••X•R
AFFIXER
INDEXER
RELAXER

XS•••••
XSANDOS

X•S••••
XYSTERS
XYSTUSI

X•••S••
XEROSES
XEROSIS
XYLOSES

X••••S•
XERXESI
XYSTUSI

X•••••S
XANADUS
XEROSES
XEROSIS
XEROXES
XIMENES
XSANDOS
XTERRAS
XYLOSES
XYSTERS

•XS••••
AXSEEDS
EXSCIND
EXSECTS
EXSERTS

•X•S•••
EXISTED

•X••S••
EXCISED
EXCISES
EXCUSAL
EXCUSAS
EXCUSED
EXCUSER
EXCUSES
EXCUSEZ
EXPOSED
EXPOSER
EXPOSES
EXPOSIT

•X•••S•
AXLROSE
EXCURSE
EXHAUST
EXOTISM
EXPANSE
EXPENSE
EXPRESS
EXTENSO
OXIDASE
OXIDISE

•X••••S
AXHEADS
AXILLAS
AXSEEDS
EXACTAS
EXARCHS
EXCEEDS
EXCEPTS
EXCIDES
EXCISES
EXCITES
EXCUSAS
EXCUSES
EXEMPTS
EXEUNTS
EXHALES
EXHORTS
EXHUMES
EXILERS
EXMATES
EXOCETS
EXONYMS
EXOTICS
EXPANDS
EXPECTS
EXPENDS
EXPERTS
EXPIRES
EXPORTS
EXPOSES
EXPRESS
EXSECTS
EXSERTS
EXTENDS
EXTENTS
EXTERNS
EXTOLLS
EXTORTS
EXWIVES
EXWORKS
EXYANKS
OXCARTS
OXFORDS
OXHIDES
OXTAILS

••XS•••
BOXSEAT
BOXSETS
BOXSTEP
BOXSTER
HEXSIGN
TAXSALE

••X•S••
BOXESIN
BOXESUP
FIXESON
FIXESUP
HEXOSES
LEXISES
LEXUSES
LEXUSGS
LEXUSGX
LEXUSIS
LEXUSLS
LEXUSLX
LEXUSRX
LEXUSSC
MIXESIN
MIXESUP
NEXUSES
SEXISTS
WAXESUP

••X••S•
BOXIEST
COXLESS
FOXIEST
LAXNESS
LEXUSSC
PIXYISH
SEXIEST
SEXLESS
TAXBASE
TAXLESS
WAXIEST

••X•••S
ANXIOUS
BOXBEDS
BOXBOYS
BOXCARS
BOXFULS
BOXSETS
BOXTOPS
COXLESS
FIXATES
FIXINGS
FOXNEWS
HEXANES

HEXNUTS
HEXOSES
LAXNESS
LEXISES
LEXUSES
LEXUSGS
LEXUSIS
LEXUSLS
LUXATES
MAXIMAS
MAXIMUS
MAXIXES
MIXTECS
NEXRADS
NEXUSES
NOXIOUS
REXCATS
SEXISTS
SEXLESS
SEXPOTS
SEXTANS
SEXTETS
SEXTONS
SIXGUNS
SIXTIES
SOXFANS
TAXCUTS
TAXLAWS
TAXLESS
TUXEDOS
WAXINGS

•••X•S•

BRUXISM
COEXIST
MARXISM
MARXIST
MINXISH
XERXESI

•••X••S

COAXERS
DIOXINS
DROXIES
ELIXIRS
EPOXIES
FAUXPAS
FLEXORS
GENXERS
HOAXERS
JINXERS
KLAXONS
PLEXORS
PREXIES
PROXIES

••••X•S

ABRAXAS
ADDAXES
ADMIXES
AFFIXES
ANNEXES
CALYXES
CULEXES
DEHEXES
DESEXES
DETOXES
DEWAXES
FEDEXES
GALAXES
HELIXES
HYRAXES
ICEAXES
IMMIXES
INBOXES
INDEXES
INFIXES
LATEXES
LUREXES
MAXIXES
PHLOXES
POBOXES
RADIXES
REBOXES
REDOXES
REFAXES
REFIXES
RELAXES
REMIXES
RETAXES
REWAXES
ROLEXES
TELEXES
THEAXIS
TIMEXES
UNBOXES
UNFIXES
UNLAXES
UNMIXES
UNTAXES
URTEXTS
VELOXES
XEROXES

XT•••••

XTERRAS

X••T•••

XANTHAN
XANTHIC
XRATING
XYSTERS
XYSTUSI

X•••T••

XEROTIC
XFACTOR

X•••••T

XAMOUNT
XINGOUT

•XT••••

EXTENDS
EXTENSO
EXTENTS
EXTERNE
EXTERNS
EXTINCT
EXTOLLS
EXTORTS
EXTRACT
EXTREME
EXTRUDE
OXTAILS

•X•T•••

EXITFEE
EXITING
EXITNOW
EXOTICA
EXOTICS
EXOTISM

•X••T••

EXACTAS
EXACTED
EXACTER
EXACTLY
EXACTOR
EXALTED
EXALTER
EXCITED
EXCITER
EXCITES
EXCITOR
EXERTED
EXERTER
EXISTED
EXMATES
EXULTED

•X•••T•

AXOLOTL
EXABYTE
EXCEPTS
EXCRETE
EXECUTE
EXEGETE
EXEMPTS
EXEUNTS
EXFACTO
EXHORTS
EXOCETS
EXPARTE
EXPECTS
EXPERTS
EXPIATE
EXPORTS
EXSECTS
EXSERTS
EXTENTS
EXTORTS
EXUDATE
OXALATE
OXCARTS
OXIDATE

•X••••T

EXCELAT
EXCERPT
EXHAUST
EXHIBIT
EXIGENT
EXPLOIT
EXPOSIT
EXTINCT
EXTRACT
OXHEART
OXIDANT

••XT•••

BOXTOPS
DEXTRAL
DEXTRIN
FIXTURE
FOXTAIL
FOXTROT
MIXTECS
MIXTURE
NEXTDAY
SAXTUBA
SEXTANS
SEXTANT
SEXTETS
SEXTONS
SIXTEEN
SIXTHLY
SIXTIES
SIXTYAD
SIXTYBC
TEXTILE
TEXTING
TEXTRON
TEXTUAL
TEXTURE

••X•T••

BOXSTEP
BOXSTER
FIXATED
FIXATES
LUXATED
LUXATES
MIXITUP

••X••T•

ANXIETY
BOXKITE
BOXSETS
HEXNUTS
REXCATS
REXROTH
SEXISTS
SEXPOTS
SEXTETS
TAXCUTS
TAXRATE

••X•••T

BOXCOAT
BOXIEST
BOXSEAT
FOXHUNT
FOXIEST
FOXTROT
SEXIEST
SEXTANT
SIXFEET
SIXFOOT
WAXIEST

•••XT••

BRAXTON

•••X•T•

BAUXITE
QUIXOTE

•••X••T

COEXIST
INEXACT
MANXCAT
MARXIST

••••XT•

URTEXTS

••••X•T

MRFIXIT

•••••XT

BATNEXT
BETWIXT
CONTEXT
PRETEXT
SUBTEXT

X•••U••

XAMOUNT
XYSTUSI

X••••U•

XANADUS
XINGOUT

X•••••U

XAVIERU

•XU••••

EXUDATE
EXUDING
EXULTED
EXUPERY
EXURBAN
EXURBIA

•X•U•••

EXCURSE
EXCUSAL
EXCUSAS
EXCUSED
EXCUSER
EXCUSES
EXCUSEZ
EXEUNTS
EXHUMED
EXHUMER
EXHUMES
EXPUNGE

•X••U••

EXCLUDE
EXECUTE
EXHAUST
EXPOUND
EXTRUDE

••XU•••

FIXUPON
LEXUSES
LEXUSGS
LEXUSGX
LEXUSIS
LEXUSLS
LEXUSLX
LEXUSRX
LEXUSSC
NEXUSES

••X•U••

BOXFULS
FIXTURE
FOXHUNT
HEXNUTS
MIXTURE
ROXBURY
SAXTUBA
SIXGUNS
TAXCUTS
TEXTUAL
TEXTURE

••X••U•

ANXIOUS
BOXEDUP
BOXESUP
FIXEDUP
FIXESUP
MAXIMUM
MAXIMUS
MIXEDUP
MIXESUP
MIXITUP
NOXIOUS
SIXFOUR
WAXEDUP
WAXESUP

••X•••U

PAXINOU

•••XU••

ASEXUAL
FLEXURE

•••X•U•

FAUXFUR

•••X••U

DREXELU

X•V••••

XAVIERU

•X••V••

EXWIVES

•X•••V•

EXCLAVE

••X••V•

SIXFIVE
TAXLEVY

••••XV•

JOHNXVI

••••X•V

JOHNXIV

•••••XV

LOUISXV

•XW••••

EXWIVES
EXWORKS

•X••••W

EXITNOW

••XW•••

MAXWELL
SIXWEEK
WAXWING
WAXWORK

••X•W••

TAXIWAY

••X••W•

FOXNEWS
TAXLAWS

X••X•••

XERXESI

X•••X••

XEROXED
XEROXES

••X•X••

MAXIXES

••X•••X

LEXUSGX
LEXUSLX
LEXUSRX

•••X••X

CHEXMIX

••••XX•

JOHNXXI

••••X•X

JOHNXIX

•••••XX

JIMFIXX

XY•••••

XYLOSES
XYSTERS
XYSTUSI

X••Y•••

XRAYING
XRAYLAB

•XY••••

EXYANKS
OXYMORA

•X••Y••

EXABYTE
EXMAYOR
EXONYMS

•X••••Y

AXIALLY
EXACTLY
EXENEMY
EXOGAMY
EXUPERY

••XY•••

PIXYISH
SIXYEAR
TAXYEAR

••X•Y••

SIXTYAD
SIXTYBC

••X••Y•

BOXBOYS

••X•••Y

ANXIETY
BUXOMLY
FIXEDLY
MIXEDLY
NEXTDAY
ROXBURY
SIXTHLY
TAXIWAY
TAXLEVY
VEXEDLY
VIXENLY

••••XY•

TUVWXYZ

•••••XY

ATARAXY
BYPROXY
STUVWXY

•X•••Z•

OXIDIZE

•X••••Z

EXCUSEZ

••XZ•••

NOXZEMA

••••X•Z

TUVWXYZ

YA•••••

YACHTED
YACHTER
YACHTIE
YAHTZEE
YAKIMAS
YAKKERS
YAKKING
YAKUTSK
YALELAW
YALEMAN
YALEMEN
YAMAHAS
YAMMERS
YANGTZE
YANKEES
YANKERS
YANKING
YANKOFF
YANKOUT
YANKSAT
YANKSON
YANKTON
YANNICK
YANQUIS
YAOMING
YAOUNDE
YAPPERS
YAPPING
YARDAGE
YARDARM
YARDERS
YARDING
YARDMAN
YARDMEN
YARNELL
YARNING
YARROWS
YASBECK
YASHICA
YASHMAK
YASMINE
YATTERS
YAWNERS
YAWNFUL
YAWNIER
YAWNING
YAWPERS
YAWPING
YAYTEAM

Y•A••••

YEAHBUT
YEAHMAN
YEAHYOU
YEANING
YEAREND
YEARNED
YEARNER
YEARNTO
YEARONE
YEASTED
YEATEAM

Y••A•••

YAMAHAS
YOGAMAT
YOLANDA
YOUANDI
YSHAPED
YSHAPES
YUCAIPA
YUCATAN
YUCATEC
YUKATAS

Y•••A••

YARDAGE
YARDARM
YEOMANS
YESMAAM
YOPLAIT
YOTEAMO
YOUMANS
YOURANG

Y••••A•

YAKIMAS
YALELAW
YALEMAN
YAMAHAS
YANKSAT
YARDMAN
YASHMAK
YAYTEAM
YEAHMAN
YEATEAM
YELLSAT
YEREVAN
YESDEAR
YESICAN
YESMAAM
YITZHAK
YOGAMAT
YTTRIAS
YUCATAN
YUKATAS
YZERMAN

Y•••••A

YASHICA
YESHIVA
YOLANDA
YUCAIPA

•YA••••

BYAHAIR
BYAMILE
BYANDBY
BYANECK
BYANOSE
CYANIDE
CYANIDS
HYALITE
HYALOID
HYANNIS
MYALGIA
MYALGIC
MYANMAR

•Y•A•••

AYEAYES
BYCATCH
BYNAMES
BYPATHS
BYTALKS
BYWAYOF
DYNAMIC
DYNAMOS
DYNASTS
DYNASTY
GYRALLY
GYRATED
GYRATES
GYRATOR
HYPATIA
HYRACES
HYRAXES
MYFAULT
MYLANTA
MYMAMMY
NYYANKS
PYRAMID
PYRAMUS
SYNAPSE
TYRANNY
TYRANTS

•Y••A••

AYNRAND
BYAHAIR
BYHEART
BYPLAYS
BYROADS
BYTRAIN
CYMBALS
DYEBATH
DYEVATS
EYEBALL
EYEBANK
EYECARE
EYEHAND
EYELASH
EYEMASK
EYEWALL
EYEWASH
GYMBAGS
GYMBALL
GYMNAST
GYMRATS
HYDRANT
HYDRATE
HYMNALS
HYMNARY
MYGIANT
MYRIADS
MYSPACE
MYSTARS
NYGIANT
RYOKANS
SYLLABI
SYRIANA
SYRIANS
TYMPANA
TYMPANI
TYNDALL
TYPEABS
WYOTANA

•Y•••A•

CYNICAL
CYPRIAN
EYEEXAM
EYEWEAR
GYROCAR
HYGELAC
HYUNDAI
LYESOAP
LYRICAL
MYANMAR
MYCENAE
MYOPIAS
MYTREAT
NYMPHAL
PYTHIAN
PYTHIAS
RYELOAF
SYNGMAN
SYNODAL
TYPICAL
WYNDHAM

•Y••••A

CYNTHIA
DYKSTRA
HYGIEIA
HYPATIA
MYALGIA
MYLANTA
PYREXIA
SYRIANA
TYMPANA
WYNONNA
WYOTANA

••YA•••

BAYAREA
BUYABLE
DRYABLE
DRYADES
DRYADIC
EXYANKS
FLYABLE
FLYAWAY
FRYABLE
KAYAKED
KAYAKER
LAYAWAY
LOYALER
LOYALES
LOYALLY
LOYALTO
LOYALTY
MAYALIN
NAYARIT
NYYANKS
PAYABLE
ROYALES
ROYALLY
ROYALTY
ROYALWE
SAYABLE
SAYAMEN
SHYAWAY
ULYANOV
VOYAGED
VOYAGER
VOYAGES

••Y•A••

AMYLASE
ANYWAYS
BOYBAND
BUYBACK
CAYMANS
CRYBABY
DAYCAMP
DAYCARE
DAYGAME
DAYMARE
DAYPACK
DAYSAIL
DRYWALL
DRYWASH
FLYBALL
FLYCAST
FLYPAST
FLYWAYS
FRYPANS
HAYBALE
HAYRACK
HAYWARD
HEYDAYS
HEYMANS
HEYWARD
INYEARS
JAYWALK
JAYWARD
JOYPADS
KEYBANK
KEYCARD
KEYCASE
KEYPADS
KEYPALS
KEYWAYS
LAYBACK
LAYBARE
MAYDAYS
MAYFAIR
MAYNARD
MAYTAGS
NAYSAID
NAYSAYS
PAYBACK
PAYCASH
PAYDAYS
PAYRATE
PSYWARS
RAYBANS
REYNARD
REYNAUD
SAYMASS
SAYSAAH
SAYSAYE
SAYWAIT
SKYCAMS
SKYCAPS
SKYJACK
SKYLARK
SKYMAPS
SKYWALK
SKYWARD
SKYWAYS
SPYCAMS
SPYWARE
TAYBACK
TOYBALL
TOYCARS
TOYCART
TOYFAIR
TOYHATS
TOYLAND
TOYPAIL
TRYHARD
TRYSAIL
WAYBACK
WAYLAID
WAYLAND
WAYLAYS
WAYWARD
WBYEATS
WHYWAIT

••Y••A•

ABYSMAL
ABYSSAL
ALYKHAN
ANYROAD
BAYEDAT
BAYLEAF
CAYUGAS
CRYSTAL

DAYSPAS
DAYSTAR
DAYWEAR
DRYHEAT
ELYSIAN
FAYWRAY
FEYDEAU
FEYNMAN
FLYAWAY
FLYLEAF
FLYTRAP
JOYCEAN
KEYSPAN
LAYAWAY
LOYOLAU
MAYORAL
PAYLOAD
PAYOLAS
RAYOVAC
ROYBEAN
RUYBLAS
SAYSAAH
SAYSNAY
SAYWHAT
SHYAWAY
SOYBEAN
SOYMEAL
STYGIAN
SZYSLAK
TOYBOAT
TOYOTAS
YAYTEAM
ZOYSIAS

••Y•••A
ALYOSHA
BAYAREA
DAYTONA
DRYIDEA
HRYVNIA
OLYMPIA
OXYMORA
REYNOSA
SOYINKA

•••YA••
ABEYANT
ADAYAGO
ALEYARD
ALIYAHS
ARMYANT
ASBYATT
BANYANS
BEEYARD
BIRYANI
BODYART
BUOYANT
DRAYAGE
ELIYALE
GOBYAIR
HALYARD
HOLYARK
KENYANS
LANYARD
LIBYANS
MAGYARS
MARYANN
MINYANS
ONEYARD
PLAYACT
QUAYAGE
RUDYARD

•••Y•A•
BABYGAP
BABYSAT
BODYBAR
BODYFAT
BOGYMAN
CITYGAL
COPYCAT
COPYMAN
CORYZAS
DRAYMAN
ECTYPAL
ELLYMAY
FREYTAG
GOBYCAB
GOBYCAR
GRAYJAY
GRAYLAG
GREYLAG
HOLYDAY
HOLYMAN
HOLYWAR
INDYCAR
INKYCAP
JULYDAY
JURYMAN
KHAYYAM
LADYDAY
LADYNAS
LILYPAD
MANYEAR
MARYKAY
MIDYEAR
NAVYMAN
NEWYEAR
OFFYEAR
ONEYEAR
PERYEAR
PLAYSAT
SIXYEAR
STAYSAT
SWAYBAR
TAXYEAR
TENYEAR
THEYSAY
TWOYEAR
VERYBAD
VERYMAD
VERYSAD
XRAYLAB

•••Y••A
ASSYRIA
CRAYOLA
DESYLVA
GOBYSEA
ILLYRIA
PHRYGIA

••••YA•
AALIYAH
ALNIYAT
ANGRYAT
ARRAYAL
BABIYAR
FIFTYAD
FORTYAD
GIDDYAP
KHAYYAM
MALAYAN
MARRYAT
MEGRYAN
NARAYAN
PAPAYAS
PITAYAS
RUFIYAA
SAROYAN
SIXTYAD
UNLOYAL
VISAYAN

••••Y•A
KOPIYKA
PALMYRA
RUFIYAA
VOTEYEA
WOJTYLA

•••••YA
IHEARYA
MONTOYA
MTKENYA
OUGUIYA
SEQUOYA

Y•B••••
YOBBISH

Y••B•••
YASBECK
YOBBISH

Y•••B••
YEAHBUT

•YB••••
BYBIRTH
CYBORGS
DYBBUKS
HYBRIDS
MYBUDDY

•Y•B•••
BYEBYES
CYMBALS
DYBBUKS
DYEBATH
EYEBALL
EYEBANK
EYEBOLT
EYEBROW
GYMBAGS
GYMBALL
RYEBEER
SYMBOLS

•Y•••B•
BYANDBY
BYTHEBY
DYEJOBS
LYINGBY
SYLLABI
TYPEABS

•Y••••B
GYMCLUB
LYNDONB

••YB•••
ANYBODY
BOYBAND
BUYBACK
CRYBABY
DAYBEDS
DAYBOOK
DRYBULB
FLYBALL
FLYBOYS
HAYBALE
JAYBIRD
KEYBANK
LAYBACK
LAYBARE
MAYBESO
MUYBIEN
PAYBACK
RAYBANS
RAYBURN
ROYBEAN
RUYBLAS
SKYBLUE
SOYBEAN
SPYBOTS
TAYBACK
TOYBALL
TOYBIKE
TOYBOAT
TOYBOOK
WAYBACK
WAYBILL

••Y•B••
BUYABLE
DRYABLE
FLYABLE
FRYABLE
PAYABLE
ROYGBIV
SAYABLE
SAYSBOO
TOYNBEE

••Y••B•
CRYBABY
DAYJOBS
HEYRUBE

••Y•••B
DRYBULB
KEYCLUB
PAYSTUB

•••YB••
BABYBOP
BODYBAR
BUSYBEE
CITYBOY
COPYBOY
GOBYBUS
JURYBOX
LADYBUG
PLAYBOY
SWAYBAR
TINYBIT
VERYBAD
VERYBIG

•••Y•B•
PLAYSBY

•••Y••B
BODYRUB
EASYJOB
GOBYCAB
XRAYLAB

••••YB•
FIFTYBC
FORTYBC
GLORYBE
HUNNYBS
ITMAYBE
SIXTYBC

•••••YB
JOHNNYB

Y•C••••
YACHTED
YACHTER
YACHTIE
YUCAIPA
YUCATAN
YUCATEC
YUCKIER

Y•••C••
YESICAN

Y••••C•
YANNICK
YASBECK
YASHICA

Y•••••C
YOUNGMC
YUCATEC

•YC••••
BYCATCH
CYCLERS
CYCLING
CYCLIST
CYCLOID
CYCLONE
CYCLOPS
LYCEUMS
MYCENAE
MYCROFT
TYCOONS

•Y•C•••
EYECARE
EYECUPS
GYMCLUB
LYOCELL
PYNCHON
SYNCHED
SYNCING
SYNCOPE

•Y••C••
CYNICAL
GYROCAR
HYRACES
LYRICAL
LYRICON
TYPICAL
ZYDECOS

•Y•••C•
BYANECK
BYCATCH
BYFORCE
CYMRICS
EYETUCK
GYMSOCK
MYSPACE
MYSTICS
SYNDICS

•Y••••C
BYRONIC
DYNAMIC
HYGELAC
MYALGIC
MYRRHIC
NYMPHIC
PYRETIC
PYRITIC
PYRRHIC
SYLPHIC
SYNODIC

••YC•••
BAYCITY
BOYCOTT
DAYCAMP
DAYCARE
DRYCELL
FLYCAST
FRYCOOK
GLYCINE
GLYCOLS
JAYCEES
JOYCEAN
KEYCARD
KEYCASE
KEYCLUB
PAYCASH
PAYCUTS
PSYCHED
PSYCHES
PSYCHIC
PSYCHOS
PSYCHUP
ROYCOHN
SKYCAMS
SKYCAPS
SPYCAMS
TOYCARS
TOYCART
WAYCOOL

••Y••C•
ANYLUCK
BEYONCE
BUYBACK
DAYPACK
DRYDOCK
HAYRACK
HAYRICK
KEYLOCK
LAYBACK
PAYBACK
PHYSICS
SHYLOCK
SKYJACK
TAYBACK
WAYBACK

••Y•••C
ACYCLIC
CRYPTIC
DRYADIC
GLYPHIC
GLYPTIC
IDYLLIC
OLYMPIC
PSYCHIC
RAYKROC
RAYOVAC
STYPTIC

•••YC••
BICYCLE
CALYCES
COPYCAT
GOBYCAB
GOBYCAR
GREYCUP
HOLYCOW
INDYCAR
INKYCAP
RECYCLE

•••Y•C•
INSYNCH
PLAYACT
POLYSCI

•••Y••C
ACRYLIC
ENZYMIC
SATYRIC
SIBYLIC
UNLYRIC
VINYLIC

••••YC•
DIPTYCH
VANDYCK
VANEYCK
VANWYCK

••••Y•C
FIFTYBC
FORTYBC
LIPSYNC
SIXTYBC

Y•D••••
YIDDISH
YODELED
YODELER

Y••D•••
YARDAGE
YARDARM
YARDERS
YARDING
YARDMAN
YARDMEN
YESDEAR
YIDDISH

Y•••D••
YESIDID
YIELDED
YIELDER
YIELDTO

Y••••D•
YAOUNDE
YOLANDA
YOUANDI

Y•••••D
YACHTED
YEAREND
YEARNED
YEASTED
YESIDID
YIELDED
YODELED
YSHAPED

•YD••••
HYDRANT
HYDRATE
HYDRIDE
HYDROUS
LYDDITE
SYDHOFF
ZYDECOS

•Y•D•••
EYEDROP
LYDDITE
LYNDONB
PYEDOGS
SYNDICS
TYNDALL
WYNDHAM

•Y••D••
BYANDBY
DYNODES
HYPEDUP
HYUNDAI
KYOODLE
MYBUDDY
SYNODAL
SYNODIC
TYPEDIN
TYPEDUP

•Y•••D•
BYROADS
BYWORDS
CYANIDE
CYANIDS
EYELIDS
HYBRIDS
HYDRIDE
HYMNODY
MYBUDDY
MYRIADS

•Y••••D
AYKROYD
AYNRAND
BYLINED
CYCLOID
DYEWOOD
EYEFOLD
EYEHAND
GYRATED
HYALOID
HYPNOID
MYRRHED
MYWORLD
PYRAMID
SYNCHED
TYPHOID

••YD•••
BUYDOWN
COYDOGS
CRYDOWN
DRYDOCK
FEYDEAU
HEYDAYS
HOYDENS
KEYDETS
LAYDOWN
MAYDAYS
PAYDAYS
PAYDIRT
SKYDIVE
SKYDOME
SPYDERS
TOYDOGS
TOYDOLL

••Y•D••
BAYEDAT
DRYADES
DRYADIC
DRYIDEA
KEYEDIN
KEYEDON
KEYEDUP
LAYODDS

••Y••D•
ANYBODY
DAYBEDS
DAYSIDE
FLYRODS
HAYRIDE
HEYJUDE
HEYMRDJ
JOYPADS
JOYRIDE
KEYPADS
LAYODDS
SAYSIDO
SPYKIDS
WAYSIDE

••Y•••D
ANYKIND
ANYROAD
BOYBAND
BOYHOOD
DAYSEND
DRYEYED
GAYLORD
HAYSEED
HAYWARD
HEYWARD
HEYWOOD
ICYWIND
JAYBIRD
JAYWARD
KAYAKED
KEYCARD
KEYWORD
LAYERED
MAYNARD
NAYSAID
PAYHEED
PAYLOAD
PLYWOOD
PSYCHED
RAYMOND
REYNARD
REYNAUD
REYOKED
SCYTHED
SKYNYRD
SKYWARD
STYMIED
THYROID
TOYLAND
TOYSLED
TRYHARD
TRYSTED
UNYOKED
VOYAGED
WAYLAID
WAYLAND
WAYWARD

•••YD••
HOLYDAY
JOEYDEE
JULYDAY
KATYDID
LADYDAY
PLAYDOH
RUBYDEE
STAYDRY
TONYDOW
VERYDRY

•••Y•D•
VERYODD

•••Y••D
ALEYARD
BEEYARD
HALYARD
KATYDID
LANYARD
LILYPAD
ONEYARD
POLYPED
POLYPOD
RETYPED
RUBYRED
RUDYARD
UNGYVED
UNTYPED
VERYBAD
VERYMAD
VERYODD
VERYOLD
VERYRED
VERYSAD

••••YD•
HOWDYDO

••••Y•D
ALLAYED
ALLOYED
ANNOYED
ARRAYED
ASSAYED
BELAYED
BIGEYED
BOGEYED
BUGEYED
CATEYED
DECAYED
DECOYED
DELAYED
DOEEYED
DRYEYED
EMBAYED
ENJOYED
ESSAYED
FIFTYAD
FORAYED
FORTYAD
HONEYED
MONEYED
MOSEYED
ONEEYED
OWLEYED
PIEEYED
PIGEYED
POPEYED
REDEYED
REKEYED
RELAYED
SADEYED
SAMOYED
SIXTYAD
SKYNYRD
SPLAYED
SPRAYED
STRAYED
TIEDYED
UNGUYED
UNHAYED
UNJOYED
UNKEYED
UNRAYED
VATDYED
WETEYED

•••••YD
AYKROYD
SAMLOYD

YE•••••
YEAHBUT
YEAHMAN
YEAHYOU
YEANING
YEAREND
YEARNED
YEARNER
YEARNTO
YEARONE
YEASTED
YEATEAM
YELLERS
YELLFOR
YELLING
YELLOUT
YELLOWS
YELLOWY
YELLSAT
YELPERS
YELPING
YELTSIN
YEMENIS
YENNING
YENSFOR
YEOMANS
YEREVAN
YERKISH
YESDEAR
YESHIVA
YESICAN
YESIDID
YESISEE
YESITIS
YESLETS
YESMAAM
YESORNO
YESSING
YESSIRE
YESVOTE
YETTIES
YEVGENY
YEWTREE

Y•E••••
YIELDED
YIELDER
YIELDTO
YZERMAN

Y••E•••
YALELAW
YALEMAN
YALEMEN
YEMENIS
YEREVAN
YODELED
YODELER
YOTEAMO
YULELOG

Y•••E••
YAKKERS
YAMMERS
YANKEES
YANKERS
YAPPERS
YARDERS
YARNELL
YASBECK
YATTERS
YAWNERS
YAWPERS
YAYTEAM
YEAREND
YEATEAM
YELLERS
YELPERS
YESDEAR
YESLETS
YEVGENY
YONKERS
YORKERS
YOTHERS
YOUREIT
YOUREON
YOWLERS

Y••••E•
YACHTED
YACHTER
YAHTZEE
YALEMEN
YANKEES
YARDMEN
YAWNIER
YEARNED
YEARNER
YEASTED
YESISEE
YETTIES
YEWTREE
YIELDED
YIELDER
YIPPIES
YODELED
YODELER
YORKIES
YOUNGER
YOUTHEN
YSHAPED
YSHAPES
YUCATEC
YUCKIER
YUMMIER
YUPPIES

Y•••••E
YACHTIE
YAHTZEE
YANGTZE
YAOUNDE
YARDAGE
YASMINE
YEARONE
YESISEE
YESSIRE
YESVOTE
YEWTREE
YOULOSE

•YE••••
AYEAYES
BYEBYES
DYEBATH
DYEJOBS
DYELOTS
DYEVATS
DYEWOOD
EYEBALL
EYEBANK
EYEBOLT
EYEBROW
EYECARE
EYECUPS
EYEDROP
EYEEXAM
EYEFOLD
EYEFULS
EYEHAND
EYEHOLE
EYEHOOK
EYELASH
EYELESS
EYELETS
EYELIDS
EYELIFT
EYELIKE
EYELINE
EYEMASK
EYEPITS
EYEROLL
EYESHOT
EYESORE
EYESPOT
EYETEST
EYETUCK
EYEWALL
EYEWASH
EYEWEAR
EYEWINK
LYESOAP
MYERSON
PYEDOGS
RYEBEER
RYELOAF

•Y•E•••
BYHEART
EYEEXAM
GYRENES
HYGELAC
HYPEDUP
HYPERON
HYPESUP
LYCEUMS
LYNETTE
LYSENKO
MYCENAE
PYRETIC
PYREXIA
SYNERGY
TYLENOL
TYPEABS
TYPEDIN
TYPEDUP
TYPESET
TYPESIN
TYPESUP
WYNETTE
WYVERNS
ZYDECOS

•Y••E••
BYANECK
BYTHEBY
CYCLERS
CYGNETS
CYPHERS
CYPRESS
EYELESS
EYELETS
EYETEST
EYEWEAR
GYPPERS
HYGIEIA
HYGIENE
HYPHENS
LYOCELL
LYONELL
MYNHEER
MYSTERY
MYTREAT
OYSTERS
RYEBEER
SYSTEMS
XYSTERS

•Y•••E•
AYEAYES
BYEBYES
BYFIVES
BYGONES
BYLINED
BYLINER
BYLINES
BYNAMES
DYNODES
GYPSIES
GYRATED
GYRATES
GYRENES
HYRACES
HYRAXES
MYNHEER
MYRRHED
MYRTLES
NYTIMES
PYGMIES
PYRITES
RYEBEER
SYNCHED
SYNFUEL
TYPESET
XYLOSES
ZYGOTES

•Y••••E
BYAMILE
BYANOSE
BYFORCE
BYPHONE
CYANIDE
CYCLONE
EYECARE
EYEHOLE
EYELIKE
EYELINE
EYESORE
GYMSHOE
HYALITE
HYDRATE
HYDRIDE
HYGIENE
KYOODLE
LYDDITE
LYNETTE
MYCENAE
MYSPACE
SYNAPSE
SYNCOPE
SYRINGE
SYSTOLE
WYNETTE

••YE•••
BAYEDAT
CAYENNE
DOYENNE
DRYEYED
DRYEYES
FAYETTE
HAYESES
INYEARS
KEYEDIN
KEYEDON
KEYEDUP
LAYERED
LAYETTE
WBYEATS
WHYEVER

••Y•E••
ANYNEWS
BAYLEAF
COYNESS
DAYBEDS
DAYSEND
DAYWEAR
DRYCELL
DRYHEAT
DRYNESS
DRYPERS
DRYWELL
ELYSEES
FEYDEAU
FEYNESS
FLYLEAF
FLYLESS
FLYNETS
GAYNESS
GEYSERS
GWYNETH
HAYSEED
HOYDENS
HUYGENS
JAYCEES
JAYLENO
JAYVEES
JOYCEAN
JOYLESS
KAYLENZ
KEYDETS
KEYLESS
KEYWEST
MAYBESO
MAYHEMS
MEYNELL
PAYHEED
PAYLESS
PAYMENT
PAYWELL
RAYLESS
RAYNELL
RHYMERS
ROYBEAN
SHYNESS
SKYLESS
SLYNESS
SOYBEAN
SOYLENT
SOYMEAL
SPYDERS
STYLERS
STYLETS
STYRENE
THYSELF
TOYLESS
WAYLESS
WRYNESS
YAYTEAM

••Y••E•
ABYSSES
ANYONES
BAYAREA
BAYONET
BAYTREE
BLYNKEN
BRYNNER
CAYUSES
COYOTES
CRYOGEN
CRYOVER
DRYADES
DRYEYED
DRYEYES
DRYIDEA
ELYSEES
FLYOPEN
FLYOVER
FLYTIER
HAYESES
HAYSEED
JAYCEES
JAYVEES
KAYAKED
KAYAKER
LAYERED
LAYOPEN
LAYOVER
LOYALER
LOYALES
MUYBIEN
ODYSSEY
PAYHEED
PEYOTES
PRYOPEN
PSYCHED
PSYCHES
REYOKED
REYOKES
ROYALES
SAYAMEN
SAYOVER
SAYSYES
SAYWHEN
SCYTHED
SCYTHES
SHYSTER
STYMIED
STYMIES
TOYNBEE
TOYSLED
TRYSTED
TRYSTER
ULYSSES
UNYOKED
UNYOKES
VOYAGED
VOYAGER
VOYAGES
WHYEVER

••Y•••E
AMYLASE
ANYHOPE
ANYMORE
ANYTIME
ANYWISE
BAYONNE
BAYTREE
BEYONCE
BOYLIKE
BUYABLE
BUYTIME
CAYENNE
DAYCARE
DAYGAME
DAYMARE
DAYSIDE
DAYTIME
DOYENNE
DRYABLE
DRYHOLE
FAYETTE
FLYABLE
FRYABLE
GLYCINE
GUYROPE
HAYBALE
HAYRIDE
HAYWIRE
HEYJUDE
HEYRUBE
IVYLIKE
JOYRIDE
KEYCASE
KEYHOLE
KEYLIME
KEYNOTE
KRYSTLE
LAYBARE
LAYETTE
MAYPOLE
MAYTIME
MAYWINE
PAYABLE
PAYMORE
PAYRATE
RAYLIKE
ROYALWE
SAYABLE
SAYMORE
SAYSAYE
SKYBLUE
SKYDIVE
SKYDOME
SKYLIKE
SKYLINE
SPYHOLE
SPYWARE
STYLISE
STYLIZE
STYRENE
THYMINE
TOYBIKE
TOYKITE
TOYLIKE
TOYNBEE
WAYSIDE

•••YE••
BOWYERS
BRAYERS
BREYERS
CORYELL
EBAYERS
FLAYERS
FTMYERS
GRAYEST
GREYEST
GRUYERE
LAWYERS
MANYEAR
MIDYEAR
NCWYETH
NEWYEAR
OBEYERS
OFFYEAR
ONEYEAR
OUTYELL
OUTYELP
PERYEAR
PLAYERS
PRAYERS
PREYERS
SAWYERS
SIXYEAR
SLAYERS
SPAYERS
SPRYEST
STAYERS
SWAYERS
TAXYEAR
TENYEAR
TWOYEAR

•••Y•E•
ARGYLES
ATTYGEN
BOGYMEN
BUSYBEE
CALYCES
CALYXES
CLAYIER
COPYMEN
DRAYMEN
ECDYSES
ECTYPES
ENZYMES
GOBYSEA
GREYHEN
HOLYMEN
HOLYSEE
JOEYDEE
JURYMEN
NAVYMEN
OOCYTES
PLAYLET
PLAYPEN
PLAYTEX
POLYMER
POLYPED
PONYKEG
RETYPED
RETYPES
RUBYDEE
RUBYRED
UNGYVED
UNTYPED
VERYFEW
VERYNEW
VERYRED
VERYWET

•••Y••E
ALCYONE
BICYCLE
BUSYBEE
GHAYOTE
DRAYAGE
EASYONE
ELIYALE
GRUYERE
HOLYJOE
HOLYOKE
HOLYONE
HOLYSEE
JOEYDEE
MARYURE
QUAYAGE
RECYCLE
RUBYDEE

••••YE•
ALLAYED
ALLAYER
ALLEYES
ALLOYED
ANNOYED
ANNOYER
ARRAYED
ARRAYER
ASSAYED
ASSAYER
AYEAYES
AZODYES
BELAYED
BELAYER
BIGEYED
BIGEYES
BOGEYED
BONEYER
BUGEYED
BYEBYES
CATEYED
COBUYER
COLLYER
DAIRYER
DECAYED
DECAYER
DECOYED
DECOYER
DELAYED
DELAYER
DOEEYED
DRYEYED
DRYEYES
EMBAYED
ENJOYED
ENJOYER
ERINYES
ESSAYED
ESSAYER
FADAYEV
FORAYED
GEMAYEL
HECKYES
HELLYES
HONEYED
INLAYER
KATAYEV
LOBBYER
MONEYED
MOSEYED
NUREYEV
ONEEYED
OWLEYED
PARTYER
PIEEYED
PIGEYED
POPEYED
POPEYES
RALLYES
REDDYES
REDEYED
REDEYES
REKEYED
RELAYED
RELAYER
RIBEYES
RITDYES
SADEYED
SADEYES
SAMOYED
SAYSYES
SCHAYES
SPLAYED
SPRAYED
SPRAYER
STRAYED
STRAYER
TIEDYED
TIEDYES
UNCOYER
UNGUYED
UNHAYED
UNJOYED
UNKEYED
UNRAYED
UNSHYER
UNSLYER
VATDYED
VATDYES
VOTEYEA
VOTEYES
WELLYES
WETEYED

••••Y•E
ACOLYTE
ANALYSE
ANALYTE
ANALYZE
ANODYNE
BIOTYPE
CAMRYLE
CARLYLE
DENTYNE
ECOTYPE
EXABYTE
FORSYTE
FTWAYNE
GENZYME
GLORYBE
INSTYLE
ITMAYBE
LEMOYNE
MARRYME
MISTYPE
NEOLYTE
OLDLYME
ONEBYTE
PRETYPE
RESTYLE
SETTYPE
SILLYME
SUBTYPE
TINTYPE
UNRHYME
VANDYKE

•••••YE
BILLNYE
BUCKEYE
CATSEYE
DEADEYE
EVILEYE
FISHEYE
GLADEYE
GOODBYE
HAIRDYE
HANDEYE
HAWKEYE
LEFTEYE
MOONEYE
OVERDYE
SAIDAYE
SAYSAYE
SHUTEYE
SOCKEYE
VOTEAYE
WALLEYE

Y•••F••
YAWNFUL
YELLFOR
YENSFOR

Y••••F•
YANKOFF
YUPPIFY

Y•••••F
YANKOFF

•YF••••
BYFIVES
BYFORCE
BYFORMS
MYFAULT

•Y•F•••
EYEFOLD
EYEFULS
SYNFUEL

•Y•••F•
EYELIFT
MYCROFT
MYSTIFY
MYTHIFY
SYDHOFF

•Y••••F
BYWAYOF
RYELOAF
SYDHOFF

••YF•••
DRYFOGS
FLYFISH
HAYFORK
MAYFAIR
SHYFROM
TOYFAIR

••Y•F••
BUYOFFS
LAYOFFS
LAYSFOR
PAYOFFS
PAYSFOR

••Y••F•
BUYOFFS
BUYSOFF
DAYSOFF
HAYLOFT
LAYOFFS
LAYSOFF
PAYOFFS
PAYSOFF

••Y•••F
BAYLEAF
BUYSOFF
CRYWOLF
DAYSOFF
FLYLEAF
LAYSOFF
PAYSOFF
SKYSURF
THYSELF

•••YF••
BODYFAT
DREYFUS
PLAYFUL
PRAYFOR
STAYFOR
TRAYFUL
VERYFEW
VERYFIT

•••Y•F•
EASYOFF
PLAYOFF
STAYOFF

•••Y••F
EASYOFF
PLAYOFF
STAYOFF

••••Y•F
BYWAYOF
DARRYLF

Y•G••••
YOGAMAT
YOGHURT
YOGIISM
YOGINIS
YOGURTS

Y••G•••
YANGTZE
YEVGENY

Y•••G••
YOUNGER
YOUNGMC
YOUNGUN

Y••••G•
YARDAGE

Y•••••G
YAKKING
YANKING
YAOMING
YAPPING
YARDING
YARNING
YAWNING
YAWPING
YEANING
YELLING
YELPING
YENNING
YESSING
YIPPING
YOURANG
YOWLING
YOYOING
YUKKING
YULELOG

•YG••••
BYGOLLY
BYGONES
CYGNETS
HYGELAC
HYGIEIA
HYGIENE
HYGINUS
MYGIANT
NYGIANT
PYGMIES
ZYGOTES

•Y•G•••
SYNGMAN

•Y••G••
BYRIGHT
LYINGBY
LYINGON
LYINGTO
LYINGUP
MYALGIA
MYALGIC
TYINGIN
TYINGON
TYINGTO
TYINGUP

•Y•••G•
BYJINGO
CYBORGS
GYMBAGS
MYOLOGY
PYEDOGS
SYNERGY
SYRINGE
ZYMURGY

•Y••••G
CYCLING
CYYOUNG
GYPPING
HYMNING
HYPOING
SYNCING
WYOMING
WYSIWYG

••YG•••
DAYGAME
FLYGIRL
HUYGENS
KEYGRIP
RAYGUNS
ROYGBIV
STYGIAN
TOYGUNS

••Y•G••
CAYUGAS
CRYOGEN
ERYNGOS
VOYAGED
VOYAGER
VOYAGES

••Y••G•
COYDOGS
DRYFOGS
FLYHIGH
HAYINGS
IFYOUGO
MAYINGS
MAYTAGS
SAYINGS
SKYHIGH
SPYINGS
TOYDOGS
WAYTOGO

••Y•••G
CYYOUNG
DAYLONG
DEYOUNG
KAYOING
KEYRING
RHYMING
SPYRING
STYLING
UNYOUNG
YOYOING

•••YG••
ATTYGEN
BABYGAP
CITYGAL
KOSYGIN
OKAYGUY
PHRYGIA
POLYGON

•••Y•G•
ADAYAGO
DRAYAGE
QUAYAGE

•••Y••G
ALAYING
ALLYING
BABYING
BELYING
BRAYING
BUOYING
BURYING
BUSYING
CLAYING
CLOYING
COPYING
COSYING
COZYING
DEFYING
DENYING
DRAYING
EDDYING
ENVYING
ESPYING
FLAYING
FRAYING
FREYTAG
GRAYING
GRAYLAG
GREYING
GREYLAG
INLYING
JURYING
JURYRIG
LADYBUG
LEVYING
OBEYING
OKAYING
PITYING
PLAYING
PONYING
PONYKEG
PRAYING

PREYING
REDYING
REFYING
RELYING
SLAYING
SPAYING
STAYING
SWAYING
TIDYING
UNDYING
UNLYING
UNTYING
UNVYING
VARYING
VERYBIG
WIFYING
XRAYING

•••••YG
WYSIWYG

Y•H••••
YAHTZEE
YSHAPED
YSHAPES

Y••H•••
YACHTED
YACHTER
YACHTIE
YASHICA
YASHMAK
YEAHBUT
YEAHMAN
YEAHYOU
YESHIVA
YOGHURT
YOOHOOS
YOTHERS

Y•••H••
YAMAHAS
YITZHAK
YOUTHEN

Y•••••H
YERKISH
YIDDISH
YOBBISH
YOUWISH

•YH••••
BYHEART

•Y•H•••
BYAHAIR
BYPHONE
BYTHEBY
CYPHERS
EYEHAND
EYEHOLE
EYEHOOK
HYPHENS
MYNHEER
MYTHIFY
PYTHIAN
PYTHIAS
PYTHONS
SYDHOFF
TYPHOID
TYPHOON

•Y••H••
CYNTHIA
EYESHOT
GYMSHOE
MYRRHED
MYRRHIC
NYMPHAL
NYMPHIC
PYNCHON
PYRRHIC
PYRRHUS
SYLPHIC
SYNCHED
WYNDHAM

•Y•••H•
BYPATHS
BYRIGHT

•Y••••H
BYBIRTH
BYCATCH
BYMOUTH
DYEBATH
EYELASH
EYEWASH

••YH•••
ANYHOPE
BOYHOOD
DAYHOPS
DRYHEAT
DRYHOLE
FLYHIGH
KEYHOLE
MAYHEMS
PAYHEED
SAYHITO
SKYHIGH
SKYHOOK
SPYHOLE
TOYHATS
TOYHOOP
TRYHARD

••Y•H••
ALYKHAN
ERYTHRO
GLYPHIC
GRYPHON
PSYCHED
PSYCHES
PSYCHIC
PSYCHOS
PSYCHUP
RHYTHMS
SAYWHAT
SAYWHEN
SCYTHED
SCYTHES
TOYSHOP

••Y••H•
ALYOSHA
ROYCOHN
SAYSWHO

••Y•••H
DRYWASH
FLYFISH
FLYHIGH
GWYNETH
PAYCASH
SAYSAAH
SKYHIGH
STYLISH
TOYWITH

•••YH••
GREYHEN
VERYHIP
VERYHOT

•••Y•H•
ALIYAHS
VERYSHY

•••Y••H
BABYISH
CLAYISH
FOGYISH
GRAYISH
GREYISH
INSYNCH
LADYISH
LAZYISH
NCWYETH
PIXYISH
PLAYDOH
TORYISH
WHEYISH
ZANYISH

••••YH•
TALLYHO

••••Y•H
AALIYAH
DIPTYCH
FORSYTH

YI•••••
YIDDISH
YIELDED
YIELDER
YIELDTO
YIPPIES
YIPPING
YITZHAK

Y••I•••
YAKIMAS
YESICAN
YESIDID
YESISEE
YESITIS
YOGIISM
YOGINIS

Y•••I••
YAKKING
YANKING
YANNICK
YAOMING
YAPPING
YARDING
YARNING
YASHICA
YASMINE
YAWNIER
YAWNING
YAWPING
YEANING
YELLING
YELPING
YENNING
YERKISH
YESHIVA
YESSING
YESSIRE
YETTIES
YIDDISH
YIPPIES
YIPPING
YOBBISH
YOGIISM
YORKIES
YORKIST
YOUWISH
YOWLING
YOYOING
YTTRIAS
YTTRIUM
YUCAIPA
YUCKIER
YUKKING
YUMMIER
YUPPIES
YUPPIFY

Y••••I•
YACHTIE
YANQUIS
YELTSIN
YEMENIS
YESIDID
YESITIS
YOGINIS
YOPLAIT
YOUREIT
YUKOLIS

Y•••••I
YOUANDI

•YI••••
LYINGBY
LYINGON
LYINGTO
LYINGUP
TYINGIN
TYINGON
TYINGTO
TYINGUP

•Y•I•••
BYBIRTH
BYFIVES
BYJINGO
BYLINED
BYLINER
BYLINES
BYRIGHT
CYNICAL
HYGIEIA
HYGIENE
HYGINUS
LYRICAL
LYRICON
LYRISTS
MYGIANT
MYRIADS
NYGIANT
NYTIMES
PYRITES
PYRITIC
SYRIANA
SYRIANS
SYRINGE
TYPICAL
TYPISTS
WYSIWYG

•Y••I••
BYAMILE
CYANIDE
CYANIDS
CYCLING
CYCLIST
CYMRICS
CYPRIAN
CYPRIOT
EYELIDS
EYELIFT
EYELIKE
EYELINE
EYEPITS
EYEWINK
GYPPING
GYPSIES
HYALITE
HYBRIDS
HYDRIDE
HYMNING
HYPOING
LYDDITE
MYOPIAS
MYSTICS
MYSTIFY
MYTHIFY
PYGMIES
PYTHIAN
PYTHIAS
SYNCING
SYNDICS
WYOMING

•Y•••I•
BYAHAIR
BYRONIC
BYTRAIN
CYCLOID
CYNTHIA
CYRUSII
DYNAMIC
GYMSUIT
HYALOID
HYANNIS
HYGIEIA
HYPATIA
HYPNOID
MYALGIA
MYALGIC
MYRRHIC
NYMPHIC
PYRAMID
PYRETIC
PYREXIA
PYRITIC
PYRRHIC
SYLPHIC
SYNODIC
TYINGIN
TYPEDIN
TYPESIN
TYPHOID

•Y••••I
CYRUSII
HYUNDAI
SYLLABI
TYMPANI
XYSTUSI

••YI•••
BUYINTO
DRYIDEA
FLYINTO
HAYINGS
KEYINON
LAYINTO
LAYITON
MAYINGS
PAYINTO
PRYINTO
SAYINGS
SOYINKA
SOYINKS
SPYINGS
TRYITON
WHYISIT

••Y•I••
ANYKIND
ANYTIME
ANYWISE
BAYCITY
BOYLIKE
BUYTIME
DAYLILY
DAYSIDE
DAYSINN
DAYTIME
ELYSIAN
ELYSIUM
FLYFISH
FLYGIRL
FLYHIGH
FLYTIER
GLYCINE
HAYRICK
HAYRIDE
HAYWIRE
ICYWIND
IDYLIST
IVYLIKE
JAYBIRD
JOYRIDE
KAYOING
KEYLIME
KEYRING
MAYTIME
MAYWINE
MUYBIEN
PAYDIRT
PHYSICS
RAYLIKE
RHYMING
RHYMIST
SAYHITO
SAYSIDO
SKYDIVE
SKYHIGH
SKYLIKE
SKYLINE
SOYMILK
SPYKIDS
SPYRING
STYGIAN
STYLING
STYLISE
STYLISH
STYLIST
STYLIZE
STYMIED
STYMIES
THYMINE
TOYBIKE
TOYKITE
TOYLIKE
TOYWITH
WAYBILL
WAYSIDE
YOYOING
ZOYSIAS

••Y••I•
ACYCLIC
CRYPTIC
DAYQUIL
DAYSAIL
DAYTRIP
DRYADIC
DRYSUIT
GLYNNIS
GLYPHIC
GLYPTIC
HRYVNIA
IDYLLIC
KEYEDIN
KEYGRIP
MAYALIN
MAYFAIR
NAYARIT
NAYSAID
OLYMPIA
OLYMPIC
PAYSLIP
PHYLLIS
PSYCHIC
ROYGBIV
SAYWAIT
STYPSIS
STYPTIC
THYROID
TOYFAIR
TOYPAIL
TRYSAIL
WAYLAID
WHYISIT
WHYWAIT

•••YI••
ALAYING
ALLYING
BABYING
BABYISH
BELYING
BRAYING
BUOYING
BURYING
BUSYING
CLAYIER
CLAYING
CLAYISH
CLOYING
COPYING
COPYIST
COSYING
COZYING
DEFYING
DENYING
DRAYING
EDDYING
ENVYING
ESPYING
FLAYING
FOGYISH
FOGYISM
FRAYING
GRAYING
GRAYISH
GREYING
GREYISH
INLYING
JURYING
LADYISH
LAZYISH
LEVYING
OBEYING
OKAYING
PITYING
PIXYISH
PLAYING
PONYING
PRAYING
PREYING
REDYING
REFYING
RELYING
SLAYING
SPAYING
STAYING
SWAYING
THEYIPS
TIDYING
TORYISH
TORYISM
UNDYING
UNLYING
UNTYING
UNVYING
VARYING
VERYILL
WHEYISH
WIFYING
XRAYING
ZANYISH
ZANYISM

•••Y•I•
ACRYLIC
ASSYRIA
BABYOIL
BABYSIT
BODYKIT
CLAYPIT
ECDYSIS
ENZYMIC
GOBYAIR
HOLYOIL
ILLYRIA
JURYRIG
KATYDID
KOSYGIN
LADYKIN
LUCYLIU
PHRYGIA
SATYRIC
SIBYLIC
STAYSIN
TINYBIT
TINYTIM
UNLYRIC
VERYBIG
VERYFIT
VERYHIP
VINYLIC

•••Y••I
BIRYANI
POLYSCI

••••YI•
CARRYIN
HENRYII
HENRYIV
LCHAYIM
MARRYIN
ROCKYII
ROCKYIV

••••Y•I
HENRYII
HENRYVI
PLATYPI
ROCKYII

•••••YI
KAROLYI
POLANYI

•YJ••••
BYJINGO

•Y•J•••
DYEJOBS

••YJ•••
DAYJOBS
HEYJUDE
SKYJACK

••Y•••J
HEYMRDJ

•••YJ••
EASYJOB
GRAYJAY
HOLYJOE

••••YJ•
SAMMYJO

Y•K••••
YAKIMAS
YAKKERS
YAKKING
YAKUTSK
YOKOONO
YUKATAS
YUKKING
YUKOLIS

Y••K•••
YAKKERS
YAKKING
YANKEES
YANKERS
YANKING
YANKOFF
YANKOUT
YANKSAT
YANKSON
YANKTON
YERKISH
YONKERS
YORKERS
YORKIES
YORKIST
YORKTON
YOUKNOW
YUCKIER
YUKKING

Y•••••K
YAKUTSK
YANNICK
YASBECK
YASHMAK
YITZHAK

•YK••••
AYKROYD
DYKSTRA
MYKONOS

•Y•K•••
RYOKANS
RYUKYUS

•Y•••K•
BYTALKS
DYBBUKS
EYELIKE
LYSENKO
NYYANKS

•Y••••K
BYANECK
EYEBANK
EYEHOOK
EYEMASK
EYETUCK
EYEWINK
GYMSOCK

••YK•••
ALYKHAN
ANYKIND
RAYKROC
SPYKIDS
TOYKITE

••Y•K••
BLYNKEN
KAYAKED
KAYAKER
REYOKED
REYOKES
UNYOKED
UNYOKES

••Y••K•
BOYLIKE
EXYANKS
IVYLIKE
NYYANKS
RAYLIKE
SKYLIKE
SOYINKA
SOYINKS
TOYBIKE
TOYLIKE

••Y•••K
ANYLUCK
BUYBACK
DAYBOOK
DAYPACK
DMYTRYK
DRYDOCK
FRYCOOK
HAYFORK
HAYRACK
HAYRICK
HEYLOOK
JAYWALK
KEYBANK
KEYLOCK
LAYBACK
PAYBACK
SHYLOCK
SKYHOOK
SKYJACK
SKYLARK
SKYWALK
SLYLOOK
SOYMILK
SZYSLAK
TAYBACK
TOYBOOK
WAYBACK

•••YK••
BODYKIT
LADYKIN
MARYKAY
PONYKEG

•••Y•K•
HOLYOKE

•••Y••K
HOLYARK
NEWYORK

••••YK•
DANEYKO
GROMYKO
KOPIYKA
VANDYKE

••••Y•K
VANDYCK
VANEYCK
VANWYCK

•••••YK
DMYTRYK
MASARYK

Y•L••••
YALELAW
YALEMAN
YALEMEN
YELLERS
YELLFOR
YELLING
YELLOUT
YELLOWS
YELLOWY
YELLSAT
YELPERS
YELPING
YELTSIN
YOLANDA
YULELOG

Y••L•••
YELLERS
YELLFOR
YELLING
YELLOUT
YELLOWS
YELLOWY
YELLSAT
YESLETS
YIELDED
YIELDER
YIELDTO
YOPLAIT
YOULOSE
YOWLERS
YOWLING

Y•••L••
YALELAW
YODELED
YODELER
YUKOLIS
YULELOG

Y••••L•
YARNELL

Y•••••L
YARNELL
YAWNFUL

•YL••••
BYLINED
BYLINER
BYLINES
MYLANTA
SYLLABI
SYLPHIC
TYLENOL
XYLOSES

•Y•L•••
BYPLAYS
CYCLERS
CYCLING
CYCLIST
CYCLOID
CYCLONE
CYCLOPS
DYELOTS
EYELASH
EYELESS
EYELETS
EYELIDS
EYELIFT
EYELIKE
EYELINE
HYALITE
HYALOID
MYALGIA
MYALGIC
MYOLOGY
RYELOAF
SYLLABI

•Y••L••
BYGOLLY
BYTALKS
GYMCLUB
GYRALLY
HYGELAC
MYRTLES

•Y•••L•
BYAMILE
BYGOLLY
CYMBALS
EYEBALL
EYEBOLT
EYEFOLD
EYEFULS
EYEHOLE
EYEROLL
EYEWALL
GYMBALL
GYRALLY
HYMNALS
KYOODLE
LYOCELL
LYONELL
MYFAULT
MYWORLD

SYMBOLS
SYSTOLE
TYNDALL

•Y••••L
CYNICAL
EYEBALL
EYEROLL
EYEWALL
GYMBALL
LYOCELL
LYONELL
LYRICAL
NYMPHAL
SYNFUEL
SYNODAL
TYLENOL
TYNDALL
TYPICAL

••YL•••
AMYLASE
ANYLUCK
ASYLUMS
BAYLEAF
BAYLORU
BAYLYNX
BOYLIKE
DAYLILY
DAYLONG
FLYLEAF
FLYLESS
GAYLORD
HAYLOFT
HEYLOOK
IDYLIST
IDYLLIC
IVYLIKE
JAYLENO
JOYLESS
KAYLENZ
KEYLESS
KEYLIME
KEYLOCK
PAYLESS
PAYLOAD
PHYLLIS
PHYLLOS
RAYLESS
RAYLIKE
SHYLOCK
SKYLARK
SKYLESS
SKYLIKE
SKYLINE
SLYLOOK
SOYLENT
STYLERS
STYLETS
STYLING
STYLISE
STYLISH
STYLIST
STYLIZE
TAYLORS
TOYLAND
TOYLESS
TOYLIKE

WAYLAID
WAYLAND
WAYLAYS
WAYLESS

••Y•L••
ACYCLIC
IDYLLIC
KEYCLUB
LAYSLOW
LOYALER
LOYALES
LOYALLY
LOYALTO
LOYALTY
LOYOLAU
MAYALIN
PAYOLAS
PAYSLIP
PHYLLIS
PHYLLOS
ROYALES
ROYALLY
ROYALTY
ROYALWE
RUYBLAS
SKYBLUE
SZYSLAK
TOYSLED

••Y••L•
BUYABLE
CRYWOLF
DAYLILY
DRYABLE
DRYBULB
DRYCELL
DRYHOLE
DRYWALL
DRYWELL
FLYABLE
FLYBALL
FLYSOLO
FRYABLE
GLYCOLS
HAYBALE
JAYWALK
KEYHOLE
KEYPALS
KRYSTLE
LOYALLY
MAYPOLE
MEYNELL
PAYABLE
PAYROLL
PAYWELL
RAYNELL
ROYALLY
SAYABLE
SKYWALK
SOYMILK
SPYHOLE
THYSELF
TOYBALL
TOYDOLL
WAYBILL

••Y•••L
ABYSMAL
ABYSSAL
CRYSTAL
DAYQUIL
DAYSAIL
DRYCELL
DRYWALL
DRYWELL
FLYBALL
FLYGIRL
MAYORAL
MEYNELL
PAYROLL
PAYWELL
RAYNELL
SOYMEAL
TOYBALL
TOYDOLL
TOYPAIL
TRYSAIL
WAYBILL
WAYCOOL

•••YL••
ACRYLIC
ARGYLES
BABYLON
DESYLVA
EMMYLOU
GRAYLAG
GREYLAG
LUCYLIU
MARYLOU
PLAYLET
SIBYLIC
VERYLOW
VINYLIC
XRAYLAB

•••Y•L•
BICYCLE
CORYELL
CRAYOLA
ELIYALE
OUTYELL
OUTYELP
RECYCLE
VERYILL
VERYOLD

•••Y••L
BABYOIL
CITYGAL
CORYELL
ECTYPAL
HOLYOIL
OUTYELL
PLAYFUL
TRAYFUL
VERYILL

••••YL•
CAMRYLE
CARLYLE
DACTYLS
DARRYLF
INSTYLE

RESTYLE
UNCOYLY
UNSHYLY
UNSLYLY
WOJTYLA

••••Y•L
ARRAYAL
GEMAYEL
UNLOYAL

Y•M••••
YAMAHAS
YAMMERS
YEMENIS
YOMTOVS
YUMMIER

Y••M•••
YAMMERS
YAOMING
YASMINE
YEOMANS
YESMAAM
YOUMANS
YUMMIER

Y•••M••
YAKIMAS
YALEMAN
YALEMEN
YARDMAN
YARDMEN
YASHMAK
YEAHMAN
YOGAMAT
YZERMAN

Y••••M•
YOTEAMO
YOUNGMC

Y•••••M
YARDARM
YAYTEAM
YEATEAM
YESMAAM
YOGIISM
YTTRIUM

•YM••••
BYMOUTH
CYMBALS
CYMRICS
GYMBAGS
GYMBALL
GYMCLUB
GYMNAST
GYMRATS
GYMSHOE
GYMSOCK
GYMSUIT
HYMNALS
HYMNARY
HYMNING
HYMNODY
MYMAMMY
NYMPHAL

NYMPHIC
SYMBOLS
SYMPTOM
TYMPANA
TYMPANI
ZYMURGY

•Y•M•••
BYAMILE
EYEMASK
PYGMIES
WYOMING

•Y••M••
BYNAMES
DYNAMIC
DYNAMOS
MYANMAR
MYMAMMY
NYTIMES
PYRAMID
PYRAMUS
SYNGMAN

•Y•••M•
BYFORMS
GYPSUMS
LYCEUMS
MYMAMMY
SYSTEMS

•Y••••M
EYEEXAM
HYPONYM
SYMPTOM
SYNONYM
WYNDHAM

••YM•••
ANYMORE
CAYMANS
DAYMARE
DRYMOPS
ETYMONS
HAYMOWS
HEYMANS
HEYMRDJ
OLYMPIA
OLYMPIC
OLYMPUS
OXYMORA
PAYMENT
PAYMORE
RAYMOND
REYMONT
RHYMERS
RHYMING
RHYMIST
SAYMASS
SAYMORE
SEYMOUR
SKYMAPS
SOYMEAL
SOYMILK
STYMIED
STYMIES
THYMINE

••Y•M••
ABYSMAL
FEYNMAN
SAYAMEN

••Y••M•
ANYTIME
ASYLUMS
BAYRUMS
BUYTIME
DAYCAMP
DAYGAME
DAYTIME
KEYLIME
MAYHEMS
MAYTIME
RHYTHMS
SKYCAMS
SKYDOME
SPYCAMS

••Y•••M
ALYSSUM
DAYROOM
ELYSIUM
SHYFROM
YAYTEAM

•••YM••
BOGYMAN
BOGYMEN
COPYMAN
COPYMEN
DRAYMAN
DRAYMEN
ELLYMAY
ENZYMES
ENZYMIC
HOLYMAN
HOLYMEN
JURYMAN
JURYMEN
NAVYMAN
NAVYMEN
POLYMER
VERYMAD

•••Y••M
FOGYISM
KHAYYAM
TIDYSUM
TINYTIM
TORYISM
ZANYISM

••••YM•
ANONYMS
EPONYMS
EPONYMY
EUONYMS
EXONYMS
GENZYME
MARRYME
OLDLYME
SILLYME
UNRHYME

••••Y•M
KHAYYAM
LCHAYIM

•••••YM
ACRONYM
ALLONYM
ANTONYM
AUTONYM
CACONYM
DEMONYM
HOMONYM
HYPONYM
PARONYM
SYNONYM
TOPONYM

Y•N••••
YANGTZE
YANKEES
YANKERS
YANKING
YANKOFF
YANKOUT
YANKSAT
YANKSON
YANKTON
YANNICK
YANQUIS
YENNING
YENSFOR
YONKERS

Y••N•••
YANNICK
YARNELL
YARNING
YAWNERS
YAWNFUL
YAWNIER
YAWNING
YEANING
YENNING
YOUNGER
YOUNGMC
YOUNGUN

Y•••N••
YAOUNDE
YEARNED
YEARNER
YEARNTO
YEMENIS
YOGINIS
YOLANDA
YOUANDI
YOUKNOW

Y••••N•
YAKKING
YANKING
YAOMING
YAPPING
YARDING
YARNING
YASMINE
YAWNING
YAWPING

YEANING
YEAREND
YEARONE
YELLING
YELPING
YENNING
YEOMANS
YESORNO
YESSING
YEVGENY
YIPPING
YOKOONO
YOUMANS
YOURANG
YOWLING
YOYOING
YUKKING

Y•••••N
YALEMAN
YALEMEN
YANKSON
YANKTON
YARDMAN
YARDMEN
YEAHMAN
YELTSIN
YEREVAN
YESICAN
YORKTON
YOUNGUN
YOUREON
YOUTHEN
YUCATAN
YZERMAN

•YN••••
AYNRAND
BYNAMES
CYNICAL
CYNTHIA
DYNAMIC
DYNAMOS
DYNASTS
DYNASTY
DYNODES
LYNDONB
LYNETTE
MYNHEER
PYNCHON
SYNAPSE
SYNCHED
SYNCING
SYNCOPE
SYNDICS
SYNERGY
SYNFUEL
SYNGMAN
SYNODAL
SYNODIC
SYNONYM
TYNDALL
WYNDHAM
WYNETTE
WYNONNA

•Y•N•••
BYANDBY
BYANECK
BYANOSE
CYANIDE
CYANIDS
CYGNETS
GYMNAST
HYANNIS
HYMNALS
HYMNARY
HYMNING
HYMNODY
HYPNOID
HYUNDAI
LYINGBY
LYINGON
LYINGTO
LYINGUP
LYONELL
MYANMAR
TYINGIN
TYINGON
TYINGTO
TYINGUP

•Y••N••
BYGONES
BYJINGO
BYLINED
BYLINER
BYLINES
BYRONIC
GYRENES
HYANNIS
HYGINUS
HYPONYM
LYSENKO
MYCENAE
MYKONOS
MYLANTA
NYYANKS
SYNONYM
SYRINGE
TYLENOL
TYRANNY
TYRANTS
WYNONNA

•Y•••N•
AYNRAND
BYPHONE
BYTURNS
CYCLING
CYCLONE
CYYOUNG
EYEBANK
EYEHAND
EYELINE
EYEWINK
GYPPING
HYDRANT
HYGIENE
HYMNING
HYPHENS
HYPOING
LYNDONB
MYGIANT
NYGIANT
PYTHONS
RYOKANS
SYNCING
SYRIANA
SYRIANS
TYCOONS
TYMPANA
TYMPANI
TYRANNY
WYNONNA
WYOMING
WYOTANA
WYVERNS

•Y••••N
BYTRAIN
CYPRIAN
HYPERON
LYINGON
LYRICON
MYERSON
PYNCHON
PYTHIAN
SYNGMAN
TYINGIN
TYINGON
TYPEDIN
TYPESIN
TYPHOON

••YN•••
ANYNEWS
BLYNKEN
BRYNNER
COYNESS
DRYNESS
ERYNGOS
FEYNESS
FEYNMAN
FLYNETS
GAYNESS
GLYNNIS
GWYNETH
KEYNOTE
MAYNARD
MEYNELL
RAYNELL
REYNARD
REYNAUD
REYNOSA
SAYNOTO
SHYNESS
SKYNYRD
SLYNESS
TOYNBEE
WRYNESS

••Y•N••
ANYONES
BAYONET
BAYONNE
BEYONCE
BRYNNER
BUYINTO
CAYENNE
DOYENNE
EXYANKS
FLYINTO
GLYNNIS
HAYINGS
HRYVNIA
KEYINON
LAYINTO
MAYINGS
NYYANKS
PAYINTO
PAYSNOW
PRYINTO
SAYINGS
SAYSNAY
SOYINKA
SOYINKS
SPYINGS
ULYANOV

••Y••N•
ANYKIND
BAYLYNX
BAYONNE
BOYBAND
CAYENNE
CAYMANS
CHYRONS
CYYOUNG
DAYLONG
DAYSEND
DAYSINN
DAYTONA
DEYOUNG
DOYENNE
DRYRUNS
ETYMONS
FRYPANS
GLYCINE
HEYMANS
HOYDENS
HUYGENS
ICYWIND
JAYLENO
KAYLENZ
KAYOING
KEYBANK
KEYRING
MAYWINE
PAYMENT
RAYBANS
RAYGUNS
RAYMOND
REYMONT
RHYMING
SKYLINE
SOYLENT
SPYRING
STYLING
STYRENE
THYMINE
TOYGUNS
TOYLAND
UNYOUNG
WAYLAND
YOYOING

••Y•••N
ALYKHAN
ANYTOWN
BLYNKEN
BUYDOWN
CRYDOWN
CRYOGEN
DAYSINN
ELYSIAN
FEYNMAN
FLYOPEN
GRYPHON
JOYCEAN
KEYEDIN
KEYEDON
KEYINON
KEYSPAN
KRYPTON
LAYDOWN
LAYITON
LAYOPEN
LAYUPON
MAYALIN
MUYBIEN
PRYOPEN
RAYBURN
ROYBEAN
ROYCOHN
SAYAMEN
SAYWHEN
SOYBEAN
SPYUPON
STYGIAN
TRYITON
WAYWORN

•••YN••
INSYNCH
LADYNAS
TRAYNOR
VERYNEW

•••Y•N•
ABEYANT
ALAYING
ALCYONE
ALLYING
ARMYANT
BABYING
BANYANS
BARYONS
BELYING
BIRYANI
BRAYING
BUOYANT
BUOYING
BURYING
BUSYING
CANYONS
CLAYING
CLOYING
COPYING
COSYING
COZYING
CRAYONS
DEFYING
DENYING
DRAYING
EASYONE
EDDYING
ENVYING
ESPYING
FLAYING
FRAYING
GRAYING
GREYING
HOLYONE
INLYING
JURYING
KENYANS
LEVYING
LIBYANS
MARYANN
MINYANS
OBEYING
OKAYING
PITYING
PLAYING
PONYING
PRAYING
PREYING
REDYING
REFYING
RELYING
SLAYING
SPAYING
STAYING
SWAYING
TIDYING
UNDYING
UNLYING
UNTYING
UNVYING
VARYING
WIFYING
XRAYING

•••Y••N
ALLYSON
ATTYGEN
AVEYRON
BABYLON
BOGYMAN
BOGYMEN
CLAYTON
COPYMAN
COPYMEN
DRAYMAN
DRAYMEN
DRAYTON
GRAYSON
GREYHEN
HOLYMAN
HOLYMEN
JURYMAN
JURYMEN
KOSYGIN
LADYKIN
LLEYTON
MARYANN
NAVYMAN
NAVYMEN
ONMYOWN
PLAYPEN
PLAYSON
POLYGON
PREYSON
SLAYTON
STAYSIN
STAYSON

••••YN•
ANODYNE BAYLYNX DENTYNE FTWAYNE LEMOYNE LIPSYNC PHARYNX

••••Y•N
CARRYIN CARRYON EARLYON HALCYON JIMRYUN MALAYAN MARRYIN MEGRYAN NARAYAN PARTYON PROCYON SAROYAN SPRAYON SUELYON TACHYON VISAYAN

•••••YN
BURSTYN CAROLYN FONTEYN GOLDWYN JERILYN JOCELYN KATHRYN MADALYN MARILYN ROSALYN TAMBLYN VANDUYN

YO•••••
YOBBISH YODELED YODELER YOGAMAT YOGHURT YOGIISM YOGINIS YOGURTS YOKOONO YOLANDA YOMTOVS YONKERS YOOHOOS YOPLAIT YORKERS YORKIES YORKIST YORKTON YOTEAMO YOTHERS YOUANDI YOUKNOW YOULOSE YOUMANS YOUNGER YOUNGMC YOUNGUN YOURANG YOUREIT YOUREON YOUTHEN YOUWISH YOWLERS YOWLING YOYOING

Y•O••••
YAOMING YAOUNDE YEOMANS YOOHOOS

Y••O•••
YESORNO YOKOONO YOYOING YUKOLIS

Y•••O••
YANKOFF YANKOUT YARROWS YEARONE YELLOUT YELLOWS YELLOWY YESVOTE YOKOONO YOMTOVS YOOHOOS YOULOSE

Y••••O•
YANKSON YANKTON YEAHYOU YELLFOR YENSFOR YOOHOOS YORKTON YOUKNOW YOUREON YULELOG

Y•••••O
YEARNTO YESORNO YIELDTO YOKOONO YOTEAMO

•YO••••
KYOODLE LYOCELL LYONELL MYOLOGY MYOPIAS RYOKANS WYOMING WYOTANA

•Y•O•••
BYFORCE BYFORMS BYGOLLY BYGONES BYMOUTH BYROADS BYRONIC BYWORDS CYBORGS CYYOUNG DYNODES GYROCAR HYPOING HYPONYM KYOODLE MYKONOS MYWORLD SYNODAL SYNODIC SYNONYM TYCOONS WYNONNA XYLOSES ZYGOTES

•Y••O••
AYKROYD BYANOSE BYPHONE BYPROXY CYCLOID CYCLONE CYCLOPS DYEJOBS DYELOTS DYEWOOD EYEBOLT EYEFOLD EYEHOLE EYEHOOK EYEROLL EYESORE GYMSOCK HYALOID HYDROUS HYMNODY HYPNOID HYSSOPS LYESOAP LYNDONB MYCROFT MYOLOGY PYEDOGS PYTHONS RYELOAF SYDHOFF SYMBOLS SYNCOPE SYSTOLE TYCOONS TYPHOID TYPHOON

•Y•••O•
BYWAYOF CYPRIOT DYEWOOD DYNAMOS EYEBROW EYEDROP EYEHOOK EYESHOT EYESPOT GYMSHOE GYRATOR HYPERON LYINGON LYRICON MYERSON MYKONOS PYNCHON SYMPTOM TYINGON TYLENOL TYPHOON ZYDECOS

•Y••••O
BYJINGO LYINGTO LYSENKO TYINGTO

••YO•••
ALYOSHA ANYONES BAYONET BAYONNE BEYONCE BUYOFFS BUYOUTS COYOTES CRYOGEN CRYOVER CYYOUNG DEYOUNG FLYOPEN FLYOVER IFYOUGO IMYOURS KAYOING LAYODDS LAYOFFS LAYOPEN LAYOUTS LAYOVER LOYOLAU MAYORAL PAYOFFS PAYOLAS PAYOUTS PEYOTES PRYOPEN RAYOVAC REYOKED REYOKES SAYOVER TOYOTAS TRYOUTS UNYOKED UNYOKES UNYOUNG YOYOING

••Y•O••
ANYBODY ANYHOPE ANYMORE ANYROAD ANYTOWN BAYLORU BOYCOTT BOYHOOD BOYTOYS BUYDOWN BUYSOFF BUYSOUT CHYRONS COYDOGS CRYDOWN CRYWOLF DAYBOOK DAYHOPS DAYJOBS DAYLONG DAYROOM DAYSOFF DAYTONA DRYDOCK DRYFOGS DRYHOLE DRYMOPS DRYROTS ETYMONS FLYBOYS FLYRODS FLYSOLO FRYCOOK GAYLORD GLYCOLS GUYROPE HAYFORK HAYLOFT HAYMOWS HEYLOOK HEYWOOD KEYHOLE KEYLOCK KEYNOTE KEYWORD LAYDOWN LAYSOFF LAYSOUT MAYPOLE OXYMORA PAYLOAD PAYMORE PAYROLL PAYSOFF PAYSOUT PLYWOOD RAYMOND REYMONT REYNOSA ROYCOHN SAYMORE SAYNOTO SEYMOUR SHYLOCK SKYDOME SKYHOOK SLYLOOK SPYBOTS SPYHOLE TAYLORS THYROID TOYBOAT TOYBOOK TOYDOGS TOYDOLL TOYHOOP TOYTOPS WAYCOOL WAYTOGO WAYWORN

••Y••O•
BOYHOOD BRYUSOV CRYPTOS DAYBOOK DAYROOM ERYNGOS FRYCOOK GRYPHON HEYLOOK HEYWOOD KEYEDON KEYINON KRYPTON LAYITON LAYSFOR LAYSLOW LAYUPON PAYSFOR PAYSNOW PHYLLOS PLYWOOD PSYCHOS RAYKROC SAYSBOO SAYSYOU SHYFROM SKYHOOK SLYLOOK SPYUPON TOYBOOK TOYHOOP TOYSHOP TRYITON ULYANOV WAYCOOL

••Y•••O
BUYINTO ERYTHRO FLYINTO FLYSOLO IFYOUGO JAYLENO LAYINTO LOYALTO MAYBESO PAYINTO PRYINTO SAYHITO SAYNOTO SAYSBOO SAYSIDO SAYSWHO WAYTOGO

•••YO••
ALCYONE BABYOIL BARYONS CANYONS CHAYOTE CRAYOLA CRAYONS EASYOFF EASYONE HOLYOIL HOLYOKE HOLYONE NEWYORK ONMYOWN PLAYOFF PLAYOUT STAYOFF STAYOUT VERYODD VERYOLD

•••Y•O•
ALLYSON AVEYRON BABYBOP BABYLON CITYBOY CLAYTON COPYBOY DRAYTON EASYJOB EMMYLOU GRAYSON HOLYCOW HOLYJOE ICKYPOO IGGYPOP JURYBOX LLEYTON MARYLOU ONLYTOO ONLYYOU PLAYBOY PLAYDOH PLAYSON POLYGON POLYPOD PRAYFOR PREYSON SLAYTON STAYFOR STAYSON TINYTOT TONYDOW TRAYNOR VERYHOT VERYLOW

•••Y••O
ADAYAGO CALYPSO ICKYPOO ONLYTOO PLAYSTO PRAYSTO

••••YO•
ARROYOS BYWAYOF CARRYON EARLYON EMBRYOS EXMAYOR HALCYON IBEGYOU IGOTYOU IOWEYOU ISEEYOU LOOKYOU LOVEYOU MISSYOU NEARYOU ONLYYOU PARTYON PROCYON SAYSYOU SPRAYON SUELYON TACHYON WILLYOU YEAHYOU

••••Y•O
APPLYTO DANEYKO GROMYKO HANDYTO HAPPYTO HOWDYDO IDSAYSO PRIVYTO RALLYTO REPLYTO SAMMYJO TALLYHO

•••••YO
THEMAYO

Y•P••••
YAPPERS YAPPING YIPPIES YIPPING YOPLAIT YUPPIES YUPPIFY

Y••P•••
YAPPERS YAPPING YAWPERS YAWPING YELPERS YELPING YIPPIES YIPPING YUPPIES YUPPIFY

Y•••P••
YSHAPED YSHAPES

Y••••P•
YUCAIPA

•YP••••
BYPATHS BYPHONE BYPLAYS BYPROXY CYPHERS CYPRESS CYPRIAN CYPRIOT GYPPERS GYPPING GYPSIES GYPSUMS HYPATIA HYPEDUP HYPERON HYPESUP HYPHENS HYPNOID HYPOING HYPONYM TYPEABS TYPEDIN TYPEDUP TYPESET TYPESIN TYPESUP TYPHOID TYPHOON TYPICAL TYPISTS

•Y•P•••
EYEPITS GYPPERS GYPPING MYOPIAS MYSPACE NYMPHAL NYMPHIC SYLPHIC SYMPTOM TYMPANA TYMPANI

•Y••P••
EYESPOT SYNAPSE

•Y•••P•
CYCLOPS EYECUPS HYSSOPS SYNCOPE

•Y••••P
EYEDROP HYPEDUP HYPESUP LYESOAP LYINGUP TYINGUP TYPEDUP TYPESUP

••YP•••
CRYPTIC CRYPTOS DAYPACK DRYPERS FLYPAST FRYPANS GLYPHIC GLYPTIC GRYPHON JOYPADS KEYPADS KEYPALS KRYPTON MAYPOLE STYPSIS STYPTIC TOYPAIL

••Y•P••
DAYSPAS FLYOPEN KEYSPAN LAYOPEN LAYUPON OLYMPIA OLYMPIC OLYMPUS PRYOPEN SPYUPON

••Y••P•
ANYHOPE DAYHOPS DRYMOPS GUYROPE SKYCAPS SKYMAPS TOYTOPS

••Y•••P
DAYCAMP DAYTRIP FLYTRAP KEYEDUP KEYGRIP PAYSLIP PSYCHUP TOYHOOP TOYSHOP

•••YP••
CALYPSO CLAYPIT ECTYPAL ECTYPES ICKYPOO IGGYPOP LILYPAD PLAYPEN POLYPED POLYPOD RETYPED RETYPES STAYPUT UNTYPED

•••Y•P•
THEYIPS

•••Y••P
BABYBOP BABYGAP BUOYSUP GREYCUP IGGYPOP INKYCAP OUTYELP PLAYSUP STAYSUP VERYHIP

••••YP•
BIOTYPE DECRYPT ECOTYPE ENCRYPT MISTYPE PLATYPI PRETYPE SETTYPE SUBTYPE TINTYPE

••••Y•P
BELLYUP BUDDYUP DIVVYUP DUMMYUP FANCYUP GIDDYAP GIDDYUP GUSSYUP HURRYUP PHONYUP TALLYUP

Y••Q•••
YANQUIS

••YQ•••
DAYQUIL

Y•R••••
YARDAGE YARDARM YARDERS YARDING YARDMAN YARDMEN YARNELL YARNING YARROWS YEREVAN YERKISH YORKERS YORKIES YORKIST YORKTON

Y••R•••
YARROWS YEAREND YEARNED YEARNER YEARNTO YEARONE YOURANG YOUREIT YOUREON YTTRIAS YTTRIUM YZERMAN

Y•••R••
YESORNO YEWTREE YOGURTS

Y••••R•
YAKKERS YAMMERS YANKERS YAPPERS YARDARM YARDERS YATTERS YAWNERS YAWPERS YELLERS YELPERS YESSIRE YOGHURT YONKERS YORKERS YOTHERS YOWLERS

Y•••••R
YACHTER YAWNIER YEARNER YELLFOR YENSFOR YESDEAR YIELDER YODELER YOUNGER YUCKIER YUMMIER

•YR••••
BYRIGHT BYROADS BYRONIC CYRUSII GYRALLY GYRATED GYRATES GYRATOR GYRENES GYROCAR HYRACES HYRAXES LYRICAL LYRICON LYRISTS MYRIADS MYRRHED MYRRHIC MYRTLES PYRAMID PYRAMUS PYRETIC PYREXIA PYRITES PYRITIC PYRRHIC PYRRHUS SYRIANA SYRIANS SYRINGE TYRANNY TYRANTS

•Y•R•••
AYKROYD AYNRAND BYPROXY BYTRAIN CYMRICS CYPRESS CYPRIAN CYPRIOT EYEROLL GYMRATS HYBRIDS HYDRANT HYDRATE HYDRIDE HYDROUS MYCROFT MYERSON MYRRHED MYRRHIC MYTREAT PYRRHIC PYRRHUS

•Y••R••
BYBIRTH BYFORCE BYFORMS BYTURNS BYWORDS CYBORGS EYEBROW EYEDROP HYPERON MYWORLD SYNERGY WYVERNS ZYMURGY

•Y•••R•
BYHEART CYCLERS CYPHERS DYKSTRA EYECARE EYESORE GYPPERS HYMNARY MYSTARS MYSTERY OYSTERS XYSTERS

•Y••••R
BYAHAIR BYLINER EYEWEAR GYRATOR GYROCAR

MYANMAR
MYNHEER
RYEBEER

••YR•••
ANYROAD
BAYRUMS
CHYRONS
DAYROOM
DRYROTS
DRYRUNS
FLYRODS
GUYROPE
HAYRACK
HAYRICK
HAYRIDE
HEYRUBE
JOYRIDE
KEYRING
PAYRATE
PAYROLL
SPYRING
STYRENE
THYROID

••Y•R••
BAYAREA
BAYTREE
DAYTRIP
DMYTRYK
FAYWRAY
FLYTRAP
HEYMRDJ
KEYGRIP
LAYERED
MAYORAL
NAYARIT
RAYKROC
SHYFROM
TOYSRUS

••Y••R•
ANYMORE
BAYLORU
DAYCARE
DAYMARE
DRYPERS
ERYTHRO
FLYGIRL
GAYLORD
GEYSERS
HAYFORK
HAYWARD
HAYWIRE
HEYWARD
IMYOURS
INYEARS
JAYBIRD
JAYWARD
KEYCARD
KEYWORD
LAYBARE
MAYNARD
OXYMORA
PAYDIRT
PAYMORE
PSYWARS
RAYBURN
REYNARD
RHYMERS
SAYMORE
SKYLARK
SKYNYRD
SKYSURF
SKYWARD
SPYDERS
SPYWARE
STYLERS
TAYLORS
TOYCARS
TOYCART
TRYHARD
WAYWARD
WAYWORN

••Y•••R
BRYNNER
CRYOVER
DAYSTAR
DAYWEAR
FLYOVER
FLYTIER
KAYAKER
LAYOVER
LAYSFOR
LOYALER
MAYFAIR
PAYSFOR
SAYOVER
SEYMOUR
SHYSTER
TOYFAIR
TRYSTER
VOYAGER
WHYEVER

•••YR••
ASSYRIA
AVEYRON
BODYRUB
ILLYRIA
JURYRIG
PAPYRUS
RUBYRED
SATYRIC
UNLYRIC
VERYRED

•••Y•R•
ALEYARD
BEEYARD
BODYART
BOWYERS
BRAYERS
BREYERS
EBAYERS
FLAYERS
FTMYERS
GRUYERE
HALYARD
HOLYARK
LANYARD
LAWYERS
MAGYARS
MARYURE
NEWYORK
OBEYERS
ONEYARD
PLAYERS
PRAYERS
PREYERS
RUDYARD
SAWYERS
SLAYERS
SPAYERS
STAYDRY
STAYERS
SWAYERS
VERYDRY

•••Y••R
BODYBAR
CLAYIER
GOBYAIR
GOBYCAR
HOLYWAR
INDYCAR
MANYEAR
MIDYEAR
NEWYEAR
OFFYEAR
ONEYEAR
PERYEAR
POLYMER
PRAYFOR
SIXYEAR
STAYFOR
SWAYBAR
TAXYEAR
TENYEAR
TRAYNOR
TWOYEAR

••••YR•
MARTYRS
PALMYRA
SKYNYRD
ZEPHYRS

••••Y•R
ALLAYER
ANNOYER
ARRAYER
ASSAYER
BABIYAR
BELAYER
BONEYER
COBUYER
COLLYER
DAIRYER
DECAYER
DECOYER
DELAYER
ENJOYER
ESSAYER
EXMAYOR
INLAYER
LOBBYER
PARTYER
RELAYER
SPRAYER
STRAYER
UNCOYER
UNSHYER
UNSLYER

YS•••••
YSHAPED
YSHAPES

Y•S••••
YASBECK
YASHICA
YASHMAK
YASMINE
YESDEAR
YESHIVA
YESICAN
YESIDID
YESISEE
YESITIS
YESLETS
YESMAAM
YESORNO
YESSING
YESSIRE
YESVOTE

Y••S•••
YEASTED
YENSFOR
YESSING
YESSIRE

Y•••S••
YANKSAT
YANKSON
YELLSAT
YELTSIN
YESISEE

Y••••S•
YAKUTSK
YERKISH
YIDDISH
YOBBISH
YOGIISM
YORKIST
YOULOSE
YOUWISH

Y•••••S
YAKIMAS
YAKKERS
YAMAHAS
YAMMERS
YANKEES
YANKERS
YANQUIS
YAPPERS
YARDERS
YARROWS
YATTERS
YAWNERS
YAWPERS
YELLERS
YELLOWS
YELPERS
YEMENIS
YEOMANS
YESITIS
YESLETS
YETTIES
YIPPIES
YOGINIS
YOGURTS
YOMTOVS
YONKERS
YOOHOOS
YORKERS
YORKIES
YOTHERS
YOUMANS
YOWLERS
YSHAPES
YTTRIAS
YUKATAS
YUKOLIS
YUPPIES

•YS••••
HYSSOPS
LYSENKO
MYSPACE
MYSTARS
MYSTERY
MYSTICS
MYSTIFY
OYSTERS
SYSTEMS
SYSTOLE
WYSIWYG
XYSTERS
XYSTUSI

•Y•S•••
DYKSTRA
EYESHOT
EYESORE
EYESPOT
GYMSHOE
GYMSOCK
GYMSUIT
GYPSIES
GYPSUMS
HYSSOPS
LYESOAP

•Y••S••
CYRUSII
DYNASTS
DYNASTY
HYPESUP
LYRISTS
MYERSON
TYPESET
TYPESIN
TYPESUP
TYPISTS
XYLOSES

•Y•••S•
BYANOSE
CYCLIST
CYPRESS
EYELASH
EYELESS
EYEMASK
EYETEST
EYEWASH
GYMNAST
SYNAPSE
XYSTUSI

•Y••••S
AYEAYES
BYEBYES
BYFIVES
BYFORMS
BYGONES
BYLINES
BYNAMES
BYPATHS
BYPLAYS
BYROADS
BYTALKS
BYTURNS
BYWORDS
CYANIDS
CYBORGS
CYCLERS
CYCLOPS
CYGNETS
CYMBALS
CYMRICS
CYPHERS
CYPRESS
DYBBUKS
DYEJOBS
DYELOTS
DYEVATS
DYNAMOS
DYNASTS
DYNODES
EYECUPS
EYEFULS
EYELESS
EYELETS
EYELIDS
EYEPITS
GYMBAGS
GYMRATS
GYPPERS
GYPSIES
GYPSUMS
GYRATES
GYRENES
HYANNIS
HYBRIDS
HYDROUS
HYGINUS
HYMNALS
HYPHENS
HYRACES
HYRAXES
HYSSOPS
LYCEUMS
LYRISTS
MYKONOS
MYOPIAS
MYRIADS
MYRTLES
MYSTARS
MYSTICS
NYTIMES
NYYANKS
OYSTERS
PYEDOGS
PYGMIES
PYRAMUS
PYRITES
PYRRHUS
PYTHIAS
PYTHONS
RYOKANS
RYUKYUS
SYMBOLS
SYNDICS
SYRIANS
SYSTEMS
TYCOONS
TYPEABS
TYPISTS
TYRANTS
WYVERNS
XYLOSES
XYSTERS
ZYDECOS
ZYGOTES

••YS•••
ABYSMAL
ABYSSAL
ABYSSES
ALYSSUM
BUYSOFF
BUYSOUT
CRYSTAL
DAYSAIL
DAYSEND
DAYSIDE
DAYSINN
DAYSOFF
DAYSPAS
DAYSTAR
DRYSUIT
ELYSEES
ELYSIAN
ELYSIUM
FLYSOLO
GEYSERS
HAYSEED
KEYSPAN
KRYSTLE
LAYSFOR
LAYSLOW
LAYSOFF
LAYSOUT
NAYSAID
NAYSAYS
ODYSSEY
PAYSFOR
PAYSLIP
PAYSNOW
PAYSOFF
PAYSOUT
PAYSTUB
PHYSICS
SAYSAAH
SAYSAYE
SAYSBOO
SAYSIDO
SAYSNAY
SAYSWHO
SAYSYES
SAYSYOU
SHYSTER
SKYSURF
SZYSLAK
THYSELF
TOYSHOP
TOYSLED
TOYSRUS
TRYSAIL
TRYSTED
TRYSTER
ULYSSES
WAYSIDE
ZOYSIAS

••Y•S••
ABYSSAL
ABYSSES
ALYOSHA
ALYSSUM
BRYUSOV
CAYUSES
HAYESES
ODYSSEY
STYPSIS
ULYSSES
WHYISIT

••Y••S•
AMYLASE
ANYWISE
COYNESS
DRYNESS
DRYWASH
FEYNESS
FLYCAST
FLYFISH
FLYLESS
FLYPAST
GAYNESS
IDYLIST
JOYLESS
KEYCASE
KEYLESS
KEYWEST
MAYBESO
PAYCASH
PAYLESS
RAYLESS
REYNOSA
RHYMIST
SAYMASS
SHYNESS
SKYLESS
SLYNESS
STYLISE
STYLISH
STYLIST
TOYLESS
WAYLESS
WRYNESS

••Y•••S
ABYSSES
ANYNEWS
ANYONES
ANYWAYS
ASYLUMS
BAYRUMS
BOYTOYS
BUYOFFS
BUYOUTS
CAYMANS
CAYUGAS
CAYUSES
CHYRONS
COYDOGS
COYNESS
COYOTES
CRYPTOS
DAYBEDS
DAYHOPS
DAYJOBS
DAYSPAS
DRYADES
DRYEYES
DRYFOGS
DRYMOPS
DRYNESS
DRYPERS
DRYROTS
DRYRUNS
ELYSEES
ERYNGOS
ETYMONS
EXYANKS
FEYNESS
FLYBOYS
FLYLESS
FLYNETS
FLYRODS
FLYWAYS
FRYPANS
GAYNESS
GEYSERS
GLYCOLS
GLYNNIS
HAYESES
HAYINGS
HAYMOWS
HEYDAYS
HEYMANS
HOYDENS
HUYGENS
IMYOURS
INYEARS
JAYCEES
JAYVEES
JOYLESS
JOYPADS
KEYDETS
KEYLESS
KEYPADS
KEYPALS
KEYWAYS
LAYODDS
LAYOFFS
LAYOUTS
LOYALES
MAYDAYS
MAYHEMS
MAYINGS
MAYTAGS
NAYSAYS
NYYANKS
OLYMPUS
PAYCUTS
PAYDAYS
PAYLESS
PAYOFFS
PAYOLAS
PAYOUTS
PEYOTES
PHYLLIS
PHYLLOS
PHYSICS
PSYCHES
PSYCHOS
PSYWARS
RAYBANS
RAYGUNS
RAYLESS
REYOKES
RHYMERS
RHYTHMS
ROYALES
RUYBLAS
SAYINGS
SAYMASS
SAYSYES
SCYTHES
SHYNESS
SKYCAMS
SKYCAPS
SKYLESS
SKYMAPS
SKYWAYS
SLYNESS
SOYINKS
SPYBOTS
SPYCAMS
SPYDERS
SPYINGS
SPYKIDS
STYLERS
STYLETS
STYMIES
STYPSIS
TAYLORS
TOYCARS
TOYDOGS
TOYGUNS
TOYHATS
TOYLESS
TOYOTAS
TOYSRUS
TOYTOPS
TRYOUTS
ULYSSES
UNYOKES
VOYAGES
WAYLAYS
WAYLESS
WBYEATS
WRYNESS
ZOYSIAS

•••YS••
ALLYSON
BABYSAT
BABYSIT
BUOYSUP
ECDYSES
ECDYSIS
GOBYSEA
GRAYSON
HOLYSEE
PLAYSAT
PLAYSBY
PLAYSON
PLAYSTO
PLAYSUP
POLYSCI
PRAYSTO
PREYSON
STAYSAT
STAYSIN
STAYSON
STAYSUP
THEYSAY
TIDYSUM
VERYSAD
VERYSHY

•••Y•S•
BABYISH
CALYPSO
CLAYISH
COPYIST
FOGYISH
FOGYISM
GRAYEST
GRAYISH
GREYEST
GREYISH
LADYISH
LAZYISH
PIXYISH
SPRYEST
TORYISH
TORYISM
WHEYISH
ZANYISH
ZANYISM

•••Y••S
ALIYAHS
ARGYLES
BANYANS
BARYONS
BOWYERS
BRAYERS
BREYERS
CALYCES
CALYXES
CANYONS
CORYZAS
CRAYONS
DREYFUS
EBAYERS
ECDYSES
ECDYSIS
ECTYPES
ENZYMES
FLAYERS
FTMYERS
GOBYBUS
KENYANS
LADYNAS
LAWYERS
LIBYANS
MAGYARS
MINYANS
OBEYERS
OOCYTES
PAPYRUS
PLAYERS
PRAYERS
PREYERS
RETYPES
SAWYERS
SLAYERS
SPAYERS
STAYERS
SWAYERS
THEYIPS

••••YS•
ANALYSE
ANALYST
IDSAYSO

••••Y•S
ALLEYES
ANONYMS
ARROYOS
AYEAYES
AZODYES
BIGEYES
BYEBYES
DACTYLS
DRYEYES
EMBRYOS
EPONYMS
ERINYES
EUONYMS
EXONYMS
HECKYES
HELLYES
HUNNYBS
KIKUYUS
MARTYRS
PAPAYAS
PITAYAS
POPEYES
RALLYES
REDDYES
REDEYES
RIBEYES
RITDYES
RYUKYUS
SADEYES
SAYSYES
SCHAYES
TIEDYES
VATDYES
VOTEYES
WELLYES
ZEPHYRS

•••••YS
AFFRAYS
AIRWAYS
ALTKEYS
ANYWAYS
BADBOYS
BADDAYS
BADGUYS
BAGBOYS
BARLEYS
BARNEYS
BATBOYS
BATDAYS
BENDAYS
BERNAYS
BETRAYS
BIGBOYS
BIGDAYS
BOXBOYS
BOYTOYS
BUGBOYS
BUSBOYS
BYPLAYS
CAMBOYS
CARBOYS
CARKEYS
CATTOYS
CONVEYS
CONVOYS
COWBOYS
DEEJAYS
DEFRAYS
DELKEYS
DELRAYS
DEPLOYS
DICKEYS
DISMAYS
DOGDAYS
DOGTOYS
DONKEYS
DORSEYS
EMPLOYS
ENDWAYS
ESTRAYS
EVERLYS
FLYBOYS
FLYWAYS
FRIDAYS
GALLEYS
GOODBYS
GOONEYS
GRAMMYS
GURNEYS
HALLEYS
HANGBYS
HARLEYS
HEYDAYS
HICKEYS
HOORAYS
HOTDAYS
HOTKEYS
HURRAYS
INTRAYS
JCPOWYS
JERSEYS
JETWAYS
JITNEYS
JOCKEYS
JOSBOYS
KEYWAYS
KIDNEYS
LACKEYS
LAZBOYS
LEAKEYS
LEEWAYS
LOWBOYS
MANDAYS
MAYDAYS
MEDLEYS

MICKEYS
MIDDAYS
MIDWAYS
MINSKYS
MISKEYS
MISLAYS
MISSAYS
MONDAYS
MONKEYS
MOTLEYS
MURPHYS
NAYSAYS
NEWTOYS
NOBODYS
OFFDAYS
OLDBOYS
OLDDAYS
OLDWAYS
ORKNEYS
OSPREYS
OUTBUYS
OUTLAYS
OUTPAYS
OUTSAYS
PARLAYS
PARLEYS
PAYDAYS
PEDWAYS
PENNEYS
PEPBOYS
PETTOYS
PHONEYS
PINBOYS
PREBUYS
PREPAYS
PULLEYS
PURVEYS
REDBAYS
REPLAYS
RICKEYS
RIDEBYS
ROBROYS
ROMNEYS
RUNWAYS
SASHAYS
SEAWAYS
SEGWAYS
SKYWAYS
SMILEYS
SMOKEYS
STMARYS
SUBWAYS
SUNDAYS
SUNRAYS
SURREYS
SURVEYS
TABKEYS
TAGDAYS
TEAPOYS
TENDAYS
TFPOWYS
THEBOYS
TOMBOYS
TURKEYS
TWODAYS
VALLEYS
VEEJAYS
VOLLEYS
WAYLAYS

YT•••••

YTTRIAS
YTTRIUM

Y•T••••

YATTERS
YETTIES
YITZHAK
YOTEAMO
YOTHERS
YTTRIAS
YTTRIUM

Y••T•••

YAHTZEE
YATTERS
YAYTEAM
YEATEAM
YELTSIN
YETTIES
YEWTREE
YOMTOVS
YOUTHEN

Y•••T••

YACHTED
YACHTER
YACHTIE
YAKUTSK
YANGTZE
YANKTON
YEASTED
YESITIS
YORKTON
YUCATAN
YUCATEC
YUKATAS

Y••••T•

YEARNTO
YESLETS
YESVOTE
YIELDTO
YOGURTS

Y•••••T

YANKOUT
YANKSAT
YEAHBUT
YELLOUT
YELLSAT
YOGAMAT
YOGHURT
YOPLAIT
YORKIST
YOUREIT

•YT••••

BYTALKS
BYTHEBY
BYTRAIN
BYTURNS
MYTHIFY
MYTREAT
NYTIMES
PYTHIAN
PYTHIAS
PYTHONS

•Y•T•••

CYNTHIA
EYETEST
EYETUCK
MYRTLES
MYSTARS
MYSTERY
MYSTICS
MYSTIFY
OYSTERS
SYSTEMS
SYSTOLE
WYOTANA
XYSTERS
XYSTUSI

•Y••T••

BYCATCH
BYPATHS
DYKSTRA
GYRATED
GYRATES
GYRATOR
HYPATIA
LYNETTE
PYRETIC
PYRITES
PYRITIC
SYMPTOM
WYNETTE
ZYGOTES

•Y•••T•

BYBIRTH
BYMOUTH
CYGNETS
DYEBATH
DYELOTS
DYEVATS
DYNASTS
DYNASTY
EYELETS
EYEPITS
GYMRATS
HYALITE
HYDRATE
LYDDITE
LYINGTO
LYNETTE
LYRISTS
MYLANTA
TYINGTO
TYPISTS
TYRANTS
WYNETTE

•Y••••T

BYHEART
BYRIGHT
CYCLIST
CYPRIOT
EYEBOLT
EYELIFT
EYESHOT
EYESPOT
EYETEST
GYMNAST
GYMSUIT
HYDRANT
MYCROFT
MYFAULT
MYGIANT
MYTREAT
NYGIANT
TYPESET

••YT•••

ANYTIME
ANYTOWN
BAYTREE
BOYTOYS
BUYTIME
DAYTIME
DAYTONA
DAYTRIP
DMYTRYK
ERYTHRO
FLYTIER
FLYTRAP
MAYTAGS
MAYTIME
RHYTHMS
SCYTHED
SCYTHES
TOYTOPS
WAYTOGO
YAYTEAM

••Y•T••

COYOTES
CRYPTIC
CRYPTOS
CRYSTAL
DAYSTAR
FAYETTE
GLYPTIC
KRYPTON
KRYSTLE
LAYETTE
LAYITON
PAYSTUB
PEYOTES
SHYSTER
STYPTIC
TOYOTAS
TRYITON
TRYSTED
TRYSTER

••Y••T•

BAYCITY
BOYCOTT
BUYINTO
BUYOUTS
DRYROTS
FAYETTE
FLYINTO
FLYNETS
GWYNETH
KEYDETS
KEYNOTE
LAYETTE
LAYINTO
LAYOUTS
LOYALTO
LOYALTY
PAYCUTS
PAYINTO
PAYOUTS
PAYRATE
PRYINTO
ROYALTY
SAYHITO
SAYNOTO
SPYBOTS
STYLETS
TOYHATS
TOYKITE
TOYWITH
TRYOUTS
WBYEATS

••Y•••T

BAYEDAT
BAYONET
BOYCOTT
BUYSOUT
DRYHEAT
DRYSUIT
FLYCAST
FLYPAST
HAYLOFT
IDYLIST
KEYWEST
LAYSOUT
NAYARIT
PAYDIRT
PAYMENT
PAYSOUT
REYMONT
RHYMIST
SAYWAIT
SAYWHAT
SOYLENT
STYLIST
TOYBOAT
TOYCART
WHYISIT
WHYWAIT

•••YT••

CLAYTON
DRAYTON
FREYTAG
LLEYTON
ONLYTOO
OOCYTES
PLAYTEX
SLAYTON
TINYTIM
TINYTOT

•••Y•T•

ASBYATT
CHAYOTE
NCWYETH
PLAYSTO
PRAYSTO

•••Y••T

ABEYANT
ARMYANT
ASBYATT
BABYSAT
BABYSIT
BODYART
BODYFAT
BODYKIT
BUOYANT
CLAYPIT
COPYCAT
COPYIST
GRAYEST
GREYEST
PLAYACT
PLAYLET
PLAYOUT
PLAYSAT
SPRYEST
STAYOUT
STAYPUT
STAYSAT
TINYBIT
TINYTOT
VERYFIT
VERYHOT
VERYWET

••••YT•

ACOLYTE
ANALYTE
APPLYTO
EXABYTE
FORSYTE
FORSYTH
HANDYTO
HAPPYTO
NEOLYTE
ONEBYTE
PRIVYTO
RALLYTO
REPLYTO

••••Y•T

ALNIYAT
ANALYST
ANGRYAT
DECRYPT
ENCRYPT
MARRYAT

YU•••••

YUCAIPA
YUCATAN
YUCATEC
YUCKIER
YUKATAS
YUKKING
YUKOLIS
YULELOG
YUMMIER
YUPPIES
YUPPIFY

Y•U••••

YOUANDI
YOUKNOW
YOULOSE
YOUMANS
YOUNGER
YOUNGMC
YOUNGUN
YOURANG
YOUREIT
YOUREON
YOUTHEN
YOUWISH

Y••U•••

YAKUTSK
YAOUNDE
YOGURTS

Y•••U••

YANQUIS
YOGHURT

Y••••U•

YANKOUT
YAWNFUL
YEAHBUT
YELLOUT
YOUNGUN
YTTRIUM

Y•••••U

YEAHYOU

•YU••••

HYUNDAI
RYUKYUS

•Y•U•••

BYTURNS
CYRUSII
MYBUDDY
ZYMURGY

•Y••U••

BYMOUTH
CYYOUNG
DYBBUKS
EYECUPS
EYEFULS
EYETUCK
GYMSUIT
GYPSUMS
LYCEUMS
MYFAULT
SYNFUEL
XYSTUSI

•Y•••U•

GYMCLUB
HYDROUS
HYGINUS
HYPEDUP
HYPESUP
LYINGUP
PYRAMUS
PYRRHUS
RYUKYUS
TYINGUP
TYPEDUP
TYPESUP

••YU•••

BRYUSOV
CAYUGAS
CAYUSES
LAYUPON
SPYUPON

••Y•U••

ANYLUCK
ASYLUMS
BAYRUMS
BUYOUTS
CYYOUNG
DAYQUIL
DEYOUNG
DRYBULB
DRYRUNS
DRYSUIT
HEYJUDE
HEYRUBE
IFYOUGO
IMYOURS
LAYOUTS
PAYCUTS
PAYOUTS
RAYBURN
RAYGUNS
SKYSURF
TOYGUNS
TRYOUTS
UNYOUNG

••Y••U•

ALYSSUM
BUYSOUT
ELYSIUM
KEYCLUB
KEYEDUP
LAYSOUT
OLYMPUS
PAYSOUT
PAYSTUB
PSYCHUP
REYNAUD
SEYMOUR
SKYBLUE
TOYSRUS

••Y•••U

BAYLORU
FEYDEAU
LOYOLAU
SAYSYOU

•••YU••

MARYURE

•••Y•U•

BODYRUB
BUOYSUP
DREYFUS
GOBYBUS
GREYCUP
LADYBUG
OKAYGUY
PAPYRUS
PLAYFUL
PLAYOUT
PLAYSUP
STAYOUT
STAYPUT
STAYSUP
TIDYSUM
TRAYFUL

•••Y••U

EMMYLOU
LUCYLIU
MARYLOU
ONLYYOU

••••YU•

BELLYUP
BUDDYUP
DIVVYUP
DUMMYUP
FANCYUP
GIDDYUP
GUSSYUP
HURRYUP
JIMRYUN
KIKUYUS
PHONYUP
RYUKYUS
TALLYUP

••••Y•U

IBEGYOU
IGOTYOU
IOWEYOU
ISEEYOU
LOOKYOU
LOVEYOU
MISSYOU
NEARYOU
ONLYYOU
SAYSYOU
WILLYOU
YEAHYOU

•••••YU

CHANOYU

Y•V••••

YEVGENY

Y••V•••

YESVOTE

Y•••V••

YEREVAN

Y••••V•

YESHIVA
YOMTOVS

•YV••••

WYVERNS

•Y•V•••

DYEVATS

•Y••V••

BYFIVES

••YV•••

HRYVNIA
JAYVEES

••Y•V••

CRYOVER
FLYOVER
LAYOVER
RAYOVAC
SAYOVER
WHYEVER

••Y••V•

SKYDIVE

••Y•••V

BRYUSOV
ROYGBIV
ULYANOV

•••YV••

UNGYVED

•••Y•V•

DESYLVA

••••YV•

HENRYVI

••••Y•V

FADAYEV
HENRYIV
KATAYEV
NUREYEV
ROCKYIV

Y•W••••

YAWNERS
YAWNFUL
YAWNIER
YAWNING
YAWPERS
YAWPING
YEWTREE
YOWLERS
YOWLING

Y••W•••

YOUWISH

Y••••W•

YARROWS
YELLOWS
YELLOWY

Y•••••W

YALELAW
YOUKNOW

•YW••••

BYWAYOF
BYWORDS
MYWORLD

•Y•W•••

DYEWOOD
EYEWALL
EYEWASH
EYEWEAR
EYEWINK

•Y••W••

WYSIWYG

•Y••••W

EYEBROW

••YW•••

ANYWAYS
ANYWISE
CRYWOLF
DAYWEAR
DRYWALL
DRYWASH
DRYWELL
FAYWRAY
FLYWAYS
HAYWARD
HAYWIRE
HEYWARD
HEYWOOD
ICYWIND
JAYWALK
JAYWARD
KEYWAYS
KEYWEST
KEYWORD
MAYWINE
PAYWELL
PLYWOOD
PSYWARS
SAYWAIT
SAYWHAT
SAYWHEN
SKYWALK
SKYWARD
SKYWAYS
SPYWARE
TOYWITH
WAYWARD
WAYWORN
WHYWAIT

••Y•W••

FLYAWAY
LAYAWAY
SAYSWHO
SHYAWAY

••Y••W•

ANYNEWS
ANYTOWN
BUYDOWN
CRYDOWN
HAYMOWS
LAYDOWN
ROYALWE

••Y•••W

LAYSLOW
PAYSNOW

•••YW••

HOLYWAR
VERYWET

•••Y•W•

ONMYOWN

•••Y••W

HOLYCOW
TONYDOW
VERYFEW
VERYLOW
VERYNEW

•Y••X••

EYEEXAM
HYRAXES
PYREXIA

•Y•••X•

BYPROXY

••Y•••X

BAYLYNX

•••YX••

CALYXES

•••Y••X

JURYBOX
PLAYTEX

••••Y•X

BAYLYNX
PHARYNX

•••••YX

APTERYX
HENDRYX

Y•Y••••

YAYTEAM
YOYOING

Y•••Y••

YEAHYOU

Y•••••Y

YELLOWY
YEVGENY
YUPPIFY

•YY••••

CYYOUNG
NYYANKS

•Y••Y••

AYEAYES
BYEBYES
BYWAYOF
RYUKYUS

•Y•••Y•

AYKROYD
BYPLAYS
HYPONYM
SYNONYM
WYSIWYG

•Y••••Y

BYANDBY
BYGOLLY
BYPROXY
BYTHEBY
DYNASTY
GYRALLY
HYMNARY
HYMNODY
LYINGBY
MYBUDDY
MYMAMMY
MYOLOGY
MYSTERY
MYSTIFY
MYTHIFY
SYNERGY
TYRANNY
ZYMURGY

••Y•Y••

BAYLYNX
DRYEYED
DRYEYES
SAYSYES
SAYSYOU
SKYNYRD

••Y••Y•

ANYWAYS
BOYTOYS
DMYTRYK
FLYBOYS
FLYWAYS
HEYDAYS
KEYWAYS
MAYDAYS
NAYSAYS
PAYDAYS
SAYSAYE
SKYWAYS
WAYLAYS

••Y•••Y

ANYBODY
BAYCITY
CRYBABY
DAYLILY
FAYWRAY
FLYAWAY
LAYAWAY
LOYALLY
LOYALTY
ODYSSEY
ROYALLY
ROYALTY
SAYSNAY
SHYAWAY

•••YY••

KHAYYAM
ONLYYOU

•••Y••Y

CITYBOY
COPYBOY
ELLYMAY
GRAYJAY
HOLYDAY
JULYDAY
LADYDAY

MARYKAY
OKAYGUY
PLAYBOY
PLAYSBY
STAYDRY
THEYSAY
VERYDRY
VERYSHY

••••Y•Y
EPONYMY
UNCOYLY
UNSHYLY
UNSLYLY

YZ•••••
YZERMAN

Y••Z•••
YITZHAK

Y•••Z••
YAHTZEE

Y••••Z•
YANGTZE

••Y••Z•
STYLIZE

••Y•••Z
KAYLENZ

•••YZ••
CORYZAS

••••YZ•
ANALYZE

•••••YZ
TUVWXYZ

ZA•••••
ZABUTON
ZACHARY
ZADKINE
ZAGAZIG
ZAGGING
ZAGNUTS
ZAIRIAN
ZAKUSKA
ZAMBEZI
ZAMBIAN
ZAMBONI
ZANETTO
ZANIEST
ZANYISH
ZANYISM
ZAPATAS
ZAPATEO
ZAPOTEC
ZAPPERS
ZAPPIER
ZAPPING
ZATOPEK

Z•A••••
ZEALAND
ZEALOTS
ZEALOUS
ZWANZIG

Z••A•••
ZAGAZIG
ZAPATAS
ZAPATEO
ZELAZNY
ZENANAS
ZIMARRA
ZOCALOS
ZONALLY

Z•••A••
ZACHARY
ZEALAND
ZEBRAIC
ZEBRASS
ZEELAND
ZERMATT
ZHIVAGO
ZIGZAGS
ZODIACS
ZONIANS
ZUMWALT
ZUNIANS

Z••••A•
ZAIRIAN
ZAMBIAN
ZAPATAS
ZENANAS
ZINNIAS
ZONULAR
ZOOIDAL
ZOYSIAS
ZWICKAU

Z•••••A
ZAKUSKA
ZENOBIA
ZIMARRA
ZOSSIMA

•ZA••••
AZALEAS
AZANIAN
CZARDAS
CZARDOM
CZARINA
CZARISM
CZARIST
IZATION
TZARINA

•Z•A•••
AZKABAN
IZZATSO

•Z••A••
AZUSACA
SZILARD

•Z•••A•
AZALEAS
AZANIAN
AZKABAN
AZOREAN
AZORIAN
AZTECAN
CZARDAS
SZYSLAK
YZERMAN

•Z••••A
AZUSACA
CZARINA
TZARINA

••ZA•••
BAZAARS
BIZARRE
BIZARRO
CEZANNE
DIZAINS
HAZANIM
HAZARDS
IZZATSO
LAZARUS
LIZARDS
MAZARIN
PIZARRO
ROZANOV
SIZABLE
SIZABLY
SUZANNE
ULZANAS
WIZARDS

••Z•A••
BAZAARS
BUZZARD
GAZZARA
GIZZARD
HAZMATS
HUZZAHS
JAZZAGE
MIZRAHI
PIZZAZZ

••Z••A•
BOZEMAN
BUZZSAW
ECZEMAS
GAZEDAT
GAZESAT
JAZZMAN
MEZUZAH
MEZUZAS
MIZUNAS
ULZANAS
VIZSLAS
WOZNIAK

••Z•••A
BAZOOKA
GAZZARA
LAZONGA
MAZEPPA
MAZURKA
MOZETTA
MOZILLA
RUZICKA

•••ZA••
BANZAIS
BENZALI
BORZAGE
BUZZARD
CHAZANS
CINZANO
CRUZADO
CRUZANS
GAZZARA
GIZZARD
GONZAGA
HUZZAHS
IBIZANS
JAZZAGE
PIZZAZZ
TARZANA
TARZANS
VANZANT
ZIGZAGS

•••Z•A•
BUZZSAW
CHAZZAN
DRUZEAN
DRUZIAN
HOLZMAN
JAZZMAN
MITZVAH
PENZIAS
PIAZZAS
YITZHAK

•••Z••A
ARIZONA
CANZONA
GAZZARA
GONZAGA
NOXZEMA
TARZANA

••••ZA•
ALCAZAR
CABEZAS
CHAZZAN
CORYZAS
ELEAZAR
KWANZAA
KWANZAS
MEZUZAH
MEZUZAS
PIAZZAS
QUETZAL
SALAZAR
STANZAS

••••Z•A
CHUTZPA
KWANZAA
VENEZIA

•••••ZA
BONANZA
CADENZA
CERVEZA
FIRENZA
FORENZA
IMPREZA
JERITZA
LEGANZA
ORGANZA
SPINOZA
VICENZA

Z•B••••
ZABUTON
ZEBRAIC
ZEBRASS
ZEBRINE
ZEBROID
ZEBULON
ZEBULUN

Z••B•••
ZAMBEZI
ZAMBIAN
ZAMBONI
ZOMBIES
ZOMBIFY

Z•••B••
ZENOBIA

•Z••B••
AZKABAN

••ZB•••
LAZBOYS

••Z•B••
GAZEBOS
JAZZBOS
JEZEBEL
SIZABLE
SIZABLY

••Z••B•
LAZENBY

•••ZB••
JAZZBOS

Z•C••••
ZACHARY
ZOCALOS

Z••C•••
ZILCHES
ZINCIFY
ZINCING
ZINCITE
ZINCKED
ZINCOUS
ZIPCODE
ZIPCUFF
ZIRCONS
ZITCOMS
ZWICKAU

Z•••C••
ZYDECOS

Z••••C•
ZIPLOCK
ZIPLOCS
ZODIACS

Z•••••C
ZAPOTEC
ZEBRAIC

•Z••C••
AZTECAN

•Z•••C•
AZUSACA

••Z•C••
BUZZCUT
RUZICKA

••Z••C•
WOZZECK

••Z•••C
ENZYMIC

•••ZC••
BUZZCUT

•••Z•C•
WOZZECK

Z•D••••
ZADKINE
ZEDILLO
ZEDONKS
ZODIACS
ZYDECOS

Z••D•••
ZIPDISK

Z•••D••
ZOOIDAL

Z••••D•
ZIPCODE

Z•••••D
ZEALAND
ZEBROID
ZEELAND
ZINCKED

•Z•D•••
AZODYES

•Z••D••
CZARDAS
CZARDOM

•Z••••D
SZILARD

••Z•D••
DAZEDLY
GAZEDAT
GAZEDON
SIZEDUP

••Z••D•
HAZARDS
LIZARDS
WIZARDS

••Z•••D
BUZZARD
COZENED
DAZZLED
DIZZIED
FIZZLED
GIZZARD
GUZZLED
MIZZLED
MUZZLED
NUZZLED
PUZZLED
RAZORED
REZONED
SIZZLED
UNZONED
VIZORED
WIZENED

•••Z•D•
CRUZADO

•••Z••D
BUZZARD
DAZZLED
DIZZIED
FIZZLED
FOOZLED
FRIZZED
GIZZARD
GUZZLED
MIZZLED
MUZZLED
NUDZHED
NUZZLED
PUZZLED
QUIZZED
SIZZLED
WHIZKID
WHIZZED

••••Z•D
BEDAZED
BLITZED
BLOWZED
BREEZED
BRONZED
FRIZZED
GLITZED
IODIZED
IONIZED
PLOTZED
QUIZZED
RESIZED
SNEEZED
SNOOZED
TWEEZED
UNDAZED
UNFAZED
UNHAZED
UNRAZED
UNSIZED
UPGAZED
UPSIZED
WALTZED
WHEEZED
WHIZZED

ZE•••••
ZEALAND
ZEALOTS
ZEALOUS
ZEBRAIC
ZEBRASS
ZEBRINE
ZEBROID
ZEBULON
ZEBULUN
ZEDILLO
ZEDONKS
ZEELAND
ZEITUNG
ZELAZNY
ZEMSTVO
ZENANAS
ZENISTS
ZENITHS
ZENOBIA
ZEPHYRS
ZEPPOLE
ZEPPOLI
ZERMATT
ZERNIKE
ZEROING
ZEROOUT
ZEROSIN
ZEROSUM
ZESTERS
ZESTFUL
ZESTIER
ZESTILY
ZESTING

Z•E••••
ZEELAND
ZIEGLER
ZIERING
ZOELLER

Z••E•••
ZANETTO
ZONEOUT
ZYDECOS

Z•••E••
ZAMBEZI
ZANIEST
ZAPPERS
ZESTERS
ZINGERS
ZIPPERS
ZITHERS
ZOOIEST

Z••••E•
ZAPATEO
ZAPOTEC
ZAPPIER
ZATOPEK
ZESTIER
ZIEGLER
ZILCHES
ZINCKED
ZINGIER
ZINKIER
ZIPPIER
ZOELLER
ZOMBIES
ZONULES
ZYGOTES

Z•••••E
ZADKINE
ZEBRINE
ZEPPOLE
ZERNIKE
ZINCITE
ZIPCODE

•ZE••••
EZEKIEL
YZERMAN

•Z•E•••
AZTECAN

•Z••E••
AZALEAS
AZOREAN
AZULEJO
OZZFEST

•Z•••E•
AZINGER
AZODYES
EZEKIEL
TZIMMES

•Z••••E
AZURITE
OZONISE
OZONIZE

••ZE•••
BOZEMAN
COZENED
COZENER
DAZEDLY
DOZENTH
DOZEOFF
ECZEMAS
GAZEBOS
GAZEDAT
GAZEDON
GAZELLE
GAZESAT
GAZESON
GAZETTE
JEZEBEL
LAZENBY
LIZETTE
LOZENGE
MAZEPPA
MOZETTA
OOZEOUT
REZEROS
ROZELLE
SIZEDUP
SIZEONE
SIZESIX
SIZESUP
SIZETEN
SIZETWO
SUZETTE
WIZENED

••Z•E••
BEZIERS
BUZZELL
BUZZERS
COZIEST
COZZENS
DOZIEST
FIZZERS
HAZIEST
JAZZERS
KUZNETS
LAZIEST
LAZZERI
MAZIEST
MIZZENS
OOZIEST
OZZFEST
VIZIERS
WOZZECK

••Z••E•
BUZZIER
COZENED
COZENER
COZUMEL
DAZZLED
DAZZLER
DAZZLES
DIZZIED
DIZZIER
DIZZIES
ENZYMES
FIZZIER
FIZZLED
FIZZLER
FIZZLES
FUZZIER
GUZZLED
GUZZLER
GUZZLES
JAZZIER
JAZZMEN
JEZEBEL
LIZZIES
MIZZLED
MIZZLES
MUZZIER
MUZZLED
MUZZLER
MUZZLES
NOZZLES
NUZZLED
NUZZLER
NUZZLES
POZOLES
PUZZLED
PUZZLER
PUZZLES
RAZORED
RAZZIES
REZONED
REZONES
SIZETEN
SIZZLED
SIZZLER
SIZZLES
TIZZIES
UNZONED
UNZONES
VIZORED
WIZENED

••Z•••E
BEZIQUE
BIZARRE
CEZANNE
GAZELLE
GAZETTE
JAZZAGE
LIZETTE
LOZENGE
ROZELLE
SIZABLE
SIZEONE
SUZANNE
SUZETTE

•••ZE••
BEEZERS
BENZELL
BENZENE
BLAZERS
BLAZEUP
BOOZERS
BRAZENS
BUZZELL
BUZZERS
COZZENS
DOOZERS
DRUZEAN
FIZZERS
FROZEUP
GEEZERS
GLAZERS
GRAZERS
JAZZERS
LAZZERI
MIZZENS
NETZERO
NONZERO
NOXZEMA
PANZERS
PATZERS
SEIZEON
SEIZERS
SUBZERO
VONZELL
WOZZECK

•••Z•E•
BOOZIER
BRAZIER
BUZZIER
CRAZIER
CRAZIES
CROZIER
DAZZLED
DAZZLER
DAZZLES
DITZIER
DIZZIED
DIZZIER
DIZZIES
DOOZIES
FIZZIER
FIZZLED
FIZZLER
FIZZLES
FOOZLED
FOOZLER
FOOZLES
FRAZIER
FRIZZED
FRIZZER
FRIZZES
FUZZIER
GAUZIER
GLAZIER
GRAZIER
GUZZLED
GUZZLER
GUZZLES
JAZZIER
JAZZMEN
KLEZMER
LIZZIES
MENZIES
MIZZLED
MIZZLES
MUZZIER
MUZZLED
MUZZLER
MUZZLES
NOZZLES
NUDZHED
NUDZHES
NUZZLED
NUZZLER
NUZZLES
PUZZLED
PUZZLER
PUZZLES
QUIZZED
QUIZZER
QUIZZES
RAZZIES
RITZIER
SCUZZES
SIZZLED
SIZZLER
SIZZLES
TIZZIES
WHIZZED
WHIZZER
WHIZZES
WOOZIER

•••Z••E
BENZENE
BORZAGE
CALZONE
CANZONE
CORZINE
DRIZZLE
ENDZONE
FANZINE
FRAZZLE
FRIZZLE
FROZONE
GENZYME
GRIZZLE
HOTZONE
JAZZAGE
MISZONE
REDZONE
RHIZOME
SEIZURE
SUBZONE
SWIZZLE
WARZONE
WEBZINE

••••ZE•
ASSIZES
BEDAZED
BEDAZES
BEDIZEN
BLITZED
BLITZEN
BLITZER
BLITZES
BLOWZED
BREEZED
BREEZES
BRONZED
BRONZER
BRONZES
CITIZEN
COETZEE
CRUTZEN
DENIZEN
ELIEZER
FREEZER
FREEZES
FRIEZES
FRIZZED
FRIZZER
FRIZZES
GLITZED
GLITZES
IODIZED
IODIZER
IODIZES
IONIZED
IONIZER
IONIZES
KLUTZES
NETIZEN
PLOTZED
PLOTZES
PRETZEL
QUINZES
QUIZZED
QUIZZER
QUIZZES
RESIZED
RESIZER
RESIZES
SARAZEN
SCUZZES
SELTZER
SLEAZES
SNEEZED
SNEEZER
SNEEZES
SNOOZED
SNOOZER
SNOOZES
SPITZES
STUTZES

SWITZER
TOPAZES
TREIZES
TWEEZED
TWEEZER
TWEEZES
UNDAZED
UNFAZED
UNHAZED
UNRAZED
UNSIZED
UPGAZED
UPGAZES
UPSIZED
UPSIZES
WALTZED
WALTZER
WALTZES
WHEEZED
WHEEZER
WHEEZES
WHIZZED
WHIZZER
WHIZZES
YAHTZEE

••••Z•E
COETZEE
DRIZZLE
FRAZZLE
FRIZZLE
GRIZZLE
SWIZZLE
YAHTZEE

•••••ZE
AGONIZE
ANALYZE
ANODIZE
ATOMIZE
BAPTIZE
BLINTZE
BRASIZE
CAPSIZE
COGNIZE
DEGLAZE
DUALIZE
EBONIZE
ELEGIZE
EMBLAZE
FIRENZE
FORSIZE
GRECIZE
HATSIZE
IDOLIZE
INADAZE
ITEMIZE
LAICIZE
LIONIZE
MANSIZE
MIDSIZE
OBELIZE
ODORIZE
ONESIZE
OUTGAZE
OUTSIZE
OXIDIZE
OZONIZE
POETIZE
REALIZE
REGLAZE
RESEIZE
SQUEEZE
STYLIZE
TRAPEZE
UNFROZE
UNISIZE
UNITIZE
UTILIZE
YANGTZE

Z•••F••
ZESTFUL

Z••••F•
ZINCIFY
ZIPCUFF
ZIPSOFF
ZOMBIFY

Z•••••F
ZIPCUFF
ZIPSOFF

•Z•F•••
OZZFEST

••ZF•••
OZZFEST

••Z••F•
BUZZOFF
DOZEOFF

••Z•••F
BUZZOFF
DOZEOFF

•••Z•F•
BUZZOFF

•••Z••F
BUZZOFF

Z•G••••
ZAGAZIG
ZAGGING
ZAGNUTS
ZIGGING
ZIGZAGS
ZYGOTES

Z••G•••
ZAGGING
ZIEGLER
ZIGGING
ZINGERS
ZINGIER
ZINGING
ZIPGUNS

Z•••G••
ZWINGLI

Z••••G•
ZHIVAGO
ZIGZAGS
ZOOLOGY
ZYMURGY

Z•••••G
ZAGAZIG
ZAGGING
ZAPPING
ZEITUNG
ZEROING
ZESTING
ZIERING
ZIGGING
ZINCING
ZINGING
ZIPPING
ZONKING
ZOOMING
ZWANZIG

•Z•G•••
AZINGER

••ZG•••
FIZGIGS

••Z•G••
FIZGIGS
HAZINGS
JAZZAGE
LAZONGA
LOZENGE

••Z•••G
BUZZING
COZYING
FIZZING
FUZZING
JAZZING
RAZZING

•••Z•G•
BORZAGE
GONZAGA
JAZZAGE
ZIGZAGS

•••Z••G
AMAZING
BLAZING
BOOZING
BRAZING
BUZZING
CRAZING
FIZZING
FUTZING
FUZZING
GLAZING
GRAZING
JAZZING
PRIZING
RAZZING
SEIZING
TENZING

••••Z•G
FUNFZIG
LEIPZIG
SECHZIG
SIEBZIG
VIERZIG
ZAGAZIG
ZWANZIG

ZH•••••
ZHIVAGO

Z•H••••
ZACHARY
ZEPHYRS
ZITHERS

Z•••H••
ZILCHES

Z••••H•
ZENITHS

Z•••••H
ZANYISH

•Z••••H
AZIMUTH

••Z•H••
HUZZAHS
MIZRAHI

••Z•••H
DOZENTH
JAZZISH
LAZYISH
MEZUZAH

•••ZH••
NUDZHED
NUDZHES
YITZHAK

•••Z•H•
HUZZAHS
MATZOHS

•••Z••H
JAZZISH
MATZOTH
MITZVAH

••••Z•H
MEZUZAH

ZI•••••
ZIEGLER
ZIERING
ZIGGING
ZIGZAGS
ZILCHES
ZILLION
ZIMARRA
ZINCIFY
ZINCING
ZINCITE
ZINCKED
ZINCOUS
ZINGERS
ZINGIER
ZINGING
ZINKIER
ZINNIAS
ZIONISM
ZIONIST
ZIPCODE
ZIPCUFF
ZIPDISK
ZIPGUNS
ZIPLOCK
ZIPLOCS
ZIPPERS
ZIPPIER
ZIPPING
ZIPSOFF
ZIPTOPS
ZIRCONS
ZITCOMS
ZITHERS

Z•I••••
ZAIRIAN
ZEITUNG
ZHIVAGO
ZWICKAU
ZWINGLI

Z••I•••
ZANIEST
ZEDILLO
ZENISTS
ZENITHS
ZODIACS
ZONIANS
ZOOIDAL
ZOOIEST
ZOSIMUS
ZUNIANS

Z•••I••
ZADKINE
ZAGGING
ZAIRIAN
ZAMBIAN
ZANYISH
ZANYISM
ZAPPIER
ZAPPING
ZEBRINE
ZERNIKE
ZEROING
ZESTIER
ZESTILY
ZESTING
ZIERING
ZIGGING
ZILLION
ZINCIFY
ZINCING
ZINCITE
ZINGIER
ZINGING
ZINKIER
ZINNIAS
ZIONISM
ZIONIST
ZIPDISK
ZIPPIER
ZIPPING
ZOMBIES
ZOMBIFY
ZONKING
ZOOMING
ZOSSIMA
ZOYSIAS

Z••••I•
ZAGAZIG
ZEBRAIC
ZEBROID
ZENOBIA
ZEROSIN
ZOOMSIN
ZWANZIG

Z•••••I
ZAMBEZI
ZAMBONI
ZEPPOLI
ZWINGLI

•ZI••••
AZIMUTH
AZINGER
SZILARD
TZIMMES

•Z•I•••
AZANIAN
AZORIAN
AZURITE
CZARINA
CZARISM
CZARIST
EZEKIEL
IZATION
OZONISE
OZONIZE
TZARINA

••ZI•••
BEZIERS
BEZIQUE
COZIEST
DOZIEST
HAZIEST
HAZINGS
LAZIEST
MAZIEST
MOZILLA
OOZIEST
RUZICKA
VIZIERS

••Z•I••
BUZZIER
BUZZING
COZYING
DIZAINS
DIZZIED
DIZZIER
DIZZIES
DIZZILY
FIZGIGS
FIZZIER
FIZZING
FUZZIER
FUZZILY
FUZZING
HAZLITT
JAZZIER
JAZZILY
JAZZING
JAZZISH
LAZYISH
LIZZIES
MAZZINI
MUZZIER
MUZZILY
RAZZIES
RAZZING
TIZZIES
WOZNIAK

••Z••I•
ADZUKIS
ENZYMIC
HAZANIM
MAZARIN
SIZESIX
SUZUKIS

••Z•••I
LAZZERI
MAZZINI
MIZRAHI

•••ZI••
AMAZING
BLAZING
BOOZIER
BOOZILY
BOOZING
BRAZIER
BRAZING
BUZZIER
BUZZING
CORZINE
CRAZIER
CRAZIES
CRAZILY
CRAZING
CROZIER
DITZIER
DIZZIED
DIZZIER
DIZZIES
DIZZILY
DOOZIES
DRUZIAN
FANZINE
FIZZIER
FIZZING
FRAZIER
FUTZING
FUZZIER
FUZZILY
FUZZING
GAUZIER
GAUZILY
GLAZIER
GLAZILY
GLAZING
GRAZIER
GRAZING
JAZZIER
JAZZILY
JAZZING
JAZZISH
LIZZIES
MAZZINI
MENZIES
MUZZIER
MUZZILY
PENZIAS
PRIZING
RAZZIES
RAZZING
RITZIER
RITZILY
SEIZING
TENZING
TIZZIES
WEBZINE
WOOZIER
WOOZILY

•••Z•I•
BANZAIS
BORZOIS
MUEZZIN
PRIZZIS
WHIZKID

•••Z••I
BELZONI
BENZALI
CANZONI
CHEZMOI
LAZZERI
MAZZINI
RONZONI

••••ZI•
BENAZIR
CHEEZIT
DWEEZIL
FUNFZIG
LEIPZIG
MUEZZIN
PRIZZIS
RENUZIT
SECHZIG
SIEBZIG
SKEEZIX
VENEZIA
VIERZIG
ZAGAZIG
ZWANZIG

••••Z•I
ABRUZZI
JACUZZI
PALAZZI

•••••ZI
ABRUZZI
ANASAZI
FABRIZI
JACUZZI
PALAZZI
SCHERZI
ZAMBEZI

•Z•••J•
AZULEJO

Z•K••••
ZAKUSKA

Z••K•••
ZADKINE
ZINKIER
ZONKING
ZONKOUT

Z•••K••
ZINCKED
ZWICKAU

Z••••K•
ZAKUSKA
ZEDONKS
ZERNIKE

Z•••••K
ZATOPEK
ZIPDISK
ZIPLOCK

•ZK••••
AZKABAN

•Z•K•••
EZEKIEL

•Z••••K
SZYSLAK

••Z•K••
ADZUKIS
SUZUKIS

••Z••K•
BAZOOKA
MAZURKA
RUZICKA

••Z•••K
WOZNIAK
WOZZECK

•••ZK••
WHIZKID

•••Z••K
WOZZECK
YITZHAK

••••ZK•
GRETZKY

Z•L••••
ZELAZNY
ZILCHES
ZILLION

Z••L•••
ZEALAND
ZEALOTS
ZEALOUS
ZEELAND
ZILLION
ZIPLOCK
ZIPLOCS
ZOELLER
ZOOLOGY

Z•••L••
ZEBULON
ZEBULUN
ZEDILLO
ZIEGLER
ZOCALOS
ZOELLER
ZONALLY
ZONULAR
ZONULES

Z••••L•
ZEDILLO
ZEPPOLE
ZEPPOLI
ZESTILY
ZONALLY
ZUMWALT
ZWINGLI

Z•••••L
ZESTFUL
ZOOIDAL

•Z•L•••
AZALEAS
AZULEJO
SZILARD

•Z••L••
SZYSLAK

•Z••••L
EZEKIEL

••ZL•••
HAZLITT

••Z•L••
DAZZLED
DAZZLER
DAZZLES
FIZZLED
FIZZLER
FIZZLES
GAZELLE
GUZZLED
GUZZLER
GUZZLES
MIZZLED
MIZZLES
MOZILLA
MUZZLED
MUZZLER
MUZZLES
NOZZLES
NUZZLED
NUZZLER
NUZZLES
POZOLES
PUZZLED
PUZZLER
PUZZLES
ROZELLE
SIZZLED
SIZZLER
SIZZLES
VIZSLAS

••Z••L•
BUZZELL
DAZEDLY
DIZZILY
FUZZILY
GAZELLE
JAZZILY
MOZILLA
MUZZILY
ROZELLE
SIZABLE
SIZABLY

••Z•••L
BUZZELL
COZUMEL
JEZEBEL

•••ZL••
DAZZLED
DAZZLER
DAZZLES
FIZZLED
FIZZLER
FIZZLES
FOOZLED
FOOZLER
FOOZLES
GUZZLED
GUZZLER
GUZZLES
MIZZLED
MIZZLES
MUZZLED
MUZZLER
MUZZLES
NOZZLES
NUZZLED
NUZZLER
NUZZLES
PUZZLED
PUZZLER
PUZZLES
SIZZLED
SIZZLER
SIZZLES

•••Z•L•
BENZALI
BENZELL
BOOZILY
BUZZELL
CRAZILY
DIZZILY
DRIZZLE
DRIZZLY
FRAZZLE
FRIZZLE
FRIZZLY
FUZZILY
GAUZILY
GLAZILY
GRIZZLE
GRIZZLY
JAZZILY
MUZZILY
RITZILY
SWIZZLE
VONZELL
WOOZILY

•••Z••L
BENZELL
BUZZELL
VONZELL

••••ZL•
DRIZZLE
DRIZZLY
FRAZZLE
FRIZZLE
FRIZZLY
GRIZZLE
GRIZZLY
SWIZZLE

••••Z•L
DWEEZIL
PRETZEL
QUETZAL

Z•M••••
ZAMBEZI
ZAMBIAN
ZAMBONI
ZEMSTVO
ZIMARRA
ZOMBIES
ZOMBIFY
ZUMWALT
ZYMURGY

Z••M•••
ZERMATT
ZOOMING
ZOOMOUT
ZOOMSIN

Z•••M••
ZOSIMUS

Z••••M•
ZITCOMS
ZOSSIMA

Z•••••M
ZANYISM
ZEROSUM
ZIONISM

•Z•M•••
AZIMUTH
TZIMMES

•Z••M••
TZIMMES
YZERMAN

•Z••••M
CZARDOM
CZARISM

••ZM•••
HAZMATS

••Z•M••
BOZEMAN
COZUMEL
ECZEMAS
ENZYMES
ENZYMIC
JAZZMAN
JAZZMEN

••Z•••M
HAZANIM

•••ZM••
CHEZMOI
HOLZMAN
JAZZMAN
JAZZMEN
KLEZMER

•••Z•M•
GENZYME
NOXZEMA
RHIZOME

Z•N••••
ZANETTO
ZANIEST
ZANYISH
ZANYISM
ZENANAS
ZENISTS
ZENITHS
ZENOBIA
ZINCIFY
ZINCING
ZINCITE
ZINCKED
ZINCOUS
ZINGERS
ZINGIER
ZINGING
ZINKIER
ZINNIAS
ZONALLY
ZONEOUT
ZONIANS
ZONKING
ZONKOUT
ZONULAR
ZONULES
ZUNIANS

Z••N•••
ZAGNUTS
ZERNIKE
ZINNIAS
ZIONISM
ZIONIST
ZWANZIG
ZWINGLI

Z••N•••
ZEDONKS
ZENANAS

Z•••N••
ZADKINE
ZAGGING
ZAMBONI
ZAPPING
ZEALAND
ZEBRINE
ZEELAND
ZEITUNG
ZELAZNY
ZEROING
ZESTING
ZIERING
ZIGGING
ZINCING
ZINGING
ZIPGUNS
ZIPPING
ZIRCONS
ZONIANS
ZONKING
ZOOMING
ZUNIANS

Z•••••N
ZABUTON
ZAIRIAN
ZAMBIAN
ZEBULON
ZEBULUN
ZEROSIN
ZILLION
ZOOMSIN

•Z•N•••
AZANIAN
AZINGER
OZONISE
OZONIZE
OZONOUS

•Z•••N•
CZARINA
TZARINA

•Z••••N
AZANIAN
AZKABAN
AZOREAN
AZORIAN
AZTECAN
IZATION
YZERMAN

••ZN•••
KUZNETS
WOZNIAK

••Z•N••
CEZANNE
COZENED
COZENER
DOZENTH
HAZANIM
HAZINGS
LAZENBY
LAZONGA
LOZENGE
MIZUNAS
REZONED
REZONES
ROZANOV
SUZANNE
ULZANAS
UNZONED
UNZONES
WIZENED

••Z••N•
BUZZING
CEZANNE
COZYING
COZZENS
DIZAINS
FIZZING
FUZZING
JAZZING
MAZZINI
MIZZENS
RAZZING
SIZEONE
SUZANNE

••Z•••N
BOZEMAN
GAZEDON
GAZESON
JAZZMAN
JAZZMEN
MAZARIN
SIZETEN

•••ZN••
QUIZNOS

•••Z•N•
AMAZING
AMAZONS
ARIZONA
BELZONI
BENZENE
BLAZING
BLAZONS
BOOZING
BRAZENS
BRAZING
BUZZING
CALZONE
CANZONA
CANZONE
CANZONI
CHAZANS
CINZANO
CORZINE
COZZENS
CRAZING
CRUZANS
ENDZONE
FANZINE
FIZZING
FROZONE
FUTZING
FUZZING
GLAZING
GRAZING
HOTZONE
IBIZANS
JAZZING
MAZZINI
MISZONE
MIZZENS
PRIZING
RAZZING
REDZONE
RONZONI
SEIZING
SUBZONE
TARZANA
TARZANS
TENZING
VANZANT
WARZONE
WEBZINE

•••Z••N
CHAZZAN
DRUZEAN
DRUZIAN
HOLZMAN
JAZZMAN
JAZZMEN
MUEZZIN
SEIZEON

••••ZN•
ZELAZNY

••••Z•N
BEDIZEN
BLITZEN
CHAZZAN
CITIZEN
CORAZON
CRUTZEN
DENIZEN
HORIZON
MUEZZIN
NETIZEN
SARAZEN
VERIZON

ZO•••••
ZOCALOS
ZODIACS
ZOELLER
ZOMBIES
ZOMBIFY
ZONALLY
ZONEOUT
ZONIANS
ZONKING
ZONKOUT
ZONULAR
ZONULES
ZOOIDAL
ZOOIEST
ZOOLOGY
ZOOMING
ZOOMOUT
ZOOMSIN
ZOSIMUS
ZOSSIMA
ZOYSIAS

Z•O••••
ZIONISM
ZIONIST
ZOOIDAL
ZOOIEST
ZOOLOGY
ZOOMING
ZOOMOUT
ZOOMSIN

Z••O•••
ZAPOTEC
ZATOPEK
ZEDONKS
ZENOBIA
ZEROING
ZEROOUT
ZEROSIN
ZEROSUM
ZYGOTES

Z•••O••
ZAMBONI
ZEALOTS
ZEALOUS
ZEBROID
ZEPPOLE
ZEPPOLI
ZEROOUT
ZINCOUS
ZIPCODE
ZIPLOCK
ZIPLOCS
ZIPSOFF
ZIPTOPS
ZIRCONS
ZITCOMS
ZONEOUT
ZONKOUT
ZOOLOGY
ZOOMOUT

Z••••O•
ZABUTON
ZEBULON
ZILLION
ZOCALOS
ZYDECOS

Z•••••O
ZANETTO
ZAPATEO
ZEDILLO
ZEMSTVO
ZHIVAGO

•ZO••••
AZODYES
AZOREAN
AZORIAN
OZONISE
OZONIZE
OZONOUS

•Z•O•••
OZONOUS

•Z•••O•
CZARDOM
IZATION

•Z••••O
AZULEJO
IZZATSO

••ZO•••
BAZOOKA
LAZONGA
POZOLES
RAZORED
REZONED
REZONES
UNZONED
UNZONES
VIZORED

••Z•O••
BAZOOKA
BUZZOFF
DOZEOFF
LAZBOYS
OOZEOUT
SIZEONE

••Z••O•
GAZEBOS
GAZEDON
GAZESON
JAZZBOS
REZEROS
ROZANOV

••Z•••O
BIZARRO
IZZATSO
PIZARRO
RIZZUTO
SIZETWO

•••ZO••
AMAZONS
ARIZONA
BELZONI
BLAZONS
BORZOIS
BUZZOFF
CALZONE
CANZONA
CANZONE
CANZONI
ENDZONE
FROZONE
HOTZONE
MAHZORS
MATZOHS
MATZOTH
MISZONE
REDZONE
RHIZOME
RONZONI
SEIZORS
SUBZONE
WARZONE

•••Z•O•
CHEZMOI
FITZROY
JAZZBOS
QUIZNOS
SEIZEON

•••Z••O
CINZANO
CRUZADO
NETZERO
NONZERO
RIZZUTO
SUBZERO

••••ZO•
CORAZON
HORIZON
KUTUZOV
MINIZOO
REBOZOS
VERIZON

••••Z•O
DAREZZO
MINIZOO
PALAZZO

•••••ZO
CARDOZO
CHORIZO
DAREZZO
LORENZO
PALAZZO
SCHERZO

Z•P••••
ZAPATAS
ZAPATEO
ZAPOTEC
ZAPPERS
ZAPPIER
ZAPPING
ZEPHYRS
ZEPPOLE
ZEPPOLI
ZIPCODE
ZIPCUFF
ZIPDISK
ZIPGUNS
ZIPLOCK
ZIPLOCS
ZIPPERS
ZIPPIER
ZIPPING
ZIPSOFF
ZIPTOPS

Z••P•••
ZAPPERS
ZAPPIER
ZAPPING
ZEPPOLE
ZEPPOLI
ZIPPERS
ZIPPIER
ZIPPING

Z•••P••
ZATOPEK

Z••••P•
ZIPTOPS

••Z•P••
MAZEPPA

••Z••P•
MAZEPPA

••Z•••P
SIZEDUP
SIZESUP

•••Z••P
BLAZEUP
FROZEUP
SNAZZUP

••••ZP•
CHUTZPA

••••Z•P
SNAZZUP

••Z•Q••
BEZIQUE

Z•R••••
ZERMATT
ZERNIKE
ZEROING
ZEROOUT
ZEROSIN
ZEROSUM
ZIRCONS

Z••R•••
ZAIRIAN
ZEBRAIC
ZEBRASS
ZEBRINE
ZEBROID
ZIERING

Z•••R••
ZIMARRA
ZYMURGY

Z••••R•
ZACHARY
ZAPPERS
ZEPHYRS
ZESTERS
ZIMARRA
ZINGERS
ZIPPERS
ZITHERS

Z•••••R
ZAPPIER
ZESTIER
ZIEGLER
ZINGIER
ZINKIER
ZIPPIER
ZOELLER
ZONULAR

•Z•R•••
AZOREAN
AZORIAN
AZURITE
CZARDAS
CZARDOM
CZARINA
CZARISM
CZARIST
TZARINA
YZERMAN

•Z•••R•
SZILARD

•Z••••R
AZINGER

••ZR•••
MIZRAHI

••Z•R••
BIZARRE
BIZARRO
HAZARDS
LAZARUS
LIZARDS
MAZARIN
MAZURKA
PIZARRO
RAZORED
REZEROS
VIZORED
WIZARDS

••Z••R•
BAZAARS
BEZIERS
BIZARRE
BIZARRO
BUZZARD
BUZZERS
FIZZERS
GAZZARA
GIZZARD
JAZZERS
LAZZERI
PIZARRO
VIZIERS

••Z•••R
BUZZIER
COZENER
DAZZLER
DIZZIER
FIZZIER
FIZZLER
FUZZIER
GUZZLER
JAZZIER
MUZZIER
MUZZLER
NUZZLER
PUZZLER
SIZZLER

•••ZR••
FITZROY

•••Z•R•
BEEZERS
BLAZERS
BOOZERS
BUZZARD
BUZZERS
DOOZERS
FIZZERS
GAZZARA
GEEZERS
GIZZARD
GLAZERS
GRAZERS
JAZZERS
LAZZERI
MAHZORS
NETZERO
NONZERO
PANZERS
PATZERS
SEIZERS
SEIZORS
SEIZURE
SUBZERO

•••Z••R
BOOZIER
BRAZIER
BUZZIER
CRAZIER
CROZIER
DAZZLER
DITZIER
DIZZIER
FIZZIER
FIZZLER
FOOZLER
FRAZIER
FRIZZER
FUZZIER
GAUZIER
GLAZIER
GRAZIER
GUZZLER
JAZZIER
KLEZMER
MUZZIER
MUZZLER
NUZZLER
PUZZLER
QUIZZER
RITZIER
SIZZLER
WHIZZER
WOOZIER

••••Z•R
ALCAZAR
BENAZIR
BLITZER
BRONZER
ELEAZAR
ELIEZER
FREEZER
FRIZZER
IODIZER
IONIZER
QUIZZER
RESIZER
SALAZAR
SELTZER
SNEEZER
SNOOZER
SWITZER
TWEEZER
WALTZER
WHEEZER
WHIZZER

Z•S••••
ZESTERS
ZESTFUL
ZESTIER
ZESTILY
ZESTING
ZOSIMUS
ZOSSIMA

Z••S•••
ZEMSTVO
ZIPSOFF
ZOSSIMA
ZOYSIAS

Z•••S••
ZAKUSKA
ZENISTS
ZEROSIN
ZEROSUM
ZOOMSIN

Z••••S•
ZANIEST
ZANYISH
ZANYISM
ZEBRASS
ZIONISM
ZIONIST
ZIPDISK
ZOOIEST

Z•••••S
ZAGNUTS
ZAPATAS
ZAPPERS
ZEALOTS
ZEALOUS
ZEBRASS
ZEDONKS
ZENANAS
ZENISTS
ZENITHS
ZEPHYRS
ZESTERS
ZIGZAGS
ZILCHES
ZINCOUS
ZINGERS
ZINNIAS
ZIPGUNS
ZIPLOCS
ZIPPERS
ZIPTOPS
ZIRCONS
ZITCOMS
ZITHERS
ZOCALOS
ZODIACS
ZOMBIES
ZONIANS
ZONULES
ZOSIMUS
ZOYSIAS
ZUNIANS
ZYDECOS
ZYGOTES

•Z•S•••
AZUSACA
SZYSLAK

•Z•••S•
CZARISM
CZARIST
IZZATSO
OZONISE
OZZFEST

•Z••••S
AZALEAS
AZODYES
CZARDAS
OZONOUS
TZIMMES

••ZS•••
VIZSLAS

••Z•S••
BUZZSAW
GAZESAT
GAZESON
SIZESIX
SIZESUP

••Z••S•
COZIEST
DOZIEST
HAZIEST
IZZATSO
JAZZISH
LAZIEST
LAZYISH
MAZIEST
OOZIEST
OZZFEST

••Z•••S
ADZUKIS
BAZAARS
BEZIERS
BUZZERS
COZZENS
DAZZLES
DIZAINS
DIZZIES
ECZEMAS
ENZYMES
FIZGIGS
FIZZERS
FIZZLES
GAZEBOS
GUZZLES
HAZARDS
HAZINGS
HAZMATS
HUZZAHS
JAZZBOS
JAZZERS
KUZNETS
LAZARUS
LAZBOYS
LIZARDS
LIZZIES
MEZUZAS
MIZUNAS
MIZZENS
MIZZLES
MUZZLES
NOZZLES
NUZZLES
POZOLES
PUZZLES
RAZZIES
REZEROS
REZONES
SIZZLES
SUZUKIS
TIZZIES
ULZANAS
UNZONES
VIZIERS
VIZSLAS
WIZARDS

•••ZS••
BUZZSAW

•••Z•S•
JAZZISH

•••Z••S
AMAZONS
BANZAIS
BEEZERS
BLAZERS
BLAZONS
BOOZERS
BORZOIS
BRAZENS
BUZZERS
CHAZANS
COZZENS
CRAZIES
CRUZANS
DAZZLES
DIZZIES
DOOZERS
DOOZIES
FIZZERS
FIZZLES
FOOZLES
FRIZZES
GEEZERS
GLAZERS
GRAZERS
GUZZLES
HUZZAHS
IBIZANS
JAZZBOS
JAZZERS
LIZZIES
MAHZORS
MATZOHS
MENZIES
MIZZENS
MIZZLES
MUZZLES
NOZZLES
NUDZHES
NUZZLES
PANZERS
PATZERS
PENZIAS
PIAZZAS
PRIZZIS
PUZZLES
QUIZNOS
QUIZZES
RAZZIES
SCUZZES
SEIZERS
SEIZORS
SIZZLES
TARZANS
TIZZIES
WHIZZES
ZIGZAGS

••••Z•S
ASSIZES
BEDAZES
BLITZES
BREEZES
BRONZES
CABEZAS
CORYZAS
FREEZES
FRIEZES
FRIZZES
GLITZES
IODIZES
IONIZES
KLUTZES
KWANZAS
MEZUZAS
PIAZZAS
PLOTZES
PRIZZIS
QUINZES
QUIZZES
REBOZOS
RESIZES
SCUZZES
SLEAZES
SNEEZES
SNOOZES
SPITZES
STANZAS
STUTZES
TOPAZES
TREIZES
TWEEZES
UPGAZES

UPSIZES
WALTZES
WHEEZES
WHIZZES

Z•T••••
ZATOPEK
ZITCOMS
ZITHERS

Z••T•••
ZEITUNG
ZESTERS
ZESTFUL
ZESTIER
ZESTILY
ZESTING
ZIPTOPS

Z•••T••
ZABUTON
ZANETTO
ZAPATAS
ZAPATEO
ZAPOTEC
ZEMSTVO
ZENITHS
ZYGOTES

Z••••T•
ZAGNUTS
ZANETTO
ZEALOTS
ZENISTS
ZERMATT
ZINCITE

Z•••••T
ZANIEST
ZERMATT
ZEROOUT
ZIONIST
ZONEOUT
ZONKOUT
ZOOIEST
ZOOMOUT
ZUMWALT

•ZT••••
AZTECAN

•Z•T•••
IZATION

•Z••T••
IZZATSO

•Z•••T•
AZIMUTH
AZURITE

•Z••••T
CZARIST
OZZFEST

••Z•T••
GAZETTE
IZZATSO
LIZETTE
MOZETTA
SIZETEN
SIZETWO
SUZETTE

••Z••T•
DOZENTH
GAZETTE
HAZLITT
HAZMATS
KUZNETS
LIZETTE
MOZETTA
RIZZUTO
SUZETTE

••Z•••T
BUZZCUT
COZIEST
DOZIEST
GAZEDAT
GAZESAT
HAZIEST
HAZLITT
LAZIEST
MAZIEST
OOZEOUT
OOZIEST
OZZFEST

•••Z•T•
MATZOTH
RIZZUTO

•••Z••T
BUZZCUT
VANZANT

••••Z•T
CHEEZIT
RENUZIT

ZU•••••
ZUMWALT
ZUNIANS

Z••U•••
ZABUTON
ZAKUSKA
ZEBULON
ZEBULUN
ZONULAR
ZONULES
ZYMURGY

Z•••U••
ZAGNUTS
ZEITUNG
ZIPCUFF
ZIPGUNS

Z••••U•
ZEALOUS
ZEBULUN
ZEROOUT
ZEROSUM
ZESTFUL
ZINCOUS
ZONEOUT
ZONKOUT
ZOOMOUT
ZOSIMUS

Z•••••U
ZWICKAU

•ZU••••
AZULEJO
AZURITE
AZUSACA

•Z••U••
AZIMUTH

•Z•••U•
OZONOUS

••ZU•••
ADZUKIS
COZUMEL
MAZURKA
MEZUZAH
MEZUZAS
MIZUNAS
SUZUKIS

••Z•U••
RIZZUTO

••Z••U•
BEZIQUE
BUZZCUT
LAZARUS
OOZEOUT
SIZEDUP
SIZESUP

•••ZU••
RIZZUTO
SEIZURE

•••Z•U•
BLAZEUP
BUZZCUT
FROZEUP
SNAZZUP

••••ZU•
SNAZZUP

•••••ZU
SHIHTZU

Z••V•••
ZHIVAGO

Z••••V•
ZEMSTVO

••Z•••V
ROZANOV

•••ZV••
MITZVAH

••••Z•V
KUTUZOV

ZW•••••
ZWANZIG
ZWICKAU
ZWINGLI

Z••W•••
ZUMWALT

••Z••W•
SIZETWO

••Z•••W
BUZZSAW

•••Z••W
BUZZSAW

••Z•••X
SIZESIX

••••Z•X
SKEEZIX

ZY•••••
ZYDECOS
ZYGOTES
ZYMURGY

Z•Y••••
ZOYSIAS

Z••Y•••
ZANYISH
ZANYISM

Z•••Y••
ZEPHYRS

Z•••••Y
ZACHARY
ZELAZNY
ZESTILY
ZINCIFY
ZOMBIFY
ZONALLY
ZOOLOGY
ZYMURGY

•ZY••••
SZYSLAK

•Z••Y••
AZODYES

••ZY•••
COZYING
ENZYMES
ENZYMIC
LAZYISH

••Z••Y•
LAZBOYS

••Z•••Y
DAZEDLY
DIZZILY
FUZZILY
JAZZILY
LAZENBY
MUZZILY
SIZABLY

•••ZY••
GENZYME

•••Z••Y
BOOZILY
CRAZILY
DIZZILY
DRIZZLY
FITZROY
FRIZZLY
FUZZILY
GAUZILY
GLAZILY
GRIZZLY
JAZZILY
MUZZILY
RITZILY
WOOZILY

••••Z•Y
DRIZZLY
FRIZZLY
GRETZKY
GRIZZLY
ZELAZNY

•••••ZY
CHINTZY
GOCRAZY
LOWEEZY
QUARTZY
TEACOZY
UNCRAZY

Z••Z•••
ZIGZAGS

Z•••Z••
ZAGAZIG
ZELAZNY
ZWANZIG

Z••••Z•
ZAMBEZI

•ZZ••••
IZZATSO
OZZFEST

•Z•••Z•
OZONIZE

••ZZ•••
BUZZARD
BUZZCUT
BUZZELL
BUZZERS
BUZZIER
BUZZING
BUZZOFF
BUZZSAW
COZZENS
DAZZLED
DAZZLER
DAZZLES
DIZZIED
DIZZIER
DIZZIES
DIZZILY
FIZZERS
FIZZIER
FIZZING
FIZZLED
FIZZLER
FIZZLES
FUZZIER
FUZZILY
FUZZING
GAZZARA
GIZZARD
GUZZLED
GUZZLER
GUZZLES
HUZZAHS
JAZZAGE
JAZZBOS
JAZZERS
JAZZIER
JAZZILY
JAZZING
JAZZISH
JAZZMAN
JAZZMEN
LAZZERI
LIZZIES
MAZZINI
MIZZENS
MIZZLED
MIZZLES
MUZZIER
MUZZILY
MUZZLED
MUZZLER
MUZZLES
NOZZLES
NUZZLED
NUZZLER
NUZZLES
PIZZAZZ
PUZZLED
PUZZLER
PUZZLES
RAZZIES
RAZZING
RIZZUTO
SIZZLED
SIZZLER
SIZZLES
TIZZIES
WOZZECK

••Z•Z••
MEZUZAH
MEZUZAS

••Z••Z•
PIZZAZZ

••Z•••Z
PIZZAZZ

•••ZZ••
CHAZZAN
DRIZZLE
DRIZZLY
FRAZZLE
FRIZZED
FRIZZER
FRIZZES
FRIZZLE
FRIZZLY
GRIZZLE
GRIZZLY
MUEZZIN
PIAZZAS
PRIZZIS
QUIZZED
QUIZZER
QUIZZES
SCUZZES
SNAZZUP
SWIZZLE
WHIZZED
WHIZZER
WHIZZES

•••Z•Z•
PIZZAZZ

•••Z••Z
PIZZAZZ

••••ZZ•
ABRUZZI
DAREZZO
JACUZZI
PALAZZI
PALAZZO

•••••ZZ
GINFIZZ
OUTBUZZ
PIZZAZZ
SCHNOZZ

Crossword Answer Glossary

A

AAA: Road-service org.
AAAA: Very narrow shoe
AAA CELL: Kind of battery
AAAUGH: Comic-strip cry
AABA: Rhyme scheme
AABBA: Rhyme scheme
AA CELL: Type of battery
AACHEN: German city
A.A. FAIR: Erle Stanley Gardner pen name
AA JUMBO: Type of egg
AA LARGE: Type of egg
AALIYAH: R&B singer
AALTO: Finnish architect
AAMCO: Transmission-repair chain
AAMES: Actor Willie
A.A. MILNE: Winnie-the-Pooh creator
A AND E: "Biography" network
A AND M: Texas school
A AND P: Grocery chain
A AND W: Root-beer brand
AAR: Swiss river
AA RATED: High-quality, as a bond
AARAU: Swiss town
AARE: Swiss river
AARGAU: Swiss canton
AARGH: Comic-strip cry
AARHUS: Danish city
AARON: Brother of Moses
AARP: Seniors' org.
AAS: Some batteries
AASE: Peer Gynt's mother
AAU: Amateur sports org.
ABA: Lawyers' org.
ABAA: Rhyme scheme
ABAB: Rhyme scheme
ABABA: Addis __, Ethiopia
ABACA: Philippine plant
ABACAB: Genesis rock album
ABACO: Bahama island group
ABAFT: Astern
ABAJO: Down: Spanish
A BAS: Down with: French
ABATIS: Barricade of trees
ABBA: Eban of Israel
ABBADO: Italian conductor
ABBAS: Eastern bishops
ABBE: French cleric
ABBIE: 1960s radical Hoffman
ABBOTT: Comedian Bud
ABBY: "Dear __" (advice column)
ABDEL: Gamal __ Nasser
ABDIEL: "Paradise Lost" angel
ABDUCE: Draw away
ABDUL: Singer Paula
ABE: Lincoln nickname
ABEAM: Nautical direction
A BEAR: Very difficult
ABED: Still sleeping
ABEL: Brother of Cain
ABELARD: French philosopher
ABELE: Poplar tree
ABEND: Evening: German
ABER: But: German
AB FAB: British sitcom, for short
ABIDJAN: Ivory Coast capital
ABIE'S: "__ Irish Rose"
ABIGAIL: First lady Adams
ABILENE: Texas city
AB INTRA: From the inside: Latin
ABIOTIC: Not involving organisms
ABITIBI: Canadian river
ABJURE: Renounce
ABLATE: Erode
ABM: Arms-treaty subj.
ABMHO: Conductance unit
ABNER: "Li'l __"
ABO: Blood group
ABOHM: Resistance unit
ABOLLA: Roman cloak
ABOMA: South American snake
ABORAL: Away from the mouth
ABOU: "__ Ben Adhem" (Hunt poem)
ABOUT IT: Everything
AB OVO: From the beginning: Latin
ABR: Shortened: Abbr.
ABRA: Cadabra preceder
ABRAHAM: Biblical patriarch
ABRAM: Biblical patriarch
ABRAMS: Vietnam War general
ABRAXAS: Santana album
ABRI: Dugout shelter
ABRIL: April: Spanish
ABRUZZI: Italian region
ABS: Belly muscles
ABSALOM: Son of King David
ABSCAM: 1970s FBI sting
ABSCISE: Cut off
ABSOLUT: Vodka brand
ABT: Dance company: Abbr.
ABU: __ Dhabi
ABUJA: Nigerian capital
ABUT ON: Lie next to
ABY: Ending for lull
ABZUG: Former Big Apple congresswoman
ACA: Here: Spanish
ACADIA: Maine national park
ACADIAN: Cajun
ACANTHI: Mediterranean plants
ACAR: Mite: Comb. form
ACARID: Mite
ACAUDAL: Tailless
ACC: IRS employee
ACCRA: Ghana capital
ACD: Sherlock's creator's monogram
AC DELCO: Auto-parts brand
ACEDIA: Laziness
ACE IT: Do extremely well
ACELA: Fast Amtrak train
ACER: Skillful server
ACERATE: Needle-shaped
ACERB: Sour
ACERBIC: Sour
ACEROLA: Cherrylike fruit
ACEROSE: Needle-shaped
ACES UP: Poker hand
ACETAL: Organic solvent
ACETO: Vinegar: Comb. form
ACETYL: Vinegar radical
ACEY: __-deucy
ACH: German exclamation
ACHEBE: Nigerian novelist
ACHENE: Strawberry part
ACHERON: Mythical river
ACHESON: Truman cabinet member
ACHIEVA: Oldsmobile model
ACHILLE: "__ Lauro" (cruise ship)
ACHT: Eight: German
ACHTUNG: Attention: German
ACIS: Galatea's love
ACK: Comic-strip cry
ACK-ACK: Antiaircraft gun
ACLU: Rights org.
ACOLYTE: Aide
ACONITE: Plant of the buttercup family
ACQUA: Water: Italian
ACR: Height: Comb. form
ACRO: Height: Comb. form
ACS: Apt. amenities
ACTA: Official proceedings
ACTAEON: Mythical hunter
ACT AS: Have the role of
ACTE: Act: French
ACTER: One-__ (type of play)
ACTH: Growth hormone: Abbr.
ACT I: Play part
ACTIFED: Cold-remedy brand
ACT II: Play part
ACT III: Play part
ACTINON: Isotope of radon
ACTIUM: Battle site of 31 B.C.
ACT IV: Play part
ACTIVA: Citroën model
ACTO: Act: Spanish
ACT V: Play part
ACU: Needle: Comb. form
ACUATE: Pointed
ACUFF: Country singer Roy
ACURA: Honda make
ACY: Noun ending
ADA: Dentists' org.
ADAH: Wife of Esau
ADAIR: Oil-rig firefighter
ADAK: Alaskan island
ADAMA: "Battlestar Galactica" role
ADAMITE: Human being
ADAMSES: 1790s First Family
ADAMSON: "Born Free" author
ADANA: City in Turkey
ADANO: "A Bell for __"
ADA, OK: Sooner State city
ADAR: Hebrew month
A DARN: The slightest amount
AD-AWARE: Protective software
AD BIZ: Madison Avenue industry
ADC: Military asst.
ADDAMS: Cartoonist Charles
ADDAX: African antelope
ADDIE: "Paper Moon" character
ADDIO: Good-bye: Italian
ADDIS: __ Ababa, Ethiopia
ADDISON: English essayist
ADDUCE: Affirm
ADDUCT: Bring together
ADE: Citrus drink
ADEEM: Revoke, in law
ADELA: "A Passage to India" character
ADELE: "Die Fledermaus" maid
ADELE H.: Isabelle Adjani role
ADELIE: Type of penguin
ADELINA: Opera singer Patti
ADELINE: "Sweet __" (old song)
ADELLE: Author Davis
ADELPHI: Long Island university
ADEN: Port of Yemen
ADENINE: DNA component
ADENO: Gland: Comb. form
ADESTE: "__ Fideles" (Christmas carol)
A DEUX: For two: French
ADHEM: "Abou Ben __" (Hunt poem)
ADHIBIT: Let in
ADIA: Sarah McLachlan tune
ADIDAS: Running-shoe brand
ADIGE: Italian river

AD IN: Tennis situation
ADIT: Mine entrance
ADJANI: Actress Isabelle
ADJT: Mil. assistant
ADJURE: Entreat
ADL: B'nai B'rith org.
ADLAI: Illinois politician Stevenson
ADLER: "Damn Yankees" composer
ADNAN: Arms merchant Khashoggi
ADNATE: Attached
ADNOUN: Adjective used as a noun
ADOBO: Mexican marinade
ADOLF: Violinist Busch
ADOLFO: Nancy Reagan's designer
ADOLPH: Brewer Coors
ADOLPHE: Actor Menjou
ADONAI: Hebrew Almighty
ADONAIS: Shelley poem
ADONIS: Handsome man
ADOREE: Actress Renée
AD OUT: Tennis situation
ADP: Payroll-processing co.
AD RATE: Classified cost
AD REM: Pertinent
ADRENO: ACTH part
AD REP: Newspaper employee
ADRIAN: Director Lyne
ADRIANA: "Comedy of Errors" character
ADRIEN: Arpel of cosmetics
A DRIVE: Computer-disk slot
ADSORB: Gather on a surface
A DUE: Together, in music
ADUST: Scorched
ADVERT: Allude (to)
ADVIL: Pain-reliever brand
AD WAR: Media battle of a sort
ADWARE: Ads integrated into software
AD WEEK: Madison Ave. magazine
ADYTUM: Inner sanctum
ADZ: Axlike tool
ADZE: Axlike tool
ADZUKI: Asian bean
AEAEA: Circe's home, in Greek myth
AEC: 1960s nuclear agcy.
AECIUM: Fungal spore sac
AEDES: Mosquito genus
AEDILE: Roman magistrate
AEF: WWI army
AEGEAN: Arm of the Mediterranean
AEGIR: Norse sea god
AEIOU: Vowel sequence
AELFRIC: Anglo-Saxon writer
AENEAS: Trojan hero
AENEID: Vergil epic poem
AEOLIA: Ancient Greek colony
AEOLUS: Greek wind god
AEON: Geologic time unit
AER: __ Lingus (Irish airline)
AEREO: Correo __ (Spanish airmail)
AERI: Atmosphere: Comb. form
AERIE: Eagle's nest
AERIO: Suzuki model
AERO: Nautical prefix
AEROBAT: Stunt flyer
AEROBE: Bacterium
AEROS: Akron baseball team
AES: JFK's UN ambassador
AESIR: Norse gods
AESOP'S: "__ Fables"
AETHER: Heavens
AETNA: Insurance company
AFARS: Nomadic Muslim people
A FAT LOT: Little, if any
AFB: Mil. outpost
AFC: Pro football grp.
AFFAIRE: __ d'honneur (duel)
AFFIANT: Notary-public user
AFFINE: In-law
AFFINED: Closely related
AFFLECK: Actor Ben
AFFRAY: Brawl
AFG.: Pak. neighbor
A FIFTH: Twenty percent
A FIG: The slightest amount
AFL: CIO partner
AFLAC: Insurance company
A.F. OF L.: Labor group, for short
AFORE: Ere
A-FRAME: Home style
AFROPOP: Music genre
AFS: Mil. branches
AFTA: Aftershave brand
AFTERS: Dessert, in Britain
AFTON: Scottish river
AFTRA: Actors' org.
AGA: Turkish title
AGADIR: Moroccan city
AGA KHAN: Islamic leader
AGAL: Arab headcord
AGAMA: Type of lizard
A-GAME: Top performance level
AGANA: Capital of Guam
AGAR: Culture medium
AGARIC: Common mushroom
AGARN: "F Troop" corporal
AGASSI: Tennis pro Andre
AGASSIZ: Zoologist Louis
AGATHA: Author Christie
AGATINE: Marblelike
AGAVE: Arizona plant
AGAWAM: Massachusetts city
AGEE: "The African Queen" screenwriter
AGENA: 1960s rocket stage
AGENCE: Bureau: French
AGENT J: Will Smith, in "Men in Black"
AGENT K: Tommy Lee Jones, in "Men in Black"
AGFA: Film brand
AGHA: Turkish title
AGI: Tax-return line: Abbr.
AGIN: Not "fer"
AGIO: Exchange premium
AGIS: Spartan king
AGITA: Heartburn
AGITATO: Excitedly, in music
AGLAIA: One of the Graces
AGLET: Shoelace tip
AGLEY: "...gang aft __": Robert Burns
AGNAIL: Finger inflammation
AGNATE: Male relative
AGNES: Actress Moorehead
AGNEW: Nixon vice president
AGNI: Hindu fire god
AGNOMEN: Nickname
AGNON: Israeli literature Nobelist
AGNUS: "__ Dei" (Christian prayer)
A GOGO: Galore
AGON: Ancient Greek contest
AGONISM: Verbal combat
AGORA: Ancient Greek marketplace
AGOROT: Israeli money
AGOSTO: August: Italian
AGOUTI: Rabbitlike rodent
AGR.: Cabinet dept.
AGRA: Taj Mahal site
AGRI: Farming: Comb. form
AGRIBIZ: Farming, familiarly
AGRIPPA: Roman general
AGRO: Soil: Comb. form
AGRON: Crop management: Abbr.
AGS.: Cabinet offs.
AGST.: Opposed to: Abbr.
AGUA: Water: Spanish
AGUE: Flu symptom
AGULHAS: African Cape
AGURA: Israeli coin
AGUTTER: Actress Jenny
AGWAY: Supermarket chain
AHAB: "Moby-Dick" captain
AH AH: "Don't do that!"
A HAIR: The slighest amount
A HANG: The slightest amount
A HASSLE: Very inconvenient
A HEAP: Considerably
AHERNE: Actor Brian
AHI: Hawaiian tuna
AHIMSA: Buddhist principle
AHMAD: Sportscaster Rashad
AHMED: "Arabian Nights" prince
AHN: Actor Philip
AHOLIC: Addict: Comb. form
A HOOT: The slightest amount
AHORA: Now: Spanish
AHORSE: On a stallion
A HOST OF: Many
AH SIN: Harte/Twain character
AH SO: Cry of acknowledgment
AIA: Architects' org.
AIC: Chemists' org.
AIDA: Verdi opera
AIDAN: Actor Quinn
AIDMAN: Army medic
AIDOO: Ghanian author
AIEA: Hawaiian city
AIELLO: Actor Danny
AIG: Insurance company
AIGLET: Shoelace tip
AIGRET: Plume
AIKEN: Poet Conrad
AIKIDO: Martial art
AIKMAN: Troy of football
AILE: Wing: French
AILEEN: Actress Quinn
AILERON: Airplane part
AILEY: Choreographer Alvin
AILUR: Cat: Comb. form
AILURO: Cat: Comb. form
AIME: Love: French
AIMEE: Actress Anouk
AIN: Own: Scottish
AINGE: Danny of basketball
AINSI: Thus: French
AIN'T HAY: Is of value, slangily
AINU: Japanese aborigine
AIOLI: Garlic-flavored mayonnaise
AIRBALL: Hoops missed shot
AIR BUD: 1997 Disney film
AIR DAM: Auto part
AIRDRIE: Scottish city
AIRE: Leeds' river
AIRES: Buenos __, Argentina
AIRFOIL: Plane wing
AIRFONE: Inflight calling service
AIRMADA: Large fleet of planes
AIRNESS: His __ (Michael Jordan nickname)
AIR POP: Prepare snack corn, perhaps
AIRPOT: Insulated coffee container
AIR-SEA: Like some Coast Guard rescues
AIR SIGN: Libra, for one
AIR TRAP: Barometer device
AIR UP: Inflate
AIRWICK: Freshener brand
AIRWOLF: 1980s TV action series
AIS: Three-toed sloths
AISHA: Wife of Muhammad
AISNE: French river
AIT: River island
AIWA: Electronics brand
AIX: __-en-Provence, France
AJA: Steely Dan album
AJACCIO: Corsican port
AJAX: Trojan War hero
A.J. FOYT: Auto racer
AJI: Chili pepper
AJIJIC: Mexican city
AJO: Garlic: Spanish
AJOWAN: Flower of India
A.J.S: Racer Foyt and novelist Cronin
A.J. SIMON: Jameson Parker TV role
AKA: Wanted-poster letters
AKAI: Car-stereo brand
AKBAR: Emperor of India
AKC: Canine grp.
AKEBONO: Hawaiian sumo wrestler
AKEEM: Olajuwon of basketball
AKELA: Cub Scout leader
AKENE: Buttercup
AKERLOF: 2001 economics Nobelist
AKERS: Singer Karen
AKIHITO: Emperor of Japan
AKIM: Actor Tamiroff
AKINS: Actor Claude
AKIN TO: Like
AKIO: Sony cofounder Morita
AKIRA: Director Kurosawa
AKITA: Japanese dog
AKRON, OH: Midwest city
AKSAKOV: Russian writer
AKU-AKU: Heyerdahl book
ALABAM': "Midnight Choo Choo" destination

ALABAMY: State, slangily
A LACK OF: No
ALADINE: "Faerie Queene" character
ALADO: Winged: Spanish
ALAE: Wings: Latin
ALAI: Jai __
ALAIN: Novelist Lesage
ALAINA: Actress __ Reed Hall
ALAIS: Russian mountain range
A LA KING: Chicken style
ALALA: Hawaiian bird
ALAMEDA: California city
ALAMEIN: El __ (Egyptian WWII battle site)
ALAMOS: Poplar trees
ALAMOSA: Colorado city
ALAN: Actor Alda
ALANA: George Hamilton ex
ALANINE: Protein component
ALANIS: Singer Morissette
ALAN JAY: Lyricist Lerner
ALANNAH: Singer Myles
AL-ANON: AA offshoot
ALAR: Winglike
ALARBUS: "Titus Andronicus" role
ALARCON: Spainish writer
ALARIC: Conqueror of Rome
ALARUM: Call to arms
ALASKAS: Baked __ (desserts)
AL-ASSAD: Former Syrian president
ALATE: Winged
ALATEEN: Kids' support group
ALAVA: Cape in Washington State
A-LAYING: "Six geese __..."
ALB: Church vestment
ALBA: Actress Jessica
ALBAN: Composer Berg
ALBANIA: European country
ALBANO: Italian lake
ALBANS: St. __ (city near London)
ALBANY: New York capital
ALBAS: Troubadour love songs
ALBEDO: Astronomer's light ratio
ALBEE: Playwright Edward
ALBEIT: Although
ALBEN: Truman vice president Barkley
ALBENIZ: Spanish composer
ALBERS: German artist
ALBERT: Victoria's husband
ALBERTA: Canadian province
ALBERT I: Belgian king
ALBERTO: Fujimori of Peru
ALBINE: "Thaïs" role
ALBINO: Pigmentless animal
ALBION: Literary term for Britain
ALBIREO: Star in Cygnus
ALBOM: "Tuesdays With Morrie" author
ALBORAK: Mohammed's horse
ALBORG: Danish city
AL B. SURE: 1980s pop singer
ALBUMEN: Egg white
ALBUMIN: Milk protein
AL BUNDY: "Married...With Children" role
ALC.: Vodka, e.g.: Abbr.
ALCAIDE: Mexican warden
ALCALDE: Mexican mayor
ALCAN: Highway to Fairbanks
AL CAPP: "Li'l Abner" cartoonist
ALCAZAR: Seville castle
ALCESTE: Gluck opera
ALCHEMY: Medieval "science"
ALCINA: Handel opera
ALCOA: Foil brand
ALCOPOP: Soft drink with liquor
ALCOR: Big Dipper star
ALCOTT: Author Louisa May
ALCS: World Series prelude: Abbr.
ALCYONE: Star in Taurus
ALD.: City official: Abbr.
ALDA: Actor Alan
AL DAVIS: Pro football Hall of Fame executive
ALDEN: "Mayflower" passenger
AL DENTE: Pasta specification
ALDER: Cabinet wood
ALDINE: Italic type
ALDISS: Author Brian
ALDO RAY: Actor
ALDOUS: Author Huxley
ALDRICH: Nelson __ Rockefeller
ALDRIN: Apollo astronaut
AL DUBIN: "Lullaby of Broadway" lyricist
ALEA: Athena epithet
ALEARDI: Italian poet
A.L. EAST: Yankees' div.
ALEC: Actor Baldwin
ALECTO: One of the Furies
ALEE: Nautical direction
ALEF: Hebrew letter
ALEGAR: Ale vinegar
ALEGRE: Pôrto __, Brazil
ALEGRIA: Joy: Spanish
A LEG UP: Assistance
ALEK: Supermodel Wek
ALE KEG: Pub delivery
ALEKSEI: Soviet leader Kosygin
ALEMAN: 1940s Mexican president
ALEMBIC: Distillery vessel
ALEN: Architect William Van __
ALENCON: French lace
ALENE: Coeur d'__, ID
ALEPH: Hebrew letter
ALEPPO: Syrian city
ALER: Oriole or Yank
ALERO: Oldsmobile model
ALETA: Prince Valiant's wife
ALE TAP: Tavern fixture
ALETTE: Building wing
ALEUT: Alaska native
ALEVE: Pain-reliever brand
A LEVEL: British school exam
ALEWIFE: North American fish
ALEX: Emcee Trebek
ALEXA: Billy Joel's daughter
ALEXAS: "Antony and Cleopatra" character
ALEXEI: "Anna Karenina" character
ALEXEY: "Anna Karenina" character
ALEXI: Cosmonaut Leonov
ALEXIA: Inability to read
ALEXIS: "Dynasty" role
ALEYARD: Pub vessel
ALF: 1936 presidential candidate Landon
ALFA: __ Romeo (auto)
ALFALFA: "Our Gang" character
ALFEROV: Russian physics Nobelist
ALFIE: Michael Caine role
ALFIERI: Italian playwright
AL FINE: Musical direction
ALFIO: "Winter of Our Discontent" character
ALFONSE: Former New York senator D'Amato
ALFONSO: Former king of Spain
ALFORJA: Saddlebag
ALFRE: Actress Woodard
ALFRED: "Batman" butler
ALFRED A.: Publisher Knopf
ALFRED E.: Neuman of "Mad" magazine
ALFREDO: Pasta sauce
ALFRED U.: NY school
ALFVEN: Swedish physics Nobelist
ALG.: H.S. math
ALGARVE: Portuguese region
ALGEDI: Star in Capricorn
ALGER: Author Horatio
ALGERIA: African country
ALGIA: Pain: Comb. form
ALGID: Chilly
ALGIEBA: Star in Leo
ALGIERS: African capital
ALGOL: Computer language
AL GORE: "Earth in the Balance" author
AL GREEN: "I'm Still in Love With You" singer
ALGREN: Author Nelson
AL HAIG: Former NATO chief
ALHENA: Star in Gemini
AL HIRT: Dixieland trumpeter
ALIA: Et __ (and others)
ALIBLE: Nourishing, old-style
ALICE: Mrs. Kramden
ALICE B.: Writer Toklas
ALICE'S: "__ Restaurant" (Guthrie tune)
ALICIA: Actress Silverstone
ALIDA: Actress Valli
ALIDADE: Surveyor's instrument
ALIENEE: Proprerty recipient
ALIENOR: One who transfers property
ALIF: Arabic letter
ALIFORM: Wing-shaped
ALIGOTE: French wine
ALII: Et __ (and others)
ALIKES: Look-__ (twins)
ALIMENT: Food
ALIOS: Inter __ (among others)
ALIOTH: Star in Ursa Major
ALIOTO: Former San Francisco mayor
ALIPED: Like a bat
ALISA: "Lucia di Lammermoor" character
ALISON: Author Lurie
A-LIST: Desirable guests
ALITO: 2006 Supreme Court appointee
ALITY: Noun suffix
ALIVE-O: "Cockles and Mussels" word
ALIVE TO: Aware of
ALIX: Actress __ Elias
ALIYAH: Synagogue ritual
ALIYOT: Synagogue rituals
ALK.: Kind of battery: Abbr.
ALKA: __-Seltzer
AL KAB: Star in Auriga
AL KAID: Star in Ursa Major
ALKENE: Ethylene, e.g.
ALKI: Washington State motto
ALKY: Hooch
ALKYD: Paint ingredient
ALKYL: Hydrocarbon radical
ALLA: __ breve (music term)
ALL AGES: Everyone
ALLAH: Islamic Almighty
ALLAIS: French economics Nobelist
ALLAN: Humorist Sherman
ALLANTE: Cadillac model
ALL-BRAN: Cereal brand
ALL CAPS: Proofreading notation
ALL-CLAD: Cookware brand
ALLE: All: German
ALL EARS: Alert
ALLEE: Path: French
ALLEGRA: Antihistimine brand
ALLEGRO: Brisk tempo
ALLELE: Form of a gene
ALL ELSE: The remainder
ALLEN: Director Woody
ALLENBY: WWI British field marshal
ALLENDE: Chilean author
ALLER: To go: French
ALLES: "Deutschland uber __"
AL LEWIS: "The Munsters" actor
ALL EYES: Attentive
ALLEYN: Fictional detective
ALLEZ: Go!: French
ALLHEAL: Curative plant
ALLIE: Kate's TV mate
ALL IN: Exhausted
ALLIS: Chalmers' business partner
ALLISON: Auto racer Bobby
ALLIUM: Garden bulb
ALL MAN: Virile
ALL-NEWS: Radio-station format
ALLO: Other: Comb. form
ALL OF ME: Steve Martin film
ALL OF US: The whole gang
ALL OK: Satisfactory
ALLONGE: Stretched, in ballet
ALLONYM: Pen name
AL LOPEZ: Baseball Hall of Fame manager
ALLOWAY: Robert Burns' birthplace
ALL-PRO: NFL designation
ALL RISE: Bailiff's command
ALLSTON: Painter Washington
ALLUVIA: River deposits
ALLYCE: Actress Beasley
ALLYL: Hydrocarbon radical
ALLYN: Actor Joslyn

ALLYSON: Actress June
ALMA: __ mater
ALMA-ATA: Kazakhstan city
ALMAAZ: Star in Auriga
ALMACH: Star in Andromeda
ALMADEN: Wine brand
ALMATY: Kazakhstan city
ALMAY: Cosmetics brand
ALMERIA: Spanish port
ALMONER: Social worker, in Britain
ALMONRY: Place where charity is distributed
A.L. MVP: Baseball honoree
ALNASL: Star in Sagittarius
ALNICO: Alloy
ALNILAM: Star in Orion
ALNITAK: Star in Orion
ALNIYAT: Star in Scorpio
A LOAD OF: Much
ALOGIA: Loss of speech
ALOHA OE: Hawaiian song
ALOIS: Arnold __ Schwarzenegger
ALOMAR: Roberto of baseball
ALONGS: Take-__
ALONSO: "The Tempest" character
ALONZO: Football coach Amos __ Stagg
ALOP: Cockeyed
ALORS: Then: French
ALOU: Moises of baseball
ALOW: In a ship's hold
ALPACA: Andes animal
ALPE: French mountain
ALPEN: Austrian mountains
ALPERT: Trumpeter Herb
ALPH: Coleridge's sacred river
ALPHARD: Star in Hydra
ALPINER: Certain skier
ALPO: Dog-food brand
ALQUIST: "R.U.R." character
AL RITZ: Comedy-trio member
AL ROKER: TV weatherman
AL ROSEN: 1953 AL MVP
ALROY: "Cakes and Ale" character
ALS: Capp and Capone
ALSAB: 1942 Preakness winner
ALSACE: French region
ALSATIA: Ancient European region
ALSHAIN: Star in Aquila
AL SMITH: 1928 presidential candidate
ALSOP: Columnist Joseph
ALSTON: 1950s Dodger manager
ALTA: Utah resort
ALTAI: Asian mountain range
ALTAIC: Eurasian language group
ALTAIR: Star in Aquila
ALTARF: Star in Cancer
ALTDORF: Home of William Tell
ALTE: "Der __" (Adenauer)
ALTHEA: Tennis star Gibson
ALTHING: Iceland legislature
ALTHORN: Brass instrument
ALTI: High: Comb. form
ALTIMA: Nissan model
ALTIUS: Higher: Latin
ALTMAN: Director Robert
ALTOIDS: Breath-mint brand
ALTON: Illinois city
ALTOONA: Pennsylvania city
ALTRIA: Fortune 500 firm
ALT TAB: Switch Windows programs
ALTUS: Oklahoma city
ALUDEL: Lab vessel
ALUDRA: Star in Canis Major
A LUI: His: French
ALUKO: Nigerian writer
ALULA: False wing
ALUMINA: Metal oxide
AL UNSER: Auto racer
ALVA: Thomas __ Edison
ALVAR: Finnish architect Aalto
ALVAREZ: 1968 physics Nobelist
ALVARO: Italian novelist
ALVEOLI: Lung cells
ALVIN: Choreographer Ailey
ALVING: "Ghosts" character
ALVINO: Bandleader Rey
ALVY: Woody, in "Annie Hall"
A.L. W.: Seattle Mariners' div.
A.L. WEST: Seattle Mariners' div.
ALWORTH: Lance of football
ALYCE: Asian clover
ALYDAR: 1970s racehorse
ALY KHAN: Rita Hayworth ex
ALYN: First film Superman
ALYOSHA: Karamazov brother
ALYSSA: Actress Milano
ALYSSUM: Plant of the mustard family
ALZADO: Lyle of football
ALZIRA: Verdi opera
AMA: Doctors' org.
AMADA: Beloved: Spanish
AMADEO: Physicist Avogadro
AMADEUS: Mozart's middle name
AMADIS: Lully opera
AMADO: Brazilian novelist
AMAH: Asian nurse
AMAHL: Menotti opera subject
AMAIN: At full force, old-style
A MAJ.: Mus. key
AMALFI: Italian town
AMALIA: "The Castle" character
AMALIE: Charlotte __, VI
AMANA: Appliance brand
AMAND: Patron saint of innkeepers
AMANDA: Actress Plummer
AMANITA: Poisonous fungus
AMANT: Lover: French
AMANTI: Kia model
AMAPA: Brazilian region
AMAPOLA: Jimmy Dorsey tune
AMARA: Soprano Lucine
AMARE: To love: Italian
AMARNA: Egypt archeological site
AMARONE: Italian wine
AMAS: You love: Latin
AMAT: He loves: Latin
AMATI: Italian violin
AMATO: Italian baritone
AMATOL: Explosive mixture
AMAZIN': The __ Mets
AM BAND: Transistor radio feature
AMBI: Both: Prefix
AMBIEN: Sleep-aid brand
AMBIENT: Surrounding
AMBIT: Boundary
AMBLIN: Spielberg production company
AMBO: Church desk
AMBOY: Perth __, NJ
AMBROSE: Writer Bierce
AMBRY: Church cupboard
AMC: Former auto make
AME: Soul: French
AMECHE: Actor Don
AMEDEE: Ionesco play
AMEDEO: Artist Modigliani
AMEER: Arab leader
AMELIA: Aviator Earhart
AMELIE: 2001 French film
AMEN-RA: Egyptian god
AMENT: Catkin
AMERADA: __ Hess (oil company)
AMERCE: Punish by fine
AMERIGO: Explorer Vespucci
AMERIKA: Kafka novel
AMERIND: Apache or Paiute
AMERY: Antarctic ice shelf
AMES: Actor Ed
AMES, IA: Midwest city
AMESLAN: Gestural speaking
AMEX: Stock-trading venue
AMF: Bowling-alley manufacturer
AMHARIC: Ethiopian language
AMHERST: Massachusetts city
AMI: Friend: French
AM I BLUE: Ethel Waters tune
AMIC: Of an ammonia compound
AMICA: Friend: Italian
AMICAL: Friendly
AMICE: Church vestment
AMICHAI: Israeli poet
AMICI: Friends: Italian
AMICK: Actress Madchen
AMICO: Friend: Italian
AMICUS: Friend: Latin
AMIDALA: "Star Wars" series princess
AMIDAS: "Faerie Queene" character
AMIDE: Ammonia derivative
AMIDOL: Film-developing chemical
AMIE: Friend: French
AMIEL: Director Jon
AMIENS: French city
AMIGA: Friend: Spanish
AMIGO: Friend: Spanish
AMII: Singer Stewart
AM I LATE: Tardy person's query
AMIN: 1970s African dictator
AMINE: Ammonia derivative
AMINO: __ acid (protein component)
AMINTA: Tasso play
AMIR: Arab leader
AMIRI: Poet Baraka
AMISTAD: Spielberg film
A MITE: Slightly
AMITIE: Friendship: French
AM LIT: Eng. Dept. course
AMMAN: Capital of Jordan
AMMETER: Current measurer
AMNERIS: "Aïda" character
AMNIA: Embryo membranes
AMNION: Embryo membrane
AMO: I love: Latin
AMOCO: British Petroleum acquisition
A MOI: Mine: French
AMOLE: Soap plant
AMON: Egyptian god
AMON-RA: Egyptian god
AMOR: Love: Spanish
AMORE: Love: Italian
AMORES: Book by Ovid
AMORET: "Faerie Queene" character
AMOROSO: Spanish sherry
AMORS: Asteroid group
AMORT: Spiritless, old-style
AMORY: Writer Cleveland
AMOS: Wally of cookies
AMOS OZ: Israeli author
AMOUR: Love: French
AMOY: Chinese island
AMPAS: Oscars org.
AMPHI: Both: Comb. form
AMPHION: Husband of Niobe
AMPHORA: Ancient storage jar
AMRAM: Father of Moses
AMREETA: Hindu nectar
AMRITA: Hindu nectar
AM SO: "Are not!" response
AMSTEL: Beer brand
AM TOO: "Are not!" response
AMTRAC: Amphibious vehicle
AMTRACK: Amphibious vehicle
AMTRAK: Railroad corporation
AMU: __ Darya (Asian river)
AMUL: Iranian city
AMUR: Asian river
AMUSE ME: "Say something funny!"
A MUST: Imperative
AMVET: Former GI
AMWAY: Home-products company
AMY: Poet Lowell
AMYAS: "Faerie Queene" character
AMYL: Organic radical
AMYLASE: Enzyme
AMYLO: Starch: Comb. form
AMY TAN: "The Joy Luck Club" author
ANA: Santa __, CA
ANACIN: Pain-reliever brand
ANADEM: Head wreath
ANAG.: Bit of wd. play
ANAHEIM: California city
ANAIS: Diarist Nin
ANAKIN: Darth Vader's real name
ANALYTE: Something being analyzed
ANANA: Pineapple
ANAND: Chessmaster of India
ANANIAS: Biblical liar
ANANKE: Moon of Jupiter
ANAPEST: Poetic foot
ANASAZI: Type of bean
ANAT.: Art sch. class
ANATASE: White pigment
ANATOLE: Writer France
ANATOLY: Chessmaster Karpov

ANATTO: Yellow-red dye
ANBESOL: Pain-reliever brand
ANC.: Very old: Abbr.
ANCE: Noun suffix
ANCHO: Chili pepper
ANCIEN: Ancient: French
ANCON: Architectural bracket
ANCY: Noun suffix
ANDAMAN: Asian sea
ANDANTE: Slow tempo
ANDERS: Astronomer Celsius
ANDIAMO: Let's go: Italian
ANDIE: Actress MacDowell
ANDIRON: Fireplace stand
AND MORE: Infomercial phrase
AND/OR: Legalese conjunction
ANDORRA: European republic
ANDOVER: Massachusetts prep school
ANDRADE: Brazilian poet
ANDRAE: Gospel singer Crouch
ANDRE: Conductor Previn
ANDREA: Singer McArdle
ANDREAS: San __ fault
ANDREI: Diplomat Gromyko
ANDRES: Guitarist Segovia
ANDRESS: Actress Ursula
ANDREW: Composer __ Lloyd Webber
ANDREWS: Actress Julie
ANDREY: "War and Peace" character
ANDRIC: Serbo-Croatian writer
ANDRO: Male: Comb. form
ANDROID: Sci-fi being
ANDROS: Bahamas island
ANDROUS: Male: Comb. form
ANDRY: Male: Comb. form
AND SO ON: Et cetera
AND SUCH: Et cetera
AND UP: Ad-sign small print
ANDY: Raggedy doll
ANDY'S: "__ Gang" (1950s kids' show)
ANE: Actress Sue __ Langdon
ANELE: Anoint, old-style
ANEMO: Wind: Comb. form
ANENT: Concerning
ANERGY: Lack of energy
ANEROID: Type of barometer
ANES: Donkeys: French
ANETO: Spanish mountain
ANG: Director Lee
ANGA: Yoga practice
ANGE: Angel: French
ANGELA: Actress Lansbury
ANGELA'S: "__ Ashes" (McCourt book)
ANGELI: Actress Pier
ANGELL: Baseball author Roger
ANGELO: "Measure for Measure" character
ANGELOU: Writer Maya
ANGELUS: Church bell
ANGIE: Actress Dickinson
ANGIO: Blood vessel: Comb. form
ANGKOR: __ Wat (Cambodian ruins site)
ANGLAIS: English: French
ANG LEE: "Crouching Tiger, Hidden Dragon" director
ANGLIA: England: Latin
ANGLIC: Old English dialect
ANGOLA: African country
ANGUS: Bovine breed
ANI: Black cuckoo
ANIGH: Near, old-style
ANIL: Indigo dye
ANILE: Doddering
ANILINE: Dye source
ANIM.: Lively, in mus.
ANIMA: Soul
ANIMATO: Lively, in music
ANIME: Japanese movie genre
ANIMES: Varnish resins
ANIMISM: Belief in souls
ANIMO: Mind: Latin
ANIMUS: Antagonism
ANION: Charged atom
ANISE: Liqueur flavoring
ANISEED: Liqueur flavoring
ANISTON: Actress Jennifer
ANITA: Singer Baker
ANITRA'S: "__ Dance" ("Peer Gynt" part)
ANJOU: Type of pear
ANKA: Singer Paul
ANKARA: Capital of Turkey
ANKE: Huber of tennis
ANKH: Egyptian cross
ANN: Author Beattie
ANNA: Author Sewell
ANNABEL: "__ Lee" (Poe poem)
ANNAKIN: Director Ken
ANNA LEE: "General Hospital" actress
ANNALES: Tacitus work
ANNAM: Part of Vietnam
ANNA MAY: Actress Wong
ANNAN: U.N. head
ANNAS: Former coins of India
ANNATTO: Yellow-red dye
ANNE: Daughter of Queen Elizabeth
ANNEAL: Toughen
ANNEE: Year: French
ANNELID: Earthworm
ANNETTE: Actress Funicello
ANNIE: Comic-strip girl
ANNIE'S: "__ Song" (John Denver tune)
ANNIKA: Golf pro Sorenstam
ANNINA: "Der Rosenkavalier" role
ANN LEE: American Shakers founder
ANNO: Part of A.D.
ANNUIT: Word on a $1 bill
ANNULAR: Ring-shaped
ANNULET: Architectural band
ANNULUS: Growth ring
ANNUM: Year: Latin
ANNUS: Year: Latin
ANNY: "Jude the Obscure" character
ANOA: Indonesian ox
ANODE: Battery terminal
ANODYNE: Pain reliever
ANOKA: Minnesota city
ANOLE: Arboreal lizard
ANOMIA: Inability to name objects
ANOMIC: Lawless
ANOMIE: Absence of societal values
ANOMY: Absence of societal values
ANONYM: Alias
ANORAK: Arctic coat
ANOSMIA: Inability to smell
ANOUILH: French playwright
ANOUK: Actress Aimee
ANOXIA: Lack of oxygen
ANSA: Vase handle
ANSARA: Actor Michael
ANSATE: Having a handle
ANSE: Faulkner character
ANSEIS: "Song of Roland" character
ANSEL: Photographer Adams
ANSELM: English saint
ANSELMO: "For Whom the Bell Tolls" character
ANSER: Duck genus
ANSON: Actor Williams
ANSONIA: Connecticut city
ANSPACH: Actress Susan
ANTA: Architectural pier
ANTAL: Conductor Dorati
ANTARES: Star in Scorpio
ANTAWN: Jamison of basketball
ANTBEAR: Aardvark
ANTCOW: Aphid
ANTERO: Colorado mountain
ANTERUS: Pope
ANTH: Flower: Comb. form
ANTHEIL: Composer George
ANTHER: Flower part
ANTHONY: Suffragist Susan B.
ANTIBES: French resort
ANTIGEN: Immunological substance
ANTIGO: Wisconsin city
ANTIGUA: West Indies island
ANTILOG: Math term
ANTIOCH: Ohio college
ANTLIA: Southern constellation
ANT LION: Insect
ANTOINE: Writer de Saint-Exupery
ANTON: Actress Susan
ANTONE: San __ (Texas city, familiarly)
ANTONIA: Cather heroine
ANTONIN: Composer Dvorák
ANTONIO: Actor Banderas
ANTONY: "Julius Caesar" character
ANTRE: Cave
ANTRIM: Irish county
ANTRON: Nylon-fiber brand
ANTRUM: Bone cavity
ANTWERP: Belgian city
ANTZ: 1998 film
ANU: Akkadian god
ANUBIS: Egyptian god
AN WANG: Computer company founder
ANWAR: Sadat of Egypt
ANYA: Author Seton
ANYON: Subatomic particle
ANY ROAD: George Harrison tune
ANYTOWN: Typical American locale
ANZAC: Australian soldier
ANZIO: Italian town
ANZUS: Alliance of 1952
AOKI: Golfer Isao
AOL: Internet service provider, for short
A OR B: Column choice
AORT: Cardiology combining form
AOSTA: Italian city
AOUDAD: African sheep
AOUT: August: French
APA: Therapists' grp.
A PAIN: Very inconvenient
APAR: Armadillo
APATITE: Calcium mineral
APEAK: Vertical, nautically
A PECK OF: Much
APE DIET: Type of vegetarian fare
APEEK: Vertical, nautically
APERCU: Brief glimpse
A PERSON: One
APFEL: Apple: German
APHAGIA: Difficulty in swallowing
APHASIA: Inability to speak
APHELIA: Orbital points
A. PHILIP: Labor leader Randolph
APHONIA: Loss of voice
API: Bee: Comb. form
APIA: Samoan city
APIAN: Of bees
APICAL: At the top
APICES: High points
A PIED: Walking: French
A PILE OF: Much
APIS: Egyptian sacred bull
APLEY: Marquand title character
APLITE: Type of granite
APNEA: Breathing anomaly
APO: GI mail abbr.
APOC.: Part of the Bible: Abbr.
APOD: Footless creature
APOGEE: Orbital point
APOLLO: Handsome man
A POP: Apiece
APOPKA: Florida city
APORT: Nautical direction
APOTHEM: Geometry term
APP: Computer program, for short
APPARAT: Political organization
APPEL: Fencing movement
APPERT: French chef
APPETIT: "Bon __!"
APPIA: Via __ (Roman road)
APPIAN: __ Way (Roman road)
APPL.: Part of N/A
APPLET: Internet program
APPLING: Luke of baseball
APPOSE: Place side by side
APRES: After: French
APRILE: April: Italian
APSE: Church area
APSIDES: Orbital points
APSIS: Orbital point
APSO: Lhasa __ (dog)
APTED: Director Michael
APTERAL: Aisleless
APTERYX: Kiwi
APU: "The Simpsons" clerk
APULIA: Italian region

APUS: Southern constellation
AQABA: Jordan port
AQUAMAN: Comics superhero
AQUAVIT: Scandinavian liquor
AQUI: Here: Spanish
AQUIFER: Water source
AQUILA: Northern constellation
AQUINAS: St. Thomas __
AQUINO: Former Philippine leader
ARA: Altar constellation
ARABICA: Kind of coffee
ARACARI: Toucan
ARACHNE: Mythical weaver
ARACHNO: Spider: Comb. form
ARAD: Romanian city
ARADO: Plowed land
ARAFAT: Former PLO leader
A RAFT OF: Much
ARAFURA: Asian sea
ARAGON: Spanish region
ARAGORN: "Lord of the Rings" character
ARAL SEA: Large Asian lake
ARAM: Composer Khatchaturian
ARAMAIC: Ancient language
ARAMARK: Fortune 500 firm
ARAME: Edible seaweed
ARAMEAN: Ancient language
ARAMID: Synthetic fiber
ARAMIS: A Musketeer
ARAN: Irish island group
ARANEID: Spider
ARANTXA: Tennis pro __ Sanchez-Vicario
A RAP: The slightest amount
ARAPAHO: Western Indian
ARARA: Brazilian macaw
ARARAT: Biblical mountain
ARAS: Armenian river
ARB: Wall Street trader
ARBACES: "Last Days of Pompeii" character
ARBELA: Assyrian city
ARBER: Swiss medicine Nobelist
ARBIL: Iraqi town
ARBOL: Tree: Spanish
ARBRE: Tree: French
ARBUS: Photographer Diane
ARBY'S: Fast-food chain
ARCA: Medieval chest
ARCADIA: California city
ARCARO: Jockey Eddie
ARC COS: Trig function
ARCHE: First: Comb. form
ARCHI: First: Comb. form
ARCHIE: Comic-book teen
ARCHIES: "Sugar, Sugar" group
ARCHON: Ancient Greek magistrate
ARCHSEE: Church district
ARCHWAY: Cookie brand
ARCHY: Fictional cockroach
ARCO: West Coast gas brand
ARC SEC: Trig function
ARC SIN: Trig function
ARC SINE: Trig function
ARC TAN: Trig function
ARCUATE: Bow-shaped
ARD: Suffix for dull
ARDECHE: French department
ARDEN: "As You Like It" locale
ARDMORE: Oklahoma city
ARECA: Asian palm
ARECIBO: Puerto Rican port
AREEL: Spinning
ARENDT: Author Hannah
ARENOSE: Gritty
ARENS: Former Israeli defense minister
ARENSKY: Russian composer
AREO: Mars: Comb. form
AREOLA: Anatomical ring
AREOLE: Anatomical ring
ARES: Greek war god
ARE SO: "Ain't!" response
ARETE: Mountain ridge
ARETHA: Singer Franklin
ARETINO: Italian dramatist
ARE TOO: "Am not!" response
AREZZO: Italian city
ARGALI: Asian sheep
ARGANTE: "Faerie Queene" character
ARGENT: Silver, in heraldry
ARGENTI: Silver: Comb. form
ARGENTO: Silver: Comb. form
ARGIVE: Greek
ARGO: Jason's ship
ARGON: Inert gas
ARGONNE: French forest
ARGOS: Ancient Greek city
ARGOSY: Abundance
ARGOT: Special vocabulary
ARGUFY: Dispute, slangily
ARGUS: Watchful one
ARGYLL: Historic Scottish county
ARHAT: Buddhist in Nirvana
ARI: Onassis nickname
ARIADNE: Daughter of Minos
ARIAL: Computer typeface
ARIAN: Adherent: Suffix
ARIANA: Actress Richards
ARIANE: French rocket
ARIARY: Madagascar money
ARICA: Chilean city
ARIE: Auto racer Luyendyk
ARIEGE: French department
ARIEL: "The Tempest" character
ARIGATO: Thank you: Japanese
ARIKARA: Dakota Indian
ARIL: Seed coat
ARION: Greek poet
ARIOSO: Melodic section
ARIOSTO: Italian poet
ARISTA: Grain beard
ARISTO: British blue blood
ARIUM: Suffix for planet
ARJUNA: "Bhagavad-Gita" hero
ARKIN: Actor Alan
ARKY: Vaughan of baseball
ARLBERG: Austrian Alps pass
ARLEDGE: Former ABC News head
ARLEN: Composer Harold
ARLENE: Actress Dahl
ARLES: French city
ARLISS: Actor George
ARLO: Singer Guthrie
ARLOVA: "Darkness at Noon" character
ARMA: First word of "The Aeneid"
ARMAGH: Irish county
ARMAH: Ghanian writer
ARMAND: Actor Assante
ARMANI: Fashion designer
ARMAS: Tony of baseball
ARME: Weapon: French
ARMEE: Army: French
ARMEN: Singer Kay
ARMENIA: Asian nation
ARMET: Armor helmet
ARMEY: Former House Democratic leader
ARMIN: Actor Mueller-Stahl
ARMONK: IBM's New York headquarters
ARN: Prince Valiant's son
ARNALL: "A Portrait of the Artist as a Young Man" character
ARNAZ: Bandleader Desi
ARNE: English composer
ARNEIS: Italian wine
ARNEL: Synthetic fiber
ARNESS: "Gunsmoke" star
ARNETT: CNN Desert Storm reporter
ARNHEM: Dutch city
ARNICA: Medicinal plant
ARNIE: "L.A. Law" character
ARNIE'S: "__ Army" (golf crowd)
ARNO: Florence's river
ARNOLD: Golfer Palmer
ARNOLD'S: "Happy Days" hangout
AROA: Venezuelan mining town
A-ROD: Baseball superstar's nickname
AROID: Calla lily
AROINT: Begone, old-style
ARON: Elvis __ Presley
A RONI: With pasta, in product names
ARONNAX: Verne character
AROO: Slangy suffix
AROUET: Voltaire's real name
AROW: In line
ARP: French painter
ARPA: Harp: Italian
ARPAD: Hungarian national hero
ARPEGE: Perfume brand
ARPEL: Adrien of cosmetics
ARPELS: Van Cleef's partner
ARRABAL: Spanish playwright
ARRACK: Mideast liquor
ARRAH: Irish exclamation
ARRAN: Scottish island
ARRAS: Tapestry
ARRAU: Chilean pianist
ARRET: Stop: French
ARRETE: Stopped: French
ARRIBA: Spanish exclamation
ARRID: Deodorant brand
ARRIERE: Back: French
ARRIS: Column ridge
ARROYO: Southwestern gulch
ARROZ: Rice: Spanish
ARS: "__ Gratia Artis" (MGM motto)
ARSENE: Fictional detective Lupin
ARSENIC: Element #33
ARSENIO: TV host Hall
ARSENO: Arsenic: Comb. form
ARSHILE: Armenian painter Gorky
ARSIS: Musical upbeat
ARTA: Greek gulf
ARTAUD: French playwright
ART CAR: Fancily decorated auto
ARTE: Comic Johnson
ARTEL: Russian cooperative
ARTEMIS: Apollo's sister
ARTEMUS: Humorist Ward
ARTERIO: Artery: Comb. form
ARTEST: Ron of basketball
ART FERN: Johnny Carson persona
ART GUM: Type of eraser
ARTHRO: Joint: Comb. form
ARTHUR: Ashe of tennis
ARTHUR C.: Author Clarke
ARTHUR M.: Historian Schlesinger
ARTHURS: 1880s First Family
ART I: Painting class
ARTIE: Bandleader Shaw
ARTIS: "Ars gratia __" (MGM motto)
ARTOIS: Former French province
ARTOO: __ Detoo ("Star Wars" character)
ART ROCK: Music genre
ARTUR: Pianist Rubinstein
ARTURO: Conductor Toscanini
ART WALL: Pro golfer
ARU: Indonesian island group
ARUBA: Antilles island
ARUGULA: Salad ingredient
ARUM: Calla lily
ARUNDEL: English town
ARUNS: "Aeneid" character
ARUSPEX: Roman seer
ARVADA: Colorado city
ARWEN: "Lord of the Rings" character
ARY: Adjective suffix
ARYAN: Indo-European
ARYE: Actor Gross
ARYL: Organic radical
ASA: King of Judah
AS A BODY: En masse
ASAGI: "Raisin in the Sun" character
ASA GRAY: Botanist
ASAHI: Japanese beer brand
AS A LARK: Facetiously
AS AM I: "Me too"
ASANA: Yoga posture
ASANTE: African people
ASARCO: Major mining company
ASBURY: __ Park, NJ
A.S. BYATT: British novelist
ASC: Cinematographers' org.
A SCALE: Piano practice
ASCAP: Music licensing org.
ASCETIC: Rigorously abstinent
ASCH: Author Sholem
ASCII: Computer data acronym
AS COLD: Comparable to ice
ASCUS: Spore sac
ASDIC: British sonar

ASE: Enzyme suffix
ASEPSIS: Absence of germs
ASE'S: "__ Death" (Grieg work)
AS EVER: Invariably
AS FAR AS: To the extent that
ASGARD: Norse gods' home
A SHADE: Slightly
A SHAME: "Too bad"
ASHANTI: R&B singer
ASHBERY: Poet John
ASHBURN: Richie of baseball
ASHBURY: San Francisco street
ASHBY: Director Hal
ASHCAKE: Corn bread
ASHDOD: Israeli town
ASHE: Arthur of tennis
ASHER: Son of Jacob
ASHFORD: Sprinter Evelyn
ASHLAND: Kentucky city
ASHLAR: Building stone
ASHLEE: Singer Simpson
ASHLEY: "Gone With the Wind" character
AS HOT: Comparable to a pistol
ASHRAM: Hindu retreat
ASHTON: Actor Kutcher
ASHUR: Assyrian war god
ASIAGO: Italian cheese
ASICS: Sneaker brand
ASIE: Asia: French
AS IF: "A likely story!"
ASIMOV: Author Isaac
ASIR: Saudi Arabian region
AS IS: Sale condition
AS I SAID: "To reiterate..."
ASK AMY: Advice column
ASL: "The Joy of Signing" subj.
ASLAK: "Peer Gynt" character
ASLAN: C.S. Lewis lion
A SLEW OF: Abundant
ASMARA: Capital of Eritrea
A SNAP: "Child's play!"
ASNER: "Lou Grant" star
AS NEW: In perfect condition
ASO: Japanese volcano
ASOK: "Dilbert" character
ASONANT: Unvoiced
AS ONE: In unison
ASONIA: Tone deafness
ASOR: Ancient Hebrew instrument
ASOSAN: Japanese volcano
A SOUL: Anyone
ASPEN: Poplar tree
ASPEN, CO: Ski resort
AS PER: According to
ASPERA: "Ad astra per __" (Kansas motto)
ASPIN: Clinton defense secretary
ASQUITH: 1910s British prime minister
ASSAD: Syrian leader
ASSAI: Allegro __ (very fast)
ASSAM: State of India
ASSANTE: Actor Armand
ASSER: Dutch peace Nobelist
ASSEZ: Enough: French
ASSISI: Home of St. Francis
ASSIZE: Legislative edict
ASST. D.A.: Prosecutorial aide: Abbr.
ASSUNTA: "Count of Monte Cristo" character
ASSYR.: From Nineveh: Abbr.
ASSYRIA: Ancient Asian empire
AST: Bermuda clock setting: Abbr.
ASTA: "The Thin Man" canine
ASTAIRE: "Swing Time" star
ASTANA: Kazakhstan capital
ASTART: Suddenly
ASTARTE: Phoenician goddess
A STEAL: "You've gotta buy this!"
ASTERIX: French comic-book hero
ASTERO: Star: Comb. form
ASTHER: Actor Nils
ASTI: Italian wine city
ASTIN: Actor Sean
ASTLEY: Rock singer Rick
AS TO: Concerning
ASTOLAT: Arthurian locale
ASTON: __ Martin (English car)
ASTOR: Fur-trading tycoon
ASTORIA: Oregon city
ASTR.: Space sci.
ASTRA: "Ad __ per aspera" (Kansas motto)
ASTRE: Pontiac model
ASTRID: Novelist Lindgren
ASTROS: 2005 World Series team
ASTROV: "Uncle Vanya" character
ASTRUD: Singer Gilberto
ASU: Tempe sch.
ASWAN: Egyptian city
AT A BOIL: Very hot
ATACAMA: Chilean desert
AT A CLIP: Without stopping
A TAD: Slightly
ATALA: Chateaubriand novel
AT ALL: In any way
ATAMAN: Cossack chief
ATAR: Perfume oil
ATARAXY: Tranquillity
ATARI: Computer-game company
AT A TIME: Simultaneously
ATATURK: Istanbul airport
ATAVIST: Genetic throwback
ATAXIA: Loss of coordination
AT BAR: Before the court
ATC: Flight coordination grp.
ATCO: 1960s record label
A.T. CROSS: Pen company
AT DEUCE: Tied, in tennis
ATE AT: Bothered
AT EIGHT: When some prime-time shows start
ATE IT: Absorbed the loss
ATELIER: Art studio
A TEMPO: Music-score marking
ATEN: Egyptian sun god
A TENTH: Tither's fraction
ATE OF: Sampled
A TERRE: Ballet position
ATES: Actor Roscoe
A TEST: Alamogordo event
ATF: Arm of the Treasury Dept.
ATHENA: Greek goddess
ATHENE: Greek goddess
A THING: Diddly-squat
ATHOL: Playwright Fugard
AT-HOME: Reception of visitors
ATHON: Elongated event: Comb. form
ATHOS: One of the Musketeers
ATHWART: Wrongly
ATI: Suffix for glitter
ATIC: Suffix for problem
ATIK: Star in Perseus
A TILE: Scrabble one-pointer
ATION: Noun suffix
ATIP: Expectantly
ATIS: Poisonous Asian plant
AT ISSUE: Being debated
AT IT: Working hard
ATIVE: Adjective suffix
ATKA: Alaskan island
ATKINS: Low-carb diet
ATLE: Tamarisk tree
ATLI: Hun king
ATMAN: Hindu soul
ATMO: Air: Comb. form
ATMOS: Clock brand
AT. NO.: Element ID
AT ODDS: Antagonistic
A TOI: Thine: French
ATOMY: Mote
ATON: Egyptian sun god
ATONIA: Muscle weakness
ATONIC: Unaccented syllable
A TON OF: Much
ATONY: Muscle weakness
ATOR: Agent: Suffix
ATORY: Adjective suffix
ATP: Chem. neurotransmitter
ATQUE: Ave __ vale (hail and farewell: Latin)
ATRA: Razor brand
A TRAIN: Subway of song
ATREUS: Father of Agamemnon
ATRI: Longfellow bell town
ATRIP: Anchor position
A TROIS: For three: French
ATROPHY: Decay
ATROPOS: One of the Fates
AT STUD: Retired, as some racehorses
ATTA: "__ girl!"
ATTAINT: Disgrace
ATTAR: Perfume oil
AT THIRD: Almost home, in baseball
ATTICA: Greek region
ATTICUS: "To Kill a Mockingbird" character
ATTILA: Hun leader
ATTLEE: 1950s British prime minister
ATTO: Quintillionth: Comb. form
ATTRIT: Wear down, as an army
ATTRITE: Worn down by rubbing
ATTU: Alaskan island
ATTUCKS: Boston Massacre victim
ATTY. GEN.: Cabinet mem.
ATV: Dune buggy: Abbr.
ATWATER: George H.W. Bush advisor
ATWOOD: Novelist Margaret
AT. WT.: Elemental stat.
AUBADE: Dawn music
AUBE: French river
AUBER: French composer
AUBERGE: French inn
AUBREY: Illustrator Beardsley
AUBURN U.: Alabama school
AUDE: French department
AUDEN: English poet
AUDI: German auto
AUDIE: WWII hero Murphy
AUDRA: Actress Lindley
AUDREY: "Little Shop of Horrors" character
AUDUBON: Bird artist
AUEL: "Clan of the Cave Bear" author
AUER: Actor Mischa
AUF: "__ wiedersehen"
AU FAIT: Expert: French
AU FOND: Fundamentally: French
AUGEAN: Difficult and unpleasant
AUGEAS: Mythical king
AUGEND: Something to be added to
AUGER: Boring tool
AUGIE: Saul Bellow character
AUGITE: Common mineral
AUGUR: Predict
AUGUSTA: Maine capital
AUGUSTE: Chef Escoffier
AUGUSTO: Former Chilean leader Pinochet
AU JUS: Menu phrase
AUK: Diving bird
AU LAIT: With milk: French
AULD: "__ Lang Syne"
AULD SOD: Nickname for Ireland
AULETTA: Author Ken
AULIS: Agamemnon's port
AULUS: "Quo Vadis?" character
AUMONT: Actor Jean-Pierre
AUNG: 1991 peace Nobelist __ San Suu Kyi
AUNT BEE: "Andy Griffith Show" character
AUNT EM: Baum character
AU PAIR: Nanny
AUR: Gold: Comb. form
AURA LEE: Song on which "Love Me Tender" is based
AURAR: Iceland money
AURATE: Golden
AUREATE: Golden
AUREOLA: Corona
AUREOLE: Corona
AURI: Gold: Comb. form
AURIC: 007 foe Goldfinger
AURICLE: Earlike part
AURIFY: Gild
AURIGA: Northern constellation
AURIST: Ear specialist
AUROUS: Containing gold
AURUM: Gold: Latin
AUS: Switz. neighbor
AUSABLE: New York river
AUSLESE: German wine
AUSPEX: Roman seer
AUSSI: Also: French

AUST.: Switz. neighbor
AUSTEN: Novelist Jane
AUSTER: South wind
AUSTIN: Texas capital
AUSTINS: British cars
AUSTR: South: Comb. form
AUSTRAL: Southern
AUSTRO: South: Comb. form
AUT: Self: Comb. form
AUTARCH: Despot
AUTARKY: Economic self-sufficiency
AUTEUR: Film creator
AUTOMNE: Autumn: French
AUTONYM: Person's own name
AUTOPEN: Script imitator
AUTOPIA: Disneyland attraction
AUTRE: Other: French
AUTRY: Cowboy singer Gene
AU VIN: With wine: French
AUX: "La Cage __ Folles"
AVA: Actress Gardner
AVAL: Grandfatherly
AVALON: Arthurian paradise
AVALONS: Toyota models
AVANT: Before: French
AVANTI: Sports car
AVAST: Nautical command
AVATAR: Hindu incarnation
AVAUNT: "Begone!", old-style
AVEC: With: French
AVEDON: Fashion photographer Richard
AVEENO: Skin-care brand
AVENA: Oat genus
AVENIDA: Avenue: Spanish
AVENUE Q: Tony Award musical
AVERELL: Diplomat Harriman
AVERILL: Earl of baseball
AVERNAL: Infernal
AVERNUS: Hades
AVERY: Murphy Brown's son
AVESTA: Zoroastrian sacred text
AVEYRON: French department
AVGAS: Airplane fuel
AVI: Bird: Comb. form
AVIA: Sneaker brand
AVIAN: Bird
AVIANCA: Colombian airline
AVIDE: Greedy: French
AVIGNON: French city
AVILA: City of Spain
AVION: Par __ (via airmail)
AVIONIC: Of cockpit devices
AVIOR: Star in Carina
AVIS: Car-rental company
AVISO: Dispatch boat
AVISON: Canadian poet
AVIV: Tel __, Israel
AVNET: Director Jon
AVO: Macao coin
AVOCET: Shorebird
AVOIR: Have: French
AVON: Shakespeare's river
AVONLEA: "Anne of Green Gables" locale
AVOUCH: Acknowledge
AVRIL: April: French
AVS: Colorado NHLers
AVULSE: Extract
AWACS: Military plane
AWAG: Active, as gossips' tongues
AWASH IN: Overwhelmed by
AW C'MON: Encouraging words
AWEIGH: "Anchors __"
A WHIT: The slightest amount
AWK: Parrot cry
AWN: Grain beard
AWOONOR: Ghanian writer
AWW: "How cute!"
AXEL: Skating jump
AXEL F: "Beverly Hills Cop" tune
AXELROD: 1970 medicine Nobelist
AXENIC: Germfree
AXIL: Leaf angle
AXILLA: Armpit
AXION: Hypothetical particle
AXISES: Asian deers
AXL ROSE: Guns N' Roses leader
AXOLOTL: Mexican salamander
AXON: Nerve-cell part
AXONE: Nerve-cell part
AXSEED: Erosion-preventing plant
AXTON: Singer Hoyt
AYAH: Asian nanny
AYAKO: Pro golfer Okamoto
AYDE: "The Invisible Man" character
A YEAR: Annually
AYEAYES: African lemurs
AYER: Yesterday: Spanish
AYERS: __ Rock (Australian landmark)
AYESHA: Wife of Mohammed
AYIN: Hebrew letter
AYKROYD: Actor Dan
AYLA: "Clan of the Cave Bear" heroine
AYME: French novelist
AYN RAND: "Atlas Shrugged" author
AYR: Scottish port
AYRES: Actor Lew
AYRTON: "Mysterious Island" character
AZAN: Muslim call to prayer
AZANIA: South Africa
AZARIA: Actor Hank
AZELMA: "Les Misérables" character
AZERA: Hyundai model
AZERI: Baku native
AZIDE: Nitrogen compound
AZIMUTH: Navigational arc
AZINGER: Golfer Paul
AZIZ: "A Passage to India" doctor
AZKABAN: Harry Potter series locale
AZO DYE: Cotton coloring
AZOIC: Kind of dye
AZOLE: Nitrogen compound
AZORES: Portuguese island group
AZORIN: Spanish novelist
AZOTH: Alchemist's mercury
AZOV: Arm of the Black Sea
AZRAEL: Smurf cat
AZT: Antiviral drug
AZTECA: Mexican airline
AZTEK: Pontiac model
AZUELA: Mexican writer
AZUKI: Kind of bean
AZUL: Blue: Spanish
AZULEJO: Ceramic tile
AZUR: Cote d'__
AZURITE: Blue gem
AZUSA, CA: Golden State city

B

BAAL: False god
BAALIM: False gods
BAB: "__ Ballads" (W.S. Gilbert work)
BABA: Rum cake
BABALU: Desi Arnaz tune
BABAR: Kid-lit elephant
BABBAGE: British mathematician
BABBITT: Sinclair Lewis novel
BABCOCK: Actress Barbara
BABENCO: Director Hector
BABETTE: Poet Deutsch
BABI YAR: Yevtushenko poem
BABKA: Polish cake
BAB-O: Cleanser brand
BABOO: Hindu gentleman
BABS: Streisand, in headlines
BABSON: Massachusetts college
BABU: Hindu gentleman
BABY BOP: Friend of Barney the dinosaur
BABY GAP: Infants' clothing brand
BABY'S: __ breath (flower)
BAC: Breathalyzers measure it: Abbr.
BACA: Colorado county
BACALL: Actress Lauren
BACARDI: Rum brand
BACCHAE: Euripides work
BACCHIC: Bacchanalian
BACCHUS: God of wine
BACH: German composer
BACHATA: Dominican Republic music
BACH IT: Live alone
BACHMAN: Stephen King pen name
BACI: Chocolate brand
BACIO: Kiss: Italian
BACKBAR: Tavern storage area
BACK BAY: Area of Boston
BACKBIT: Slandered
BACKUS: Actor Jim
BACOS: Crunchy salad toppers
BACTRIA: Ancient Asian country
BAD CALL: Why an ump may be booed
BAD COP: Half a police pair
BADD: Color Me __ (rap group)
BAD EMS: German spa
BADEN: German region
BADENOV: Bullwinkle foe
BADER: Justice Ruth __ Ginsburg
BADHAM: Director John
BAD HAT: Rascal
BAD LIE: Golf woe
BAD LOT: Crooked bunch
BAD LOVE: Jonathan Kellerman novel
BADU: Singer Erykah
BAD 'UN: Rogue
BAEDA: English historian
BAER: Boxer Max
BAERGA: Carlos of baseball
BAEYER: German chemist Adolf von __
BAEZ: Singer Joan
BAEZA: Jockey Braulio
BAFF: Bad golf shot
BAFFIN: Arctic Ocean bay
BAFFY: Golf club
BAG BOY: Supermarket employee
BAGDAD: Capital of Iraq
BAGEHOT: English economist
BAG END: Bilbo's home
BAGGINS: "Lord of the Rings" character
BAG GIRL: Supermarket employee
BAGHDAD: Capital of Irag
BAG IT: Abdicate
BAG JOB: Break-in
BAGMAN: Dishonest official
BAGNIO: Turkish bathhouse
BAGNOLD: Author Enid
BAGWELL: Jeff of baseball
BAHA'I: Iranian religion
BAHAMA: Grand __ Island
BAHA MEN: Rock group
BAHIA: Brazilian port
BAHN: German road
BAHNEN: German roads
BAHRAIN: Mideast nation
BAHREIN: Mideast nation
BAHT: Thai money
BAIE: Bay: French
BAIKAL: Russian lake
BAILEE: Custodian of goods
BAILEY: Singer Pearl
BAIL ON: Leave in the lurch
BAILOR: Surety poster
BAIN: Actress Barbara
BAINES: Lyndon __ Johnson
BAINTER: Actress Fay
BAIO: Actor Scott
BAIRD: Alaskan mountain range
BAIRN: Child: Scottish
BAISA: Oman coin
BAIT CAR: Cops' auto-thief lure
BAIUL: Ukrainian skater
BAIZA: Coin of Oman
BAIZE: Billiard table cloth
BAJA: Mexican region
BAJER: 1908 peace Nobelist
BAJO: Low: Spanish
BAKER ST.: Sherlock Holmes' home
BAKKER: Onetime televangelist
BAKLAVA: Mideast dessert
BAKR: Abu-__ (Mohammed's successor)
BAKSHI: Director Ralph
BAKST: Russian painter
BAKU: Capital of Azerbaijan
BAKULA: Actor Scott
BAL: Formal dance: French
BALA: Book of the Douay Bible
BALAAM: Biblical prophet
BALABAN: Actor Bob

BALAS: Red gemstone
BALATA: Golf-ball cover material
BALATON: Hungarian lake
BALBO: Italian aviator
BALBOA: Spanish explorer
BALBOAS: Panama coins
BALCH: 1946 peace Nobelist
BALDIE: Saltless pretzel
BALDRIC: Ornamented belt
BALDUR: Son of Odin
BALDWIN: Actor Alec
BALEEN: Whalebone
BALFOUR: "Kidnapped" character
BALI: Indonesian island
BALI HAI: "South Pacific" song
BALIN: Actress Ina
BALINE: Irving Berlin's real last name
BALKI: "Perfect Strangers" role
BALLADE: Chopin work
BALLARD: Actress Kaye
BALLIN': "__ the Jack" (old song)
BALLIOL: College of Oxford
BALLMER: Microsoft bigwig
BALLO: "Un __ in Maschera" (Verdi opera)
BALLON: Grace, in ballet
BALL ONE: Ump's call
BALLOU: Jane Fonda film role
BALL ST.: Indiana univ.
BALLUET: French peace Nobelist
BALL UP: Make a mess of
BALLY: Pinball brand
BALLY'S: Las Vegas casino
BALMAIN: French fashion designer
BALMER: "When Worlds Collide" author
BALON: Grace, in ballet
BALOO: "The Jungle Book" bear
BALPH: "Atlas Shrugged" character
BALT: Estonian or Lithuanian
BALTO: 1995 animated film
BALZAC: French writer
'BAMA: Southern school, for short
BAMAKO: Capital of Mali
BAMBA: "La __" (Valens tune)
BAMBI: Disney deer
BAMBI II: 2006 Disney film
BAMBINA: Little girl: Italian
BAMBINO: Little boy: Italian
BAMMY: West Indies pancake
BANACEK: Peppard TV role
BANANE: Banana: French
BANBURY: British town
BANC: Bench: French
BANCA: Bank: Italian
BANCO: Baccarat announcement
BANDA: Asian sea
B AND B: Type of inn
BANDEAU: Headband
BANDERA: Flag: Spanish
B AND O: Monopoly railroad
B AND W: Not in color
BANFF: Alberta city
BANGOR: Maine city
BANGUI: Central African Republic capital
BANI: __-Sadr (Iranian leader)
BANJUL: Capital of Gambia
BANKIT: Raised sidewalk
BANK ONE: Credit-card issuer
BANKY: Valentino co-star
BAN-LON: Synthetic fabric
BANNEN: Actor Ian
BANNS: Betrothal announcement
BANO: Bath: Spanish
BANON: French cheese
BANQUE: Bank: French
BANQUO: Ghost in "Macbeth"
BANTA: "Taxi" role
BANTING: Insulin discoverer
BAO: __ Dai (Vietnamese leader)
BAOBAB: African tree
BAP.: Christian denom.
BARA: Actress Theda
BARACK: Senator Obama
BARACUS: "The A-Team" character
BARADA: Damascus' river
BARAK: Ehud of Israel
BARAKA: Writer Imamu
BARANOF: Alaskan island
BARANY: Austrian medicine Nobelist
BARATA: Sale: Spanish
BARATO: Cheap: Spanish
BARBA: Beard: Spanish
BARBAN: "Tender Is the Night" character
BARBARY: African region
BARBATE: Bearded
BARBEAU: Actress Adrienne
BARBERA: Hanna's animation partner
BARBET: Tropical bird
BARBI: Actress Benton
BARBRA: Singer Streisand
BARBUDA: West Indies island
BARBULE: Thorn
BARCA: Hannibal's family name
BARCLAY: British banking name
BARCO: Boat: Spanish
BARDEEN: Physics Nobelist
BARDOT: French actress
BAREGE: Veil fabric
BAREGES: French ski resort
BARENTS: Arctic explorer
BARETTA: Robert Blake TV role
BARFY: "Family Circus" canine
BARGE IN: Arrive abruptly
BARI: Italian port
BARIC: Of air pressure
BARISTA: Starbucks clerk
BARIT.: Voice range: Abbr.
BARIUM: Element #56
BARKIN: Actress Ellen
BARKLA: British physics Nobelist
BARKLEY: Truman vice president
BARLICK: Baseball Hall of Fame umpire
BARLOW: Poet Joel
BARM: Brewers' yeast
BARNABY: TV sleuth Jones
BARNARD: New York college
BARNES: Noble's partner
BARNET: Big Band leader Charlie
BARNEY: Argument
BAR NONE: All included
BARNUM'S: __ Animals (cookie brand)
BARO: Pressure: Comb. form
BAROJA: Spanish novelist
BAROLO: Italian wine
BARONE: "Everybody Loves Raymond" surname
BARONI: "A Night at the Opera" role
BARQ'S: Root-beer brand
BARQUE: Sailing vessel
BARR: Actress Roseanne
BARRE: Ballet rail
BARRET: Medieval cap
BARRETT: Elizabeth __ Browning
BARRIE: "Peter Pan" author
BARRIO: Hispanic neighborhood
BARRIS: "The Gong Show" host
BARRON'S: Business publication
BARSTOW: California city
BART: "Simpsons" kid
BARTEL: Actor Paul
BARTH: Novelist John
BARTLE: "Adam Bede" character
BARTLES: Jaymes partner
BARTLET: "The West Wing" role
BARTOK: Hungarian composer
BARTOLO: "The Barber of Seville" role
BARTON: Red Cross founder
BAR TRAY: Pub server
BARTY: Actor Billy
BARUCH: Financier Bernard
BARYON: Subatomic particle
BARZUN: Historian Jacques
B.A.S: Undergrad degs.
BASALT: Igneous rock
BASEL: City in Switzerland
BASENJI: Dog breed
BASF: Audiotape brand
BASHO: Japanese poet
BASIA: Polish singer
BASIAL: Of a cranial point
BASIE: Pianist/bandleader
BASIFY: Make alkaline
BASILIO: "Barber of Seville" role
BASKETT: "Song of the South" actor
BASKIN: Robbins' partner
BASLE: City in Switzerland
BASMATI: Aromatic rice
BASOV: Russian physics Nobelist
BASQUE: Pyrenees resident
BASRA: Iraqi city
BASRAH: Al __, Iraq
BAS-RHIN: French department
BASS ALE: Pub order
BASSANI: Italian novelist
BASSANO: Italian painter
BASSE: __-Terre (capital of Guadeloupe)
BASSETT: Actress Angela
BASSEY: "Goldfinger" singer
BAST: Cord fiber
BASTA: Enough: Italian
BASTIA: Corsican seaport
BATAAN: Philippine peninsula
BATAVIA: Illinois city
BATEAU: Riverboat
BATEMAN: Actress Justine
BATHO: Depth: Comb. form
BATHOS: Schmaltz
BATHY: Depth: Comb. form
BATIK: Hand-dyed fabric
BAT IN: Bring home a runner
BATISTA: Castro preceder
BATISTE: Sheer fabric
BATLEY: Yorkshire town
BATMEN: British aides-de-camp
BATNA: Algerian city
BATOR: Ulan __, Mongolia
BATSON: Captain Marvel alter ego
BATT: Sheet of fabric
BATTEN: Fasten down
BATU: African mountain
BAT YAM: Israeli city
BAUD: Data transfer measure
BAUER: Hank of baseball
BAUGH: Sammy of football
BAUHAUS: German architecture school
BAULK: Be obstinate
BAUM: "The Wizard of Oz" author
BAUMAN: Sha Na Na leader
BAUME: French chemist
BAUMER: "All Quiet on the Western Front" hero
BAUSCH: __ and Lomb
BAUXITE: Aluminum ore
BAV.: Ger. state
BAVIER: Actress Frances
BAX: English composer
BAXTER: Actress Anne
BAYAR: 1950s Turkish president
BAYARD: Legendary horse
BAY AREA: San Francisco's environs
BAY CITY: Michigan metropolis
BAYER: Aspirin brand
BAYERN: Bavaria: German
BAYES: Vaudevillian Nora
BAYEUX: French town
BAYH: Indiana political surname
BAYLE: French philosopher
BAYLOR: Texas university
BAYONNE: New Jersey city
BAZOO: Mouth, slangily
BBA: Bus. school degree
B-BALL: Hoops sport
BBB: Bond rating
B.B. KING: Blues guitarist
BBL.: OPEC unit
B-BOY: Rap music fan
BCC: E-mail abbr.
BCE: Bridge builder's deg.
B CELL: Type of lymphocyte
B.C. LIONS: CFL team
B DALTON: Bookstore chain
B-DAY: Age celebration, for short
BD. FT.: Lumber meas.
BDL.: Pkg.
BDRM.: Apt. feature
BDS.: Chairpersons' concerns: Abbr.
BEA: Actress Arthur
BEACHAM: Actress Stephanie
BEADER: Certain craftsperson
BEADLE: Parish officer

BEAH: Actress Richards
BE A HERO: Do something courageous
BEALE: "__ Street Blues"
BE A LION: "The Wiz" song
BE-ALL: Ultimate aim
BEALS: Actress Jennifer
BE A MAN: Macho exhortation
BEAME: Former Big Apple mayor
BEAMON: 1968 Summer Olympics star
BEANO: Game like bingo
BEANY: Cecil's TV buddy
BE A PAL: Pleader's phrase
BEAR OFF: Steer away, nautically
BEARSE: Actress Amanda
BEART: Actress Emmanuelle
BEASLEY: "Blondie" mailman
BEATBOX: Electronic drum machine
BEATIFY: Bless
BEATRIX: Author Potter
BEATTIE: Author Ann
BEATTY: Actor Warren
BEATY: Shirley MacLaine's real surname
BEAV: Wally Cleaver's brother
BEAVIS: MTV toon
BE BAD: Misbehave
BEBE: Actress Neuwirth
BEBOP: Jazz style
BE BRAVE: Words of encouragement
BEC: Beak: French
BECALM: Deprive of wind
BECCA: "Life Goes On" role
BECH: Updike character
BECHET: Jazz clarinetist
BECKER: Boris of tennis
BECKET: "A Man for All Seasons" subject
BECKETT: Irish playwright
BECKHAM: Soccer superstar
BECKY: Tom Sawyer's girlfriend
BED BATH: Home-goods chain, for short
BEDDY: __-bye (sleep)
BEDE: George Eliot character
BEDELIA: Actress Bonnie
BEDFORD: "Henry IV" duke
BEDIZEN: Adorn
BEDLOE'S: __ Island (Liberty Island, formerly)
BEDNORZ: 1987 physics Nobelist
BEDNY: Russian poet
BEDSIT: Room in a flat
BEDWIN: "Oliver Twist" character
BEEB: BBC nickname
BEEBE: Bathysphere designer
BEECHAM: British conductor
BEECHER: Harriet __ Stowe
BEEFALO: Hybrid bovine
BEEF TEA: Bouillon, in Britain
BEEGEES: Australian trio
BEEM: Pro golfer Rich
BEEMER: Yuppie auto
BEENE: Designer Geoffrey
BEENS: Has-__
BEE TREE: Hive location
BEEVES: Cattle
BEEYARD: Apiary
BEEZER: Nose, slangily
BE FOR: Favor
BEGA: MTV mambo artist
BEGAY: Pro golfer Notah
BEGLEY: Actor Ed
BEGORRA: Irish exclamation
BEHAIM: German geographer
BEHAN: Irish playwright
BEHAR: Comic Joy
BEHOOF: Advantage
BEHRENS: German architect
BEHRING: German bacteriologist
BEHRMAN: Playwright S.N.
BEI: "__ Mir Bist Du Schön"
B EIGHT: Bingo call
BEIGNE: French donut
BEIGNET: French donut
BE-IN: Hippie happening
BE IN ON: Know about
BEIRA: Mozambique seaport
BEJART: French choreographer
BEKAA: __ Valley, Lebanon
BEL: Loudness unit
BELA: Actor Lugosi
BEL AIR: Chevy model
BELARUS: Minsk locale
BELASCO: Playwright David
BELAU: Pacific island republic
BELBY: "Forsyte Saga" character
BELDAM: Crone
BELDAME: Crone
BELEM: Brazilian port
B ELEVEN: Bingo call
BELFAST: Capital of Northern Ireland
BELFORT: French city
BELGAE: "Faerie Queene" character
BELIAL: Satan
BELINDA: Singer Carlisle
BELIZE: Central American nation
BELLA: Congresswoman Abzug
BELLAMY: Actor Ralph
BELLAY: French poet
BELLEAU: __ Wood (French forest)
BELLEEK: Irish porcelain
BELLI: Attorney Melvin
BELLINI: Italian painter
BELL LAP: Race finale
BELLO: Venezuelan poet
BELLOC: English essayist
BELLOW: Author Saul
BELLSON: Jazz drummer
BELLUM: War: Latin
BELMONT: Triple Crown horse race
BELO: 1996 peace Nobelist
BELOIT: City in Wisconsin
BELON: Type of oyster
BELTANE: Celtic May Day
BELTON: Missouri city
BELTRAN: Actor Robert
BELUSHI: "Animal House" star
BELVA: Author Plain
BELVOIR: Virginia army base
BELVOUR: King Arthur knight
BELY: Russian writer
BELZER: Comedian Richard
BELZONI: Italian egyptologist
BEM: Grotesque ET
BEMA: Altar area
BEMAN: Golf pro Deane
BEMATA: Altar areas
BENARES: City of India
BENATAR: Singer Pat
BENAZIR: Pakistani leader Bhutto
BENBEN: Actor Brian
BEN BLUE: Canadian comedian
BEN BOVA: Sci-fi author
BENBOW: Admiral __ Inn ("Treasure Island" locale)
BEN DAY: Photographic technique
BENDIX: "Life of Riley" actor
BENE: Well: Latin
BENEKE: Jazz saxophonist
BENELUX: European alliance
BENES: "Seinfeld" character
BENET: Poet Stephen Vincent
BENGAY: Liniment brand
BEN GUNN: "Treasure Island" character
BEN-HUR: Charlton Heston film
BENI: Blessed: French
BENICIA: California city
BENICIO: Actor Del Toro
BENIGNI: Actor Roberto
BENIGNO: Philippine statesman Aquino
BENIN: African country
BENING: Actress Annette
BENISON: Blessing
BENITO: Mexican statesman Juarez
BENJI: Film dog
BENNETT: Singer Tony
BENNIE: "__ and the Jets" (Elton John tune)
BENNING: Georgia army base
BENNY: Comic Hill
BENOIT: Marathoner Joan
BENOTE: Annotate excessively
BENSEY: "Tobacco Road" character
BENSON: "Soap" spin-off
BENTHAM: British philosopher
BENTHOS: Lake bottom
BENTLEY: British auto
BENTO: Japanese boxed meal
BENTON: Painter Thomas Hart __
BENTSEN: Clinton treasury secretary
BENZ: German auto pioneer
BENZALI: Actor Daniel
BENZELL: Singer Mimi
BENZOL: Petroleum byproduct
BE OFF: "Scram!"
BEOGRAD: Belgrade, to Serbians
BEOWULF: English epic poem
BEPPE: "I Pagliacci" role
BEPPO: Italian clown
BERBICK: Boxer Trevor
BERCEO: Spanish poet
BERCY: French sauce
BEREA: Ohio city
BERENDT: "Midnight in the Garden..." author
BERETTA: Chevy model
BERGAMO: City in Italy
BERGEN: Actress Candice
BERGER: Novelist Thomas
BERGERE: Folies __
BERGIUS: German chemist
BERGMAN: Actress Ingrid
BERGSON: French philosopher
BERIA: Stalin minister
BERIGAN: Jazz trumpeter
BERING: Danish explorer
BERKLEY: Michigan city
BERKNER: Antarctic island
BERKOW: Sportswriter Ira
BERKS: British county
BERLE: "Mr. Television"
BERLIOZ: French composer
BERLITZ: Language-school name
BERM: Road shoulder
BERMAN: Sportscaster Len
BERNARD: Financier Baruch
BERNAYS: Public-relations pioneer
BERNI: Italian poet
BERNIE: Lyricist Taupin
BERNINA: Swiss Alp
BERNINI: Italian sculptor
BERNSEN: Actor Corbin
BEROWNE: "Love's Labour's Lost" character
BERRA: Yogi of baseball
BERSUNT: King Arthur knight
BERT: "Sesame Street" character
BERTA: "Barber of Seville" role
BERTHA: Lace collar
BERTHE: "Madame Bovary" character
BERTIE: Wodehouse character
BERTOLT: Dramatist Brecht
BERTRAM: "All's Well That Ends Well" character
BERVOIX: "La Traviata" role
BERWICK: British city
BERWYN: Illinois city
BERYL: Gemstone
BES: Hebrew letter
BESAME: Kiss me: Spanish
BESANT: British philosopher
BESO: Kiss: Spanish
BESOM: Broom
BE SORE: Hold a grudge
BESS: Porgy's love
BESSEL: German astronomer
BESSELL: Actor Ted
BESSER: One of the Three Stooges
BESSIE: Blues singer Smith
BESSON: French director
BEST BOY: Film-crew member
BEST BUD: Pal
BEST CUT: Butcher's prize
BESTER: Sci-fi author Alfred
BETA: Greek letter
BETAKE: Cause to go
BETAMAX: VCR format
BETA RAY: Electron stream
BETCHA: "You __!"
BETE: Beast: French
BETEL: Asian palm
BETH: Hebrew letter
BETHANY: Lazarus' home
BETHEL: Church for sailors

BE THERE: Invitation phrase
BETHINK: Bear in mind
BETHUNE: Educator Mary McLeod __
BETIDE: Come to pass
BETIMES: Early
BET ON: Back, as a horse
BETONY: Medicinal plant
BETSEY: "David Copperfield" character
BETSY: Flagmaker Ross
BETSY'S: "__ Wedding" (1990 film)
BETTA: Fighting fish
BETTANY: Actor Paul
BETTE: Singer Midler
BETTGER: Actor Lyle
BETTI: Italian playwright
BETTY: Actress Grable
BETTYE: Actress Ackerman
BETZ: Actor Carl
BEULAH: 1950s sitcom
BEURRE: Butter: French
BEV.: Drink: Abbr.
BEVANS: Actor Clem
BEVERLY: Massachusetts city
BEVIN: British labor leader
BE WELL: Parting words
BEXAR: San Antonio's county
BEY: Ottoman official
BEYLE: Stendhal's real name
BEYMER: Actor Richard
BEYONCE: Singer Knowles
BEZEL: Watch part
BEZIERS: French city
BEZIQUE: Card game
BEZOS: Amazon.com founder
BFA: Art deg.
B FIVE: Bingo call
B FOUR: Bingo call
B-GIRL: Bar employee
B'GOSH: OshKosh __ (clothing brand)
B.G.S: "One-star" offs.
BHA: Food additive
BHAER: "Little Women" character
BHANG: Hemp
BHAT: Bard, in India
BHOPAL: City of India
BHT: Food additive
BHUTAN: Asian kingdom
BHUTTO: Former Pakistani leader
BIAFRA: Former Nigerian secessionist state
BIALIK: Hebrew poet
BIALY: Bagel relative
BIANCA: White: Italian
BIANCHI: Actress Daniela
BIANCO: White: Italian
BIAO: Lin __ (1960s Chinese leader)
BIAS-PLY: Type of tire
BIBB: Lettuce variety
BIBBER: Tippler
BIBBIDI: "__ Bobbidi Boo"
BIBCOCK: Kind of faucet
BIBELOT: Curio
BIBI: Actress Andersson
BIBL.: Back-of-bk. listing
BIBLIO: Book: Comb. form
BIC: Pen brand
BICHON: Dog breed, for short
BICORN: Napoleon's hat
BICORNE: Napoleon's hat
BIDEN: Delaware senator
BID FAIR: Seem likely
BID IN: Try to buy your own stuff, at auction
BIDU: Soprano Sayao
BIEBER: Former UAW head
BIEHN: Actor Michael
BIEL: Actress Jessica
BIEN: Well: Spanish
BIENTOT: Soon: French
BIERCE: Journalist Ambrose
BIERE: Beer: French
BIERI: Actor Ramon
BIFF: Punch
BIFID: Cleft
BIG A: Aqueduct Racetrack, familiarly
BIG AIR: High jump in sports
BIG BAD: Like a toon wolf
BIG BEAR: California lake
BIG BEAT: Music genre
BIG BEND: Texas national park
BIG BIRD: "Sesame Street" character
BIG BLUE: IBM nickname
BIG BOI: Rap artist
BIG BOX: Very large store
BIG D: Dallas nickname
BIG DIG: Major archaeological project
BIG EAST: College football conference
BIG EASY: New Orleans nickname
BIGELOW: Tea brand
BIG END: Engine part
BIGEYE: Tropical fish
BIG FIVE: Post-WWII alliance
BIG FOUR: WWII alliance
BIGGERS: Charlie Chan creator
BIGGITY: Self-important
BIGGS: British organist
BIG GULP: 7-Eleven drink
BIGHT: Bay
BIG JAKE: John Wayne film
BIG JOE: Blues singer Turner
BIG JOHN: Shirelles tune
BIG LOTS: Retail closeout chain
BIG LOVE: HBO series
BIG MAMA: "Cat on a Hot Tin Roof" character
BIG MO: Battleship's nickname
BIG O: Oscar Robertson's nickname
BIG OIL: ExxonMobil, Shell, etc.
BIG ON: Enthused about
BIG RED: Cornell team
BIGS: Major leagues
BIG SKY: Montana nickname
BIG SUR: California region
BIG TEN: College football conference
BIG TENT: Political-party concept
BIG UNIT: Randy Johnson's nickname
BIJOU: Jewel
BIKEL: Actor Theodore
BIKILA: Ethiopian runner
BIKO: Anti-apartheid activist
BIL: Cartoonist Keane
BILBAO: Spanish port
BILBO: "The Hobbit" character
BILDAD: "Moby-Dick" character
BILIOUS: Cranky
BILKO: Phil Silvers TV role
BILL G.: Microsoft head, familiarly
BILLIE: Actress Burke
BILLIS: "South Pacific" character
BILL NYE: "Science Guy" of TV
BILL W.: AA founder
BILLY: Police club
BILOBED: Type of leaf
BILOXI: Mississippi city
BILT: Constructed, in brand names
BIMBO: Knucklehead
BIMINIS: Bahama islands
BINACA: Breath-freshener brand
BINCHY: Author Maeve
BINDLE: Hobo's goods
BINE: Twining stem
BINET: IQ test developer
BINGHAM: Actress Traci
BINGLE: Base hit
BINNEY: Smith's crayon-making partner
BINNIE: Actress Barnes
BINNIG: 1986 physics Nobelist
BINOCHE: Actress Juliette
BINYON: British poet
BIOCHIP: Experimental circuit
BIOCIDE: Poison
BIODATA: Personal information
BIOFUEL: Ethanol, e.g.
BIOGAS: Fuel derived from garbage
BIOLITE: Organic rock
BIOMASS: Energy source
BIOME: Ecological community
BIONDI: Olympic swimmer Matt
BIONIC: Like The Six Million Dollar Man
BIONT: Organism
BIORE: Skin-care brand
BIOT: French physicist
BIOTA: Ecological group
BIOTECH: Environmental science
BIOTIN: B vitamin
BIOTITE: Mica
BIP: Marcel Marceau character
BIPOD: Rifle stand
BIPPY: "You bet your sweet __!"
BIREME: Ancient ship
BIRETTA: Clerical cap
BIRGIT: Opera singer Nilsson
BIRIANI: Indian dish
BIRL: Spin a floating log
BIRMAN: Cat breed
BIRNEY: Actor David
BIRO: Pen brand
BIRR: Whirr
BIRRA: Beer: Italian
BIRSE: Anger: Scottish
BIRYANI: Indian dish
BIS: Encore
BISBEE: Arizona city
BISCAY: European bay
BISHKEK: Capital of Kirghizia
BISMUTH: Element #83
BISSAU: African capital
BISSELL: Vacuum brand
BISSET: Actress Jacqueline
BIST: "Bei Mir __ Du Schön"
BITMAP: Computer display
BITNET: Network of educational sites
BITT: Mooring post
BITTE: Please: German
BITTERN: Marsh bird
BIV: ROY G. __ (spectrum mnemonic)
BIWA: Japanese lake
BIX: Biederbecke of jazz
BIXBY: Actor Bill
BIZARRO: Newspaper cartoon
BIZET: French composer
BIZKIT: Limp __ (rock group)
BJORK: Icelandic singer
BJORN: Borg of tennis
BJ'S: Warehouse-club chain
B. KLIBAN: Cat cartoonist's signature
BKPG.: Acct.'s job
BKPR.: Ledger worker: Abbr.
BLACKIE: Boston __ (fictional detective)
BLACULA: 1972 film
BLAFF: West Indian stew
BLAINE: 1884 presidential candidate
BLAIR: Actress Linda
BLAIS: Canadian poet
BLAISE: Philosopher Pascal
BLAKE: English poet
BLAKELY: Actress Susan
BLAKEY: Jazz drummer
BLAKLEY: Actress Ronee
BLALOCK: Actress Jolene
BLAM: Explosion sound
BLANC: French Alp
BLANCA: White: Spanish
BLANCHE: "Streetcar" character
BLANCO: White: Spanish
BLANDA: George of football
BLANE: Composer Ralph
BLANTON: Jazz bassist
BLAS: "Gil __" (Lesage novel)
BLASS: Designer Bill
BLAT: Blurt out
BLATHER: Baloney
BLATTY: "The Exorcist" author
BLATZ: Beer brand
BLAU: Blue: German
BLAUBOK: African antelope
BLAZON: Coat of arms
BLE: Wheat: French
BLEB: Air bubble
BLEDSOE: Actress Tempestt
BLEETH: Actress Yasmine
BLENCH: Cower
BLENDE: Zinc mineral
BLERIOT: French aviator
BLEU: Blue: French
BLIFIL: "Tom Jones" character
BLIGE: Singer Mary J. __

BLIGH: "Bounty" captain
BLIGHTY: England, to Brits
BLIMEY: British exclamation
BLIMPIE: Sandwich-shop chain
BLIN: Buckwheat pancake
BLING: Jewelry, slangily
BLINI: Russian pancakes
BLINIS: Russian pancakes
BLISH: Sci-fi author James
B-LIST: Secondary choices
B. LIT.: English deg.
B. LITT.: English deg.
BLITZEN: Santa reindeer
BLIXEN: Isak Dinesen's real name
BLOBEL: 1999 medicine Nobelist
BLOCH: Composer Ernest
BLOG: Web diary
BLOIS: French city
BLOK: Russian poet
BLOOEY: Awry
BLOOIE: Awry
BLORE: Actor Eric
BLOTTO: Besotted
BLOUNT: "Kenilworth" character
BLOW POP: Lollipop brand
BLOWSY: Bedraggled
BLOWZED: Bedraggled
BLOWZY: Bedraggled
BLS: CPI agency
BLU: Blue: Italian
BLUDGE: Avoid work
BLUE BOY: Gainsborough painting
BLUEFIN: Large tuna
BLUE FLU: Police sickout
BLUE HEN: University of Delaware mascot
BLUE ICE: Glacier layer
BLUE OX: Paul Bunyan's Babe
BLUE-RED: Purplish
BLUE SUN: O star
BLUET: Low-growing flower
BLUE TIT: Small bird
BLUM: 1940s French leader
BLUME: Novelist Judy
BLUNDEN: British writer
BLUSH-ON: Type of cosmetic
BLUTH: Director Don
BLUTO: Popeye foe
BLY: Globetrotting journalist Nellie
BLYDEN: Actor Larry
BLYNKEN: Sailor of rhyme
BLYTH: Actress Ann
BLYTHE: Bill Clinton's original last name
BLYTON: Author Enid
BME: Engr. degree
BMI: Music-licensing org.
BMOC: Campus VIP
B MOVIE: Low-budget film
BMT: NYC subway
B. MUS.: Conservatory deg.
BMW: German auto
BMX: Type of motorcycle race
BNAI: __ B'rith
B NEG: Blood type: Abbr.
B NINE: Bingo call
BOAC: Airline's former name
BOATEL: Waterside lodging
BOAZ: Husband of Ruth
BOBA TEA: Frothy Chinese drink
BOBBIDI: "Bibbidi __ Boo"
BOBBIE: Country singer Gentry
BOBBSEY: Kid-lit twin
BOBBY: London cop
BOBBY'S: "__ Girl" (1962 tune)
BOB DOLE: Former Kansas senator
BOB GOEN: Former "Wheel of Fortune" host
BOB HOPE: Beloved comedian
BOB KANE: Batman creator
BOBO: Mrs. Winthrop Rockefeller
BOB TWAY: Pro golfer
BOB VILA: Home-repair guru
BOB WEIR: Grateful Dead member
BOCA: Mouth: Spanish
BOCCE: Italian bowling
BOCCI: Italian bowling
BOCCIE: Italian bowling
BOCELLI: Tenor Andrea
BOCHCO: "N.Y.P.D. Blue" creator
BOCHNER: Actor Hart
BOCHSA: French composer
BOCHY: Baseball manager Bruce
BODDY: Victim in Clue
BODEGA: Hispanic grocery
BODEL: French poet
BO DEREK: "10" actress
BODETT: Motel 6 spokesperson
BODINE: Auto racer Geoff
BODKIN: Hairpin
BODLEY: British architect
BO DUKE: Hazzard County guy
BODY ART: Tattoos
BODY BAR: Sort of soap
BODY KIT: Auto-decoration gear
BOEING: Aircraft brand
BOER: Dutch South African
BOER WAR: 1899-1902 event
BOESKY: Financier Ivan
BOEUF: Beef: French
BOFF: Belly laugh
BOFFIN: Scientist, in Britain
BOFFO: Box-office hit
BOFFOLA: Box-office hit
BOGAN: Poet Louise
BOGARDE: Actor Dirk
BOGART: "Casablanca" star
BOGARTS: Monopolizes
BOGGS: Wade of baseball
BOGGUSS: Country singer Suzy
BOGIE: Evil spirit
BOGLE: Evil spirit
BOGOTA: Colombian capital
BOGY: Evil spirit
BOHAY: Actress Heidi
BOHEA: Black tea
BOHEME: "La __" (Puccini opera)
BOHEMIA: Czech region
BOHM: Austrian conductor
BOHO: Bohemian
BOHR: Danish physicist
BOHRER: Actress Corinne
BOHRIUM: Element #107
BOIARDO: Italian poet
BOING: Cartoon sound effect
BOINGO: Oingo __ (rock band)
BOIRE: To drink: French
BOIS: Forest: French
BOISE, ID: Northwest city
BOITANO: Figure skater Brian
BOITE: Cabaret
BOITO: Italian composer
BOJER: Norwegian novelist
BOK CHOY: Chinese cabbage
BOKHARA: Valuable rug
BOKKEN: Japanese martial-arts sword
BOL: Manute of basketball
BOLA: Gaucho's weapon
BOLAR: Clayey
BOLA TIE: Arizona neckwear
BOLCOM: Pianist William
BOLDEN: Jazz cornetist
BOLE: Tree trunk
BOLENA: "Anna __" (Donizetti opera)
BOLERO: Spanish dance
BOLET: Cuban pianist
BOLEYN: Wife of Henry VIII
BOLGER: Dancer Ray
BOLIDE: Fireball
BOLIVAR: South American liberator
BOLIVIA: South American nation
BOLL: Cotton capsule
BOLLA: Italian wine brand
BOLLING: D.C. Air Force base
BOLO: Army machete
BOLO TIE: Arizona neckwear
BOLSHOI: Russian ballet company
BOLSHY: Lenin supporter
BOLTON: Singer Michael
BOLUS: Large pill
BOLYAI: Hungarian mathematician
BOM: Good: Portuguese
BOMBA: "Jungle Boy" of films
BOMBAL: Chilean writer
BOMBAY: Indian city's former name
BOMBE: Frozen dessert
BOMBECK: Humorist Erma
BON: Good: French
BONA: __ fide
BONACI: Marine fish
BONAIRE: Netherlands Antilles island
BON AMI: Cleanser brand
BONAR: 1920s British prime minister Law
BONARIO: "Volpone" character
BONDI: Actress Beulah
BONE ASH: Ceramics ingredient
BONERZ: Actor Peter
BONESET: Folk-medicine plant
BONET: Actress Lisa
BONHAM: Actress Helena __ Carter
BONHEUR: French painter
BONIATO: Sweet potato
BONILLA: Bobby of baseball
BONITA: Pretty: Spanish
BONITO: Type of tuna
BONJOUR: French greeting
BON JOVI: Rock group
BON MOT: Witty remark
BONN: German city
BONNARD: French painter
BONNE: Good: French
BONNER: Russian activist Yelena
BONNES: French maids
BONNEY: Billy the Kid's surname
BONNIE: Actress Bedelia
BONO: Good: Italian
BONSAI: Dwarf tree
BONSOIR: Good evening: French
BONT: Director Jan de __
BON TON: Chic
BONUM: Good: Latin
BONZ: Dog-treat brand
BONZE: Buddhist monk
BONZO: Chimp of films
BOOBIRD: Disapproving fan
BOOBY: Dunce
BOOCOO: Abundance
BOOG: Powell of baseball
BOOHBAH: PBS kids' show
BOO HISS: Audience disapproval
BOOJUM: Lewis Carroll creature
BOOK 'EM: "Hawaii Five-O" catchphrase
BOOKER T.: Educator Washington
BOOK I: Part of a literary set
BOOK II: Part of a literary set
BOOK III: Part of a literary set
BOOK IV: Part of a literary set
BOOK IX: Part of a literary set
BOOK V: Part of a literary set
BOOK VI: Part of a literary set
BOOK VII: Part of a literary set
BOOK X: Part of a literary set
BOOLA: College cheer
BOOLE: English mathematician
BOOLEAN: Branch of algebra
BOOMCAR: Auto with a powerful audio system
BOONE: Singer Pat
BOONIES: Backwoods
BOOP: Cartoon girl Betty
BOOPSIE: "Doonesbury" character
BOORMAN: Director John
BOOSLER: Comic Elayne
BOOT-CUT: Flared slightly, as jeans
BOOTER: Soccer player
BOOTES: Northern constellation
BOOTHE: Clare __ Luce
BOOTHIA: Canadian peninsula
BOOT IT: Make an error
BOOT UP: Start a computer
BOP: Jazz style
BO PEEP: Nursery-rhyme girl
BOPHA: Danny Glover film
BOPP: Comet Hale-__
BOR.: Part of NYC
BORA: Adriatic wind
BORAH: Former Idaho senator
BORAX: Cleanser powder
BORAXO: Soap brand
BORDEN: Condensed milk inventor
BORDET: 1919 medicine Nobelist
BORDONI: Actress Irene
BOREAL: Of the north wind
BOREAS: North wind personified
BOREL: French mathematician
BOREN: Former Oklahoma senator
BORG: Bjorn of tennis

BORGE: Danish comic pianist
BORGES: Argentina writer
BORGIAS: Historic Italian family
BORGLUM: Mount Rushmore sculptor
BORGS: "Star Trek" villains
BORIS: Actor Karloff
BORK: 1987 Supreme Court nominee
BORKS: Attacks a candidate in the media
BORLAUG: 1970 peace Nobelist
BORMAN: Apollo astronaut
BORNEO: Malay island
BORO: Part of NYC
BORODIN: Russian composer
BOROMIR: "Lord of the Rings" character
BORON: Element #5
BORS: King Arthur knight
BORSA: "Rigoletto" character
BORSTAL: "__ Boy" (Behan story)
BORU: Brian __ (Irish hero)
BORZAGE: Director Frank
BORZOI: Dog breed
BOS: MA city
BOSCAGE: Mass of trees
BOSCH: Dutch artist
BOSCO: Chocolate syrup brand
BOSE: Audio-system brand
BOSLEY: Actor Tom
BO'S'N: Ship officer
BOSNIA: European nation
BOSON: Subatomic particle
BOSOX: A.L. team
BOSSA: __ nova (Brazilian dance)
BOSSON: Actress Barbara
BOSTONS: Waltzlike dances
BOSUN: Naval officer
BOSWELL: Scottish author
BOT: Automated Web-site assistant
BOTEL: Waterside lodging
BOTHA: South African statesman
BOTHE: German physics Nobelist
BOTHNIA: Baltic gulf
BOTOX: Wrinkle remover
BO TREE: Sacred fig of india
BOTTEGA: Art-studio cooperative
BOTTS: __ dots (highway-lane reflectors)
BOUCHE: Mouth: French
BOUCHER: French painter
BOUDIN: French sausage
BOUFFE: Comic opera
BOULE: Metal ball
BOULEZ: French composer
BOULT: English conductor
BOURG: French market town
BOURGET: French writer
BOURKE: Photographer Margaret __-White
BOURNE: "The __ Identity" (Ludlum novel)
BOURSE: European stock exchange
BOUSONO: Spanish poet
BOUTON: Jim of baseball
BOUTROS: First name at the U.N.
BOUVIER: Jackie Kennedy's maiden name
BOVA: Sci-fi author Ben
BOVARY: Flaubert character
BOVET: Italian medicine Nobelist
BOVID: Cow
BOWA: Larry of baseball
BOWDLER: English expurgator
BOWDOIN: Maine college
BOWE: Boxer Riddick
BOW ECHO: Storm's radar signature
BOWEN: English author
BOWES: "Amateur Hour" radio host
BOWFIN: Atlantic fish
BOWHEAD: Type of whale
BOWIE: Rock singer David
BOWLES: Camilla Parker-__
BOWLINE: Nautical rope
BOW OAR: Rower
BOWSHOT: Archery distance
BOWYER: Archer supplier
BOWZER: Sha Na Na leader
BOXBALL: Street game
BOX SET: Stage area
BOXSTER: Porsche model
BOYD: Hopalong Cassidy portrayer
BOYER: Actor Charles
BOYLE: Actor Peter
BOYLE'S: __ law (physics principle)
BOYO: Australian lad
BOY TOY: Date, to Madonna
BOYZ: __ II Men (rap group)
BOZ: Dickens pen name
BOZEMAN: Montana city
BPI: Computer-tape density meas.
BPOE: Fraternal lodge: Abbr.
BPS.: Church dignitaries: Abbr.
BRAC: Bric-a-__
BRACCO: Actress Lorraine
BRACERO: Migrant worker
BRACH'S: Candy brand
BRACK: "Hedda Gabler" character
BRACKEN: Actor Eddie
BRACT: Leaflike part
BRAD: Thin nail
BRADLEE: Former Washington Post exec
BRADLEY: Former New Jersey senator
BRADY: Civil War photographer
BRAE: Scottish hillside
BRAEDEN: Actor Eric
BRAGA: Actress Sonia
BRAGG: Confederate general
BRAGH: "Erin go __!"
BRAHE: Danish astronomer
BRAHMA: Bull breed
BRAHMAN: Hindu priest
BRAHMIN: Boston bigwig
BRAHMS: German composer
BRAILLE: Alphabet inventor
BRAINER: No-__ (easy decision)
BRAM: Author Stoker
BRAMAH: English inventor
BRAMLEY: Apple variety
BRANAGH: Actor Kenneth
BRANCA: Ralph of baseball
BRANDI: Soccer star Chastain
BRANDO: Actor Marlon
BRANDON: "Beverly Hills 90210" role
BRANDT: 1970s German leader
BRAND X: Unnamed product
BRANG: Fetched, to a hillbilly
BRANIFF: Former airline
BRANSON: Missouri city
BRANT: Arctic goose
BRAQUE: French artist
BRASCO: Johnny Depp role
BRASIER: Charcoal grill
BRASIL: South American land, to natives
BRASOV: Romanian city
BRASSIE: Golf club
BRATSK: Russian city
BRATT: Actor Benjamin
BRATTLE: Scamper noisily
BRAUN: Wernher von __
BRAVADA: Oldsmobile model
BRAWLEY: California city
BRAXTON: Singer Toni
BRAZ.: S.A. country
BRAZIER: Charcoal grill
BRAZO: Arm: Spanish
BRAZOS: Texas river
BRAZZA: French explorer of Africa
BRAZZI: Actor Rossano
BREA: California city
BREAM: Freshwater fish
BRECA: "Beowulf" character
BRECHT: German playwright
BRECK: Shampoo brand
BREDA: Dutch city
BREDE: Braid, old-style
BREE: Broth: Scottish
BREEDY: Prolific
BREEN: Actor Bobby
BREI: Matzo __ (Passover meal)
BREL: French composer
BREMEN: German city
BREMER: Actress Lucille
BREN: British gun
BRENDA: "Beverly Hills 90210" character
BRENDAN: Actor Fraser
BRENDEL: Austrian pianist
BRENDON: Actor Nicholas
BREN GUN: British firearm
BRENLY: Baseball manager Bob
BRENNAN: Actor Walter
BRENNER: Comedian David
BRENT: Sportscaster Musburger
BRER FOX: Uncle Remus character
BRESCIA: Italian city
BRESLIN: Columnist Jimmy
BREST: French port
BRET: Author Harte
BRETON: Native of Brittany
BRETT: George of baseball
BRETTON: __ Woods, NH
BREUER: Hungarian furniture designer
BREVE: Vowel mark
BREVET: Honorary promotion
BREVI: Short: Comb. form
BREVIS: "Ars longa, vita __"
BREYER: Clinton Supreme Court appointee
BREYER'S: Ice-cream brand
BRIAN: Director De Palma
BRIANA: "Faerie Queene" character
BRIAND: French statesman
BRIARD: Dog breed
BRIC: __-a-brac
BRICE: "Funny Girl" subject
BRICKLE: Easily broken
BRIDGER: Old West mountain man
BRIDGET: Actress Fonda
BRIENZ: Swiss lake
BRIGAND: Bandit
BRIGHAM: Mormon leader Young
BRIGID: Patron saint of Ireland
BRIGIT: Patron saint of Ireland
BRILL: Comic Charlie
BRILLIG: "Jabberwocky" word
BRILLO: Soap-pad brand
BRIMLEY: Actor Wilford
BRINDLE: Kind of cat
BRING IN: Acquire
BRING IT: Throw a fastball
BRINKER: Fictional skater
BRIO: Allegro con __
BRIOCHE: French roll
BRISE: Ballet leap
BRISTOL: British port
BRITCOM: British sitcom
BRITE: Shiny, in product names
BRITH: B'nai __
BRITNEY: Singer Spears
BRITPOP: Rock music genre
BRITT: Actress Ekland
BRITTEN: English composer
BRITTON: Actress Barbara
BRITZ: Golfer Jerilyn
BRIX: Tarzan portrayer
BRN.: Eye color: Abbr.
BRNO: Czech city
BROAD A: Vowel sound
BROCA: French anthropologist
BROCA'S: "__ Brain" (Sagan book)
BROCK: Lou of baseball
BRODIE: Daredevil leap
BRODKEY: Author Harold
BRODSKY: Former U.S. poet laureate
BRODY: Actor Adrien
BROKAW: Former NBC anchorman
BROLIN: Actor James
BROLLY: Umbrella, in Britain
BROM: Washington Irving character
BROMINE: Element #35
BROMO: Bromine: Comb. form
BRON: Actress Eleanor
BRONKO: Football great Nagurski
BRONSON: Actor Charles
BRONTE: "Jane Eyre" author
BRONTES: Literary sisters
BRONWEN: "How Green Was My Valley" character
BRONX: Big Apple borough
BROOKE: Actress Shields
BROPHY: British writer
BROR: "Out of Africa" character
BROSNAN: Actor Pierce

BROSSE: Brush: French
BROT: Bread: German
BROUD: "Clan of the Cave Bear" character
BROUGH: Louise of tennis
BROUN: Writer Heywood
BROVIK: "The Master Builder" role
BROWARD: Ft. Lauderdale's county
BROWNE: Cartoonist Dik
BROWN U.: Rhode Island school
BROW WAX: Spa service
BROZ: Tito's real surname
BRR: "It's cold!"
BRRR: "It's cold!"
BRS.: Apartment ad abbr.
BRUBECK: Jazz pianist
BRUCE: Comic Lenny
BRUCH: German composer
BRUDER: Brother: German
BRUEGEL: Flemish painter
BRUGES: Belgian city
BRUHL: "Deathtrap" character
BRUHN: Danish ballet dancer
BRUIT: Spread the news
BRULE: Burnt: French
BRULEE: Burnt: French
BRUMAL: Wintry
BRUME: Fog
BRUMEL: Russian high jumper
BRUMMEL: Beau __
BRUN: "Clan of the Cave Bear" character
BRUNEI: Asian country
BRUNI: Supermodel Carla
BRUNO: Shoe designer Magli
BRUNOR: King Arthur knight
BRUT: Very dry, as wine
BRUTUS: "Julius Caesar" character
BRUX: Grind one's teeth
BRUXISM: Teeth grinding
BRYAN: Orator William Jennings __
BRYANT: Poet William Cullen __
BRYCE: __ Canyon National Park
BRYN: __ Mawr College
BRYNNER: Actor Yul
BRYNZA: Sharp cheese
BRYSON: Singer Peabo
BRYUSOV: Russian poet
BSA: Scouting org.
B SCALE: Piano practice
B SCHOOL: MBA offerer
B SEVEN: Bingo call
BSH.: Farmer's meas.
BSHARP: C alias
B SIDE: Record surface
B SIX: Bingo call
BSMT.: Real-estate ad abbr.
B.S.S: Four-year degs.
B STAR: Spectral type
B TEAM: Athletic substitutes
B TEN: Bingo call
BTFSPLK: "Li'l Abner" character
B THREE: Bingo call
B TILE: Scrabble three-pointer
B TO B: Type of Yellow Pages
BTU: Heat unit: Abbr.
BTW: Incidentally, in cyber-shorthand
B TWELVE: Bingo call
B TWO: Bingo call
BUBBA: Good ole boy
BUBER: Jewish philosopher
BUBKA: Ukrainian pole vaulter
BUBKES: Nada
BUC: Tampa Bay footballer
BUCCAL: Oral
BUCCO: "The Sopranos" role
BUCHAN: Scottish novelist
BUCHMAN: "Mad About You" surname
BUCHNER: 1907 chemistry Nobelist
BUCKEYE: Ohioan
BUCKLEY: Conservative commentator
BUCKNER: Bill of baseball
BUCKO: British fellow
BUCKRAM: Bookbinding fabric
BUCKY: Dent of baseball
BUCO: Osso __
BUDA: City that merged with Pest
BUDD: Melville character
BUDGIE: Parakeet
BUELL: "Little Lulu" cartoonist
BUELLER: Matthew Broderick role
BUENA: Good: Spanish
BUENAS: "__ noches"
BUENO: Good: Spanish
BUENOS: "__ días"
BUFFA: Comic opera
BUFFAY: "Friends" role
BUFFETT: Singer Jimmy
BUFFO: Comic-opera role
BUFFON: French naturalist
BUFFY: "__ the Vampire Slayer"
BUGAKU: Japanese dance
BUGALOO: Fast dance
BUGATTI: Italian auto
BUGBEAR: Persistent problem
BUGBOY: Apprentice jockey
BUGGLES: "Video Killed the Radio Star" group
BUGSY: Warren Beatty film
BUICK: GM auto
BUISSON: 1927 peace Nobelist
BUITONI: Pasta brand
BUJOLD: Actress Genevieve
BUJONES: Cuban ballet dancer
BUKAVU: Congo city
BUKHARA: Fine rug
BULBA: "Taras __" (Gogol novel)
BULDEO: "Jungle Book" character
BULG.: Balkan land: Abbr.
BULGARI: Italian retail chain
BULGHUR: Type of wheat
BULGUR: Type of wheat
BULLA: Papal seal
BULLINS: Playwright Ed
BULLITT: Steve McQueen film
BULLOCK: Actress Sandra
BULL RUN: Civil War battle
BULOVA: Watch brand
BULOW: Claus von __
BULWER: Author Edward __-Lytton
BUMBRY: Opera singer Grace
BUMPPO: "The Deer Slayer" character
BUM-RUSH: Crash
BUNCHE: 1950 peace Nobelist
BUNCO: Swindle
BUND: Political society
BUNDT: Kind of cake
BUNDY: "Married...With Children" surname
BUNGAY: "Tono-__" (H.G. Wells novel)
BUNIN: Russian poet
BUNNING: Jim of baseball
BUNRAKU: Japanese puppet theater
BUNSEN: German chemist
BUNTON: One of the Spice Girls
BUNUEL: Spanish director
BUNUELO: Mexican pastry
BUNYAN: Legendary lumberjack
BUON: Good: Italian
BUONA: Good: Italian
BUONO: Actor Victor
BUPKES: Nada
BUPKIS: Nada
BUPKUS: Nada
BUQSHA: Money of Yemen
BURANA: "Carmina __" (Orff work)
BURBAGE: Shakespeare associate
BURBANK: California city
BURBOT: Freshwater cod
BURDICK: Novelist Eugene
BUREN: Martin Van __
BURET: Lab tube
BURETTE: Chemist's tube
BURGEE: Yacht flag
BURGESS: Actor Meredith
BURGH: Scottish town
BURGOO: Highly seasoned stew
BURGOS: City in Spain
BURIN: Ancient chisel
BURKA: Muslim woman's garment
BURKE: Actress Billie
BURKINA: __ Faso (African nation)
BURL: Tree knot
BURLEY: Type of tobacco
BURMA: Myanmar's former name
BURNABY: British Columbia city
BURNET: Australian medicine Nobelist
BURNETT: Comedienne Carol
BURNEY: British writer
BURNIE: Glen __, MD
BURNLEY: English city
BUR OAK: Acorn producer
BURPEE: Seed merchant
BURR: Scottish accent
BURSA: Anatomical sac
BURSTYN: Actress Ellen
BURT: Actor Lancaster
BURTON: Actor Richard
BURUNDI: African nation
BUSBY: Military hat
BUSCEMI: Actor Steve
BUSCH: Anheuser-__
BUSEY: Actor Gary
BUSHER: Minor leaguer
BUSHHOG: Land-clearing device
BUSHIDO: Samurai code
BUSHWA: Baloney
BUSHWAH: Baloney
BUSK: Entertain on the street
BUSMAN'S: __ holiday
BUSON: Japanese poet
BUSONI: Italian composer
BUSTA: __ Rhymes (rap artist)
BUSTARD: Australian bird
BUSTIER: Kind of blouse
BUTCH: Short haircut
BUTENE: Flammable hydrocarbon
BUTEO: Buzzard
BUTKUS: Dick of football
BUT NO: Belushi catchphrase
BUTTE, MT: Northwestern city
BUTTRAM: Actor Pat
BUTUT: Gambian coin
BUTYL: Kind of alcohol
BUTZ: Nixon cabinet member
BUYDOWN: Mortgage prepayment
BUZ: Sawyer of the comics
BUZZELL: Director Edward
BUZZI: Comic Ruth
BVD: Underwear brand
BWANA: Boss, in Africa
BWAY: NYC theater district
BWI: Caribbean island grp.
BYAM: "Mutiny on the Bounty" character
BYATT: British novelist
BYCATCH: Mistakenly caught marine animals
BYFORM: Linguistic variant
BY ME: Poker phrase
BYNER: Comedian John
BYNG: Lady __ Memorial Trophy (NHL award)
BYO: Invitation letters
BYOB: Invitation letters
BYRD: Polar explorer
BYRDS: 1960s folk-rock band
BYRNE: Actor Gabriel
BYRNES: Truman cabinet member
BYRON: British poet
BYSSHE: Percy __ Shelley
BY TENS: One way to count
BYU: Utah sch.

C

CAA: Presidential monogram
CAAN: Actor James
CABALA: Ancient occultism
CABALLE: Spanish soprano
CABBALA: Ancient occultism
CABELL: Enos of baseball
CABER: Scottish pole
CABEZA: Head: Spanish
CABLET: Nautical rope
CABLE TV: Antenna alternative
CABO: __ San Lucas (Mexican resort)
CABOB: Skewered dish
CABOT: Italian explorer
CABRAL: Portuguese explorer
CABRINI: Canonized nun
CABRIO: Volkswagen model
CAC: Bad: Comb. form

CACHACA: Brazilian rum
CACIQUE: Tropical oriole
CACO: Bad: Comb. form
CACONYM: Misnomer
CADBURY: Candy brand
CADE: Procession: Comb. form
CADEAU: Gift: French
CADENT: Having rhythmic flow
CADENZA: Concerto part
CADETTE: Girl Scout member
CADGE: Be a moocher
CADI: Islamic judge
CADIZ: Spanish port
CADMIC: Of element #48
CADMIUM: Element #48
CADMUS: Phoenician prince
CADUCEI: Medical symbols
CADY: Elizabeth __ Stanton
CAEN: French city
CAESURA: Pause
CAFFE: Coffee: Italian
CAGNEY: "White Heat" star
CAGUAS: Puerto Rican city
CAHIER: French notebook
CAHILL: "__ - United States Marshal" (John Wayne film)
CAHN: Lyricist Sammy
CAHOKIA: Illinois city
CAICOS: Bahamas island group
CAILLOU: Kiddie cartoon character
CAIMAN: Crocodile
CAINE: Actor Michael
CAIN'T: "I __ Say No" ("Oklahoma!" tune)
CAIRENE: Cairo native
CAIRN: Stone landmark
CAISSON: Ammo wagon
CAIUS: __ Julius Caesar
CAJON: El __, CA
CAL: Presidential nickname
CALABRO: Actor Thomas
CALAF: "Turandot" role
CALAIS: French port
CALAMAR: Squid
CALANDO: Becoming slower and softer: Mus.
CALASH: Horse-drawn carriage
CALCIFY: Become bony
CALCITE: Chalk or marble
CALCIUM: Element #20
CALCULI: Tooth deposits
CALDER: Mobile artist
CALDERA: Volcano crater
CALE: Auto racer Yarborough
CALEB: Author Carr
CALENDS: First of a Roman month
CALGARY: Alberta city
CALGON: Detergent brand
CALHOUN: John Quincy Adams vice president
CALI: Colombian city
CALIBAN: "The Tempest" character
CALICES: Church cups
CALIFS: Ottoman rulers
CALIPH: Ottoman ruler
CALISTA: Actress Flockhart
CALIX: Church cup
CALKINS: Philosopher Mary
CALLAN: Actor Michael
CALLAO: City in Peru
CALLAS: Soprano Maria
CALLBOY: Certain stagehand
CALLE: Street: Spanish
CALLI: Beautiful: Comb. form
CALL IT: Make an accurate prediction
CALME: Calm: French
CAL-MEX: Spicy cuisine
CALOR: Heat: Spanish
CALOTTE: Priest's skullcap
CAL POLY: Engineering school, for short
CAL TECH: Engineering school, for short
CALVARY: New Testament locale
CALVERT: Maryland founder
CALVET: Actress Corinne
CALVIN: French theologian
CALVINO: Italian writer
CALX: Ashy residue
CALYCES: Flower parts
CALYX: Flower part
CALZONE: Italian turnover
CAMA: Bed: Spanish
CAMACHO: Boxer Hector
CAMARO: Chevy model
CAMAY: Soap brand
CAMBER: Arch slightly
CAM BOY: Internet self-photographer
CAMBRIA: Ancient name of Wales
CAMBRIC: Cotton fabric
CAMBS: English county
CAMDEN: New Jersey city
CAMERAE: Judges' chambers
CAMERON: "Titanic" director
CAM GIRL: Internet self-photographer
CAMILLA: Prince Charles' second
CAMILLE: Composer Saint-Saëns
CAMINO: Road: Spanish
CAMION: Army truck
CAMISE: Loose shirt
CAMMIE: Camouflage
CAMO: Army wear
CAMOES: Portuguese poet
CAMPARI: Italian aperitif
CAMPION: Director Jane
CAMPO: Argentina plain
CAMP UP: Overact
CAMRY: Toyota model
CAMRY LE: Toyota model
CAMRYN: Actress Manheim
CAMUS: French novelist
CANA: Biblical miracle site
CANAAN: Biblical land
CANBY: Critic Vincent
CANCHA: Jai alai court
CANCUN: Mexican resort
CANDACE: Author Bushnell
CANDELA: Luminosity unit
CANDENT: White-hot
CANDIA: Cretan port
CANDICE: Actress Bergen
CANDIDA: Tony Orlando and Dawn tune
CANDIDE: Voltaire novel
CAN-DO: Enthusiastic
C AND W: Music genre
CANEA: Capital of Crete
CANEM: Dog: Latin
CANETTI: Author Elias
CANID: Dog
CANIDAE: Dog family
CANIFF: Cartoonist Milton
CANIO: "I Pagliacci" role
CANIS: Astronomical dog
CAN IT: "Be quiet!"
CANKER: Mouth sore
CANLIT: North-of-the-border writings
CANNA: Tropical plant
CANNEL: Form of coal
CANNELL: "Rockford Files" creator
CANNES: French resort
CANNOCK: English town
CANNOLI: Italian dessert
CANNULA: Medical tube
CANOPUS: Bright star
CANOVA: Actress Judy
CANSECO: Jose of baseball
CANTAB: Cambridge student
CANTAL: French cheese
CANTINO: Violin string
CANTLE: Saddle part
CANTON: Swiss state
CANTRIP: Magic spell
CAN'T SAY: "I'm not sure"
CANTY: "Prince and the Pauper" character
CANUCKS: NHL team
CANULA: Medical tube
CANUTE: Danish king
CANZONA: Italian ode
CANZONE: Italian ode
CAPA: Bullfighter's cloak
CAPADES: Ice __ (skating show)
CAP-A-PIE: From head to foot
CAPE ANN: Massachusetts peninsula
CAPEESH: "Understand?"
CAPEK: Czech writer
CAPELLA: Star in Auriga
CAPE MAY: New Jersey city
CAPET: French king
CAPITA: Heads: Latin
CAPITAN: El __ (Yosemite peak)
CAPNUT: Bolt cover
CAPO: Guitar device
CAPONE: Eliot Ness adversary
CAPONI: Golfer Donna
CAPOTE: Author Truman
CAPOTES: Long cloaks
CAPP: "Li'l Abner" cartoonist
CAPRA: Director Frank
CAPRI: Italian island
CAPRID: Goatish
CAPRINE: Goatish
CAPRIS: Women's pants
CAPSHAW: Actress Kate
CAPSTAN: Machine part
CAPTIVA: Florida island
CAPUANA: Italian author
CAPUCHE: Monk's hood
CAPULET: Juliet's family name
CAPUT: Head: Latin
CARA: Singer Irene
CARABOO: "Princess __" (1994 film)
CARACAS: Capital of Venezuela
CARAMBA: Spanish exclamation
CARA MIA: Darling: Italian
CARAY: Sportscaster Harry
CARBOY: Glass bottle
CAR BRA: Auto-grille protector
CARDI: Heart: Comb. form
CARDIA: Heart: Comb. form
CARDIFF: Capital of Wales
CARDIN: Designer Pierre
CARDIO: Heart: Comb. form
CARDIUM: Heart: Comb. form
CARDOZO: FDR Supreme Court appointee
CAREW: Rod of baseball
CAREY: Singer Mariah
CARFREE: Like pedestrian malls
CARIB: Antilles Indian
CARIBE: Piranha
CARIBOO: Mountains of British Columbia
CARIES: Tooth decay
CARINA: Bird bone
CARIOCA: Brazilian dance
CARIOLE: One-horse vehicle
CARIOU: Actor Len
CARIOUS: Decayed
CARL: Author Sagan
CARLA: "Cheers" character
CARLE: Composer Frankie
CARLENE: Singer Carter
CARLIN: Comic George
CARLING: Nautical beam
CARLO: Monte __, Monaco
CARLOS: Guitarist Santana
CARLOTA: Empress of Mexico
CARLOW: Irish county
CARLSON: Photocopier inventor
CARLTON: Steve of baseball
CARLY: Singer Simon
CARLYLE: Scottish historian
CARME: Moon of Jupiter
CARMEL: California town
CARMELA: "The Sopranos" role
CARMEN: Bizet opera
CARMINA: "__ Burana" (Orff work)
CARNABY: Fashionable 1960s London street
CARNAC: Johnny Carson alter ego
CARNAP: German philosopher
CARNE: Meat: Spanish
CARNER: Golfer JoAnne
CARNERA: 1930s boxing champ
CARNES: Singer Kim
CARNET: Travel document
CARNEY: Actor Art
CARO: LBJ biographer
CAROLE: Actress Lombard
CAROL I: King of Romania
CAROL II: King of Romania
CAROLL: Big Bird portrayer Spinney
CAROLYN: Actress Jones
CARON: Actress Leslie
CARONI: Trinidad river

CAROTIN: Vitamin A source
CAR PARK: Auto lot, in Britain
CARP AT: Censure
CARPE: "__ diem"
CARPEL: Flower part
CARPO: Fruit: Comb. form
CARPOUS: Fruited: Comb. form
CARPUS: Wrist bone
CARR: Singer Vikki
CARRARA: Italian city
CARRE: Novelist John le __
CARREL: Library desk
CARRERA: Actress Barbara
CARRERE: Actress Tia
CARREY: Actor Jim
CARRIE: Stephen King novel
CARROL: Actor J. __ Naish
CARROLL: Actor O'Connor
CARSEY: TV producer Marcy
CARSON: Author Rachel
CARTA: Magna __
CAR TALK: NPR series
CARTIER: French explorer
CARUSO: Italian tenor
CARVEL: Spanish ship
CARVEY: Comic Dana
CARY: Actor Grant
CAS: Case: French
CASA: House: Spanish
CASALS: Spanish cellist
CASAVA: Tapioca source
CASBAH: Algiers section
CASBY: "Little Dorrit" character
CASCA: "Julius Caesar" character
CASCO: Bay of Maine
CASEATE: Turn to cheese
CASEFY: Turn to cheese
CASEIN: Milk protein
CASELLA: Italian composer
CASE LOT: Wholesale quantity
CASEOUS: Like cheese
CASERN: Barracks
CASERNE: Barracks
CASERTA: Italian city
CASEY: Stengel of baseball
CASIMIR: Revolutionary War general Pulaski
CASIO: Watch brand
CASITA: Bungalow
CASPAR: One of the Magi
CASPARY: Author Vera
CASPER: Ghost of cartoons
CASPIAN: Asian sea
CASQUE: Medieval helmet
CASS: Mama __ Elliott
CASSATT: Painter Mary
CASSAVA: Tapioca source
CASSIA: Chinese cinnamon
CASSIDY: Western outlaw Butch
CASSIE: "A Chorus Line" role
CASSIM: Ali Baba's brother
CASSIN: French peace Nobelist
CASSINI: Designer Oleg
CASSINO: Italian town
CASSIO: "Othello" role
CASSIS: French brandy
CASSIUS: "Julius Caesar" character
CASSOLA: Italian author
CASTA: "__ diva" (Bellini aria)
CASTEL: __ Gandolfo, Italy
CASTILE: Former Spanish kingdom
CAST ON: Start knitting
CASTOR: Mythical twin
CASTROL: Motor-oil brand
CASUIST: Logician
CASUS: Occurrence: Latin
CASY: "The Grapes of Wrath" character
CATALAN: Romance language
CATALO: Bovine hybrid
CATALPA: Southern tree
CATANIA: City of Sicily
CATANO: Puerto Rican city
CATAWBA: White wine
CATBERT: "Dilbert" character
CAT CHOW: Purina product
CATE: Actress Blanchett
CATENA: Chain
CATERA: Cadillac model
CATES: Actress Phoebe
CATHAY: China, old-style
CATHEAD: Nautical beam
CATHER: Author Willa
CATHODE: Battery part
CATHY: Guisewhite comic strip
CATHY'S: "__ Clown" (Everly Brothers tune)
CATION: Charged atom
CATKIN: Willow flower
CATLIN: Painter George
CAT MAN: Lion tamer
CATMINT: Catnip, in Britain
CATO: Roman censor
CATORCE: 14: Spanish
CAT RIG: Boat mast
CAT SUIT: Jumpsuit, in Britain
CATT: Suffragist Carrie
CATTALO: Bovine hybrid
CATTON: Historian Bruce
CATV: Cable syst.
CAUCHY: French mathematician
CAUD: Tail: Comb. form
CAUDAD: Toward the tail
CAUDAL: At the tail
CAUDATE: Tailed
CAUDI: Tail: Comb. form
CAUDO: Tail: Comb. form
CAUL: Stalk: Comb. form
CAUTHEN: Jockey Steve
CAV: Cleveland NBAer
CAVA: Vena __
CAVAE: Venae __
CAVAFY: Greek poet
CAVAN: Irish county
CAVELL: Heroic nurse of WWI
CAVETT: Talk-show host Dick
CAVY: Guinea pig
CAWDOR: Macbeth, Thane of __
CAY: Small island
CAYCE: "The Sleeping Prophet"
CAYMAN: __ Islands (Caribbean group)
CAYUGA: Iroquois Indian
CAYUSE: Indian pony
CAZALE: Actor John
CBC: North-of-the-border network
CBER: Certain trucker
CCC: New Deal agcy.
CCCP: USSR, to Russians
CC'ED: Sent a duplicate to
C CELL: Type of battery
CCH: Actress Pounder
C-CLAMP: Carpenter's tool
C CLEF: Treble marking
CCNY: Big Apple sch.
CCR: "Proud Mary" band, for short
C.C. RIDER: R&B song
CCU: Hosp. ward
CDC: Federal health agcy.
CDR.: Naval off.
CD RACK: Music holder
CD RATE: Bank posting
CD ROM: Computer disk
C.D.T.: Summer clock setting in Chicago: Abbr.
CEA: Pres. council
CEARA: Brazilian port
CEBU: Philippine island
CECE: Singer Winans
CECI: Chickpeas
CECIL B.: Director DeMille
CECILE: One of the Dionnes
CECILIA: "Last Tycoon" character
CECUM: Part of the intestine
CEDI: Ghana money
CEDILLA: "Garçon" feature
CEDRIC: Actor Hardwicke
CEIBA: Kapok
CEL: Animation frame
CELA: Spanish writer
CELADON: Chinese porcelain
CELAENO: "Aeneid" character
CELEBES: Indonesian island
CELEBRE: Cause __
CELESTA: Musical instrument
CELESTE: Actress Holm
CELIA: "As You Like It" character
CELICA: Toyota model
CELIE: "The Color Purple" role
CELINE: Singer Dion
CELLA: Classical temple's center
CELLE: That: French
CELLINI: Italian sculptor
CELOTEX: Insulation material
CELT: NBAer
CELTIC: NBAer
CEMBALO: Harpsichord
CENA: Dinner: Spanish
CENACLE: Retreat house
CENE: Geologist's combining form
CENO: New: Comb. form
CENSE: Add aroma to
CENTAI: Lithuanian coins
CENTAL: Hundredweight
CENTARE: Square meter
CENTAS: Lithuanian coin
CENTI: Hundred: Comb. form
CENTIME: Former French coin
CENTIMO: Former Spanish coin
CENTO: Literary work
CENTR: Middle: Comb. form
CENTRI: Middle: Comb. form
CENTRO: Middle: Comb. form
CENTRUM: Hundred: Latin
CENTU: Lithuanian coins
CENTUM: Hundred
CEORL: Anglo-Saxon freeman
CEP: Edible mushroom
CEPE: Edible mushroom
CEPEDA: Orlando of baseball
CEPHAL: Head: Comb. form
CEPHALO: Head: Comb. form
CEPHALY: Head: Comb. form
CEPHEUS: Northern constellation
CER: Wax: Comb. form
CERA: Wax: Latin
CERAM: Indonesian island
CERAT: Horn: Comb. form
CERATE: Ointment
CERATED: Covered with wax
CERATO: Horn: Comb. form
CERE: Part of a bird's beak
CEREBR: Brain: Comb. form
CEREBRO: Brain: Comb. form
CERES: Agriculture goddess
CEREUS: Cactus
CERF: Random House cofounder
CERIA: Ceramics compound
CERIC: Containing cerium
CERIUM: Element #58
CERNAN: Apollo astronaut
CERO: Mackerel
CERRO: Hill: Spanish
CERT.: Part of CD
CERTS: Breath-mint brand
CERUMEN: Ear wax
CERVEZA: Beer: Spanish
CERVID: Deer
CERVINE: Like deer
C.E.S: Bridge designers: Abbr.
CESAIRE: West Indian poet
CESAR: Composer Franck
CESARE: Basso Siepi
CESARS: French Oscars
CESIUM: Element #55
CESS: Tax, in Britain
CESSNA: Small-plane brand
CESSPIT: Refuse receptacle
C'EST: "__ la vie!"
CESTA: Jai alai basket
C'EST MOI: "Camelot" tune
CESTUS: Ancient Greek belt
CET: Whale: Comb. form
CETA: Govt. job-training program
CETANE: Hydrocarbon
CETE: Group of badgers
CETERA: Others: Latin
CETERIS: __ paribus (other things being equal)
CETO: Whale: Comb. form
CETTE: That: French
CETUS: Whale constellation
CEUTA: Port of Spain
CEVICHE: Raw-fish appetizer
CEY: Ron of baseball
CEYLON: Sri Lanka's former name
CEZANNE: French painter
CFA: Wall St. analyst's designation
CFC: Banned pollutant: Abbr.
CFL: North-of-the-border sports league: Abbr.
CFO: Business VIP

CFS: Baseball positions: Abbr.
CGM.: Metric wt.
CGS: Metric measurement syst.
CHA: Chinese tea
CHABLIS: White wine
CHACEL: Spanish writer
CHACHI: "Happy Days" role
CHACHKA: Knickknack
CHACO: South American region
CHACUN: Each: French
CHAD: African nation
CHADS: Punch-card ballot parts
CHAFER: Type of beetle
CHAFF: Tease
CHAFFEE: Skier Suzy
CHAFFER: Haggle
CHAGALL: Russian painter
CHAI: Jewish pendant
CHAIM: Author Potok
CHAINE: Ballet movement
CHAKA: Singer Khan
CHAKRA: Yoga power point
CHALCIS: Greek city
CHALLAH: Braided loaf
CHALONS: French city
CHALUPA: Fried tortilla
CHAMBRE: Room: French
CHAMFER: Carpenter's cut
CHAN: Fictional detective
CHANCEL: Church area
CHANDU: Magician of old radio
CHANEL: Perfume brand
CHANEY: Actor Lon
CHANG: Michael of tennis
CHANGO: "Presto __!"
CHANOYU: Japanese tea ceremony
CHANSON: Song: French
CHANTE: Jazz singer Moore
CHANTRY: Chapel
CHAO: Actress Rosalind
CHAPALA: Mexican lake
CHAPATI: Indian bread
CHAPEAU: Hat: French
CHAPIN: Singer Harry
CHAPLET: Head wreath
CHAPLIN: "Modern Times" star
CHAPMAN: Peddler, in Britain
CHARCOT: French explorer
CHARING: __ Cross Road (London street)
CHARLEY: __ horse (sore spot)
CHARLY: Cliff Robertson film
CHARMAN: Janitor
CHARMIN: Tissue brand
CHARNIN: "Annie" lyricist
CHARO: Spanish guitarist
CHARON: Moon of Pluto
CHARPAK: 1992 physics Nobelist
CHARRO: Mexican cowboy
CHARTA: Magna __
CHARVET: Actor David
CHAS.: Cartoonist Addams
CHASSE: Ballet step
CHAST: Cartoonist Roz
CHATHAM: English city
CHATTEL: Piece of property, in law
CHATWIN: British novelist
CHAUCER: "Canterbury Tales" author
CHAUD: Hot: French
CHAVA: "Fiddler on the Roof" character
CHAVEZ: Mexican composer
CHAYOTE: Tropical fruit
CHAZAN: Synagogue cantor
CHAZZ: Actor Palminteri
CHAZZAN: Synagogue cantor
CHE: Guerrilla Guevara
CHEADLE: Actor Don
CHEATIN': "Your __ Heart"
CHECHEN: Muslim people
CHEDER: Hebrew school
CHEE: Kim __ (Korean cabbage)
CHEECH: Comic Marin
CHEETOS: Snack-food brand
CHEEVER: Novelist John
CHEEZ: __ Whiz (snack-food brand)
CHEEZ-IT: Snack-food brand
CHEKA: Soviet secret police
CHEKHOV: Russian playwright
CHEKOV: "Star Trek" officer
CHELA: Crab claw
CHELSEA: 1990s First Daughter
CHELY: Country singer Wright
CHEMIC: Of alchemy
CHEMIN: __ de fer (gambling game)
CHEMO: Chemical: Comb. form
CHEN: Actress Joan
CHENEY: Al Gore successor
CHENIER: French poet
CHENIN: __ Blanc (wine grape)
CHEOPS: Egyptian pharaoh
CHER: "Moonstruck" star
CHERE: Beloved: French
CHERI: Sweetheart: French
CHERIE: Sweetheart: French
CHERT: Quartz rock
CHERVIL: Aromatic herb
CHERYL: Actress Ladd
CHESTER: English city
CHET: Guitarist Atkins
CHETA: Tarzan's chimp
CHETRUM: Bhutan money
CHEVAL: Horse: French
CHEVAUX: Horses: French
CHEVET: Cathedral apse
CHEVIOT: Sheep breed
CHEVON: Goat meat
CHEVRE: Goat's-milk cheese
CHEVRET: Goat's-milk cheese
CHEW TOY: Pup's plaything
CHEX: Cereal brand
CHEX MIX: Party-snack brand
CHEXX: Table-hockey game
CHEZ MOI: At my home: French
CHI: Greek letter
CHIA: Mexican plant
CHIANG: Mao opponent
CHIANTI: Italian wine
CHIAPAS: State of Mexico
CHIA PET: Ceramic/plant gift
CHICA: Girl: Spanish
CHICANA: Hispanic woman
CHICANE: Deceive
CHICANO: Hispanic man
CHICHA: South American beer
CHICHEN: __ Itzá (Mayan city)
CHICHI: Pretentious
CHI-CHI'S: Mexican restaurant chain
CHICLET: Gum brand
CHICO: Boy: Spanish
CHIEN: Dog: French
CHIGGER: Parasitic bug
CHIGNON: Hair bun
CHIGOE: Flea
CHILCAT: Alaska Indian
CHILDE: "__ Harold's Pilgrimage" (Byron poem)
CHILES: Actress Lois
CHILIAD: Group of a thousand
CHILKAT: Alaska Indian
CHILLUM: Maryland city
CHIM: "Mary Poppins" song-title word
CHIMERA: Idle fancy
CHI MINH: Ho of Vietnam
CHINCH: Grain-eating bug
CHINE: Backbone
CHING: "I __" (ancient Chinese text)
CHINO: California city
CHINOIS: Cone-shaped sieve
CHINOOK: Warm wind
CHINUA: Author __ Achebe
CHINWAG: Gossip
CHIOS: Aegean isle
CHIRAC: French statesman
CHI-RHO: Vestment monogram
CHIRICO: Italian painter
CHIRO: Hand: Comb. form
CHIRON: Mythical centaur
CHIRR: Cicada sound
CHIRRUP: Bird call
CHISOX: A.L. team
CHISUM: John Wayne film
CHITA: Actress Rivera
CHITLIN: Pig product
CHITON: Ancient Greek garment
CHI-TOWN: Chicago nickname
CHITRA: Tagore work
CHITTER: Twitter
CHITTY: Start of an Ian Fleming book title
CHIVAS: Scotch brand
CHIVY: Chase, in Britain
CHLOE: Lover of Daphnis
CHLOR: Green: Comb. form
CHLORO: Green: Comb. form
CHM.: CEO, often
CHMN.: CEO, often
CHO: Comic Margaret
CHOATE: Connecticut prep school
CHOCK: Wheel wedge
CHOCTAW: Oklahoma Indian
CHOL: Bile: Comb. form
CHOLE: Bile: Comb. form
CHOLINE: B vitamin
CHOLLA: Cactus
CHOLO: Mexican gang member
CHOMSKY: Linguist Noam
CHON: North Korean money
CHONG: Actress Rae Dawn
CHOO: Sneeze sound
CHOPIN: Polish composer
CHOPINE: Old European shoe
CHOPRA: Author Deepak
CHOREO: Dance: Comb. form
CHORINE: Chorus girl
CHORIO: Dance: Comb. form
CHORIZO: Spanish sausage
CHORO: Brazilian dance band
CHOU: Chinese leader __ En-lai
CHOUGH: Crowlike bird
CHOY: Bok __ (Chinese cabbage)
CHRIS: Evert of tennis
CHRISM: Consecrated oil
CHRISOM: Baptismal robe
CHRISTA: Astronaut McAuliffe
CHRISTI: Corpus __, TX
CHRISTO: Bulgarian artist
CHRISTY: New __ Minstrels
CHROM: Color: Comb. form
CHROMA: Purity of color
CHROMAT: Color: Comb. form
CHROMO: Color: Comb. form
CHROMY: Coloring: Comb. form
CHRON.: O.T. book
CHRONO: Time: Comb. form
CHUB: Freshwater fish
CHUBB: Insurance company
CHUCKY: "Child's Play" villain
CHUFF: Locomotive sound
CHUFFY: Churlish
CHU HSI: Chinese philosopher
CHUKKER: Polo period
CHULA: __ Vista, CA
CHUMASH: California Indian
CHUNG: TV anchor Connie
CHUNNEL: England-France connector
CHUPPA: Jewish wedding canopy
CHUPPAH: Jewish wedding canopy
CHURRO: Mexican pastry
CHUTZPA: Effrontery
CHYNNA: Singer Phillips
CHYRON: Electronic TV caption
CIANO: 1940s Italian foreign minister
CIARDI: Poet John
CIA SPY: Government agent
CIB.: Prescription abbr.
CIBBER: British poet laureate
CIBOLA: Legendary treasure cities
C.I.C.: Pres. title
CICCONE: Madonna's last name
CICELY: Actress Tyson
CICERO: Roman orator
CICHLID: Aquarium fish
CID: El __ (Spanish hero)
CIDE: Anti-pest suffix
CIE.: Company: French abbr.
CIEL: Sky: French
CIELO: Sky: Spanish
CIEN: Cadillac model
CIERA: Oldsmobile model
CIGNA: Insurance company
CILENTO: Actress Diane
CILIA: Eyelashes
CILLA: Singer Black
CIMABUE: Italian painter
CIMINO: "The Deer Hunter" director
C. IN C.: Pres. title
CINCO: Five: Spanish
CINDY: Supermodel Crawford

CINEMAX: Cable film channel
CINEOL: Eucalyptus oil
CINEOLE: Eucalyptus oil
CINERGY: Fortune 500 firm
CINESIA: Motion: Comb. form
CINNA: "Julius Caesar" character
CINQ: Five: French
CINQUE: Five, in dice
CINZANO: Vermouth brand
CIO: Union merger partner
CION: Plant shoot
CIR.: About: Abbr.
CIRCE: Mythical sorceress
CIRCUM: Around: Comb. form
CIRE: Glazed fabric
CIRQUE: Circus: French
CIRRATE: Wispy
CIRRO: Cloud combining form
C.I.S.: USSR successor
CISCO: Whitefish
CISEAUX: Ballet leap
CISKEI: South African territory
CISSY: Singer Houston
CIST: Ancient box
CIT.: Footnote abbr.
CITGO: Gas-station brand
CITIUS: Faster: Latin
CITO: Baseball manager Gaston
CITRI: Citrus: Comb. form
CITRIC: Acid in lemons
CITRIN: Bioflavonoid source
CITRINE: Lemon-colored
CITRO: Citrus: Comb. form
CITROEN: French auto
CITRON: Yellow fruit
CIUDAD: City: Spanish
CIVET: Catlike mammal
CIXOUS: French writer
CLABBER: Curdle
CLACK: Cackle
CLACTON: English town
CLAD IN: Wearing
CLAES: Sculptor Oldenburg
CLAIR: Light: French
CLAIRE: Actress Danes
CLAIROL: Hair-care brand
CLAMANT: Noisy
CLAMATO: Juice brand
CLAMBER: Ascend
CLAMMA: Soprano Dale
CLANCY: Author Tom
CLANTON: Earp opponent
CLAPTON: Guitarist Eric
CLAQUE: Group of toadies
CLAR.: Orch. instrument
CLARA: Nurse Barton
CLARE: Irish county
CLARET: Red wine
CLARICE: "The Silence of the Lambs" role
CLARK: "American Bandstand" host
CLARKE: Author Arthur C.
CLARO: Mild cigar
CLARY: Actor Robert
CLASE: Mineral combining form
CLASS A: First-rate
CLASSE: Class: French
CLASSON: Subatomic particle
CLAUDE: Composer Debussy
CLAUDEL: French writer
CLAUDIA: Actress Cardinale
CLAUDIO: Conductor Abbado
CLAVATE: Club-shaped
CLAVE: Musical stick
CLAVELL: "Shogun" novelist
CLAVIER: Keyboard instrument
CLAVIN: "Cheers" mailman
CLAYTON: Adam __ Powell
CLE: Key: French
CLEA: Durrell novel
CLEANTE: "Tartuffe" character
CLEARY: Author Beverly
CLEAVON: Actor Little
CLEEF: Actor Lee Van __
CLEEK: Golf club
CLEESE: Monty Python member
CLEM: Red Skelton character
CLEMENS: Twain's real name
CLEMSON: South Carolina school
CLEO: "Pinocchio" goldfish
CLEON: Jones of baseball
CLEPT: Named, old-style
CLERISY: Literati
CLETE: Boyer of baseball
CLEVE.: OH city
CLEVES: Anne of __ (wife of Henry VIII)
CLEW: Ball of thread
CLIBURN: Pianist Van
CLICHY: French city
CLIFT: Actor Montgomery
CLIFTON: New Jersey city
CLIMAT: Mood: French
CLINE: Country singer Patsy
CLINT: Actor Eastwood
CLIO: Advertising award
CLIVE: Author Barker
CLK.: Judge's asst.
CLOCHE: Bell-shaped hat
CLOETE: South African novelist
CLOONEY: Actor George
CLORETS: Breath-mint brand
CLORIS: Actress Leachman
CLOROX: Bleach brand
CLOTHO: One of the Fates
CLOTURE: Debate-limiting rule
CLOUGH: English poet
CLOVIS: California city
CLOWDER: Group of cats
CLR: Calculator key
CLU: Actor Gulager
CLUB MED: Vacation resort
CLUB UP: Act in concert
CLUEFUL: Well-informed
CLUNY: French town
CLWYD: Welsh county
CLY: "Tale of Two Cities" character
CLYDE: Inept one
CLYM: "Return of the Native" character
C MAJ.: Mus. key
CMD.: Mil. authority
CMDG.: In charge: Abbr.
CMDR.: Nav. rank
C'MON: "Let's go!"
CMT: Nashville cable network
CMTE.: Congressional grp.
CNBC: Cable network
C.N.O.: Navy VIP
CNOSSUS: Ancient city in Crete
C-NOTE: $100 bill
CNS: Brain and spinal cord: Abbr.
CN TOWER: Toronto attraction
CNUT: Ancient English king
C.O.A.: USPS form
COAPT: Bring close
COASE: British economics Nobelist
COATEE: Short coat
COATES: Actress Phyllis
COATI: Tropical carnivore
COBAIN: Rock singer Kurt
COBALT: Chevy model
COBB: Actor Lee J.
COBH: Irish port
COBHAM: Model for Falstaff
COBLENZ: German city
COBO: Detroit arena
COBOL: Computer language
COBRAND: Collaborate in business
COBURG: German city
COBURN: Actor James
COCA: Comic Imogene
COCAS: Andean shrubs
COCCOID: Globular, in zoology
COCCYX: Spinal bone
COCHISE: Apache leader
COCHLEA: Inner-ear part
COCHRAN: Aviator Jacqueline
COCKADE: Ribbon badge
COCO: Designer Chanel
COCOS: Australilan island group
COCTEAU: French director
CODE RED: Emergency status
CODEX: Ancient book
CODICES: Ancient books
CODON: RNA triplet
CODY: "Wild West" showman
CODY, WY: Buffalo Bill Historical Ctr. locale
COE: Track star Sebastian
COELIA: "Faerie Queene" character
COEN: Director Joel
COEPTIS: Word on a $1 bill
COETZEE: South African author
COEUR: Heart: French
COEVAL: Contemporary
C. OF C.: Business-promoting org.
C. OF S.: Sr. presidential aide
COGBURN: "Rooster __" (John Wayne movie)
COGGLE: Ceramics tool
COGHLAN: Irish runner Eamonn
COGITO: "__ ergo sum"
COGNIZE: Perceive
COHAN: "Over There" composer
COHEN: Skater Sasha
COHN: Columbia Pictures cofounder
COHO: Salmon
COHOES: New York city
COIGN: Cornerstone
COIGNE: Cornerstone
COIN-OP: Vending machine
COIR: Coconut fiber
COIT: San Francisco tower
COKIE: TV reporter Roberts
COLADA: Piña __
COLBERT: Actress Claudette
COLBY: Mild cheese
COLCHIS: Golden Fleece land
COLD ONE: Glass of beer
COLE: Composer Porter
COLECO: Former toy company
COLEMAN: Actor Dabney
COLES: Tap dancer Honi
COLETTE: "Gigi" author
COLEUS: Houseplant
COLFAX: Grant's vice president
COLGATE: Toothpaste brand
COLI: E. __ (rod-shaped bacteria)
COLIMA: State of Mexico
COLIN: General Powell
COLLAT.: Bank-loan need: Abbr.
COLLET: Jewel's enclosing rim
COLLIER: Coal miner
COLLINE: "La Bohème" character
COLLINS: Singer Judy
COLLODI: "Pinocchio" author
COLLOID: Gel
COLLOP: Slice of bacon
COLLOQ.: Dictionary abbr.
COLLUDE: Conspire
COLLYER: Game-show host Bud
COLM: Actor Meaney
COLMAN: Actor Ronald
COLMAR: French city
COLOMBO: Sri Lanka capital
COLONES: Costa Rica money
COLONNA: Comedian Jerry
COLONUS: Roman serf
COLSON: Chuck of Watergate
COLTER: Country singer Jessi
COLTON: California city
COLUM: Irish playwright
COLUMBA: Dove constellation
COLUMBO: Peter Falk role
COM: Dot-__ (Internet company)
COMAE: Comet heads
COMATE: Hairy
COMBIEN: How much: French
COMCAST: Cable TV company
COMDEN: Lyricist Betty
COMDEX: Big computer trade show
COMDR.: Nav. rank
COME AS: Impersonate at a Halloween party
COME AT: Approach
COMEDIA: Comedy: Spanish
COMEDIE: Comedy: French
COMETH: "The Iceman __"
COMEX: Financial market
COMFIT: Kind of candy
COMICE: Type of pear
COMIDA: Meal: Spanish
COMIN': "__ Thro' the Rye"
COMIQUE: Comic: French
COMITY: Amity
COMIX: Cartoons
COMM.: Cabinet dept.
COMME: How: French
COMMISH: City official, informally
COMMOVE: Agitate
COMO: Singer Perry

COMOROS: Indian Ocean island group
COMPAQ: Computer company
COMPART: Subdivide
COMPAS: Haitian music
COMPEND: Epitome
COMPLIN: Canonical hour
COMPOS: Non __ mentis
COMPOZ: Sleep-aid brand
COMPTON: California city
COMSAT: Communications satellite
COMTE: French noble
COMTISM: Positivist's philosophy
COMTREX: Cold-remedy brand
COMUS: Thomas Arne work
CONAGRA: Fortune 500 firm
CON AIR: Nicolas Cage film
CONAKRY: Capital of Guinea
CONAN: Schwarzenegger role
CONANT: Former Harvard president
CON BRIO: Musical direction
CONC.: Like some OJ
CONCHA: Outer ear
CONCHO: Shell: Comb. form
CONCHOS: Mexican river
CONCUSS: Agitate
COND.: RR employee
CONDE: Magazine publisher Nast
CONDI: Rice's nickname
CONDIGN: Well-deserved
CONDOLE: Commiserate
CONDUCE: Gravitate
CONEY: __ Island, NY
CONEYS: Rabbits
CONF.: Meeting: Abbr.
CONFECT: Put together
CONFIT: Cooked duck
CONFREY: Composer Zez
CONFUTE: Disprove
CONGE: Leave-taking
CONGER: Marine eel
CONGOU: Black tea
CONKER: Horse chestnut
CONKLIN: Silents actor Chester
CONLAN: Baseball Hall of Fame umpire
CON MOTO: Musical direction
CONN: Steer a ship
CONNATE: Inborn
CONNEE: Singer Boswell
CONNERY: Actor Sean
CONNICK: Singer Harry
CONNIE: Actress Sellecca
CONNIFF: Orchestra leader Ray
CONNOR: America's Cup victor Dennis
CONNORS: Actor Chuck
CONOCO: Oil company
CONOID: Cone shape
CONON: Pope
CONRACK: Jon Voight film
CONRAD: "Lord Jim" author
CONRIED: Actor Hans
CONROY: Author Pat
CONST.: U.S. document
CONT.: Eur. or N.A.
CONTAC: Cold-remedy brand
CONTE: Italian noble
CONTEMN: Treat with scorn
CONTI: Film composer Bill
CONTR.: Legal doc.
CONTRA: Nicaraguan guerrilla
CONTRE: Against: French
CONTUSE: Bruise
CONURE: Parrot
CON. U.S.: Mainland Amer.
CONV.: Annual business mtg.
CONVY: TV host Bert
CONWAY: Comic Tim
CONY: Rabbit fur
COODER: Guitarist Ry
COODY: Golfer Charles
COOEE: Aborigine call
COOGAN: Actor Jackie
COOKE: TV host Alistair
COOLEY: "Dick Van Dyke Show" role
COOLIO: Rap artist
COOLMAX: Sportswear fabric
COOLPIX: Nikon brand
COONCAN: Card game
COONEY: Boxer Gerry
COOPER: Barrel maker
COOPT: Assimilate
COORS: Beer brand
COOSA: Georgia river
COOTE: Actor Robert
COOTER: Aquatic turtle
COPA: "At the __" (Manilow tune)
COPAL: Varnish ingredient
COPIA: Plenty: Latin
COP IT: Get beaten
COPLAND: Composer Aaron
COPLEY: Painter John Singleton __
COPPICE: Thicket
COPPOLA: "The Godfather" director
COPRA: Coconut meat
COPSE: Thicket
COP SHOP: Police station
COPT: Egyptian Christian
COP TO: Admit
COPULA: Linking verb
COQ: Rooster: French
COQUI: Puerto Rican tree frog
COQUINA: Kind of clam
COR: English horn
CORA: "Blondie" character
CORACI: Director Frank
CORACLE: Welsh boat
CORAZON: Heart: Spanish
CORBEL: Stone bracket
CORBETT: Boxer Jim
CORBIN: Actor Bernsen
CORBY: Actress Ellen
CORDA: String, in music
CORDATE: Heart-shaped
CORDAY: French Revolution figure
CORDELL: FDR secretary of state Hull
CORDERO: Jockey Angel
CORDIA: Mitsubishi model
CORDITE: Explosive
CORDOBA: Spanish city
COREA: Jazz pianist
CORELLI: Italian composer
CORETTA: __ Scott King
COREY: Actor Wendell
CORFAM: Synthetic leather
CORFU: Greek island
CORI: 1947 medicine Nobelist
CORINNE: Actress Calvet
CORINTH: Ancient Greek city
CORIUM: Skin
CORM: Plant-stem base
CORMACK: 1979 medicine Nobelist
CORMAN: Director Roger
CORNEL: Actor Wilde
CORNELL: Ivy League school
CORNING: Glass brand
CORNISH: Chicken breed
CORNO: French horn
CORNU: Horn
CORNUTE: Horn-shaped
COROLLA: Toyota model
COROT: French painter
CORPORA: Writing collections
CORPUS: Body of work
CORRADE: Rub away
CORREO: Mail: Spanish
CORRI: Actress Adrienne
CORRIDA: Bullfight
CORSA: Opel model
CORSAIR: Pirate
CORSICA: Mediterranean island
CORSO: Beat poet Gregory
CORT: Actor Bud
CORTES: Aztec conqueror
CORTEZ: Aztec conqueror
CORTICO: Cortex: Comb. form
CORTINA: 1956 Winter Olympics site
CORTOT: Pianist Alfred
CORVAIR: Chevy model
CORVEE: Feudal worker
CORVID: Crow
CORVINA: Game fish
CORVINE: Like a crow
CORVO: Italian wine
CORVUS: Crow constellation
CORWIN: Brown of football
CORY: Robinson poem subject
CORYELL: Detective novelist
CORYZA: Common cold
CORZINE: New Jersey politician
COS: Romaine lettuce
COSA: __ Nostra
COSBY: Bill of sitcoms
COSEC: Trig function
COSELL: Sportscaster Howard
COSET: Math group
COSETTE: "Les Misérables" character
COSH: Hit on the head, in Britain
COSHER: Pamper
COSI: "__ fan tutte" (Mozart opera)
COSINE: Trig function
COSM: World: Comb. form
COSMAS: Patron saint of barbers
COSMO: Women's mag
COSSET: Pamper
COSTA: Rib
COSTAIN: "The Silver Chalice" author
COSTARD: English apple
COSTAS: Sportscaster Bob
COSTATE: Having ribs
COSTCO: Warehouse-club chain
COSTIVE: Uncommunicative
COSTNER: Actor Kevin
COSY UP: Snuggle
COTAN: Trig function
COTE D'OR: French department
COTLER: Actress Kami
COTTA: Church vestment
COTTEN: Actor Joseph
COTTER: Machine wedge
COTY: 1950s French president
COUE: French psychotherapist
COULDA: "I __ been a contender!"
COULEE: Deep ravine
COULOMB: French physicist
COULTER: Plow attachment
COUNTEE: Poet Cullen
COUNT 'EM: "Look at how many!"
COURANT: Au __ (up to date)
COURBET: French painter
COURIC: TV host Katie
COURT TV: Cable channel
COURU: Running, in ballet
COUSINE: French relative
COUSY: Bob of basketball
COUTER: Elbow armor
COVENT: London's __ Garden
COVER ME: Western-film gunfight line
COVINA: California city
COWBANE: Poisonous plant
COWENS: Dave of basketball
COWES: Isle of Wight resort
COWLEY: English poet
COWPER: English poet
COWRIE: Seashell
COWRY: Seashell
COX: Comedian Wally
COXA: Hip joint
COXCOMB: Conceited dandy
COXES: Steers a racing shell
COYDOG: Canine hybrid
COYPU: Aquatic rodent
COZ: Cousin, informally
COZEN: Deceive
COZUMEL: Mexican resort
COZZENS: Novelist James Gould
C.P.E. BACH: German composer
C.P.I.: Inflation meas.
CPL.: NCO
C.P.O.: Nav. rank
C.P. SNOW: English novelist
CPT.: Army rank: Abbr.
C.P.U.: Computer brain: Abbr.
CRABBE: Actor Buster
CRACK'D: "The Mirror __" (Christie novel)
CRACOW: Polish city
CRACY: Government: Comb. form
CRAFTSY: Artsy-__
CRAIG: Diet guru Jenny
CRAIGIE: Scottish lexicographer
CRAIG T.: Actor Nelson
CRAIK: Canadian town
CRAIN: Actress Jeanne
CRAIN'S: Business magazine

CRAISIN: Dried cranberry
CRAKE: Short-billed bird
CRAMBO: Rhyming game
CRAMER: Pianist Floyd
CRAMPON: Climber's gear
CRAN: Berry starter
CRANI: Skull: Comb. form
CRANIO: Skull: Comb. form
CRANMER: Protestant Reformation leader
CRAPPIE: Small fish
CRASHAW: English poet
CRASSUS: Roman general
CRAT: Ruler: Comb. form
C RATION: GI meal
CRAWLEY: English town
CRAY: Supercomputer brand
CREB: "Clan of the Cave Bear" character
CRECY: Garnished with carrots
CRED: Street __ (believability)
CREE: Canadian Indian
CREELEY: Poet Robert
CREMA: Cream: Italian
CREMER: British peace Nobelist
CREMINI: Type of mushroom
CREMONA: Italian city
CREMORA: Coffee additive brand
CRENATE: Having a notched edge
CRENEL: Battlement feature
CRENNA: Actor Richard
CREO: I believe: Spanish
CREON: King of Thebes
CREOSOL: Coal-tar derivative
CRESC.: Incr. volume, in music
CRESOL: Coal-tar derivative
CRESPIN: French soprano
CRESSET: Ancient torch
CRESTON: Composer Paul
CRETIN: Blockhead
CREUSA: Wife of Aeneas
CREUSE: French department
CREVE: __ Coeur, MO
CRI: Dernier __ (latest thing)
CRIKEY: Shout of surprise
CRIMEA: Ukraine region
CRIMINY: Exclamation of anger
CRIN: Cotton fabric, for short
CRISCO: Cooking-oil brand
CRISPIN: Patron saint of shoemakers
CRISPIX: Cereal brand
CRISPUS: 1770 patriot Attucks
CRIST: Film critic Judith
CRISTO: "The Count of Monte __"
CRIT: Review, for short
CRITIAS: Plato work
CRIUS: One of the Titans
CRO: __-Magnon man
CROATIA: European country
CROCE: "Bad, Bad Leroy Brown" singer
CROCKED: Tipsy
CROCKER: General Mills symbol
CROCKET: Leaf-shaped ornament
CROESUS: Legendary wealthy king
CROFT: Small farm, in Britain
CROIRE: To believe: French
CROIX: Cross: French
CRONE: Witch
CRONIN: Author A.J.
CRONUS: Father of Zeus
CRONYN: Actor Hume
CROOKES: British physicist
CROP TOP: Type of blouse
CROQUIS: Rough drawing
CRORE: 10,000,000 rupees, in India
CROSBY: Singer Bing
CROSIER: Abbot's staff
CROSSE: Field-sport equipment
CROTON: Tropical plant
CROUP: Childhood malady
CROUSE: Playwright Russel
CROUTE: Crust: French
CROWE: Director Cameron
CROWELL: "Our Town" character
CROWLEY: Actress Pat
CROWNE: __ Plaza (hotel chain)
CROZIER: Abbot's staff
CRS.: Acct. entries
C.R.T.: Computer screen: Abbr.
CRU: French vineyard
CRUCES: Las __, NM
CRUD UP: Besmirch
CRUE: Motley __ (rock band)
CRUELLA: Disney villainess
CRUGUET: Triple Crown jockey
CRUMBUM: Ne'er-do-well
CRUMP: Crunch
CRUOR: Coagulation
CRUPPER: Saddle strap
CRURA: Shanks
CRURAL: Of the leg
CRUS: Shank
CRUSE: Earthen pot
CRUTZEN: Dutch chemistry Nobelist
CRUZ: Vera __, Mexico
CRUZADO: Brazilian money
CRUZAN: St. Croix native
CRV: Honda model
CRWTH: Celtic instrument
CRYO: Cold: Comb. form
CRYOGEN: Freezing mixture
CRYPTO: Secret member
C.S.A.: Civil War side: Abbr.
CSARDAS: Hungarian dance
C SCALE: Piano practice
C.S.E.A.: Gov't workers' org.
CSI: CBS police series
CSI NY: CBS police series
C.S. LEWIS: British author
CSONKA: Larry of football
CSPAN: Congressional cable channel
C SPOT: $100 bill
C.S.T.: Chicago clock setting: Abbr.
C STAR: Spectral type
C.S.U.: Ft. Collins campus
CTEN: Comb: Comb. form
CTENO: Comb: Comb. form
CTENOID: Comblike
C TILE: Scrabble three-pointer
CTO.: Orchestral work: Abbr.
CTRL: Computer key
CT SCAN: Med. test
CUAL: Which: Spanish
CUANDO: When: Spanish
CUANTO: How much: Spanish
CUATRO: Four: Spanish
CUBAGE: Volume
CUBBINS: Dr. Seuss character
CUBEB: Spicy fruit of India
CUBIT: Old length measure
CUBITUS: Foot bone
CUBOID: Foot bone
CUDAHY: California city
CUDDY: Boat pantry
CUE BID: Bridge term
CUESTA: Low ridge
CU. FT.: 3-D meas.
CUGAT: Bandleader Xavier
CUI: Russian composer
CUI BONO: For whose benefit: Latin
CUICA: Samba drum
CU. IN.: 3-D meas.
CUIRASS: Armor plate
CUIRE: To cook: French
CUJO: Stephen King novel
CUKOR: Director George
CUL: __-de-sac
CULCH: Oyster bed
CULE: Diminutive suffix
CULET: Armor piece
CULKIN: Actor Macaulay
CULLEN: Game-show host Bill
CULLET: Broken glass
CULLIS: Roof gutter
CULLUM: Actor John
CULLY: Cheat
CULP: "I Spy" star
CULPA: Mea __
CULTCH: Oyster bed
CULT JAM: 1980s rock band
CULTUS: Sect
CULVERT: Water channel
CUM: Summa __ laude
CUMBIA: Latin dance
CUMBRIA: English county
CUME: College average, for short
CUMSHAW: Gratuity
CUMUL: Heap: Comb. form
CUMULI: Heap: Comb. form
CUMULO: Heap: Comb. form
CUNARD: Cruise line
CUNEAL: Wedge shaped
CUNEATE: Wedge-shaped
CUNEO: City in Italy
CUNY: Brooklyn Coll. is part of it
CUOMO: Former New York governor
CUORE: Daihatsu model
CUPEL: Assay
CUPPA: Tea, in Britain
CUPR: Copper: Comb. form
CUPRI: Copper: Comb. form
CUPRIC: Containing copper
CUPRITE: Copper ore
CUPRO: Copper: Comb. form
CUPROUS: Containing copper
CUPULE: Acorn cap
CURACAO: Netherlands Antilles island
CURAD: Bandage brand
CURARE: Arrow poison
CUREL: Skin-lotion brand
CURET: Surgical scoop
CURETTE: Surgical scoop
CURIA: Papal court
CURIAE: Amicus __
CURIE: Polish physicist
CURIES: Radioactivity units
CURIOSA: Books on unusual subjects
CURITE: Uranium ore
CURIUM: Element #96
CURLEW: Shorebird
CURLEY: "Of Mice and Men" character
CURNOW: New Zealand poet
CURR: Purr
CURRIER: __ and Ives
CURSA: Star in Eridanus
CURTATE: Shortened
CURTIN: Comic Jane
CURTIS: Actress Jamie Lee
CURTISS: Aviator Glenn
CURTIZ: Director Michael
CURVET: Dressage leap
CURVI: Bent: Comb. form
CURZON: British pianist
CUS: Boxing trainer D'Amato
CUSACK: Actress Joan
CUSEC: Unit of flow
CUSH: Ancient African kingdom
CUSHAW: Squash variety
CUSHING: Former Boston cardinal
CUSK: Marine fish
CUSSLER: Author Clive
CUSTER: Civil War general
CUSTER'S: __ Last Stand
CUSTIS: Martha Washington's first husband
CUTEX: Nail-polish brand
CUTIS: Skin
CUTLER: Knife merchant
CUT TIME: Music term
CUTTY: "__ Sark" (historic ship)
CUTWORK: Type of embroidery
CUVEE: Blended wine
CUVETTE: Lab vessel
CUVIER: French naturalist
CU. YD.: Volume meas.
CUYLER: Kiki of baseball
CUZ: Since, informally
CUZCO: City in Peru
CVS: Drugstore chain
CWM: Mountain basin
C.W.O.: Nav. rank
CWP: Crossword: Abbr.
C.W. POST: Long Island college
CWT.: Hundredweight: Abbr.
CYAN: Blue shade
CYANO: Blue: Comb. form
CYBER: Computer: Comb. form
CYBILL: Actress Shepherd
CYBORG: Sci-fi character
CYCAD: Palmlike tree
CYCL: Ring: Comb. form
CYCLO: Rickshaw
CYD: Actress Charisse
CYDER: British beverage
CYGNI: Swans: Latin
CYGNUS: Swan constellation

CYMA: Cornice molding
CYME: Flower cluster
CYMRIC: Welsh
CYMRY: Welsh people
CYNDI: Singer Lauper
CYNO: Dog: Comb. form
CYNTHIA: Cindy Crawford's real first name
C.Y.O.: Christian youth grp.
CYPHER: Code, in Britain
CYPRIOT: Cyprus native
CYPRUS: Mediterranean island
CYRANO: Rostand hero
CYRIL: Actor Ritchard
CYRUS: Singer Billy Ray
CYRUS II: Persian king
CYS: Coleman and Young
CYTE: Cell: Comb. form
CYTO: Cell: Comb. form
CY YOUNG: Baseball great
CZARDAS: Hungarian dance
CZERNY: Austrian composer

D

DABA: "The Aba __ Honeymoon"
DAB AT: Sponge gently
DABBA: "Yabba __ doo!"
DAB HAND: Skillful one
DABIH: Star in Capricorn
DABNEY: Actor Coleman
D'ABO: Actress Olivia
DAB ON: Apply in small amounts
DA BRAT: Rap artist
DA CAPO: Repeated musical passage
DACCA: Bangladesh capital
DACE: Freshwater fish
DACHA: Russian villa
DACHE: Hollywood hat designer
DACIA: Ancient Romania
DA COSTA: Director Morton
DACTYL: Poetic foot
DADA ART: Duchamp works
DADDY'S: "__ Gone A-Hunting" (1969 film)
DADE: Miami-__ County
DADO: Pedestal part
DAE: Kim __ Jung (former South Korean leader)
DAEDAL: Clever
DAEMON: Archfiend
DAEWOO: Korean auto
DAFOE: Actor Willem
DAG: Statesman Hammarskjöld
DA GAMA: Portuguese explorer
DAGAN: Mesopotamian earth god
DAGGOO: "Moby-Dick" character
DAGMAR: "Broadway Open House" regular
DAGWOOD: Blondie's husband
DAH: Morse code syllable
DAHL: Actress Arlene
DAHOMEY: Benin's former name
DAI: Bao __ (1950s Vietnamese leader)
DAIL: Dublin legislature
DAILEY: Actor Dan
DAIMLER: German auto
DAIN: "The __ Curse" (Hammett novel)
DAIWA: Japanese sporting goods company
DAK: Former U.S. terr.
DAKAR: Senegal capital
DAKTARI: 1960s TV series
DAL: Sauce of India
DALAI: The __ Lama
DALAND: "The Flying Dutchman" character
DALASI: Gambia money
DALEN: 1912 physics Nobelist
D'ALENE: Coeur __, ID
DALET: Hebrew letter
DALETH: Hebrew letter
DALEY: Chicago mayor
DALI: Spanish artist
DALLES: Rapids
DALTON: British chemist
DALTONS: Old West gang
DALTREY: Leader of The Who
DALY: Actress Tyne
DAMA: Lady: Spanish
DAMASUS: Pope
D'AMATO: Former New York senator
DAMEN: Ladies: German
DAMIEN: Belgian missionary
DAMIS: "Tartuffe" character
DAMITA: Actress Lili
DAMME: Actor Jean-Claude Van __
DAMON: Actor Matt
DAMONE: Singer Vic
D'AMORE: Oboe __
DAMOSEL: Medieval maiden
D'AMOUR: "Melodie __" (Ames Brothers tune)
DAMP-DRY: Prepare laundry for ironing
DAMSON: Type of plum
DAN: Newsman Rather
DANA: Comic Carvey
DANAE: Mother of Perseus
D'ANANAS: Crème __ (pineapple liqueur)
DANANG: Vietnam port
DANBURY: Connecticut city
DANCIN': Fosse musical
D AND D: Role-playing game, informally
DANDIE: __ Dinmont terrier
DANDLE: Pamper
DANELAW: Ancient legal code
DANEYKO: Ken of hockey
D'ANGELO: Actress Beverly
DANG ME: Roger Miller tune
DANIA: Florida city
DANIEL: Writer Defoe
DANIELA: Actress Bianchi
DANIEL J.: Actor Travanti
DANIELS: Actor Jeff
DANIKEN: Author Erich Von __
DANILO: "The Merry Widow" role
DANIO: Fish of India
DANITE: Hebrew tribesman
DANKE: Thanks: German
DAN'L: Boone's nickname
DANNAY: Author Frederic
DANNER: Actress Blythe
DANNING: Actress Sybil
DANNO: "Hawaii Five-O" character
DANNON: Yogurt brand
DANNY: Comedian Kaye
DANNY'S: "__ Song" (Kenny Loggins tune)
DANO: Actress Linda
DANOVA: Actor Cesare
DANS: Martial-arts levels
DANSE: Dance: French
DANSON: "Cheers" star
DANTE: "Inferno" writer
DANTE I: NASA robot
DANTE II: NASA robot
DANTES: Count of Monte Cristo
DANTON: French Revolution leader
DANUBE: Vienna's river
DANVERS: Massachusetts city
DANZA: Actor Tony
DANZIG: Baltic gulf
D'AOSTA: Valle __ (Italian region)
DAP: Bob bait lightly
DAPHNE: European shrub
DAPHNIA: Crustacean genus
DAPHNIS: Lover of Chloe
DAR: Patriotic org.
DARA: Olympic swimmer Torres
DARBY: Actress Kim
D'ARC: Ste. Jeanne __
DARCEL: Actress Denise
DARCI: Ballerina Kistler
DARCY: "Pride and Prejudice" character
DARDY: Lardy-__
DARE ME: Challenging words
D'AREZZO: Italian music theorist
DARIA: MTV teen toon
DARIEN: Connecticut city
DARIN: Singer Bobby
DARIO: Nicaraguan poet
DARIUS I: King of Persia
DARKLE: Become gloomy
DARKMAN: Liam Neeson film
DARLA: "Our Gang" girl
DARLEEN: Actress Carr
DARLENE: 1950s Mouseketeer
DARLIN': "Little __" (1950s tune)
DARNAY: "A Tale of Two Cities" character
DARNELL: Actress Linda
DARREN: Actor McGavin
DARRIN: "Bewitched" husband
DARROW: Lawyer Clarence
DARRYL: Actor Hickman
DARRYL F.: Film producer Zanuck
D'ARTE: "Vissi __" (Puccini aria)
DARTH: __ Vader
DARTLE: Shoot forth
DARWELL: Actress Jane
DARWIN: Evolution theorist
DARYA: Amu __ (Asian river)
DARYL: Actress Hannah
DAS BOOT: 1981 film
DASCHLE: Former South Dakota senator
DASH DOT: N, in Morse code
DASHI: Japanese soup stock
DASHIKI: African garment
DASH IT: "Darn!"
DASHPOT: Machine part
DASHY: Stylish
DA SILVA: Actor Howard
DASN'T: Nonstandard contraction
DASSIN: "Never on Sunday" director
DASTARD: Bad guy
DAT: "Can't Help Lovin' __ Man"
DATA BUS: Computer part
DATARY: Church official
DATHAN: "The Ten Commandments" role
DATIVE: Verb case
DATO: Malay chief
DATRIL: Pain-reliever brand
DATSUN: Japanese auto
DAU.: Fam. member
DAUBE: French stew
DAUDET: French novelist
DAUMIER: French painter
DAUPHIN: Eldest son of a French king
DAUSSET: French medicine Nobelist
D.A.V.: Grp. of former GIs
DAVAO: Philippines gulf
DAVE KOZ: Jazz saxophonist
DAVEN: Pray in a synagogue
DAVEY: Lopes of baseball
DAVI: Actor Robert
DAVID E.: TV producer Kelley
DAVID I: King of Scotland
DAVID L.: Film producer Wolper
DAVID O.: Film producer Selznick
DAVIE: Florida city
DAVIES: Canadian writer
DA VINCI: "The Last Supper" painter
DAVIS: Jazz trumpeter Miles
DAVISON: Actor Bruce
DAVIT: Nautical crane
DAVOS: Swiss ski resort
DAVY: __ Jones's locker
DAW: Black bird
DAWBER: Actress Pam
DAWES: Coolidge vice president
DAWG: "Hi and Lois" canine
DAWKINS: Darryl of basketball
DAWNN: Actress Lewis
DAWSON: "Family Feud" host
DAX: "Deep Space Nine" character
DAYAN: Former Israeli defense minister
DAY-GLO: Bright paint
DAYHOP: Short trip
DAYNE: Singer Taylor
DAY-O: Belafonte tune
DAYPACK: Student's bag
DAYQUIL: Cold-remedy brand
DAY SAIL: Short cruise
DAYS INN: Motel chain
DAY SPA: Massage milieu
DAYTON: Ohio city
DAYTONA: Auto race site
DAZS: Häagen-__ (ice-cream brand)
D'AZUR: Côte __ (French Riviera)

DAZZY: Vance of baseball
D.B.A.: AKA, in business
D-BACK: NL player
DBL.: Duplicate: Abbr.
D.C. AREA: Inside the Beltway
D.C. CAB: Mr. T film
D CELL: Battery type
D.C.M.: Brit. decoration
D-CON: Insecticide brand
DDE: Presidential monogram
DDMMYY: British date format
D.D.S.: Dentist's deg.
DDT: "Silent Spring" subject
DEA: Goddess: Latin
DEAD AIR: Broadcast silence
DEADEYE: Sharpshooter
DEAD ON: Precise
DE-AIR: Remove air from
DEAL TO: Present with a hand
DEANA: Country singer Carter
DEANE: Colonial patriot Silas
DEANERY: Church jurisdiction
DEANNA: Actress Durbin
DEARDEN: Director Basil
DEARE: "The Wreck of the Mary __" (1959 film)
DEAR GOD: Greg Kinnear film
DEAR ONE: Sweetheart
DEASIL: Clockwise
DEBAKEY: Artificial-heart pioneer
DEBAR: Exclude
DEBARGE: 1980s singing group
DEBBE: Actress Dunning
DEBBI: Cookie mogul Fields
DEBBIE: Actress Reynolds
DEBBY: Singer Boone
DE BEERS: Big name in diamonds
DEBI: Gymnast Thomas
DEBLUR: Clear up
DEBOITE: Ballet step
DE BONT: Director Jan
DEBORAH: Actress Kerr
DEBOULE: Ballet turn
DEBRA: Actress Messing
DEBRAH: Actress Farentino
DEBRAY: "Count of Monte Cristo" character
DEBRETT: British peerage expert
DEBREU: 1983 economics Nobelist
DE BURGH: Singer Chris
DEBUSSY: French composer
DEBYE: 1936 chemistry Nobelist
DECA: Ten: Comb. form
DECAD: Group of ten
DECALOG: Ten Commandments
DECAPOD: Crab or lobster
DECARE: 1,000 square meters
DE CARLO: Actress Yvonne
DECATUR: Illinois city
DECCA: Record label
DECEM: Ten: Comb. form
DECI: Ten: Comb. form
DECIARE: 10 square meters
DECILE: Statistical unit
DECIR: To say: Spanish
DECIUS: Roman emperor
DECKER: Double-__
DECKLE: Paper edge
DECO: Art __ (1920s style)
DECOCT: Boil down
DECRYPT: Break a code
DECUPLE: Tenfold
DEDALUS: "Ulysses" hero
DEDANS: Tennis gallery
DEDE: "__ Dinah" (Avalon tune)
DEDHAM: Massachusetts town
DEDINI: Cartoonist Eldon
DEDO: Finger: Spanish
DE DUVE: Belgian medicine Nobelist
DEEDBOX: Valuables container
DEEDEE: Clinton spokesperson Myers
DEENIE: Judy Blume book
DEEPAK: Author Chopra
DEEP-SKY: Beyond the solar system
DEERE: Farm machinery brand
DEET: Bug repellent
DEEVER: Kipling characer
DEF: 3, on a phone
DE FACTO: Actual
DE FALLA: Spanish composer
DEFARGE: "A Tale of Two Cities" character
DEFCON: Military alert status
DEF JAM: Hip-hop music label
DEFOE: "Robinson Crusoe" author
DEFORD: Sports author Frank
DEFORE: Actor Don
DEFUND: Stop backing
DEGAGE: Unemotional
DEGAS: French artist
DEGAUSS: Demagnetize
DEGUST: Savor
DEHAVEN: Actress Gloria
DEHISCE: Burst open
DEHMEL: German poet
DEHMELT: 1989 physics Nobelist
DEI: "Agnus __" (prayer)
DEIDRE: Actress Hall
DEIL: Devil: Scottish
DEIMOS: Moon of Mars
DEION: Sanders of football
DEIRDRE: Heroine of Irish legend
DEISM: Religious belief
DE JURE: According to law
DEK: Ten: Comb. form
DEKA: Ten: Comb. form
DEKALB: Revolutionary War general
DEKE: Astronaut Slayton
DEKES: Fakes, in sports
DEKKER: Actor Albert
DEKKO: Glimpse, in Britain
DE KLERK: South African statesman
DEL.: Penna. neighbor
DELAND: Florida city
DELANEY: "A Taste of Honey" playwright
DELANO: Part of FDR
DELANY: Actress Dana
DELARUE: British astronomer
DELBERT: Director Mann
DEL CITY: Oklahoma city
DELCO: Battery brand
DELE: Manuscript marking
DELEDDA: Italian novelist
DELFT: Type of pottery
DELHI: City of India
DELIA: Novelist Ephron
DELIAN: League of ancient Greece
DELIBES: French composer
DELICT: Misdemeanor
DELICTI: Corpus __
DELICTO: In flagrante __
DE LILLO: Author Don
DELI MAN: Corned-beef expert
DELISH: Tasty, slangily
DELIUS: British composer
DEL KEY: PC striker
DELLA: Singer Reese
DELLO: Composer Norman __ Joio
DEL MAR: California racetrack
DELMONT: Oldsmobile model
DELMORE: Poet Schwartz
DELON: Actor Alain
DELORIS: Whoopi's "Sister Act" role
DELORME: French architect
DELOS: Aegean island
DELPHI: Ancient Greek city
DELPHIC: Obscure
DELPY: Actress Julie
DELRAY: Chevrolet model
DEL REY: Sci-fi author Lester
DEL RIO: Actress Dolores
DELROY: Actor Lindo
DEL RUTH: Director Roy
DEL SOL: Honda model
DELT: Shoulder muscle
DELTOID: Shoulder muscle
DELTONA: Florida city
DEL TORO: Actor Benicio
DE LUGG: Bandleader Milton
DE LUISE: Comedian Dom
DEM.: GOP opponent
DEMAGOG: Inciter
DEMAIN: Tomorrow: French
DE MARCO: Johnny Depp role
DEMARET: Golfer Jimmy
DEMAST: Strip down, as a ship
DEM BUMS: Brooklyn Dodgers, affectionately
DEME: Greek district
DEMENTO: Novelty-record "Doctor"
DEMEROL: Sedative
DEMESNE: Estate
DEMETER: Agriculture goddess
DEMI: Actress Moore
DE MILLE: "The Ten Commandments" director
DE MILO: Venus __
DEMISE: Transfer legally
DEMIT: Resign
DEMME: Director Jonathan
DEMOB: Disband
DEMODE: Out of date
DEMOLAY: Teen service organization
DEMOND: Actor Wilson
DEMONYM: "New Yorker" or "Norwegian"
DEMOTIC: Vernacular
DEMPSEY: Boxer Jack
DEMY: Paper size
DENA: Actress Dietrich
DE NADA: You're welcome: Spanish
DENALI: Alaska national park
DENAR: Macedonian money
DENARI: Macedonian money
DENARII: Ancient Roman coins
DENARY: Tenfold
DENCH: Actress Judi
DENDR: Tree: Comb. form
DENDRA: Nerve branches
DENDRI: Tree: Comb. form
DENDRO: Tree: Comb. form
DENDRON: Nerve branch
DENE: Sand hill, in Britain
DENEB: Star in Cygnus
DENEUVE: French actress
DENG: 1980s Chinese leader
DEN HAAG: Dutch city, to natives
DENHAM: "King Kong" character
DENIECE: Singer Williams
DE NIRO: "Raging Bull" star
DENIS: Patron saint of France
DENISE: "Cosby Show" daughter
DENISON: Texas city
DENIZEN: Dweller
DEN MOM: Girl Scout leader
DENNEHY: Actor Brian
DENNIS: Actor Hopper
DENNY: Actor Reginald
DENNY'S: Restaurant chain
DENOM.: Religious grp.
DE NOVO: Anew: Latin
DENTATE: Having teeth
DENTE: Al __ (pasta order)
DENTI: Tooth: Comb. form
DENTIN: Tooth part
DENTINE: Tooth part
DENTO: Tooth: Comb. form
DENTON: Texas city
DENTONS: Doctor __ (kids' sleepwear)
DENTYNE: Gum brand
DENYS: Patron saint of France
DENZEL: Actor Washington
DEO: God: Latin
DEODAR: Asian cedar
DEODATO: 1974 Grammy winner
DEOXY: Part of DNA
DEP.: Arr. opposite
DE PALMA: Director Brian
DEPAUL: Illinois university
DEPAUW: Indiana university
DEPECHE: __ Mode (rock band)
DE PERE: Wisconsin city
DEPEW: Buffalo suburb
DEPONE: Testify
DEPP: Actor Johnny
DER: German article
DERAIN: French painter
DER ALTE: Adenauer's nickname
DERAT: Emulate the Pied Piper
DERE: "__ Mable" (Streeter book)
DERECHO: Storm system
DEREK: Actress Bo
DE RITA: Curly Joe of The Three Stooges
DERM: Skin: Comb. form
DERMA: Skin layer

DERMAT: Skin: Comb. form
DERMATO: Skin: Comb. form
DERMIS: Skin layer
DERMO: Skin: Comb. form
DERMOT: Actor Mulroney
DERN: Actress Laura
DERNIER: Latest: French
DERONDA: George Eliot character
DE ROSE: "Deep Purple" composer
DERR: Author Earl __ Biggers
DERREK: Lee of baseball
D'ERRICO: Actress Donna
DERRIDA: French philosopher
DERRING: __-do (heroism)
DERRY: County of Northern Ireland
DERVISH: Muslim ascetic
DERWENT: British river
DES: __ Moines, IA
DE SADE: Infamous marquis
DESAI: Indian novelist
DESC.: Genealogy abbr.
DESCANT: Comment
DESCRY: Catch a glimpse of
DESDE: Since: Spanish
DESE: Brookynese pronoun
DESERET: Utah's former name
DE SETA: Italian director
DESI: Arnaz of TV
DE SICA: Italian director
DESILU: "I Love Lucy" production company
DESIREE: Brando film
DESK SET: Tracy/Hepburn film
DESKTOP: Kind of computer
DESMOND: Bishop Tutu
DESNA: Russian river
DESNOS: French poet
DESOTO: Erstwhile auto
DESPINA: "Così fan tutte" role
DESPOND: Languish
DES'REE: British pop singer
DESSAU: German city
DE STAEL: Swiss author
D'ESTE: Villa __ (Tivoli palace)
DESTINO: "La Forza del __" (Verdi opera)
DESTRY: "__ Rides Again" (1939 film)
DE SYLVA: Songwriter Buddy
DET.: Police rank: Abbr.
D'ETAT: Coup __
DETECTO: Scale brand
DETENT: Machine part
DETENTE: Political thaw
DETERGE: Cleanse
DETMER: 1990 Heisman Trophy winner
DETOO: Artoo-__
DE TOTH: "House of Wax" director
D'ETRE: Raison __
DE TROP: Too much: French
DETRUDE: Force down
DETTE: Debt: French
DETUNE: Make sharp or flat
DEUCY: Acey-__
DEUEL: Actor Peter
DEUM: Te __ (Latin hymn)
DEUS: God: Latin
DEUT.: O.T. book
DEUTCH: Former CIA director
DEUTER: Second: Comb. form
DEUTERO: Second: Comb. form
DEUTO: Second: Comb. form
DEUTSCH: German, in German
DEUX: Two: French
DEV.: Growth: Abbr.
DEVA: Hindu god
DEVANE: Actor William
DE VEGA: Spanish playwright
DEVEIN: Prepare shrimp
DEVERE: Actress Trish Van __
DEVERS: Olympic runner Gail
DEVEST: Take away, in law
DEVI: Hindu goddess
DEVICQ: Actress Paula
DEVILLE: Cadillac model
DEVINE: Comedian Andy
DEVISEE: Heir
DE VITO: Actor Danny
DEVO: Rock group
DEVOIR: Act of respect
DE VOL: Orchestra leader Frank
DEVOLVE: Delegate
DEVON: English county
DEVORE: Velvet fabric
DE VOTO: Writer Bernard
DE VRIES: Dutch botanist
DEVRY: Career-training college
DE WAART: Dutch conductor
DEWAR: Scottish chemist
DEWAR'S: Scotch brand
DEWATER: Parch
DEWCLAW: Pig hoof
DEWEY: 1948 presidential candidate
DE WILDE: Actor Brandon
DE WITT: Actress Joyce
DEWLAP: Anatomical fold
DEW LINE: Arctic radar system
DE WOLF: Actor Hopper
DEX: "Dynasty" role
DEXTER: Saxophonist Gordon
DEXTR: Clockwise: Comb. form
DEXTRAL: Right-handed
DEXTRIN: Thickening agent
DEXTRO: Clockwise: Comb. form
DEY: Actress Susan
DEYOUNG: Lead singer of Styx
D.F.C.: Air Force medal: Abbr.
D FLAT: C sharp alias
D.F.M.: British mil. award
DHA: Omega-3 fatty acid
DHABI: Abu __
DHAKA: Bangladesh capital
DHAL: Arabic letter
DHARMA: Hindu virtue
DHEIGH: Actor Khigh
DHL: FedEx rival
DHOLE: Asian wild dog
D'HOTE: Table __
D'HOTEL: Maître __
DHOTI: Cotton fabric
DHOW: Arab boat
DHS: Amer. League specialists
DHU: "Lady of the Lake" character
DHURRIE: Indian rug
DIA: Day: Spanish
DIABLE: Devil: French
DIABLO: Devil: Spanish
DIABOL: Devil: Comb. form
DIABOLO: Devil: Comb. form
DIADEM: Crown
DIAHANN: Actress Carroll
DIAL O: Seek information, perhaps
DIAN: Gorilla studier Fossey
DIANA: Singer Ross
DIANE: "Cheers" character
DIANNE: Actress Wiest
DIAPHAN: Transparent: Comb. form
DIARIO: Newspaper: Spanish
DIATOM: Type of alga
DIAVOLO: Lobster Fra __
DIAZ: Actress Cameron
DIBBLE: Garden tool
DICHO: Apart: Comb. form
DICHTER: Pianist Misha
DICILLO: Director Tom
DICKENS: "A Christmas Carol" author
DICKEY: Detachable collar
DICKIE: Detachable collar
DICKORY: "Hickory, __, dock"
DICKSON: Band-Aid inventor
DICKY: Detachable collar
DICOT: Flowering plant
DICTU: Mirabile __ (strange to say: Latin)
DIDACT: Instructor
DID BY: Dealt with
DIDDLE: Cheat
DIDDLEY: Blues guitarist
DIDDLY: Minimal amount
DIDEROT: French philosopher
DIDI: Actress Conn
DIDION: Author Joan
DIDO: Prank
DID OK: Performed satisfactorily
DIDY: Baby's wear
DIEBOLD: ATM manufacturer
DIECI: Ten: Italian
DIEGO: Artist Rivera
DIELS: Germany chemistry Nobelist
DIEM: Per __ worker
DIEMEN'S: Van __ Land (Tasmania, once)
DIEN: Actor Casper Van __
DIENE: Chemical compound
DIEPPE: French port
DIESIS: Printer's mark
DIETE: Diet: French
DIETZ: "That's Entertainment" lyricist
DIEU: God: French
DIEUX: Gods: French
DIEZ: Ten: Spanish
DIF: "What's the __?"
DIGAMY: Remarriage
DIGBY: British writer
DI-GEL: Antacid brand
DIG 'EM: Kellogg's toon frog
DIGGITY: "Hot __ dog"
DIGGORY: "Return of the Native" character
DIGGS: Actor Taye
DIGICAM: Modern picture taker
DIGIPET: Electronic toy
DIGLOT: Bilingual book
DIGRAM: Two-letter sequence
DIGRAPH: Two-letter sequence
DIJON: French city
DIK: Cartoonist Browne
DIK-DIK: African antelope
DIKTAT: Decree
DIL.: Water down: Abbr.
DILBERT: Scott Adams comic strip
DILI: East Timor capital
DILLAR: "A __, a dollar..."
DILLARD: Author Annie
DILLER: Comedienne Phyllis
DILLMAN: Actor Bradford
DILLON: "Gunsmoke" marshal
DILSEY: Faulkner character
DILUENT: Paint thinner, e.g.
DI MAG: Yankee great's nickname
DIMAGE: Minolta camera brand
DIMAS: San __, CA
DIMED: Nickel-and-__
DIMETER: Line of two feet
DIMIN.: Decrease: Abbr.
DIMITRI: Film composer Tiomkin
DIMITY: Cotton fabric
DIM SUM: Chinese appetizer
DINA: Actress Merrill
DINADAM: King Arthur knight
DINAH: "Alice in Wonderland" cat
DINAR: Iran money
DINARIC: Range of the Alps
D'INDY: French composer
DINESEN: "Out of Africa" author
DINGE: Shabby state
DINGLE: Narrow valley
DINGO: Wild dog of Australia
DINGUS: Doodad
DINH: Ngo __ Diem (1960s Vietnamese leader)
DINK: Two-worker couple
DINKA: African people
DINKUM: Authentic, in Australia
DINMONT: Dandie __ terrier
DINNY: Alley Oop's dinosaur
DINO: Flintstones' pet
DINO'S: "77 Sunset Strip" restaurant
DINTY: __ Moore (canned stew brand)
DIO: God: Italian
DIOMED: "Last Days of Pompeii" character
DIOMEDE: Alaska's Little __ Island
DION: Singer Celine
DIONE: Moon of Saturn
DIONNE: Canadian quintuplets' surname
DIOPTER: Eyeglass prescription measurement
DIOR: Designer Christian
DIORITE: Igneous rock
DIOS: God: Spanish
DIOTIMA: Asteroid
DIOXIN: Toxic compound
DIPL: Double: Comb. form
DIPLEX: Type of radio channel
DIPLO: Double: Comb. form
DIPNET: Fishing device
DIPODY: Two-foot meter

DIPOLE: Antenna type
DIPSY: One of the Teletubbies
DIPTYCH: Hinged pair of pictures
DIR.: Film-set VIP
DIRAC: 1933 physics Nobelist
DIRAE: Roman Furies
DIRAM: Tajikistan money
DIRECTV: Satellite service provider
DIRHAM: Libyan money
DIRIGE: Church service
DIRIGO: Maine motto
DIRK: Scottish dagger
DIRKSEN: 1960s Illinois senator
DIRNDL: Alpine dress
DIRTBAG: Sleazy one
DIS: Insult, slangily
DISANT: Soi-__ (self-styled)
DISCI: Recording: Comb. form
DISCMAN: Sony CD player
D'ISERE: Val __ (French ski resort)
DISEUR: Monologist
DISHY: Gossipy
DISKO: "Captains Courageous" character
DISMAS: Patron saint of thieves
DISME: Former U.S. coin
DISS: Insult, slangily
DISSERT: Discourse formally
DIST.: Congressman's concern: Abbr.
DISTAL: Terminal
DISTICH: Rhyming couplet
DISTRO: Web-mag seller
DIT: Bit of Morse code
DITALI: Tubular pasta
DITAT: __ Deus (Arizona motto)
DITH: "The Killing Fields" character
DITKA: Mike of football
DITZ: Scatterbrain
DIU: Former Portuguese colony
DIURNAL: Daily
DIVAC: Vlade of basketball
DIVULSE: Tear away
DIX: New Jersey fort
DIXIT: Utterance
DIXON: Mason-__ line
DIXY: __ Lee Ray (former Washington governor)
D.I.Y.: Home repair: Abbr.
DIZAIN: French poem
DJEBAR: Algerian writer
D.J.I.A.: Stock index: Abbr.
DJILAS: Yugoslavian author
DJIN: Genie
DJINN: Genie
DJINNI: Genie
DJUNA: Feminist author Barnes
DKG.: Metric wt.
DKL.: Metric liquid meas.
DKM.: Metric length meas.
DKNY: Fashion initials
D LAYER: Ionosphere part
D. LIT.: Advanced Eng. degree
D.L.O.: P.O. limbo
DLR.: Retailer: Abbr.
D.L.S.: Librarian's deg.
D MAJOR: Musical key
D-MARK: Former German money
DMC: Run-__ (rap group)
D.M.D.: Dentist's deg.
D MINOR: Musical key
DMITRI: Karamazov brother
DMITRY: Composer Shostakovich
D. MUS.: Graduate deg.
D.M.V.: State auto agcy.
DMYTRYK: Director Edward
D.M.Z.: Truce sector: Abbr.
DNAASE: Genetic enzyme
DNASE: Genetic enzyme
DNEPR: Kiev's river
D NET: Plankton-collecting device
DNIEPER: Kiev's river
D.O.A.: Edmond O'Brien film
DOAK: Walker of football
DOAKES: Typical Joe
DOANE: "Babbitt" character
DOAN'S: Back-pill brand
DO A SET: Perform while onstage
DO AS I DO: "Follow my example"
DOATS: "Mairzy __" (old song)
D.O.B.: Driv. lic. stat
DO BAD: Transgress
DOBBS: Lou of CNN
DO BEE: "Romper Room" role model
DOBIE: Fictional Gillis
DOBLE: Paso __ (Spanish dance)
DOBLIN: German novelist
DOBRO: Country music guitar
DO BY: Deal with
DOBYNS: Poet Stephen
DOC BOY: "Garfield" character
DOCE: 12: Spanish
DOCENT: Tour guide
DOCOMO: Japanese cell-phone company
DOCU: Prefix for drama
D.O.D.: Cabinet dept.
DODD: Connecticut political surname
DODEC: 12: Comb. form
DODECA: 12: Comb. form
DODGEM: Bumper-car ride
DODGSON: Lewis Carroll's real last name
DODICI: 12: Italian
DODIE: Singer Stevens
DO DO DO: Gershwin song
DODOMA: Tanzanian capital
DODY: Actress Goodman
DOERR: Bobby of baseball
DOESKIN: Glove leather
DOEST: Biblical verb
DOETH: Biblical verb
D'OEUVRE: Chef-__ (masterpiece)
DOG APE: Baboon
DOGBERT: Comics canine
DOGCHEW: Pet-shop purchase
DOGE: Former Venetian ruler
DOG-EAR: Paper fold
DOGFACE: G.I.
DOGGETT: Jazz pianist
DOGGO: Out of sight
DOGIE: Calf
DOG IT: Avoid work
DOGLEG: Golf-course bend
DOGON: African people
DO GOOD: Be philanthropic
DOGPILE: Internet search engine
DO GREAT: Succeed
DOG'S AGE: Very long time
DOG'S-EAR: Paper fold
DOH: Homer Simpson shout
DOHA: Qatar capital
DOHERTY: Actress Shannen
DO I: "Absolutely!"
DO I DO: Stevie Wonder tune
DOIN': "How'm I __?"
DOIS: Two: Portuguese
DOISY: 1943 medicine Nobelist
DO IT: Succeed
DOITS: Old Dutch coins
DO IT UP: Accomplish, so to speak
D.O.J.: Cabinet dept.
DOJO: Karate school
DOKE: Okey-__
DOKEY: Okey-__
DOKKEN: Heavy-metal rock band
DOKTOR: Physician: German
DO LAPS: Run around a track
DOLBY: Theater sound system
DOLCE: "La __ Vita"
DOLCI: Sweets: Italian
DOLENZ: One of the Monkees
DO LIKE: Emulate
DOLIN: Ballet star Anton
DOLLEY: First Lady Madison
DOLMA: Stuffed grape leaf
DOLMAN: Woman's cape
DOLON: "The Faerie Queene" character
DOLOR: Sorrow
DOLORE: Sorrow: Italian
DOLORES: "__ Claiborne" (Stephen King novel)
DOLPH: Actor Lundgren
DOLTON: Illinois city
DO LUNCH: Eat
DOM: Monk's title
DOMAINE: French vineyard
DOMANI: Tomorrow: Italian
DOMBEY: Dickens character
DOME CAR: Sightseeing train feature
DOMICIL: Abode
DOMINE: Master: Latin
DOMINGO: Sunday: Spanish
DOMINI: Anno __
DOMINIC: Spanish saint
DOMINO'S: Pizza chain
DOMINUS: God: Latin
DOMO: Major-__ (butler)
DOM. REP.: Caribbean country, for short
DONA: Lady: Spanish
DONAHUE: TV talk-show host
DONALD: Trump of real estate
DONAT: "Goodbye, Mr. Chips" star
DONATH: Actor Ludwig
DONATUS: Roman grammarian
DONAU: Danube: German
DONC: Thus: French
DONDE: Where: Spanish
DONDER: One of Santa's reindeer
DONDI: Adoptee of the comics
DONEGAL: Irish county
DONEGAN: Singer Lonnie
DONEN: Director Stanley
DONETS: Russian river
DONETSK: Ukraine city
DONGLE: Computer device
DON HO: Hawaiian crooner
DON IMUS: Radio personality
DONITZ: WWII German admiral
DONJON: Castle tower
DON JOSE: "Carmen" role
DON KING: Boxing promoter
DONLEVY: Actor Brian
DONN: Clendenon of baseball
DONNA: Actress Reed
DONNALL: 1990 medicine Nobelist
DONNE: English poet
DONNER: "Superman" director
DONNIE: "__ Brasco" (Johnny Depp film)
DONNISH: Bookish
DONNY: Singer Osmond
DONOHOE: Actress Amanda
DONORA: Pennsylvania city
DONOSO: Chilean writer
DONOVAN: 1960s pop singer
DO NOW: Teacher's assignment
DONRUSS: Baseball card company
DON'T BEE: "Romper Room" non-role model
DONUS: Pope
DOO: "Inka Dinka __"
DOOD: "I __ It" (Skelton film)
DOO-DAH: "Camptown Races" word
DOODY: Howdy __
DOOFUS: Dolt
DOOGIE: Dr. Howser of TV
DOOHAN: "Star Trek" star
DO OK: Manage fine
DOOLEY: "Tom __" (Kingston Trio tune)
DOOLIE: Air Force Academy freshman
DOON: Scottish river
DOONE: "Lorna __"
DO ONE IN: Mess up a person
DO-OR-DIE: All-out
DOORN: Dutch town
DOOS: Ski-__ (snowmobiles)
DO OUT OF: Rob
DO-OVER: Second chance
DOO-WOP: Harmonizing style
DOOZER: Lulu
DOPA: Amino acid
DOPPLER: Weather radar
D'OR: Golden: French
DORA: Mrs. Copperfield
DORADO: El __ (legendary treasure city)
DO-RAG: Kerchief
DORAL: PGA tournament site
DORAN: Actress Ann
DORATI: Hungarian conductor
DORCAS: Biblical seamstress
DORE: French painter
DOREEN: 1950s Mouseketeer
DO RE MI: "The Sound of Music" song
DOREN: Writer Carl Van __

DORFF: Actor Stephen
DORFMAN: "Animal House" role
DORIA: "Andrea __" (ill-fated ship)
DORIAN: Oscar Wilde character
DORIC: Column order
DO-RIGHT: Cartoon Mountie
DORINE: "Tartuffe" character
DORIS: Actress Day
DORITOS: Snack-chip brand
DORK: Social misfit
DORMER: Type of window
DORMIE: Golf term
DORMY: Golf term
DORN: "Star Trek: The Next Generation" actor
D'ORO: Golden: Italian
DOROTHY: "Wizard of Oz" girl
DORP: Hamlet
DORRIT: Dickens character
DORS: Actress Diana
DORSAD: Toward the back
D'ORSAY: Actress Fifi
DORSET: English county
DORSETT: Tony of football
DORSEY: Big Band brother
DORSI: Back: Comb. form
DORSO: Back: Comb. form
DORSUM: Animal's back
DORY: Flat-bottom boat
DOS: Two: Spanish
DO-SA-DO: Square-dance call
DOS-A-DOS: Square-dance call
DO SAY: "Indeed!"
DO SHOTS: Drink at a bar
DO-SI-DO: Square-dance call
DO SO: Accomplish it
DOSS: Sleep, in Britain
DOSSAL: Altar cloth
DOST: Shakespearean verb
DO SUMS: Find a total
DOTAL: Of a dowry
DOTBOMB: Failed Internet company
DOT-COM: Internet company
DOT DASH: A, in Morse code
DOT DOT: I, in Morse code
DO TELL: "Go on!"
DOT GOV: Federal Web-site ending
DOTH: "How __ the busy bee..."
DOTHAN: Alabama city
DO TIME: Serve a sentence
DO TO: Inflict upon
DO TO A T: Perform perfectly
DO TO DO: Scale range
DOT ORG: Nonprofit Web-site ending
DOTRICE: Actress Karen
DOTTIE: Country singer West
DOTTLE: Pipe ash
DOTTO: 1950s game show
DOUAI: French city
DOUANE: Customs house: French
DOUAY: Bible edition
DOUBS: French river
DOUCE: Gentle: French
DOUCEUR: Gratuity
DOUD: Mamie Eisenhower's maiden name
DOUG: Flutie of football
DOUGAL: Little Lord Fauntleroy's dog
DOUGHTY: Valiant
DOUGLAS: Type of fir
DOULA: Pregnancy coach
DO UP: Arrange
DOURIF: Actor Brad
DOURO: Iberian river
DOUTE: Doubt: French
DOUW: Dutch painter
DOUX: Billet-__ (love letter)
DOUZE: 12: French
DOVE BAR: Ice-cream brand
DOVECOT: Pigeon coop
DOVER, DE: Eastern capital
DOVEY: Lovey-__
DOW: Jones' partner
DOWD: "Harvey" character
DOWDY: Old-fashioned
DOWEL: Wooden pin
DO WELL: Succeed
DOWERY: Bride bestowal
DO WITH: Make out
DOWLING: Long Island college
DOWNBOW: Violinist's direction
DOWNES: Music critic Olin
DOWNEY: Actress Roma
DOWSE: Search for water
DOWSON: English poet
DOXIE: Dog breed, for short
DOXY: Dog breed, for short
DOYCE: "Little Dorrit" character
DOYEN: Senior member
DOYENNE: High-ranking woman
DOYLE: "A Study in Scarlet" author
D'OYLY: Theater producer Richard __ Carte
DOZO: Please: Japanese
D.P.I.: Laser-printer stat.
DPL.: UN license plate abbr.
D.P.M.: Foot doctor's deg.
D.P.S: Baseball plays: Abbr.
DPT.: Corp. unit
D.P.W.: Local building agcy.
DRABBLE: British author
DRABEK: Doug of baseball
DRABS: Dribs and __
DRACHMA: Former Greek coin
DRACO: Dragon constellation
DRAGEE: Sugar-coated candy
DRAGGLE: Besmear
DRAGO: Rocky Balboa opponent
DRAGOON: Former cavalryman
DRAGOTI: Director Stan
DRAKE U.: Des Moines sch.
DRAM: Ounce fraction
DRAMADY: Funny/serious work
DRAMEDY: Funny/serious work
DRANCY: French city
DRANG: Sturm und __
DRANO: Liquid-Plumr alternative
DRAVA: Danube feeder
DRAWBAR: Tractor attachment
DRAWMAN: Plastics worker
DRAW TO: Try for, as an inside straight
DRAX: 007 foe
DRAY: Strong cart
DRAYTON: British poet
DR. BROWN: "Back to the Future" scientist
DR. CHAOS: Nintendo game
DR. CLAW: "Inspector Gadget" villain
DR. DOOM: Comics supervillain
DR. DRE: Rap artist
DREA: Actress de Matteo
DREAMIN': "California __" (1966 tune)
DREAR: Gloomy
DREBIN: Leslie Nielsen role
DRECK: Rubbish
DRED: Stowe novel
DREDD: Comic-book judge
DREFT: Detergent brand
D REGION: Lower ionosphere
DREI: Three: German
DREIDEL: Chanukkah top
DREISER: "An American Tragedy" writer
DREK: Rubbish
DRESDEN: German city
DRESS AS: Emulate
DRESS IN: Wear
DR. EVIL: Austin Powers foe
DREW U.: NJ school
DREXEL: Pennsylvania school
DREXLER: Clyde of basketball
DREYER: Danish director
DREYFUS: Zola subject
DR. FREUD: Austrian psychiatrist
DR. FRIST: Senate leader, formally
DR. HOOK: 1970s rock group
DR. HUG: Leo Buscaglia's nickname
DRIAM: King Arthur knight
DRIESCH: German philosopher
DRIGO: Italian conductor
DRIN: Adriatic Sea feeder
DRINA: Serbian river
D-RING: Strap closure
DRINK ME: "Alice in Wonderland" bottle label
DR. I.Q.: Radio quiz show
DR. I.Q. JR.: Radio quiz show
DRISTAN: Cold medicine
DRIVIN': "__ My Life Away" (Eddie Rabbitt tune)
DR. J: Julius Erving nickname
DR. JUNG: Swiss psychiatrist
DR. K: Dwight Gooden nickname
DR. KING: Civil-rights leader
DR. KOOP: Former Surgeon General
DR. LAO: Tony Randall role
DR. LAURA: Radio psychologist
DR. MARIO: Nintendo game
DR. MCCOY: "Star Trek" character
DR. MELFI: "Sopranos" psychiatrist
DR. NO: 007 film
DROGUE: Type of parachute
DROID: "Star Wars" character
DROIT: Right: French
DROLE: Funny: French
DROME: Course: Comb. form
DROMIO: "Comedy of Errors" character
DROOD: Dickens character
DROP CAP: Chapter-starting typesetting character
DROP NET: Fishing gear
DROPO: Walt of baseball
DROPSY: Fish ailment
DROPT: Let fall, poetically
DROP TOP: Convertible type
DROUET: "Sister Carrie" character
DROXIES: Oreos competitor
DR. PHIL: TV psychologist
DR. QUINN: Jane Seymour TV role
DR. RICE: Bush adviser, formally
DR. RUTH: Westheimer of talk shows
DR. SEUSS: Cat in the Hat creator
DR. SLOAN: "Diagnosis: Murder" sleuth
DR. SPOCK: "Baby and Child Care" author
DR. T: "The 5,000 Fingers of __" (1953 film)
DR. TEETH: Muppet pianist
DRU: Actress Joanne
DRUCKER: Management guru
DRUID: Ancient Celt
DRUMLIN: Narrow hill
DRUON: "The Faerie Queene" character
DRUPE: Type of fruit
DRURY: "Advise and Consent" author
DRUSE: Certain Syrian
DRUZE: Certain Syrian
DR. VEGAS: Rob Lowe film
DR. WELBY: Robert Young TV role
DR. WHO: BBC sci-fi character
DR. X: 1939 Bogart title role
DRYAD: Forest nymph
DRY BULB: Type of thermometer
DRYDEN: English poet
DRY FLY: Fishing lure
DRY IDEA: Deodorant brand
DRYPERS: Diaper brand
DRYS: Prohibition supporters
DRY SUIT: Diver's outfit
D.S.C.: Army medal: Abbr.
D SCALE: Piano practice
DSL: Internet serv.
D.S.M.: Brit. war award
D.S.O.: British medal: Abbr.
D.S.T.: "Spring forward" abbr.
D.S.U.: Dover sch.
D. TH.: Theology deg.
D TILE: Scrabble two-pointer
DTS: Sot's symptoms
DUAD: Couple
DUANE: Guitarist Eddy
DUARTE: 1980s Salvadoran leader
DUBAI: Arab emirate
DU BARRY: Friend of Louis XV
DUBCEK: 1960s Czech leader
DUBHE: Star in Ursa Major
DUBIETY: Mistrust
DUBIN: "42nd Street" lyricist
DUBNIUM: Element #105
DUBOIS: "Streetcar" character
DU BOSE: Author Heyward

DUBUQUE: Iowa city
DUBYA: Presidential nickname
DUC: Duke: French
DUCAT: Admission ticket
DUCE: Dictator
DUCHAMP: French artist
DUCHIN: Pianist Peter
DUCO: Glue brand
DUDDLE: Fuddle-__
DUDDY: Fuddy-__
DUDEK: Canadian poet
DUDGEON: Anger
DUDLEY: Actor Moore
DUELLO: Art of dueling
DUENA: Landlady: Spanish
DUENNA: Chaperone
DUENO: Landlord: Spanish
DUER: Poet Alice __ Miller
DUESSA: "The Faerie Queene" character
DUETTO: Song for two
DUE UP: Next to bat
DUFAY: French composer
DUFF: Actor Howard
DUFFER: Bad golfer
DUFFY: Actress Julia
DUFFY'S: Tavern of old-time radio
DUFUS: Dolt
DUFY: French artist
DUGALD: Scottish philosopher Stewart
DUGAN: "Max __ Returns" (1983 film)
DU GARD: French literature Nobelist
DUGONG: Aquatic mammal
DUH: "Silly me!"
DUHAMEL: French writer
D.U.I.: MADD concern
DUINO: "The __ Elegies" (Rilke book)
DUKAKIS: "Moonstruck" star
DUKAS: "Sorcerer's Apprentice" composer
DULCE: Sweet: Spanish
DULLEA: Actor Keir
DULLES: D.C.-area airport
DULUTH: Minnesota city
DUM: While: Latin
DUMA: Russian parliament
DUMAS: "Three Musketeers" author
DUMBO: Disney elephant
DUMBOS: Dolts
DUMONT: "Duck Soup" actress
DUMPISH: Sad
DUMP ON: Torment
DUMPTY: Humpty-__
DUN: Press for payment
DUNA: Danube in Hungary
DUNANT: 1901 peace Nobelist
DUNAWAY: Actress Faye
DUNBAR: Poet Paul
DUNCAN: Dancer Isadora
DUNDALK: Irish port
DUNDAS: Town in Ontario
DUNDEE: Scottish port
DUNEDIN: Florida city
DUNHAM: Choreographer Katherine
DUNKIN': __ Donuts
DUNKIRK: French city
DUNLAP: Grosset partner
DUNLIN: Sandpiper
DUNLOP: Tire brand
DUNN: Nora of "Saturday Night Live"
DUNNAGE: Personal effects
DUNNE: Actress Irene
DUNNING: Actress Debbe
DUNNO: "I __!" ("Search me!")
DUNST: Actress Kirsten
DUNSTAN: British saint
DUODENA: Intestine sections
DUOMO: Italian cathedral
DUOPOLY: Two-seller situation
DUP: Copy, for short
DUPIN: Poe detective
DUPLE: Two-part
DUPLO: Kiddie-block brand
DUPONT: Chemical giant
DUPRE: French painter
DURA: __ mater (brain covering)
DURAN: Boxer Roberto
DURANCE: Imprisonment
DURANGO: Colorado city
DURANT: Historian Will
DURANTE: Comedian Jimmy
DURAS: French writer
DURBAN: South African port
DURBIN: Actress Deanna
DURC: "Clan of the Cave Bear" character
DUREN: Ryne of baseball
DURER: German engraver
D'URFEY: English playwright
DURHAM: North Carolina city
DURNING: Actor Charles
DURN IT: "Rats!"
DURO: Old Spanish coin
DUROC: Hog breed
DURRA: Grain sorghum
DURRELL: British novelist
DURST: Dared, old-style
DURWARD: TV host Kirby
DURWENT: Australian river
DURYEA: Actor Dan
DUSE: Actress Eleonora
DUSTIN: Actor Hoffman
DUSTMAN: British trash collector
DUSTUP: Quarrel
DUTTON: Actor Charles
DUUMVIR: Roman official
DUUN: Norwegian writer
DUVAL: Golfer David
DUVALL: Actor Robert
DUVE: 1974 medicine Nobelist
DUVET: Bed cover
DUZ: Detergent brand
DVINA: Baltic Sea feeder
D.V.M.: Veterinarian deg.
DVORAK: Czech composer
DWAN: Director Allan
DWAYNE: Actor Hickman
DWEEB: Nerd
DWEEZIL: Guitarist Zappa
D.W.I.: MADD concern
DWIGHT D.: President Eisenhower
DWINDLE: Abate
DWT.: Jeweler's meas.
DYAD: Pair
DYAN: Actress Cannon
DYBBUK: Hebrew demon
DYCE: Scottish painter
DYCK: Flemish painter Van __
DYESS: Texas Air Force base
DYKE: Dick Van __
DYKER: Name meaning "mason"
DYKSTRA: Len of baseball
DYLAN: Folk-rock singer
DYNA: Power: Comb. form
DYNAST: Czar
DYNE: Unit of force
DYNEL: Synthetic fabric
DYNODE: Electrical conductor
DYO: Two: Comb. form
DYS: Bad: Comb. form
DYSART: Actor Richard
DYSON: Physicist Freeman

E

EAD.: Prescription abbr.
EADGILS: "Beowulf" character
EADIE: "Embraced by the Light" author
EADS: Bridge engineer
EAGAN: "The Secret Garden" Tony winner
EAGRE: Tidal flood
EAKINS: Painter Thomas
EALING: London borough
EAMES: Chair designer
EAMON: De Valera of Ireland
EAMONN: Miler Coghlan
EANMUND: "Beowulf" character
E. ANNIE: Author Proulx
E.A.P.: Literary monogram
E.A. POE: Literary signature
EARBUD: Small earphone
EARHART: Aviator Amelia
EARING: Sprouting corn
EARLAP: Cap part
EARLE: "College Bowl" host
EARLESS: Like some seals
EARLOCK: Certain hair
EARLY ON: Almost from the start
EARNIE: Boxer Shavers
EARN IT: Deserve one's pay
EARTAB: Cap part
EARTHA: Singer Kitt
EARVIN: Magic Johnson's first name
EARWIG: Nocturnal insect
EASE BY: Pass slowly
EASE ON: Travel casually
EASLEY: South Carolina city
EAST EGG: "Great Gatsby" locale
EAST END: London area
EASTHAM: Cape Cod town
EASTING: Nautical direction
EAST L.A.: "Chico and the Man" setting
EASTMAN: Kodak creator
EASTON: Singer Sheena
EASY A: Cushy class
EASY-GO: Not here long
EASY OFF: Oven-cleaner brand
EASY ONE: It's not difficult
EAT HERE: Diner sign
EAT IT: Yankovic parody
EAT IT UP: Enjoy something a lot
EAT ME: Carroll cake inscription
EAT OF: Ingest
EATON: Iacocca's successor at Chrysler
EAU: __ de Cologne
EAUX: Waters: French
EAVAN: Poet Boland
EAZY-E: Rap artist
EBAN: Israeli diplomat
E-BANK: Internet S&L
EBATES: Internet cash-back site
EBAY: Internet auction site
EBBETS: Brooklyn Dodgers' home
EBEL: Watch brand
EBEN: "Desire Under the Elms" role
EBERLE: Singer Ray
EBERLY: Singer Bob
EBERT: Film reviewer of TV
EBN: Nautical dir.
E BOAT: WWII vessel
EBOLA: Congo river
EBOLI: "Christ Stopped at __"
EBON: Black, in poems
E BOND: Type of government investment
EBONICS: African-American vernacular
EBONITE: Bowling-ball material
E-BOOK: Digitized publication
EBRO: River of Spain
EBSEN: "Barnaby Jones" actor
E BUZZ: "Poltergeist" dog
E.B.W.: Literary monogram
E.B. WHITE: "Charlotte's Web" author
E-CARD: High-tech greetings
ECARTE: Card game
E-CASH: Internet payment method
ECCE: Behold: Latin
ECCL.: O.T. book
ECCLES: Australian medicine Nobelist
ECCLESI: Church: Comb. form
ECCO: Behold: Italian
ECDYSIS: Molting
ECESIS: Plant process
ECG: Heart chart: Abbr.
ECHAPPE: Ballet leap
ECHIDNA: Australian animal
ECHOS: Communications satellites
ECHT: Genuine: German
ECK: German theologian
ECKART: German theologian
ECKERD: Drugstore chain
ECKHART: German theologian
E CLASS: Mercedes-Benz category
ECLAT: Acclaim
ECLOGUE: Pastoral poem
ECO: Earth-friendly prefix
ECOCIDE: EPA concern
ECOL.: Earth sci.
ECOLAB: Cleaning-supply company
ECOLAW: Environment-related regulations

ECOLE: School: French
E COLI: Dangerous bacteria
ECON.: Social sci.
ECONO: Low-budget, in brand names
ECORSE: City near Detroit
ECOTAGE: Environmental vandalism
ECOTEUR: Environmental vandal
ECOTRIN: Pain-reliever brand
ECOTYPE: Adaptable subspecies
ECRU: Brown shade
ECT: Outer: Comb. form
ECTAD: Outward, in anatomy
ECTAL: Exterior, in anatomy
ECTO: Outer: Comb. form
ECTOMY: Excision: Comb. form
ECTOR: Texas county
ECTYPE: Copy
ECU: Former French coin
ECUA.: Andean land: Abbr.
ECUELLE: Two-handed soup bowl
ECZEMA: Itching condition
EDA: Author Le Shan
EDACITY: Hunger
EDAM: Dutch cheese
ED AMES: "Daniel Boone" actor
ED ASNER: "Lou Grant" actor
ED. B.: Teacher's deg.
EDBERG: Stefan of tennis
ED. D.: Teacher's deg.
EDDA: Icelandic literary work
EDDO: Taro root
EDE: Dutch city
EDEL: Author Leon
EDEMA: Plant swelling
EDEMATA: Plant swellings
EDENIC: Blissful
EDER: Singer Linda
EDERLE: 1920s English Channel swimmer
EDESSA: Ancient Turkish city
EDGAR: Mystery writer's award
EDGARD: Composer Varese
EDGARDO: "Lucia di Lammermoor" character
EDH: Anglo-Saxon letter
EDIE: Singer Adams
EDILE: Ancient Roman magistrate
EDINA, MN: Minneapolis suburb
EDIPO: Mussorgsky work
EDIRNE: City near Istanbul
EDITH: Mrs. Bunker
EDITIO: Edition: Latin
ED KOCH: Former New York mayor
ED. M.: Teacher's deg.
EDMAR: Chessmaster Mednis
ED MEESE: Reagan advisor
EDMOND: Actor O'Brien
EDMONDS: "Drums Along the Mohawk" author
EDMUND: Mountaineer Hillary
EDMUND I: English king
EDMUNDS: Singer Dave
EDNA: Author Ferber
EDNA MAY: Actress Oliver
EDO: Tokyo's former name
EDOM: Ancient Biblical country
EDOMITE: Descendant of Esau
EDOUARD: Painter Manet
E.D.P.: Company's computer dept.
EDRED: English king
EDSEL: 1950s Ford
EDSON: Comic-strip artist Gus
E.D.T.: NY summer clock setting
EDTA: Food preservative
EDTV: Ron Howard film
EDU: College Web site suffix
EDUARD: Czech statesman Benes
EDUARDO: Argentine novelist Mallea
EDUC.: Cabinet dept.
EDUCE: Draw forth
EDUCT: Chemical extract
EDVARD: Composer Grieg
EDWARD G.: Actor Robinson
EDWARD I: English king
EDWARD R.: TV journalist Murrow
EDWARDS: "ER" star
EDWARD V: English king
EDWIN: Actor Booth
EDWINA: Author Currie
ED WOOD: Johnny Depp film
ED WYNN: Old-time radio comedian
EDY: Actress Williams
EDY'S: Ice-cream brand
EEC: Common Market: Abbr.
EEE: Shoe width
EEEE: Shoe width
EEG: Brain scan: Abbr.
EEK: "A mouse!"
EELPOT: Fish trap
EELPOUT: European fish
EELY: Hard to hold
E'EN: Poetic dusk
EENSIE: __-weensie
EENSY: __-weensy
EENY: Counting-rhyme starter
E.E.O.: Anti-discrimination prog.
E.E.O.C.: Anti-discrimination agcy.
E'ER: Poetic adverb
EERO: Architect Saarinen
E.E.S: Cal Tech degrees
EEYORE: "Winnie-the-Pooh" donkey
EFAX: Computer message service
EFFABLE: Utterable
EFFACE: Blot out
EFFENDI: Turkish title
EFFETE: Decadent
EFFIE: Edgar Bergen dummy
EFFLUX: Outward flow
EFFUSE: Disseminate
EFIK: African people
E-FILE: Submit taxes via the Web
EFREM: Actor Zimbalist
EFS: Gee preceders
EFT: Newt
EGA: Video-screen format: Abbr.
EGADI: Islands off Sicily
EGAL: Equal: French
EGALE: Equal: French
EGALITE: "Liberté, __, fraternité"
EGAN: Actor Richard
EGBDF: Clef letters
EGBERT: English king
EGDON: __ Heath (Thomas Hardy setting)
EGER: City in Hungary
EGERIA: Female adviser
EGEST: Cast off
EGESTA: Discharged matter
EGEUS: "A Midsummer Night's Dream" character
EGGAR: Actress Samantha
EGGER: Tent caterpillar
EGGERT: Actress Nicole
EGGLER: British dairy merchant
EGGO: Frozen-waffle brand
EGHAM: Town in Surrey
EGIS: Shield
EGLI: He: Italian
EGLIN: Florida Air Force base
EGLISE: Church: French
EGMONT: Beethoven overture
EGOISTE: Chanel fragrance
EGON: "Ghostbusters" character
EGOSURF: Search the Web for your own name
EGOYAN: Director Atom
EGRESS: Barnum "attraction"
EGUREN: Peruvian poet
EHLE: Actress Jennifer
EHLO: Craig of basketball
EHRE: Honor: German
EHREN: Honors: German
EHRLICH: German immunologist
EHUD: Barak of Israel
EID: Islamic holiday
EIDETIC: Kind of memory
EIDOLA: Apparitions
EIDOLIC: Eerie
EIDOLON: Apparition
E-I-E-I-O: "...had a farm, __"
EIER: Eggs: German
EIGEN: 1967 chemistry Nobelist
EIGER: "The __ Sanction" (Eastwood film)
EIGG: Inner Hebrides isle
EIGHT A: Shoe size
EIGHT B: Shoe size
EIGHT C: Shoe size
EIGHT D: Shoe size
EIGHT E: Shoe size
EIGHT EE: Shoe size
EIJKMAN: Dutch medicine Nobelist
EIK: Apt. feature
EILAT: Israeli port
EILE: Haste: German
EILEEN: Actress Brennan
EILERS: Actress Sally
EILERT: "Hedda Gabler" character
EIMI: e.e. cummings book
EIN: A: German
EINE: "__ kleine Nachtmusik"
EINEN: Unite: German
EINER: One: German
EINES: One: German
EINS: One: German
EIRENE: Aristophanes comedy
EIS: Ice: German
EISELE: Apollo astronaut
EISEN: Iron: German
EISLEY: Actor Anthony
EISNER: Cartoonist Will
EJECTA: Lava, e.g.
EJEMPLO: Example: Spanish
EJIDO: Mexican farm
EKBERG: Actress Anita
EKCO: Cookware manufacturer
EKE: Supplement, with "out"
EKELOF: Swedish poet
EKG: Heart chart: Abbr.
EKISTIC: Of city planning
EKLAND: Actress Britt
EKUELE: Equatorial Guinea money
EKWENSI: Nigerian writer
E LA: Guido's high note
EL AAIUN: Western Sahara capital
ELADIO: "For Whom the Bell Tolls" character
ELAINE: Actress Stritch
ELAINE'S: Big Apple restaurant
EL AL: Israeli airline
ELAM: Actor Jack
ELAMITE: Ancient Babylonian
ELAN: Ardor
ELANCE: Ballet movement
ELAND: African antelope
ELANET: Small bird
ELANTRA: Hyundai model
ELAPID: Cobra
ELARA: Moon of Jupiter
ELAS: WWII Greek underground org.
ELASTIN: Tissue protein
ELAT: Israeli port
ELATER: Type of beetle
ELATH: Israeli port
E LAYER: Ionosphere part
ELAYNE: Comic Boosler
ELBA: Napoleon exile isle
ELBE: German river
ELBERT: Colorado mountain
ELBERTA: Type of peach
ELBRUS: Caucasus mountain
ELBURZ: Iran mountain range
EL CAJON: California city
EL CAMPO: Latin American plain
ELCAR: Actor Dana
EL CID: Spanish national hero
ELD: Antiquity, old-style
ELDIN: "Murphy Brown" housekeeper
ELDON: Cartoonist Dedini
ELDRICH: Unearthly
ELDRICK: Tiger Woods' first name
ELEA: Ancient Greek City
ELEAZAR: Son of Aaron
ELECTRA: Daughter of Agamemnon
ELECTRO: Prefix for magnetic
ELEGIAC: Doleful
ELEGIT: Type of writ
ELEISON: "Kyrie __" (Mass section)
ELEKTRA: Asteroid
ELEM.: Periodic-table entry: Abbr.
ELEMI: Fragrant resin
ELENA: Actress Verdugo
ELENI: Kate Nelligan film
ELENIAK: Actress Erika
ELEVE: Student: French
ELEVEN A: Shoe size
ELEVEN B: Shoe size
ELEVEN C: Shoe size

ELEVEN D: Shoe size
ELEVEN E: Wide shoe
ELEVON: Airplane part
ELFLOCK: Tangled curl
ELFMAN: Actress Jenna
ELF OWL: Small bird
E.L. FUDGE: Cookie brand
ELG: Actress Taina
EL GALLO: "The Fantasticks" character
ELGAR: "The Planets" composer
ELGART: Bandleader Larry
ELGIN: Baylor of basketball
EL GRECO: Spanish artist
ELHI: Grades K-6
ELI: Inventor Whitney
ELIA: British essayist
ELIAS: Inventor Howe
ELIDE: Omit in pronunciation
ELIE: Author Wiesel
ELIEL: Architect Saarinen
ELI ELI: Yom Kippur song
ELIEZER: Son of Moses
ELIGIUS: Patron saint of jewelers
ELIHU: 1912 peace Nobelist Root
ELIJAH: Biblical prophet
ELINOR: Novelist Glyn
ELIO: Director Petri
ELION: 1988 medicine Nobelist
ELIOT: Writer T.S.
ELIS: Yale students
ELISA: "Aeneid" queen
ELISE: "Für __" (Beethoven piece)
ELISEO: Cuban poet Diego
ELISHA: Inventor Otis
ELISION: Omission
ELISSA: Actress Landi
E-LIST: Direct-mail database
ELI YALE: University benefactor
ELIZ.: 16th-c. queen
ELIZA: "My Fair Lady" heroine
ELKE: Actress Sommer
ELKHART: Indiana city
ELKIN: Novelist Stanley
ELKO, NV: Silver State city
ELKTON: Maryland city
ELL: Pipe joint
ELLA: Singer Fitzgerald
ELLA MAE: Singer Morse
ELLE: Fashion mag
ELLEN: Actress Barkin
ELLER: "Oklahoma!" aunt
ELLERY: Author Queen
ELLES: They: French
ELLICE: __ Islands (former name of Tuvalu)
ELLIE: "Dallas" character
ELLIN: Author Stanley
ELLIO'S: Frozen-pizza brand
ELLIOT: "Mama" Cass
ELLIOTT: Actor Sam
ELLIS: Island near Manhattan
ELLISON: "Invisible Man" author
ELLMANN: Author Richard
ELLORA: Archaeological site in India
ELLOS: They: Spanish
ELLY MAY: "Beverly Hillbillies" character
ELMAN: Violinist Mischa
ELMAR: Violinist Oliveira
ELM CITY: New Haven nickname
ELMER: Bugs Bunny's pursuer
ELMER'S: Glue brand
ELMIRA: New York city
ELMIRE: "Tartuffe" character
EL MISTI: Volcano of Peru
ELMO: "Blondie" boy
ELMONT: Long Island town
EL MONTE: California city
ELMORE: Author Leonard
ELMOS: St. __ fire
ELM ST.: "Nightmare" place
EL MUNDO: Madrid newspaper
ELMWOOD: __ Park, IL
ELNATH: Star in Taurus
EL NINO: Weather-affecting current
ELNORA: Indiana city
EL NORTE: U.S.A., to Mexicans
ELO: Rock band
ELOCUTE: Declaim
ELODEA: Aquarium plant
ELOGE: Praise: French
ELOI: "Time Machine" race
ELOISA: "__ to Abelard" (Pope work)
ELOISE: Fictional Plaza Hotel girl
ELON: North Carolina college
EL ORO: Gold: Spanish
EL PAIS: Newspaper of Spain
ELPIS: Asteroid
EL PRADO: Madrid museum
EL RENO: Oklahoma city
EL REY: King: Spanish
ELROY: Youngest Jetson
ELS: Chicago trains
ELSA: "Born Free" lioness
ELSA'S: "__ Dream" (Wagner aria)
ELSIE: Borden cow
EL SOL: Mexico City daily
ELSTON: 1960s Yankee __ Howard
ELTON: Sir __ John
EL TORO: Matador adversary
EL TRAIN: Chicago transport
ELU: Elected: French
ELUANT: Solvent
ELUARD: French poet
ELUATE: Solvent
ELUL: Hebrew month
ELURA: Canon camcorder brand
ELUTE: Remove by dissolving
ELUVIUM: Wind-deposited soil
ELVER: Young eel
ELVIN: Hayes of basketball
ELVIRA: "__ Madigan"
ELWAY: Quarterback John
ELWES: "The Princess Bride" star
ELWOOD: "Harvey" character
ELY: TV Tarzan
ELY, NV: Silver State city
ELYOT: "Private Lives" character
ELYRIA: Ohio city
ELYSE: "Family Ties" mom
ELYSEE: Paris' __ Palace
ELYSEES: Paris' Champs __
ELYSIAN: Blissful
ELYSIUM: Paradise
ELYTIS: Greece literature Nobelist
E-MAG: On-line 'zine
E MAJ.: Mus. key
E-MALL: Internet shopping site
EMANUEL: Pianist Ax
EMB.: Ambassador's res.
EMBANK: Build a dam
EMBAR: Block
EMBAY: Enclose in an inlet
EMBOG: Become mired
EMBOITE: Ballet step
EMBOSOM: Cherish
EMBOWER: Hide in trees
EMBROWN: Darken
EMBRUE: Defile
EM DASH: Bit of punctuation
EMDEN: German city
EME: Uncle: Scottish
EMEER: Mideast ruler
EMER.: Part of EMT
EMERIC: Director Pressburger
EMERIL: TV chef
EMERITA: Honorary title
EMERSED: Like a lotus
EMERSON: Poet/essayist
EMESA: Ancient Syrian city
EMETIC: Ipecac, e.g.
EMEU: Australian bird
EMEUTE: Riot: French
EMF: Voltage meas.
EMI: British record label
EMIA: Blood: Comb. form
EMIGRE: Asylum seeker
EMIGREE: Asylum seeker
EMIL: Czech runner Zatopek
EMILE: Novelist Zola
EMILIA: "Othello" character
EMILIE: One of the Dionnes
EMILIO: Actor Estevez
EMILY: "Our Town" heroine
EMILY'S: __ List (female-candidate PAC)
EMINEM: Rap artist
EMIR: Mideast ruler
EMIRATE: Abu Dhabi, e.g.
EMK: Mass. senator's monogram
EMLEN: Tunnell of football
EM'LY: "David Copperfield" girl
EMLYN: Playwright Williams
EMMA: Poet Lazarus
EMMAUS: Pennsylvania town
EMME: "Plus-size" supermodel
EMMER: Type of wheat
EMMET: Ant
EMMETT: "Dixie" composer
EMMITT: Smith of football
EMMUSKA: Baroness __ Orczy ("The Scarlet Pimpernel" author)
EMMYLOU: Country singer Harris
EMO: Comic Philips
EMORY U.: Coll. in Atlanta
EMP.: Akihito, e.g.: Abbr.
EMPALE: Pierce
EMPATH: Reader of another's feelings
EMPERY: Absolute dominion
EMPIRIC: Experiential
EMPIRIN: Headache remedy brand
EMPRISE: Adventure
EMPSON: British poet
EMPTOR: Buyer: Latin
EM QUAD: Printer measure
E.M.T.: CPR expert
EMU: Australian bird
ENA: "Bambi" aunt
EN AMI: As a friend: French
ENARBOR: Surround with trees
ENARE: Finnish lake
ENARM: Equip with weapons
ENATE: Mother's-side relative
EN BANC: Sitting, as a court
EN BAS: Ballet position
ENBERG: Sportscaster Dick
EN BLOC: As a whole: French
ENC.: Ref. book set
EN CARRE: Roulette bet
ENCARTA: Microsoft's dictionary
ENCHASE: Decorate with engraving
ENCINA: California oak
ENCINO: L.A. suburb
ENCL.: Env. contents
ENCOMIA: Praises
ENCRE: Ink: French
ENCY.: Ref. set
ENCYC.: Ref. set
ENCYCL.: Ref. set
END-ALL: Ultimate goal
EN DASH: Typesetting character
END CUT: Beef portion
ENDE: "The NeverEnding Story" author
ENDEMIC: Indigenous
ENDER: Bitter-__ (diehard)
ENDERBY: __ Land (Antarctic region)
END GAME: Area of chess study
END IN: Conclude with
END IT: Stop
END LEAF: Book page
END LINE: Football marker
ENDLONG: Lengthwise, old-style
END MAN: Minstrel-show participant
ENDNOTE: Article afterthought
ENDO: Inner: Comb. form
END ON: Conclude with
ENDOR: Home of a Biblical witch
ENDORA: "Bewitched" mother
ENDPIN: Cello part
ENDPLAY: Bridge game maneuver
END RUN: Evasive maneuver
ENDUE: Assume
ENDURO: Auto race
ENDWAYS: Lengthwise
ENDWISE: Lengthwise
ENE: Compass pt.
ENERO: January: Spanish
ENESCO: Romanian composer
ENFACE: Write on the front
EN FAIT: As a matter of fact: French
ENFANT: Child: French
ENFIELD: Connecticut town
ENFIN: At last: French
ENGEL: "Mary Tyler Moore Show" actress
ENGELS: Karl Marx collaborator

ENGILD: Brighten
ENGLE: Poet Paul
ENG. LIT.: College course, for short
ENGLUND: Freddy Krueger portrayer
ENGLUT: Gulp down
ENGR.: MIT grad
ENGRAM: Memory trace
EN HAUT: Ballet position
ENIAC: 1940s computer
ENID: Arthurian woman
ENID, OK: Sooner State city
ENIF: Star in Pegasus
ENISLE: Isolate
ENKE: Elizabeth __ (Edie Adams' real name)
ENL.: Blow up: Abbr.
EN-LAI: Chou __ of China
ENNA: City in Italy
ENNE: Feminine suffix
ENNEA: Nine: Comb. form
ENNEAD: Group of nine
ENNIO: Film composer Morricone
ENNIS: "Brokeback Mountain" role
ENNIUS: Roman poet
ENNS: Austrian town
ENNUI: Boredom
ENO: Rock producer Brian
ENOCH: Fictional Arden
ENOIL: Anoint, old-style
ENOKI: Japan mushroom
ENOL: Organic compound
ENOLA: "__ Gay" (WWII plane)
ENOLOGY: Study of winemaking
ENON: __ Valley, PA
ENORM: Huge, old-style
ENORME: Huge: French
ENOS: Son of Seth
E-NOTE: High-tech message
ENOW: Sufficient, old-style
EN PRISE: In danger, in chess
EN QUAD: Printer measure
ENRICO: Physicist Fermi
ENRIGHT: "Quiz Show" character
ENRIQUE: Singer Iglesias
ENRON: Embattled energy company
'ENRY: "Just You Wait, __ 'iggins"
ENS: Nav. rank
ENSATE: Sword-shaped
ENSE: Massachusetts motto starter
ENSILE: Store fodder
ENSKY: Exalt
ENSLER: Playwright Eve
ENSOR: Belgian artist
ENSUITE: Afterwards: French
E.N.T.: Med. specialty
ENTAD: Inward
ENTEBBE: Ugandan city
ENTENTE: Accord
ENTERIC: Intestinal
ENTER IN: Join
ENTERO: Intestine: Comb. form
ENTER ON: Begin
ENTIAL: Adjective suffix
ENTO: Inner: Comb. form
ENTOM.: Bug sci.
ENTOMO: Insect: Comb. form
ENTR: __'acte
ENTRADA: Doorway: Spanish
ENTRE: Between: French
ENTREZ: Come in: French
ENTROPY: Chaos
ENTS: "Lord of the Rings" creatures
ENUF: Adequate, informally
ENURE: Become accustomed
ENVENOM: Embitter
ENVER: __ Pasha (Turkish statesman)
ENVIRO: Ecology-minded person
EN VOGUE: Fashionable: French
ENVOI: Ballade conclusion
ENYA: Irish singer
ENYO: Greek war goddess
ENZ: Split __ (rock group)
ENZO: Auto designer Ferrari
EOAN: Of the dawn
EOCENE: Geological epoch
E.O.E.: Help-wanted abbr.
EOFOR: "Beowulf" character
EOLA: Texas town
EOLIA: Kentucky town
EOLIAN: Borne by the wind
EOLIC: Ancient Greek dialect
EOLITH: Ancient flint
EOLUS: Colorado mountain
E.O.M.: Acctg. term
EONIAN: Boundless
E ONLINE: Cable network Web site
EOS: Dawn goddess
EOSIN: Red dye
EOUS: Adjective suffix
EPA: Ecology agcy.
EPACT: Astronomy term
EPARCH: Bishop
EPCOT: Orlando attraction
EPERGNE: Centerpiece
EPERNAY: French town
EPH.: N.T. book
EPHA: Biblical bushel
EPHAH: Biblical bushel
EPHEBUS: Youth of ancient Greece
EPHEDRA: Dry-climate plant
EPHESUS: Temple of Artemis site
EPHOD: Biblical vestment
EPHOR: Ancient magistrate
EPHRAIM: Son of Joseph
EPHRON: Director Nora
EPI: Center starter
EPICARP: Fruit peel
EPICENE: Feeble
EPIDERM: Skin layer
EPIDOTE: Crystalline mineral
EPIGONE: Inferior artist
EPIGRAM: Aphorism
EPILADY: Shaver brand
EPILATE: Remove hair
EPINAL: French city
EPIS.: Prot. branch
EPISC.: Prot. branch
EPODE: Lyric poem
EPONINE: "Les Miz" character
EPONYM: Samuel Maverick, e.g.
EPOPEE: Epic poem
EPOQUE: Epoch: French
EPOS: Epic poem
E. POWER: Organist Biggs
EPPA: Baseball Hall of Famer Rixey
EPPERLY: Antarctic mountain
EPPIE: "Silas Marner" character
EPPING: England's __ Forest
EPPS: Actor Omar
EPROM: Computer memory
E.P.S.: Wall Street abbr.
EPSILON: Greek letter
EPSOM: British track site
EPSON: Computer printer brand
EPSTEIN: British sculptor
EQUERRY: Horse handler
EQUIANO: Nigerian writer
EQUIFAX: Credit-reporting agency
EQUIS: Dos __ (Mexican beer)
EQUOID: Of horses
EQUUS: Horse genus
ERAL: Of an age
ERASMUS: Dutch theologian
ERASTUS: German theologian
ERAT: Part of QED
ERATO: Muse poetry
ERBIL: Iraq city
ERBIUM: Element #68
ERDA: "Das Rheingold" role
ERDE: "Das Lied von der __"
ERDMAN: Business writer Paul
ERDOS: Hungarian-born mathematician
ERDRICH: Native American author
ERE: Before, in poems
EREBUS: Antarctic mountain
ERECTUS: Homo __ (human ancestor)
EREDE: Conductor Alberto
ERELONG: Soon
EREMITE: Loner
ERENOW: Before
ERES TU: Song of 1974
ERETZ: Land: Hebrew
EREV: Eve of a Jewish holiday
EREVAN: Capital of Armenia
EREWHON: Butler novel
ERFURT: German city
ERG: Unit of work
ERGO: Therefore
ERGOT: Plant malady
ERGY: Effect: Comb. form
ERHARD: 1960s German leader
ERI: "__ tu" (Verdi aria)
ERIA: Assam silkworm
ERIC: Norse explorer
ERICA: Author Jong
ERICAS: Evergreen shrubs
ERICH: Director Von Stroheim
ERICK: Oklahoma town
ERICSON: Norse explorer
ERIE, PA: Keystone State city
ERIES: Erstwhile Iroquoians
ERIGENA: Irish philosopher
ERIK: Actor Estrada
ERIKA: Actress Eleniak
ERIKSON: "Childhood and Society" author
E-RING: NBC series
ERINNA: Ancient Greek poet
ERINYES: Greek goddesses
ERINYS: Greek goddess
ERIQ: Actor La Salle
ERIS: Goddess of discord
ERISA: Pension-act acronym
ERISTIC: Controversial
ERITREA: African nation
ERI TU: Verdi aria
ERIVAN: Armenian capital
ERL: "The __-King" (Goethe work)
ERLANG: Unit of traffic intensity
ERLE: Author __ Stanley Gardner
ERMA: Author Bombeck
ERMA'S: "Aunt __ Cope Book"
ERMINIA: Tasso heroine
ERN: Sea eagle
ERNA: Opera singer Berger
ERNANI: Verdi opera
ERNE: Sea eagle
ERNESTA: One of TV's Snoop Sisters
ERNESTO: Che Guevara's first name
ERNIE: Comedian Kovacs
ERNO: Cube inventor Rubik
ERNST: Director Lubitsch
ERO: "__ e Leandro" (opera)
'EROES: Kipling's "Thin red line of __"
EROICA: Beethoven's Third
EROO: Slangy suffix
EROS: Greek war god
EROSE: Uneven
ERRARE: __ humanum est
ERROL: Actor Flynn
ERROLL: Pianist Garner
ERS: Hosp. areas
ERSATZ: Artificial
ERSE: Scots Gaelic
ERSKINE: Author Caldwell
ERST: Prefix for while
ERSTAD: Darren of baseball
ERTE: Art Deco artist
ERTEGUN: Atlantic Records founder
ERUCT: Belch
ERVIN: Watergate hearings senator
ERVING: Julius of basketball
ERWIN: Actor Stu
ERY: Noun suffix
ERYKAH: Singer Badu
ERYNGO: Sea holly
ERYTHRO: Red: Comb. form
ESA: That: Spanish
ESAI: Actor Morales
ESAKI: 1973 physics Nobelist
ESALEN: __ Institute (self-improvement group)
ESAR: "Comic Dictionary" author
ESAS: Those: Spanish
ESAU: Jacob's twin
ESBAT: Convocation of witches
ESC: Computer key
E SCALE: Piano practice
ESCALOP: Bake, in a way
ESCALUS: "Measure for Measure" character
ESCARP: Cliff
ESCAUT: French river
ESCE: Verb suffix
ESCENCE: Noun suffix

ESCENT: Adjective suffix
ESCHEAT: Confiscate
ESCHER: Dutch artist
ESCHEW: Avoid
ESCUDO: Former Portugese coin
ESCUELA: School: Spanish
ESD.: Apocrypha bk.
ESDRAS: Apocrypha book
ESE: Language suffix
ESEL: Donkey: German
ESENIN: Russian poet
E.S.G.: Perry Mason author's monogram
ESHKOL: 1960s Israeli leader
ESIASON: Boomer of football
ESIS: Process: Suffix
ES IST: It is: German
ESK.: Certain Alaskan: Abbr.
ESKER: Geological ridge
E.S.L.: Adult ed. subj.
ESME: Salinger character
ESNE: Feudal laborer
ESO: That: Spanish
ESO BESO: Paul Anka tune
ESOP: Job-perk acronym
ESOS: Those: Spanish
ESOTERY: Arcane things
ESPANA: Spain: Spanish
ESPANOL: Spanish, in Spanish
ESPARTO: African grass
ESPIO: Pentax camera brand
ESPN: Sports cable network
ESPNEWS: Sports cable channel
ESPO: Hockey great's nickname
ESPOO: Finnish city
ESPOSA: Wife: Spanish
ESPOSO: Husband: Spanish
ESPYS: Annual sports awards
ESQ.: Atty.'s title
ESQUE: -ish relative
ESQUIRE: Attorney title
ESSA: Italian pronoun
ESSAI: Attempt: French
ESSE: To be: Latin
ESSEN: German city
ESSENE: Ancient ascetic
ESSEX: Friend of Elizabeth I
ESSI: They: Italian
ESSIE: "Ah, Wilderness!" character
ESSO: Exxon's former name
EST: Superlative suffix
ESTA: Are: Spanish
ESTAB.: Founded: Abbr.
ESTADO: State: Spanish
ESTAMIN: Worsted fabric
ESTAN: They are: Spanish
ESTAR: To be: Spanish
ESTAS: These: Spanish
ESTD.: Founded: Abbr.
ESTE: East: Spanish
ESTEBAN: Stephen: Spanish
ESTEE: Lauder of cosmetics
ESTEFAN: Singer Gloria
ESTELLA: "Great Expectations" character
ESTELLE: Actress Parsons
ESTER: Organic compound
ESTES: 1950s senator Kefauver
ESTEVEZ: Actor Emilio
ESTH.: O.T. book
ESTHER: Biblical queen
ESTHETE: Art lover
ESTHS: Eastern Europeans
ESTIME: Guess: French
ESTIVAL: Of summer
ESTLIN: Edward __ Cummings
ESTO: This: Spanish
ESTOC: Sword of yore
ESTONIA: Baltic nation
ESTOP: Hinder legally
ESTORIL: Portuguese resort
ESTOS: These: Spanish
ESTRADA: "CHiPs" star
ESTRAY: Wanderer
E STRING: Guitar part
ESTUARY: Arm of the sea
ESV: Cadillac model
ETA: Greek vowel
ETAGE: Floor: French
ETAGERE: Bric-a-brac stand
ETAH: Arctic explorer's base
E-TAIL: Internet commerce
ET AL.: Footnote abbr.
ET ALIA: And others: Latin
ET ALIBI: And elsewhere: Latin
ET ALII: And others: Latin
ETAMINE: Cotton fabric
ETAOIN: __ shrdlu (typesetting placeholder)
ETAPE: Day's march
ETAT: State: French
ETC. ETC.: "And blah blah blah"
ETD: Airport abbr.
ETE: Summer: French
ETERNE: Ageless, old-style
ETESIAN: Annual, as some winds
ETH: Ordinal suffix
ETHAN: Fictional Frome
ETHANE: A flammable gas
ETHANOL: Alternative fuel
ETHEL: Singer Merman
ETHENE: Anesthetic gas
ETHERIC: Airy
ETHIOP: East African, old-style
ETHMOID: Head bone
ETHN: Culture: Comb. form
ETHNO: Culture: Comb. form
ETHNOS: Cultural group
ETHOS: Spirit of a culture
ETHYL: Antiknock fluid
ETI: Life in outer space: Abbr.
ETIC: Adjective suffix
E-TICKET: Airline Web site offering
ETIENNE: Steven: French
E TILE: Scrabble one-pointer
ET MOI: Me too: French
ETNA: Sicilian volcano
ETNAS: Alcohol burners
ETO: WWII arena
ETOILE: Ballet star
ETON: British prep school
ETONIC: Sports-shoe brand
ETONS: Types of jackets
E-TRADE: Internet brokerage service
ETRE: To be: French
ETRES: Beings: French
ETRURIA: Ancient Italian region
E.T.S: Sci-fi characters: Abbr.
ET SEQ.: And the following: Abbr.
ET SEQQ.: And those following: Abbr.
ETTA: Sundance Kid's girlfriend
ETTING: Singer Ruth
ETTORE: Automaker Bugatti
ET TU: "Julius Caesar" phrase
ETUDE: Chopin piece
ETUI: Needle case
ETUM: Garden: Comb. form
ETV: Instructional broadcast
ET VOILA: French chef's shout
ETYM.: Dictionary abbr.
ETYMA: Root words
ETYMOL: Linguistic sci.
ETYMON: Root word
EUBANKS: "Newlywed Game" host
EUBIE: Composer Blake
EUBOEA: Greek island
EUCERIN: Skin-care brand
EUCHRE: Cheat
EUCKEN: German philosopher
EUCLID: Greek mathematician
EUDEMON: Benevolent spirit
EUDORA: Author Welty
EUELL: Natural-diet proponent Gibbons
EUER: Your: German
EUGENE: Playwright Ionesco
EUGENIA: Asteroid
EUGENIC: Of good breeding
EUGENIE: An empress of France
EUGLENA: Protozoa genus
EULA: Faulkner character
EULABUS: Pope
EULER: Swiss mathematician
EULESS: Texas city
EUNICE: Sister of JFK
EUNOMIA: One of the Horae
EUONYM: Appropriate name
EUPHONY: Pleasant sound
EUPNEA: Breath
EURAIL: Overseas train pass
EURASIA: Two continents combined
EURE: French department
EUREKA: California motto
EURO: French money
EUROPA: Moon of Jupiter
EUROPOP: Music genre
EUROVAN: Volkswagen model
EURUS: East wind
EUSDEN: British poet
EUSTACE: Name meaning "steadfast"
EUSTIS: Florida city
EUTAXY: Good order
EUTERPE: Muse of music
EUWE: Dutch chessmaster
EVA: Actress Gabor
EVAH: "Well, Did You __!" (Porter tune)
EVAL.: Assessment: Abbr.
EVA LUNA: Isabel Allende novel
EVAN: Author Hunter
EVANDER: Boxer Holyfield
EVANGEL: Good tidings
EVANISH: Disappear
EVANS: Mrs. Roy Rogers
EVAP.: Turn to steam: Abbr.
EVEL: Daredevil Knievel
EVELONG: From sunset on
EVELYN: Writer Waugh
EVEN AS: While
EVERDUR: Type of alloy
EVERETT: Actor Chad
EVERLYS: Singing brothers
EVERS: Civil-rights leader Medgar
EVER SO: Exceedingly
EVERT: Chris of tennis
EVERTOR: Type of muscle
EVIAN: Bottled-water brand
EVIE: "Howards End" role
EVIL ONE: Archfiend
EVINCE: Prove
EVITA: Lloyd Webber musical
EVITE: E-mailed invitation
EVOE: Greek reveler's utterance
EVOLUTE: Geometry term
EVONNE: Goolagong of tennis
EVORA: City in Portugal
EV'RY: "Climb __ Mountain"
EVS: Units of energy: Abbr.
EVULSE: Extract
EWA: Actress Aulin
EWAINE: King Arthur knight
EWALD: Danish writer
EWAN: Actor McGregor
EWART: Gladstone's middle name
EWBANK: Football coach Weeb
EWEEK: Technology Web magazine
EWEN: Musicologist David
EWENECK: Horse feature
EWER: Water pitcher
EWERY: Place for water pitchers
EWINGS: "Dallas" clan
EWOK: "Return of the Jedi" beast
EWR: Airport serving NYC
EWW: "That's gross!"
EXA: Quintillion: Comb. form
EXACTA: Track bet
EX ANIMO: Sincerely: Latin
EXARCH: Bishop
EXC.: Ambassador title: Abbr.
EXCIDE: Cut out
EXCL.: Not incl.
EXCLAVE: Alaska, for instance
EXCURSE: Ramble
EXCUSA: Excuse: Spanish
EXCUSEZ: __-moi (pardon me: French)
EX DIV.: Stock listing abbr.
EXE: British river
EXEDRA: Outdoor bench
EXEGETE: Bible expert
EXEL: Nick Van __ of basketball
EXEMPLA: Parables
EXETER: New Hampshire town
EXEUNT: Shakespeare stage direction
EX FACTO: Actually: Latin
EX-GI: VFW member
EXHEDRA: Outdoor bench
EXIGENT: Acute

EXIT NOW: Highway billboard phrase
EXITUS: Departure: Latin
EX LIB.: Bookplate abbr.
EXMOOR: "Lorna Doone" locale
EX MORE: According to custom: Latin
EXO: Outer: Comb. form
EXOCARP: Fruit peel
EXOCET: French missile
EXOD.: O.T. book
EXOGAMY: Marriage outside a tribe
EXON: Yeoman of the guard
EXONYM: Name for natives used by outsiders
EXORDIA: Introductions
EXP.: No longer valid: Abbr.
EX PARTE: Legal term
EXPAT: Citizen abroad
EXPIATE: Atone for
EXPOSIT: Put forth
EX POST: After the fact
EXPT.: Lab work: Abbr.
EXPUNGE: Abolish
EX'S: "All My __ Live in Texas"
EXSCIND: Cut out
EXSECT: Cut out
EXSERT: Thrust out
EXT.: Office phone: Abbr.
EXTANT: Alive
EXTENSO: In __ (at full length: Latin)
EXTERN: Nonresident doctor
EXTERNE: Nonresident doctor
EXTRO: Outside: Comb. form
EXTRUDE: Eject
EXUMA: Bahama island
EXUPERY: Saint-__ (French writer)
EXURB: Bedroom community
EX-WORKS: Direct from the factory
EXXON: Mobil merger partner
EYCK: Painter Jan van __
EYDIE: Singer Gormé
EYEBOLT: Fastener for a hook
EYE-HAND: Type of coordination
EYELESS: "__ in Gaza" (Huxley novel)
EYELET: Small hole
EYEPIT: Ocular socket
EYEROLL: "Here we go again" look
EYESHOT: Field of view
EYESPOT: Peacock tail feature
EYE UP: Examine, slangily
EYEWALL: Hurricane area
EYRA: Wild cat
EYRE: Brontë heroine
EYRIE: Eagle nest
EYRIR: Iceland money
EYVIND: Swedish writer Johnson
EZEK.: O.T. book
EZEKIEL: Biblical prophet
EZER: Israeli statesman Weizman
E-ZINE: Internet mag
EZIO: Opera singer Pinza
EZ PASS: Toll-paying convenience
EZR.: O.T. book
EZRA: Biblical prophet
EZZARD: Boxer Charles

F

F.A.A.: Airplane agcy.
FAB: "Groovy!"
FABARES: Actress Shelley
FABER: "Animal House" college
FABERGE: Perfume brand
FAB FOUR: Beatles' nickname
FABI: Auto racer Teo
FABIAN: 1950s pop singer
FABIO: Italian supermodel
FABRAY: Actress Nanette
FABRE: French entomologist
FABRIZI: Actor Aldo
FAC.: Copy: Abbr.
FACE IT: Be realistic
FACE ON: Be situated in front of
FACIA: British dashboard
FACIE: Prima-__ evidence
FACIES: Appearance
FACIL: Easy: Spanish
FACILE: Fluent
FACONNE: Patterned fabric
FACP: M.D.'s designation
FACS: M.D.'s designation
FACTA: Statements in a legal case
FACTO: De __ (in reality)
FACTOID: Bit of trivia
FACTUM: Post __ (after the fact)
FACULA: Bright spot on the sun
FADAYEV: Russian writer
FAD DIET: Atkins or Scarsdale
FADDLE: Fiddle-__ (nonsense)
FADIMAN: Author Clifton
FADO: Portuguese folk song
FAENA: Bullfight part
FAERIE: "The __ Queene" (Spenser work)
FAEROE: Danish islands
FAFNER: "Das Rheingold" character
FAFNIR: Dragon in Norse myth
FAG END: Remnant
FAGIN: "Oliver Twist" character
FAGINS: Instructors in crime
FAGOT: Bundle of sticks
FAHD: Saudi king
FAHEY: Actor Jeff
FAHR.: Temp. scale
FAIENCE: Earthenware
FAILLE: Soft fabric
FAIM: Hunger: French
FAIMAN: Director Peter
FAIN: Willing
FAIRE: Laissez-__
FAIRED: Aligned
FAIRFAX: Virginia city
FAIR OFF: Become clear
FAIR SEX: Women, quaintly
FAIR UP: Align
FAIR USE: Copyright law concept
FAISAL I: Iraqi king
FAIT: __ accompli
FAITES: __ vos jeux (place your bets: French)
FAJA: Spanish sash
FAJITA: Mexican beef dish
FAKE ID: Forged document
FAKIR: Indian ascetic
FALA: FDR's dog
FALAFEL: Chickpea croquette
FA LA LA: "Deck the Halls" syllables
FALANA: Entertainer Lola
FALCATE: Crescent-shaped
FALCO: "The Sopranos" actress
FALDO: Golfer Nick
FALINE: "Bambi" character
FALK: "Columbo" star
FALKE: "Die Fledermaus" role
FALKIRK: Scottish city
FALLA: Spanish composer
FALLAL: Bit of finery
FALL ON: Assail
FALUDI: Feminist Susan
FALWELL: Evangelist Jerry
FAM.: Relatives: Abbr.
FAMA: Roman goddess of rumor
FAMER: Hall of __
FAMICOM: Nintendo game system
FAMILIA: Family: Spanish
FAMILLE: Family: French
FAMKE: Actress Janssen
FAMULUS: Magician's assistant
FANE: Temple
FANEUIL: Boston's __ Hall
FANFEST: Pro-sports promo event
FANFIC: Amateur pop-culture story
FANFOLD: Invoice pad
FANGIO: Auto racer Juan
FANION: Small flag
FANNIE: Author Flagg
FANNY: "Funny Girl" role
FANON: Papal vestment
FANSLER: Fictional sleuth Kate
FANTA: Soda brand
FAN-TAN: Card game
FANTINE: "Les Misérables" character
FANTODS: Nervous state
FANZINE: Amateur mag
FAO: Schwarz of toydom
FAQ: Web site info
FAQIR: Hindu ascetic
FARACY: Actress Stephanie
FARAD: Unit of capacitance
FARADAY: British physicist
FARAH: Slacks brand
FARCI: Stuffed, in cookery
FARFEL: Jewish cooking staple
FARGO, ND: Northwest city
FARIS: Actress Anna
FARLEY: FDR cabinet member
FARLOW: Keel's "Dallas" role
FARM AID: Willie Nelson cause
FARNUM: Actor Dustin
FARO: Gambling game
FAROES: Danish islands
FARON: Country singer Young
FAROUK I: Egyptian king
FARR: Jamie of "M*A*S*H"
FARRAGO: Hodgepodge
FARRAH: Actress Fawcett
FARRAR: Opera singer Geraldine
FARRELL: "Studs Lonigan" author
FARRIER: Horseshoer
FARRIS: Singer Dionne
FARROW: Litter of pigs
FARSI: Iranian language
FAR SIDE: Gary Larson domain
FARTLEK: Exercise regimen
FARUK I: Egyptian king
FAS: Scale notes
FASCES: Roman emblem of power
FASCIA: Hair band
FASO: Burkina __ (African nation)
FASTNET: Web service provider
FAST ONE: Scam
FATA: __ Morgana (mirage)
FATALE: Femme __
FATBACK: Pork cut
FAT CITY: Comfortable circumstances
FAT FARM: Sort of resort
FATH.: Length meas.
FATHA: Earl "__" Hines
FATIDIC: Prophetic
FATIMA: Daughter of Mohammed
FATLING: Young ranch animal
FATMAN: "Jake and the __" (TV series)
FAT ONE: Easy pitch to hit
FATOUSH: Mideast salad
FATS: Singer Domino
FATSIS: "Word Freak" author
FATSO: Dom De Luise film
FATWA: Muslim decree
FAUN: Woodland deity
FAUNA: Animals of a region
FAUNUS: "The Faerie Queene" character
FAURE: French composer
FAUSS: "Little __ and Big Halsy" (Redford film)
FAUST: Goethe character
FAUSTUS: Marlowe title character
FAUT: "Comme il __" (fittingly: French)
FAUTE: Error: French
FAUVE: French art style
FAUX: Artificial
FAUX PAS: Minor mistake
FAVA: Type of bean
FAVE: Preference
FAVRE: Brett of football
FAWCETT: Actress Farrah
FAWKES: Guy __ Day
FAWLTY: "__ Towers" (British sitcom)
FAXLORE: Type of urban legend
FAY: Former baseball commissioner Vincent
FAYARD: Tap dancer __ Nicholas
FAYE: Actress Dunaway
FAYETTE: County in 11 states
FAYLEN: Actor Frank
FAYS: Fairies
FAY WRAY: "King Kong" star
FAZOOL: Pasta __ (Italian soup)
FBS: Football positions: Abbr.
F CLEF: Music notation
FDNY: Big Apple's "Bravest"
F.D.S: Blaze-fighting orgs.
FEALTY: Allegiance
FEBRERO: February: Spanish

FEBRILE: Feverish
F.E.C.: Govt. voting agency
FECHNER: German physicist
FECUND: Productive
FEDDERS: Air-conditioner brand
FEDERKO: Bernie of hockey
FED EX: Delivery service
FEDOROV: Sergei of hockey
FEDS: Govt. agents
FEEB: Wimp
FEEBATE: Energy-efficiency reward
FEEDLOT: Livestock area
FEED ON: Consume
FEE-FREE: Like some credit cards
FEEJEE: __ Mermaid (Barnum hoax)
FEELY: Touchy-__
FEET'S: "Your __ Too Big" (Fats Waller tune)
FEH: Exclamation of disgust
FEHR: Baseball union boss
FEIFFER: Cartoonist Jules
FEIN: Ireland's Sinn __
FELDMAN: "Silent Movie" actor
FELDON: "Get Smart" actress
FELICE: Name that means "happy"
FELICIA: Actress Farr
FELID: Cat
FELIPE: Alou of baseball
FELIS: Cat: Latin
FELIX: Cartoon cat
FELIX I: Pope
FELIX V: Pope
FELIZ: Happy: Spanish
FELLAH: Egyptian peasant
FELLINI: "La Dolce Vita" director
FELS: Philadelphia planetarium
FELSON: "The Hustler" character
FELT HAT: Haberdashery item
FEMA: Disaster relief org.
FEMBOT: "Austin Powers" character
FEME: Woman, in law
FEMINUM: Metal in Wonder Woman's bracelets
FEMME: Woman: French
FEMORA: Leg bones
FEMORIS: Biceps __ (leg muscle)
FEMTO: Quadrillionth: Comb. form
FEMUR: Leg bone
FENDI: Italian designer
FENELON: French theologian
FENETRE: Window: French
FENG: __ shui (Chinese art)
FENN: Actress Sherilyn
FENNER: Merrill Lynch partner
FENWAY: Red Sox home
FEODOR: "Boris Godunov" role
FEODOR I: Russian czar
FEOFF: Invest in a feudal estate
FER: Not "agin"
FERAL: Untamed
FERBER: Author Edna
FERDE: Composer Grofé
FERDIE: Mickey Mouse nephew
FERENC: Author Molnár
FERGIE: Prince Andrew ex
FERIA: Spanish festival
FERITY: Savagery
FERMAT: French mathematician
FERMATA: Music marking
FERMATE: Music markings
FERMAT'S: __ last theorem
FERMI: 1938 physics Nobelist
FERMION: Subatomic particle
FERMIS: Units of nuclear distances
FERMIUM: Element #100
FERNAND: Painter Léger
FERNAO: Portuguese historian Lopes
FERN BAR: Stylish tavern
FEROUS: Containing: Comb. form
FERRARA: City in Italy
FERRARE: Supermodel Cristina
FERRARI: Italian auto
FERRARO: 1984 vice presidential candidate
FERRER: Actor Mel
FERRI: Iron: Comb. form
FERRIS: Playground wheel inventor
FERRO: Iron: Comb. form
FERRULE: Pencil part
FERULE: Punishing rod
FESCUE: Lawn grass
FESS: Actor Parker
FESTA: Holiday
FESTE: "Twelfth Night" clown
FESTER: "Addams Family" uncle
FESTINA: __ lente (make haste slowly: Latin)
FESTIVA: Ford model
FESTOON: Adorn
FESTOSO: Merry, in music
FESTUS: "Gunsmoke" deputy
FETID: Foul-smelling
FETISH: Amulet
FETLOCK: Part of a horse's leg
FETOR: Stink
FETT: Boba __ ("Star Wars" character)
FEU: Fire: French
FEUER: Fire: German
FEUX: Fires: French
FEVRIER: February: French
FEY: Whimsical
FEYDEAU: French playwright
FEYNMAN: 1965 physics Nobelist
FFF: Very loudly, in music
F FLAT: E alias
F.G.S: NFL three-point plays
FHA LOAN: Type of mortgage
F-HOLE: Cello feature
FIACRE: Horse-drawn carriage
FIAT: Edict
FIAT LUX: Let there be light: Latin
FIBIGER: Danish medicine Nobelist
FIBRIN: Coagulating protein
FIBRO: Filament: Comb. form
FIBULA: Leg bone
FIC: Causing: Comb. form
FICA: Pay-stub acronym
FICHE: Document storage medium
FICHTE: German philosopher
FICHU: Shawl
FICT.: Bk. category
FICTILE: Moldable
FICTIVE: Imaginary
FICUS: Tropical tree
FID: Nautical bar
FIDE: Bona __
FIDELES: "Adeste __"
FIDELIA: "The Faerie Queene" character
FIDELIO: Beethoven opera
FIDELIS: "Semper __" (Marines motto)
FIDLER: Hollywood columnist Jimmy
FIDO: Dog name
FIE: Old-time oath
FIEDLER: Onetime Boston Pops conductor
FIEF: Feudal land
FIENNES: Actor Ralph
FIERO: Oldsmobile model
FIERS: "The Cherry Orchard" character
FIERY: Ablaze
FIEVEL: "An American Tail" mouse
FIFI: French poodle name
FIFO: Accounting abbr.
FIGARO: Operatic barber
FIG BAR: Fruit snack
FIL: Mideast coin
FILA: Running-shoe brand
FILAR: Of threads
FILBERT: Type of nut
FILE BY: March
FILENE'S: Retail-store chain
FILI: Thread: Comb. form
FILIAL: Of a child
FILIBEG: Kilt
FILIPPO: Italian painter Lippi
FILLE: Girl: French
FILLIP: Strike smartly
FILO: Mideast pastry
FILOFAX: Personal-organizer brand
FILOSE: Threadlike
FILUM: Fine thread
FINA: Fine: Spanish
FINBACK: Type of whale
FINCA: South American ranch
FINDLAY: Ohio city
FINDLEY: Canadian writer
FINGAL'S: __ Cave (Hebrides locale)
FINI: Done: French
FINIAL: Furniture ornament
FINIAN'S: "__ Rainbow" (Astaire film)
FINIS: End
FINISH'D: O'er
FINITO: Done
FINKEL: Actor Fyvush
FINK ON: Betray
FINLEY: Onetime Oakland A's owner
FINNAIR: SAS competitor
FINNAN: __ haddie (Scottish seafood)
FINNEY: Actor Albert
FINNIC: European language group
FINNO: Finnish: Comb. form
FINO: Spanish sherry
FINSEN: Danish medicine Nobelist
FIONA: "Brigadoon" role
FIORE: Flower: Italian
FIORI: Flowers: Italian
FIORINA: Former Hewlett-Packard head
FIPPLE: Flute part
FIRBANK: British writer
FIRE ANT: Tropical insect
FIREARM: Automatic
FIRE AT: Strafe
FIREFOX: Web browser
FIRE ICE: Clive Cussler novel
FIRENZA: Oldsmobile model
FIRENZE: City in Italia
FIRKIN: Small barrel
FIRMA: Terra __
FIRN: Granular snow
FIRPO: Jack Dempsey foe
FIRST R: Reading
FIRTH: Scottish bay
FISC: Royal treasury
FISCHER: Chessmaster Bobby
FISHEYE: Type of lens
FISK: Carlton of baseball
FISKE: 1940s Chief Justice Harlan __ Stone
FISSILE: Cleavable
FISTIC: Of boxing
FITCH: Abercrombie partner
FIT ON: Suit well, as clothing
FITZROY: 18th-century British prime minister
FIVE A: Shoe size
FIVE AA: Shoe size
FIVE AAA: Shoe size
FIVE B: Shoe size
FIVE C: Shoe size
FIVE D: Shoe size
FIVE E: Shoe size
FIVE EE: Shoe size
FIVE EEE: Shoe size
FIVE NO: Bridge bid, briefly
FIVE-O: "Hawaii __" (TV series)
FIVE ONE: 61 inches tall
FIVE PIN: Alley target
FIVE SIX: 66 inches tall
FIVE TEN: 70 inches tall
FIVE TWO: 62 inches tall
FIVE W'S: Journalist's list
FIXE: Prix-__ dinner
FIXIN'S: Ingredients, informally
FIXIT: Mr. __ (repairman)
FIXITY: Permanence
FIX ON: Choose
FIX UPON: Choose
FIXX: "Complete Book of Running" author
FIZGIG: Firework
FLACK: Press agent
FLACON: Small bottle
FLAGG: Author Fannie
FLAGON: Large bottle
FLAM: Deception
FLAN: Custard dessert
FLANEUR: Idler: French
FLANKEN: Cut of meat
FLANN: Novelist O'Brien
FLASH ON: Recall
FLAT-HAT: Hedgehop

FLATLET: Small British apartment
FLATT: Guitarist Lester
FLAT TAX: 1996 campaign issue
FLATTOP: Aircraft carrier
FLAUTA: Tortilla dish
FLAVA: Taste, to a rapper
FLAVIA: "Prisoner of Zenda" character
FLAVIUS: "Julius Caesar" character
F LAYER: Ionosphere part
FLD.: Liquid: Abbr.
FLEA DIP: Pet grooming service
FLEANCE: "Macbeth" role
FLEAPIT: Shabby establishment
FLECHE: Arrow: French
FLEDGE: Cover with feathers
FLEEGLE: Evil-Eye __ ("Li'l Abner" character)
FLEER: Mock
FLEM: Faulkner character
FLEMING: Skater Peggy
FLEMISH: Belgian language
FLENSE: Cut blubber from
FLETCH: Chevy Chase film
FLEUR: Flower: French
FLEURON: Floral ornament
FLEXILE: Pliable
FLEXION: Joint exercise
FLEXNER: "I Hear America Talking" author
FLEXOR: Bending muscle
FLEXURE: Bending
FLIC: Policeman: French
FLICKA: Horse of fiction
FLIM: "The __-Flam Man" (Scott film)
FLINT, MI: City near Detroit
FLINTY: Stubborn
FLIPPEN: Actor Jay C.
FLIR: Electronic heat sensor
FLIVVER: Car, slangily
FLIX: Cable film channel
FLO: Impresario Ziegfeld
FLO-JO: Sprinter's nickname
FLON: Flin __, Manitoba
FLOOEY: Amiss
FLOOR IT: Step on the gas
FLOPIT: "Seventeen" dog
FLOPSY: Beatrix Potter rabbit
FLOR: Flower: Spanish
FLOREAL: French Revolution calendar month
FLOREK: Actor Dann
FLORENZ: Impesario Ziegfeld
FLORET: Bit of broccoli
FLOREY: 1945 medicine Nobelist
FLORI: Flower: Comb. form
FLORIAN: Patron saint of firefighters
FLORIN: Former Dutch coin
FLORIO: Former New Jersey governor
FLORY: 1974 chemistry Nobelist
FLOSSIE: Bobbsey twin
FLOTAGE: Buoyancy
FLOUNCE: Frill
FLOY: "__ Joy" (Supremes song)
FLOYD: Aviator Bennett
FL. OZ.: Liquid meas.
FLUBBER: "Absent-Minded Professor" substance
FLUBDUB: Nonsense
FLU BUG: Winter malady
FLUME: Amusement park ride
FLUMMOX: Confuse
FLUOR: Fluorine: Comb. form
FLUORO: Fluorine: Comb. form
FLUSHER: Four-__ (cheater)
FLUTIE: Doug of football
FLUTING: Groove
FLUVIAL: Of a river
FLY ASH: Furnace product
FLYCAST: One way to fish
FLYLEAF: Book page
FLYMAN: Stagehand
FLY ME: National Airlines slogan
FLYNN: Actor Errol
FLY ON: Patronize, as an airline
FLYROD: Fishing gear
FLYTIER: Fishing-lure hobbyist
F MAJ.: Mus. key
F. MURRAY: Actor Abraham
FNMA: Home loan org.
FNS.: Thesis citations: Abbr.
F NUMBER: Camera setting
FOB: Watch pocket
FOB OFF: Pass as valuable
FOCH: Actress Nina
FO'C'S'LE: Ship section
FOCUS ON: Highlight
FODOR: Violinist Eugene
FODOR'S: Travel-guide name
FOETID: Foul-smelling
FOGBOW: Post-shower sight
FOG CITY: San Francisco nickname
FOGDOG: Weather phenomenon
FOGEL: 1993 economics Nobelist
FOGERTY: Creedence Clearwater Revival leader
FOGG: "Around the World in 80 Days" hero
FOG IN: Keep from flying, perhaps
FOHN: Alpine wind
FOI: Faith: French
FOIE: Liver: French
FOKINE: Russian choreographer
FOKKER: WWI German warplane
FOL.: Coming after: Abbr.
FOLATE: B vitamin
FOLENGO: Italian poet
FOLEY: Film sound effects
FOLGER'S: Coffee brand
FOLIAR: Leaf-like
FOLIATE: Having leaves
FOLIC: __ acid (B vitamin)
FOLIES: __ Bergère
FOLIO: Sheet of paper
FOLIOSE: Leafy
FOLIUM: Thin layer
FOLKIE: Pete Seeger, e.g.
FOLKWAY: Unwritten rule
FOLLETT: Novelist Ken
FOLSOM: California prison
FONDANT: Kind of candy
FONDAS: Filmdom family
FONG: Onetime Hawaii senator
FONTANA: California city
FONTANE: German poet
FONTEYN: British ballet dancer
FONTINA: Italian cheese
FONZ: "Happy Days" character
FONZIE: "Happy Days" character
FOO: Egg __ yung
FOODIE: Epicure
FOOD WEB: Ecological cycle
FOOTBAG: Pellet-filled plaything
FOOTE: Historian Shelby
FOOT IT: Walk
FOOTLE: Talk nonsense
FOOTLET: Low sock
FOOTPAD: Robber
FOOT UP: Add
FOOZLE: Blunder
FOOZY: Friend of Alley Oop
FOP: Vain man
FOR A BIT: Awhile
FOR A SEC: Temporarily
FORBAD: Did not permit
FORBES: Business magazine
FORBORE: Desisted from
FORBUSH: "South Pacific" heroine
FORCHE: Poet Carolyn
FORD GT: Sports car
FORDHAM: Bronx university
FORD LTD: Former luxury car
FORDO: Destroy
FOR EACH: Per
FOREBAY: Waterwheel reservoir
FORENZA: Suzuki model
FORETOP: Nautical platform
FORFEND: Forbid
FORINT: Hungarian coin
FOR JOY: How some jump
FORLANI: Actress Claire
FORMA: Pro __ (accounting term)
FORMAN: Director Milos
FORMIC: Of ants
FORNAX: Southern constellation
FOR NOW: In the meantime
FOR ONE: Each
FORREST: Fictional Gump
FORS: "Yes" voters
FOR SIZE: Why to try something on
FORSOOK: Abandoned
FORSTER: "Howards End" author
FORSYTE: "The __ Saga"
FORSYTH: Director Bill
FORTAS: 1960s Supreme Court justice
FORT DIX: New Jersey army base
FORTIS: Phonetics term
FORTIUS: Stronger: Latin
FORT LEE: New Jersey city
FORT ORD: Former California army base
FORTRAN: Computer language
FORTUNA: Roman goddess
FORWHY: Wherefore
FOR YOU: Gift-card phrase
FORZA: "La __ del destino" (Verdi opera)
FOSCOLO: Italian poet
FOSDICK: "Li'l Abner" character
FOSS: Conductor Lukas
FOSSA: Bone cavity
FOSSAE: Anatomical cavities
FOSSE: "All That Jazz" director
FOSSES: Defensive ditches
FOSSEY: "Gorillas in the Mist" author
FOTO: Part of some film-lab names
FOTOMAT: Former film-developing company
FOU: Foolish: French
FOUDRE: Wine cask
FOUETTE: Ballet move
FOULARD: Tie fabric
FOUL TIP: Baseball call
FOUR A: Shoe size
FOUR AA: Shoe size
FOUR AAA: Shoe size
FOUR A.M.: A wee hour
FOUR B: Shoe size
FOUR C: Shoe size
FOUR D: Shoe size
FOUR E: Shoe size
FOUR EE: Shoe size
FOUR EEE: Shoe size
FOUR-F: Draft classification
FOUR-H: Agricultural club
FOURIER: French mathematician
FOUR-MAN: Like bobsled teams
FOUR NO: Bridge bid, briefly
FOUR PIN: Alley target
FOUTS: Dan of football
FOWLER: Bird hunter
FOWLES: British novelist
FOWLING: Bird-shooting sport
FOXBORO: Massachusetts town
FOXFIRE: Joyce Carol Oates book
FOX NEWS: CNN rival
FOX TV: Broadcast network
FOXX: Ray Charles portrayer
FOY: Vaudevillian Eddie
FOYLE: Ginger Rogers Oscar role
FOYT: Auto racer A.J.
FOZZIE: Muppet bear
F.P.A.: "Conning Tower" monogram
FPL.: Real-estate ad abbr.
FRA: Monk title
FRACTAL: Geometric pattern
FRACTO: Broken: Comb. form
FRAE: From: Scottish
FRAGGLE: "__ Rock" (kids' TV series)
FRAICHE: Fresh: French
FRAIDY: __-cat
FRAIS: Fresh: French
FRAISE: Strawberry: French
FRAKES: "Star Trek: The Next Generation" actor
FRAM: Auto-parts brand
FRAN: "Kukla, __ and Ollie"
FRANC: Former French money
FRANCA: Brazilian city
FRANCES: Pulitzer author FitzGerald
FRANCHI: Singer Sergio
FRANCIS: Novelist Dick
FRANCK: French composer
FRANCO: Former Spanish leader
FRANKEN: Comedian Al
FRANKIE: Singer Avalon

FRANK OZ: Voice of Miss Piggy
FRANN: "Newhart" actress
FRANNY: Salinger character
FRANS: Dutch painter Hals
FRANTZ: Writer Fanon
FRANZ: Composer Liszt
FRASER: Actor Brendan
FRASIER: Kelsey Grammer role
FRATER: Comrade
FRAU: Wife: German
FRAUEN: Wives: German
FRAUGHT: Brimming
FRAWLEY: "I Love Lucy" actor
FRAYN: British playwright
FRAZER: Scottish anthropologist
FRAZIER: Boxer Joe
F.R.B.: Greenspan's former grp.
FREBERG: Humorist Stan
FRED: Mr. Flintstone
FREDA: Singer Payne
FREDDIE: __ and the Dreamers (1960s rock group)
FREDDY: Elm Street villain
FRED EBB: "Cabaret" lyricist
FREDO: "The Godfather" character
FREDRIC: Actor March
FREDRO: Polish playwright
FREE AIR: Former gas-station amenity
FREEH: Former FBI director
FREESIA: Fragrant flower
FREE TO: Complimentary for
FREE TOY: Cereal-box bonus
FREI: Free: German
FREIA: Asteroid
FREITAG: Friday: German
FRELENG: Cartoon animator Friz
FREMONT: California city
FRENCH I: Language course
FRENCH'S: Mustard brand
FRENEAU: Poet Philip
FRENEMY: False friend
FRENESI: Artie Shaw tune
FRENI: Soprano Mirella
FRENUM: Tongue part
FREON: Refrigerant
FREQ.: 90.1 FM, e.g.
FRERE: Brother: French
FRESCA: Soft-drink brand
FRESHET: Flash flood
FRESNEL: Spotlight lens
FRESS: Eat, slangily
FRETSAW: Carpenter's tool
FREUND: German philologist
FREWER: "Max Headroom" actor
FREY: Norse god
FREYA: Norse goddess
FREYTAG: German playwright
FRIA: Cold: Spanish
FRIABLE: Brittle
FRIBBLE: Trifle
FRICK: Art gallery philanthropist
FRICKA: "Das Rheingold" character
FRICKE: Country singer Janie
FRICKER: "My Left Foot" actress
FRID: "Dark Shadows" actor
FRIDA: Painter Kahlo
FRIDLEY: Minnesota city
FRIEDA: "The Castle" character
FRIEDAN: Feminist Betty
FRIEL: Irish dramatist
FRIELS: Actor Colin
FRIEZE: Architectural decoration
FRIG: Appliance, for short
FRIGG: Norse goddess
FRIJOL: Mexican bean
FRIJOLE: Mexican bean
FRIML: Composer Rudolf
FRIO: Cold: Spanish
FRISCH: 1969 economics Nobelist
FRISE: Curly: French
FRISEE: Curly: French
FRISES: Upholstery fabrics
FRISEUR: Hairdresser: French
FRISIAN: Germanic language
FRISSON: Thrill
FRIST: Tennessee senator
FRIT: Glassmaking material
FRITA: Fried: Spanish
FRITAS: Papas __ (French fries: Spanish)
FRITE: Fried: French
FRITES: French fries
FRITO: Fried: Spanish
FRITOS: Corn-chip brand
FRITTA: Fried: Italian
FRITTO: Fried: Italian
FRITZ: Mondale nickname
FRITZI: Nancy's aunt
FRIVOL: Trifle
FRIZ: Cartoon animator Freleng
FRIZZLE: Fry
FROBE: Goldfinger portrayer
FRODING: Swedish poet
FRODO: "The Lord of the Rings" character
FROE: Cleaver
FROEBEL: German educational reformer
FROGGER: 1980s video game
FROH: "Das Rheingold" character
FROID: Cold: French
FROMAGE: Cheese: French
FROME: Wharton character
FROMM: "The Art of Loving" author
FROMMER: Travel-guide name
FROND: Fern feature
FRONTON: Jai alai court
FROOGLE: Price-comparison Web site
FROOT: __ Loops (cereal brand)
'FROS: Big hairdos
FROW: Cleaver
FROWARD: Disobedient
FROWZY: Slovenly
FRO-YO: Frozen yogurt
FROZONE: "The Incredibles" character
F.R.S.: Greenspan's former org.
FRT.: Transp. chge.
FRUCT: Fruit: Comb. form
FRUCTI: Fruit: Comb. form
FRUG: 1960s dance
FRUMP: Dowdy one
FRUNZE: Capital of Kirghizia
FRUSTUM: Curtailed cone, in geometry
FRUTTI: Tutti-__
FRYE: Impressionist David
F SCALE: Piano practice
F. SCOTT: Author Fitzgerald
FSLIC: Bank acct. insurer
F STAR: Spectral type
F-STOP: Camera setting
F.S.U.: Seminoles sch.
FT. BLISS: Texas army base
FT. BRAGG: North Carolina army base
F.T.C.: Ad regulating agcy.
F.T.D.: 1-800-FLOWERS rival
FT. DIX: New Jersey army base
FT. DODGE: Iowa city
FT. HENRY: Ontario historic site
F TILE: Scrabble four-pointer
FT. KNOX: Bullion site
FT. LB.: Work unit: Abbr.
FT. LEE: New Jersey city
FT. MEADE: Maryland army base
FT. MYERS: Florida city
FTO: Mitsubishi model
FT. ORD: Former California army base
FT. RILEY: Kansas army base
F TROOP: 1960s sitcom
FT. WAYNE: Indiana city
FT. WORTH: Texas city
FUAD I: Egyptian king
FUBSY: Short and stout
FUBU: Clothing brand
FUCA: Juan de __ Strait
FUCHS: British geologist
FUCHSIA: Garden flower
FUDD: Bugs Bunny pursuer
FUDDIES: Fussy ones
FUDDY: __-duddy
FUEGO: Fire: Spanish
FUEL ROD: Reactor cylinder
FUENTES: Mexican author
FUGARD: South African playwright
FUGATO: Music section
FUGE: Repeller: Comb. form
FUGIT: Tempus __
FUGU: Puffer fish
FUGUE: Bach piece
FUISSE: Pouilly-__ (white wine)
FUJI: Camera brand
FUJISAN: Japanese volcano
FUJITSU: Computer company
FUL: Adjective suffix
FULCRUM: Lever support
FULDA: German river
FULGENT: Dazzling
FULGHUM: Author Robert
FULL LOT: Parker's problem
FULMAR: Sea bird
FULSOME: Overdone
FULTON: Steamboat creator
FUM: "Fe fi fo __!"
FUME AT: Be angry with
FUMET: Sauce flavoring
FUNDY: Canada's Bay of __
FUNF: Five: German
FUN FAIR: Amusement park
FUNFZIG: Fifty: German
FUNGO: Baseball practice shot
FUNK: Dejected mood
FUNPLEX: Indoor amusement park
FUNSTER: Comedian
FUNT: "Candid Camera" creator
FUOCO: Fire: Italian
FURBY: Hasbro toy
FURCATE: Branch out
FURIE: Director Sidney
FURILLO: "The Boys of Summer" subject
FURIOSO: Forceful, in music
FURLONG: Horse-race unit
FURMAN: South Carolina university
FURNESS: Consumer advocate Betty
FURO: Japanese bathtub
FURST: Actor Stephen
FURTADO: Singer Nelly
FURZE: Spiny shrub
FUSEE: Railroad flare
FUSIL: Musket
FUSILE: Formed by melting
FUSILLI: Type of pasta
FUSS AT: Chide
FUST: Gutenberg partner
FUSTIAN: Worthless
FUSTY: Moldy
FUSUMA: Japanese partition
FUTHARK: Runic alphabet
FUTUNA: Pacific islands
FUTURA: Ford model
FUTZ: Fool (around)
F.W.D.: ATV feature
FWIW: Chat-room letters
F.Y.I.: "Read this"
FYN: Danish island
FYODOR: Author Dostoyevsky
FYVUSH: Actor Finkel

G

GABBANA: Dolce & __ (Italian fashion house)
GABBLE: Chatter
GABBRO: Igneous rock
GABE: Comic Kaplan
GABEL: Actor Martin
GABIN: Actor Jean
GABLER: "Hedda __" (Ibsen play)
GABON: African country
GABOR: Actress Eva
GABRIEL: Archangel
GABY: Actress Hoffmann
GADDI: Italian painter
GADDIS: Author William
GADSDEN: __ Purchase (1853 U.S. acquisition)
GAE: Go: Scottish
GAEA: Greek earth goddess
GAEL: Celt
GAETA: Italian city
GAETANO: Composer Donizetti
GAF: Film manufacturer
GAFF: Cheat, slangily
GAFFER: Film-set electrician

GAGARIN: Russian cosmonaut
GAGE: Pledge, old-style
GAG REEL: Frequent DVD extra
GAHAGAN: Actress Helen __ Douglas
GAHAN: Cartoonist Wilson
GAI: Gay: French
GAIA: Greek earth goddess
GAIJIN: Foreigner: Japanese
GAIL: Author Sheehy
GAINES: "Mad" magazine founder
GAINSAY: Deny
GAITER: Ankle covering
GAIUS: Roman jurist
GALAHAD: King Arthur knight
GALANOS: Fashion designer James
GALANT: Mitsubishi model
GALATEA: Mythical sea nymph
GALATIA: Ancient Asia Minor country
GALAX: Beetleweed
GALAXIE: Ford model
GALBA: Roman emperor
GALEA: Helmet-shaped part
GALEAO: Rio de Janeiro airport
GALEATE: Helmet-shaped
GALEN: Greek physician
GALENA: Lead ore
GALENTO: Boxer Tony
GALETTE: Type of cake
GALICIA: Region of Spain
GALILEE: Sea of Israel
GALILEI: Italian astronomer
GALILEO: Italian astronomer
GALLI: Soprano Amelita __-Curci
GALLIA: Gaul: Latin
GALLIC: French
GALLICO: Writer Paul
GALLIUM: Element #31
GALLO: Wine brand
GALLUP: Pollster George
GALOIS: French mathematician
GALOP: Lively dance
GALT: "Atlas Shrugged" character
GALTON: British scientist
GALUMPH: Move heavily
GALVANI: Italian physicist
GALVANO: Current: Comb. form
GALWAY: Irish city
GAM: Group of whales
GAMA: Explorer Vasco da __
GAMAL: __ Abdel Nasser
GAMAY: Beaujolais grape
GAMBA: Viola da __
GAMBADO: Caper
GAMBIA: African country
GAMBIER: French Polynesian island group
GAMEBAG: Hunter's tote
GAME BOY: Nintendo product
GAMELAN: Indonesian orchestra
GAMETE: Reproductive cell
GAMGEE: "Lord of the Rings" character
GAMIN: Urchin
GAMINE: Urchin
GAMMON: Nonsense
GAMOUS: Marriage: Comb. form
GAMOW: Physicist George
GAMP: Umbrella, in Britain
GANCE: Director Abel
GANDALF: Tolkien wizard
GANDHI: Leader of India
G. AND T.: Gin and tonic
GANDY: __ dancer (railroad worker)
GANEF: Thief
GANGES: River of India
GANGLIA: Nerve-tissue mass
GANGSTA: Rap-music variety
GANGTOK: Capital of Sikkim
GANN: Writer Ernest K. __
GANNET: Large seabird
GANNETT: Newspaper publisher
GANNON: "Dragnet" character
GANSU: Chinese province
GANT: "Look Homeward, Angel" character
GANTLET: Armor glove
GANTRY: Rocket scaffold
G.A.O.: General Accounting Office: Abbr.
GAOL: British jail
GAP KIDS: Children's clothing store
GAR: Long-jawed fish
GARBER: Actor Victor
GARBO: Actress Greta
GARCIA: Rock guitarist Jerry
GARCON: Waiter: French
GARD: French department
GARDA: Italian lake
GARDE: Avant-__
GARDENA: California city
GARDNER: Writer Erle Stanley __
GARE: Depot: French
GARETH: King Arthur knight
GARGAN: Actor William
GARLITS: Drag racer Don
GARN: Former Utah senator
GARNEAU: Canadian historian
GARNETT: Singer Gale
GARNI: Garnished: French
GARO: Football kicker Yepremian
GARONNE: French river
GAROU: Loup-__ (werewolf)
GARP: John Irving hero
GARPIKE: Long-jawed fish
GARR: Actress Teri
GARRETT: Old West lawman Pat
GARRICK: Actor David
GARRY: TV host Moore
GARSON: Actress Greer
GARTH: Country singer Brooks
GARVEY: Steve of baseball
GARY: Actor Coleman
GARY, IN: Midwest city
GASCON: Boaster
GASCONY: Region of France
GASKELL: British novelist
GAS OIL: Commodity futures listing
GASOL: NBA star from Spain
GASPAR: One of the Magi
GASPARD: "Count of Monte Cristo" character
GASPE: Region of Canada
GASSMAN: Actor Vittorio
GASTER: Stomach: Comb. form
GASTERO: Stomach: Comb. form
GASTON: "Beauty and the Beast" villain
GASTONE: "La Traviata" role
GASTR: Stomach: Comb. form
GASTRO: Stomach: Comb. form
GAS-X: Stomach-remedy brand
GAT: Pistol
GATEAU: French cake
GATE-LEG: Type of table
GATLIN: Singing brothers' surname
GATLING: Gun inventor
GATO: Cat: Spanish
GATSBY: Fitzgerald character
GATT: General Agreement on Tariffs and Trade: Abbr.
GATTACA: Ethan Hawke film
GATTO: Cat: Italian
GATUN: Panamanian lake
GATWICK: London airport
GAUD: Trinket
GAUDENS: Sculptor Augustus Saint-__
GAUDI: Spanish architect
GAUGUIN: French artist
GAUL: Frenchman
GAULLE: Charles de __
GAUR: Wild ox
GAUSS: Magnetic unit
GAUTAMA: Buddha
GAUTIER: Actor Dick
GAVIAL: Crocodile
GAVILAN: 1950s welterweight champ
GAVIN: Actor MacLeod
GAVOT: Old French dance
GAVOTTE: Old French dance
GAVRAS: Director Costa-__
GAWAIN: King Arthur knight
GAWP: Gape
GAYE: Singer Marvin
GAYLE: Singer Crystal
GAYLORD: Gymnast Mitch
GAYNES: Actor George
GAYNOR: Actress Janet
GAZA: __ Strip (Mideast region)
GAZZARA: Actor Ben
G.B.E.: U.K. honor
G.B.S.: Shaw monogram
GDANSK: Polish port
G'DAY: Aussie greeting
G.D.R.: East Germany: Abbr.
GDS.: Merchandise: Abbr.
GEARY: Actor Anthony
G.E.D.: General equivalency diploma: Abbr.
GEDDES: Actress Barbara Bel __
GEDRICK: Actor Jason
GEEGAW: Trinket
GEEKED: Enthusiastic
GEENA: Actress Davis
GEEP: Goat-sheep hybrid
GEER: Actor Will
GEES: Turns to the right
GEESON: Actress Judy
GEEZ: Frustration exclamation
GEFFEN: Media mogul David
GEFILTE: Deli fish
GEHENNA: Place of torment
GEHRIG: Lou of baseball
GEICO: Insurance company
GEIGER: German physicist
G EIGHT: Top economic countries
GEISEL: Dr. Seuss' real surname
GEIST: Spirit: German
GEKKO: "Wall Street" role
GELATE: Harden
GELATI: Italian ice cream
GELATO: Italian ice cream
GELCAP: Type of medicine pill
GELDOF: Live Aid organizer
GELEE: Aspic
GELETT: Humorist Burgess
GELID: Very cold
GELL: Physics Nobelist __-Mann
GELLAR: Actress Sarah Michelle
GELLER: Mentalist Uri
GEL PEN: Writing implement
GELSEY: Ballerina Kirkland
GELT: Money
GELUSIL: Antacid brand
GEMARA: Talmud section
GEMAYEL: Former Lebanese leader
GEMELLI: Rod-shaped pasta
GEMMA: Botanist's bud
GEMSBOK: African antelope
GENA: Actress Rowlands
GENERA: Biological categories
GENERIS: Sui __ (one of a kind)
GENESEE: New York river
GENET: Spotted carnivore
GENEVA: Swiss city
GENEVE: Swiss city
GENF: Swiss city, to natives
GENGHIS: Conqueror Khan
GENIC: Causing: Comb. form
GENITOR: Parent
GENLOCK: Video synchronizer
GENNAIO: January: Italian
GENNARO: Choreographer Peter
GENO: Race: Comb. form
GENOA: Italian port
GENOAS: Racing jibs
GENOISE: Sponge cake
GENOME: Set of chromosomes
GENOVA: Italian city, to natives
GENTE: People: Spanish
GENTIAN: Blue flower
GENTILE: Non-Jewish
GENU: Knee: Latin
GENUAL: Of the knee
GEN-X: Baby boomer's offspring
GENZYME: Biotech company
GEO: Chevy model
GEOCODE: Neighborhood demographics
GEODE: Crystalline rock
GEODESY: Science of earth measurement
GEODUCK: Large clam
GEORDI: "Star Trek: The Next Generation" character
GEORG: Conductor Solti
GEORGE C.: Actor Scott
GEORGE I: British king
GEORGE M.: Composer Cohan

GEORGES: French statesman Clemenceau
GEORGE V: British king
GEORGE W.: President Bush
GEORGI: 1950s Russian leader Malenkov
GEORGIC: Agricultural
GEORGIE: "__ Porgie"
GEORGY: "__ Girl" (1966 film)
GERAINT: King Arthur knight
GERALD: President Ford
GERALDO: TV host Rivera
GERARD: "The Fugitive" role
GERBER: Baby-food brand
GERE: Actor Richard
GERENT: Ruler
GERI: Pop singer Halliwell
GERITOL: Tonic brand
GERMAIN: French mathematician
GERRY: James Madison vice president
GERSHON: Actress Gina
GERT: Actor Frobe
GERTIE: Gravel __ ("Dick Tracy" character)
GERTZ: Actress Jami
GERVAIS: French cheese
GERVIN: George of basketball
G.E.S: Some home appliances
GESSO: Plaster of Paris
GEST: Adventure
GESTAE: Res __ (accomplishments: Latin)
GESTALT: Psychology school
GESTE: Adventure
GESTIC: Of body movement
GETA: Japanese sandal
GET BENT: Bart Simpson exclamation
GET GOOD: Obtain vengeance on
GET THIS: "Listen..."
GETTIN': "__ Jiggy Wit It" (Will Smith song)
GETTY: Oil magnate
GETZ: Jazz saxophonist
G FIFTY: Bingo call
G. GORDON: Liddy of Watergate
GHAIN: Arabic letter
GHALI: Former U.N. head Boutros-__
GHANA: African country
GHAT: Mountain pass of India
GHAZI: Muslim soldier
GHEE: Indian butter
GHENT: Belgian city
GHIA: Karmann __ (German auto)
GHIRSH: Saudi Arabian coin
GHWB: Presidential initials
GHZ: CPU speed unit
GIA: Actress Scala
GIACOMO: Composer Puccini
GIAMBI: Jason of baseball
GIAN: Composer __ Carlo Menotti
GIANNI: Designer Versace
GIAUQUE: 1949 chemistry Nobelist
GIB: Male cat
GIBB: Bee Gees' surname
GIBBER: Chatter
GIBBOUS: Humpbacked
GIBBS: Singer Georgia
G.I. BILL: Vets' boon
G.I. BLUES: Elvis film of 1960
GIBRAN: "The Prophet" author
GIBSON: Martini with an onion
GIBUS: Opera hat
GIDE: French novelist
GIDEON: Biblical judge
GIDEONS: Bible distributor
GIDGET: Sally Field role
GIE: Give: Scottish
GIELGUD: Actor John
GIF: Computer graphics format: Abbr.
GIFFORD: Frank of football
GIGA: Billion: Prefix
GIG BAG: Guitar case
GIGI: Leslie Caron role
GIGIO: Topo __ (Ed Sullivan regular)
GIGLI: Jennifer Lopez film
GIGO: Garbage in, garbage out: Abbr.
GIGOT: Leg of lamb
GIGUE: Fast dance
G.I. JANE: Demi Moore film
G.I. JOE: Action figure
GIL: Hodges of baseball
GILA: Southwest lizard
GILBERT: Sullivan collaborator
GIL BLAS: Le Sage novel
GILDA: Actress Radner
GILEAD: Mountain of Jordan
GILELS: Pianist Emil
GILES: John Barth character
GILFORD: Actor Jack
GILLAN: Rock singer Ian
GILLEY: Singer Mickey
GILLIAM: Monty Python member
GILLIAN: Actress Anderson
GILLIS: Dwayne Hickman TV role
GILLMAN: Creature from the Black Lagoon
GILMAN: Author Dorothy
GILMORE: Artis of basketball
GILPIN: Actress Peri
GILROY: California garlic center
GIMBAL: Compass holder
GIMBEL'S: Macy's former rival
GIMEL: Hebrew letter
GIMLI: "Lord of the Rings" character
GIMMIE: Conceded putt
GINA: Actress Lollobrigida
GINGIVA: Gum
GINGOLD: Actress Hermione
GINNIE: __ Mae (mortgage agency)
GINO: Singer Vannelli
GINSU: Knife brand
GIN UP: Enliven
GINZA: Tokyo district
GIOCOSO: Playful, in music
GIONO: French novelist
GIORGIO: Designer Armani
GIORGOS: Literature Nobelist Seferis
GIORNO: Day: Italian
GIOTTO: Florentine painter
GIPP: Reagan film role
GIPPER: "Win one for the __!"
GIRASOL: Type of opal
GIRL SHY: Harold Lloyd film
GIRO: Copter relative
GIROLLE: Type of mushroom
GIRONDE: French department
GIRSH: Saudi Arabian money
GISCARD: Former French leader Valéry __ D'Estaing
GISELE: Singer MacKenzie
GISELLE: Ballerina role
GISH: Actress Lillian
GISSING: British novelist
GITA: "Bhagavad-__" (sacred Hindu text)
GITANO: Jeans brand
GITGO: Beginning
GITMO: Guantánamo, to GIs
GIUGNO: June: Italian
GIVE ON: Relent with
GIZA: Sphinx site
GJETOST: Norwegian cheese
GLACE: Candied
GLACIS: Gentle slope
GLAD EYE: Friendly glance
GLADYS: Singer Knight
GLARUS: Swiss canton
GLASER: Actor Paul Michael __
GLASGOW: Scottish city
GLASHOW: 1979 physics Nobelist
GLATT: __ kosher
GLAVINE: Tom of baseball
GLAXO: Drug manufacturer
GLC: Mazda model
GLEASON: Comedian Jackie
GLEEM: Toothpaste brand
GLEEMAN: Minstrel
GLEN COE: Scottish region
GLENDA: Actress Jackson
GLENN: Mercury astronaut
GLENNE: Actress Headly
GLESS: Actress Sharon
GLIA: Nerve network
GLICK: Martin Short character
GLIERE: Russian composer
GLIM: Lamp
GLINDA: "Wizard of Oz" character
GLINKA: Russian composer
GLISTER: Shine
GLO: Day-__ paint
GLOAM: Twilight, old-style
GLOAMIN': "Roamin' in the __" (Scottish song)
GLOBIN: Blood protein
GLOCK: Austrian pistol
GLOGG: Hot drink
GLORIA: Halo
GLOSSA: Tongue
GLOSSO: Speech: Comb. form
GLOT: Language: Comb. form
GLOTT: Language: Comb. form
GLOTTIS: Larynx opening
GLOTTO: Language: Comb. form
GLOUCS: English county
GLOVER: Actor Danny
GLUC: Sugar: Comb. form
GLUCK: Soprano Alma
GLUCO: Sugar: Comb. form
GLUNK: Dr. Seuss character
GLUON: Subatomic particle
GLURGE: Web-based sentimental writing
GLUTEN: Flour ingredient
GLYC: Sugar: Comb. form
GLYCINE: Amino acid
GLYCO: Sugar: Comb. form
GLYCOL: Antifreeze
GLYN: Author Elinor
GLYNIS: Actor Johns
GLYNNIS: Actress O'Connor
GLYPH: Pictograph
GLYPT: Carved: Comb. form
GLYPTIC: Of gem carving
GLYPTO: Carved: Comb. form
GMA: ABC morning show
GMAC: Car-loan source: Abbr.
GMAT: Coll. seniors' test
GMC: Truck make
GMS: General managers: Abbr.
G.M.T.: Greenwich Mean Time: Abbr.
GNAR: Snarl
GNC: Vitamin-store chain
GNEISS: Metamorphic rock
GNMA: Home-loan source: Abbr.
GNOCCHI: Italian dumplings
GNOMON: Sundial part
GNOMY: Knowledge: Comb. form
GNOSIS: Mystical knowledge
GNOSSUS: Cretan city
GNOSTIC: Of knowledge
G.N.P.: Economic stat.
GNU: African antelope
GOA: Tibetan gazelle
GOALBY: Golfer Bob
GO ASK: Consult
GO AT IT: Battle
GOBANG: Japanese board game
GOBAT: 1902 peace Nobelist
GOBEL: Comic George
GOBELIN: French tapestry
GOBI: Mongolian desert
GOBIES: Small fish
GOBO: Camera-lens shield
GOBOT: 1980s toy fad
GO BY: Elapse
GO COED: Start accepting both sexes
GODARD: Director Jean-Luc
GODDARD: Actress Paulette
GODEL: Mathematician Kurt
GODET: Dressmaker insert
GO-DEVIL: Logging sled
GODEY'S: "__ Lady's Book" (old magazine)
GODFREY: Comic Cambridge
GODIVA: Chocolate brand
GODOT: "Waiting for __" (Beckett play)
GODTHAB: Capital of Greenland
GODUNOV: Russian czar
GODWIN: Writer Gail
GODWIT: Shorebird
GOEN: TV host Bob
GOETHE: German writer
GOFFIN: Lyricist Gerry

GO FISH: Card game
GOG: Armageddon nation
GO GET: Fetch
GO GET 'EM: Encouraging words
GOGH: Vincent van ___
GOGI: Singer Grant
GO-GIRL: Young active woman
GO-GO: Full of vitality
GOGOL: Russian novelist
GO-GO'S: All-girl rock group
GO IN: Enter
GO IRISH: Notre Dame cheer
GOITER: Sign of iodine deficiency
GOLA: Tom of basketball
GOLAN: ___ Heights (Mideast region)
GOLDA: Israeli leader Meir
GOLDE: Tevye's wife
GOLDIE: Actress Hawn
GOLDING: British novelist
GOLDMAN: Anarchist Emma
GOLDONI: Italian dramatist
GOLD'S: Gym chain
GOLDWYN: Producer Samuel
GOLEM: Automaton
GOLETA: California city
GOLGI: 1906 medicine Nobelist
GOLINO: Actress Valeria
GOLLUM: "Lord of the Rings" character
GOMER: Jim Nabors role
GOMERS: Enemy aviators
GOMEZ: "Addams Family" role
GOMPERS: Union leader Samuel
GON: Angled: Suffix
GONERIL: Daughter of King Lear
GONGORA: Spanish poet
GO/NO-GO: NASA decision
GO NOW: Moody Blues tune
GONY: Generation: Comb. form
GONZAGA: Spokane school
GONZO: Bizarre
GOOCH: "Auntie Mame" character
GOODALL: Chimp studier Jane
GOODBAR: "Looking for Mr. ___" (1977 film)
GOODE: "Johnny B. ___" (Chuck Berry tune)
GOODEN: Dwight of baseball
GOODER: Do-___
GOODING: Actor Cuba
GOODMAN: Bandleader Benny
GOODNIK: No-___ (bad guy)
GOOD-OH: British approval
GOODSON: Game-show producer Mark
GOODWIN: Nero Wolfe's assistant
GOOFUS: Foolish one
GOOGLE: Web-search site
GOOGLY: Cricket ball
GOOGOL: Very large number
GOOMBAH: Older friend
GOOMBAY: Calypso music
GO ON: Continue
GOONEY: Albatross
GOONIE: Albatross
GO ON IN: Enter
GOOSEN: Golfer Retief
GOPIK: Azerbaijan money
GOR: British oath
GORAN: Ivanisevic of tennis
GORBY: Gorbachev, in headlines
GORCEY: Actor Leo
GORDIAN: ___ knot
GORDIE: Howe of hockey
GORDITA: Cornmeal concoction
GORDIUS: Father of Midas
GORDO: Fat: Spanish
GORDON: Actress Ruth
GORDY: Berry of Motown
GOREN: Bridge expert Charles
GORE-TEX: Water-repellent fabric
GOREY: Illustrator Edward
GORGON: Greek mythical monster
GORHAM: Chinaware brand
GORIOT: "Père ___" (Balzac work)
GORKI: Russian author
GORKY: Russian author
GORM: Smear
GORME: Singer Eydie
GORO: "Madama Butterfly" character
GORP: Trail mix
GORSE: Spiny shrub
GORT: "The Day the Earth Stood Still" robot
GORTNER: Preacher Marjoe
GOSDEN: Amos portrayer Freeman
GOSFORD: "___ Park" (2001 film)
GOSHAWK: Short-winged bird
GOSHEN: Land of plenty
GO SIT: Words to a bad kid
GOSLIN: Goose of baseball
GOSS: CIA director
GOSSAGE: Goose of baseball
GOSSE: British poet
GOSSETT: Actor Lou
GOTAMA: Buddha
GOTH: Germanic invader
GOTHA: German city
GOTHAM: Manhattan, in journalese
GOTHIKA: Halle Berry film
GO-TO GAL: Reliable one
GO-TO GUY: Reliable one
GOTT: God: German
GOTTA GO: Rushed one's comment
GOTTI: "The Dapper Don"
GOUACHE: Painting technique
GOUDY: Printing font
GOULD: Actor Elliott
GOULET: Singer Robert
GOUNOD: French composer
GOURAMI: Aquarium fish
GOURDE: Haitian money
GOWDY: Sportscaster Curt
GOWER: Director Champion
GOYA: Spanish painter
GOYEN: Dutch painter
GOZZI: Italian playwright
G.P.A.: Grade point average: Abbr.
G.P.O.: General Post Office: Abbr.
G.P.S: Some MDs
GQ MODEL: Hunky poser, perhaps
GRAAFF: Van de ___ generator
GRABLE: Actress Betty
GRACIE: Comic Allen
GRACILE: Slender
GRACKLE: Black bird
GRAECO: Greek: Comb. form
GRAF: Steffi of tennis
GRAFF: Actress Ilene
GRAFTON: Writer Sue
GRAHAM: Kind of cracker
GRAHAME: Scottish author
GRAIG: Nettles of baseball
GRAMM: Texas politician Phil
GRAMMER: Actor Kelsey
GRAMMES: Metric weights, in England
GRAMMY: Music award
GRAMPUS: Large dolphin
GRANADA: Spanish city
GRANBY: Canadian city
GRAND AM: Pontiac model
GRANDE: Large: Spanish
GRANDEE: Spanish nobleman
GRANDY: "Love Boat" actor
GRANI: Grain: Comb. form
GRANIT: Finnish medicine Nobelist
GRANITA: Fruit-ice dessert
GRAPHO: Writing: Comb. form
GRAPHY: Drawing: Comb. form
GRAPNEL: Small anchor
GRAPPA: Italian brandy
GRAS: Mardi ___
GRASSLE: Actress Karen
GRASSO: Former Connecticut governor
GRATA: Persona non ___
GRATAE: Personae non ___
GRATIA: "Ars ___ artis" (MGM motto)
GRATIAS: Deo ___ (Thanks be to God: Latin)
GRATIN: Au ___ (potato style)
GRAU: Grey: German
GRAUMAN: Chinese Theatre owner
GRAVAS: "Taxi" character
GRAVI: Heavy: Comb. form
GRAVID: Pregnant
GRAVLAX: Cured salmon
GRAVURE: Printing method
GRAYLAG: European goose
GRAYSON: Robin's secret identity
GRAZ: Austrian city
GRAZIE: Thanks: Italian
GR. BR.: The U.K.
G.R.E.: Coll. seniors' test
GREAVE: Leg armor
GREBE: Diving bird
GRECO: Dancer José
GREELEY: Writer Andrew
GREENE: Actor Lorne
GREER: Actress Garson
GREG: Actor Kinnear
GREGG: Singer Allman
GREGOR: "Metamorphosis" role
GREGORY: Dancer Hines
GREIST: Actress Kim
GRENADA: Windward Island
GRENDEL: "Beowulf" beast
GRESHAM: British financier
GRETA: Actress Garbo
GRETE: Marathoner Waitz
GRETNA: ___ Green (elopers' locale)
GRETZKY: Hockey great Wayne
GREY CUP: Canadian football trophy
GREYLAG: European goose
G.R.F.: Presidential monogram
G-RIDE: Stolen car
GRIECO: Actor Richard
GRIEG: Norwegian composer
GRIER: Actress Pam
GRIESE: Bob of football
GRIFFEY: Ken of baseball
GRIFFON: Belgian dog
GRIFT: Swindle
GRIG: Young eel
GRIGRI: African amulet
GRIMKE: Abolitionist Angelina
GRIMM'S: "___ Fairy Tales"
GRIMMY: Comics dog
GRIMSBY: English port
GRINCH: Dr. Seuss character
GRINDL: Imogene Coca sitcom
GRINGO: Yankee
GRINKOV: Figure skater Sergei
GRINT: Actor Rupert
GRIOT: African storyteller
GRIPPE: Flu
GRIS: Spanish painter
GRISE: Gray: French
GRISHA: "Anna Karenina" character
GRISHAM: Author John
GRISLET: King Arthur knight
GRIS-NEZ: French cape
GRISSOM: Astronaut Gus
GRITTI: Venice's ___ Palace
GRO: Miracle-___ (plant-food brand)
GROAT: Old English coin
GROBAN: Singer Josh
GRODIN: Actor Charles
GRODY: Sleazy
GROFE: Composer Ferde
GROH: Actor David
GROIN: Vault intersection
GROK: Understand
GROLIER: Encyclopedia publisher
GROMIT: British toon
GROMMET: Eyelet
GROMYKO: Former Russian ambassador
GROOVIN': Young Rascals tune
GROPIUS: German architect
GROS: ___ point (embroidery stitch)
GROSSE: ___ Pointe, MI
GROSSO: Concerto ___
GROSZ: Polish money
GROSZY: Polish money
GROT: Cave
GROTE: Jerry of baseball
GROTIUS: Dutch statesman
GROTON: Connecticut town
GROTTY: Seedy
GROUCHO: One of the Marx brothers
GROUTY: Surly
GROVER: President Cleveland
GROVER'S: ___ Corners ("Our Town" town)
GROZA: Lou of football
GROZNY: Chechen city
GRRL: Independent young woman
GRRRL: Independent young woman
GRUCCI: Fireworks-show name

GRUE: Shudder
GRUMIO: "Taming of the Shrew" character
GRUMMAN: Plane builder Leroy
GRUN: Green: German
GRUNDY: Prissy Mrs.
GRUNGER: Certain rock-music fan
GRUNION: Small fish
GRUS: Southern constellation
GRUYERE: French cheese
GR. WT.: Gross weight: Abbr.
GRYPHON: Griffin
G.S.A.: General Services Administration: Abbr.
G SCALE: Piano practice
G SEVEN: Top economic countries
G SIXTY: Bingo call
G.S.O.: Mil. aide
GSTAAD: Swiss resort
G STAR: Spectral type
G-SUIT: Astronaut's wear
GT. BR.: Part of the U.K.
GTD.: Guaranteed: Abbr.
GTE: Verizon merger partner
GTI: Volkswagen model
G TILE: Scrabble two-pointer
GTO: 1960s sports car
GTV: Alfa Romeo model
GTX: Plymouth model
GUANACO: Andes ruminant
GUANINE: DNA constituent
GUANO: Type of fertilizer
GUAPA: Good-looking: Spanish
GUAPO: Good-looking: Spanish
GUAR: Legume
GUARANI: Paraguay money
GUARE: "Six Degrees of Separation" playwright
GUAR GUM: Ice-cream ingredient
GUCCI: Designer Aldo
GUCK: Slime
GUDGEON: Bait fish
GUELPH: Canadian city
GUERDON: Reward
GUERRE: War: French
GUEVARA: Cuban revolutionary
GUGINO: Actress Carla
GUIANA: South American region
GUIDO: Italian painter Reni
GUIDRY: Ron of baseball
GUIGNOL: Grand __ (horror drama)
GUILDER: Former Dutch coin
GUINAN: "Star Trek: The Next Generation" character
GUINEA: Old British coin
GUITRY: French playwright
GUJARAT: State of India
GULAG: Russian prison camp
GULDEN'S: Mustard brand
GULF OIL: Gas company
GULLAH: Creolized English
GUMBEL: TV host Bryant
GUMBY: Clay character
GUMEE: Gitchee __ (Hiawatha's lake)
GUMM: Judy Garland's real surname
GUMMI: __ Bears (candy brand)
GUMMO: One of the Marx brothers
GUMP: Hanks Oscar role
GUND: Cleveland arena
GUNG: __-ho
GUNGA: "__ Din" (Kipling poem)
GUN IT: Floor the accelerator
GUNITE: Cement mixture
GUN LAP: Race finale
GUNN: 1960s TV detective
GUNNAR: Economics Nobelist Myrdal
GUNNY: Sack material
GUNSEL: Armed thug
GUNTER: Author Grass
GUNTHER: "Inside U.S.A." author
GUNWALE: Boat part
GURDY: Hurdy-__
GURION: David Ben-__
GURKHA: Nepalese soldier
GURLEY: Helen __ Brown
GURNEE: Illinois town
GURSH: Saudi Arabian coin
GUS: Astronaut Grissom
GUSSET: Shirt insert
GUSTAV: Composer Mahler
GUSTAVE: Novelist Flaubert
GUTE: Good: German
GUTEN: Good: German
GUTHRIE: Singer Arlo
GUTMAN: "Maltese Falcon" character
GUTZON: Sculptor Borglum
GUV: British term of address
GUVNOR: Boss, in Britain
GUYANA: South American country
GUYED: Secured with a rope
GUYON: "The Faerie Queene" character
GUY ROPE: Cable
GUZMAN: Mexican novelist
G.V.W.: Truck stat.
GWEN: Dancer Verdon
GWENN: Actor Edmund
GWTW: Mitchell novel, for short
G.W.U.: D.C. school
GWYN: Actress Nell
GWYNETH: Actress Paltrow
GWYNN: Tony of baseball
GWYNNE: Actor Fred
GYMNO: Bare: Comb. form
GYM RAT: Perpetual exerciser
GYN: Female: Comb. form
GYNE: Female: Comb. form
GYNEC: Female: Comb. form
GYNECO: Female: Comb. form
GYNOUS: Female: Comb. form
GYNT: Ibsen character
GYNY: Female: Comb. form
GYOZA: Japanese dumpling
GYR: Circle: Comb. form
GYRE: Revolve
GYRENE: U.S. Marine
GYRO: Greek sandwich
GYROCAR: Two-wheeled auto

H

HAAA: "They're Coming To Take Me Away, Ha-__!"
HAAG: Den __ (Dutch city, to natives)
HAAGEN: __-Dazs
HAAKON: King of Norway
HAARLEM: Dutch city
HAAS: Actor Lukas
HAB.: Bk. before Zephaniah
HABANA: Cuban capital, to natives
HABER: German chemistry Nobelist
HABIB: Arabic name meaning "beloved"
HABILE: Adept
HABILIS: Homo __ (human ancestor)
HABLA: "Se __ español"
HABLAR: To speak: Spanish
HABS: Montreal Canadiens, familiarly
HACEK: Diacritical mark
HACKETT: Comic Buddy
HACKL: "Hello, Dolly!" character
HACKLE: Bird feather
HACKLY: Jagged
HACKMAN: Actor Gene
HACKY: __ Sack (toy beanbag)
HAD A ROW: Went at it
HADDEN: "Time" co-founder
HADDIE: Finnan __ (Scottish seafood)
HADDIX: Harvey of baseball
HADES: Greek underworld
HADJ: Islamic pilgrimage
HADJI: Islamic pilgrim
HADRIAN: Roman emperor
HADRON: Subatomic particle
HAE: Have: Scottish
HAEC: This: Latin
HAECKEL: German biologist
HAEMA: Blood: Comb. form
HAFIZ: Persian poet
HAFNIUM: Element #72
HAGAR: Cartoon Viking
HAGEN: Actress Jean
HAGERTY: Actress Julie
HAGGAI: Bible book
HAGGIS: Scottish pudding
HAGI: Holy: Comb. form
HAGIO: Holy: Comb. form
HAGLER: Boxer Marvin
HAGMAN: Actor Larry
HAHN: German chemistry Nobelist
HAHNIUM: Element #105
HAI: "Bali __"
HAID: Actor Charles
HAIDA: Alaska Indian
HAIDEE: "Count of Monte Cristo" character
HAIFA: Israeli port
HAIG: Reagan secretary of state
HAIGHT: San Francisco street
HAIK: Arab garment
HAIKAI: Japanese verse
HAIKU: Japanese poem
HAILE: Ethopian emperor __ Selassie
HAILEY: Novelist Arthur
HAIM: Actor Corey
HAIMISH: Unpretentious
HAINES: Director Randa
HAING: Actor __ S. Ngor
HAISE: Apollo 13 astronaut
HAJ: "The __" (Uris book)
HAJE: Actress Khrystyne
HAKE: North Atlantic fish
HAKEEM: Olajuwon of basketball
HAKIM: Muslim physician
HAL: "2001" computer
HALAL: Islamic dietary laws
HALALA: Saudi Arabian coin
HALAS: NFL coach George
HALAVAH: Turkish candy
HALDANE: British biochemist
HALEN: Rock singer Eddie Van __
HALEVY: French composer
HALEY: Tin Man portrayer
HALF-ROD: 8+ feet
HALI: Salt: Comb. form
HALIFAX: Canadian city
HALLAM: British historian
HALLE: Actress Berry
HALLEL: Hanukkah prayer
HALLEY: British astronomer
HALLEY'S: __ Comet
HALLIE: Actress Foote
HALLO: Fox-hunt shout
HALLOO: Fox-hunt shout
HALLUX: Big toe
HALOP: Actor Billy
HALPIN: Actor Luke
HALS: Dutch artist
HALSEY: WWII admiral
HALSTON: Designer name
HALVA: Turkish candy
HALVAH: Turkish candy
HAMA: Syrian city
HAMACHI: Sushi fish
HAMAN: Old Testament villain
HAMAS: Mideast group
HAMATE: Hook-shaped
HAMBURG: German city
HAMDEN: Connecticut city
HAME: Harness part
HAMEL: Actress Veronica
HAMELIN: German city
HAMELN: German city
HAMER: Actor Rusty
HAMILL: Actor Mark
HAMITE: Egyptian ancestor
HAMLIN: Lincoln vice president
HAMLINE: University in St. Paul
HAMM: Soccer star Mia
HAMMETT: Author Dashiell
HAMMOND: Indiana city
HAMM'S: Beer brand
HAMP: Vibraphonist Lionel's nickname
HAMPTON: Vibraphonist Lionel
HAMSUN: Norwegian novelist
HAMULUS: Small hook
HANA: Tennis pro Mandlikova
HANAPER: Wicker receptacle
HANDEL: German composer
HAND-EYE: __ coordination
HANDI: __-Wipes (kitchen product)
HANDKE: Austrian novelist
HANDLIN: Historian Oscar
HANDSEL: Good-luck gift

HANES: Pantyhose brand
HANEY: "Green Acres" role
HANFF: Author Helene
HANG-BY: Hanger-on
HANGUL: Korean alphabet
HANK IBA: Basketball Hall of Famer
HANLEY: Novelist James
HANLON: Baseball Hall of Fame manager
HANNA: Barbera's animation partner
HANNAH: Actress Daryl
HANOI: Vietnamese city
HANOVER: British royal house
HANS: Physicist Geiger
HANSA: Medieval guild
HANS ARP: French artist
HANSE: Medieval guild
HAN SOLO: Harrison Ford role
HANSON: Composer Howard
HANTS: English county
HANYA: Choreographer Holm
HAO: Vietnamese coin
HAOLE: Hawaiian non-native
HAP: Accident, old-style
HA'PENNY: Old British coin
HAPKIDO: Martial art
HAPLOID: Single
HAPLY: By chance, old-style
HAPTICS: Branch of psychology
HAR: Mock laugh
HARA: __-kiri
HARALD: Norwegian king
HARARE: Capital of Zimbabwe
HARBACH: Lyricist Otto
HARBIN: Chinese city
HARBURG: Lyricist E.Y.
HARDEE'S: Fast-food chain
HARDIN: Actor Ty
HARDING: 29th president
HARD SIX: Dice roll
HARD TEN: Dice roll
HARI: Mata __
HARICOT: Lamb stew
HARKER: "Dracula" character
HARLAN: Eisenhower Supreme Court appointee
HARLAND: Colonel Sanders
HARLEY: Motorcycle brand
HARLIN: Director Renny
HARLINE: Composer Leigh
HARLOW: Actress Jean
HARMON: Actor Mark
HARNEY: Black Hills mountain
HARNICK: Lyricist Sheldon
HAROLD: Composer Arlen
HAROLD I: English king
HARPER: Actress Valerie
HARPER'S: Monthly magazine
HARPO: Oprah's company
HARRAD: "The __ Experiment" (Rimmer novel)
HARRAH: Toby of baseball
HARRAH'S: Vegas casino
HARRIET: Abolitionist Tubman
HARRIS: Writer Joel Chandler
HARROD'S: London department store
HARROLD: Actress Kathryn
HARRY-O: David Janssen TV series
HARRY S: President Truman
HART: Poet Crane
HARTACK: Jockey Bill
HARTE: Author Bret
HARTLEY: Actress Mariette
HARTMAN: Actress Lisa
HARTMUT: German chemistry Nobelist Michel
HARUM: Rock group Procol __
HARVEY: Blood-circulation discoverer
HARWELL: Sportscaster Ernie
HARZ: German mountain range
HAS A SET: Completes the collection
HASBRO: Toy company
HASEK: Hockey pro Dominik
HASID: Certain Jew
HASIDIM: Certain Jews
HASKELL: "Leave It to Beaver" character
HASP: Door fastener
HASSAM: Artist Childe __
HASSAN: King of Morocco
HASSEL: Norwegian chemistry Nobelist
HASSID: Certain Jew
HASSIUM: Element #108
HASSO: Actress Signe
HASTA: Until: Spanish
HASTERT: House speaker Dennis
HATARI: John Wayne film
HATCHER: Actress Teri
HATHA: __-yoga
HATHI: "Jungle Books" character
HATHOR: Egyptian goddess
HATLO: Cartoonist Jimmy
HATS OFF: Phrase of praise
HATTIE: Actress McDaniel
HAUER: Actor Rutger
HAUS: House: German
HAUT: High: French
HAUTBOY: Oboe
HAUTE: __ couture (high fashion)
HAUTEUR: Arrogance
HAVA: "__ Nagila" (Jewish song)
HAVARTI: Kind of cheese
HAVASU: Lake __ City, AZ
HAVEL: Czech playwright
HAVENER: Harbor master
HAVER: Actress June
HAVRE: Le __, France
HAW: "Hee __"
HAWG: Motorcycle, slangily
HAWKE: Actor Ethan
HAWKEYE: Iowa native
HAWKINS: Jazz saxophonist
HAWKMAN: Comics superhero
HAWN: Actress Goldie
HAWORTH: Actress Jill
HAWSE: Anchor cable hole
HAWSER: Anchor cable
HAYDEN: Former Arizona senator
HAYDN: Austrian composer
HAYEK: Actress Salma
HAYES: Actress Helen
HAYESES: 1870s First Family
HAYLEY: Actress Mills
HAYMES: Singer Dick
HAYNES: Director Todd
HAYNIE: Golfer Sandra
HAYWARD: California city
HAZAN: Cantor
HAZANIM: Cantors
HAZLITT: British essayist
HAZMAT: Hazardous material: Abbr.
H-BAR: Construction beam
H-BEAM: Girder
H.C.H.: FDR predecessor
HCL: Strong acid
HDBK.: Instruction manual: Abbr.
HDG.: Ship's course: Abbr.
H.D.L.: "Good" cholesterol
HDS.: Bosses: Abbr.
HDTV: High-definition TV: Abbr.
HEADEND: Communication center
HEADOFF: Avert
HEADPIN: Alley target
HEAL-ALL: Medicinal plant
HEALD: Actor Anthony
HEALEY: Austin-__ (British auto)
HEALY: Sportscaster Fran
HEANEY: Irish poet
HEARN: Actor George
HEARNS: Boxer Thomas
HEARST: Publisher William Randolph
HEARTED: Big-__ (generous)
HEATON: Actress Patricia
HEAT RAY: Sci-fi weapon
HEATTER: Radio newsman Gabriel
HEB.: Old Testament book: Abbr.
HEBB: Singer Bobby
HEBBEL: German poet
HEBE: Greek goddess
HEBR.: Israeli language: Abbr.
HEBRON: Ancient city of Palestine
HEC: "__ Ramsey" (1970s western)
HECATE: Greek goddess
HECHE: Actress Anne
HECHT: Dramatist Ben
HECKART: Actress Eileen
HECKMAN: Economics Nobelist
HECT: Hundred: Comb. form
HECTARE: 10,000 square meters
HECTO: Hundred: Comb. form
HECUBA: Wife of King Priam
HEDDA: "__ Gabler" (Ibsen play)
HEDIN: Swedish explorer
HEDISON: Actor David
HEDLEY: "Doonesbury" character
HEDONIC: Of pleasure
HEDRAL: Faced: Comb. form
HEDREN: Actress Tippi
HEDRON: Face: Comb. form
HEDY: Actress Lamarr
HEE: "__ Haw"
HEEBIE: __-jeebies
HEEGER: Chemistry Nobelist
HEEP: "David Copperfield" character
HEER: Mister: Dutch
HEET: Liniment brand
HEF: "Playboy" founder, familiarly
HEFLIN: Actor Van
HEFNER: Publisher Hugh
HEFTI: Composer Neal
HEGEL: German philosopher
HEGGEN: "Mister Roberts" author
HEGYES: Actor Robert
HEIDEN: Olympic skater Eric
HEIDT: Bandleader Horace
HEIFETZ: Violinist Jascha
HEIGH-HO: "Snow White" song
HEIGL: Actress Katherine
HEIN: Football Hall of Famer Mel
HEINE: German poet
HEINIE: Baseball Hall of Famer Manush
HEINSE: German author
HEINZ: Ketchup brand
HEISMAN: Football trophy
HEISS: Olympic skater Carol
HEL: Norse goddess
HELENA: Montana capital
HELENE: Author Hanff
HELENS: Mt. St. __, WA
HELGA: Hägar's wife
HELI: Sun: Comb. form
HELIC: Spiral: Comb. form
HELICAL: Coiled
HELICO: Spiral: Comb. form
HELICON: Type of tuba
HELIO: Sun: Comb. form
HELIOS: Greek sun god
HELLAS: Ancient Greece
HELLBOY: Ron Perlman film
HELLENE: Greek
HELLENO: Greek: Comb. form
HELLER: Novelist Joseph
HELLMAN: Playwright Lillian
HELMER: "A Doll's House" character
HELMOND: Actress Katherine
HELMUT: German leader Kohl
HELO: Copter
HELOISE: Abélard's beloved
HELOT: Ancient serf
HELSING: Van __ ("Dracula" character)
HELTER: __-skelter
HEMA: Blood: Comb. form
HEMAL: Of blood
HEMAT: Blood: Comb. form
HEMATIC: Of blood
HEMATIN: Blood pigment
HEMATO: Blood: Comb. form
HEME: Blood pigment
HEMET: California city
HEMI: Half: Comb. form
HEMIC: Of blood
HEMO: Blood: Comb. form
HEMON: Canadian novelist
HEMSLEY: Actor Sherman
HENBANE: Poisonous plant
HENBIT: Common weed
HENCH: Medicine Nobelist
HENDEC: 11: Comb. form
HENDECA: 11: Comb. form
HENDRIX: Guitarist Jimi
HENDRY: Actor Ian
HENDRYX: Soul singer Nona
HENGE: Neolithic monument
HENIE: Skater Sonja
HENLEY: British regatta site

HENN: Actress Carrie
HENNER: Actress Marilu
HENNY: Comic Youngman
HENREID: "Casablanca" actor
HENRI: Artist Matisse
HENRICH: Tommy of baseball
HENRIES: Units of inductance
HENRIK: Playwright Ibsen
HENRY I: English king
HENRY II: English king
HENRY IV: English king
HENRYK: Novelist Sienkiewicz
HENRY V: English king
HENRY VI: English king
HENSLEY: Actress Pamela
HENSON: Muppets creator
HENTOFF: Columnist Nat
HENZE: German composer
HEPARIN: Anticoagulant
HEPAT: Liver: Comb. form
HEPATIC: Of the liver
HEPATO: Liver: Comb. form
HEPBURN: Actress Audrey
HEPT: Seven: Comb. form
HEPTA: Seven: Comb. form
HERA: Greek goddess
HERAT: Afghan city
HERBART: German philosopher
HERBAUT: "Count of Monte Cristo" character
HERBE: French seasoning
HERBERT: Composer Victor
HERBIE: "The Love Bug" car
HERCULE: Agatha Christie detective
HEREDIA: Cuban-born poet
HEREK: Actor Stephen
HERITOR: Heir
HERKY: __-jerky
HERMAN: Author Melville
HERMANA: Sister: Spanish
HERMANN: Novelist Hesse
HERMANO: Brother: Spanish
HERMAN'S: __ Hermits (rock group)
HERMES: Greek messenger god
HERMON: Syrian mountain
HERMOSA: Beautiful: Spanish
HERMOSO: Beautiful: Spanish
HERNAN: Explorer Cortez
HERNANI: Victor Hugo work
HERNDON: Lincoln's law partner
HERNE: German city
HER NIBS: Georgia Gibbs nickname
HERPET: Reptile: Comb. form
HERPETO: Reptile: Comb. form
HERR: Mister: German
HERREN: Gentlemen: German
HERRICK: British poet
HERRIOT: British writer/veterinarian
HERSEY: "A Bell for Adano" writer
HERSH: Writer Seymour
HERSHEY: Chocolate magnate
HERTS: English county
HERTZ: Avis competitor
HERVE: Actor Villechaize
HERVEY: Actress Irene
HERZL: Zionism founder
HERZOG: Saul Bellow novel
HE/SHE: Politically correct pronoun
HESHVAN: Hebrew month
HESIOD: Ancient Greek poet
HE'S ON: Sportscaster's call
HE'S OUT: Sportscaster's call
HESS: British pianist
HE'S SAFE: Sportscaster's call
HESSE: German author
HEST: Command, old-style
HESTER: "Scarlet Letter" character
HESTIA: Greek goddess of the hearth
HESTON: Actor Charlton
HET: __ up (agitated)
HETER: Different: Comb. form
HETERO: Different: Comb. form
HETH: Hebrew letter
HETTY: "Adam Bede" character
HEUER: TAG __ (Swiss watch brand)
HEURE: Hour: French
HEURIGE: Austrian wine
HEUSEN: Composer James Van __
HEWISH: British physics Nobelist
HEWITT: "60 Minutes" producer
HEWLETT: Packard's computer partner
HEXA: Six: Comb. form
HEXANE: Organic solvent
HEXAPOD: Insect
HEXOSE: Simple sugar
HEX SIGN: Barn symbol
HEYER: Romance novelist
HEY JUDE: Beatles song
HEY MAN: Attention getter
HEYMANS: Belgian medicine Nobelist
HEY MR. DJ: Backstreet Boys tune
HEY RUBE: Circus distress signal
HEYSE: German literature Nobelist
HEYWARD: Writer DuBose
HEYWOOD: Writer Broun
HGT.: Alt.
HGTV: Cable network for remodelers
H.G.W.: "The Time Machine" monogram
H.G. WELLS: British novelist
H.H.H.: LBJ's vice president
H.H. MUNRO: Saki's real name
H.H.S.: Cabinet dept.
HIALEAH: Florida city
HIBBING: Minnesota city
HIBBLER: Jazz singer Al
HIBERNO: Irish: Comb. form
HICKAM: Pearl Harbor Air Force base
HICKEY: Kiss mark
HICKMAN: Actor Darryl
HICKOK: Wild Bill of westerns
HIDALGO: Spanish gentleman
HI-DE-HO: Cab Calloway catchphrase
HIDEKI: Irabu of baseball
HIDEO: Nomo of baseball
HIDEY: __-hole (place of concealment)
HIEMAL: Wintry
HIER: Yesterday: Spanish
HIERO: Sacred: Comb. form
HIGGINS: "Pygmalion" professor
HIGGLE: Bargain
HIGH DAY: Feast day
HIGH-RES: Like some computer monitors
HIGH-TOP: Big sneaker
HI-HAT: Set of cymbals
HI, HI, HI: McCartney tune
HI HOS: Cracker brand
HIJA: Daughter: Spanish
HIJO: Son: Spanish
HIKEN: "Car 54, Where Are You?" creator
HILAIRE: Author Belloc
HILARY: Actress Swank
HILBERT: German mathematician
HILDA: "Broom-__" (comic strip)
HILLARY: Everest conqueror
HILLEL: B'nai B'rith offshoot
HILLER: Director Arthur
HILO: Hawaiian city
HILUM: Seed scar
HIMALIA: Moon of Jupiter
HIMES: Novelist Chester
HIMMEL: Heaven: German
HI MOM: TV greeting
HINES: Dancer Gregory
HINGIS: Tennis pro Martina
HINGLE: Actor Pat
HINKLE: Golfer Lon
HINKY: Dishonest
HINNY: Horse/donkey hybrid
HINTON: Author S.E.
HIP-HOP: Music style
HIPPITY: __-hop
HIPPUS: Horse: Comb. form
HI-Q: Jumping-peg game
HIRAM: General Grant's original first name
HIRCINE: Goatish
HIRSCH: Actor Judd
HIRSUTE: Hairy
HIRT: Trumpeter Al
HIS'N: Nonstandard pronoun
HIS NIBS: Big shot
HISPANO: Spain: Comb. form
HI-SPEED: Fast, informally
HIST.: High school subject: Abbr.
HISTO: Tissue: Comb. form
HITACHI: Electronics brand
HITE: Sociologist Shere
HI-TEST: Gasoline grade
HIT-IN: Polo play
HIT INTO: Cause, as a double play
HIT IT: "Start playing!"
HIT ME: Blackjack phrase
HIT ONE: Knock a homer
HITTITE: Ancient Asian
HIVA: "Fatu __" (Thor Heyerdahl book)
HIVA OA: French Polynesian island
HIVE OFF: Separate from a group
HIX: "The Music Man" character
HI Y'ALL: Southern greeting
HI-YO: Lone Ranger exclamation
HJALMAR: Swedish playwright Bergman
H.J. HEINZ: Food company
H.L. HUNT: Texas oilman
HMONG: Chinese people
H.M.S.: British ship designation
HOAD: Tennis pro Lew
HOAG: Novelist Tami
HOAGIE: Long sandwich
HOAGY: Composer Carmichael
HOAR: Frost
HOARE: British statesman
HOB: Fireplace shelf
HOBAN: White House architect
HOBART: Australian city
HOBBES: British philosopher
HOBBIT: Tolkien character
HOBBS: "The Natural" hero
HOBE: __ Sound, FL
HOBEY: Hockey great Baker
HOBIE: __ Cat (personal watercraft)
HOBOKEN: New Jersey city
HOBSON'S: __ choice (no choice)
HOC: This: Latin
HOCH: Golfer Scott
HOCUS: Play a trick on
HOD: Brick carrier
HO-DAD: Poor surfer
HO-DADDY: Poor surfer
HODDING: Journalist Carter
HODGES: Gil of baseball
HODIAK: Actor John
HOEST: Cartoonist Bill
HOF: Court: German
HOFBRAU: German tavern
HOFF: Cartoonist Syd
HOFFA: Former Teamsters leader
HOFFER: Writer Eric
HOFFMAN: Actor Dustin
HOFMANN: Pianist Josef
HOFSTRA: Long Island university
HOGAN: Navajo dwelling
HOGARTH: British painter
HOGBACK: Crested ridge
HOGG: "Dukes of Hazzard" boss
HOGNOSE: Harmless snake
HOGNUT: Hickory tree
HOHNER: Harmonica brand
HO-HOS: Snack-cake brand
HOI: __ polloi (common people)
HOISIN: Chinese sauce
HOITY: __-toity
HOJO: Restaurant chain, for short
HOKIE: Virginia Tech athlete
HOL.: Day off: Abbr.
HOLA: Hello: Spanish
HOLBEIN: German artist
HOLBERG: Danish playwright
HOLD 'EM: Poker variety
HOLDEN: Actor William
HOLE OUT: Finish on the green
HOLIC: Addict: Comb. form
HOLIST: New Age practitioner
HOLLEY: Medicine Nobelist
HOLLIS: Pro golfer Stacy
HOLM: Actress Celeste
HOLMAN: Basketball Hall of Famer Nat
HOLMIUM: Element #67
HOLMS: River islands
HOLO: Whole: Comb. form

HOLST: "The Planets" composer
HOLT: Novelist Victoria
HOLTZ: Football coach Lou
HOLY ARK: Synagogue cabinet
HOLY JOE: Chaplain, slangily
HOLYOKE: Massachusetts city
HOLY SEE: The Vatican
HOLZMAN: Basketball coach Red
HOM: Alike: Comb. form
HOMAGER: Vassal
HOME EC: High-school class
HOME ICE: Hockey team locale
HOMEIER: Actor Skip
HOME LAB: Type of computer setup
HOMEO: Similar: Comb. form
HOMEYS: Close friends
HOMIE: Close friend
HOMINID: Human, for one
HOMME: Man: French
HOMO: __ sapiens
HONALEE: Dragon's home, in song
HONAN: Chinese province
HOND.: Central Amer. country
HONDA: Auto make
HONDO: John Wayne film
HONG: __ Kong
HONI: Hägar the Horrible's daughter
HONIARA: Solomon Islands capital
HONKY: __-tonk
HONORE: Author Balzac
HONSHU: Japanese island
HONUS: Baseball great Wagner
HOO: "Yoo-__!"
HOODIE: Sort of sweatshirt
HOODOO: Hex
HOODY: Sort of sweatshirt
HOOEY: Baloney
HOOF IT: Walk
HOOKA: Water pipe
HOOKAH: Water pipe
HOOKE: British physicist
HOOPLE: Comic-strip Major
HOOPMAN: Basketball player
HOOPOE: Crested bird
HOOSAC: Massachusetts mountain range
HOOSIER: Indiana native
HOOTCH: Alcohol
HOOTIE: Blowfish bandmate
HOOVER: Vacuum brand
HOPEH: Chinese province
HOPI: Arizona Indian
HOPKIN: 1960s singer Mary
HOPKINS: British poet
HOPLITE: Ancient Greek soldier
HOPPE: Billiards champ Willie
HOP SING: "Bonanza" cook
HOR.: Not vert.
HORA: Bar mitzvah dance
HORACE: Roman poet
HORAE: Goddesses of the seasons
HORAL: Hourly
HORATIO: Admiral Nelson
HOREB: Biblical mountain
HORGAN: Pulitzer author Paul
HORMEL: Spam producer
HORMUZ: Persian Gulf strait
HORNBY: Twiggy's surname
HORNE: Singer Lena
HORNER: Pie eater of rhyme
HORNISH: Auto racer Sam
HORNSBY: Baseball great Rogers __
HORNUNG: Football Hall of Famer Paul
HORS: __ d'oeuvres
HORSLEY: Actor Lee
HORST: Actor Buchholz
HORT.: Plant sci.
HORTON: Dr. Seuss character
HORUS: Egyptian god
HORVITZ: Medicine Nobelist
HOS.: Bk. before Joel
HO SCALE: Model-railroad standard
HOSEA: Biblical prophet
HOSEL: Golf-club part
HOSEN: Breeches: German
HOSER: Con man, slangily
HOSKINS: Actor Bob
HOSNI: Egyptian statesman Mubarak
HOSTA: Plantain lily
HOSTLER: Horse groom
HOTBOT: Internet search engine
HOT CAP: Plant protector
HOTE: Table d'__
HOTH: "The Empire Strikes Back" planet
HOT LICK: Jazz phrase
HOT LIPS: "M*A*S*H" character
HOTMAIL: Web service provider
HOT PACK: Pain reliever
HOTSPUR: Reckless one
HOTSY: __-totsy
HOTTIE: Attractive one
HOT TUNA: Rock band
HOUDINI: Legendary magician
HOUDON: French sculptor
HOUGH: Novelist Emerson
HOUK: Baseball manager Ralph
HOUMA: Louisiana city
HOURI: Beautiful woman
HOUSMAN: Poet A.E.
HOUSSAY: Argentine physiology Nobelist
HOVEY: Poet Richard
HOVIS: Actor Larry
H.O.V. LANE: Carpooler's strip
HOWAR: Author Barbara
HOWARD K.: TV newsman Smith
HOWARDS: "__ End" (Emma Thompson film)
HOWARD U.: D.C. school
HOWBEIT: Nevertheless
HOWDAH: Elephant saddle
HOWE: Inventor Elias
HOWELL: Bell & __ (film-equipment maker)
HOWELLS: Author William Dean
HOWES: Actress Sally Ann
HOWIE: Actor Mandel
HOWLIN': __ Wolf (blues singer)
HOW'M: "__ I doin'?"
HOWSER: "Doogie __, M.D." (sitcom)
HOXHA: Former Albanian leader
HOY: Today: Spanish
HOYA: Georgetown athlete
HOYDEN: Tomboy
HOYLE'S: "__ Rules of Games"
HOYT: Pitcher Wilhelm
HPS: Some computer printers: Abbr.
HQS: Bases: Abbr.
H. RAP: 1960s militant Brown
HRBEK: Kent of baseball
H.R.E: Charlemagne's domain: Abbr.
HRETHEL: "Beowulf" character
H.R.H.: Royal letters
H. RIDER: Author Haggard
H. ROSS: Computer magnate Perot
HRYVNA: Ukrainian money
HRYVNIA: Ukrainian money
HSI: Chinese river
HSIA: Chinese dynasty
HSN: Cable shopping channel
H.S.T.: FDR successor
H-TEST: 1950s experiment
H TILE: Scrabble four-pointer
HTML: Internet programming language
HTTP: Web-address start
HUA: 1970s Chinese premier
HUAC: 1950s anti-subversive grp.
HUANGHE: Yellow River
HUANG TI: First emperor of China
HUBBARD: Nursery-rhyme mother
HUBBELL: Baseball great Carl
HUBBLE: Space telescope
HUBEL: Medicine Nobelist
HUBER: German chemistry Nobelist
HUBERT: Senator Humphrey
HUBIE: Brooks of baseball
HUBLEY: Actress Season
HUBRIS: Excessive pride
HUCK: Twain kid
HUD: Paul Newman film
HUDDIE: Folk singer Ledbetter
HUDSON: New York river
HUEVO: Egg: Spanish
HUEY: Military copter
HUFFMAN: Actress Felicity
HUGGIES: Diaper brand
HUGGINS: Babe Ruth manager
HUGH: TV host Downs
HUGHES: Skater Sarah
HUGHIE: Eugene O'Neill play
HUGO: Author Victor
HUGOS: Sci-fi writing awards
HUIS: Sartre's "__ Clos"
HUIT: Eight: French
HULCE: "Amadeus" star
HULLO: Hello, in Britain
HULLY: __ gully (1960s dance)
HULME: British author
HULOT: Tati film role
HUMANUM: __ est errare
HUMBARD: Evangelist Rex
HUMBER: British river
HUMBERT: "Lolita" character
HUME: Actor Cronyn
HUMERUS: Arm bone
HUMIDEX: Uncomfortableness measure
HUMMEL: Collectible figurine
HUMMUS: Mideast dip
HUMORAL: Of bodily fluids
HUMPHRY: Chemist Davy
HUMPTY: __ Dumpty
HUMUS: Compost material
HUMVEE: Jeep relative
HUNAN: Chinese cuisine
HUND: Dog: German
HUNH: "What?"
HUNLEY: Actress Leann
HUNNY BS: Kellogg cereal
HUNTLEY: TV newsman Chet
HUNTZ: Actor Hall
HUP: Marching syllable
HUPPAH: Jewish wedding canopy
HUPPERT: Actress Isabelle
HUR: "Ben-__"
HURDY: __-gurdy
HURLEY: Actress Elizabeth
HURLY: __-burly (commotion)
HUROK: Impresario Sol
HURON: Canadian Indian
HURST: Novelist Fannie
HURSTON: Novelist Zora Neale
HUS: Czech religious reformer
HUSAK: Former Czech president
HUSING: Pioneer sportscaster Ted
HUSSAR: Hungarian cavalryman
HUSSEIN: Jordanian monarch
HUSSERL: German philosopher
HUSSEY: Actress Olivia
HUSSITE: Bohemian religious reformer
HUSTON: Actress Anjelica
HUT ONE: Quarterback call
HUTT: Jabba the __ ("Star Wars" series villain)
HUTTO: "The Yearling" character
HUTTON: Model Lauren
HUT TWO: Quarterback call
HUTU: African people
HUXLEY: Author Aldous
HUYGENS: Dutch astronomer
HYADES: Star cluster
HYALITE: Colorless opal
HYALOID: Glassy
HYAMS: Director Peter
HYANNIS: Massachusetts town
HYATT: Big name in hotels
HYDE: London park
HYDR: Water: Comb. form
HYDRA: Freshwater creature
HYDRO: Seaplane
HYDROX: Former cookie brand
HYDRUS: Water Snake constellation
HYER: Actress Martha
HYET: Rain: Comb. form
HYETAL: Rainy
HYETO: Rain: Comb. form
HYGELAC: "Beowulf" character
HYGIEIA: Goddess of health
HYGINUS: Pope
HYGRIC: Of moisture
HYGRO: Moist: Comb. form
HYKSOS: Ancient Egyptians
HYLA: Tree frog
HYMAN: Admiral Rickover
HYNDE: Singer Chrissie

HYOID: Tongue bone
HYP.: Rt.-triangle side
HYPATIA: Greek philosopher
HYPERON: Subatomic particle
HYPN: Sleep: Comb. form
HYPNO: Sleep: Comb. form
HYPNOID: Of sleep
HYPNOS: Greek god of sleep
HYPONYM: Subcategory name
HYRAX: African mammal
HYSER: Actress Joyce
HYSON: Green tea
HYSSOP: Aromatic herb
HYUNDAI: Korean automaker

I

IACOCCA: Former Chrysler head
IAGO: "Othello" villain
IAL: Adjective suffix
I AM: Decartes' conclusion
IAMB: Poetic foot
IAMBI: Poetic feet
I AM LOVE: Jackson 5 song
IAMS: Dog-food brand
I AM SAM: Sean Penn film
IAN: Author Fleming
IANA: Bibliography suffix
IAN HOLM: "Chariots of Fire" actor
IAPETUS: Moon of Saturn
IASI: Romanian city
IATRIC: Curative
IATRICS: Healing: Comb. form
IATRO: Healer: Comb. form
IATRY: Healing: Comb. form
IBA: Basketball Hall of Fame coach
IBADAN: Nigerian city
IBANEZ: Spanish novelist Blasco __
IBAR: Construction beam
IBARRA: Mexican chocolate brand
I-BEAM: Building support
IBERT: French composer
IBEW: Wirers' org.
IBEX: Wild goat
IBICES: Wild goats
IBID.: Footnote abbr.
IBIDEM: Footnote notation
IBILITY: Capacity suffix
IBIS: Wading bird
IBIZA: One of the Balearic Islands
IBLE: Adjective suffix
IBLY: Adverb suffix
IBM: Computer company
IBM PC: Desktop machine
IBN: Son of: Arabic
IBN SAUD: Onetime Arab ruler
IBO: African people
IBOOK: Apple computer
IBSEN: Norwegian dramatist
ICAHN: Corporate financier Carl
ICAL: Adjective suffix
I CALL: Poker phrase
ICALLY: Adverb suffix
I CAME: Start of Caesar's boast
ICARIA: Aegean island
ICARUS: Mythical flier
I.C.C.: Freight agcy.
ICE AX: Alpine tool
ICE BATH: Cold-shower alternative
ICE DAM: Roof-water blocker
ICEE: Frozen confection brand
ICEFALL: Glacial matter
ICE IN: Make housebound, perhaps
ICE IT: "That's enough!"
ICEL.: N. Atlantic island
ICELINE: Arctic map boundary
ICENI: Ancient British Celts
ICE OUT: Ban
ICE RUN: Rapid river thaw
ICE-T: Rap artist
ICH: I: German
ICHABOD: Washington Irving character
ICH DIEN: Prince of Wales' motto
I CHING: Divination book
ICHIRO: Suzuki of baseball
ICHOR: Blood of the gods
ICHTHY: Fish: Comb. form
ICI: Here: French
I.C.J.: U.N. judicial body
ICK: "Disgusting!"
ICKES: FDR interior secretary
ICON: Computer-screen picture
ICONO: Image: Comb. form
ICOS: Twenty: Comb. form
ICOSA: Twenty: Comb. form
ICOSI: Twenty: Comb. form
ICS: "Science of" ending
ICTERUS: Jaundice
ICTINUS: Parthenon designer
ICTUS: Metrical stress
I.C.U.: Hosp. area
IDA: Author Tarbell
IDAE: Zoological suffix
IDA RED: Type of apple
IDE: Chemical suffix
ID'ED: Fingered
IDEE: Notion: French
IDEM: Footnote word
IDENT.: Birth cert., e.g.
IDENTI: __-Kit (detective tool)
IDENTIC: Same
IDEO: Notion: Comb. form
IDES: March 15th
ID EST: That is: Latin
IDI AMIN: Former Ugandan leader
IDIO: Peculiar: Comb. form
IDLESSE: Do-nothing's state
I DO, I DO: 1960s Broadway musical
IDOLUM: Fallacy
I DOOD IT: Red Skelton's admission
I DOTTER: Meticulous one
I DUNNO: "Beats me!"
I'D'VE: "If I Knew You Were Comin' __ Baked a Cake"
IDY: Charley Weaver's Mount __
IDYL: Pastoral poem
IDYLL: Pastoral poem
I-EIGHT: Highway through Yuma
I-EIGHTY: Major east-west highway
IEOH: Architect __ Ming Pei
IER: Comparative suffix
IERI: Yesterday: Italian
IEST: Superlative suffix
IF I FELL: Beatles tune
IFILL: Telejournalist Gwen
IF IT DIE: Gide autobiography
IF IT IS: "In that case..."
I-FIVE: Highway through Sacramento
IFNI: Moroccan region
I FOLD: Poker comment
I-FORTY: Highway through Memphis
I-FOUR: Highway through Tampa
IFS: Preconditions
IF SAY: Words starting a supposition
I.F. STONE: Investigative journalist
IF-THEN: Kind of proposition, in logic
IFY: Verb suffix
IF YOU GO: Travel-article header
IGA: Grocery chain
IGBY: Title character of a 2002 film
IGER: Eisner's Disney successor
IGG: Ignore
'IGGINS: Eliza's mentor
IGGY POP: Punk-rock singer
IGN.: Car-key place: Abbr.
IGNACE: Pianist Paderewski
IGNARRO: 1998 medicine Nobelist
IGNATOW: Poet David
IGNATZ: "Krazy Kat" mouse
IGNEOUS: Type of rock
IGNES: __ fatui (will-o'the-wisps)
IGNIS: Fire: Latin
IGOR: Composer Stravinsky
IGOROT: Philippines people
IGRAINE: King Arthur's mother
IGUANID: Type of lizard
IGUASSU: Argentina waterfall
IGY: 1957-58, to scientists: Abbr.
IHN: It: German
IHOP: Restaurant franchise
IHR: It: German
IHRE: Her: German
IHS: Christian letters
IIII: Sundial numeral
III JOHN: N.T. book
II JOHN: N.T. book
II KINGS: O.T. book
II PETER: N.T. book
I JOHN: N.T. book
IJSSEL: Branch of the Rhine
IKEA: Furniture-store chain
IKEBANA: Japanese art
I KINGS: O.T. book
IKO IKO: Dixie Cups tune
ILA: Dock grp.
ILE: Island: French
ILEAC: Of the small intestine
ILEAL: Of the small intestine
ILEANA: Diva Cotrubas
ILENE: Actress Graff
ILER: Actor Robert
ILEUM: Small intestine
ILEX: Evergreen oak
ILGWU: Labor org.
ILIA: Hipbone parts
ILIAC: "Sacro" ending
ILIAD: Homeric epic
ILIAMNA: Alaskan volcano
ILICH: Peter __ Tchaikovsky
ILIE: Nastase of tennis
ILIESCU: Former Romanian leader
ILION: Ancient Troy
ILIUM: Ancient Troy
ILK: Variety
ILKA: Actress Chase
ILLA: That one: Latin
I'LL BE: "Son of a gun!"
I'LL CALL: Poker phrase
I'LL DRY: Offer to help in the kitchen
ILLE: "Winnie __ Pu"
ILLEANA: Actress Douglas
ILLIN': Foolish
ILLINI: Big Ten team
I'LL KNOW: "Guys and Dolls" tune
ILL-LIT: Dark
I'LL LIVE: "Don't worry about me"
ILL-OFF: Bankrupt
ILL-SET: Poorly placed
I'LL TELL: Kid's threat
ILLUDE: Deceive
ILLUME: Brighten
ILLUS.: Like some bks.
ILL-USE: Maltreat
ILLYA: "The Man From U.N.C.L.E." character
ILLYRIA: "Twelfth Night" setting
I.L.M.: Lucas special effects co.
I.L.O.: Worldwide workers' org.
ILOCANO: Philippines people
ILOILO: Philippines port
ILONA: Actress Massey
I LOVE: What "amo" means
I LOVE L.A.: Randy Newman song
ILS: They: French
ILSA: "Casablanca" character
ILUS: Founder of Troy
ILYA: Author Ehrenburg
IMA: Philanthropist Hogg
IMAC: Apple computer
I'M A COP: Sgt. Friday declaration
IMAGISM: Poetic style
IMAGO: Adult insect
IMA HOGG: Texas philanthropist
IMAM: Muslim title
I'M A MAN: Yardbirds tune
IMAMU: Poet Baraka
IMAN: Model from Somalia
IMARET: Turkish inn
IMARI: Japanese porcelain
IMAX: Big-screen theater
IMBRUE: Defile
IMBUE: Inspire
I'M EASY: Tune from "Nashville"
IMELDA: Mrs. Marcos
I ME MINE: Beatles song
I.M.F.: "Mission: Impossible" org.
IMHO: Chat-room letters
IMHOTEP: Boris Karloff, in "The Mummy"
IMIDE: Ammonia compound
I'M IN: Poker phrase
IMINE: Organic compound
IMIT.: Not an orig.
I'M LATE: White Rabbit's admission
I'M LIKE: Teen phrase
IMMERGE: Plunge
IMMIE: Playing marble
IMMIX: Blend
IMMUNO: Medical comb. form
IMMURE: Confine

IMOGEN: "Cymbeline" heroine
IMOGENE: Comic Coca
I'M OK: "Don't worry about me"
IMPASTO: Thickly laid paint
IMPAVID: Bold
I.M. PEI: Chinese-born architect
IMPERF.: With flaws: Abbr.
IMPF.: Verb tense: Abbr.
IMPLEAD: Sue in court
IMPOST: Customs duty
IMPREST: Advance of money
IMPREZA: Subaru model
IMPROV: Ad-lib comedy
IMRE: Hungarian leader Nagy
IMS: AOL exchanges
I'M THERE: "Count me in!"
IMU: Luau cooking pit
IMUS: Radio deejay Don
INA: Actress Claire
IN A FUNK: Feeling blue
IN AGE: Years old
IN AGES: Since way back when
IN A JIFF: Very quickly
IN A MOOD: Sulking
IN A PET: Irate
IN A PIE: Blackbirds' place
IN A POD: Peas' place
IN A POEM: Robert Frost work
IN A POKE: Hidden, as a pig
INA RAY: Bandleader Hutton
INARCH: Graft a tree branch
INARI: Finnish lake
IN A RUG: Bug's place
IN A SHOE: Where the Old Woman lived
IN A TUB: Place for a male trio
IN A VALE: Robert Frost poem
IN BAD: Needing rescue
IN BIG: Heavily involved
INBOARD: Kind of boat motor
IN-BUILT: Natural
INCE: Silents director Thomas
INCENT: Encourage
INCEPT: Eat
INCHON: Korean seaport
INCL.: Comprehensive: Abbr.
INCOG: Disguised, for short
INCR.: Augment: Abbr,
INCUBUS: Evil spirit
INCUDES: Ear bones
INCULT: Rude
INCUS: Ear bone
INCUSE: Stamp
IN-DASH: Type of auto DVD player
INDEF.: Like some articles: Abbr.
INDIC: Asian language group
INDICIA: Bulk-mailing markers
INDIE: Freelance, informally
INDIGEN: Native
INDIO: California city
INDIRA: Gandhi of India
INDITE: Write
INDIUM: Element #49
INDIV.: Single: Abbr.
INDO: __-European languages
INDRA: Chief Vedic god
IN-DRAWN: Reserved
INDRE: French department
INDUE: Assume
INDUS: Asian river
INDWELL: Reside
INEDITA: Unpublished works
INEE: Arrow poison
INES: Don Juan's mother
IN ESSE: Actually: Latin
I NEVER: Aghast one's comment
INEZ: Don Juan's mother
INF.: Verb form: Abbr.
IN FAITH: Devoutly
INFANTA: Spanish princess
INFANTE: Spanish prince
IN FIVES: How change may be asked for
IN FOR: Bound to get
INFRACT: Breach
ING: Gerundial ending
INGA: Actress Swenson
INGALLS: "Little House" family name
INGATE: Molten metal channel
INGE: Playwright William
INGELS: Comedian Marty
INGEMAR: Boxer Johansson
INGER: Actress Stevens
INGESTA: Food
INGLE: Fireplace
INGLES: English: Spanish
INGLESE: English: Italian
INGMAR: Director Bergman
INGO: Movie producer Preminger
IN-GOAL: Rugby area
IN GOOD: Fitting well
INGRAM: Pop singer James
INGRES: French painter
INGRESS: Access
INGRID: Actress Bergman
INHERE: Belong intrinsically
IN HOC: With respect to this: Latin
INHUME: Bury
INIGO: Architect Jones
INIKI: Hurricane of 1992
I-NINETY: Highway through Cleveland
INION: Skull bone
IN IRONS: Manacled
INIT.: Monogram part: Abbr.
INITIO: Ab __ (from the beginning)
INJUN: __ Joe (Twain character)
INKA: "__ Dinka Doo"
IN KEY: Euphonious
INK IN: Color a comic strip
IN-KIND: Reciprocal
INK-JET: Type of computer printer
INKLE: Linen tape
IN KNOTS: All tied up
INKSAC: Cuttlefish organ
INKSTER: Golfer Juli
INKY CAP: Kind of mushroom
IN LEAF: Covered with foliage
INLY: Deeply
INNAGE: Container contents
INNERVE: Animate
INNES: "ER" actress
INNESS: Painter George
INNIE: Navel variety
INNIS: CORE leader
INNY: Navel variety
INO: Mythical sea goddess
INOCULA: Flu-shot substances
IN ON: A part of
IN ONES: How change may be asked for
INONU: 1940s Turkish president
INORG.: Branch of chemistry: Abbr.
INOUYE: Hawaii senator
IN POINT: Applicable
INQ.: Ask: Abbr.
IN RE: Concerning
IN REM: Against a thing, in law
INRI: Crucifix letters
INRO: Small Japanese box
INRUN: Ski-jump ramp
INSANA: Ron of CNBC
INSECTA: Class of animals
INSIGNE: Badge
IN SITU: As found: Latin
INSOFAR: Legalese adverb
INSP.: Police rank: Abbr.
INSPAN: Harness
INST.: Part of MIT
INSTR.: Teacher: Abbr.
INSWEPT: Narrowing at the front
INT.: Bank acct. payment
IN TAILS: Dressed formally
IN TASTE: With class
INTEGRA: Acura model
INTEL: Computer-chip company
IN TENS: How change may be asked for
INTERJ.: Pt. of speech
INTER SE: Among themselves: Latin
IN THERE: Baseball broadcaster's call
IN THING: Craze
INTL.: Worldwide: Abbr.
INTO IT: Enjoying an activity
IN TOTO: All
INTR.: Like some vbs.
IN-TRAY: Place for some memos
INTROIT: Psalm part
INTUIT: Have a hunch
INU: Shiba __ (Japanese dog)
INUIT: Alaska native
INULASE: Enzyme
INUPIK: Alaska native
INURE: Acclimate
IN UTERO: Unborn
INUTILE: Of no value
INV.: Bill: Abbr.
IN VACUO: Isolated: Latin
INVEIGH: Protest
INVER: __ Grove Heights, IL
INVICTA: Watch brand
IN VITRO: From a lab
IN VIVO: Not outside the body
INXS: Rock band
IN YEARS: For a long time
INYO: California county
I.O.C.: Olympics org.
IODO: Iodine: Comb. form
IOLA: City in Kansas
IOLANI: Honolulu's __ Palace
IOLE: Captive of Hercules
IOMEGA: Computer hardware maker
IO MOTH: Showy insect
IONA: New York college
IONE: Actress Skye
IONESCO: French playwright
IONIA: Ancient Asia Minor region
IONIAN: Arm of the Mediterranean
IONIC: Column order
IONICS: Poetic feet
IONIUM: Isotope of thorium
IONO: Ion: Comb. form
IONONE: Perfume ingredient
I.O.O.F.: Fraternal org.
IOR: Adjective suffix
IOS: Aegean island
IOWAS: Midwest Indians
IOWA U.: Hawkeye coll.
IOWAY: Hawkeye's home, humorously
IPA: Phonetic alphabet
IPANA: 1950s toothpaste
IPANEMA: Rio district
IPCRESS: Len Deighton's "The __ File"
IPECAC: Medicinal root
I PETER: N.T. book
I.P.O.: Wall St. debut
IPOD: Digital song player
IPOH: Malaysian city
I.P.S.: Tape-speed meas.
IPSA: Itself: Latin
IPSE: __ dixit
IPSO: __ facto
IPSWICH: Massachusetts city
IQBAL: Pakistani poet
IRA: Lyricist Gershwin
IRABU: Hideki of baseball
IRAE: "Dies __" (Latin hymn)
I RAISE: Poker phrase
IRENA: "The Faerie Queene" character
IRENE: Actress Dunne
IRENIC: Peaceful
IRENICS: Branch of theology
IRID: Certain plant
IRIDES: Eye parts
IRIDIC: Of element #77
IRIDIUM: Element #77
IRIDO: Iris: Comb. form
IRINA: Chekhov character
IRIS-IN: Movie-camera technique
IRIS-OUT: Movie-camera technique
IRITIS: Eye inflammation
IRKUTSK: Russian city
IRLENE: A Mandrell sister
IRMA: "My Friend __"
I.R.O.: Displaced people's grp.
I, ROBOT: Asimov novel
IROC: Auto race
IRON-ON: Type of patch
IRR.: Not first-quality: Abbr.
IRRA: Akkadian god
IRREAL: Imaginary
IRRUPT: Break in
I.R.T.: New York subway
IRTYSH: Asian river
IRUS: "Odyssey" beggar
IRV: Sportscaster Cross
IRVIN: Monte of baseball

IRVINE: California city
IRVING: Actress Amy
IRWIN: Author Shaw
ISAAC: Sir __ Newton
ISAACS: Novelist Susan
ISAAK: Singer Chris
ISABEAU: Mascagni opera
ISABEL: Actress Sanford
ISADORA: Dancer Duncan
ISADORE: Animator Freleng
ISAIAH: Biblical prophet
ISAIAN: Of a prophet
ISAK: Author Dinesen
ISAMU: Sculptor Noguchi
ISANTI: Minnesota county
ISAO: Aoki of golf
ISAR: Bavarian river
I SAY: Brit's exclamation
I.S.B.N.: Book ID
ISCHIUM: Hip bone
ISE: British verb ending
I SECOND: Parliamentary phrase
ISELIN: New Jersey city
ISER: Czech river
ISERE: French river
I SERVE: Prince Charles's motto
ISEULT: Tristan's beloved
ISFAHAN: Irani city
ISH: Adjective suffix
ISHAM: Bandleader Jones
ISHMAEL: "Moby-Dick" narrator
ISHTAR: Babylonian goddess
ISIAH: Thomas of basketball
ISIDOR: Physicist Rabi
ISIDORE: Saint of Seville
ISIDRO: Spanish saint
IS INTO: Loves
ISIS: Egyptian goddess
IS IT A GO: "Can we do it?"
ISLA: Island: Spanish
ISLEY: Singing brothers' surname
ISLIP: Long Island town
ISM: Doctrine
ISMAIL: "Rocket" of football
ISMENE: Daughter of Oedipus
ISO: Equal: Comb. form
ISOGON: Equal-angled figure
ISOGRAM: Weather-map line
ISOHEL: Weather-map line
ISOLA: "87th Precinct" novels' setting
ISOLATO: Hermit
ISOLDA: Tristan's love
ISOLDE: Tristan's love
ISOLINE: Weather-map feature
ISOLT: "Idylls of the King" character
ISONOMY: Equality of rights
ISOPOD: Marine crustacean
ISOTONE: Atom variant
I.S.P.: AOL, for one
I SPY: 1960s Cosby show
ISR.: Neighbor of Leb.
ISRAFEL: Poe poem
ISRAIR: Mideast airline
ISS.: Copy of a mag.
ISSEI: Japanese-American
ISSEL: Basketball Hall of Famer
ISSUANT: Heraldic term
ISSUE AD: Political commercial
ISSUS: Where Alexander beat Darius
ISSY: French city
IST: Adherent's suffix
ISTH.: Atlas abbr.
ISTIC: Adjective suffix
ISTLE: Carpet fiber
IS TO: Ratio phrase
ISTOMIN: Pianist Eugene
IS TOO: Playground retort
ISTRES: French town
ISTRIA: Adriatic peninsula
I.S.U.: Ames coll.
ISUZU: Imported auto
ITA: Spanish diminutive suffix
ITAL.: Emphatic type: Abbr.
ITALIA: Napoli locale
ITALO: Writer Calvino
ITAR: __-TASS (Russian news agency)
ITASCA: Minnesota lake
IT'D: "__ be a pleasure"
ITE: "Follower" suffix
ITEA: Virginia willow
I-TEN: Coast-to-coast highway
ITER: Roman road
IT GIRL: Clara Bow's nickname
IT GIRLS: Socialite celebrities
ITHACA: Cornell's locale
I-THIRTY: Highway through Little Rock
ITIC: Adjective suffix
I TILE: Scrabble one-pointer
I, TINA: Singer Turner's autobiography
ITIOUS: Adjective suffix
ITIS: Medical suffix
IT'LL: "__ never work"
ITO: Spanish diminutive suffix
ITOL: Chemical suffix
I TOO: Langston Hughes poem
IT'S GONE: Sportscaster's phrase
IT'S LOVE: "Wonderful Town" tune
IT'S ON ME: Treater's words
IT'S OPEN: "Come on in!"
IT'S PAT: Julia Sweeney film
ITSY: __-bitsy
IT'S YOU: Dress-shop comment
ITT: "Addams Family" cousin
ITTY: __-bitty
ITURBI: Pianist José
ITV: BBC competitor
I-TWELVE: Highway through Baton Rouge
I-TWENTY: Highway through Atlanta
ITY: Noun suffix
ITZA: Chichen-__
ITZHAK: Violinist Perlman
IUM: Element ending
IUS: Vitamin A amts.
IVA: "The Maltese Falcon" character
IVAN: Typical Russian
IVANA: Trump ex
IVANHOE: Walter Scott novel
IVAN I: Old Russian ruler
IVAN III: Russian czar
IVAN IV: "Terrible" czar
IVANKA: Donald Trump's daughter
IVANOV: Russian playwright
IVANOVO: Russian city
IVAN V: Russian czar
IVAN VI: Russian czar
IVAR: Physics Nobelist Giaever
IVERSON: Allen of basketball
IVES: Currier's partner
IVEY: Actress Judith
IVIE: Singer Anderson
IVINS: Author Molly
IVO: Literature Nobelist Andric
IVOR: Composer Novello
IVORIAN: Abidjan resident
IVORINE: Piano-key material
IWO JIMA: 1945 battle site
IWW: Debs' org.
IXIA: Corn lily
IXION: King of myth
IX-NAY: Slangy refusal
IYAR: Hebrew month
IZA: "Clan of the Cave Bear" character
IZAAK: "The Compleat Angler" writer Walton
IZATION: Noun suffix
IZE: Verb ending
IZMIR: Aegean gulf
IZOD: Men's shirt brand
IZZ: "Tess of the d'Urbervilles" character
IZZATSO: "Oh yeah?"
IZZY: Atlanta Olympics mascot

J

JABBA: __ the Hutt
JABBAR: Hoopster Kareem Abdul-__
JABOT: Blouse ruffle
JAC: Outerwear, for short
JACAL: Mexican hut
JACAMAR: Tropical bird
J'ACCUSE: Zola book
JACET: Hic __ (here lies: Latin)
JACEY: "The Music Man" character
JACINTH: Reddish-orange
JACINTO: San __ Day (Texas holiday)
JACKDAW: Black bird
JACKIE O: Former first lady, for short
JACKO: "Thriller" singer's nickname
JACK SOO: "Barney Miller" actor
JACK-TAR: Sailor
JACKY: British gin
JACLYN: Actress Smith
JACOBI: "I, Claudius" star
JACOBIN: French revolutionary
JACOBY: Bridge expert Oswald
JACONET: Cotton fabric
JACQUES: Chirac of France
JADA: Actress __ Pinkett Smith
JAECKEL: Actor Richard
JAEGER: Seabird
JAFAR: "Aladdin" genie
JAFFA: Israeli city
JAFFE: Author Rona
JAFFEE: "Mad" cartoonist Al
JAGGER: Rolling Stones leader
JAGGIES: Computer-display effect
JAGLOM: Director Henry
JAGR: Jaromir of hockey
JAHAN: Shah of old Persia
JAHR: Year: German
JAHRE: Years: German
JAI: __ alai
JAI ALAI: Game from Spain
J'AIME: I love: French
JAINISM: Hindu creed
JAIPUR: City of India
JA JA: German's emphatic agreement
JAKARTA: Capital of Indonesia
JAKE: Boxer LaMotta
JAKES: "North and South" novelist
JAKOB: Bob Dylan's son
JAL: Airline to Tokyo
JALAPA: Capital of Veracruz
JALISCO: State of Mexico
JALPA: Lamborghini model
JAMA: Journal for MDs
JAMAAL: Name meaning "beauty"
JAMAIS: Never: French
JAMBA: __ Juice (fruit-drink chain)
JAM BAND: Improvisational music group
JAMBE: Leg: French
JAMBEAU: Leg armor
JAMCAM: Traffic video source
JAMES A.: President Garfield
JAMES I: British king
JAMES J.: Boxer Braddock
JAMES K.: President Polk
JAMES M.: Author Cain
JAMESON: Actor __ Parker
JAMES'S: The Court of St. __
JAMES T.: Author Farrell
JAMES V: Scottish king
JAMES VI: Son of Mary Stuart
JAMI: Actress Gertz
JAMIE: Actor Farr
JAM IN: Cram
JAMISON: Hoopster Antawn
JAMMIES: Nightclothes
JAMOCA: Ice-cream flavor
JAMOKE: Coffee
JAMON: Ham: Spanish
JANA: Tennis pro Novotna
JANACEK: Czech composer
J AND B: Liquor brand
J. AND J.: Band-Aid maker, for short
JANEANE: Actress Garofalo
JANE DOE: Anonymous woman
JANEIRO: Rio de __
JANET: Actress Leigh
JANEWAY: Economist Eliot
JAN HUS: Czech religious reformer
JANICE: "Star Trek" yeoman
JANIE: Country singer Fricke
JANINE: Actress Turner
JANIS: Singer Ian
JANKLOW: Literary agent Morton
JANN: "Rolling Stone" founder Wenner

JANNEY: Actress Allison
JANOS: Hungarian leader Kádár
JANSEN: Dutch theologian
JANSSEN: "The Fugitive" star
JANSSON: Scandinavian author Tove
JANUAR: January: German
JANUS: Two-faced god
JANVIER: January: French
JANZEN: Golfer Lee
JAPANS: Applies a lacquer
JAPE: Jest
JAPHETH: Son of Noah
JAQ: "Cinderella" mouse
JARABE: __ tapatio (Mexican dance)
JARDIN: Garden: French
JARDINE: Rock guitarist Alan
JARED: Actor __ Martin
JAR JAR: "Phantom Menace" character
JAROMIR: Jagr of hockey
JARRE: Film composer Maurice
JARRELL: Poet Randall
JARRETT: Auto racer Dale
JARROTT: Director Charles
JA RULE: Rap star
JARVIK: Artificial heart developer
JAS.: N.T. book
JASCHA: Violinist Heifetz
JASMIN: French poet
JASON: "Argo" captain
JASPER: Artist Johns
JASPERS: German philosopher
JATO: Jet-assisted takeoff
JAUN: "Finnegans Wake" character
JAUNE: Yellow: French
JAURES: French writer
JAVA MAN: Famous fossil
JAVERT: "Les Misérables" character
JAVIER: __ Pérez de Cuellar
JAVITS: New York convention center
JAW AT: Speak abusively to
JA WOHL: German agreement
JAX: Florida city, for short
JAYCEE: Civic booster
JAYE: Actor Davidson
JAY LENO: Letterman rival
JAYMES: Bartles' partner
JAYNE: Ice dancer Torvill
JAY WARD: Bullwinkle creator
JAY-Z: Rap artist
JAZZ AGE: Roaring Twenties
JAZZBO: Certain music fan
JAZZ UP: Enliven
J-BAR: Ski lift
J. CARROL: Actor Naish
J CLOTH: Towel brand
J.C. POWYS: Welsh author
J. CREW: Clothing brand
J.C.S: Two-yr. schools
JCT.: Crossroads: Abbr.
J.D. POWER: Auto-survey company
J.D.S: Law degs.
JEAN ARP: French artist
JEANE: Former ambassador Kirkpatrick
JEANIE: Girl in a Foster song
JEAN-LUC: Director Godard
JEANNE: __ d'Arc
JEANNIE: Actress Berlin
JEANNOT: Director Szwarc
JEB BUSH: Florida governor
J.E.C.: Presidential monogram
JECKLE: Cartoon magpie
JED: "Beverly Hillbillies" character
J. EDGAR: Hoover of the FBI
JEDI: "Star Wars" knight
JEEBIES: Heebie-__
JEETER: "Tobacco Road" character
JEEVES: Fictional butler
JEEZ: "Good grief!"
JEFE: Chief: Spanish
JEFF: Mutt's partner
JEFFERS: Poet Robinson __
JEFFREY: Media mogul Katzenberg
JEFFY: "Family Circus" character
JEHAN: Persian shah
JEHU: Fast driver
JEJUNE: Arid
JEJUNUM: Intestine part
JEKYLL: Stevenson character
JELL: Congeal
JEMIMA: Aunt on syrup labels
JEMISON: Astronaut Mae
JEN: "Dawson's Creek" character
JENA: 1806 battle
JENKINS: Pitcher Ferguson __
JENNA: Actress Elfman
JENNER: Smallpox vaccine discoverer
JENNET: Female donkey
JENNEY: Skyscraper architect
JENNIE: Actress Garth
JENNY: Actress Agutter
JENO'S: Frozen pizza brand
JENS: Actress Salome
JENSEN: German physics Nobelist
JEON: South Korean money
JEPHTHA: Handel oratorio
JER.: O.T. book
JERBOA: African rodent
JEREMY: Actor Irons
JEREZ: City of Spain
JERGENS: Actress Adele
JERI: Actress Ryan
JERICHO: Ancient city of Palestine
JERILYN: Golfer Britz
JERITZA: Soprano Maria
JERKIN: Close-fitting jacket
JERNE: Danish medicine Nobelist
JEROME: Composer Kern
JERRY: Comedian Lewis
JERZY: Author Kosinski
JESS: Boxer Willard
JESSE: Reverend Jackson
JESSEL: "The Toastmaster General"
JESSICA: Actress Tandy
JESSY: Sally __ Raphael
JESSYE: Opera singer Norman
JESU: "__, Joy of Man's Desiring"
JESUIT: Loyola follower
JESUS: Alou of baseball
JETE: Ballet leap
JETER: Derek of baseball
JETFIRE: Oldsmobile model
JETFOIL: Fast boat
JET GUN: Immunization device
JETHRO: "Beverly Hillbillies" role
JET LI: Martial-arts actor
JET PACK: Sci-fi device
JETSKI: Water vehicle
JETSONS: Cartoon family
JETSTAR: Oldsmobile model
JETT: Rock singer Joan
JETTA: Volkswagen model
JETTY: Pier
JET WASH: Plane-engine phenomenon
JETWAY: Bridge to an aircraft
JEU: Game: French
JEUDI: Thursday: French
JEUNE: Young: French
JEUX: Games: French
JEVONS: British economist
JEWETT: Writer Sarah Orne __
JEWISON: "Fiddler on the Roof" director
JEZEBEL: Bette Davis film
J.F.K. JR.: 1960s First Son
J.H.S.: Educ. institution
JIANG: __ Qing (Mao's wife)
JIB BOOM: Nautical spar
JIBE: Agree
JIBE AT: Belittle
JICAMA: Edible root
JIDDA: Saudi Arabian city
JIF: Peanut butter brand
JIGGERY: __-pokery
JIGGS: "Bringing Up Father" father
JIGGY: Uninhibited
JIG TIME: Certain dance tempo
JIHAN: Mrs. Sadat
JILL: Actress Eikenberry
JILLIAN: Actress Ann
JILLIE: Actress Mack
JILLION: Large number
JIMA: Iwo __
JIM BEAM: Liquor brand
JIM BOB: "The Waltons" son
JIM CHEE: Tony Hillerman sleuth
JIM DALE: Barnum on Broadway
JIM DIAL: "Murphy Brown" anchorman
JIMENEZ: Bill Dana character
JIM FIXX: "The Complete Book of Running" author
JIM HOGG: Texas county
JIMI: Guitarist Hendrix
JIMINEZ: Director Neal
JIMINY: Mild oath
JIMJAMS: Jitters
JIM KAAT: Baseball pitcher
JIMMIE: Baseball great Foxx
JIM RICE: 1980s Red Sox star
JIM RYUN: 1960s miler
JIMSON: Poisonous weed
JINGO: Chauvinist
JINKS: Pranks
JINN: Islamic spirit
JINNI: Islamic spirit
JIP: David Copperfield's dog
JIRASEK: Czech writer
JITNEY: Airport vehicle
J.K.P.: President Polk's initials
J. LO: Jennifer Lopez nickname
J.M.W.: British artist Turner
JOACHIM: Hungarian violinist
JOADS: "The Grapes of Wrath" family
JOAN: Actress Cusack
JOANIE: "Happy Days" girl
JOANNA: Actress Cassidy
JOANNE: Golfer Carner
JOANOU: Director Phil
JOAQUIN: California's San __ Valley
JO BETH: Actress Williams
JOB HOP: Change employment frequently
JOB JAR: Household-task holder
JOB LOCK: Inability to leave one's employer
JOB LOT: Wholesale quantity
JOB ONE: Top priority
JOB SHOP: Small, specialized manufacturer
JOBSON: Hobson-__
JOBYNA: Actress Ralston
JOCASTA: Wife of Oedipus
JOCELYN: Former surgeon general Elders
JOCK: Athlete
JOCKO: Chimp
JOCULAR: Amusing
JOCUND: Cheerful
JODHPUR: Ankle-length footwear
JODIE: Actress Foster
JODRELL: __ Bank Observatory
JODY: Singer Watley
JOE BLOW: Average guy
JOE BUCK: "Midnight Cowboy" character
JOE CAMP: "Benji" director
JOE COOL: Snoopy persona
JOE D: DiMaggio nickname
JOE DON: Actor Baker
JOE E.: Comedian Brown
JOE HILL: Legendary labor organizer
JOE KIDD: Eastwood film
JOEL: Pop singer Billy
JOE ROTH: "America's Sweethearts" director
JOE TEX: Soul singer
JOEY: Baby kangaroo
JOEY DEE: "Peppermint Twist" singer
JOFFE: Director Roland
JOFFRE: French WWI general
JOFFREY: Ballet company
JOG: Activate
JOG BRA: Runner's wear
JOG TROT: Humdrum routine
JOHAN: Tennis pro Kriek
JOHANN: Composer Strauss
JOHANNA: Author Spyri
JOHN BOY: "The Waltons" character
JOHN C.: Jackson vice president Calhoun
JOHN D.: Tycoon Rockefeller
JOHN DOE: Anonymous man

JOHN F.: President Kennedy
JOHN GAY: "Beggar's Opera" author
JOHN I: Pope
JOHN II: Pope
JOHN III: Pope
JOHN IV: Pope
JOHN IX: Pope
JOHN J.: Bird artist Audubon
JOHN JAY: First chief justice
JOHN L.: Boxer Sullivan
JOHN LAW: Policeman, slangily
JOHN LEE: Blues singer Hooker
JOHNNIE: Attorney Cochran
JOHNNY B.: Mr. Goode of song
JOHN P.: Novelist Marquand
JOHN Q.: __ Public (average person)
JOHNS: Philanthropist Hopkins
JOHN V: Pope
JOHN VI: Pope
JOHN VII: Pope
JOHN WOO: "Broken Arrow" director
JOHN X: Pope
JOHN XI: Pope
JOHN XII: Pope
JOHN XIV: Pope
JOHN XIX: Pope
JOHN XV: Pope
JOHN XVI: Pope
JOHN XX: Pope
JOHN XXI: Pope
JOI: Actress Lansing
JOIE: __ de vivre
JOINDER: Act of uniting
JOINERY: Some woodwork
JOIST: House beam
JOJO: Skater Starbuck
JOJOBA: Cosmetic oil
JOLENE: Actress Blalock
JOLI: Pretty: French
JOLIE: Actress Angelina
JOLIET: Canadian explorer
JOLIOT: Irène __-Curie
JOLLA: La __, CA
JOLLEY: Australian writer
JOLLIET: Canadian explorer
JOLSON: "Swanee" singer
JOLTIN': __ Joe DiMaggio
JO MARCH: "Little Women" girl
JOMO: Kenyatta of Kenya
JON: "Garfield" character
JONAH: Jinx
JONAS: Dr. Spock
JON ERIK: Actor Hexum
JONESED: Craved
JONESES: Family to "keep up with"
JONES'S: "Bridget __ Diary" (Zellweger film)
JONESY: "Alien" cat
JONG: "Fear of Flying" novelist
JONGG: Mah-__
JON HALL: "Ramar of the Jungle" star
JONI: Singer Mitchell
JONNY: Cartoon kid Quest
JONQUIL: Garden flower
JONSON: "The Alchemist" dramatist
JONZE: Director Spike
JOON: "Benny & __" (1993 film)
JOOSS: German ballet dancer
JOPLIN: Missouri city
JOPPOLO: "A Bell for Adano" character
JORDANA: Actress Brewster
JOR-EL: Superman's father
JORGE: Author Amado
JORUM: Large bowl
JORY: Actor Victor
JOS: Sweethearts
JO'S BOYS: Alcott novel
JOSE: Singer Feliciano
JOSEF: Painter Albers
JOSEPHA: Sarah __ Hale
JOSEPH I: Holy Roman emperor
JOSEY: "The Outlaw __ Wales" (Eastwood film)
JOSHUA: Moses' successor
JOSIAH: King of Judah
JOSIE: "__ and the Pussycats" (TV cartoon)
JOSIP: Tito's real first name
JOSS: Chinese idol
JOTA: Castanet dance
JOTTO: Word game
JOUHAUX: French peace Nobelist
JOULE: Unit of work
JOUNCE: Bounce
JOUR: Day: French
JOURDAN: Actor Louis
JOURNEE: Day: French
JOURNO: Reporter, slangily
JOUVE: French writer
JOVAN: Fragrance brand
JOVE: Jupiter alias
JOVI: Rock band Bon __
JOVIAN: Of Jupiter
JOYCE: "Finnegans Wake" author
JOYCEAN: Like "Ulysses"
JOYNER: Jackie __-Kersee
JOYPAD: Computer-game device
JOZSEF: Hungarian author Attila
J. PAUL: Oil tycoon Getty
JPEG: Computer-screen image
JPG: Computer-screen image
J.P.S: Elopers' officials: Abbr.
J.Q.A.: Presidential monogram
J.R. EWING: "Dallas" villain
J. ROBERT: Physicist Oppenheimer
JROTC: High-school military org.
J.R.R: Writer Tolkien
J.S. BACH: Baroque composer
J-STROKE: Canoeing motion
J TILE: Scrabble eight-pointer
J.T. MONEY: Hip-hop artist
JUAB: Utah county
JUAN: San __, PR
JUANO: "West Side Story" character
JUAREZ: "The Mexican Washington"
JUBAL: Confederate general Early
JUCO: Junior college
JUD: "Oklahoma!" role
JUDAEA: Biblical kingdom
JUDAH: Ben-Hur's first name
JUDAS: One of the Apostles
JUDASES: Traitors
JUDD: Singer Naomi
JUDDS: Country music duo
JUDE: New Testament book
JUDEA: Biblical kingdom
JUDE LAW: "Alfie" actor
JUDEO: __-Christian
JUDE'S: St. __ (children's hospital)
JUD FRY: "Oklahoma!" villain
JUDI: Actress Dench
JUDIT: Chessmaster Polgar
JUDITH: Dame __ Anderson
JUDOKA: Martial-arts expert
JUDSON: Buntline's real name
JUEGO: Game: Spanish
JUEVES: Thursday: Spanish
JUGAL: Cheekbone
JUG BAND: Blues group
JUGHEAD: Archie's friend
JUICE UP: Activate
JUILLET: July: French
JUIN: June: French
JUJU: African amulet
JUKE: Football feint
JULE: Composer Styne
JULES: Author Verne
JULEY: "Howards End" character
JULI: Golfer Inkster
JULIA: Actress Roberts
JULIAN: John Lennon's son
JULIANA: Former Dutch queen
JULIE: Actress Andrews
JULIEN: Novelist Green
JULIO: Winemaker Gallo
JULIUS: __ Caesar
JUMADA: Islamic month
JUMANJI: Robin Williams film
JUMBUCK: Australian sheep
JUMNA: Agra's river
JUMP AT: Accept eagerly
JUMP BID: Bridge term
JUMP CUT: Film discontinuity
JUNC.: Crossroads: Abbr.
JUNCO: Snowbird
JUNG: Swiss psychologist
JUNGER: German author
JUNI: June: German
JUNIO: June: Spanish
JUNIUS: Actor Booth
JUNO: Roman goddess
JUNTA: Bloc
JUNTO: Cabal
JURA: French department
JURADO: Actress Katy
JURAL: Legal
JURAN: Director Nathan
JURE: Law: Latin
JURGENS: Actor Curt
JURIDIC: Legal
JURIS: J.D. part
JUS: Roast beef au __
JUSQUE: Until: French
JUST AS: While
JUSTE: Equitable: French
JUST IN: Recently arrived
JUSTINE: Alexandria Quartet book
JUST ONE: Small sample
JUSTY: Subaru model
JUTE: Rope fiber
JUTLAND: Danish peninsula
JUVENAL: Roman poet
JVC: TV brand
J.V.S: H.S. teams

K

KAA: "Jungle Book" python
KAAT: Pitcher Jim
KABA: Mecca shrine
KABBALA: Secret doctrine
KABOOM: Explosion sound
KABUKI: Japanese drama
KABUL: Afghan capital
KACHINA: Hopi doll
KA-CHING: Cash-register sound
KADAR: Former Hungarian leader
KADDISH: Synagogue prayer
KADEEM: Actor Hardison
KADETT: Opel model
KAEL: Critic Pauline
KAETHE: "Tender Is the Night" character
KAF: Arabic letter
KAFKA: Austrian novelist
KAGAWA: Japanese social reformer
KAHLIL: Writer Gibran
KAHLO: Artist Frida
KAHLUA: Kind of liqueur
KAHN: Actress Madeline
KAHN'S: Hot-dog brand
KAHUNA: Hawaiian hotshot
KAIA: "The Master Builder" character
KAILUA: Hawaiian city
KAI-SHEK: Chiang of China
KAKAPO: New Zealand parrot
KAKI: Actress Hunter
KAKURO: Cross-sums puzzle
KALB: Newscaster Bernard
KAL-EL: Superman's birth name
KALI: Wife of Shiva
KALINE: Al of baseball
KALININ: 1920s Soviet president
KAL-KAN: Dog-food brand
KALKI: Gore Vidal book
KALLEN: Singer Kitty
KALMAR: Lyricist Bert
KAM: Actor Fong
KAMA: "__ Sutra"
KAMALI: Designer Norma
KAMEN: Comedian Milt
KAMERAD: Ally: German
KAM FONG: "Hawaii Five-O" actor
KAMI: Actress Cotler
KAMPALA: Uganda capital
KAN.: Topeka's loc.
KANA: Japanese script
KANAKA: Hawaii native
KANALY: Actor Steve
KANAR: Thriller writer Stephen
KANATA: Canadian city
KANAWA: Soprano Kiri te __
KANDEL: Austrian medicine Nobelist
KANDER: "Cabaret" composer
KANDY: Sri Lanka city
KANE: Orson Welles role

KANEOHE: Hawaiian city
KANG: Chinese sleeping platform
KANGA: Milne character
KANIN: Author Garson
KANJI: Japanese writing
KANS.: Topeka's loc.
KANSA: Oklahoma Indian
KANT: German philosopher
KANTOR: Novelist MacKinlay
KANYE: Rap star West
KAOLIN: Porcelain ingredient
KAON: Subatomic particle
KAOS: "Get Smart" foe
KAPELL: Pianist William
KAPH: Hebrew letter
KAPITAL: "Das __"
KAPITSA: Russian physics Nobelist
KAPLAN: Author Justin
KAPOK: Tropical tree
KAPPA: Greek letter
KAPTURE: Actress Mitzi
KAPUTT: Broken: German
KARA: Arctic sea
KARACHI: Pakistan port
KARAJAN: Austrian conductor
KARA KUM: Asian desert
KARAN: Designer Donna
KARAOKE: Bar attraction
KARAS: Composer Anton
KARA SEA: Arctic Ocean arm
KAREEM: Abdul-Jabbar of basketball
KAREL: Author Capek
KAREN: Actress Black
KARI: Actress Michaelson
KARINA: Actress Lombard
KARKOV: "For Whom the Bell Tolls" character
KARL: Actor Malden
KARLA: Singer Bonoff
KARLE: Chemistry Nobelist
KARLEN: Actor John
KARLOFF: Actor Boris
KARLOVY: __ Vary (Czech city)
KARLSON: Director Phil
KARN: "Home Improvement" actor
KARNAK: Egypt archeological site
KARNS: Actor Roscoe
KARO: Corn-syrup brand
KAROL: John Paul II's first name
KAROLYI: Gymnastics coach Bela
KARPOV: Russian chessmaster
KARRAS: Actor Alex
KARRER: Swiss chemistry Novelist
KARRIE: Golfer Webb
KARSH: Photographer Yousuf
KARST: Limestone rock formation
KART: Go-__
KARUS: "Bambi" character
KARYN: Pop singer White
KASBAH: Algiers area
KASDAN: Director Jake
KASEM: DJ Casey
KASHA: Buckwheat dish
KASHI: Cereal brand
KASHMIR: Former Asian nation
KASI: Actress Lemmons
KASTLER: French physics Nobelist
KAT: "Krazy __"
KATA: Judo warm-up
KATAYEV: Russian writer
KATE: "Kiss Me __"
KATEY: Actress Sagal
KATHE: German painter Kollwitz
KATHIE: __ Lee Gifford
KATHRYN: Director Bigelow
KATHY: Actress Bates
KATIE: Couric of TV
KATISHA: "The Mikado" character
KATMAI: Alaskan volcano
KATO: Green Hornet's assistant
KATRIN: "I Remember Mama" role
KATRINA: Hurricane of 2005
KATRINE: Scottish lake
KATT: Actor William
KATY: Actress Jurado
KATYDID: Grasshopper
KATZ: Medicine Nobelist
KATZE: Cat: German
KATZEN: Cats: German
KAUAI: Hawaiian island
KAUFMAN: Playwright George S.
KAUNAS: Lithuanian city
KAUNDA: Former Zambian president
KAVA: Polynesian beverage
KAVNER: Actress Julie
KAYE: Actress Ballard
KAY LENZ: David Cassidy ex
KAY YOW: Basketball Hall of Famer
KAZAN: "East of Eden" director
KAZIN: Literary critic Alfred
KCAL: Heat meas.
K-CAR: 1980s Chrysler product
K.C. JONES: Basketball Hall of Famer
KCL: Sodium chloride
K.C. STAR: Midwest paper, for short
KDKA: Pittsburgh radio station
K.D. LANG: Pop singer
K-DOE: R&B singer
KEA: New Zealand parrot
KEACH: Actor Stacy
KEAN: Actor Edmund
KEANE: "Family Circus" cartoonist
KEANU: Actor Reeves
KEAR: "Cakes and Ale" character
KEARNEY: Nebraska city
KEARNS: Actor Joseph
KEARNY: New Jersey city
KEATON: Actress Diane
KEATS: British poet
KEDGE: Small anchor
KEDROVA: Actress Lila
KEDS: Sneaker brand
KEEBLER: Cookie brand
KEEFE: Actor Brasselle
KEELER: Actress Ruby
KEELY: Singer Smith
KEENAN: Actor Wynn
KEENE: Nancy Drew byline
KEENEN: Actor __ Ivory Wayans
KEENE, NH: New Eng. city
KEENER: Actress Catherine
KEESHAN: Captain Kangaroo portrayer
KEESLAR: Actor Matt
KEESLER: Mississippi Air Force base
KEFIR: Dairy product
KEGGER: Beer party
KEILLOR: Lake Wobegon creator
KEINO: Kenyan runner
KEIR: Actor Dullea
KEIRA: Actress Knightley
KEITEL: Actor Harvey
KEITH: "Partridge Family" role
KEL: "Kenan & __" (TV series)
KELL: George of baseball
KELLER: Author Helen
KELLEY: Actor De Forest
KELLI: Actress Williams
KELLIE: Actress Martin
KELLJAN: Director Bob
KELLOGG: Cereal name
KELLY: "Pogo" cartoonist
KELLY'S: "__ Heroes" (Eastwood film)
KELOWNA: British Columbia city
KELPIE: Australian dog
KELSEY: Actor Grammer
KELSO: 1960s racehorse
KELTON: Actress Pert
KELVIN: British physicist
KELVINS: Units of temperature
KEMAL: Ataturk of Turkey
KEMBLE: Actress Fanny
KEMIDOV: "The Maltese Falcon" character
KEMO: __ Sabe (Tonto's friend)
KEMP: 1996 vice presidential candidate
KEMPIS: Author Thomas à __
KEMPT: Fastidious
KEMPTON: Writer Murray
KEN: Author Follett
KENAI: Alaska city
KENDALL: Medicine Nobelist
KENDO: Bamboo fencing
KEN DOLL: Mattel product
KENDREW: British chemistry Nobelist
KENICHI: Chemistry Nobelist Fukui
KENMORE: Appliance brand
KENN: "The Mill on the Floss" character
KENNAN: Diplomat/author George
KENNER: Old toy brand
KENNETH: Designer Cole
KENNY: Singer Rogers
KENNY G: Jazz saxophonist
KENOBI: Obi-Wan __
KEN OLIN: "Thirtysomething" star
KENOSHA: Wisconsin city
KENSIT: Actress Patsy
KENT: "Daily Planet" reporter
KENTISH: Of a British county
KENTON: Bandleader Stan
KEN WAHL: "Wiseguy" star
KENYON: Ohio college
KEOGHAN: "Amazing Race" host
KEOKUK: Iowa city
KEOS: Aegean island
KEPI: Military cap
KEPLER: German astronomer
KER: Plunk preceder
KERALA: Indian state
KERATIN: Hair protein
KERB: British road edge
KERF: Carpenter's notch
KERI: Actress Russell
KERMIT: Frog Muppet
KERN: Composer Jerome
KERNE: Irish peasant
KERNS: "Growing Pains" star
KEROUAC: Author Jack
KERR: Actress Deborah
KERRI: Gymnast Strug
KERRY: 2004 presidential candidate
KERSEE: Olympian Jackie Joyner-__
KERSH: Country singer David
KERSHAW: Singer Nik
KERT: Larry of Broadway
KERTESZ: Hungarian literature Nobelist
KERWIN: Actor Brian
KES: "Star Trek: Voyager" character
KESEY: Author Ken
KESHIA: Actress __ Knight Pulliam
KESTREL: Falcon
KETCH: Sailboat
KETCHAM: Cartoonist Hank
KETCHUM: Idaho town
KETONE: Organic compound
KETT: Etta __ of comics
KETTI: Dramatist Frings
KETTY: Singer Lester
KEV: Electrical unit: Abbr.
KEVIN: "Home Alone" kid
KEVLAR: Bulletproof vest material
KEVON: Singer Edmonds
KEW: __ Gardens, London
KEWPIE: Kind of doll
KEY BANK: Financial services company
KEYDETS: VMI athletes
KEYE: Actor Luke
KEYES: Actress Evelyn
KEY GRIP: Chief stagehand
KEYNES: British economist
KEYPAL: E-mail friend
KEYSER: West Virginia town
KEYSPAN: New York utility company
KEYWAY: Lock part
KFC: Fast-food letters
KGB: Russian spy agcy.
KHA: Arabic letter
KHALID: Former Saudi king
KHAN: Mongol conqueror
KHANATE: Mongol empire
KHARKOV: Ukraine city
KHATAMI: Iranian statesman
KHAYYAM: Persian poet
KHEDIVE: Turkish viceroy in Egypt
KHMER: Cambodian
KHOUMS: Mauritania money
KHUFU: Egyptian pharaoh
KHYBER: Mountain pass into India
KHZ.: Freq. unit
KIA: Korean auto

KIAM: Victor of shaving commercials
KIA RIO: Imported auto
KIBBEE: Actor Guy
KIBBUTZ: Israeli community
KIBITZ: Advise at cards
KIBOSH: Put the __ on (stop)
KICKUP: Commotion
KIDCOM: TV cartoon
KIDD: Legendary pirate
KIDEO: Children's TV
KIDLIT: Children's books
KIDMAN: Actress Nicole
KID ORY: Jazz trombonist
KID ROCK: Rap artist
KIDS R US: Retail chain
KIDULT: One with Peter Pan syndrome
KIDVID: Children's TV
KIEFER: Actor Sutherland
KIEFFER: Type of pear
KIEL: German city
KIERAN: Actor Culkin
KIERON: Actor Moore
KIEV: Ukraine capital
KIGALI: Rwanda capital
KIIL: "An Enemy of the People" character
KIKI DEE: Pop singer
KIKUYU: African grass
KIL.: .621 mi.
KILAUEA: Hawaiian volcano
KILBY: Physics Nobelist
KILDARE: 1960s TV doctor
KILEY: Actor Richard
KILIM: Persian rug
KILLEEN: Texas city
KILL FEE: Cancellation payment
KILLY: French skier
KILMER: "Trees" poet
KILN: Oven
KILOBAR: Pressure unit
KILOBIT: Data storage unit
KILROY: Mythical GI who "was here"
KILTER: Good condition
KILTIE: Certain Scot
KIM: Actress Basinger
KIMBA: Cartoon lion
KIMBALL: Organ maker
KIMBLE: "The Fugitive" role
KIMCHEE: Korean dish
KIMCHI: Korean dish
KIMPO: Seoul's airport
KINA: Papua New Guinea currency
KINCAID: "Law & Order" character
KINDA: In a way
KINE: Action: Comb. form
KINER: Ralph of baseball
KINESIS: Movement
KINGLET: Small bird
KINGMAN: Arizona city
KING ME: Checkers order
KING RAT: Clavell novel
KINISON: Comedian Sam
KINKAID: WWII admiral
KINKO'S: Copy-center chain
KINMONT: Actress Kathleen
KINNAN: Author Marjorie __ Rawlings
KINNEAR: Actor Greg
KINNELL: Poet Galway
KINS: Diminutive suffix
KINSEY: Liam Neeson role
KINSKI: "Tess" star
KINTE: "Roots" surname
KIOWA: Southwestern Indian
KIP: Laotian money
KIPLING: "Kim" novelist
KIPPER: Smoked herring
KIPPUR: Yom __
KIR: Wine drink
KIRBY: Puckett of baseball
KIRI: Opera star __ Te Kanawa
KIRIN: Beer brand
KIRK: "Star Trek" captain
KIRKS: Scottish churches
KIRKUK: Iraq city
KIRMAN: Persian carpet
KIROV: Russian ballet
KIRSCH: Cherry: German
KIRSTEN: Actress Dunst
KIRSTIE: Actress Alley
KISER: Actor Terry
KISHKA: Stuffed deli item
KISHKE: Stuffed deli item
KISKA: Aleutian island
KISLEV: Hebrew month
KISSEL: 1920s auto
KISSIN': __ cousins
KIST: Star-__ tuna
KITAEN: Actress Tawny
KITH: Acquaintances
KITHARA: Ancient harplike instrument
KITKAT: Candy brand
KITT: Singer Eartha
KITTERY: Maine town
KITTS: St. __ (Caribbean island)
KIVA: Pueblo chamber
KIWANIS: Civic group
KIWI: New Zealand bird
KIX: Cereal brand
KJELLIN: Actor Alf
K.J.V.: Bible edition: Abbr.
K-K-K-KATY: Song of 1918
KLAATU: "The Day the Earth Stood Still" character
KLAMATH: __ Falls, OR
KLAMM: "The Castle" character
KLAMMER: Austrian skier
KLATCH: Coffee __
KLATSCH: Coffee __
KLAUS: Actor Kinski
KLAXON: Harsh horn
KLEE: Swiss artist
KLEIBER: Austrian conductor
KLEIN: "Primary Colors" author
KLEINE: "Eine __ Nachtmusik"
KLEISER: Director Randal
KLEIST: German writer
KLEM: Baseball Hall of Fame umpire
KLENSCH: Fashion reporter Elsa
KLEZMER: Jewish music
KLIBAN: Cat cartoonist
KLICK: Kilometer, slangily
KLIEG: Film light
KLIMT: Austrian painter
KLINE: Actor Kevin
KLINGER: "M*A*S*H" role
KLINGON: "Star Trek" alien
KLINK: "Hogan's Heroes" role
KLINKER: Bergen dummy
KLISTER: Ski wax
KLM: European airline
KLUDGE: Clumsy fix
KLUGH: Jazz guitarist
KLUGMAN: "The Odd Couple" star
KLUM: Supermodel Heidi
KLUMP: "Nutty Professor" role
KLUTE: Donald Sutherland film
K MESON: Subatomic particle
KNAG: "Nicholas Nickleby" character
KNAP: Sack starter
KNAR: Tree knot
KNEBEL: Author Fletcher
KNEES-UP: British dance party
KNESSET: Israeli parliament
KNICK: NBA player
KNIEVEL: Daredevil Evel
KNISH: Baked turnover
KNOPF: Publisher Alfred
KNORR: Soup brand
KNOSSOS: Ancient city in Crete
KNOTT: Berry Farm founder
KNOTTS: Comedian Don
KNOUT: Kind of whip
KNOWLES: Singer Beyoncé
KNOX: Fort __, KY
KNT.: Titled Brit.
KNUR: Bump on a log
KNURL: Button ridge
KNUT: Author Hamsun
KNUTE: Football coach Rockne
KOA: Hawaiian tree
KOAN: Zen paradox
KOB: African antelope
KOBE: Japanese city
KOBLENZ: German city
KOBO: Nigerian coin
KOBOLD: Elf
KOCH: Former New York mayor
KOCHEL: Mozart cataloguer
KOCHER: Swiss medicine Nobelist
KO'D: Bested in the ring
KODALY: Hungarian composer
KODEL: Synthetic fabric
KODES: Czech tennis pro
KODIAK: Alaska bear
KOEHLER: Harold Arlen collaborator
KOENIG: "Star Trek" actor
K. OF C.: Fraternal org.
KOFI: Annan of the U.N.
K. OF P.: Fraternal org.
KOH: Potassium hydroxide
KOHL: Former German leader
KOHLER: German medicine Nobelist
KOHL'S: Department store
KOI: Japanese carp
KOJAK: Savalas role
KOJI: Soy-sauce ingredient
KOKO: Cartoon clown
KOKOMO: Indiana city
KOL: "__ Nidre" (Jewish prayer)
KOLA: African tree
KOLA NUT: Soft-drink ingredient
KOLKATA: City of India
KOLN: German city
KOMATSU: Construction machine brand
KOMBAT: Mortal __ (video game)
KOMBU: Japanese cooking ingredient
KOMODO: __ dragon (large reptile)
KON: "__-Tiki" (Heyerdahl craft)
KONA: Hawaiian wind
KONG: Ape of films
KONICA: Camera brand
KONRAD: German statesman Adenauer
KON-TIKI: Heyerdahl craft
KOO: Chinese statesman
KOOKIE: Edd Byrnes role
KOOL: __ & the Gang (R&B group)
KOOL-AID: Drink-mix brand
KOONING: Painter Willem de __
KOONTZ: Novelist Dean
KOOP: Former surgeon general
KOOSH: Brand of kid's ball
KOP: Keystone character
KOPECK: Russian money
KOPEK: Russian money
KOPELL: Actor Bernie
KOPF: Head: German
KOPFE: Heads: German
KOPH: Hebrew letter
KOPIT: Playwright Arthur
KOPIYKA: Ukrainian money
KOPJE: South African hill
KOPPEL: TV newsman Ted
KORAT: Cat breed
KORBUT: Gymnast Olga
KORDA: Author Michael
KORDELL: Stewart of football
KORMAN: Comedian Harvey
KORN: "Hee Haw" radio station
KORS: Fashion designer Michael
KORUNA: Czech money
KOSAR: Bernie of football
KOSCINA: Actress Sylva
KOSHIBA: Japanese physics Nobelist
KOSOVAR: Certain European
KOSOVO: European region
KOSS: Headphone brand
KOSSEL: German medicine Nobelist
KOSSUTH: Hungarian statesman
KOSTER: Director Henry
KOSYGIN: 1960s Russian leader
KOTCH: Matthau film
KOTO: Japanese zither
KOTTER: Gabe Kaplan character
KOTTKE: Guitarist Leo
KOTTO: Actor Yaphet
KOUFAX: Sandy of baseball
KOVACS: Comedian Ernie
KOVIC: "Born on the Fourth of July" subject
KOWLOON: Chinese peninsula
KOZ: Sax player Dave
K-PAX: Kevin Spacey film
K.P. DUTY: Mil. assignment
K.P.H.: Metric velocity meas.
KRA: Malay isthmus

KRAAL: African cattle enclosure
KRACKEL: Chocolate-bar brand
KRAFT: Food conglomerate
KRAIT: Asian snake
KRAKEN: Norwegian sea monster
KRAKOW: City in Poland
KRAMDEN: "The Honeymooners" surname
KRAMER: Director Stanley
KRAMNIK: Russian chessmaster
KRANTZ: Author Judith
KRASNA: Screenwriter Norman
KRASNER: Artist Lee
K RATION: Army meal
KRAUS: Austria writer
KRAUSS: Country singer Alison
KRAUT: Hot-dog topper
KRAVIS: Financier Henry
KRAZY: "__ Kat"
KREBS: Dobie Gillis pal
KREME: Krispy __
KRENEK: Composer Ernst
KREPS: Carter cabinet member
KRESGE: Department-store magnate
KRESKIN: "Amazing" mentalist
KRESS: Dime-store magnate
KREUK: Actress Kristin
KREWE: New Orleans social club
KRIEG: War: German
KRIGE: Actress Alice
KRILL: Whale food
KRINGLE: Santa alias
KRIPS: Austrian conductor
KRIS: Singer Kristofferson
KRISHNA: Avatar of Vishnu
KRISPY: __ Kreme
KRISS: Mr. Kringle
KRISTI: Skater Yamaguchi
KRISTIN: Actress __ Scott Thomas
KROC: McDonald's founder
KROCK: Pulitzer journalist Arthur
KROEMER: Physics Nobelist Herbert
KROFFT: Kids' TV producer
KROFT: Steve of "60 Minutes"
KROGER: Supermarket chain
KROGH: Danish medicine Nobelist
KRONA: Swedish money
KRONE: Danish money
KRONER: Norwegian money
KRONOR: Swedish money
KRONUR: Icelandic money
KROON: Estonian money
KROTO: British chemistry Nobelist
KRUEGER: Elm Street terrorizer
KRUGER: South African statesman
KRUK: John of baseball
KRULL: Thomas Mann character
KRUPA: Drummer Gene
KRUPP: German industrialist
KRUPS: German appliance brand
KRUSTY: "The Simpsons" clown
KRYLON: Spray-paint brand
KRYLOV: Russian fable writer
KRYPTO: Superman's dog
KRYPTON: Superman's birthplace
KRYSTLE: "Dynasty" role
K STAR: Spectral type
K.S.U.: Big Twelve sch.
K-SWISS: Tennis-shoe brand
K-TEL: Informercial company
K TILE: Scrabble five-pointer
K.T. OSLIN: Country singer
KTS.: Jeweler's measures: Abbr.
K TWO: Himalayan peak
KUALA: __ Lumpur, Malaysia
KUBEK: Tony of baseball
KUBELIK: Czech conductor
KUBLA: "__ Khan" (Coleridge poem)
KUBLAI: Genghis' grandson
KUBLER: Author Elisabeth __-Ross
KUBRICK: Director Stanley
KUCHEN: German cake
KUDO: Accolade
KUDROW: "Friends" actress
KUDU: African antelope
KUDZU: Chinese vine
KUGEL: Jewish casserole
KUHN: Former baseball commissioner
KUKLA: Dragon of kids' TV
KULAK: Russian peasant
KULIK: Director Buzz
KULP: Actress Nancy
KUMIN: Poet Maxine
KUMMEL: German liqueur
KUN: Former Hungarian leader
KUNDERA: Czech author
KUNDRY: "Parsifal" character
KUNG FU: Martial art
KUNITZ: Poet Stanley
KUNTA: "Roots" character
KUNZEL: Conductor Erich
KUPRIN: Russian novelist
KURALT: CBS newsman
KURD: Certain Asian
KURILE: Japanese island group
KURT: Actor Russell
KURTZ: Actress Swoosie
KURUS: Turkish money
KURYS: Director Diane
KUSCH: 1955 Physics Nobelist
KUTCHER: Actor Ashton
KUTUZOV: Russian military leader
KUVASZ: Hungarian dog
KUZNETS: 1971 economics Nobelist
KVACK: Hägar the Horrible's duck
KVASS: Russian beer
KVELL: Burst with pride
KWA: African language
KWACHA: Malawi money
KWAI: "The Bridge on the River __"
KWAME: Nkrumah of Ghana
KWAN: Suzie Wong portrayer
KWANZA: Angolan coin
KWANZAA: African-American festival
KWEISI: Mfume of the NAACP
KWH: Elec. meas.
KWON: Tae __ do (martial art)
KYAT: Myanmar money
KYD: British dramatist
KYLE: Actor MacLachlan
KYLIE: Singer Minogue
KYOODLE: Bark
KYOTO: Japanese city
KYRA: Actress Sedgwick
KYRIE: "__ eleison" (Mass section)
KYSER: Bandleader Kay
KYUSHU: Japanese island
KYZYL: __ Kum (Asian desert)

L

LAA-LAA: One of the Teletubbies
LA BAMBA: Ritchie Valens tune
LABAN: Father of Rachel
LABATT'S: Canadian beer brand
LA BELLE: Singer Patti
LABIALS: Some consonants
LABILE: Changeable
LABINE: "The Boys of Summer" subject
LABIUM: Lip
LABOR AT: Overplay
LAB RAT: Maze runner
LA BREA: Tar: Spanish
LAB TECH: Hospital worker
LAC: Varnish ingredient
LA CAGE: Broadway musical, for short
LA CASA: House: Spanish
LA CAVA: Director Gregory
LACERTA: Lizard constellation
LACEY: "Alfie" character
LACHEY: Pop singer Nick
LA CHOY: Chinese food brand
LACIE: Lewis Carroll character
LACKWIT: Fool
LACLOS: "Dangerous Liaisons" author
LACONIA: New Hampshire city
LACOSTE: French tennis pro
LACRIMO: Fashion designer Christian
LACT: Milk: Comb. form
LACTAID: Dairy product substitute
LACTASE: Enzyme
LACTEA: Via __ (Milky Way)
LACTEAL: Milky
LACTI: Milk: Comb. form
LACTIC: Acid from milk
LACTO: Milk: Comb. form
LACTOSE: Milk sugar
LACUNA: Gap
LA CUREE: Zola work
LADA: Russian auto
LAD A DOG: Terhune novel
LADD: Actor Alan
LA-DI-DA: Pretentious exclamation
LADINO: Wild horse
LADOGA: Largest lake in Europe
LA DOUCE: Irma's epithet
LADRONE: Southwestern bandit
LADUKE: Native American author
LADY DAY: Billie Holiday's nickname
LADY DI: 1981 royal bride
LADY L: Sophia Loren film
LADYNAS: King Arthur knight
LADY'S: "The __ Got Potential" ("Evita" tune)
LAE: New Guinea port
LAEMMLE: Universal Studios founder
LAENNEC: Stethoscope inventor
LAERTES: "Hamlet" role
LA FARGE: Novelist Oliver
LA FEMME: Churchy __ ("Pogo" character)
LA FEU: "All's Well That Ends Well" character
LAFF: Gag reaction, informally
LAFFER: Economist Arthur
LAFITTE: French pirate
LAFLEUR: Guy of hockey
LAGASSE: Food Network chef
L.A. GEAR: Shoe brand
LAGO: Lake: Spanish
LAGOS: Nigerian city
LAGUNA: Inlet
LAH: __-di-dah
LAHAINA: Maui city
LAHORE: City in Pakistan
LAHR: Cowardly Lion portrayer
LAHTI: Actress Christine
LAI: Medieval French poem
LAIC: Not of the clergy
LAIKA: Russian space dog
LAILA: Boxer Ali
LAINE: Singer Frankie
LAING: British psychiatrist
LAINIE: Singer Kazan
LAIRD: Nixon defense secretary
LAIRDS: Scottish landowners
LAISSEZ: __-faire
LAIT: Café au __
LAIUS: Father of Oedipus
LAJOIE: Napoleon of baseball
LA JOLLA: City near San Diego
LAK': "Mighty __ a Rose" (old song)
LAKIST: Wordsworth or Coleridge
LAKME: Delibes opera
LAKOTA: Western Indian
LAKSHMI: Hindu goddess
LAL: Indian statesman Shastri
L.A. LAKER: Basketball pro
LA LANNE: Fitness guru Jack
L.A. LAW: 1980s NBC drama
LALIA: Speech: Comb. form
LALIQUE: French glass designer
LALL: Pronounce R's incorrectly
LALLA: "__ Rookh" (Moore poem)
LALO: Composer Schifrin
LA LOOSH: "Bull Durham" character
LAMAR: Truman birthplace
LAMARCK: French naturalist
LAMARR: Actress Hedy
LAMAS: Actor Fernando
LAMAZE: Birthing training
LAMBADA: 1990s fad dance
LAMBDA: Greek letter
LAMBEAU: Football coach Curly
LAMBENT: Glowing
LAMBERT: St. Louis airport
LAMBETH: Borough of London
LAMED: Hebrew letter
LA MESA: California city
LAMIA: Female demon
LAMINA: Thin layer

LAM INTO: Hit hard
LAM IT: Flee
LAMONT: The Shadow's secret identity
LA MOTTA: "Raging Bull" subject
LAMOTTE: "The Forsyte Saga" character
LAMOUR: Costar of Hope and Crosby
LAMPERT: Actress Zohra
LAMPREY: Type of eel
LAN: Office computer system: Abbr.
LANA: Actress Turner
LANAI: Hawaiian veranda
LANARK: Historic Scottish county
LANATE: Woolly
LANCET: Small knife
LANCIA: Italian auto
LANCIE: Actor John de __
LANCOME: Cosmetics brand
LANDAU: Actor Martin
LANDAUS: Types of carriages
LANDERS: Advice columnist
LANDI: Actress Elissa
LANDINI: Italian composer
LANDIS: "Animal House" director
LANDLER: Austrian dance
LANDMAN: Compatriot
LANDO: "Return of the Jedi" character
LANDON: "Bonanza" actor
LANDOR: British poet
LANDRY: Football coach Tom
LANDSAT: Map-making Earth orbiter
LANDTAG: German parliament
LANDUS: Pope
LANFORD: Playwright Wilson
LANG: Singer k.d.
LANGDON: Silents comedian Harry
LANGE: Actress Jessica
LANGER: Golfer Bernhard
LANGHAM: Actor Wallace
LANGLEY: CIA headquarters
LANGTON: British theologian
LANGTRY: Actress Lillie
LANGUID: Sluggish
LANGWAY: Rod of hockey
LANI: 1988 Miss America Kaye __ Rae Rafko
LANIER: Bob of basketball
LANIN: Bandleader Lester
LA NINA: The girl: Spanish
LANKA: Sri __
LANNY: Golfer Wadkins
LANO: Wool: Comb. form
LANOLIN: Shampoo ingredient
LANOS: Daewoo model
LANOSE: Woolly
LA NOTTE: 1961 Italian film
LANSING: Michigan capital
LANSKY: Crime boss Meyer
LANSON: Singer Snooky
LANTANA: Florida city
LANTOS: California congressman
LANTZ: Woody Woodpecker creator
LANVAL: King Arthur knight
LANVIN: Perfume brand
LANYARD: Nautical rope
LANZA: Opera singer Mario
LAO: Southeast Asian
LAOCOON: Priest of Troy
LAO-TSE: Chinese philosopher
LAO-TZU: Chinese philosopher
LA PALMA: California city
LAP AT: Wash against
LA PAZ: Bolivian city
L.A.P.D.: "Dragnet" org.
LA PERI: Dukas ballet
LAPERM: Cat breed
LAPHAM: Fictional Silas
LAPIN: Rabbit fur
LAPIS: __ lazuli
LA PLACA: Actress Alison
LAPLACE: French astronomer
LAPLAND: Norwegian region
LA PLATA: Argentina city
LA PORTE: Indiana city
LAPPET: Garment flap
LAP ROBE: Outdoor blanket
LAPSANG: Chinese tea
LAPSUS: Error
LAPTEV: Asian sea
LAPUTA: "Gulliver's Travels" land
LAPWARE: Computer games for infants
LAPWING: European bird
LAR: Malay gibbon
LARA: "Doctor Zhivago" character
LARAINE: Actress Day
L.A. RAM: Former NFL player
LARAMIE: Wyoming city
LARA'S: "__ Theme" ("Doctor Zhivago" tune)
LA RAZA: Mexican-Americans
L'ARC: __ de Triomphe
LARCH: European tree
LARDER: Cupboard
LARDNER: Author Ring
LARDON: Chef's fat strip
LAREDO: Texas city
LAREDOS: Jeep models
LAREE: Maldives coin
LARES: Guardian spirits
LARGENT: Steve of football
LARGE O.J.: Breakfast order
LARGESS: Generosity
LARGO: Slow, in music
LARI: Maldives coin
LARINE: Gull-like
LARKIN: "Atlas Shrugged" character
LARMEN: Japanese noodles
LARMOR: British mathematician
LAROCHE: French designer
LA ROSA: Singer Julius
LARRUP: Thrash
LARRY: One of the Stooges
LARS: Swedish form of Lawrence
LARSEN: Jack London character
LARSON: Singer Nicolette
LARTER: Actress Ali
LARTET: French anthropologist
LARUE: Film cowboy Lash
LA RUSSA: Baseball manager Tony
LARVA: Caterpillar
LARY: Football great Yale
LA SALLE: French explorer
LA SCALA: Milan opera house
LASCAR: Sailor of India
LASCAUX: French site of prehistoric art
LASE: Emit coherent light
LASHUP: Improvisation
LASIK: Vision-correction procedure
LASKER: German chessmaster
LASKI: British political scientist
LASKY: Pioneer Hollywood producer
LASORDA: Baseball manager Tommy
LASSE: Finnish runner Viren
LASSEN: California volcano
LASSER: Income-tax book author
LAST DON: Puzo title character
LASTEX: Stretchable thread
LAST GAS: Service-station sign
LAST ONE: Rotten egg, perhaps
L.A. STORY: Steve Martin film
LASZLO: "Casablanca" role
LAT: Back muscle, for short
LATEEN: Type of sail
LA TENE: Iron Age culture
LATE OF: Recently from
LATE ON: Slow to swing at, as a pitch
LATERAN: Church of Rome
LATERI: Side: Comb. form
LATERO: Side: Comb. form
LATE TAG: Infielder's woe
LATH: Wooden strip
LATHEN: Whodunit author Emma
LATHY: Long and thin
LATICES: Rubbery liquids
LATIFAH: Actress Queen
LATIGO: Saddle strap
L.A. TIMES: California daily
LATIN I: Language course
LATIN II: Language course
LATINUS: "The Aeneid" character
LATKA: "Taxi" character
LATKE: Potato pancake
LA TOSCA: Sardou play
LA TOUR: French painter
LA TOYA: Singer Jackson
LATRELL: Sprewell of basketball
LATRIA: Form of worship
LATROBE: Psnnsylvania town
LATTE: Coffeehouse order
LATVIA: European nation
LAU: Charlie of baseball
LAUDA: Auto racer Niki
LAUDE: Magna cum __
LAUE: 1914 physics Nobelist
LAUER: "Today" cohost
LAUGH-IN: 1960s TV series
LAU LAU: Luau dish
LAUPER: Singer Cyndi
LAURA: Jenna Bush's mom
LAUREN: Actress Bacall
LAURENT: Yves Saint __
LAUREY: "Oklahoma!" character
LAURIA: Actor Dan
LAURIC: Acid in soaps
LAURIE: "Annie __" (old poem)
LAURITZ: Tenor Melchior
LAURO: "Achille __" (cruise ship)
LAURYL: __ alcohol (detergent ingredient)
LAURYN: Singer Hill
LAUTER: Actor Ed
LAUTREC: Toulouse-__
LAV: Washroom, for short
LAVABO: Washbowl
LAVACHE: "All's Well That Ends Well" character
LAVAGE: Washing
LAVAIN: King Arthur knight
LAVAINE: "Idylls of the King" character
LAVAL: Canadian city
LA VALSE: Ravel ballet
LAVE: Wash
LAVELLI: Dante of football
LAVER: Rod of tennis
LAVERAN: French medicine Nobelist
LAVERN: Singer Baker
LAVERNE: Andrews sister
LAVERS: Water bowls
LAVI: Actress Dahlia
LA VIDA: Life: Spanish
LA VIE: Life: French
LAVIN: "Alice" star
LAVINIA: "The Aeneid" character
LAVORIS: Mouthwash brand
LA WANDA: Actress Page
LAWD: "Green Pastures" character
LAWES: Sing Sing warden
LAWFORD: Actor Peter
LAWSON: Actress Twiggy
LAWTON: Oklahoma city
LAXALT: Former Nevada senator
LAYLA: Eric Clapton tune
LAYNE: Bobby of football
LAZAR: Agent Swifty
LAZARUS: Poet Emma
LA-Z-BOY: Recliner brand
LAZENBY: 007 portrayer
LAZONGA: Dance teacher of song
LAZULI: Lapis __
LAZZERI: Tony of baseball
L BAR: Girder
L BEAM: Girder
LBJ: JFK successor
LBO: Wall St. deal
L.C.D.: Math. term
L'CHAIM: Hebrew toast
L'CHAYIM: Hebrew toast
L.C.M.: Math. term
LDL: "Bad" cholesterol
L-DOPA: "Awakenings" drug
LDR.: CEO, e.g.
L.D.S.: Mormon church: Abbr.
LEACH: Dissolve out
LEACOCK: Canadian humorist
LEADETH: Lord's Prayer verb
LEAD ORE: Galena
LEAF OUT: Burgeon
LEAH: Wife of Jacob
LEAHY: WWII admiral
LEAKE: British topographer
LEAKEYS: Anthropologist family
LEAL: Faithful: Scottish

LEANDER: Lover of Hero
LEANN: Singer Rimes
LEANNE: Author Banks
LEAR: Shakespearian king
LEAR'S: Former women's magazine
LEARY: Counterculture guru
LEAUD: Actor Jean-Pierre
LEAVEN: Add yeast to
LEAWOOD: Kansas town
LEB.: Neighbor of Isr.
LE BARON: Chrysler model
LE BEAU: "Hogan's Heroes" role
LEBLANC: Actor Matt
LEBRET: Friend of Cyrano
LE BROCK: Actress Kelly
LEBRON: James of basketball
LEBRUN: 1930s French president
LECAIN: Artist Errol
LE CAR: 1970's auto
LE CARRE: Spy novelist
LECH: Walesa of Poland
LECHE: Milk: French
LECHER: Libertine
LE CID: French drama about a Spanish hero
LECKY: Irish essayist
LECON: Lesson: French
LECONTE: French poet __ de Lisle
LECT.: Coll. class
LECTER: "Silence of the Lambs" villain
LECTOR: College teacher
LECTRIC: __ Shave (pre-shave lotion)
LECUONA: Cuban composer
LEDA: Mother of Helen
LEDEE: Ricky of baseball
LEDER: Director Mimi
LEDERER: Ann Landers's real surname
LEDOUX: French architect
LEDS: Watch displays
LEE ANN: Singer Womack
LEECH: Parasite
LEECHEE: Chinese tree
LEEDS: Yorkshire city
LEEFORD: "Oliver Twist" character
LEE J.: Actor Cobb
LEEKIE: Cock-a-__ (Scottish soup)
LEELEE: Actress Sobieski
LEE MAY: 1970s baseballer
LEEVES: Actress Jane
LEEZA: TV host Gibbons
LE FAY: King Arthur sorceress
LE FREAK: 1978 disco tune
LEGANZA: Daewoo model
LEG ART: High-fashion hosiery
LEGATE: Envoy
LEGATEE: Beneficiary
LEGATO: Smooth musical passage
LEGATOR: One who bequeaths
LEGER: French artist
LEGG: Mason's Wall Street partner
L'EGGS: Hosiery brand
LEGHORN: Chicken breed
LEG IRON: Manacle
LEGIST: Attorney
LEGNO: Col __ (music term)
LEGO: Kids block brand
LEGOLAS: "Lord of the Rings" character
LEG-PULL: Comical hoax
LEGRAND: Composer Michel
LEGREE: Fictional Simon
LEG REST: Recliner part
LEG-ROPE: Surfboard attachment
LEGROS: Actor James
LEGS IT: Walks
LE GUIN: Author Ursula
LEG UP: Advantage
LEHAR: "Merry Widow" composer
LE HAVRE: French port
LEHI: Utah city
LEHIGH: Allentown's river
LEHIGH U.: Pennsylvania school
LEHMAN: Golfer Tom
LEHMANN: German soprano
LEHN: French chemistry Nobelist
LEHNEN: Lean: German
LEHR: Glass oven
LEHRER: Satirist Tom
LEHUA: Hawaiian flower
LEIA: "Star Wars" heroine
LEIBNIZ: German mathematician
LEICA: Camera brand
LEIDEN: Dutch city
LEIF: Explorer Ericson
LEIGH: Actress Janet
LEILA: Bizet opera character
LEIPZIG: German city
LEISEN: Director Mitchell
LEISTER: Fish spear
LEITER: 007 ally
LEITH: Scottish port
LEITRIM: Irish county
LEIX: Irish county
LEJEUNE: North Carolina Marine base
LEK: Albanian coin
LELA: Actress Rochon
LELAND: Charles Foster Kane aide
LELIA: George Sand novel
LELOIR: Argentine chemistry Nobelist
LELOUCH: French director
LELY: Dutch painter
LEM: Project Apollo vehicle
LEMA: Golfer Tony
LEMAN: Sweetheart, old-style
LE MANS: French auto race
LE MAT: "Melvin and Howard" actor
LE MAY: 1960s Air Force chief of staff
LEMIEUX: Mario of hockey
LEMMA: Proposition in logic
LEMMATA: Propositions in logic
LEMME: Slangy demand
LEMMING: Mouselike rodent
LEMMON: Actor Jack
LEMNOS: Aegean island
LE MOKO: Charles Boyer role
LEMOND: Bike racer Greg
LE MONDE: French newspaper
LEMOYNE: Syracuse college
LEMPIRA: Honduras money
LEMUEL: Gulliver's first name
LEMUR: African primate
LEN: Author Deighton
LENA: Singer Horne
LENAIN: French painter
LENAPE: Delaware Indian
LENARD: Acrtor Mark
LENDL: Ivan of tennis
LENES: Certain consonants
L'ENFANT: Designer of Washington, D.C.
L'ENGLE: "A Wrinkle in Time" author
LENGUA: Tongue: Spanish
LENI: Director Riefenstahl
LENINA: "Brave New World" character
LENIS: Certain consonant
LENITY: Gentleness
LENNI: __ Lenape (Delaware Indian)
LENNIE: "Of Mice and Men" character
LENNON: One of the Beatles
LENNONS: Singing sisters
LENNOX: Air-conditioner brand
LENNY: Singer Kravitz
LENO: "Tonight Show" host
LENORE: Woman in a Poe poem
LENOS: Woven fabrics
LENOVO: Computer brand
LENOX: Chinaware brand
LENSMAN: Photographer
LENTE: Slow: French
LENTIGO: Freckle
LENTO: Musical tempo
LENYA: Singer Lotte
LENZ: Actress Kay
LEO G.: Actor Carroll
LEO GENN: British actor
LEO I: Pope
LEO II: Pope
LEO III: Pope
LEO IV: Pope
LEO IX: Pope
LEON: Boxer Spinks
LEONA: Hotelier Helmsley
LEONARD: Film critic Maltin
LEONATO: "Much Ado About Nothing" character
LEON DAY: Baseball Hall of Famer
LEONE: Sierra __
LEONI: Actress Téa
LEONIA: New Jersey city
LEONID: Russian leader Brezhnev
LEONIDS: Meteor shower
LEONINE: Like a lion
LEONORA: "Fidelio" heroine
LEONORE: Beethoven overture
LEOPOLD: Mozart's father
LEORA: "Arrowsmith" wife
LEO V: Pope
LEO VI: Pope
LEO VII: Pope
LEO VIII: Pope
LEO X: Pope
LEO XI: Pope
LEO XII: Pope
LEO XIII: Pope
LEPANTO: Greek port
LE PEN: French politician
LEPER: Outcast
LE PEW: Cartoon skunk
LEPIDUS: Roman general
LEPKE: Tony Curtis film
LEPPARD: Def __ (rock group)
LEPTON: Subatomic particle
LEPUS: Hare constellation
LER: Celtic sea god
LERIDA: Spanish city
LERNER: "Brigadoon" lyricist
LEROI: Poet Jones
LEROS: Greek island
LEROUX: French novelist
LEROY: Composer Anderson
LES: Bandleader Brown
LE SABRE: Buick model
LESAGE: "Gil Blas" author
LESBOS: Aegean island
LESCAUT: "Manon" role
LESE: __ majesty (high crime)
LE SHAN: Author Eda
LESLEY: Singer Gore
LESLIE: Actor Nielsen
LES MIZ: Broadway musical, for short
LESOTHO: African country
LES PAUL: Electric guitar pioneer
LESSEPS: Suez Canal engineer
LESSING: British novelist
LESS TAR: Cigarette ad claim
LEST: "__ we forget"
LESTAT: Anne Rice vampire
LESTER: Canadian statesman Pearson
LESTOIL: Household cleaner brand
LET 'EM IN: Wings tune
LET GO OF: Give up
LETHE: Mythical river
LET IT BE: Beatles tune
LETITIA: Etiquette expert Baldrige
LETO: Actor Jared
LE TOUR: French bike race, for short
LET'S EAT: "Dig in!"
LET'S SEE: "Hmm..."
LETT: Latvian
LETTISH: Latvian
LETTRE: Letter: French
LETTY: Feminist __ Cottin Pogrebin
LEU: Romanian coin
LEUCINE: Amino acid
LEUKO: White: Comb. form
LEUMI: Bank __ (Israeli bank)
LEUR: Their: French
LEURS: Their: French
LEUTZE: "Washington Crossing the Delaware" painter
LEV: Bulgarian coin
LEVA: Bulgaria coins
LEVADE: Dressage movement
LEVANT: Pianist Oscar
LE VAR: Actor Burton
LEVATOR: Type of muscle
LEVENE: Actor Sam
LEVERET: Young hare
LEVERT: Singer Gerald
LEVI: Strauss of jeans
LE VILLI: Puccini opera

LEVIN: "Deathtrap" author
LEVINE: Film producer Joseph E.
LEVIT.: O.T. book
LEVITE: Ancient Hebrew
LEVITT: 1940s housing innovator
LEVO: Counterclockwise: Comb. form
LEVON: Elton John tune
LEVU: Vanua __ (Fiji island)
LEW: Author Wallace
LEWES: British author
LEW HOAD: Australian tennis pro
LEWIS: "Arrowsmith" author
LEX: Superman foe Luthor
LEXAN: Shatterproof window material
LEXICAL: Word-related
LEXIS: Vocabulary
LEXMARK: Computer-printer brand
LEXUS: Luxury auto
LEXUS GS: Luxury auto model
LEXUS GX: Luxury auto model
LEXUS IS: Luxury auto model
LEXUS LS: Luxury auto model
LEXUS LX: Luxury auto model
LEXUS RX: Luxury auto model
LEXUS SC: Luxury auto model
LEY: Romanian coins
LEYDEN: Dutch cheese
LEYTE: Philippine island
L. FRANK: Author Baum
LGA: NYC airport
LGE.: T-shirt size: Abbr.
L.G.S: NFL positions
LGTH.: One-dimensional meas.
LHASA: Capital of Tibet
LHB: NFL position
L.H.D.: Honorary deg.
LHOTSE: Himalayan peak
LIAISE: Be a go-between
LIAM: Actor Neeson
LIANA: Amazon vine
LIANE: Amazon vine
LIANG: Chinese weight
LIAO: Chinese dynasty
LIAT: "South Pacific" child
LIB: Ad __
LIBBED: Ad-__
LIBBER: Activist of a sort
LIBBY: 1960 chemistry Nobelist
LIBBY'S: Vegetable brand
LIBER: Book of public records
LIBERIA: African nation
LIBERTE: Part of France's motto
LIBIDO: Freudian concept
LIBRAE: Pounds: Latin
LIBRE: Free: Spanish
LIBRI: Books: Latin
LIBRIS: Bookplate word
LIBRO: Book: Spanish
LIBYA: African country
LIC: Driv. __
LICHEE: Chinese nut
LICHT: Light: German
LICIA: Opera singer Albanese
LICKETY: __-split
LIDA: "__ Rose" ("Music Man" song)
LIDAR: Laser radar
LIDDY: G. Gordon of Watergate
LIDO: Beach resort
LIDWINA: Patron saint of skaters
LIE-ABED: Late riser
LIEB: Beloved: German
LIEBE: Love: German
LIEBER: "Ach du __!"
LIEBIG: German chemist
LIE-BY: British road shoulder
LIEDER: Songs: German
LIEF: Willing, old-style
LIEGE: Feudal lord
LIENEE: One with a mortgage
LIESL: "The Sound of Music" character
LIEST: Biblical verb
LIE TEST: Polygraph exam
LIEV: Actor Schreiber
LIEVIO: Ring-a-__
LIFAR: Russian ballet dancer
LIFE IS: Kander and Ebb song
LIFE NET: Firefighter gear
LIFO: Accounting abbr.
LIGAND: Antibody
LIGATE: Bind
LIGEIA: Poe short story
LIGER: Big-cat hybrid
LIGETI: Hungarian composer
LIGGETT: Myers' business partner
LIGHT ON: Discover
LIGN: Wood: Comb. form
LIGNE: Watchmaker length unit
LIGNI: Wood: Comb. form
LIGNIFY: Turn to wood
LIGNIN: Constituent of wood
LIGNITE: Form of coal
LIGNO: Wood: Comb. form
LIGNUM: Wood: Latin
LIGURIA: Italian region
LIKE SO: This way
LIKUD: Israel political party
LIKUTA: Zaire money
LI'L: "__ Abner"
LILA: Actress Kedrova
LILA LEE: Valentino co-star
LIL E. TEE: 1992 Kentucky Derby winner
LILI: Leslie Caron film
LILIA: Gymnast Popkopayeva
LILIAN: Novelist __ Jackson Braun
LILINAU: "Evangeline" character
LILIOM: Molnár work
LILITH: Adam's first wife
LIL' KIM: Rap artist
LILLE: French city
LILLI: Actress Palmer
LILLIAN: Jimmy Carter's mother
LILLIE: Actress Langtry
LILLIS: Bing Crosby's middle name
LILLY: Bob of football
LILO: "__ & Stitch" (2002 film)
LIM.: Bound: Abbr.
LIMA: Peru's capital
LIMACON: Geometric shape
LIMBIC: Marginal
LIMBURG: Dutch province
LIMINAL: Barely perceptible
LIMN: Clearly outline
LIMNITE: Iron ore
LIMOGES: French porcelain
LIMON: Mexican choreographer
LIMPET: Shellfish
LIMPID: Transparent
LIMPOPO: African river
LIN: Author Yutang
LINA: Director Wertmuller
LIN BIAO: 1960s Chinese defense minister
LINC.: Luxury car, for short
LIND: Singer Jenny
LINDA: Singer Ronstadt
LINDEN: Shade tree
LINDER: Actress Kate
LINDNER: "A Raisin in the Sun" character
LINDO: Pretty: Spanish
LINDORF: "Tales of Hoffman" character
LINDROS: Eric of hockey
LINDSAY: Actress Wagner
LINDSEY: Goober Pyle portrayer
LINDT: Swiss chocolatier
LINDY: 1930s dance
LINE A: Tax-form entry
LINEAR A: Ancient writing system
LINEAR B: Ancient writing system
LINE B: Tax-form entry
LINE C: Tax-form entry
LINE CUT: Kind of engraving
LINE DRY: One way to handle the laundry
LIN. FT.: Lumber meas.
LING: European fish
LINGCOD: Game fish
LINGLE: Pitcher Van __ Mungo
LINGU: Tongue: Comb. form
LINGUA: Language: Latin
LINGULA: Tongue-shaped object
LINGUS: Aer __ (Irish airline)
LINN: Actor Mark __-Baker
LINNET: Small bird
LINNEY: Actress Laura
LINO: Brit's floor covering
LIN PIAO: 1960s Chinese defense minister
LINSEED: Flax-oil source
LINTEL: Architectural support
LINTER: Fuzz-removing machine
LINTON: Anthopologist Ralph
LINUX: Computer operating system
LINZ: Austrian city
LINZER: __ torte
LIONEL: Toy-train brand
LIONELL: King Arthur knight
LIOTTA: Actor Ray
LIPARI: Island group off Sicily
LIPASE: Digestive enzyme
LI PENG: 1990s Chinese leader
LIPID: Fatty compound
LIPMANN: 1953 medicine Nobelist
LI PO: Chinese poet
LIP OFF: Talk without thinking
LIP OUT: Golf term
LIPP: Soprano Wilma
LIPPI: Italian painter
LIPPO: Fra __ Lippi
LIPTON: Tea brand
LIQUATE: Heat metal
LIRA: Turkish money
LIRE: Former Italian money
LIRR: A way to the Hamptons: Abbr.
LIS: Fleur-de-__
LISA: Actress Kudrow
LISA GAY: Actress Hamilton
LISBETH: "Adam Bede" character
LISBOA: European capital, to natives
LISENTE: Lesotho coins
LISI: Actress Virna
LISSE: Gauze fabric
LISSOME: Supple
LISTON: Boxer Sonny
LISZT: Hungarian composer
LITA: Singer Ford
LIT. B.: College deg.
LITCHI: Chinese nut
LIT CRIT: Novel analysis, for short
LIT. D.: College deg.
LITE: Lo-cal
LITEL: Actor John
LITH: Stone: Comb. form
LITHGOW: Actor John
LITHIC: Rocky
LITHIUM: Element #3
LITHO: Art print
LITHOID: Stony
LIT. M.: College deg.
LITMUS: Acid-test need
LIT ON: Discovered
LITOTES: Figure of speech
LITOVSK: Treaty of Brest-__
LITS: Beds: French
LITT. B.: College deg.
LITT. D.: College deg.
LITTRE: French philosopher
LITVAK: Director Anatole
LIU: Actress Lucy
LIV: Actress Tyler
LIVE AID: 1985 benefit rock concert
LIVE FOR: Like very much
LIVE ONE: Gullible sort
LIVERED: Lily-__ (scared)
LIVE SET: Concert recording
LIVESEY: Actor Roger
LIVETH: Biblical verb
LIVIA: "The Sopranos" mother
LIVIN': "Summertime and the __ is easy"
LIVORNO: Italian port
LIVRE: Book: French
LIVY: Roman historian
LIZ: Designer Claiborne
LIZA: Singer Minnelli
LIZA LU: "Tess of the d'Urbervilles" character
LIZETTE: Poet Reese
LIZZI: "Ship of Fools" character
LIZZIE: Tin __ (old auto)
LLADRO: Porcelain brand
LLANERO: Spanish cowboy
LLANO: Plain: Spanish
LL. B.: Law deg.
L.L. BEAN: Maine clothing merchant
LLC: Inc. kin

LL COOL J: Rap artist
LL. D.: Law deg.
LLEYTON: Hewitt of tennis
LL. M.: Law deg.
LLOSA: Author Mario Vargas __
LLOYD: Actor Bridges
LLOYD'S: British insurance association
L.M.A.: "Little Women" monogram
L.N.G.: Compressed fuel: Abbr.
LOA: Mauna __
LOAM: Rich soil
LOBAR: Like lungs
LOBATE: Like lungs
LOBO: Timber wolf
LOBULE: Small lobe
LOC: __ cit. (footnote abbr.)
LOCA: "Livin' La Vida __"
LOCANE: Actress Amy
LOCARNO: Swiss resort
LOC. CIT.: Footnote abbr.
LOCH: __ Ness monster
LOCHER: Pulitzer cartoonist Dick
LOCKA: Opa-__, FL
LOCKE: British philosopher
LOCKLIN: Country singer Hank
LOCO: Plumb __
LOCULUS: Altar compartment
LOCUM: Place: Latin
LOD: Israeli airport
LODEN: Thick fabric
LODER: MTV newsman
LODI, NJ: Garden State city
LODZ: Austrian city
LOEB: Singer Lisa
L'OEIL: Trompe __
LOESS: Windborne soil
LOESSER: "Guys and Dolls" composer
LOEW: MGM cofounder
LOEWE: "Brigadoon" composer
LOEWI: German medicine Nobelist
LOEW'S: Cinema chain
LOEWY: NASA interior designer
LO-FAT: Good for dieters
LOFTON: Kenny of baseball
LOFTUS: Man O'War jockey
LOGAN: Boston airport
LOGAN'S: "__ Run" (1976 film)
LOGAN, UT: Beehive State city
LOGGIA: Actor Robert
LOGGIAS: Open-air galleries
LOGGINS: Rock singer Kenny
LOGIA: Religious sayings
LOG IN: Access a computer network
LOG ON: Access a computer network
LOGROLL: Do some politicking
LOGUE: Communication: Comb. form
LOGY: Sluggish
LOHAN: Actress Lindsay
LOI: Law: French
LOID: Burglar's device
LOIRE: French river
LOIRET: French department
LOIS: "Daily Planet" name
LOKI: Norse god
LOL: Chat-room guffaw
LOLA: Entertainer Falana
LOLICH: Mickey of baseball
LOLITA: Nabokov novel
LOLLARD: Wycliffe follower
LOM: "Pink Panther" films actor
LOMA: Southwestern ridge
LOMAN: Arthur Miller character
LOMAX: Music folklorist
LOMB: Bausch's partner
LOMBARD: Actress Carole
LOME: Capital of Togo
LO MEIN: Chinese noodles
LOMOND: Scottish loch
LOMPOC: California city
LON: Actor Chaney
LONBORG: Jim of baseball
LONDRES: British capital, in Paris
LONETTE: Actress McKee
LONGA: "Ars __, vita brevis"
LONG BED: Truck feature
LONGDEN: Triple Crown jockey
LONG E: Vowel sound
LONGES: Horse-guiding ropes
LONGET: Actress Claudine
LONG I: Vowel sound
LONGIES: Winter underwear
LONG O: Vowel sound
LONG TOM: WWII cannon
LONG TON: 2,240 pounds
LONG U: Vowel sound
LONGUE: Chaise __
LONI: Actress Anderson
LONIGAN: Studs of fiction
LONNIE: Singer Donegan
LON NOL: 1970s Cambodian leader
LOO: Card game
LOOBY: Awkward one
LOOEY: Sarge's superior
LOOFA: Bath sponge
LOOFAH: Bath sponge
LOOIE: Sarge's superior
LOOKISM: Sort of discrimination
LOOK MA: Attention-getting phrase
LOOMPAS: Oompa __ (Wonka employees)
LOONEY: __ Tunes (Warner Bros. cartoons)
LOONIE: Canadian coin
LOOS: Author Anita
LOOSEY: Goosey __
LOPAT: Eddie of baseball
LOPEZ: Actress Jennifer
LOQUAT: Chinese fruit
LORAIN: Ohio city
LORAN: Air navigation system
L'ORANGE: Duck à __
LORAX: Dr. Seuss character
LORCA: Spanish poet García __
LORD IT: Domineer
LORD JIM: Conrad novel
L'OREAL: Hair-coloring brand
LORELAI: "Gilmore Girls" mother
LORELEI: Rhine maiden
LOREN: Actress Sophia
LORENE: Mime Yarnell
LORENTZ: Dutch physicist
LORENZ: Lyricist Hart
LORENZO: Actor Lamas
LORETTA: Actress Swit
LORGNON: Opera glasses
LORI: Actress Petty
LORIENT: French port
LORIN: Conductor Maazel
LORING: Singer Gloria
LORIS: Lemur of India
LORNA: "__ Doone"
LORNE: Actor Greene
LORRE: "Casablanca" actor
LORRIE: Country singer Morgan
LORRY: Truck, in Britain
LORUS: Watch brand
LORY: Australian parrot
LOS DOS: Both, in Bolivia
LOSEY: Director Joseph
LOSIN': "__ It" (Tom Cruise film)
LOTET: __-Garonne (French department)
LOTHAIR: Holy Roman emperor
LOTHAR: Mandrake the Magician's assistant
LOTHIAN: Region in Scotland
LOTHROP: Children's author Harriet
LOTI: French author
LOT NO.: Auction ID
LOTOS: "The __ Eaters" (Tennyson poem)
LOTSA: "__ luck!"
LOTT: Former Senate majority leader
LOTTA: "Little" girl of comics
LOTTE: Singer Lenya
LOU: Comic Costello
LOU ANN: Gomer Pyle's girlfriend
LOUCHE: Disreputable
LOUDON: Actress Dorothy
LOUELLA: Gossip columnist Parsons
LOUIE: Sarge's superior
LOUISA: __ May Alcott
LOUIS B.: Mayer of MGM
LOUISE: Canadian lake
LOUIS I: French king
LOUIS II: French king
LOUIS IV: French king
LOUIS IX: French saint
LOUIS V: French king
LOUIS VI: French king
LOUIS X: French king
LOUIS XI: French king
LOUIS XV: French king
LOUMA: Armenian money
LOUP: Cloth mask
LOUPE: Jeweler's eyepiece
LOUR: Frown
LOURDES: French city
LOU REED: "Walk on the Wild Side" singer
LOURY: Gloomy
LOUTH: Irish county
LOUVIN: Country singer Charlie
LOUVRE: Paris museum
LOV: "Tobacco Road" character
LOVAGE: European herb
LOVE BUG: Herbie, in Disney films
LOVE-IN: Hippie gathering
LOVEJOY: Actor Frank
LOVELL: Apollo 13 astronaut
LOVE SET: Tennis shutout
LOVETT: Singer Lyle
LOVIN': "After the __" (Humperdinck tune)
LOWBOY: Chest of drawers
LOWCHEN: Dog breed
LOWE: Actor Rob
LOWEEZY: Snuffy Smith's wife
LOWELL: Poet Robert
LOWERY: Gloomy
LOWE'S: Home Depot competitor
LOW IQ: Barrier to Mensa
LOW ON: Running out of
LOW PH: Acid-test finding
LOW POST: Basketball-court area
LOW-RES: Not highly detailed, as a computer screen
LOWRY: Novelist Malcolm
LOW-SET: Stocky
LOW-TOP: Type of sneaker
LOXY: Foxy __
LOY: Actress Myrna
LOYALE: Subaru model
LOYD: Puzzlemaster Sam
LOYOLA: Chicago university
L.P.G.: Camper fuel: Abbr.
L.P.G.A.: Sorenstam org.
L.P. GAS: Bottled fuel
L.P.N.: Hosp. worker
L. RON: Author Hubbard
L.S.A.T.: Aspiring atty.'s exam
L.S.D.: Hallucinogen: Abbr.
L-SHAPED: "The __ Room" (Caron film)
L.S.T.: D-Day craft
L.S.U.: Baton Rouge sch.
L.T.A.: Like hot-air balloons: Abbr.
LT. COL.: Army rank: Abbr.
LT. COM.: Navy rank: Abbr.
LTD: Ford model
LT. GEN.: Army rank: Abbr.
LT. GOV.: State official: Abbr.
L TILE: Scrabble one-pointer
LT. J.G.: Navy rank: Abbr.
LT. KOJAK: Savalas TV role
LTS.: Army ranks: Abbr.
LT. SULU: "Star Trek" role
LT. YR.: Astronomy dist.
LUA: "Back to Methuselah" character
LUANA: Actress Anders
LUANDA: Capital of Angola
LUANG: __ Prabang (city in Laos)
LUANN: Greg Evans comic strip
LUB.: Auto job: Abbr.
LUBBER: Awkward one
LUBBOCK: Texas city
LUBECK: German city
LUBIN: Director Arthur
LUBLIN: Polish city
LUC: Director Jean-__ Godard
LUCAN: Roman poet
LUCANIA: Region of Italy
LUCARNE: Dormer window
LUCAS: "Star Wars" director
LUCCA: City of Italy
LUCCI: "All My Children" actress

LUCE: Cofounder of "Time"
LUCENT: Shining
LUCERNE: Swiss lake
LUCETTA: "Two Gentlemen of Verona" character
LUCHINO: Director Visconti
LUCI: 1960s First Daughter
LUCIA: "__ di Lammermoor"
LUCIAN: Greek satirist
LUCIANA: "Comedy of Errors" character
LUCIANO: Opera star Pavarotti
LUCIDA: Brightest star in a constellation
LUCIE: "A Tale of Two Cities" character
LUCIEN: "Count of Monte Cristo" character
LUCILE: Actress Watson
LUCILLE: Desi ex
LUCINDA: Choreographer Childs
LUCINE: Soprano Amara
LUCIO: "Measure for Measure" character
LUCITE: Kind of plastic
LUCIUS I: Pope
LUCKMAN: Sid of football
LUCKNOW: City of India
LUCRE: "Filthy" money
LUCY: Desi ex
LUCY LIU: "Charlie's Angels" star
LUDDEN: "Password" host
LUDDITE: Technology hater
LUDEN'S: Cough-drop brand
LUDIC: Playful
LUDLOW: Massachusetts town
LUDLUM: "The Bourne Identity" author
LUDWIG: Composer Beethoven
LUEGO: "Hasta __!"
LUELLA: Designer Bartley
LUFF: Sail into the wind
LUFT: Actress Lorna
LUGAR: Indiana senator
LUGLIO: July: Italian
LUGOSI: Dracula portrayer
LUI: Him: French
LUIGI: Playwright Pirandello
LUIS: "The Bridge of San __ Rey"
LUISA: "The Fantasticks" character
LUISE: Actress Rainer
LUIZ: "The Gondoliers" role
LUJAN: 1990s interior secretary
LUKA: "The Inspector General" character
LUKAS: Actor Haas
LUKE: Gospel writer
LUKICH: "The Inspector General" character
LUKS: Painter George
LULA: "Be-Bop-A-__"
LULEA: Swedish city
LULLY: French composer
LUM: Abner's radio friend
LUMA: Armenian money
LUMAN: Country singer Bob
LUMBAR: Kind of vertebra
LUMEN: Brightness unit
LUMET: Director Sidney
LUMIERE: French movie-camera inventor
LUMINA: Chevy model
LUMLEY: Actress Joanna
LUMPEN: Uprooted
LUMP IT: Don't accept a situation
LUMPUR: Kuala __, Malaysia
LUNA: Type of moth
LUNATE: Wrist bone
LUNCHY: Dull-witted
LUND: "Casablanca" character
LUNDEN: Former "Good Morning America" host
LUNDI: Monday: French
LUNDY: British island
LUNE: Moon: French
LUNEDI: Monday: Italian
LUNER: Actress Jamie
LUNESTA: Sleep-aid brand
LUNETTE: Crescent
LUNIK: Russian spacecraft
LUNKER: Big fish
LUNN: Sally __ (teacake)
LUNT: Actor Alfred
LUN THA: "The King and I" character
LUNTS: Distinguished acting couple
LUNULA: Fingernail crescent
LUPE: Actress Velez
LUPIN: Fictional detective
LUPINE: Wolflike
LUPINES: Tall flowers
LUPINO: Actress Ida
LU PONE: "Evita" Tony winner
LUPTON: Actor John
LUPUS: "Mission: Impossible" actor
LURAY: Virginia caverns
LURENE: Actress Tuttle
LUREX: Metallic yarn
LURIA: 1969 medicine Nobelist
LURIE: Author Alison
LURKEY: Turkey __
LURLEEN: Former Alabama governor Wallace
LUSAKA: Zambia capital
LUSTRUM: Half a decade
LUTECE: Big Apple restaurant
LUTETIA: Ancient name of Paris
LUTH.: Prot. denomination
LUTHER: Reformation figure
LUTHIER: Violin maker
LUTHOR: Superman foe
LUTHULI: 1960 peace Nobelist
LUTSK: Ukraine city
LUTZ: Figure-skating jump
LUV: Schisgal play
LUVS: Diaper brand
LUX: Illumination unit
LUXATE: Dislocate
LUXE: Class
LUXOR: Egyptian town
LUZ: Light: Spanish
LUZON: Philippine island
L.V.B.: Beethoven monogram
LVOV: Ukraine city
L WAVE: Seismograph reading
LWEI: Angolan money
LWOFF: 1965 medicine Nobelist
LYCEE: French school
LYCEUM: Academy
LYCO: Wolf: Comb. form
LYCOS: Internet search engine
LYCRA: Elastic material
LYDDITE: High explosive
LYDIA: Tattooed lady of song
LYDIAN: Church music mode
LYDON: Actor Jimmy
LYELL: British geologist
LYGIA: "Quo Vadis?" character
LYIN': "__ Eyes" (Eagles tune)
LYLE: Singer Lovett
LYLY: British playwright
LYMAN: __ Frank Baum
LYME: Old __, CT
LYMON: Singer Frankie
LYN: Reagan advisor Nofziger
LYNCH: Director David
LYND: "Middletown" author
LYNDA: Actress Carter
LYNDE: "Hollywood Squares" regular
LYNDON B.: President Johnson
LYNE: Director Adrian
LYNEN: 1964 medicine Nobelist
LYNETTE: "Idylls of the King" character
LYNG: Reagan cabinet member
LYNLEY: Actress Carol
LYNN: Actress Redgrave
LYNNE: Actress Thigpen
LYNX: Wildcat
LYNYRD: __ Skynyrd (rock group)
LYOCELL: Synthetic carpet fiber
LYON: French city
LYONELL: King Arthur knight
LYONNE: Actress Natasha
LYONS: French city
LYRA: Northern constellation
LYRAS: Glockenspiels
LYRICON: Electronic instrument
LYRID: Meteor shower
LYS: Belgian river
LYSE: Destroy, as cells
LYSENKO: Russian biologist
LYSINE: Amino acid
LYSIS: Cell breakdown
LYSOL: Household cleaner brand
LYTE: Fossil: Comb. form
LYTTON: British author Bulwer-__

M

MAA: Barnyard bleat
MAALOX: Antacid brand
MA AND PA: The folks
MAARTEN: Sint __ (Caribbean island)
MAAS: "Serpico" author
MAAZEL: Conductor Lorin
MAB: Fairy queen
MABEL: "Pirates of Penzance" heroine
MA BELL: Big name in telephony
MABLEY: Comic Moms
MACACO: African lemur
MACAO: Port near Hong Kong
MACAPA: Brazilian city
MACAQUE: Short-tailed monkey
MACDUFF: "Macbeth" role
MACEDON: Home of Alexander the Great
MACER: Ceremonial staff bearer
MACGRAW: Actress Ali
MACHAON: "Iliad" character
MACHE: Papier-__
MACHINA: Deus ex __ (literary device)
MACH ONE: The speed of sound
MACHREE: "Mother __" (Irish-American tune)
MACHU: __ Picchu (Incan city)
MACHY: Warfare: Comb. form
MACKE: German painter
MACKIE: Fashion designer Bob
MACLE: Twin crystal
MACLEAN: Novelist Alistair
MACLEN: Beatles music company
MACLEOD: Insulin discoverer
MACNEE: Actor Patrick
MACNEIL: PBS newscaster
MACOMB: Illinois city
MACON: French wine
MACON, GA: Southern city
MACOUN: Type of apple
MACR: Large: Comb. form
MACRAE: Actor Gordon
MACRON: Diacritical mark
MACULA: Skin spot
MAC USER: Apple Computer patron
MACY'S: Department store chain
MADALYN: Atheist O'Hair
MADAMA: "__ Butterfly"
MADAME X: Lana Turner film
MADCHEN: Actress Amick
MADD: Anti-DWI org.
MADDERS: Reddish dyes
MADDIE: "Moonlighting" role
MADDOX: Garry of baseball
MADDUX: Greg of baseball
MADEIRA: Portuguese wine
MADELON: "The Sin of __ Claudet" (Helen Hayes film)
MADERA: California city
MADERO: Mexican revolutionary
MADGE: TV-ad manicurist
MADIGAN: Actress Amy
MADISON: Wisconsin city
MAD-LIBS: Party word game
MADLOCK: Bill of baseball
MADLYN: Actress Rhue
MAD MAX: Mel Gibson role
MADOC: Southey epic poem
MADOX: Ford __ Ford (British writer)
MADRAS: Bay of Bengal city
MADRE: Mother: Spanish
MADRID: Capital of Spain
MADSEN: Actress Virginia
MAD TV: Fox comedy series
MADURO: Strong cigar
MADVIG: "The Glass Key" character
MAE: Ginnie __ (mortgage agency)

MAENAD: Dionysian priestess
MAEVE: Author Binchy
MAE WEST: "My Little Chicakdee" star
MAGALOG: Magazine/catalog
MAGDA: Gabor sister
MAGE: Ancient wizard
MAGEE: Actor Patrick
MAGGIE: Jiggs' wife
MAGGIO: Sinatra Oscar role
MAGILLA: Cartoon ape
MAGINOT: __ line (French fortification)
MAGLEV: High-speed train
MAGLIE: Sal of baseball
MAGMA: Molten rock
MAGNA: __ cum laude
MAGNANI: Actress Anna
MAGNOL: French botanist
MAGNON: Cro-__ man
MAGNUS: Great: Latin
MAGOG: Armageddon nation
MAGOO: Nearsighted toon
MAGUA: "Last of the Mohicans" character
MAGUIRE: Tom Cruise film role
MAGUS: Ancient sorcerer
MAGYAR: Hungarian
MAH: __-jongg
MAHAL: Taj __
MAHALIA: Singer Jackson
MAHALO: Thank you: Hawaiian
MAHAN: Naval historian
MAHARIS: Actor George
MAHATMA: Hindu sage
MAHDI: Muslim prophet
MAHER: "Politically Incorrect" host
MAHFOUZ: Egyptian literature Nobelist
MAHI: Hawaiian fish, on menus
MAHLER: German composer
MAHON: Minorca city
MAHONEY: Jerry __ (Paul Winchell dummy)
MAHOUT: Elephant driver
MAHRE: Olympic skier Phil
MAHZOR: Jewish prayer book
MAI: May: French
MAIA: Mother of Hermes
MAIGRET: Fictional detective
MAILLOL: French sculptor
MAILLOT: Type of swimsuit
MAIL TO: Shipping-label words
MAIMITI: "Mutiny on the Bounty" character
MAIN MAN: Best friend
MAIN ST.: Anytown, USA address
MAINTOP: Ship platform
MAINZ: German city
MAIO: May: Portuguese
MAIRE: Mayor: French
MAIRZY: "__ Doats" (old song)
MAIS: But: French
MAISIE: Henry James character
MAISON: House: French
MAIS OUI: Of course: French
MAI TAI: Rum drink
MAJA: Goya subject
MAJESTE: Lèse __ (high crime)
MAJEURE: Force __ (unexpected event)
MAJ. GEN.: Army rank: Abbr.
MAJLIS: Islamic parliament
MA JOAD: Steinbeck character
MAJORCA: Balearic Island
MAKEBA: Singer Miriam
MAKEM: Irish singer Tommy
MAKIN': "__ Whoopie" (old song)
MAKO: Type of shark
MAKSIM: Author Gorki
MAKUTA: Zaire money
MAL: __ de mer (seasickness)
MALA: __ fide (bad faith)
MALABAR: Coastal region of India
MALABO: African capital
MALACCA: Cane
MALACHI: Old Testament book
MALAGA: Spanish wine
MALAMUD: Author Bernard
MALAR: Cheekbone
MALAWI: Nyasaland, formerly
MALAY: Indonesia native
MALAYA: Asian peninsula
MALCOLM: "__ X" (Spike Lee film)
MALDEN: Actor Karl
MALDIVE: __ Islands (Indian Ocean nation)
MALEFIC: Evil
MALEIC: Acid used in fabric dyes
MALEV: Hungarian airline
MALI: African country
MALIBU: California beach
MALIC: Acid in apples
MALICK: Actress Wendie
MALLE: Director Louis
MALLEUS: Ear bone
MALLIKA: "Lakmé" role
MALLON: Pro golfer Meg
MALLOW: Okra family
MALMO: Swedish port
MALMSEY: Sweet wine
MALO: Bad: Spanish
MALONE: "Cheers" bar owner
MALORY: "Le Morte d'Arthur" author
MALOTI: Lesotho money
MALPASO: Eastwood production company
MALPH: "Happy Days" character
MALRAUX: French novelist
MALTA: Island near Sicily
MALTASE: Digestive enzyme
MALTBIE: Pro golfer Roger
MALTBY: Broadway lyricist Richard
MALTHUS: British economist
MALTIN: Film critic Leonard
MALTOSE: Type of sugar
MALVINA: Sculptor Hoffman
MALWARE: Malicious software
MAM: Mother
MAMA MIA: Italian exclamation
MAMBA: African snake
MAME: Broadway musical
MAMET: Playwright David
MAMIE: Mrs. Eisenhower
MAMMON: Material wealth
MANAGUA: Capital of Nicaragua
MANAMA: Capital of Bahrain
MANAOS: Brazilian city
MAN-APE: Missing link, perhaps
MANAT: Azerbaijan money
MANCHA: La __ (Don Quixote's home)
MANCHE: French department
MANCHU: Chinese dynasty
MANCINI: Film composer Henry
MANCUSO: Actor Nick
MANCY: Divination: Comb. form
MANDALA: Symbol of the universe
MANDAN: North Dakota Indian
MANDEL: Actor Howie
MANDELA: Former South African leader
M AND M'S: Candy brand
MANDOKI: Director Luis
MANDREL: Machine spindle
MANDY: Barry Manilow tune
MANEGE: Riding school
MANERO: "Saturday Night Fever" hero
MANET: French painter
MANETTE: "Tale of Two Cities" character
MANFRED: Byron poem
MANGA: Japanese graphic novel
MANGANO: Actress Silvana
MANHEIM: Actress Camryn
MANILOW: Singer Barry
MANIPLE: Church vestment
MANIPUR: State in India
MANKATO: Minnesota city
MANLEY: Poet Gerard __ Hopkins
MANN: German author
MANNE: Jazz drummer Shelly
MANNIES: Male nannies
MANNIX: TV sleuth
MANNON: "Mourning Becomes Electra" character
MANNY: Trillo of baseball
MANO: Hand: Spanish
MANOFF: Actress Dinah
MANOLIN: "Old Man and the Sea" character
MANON: Massenet opera
MAN O'WAR: Famous racehorse
MANQUE: Unsuccessful
MAN RAY: Dada artist
MANRICO: "Il Trovatore" hero
MANROPE: Gangplank handrail
MANSARD: Type of roof
MANSE: Minister's house
MAN'S MAN: Valet
MANTA: Devilfish
MANTECA: California town
MANTEE: Bogart in "The Petrified Forest"
MANTIC: Of prophesy
MANTLET: Short cape
MAN-TRAP: Dangerous female
MANTUA: Italian city
MANUEL: Composer de Falla
MANUMIT: Release
MANUS: Hand: Latin
MANUSH: Baseball great Heinie
MANUTE: Bol of basketball
MANX: Tailless cat
MANXMAN: Certain Brit
MANZON: Italian novelist
MAO: Former Chinese leader
MAO II: Don DeLillo novel
MAORI: New Zealand native
MAO SUIT: Beijing outfit
MAO-TAI: Chinese liquor
MAPES: Author Mary __ Dodge
MAPPLE: "Moby-Dick" character
MAPUTO: Capital of Mozambique
MAQUI: Evergreen shrub
MARA: NFL Giants owner
MARANTZ: Sound-system brand
MARAT: French Revolution figure
MARC: Painter Chagall
MARCA: __ registrada (Spanish trademark)
MARCATO: Musical direction
MARCEAU: French mime Marcel
MARCEL: Author Proust
MARCELS: "Blue Moon" performers
MARCHE: Bon __ (inexpensive: French)
MARCIA: Actress Strassman
MARCIE: "Peanuts" girl
MARCIL: Actress Vanessa
MARCI X: Lisa Kudrow film
MARCO: Italian explorer Polo
MARCONI: Radio inventor
MARCOS: Former Philippine leader
MARCUS: __ Aurelius (Roman emperor)
MARCUSE: German-born philosopher
MARCY: Adirondacks mountain
MARDEN: Painter Brice
MARDI: __ Gras
MARDIAN: "Antony and Cleopatra" role
MAREK: "My Antonia" character
MARENGO: Napoleon victory site
MARG: Actress Helgenberger
MARGATE: British resort
MARGAUX: Actress Hemingway
MARGE: Mrs. Homer Simpson
MARGERY: Daw of nursery rhymes
MARGIE: "My Little __" (sitcom)
MARGO: "Lost Horizon" star
MARGOT: Dancer Fonteyn
MARGRET: Actress Ann-__
MARGY: "State Fair" role
MARHAUS: King Arthur knight
MARI: Spouse: French
MARIA: "Ave __"
MARIAH: Singer Carey
MARIAN: Contralto Anderson
MARIANA: "Measure for Measure" character
MARIANO: Rivera of baseball
MARIAS: Black __ (police vans)
MARIDA: Wife: Spanish
MARIDO: Husband: Spanish
MARIE: Singer Teena
MARIEL: Actress Hemingway
MARIKO: "Shogun" character
MARILLA: "Anne of Green Gables" character

MARILU: Actress Henner
MARILYN: Actress Monroe
MARIN: California county
MARINO: Dan of football
MARIO: Author Puzo
MARION: Revolutionary War general
MARIS: Roger of baseball
MARISA: Actress Tomei
MARIST: New York college
MARJOE: Evangelist Gortner
MARKA: Bosnian money
MARKEY: Actress Enid
MARKHAM: Poet Edwin
MARK I: Early computer
MARKIE: Actress Post
MARK II: Early computer
MARK III: Early computer
MARK IV: Early computer
MARK IX: Jaguar model
MARKKA: Former Finnish coin
MARKKAA: Former Finnish coins
MARKOV: Russian mathematician
MARKOVA: Ballerina Alicia
MARK V: Lincoln model
MARK VI: Lincoln model
MARK VII: Lincoln model
MARL: Clay fertilizer
MARLA: Actress Gibbs
MARLEE: Actress Matlin
MARLENE: Actress Dietrich
MARLEY: Scrooge's partner
MARLO: Actress Thomas
MARLON: Actor Brando
MARLOWE: British playwright
MARM: Frontier schoolteacher
MARMARA: Turkish sea
MARMEE: "Little Women" role
MARMION: Sir Walter Scott epic poem
MARMOT: Type of rodent
MARNE: French river
MARNER: George Eliot character
MARNI: Singer Nixon
MARNIE: Hitchcock film
MARNIER: Grand __ (liqueur)
MAROT: French poet
MARPLE: Agatha Christie sleuth
MARQUE: Car model
MARQUEZ: Colombian novelist Gabriel Garcia __
MARRON: Chestnut
MARRYAT: British novelist
MARRYIN': __ Sam ("Li'l Abner" character)
MARSALA: Italian wine
MARS BAR: Chocolate brand
MARSDEN: Pop singer Gerry
MARSHA: Playwright Norman
MARSTON: British playwright
MARTA: "I Remember Mama" mama
MARTEL: Charlemagne's grandfather
MARTEN: Weasel relative
MARTES: Tuesday: Spanish
MARTHA: First first lady
MARTHE: Actress Keller
MARTI: Cuban patriot
MARTINA: Tennis pro Navratilova
MARTINO: Singer Al
MARTINS: Choreographer Peter
MARTINU: Czech composer
MARTIN V: Pope
MARTIUS: "Titus Andronicus" role
MARTY: Singer Robbins
MARU: Japanese ship designation
MARULLO: "Rigoletto" character
MARUSJA: "The Magic Mountain" character
MARV: Sportscaster Albert
MARVELL: British poet
MARVIN: Soul singer Gaye
MARVIS: Boxer Frazier
MARX: German philosopher
MARXES: "Animal Crackers" family
MARYA: "The Inspector General" character
MARYAM: Actress D'Abo
MARY ANN: "Gilligan's Island" character
MARY I: English queen
MARY II: English queen
MARY J.: Singer Blige
MARY JO: Poet Salter
MARY KAY: Cosmetics brand
MARY LOU: Gymnast Retton
MARY'S: "The Bells of St. __"
MARY URE: British actress
MARZ: March: German
MARZO: March: Italian
MASA: Tortilla flour
MASADA: Ancient Israeli fortress
MASAI: African people
MASALA: "Mississippi __" (Denzel Washington film)
MASARYK: Czech statesman
MASER: Wave amplifier
MASERU: Capital of Lesotho
MASHA: Chekhov character
MASHIE: Golf club
MASLIN: Film critic Janet
MASQUE: Masked ball
MASSA: Italian city
MASSE: Billiards stroke
MASSEY: Actor Raymond
MASSIF: Mountain-range portion
MASSINE: Russian-born choreographer
MASSON: Vintner Paul
MASSYS: Flemish painter
MASTER P: Rap artist
MASTIC: Varnish ingredient
MASTOID: Bone near the ear
MASUR: Conductor Kurt
MATA: __ Hari
MATALIN: Political commentator Mary
MATEO: San __, CA
MATER: Mother, in Britain
MATEWAN: John Sayles film
MATHER: Clergyman Cotton
MATHERS: Beaver Cleaver portrayer
MATHEW: Photographer Brady
MATHEWS: Baseball great Eddie
MATHIAS: Track star Bob
MATHIEU: French painter
MATHIS: Singer Johnny
MATHS: Brit's school subject
MATILDA: "Waltzing __"
MATIN: Morning: French
MATINAL: Of morning
MATISSE: French painter
MATJES: Type of herring
MATLIN: Actress Marlee
MATLOCK: Andy Griffith TV series
MAT MAN: Wrestler
MATO: __ Grosso (state of Brazil)
MATR: Mother: Comb. form
MATRI: Mother: Comb. form
MATRO: Mother: Comb. form
MATSON: Football great Ollie
MATSU: Island off China
MATSUI: Hideki of baseball
MATSUO: Japanese poet Basho
MATT: Actor Dillon
MATTEA: Country singer Kathy
MATTEL: Toy maker
MATTHAU: Actor Walter
MATTHEW: Poet Arnold
MATTIE: "Ethan Frome" character
MATTOCK: Farming tool
MATTY: Alou of baseball
MATZOTH: Unleavened bread
MAUD: Actress Adams
MAUDE: Bea Arthur sitcom
MAUGHAM: British author
MAUI: Hawaiian island
MAULDIN: Cartoonist Bill
MAU MAU: Kenyan revolutionary
MAUMEE: Ohio river
MAUNA: __ Loa
MAUNDER: Babble
MAUNDY: __ Thursday (Holy Week day)
MAUPRAT: George Sand novel
MAURA: Irish form of Mary
MAUREEN: Actress Stapleton
MAURIAC: French novelist
MAURIAT: French orchestra leader
MAURICE: Actor Chevalier
MAUROIS: French novelist
MAURY: TV host Povich
MAUS: Mouse: German
MAUSER: German pistol
MAUVAIS: Bad: French
MAV: Dallas NBAer
MAVIS: Thrush
MAWR: Bryn __, PA
MAWSON: Antarctica explorer
MAX BAER: 1930s boxer
MAX BORN: Physics Nobelist
MAXELL: Audiotape brand
MAXENE: Andrews sister
MAXIE: Boxer Rosenbloom
MAXILLA: Jawbone
MAXIMA: Nissan model
MAXIMUS: Circus __
MAXINE: Testy cartoon character
MAXIXE: Ballroom dance
MAXSON: "Fences" character
MAXWELL: Scottish physicist
MAXX: T.J. __ (clothing-store chain)
MAYA: Ancient Mexican
MAYA LIN: Vietnam Memorial architect
MAYER: MGM mogul
MAYFAIR: London neighborhood
MAYHAP: Perhaps
MAYING: Spring celebration
MAYLE: "A Year in Provence" author
MAYNARD: Dobie Gillis' pal
MAYPO: Hot-cereal brand
MAYRON: Actress Melanie
MAYTAG: Appliance brand
MAZ: 1960 World Series hero, familiarly
MAZAR: Actress Debi
MAZARIN: Louis XIV minister
MAZDA: Imported auto
MAZEL: __ tov
MAZEPPA: Tchaikovsky opera
MAZO: Author de la Roche
MAZOLA: Cooking-oil brand
MAZUMA: Money
MAZURKA: Polish dance
MAZZINI: Italian patriot
MBABANE: Capital of Swaziland
M.B.E.: U.K. honor
MBEKI: South African leader
MCA: Record label
MCADAMS: Actress Rachel
MCADOO: Wilson's Secretary of State
MCAFEE: Antivirus software brand
MCALLEN: Texas city
MCAN: Thom of shoe stores
MCARDLE: Singer Andrea
MCAT: Would-be MD's exam
MCAVOY: Actress May
MCBAIN: Mystery writer Ed
MCBEAL: TV lawyer Ally
MCBRIDE: Country singer Martina
MCCABE: "__ and Mrs. Miller" (Beatty film)
MCCAIN: Arizona senator
MCCALL'S: Women's magazine
MCCANN: Comic Chuck
MCCAREY: Director Leo
MCCLOUD: Dennis Weaver role
MCCLURE: Actor Doug
MCCLURG: Actress Edie
MCCOO: Singer Marilyn
MCCORD: Actor Kent
MCCOURT: Actor Frank
MCCOVEY: Baseball great Willie
MCCOWEN: Actor Alec
MCCOY: "Star Trek" physician
MCCRAE: Canadian poet
MCCRARY: Radio host Tex
MCCREA: Actor Joel
MCCRUMB: Author Sharyn
MCDUCK: Disney character Scrooge
MCENROE: Tennis pro John
MCEWAN: British novelist
MCEWEN: TV weatherman Mark
MCFLY: "Back to the Future" kid
MC G: "Charlie's Angels" director
MCGAVIN: Actor Darren
MCGEE: Fibber of old-time radio
MCGILL: Canadian university
MCGRAW: Cartoon horse Quick Draw
MCGREW: "The Shooting of Dan __"

MCGRIFF: Fred of baseball
MCGRORY: Columnist Mary
MCGRUFF: Crime prevention dog
MCGUIRE: Basketball great Dick
MCGWIRE: Mark of baseball
MCHALE'S: "__ Navy" (sitcom)
MCHARG: "You Can't Go Home Again" character
MCHENRY: Maryland fort
MCHUGH: Songwriter Jimmy
MCJOB: Tame occupation
MCKAY: ABC sportscaster
MCKEAN: Actor Michael
MCKEE: Actress Lonette
MCKENNA: Actress Siobhan
MCKEON: Actor Doug
MCKERN: Actor Leo
MCKIM: Architect Charles
MCKUEN: Poet Rod
MCLAIN: Denny of baseball
MCLEAN: Singer Don
MCLUHAN: Writer Marshall
MCMAHON: TV host Ed
MCMURDO: __ Sound (Antarctic inlet)
MCNAB: "The Pathfinder" character
MCNABB: Donovan of football
MCNAIR: Singer Barbara
MCNALLY: Rand's mapmaking partner
MCNEIL: Newscaster Robin
MCNEILL: Painter James __ Whistler
M.C.P.: Feminist's bane: Abbr.
MCPAPER: "USA Today," unflatteringly
MCPHEE: "Nanny __" (2005 film)
MCQ: John Wayne film
MCQUEEN: Actor Steve
MCRAE: Jazz singer Carmen
MCRANEY: Actor Gerald
MCRIBS: McDonald's offering
MCSHANE: Actor Ian
MCSWINE: "Li'l Abner" character
MCVIE: Singer Christine
M.D.T.: Denver summer clock setting: Abbr.
MEA: __ culpa
MEAD: Fermented honey drink
MEADE: Gettysburg victor
MEADER: JFK parodist Vaughn
MEAGLES: "Little Dorrit" character
MEALIE: South African corn
MEAN AGE: Demographer's stat
MEANEY: Actor Colm
MEAN IT: Be serious
MEAN JOE: Greene of football
MEARA: Actress Anne
MEARS: Auto racer Rick
MEATH: County in Ireland
MEATUS: Bone opening
MECH.: Physical sci.
MECHLIN: Fine lace
MECUM: Vade __ (handbook)
MEDAKA: Aquarium fish
MEDAWAR: British medicine Nobelist
MEDE: Ancient Persian
MEDEA: Wife of Jason
MEDEE: Corneille work
MEDEVAC: Hospital helicopter
MEDFORD: Oregon city
MEDGAR: Civil rights activist Evers
MEDI: Prefix for care
MEDIANT: Tone of a musical scale
MEDIAS: In __ res (in the middle of things)
MEDICA: Materia __ (study of drugs)
MEDICI: Noted Florentine surname
MEDIGAP: Supplemental health insurance
MEDINA: Saudi Arabian city
MEDIO: Half: Spanish
MEDIUS: Middle finger
MEDIVAC: Hospital helicopter
MEDNIS: Chessmaster Edmar
MEDOC: Bordeaux wine
MEDULLA: Brain part
MEDWICK: Baseball great Joe
MEEBER: "Sister Carrie" character
MEEMIES: Screaming-__ (nervousness)
MEENY: Counting-out word
MEER: Painter Jan van der __
MEERKAT: Mongoose relative
MEESE: Reagan advisor
MEG: Computer memory unit
MEGA: Large: Comb. form
MEGAERA: One of the Furies
MEGALO: Very large: Comb. form
MEGALON: Godzilla foe
MEGAN: Actress Gallagher
MEGANE: Renault model
MEGILLA: Lengthy account
MEGREZ: Big Dipper star
MEGRIM: Headache
MEG RYAN: "Sleepless in Seattle" star
MEHTA: Conductor Zubin
MEIER: Getty Center architect
MEI FUN: Chinese noodles
MEIJI: Japanese emperor
MEIN: Chow __
MEINE: My: German
MEIOSIS: Cell division
MEIR: Former Israeli leader
MEISSEN: Fine porcelain
MEISTER: Expert: Comb. form
MEITNER: Austrian physicist
MEJICO: Mexico: Spanish
MEKHI: Actor Phifer
MEKKA: Actor Eddie
MEKONG: Asian river
MEL: Singer Torme
MELAMED: Talmud teacher
MELANIA: Third Mrs. Trump
MELANIE: Actress Griffith
MELANIN: Skin pigment
MELBA: __ toast
MELETE: Muse of meditation
MELFI: "The Sopranos" role
MELIC: Of song
MELINA: Actress Mercouri
MELINDA: Actress Dillon
MELIS: Jack Paar's bandleader
MELISMA: Song phrase
MELISSA: Singer Etheridge
MELITTA: Coffee brand
MELL: Cartoonist Lazarus
MELLO: __ Yello (soft drink)
MELLON: Philanthropist Andrew
MELMAC: Dinnerware plastic
MELO: Black: Comb. form
MELODIA: Organ stop
MELOS: Greek island
MELOT: "Tristan und Isolde" role
MEL OTT: Baseball Hall of Famer
MELROSE: "__ Place" (TV series)
MEL'S: "Alice" diner
MELTON: Actor Sid
MELVIL: Librarian Dewey
MELVIN: Attorney Belli
MELVYN: Actor Douglas
MEM: Hebrew letter
MEME: Same: French
MEMLING: German painter
MEMOIRE: Aide-__ (summary note)
MEMOREX: Audiotape brand
MEMPHIS: Tennessee city
MENA: Actress Suvari
MENAS: "Antony and Cleopatra" character
MENCIUS: Chinese philosopher
MENCKEN: Writer H.L.
MENDEL: Austrian botanist
MENDEL'S: __ law (genetics axiom)
MENDES: Bandeader Sergio
MENE: "Handwriting on the wall" word
MENES: First Egyptian king
MENISCI: Convex curves
MENJOU: Actor Adolphe
MENKEN: Broadway composer Alan
MENLO: __ Park, NJ
MENNEN: After-shave brand
MENNIN: Composer Peter
MENORAH: Hanukkah candelabrum
MENORCA: Balearic Island
MENOS: Less: Spanish
MENOTTI: Composer Gian Carlo
MENSA: High-IQ group
MENSAL: Monthly
MENSCH: Good guy
MENT: Noun suffix
MENTEE: One being mentored
MENTHE: Creme de __
MENTIS: Non compos __
MENTOS: Candy brand
MENU BAR: Web-browser feature
MENUDO: Spicy Mexican soup
MENUHIN: Violinist Yehudi
MENZIES: Actress Heather
MEOW MIX: Cat-food brand
MER: Sea: French
MERC: Ford auto, for short
MERCADO: Market: Spanish
MERCE: Choreographer Cunningham
MERCED: California city
MERCER: Lyricist Johnny
MERCERS: Textile dealers
MERCI: Thank you: French
MERCK: Pharmaceutical company
MERCKX: Bicyclist Eddy
MERCURE: Erik Satie work
MERDLE: "Little Dorrit" character
MERES: Mothers: French
MERIDA: Mexican city
MERIDEN: Connecticut city
MERIMEE: French novelist
MERINO: Sheep breed
MERKEL: German leader Angela
MERL: Blackbird
MERLE: Singer Haggard
MERLIN: Arthurian wizard
MERLINS: Small falcons
MERLOT: Red wine
MERM: "La __" (brassy singer's nickname)
MEROE: Ancient Ethiopian city
MEROPE: Pleiades star
MEROPS: "Iliad" seer
MERRIAM: Dictionary name
MERRICK: Broadway producer David
MERRILL: Lynch's Wall Street partner
MERSEY: River in England
MERTON: Sociologist Robert
MERTZ: "I Love Lucy" landlord
MERV: TV host Griffin
MERVYN: Director LeRoy
MERYL: Actress Streep
MERYLL: "Yeoman of the Guard" role
MES: Month: Spanish
MESA, AZ: Southwestern city
MESABI: Minnesota iron range
MES AMIS: My friends: French
MESCAL: Agave liquor
MESEEMS: I think, old-style
MESHACH: Companion of Daniel
MESHUGA: Loopy
MESIAL: Central
MESMER: Austrian hypnotist
MESNE: Feudal lord
MESO: Middle: Comb. form
MESON: Subatomic particle
MESSALA: "Ben-Hur" character
MESSE: Mass: French
MESSICK: Cartoonist Dale
MESSINA: Sicilian city
MESSRS: Plural of Mr.
MESTA: Hostess Perle
META: Beyond: Comb. form
METATE: Mexican grinding stone
METCALF: Actress Laurie
METH.: Prot. church
METHYL: Chemical prefix
METIER: Field of work
METIS: Moon of Jupiter
MET LIFE: Insurance company
METRIST: Expert in poetry
METRY: Measuring: Comb. form
METZ: French city
MEUM: Mine: Latin
MEUSE: Belgian river
MEYER: Mobster Lansky
MEYERS: Actress Ari
MEYNELL: British poet
MEZUZAH: Jewish parchment scroll
MEZZO: Certain soprano

M.F.A.: Painter's degree: Abbr.
MFD.: Built in a factory: Abbr.
MFG.: Factory work: Abbr.
MFR.: Builder: Abbr.
MFUME: Former NAACP leader
MGB: British auto
MGS: British autos
MHO: Conductance unit
MIA: Rambo rescuee
MIA HAMM: Soccer star
MIAMI, FL: Southeast city
MIAMIS: Midwest Indians
MIAMI U.: Ohio school
MIAOU: Cat call
MIAOW: Cat call
MIA SARA: "Timecop" actress
MIATA: Mazda model
MIB: Playing marble
MIC: Cassette-recorder jack
MICAELA: "Carmen" role
MICAH: Biblical prophet
MICH.: Detroit locale
MICHAUX: French poet
MICHEL: Composer Legrand
MICK: Rocker Jagger
MICKEY: Knockout drink
MICKY: Dolenz of the Monkees
MICMAC: Canadian Indian
MICR: Small: Comb. form
MICRA: Meter fractions
MICRON: Meter fraction
MIDAS: Mythical king
MIDASES: Wealthy ones
MIDCAP: Medium-size company
MIDDIE: Annapolis student
MIDDLE C: Piano key
MIDDY: Annapolis student
MIDGE: Gnat
MIDI: South of France
MIDIAN: Son of Abraham
MIDIRON: Golf club
MIDLER: Actress Bette
MIDLIST: Part of a publisher's catalog
MID-OFF: Cricket position
MID-ON: Cricket position
MIDORI: Figure skater Ito
MIDRIB: Leaf vein
MIEL: Honey: French
MIELE: Vacuum-cleaner brand
MIERS: George W. Bush advisor
MIES: Architect __ van der Rohe
MIEUX: Better: French
MIFFLIN: Houghton's publishing partner
MIFUNE: Actor Toshiro
MIG: Russian fighter plane
MIGENES: Soprano Julia
MIGUEL: Author __ de Cervantes
MIKADO: Japanese emperor
MIKAN: Basketball great George
MIKASA: Chinaware brand
MIKEY: Boy in Life cereal ads
MIKHAIL: Soviet leader Gorbachev
MIKITA: Hockey great Stan
MILA: "__ 18" (Uris novel)
MILAGRO: "The __ Beanfield War" (Redford film)
MILAN: Italian city
MILANO: Actress Alyssa
MILANS: Mercury models
MILDRED: "__ Pierce" (Joan Crawford film)
MILHAUD: French composer
MILHOUS: Nixon's middle name
MILK DUD: Candy brand
MILLAGE: Property tax rate
MILLAIS: British painter
MILLAND: Actor Ray
MILLARD: President Fillmore
MILLAY: Poet Edna St. Vincent
MILLE: Thousand: French
MILL END: Fabric remnant
MILLET: Cereal grass
MILLETT: Feminist Kate
MILLI: Thousand: Comb. form
MILLIE: 1980s White House dog
MILLIME: Coin of Tunisia
MILLO: Diva Aprile
MILNE: British author
MILNER: Actor Martin
MILNES: Baritone Sherrill __
MILO: Venus de __
MILOS: Director Forman
MILOSZ: Polish-born literature Nobelist
MILSAP: Country singer Ronnie
MILT: Cartoonist Caniff
MILTIE: Uncle __ (Berle)
MILTON: British poet
MIM: Arabic letter
MIMESIS: Mimicry
MIMI: "La Bohème" role
MIMIEUX: Actress Yvette
MIMOSA: Champagne cocktail
MIMSY: "Jabberwocky" word
MINA: Talking bird
MINDEN: Louisiana city
MINDORO: Philippine island
MINDY: Mork's girlfriend
MINEO: Actor Sal
MINEOLA: Long Island town
MINERVA: Roman goddess
MINETA: George W. Bush cabinet member
MINEY: Counting-out word
MING: Chinese dynasty
MINGUS: Jazz bassist Charlie
MINGY: Mean and stingy
MINH: Ho Chi __ (Vietnamese leader)
MINHO: Portuguese river
MINIKIN: Tiny object
MINIM: Pharmacist's measure
MINIMAX: Game-theory strategy
MINI ME: "Austin Powers" character
MINIMUS: Little toe
MINI TV: Small set
MINIVER: Greer Garson role
MINNIE: Actress Driver
MINOAN: Cretan of old
MINOGUE: Singer Kylie
MINOLTA: Camera brand
MINORCA: Balearic Island
MINOS: King of Crete
MINOSO: Minnie of baseball
MINOT, ND: Midwest city
MINOW: Former FCC head
MINSK: Belarus capital
MINSKY'S: Memorable burlesque theater
MINSTER: Large church
MINUEND: Number in subtraction
MINUIT: Dutch buyer of Manhattan
MINYAN: Synagogue quorum
MIO: "O Sole __"
MIOCENE: Tertiary epoch
MIPS: Computer speed unit
MIR: Russian space station
MIRA: Actress Sorvino
MIRABEL: Montreal airport
MIRADA: Dodge model
MIRADOR: Spanish balcony
MIRAMAR: Florida city
MIRAMAX: Movie studio
MIRANDA: "The Tempest" character
MIRIAM: Singer Makeba
MIRIN: Rice wine
MIRISCH: Film producer Walter
MIRO: Spanish painter
MIRREN: Actress Helen
MIRRO: Cookware brand
MIRS: Russian communes
MIRV: Ballistic missile
MISCHA: Actor Auer
MISE: __ en scene (stage setting)
MISHA: Pianist Dichter
MISHIMA: Japanese novelist
MISHNAH: Judaic laws
MISKOLC: Hungarian city
MISO: Japanese soup flavoring
MISSA: Latin mass
MISSISH: Prim
MISS M: Bette Midler nickname
MISSY: Young girl's address
MISTBOW: Fog phenomenon
MISTI: El __ (Peruvian volcano)
MISTRAL: Chilean literature Nobelist
M.I.T.: Univ. near Harvard
MITA: Copier brand
MITCH: Sing-along leader Miller
MITCHUM: Actor Robert
MITFORD: British novelist
MITHRAS: Persian sun god
MITLA: "__ Pass" (Uris book)
MITOSIS: Cell division
MITRAL: Heart valve
MITSOU: Colette novel
MITTAG: Noon: German
MITTY: Thurber character
MITYA: Karamazov brother
MITZI: Actress Gaynor
MITZVAH: Bar __ (Jewish ritual)
MIXTEC: Mexican Indian
MIZ: "Les __" (Broadway musical)
MIZAR: Star in Ursa Major
MIZE: Johnny of baseball
MIZRAHI: Designer Isaac
MIZUNA: Japanese mustard
MIZZEN: Ship sail
MIZZLE: Fine rain
MKTG.: Business school subj.
M.L.B.: Big leagues: Abbr.
MLIFE: Cell-phone service
M.L.K.: "I have a dream" initials
M.L.S.: Librarian's deg.
MMDDYY: Date format
MMM: "Delicious!"
MMMBOP: Hanson song of 1997
MMMM: "Delicious!"
MNEM: Memory: Comb. form
MNEME: Muse of memory
MNEMO: Memory: Comb. form
MOA: Extinct bird
MOAB: Ancient Mideast kingdom
MOBERG: Swedish author
MOBIL: Gas brand
MOBIUS: __ strip (one-sided surface)
MOBLEY: Actress Mary Ann
MOBUTU: Former African leader
MOBY: "__-Dick"
MOCHRIE: Colin of "Who's Line Is It Anyway?"
MODAL: Auxiliary verb
MODEL A: Antique Ford
MODEL B: Antique Ford
MODEL T: Antique Ford
MODENA: Italian city
MODERNE: Pretentiously new
MODESTO: California city
MODI: __ operandi
MODINE: Actor Matthew
MODISTE: Fashion designer
MODRED: Arthurian villain
MODULO: Math term
MODULUS: Math term
MODUS: __ operandi
MOE: One of the Stooges
MOE BERG: "Catcher Was a Spy" subject
MOEN: Faucet brand
MOERAE: The Fates
MOE'S: "The Simpsons" bar
MOESHA: Brandy sitcom role
MOET: Champagne name
MOFFO: Soprano Anna
MOGADOR: Necktie fabric
MOGAMBO: Clark Gable movie
MOGEN: __ David (wine brand)
MOHAVE: Arizona Indian
MOHEGAN: New England Indian
MOHICAN: New England Indian
MOHS: Hardness scale
MOI: Me: French
MOIETY: Half
MOIL: Work hard
MOINES: Des __, IA
MOIRA: Ballerina Shearer
MOIRE: Watered silk
MOIS: Month: French
MOISES: Alou of baseball
MOISSAN: French chemistry Nobelist
MOJAVE: Arizona Indian
MOJITO: Cuban cocktail
MOJO: Amulet
MOKO: Pepe Le __ (Charles Boyer role)
MOL.: Grp. of atoms
MOLDAU: Czech river
MOLDOVA: European region

MOLE RAT: African rodent
MOLIERE: French playwright
MOLINA: Actor Alfred
MOLINE: Illinois city
MOLITOR: Paul of baseball
MOLLIE: Aquarium fish
MOLLOY: Samuel Beckett novel
MOLLY: Aquarium fish
MOLNAR: Hungarian playwright
MOLOKAI: Hawaiian island
MOLOTOV: Former Russian foreign minister
MOLSON: Beer brand
MOLTKE: WWI German general
MOLTO: Very, in music
MOLUCCA: Indonesian islands
MOLY: "Holy __!"
MOMA: NYC art gallery
MOMBASA: Kenyan city
MOME: "Jabberwocky" word
MOMMSEN: German literature Nobelist
MO' MONEY: Damon Wayans film
MOMUS: Faultfinder
MONA: "__ Lisa"
MONAD: Single unit
MON AMI: My friend: French
MONCTON: Canadian city
MONDALE: Carter's vice president
MONDAVI: Wine brand
MONDE: World: French
MONDESI: Raul of baseball
MONDIAL: Ferrari model
MON DIEU: French expletive
MONDO: Huge, slangily
MONDOS: Zen questions
MONEL: Nickel alloy
MONET: French painter
MONETA: Italian peace Nobelist
MONGER: Sell
MONGKUT: "The King and I" king
MONGO: Ming the Merciless' planet
MONGOS: Mongolian money
MONIC: First-degree, in math
MONICA: Tennis pro Seles
MONISM: Philosophical theory
MONIZ: Portuguese medicine Nobelist
MONKEES: 1960s rock group
MONNET: French economist
MONOD: French chemist
MONODY: Lament
MONOMER: Polymer component
MONOSKI: Snowboard cousin
MONRO: Singer Matt
MONROE: "Bus Stop" star
MONROES: 1820s First Family
MONSTRO: "Pinocchio" whale
MONT: French peak
MONTAG: Monday: German
MONTAGU: British author
MONTALE: Italian poet
MONTANO: "Othello" character
MONTAUK: Long Island town
MONTE: "The Count of __ Cristo"
MONTEGO: __ Bay, Jamaica
MONTEL: Talk-show host Williams
MONTERO: Mitsubishi model
MONTEUX: Conductor Pierre
MONTEZ: Dancer Lola
MONTOYA: Guitarist Carlos
MONTUNO: Rumba passage
MONTY: Game-show host Hall
MONY: Insurance company
MONZA: Chevy model
MOODY'S: Bond-rating service
MOOG: Electronic instrument
MOOKIE: Wilson of baseball
MOON DOG: Lunar halo spot
MOONEY: "Lucy Show" character
MOONEYE: Herringlike fish
MOONIE: Unification Church member
MOONIER: More absent-minded
MOONISH: Fickle
MOON PIE: Chocolaty snack
MOORE: Actress Demi
MOPHEAD: One with a Beatle haircut
MOPSY: Kid-lit rabbit
MOP TOP: Beatle haircut
MOR.: North Afr. nation
MORA: NFL coach Jim
MORAINE: Glacial debris
MORAN: Actress Erin
MORANIS: Actor Rick
MORANT: "Breaker __" (1979 film)
MORANTE: Italian novelist
MORATH: Ragtime pianist Max
MORAVIA: Czech region
MORCERF: "Count of Monte Cristo" character
MORDENT: Melodic embellishment
MORDRED: Arthurian villain
MOREAU: Actress Jeanne
MOREEN: Heavy fabric
MOREL: Edible mushroom
MORELLA: Poe story
MORELLO: Sour cherry
MORELOS: Mexican state
MORENO: Actress Rita
MORES: "O tempora! O __!"
MORESBY: Port __ (Papua New Guinea capital)
MORETTI: "A Farewell to Arms" character
MOREY: Comic Amsterdam
MORGAN: Banker J.P.
MORGANA: Fata __ (mirage)
MORGANS: Saddle horses
MORGEN: Morning: German
MORISOT: French painter
MORITA: Actor Pat
MORITZ: St. __, Switzerland
MORK: Robin Williams TV role
MORLEY: Safer of "60 Minutes"
MORLOCK: "The Time Machine" character
MORNAY: White sauce
MORO: Philippine Muslim
MOROLT: King Arthur knight
MORONI: Comoro Islands capital
MOROSS: Film composer Jerome
MORPH: Change gradually
MORPHIC: Shape: Comb. form
MORPHIN: Mighty __ Power Rangers
MORPHO: Structure: Comb. form
MORRA: "How Are Things in Glocca __?"
MORREL: "Count of Monte Cristo" character
MORRIE: "Tuesdays With __" (1990s bestseller)
MORRIS: Cat in commercials
MORRO: __ Castle (Havana landmark)
MORT: Humorist Sahl
MORTE: "Le __ d'Arthur" (Malory work)
MORTEN: "An Enemy of the People" character
MORTICE: Carpentry notch
MORTISE: Carpentry notch
MORTON: Jazz pianist Jelly Roll
MORTON'S: Steakhouse chain
MORTY: Mickey Mouse nephew
MOSCATO: Italian wine
MOSCONI: Pool champ Willie
MOS DEF: Rap star
MOSE: Jazz pianist Allison
MOSEL: River in France
MOSELLE: River in France
MOSH: 1990s dance
MOSHAV: Israeli cooperative
MOSHE: Israeli general Dayan
MOSKVA: Moscow: Russian
MOSLEY: Actor Roger E.
MOSSAD: Israeli spy agency
MOSSO: Brisk, in music
MOSTEL: Actor Zero
MOSUL: Iraqi city
MOTA: Manny of baseball
MOTET: Choral composition
MOTHRA: Godzilla foe
MOTO: Lorre film role
MOTRIN: Pain-reliever brand
MOTT: Feminist Lucretia
MOTT'S: Apple-juice brand
MOTT ST.: Thoroughfare in NYC's Chinatown
MOUCH: "Atlas Shrugged" character
MOUE: Grimace
MOULAGE: Plaster mold
MOULIN: __ Rouge (French nightclub)
MOVADO: Watch brand
MOVIN': "__ On Up" ("Jeffersons" theme)
MOWAT: Canadian novelist
MOWBRAY: Actor Alan
MOWEN: "Atlas Shrugged" character
MOWGLI: "Jungle Book" character
MOWIS: "Evangeline" character
MOXIE: Nerve
MOYERS: LBJ press secretary
MOZETTA: Papal cape
MOZILLA: Internet software suite
MOZO: Southwestern waiter
M.P.A.A.: Film-rating org.
MPEG: Video-file format
MP THREE: Digital audio format
MPV: Mazda model
MR. B.: Hazel's boss
MR. BEAN: Rowan Atkinson character
MR. BILL: "Saturday Night Live" clay figure
MR. BLISS: Tolkien children's book
MR. BLUE: Fleetwoods tune
MR. BODDY: "Clue" victim
MR. BOND: 007, to Goldfinger
MR. BONES: Minstrel-show figure
MR. BROWN: Tarantino, in "Reservoir Dogs"
MR. BURNS: Homer Simpson's boss
MR. BUTTS: "Doonesbury" character
MR. C.: "Happy Days" dad, informally
MR. CHIPS: James Hilton's schoolmaster
MR. CLEAN: Cleaner brand
MR. CUB: Ernie Banks' nickname
MR. DARCY: "Pride and Prejudice" character
MR. DEEDS: Gary Cooper title role
MR. DICK: "David Copperfield" character
M.R.E.: Army chow: Abbr.
MR. ED: Sitcom horse
MR. FOX: Roald Dahl character
MR. GREEN: "Clue" suspect
MR. HANEY: "Green Acres" character
MR. HEX: Bowery Boys film
MR. HOBBS: James Stewart title role
MR. HORSE: "Ren and Stimpy" character
MR. HULOT: Tati title role
MR. HYDE: Jekyll's alter ego
MRI: X-ray cousin
MR. JINX: "Meet the Parents" cat
MR. JONES: Richard Gere film
MR. LEE: Tune of 1957
MR. LUCKY: Cary Grant title role
MR. MACHO: He-man
MR. MAGOO: Jim Backus voice
MR. MARCH: Alcott character
MR. MET: Shea Stadium mascot
MR. MOM: Michael Keaton film
MR. MOOSE: "Captain Kangaroo" puppet
MR. MOTO: Peter Lorre role
MR. MUSIC: George Gershwin nickname
MR. NANNY: Hulk Hogan film
MR. NORTH: Old-time radio detective
MR. NOVAK: 1960s TV series
MR. PADRE: Tony Gwynn nickname
MR. PAWS: "Harry Potter" series cat
MR. PIBB: Soft-drink brand
MR. QUILP: "Old Curiosity Shop" character
MRS. BASS: "...Unfortunate Events" teacher
MRS. C.: "Happy Days" mom, informally
MR. SCOTT: "Star Trek" engineer
MR. SLATE: Flintstone's boss

MR. SMITH: James Stewart title role
MRS. MUIR: Gene Tierney film role
MRS. PAUL: Fish-stick name
MRS. PEEL: Diana Rigg role
MR. SPOCK: "Star Trek" role
MR. SULU: "Star Trek" officer
MR. T: "The A-Team" star
MR. TIBBS: Sidney Poitier film role
MR. TIGER: Al Kaline nickname
MR. WONG: Boris Karloff film role
MR. WORDS: Ira Gershwin nickname
MR. X: Unknown man
MR. YUK: Poison-label cartoon character
MS-DOS: Computer operating system
MSEC: Very brief time
M.S. ED.: Teacher's deg.
M.S.G.: Flavor-enhancer initials
MSGR.: Cath. offficial
M.SGT.: NCO
M'SIEUR: French fellow, for short
MSN: AOL competitor
MSNBC: Cable network
M SQUAD: Lee Marvin TV series
M.S.R.P.: Car's full price: Abbr.
MSS.: Author's submissions: Abbr.
M.S.T.: Denver hrs.
M STAR: Spectral type
M.S.U.: Big Ten sch.
MTA: Kingston Trio tune
MT. ADAMS: New Hampshire peak
MT. AIRY: North Carolina city
MT. APO: Philippine peak
MT. ATHOS: Greek peak
MT. BALDY: Peak near L.A.
MT. BLANC: French peak
MT. COOK: New Zealand peak
MT. ELY: Nevada peak
MT. ETNA: Volcano in Sicily
MT. EVANS: Peak near Denver
MT. FUJI: Volcano in Japan
MTG.: Appt.
MTGE.: House lien: Abbr.
MT. HOOD: Cascades peak
MT. IDA: Crete peak
MT. IDY: Charley Weaver's hometown
M TILE: Scrabble three-pointer
MT. KENYA: Second-highest African peak
MT. LOGAN: Canada's highest peak
MTM: "Hill Street Blues" production co.
MT. MARCY: Highest of the Adirondacks
MT. OSSA: Greek peak
MT. PELEE: Martinique volcano
MT. SINAI: Biblical peak
MTV VJ: Cable-network employee
MTWTF: Calendar run
MUAMMAR: Libyan leader Khadafy
MUBARAK: Egyptian president
MUCHAS: "__ gracias!"
MUDCAT: Whiskery fish
MUDD: TV newsman Roger
MUDDER: Certain horse
MUD EEL: Salamander
MUD FLAT: Dry lake bed
MUELLER: Swiss medicine Nobelist
MUESLI: Breakfast cereal
MUESLIX: Cereal brand
MUEZZIN: Minaret crier
MUFASA: "The Lion King" character
MUFTI: Civilian attire
MUGABE: Zimbabwean leader
MUGGLE: Non-magical person in "Harry Potter" books
MUGGS: "Today Show" chimp
MUGWUMP: Neutral party
MUIR: Naturalist John
MUJER: Woman: Spanish
MUKLUK: Eskimo boot
MULAN: 1998 Disney film
MULCAHY: "M*A*S*H" priest
MULCT: Swindle
MULDAUR: Actress Diana
MULDER: "X-Files" character
MULDOON: "Car 54, Where Are You?" cop
MULETA: Matador's cloth
MULEY: Dehorned bull
MULGREW: Actress Kate
MULHARE: Actor Edward
MULLA: Islamic teacher
MULLAH: Islamic teacher
MULLET: Food fish
MULLIN: Sports caricaturist Willard
MULLINS: "Moon __" (comic strip)
MUMBAI: City in India
MUMBLY: __-peg (kid's game)
MUMBO: __-jumbo
MU MESON: Subatomic particle
MUMFORD: Social scientist Lewis
MUMMER: Parade pantomimist
MUMM'S: Champagne brand
MUMMY'S: "The __ Hand" (1940 film)
MUN.: Of a city: Abbr.
MUNCHEN: Munich, to natives
MUNCIE: Indiana city
MUNDI: "Sic transit gloria __"
MUNERA: "The Faerie Queene" character
MUNG: Type of bean
MUNI: Investment bond
MUNICH: German city
MUNRO: Saki's real surname
MUNROE: Fawcett, on "Charlie's Angels"
MUNSTER: Kind of cheese
MUON: Subatomic particle
MUR: Wall: French
MURANO: Nissan model
MURAT: Turkish river
MURCIA: Spanish city
MURDOCH: Newspaper mogul
MURES: Romanian river
MURIEL: Mrs. Hubert Humphrey
MURIEL'S: "__ Wedding" (1994 film)
MURILLO: Spanish painter
MURINE: Eyedrops brand
MURPHY: WWII hero Audie
MURPHY'S: __ Law (pessimist's maxim)
MURRAY: Dance teacher Arthur
MURRE: Diving bird
MURROW: "Person to Person" moderator
MUS: Greek letters
MUSANTE: Actor Tony
MUSCA: Fly constellation
MUSCAT: Raisin grape
MUSCIDA: Star in Ursa Major
MUSEE: Museum: French
MUSEO: Museum: Spanish
MUSETTA: " La Boheme" character
MUSETTE: Woodwind instrument
MU SHU: Chinese dish
MUSIAL: Stan of baseball
MUSICK: Compose for
MUSIGNY: Red wine
MUSIL: Austrian writer
MUSKEGO: Wisconsin city
MUSKIE: Carter secretary of state
MUSKIES: Game fish
MUSKOX: Arctic bovine
MUSSET: French poet
MUSTAFA: Turkish leader Kemal
MUTABLE: Inconstant
MUTAGEN: Agent of change
MUTI: Conductor Riccardo
MUTIUS: "Titus Andronicus" role
MUTON: DNA unit
MUTUEL: Pari-__ betting
MUUMUU: Loose garment
MUY BIEN: Very good: Spanish
MUZAK: Elevator music
MUZZY: Confused
MVP: Sports award
MYALGIA: Muscle pain
MYANMAR: Asian nation
MY BABY: Temptations song
MY BAD: Informal apology
MY BUDDY: Gus Kahn song
MYCENAE: Ancient Greek city
MYCIN: Fungus: Comb. form
MYCO: Fungus: Comb. form
MYCROFT: Sherlock Holmes' brother
MY DAD: Paul Petersen tune
MY DAY: Eleanor Roosevelt's column
MYERS: Austin Powers portrayer
MYERSON: Consumer advocate Bess
MY GIANT: Billy Crystal film
MY GIRL: Temptations tune
MY GUY: Mary Wells tune
MYKONOS: Aegean island
MY LADY: Noblewoman's address
MYLANTA: Antacid brand
MYLAR: Balloon material
MYLES: Singer Alannah
MY LIFE: Billy Joel tune
MY LORD: English judge's address
MY LOVE: McCartney/Wings song
MY MAMMY: Jolson tune
MYNHEER: Sir: Dutch
MYO: Muscle: Comb. form
MYOB: Advice column abbr.
MYOLOGY: Study of muscles
MYOPE: Nearsighted one
MYOPIA: Nearsightedness
MYOSIN: Muscle protein
MYOSIS: Pupil contraction
MYRA: Pianist Hess
MYRDAL: Swedish peace Nobelist
MYRIA: 10,000: Comb. form
MYRNA: Actress Loy
MYRON: Economist Scholes
MY SIN: Perfume brand
MYSORE: City of India
MYSPACE: Networking Web site
MYST: Video game
MYTHOS: Belief system
MY TURN: Nancy Reagan book
MYUNG: Sun __ Moon (Unification Church founder)
MY WAR: Andy Rooney book
MY WAY: Sinatra tune
MY WORLD: Bee Gees tune

N

NABE: Local cinema
NABI: Muslim prophet
NABOB: Powerful person
NABOKOV: "Lolita" author
NABOO: "The Phantom Menace" planet
NABORS: Actor Jim
NABUCCO: Verdi opera
NACELLE: Aircraft enclosure
NACHAS: Pride in another's success
NACHO: Mexican snack
NACHT: Night: German
NACIO: Songwriter __ Herb Brown
NACION: Country: Spanish
NACL: Salt, to chemists
NACRE: Mother-of-pearl
NADER: Consumer advocate Ralph
NADIA: Gymnast Comaneci
NADINE: Chuck Berry tune
NADIR: Low point
NADJA: Peter Fonda film
NADSAT: "Clockwork Orange" teen slang
NAE: No: Scottish
NAFTA: 1990s trade pact
NAGANO: 1998 Winter Olympics site
NAG AT: Bother
NAGEL: Actor Conrad
NAGOYA: Japanese city
NAGY: Hungarian statesman
NAHA: Capital of Okinawa
NAHUATL: Aztec
NAHUM: Minor Prophet
NAIAD: Aquatic nymph
NAIF: Artless one
NAIL IN: Fasten down
NAIL IT: Perform something perfectly
NAIL KEG: Old hardware-store fixture
NAIL SET: Carpenter's tool
NAIMA: John Coltrane ballad
NAINA: Mrs. Yeltsin
NAIPAUL: British literature Nobelist

NAIR: Director Mira
NAIRA: Money of Nigeria
NAIROBI: Kenyan capital
NAISH: Actor J. Carrol
NAJIMY: Actress Kathy
NAKFA: Eritrean money
NAL: Paperback-publisher initials
NALA: "The Lion King" lion
NALDI: Actress Nita
NAM: "Apocalypse Now" setting
NAMATH: "Broadway Joe"
NAMBY: __-pamby
NAME DAY: When a saint is honored
NAMIB: African desert
NAMIBIA: African country
NAMPA: Idaho city
NAMU: Killer whale of film
NAMUR: Belgian province
NAN: A Bobbsey twin
NANA: "Peter Pan" dog
NANAIMO: British Columbia city
NANAK: Sikh founder
NANCE: FDR V.P. John __ Garner
NANCI: Singer Griffith
NANETTE: Actress Fabray
NANG: Da __, Vietnam
NANINE: Camille's maid
NANJING: Chinese city
NANKI: __-Poo ("Mikado" character)
NANKING: Chinese city
NANNA: Granny
NANNIE: Granny
NANNO: Billionth: Comb. form
NANO: Billionth: Comb. form
NANON: George Sand work
NANOOK: "__ of the North"
NANSEN: Arctic explorer
NANTES: French city
NANTZ: Sportscaster Jim
NANU: Orkan greeting
NAOH: Sodium hydroxide
NAOMI: Ruth's mother-in-law
NAOS: Ancient Greek temple
NAPA, CA: W. Coast wine region
NAPE: Back of the neck
NAPERY: Linen
NAPHTA: "The Magic Mountain" character
NAPHTHA: Mothball compound
NAPIER: Inventor of logarithms
NAPIER'S: __ bones (early calculator)
NAPLES: Italian city
NAPLESS: Like some carpet
NAPPE: Half a cone, in geometry
NAPPIE: Diaper, in Britain
NAPPY: Downy
NAPSTER: Internet music site
NAR.: Not wide: Abbr.
NARA: Japanese city
NARADA: New Age record label
NARAS: Grammy org.
NARAYAN: Indian writer
NARCO: Antidrug cop
NARD: Ancient ointment
NARDA: Mandrake the Magician's girlfriend
NARDO: "Taxi" character
NARES: Nostrils
NARIAL: Of nostrils
NARIC: Of nostrils
NARINE: Of nostrils
NARIS: Nostril
NARITA: Tokyo airport
NARK: British informer
NARNIA: C.S. Lewis locale
NARTHEX: Church area
NARVAEZ: Florida explorer
NARVIK: Norway city
NARWHAL: Arctic whale
NARZ: Game-show host Jack
N.A.S.: "Emerald Point __"
NASALS: Speech sounds
NASBY: Satirist Petroleum V. __
NASCENT: Beginning
NASD: Wall Street org.
NASDAQ: AMEX alternative
NASEBY: English village
NASH: Poet Ogden
NASHE: British playwright
NASHES: Defunct autos
NASHUA: New Hampshire city
NASI: Nose: Comb. form
N.A.S.L.: Former soccer org.
NASO: Nose: Comb. form
NASSAU: Bahamas capital
NASSER: Former president of Egypt
NAST: Boss Tweed's nemesis
NASTASE: Ilie of tennis
NAT: Singer Cole
NATAL: Birth-related
NATALE: Christmas: Italian
NATALIA: Ballet star Makarova
NATALIE: Singer Cole
NATAN: Russian author Sharansky
NATANT: Afloat
NATASHA: Bullwinkle foe
NATATOR: Swimmer
NATCH: Slangy agreement
NATCHEZ: Mississippi city
NATE: Archibald of basketball
NATHAN: Actor Lane
NATHAN'S: Coney Island restaurant
NATICK: Massachusetts city
NATL.: Part of NAACP
NATR: Sodium: Comb. form
NATRIUM: Former name for sodium
NATRO: Sodium: Comb. form
NATRON: Means of football
NATS: Washington baseballers
NATSUME: Japanese novelist
NATTA: Italian chemistry Nobelist
NATUREL: Au __ (bare)
NATWICK: Actress Mildred
NAURU: Pacific island nation
NAUSEAM: Ad __ (excessively)
NAUT.: Of the sea: Abbr.
NAUTES: "Aeneid" character
NAUTICA: Tommy Hilfiger competitor
NAUTILI: Sea creatures
NAV.: Seagoing force: Abbr.
NAVAID: Helm device
NAVARRE: Onetime Basque kingdom
NAVE: Church area
NAVEE: "Ruler of the Queen's __"
NAVIDAD: Christmas: Spanish
NAVIG.: Nautical sci.
NAVIS: Ship: Latin
NAXOS: Greek island
NAYA: Bottled-water brand
NAYARIT: State of Mexico
NAZI: Indiana Jones foe
NBAER: Pro hoopster
NBA LIVE: Popular video game
NBC BLUE: Old-time radio network
NBC RED: Old-time radio network
NBW: Helm dir.
NCAA: "Final Four" letters
N. CAR.: Va. neighbor
NCC: U.S.S. Enterprise letters
N.C.O.: Sgt., e.g.
NCR: ATM manufacturer
N.C. WYETH: Artist from Pa.
N. DAK.: Bismarck's st.
N. DAKOTA: Bismarck's st.
N.D.U.: South Bend sch.
N.E.A.: Teachers' org.
NEAL: Actress Patricia
NEALE: Football coach "Greasy"
NEALON: Comedian Kevin
NEALY: "Atlas Shrugged" character
NEAME: "The Poseidon Adventure" director
NEAP: Type of tide
NEAR PAR: Like some bond prices
NEAR TO: Close by
NEAR YOU: Berle's theme
'NEATH: Opposite of o'er
NEATNIK: Felix Unger, for one
NEATO: "Cool!"
NEAT'S: __-foot oil
NEB: Pen point
NEBBISH: Luckless one
NEBO: Biblical mount
NEBR.: Omaha's st.
NEBULA: Astronomical cloud
NEC: Computer co.
NECKLET: Fur piece, e.g.
NECTARY: Bee's target
NED: Actor Beatty
NEDDA: "Pagliacci" soprano
NED LAND: "Twenty Thousand Leagues..." character
NEDRA: Actress Volz
NEE: Born: French
NEED BE: Required
NEEDHAM: Boston suburb
NEEL: French physicist
NEELIX: "Star Trek: Voyager" role
NEELY: "Valley of the Dolls" character
NEEME: Conductor Jarvi
NEENAH: Wisconsin city
NEESON: Actor Liam
NEET: Nair competitor
NEFF: Actress Hildegarde
NEFUD: Arabian desert
NEG.: Battery term.
NEGEB: Region of Israel
NEGEV: Region of Israel
NEGRI: Actress Pola
NEGRO: Amazon tributary
NEGRONI: Vermouth cocktail
NEGUS: Hot wine drink
NEH.: Bib. book
NEHER: Medicine Nobelist Erwin
NEHI: "M*A*S*H" beverage
NEHRU: Gandhi colleague
NEHRUS: Jackets of the 1960s
NEI: Estonian chess master
NEIGE: Snow: French
NEILL: Actor Sam
NEIMAN: Marcus' retail partner
NEIN: No: German
NEISSE: Czech river
NEJD: Saudi Arabian region
NEL: "__ Blu Dipinto Di Blu"
NELL: Singer Carter
NELLE: Reagan's mother
NELLIE: "South Pacific" heroine
NELLIS: Nevada Air Force base
NELLO: "Romola" character
NELLY: Singer Furtado
NELS: "I Remember Mama" role
NELSE: "O Pioneers!" character
NELSON: Singer Willie
NELSONS: 1950s TV family
NEMAN: Baltic feeder
NEMEA: Hercules labor site
NEMEAN: Like Hercules's lion
NEMEC: Actor Corin
NEMEROV: Poet Howard
NEMO: Verne captain
NEMOS: On-site TV showings
NEN: Robb of baseball
NENA: "99 Luftballons" group
NENE: Hawaiian goose
NENEH: Singer Cherry
N. ENG.: RI, MA, VT, etc.
NENNIUS: Welsh historian
NEO: Recent: Prefix
NEOCENE: Geologic period
NEOCON: One on the right wing
NEOGENE: Geologic period
NEOLITH: Cro-Magnon tool
NEOLOGY: New word
NEOLYTE: Shoe-sole material
NEONATE: Baby
NEON GAS: Light medium
NEOS: Modernists
NEOSHO: Kansas river
NEPEAN: Canadian city
NEPHR: Kidney: Comb. form
NEPHRIC: Renal
NEPHRO: Kidney: Comb. form
NEPOS: Roman historian
NER: Abner's father
NERA: Italian river
NEREID: Daughter of Neptune
NERF: Brand of soft ball
NERI: St. Philip __
NERISSA: "The Merchant of Venice" maid
NERMAL: "Garfield" kitten
NERNST: German chemist
NEROL: Orange-blossom oil
NEROLI: Orange-blossom oil
NERONE: Mascagni opera

NERTS: "Baloney!"
NERTZ: "Baloney!"
NERUDA: Chilean literature Nobelist
NERVA: Roman emperor
NERVINE: Soothing medicine
NERVO: Mexican poet
NES: Computer-game initials
NESBIT: "Of Human Bondage" character
NESBITT: Actress Cathleen
NESCAFE: Folger's rival
NESIA: Island: Comb. form
NESMITH: One of the Monkees
NESQUIK: Drink-mix brand
NESS: "The Untouchables" hero
NESSEN: Ford press secretary
NESSES: Capes
NESSIE: Legendary monster
NESSMAN: WKRP anchorman
NESSUS: Centaur of myth
NESTEA: Bigelow competitor
NEST IN: Occupy, as birds
NESTOR: Wise counselor
NET BALL: Tennis call
NET CAFE: Surfer's hangout
NETFLIX: DVD mail service
NET GAME: Tennis technique
NETH.: Belg. neighbor
NETHER: Below
NETHOU: Pic de __ (Pyrenees peak)
NETIZEN: Web user
NETMAN: Tennis player
NETSTER: Tennis player
NETSUKE: Japanese figurine
NETSURF: Browse online
NET TON: 907 kilograms
NETWARE: Networking software
NET WT.: Cereal box abbr.
NETZERO: Internet service provider
NEU: Modern: German
NEUE: Modern: German
NEUF: Nine: French
NEUILLY: Suburb of Paris
NEUMAN: Mad magazine mascot
NEUMANN: Mathematician John von __
NEUN: Nine: German
NEUR: Nerve: Comb. form
NEURO: Nerve: Comb. form
NEUROL.: Anatomical sci.
NEURON: Nerve cell
NEURONE: Nerve cell
NEUSS: City near Düsseldorf
NEUT.: Not masc. or fem.
NEVA: Russian river
NEVE: Actress Campbell
NEVERS: City southeast of Orléans
NEVES: Granular snows
NEVI: Birthmarks
NEVIL: Author Shute
NEVILL: Nobel physicist Mott
NEVILLE: British prime minister Chamberlain
NEVIN: "Mighty Lak' a Rose" composer
NEVINS: Historian Allan
NEVIS: Leeward Island
NEVSKI: Russian saint
NEVSKY: Russian saint
NEVUS: Birthmark
NEW AGE: Music genre
NEW AT: Unfamiliar with
NEW BERN: North Carolina city
NEWBERY: Children's book award
NEWBIE: Beginner
NEWBOLT: "Admirals All" author
NEWBURG: Lobster style
NEW DEAL: F.D.R. program
NEWEL: Banister post
NEWELL: Director Mike
NEW ERA: Fresh start
NEWF.: Can. province
NEWGATE: British prison
NEW HAND: Beginner
NEWHART: 1980s sitcom
NEW HOPE: Minnesota city
NEWIE: Apprentice
NEW-LAID: Fresh, as eggs
NEW LEAF: Something turned over
NEW LEFT: 1960s-1970s political movement
NEWLEY: Actor Anthony
NEW LINE: Hollywood studio
NEW LOOK: Dior style
NEWLOVE: Canadian poet
NEWMADE: Fresh, as bread
NEWMAN: Actor Paul
NEWMAN'S: __ Own (pasta sauce brand)
NEWMAR: Actress Julie
NEW MATH: School subject
NEW-MINT: Create afresh
NEWMONT: Mining company
NEW RICH: Upstarts, maybe
NEWSDAY: Long Island paper
NEWSOM: Bobo of baseball
NEWSOME: "Our Town" character
NEWS PEG: Journalist's angle
NEWT: Salamander
NEW TO: Not familiar with
NEWTONS: Units of force
NEW TOWN: Planned community
NEW ULM: Minnesota city
NEXIS: Internet database
NEXO: Danish writer
NEXRAD: Storm-system tracker
NEXTEL: Cell-phone company
NEXT UP: On deck
NEXUS: Link
NEY: Napoleonic marshal
NEZ: Nose: French
NFC: Pro gridiron div.
NFD.: Can. province
NFL: Gridiron org.
NFLD.: Can. province
NFLER: Pro footballer
N FORTY: Bingo call
NGAIO: Author Marsh
NGANA: "South Pacific" character
NGO: Former Vietnamese leader __ Dinh Diem
NGOR: "The Killing Fields" actor
NGUYEN: Vietnamese name
NGWEE: Zambian money
NHA: Shelter org.
NHAT: Author Thich __ Hanh
N. HEB.: Vanuatu's former name: Abbr.
N.H.L.: Icemen's org.
NHLER: Pro hockey player
N.H.R.A.: Auto racing org.
NHU: Madame __ of Vietnam
NIA: Actress Peeples
NIA LONG: "Alfie" actress
NIAMEY: Niger capital
NIANTIC: Connecticut town
NIB: Pen point
NIBLET: Canned corn morsel
NIBLICK: Golf club
NIBLO: Silents director Fred
NIC: Kidman, to friends
NIC CAGE: Film star, for short
NICCOLO: Writer Machiavelli
NICE JOB: Encouraging words
NICENE: Ancient creed
NICE ONE: "Good going!"
NICHOLS: "The Graduate" director
NICHT: Not: German
NICIAS: "Thaïs" role
NICK JR.: Pre-school cable programming
NICKLES: Oklahoma politician
NICKY: Liz Taylor ex
NICOBAR: Bay of Bengal islands
NICOISE: Salad style
NICOL: Actor Williamson
NICOLA: Actress Pagett
NICOLAS: Actor Cage
NICOLE: Actress Kidman
NICOLET: Discoverer of Lake Michigan
NICOLLE: French medicine Nobelist
NICOLO: Violin maker Amati
NICOSIA: Capital of Cyprus
NICTATE: Blink
NIDE: Brood of pheasants
NIDETCH: Jean of Weight Watchers
NIDI: Insect nests
NIDIFY: Build a nest
NIDRE: Kol __ (synagogue prayer)
NIDUS: Insect nest
NIE: Never: German
NIEBUHR: German historian
NIEKRO: Phil of baseball
NIELLO: Metal ornamental work
NIELS: Physicist Bohr
NIELSEN: TV ratings name
NIENTE: Nothing: Italian
NIETA: Granddaughter: Spanish
NIETO: Grandson: Spanish
NIEUW: __ Amsterdam (early European colony)
NIEVE: Snow: Spanish
NIGEL: Actor __ Bruce
NIGER: African nation
NIGGLE: Criticize
NIGH ON: Nearly
N.I.H.: Biomedical research agcy.
NIHIL: Nothing: Latin
NIHILO: Nothing: Latin
NIHON: Japan
NIIHAU: Hawaiian island
NIK: Russian suffix
NIKA: "Doctor Zhivago" character
NIKE: Reebok rival
NIKE AD: Frequent sports-show commercial
NIKITA: Russian leader Khrushchev
NIKKEI: Japanese stock index
NIKKI: Actress Cox
NIKOLA: Inventor Tesla
NIKOLAI: Composer Rimski-Korsakov
NIKOLAY: Russian poet Nekrasov
NIKON: Camera brand
NILES: "Frasier" character
NILES, OH: McKinley's birthplace
NILLA: __ Wafers (cookie brand)
NILLY: Willy-__
NILS: Actor Asther
NILSSON: "Everybody's Talkin'" composer
NIM: Counting game
NIMBY: Suburban protester's acronym
NIMES: French city
NIMH: "The Secret of __" (children's film)
NIMIETY: Excess
NIMINY: __-piminy
NIMITZ: WWII admiral
NIMOY: Mr. Spock portrayer
NIMROD: Hunter
NIMS: Poet John Frederick
NIN: French diarist
NINAS: They're hidden in Hirschfeld drawings
NINE A: Shoe size
NINE B: Shoe size
NINE C: Shoe size
NINE D: Shoe size
NINE E: Shoe size
NINE EE: Shoe size
NINE EEE: Shoe size
NINE PIN: Alley target
NINER: California footballer
NINEVEH: Capital of Assyria
NINGBO: Chinese seaport
NINO: Boy: Spanish
NINON: Drapery fabric
NIOBE: Mythical weeper
NIOBIC: Of element #41
NIOBIUM: Element #41
NIORT: French city
NIPA: Asian palm
NIP AT: Almost catch
NIPIGON: Ontario lake
NIPMUCK: Massachusetts Indian
NIPPON: Japan
NIPSEY: Comic Russell
NIP-UP: Acrobatic move
NIRO: Robert De __
NIRVANA: Buddhist state
NISAN: Hebrew month
NISEI: Japanese-American
NISSAN Z: Sports car
NISSEN: __ hut (Army dwelling)
NISUS: "Aeneid" character

N.I.T.: Coll. hoops tourney
NITA: Actress Naldi
NITER: Gunpowder ingredient
NITID: Bright
NITON: Former name of radon
NITRATE: Fertilizer ingredient
NITRE: British fertilizer
NITTANY: __ Lions (Penn State team)
NITTI: "The Untouchables" role
NIUE: Pacific island
NIVAL: Of snow
NIVEA: Skin-lotion brand
NIVEN: Actor David
NIVEOUS: Snow-white
NIXIE: Undeliverable letter
NIXONS: 1970s First Family
NIZER: "My Life in Court" author
NKRUMAH: Ghana's first president
NKVD: KGB predecessor
N. LAT.: Gazetteer abbr.
NLC: Astros div.
NLCS: World Series prelim
NLE: Braves div.
N.L. EAST: Braves div.
NLER: Cardinal or Giant
N.L.F.: South Vietnam rebel org.
N.L. MVP: Baseball honoree
N.L.R.B.: Agcy. dealing with unions
NLW: Diamondbacks div.
N.L. WEST: Diamondbacks' div.
N. MEX.: Ariz. neighbor
N.M.I.: No middle initial: Abbr.
NNE: Compass pt.
NNW: Compass pt.
N.O.A.A.: Commerce Dept. agency
NOAM: Linguist Chomsky
NO ANGEL: Bad kid
NOB: __ Hill (San Francisco area)
NO-BAKE: Sort of dessert
NO BALL: Cricket violation
NOBBY: Chic, in Britain
NO BET: Poker declaration
NOB HILL: San Francisco area
NO-BID: Like some contracts
NOBILE: Arctic explorer
NOBIS: "Dona __ pacem"
NOBODY'S: __ fool (not naive)
NOBS: Cribbage pieces
NO-CAL: Like some colas
NO CATCH: Football ref's decision
NOCENT: Harmful
NOCHE: Night: Spanish
NOCK: Arrow notch
NO CLASS: Boor's quality
NO-COUNT: Worthless
NOCT: Night: Comb. form
NOCTI: Night: Comb. form
NOCUOUS: Harmful
NO-CUT: Like some athletes' contracts
NODDY: Fool
NODI: Central points
NODOSE: Knobby
NODOUS: Knotty
NO DOZ: Alertness aid
NO DUH: "Silly me!"
NODUS: Central point
NOE: Douay Bible shipbuilder
NO EAR: Lack of musical talent
NOEMON: "Odyssey" character
NO ENTRY: Highway sign
NOESIS: Cognition
NOETIC: Of the intellect
NOETICS: Reasoning
NO EXIT: Sartre drama
NO-FAULT: Like some insurance
NO-FEE: Kind of checking account
NOGALES: Arizona town
NO GAS: Shortage sign of 1973
NOGGS: "Nicholas Nickleby" character
NO GIFTS: Invitation request
NO-GO: NASA cancellation
NOGUCHI: Sculptor Isamu
NOH: Japanese theater
NOHANT: George Sand work
NO HIT: Pitch very well
NOHO: Manhattan neighborhood
NOIA: Thought: Comb. form
NO ID: Admittance obstacle
NOIL: Cotton fiber
NOIR: Black: French
NOIRE: Black: French
NOIRET: Actor Philippe
NO-IRON: Drip-dry
NOISOME: Harmful
NO JIVE: "Seriously!"
NOK: __-Hockey (table game)
NOKIA: Cell-phone brand
NO-KNOCK: Kind of police raid
NOKOMIS: Grandmother of Hiawatha
NOL: Lon of Cambodia
NOLA: Vincent Lopez's theme
NOLAN: Pitcher Ryan
NOLDE: German painter
'NOLE: Florida footballer
NO LEAD: Fuel choice
NOLI: Do not: Latin
NO LIMIT: Type of poker
NOLL: Football coach Chuck
NOLLE: __ prosequi
NOLO: Court plea, for short
NO-LOAD: Kind of mutual fund
NO-LOSE: Guaranteed
NO LOSS: "Don't sweat it"
NOLTE: Actor Nick
NOM: __ de plume
NO MA'AM: Polite denial
NOMAR: Garciaparra of baseball
NO MAS: Enough: Spanish
NO MAYO: Diner request
NOMBRE: Name: Spanish
NOME, AK: Iditarod ending
NO MEAT: Vegetarian restriction
NOMEN: Name: Latin
NO MERCY: Pop-music trio
NO MERGE: Highway sign
NOMIAL: Math suffix
NOMO: Pitcher Hideo
NO MSG: Chinese menu words
NOMY: Arrangement: Comb. form
NONAGE: Adolescence
NO-NAME: Generic
NONARY: Nine-part
NONCE: Present time
NONEGO: External world, in philosophy
NONES: Canonical hour
NONET: Group of nine
NO NEVER: Emphatic denial
NONGOGO: Fugard play
NON-NET: Including tax
NONNO: Grandfather: Italian
NONS: French denials
NON-U: Bourgeois
NO NUKES: Peacenik slogan
NONUPLE: Music term
NOODGE: Annoy
NOOGIE: Playful poke
NO OIL: Automobile problem
NOONAN: Bush speechwriter
NO ONE: Nary a soul
NOONER: Midday activity
NO ONE'S: Up for grabs
NOONING: Lunch
NOOR: Former Queen of Jordan
NOORT: Flemish painter Adam van __
NO OTHER: The one and only
NOOTKA: West Coast Indian
NOPAL: Cactus
NO-PAR: Kind of bond
NO PROB: "Piece of cake!"
NORA: Hammett character
NORAD: Defense org.
NORAH: Singer Jones
NORBERT: Computer pioneer Wiener
NORD: North: French
NORDIC: Aryan
NORDICA: Soprano Lillian
NORDOFF: Novelist Charles
NOREEN: Corcoran of "Bachelor Father"
NORELCO: Shaver brand
NORELL: Designer Norman
NOREN: Irv of baseball
NO RENT: Super's perk
NORGAY: Everest conqueror
NORGE: Appliance brand
NOR I: "Me neither!"
NORIA: Water wheel
NORIEGA: Former leader of Panama
NORIS: Edible seaweeds
NO-RISK: Guaranteed
NORITE: Igneous rock
NORMA: Actress Shearer
NORMAN: "Psycho" role
NORMAND: Chaplin costar
NORMANS: 1066 conquerors
NORN: Scandinavian goddess
NORRIS: Actor Chuck
NORRISH: British chemistry Nobelist
NORSK: From Oslo, to natives
NORTE: North: Spanish
NORTHER: Texas wind
NORTON: "The Honeymooners" role
NORTONS: Kramdens' neighbors
NO-RUN: Kind of ball game
NO RUNS: Inning recap part
NORVAL: Dr. Seuss character
NORVO: Jazz musician Red
NORW.: Eur. country
NORWALK: Connecticut city
NORWICH: City in England
NORWOOD: Brandy's last name
NO SALE: Cash-register button
NO SCORE: Sportscaster's phrase
NO SEATS: Sellout situation
NOSE BRA: Auto accessory
NO-SEE-UM: Gnat
NOSE OUT: Barely beat
NOSER: High wind
NOSE UP: Take off, as a plane
NO-SHOW: AWOL
NO SOAP: "Can't do it"
NO STARS: Bad review
NO STEP: Plane-wing warning
NOSTER: Pater __
NOSTRA: Cosa __
NOSTRUM: Quack medicine
NOTA: __ bene
NOTAH: Golfer Begay
NO TAIL: Manx cat feature
NOT ALL: Less than 100%
NO TASTE: Blandness
NOTH: Actor Christopher
NOTHIN': "__ doin'!"
NOTHIN'S: "Sweet __" (Brenda Lee tune)
NO TIE: Casual-dress phrase
NOT ILL: Healthy
NO TIP: Bad-service result
NOT IT: "Tag" shout
NOT OK: Prohibited
NO-TOLL: Like some highways
NOT ON: Off
NOT ONCE: Never
NO-TRADE: Type of sports contract
NO-TRUMP: Bridge bid
NOTS: Have-__ (indigents)
NOTTE: Night: Italian
NOTTING: "__ Hill" (1999 movie)
NOT TO BE: Hamlet choice
NOT TOO: Minimally
NOTUS: Son of Eos
NOT USED: Idle
NO TV: Teen punishment
NOT WELL: Ailing
NOT WITH: Against
NOUMEA: New Caledonia capital
NOURI: Actor Michael
NOUS: Entre __
NO USE: Pointless
NO U-TURN: Highway sign
NOUVEAU: Art __
NOVAK: Actress Kim
NOVALIS: German poet
NOVARRO: Actor Ramón
NOVATO: California city
NOVE: Nine: Italian
NOVELA: Spanish soap opera
NOVEM: Nine: Latin
NOVENA: Catholic devotion
NOVIA: Fiancée: Spanish
NOVIO: Fiancé: Spanish
NOVI SAD: City on the Danube
NOVO: De __ (again)
NO VOTE: Nay

NOVOTNY: Former Czech president
NOVUS: Word on the Great Seal
NO WAIT: "Hold it!"
NO-WIN: Kind of situation
NO-WISE: Au contraire
NOW I SEE: "Aha!"
NO WISER: Still clueless
NOWLAN: Canadian poet
NO WORSE: Just as good
NOXZEMA: Lotion brand
NOYCE: Director Phillip
NOYES: British poet
NOYORI: Japan chemistry Nobelist
N.P.R.: "All Things Considered" network
N.P.S: Document attestors: Abbr.
N.R.A.: New Deal org.
N.R.C.: AEC successor
N.R.O.T.C.: Would-be sailors' org.
N.S.A.: Hush-hush org.
N.S.C.: Presidential advisory grp.
N.S.F.: Abbr. on an overdrawn account
N STAR: Spectral type
N.S.W.: Austr. state
NSX: Acura model
NSYNC: Rock band
N-TEST: Atomic experiment
N TILE: Scrabble one-pointer
N.T.S.B.: Accident investigation agcy.
N-TUPLE: Math term
NT. WT.: Food label abbr.
NUBBER: Weakly hit baseball
NUBBIN: Pencil stub
NUBBLE: Small piece
NUBIA: Ancient African land
NUBIAN: African desert
NUBILE: Marriageable
NUBIRA: Daewoo model
NUCHA: Back of the neck
NUCLEO: Nucleus: Comb. form
NUCLEON: Part of an atom
NUDNIK: Pest
NUDZH: Pester
NUECES: Corpus Christi county
NUESTRA: Our: Spanish
NUESTRO: Our: Spanish
NUEVA: New: Spanish
NUEVE: Nine: Spanish
NUEVO: New: Spanish
'NUFF: "__ said!"
NUFLO: "Green Mansions" character
NUGENT: Rock guitarist Ted
NUI: Rapa __ (Easter Island)
NUIT: Night: French
NULLA: Nothing: Italian
NULLO: Bid to take no tricks
NUMAN: British singer Gary
NUMBAT: Australian marsupial
NUMEN: Divine power
NUMERO: Number: Spanish
NUMIC: Comanche language family
NUMINA: Divine powers
NUM LOCK: Keyboard key
NUNAVUT: Canadian territory
NUNC: Now: Latin
NUNCA: Never: Spanish
NUNCIO: Papal representative
NUNEZ: Vasco __ de Balboa
NUNG EN: "The Good Earth" character
NUNG WEN: "The Good Earth" character
NUNN: Former Georgia senator
NUNZIO: "Dharma & Greg" dog
NUOVA: New: Italian
NUOVO: New: Italian
NUR: Only: German
NUREYEV: Russian ballet star
NURMI: Finnish runner
NUS: Greek letters
NUTATE: Nod the head
NUTKIN: Beatrix Potter's squirrel
NUT OIL: Frying medium
NUTRIA: Beaverlike fur
NUTRO: Dog-food brand
NUYEN: Actress France
NUYS: Van __, CA
NWAPA: Nigerian writer
N.W.S.: Govt. meteorology org.
NWT: Alta. neighbor
NYACK: City on the Hudson
NYAD: Swimmer Diana
NYALA: African antelope
NYASA: African lake
NYBY: Director Christian
NYCT: Night: Comb. form
NYCTI: Night: Comb. form
NYCTO: Night: Comb. form
NYDIA: "Last Days of Pompeii" character
NYE: Comedian Louis
NYET: No: Russian
N.Y. GIANT: NFLer
N.Y. JET: NFL player
NYM: Friend of Falstaff
NYMAN: Actress Lena
N.Y. MET: National Leaguer
NYNEX: Former Baby Bell
N.Y., N.Y.: Big Apple: Abbr.
NYPD: "__ Blue"
N.Y. POST: Big Apple paper
NYQUIL: Cold-remedy brand
NYRO: Songwriter Laura
N.Y.S.: Where Albany is cap.
N.Y.S.E.: Wall Street letters
N.Y.T.: Big Apple newspaper, for short
N.Y. TIMES: Big Apple newspaper
NYTOL: Sleep-aid brand
NYU: Greenwich Village sch.
NYUK: Curly chuckle
NYX: Greek night goddess
NYY: Yankees, on scoreboards
N.Y. YANK: American Leaguer

O

OAKES: Actress Randi
OAKIE: Actor Jack
OAK LAWN: Illinois city
OAKLEY: Sharpshooter Annie
OAKMOSS: Lichen
OAK PARK: Illinois city
OAKTAG: Poster material
OAKUM: Caulking material
O.A.S.: U.S. alliance
OASAL: Of an oasis
OAST: Hops kiln
OATER: Western
OATES: Author Joyce Carol __
O.A.U.: Organization of African Unity: Abbr.
OAXACA: Mexican city
OBAD.: Bk. after Amos
OBADIAH: Book after Amos
OBAMA: Illinois senator Barack
OBAN: Scottish port
O.B.E.: U.K. honor
OBEAH: West Indies sorcery
OBELUS: Dagger, in printing
OBENTO: Japanese boxed meal
OBER: Upper: German
OBERLIN: Ohio college
OBERON: Fairy king
OBERTO: Verdi opera
OB-GYN: Med. specialty
OBI: Japanese sash
OBIE: "Village Voice" award
OBISPO: San Luis __, CA
OBITER: __ dictum (passing remark)
OBI-WAN: "Star Wars" character
OBJET: __ d'art
OBL.: Oblong: Abbr.
OB-LA-DI: "__, Ob-La-Da"
OBLAST: Russian province
OBLATE: Catholic layperson
OBLOQUY: Censure
OBOL: Ancient Greek coin
OBOLER: Radio writer Arch
OBOLUS: Greek weight
OBOTE: Former Ugandan president
OBRA: Work: Spanish
O'BRIAN: Actor Hugh
O'BRIEN: Author Edna
OBS.: Obsolete: Abbr.
OBSCURA: Camera __
OBTEST: Beseech
OBTRUDE: Thrust forth
OBTUND: Make blunt
OBV.: Front of a coin: Abbr.
OBVERSE: Front of a coin
OBVERT: Turn
OBVIATE: Make unnecessary
OCA: Andean tuber
OCALA, FL: Sunshine State city
O CANADA: National anthem
OCASEK: Rock singer Ric
O'CASEY: Irish playwright
OCC.: Profession: Abbr.
OCCAM: English philosopher
OCCAM'S: __ razor (maxim in logic)
OCCIPUT: Back of the head
OCEANIA: Pacific region
OCEANID: Sea nymph
OCEANUS: One of the Titans
O'CEDAR: Mop brand
OCELLUS: Eyelike spot
OCH: Scottish cry of disapproval
OCHENTA: Eighty: Spanish
OCHO: Eight: Spanish
OCHOA: Medicine Nobelist Severo
OCHS: Publisher Adolph
OCICAT: Feline breed
OCK: Diminutive suffix
OCONEE: Georgia river
O'CONNOR: Author Flannery
O.C.R.: Optical character recognition: Abbr.
OCRAT: Advocate: Comb. form
O.C.S.: Officer Candidate School: Abbr.
OCTAN: Every eighth day
OCTANS: Southern constellation
OCTANT: Navigator's instrument
OCTAVIA: Wife of Nero
OCTAVIO: Mexican writer Paz
OCTAVO: Book size
OCTOBRE: October: French
OCTOOT: P.D.Q. Bach work
OCTROI: Old French tax
OCTUBRE: October: Spanish
OCUL: Eye: Comb. form
OCULUS: Eye
ODA: Harem room
ODA MAE: Whoopi Oscar role
O'DAY: Singer Anita
ODD DUCK: Weird one
ODEA: Theaters
OD'ED ON: Had too much of
O'DELL: Author Scott
ODENSE: Danish seaport
ODEON: Concert hall
ODER: German river
ODESA: Ukrainian city
ODESSA: Ukrainian city
ODETS: Dramatist Clifford
ODETTA: 1960s folk singer
ODETTE: "Swan Lake" role
ODEUM: Theater
ODIE: "Garfield" canine
ODILE: "Swan Lake" role
ODIN: Norse war god
OD'ING ON: Having too much of
ODO: "Deep Space Nine" character
ODOM: "Blue Moon" of baseball
OD ON: Have too much of
ODONT: Tooth: Comb. form
ODONTIA: Tooth-care: Suffix
ODONTO: Tooth: Comb. form
O'DOUL: Lefty of baseball
O'DOUL'S: Nonalcoholic beer
ODRA: Polish river
ODS: "__ bodkins!"
O.E.D.: Oxford English Dictionary: Abbr.
OEDIPUS: Mythical king
OEIL: Eye: French
O.E.M.: Original equipment manufacturer: Abbr.
OEN: Wine: Comb. form
OENO: Wine: Comb. form
OENONE: Wife of Paris
O.E.O.: Office of Economic Opportunity: Abbr.
O'ER: "...__ the fields we go..."
OERSTED: Danish physicist
OERTER: Discus thrower Al
OESTE: West: Spanish
OEUF: Egg: French

OEUVRE: Artistic work
OFFAL: Garbage
OFFALY: Irish county
OFFCAST: Discarded
OFFICIO: Ex __ member
OFF OF: No longer using
OFF RAMP: Exit
OFFUTT: Nebraska Air Force base
OGA: "Clan of the Cave Bear" character
OGAM: Old Irish script
O GAUGE: Model-railroad scale
OGDEN, UT: Western city
OGDOAD: Group of eight
OGEE: Double curve
OGGI: Today: Italian
OGHAM: Old Irish script
OGIER: "Song of Roland" character
OGIVE: Pointed arch
OGLALA: Dakota Indian
O GOD: Hymn start
OGPU: KGB predecessor
O'GRADY: Rosie of song
OGRO: Monster: Spanish
O'HAIR: Atheist Madalyn Murray __
O'HANLON: Virginia of Santa Claus letter fame
O'HARA: "Gone With the Wind" surname
O'HARE: Chicago airport
OHAYO: Good morning: Japanese
OH CAROL: Neil Sedaka tune
O. HENRY: Short-story writer
OH GOD: George Burns film
OHIO ART: Etch-A-Sketch company
OHIO U.: Midwest school
OH KAY: Gershwin musical
OHLIN: Swedish economics Nobelist
OHM'S LAW: Physics formula
OHNE: "Die Frau __ Schatten" (Strauss opera)
OH OK: "I get it now"
OHR: Ear: German
OHRE: Czech river
OH ROB: "Dick Van Dyke Show" catchphrase
OH SO: Very
OIC: Acid suffix
OID: Resembling: Suffix
OIDAL: Looking like: Suffix
OIE: Goose: French
OIL-BASE: Type of paint
OIL CAKE: Livestock food
OIL-LIT: Type of lamp
OIL RING: Auto part
OINGO: __ Boingo (rock band)
OIR: Listen: Spanish
OISE: French river
OISEAU: Bird: French
OITA: Japanese city
OJAI, CA: Golden State city
OJAYS: "Love Train" group
OJEDA: Bobby of baseball
OJIBWA: Canadian Indian
OJIBWAY: Canadian Indian
OJO: Eye: Spanish
OKA: Russian river
OKAPI: Giraffe relative
OKARA: Nigerian poet
OKE: All right, informally
O'KEEFE: Actor Dennis
O'KEEFFE: Painter Georgia
O'KELLEY: 1950s Irish president
OKEMO: Vermont ski resort
OKEY: "__-doke!"
OKHOTSK: Russian sea
OKIE: "Dust Bowl" migrant
OKINAWA: Japanese island
OKSANA: Figure skater Baiul
OK SHOOT: "Let's hear it!"
OKTOBER: October: German
OLA: Wave: Spanish
OLAF I: Norwegian king
OLAF II: Norwegian king
OLAF III: Norwegian king
OLAF IV: Norwegian king
OLAF V: Norwegian king
OLAH: Chemistry Nobelist George
O'LAKES: Land __ (butter brand)
O-LAN: "The Good Earth" heroine
OLAND: Charlie Chan portrayer
OLATHE: Kansas city
OLAV: Norwegian king
OLAV I: Norwegian king
OLAV II: Norwegian king
OLAV III: Norwegian king
OLAV IV: Norwegian king
OLAV V: Norwegian king
OLAY: Oil of __
OLD BLUE: "No Time for Sergeants" dog
OLD CITY: Jerusalem area
OLDE: Ye __ Shoppe
OLD ELI: Yale nickname
OLD GOLD: Yellowish hue
OLDHAM: English city
OLD LYME: Connecticut city
OLD NAVY: Clothing brand
OLD NICK: Satan
OLD ROSE: Grayish red
OLDS: Former GM make
OLDUVAI: Tanzanian dig site
OLD VIC: London theater
OLEA: Olive genus
OLEANNA: David Mamet play
OLEAN, NY: Empire State city
O'LEARY: Legendary cow owner
OLEATE: Ointment chemical
OLE BULL: Norwegian violinist
OLEFIN: Synthetic fiber
OLEG: Designer Cassini
OLEIN: Vegetable-oil part
OLE MISS: Southern school
OLEN: Author Robert __ Butler
OLE OLE: World Cup chant
OLEO OIL: Margarine ingredient
OLERUD: John of baseball
OLESHA: Russian writer
OLESON: "Little House on the Prairie" character
OLESTRA: Dietary fat substitute
OLETA: Singer Adams
OLEUM: Oil, to a pharmacist
O LEVEL: British school exam
OLGA: Gymnast Korbut
OLIC: Acid suffix
OLICOOK: Donut
OLID: Fetid
OLIG: Few: Comb. form
OLIGO: Few: Comb. form
OLIN: Actress Lena
OLINDA: Brazilian city
OLIO: Miscellany
OLIVA: Tony of baseball
OLIVER: Director Stone
OLIVIA: Singer Newton-John
OLIVIER: Actor Laurence
OLIVINE: Green mineral
OLLA: Earthenware jar
OLLIE: Comic Hardy
OLMEC: Ancient Mexican
OLMERT: Israeli leader Ehud
OLMOS: Actor Edward James __
OLMSTED: Architect Frederick
OLOF: Swedish statesman Palme
OLOGY: Scientific study
OLOR: Scent: Spanish
OLOROSO: Spanish sherry
OLPE: Greek jug
OLSEN: Merlin of football
OLSON: Game-show announcer Johnny
OLYMPIA: Washington capital
OMA: Medical suffix
OMAHA, NE: Midwest city
OMAHAS: Midwest Indians
O'MALLEY: Former Dodgers owner
OMAN: Arabian sultanate
OMAR: Actor Sharif
OMARR: Astrologer Sydney
OMASUM: Cow stomach
OMAT: Self-service suffix
O.M.B.: Fed. budget agcy.
OMBER: Card game
OMBRE: Card game
'OME: Cockney residence
O'MEARA: Golfer Mark
OMEI: Buddhist sacred mountain
OMER: Hebrew measure
OMERTA: Code of silence
OMI: Japanese lake
OMICRON: Greek letter
OMN: All: Comb. form
OMNES: "Exeunt __"
OMNI: All: Comb. form
OMNIA: All: Latin
OMNIMAX: Mega movie theater
OMNIS: All: Latin
OMNIUM: __-gatherum (miscellany)
OMOO: Melville novel
OMPHAL: Navel: Comb. form
OMPHALO: Navel: Comb. form
OMRI: Biblical king
OMS: Chanting syllables
OMSK: Russian city
ONA: Actress Munson
ONAGER: Ancient catapult
ON A JAG: Binging
ON A LEAD: Tethered
ON A LINE: Level
ONAN: Son of Judah
ONASSIS: Mogul Aristotle
ONATE: Explorer Juan de __
ON AUTO: Not human-controlled
ON CD: Like much recorded music
ONCLE: Uncle: French
ONDA: Wave: Spanish
ONDE: Wave: French
ON DIT: Bit of gossip
ONE-A: Highest draft rating
ONE-A-CAT: Ball game
ONE A DAY: Vitamin brand
O'NEAL: Actor Ryan
ONE ALL: Game score
ONE ARM: Slot-machine feature
ONE B: Apartment number
ONE-BASE: __ hit (single)
ONE C: Apartment number
ONE D: Apartment number
ONE E: Shoe size
ONE EE: Shoe size
ONE EEE: Shoe size
ONE EEEE: Shoe size
ONE F: Apartment number
ONEFOLD: Complete
ONE G: $1000
ONEGA: Russian lake
ONEGIN: Pushkin hero
ONE H: Apartment number
ONE-HIT: __ wonder
ONEIDA: New York Indian
O'NEIL: Buck of baseball
O'NEILL: Playwright Eugene
ONEIR: Dream: Comb. form
ONEIRIC: Of dreams
ONEIRO: Dream: Comb. form
ONE-K: Runner's distance
ONE-L: Law student
ONELA: "Beowulf" character
ONE LB.: Sixteen oz.
ONE MEG: 1,000,000+ bytes
ONE NO: Bridge bid
ONE-O'-CAT: Ball game
ONE-OFF: Something not repeated
ONE ON: Baseball situation
ONEONTA: New York city
ONER: Unique thing
ONERA: Burdens: Latin
ONE WOOD: Driver
ONEY: Johnny Cash tune
ON HIRE: Ready for work
O.N.I.: Office of Naval Intelligence: Abbr.
ONIC: Acid suffix
ONKYO: Japanese electronics company
ONLAY: Dental work
ONLY TOO: Extremely
ONLY YOU: 1955 tune
ON-MIKE: Amplified
ON MY OWN: Eleanor Roosevelt book
ONNA: Choreographer White
ONNES: Dutch physics Nobelist
ONO: Yoko __
ON ONE: Football-huddle phrase
ONORATI: Actor Peter
ONS: Switch positions
ONSAGER: Chemistry Nobelist Lars
ONSTAR: Auto navigation system
ONT.: Canadian prov.

ON THE D.L.: Injured, as a baseballer
ON THREE: Football-huddle phrase
ONTKEAN: Actor Michael
ON TWO: Football huddle phrase
ONYM: Name: Comb. form
OOBLECK: Dr. Seuss goo
OOCYTE: Immature egg
OOID: Egg-shaped
OOKY: Like the Addams family
OOLA: "Return of the Jedi" girl
OOLITE: Egg stone
OOLOGY: Study of eggs
OOLONG: Tea variety
OOM: __ pah pah
OOMPA: __ Loompas (Wonka employees)
OOMPAH: Tuba sound
OON: Bass ending
OONA: Eugene O'Neill's daughter
OOO: "Hollywood Squares" win
OOOLA: Alley Oop's girlfriend
OOOO: Goose eggs
OOOOO: Goose eggs
OOP: "Alley __!"
OOPOD: Part of an insect stinger
OORT: Dutch astronomer
OOTID: Egg cell
OOX: "Hollywood Squares" non-win
OPA: __-Locka, FL
OPAH: Aquarium fish
OP ART: 1960s artistic genre
OP. CIT.: Bibliographical abbr.
OPE: Open, in verse
OPEC: Oil cartel
OP-ED: Newspaper page
OPEL: German auto
OPEN NET: Ice-hockey situation
OPER: Phone button
OPERE: Part of op. cit.
OPEROSE: Industrious
OPHELIA: "Hamlet" character
OPHIR: Biblical country
OPHULS: Director Marcel
OPIA: Sight: Comb. form
OPIE: "Andy Griffith Show" kid
OPIS: "The Aeneid" character
OPORTO: Portuguese city
OPPER: "Happy Hooligan" cartoonist
OPPUGN: Assail
OPRAH: TV host Winfrey
OPRAH'S: __ Book Club
OPRY: Grand Ole __
OPS: Goddess of plenty
OPTICKS: Isaac Newton book
OPTIMAS: Kia models
OPTIMO: Best: Spanish
OPTO: Eye: Comb. form
OPUNTIA: Type of cactus
ORA: Anglo-Saxon coin
ORACH: Spinachlike plant
ORACY: Ability to express oneself
ORAD: Toward the mouth
ORAJEL: Toothache-soother brand
ORAL-B: Toothbrush brand
ORALE: Church vestment
ORALIST: Lip reader
ORAMA: Display: Comb. form
ORAN: Algerian city
ORANT: Prayer figure
ORANTES: Tennis pro Manuel
ORARION: Church stole
ORARIUM: Church stole
ORBACH: Actor Jerry
ORBISON: Singer Roy
ORC: Tolkien creature
ORCA: Killer whale
ORCUS: Roman underworld
ORCZY: "The Scarlet Pimpernel" author
ORD: Former California fort
ORDINES: Church calendars
ORDO: Church calendar
ORDONEZ: Magglio of baseball
OREAD: Mountain nymph
ORECK: Vacuum-cleaner brand
ORECTIC: Of desire
OREE: Camp suffix
ORE-IDA: Frozen-potatoes brand
O'REILLY: Radar's last name
OREL: Pitcher Hershiser
OREM: Utah city
OREN: Opera conductor Daniel
ORENA: Former name of an Orlando stadium
ORENSE: City in Spain
OREO O'S: Breakfast cereal
ORESTES: Agamemnon's son
OREXIA: Appetite: Comb. form
OREXIS: Appetite, in psychology
ORFE: Aquarium fish
ORFEO: "__ ed Euridice"
ORFF: German composer
ORG.: Organization: Abbr.
ORGANA: "Star Wars" princess Leia __
ORGANDY: Cotton fabric
ORGANZA: Sheer fabric
ORGEAT: Almond drink
ORGON: "Tartuffe" character
ORI: Mouth: Comb. form
ORIANA: Author Fallaci
ORIANI: Italian author
ORIBI: African antelope
ORIEL: Bay window
ORIENTE: East: Spanish
ORIGEN: Christian theologian
ORIGINE: Ab __ (from the beginning)
ORIN: "Little Shop of Horrors" dentist
O-RING: Gasket
ORINOCO: Venezuelan river
ORION: Hunter of myth
ORION'S: __ Belt
ORISON: Prayer
ORISSA: State of India
ORIUM: Place: Comb. form
ORK: Mork's planet
ORKIN: Exterminator company
ORKNEYS: Islands off Scotland
ORLANDO: Florida city
ORLE: Heraldic border
ORLEANS: French city
ORLO: Pedestal part
ORLOP: Ship deck
ORLY: Paris airport
ORMAN: Suze of personal finance
ORMANDY: Conductor Eugene
ORMOLU: Copper alloy
ORMOND: Actress Julia
ORNE: Novelist Sarah __ Jewett
ORNETTE: Saxophonist Coleman
ORNIS: Birds of a region
ORNITH: Bird: Comb. form
ORO: Gold: Spanish
OROGENY: Mountain-making process
OROLOGY: Study of mountains
O ROMEO: Words from Juliet
ORONO: University of Maine town
O'RORY: "The Glass Key" character
OROSCO: Jesse of baseball
OROTUND: Pompous
O'ROURKE: Satirist P.J.
OROZCO: Mexican painter
ORPAH: Naomi's daughter-in-law
ORPHANT: "Little __ Annie" (Riley poem)
ORPHEUM: Theater name
ORPHEUS: Lyrist of myth
ORPHIC: Mystic
ORR: Hockey great Bobby
ORRA: Odd: Scottish
ORREN: "Atlas Shrugged" character
ORRERY: Planetarium
ORRIN: Utah senator Hatch
ORRIS: Aromatic root
ORSAY: Quai d'__ (Paris street)
'ORSE: Cockney steed
ORSER: Figure skater Brian
ORSINI: Italian noble surname
ORSINO: "Twelfth Night" duke
ORSK: Russian city
ORSON: Director Welles
ORT: Scrap of food
ORTEGA: Former Nicaraguan president
ORTEGAL: Spanish Cape
ORTH: Straight: Comb. form
OR THEN: Otherwise
ORTHO: Right: Comb. form
ORTIZ: 1930s president of Argentina
ORTOLAN: Bobolink
ORTON: Dramatist Joe
ORTRUD: "Lohengrin" role
ORURO: Bolivian city
O.R.V.: Off-road vehicle: Abbr.
ORVAL: Arkansas politician Faubus
ORVIETO: Italian wine
ORVILLE: Inventor Wright
ORVIS: Fishing-gear brand
ORWELL: "1984" author
ORY: Jazz trombonist
ORYX: African antelope
ORZO: Ricelike pasta
OSA: Female bear: Spanish
OSAKA: Japanese city
OSAR: Gravel ridges
OSBERT: "Auntie Mame" character
OSBORN: Playwright Paul
OSBORNE: "Look Back in Anger" playwright
OSCAN: Ancient Italian
OSCEOLA: Seminole chief
OSCINE: Songbird
OSCULAR: Of kissing
OSCULE: Sponge hole
OSE: Sugar: Suffix
OSEE: Douay Bible prophet
OSETRA: Type of caviar
OSGOOD: TV host Charles
OSH: Kirghizia city
OSHA: Workplace safety org.
OSHAWA: Canadian city
O'SHAY: "Rick __" (western comic strip)
O'SHEA: Actor Milo
OSHKOSH: Wisconsin city
OSI: "Six Million Dollar Man" org.
OSIER: Willow tree
OSIP: Poet Mandelstam
OSIRIS: Ancient Egyptian god
OSIS: Condition: Suffix
OSKAR: Actor Werner
OSLER: Canadian physician
OSLIN: Country singer K.T.
OSLO: Norway's capital
OSMAN: Ottoman Empire founder
OSMATIC: Of smell
OSMIC: Of element #76
OSMICS: Science of smell
OSMIUM: Element #76
OSMONDS: Singing family
OSMUND: Type of fern
OSO: Bear: Spanish
OSPREY: Bird of prey
OSRIC: "Hamlet" character
O.S.S.: CIA predecessor
OSSA: Greek peak
OSSEO: Bone: Comb. form
OSSEOUS: Bony
OSSET: Caucasus native
OSSETRA: Type of caviar
OSSI: Bone: Comb. form
OSSIA: Or else, in music
OSSIAN: Legendary Gaelic hero
OSSICLE: Small bone
OSSIE: Actor Davis
OSSIFY: Become inflexible
OSSIPEE: New Hampshire town
OSSO: __ buco (veal dish)
OSSUARY: Place for bones
OST: East: German
O STAR: Spectral type
OSTE: Bone: Comb. form
OSTEND: Belgian city
OSTEO: Bone: Comb. form
OSTER: Appliance brand
OSTIA: Port of ancient Rome
OSTIARY: Church doorkeeper
OSTLER: Horse handler
OSTMARK: East German currency
OSTOSIS: Formation of bone
OSTRAVA: Czech city
OSTWALD: German chemistry Nobelist
OSU: Columbus sch.
OSWALD: "King Lear" character
OSWEGO: New York port
OTA: Taxonomic suffix
OTALGIA: Earache

OTARU: Japanese city
OTARY: Eared seal
OTAY: "Our Gang" affirmative
OTB: Off-track betting: Abbr.
O.T.C.: Over-the-counter: Abbr.
OTE: Native of: Suffix
OTEA: Great Barrier Island
OTELLO: Verdi opera
OTERI: Cheri of "Saturday Night Live"
OTERO: New Mexico county
OTHELLO: Shakespeare play
OTHMAR: "Peanuts" teacher
OTHO: Roman emperor
OTHON: "Song of Roland" character
OTIC: Of the ear
O TILE: Scrabble one-pointer
OTIOSE: Idle
OTIS: Singer Redding
OTITIS: Ear inflammation
OTO: Oklahoma Indian
OTOE: Oklahoma Indian
OTOLOGY: Study of the ear
OTOMI: Mexican Indian
OTOÑO: Autumn: Spanish
O'TOOLE: Actor Peter
OTOSIS: Mishearing
O-TOWN: Male vocal group
OTRA: Other: Spanish
OTRANTO: Adriatic strait
OTS: Overtimes: Abbr.
OTSEGO: New York lake
OTT: Mel of baseball
OTTAVA: __ rima (Italian stanza)
OTTAVIO: "Don Giovanni" character
OTTAWA: Canadian capital
OTTAWAS: Canadian Indians
OTTIS: Anderson of football
OTTO: Director Preminger
OTTO I: Holy Roman Emperor
OTTO II: Holy Roman Emperor
OTTO III: Holy Roman Emperor
OTTO IV: Holy Roman Emperor
OTTONE: Handel opera
OTTUMWA: Iowa city
OTWAY: English playwright
OUD: Arab lute
OUEST: West: French
OUGUIYA: Mauritanian money
OUI: Yes: French
OUIDA: "A Dog of Flanders" author
OUIJA: Spiritualist's board
OUIMET: Golfer Francis
OULU: Finnish city
OURAY: Colorado city
OUR GANG: Spanky's group
OUR TOWN: Thornton Wilder play
OUS: Full of: Suffix
OUSE: English river
OUSEL: Diving bird
OUTFOOT: Run faster than
OUTIE: Belly-button variety
OUTKAST: Hip-hop group
OUTPORT: Place of departure
OUTSERT: Sheet around a newspaper
OUTTA: "I'm __ here!"
OUTWIND: Lose one's breath
OUTWITH: Beyond the limit of
OUZEL: Diving bird
OUZO: Greek liqueur
OVA: Eggs: Latin
OVATE: Almost round
OVERDOG: One with an advantage
OVERS: Cricket rounds
OVETA: First H.E.W. Secretary __ Culp Hobby
OVETT: Runner Steve
OVI: Egg: Comb. form
OVID: Roman poet
OVIEDO: Spanish city
OVIFORM: Egg-shaped
OVINE: Sheep
OVIPARA: Egg-laying animals
OVIS: Sheep: Latin
OVISAC: Egg capsule
OVITZ: Former Disney president
OVO: Ab __ (from the beginning)
OVOLO: Convex molding
OVULAR: Egg-shaped
OVULE: Botanical seed
OVUM: Egg: Latin
OWEN: Actor Wilson
OWENS: Track star Jesse
O.W.I.: Office of War Information: Abbr.
OWIE: Bruise, to a tot
OWN GOAL: Soccer term
OWOSSO: Michigan city
OXALATE: Chemical in spinach
OXALIC: Cleanser acid
OXALIS: Wood sorrel
OXANA: Pianist Yablonskaya
OXBLOOD: Dark red
OXBOW: River bend
OXES: Clumsy ones
OXEYE: Daisylike flower
OXFAM: British charity
OXHEART: Cherry variety
OXLIP: Eurasian primrose
OXNARD: California city
OXO: Tic-tac-toe nonwinner
OXON: English county
OXONIAN: Oxford student
OXUS: Asian river
OXX: Tic-tac-toe nonwinner
OXY: Sharp: Comb. form
OXYDOL: Detergent brand
OYE: "__ Como Va" (Santana tune)
OYER: Court hearing
OYEZ: Courtroom cry
OYL: Popeye's girlfriend
OYS: Yiddish exclamations
OY VEY: Cry of dismay
OZAWA: Conductor Seiji
OZICK: Writer Cynthia
OZMA: Baum princess
OZZFEST: Heavy-metal rock tour
OZZIE: Actor Nelson
OZZY: Rock singer Osbourne

P

PAANGA: Money in Tonga
PAAR: Johnny Carson predecessor
PAAVO: Finnish runner Nurmi
PABA: Sunscreen ingredient
PABLO: Artist Picasso
PABLUM: Cereal brand
PABST: Beer brand
PABULUM: Nutrition
PAC: Contributor to Congress: Abbr.
PACA: South American rodent
PAC BELL: Former phone company
PACE LAP: Auto racer's warmup
PACEM: Peace: Latin
PACEY: Fast
PA CHIN: Chinese writer
PACHISI: Board game
PACHY: Thick: Comb. form
PACINO: Actor Al
PACKARD: Antique auto
PACK ICE: Arctic mass
PAC-MAN: 1980s video game
PACO: Fashion designer Rabanne
PACQUIN: Skin-cream brand
PAC TEN: College football conference
PACULA: Actress Joanna
PADGETT: Author Lewis
PADOVA: Italian city, to natives
PADRAIC: Author Colum
PADRONE: Boss
PADSITE: Lot near a mall
PADUA: "Taming of the Shrew" locale
PADUCAH: Kentucky city
PAEAN: Hymn of praise
PAESE: Bel __ cheese
PAGE SIX: Newspaper gossip locale
PAGET: Actress Paget
PAGE UP: Computer key
PAGLIA: Straw: Italian
PAGNOL: French playwright
PAGO: Half a Samoan city's name
PAH: Oom-__ band
PAHLAVI: Shah surname
PAHS: Disgusted exclamations
PAI: Father: Portuguese
PAID AD: Infomercial, e.g.
PAIGE: Actress Janis
PAINE: "Common Sense" writer
PAIS: Country: Spanish
PAISA: Bangladesh money
PAISAN: Buddy
PAISANO: Buddy
PAISE: Bangladesh money
PAIUTE: Western Indian
PAIX: Peace: French
PA JOAD: "Grapes of Wrath" character
PAK.: India neighbor: Abbr.
PAKULA: Director Alan
PALABRA: Word: Spanish
PALADE: 1974 medicine Nobelist
PALADIN: Heroic champion
PALAIS: Palace: French
PALAMAS: Greek poet
PALANCE: Actor Jack
PALAR: Like a stake
PALAU: Pacific island group's former name
PALEA: Botanical bract
PALE ALE: Pub serving
PALEMON: "Thaïs" role
PALEO: Ancient: Comb. form
PALERMO: City in Sicily
PALEY: CBS founder
PALFREY: Riding horse
PALI: Buddhist scriptures language
PALIN: Monty Python member
PALINGS: Fence stakes
PAL JOEY: Rodgers and Hart musical
PALLAS: Epithet for Athena
PALMA: Majorca city
PALMAR: Of the palm
PALMARY: Praiseworthy
PALMAS: Las __, Canary Islands
PALMATE: Web-footed
PALME: Swedish statesman
PALMER: Golfer Arnold
PALMERS: Pilgrims
PALMTOP: Small computer
PALMYRA: Ancient Syrian city
PALO: __ Alto, CA
PALOMA: Dove: Spanish
PALOMAR: California observatory
PALOOKA: Big ape
PALOS: Spanish seaport
PALP: Animal feeler
PALPATE: Examine by touch
PALSY: __-walsy
PALTER: Equivocate
PALTROW: Actress Gwyneth
PALUDAL: Swampy
PAM: Country singer Tillis
PAMBY: Namby-__
PAMELA: Actress Anderson
PAMINA: "The Magic Flute" role
PAMIRS: Highlands of India
PAMLICO: Sound of North Carolina
PAMPA: Argentine plain
PANADA: Thick sauce
PAN AM: Former international airline
PANAMAS: Types of hats
PANAY: Philippine island
PANCHAX: Tropical fish
PANCHO: Tennis pro Gonzales
PANCKS: "Little Dorrit" character
PANDIT: Wise man of India
P. AND L.: Accounting statement
PANDORA: Box opener of myth
PANETTA: Clinton chief of staff
PANGAEA: Hypothetical supercontinent
PANGRAM: Sentence using every letter
PANICLE: Flower cluster
PANIER: Large basket
PAN IN: Prepare for a closeup
PANINI: Italian sandwich
PANINO: Italian sandwich
PANIS: Bread: Latin
PANKY: Hanky-__
PANNE: Velvet fabric
PANNIER: Large basket
PANOPE: "Faerie Queene" character
PANOPLY: Impressive array
PANTA: All: Comb. form
PANTENE: Shampoo brand

PANTERA: Italian auto
PANTILE: Roofing tile
PANTO: British pantomime
PANTONE: Color control system
PANURGE: Pantagruel's companion
PANZA: Cervantes character
PANZER: WWII tank
PAO: Kung __ chicken
PAOLI: Philadelphia suburb
PAOLO: Painter Veronese
PAON: Peacock blue
PAPA DOC: Duvalier nickname
PAPAGO: Arizona Indian
PAPAW: North American tree
PAPEETE: City in Tahiti
PAPEL: Paper: Spanish
PAPIER: Paper: French
PAPILLA: Part of the tongue
PAPP: "A Chorus Line" producer
PAPPAS: TV reporter Ike
PAPUA: Coral Sea inlet
PAQUIN: Actress Anna
PARADOR: Spanish inn
PARAIBA: State of Brazil
PARAMUS: New Jersey city
PARANA: Argentine city
PARAPH: Signature flourish
PARAS: Plane jumpers, for short
PARASKI: Hit the slopes with a sail
PARATUS: Ready: Latin
PARBAKE: Bake partially
PARC: Park: French
PARCA: Roman goddess of destiny
PARDO: "Saturday Night Live" announcer
PARETO: Italian sociologist
PAREU: Polynesian dress
PAREVE: Containing no meat or milk
PARFUM: French perfume
PARGE: Coat with plaster
PARI: Equal: Comb. form
PARIBUS: Ceteris __ (other things being equal)
PARINI: Italian poet
PARKADE: Canadian garage
PARK AVE.: Manhattan addr.
PARKAY: Margarine brand
PARKES: British inventor
PARKINS: Actress Barbara
PARK IT: Have a seat
PARKMAN: Historian Francis
PARLE: "Ici on __ français"
PARLEZ: "__-vous français?"
PARLOUS: Dangerous
PARMA: Italian city
PARNIS: Fashion designer Mollie
PAROL: Spoken statement
PARONYM: Word with the same root
PAROO: "The Music Man" character
PAROS: Greek island
PAROTID: Salivary gland
PARR: Henry VIII's sixth wife
PARRA: Chilean poet
PARRIS: South Carolina island
PARRISH: Painter Maxfield
PARRS: Young salmons
PARSEC: 3.26 light years
PARSEE: Zoroastrian
PARSI: Zoroastrian
PART A: First section
PARTE: Ex __ (from one side only)
PART I: Book section
PART II: Book section
PART III: Book section
PARTITA: Bach work
PART IV: Book section
PARTON: Singer Dolly
PART ONE: First section
PART V: Book section
PARTY ON: Reveler's exclamation
PARTY'S: "The __ Over"
PARURE: Matching set of jewels
PARVENU: Johnny-come-lately
PAS: Faux __
PASA: "Qué __?"
PAS ALLE: Ballet step
PASCAL: French philosopher
PASCH: Easter
PASCO: City in Washington
PASCOLI: Italian poet
PASCUA: Easter: Spanish
PASDAR: Actor Adrian
PASE: Bullfighter maneuver
PASEO: Spanish avenue
PASH: Ardor in Tin Pan Alley
PASHA: Turkish title
PASHTO: Afghan language
PAS MOI: French denial
PASO: El __, TX
PASOS: __ dobles (Spanish dances)
PASSADE: Equestrian move
PASSADO: Fencing maneuver
PASSAIC: New Jersey city
PASSANT: En __ (chess term)
PASS AS: Be mistaken for
PASSAT: Volkswagen model
PAS SEUL: Ballet solo
PASS GO: Collect $200 in Monopoly
PASSIM: Here and there
PASS ON: Decline
PASSOS: Author John Dos __
PASSU: Pari __ (equably)
PASSY: French peace Nobelist
PASTERN: Part of a horse's hoof
PASTEUR: French chemist
PASTINA: Tiny pasta
PASTIS: Liqueur
PAST IT: Over the hill
PASTO: Meal: Italian
PATACA: Money of Macao
PATAKI: Mario Cuomo's successor
PAT CASH: 1987 Wimbledon winner
PATCHEN: Poet Kenneth
PATCO: Former traffic controllers' union
PAT DAY: Derby-winning jockey in 1992
PATED: Ending for addle
PATEK: __ Philippe (fancy watch)
PATEN: Altar plate
PATER: Father, in Britain
PATERNO: Penn State football coach
PATHAN: Afghan
PAT HAND: Full house, e.g.
PATHE: Newsreel maker
PATHIC: Practicing: Comb. form
PATHO: Feeling: Comb. form
PATHY: Feeling: Comb. form
PATINE: Copper coating
PATMOS: Greek island
PATNA: City of India
PATO: Duck: Spanish
PATON: South African novelist
PATR: Father: Comb. form
PATRI: Father: Comb. form
PATRIA: Country: Latin
PATRIC: Actor Jason
PATRICE: Opera singer Munsel
PATRIE: Country: French
PATRO: Father: Comb. form
PATROON: Colonial landowner
PATTEN: Actor Dick Van __
PATTI: Singer Page
PATTON: WWII general
PATZER: Bad chess player
PAUCITY: Lack
PAULA: Singer Abdul
PAULEY: TV host Jane
PAULI: Austrian physicist
PAUL II: Pope
PAUL III: Pope
PAULINA: Model Porizkova
PAULINE: "Perils" girl
PAULING: Chemist Linus
PAULIST: Certain missionary
PAUL IV: Pope
PAULO: Sao __, Brazil
PAUL PRY: Busybody
PAULSEN: Comic Pat
PAUL V: Pope
PAUL VI: Pope
PAVANE: French dance
PAVEL: Paul: Russian
PAVESE: Italian novelist
PAVIA: Italian city
PAVID: Afraid
PAVIN: Pro golfer Corey
PAVIOR: Building brick
PAVLOV: Russian medicine Nobelist
PAVLOVA: Russian ballerina
PAVO: Peacock constellation
PAWL: Machine part
PAWNEE: Oklahoma Indian
PAWPAW: North American tree
PAX: Cable channel
PAXINOU: Actress Katina
PAXOS: Greek island
PAXTON: Actor Bill
PAYNE: Singer Freda
PAYPAL: Internet payment service
PAYSON: Author Albert __ Terhune
PAYT.: Remittance: Abbr.
PAY TO: Check instruction
PAYTON: Walter of football
PAZ: Peace: Spanish
P.B.A.: Keglers' org.
P.B. AND J.: Sandwich, for short
P.B.J.: Sandwich, for short
P-BOOK: Book printed on paper
PBS: "Antiques Roadshow" network
PBX: Office phone syst.
P.C.B.: Water pollutant: Abbr.
PC CLONE: Type of computer
PC LAB: College computer center
PCP: Illicit drug: Abbr.
PCS: Some computers: Abbr.
PC USER: Certain computer owner
PCV: __ valve (auto part)
PC WORLD: Computer magazine
P.D.A.: Hand-held computer: Abbr.
PDF: Computer print-file format
P. DIDDY: Rap star
P.D.J.: Literary monogram
P.D. JAMES: British author
P.D.Q. BACH: "Oedipus Tex" composer
P.D.R.: Doctor's reference bk.
P.D.S: APB broadcasters
P.D.T.: L.A. summer clock setting
PEABO: Singer Bryson
PEABODY: Massachusetts city
PEACHED: Betrayed
PEALE: Positive thinking proponent
PEALES: Family of artists
PEANO: Italian mathematician
PEARCE: Actress Alice
PEARLE: Eyeglass-store chain
PEARSON: 1960s Canadian leader
PEARY: Arctic explorer
PEASE: "__ Porridge Hot"
PEAU: __ de soie (silk cloth)
PEBA: Armadillo
PEC: Chest muscle
PECCANT: Wrong
PECCARY: Piglike mammal
PECCAVI: Confession of guilt
PECHE: Peach: French
PECKISH: Irritable, in Britain
PECOS: Texas river
PECTIN: Jelly ingredient
PED.: Walker, for short
PEDATE: Having feet
PEDE: Footed: Comb. form
PEDER: "Giants in the Earth" character
PEDI: Foot: Comb. form
PEDICAB: Foot-powered taxi
PEDO: Child: Comb. form
PEDRO: Director Almodóvar
PEDWAY: Urban walker's route
PEEBLES: Director Mario Van __
PEE DEE: Carolina river
PEELE: British playwright
PEEN: Ball-__ hammer
PEEPLES: Actress Nia
PEERCE: Opera singer Jan
PEET: Actress Amanda
PEETE: Golfer Calvin
PEG AWAY: Work hard
PEGBOX: Violin part
PEGEEN: "Auntie Mame" character
PEGGY: Singer Lee
PEGLER: Journalist Westbrook
PEGTOPS: Narrow-ankle trousers
PEGUY: French poet
PEI: Chinese architect
PEIPING: Beijing's former name
PEIRCE: Philosopher Charles
PEKE: Small dog
PEKEPOO: Dog breed

PEKIN: Illinois city
PEKKA: Conductor Esa-__ Salonen
PELAGE: Animal fur
PELAGIC: Of the sea
PELE: Soccer great
PELEE: Martinique volcano
PELEG: "Moby-Dick" character
PELEUS: Father of Achilles
PELF: Ill-gotten gains
PELHAM: Bulwer-Lytton work
PELION: Greek mountain
PELISSE: Woman's cloak
PELL: Former Rhode Island senator
PELLA: City of ancient Greece
PELLAM: "Idylls of the King" character
PELLE: "__ the Conqueror" (1988 film)
PELLEAS: King Arthur knight
PELLI: Architect César
PELOSI: House Democratic leader
PELOTA: Jai alai ball
PELOTON: Bike-race riders
PELTATE: Shield-shaped
PELTRY: Fur skins
PEMBA: Island north of Zanzibar
PENA: Clinton cabinet member
PENATES: Household gods
PENCHE: Leaning forward, in ballet
PENDENT: Dangling
PENG: Chinese premier Li __
PENGPU: Chinese city
PENH: Phnom __, Cambodia
PENICK: Golf teacher Harvey
PEN IN: Corral
PENNATE: Feathered
PENNE: Tubular pasta
PENNEY'S: Retail chain
PENNI: Old Finnish coin
PENNIA: Old Finnish coins
PENNINE: Range of the Alps
PENNOCK: Herb of baseball
PENNON: Flag
PENROD: Booth Tarkington boy
PENROSE: Stephen Hawking colleague
PENSEE: Thought: French
PENS IN: Corrals
PENTAD: Group of five
PENTANE: Bottled gas
PENTAX: Camera brand
PENTE: Board game
PENTEL: Pen brand
PENTIUM: Computer chip
PENUCHE: Fudgelike candy
PENULT: Next-to-last syllable
PENZIAS: 1978 physics Nobelist
PEPA: Rappers Salt-N-__
PEP BOYS: Auto-parts store chain
PEPCID: Antacid brand
PEPE: Cartoon skunk
PEPIN: Charlemagne's father
PEPINO: "The Real McCoys" character
PEPITA: Pumpkin seed
PEPLUM: Short skirt
PEPO: Gourd
PEPPARD: Actor George
PEPPINO: "Count of Monte Cristo" character
PEPSICO: Food/drink conglomerate
PEPSIN: Enzyme
PEPTIC: Digestive
PEPTIDE: Amino-acid derivative
PEPTO: __-Bismol
PEPTONE: Protein derivative
PEPYS: British diarist
PEQUOD: "Moby-Dick" ship
PEQUOT: Eastern Indian
PERA: Pear: Spanish
PERAHIA: Pianist Murray
PER AN,: By the yr.
P.E. RATIO: Investor's stat.
PERC: Job benefit
PERCE: Nez __ Indians
PERCEPT: Something seen
PERCHA: Gutta-__ (golf-ball material)
PERCHIK: "Fiddler on the Roof" character
PERCUSS: Tap firmly
PERCY: Orchestra leader Faith
PERDIDO: Pyrenees peak
PERDITA: "101 Dalmatians" dog
PERDU: Hidden
PERDUE: Chicken brand
PERDURE: Continue
PERE: Father: French
PERES: Shimon of Israel
PERETTI: Italian jewelry designer
PEREZ: Javier __ de Cuellar
PERF: Postage-stamp feature, for short
PERFIDY: Bad faith
PERFUSE: Overspread with color
PERGOLA: Arbor
PERI: Persian sprite
PERIAPT: Amulet
PERIDOT: August birthstone
PERIGEE: Orbital point
PERINE: "Maltese Falcon" character
PERISSA: "Faerie Queene" character
PERITUS: Expert theologian
PERKIN: British chemist
PERKINS: FDR labor secretary
PERLE: Hostess Mesta
PERLEA: Romanian conductor
PERLITE: Glassy rock
PERLMAN: Israeli violinist
PERMA: Prefix for frost
PERMIAN: Paleozoic period
PERNOD: Anise liqueur
PERO: But: Spanish
PERON: "Evita" role
PERORAL: Through the mouth
PEROT: 1992 presidential candidate
PERP: Crook, to a cop
PERREAU: Actress Gigi
PERRIER: Water brand
PERRIN: French physics Nobelist
PERRINE: Actress Valerie
PERRINS: Steak-sauce name
PERRO: Dog: Spanish
PERRY: Actor Matthew
PERS.: Type of pronoun: Abbr.
PER SE: Intrinsically
PERSEID: Annual meteor shower
PERSEUS: Northern constellation
PERSIA: Iran, formerly
PERSIS: Actress Khambatta
PERSIUS: Roman satirist
PERSOFF: Actor Nehemiah
PERSSON: Swedish singer
PERTH: Australian city
PERUGIA: Italian city
PERUKE: Hairpiece of yore
PERUTZ: 1962 chemistry Nobelist
PES: Anatomical foot
PESACH: Jewish holiday
PESADE: Equestrian maneuver
PESANTE: Heavily, in music
PESCE: Fish: Italian
PESCI: Actor Joe
PESCOW: Actress Donna
PESETA: Former Spanish coin
PESEWA: Ghana coin
PETA: Animal rights org.
PETAIN: 1940s French leader
PETALE: Petal: French
PETARD: Detonating device
PETCO: Pet-store chain
PETCOCK: Faucet
PETE: Sampras of tennis
PETEMAN: Safecracker
PETER I: Czar
PETER II: Czar
PETERS: Actress Bernadette
PETE'S: "For __ sake!"
PETEY: "Our Gang" dog
PETIOLE: Leaf stalk
PETIPA: French ballet dancer
PETIT: Small: French
PETNAP: Steal a dog
PETO: Mackerel
PETRA: Ancient city of Jordan
PETRE: Schwarzkopf biography collaborator
PETRI: __ dish (lab item)
PETRIE: "Dick Van Dyke Show" family name
PETRO: Rock: Comb. form
PET ROCK: 1970s fad
PETROL: British gasoline
PETROUS: Rocky
PET SCAN: Diagnostic procedure
PETTET: Actress Joanna
PETTI: Undergarment, for short
PETTISH: Grumpy
PETTIT: Basketball Hall of Famer
PETULA: Singer Clark
PETULIA: Julie Christie film
PEU: Little bit: French
PEUGEOT: French auto
PEUR: Fear: French
PEUT: __-être (perhaps: French)
PEVNEY: Director Joseph
PEWEE: European bird
PEWIT: European bird
PEYOTE: Mexican cactus
PEYTON: "__ Place" (Metalious novel)
PEZ: Candy brand
P.F.C.: Army rank: Abbr.
PFD.: Adj. for some stock
PFENNIG: Former German coin
PFERD: Horse: German
PFFFT: Fizzling sound
PFFT: Fizzling sound
PFIZER: Drug company
PFLUG: Actress Jo Ann
PFUI: "Rats!"
PGA TOUR: Golf pros' circuit
PG-RATED: Like some movies
PHAEDRA: Wife of Theseus
PHAETON: Antique auto
PHAG: Eater: Comb. form
PHAGE: Eater: Comb. form
PHAGIA: Eating: Comb. form
PHAGO: Eating: Comb. form
PHAGY: Eating: Comb. form
PHAIR: Singer Liz
PHALANX: Battalion
PHANY: Appearance: Comb. form
PHAR LAP: 1983 film
PHAROS: Ancient lighthouse
PHARYNX: Throat
PHASER: Sci-fi weapon
PHAT: Excellent, slangily
PHEBE: "As You Like It" character
PHEDRE: Racine play
PHELPS: "Mission: Impossible" role
PHEMIUS: "Odyssey" character
PHEN: Appearing: Comb. form
PHENO: Appearing: Comb. form
PHENOL: Benzene derivative
PHEW: "That was close!"
PHFFFT: Jack Lemmon film
PHFFT: Fizzling sound
PHI: Greek letter
PHIAL: Ampule
PHIDIAS: Greek sculptor
PHIL: TV host Donahue
PHILBIN: TV host Regis
PHILBY: British spy
PHILCO: Old radio brand
PHILE: Lover: Comb. form
PHILEAS: Verne hero
PHILIC: Loving: Comb. form
PHILIP: Prince Charles' dad
PHILIP K.: Author Dick
PHILIPS: TV brand
PHILIP V: King of Spain
PHILLIE: National Leaguer
PHILLIP: "Sleeping Beauty" prince
PHILLY: Eastern city's nickname
PHILO: Fictional sleuth Vance
PHILOUS: Loving: Comb. form
PHILTER: Magic potion
PHINEAS: Showman Barnum
PHISH: Work an e-mail scam
PHIZ: Dickens illustrator
PHLEB: Vein: Comb. form
PHLEBO: Vein: Comb. form
PHLOEM: Plant tissue
PHLOX: Showy flower
PHNOM: __ Penh, Cambodia
PHOBE: Fearer: Comb. form
PHOBO: Fear: Comb. form
PHOBOS: Moon of Mars
PHOEBE: Songbird
PHOEBUS: Sun personified

PHON: Unit of loudness
PHONEME: Linguistics unit
PHONE NO.: Addr. book entry
PHOT: Unit of light
PHOTIC: Of light
PHOTICS: Science of light
PHOTO ID: Security badge
PHOTON: Bit of light
PHOTO OP: Media event
PHR.: Group of wds.
PHRENIC: Of the mind
PHRYGIA: Ancient country of Asia Minor
PHS: Acidity measures
PHU: Dien Bien __, Vietnam
PHYFE: Cabinetmaker Duncan
PHYLL: Leaf: Comb. form
PHYLLIS: "The Mary Tyler Moore Show" spin-off
PHYLLO: Greek pastry layer
PHYLO: Race: Comb. form
PHYLUM: Biological subdivision
PHYS. ED.: Coll. course
PHYSIC: Cure
PHYSIO: Nature: Comb. form
PHYT: Plant: Comb. form
PHYTE: Plant: Comb. form
PHYTO: Plant: Comb. form
PIA: Actress Zadora
PIAF: French singer
PIAFFE: Dressage trot
PIAGET: Swiss psychologist
PIANI: "Farewell to Arms" character
PIANOLA: Player piano
PIAO: Lin __ (Mao opponent)
PIASTER: Coin of Egypt
PIASTRE: Coin of Egypt
PIAUI: Brazilian state
PIAVE: Italian cheese
PIAZZA: Public square
PIAZZI: Italian astronomer
PIBB: Mr. __ (soft-drink brand)
PICA: Printing measure
PICABO: Olympic skier Street
PICADOR: Bullfight participant
PICANTE: Spicy, as sauces
PICARA: Adventuress
PICARD: "Star Trek: The Next Generation" captain
PICARDO: Actor Robert
PICARDY: French region
PICARO: Rogue
PICASSO: Spanish artist
PICCARD: Swiss physicist
PICCATA: Veal serving
PICCHU: Machu __ (Inca city)
PICE: Money of India
PICEOUS: Like tar
PICHEL: Director Irving
PICKENS: Actor Slim
PICKETT: Soul singer Wilson
PICO: Trillionth: Comb. form
PICON: Actress Molly
PICONE: Evan-__ (designer label)
PICOT: Decorative loop
PICRIC: Acid used in explosives
PICT: Ancient Brit
PICTO: Graphic prefix
PICTOR: Southern constellation
PIDGEON: Actor Walter
PIEBALD: Kind of horse
PIEDS: Feet: French
PIEL: Skin: Spanish
PIELS: Old beer brand
PIERCE: "M*A*S*H" captain
PIERIA: Greek region
PIERIAN: Of the Muses
PIERRE: South Dakota capital
PIERROT: Buffoon
PIE SAFE: Amish furniture
PIET: Artist Mondrian
PIETA: Religious sculpture
PIETER: Flemish painter Breughel
PIETOSO: Tenderly, in music
PIETRO: Peter: Italian
PIG IT: Live in squalor
PIK: Water __ (dental appliance)
PIKA: Rabbitlike mammal
PILAR: "For Whom the Bell Tolls" character
PILATE: New Testament character
PILATES: Exercise method
PILATUS: Swiss Alp
PILCROW: Paragraph mark
PILEATE: Crested
PILEGGI: Author Nicholas
PILEOUS: Hairy
PILEUM: Top of a bird's head
PILEUS: Mushroom cap
PILLION: Biker's cushion
PILO: Hair: Comb. form
PILON: Sculptor Germain
PILOSE: Hairy
PILOUS: Hairy
PILSNER: Lager beer
PILUS: Hair
PIM: "Mr. __ Passes By" (Milne work)
PIMA: Arizona Indian
PIMEN: "Boris Godunov" role
PI MESON: Subatomic particle
PIMINY: Niminy-__
PIMLICO: Preakness site
PINA: __ colada
PINATA: Birthday-party item
PINCAY: Jockey Laffit
PINCE: __-nez glasses
PINCHAS: Violinist Zuckerman
PINCHOT: Actor Bronson
PINDAR: Greek poet
PINDUS: Greek mountain range
PINEAL: Endocrine gland
PINERO: British playwright
PINE-SOL: Household cleaner brand
PINETOP: Arizona town
PINETUM: Conifer arbor
PINFOLD: Pound for stray animals
PINGUID: Oily
PINKETT: Actress Jada __ Smith
PINKHAM: Patent-medicine maker
PINNA: Winglike part
PINNACE: Sailing ship
PINNATE: Featherlike
PINON: Pine tree
PINOT: Wine grape
PINOTTA: Mascagni opera
PIN SEAL: Type of leather
PINSK: Belarus city
PINSON: Vada of baseball
PINTER: Dramatist Harold
PINWALE: Type of corduroy
PINYIN: Chinese transliteration system
PINZA: Basso Ezio
PINZON: Navigator with Columbus
PIO: "Bridge of San Luis Rey" character
PIOLET: Ice ax
PION: Subatomic particle
PIP CARD: Card lower than a jack
PIPET: Lab tube
PIPETTE: Lab tube
PIPIT: Small songbird
PIPP: Gehrig replaced him
PIPPA: "__ Passes" (Browning poem)
PIPPET: "Jaws" dog
PIPPI: Fictional Longstocking
PIPPIN: 1972 Broadway musical
PIPPINS: Types of apples
PIP-PIP: So long, in Britain
PIQUET: Card game
PIRAEUS: Greek city
PIRE: 1958 peace Nobelist
PIRELLI: Tire brand
PIRN: Bobbin, in Britain
PIROGEN: Russian pastry
PIROGUE: Canoelike boat
PIRRIP: "Great Expectations" character
PIS: Greek letters
PISA: Italian city
PISANIO: "Cymbeline" character
PISANO: Italian sculptor
PISARRO: French artist
PISCI: Fish: Comb. form
PISCINE: Fishlike
PISCOPO: Comic Joe
PISGAH: Mideast mountain
PISH: "Nonsense!"
PISMIRE: Ant
PISMO: Large clam
PISTE: Ski run
PISTIL: Blossom part
PISTOLE: Old Spanish coin
PISTOU: French sauce
PITAYA: Southwestern cactus
PITH: Basic idea
PITHEAD: Mine entrance
PITILLO: Actress Maria
PITKIN: Aspen's county
PITMAN: Coal miner
PITNEY: Singer Gene
PITON: Climbing spike
PITOT: Velocity-measuring tube
PIT ROW: NASCAR service area
PITT: Actor Brad
PITTI: Florence palace
PITTMAN: Cicely Tyson role
PITTS: Actress ZaSu
PITY'S: "For __ sake!"
PIU: More, in music
PIUS I: Pope
PIUS II: Pope
PIUS III: Pope
PIUS IV: Pope
PIUS IX: Pope
PIUS V: Pope
PIUS VI: Pope
PIUS VII: Pope
PIUS X: Pope
PIUS XI: Pope
PIUS XII: Pope
PIUTE: Western Indian
PIVEN: Actor Jeremy
PIXAR: Computer-animation studio
PIXEL: Computer image bit
PIZARRO: Inca conqueror
PIZZ.: Plucked, in mus.
PKG.: UPS delivery
PLACIDO: Tenor Domingo
PLACKET: Skirt slit
PLAGE: Resort beach
PLAICE: European fish
PLAINES: Des __, IL
PLAISIR: Pleasure: French
PLAKAT: Siamese fighting fish
PLAN A: First strategy
PLANAR: Two-dimensional
PLAN B: Alternate strategy
PLANCK: German physicist
PLANI: Flat: Comb. form
PLANO: Texas city
PLANTAR: Of the sole
PLANTE: Jacques of hockey
PLAN TO: Shall
PLASH: Splash gently
PLASM: Tissue: Comb. form
PLASMO: Blood fluid: Comb. form
PLAST: Cell: Comb. form
PLAT: Land map
PLATA: Silver: Spanish
PLATEN: Typewriter part
PLATH: Poet Sylvia
PLATO: Greek philosopher
PLATO'S: "__ Republic"
PLATT: Actor Oliver
PLATTE: Nebraska river
PLATY: Aquarium fish
PLAUTUS: Roman playwright
PLAX: Mouth-rinse brand
PLAYA: Shore: Spanish
PLAY-DOH: Kids' clay
PLAY IT: Rick's order to Sam
PLAYTEX: Lingerie brand
PLEB: Academy freshman
PLEBE: Academy freshman
PLECTRA: Guitar pluckers
PLEIAD: Daughter of Atlas
PLENARY: Complete
PLENUM: Full assembly
PLEURA: Lung membrane
PLEX: Movie-theater suffix
PLEXOR: Medical hammer
PLEXUS: Nerve network
PLICATE: Folded like a fan
PLIE: Ballet bend
PLINTH: Column base
PLINY: Roman writer
PLISSE: Lightweight fabric
P.L.O.: U.N. observer grp.

PLOCE: Repetition for rhetorical effect
PLOESTI: Romanian city
PLOMER: South African author
PLOSION: Phonetics term
PLOTZ: Collapse
PLOVDIV: Bulgarian city
PLOVER: Shore bird
PLS.: Kindly, in bus. memos
PLU.: Not singular: Abbr.
PLUGOLA: Promotional praise
PLUIE: Rain: French
PLUMBIC: Containing lead
PLUMBO: Lead: Comb. form
PLUMBUM: Lead
PLUMCOT: Hybrid tree
PLUMMER: Actress Amanda
PLUMOSE: Feathered
PLUM PIE: Fruity dessert
PLUMR: Liquid-__ (drain-cleaner brand)
PLUMULE: Feather
PLURI: Many: Comb. form
PLUS ONE: Golf-scoreboard notation
PLUT: Wealth: Comb. form
PLUTON: Igneous rock
PLUTUS: Aristophanes play
PLUVI: Rain: Comb. form
PLUVIA: Rain: Comb. form
PLUVIAL: Rainy
PLUVIO: Rain: Comb. form
PLZEN: Czech city
PMK.: Stamp cancellation: Abbr.
PMT.: Remittance: Abbr.
PNEUM: Lung: Comb. form
PNEUMA: Vital spirit
PNEUMAT: Air: Comb. form
PNEUMO: Air: Comb. Form
PNEUMON: Lung: Comb. form
PNIN: Nabokov novel
PNOM: __ Penh, Cambodia
P.O.B.: Addr. part
POBLANO: Chili pepper
P.O. BOX: Address part
PO' BOY: Hero sandwich
POBRE: Poor: Spanish
P.O.C.: Cruise-ship stop: Abbr.
POCO: A little, in music
POCONOS: Pennsylvania mountains
POCUS: Hocus-__
PODA: Feet: Comb. form
PODAL: Of the foot
PODCAST: Type of digital recording
PODO: Foot: Comb. form
PODOUS: Footed: Comb. form
PODRIDA: Olla __ (miscellany)
PODUNK: Tiny town
POEANA: "Faerie Queene" character
POEME: Poem: French
POESY: Art of poetry
POETE: Poet: French
POETICA: "Ars __" (Horace work)
POG: 1990s fad disk
POGNER: "Die Meistersinger" role
POGO: Comics possum
POHL: Sci-fi author Frederik
POI: Luau side dish
POILU: French soldier
POINT A: Starting place
POINT B: Ending place
POINTE: Ballet position
POIRE: Pear: French
POIRET: French fashion designer
POIROT: Christie sleuth
POIS: Peas: French
POISHA: Bangladesh money
POISSON: Fish: French
POITIER: Actor Sidney
POITOU: French region
POIVRE: Pepper: French
POKEMON: Japanese game character
POKERY: Jiggery-__ (monkey business)
POLA: Actress Negri
POLANER: Jelly brand
POLANYI: 1986 chemistry Nobelist
POLARA: Dodge model
POLARIS: North Star
POLE CAR: Indy time-trials winner
POLENTA: Cornmeal concoction
POLGAR: Chess whiz Judit
POLI: __ sci (college course)
POLIS: Ancient Greek city-state
POLITY: Form of government
POLK: 11th president
POLKS: 1840s First Family
POLLACK: Director Sydney
POLLAK: Actor Kevin
POLLARD: Actor Michael J.
POLLERA: Fiesta costume
POLLEX: Thumb
POLLO: Chicken: Spanish
POLLOCK: Artist Jackson __
POLLOI: Hoi __
POLLUX: Mythical twin
POLONIA: Poland: Spanish
POL POT: 1970s Cambodian leader
POLSKA: Poland, in Polish
POLTAVA: Ukraine city
POLYGON: Closed figure
POLYMER: Organic compound
POLYP: Tentacled creature
POLYPED: Having many legs
POLY SCI: College course
POMMARD: French wine
POMME: Apple: French
POMMEL: Saddle knob
POMO: California Indian
POMONA: California city
POMPANO: __ Beach, FL
POMPEIA: Wife of Julius Caesar
POMPEII: Ancient Roman city
POMPEO: Actress Ellen
POMPEY: Julius Caesar opponent
PONCA: Oklahoma Indian
PONCE: Puerto Rico city
PONCH: "CHiPs" role
PONG: 1970s video game
PONGEE: Cotton fabric
PONGID: Great ape
PONGO: "101 Dalmatians" dog
PONGS: Ping-__ (bounces)
PONIARD: Dagger
PONS: Opera singer Lily
PONT: Bridge: French
PONTA: __ Delgada (Azores capital)
PONTANO: Italian poet
PONTE: Bridge: Italian
PONTI: Italian film producer
PONTIAN: Pope
PONTIUS: __ Pilate
PONY KEG: Small beer barrel
PONZI: Investment scheme
PONZU: Japanese dipping sauce
POO: Cutesy-__
POOCHIE: "Nancy" dog
POOH-BAH: Bigwig
POOLE: Dorset town
POONA: City of India
POORI: Bread of India
POOR'S: Standard & __
POOR TAX: Monopoly payment
POPE A.F.B.: N.C. mil. post
POPEIL: Informercial king
POPE LEO: Attila-era pontiff
POPEYE'S: Fast-food chain
POPI: Alan Arkin film
POPLE: 1998 chemistry Nobelist
POPOV: Vodka brand
POPP: Austrian soprano
POPPINS: Julie Andrews role
POPPLE: Move like boiling water
POP ROCK: Music genre
POP-TART: Breakfast-food brand
POPULI: Vox __
POP-UP AD: Web-site "commercial"
POP WINE: Fruit-flavored beverage
POR: __ favor (please: Spanish)
PORC: Pig: French
PORGY: Atlantic fish
PO RIVER: It flows through Italy
PORKPIE: Flat hat
PORKY'S: Film of 1981
POROSE: Full of holes
PORSENA: Etruscan king
PORTA: Prefix for crib
PORTE: Door: French
PORTHOS: A Musketeer
PORTIA: "Merchant of Venice" character
PORTMAN: Actress Natalie
PORTNOY: Philip Roth character
PORTO: City of Portugal
POSADA: Spanish inn
POSEUR: Charlatan
POSEUSE: Con woman
POSEY: Actress Parker
POSOLE: Thick soup
POSSLQ: Housemate, perhaps
POSTDOC: Advanced degree
POSTE: Mail: French
POSTERN: Back door
POSTHOC: Afterward: Latin
POSTIE: Letter carrier
POSTON: Actor Tom
POST-OP: Hospital area
POSTUM: Breakfast beverage
POTAMUS: Peter __ (toon hippo)
POTBOIL: Write bad fiction
POTEEN: Irish moonshine
POTHER: Annoy
POTHOS: Climbing plant
POTOK: "The Chosen" author
POTOSI: Bolivian city
POTSDAM: 1945 Allied conference site
POTSIE: "Happy Days" character
POTSY: Kids' game
POTTO: African primate
POTTS: Actress Annie
POTUS: One in the White House: Abbr.
POTVIN: Denis of hockey
POUDRE: Powder: French
POUF: Hairdo
POULE: Hen: French
POULENC: French composer
POULT: Young fowl
POUPON: Grey __ (mustard brand)
POUSSE: __-café (after-dinner drink)
POUSSIN: French painter
P.O.V.: Camera shot: Abbr.
POVICH: TV host Maury
POWAY: California city
POWELL: Former secretary of state
POWYS: British author
POYSER: "Adam Bede" character
POZNAN: Polish city
POZOLE: Thick soup
POZZO: "Waiting for Godot" character
PPD.: Mail-order ad abbr.
P.P.M.: Air-pollution meas.
P.P.O.: Employee health plan: Abbr.
PPP: Very softly, in music
P.P.V.: Cable-TV service: Abbr.
PRACTIC: Sensible
PRADA: Italian designer label
PRADESH: Uttar __, India
PRADO: Madrid museum
PRAETOR: Roman official
PRAGUE: Czech capital
PRAHA: Czech capital, to natives
PRAIA: Cape Verde capital
PRALINE: Almond confection
PRAM: British baby carriage
PRAN: "The Killing Fields" character
PRANA: Buddhist energy
PRAT: Fall preceder
PRATO: Italian city
PRATT: Brooklyn institute
PRAVDA: Russian newspaper
PRAWER: Author Ruth __ Jhabvala
PRAXIS: Custom
P.R.C.: Beijing's loc.
PREAMP: Hi-fi component
PRED.: Pt. of a sentence
PREEMIE: Early baby
PREFECT: Authority figure
PREGL: Austrian chemistry Nobelist
PREGO: Pasta-sauce brand
PRE-K: Nursery school
PRELL: Shampoo brand
PRELOG: 1975 chemistry Nobelist
PREM.: Ins. payment
PREMIE: Early baby
PRENUP: Marriage contract, for short

PRESA: Music marking
PRESE: Music markings
PRESQUE: __ Isle, ME
PRESSEL: LPGA golfer Morgan __
PRESTON: "The Music Man" star
PRET.: A past tense: Abbr.
PRETER: Beyond: Comb. form
PRETOR: Roman magistrate
PREVERB: Verb prefix
PREVERT: French poet
PREVIA: Toyota model
PREVIN: Conductor André
PREVOST: French novelist
PREWITT: "From Here to Eternity" character
PREX: Business leader, for short
PRIAM: "Iliad" king
PRIE: __-dieu (prayer bench)
PRIMA: __ donna
PRIMERA: First: Spanish
PRIMERO: First: Spanish
PRIMUS: Scottish bishop
PRINE: Folk singer John
PRINGLE: Actress Aileen
PRINK: Deck out
PRINZE: Actor Freddie
PRIORI: A __
PRITHEE: Please, old-style
PRIUS: Toyota model
PRIX: Prize: French
PRIZM: Chevy model
PRIZZI'S: "__ Honor" (Huston film)
P.R.N.: Prescription abbr.
PRNDL: Gearshift sequence
PROA: Indonesian boat
PRO-AM: Type of tournament
PRO BALL: Major leagues, e.g.
PROBIE: Provisional employee
PRO BONO: Free
PRO BOWL: Annual football game
PROBST: "Survivor" host
PROCLUS: Greek philosopher
PROCOL: __ Harum (rock group)
PROCTER: __ and Gamble
PROCYON: Star in Canis Minor
PROEM: Foreword
PROJET: Project: French
PRO KEDS: Sneaker brand
PROLATE: Drawn out at the poles
PROLE: Average worker
PROLIX: Wordy
PROM BID: School-dance ticket
PRONATE: Rotate, as an extremity
PROPONE: Tell to a judge
PROPRE: Amour-__ (self-esteem: French)
PROPYL: __ alcohol
PROSCAN: TV brand
PROSIT: "To your health!"
PROSKY: Actor Robert
PROSODY: Science of verse
PROSS: "Tale of Two Cities" character
PROST: Auto racer Alain
PROTEA: Shrub genus
PROTEUS: Sea god
PROTIST: Amoeba or paramecium
PROTO: First: Comb. form
PROULX: Author E. Annie
PROUST: French novelist
PROVINE: Actress Dorothy
PROVO: Utah city
PROWAR: Hawkish
PROWSE: Dancer Juliet
PROXIMA: __ Centauri
PROXIMO: During the next month
PROYAS: Director Alex
PROZAC: Antidepressant drug
PRS: 7 on a phone
PRU: Boston skyscraper, for short
PRUDHOE: Alaska bay
PRUETT: Country singer Jeanne
PRUSSIA: Former German state
PRYCE: Actor Jonathan
PRYNNE: "The Scarlet Letter" character
PRYOR: Comedian Richard
P.S.A.: Free TV spot
PSALTER: Prayer book
PS AND QS: Things to watch
P.S.C.: Util. regulator
PSEUDS: Intellectual fakers
P.S.F.: Pressure meas.
PSHAW: Old-time oath
PSI: Greek letter
PSST: "Ahem!"
P.S.T.: L.A. clock setting
P.S.U.: Big Ten school
PTAH: Egyptian god
PTER: Feather: Comb. form
PTERO: Wing: Comb. form
PTEROUS: Winged: Comb. form
P TILE: Scrabble three-pointers
P.T.L.: Bakkers' ministry
P.T.O.: End-of-page abbr.
PTOLEMY: Ancient astronomer
PTOOEY: Spitting sound
P TRAP: Sink pipe
PTUI: Spitting sound
PUBLIUS: "Federalist Papers" pseudonym
PUBLIX: Supermarket chain
PUCCI: Italian designer
PUCCINI: Italian composer
PUCKETT: Kirby of baseball
PUDDY: "...taw a __ tat!"
PUDENCY: Modesty
PUEBLA: State of Mexico
PUENTE: Bandleader Tito
PUENZO: Actor Luis
PUER: Boy: Latin
PUF: Sta-__ (fabric-softener brand)
PUFFIN: Sea bird
PUGET: Northwestern sound
PUGGLE: Dog breed
PUGH: Exclamation of disgust
PUGSLEY: "Addams Family" character
PUIG: "Kiss of the Spider Woman" author
PUJOLS: Albert of baseball
PUKA: Hawaiian necklace shell
PUKKA: Authentic
PUL: Afghani coin
PULA: Botswana money
PULASKI: Revolutionary War general
PULI: Hungarian dog
PULIK: Hungarian dogs
PULL-INS: Roadside eateries, in Britain
PULMO: Lung: Comb. form
PULMON: Lung: Comb. form
PULMONI: Lung: Comb. form
PULMONO: Lung: Comb. form
PULVER: "Mister Roberts" character
PUNG: Boxlike sleigh
PUNIC: Of Carthage
PUNJAB: State of India
PUNKA: Ceiling fan of India
PUNKER: Rock musician
PUNKIE: Gnat
PUNTA: Point: Spanish
PUPA: Insect stage
PUPIN: Hungarian-born physicist
PUPKIN: De Niro, in "King of Comedy"
PUPP: "Krazy Kat" policeman
PUPU: Chinese appetizer
PURA: Pure: Latin
PURCELL: British composer
PURDUE: Big Ten school
PURDY: Canadian poet
PUREX: Detergent brand
PURFLE: Adorn
PURIM: Jewish festival
PURINA: Pet-food brand
PURLIE: 1970 Ossie Davis musical
PURLIEU: Area
PURO: Pure: Spanish
PUSAN: Korean port
PUSH IT: Be persistent
PUSHKIN: Russian poet
PUSHROD: Auto part
PUT 'EM UP: Fighting words
PUTNAM: Revolutionary War general
PUTNEY: Vermont town
PUT-PUT: Boat engine sound
PUTSCH: Revolt
PUTTEE: Leg covering
PUTTIN': "__ on the Ritz"
PU-YI: Last emperor of China
PUZO: Author Mario
P.V.C.: Pipe plastic
P.W.A.: New Deal org.
P.W. BOTHA: South African statesman
PWT.: Jeweler's meas.
P.X.S: G.I. stores
PYA: Myanmar money
PYE: British poet laureate
PYE-DOG: Cur
PYKE: "Nicholas Nickleby" character
PYLE: WWII reporter
PYM: British writer
PYNCHON: Author Thomas
PYNE: 1960s TV talk show host
PYR: Fire: Comb. form
PYRAMUS: Thisbe's love
PYRETIC: Feverish
PYREX: Baking-dish brand
PYREXIA: Fever
PYRHHO: Greek philosopher
PYRITE: Fool's gold
PYRO: Fire: Comb. form
PYRRHIC: __ victory
PYRRHUS: Mythical king
PYT: Michael Jackson tune
PYTHIAN: Lodge member
PYTHIAS: Damon's friend
PYX: Eucharist box

Q

QABALA: Secret doctrine
QABALAH: Secret doctrine
QADDAFI: Libyan leader
QAF: Arabic letter
QAID: Muslim judge
Q. AND A.: Press conference, for short
QANTAS: Australian airline
QAT: Arabian evergreen
QATAR: Arab League member
QATARI: Certain Arab
QBERT: 1980s video game
QBS: Football positions: Abbr.
QB SNEAK: Football ploy, for short
QB VII: Uris novel
Q.E.D.: Math-proof letters
QE II: Retired ocean liner, for short
Q.I.D.: Prescription abbr.
QIN: Chinese dynasty
QINTAR: Albania money
QIRSH: Saudi Arabian money
QOM: City of Iran
QOPH: Hebrew letter
Q-RATIO: Corporate asset replacement calculation
Q SCHOOL: PGA Tour hopefuls' academy
Q TILE: Scrabble 10-pointer
QTIP: Ear cleaner
QTO.: Book size: Abbr.
QTR.: 15 min. of football
QTS.: Amts. of oil
QTY.: Amount: Abbr.
QUA: As
QUAD: Campus area
QUADR: Four: Comb. form
QUADRI: Four: Comb. form
QUADRIC: Second-degree, in math
QUAE: Which: Latin
QUAG: Bog
QUAGGA: Extinct African beast
QUAGGY: Swampy
QUAHOG: Kind of clam
QUAI: Dock: French
QUAID: Actor Dennis
QUAILED: Flinched
QUAKIE: Aspen tree
QUALES: "Rich Man, Poor Man" role
QUAM: Esse __ videri (North Carolina motto)
QUAND: When: French
QUANG: __ Tri, Vietnam
QUANT: Designer Mary
QUANTA: Amounts
QUANTUM: "__ Leap"
QUAPAW: Oklahoma Indian
QUAR.: 25 pct.

QUARE: "The __ Fellow" (Behan play)
QUARK: Subatomic particle
QUARLES: British poet
QUARTAN: Every four days
QUARTE: Fencing position
QUARTIC: Fourth-degree, in math
QUARTO: Book size
QUASAR: Astronomical object
QUAT: Four, in prescriptions
QUATRE: Four: French
QUATTRO: Audi model
QUAXO: "Cats" role
QUAY: Wharf
QUAYLE: Bush vice president
QUE: What: Spanish
QUECHUA: Inca language
QUEEG: "Caine" captain
QUEENE: "The Faerie __"
QUEENED: Cashed a pawn, in chess
QUEENIE: Dog name
QUEEN IT: Be arrogant
QUEIROS: Brazilian writer
QUEL: What: French
QUELER: Conductor Eve
QUELQUE: Some: French
QUEM: Which: Latin
QUEMOY: Chinese island
QUENEAU: French poet
QUENTIN: San __ prison
QUE PASA: "What's happening?" in Spanish
QUERIDA: Spanish sweetheart
QUERIDO: Spanish sweetheart
QUES.: Inquiry: Abbr.
QUE SERA: What will be: Spanish
QUESNAY: French economist
QUESO: Cheese: Spanish
QUETZAL: Central American bird
QUEZON: __ City (Philippines metropolis)
QUI: Who: Latin
QUID: British pound
QUIDDE: 1927 Peace Nobelist
QUIEN: Who: Spanish
QUIETUS: Finishing stroke
QUIGLEY: Selleck film role
QUIK: Nestlé product
QUILLER: British writer Sir Arthur __-Couch
QUILP: "Old Curiosity Shop" character
QUINARY: In groups of five
QUINATE: In groups of five
QUINCE: Fruit tree
QUINCEY: British writer Thomas De __
QUINCY: Massachusetts city
QUINE: Actor Richard
QUINELA: Track bet
QUINION: "David Copperfield" character
QUINLAN: Actress Kathleen
QUINN: Actor Anthony
QUINO: Argentine artist
QUINQU: Five: Comb. form
QUINQUE: Five: Comb. form
QUINTA: Portuguese inn
QUINTAL: Hundredweight
QUINTE: Fencing position
QUINTI: Fifth: Comb. form
QUINTIC: Fifth-degree, in math
QUINTON: Ernest, in "McHale's Navy"
QUINTUS: "Ben-Hur" character
QUINZE: 15: French
QUIPU: Inca counting device
QUIRE: 24 sheets
QUIRT: Riding whip
QUISP: Cereal brand
QUITO: Capital of Ecuador
QUI VIVE: French sentry's query
QUIXOTE: Cervantes character
QUIZNOS: Sandwich-shop chain
QUM: City in Iran
QUO: "__ Vadis?"
QUOD: Part of Q.E.D.
QUOI: What: French
QUOIN: Cornerstone
QUOIT: Ring of rope
QUOITS: Throwing game
QUONDAM: Bygone
QUONSET: Certain hut
QUOQUE: Also: Latin
QUOT.: Bartlett's entry: Abbr.
QUOTH: "__ the raven..."
QURAN: Muslim Bible
QVC: Cable channel
QWERTY: Keyboard sequence
QWEST: Telephone company

R

RAABE: German novelist
RAAF: Aussie pilots: Abbr.
RABAT: Morocco capital
RABBET: Carpenter's joint
RABBITT: Singer Eddie
RABE: Playwright David
RABI: 1944 physics Nobelist
RABIN: Former Israeli leader
RACEME: Flower part
RACHAEL: Actress __ Leigh Cook
RACHEL: Wife of Jacob
RACINE: Wisconsin city
RACINO: Track that has slot machines
RACK OUT: Go to sleep
RAD: Teen's exclamation
RADAMES: "Aïda" role
RADER: Writer Dotson
RADFORD: Actor Basil
RADIAN: Circle measure
RADICLE: Root
RADIX: Base of a number system
RADLEY: "To Kill a Mockingbird" character
R. ADM.: Nav. rank
RADNER: Comic Gilda
RADNOR: Pennsylvania city
RADO: "Hair" lyricist
RADOME: Antenna housing
RADON: Element #86
RADS: X-ray units
RAE: Actress Charlotte
RAEBURN: Scottish painter
RAE DAWN: Actress Chong
RAF: Brit. fliers
RAFAEL: San __, CA
RAFER: 1960 Olympian Johnson
RAFF: Commoners
RAFFI: Children's singer
RAFFIA: African palm tree
RAFFIN: Actress Deborah
RAFFISH: Bohemian
RAFKO: 1988 Miss America
RAGA: Music of India
RAGBAG: Conglomeration
RAGHIB: Ismail of football
RAGLAN: Type of overcoat
RAGMAN: Cloth dealer
RAGMAN'S: "The __ Son" (Kirk Douglas book)
RAGNAR: "Atlas Shrugged" character
RAG ON: Tease
RAGOUT: French stew
RAG SHOP: Fabric-store chain
RAGTAG: Disheveled
RAGTOP: Convertible
RAGU: Pasta-sauce brand
RAGUSA: "Laverne and Shirley" character
RAHAL: Auto racer Bobby
RAHWAY: New Jersey city
RA I: Heyerdahl craft
RA II: Heyerdahl raft
RAIMI: "Spider-Man" director
RAINE: British poet
RAINER: Actress Luise
RAINES: Actress Ella
RAINEY: "Mother of the Blues"
RAIN MAN: Dustin Hoffman film
RAIN ON: Spoil, in a way
RAIPUR: City in India
RAISA: Mrs. Gorbachev
RAISON: Reason: French
RAITA: Indian salad
RAITT: Singer Bonnie
RAJ: British rule in India
RAJAB: Islamic month
RAJA RAO: Indian author
RAJIV: Gandhi of India
RAKU: Japanese earthenware
RAL.: N.C. capital
RALE: Breathing sound
RALEIGH: North Carolina capital
RALL.: Gradually slower, in mus.
RALLYE: Road race
RALPH: Actor Bellamy
RALPHIE: Kramden, to Norton
RALPH J.: Diplomat Bunche
RALSTON: Cereal brand
RAMA: Avatar of Vishnu
RAMADA: Arbor
RAMADAN: Islamic month
RAMAN: 1930 physics Nobelist
RAMAPO: Appalachian range
RAMAR: "__ of the Jungle" (1950s TV show)
RAMATE: Branched
RAMBLIN': "__ Man" (1973 song)
RAMBO: Stallone role
RAMBOS: Fanatical militants
RAMEAU: French composer
RAMEKIN: Baking dish
RAMEN: Japanese noodles
RAMESES: Egyptian king
RAMET: Clone unit
RAMEY: Opera singer Samuel
RAMFIS: "Aïda" character
RAMIE: Asian shrub
RAMIFY: Spread out
RAMIREZ: Manny of baseball
RAMIS: Director Harold
RAMON: Actor Novarro
RAMONA: Helen Hunt Jackson heroine
RAMONES: Punk-rock group
RAMOS: __ gin fizz
RAMOSE: Arboreal
RAMPAL: French flutist
RAMP UP: Accelerate
RAMSAY: British chemistry Nobelist
RAMSES I: King of Egypt
RAMSEY: Actress Anne
RAMSON: Type of garlic
RAMUS: Branch
RAMUZ: Swiss writer
RANA: Indian prince
RAND: Author Ayn
RANDA: Director Haines
RANDAL: Director Kleiser
RANDALL: "The Odd Couple" star
R. AND B.: Music genre
R. AND D.: Corporate department
RANDI: "Amazing" magician
R. AND R.: Time off
RAN DRY: Became waterless
RANDY: Actor Quaid
RANEE: Indian princess
RANGEL: New York congressman
RANGO: Tim Conway TV series
RANGOON: Capital of Burma
RANI: Indian princess
RANID: Frog
RANINE: Froglike
RANKE: Historian Leopold von __
RANKIN: First elected Congresswoman
RANKINE: Scottish physicist
RANN: "Adam Bede" character
RANS: Also-__
RANT AT: Assault verbally
RAO: 1990s prime minister of India
RAOUL: Director Walsh
RAPALLO: Italian port
RAPA NUI: Easter Island
RAPEE: Hungarian composer
RAPH: Jazz trombonist
RAPHAEL: Italian painter
RAPIDAN: Virginia river
RAPIDO: Speedy: Spanish
RAPINE: Plunder
RAPINI: Turnip leaves
RAPPEL: Climber's descent
RAPTUS: Ecstasy
RAQUEL: Actress Welch
RARA: __ avis
RARAE: __ aves

RAREE: Carnival
RAREFY: Make less dense
RARE GAS: Argon or neon
RARING: __ to go
RARITAN: New Jersey river
RAS: Abyssinian prince
RASA: Tabula __ (blank slate)
RASAE: Tabulae __
RASBORA: Aquarium fish
RASCHE: Actor David
RASE: Demolish
RASHAD: "Cosby Show" co-star
RASHI: French Hebrew scholar
RASHID: Designer Karim
RASHIDA: Actress Jones
RASHT: City in Iran
RASKIN: Author Ellen
RASPA: Mexican dance
RASPE: "Baron Munchausen" author
RASSE: Chinese civet
RASTA: Dreadlocks wearer
RASTER: Computer-screen lines
RASURE: Obliteration
RATA: Pro __ (proportionally)
RATAFIA: Liqueur
RATBERT: Comic-strip rodent
RATED G: Like some films
RATED PG: Like some films
RATED R: Like some films
RATED X: Like some films
RATEL: African weasel
RATHS: "And the mome __ outgrabe"
RATINE: Loosely woven fabric
RATITE: Ostrich or emu
RATLIN: Nautical rope
RATLINE: Nautical rope
RATNER: Director Brett
RATOFF: Director Gregory
RATON: Boca __, FL
RATSO: "Midnight Cowboy" character
RATTAIL: Type of cactus
RAT-TAT: Drum sound
RAU: Author Santha Rama __
RAUL: Actor Julia
RAVELOE: Silas Marner's home
RAVENAL: "Show Boat" character
RAVENNA: Italian city
RAVE ON: Buddy Holly song
RAVE-UP: Party, in Britain
RAVI: Sitarist Shankar
RAW BAR: Place for seafood
RAWDON: "Vanity Fair" character
RAWHIDE: TV western
RAWIST: Cooked-food avoider
RAWLINS: Walter Mosley sleuth
RAWLS: Singer Lou
RAX: Stretch: Scottish
RAYBAN: Sunglasses brand
RAYBURN: Game-show host Gene
RAYE: Actress Martha
RAY KROC: McDonald's founder
RAYMOND: Actor Massey
RAYNELL: "Fences" character
RAYOVAC: Battery brand
RAZAF: Eubie Blake collaborator
RAZZIE: Bad-film award
RAZZLE: __-dazzle
R.B.C.: Erythrocyte: Abbr.
RBI: Baseball stat
RCA: "His Master's Voice" co.
RCA DOME: Indianapolis arena
RCAF: Can. fliers
R.C. COLA: Coke competitor
RCD.: Obtained: Abbr.
R.C.M.P.: Mounties' org.
R.C.N.: Canadian sailors: Abbr.
RCPT.: "Bill paid" paper: Abbr.
R. CRUMB: Underground cartoonist
RCT.: Army rookie: Abbr.
R.D.A.: Nutrition-label abbr.
R.D. LAING: British psychiatrist
REA: Actor Stephen
READE: British author
REAGANS: 1980s First Family
REAGENT: Analyst's chemical
REALES: Old Spanish coins
REALIA: Teaching aids
REALS: Non-imaginary numbers
REAO: Polynesian island
REARDON: "Atlas Shrugged" character
REATA: Lasso
REATTA: Buick model
REAUMUR: French physicist
REAVE: Rob, old-style
REB: Confederate soldier
REBA: Country singer McEntire
REBAR: Concrete reinforcement
REBBE: Yeshiva teacher
REBBIE: Singer Jackson
REBEC: Renaisssance fiddle
REBECCA: Sunnybrook Farm girl
REBEKAH: Wife of Isaac
REBER: Astronomer Grote
REBOANT: Big-voiced
REBOOT: Computer verb
REBOP: 1940s jazz style
REBOTE: Jai alai wall
REBOZO: Mexican scarf
REC: VCR remote button
RECD.: Accepted: Abbr.
REC HALL: Place to play pool
RECIFE: Brazilian city
RECIP.: 1/4, to four: Abbr.
RECK: Care, old-style
RECLAME: Notoriety
REC ROOM: Basement area
RECT.: 4-sided fig.
RECTA: Cyma __ (molding)
RECTI: Straight: Comb. form
RECTO: Book page
RECTUS: Abdomen muscle
RECUSE: Disqualify (oneself)
RED A: Hester Prynne's mark
RED ACE: Certain playing card
REDACT: Edit
RED ALGA: Type of seaweed
REDAN: Battle-line projection
RED ANT: Biting insect
RED ARMY: Soviet soldiers
RED BAY: Evergreen
REDBONE: Hunting hound
REDBOOK: Women's magazine
REDBUD: Oklahoma state tree
RED CHIP: Hong-Kong based company
REDCOAT: 1776 soldier
RED COD: New Zealand fish
REDD: Comic Foxx
RED DAWN: 1984 film
REDDI: __ Wip
REDDIN: Playwright Keith
REDDING: Singer Otis
RED-DOG: Charge the quarterback
RED DUST: Clark Gable film
REDDY: Singer Helen
REDE: Advise, in Britain
REDFERN: "Look Back in Anger" character
REDFIN: Minnow
REDFORD: "The Way We Were" star
REDHAWK: Miami of Ohio athlete
RED HEAT: Schwarzenegger film
REDI: "Handy" product-name prefix
RED INK: Business loss
REDLEG: Cincinnati baseballer, formerly
RED LINE: Ice-hockey area
REDMOND: Microsoft's headquarters
RED OAK: Acorn bearer
REDON: French painter
REDONDO: __ Beach, CA
REDOUBT: Defensive position
REDOUND: Accrue
RED-OUT: Astronaut's vision problem
REDOX: Chemical reaction
REDPOLL: Small bird
RED PONY: Steinbeck title animal
RED RAG: Bull teaser
RED ROBE: Papal vestment
REDROOT: North American plant
REDRUM: "The Shining" word
REDSKIN: NFL player
RED SKY: Sailor's omen
RED SOX: 2004 World Series winners
RED SPOT: Jupiter feature
RED TAB: Levi's feature
REDTAIL: North American hawk
REDTOP: Lawn grass
REDUX: Brought back
RED WING: NHL player
REE: Dakota Indian
REEBOK: Sneakers brand
REECE: Model Gabrielle
REEDMAN: Saxophonist, e.g.
REEFER: Short jacket
REEGE: Former "Millionaire" host, to fans
REENIE: "The Dark at the Top of the Stairs" character
REES: Actor Roger
REESE: Pee Wee of baseball
REESE'S: Candy brand
REET: "__ Petite" (Jackie Wilson song)
REEVE: "Canterbury Tales" character
REEVED: Fastened, nautically
REEVES: Actor Keanu
REFI: Second mortgage, to brokers
REFL.: Mirror image: Abbr.
REFLATE: Blow up again
REFLUX: Ebb
REFT: Broken, old-style
REG: Bylaw, for short
REGAN: Daughter of King Lear
REGD.: Like some mail: Abbr.
REGER: German composer
REGES: Kings: Latin
REGGIE: Jackson of baseball
REGIA: Aqua __ (gold dissolver)
REGINA: Queen
REGIS: TV host Philbin
REGIUS: Of kings
REGLE: Sliding-door groove
REGNARD: French playwright
REGNAT: "__ populus" (Arkansas motto)
REGNIER: French poet
REGNUM: Dominion
REGO: __ Park, NY
REGT.: Army grp.
REGULUS: Star in Leo
REHAN: Actress Ada
REI: Defendants, in law
REICH: Clinton cabinet member
REID: Actor Tim
REIFY: Regard as real
REIGER: "Taxi" driver
REILLY: Comic Charles Nelson __
REIMS: French city
REINA: Queen: Spanish
REINE: Queen: French
REINER: Director Carl
REISER: "Mad About You" star
REISZ: Director Karel
REIT: Type of mutual fund: Abbr.
REITER: Rider: German
REITMAN: Director Ivan
REJIG: Adjust
REL.: Fam. member
R.E. LEE: Douglas Freeman biography
RELEVE: Ballet movement
RELICT: Survivor
RELLENO: Chili serving
RELO: Transferred employee's need, for short
RELUCT: Struggle
RELUME: Light up again
REM: Sleep phenomenon
REMAND: Send back
REMAX: Real-estate company
REMI: Ancient people of Gaul
REMICK: Actress Lee
REMINI: Actress Leah
REMISE: Cede claim to
REMO: San __, Italy
REMORA: Type of fish
REMSEN: Chemist Ira
REMUS: Storytelling uncle of fiction
REMY: __ Martin (cognac brand)
REN: Cartoon Chihuahua
RENA: Actress Sofer
RENAL: Of the kidneys
RENALDO: Actor Duncan

RENAN: French historian
RENARD: French author
RENATA: Opera singer Tebaldi
RENATO: 1975 medicine Nobelist Dulbecco
RENAULT: French auto
RENAY: Singer Diane
RENDELL: Mystery novelist Ruth
RENE: Actress Russo
RENEE: Actress Zellweger
RENFREW: Historic Scottish county
RENFRO: Actor Brad
RENGA: Japanese verse
RENI: Italian artist
RENIN: Kidney enzyme
RENNES: French city
RENNET: Cheese ingredient
RENNIE: Actor Michael
RENNIN: Cheese-making enzyme
RENNY: Director Harlin
RENOIR: French painter
RENO, NV: Silver State city
RENTE: Revenue: French
RENTIER: One on a fixed income: French
RENTON: Washington city
RENUZIT: Air-freshener brand
RENVOI: Expulsion from a country
RENWICK: Smithsonian designer
REO: 1920s auto
REPINE: Complain
REPL.: Substitute: Abbr.
REPO: Auto takeback
REPO MAN: 1984 film
REPOSIT: Put back
REPP: Tie fabric
REPROVE: Admonish
REPT.: CNN offering: Abbr.
REPUGN: Oppose
REQD.: Necessary: Abbr.
REQUITE: Avenge
REREDOS: Altar screen
RES: Scale notes
RESEAU: Network
RESECT: Cut
RESEDA: California city
RESH: Hebrew letter
RESHT: City in Iran
RESIDUA: Leftovers
RESILE: Spring back
RESNAIS: Director Alain
RESNIK: Soprano Regina
RESOJET: Type of plane engine
RESORB: Soak up again
RESP.: Ans.
RESTE: Remainder: French
RESTON: Columnist James
RET.: No longer working: Abbr.
RETA: Actress Shaw
RETABLE: Altar part
RETD.: Sent back: Abbr.
RETE: Anatomical network
RETIA: Anatomical networks
RETICLE: Cross hairs
RETIEF: Golfer Goosen
RETINOL: Vitamin A
RETRAL: Toward the back
RETS: Soaks flax
RETSINA: Greek wine
RETTIG: Actor Tommy
RETTON: 1984 Olympics star
RETTY: "Tess of the d'Urbervilles" character
REUBEN: Deli sandwich
REUEL: Part of J.R.R. Tolkien
REUNE: What alumni do
REUP: Go back into the army
REUS: Defendant, in law
REUSS: Jerry of baseball
REUTER: News agency founder
REUTERS: News agency
REUTHER: Former auto-union head
REVA: Actress Rose
REVE: Dream: French
REVERDY: French poet
REVERS: Garment part
REVERSA: Cyma __ (type of molding)
REVET: Face an embankment
REVLON: Cosmetics brand
REVOIR: Au __ (French farewell)
REVSON: Cosmetics magnate
REW: VCR button
REX: Cat breed
REXALL: Drugstore chain
REX REED: Film critic
REXROTH: Poet Kenneth
REY: King: Spanish
REYLES: Uruguayan novelist
REYMONT: Poland literature Nobelist
REYNARD: Fox of fable
REYNAUD: 1940s French premier
REYNOSA: Mexican city
REZA: Iran royal name
REZIA: "Mrs. Dalloway" character
RFB: NFL position
R.F.D.: Former P.O. service
R.F.K.: 1960s Atty. Gen.
R.F.S: Baseball positions: Abbr.
R.G.S: NFL positions
RGT.: Army grp.
RHAMES: Actor Ving
RHAP.: Mus. composition
RHB: NFL position
RHE: Baseball scoreboard heading
RHEA: South American bird
RHEBOK: African antelope
RHEE: 1950s South Korean president
RHEEM: Air-conditioner brand
RHEIMS: French city
RHEIN: German river
RHEME: Linguistic comment
RHENISH: Of a German river
RHENIUM: Element #75
RHEO: Current: Comb. form
RHES: Fluidity units
RHESUS: Type of monkey
RHET.: Art of prose: Abbr.
RHETOR: Orator
RHETT: "Gone With the Wind" character
RHEUM: Common cold
RHIN: Nose: Comb. form
RHINAL: Nasal
RHINE: German river
RHIZOME: Rootlike stem
RHO: Greek letter
RHOD: Rose: Comb. form
RHODA: "The Mary Tyler Moore Show" spin-off
RHODES: British diamond king
RHODIAN: Of an Aegean island
RHODIUM: Element #45
RHODO: Rose: Comb. form
RHODY: Aunt of an old folk song
RHOECUS: Greek sculptor
RHOMB: Diamond shape
RHOMBI: Diamond shapes
RHOMBUS: Diamond shape
RHONDA: Actress Fleming
RHONE: French river
RHUE: Actress Madlyn
RHUM: Baba au __
RHUMB: Compass point
RHYS: Novelist Jean
RIA: Inlet
R.I.A.A.: Music-business org.
RIAL: Iranian coin
RIALTO: Theater district
RIANT: Smiling
RIATA: Lasso
RIBAND: Ribbon
RIBBIT: Frog sound
RIBBY: Baseball stat, familiarly
RIB CUT: Kind of pork chop
RIBERA: Spanish painter José de __
RIBISI: Actor Giovanni
RIBO: Part of RNA
RIBOSE: RNA sugar
RIB PAD: Footballer's protection
RIC: Rock singer Ocasek
RICA: Costa __
RICARDO: "I Love Lucy" family name
RICCI: Designer Nina
RICE U.: Houston sch.
RICHE: Wealthy: French
RICHET: French medicine Nobelist
RICHIE: Singer Lionel
RICH IN: Abounding with
RICHLER: Canadian novelist
RICHTER: Seismologist Charles
RICK: "Casablanca" role
RICKEY: Bar order
RICKI: Talk-show host Lake
RICKIE: Singer __ Lee Jones
RICKLES: Comedian Don
RICKMAN: Actor Alan
RICK'S: "Casablanca" cafe
RICKY: "I Love Lucy" character
RICO: Puerto __
RICOH: Copier brand
RICOLA: Cough-drop brand
RICOTTA: Italian cheese
RICRAC: Dress trim
RICTAL: Gaping
RIDD: "Lorna Doone" character
RIDDER: Knight's publishing partner
RIDDICK: Boxer Bowe
RIDDLER: Batman foe
RIDENT: Cheerful
RIDGWAY: Korean War general
RIDI: "__ Pagliaccio"
RIDLEY: Director Scott
RIDOTTO: Masquerade ball
RIEGERT: Actor Peter
RIEL: Cambodian money
RIEMANN: German mathematician
RIEN: Nothing: French
RIENZI: Roman orator
RIESEN: Candy brand
RIESMAN: Sociologist David
RIESSEN: Tennis pro Marty
RIETI: Italian-born composer
RIF: Region of Morocco
RIFF: Jazz phrase
RIFKIN: Actor Ron
RIFS: Layoffs, for short
RIGA: Latvian capital
RIGATI: Ridged pasta
RIGBY: "Eleanor __" (Beatles song)
RIGEL: Star in Orion
RIGG: Actress Diana
RIGGS: Bobby of tennis
RIGUEUR: De __ (required)
RIG-VEDA: Hindu hymn collection
RIIS: Journalist Jacob
RIJEKA: Croatian city
RIJN: Dutch river
RIJO: Jose of baseball
RIK: Smits of basketball
RIKER: "Star Trek: The Next Generation" character
RIKERS: Island off Manhattan
RIKKI: "__-tikki-tavi"
RIKSDAG: Swedish parliament
RILEY: Hoosier poet
RILIEVO: Raised, in sculpture
RILKE: Austrian poet
RILL: Brook
RILLE: Lunar valley
RILLET: Small stream
RIMA: "Green Mansions" girl
RIMATE: Fissured
RIMBAUD: French poet
RIME: Frost
RIMER: Bard
RIMES: Country singer LeAnn
RIMINI: Italian city
RIMOSE: Cracked
RIMOUS: Cracked
RIMPLE: Furrow
RIMROCK: Canyon edge
RIMSHOT: Drummer's sound
RIMSKY: Composer __-Korsakov
RIN: __ Tin Tin
RINA: "The Carpetbaggers" character
RINALDO: "All's Well That Ends Well" character
RINGO: One of the Beatles
RINK RAT: Hockey buff
RINKY: __-dink
RINSO: Detergent brand
RINTY: Film dog, familiarly
RIO: River: Spanish
RIOJA: Spanish wine
RIO LOBO: John Wayne film
RIO MUNI: Part of Equatorial Guinea

RIOPAN: Antacid brand
RIORDAN: Former L.A. mayor
RIO RITA: Abbott and Costello film
RIPA: Philbin cohost
RIPIENO: All, musically
RIPKEN: Cal of baseball
RIPLEY: "Believe It or Not" writer
RIP ON: Tease
RIPRAP: Wall of stones
RIPS ONE: Hits a ball hard
RIPSTOP: Type of nylon
RIP TORN: "Men in Black" actor
RIRE: To laugh: French
RIS: Laugh: French
RISHI: Hindu sage
RISIBLE: Comic
RISOTTO: Rice dish
RISSOLE: French pastry
RIT.: Slow down, in mus.
RITA: Actress Moreno
RITA GAM: "King of Kings" actress
RITALIN: Hyperactivity medication
RITA MAE: Author Brown
RITARD: Slow down, in music
RITCHIE: "Dick Van Dyke Show" kid
RIT DYE: Clothing-coloring brand
RITE AID: Drugstore chain
RITSOS: Greek poet
RITT: Director Martin
RITTER: Singer Tex
RITZ: Ostentation
RIV: "6 Rms __ Vu"
RIVA: 1972 Derby winner __ Ridge
RIVE: Tear
RIVERA: Mexican painter
RIVER PO: It flows through Italy
RIVIERE: Diamond necklace
RIVOLI: Rue de __ (Paris street)
RIVULET: Stream
RIXEY: Baseball Hall of Famer
RIYADH: Saudi Arabian capital
RIYAL: Qatar money
RIZAL: Philippine novelist
RIZZO: "Midnight Cowboy" role
RIZZUTO: Phil of baseball
RJR: Nabisco partner
R. KELLY: R&B singer
RKO: "King Kong" studio
RKOS: Bygone theaters
R-LESS: Like bad months for oyster-eating
R.L.S.: "Kidnapped" monogram
R.L. STINE: "Goosebumps" series author
R.M.A.: Sandhurst sch.
RMDR.: Div. leftover
R.M.N.: Presidential monogram
RMS.: "6 __ Riv Vu"
RNA: Single-helix molecule
RNAASE: Genetic enzyme
RNASE: Genetic enzyme
R.N.C.: GOP fund-raising org.
RND.: Ammo unit: Abbr.
R.N.S: Hosp. workers
R.O.A.: Bookkeeper's abbr.
ROADEO: Trucker's competition
ROADER: Middle-of-the-__
ROADIE: Rock-tour worker
ROALD: Explorer Amundsen
ROAMIN': "__ in the Gloamin'" (Scottish song)
ROAN: Kind of horse
ROANOKE: Virginia city
ROARK: "The Fountainhead" character
ROBARDS: Actor Jason
ROBB: LBJ in-law
ROBBE: French writer Alain __-Grillet
ROBBIA: Italian sculptor
ROBBIE: "My Three Sons" son
ROBBINS: Country singer Marty
ROBB NEN: Baseball pitcher
ROBBY: 1950s film robot
ROBERTA: Jerome Kern musical
ROBERT E.: General Lee
ROBERT F.: One of the Kennedy brothers
ROBERT H.: Rocketeer Goddard
ROBERT I: King of France
ROBERTO: Clemente of baseball
ROBERTS: Actress Julia
ROBESON: Opera singer Paul
ROBLE: California oak
ROB LOWE: "The West Wing" actor
ROBOCOP: Sci-fi film of 1990
ROB ROY: Scotch cocktail
ROBSART: "Kenilworth" character
ROBSON: Actress Flora
ROBT.: Gen. __ E. Lee
ROBUSTA: Kind of coffee
ROBUSTO: Strong: Italian
ROBYN: Actress Douglass
ROC: "Arabian Nights" bird
ROCA: Portuguese cape
ROCCO: "Fidelio" role
ROCHAT: Director Eric
ROCHE: Tony of tennis
ROCHET: Priestly vestment
ROCHON: Actress Lela
ROCKERY: Type of garden
ROCKIE: Coors Field player
ROCKIN': "__ Around the Christmas Tree" (1960 song)
ROCK IT: Herbie Hancock tune
ROCKNE: Memorable Notre Dame football coach
ROCK OIL: Petroleum
ROCKOON: High-altitude sounding device
ROCKY II: Stallone film
ROCKY IV: Stallone film
ROCKY V: Stallone film
ROCOCO: Art genre
RODALE: "Prevention" publisher
RODAN: Flying monster of film
RODD: Actress Marsha
RODDER: Hot __ (fast driver)
RODDICK: Andy of tennis
RODDY: Actor McDowall
RODGERS: "Sound of Music" composer
RODHAM: Hillary __ Clinton
RODIN: French sculptor
RODINO: Nixon impeachment chairman
RODION: "Crime and Punishment" character
RODMAN: Surveyor's employee
RODNEY: Comic Dangerfield
RODOLFO: "La Bohème" character
RODRIGO: "Don Carlos" role
RODYA: "Crime and Punishment" character
ROEG: "Insignificance" director
ROEPER: Film reviewer of TV
ROETHKE: Poet Theodore
ROGAINE: Hair-growing treatment
ROGER E.: Actor Mosley
ROGERS: Astaire's dancing partner
ROGET'S: Popular thesaurus
ROH: __ Tae Woo (South Korean leader)
ROHE: Architect Ludwig Mies van der __
ROHMER: Fu Manchu creator
ROHRER: 1986 physics Nobelist
ROI: King: French
ROISTER: Revel
ROJA: Red: Spanish
ROJAS: Cookie of baseball
ROJO: Red: Spanish
ROK: Korean soldier
ROKER: "Today" forecaster
ROLAIDS: Antacid brand
ROLAND: Actor Gilbert
ROLEN: Scott of baseball
ROLEO: Birling match
ROLEX: Watch brand
ROLF: Deep massage
ROLFE: Husband of Pocahontas
ROLLAND: French novelist
ROLLBAR: Auto part
ROLLE: Actress Esther
ROLLEI: Camera brand
ROLLIE: Fingers of baseball
ROLLINS: Actor Howard
ROLLO: "Nancy" boy
ROLLWAY: Lumberjack slide
ROLO: Candy brand
ROLONDA: Talk-show host Watts
ROLVAAG: Norwegian-born novelist
ROLY: __-poly
ROM.: N.T. book
ROMAIC: Of modern Greece
ROMAIN: French novelist Gary
ROMAINS: French novelist
ROMAJI: Japanese writing
ROMANI: Gypsy
ROMANO: Italian cheese
ROMANOV: Russian czar surname
ROMANSH: Swiss language
ROMANUS: Pope
ROMANY: Gypsy
ROMBERG: Composer Sigmund
ROMCOM: Romantic comedy
ROMERO: Actor Cesar
ROMES: Apple varieties
ROMIJN: Actress Rebecca
ROMMEL: "Patton" character
ROMNEY: Sheep breed
ROMOLA: George Eliot work
ROMS: CD-__
ROMULAN: "Star Trek" alien
ROMULO: Philippine diplomat
ROMULUS: Mythical twin
ROMY: Actress Schneider
RON: Director Howard
RONA: Author Jaffe
RONAN: Legendary Irish king
RON CEY: "Penguin" of baseball
RONCO: Informercial company
RONDE: Typeface resembling handwriting
RONDEAU: Type of poem
RONDEL: Type of poem
RONDO: Sonata movement
RONDURE: Graceful curve
RONEE: Actress Blakley
RON ELY: Former Miss America host
RONETTE: "Little Shop of Horrors" character
RONI: Pasta, in brand names
RONIN: 1998 De Niro film
RON MIX: Pro football Hall of Famer
RONNIE: Country singer Milsap
RONNY: Actor Cox
RONSARD: French poet
RONSON: Lighter brand
RONTGEN: X-ray discoverer
RON WOOD: Rolling Stones member
RONZONI: Pasta brand
ROO: Aussie beast
ROOD: Crucifix
ROOKER: Actor Michael
ROOKERY: Dilapidated tenement
ROOMBA: Robotic vacuum
ROONE: TV exec Arledge
ROONEY: "60 Minutes" regular
ROOSA: Apollo 14 astronaut
ROOTCAP: Plant protector
ROOTIE: __ Kazootie (1950s TV puppet)
ROOTIN': __-tootin'
ROOTLE: Dig, as a pig
ROOTSY: Down-to-earth, as music
ROPA: Clothing: Spanish
ROQUE: Croquet variation
RORAIMA: State of Brazil
ROREM: Composer Ned
RORQUAL: Type of whale
RORY: Actor Calhoun
ROS: Bandleader Edmundo
ROSA: Parks of civil rights
ROSABUD: "Mystery of Edwin Drood" character
ROSALIA: Patron saint of Palermo
ROSALIE: Cole Porter musical
ROSALYN: Medicine Nobelist Yalow
ROSANNA: Actress Arquette
ROSANNE: Singer Cash
ROSARIO: Actress Dawson
ROSCOE: Gangster's gun
ROSEATE: Promising
ROSEAU: Capital of Dominica
ROSEBAY: Type of rhododendron
ROSE HIP: Certain shrub's fruit
ROSELLA: Ballerina Hightower
ROSELLE: New Jersey city
ROSEN: 1953 A.L. MVP

ROSEOLA: German measles
ROSE RED: Pinkish hue
ROSERY: Garden section
ROSETTA: Town in Egypt
ROSETTE: Architectural ornament
ROSEY: Grier of football
ROSH: Beginning: Hebrew
ROSHI: Zen master
ROSIE: TV host O'Donnell
ROSIE'S: "M*A*S*H" bar
ROSINA: "Barber of Seville" role
ROSITA: "Sesame Street" Muppet
ROSLYN: Singer Kind
ROSS: "Friends" character
ROSSA: Red: Italian
ROSSANO: Singer Brazzi
ROSSEN: Director Robert
ROSSET: Swiss tennis pro
ROSSI: "Lou Grant" character
ROSSINI: "William Tell" composer
ROSSNER: Author Judith
ROSSO: Red: Italian
ROSS SEA: Antarctic Ocean arm
ROSSUM: Capek character
ROSTAND: French playwright
ROSTEN: Yiddish expert Leo
ROSTOCK: German city
ROSTOV: Russian port
ROSWELL: New Mexico city
ROTA: "The Godfather" composer
ROTAS: Church tribunals
ROTBLAT: 1995 peace Nobelist
ROTELLE: Spiral pasta
ROTGUT: Inferior liquor
ROTH: "Goodbye, Columbus" novelist
ROTH I.R.A.: Type of nest egg
ROTHKO: Russian-born artist
ROTI: Roast: French
ROTIFER: Microscopic animal
ROTINI: Corkscrew pasta
ROTL: Islamic weight
ROTO: Newspaper section
ROUAULT: French painter
ROUBAIX: French city
ROUE: Cad
ROUEN: French city
ROULADE: Meat dish
ROULEAU: Roll of coins
ROUNDEL: Small window
ROUND ON: Attack
ROURKE: Actor Mickey
ROUS: 1966 medicine Nobelist
ROUSH: Baseball Hall of Famer Edd
ROUX: Chef's thickener
ROVETTA: Italian playwright
ROW A: Orchestra locale
ROWAN: Ash tree
ROW B: Orchestra locale
ROW C: Orchestra locale
ROW D: Orchestra locale
ROWE: British poet
ROWEL: Boot wheel
ROWEN: Aftermath
ROWENA: "Ivanhoe" character
ROW F: Orchestra locale
ROW G: Orchestra locale
ROW H: Orchestra locale
ROW I: Orchestra locale
ROW J: Orchestra locale
ROW K: Orchestra locale
ROW L: Orchestra locale
ROWLAND: Columnist Evans
ROWLEY: British playwright
ROWLF: Muppet pianist
ROWLING: Harry Potter creator
ROW M: Orchestra locale
ROW N: Orchestra locale
ROW O: Orchestra locale
ROW P: Orchestra locale
ROW Q: Orchestra locale
ROW R: Orchestra locale
ROWSE: British poet
ROW T: Orchestra locale
ROW U: Orchestra locale
ROW V: Orchestra locale
ROW W: Orchestra locale
ROW X: Orchestra locale
ROW Y: Orchestra locale
ROW Z: Orchestra locale
ROX: "L.A. Law" character
ROXANA: Defoe novel
ROXANE: Cyrano's beloved
ROXANNE: Steve Martin film
ROXBURY: Boston neighborhood
ROXIE: "Chicago" role
ROXY: 1930s cinema impresario
ROY: Singer Orbison
ROYALE: Molded custard
ROYAL WE: Formal pronoun
ROY BEAN: Old West judge
ROYCE: Rolls-__
ROY COHN: McCarthy aide
ROY G. BIV: Spectrum mnemonic
ROYKO: Columnist Mike
ROZ: "Frasier" character
ROZANOV: Russian writer
ROZELLE: Former NFL commissioner
R.P.I.: N.Y. engineering school
R.P.S.: Engine meas.
RPT.: Off. work
R-RATED: Like most violent films
RRHEA: Flow: Comb. form
RRR: Basic education
RRS: Train lines: Abbr.
R.S.A.: Botha's country: Abbr.
R.S.F.S.R.: Largest part of the USSR
RSS: Feed format used in blogs
R.S.V.: Bible edition: Abbr.
RSX: Acura model
R TILE: Scrabble one-pointer
RT. REV.: Church official: Abbr.
RTS.: ACLU concerns
R.T.W.: Off-the-rack clothing: Abbr.
RUANDA: African people
RUARK: "Something of Value" author
RUB-A-DUB: Drum-beating sound
RUBATO: Expressive musical phrase
RUBBIA: 1984 physics Nobelist
RUBE: Cartoonist Goldberg
RUBEL: Belarus money
RUBELLA: German measles
RUBEN: Actor Blades
RUBENS: Flemish painter
RUBEOLA: Measles
RUBICON: River crossed by Caesar
RUBIFY: Redden
RUBIK'S: __ Cube (1980s fad)
RUBIN: Clinton cabinet member
RUBIOUS: Red-colored
RUBLE: Russian money
RUBLEV: Russian iconographer
RUB RAW: Abrade badly
RUBRIC: Chapter heading
RUBY DEE: "A Raisin in the Sun" actress
RUCHE: Collar lace
RUCK: Crease
RUCKER: Alabama army fort
RUCKERT: German poet
RUCK UP: Pucker
RUCTION: Quarrel
RUDD: 1960s revolutionary Mark
RUDEL: Austrian conductor
RUDGE: Dickens character
RUDI: Joe of baseball
RUDKIN: British playwright
RUDKUS: "The Jungle" character
RUDMAN: Former New Hampshire senator
RUDNER: Comic Rita
RUDOLF I: Holy Roman emperor
RUDOLPH: Reindeer of song
RUDY: Singer Vallee
RUDYARD: Writer Kipling
RUEHL: Actress Mercedes
RUFF: "Dennis the Menace" dog
RUFFALO: Actor Mark
RUFFING: Baseball Hall of Fame pitcher
RUFIYAA: Maldives money
RUFOUS: Reddish
RUFUS: Groucho in "Duck Soup"
RUGGLES: Actor Charles
RUG RAT: Baby
RUHR: German region
RULA: Actress Lenska
RULETH: Biblical verb
RULFO: Mexican novelist
RUMAKI: Hawaiian appetizer
RUMAN: Actor Sig
RUMER: Author Godden
RUMFORD: Maine town
RUMMER: Large glass
RUMP END: Cut of beef
RUMPOLE: "__ of the Bailey" (British TV series)
RUNCIE: Former Archbishop of Canterbury
RUNDLE: Ladder rung
RUN-DMC: Rap group
RUNE: Ancient alphabetic symbol
RUNLET: Brook
RUNNEL: Brook
RUNNETH: "My cup __ over"
RUNYON: Author Damon
RUPEE: Money of India
RUPERT: Media mogul Murdoch
RUPIAH: Indonesian money
RUR: Robot play
RURIK: Founder of the Russian monarchy
RUS: Ukr. neighbor
RUSHDIE: "Satanic Verses" author
RUSHEE: Would-be frat member
RUSK: 1960s Secretary of State
RUSKA: 1986 physics Nobelist
RUSKIN: British author
RUSKS: Crisp breads
RUSS: Actor Tamblyn
RUSSA: Baseball manager Tony La __
RUSSE: Charlotte __ (sponge-cake dessert)
RUSSEL: Playwright Crouse
RUSSELL: English philosopher
RUSSERT: "Meet the Press" moderator
RUSSET: Brown shade
RUSSLAN: "__ and Ludmilla" (Glinka opera)
RUSSO: Actress Rene
RUTA LEE: "High Rollers" hostess
RUTGER: Actor Hauer
RUTGERS: New Jersey school
RUTH: Old Testament book
RUTH ANN: Soprano Swenson
RUTHFUL: Compassionate
RUTHIE: "Grapes of Wrath" character
RUTILE: Titanium ore
RUTIN: A bioflavonoid
RUTLAND: Vermont city
RUTTAN: Actress Susan
RUTTER: Type of plow
RUXPIN: Teddy __ (animatronic teddy bear)
RUY: __ Lopez (chess opening)
RUY BLAS: Victor Hugo play
RUZICKA: Swiss chemistry Nobelist
R-VALUE: Insulation measure
RVER: Camper driver
RV'ING: Traveling by motor home
RWANDA: African nation
R.W.E.: Essayist's monogram
R.W.R.: Presidential monogram
RWY.: Train line: Abbr.
RXS: Prescriptions
RYA: Scandinavian rug
RYAL: Old Scottish coin
RYAN: Author Cornelius
RYANS: "Von __ Express" (Sinatra film)
RYDELL: Pop singer Bobby
RYDER: Actress Winona
RYENCE: King Arthur knight
RYLE: British astronomer
RYN: Painter Rembrandt van __
RYNE: Sandberg of baseball
RYOKAN: Japanese inn
RYUKYUS: Japanese island chain
RYUN: Former mile-run record holder
RZA: Rap-music producer

S

SAAB: Swedish auto
SAAR: German industrial region
SAATCHI: Ad-agency founder

SAB.: Day of rest: Abbr.
SABA: Antilles island
SABADO: Saturday: Spanish
SABAL: Tropical tree
SABATO: Actor Antonio
SABE: Kemo __ (Lone Ranger)
SABENA: Belgian airline
SABIN: Polio vaccine developer
SABINA: "Skin of Our Teeth" character
SABINE: Ancient Italian
SABO: Chris of baseball
SABOT: Wooden shoe
SABRA: Israel native
SABRE: Buffalo hockey pro
SABRINA: Audrey Hepburn film
SABU: Actor from India
SACCADE: Rein pull
SACCO: 1920s anarchist
SAC FLY: Baseball term
SACHEM: Tribal chief
SACHER: Rich torte
SACHS: Goldman's Wall Street partner
SACO: Maine river
SACQUE: Loose dress
SACRA: Pelvic bones
SACRE: "__ bleu!" (French oath)
SACRO: Iliac preceder
SACRUM: Pelvic bone
SADA: Actress Thompson
SADAT: Former Egyptian president
SAD CAFE: Carson McCullers locale
SADD: Anti-DWI grp.
SADDAM: Hussein of Iraq
SADE: Marquis de __
SADHE: Hebrew letter
SADHU: Hindu ascetic
SADIE: Maugham character
SADLER: Auto racer Elliott
SADO: Cruel prefix
SADR: Bani-__ (Irani politician)
SAD SACK: Army cartoon character
S.A.E.: Manuscript encl.
SAENS: Saint-__ (French composer)
SAFAR: Islamic month
SAFECO: Insurance company
SAFEWAY: Supermarket chain
SAFFI: Moroccan port
SAFIN: Tennis pro Marat
SAFIRE: Columnist on language
SAGAL: "Married...With Children" star
SAGAN: Astronomer Carl
S.A.G. CARD: Actor's ID
SAGET: TV host Bob
SAGINAW: Michigan city
SAGO: Palm starch
SAGUARO: Tall cactus
SAHEL: North African region
SAHL: Humorist Mort
SAIGON: Vietnamese city
SAINTE: French holy woman
SAINT LO: Normandy town
SAIPAN: One of the Marianas
SAIRY: "Grapes of Wrath" character
SAIS: Je ne __ quoi (indefinable quality)
SAISON: Season: French
SAITEK: Electronic game company
SAITH: Says, old-style
SAJAK: Game-show host Pat
SAKAI: Japanese port
SAKI: Rice wine
SAKS: Fifth Avenue store
SAL: Actor Mineo
SALA: Room: Spanish
SALAAM: Low bow
SALADA: Tea brand
SALADE: Salad: French
SALADIN: Crusaders' foe
SALAZAR: Former Portuguese leader
SALCHOW: Skating jump
SALEM, OR: Western capital
SALEP: Dried orchid tuber
SALERNO: Italian port
SALIC: Of the Franks
SALIERI: "Amadeus" antagonist
SALIFY: Add NaCl to
SALINA: Kansas city
SALINAS: California city
SALINE: Brackish
SALINES: Briny solutions
SALISH: British Columbia Indian
SALK: Polio vaccine developer
SALLE: Room: French
SALLIE: __ Mae (student-loan agency)
SALMA: Actress Hayek
SALMAN: Author Rushdie
SALMI: Pheasant stew
SALMON P: Chase of Lincoln's Supreme Court
SALOME: Biblical dancer
SALOMON: __ Smith Barney (investment firm)
SALONGA: "Miss Saigon" Tony winner
SALOP: English county
SAL'S: "Do the Right Thing" pizzeria
SAL SODA: Bleach ingredient
SALTANT: Leaping
SALTBOX: New England house
SALTEN: "Bambi" author
SALT I: Arms treaty
SALT II: Arms treaty
SALTON: California "sea"
SALUD: Spanish toast
SALUKI: Dog breed
SALUT: French toast
SALUTO: Frozen-pizza brand
SALVER: Tray
SALVOR: Salvager
SALYUT: Soviet space station
SAMAR: Philippine island
SAMARA: Maple seed
SAMARIA: Ancient Mideast kingdom
SAMBA: Ballroom dance
SAM BASS: Western outlaw
SAMBORA: Bon Jovi lead guitarist
SAMBUCA: Type of liqueur
SAME-DAY: Kind of service
SAMEDI: Saturday: French
SAMEKH: Hebrew letter
SAM HILL: Euphemistic name
SAM HUFF: Football Hall of Famer
SAMI: Laplander
SAM I AM: Seuss character
SAMISEN: Geisha's guitar
SAML.: Heb. judge
SAMLET: Young salmon
SAM LOYD: Puzzlemaster of old
SAMMI: Country singer Smith
SAMMS: Actress Emma
SAMMY: Bandleader Kaye
SAMMY JO: "Dynasty" character
SAM NUNN: Former Georgia senator
SAMOA: South Pacific island group
SAMOS: Aegean island
SAMOSA: Indian turnover
SAMOSET: Pilgrims' Indian friend
SAMOVAR: Tea urn
SAMOYED: Dog breed
SAMP: Coarsely-ground corn
SAMPAN: Chinese boat
SAMPRAS: Tennis pro Pete
SAMPSON: Ralph of basketball
SAM'S: __ Club (warehouse-store chain)
SAMSA: Kafka hero
SAMSON: Delilah's wooer
SAMSONS: Strongmen
SAMSUNG: Electronics company
SAMUEL: Diarist Pepys
SAMUEL L.: Actor Jackson
SAMWISE: "Lord of the Rings" character
SAN'A: Capital of Yemen
SANAA: Capital of Yemen
SAN BLAS: Panamanian gulf
SANBORN: Chase's coffee partner
SANCHO: Cervantes character
SANCTA: Holy places
SANCTUM: Holy place
SANCTUS: Hymn of praise
SAND DAB: Flounderlike fish
SANDE: Triple Crown jockey Earl
S. AND H.: Green-stamp company
SANDHOG: Construction worker
SANDIA: New Mexico peak
S. AND L.: CD source
SANDLER: Actor Adam
S. AND P.: Stock-rating co.
SANDRA: Actress Dee
SANDRO: Painter Botticelli
SANFORD: Redd Foxx role
SANGER: Activist Margaret
SANGRE: Blood: Spanish
SANI: __-Flush (cleaner brand)
SANIBEL: Florida island
SAN JOSE: California city
SAN JUAN: Capital of Puerto Rico
SANKA: Coffee brand
SAN REMO: Italian resort
SANS: Without: French
SANSEI: Japanese American
SANT: Director Gus Van __
SANTA FE: New Mexico capital
SANTANA: Spanish rock band
SANTE: Health: French
SANTEE: Carolina river
SANTHA: __ Rama Rau (Indian writer)
SANTINI: Duvall role
SANTO: Saint: Spanish
SANTOS: Brazilian port
SANYO: Electronics brand
SAO: __ Paulo, Brazil
SAONE: French river
SAO TOME: Island off western Africa
SAPID: Flavorful
SAPIENS: Homo __ (human species)
SAPIENT: Wise
SAPOR: Flavor
SAPP: Warren of football
SAPPER: Military engineer
SAPPHO: Greek poet
SAPPORO: Japanese city
SAPSAGO: Green cheese
S.A.R.: Colonial descendants org.
SARA: Author Paretsky
SARACEN: Crusaders' foe
SARAH: Actress Bernhardt
SARAI: Wife of Abram
SARA LEE: Cake brand
SARAN: Food wrap
SARANAC: Adirondack lakes
SARAWAK: Borneo region
SARAZEN: Golfer Gene
SARD: Orange-red mineral
SARDI'S: Big Apple restaurant
SARDOU: French dramatist
SAREE: Hindu attire
SAREK: Mr. Spock's father
SARG: Puppeteer Tony
SARGENT: Painter John Singer
SARGON: Ancient Assyrian king
SARI: Hindu attire
SARK: English Channel island
SARNIA: Ontario port
SARNOFF: Former RCA head
SAROS: Aegean gulf
SAROYAN: Novelist William
SARTO: Painter Andrea del __
SARTON: Poet May
SARTOR: Tailor, humorously
SARTRE: French writer
SARUMAN: "Lord of the Rings" wizard
SAS: European airline
SASEBO: Japanese port
SASHA: "Peter and the Wolf" bird
SASHIMI: Raw-fish appetizer
SASK.: Canadian province: Abbr.
SASSON: Jeans brand
SASSOON: Hair stylist Vidal
SATAY: Asian kebab
S.A.T.B.: For full chorus: Abbr.
SATCH: Pitcher Paige's nickname
SATCHMO: Armstrong's nickname
SATCOM: Communications satellite
SAT I: H.S. exam
SATIE: Composer Erik
SAT II: H.S. exam
SATINET: Light fabric
SAT IN ON: Audited
SATO: Japanese peace Nobelist
SATORI: Breakthrough in meditation

SATRAP: Petty tyrant
SATRAPY: Despot's domain
SATSUMA: Japanese porcelain
SATURN: GM car
SAUCONY: Sneaker brand
SAUD: Mideast king
SAUK: Oklahoma Indian
SAUL: Author Bellow
SAULT: __ Ste. Marie, MI
SAUR: Reptile: Comb. form
SAURIAN: Lizard
SAURO: Reptile: Comb. form
SAURON: "Lord of the Rings" villain
SAURUS: Reptile: Comb. form
SAV: Part of a discount-store name
SAVAII: Samoan island
SAVALAS: Actor Telly
SAVANA: GMC van model
SAVANT: Learned one
SAVARIN: Coffee brand
SAVATE: French kickboxing
SAVE AS: Word-processor command
SAVE FOR: Except
SAVE ME: Damsel's cry
SAVOIE: French department
SAVOIR: __-faire
SAVOY: Historic region of France
SAWATCH: Colorado range
SAWCHUK: Hockey Hall of Famer
SAW II: 2005 film
SAWYER: Twain character
SAWYERS: Woodworkers
SAXE: Old German duchy
SAXON: Ancient Brit
SAXONY: Kind of carpet
SAY HEY: Willie Mays' nickname
SAYLES: Director John
S.B.A.: Entrepreneurs' agcy.
SBARRO: Italian restaurant chain
SCAASI: Fashion designer Arnold
SCACCHI: Actres Greta
SCAGGS: Rock singer Boz
SCALA: La __ (Milan opera house)
SCALAGE: Loss allowance
SCALAR: Ladderlike
SCALENE: Type of triangle
SCALIA: Supreme Court Justice
SCAMPI: Shrimp dish
SCAPA: __ Flow (Orkney Islands basin)
SCAPULA: Shoulder blade
SCARAB: Pharoah's amulet
SCAREDY: __-cat
SCARIFY: Scratch
SCARNE: Card-game expert John
SCARP: Line of cliffs
SCARRY: Kid-lit author Richard
SCARUM: Harum-__ (reckless)
SCARWID: Actress Diana
SCATHE: Criticize
SCATMAN: Actor Crothers
SCENA: Extended aria
SCH.: Coll. or univ.
SCHAAP: Sports reporter Dick
SCHAV: Chilled soup
SCHAYES: Basketball Hall of Famer
SCHEIB: Earl of car-painting fame
SCHELDT: Belgian river
SCHELL: Actor Maximilian
SCHEMA: Conceptual framework
SCHERZO: Music movement
SCHICK: Razor brand
SCHIRRA: Apollo 7 astronaut
SCHIST: Crystalline rock
SCHLEP: Lug
SCHLEPP: Lug
SCHLITZ: Beer brand
SCHLOCK: Cheap
SCHLUB: Dolt
SCHLUMP: Dull one
SCHMEAR: Bribe
SCHMEER: Bribe
SCHMIDT: Former German leader
SCHMITT: Apollo 17 astronaut
SCHMO: Hapless type
SCHNAPS: Strong liquor
SCHNOOK: Dupe
SCHOLES: Economics Nobelist
SCHOLL: Shoe-accessory doctor
SCHON: "Bei Mir Bist du __"
SCHORR: Telejournalist Daniel
SCHTICK: Show-biz routine
SCHULTZ: "Hogan's Heroes" character
SCHULZ: "Peanuts" cartoonist
SCHUMER: New York senator
SCHUSS: Ski run
SCHWA: Vowel sound
SCHWAB: Broker Charles
SCHWANN: Recorded-music catalog
SCHWINN: Bike brand
SCI: __-fi
SCIATIC: Kind of nerve
SCIORRA: Actress Annabella
SCIPIO: Defeater of Hannibal
SCIRE: __ facias (judicial writ)
SCI-TECH: Scientific/technical
SCLAFF: Hit a golf ball badly
S.C.L.C.: Civil rights org.
SCLERA: Eyeball coat
SCOLARI: Actor Peter
SCONCE: Candle bracket
SCOOBA: Robotic floor washer
SCOOBY: __-Doo (cartoon canine)
SCORIA: Type of lava
SCOTER: Diving duck
SCOTIA: Nova __, Canada
SCOTT: "Ivanhoe" author
SCOTTO: Soprano Renata
SCOTT'S: Lawn-care brand
SCOTTY: "Star Trek" engineer
S COUPE: Type of auto body
SCRAG: Skinny one
SCRAT: "Ice Age" squirrel
SCREAK: Shrill cry
SCREE: Loose rock
SCREED: Diatribe
SCRIBER: Carpentry tool
SCRIM: Stage backdrop
SCRIP: Cash substitute
SCRIPPS: Newspaper publisher
SCROD: New England seafood
SCRUGGS: Country banjoist Earl
SCRUM: Rugby huddle
SCTV: John Candy's old show
SCUD: Gulf War missile
SCUDDER: Mutual-fund company
SCULLY: "X-Files" character
SCUP: Food fish
SCUPPER: Boat-deck drain
SCURFY: Scaly
S-CURVE: Winding turn
SCUSA: Excuse: Italian
'SCUSE ME: "Pardon," slangily
SCUSI: Pardon me: Italian
SCUT: Deer tail
SCUTTLE: Coal bucket
SCUZZ: Gross thing
SCYLLA: "Odyssey" menace
S. DAK.: Pierre's st.
S. DAKOTA: Pierre's st.
S.D.I.: Reagan defense pgm.
S.D.S.: 1960s campus org.
SEABEE: Navy builder
SEABORG: Chemistry Nobelist Glenn
SEA CALM: Langston Hughes poem
SEACAT: Type of ferryboat
SEA COW: Manatee
SEA DOG: Sailor
SEA FOX: Type of shark
SEAGAL: Actor Steven
SEA GATE: Navigable channel
SEAGIRT: Surrounded by the ocean
SEAGRAM: Liquor company
SEAGREN: 1968 Olympic pole-vault champ
SEA HAG: "Little Mermaid" villainess
SEAHAWK: NFL player
SEA HUNT: Lloyd Bridges TV series
SEALE: Black Panthers leader
SEA LEGS: Sailor's asset
SEALIFT: Transport via ship
SEALY: Mattress brand
SEA MOSS: Red algae
SEAMUS: Irish poet Heaney
SEAN: Actor Connery
SEANN: Actor __ William Scott
SEA RACE: Yachting event
SEARLE: Cartoonist Ronald
SEA STAR: Beach find
SEA-TAC: Washington State airport
SEATO: Former Asian alliance
SEATON: Director George
SEA TRIP: Cruise
SEATTLE: Puget Sound port
SEAU: Junior of football
SEAVER: Pitcher Tom
SEA WOLF: Pirate
SEBERG: Actress Jean
SEBRING: Chrysler model
SECADA: Singer Jon
SECANT: Line crossing a circle
SECHS: Six: German
SECHZIG: Sixty: German
SECKEL: Type of pear
SECO: Dry: Spanish
SECONDO: Piano-duet part
SECOND R: Writing
SED: Thirst: Spanish
SEDAKA: Singer Neil
SEDALIA: Missouri city
SEDER: Passover dinner
SEDGE: Marsh grass
SEDICI: Sixteen: Italian
SEDLEY: "Vanity Fair" character
SEDONA: Arizona art colony
SEDONAS: Kia models
SEDUM: Garden plant
SEE ALSO: Dictionary notation
SEE AS: Take to be
SEEGER: Folk singer Pete
SEE ME: Boss' request
SEE PAST: Ignore, as faults
SEEST: Biblical verb
SEETH: Biblical verb
SEFERIS: Greek literature Nobelist
SEG.: Div.
SEGA: Computer-game name
SEGAL: Actor George
SEGAR: "Popeye" cartoonist
SEGER: Singer Bob
SEGNO: Musical notation
SEGO: Western lily
SEGOVIA: Spanish guitarist
SEGRE: Italian physics Nobelist
SEGURA: Tennis great Pancho
SEGWAY: Modern scooter
SEHR: Very: German
SEI: Six: Italian
SEIJI: Conductor Ozawa
SEIKO: Watch brand
SEIN: "__Language" (1990s bestseller)
SEINE: Paris river
SEINES: Fishing nets
SEIS: Six: Spanish
SEISM: Earthquake
SEISMO: Earthquake: Comb. form
SEJM: Polish legislature
SEKO: Zairian despot
SEL: Salt: French
SELA: Actress Ward
SELAH: Psalm word
SELENA: Tejano singer
SELENE: Greek moon goddess
SELENIC: Containing element 34
SELES: Tennis pro Monica
SELIG: Baseball commissioner
SELKIRK: Robinson Crusoe prototype
SELL BY: Product-label phrase
SELLECK: Actor Tom
SELL IT: Do a convincing job
SELMA, AL: Southern city
SELTEN: German economics Nobelist
SELVAGE: Stamp-sheet edge
SEM.: School yr. part
SEMANA: Week: Spanish
SEMELE: Mother of Dionysus
SEMILOG: Type of graph paper
SEMINAL: Formative
SEMITE: Hebrew, e.g.
SEMPER: Always: Latin
SEMPLE: Evangelist Aimee __ McPherson
SEMPRE: Always, in music

SEN.: D.C. VIP
SENARY: Six-part
SENAT: French legislature
SENDAK: Children's author Maurice
SEND-UP: Spoof
SENE: Coin of Western Samoa
SENECA: New York Indian
SENEGAL: African nation
SENESCE: Get older
SENG: Hang __ (Hong Kong stock index)
SENGI: Zaire monetary unit
SENHOR: Sir: Portuguese
SENHORA: Lady: Portuguese
SENITI: Tonga coin
SENNA: Medicinal plant
SENNETT: "Keystone Kops" producer
SENOR: Sir: Spanish
SENORA: Lady: Spanish
SENSATE: Able to feel
SENSEI: Karate instructor
SEN-SEN: Breath-mint brand
SENTA: Actress Berger
SENTE: Lesotho coin
SENTRA: Nissan model
SEOUL: Korean city
SEPAL: Flower part
SEPHIA: Kia model
SEPIA: Brown pigment
SEP-IRA: Type of nest egg
SEPOY: Soldier of India
SEPTA: Biological partitions
SEPTIC: Infected
SEPTUM: Biological partition
SEQ.: Follow-up: Abbr.
SEQUOYA: Cherokee scholar
SER.: Sun. speech
SERA: Evening: Italian
SERAC: Glacial ridge
SERAI: Arabian inn
SERAL: Ecological adjective
SERAPH: Angel
SERAPIS: Ship captured by John Paul Jones
SERBIA: Balkan nation
SERBO: __-Croatian
SERE: Dried up
SERENA: Tennis pro Williams
SERGE: Suit material
SERGEI: Composer Prokofiev
SERGIO: Director Leone
SERIA: Opera __ (dramatic opera)
SERIATE: Arranged in order
SERIES E: Savings-bond category
SERIES F: Savings-bond category
SERIES G: Savings-bond category
SERIES H: Savings-bond category
SERIES I: Savings-bond category
SERIES J: Savings-bond category
SERIES K: Savings-bond category
SERIF: Typeface detail
SERIN: Canarylike bird
SERIO: __-comic (play type)
SE RI PAK: Korean golfer
SERKIN: Pianist Rudolf
SERKIS: Actor Andy
SERLING: "Twilight Zone" host
SEROUS: Watery
SERPENS: Snake constellation
SERPICO: Pacino film
SERRA: California mission founder
SERRATE: Notched
SERT: Spanish muralist
SERTA: Mattress brand
SERVE AS: Be
SERVO: Control mechanism
SES: His: French
SESE: Mobutu __ Seko (Zairian despot)
SESQUI: One and a half: Comb. form
SESS.: Conference: Abbr.
SESSILE: Permanently attached
SESSUE: Actor Hayakawa
SESTINA: Type of poem
SETA: Bristle
SET AT: Rip into
SETENTA: Seventy: Spanish
SETH: Clockmaker Thomas
SETI: "X-Files" grp.
SET INTO: Embed
SET ON: Attack
SETOSE: Bristly
SET PLAY: Prearranged maneuver in sports
SET SHOT: Basketball throw
SETT: Paving stone
SETTE: Seven: Italian
SETTLOR: Legal term
SETZER: Bandleader Brian
SEUL: Alone: French
SEULE: Alone: French
SEURAT: French painter
SEUSS: Grinch creator
SEVE: Golfer Ballesteros
SEVEN A: Shoe size
SEVEN B: Shoe size
SEVEN C: Shoe size
SEVEN D: Shoe size
SEVEN E: Shoe size
SEVEN EE: Shoe size
SEVEN NO: Bridge bid, for short
SEVEN-UP: Card game
SEVERN: English river
SEVERUS: Roman emperor
SEVIGNY: Actress Chloë
SEVILLA: Spanish city, to natives
SEVILLE: Spanish city
SEVRES: French porcelain
SEWARD: Lincoln cabinet member
SEWARD'S: "__ Folly" (Alaska)
SEWELL: "Black Beauty" author
SEWIST: Tailor
SEXER: Baby chick classifier
SEXTANS: Southern constellation
SEXTANT: Navigational instrument
SEXTON: Bell ringer
SEYMOUR: Actress Jane
SEZ: "Oh yeah, __ who?"
SFAX: Tunisian port
S.F. BAY: Golden Gate loc.
S.F.C.: Mil. rank
SFO: Calif. airport
SFORZA: Italian noble surname
S.F.P.D.: Dirty Harry's employer: Abbr.
SGT.: Mil. rank
SGT. MAJ.: Mil. rank
SHA: __ Na Na (singing group)
SHABBAT: Hebrew Sabbath
SHAD: Food fish
SHAD ROE: Caviar variety
SHAEF: DDE command
SHAFFER: Playwright Peter
SHAHN: Painter Ben
SHAKIN': "Whole Lot of __ Going On"
SHAKIRA: Latin pop singer
SHAKO: Military cap
SHAKUR: Rapper Tupac
SHALALA: Clinton cabinet member
SHALIT: Film critic Gene
SHALLOT: Onion relative
SHALLY: Shilly-__ (vacillate)
SHALOM: Hebrew greeting
SHALT: Biblical verb
SHAMIR: Former Israeli leader
SHAMMY: Soft leather
SHAMU: SeaWorld Whale
SHAMUS: Gumshoe
SHAN: Myanmar people
SHANA: Journalist Alexander
SHA NA NA: Singing group
SHANDY: Beer/lemonade drink
SHANE: Alan Ladd film
SHANG: Chinese dynasty
SHANGRI: __-la (paradise)
SHANIA: Singer Twain
SHANKAR: Sitar player Ravi
SHANNEN: Actress Doherty
SHANNON: Irish river
SHANTER: Tam-o'-__ (cap)
SHANTY: Crude hut
SHAPIRO: Simpson trial attorney
SHAQ: O'Neal of basketball
SHAR: __-Pei (Chinese dog)
SHARD: Pottery fragment
SHARI: Puppeteer Lewis
SHARIF: Actor Omar
SHARKEY: Don Rickles TV role
SHARON: Actress Stone
SHARONA: "My __" (1979 tune)
SHARPE: Shannon of the NFL
SHARPED: Raised in pitch, in music
SHAR-PEI: Chinese dog
SHARYN: Author McCrumb
SHASTA: California peak
SHASTRI: Former leader of India
SHATNER: Captain Kirk portrayer
SHATT: __ al Arab (Iraqi river)
SHAUN: Singer Cassidy
SHAVIAN: Of playwright George Bernard
SHAVUOT: Jewish festival
SHAW: Playwright George Bernard
SHAWN: Former "New Yorker" editor
SHAWNEE: Oklahoma Indian
SHAY: Open carriage
SHAYNE: Fictional gumshoe Mike
SHAZAM: Captain Marvel's magic word
SH-BOOM: Tune of 1954
SHEA: New York Mets ballpark
SHEAN: Gallagher's vaudeville partner
SHEB: Singer Wooley
SHEBA: Ancient Yemen
SHEBAT: Hebrew month
SHE BOP: Cyndi Lauper tune
SHECKY: Comic Greene
SHE-CRAB: Seafood soup
SHEDD'S: Margarine brand
SHED ON: Litter with fur
SHEEDY: Actress Ally
SHEEHAN: Golfer Patty
SHEEHY: Writer Gail
SHEENA: Singer Easton
SHEESH: "Gimme a break!"
SHEFFER: Actor Craig
SHEILA: Aussie gal
SHEILA E: Pop singer
SHEK: Chiang Kai-__ (Mao opponent)
SHEKEL: Israeli coin
SHEL: Writer Silverstein
SHELBY: Chess expert Lyman
SHELDON: Author Sidney
SHELLEY: British poet
SHELTIE: Sheepdog
SHELTY: Sheepdog
SHEM: Son of Noah
SHEMP: One of the Stooges
SHEP: Herding dog name
SHEPARD: Astronaut Alan
SHE-RA: "Masters of the Universe" heroine
SHERE: __ Khan (Kipling tiger)
SHEREE: Actress North
SHERM: Colonel Potter, familiarly
SHERMAN: Actor Hemsley
SHERPA: Himalayan guide
SHERRI: Pro golfer Steinhauer
SHERWIN: Williams' paint partner
SHERYL: Singer Crow
SHEVAT: Hebrew month
SHEW: What Ed Sullivan called his program
SHIATSU: Japanese massage
SHIH TZU: Tibetan dog
SHIISM: Muslim belief
SHIKOKU: Japanese island
SHILLY: __-shally (vacillate)
SHILOH: Civil War battle
SHIMON: Israeli leader Peres
SHINDY: Rumpus
SHINNY: Climb a rope
SHINOLA: Shoe-polish brand
SHIN PAD: Catcher's gear
SHINTO: Japanese religion
SHIP TO: Invoice phrase
SHIRAZ: Irani city
SHIRE: English county
SHIRER: Third Reich historian
SHIRLEY: Actress Temple
SHIRR: Bake eggs
SHISH: __ kebab
SHIV: Switchblade
SHIVA: Hindu god
SHLEP: Lug

SHLOCK: Cheap goods
SHMO: Jerk
SHMOO: "Li'l Abner" critter
SHNOOK: Gullible one
SHO: "__ 'nuff!"
SHOAT: Young pig
SHOEPAC: Heavy boot
SHOFAR: Synagogue ram's horn
SHOGI: Japanese board game
SHOGUN: Old Japanese ruler
SHOJI: Japanese screen
SHOLEM: Novelist Asch
SHOLOM: Author Aleichem
SHO' 'NUFF: Cowboy assent
SHOOFLY: Molasses pie
SHOPKO: Department-store chain
SHOPNBC: Cable channel
SHOR: Restaurateur Toots
SHORT A: "Pat" has one
SHORT E: "Pet" has one
SHORT I: "Pit" has one
SHORT O: "Pot" has one
SHORT U: "Put" has one
SHORTZ: NPR puzzlemaster
SHOULDA: Hindsight word
SHR.: NYSE unit
SHREK: Cartoon ogre
SHREVE: Author Anita
SHRIFT: Make short __ of
SHRIKE: Songbird
SHRINER: Fez wearer
SHRIVE: Impose penance on
SHRIVER: Mrs. Schwarzenegger
SHROVE: __ Tuesday (Lent preceder)
SHS: Library warnings
SHTETL: Jewish village
SHTICK: Show-biz routine
SHU: Moo __ pork
SHUBERT: Big name in theaters
SHUE: Actress Elizabeth
SHUI: Feng __ (harmonious placement)
SHUL: Synagogue
SHULA: Football coach Don
SHULMAN: Writer Max
SHULTZ: Reagan cabinet member
SHUMAI: Japanese dumplings
SHUSTER: Superman co-creator
SHUTE: Author Nevil
SHYLOCK: Loan shark
SHY OF: Less than
SHYSTER: Shady lawyer
SIAL: Earth's crust layer
SIAM: Thailand's former name
SIAN: Chinese city
SIBYL: Oracle
SICA: Director Vittorio De __
SIC 'EM: Angry dog owner's command
SICILIA: Italian island, to natives
SICILY: Italian island
SICK BAY: Ship hospital
SICKOUT: Employee protest
SID: Comedian Caesar
SIDDONS: Actress Sarah
SIDDUR: Jewish prayer book
SIDE A: 45 record surface
SIDE B: 45 record surface
SIDEMAN: Jazz-band member
SIDEWAY: Aslant
SIDIOUS: "Star Wars" series villain
SIDNEY: Author Sheldon
SIDON: Phoenician city
SIE: You: German
SIEBEN: Seven: German
SIEBZIG: Seventy: German
SIECLE: Fin de __ (end of century: French)
SIEG: Victory: German
SIEGEL: Gangster Bugsy
SIEMENS: Electronics company
SIENA: Italian city
SIENESE: Certain Italians
SIENNA: Reddish-brown
SIERRA: Mountain chain
SIETE: Seven: Spanish
SIG.: Autograph, for short
SIGIL: Official seal
SIGLER: Actress Jamie-Lynn
SIGMA: Greek letter
SIGMOID: S-shaped
SIGMUND: Dr. Freud
SIGNE: Actress Hasso
SIGNET: Finger-ring seal
SIGNOR: Sir: Italian
SIGNORA: Lady: Italian
SIGNORE: Sir: Italian
SIGURD: Norse myth hero
SIKA: Asian deer
SIKES: "Oliver Twist" villain
SIKH: Certain Hindu
SIKKIM: Himalayan kingdom
S'IL: Part of RSVP
SILAS: Fictional miser Marner
SILESIA: European region
SILEX: Proctor-__ (appliance brand)
SILICA: Mineral in quartz
SILICON: Element #14
SILVA: Forest
SILVERS: Comedian Phil
SIM: Actor Alastair
SIMA: Earth's crust layer
SIMBA: Lion, to Tarzan
SIM CITY: Video game
SIMENON: French novelist
SIMEON: San __ (Hearst Castle site)
SIMI: __ Valley, CA
SIMIAN: Ape
SIMILAC: Baby-formula brand
SIMMONS: Mattress brand
SIMMS: Phil of football
SIMON: Songwriter Paul
SIMONE: Actress Signoret
SIMONIZ: Car-wax brand
SIMP: Airhead
SIMPLEX: One-floor apartment
SIMPSON: Duchess of Windsor's surname
SIMS: Zoot of jazz
SINBAD: "Arabian Nights" hero
SIN CITY: 2005 film
SINDBAD: "Arabian Nights" hero
SINE: Trig function
SINEAD: Singer O'Connor
SINE DIE: Indefinitely: Latin
SINEX: Nasal-spray brand
SINGH: Golfer Vijay
SINGIN': "__ in the Rain"
SINGLET: Athletic jersey
SINH: Trig function
SINISE: Actor Gary
SINN: __ Fein (Irish movement)
SINO: Chinese: Comb. form
SINUATE: Coil
SINUOUS: Winding
SINUTAB: Cold-remedy brand
SIOBHAN: British actress McKenna
SION: Noun suffix
SIPE: Brian of football
SIR BEN: Actor Kingsley, formally
SIR DUKE: Stevie Wonder tune
SIREE: "No __!"
SIRICA: Watergate judge
SIRIUS: Dog Star
SIR KAY: King Arthur knight
SIROCCO: Hot desert wind
SIRRAH: Buster, old-style
SIRREE: "No __!"
SIRUP: Waffle topper
SISAL: Rope fiber
SI, SENOR: Spanish assent
SISKEL: Film critic Gene
SISLER: Baseball great George
SISLEY: French painter
SISQO: Rap star
SISS: Greeting for the villain
SISSLE: Eubie Blake collaborator
SISTINE: Vatican chapel
SITE MAP: Internet table of contents
SITKA: Alaskan city
SIT ON IT: "Happy Days" catchphrase
SITTIN': "__ on the dock of the bay"
SITU: In __ (as found)
SITWELL: British poet
SITZ: Bath prefix
SIVA: Hindu god
SIVAN: Hebrew month
SIX A: Shoe size
SIX B: Shoe size
SIX C: Shoe size
SIX D: Shoe size
SIX E: Shoe size
SIXED: Deep-__ (discarded)
SIX EE: Shoe size
SIX EEE: Shoe size
SIX EEEE: Shoe size
SIXER: Philadelphia NBAer
SIX NO: Bridge bid, for short
SIX PIN: Alley target
SIXTUS: Pope
SIZER: Measuring device
SKA: Jamaican music
SKAGGS: Country singer Ricky
SKAGWAY: Alaskan city
SKALD: Ancient Norse bard
SKANK: Sleaze
SKAT: Three-handed card game
SKED: Timetable, informally
SKEE: __-Ball (arcade game)
SKEETER: Biting insect, informally
SKEEZIX: "Gasoline Alley"character
SKEG: Keel extension
SKELTER: Helter-__
SKELTON: Comedian Red
SKIBOB: Snow vehicle
SKIDDY: Apt to slide
SKID,LID: Helmet, slangily
SKIFFLE: Music genre
SKIL: Power-tool brand
SKILFUL: Adept, in Britain
SKINK: Lizard
SKIPPY: Peanut-butter brand
SKIRL: Play the bagpipes
SKITCH: Bandleader Henderson
SKITTLE: British bowling pin
SKNXX: Dagwood's snore
SKNXXX: Dagwood's snore
SKOAL: Scandinavian toast
SKOKIE: Chicago suburb
SKOPJE: Macedonian capital
SKORT: Women's casual attire
SKU: Merchandise ID
SKUA: Diving bird
SKULLED: Thick-__ (doltish)
SKY DOME: Toronto stadium
SKYE: Type of terrier
SKYEY: Azure
SKYHOOK: Copter device
SKYLAB: NASA space station
SKYMAN: Aviator
SKYNYRD: Lynyrd __ (rock group)
SKYPE: Internet telephone service
SKY'S: "The __ the limit!"
SKYTEL: Paging service
S.L.A.: Patty Hearst kidnappers
SLADE: Playwright Bernard
SLAPPY: Comedian White
SLATER: Actor Christian
SLATKIN: Conductor Leonard
SLAVER: Drool
SLAYTON: Astronaut Deke
SLEIGHT: Adeptness
SLEY: Loom part
SLEZAK: Actress Erika
SLIGO: Irish county
SLIM JIM: Lock-picking tool
SLIPPY: Slippery
SLITHY: Jabberwocky word
SLIWA: Guardian Angels founder
SLO: Road-sign word
SLOAN: Painter John
SLOANE: Actor Everett
SLOE: Wild plum
SLO-MO: Instant-replay technique
SLOOPY: "Hang on __" (1965 song)
SLOPER: Sewing pattern
SLOT CAR: Toy racer
SLOUGH: Shed, as a snake
SLOVENE: Eastern European
S.L.R.: Kind of camera: Abbr.
SLUE: Swing around
SLUGGO: Nancy's comics pal
SLURPEE: 7-Eleven drink
SLURRY: Thin cement
SLX: Acura model
SLYE: Roy Rogers's real surname
SLYKE: Novelist Helen Van __
SMA: Little: Scottish
SMALL O.J.: Breakfast order

SMARM: False flattery
SMATTER: Dabble in
SMAUG: "Lord of the Rings" dragon
SMAZE: Air pollution
SMEAGOL: "Lord of the Rings" character
SMEAL: Feminist Eleanor
SMEE: "Peter Pan" pirate
SMEES: Pintail ducks
SMERSH: 007 foe
SMETANA: Czech composer
SMEW: Kind of duck
SMILEY'S: "__ People" (le Carré novel)
SMILLA'S: "__ Sense of Snow" (Julia Ormond film)
SMIRNOV: Vodka brand
SMITS: Actor Jimmy
SMITTY: Comic strip of yore
S.M.L.: T-shirt size choices: Abbr.
SMOKEY: Highway cop
SMOKIES: Appalachian range
SMOLT: Young salmon
SMOOSH: Squash
SMOOT: Tariff act co-sponsor
SMORE: Campfire treat
S.M.U.: Dallas sch.
SMUCKER: Jelly company
SMURF: Blue cartoon character
SMUSH: Compress
SMYRNA: Type of fig
SMYTH: Rock singer Patty
SNA: Snow: Scottish
SNAPPLE: Soft-drink brand
SNARF: Eat greedily
SNARK: Lewis Carroll beast
SNARKY: Testy
SNATH: Scythe handle
SNAX: Noshes, in ads
SNAZZ UP: Make fancier
S.N.C.C.: 1960s civil rights grp.
SNEAD: Golf great Sam
SNEE: Old dagger
SNEETCH: Dr. Seuss character
SNELL: Fishhook attachment
SNELLEN: Eye-chart inventor
SNERD: Edgar Bergen dummy
SNERT: Hägar the Horrible's dog
SNEVA: Auto racer Tom
SNICK: Small cut
SNICKET: Kid-lit author Lemony
SNIDER: Baseball great Duke
SNIFTER: Brandy glass
SNIGLET: Comical word coinage
S.N.L.: NBC skit show
SNO: __-Cone (icy treat)
SNO BALL: Hostess snack
SNOBOL: Computer language
SNO-CAPS: Candy brand
SNO-CAT: Winter vehicle
SNO-CONE: Icy treat
SNOOD: Hairnet
SNOOK: Ocean fish
SNOOKER: Variety of pool
SNOOKS: Fanny Brice character
SNOPES: Faulkner family name
SNORRI: Icelandic historian Sturluson
SNOWCAT: Winter vehicle
SNOWDON: Welsh peak
SNOWE: Maine senator
SNR.: H.S. student
SNUFFY: Smith of comic strips
SNUGLI: Baby-carrier brand
SNYDER: TV host Tom
SOAPNET: Cable channel
SO AS: In order (to)
SO AS TO: In order that
SOAVE: White wine
SOBA: Japanese noodle
SO BAD: Paul McCartney tune
SO BIG: Ferber novel
SOC.: Assn.
SOCA: Caribbean music
SO. CAL.: UCLA rival
SOCIO: Economic prefix
SOCKEYE: Red salmon
SOCLE: Column base
SOEUR: Sister: French
SOFER: Actress Rena
SO FEW: RAF, to Churchill
SOFFIT: Underside of a beam
SOFIA: Capital of Bulgaria
SOFIE: Opera singer Anne __ von Otter
SO FINE: Tune of 1959
SOFTGEL: Type of vitamin capsule
SOFT-TOP: Kind of auto
SOHO: London district
SOI: __-disant (self-styled)
SOIE: Silk: French
SOIGNE: Well-groomed
SOIGNEE: Well-groomed
SOIR: Evening: French
SO I SEE: "Aha!"
SO IT IS: "Aha!"
SOLA: Alone, on stage
SOLAN: Kind of goose
SOLANO: Northern California county
SOLARA: Camry model
SO LA TI: Scale trio
SOLDO: Old Italian coin
SOLEA: Roman sandal
SOLEDAD: O'Brien of CNN
SOLEIL: Sun: French
SOLEUS: Calf muscle
SOLFEGE: Voice exercise
SOLI: Arias
SOL LA: Scale pair
SOL LA TI: Scale trio
SOLNESS: "Master Builder" character
SOLON: Wise lawgiver
SOLTI: Conductor Sir Georg
SOLUTE: Dissolved substance
SOMA: Body of an organism
SOMALI: East African people
SOMALIA: African nation
SOMAT: Body: Comb. form
SOMATA: Bodies of an organism
SOMERS: Actress Suzanne
SOMINEX: Sleep-aid brand
SOMME: French river
SOMMER: Actress Elke
SOMNI: Sleep: Comb form
SOMONI: Tajikistan money
SONAL: Of sound
SONANCE: Sound
SONANT: Audible
SONDE: Atmospheric balloon
SONDRA: Actress Locke
SONE: Loudness unit
SONIA: Actress Braga
SONICS: NBA team
SONJA: Skater Henie
SONOMA: Northern California county
SONORA: Mexican state
SONTAG: Author Susan
SONY: Electronics company
SONYA: "Crime and Punishment" character
SOO: Great Lakes canal
SOOEY: Hog call
SOONERS: Oklahomans
SOON-YI: Woody Allen's wife
SOOTH: Truth, old-style
SOPH: Second-yr. student
SOPHIA: Actress Loren
SOPHIE: Singer Tucker
SOPHIE'S: "__ Choice" (Streep film)
SOPHISM: False argument
SOPOR: Deep sleep
SOPWITH: British aircraft designer
SOR.: Campus org.
SORA: Marsh bird
SORB: European tree
SORBATE: Food preservative
SORBIC: Preservative acid
SORBO: Actor Kevin
SORDINO: Trumpet mute
SOREL: Stendhal hero
SOREN: Philosopher Kierkegaard
SORENTO: Kia model
SORGHUM: Cereal grass
SORIANO: Alfonso of baseball
SORORAL: Sisterly
SOROS: Hungarian-born financier
SORREL: Reddish-brown horse
SORRELL: Actor Booke
SORTIE: Raid
SORVINO: Actress Mira
SOSA: Sammy of baseball
S.O.S. PAD: Steel-wool brand
SOTHEBY: London auctioneer
SOTHERN: Actress Ann
SOTO: Explorer de __
SOTTO: __ voce (softly)
SOT-WEED: "The __ Factor" (Barth book)
SOU: Former French coin
SOUBISE: Oniony sauce
SOUCI: Sans __ (carefree)
SOUL MAN: Sam and Dave tune
SOUNDER: Cicely Tyson film
SOUPCON: Trace
SOUPER: Pea-__ (dense fog)
SOUP'S ON: "Come and get it!"
SOUR ALE: Pub serving
SOUSA: March composer
SOUTER: Supreme Court Justice
SOUTHEY: British poet
SOV.: Monarch: Abbr.
SOWETO: South African region
SOX: Boston Red __
SOY INK: Printer's purchase
SOYINKA: Nigerian literature Nobelist
SOYLENT: "__ Green" (Heston film)
SOYUZ: Soviet spacecraft
SPAAK: Belgian statesman
SPACEK: Actress Sissy
SPACELY: George Jetson's boss
SPACEY: Actor Kevin
SPAD: WWI French plane
SPAGO: L.A. restaurant
SPAHN: Warren of baseball
SPAKE: Said, old-style
SPAMBOT: Automated junk e-mail sender
SPANAIR: European airline
SPANDEX: Elastic fabric
SPANG: Directly
SPANKER: Type of sail
SPANKY: "Little Rascals" kid
SPANNER: Wrench
SPANO: Actor Joe
SPARKY: Baseball manager Anderson
SPARTA: Ancient Greek city
SPASSKY: Russian chessmaster
SPATHE: Flower bract
S.P.C.A.: Pet protection org.
SPEARE: Novelist Elizabeth George __
SPECIE: Coin
SPECTOR: Rock singer Ronnie
SPEE: WWI German admiral
SPEEDO: Swimsuit brand
SPEER: "Inside the Third Reich" author
SPEKE: British explorer
SPELUNK: Explore caves
SPENCE: Attorney Gerry
SPENCER: British philosopher
SPENDY: Expensive
SPENSER: British poet Edmund
SPERO: "Dum spiro, __" (South Carolina motto)
SPERRY: Gyrocompass inventor
SPET: Barracuda
SPEX: Glasses, in ads
S.P.F.: Tanning lotion no.
SPHYNX: Cat breed
SPIC: __ and Span (cleaner brand)
SPICA: Star in Virgo
SPIDEY: Comics hero, familiarly
SPIEGEL: Former cataloguer
SPIKE TV: Cable channel
SPILE: Sap spout
SPINEL: Crystalline gem
SPINER: Actor Brent
SPINKS: Boxer Leon
SPINNEY: Big Bird portrayer Caroll
SPINOZA: Dutch philosopher
SPIREA: Flowering shrub
SPIRO: Vice president Agnew
SPITZ: Type of dog
SPIVAK: 1970s "Meet the Press" host
SPLENDA: Sweetener brand
SPLINE: Thin strip

SPLOSH: Bathtub sound
SPOCK: "Star Trek" character
SPODE: Fine china
SPOKANE: City in Washington
SPONDEE: Metrical foot
SPOONER: Word-mangling reverend
SPOONY: Foolish
SPOOR: Animal track
SPORK: Hybrid eating utensil
SPORRAN: Kilt pouch
SPORTIN': __ Life ("Porgy and Bess" character)
SPOSA: Wife: Italian
S'POSE: Slangy "what if"
SPOSO: Husband: Italian
SPOT-ON: Precise
SPOT TV: Network ad production
SPQR: Roman inscription
SPR.: Time of yr.
SPRACH: "Also __ Zarathustra" (Nietzsche work)
SPRIT: Ship pole
SPRITZ: Dash of seltzer
SPT.: Seaport: Abbr.
SPUTNIK: Russian satellite
SPYBOT: Destructive-software remover
SPYDER: Mitsubishi model
SPY HOLE: Front-door feature
SPY KIDS: Antonio Banderas film
SPYRI: "Heidi" author
SPYRO: __ Gyra (pop-jazz band)
SPYS: Donald Sutherland film
SPYWARE: Intrusive computer programs
SQ. FT.: Area meas.
SQ. IN.: Area meas.
SQ. MI.: Area meas.
SQR.: Plaza: Abbr.
SQS.: Plazas: Abbr.
SQUANTO: Pilgrims' Indian friend
SQUAW: __ Valley, CA
SQUEERS: "Nicholas Nickleby" character
SQUIB: Short news story
SQUIBB: Drug company
SQUINCH: Crouch down
SQ. YD.: Area meas.
SRA.: Mrs.: Spanish
SRI: __ Lanka
SRIS: Hindu honorifics
SRS.: AARP members
SRTA.: Miss: Spanish abbr.
SRX: Cadillac model
S.S.A.: Org. for retirees
SSE: Compass dir.
SSGT.: NCO
SSH: "Quiet!"
S.S.I.: Govt. stipend
S.S.N.: 9-digit ID
S.S.R.: Soviet div.
S.S.S.: Draft org.
SSSS: Flat-tire sound
SSSSSSS: Snake film of 1973
S STAR: Spectral type
SSW: Compass pt.
STA.: Depot: Abbr.
STABAT: "__ Mater" (hymn)
STABILE: Abstract sculpture
STAC.: Disconnected, in music: Abbr.
STACEY: Actress Dash
STACY: Actor Keach
STAD: South African village
STADE: Frederica von __ (opera singer)
STADLER: Golfer Craig
STADT: Town: German
STAEL: Writer Madame de __
STAGG: Football coach Amos Alonzo
STAGGED: Went without a date
ST. AGNES: Patron of gardeners
STAHL: TV reporter Lesley
STAHR: "Last Tycoon" title character
STALAG: "Hogan's Heroes" locale
STALIN: WWII Soviet leader
STAMOS: Actor John
STAN: Saxophonist Getz
STANG: Actor Arnold
STANINE: Aptitude-test score
STAN LEE: Spider-Man creator
STANLEY: Dr. Livingstone's finder
STANNIC: Containing tin
STANNUM: Tin: Latin
STANS: Nixon cabinet member
STANTON: Lincoln cabinet member
STAPES: Ear bone
STAPH: Type of bacteria
STA-PUF: Fabric-softener brand
STAR IN: Head the cast of
STARION: Mitsubishi model
STARKEY: Ringo's real last name
STARLOG: Sci-fi film mag
STARMAN: Jeff Bridges film
STARR: Drummer Ringo
STARSKY: TV cop
STARZ: Cable channel
STARZZ: WNBA team
STASI: East German secret police
STASIS: Condition of equilibrium
STASSEN: 1950s presidential contender
STATEN: __ Island, NY
STATER: Ancient Greek coin
STATICE: Garden flower
STATICS: Branch of physics
STATIN: Cholesterol-reducing drug
STATIST: Advocate of central government
STATLER: Country music brothers' surname
STATOR: Machine part
STAUB: Rusty of baseball
S.T.B.: Seminary deg.
ST. BARTS: Caribbean island, for short
ST. BASIL: Russian saint
ST. BEDE: "Venerable" monk
ST. CLOUD: Minnesota city
ST. CROIX: Antilles island
STD.: Norm: Abbr.
ST. DENIS: Patron of France
STE.: Fr. holy woman
STE. ANNE: Quebec's patron
STEARIC: Fatty acid
STEARIN: Candle ingredient
STEARNS: The "S" in T.S. Eliot
STEELE: British essayist
STEELER: Pittsburgh NFLer
STEEN: Dutch painter
STEEVE: Fill the hull
STEFAN: Tennis pro Edberg
STEFANI: Singer Gwen
STEFFI: Tennis pro Graf
STE.-FOY: Canadian city
STEIG: "New Yorker" cartoonist
STEIGER: Actor Rod
STEINEM: Feminist Gloria
STEINER: Film composer Max
STELA: Stone monument
STELE: Stone monument
ST. ELIAS: Canadian peak
STELLA: "Streetcar..." character
ST. ELMO: Patron of sailors
STEMPEL: "Quiz Show" character
STEN: British gun
STENGEL: Baseball manager Casey
STEN GUN: British weapon
STENNIS: Former Mississippi senator
STENT: Artery implant
STENTOR: Loud talker
STEPHEN: Novelist King
STEPPE: Treeless plain
STER: Occupational suffix
STERE: Cubic meter
STERIC: Two-dimensional
STERNE: British novelist
STERNO: Barbecue fuel
STERNUM: Breastbone
STEROL: Solid alcohol
STERTOR: Heavy snoring
STET: Proofer's notation
STETHO: Chest: Comb. form
STEUBEN: Art-glass brand
STEVE: Actor McQueen
STEVEN: Director Spielberg
STEVENS: Singer Cat
STEVIE: Singer Wonder
STEWART: Singer Rod
STEWIE: "Family Guy" character
STICH: Tennis pro Michael
STICK IN: Add
ST. IDES: Malt-liquor brand
STIEB: Dave of baseball
STIERS: Actor David Ogden __
STIFFEL: Lamp brand
STILLE: "__ Nacht" (Christmas carol)
STILTON: Type of cheese
STIMPY: Cartoon cat
STIMSON: FDR cabinet member
STINE: Kid-lit author R.L.
STIPE: Rock singer Michael
STIPES: Mushroom stalks
STIVIC: "All in the Family" character
ST. JAMES: Monopoly property
ST. JOAN: Shaw heroine
ST. JOE: Missouri city, informally
ST. JOHN: Actress Jill
ST. JOHN'S: New York university
ST. JUDE: Patron of lost causes
STK.: Wall St. commodity
ST. KITTS: West Indies island
STL: St. Louis: Abbr.
ST. LEO: 5th-century pope
ST. LO: Normandy town
ST. LUCIA: West Indies island
ST. LUKE: Gospel writer
ST. LUKE'S: Hospital name
ST. MALO: French port
ST. MARK: Gospel writer
ST. MARK'S: Venice cathedral
ST. MARY'S: River to Lake Huron
STN.: RR stop
STO: Pou __ (vantage point)
STOA: Greek portico
STOAT: Brown ermine
STODGE: Stuff oneself
STOJKO: Canadian figure skater
STOKELY: Activist Carmichael
STOL: Mil. plane
STOLA: Roman tunic
ST. OLAF: Patron of Norway
STOLI: Vodka brand
STOLLE: Tennis pro Fred
STOLLEN: German bread
STOLON: Plant runner
STOLTZ: Actor Eric
STOMA: Botanical opening
STOMATA: Botanical openings
STOMPIN': "__ at the Savoy"
STOOKEY: Folk singer Paul
STOPPLE: Bottle plug
STORCH: Comedian Larry
STORRS: Connecticut town
STOTIN: Slovenian money
STOVER: Russell __ (chocolate brand)
STOWE: Vermont ski resort
STP: Motor-oil additive
ST. PAT: Mar. honoree
ST. PAT'S: March 17, informally
ST. PAUL: Capital of Minnesota
ST. PAUL'S: London cathedral
ST. PETE: City near Tampa
ST. PETER: An apostle
ST. PIUS I: Canonized pope
ST. PIUS V: Canonized pope
ST. PIUS X: Canonized pope
STR.: Atlas abbr.
STRAD: Valuable violin
STRADA: Road: Italian
STRAM: Football coach Hank
STRASSE: Street: German
STRAT: Guitar brand, familiarly
STRATAS: Diva Teresa
STRATI: Layer: Comb. form
STRATO: Layer: Comb. form
STRAUB: Novelist Peter
STRAUSS: "The Waltz King"
STREEP: Actress Meryl
ST. REGIS: Fancy hotel chain
STREP: Throat bug
STRETTO: Fugue feature
STRIA: Narrow groove
STRIATE: Furrowed
STRIPY: Banded
STRITCH: Actress Elaine
STROH'S: Beer brand
STROM: Senator Thurmond
STROPHE: Poem section

'STROS: Houston baseballers, for short
STROUD: Birdman of Alcatraz
STROUSE: Broadway composer Charles
STRUG: Gymnast Kerri
STRUNK: "The Elements of Style" coauthor
ST. SIMON: An apostle
STU: Actor Erwin
STUART: British royal house
STUARTI: Singer Enzo
STUBBY: Comic Kaye
STUBING: "Love Boat" captain
STUDLY: Attractive, slangily
STUKA: WWII plane
STUPA: Buddhist shrine
STURGES: Director Preston __
STURM: __ und Drang (turmoil)
STUTZ: Vintage auto
STYE: Eye annoyance
STYGIAN: Dark
STYLET: Dagger
STYLUS: Phonograph needle
STYNE: Songwriter Jule
STYPSIS: Astringent usage
STYRENE: Synthetic rubber component
STYRO: Prefix for foam
STYRON: Author William
STYX: Mythical river
SUASION: Art of coaxing
SUBARU: Japanese auto
SUBBASS: Organ stop
SUBDEB: Society teen
SUBDUCT: Take away
SUBGUM: Chinese dish
SUBIC: Philippine bay
SUBITO: Abruptly, in music
SUBJOIN: Append
SUBORN: Bribe
SUB ROSA: Secretly
SUBSUME: Contain
SUBTEND: Be opposite to
SUBVENE: Come to help
SUCCOR: Aid
SUCCOTH: Jewish holiday
SUCRASE: Sugar-digesting enzyme
SUCRE: Ecuador coin
SUD: South: French
SUDAFED: Decongestant brand
SUDAN: African nation
SUDBURY: Canadian city
SUDOKU: Numbers game
SUDSER: Soap opera
SUE ANE: Actress Langdon
SUE ANN: "Mary Tyler Moore Show" character
SUELLEN: Sister of Scarlett
SUE LYON: "Lolita" star
SUENO: Dream: Spanish
SUEY: Chop __
SUEZ: Mideast canal site
SUFFOLK: British county
SUFFUSE: Overspread
SUFI: Muslim mystic
SUHARTO: Former Indonesian leader
SUI: __ generis (unique)
SUISSE: Switzerland: French
SUK: Arab bazaar
SUKARNO: Former Indonesian leader
SUKKOTH: Jewish holiday
SULA: Toni Morrison novel
SULFA: Drug family
SULFUR: Element #16
SULKIES: Harness-racing vehicles
SULLA: Roman general
SULTANA: Seedless raisin
SULU: "Star Trek" character
SULU SEA: Waters off Borneo
SUMATRA: Indonesian island
SUMER: Ancient Asian region
SUMMA: __ cum laude
SUMMAND: Part of a total
SUMNER: Sting's real last name
SUMP: Cesspool
SUMTER: Carolina fort
SUNBIRD: Pontiac model
SUN BOWL: Postseason football game
SUN CITY: Arizona town
SUNDA: Indonesian island group
SUNDOG: Incomplete rainbow
SUNFAST: Unlikely to fade
SUNFIRE: Pontiac model
SUNGLOW: Haze phenomenon
SUNKIST: Orange-juice brand
SUN-MAID: Raisin brand
SUNNA: Islamic law
SUNNI: Certain Muslim
SUNOCO: Oil company
SUNUNU: Bush chief of staff
SUNY: Empire St. schools
SUOMI: Finland, to Finns
SUPE: Movie extra
SUPER G: Skiing event
SUPPE: Soup: German
SUPRA: Toyota model
SUPT: Apt. building employee
SUR: Big __, CA
SURA: Koran chapter
SURAH: Koran chapter
SURETE: French FBI
SURFEIT: Excess
SURFIN': "__ U.S.A." (Beach Boys tune)
SURG.: OR staffer
SURIMI: Japanese imitation shellfish
SURINAM: South American nation
SURREY: Horse-drawn carriage
SUSAN: Writer Sontag
SUSAN B.: Feminist __ Anthony
SUSANN: Author Jacqueline
SUSANNA: Figaro's love
SUSANNE: Philosopher Langer
SUSIE: "Calvin and Hobbes" girl
SUSSEX: Anglo-Saxon kingdom
SUSS OUT: Investigate
SUTRA: Kama __
SUTRAS: Buddhist sermons
SUTTER: Gold-rush mill owner
SUTTON: Bank robber Willie
SUU KYI: Myanmar Peace Nobelist
SUVA: Capital of Fiji
SUVARI: Actress Mena
SUZANNE: Actress Somers
SUZE: Orman of personal finance
SUZETTE: Crêpe __
SUZI: Rock singer Quatro
SUZIE: "The World of __ Wong"
SUZIE Q: Creedence Clearwater tune
SUZUKI: Motorcycle maker
SUZY: Country singer Bogguss
SUZY Q: Snack-cake brand
SVEDKA: Vodka brand
SVEN: Explorer Hedin
SVERIGE: Sweden, to Swedes
SVX: Subaru model
S.W.A.: Namibia, once: Abbr.
SWABBY: Sailor
SWADDLE: Bandage
SWAGMAN: Aussie hobo
S.W.A.K.: Love-letter abbr.
SWALE: Low-lying land
SWANEE: Gershwin tune
SWANN: Lynn of football
SWANN'S: "__ Way" (Proust novel)
SWANSEA: Welsh port
SWANSON: Actress Gloria
SWARD: Turf
SWARTHY: Dark
SWASH: Swagger
SWATHE: Bandage
SWAY BAR: Car safety feature
SWAYZE: Actor Patrick
SWAZI: African language
SWE.: Scand. country
SWED.: Scand. nation
SWEENEY: Todd of a Sondheim musical
SWEE'PEA: Popeye's kid
SWELTRY: Sizzling
SWENSON: Actress Inga
SWF: Personal ad abbr.
SWIGERT: Apollo 13 astronaut
SWING IT: Manage
SWINTON: Actress Tilda
SWIRLZ: Mini __ (Kellogg's cereal)
SWIT: Actress Loretta
SWITZER: Football coach Barry
SWIVET: Anxious state
SWM: Personal ad abbr.
SWOOSIE: Actress Kurtz
SYBIL: Sally Field Emmy role
SYD: 2000 Olympics mascot
SYD HOFF: "New Yorker" cartoonist
SYDNEY: Australian city
SYDOW: Actor Max von __
SYL.: Part of a wd.
SYLL.: Part of a wd.
SYLPH: Graceful woman
SYLVAN: Wooded
SYLVIA: Poet Plath
SYM.: Orch. piece
SYMS: Actress Sylvia
SYN.: Alternative wd.
SYNAPSE: Nerve junction
SYNC: Harmonize
SYNCH: Harmonize
SYNCOPE: Fainting spell
SYNDIC: Business agent
SYNE: "Auld Lang __"
SYNERGY: Combined action
SYNFUEL: Coal extract
SYNGE: Irish playwright
SYNGMAN: Former Korean leader Rhee
SYNOD: Church assembly
SYNTH: Moog, familiarly
SYR.: Neighbor of Isr.
SYRIANA: George Clooney film
SYS.: Method: Abbr.
SYSCO: Food-service company
SYSOP: Computer administrator
SYST.: Method: Abbr.
SYSTOLE: Blood-pressure factor
SYZYGY: Astronomical alignment
SZELL: Hungarian conductor
SZILARD: Physicist Leo
SZYSLAK: "Simpsons" tavern owner

T

TAAL: The __ (South African language)
TABARD: Knight's cloak
TABARET: Upholstery fabric
TABI: Japanese sock
TABITHA: "Bewitched" baby
TABLA: Drum of India
TABOR: Small drum
TABORET: Small drum
TABOULI: Mideast salad
TABRIZ: Iranian city
TAB SET: Typewriter feature
TABULA: __ rasa (clean slate)
TAC: Tic-__-toe
TACET: "Be silent," in music
TACH: RPM gauge
TACHO: Speed: Comb. form
TACHYON: Hypothetical particle
TACITUS: Roman historian
TACOMA: Washington city
TACOMAS: Toyota models
TACONIC: New England range
TACTEL: Synthetic fiber
TACTUAL: Touch-related
TA-DA: Shout of triumph
TAE: Menlo Park monogram
TAE BO: Martial-arts exercise
TAEGU: Korean city
TAEL: Asian weight
TAFTS: 1910s First Family
TAGALOG: Philippine language
TAGAMET: Heartburn remedy
TAG DAY: Charity event
TAGGANT: Product-tracing substance
TAG ON: Add
TAGORE: Indian literature Nobelist
TAG-OUT: Pick-off play
TAG TEAM: Wrestling pair
TAG UP: Advance after a catch
TAGUS: Portuguese river
TAHINI: Mideast paste
TAHNEE: Actress Welch

TAHOE: California/Nevada lake
TAHOES: Chevy models
TAI: Mai __ (rum drink)
TAI CHI: Martial art
TAIGA: Subarctic forest
TAIL FIN: 1950s car feature
TAIL PIN: Cello part
TAINA: Actress Elg
TAI-PAN: Clavell novel
TAIPEI: Capital of Taiwan
TAITO: Video-game name
TAIWAN: Asian nation
TAJ: __ Mahal
TAJO: Spanish river
TAKA: Bangladesh coin
TAKEI: Sulu, on "Star Trek"
TAKE-INS: Deceptions
TAKIN': "__ Care Of Business"
TAL: Russian chess champion
TALA: Samoan money
TALARIA: Mercury's winged sandals
TALER: Old German coin
TALESE: Author Gay
TALI: Anklebones
TALIA: Actress Shire
TALIBAN: Afghan group
TALISA: Actress Soto
TALKIE: Walkie-__
TALKIN': "Jive __" (Bee Gees tune)
TALLINN: Capital of Estonia
TALLITH: Jewish prayer shawl
TALL ONE: Bar serving
TALMUD: Jewish law
TALTOS: Anne Rice novel
TALUS: Anklebone
TAMA: Author Janowitz
TAMAR: Daughter of King David
TAMARA: Skier McKinney
TAMARAC: Florida city
TAMAYO: Mexican painter
TAMBALA: Malawi coin
TAMBLYN: Actor Russ
TAMBOR: Actor Jeffrey
TAM GLEN: Robert Burns poem
TAMI: Author Hoag
TAMIAMI: __ Trail (Everglades road)
TAMIL: Sri Lankan people
TAMMANY: Onetime LaGuardia target
TAMMI: Singer Terrell
TAMMUZ: Hebrew month
TAMMY: Singer Wynette
TAMP: Push down
TAMPA, FL: Southeast city
TAMPICO: Mexican port
TAM-TAM: Gong
TANA: Blue Nile source lake
TANAGER: Songbird
TANAKA: Godzilla creator
TANANA: Alaskan river
TANBARK: Type of oak
TANDOOR: Clay oven of India
TANDY: Actress Jessica
TANEY: 1800s Chief Justice
TANGRAM: Chinese puzzle
TANGUY: French painter
TANH: Trig function
TANIA: Patty Hearst alias
TANIS: Ancient Egyptian city
TANKA: Japanese poem
TANKINI: Type of swimsuit
TANNA: "Vega$" role
TANNIC: Acid in tea
TANNIN: Compound in wine
TANSY: Aromatic herb
TANTARA: Trumpet blast
TANTE: Aunt: French
TANTIVY: At full gallop
TANTO: So much, in music
TANTRA: Buddhist philosophy
TANYA: Singer Tucker
TAO: Chinese virtue
TAOISM: Chinese philosophy
TAOS, NM: Southwest town
TAPA: Spanish appetizer
TAPEMAN: Surveyor's assistant
TAP-IN: Short putt
TAP INTO: Access
TAPIR: Piglike mammal
TAPIS: Old wall covering
TAP OFF: Remove beer from a keg
TAPPAN: Appliance brand
TAPPET: Engine part
TAPSTER: Bartender
TARA: "Gone With the Wind" estate
TARANTO: Italian city
TARAS: "__ Bulba" (Gogol novel)
TARAWA: Pacific island
TAR BABY: Toni Morrison work
TARBELL: Muckraker Ida
TARDE: Afternoon: Spanish
TARDO: Slow, in music
TARE: Weight allowance
TARGA: Porsche model
TAR HEEL: North Carolinian
TARIQ: Aziz of Iraq
TARLEK: "WKRP in Cincinnati" role
TARN: Mountain lake
TARO: Poi base
TAR OIL: Coal product
TARPON: Florida game fish
TARSAL: Foot bone
TARSO: Ankle: Comb. form
TARSUS: Foot bone
TARTE: Tart: French
TARTU: Estonian city
TART UP: Make gaudy
TARZANA: California city
TARZAN'S: "__ New York Adventure" (1942 film)
T.A.S: Prof.'s aides
TASHI: __ Lama (Tibetan monk)
TASHLIN: Director Frank
TASKBAR: Computer-screen control panel
TASKET: "A-Tisket, A-__"
TASM.: Australian isl.
TASMAN: Dutch explorer
TASS: Soviet news agency
TASSE: Cup: French
TASSO: Italian poet
TASTEE: __-Freez (ice-cream brand)
TAT: Make lace
TATAMI: Japanese mat
TATAR: Crimean people
TATE: London art gallery
TATES: "Soap" family
TATI: French actor
TATIANA: Mezzo-soprano Troyanos
TATIS: Fernando of baseball
TATLER: Addison/Steele periodical
TATRA: Carpathians range
TATUM: Actress O'Neal
TAU: Greek letter
TAUNTON: Massachusetts city
TAUON: Subatomic particle
TAUPIN: Lyricist Bernie
TAUR: Bull: Comb. form
TAURI: Bull: Comb. form
TAURO: Bull: Comb. form
TAUROG: Director Norman
TAUTO: Same: Comb. form
TAV: Hebrew letter
TAVEL: French wine
TAVERNA: Athens eatery
TAVI: "Rikki-Tikki-__" (Kipling work)
TAVIS: PBS talk host Smiley
TAVIST: Antihistamine brand
TAW: Playing marble
TAWT: Verb for Tweety
TAXA: Biological classes
TAXCO: Mexican city
TAXO: Arrangement: Comb. form
TAXOL: Medicine from yews
TAXON: Biological category
TAXY: Arrangement: Comb. form
TAY: Scottish river
TAYBACK: Actor Vic
TAYE: Actor Diggs
TAYLOR: Actress Elizabeth
TAYLORS: 1840s First Family
TAZ: Bugs Bunny adversary
TBA: Schedule abbr.
T-BALL: Beginners' baseball
T-BAR: Ski lift
TBILISI: Capital of Georgia
T-BILL: Government security
T-BIRD: Ford model
T-BOND: Government security
T. BOONE: Corporate takeover artist Pickens
TBS.: Kitchen meas.
TBSP.: Kitchen meas.
TCBY: Frozen-dessert chain
T CELL: Immune-system part
TCHR.: NEA member: Abbr.
TCI: Former cable TV giant
TCM: Cable channel
T.C.U.: Fort Worth sch.
TDK: Audiotape brand
TDS.: NFL scores
TEA ACT: 1773 Boston irritant
TEAC: Sound-system brand
TEACH-IN: Peaceful protest
TE AMO: I love you: Spanish
TEAM USA: Olympic competitor
TEANECK: New Jersey city
TEAPOY: Three-legged table
TEASEL: Prickly flower
TEATRO: Theater: Spanish
TEBALDI: Diva Renata
TEBET: Hebrew month
TEC: Gumshoe
TECATE: Mexican beer brand
TECHIE: Computer expert
TECHNO: Form of electronic music
TECH TV: Former cable channel
TE DEUM: Latin hymn
TED KEY: "Hazel" cartoonist
TED MACK: "Amateur Hour" host
TEE BOX: Golf starting point
TEENA: Singer __ Marie
TEENSIE: __-weensie
TEER: Golfer, at times
TEGRIN: Shampoo brand
TEHERAN: Capital of Iran
TEHRAN: Capital of Iran
TEICHER: Pianists Ferrante & __
TEJANA: Mexican in Texas
TEJANO: Spanish music style
TEKEL: "Handwriting on the wall" word
TEKKIE: Computer expert
TEK WAR: Shatner novel
TELAR: Of tissue
TEL AVIV: Israeli city
TEL. CO.: Phone-serv. provider
TELEPIC: TV movie
TELERAN: Air-traffic control system
TELESTO: Moon of Saturn
TELEX: Fax predecessor
TELIC: Purposeful
TELMA: Actress Hopkins
TELNET: Web software
TELSTAR: 1960s communications satellite
TEM: President pro __
TEMA: Musical motif
TEMBLOR: Earthquake
TEMPE, AZ: Southwest city
TEMPEH: Soybean cake
TEMPERA: Type of paint
TEMPLAR: Fictional detective
TEMPORE: President pro __
TEMPUS: __ fugit
TEN A: Shoe size
TENACE: Bridge holding
TEN B: Shoe size
TEN C: Shoe size
TENCH: Freshwater fish
TEN CODE: CBers' numerical system
TENDRIL: Plant offshoot
TENDU: Held, in ballet
TEN E: Shoe size
TEN EE: Shoe size
TEN EEE: Shoe size
TEN EEEE: Shoe size
TENG: Former Chinese leader
TENGE: Kazakhstan money
TENGO: I have: Spanish
TEN-HUT: Drill sergeant's command
TEN-K RUN: Long race
TEN LB.: Flour sack weight
TENLEY: Skater Albright
TENNANT: Actress Victoria
TENNECO: Auto-parts giant
TENNER: Sawbuck
TENNIEL: British illustrator
TENNIES: Sneakers
TENON: Carpentry joint

TEN-ONE: Receiving poorly, in CB-talk
TENSOR: Body muscle
TEN-TWO: Receiving well, in CB-talk
TENUTA: Comic Judy
TENUTO: Sustained, in music
TENZING: Everest conqueror Norgay
TEO: Car racer Fabi
TER: Three: Comb. form
TERA: Trillion: Comb. form
TERAOHM: Electrical unit
TERAT: Monster: Comb. form
TERATO: Monster: Comb. form
TERBIC: Of element #65
TERBIUM: Element #65
TERCE: Canonical hour
TERCEL: Toyota model
TERENCE: Roman playwright
TERESA: Avila saint
TERETE: Cylindrical
TERHUNE: Author Albert Payson
TERI: Actress Hatcher
TERIA: Self-service: Comb. form
TERKEL: Author Studs
TERME: Semester: French
TERN: Aquatic bird
TERNARY: Triple
TERNATE: Triple
TERNE: Lead/tin alloy
TERO: Mr. T.'s surname
TERP: Maryland athlete
TERR.: District: Abbr.
TERRA: __ firma
TERRAN: Earthling
TERRE: Land: French
TERRELL: Singer Tammi
TERRENE: Earthly
TERRET: Harness ring
TERRI: Country singer Clark
TERRINE: Casserole dish
TERRIS: "Pacem in __" (Papal encyclical)
TERROIR: Wine's natural environment
TERZA: __ rima (Italian verse form)
TES: Your: French
TESH: New Age composer John
TESLA: Unit of magnetic induction
TESS: Thomas Hardy heroine
TESSA: "The Gondoliers" girl
TESSERA: Piece of mosaic
TESSIE: Actress O'Shea
TESSIO: "The Godfather" character
TESTA: Seed coat
TESTATE: Having made a will
TEST BED: Experiment environment
TET: Lunar new year
TETCHY: Irritable
TETE: Head: French
TETH: Hebrew letter
TETHYS: Moon of Saturn
TETLEY: Tea brand
TETON: Wyoming range
TETR: Four: Comb. form
TETRA: Aquarium fish
TETRAD: Foursome
TETRI: Money of Georgia
TETRIS: Computer game
TETRODE: Electron tube
TETZEL: Martin Luther foe
TEUT.: German: Abbr.
TEUTON: German
TEVERE: Rome's river, to natives
TEVET: Hebrew month
TEVYE: "Fiddler on the Roof" father
TEWA: New Mexico Indian
TEWES: Lauren of "Love Boat"
TEXACO: Oil company
TEXTRON: Defense contractor
TEY: Mystery novelist Josephine
T.F. POWYS: British author
TFR.: Bank transaction: Abbr.
THA: Arabic letter
THAD: Senator Cochran
THAE: Those: Scottish
THALER: Old German coin
THALES: Greek philosopher
THALIA: Muse of comedy
THAMES: London river
THANDIE: Actress Newton
THANE: "Macbeth" title
THANT: U __ (Former U.N. leader)
THANX: Gratitude, slangily
THAR: "__ she blows!"
THARP: Choreographer Twyla
THAYER: "Casey at the Bat" poet
TH.D.: Seminary deg.
THE ACT: Liza Minnelli Broadway musical
THE AGE: Melbourne newspaper
THE AGES: All history
THE ALPS: European mountains
THE APE: Karloff horror film
THE A'S: A.L. team
THE ASP: "Little Orphan Annie" character
THE AX: Dismissal, so to speak
THE AXIS: WWII foe
THE BABE: Ruth's nickname
THE BAND: Bob Dylan back-up group
THE BAR: Lawyers
THE BARD: Shakespeare
THE BAY: Canadian retail chain
THE B.B.C.: U.K. shortwave service
THEBE: Moon of Jupiter
THE BEAR: Faulkner story
THE BEE: Sacramento newspaper
THE BELL: Iris Murdoch novel
THEBES: Ancient Egyptian city
THE BEST: Tops
THE BIG A: Anaheim stadium, familiarly
THE BLOB: 1958 sci-fi movie
THE BOBO: Peter Sellers film
THE BODY: Jesse Ventura nickname
THE BOMB: Nuclear capability, so to speak
THE BOSS: Springsteen nickname
THE BOYS: One's male friends
THE BRAT: McEnroe nickname
THE BUSH: Australian rural region
THE CAN: Hoosegow
THE CAPE: Launch locale
THE CAR: James Brolin film
THE CARS: 1980s pop group
THE CAVS: NBA team
THE C.I.A.: Spy org.
THE CID: Spanish national hero
THE CITY: Manhattan, to suburbanites
THE CRAB: Sign of summer
THE CROW: Brandon Lee film
THE CUBS: Chicago team
THEDA: Silents actress Bara
THE DEEP: Peter Benchley thriller
THE DELL: Farmer's place
THE DIET: Japanese legislature
THE DOLE: Welfare, slangily
THE DOW: Stock index, familiarly
THE DUKE: John Wayne nickname
THE EAST: Orient
THE EDGE: Dick Francis novel
THE E.P.A.: Clean-air agcy.
THE EYE: Renée Zellweger film
THE FALL: Albert Camus work
THE FAN: Robert De Niro film
THE F.B.I.: G-men's org.
THE FED: Interest-rate setter
THE FEDS: Government cops
THE FIRM: John Grisham novel
THE FIVE: Group of Russian composers
THE FLEA: John Donne work
THE FLOP: First three face-up cards, in hold 'em
THE FLY: Sci-fi movie of 1958
THE FOG: John Carpenter film
THE FONZ: "Happy Days" character
THE FOOL: Tarot card
THE FOX: D.H. Lawrence novel
THE FRUG: 1960s fad dance
THE GAME: Michael Douglas film
THE GANG: One's pals
THE GAP: Clothing store chain
THE GIFT: Danielle Steel novel
THE GOLD: First place, so to speak
THE HAJ: Leon Uris novel
THE HEAT: Miami team
THE HELP: Servants
THE HERO: Somerset Maugham work
THE HILL: U.S. Congress, slangily
THE HOGS: Arkansas football team
THE HOOD: One's home
THE HOPE: Herman Wouk work
THE HUB: Boston nickname
THE HULK: Green superhero
THE IDEA: "Some nerve!"
THEISM: Belief in a god
THE JERK: Steve Martin film
THE JETS: NFL team
THE KID: Chaplin film
THE KING: Presley nickname
THE KISS: Rodin sculpture
THE LAMB: William Blake poem
THE LARK: Jean Anouilh work
THE LAW: Long-armed entity
THE LEFT: Labour Party, in England
THE LIKE: Similiar things
THE LIP: Leo Durocher nickname
THELMA: "__ & Louise" (1991 film)
THE LOOK: Lauren Bacall nickname
THE LOOP: Downtown Chicago
THE LOT: All
THEMA: Recurring melody
THE MAGI: Bethlehem trio
THE MALL: D.C. green spot
THE MAN: Stan Musial nickname
THE MASK: Jim Carrey film
THE MAVS: NBA team
THE MET: Big Apple opera house
THE METS: National League team
THE MICK: Mantle nickname
THE MOB: Organized crime
THE MOON: Project Apollo destinatión
THE MOST: More than anything else
THE MRS.: One's wife
THEM'S: "__ fightin' words!"
THE N.B.A.: Basketball org.
THE NET: World Wide Web
THE NETS: NBA team
THE NEWS: Prime-time follower
THE N.F.L.: Gridiron org.
THE N.H.L.: Hockey org.
THE N.R.A.: Gun owner's org.
THEO: Kojak's first name
THE OATH: Elie Wiesel novel
THE O.C.: Fox Network series
THEODOR: Dr. Seuss' first name
THE O.K.: Permission
THEOL.: Seminary subject: Abbr.
THE OMEN: 1976 Peck/Remick film
THE OMNI: Former Atlanta arena
THE ONE: Elton John tune
THE PIPS: Gladys Knight's backup
THE PIT: Casino area
THE PITS: Awful
THE PO: Italian river
THE POND: Atlantic Ocean, to Brits
THE POOH: Milne moniker
THE POPE: Vatican VIP
THE POST: D.C. paper
THE PRU: Boston skyscraper, familiarly
THE PUMP: Reebok sneaker
THERA: Aegean island
THE RAM: Aries
THE RAMS: N.F.L. team
THE RAP: Blame, so to speak
THE RAT: Günter Grass book
THE RED: Norse explorer's nickname
THE REDS: National League team
THE REF: Denis Leary film
THE RENT: Monthly payment
THERESA: Spanish saint
THERIAC: Molasses
THE RING: Boxing magazine
THE RINK: Kander and Ebb musical
THE RITZ: Paris hotel
THERM: Gas-bill unit
THERMIC: Of heat
THERMO: Heat: Comb. form
THERMOS: Vacuum bottle
THE ROBE: Richard Burton film
THE ROCK: Alcatraz nickname
THE ROD: Punishment, so to speak
THERON: Actress Charlize

THE ROOM: Harold Pinter work
THE ROPE: Eugene O'Neill work
THE ROSE: Bette Midler song
THEROUX: Writer Paul
THE RULE: Customary
THES.: Dict. companion
THE SACK: Dismissal, so to speak
THE SAME: "Ditto!"
THE SEA: Debussy work
THE SELF: Freud concern
THESEUS: Minotaur slayer
THE SHOW: Major leagues, slangily
THE SIMS: Computer game
THE SON: Trinity member
THE SOX: Chicago or Boston team
THESP: Actor
THESPIS: Greek poet
THE SPY: James Fenimore Cooper work
THE STAR: Tarot card
THE SUN: Sol
THE SUNS: Phoenix team
THE SWAN: Molnár work
THE T: Boston's subway, familiarly
THETA: Greek letter
THE TED: Atlanta stadium's nickname
THETIS: Achilles' mother
THE TOP: #1 position
THE TOUR: French bike race, familiarly
THE TOY: Richard Pryor film
THE TREE: John Fowles book
THE TRIB: Chicago paper, for short
THE TUBE: London subway
THE TURN: Fourth face-up card in hold 'em
THE U.N.: Annan's org.
THE U.S.A.: America
THE U.S.S.R.: Cold War principal
THE VET: Former Philly ballpark
THE VIEW: ABC talk show
THE VIPS: Elizabeth Taylor film
THEW: Beefiness
THE WALL: Vietnam Memorial, familiarly
THE WAVE: Sports spectators' ritual
THE WAY: Tao, literally
THE WB: TV network
THE WEB: Cybersurfer's milieu
THE WHO: Rock band
THE WIND: Power source
THE WIZ: "Ease on Down the Road" musical
THEWS: Physical strength
THE YIPS: Golfer's nervousness
THI: Uncomfortability measure: Abbr.
THIAMIN: Vitamin B-1
THICKE: Actor Alan
THIERRY: Château-__ (WWI battle site)
THIEU: Nguyen Van __ (former Vietnamese leader)
THIGPEN: Actress Lynne
THILL: Wagon shaft
THIMPHU: Bhutanese capital
THIN MAN: Hammett title character
THIRD R: 'Rithmetic
THISBE: Pyramus' love
THIS ONE: The item here
THO': Even if, for short
THOLE: Oar pin
THOM: McAn of shoes
THOMAS: Inventor Edison
THOMSON: British physics Nobelist
THON: Endurance event: Comb. form
THOR: Norse god
THORA: Actress Birch
THORAX: Chest
THOREAU: Writer Henry David
THORIC: Of element #90
THORIUM: Element #90
THORO: Complete, for short
THORON: Radon isotope
THORPE: Football great Jim
THORSON: Actress Linda
THOS.: Pres. Jefferson
THRACE: Balkan region
THRALL: Slave
THREE A: Shoe size
THREE B: Shoe size
THREE C: Shoe size
THREE D: Shoe size
THREE E: Shoe size
THREE EE: Shoe size
THREE NO: Bridge bid, for short
THREE R'S: School basics
THRILLA: "__ in Manila" (historic boxing match)
THRO': "Comin' __ the Rye"
THRUM: Play the guitar
THRUPUT: Computer's work
THULE: Greenland air base
THULIUM: Element #69
THUNK: Dull sound
THURBER: Walter Mitty creator
THURGAU: Swiss canton
THURMAN: Actress Uma
T.H. WHITE: "The Once and Future King" author
THX: "__ 1138" (Lucas film)
THYMINE: DNA component
THYMUS: Small gland
TIA: Aunt: Spanish
TIAGO: Sao __ (Cape Verde Island)
TI AMO: I love you: Italian
TIANT: Luis of baseball
TIBBETT: Baritone Lawrence
TIBBS: Poitier role
TIBER: Rome's river
TIBET: Dalai Lama's land
TIBIA: Leg bone
TIBURON: Hyundai model
TICAL: Old Siamese coin
TICINO: Swiss canton
TICKY: __-tacky (shoddy)
TICO: Costa Rican
TICOTIN: Actress Rachel
TIC-TAC: Mint brand
T.I.D.: Prescription abbr.
TIDERIP: Dangerous current
TIEBACK: Curtain accessory
TIE BEAM: Structural timber
TIEGS: Model Cheryl
TIE LINE: Phone-system service
TIEMPO: Time: Spanish
TIENDA: Store: Spanish
TIENE: Has: Spanish
TIEPOLO: Italian painter
TIERCE: Fencing position
TIERNEY: Actress Gene
TIE ROD: Auto part
TIERRA: Land: Spanish
TIF: Graphic file format
TIFFANY: Stained-glass lamp
TIFFIN: Lunch, in Britain
TIGE: Buster Brown's dog
TIGGER: Pal of Pooh
TIGLON: Big-cat hybrid
TIGON: Big-cat hybrid
TIGRE: Tiger: Spanish
TIGRIS: Fertile Crescent river
TIJUANA: Baja border town
TIKI: Polynesian carving
TIKKA: Indian shish kebab
TIKKI: "Rikki-__-Tavi" (Kipling work)
TIKRIT: Iraqi town
TILAK: Hindu forehead mark
TILDA: Actress Swinton
TILDE: Diacritical mark
TILDEN: 1876 loser to Hayes
TILEX: Bathroom-cleaner brand
TIL HIM: "The Producers" tune
TILLAGE: Cultivated soil
TILLET: Glazed fabric
TILLEY: "The New Yorker" mascot
TILLIE: Comic-strip toiler
TILLIS: Country singer Mel
TILLY: Actress Meg
TILSIT: Type of cheese
TILSON: Conductor Michael __ Thomas
TILTH: Cultivated soil
TILTON: Actress Charlene
TILT-TOP: Type of table
TIM: "A Christmas Carol" boy
TIMBAL: Kettledrum
TIMBALE: Pastry shell
TIMBRE: Voice quality
TIMECOP: Van Damme film
TIME WAS: In the old days
TIMEX: Watch brand
TIM HOLT: Oater star
TIMMINS: Ontario city
TIMMY: Lassie's master
TIMON: Shakespeare's Athenian
TIMOR: Indonesian island
TIMOTHY: Actor Dalton
TIMPANI: Kettledrums
TIM REID: "WKRP" actor
TIM RICE: Lloyd Webber lyricist
TIM ROTH: "Pulp Fiction" actor
TINA: Singer Turner
TINA FEY: "Saturday Night Live" regular
TINAMOU: Partridgelike bird
TINCT: Color slightly
TIN CUP: Costner film
TINE: Prong
TINEA: Fungal infection
TIN FISH: Torpedo, slangily
TIN GOD: Dictatorial one
TIN HAT: Soldier's helmet
TINIAN: Marianas island
TINK: "Peter Pan" character, familiarly
TIN MAN: Oz visitor
TIN MEN: Danny DeVito film
TINO: Martinez of baseball
TIN-PAN: Harsh-sounding
TIN-POT: Shoddy
TIN STAR: Sheriff's badge
TINTERN: "__ Abbey" (Wordsworth poem)
TIO: Uncle: Spanish
TIOGA: New York river
TIOMKIN: Film composer Dimitri
TION: Noun suffix
TIOUS: Adjective suffix
TIPCART: Wheelbarrow relative
TIPI: Indian abode
TIPIN: Easy basket
TIP LINE: Crime reporter's link
TIPPET: Fur scarf
TIPPI: Actress Hedren
TIRANA: Capital of Albania
TIRANE: Capital of Albania
TIRIAC: Tennis pro Ion
TIRO: Beginner
TIROL: Austrian region
TIRPITZ: WWI German admiral
TISANE: Herb tea
TISCH: Former CBS chairman
TISH: Addams family nickname
TISHA: Actress Campbell
TISHRI: Hebrew month
TISKET: "A __, A-Tasket"
TISSOT: Watch brand
TIT: Songbird
TITAN A.E.: Matt Damon film
TITANIA: Fairy queen
TITER: Lab solution strength
TITI: South American monkey
TITIAN: Italian painter
TITO: Former Yugoslav leader
TITOV: Russian cosmonaut
TITRATE: Test solution strength
TITTLE: Dot on an i
TITULAR: Honorary
TITUS: "__ Andronicus" (Shakespeare play)
TIU: Teutonic war god
TIVO: TV-show digitizer
TIVOLI: Copenhagen park
TIWA: New Mexico Indian
T.J. MAXX: Clothing-store chain
TKT.: Box office purchase: Abbr.
TLA: Three-letter acronym: Abbr.
T.L.C.: RN's specialty
TLINGIT: Alaskan people
T-MAN: Treasury agent
TMAX: Kodak film brand
TMC: Cable film channel
TMESIS: Word interpolation
T.M.I.: PA nuclear accident site
T MINUS: NASA countdown term
T-MOBILE: Cell-phone service provider
TMS.: Logos: Abbr.
TNN: Former C&W cable channel
T-NOTE: Government security

TNPK.: Toll rd.
TNS.: Heavy wts.
T-NUT: Bolt holder
TO A HAIR: Precisely
TO A MAN: Everybody
TO A T: Exactly
TO A TEE: Exactly
TO A TURN: Perfectly
TOBAGO: Island off Venezuela
TO BE: Basic infinitive
TO BE HAD: Up for grabs
TOBEY: Actor Maguire
TOBIAS: Author Smollett
TOBIT: Apocrypha book
TO BITS: In little pieces
TO BURN: In abundance
TOBY: Drinking mug
TOCCATA: Bach piece
TO CELIA: Ben Jonson poem
TOCK: Clock sound
TO COME: In the future
TOCSIN: Alarm
TOD: Director Browning
TODD: Mary __ Lincoln
TODD-AO: Wide-screen film process
TODI: Italian town
TODMAN: Game-show producer Bill
TODS: Wool weights
TOEA: Papua New Guinea coin
T.O.E.F.L.: Exam for immigrants: Abbr.
TOE-IN: Wheel adjustment
TOE LOOP: Skater's leap
TOE PICK: Part of a skater's shoe
TOFF: Dandy, in Britain
TOFFLER: Author Alvin
TOFT: Homestead, in Britain
TOFUTTI: Soy-based cheese substitute
TOG OUT: Get dressed
TOGUE: Lake trout
TOG UP: Get dressed
TO HEART: Personally
TO HEEL: Close behind
TO HELEN: Poe poem
TO HOMER: John Keats poem
TO HORSE: Equestrian's cry
TOI: You: French
TOILE: Thin fabric
TOITY: Hoity-__
TOJO: Axis leader
TOKAY: Hungarian wine
TOKE: Casino gratuity
TOKLAS: Author Alice B.
TOKO-RI: Movie bridges locale
TOL': "My mama done __ me"
TOLAR: Slovenian money
TO LAST: Durably
TOLE: Decorated metalware
TO LEASE: Available, as an apartment
TOLEDO: Ohio city
TOLEDOS: Fine swords
TOLER: Charlie Chan portrayer
TO LET: "For Rent" sign
TO LIFE: "Fiddler on the Roof" tune
TOLKIEN: Hobbit creator
TOLSTOI: Russian novelist
TOLSTOY: Russian novelist
TOLTEC: Ancient Mexican
TOLUENE: Part of TNT
TOMA: 1970s TV detective
TOMAR: To take: Spanish
TOMAS: __ de Torquemada
TOMBA: Skier Alberto
TOMBE: Ballet step
TOMEI: Actress Marisa
TOM GOLA: Basketball Hall of Famer
TOM JOAD: Henry Fonda film role
TOM KITE: Pro golfer
TOMLIN: Comedienne Lily
TOMMIE: Agee of baseball
TOM MIX: Oater actor
TOMMY: Designer Hilfiger
TOMSK: Russian city
TOM T.: Country singer Hall
TOMTIT: Small bird
TONDO: Round painting
TONE ARM: Phonograph part
TONE LOC: Rap artist
TONEME: Phonetics unit
TONE ROW: Music term
TONETTE: Simple flute
TONGA: Polynesian kingdom
TONI: Author Morrison
TONIO: "I Pagliacci" clown
TONITE: This evening, informally
TONK: Honky-__
TONKA: Toy-truck brand
TONKIN: South China Sea gulf
TONNE: Metric weight
TONNEAU: Auto body
TONO: "__-Bungay" (Wells novel)
TO NOW: So far
TONS OF: Umpteen
TONTINE: Annuity scheme
TONTO: Lone Ranger sidekick
TONUS: Muscle quality
TONY: Drama award
TONYA: Skater Harding
TONY DOW: "Leave It to Beaver" actor
TOODLE: "__-oo!"
TOODLES: Informal farewell
TOODY: "Car 54, Where Are You?" cop
TOOER: Me-__ (copycat)
TOOLBAR: Computer desktop accessory
TOOLE: Actor Peter O'__
TOOMEY: 1968 Olympic decathlon champ
TOONIE: Canadian coin
TO ORDER: Custom-made
TOO TALL: Pro footballer Jones
TOOT AT: Acknowledge, on the road
TOOTIE: "The Facts of Life" character
TOOTIN': "Yer darn __!"
TOOTSIE: Dustin Hoffman film
TOP CAT: Cartoon feline
TOPE: Drink too much
TOPEE: Pith helmet
TOPEKA: Kansas city
TOP-HOLE: First-rate, in Britain
TOPI: Pith helmet
TOPIARY: Hedge sculpture
TOPKAPI: Ustinov film
TOP KICK: First sergeant
TOPMAST: Rigging support
TOPO: __ Gigio ("Ed Sullivan Show" mouse)
TOPOG.: Mapping science: Abbr.
TOPOL: "Fiddler on the Roof" star
TOPONYM: Place name
TOP OUT: Peak
TOPPS: Baseball-card company
TOPSIDE: On deck
TOPSPIN: Tennis-ball rotation
TOPSY: __-turvy
TOP UP: Keep full
TOQUE: Brimless hat
TOR: Rocky pinnacle
TORA: Synagogue scroll
TORAH: Synagogue scroll
TORBAY: British seaside resort
TORERO: Bullfighter
TORI: Actress Spelling
TORIC: Donut-shaped
TORII: Shinto temple gate
TORINO: Ford model
TORK: Peter of the Monkees
TORME: Singer Mel
TORO: Bull: Spanish
TOROID: Doughnut shape
TORONTO: Canadian city
TORR: Unit of pressure
TORRE: Baseball manager Joe
TORREFY: Scorch
TORRES: Towers: Spanish
TORREY: __ Pines (PGA tour site)
TORT: Legal wrong
TORTA: Pie: Spanish
TORTE: Rich cake
TORTOLA: West Indies island
TORTUGA: Island off Haiti
TORUS: Doughnut shape
TORVALD: "A Doll's House" character
TORVILL: Skaters __ and Dean
TORY: British conservative
TOS: Lean-__ (sheds)
TOSCA: Puccini opera
TO SEA: Out of port
TOSH: Nonsense, in Britain
TOSHIBA: Electronics brand
TOSHIRO: Actor Mifune
TOSTADA: Mexican menu item
TO START: At first
TO TERM: Until the end
TOTIE: Comic Fields
TOTINO'S: Frozen pizza brand
TOTO: Oz dog
TOTO TOO: Memorable "Wizard of Oz" line
TOTSY: Hotsy-__
TOTTED: Added up
TOUAREG: Volkswagen model
TOULON: French port
TOURO: New York college
TOUTE: All: French
TOV: "Mazel __!"
TOVAH: Actress Feldshuh
TOVE: Lewis Carroll's "slithy" thing
TO WAR: Into battle
TOWHEE: Long-tailed finch
TO WIT: Namely
TOWN CAR: Lincoln model
TOWNE: Screenwriter Robert
TOWNER: Out-of-__ (tourist)
TOWNIE: Local citizen
TOWPATH: Canal route
TOX: Poison: Comb. form
TOXO: Poison: Comb. form
TOYA: Singer La__ Jackson
TOYAMA: Japanese city
TOYNBEE: British historian
TOYO: Tire brand
TOYON: Evergreen shrub
TOYOTA: Japanese auto
TO YOU: Gracious toast
TOYS R US: Toy-store chain
TPK.: Toll rd.
TPKE.: Toll rd.
TPS.: Military grps.
TRA: Singing syllable
TRABERT: Tennis pro Tony
TRAC: Farm machine
TRACEY: Actress Ullman
TRACHE: Windpipe: Comb. form
TRACHEA: Windpipe
TRACI: Actress Bingham
TRAC II: Razor brand
TRADUCE: Defame
TRAGG: "Perry Mason" cop
TRAGUS: Ear part
TRAJAN: Roman emperor
TRALEE: Irish city
TRAMMEL: Fetter
TRAMPAS: "The Virginian" role
TRANE: Air-conditioner brand
TRANNY: Auto part, informally
TRANS AM: Pontiac model
TRAP GUN: Skeet weapon
TRAPP: Maria Von __ ("Sound of Music" role)
TRASK: "East of Eden" surname
TRAUBEL: Soprano Helen
TRAVE: Crossbeam
TRAVEN: "Treasure of the Sierra Madre" author
TRAVERS: "Mary Poppins" author
TRAVIS: Country singer Randy
TRAX: Recordings, MTV-style
TRAYNOR: Baseball Hall of Famer
TRE: Three: Italian
TREACLE: Excessive sentimentality
TREAD ON: Trample
TREAS.: Cabinet dept.
TREBEK: TV host Alex
TRECE: Thirteen: Spanish
TREDIA: Mitsubishi model
TREEN: Made of wood
TREF: Not kosher
TREFOIL: Clover
TREINTA: Thirty: Spanish
TREIZE: Thirteen: French
TREKKIE: "Star Trek" fan
TREMOLO: Vibrating effect
TRENARY: Figure skater Jill
TRENT: British river

TRENTA: Thirty: Italian
TRENTE: Thirty: French
TRENTO: Italian city
TRENTON: New Jersey capital
TREPAN: Drilling tool
TREPID: Fearful
TRES: Very: French
TRET: Waste allowance
TREVI: Fountain in Rome
TREVINO: Golfer Lee
TREVOR: Actress Claire
TREWS: Scottish trousers
T-REX: "Jurassic Park" menace
TREY: Playing card
TRIAGE: "M*A*S*H" procedure
TRIB: Newspaper nickname
TRIBBLE: "Star Trek" animal
TRIBECA: Manhattan neighborhood
TRIBORO: Big Apple bridge
TRICIA: Nixon daughter
TRICORN: Minuteman's hat
TRIESTE: Italian port
TRIFFID: 1960s sci-fi film monster
TRIGON: Three-sided figure
TRIGRAM: Three-letter sequence
TRIJET: Type of plane
TRILBY: Du Maurier novel
TRILLIN: Essayist Calvin
TRILLO: Manny of baseball
TRIM TAB: Airplane stabilizer
TRINA: "I Remember Mama" aunt
TRINAL: Threefold
TRINARY: Three-part
TRINE: Group of three
TRINI: Singer Lopez
TRIODE: Vacuum tube
TRIOLET: Eight-line verse
TRIPLE A: Driver's org.
TRIPOLI: Capital of Libya
TRIPP: "Tubby the Tuba" writer
TRIPPET: Machine part
TRIREME: Ancient galley
TRIS: Speaker of baseball
TRISH: Actress Van Devere
TRISHA: Country singer Yearwood
TRISTAN: Round Table knight
TRI-STAR: Lockheed plane
TRISTE: Sad: French
TRITIUM: Hydrogen isotope
TRITON: Spiral seashell
TRITONE: Musical interval
TRITT: Country singer Travis
TRIUNE: Three-in-one
TRIVIOT: Factoid collector
TRIVIUM: Medieval academic division
TRIX: Cereal brand
TRIXIE: "Hi and Lois" baby
TROCHE: Cough drop
TROCHEE: Two-syllable foot
TROGGS: "Wild Thing" rock group
TROI: "Star Trek: The Next Generation" character
TROIKA: Russian sleigh
TROILUS: Lover of Cressida
TROIS: Three: French
TROLLOP: Slattern
TROMPE: __ l'oeil (art technique)
TRON: 1982 Jeff Bridges film
TROON: Scottish golf mecca
TROP: Too much: French
TROPE: Figure of speech
TROPEZ: Saint-__ (Riviera resort)
TROPISM: Botanical orientation
TROPO: Prefix for sphere
TROPPO: Adagio non __
TROTSKY: Russian revolutionary
TROUP: Actor Bobby
TROW: Believe, old-style
T. ROWE: Mutual-fund seller Price
TROYER: Actor Verne
TROY, NY: Empire State city
TRS: __-80 (classic Radio Shack computer)
TRU: Play about Capote
TRUCKEE: Nevada river
TRUDEAU: "Doonesbury" cartoonist
TRUDGEN: Swimming stroke
TRUDY: Jerry Marcus comic strip
TRUK: Pacific island group
TRUMAN: Author Capote
TRUMANS: 1940s First Family
TRUMBO: Screenwriter Dalton
TRUNDLE: Roll along
TRURO: Cape Cod town
TRW: Credit-file co.
TRYGVE: First U.N. head Lie
TRYLON: 1939 World's Fair symbol
TSADE: Hebrew letter
TSADI: Hebrew letter
TSAVO: Kenya national park
TSE: Mao __-tung
T.S. ELIOT: British poet
TSETSE: African fly
TSE-TUNG: Mao's given name
T.S. GARP: John Irving hero
T.SGT.: Air Force NCO
TSONGAS: 1992 presidential contender
TSO'S: General __ chicken (Chinese dish)
TSOTSI: 2005 foreign-film Oscar winner
TSOURIS: Aggravation
TSP.: Recipe amt.
T-SQUARE: Drafting tool
TSR: Dungeons & Dragons company
T-STOP: Camera setting
T-STRAP: Woman's shoe style
T.S.U.: Nashville sch.
TSURIS: Aggravation
TSX: Acura model
T TILE: Scrabble one-pointer
T-TOP: Pseudo-convertible
T.T.U.: Lubbock sch.
TUBATE: Tubular
TUBB: Country singer Ernest
TUBBS: "Miami Vice" cop
TUBIST: Tuba player
TUBMAN: Abolitionist Harriet
TUCANA: Southern constellation
TUCCI: Actor Stanley
TUCHMAN: Historian Barbara
TUCSON: Arizona city
TUCSONS: Hyundai models
TUDE: Noun suffix
TUDOR: Home style
TUFTS U.: Massachusetts school
TUGRIK: Mongolian money
TUI: New Zealand bird
TUILLE: Thigh armor
TULA: Toltec ruins site
TULANE: New Orleans university
TULARE: California city
TULE: Bulrush
TULL: Jethro __ (rock band)
TULLE: Ball-gown fabric
TULLY: Alice __ Hall (Lincoln Center theater)
TULSA, OK: Midwest city
TUM: Rum __ Tugger ("Cats" cat)
TUMBREL: Farm cart
TUMEFY: Become swollen
TUMESCE: Become swollen
TUMID: Swollen
TUMMLER: Catskills resort employee
TUMS: Antacid brand
TUN: Large cask
TUNG OIL: Varnish ingredient
TUNICLE: Church vestment
TUNIS: African capital
TUNISIA: African country
TUNNEY: Boxer Gene
TUP: Male sheep, in Britain
TUPAC: Rapper __ Shakur
TUPELO: Swamp tree
TUPOLEV: Russian aircraft designer
TUPPER: Kitchenware inventor
TUPTIM: "The King and I" character
TUQUE: Stocking cap
TURBO: Airplane engine
TURBOT: Flatfish
TURCO: Turkish: Comb. form
TURFMAN: Horse-racing fan
TURF SKI: Elongated skateboard
TURF TOE: Sports injury
TURGID: Swollen
TURHAN: Actor Bey
TURIN: Italian city
TURING: British mathematician
TURISMO: Part of GTO
TURISTA: Tourist: Spanish
TURKIC: Language subfamily
TURKU: Finnish port
TURNERY: Lathe work
TURNUPS: Trouser cuffs
TUROW: Novelist Scott
TURPIN: Silents comedian Ben
TURVY: Topsy-__
TUSCANY: Italian region
TUSHERY: Pretentious writing
TUSSAL: Of coughs
TUSSAUD: Madame of waxworks
TUSSIVE: Of coughs
TUSSOCK: Clump of grass
TUT: Disapproving sound
TUTELAR: Acting as guardian
TUTSI: Rwandan people
TUTTE: "Così fan __" (Mozart opera)
TUTTI: __-frutti
TUTTIS: Musical passages
TUTTO: All, in music
TUTUILA: Pago Pago's island
TUVALU: Pacific island nation
T.V.A.: Hydroelecric power agcy.
TVG: Prime-time rating
TV LAND: Cable channel
TVMA: Prime-time rating
TV MAN: Appliance repairer
TVPG: Prime-time rating
TV/VCR: Combo appliance
TVY: Kiddie-show rating
TWA: Erstwhile airline
TWAIN: Huck Finn creator
TWAINS: Couples
TWAY: Pro golfer Bob
TWEE: Dainty, in Britain
TWEEDLE: Imitate a chirp
TWEEN: Preadolescent
TWEENER: Preadolescent
TWEENY: Preadolescent
TWEETY: Cartoon canary
TWELVE A: Shoe size
TWELVE B: Shoe size
TWELVE C: Shoe size
TWELVE D: Shoe size
TWELVE E: Shoe size
TWI: Prefix for light
TWINKIE: Snack-cake brand
TWIN SET: Pair of sweaters
TWITTY: Country singer Conway
TWIX: Candy-bar brand
TWO A: Apartment number
TWO B: Apartment number
TWO-BASE: __ hit (double)
TWO C: Apartment number
TWO D: Apartment number
TWO E: Shoe size
TWO EE: Shoe size
TWO EEE: Shoe size
TWO EEEE: Shoe size
TWO-EM: Long dash
TWO-FACE: Batman foe
TWO ON: Baseball situation
TWOONIE: Canadian coin
TWO PIN: Alley target
TWO-SPOT: Deuce
TWO-UNIT: Duplex
TWP.: County div.
TWYLA: Choreographer Tharp
TWYMAN: Basketball Hall of Famer
TYBALT: Juliet's cousin
TYCHE: Greek goddess of fortune
TYCHO: Astronomer Brahe
TYCO: Electronics company
TY COBB: Baseball great
TY-D-BOL: Household cleaner brand
TYE: Ship rope
TYEE: Chinook salmon
TYGER: William Blake animal
TYIYN: Kyrgyzstan money
TYLENOL: Pain-reliever brand
TYLER: Actress Liv
TYLERS: 1840s First Family
TYLO: Actress Hunter __
TYMPANA: Eardrums
TYMPANI: Kettledrums
TYNAN: Theater critic Kenneth
TYNDALL: Sierra Nevada peak
TYNE: Actress Daly
TYNER: Jazz pianist McCoy

TYP.: Art of printing: Abbr.
TYPAL: Representative
TYPE A: Tense personality
TYPE AB: Blood-bank category
TYPE B: Laid-back personality
TYPEE: Melville novel
TYPE O: Blood-bank category
TYPHOID: __ Mary
TYR: Norse war god
TYRA: Model Banks
TYRE: Phoenician port
TYRES: Tires, in Britain
TYROL: Alpine region
TYRONE: Actor Power
TYRUS: Baseballer Cobb's first name
TYS: Cobb and Hardin
TYSON: Actress Cicely
TYSON'S: __ Corner, VA
TYUS: Olympic runner Wyomia
TYVEK: House-siding brand
TZARA: Dadaist poet Tristan
TZE: Chinese philosopher Mo-__
TZIMMES: Vegetable stew
TZU: Tao author Lao-__
TZUS: Shih __ (Tibetan dogs)

U

U.A.E.: Abu Dhabi's country: Abbr.
U.A.L.: Delta competitor
U.A.R.: 1950s Mideast country: Abbr.
U.A.W.: AFL-CIO constituent
UBANGI: African river
UBI: Where: Latin
UBIETY: Presence
U-BOAT: WWII sub
U BOLT: Axle holder
UBS: Network in "Network"
UBU ROI: Alfred Jarry play
U. CAL.: West Coast sch.
UCCELLO: Italian painter
UCLAN: Bruin
U. CONN: Nutmeg State sch.
UDALL: 1960s Interior Secretary
UDE: Suffix for quiet
UDINE: Italian city
UDO: Japanese vegetable
UECKER: "Mr. Belvedere" star
UELE: African river
UEY: 180-degree turn
U.F.T.: Educational grp.
UFW: United Farm Workers: Abbr.
UGARTE: "Casablanca" role
UGGAMS: Singer Leslie
UGLI: Jamaican fruit
UGO: Actor Tognazzi
UGOLINO: Rodin work
UGRIC: Finno-__ (language group)
UGSOME: Horrid: Scottish
UHF: Broadcast band
UHLAN: Polish lancer
UHNAK: Novelist Dorothy
UHRY: "Driving Miss Daisy" playwright
UHURA: "Star Trek" character
UHURU: Ruark novel
UINTA: Utah mountain range
UJIJI: Tanzanian city
UKA: "The Clan of the Cave Bear" character
UKASE: Edict
UKIAH: California city
UKR.: Ukraine: Abbr.
ULA: Diminutive suffix
ULALUME: Poe poem
ULAN: __ Bator, Mongolia
ULANOVA: Ballerina Galina
ULAN-UDE: Siberian city
ULAR: Adjective suffix
ULE: Diminutive suffix
ULEE'S: "__ Gold" (Peter Fonda film)
ULENE: TV doctor Art
ULENT: Adjective suffix
ULF: Samuelsson of hockey
ULLA: "The Producers" role
ULLAGE: Empty portion of a bottle
ULLMAN: Actress Tracey
ULLMANN: Actress Liv
ULM: German city
ULNA: Arm bone
ULOUS: Adjective suffix
ULRIC: Actress Lenore
ULRICH: Actor Skeet
ULSTER: Overcoat
ULT.: Final: Abbr.
ULTIMA: Final syllable
ULTIMO: In the prior month
ULU: Eskimo knife
ULULATE: Howl
ULYANOV: Lenin's real surname
ULZANA'S: "__ Raid" (Lancaster film)
UMA: Actress Thurman
U. MASS: New England sch.
UMBEL: Flower cluster
UMBER: Brown shade
UMBERTO: Author Eco
'UMBLE: Heep's word for himself
UMBRA: Shadow
UMBRAGE: Anger
UMBRIA: Italian region
UMBRIEL: Moon of Uranus
UMEKI: Actress Miyoshi
UMIAK: Alaskan boat
UMPH: Annoyance exclamation
UMS: Conversation fillers
UMTATA: Capital of Transkei
U.M.W.: United Mine Workers: Abbr.
UNA: Actress Merkel
UNAMI: Algonquin tribe
UNAMUNO: Writer Miguel de __
UNARY: Having a single element
UNAU: Two-toed sloth
UN BEL DI: Puccini aria
UNBLENT: Not mixed
UNBOSOM: Confide all
U.N.C.: Tar Heels sch.
UNCA: Donald Duck, to his nephews
UNCAS: Cooper hero
UNCIAL: Capital letter
UNCLAY: T.F. Powys work
UNCOLA: 7-Up nickname
UNCTION: Anointment
UND: And: German
U.N. DAY: October 24th
UNDEAD: Like a zombie
UNDEC: Eleven: Comb. form
UNDICI: Eleven: Italian
UNDINE: Female water spirit
UNDSET: Norwegian literature Nobelist
UNE: One: French
UNES: Ones: French
UNESCO: Intl. cultural org.
UNFERTH: "Beowulf" character
UNGAR: "The Odd Couple" role
UNGAVA: Canadian bay
UNGER: "The Odd Couple" role
UNGUAL: Like a claw
UNGUENT: Ointment
UNGUES: Hooves
UNGUIS: Hoof
UNGULA: Hoof
U.N.H.: New England sch.
UNH-UNH: Slangy denial
UNIAT: Eastern Catholic
UNIATE: Eastern Catholic
UNIBALL: Pen brand
UNIBODY: Type of auto-frame construction
UNICEF: Intl. relief agency
UNICODE: Computer character encoding system
UNIE: Combined: French
UNIPED: Having a single foot
UNIPLEX: One-screen theater
UNIPOD: Camera support
UNIS: Les États-__
UNISOM: Sleep-aid brand
UNISYS: Computer company
UNITA: Angolan rebel org.
UNITARD: Bodysuit
UNITAS: Football great Johnny
UNIVAC: Early computer
UNIX: Computer operating system
UNLAX: Rest
UNLAY: Separate rope strands
U.N.L.V.: Western sch.
U.N.M.: Albuquerque sch.
UNMEET: Not fitting
UNMEW: Set free
UNMITER: Depose a bishop
UNO: One: Spanish
UNOCAL: Fortune 500 firm
UN-P.C.: Improper
'UNS: Young __ (kids)
UNSELD: Basketball great Wes
UNSER: Auto racer Al
UNTER: Below: German
U NU: Burmese leader
UNUM: E pluribus __
U. OF M.: Minneapolis sch.
UOMO: Man: Italian
UOUS: Adjective suffix
UOVO: Egg: Italian
UP AND IN: Like a beanball
U.P.C. CODE: Scanner ID
UP CURVE: Rising arc
UPDIKE: Author John
U. PENN: Philadelphia sch.
UPHERE: "Yoo-hoo!"
U.P.I.: News serv.
UPJOHN: Drug company
UP LAST: Like the pitcher, usually
UPN: Cable channel
UPOLU: Samoan island
UP-OR-OUT: Type of employment system
UPPSALA: Swedish city
UP QUARK: Subatomic particle
UPS: FedEx competitor
UPSA: __-daisy
UPSALA: Swedish city
UPSHAW: Soprano Dawn
UPSILON: Greek letter
UPSY: __-daisy
UPTON: Author Sinclair
U QUARK: Subatomic particle
URACIL: RNA component
URAEUS: Asp
URALIC: European language group
URALS: Russian mountain range
URALSK: Kazakhstan city
URAN: Heaven: Comb. form
URANIA: Muse of astronomy
URANO: Heaven: Comb. form
URAWA: Japanese city
URBANA: Illinois city
URBAN I: Pope
URBAN II: Pope
URBAN IV: Pope
URBAN V: Pope
URBAN VI: Pope
URDU: Pakistani language
URE: Actress Mary
UREA: Plastic component
UREY: Chemistry Nobelist
URGY: Art: Comb. form
URI: Swiss canton
URIAH: Dickens character
URICH: "Spenser: For Hire" star
URIEL: "Paradise Lost" angel
URIS: Novelist Leon
URKEL: "Family Matters" role
URL: Web-site ID
URNE: Ballot box: French
URO: Tail: Comb. form
UROUS: Adjective suffix
URSA: __ Major
URSAE: Alpha __ Majoris
URSID: Bear
URSINE: Bearish
URSINUS: Pope
URSO: Violinist Camilla
URSULA: Actress Andress
URSULA K.: Author Le Guin
URSUS: Bear: Latin
URTEXT: Composition's original form
URU.: Argentina neighbor: Abbr.
U.S.A.F.A.: Colorado Springs sch.
U.S. AIR: Airline's former name
USANCE: Grace period
U.S.A.R.: Mil. branch
USA USA: Olympics chant
USB: Computer port
U.S.C.: L.A. school
U.S.C.G.: S.O.S. responder

U.S.C.G.A.: New London sch.
U.S.D.: Coyote State sch.
USDA: Cabinet dept.
USDT: Cabinet dept.
USEE: Lawsuit beneficiary
USE ME: Bill Withers tune
USENET: Newsgroup system
U.S.F.L.: Defunct gridders' org.
U.S.G.: Presidential monogram
U.S.G.A.: Golf org.
U.S. GRANT: Civil War general
USH: Accompany to a seat
U.S.I.A.: Voice of Amer. overseer
U.S.L.T.A.: Tennis org.
U.S.M.: Mil. branch
U.S.M.A.: West Point sch.
U.S.M.C.: Mil. branch
U.S.N.: Mil. branch
U.S.N.A.: Annapolis sch.
U.S. NEWS: "Time" rival
U.S.N.R.: Mil. branch
U.S.O.C.: Amateur sports org.
U.S. ONE: Maine-to-Fla. highway
U.S.P.S.: Stamp seller: Abbr.
U.S. R.D.A.: Vitamin std.
USS: Battleship letters
U.S.T.A.: Court org.
USTED: "¿Cómo está __?"
USTEDES: You: Spanish
U.S. TEN: Road through St. Paul
USTINOV: Actor Peter
U.S. TOUR: 1964 Beatles event
USX: U.S. Steel stock symbol
UTA: Actress Hagen
UTE: Western Indian
U.T.E.P.: Texas sch.
U THANT: 1960s U.N. head
UTHER: Arthur's father
UTICA, NY: Empire State city
UTILE: Useful
UTLEY: TV reporter Garrick
UTNE: Eclectic publication
UTO: __-Aztecan languages
UTRECHT: Netherlands city
UTRILLO: French artist
UTS: Scale notes
UTTAR: __ Pradesh, India
UTU: Sumerian sun god
U TUBE: Lab item
U TWO: 1960s spy plane
U. VA.: Charlottesville sch.
UVALDE: Texas city
U-VALUE: Insulation measure
UVEA: Eye part
UVULA: Tonsil neighbor
UWE: Krupp of hockey
UXMAL: Mayan city
UXOR: Wife: Latin
UXORIAL: Of wives
UZBEK: Asian language
UZI: Commando weapon

V

VAC: Appliance, for short
VACA: Cow: Spanish
VACCARO: Actress Brenda
VACHE: Cow: French
VACHEL: Poet Lindsay
VACLAV: Czech statesman Havel
VACUA: Empty spaces
VACUOLE: Cell cavity
VADE: __ mecum (handbook)
VADER: Darth __
VADIM: Director Roger
VADIS: "Quo __?"
V. ADM.: High naval off.
VADUZ: Liechtenstein capital
VAG: Hobo
VAGUS: Cranial nerve
VAIL, CO: Ski resort
VAL: Actor Kilmer
VALADON: French painter
VALAIS: Swiss canton
VALANCE: Bed ruffle
VALDEZ: Alaska city
VALE: Singer Jerry
VALENCE: Elemental stat
VALENE: "Knots Landing" character
VALENS: Pop singer Ritchie
VALENT: Combinable chemically
VALENTE: Singer Caterina
VALENTI: Former film-rating czar
VALERA: Eamon De __ (Irish statesman)
VALERE: "Tartuffe" character
VALERIE: Actress Harper
VALERO: Gas-station company
VALERY: __ Giscard D'Estaing
VALID ID: Security requirement
VALINE: Amino acid
VALIUM: Calming drug
VALJEAN: Hugo character
VALLE: Valley: Italian
VALLEE: Singer Rudy
VALLEJO: California city
VALLI: Singer Frankie
VALLONE: Actor Raf
VALMIKI: Hindu poet
VALO: Elmer of baseball
VALOIS: French royal house
VALOREM: Ad __ tax
VALOTTE: Julian Lennon song
VALOVA: Skater Elena
VALSE: Waltz: French
VAMOOSE: "Get lost!"
VAMOS: Let's go: Spanish
VAMP: Theda Bara persona
VAMPA: "Count of Monte Cristo" character
VAMPIRA: Actress in Ed Wood movies
VAMPY: Impromptu
VANADIC: Of element #23
VAN ARK: Actress Joan
VAN CAMP: Baked-beans maker
VANCE: "I Love Lucy" actress
VAN DIEN: Actor Casper
VAN DINE: Mystery writer S.S.
VANDURA: GMC model
VAN DUYN: Poet Mona
VAN DYCK: Flemish painter
VAN DYKE: Pointy beard
VANESSA: Actress Redgrave
VAN EXEL: Nick of basketball
VAN EYCK: Flemish painter
VAN GOGH: Dutch painter
VANIER: Ontario city
VANILLI: Milli __ (pop duo)
VANNA: White of "Wheel of Fortune"
VANNES: French city
VANOCUR: TV newsman Sander
VAN OWEN: "L.A. Law" character
VAN PELT: Linus of "Peanuts"
VAN POOL: Commuter arrangement
VAN RIJN: Painter Rembrandt
VAN RYN: Painter Rembrandt
VAN SANT: Director Gus
VANUA: __ Levu (Fiji island)
VANUATU: Pacific island group
VAN VOGT: Sci-fi author A.E.
VANWARD: Toward the front
VAN WYCK: Historian Brooks
VANYA: Chekhov uncle
VAN ZANT: Rock singer Ronnie
VAPORUB: Cold-remedy brand
VAQUERO: Cowboy
VAR.: Dictionary abbr.
VARDA: Director Agnes
VARDEN: Dolly __ trout
VARESE: French-born composer
VARGAS: Pinup painter
VARIA: Literary miscellany
VARIG: Brazilian airline
VARITEK: Jason of baseball
VARLAAM: "Boris Godunov" role
VARLET: Cad
VARMUS: Medicine Nobelist Harold
VARNA: Hindu caste
VARNEY: Ernest Worrell portrayer
VARO: Spanish Surrealist
VARRICK: Matthau film role
VARRO: Roman scholar
VARSI: Actress Diane
VARYA: "Cherry Orchard" character
VAS: Anatomical duct
VASA: Anatomical ducts
VASCO: Explorer da Gama
VASHTI: Biblical queen
VASILY: Chessmaster Smyslov
VASLAV: Dancer Nijinsky
VASO: Blood vessel: Comb. form
VASQUEZ: Francisco __ de Coronado
VASSAL: Feudal worker
VASSAR: New York college
VASTS: Immense expanses
VASTUS: Leg muscle
VASTY: Immense
VATER: Father: German
VATIC: Prophetic
VATICAL: Prophetic
VATU: Vanuatu coin
VAUD: Swiss canton
VAUDOIS: Certain Swiss native
VAUGHAN: Singer Sarah
VAUGHN: Actor Robert
VAULTY: Arching
VAUNT: Be boastful
VAUX: Central Park designer
VAV: Hebrew letter
VAX: 1970s minicomputer
VAYA: __ con Dios (Spanish farewell)
V-BLOUSE: Woman's garment
VBS.: Action wds.
V-CHIP: TV censoring device
VCR: TV adjunct
V-DAY: War ender
V.D.T.: Computer screen: Abbr.
VEADAR: Hebrew month
VEALE: Pitcher Bob
VEAU: Veal: French
VEBLEN: Economist Thorstein
VECHTEN: Writer Carl Van __
VECTRA: Opel model
VEDA: Hindu holy work
V-E DAY: May 8, 1945
VEDDER: Rock singer Eddie
VEDETTE: Navy boat
VEDIC: Sanskrit language
VEDIST: Hindu scripture scholar
VEECK: Baseball Hall of Fame executive
VEEJAY: MTV employee
VEE NECK: Shirt feature
VEERY: Thrush
VEG: Act the couch potato
VEGA: Star in Lyra
VEGAN: Animal-product eschewer
VEG OUT: Emulate a couch potato
VEH.: Part of RV
VEIDT: Actor Conrad
V-EIGHT: Automobile motor
VEINTE: Twenty: Spanish
VEL.: Speed: Abbr.
VELA: Sail constellation
VELAR: Consonant sound
VELD: African grassland
VELDA: Mike Hammer's assistant
VELDT: African grassland
VELEZ: Actress Lupe
VELLUM: Fine paper
VELMA: "Chicago" character
VELO: Drome starter
VELOCE: Fast, in music
VELOUTE: White sauce
VELOX: Photographic print
VELSEN: Dutch seaport
VELTMAN: Dutch physics Nobelist
VELUM: Soft palate
VELURE: Hat fabric
VELVA: Aqua __ (after-shave brand)
VEN.: Italian city: Abbr.
VENA: __ cava
VENABLE: Actress Evelyn
VENAL: Bribable
VENATIC: Of hunting
VENDEE: Buyer
VENDOME: French general
VENDUE: Public auction
VENEMAN: George W. Bush cabinet member
VENERA: Russian space probe
VENETO: Italian region
VENEZ.: S. Amer. country
VENEZIA: City in Italia
VENI: I came: Latin
VENIAL: Allowable
VENIN: Snake toxin

VENIRE: To come: Latin
VENISON: Deer meat
VENITE: 95th Psalm
VENLO: Dutch city
VENN: Circle diagram developer
VENNER: "House of the Seven Gables" character
VENO: Arterio- counterpart
VENORA: Actress Diane
VENOSE: Of veins
VENOUS: Of veins
VENTA: Sale: Spanish
VENTAGE: Flute hole
VENTI: Wind: Comb. form
VENTNOR: Monopoly avenue
VENTO: Wind: Comb. form
VENTRAD: Toward the belly
VENTRAL: Anterior
VENTRIS: British architect
VENTURA: California city
VENTURI: Golfer Ken
VENULE: Small vein
VENUTI: Jazz violinist Joe
VER.: Bib. edition
VERA: "Alice" waitress
VERBENA: Garden flower
VERBID: Infinitive
VERDE: Green: Spanish
VERDELL: "As Good as It Gets" dog
VERDI: Italian composer
VERDIN: Southwestern bird
VERDON: Actress Gwen
VERDOUX: Chaplin role
VERDUGO: Actress Elena
VERDUN: 1916 battle site
VERDURE: Foliage
VERE: "Billy Budd" captain
VEREEN: "Pippin" Tony winner
VEREIN: German union
VEREINE: German unions
VERGER: Church attendant
VERGIL: "The Aeneid" author
VERIDIC: Correct
VERIEST: Utmost
VERISM: Art theory
VERISMO: Use of everyday life in art
VERITAS: "In vino __"
VERITE: Cinéma __
VERIZON: Phone company
VERJEE: CNN reporter Zain
VERMEER: Dutch painter
VERMEIL: Red shade
VERMI: Worm: Comb. form
VERN: "My Little Margie" dad
VERNA: Actress Bloom
VERNAL: Of the spring
VERNE: French author
VERNET: French painter
VERNIER: Measurement scale
VERNON: Dancer Castle
VERO: __ Beach, FL
VERONA: "Romeo and Juliet" locale
VERONIA: Blue flower
VERRE: Glass: French
VERRUCA: Wart
VERS: Toward: French
VERSA: Vice __
VERSACE: Italian designer
VERSANT: Mountain slope
VERSET: Brief poem
VERSO: Book page
VERST: Russian length measure
VERT: Green: French
VERTE: Green: French
VERTIGO: Hitchcock film
VESCO: Fugitive financier
VESICLE: Small sac
VESPA: "Spaceballs" princess
VESPAS: Italian motor scooters
VESPER: Evening star
VESPERS: Evening service
VESPID: Wasp or hornet
VESTA: Large asteroid
VESTAL: Chaste
VESTAS: British matches
VESTEE: Jacket insert
VESTI: "__ la giubba"
VESTRAL: Of a church room
VESTRON: 1980s video distributor
VESTRY: Church area
VESTURE: Accouterments
VETA: "Harvey" character
VETCH: Climbing plant
'VETTE: Chevy model
VEY: "Oy __!"
VEZ: Occasion: Spanish
VEZINA: NHL annual trophy
V-FOUR: Automobile motor
V.F.W.: Ex-G.I.'s org
V.G.A.: Computer monitor: Abbr.
V.H.F.: TV band
VH ONE: Cable channel
VHS: Camcorder format
VIACOM: Broadcasting giant
VIADENT: Toothpaste brand
VIAGRA: Drug in the news
VIAND: Article of food
VIATICA: Money for travel
VIATOR: Traveler
VIBIST: Certain percussionist
VIBRAM: Boot-sole brand
VIBRATO: Singer's effect
VIC: Singer Damone
VIC DANA: "Red Roses for a Blue Lady" singer
VICENTE: Sao __, Brazil
VICENZA: City in Italy
VICHY: City in France
VICI: "Veni, vidi, __"
VICINAL: Neighboring
VICKERS: Sinclair Lewis character
VICKI: Actress Lawrence
VICKREY: Canadian economics Nobelist
VICKS: Cold remedy name
VICKY: Tiny Tim ex
VICO: Philosopher Giambattista
VICOMTE: French noble
VICTRIX: Successful woman
VICTUAL: Supply with food
VID: Film, for short
VIDA: Life: Spanish
VIDAL: Author Gore
VIDALIA: Sweet onion
VIDE: Part of q.v.
VIDERI: Part of North Carolina's motto
VIDETTE: Mounted sentry
VIDI: I saw: Latin
VIDICON: TV camera part
VIDIOT: Boob-tube addict
VIDOR: Director King
VIEIRA: TV host Meredith
VIEJA: Old: Spanish
VIEJO: Mission __, CA
VIELLE: Hurdy-gurdy
VIENNE: French department
VIERNES: Friday: Spanish
VIERZIG: Forty: German
VIET: __ Cong
VIEUX: Old: French
VIEWY: Visionary
VIG: Interest, to a usurer
VIGGO: Actor Mortensen
VIGIA: Navigational hazard
VIGNOLA: Italian architect
VIGNY: French poet
VIGO: City of Spain
VIGODA: Actor Abe
VIHARA: Buddhist monastery
VIJAY: Amritraj of tennis
VIKES: NFL team, for short
VIKKI: Singer Carr
VIKTOR: Russian author Nekrasov
VIL: Cruella De __
VILA: Bob of home improvement
VILAS: Guillermo of tennis
VILLARD: Publisher Henry
VILLARI: Italian physicist
VILLE: City: French
VILLEIN: Feudal serf
VILLI: Fruit hairs
VILLON: French painter
VILMA: Actress Banky
VILNA: Capital of Lithuania
VILNIUS: Capital of Lithuania
VIMINAL: One of Rome's hills
VIN: Wine: French
VINA: Stringed instrument of India
VINCE: Actor Edwards
VINCI: Leonardo da __
VINCIT: Amor omnia __
VINCULA: Math markings
VINCY: "Middlemarch" character
VINER: Pea-picking machine
VINERY: Grape arbor
VING: Actor Rhames
VINGT: 20: French
VINI: Wine: Comb. form
VINIC: Winy
VINIFY: Produce, as champagne
VINLAND: Norse colony
VINNIE: "Welcome Back, Kotter" character
VINNY: "My Cousin __"
VINO: Wine: Italian
VINOUS: Wine-colored
VIN ROSE: French wine
VINSON: 1940s Chief Justice
VINTON: Singer Bobby
VIOLONE: Double bass
VIORST: Poet Judith
VIR: Man: Latin
VIRAGO: Shrew
VIRDON: Bill of baseball
VIREO: Songbird
VIRGA: Rain that doesn't reach the ground
VIRGATE: Rod-shaped
VIRGIL: "Aeneid" author
VIRGULE: Slash mark
VIRID: Green
VIRNA: Actress Lisi
VIRTU: Objets d'art
VIS: Strength: Latin
VISALIA: California city
VIS-A-VIS: Against
VISAYAN: Indonesian language
VISC.: British noble: Abbr.
VISCERA: Guts
VISCID: Sticky
VISCOUS: Adhesive
VISCUSO: Actor Sal
VISHNU: Hindu god
VISINE: Eye-drops brand
VISTEON: Auto-parts company
VISTULA: Baltic feeder
VIT.: A or C: Abbr.
VITA: Life: Latin
VITALE: Sportscaster Dick
VITALIS: Hair-care brand
VITAM: Ad __ (for life)
VITARA: Suzuki model
VITAS: Gerulaitis of tennis
VITE: Quickly, in music
VITEBSK: Belarus city
VITI: Vine: Comb. form
VITO: "Godfather" character
VITORIA: Spanish city
VITR: Glass: Comb. form
VITRI: Glass: Comb. form
VITRIC: Glassy
VITRICS: Glass production
VITRIFY: Turn to glass
VITRINE: Glass case
VITRIOL: Severe criticism
VITRO: Glass: Comb. form
VITTLES: Food
VITUS: Explorer Bering
VIV: Lucy's pal
VIVA: "__ Las Vegas"
VIVACE: Lively, in music
VIVALDI: Italian composer
VIVANT: Bon __
VIVARIA: Ant farms, e.g.
VIVE: "__ la France!"
VIVECA: Actress Lindfors
VIVENDI: Modus __
VIVI: Alive: Comb. form
VIVIAN: Actress Vance
VIVICA A.: Actress Fox
VIVIEN: Actress Leigh
VIVITAR: Camera brand
VIVO: In __ (occurring naturally)
VIVRE: Joie de __
VIZ.: Namely: Abbr.
VIZIER: Old Muslim minister
VIZIR: Old Muslim minister
VIZSLA: Hungarian dog
V-J DAY: May 15, 1945
VJS: MTV hosts

VLAD: "The Impaler"
VLADE: Divac of basketball
VLASIC: Pickle brand
VLECK: Physicist John van __
V.L.F.: Radio band: Abbr.
V.M.I.: Cadet sch.
V NECK: Blouse feature
V.O.A.: U.S. shortwave service
VOCAB.: Dict. content
VOCABLE: Word
VOCE: Sotto __
VOCODER: Speech synthesizer
VOGEL: Bird: German
VOGUED: Struck a pose
VOGUER: Model emulator
VOICI: Here: French
VOIGHT: Actor Jon
VOILA: "There you are!"
VOILE: Sheer fabric
VOIP: Internet telephone company
VOIR: See: French
VOIT: AMF competitor
VOITURE: Wheeled vehicle
VOIX: Voice: French
VOL.: Bk.
VOLANS: Southern constellation
VOLANT: Airborne
VOLANTE: Musical direction
VOLAR: Of the palm
VOLARE: Song of 1958
VOLCKER: Former Federal Reserve head
VOLE: Ratlike rodent
VOLENTE: Deo __ (God willing)
VOLGA: Russian river
VOLK: People: German
VOLPE: Nixon cabinet member
VOLPONE: Ben Jonson work
VOLTA: African river
VOLTAIC: Battery type
VOLTE: __-face (reversal)
VOLTORE: "Volpone" character
VOLUBLE: Talkative
VOLUTE: Spiral object
VOMER: Skull bone
VON BAER: German embryologist
VONDA: Singer Shepard
VON LAUE: German physics Nobelist
VON OPEL: German automaker
VON ZELL: Radio announcer Harry
VOO: "Hinky Dinky Parlay __"
VOOM: "Va-va-__!"
VORA: Eaters: Comb. form
VORE: Eater: Comb. form
VORLAGE: Skiing stance
VOROUS: Eating: Comb. form
VORPAL: "The __ blade went snicker-snack!"
VORSTER: Former South African president
VORTEX: Eddy
VOS: Columnist Marilyn __ Savant
VOSGES: French department
VOSKHOD: Russian spacecraft
VOSS: TV meteorologist
VOSTOK: Russian spacecraft
VOTARY: Advocate
VO-TECH: Like many night schools
VOTIVE: Church candle
VOTRE: Your: French
VOUS: You: French
VOUVRAY: French wine
VOX: Voice: Latin
VOX POP: Public opinion, for short
V.P.I.: Blacksburg sch.
VRAI: True: French
VRONSKY: "Anna Karenina" character
VROOM: Motorcycle sound
V SIGN: Churchill trademark
V-SIX: Auto engine
VSO: Brandy designation
VSOP: Brandy designation
VSS: Bible editions: Abbr.
V-TEN: Auto motor
V TILE: Scrabble four-pointer
VTOL: Type of aircraft
V-TYPE: Kind of engine
VUE: Saturn model
VUG: Rock cavity
VUITTON: French fashion designer
VUL.: Lat. version of the Bible
VULCAN: Roman god
VULCANS: Mr. Spock's people
VULG.: Lat. version of the Bible
VULGATE: Bible edition
VULGUS: Common people
VULPINE: Crafty
VU METER: Recording-studio device
VW BUG: Disney's Herbie
VWS: German autos
VYE: "Return of the Native" character
VYSE: "A Room With a View" character

W

WAAC: WWII female
WAALS: Physics Nobelist Johannes van der __
WAART: Conductor Edo de __
WABASHA: Minnesota city
WABBIT: Fudd's bunny
WABE: "...gyre and gimble in the __"
WAC: WWII female
WACE: Poet Robert
WACK: Crackpot
WACO, TX: Lone Star city
WADDELL: Baseball Hall of Fame pitcher
WADENA: Minnesota county
WADI: African gully
WADKINS: Golfer Lanny
WAF: Female flier: Abbr.
WAGNER: German composer
WAH: Baby's cry
WAHINE: Hawaiian girl
WAHL: Actor Ken
WAHLOO: Swedish writer
WAHOO: Exuberant cry
WAHR: True: German
WAH-WAH: Guitar effect
WAIKATO: New Zealand river
WAIN: Farm cart
WAITE: Actor Ralph
WAITRON: Server
WAITZ: Runner Grete
WAJDA: Polish director
WAKA: Japanese poem
WAKAME: Brown seaweed
WAKKO: "Animaniacs" brother
WAKSMAN: Microbiologist Selman
WAL: __-Mart
WALCOTT: Playwright Derek
WALD: Forest: German
WALDORF: Hotel name
WALE: Fabric ridge
WALESA: Polish statesman
WALKEN: Actor Christopher
WALKIE: __-talkie
WALKURE: "Die __" (Wagner opera)
WALLA: Half a Washington city name
WALLABY: Australian jumper
WALLACE: "Ben-Hur" author
WALLACH: Actor Eli
WALLER: "Ain't Misbehavin'" composer
WALLEYE: Fish
WALLIS: "Casablanca" producer
WALLOON: Belgian native
WALL ST.: N.Y.S.E. address
WALLY: Astronaut Schirra
WALPOLE: British prime minister
WALSTON: Actor Ray
WALSY: Palsy-__
WALTER: Newsman Cronkite
WALTERS: TV interviewer Barbara
WALTHAM: Massachusetts city
WALTHER: "Die Meistersinger" role
WALTON: Retail-store magnate
WALTONS: 1970s TV family
WAMBLE: Move unsteadily
WAMPUM: Money
WANDA: "A Fish Called __"
WANER: Baseball Hall of Famer Paul
WANG: Computer pioneer An __
WANKEL: Car engine
WANNABE: Arriviste
WANTAGH: Long Island town
WANY: Decreasing
WAPITI: Elk
WAPNER: "People's Court" judge
WAPSHOT: John Cheever title word
WARBURG: German medicine Nobelist
WARE: Piece of merchandise
WARHOL: Artist Andy
WARING: Bandleader Fred
WARKS: County in England
WARLOCK: Male witch
WARNER: __ Bros. (Hollywood studio)
WARNES: Actress Jennifer
WARREN: Rabbit burrow
WARREN G.: President Harding
WARWICK: Singer Dionne
WASABI: Japanese horseradish
WASATCH: Idaho mountain range
WASCO: California city
WASECA: Minnesota county
WASH ME: Message on a dirty car
WASHO: California Indian
WASHOE: Nevada county
WASHY: Wishy-__
WAS I: "Able __ ere I saw Elba"
WASS: Actor Ted
WASSER: Water: German
WASSILY: Russian painter Kandinsky
WAST: Biblical verb
WAT: Angkor __ (Cambodian temple)
WATFORD: British city
WATKINS: __ Glen, NY
WATNEY: Ale maker
WATS: Bulk-rate phone line
WATSON: Holmes' assistant
WATTEAU: French painter
WATTLE: Interweave
WATUSI: 1960s dance
WAUGH: British novelist
WAUSAU: Wisconsin city
WAVICLE: Subatomic particle
WAW: Arabic letter
WAWA: Trumpet sound
WAXWING: Songbird
WAXWORK: Madame Tussaud creation
WAYANS: Actor Keenen Ivory __
WAYLAND: Massachusetts city
WAYLON: Singer Jennings
WAYNE'S: "__ World" (1992 film)
WBA: Boxing org.
WBC: Boxing org.
W.B. YEATS: Irish poet
W.C. HANDY: Blues composer
WCS: Restrooms
W.C.T.U.: "Dry" grp.
WEAKON: Subatomic particle
WEAL: Prosperity
WEALD: Uncultivated country
WEB AD: Banner
WEBB: "Dragnet" star
WEBBER: Paine's Wall Street partner
WEBER: Magnetic flux unit
WEBERN: Austrian composer
WEB-FED: Type of printing press
WEBSTER: Lexicographer Noah
WEB-TOED: Like the platypus
WEB-TV: AOL competitor
WEBZINE: E-mag
WEDDELL: Antarctic sea
WEDEL: One way to ski
WEDELN: Skiing technique
WEDGIE: Type of shoe
WEEB: Football coach Ewbank
WEEMS: Washington biographer
WEENA: "The Time Machine" girl
WEENIE: Hot dog
WEENSY: Teensy-__
WEENY: Teeny-__
WEE UN: Tyke
WEEZER: Rock band
WEFT: Woven fabric
WEGENER: German geophysicist
WEI: Chinese dynasty
WEIDER: Fitness expert Joe

WEIDMAN: Author Jerome
WEIL: Author Simone
WEILL: Composer Kurt
WEIMAR: German city
WEIN: Wine: German
WEIR: Small dam
WEIRD AL: Parodist Yankovic
WEIRTON: West Virginia city
WEIS: Director Don
WEISS: "Marat/Sade" author
WEISZ: Actress Rachel
WEITZ: Director Paul
WELBY: Robert Young TV role
WELCH: Actress Raquel
WELCH'S: Jelly brand
WELDON: Author Fay
WELK: Bandleader Lawrence
WELLA: Shampoo brand
WELLAND: Canadian city
WELLER: Actor Peter
WELLES: Director Orson
WELLMAN: Director William
WELTER: Certain boxer
WELTY: Author Eudora
WELU: Bowler Billy
WEMBLEY: Borough near London
WENCES: Ventriloquist Señor __
WENDELL: Poet Berry
WENDERS: Director Wim
WENDIE: Actress Malick
WENDKOS: Director Paul
WENDT: Actor George
WENDY: "Peter Pan" girl
WENDY'S: Fast-food chain
WENG: Puzzle editor Will
WENNER: "Rolling Stone" founder
WERFEL: Austrian novelist
WERKER: Director Alfred
WERNER: Chemistry Nobelist Alfred
WERNHER: Rocket scientist __ von Braun
WERT: "Bird thou never __"
WERTHER: Goethe hero
WES: Director Craven
WESCOTT: Writer Glenway
WESER: German river
WESKER: Playwright Arnold
WESKIT: Vest
WESLEY: Actor Snipes
WESSEX: Anglo-Saxon kingdom
WESSON: Cooking-oil brand
WEST EGG: "Great Gatsby" locale
WESTIE: Type of terrier
WESTIN: Hotel chain
WESTON: Actor Jack
WET KISS: Amaretto cocktail
WET-NAPS: Sanitary cloth brand
WETTIG: Actress Patricia
WETWARE: Computer operator
WEXFORD: Irish county
WEZEN: Star in Canis Major
W.F.U.: North Carolina sch.
W.G.H.: Presidential initials
WGN: Chicago superstation
WHA: "Huh!?"
WHALEY: Actor Frank
WHALLEY: Actress Joanne
WHAMMO: Sound of a collision
WHAM-O: Frisbee company
WHANG: Bash
WHARTON: Author Edith
WHAT AM I: Riddle phrase
WHAT'D: "__ I Say" (Ray Charles tune)
WHAT'LL: "__ I Do"
WHAT SAY: "Come again?"
WHAT THE: Cry of surprise
W.H. AUDEN: British poet
WHEATON: Maryland city
WHELAN: Actress Jill
WHELK: Big snail
WHELM: Engulf
WHELP: Give birth
WHEN'S: "__ dinner?"
WHERRY: Rowboat
W.H.H.: Presidential initials
WHIGS: 19th-century party
WHIP IN: Keep together
WHIPPLE: Grocer in Charmin ads
WHISKAS: Cat-food brand
WHIST: Card game
WHITBY: Canadian city
WHITEY: Pitcher Ford
WHITING: Singer Margaret
WHITMAN: Poet Walt
WHITNEY: California peak
WHITSUN: Pentecost
WHITTY: Actress May
WHIZZY: Marvelous
WHO DAT: Rapper's query
WHO'LL: "__ Stop The Rain"
WHOOPI: Actress Goldberg
WHOOPIE: __ cushion
WHOOSIS: Whatchamacallit
WHORL: Fingerprint ridge
WHO SAID: Attribution request
WHO'S IN: Poker question
WHO'S OUT: Poker question
WHOS WHO: Directory
W.H.T.: Presidential initials
WH-WORD: Interrogative
WHYTE: Author William H.
WICCA: Good witchcraft
WICHITA: Kansas city
WICKIUP: Indian hut
WICKLOW: Irish county
WIDDER: "Young __ Brown" (old-time radio series)
WIDGEON: Type of duck
WIDMARK: Actor Richard
WIE: Golf pro Michelle
WIEBE: Canadian writer Rudy
WIELAND: German poet
WIEMAN: Physics Nobelist Carl
WIEN: Vienna: German
WIESEL: Novelist Elie
WIEST: Actress Dianne
WIFEY: Judy Blume work
WIFFLE: __ Ball (kid's toy)
WIFI: Wireless computer network
WIGAND: "The Insider" subject
WIGGIN: "Rebecca of Sunnybrook Farm" author
WIGHT: Britain's Isle of __
WIGHTS: Human beings
WIGNER: Physics Nobelist Eugene
WII: Nintendo game console
WIKI: Collaborative Web site
WIL: Actor Wheaton
WILBERT: Singer Harrison
WILBUR: Wright brother
WILBY: "The __ Conspiracy" (1975 film)
WILCO: Radioer's assent
WILCOX: Poet Ella
WILDE: Author Oscar
WILDING: Husband of Liz Taylor
WILD ONE: Bobby Rydell tune
WILE E.: Cartoon coyote
WILEY: Aviator Post
WILFORD: Actor Brimley
WILFRED: Director Jackson
WILHELM: German kaiser
WILKENS: Lenny of basketball
WILKES: John __ Booth
WILKIE: British novelist Collins
WILKINS: Medicine Nobelist Maurice
WILLA: Novelist Cather
WILLARD: TV weatherman Scott
WILLEM: Actor Dafoe
WILLIE: Baseball great Mays
WILLIES: Jitters
WILLIS: Actor Bruce
WILLKIE: FDR's 1940 opponent
WILLSON: Composer Meredith
WILLY: Whale of films
WILLYS: Old-time auto make
WILMA: Mrs. Flintstone
WILMUT: Cloner scientist Ian
WILSON: Soul singer Pickett
WILSONS: 1910s First Family
WILTON: Connecticut city
WIM: Director Wenders
WIMMER: Actor Brian
WIMMIN: Females, to Popeye
WIMOWEH: "The Lion Sleeps Tonight" word
WIMPLE: Nun's headcloth
WIMPOLE: "The Barretts of __ Street"
WIMSEY: Fictional detective
WINANS: Gospel singer CeCe
WINDAUS: German chemistry Nobelist
WINDEX: Glass-cleaner brand
WINDIGO: Folklore giant
WINDOM: Actor William
WINDOM'S: "__ Way" (1957 film)
WINDSOR: Canadian city
WIND TEE: Airfield weather vane
WINESAP: Type of apple
WINFREY: TV talk-show host
WINGMAN: Hockey position
WINKIE: Wee Willie __
WINKLER: Actor Henry
WINN: __-Dixie (supermarket chain)
WINNIE: Milne character
WINONA: Actress Ryder
WINSLET: Actress Kate
WINSLOW: Arizona city
WINSOME: Charming
WINSOR: Cartoonist McCay
WINSTON: Sir __ Churchill
WINWOOD: Actress Estelle
WIRE IN: Send a telegram
WIRTH: Sociologist Louis
WIS.: Minn. neighbor
WISC.: Minn. neighbor
WISHIN': "__ and Hopin'"
WISHY: __-washy
WISK: Detergent brand
WISTER: "The Virginian" author
WITE-OUT: Correction-fluid brand
WITHAL: Besides
WITH US: Alive
WITLING: Would-be wag
WITT: Figure-skater Katarina
WITTE: Dutch artist Emanuel de __
WITTER: Dean __ (former Wall St. firm)
WITTIG: German chemistry Nobelist
WIZEN: Desiccate
W.J.C.: Presidential initials
WJM: "Mary Tyler Moore Show" station
WKLY.: Like some mags.
WKRP: 1970s-1980s sitcom
WLS: Chicago radio station
WNBA: Female hoops grp.
WNW: Compass pt.
WOAD: Blue dye
WOBEGON: Keillor's fictional lake
WOBURN: Massachusetts city
WODEN: Anglo-Saxon god
WO FAT: "Hawaii Five-O" arch-criminal
WOHLER: German chemist
WOJO: "Barney Miller" character
WOJTYLA: John Paul II's surname
WOLE: Literature Nobelist Soyinka
WOLFE: "The Right Stuff" author
WOLFF: Author Tobias
WOLF GAL: Dogpatch denizen
WOLFRAM: Tungsten
WOLPER: TV producer David L.
WOLSEY: British cardinal
WOMACK: Singer Bobby
WOMAN'S: "__ Day" (supermarket mag)
WOMBAT: Marsupial
WOMYN: Feminist females
WONG: Actress Anna May
WONK: Bookworm
WONKA: Fictional candy maker
WONTED: Accustomed
WON TON: Chinese dumpling
WOODARD: Actress Alfre
WOODIE: Old-style station wagon
WOODLEY: Bumstead neighbor
WOODROW: President Wilson
WOODSON: Historian Carter
WOOGIE: Boogie-__
WOOKIEE: "Star Wars" beast
WOOLERY: TV host Chuck
WOOLEY: Singer Sheb
WOOLF: Author Virginia
WOOL FAT: Lanolin
WOOLITE: Detergent brand
WOOLLEY: Actor Monty
WOOLSEY: Former CIA director
WOOSNAM: Golfer Ian

WOOSTER: Ohio city
WOOTSY: Tootsy-___
WOPAT: Actor Tom
WORF: "Star Trek: The Next Generation" role
WORLEY: Comedienne Jo Anne
WORRELL: Jim Varney persona
WORSLEY: Hockey great Gump
WORT: Beer in the making
WOTAN: German god
WOUK: "The Caine Mutiny" novelist
WOULDA: Hindsight word
WOW 'EM: Do a great job
WOZ: Apple co-founder, for short
WOZNIAK: Apple Computer co-founder
WOZZECK: Alban Berg opera
WPA: New Deal agcy.
WPM: Typing-speed stat.
WRANGEL: Arctic Ocean island
WRASSE: Tropical fish
WRAY: Actress Fay
WRIGHT: Craftsperson
WRIGLEY: Chicago Cubs' field
WROCLAW: Polish city
WROTH: Angry
WRX: Subaru model
W.S.J.: Financial newspaper: Abbr.
WSW: Compass pt.
W TILE: Scrabble four-pointer
W-TWO: Tax filer's form
WUHAN: Chinese city
WUHL: Actor Robert
WUNDT: German psychologist
WURST: Sausage
WUSA: Paul Newman film
WUSHU: Chinese martial arts
WUSS: Wimp
WUXIA: Martial-arts film genre
WUZ: "We ___ robbed!"
W. VA.: Md. neighbor
W.V.U.: Morgantown sch.
WWE: Wrestling org.
WWF: Former wrestling org.
WWW: World Wide Web: Abbr.
WYATT: Marshal Earp
WYE: 25th letter
WYETH: Painter Andrew
WYLE: Actor Noah
WYLER: Director William
WYLER'S: Drink-mix brand
WYLIE: Author Philip
WYMAN: Rolling Stones member
WYNDHAM: Hotel chain
WYNETTE: Singer Tammy
WYNKEN: Blynken shipmate
WYNN: Actor Keenan
WYNNE: Crossword inventor
WYNONNA: Singer Judd
WYNTER: Actress Dana
WYNTON: Trumpeter Marsalis
WYO.: Colo. neighbor
WYOTANA: Northwest region
WYSIWYG: What you see is what you get: Abbr.
WYSS: "Swiss Family Robinson" author
WYSTAN: ___ Hugh Auden
WYTHE: Declaration signer
WYVERN: Heraldic dragon

X

X-ACTO: Craft-knife brand
X AMOUNT: Unknown quantity
XANADU: Luxurious locale
X AND O: Tic-tac-toe symbols
X AND Y: Standard axes
XANTHAN: ___ gum (ice-cream ingredient)
XANTHIC: Yellow
XAVIER: Bandleader Cugat
XAVIER U.: Cincinnati school
X-AXIS: Graph line
XBOX: Microsoft gaming product
X'D IN: Marked, as a ballot
X-DIV: Wall Street abbr.
X'D OUT: Crossed through
XEBEC: Pirate vessel
XED IN: Marked, as a ballot
XEMEX: Swiss watch brand
XENA: TV's "Warrior Princess"
XENIA: "Boris Godunov" role
XENIA, OH: City near Dayton
XENICAL: Weight-control drug
XENO: Alien: Comb. form
XENON: Inert gas
XEON: Intel microprocessor
XER: Arid: Comb. form
XERIC: Having a dry environment
XERO: Arid: Comb. form
XEROSIS: Abnormal dryness
XEROTIC: Very dry
XEROX: Copier brand
XERXES I: King of Persia
XES IN: Marks, as a ballot
XES OUT: Deletes
X-FACTOR: Comic-book series
XFILE: Alien investigation
X-GAMES: ESPN event
XHOSA: African people
XIAN: Chinese city
XIMENES: Spanish cardinal
X IN: Mark, as a ballot
XING: PED ___
XINHUA: Chinese news agency
XIPHOID: Sword-shaped
XIS: Greek letters
XIXO: "The Gods Must Be Crazy" character
XJS: Jaguar model
XKE: Jaguar model
XKR: Jaguar model
X-LARGE: Shirt size
XLS: Suit sizes: Abbr.
X-MEN: Comic book heroes
XM RADIO: Satellite broadcasting service
XOO: "Hollywood Squares" non-winner
X OR Y: Chromosome choice
X-OUT: Deletion
XOX: "Hollywood Squares" non-winner
XOXOX: Love and kisses, in a letter
XOXOXO: Love and kisses, in a letter
X PRIZE: Civilian rocket-building award
X-RATED: Like some films
X'S AND O'S: Tic-tac-toe symbols
XSARA: Citroën model
X'S OUT: Deletes
XTC: British rock group
XTERRA: Nissan model
X TILE: Scrabble eight-pointer
XTRA: Additional, in ads
X-TYPE: Jaguar model
XXO: "Hollywood Squares" non-winner
XXXX: Confectioners' sugar symbol
X Y AND Z: 3-D graph axes
XYLEM: Plant tissue
XYLO: Wood: Comb. form
XYLOID: Woody
XYLOSE: Sugar from straw
XYST: Ancient portico
XYSTER: Surgical instrument
XYSTUS I: Pope
XZIBIT: Rap star

Y

YABBA: Start of a Flintstone cheer
YACHTIE: Certain mariner
YAD: Torah place marker
YADA: "And so on," when tripled
YADDA: "And so on," when tripled
YADIM: Torah place markers
YAH: Exclamation of impatience
YAHTZEE: Dice game
YAKIMA: Washington city
YAKIMAS: Northwest Indians
YAKOV: Comedian Smirnoff
YAKUT: Russian people
YAKUTSK: Russian city
YAKUZA: Japanese gangster group
YALE LAW: Clinton alma mater
YALE U.: Conn. school
YALIE: Ivy Leaguer
Y'ALL: Dixie contraction
YALOW: Physicist Rosalyn
YALTA: "Big Three" conference site
YALU: Asian river
YAMAHA: Motorcycle make
YAMANI: Former OPEC minister
YAMUNA: Agra's river
YAN: "___ Can Cook" (PBS show)
YANCY: "___ Derringer" (1950s TV western)
YANG: Chinese principle
YANGON: Myanmar capital
YANGTZE: Chinese river
YANKTON: South Dakota city
YANNI: New Age performer
YANNICK: Noah of tennis
YANQUI: American, in Mexico
YAO MING: NBA star
YAOUNDE: Cameroon capital
YAPHET: Actor Kotto
YAQUI: Mexican Indian
YAR: "Babi ___" (Yevtushenko poem)
YARDARM: Sail support
YARDMAN: Train employee
YARE: Agile
YARNELL: Mime Lorene
YARRA: Melbourne's river
YARROW: Fernlike plant
YAS: Slangy affirmatives
YASBECK: Actress Amy
YASGUR: Owner of the Woodstock site
YASHA: "The Cherry Orchard" character
YASHICA: Camera brand
YASHIN: Russian writer
YASHMAK: Muslim veil
YASIR: Mr. Arafat
YASMIN: Rita Hayworth's daughter
YASMINE: Actress Bleeth
YASSER: Mr. Arafat
YAT: Sun ___-sen
YA-TA-TA: Empty talk
YATES: "Breaking Away" director
YAT-SEN: Sun ___ (Chinese statesman)
YATTER: Idle talk
YAWKEY: Onetime Red Sox owner
YAWL: Small boat
YAWP: Bawl
Y-AXIS: Graph line
YAY: "Hurray!"
YA-YA'S: "Get Yer ___ Out" (Rolling Stones album)
YAY ME: Self-congratulatory cry
YAY TEAM: Cheering words
YAZ: Baseball great's nickname
YAZOO: Mississippi feeder
YBOR: ___ City (Tampa district)
Y-CLEPT: Called, old-style
YEA BIG: Size indicator, slangily
YEAGER: "The Right Stuff" role
YEAN: Bear a goat
YEATS: Irish poet
YECCH: "Gross!"
YECH: "Ugh!"
YEEHAW: ___ Junction, FL
YEGG: Safecracker
YE GODS: Old oath
YEHUDI: Violinist Menuhin
YELENA: Russian activist Bonner
YELLO: Mello ___ (soft-drink brand)
YELTSIN: Russian statesman Boris
YEMANA: "Barney Miller" role
YEN SID: "Fantasia" sorcerer
YENTA: Busybody
YENTE: "Fiddler on the Roof" role
YENTL: Streisand film
YEO.: Nav. petty officer
YEOH: Actress Michelle
YE OLDE: Shoppe-sign words
YEOMAN'S: ___ service (loyal support)
YEOW: "That hurts!"
YER: "So's ___ old man!"
YERBA: ___ Buena (California island)
YEREVAN: Armenian capital
YERKES: Wisconsin observatory
YERKISH: Ape-communication language

YERTLE: Dr. Seuss character
YES DEAR: CBS sitcom
YESHIVA: Hebrew school
YES I CAN: Sammy Davis book
YES IT IS: Beatles song
YES LET'S: "Shall we?" response
YES'M: Informal assent
YES-NO: Kind of answer
YES OR NO: "Make up your mind!"
YES SIRE: Response to a king
YESTER: Day or year starter
YETI: Abominable Snowman
YETTA: Broadway role for Barbra
YETTIE: Young Web worker
YEUX: Eyes: French
YEVGENY: Russian poet Yevtushenko
YGOR: "Son of Frankenstein" character
YIDDISH: Shalom Aleichem's language
YIN: Chinese principle
YIPPIE: 1960s activist
YITZHAK: Israeli statesman Rabin
YLD.: Bond stat.
YLEM: Protomatter of the universe
Y-LIKE: Slingshot-shaped
YMA: Singer Sumac
YMIR: Giant of Norse mythology
YNEZ: Santa __ Valley, CA
YOAKAM: Country singer Dwight
YOB: Hooligan, in Britain
YOCTO: Septillionth: Comb. form
YOD: Hebrew letter
YODA: "Return of the Jedi" role
YODH: Hebrew letter
YO DUDE: Slangy greeting
YOGA MAT: Hindu worshiper's accessory
YOGHURT: Milk product
YOGIISM: Berra quotation
YOGINI: Yoga practicer
YOICKS: Fox-hunting exclamation
YOKO ONO: Sean Lennon's mother
YOKUM: Dogpatch surname
YOLANDA: "__ and the Thief" (Astaire film)
YOM: Day: Hebrew
YOM TOV: Hebrew holiday
YOND: "__ Cassius has a lean..."
YONEX: Sports-gear brand
YONG: Egg foo __
YONKERS: New York city
YONNE: French department
YOO: Hoo preceder
YOPLAIT: Yogurt brand
YORBA: __ Linda, CA
YORICK: Friend of Hamlet
YORKIE: Small dog
YORKIN: Director Bud
YORKIST: Wars of the Roses combatant
YORK, PA: Keystone State city
YORKS: County of England
YORKTON: Saskatchewan city
Y OR N: Questionnaire choices
YORTY: One-time L.A. mayor
YOS: Attention-getting calls
YOSANO: Japanese poet
YO SOY: I am: Spanish
YOST: Eddie of baseball
YO TE AMO: I love you: Spanish
YOTHERS: Actress Tina
YOTTO: Septillion: Comb. form
YOUMANS: "Tea for Two" songwriter
YOUNG MC: Rap artist
YOUNT: Robin of baseball
YOU'RE IT: Cry after "Tag!"
YOU'RE ON: Bet taker's response
YOURN: Backwoods possessive
YOUSE: Brooklynese pronoun
YOUSUF: Photographer Karsh
YOW: "That hurts!"
YOWIE: "That hurts!"
YOWL: Bawl
YOWZA: Absolutely
YOWZAH: Absolutely
YO-YO MA: Cellist
YPRES: 1914 battle site
YREKA: California city
YSAYE: Belgian violinist
YSER: North Sea feeder
YSIDRO: San __, CA
YSL: Couture letters
Y.T.D.: Since 1/1: Abbr.
Y TILE: Scrabble four-pointer
YTTRIA: Rare-earth oxide
YTTRIC: Of element #39
YTTRIUM: Element #39
YUAN: Chinese coin
YUBA: __ City, CA
YUBAN: Coffee brand
YUCAIPA: California town
YUCATAN: Mexican peninsula
YUCATEC: Mexican Indian
YUGO: European car
YUK: Chuckle
YUKATA: Japanese robe
YUKAWA: Japanese physics Nobelist
YUKIO: Japanese author Mishima
YUKONS: GMC truck models
YUKOS: Russian oil company
YUL: Actor Brynner
YULIN: Actor Harris
YULKA: "My Antonia" character
YUMA, AZ: City on the Colorado
YUNG: Egg foo __
YUPPIE: Affluent one
YURI: Astronaut Gagarin
YURT: Mongol tent
YUTANG: Lin __ (Chinese writer)
YUTZ: Dolt
YVAIN: King Arthur knight
YVES: Actor Montand
YVETTE: Actress Mimieux
YVONNE: Actress De Carlo
YWAIN: King Arthur knight
YZERMAN: Steve of hockey

Z

ZABRZE: City in Poland
ZABUTON: Japanese cushion
ZAC: Rock singer Hanson
ZACH: "A Chorus Line" character
ZACHARY: President Taylor
ZACK: Baseball Hall of Famer Wheat
ZADAR: Croatian port
ZADDIK: Hasidic leader
ZADIE: Novelist Smith
ZADIG: Voltaire novel
ZADKINE: Russian sculptor
ZADORA: Actress Pia
ZAFTIG: Full-bodied
ZAFU: Meditation cushion
ZAG: Turn sharply
ZAGAT: Restaurant-guide author
ZAGAZIG: City in Egypt
ZAGNUT: Candy-bar brand
ZAGREB: Balkan capital
ZAHN: TV journalist Paula
ZAHND: Rock singer Ricky
ZAIRE: Former name of an African nation
ZAIRES: Former African money
ZAK: Ringo Starr's son
ZAKUSKA: Russian hors d'oeuvre
ZAL: Actress Roxana
ZALE: Boxer Tony
ZALES: Jewelry store
ZAMBEZI: African river
ZAMBIA: African country
ZAMBONI: Hockey-rink machine
ZAMORA: Former Mexican president
ZANE: Author Grey
ZANETTO: Mascagni opera
ZANONI: Bulwer-Lytton work
ZANT: Rock singer Ronnie Van __
ZANTAC: Heartburn drug
ZANUCK: Film producer Darryl
ZAPATA: Mexican revolutionary
ZAPATAS: Shoes: Spanish
ZAPATEO: Cuban dance
ZAPOTEC: Mexican Indian
ZAPPA: Mothers of Invention leader
ZAPPY: Sprightly
ZARA: Princess Anne's daughter
ZARF: Coffee cup
ZARKOV: Flash Gordon colleague
ZAS: Italian pies, for short
ZASU: Actress Pitts
ZATOPEK: Czech runner Emil
ZAX: Dr. Seuss character
Z-AXIS: 3-D graph line
ZAYAK: Skater Elaine
ZAYIN: Hebrew letter
ZAZA: "La Cage aux Folles" character
ZAZEN: Seated meditation
Z-BAR: Construction piece
ZEALAND: Copenhagen's island
ZEBRASS: Hybrid equine
ZEBROID: Equine hybrid
ZEBU: Cattle of India
ZEBULON: Explorer Pike
ZEBULUN: Son of Jacob
ZECH.: O.T. book
ZED: Last British letter
ZEDILLO: Former Mexican president
ZEDONG: Mao __
ZEDONK: Equine hybrid
ZEELAND: Dutch province
ZEEMAN: 1902 Physics Nobelist Pieter
ZEENA: "Ethan Frome" character
ZEHN: Ten: German
ZEILE: Todd of baseball
ZEISS: Optical lens manufacturer
ZEIST: Dutch city
ZEIT: Time: German
ZEITUNG: Newspaper: German
ZEKE: Bert Lahr's Kansas role
ZELAZNY: Sci-fi author Roger
ZELDA: Mrs. Fitzgerald
ZELIG: Woody Allen film
ZELL: Harry Von __ (old-time radio announcer)
ZEMSTVO: Czarist council
ZEN: Meditative sect
ZENANA: Harem
ZEND: Zoroastrian Bible
ZENDA: "The Prisoner of __"
ZENDO: Zen meditation room
ZENER: __ cards (ESP testers)
ZENGER: Early American publisher John Peter
ZENIC: Of a meditative sect
ZENO: Greek philosopher
ZENOBIA: "Ethan Frome" character
ZENO'S: __ paradox
ZEPH.: O.T. book
ZEPHYR: Gentle breeze
ZEPPO: Marx brother
ZEPPOLE: Italian pastry
ZEPTO: Sextillionth: Comb. form
ZERBE: Actor Anthony
ZERMATT: Swiss resort
ZERNIKE: Dutch physics Nobelist
ZERO-G: Like a weightless atmosphere
ZERO-SUM: Kind of game
ZESTA: Cracker brand
ZESTER: Kitchen device
ZETA: Greek letter
ZETTA: Sextillion: Comb. form
ZEUS: Chief Greek god
ZEUXIS: Greek painter
ZEVON: Rock singer Warren
ZEZ: Composer Confrey
ZHIVAGO: Pasternak hero
ZHLOB: Dolt
ZHLUB: Dolt
ZHOU: __ En-lai
ZHUKOV: Russian marshal
ZIA: Former Pakistani president
ZIEFF: Director Howard
ZIEGLER: Nixon press secretary
ZIERING: Actor Ian
ZIFF: Magazine publisher __-Davis
ZIFFEL: "Green Acres" character
ZIGGY: Trumpeter Elman
ZIL: Russian limo
ZILL: Finger cymbal
ZILLA: "Babbitt" character
ZILLION: Huge number
ZIMA: Coors brand
ZIMARRA: Catholic cassock
ZIMMER: Don of baseball

ZIN: California wine, familiarly
ZINA: Garrison of tennis
ZINE: Amateur mag
ZIO: Uncle: Italian
ZION: Utah national park
ZIONIST: Champion of Israel
ZIPCUFF: Temporary handcuff
ZIP DISK: Data storage medium
ZIPGUN: Crude weapon
ZIP IT: Shut up
ZIPLOC: Food storage brand
ZIPLOCK: Type of plastic bag
ZIPPO: Lighter brand
ZIRA: "Planet of the Apes" role
ZITCOM: Sitcom for teens
ZITHER: Stringed instrument
ZITO: Barry of baseball
ZIZITH: Rabbi's tassels
ZIZZ: Nap, slangily
ZLOTY: Polish money
ZMED: Actor Adrian
ZOA: Animals: Comb. form
ZOCALO: Mexican plaza
ZOD: Horoscope concern: Abbr.
ZOE: Actress Caldwell
ZOELLER: Pro golfer Fuzzy
ZOG I: One-time Albanian king
ZOIC: Geologic-era suffix
ZOLA: Author Emile
ZOLTAN: Composer Kodaly
ZOMBIE: Rum drink
ZOMBIFY: Turn into a sci-fi creature
ZONA: Author Gale
ZONE OUT: Daydream
ZONIAN: Certain Panama resident
ZONK: "Let's Make a Deal" prize
ZONKER: "Doonesbury" character
ZONK OUT: Fall asleep
ZONULE: Small belt
ZOOEY: Salinger title character
ZOOID: Animal organism
ZOOL.: Animal sci.
ZOOT: Sims of jazz
ZORA: Author __ Neale Hurston
ZORBA: "__ the Greek"
ZOR-EL: Supergirl's father
ZORI: Japanese footwear
ZORINA: Actress Vera
ZORN: Swedish painter
ZORRO: Fictional swordsman
ZOSIMUS: Pope
ZOSMA: Star in Leo
ZOSSIMA: Dostoevsky character
ZOT: "B.C." sound effect
ZOTZ: 1962 film
ZOUK: Caribbean dance music
ZOUNDS: "Egad!"
ZOWIE: "Ooh-la-la!"
ZOYSIA: Lawn grass
Z.P.G.: Demographer's abbr.
ZSA ZSA: Actress Gabor
Z TILE: Scrabble 10-pointer
ZUBIN: Conductor Mehta
ZUCCO: Actor George
ZUCKER: Director Jerry
ZUG: Swiss canton
ZUKOR: Film producer Adolph
ZULU: Bantu language
ZUMWALT: Admiral Elmo
ZUNI: New Mexico Indian
ZUNIGA: Actress Daphne
ZUPPA: Soup: Italian
ZUT: French exclamation
ZWANZIG: Twenty: German
ZWEI: Two: German
ZWEIG: German writer Arnold
ZWICK: Film producer Edward
ZWICKAU: German city
ZWINGLI: Swiss religious reformer
ZWOLF: Twelve: German
ZYDECO: Cajun music
ZYGOMA: Face bone
ZYGOTE: Type of cell
ZYMASE: Yeast fermentation agent
ZYMURGY: Brewery science
ZYRA: "When Worlds Collide" planet
ZZ TOP: 1980s rock group
ZZZ: Dozing sound